Fuster and Hurst's
The Heart

Fuster and Hurst's The Heart, Fifteenth Edition

1 2 3 4 5 6 7 8 9   LWI   27 26 25 24 23 22

ISBN 978-1-264-25756-0
MHID 1-264-25756-2

This book was set in Minion Pro by KnowledgeWorks Global Ltd.
The editors were Timothy Y. Hiscock and Peter J. Boyle.
The production supervisor was Catherine H. Saggese.
Project management was provided by Nitesh Sharma, KnowledgeWorks Global Ltd.
The text designer was Mary McKeon.

This book is printed on acid-free paper.

Library of Congress Control Number: 2022932258

Fuster and Hurst's The Heart

Fifteenth Edition

EDITORS

Valentin Fuster, MD, PhD
Physician-in-Chief, The Mount Sinai Hospital
Director, Mount Sinai Heart
Ricard Gorlin, M.D. Heart Foundation Professor
  of Cardiology
New York, New York
General Director
Centro Nacional de Investigaciones Cardiovasculares
Madrid, Spain

Jagat Narula, MD, PhD
Philip J. and Harriet L. Goodhart Chair of Medicine
Professor of Medicine, Radiology, and Health
  System Design and Global Health
Chief, Division of Cardiology
Mount Sinai Morningside
Associate Dean for Global Health
Icahn School of Medicine at Mount Sinai
New York, New York

Prashant Vaishnava, MD, FACC
Senior Medical Director; Cardiovascular Care
Biofourmis
Boston, Massachusetts
Assistant Professor of Medicine
Columbia University Irving Medical Center
Attending Physician, New York Presbyterian Hospital
Attending Cardiologist, New York City Health and
  Hospital Commission Harlem Hospital
New York, New York

Martin B. Leon, MD
Mallah Family Professor of Cardiology
Columbia University Irving Medical Center
New York Presbyterian Hospital
New York, New York

David J. Callans, MD
Professor of Medicine
Perelman School of Medicine
Associate Director of Electrophysiology
University of Pennsylvania
Philadelphia, Pennsylvania

John S. Rumsfeld, MD, PhD
Professor of Medicine
University of Colorado School of Medicine
Aurora, Colorado

Athena Poppas, MD
Chief, Cardiology Division, and Director
Lifespan Cardiovascular Institute
Director, Echocardiography Laboratory
Rhode Island, The Miriam, and Newport Hospitals
Providence, Rhode Island

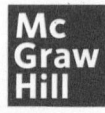

New York   Chicago   San Francisco   Athens   London   Madrid   Mexico City
Milan   New Delhi   Singapore   Sydney   Toronto

Contents

Contributors

Nina Ajmone Marsan, MD, PhD
Associate Professor in Cardiology, Department of Cardiology, Leiden University Medical Center, Leiden, The Netherlands
Chapter 30

Yousaf Ali, MD
Chief, Division of Rheumatology, Mount Sinai West/St Luke's Hospital, Professor of Medicine, Icahn School of Medicine at Mount Sinai, New York, New York
Chapter 76

Ziad Ali, MD, DPhil
Associate Professor of Medicine, Cardiology, Columbia University Irving Medical Center; Director, Angiographic Core Laboratory, Cardiovascular Research Foundation, New York, New York
Chapter 21

Robert Allman, MD
Senior Resident, Department of Surgery, ECU Department of Surgery, Medical School Annex, Greenville, North Carolina
Chapter 79

Rafael Alonso-Gonzalez, MD, MSc
Assistant Professor of Medicine, Peter Munk Cardiac Centre; Director of the ACHD Fellowship Program, University of Toronto, Toronto, Ontario, Canada
Chapter 70

Daniel Alyesh, MD
Cardiac Electrophysiologist, South Denver Cardiology, The South Denver Heart Center, Littleton, Colorado
Chapter 72

Charles Antzelevitch, PhD
Professor and Executive Director of Cardiovascular Research, Lankenau Institute for Medical Research and Lankenau Heart Institute, Wynnewood, Pennsylvania; Professor of Medicine and Pharmacology Division of Cardiology, Sidney Kimmel Medical College, Thomas Jefferson University, Philadelphia, Pennsylvania
Chapter 34

Hugo J. Aparicio, MD, MPH
Assistant Professor of Neurology, Department of Neurology, Boston University School of Medicine, Boston, Massachusetts
Chapter 25

Eloisa Arbustini, MD
Director, Center for Inherited Cardiovascular Diseases, Fondazione IRCCS Policlinico San Matteo, Pavia, Italy
Chapters 40, 41, 44, 45, 56

Edgar Argulian, MD, MPH
Associate Professor of Medicine, Mount Sinai Morningside and Mount Sinai West, The Mount Sinai Hospital, New York, New York
Chapter 43

Jeffrey Arkles, MD
Assistant Professor, Hospital of the University of Pennsylvania, Philadelphia, Pennsylvania
Chapter 38

Omar Baber, MD
Fellow, Cardiovascular Diseases, Department of Medicine (Cardiology), University of Oklahoma College of Medicine, Oklahoma City, Oklahoma
Chapter 75

Usman Baber, MD, MS
Associate Professor of Medicine (Cardiology), University of Oklahoma Health Sciences Center, Oklahoma City, Oklahoma
Chapters 18, 75

Luigi P. Badano, MD, PhD
Professor of Cardiology, Department of Medicine and Surgery, University Milano-Bicocca; Director, Cardiovascular Imaging Unit, Istituto Auxologico Italiano, IRCCS, Department of Cardiac, Neurologic and Metabolic Sciences, San Luca Hospital, Milan, Italy
Chapter 31

Vinay K. Bahl, MBBS, MD, DM
Dean (Academic), Chief, Cardio-Thoracic Centre; Professor and Head, Department of Cardiology, All India Institute of Medical Sciences, New Delhi, India
Chapter 32

Sripal Bangalore, MD, MHA
Professor of Medicine, Director, Cardiac Catheterization Laboratory, Bellevue, NYU Grossman School of Medicine, New York, New York
Chapter 21

Elvera L. Baron, MD, PhD
Assistant Professor, Department of Anesthesiology, Perioperative and Pain Medicine, Department of Medical Education, Icahn School of Medicine at Mount Sinai, New York, New York
Chapter 73

Eric R. Bates, MD
Professor of Internal Medicine, Division of Cardiovascular Medicine, Department of Internal Medicine, University of Michigan, CVC Cardiovascular Medicine, Ann Arbor, Michigan
Chapter 19

Jeroen J. Bax, MD, PhD
Professor in Cardiology, Director of Non-Invasive Cardiovascular Imaging, Department of Cardiology, Leiden University Medical Center, Leiden, The Netherlands
Chapter 30

Tina Baykaner, MD, MPH
Clinical Instructor, Department of Medicine, Cardiovascular Institute, Stanford University Medical Center, Stanford, California
Chapter 36

Neal L. Benowitz, MD
Professor of Medicine Emeritus, University of California San Francisco, Zuckerberg San Francisco General Hospital, San Francisco, California
Chapter 8

Catherine P. Benziger, MD, MPH
Medical Director of Heart and Vascular Research, Essentia Health; Adjunct Assistant Professor, University of Minnesota Medical School, Duluth Campus, Duluth, Minnesota
Chapter 1

Benjamin Bier, MD
Chief Cardiovascular Fellow, Icahn School of Medicine at Mount Sinai, New York, New York
Chapter 62

Ann F. Bolger, MD
Professor of Medicine, Emeritus, University of California, San Francisco, California
Chapter 33

Barry A. Borlaug, MD
Professor of Medicine, Department of Cardiovascular Medicine, Mayo Clinic and Foundation, Rochester, Minnesota
Chapter 57

Jason S. Bradfield, MD
Associate Professor of Medicine, Director, Specialized Program for Ventricular Tachycardia, UCLA Cardiac Arrhythmia Center, David Geffen School of Medicine at UCLA, Los Angeles, California
Chapter 37

Darryl J. Burstow, MBBS, FRACP
Associate Professor of Medicine, The Prince Charles Hospital, Brisbane, Queensland, Australia
Chapter 54

Javed Butler, MD, MPH, MBA
Professor and Chairman of Medicine, Department of Medicine, University of Mississippi Medical Center, Jackson, Mississippi
Chapters 48, 49

Hugh Calkins, MD
Professor of Medicine, Johns Hopkins University School of Medicine; Director of Electrophysiology, Division of Cardiology and Electrophysiology, Johns Hopkins Hospital, Baltimore, Maryland
Chapter 35

David J. Callans, MD, FHRS
Professor of Medicine, Perelman School of Medicine at the University of Pennsylvania; Associate Director of Electrophysiology, University of Pennsylvania Health System, University of Pennsylvania, Philadelphia, Pennsylvania
Chapter 38

Jonathan R. Carapetis, AM, MBBS, FRACP, PhD
Professor, UWA Centre for Child Health Research, University of Western Australia; Co-Director, REACH; Director, Telethon Kids Institute; Head, Strep A and Rheumatic Heart Disease Team Perth Children's Hospital, Nedland, Western Australia, Australia
Chapter 27

Emily Carroll, MD
Clinic Fellow, Division of Rheumatology, Icahn School of Medicine at Mount Sinai, New York, New York
Chapter 76

Ari M. Cedars, MD
Associate Professor of Medicine and Pediatrics, Johns Hopkins University, Baltimore, Maryland
Chapter 66

Marie-A. Chaix, MD, MSc
Clinical Assistant Professor of Medicine, Université de Montréal, Montreal Heart Institute Adult Congenital Center, Montreal Heart Institute, Montreal, Quebec, Canada
Chapter 69

Jaya Chandrasekhar, MBBS, MS, PhD
Associate Professor, Department of Cardiology, Box Hill Hospital and Eastern Health Clinical School, Melbourne, Victoria, Australia
Chapter 20

Peng-Sheng Chen, MD
Staff Physician III, Department of Cardiology, Cedars-Sinai Medical Center, Los Angeles, California
Chapter 34

Alexandra Chitroceanu, MD
Cardiology Resident, Department of Cardiology, University of Liége Hospital, Liége, Belgium
Chapter 29

Marie-Annick Clavel, DVM, PhD
Institut Universitaire de Cardiologie et de Pneumologie, Université Laval, Quebec, Canada
Chapter 28

Jennifer Cohen, MD
Assistant Professor of Pediatrics, Division of Pediatric Cardiology, Icahn School of Medicine at Mount Sinai; Director of Pediatric/Congenital Cardiac Computed Tomography, Mount Sinai Kravis Children's Heart Center, New York, New York
Chapter 68

Andrew Constantine, MBBS, MA, MRCP
CHAMPION PhD Research Fellow, The National Heart and Lung Institute, Imperial College London, Adult Congenital Heart Centre, Royal Brompton and Harefield NHS Foundation Trust, London, United Kingdom
Chapter 67

Anna Csiszar, MD, PhD
Professor, Center for Geroscience and Healthy Brain Aging, Department of Biochemistry and Molecular Biology, University of Oklahoma Health Sciences Center, Oklahoma City; International Training Program in Geroscience, Department of Translational Medicine, Semmelweis University, Budapest, Hungary
Chapter 82

Anne B. Curtis, MD
SUNY Distinguished Professor, Charles and Mary Bauer Professor and Chair, Jacobs School of Medicine and Biomedical Sciences, University at Buffalo, Buffalo General Medical Center, Buffalo, New York
Chapter 36

Dao-Fu Dai, MD, PhD
Assistant Professor, Department of Pathology, University of Iowa, Iowa City, Iowa
Chapter 82

James P. Daubert, MD
Senior Vice Chief, Cardiology, Professor of Medicine, Duke University School of Medicine, Duke Clinical Research Institute, Durham, North Carolina
Chapter 63

Michele DeBonis, MD
Associate Professor of Cardiac Surgery, Chief of Cardiac Surgery, Innovation and Research, San Raffaele University Hospital; Director Postgraduate School in Cardiac Surgery, Vita-Salute San Raffaele University, Milan, Italy
Chapter 30

G. William Dec, MD
Roman W. DeSanctis Professor of Medicine, Chief Emeritus, Cardiology Division, Harvard Medical School, Massachusetts General Hospital, Boston, Massachusetts
Chapters 41, 44, 47

Victoria Delgado, MD, PhD
Associate Professor in Cardiology, Department of Cardiology, Leiden University Medical Center, Leiden, The Netherlands
Chapter 30

Adam D. DeVore, MD, MHS
Associate Professor of Medicine, Medical Director, Cardiac Transplant Program, Division of Cardiology and the Duke Clinical Research Institute, Durham, North Carolina
Chapter 52

Konstantinos Dimopoulos, MD, MSc, PhD
Senior Consultant Cardiologist, and Professor of Practice in Adult Congenital Heart Disease and Pulmonary Hypertension, The National Heart and Lung Institute, Imperial College London, Adult Congenital Heart Centre and National Centre for Pulmonary Hypertension, Royal Brompton and Harefield NHS Foundation Trust, London, United Kingdom
Chapter 67

Alessandro Di Toro, MD
Physician Researcher, Center for Inherited Cardiovascular Diseases, Fondazione IRCCS Policlinico San Matteo, Pavia, Italy
Chapters 41, 44, 45, 46

Ashish Doshi, MD, PhD
Post-Doctoral Fellow, Alliance for Cardiovascular Diagnostic and Treatment Innovation (ADVANCE), Trayanova Lab, Whiting School of Engineering, Johns Hopkins University, Baltimore, Maryland
Chapter 66

Raluca Dulgheru, MD, PhD
Cardiologist, Department of Cardiology, University of Liége Hospital, Liége, Belgium
Chapter 29

Marc R. Dweck, MD, PhD
British Heart Foundation Centre for Cardiovascular Sciences,
University of Edinburgh, Edinburgh, United Kingdom
Chapter 28

Kim A. Eagle, MD
Albion Walter Hewlett Professor of Internal Medicine; Director,
Cardiovascular Center, University of Michigan Health System,
Ann Arbor, Michigan
Chapter 72

Katherine E. Economy, MD, MPH
Co-Director, Pregnancy and Cardiovascular Disease Program,
Department of Obstetrics and Gynecology, Division of
Maternal Fetal Medicine, Brigham and Women's Hospital,
Harvard Medical School, Boston, Massachusetts
Chapter 78

John A. Elefteriades, MD
William W.L. Glenn Professor of Surgery, Founding Director,
Aortic Institute at Yale-New Haven, Aortic Institute at Yale-
New Haven, New Haven, Connecticut
Chapter 23

Uri Elkayam, MD
Professor of Medicine; Professor of Obstetrics and Gynecology;
Director, Maternal Cardiology, Department of Medicine,
Division of Cardiology, Department of Obstetrics and
Gynecology, University of Southern California, Keck School of
Medicine, Los Angeles, California
Chapter 51

Perry M. Elliott, MBBS, MD, FRCP
Professor and Chair of Cardiovascular Medicine, University
College London; Head of Clinical Research, UCL Institute of
Cardiovascular Science; Consultant Cardiologist, Barts Heart
Centre, St Bartholomew's Hospital, London, United Kingdom
Chapter 42

Mark Engel, MPH, PhD
Associate Professor of Medicine, Department of Medicine,
University of Cape Town, Cape Town, South Africa
Chapter 27

David Ezon, MD
Assistant Professor of Pediatrics, Division of Pediatric
Cardiology, Jack and Lucy Clark Department of Pediatrics,
Icahn School of Medicine at Mount Sinai; Director of
Technology and Innovation for Education, Mount Sinai Kravis
Children's Heart Center, New York, New York
Chapter 68

Michael E. Farkouh, MD, MSc
Professor and Vice-Chair, Research, Department of Medicine,
The University of Toronto; Peter Munk Chair in Multinational
Clinical Trials at the Peter Munk Cardiac Centre; Director,
Heart and Stroke/Richard Lewar Centre of Excellence in
Cardiovascular Research, Toronto, Ontario, Canada
Chapter 7

T. Bruce Ferguson, Jr, MD
Former Professor and Inaugural Chair, Department of CV
Sciences, East Carolina Heart Institute, East Carolina Diabetes
and Obesity Institute, Brody School of Medicine at ECU; Chief
Visiting Scientist, RFPi, Inc., Greenville, North Carolina
Chapter 79

João Pedro Ferreira, MD, PhD
Professor of Medicine, Clinical Investigation Multidisciplinary
Canter Pierre Drouin, University of Lorraine, Vandoeuvre-Les-
Nancy, France
Chapter 49

Valentin Fuster, MD, PhD
Physician-in-Chief, The Mount Sinai Hospital; Director,
Mount Sinai Heart; Ricard Gorlin, M.D. Heart Foundation
Professor of Cardiology
New York, New York
General Director
Centro Nacional de Investigaciones Cardiovasculares
Madrid, Spain
Chapters 16, 17, 18

Inés García-Lunar, MD, PhD
Centro Nacional de Investigaciones Cardiovasculares (CNIC),
CIBER de Enfermedades Cardiovasculares (CIBERCV) and
Cardiology Department, Hospital Universitario Ramón y
Cajal, Madrid, Spain
Chapter 18

W. Timothy Garvey, MD
Professor of Medicine and Chair, Department of Nutrition
Sciences, University of Alabama at Birmingham, Birmingham,
Alabama
Chapter 6

Morie A. Gertz, MD
Seidler Jr. Professor of the Art of Medicine, Mayo Alix School
of Medicine, Rochester, Minnesota
Chapter 43

Umesh Gidwani, MD, MS
Chief, Cardiac Critical Care, Associate Professor of Medicine,
Icahn School of Medicine at Mount Sinai, New York, New York
Chapter 62

Lorenzo Giuliani, MSc
Cardiovascular Physiologist/Sonographer, Center for Inherited Cardiovascular Diseases, Fondazione IRCCS Policlinico San Matteo, Pavia, Italy
Chapters 41, 44, 45

Gennaro Giustino, MD
Cardiovascular Medicine Fellow, Zena and Michael A. Wiener Cardiovascular Institute/Marie-Josée and Henry R. Kravis Center for Cardiovascular Health, Icahn School of Medicine at Mount Sinai, New York, New York
Chapter 84

Zachary D. Goldberger, MD
Associate Professor of Medicine Division Cardiovascular Medicine/Electrophysiology, University of Wisconsin-Madison School of Medicine and Public Health, Clinical Science Center, Madison, Wisconsin
Chapter 39

Kevin L. Greason, MD
Associate Professor of Surgery, Division of Cardiovascular Surgery, Mayo Clinic, Rochester, Minnesota
Chapter 55

Jasmine Grewal, MD, FRCPC
Director, Pacific Adult Congenital Heart Program; Director, Cardiac Obstetrics Program; Associate Director, Echocardiography Program, St. Paul's Hospital; Clinical Associate Professor, University of British Columbia, Vancouver, British Columbia, Canada
Chapter 65

Blair P. Grubb, MD
Distinguished University Professor of Medicine and Pediatrics; Director, Cardiac Electrophysiology Program, University of Toledo, Heart and Vascular Center, Toledo, Ohio
Chapter 39

Marta Guasch-Ferré, PhD
Research Scientist, Department of Nutrition, Harvard TH Chan School of Public Health, Instructor in Medicine, Channing Division of Network Medicine, Department of Medicine, Brigham and Women's Hospital and Harvard Medical School, Boston, Massachusetts
Chapter 13

Rajeev Gupta, MD, PhD
Chair, Preventive Cardiology and Internal Medicine, Eternal Heart Care Centre and Research Institute; Chair, Academic Research Development Unit, Rajasthan University of Health Sciences, Jaipur, India
Chapter 15

Michael B. Hadley, MD, MPH
Cardiology Fellow, Zena and Michael A. Wiener Cardiovascular Institute, Icahn School of Medicine at Mount Sinai, New York, New York
Chapter 9

John E. Hall, PhD
Arthur C. Guyton Professor and Chair, Department of Physiology and Biophysics; Director, Mississippi Center for Obesity Research, University of Mississippi Medical Center, Jackson, Mississippi
Chapter 5

Michael E. Hall, MD, MS
Associate Professor, Department of Medicine; Associate Division Director, Division of Cardiovascular Diseases; Director of Clinical and Population Studies, Mississippi Center for Clinical and Translational Research, University of Mississippi Medical Center, Jackson, Mississippi
Chapter 5

Jonathan L. Halperin, MD
Robert and Harriet Heilbrunn Professor of Medicine (Cardiology), Icahn School of Medicine at Mount Sinai, The Cardiovascular Institute, Mount Sinai Medical Center, New York, New York
Chapter 18, 23

Dan G. Halpern, MD
Director, Adult Congenital Heart Disease Program, The Leon H. Charney Division of Cardiology, New York University Langone Health; Assistant Professor of Medicine, New York University Grossman School of Medicine, New York, New York
Chapter 78

Justin Hayase, MD
Cardiac Electrophysiology Fellow, UCLA Cardiac Arrhythmia Center, David Geffen School of Medicine at UCLA, Los Angeles, California
Chapter 37

Rosalba Hernandez, PhD
Associate Professor, School of Social Work, University of Illinois at Urbana-Champaign, Urbana, Illinois
Chapter 11

Robert A. Hegele, MD, FRCPC
Distinguished University Professor of Medicine and Biochemistry, Western University; Director, London Regional Genomics Centre, Robarts Research Institute, London, Ontario, Canada
Chapter 10

Siew Yen Ho, PhD
Emeritus Professor, Cardiac Morphology, National Heart & Lung Institute, Imperial College London, London, United Kingdom
Chapter 34

Jared Hooker, MD
Fellow, Cardiovascular Diseases, Department of Medicine (Cardiology), University of Oklahoma College of Medicine, Oklahoma City, Oklahoma
Chapter 75

Frank Hu, MD, PhD
Fredrick J. Stare Professor of Nutrition and Epidemiology, Chair, Departments of Nutrition and Epidemiology, Harvard TH Chan School of Public Health, Channing Division of Network Medicine, Department of Medicine, Brigham and Women's Hospital and Harvard Medical School, Boston, Massachusetts
Chapter 13

Borja Ibanez, MD, PhD
Full Professor and Director of Clinical Research Department, National Centre for Cardiovascular Research CNIC, Fundacion Jimenez Diaz Hospital, Madrid, Spain
Chapters 16, 17, 18

Bernard Iung, MD
Professor in Cardiology; Director of Echocardiography, Bichat Hospital/Université de Paris, Paris, France
Chapter 30

Ali Javaheri, MD, PhD
Assistant Professor, Department of Medicine, Washington University School of Medicine, Division of Cardiology, Advanced Heart Failure and Transplant, Saint Louis, Missouri
Chapter 60

Shahrokh Javaheri, MD,
Adjunct Professor, Department of Internal Medicine, Division of Cardiology, Ohio State University; Emeritus Professor of Medicine, University of Cincinnati, College of Medicine; Sleep Physician, Bethesda Montgomery Sleep Laboratory, Division of Pulmonary and Sleep Disorders, Bethesda North Hospital, Cincinnati, Ohio
Chapter 60

Hillary Johnston-Cox, MD, PhD
Interventional Cardiology Fellow, Cardiovascular Medicine Division, University of Pennsylvania, Perelman Center for Advanced Medicine, Philadelphia, Pennsylvania
Chapters 26, 56

Philip Joseph, MD
Associate Professor, McMaster University, Population Health Research Institute, Hamilton, Ontario, Canada
Chapter 15

Daniella Kadian-Dodov, MD
Assistant Professor of Medicine, Zena and Michael A. Wiener Cardiovascular Institute, Icahn School of Medicine at Mount Sinai, New York, New York
Chapters 26, 56

Sara Kalkhoran, MD, MAS
Assistant Professor of Medicine, Harvard Medical School, Massachusetts General Hospital, Boston, Massachusetts
Chapter 8

Garvan C. Kane, MD, PhD
Professor of Medicine, Chair, Division of Cardiovascular Ultrasound, Department of Cardiovascular Medicine, Rochester, Minnesota
Chapter 54

Joel A. Kaplan, MD
Professor of Anesthesiology, University of California at San Diego, San Diego, California; Dean Emeritus, School of Medicine, University of Louisville, Louisville, Kentucky
Chapter 73

Paul Khairy, MD, PhD
Professor of Medicine, Université de Montréal, Montreal Heart Institute Adult Congenital Center, Montreal Heart Institute, Montreal, Quebec, Canada
Chapter 69

Muhammad Shahzeb Khan, MD, MSc
Assistant Professor of Medicine, Department of Medicine, University of Mississippi Medical Center, Jackson, Mississippi
Chapter 48

Michelle M. Kittleson, MD, PhD
Professor of Medicine; Director, Advanced Heart Disease Fellowship Program, Department of Cardiology and the Cedars-Sinai Smidt Heart Institute, Los Angeles, California
Chapter 52

Jon Kobashigawa, MD
Professor of Medicine; Director, Advanced Heart Disease Division, Department of Cardiology and the Cedars-Sinai Smidt Heart Institute, Los Angeles, California
Chapter 52

Nitin Kondamudi, MD
Research Fellow, Division of Cardiology, Department of Internal Medicine, University of Texas Southwestern Medical Center, Clinical Heart and Vascular Center, Dallas, Texas
Chapter 12

Jayanthi N. Koneru, MBBS
Assistant Professor of Medicine, Division of Cardiology and Cardiac Electrophysiology, Medical College of Virginia and VCU School of Medicine, Richmond, Virginia
Chapter 38

Marlys L. Koschinsky, PhD
Scientist, Robarts Research Institute; Professor, Department of Physiology and Pharmacology, Schulich School of Medicine & Dentistry, Western University, London, Ontario, Canada
Chapter 10

Harlan M. Krumholz, MD, SM
Harold H. Hines, Jr. Professor of Medicine, Yale University; Director, Center for Outcomes Research and Evaluation, Yale New Haven Hospital, New Haven, Connecticut
Chapter 83

Shelby Kutty, MD, MS, PhD
The Helen B. Taussig Professor; Director, Helen B. Taussig Heart Center; Director, Pediatric and Congenital Cardiology, Johns Hopkins University, Baltimore, Maryland
Chapter 66

Darwin R. Labarthe, MD, MPH, PhD
Professor of Preventive Medicine, Department of Preventive Medicine, Feinberg School of Medicine, Northwestern University, Chicago, Illinois
Chapter 11

Anuradha Lala, MD
Assistant Professor of Medicine, Cardiology and Population Health Science and Policy, Zena and Michael A. Wiener Cardiovascular Institute, The Mount Sinai Hospital, The Lauder Family Cardiovascular Ambulatory Center, New York, New York
Chapter 50

Patrizio Lancellotti, MD, PhD
Professor of Cardiology and Director, Interdisciplinary Cluster for Applied Genoproteomics, Cardiovascular Science Unit, University of Liége, Liége, Belgium; Head, Department of Cardiology, University of Liége Hospital, Liége, Belgium; Gruppo Villa Maria Care and Research, Anthea Hospital, Bari, Italy
Chapter 29

Carl J. Lavie, Jr, MD
Professor of Medicine; Medical Director Cardiac Rehabilitation and Prevention; Director Exercise Laboratories, John Ochsner Heart and Vascular Institute, Ochsner Clinical School-The University of Queensland School of Medicine, New Orleans, Louisiana
Chapter 12

Charlotte Lee, MD
Clinical Fellow in Medicine, Harvard Medical School, Massachusetts General Hospital, Boston, Massachusetts
Chapter 47

Martin B. Leon, MD
Mallah Family Professor of Cardiology
Columbia University Irving Medical Center
New York Presbyterian Hospital
New York, New York
Chapter 28

Vasileios Lioutas, MD
Assistant Professor of Neurology, Department of Neurology, Beth Israel Deaconess Medical Center, Harvard Medical School, Boston, Massachusetts
Chapter 25

James W. Lloyd, MD
Fellow, Department of Cardiovascular Medicine, Mayo Clinic, Rochester, Minnesota
Chapter 53

Massimiliano Lorenzini, MD, PhD
Barts Heart Centre, St Bartholomew's Hospital, London, United Kingdom
Chapter 42

Sushil Allen Luis, MBBS
Associate Professor of Medicine; Co-Director, Pericardial Diseases Clinic, Department of Cardiovascular Medicine, Mayo Clinic, Rochester, Minnesota
Chapters 53, 54

Kiran Mahmood, MD
Assistant Professor of Medicine, Zena and Michael A. Wiener Cardiovascular Institute, Mount Sinai Morningside, New York, New York
Chapter 50

Pravin Manga, MBBC, PhD
Emeritus Professor, Department of Internal Medicine, School of Clinical Medicine, Faculty of Health Sciences, University of Witwatersrand, Johannesburg, South Africa
Chapter 77

Barry J. Maron, MD
Director, Clinical Research, Hypertrophic Cardiomyopathy Center, Professor, Tufts University School of Medicine, Boston, Massachusetts
Chapter 40

Thomas H. Marwick, MBBS, PhD, MPH
Professor, Director and Chief Executive, Head of Imaging Research, Baker Heart and Diabetes Institute, Melbourne, Victoria, Australia
Chapter 3

Danielle Massarella, MD
Fellow in Adult Congenital Heart Disease, Peter Munk Cardiac Centre, Toronto, Ontario, Canada
Chapter 70

Ravi S. Math, MBBS, MD, DM
Associate Professor of Cardiology, Department of Cardiology, Sri Jayadeva Institute of Cardiovascular Sciences and Research, Bangalore, India
Chapter 32

Keir McCutcheon, MBBCH, MSc, PhD
Assistant Professor, Department of Cardiovascular Sciences, Katholieke Universiteit Leuven, Leuven, Belgium
Chapter 77

Jeffrey I. Mechanick, MD
Professor of Medicine and Medical Director, Marie-Josée and Henry R. Kravis Center for Cardiovascular Health/Zena and Michael A. Wiener Cardiovascular Institute; Director of Metabolic Support, Division of Endocrinology, Diabetes and Bone Disease, Icahn School of Medicine at Mount Sinai, New York, New York
Chapters 6, 7, 84

Venu Menon, MD
Mehdi Razavi Endowed Chair and Professor of Medicine, Cleveland Clinic Lerner College of Medicine; Director, Cardiac Intensive Care Unit, Cleveland Clinic Department of Cardiovascular Medicine; Section Head, Clinical Cardiology, Robert and Suzanne Tomisch Department of Cardiovascular Medicine, Sydell and Arnold Miller Family Heart, Vascular & Thoracic Institute, Cleveland, Ohio
Chapters 61, 64

George A. Mensah, MD
Director of the Center for Translation Research and Implementation Science, National Heart, Lung, and Blood Institute, National Institutes of Health, Bethesda, Maryland
Chapter 1

Bela Merkely, MD, PhD, DSc
Professor and Chair, Heart and Vascular Center, Semmelweis University, Budapest, Hungary
Chapter 82

Carmelo A. Milano, MD
Professor of Surgery, Chief, Section of Adult Cardiac Surgery and Surgical Director of the Left Ventricular Assist Device Program, Duke University Medical Center, Durham, North Carolina
Chapter 52

William R. Miranda, MD
Assistant Professor of Medicine, Division of Cardiovascular Diseases, Mayo Clinic College of Medicine, Rochester, Minnesota
Chapters 2, 55

Sumeet S. Mitter, MD
Assistant Professor of Medicine, The Mount Sinai Hospital, The Lauder Family Cardiovascular Ambulatory Center, New York, New York
Chapter 43

David J. Moliterno, MD
Professor of Medicine and Chairman, Department of Internal Medicine, University of Kentucky College of Medicine, Lexington, Kentucky
Chapter 19

Philip Moons, PhD, RN
Professor, Department of Public Health and Primary Care, Faculty of Medicine, KU Leuven, Leuven, Belgium
Chapter 71

Andrew E. Moran, MD, MPH
Associate Professor of Medicine, Columbia University Irving Medical Center, New York, New York
Chapter 1

Bobak J. Mortazavi, PhD
Assistant Professor Adjunct, Center for Outcomes Research and Evaluation, Yale School of Medicine, Yale University, New Haven, Connecticut; Assistant Professor, Department of Computer Science and Engineering, Texas A&M University, College Station, Texas
Chapter 83

Denisa Muraru, MD, PhD
Assistant Professor, Department of Medicine and Surgery, University Milano-Bicocca, Cardiologist, Istituto Auxologico Italiano, IRCCS, Department of Cardiac, Neurologic and Metabolic Sciences, San Luca Hospital, Milan, Italy
Chapter 31

Sanjiv M. Narayan, MD, PhD
Co-Director, Stanford Arrhythmia Center; Professor, Department of Medicine, Cardiovascular Institute, Stanford University Medical Center, Stanford, California
Chapters 36, 63

Jagat Narula, MD, PhD
Philip J. and Harriet L. Goodhart Chair of Medicine, Professor of Medicine, Radiology, and Health System Design and Global Health; Chief, Division of Cardiology, Mount Sinai Morningside; Associate Dean for Global Health, Icahn School of Medicine at Mount Sinai, New York, New York
Chapters 3, 22, 27, 40, 41, 43, 44, 46

Navneet Narula, MD
Professor, Dept of Pathology, NYU Grossman School of Medicine, NYU Pathology Associates, New York, New York
Chapters 16, 40

Nupoor Narula, MD
Assistant Professor of Medicine, Cardiology, Physician-Investigator, Weill Cornell Medical College Cardiology at Weill Cornell Medical Center, New York, New York
Chapter 45

Thanh N. Nguyen, MD, FRCPC
Professor, Departments of Neurology, Neurosurgery, and Radiology, Boston University School of Medicine, Boston, Massachusetts
Chapter 25

Rick A. Nishimura, MD
Judd and Mary Morris Leighton Professor of Cardiovascular Diseases and Hypertension, Division of Cardiovascular Diseases, Mayo Clinic College of Medicine, Rochester, Minnesota
Chapter 2

Børge G. Nordestgaard, MD, DMSc
Professor, University of Copenhagen, Copenhagen University Hospital; Chief Physician, Department of Clinical Biochemistry, Herlev and Gentofte Hospital, Herlev, Denmark
Chapter 10

Jac K. Oh, MD
Samsung Professor in Cardiovascular Diseases, Director, Pericardial Diseases Clinic, Department of Cardiovascular Medicine, Mayo Clinic, Rochester, Minnesota
Chapters 53, 54, 55

Jeffrey W. Olin, DO
Professor of Medicine (Cardiology); Director, Vascular Medicine and Vascular Diagnostic Laboratory, Zena and Michael A. Wiener Cardiovascular Institute and Marie-Josée and Henry R. Kravis Center for Cardiovascular Health, Icahn School of Medicine at Mount Sinai, New York, New York
Chapters 26, 56

Alexander R. Opotowsky, MD, MMSc
Director, Adult Congenital Heart Disease Program; Co-Director, Exercise Laboratory; Co-Director, The Heart Institute Research Core; Professor, Department of Pediatrics, Cincinnati Children's Hospital, University of Cincinnati College of Medicine, Cincinnati, Ohio
Chapter 65

Ambarish Pandey, MD, MSCS
Assistant Professor of Internal Medicine, Division of Cardiology, Department of Internal Medicine, University of Texas Southwestern Medical Center, Clinical Heart and Vascular Center, Dallas, Texas
Chapter 12

Ana Pardo, MD
Cardiologist, Department of Cardiology, Ramón y Cajal University Hospital, Madrid, Spain
Chapter 31

Jignesh K. Patel, MD, PhD
Professor of Medicine; Medical Director, Cardiac Transplant Program, Department of Cardiology and the Cedars-Sinai Smidt Heart Institute, Los Angeles, California
Chapter 52

Manesh R. Patel, MD
Professor of Medicine, Richard Sean Stack, M.D. Distinguished Professor; Chief, Division of Clinical Pharmacology, Chief, Division of Cardiology, Department of Medicine; Duke University School of Medicine, Durham, North Carolina
Chapters 18, 19

Dirk Pevernagie, MD
Associate Professor, Department of Internal Medicine and Pediatrics, Ghent University Senior Staff Member, Department of Respiratory Diseases and Sleep Medicine Centre, Ghent University Hospital, Ghent, Belgium
Chapter 60

Philippe Pibarot, DVM, PhD
Institut Universitaire de Cardiologie et de Pneumologie, Université Laval, Quebec, Canada
Chapter 28

Sean Pinney, MD
Director, Advanced Heart Failure & Cardiac Transplantation; Director, Richard P. Parrillo Family Center for Clinical and Translational Cardiology; Professor of Medicine, University of Chicago, Chicago, Illinois
Chapters 46, 84

Jena Pizula, MD
Cardiology Fellow, Department of Medicine, Division of Cardiology, University of Southern California, Keck School of Medicine, Los Angeles, California
Chapter 51

Adriana Postolache, MD, PhD
Cardiologist, Department of Cardiology, University of Liége Hospital, Liége, Belgium
Chapter 29

Bernard Prendergast, BMedSci, BM, BS, MD
Professor in Cardiology; Director, Cardiac Structural Intervention Programme, Guy's and St Thomas' NHS Foundation Trust, St Thomas' Hospital, London, United Kingdom
Chapter 30

Silvia G. Priori, MD, PhD
Scientific Director, Molecular Cardiology, Istituti Clinici Scientifici Maugeri IRCCS, Pavia, Italy; Professor of Cardiology, Department of Molecular Medicine, University of Pavia, Pavia, Italy; Professor and Director of Molecular Cardiology Laboratories, Centro de Investigaciones Cardiovasculares Carlos III, Madrid, Spain
Chapter 34

John Puskas, MD
Professor of Cardiovascular Surgery, Icahn School of Medicine at Mount Sinai; Chairman, Department of Cardiovascular Surgery, Mount Sinai Morningside, New York, New York
Chapter 21

Sanjay Rajagopalan, MD
Director, Case Cardiovascular Research Institute; Professor, Department of Medicine, Case Western Reserve University School of Medicine, Harrington Heart and Vascular Institute, University Hospitals, Cleveland, Ohio
Chapter 9

Penelope Rampersad, MD, MSc, FRCPC
Quality Improvement Officer, Section of Clinical Cardiology & Cardiac Critical Care, Cleveland Clinic Department of Cardiovascular Medicine, Sydell and Arnold Miller Family Heart, Vascular, and Thoracic Institute, Cleveland, Ohio
Chapter 61

Yogesh N. V. Reddy, MD, MSc
Assistant Professor of Medicine, Department of Cardiovascular Medicine, Mayo Clinic and Foundation, Rochester, Minnesota
Chapter 57

Harmony Reynolds, MD
Associate Professor; Director, Sarah Ross Soter Center for Women's Cardiovascular Research; Associate Director, Cardiovascular Clinical Research Center, Leon H. Charney Division of Cardiology, Department of Medicine, NYU Grossman School of Medicine, New York, New York
Chapter 20

June-Wha Rhee, MD
Instructor, Department of Medicine, Division of Cardiology, Stanford University School of Medicine, Stanford Cardiovascular Institute, Palo Alto, California
Chapter 4

David L. Reich, MD
President and Chief Operating Officer, The Mount Sinai Hospital, Professor of Anesthesiology, Perioperative and Pain Medicine, Icahn School of Medicine at Mount Sinai, New York, New York
Chapter 73

Paul M. Ridker, MD, MPH
Divisions of Cardiovascular Medicine and Preventive Medicine, Department of Medicine, Harvard Medical School, Center for Cardiovascular Disease Prevention, Brigham and Women's Hospital, Boston, Massachusetts
Chapter 14

Nancy A. Rigotti, MD
Professor of Medicine, Harvard Medical School, Massachusetts General Hospital, Boston, Massachusetts
Chapter 8

Austin Rogers, MD
Senior Resident, Department of Surgery, ECU Department of Surgery, Medical School Annex, Greenville, North Carolina
Chapter 79

Joseph G. Rogers, MD
Professor of Medicine, Division of Cardiology and the Duke Clinical Research Institute, Durham, North Carolina
Chapter 52

Annika Rosengren, MD, PhD
Professor of Medicine, University of Gothenburg and Sahlgrenska University Hospital, Göteborg, Sweden
Chapter 15

Robert S. Rosenson, MD
Professor of Medicine (Cardiology), Icahn School of Medicine at Mount Sinai; Director of Metabolism and Lipids, Mount Sinai Health System, The Lauder Family Cardiovascular Ambulatory Center, New York, New York
Chapter 10

Gregory A. Roth, MD, MPH
Associate Professor of Medicine-Cardiology; Adjunct Associate Professor of Global Health and Health Metrics Science, Division of Cardiology, Department of Medicine, University of Washington and Institute for Health Metrics and Evaluation, Seattle, Washington
Chapter 1

Alan Rozanski, MD
Director, Nuclear Cardiology; Executive Director, Cardiology Fellowships; Chief Academic Officer, Division of Cardiology, Mount Sinai Morningside Hospital; Professor of Medicine, Icahn School of Medicine at Mount Sinai, New York, New York
Chapter 22

Lewis J. Rubin, MD
Professor Emeritus of Medicine, University of California, San Diego School of Medicine, California; Adjunct Professor of Medicine, College of Physicians and Surgeons, Columbia University, New York, New York
Chapter 59

John S. Rumsfeld, MD, PhD
Professor of Medicine, University of Colorado School of Medicine, Aurora, Colorado
Chapter 83

Mohammed Ruzieh, MD
Assistant Professor of Medicine, Division of Cardiovascular Medicine, University of Florida, Gainsville, Florida
Chapter 39

Amy Sarma, MD
Instructor in Medicine, Department of Medicine, Division of Cardiology, Massachusetts General Hospital, Harvard Medical School, Boston, Massachusetts
Chapter 78

Jacqueline Saw, MD, FRCPC
Clinical Professor, University of British Columbia, Division of Cardiology (Interventional Cardiology), Vancouver General Hospital, Vancouver, British Columbia, Canada
Chapter 20

Alessandra Serio, MD
Cardiologist, Center for Inherited Cardiovascular Diseases, IRCCS Foundation, University Hospital Policlinico San Matteo, Pavia, Italy
Chapter 45

Gregory Serrao, MD, MSE
Assistant Professor of Medicine, Icahn School of Medicine at Mount Sinai, New York, New York
Chapter 62

Sudha Seshadri, MD
Robert R. Barker Distinguished University Professor of Neurology, Psychiatry and Cellular and Integrative Physiology, University of Texas Health Sciences Center, San Antonio, Texas
Chapter 25

Saman Setareh-Shenas, MD, MS
Department of Cardiology, Mount Sinai Morningside Hospital, Mount Sinai Heart and the Icahn School of Medicine at Mount Sinai, New York, New York
Chapter 22

Kavita Sharma, MD
Professor of Medicine; Director, Heart Failure and Cardiac Transplantation, Division of Cardiology, Heart and Vascular Institute, The Johns Hopkins University School of Medicine, Baltimore, Maryland
Chapter 49

Leslee J. Shaw, PhD
Professor and Endowed Chair, Weill Cornell College of Medicine, New York, New York
Chapter 80

Kalyanam Shivkumar, MD, PhD
Professor of Medicine (Cardiology), Radiology and Bioengineering; Director, UCLA Cardiac Arrhythmia Center & EP Programs, UCLA Cardiac Arrhythmia Center, David Geffen School of Medicine at UCLA, Los Angeles, California
Chapter 37

Hasan K. Siddiqi, MD, MSCR
Divisions of Cardiovascular Medicine and Preventive Medicine, Department of Medicine, Harvard Medical School, Brigham and Women's Hospital, Harvard Medical School, Boston, Massachusetts
Chapter 14

Simona Sperlongano, MD
Cardiology Resident, Department of Cardiology, University of Liége Hospital, Liége, Belgium
Chapter 29

David Spragg, MD
Associate Professor, Division of Cardiology and Electrophysiology, Johns Hopkins Hospital, Baltimore, Maryland
Chapter 35

Kenan Stern, MD
Assistant Professor of Pediatrics and Radiology, Division of Pediatric Cardiology, Icahn School of Medicine at Mount Sinai and Mount Sinai Kravis Children's Hospital; Director of Non-Invasive Imaging and Director of Pediatric/Congenital Cardiac MRI, Mount Sinai Kravis Children's Heart Center, New York, New York
Chapter 68

Gregg W. Stone, MD
Director of Academic Affairs for the Mount Sinai Heart Hospital; Professor of Medicine (Cardiology); Professor of Population Health Sciences and Policy, The Zena and Michael A. Wiener Cardiovascular Institute, Icahn School of Medicine at Mount Sinai, New York, New York
Chapter 21

John M. Stulak, MD
Professor of Surgery, Division of Cardiovascular Surgery, Mayo Clinic, Rochester, Minnesota
Chapter 55

Victor F. Tapson, MD
Professor of Medicine; Director, Clinical Research for the Women's Guild Lung Institute; Director, Venous Thromboembolism and Pulmonary Vascular Disease Research Program; Associate Director, Pulmonary and Critical Care Division, Pulmonary Hypertension Clinic, Cedars-Sinai Medical Center, Los Angeles, California
Chapter 58

Viviany R. Taqueti, MD, MPH
Assistant Professor of Medicine, Brigham and Women's Hospital, Harvard Medical School, Boston, Massachusetts
Chapter 80

Hendrik Treede, MD
Professor in Cardiothoracic Surgery; Director of the Department of Cardiac Surgery at Mid-German Heart Center University Hospital Halle (Saale), Germany
Chapter 30

Nqoba Tsabedze, MBBCH, MMed
Head, Division of Cardiology, Department of Medicine, School of Clinical Medicine, Faculty of Health Sciences, University of Witwatersrand, Johannesburg, South Africa
Chapter 77

Zoltan Ungvari, MD, PhD
Professor, Center for Geroscience and Healthy Brain Aging, Department of Biochemistry and Molecular Biology, University of Oklahoma Health Sciences Center, Oklahoma City, Oklahoma
Chapter 82

Mario Urtis, MSc
Research Scientist, Bioinformatics Engineer, Fondazione IRCCS Policlinico San Matteo, Pavia, Italy
Chapters 41, 46

Muthiah Vaduganathan, MD, MPH
Instructor of Medicine, Division of Cardiovascular Medicine, Brigham and Women's Hospital and Harvard Medical School, Boston, Massachusetts
Chapter 48

Prashant Vaishnava, MD, FACC
Senior Medical Director
Cardiovascular Care
Biofourmis
Boston, Massachusetts
Assistant Professor of Medicine
Columbia University Irving Medical Center
Attending Physician, New York Presbyterian Hospital
Attending Cardiologist, New York City Health and Hospital Commission Harlem Hospital
New York, New York
Chapter 72

Anne Marie Valente, MD
Director, Boston Adult Congenital Heart Disease Program; Co-Director, Pregnancy and Cardiovascular Disease Program, Department of Medicine, Division of Cardiology, Brigham and Women's Hospital, Harvard Medical School, Department of Cardiology, Boston Children's Hospital, Boston, Massachusetts
Chapter 78

Pieter van der Bijl, MD, PhD
Associate Professor in Cardiology, Department of Cardiology, Leiden University Medical Center, Leiden, The Netherlands
Chapter 30

Eric J. Velazquez, MD
Robert W. Berliner Professor of Medicine, Chief, Cardiovascular Medicine, Yale School of Medicine, Physician-in-Chief, Heart and Vascular Center, Yale New Haven Health, New Haven, Connecticut
Chapter 50

Pugazhendhi Vijayaraman, MD
Professor of Medicine, Geisinger Commonwealth School of Medicine, Program Director, Clinical Cardiac Electrophysiology, Geisinger Heart Institute, Wilkes Barre, Pennsylvania
Chapter 38

Gemma Vilahur, DVM, PhD
Senior I3P Researcher, Catalan Institute of Cardiovascular Sciences (ICCC), IR-Hospital de la Santa Creu i Sant Pau, Barcelona, Spain
Chapter 17

Renu Virmani, MD
Clinical Professor of Pathology, Georgetown University, Washington DC; University of Maryland, Baltimore; George Washington University, Washington DC; Vanderbilt University, Nashville, Tennessee; and President and Medical Director, CVPath Institute, Gaithersburg, Maryland
Chapter 16

Nanette K. Wenger, MD
Professor of Medicine, Division of Cardiology, Emory University School of Medicine, Atlanta, Georgia
Chapter 80

Paul K. Whelton, MB, MD, MSc
Show Chwan Professor of Global Public Health, Department of Epidemiology, Tulane University School of Public Health and Tropical Medicine, New Orleans, Louisiana
Chapter 5

Christopher J. White, MD
Professor and Chairman of Medicine, The Ochsner Clinical School, University of Queensland, Australia; System Chairman of Cardiovascular Diseases, Ochsner Health, New Orleans, Louisiana
Chapter 24

Joseph C. Wu, MD, PhD
Simon H. Stertzer, MD, Professor of Medicine and Radiology, Department of Medicine, Division of Cardiology and Department of Radiology, Stanford University School of Medicine, Palo Alto, California
Chapter 4

Clyde W. Yancy, MD, MSc
Vice Dean, Diversity & Inclusion, Magerstadt Professor of Medicine; Professor, Medical Social Sciences; Chief, Division of Cardiology Northwestern University, Feinberg School of Medicine; Associate Director, Bluhm Cardiovascular Institute Northwestern Memorial Hospital, Chicago, Illinois
Chapter 81

Zi Ye, MD, PhD
Research Associate, Department of Cardiovascular Medicine, Mayo Clinic, Rochester, Minnesota
Chapter 53

Edward T. H. Yeh, MD
Chair, Department of Internal Medicine and Nolan Family Distinguished Chair in Internal Medicine, College of Medicine at the University of Arkansas for Medical Sciences, Little Rock, Arkansas
Chapter 74

Salim Yusuf, MBBS, DPhil
Distinguished University Professor of Medicine, McMaster University; Executive Director, Population Health Research Institute, Hamilton Heath Sciences and McMaster University, Hamilton, Ontario, Canada
Chapter 15

Ali N. Zaidi, MD
Director, Mount Sinai Adult Congenital Heart Disease Center, Mount Sinai Cardiovascular Institute & The Children's Heart Center, Mount Sinai Kravis Children's Hospital; Director, Academic Affairs, Children's Heart Center, Mount Sinai Kravis Children's Hospital; Director, Transition Program, Children's Heart Center, Mount Sinai Kravis Children's Hospital; Associate Professor, Internal Medicine and Pediatrics, Icahn School of Medicine at Mount Sinai, New York, New York
Chapter 68

Sarah Zaman, MD
Associate Professor, Department of Cardiology, Westmead Hospital, Westmead Applied Research Centre, University of Sydney, Sydney, New South Wales, Australia
Chapter 20

Jose Louis Zamorano, MD
Professor of Medicine, University Complutense, Head of Cardiology, Ramón y Cajal University Hospital, Madrid, Spain
Chapter 31

Bulat A. Ziganshin, MD
Aortic Institute at Yale-New Haven, New Haven, Connecticut
Chapter 23

Liesl Zühlke, MBChB, DCH, MPH, PhD
Professor, University of Cape Town; Director of the Children's Heart Disease Research Unit, Red Cross Children's Hospital, Cape Town, South Africa
Chapter 27

Preface

The 15th edition of *The Heart* is a milestone in the publication of this iconic textbook, which has been the lighthouse for every cardiologist since the publication of its first edition in 1966. The first and second editions of *The Heart* were edited by J. Willis Hurst and R. Bruce Logue. Dr Hurst remained the editor through the 7th edition and in the year 1994, in its 8th edition, it was deservingly named *Hurst's The Heart*, paying homage to the inaugural editor of this enduring series. Valentin Fuster took over as Editor-in-Chief for the 10th edition, published in 2000, and has devotedly, and meticulously steered a textbook that is a landmark in the field of cardiovascular medicine nationally and internationally, for all levels of learners from medical students to seasoned cardiologists. It is an honor for the editors and the McGraw Hill publishing team to pay tribute to the legacy of both these giants in cardiology and rename the book *Fuster and Hurst's The Heart*.

Much has changed since the publication of the first edition of *The Heart*. However, advances in science have not changed that caring for the heart is motivated by compassion. Dr Hurst's final publication before his passing in 2011 was an inspiring reflection on his interactions with trainees from Emory University and how, during one of these encounters, he shared one of the many invaluable teachings of Dr Francis Weld Peabody:

> "One of the essential qualities of the physician is interest in humanity, for the secret of care of the patient is in caring for the patient."

There is a clinical focus throughout the entire 15th edition, with most chapters including sections specifically devoted to commonly encountered scenarios or dilemmas in clinical practice. Content from chapters that had previously been devoted exclusively to imaging or procedural techniques has been assimilated throughout the text to more closely align with corresponding clinical content. Section 2 of the book is devoted entirely to "Risk Factors for Cardiovascular Disease," with each of the 11 chapters addressing a single component of the risk factor profile and proven, practical lifestyle changes. A new section on cardiovascular critical care recognizes the expanding role of this field as its own entity in a cardiac population that is sustainable owing to incrementally sophisticated interventions. The final chapter in the book, "Cardiovascular Manifestations of COVID-19," is, of course, the most-timely treatise on the protean cardiovascular manifestations of SARS-CoV-2 infection, and emerging trends in management and prevention.

Although *Fuster and Hurst's The Heart* was curated with focus on the patient, the idea of the lifelong learning was just as much of a cornerstone in creating this new edition. Chapter summaries and Central Illustrations are provided to give the reader a quick but comprehensive overview of what is covered in each chapter, and diagrams, graphs, tables, and algorithms serve to coalesce large amounts of content. Reference lists have been truncated and updated to provide practical reading suggestions. The latest guidelines, across international societies, are incorporated into the text.

Continuing in the tradition of the 14th edition and complementing the print edition, the 15th edition has a prominent online presence, aligned with contemporary needs that rely on multiple digital formats available at the point of care. The online platform allows for timely release of updates of the latest science from meetings of the American Heart Association, American College of Cardiology, and European Society of Cardiology.

An undertaking like the 15th edition is the combined effort of so many individuals to whom we extend much gratitude. First and foremost, the authors of this edition, many of whom faced challenges during the COVID-19 pandemic or were ill themselves. Authors spanning generations of cardiologists and disciplines and interests, all united by a common thread to maintain the legacy of this landmark textbook more than half a century after its inception. We thank the editors' families who stood with us, offering their unrelenting support—their spouses Maria Fuster, Navneet Narula, Shobi Rajasekaran, Linda Leon, Melissa Callans, Christina Johnson, and Philip Gould. The 15th edition could simply not have come to fruition without the tireless and undivided devotion of Bryony Mearns and Alexandra Roberts. We especially acknowledge Dr. Ali Zaidi for his devotion and assistance with revamping the section on Congenital Heart Disease. Administrative support from Robinson Santana, Alfred Kemp, Alanur Inal-Veith, and Shondra Rushing was invaluable. We are indebted to our partners at McGraw Hill Professional, particularly Scott Grillo, James Shanahan, Jason Malley, and their associates Karen Edmonson, Andrew Moyer, Tim Hiscock, and Peter Boyle for their immense energy, commitment, and passion.

SECTION I

INTRODUCTION

1

The Global Burden of Cardiovascular Diseases

Catherine P. Benziger, Andrew E. Moran, Gregory A. Roth, and George A. Mensah

CHAPTER OUTLINE

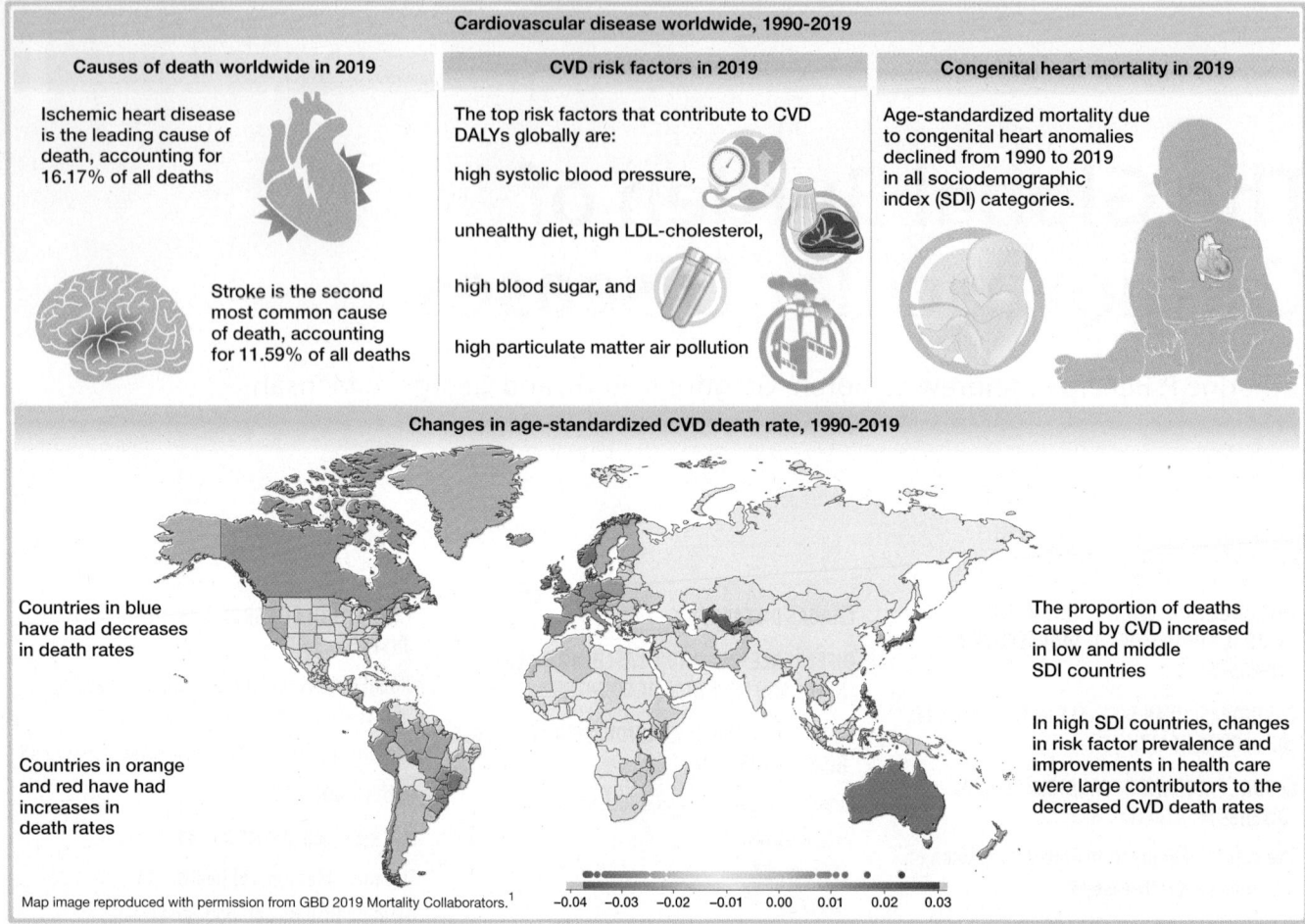

Chapter 1 Fuster and Hurst's Central Illustration. Trends in risk factors for cardiovascular diseases (CVD) and deaths caused by CVD, from 1990 through 2019.

CHAPTER SUMMARY

This chapter highlights the global burden of cardiovascular disease (CVD) using comparable health metrics from the Global Burden of Disease (GBD) 2019 study. It discusses cause- and region-specific trends, from 1990 through 2019, in the major CVDs, including ischemic heart disease, stroke, abdominal aortic aneurysm, atrial fibrillation, congenital heart disease, infective endocarditis, and valvular heart disease (see Fuster and Hurst's Central Illustration). Despite a decline in age-specific death rates, CVD prevalence and mortality have increased since 1990, to more than 18.6 million deaths in 2019, largely the result of population growth and aging. About 60% of these deaths occur in low, low-middle, and middle sociodemographic index (SDI) countries, and nearly half of the deaths are in women. Age-standardized mortality from CVD declined significantly (52.8%) in high-SDI countries; however, global CVD deaths did not change. The chapter explores modifiable and nonmodifiable risk factor trends, COVID-19, pregnancy-related cardiovascular risk factors, air pollution, mental illness, human immunodeficiency virus (HIV) infection, and social determinants of health. Modeling studies suggest that significant reductions in premature CVD are possible by 2025 if multiple risk factor targets are achieved; however, given current trends, the probability of dying prematurely from CVD is projected to remain unchanged in many of the world's most populous regions.

INTRODUCTION: WHAT'S NEW IN THE GLOBAL BURDEN OF CARDIOVASCULAR DISEASES?

The rich history of cardiac diseases and the development of cardiovascular medicine as a specialty highlight many of the remarkable advances made in the prevention, detection, treatment, and control of cardiovascular disease (CVD) worldwide. Despite these advances, the global burden of CVDs remains large and is increasing. For example, CVDs continue to be the leading cause of mortality and accounted for 18.6 million deaths worldwide in 2019 alone.[1] They are also a major contributor to premature death, disability, health care expenditures, and lost productivity globally. CVDs contribute nearly half of the estimated $47 trillion in economic output that would be lost due to noncommunicable diseases by 2030.[2] Projections for the United States alone suggest that the costs of CVD will skyrocket from $555 billion in 2016 to $1.1 trillion by 2035.[3]

This chapter is aimed at health care providers and students, public health researchers, epidemiologists, and policymakers seeking a better understanding of the field. This overview emphasizes cause-specific and region-specific trends of CVDs and related risk factors as estimated for the Global Burden of Disease 2019 (GBD 2019) study.[1,4,5] The chapter begins with an overview of CVD in the context of global health and then addresses important global and regional patterns of cardiovascular mortality as well as the implications of population growth and aging. It then provides updated estimates of summary measures of health for ischemic heart disease (IHD), stroke, three other acquired CVDs, congenital heart disease, valvular heart disease, and two common endemic diseases—rheumatic heart disease (RHD) and Chagas disease. In addition to addressing these two neglected diseases of poverty, the chapter highlights the significant variation in the patterns and trends of CVD in countries with a higher sociodemographic index (SDI) compared with those with a lower SDI, findings that are often masked by discussions of global trends in CVD.

The chapter also discusses the global burden and trends for CVD risk factors and provides updated estimates of the effect of the metabolic, environmental, and behavioral risk factors on total burden of disease. The burden of CVD and risk factors in people living with HIV is addressed. The impact of mental illness on the global burden of CVD and risk factors is also addressed. The chapter then presents an overview of the relevance of these global burden data to the prevention and control of CVD and risk factors and the worldwide efforts in the use of global targets to monitor progress in CVD prevention. In this light, we also consider efforts to forecast the global burden of CVDs into the future. A summary of GBD methods, including data sources and case definitions relevant to CVD, is provided at the end of the chapter.

New in this chapter are the sections on nonrheumatic degenerative mitral and aortic valve diseases; pregnancy-related hypertensive disorders; congenital heart diseases; and the cardiovascular implications of the COVID-19 pandemic and its impact on the incidence and burden of other CVD, such as the incidence of acute myocardial infarction.[6] Also new is a discussion of the availability and affordability of essential cardiovascular medicines and their impact on the global burden of CVD and of the emerging role, challenges, and opportunities of large-scale genomic biobanks on the global burden and the prevention, detection, treatment, and control of CVD.[7,8]

CARDIOVASCULAR DISEASES IN THE CONTEXT OF GLOBAL HEALTH

Although there had been a steady and dramatic decrease in mortality rates for CVDs beginning in the last third of the 20th century in high-income countries, many low- and middle-income countries (LMICs) have not benefited similarly from this favorable trend. As a result, more than 18.6 million (95% uncertainty interval [UI], 17.1-19.7 million) people died from CVDs in 2019, and as a consequence of the large populations in many LMICs, nearly 60% of global CVD deaths occurred in low-, low-middle–, and middle-SDI countries and 48% were in women.[4] CVDs account for 44% of all noncommunicable disease (NCD) deaths in the world each year[1] and represent a significant threat to sustainable development.[9-11] On average, CVDs are also the leading cause of death in every region of the world, with the exceptions of low-SDI countries, particularly those in southern sub-Saharan Africa, where infectious diseases are still the leading cause of death.[1] However, this rank ordering of CVD is not always true for specific countries or regions within countries; in some regions, NCDs, such as Alzheimer disease (Japan), diabetes (Cook Islands, Fiji), maternal and neonatal disorders (Angola, Pakistan, Ethiopia, Mali, Nigeria, Senegal, South Sudan, Uganda, Tanzania), or chronic obstructive pulmonary disease (COPD) (Nepal), are leading causes of death, and in other regions, infectious diseases, such as lower respiratory infections (Somalia, Peru, Guatemala), HIV/AIDS (Botswana, Cameroon, Djibouti, Equatorial Guinea, Eswatini, Gabon, Kenya, Lesotho, Malawi, Mozambique, Namibia, South Africa, Zambia, Zimbabwe), or neglected tropical diseases and malaria (Burkina Faso, Benin, Congo, Cote d'Ivoire, Ghana, Mauritania, Sierra Leone), are estimated to be leading causes of death.[1]

These global, regional, and national comparisons in the patterns of disease burden are possible because of advances in the science of health metrics and evaluation that enable a systematic, comprehensive, and comparative quantification of health loss due to diseases and injuries by age, sex, and location over time.[12] For example, the disability-adjusted life-year (DALY) is a core summary measure of health that represents the gap between a population's actual health and an ideal standard (GBD methods are summarized at the end of this chapter). Between 1990 and 2019, the number of global DALYs decreased from 2.59 billion (95% UI, 2.44–2.78 billion) to 2.54 billion (2.29–2.81 billion)[5] (**Fig. 1–1**). There were large increases in disease burden for HIV and Alzheimer disease, with smaller increases for road injuries and a wide range of NCDs, including musculoskeletal disorders, IHD, depression,

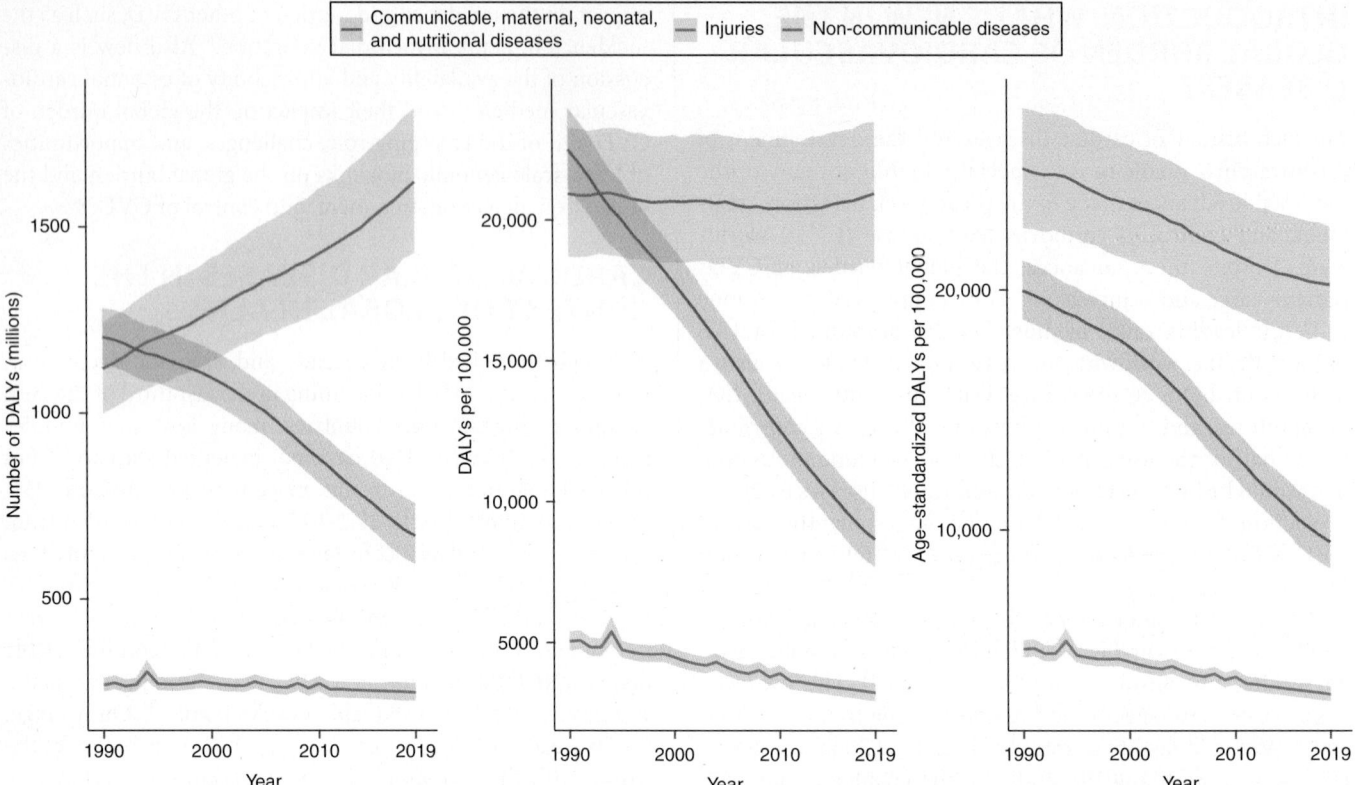

Figure 1–1. **Total disability-adjusted life-years (DALYs), crude DALY rates, and age-standardized DALY rates from 1990 to 2019.** Changes in global DALYs caused by communicable, maternal, neonatal, and nutritional disorders; noncommunicable diseases; and injuries shown in terms of numbers of DALYs (**A**), DALY rates per 100,000 people (**B**), and age-standardized DALY rates per 100,000 people (**C**). The difference in trends between **A** and **B** is caused by population growth, and the difference between **B** and **C** exists because of changes in the percentage distribution of the population by age. Shaded areas show 95% uncertainty intervals. Data from Global Burden of Disease, 2019 (GBD).

anxiety, lung cancer, and chronic kidney disorders (**Fig. 1–2**). Most DALY increases from 1990 to 2019 were caused by aging of the population and population growth.[5]

The 30-year trends in age-standardized DALY rates for leading categories of disease are shown in **Fig. 1–3**. There were significant reductions in certain infectious diseases, such as measles, meningitis, malaria, and tuberculosis; however, the disease burden from HIV substantially increased. Overall, the age-standardized DALY rates for neonatal disorders, IHD, lower respiratory infections, and stroke declined, although not sufficient for these conditions to be replaced as the leading causes of disease burden worldwide. Diabetes, low back and neck pain, road injuries, and COPD have all increased in rank. However, the overall age-standardized rates decreased significantly for 20 of the 25 leading causes of DALYs in 2019.[1]

GLOBAL PATTERNS IN CARDIOVASCULAR DISEASE MORTALITY

CVD was the primary cause of 18.56 million deaths in 2019,[4] with an estimated total economic cost of US $11.3 trillion (including treatment costs) of estimated lost gross domestic product (GDP) between 2015 and 2050 in the United States.[13] **Table 1–1** shows the total estimated CVD-related deaths for each cause in 2019. The leading cause of CVD-related death was IHD, accounting for more than 9 million deaths (95% UI, 8.4–9.7 million), followed by stroke, with more than 6.5 million deaths (95% UI, 3.0–3.5 million for ischemic stroke; 95% UI, 2.6–3.1 million for intracerebral hemorrhage; and 95% UI, 0.3–0.4 million for subarachnoid hemorrhage).[4] RHD, although not the leading cause of death, was a significant contributor to the global burden and a leading cause of highly preventable death, with approximately 305,651 deaths in 2019 (95% UI, 259,220–340,486)[4] (see Table 1–1). The age-standardized death rates due to CVD are shown by country on the map in **Fig. 1–4**. Globally, the death rate as a result of CVD was 225.6 per 100,000 people (95% UI, 213.7–234.6) in 1990 and fell 6.3% to 239.9 per 100,000 (95% UI, 220.7–254.9) by 2019.[4] However, there are regional variations, with the highest CVD mortality in Central Asia and Eastern Europe and the lowest rates in some high-income countries. In addition, males have higher age-standardized death rates than females (**Fig. 1–5**). Despite the steady decrease in death rate for both sexes over the past 30 years, the total number of deaths is increasing as a result of population growth and aging, which disproportionately affect low- and middle-SDI countries (**Fig. 1–6**). Globally, the total number of CVD deaths increased from 12.1 million (95% UI, 11.4–12.6 million) in 1990 to 18.6 million (95% UI, 17.1–19.7 million) in 2019, a 53.8% increase.[4]

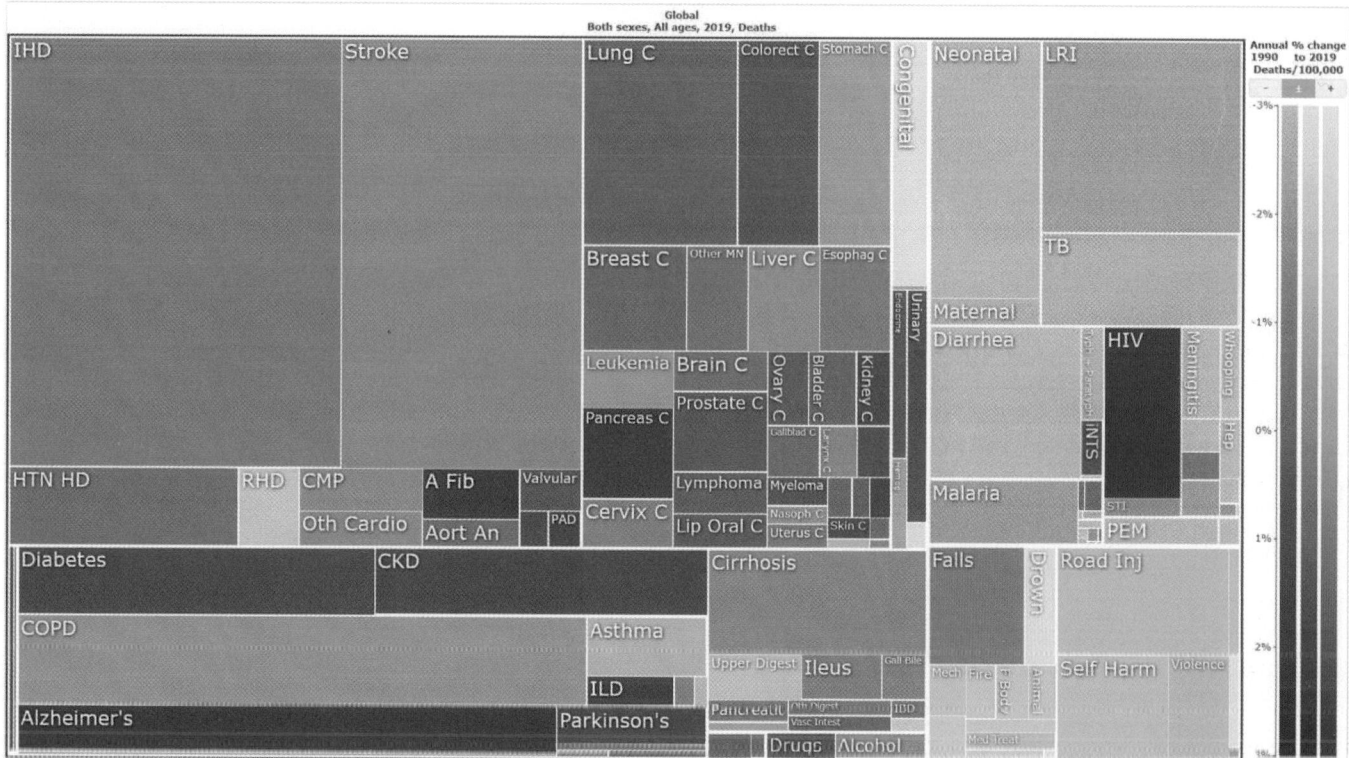

Figure 1–2. Global deaths for Global Burden of Disease level three causes from 2019. Within this tree map, the size of the rectangle for each cause is proportional to the magnitude of the deaths for each cause. Dark shading shows statistically significant changes, and light shading shows changes that are not significant. A Fib, atrial fibrillation, and flutter; Alcohol, alcohol use disorders; Alzheimer's, Alzheimer disease and other dementias; Animal, animal contact; Aort An, aortic aneurysm; Bladder C, bladder cancer; Brain C, brain cancer; Breast C, breast cancer; Cervix C, cervical cancer; Cirrhosis, cirrhosis and other chronic liver diseases; CKD, chronic kidney disease; CMP, cardiomyopathy and myocarditis; Colorect C, colon and rectum cancer; Congenital, congenital birth defects; COPD, chronic obstructive pulmonary disease; Diabetes, diabetes mellitus; Diarrhea, diarrheal diseases; Drown, drowning; Drugs, drug use disorders; Endocrine, endocrine, metabolic, blood, and immune disorders; Esophag C, esophageal cancer; F body, foreign body; Fire, fire, heat, and hot substances; Gall Bile, gallbladder and biliary diseases; Gallblad C, gallbladder and biliary tract cancer; Hemog, hemoglobinopathies and hemolytic anemias; Hep, acute hepatitis; HIV, HIV/AIDS; HTN HD, hypertensive heart disease; IBD, inflammatory bowel disease; IHD, ischemic heart disease; ILD, interstitial lung disease and pulmonary sarcoidosis; Ileus, paralytic ileus and intestinal obstruction; iNTS, invasive nontyphoidal salmonella (iNTS); Kidney C, kidney cancer; Larynx C, larynx cancer; Lip Oral C, lip and oral cavity cancer; Liver C, liver cancer; LRI, lower respiratory infections; Lung C, tracheal, bronchus, and lung cancer; Lymphoma, non-Hodgkin lymphoma; Maternal, maternal disorders; Mech, exposure to mechanical forces; Med Treat, adverse effects of medical treatment; Myeloma, multiple myeloma; Nasoph C, nasopharynx cancer; Neonatal, neonatal disorders; Oth Cardio, other cardiovascular and circulatory diseases; Oth Digest, other digestive diseases; Other MN, other malignant neoplasms; Ovary C, ovarian cancer; PAD, peripheral artery disease; Pancreas C, pancreatic cancer; Pancreatit, pancreatitis; Parkinson's, Parkinson disease; PEM, protein-energy malnutrition; Prostate C, prostate cancer; RHD, rheumatic heart disease; Road Inj, road injuries; Skin C, nonmelanoma skin cancer; STI, sexually transmitted infections excluding HIV; Stomach C, stomach cancer; TB, tuberculosis; Typh + Paratyph, typhoid and paratyphoid; Upper Digest, upper digestive system diseases; Urinary, urinary diseases and male infertility; Uterus C, uterine cancer; Valvular, nonrheumatic valvular heart disease; Vasc Intest, vascular intestinal disorders; Violence, interpersonal violence; Whooping, whooping cough. Data from Global Burden of Disease, 2019 (GBD).

Figure 1–7 shows the percentage of deaths as a result of CVD in 1990 and 2019 by sex. The high-SDI countries saw a significant (52.8%) decline in the age-standardized death rate for males and females. However, the number of CVD-related deaths did not change significantly (2.85 million [95% UI, 2.66-2.95 million] in 1990 to 2.82 million [95% UI, 2.45-3.01 million] in 2019).[4] There is an increased proportion of deaths caused by CVD in low- and middle-SDI countries (see Fig. 1–7). Therefore, the burden of CVD deaths is disproportionately affecting those in low- and middle-SDI countries. Globally, there are complex interactions between environmental exposures, demographic changes, cardiometabolic risk factors, and access to quality health care.[7] In high-SDI countries, changes

in risk factor prevalence and improvements in health care were large contributors to the decreased CVD death rates; in most countries, significant population growth and aging of the population contribute to this trend.[6]

The Impact of Population Growth and Aging on Cardiovascular Disease

Despite an overall decrease in the global age-specific CVD death rate, a continued increase in the number of CVD deaths is expected as a result of demographic changes. The United Nations estimated that the global population in 2019 was 7.7 billion and will increase to a total of 9.7 billion by 2050 with one in six people in the world over the age of 65 (16%) up from

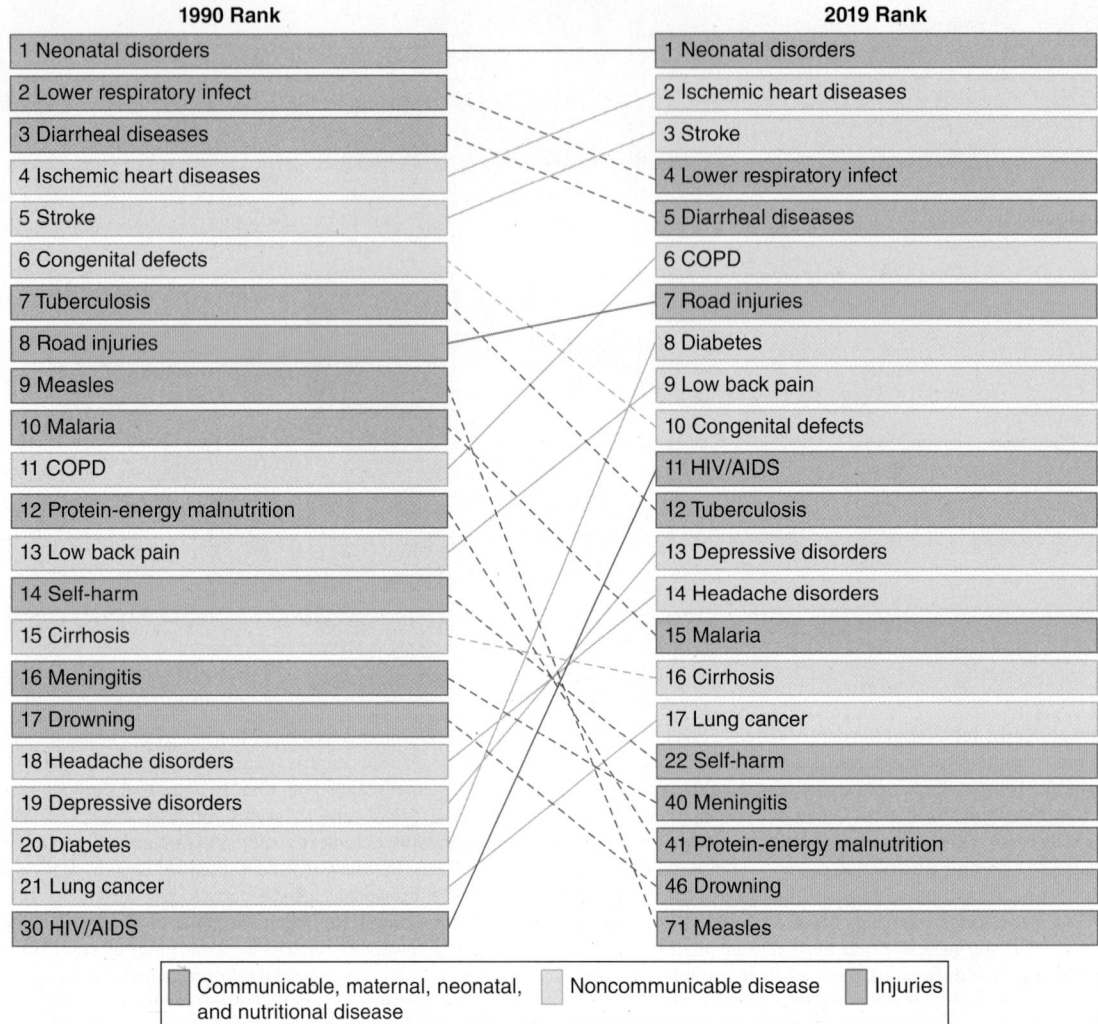

**Global
Both sexes, All ages, DALYs**

1990 Rank

| 1 Neonatal disorders |
| 2 Lower respiratory infect |
| 3 Diarrheal diseases |
| 4 Ischemic heart diseases |
| 5 Stroke |
| 6 Congenital defects |
| 7 Tuberculosis |
| 8 Road injuries |
| 9 Measles |
| 10 Malaria |
| 11 COPD |
| 12 Protein-energy malnutrition |
| 13 Low back pain |
| 14 Self-harm |
| 15 Cirrhosis |
| 16 Meningitis |
| 17 Drowning |
| 18 Headache disorders |
| 19 Depressive disorders |
| 20 Diabetes |
| 21 Lung cancer |
| 30 HIV/AIDS |

2019 Rank

| 1 Neonatal disorders |
| 2 Ischemic heart diseases |
| 3 Stroke |
| 4 Lower respiratory infect |
| 5 Diarrheal diseases |
| 6 COPD |
| 7 Road injuries |
| 8 Diabetes |
| 9 Low back pain |
| 10 Congenital defects |
| 11 HIV/AIDS |
| 12 Tuberculosis |
| 13 Depressive disorders |
| 14 Headache disorders |
| 15 Malaria |
| 16 Cirrhosis |
| 17 Lung cancer |
| 22 Self-harm |
| 40 Meningitis |
| 41 Protein-energy malnutrition |
| 46 Drowning |
| 71 Measles |

Communicable, maternal, neonatal, and nutritional disease   Noncommunicable disease   Injuries

Figure 1–3. Top 20 most common Global Burden of Disease (GBD) level three causes of global disability-adjusted life-years (DALYs) for both sexes combined, 1990 and 2019. Ranks are based on the number of DALYs. Communicable, maternal, neonatal, and nutritional disorders causes are shown in red, noncommunicable causes in blue, and injuries in green. COPD, chronic obstructive pulmonary disease; HIV/AIDS, human immunodeficiency virus/acquired immunodeficiency syndrome. Adapted with permission from GBD 2017 DALYs and HALE Collaborators. Global, regional, and national disability-adjusted life-years (DALYs) for 359 diseases and injuries and healthy life expectancy (HALE) for 195 countries and territories, 1990-2017: a systematic analysis for the Global Burden of Disease Study 2017. *Lancet.* 2018 Nov 10;392(10159):1859-1922.

9% today.[14] When population growth slows down as a result of a reduction in fertility, the population ages and the proportion of older persons increases over time. In 2019, 9% of the population was aged 65 years or older, and the number of adults in this age group is projected to more than double by 2050 and more than triple by 2100, with more than two-thirds of these older adults residing in LMICs. The number of persons aged 80 years or over is projected to triple from 143 million in 2019 to 426 million in 2050.[14,15]

There are regional variations in the contribution of population growth and population aging to trends in the burden of CVD. Demographic changes over the past three decades can be classified into one of six general categories, shown in **Table 1–2**. Categories 1, 2, and 3 represent regions in which population aging and population growth served to drive relative increases in the number of CVD-related deaths. Categories 4, 5, and 6 represent regions in which gains in cardiovascular

health, represented by declines in the age-specific CVD-related death rate, appear to have partially or completely negated the increase in CVD-related deaths caused by population growth and aging. The joint effects of population growth, population aging, and age-specific CVD death rate are also illustrated in **Fig. 1–8**. There is substantial variation in each geographical region, with only Central and Western Europe showing substantial decreases in CVD deaths caused by improvements in cardiovascular health (see Fig. 1–8).[16] Some regions, such as southern Latin America, Australasia, and high-income North America, had no detectable change in the number of deaths because demographic changes balanced out declines in age-specific death rates. Only one region, western sub-Saharan Africa, had an increase in cardiovascular deaths due largely to epidemiologic changes. The high-income Asia-Pacific region has had a rapidly aging population, but the increase in cardiovascular mortality was offset by a significant decline in

TABLE 1–1. Total Estimated Cardiovascular Disease-Related Deaths for Each Cause in 2019

Cause	Deaths in 2019	95% Uncertainty Interval
Ischemic heart disease	9,137,791	(8,395,682–9,743,550)
Stroke	6,552,725	(5,995,200–7,015,139)
Hypertensive heart disease	1,156,733	(859,826–1,278,563)
Cardiomyopathy and myocarditis	340,349	(284,904–371,305)
Atrial fibrillation and flutter	315,337	(267,964–361,014)
Rheumatic heart disease	305,651	(259,220–340,486)
Other cardiovascular and circulatory diseases	276,989	(252,564–301,330)
Aortic aneurysm	172,427	(157,357–182,899)
Non-rheumatic valvular heart disease	164,125	(140,082–179,558)
Peripheral artery disease	74,063	(41,183–128,164)
Endocarditis	66,322	(46,209–75,862)

Data from Roth GA, Mensah GA, Johnson CO, et al. Global Burden of Cardiovascular Diseases and Risk Factors, 1990-2019. Update From the GBD 2019 Study. *J Am Coll Cardiol.* 2020 Dec 22;76(25):2982-3021.

age-specific cardiovascular death rates since 1990. South Asia showed a worrisome pattern, with a dramatic rise in CVD deaths without a significant decline in deaths caused by epidemiologic changes. North Africa and the Middle East offset a similar trend in population growth and aging with a significant reduction in age-specific death rates.[16]

ISCHEMIC HEART DISEASE

IHD is the leading cause of death worldwide and accounted for 9.1 million (95% UI, 8.4–9.7 million) deaths globally in 2019.[4] IHD encompasses myocardial infarction and all other acute coronary syndromes as well as long-term sequelae of coronary heart disease, including angina pectoris and ischemic cardiomyopathy, as well as surgical or percutaneous revascularization and the need for chronic medical therapy when available. Measuring the global burden of IHD is difficult given the challenge of collecting information not only on acute events but also chronic disease that may often go undiagnosed.

Efforts to track international patterns of IHD epidemiology began with the Seven Countries Study starting in the late 1950s and the Monitoring of Trends and Determinants in Cardiovascular Disease (MONICA) studies starting in the 1980s.[17,18] It is difficult to accurately measure IHD prevalence.[19] Efforts to apply standard provocative diagnostic testing, such as exercise treadmill tests, in population-based surveys have been uncommon and have rarely been repeated since the heyday of cardiovascular epidemiology in the late 1970s. Furthermore, nonfatal IHD incidence and prevalence do not always correlate with IHD mortality. For example, one population may have improved acute and chronic IHD treatments, which may

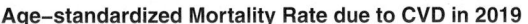
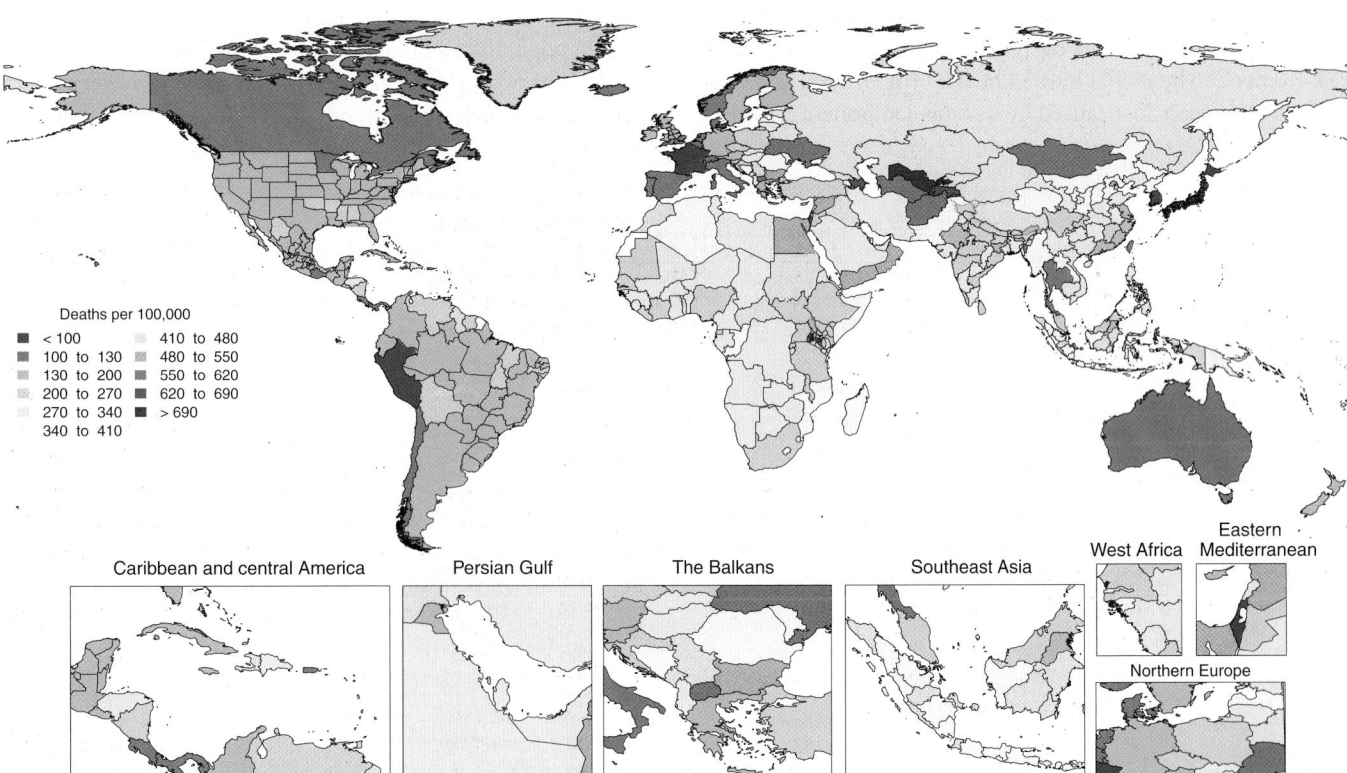

Figure 1–4. Map of age-standardized death rates attributable to cardiovascular disease (CVD), 2019. Countries in blue and green have the lowest death rates, whereas those in orange and red have the highest. Adapted with permission from GBD 2017 DALYs and HALE Collaborators. Global, regional, and national disability-adjusted life-years (DALYs) for 359 diseases and injuries and healthy life expectancy (HALE) for 195 countries and territories, 1990-2017: a systematic analysis for the Global Burden of Disease Study 2017. *Lancet.* 2018 Nov 10;392(10159):1859-1922.

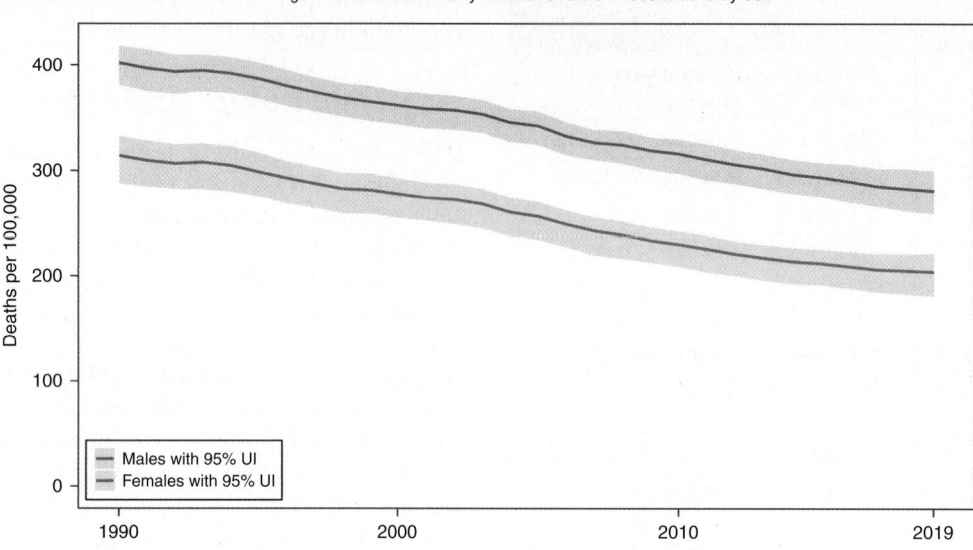

Figure 1–5. Age-standardized death rates for cardiovascular disease (CVD) stratified by sex, 1990 to 2019. UI, uncertainty interval. Data from Global Burden of Disease, 2019 (GBD).

lead to decreased IHD mortality with a growing population of chronic IHD survivors, whereas another population may have a high IHD incidence with a high case fatality rate that may lead to a relatively low prevalence. Furthermore, stable angina prevalence is based on self-reported symptoms and does not necessarily correlate directly with acute coronary syndrome event incidence; in fact, in many surveys, stable angina prevalence is higher in women, despite the higher acute IHD event risk in men.[20] The global burden of IHD (in DALYs) is dominated by life-years lost caused by its fatal component, whereas

disability from nonfatal IHD, including acute nonfatal acute coronary syndromes, makes a smaller contribution.[5]

Globally, the age-standardized IHD incidence decreased from 1990 to 2019, from 405.3 per 100,000 to 333.5 in males and from 239.9 per 100,000 to 198.5 in females.[4] However, an IHD epidemic has emerged in certain regions. For example, in Eastern Europe, there was an increased IHD incidence (100 per 100,000 population in males and 53 per 100,000 population in females), as well as increased IHD mortality, between 1990 and the mid-2000s. This trend was correlated with changing

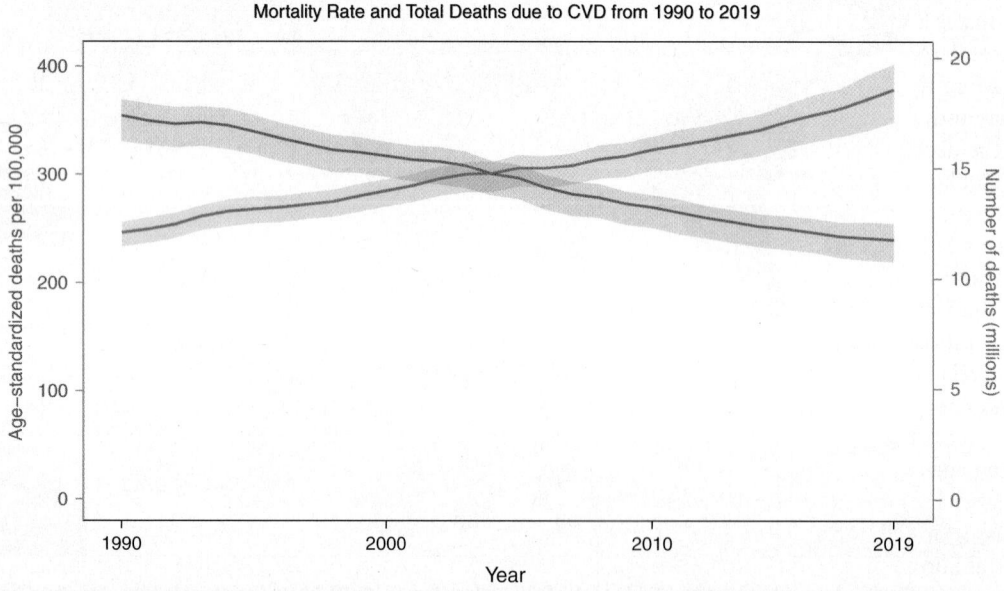

Figure 1–6. Change in age-standardized cardiovascular disease (CVD) death rate and total number of CVD deaths, 1990 to 2019. Data from Global Burden of Disease, 2019 (GBD).

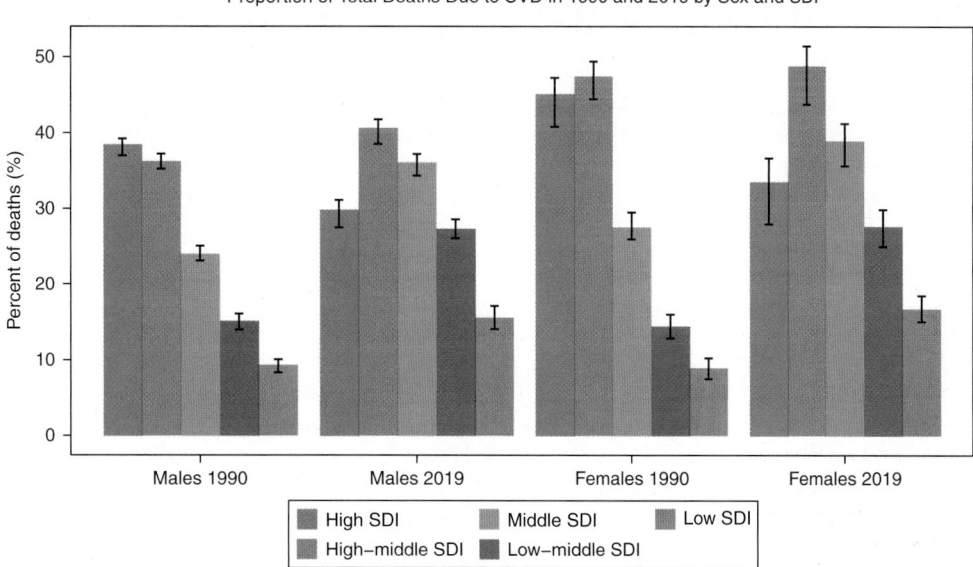

Figure 1–7. Proportion of total deaths attributable to cardiovascular disease (CVD) by sociodemographic index (SDI) stratified by sex, 1990 to 2019. Data from Global Burden of Disease, 2019 (GBD).

sociopolitical circumstances after the breakup of the Soviet Union in the early 1990s.[4] The reason for this increased incidence is controversial but may be due in part to unhealthy patterns of alcohol consumption, smoking, and hypertension, as peak IHD death rates coincided with economic downturns and societal unrest, with the largest fluctuations in the non–myocardial infarction portion of IHD deaths.[21,22] Central and Eastern Europe and Central Asia experienced a combined 26.3 million years of life lost (YLLs) in 2019 because of IHD, third only to Southeast Asia, East Asia, and Oceania and to South Asia despite having less than a fifth and a fourth of the population, respectively (**Table 1–3**).[4]

Since 1990, Australasia, Western Europe, and North America have seen dramatic declines in the age-standardized IHD mortality in both males and females.[4] In 2019, there was wide variation in age-standardized IHD mortality rates across the globe (**Fig. 1–9**). More recently, North Africa and the Middle East, Central Asia, and Eastern Europe have also started to decline. Globally, the decline in age-standardized deaths attributable to IHD is similar for males (30% decline) and females (33% decline).[4] However, this dramatic decline in IHD mortality has stalled in several high-income countries.[23,24] Since 2015, increasing age-standardized IHD DALYs have been seen in Canada, parts of the United States, the United Kingdom, and New Zealand.[4] IHD mortality has actually increased in Oceania and East Asia and is relatively unchanged in Southeast Asia, sub-Saharan Africa, and South Asia, leading to an increased burden of disease in these areas. The large population in these regions and relatively young age at IHD death leads to more YLLs per fatal case and a higher DALY burden. Percentages of YLLs due to premature disease for IHD are highest in Eastern Europe, Central Asia, Central Europe, and North Africa, and the Middle East. Current estimates suggest over half of global IHD DALYs occurred in low-middle– and middle-SDI countries.[4] There is

significant variation in age-standardized DALYs within regions, with the most variation in middle-SDI countries and lowest variation in high-SDI countries. Although IHD burden falls largely on those aged older than 70 years in high-SDI regions, the age of IHD deaths is much younger in other regions (**Fig. 1–10**). Although the age-standardized IHD DALYs have decreased in most countries, the DALYs for Oceania have increased.[4]

As more patients with IHD survive their initial event, the IHD death rate and case fatality will no longer be the sole public health benchmark for success; improved symptom control and overall quality of life and access to adequate treatment will be important secondary outcomes. The mainstays of treatment include standard, low-cost medications that are insufficiently used in low- and middle-SDI countries. The Prospective Urban Rural Epidemiological (PURE) study found that only 11% of patients from high-income countries were not taking standard secondary prevention medications, whereas 80% of low-income region patients were taking none of the recommended medications.[25,26] Overall, the availability of guideline-recommended medications is low and often not affordable, resulting in few essential CVD medicines meeting the World Health Organization (WHO) target in low- and middle-SDI countries.[27,28] Prevention of risk factors and improved access to essential medications that are not only available but also affordable remain key to reversing both the IHD and stroke pandemics globally. In addition, universal access to organized acute coronary syndrome and acute stroke services remains a priority, especially in the poorest areas.[9,29]

STROKE

Global stroke burden continues to rise, with low-, low-middle–, and middle-SDI countries contributing 86% of incident cases, 89% of deaths, and 91% of stroke-related DALYs.[4] Stroke is the

TABLE 1–2. Patterns of Demographic and Epidemiologic Changes in Cardiovascular Mortality

Category	Change in Cardiovascular Deaths, 1990–2013	Effect of Population Growth	Effect of Population Aging	Effect of Age-Specific Cardiovascular Death Rate	Regions
Category 1—Population growth and aging: Regions with large and continuous increases in the number of cardiovascular deaths due to population growth or aging but little change in age-specific rates of death	Increase	Large (≥20%)	Large (>30%)	Small (decline <30%)	Oceania, South Asia, Southeast Asia, Caribbean
Category 2—Population growth: Regions with increases in deaths due mostly to population growth	Increase	Large (>80%)	Small (<10%)	Small (decline <30%)	Central sub-Saharan Africa, Western sub-Saharan Africa, Eastern sub-Saharan Africa
Category 3—Population aging: Regions in which cardiovascular deaths rose and then fell during the preceding 20 years, resulting in a net increase in deaths due to population aging and only a small decrease in age-specific rates of cardiovascular death	Increase then decrease	Very small (<20%)	Moderate (>20%)	Very small (decline <15%)	Eastern Europe, Central Asia
Category 4—Improved health moderating effect of population aging: Regions in which large increases in the number of cardiovascular deaths due to population aging were moderated by a fall in age-specific rates of death	Increase	Small (<30%)	Very large (>70%)	Large (decline >30%)	High-income Asia-Pacific, East Asia
Category 5—Improved health moderating effect of population growth and aging: Regions with large relative increases in the number of cardiovascular deaths due to both population growth and aging that were moderated by a fall in age-specific rates of death	Increase	Large (>30%)	Large (>30%)	Large (decline >30%)	Central Latin America, Tropical Latin America, Andean Latin America, Southern sub-Saharan Africa, North Africa and Middle East
Category 6—Improved health exceeding effect of population growth and aging: Regions in which large declines in age-specific cardiovascular death rates have led to only small increases or even a decline in the number of cardiovascular deaths despite the large effects of an aging population	Small increase or decrease	Small (<40%)	Large (>30%)	Large (decline >30%)	Southern Latin America, Australasia, high-income North America, Central Europe, Western Europe

Reproduced with permission from Roth GA, Forouzanfar MH, Moran AE, et al. Demographic and epidemiologic drivers of global cardiovascular mortality. *N Engl J Med.* 2015 Apr 2;372(14):1333-1341.

leading cause of death in high-income Asia-Pacific, Southeast Asia, East Asia, and sub-Saharan Africa.[1] Since 1990, there have been significant increases in (1) the absolute number of DALYs caused by ischemic stroke (IS); (2) deaths from IS, intracerebral hemorrhage, and subarachnoid hemorrhage; and therefore, (3) survivors and incident events for all causes of stroke.[4]

Overall, the age-standardized rates of stroke mortality have decreased worldwide in the past three decades. However, similar to IHD, the absolute number of people living with stroke is increasing. In 2019, there were an estimated 101 million stroke survivors (73% with IS), 6.6 million deaths from stroke (50% died from IS), 143 million DALYs caused by stroke (44% as a result of IS), and 12.2 million new strokes (62% IS).[4]

Figure 1–11 represents the incidence rates of stroke broken down into 5-year age bands for males and females in 2019. Overall, the age-adjusted incidence rate of stroke decreased over the 30-year period in both males and females. IS prevalence rates were significantly higher for females compared with males in both 1990 and 2019. The increase in number of prevalent cases of IS between 1990 and 2019 despite significant declines in incident stroke is consistent with change caused by population growth, population aging, and, for some regions, decreases in stroke-related mortality.[4,30] As stroke survival improves, there is a greater need for secondary prevention and rehabilitation.[31] While the incidence of stroke is decreasing globally, the age-standardized prevalence rates for stroke have not changed significantly globally (IS: 969 per 100,000 in 1990 vs 951 per 100,000 in 2019; intracerebral hemorrhage: 299 per 100,000 in 1990 vs 249 per 100,000 in 2019; subarachnoid hemorrhage: 117 per 100,000 in 1990 vs 102 per 100,000 in 2019).[4] Between 1990 and 2019, small downward trends in prevalence were seen in Eastern Europe and Central Asia, as well as Latin America.[4]

As with IHD, there was significant regional variation in the age-adjusted incidence, prevalence, and mortality of IS, intracerebral hemorrhage, and subarachnoid hemorrhage. The highest age-standardized prevalence of IS (1080 per 100,000)

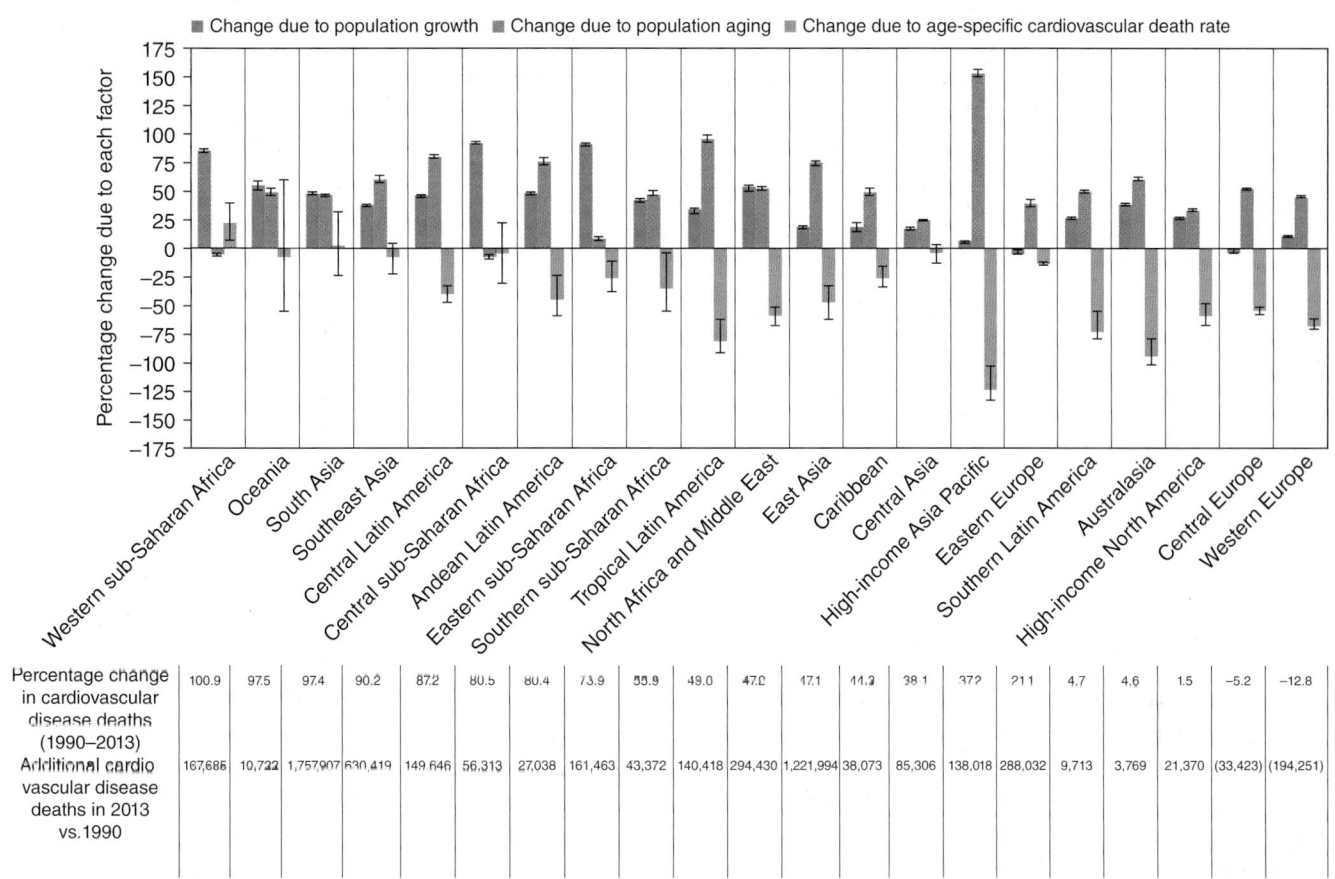

	Western sub-Saharan Africa	Oceania	South Asia	Southeast Asia	Central Latin America	Central sub-Saharan Africa	Andean Latin America	Eastern sub-Saharan Africa	Southern sub-Saharan Africa	Tropical Latin America	North Africa and Middle East	East Asia	Caribbean	Central Asia	High-income Asia Pacific	Eastern Europe	Southern Latin America	Australasia	High-income North America	Central Europe	Western Europe
Percentage change in cardiovascular disease deaths (1990–2013)	100.9	97.5	97.4	90.2	87.2	80.5	80.4	73.9	53.9	49.0	47.0	17.1	14.3	38.1	37.2	21.1	4.7	4.6	1.5	−5.2	−12.8
Additional cardiovascular disease deaths in 2013 vs.1990	167,686	10,722	1,757,907	630,419	149,646	56,313	27,038	161,463	43,372	140,418	294,430	1,221,994	38,073	85,306	138,018	288,032	9,713	3,769	21,370	(33,423)	(194,251)

Figure 1–8. Contribution of changes in population growth, population aging, and rates of age-specific cardiovascular death to changes in cardiovascular mortality, 1990 to 2013. Reproduced with permission from Roth GA, Forouzanfar MH, Moran AE, et al. Demographic and epidemiologic drivers of global cardiovascular mortality. *N Engl J Med.* 2015 Apr 2;372(14):1333-1341.

was found in middle-SDI countries, with the lowest (756 per 100,000) in low- and low-middle–SDI countries (**Fig. 1–12**). The highest IS mortality (from 133 to 206 per 100,000 person-years) was observed in Serbia, Bulgaria, and North Macedonia, with the lowest (≤20 per 100,000 person-years) seen in Australasia, Andean and Central Latin America, and high-income Asia-Pacific and North America. Prevalence of intracerebral hemorrhage was highest (664–972 per 100,000) in Oceania, Mongolia, Papua New Guinea, Indonesia, and Kiribati and lowest (<100 per 100,000) in Canada, Slovenia, Australasia, and parts of Western Europe. Intracerebral hemorrhage death rates were highest (178–215 per 100,000 person-years) in Mongolia and Solomon Islands and lowest (<10 per 100,000) in high-income Asia-Pacific and North America, most parts of Western Europe, and Australasia. The highest age-standardized prevalence of subarachnoid hemorrhage was observed in Japan (373 per 100,000), and the lowest (<50 per 100,000) was observed in several countries in sub-Saharan Africa and Iran. Mortality of subarachnoid hemorrhage was highest (>14 per 100,000 person-years) in Georgia, Mongolia, Kiribati, and the Solomon Islands and lowest (<1.7 per 100,000 person-years) in parts of Africa and Malta.[4]

IS incidence and prevalence in high-SDI countries were greater and demonstrated a steeper increase with age than those in low- and middle-SDI countries at younger ages, whereas IS death rates after the age of 49 years were greater in low- and middle-SDI countries (see Fig. 1–11). The age-related patterns of increase in IS mortality were similar across SDI.[4] The prevalence of intracerebral hemorrhage and the age-specific incidence and mortality of intracerebral hemorrhage were statistically significantly greater in low- and high-SDI countries in younger individuals, but there was no statistically significant difference in the age-specific prevalence between low- and high-SDI countries after 74 years of age.[4]

Stroke was the second largest contributor to DALYs globally and in high-, high-middle–, middle-, and low-middle–SDI countries, whereas it was the fifth largest contributor in low-SDI countries, with significant regional variation in disease burden.[4] There is a diverging trend between countries with middle SDI and high SDI, with a significant increase in stroke DALYs and deaths in middle-SDI countries and no measurable change in the proportional contribution of DALYs and deaths from stroke in high-SDI countries.[4] Globally, the proportional contribution of stroke-related DALYs as a proportion of all diseases increased from 4.2% (95% UI, 3.9%–4.5%) in 1990 to 5.7% (95% UI, 5.1%–6.2%) in 2019. The deaths caused by stroke also increased from 9.8% (95% UI, 9.3%–10.5%) in 1990 to 11.6% (95% UI, 10.8%–12.2%) in 2019.[5]

TABLE 1–3. Years of Life Lost Owing to Ischemic Heart Disease in the Global Burden of Disease 2019 Study, Males and Females, by 21 Regions, 1990 and 2019

Region	Number of YLLs, 1990	Lower 95% UI, 1990	Upper 95% UI, 1990	Number of YLLs, 2019	Lower 95% UI, 2019	Upper 95% UI, 2019
Central Asia	2,632,445	2,545,455	2,698,237	4,193,060	3,805,733	4,622,856
Central Europe	7,270,913	7,051,268	7,393,524	5,280,417	4,631,978	5,933,738
Eastern Europe	14,878,036	14,350,993	15,222,300	16,786,349	15,092,893	18,434,645
Australasia	704,544	674,658	721,943	441,285	398,681	467,806
High-income Asia Pacific	2,712,332	2,589,329	2,782,838	2,239,019	1,939,844	2,424,060
High-income North America	11,062,923	10,536,525	11,337,415	9,353,953	8,728,741	9,850,719
Southern Latin America	1,241,317	1,199,916	1,270,908	1,035,084	970,219	1,088,501
Western Europe	15,085,392	14,470,352	15,416,043	8,691,020	7,955,168	9,190,341
Andean Latin America	407,027	363,300	455,448	614,242	505,102	743,726
Caribbean	881,746	839,646	926,212	1,209,969	1,039,946	1,398,484
Central Latin America	1,955,852	1,888,099	2,012,590	4,010,034	3,492,323	4,655,449
Tropical Latin America	2,782,579	2,690,515	2,864,504	3,668,963	3,458,456	3,837,518
North Africa and Middle East	10,719,667	9,921,716	11,566,815	17,643,805	15,257,317	20,451,537
South Asia	20,700,892	18,562,073	22,694,676	45,278,458	39,855,937	51,203,327
East Asia	14,662,303	12,914,367	16,487,010	33,868,197	29,134,539	38,785,107
Oceania	138,465	111,278	176,965	350,871	277,524	449,402
Southeast Asia	6,101,820	5,562,728	6,630,373	13,418,090	12,052,526	14,853,182
Central Sub-Saharan Africa	587,452	485,898	719,928	1,163,465	891,503	1,522,189
Eastern Sub-Saharan Africa	1,475,830	1,265,481	1,702,935	2,820,152	2,284,074	3,388,301
Southern Sub-Saharan Africa	493,341	447,998	541,753	936,492	846,161	1,033,831
Western Sub-Saharan Africa	1,904,550	1,565,984	2,399,205	3,631,991	2,974,717	4,360,995

Abbreviations: UI, uncertainty interval; YLLs, years of life lost.
Data from Roth GA, Mensah GA, Johnson CO, et al. Global Burden of Cardiovascular Diseases and Risk Factors, 1990-2019: Update From the GBD 2019 Study. *J Am Coll Cardiol.* 2020 Dec 22;76(25):2982-3021.

ABDOMINAL AORTIC ANEURYSM

Abdominal aortic aneurysm (AAA) is a focal dilatation of the abdominal aorta of at least 1.5 times the normal diameter or an absolute value of 3.0 cm or greater. Risk factors include male sex, smoking, hypertension, atherosclerosis, and history of AAA in a first-degree relative. Mortality is high for those previously undiagnosed, and up to 90% die if rupture occurs outside the hospital. The global age-specific prevalence and incidence rates increase with age, are higher in males than females, are higher in developed countries than developing countries, and were higher in 1990 than they are today.

In 2010, the age-specific prevalence per 100,000 ranged from 7.9 (95% CI, 6.54–9.59) to 2274 (95% CI, 2149.77–2410.17). Prevalence was higher in developed versus developing nations. The age-specific annual incidence per 100,000 also ranged from 0.83 (95% CI, 0.61–1.11) to 164.6 (95% CI, 152.20–178.78). The highest prevalence was in Australasia at 310.27 (95% CI, 289.01–332.94).[32] The associated death rates declined in the early 2000s in high-SDI countries but then started to rise again over the past 10 years. While global death rate trends remained constant over the past 30 years, DALYs have increased from 2.0 million (95% UI, 1.8–2.2 million) in 1990 to 3.3 million (95% UI, 3.1–3.5 million) in 2019 with significant regional variations.[5] Tropical Latin America has the highest age-standardized death rate, followed by Asia-Pacific high-income countries.[1] Reducing the burden of AAA will require significant risk factor reduction, especially smoking, as well as improvements in diagnosis, treatment, and overall disease surveillance.

PERIPHERAL ARTERIAL DISEASE

Peripheral arterial disease (PAD) is a circulatory problem in which narrowed arteries reduce blood flow to the limbs and cause symptoms of leg pain with walking (claudication). PAD is defined as ankle-brachial index (ABI) lower than or equal to 0.90. Globally, the burden of PAD is increasing. Between 1990 and 2019, prevalent cases increased from 65.8 million (95% UI, 57.2–74.5 million) to 113.4 million (95% UI, 99.2–128.4 million). Of the 113.4 million people living with PAD in 2019, 29.6 million live in East Asia with a significant portion under the age of 50 years[4] (**Fig. 1–13**). The burden of PAD has steadily increased over time, but the rate of change is lowest in

Age–standardized Mortality Rate due to Ischemic Heart Disease in 2019

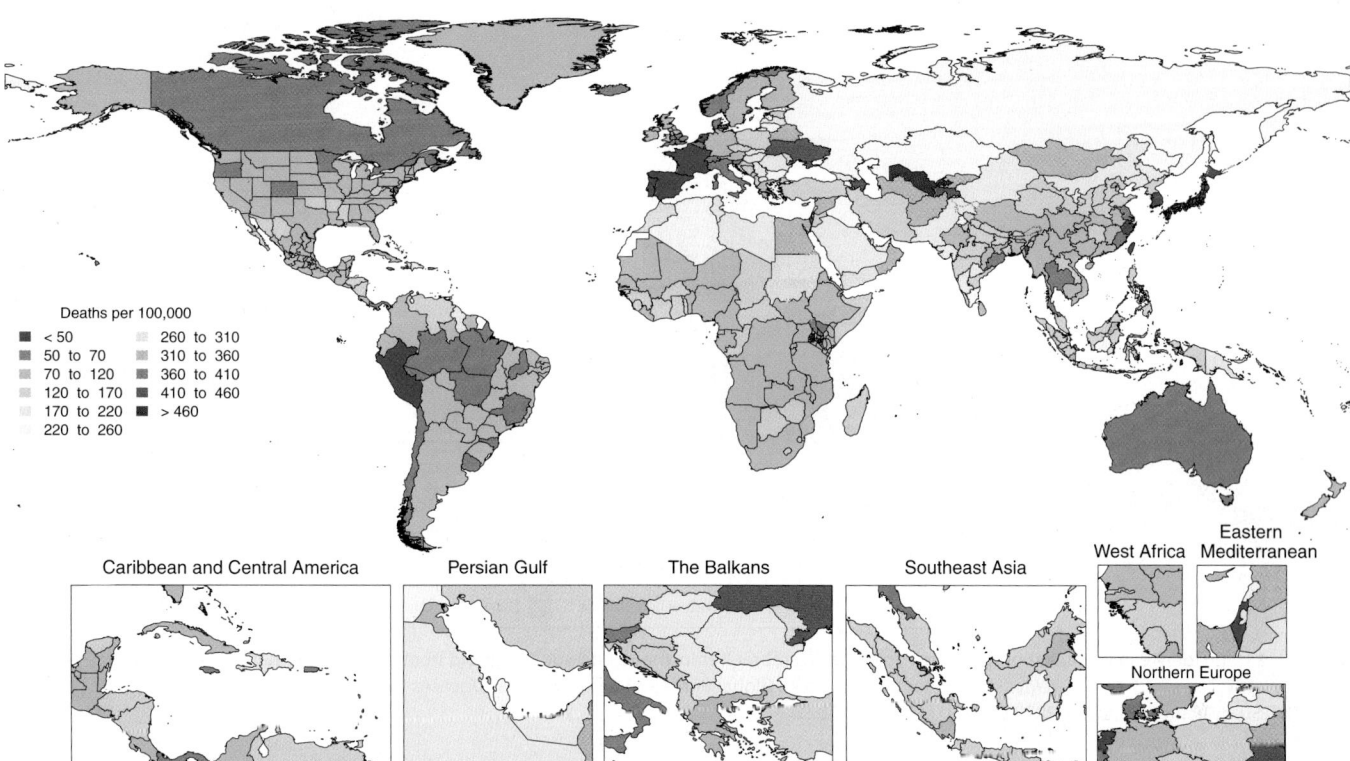

Deaths per 100,000
- ■ < 50
- ■ 50 to 70
- ■ 70 to 120
- ■ 120 to 170
- ■ 170 to 220
- ■ 220 to 260
- ■ 260 to 310
- ■ 310 to 360
- ■ 360 to 410
- ■ 410 to 460
- ■ > 460

Caribbean and Central America   Persian Gulf   The Balkans   Southeast Asia   West Africa   Eastern Mediterranean

Northern Europe

Figure 1–9. Map of age-standardized ischemic heart disease mortality rate per 100,000 persons in 21 world regions in 2019, according to the Global Burden of Disease 2019 Study. Data from Global Burden of Disease, 2019 (GBD).

high- and high-middle–SDI countries (the number of individuals with PAD between 1990 and 2019 increased by 126% in low-SDI countries vs 20% in high-SDI countries).[4]

The age distribution varies by region. In high-SDI countries, among adults age 50 to 69 years, the prevalence was similar for males and females (4.0% for males vs 5.3% for females) in 2019.

The prevalence increases to around 16.6% for males and 23.6% for females in those aged over 80 years. In middle-SDI countries, in the same age groups, the prevalence is around 4.5% for females and 2.2% for males and increases to 16.8% in females and 8.6% in males.[4] In high-SDI countries, notably Europe and North America, the largest age group with PAD was more than

Number of Ischemic Heart Disease Deaths in 2019 by Age

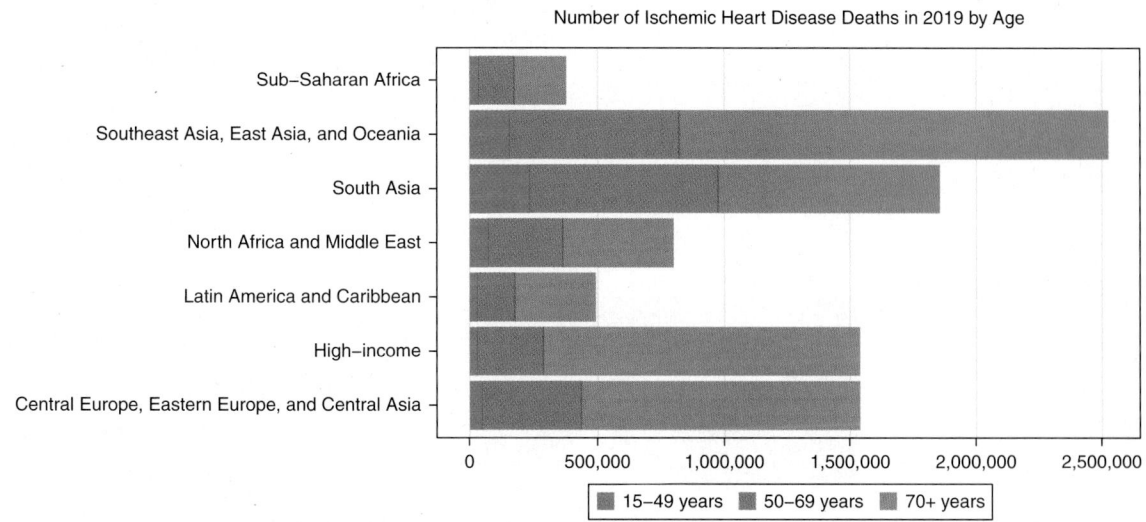

- Sub–Saharan Africa
- Southeast Asia, East Asia, and Oceania
- South Asia
- North Africa and Middle East
- Latin America and Caribbean
- High–income
- Central Europe, Eastern Europe, and Central Asia

0   500,000   1,000,000   1,500,000   2,000,000   2,500,000

■ 15–49 years   ■ 50–69 years   ■ 70+ years

Figure 1–10. Age composition of absolute numbers of ischemic heart disease deaths in 2019, by super-region, the Global Burden of Diseases, Injuries, and Risk Factors 2019 study. Data from Global Burden of Disease, 2019 (GBD).

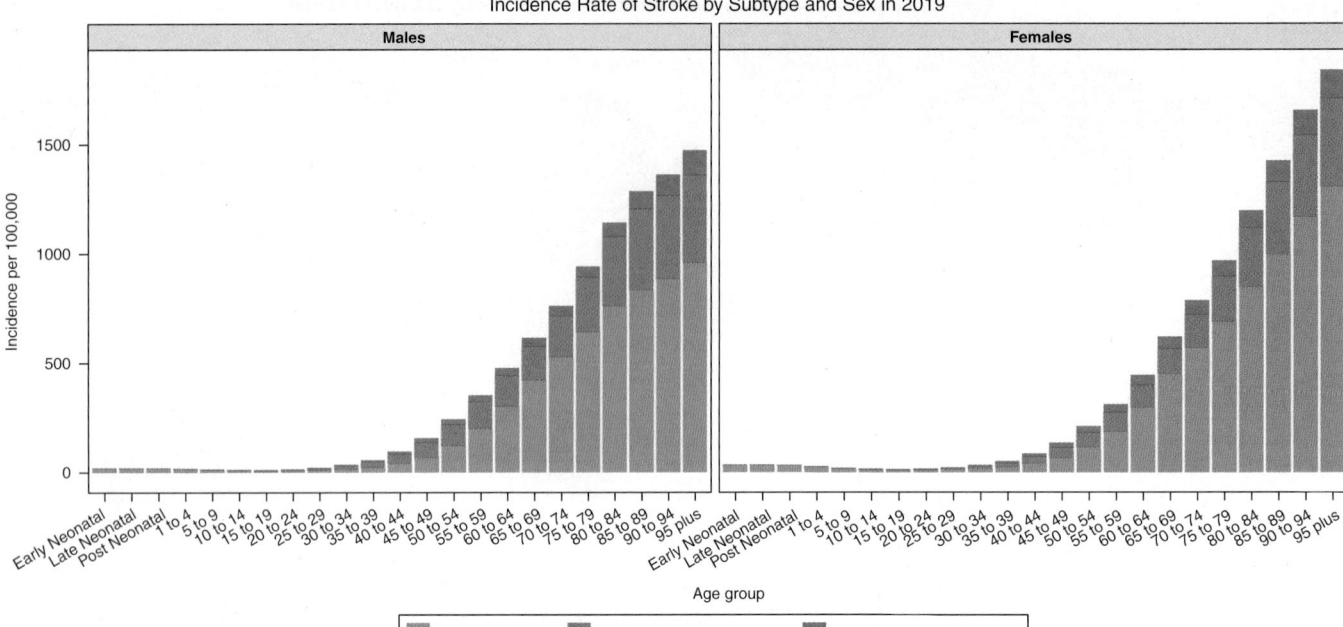

Figure 1–11. Incidence per 100,000 of ischemic stroke, intracerebral hemorrhage and subarachnoid hemorrhage in females and males by 5-year age bands in 2019. Data from Roth GA, Mensah GA, Johnson CO, et al. Global Burden of Cardiovascular Diseases and Risk Factors, 1990-2019: Update From the GBD 2019 Study. *J Am Coll Cardiol.* 2020 Dec 22;76(25):2982-3021.

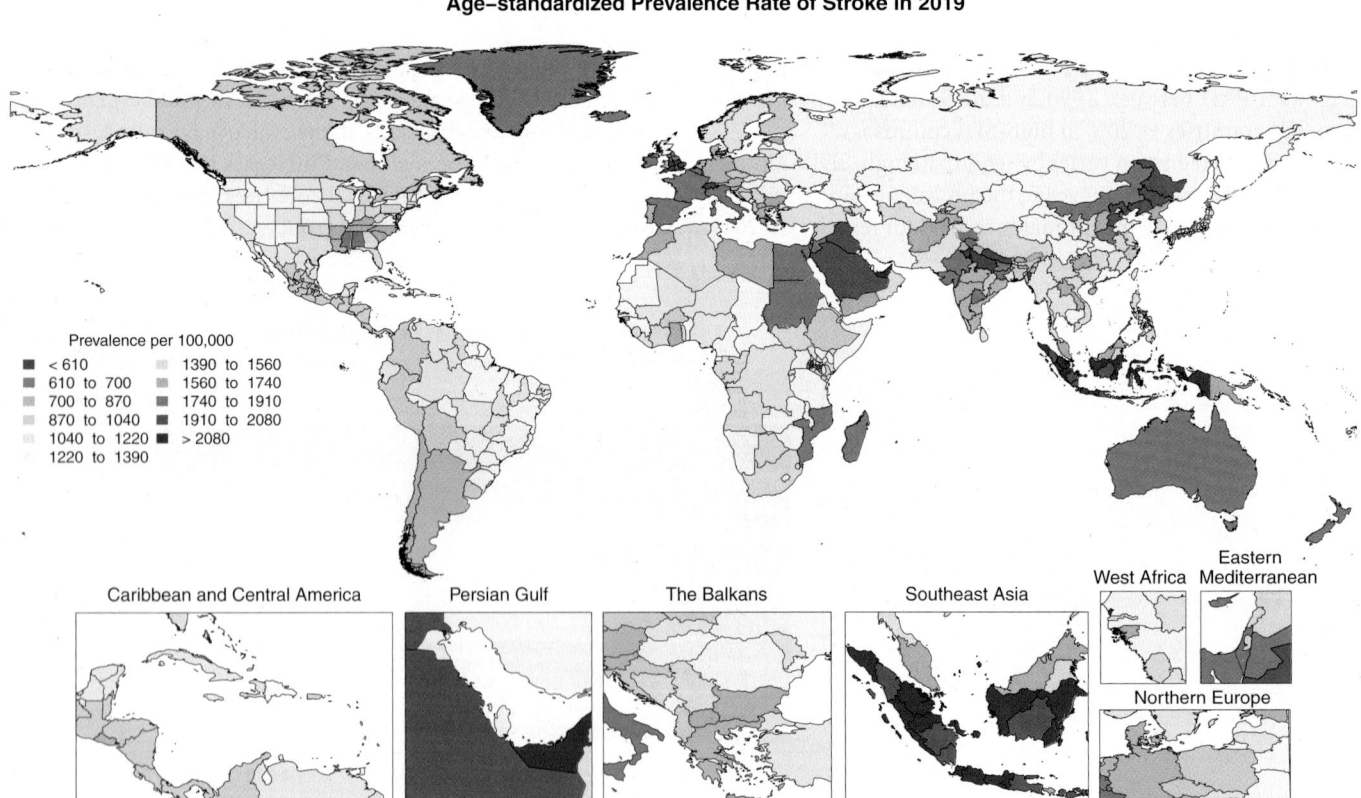

Figure 1–12. Age-standardized prevalence (A) and mortality (B) of stroke per 100,000 person-years in various regions in 2019. Reproduced with permission from Roth GA, Mensah GA, Johnson CO, et al. Global Burden of Cardiovascular Diseases and Risk Factors, 1990-2019: Update From the GBD 2019 Study. *J Am Coll Cardiol.* 2020 Dec 22;76(25):2982-3021.

Age–standardized Mortality Rate due to Stroke in 2019

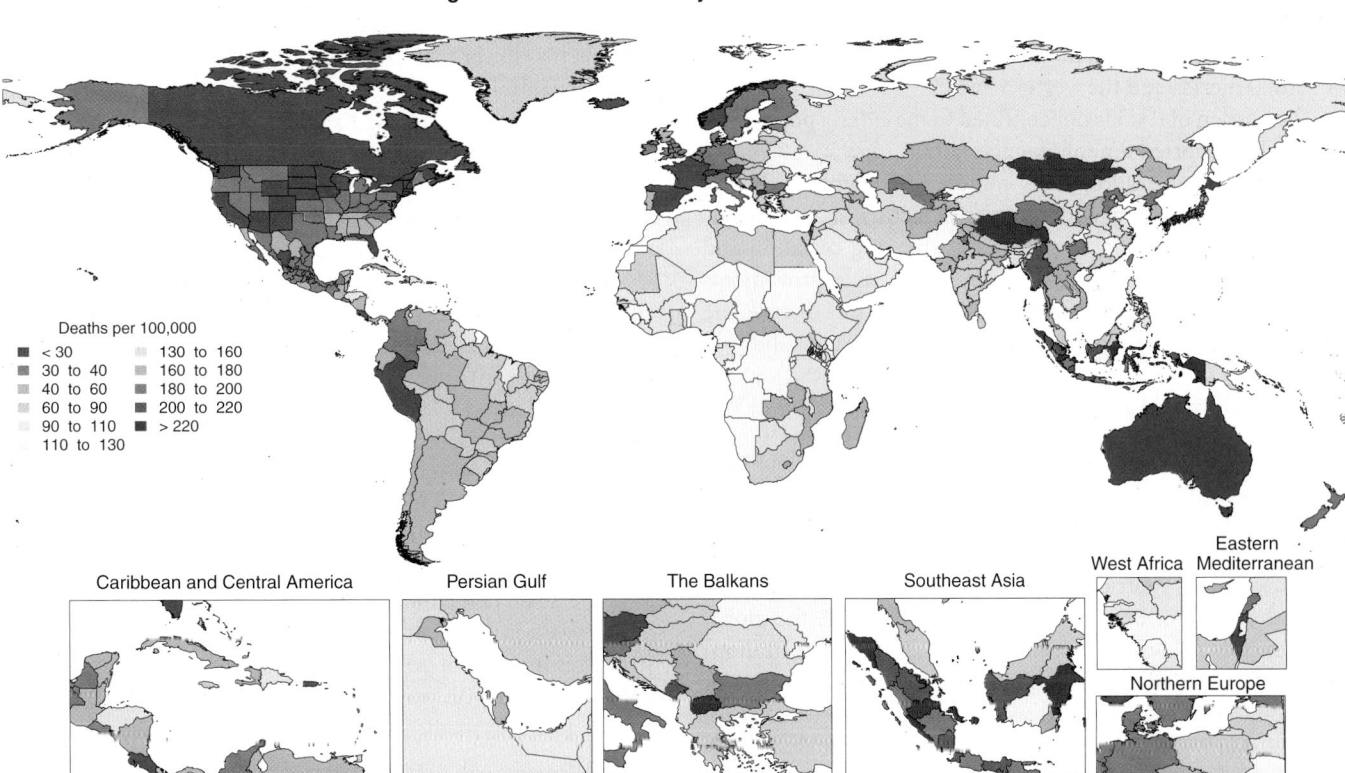

Deaths per 100,000
- < 30
- 30 to 40
- 40 to 60
- 60 to 90
- 90 to 110
- 110 to 130
- 130 to 160
- 160 to 180
- 180 to 200
- 200 to 220
- > 220

Caribbean and Central America   Persian Gulf   The Balkans   Southeast Asia   West Africa   Eastern Mediterranean

Northern Europe

Figure 1–12. (Continued)

55 years of age, compared to western Pacific and Southeast Asia regions where the majority of cases were in people younger than 55 years.

Smoking is an important risk factor, with an odds ratio for current smoking of 2.72 (95% confidence interval [CI],

2.39–3.09) in high-income countries and 1.42 (95% CI, 1.25–1.62) in LMICs; diabetes, hypertension, and hypercholesterolemia are other significant risk factors.[33]

Disability and mortality associated with PAD have increased over the past 30 years, with 74,063 (95% UI, 41,183–128,164)

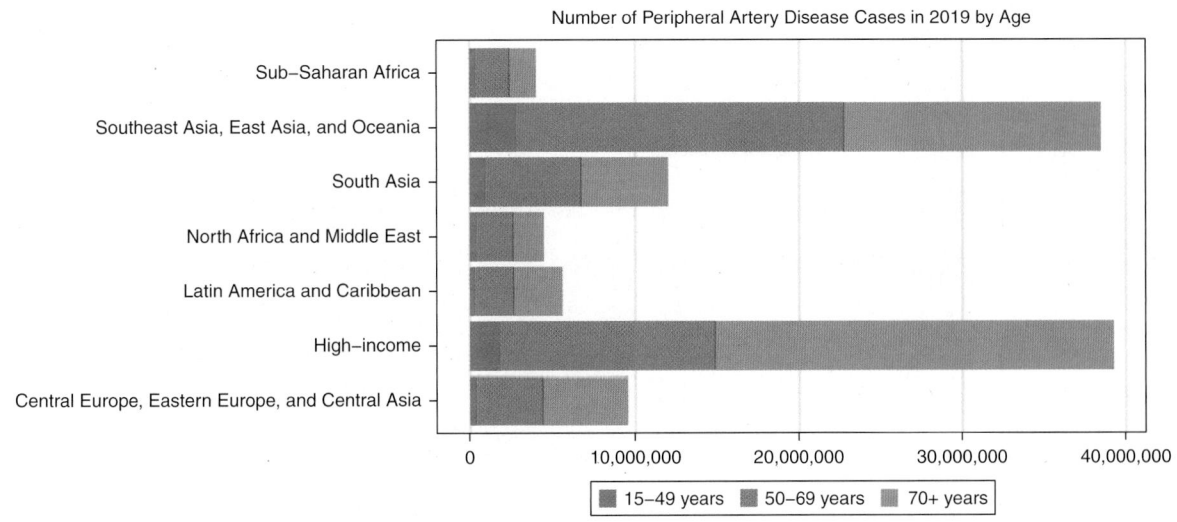

Number of Peripheral Artery Disease Cases in 2019 by Age

Legend: 15–49 years, 50–69 years, 70+ years

Figure 1–13. **Estimate of the number of cases of peripheral arterial disease, and contributing age groups, by super regions in 2019.** Data from Roth GA, Mensah GA, Johnson CO, et al. Global Burden of Cardiovascular Diseases and Risk Factors, 1990-2019: Update From the GBD 2019 Study. *J Am Coll Cardiol.* 2020 Dec 22;76(25):2982-3021.

deaths in 2019, and this increase in burden has been greatest among women in the high-income Asia-Pacific region.[4] While Europe has the largest number of deaths, DALYs are increasing in Latin America and the western Pacific.[1]

The burden of PAD is not confined to the elderly population and is also reported among younger adults (age 50–69 years), especially in high-middle– and middle-SDI countries. Multi-faceted approaches that address the risk factors, such as avoiding smoking initiation and promoting smoking cessation and promoting exercise and healthful diet, as well as improvements in the diagnosis, treatment, and prevention of this disease, are all urgently needed to reduce the burden of PAD globally.[4]

ATRIAL FIBRILLATION

Atrial fibrillation (AF) and atrial flutter are irregular heart rhythms that often cause a rapid heart rate and can increase the risk of stroke, heart failure, and other heart-related complications. During AF, the atria beat chaotically and out of "sync" with the ventricles. Symptoms include heart palpitations, shortness of breath, and weakness. In 2019, the global prevalence of AF was 59.7 million (95% UI, 45.7–75.3 million) with over 15 million patients (95% UI, 11.2–19.4 million) over the age of 80 years. The DALYs have rapidly increased from 3.8 million (95% UI, 3.0–4.8 million) in 1990 to 8.4 million (95% UI, 6.7–10.5 million) in 2019.[5] The death rate has increased slightly since 1990 to 4.1 per 100,000, but because of population aging, the number of deaths due to AF has increased 169% from 117,038 (95% UI, 103,695–138,452) in 1990 to 315,337 (95% UI, 267,964–361,014) in 2019.[1] Overall, there is a significantly lower estimated AF prevalence rate and death rate in low- and low-middle–SDI countries compared to high- and high-middle–SDI countries; AF is rapidly increasing in the 50- to 60-year age group in middle-SDI countries.[4] It is unclear whether the significantly lower estimated burden of AF in lower SDI countries represents less AF due to fewer risk factors, such as lower rates of obesity and obstructive sleep apnea, or lower rates of detection caused by less awareness of the condition or decreased access to diagnostic technology such as electrocardiograms. AF in low-SDI countries is more likely to be valvular in nature, caused by RHD, compared with the non-valvular AF most commonly seen in high-SDI countries. As a result, AF may be less recognized as a separate condition and less reported as an underlying cause of death in some low-SDI countries.

In 2019, the estimated age-standardized DALYs resulting from AF were 107 per 100,000 population (95% UI, 86–134); DALY burden was higher in males (114 per 100,000; 95% UI, 90–144) compared to females (101 per 100,000; 95% UI, 81–126)[4] with variation in sex by SDI (**Fig. 1–14**). A rapid rise in AF has been observed in death records in the United States since the year 2010 despite little evidence for significant changes in AF incidence or survival in that country.[34,35] There is increased awareness and detection of AF, and improved treatment of IHD has allowed individuals to reach older ages at which embolic stroke, as a result of AF, is more common. Higher burden in men compared with women may reflect actual disease rates or poorer access to medical care among women in resource-poor settings.

CONGENITAL HEART DISEASE

Congenital heart disease (CHD) is a group of birth defects that range in severity from mild to severe. Estimates for GBD were generated for an aggregate of five subcategories of CHD (single ventricle and single ventricle pathway congenital heart anomalies; severe congenital heart anomalies excluding single ventricle heart defects; critical malformations of great vessels,

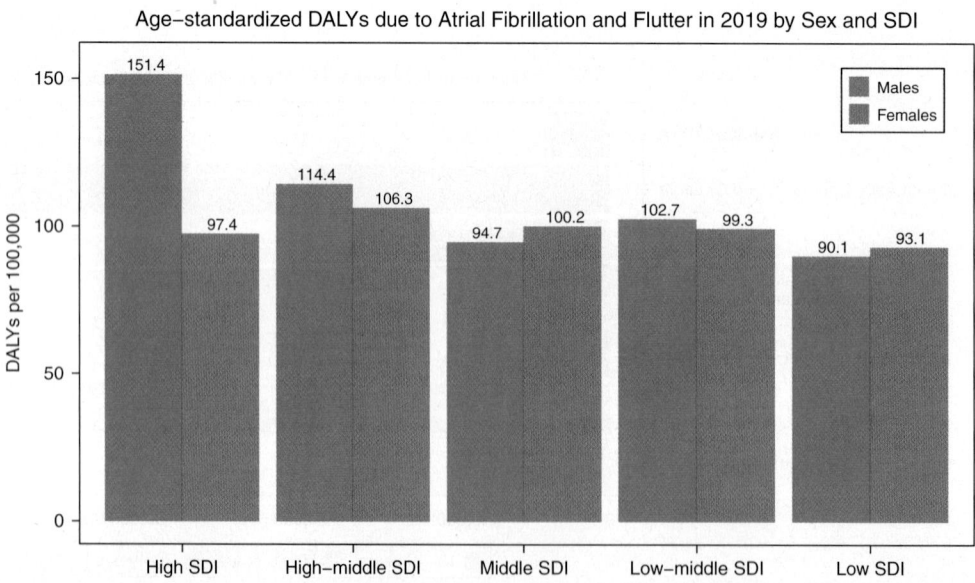

Figure 1–14. **Age-standardized disability-adjusted life-year (DALY) rates of atrial fibrillation for men and women by sociodemographic index (2019).** SDI, sociodemographic index. Data from Roth GA, Mensah GA, Johnson CO, et al. Global Burden of Cardiovascular Diseases and Risk Factors, 1990-2019: Update From the GBD 2019 Study. *J Am Coll Cardiol.* 2020 Dec 22;76(25):2982-3021.

congenital valvular heart disease, and patent ductus arteriosus; ventricular septal defect and atrial septal defect; and other congenital heart anomalies).[5,36]

The incidence of CHD is higher in low-SDI countries compared to high-SDI countries, and therefore, the burden of supporting CHD patients falls more heavily on lower SDI countries. Despite a global decline in age-standardized death rates for CHD, the lower SDI countries typically have higher fertility rates and therefore have higher proportion of deaths due to CHD as well (**Fig. 1–15**).[36] The prevalence rates of CHD at birth changed

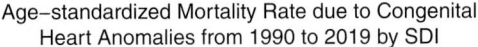
Age–standardized Mortality Rate due to Congenital Heart Anomalies from 1990 to 2019 by SDI

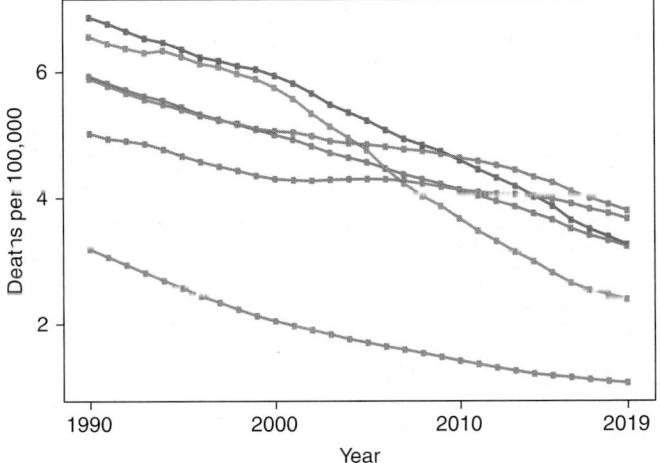

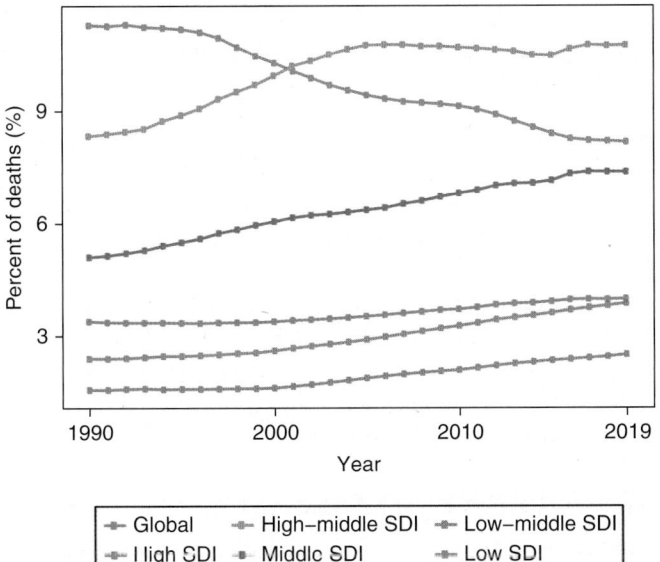
Proportion of Deaths Due to Congenital Heart Anomalies Among Children <1 Year from 1990 to 2019 by SDI

Legend: Global, High–middle SDI, Low–middle SDI, High SDI, Middle SDI, Low SDI

Figure 1–15. Trends in prevalence of congenital heart disease from 1990 to 2017. Data are prevalence (95% UI). (**A**) All-age prevalence and (**B**) age-standardized prevalence by sociodemographic index (SDI) and congenital heart defect subcategory with 95% uncertainty intervals. Reproduced with permission from GBD 2017 Congenital Heart Disease Collaborators. Global, regional, and national burden of congenital heart disease, 1990-2017: a systematic analysis for the Global Burden of Disease Study 2017. *Lancet Child Adolesc Health.* 2020 Mar;4(3):185-200.

little temporally or by SDI, resulting in 13.3 million (95% UI, 11.5–15.4 million) people living with CHD globally, a 28% increase from 1990 to 2019, and causing a total of 590,881 (95% UI, 285,913–980,683) years lived with disability (**Fig. 1–16**). Globally in 2019, CHD caused 216,896 deaths (95% UI, 177,353–261,746), a 42.7% decline since 1990, with 174,442 deaths (95% UI, 138,090–219,702) being among those aged less than 5 years[1,5] (**Fig. 1–17**). Strategies to improve survival and quality of life of patients with CHD will require improving local health services and controlling infectious diseases (eg, diarrheal diseases, rheumatic fever, measles), while improving maternal education and interventions aimed at reducing poverty and reducing birth rates may have the largest impact.[37–40]

INFECTIVE ENDOCARDITIS

Infective endocarditis (IE) is an infection caused by bacteria, or other infectious pathogens, that enter the bloodstream and cause inflammation in the heart tissues, often on a valve. Because of the lack of direct blood supply, the heart valves are particularly susceptible to bacterial colonization and are neither protected by the typical immune response nor easily reached by antibiotics. Due to a rising opioid epidemic in North America, between 1999 and 2019, there was a staggering rise in age-adjusted rate of overdose deaths from intravenous (IV) drug use.[41] The increasing rate of drug overdose death has been accompanied by an increase in incidence of IV drug–associated IE.[42] The highest prevalence of drug use is in the United States (3.26%; 95% UI, 2.85%–3.76%).[5] DALYs due to drug use are also highest in the United States and twice as high as the next highest countries, Estonia and Canada. South Africa peaked in the mid-2000s and has seen a steady decline since then.[5]

IE is a serious illness with up to 22% in-hospital and 40% 5-year mortality.[43] Valve surgery, either by replacement or repair, may be lifesaving and reduce embolic events. Despite evidence of a benefit of surgery during the index hospitalization for IE, especially for cases with left-sided native or prosthetic valve IE complicated by heart failure, severe valvular regurgitation, abscess, or large vegetation, the timing and outcome of surgery vary.[44-46]

The age-standardized incidence of IE is low at 13.8 per 100,000 (95% UI, 11.6–16.3) in 2019 and ranges between 5.7 and 35.8 cases per 100,000 population.[4] The highest incidence is in the Caribbean and Latin America, but incidence has been rising fastest in Brazil and Chile (up to 16% per year) since 1990. Death rate and DALYs are rising fastest in Taiwan, Italy, the Netherlands, the United States, the United Kingdom, the Philippines, and Switzerland. Although China and the Republic of Korea have seen a decrease in DALY rates over time, the number of DALYs remains high given their population size.[4]

A global collaboration was formed to assess the current characteristics of patients with IE via a large, prospective multicenter registry, called the International Collaboration on Endocarditis (ICE) between 2000 and 2006 and then ICE-plus from 2008 to 2012.[47] ICE found that contemporary IE is most often an acute disease with a high rate of infection with

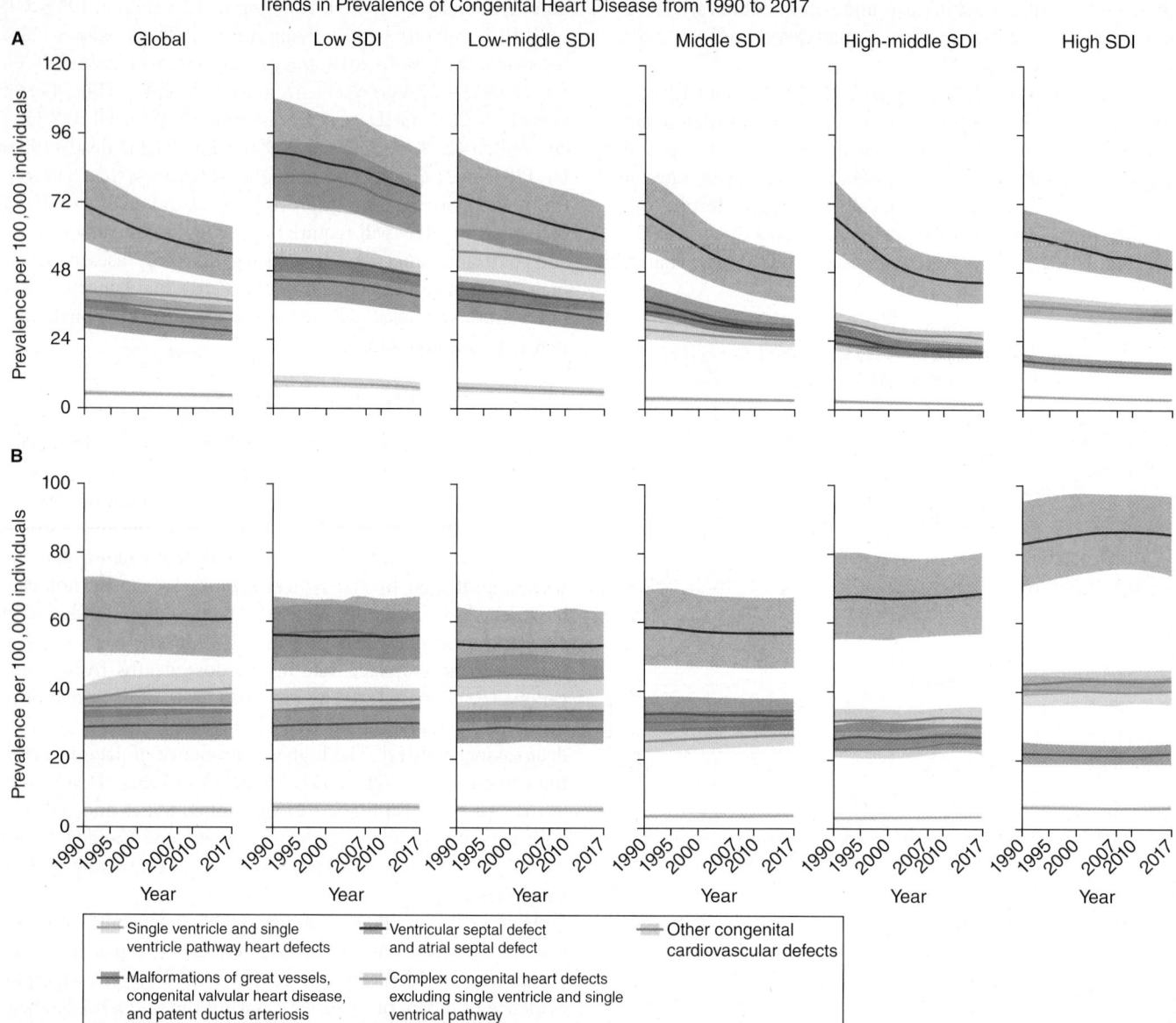

Trends in Prevalence of Congenital Heart Disease from 1990 to 2017

Figure 1–16. Map of under 5 mortality for congenital heart disease in 2019. Data from Global Burden of Disease, 2019 (GBD).

Staphylococcus aureus and involving the mitral valve (41.1%) and aortic valve (37.6%). Common complications included stroke (16.9%), embolization other than stroke (22.6%), heart failure (32.3%), and intracardiac abscess (14.4%); these often required surgical intervention (48.2%). In-hospital and 6-month mortality remains high, with those having *Staphylococcus* infection and abscess having an increased risk of death.[44,48] Unfortunately, there were few sites in Asia and Africa included in the registry, which limits the ability to assess geographic differences in patient and microbiologic characteristics in these areas. Deaths due to IE have increased 131% since 1990, with an estimated 66,322 deaths (95% UI, 46,209–75,862) and 1.7 million DALYs (95% UI, 1.4-1.9 million) in 2019.[4] The highest number of DALYs is in India (214,669) followed by the United States (148,628); yet, the United States leads the world

in deaths due to IE (8363 deaths [95% UI, 4073–10,257] in 2019), with Florida and California having the highest number of cases. Decreased opiate and IV drug use, as well as improved treatment of mental health disorders, may prevent infections and reduce burden of IE over time.

VALVULAR HEART DISEASE

Calcific Aortic Valve Disease and Degenerative Mitral Valve Disease

Calcific aortic valve disease (CAVD) and nonrheumatic degenerative mitral valve disease (DMVD) are increasingly prevalent worldwide. While there is a decreasing trend in global deaths due to RHD, there is an increase in CAVD and DMVD morbidity and mortality (**Fig. 1–18**). In CAVD, the aortic valve leaflets

Mortality Rate due to Congenital Heart Anomalies Among Children Under 5 in 2019

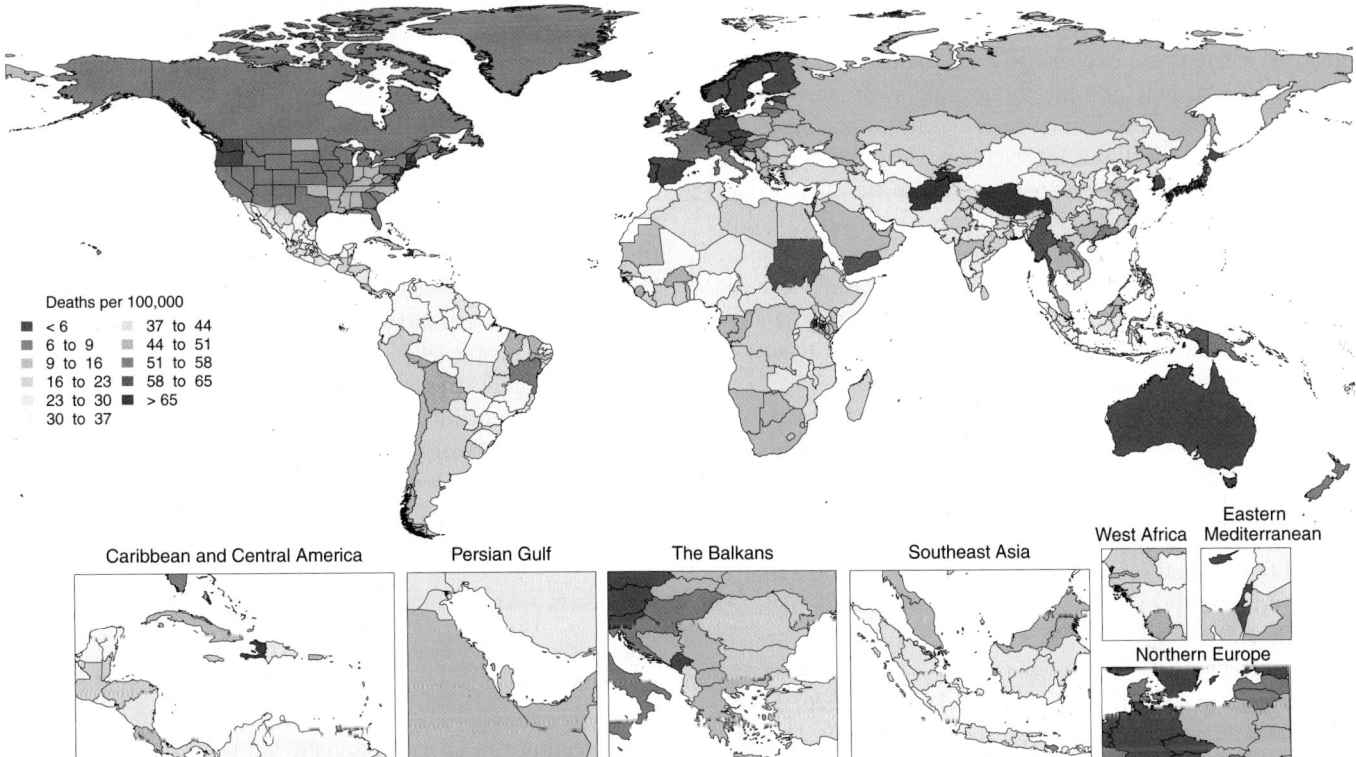

Figure 1–17. Mortality of congenital heart disease in children under 1 year of age, 1990 to 2019. (A) Mortality per 100,000 infants by country in 2019 and **(C)** by SDI from 1990 to 2019. **(B)** Proportion of infant deaths by country in 2019 and **(D)** by SDI from 1990 to 2019. Subnational data are available for Brazil, China, India, Indonesia, Japan, Kenya, Mexico, the United Kingdom, and the United States. SDI, sociodemographic index; TLS, Timor-Leste; TTO, Trinidad and Tobago; VCT, Saint Vincent and the Grenadines. Data from Global Burden of Disease, 2019 (GBD).

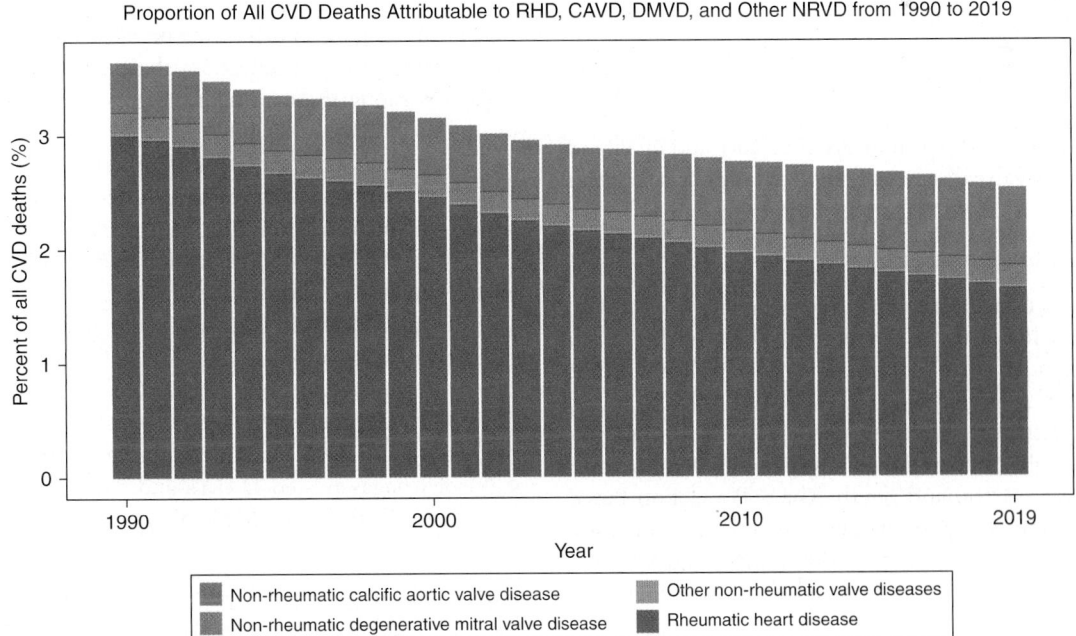

Figure 1–18. Proportion of all cardiovascular disease (CVD) deaths attributable to rheumatic heart disease (RHD), calcific aortic valve disease (CAVD), degenerative mitral valve disease (DMVD), and other nonrheumatic valve disease (NRVD) from 1990 to 2019. The colored area represents the proportion of all CVD deaths attributable to each respective disease. RHD contributes the largest proportion of deaths attributable to these diseases and has declined over time. The proportion of CVD deaths attributable to CAVD has increased slightly over time, and the proportions attributable to DMVD and other NRVD have remained comparatively small. Data from Roth GA, Mensah GA, Johnson CO, et al. Global Burden of Cardiovascular Diseases and Risk Factors, 1990-2019: Update From the GBD 2019 Study. *J Am Coll Cardiol.* 2020 Dec 22;76(25):2982-3021.

become thick, stiff, scarred, and calcified, often covered with nodules on the surface facing the aorta. In general, symptoms of CAVD are minimal even as the valve narrows into aortic stenosis, where pressure overload leads to progressive left ventricular hypertrophy and life-threatening symptoms—angina and/or syncope. This hemodynamic catastrophe results in heart failure and, without intervention, death. The mainstay of treatment for CAVD is either surgical aortic valve replacement (AVR) with a mechanical or bioprosthetic valve or, more recently, the less invasive transcatheter aortic valve replacement (TAVR). The major cause of DMVD is mitral valve prolapse. Untreated, this can lead to chronic mitral regurgitation, AF, and heart failure. DMVD can also be treated with surgical or transcatheter therapies.

Globally, the number of DALYs increased for CAVD between 1990 and 2019 by 88% (95% UI, 72%–107%). In 2019, CAVD caused 126,827 (95% UI, 105,603–141,390) deaths with over 9.4 million (95% UI, 8.1–10.9 million) prevalent cases.[4,49] There is significant geographic variation in the prevalence, mortality rate, and overall burden of CAVD, with the highest age-standardized DALY rates of CAVD estimated for high-SDI countries.[4,49]

The total number of DALYs due to DMVD has increased since 1990, reaching 883,362 (95% UI, 754,183–1,091,526) DALYs and 34,171 (95% UI, 28,272–43,320) deaths in 2019. The GBD 2019 study estimated 24.2 million (95% UI, 23.1–25.4 million) prevalent cases of DMVD in 2019.[4,49] For all age groups, DMVD DALYs were higher in women than men.[4] While total number of cases has increased, the age-standardized rates for DALYs, deaths, and prevalent cases of DMVD have declined over this time period, suggesting the global increases in DMVD have been due to population growth and aging.

Despite overall decreasing age-standardized rates for both CAVD and DMVD, health systems should also focus on improving access to diagnostic imaging and surgical and percutaneous interventions that improve mortality and quality of life for those with valve disease and prevent long-term sequelae of untreated valve disease as the population ages.

Rheumatic Heart Disease

RHD is sequela of acute rheumatic fever and is typically an endemic disease in settings of poverty with overcrowding, poor sanitation, and other social determinants of poor health.[46] It is caused by group A *Streptococcus* infection and leads to mitral stenosis and premature mortality, particularly in young, predominantly female, poorer individuals living in Oceania, central sub-Saharan Africa, and South Asia.[50] Population-based screening programs of children aged 5 to 14 years suggest a prevalence of 0.3 to 5.7 cases per 1000 individuals, with the highest values from studies that included echocardiographic screening.[4,51]

RHD can progress to cause moderate to severe multivalvular disease, leading to heart failure, pulmonary hypertension, or AF. Many patients in low-SDI countries are first diagnosed with advanced disease, at a stage when the chance of a good outcome is unlikely in the absence of surgical intervention.

RHD is at least as severe in low-SDI countries as it is in middle-SDI countries; yet, only 11% of surgical interventions occurred in low-income countries compared with 61% in high-income countries.[50] Overall, treatment with oral anticoagulants, secondary antibiotic prophylaxis, and contraception is often indicated in RHD patients, but these are often underprescribed. Even when these treatments are prescribed, they are often inadequately dosed.[52,53]

Globally in 1990, there were an estimated 362,160 deaths (95% UI, 326,259–408,222) from RHD; this number decreased by 16% (95% UI, –30%--2%) to 305,651 deaths (95% UI, 259,220–340,486) in 2019. In 2019, RHD affected more than 40.5 million people (95% UI, 32.1–50.1 million) and resulted in 10.7 million DALYs lost per year (95% UI, 9.2–12.1 million), almost all in endemic countries.[4] Most DALYs due to RHD were the result of years of life lost (81.4%), which indicated that premature death was a larger driver of total health loss from RHD than was years of life lived with disability.[5]

CHAGAS DISEASE

Chagas disease is a disease of poverty and is localized to Latin America because it is primarily transmitted through bites from the insect *Triatoma infestans*, which is endemic to this region. The infection can be asymptomatic but can eventually lead to premature morbidity and mortality, especially in young women of childbearing age. There are rapid diagnostic tests that can detect the causative parasite, *Trypanosoma cruzi*, in serum and diagnose chronic infections. Between 5 and 18 million people are currently infected, and the infection is estimated to cause more than 10,000 deaths annually.[1] The burden of Chagas disease is challenging to determine because it requires estimating the prevalence of the infection, the prevalence of each of its sequelae among those with the infection, and the number of deaths attributable to the infection. Prevalence had been limited to Central and South America, but increased immigration has expanded the prevalence to Latin American immigrant populations in North America, Europe, Australia, and Japan.[54,55] The Pan-American Health Organization's country-level seroprevalence estimates ranged from less than 1 per 10,000 (0.01%) in Panama to nearly 7% in Bolivia in 2005. In 2019, Chagas disease prevalence was 6.5 million (95% UI, 5.7–7.4 million), and the disease was estimated to cause 275,377 (95% UI, 184,453–459,354) DALYs, driven mostly by YLLs (79% of DALYs), with significant regional variation in Latin America[4] (**Fig. 1–19**). Approximately 4.2% of Chagas-related DALYs and 21.7% of Chagas-related health care costs occur outside of Latin America.[56]

DIFFERENCES IN CARDIOVASCULAR DISEASE IN HIGH- AND LOW-INCOME COUNTRIES

There is significant variation in the patterns of CVD around the world, a fact often obscured by discussions of global trends in CVD. The variation occurs both between large

Age–standardized DALYs due to Chagas Disease in 2019

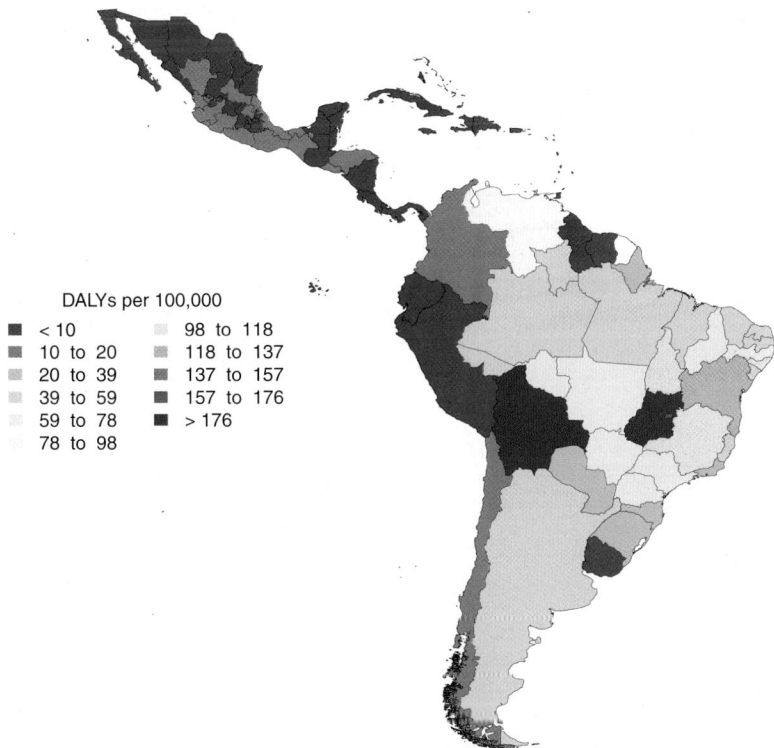

Figure 1–19. **Disability-adjusted life years (DALYs) attributable to Chagas disease, per 100,000 people, for 2019 by country.** Data from Roth GA, Mensah GA, Johnson CO, et al. Global Burden of Cardiovascular Diseases and Risk Factors, 1990-2019: Update From the GBD 2019 Study. *J Am Coll Cardiol.* 2020 Dec 22;76(25):2982-3021.

regions but is also striking among even adjacent countries. This profound heterogeneity extends even within countries and has been shown among states and provinces, counties, cities, and even neighborhoods.[57] **Figure 1–20** shows the relationship between age-standardized mortality rates for CVD by SDI and region over time for males and females. Regions with the lowest SDI have seen the smallest change in age-standardized mortality rates from 1990 to 2019. **Figure 1–21** shows the global burden of DALYs and DALY rates disaggregated into YLLs and years lived with disability (YLDs) by 5-year age groups in the poorest billion.[29] Although the DALY rates for NCDs increase with age (particularly for CVD), 50% of all-age DALYs accrue before the age of 40 years in the youth of the poorest billion. Conversely, in high-income populations, only 19% of all-age NCD DALYs accrue before the age of 40 years, although the pattern of rates by age group is similar.[29] Some regions, led by Central Asia, face high rates of premature death from IHD, whereas sub-Saharan Africa and Asia suffer disproportionately from deaths caused by stroke[1] (**Fig. 1–22**). Figure 1–22 illustrates the YLLs for the top causes of CVD in each region. Cardiomyopathy (in light green) is more common in sub-Saharan Africa and Eastern Europe than elsewhere. Stroke (in green) dominates over IHD (in light blue) as the leading cause of death in East and Southeast Asia. Understanding these global trends and regional variation is important in order to help create policies and health interventions that can

be tailored and scaled for a broad range of local conditions with the ultimate goal of improving cardiovascular health.

There are large differences in the mortality for CVD in high-SDI countries, with Japan (77 per 100,000; 95% UI, 64.4–84.0) having the lowest age-standardized rates in 2019.[4] In Western Europe, France, Israel, Spain, Switzerland, Iceland, the Netherlands, Norway, and Andorra have similarly low rates, as do Australia and Canada. Cyprus, Greece, Finland, and Germany have some of the highest death rates in Western Europe (159 per 100,000; 95% UI, 143–168), likely due to the higher risk factor burden in these countries.[4] CVD mortality in other high-income countries, including Brunei Darussalam, Greenland, Argentina, and Uruguay, is higher than in Western Europe, possibly because of their specific dietary patterns and other risk factors, as well as quality of health care services.[1]

The lowest SDI countries have many challenges to overcome in reducing CVD burden. These challenges include their persistent "double burden" related to infectious disease, including HIV, tuberculosis, and malaria; limited availability of data on CVD and risk factors; inadequate primary health care infrastructure and access to medical care and medications; financial constraints on the individual and country level; inadequate training and retention of health professionals; and limited awareness of CVD and risk factors. The sub-Saharan Africa region has experienced the lowest levels of CVD burden over the past 30 years (only 5.1% of the global

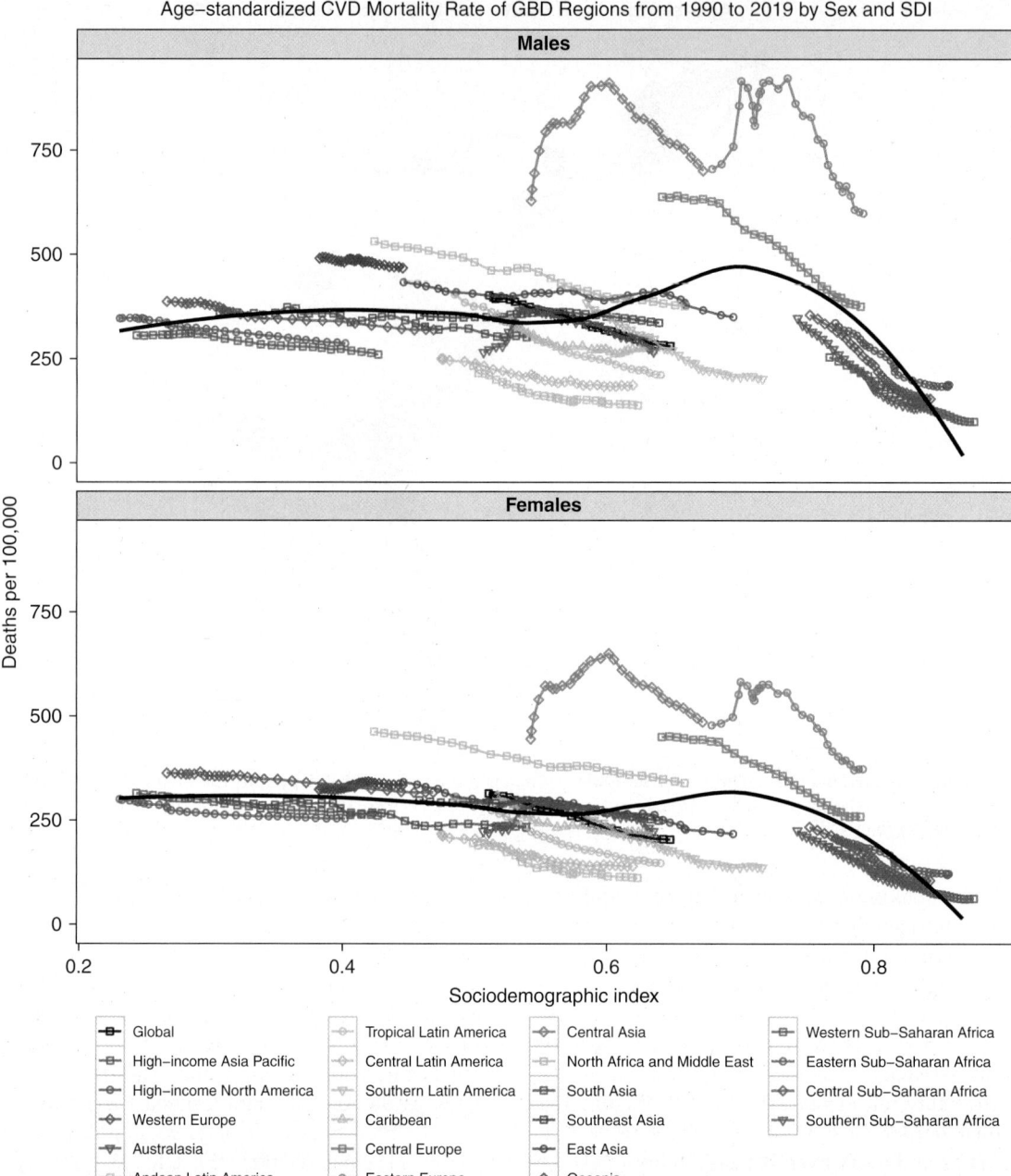

Age–standardized CVD Mortality Rate of GBD Regions from 1990 to 2019 by Sex and SDI

Figure 1–20. **Relationship between age-standardized mortality rate for cardiovascular disease (CVD) and sociodemographic index (SDI) over time.** Each colored line represents a time trend of the relationship for the specified region. Each point represents a specific year for that region. The black line represents the overall global trend for age-standardized death rate of cardiovascular disease in relation to SDI. GBD, Global Burden of Disease. Data from Global Burden of Disease, 2019 (GBD).

CVD deaths), but the number of CVD deaths is rising as the adult population grows rapidly.[58] In 2019, CVD caused over 1 million deaths in sub-Saharan Africa, constituting 36.9% of NCD deaths and 13.1% of deaths from all causes in that region.[1,4] Accurate estimates are limited as a result of scarce data available throughout the region and reflect, among other sources, verbal autopsy surveys showing 9% to 13% of deaths attributable to CVD, especially stroke.

Contrary to trends in high-SDI regions, the age-adjusted mortality for CVD in sub-Saharan Africa has not declined as rapidly as in other regions. The age-standardized CVD mortality was 314.3 per 100,000 (95% CI, 281.9–347.9) in 1990 and 269.1 per 100,000 (95% CI, 240.2–297.4) in 2019, representing only a 14% decrease in nearly three decades.[4]

Hypertensive heart disease and cardiomyopathy represent a much larger proportion of total death in sub-Saharan Africa

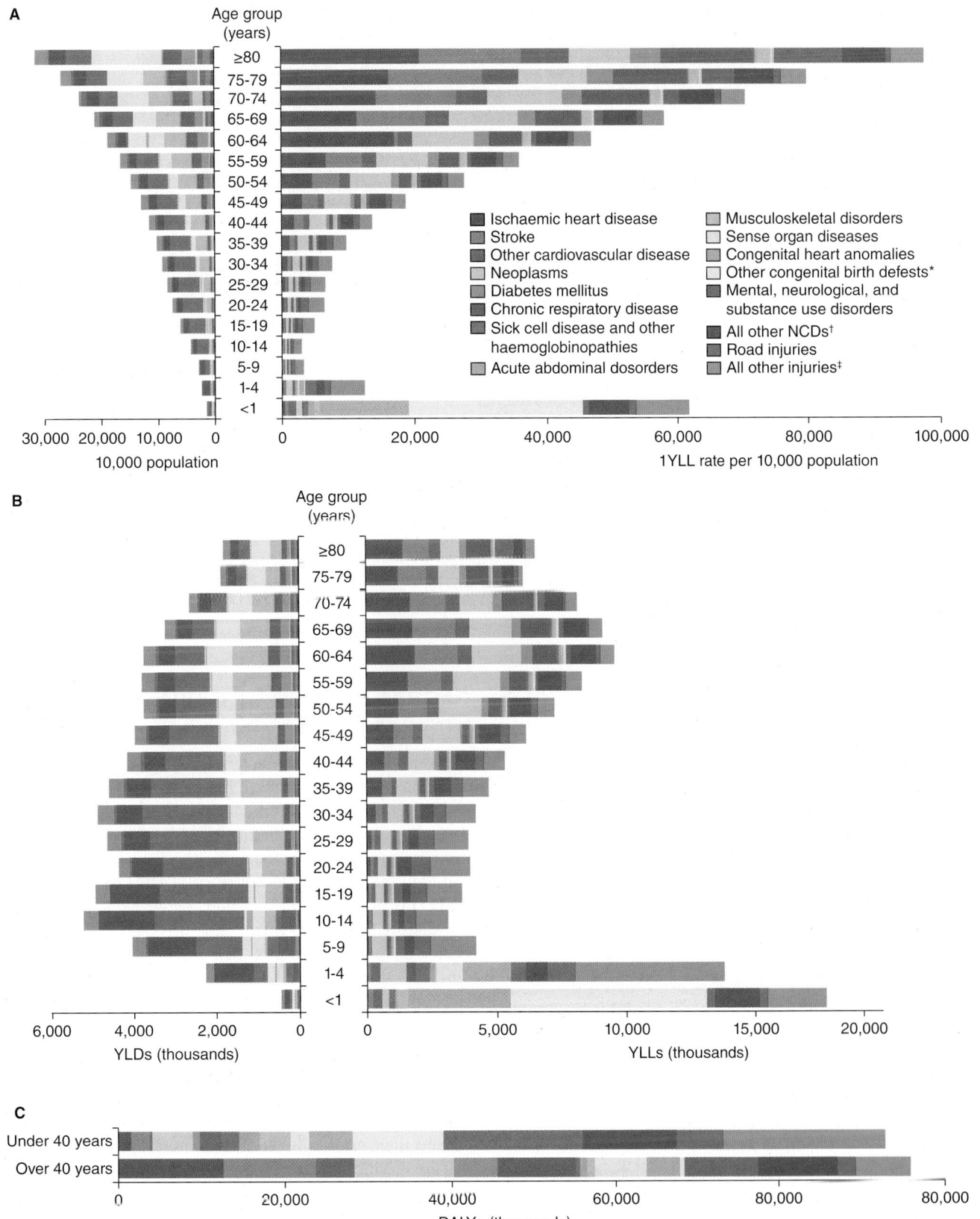

A

Age group (years): ≥80, 75-79, 70-74, 65-69, 60-64, 55-59, 50-54, 45-49, 40-44, 35-39, 30-34, 25-29, 20-24, 15-19, 10-14, 5-9, 1-4, <1

Legend:
- Ischaemic heart disease
- Stroke
- Other cardiovascular disease
- Neoplasms
- Diabetes mellitus
- Chronic respiratory disease
- Sick cell disease and other haemoglobinopathies
- Acute abdominal dosorders
- Musculoskeletal disorders
- Sense organ diseases
- Congenital heart anomalies
- Other congenital birth defests*
- Mental, neurological, and substance use disorders
- All other NCDs†
- Road injuries
- All other injuries‡

Left axis: 30,000 20,000 10,000 0 — 10,000 population
Right axis: 0 20,000 40,000 60,000 80,000 100,000 — 1YLL rate per 10,000 population

B

Age group (years): ≥80, 75-79, 70-74, 65-69, 60-64, 55-59, 50-54, 45-49, 40-44, 35-39, 30-34, 25-29, 20-24, 15-19, 10-14, 5-9, 1-4, <1

Left axis: 6,000 4,000 2,000 0 — YLDs (thousands)
Right axis: 0 5,000 10,000 15,000 20,000 — YLLs (thousands)

C

Under 40 years
Over 40 years

0 20,000 40,000 60,000 80,000 80,000 — DALYs (thousands)

Figure 1–21. The global burden of disability-adjusted life-years (DALYs) and DALY rates disaggregated into years life lost and years lived with disability by 5-year age groups in the poorest billion. Reproduced with permission from Bukhman G, Mocumbi AO, Atun R, et al. The Lancet NCDI Poverty Commission: bridging a gap in universal health coverage for the poorest billion. *Lancet.* 2020 Oct 3;396(10256):991-1044.

YLLs due to CVD by Region, All Ages and Both Sexes in 2019

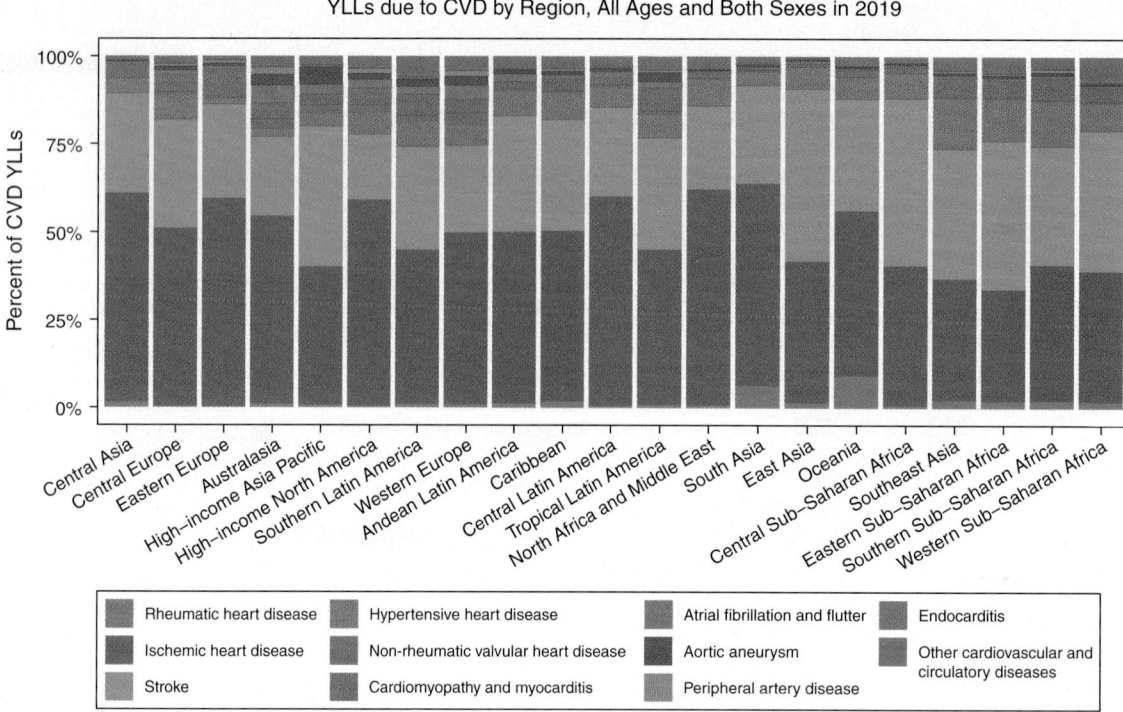

Figure 1–22. **Proportion of years of life lost (YLLs) because of cardiovascular disease (CVD) stratified by global region, 2019.** YLL is a measure of premature mortality calculated by using a normative goal for survival computed from the lowest observed death rate across countries. Data from Roth GA, Mensah GA, Johnson CO, et al. Global Burden of Cardiovascular Diseases and Risk Factors, 1990-2019: Update From the GBD 2019 Study. *J Am Coll Cardiol.* 2020 Dec 22; 76(25):2982-3021.

than in other regions and are suspected to represent untreated hypertension and rheumatic disease. Endomyocardial fibrosis, an uncommon idiopathic disease of heart muscle tissue, has become rare in communities where it used to be common, and its etiology continues to be elusive.[58] The average age of death caused by IHD in sub-Saharan Africa was the youngest in the world in 2019, at 64.9 years (95% UI, 64.4–65.4 years) compared with 67.6 to 81.2 years for the rest of the world, reflecting the higher all-cause mortality and shorter life span in this region.[59]

Although CVDs are not the leading causes of death in sub-Saharan Africa, they represent a significant number of deaths caused by population growth, aging, and the epidemiologic transition from infectious diseases to NCDs, with increasing prevalence of risk factors for CVD.[60,61] This transition is faced not only in sub-Saharan Africa but also across many rapidly developing middle-income countries, such as India, Brazil, Indonesia, and China. Promotion of cardiovascular health and CVD prevention, treatment, and control is needed, as are investments in human resources, infrastructure, technical capacity, and funding. Efforts are needed to improve data collection via household surveillance studies, death certification, and burden of disease estimates; in addition, increased data are needed on health care capacity and quality, adherence to medications, and microeconomic costs experienced by patients and their families.[29] Such costs include catastrophic spending on health, distress financing, and other measures of financial risk associated with disease.[9]

GLOBAL BURDEN OF CARDIOVASCULAR DISEASE RISK FACTORS

Exposure to known risk factors for CVD remains alarmingly common and presents one of the largest barriers to improved global health. Most CVD premature deaths are linked to these common risk factors, including high blood pressure, high body mass index, tobacco use, and unhealthy diet with low fruit intake and high sodium.[4] The top three risk factors that contribute to CVD DALYs globally include high systolic blood pressure, high low-density lipoprotein (LDL) cholesterol, and high particulate matter air pollution (**Fig. 1–23**). Among the most important observations, we can make from this assessment of risk factors is that the vast majority of CVD is a result of the combination of preventable behavioral and metabolic risk factors. Globally, CVD prevention emphasizes healthy lifestyle behaviors (not smoking, ideal body weight, adequate physical activity, and healthy diet) and optimal biologic factors (control of blood pressure, cholesterol, and glucose). However, certain regions may need to expand their priority list to include nontraditional risk factors that are specific to their region, such as air pollution in South and East Asia and infectious risks in sub-Saharan Africa.[62,63]

Modifiable Cardiovascular Risk Factors

Hypertension

Elevated blood pressure is estimated to be the single largest contributor to the global burden of disease and global mortality. In high-SDI countries, it is estimated to be responsible for

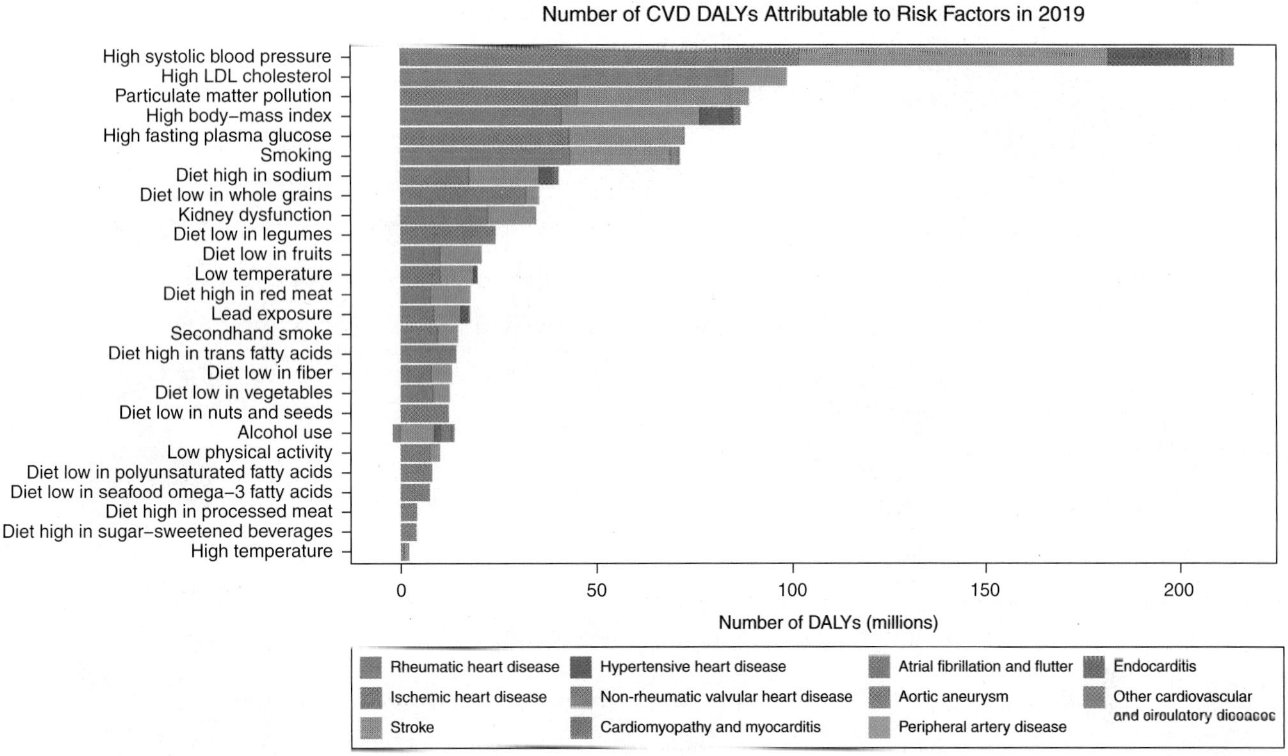

Number of CVD DALYs Attributable to Risk Factors in 2019

Figure 1–23. Number of cardiovascular disease disability-adjusted life-years (DALYs) attributable to avoidable risk factors in 2019, by cardiovascular disease subtype. LDL, low-density lipoprotein. Data from Roth GA, Mensah GA, Johnson CO, et al. Global Burden of Cardiovascular Diseases and Risk Factors, 1990-2019: Update From the GBD 2019 Study. *J Am Coll Cardiol.* 2020 Dec 22;76(25):2982-3021.

45% of deaths from stroke, 49% of deaths from IHD, and 17% of all global deaths.[1] Screening is key to diagnosis as it is largely an asymptomatic condition. The development of hypertension is associated with dietary exposures, such as high-sodium diet, low physical activity, and low intake of fruit and vegetables.[64] There are gaps in the awareness, treatment, and control of hypertension globally. High blood pressure tends to occur in tandem with economic development, but notably in the highest SDI countries, individuals with lower socioeconomic status and younger individuals are most likely to be untreated.[65] Over the past 5 years, a concerning trend has emerged in the United States, with blood pressure control decreasing among those with hypertension.[65]

The age-standardized mean systolic blood pressure (SBP) worldwide was 129.4 mm Hg (95% UI, 128.6–130.2) in males and 125.8 mm Hg (95% UI, 124.8–126.8) in females.[5] In 2019, the prevalence of high blood pressure (SBP ≥140 mm Hg or diastolic blood pressure ≥90 mm Hg) was 28.3% (95% UI, 25.9%–30.6%) in males and 27.5% (95% UI, 25.0%–30.0%) in females.[66] There were 235.4 million DALYs (95% UI, 211.1–260.6 million) and 10.8 million deaths (95% UI, 9.5–12.1 million) in 2019 attributable to high blood pressure[5] (**Fig. 1–24**). DALYs and deaths have increased since 1990 (DALYs in 1990: 153.7 million [95% UI, 138.7–169.5 million]; deaths in 1990: 6.8 million [95% UI, 6.1–7.5 million]), as has the number of people living with uncontrolled hypertension.[4]

Overall, there has been a decreasing trend in population mean SBP over the past 30 years, with the highest reductions in high-income North America for males and Western Europe and Australasia for both males and females. However, mean SBP rose in certain regions with variations in urban and rural areas, including Oceania, East Africa, and South and Southeast Asia for both sexes and in West Africa for women.[4,66]

Obesity

There has been a global rise in obesity among adults, as well as adolescents and children, with little success over the past 30 years to modify the upward trend. Overweight is defined as a body mass index (BMI) greater than or equal to 25 kg/m², and obesity is defined as a BMI greater than or equal to 30 kg/m². The prevalence of obesity is higher in high-SDI countries than low-SDI countries, and there are age and sex differences by region[67] (**Fig. 1–25**). The summary exposure value of overweight and obesity was 10.5 (95% UI, 7.7–14.3) in 1990 and increased 87% to 19.7 (95% UI, 15.7–24.9) in 2019.[4] It was higher in males than females in high-SDI countries, whereas in low- and middle-SDI countries, females have higher rates of overweight and obesity than males. Only one country has had a decrease in prevalence of obesity since 1990—Somalia—possibly related to severe drought, internal conflict, and the famine in 2011.[67]

Research has shown that the peak age of obesity is slightly older in females than males in high-SDI countries, with nearly 30.2% of men and 31.7% of women being obese. In low-SDI countries, the prevalence is much lower (9.5% in males and 13.2% in females).[67] In high-SDI countries, overweight and obesity peaked in men at about 55 years of age, with two of three

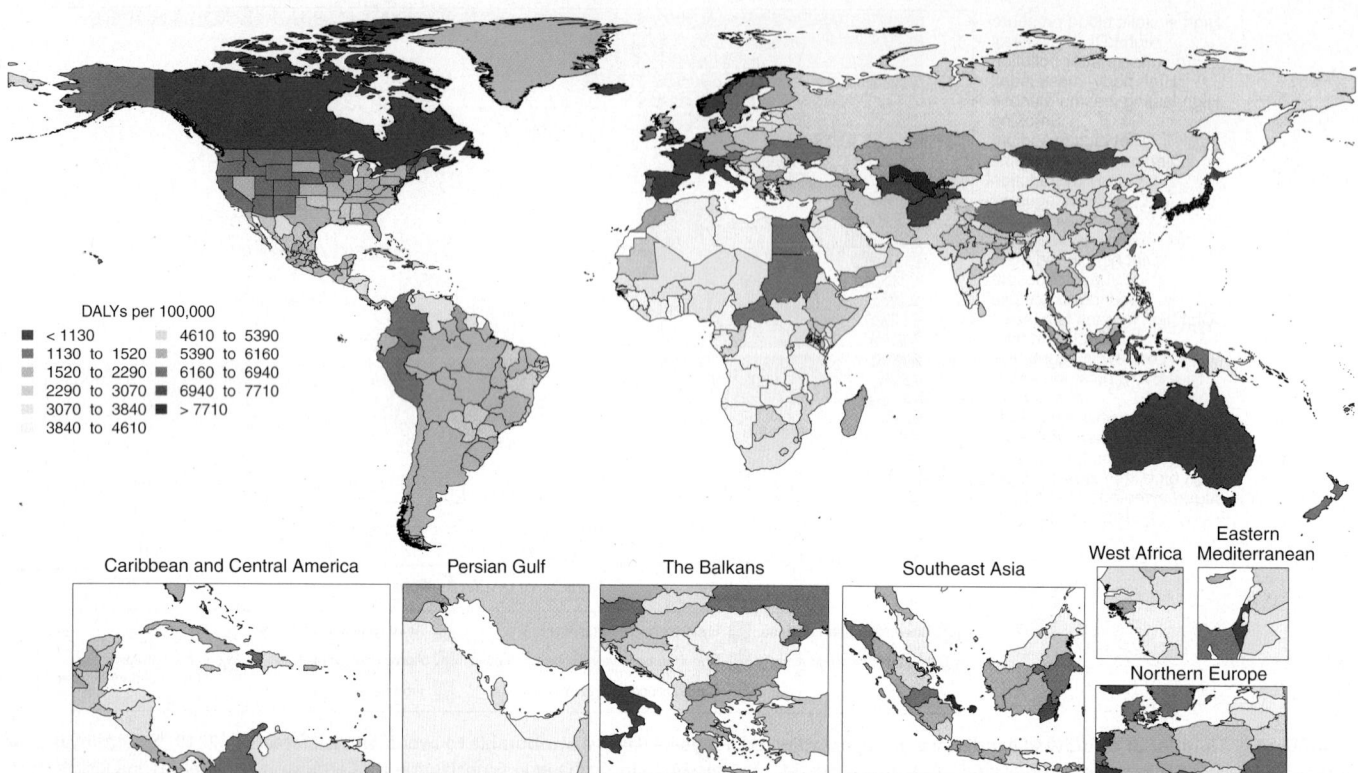

Figure 1–24. Map of age-standardized rate of disability-adjusted life-years (DALYs) of high systolic blood pressure in 2019, according to the Global Burden of Disease 2019 Study. Modified with permission from GBD 2019 Risk Factors Collaborators. Global burden of 87 risk factors in 204 countries and territories, 1990-2019: a systematic analysis for the Global Burden of Disease Study 2019. *Lancet.* 2020 Oct 17;396(10258):1223-1249.

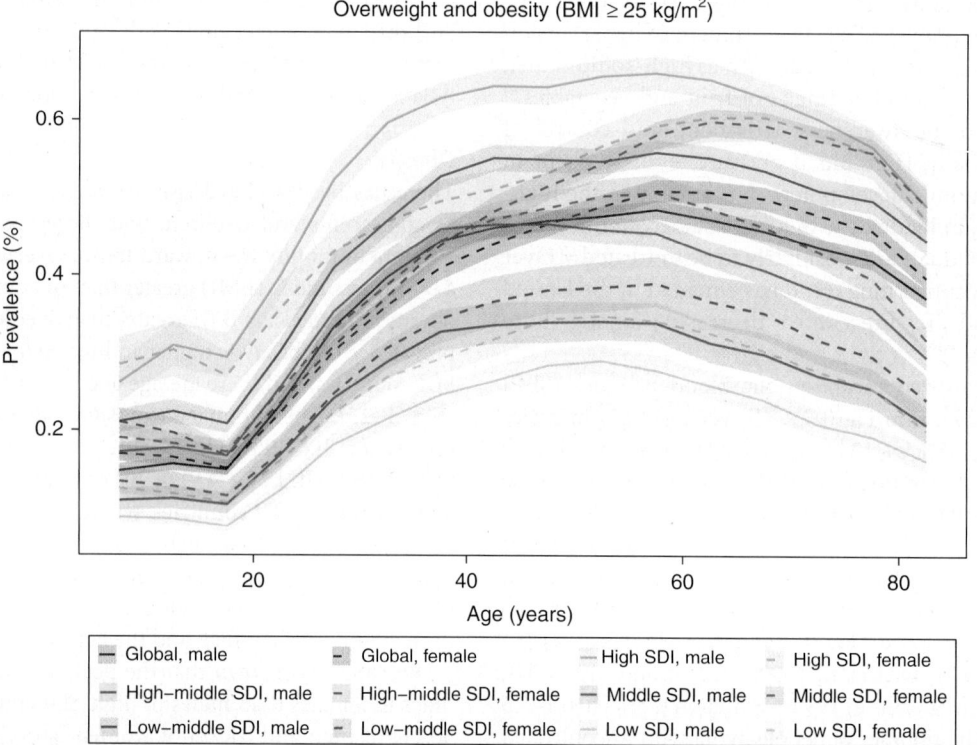

Figure 1–25. Prevalence of obesity at the global level by age and sex and sociodemographic index, Global Burden of Disease 2019 Study. Male; solid line. Female; dashed line. BMI, body-mass index. Data from Roth GA, Mensah GA, Johnson CO, et al. Global Burden of Cardiovascular Diseases and Risk Factors, 1990-2019: Update From the GBD 2019 Study. *J Am Coll Cardiol.* 2020 Dec 22;76(25):2982-3021 and GBD 2015 Obesity Collaborators, Afshin A, Forouzanfar MH, et al: Health Effects of Overweight and Obesity in 195 Countries over 25 Years, *N Engl J Med* 2017 Jul 6;377(1):13-27.

men overweight and one in four obese; for women, the peak age was closer to 60 years, with 31.3% (95% UI, 28.9%–33.8%) obese and 64.5% (95% UI, 62.5%–66.5%) overweight or obese.[67] The age-standardized global death rate due to high BMI has stayed largely unchanged since 1990 at 62.6 per 100,000 (95% UI, 39.9–89.1), but the number of deaths has increased to 5.0 million (95% UI, 3.2–7.1 million) in 2019, largely due to increases in BMI in middle-SDI countries, such as China and India. DALYs also increased over time, with 160.3 million DALYS (95% UI, 106.0–218.9 million) in 2019. The highest rates of change of age-standardized deaths attributable to high BMI are in Equatorial Guinea (208.1%), Mozambique (180.4%), Ghana (176.6%), and Nepal (176.4%).[5]

Diet

Ideal diet, as defined by the American Heart Association (AHA), involves eating a balanced diet that includes at least a variety of fruits and vegetables daily; whole grains; fat-free and low-fat dairy products; fish, legumes, poultry, and lean meats; and limited intake of salt (sodium chloride <5 g/d), alcohol (no more than one drink per day for women and two drinks per day for men), and saturated fats and cholesterol.[68] The goal of the AHA dietary guidelines is to assist individuals in achieving and maintaining cardiovascular and overall health, and they are designed for the general population. Increasingly, dietary guidelines are being developed for specific regions that are tailored to local diet and culture. Low fruit intake and high sodium intake are significant contributors to overall CVD deaths, accounting for 1.09% and 1.77% of total global DALY in 2019, respectively.[5,69] The burden of high dietary sodium, estimated as above approximately 5 g/d, is highest in China and Eastern Europe, with 7.9% of total DALYs in Bulgaria and 5.5% in China.[5] Men are more affected than women. Other dietary risk factors for CVD include low consumption of whole grains, low legumes, low vegetables, high red meat, low nuts and seeds, low omega-3 and polyunsaturated fats, low fiber, high processed meats, and high trans fats.[4,70]

Dyslipidemia

Excessive levels of serum cholesterol contributed to 3.9% of total global DALYs (95% UI, 3.2%–4.7%) in 2019. The total DALYs attributable to high LDL cholesterol (LDL-c) was 69.7 million (95% UI, 58.5–83.3 million) in 1990 and increased 41% to 98.6 million (95% UI, 80.3–119.0 million) in 2019. Deaths attributable to high LDL-c also increased over this time from 3.0 million (95% UI, 2.4–3.8 million) in 1990 to 4.4 million (95% UI, 3.3–5.7 million) in 2019 with significant increases seen in middle-SDI countries, such as China and India. The highest DALY burden of high LDL-c is in Eastern Europe, with up to 12% of total DALYs related to this risk in Ukraine and Belarus, whereas sub-Saharan Africa has the lowest burden of DALYs for high LDL-c.[4,5] Research has shown that the peak age of high cholesterol was slightly older in females than males in high-SDI countries, with an estimated summary exposure value of 30.9 per 100 (95% UI, 28.0–34.1) for men and 34.1 per 100 (95% UI, 31.2–37.2) for women having high cholesterol.[5] Cholesterol guidelines highlight target LDL-c levels for primary and secondary prevention.[71-74] Poor adherence to these guidelines in high-SDI countries has contributed to the high burden of CVD.[75] Furthermore, population-based genetic testing, such as

23andMe and the National Institutes of Health All of Us Research program (primarily in high-SDI countries), has increased the diagnosis of familial hypercholesterolemia. The awareness, treatment, and control of levels for hypercholesterolemia mirror the suboptimal patterns for poor diet as well as access to treatment with effective therapy such as statins, ezetimibe, and proprotein convertase sutilisin/kexin type 9 (PCSK9) inhibitor medications.

Tobacco and Smoking

Tobacco caused 8.7 million deaths, 11.6% of YLLs, and 9.1% of DALYs in 2019.[76] The YLLs decreased in high-SDI countries but are increasing in all other SDI groups. The use of daily cigarettes has declined significantly since 1980, from a high of 41.2% (95% UI, 40.4%–42.6%) for males and 10.6% (95% UI, 10.2%–11.1%) for females. Since 1990, the annualized rate of change is approximately 1% lower per year (annualized rate of change between 1990-2019 is 0.99%, 95% UI, –1.04% to –0.94%).[76] The summary exposure value has decreased from 23.1 per 100 (95% UI, 20.5–25.9) in 1990 to 18.7 per 100 (95% UI, 16.6–21.0) in 2019 for males and from 6.1 per 100 (95% UI, 5.4–6.9) in 1990 to 4.1 per 100 (95% UI, 3.6–4.6) in 2019 for females.[5,76] While encouraging, the number of daily smokers increased significantly. In 2015, there were 933.1 million (95% UI, 831.3–1054.3 million) daily smokers in the world, 82.3% of whom were men (768.1 million [95% UI, 690.1–852.2 million]). The 10 countries with the largest number of smokers together accounted for 63.6% of the world's daily smokers (see red and orange countries in **Fig. 1–26**).[76]

The prevalence rates of tobacco use, and specifically daily cigarette use, vary greatly by age, sex, and region, with summary exposure values for tobacco use below 8% for males in some African countries to more than 32% for males in Eastern Europe, Russia, and North Africa (**Fig. 1–27**). For females, estimated prevalence rates ranged from more than 35% in Palestine, Lebanon, Jordan, Kyrgyzstan, and Montenegro, to less than 6% in a number of countries, such as Ethiopia, Sao Tome and Principe, and Congo. There are also large variations within regions, with Chile, Argentina, and Uruguay having a much higher estimated prevalence than other Latin American countries.[76] Estimated age-standardized prevalence of daily smoking in males was only weakly correlated with that in females (r = 0.38), with prevalence in males exceeding that in females in all countries except Sweden.[76] Interestingly, the number of cigarettes per smoker per day varies widely across countries and is not correlated with prevalence.

Diabetes

Hyperglycemia and diabetes mellitus are significant contributors to CVD worldwide. Unlike blood pressure, age-standardized mean fasting plasma glucose has continued to rise for males and females over the past 30 years, with no country having a meaningful decrease in fasting plasma glucose.[5,77,78] In 2019, the summary exposure value of elevated blood glucose was 12.5% (95% UI, 11.2%–13.8%) for males and 11.2% (10.1%–12.3%) in females, which corresponds to an 189.6% increase in the number of people living with diabetes today compared with 1990 (**Fig. 1–28**).[5,79] Nearly 40% of these individuals reside in China and India (~177 million), with another 10% (~46 million) in

Age–standardized Summary Exposure Value of Smoking in 2019, Females

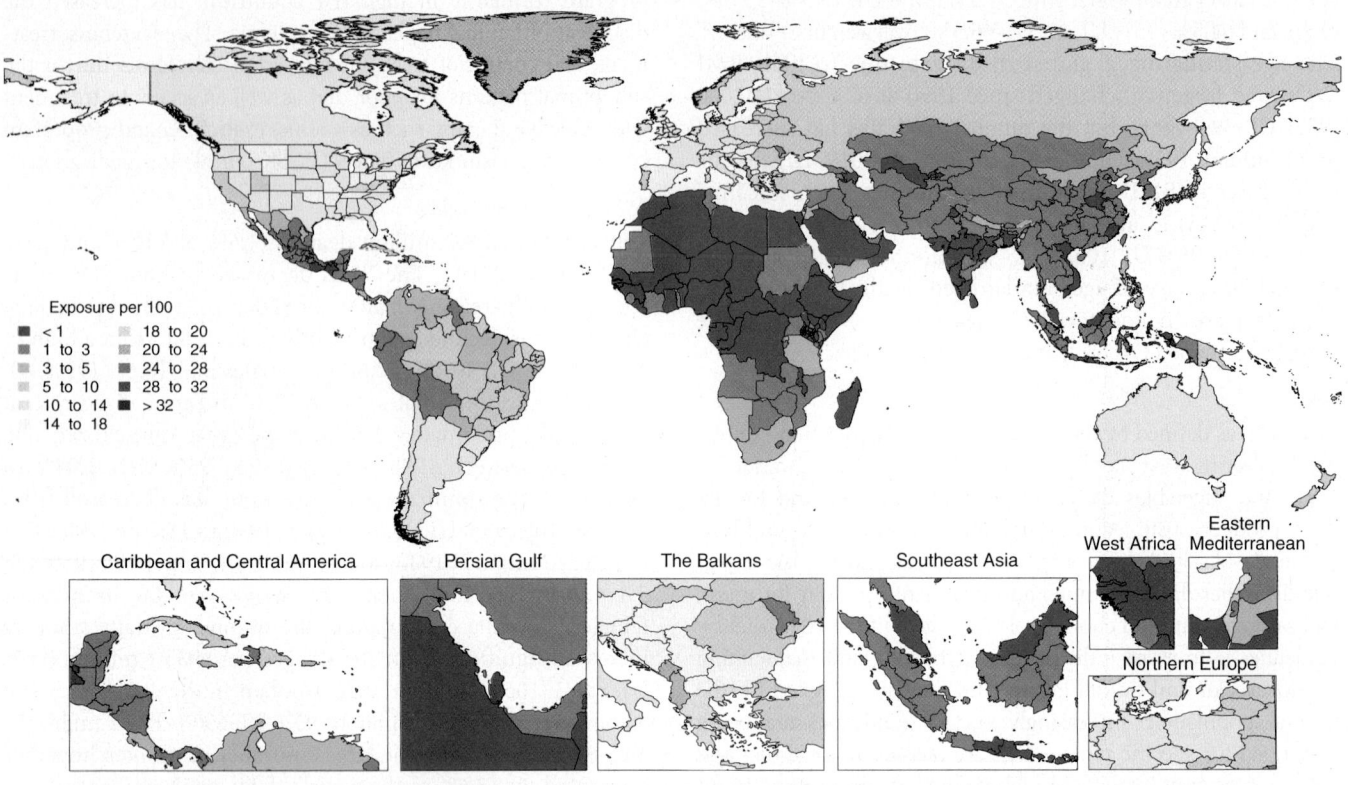

Exposure per 100
- < 1
- 1 to 3
- 3 to 5
- 5 to 10
- 10 to 14
- 14 to 18
- 18 to 20
- 20 to 24
- 24 to 28
- 28 to 32
- > 32

Caribbean and Central America   Persian Gulf   The Balkans   Southeast Asia   West Africa   Eastern Mediterranean

Northern Europe

Age–standardized Summary Exposure Value of Smoking in 2019, Males

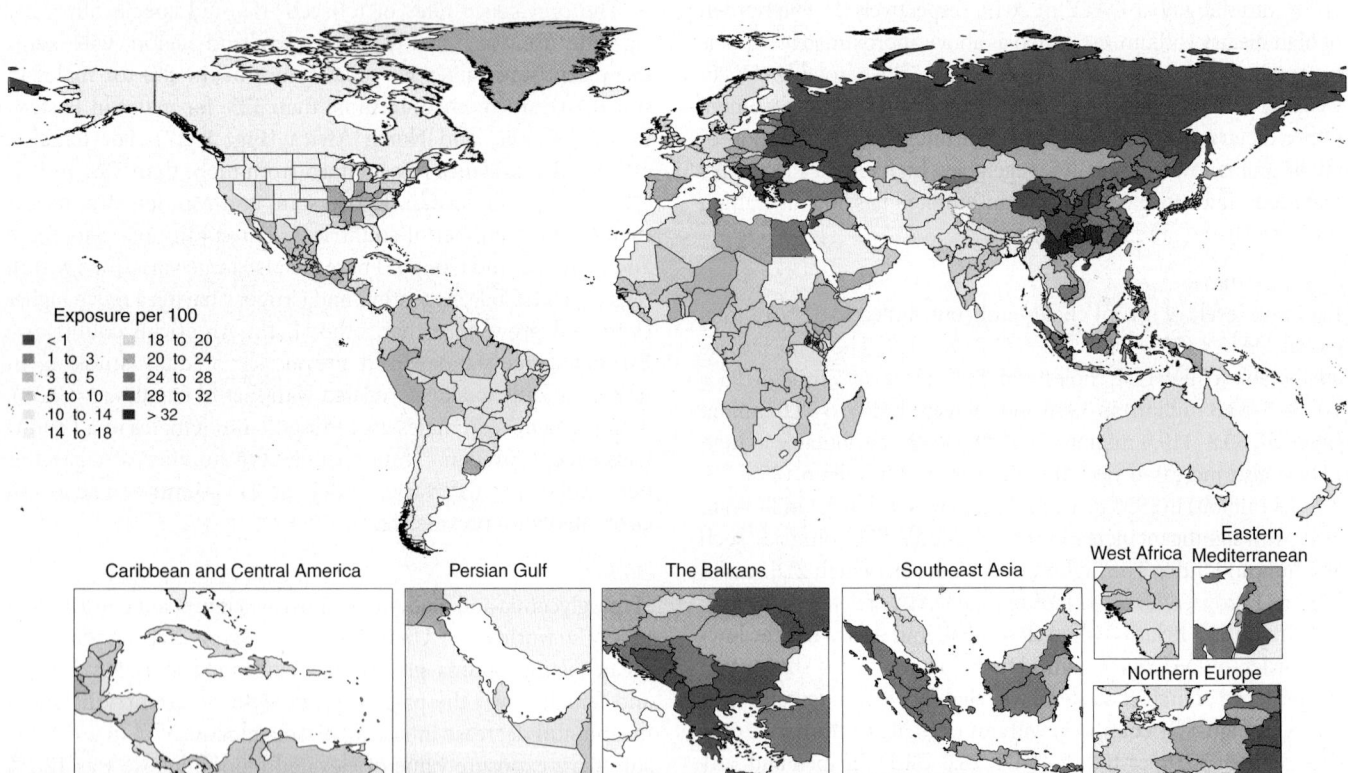

Exposure per 100
- < 1
- 1 to 3
- 3 to 5
- 5 to 10
- 10 to 14
- 14 to 18
- 18 to 20
- 20 to 24
- 24 to 28
- 28 to 32
- > 32

Caribbean and Central America   Persian Gulf   The Balkans   Southeast Asia   West Africa   Eastern Mediterranean

Northern Europe

Figure 1–26. Map of global estimated age-standardized summary exposure value of daily smoking in (A) women and (B) men in 2019. Modified with permission from GBD 2019 Risk Factors Collaborators. Global burden of 87 risk factors in 204 countries and territories, 1990-2019: a systematic analysis for the Global Burden of Disease Study 2019. *Lancet*. 2020 Oct 17;396(10258):1223-1249.

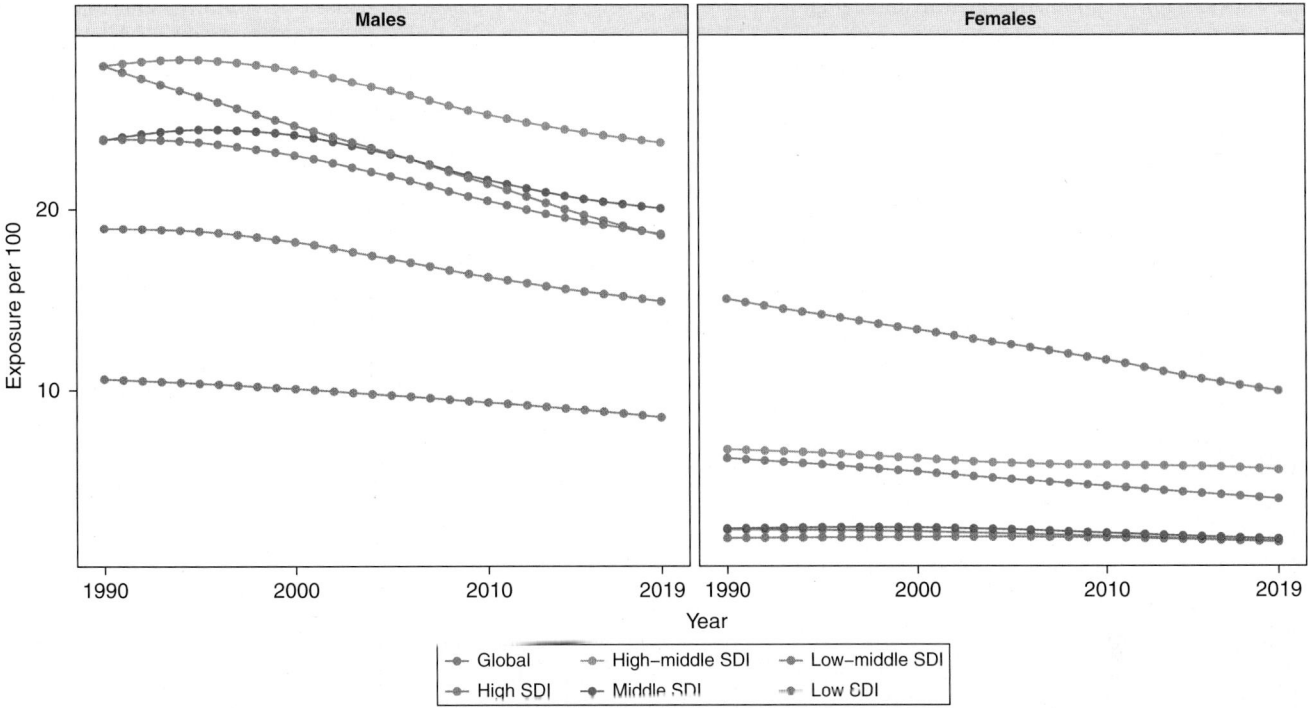

Figure 1–27. **Estimated age-standardized summary exposure value of daily smoking by sex over time by sociodemographic index (SDI), 1990 to 2019.** Data from Roth GA, Mensah GA, Johnson CO, et al. Global Burden of Cardiovascular Diseases and Risk Factors, 1990-2019: Update From the GBD 2019 Study. *J Am Coll Cardiol.* 2020 Dec 22;76(25):2982-3021.

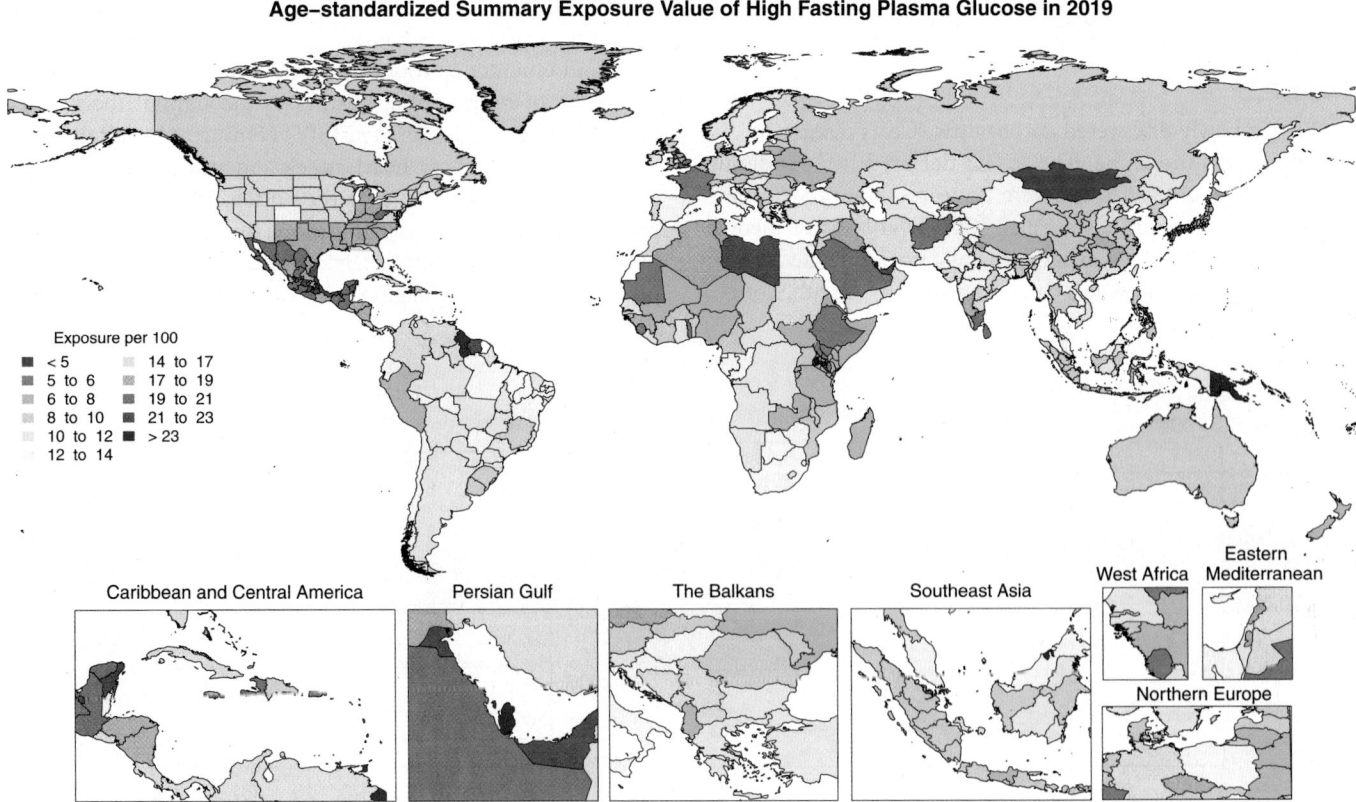

Figure 1–28. **Map of age-standardized summary exposure value (SEV) of high fasting plasma glucose in 2019, according to the Global Burden of Disease 2019 Study.** Countries in orange and red have a SEV of >20%. Modified with permission from GBD 2019 Risk Factors Collaborators. Global burden of 87 risk factors in 204 countries and territories, 1990-2019: a systematic analysis for the Global Burden of Disease Study 2019. *Lancet.* 2020 Oct 17; 396(10258):1223-1249.

the United States and Russia.[5] The change in the past 30 years is largely attributable to population growth and aging, but approximately 30% is attributable to a rise in age-specific prevalence. The trends over time ranged from an increase in age-standardized diabetes prevalence of 16% in tropical Latin America to a substantial increase of 86% and 90% for North Africa and Middle East and for Central Asia, respectively. Ethiopia has had no increase in prevalence of diabetes, whereas population aging and population growth have caused the number of diabetics in the rest of North Africa and Southeast Asia to continue to rise. In the past 10 years, the DALYs have been rising fastest in the United Arab Emirates and Qatar (nearly +8%/year), likely partly attributable to the rapid rise in obesity in this region.[5]

Physical Inactivity

Physical inactivity has become a leading risk factor for CVD globally. There is an increased risk of death associated with low physical inactivity, contributing to 0.6% of total DALYs in 2019,[5] much of which appears to be via its contribution to increased body weight and abdominal fat deposition. This risk is estimated to begin as early as 25 years of age. The WHO adopted a Global Strategy on Diet, Physical Activity, and Health, which specifically aims to promote physical activity and reduce sedentary behavior; ensure locations for physical activity are attractive; allow for a safely built environments; promote accessible public spaces and infrastructure; and provide equal opportunities for physical activity, regardless of gender, age, income, education, ethnicity, or disability. Low physical activity levels are common in most high-SDI countries, as well as in North Africa and the Middle East, tropical Latin America, and the Pacific Islands.[4,5]

COVID-19 and Cardiovascular Disease

In 2019, a newly discovered coronavirus (CoV) disease spread rapidly across the globe. The WHO declared it a pandemic in early 2020 and called it severe acute respiratory syndrome (SARS)-CoV-2 virus, also called COVID-19. Most people infected with the virus experience mild to moderate flu-like symptoms, including fever, chills, shortness of breath, cough, fatigue, muscle or body aches, headache, loss of taste or smell, sore throat, congestion, nausea or vomiting, and diarrhea. As of September 2021, there were over 4.6 million death reported worldwide due to due COVID-19 with over 659,000 deaths in the United States alone. The number of confirmed cases is over 224 million and continues to rise.[80,81] Predictors of death in COVID-19 are older age, cardiovascular comorbidities, and elevated troponin. SARS-CoV-2 enters the cell on the ACE2 receptor, which is widely expressed in the heart and on endothelial cells and is linked to inflammatory activation. While development of acute respiratory distress syndrome is a common pathology seen in severe illness, vascular inflammation is not commonly seen. Myocardial injury has been described, with elevated troponin found in up to 30% of symptomatic cases; however, evidence that COVID-19 causes myocarditis is less well established.[82] There are data to suggest that most COVID-19 cardiac injury is related to stress or high circulating cytokine levels and not the virus itself. ST-segment elevation myocardial infarction (STEMI)-like patterns have been seen and are often associated with normal epicardial coronary arteries. As a result, most STEMI activations were no longer brought directly to the cardiac catheterization laboratory but were screened for COVID-19 infection first so as to not unnecessarily expose the catheterization lab staff to an infected patient without appropriate protective equipment.

Besides the direct mortality associated with COVID-19, the indirect CVD mortality will be significant. Besides increase in stress and mental health disorders during the pandemic, there were significant delays in health care–seeking behavior, including decrease in routine primary care, cardiovascular care, and emergency room utilization, due to the widespread shutdown of nonessential businesses throughout the world[83] (**Fig. 1–29**). Patients were fearful of coming to hospitals when they had symptoms of heart attack and stroke due to fear of contracting the virus, and so they often presented later with more advanced disease. Furthermore, limited clinic access also led to delays in patients receiving medications and obtaining outpatient elective imaging and cardiovascular procedures.

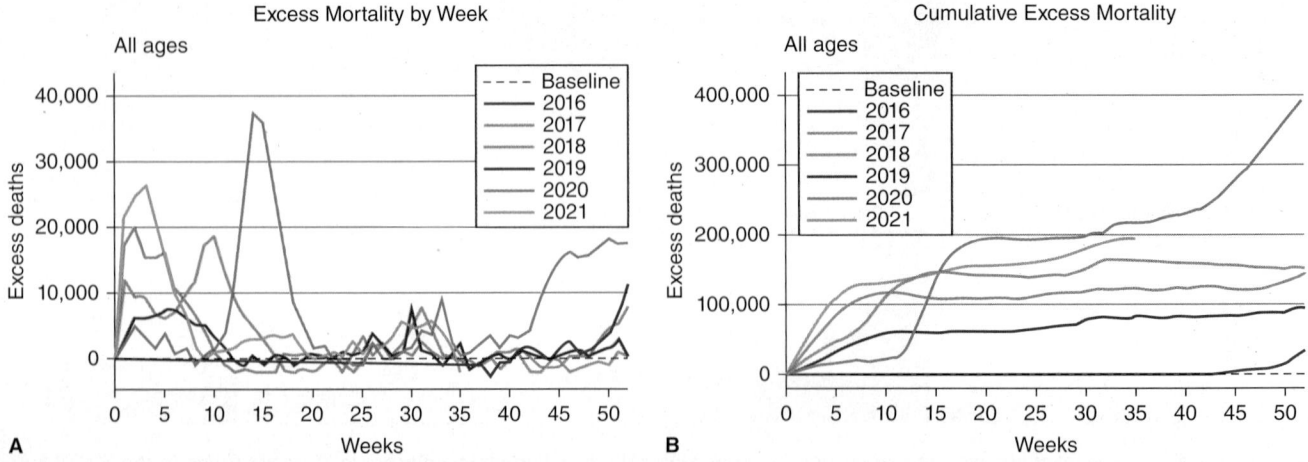

Figure 1–29. EuroMOMO pooled estimates of excess all-cause mortality by week in 2016 to 2020. For reference, the novel coronavirus, COVID-19, pandemic was declared by the World Health Organization on January 30, 2020.[83]

The long-term impact of these delays and associated morbidity and mortality such as heart failure and stroke due to untreated AF, hypertension, and coronary artery disease are yet to be seen. In addition, temporary closure of many clinics that provide suboxone and other opioid treatments for substance abuse may have caused an increase in IV drug use and subsequent increase in endocarditis. Better modeling to accurately determine the impact of COVID-19 on CVD is needed. Future research efforts are underway to better define the effect of COVID-19 on CVD.[84]

Pregnancy-Related Cardiometabolic Risk Factors

There is increasing evidence that the physiologic changes that occur with pregnancy affect a women's cardiovascular system, immune system, and metabolic function. Often referred to as an early "stress test," pregnancy can unmask susceptibility for developing cardiometabolic disorders. Specifically, women with a history of gestational diabetes mellitus, gestational hypertension, preeclampsia, eclampsia, spontaneous preterm birth, and delivery of a small gestational age baby (<2500 g) have twice the risk of future CVD events.[85,86] An estimated 10% to 15% of women have hypertensive disorders of pregnancy in high-SDI countries, which corresponded to an estimated 228,558 cases (95% UI, 146,155–323,927) in high-SDI countries in 2019[5]; however, the largest burden of premature deaths due to CVD complications of pregnancy disproportionately occurs in low-, low-middle–, and middle-SDI countries due to higher fertility rates. Accurate estimates are lacking in these countries due to lack of diagnostic tools, but the GBD 2019 study estimated a prevalence of 3.5 million (95% UI, 2.2–4.9 million) cases in 2019. The age-standardized death rate for females for maternal hypertensive disorders decreased over time, from 1.43 per 100,000 (95% UI, 1.29–1.57) in 1990 to 0.71 per 100,000 (95% UI, 0.62–0.81) in 2019, possibly due to improved global prenatal and peripartum care.[1] Yet, women in rural areas are disadvantaged due to limited access to health care infrastructure, poverty, and educational and sociocultural barriers and may be at increased risk.

Globally, the number of DALYs due to maternal hypertensive disorders decreased over time from 2.6 million (95% UI, 2.3–2.8 million) in 1990 to 1.8 million (95% UI, 1.6–2.1 million) in 2019, as did total deaths (from 39,790 deaths [95% UI, 36,106–43,783] in 1990 to 27,834 [95% UI, 24,296–31,560] in 2019).[5] Still, an estimated 20.56 maternal deaths per 100,000 live births in 2019 (95% UI, 17.95–23.32) were attributable to maternal hypertensive disorder. The long-term CVD consequences of this condition on women later in life are currently being investigated. Mobile health technologies have the potential to increase equity, quality, and efficiency of service delivery in low- and middle-SDI countries, but outcomes on mortality and CVD events are lacking. Measurement of blood pressure, lipids, and glucose is recommended annually to every 5 years after delivery to identify those at risk; however, most women with a complicated pregnancy do not routinely receive postpartum follow-up. Future integration of antenatal and postpartum care and screening for CVD risk throughout the life course is one way in which women may be more engaged in the health system and improve CVD prevention.

Air Pollution and Cardiovascular Disease

Multiple mechanisms have been considered as the cause for the association between air pollution and CVD, including inflammation, autonomic nervous system imbalance, changes in vascular responsiveness and compliance, and altered cardiac structure and promotion of atherosclerosis (**Fig. 1–30**). Air pollution has now been shown to increase preclinical risk factors such as atherosclerosis, endothelial dysfunction, and hypertension. Particulate matter (PM) is generally used to describe types of air pollution and is classified by size into PM_{10} (<10 μm mean aerodynamic diameter), coarse (<10 μm and >2.5 μm diameter), fine ($PM_{2.5}$; <2.5 μm diameter), and ultrafine (<0.1 μm diameter) fractions (**Fig. 1–31**). Air pollution includes not only ambient PM but also household indoor air pollution from solid fuels as well as ambient ozone pollution. High levels of $PM_{2.5}$ can occur with domestic combustion of biomass, coal, or kerosene for cooking and heating and is predominantly seen in low-SDI countries.[63] Upon inhalation, particles less than 10 μm diameter can deposit in the airways and lungs, with smaller particles effectively reaching the alveolar periphery. The deposited particles can activate sensory receptors, induce inflammatory and stress responses, or cross the permeable epithelial barrier into the systemic circulation.

Billions of people are exposed to indoor and outdoor air pollution, and such pollution ranks as the largest single environmental health risk factor, with more than 4.1 million (95% UI, 3.5–4.8 million) total deaths attributed to outdoor air pollution and 2.3 million (95% UI, 1.6–3.1 million) deaths attributed to indoor air pollution in 2019.[1] The age-standardized death rate due to indoor air pollution has decreased by 69.9% since 1990 due to initiatives to provide clean cook stoves to low-SDI countries; however, ambient outdoor air pollution has only decreased 0.9%, predominantly increasing in the same population previously affected by indoor air pollution—those in low- and low-middle–SDI countries. Only recently has outdoor air pollution started to decrease in middle-SDI countries, such as China. The total global DALY burden due to air pollution decreased 24% over time but still caused 213.3 million (95% UI, 188.9–239.5 million) DALYs in 2019.[5] The estimated excess risk of cardiovascular mortality rises 11% per 10 μg/m³ rise in levels of PM,[87] with no threshold level below which long-term exposure to urban air pollution had no ill effect on cardiovascular health.[63] The strongest associations between air pollution are with IHD, heart failure, and stroke, as well as contributions to obesity and type 2 diabetes. Data suggest that both short-term exposures to elevated levels of air pollutants and long-term exposure trigger CVD in susceptible populations.[88,89]

Mental Illness and Its Impact on Cardiovascular Disease

The relationship between mental health disorders and CVD is complex but receiving increasing attention as an important comorbid condition. Those with CVD are at higher risk for developing depression, while simultaneously, those with mental disorders are at greater risk for developing risk factors, as well as CVDs.[90] There is evidence for a causal association

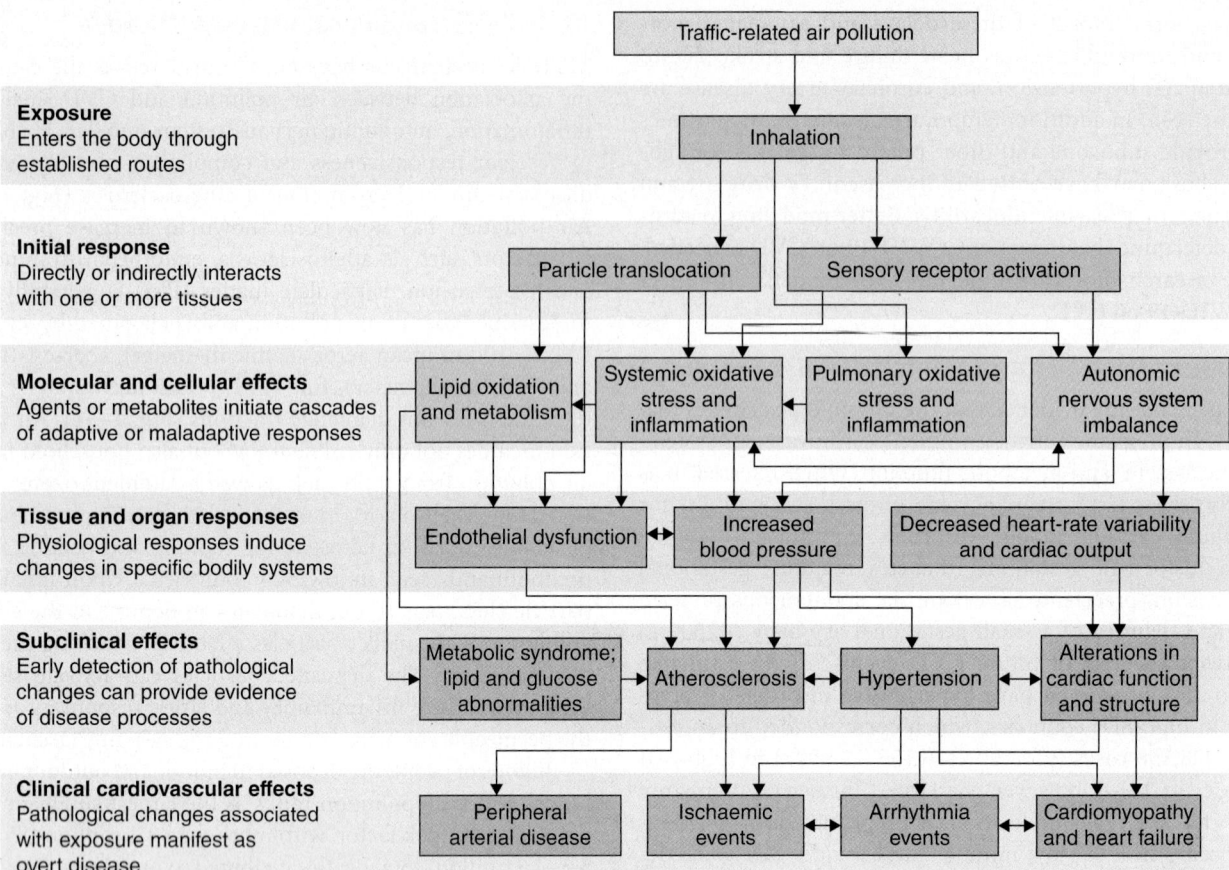

Figure 1–30. Cardiovascular effects and proposed mechanisms of chronic exposure to traffic-related air pollution. Inhaled pollutants can activate receptors in the lung or potentially cross at the alveolar level to enter the systemic circulation. Molecular and cellular effects lead to responses in various tissues and organs, to subclinical effects, and eventually to clinical cardiovascular effects. Reproduced with permission form Cosselman KE, Navas-Acien A2, Kaufman JD. Environmental factors in cardiovascular disease. *Nat Rev Cardiol.* 2015 Nov;12(11):627-642.

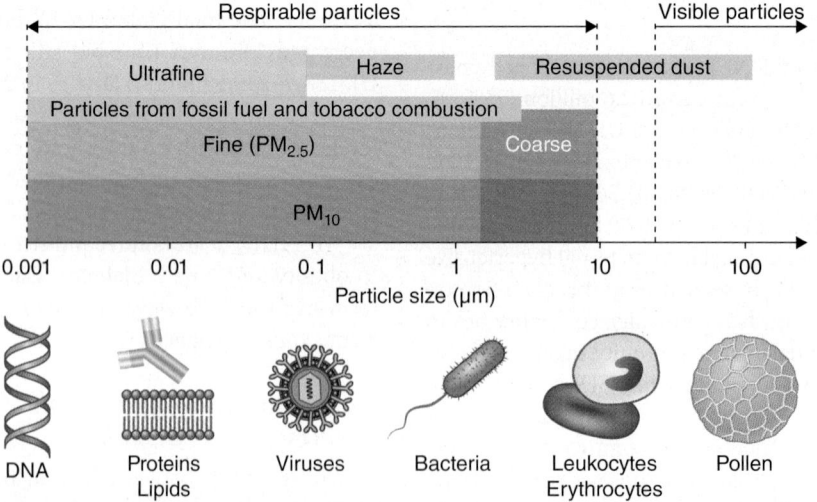

Figure 1–31. Size categorization of airborne pollutants. The particulate matter (PM) that contributes to airborne pollution is categorized according to the mean aerodynamic diameter of the particles. The broadest category (PM$_{10}$) includes all particles less than 10 μm diameter. This category is subdivided into coarse, fine, and ultrafine particles. Fine particles less than 2.5 μm diameters are also known as PM$_{2.5}$. Biological entities representative of this range of sizes are also shown. Reproduced with permission form Cosselman KE, Navas-Acien A2, Kaufman JD. Environmental factors in cardiovascular disease. *Nat Rev Cardiol.* 2015 Nov;12(11):627-642.

between depression and CVD even after adjustment for traditional CVD risk factors.[91]

The estimated global prevalence in the prior 12 months of any mental health disorder is high, estimated at 12.5% (95% UI, 11.6%–13.5%) in 2019. Globally, mental health disorders accounted for approximately 14.6% of the total global burden of disability (YLDs) in 2019, with a 55.1% increase in the number of YLDs between 1990 and 2019.[5] The prevalence of mental disorders has regional variation and is higher in Iran, Portugal, Australia, New Zealand, and Spain and lowest in high-income Asia-Pacific, Central Asia, Central Europe, and Southeast Asia.[5] In studies that assumed the association between depression and CVD to be causal, an estimated 4 million, or 3%, of IHD DALYs were attributable to major depression.[91] However, no randomized trials have demonstrated that treating depression reduces IHD risk. There is significant heterogeneity in the epidemiologic studies in this area, as well as a lack of data from many low-SDI countries.[5]

Cardiovascular Disease in the HIV-Infected Population

CVD has become more common among individuals with HIV, as survival improves as a result of highly active antiretroviral treatment. HIV can increase the risk of myocardial infarction, stroke, heart failure, and hypertension.[92-94] Antiretroviral drugs may induce dyslipidemias, reduce insulin sensitivity, and promote body fat redistribution, which contribute to CVD risk. Sustained HIV suppression reduced systemic inflammatory markers and is associated with a moderate reduction in CVD events.

The prevalence of HIV continues to increase globally, with the highest prevalence in South Africa, Botswana, Lesotho, and Eswatini (up to 20% of the population) in 2019 (**Fig. 1–32**). The

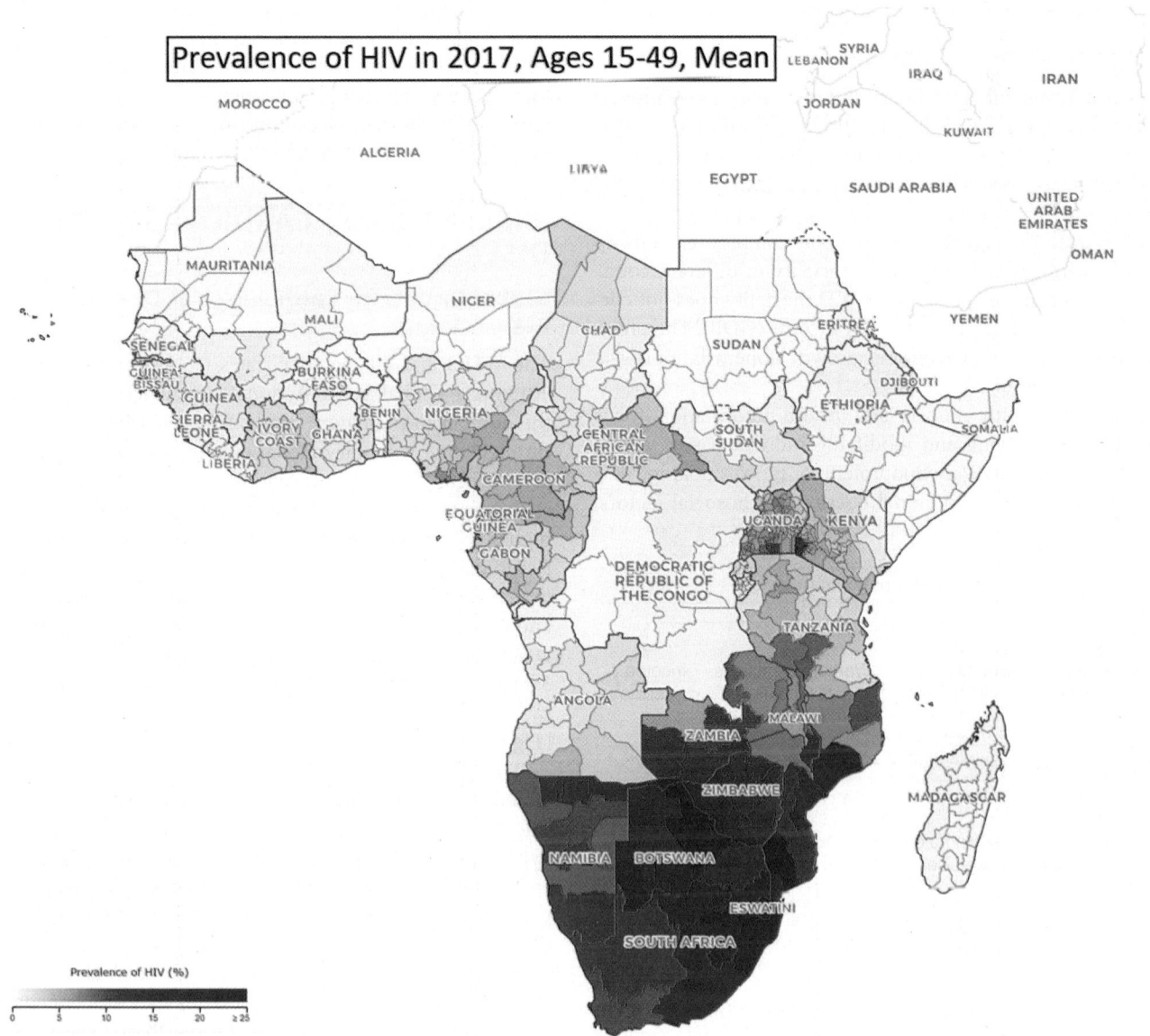

Figure 1–32. Local burden of disease for HIV in Africa. Reproduced with permission from Institute for Health Metrics and Evaluation (IHME). *Local Burden of Disease for HIV*. Seattle, WA: IHME, University of Washington; 2020. Available from https://vizhub.healthdata.org/lbd/hiv (Accessed September 28, 2020).

death rate and DALYs due to HIV peaked in the mid-2000s and have shown a steady decreasing trend, likely due to improved treatment and decreasing YLLs as more HIV-infected people live with the disease. Global deaths due to HIV in 2019 were 863,837 (95% UI, 786,075–996,045).[5] The crude rate of CVD in HIV is estimated at 61.8 (95% CI, 45.8–83.4) per 10,000 person-years.[94] Compared to individuals without HIV, the risk ratio for CVD is 2.16 (95% CI, 1.68–2.77). Over the past two decades, the global population-attributable fraction from CVD due to HIV increased from 0.36% (95% CI, 0.21%–0.56%) to 0.92% (95% CI, 0.55%–1.41%) and DALYs increased from 0.74 million (95% CI, 0.44–1.16 million) to 2.57 million (95% CI, 1.53–3.92 million).[94] Globally, the population-attributable fraction for CVD associated with HIV infection increased from 0.36% (95% CI, 0.21%–0.56%) in 1990 to 0.92% (95% CI, 0.55%–1.41%) in 2015.[95] This was associated with a greater than three-fold increase in DALYs from HIV-associated CVD from 0.74 million (95% CI, 0.44–1.16 million) in 1990 to 2.57 million (95% CI, 1.53–3.92 million) in 2015.[94]

Social Determinants of Health

While improvements in primary and secondary prevention of CVD have occurred over the past 30 years, significant inequalities remain. Although most countries have seen an increased national income per capita over this time, the decrease in the number of CVD deaths cannot be entirely explained by economic growth.[96,97] **Figure 1–33** shows the complex relationship between national SDI and CVD mortality in different countries. The decline in age-specific CVD mortality does not correlate well with increases in country income (GDP). Therefore, it appears unlikely that economic growth alone will improve a country's burden of CVD.

Currently, health models and health information focus mainly on identifying and modifying individual risk factors (eg, apolipoprotein B/apolipoprotein A ratio, smoking, diabetes, hypertension, abdominal obesity, psychosocial factors,

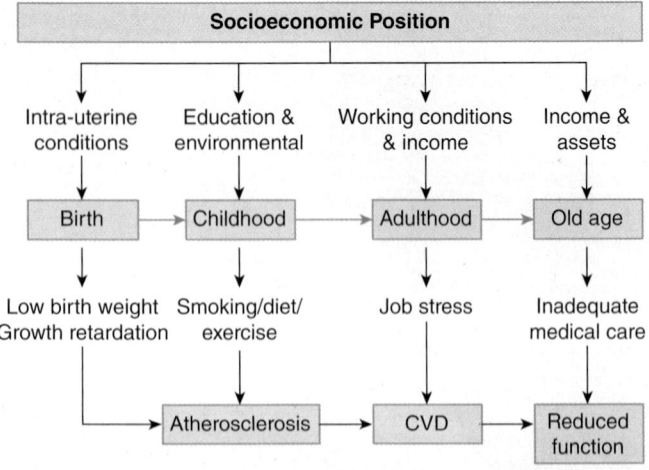

Figure 1–33. Socioeconomic influences on cardiovascular disease (CVD) across the life course. Reproduced with permission from Berkman LF, Kawachi I. *Social Epidemiology.* New York, NY: Oxford University Press; 2000.

fruit/vegetable consumption, physical activity, and alcohol consumption), which account for 90% of the population-attributable risk for myocardial infarction as demonstrated in the INTERHEART study.[98] However, some of the most important determinants of health are likely beyond the control of most individuals. Understanding the social determinants of health is critical to assess the impact of the social environment on health. This dynamic relationship can change over time, and imbalances in these social determinants of health have been attributed to the inequities in health observed both between and within countries. For example, socioeconomic circumstances at birth can still contribute to CVD even after accounting for traditional risk factors. Social determinants such as education, occupation, social norms, culture, geography, policy, economic factors, and environment factors are just a few of the influences on CVD from a life-course perspective (Fig. 1–33).[99] These social determinants of health help illuminate how social processes interact with CVD health on a global, national, and individual level. Specifically, if disadvantaged groups can be identified, intervention strategies can then be tailored at an early stage before the individual exhibits the traditional risk factors, thereby improving population cardiovascular health and reducing the burden placed on limited health care resources, especially in low- and middle-SDI countries.

PREVENTION OF CARDIOVASCULAR DISEASE

Global Targets for Cardiovascular Disease Prevention

The WHO and all member states (194 countries) agreed in 2013 to a Global NCD Action Plan, which aims to reduce the number of premature deaths from NCDs by 25% by 2025 through nine voluntary global targets. Two of the global targets directly focus on preventing and controlling CVD. The sixth target calls for a global reduction in the prevalence of high blood pressure by 25%. The seventh target calls to halt the rise in diabetes and obesity. The eighth target in the plan states that at least 50% of eligible people should receive drug therapy and counseling (including glycemic control) to prevent heart attacks and strokes. While sustainable development goal (SDG) 3.4 aims for a 30% reduction in premature deaths due to NCDs by 2030, achieving many of the other SDGs can impact CVD (**Fig. 1–34**).[10]

The World Heart Federation proposed nine roadmap plans aimed at reducing premature CVD mortality 25% by 2025. The first two roadmaps—on secondary prevention and on hypertension—are primarily focused on health system issues and identify roadblocks on the care pathway for patients with prevalent CVD or raised blood pressure[100,101] (**Fig. 1–35**). The third roadmap, on tobacco, summarizes key elements of the Framework Convention on Tobacco Control and its guidelines, describes the main roadblocks for their implementation, and proposes strategies for overcoming them. The roadmaps are developed with experts from around the world to simplify

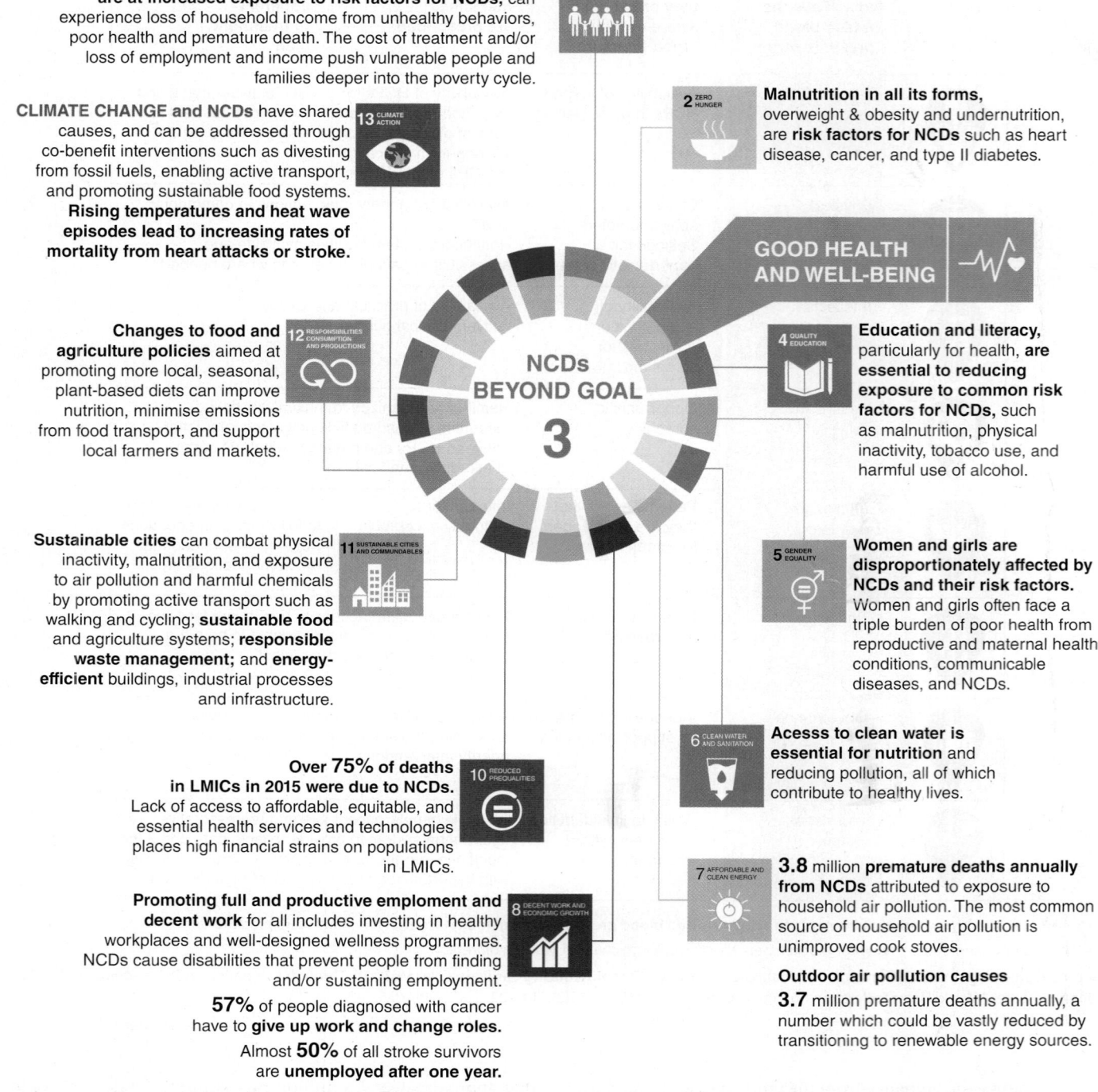

Populations in low- and middle-income countries (LMICs) are at increased exposure to risk factors for NCDs, can experience loss of household income from unhealthy behaviors, poor health and premature death. The cost of treatment and/or loss of employment and income push vulnerable people and families deeper into the poverty cycle.

CLIMATE CHANGE and NCDs have shared causes, and can be addressed through co-benefit interventions such as divesting from fossil fuels, enabling active transport, and promoting sustainable food systems. **Rising temperatures and heat wave episodes lead to increasing rates of mortality from heart attacks or stroke.**

Changes to food and agriculture policies aimed at promoting more local, seasonal, plant-based diets can improve nutrition, minimise emissions from food transport, and support local farmers and markets.

Sustainable cities can combat physical inactivity, malnutrition, and exposure to air pollution and harmful chemicals by promoting active transport such as walking and cycling; **sustainable food and agriculture systems; responsible waste management; and energy-efficient** buildings, industrial processes and infrastructure.

Over 75% of deaths in LMICs in 2015 were due to NCDs. Lack of access to affordable, equitable, and essential health services and technologies places high financial strains on populations in LMICs.

Promoting full and productive emploment and decent work for all includes investing in healthy workplaces and well-designed wellness programmes. NCDs cause disabilities that prevent people from finding and/or sustaining employment.

57% of people diagnosed with cancer have to **give up work and change roles.**

Almost **50%** of all stroke survivors are **unemployed after one year.**

Malnutrition in all its forms, overweight & obesity and undernutrition, are **risk factors for NCDs** such as heart disease, cancer, and type II diabetes.

GOOD HEALTH AND WELL-BEING

NCDs BEYOND GOAL 3

Education and literacy, particularly for health, **are essential to reducing exposure to common risk factors for NCDs,** such as malnutrition, physical inactivity, tobacco use, and harmful use of alcohol.

Women and girls are disproportionately affected by NCDs and their risk factors. Women and girls often face a triple burden of poor health from reproductive and maternal health conditions, communicable diseases, and NCDs.

Acesss to clean water is essential for nutrition and reducing pollution, all of which contribute to healthy lives.

3.8 million **premature deaths annually from NCDs** attributed to exposure to household air pollution. The most common source of household air pollution is unimproved cook stoves.

Outdoor air pollution causes

3.7 million premature deaths annually, a number which could be vastly reduced by transitioning to renewable energy sources.

Figure 1–34. NCDs across the SDGs A call for an integrated approach. Noncommunicable diseases (NCDs) across the sustainable development goals (SDGs): a call for an integrated approach. Reproduced with permission from NCD Alliance. NCDs across the SDGs: A call for an integrated approach, 2017 https://ncdalliance.org/resources/ncds-across-sdgs-a-call-for-an-integrated-approach.

		Actions needed to achieve the raised blood pressure target	Individuals aware they are at risk/ aware of their blood pressure	Priority medicines* are prescribed	Patients are adherent to treatment plan
		Human resources	Availability of trained HCPs to do screening	Availability of HCPs to prescribe recommendations at diagnosis and for long-term education of HCPs on guidelines	HCPs aware that blood pressure treatment is nearly always for life
		Physical resources	Calibrated sphygmometers Settings for opportunistic screening	Availability of priority interventions at community level* Healthcare-system facilities available and accessible to patients when and where needed	
		Intellectual resources	Availability of standardized guidelines for screening	Availability of practical and locally relevant clinical guidelines	
		Healthcare delivery	Opportunistic screening	Healthcare organized to maximize existing resources to ensure efficiency in the interaction between HCPs and patients. Adequate supply of affordable medications	
		Healthcare recipient	Patients aware that they are at risk/open to screening	Interventions culturally acceptable	Patients aware and willing to follow recommendations. Patients understand that recommendations are for life
		Financing	Free availability of screening	Patients can afford access to healthcare facilities Priority interventions are affordable to both the healthcare system and the patient	
		Governance	Adequate governance to support screening	Adequate political and regulatory framework supporting the stategy to implement and maintain priority interventions	
		Information system	Ability to link identified individuals with treatment	A simple, timely, acceptable and representative information system to provide reliable data about the incidence, prognosis and quality of care of patients with hypertension or at high-risk of hypertension	

Figure 1–35. **Health-system requirements to achieve raised blood pressure management targets.** HCP, health care practitioner.

*ACE inhibitor or angiotensin receptor blocker; beta blocker; calcium channel blocker; diuretic.

Reproduced with permission from Adler AJ, Prabhakaran D, Bovet P, et al. Reducing Cardiovascular Mortality Through Prevention and Management of Raised Blood Pressure: A World Heart Federation Roadmap. *Glob Heart.* 2015 Jun;10(2):111-122.

and synthesize the guidance from the guidelines and overcome potential barriers.[102] Subsequently, concrete examples of other roadmaps for improved global cardiovascular health have been described using a similar process (**Fig. 1–36**) for heart failure,[103] CVD and diabetes,[78] AF,[104] RHD,[105] cholesterol,[74] and Chagas disease.[54]

The Future of Global Cardiovascular Disease

Most modeling studies on the future of the CVD burden do not portend good news. In the United States, current projections suggest that nearly half of the population will have some form of CVD by 2035.[3] At the global level, Roth et al[106] estimated

that approximately 7.8 million premature CVD deaths would occur in 2025 if current risk factor trends continue unchanged. However, these premature CVD deaths would be reduced to 5.7 million if risk factors targets were achieved as a result of a 26% reduction for men and a 23% reduction for women in the global risk of premature CVD death.[106]

Other modeling studies have also shown that significant reductions in premature CVD are possible by 2025 if multiple risk factor targets are achieved. For example, in the British Isles, where CVD mortality is still among the highest in Europe, modeling estimates suggest that reducing four selected risk factors could substantially lead to CHD mortality reduction between

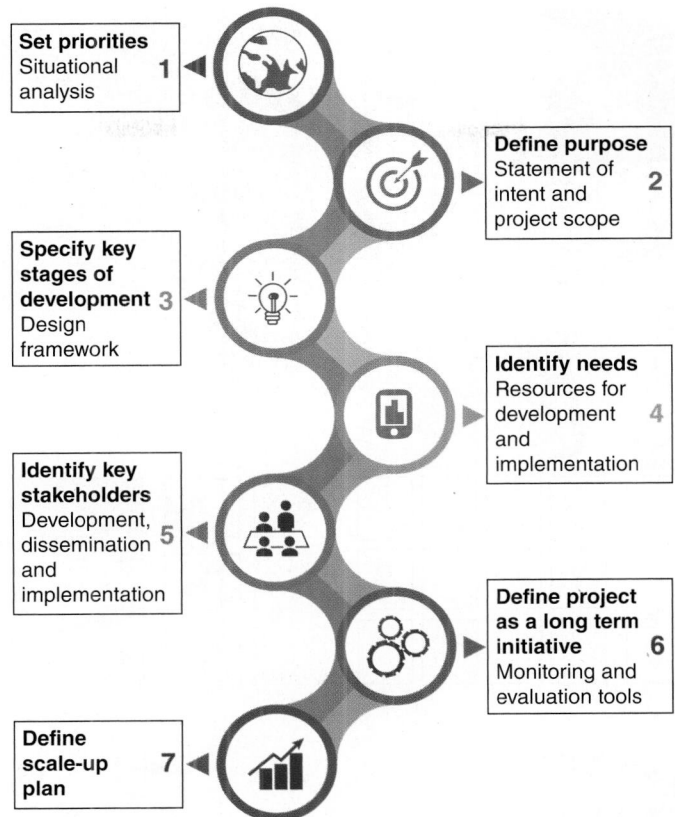

Set priorities 1
Situational
analysis

Define purpose 2
Statement of
intent and
project scope

**Specify key
stages of
development** 3
Design
framework

Identify needs 4
Resources for
development
and
implementation

**Identify key
stakeholders** 5
Development,
dissemination
and
implementation

**Define project
as a long term
initiative** 6
Monitoring and
evaluation tools

**Define
scale-up
plan** 7

Figure 1–36. The World Heart Federation Roadmap initiative. An implementation toolkit. Reproduced with permission from Mitchell S, Malanda B, Damasceno A, et al. A Roadmap on the Prevention of Cardiovascular Disease Among People Living With Diabetes. *Glob Heart.* 2019 Sep;14(3):215-240.

9% (modest scenarios) and 24% (ideal scenarios).[107] If current trends continue, the probability of dying prematurely from CVD is projected to remain unchanged in some of the world's most populous regions. Trends in tobacco use, diabetes mellitus, obesity, and blood pressure are projected to lead to a rise in premature CVD deaths from 5.9 million in 2013 to an estimated 7.8 million in 2025 with no significant change in the global probability of premature CVD deaths. Achieving these four risk factor targets would result in only 5.7 million deaths, with a 26% reduction for males and a 23% reduction for females in the global risk of premature CVD death[106] (**Fig. 1–37**).

Certain regions account for a larger burden of premature CVD death, including South Asia, East Asia, and Southeast Asia (together accounting for 60% of these deaths). The risk of a premature CVD death in 2025 would be highest for males in Central Asia and Eastern Europe (both 0.28; 95% UI, 0.26-0.30 and 0.27-0.29, respectively) and for females in Oceania (0.19; 95% UI, 0.13-0.26).[106] Western Europe, high-income Asia-Pacific regions, and Australasia would have the lowest risk (0.03 for males and 0.01 for females). Premature death and disability are not only devastating to families, but the resulting lost productivity can drag down progress and productivity in economically developing countries. Globally, the risk factor change that would lead to the largest reduction in premature mortality would be the decreased prevalence of

hypertension, followed by tobacco smoking prevalence for men and obesity for women. Results vary by region because of differences in risk factor and disease trends. Tobacco smoking would contribute the most reductions for men in North Africa and the Middle East, Central Asia, and Central sub-Saharan Africa and for women in high-income Asia-Pacific and Western Europe.[106]

Regions that have already experienced rapid declines in CVD mortality will see a relatively small benefit from proportional reductions in risk factor levels. However, for many low- and middle-income regions, a 25% reduction in premature CVD mortality would occur only in a scenario in which multiple risk factor targets are achieved.[106]

CONCLUSION

CVD continues to account for the largest loss of health globally, with the majority of premature deaths occurring in low- and middle-SDI countries. Past declines in age-standardized rates of CVD in many high-income regions were a result of improved prevention and treatment of CVD, as well as improved health care systems, but alarmingly, these rates are now rising again. The number of people in the world with CVD is increasing steadily as a result of population growth and aging, a trend that is increasingly burdening low- and

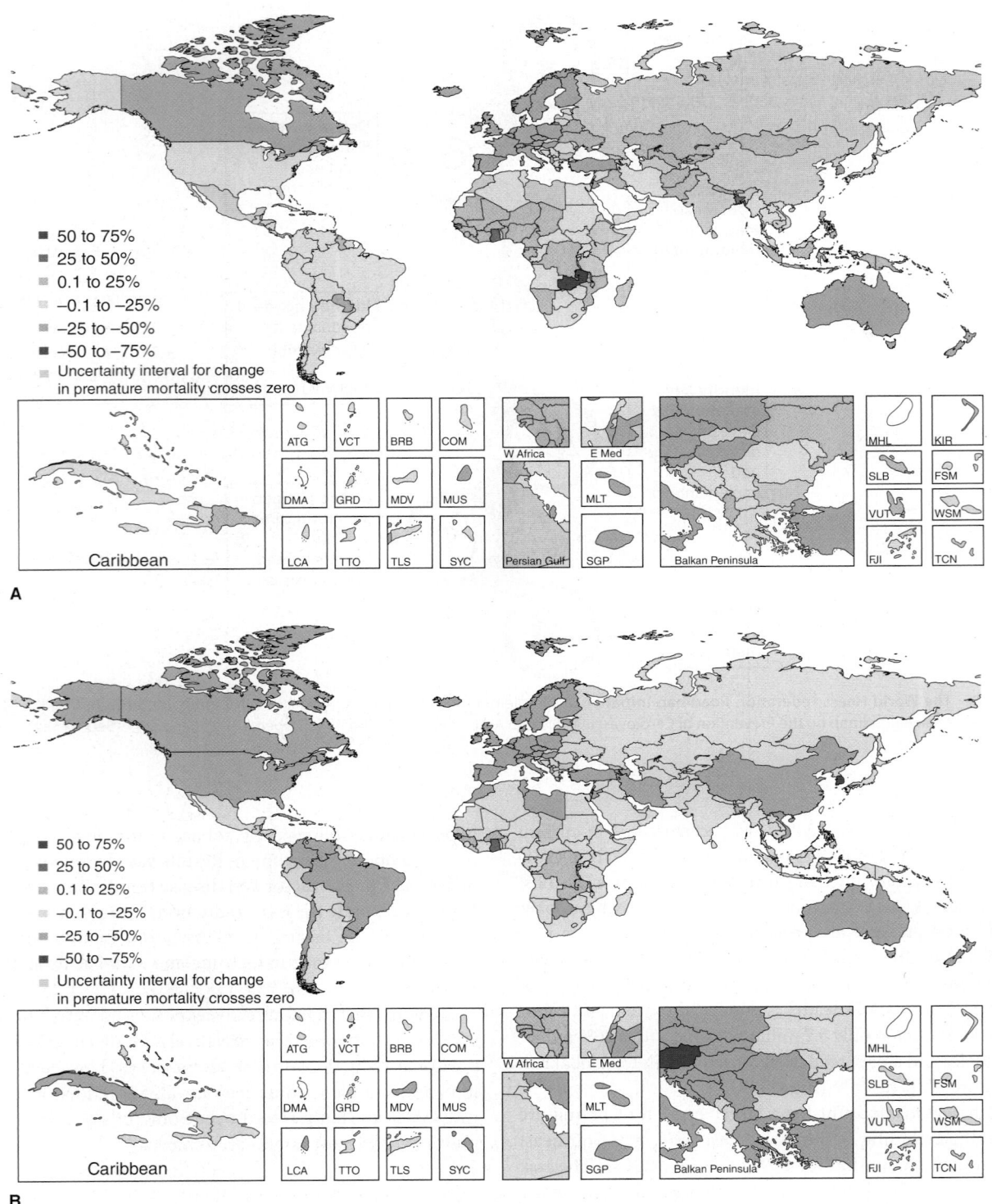

Figure 1–37. **A. Global map of percentage change in premature cardiovascular mortality from 2013 to 2025 if risk factors continue the current trend. B. Global map of percentage change in premature cardiovascular mortality from 2013 to 2025 if all risk factor targets are achieved in 2025.** Reproduced with permission from Roth GA, Nguyen G, Forouzanfar MH, et al. Estimates of global and regional premature cardiovascular mortality in 2025. *Circulation.* 2015 Sep 29;132(13):1270-1282.

middle-SDI countries and their developing health care systems. IHD remains a significant cause of death globally, and the patterns of CVD are complex and reflect regional differences in both risk factors and disease incidence.[1] Both stroke and endemic CVDs, such as Chagas disease and RHD, have varied geographic and demographic distributions.[4] Understanding the regional variations in traditional risk factors, such as high blood pressure and cholesterol, tobacco, unhealthy diet, and low physical activity, as well as nontraditional risk factors, such as air pollution, mental health disorders, and HIV, is important for determining priorities for prevention of atherosclerotic vascular diseases. Novel risk factors, such as pregnancy-related hypertensive disorders and COVID-19, warrant further investigation as the direct and indirect impact of these diseases is yet to be determined. Finally, the social determinants of health are critical to improve the social factors that determine neighborhood and environmental exposures, access to healthful diet, and physical activity and access to adequate medical care.

Achieving the four primary risk factor targets outlined by the WHO would likely result in more than a 20% reduction in the global risk of premature CVD death by 2025. However, to achieve a large-scale reduction in the global burden of CVDs, evidence-based clinical and population-level interventions that address all known health risks for CVD will need to be broadly adopted. Efforts to improve health education early in life, access to primary health care and essential medications, and access to healthy foods are likely to form the foundation of such efforts. To be sustained and successful, these efforts will require a much broader recognition of the massive impact of CVD on global health and the creation of supportive policies and the budgetary commitments to support their implementation across all sectors of society.[108,109]

METRICS AND METHODS

Summary Measures of Health

The DALY is a core summary measure of health that represents the gap between a population's actual health and an ideal standard. DALYs combine information regarding premature death (YLLs) and disability caused by the condition (YLDs). YLLs are calculated by multiplying observed deaths for a specific age in the year of interest by the age-specific reference life expectancy estimated by the use of life table methods (eg, 84.9 years at birth as the longest observed life expectancy in Singapore).[5] YLDs are calculated by multiplying disease prevalence (in number of cases for a year) by a health state–specific disability weight representing a degree of lost functional capacity. One DALY corresponds to 1 lost year of health, either caused by death or disability, and is the sum of a number of YLLs plus a number of YLDs.[5] YLLs and YLDs can be reported for specific diseases and, as cause-specific DALYs, serve as a useful tool for comparing health loss among disparate conditions. Just as with mortality, both crude and age-standardized DALY rates can be calculated by dividing the annual number of DALY by the population at risk in a given year. The summary exposure

value is a measure of a population's exposure to a particular risk factor taking into account both the level of that risk and the severity of the associated diseases. It can be interpreted as a risk-weighted prevalence. The summary exposure value is 0 when no excess risk for a population exists and 1 when the population is at the highest measured level of risk.

Defining Disease Categories

Any consistent evaluation of CVD requires the adoption of case definitions. In the GBD study, CVD is estimated separately for the 11 most common causes of CVD-related death as well as an "other" category for less common causes[4] (see Table 1–1). These causes are IHD, stroke, AF, aortic aneurysm, peripheral artery disease, hypertensive heart disease, endocarditis, cardiomyopathy, nonrheumatic valvular heart disease, RHD, and a category for other CVD conditions.[4] Congenital heart defect is also considered an NCD but is not grouped within the CVD category in GBD 2019.[5] Death is defined following international standards governing the reporting of death certificates.[1] For example, IHD is defined as an underlying cause of death across International Classification of Diseases (ICD) revisions (most recently ICD-10 I20-I25, ICD-9 410-414).[4] A proportion of deaths are erroneously assigned on death certificates to either nonfatal ICD conditions (eg, "senility") or conditions not defined as an underlying cause of death (eg, heart failure or hypertension). The GBD study developed methods for systematically reallocating these undefined or erroneously assigned deaths to CVD causes based on the total distribution of actual causes of death by country, sex, age, and year.[1,5]

Prevalent cases of IHD represent estimates of four distinct disease states: acute myocardial infarction, chronic stable angina, chronic IHD, and heart failure caused by IHD (eg, ischemic cardiomyopathy). The definition for myocardial infarction follows the WHO definition, based on the case-finding approach from the MONICA studies, which includes out-of-hospital sudden cardiac death and does not require a troponin level.[4,17] Stroke case definitions also follow the WHO and represents acute IS, hemorrhagic stroke, and subarachnoid hemorrhage and chronic disability following a stroke.[4] Peripheral artery disease is considered as an ABI less than 0.9, with disability attributed only to those reporting claudication. Prevalent AF is defined electrocardiographically, assumes either a paroxysmal or permanent state, and included atrial flutter as well as AF. Hypertensive heart disease is considered to be symptomatic heart failure as a result of hypertension (eg, New York Heart Association class II or greater). Endocarditis and RHD are diagnosed clinically, which includes cases identified either by auscultation or standard echocardiographic criteria for definite disease. For example, valve disease on a screening echocardiogram consistent with only "possible" rheumatic disease is not included; however, definite valvular disease confirmed by a clinician is included. Nonrheumatic valve disease includes both calcific aortic stenosis and DMVD, including mitral valve prolapse and mitral regurgitation.

Cardiomyopathy is an umbrella category that includes cardio-myopathy due to alcohol, myocarditis, or other causes. Maternal hypertensive disorders are defined as blood pressure greater than 140/90 mm Hg in the absence of a hypertension diagnosis prior to pregnancy, and preeclampsia and eclampsia follow standard clinical definitions. Congenital heart defects is a parent category that includes single ventricle and single ventricle pathway heart defects, malformations of great vessels, valvular heart disease and patent ductus arteriosus, ventricular septal defect and atrial septal defect, and complex congenital heart defects excluding single ventricle and single ventricle pathway.[4]

Data Sources and Analytic Methods

In brief, the most recent GBD 2019 study used all available data, including country-level surveillance, verbal autopsy, vital registration, published and unpublished disease registries, and published scientific literature.[1] These data sources are available online via the Global Health Data Exchange (http://ghdx.healthdata.org/). Regional income, metabolic and nutritional risk factors, and other covariates were estimated from surveys and published systematic reviews. Statistical approaches were used to produce estimates for all countries, including the small number without available data. Analysis of mortality adopted an ensemble model approach that includes covariates such as the levels of CVD risk factor exposures and national income while borrowing strength across space, time, and age groups.[110] Analysis of disease prevalence used custom disease modeling software, DisMod-MR, which accounts for study-level differences in measurement method and standard assumptions about the interrelationships among disease-specific incidence, prevalence, case fatality, and mortality.[1,111]

Regions of the World

GBD 2019 reported results for 21 world regions as well as 205 countries. In some sections, we collapse these regions into seven "super regions": high-income, Southeast Asia/East Asia/Oceania, North Africa/Middle East, sub-Saharan Africa, Latin American/Caribbean, Central Europe/Eastern Europe/Central Asia, and South Asia. GBD 2019 high-income regions were high-income North America, Southern Latin America, Western Europe, Australasia (Australia and New Zealand), and high-income Asia-Pacific (Japan, South Korea, Brunei, and Singapore); the remainder of countries were grouped into regions by geographic proximity and broadly similar epidemiologic patterns. A sociodemographic index was calculated for each country and divided into quintiles (high, high-middle, middle, low-middle, and low) for comparison.[1]

REFERENCES

1. GBD 2019 Diseases and Injuries Collaborators. Global burden of 369 diseases and injuries, 1990-2019: a systematic analysis for the Global Burden of Disease Study 2019. *The Lancet.* 17 October 2020. doi:10.1016/S0140-6736(20)30925-9.

2. Bloom D, Cafiero E, Jané-Llopis E, Abrahams-Gessel S, Bloom L, Fathima S. *The Global Economic Burden of Non-communicable Diseases, 2011.* Geneva, Switzerland: World Economic Forum; 2012.

3. American Heart Association. Cardiovascular disease: A costly burden for America, projections through 2035. 2017. http://www.heart.org/idc/groups/heart-public/@wcm/@adv/documents/downloadable/ucm_491543.pdf. Accessed September 12, 2020.

4. Roth GA, Mensah GA, Johnson CO, et al. Global burden of cardiovascular diseases and risk factors, 1990-2019: update from the GBD 2019 study. *J Am Coll Cardiol.* 2020;76(25):2982-3021.

5. GBD 2019 Demographics Collaborators. Global age-sex-specific fertility, mortality, healthy life expectancy (HALE), and population estimates in 204 countries and territories, 1950-2019: a comprehensive demographic analysis for the Global Burden of Disease Study 2019. *The Lancet.* 17 October 2020. doi:10.1016/S0140-6736(20)30977-6.

6. Akuze J, Blencowe H, Waiswa P, et al. Randomised comparison of two household survey modules for measuring stillbirths and neonatal deaths in five countries: the Every Newborn-INDEPTH study. *Lancet Glob Health.* 2020;8(4):e555-e566.

7. Small AM, O'Donnell CJ, Damrauer SM. Large-scale genomic biobanks and cardiovascular disease. *Curr Cardiol Rep.* 2018;20(4):22.

8. Iacoviello L, De Curtis A, Donati MB, de Gaetano G. Biobanks for cardiovascular epidemiology and prevention. *Future Cardiol.* 2014;10(2): 243-254.

9. GBD 2019 Universal Health Coverage Collaborators. Measuring universal health coverage based on an index of effective coverage of health services in 204 countries and territories, 1990-2019: a systematic analysis for the Global Burden of Disease Study 2019. *Lancet.* 2020;396(10258): 1250-1284.

10. NCD Alliance. NCDs across the SDGs: A call for an integrated approach. 2017. https://ncdalliance.org/news-events/news/infographic-ncds-across-s-dgs-a-call-for-an-integrated-approach. Accessed April 22, 2021.

11. Huffman MD, Rao KD, Pichon-Riviere A, et al. A cross-sectional study of the microeconomic impact of cardiovascular disease hospitalization in four low- and middle-income countries. *PLoS One.* 2011;6:e20821.

12. Murray CJ, Frenk J. Health metrics and evaluation: strengthening the science. *Lancet.* 2008;371(9619):1191-1199.

13. Chen S, Kuhn M, Prettner K, Bloom DE. The macroeconomic burden of noncommunicable diseases in the United States: estimates and projections. *PloS One.* 2018;13(11):e0206702.

14. United Nations, Department of Economic and Social Affairs, Population Division. *World Population Prospects 2019: Highlights (ST/ESA/SER.A/423).* Geneva, Switzerland: United Nations; 2019.

15. Chang AY, Skirbekk VF, Tyrovolas S, Kassebaum NJ, Dieleman JL. Measuring population ageing: an analysis of the Global Burden of Disease Study 2017. *Lancet Public Health.* 2019;4(3):e159-e167.

16. Roth GA, Forouzanfar MH, Moran AE, et al. Demographic and epidemiologic drivers of global cardiovascular mortality. *N Engl J Med.* 2015;372(14):1333-1341.

17. Tunstall-Pedoe H, Kuulasmaa K, Amouyel P, Arveiler D, Rajakangas AM, Pajak A. Myocardial infarction and coronary deaths in the World Health Organization MONICA Project. Registration procedures, event rates, and case-fatality rates in 38 populations from 21 countries in four continents. *Circulation.* 1994;90:583-612.

18. Keys AE. Coronary heart disease in seven countries. *Circulation.* 1970;41:1-211.

19. Moran A, Shen A, Turner-Lloveras D, et al. Utility of self-reported diagnosis and electrocardiogram Q-waves for estimating myocardial infarction prevalence: an international comparison study. *Heart.* 2012;98(22):1660-1666.

20. George J, Rapsomaniki E, Pujades-Rodriguez M, et al. How does cardiovascular disease first present in women and men? Incidence of 12 cardiovascular diseases in a contemporary cohort of 1,937,360 people. *Circulation.* 2015;132(14):1320-1328.

21. Zaridze D, Brennan P, Boreham J, et al. Alcohol and cause-specific mortality in Russia: a retrospective case–control study of 48 557 adult deaths. *Lancet.* 2009;373:2201-2214.

22. Murphy A, Johnson CO, Roth GA, et al. Ischaemic heart disease in the former Soviet Union 1990-2015 according to the Global Burden of Disease 2015 Study. *Heart.* 2018;104(1):58-66.

23. Sidney S, Quesenberry CP Jr, Jaffe MG, et al. Recent trends in cardiovascular mortality in the United States and public health goals. *JAMA Cardiol.* 2016;1(5):594-599.

24. Mensah GA, Wei GS, Sorlie PD, et al. Decline in cardiovascular mortality: possible causes and implications. *Circ Res.* 2017;120(2):366-380.

25. Gupta R, Islam S, Mony P, et al. Socioeconomic factors and use of secondary preventive therapies for cardiovascular diseases in South Asia: the PURE study. *Eur J Prev Cardiol.* 2015;22(10):1261-1271.

26. Yusuf S, Islam S, Chow CK, et al. Use of secondary prevention drugs for cardiovascular disease in the community in high-income, middle-income, and low-income countries (the PURE Study): a prospective epidemiological survey. *Lancet.* 2011;378(9798):1231-1243.

27. Ewen M, Zweekhorst M, Regeer B, Laing R. Baseline assessment of WHO's target for both availability and affordability of essential medicines to treat non-communicable diseases. *PloS One.* 2017;12(2):e0171284.

28. Khatib R, McKee M, Shannon H, et al. Availability and affordability of cardiovascular disease medicines and their effect on use in high-income, middle-income, and low-income countries: an analysis of the PURE study data. *Lancet.* 2016;387(10013):61-69.

29. Bukhman G, Mocumbi AO, Atun R, et al. The Lancet NCDI Poverty Commission: bridging a gap in universal health coverage for the poorest billion. *Lancet.* 2020;396(10256):991-1044.

30. Virani SS, Alonso A, Benjamin EJ, et al. Heart disease and stroke statistics-2020 update: a report from the American Heart Association. *Circulation.* 2020;141(9):e139-e596.

31. Feigin VL, Vos T, Nichols E, et al. The global burden of neurological disorders: translating evidence into policy. *Lancet Neurol.* 2020;19(3):255-265.

32. Sampson UK, Norman PE, Fowkes FG, et al. Estimation of global and regional incidence and prevalence of abdominal aortic aneurysms 1990 to 2010. *Glob Heart.* 2014;9(1):159-170.

33. Fowkes FGR, Rudan D, Rudan I, et al. Comparison of global estimates of prevalence and risk factors for peripheral artery disease in 2000 and 2010: a systematic review and analysis. *Lancet.* 2013;382:1329-1340.

34. Chamberlain AM, Gersh BJ, Alonso A, et al. Decade-long trends in atrial fibrillation incidence and survival: a community study. *Am J Med.* 2014;128(3):260-267.e261.

35. Schnabel RB, Yin X, Gona P, et al. 50 year trends in atrial fibrillation prevalence, incidence, risk factors, and mortality in the Framingham Heart Study: a cohort study. *Lancet.* 2015;386(9989):154-162.

36. GBD 2017 Congenital Heart Disease Collaborators. Global, regional, and national burden of congenital heart disease, 1990-2017: a systematic analysis for the Global Burden of Disease Study 2017. *Lancet Child Adolesc Health.* 2020;4(3):185-200.

37. Graetz N, Friedman J, Osgood-Zimmerman A, et al. Mapping local variation in educational attainment across Africa. *Nature.* 2018;555(7694):48-53.

38. Gakidou E, Cowling K, Lozano R, Murray CJ. Increased educational attainment and its effect on child mortality in 175 countries between 1970 and 2009: a systematic analysis. *Lancet.* 2010;376(9745):959-974.

39. Hoffman J. The global burden of congenital heart disease. *Cardiovasc J Afr.* 2013;24(4):141-145.

40. Frenk J. Bridging the divide: global lessons from evidence-based health policy in Mexico. *Lancet.* 2006;368(9539):954-961.

41. GBD 2016 Alcohol and Drug Use Collaborators. The global burden of disease attributable to alcohol and drug use in 195 countries and territories, 1990-2016: a systematic analysis for the Global Burden of Disease Study 2016. *Lancet Psychiatry.* 2018;5(12):987-1012.

42. Cook CC, Rankin JS, Roberts HG, et al. The opioid epidemic and intravenous drug-associated endocarditis: a path forward. *J Thorac Cardiovasc Surg.* 2020;159(4):1273-1278.

43. Bannay A, Hoen B, Duval X, et al. The impact of valve surgery on short- and long-term mortality in left-sided infective endocarditis: do differences in methodological approaches explain previous conflicting results? *Eur Heart J.* 2011;32(16):2003-2015.

44. Wang A, Chu VH, Athan E, et al. Association between the timing of surgery for complicated, left-sided infective endocarditis and survival. *Am Heart J.* 2019;210:108-116.

45. Wang CY, Wang YC, Yang YS, et al. Microbiological features, clinical characteristics and outcomes of infective endocarditis in adults with and without hemodialysis: a 10-year retrospective study in northern Taiwan. *J Microbiol Immunol Infect.* 2020;53(2):336-343.

46. Wang A. Statement from the International Collaboration on Endocarditis on the current status of surgical outcome in infective endocarditis. *Ann Cardiothorac Surg.* 2019;8(6):678-680.

47. Chu VH, Park LP, Athan E, et al. Association between surgical indications, operative risk, and clinical outcome in infective endocarditis: a prospective study from the International Collaboration on Endocarditis. *Circulation.* 2015;131(2):131-140.

48. Murdoch DR. Clinical presentation, etiology, and outcome of infective endocarditis in the 21st century: the International Collaboration on Endocarditis-Prospective Cohort Study. *Arch Intern Med.* 2009;169:463-473.

49. Yadgir S, Johnson CO, Aboyans V, et al. Global, regional, and national burden of calcific aortic valve and degenerative mitral valve diseases, 1990-2017. *Circulation.* 2020;141(21):1670-1680.

50. Watkins DA, Johnson CO, Colquhoun SM, et al. Global, regional, and national burden of rheumatic heart disease, 1990-2015. *N Engl J Med.* 2017;377(8):713-722.

51. Carapetis JR, Steer AC, Mulholland EK, Weber M. The global burden of group A streptococcal diseases. *Lancet Infect Dis.* 2005;5:685-694.

52. Zuhlke L, Engel ME, Karthikeyan G, et al. Characteristics, complications, and gaps in evidence-based interventions in rheumatic heart disease: the Global Rheumatic Heart Disease Registry (the REMEDY study). *Eur Heart J.* 2015;36(18):1115-1122a.

53. Watkins DA, Zuhlke LJ, Narula J. Moving forward the RHD agenda at global and national levels. *Glob Heart.* 2017;12(1):1-2.

54. Echeverria LE, Marcus R, Novick G, et al. WHF IASC roadmap on Chagas disease. *Glob Heart.* 2020;15(1):26.

55. Stanaway JD, Roth G. The burden of Chagas disease. *Glob Heart.* 2015;10:139-144.

56. Lee BY, Bacon KM, Bottazzi ME, Hotez PJ. Global economic burden of Chagas disease: a computational simulation model. *Lancet Infect Dis.* 2013;13(4):342-348.

57. Kershaw KN, Osypuk TL, Do DP, De Chavez PJ, Diez Roux AV. Neighborhood-level racial/ethnic residential segregation and incident cardiovascular disease: the multi-ethnic study of atherosclerosis. *Circulation.* 2015;131(2):141-148.

58. Mensah GA, Roth GA, Sampson UK, et al. Mortality from cardiovascular diseases in sub-Saharan Africa, 1990-2013: a systematic analysis of data from the Global Burden of Disease Study 2013. *Cardiovasc J Afr.* 2015;26(2 suppl 1):S6-10.

59. Moran A, Forouzanfar M, Sampson U, Chugh S, Feigin V, Mensah G. The epidemiology of cardiovascular diseases in sub-Saharan Africa: the Global Burden of Diseases, Injuries and Risk Factors 2010 Study. *Prog Cardiovasc Dis.* 2013;56:234-239.

60. Institute for Health Metrics and Evaluation Human Development Network, The World Bank. *Generating Evidence, Guiding Policy: Sub-Saharan Africa Regional Edition.* Seattle, WA: Institute for Health Metrics and Evaluation; 2013.

61. Mensah GA. Tackling noncommunicable diseases in Africa: caveat lector. *Health Educ Behav.* 2016;43(1 Suppl):7S-13S.

62. GBD Chronic Respiratory Disease Collaborators. Prevalence and attributable health burden of chronic respiratory diseases, 1990-2017: a systematic analysis for the Global Burden of Disease Study 2017. *Lancet Respir Med.* 2020;8(6):585-596.

63. Dzudie A, Rayner B, Ojji D, et al. Roadmap to achieve 25% hypertension control in Africa by 2025. *Glob Heart.* 2018;13(1):45-59.

64. Plante TB, Koh I, Judd SE, et al. Life's simple 7 and incident hypertension: the REGARDS study. *J Am Heart Assoc.* 2020;9(19):e016482.

65. Muntner P, Hardy ST, Fine LJ, et al. Trends in blood pressure control among US adults with hypertension, 1999-2000 to 2017-2018. *JAMA.* 2020;324(12):1190-1200.

66. Danaei G, Finucane MM, Lin JK, et al. National, regional, and global trends in systolic blood pressure since 1980: systematic analysis of health examination surveys and epidemiological studies with 786 country-years and 5·4 million participants. *Lancet.* 2011;377:568-577.

67. Afshin A, Forouzanfar MH, Reitsma MB, et al. Health effects of overweight and obesity in 195 countries over 25 years. *N Engl J Med.* 2017;377(1):13-27.

68. Mozaffarian D, Afshin A, Benowitz NL, et al. Population approaches to improve diet, physical activity, and smoking habits: a scientific statement from the American Heart Association. *Circulation.* 2012;126(12):1514-1563.

69. Mozaffarian D, Fahimi S, Singh GM, et al. Global sodium consumption and death from cardiovascular causes. *N Engl J Med.* 2014;371(7):624-634.

70. Schwingshackl L, Knuppel S, Michels N, et al. Intake of 12 food groups and disability-adjusted life years from coronary heart disease, stroke, type 2 diabetes, and colorectal cancer in 16 European countries. *Eur J Epidemiol.* 2019;34(8):765-775.

71. Mach F, Baigent C, Catapano AL, et al. 2019 ESC/EAS Guidelines for the management of dyslipidaemias: lipid modification to reduce cardiovascular risk. *Eur Heart J.* 2020;41(1):111-188.

72. Grundy SM, Stone NJ, Bailey AL, et al. 2018 AHA/ACC/AACVPR/AAPA/ABC/ACPM/ADA/AGS/APhA/ASPC/NLA/PCNA guideline on the management of blood cholesterol: executive summary: a report of the American College of Cardiology/American Heart Association Task Force on Clinical Practice Guidelines. *Circulation.* 2019;139(25):e1046-e1081.

73. Wilson PWF, Polonsky TS, Miedema MD, Khera A, Kosinski AS, Kuvin JT. Systematic review for the 2018 AHA/ACC/AACVPR/AAPA/ABC/ACPM/ADA/AGS/APhA/ASPC/NLA/PCNA guideline on the management of blood cholesterol: a report of the American College of Cardiology/American Heart Association Task Force on Clinical Practice Guidelines. *Circulation.* 2019;139(25):e1144-e1161.

74. Murphy A, Faria-Neto JR, Al-Rasadi K, et al. World Heart Federation cholesterol roadmap. *Glob Heart.* 2017;12(3):179-197.e175.

75. Bruckert E, Parhofer KG, Gonzalez-Juanatey JR, et al. Proportion of high-risk/very high-risk patients in europe with low-density lipoprotein cholesterol at target according to european guidelines: a systematic review. *Adv Ther.* 2020;37(5):1724-1736.

76. GBD 2019 Risk Factors Collaborators. Global burden of 87 risk factors in 204 countries and territories, 1990-2019: a systematic analysis for the Global Burden of Disease Study 2019. The *Lancet.* 2020. https://www.thelancet.com/journals/lancet/article/PIIS0140-6736(20)30752-2/fulltext.

77. Danaei G, Finucane MM, Lu Y, et al. National, regional, and global trends in fasting plasma glucose and diabetes prevalence since 1980: systematic analysis of health examination surveys and epidemiological studies with 370 country-years and 2·7 million participants. *Lancet.* 2011;378:31-40.

78. Mitchell S, Malanda B, Damasceno A, et al. A roadmap on the prevention of cardiovascular disease among people living with diabetes. *Glob Heart.* 2019;14(3):215-240.

79. GBD 2013 Risk Factors Collaborators, Forouzanfar MH, Alexander L, et al. Global, regional and national comparative risk assessment of 79 behavioural, environmental/occupational and metabolic risks or clusters of risks in 188 countries 1990-2013: a systematic analysis for the GBD 2013. *Lancet.* 2015;386(10010):2287-323.

80. Johns Hopkins University. Coronavirus Resource Center: Tracking. https://coronavirus.jhu.edu/data. Accessed April 22, 2021.

81. Institute for Health Metrics and Evaluation. *COVID-19 Mortality, Infection, Testing, Hospital Resource Use, and Social Distancing Projections.* Seattle, WA: Institute for Health Metrics and Evaluation, University of Washington; 2020.

82. Lang JP, Wang X, Moura FA, Siddiqi HK, Morrow DA, Bohula EA. A current review of COVID-19 for the cardiovascular specialist. *Am Heart J.* 2020;226:29-44.

83. Vestergaard LS, Nielsen J, Richter L, et al. Excess all-cause mortality during the COVID-19 pandemic in Europe: preliminary pooled estimates from the EuroMOMO network, March to April 2020. *Euro Surveill.* 2020;25(26):2001214.

84. Norton A, Mphahlele J, Yazdanpanah Y, Piot P, Bayona MT. Strengthening the global effort on COVID-19 research. *Lancet.* 2020;396(10248):375.

85. Nagraj S, Kennedy SH, Norton R, et al. Cardiometabolic risk factors in pregnancy and implications for long-term health: identifying the research priorities for low-resource settings. *Front Cardiovasc Med.* 2020;7:40.

86. Hauspurg A, Ying W, Hubel CA, Michos ED, Ouyang P. Adverse pregnancy outcomes and future maternal cardiovascular disease. *Clin Cardiol.* 2018;41(2):239-246.

87. Cosselman KE, Navas-Acien A, Kaufman JD. Environmental factors in cardiovascular disease. *Nat Rev Cardiol.* 2015;12(11):627-642.

88. Gill EA, Curl CL, Adar SD, et al. Air pollution and cardiovascular disease in the Multi-Ethnic Study of Atherosclerosis. *Prog Cardiovasc Dis.* 2011;53(5):353-360.

89. Yin P, Brauer M, Cohen AJ, et al. The effect of air pollution on deaths, disease burden, and life expectancy across China and its provinces, 1990-2017: an analysis for the Global Burden of Disease Study 2017. *Lancet Planet Health.* 2020;4(9):e386-e398.

90. Mensah GA, Collins PY. Understanding mental health for the prevention and control of cardiovascular diseases. *Glob Heart.* 2015;10(3):221-224.

91. Charlson FJ, Moran AE, Freedman G, et al. The contribution of major depression to the global burden of ischemic heart disease: a comparative risk assessment. *BMC Med.* 2013;11:250.

92. Rosenson RS, Hubbard D, Monda KL, et al. Excess risk for atherosclerotic cardiovascular outcomes among US adults with HIV in the current era. *J Am Heart Assoc.* 2020;9(1):e013744.

93. Fahme SA, Bloomfield GS, Peck R. Hypertension in HIV-infected adults: novel pathophysiologic mechanisms. *Hypertension.* 2018;72(1):44-55.

94. Shah ASV, Stelzle D, Lee KK, et al. Global burden of atherosclerotic cardiovascular disease in people living with HIV: systematic review and meta-analysis. *Circulation.* 2018;138(11):1100-1112.

95. Paisible AL, Chang CC, So-Armah KA, et al. HIV infection, cardiovascular disease risk factor profile, and risk for acute myocardial infarction. *J Acquir Immune Defic Syndr.* 2015;68(2):209-216.

96. Roger VL. Medicine and society: social determinants of health and cardiovascular disease. *Eur Heart J.* 2020;41(11):1179-1181.

97. Havranek EP, Mujahid MS, Barr DA, et al. Social determinants of risk and outcomes for cardiovascular disease: a scientific statement from the American Heart Association. *Circulation.* 2015;132(9):873-898.

98. Yusuf S, Hawken S, Ounpuu S, et al. Effect of potentially modifiable risk factors associated with myocardial infarction in 52 countries (the INTERHEART study): case-control study. *Lancet.* 2004;364:937-952.

99. Berkman LF. Social support, social networks, social cohesion and health. *Soc Work Health Care.* 2000;31(2):3-14.

100. Perel P, Avezum A, Huffman M, et al. Reducing premature cardiovascular morbidity and mortality in people with atherosclerotic vascular disease: the World Heart Federation roadmap for secondary prevention of cardiovascular disease. *Glob Heart.* 2015;10(2):99-110.

101. Adler AJ, Prabhakaran D, Bovet P, et al. Reducing cardiovascular mortality through prevention and management of raised blood pressure: a World Heart Federation roadmap. *Glob Heart.* 2015;10(2):111-122.

102. Grainger Gasser A, Welch C, Arora M, et al. Reducing cardiovascular mortality through tobacco control: a World Heart Federation roadmap. *Glob Heart.* 2015;10(2):123-133.

103. Ferreira JP, Kraus S, Mitchell S, et al. World Heart Federation roadmap for heart failure. *Glob Heart.* 2019;14(3):197-214.

104. Murphy A, Banerjee A, Breithardt G, et al. The World Heart Federation roadmap for nonvalvular atrial fibrillation. *Glob Heart.* 2017;12(4):273-284.

105. Palafox B, Mocumbi AO, Kumar RK, et al. The WHF roadmap for reducing CV morbidity and mortality through prevention and control of RHD. *Glob Heart.* 2017;12(1):47-62.

106. Roth GA, Nguyen G, Forouzanfar MH, Mokdad AH, Naghavi M, Murray CJ. Estimates of global and regional premature cardiovascular mortality in 2025. *Circulation.* 2015;132(13):1270-1282.

107. Hughes J, Kabir Z, Bennett K, et al. Modelling future coronary heart disease mortality to 2030 in the British Isles. *PloS One.* 2015;10(9):e0138044.

108. World Health Federation. The Mexico Declaration for Circulatory Health: Improving Circulatory Health for All People. 2016. https://www.world-heart-federation.org/wp-content/uploads/2017/07/The-Mexico-Declaration-Circulatory-Health-for-All-People.pdf. Accessed April 22, 2021.

109. Sixty-Sixth World Health Assembly. Follow-up to the Political Declaration of the High-level Meeting of the General Assembly on the Prevention and Control of Non-communicable Diseases. Nations U2013. https://apps.who.int/gb/ebwha/pdf_files/WHA66/A66_R10-en.pdf?ua=1. Accessed April 22, 2021.

110. Foreman KJ, Lozano R, Lopez AD, Murray CJ. Modeling causes of death: an integrated approach using CODEm. *Popul Health Metr.* 2012;10:1.

111. Flaxman A, Vos T, Murray CJ. *An Integrative Meta-Regression Framework for Descriptive Epidemiology.* Seattle, WA: University of Washington Press; 2015.

Clinical Cardiovascular Examination

William R. Miranda and Rick A. Nishimura

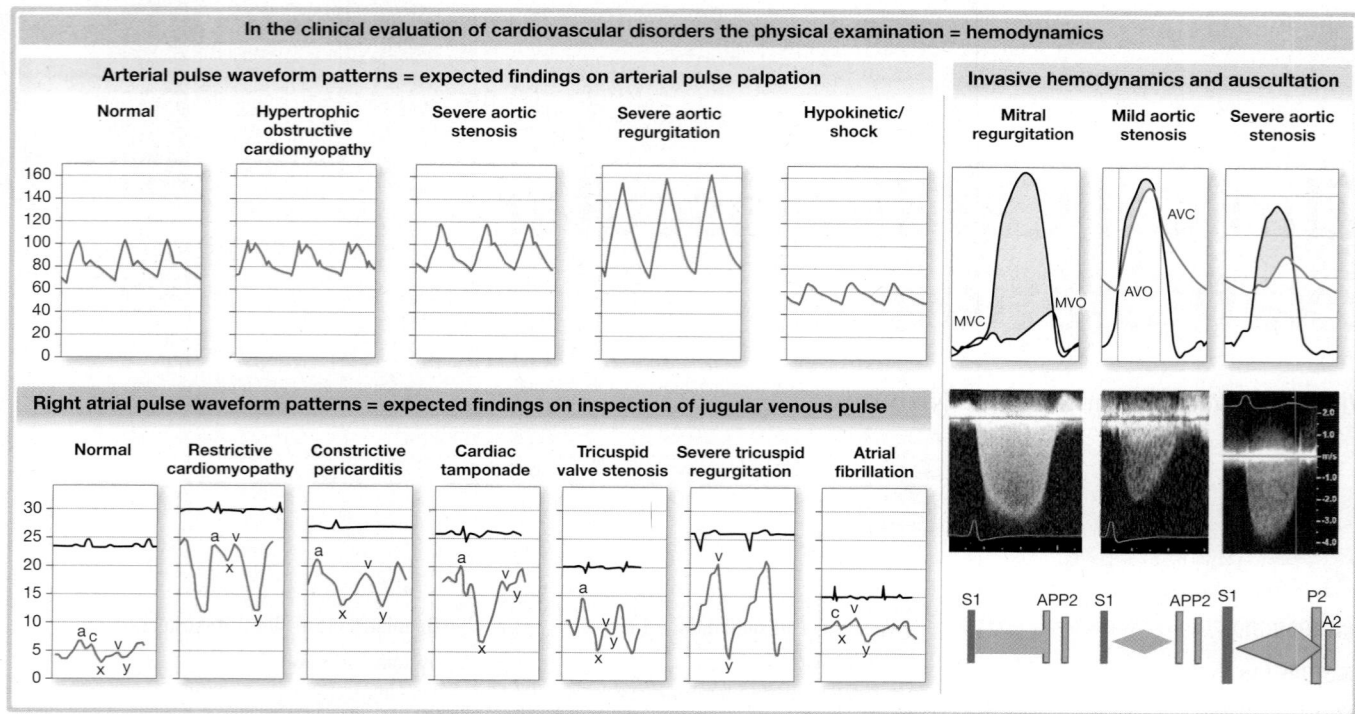

In the clinical evaluation of cardiovascular disorders the physical examination = hemodynamics

Arterial pulse waveform patterns = expected findings on arterial pulse palpation

Normal | Hypertrophic obstructive cardiomyopathy | Severe aortic stenosis | Severe aortic regurgitation | Hypokinetic/shock

Invasive hemodynamics and auscultation

Mitral regurgitation | Mild aortic stenosis | Severe aortic stenosis

Right atrial pulse waveform patterns = expected findings on inspection of jugular venous pulse

Normal | Restrictive cardiomyopathy | Constrictive pericarditis | Cardiac tamponade | Tricuspid valve stenosis | Severe tricuspid regurgitation | Atrial fibrillation

Chapter 2 Fuster and Hurst's Central Illustration. Findings on palpation, inspection, and auscultation are reflective of underlying hemodynamics. A well-performed physical examination is necessary to provide an initial clinical impression of the type and severity of cardiac disease as well as its effect on the patient. The subsequent diagnostic studies should then be used to confirm or refute this initial impression, and the final diagnosis can only be made if there is a concordance of the two. In the upper left panel, a normal arterial pulse waveform and abnormal arterial waveform patterns seen in various disease states are shown. These arterial waveforms illustrate the expected findings on arterial pulse palpation. In the lower left panel, a normal right atrial waveform and abnormal right atrial pulse waveform patterns seen in various disease states are shown. The right atrial waveform correlates with the expected findings on inspection of the jugular venous pulse. In the right panel, hemodynamic tracings showing simultaneous aortic, left ventricular and left atrial pressure, echo-Doppler, and auscultatory findings are shown for mitral regurgitation, mild stenosis, and severe aortic stenosis. AVC, aortic valve closure; AVO, aortic valve opening; HSM, holosystolic murmur; MVC, mitral valve closure; MVO, mitral valve opening; SEM, systolic ejection murmur.

CHAPTER SUMMARY

This chapter presents a modern approach to physical examination in cardiovascular disease (CVD), correlating bedside findings with echo-Doppler-derived and invasive hemodynamics. The patient's history and a physical examination have always been the central component of the clinical evaluation of CVD. Findings on palpation, inspection, and auscultation are reflective of the underlying hemodynamics (see Fuster and Hurst's Central Illustration). Although there have been tremendous advances in noninvasive testing over the past 50 years, history-taking and physical examinations are still essential in providing the pretest probability for subsequent diagnostic testing. A final diagnosis will be made only when there is agreement between the clinical assessment and test results; when discordance is present, further assessment is needed.

We are in danger of losing our clinical heritage and pinning too much faith in figures thrown up by machines. Medicine will suffer if this tendency is not checked. —Paul Wood (1950)[1]

INTRODUCTION

The history and physical examination have always been the cornerstone of the evaluation of the patient with known or suspected cardiovascular disease. In the past five decades, there has been unprecedented development and implementation of cardiovascular diagnostic modalities that provide high-resolution, real-time images of cardiac structure and measurements of cardiac function. The new generation of cardiovascular specialists is now relying more and more on the results of these tests to make clinical decisions, with decreasing emphasis on teaching and performing a proper history and physical examination. However, optimal patient care should involve cardiovascular testing to confirm and supplement the clinical impression based on the history and examination—not replace it.

The initial interview with the patient is a necessity that has not changed over the decades. A properly taken history not only provides the richest source of clinical information regarding a patient's illness but is key to understanding the effect of the illness on the patient and family as well as individual needs and preferences. This knowledge, as well as the compassion and empathy that the physician can extend to the patient and family during this initial interaction, is of great importance not only in the clinical decision-making but also in forming a trustful patient–physician relationship. It is important to always listen to patients. There are frequently subtle clues to the diagnosis that may be revealed by careful interrogation. However, many times, other clues are spontaneously brought forth by patients. Finally, patients now present with multiple medical problems in addition to the cardiovascular problem, and a thorough history will provide insight into any contribution of noncardiac causes to the new onset or exacerbation of symptoms.

With the widespread availability of cardiac imaging, there has been an evolution in the detail and focus of the physical examination. It is no longer necessary to be able to obtain all the necessary information from the examination because the imaging modalities will provide diagnostic and hemodynamic results with a greater degree of certainty and accuracy than even a master clinician can achieve. For instance, maneuvers performed on a patient with a diastolic rumble to differentiate mitral stenosis from an Austin-Flint murmur are no longer relevant; the question is easily answered from a comprehensive two-dimensional and Doppler echocardiogram. The severity of mitral stenosis is more accurately determined from a transmitral Doppler gradient as opposed to the subjective assessment of the A2-opening snap interval on the examination.

However, a well-performed physical examination is necessary to provide an initial clinical impression of the type and severity of cardiac disease, as well as its effect on the patient. The subsequent diagnostic studies should then be used to confirm or refute this initial impression, and the final diagnosis can only be made if there is a concordance of the two. No test is 100% reliable, and many results are dependent on the performance of the test and interpretation of the data. The history and examination should be used to determine a "pretest probability" to which the results of the test can be applied.[2] For instance, a patient with symptoms and physical examination findings consistent with severe aortic stenosis but a low transaortic gradient on Doppler echocardiography represents discordant data. The clinician must be aware of the limitations of echocardiography, such as when a Doppler beam is not well aligned with the velocity jet, resulting in underestimation of the severity of stenosis. In this case, the results from the echocardiogram should be questioned, and further testing with transesophageal echocardiography, computerized tomography, or cardiac catheterization is required. Alternatively, a patient with nonischemic cardiomyopathy may have the diagnosis of severe mitral regurgitation due to a large jet of mitral regurgitation on color flow imaging; however, a barely audible apical murmur on physical examination will refute this diagnosis.

Several books dedicated to physical examination have been published, and our intent is not to replicate this information. We wish to present an approach to the physical examination of correlating relevant findings on examination with key findings from our newer diagnostic modalities. It is essential to understand the underlying pathophysiology of the cardiac disease to guide optimal patient care. The findings on a well-performed physical examination provide not only diagnostic information but are also a window to normal and abnormal hemodynamics. The components of the examination, when coupled with direct hemodynamic assessment by either Doppler echocardiography or cardiac catheterization, provide the clinician with a tremendous overview of the hemodynamic effect of the disease on the cardiovascular system. When one hears a third heart sound at the bedside in a patient with heart failure, a high E velocity on a transmitral Doppler velocity curve or a rapid filling wave on left ventricular invasive catheterization hemodynamic tracings should be expected. The paradoxical splitting of the second heart sound in a patient with hypertrophic cardiomyopathy should match the marked prolongation of ejection time produced by a pressure overload on the left ventricle from the dynamic obstruction. Only with a multimodality approach combined with clinical observations can correlations between concordant/discordant clinical/imaging findings be made to provide optimal patient care.[3] Our goal in this chapter is to provide a practical, contemporary approach to history-taking and physical examination, correlating the findings to hemodynamic and imaging data from echocardiography and cardiac catheterization.

HISTORY

Overview

The clinical history is the cornerstone of the evaluation of patients with cardiovascular disease. However, like any other skill, taking a proper history requires practice and a methodology. Several things should be avoided. First, patients should always be allowed to speak. Clinicians tend to interrupt their patients only minutes into the interview; this limits the amount of information a patient can provide and compromises the patient–provider relationship. Second, open-ended questions should be used initially ("how would you describe your chest pain?" vs "is the pain sharp?") and then directed questions used afterward to avoid influencing the patient's response. Third, the examiner must confirm interpretation of the patient's description of symptoms. For example, angina pectoris due to myocardial ischemia can have multiple descriptions, such as pain, pressure, tightness, ache, burning, shortness of breath, or even an "uncomfortable feeling." The basic characteristics of each symptom should also be recorded: quality, location, severity, tempo (onset and progression), and aggravating or alleviating factors including response to medications. Last, watch for gestures or body language to provide ancillary data; a classic example is the *Levine sign*—the clinched fist over the precordium suggesting angina as the cause of the chest pain.

Here, we briefly review the approach to the cardiac history. However, a comprehensive history should include past medical history (including pregnancy history), prior surgeries (extremely important in patients with valvular or congenital heart disease), social history (smoking, illicit drug use, and alcohol use), and family history (familial cardiomyopathies, sudden death, aortopathies, and aortic dissection). An important pertinent aspect of a patient's history should include the status of dental care, especially in patients being considered for intervention using prosthetic valves or material. Finally, it is of great importance to determine patients' emotional and physical reaction to their cardiac disease and how it is affecting their lives and their family's lives.

Specific Symptoms

Chest Pain

Assessment of the etiology of chest pain is one of the most difficult tasks in the practice of cardiology. Given the adverse cardiovascular events associated with coronary artery disease, the clinician's main concern is to rule in or rule out myocardial ischemia as the underlying cause. If details regarding the patient's pain (or discomfort) are not properly gathered, overtesting is frequently performed (biomarkers, exercise/pharmacologic stress testing, or even coronary angiography) or other equally life-threatening entities might be missed (such as pulmonary embolus or aortic dissection). Not uncommonly, clinicians forego the description of patient symptoms, essentially jumping from the chief complaint ("chest pain") to laboratory testing and imaging.

The duration of the symptoms is important in patients with chest pain. Angina typically lasts less than 5 minutes and will improve after exertion is discontinued or nitroglycerin taken. Symptoms should not last more than 30 minutes unless coronary thrombosis with myocardial infarction has occurred. The chest pain in these patients with stable exertional angina occurs in response to an increase in myocardial oxygen demand. Consequently, it is precipitated by exertion, emotion, and cold temperature and is worse after heavy meals. Rarely, patients will report that angina improves with continued exercise (ie, walk-through angina). Chest pain that lasts hours and days without

signs of myocardial injury/ischemia (troponin elevation or electrographic changes) significantly argues against angina. There is usually a progression in patients with coronary artery disease, with gradually increasing frequency of angina pectoris brought on by less and less exertion. However, plaque rupture will occur on top of hemodynamically insignificant lesions,[4] with the abrupt onset of rest discomfort in the absence of a recent progression of symptoms or even in the absence of a prior history of angina or cardiac disease.

Diamond and Forrester[5] categorized chest pain into *typical angina* (all three criteria were present), *atypical angina* (two criteria), and *noncardiac chest pain* (only one criterion). They based this classification on whether the pain (1) was substernal and pressure like, (2) was precipitated by exertion or emotional stress, and (3) was relieved by rest or nitroglycerin and lasted less than 30 minutes. In certain patient populations (eg, older men), this approach yielded such a high pretest probability of coronary artery disease that stress testing was unnecessary for the diagnosis of coronary atherosclerosis. This continues to be of value in clinical practice, particularly for male patients. It is commonly stated that women often present with atypical symptoms, and the diagnosis of myocardial ischemia may be missed using these classic criteria. However, data suggest that anginal symptoms might be similar in men and women and that the concept of females frequently presenting with atypical symptoms might be misleading.[6] It is important to remember that there are many patients who will not use the term "pain" when describing their angina. Instead, they may describe their symptoms in other terms such as "pressure, ache, discomfort, uneasy feelings." These sensations may not always be substernal but often are felt in the neck, lower jaw, shoulder, and arm down to the wrist.

There are other etiologies of chest pain that require urgent diagnosis and intervention. These include, but are not limited to, aortic dissection, penetrating aortic ulcers, and pulmonary embolism. **Table 2–1** provides specific characteristics of chest pain history according to the different etiologies. These are generalizations and may not apply to an individual patient; however, application of these criteria is helpful in forming an initial impression of the etiology of the pain and can then direct the clinician to further targeted testing.

Dyspnea

The onset, progression, and triggers of dyspnea, or breathlessness, should be recorded. Shortness of breath that is cardiac in nature is usually exertional, and continuous dyspnea at rest is usually noncardiac unless there is severe New York Heart Association class IV heart failure with signs on physical examination of severe fluid overload. Patients may describe a need to take deep breaths at rest; that symptom is rarely cardiac in origin. Pulmonary symptoms such as cough, wheezing, and sputum production suggest a noncardiac etiology. This is also suggested by very intermittent worsening or oscillation of symptoms ("good days and bad days"). However, fluid congestion from a cardiac etiology can result in features of bronchospasm as the initial manifestation.

Positional changes are important to document. Orthopnea and paroxysmal nocturnal dyspnea suggest heart failure as the

TABLE 2–1. Characteristics of Chest Pain According to Different Etiologies

Etiology	Quality/Precipitating and Relieving Factors	Onset/Duration	Location/Radiation
Angina	Pressure, heaviness, tightness; precipitated by exertion or emotional stress; relieved by rest or nitroglycerin	Duration less than 10 minutes, typically 2 to 5 minutes; concern for myocardial infarction if it lasts more than 30 minutes	Substernal; typically radiates to arms and shoulders (left more commonly than right), jaw, or neck
Pericarditis	Sharp, pleuritic, positional; relieved by sitting or leaning forward	Insidious onset; lasts hours or days	Substernal; might radiate to left shoulder
Aortic dissection	Tearing, ripping; typically severe at onset	Sudden onset	Anterior chest; radiates to the back or interscapular area
Pulmonary embolism	Sharp, pleuritic	Sudden onset	Typically ipsilateral to the involved lung
Costochondritis	Dull, occasionally sharp; may be reproduced by local pressure	Insidious onset; might last for days	Sternal/parasternal
Gastroesophageal reflux	Burning, worse in the supine position; relieved by antacids	Typically 10 to 60 minutes in duration, often postprandial	Substernal, epigastric
Esophageal spasm	Pressure, tightness; might improve with nitroglycerin	Sudden onset; duration less than 30 minutes	Substernal
Psychiatric	Vague, may simulate angina; often associated with anxiety	Variable duration and onset; might last hours or days	Variable; might be substernal

cause of the patient's dyspnea. True paroxysmal nocturnal dyspnea occurs several hours after a patient lays down because there is redistribution of fluid from the venous capacitance vessels into the central circulation. Patients will feel agitated, need to sit up, and seek cold fresh air, with the dyspnea taking 10 to 15 minutes to subside. Patients who wake up at night feeling short of breath but are better within seconds after a few deep breaths do not have paroxysmal nocturnal dyspnea. Platypnea-orthodeoxia[7] (worsening dyspnea and hypoxia in the sitting position) can be seen in patients with intracardiac shunting (either through an atrial septal defect or patent foramen ovale[8]), pulmonary arteriovenous malformations, or in hepatopulmonary syndrome. Bendopnea is a recently described symptom of heart failure and represents dyspnea that is precipitated by bending over.[9]

Syncope

A thorough history is vital in the evaluation of patients with syncope and, perhaps, is the best diagnostic tool for the evaluation of those patients. The circumstance of the syncopal spell (how the patient was feeling earlier that day or the day before) as well as warning and/or postictal symptoms should be noted. The combination of diaphoresis, nausea, prolonged standing, and exposure to warm places suggests a vasovagal etiology. Situational causes of syncope should be sought, such as micturition or bowel movements. Positional changes, in particular, orthostatic changes that lead to syncope are important and suggest orthostatic hypotension as the underlying cause; this is particularly important in older adults. Exertional syncope is usually due to a structural abnormality with obstruction to outflow (aortic stenosis, hypertrophic cardiomyopathy), especially when the syncope occurs just after the cessation of exertion. Exertional syncope in pulmonary hypertension is rare but it is a very ominous sign, typically seen in young females. Syncopal spells without any warning unrelated to exertion are particularly concerning for a cardiac arrhythmia and are of high concern in patients with diseases such as hypertrophic cardiomyopathy in which there is an underlying substrate for ventricular arrhythmias.

Palpitations

For palpitations, the duration, onset and offset, and associated symptoms (presyncope, chest discomfort) should be recorded. Concomitant neck pulsations are classic for atrioventricular reentrant tachycardia. Potential triggers, such as caffeine, alcohol, or dehydration, are important for diagnosis and management. It is helpful to ask the patient to reproduce the cadence by tapping their fingers. A fast, irregular pattern suggests atrial fibrillation, whereas single, forceful taps suggest ectopic beats. It is important to remember that in patients with underlying structural heart disease, the onset of arrhythmias may indicate underlying hemodynamic deterioration.

Other Symptoms

Lower extremity edema is a common complaint in patients with heart disease. The distinction between edema from right heart failure and venous insufficiency can be difficult to establish by history, and both may coexist; edema that occurs only at the end of the day suggests a primary venous etiology. Abdominal swelling due to ascites might be present in patients with severe heart failure, severe tricuspid regurgitation, or constrictive pericarditis but needs to be differentiated from primary liver disease. Ascites and edema are the most prominent symptoms of patients with constrictive pericarditis.

Fatigue and weakness are nonspecific symptoms and can be secondary to either cardiac or noncardiac issues; therefore, ascertaining that fatigue is a manifestation of a cardiac etiology is challenging. Fatigue as a cardiac symptom is common in patients with right ventricular failure or severe tricuspid

TABLE 2-2. Canadian Cardiovascular Society Classification of Angina

Class I	Angina not induced by ordinary physical activity (walking or climbing stairs); develops only during strenuous, rapid, and/or prolonged exercise
Class II	Slight limitation of ordinary activities is present and is induced by the following: walking or climbing stairs rapidly, walking uphill, walking or climbing stairs postprandially, emotional stress, walking more than two blocks or climbing more than one flight of stairs at normal pace
Class III	Marked limitations of ordinary physical activity; angina develops on walking one or two blocks and climbing a single flight of stairs
Class IV	Inability to carry on any physical activity without developing angina; rest angina

regurgitation and constrictive pericarditis. Polypharmacy is common in cardiac and older patients, and fatigue might be a medication side effect (such as from β-blockers) or a sign of medication-induced hypotension.

Systemic symptoms such as fever, chills, and malaise might be seen in the setting of infective endocarditis. Rarely, hoarseness and dysphagia are caused by compression of contiguous structures in the setting of aortic aneurysm or severe left atrial enlargement (as in advanced mitral stenosis).

Functional Capacity

Assessment of functional capacity should be documented for management and follow-up purposes. The Canadian Cardiovascular Society[10] (**Table 2-2**) and the New York Heart Association[11] scales (**Table 2-3**) are widely used tools. In our experience, even a simple 1 (bedridden) to 10 (no physical limitations) Likert scale is helpful in the longitudinal assessment of patients and tends to correlate well with objective exercise capacity (exercise maximal oxygen consumption). In some diseases, there is such a gradual hemodynamic impairment that patients may not perceive a functional limitation; they will slowly decrease their activity level. Information obtained from a spouse or other close observer regarding activity level over the years may be of value.

TABLE 2-3. New York Heart Association Functional Classification

Class I	No limitation of physical activity; physical activity does not cause fatigue, palpitation, dyspnea, or angina
Class II	Slight limitation of ordinary activities; comfortable at rest; ordinary physical activity results in fatigue, palpitation, dyspnea, or angina
Class III	Marked limitations of physical activity; comfortable at rest; less than ordinary activities causes fatigue, dyspnea, or angina
Class IV	Inability to carry on any physical activity without symptoms; symptoms of heart failure of anginal might be present at rest If any activity is undertaken, discomfort is increased

With the aging population, it is important to assess the presence and extent of frailty in patients being considered for interventions. Frailty indices have been shown to be predictive of survival in this population.[12] The ability to perform activities of daily living is a necessary component of the frailty assessment. The degree of independence and interaction with family will be useful information for decision-making regarding interventions in the older frail patient.

PHYSICAL EXAMINATION: INSPECTION, BLOOD PRESSURE, AND PALPATION

General Examination and Inspection

A thorough general examination, including a funduscopic examination, should always be performed and signs of other comorbidities (such as cirrhosis, obstructive lung disease, or stroke) should be sought. Attention to the patient's dentition is of major importance, in particular, in patients with valve disease or for those undergoing preoperative evaluation. Visible pulsations should be noted, with respect to location and origin (arterial vs venous). Details regarding the noncardiovascular and eye examinations are, however, beyond the scope of this chapter.

Our patient population is aging, and frailty assessment should also be included as part of the physical examination. Gait speed (15-foot walk), handgrip strength, and muscle wasting should be recorded; multiple scores[13,14] have also been developed. This assessment should be a standard part of clinical evaluation and should be performed in patients undergoing catheter-based interventions or surgical treatment.

Several syndromes have been associated with cardiovascular disease, including aortopathies, hypertrophic cardiomyopathy, congenital heart disease, and even cardiac tumors. Careful inspection of the facies, body habitus, and extremities is necessary in order to suspect the presence of a syndrome. Although these syndromes are rare, their identification can lead to the initial suspicion of the cardiac diagnosis, which may have life-saving implications for patients and their families. Some of those findings are illustrated in the **Table 2-4**.

Blood Pressure Measurement

Blood Pressure: Technique

Although vital signs are frequently recorded by the ancillary staff prior to the encounter with the provider, we recommend that the measurements be repeated during physical examination by the clinician. This prevents abnormalities from being "missed" due to time constraints and also forces the examiner to certify that all the necessary steps for the measurement of blood pressure have been done (eg, that both arms are checked); this is particularly important during the patient's initial evaluation.

Blood pressure should be measured at rest (a common mistake is to measure it immediately after the patient has just walked into the room), and the appropriate cuff size should be used (the width of the inflatable bladder should correspond to 40% of the arm circumference). Smoking and caffeine should be avoided prior to blood pressure measurement. During

TABLE 2–4. Genetic Syndromes and Associated Physical Examination Findings

Syndrome	Physical Examination Findings	Cardiovascular Features
Ehlers-Danlos	Joint hypermobility, scoliosis, lax thin skin; variable according to disease type	Arterial aneurysms, mitral valve prolapse
Fabry	Angiokeratomas	Infiltrative cardiomyopathy (may resemble hypertrophic cardiomyopathy), conduction abnormalities
Holt-Oram	Upper limb deformity due to aplasia or hypoplasia or radial and carpal bones	Congenital heart defects, most commonly atrial septal defects and ventricular septal defect
Loeys-Dietz	Hypertelorism, bifid uvula; dolichocephaly, enophthalmos, down-slanting palpebral fissures, retrognathia, pectus carinatum, arachnodactyly, increased arm span	Aortopathy, vasculopathy, mitral valve prolapse
Marfan	Increased height, pectus excavatum, dolichocephaly, high-arched palate, flat feet, increased arm span, arachnodactyly, *thumb* and *wrist* signs	Aortopathy, mitral valve prolapse
Noonan	Short stature, strabismus, low-set ears, low hair line, shield-shaped chest, hypertelorism	Pulmonary valve stenosis, atrial septal defect, hypertrophic cardiomyopathy
Turner	Short stature, webbed neck, cubitus valgus	Bicuspid aortic valve, aortopathy, aortic coarctation
Williams	"Elfin face," with broad forehead, short nose, wide mouth, flat nasal bridge	Supravalvular aortic stenosis, branch pulmonary artery stenosis

initial assessment, blood pressure should be measured in both arms; differences in systolic blood pressure between arms are typically less than or equal to 20 mm Hg (usually higher in the right arm). This is a mandatory step prior to bypass surgery and in patients with internal mammary grafts who present with angina. A simple blood pressure check might be sufficient to diagnose subclavian stenosis.

Additional steps should be taken according to the clinical scenario. In patients who complain of syncope or presyncope, measurements in the supine, sitting, and standing positions must be performed. Systolic blood pressure should not fall more than 20 mm Hg upon standing; diastolic blood pressure typically rises. Mild reflex tachycardia is common, but rates above 100 beats/min should not be expected. Newly hypertensive patients or patients with known bicuspid valve should have blood pressures measured in the lower extremity since coarctation of the aorta might be present. A large cuff should be applied to the patient's thigh and the popliteal artery auscultated. Alternatively, a smaller cuff can be applied to the calf and the stethoscope applied to the dorsalis pedis artery (or palpation of this artery with documentation of the systolic reading). Normally, the lower extremity blood pressure tends to be 10 to 20 mm Hg higher than in the upper extremities.

Digital blood pressure cuffs have been shown to be reliable and accurate in most situations; however, major abnormalities might be missed if manual blood pressure measurement is not performed. Digital blood pressure cuffs may not be accurate in assessing pulse pressure in patients with aortic regurgitation or high output states. Digital cuffs cannot be used to determine the presence of a pulsus paradox or pulsus alternans. Therefore, we recommend that manual blood pressure measurement *always* be performed. With the stethoscope's diaphragm applied to the brachial artery, the ipsilateral radial pulse is palpated and the cuff inflated to 20 to 30 mm Hg above the level required to obliterate the pulse; the cuff should be then deflated slowly. Systolic blood pressure corresponds to the appearance of Korotkoff sounds (phase I), and diastolic blood pressure corresponds to the level where the Korotkoff sounds entirely disappear (phase V). In some patients, the Korotkoff sounds might disappear and become audible again at lower pressures (ie, the *auscultatory gap*). This is a common finding in older patients, and simultaneous palpation of the radial artery, while the cuff is inflated, prevents underestimation of the blood pressure. In hypotensive patients, Korotkoff sounds might not be audible; blood pressure should be determined by palpation of the radial artery.

Heart rate and cardiac rhythm (regular, regularly irregular, or irregularly irregular) should also be recorded. Other vital signs (temperature and respiratory rate) and their abnormalities should be noted.

Blood Pressure Abnormalities

Pulse pressure (the difference between systolic and diastolic blood pressure levels) should be noted. A narrow pulse pressure is seen in shock and hypotension; the arterial pulse usually shows low amplitude. A wide pulse pressure is seen in hypertension (commonly in the older adults due to noncompliant arteries), severe aortic regurgitation (secondary to lower diastolic blood pressure), and arteriovenous shunting (such as patent ductus arteriosus or dialysis fistula).

Pulsus alternans (**Fig. 2–1**) corresponds to beat-to-beat changes in systolic blood pressure (or the intensity of Korotkoff sounds); this can be detected both by auscultation and by palpation, during which time the patient should be instructed to breathe calmly. Pulsus alternans is a sign of severe left ventricular systolic dysfunction.

Pulsus paradoxus (**Fig. 2–2**) corresponds to respirophasic changes in blood pressure. "Paradox" is a misnomer because minor drops in blood pressure with inspiration are normal. In pathologic situations, there is an exaggeration of this phenomenon. Normally, systolic blood pressure should not fall more than

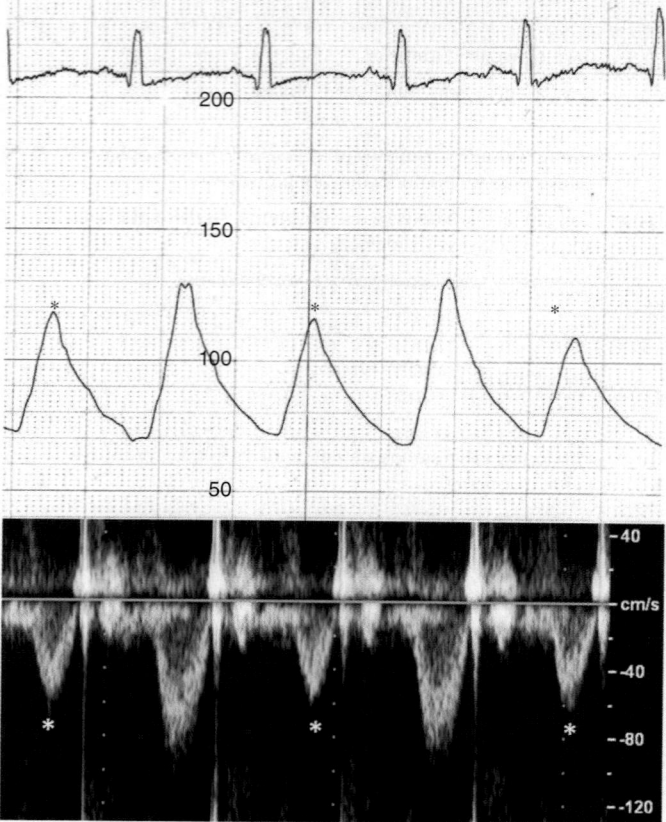

Figure 2–1. Pulsus alternans in a patient with severe left ventricular systolic dysfunction. Invasive aortic pressure tracing (*upper*) and left ventricular outflow tract pulsed-wave Doppler (*lower*) showing marked beat-to-beat reduction (*asterisk*) in left ventricular stroke volume.

10 mm Hg on inspiration. The presence of "pulsus" is a subtle finding and requires that proper technique be applied. The examiner should inflate the blood pressure cuff 15 to 20 mm Hg above the systolic blood pressure (determined by palpation and auscultation). The cuff should then be slowly deflated and the Korotkoff sounds auscultated while the patient breathes normally. The sounds will show respirophasic changes, decreasing or disappearing with inspiration. Eventually, those respirophasic changes will not be noticeable, and expiratory and inspiratory Korotkoff sounds will have similar intensities. The "pulsus" will be the difference between the peak systolic blood pressure levels measured during expiration and inspiration; greater than 10 mm Hg is abnormal. Pulsus paradoxus is classically described as a sign of cardiac tamponade or constrictive pericarditis due to the enhanced ventricular interdependence seen on those two entities (with inspiration, right ventricular stroke volume increases while left ventricular stroke volume falls; this is secondary to pericardial restraint). Pulsus paradoxus can also be seen in morbid obesity and in lung disease as a result of major changes in intrathoracic pressures.

Percussion

In the past, some authors have recommended the use of percussion for the determination of cardiac position (levocardia vs dextrocardia) and its relation to abdominal viscera (situs solitus or inversus, based on gastric tympanic sounds). Today, this can be easily determined with chest radiography and echocardiography. Thus, cardiac percussion is not necessary in current practice.

Palpation

Palpation is perhaps the most underemphasized part of the cardiovascular examination, both in medical education and bedside assessment. Proper technique includes palpation of the left and right ventricles as well as palpation of the cardiac base (great vessels). Via "simple" palpation, assessments of ventricular size, cardiac valve function, diastolic function (when third or fourth sounds are palpable), and pulmonary hypertension can be suspected. Masters of physical examination advocate that auscultation "merely" serves to confirm inspection and palpation findings.

Palpation of the great vessels is part of a comprehensive cardiovascular physical examination and should be performed over the second right intercostal space (aortic area) and left intercostal space (pulmonic area), best felt in the sitting position. A detectable pulsation represents palpable and, therefore, increased aortic (A2) or pulmonic (P2) components of the second heart sound. A palpable A2 component is rare. A palpable P2, however, is a critical finding because it suggests severe pulmonary hypertension, which can be due to either etiologies associated with increased pulmonary vascular resistance or left-sided diseases.

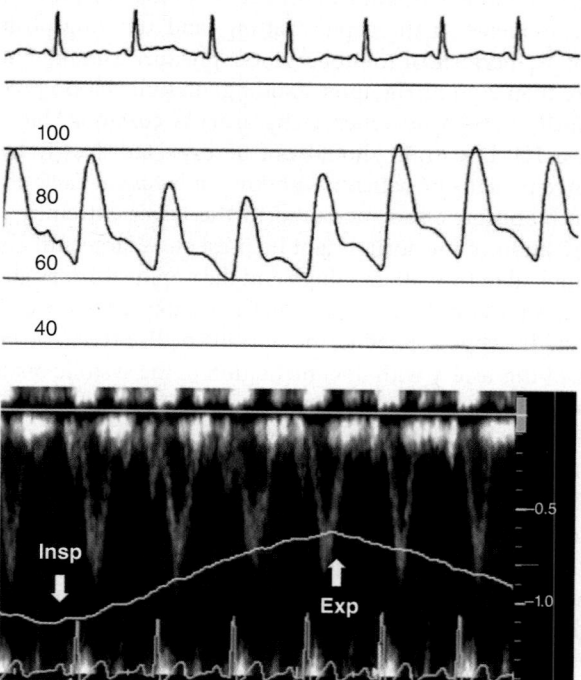

Figure 2–2. Pulsus paradoxus in a patient with cardiac tamponade. Invasive aortic pressure tracing (*upper*) and left ventricular outflow tract pulsed-wave Doppler (*lower*) with simultaneous respirometer tracing confirm marked decrease in left ventricular stroke volume with inspiration (Insp). Exp, expiration.

Attention should be turned to the presence of *thrills*, palpable murmurs that have a marked increase in the degree of turbulence. Thrills can be present at the apex, left lower sternal border, cardiac base, suprasternal notch/neck, and the posterior chest. When present, the location, timing, and radiation of a thrill should be described. Diastolic thrills are very rare. In current practice, the most common source of a thrill is a ventricular septal defect, which manifests as a systolic thrill at the left lower sternal border. A systolic thrill at the left upper sternal border is usually indicative of critical aortic stenosis. It should be emphasized that the presence of a thrill is not diagnostic of a specific cardiac lesion, and the diagnosis should be made on the basis of the constellation of findings observed on examination.

Cardiac palpation should proceed with evaluation of the apical impulse. We recommend the term *apical impulse* instead of *point of maximal impulse* because patients with significantly enlarged right ventricles might have parasternal lifts that are more prominent than the left ventricular apical impulse. The apical impulse might be visible, facilitating its localization; therefore, inspection should precede palpation. In addition, some other palpable abnormalities may also be visible (eg, a rapid filling wave that corresponds to a third heart sound). Palpation (and auscultation) must be performed directly over the skin. Thus, patients should *always* be offered an examination gown and a sheet used to preserve the patient's privacy. Examination of the patient in his or her clothes compromises the quality of the examination and is discouraged.

With the patient in the supine position, if not visible, the examiner should look for the apical impulse using the entire right hand starting at the inframammary area. In patients with large breasts, the examiner's left hand should be used to mobilize the breast to locate the apex. Once a palpable pulsation is identified, the finger pads should be used for analysis (**Fig. 2-3**). If the apical impulse cannot be palpated, the patient should be positioned in the left lateral decubitus position and asked to place his or her left hand underneath the pillow; slight elevation of the head of the bed (30°) might also be helpful. Both maneuvers facilitate expansion of the thorax, increasing

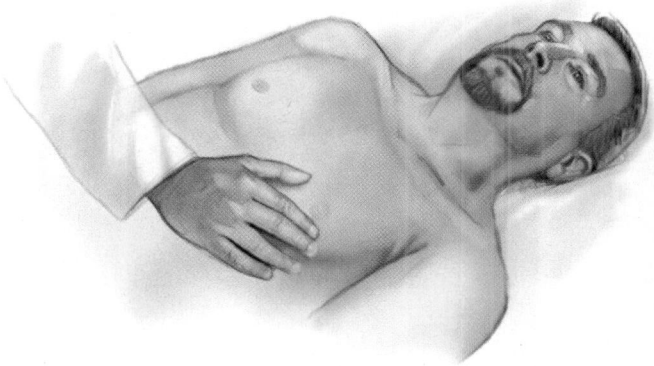

Figure 2-3. Palpation of the apical impulse. Once the apical impulse has been located, the finger pads of the right hand are used to assess apical size, location, and contour.

the space between the ribs. Held expiration may also facilitate cardiac palpation. The apical impulse should be palpable in the majority of patients, even in individuals with normal hearts.

Once the apical impulse is identified, the examiner should assess its location, size, and quality/contour. The apical impulse is usually located at the fifth intercostal space in the midclavicular line. With left ventricular enlargement, the apical impulse is deviated laterally and inferiorly while right ventricular enlargement displaces the apex laterally. Moving the patient from supine to a left lateral decubitus position aids in bringing out the contour of the impulse and shifting the apical impulse laterally by 2 to 3 cm.

When the left ventricular size is normal, the apical impulse occupies an area of 3 cm or less in diameter; the size of the apical impulse should be described in centimeters rather than fingerbreadths because it is more precise. An increase in the area occupied by the apical impulse suggests left ventricular dilatation, described as a *diffuse* apical impulse (as opposed to *localized*). Isolated left ventricular hypertrophy typically does not cause enlargement of the apical impulse; hypertrophy is associated with a sustained impulse. An enlarged apical impulse suggests an enlarged left ventricle due to a myopathic process or volume overload, as seen in severe aortic or mitral regurgitation.

The contour of the apical impulse should also be determined. Isovolumic contraction moves the apex closer to chest wall, allowing its palpation. As a consequence, the impulse is usually only palpable during the first two-thirds of ventricular systole (**Fig. 2-4**). Although simultaneous auscultation can help quantify the duration of the apical impulse, in practical terms, the determination of a normal versus prolonged (described as *sustained*) apical impulse comes with experience. It is extremely important, therefore, for the clinician to perform cardiac palpation in every patient, including those with known normal hearts, so that a sense of normality can be developed.

A *sustained* apical impulse can be found when ventricular mass is increased (ventricular hypertrophy or dilation) or when there is obstruction to left ventricular ejection (as observed in aortic stenosis or hypertrophic cardiomyopathy). Not only the duration but also the amplitude should be noted. In hypertrophy and obstruction to flow, the apical impulse is rather forceful, "pushing" the examiner's hands. Conversely, in patients with severe left ventricular dysfunction, the impulse can be quite feeble. In sinus tachycardia (eg, after exercise or related to infection), the apical impulse can be hyperdynamic. In patients with mitral stenosis and a pliable mitral valve, apical palpation results in a unique tactile (shock-like) sensation due to a prominent first heart sound—the so-called tapping apical impulse—that is essentially pathognomonic for rheumatic mitral stenosis. Patients with hypertrophic obstructive cardiomyopathy might also have a classic apical impulse—the so-called triple ripple (see Fig. 2-4). This corresponds to the presence of palpable systolic impulse in early and midsystole, separated by withdrawal of the apical impulse related to dynamic outflow obstruction; a palpable atrial contraction corresponds to the third impulse.

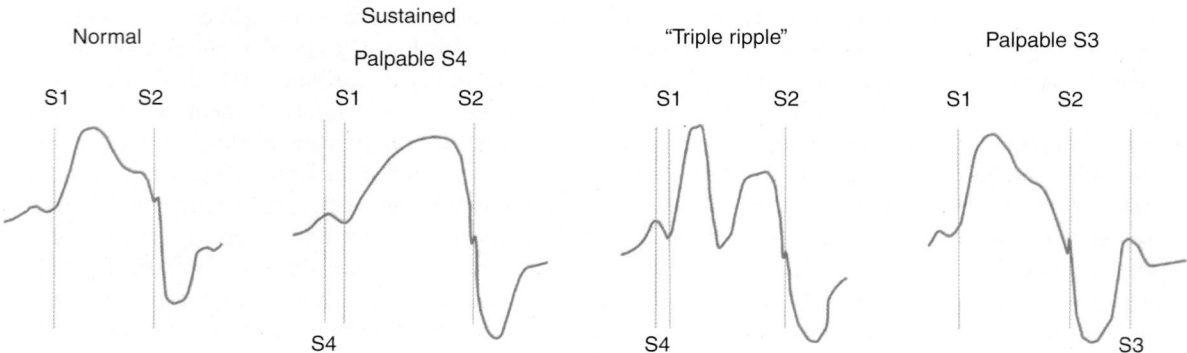

Figure 2–4. Apical impulse contour in a normal person and in various disease states. S1, first heart sound; S2, second heart sound; S3, third heart sound; S4, fourth heart sound.

A palpable third or fourth heart sound may be suspected by inspection (sometimes placing the tip of a pen over the apical impulse and watching the motion of the pen can be helpful). A palpable fourth heart sound follows atrial contraction and will be felt as a presystolic palpable impulse (preceding the rise of the apical impulse); the fourth heart sound tends to be more easily palpated than auscultated. A palpable third heart sound corresponds to the ventricular diastolic rapid filling phase and will occur in early diastolic; it can be felt as the apical impulse retracts. The third heart sound is usually more easily auscultated than palpated. Although systolic clicks and some diastolic sounds can be palpable, they are rarely felt.

Given its anterior position within the chest, an enlarged right ventricle can be palpated as a *parasternal lift* (or *heave*). It should be noted that in thin patients or patients with abnormalities of the sternum (such as *pectus excavatum*), a parasternal lift can be present in the setting of a normal right ventricular size. The right ventricle can be palpated in several ways (**Fig. 2–5**), being performed with patient in the supine position. The examiner should gently place his or her thenar/hypothenar surfaces on the patient's left lower sternal border. The right ventricle can also be palpated by placing the examiner's index, middle, and fourth fingers over the third, fourth, and fifth intercostal spaces, respectively,

at the left parasternal line. A third form of palpation is to place the right hand in the subxiphoid area. This maneuver is particularly helpful in patients with obstructive lung disease. Abnormalities in the contour of the right ventricular impulse can be appreciated but are much less prominent than apical ones. Pulmonary stenosis can give rise to a sustained parasternal lift; presystolic and early diastolic waves can also be appreciated on occasion.

PHYSICAL EXAMINATION: ARTERIAL AND VENOUS PULSE

Arterial Pulse Examination

Technique

The arterial pulse can be examined by palpating the carotid and/or brachial arteries. We encourage the examiner to be familiar with palpation of the brachial arteries, which can be particularly helpful in patients with increased neck circumference, previous cervical radiation, or in the presence of carotid disease. The brachial arteries can be palpated by resting the patient's elbow on the examiner's right palm, with palpation of the vessel being exerted with the right thumb; the brachial pulse is usually deeper than others. The examiner's left hand should gently extend/flex the patient's arm in order to improve palpation of the vessel. Alternatively, the examiner can perform

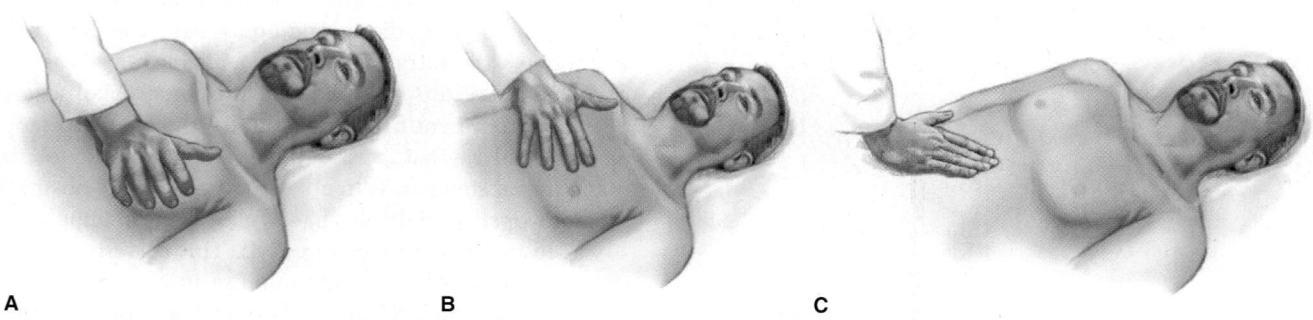

Figure 2–5. Palpation of the right ventricle. Palpation of the right ventricle can be performed using the following approaches: the thenar/hypothenar surfaces of the examiner's right hand are placed on the patient's left lower sternal border (**A**); the examiner's right second, third, and fourth fingers are placed over the patient's right third, fourth, and fifth intercostal spaces (**B**); or the examiner palpates the patient's right ventricle from the subxiphoid area (**C**).

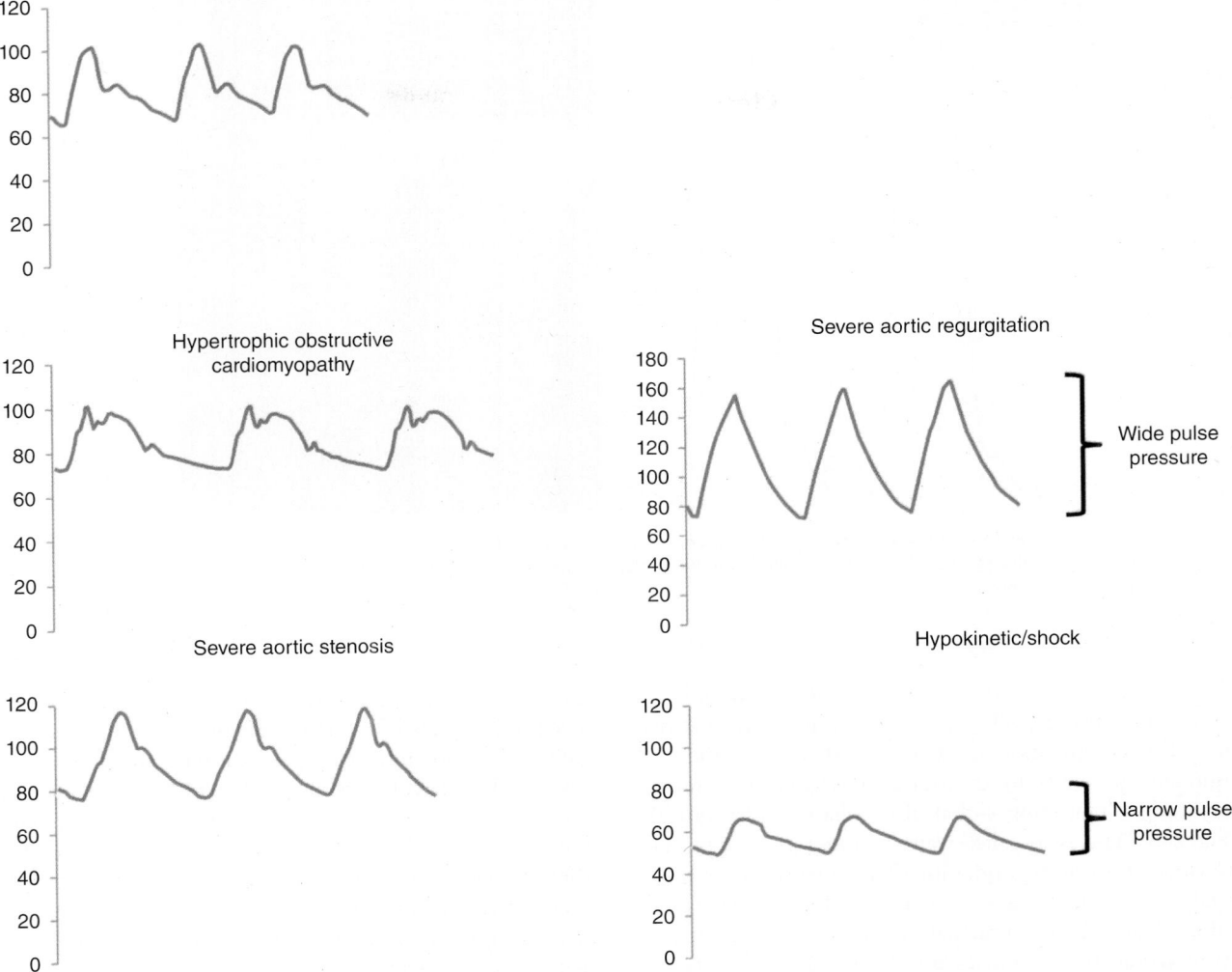

Figure 2–6. Normal arterial pulse waveform and abnormal arterial pulse waveform patterns seen in various disease states. These arterial pulse waveforms illustrate the expected findings on arterial pulse palpation.

palpation directly with his or her left finger pads, with the right fingers being used for extra pressure, if needed. The carotid arteries should be palpated with the right finger pads; the sternocleidomastoid muscle should be mobilized laterally to optimize palpation of the vessel. Once the artery has been properly identified, attention should to paid to the amplitude and contour of the arterial pulse (**Fig. 2–6**), as described below. Palpation of the other upper and lower extremity pulses is part of a comprehensive cardiovascular examination and should always be performed, particularly with simultaneous palpation of the radial and femoral pulse in patients with suspected coarctation of the aorta.

Abnormalities of Arterial Pulse

The classic arterial pulse contour described in *severe aortic stenosis* is tardus (slurred upstroke and delayed peak) and parvus (reduced in amplitude) (see Fig. 2–6). The degree of tardus (graded as 1+ to 4+) is a measure of the severity of the stenosis and reflected in the late-peaking continuous-wave velocity contour on Doppler echocardiography as well as the delayed

upstroke on the central aortic pressure at cardiac catheterization (**Fig. 2–7**). Although frequently described in textbooks as one single pattern, one of the two components might prevail (for example, more tardus than parvus), and they should be graded separately. Typically found in valvular aortic stenosis, it should be noted that the parvus and tardus pulse also accompany other forms of fixed left ventricular outflow obstruction (eg, subvalvular stenosis in the setting of subaortic membrane or supravalvular aortic stenosis). In this case, however, a normal aortic component of the second heart sound will indicate that the aortic valve is spared. In dynamic left ventricular outflow obstruction (hypertrophic cardiomyopathy), the arterial pulse is usually of normal amplitude but has brisk upstroke secondary to an unopposed forceful contraction in early systole (before obstruction develops) by the hypertrophied ventricle. Hypertrophic cardiomyopathy with obstruction is a cause of a *bifid* pulse, caused by the occurrence of obstruction starting in mid-systole. This is seen as a spike-and-dome pattern on aortic pressure (see Fig. 2–6) tracings, but the presence of this finding on examination is uncommon.

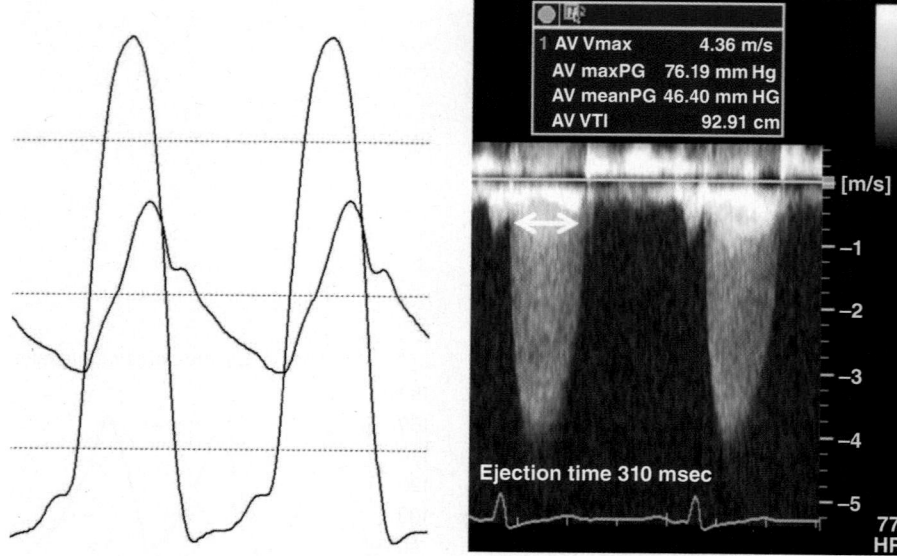

Figure 2–7. Arterial pulse waveform in severe aortic valve stenosis. Aortic and left ventricular pressure tracings (*left*) show the "parvus and tardus" pattern in a patient with severe aortic valve stenosis. The *right panel* illustrates the prolonged systolic ejection time and severely increased systolic mean gradient noted by aortic continuous-wave Doppler.

In *severe aortic regurgitation*, the associated volume overload and left ventricular dilatation cause an increase in stroke volume. The combination of increased stroke volume and regurgitation gives rise to an arterial pulse that is increased in amplitude—"bounding"—that also collapses very quickly (see Fig. 2–6). This is so-called water hammer pulse, typical of severe isolated aortic regurgitation. This phenomenon is not only palpable but might also be manifested as visible arterial pulsations (carotids and brachial arteries, most commonly). When mixed aortic valve disease is present and aortic regurgitation is the predominant lesion, an arterial contour with increased amplitude and two palpable systolic peaks can be present—the *bisferiens pulse*.

Other described abnormalities of the arterial contours include the *anacrotic pulse* of aortic stenosis,[15] where a positive inscription can be palpated on the ascending limb of the aortic contour, or the *dicrotic pulse*, when there is an exaggeration of the dicrotic notch (palpated on the descending limb of the aortic pulse), typically seen in shock and severe peripheral vasoconstriction. Hypotension and narrow pulse pressure are also usually present (see Fig. 2–6). In patients with severe left ventricular systolic dysfunction, *pulsus alternans* might be present, where the amplitude of the arterial pulse will vary with every heartbeat. In some cases, the amplitude might be so diminished that only every other beat can be palpated. As opposed to *pulsus paradoxus* (previously described in the blood pressure section), these variations in amplitude are not respirophasic. The presence of *pulsus alternans* is an ominous sign, suggesting very profound severe ventricular systolic dysfunction. These abnormalities can be easily noted invasively by arterial pulse recording or an ascending aortic pressure (see Figs. 2–1 and 2–2).

The examiner should also assess the amplitude of the arterial pulse as an indirect measurement of cardiac output; arterial pulse amplitude tends to be proportional to stroke volume. The presence of a low amplitude pulse in the absence of aortic stenosis should suggest reduced cardiac output, such as with severe left ventricular systolic dysfunction, severe mitral stenosis, or constrictive pericarditis. Conversely, the combination of bounding pulses, left ventricular enlargement, and heart failure should suggest high-output failure, patent ductus arteriosus, or other arteriovenous fistulae. In shock, the arterial pulse is of decreased amplitude but also hyperdynamic as the result of accompanying tachycardia.

Venous Pulse Examination

Inspection

The first step in analyzing the venous pressure and the venous waveform contour is to ascertain that the visible pulsation is indeed venous. A carotid arterial pulsation seen below the angle of the jaw might be mistaken for severe elevation in venous pressure. Inspection of the internal, instead of the external, jugular vein has been traditionally preferred to determine the contour of the venous pulsations. Because it emanates from a low-pressure system, venous pulsations should disappear when light pressure is applied proximally (eg, above the clavicle), whereas arterial pulsation cannot be compressed and should "push" the examiner's fingers. In normal circumstances, the venous contour has two upstrokes and the arterial waveform has a single one. This feature, however, should not be used in isolation because rhythm abnormalities (such as atrial fibrillation with loss of the *a* wave) or severe tricuspid regurgitation will lose the double venous upstroke. Lastly, venous waveforms show respirophasic changes with their waveforms becoming more prominent on inspiration, although the venous pressure itself might drop slightly or remain unchanged.

Estimation of Venous Pressure

The proper technique used to estimate central venous pressure is often confusing to the novice examiner. Estimation of central venous pressure is a crucial part of the physical examination; not only cardiologists but all clinicians should be very familiar with the method. Its importance in the diagnosis and management of patients is clearly stated in the American College of Cardiology/American Heart Association heart failure guidelines.[16] An elevated venous pressure is the equivalent of a dilated inferior vena cava on echocardiography that does not collapse with inspiration and is the first clue to hemodynamic decompensation.

Estimated central venous pressure is measured in centimeters of water (H_2O) because it represents the height of a column of fluid. Thus, the venous pressure in centimeters of H_2O does not equal the right atrial measured in mm Hg at catheterization (1 cm of H_2O = 0.74 mm Hg). Central venous pressure is recognized on physical examination as the *vertical* distance from the highest point of the visible jugular venous pulsation to the right atrium. The internal jugular vein is typically the one analyzed. The sternal angle, or angle of Louis, which corresponds to the manubriosternal junction, has been shown to lay 5 cm above the level of the mid–right atrium (**Fig. 2–8**). Therefore, estimated central venous pressure equals the vertical distance of the maximum visible jugular venous pulse to the angle of Louis plus 5 cm. The head of the bed should be adjusted in order to optimize analysis of the venous pulsations so that the *highest point* where venous pulsations can be identified is used as the reference point.

In patients with very elevated central venous pressures, such as seen in constrictive pericarditis, the top of the venous pulse might not be seen until the patient is standing. Conversely, in patients with low central venous pressures, the patient might be almost supine before venous pulsations can be appreciated. Thus, failure to perform inspection of the neck in different positions might lead to misinterpretation of central venous pressure.

There are two simple and practical ways to estimate central venous pressures at the beginning of the physical examination while the patient is sitting. At 90°, the lack of a visible pulsation typically corresponds to a normal venous pressure of less than 8 cm of H_2O, a visible venous pulsation at the level of the clavicle corresponds to 10 cm of H_2O, midneck 15 cm of H_2O, and angle of jaw 20 cm of H_2O. Another method is to simply report out the height of the venous pulsation (in centimeters) above the angle of Louis at 45°. In the normal patient without cardiac disease, the venous pressure is less than 3 cm above the angle of Louis. If pulsations cannot be visualized, the venous pressure is most likely normal. However, it is necessary to lower the head of the bed until a pulsation is seen to ensure that the venous pressure is not so high that pulsations cannot be seen.

Although the terms *jugular venous distention* and *elevated central venous pressure* are frequently used interchangeably, the central venous pressure should always be quantitated objectively. Jugular venous distention might be seen in primary venous disorders (eg, in superior vena cava syndrome).

Normal Venous Pulse

After central venous pressure has been estimated, the examiner should focus on the venous contour. Similar to the technique used to estimate venous pressure, the head of the bed should be adjusted to provide optimal visualization of the venous pulsations. The normal jugular venous contour has two upstrokes—*a* and *v* waves—and two downstrokes—*x* and *y* descents (**Fig. 2–9**). A third positive wave—the *c* wave—is seen on right atrial pressure tracings but is not usually visualized on the neck veins.

Positive waves are typically more easily appreciated on inspection than the descents. The *a* wave corresponds to atrial systole and is followed by *x* descent, which is the result of two phenomena—atrial diastole and apical displacement of the tricuspid annulus during ventricular systole. The origin of the *c* wave had been controversial, but it is believed that the inflection seen on the jugular wave recordings results from

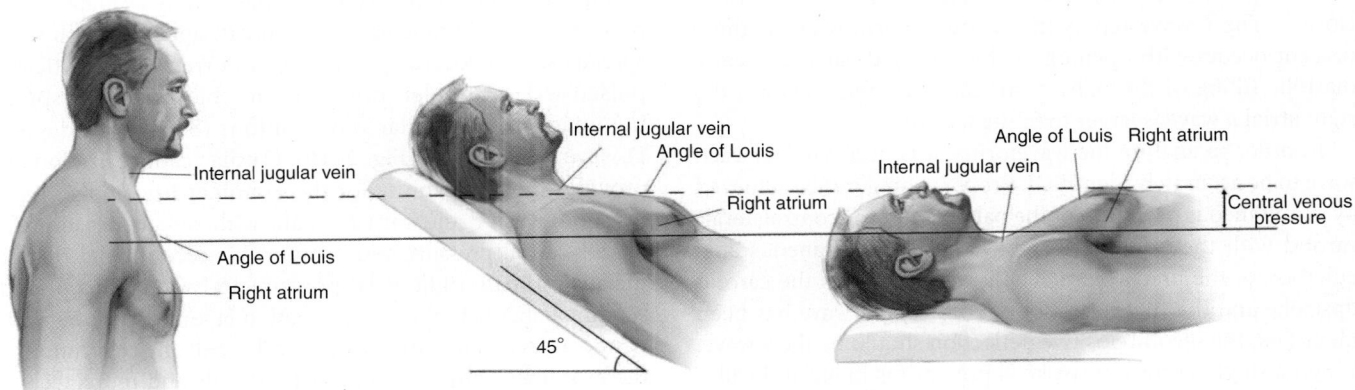

Figure 2–8. Estimation of central venous pressure. The central venous pressure corresponds to the vertical distance from the highest point of the visible jugular venous pulsation to the right atrium, irrespective of the angle at which the patient is examined. The examiner should adjust the head of the bed in order to optimize visualization of the jugular pulsations. In patients with low or normal right filling pressures, the venous pulsation might be hidden behind the sternum at higher angles. Conversely, in patients with very elevated central venous pressures, jugular pulsations might not be seen unless the patient is sitting upright or standing up.

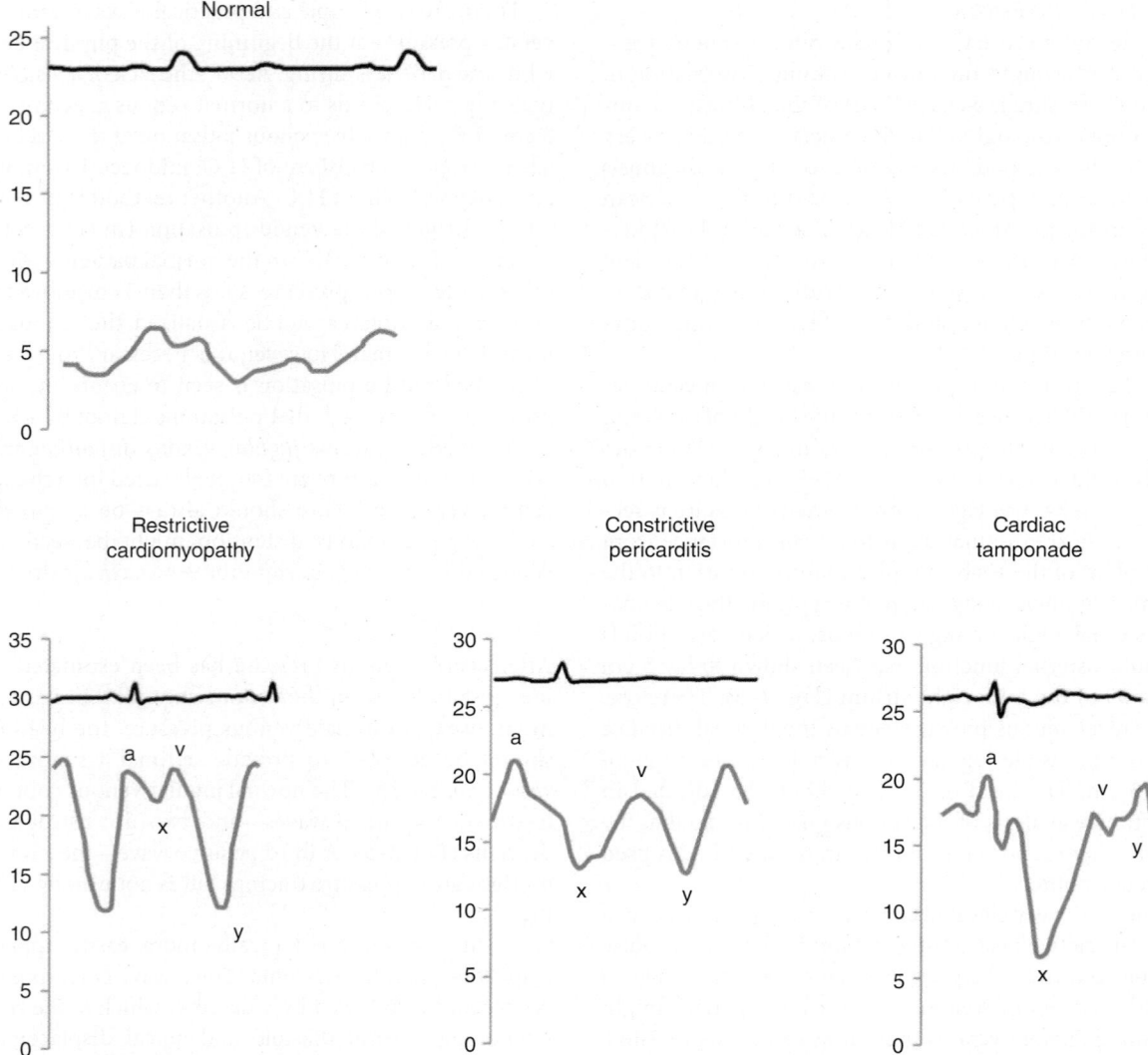

Figure 2–9. Normal right atrial pulse waveform and abnormal patterns seen in various disease states. The right atrial waveform correlates with the expected findings on inspection of the jugular venous pulse.

the contiguous carotid pulsations rather than tricuspid valve closure. The *v* wave represents venous return, whereas the *y* descent occurs with opening of the tricuspid valve and early diastolic filling of the right ventricle. In normal persons, the right atrial *a* wave is larger than the *v* wave.

In order to analyze the waveforms, it is necessary for each wave to be accurately identified. Proper timing can be achieved by simultaneous palpation of the patient's left (or contralateral) carotid with the examiner's right hand or simultaneous auscultation of the precordium. The *a* wave precedes the carotid upstroke and the first heart sound; once the *a* wave has been identified, the second positive deflection should be the *v* wave. When a single venous upstroke is present (as in atrial fibrillation), only a positive wave (*v* wave) following carotid upstroke will be noted. The radial pulse should not be used as the pulse reference because there is a small delay between the radial and carotid upstrokes, which can lead to inaccurate conclusions, especially when tachycardia is present.

Jugular venous wave recording was readily available in the past, but the technique has essentially disappeared with widespread use of echocardiography. In the current era, hepatic vein pulsed-wave Doppler provides an objective corresponding image of the jugular wave contour (S wave = *x* descent; D wave = *y* descent) (**Fig. 2–10**). Cardiac catheterization also provides the opportunity for the examiner to compare his or her noninvasive and invasive data with direct measurement of right atrial pressure and contour. We recommend that clinicians estimate right atrial pressure and waveforms prior to sending patients to the catheterization laboratory for hemodynamic assessment. This process will result in "calibration" of the examiner's physical examination skills and more accurate appreciation of the findings.

Abnormal venous pulse

Abnormalities of the *a* wave: Abnormalities of the *a* wave can result from primary right-sided valvular disease,

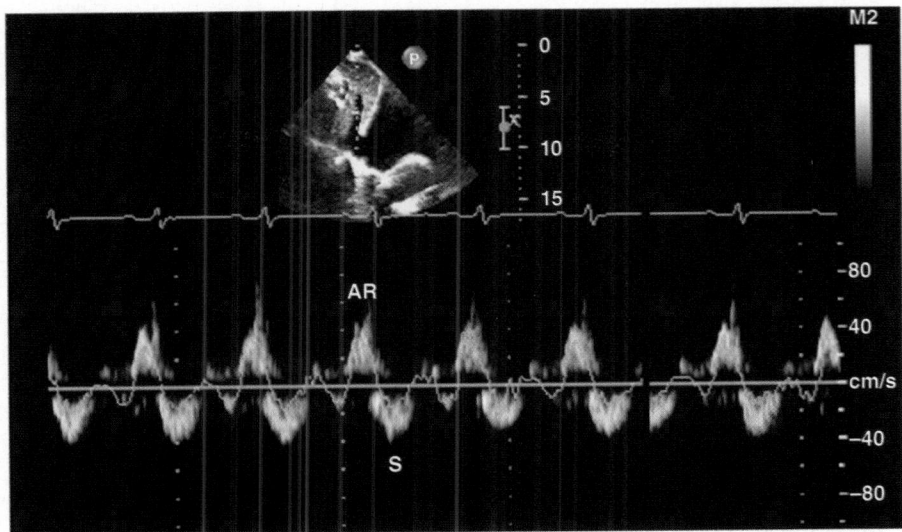

Figure 2–10. Simultaneous right atrial pressure tracings (*green*) and hepatic vein Doppler in a patient with pulmonary hypertension. The increased *a* wave is simultaneously reflected on the hepatic vein Doppler tracing as a prominent atrial reversal (AR). There are also prominent *x* descents with prominent systolic (S) waves. Hepatic vein Doppler findings mirror right atrial pressure tracings and can be used to confirm jugular venous examination findings.

hemodynamic abnormalities of the right ventricle, or heart rhythm abnormalities. An increase in the amplitude of the *a* wave is seen in situations where there is increased contribution of atrial contraction to ventricular diastolic filling. An elevated atrial reversal velocity on the hepatic vein Doppler tracing corresponds to a large *a* wave. This can occur in the setting of right ventricular diastolic dysfunction and is typically seen in pulmonary hypertension, pulmonary stenosis, or, less frequently, in restrictive cardiomyopathies. Classically described in rheumatic tricuspid stenosis, very enlarged *a* waves—*giant a waves*—will be present secondary to atrial contraction against a stenotic tricuspid valve (**Fig. 2–11**). Currently, the occurrence of very large *a* waves is primarily encountered in patients being evaluated for tricuspid prosthesis obstruction with an elevated diastolic gradient.

Atrial fibrillation is characterized by the absence of organized atrial contraction; thus, in patients with atrial fibrillation, the *a* wave will be absent (**Fig. 2–12**). In atrial flutter, small, regular flutter waves can be seen instead of *a* waves. Initially described as a delay between *a* and *v* waves on the jugular venous pulse, the diagnosis of first-degree atrioventricular block or Wenckebach phenomenon features on neck veins is of historical interest. The presence of brisk, extremely prominent *a* waves, the so-called cannon *a* waves, are still valuable in clinical practice. These are the result of atrial contraction against a closed tricuspid valve. Variable cannon *a* waves suggest the diagnosis of complete heart block in patients with new-onset bradycardia, and their occurrence in wide complex tachycardia is diagnostic of ventricular tachycardia rather than aberrancy.

Abnormalities of the *x* descent: The most common abnormality observed in clinical practice is the blunting of *x* descent that is seen in atrial fibrillation. Atrial fibrillation results in a loss of atrial contraction as well as atrial relaxation, leading to this abnormality. The corresponding finding is a reduced or absent systolic forward flow (S wave) on the hepatic vein Doppler tracing (see Fig. 2–12). In patients with myopathic diseases, annular motion can be markedly reduced, as evidenced by low tissue Doppler velocities, and thus the *x* descent will be blunted (see Fig. 2–9). Last, in patients with tricuspid regurgitation, a positive *v* wave will take the place of the *x* descent. Increased amplitude of *x* descents—*deep x* descents—are classically seen in constrictive pericarditis (see Fig. 2–6) as the result of both enhanced annular descent and preserved atrial relaxation.

Abnormalities of the *v* wave: In severe tricuspid regurgitation, right atrial pressure rises as the tricuspid regurgitant volume enters the right atrium. This leads to two abnormalities of the *v* wave—an increase in its *amplitude* and a more premature inscription of its upstroke (see Fig. 2–12). The large *v* wave occurs throughout systole and, thus, should be timed with the carotid pulsation. The most extreme example of this phenomenon is the occurrence of a single, large, positive *v* wave, described as *ventricularization* of right atrial pressure tracings. This will manifest as a systolic reversal of flow on the hepatic vein Doppler tracing.

Abnormalities of the *y* descent: Increased amplitude of the *y* descent can be seen in any disease that leads to prominent rapid filling of the right ventricle in early diastole. This can be seen in tricuspid regurgitation with or without elevation in right heart filling pressures but also in abnormalities of right ventricular diastolic function, such as restrictive cardiomyopathy or constrictive pericarditis (see Fig. 2–9). The early rapid filling is seen as a prominent early diastolic forward flow on the hepatic vein Doppler velocity curve with a high initial E velocity and short deceleration time on the tricuspid inflow Doppler signal.

Conversely, in cardiac tamponade, there is blunting of the *y* descent given the impaired ventricular filling due to elevated

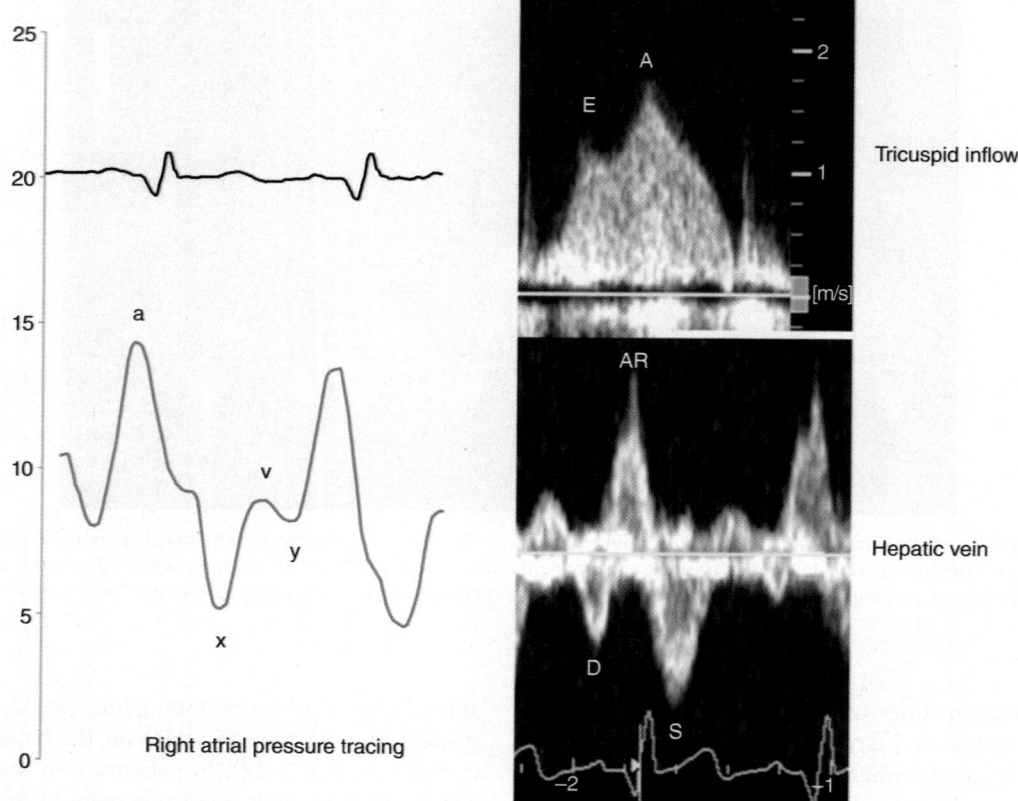

Figure 2–11. Giant *a* waves seen in tricuspid valve stenosis. Right atrial pressure tracings (*left*) showing very large *a* waves, which are also appreciated by hepatic vein pulsed-wave Doppler (large atrial reversals [AR]; *right lower*). Continuous-wave Doppler across the tricuspid valve confirmed the diagnosis of tricuspid stenosis (*right upper*). A, *A* wave; D, diastole; E, *E* wave; S, systole.

intrapericardial pressures preventing early rapid filling (see Fig. 2–8). Reduction in amplitude and slope of the *y* descent is seen in tricuspid valve native or prosthetic stenosis.

Kussmaul Sign: The Kussmaul sign is characterized by an increase in jugular venous pressure associated with inspiration as opposed to the usual drop that is seen in normal individuals (**Fig. 2–13**). Although described in constrictive pericarditis, the sign can be present in any disease associated with severe elevation in right-sided filling pressures.

Abdominojugular Reflux: Also known as *hepatojugular reflux,* the term *abdominojugular reflux* better describes the maneuver when the examiner applies gentle pressure to the center of the patient's abdomen (around the umbilicus). As abdominal pressure is applied, there is a transient, minor increase in jugular (central) venous pressure and an accentuation of jugular venous waveforms. The patient should be made aware of the maneuver in order to avoid sudden abdominal muscle tensioning and an elevation in intrathoracic pressures (similar to the ones seen with the Valsalva maneuver). Normally, these changes will only last a few beats (around 5 seconds) despite continued pressure, and the venous pressure will return to baseline. A sustained response (lasting more than 10–15 seconds)[17] (**Fig. 2–14**) suggests elevated right-sided filling pressures.

PHYSICAL EXAMINATION: AUSCULTATION HEART SOUNDS

Technique

Proper technique must be reviewed prior to discussing auscultatory findings; this involves patient positioning, areas of auscultation, and the stethoscope. In order to avoid missing subtle findings, cardiac auscultation must be performed with the patient in three positions: sitting, supine, and left lateral decubitus. The sitting position is important for auscultation of sounds that emanate from the base of heart and great vessels as well as pericardial rubs and some tricuspid murmurs. Although most standard cardiac auscultation is performed with the patient supine, auscultation over the apex with the patient in the left lateral decubitus position brings out mitral murmurs and low-pitched cardiac sounds that might not otherwise be appreciated.

Five *areas* of auscultation have been classically described (**Fig. 2–15**)—*mitral* (over the apical impulse), *tricuspid* (fifth intercostal space at the left parasternal line), *pulmonic* (second intercostal space at the left parasternal line), *aortic* (second intercostal space at the right parasternal line), and *accessory aortic area* (third intercostal space at the left parasternal line); however, the stethoscope should not "jump" from one area to the other. Instead, the examiner should march the stethoscope from the apex toward the sternum, then up along the parasternal line,

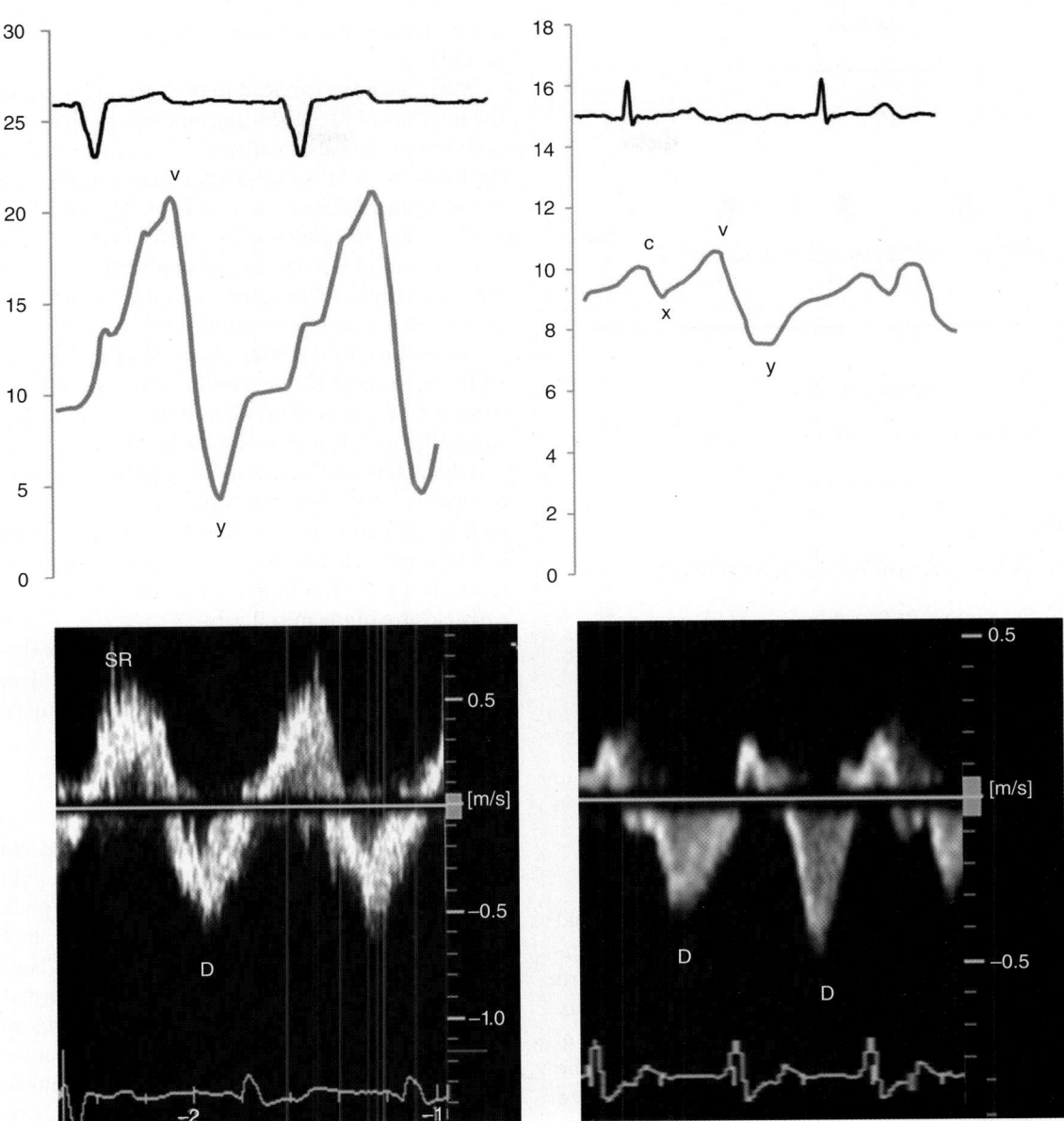

Figure 2–12. Right atrial pressure tracings in severe tricuspid regurgitation and atrial fibrillation. Right atrial pressure tracings show large *v* waves and prominent *y* descents in a patient with severe tricuspid regurgitation (*left upper*). Large systolic reversals (SR) and prominent diastolic (D) waves are also seen on hepatic vein pulsed-Doppler (*left lower*). In atrial fibrillation, right atrial tracings (*right upper*) show loss of *a* waves with blunting of the *x* descent. This is also illustrated by hepatic vein Doppler (*right lower*), which shows absence of systolic (S) waves and prominent diastolic (D) waves.

ending at the right parasternal area at the level of the second intercostal space. With the patient sitting, the opposite is then performed, using the right upper border as the starting point. This meticulous process ensures that abnormal auscultatory finding heard over a very localized area will not be missed as they might if only the five main areas are auscultated. When indicated, auscultation should also be extended to areas where murmurs typically radiate, such as the left axilla, neck, suprasternal notch, right infraclavicular area, and back. In each area, careful attention must be paid to each heart sound, systole, and diastole.

The examiner should always take full advantage of the two parts of the stethoscope: the bell and the diaphragm. The bell is designed for auscultation of low-pitched sounds (third and fourth heart sounds, diastolic rumble, vascular bruits), whereas the diaphragm should be used for most heart sounds and murmurs. The bell should be gently applied to the bare chest; if excessive pressure is exerted, the bell works as a diaphragm. The examiner, however, should also use this property in his or her favor. For example, in a patient with mitral stenosis, variable stethoscope pressure should be used to focus on the rumble (bell) or the opening snap (diaphragm).

First Heart Sound

Normal First Heart Sound

The first heart sound (S1) corresponds to closure of the atrioventricular valves and, therefore, marks the end of diastole

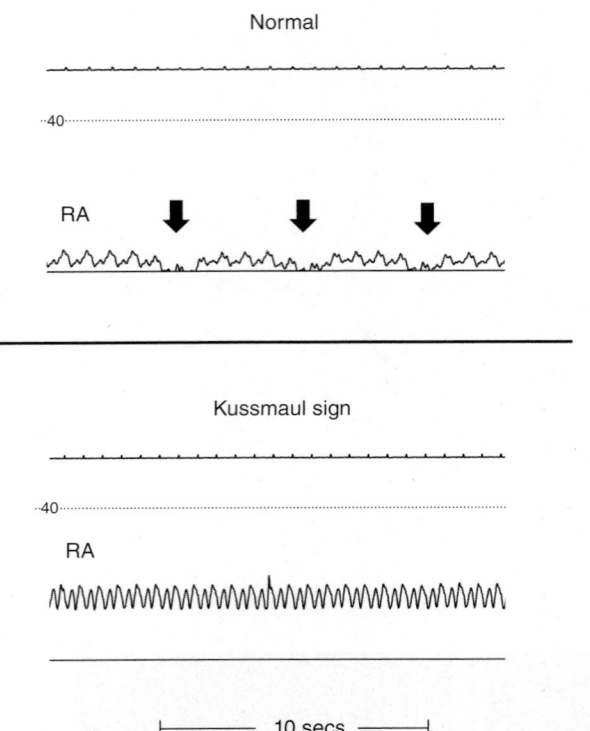

Figure 2-13. The Kussmaul sign. Right atrial (RA) pressure tracings in a normal individual (*upper*) showing drops in mean right atrial pressure associated with inspiration (*arrows*). The Kussmaul sign (*lower*) corresponds to failure of mean right atrial pressure to drop on inspiration, as observed in this patient with constrictive pericarditis.

(**Fig. 2–16**). It has two components—mitral (M1) and tricuspid (T1), with the latter following the former in normal circumstances. In most patients, M1 overshadows T1, and S1 is heard as a single sound. Sometimes, however, both components can be heard over the left lower sternal border, causing *splitting of S1*; this is a normal finding. Both components should have the same pitch and intensity and should be easily differentiated from a right-sided fourth heart sound (lower pitched) and an early systolic click (higher pitched and usually auscultated in a much wider area). Splitting of S1 might be slightly more prominent in patients with a right bundle branch block.

Abnormalities of the First Heart Sound
An increase in the intensity of the S1 can be encountered in situations where the PR interval is short, such as preexcitation or tachycardia. Sinus tachycardia associated with a hyperdynamic

left ventricle is the most common cause of a loud S1 in clinical practice.

Mitral stenosis can lead to both an increase and decrease in the intensity of S1, depending on the degree of calcification and mobility of the valve leaflets. When mitral leaflets are pliable, the intensity of S1 is increased, and this might be the only sign of rheumatic involvement of the mitral valve. The finding of a loud S1 also has therapeutic implications because it suggests that the patient is likely a good candidate for percutaneous balloon valvuloplasty. In cases where the leaflets are calcific and immobile, the first heart sound becomes soft.

A decrease in the intensity of S1 is recognized in patients with a prolonged PR interval or after long R-R intervals (diastolic periods) in patients with atrial fibrillation. Given the wide variability of R-R intervals in atrial fibrillation, S1 usually has variable intensity. Decreased S1 amplitude is also recognized in myopathic processes and in patients with severe reduction in systolic function due to a poorly contractile ventricle. Last, a soft S1 might also be observed in acute aortic regurgitation due to marked elevation in left ventricular diastolic pressures and early closure of the mitral valve.

Most clinical abnormalities alter intensity of the M1 component of the first heart sound. An exception is the patient with Ebstein anomaly when the large, sail-like anterior tricuspid leaflet gives rise to a loud T1 component.

Second Heart Sound

Normal Second Heart Sound
The second heart sound (S2) corresponds to closure of the semilunar valves and has an aortic (A2) and a pulmonary (P2) component (Fig. 2–16). The S2 sound is high pitched and best heard with the diaphragm. As opposed to S1, its two components are audible in the majority of patients. The S2 intensity and timing carry very valuable diagnostic information.

In order for the examiner to describe specific abnormalities of A2 and P2 (or to ensure that normality is indeed present), it is *mandatory* that both components are simultaneously auscultated and actively sought. P2 is typically audible in a limited area over the second left intercostal space and is sometimes only appreciated with the patient sitting. Therefore, one can only state that a *single S2* is present if appropriate auscultatory maneuvers are taken and a single component remains audible. In normal circumstances, both A2 and P2 should have similar intensities when auscultated simultaneously in the pulmonic position. A P2 should not be audible at other positions unless pulmonary hypertension is present.

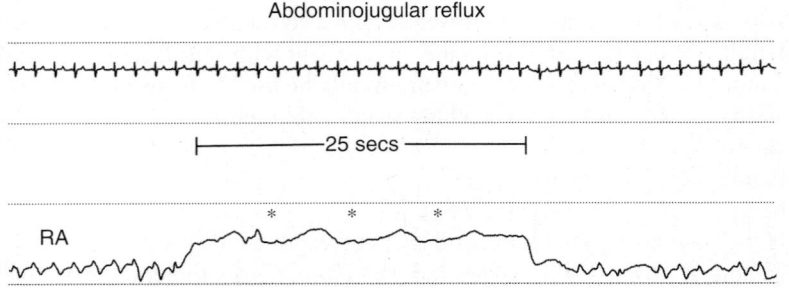

Figure 2-14. Abnormal abdominojugular reflux response in patient with heart failure. Right atrial (RA) pressure tracings illustrate the abnormal, sustained elevation in right filling pressures while pressure is applied to the patient's abdomen. The patient should be instructed to breathe normally during the maneuver as illustrated here (inspiration marked by *asterisk*).

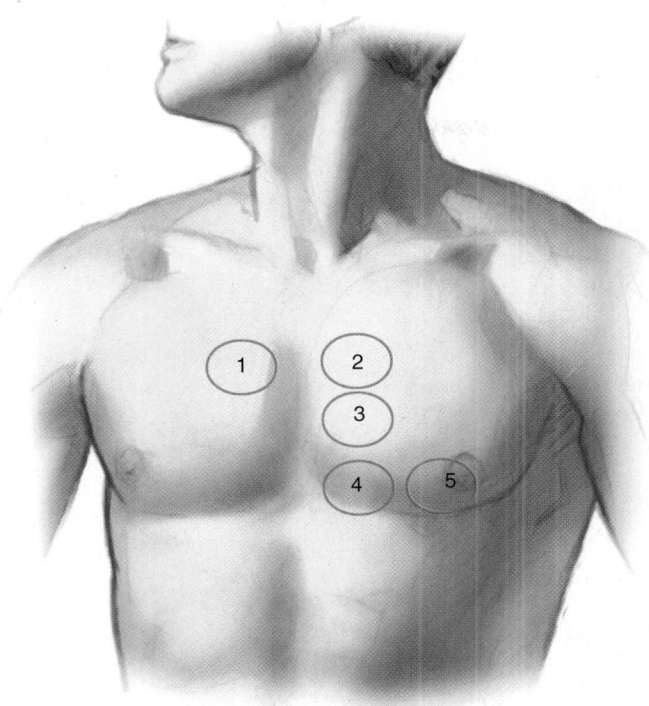

Figure 2-15. Areas of auscultation. The five classic areas of cardiac auscultation: (1) aortic (second intercostal space at the right parasternal line), (2) pulmonic (second intercostal space at the left parasternal line), (3) accessory aortic area (third intercostal space at the left parasternal line), (4) tricuspid (fifth intercostal space at the left parasternal), and (5) mitral (over the apical impulse).

Physiologic Splitting of S2

During normal inspiration, there is enhanced venous return to right-sided cardiac chambers as well as increased capacitance in pulmonary vasculature. The combination of these two phenomena leads to an increase in right ventricular ejection time with inspiration and delay in closure of the pulmonary valve following inspiration. The normal lack of significant respirophasic change in left ventricular ejection time results in a single audible S2 during expiration (P2 occurring simultaneously with A2) and two distinct components on inspiration (with P2 following A2), the so-called physiologic splitting of S2 (**Fig. 2–17**).

Abnormal Splitting of S2

Nonphysiologic splitting of S2 can be categorized as paradoxical, persistent, or fixed (see Fig. 2–17). The abnormalities can be secondary to hemodynamic or conduction derangements. In *paradoxical splitting* of S2, there is a delay in aortic valve closure, with P2 preceding A2. S2 is split during expiration and becomes single during inspiration as P2 becomes closer to A2; hence, the paradox (ie, the opposite of normal). This delay in A2 is secondary to a prolongation of left ventricular ejection time, which can be due to an increase in afterload or nonuniform contraction of the left ventricle (conduction abnormalities). The long ejection time can be measured from the duration of flow through the left ventricular outflow tract or

across the aortic valve by Doppler echocardiography; it usually exceeds 300 milliseconds in these instances.

Although classically described in valvular aortic stenosis, paradoxical splitting of the S2 is more common in obstructive hypertrophic cardiomyopathy, suggesting severe dynamic left ventricular outflow obstruction. In severe aortic stenosis, the A2 component is either absent or diminished, and splitting of S2 is rarely appreciated. In left bundle branch block, activation of the left ventricular lateral wall is delayed, also prolonging the ejection period. This is a sign of left ventricular dyssynchrony. In our experience, patients with decreased left ventricular systolic function and paradoxical splitting of S2 appear to respond favorably to cardiac resynchronization therapy. Right ventricular pacing also promotes delayed activation of the left ventricle and paradoxical spitting of S2.

In *persistent splitting*, S2 is widely split at baseline (both A2 and P2 can be heard); however, with inspiration, the A2-P2 interval becomes longer. This is secondary to an underlying delay in the occurrence of P2. Wide splitting of S2, therefore, reflects abnormal right ventricular ejection hemodynamics. The most common cause in clinical practice is right bundle branch block, although a severe increase in afterload resulting from pulmonary hypertension can also lead to wide splitting of S2.

Fixed splitting of S2 is classically found in ostium secundum atrial septal defect, where wide splitting of S2 is present at baseline with minimal or no change in the A2-P2 interval during inspiration. The wide S2 splitting on expiration is related to increased pulmonary vascular capacitance associated with

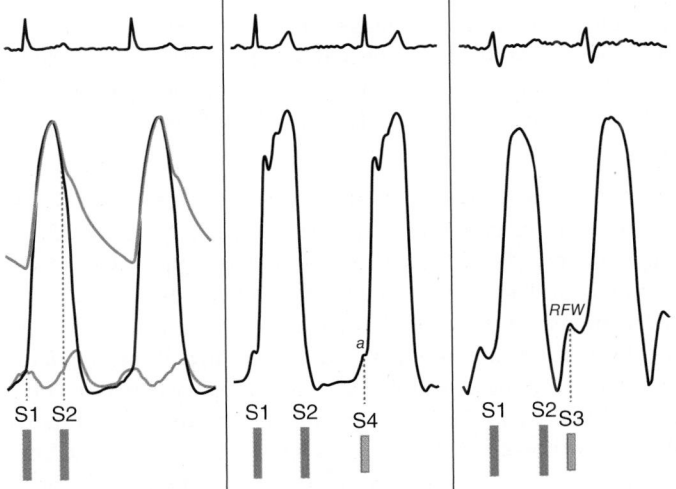

Figure 2–16. Heart sounds. Normal heart sounds depicted in the left panel. The first heart sound (S1) occurs when left ventricular pressure (black tracing) exceeds left atrial pressure (blue tracing), resulting in closure of the mitral valve. In contrast, the second heart sound (S2) occurs when left ventricular pressure falls below aortic pressure, leading to closure of the aortic valve. The fourth heart sound (S4; middle panel) is heard in late diastole and corresponds to forceful left atrial contraction into a noncompliant left ventricle. Note the large atrial wave (*a*) seen on the ventricular tracings of a patient with hypertrophic cardiomyopathy. In contrast, the third heart sound (S3; right panel) originates from early, rapid ventricular filling during diastole. Note the prominent rapid filling wave (RFW) present on the left ventricular tracings of a patient with restrictive cardiomyopathy.

Physiologic splitting

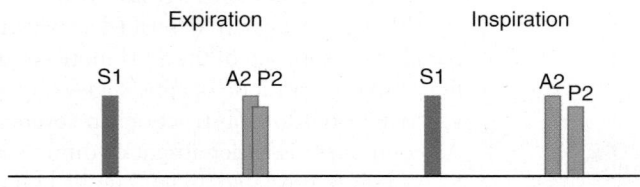

Abnormal splitting

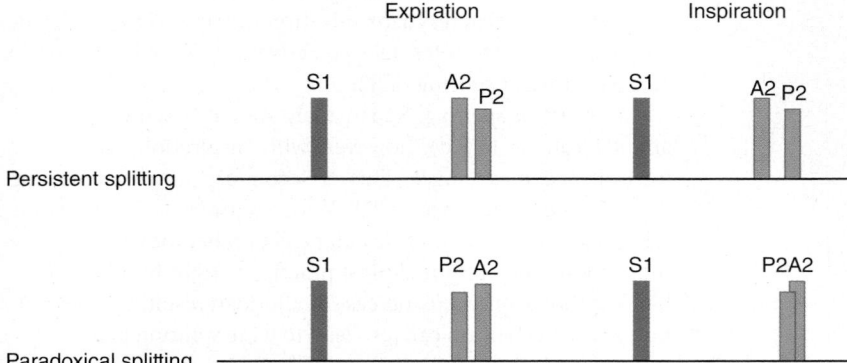

Persistent splitting

Paradoxical splitting

Figure 2–17. Respirophasic A2-P2 intervals in physiologic and abnormal splitting of second heart sound.

increased pulmonary blood flow, delaying the P2 component. As a result of the atrial communication, the decrease in venous return during expiration is compensated by an increase in left-to-right shunt without changes in right ventricular preload. The lack of significant respirophasic changes in both preload and afterload results in no change in the right ventricular ejection period and, therefore, a fixed A2-P2 interval.

Abnormalities of S2 Components

A *loud P2* is a sign of pulmonary arterial hypertension; in severe cases of pulmonary hypertension, P2 is palpable. P2 is generally heard over a small area in the left upper chest. A P2 component that can be auscultated in other areas is a clue that P2 is increased. In general, a P2 heard at the left lower sternal border indicates moderate pulmonary hypertension and, if audible at the apex, indicates severe pulmonary hypertension.

A *diminished P2* is noted in patients with increased anteroposterior thoracic distance. The opposite is also true. Patients with diminished anteroposterior thoracic dimension, such as patients with pectus excavatum, can have an abnormally loud P2. In patients with obstructive lung disease, increased lung volume contributes to a decrease in P2, this being the most common cause for a single S2 in practice. A diminished or absent P2 is also noted in patients with severe valvular pulmonary stenosis. Last, a single (and loud) S2 is a characteristic clinical finding in patients with congenitally corrected transposition, where the posterior location of the pulmonary valve prevents auscultation of the P2 component.

A *loud A2* is expected in patients with severe systemic arterial hypertension. A very loud A2—*tambour like*—was also described in syphilitic aortitis, but the disease is rarely encountered today.

A *diminished A2* is a classic finding of valvular calcific aortic stenosis and is also an important marker of disease severity, especially when the A2 component is absent. The presence of a normal A2 component in a patient with "severe aortic stenosis" and echo-Doppler findings of fixed obstruction should prompt investigation for subaortic or supravalvular obstruction.

Fourth Heart Sound

In the early phases of diastolic dysfunction, abnormal (prolonged) ventricular relaxation impairs early diastolic ventricular filling, decreasing the amount of filling in early diastole with a compensatory enhanced atrial contribution of diastolic filling.[18] An audible left fourth heart sound (S4) represents this prominent, forceful left atrial contraction into a noncompliant left ventricle (Fig. 2–16). It occurs, therefore, in late diastole (presystole) and is never present in atrial fibrillation. A left-sided S4 is a low-pitched sound, typically only heard at the apex with the bell and easily missed if auscultation in the left lateral decubitus position is not performed.

Doppler echocardiographic findings that correlate with the presence of an audible S4 are those of an abnormal relaxation pattern (grade I diastolic dysfunction) (**Fig. 2–18**) on the transmitral flow velocity curve and include a low E:A ratio and a prolonged deceleration time with a shortened duration of the A wave. There are also increased atrial reversal velocities on pulmonary vein Doppler profiles. Left ventricular tracings will show a slow rate of fall of left ventricular pressure during

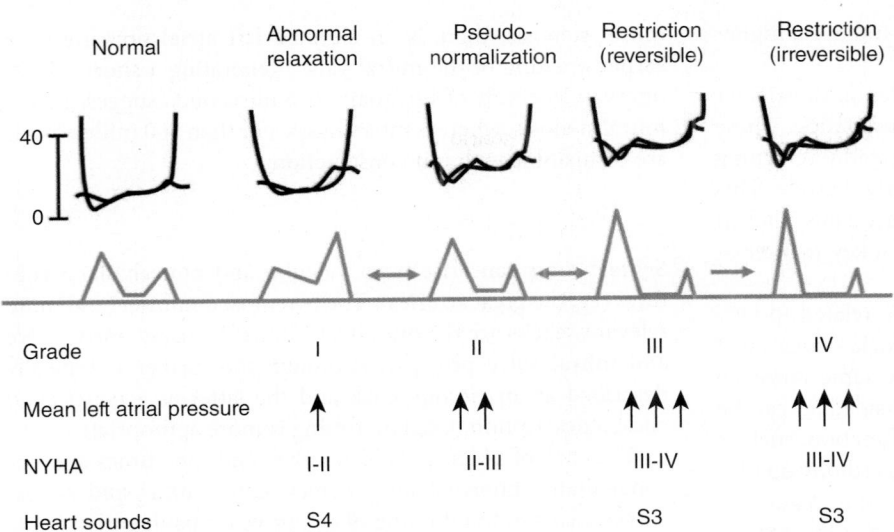

	Normal	Abnormal relaxation	Pseudo-normalization	Restriction (reversible)	Restriction (irreversible)
Grade		I	II	III	IV
Mean left atrial pressure		↑	↑↑	↑↑↑	↑↑↑
NYHA		I-II	II-III	III-IV	III-IV
Heart sounds		S4		S3	S3

Figure 2–18. Auscultation findings in different stages of diastolic dysfunction. Left ventricular and left atrial pressure tracings (*black*) as well as mitral inflow Doppler pattern (*blue*) in different degrees of left atrial pressure elevation and diastolic dysfunction. Cardiac auscultation will reflect hemodynamic abnormalities and allows longitudinal assessment of filling pressures. NYHA, New York Heart Association functional class.

isovolumic relaxation (reduced negative dP/dt), lack of rapid filling waves, and prominent *a* waves. Patients with impaired ventricular relaxation typically have normal mean left atrial pressures and thus are not in heart failure at rest but will develop shortness of breath with exertion as the diastolic filling period shortens. These patients rely on atrial contraction for diastolic filling, and therefore loss of organized atrial contraction is generally poorly tolerated.

Abnormal ventricular relaxation occurs most frequently with left ventricular hypertrophy due to aortic stenosis, hypertrophic cardiomyopathy, and systemic hypertension. It also occurs with ongoing myocardial ischemia and is frequently observed as part of aging. Thus, an audible S4 is expected in all of those entities but should not be observed in young adults since myocardial relaxation is normal in that age group.

A *right-sided S4* is usually associated with right ventricular pressure overload as seen in pulmonary hypertension, pulmonary stenosis, and early phases of restrictive cardiomyopathy. A right-sided S4 is usually heard at the left lower sternal border and increases with inspiration.

Third Heart Sound

A third heart sound (S3) will occur when there is prominent early rapid ventricular filling during diastole (Fig. 2–16). It is a low-pitched sound heard in early diastole, most likely due to tensing of the chordae as the left ventricle rapidly expands from the early filling. An S3 is best heard at the apex with the bell lightly placed and the patient in a left lateral decubitus position. It occurs 100 to 150 milliseconds after S2. This sound correlates with a high initial E velocity, an increased E:A ratio, and short deceleration time on the transmitral flow velocity curve.

There are a number of etiologies for the generation of an S3. The most common is in a patient with an abnormal stiffness of the myocardium coupled with high filling pressures. The high left atrial pressure produces high driving pressure across the mitral valve to account for the early rapid filling, which is followed by a rapid increase in left ventricular diastolic pressure.[15]

This is manifested as a steep rapid filling wave on left ventricular pressure tracing and large left atrial *v* waves (reflecting the pressure rise as pulmonary venous blood enters an overloaded left atrium). An S3 can be a dynamic finding and is usually dependent on the volume status of the patient. If there is severe elevation of left atrial pressure, there will be an S3 on auscultation with a restrictive pattern on the transmitral flow velocity curve (high E:A ratio and short deceleration time) (see Fig. 2–17). However, with diuresis and lowering of left atrial pressure, the transmitral flow pattern will change from restrictive (grade III pattern) to pseudonormal (grade II pattern) and even delayed relaxation (grade I pattern) with disappearance of the S3 on examination. A persistent S3 despite treatment indicates the end stage of diastolic dysfunction (grade IV pattern) caused by severe irreversible fibrosis of the myocardium.

There are other etiologies for an S3 on examination, all of which reflect rapid early diastolic filling. Rapid early diastolic filling occurs in young healthy hearts due to vigorous ventricular relaxation, which "sucks" the blood in from the left atrium to the left ventricle in early diastole, allowing for a higher preload while maintaining low to normal pressures. The transmitral Doppler velocity curve will have the same appearance as a restrictive filling pattern (high E:A ratio and short deceleration time). However, the mitral annular motion will be enhanced, seen as high medial and lateral e′ velocities on tissue Doppler. Thus, an S3 is often noted in young individuals, athletes, and pregnant patients. Conversely, it is rarely observed in patients aged above 40 years; the presence of an S3 in patients aged above 40 years suggests organic heart disease.

Constrictive pericarditis is also a form of severe diastolic heart failure, where the scarred, inelastic pericardium significantly impairs ventricular diastolic filling. Rapid filling waves on right and left ventricular hemodynamic tracings were some of the earliest hemodynamic signs of constrictive pericarditis described by cardiac catheterization. This prominent early diastolic filling is responsible for the *pericardial knock* heard in constrictive pericarditis. The knock tends to happen slightly earlier than the typical S3 and tends to have a higher pitch.

High E wave velocities and rapid filling waves on ventricular tracings can also be seen in severe mitral regurgitation. These are secondary to the large volume of blood rapidly returning from the left atrium to the left ventricle in early diastole. This increased rapid early diastolic filling can produce a low-pitched "filling sound" in mitral regurgitation and is a key marker of severe mitral regurgitation.

Although the findings described so far are related to left-sided etiologies (except for the pericardial knock, which most likely originates from the right ventricle), the same rationale can be applied to right-sided lesions. A right-sided S3 can be heard in severe right ventricular diastolic dysfunction, such as severe right-sided heart failure and restrictive cardiomyopathy. Filling sounds can also be heard in severe tricuspid regurgitation and may be the only finding on auscultation as the systolic murmur can be barely audible due to equalization of the right atrial and right ventricular pressures during systole. Inspiration will enhance the intensity of a right-sided S3 and S4.

Gallops

When tachycardia is present in conjunction with an S3 or an S4, a *gallop rhythm* is said to be present. If both are present and diastolic periods are markedly diminished (due to faster heart rates), S3 and S4 will occur at the same time—a *summation gallop*. This physical finding is analogous to the presence of fused E and A waves on mitral inflow echo-Doppler.

Opening Snap of Mitral Stenosis

The opening snap of rheumatic mitral stenosis is an early diastolic, high-pitched sound that originates from sudden tensing of abnormal leaflets and the subvalvular apparatus during valve opening (equivalent of the "hockey stick deformity" on two-dimensional echocardiography). The finding of an opening snap has important clinical implications and deserves meticulous assessment. Because of its high pitch, the opening snap has a much wider area of radiation than the associated diastolic rumble of mitral stenosis; it can be heard at the left sternal border and even at the base of the heart in the aortic position. An opening snap has a much higher pitch than an S3, which is low pitched and heard only at the apex. It may be difficult to differentiate an opening snap from a loud P2, but a P2 should not be heard at the aortic position unless there are systemic levels of pulmonary hypertension.

The presence of a crisp opening snap suggests that the mitral leaflets are mobile and pliable and hence amenable to percutaneous balloon valvotomy. With more severe calcification and immobility of the leaflets, the opening snap becomes softer or disappears. The opening snap also allows the assessment of left atrial pressures and severity of the mitral stenosis. The mitral valve will open when left ventricular pressure drops below left atrial pressure. With mild degrees of stenosis, left atrial pressure is not severely elevated and mitral valve opening occurs late. The result is a long A2 (aortic valve closure) to opening snap (mitral valve opening) interval. With severe mitral stenosis, there is an elevated left atrial pressure with earlier opening of the mitral valve, generating a short A2-OS interval. Intervals of less than 70 milliseconds suggest severe mitral stenosis, whereas intervals greater than 100 milliseconds are compatible with mild obstruction.

Systolic Clicks

Systolic clicks can arise from valvular and nonvalvular structures (eg, the great arteries). The two most common (and more relevant) clicks are the ones heard in the bicuspid aortic valve and mitral valve prolapse. Although the former is typically described as an *ejection* click and the latter as a *nonejection* click, a description based on timing is more appropriate.

The click of a bicuspid aortic valve (and sometimes of other congenitally abnormal aortic valves such as unicuspid valves) is secondary to the doming of the valve cusps in early systole as the aortic valve opens. The sound is high pitched (higher than S1) and sometimes quite loud; it should not be confused with a loud split S1 (two components with the same pitch and intensity) or an S4 (low-pitched sound that vanishes if the bell is firmly pressed against the skin).

Doming of the cusps is also seen in valvular pulmonary stenosis, and an early systolic click is also typical. As with the bicuspid aortic valve, the click of pulmonary stenosis introduces the systolic murmur. However, the click noted in pulmonary stenosis has a unique and important characteristic—it decreases in intensity with inspiration and moves closer to S1. This is the *only* right-sided auscultatory finding that diminishes with inspiration. As a result of increased venous return and increased right ventricular filling on inspiration, the pulmonary cusps acquire a more cephalad configuration. There is less cusp excursion during systole and a softer click.

Early systolic clicks can also arise from dilated great vessels (aorta or pulmonary artery). These are difficult to discern from the clicks associated with dysplastic or congenitally abnormal semilunar valves at the bedside. Another rare source of systolic clicks is an atrial septal aneurysm, arising from the motion of a very redundant valve of the fossa ovalis. These less common abnormalities should also be looked for when echocardiography studies are ordered for the evaluation of systolic clicks.

The systolic click(s) associated with mitral valve prolapse usually occurs in mid to late systole when there is full excursion of the prolapsed mitral leaflet(s) into the left atrium. The click can be single or multiple (*salvo* of clicks). The timing of the click of mitral valve prolapse occurring later in systole helps to differentiate it from clicks that arise from semilunar valves. With increased preload (squatting, supine), the click occurs later in systole, whereas decreased preload (Valsalva maneuver, standing) has the opposite effect. Single or multiple systolic clicks can also be heard in patients with Ebstein anomaly.

Miscellaneous

Pericardial rubs may have three components, one systolic and two diastolic. Systolic and presystolic sounds are most commonly present. The pericardial rubs are described as "scratchy," with a high pitch. Although the presence of pericardial rubs can be intermittent, the practitioner should optimize the patient's position in order to better detect the rub. Pericardial rubs are generally best heard with the patient sitting, leaning forward with held expiration.

There are extracardiac sounds that can be heard on auscultation of the heart. A mediastinal "crunch" is caused by inflammation or air in the mediastinum that is of high pitch and has a rhythm that corresponds to the cardiac contraction within the mediastinum; this sound is markedly enhanced during inspiration. Pleural rubs may be mistaken for cardiac sounds, particularly in the patient who has tachypnea. Auscultation during held respiration is required to differentiate this sound from a cardiac etiology. Pacemaker wires can produce clicks and high-pitched "squeaks" that result from excessive motion of the wires during the cardiac cycle.

Prosthetic Heart Valves

Auscultation of prosthetic heart valves is an important component of the physical examination. All mechanical valves should produce a crisp, high-pitched sound during valve closure, irrespective of the type of valve. The older-generation valves, such as a ball–cage prosthesis and some of the tilting disk prostheses, will produce a click during valve opening. However, the newer-generation floating disk and bileaflet valves are usually silent with valve opening. In some patients, the closing sound of a semilunar bioprosthesis (particularly in the pulmonary position) is audible, and a well-demarcated closing sound suggests a normally functioning prosthesis. This finding can also be used longitudinally to assess for prosthesis deterioration.

There is always an intrinsic degree of obstruction with any prosthesis, that produces a short systolic ejection murmur in the aortic or pulmonic position and may produce a diastolic rumble in the mitral or tricuspid valve position. However, murmurs of prosthetic valve regurgitation indicate pathology, due to paravalvular leaks, abnormal motion of the disc(s) of a mechanical prosthesis, or degenerated bioprosthetic leaflets.

PHYSICAL EXAMINATION: AUSCULTATION MURMURS

A murmur is the auscultatory equivalent of nonlaminar flow through an anatomic structure (eg, a cardiac valve or intracardiac shunt). When similar sounds originate from peripheral vessels, by convention, a *bruit* is described. In echocardiography, nonlaminar flow is manifest by turbulent high-velocity flow and assessed by continuous-wave Doppler echocardiography. Although other factors play a role (eg, the size of an ventricular communication, the effective orifice area in a regurgitant atrioventricular valve, or blood viscosity), murmurs tend to reflect the pressure difference between structures from which the murmur originates. The diastolic murmur from a stenotic atrioventricular valve (mitral or tricuspid) tends to be low pitched and quiet because atrial and ventricular diastolic pressures are typically low. The murmur of aortic regurgitation is a high-pitched "cooing" sound that result from the high pressure difference between the aorta and left ventricular pressures during diastole.

TABLE 2–5. Grading of Murmurs	
Grade I	Faint murmur; heard only after a few seconds of auscultation
Grade II	Moderately loud murmur; heard immediately
Grade III	Loud murmur; not associated with a thrill
Grade IV	Loud murmur; associated with a thrill
Grade V	Very loud murmur; can be heard if only the edge of the stethoscope is in contact with the skin
Grade VI	Loudest murmur possible; can be heard with stethoscope just removed from the chest and not touching the skin

When a murmur is identified, several characteristics need to be analyzed and described; these include timing (systolic, diastolic, or continuous), pitch, intensity ("loudness"), contour (or shape, eg, crescendo vs decrescendo), and radiation. Dynamic changes, such as respirophasic or postextrasystolic changes, and response to maneuvers should also be noted. The intensity of systolic murmurs should be graded from I to VI (**Table 2–5**). Diastolic murmurs are best graded from I to IV.

"Drawing" physical examination findings used to be part of clinical documentation, perhaps best exemplified in Paul Wood's legendary index cards. Although electronic clinical notes do not allow these features to be incorporated into patients' charts, we recommend trainees go through the exercise of drawing murmurs. These exercises force the examiner to critically review the auscultatory findings, which include the timing of onset and cessation of the murmur, the contour of the murmur, and the murmur's relationship to normal and abnormal heart sounds.

Systolic Murmurs

General Principles

The most commonly encountered systolic murmurs originate from regurgitant atrioventricular valves or from accelerated flow across semilunar valves. The shapes of those murmurs will reflect the differences in hemodynamics as well as dynamic changes in the valvular and subvalvular apparatus. These differences in timing of onset and cessation are reflected in the continuous-wave Doppler traces of the atrioventricular valve regurgitation and semilunar valve obstruction.

In typical atrioventricular regurgitation, the murmur starts at atrioventricular valve closure and extends to the atrioventricular valve opening (**Fig. 2–19**). As a result, the murmur will have its onset immediately after the first heart sound and will extend through the S2—*holosystolic*. Given the high pressure differences between ventricles and atria throughout systole, the murmur is high pitched and does not change in contour, hence, the term *plateau murmur*. An analogous process happens in ventricular septal defects, where the pressure gradient between left and right ventricles also extends from mitral valve closure (S1) to mitral valve opening.

Semilunar valves open when the ventricular pressure exceeds the pressure in the great vessels. Thus, these murmurs will start after S1 occurs (see Fig. 2–19). The shape of these murmurs will reflect the changes in ejection hemodynamics throughout systole, giving rise to its diamond shape, where the

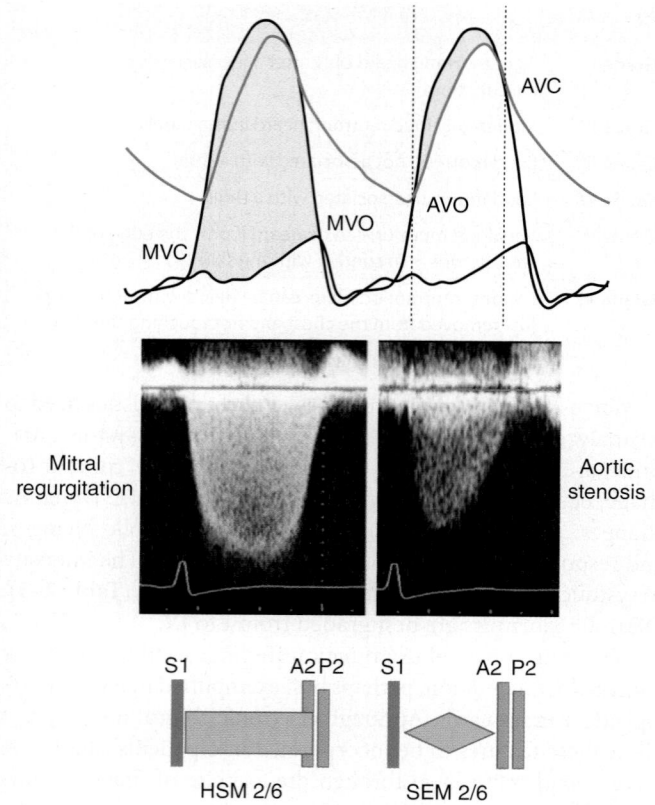

Figure 2–19. Auscultation findings in mitral regurgitation versus aortic stenosis. In mitral regurgitation (*left*), the murmur extends from mitral valve opening (MVO) to mitral valve closure (MVC) (*left upper*), which is appreciated by echo-Doppler (*left middle*). Note that the murmur encompasses A2 (*left lower*). In aortic stenosis (*right*), the murmur will start at the end of isovolumic contraction (aortic valve opening [AVO], *right upper*) and terminate as isovolumic relaxation starts (aortic valve closure [AVC]). Echo-Doppler (*right middle*) also illustrates the shorter duration of aortic stenosis compared with mitral regurgitation. Note the murmur is ejection quality and does not encompass A2 (*right lower*). HSM, holosystolic murmur; SEM, systolic ejection murmur.

murmur increases and then decreases in intensity (*crescendo-decrescendo*). These systolic ejection murmurs have a harsher quality than the regurgitant murmurs.

Atrioventricular Valve Regurgitation: Holosystolic Murmurs
Mitral regurgitation murmurs are typically best heard over the cardiac apex, but radiation will vary depending on the underlying disease. When the mitral regurgitation jet is anteriorly directed (toward the aorta), as noted in patients with prolapse or a flail segment of the posterior mitral leaflet, the murmur radiates to the left sternal border. In posteriorly directed mitral regurgitation jets caused by prolapse or flail of the anterior mitral leaflet, the murmur radiates to the left axilla, back, and thoracic spine.

Although typically described as holosystolic and plateau in quality, *mitral regurgitation* murmurs will vary according to the underlying pathology. In regurgitation that results from rheumatic mitral valve or flail mitral leaflet, the murmur will be holosystolic. In mitral valve prolapse with an intact chordal

apparatus, the regurgitation starts after the leaflet has prolapsed into the left atrium; a gap between S1 and the murmur is then present, which frequently starts after a midsystolic click. The late occurrence of a murmur in mitral valve prolapse is of great diagnostic importance. First, it suggests that the tendinous cords are intact and no flail segment is present. Second, it suggests that the regurgitation is not severe; late (ie, nonholosystolic) murmurs are rarely severe. Doppler echocardiography will clearly demonstrate the difference between a holosystolic murmur and a late systolic regurgitation both on color flow imaging and continuous-wave Doppler velocity curves (**Fig. 2–20**).

In secondary mitral regurgitation (the mitral regurgitation results from a disease of the ventricle and not the valve), the murmur can be soft and underwhelming despite the presence of severe regurgitation. This is likely due to a combination of reduced ventricular contraction and a large regurgitant orifice. If the mechanism is annular dilation, the murmur tends to be holosystolic, whereas in ischemic mitral regurgitation, the murmur may be late peaking. Ischemic mitral regurgitation can also be dynamic, with variation in the physical examination findings depending on the presence or absence of ischemia.

In *acute severe mitral regurgitation* secondary to papillary muscle rupture or mitral valve dehiscence, the left atrium is not accustomed to the severe volume overload. A very large *v* wave is generated because of lack of atrial compliance, and left ventricular and left atrial pressures essentially equalize in systole (**Fig. 2–21**). The auscultatory result is a very short, early systolic murmur or even absence of a murmur. Accordingly, color-flow and continuous-wave Doppler findings are also often very brief, making the diagnosis of acute mitral regurgitation challenging. Thus, a high clinical index of suspicion is needed. Patients with acute severe mitral regurgitation are in frank pulmonary edema and therefore sitting upright, whereas patients with post-myocardial infarction ventricular septal defect can tolerate the supine position.

Tricuspid regurgitation is usually secondary to dilatation of the tricuspid valve annulus and manifested as a holosystolic murmur, best heard at the left lower sternal border. The murmur can be very subtle, rarely greater than grade II in intensity. Although described as a classic sign in tricuspid regurgitation, an increase in the intensity of the holosystolic murmur (Carvallo sign) is not a sensitive sign. The clinical suspicion of severe tricuspid regurgitation is based more on the basis of a large *v* wave in the jugular venous contour rather than the presence of a murmur.

Ventricular septal defects can also present as holosystolic murmurs. Small ventricular septal defects are usually associated with a loud murmur, frequently accompanied by a thrill and best heard at the left lower sternal border. If there is a large septal defect, the murmur can be soft or even absent, particularly when an Eisenmenger's physiology is present.

Systolic Ejection Murmurs
In *aortic stenosis*, a diamond-shaped murmur can be auscultated at the third left intercostal space, second right intercostal space, or supraclavicular region, usually radiating to the

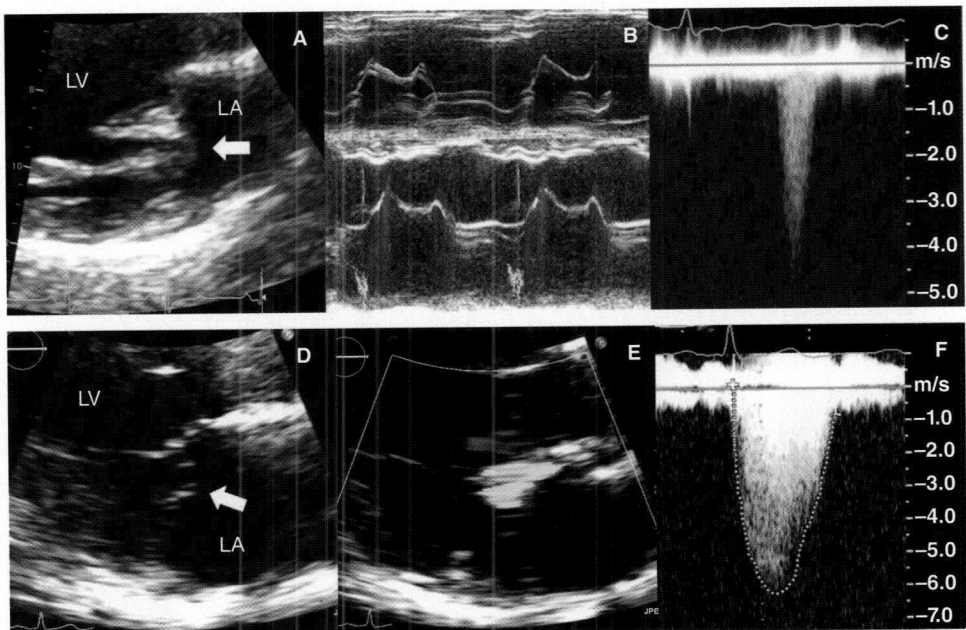

Figure 2–20. Echocardiographic findings in two patients with posterior mitral valve leaflet prolapse (arrow) and left ventricular enlargement. *Upper* panels show two-dimensional (**A**), color M-mode (**B**), and continuous-wave Doppler (**C**) echocardiography findings in a patient with mild mitral regurgitation. Auscultation revealed a late systolic murmur, consistent with mild mitral regurgitation. *Lower* panels show two-dimensional (**D**) and color Doppler (**E**) on a separate patient. Because of the eccentric jet, quantification of the severity of mitral regurgitation could not be performed by echocardiography. Physical examination, however, revealed a loud holosystolic murmur, suggestive of severe mitral regurgitation. The holosystolic nature of the murmur can also be appreciated by continuous-wave Doppler signal (**F**). LA, left atrium; LV, left ventricle.

carotids. In young patients with bicuspid valve–related aortic stenosis, the murmur is often quieter over the precordium and best heard toward the suprasternal notch. The murmur of aortic stenosis can radiate and, in fact, increase in intensity toward

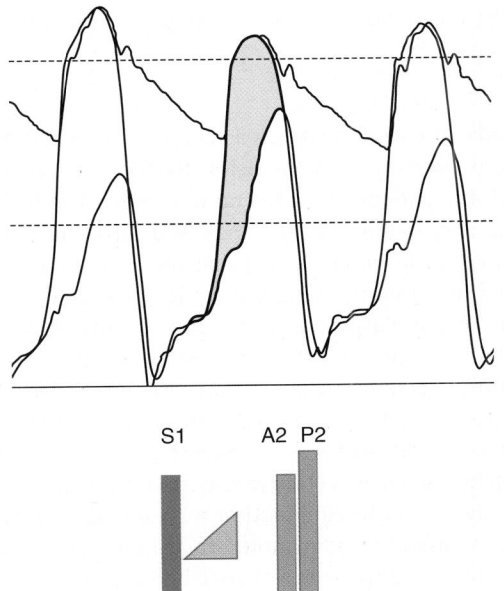

Figure 2–21. Acute mitral regurgitation. Aortic, left ventricular, and left atrial pressure tracings showing very large *v* waves in the setting of torrential, acute mitral regurgitation (*upper*). The murmur is short because of rapid equalization of pressures between the left ventricle and left atrium.

the apex—the *Gallavardin phenomenon*.[19] As the disease progresses, the peak of murmur occurs later in systole; it has an early systolic peak in mild and moderate aortic stenosis and a late peak in severe aortic stenosis (**Fig. 2–22**). The duration of the murmur becomes longer as the severity increases, so that in severe aortic stenosis, the murmur extends to the second heart sound. The pitch of the murmur also tends to change with more severe stages, when the murmur acquires a high-pitched, musical characteristic, also suggesting marked calcification of the valve. The severity of aortic stenosis based on the quality of the murmur is reflected in the continuous-wave Doppler velocity curves, with early peaking velocities in mild stenosis and mid to late peak (longer acceleration time) in more severe aortic stenosis.[20] The more severe the stenosis, the longer the ejection time on the continuous-wave Doppler tracing.

Pulmonic stenosis is less common than aortic stenosis. There will be a systolic ejection murmur heard best in the pulmonic position at the left sternal border that radiates to the left clavicle. Early ejection clicks and abnormalities of S2 are frequently present, as described previously.

In obstructive hypertrophic cardiomyopathy, two distinct systolic murmurs are audible. The harsh murmur related to subaortic obstruction is generally best heard at the left sternal border and will have a crescendo-decrescendo contour with a midsystolic peak. A separate murmur is heard best at the apex and starts in midsystole. It is caused by the secondary mitral regurgitation from distortion of the mitral valve apparatus related to systolic anterior motion of the mitral valve. This is of clinical importance because relief of the outflow obstruction will also reduce the mitral regurgitation. Both murmurs

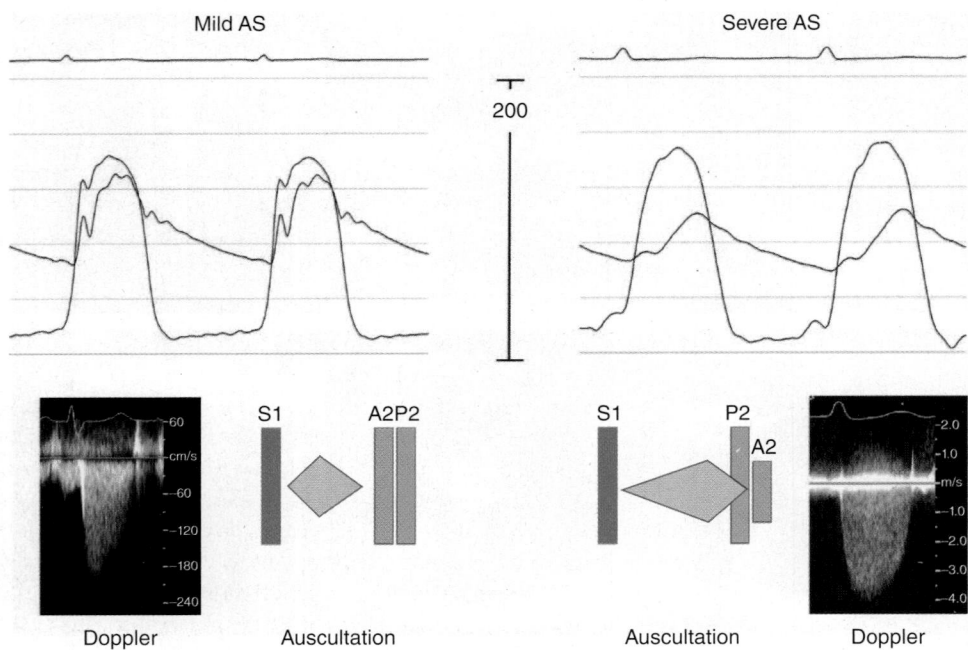

Figure 2–22. Invasive hemodynamic, echo-Doppler, and auscultatory findings in mild versus severe aortic valve stenosis (AS). In mild AS, the peak aortic pulse occurs early in systole, as illustrated by cardiac catheterization (*left upper*) and echo-Doppler (*left lower*). At the bedside, this will be appreciated as an early peaking systolic ejection murmur (*left lower*). In severe AS (*right*), the prolonged ejection time will result in late peaking of the aortic pressure tracing and continuous-wave Doppler signal (*right lower*).

will increase in intensity during the strain phase of the Valsalva maneuver, upon standing and follow premature ventricular beats. Both murmurs will also decrease with squatting. It is also important to note the dynamic changes in the apical murmur (in addition to the murmur associated with the left outflow tract obstruction) during maneuvers, particularly with squatting. If the apical murmur does not change, a primary mitral valve problem (such as a flail leaflet) should be suspected.

Pathologic murmurs should be differentiated from *innocent* or *benign* murmurs. Benign murmurs arise from increased flow through a semilunar valve and thus have a diamond shape. However, they typically peak in early systole, are usually grade II or less in intensity, and end before S2. Innocent murmurs change according to position, being more prominent in the supine compared with the sitting position. In childhood, an innocent murmur is usually caused by increased flow across the pulmonic valve and is heard best in the pulmonic position at the upper left sternal border. In older age, aortic valve sclerosis occurs because of mild thickening of the aortic valve cusps, and a soft ejection murmur is heard at the aortic position in the upper right sternal border. In both of these cases, a normal carotid upstroke and normal components of S2 are used to help in differentiating these from pathological murmurs. *Functional* murmurs result from increased forward flow across a normally functioning semilunar valve. These murmurs can be observed in pregnancy, a high-output state, or anemia. The high-output state associated with an arteriovenous fistula in patients with chronic renal failure is commonly associated with a loud functional murmur that will decrease in intensity with temporary occlusion of the fistula.

Diastolic Murmurs

General Principles

Diastolic murmurs can arise from atrioventricular valve stenosis and semilunar valve regurgitation. The timing and quality of the murmurs are based on the pressure differences across the abnormal valves, which are reflected in the continuous-wave Doppler velocity curves of these valve abnormalities. It is primarily the pitch and location of diastolic murmurs that define the etiology.

Diastolic Rumbles

The *rumble of mitral stenosis* is a subtle, low-pitched murmur, best heard over the apex; occasionally the murmur is heard only with the patient in left lateral decubitus. The bell should be placed very lightly over the apex, and the examiner should concentrate on listening during diastole. The duration of the murmur (early-mid to holodiastolic) tends to be directly proportional to the diastolic gradient and severity of stenosis. If sinus rhythm is present, the murmur increases during atrial contraction—*presystolic accentuation*. Because diastolic mean gradients are also directly related to heart rate, maneuvers that increase heart rate (sit-ups or phantom bicycling) facilitate detection of the murmur. Native tricuspid valve stenosis is rare and usually occurs in conjunction with mitral stenosis. Faint diastolic rumbles are often noted in patients with prosthetic mitral or tricuspid tissue prostheses; however, the presence of a loud diastolic murmur in a patient with a mitral or tricuspid prosthesis should raise concern for dysfunction or thrombosis.

Functional diastolic rumbles can occur with increased forward flow across the atrioventricular valves. A flow rumble is noted due to increased flow across the tricuspid valve related to the atrial level left-to-right shunt, whereas a mitral rumble can be heard in the presence of significant ventricular level shunt. A diastolic flow murmur is also heard in patients with severe mitral or tricuspid regurgitation caused by increased return flow across the valve. A mid-diastolic rumble—*the Austin-Flint murmur*—may be heard in aortic regurgitation when an eccentric jet hits the anterior leaflet of the mitral valve, causing it to reverberate and generating the apical rumble.

Diastolic Decrescendo Murmurs

The murmur of *aortic regurgitation* is a diastolic decrescendo, high-pitched blowing murmur, usually heard best at the left intercostal border. It is best heard using the diaphragm placed firmly in the sitting position. To hear a soft murmur, the patient should lean forward with a breath held. The duration as well as the intensity of the murmur are generally related to the severity of the regurgitation. In mild regurgitation, the murmur is early diastolic, whereas a holodiastolic murmur suggests more severe regurgitation. However, it is the peripheral signs of a wide pulse pressure that are most indicative of severe aortic regurgitation. Aortic regurgitation murmurs heard over the second right intercostal space result from annular dilatation (ie, aortic root enlargement), whereas murmurs heard over the third left intercostal space result from a valvular process.

The murmur associated with pulmonary regurgitation is typically heard over the second left intercostal space, has a low pitch, and can be difficult to hear. The bell of the stethoscope is generally used. The murmur typically increases with inspiration, allowing its differentiation from aortic regurgitation. In very severe cases of pulmonary regurgitation, there is equalization of right ventricular and pulmonary artery diastolic pressures in early to mid-diastole, rendering a rather short murmur. Functional pulmonary regurgitation can also be present when there is severe pulmonary hypertension—the *Graham-Steel murmur*. This murmur has a high pitch compared with primary pulmonary regurgitation and follows a loud pulmonary component of the second heart sound, suggesting the underlying association.

Continuous Murmurs

The continuous murmur is characterized by a "to-and-fro" sound with no interruption between systole and diastole. The pitch should be similar, but the intensity can vary throughout the cardiac cycle. By definition, the continuous murmur envelops the heart sounds. This is distinctly different than a systolic and diastolic murmur, as noted in mixed aortic valve disease. In that case, one will hear a harsh, diamond-shaped systolic murmur, a second heart second (which might be single), and a diastolic murmur. These murmurs will have two distinctly different pitches.

The most common continuous murmur seen in current practice is secondary to iatrogenic arteriovenous fistulas (for hemodialysis), which is generally appreciated in the region of the clavicle on the respective side. Other causes of continuous murmurs are rare and include patent ductus arteriosus (best heard over the left infraclavicular area), a ruptured sinus of Valsalva aneurysm, coronary fistula, intrathoracic arteriovenous fistulae, severe coarctation of the aorta, and a surgically created shunt (eg, Blalock-Taussig, Potts, Waterston).

The venous hum is a continuous murmur heard on auscultation of the neck. It results from a high flow in the internal jugular vein, which most likely causes a vibration of the venous wall. It is most commonly heard in young, otherwise healthy individuals and is not associated with pathology. The venous hum will disappear when in the supine position or with compression of the vein itself.

Dynamic Auscultation

Dynamic auscultation should play an integral role in differentiating the etiology of systolic murmurs. It should also be performed during examination of young individuals engaged in competitive sports in whom a latent obstruction from obstructive hypertrophic cardiomyopathy could be missed if maneuvers are not performed. Dynamic auscultation includes respirophasic changes and changes in murmur intensity on postectopic beats, as well as changes induced by specific maneuvers.

Inspiration increases venous return to the right cardiac chambers, augmenting right-sided murmurs and diastolic sounds. The exception to the rule is the systolic click of pulmonary stenosis, which diminishes with inspiration. Typically described as a classic sign of tricuspid regurgitation (vs other systolic murmurs) is the Carvallo sign: an increase in the intensity of the murmur with inspiration. Negative intrathoracic pressures generated by inspiration lead to an increase in left ventricular afterload; therefore, the dynamic left ventricular outflow tract systolic murmur of hypertrophic cardiomyopathy will decrease on inspiration (**Fig. 2–23**).

In patients with systolic murmur, attention should be paid to the change in intensity of the murmur on the postectopic beats. There is an increase in ventricular contractility and a decrease in afterload on the postectopic beat; thus, there will be an increase in the intensity of the murmur with both fixed (aortic stenosis) and dynamic (hypertrophic cardiomyopathy) left ventricular outflow tract obstruction. This response is much more striking in the setting of obstructive hypertrophic cardiomyopathy because there is also an increase in the degree of obstruction (**Fig. 2–24**). Alternatively, in patients with mitral regurgitation, there is no change in the intensity of the murmur on the postectopic beat due to the decrease in afterload.

The *Valsalva maneuver* consists of expiration against a closed glottis, generating an increase in intrathoracic pressure of 30 to 40 mm Hg for a least 10 seconds. It is a method by which systolic murmurs may be differentiated. A simple way of performing the maneuver is to place the examiner's hand over the patient's abdomen and ask the patient to push against it. The normal response to the maneuver consists of four phases[21]: phase I, a transient increase in systemic blood pressure during the strain phase secondary to the elevation in intrathoracic pressures; phase II, a decrease in pulse pressure and stroke volume to decreased venous return, which results in reflex tachycardia (the so-called active phase); phase III, a further decrease in blood pressure due to the initial release of the

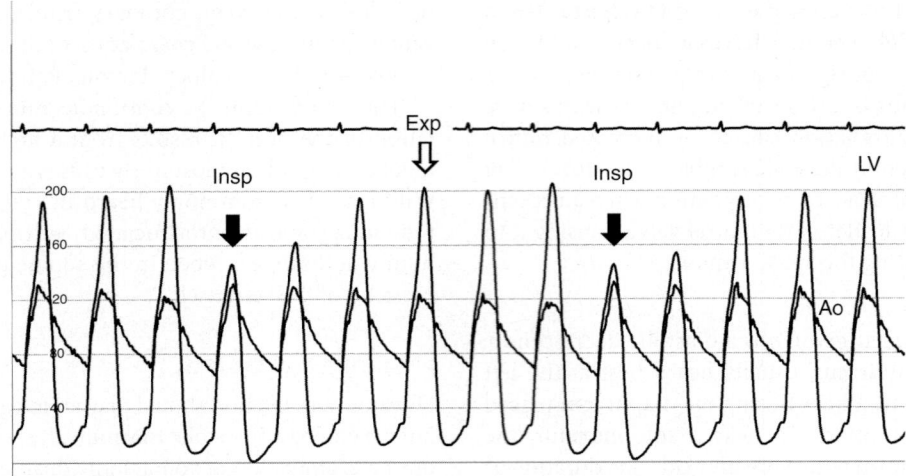

Figure 2–23. Respirophasic hemodynamic changes observed in hypertrophic obstructive cardiomyopathy. Inspiration (Insp) leads to increased left ventricular afterload. As a result, the systolic gradient between the left ventricle (LV) and aorta (Ao) decreases with inspiration. At the bedside, this is manifested by a decrease in the systolic ejection murmur noted with inspiration. The presence of this finding suggests dynamic instead of fixed outflow tract obstruction as the source of the murmur. Exp, expiration.

straining phase; and phase IV, an overshot of blood pressure levels over the ones observed at baseline. Each phase is associated with changes in heart rate; the most important ones are the reflex tachycardia observed in phase II and reflex bradycardia in phase IV as blood pressure increases (**Fig. 2–25**).

Given the reduction in stroke volume that occur during phase II of the maneuver, most systolic murmurs will decrease during that phase; the exceptions are the murmurs of mitral valve prolapse and hypertrophic cardiomyopathy. In mitral valve prolapse, there is further atrial displacement of the leaflets during phase II as left ventricular size decreases, resulting in an earlier click and longer and typically louder murmur. In hypertrophic cardiomyopathy, the smaller ventricular cavity will lead to more severe subaortic obstruction and a louder murmur. Of note, these changes tend to be more pronounced if the patient is sitting or upright. It is important to document the change in intensity of the murmur only after at least six to eight beats

during the strain phase because this is the time period during which the change in blood volume must circulate through the pulmonary circulation to reach the left side of the heart. The examiner should also note the changes in heart rate through phase II of the maneuver. If tachycardia is not present during phase II, there is autonomic dysfunction, autonomic blockade (eg, β-blockers), or high left-sided filling pressures (**Fig. 2–26**). In these cases, the response of a murmur will not be useful. During phase IV, all murmurs usually increase, except with hypertrophic cardiomyopathy.

The stand-to-squat-to-stand maneuver is particularly helpful in patients with hypertrophic cardiomyopathy and mitral valve prolapse. Squatting increases both preload and afterload. As a result, squatting significantly diminishes (or even abolishes) the intensity of the murmur of obstructive cardiomyopathy. This is also true for mitral regurgitation that is secondary to systolic anterior motion of the mitral valve. In mitral valve

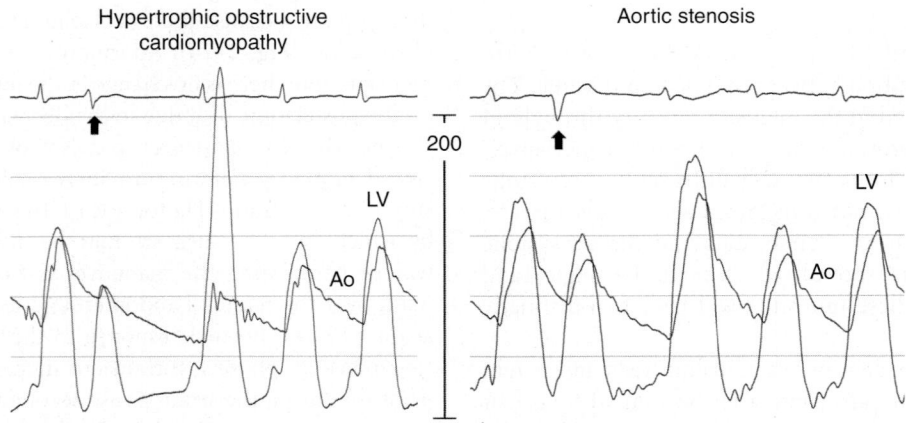

Figure 2–24. Postextrasystolic response in hypertrophic obstructive cardiomyopathy versus aortic valve stenosis. Aortic (Ao) and left ventricular (LV) pressure tracings illustrate the post ectopic beat (*arrow*) response in dynamic outflow tract obstruction (*left*) versus fixed aortic stenosis (*right*). Although systolic gradients increase in both diseases, the response is much more exuberant in hypertrophic cardiomyopathy. This phenomenon can also be appreciated at the bedside. The murmur of hypertrophic cardiomyopathy will become much louder compared with the murmur of aortic stenosis after a premature beat.

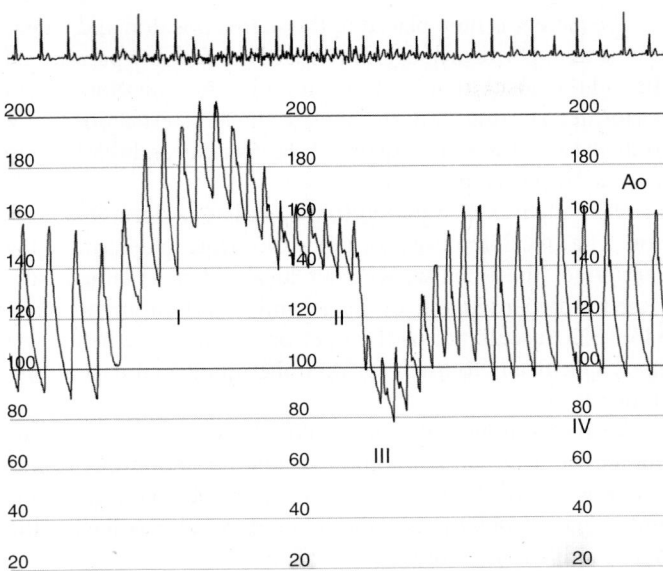

Figure 2–25. Valsalva maneuver. The normal hemodynamic changes during the four phases of the Valsalva maneuver are shown: phase I, transient increase in aortic pressure during the strain phase; phase II, decrease in pulse pressure with reflex tachycardia; phase III, further decrease in aortic pressure after the initial release of the strain phase; and phase IV, overshoot of the aortic pressure levels above baseline. Ao, aorta.

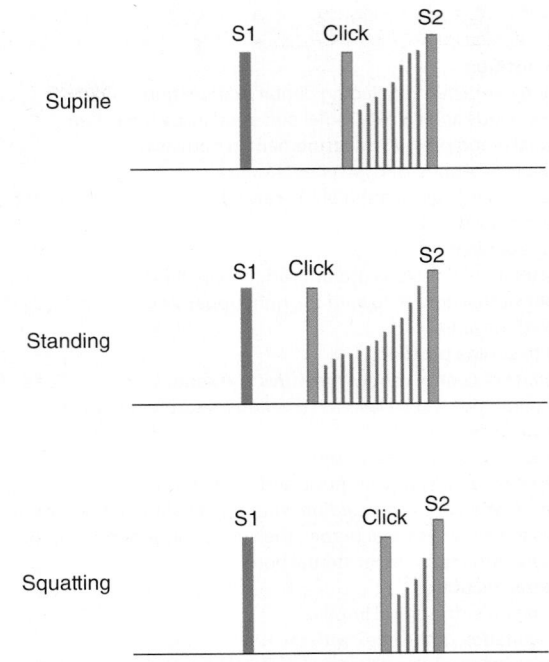

Figure 2–27. Positional changes in the systolic click and murmur of mitral valve prolapse. S1, first heart sound; S2, second heart sound.

prolapse, the systolic click occurs later in systole and the murmur becomes shorter (**Fig. 2–27**). All other murmurs will have either an increase in intensity or no change in intensity with squatting. On standing, there is an immediate decrease in afterload followed by a decrease in venous return after several beats. Thus, there will be an immediate and then progressive increase in the intensity of the dynamic outflow murmur of hypertrophic cardiomyopathy.

In instances where there are very soft murmurs that are out of proportion to the presenting symptoms, a reexamination

after exercise may reveal a significant change in the murmur's intensity and characteristic. This is important in patients with hypertrophic cardiomyopathy and labile outflow tract obstruction and in patients with mitral stenosis. Exercise can involve sit-ups on the examining table, step-ups on the bench, or even walking up and down hallways and stairwells. These exercise maneuvers are also useful to bring out an S3 if absent at rest. Handgrip isometric exercise to increase afterload and amyl nitrate to decrease afterload have been used to differentiate the rumble of mitral stenosis from an Austin-Flint murmur but they are no longer necessary with the advent of echocardiography.

PHYSICAL EXAMINATION: STEPWISE APPROACH TO THE PATIENT

Each clinician needs to develop his or her own stepwise approach to the cardiovascular examination. We wish to present our own approach (**Table 2–6**), which we apply in a general fashion to the majority of patients who present with cardiovascular disease, understanding that the examination is always then focused on the patient's specific problem. We feel that the initial history should be taken with the patient fully dressed to allow a one-to-one relationship to be built. However, for a comprehensive physical examination, it is necessary for the patient to be undressed with an appropriate gown or cover-up. An examination should never be done placing the stethoscope under a shirt or blouse, and full inspection of the chest and extremities is always necessary.

We approach the patient in the sitting position, looking at the overall appearance to determine if there are unusual features that may suggest a syndrome. Shaking hands will help in

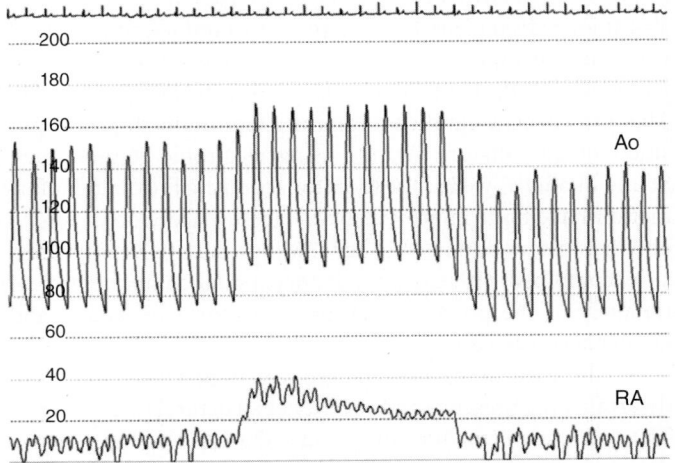

Figure 2–26. Valsalva maneuver in patient with increased left atrial pressure. Note the lack of tachycardia during the Valsalva maneuver. Although this response can be seen in elevated left-sided filling pressures, beta-blocker use or autonomic dysfunction might result in a similar response. Ao, aorta; RA, right atrium.

TABLE 2–6. Basics Steps of the Cardiovascular Examination

Sitting position
1. General inspection, including dental examination
2. Shake hands and palpate radial pulse and inspect nail bed
3. Manual blood pressure measurement in both arms
4. Inspection of chest and lower extremities
5. Palpation and auscultation of the carotids
6. Palpation of the chest
7. Lung examination
8. Auscultation of the precordium with the diaphragm: start at the right upper sternal border, toward the right upper sternal, and finally down toward the apex

Sitting to supine position
9. Estimate of central venous pressures and venous contour (head of the bed might need to be lowered if venous pressure is normal)

Supine position
10. Inspection of the precordium
11. Palpation of the apical impulse and right ventricle
12. Auscultation of the precordium with the diaphragm from the apical area toward the sternal border, then up to the left upper border, and finally at the right upper sternal border

Left lateral decubitus
13. Palpation of the apical impulse
14. Auscultation of the apex with the bell

Remaining parts of the general examination with particular attention to liver size, presence of ascites, leg edema, and vascular examination

a frailty assessment as well as in determining tissue perfusion. Palpating the radial pulse in both wrists will provide the heart rate and rhythm and any blood pressure differences in the two upper extremities. Looking at the nail beds is important for the presence of clubbing, cyanosis, or high pulse pressures. Then, blood pressure is taken by cuff in both arms.

Inspection of the rest of the chest and extremities will identify skin lesions, skin infections, or prior surgical scars that may influence the diagnosis and decision-making. Examining the venous pulsations in the sitting position will provide an initial clue as to whether there is elevation of venous pressure. Palpation of the carotid and brachial arteries is then performed, listening first for bruits. Palpation of the chest for thrills and palpable heart sounds is done next, followed by auscultation of the lungs.

Auscultation of heart sounds in the sitting position should be performed using the diaphragm, starting at the base of the heart, inching across to the left sternal border, then inferiorly to the lower left sternal border, and finally to the apex. In each position, one should listen to S1, S2, systole, and diastole. In particular, the splitting of S2 should be evaluated in the sitting position. Aortic and pulmonary outflow murmurs should be evaluated. Aortic and pulmonic regurgitant murmurs should be sought with the patient leaning over with breath held at end expiration. Pericardial rubs are best heard in this position.

Following auscultation in the sitting position, an examination of the venous pressure and venous contour should be done, with a gradual change in the position of the patient from sitting at 90° down to the supine position until the venous pulsations are visible in the internal jugular vein. Once the top of the pulsations is established, the height of the venous pressure is estimated, usually at 45° or less.

The patient is then placed in the supine position and palpation is then performed again, primarily to feel any parasternal lift and the position of the apical impulse. Auscultation is then performed starting from the apex to the left sternal border up to the base of the heart. Again, S1, S2, systole, and diastole are listened to at each position.

The patient is then placed in the left lateral decubitus position. The apical impulse is palpated, this time to determine the contour of the impulse, whether localized or enlarged, sustained or hyperdynamic or feeble, and to feel for any palpable S4 or S3. Auscultation is then performed with the bell at the apex, specifically to listen for diastolic filling sounds and diastolic rumbles.

Finally, examination of the abdomen is performed, palpating for the liver and aorta and listening for abdominal bruits. Examination of the lower extremities for edema and lesions and palpation of all pulses should be done, always feeling the radial and femoral pulses simultaneously.

Additional focused parts of the examination should be performed depending on the clinical scenario. In patients with suspected constrictive pericarditis, a more detailed evaluation of the venous pressure and contour is required. In patients who present with exertional dyspnea and no significant findings on initial examination, a repeat of auscultation during exercise may elicit an S3 or diastolic rumble. Patients with hypertrophic cardiomyopathy should always undergo further dynamic auscultation with the Valsalva maneuver, stand-to-squat-to-stand, and even exercise to further evaluate a dynamic obstruction. **Table 2–7** outlines the important physical findings for each individual cardiac lesion that aid in diagnosis and determination of severity.

PHYSICAL EXAMINATION: THE FUTURE

It is clear that the history and physical examination play a critical role in evaluation of the patient with cardiovascular disease. It is hoped that advanced technology will capitalize on the valuable information gained from a proper examination in several ways. Increasingly, telemedicine is being used to interact with patients, providing efficiencies for both provider and patient. There has been a significant improvement in the digital acquisition of auscultatory sounds using electronic stethoscopes. Sound quality as well as the tools for acquiring the digital information have both improved. Non–face-to-face video visits to obtain a history and inspect key findings, such as venous pressure, combined with the auscultatory digital components sent remotely to the provider may provide more convenient and greater access to care.

Machine learning has been used with digital heart sounds to determine the presence and severity of structural heart disease. The subtle abnormalities in the auscultatory findings that are detected by experienced clinicians may be the basis of artificial intelligence algorithms for digital heart sounds that could then be used for more universal screening of patients by all providers. This could result in earlier detection of valve disease with more rapid pathways to treatment.[22]

TABLE 2-7. Summary of Physical Examination Findings According to the Lesions[a]

	Jugular Venous Examination	Arterial Pulse	Palpation	Auscultation
Mitral regurgitation	Usually normal; increased *a* wave if pulmonary hypertension is present	Usually normal; sometimes brisk but low amplitude	Displaced and diffuse apical impulse	Soft S1; **loud P2**; holosystolic or mid-late murmur (if so, hardly ever severe); **diastolic rumble** (flow murmur); **diastolic filling sound (S3)**
Mitral stenosis	Usually normal; increased *a* wave if pulmonary hypertension is present	Low amplitude	Normal or small apical impulse; tapping apical impulse; **parasternal lift**	Loud or soft S1; **loud P2**; opening snap **(A2-OS interval <60–70 ms in severe cases)**; diastolic rumble with/without presystolic accentuation
Aortic stenosis	Usually normal	**Parvus and tardus**	Localized, sustained with a palpable S4	**Single S2; paradoxical splitting of S2; S4;** crescendo-decrescendo systolic murmur **(late peaking and louder [≥grade III] if severe)**
Aortic regurgitation	Usually normal	**Bounding; bisferiens; wide pulse pressure (diastolic blood pressure typically 60 mm Hg or less)**	Displaced, diffuse, and sustained apical impulse	Soft S1; S3, diastolic decrescendo murmur **(mid-to-late and late diastolic murmurs if severe)**; diastolic rumble, systolic flow murmur
Tricuspid regurgitation	**Elevated central venous pressure; large *v* wave**	Low-amplitude pulses	Parasternal lift	Holosystolic murmur (left lower sternal border); **right-sided filling sound; diastolic rumble** (flow murmur)
Obstructive hypertrophic cardiomyopathy	Usually normal; elevated venous pressure suggests an alternative diagnosis	Brisk pulses	Sustained apical impulse; palpable S4; "triple-ripple"	S4, **paradoxical splitting of S2**, crescendo-decrescendo systolic murmur (mid-peaking; **loud murmurs when severe**)
Constrictive pericarditis	Elevated central venous pressures; brisk *x* and *y* descents; Kussmaul sign	Low-amplitude pulse	Usually normal; pulsus paradoxus	Pericardial knock; friction rub if ongoing inflammation is present
Decompensated HFrEF	Elevated venous pressure, brisk *y* descents; hepatojugular reflux	Normal or low amplitude pulse; pulsus alternans in severe cases	Displaced and diffuse apical impulse; parasternal heave; left-sided	Soft S1; loud P2; holosystolic or mid-late murmur (if functional mitral regurgitation is present); S3
Compensated HFrEF	Normal venous pressure	Normal or low amplitude pulse	Displaced and diffuse apical impulse; parasternal heave; left-sided S4	Soft S1; normal P2; S4; holosystolic or mid-late murmur (if functional mitral regurgitation is present
HFpEF	Normal or mildly elevated; hepatojugular reflux	Normal	Sustained apical impulse; S4	Loud P2; S4

[a]For valvular lesions, signs of severity are marked in bold.
Abbreviations: HFpEF, heart failure with preserved ejection fraction; HFrEF, heart failure with reduced ejection fraction.

REFERENCES

1. Wood PH. *Diseases of the Heart and Circulation.* London, UK: Eyre & Spottiswoode; 1950.
2. Nishimura RA, Carabello B. Operationalizing the 2014 ACC/AHA Guidelines for Valvular Heart Disease: a guide for clinicians. *J Am Coll Cardiol.* 2016;67:2289-2294.
3. Fuster V. The stethoscope's prognosis: very much alive and very necessary. *J Am Coll Cardiol.* 2016;67(9):1118-1119.
4. Ambrose JA, Tannenbaum MA, Alexopoulos D, et al. Angiographic progression of coronary artery disease and the development of myocardial infarction. *J Am Coll Cardiol.* 1988;12(1):56-62.
5. Diamond GA, Forrester JS. Analysis of probability as an aid in the clinical diagnosis of coronary-artery disease. *N Engl J Med.* 1979;300(24):1350-1358.
6. Kreatsoulas C, Shannon HS, Giacomini M, Velianou JL, Anand SS. Reconstructing angina: cardiac symptoms are the same in women and men. *JAMA Intern Med.* 2013;173(9):829-831.
7. Seward JB, Hayes DL, Smith HC, et al. Platypnea-orthodeoxia: clinical profile, diagnostic workup, management, and report of seven cases. *Mayo Clin Proc.* 1984;59(4):221-231.
8. Knapper JT, Schultz J, Das G, Sperling LS. Cardiac platypnea-orthodeoxia syndrome: an often unrecognized malady. *Clin Cardiol.* Oct 2014;37(10):645-649.
9. Thibodeau JT, Turer AT, Gualano SK, et al. Characterization of a novel symptom of advanced heart failure: bendopnea. *J Am Coll Cardiol Heart Fail.* 2014;2:24-31.
10. Campeau L. Letter: grading of angina pectoris. *Circulation.* 1976;54(3):522-523.
11. Criteria Committee of the New York Heart Association. *Nomenclature and Criteria for Diagnosis of Diseases of the Heart and Great Vessels.* 9th ed. Boston, MA: Little, Brown & Co; 1994:253-256.
12. Kiani S, Stebbins A, Thourani VH, et al. The effect and relationship of frailty indices on survival after transcatheter aortic valve replacement. *J Am Coll Cardiol Cardiovasc Interv.* 2020;13:219-231.
13. Katz S, Ford AB, Moskowitz RW, Jackson BA, Jaffe MW. Studies of illness in the aged. The index of ADL: a standardized measure of biological and psychosocial function. *JAMA.* 1963;185:914-919.
14. Searle SD, Mitnitski A, Gahbauer EA, Gill TM, Rockwood K. A standard procedure for creating a frailty index. *BMC Geriatr.* 2008;8:24.
15. Eleid MF, Nishimura RA. Aortic stenosis and the pulse contour: a true marker of severity? *Catheter Cardiovasc Interv.* 2020;95:1235-1239.

16. Yancy CW, Jessup M, Bozkurt B, et al. 2013 ACCF/AHA guideline for the management of heart failure: a report of the American College of Cardiology Foundation/ American Heart Association Task Force on Practice Guidelines. *J Am Coll Cardiol.* 2013;62(16):e147-e239.

17. Sochowski RA, Dubbin JD, Naqvi SZ. Clinical and hemodynamic assessment of the hepatojugular reflux. *Am J Cardiol.* 1990;66(12):1002-1006.

18. Nishimura RA, Tajik AJ. Evaluation of diastolic filling of left ventricle in health and disease: Doppler echocardiography is the clinician's Rosetta Stone. *J Am Coll Cardiol.* 1997;30(1):8-18.

19. Giles TD, Martinez EC, Burch GE. Gallavardin phenomenon in aortic stenosis. A possible mechanism. *Arch Intern Med.* 1974;134(4):747-749.

20. Gamaza-Chulian S, Camacho-Freire S, Toro-Cebada R, Giraldez-Valpuesta A, Benezet-Mazuecos J, Vargas-Machuca JC. Ratio of acceleration time to ejection time for assessing aortic stenosis severity. *Echocardiography.* 2015;32(12):1754-1761.

21. Nishimura RA, Tajik AJ. The Valsalva maneuver and response revisited. *Mayo Clin Proc.* 1986;61(3):211-217.

22. Amiriparian S, Schmitt M, Cummins N, Qian K, Dong F, Schuller B. Deep unsupervised representation learning for abnormal heart sound classification. *Conf Proc IEEE Eng Med Biol Soc.* 2018;2018:4776-4779.

Cardiovascular Imaging

Thomas H. Marwick and Jagat Narula

CHAPTER OUTLINE

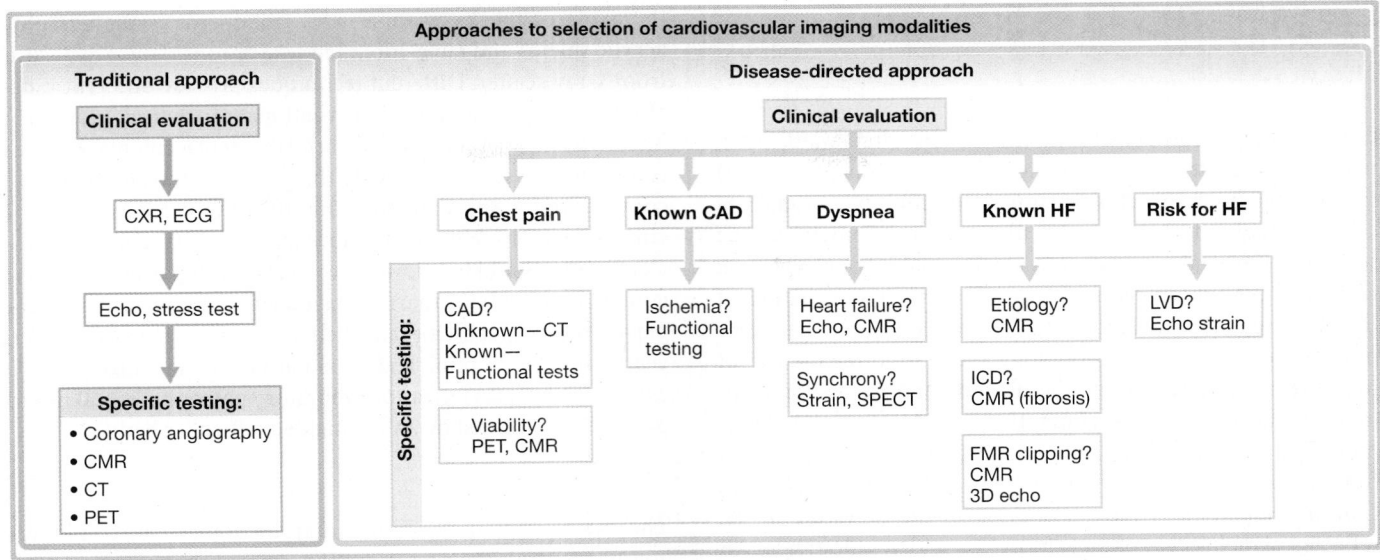

Chapter 3 Fuster and Hurst's Central illustration. Many imaging techniques are able to measure the same parameters (eg, ejection fraction). A disease-directed approach identifies the primary clinical question and optimizes test selection to address the question. By contrast, the traditional approach risks duplication, as tests are "layered" to address progressively more complex questions. CAD, coronary artery disease; CMR, cardiac magnetic resonance; CT, computed tomography; HF, heart failure; ICD, implantable cardioverter-defibrillators; LVD, left ventricular dysfunction; PET, positron emission tomography; SPECT, single-photon emission computerized tomography.

CHAPTER SUMMARY

The modern era of cardiovascular disease management is based on imaging. This chapter seeks to introduce the common imaging modalities—addressing the fundamental imaging considerations of temporal, spatial, and contrast resolution, as well as the underlying pathophysiology examined by each test—and provide the methodology and applications of each technique. Details of test performance are provided in the relevant chapters about disease entities. The main goals of cardiac imaging are the anatomic and functional assessment of the cardiac chambers, valves, great vessels, and coronary arteries. Multiple methodologies are now able to address each one of these goals. We thus risk duplication if we employ the approach of layering multiple tests, particularly when testing begins with a "generic" test, such as a chest x-ray, echocardiogram, or functional test for ischemia. Of course, in a patient with undifferentiated symptoms, this approach is unavoidable. However, given that most cardiovascular diseases are chronic and recurrent, specific questions may arise at particular times. In these settings, selecting a more advanced test that also provides generic information is desirable (see Fuster and Hurst's Central Illustration).

GENERAL CONSIDERATIONS

Test Selection

Techniques

Cardiac imaging is performed with x-ray, ultrasound, light, nuclear medicine, and magnetic resonance imaging (MRI) techniques. In many clinical situations, multiple modalities can be brought to answer a particular question. Sometimes, the selection of modality pertains to local availability or expertise. However, everything else being equal, the inherent nature of the imaging modalities should be matched to the clinical question. For any imaging methodology, there are three metrics of image resolution: spatial, temporal, and contrast. Spatial resolution is the ability to discriminate small objects and is determined in *axial* (parallel to the imaging direction; primarily a function of wavelength) or *lateral* (perpendicular to the beam). *Contrast resolution* is the distribution of the grayscale of the reflected signal and is often referred to as dynamic range. An image of low dynamic range appears as black and white with a few levels of gray; images at high *dynamic range* are often softer. *Temporal resolution* relates to the ability to distinguish events in time. For example, the assessment of myocardial dyssynchrony or contractile dispersion should be done with the highest temporal resolution technique, which is generally ultrasound. On the other hand, the interpretation of the status of atherosclerotic plaque requires very high spatial resolution, and optical coherence tomography (OCT) is more likely to provide this than intravascular ultrasound (IVUS).

Indications

The indications for imaging techniques include diagnosis, prognostic assessment, and management decisions. The aspects of the technique that make it desirable for one of these indications may not be the most important in another setting. For example, management decisions may require sequential testing, wherein the test-retest reproducibility of an investigation may become the dominant consideration, perhaps exceeding the importance of accuracy.

Radiation Safety

Many cardiac and imaging examinations require the use of ionizing radiation, including x-ray, computed tomography (CT), and nuclear imaging. These examinations are often repeated, making considerations about radiation safety even more important. There are four basic principles of radiation protection:

1. The less exposure, the less chance there is of absorbed energy biologic interaction.
2. No known level of ionizing radiation is a permissible dose or absolutely safe.
3. Radiation exposure is cumulative. There is no washout phenomenon.
4. All participants are obliged to minimize and reduce risks to other personnel and themselves.

All subjects are exposed to radiation in a dose geometrically inverse to the distance from the source. Radiation scatter occurs in all directions and in angiography, it is increased when the angle of the x-ray tube is set obliquely. In angiography, acrylic shields and table-mounted lead aprons reduce exposure from x-ray scatter. Different techniques provide different radiation exposures. Complex interventional procedures (coronary interventions, percutaneous heart valve replacements, or electrophysiology studies) provide the greatest exposure. Fluoroscopy generates approximately one-fifth the x-ray exposure of cineangiography. No dose of more than 3 rem (roentgen equivalent man) should be allowed over a 3-month period. The eyes, gonads, and red bone marrow have a whole-body limit of 5 rem per year; any specific organ, such as the thyroid or skin, has a yearly limit of 15 rem. The maximal permissible dose, or *safe* exposure, for catheterization laboratory personnel is 100 mrem per week monitored by an unshielded left collar badge.

Interpretation

The interpretation of studies may be subjective, computer-assisted, or fully automated. While an automated approach would be desirable, the artificial intelligence solutions to perform this optimally are still being developed. Part of the challenge is that many categories are not distinct—for example, there is limited consistency in the distinction of regional motion as (1) *hypokinesia,* a diminished but not absent motion of one part of the left ventricular (LV) wall; (2) *akinesia,* total lack of motion of a portion of the LV wall; and (3) *dyskinesia,* paradoxical systolic motion or expansion of one part of the LV wall (ie, an abnormal bulging outward during systole). In fact, the expert assessment of these entities does not merely involve endocardial excursion but also timing (late systolic "pseudomotion" may occur because of torsional and translational movement when the actual segment is akinetic).

The increasing workload of the modern imaging environment risks an exclusive focus on the problem at hand. Most imaging modalities—especially the chest radiogram and echocardiography—provide an opportunity to identify previously unknown or unrecognized problems. A systematic search of any imaging modality, independent of clinical and other imaging information, is often key to recognition of unexpected findings, which may be missed in a search directed by symptoms and medical history. However, clinical integration remains an invaluable component of all imaging evaluation, so the *final* imaging diagnosis should be made only after correlating the radiographic findings with clinical information and other laboratory data

Quality Control

Defining that imaging technologists and physicians should be appropriately trained for their tasks is something that is done well, but in contrast, quality control receives insufficient attention in cardiovascular imaging. Our patients and referring physicians should feel confident that in a stable patient, a test result from Tuesday will be the same as one done on Friday, and that the interpretation of a phenomenon (eg, ejection fraction [EF]) should at least be similar, however, that measurement is obtained. Unfortunately, many laboratories and practices would be unable to show data to prove consistency.

The results of a test may be measured by validity, reliability, and precision. Validity relates to the ability to represent the characteristic of interest—expressed as accuracy (the ability to recognize a particular phenomenon, for example, defined by another investigation) or, by extension, prognostic value (the ability to predict outcome). Relevant parameters are sensitivity, specificity, normalcy, and predictive value. Imaging techniques should be as quantitative as possible, and the interpretation of numerical parameters requires reliability and precision. Reliability pertains to the ability to recognize true differences, rather than differences within the technique or those measuring the test. Relevant parameters are normal ranges (and how these are established), inter- and intraobserver variation. Precision pertains to the ability to consistently measure a parameter in time, measured as test-retest variation, mean difference, least measurable difference, limits of agreement, and markers of association such as intraclass correlation coefficient.

CHEST RADIOGRAPHY

The chest radiograph has less importance for primary cardiac assessment now than it did in the past. Nevertheless, it remains ubiquitous and inexpensive, readily accessible in acute settings and after device implantation (eg, for detection of hemorrhage and pneumothorax), and may facilitate selection for definitive testing with advanced imaging techniques. The radiographic examination for heart disease consists of four major steps: (1) radiographic examination for anatomy, (2) comparison to prior studies, (3) clinical correlation, and (4) conclusion and recommendations.[1,2]

Visual Search and Characterization of Abnormalities

Overview

Although in the setting of cardiac disease, it is tempting to principally focus on the heart, cardiac conditions can be manifest in noncardiac structures. For instance, a right-sided stomach with an absent inferior vena cava (IVC) margin suggests congenital interruption of the IVC with azygos continuation[3] (**Fig. 3–1A**). A narrowed anteroposterior (AP) diameter of the thorax can be the cause of an innocent murmur.[4]

Devices

In the outpatient setting, these devices include pacemakers (**Fig. 3–1B**), implantable cardioverter-defibrillators (ICDs), and cardiac assist devices (**Fig. 3–1C**). Inpatients may also have central venous and pulmonary arterial catheters or temporary venous pacemakers. A detailed assessment of the positioning and integrity of these devices is critical to the interpretation of cardiac radiography. This should include an assessment of lead integrity, which requires both a well-penetrated radiograph and a disciplined search to maximize the likelihood that lead fractures will be recognized.[5]

Cardiac assist devices represent a diverse set of short- and long-term solutions to compensate for ventricular failure. Short-term devices include intra-aortic balloon pump, extracorporeal membrane oxygenation, and a growing list of percutaneous or surgically inserted devices. Long-term devices, which traditionally served as a bridge to cardiac transplantation, are increasingly considered to be long-term solutions for patients with severe heart failure and for whom cardiac transplantation is not a viable option. Familiarity with the

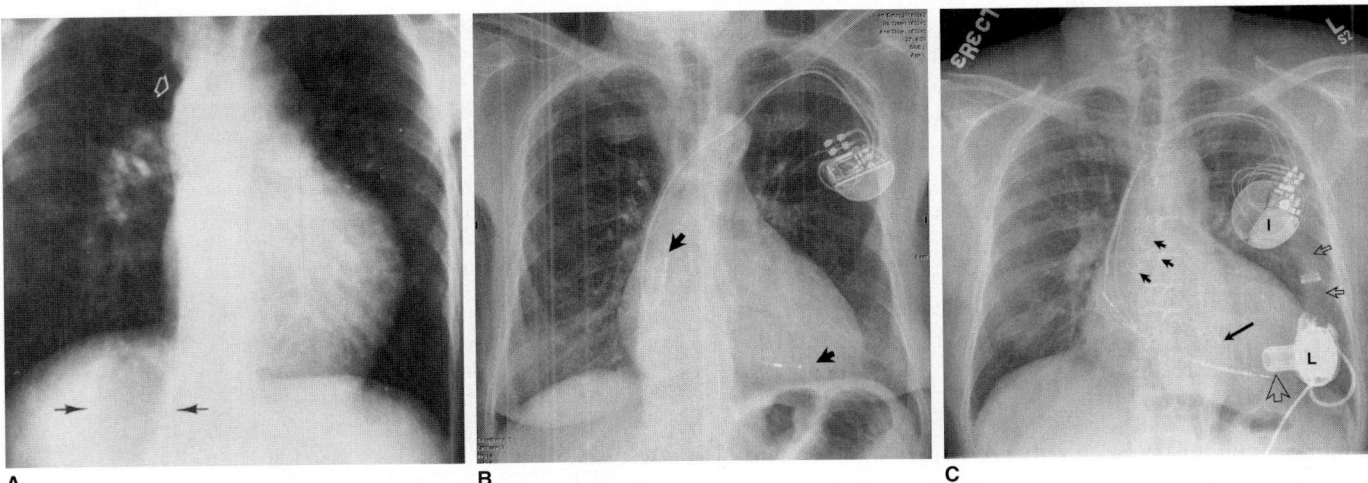

A   **B**   **C**

Figure 3–1. Visual search and characterization. (A) Patient with situs ambiguus, interruption of the inferior vena cava (IVC), ventricular septal defect, and polysplenia. The posteroanterior view shows that the aortic arch and the heart are left sided and the stomach (*lower arrows*) is right sided. The azygos vein (*upper arrow*) is markedly enlarged. The heart is mildly enlarged, and there is a moderate increase in pulmonary vascularity. **(B)** Left-sided subcutaneous pacemaker. Frontal radiograph illustrating right atrial and right ventricular leads (*arrows*) from a. **(C)** Frontal radiograph in a patient post–coronary artery bypass grafting with an implantable cardioverter-defibrillator (ICD) and left ventricular assist device (LVAD). The inflow cannula (*wide open arrow*) is engaged within the left ventricle, and the outflow cannula and barely visible conduit (*small open arrows*) carries the outflow to the aorta. Three coronary ostial ring markers (*short arrows*) are visible as well the LVAD (L) and ICD (I). In addition to the leads within the right atrium and right ventricle that contain the electrodes for defibrillation, a pacing lead is present within the coronary sinus (*long arrow*). B, Reproduced with permission from Matthew Cham, MD. The Icahn School of Medicine at Mount Sinai.

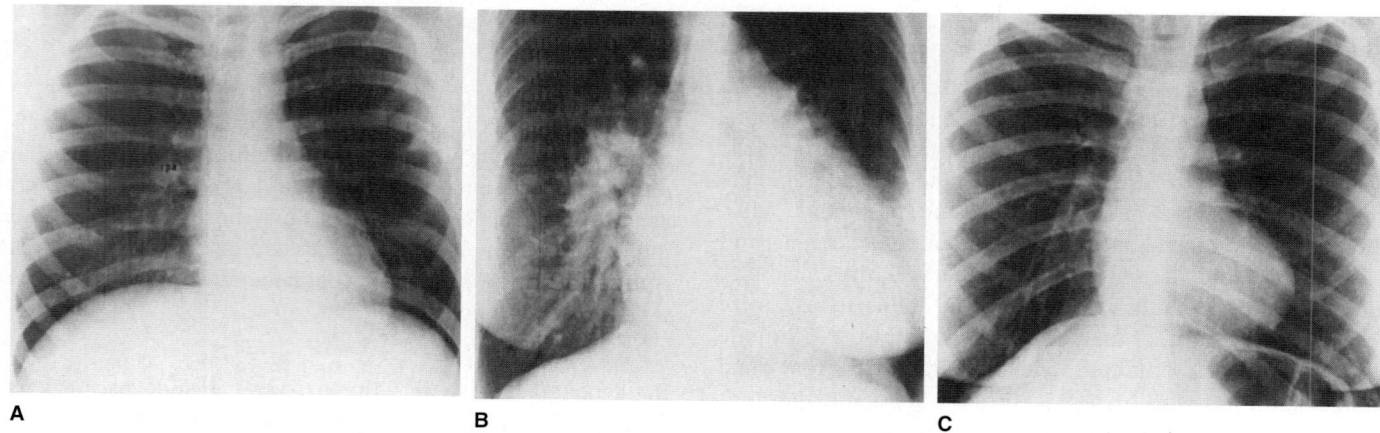

Figure 3–2. **Radiographic assessment of the volume of pulmonary blood flow (PBF).** (**A**) Normal PBF. There is caudalization of the pulmonary vascularity because of gravity. The right descending pulmonary artery measures 13 mm in diameter in this young man. (**B**) Increased PBF. Patient with a secundum atrial septal defect showing uniform increase in pulmonary vascularity bilaterally. The right descending pulmonary artery is markedly enlarged, measuring 27 mm. (**C**) Decreased PBF. Patient with tetralogy of Fallot showing a boot-shaped heart and uniform decrease in pulmonary vascularity. The right descending pulmonary artery is much smaller than normal, measuring 6 mm in diameter.

appearance and proper placement of these devices is critical to their correct radiographic assessment.[6]

Pulmonary Vasculature

The lung can often reflect the underlying pathophysiology of the heart. For example, if uniform dilatation of all pulmonary vessels is present, the diagnosis of a left-to-right shunt (**Fig. 3–2**) is more likely than a left-sided obstructive lesion. The latter typically shows a cephalic pulmonary blood flow (PBF) pattern.

Normal Pulmonary Vascularity

The normal radiographic appearance of the pulmonary vasculature of an upright human is typified by a caudal flow pattern because of gravity. The pressure differential between the apex and the base of the lung is approximately 22 mm Hg in adults in the upright position.[7] Therefore, more flow under higher distending pressure is expected in the lower lobe vessels than in the upper. Normally, whereas one sees very little vascularity above the hilum, more and larger vessels are found below the hilum. Because the pulmonary resistance is normal, all vessels taper gradually in a tree-like manner from the hilum toward the periphery of the lung. The right descending pulmonary artery measures 10 to 15 mm in diameter in males and 9 to 14 mm in females[8] (see Fig. 3–2).

Abnormal Pulmonary Vascularity

Abnormal pulmonary vascularity is classified into two categories: terms of volume or terms of distribution[9] (**Table 3–1**).

Abnormalities in Volume: In the evaluation of pulmonary vasculature, the caliber of the vessels is more important than the length or the number. As long as the PBF pattern (base > apex) remains normal, the volume of the flow is proportional to the caliber of the pulmonary arteries (see **Fig. 3–3**). Pulmonary blood volume can be assessed by measuring the right descending pulmonary artery, or comparing the size of the pulmonary

artery with that of the accompanying bronchus when these structures are viewed on end, expressed as the arterial-bronchial diameter ratio (ABR). In the normal erect subject, upper lung arteries may be slightly larger than, equal in size to, or smaller than their accompanying bronchi, whereas the lower lung arteries are almost always larger than their accompanying bronchi (ABR: mean ± standard deviation, 1.34 ± 0.25). With progressive pulmonary venous hypertension, the ABR relationship between upper and lower lungs equalizes and then reverses such that upper lung ABR exceeds lower lung ABR in decompensated congestive heart failure.[10]

Increased pulmonary blood flow: In the case of mild-to-moderate left-to-right shunts, for example, the vessels dilate in proportion

TABLE 3–1. Pulmonary Vascularity
Normal
Caudal PBF pattern in upright position (PBF controlled by gravity)
Gradual branching, treelike
RDPA = 10–15 mm in men
RDPA = 9–14 mm in women
A/B ratio = 1
Abnormal
Volume with normal PBF pattern (distribution)
Increased, larger vessels (eg, ASD)
Decreased, smaller vessels (eg, ToF)
Distribution with abnormal PBF pattern
Cephalic (eg, MS)
Centralized (eg, Eisenmenger syndrome)
Lateralized (eg, Westermark sign)
Localized (eg, pulmonary AV fistulas)
Collateralized (eg, severe ToF)
Combined
Decreased volume and cephalization (eg, critical MS)
Lateralization and localization (eg, Scimitar syndrome)

Abbreviations: A/B, arterial/bronchial; ASD, atrial septal defect; AV, arteriovenous; MS, mitral stenosis; PBF, pulmonary blood flow; RDPA, right descending pulmonary artery; ToF, tetralogy of Fallot.

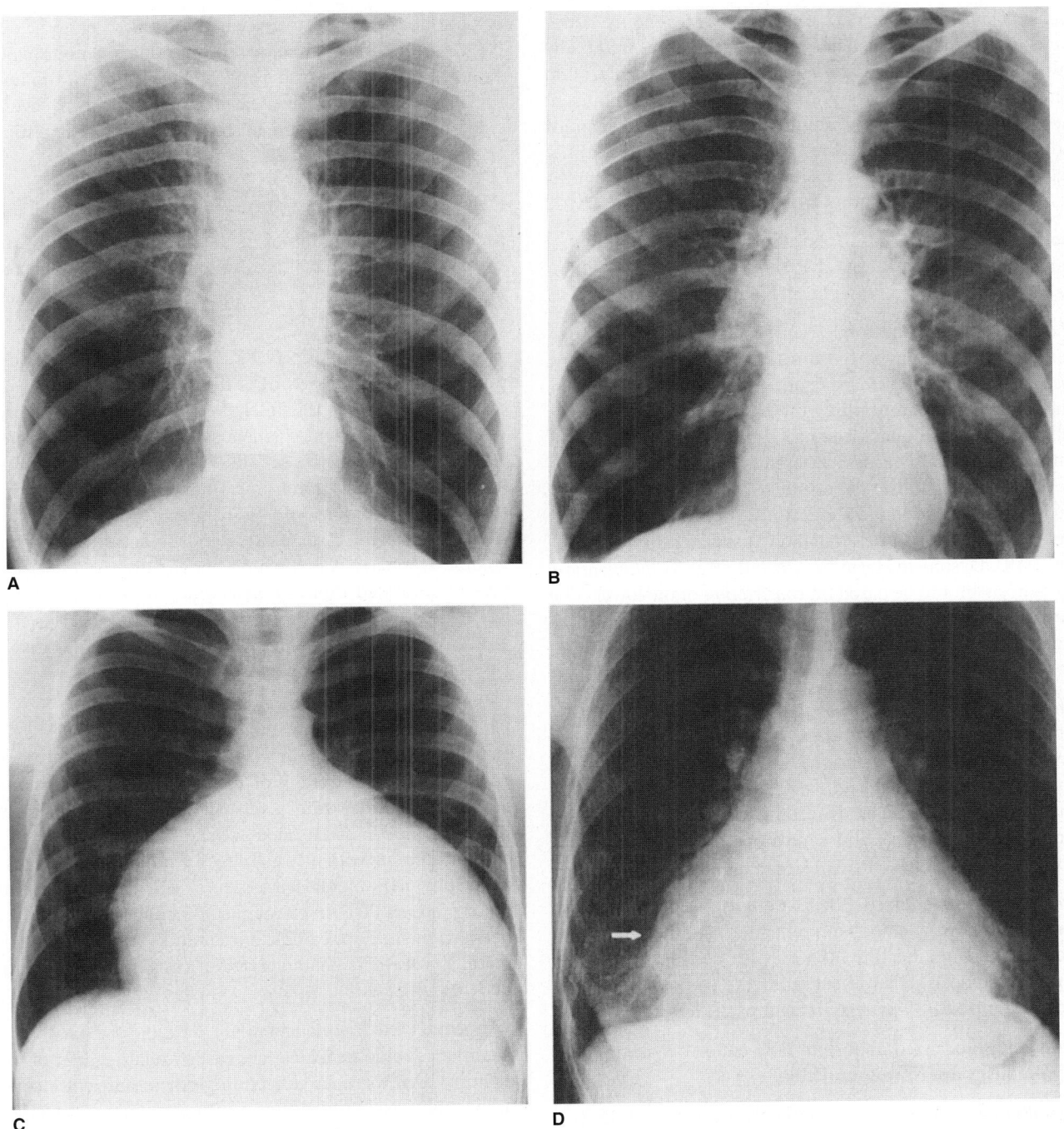

Figure 3–3. Radiographic appearance of right-sided heart failure. (A) A patient with severe obstructive emphysema showing overaeration of the lungs, centralized flow pattern, and a small heart size. **(B)** Three years later, the patient was in frank right-sided heart failure. Note that the heart enlarged as his emphysema worsened. The centralized flow pattern became more severe. **(C)** Patient with Ebstein anomaly showing gross cardiomegaly with severe decrease in pulmonary vascularity. The right cardiac border represents the huge right atrium, and the left cardiac border represents the giant right ventricle. **(D)** Patient with mitral stenosis showing a giant right atrium *(arrow)* representing severe functional tricuspid regurgitation caused by unrelenting left-sided failure. The pulmonary venous congestion had improved after the onset of right-sided heart failure.

to the increased flow with no significant change in pressure, resistance, or flow pattern. This phenomenon is also called *shunt vascularity* or *equalization.* Equalization of the PBF between the upper and lower lung zones is only apparent rather than real; however, the lower lobes still receive a great

deal more blood than the upper lobes, although the ratio of PBF between the two zones has changed—for example, from 5:1 to 4:1 or 3:1. A mild increase in pulmonary vascularity with slight cardiomegaly is commonly found in pregnant women and trained athletes with increased cardiac output.

Decreased pulmonary blood flow: Patients with pulmonic stenosis and associated ventricular septal defect (VSD) frequently show decreased pulmonary vascularity with smaller and shorter pulmonary arteries and veins and more radiolucent lungs (see Fig. 3–3). Marked reduction in PBF is also encountered in patients with isolated right-sided heart failure without a right-to-left shunt (Fig. 3–3). This is attributed to the significant decrease in cardiac output from the right ventricle (RV).

Abnormalities in Distribution: An abnormal distribution of PBF (or an abnormal PBF pattern) always reflects a changed pulmonary vascular resistance, either locally or diffusely (**Fig. 3–4**).

Cephalization: When the total intravascular pressure in post-capillary pulmonary hypertension (PH), exceeds the oncotic pressure of the blood, fluid leaks out of the vessels and collects in the interstitium before filling the alveoli. Alveolar hypoxia, resulting from pulmonary edema, leads to pulmonary vaso-constriction. As this occurs preferentially in the lung bases, flow predominates in the upper lobes. This occurs in (1) left-sided obstructive lesions—for example, mitral stenosis; (2) increased LV diastolic pressure; and (3) severe mitral regurgitation (MR). Despite the terms *redistribution* and *cephalization*, the diagnosis should be based on *constriction* of the lower-lobe vessels. Dilatation of the upper lobe vessels can be found without narrowing of the basilar vessels in a number of entities, most noticeably left-to-right shunts.

Centralization: In precapillary PH, the pulmonary trunk and central pulmonary arteries dilate, and the distal pulmonary arteries constrict from the periphery toward the lung hilum—a phenomenon called *centralization*. This occurs in patients with primary PH, Eisenmenger syndrome, recurrent pulmonary thromboembolic disease, and severe obstructive emphysema (see **Figs. 3–4A** and **3–4B**).

Lateralization: A lateralized PBF pattern is a sign of massive unilateral pulmonary embolism, reflecting blood being forced to flow through the healthy lung only. In congenital valvular pulmonary stenosis, a jet effect from the stenotic valve can cause a lateralized PBF pattern in favor of the left side.

Localization: A localized abnormal flow pattern is exemplified by a pulmonary arteriovenous fistula.

Collateralization: Patients with markedly decreased PBF (eg, pulmonic stenosis) tend to show numerous small, tortuous bronchial arterial collaterals in the upper medial lung zones near their origin from the descending aorta.

Combined Abnormalities: Abnormal pulmonary vascularity is often mixed, with a great variety of possible combinations—for example, cephalization plus decreased flow in severe mitral stenosis (MS) or centralization with increased PBF in Eisenmenger atrial septal defect (ASD).

Lung Parenchyma

With right-sided heart failure, the lungs become unusually radiolucent because of decreased PBF. Conversely, significant left-sided heart failure is characterized by the presence of pulmonary edema, a cephalic blood flow pattern, or both (**Fig. 3–5**). Long-standing, severe pulmonary venous hypertension can lead to hemosiderosis or ossification of the lung (or both).[11] When right-sided heart failure results from severe left-sided heart failure, the preexisting pulmonary congestion can improve because of the decreased PBF.

Cardiomediastinal Silhouette

Radiographic evaluation of the heart focuses on assessment of cardiac size, cardiac contour, abnormal opacities or lucencies, and cardiac position.[12]

Cardiac Size

The cardiothoracic ratio (CTR, normally ≤0.5 on the upright posteroanterior radiograph) is the simplest assessment of cardiac size. However, it is neither specific (mild cardiomegaly may reflect the chamber enlargement associated with low heart rates in athletes) nor sensitive (a CTR >0.42 is associated with worse in-hospital and long-term clinical outcome in patients with acute myocardial infarction [MI]).[13] The specific radiographic appearance can help to distinguish diagnostic entities—for example, volume overload produces a greater degree of cardiomegaly than pressure overload alone, in the absence of heart failure (ie, with a normal PBF pattern). A smaller-than-average heart is encountered in chronic obstructive pulmonary disease, Addison disease, anorexia nervosa, and starvation.

Cardiac Contour

Changes in the cardiac silhouette can be a useful diagnostic clue.[19] For instance, *coeur en sabot*, a "boot-shaped heart," is characteristic of tetralogy of Fallot (ToF). A bulge along the left cardiac border with a retrosternal double density is virtually diagnostic of LV aneurysm. A markedly widened right cardiac contour with a straightened left cardiac border is seen frequently in patients with severe MS leading to tricuspid regurgitation (TR). An elevated cardiac silhouette with lucency between the inferior cardiac border and the left hemidiaphragmatic silhouette is characteristic of congenital absence of the pericardium.

Abnormal Opacity or Lucency

Familiar "double densities" are cast by enlargement of the left atrium (LA), tortuous descending aorta, aortic, or coronary artery aneurysms.[2] Any radiologically detectable calcification in the heart may be clinically important. Mitral annular calcification is common in the elderly, and in addition to its association with increased risk of atherosclerotic cardiovascular disease[15] (perhaps both associated with inflammation), extension onto the mitral valve leaflets is an increasingly important cause of mitral stenosis.[16] The extent of valvular calcification tends to be proportionate to the severity of the valve stenosis regardless of the other radiographic signs of the disease. Calcification of the coronary artery is almost always atherosclerotic in nature.[17]

The abnormal lucent areas in and about the heart include displaced subepicardial fat stripes caused by effusion or thickening of the pericardium, pneumopericardium, and pneumomediastinum.

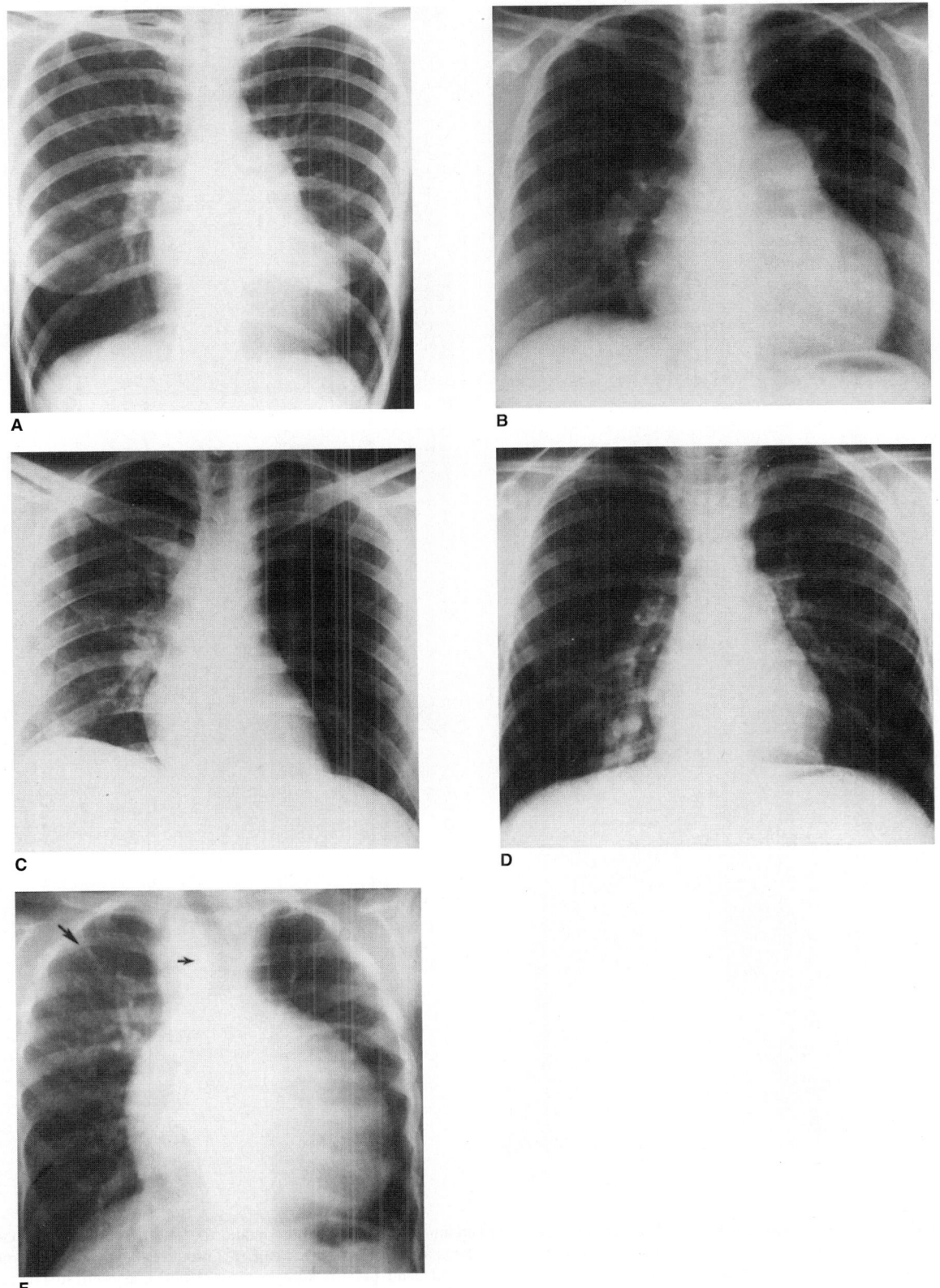

Figure 3–4. Abnormal pulmonary blood flow (PBF) patterns. (A) Cephalization. Patient with severe mitral stenosis showing dilatation of the upper vessels with constriction of the lower vessels. **(B)** Centralization. Patient with primary pulmonary hypertension showing marked dilatation of the pulmonary trunk and the central segments of both pulmonary arteries with pruning of the peripheral branches. **(C)** Lateralization. Patient with massive pulmonary embolism obstructing the left main pulmonary artery. Note the uneven distribution of PBF between the two lungs in favor of the right. **(D)** Localization. A cyanotic child showing localized vascular changes representing a large pulmonary arteriovenous fistula in the right lower lobe. **(E)** Collateralization. A child with pseudotruncus arteriosus with cardiomegaly and a right aortic arch (*small arrow*). Note severe pulmonary oligemia with numerous small tortuous vessels (*large arrow*) in the upper medial lung zones, representing bronchial arterial collaterals.

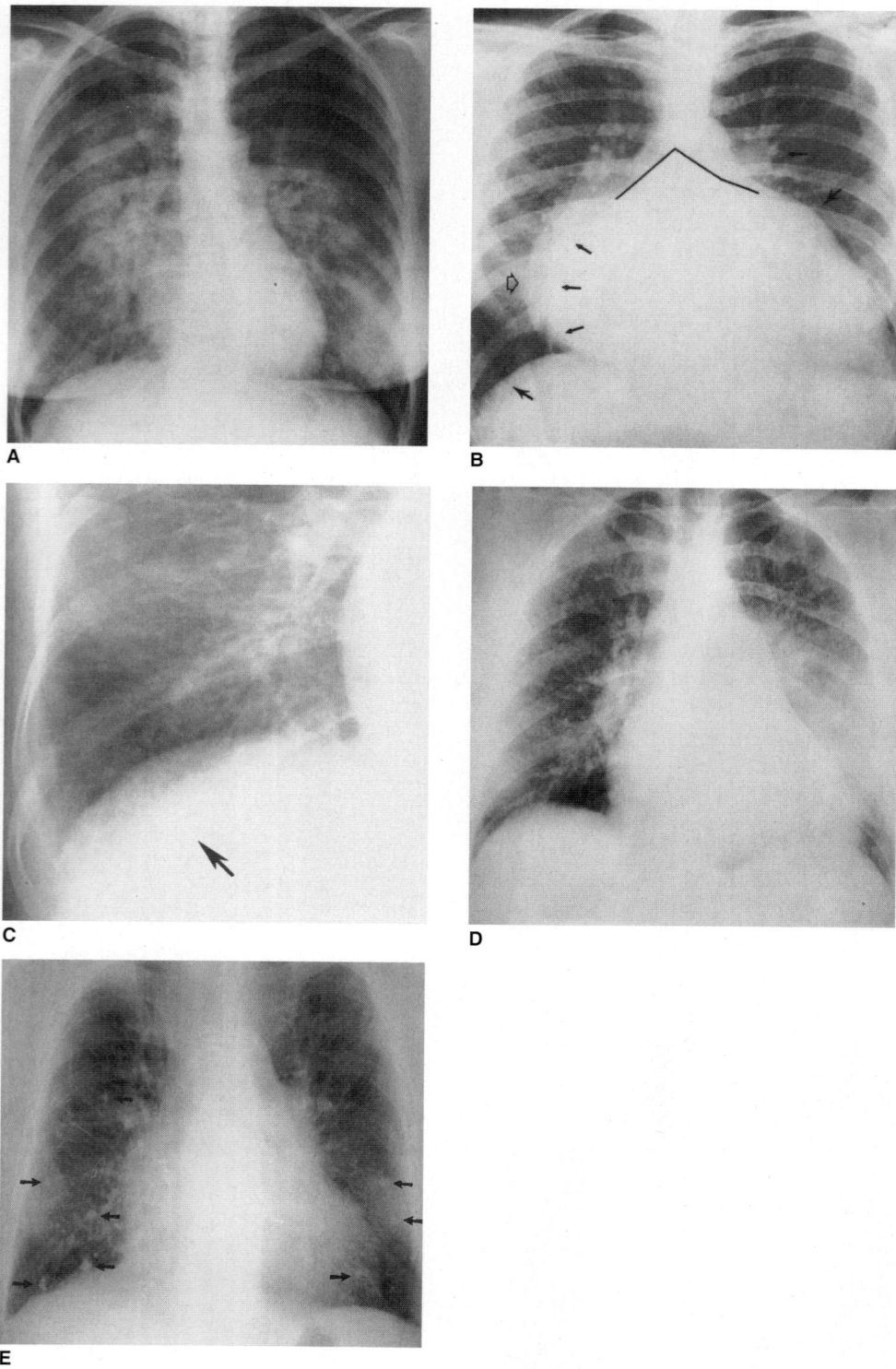

Figure 3–5. Radiographic appearance of left-sided heart failure. (A) Acute. Patient with acute mitral regurgitation because of rupture of chordae tendineae showing the "bat-wings" appearance of a severe alveolar type of pulmonary edema and a normal-sized heart. **(B)** Chronic. Patient with severe mitral and tricuspid regurgitation and mild aortic regurgitation. This is a predominantly left-sided failure pattern. Note the gross cardiomegaly with striking cephalization and interstitial pulmonary edema. The giant left atrium forms the right cardiac border (*open arrow*), makes its appendage bulge outward on the left side (*upper large arrow*), and splays the mainstem bronchi wide apart (*solid lines*). The huge right atrium forms a double density within the right cardiac border (*three small arrows*). The *small upper arrow* marks the peribronchial cuffing of edema fluid. The *large lower arrow* points to multiple Kerley B lines. **(C)** Magnified view of right costophrenic sulcus showing multiple Kerley B lines (*arrow*). **(D)** A 44-year-old woman with severe mitral stenosis (MS). The radiograph shows a diffuse stippling with fine nodules representing hemosiderosis. Hemosiderin-laden macrophages were found in her sputa. **(E)** Posteroanterior radiograph of a 63-year-old man with severe MS, status post–mitral valve replacement, shows multiple scattered bony nodules (*arrows*) 2 to 10 mm in diameter throughout the lower two-thirds of both lungs, compatible with pulmonary ossification.

Cardiac Malpositions

Cardiac malpositions are diagnosed when either the heart or the stomach is out of the normal left-sided position.

Dextrocardia is used to indicate any congenital right-sided heart regardless of the position of abdominal viscera. *Dextrocardia with situs inversus*, the mirror image of normal, is associated with a 5% prevalence of congenital heart disease, a 9-fold increase over the general population.

Dextrocardia with situs solitus comprises a right-sided heart with normal situs (ie, aortic arch, abdominal viscera and the atria are in the normal positions). Under these circumstances, abnormal relationships between the ventricles and the rest of the cardiovascular structures are bound to develop, and the prevalence of congenital heart disease is 98%. More than 80% have congenitally corrected (or L loop) transposition of great arteries. The next most common lesions are a combination of VSD and pulmonary stenosis, a tetralogy-like pathophysiology.

Levocardia with situs inversus is a mirror image of dextrocardia with situs solitus, and it is associated with nearly a 100% prevalence of cyanotic congenital cardiac lesions similar to those seen in dextrocardia with situs solitus.

In *cardiac malpositions with situs ambiguus,* the patient's heart can be on either the left or right side. The site is ambiguous because the aortic arch and the stomach are not on the same side. Under these circumstances, the patient has either asplenia or polysplenia syndrome. Patients with polysplenia syndrome tend to be acyanotic and frequently survive into adulthood. The associated lesions are bilateral left-sidedness, interruption of the IVC with azygos continuation, polysplenia, and a left-to-right shunt, most frequently an atrioventricular septal defect. Patients with asplenia tend to be cyanotic and critically ill and die in infancy.

Heart and Pulmonary Vasculature in Heart Failure

Chest radiography has historically been an important tool for assessing patients with heart failure. However, handheld ultrasound provides a more accurate means of assessing chamber dimensions, and lung ultrasound has overcome some of the traditional limitations of ultrasound imaging of pulmonary congestion and effusions.[18,19]

Acute Left-Sided Heart Failure

The pulmonary vascular changes associated with acute LV failure are usually not discernible because the resulting severe pulmonary edema obscures the pulmonary vasculature, and the redistribution of PBF secondary to acute left-sided heart failure is usually relatively mild. Acute left-sided heart failure presents with a combination of alveolar pulmonary edema and a normal-sized heart; interstitial fluid may distribute in a classical butterfly pattern.

Chronic Left-Sided Heart Failure

Typically characterized by gross cardiomegaly, striking cephalization of the pulmonary vasculature, and interstitial pulmonary edema or fibrosis with multiple distinct Kerley B lines.

Acute Right-Sided Heart Failure

This may result from massive pulmonary embolism. The typical radiographic signs are rapidly developing centralization of the pulmonary vasculature and dilatation of the right-sided cardiac chambers and vena cava. In addition, the lungs may show localized or lateralized oligemia.

Chronic Right-Sided Heart Failure

Associated with diffusely decreased pulmonary vascularity with unusually lucent lungs in right-sided heart failure without PH, a centralized PBF pattern when the right-sided heart failure is secondary to precapillary PH, or a cephalized flow pattern with lucent lungs in patients with right-sided heart failure secondary to long-standing severe left-sided heart failure

Other Abnormalities

Great Vessels

The radiographic appearance of the great vessels often provides valuable information for the diagnosis of heart disease.[2,3,20] For example, whereas selective dilatation of the ascending aorta is the hallmark of valvular aortic stenosis (AS), generalized dilatation of the entire thoracic aorta suggests aortic regurgitation (AR), systemic hypertension, or both, depending on the size of the LV. In ASD and MS, the pulmonary trunk may be enlarged, and the aortic knob is usually small. A leftward cardiac rotation occurs when an enlarged RV coexists with a normal-sized LV. When the heart rotates to the left, the aorta folds on itself in the midline and becomes inconspicuous. Meanwhile, the pulmonary trunk is brought laterally and looks larger than it actually is. Aortic aneurysm and dissection are frequently associated with hypertensive and atherosclerotic disease; heavy calcification of an ascending aortic aneurysm is suggestive of "luetic" aortitis secondary to syphilis.

Prominence of the pulmonary trunk is a reliable secondary sign of RV enlargement, with the following exceptions: (1) ToF with RV hypertrophy but pulmonary trunk hypoplasia; (2) idiopathic dilatation of the pulmonary artery; (3) patent ductus arteriosus with dilated pulmonary trunk but normal RV; and (4) straight-back syndrome, pectus excavatum, and scoliosis with narrowed AP diameter of the chest. Under the latter conditions, the heart is compressed, displaced, and rotated to the left, giving rise to a falsely enlarged pulmonary artery.

In coarctation of the aorta, the engorged aortic knob and the poststenotic dilatation of the descending aorta can cause a *3 sign* on the aorta and an *E sign* on the barium-filled esophagus, both depicting the site of coarctation.

The abnormal size and distribution of both the pulmonary and systemic veins are important clues to the presence of certain conditions—for example, anomalous pulmonary venous connections, pulmonary arteriovenous fistulas, pulmonary varix, persistent left superior vena cava (SVC), and interruption of IVC with azygos continuation.

Mediastinal Structures

The mediastinal organs are frequently affected by the cardiovascular structures because of their close spatial interrelationships. An enlarged LA not only displaces the esophagus and the descending aorta but also elevates and compresses the left mainstem bronchus. A double aortic arch can compress both the trachea and the esophagus. Also, malignant processes can invade the heart and great vessels, causing cardiac tamponade or the SVC syndrome. Usually, these mediastinal changes are evident on the chest radiograph and should be recognized promptly.

Pleura

A right-sided pleural effusion is often present with left-sided heart failure. A bilateral hydrothorax suggests biventricular heart failure or a noncardiac etiology of the effusion. Heart failure is also known to be associated with a pseudotumor or *vanishing* tumor, representing an interlobar collection of pleural fluid. As heart failure improves, the *pseudotumor* disappears.

Bones and Joints

Rib notching (see Fig. 3–12) provides important clues to the diagnosis of coarctation of the aorta.[3,21] Notching of the ribs has many origins—any of the three major intercostal structures can enlarge, compress, and erode the lower borders of the ribs, producing areas of notching. They are intercostal arteries, veins, and nerves. Coarctation of the aorta represents the most common cause of rib notching as a result of dynamic dilatation and tortuosity of the arteries. SVC syndrome can produce a similar radiographic appearance, albeit through long-standing venous dilation. Neurofibromatosis can also produce rib notching through the compressive effect of numerous intercostal neurofibromas.

Soft Tissues over the Chest

Severe edema in the soft tissues over the chest can be seen on radiographs in a setting of generalized anasarca.

Comparison of Serial Studies

To appreciate the acuteness or chronicity of a disease process or its response to therapy, one must carefully compare serial radiographs. An enlarging heart with normal pulmonary vascularity is highly suggestive of pericardial effusion. Conversely, a shrinking heart in the presence of normal vascularity is compatible with resolution of a pericardial effusion.

Cardiac Fluoroscopy

Cardiac fluoroscopy explores the dynamic features of the organ that are discernible only in motion. However, it has been largely displaced by other imaging techniques, particularly two-dimensional (2D) echocardiography, MRI, and CT, and its use is limited to the cardiac catheterization laboratory, where it can assess the function of radiodense and echodense prosthetic valves and can guide the positioning of pacemakers or ICDs. With the emergence of transcatheter aortic valve replacement therapy, cardiac fluoroscopy has experienced a resurgence at some centers.

The bileaflet St. Jude valve is used in both mitral and aortic positions. The valve is difficult to see radiographically but is readily detected under the fluoroscope or with CT. When the leaflets move sluggishly, valve thrombosis should be suspected. Rarely, one leaflet can dislodge and embolize distally, causing acute valvular regurgitation.

The position of a pacemaker or ICD can be determined promptly under the fluoroscope during initial insertion and recorded on film. The subepicardial fat line overlies the myocardium and underlies the pericardium. If the pacing catheter is found within the fat stripe, it may have passed through the coronary sinus and entered one of the major cardiac veins. If the tip of the catheter is seen outside the fat stripe, however, it may have perforated the myocardium and thus be lying within the pericardium or beyond. Although the wires and electrodes of a transmediastinal pacemaker may look normal on the radiographs, minor breakage may be appreciated only in ventricular systole with the aid of fluoroscopy.

Summary

Cardiac disease presents a broad array of manifestations on the chest radiograph. Despite the proliferation of other cardiac imaging modalities that offer superior anatomic assessment through tomographic acquisition and display, the knowledgeable and disciplined observer can glean tremendous insights into altered anatomy and physiology. The widespread availability, low cost, and ease of acquisition makes the use of cardiac radiography logical within an initial cardiac assessment, for assessing the status of assistive devices, and for monitoring dynamic processes during treatment, particularly when they result in altered pulmonary vascular physiology.

CARDIAC CATHETERIZATION AND CARDIAC ANGIOGRAPHY

Indications and Contraindications

Cardiac angiography images not only diagnose coronary artery disease (CAD) but are used to visualize abnormalities of the aorta as well as the pulmonary and peripheral vessels **Table 3–2**. Relative contraindications to cardiac catheterization include fever, anemia, electrolyte imbalance (especially hypokalemia predisposing to arrhythmias), or other systemic illnesses needing stabilization (**Table 3–3**).

Techniques and Equipment

The safety and speed of modern catheterization are a product of technological developments in imaging systems, monitors, pressure transducer systems, and a variety of disposable catheters, manifolds, and equipment.

Generation of the X-Ray Image

Cardiac angiography uses a complex series of radiographic x-ray elements, transforming energy into a visual image. The x-ray image generation chain can be simplified into three major components: (1) the x-ray generator, (2) the x-ray tube, and (3) the image intensifier. The details of x-ray equipment should be familiar to all personnel working in a catheterization laboratory.

The generator provides the power source necessary to accelerate the electrons through the x-ray tube. The duration of x-ray exposure is similar to the shutter speed on a regular camera. The exposure usually is set fast enough to stop blurring as a result of heart movement. During selective coronary arteriography, the shorter the exposure time, the better the image.

TABLE 3–2. Indications for Cardiac Catheterization

Indications	Procedures
Suspected or known coronary artery disease	
Angina: New onset, unstable, stable refractory to medical treatment, atypical	LV, COR
Ischemia: positive stress test, evaluation before major surgery,	LV, COR, ERGO
Atypical chest pain of coronary spasm	
Myocardial infarction, unstable angina postinfarction, failed thrombolysis	LV, COR, RH
Shock	LV, COR, RH
Mechanical complications (ventricular septal defect, rupture of wall, or papillary muscle)	LV, COR, RH
Sudden cardiovascular death	LV, COR, R + L
Valvular heart disease	LV, COR, R + L, AO
Congenital heart disease (before anticipated corrective surgery)	LV, COR, R + L, AO
Aortic dissection	AO, COR
Pericardial constriction or tamponade	LV, COR, R + L
Cardiomyopathy	LV, COR, R + L, BX
Initial and follow-up assessment for heart transplant	LV, COR, R + L, BX

Abbreviations: AO, aortography; BX, endomyocardial biopsy; COR, coronary angiography; ERGO, ergonovine provocation of coronary spasm; LV, left ventriculography; RH, right heart oxygen saturations and hemodynamics (eg, placement of Swan-Ganz catheter); R + L, right and left heart hemodynamics.

Exposure times of 3 to 6 milliseconds reduce movement blur. Most modern generators are capable of delivering adequate power while providing precise and automatically adjusted exposure timing. Current generators are equipped with either multiple-phase (alternating on/off) or short/long pulse widths that are automatically adjusted for correct exposure. Manual settings, which are operator selected, are limited to film frame rates (eg, 15, 30, or 60 frames per second).

X-Ray Tubes: The x-ray tube converts electrical energy, provided from the generator, to an x-ray beam. Electrons emitted from a heated filament (cathode) are accelerated toward a rapidly rotating disk (anode) and at contact undergo conversion to x-radiation. This process generates extreme heat. The heat capacity of an x-ray tube is a major limiting factor in the design

TABLE 3–3. Relative Contraindications to Cardiac Catheterization

Acute gastrointestinal bleeding or anemia
Anticoagulation (or known uncontrolled bleeding diathesis)
Electrolyte imbalance
Infection/fever
Medication intoxication (eg, digitalis)
Pregnancy
Recent cerebral vascular accident (>1 month)
Renal failure
Uncontrolled congestive heart failure, high blood pressure, arrhythmias
Uncooperative patient

of x-ray tubes. Only 0.2% to 0.6% of the electrical energy provided to the tube eventually is converted to x-rays. In addition to the exposure times (controlled by the generator system) and the size of the imaging field (controlled by the x-ray tube), two other factors of the x-ray determine the quality of x-ray for proper image exposures: electrical current and level of kilovoltage.

Electrical current: This determines the number of photons (electrical particles) generated per unit of time. The greater the electrical current, the greater the number of photons delivered, resulting in improved image resolution. However, the current level is limited by the heat capacity of the x-ray tubes as well as radiation exposure and scatter.

Level of kilovoltage: This determines the energy spectrum (wavelength) of the x-ray beam. The higher the level of kilovoltage, the shorter the wavelength of radiation and the greater the ability of x-rays to penetrate target tissue. Increased kilovoltage is especially important in obese patients. To obtain better images through more tissue, a higher kilovolt level is required. Unfortunately, a high kilovolt level also will produce lower resolution because of wide scatter. There is also greater radiation exposure to patients and laboratory personnel. Modern radiographic equipment allows for variability of the amperage and voltage to attain optimal quality radiographic images. An automatic exposure control system sets exposure times to incorporate changes in voltage (kV) and amperage (mA), providing the desired images at the best exposures possible.

Image Intensifier and Detector: After the x-rays have penetrated the body, the partially absorbed beams are cast as a shadow on the input screen of the image intensifier or flat panel detector. The image intensifier converts the invisible x-ray image into a visual image. Each x-ray photon hits the phosphorus-covered plate of the intensifier, resulting in a light particle that is detected, the position and intensity of which are noted. The sum of all events produces an image for video. Image intensifiers are equipped with various-sized image fields that alter the image resolution. In general, the smaller the image field size, the sharper the resolution, but the higher the radiation dose. Smaller input screen diameters of 13 to 18 cm (5- to 7-inches) are better suited for coronary angiography because of their enhanced resolution. For more detailed work, such as percutaneous transluminal coronary angioplasty and other coronary interventions, 13-cm (5-inch) fields are commonly used. In contrast, for large-area examinations (ie, left ventriculography, aortography, or peripheral angiography), field diameters of 23 to 28 cm (9 to 11 inches) are used, with the known trade-off of loss of resolution for small structures.

Modern image intensifiers are predominantly of a flat panel construction, eliminating many of the artifacts associated with tube-like intensifiers used in earlier x-ray systems. The x-ray image is now generated in a digital format, which lends itself to easier analysis. Digital angiography converts the x-ray image into a quantitative information format for storage and display on a computer. Digital imaging permits the contrast image to be amplified or enlarged or contrast adjusted. One image can be subtracted from another.

Catheters

The choice of catheters for coronary angiography depends on the approach (radial or femoral access) and physician preferences. Numerous shapes and sizes of catheters are available. Basic, routine catheters that are preshaped for normal anatomy are useful for both the radial and femoral approaches. There is an array of unique "universal" (one catheter for both left and right coronary artery) shapes for the radial approach, designed to aid the angiographer through difficult aortic anatomy.[22]

Every cardiovascular laboratory is equipped with an emergency crash cart containing emergency drugs, oxygen, airways, suction apparatus, and other emergency equipment. A defibrillator should be charged and ready for use during a procedure.

In recent years, most laboratories routinely have used radial artery access as their preferred diagnostic and interventional approach because of significantly fewer access-related complications and better late outcomes than the previously-standard femoral approach. A high-pressure contrast media injector is needed to administer a large bolus (20–50 mL) of contrast media into the LV at a rate of 12 to 15 mL/s; PAs at 10 to 25 mL/s; or aortic arch, at 20 to 30 mL/s.

Contrast Media and Complications

All contrast media contain three iodine molecules attached to a fully substituted benzene ring. Traditional high-osmolar contrast agents (>1400 mOsm) were ionic monomers with sodium or meglumine as the cation. These were frequently (10%) associated with peripheral arterial vasodilatation, transient myocardial dysfunction, and osmotic diuresis resulting in reduced circulating volume and blood pressure, and are now rarely used. Modern radiographic contrast media include nonionic monomeric agents (and one ionic dimeric agent), which have approximately the same viscosity and iodine concentration but less than 50% of the osmolality of the high-osmolar agents. The advantages of the nonionic, low-osmolar agents include less hemodynamic loading, patient discomfort, binding of ionic calcium, depression of myocardial function and blood pressure, and fewer anaphylactoid reactions. Currently, nonionic, low-osmolar agents are routine for nearly all patients, and are especially helpful in patients with poor LV function, renal disease, diabetes, or prior reactions to contrast media. All media are excreted predominantly by glomerular filtration with a normal half-time of excretion of 20 minutes.

There are three types of contrast allergies (**Table 3–4**): (1) minor cutaneous and mucosal manifestations, (2) smooth muscle and minor anaphylactoid responses, and (3) major cardiovascular and anaphylactoid responses. Major reactions involving laryngeal or pulmonary edema often are accompanied by minor or less severe reactions. Although some reactions to a pretest contrast dose may be violent (but rarely life-threatening), pretesting has been found to be of no value in determining who will have an adverse reaction. Although definitive data are lacking on the true effectiveness of premedication to prevent allergic reactions, patients reporting allergic

TABLE 3–4. Reactions to Contrast Medium

Cutaneous and mucosal
Angioedema
Flushing
Laryngeal edema
Pruritus
Urticaria
Smooth muscle
Bronchospasm
Gastrointestinal spasm
Uterine contraction
Cardiovascular
Arrhythmia
Hypotension (shock)
Vasodilatation

reactions to contrast media should be pretreated with prednisone and diphenhydramine. The routine for the laboratories may vary, but common dosages include 60 mg of prednisone the night before and 60 mg of prednisone the morning of, along with 50 mg of oral diphenhydramine given at the time of call to the catheterization laboratory.

Dehydrated patients or those with diabetes or renal insufficiency are at risk for contrast-induced nephropathy (CIN). Advanced precautions to limit CIN include hydration, minimizing contrast delivered, and maintenance of large-volume urine flow (>200 mL/h). These patients should be hydrated intravenously the night before the procedure. After the contrast study, intravenous fluids should be liberally continued unless intravascular volume overload is a problem. No pharmacologic regimen has been demonstrated to perform better than volume loading with normal saline. A decreased urine output after the procedure that is unresponsive to increased intravenous fluids indicates that renal insufficiency is probable. All types of contrast agents (ionic, nonionic, low-osmolar, iso-osmolar) are associated with a similar incidence of CIN.[23]

Complications of Cardiac Catheterization

For diagnostic catheterization, analysis of the complications in more than 200,000 patients indicates the incidence of risks as follows: death (<0.2%), MI (<0.05%) stroke (<0.07%), serious ventricular arrhythmia (<0.5%), and major vascular complications (thrombosis, bleeding requiring transfusion, or pseudoaneurysm; <1%)[24] (**Table 3–5**). Certain patient groups are at higher risk for complications (**Table 3–6**).

Complications of right heart catheterization may arise from access, sepsis, or damage to cardiac or vascular structures (**Table 3–7**). Significant but transient ventricular arrhythmias occur in more than 30% of patients undergoing right heart catheterization and are terminated when the catheter is readjusted. Sustained ventricular arrhythmias have been reported, especially in unstable patients or those with electrolyte imbalance, acidosis, or concurrent myocardial ischemia.

Cardiac Angiography and Coronary Arteriography

Angiography is the primary method of defining coronary anatomy in patients, providing an anatomic map of the site, severity,

TABLE 3–5. Complications of Cardiac Catheterization

Percent	
Death	0.11
Myocardial infarction	0.05
Neurologic (eg, stroke)	0.07
Arrhythmia (ventricular tachycardia, fibrillation, heart block, asystole, Supraventricular tachyarrhythmia, atrial fibrillation)	0.38
Vascular—Aortic dissection, pseudoaneurysm, hemorrhage (local, retroperitoneal, pelvic)	0.43
Contrast (contrast reaction/anaphylaxis/nephrotoxicity)	0.37
Hemodynamic (congestive heart failure)	0.26
Perforation, tamponade	0.03
Other (infection, protamine reaction, vasovagal reaction)	0.28
Total (patients)	1.98

Data from Noto TJ, Johnson LW, Krone R, et al. Cardiac catheterization 1990: a report of the Registry of the Society for Cardiac Angiography and Interventions (SCA&I). *Cathet Cardiovasc Diagn.* 1991;24:75-83 and Uretzky BF, Weinert HH. *Cardiac Catheterization: Concepts, Techniques, and Applications.* Walden: Blackwell; 1997.

and the shape and distribution of stenotic coronary lesions. In addition, the vessel size or diameter, presence of intracoronary thrombus, and extent of diffuse atherosclerotic diseases can be assessed. By using provocative maneuvers, the presence of coronary spasm can be ascertained. The functional significance of a coronary stenosis can be assessed by measuring coronary flow or pressure directly, using information obtained both at rest and during maximal coronary vasodilatation.

Left ventriculography is often part of a coronary angiographic study, but may be foregone in the context of more accurate noninvasive methods for assessing volumes, EF, and regional function.

Successful angiography requires a completed chain of actions beginning with the positioning of the patient on the table, acquiring the angiographic image, recording and storing the digital image data, and finally displaying the images for review and analysis. The nomenclature of coronary angiographic imaging is based on the position of the image

TABLE 3–6. Conditions of Patients at Higher Risk for Complications of Catheterization

Acute myocardial infarction
Advanced age (>75 y)
Aortic aneurysm
Aortic stenosis
Congestive heart failure
Diabetes
Extensive three-vessel coronary artery disease
Left ventricular dysfunction (left ventricular ejection fraction <35%)
Obesity
Prior cerebral vascular accident
Renal insufficiency
Suspected or known left main coronary stenosis
Uncontrolled hypertension
Unstable angina

TABLE 3–7. Complications of Right Heart (Pulmonary Artery) Catheterization

	Major	Minor
Access	Pneumothorax	Hematoma
	Hemothorax	Thrombosis
	Tracheal perforation (subclavian route)	
Sepsis	Cellulitis	
Cardiac/vascular	Right ventricular perforation	Ventricular arrhythmia
	Heart block (right bundle branch block)	
	Pulmonary rupture	
	Pulmonary infarction Tricuspid regurgitation Dislodgement of pacemaker leads	

intensifier relative to the patient. The image intensifier is directly over the patient collecting the x-rays from the source under the patient (**Fig. 3–6**). The x-ray source and image intensifier are connected on a C-shaped armature and move in unison in opposite directions around the patient. The body surface of the patient that faces the observer determines the specific view. This relationship holds true whether the patient is supine, standing, or rotated.

Left Coronary Artery

The ostium of the left coronary artery originates from the left sinus of Valsalva near the sinotubular ridge. The left anterior descending artery (LAD) is usually best visualized in a cranially angulated right anterior oblique (RAO) view. If the orientation of the LAD is unusually superior, a caudally angulated left anterior oblique (LAO) view or a straight lateral view may be helpful. The circumflex coronary artery travels in the atrioventricular (AV) groove, after its right-angle origin from the LAD. Its course is quite variable. The artery may terminate in one or more large, obtuse marginal branches coursing over the lateral to posterolateral LV free wall. The circumflex may continue as a large artery in the interventricular groove. In 10% to 15% of cases, the circumflex gives rise to a posterior descending artery (**Fig. 3–7**). The artery that supplies the major posterior descending artery is commonly referred to as the dominant artery. The circumflex artery in the AV groove is best seen in either caudally angulated LAO or RAO views (see Fig. 3–17).

Right Coronary Artery

The right coronary artery (RCA) ostium normally is located in the right sinus of Valsalva. It may be high near the sinotubular ridge or above it, in the midsinus, or occasionally low near the aortic valve. The artery commonly courses upward from the plane of the aortic valve and then travels in the right AV groove to reach the posterior LV wall (**Fig. 3–8**). Along the way, several vessels arise. The conus branch and sinus node arteries branch first, followed by small RV branches, then a large branch that courses over the RV. The RCA continues to become the posterior descending artery before reaching the crux of the

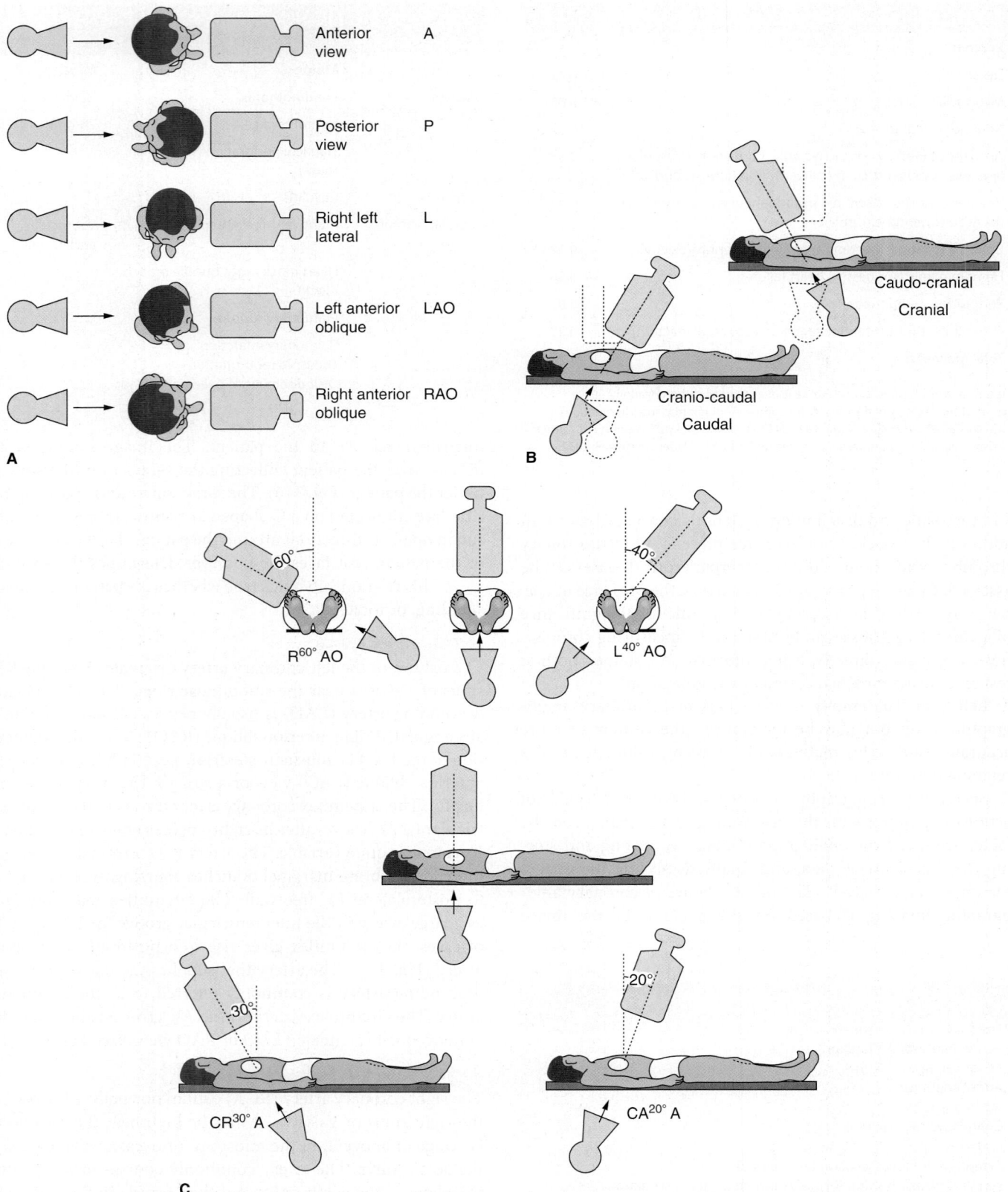

Figure 3–6. Nomenclature for radiographic projections. The *small black arrowheads* show the direction of the x-ray beam. (**A**) Anterior (*A*), posterior (*P*), lateral (*L*), and oblique (*O*). (**B**) If the intensifier is tilted toward the feet of the patient, a caudal (CA) view is produced. If the intensifier is tilted toward the head of the patient, a cranial (CR) view is produced. (**C**) CR and CA oblique views. Reproduced with permission from Paulin S. Terminology for radiographic projections in cardiac angiography. *Cathet Cardiovasc Diagn.* 1981;7(3):341-344.

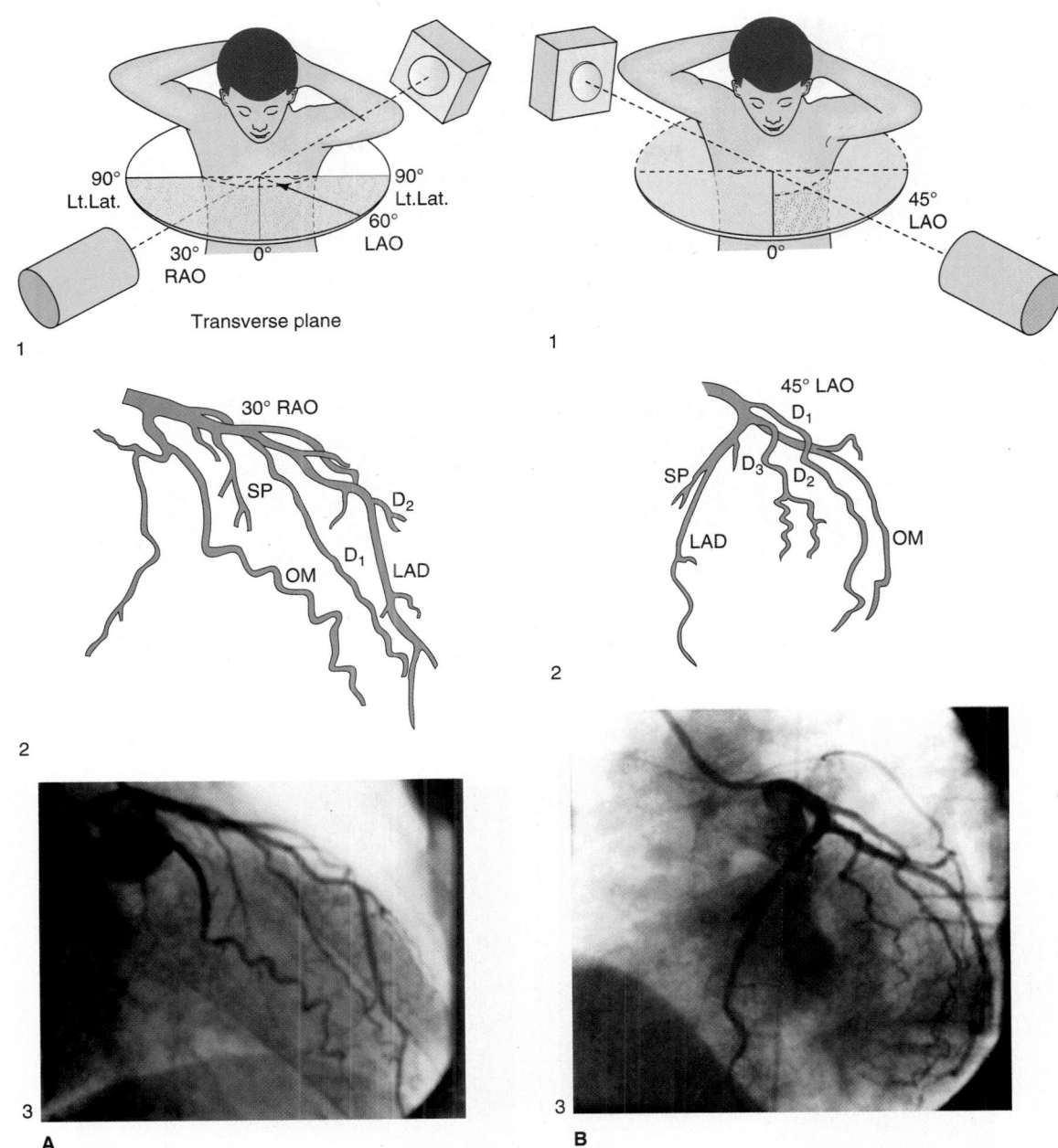

Figure 3–7. Diagrammatic representations of the standard right anterior oblique (RAO) and left anterior oblique (LAO) views (**A**) without cranial angulation and (**B**) with cranial angulation of the left coronary artery, the direction of the x-ray beam, and the position of the overhead image intensifier. In the RAO view, most of the left coronary artery is well visualized in this projection, but there is considerable overlap of the middle LAD and the diagonal branches (**D**). When the left main, circumflex, and diagonal branches have a leftward initial course, the long axis of these arterial segments is projected away from the image intensifier, preventing optimal visualization from the RAO view. The image intensifier is placed anteriorly in an RAO position relative to the patient. Diagrammatic representation of the LAO left coronary angiogram and the direction of the x-ray beam in this view. The value of this view depends in large part on the orientation of the long axis of the heart. When the heart is relatively horizontal, the LAD and diagonal branches are seen end-on throughout much of the course. In this illustration, the longitudinal axis is an intermediate position and there is moderate foreshortening of the LAD and diagonal branches in their proximal portions. The LAO projection is frequently inadequate to visualize the proximal LAD and its branches: the left main segment, which is directed toward the image tube and therefore foreshortened, and the proximal circumflex coronary artery, which may be obscured by overlapping vessels, as in this illustration. The LAO projection is frequently used to visualize the distal LAD and its branches, the midcircumflex coronary artery in the arteriovenous groove, and the distal right coronary artery that is filling via collaterals from the left coronary artery. The image intensifier is above the patient in an LAO position. The left coronary angiogram in the 45-degree LAO with 30 degrees of cranial angulation and the direction of the x-ray beam used to produce this view. This is the most valuable view of the left coronary artery in most patients. Foreshortening of the left main and proximal LAD and diagonal branches present in the LAO view is usually overcome by cranial angulation of the image intensifier. OM, obtuse marginal; SP, septal perforator.

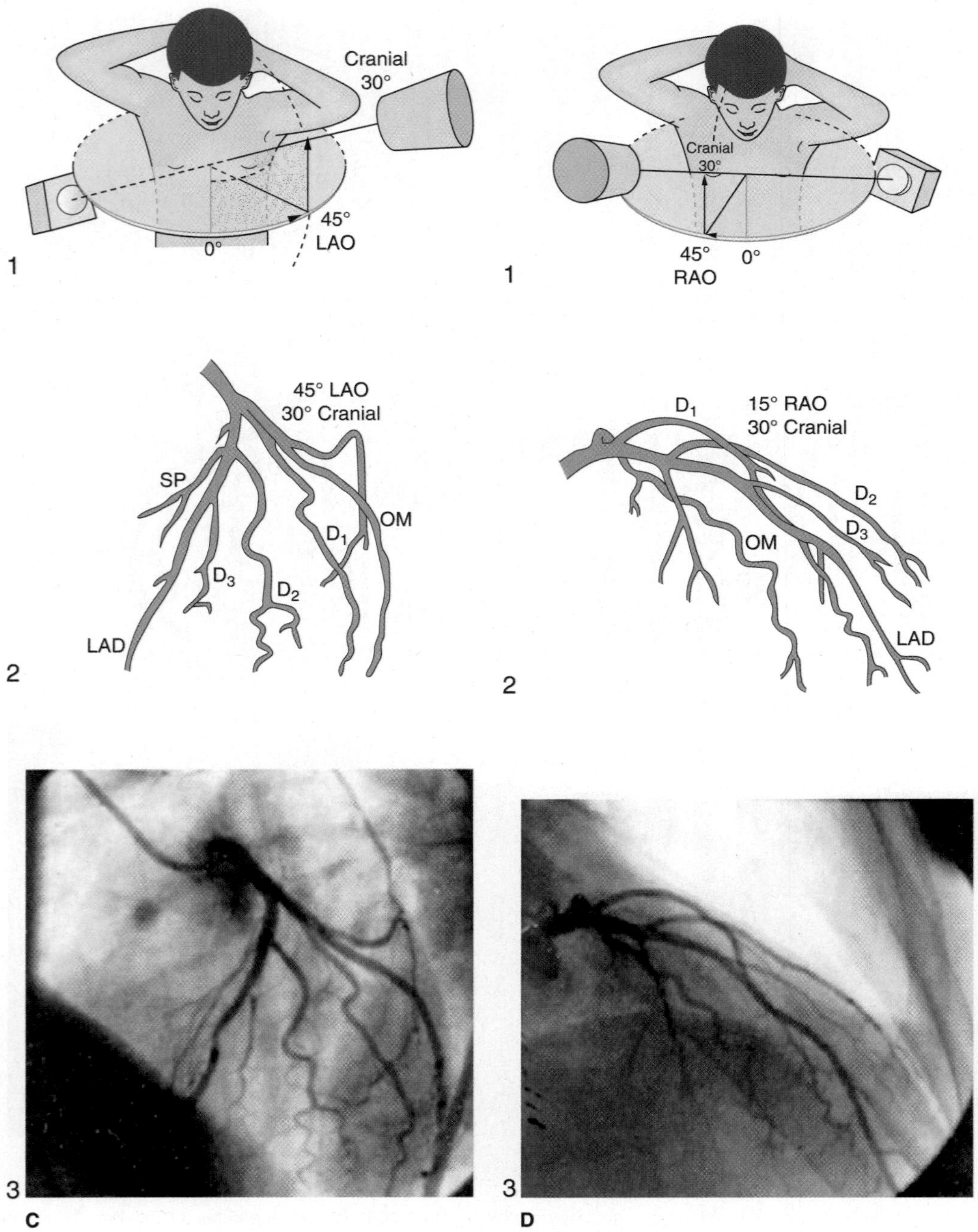

Figure 3–7. (Continued)

heart (junction of the interventricular and interatrial septa). The posterior descending artery sends branches at right angles into the posterior interventricular groove, providing the perforating branches to the basal and posterior one-third of the septum. An RCA that supplies the major posterior descending branch has been referred to as a *dominant RCA*. The posterior descending artery usually stops before reaching the apex, but it may curl around the apex in association with a short anterior descending artery. After giving rise to the posterior descending artery, the RCA becomes intramyocardial at the crux, giving rise to the AV node artery. The LV branches of the RCA are variable and cover the same area as the posterolateral branches of a large circumflex system. The proximal portion of the RCA is well seen in standard RAO and LAO views. However, because of its horizontal orientation, the origin and length of the posterior descending artery, well seen in the RAO view, is foreshortened in the LAO view. Thus, cranial angulation provides a better view of the patent ductus arteriosus.

Angiographic Interpretation
Qualitative and Quantitative Assessment

Every coronary arteriogram should be reviewed in a systematic fashion. The entire LV surface and septum should be adequately supplied with vessels. No gaps should exist. If significant

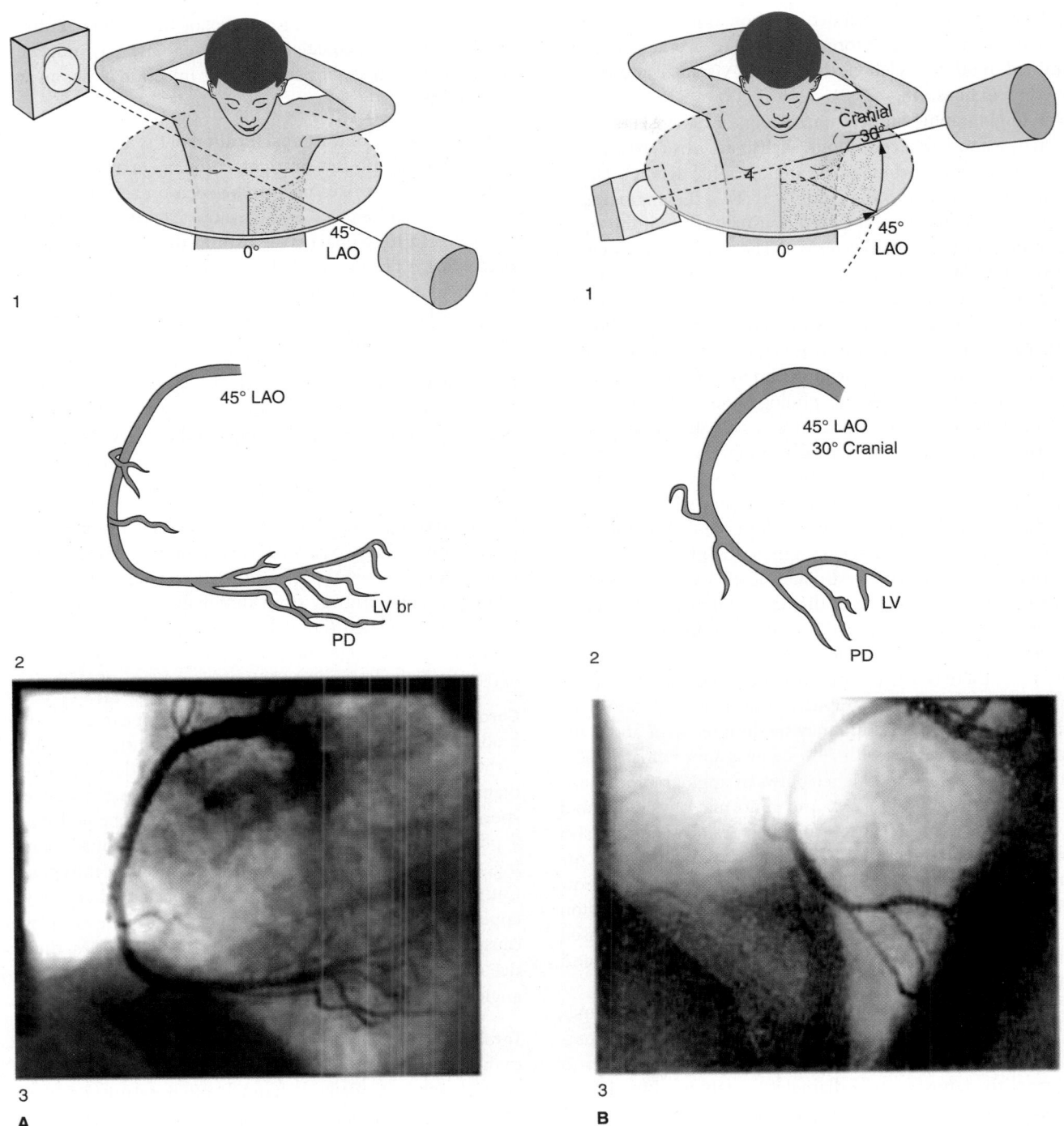

Figure 3–8. Diagrammatic illustration of the direction of the x-ray beam and the right coronary artery in the 45-degree left anterior oblique (LAO) projection. This view is excellent for visualizing the proximal mid- and distal-right coronary artery in the atrioventricular groove, because the direction of the x-ray beam is perpendicular to these arterial segments. Ostial lesions of the right coronary artery are now well visualized if the proximal right coronary artery takes an anterior direction from the aorta and therefore originates in a direction parallel to the x-ray beam. This usually can be overcome by turning to a more severe left oblique projection. The posterior descending (PD) and left ventricular (LV) branches of the right coronary artery, which pass down the posterior aspect of the heart toward the apex, are severely foreshortened because the long axis of these vessels is in the same direction as the x-ray beam. The proximal PD branches can be visualized by cranial angulation of the overhead intensifier or from a right oblique view. The image intensifier is in the standard LAO position. Lesions in the PD or LV branches can be well visualized. When the right coronary artery originates anteriorly from the aorta, the proximal portion of the vessel is frequently well seen in this projection.

vessels are missing, an occluded or anomalous artery should be suspected. Vessels with foreshortening or overlap should be examined in other angled views to better visualize and resolve the region in question.

An angiographic lumen narrowing or stenosis may be caused by a number of conditions, such as atherosclerosis, vasospasm, dissection, thrombus, or angiographic artifact. Unlike computed tomographic angiography (CTA), the angiogram is a lumenogram and does not permit visualization of the vessel wall to demonstrate atherosclerosis. The grading of a stenosis is most commonly reported as the percentage reduction in the diameter of the narrowed vessel site compared to the adjacent unobstructed vessel segment. Although the diameter stenosis is calculated in the projection where the greatest narrowing is seen, an exact percent narrowing is impossible because many stenoses have an eccentric morphology and a 2D image does not accurately reflect the importance of only the worst luminal dimension. Comparison with nearby unobstructed lumen may be complicated that this is ectatic or diffusely narrowed and thus appears *angiographically* normal but may still be diseased. In addition, angiographically *normal* adjacent proximal segments may be larger than distal segments, explaining the large disparity between observer estimates of stenosis severity. Area stenosis is always greater than diameter stenosis and assumes the lumen is circular, whereas in reality the lumen is usually eccentric. Because of the subjective nature of visual lesion assessment, there is a ±20% variation between readings of two or more experienced angiographers, especially for lesions narrowed by 40% to 70%. There may be disagreement about the number of major vessels with 70% stenosis approximately 30% of the time. The correspondence between angiographic diameter narrowings of 40% to 75% and abnormal physiology and myocardial ischemia is poor. For such lesions, noninvasive (stress testing) or direct physiologic measurements (intracoronary pressure or flow, specifically at this time fractional flow reserve [FFR]) of impaired. Other features of a coronary lesion (eg, eccentricity, distribution of calcifications, true diseased segment length) may not be appreciated by angiography and require IVUS or OCT imaging.

The degree of coronary stenosis is usually a visual estimation of the percentage of diameter narrowing using the proximal assumed normal arterial segment as a reference. The ratio of normal-to-stenosis artery diameter, widely used in clinical practice, is inadequate for a true quantitative methodology. The intraobserver variability may range between 40% and 80%, and there is frequently a range as wide as 20% on interobserver differences. Quantitative methodologies include digital calipers, automated or manual edge detection systems, or densitometric analysis with digital angiography and are principally used for research where consistency of imaging is required.

Pitfalls and Artifacts

There are a number of pitfalls and artifacts that make the performance and interpretation of coronary arteriography unreliable.

Short Left Main: When the left main orifice is very short or absent, the LAD or circumflex artery may be selectively injected. The absence of circumflex or LAD filling, either primarily or through collaterals from the RCA, may indicate that the artery was missed by subselective injection or has an anomalous location.

Ostial Lesions: Contrast opacification of the aorta may obscure the origins of the left or right coronary artery ostium. The aortocoronary orifices need to be seen on a tangent with the opacified aortic sinuses. Some contrast reflux from the orifices is needed to fully opacify the ostium to see whether an ostial narrowing is present. Catheter pressure damping may indicate that there an ostial stenosis but may reflect the acute upward angle of the catheter into the wall of the coronary artery with transient tip occlusion.

Myocardial Bridges: The LAD, diagonal, and marginal branches occasionally run an intramyocardial course. The overlying myocardium may compress the artery during systole. If the coronary artery is not viewed carefully in diastole, this bridging may give the appearance of a stenosis.

Foreshortening: Foreshortening is the viewing of a vessel in plane with its long axis. Vessels seen on end cannot display a lesion along its length. When possible, arteries that are seen coming toward or away from the image intensifier should be viewed in angulated (cranial/caudal) views. The dense opacification of vessel segments seen end-on-end may produce the appearance of a lesion in an intervening segment.

Coronary Spasm: Coronary spasm can appear as an angiographic narrowing, provoked by mechanical stimulation, acetylcholine, cold pressor testing, or hyperventilation. Definitive diagnosis is demonstrated by relief of the narrowing either spontaneously or by nitrate administration. The end point of a pharmacologic provocative test is focal coronary narrowing, which can be reversed with intracoronary nitroglycerin. Catheter-induced spasm should be suspected when the vessel appears normal except at a location near the catheter tip, which causes mechanical stimulation. In most laboratories, the practice of giving intracoronary nitroglycerin (100–200 μg) before angiography is used to eliminate catheter-related spasm.

Totally Occluded Arteries or Vein Grafts: Absence of vascularity in a portion of the heart may indicate total occlusion of its arterial supply. Collateral channels often permit visualization of the distal occluded artery. Vessels filled solely by collaterals are under low pressure and may appear smaller than their actual lumen size. This finding should not exclude the possibilities for surgical anastomosis.

Collateral Circulation: The opacification of a totally or subtotally (99%) occluded vessel from antegrade or retrograde filling is defined as *collateral filling*. Advances in the ability to open chronically occluded total occlusions have made the appreciation and visualization of collateral pathways a key to the success of this new approach. It is useful but difficult to establish the size of the recipient vessel exactly, whether the collateral circulation is ipsilateral (eg, same side filling, proximal RCA to distal RCA collateral supply) or contralateral (eg, opposite side filling, LAD to distal RCA collateral supply). Identification of exactly which region is affected by collateral supply will influence decisions regarding management of stenoses in the artery feeding the collateral supply. Collateral vessel evaluation is important for making decisions regarding which vessels might be protected or lost during coronary angioplasty.

Anomalous Coronary Arteries: Coronary arteries may arise from anomalous locations, or a single coronary artery may be present. Only by ensuring that the entire epicardial surface has an adequate arterial supply can one be confident that all branches have been visualized. Misdiagnosis of unsuspected anomalous origin of the coronary arteries is a potential problem for any angiographer. Because the natural history of a patient with an anomalous origin of a coronary artery may be dependent on the initial course of the anomalous vessel, it is the angiographer's responsibility to define accurately the origin and course of the vessel. It is an error to assume that a vessel is occluded when in fact it has not been visualized because of an anomalous origin. It is often difficult even for experienced angiographers to delineate the true course of an anomalous vessel. Alternative imaging modalities such as MRI angiography or CTA can provide information on the course of anomalous coronary arteries and their relationship to surrounding structures.

Measurements of Coronary Blood Flow and Pressure

The next section (Intravascular Imaging) summarizes coronary imaging modalities that can be used in the catheterization laboratory today (**Fig. 3–9**). However, the rationale for measuring coronary blood flow and pressure arises from the failure of angiographic or any anatomic imaging modality to accurately predict the ischemic potential of a stenosis. For the intermediately narrowed angiographic stenosis (30%–80% diameter stenosis), the visual identification of whether a lesion is flow-limiting is guesswork. This limitation of angiography has been documented repeatedly by poor correlations to stress testing (approximately 60% accuracy) and is attributable to the anatomic complexity of the atherosclerotic lumen.

Coronary angiography produces a 2D silhouette image of the 3D vascular lumen. Angiography does not provide vascular wall detail sufficient to characterize plaque size, length, and eccentricity. The eccentric lumen produces conflicting degrees of angiographic narrowing when viewed from different angulations, causing uncertainty related to lumen size and its impact on coronary blood flow. Moreover, there are at least six morphologic features that determine resistance to flow, most of which cannot be measured with the angiogram or even IVUS (**Fig. 3–10**).

Angiographically Estimated Coronary Blood Flow

The initial angiographic assessment of flow was inexact. Myocardial blood flow can be assessed angiographically using the thrombolysis in myocardial infarction (TIMI) score for qualitative grading of coronary flow into grades 0 to 3. In acute MI trials, TIMI grade 3 flows have been associated with improved clinical outcomes. Based on cineangiography with 6-Fr catheters and filming at 30 frames per second, the four grades of flow are described as follows:[25]

1. Flow equal to that in noninfarct arteries (TIMI-3)
2. Distal flow in the artery less than noninfarct arteries (TIMI-2)
3. Filling beyond the culprit lesion but no antegrade flow (TIMI-1)
4. No flow beyond the total occlusion (TIMI-0)

The TIMI frame count can further be quantitated for the length of the LAD relative to the two other major arteries; this is called the corrected TIMI frame count.

Coronary Blood Flow and Resistance

In contrast to the anatomic approach, a physiologic approach to lesion assessment examines the specific hemodynamic responses of flow across a stenosis. Such an approach has now been determined in clinical trials to improve outcomes after percutaneous coronary intervention (PCI), making physiologic lesion assessment a best practice to support the decision to proceed with PCI. There are two coronary physiologic tools

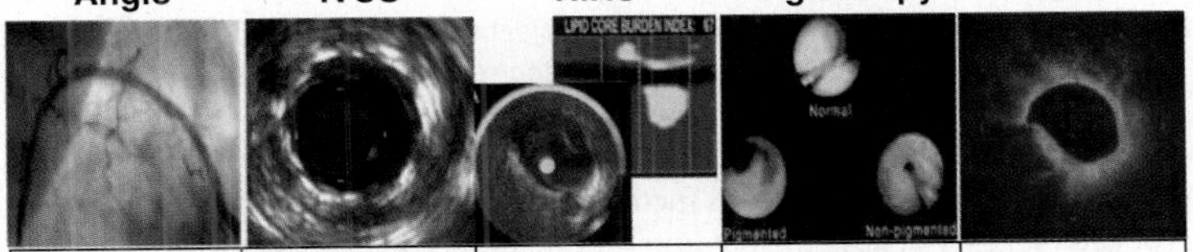

	Angio	IVUS	NIRS	Angioscopy	OCT
Resolution (μm)	100–200	80–120	=	< 200	10–15
Probe size (μm)	N/A	700	1000	800	140
Contact	No	Yes	Yes	Yes	Yes
Ionizing radiation	Yes	No	No	No	No
Other	Lumen only	N/A	N/A	Surface only	Plaque character

Figure 3–9. Comparison of coronary imaging devices in the catheterization laboratory. Angio, coronary angiography; IVUS, intravascular ultrasound imaging; NIRS, near infrared spectroscopy; OCT optical coherence tomography. Reproduced with permission from Kern MJ. *The Interventional Cardiac Catheterization Handbook,* 3rd ed. Philadelphia, PA: Elsevier; 2013.

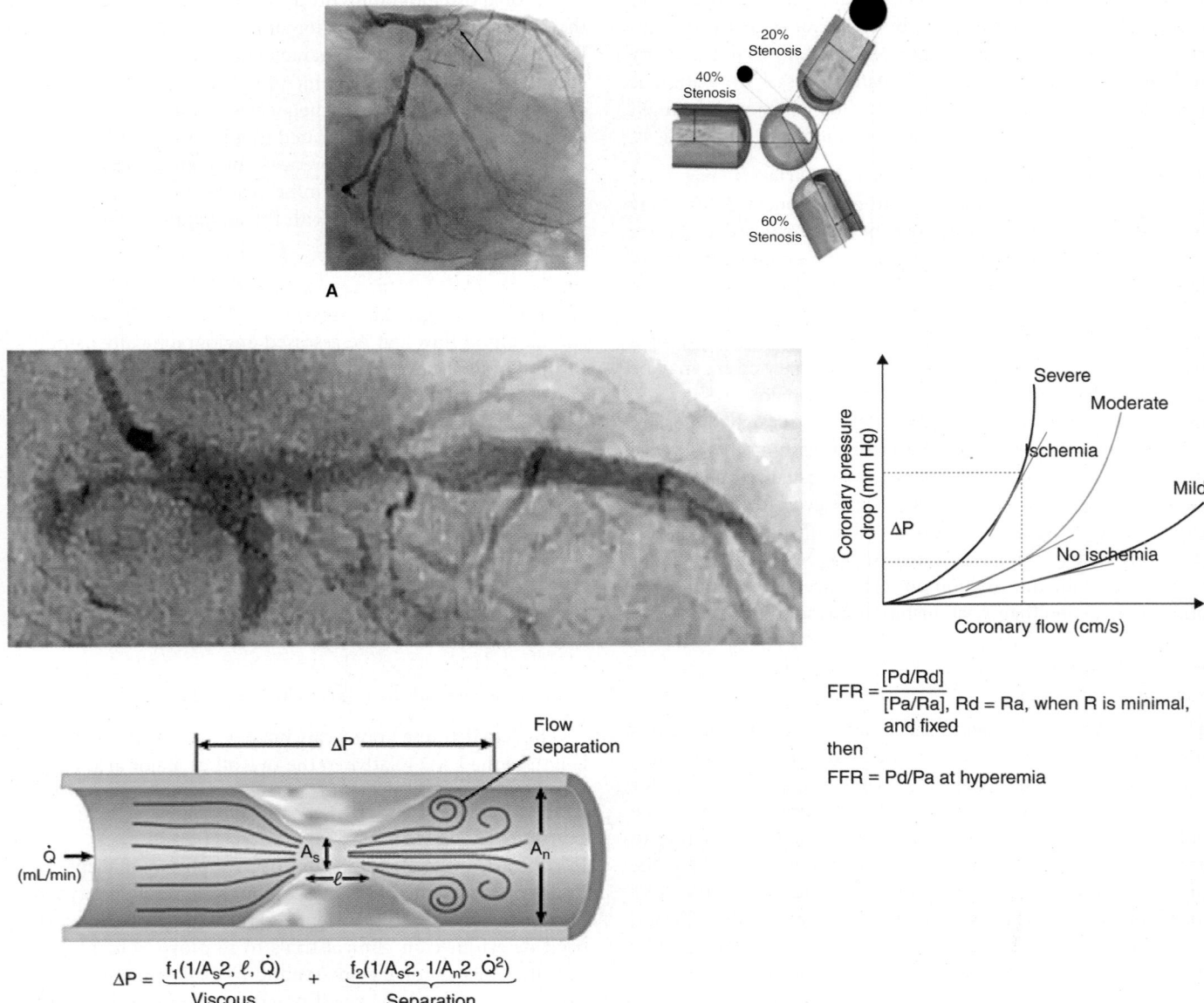

Figure 3–10. (**A**) *Left*, cineangiographic frame showing the left coronary artery with a severe lesion in the circumflex artery (*red arrow*) and moderate lesion in the left anterior descending coronary artery (*black arrow*). *Right*, diagram of eccentric lesion with three different angiographic projections in which the lumen may be assessed as mild, moderate, or severe depending on which projection is accepted. Because of the two-dimensional image projection, the severity of some lesions, especially those in the intermediate range, do not reflect the flow impairment and thus require fractional flow reserve (FFR) for accurate assessment. (**B**) Coronary pressure and flow measurements and the relationship determines the ischemic potential of a stenosis. *Top left*, cineangiogram frame showing stenosis. There are seven features that contribute to resistance to flow, length being only one. *Bottom left*, diagram of a stenosis and factors that equate the change in pressure to two factors of viscous friction and energy loss due to flow separation, right translesional pressure drop compared to change in flow (horizontal). For each severity of flow, the pressure-flow relationship becomes steeper.

available in the catheterization laboratory: (1) coronary pressure wire and microcatheter systems and (2) Doppler and thermodilution flow wires (which are principally research tools to study the microcirculation).[26,27]

Coronary blood flow can increase from a resting level to a maximum depending on increases in myocardial oxygen demand or in response to neurogenic or pharmacologic hyperemic stimuli. The ratio of maximal-to-basal flow is coronary flow reserve (CFR), or coronary vasodilatory reserve (CVR).

Resistance to flow increase occurs at three levels: epicardial conduits (R1), precapillary arterioles (R2), and intramyocardial resistance (R3). Normally, large epicardial vessel resistance (R1) is trivial. Most coronary flow is regulated by the myocardial precapillary arteriolar resistance vessels (R2). In a normal artery supplying normal myocardium, CFR can exceed three. However, several conditions, including LV hypertrophy (LVH), myocardial ischemia, and diabetes, can affect the microcirculatory resistance R3, blunting the maximal absolute increase in

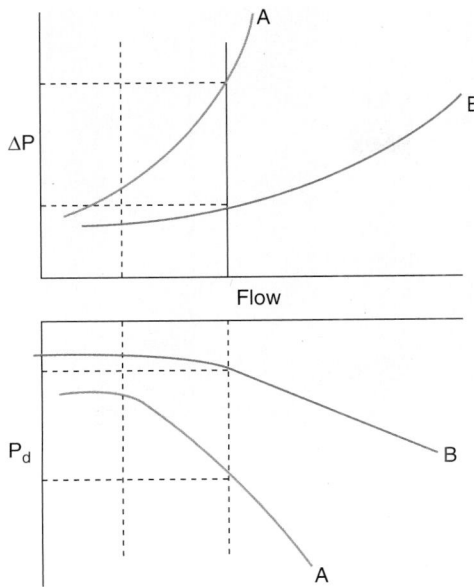

Figure 3–11. Coronary pressure-flow relationships for two stenoses of the same angiographic severity. *Top,* pressure gradient (aortic-distal coronary pressure; ΔP) versus coronary flow. *Bottom,* Absolute distal coronary pressure (P_d) versus flow. Increasing flow produces marked loss of P_d as well as an increase in ΔP. The loss of P_d in absolute terms determines myocardial perfusion pressure (P_d venous pressure) and the potential for inducible ischemia.

coronary flow. Increased R3 resistance may also be associated with increased resting flow above the expected level for myocardial oxygen demand at rest, also resulting in reduced CFR.

Significant atherosclerotic stenosis produces epicardial conduit resistance. In parallel with resistance to flow, viscous friction, flow separation forces, and flow turbulence at the site of the stenosis produce pressure loss at the stenosis. The pressure loss increases with increasing coronary flow along an exponential pressure–flow relationship of the specific coronary stenosis resistance[26] (**Fig. 3–11**). In response to the loss of perfusion pressure and flow to the distal microcirculation bed, precapillary resistance vessels (R2) dilate to maintain satisfactory basal flow appropriate for myocardial oxygen demand. However, there exists an absolute poststenotic myocardial perfusion pressure threshold below which myocardial ischemia occurs. The hemodynamic significance of a given stenosis can be measured by the pressure–flow relationship using sensor angioplasty guidewires.[27]

Pressure-Derived Fractional Flow Reserve

FFR is the preferred method for in-laboratory coronary stenosis assessment (**Fig. 3–12**). This pressure-derived ratio is an easily measured surrogate of coronary blood flow and has proven to be the most useful adjunctive test in the catheterization laboratory. It is derived from fairly straightforward principles. Myocardial perfusion is primarily dependent on coronary blood flow as determined by the interaction between the driving pressure and the three major coronary vascular resistances, based on the equation Flow = ΔPressure/Resistance

Pijls et al.[28] and De Bruyne et al.[29] defined the FFR as the ratio of coronary blood flow through a stenotic artery compared with the normal blood flow in the theoretical absence of

the stenosis. Stated another way, FFR represents that fraction of normal maximum flow that remains despite the presence of an epicardial lesion.

$$FFR = \text{Myocardial flow } (Q_s) \text{ across stenosis/Myocardial flow } (Q_n) \text{ without stenosis}$$

$$FFR = Q_s/Q_n = (P_d - P_v/R_s)/(P_a - P_v/R_n)$$

If the myocardial bed resistances are induced pharmacologically to maximal hyperemia and remain constant, then the resistances of the vessels become equivalent. The poststenotic hyperemic coronary artery pressure is linearly related to flow and represents the maximal achievable perfusion available in that vessel.

$$FFR = (P_d - P_v)/(P_a - P_v)$$

where P_a = mean aortic pressure, P_d = mean distal coronary pressure, and P_v = mean venous or RA pressure. For daily clinical practice, assuming P_v is negligible relative to P_a, FFR can be easily estimated by a simplified ratio of pressures and expressed as:

$$FFR = P_d - P_a$$

An FFR value of 0.6 means that the maximum myocardial flow across the stenosis is only 60% of what it should be without the stenosis. An FFR of 0.9 after PCI means that the maximum flow to the myocardium is 90% of a completely normal vessel.

Unlike most other physiologic indexes, FFR has a normal value of 1.0 for every patient and every coronary artery. Despite findings in animal studies defining an effect of heart rate and arterial pressure, human studies did not show significant changes in FFR with changes in heart rate, blood pressure, or contractility. FFR has a high reproducibility and low intraindividual variability. Moreover, FFR, unlike CFR, is independent of sex or CAD risk factors such as hypertension and diabetes, and has less variability with common doses of adenosine. FFR reflects both antegrade and collateral myocardial perfusion rather than merely transstenotic pressure loss (ie, a stenosis pressure gradient). Because it is calculated only at peak hyperemia, FFR is also differentiated from CFR by being largely independent of basal flow, driving pressure, heart rate, systemic blood pressure, or status of the microcirculation. The FFR, but not the resting pressure or hyperemic pressure gradient, is strongly related to provocable myocardial ischemia, demonstrated by comparisons to different clinical stress testing modalities in patients with stable angina.

Coronary Flow Velocity Reserve

Coronary flow velocity reserve is used to study the microcirculation. Because CFR is the result of flow through both the conduit and the microvascular bed, CFR is useful for coronary lesion assessment only when normal. For this reason, FFR is the preferred in-laboratory technique for physiologic lesion assessment.

CFR measures the capacity of the two-component system of the R1 coronary artery resistance and the R2 vascular resistance to achieve maximal blood flow in response to a given hyperemic stimulation. Normal CFR in young patients with IVUS-demonstrated normal arteries commonly exceeds 3.0.

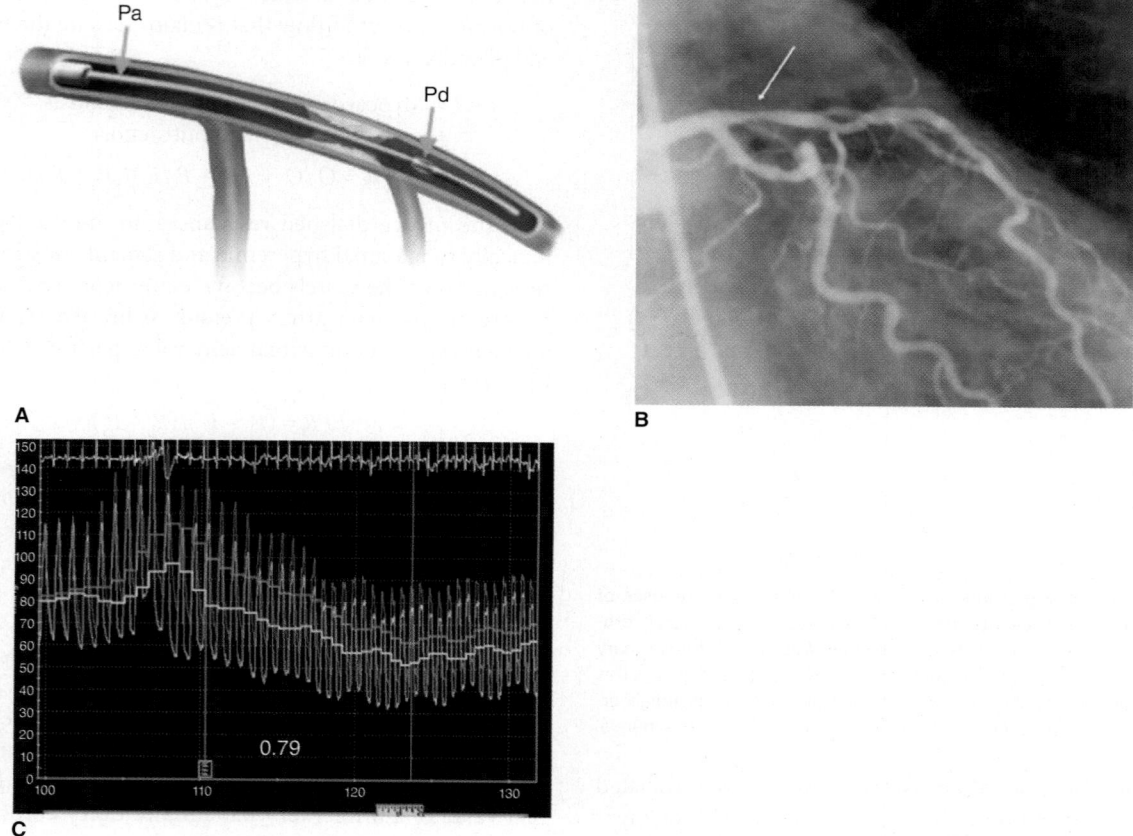

Figure 3–12. Method of measuring fractional flow reserve (FFR). (A) Diagram of coronary artery and pressure wire across stenosis **(B)**. **(C)** FFR tracing phasic and mean pressure signals used to measure FFR, calculated as the ratio of distal coronary pressure (Pd) to aortic pressure (Pa) at maximal hyperemia, which is equal to 0.79, the point of lowest Pd/Pa ratio.

In patients with chest pain undergoing cardiac catheterization with angiographically normal vessels, the normal CFR is 2.7 ± 0.6,[30] suggesting some degree of patient-to-patient variability and distal microvascular disease. The values for CFR associated with nonobstructed coronary arteries in patients with chest pain syndromes, in patients with transplanted hearts, and in normal arteries in patients with obstructive CAD elsewhere are 2.8 ± 0.6, 3.1 ± 0.9, and 2.5 ± 0.95, respectively.[30] The incidence of impaired coronary vasodilatory reserve of less than 2.0 in 450 angiographically normal coronary arteries from 220 patients undergoing evaluation for chest pain or cardiac transplant follow-up angiography is approximately 12%.[30]

Unlike FFR, CFR is subject to variations in hemodynamics that may alter resting flow and limit maximal hyperemic flow. Tachycardia increases basal flow; therefore, CFR is reduced by 10% for every 15 heart beats. Increasing mean arterial pressure reduces maximal vasodilatation, thus reducing hyperemia with less alteration in basal flow. CFR may be reduced in patients with essential hypertension or AS. Vasoconstrictor, neurologic, or humoral influences, endothelial dysfunction, and extracardiac vasoconstrictor stimuli may produce dynamic or episodic ischemia-related symptoms with activities of daily life, such as exercise, emotional stress, or adrenergic stimulation.

The variability in CFR in nonobstructed arteries may also be due to age.[25] **Table 3–8** lists pathologies associated with impairment of the microcirculation.

Ventriculography and Angiographic Studies

Left Ventriculography

Left ventriculography is the standard method for evaluating LV function in the cardiac catheterization laboratory. Standard left

TABLE 3–8. Pathologies Impairing the Microcirculation
Abnormal vascular reactivity
Abnormal myocardial metabolism
Abnormal sensitivity toward vasoactive substances
Coronary vasospasm
Myocardial infarction
Hypertrophy
Vasculitis syndromes
Hypertension
Diabetes
Recurrent ischemia

Reproduced with permission from Baumgart D, Haude M, Liu F, et al. Current concepts of coronary flow reserve for clinical decision making during cardiac catheterization. *Am Heart J.* 1998 Jul;136(1):136-149.

Left ventriculogram—wall segments

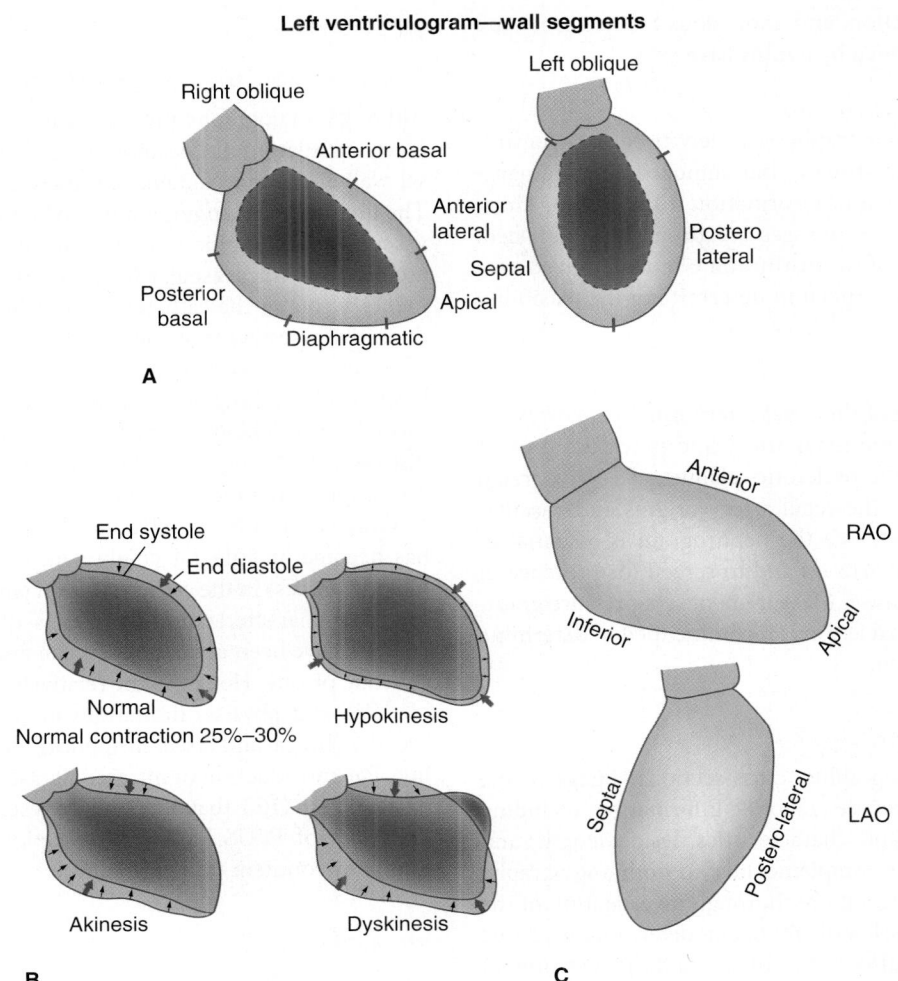

Figure 3–13. (**A**) Left ventricular wall silhouette in right anterior oblique (RAO) and left anterior oblique (LAO) views. (**B**) Types of ventricular asynergy. (**C**) Diagrammatic representation of the zones of the left ventricular inner wall in the RAO (above) and LAO (below) left ventriculograms.

ventriculographic views are (1) a 30-degree RAO that visualizes the high lateral, anterior, apical, and inferior LV walls and (2) a 45- to 60-degree LAO, 20 degrees of cranial angulation that best identifies the lateral and septal LV walls. Because the left ventriculographic is a 2D silhouette, visibility is limited to five RAO segments and two LAO LV segments (**Fig. 3–13**). The LAO with cranial angulation provides a view of the interventricular septum, projected on edge and tilted downward to give the best view of VSDs and septal wall motion. An elongated RAO view, which is useful for seeing the RV infundibulum and supracristal VSD, is obtained by a 30-degree axial RAO and 40 degrees of cranial angulation. The main PA and its bifurcation are seen in the frontal position with 30 degrees of cranial angulation; a steep LAO position with marked cranial angulation is also used.

Although mitral and aortic regurgitation can be qualitatively assessed by contrast opacification of the LV and aortic root, respectively, better noninvasive tools have superseded quantification by these methods.

Right Ventriculography

Indications for right ventriculography (including documentation of tricuspid regurgitation, RV dysplasia for arrhythmias, pulmonary stenosis, abnormalities of pulmonary outflow tract, and RV-to-LV shunts) have largely been taken over by noninvasive techniques.

Ascending and Abdominal Aortography

For abdominal aneurysms, a lateral projection is commonly needed, especially if stent graft repair of abdominal aortic aneurysm is being considered. Evaluation of peripheral lower extremity disease requires identification of iliac bifurcation and common FA patency before selective injections. The contraindications of abdominal aortography are the same as those of thoracic aortography.

Pulmonary Angiography

Visualization of vascular abnormalities of the lung vessels (eg, intraluminal defects representing pulmonary emboli, shunts, stenosis, AV malformation, and anomalous connections), are now more readily obtained by noninvasive tests.

Peripheral Vascular Angiography

Digital subtraction angiography is widely used for identifying peripheral vascular disease, but standard cineangiography can provide satisfactory information if the filming time, frame rates, and contrast dosages are properly established. Determining the level of reconstitution of collateralized vessels and distal runoff is crucial in determining the feasibility of revascularization.

Renal Arteriography

Atherosclerotic disease of the renal artery usually involves the proximal one-third of the renal artery and is seldom present without abdominal atherosclerotic plaques. Selective renal arteriography evaluates the renal artery origins and vasculature. Delayed imaging to see the nephrogram is essential to exclude accessory renal arteries and to screen for presence of severe parenchymal disease. Measurement of a pressure gradient across ostial proximal lesion is recommended to determine the need for intervention.

Other Coronary Imaging

IVUS generates a tomographic, cross-sectional image of the vessel and lumen, to provide anatomic information, including plaque quantification and characteristics, lesion length, and lumen dimensions. It is complementary to both angiography and physiology, allowing a more thorough investigation of the disease within the vessel wall. By better determining plaque characteristics, IVUS also is useful in guiding selection of interventional equipment.

Intracoronary OCT is a catheter-based optical imaging modality employing near-infrared light, providing high-resolution (10- to 20-mcm) cross-sectional images of the coronary wall. The OCT catheter is nearly identical to an IVUS catheter except that the fiberoptic imaging core replaces the ultrasound imaging core. Compared to IVUS, OCT has superior resolution to evaluate certain features of the vulnerable plaque, such as plaque rupture, intracoronary thrombus, thin-capped fibroatheroma, and macrophages within the fibrous caps. For stent placement, OCT can visualize stent malapposition and tissue protrusion after stenting and neointimal hyperplasia at late follow-up. One drawback of OCT in comparison to IVUS is its shallow depth of penetration (1–2 mm), limiting assessment of plaque composition.

Summary—Cardiac Catheterization

Measurements of coronary physiology strongly complement coronary luminography and permit exploration of the coronary microcirculation, collateral flow, MI physiology, and mechanisms of interventions for CAD. The evaluation of CAD in the cardiac catheterization laboratory necessitates that the operator defines ischemia-producing coronary lesions. Angiography alone is often insufficient and not specific enough to characterize an individual coronary stenosis.

INTRAVASCULAR IMAGING

Rationale for Intravascular Imaging

Although angiography provides a quick road map of the coronary circulation, it does not provide visualization of the vessel wall and is not suitable for assessment of atherosclerosis. The limitations of angiography can be minimized by the intravascular tomographic visualization of lumen and vessel wall architecture. Intravascular imaging plays an essential complementary role in the catheterization laboratory, enabling more definitive assessment of angiographically intermediate disease, of vessels with aneurysmal dilatation, ostial stenoses, or disease located at branching points or in the left main artery, as well as tortuous or calcified segments and eccentric plaques, complex disease morphology, intraluminal filling defects, thrombus, dissection, and lumen dimensions after coronary intervention.

Grayscale IVUS was introduced more than 25 years ago and has become an integral component of the clinical decision-making process in the catheterization laboratory. Features such as tissue characterization by means of radiofrequency data analysis have been added to facilitate evaluation of the atherosclerotic plaque. However, the relatively poor image resolution of IVUS and physical limitations of sound have hampered a broader clinical and research application of intravascular imaging. The introduction of infrared light-based imaging technologies such as OCT that offers image resolution 10 times greater than that of IVUS has allowed exploration of the vascular microenvironment for the first time.

Intravascular Ultrasound

Basic Principles

The final graphic image display of IVUS is a result of reflected ultrasound waves that are converted to electrical signals and sent to an external processing system for amplification, filtering, and scan conversion. The axial resolution of IVUS is approximately 100 μm, and lateral resolution reaches 200 to 250 μm in conventional IVUS systems (20–45 MHz).

IVUS equipment consists of a catheter incorporating a miniaturized transducer and a console to reconstruct and display the image (lately, these consoles have been incorporated into catheterization laboratory equipment for easier operation). Current catheters range from 2.6 to 3.2 Fr in size and can be introduced through conventional 6-Fr guide catheters. Rotational, mechanical IVUS catheters operate at frequencies between 30 and 45 MHz, and provide better image resolution than electronic phased-array systems operating at a frequency of approximately 20 MHz. In general, mechanical probes offer superior image quality and have a better crossing profile, but electronic catheter designs are slightly easier to set up and use.

Spectral analysis of IVUS backscattered data has been incorporated into conventional IVUS systems to facilitate image interpretation of different tissue components (**Fig. 3–14**). This function displays different plaque components in a color-coded scheme according to tissue signal properties (necrotic core in red, dense calcium in white, fibrous in dark green,

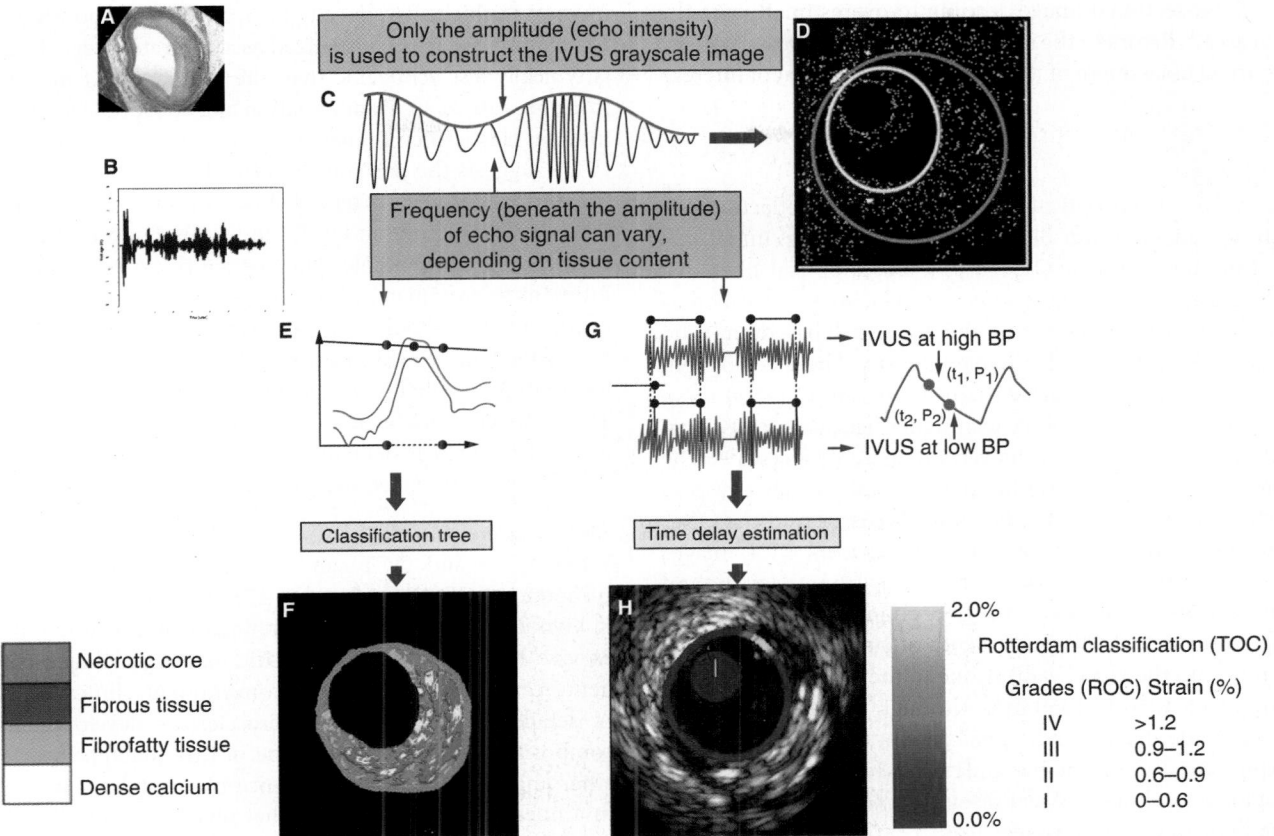

Figure 3–14. The ultrasound signal is generated in a piezoelectric crystal that transmits and receives sound waves (A). Ultrasound reflected by the tissue deforms crystal generating radiofrequency (RF) signal (B). Grayscale intravascular ultrasound (IVUS) is derived from the amplitude of RF signal, discarding information beneath the peaks of the signal (C). Changes in the electric field of the piezoelectric crystal caused by ultrasound reflection is used to generate a gray image (D). IVUS RF analysis uses several additional spectral parameters to identify four plaque components (E). Plaque components that are identified are dense calcium (*white*), fibrous (*green*), fibrofatty (*greenish-yellow*), and necrotic core (*red*) (F). IVUS palpography takes advantage of RF signals generated by the artery being deformed by blood pressure (BP). Using analysis of RF signals at "low" and "high" BP, the strain (deformation) in the inner layer of atheroma is determined (G). This strain is quantified and superimposed on the IVUS image at the lumen–vessel wall boundary (H). Note that high strain (*yellow*) is found at the shoulders of the eccentric plaque.

and fibrofatty in light green).[31] IVUS-VH (virtual histology) imaging has been extensively used in clinical trials to monitor progression of atherosclerosis and to predict plaque growth, providing for the first time evidence that plaque composition carries significant prognostic information.[32] IVUS palpography provides insight into the mechanical properties of plaque, based on deformability using the analysis of radiofrequency signals at different diastolic pressure levels. Although the resulting "strain" image allows detection of vulnerable plaques, this may not be prognostically important.[34]

Safety

IVUS has been performed safely in research studies, with no apparent increase in the incidence of adverse effects. In 2207 patients from 28 centers, 63 patients (2.9%) had transient vasospasm, and 9 (0.4%) had complications were judged to be related to the IVUS procedure (occlusion, dissection, and embolism). The complication rate was higher in patients with unstable angina or acute MI and in patients undergoing intervention compared with diagnostic IVUS.[35] In these high-risk populations, the complications caused by IVUS imaging were

1.6% in the PROSPECT study and only 0.6% in the PREDICTION study.[36,37]

Limitations and Image Artifacts

The similar appearance of different materials represents an inherent limitation of all grayscale IVUS systems. For example, an echolucent intraluminal image may represent thrombus, atheroma with a high lipid content, retained contrast, or an air bubble. Most mechanical limitations of IVUS imaging are specific to the design of each system.[38] The *ring-down* artifact is specific to electronic systems and is caused by transducer oscillations that obscure the near-field image. The *side lobe* artifact is an intense reflection that comes from strong reflectors, such as calcium and stent struts. This usually follows the circumferential sweep of the beam. The presence of the side lobes may mask the actual lumen edge or may also be taken as tissue prolapse or dissection flaps. *Reverberation* is another artifact that comes from strong reflectors and is concentric repetitions at equidistant locations of the same image. Eccentric or nonperpendicular position of the IVUS catheter can produce geometric distortions and an artificially elliptical appearance of the cross-sectional image, leading to overestimation of the lumen area.[38] Errors in the speed of catheter pullback may lead to incorrect assessment of the length of the segment of interest.

Optical Coherence Tomography

Basic Principles

OCT evolved from optical 1D, low-coherence reflectometry, which was adapted into B-scans and 2D imaging, initially of the retina. Intravascular OCT uses a single optical fiber that both emits and records light reflection. The image is formed by the backscattering of light from the vessel wall based on "echo time delay" with measurable signal intensity. The speed of light (3×10^8 m/s) is much faster than that of sound (1500 m/s), thus requiring interferometry techniques because direct signal quantification cannot be achieved on such a time scale. The interferometer uses a fiberoptic coupler similar to a beam splitter, which directs half of the beam to the tissue and the other half to the reference arm, used for comparison. OCT images are formed by the reflected signal returning from the tissue and reference arms "interferes" in the fiber coupler and are detected by a photodetector. The image depth of current OCT systems (1–3 mm into the vessel wall) is due to the use of wavelengths ranging from 1250 to 1350 nm. Although longer wavelengths would provide deeper tissue penetration, they are limited by absorption and the refractive index caused by protein, water, hemoglobin, and lipids. Axial resolution, which is determined by the light wavelength, ranges from 12 to 20 μm. The lateral resolution in catheter-based OCT is typically 20 to 90 μm.

Safety

Safety concerns are mainly dependent on mechanical properties and need for blood clearance for image acquisition. Transient chest pain and QRS widening or ST-segment depression or elevation are quite common, but major complications are rare.[39]

Limitations and Image Artifacts

Image artifacts are common to both OCT and IVUS, including focal image loss and shape distortion. Residual blood produces light attenuation and may defocus the beam if the red blood cell density is high. This reduces the brightness of the vessel wall.

Other Techniques

Near-infrared spectroscopy (NIRS) has enabled more reliable assessment of plaque composition and detection of the lipid component. Other emerging invasive imaging techniques, such as Raman spectroscopy photoacoustic imaging, near-infrared fluorescence imaging, and time-resolved fluorescence spectroscopy, are currently under development (**Fig. 3–15**).

Imaging of Coronary Artery Structure

Normal

The normal coronary architecture can be assessed using intravascular imaging. The circulating blood elements may assist IVUS image interpretation and differentiate the lumen from the vessel wall because these produce characteristic speckles in the image. The reported normal value for intimal thickness in young subjects is typically 0.15 ± 0.07 mm, poorly reflects ultrasound and is not visualized as a separate layer. The media is typically less echogenic than the intima, but it may appear thick because of signal attenuation and weak reflectivity of the internal elastic membrane (IEM). A trilayered appearance by IVUS suggests the presence of intimal thickening. In contrast, the normal coronary artery wall (<1.5 mm thick) appears as a three-layer structure on OCT, but imaging beyond the adventitial layer is not possible. The normal thickness of the tunica intima is approximately 4 μm (beyond the resolution capacity of current OCT systems) so the first visualized layer is the internal elastic lamina (IEL) (not seen by IVUS), which despite its less than 3-μm thickness, generates a 20-μm signal-rich band. The relatively thick media (>100 μm) can be visualized easily by OCT,[40] which is depicted as a low-intensity band between the IEL and external elastic lamina (EEL).

Atheroma

While IVUS and OCT can differentiate coronary atheroma components (**Figs. 3–16** and **3–17**), it should be stressed that in vivo intravascular imaging is fundamentally different from ex vivo histology and that specific histologic plaque components cannot be assessed by conventional clinical imaging. A detailed description of atherosclerosis development and composition is beyond the scope of this chapter. In brief, an atheroma is formed by a sequence of events, not necessarily in a linear chronologic order, that involves extracellular lipid accumulation, endothelial dysfunction, leukocyte recruitment, intracellular lipid accumulation (foam cells), smooth muscle cell migration and proliferation, expansion of extracellular matrix, neoangiogenesis, tissue necrosis, and mineralization at later stages. The ultimate characteristic of an atherosclerotic plaque at any given time depends on the relative contribution of each of these features.[41] Pathologic intimal thickening (PIT) is rich in proteoglycans and lipid pools, but no trace of necrotic core is seen. The earliest lesion with a necrotic core is fibroatheroma (FA), and this is the precursor lesion that may give rise to symptomatic heart disease. Thin-cap fibroatheroma (TCFA) is a lesion characterized by a large necrotic core containing cholesterol clefts. The overlying fibrous cap is thin and rich in inflammatory cells, macrophages, and T lymphocytes, with few smooth muscle cells. A cutoff value for cap thickness of less than 65 μm has been suggested by histology studies to define a thin cap vulnerable coronary plaque.[42]

Based on tissue echogenicity, not necessarily histologic composition, atheromas have been classified into four categories by grayscale IVUS: (1) soft plaque (lesion echogenicity less than the surrounding adventitia), (2) fibrous plaque (intermediate echogenicity between soft [echolucent] atheromas and highly echogenic calcified plaques), (3) calcified plaque (echogenicity higher than the adventitia with acoustic shadowing), and (4) mixed plaques (no single acoustical subtype represents >80% of the plaque)[38] (see Fig. 3–29).

IVUS-VH can potentially identify all of the previously mentioned plaque types.[43] **Figure 3–18** outlines the VH plaque and lesion types that are proposed based on the histological data. Intravascular ultrasound-derived thin-cap fibroatheroma

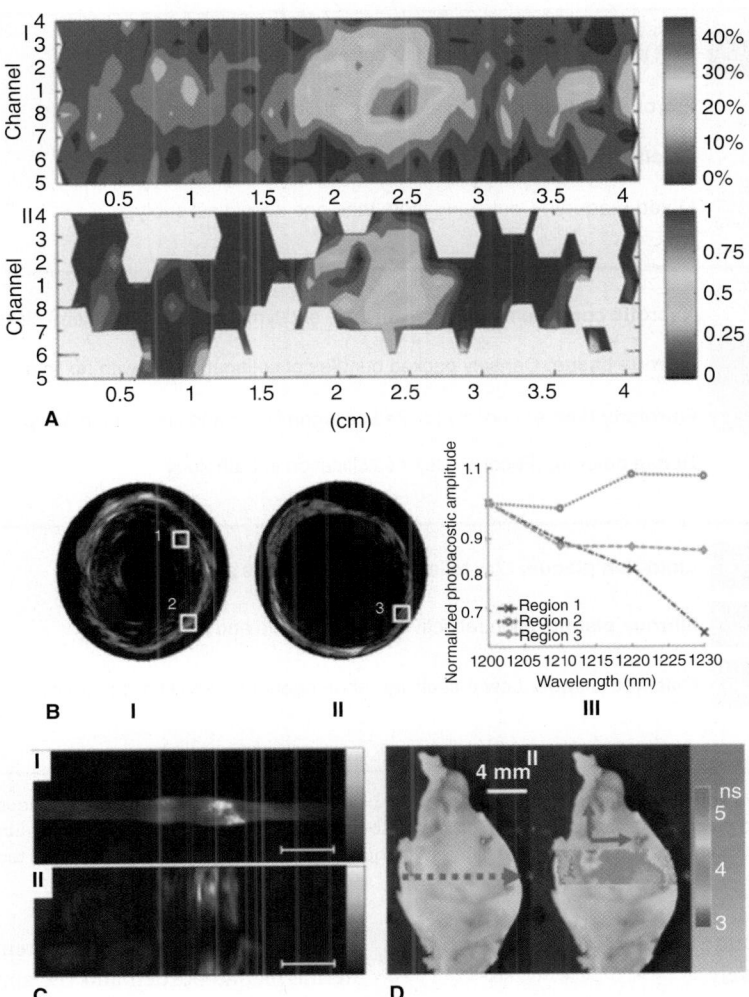

Figure 3–15. Emerging intravascular imaging techniques. (A) Spread-out plots of the compositional characteristics of the plaque estimated by an intravascular Raman spectroscopy catheter. The first panel portrays the distribution of the total cholesterol (in *y*-axis the number of the sensors used to scan the vessel); the *yellow-red* color corresponds to increased cholesterol. The second panel provides estimation of the nonesterified cholesterol, which was measured when the total cholesterol was greater than 5%. **(B)** Intravascular photoacoustic images of a diseased (I) and a normal (II) aorta. The unique photoacoustic characteristics of different tissues (eg, lipid tissue [1], normal vessel wall [2], and media-adventitia [3]) allow identification of the plaque's composition (III). **(C)** Fluorescence reflectance imaging (I) and near-infrared fluorescence (NIRF) images obtained by an intravascular NIRF catheter in a stented rabbit aorta (II). An activatable NIRF agent has been used to mark the cysteine protease activity before pullback. An increased activity was noted at the edges of the stent (indicated with a *white-yellow* color), suggesting inflammation of the vessel wall. **(D)** A carotid atherosclerotic plaque assessed by time-resolved spectroscopy (TRFS) imaging. TRFS allows evaluation of the biochemical composition of superficial plaque that is portrayed in a color-coded map (red corresponds to fibrotic plaque, the *yellow* color to fibrolipid and the cyan to normal endothelium) (II). Reproduced with permission from Bourantas CV, Garcia-Garcia HM, Naka KK, et al. Hybrid intravascular imaging: current applications and prospective potential in the study of coronary atherosclerosis. *J Am Coll Cardiol.* 2013 Apr 2;61(13):1369-1378.

(IDTCFA) using IVUS-VH has been defined as a lesion fulfilling the following criteria in at least three consecutive frames: (1) necrotic core of 10% or more (2) without evident overlying fibrous tissue, and (3) plaque burden of 40% or more. Here, thin cap is defined as all fibrous caps of less than 200 microns, which is the limit of IVUS resolution. IDTCFA is more common in acute coronary syndrome (ACS) than in stable patients, and two-thirds are seen within the first 2 cm of each artery.[44] The plaque burden and the mean necrotic core areas of the IDTCFAs detected by IVUS-VH are also similar to previously reported histopathologic data (55.9% vs 59.6% and 19% vs 23%, respectively).[45]

OCT may be superior to conventional and integrated backscatter IVUS for characterization of coronary atherosclerotic plaque composition, even though the 2-mm imaging depth of OCT limits the ability of this method to assess deeper arterial wall structures such as the adventitia.[46] Nonetheless, studies comparing OCT with histopathology show variable results, with reports of >40% plaque misclassification (mostly caused by a combination of incomplete image penetration and the inability to distinguish calcium deposits from lipid pools),[47] and other studies showing sensitivities and specificities of 71% to 79% and 97% to 98% for fibrous plaques; 95% to 96% and

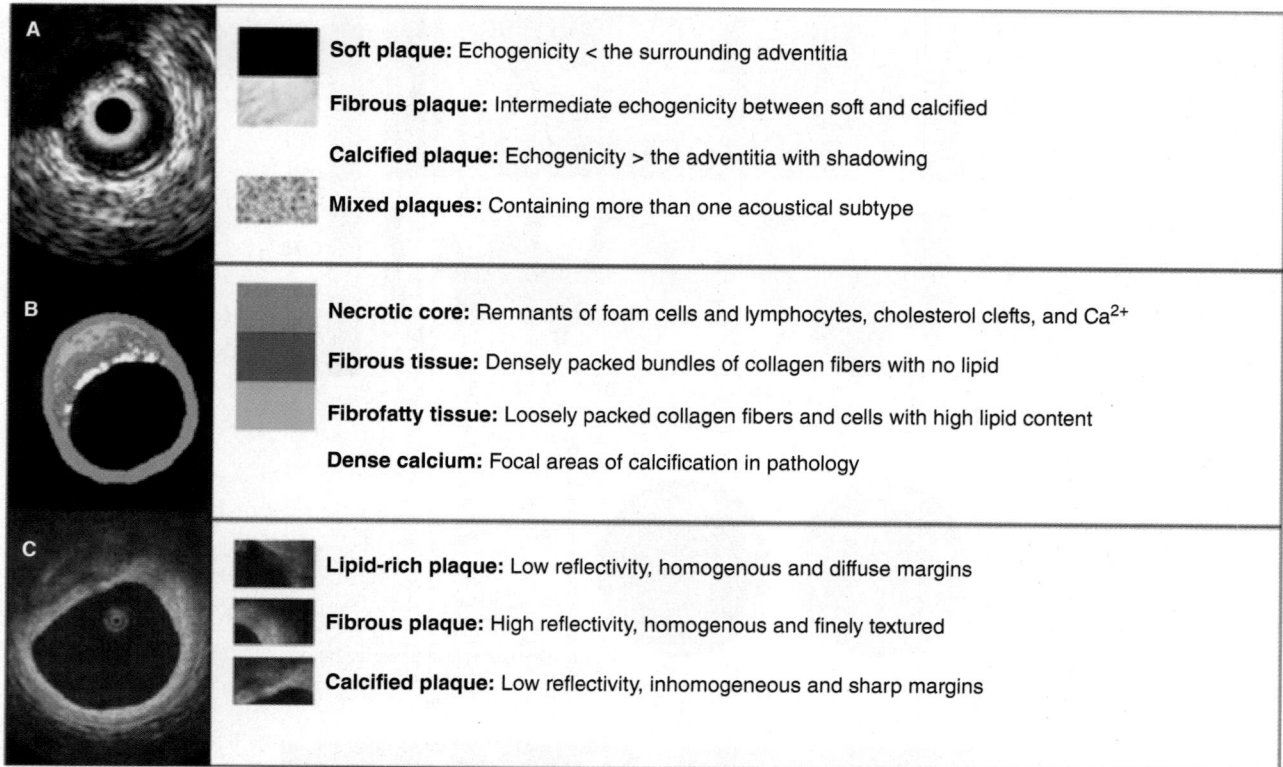

Figure 3–16. (**A**), (**B**), and (**C**) are corresponding images of the same coronary plaque. By grayscale, atherosclerotic plaque can be classified into four categories: soft, fibrous, calcified, and mixed plaques (**A**). Virtual histology (**B**) is able to detect four tissue types: necrotic core, fibrous, fibrofatty, and dense calcium. At the bottom, optical coherence tomography (**C**) is showing the different plaque types that can be detected with this technique.

97% for fibrocalcific plaques; and 90% to 94% and 90% to 92% for lipid-rich plaques, respectively.[48]

Calcification

On IVUS, calcium appears as bright echoes that obstruct the penetration of ultrasound (acoustic shadowing) (see Fig. 3–29). IVUS detects only the leading edge of calcium and cannot determine its thickness, so calcification on IVUS is usually described based on its circumferential angle (arc) and longitudinal length, rather than depth. Calcification can be located deeper in the arterial wall or in the surface of the plaque in close contact with the lumen wall interface. IVUS has shown significantly higher sensitivity than fluoroscopy in the detection of coronary calcification, and VH has a predictive accuracy of 96.7% compared with histology for detection of dense calcium.[31]

In contrast, light penetrates calcium well, and OCT can depict calcification within plaques as well-delineated, low-backscattering heterogeneous regions (see Figs. 3–29 and 3–30), so OCT can quantify calcium burden. Superficial microcalcifications can also be identified on OCT images as small calcific deposits separated from the lumen by a thin tissue layer. OCT has a sensitivity of 96% and specificity of 97% to detect calcified nodules by compared with histology.[48]

Arterial Remodeling

Arterial remodeling refers to a continuous process involving positive or negative changes in vessel size measured by the external elastic membrane (EEM) cross-sectional area (CSA).

Detection of remodeling is extremely important during PCI to define plaque burden and the appropriate size of devices. The magnitude and direction of remodeling can be expressed by the following index: EEM CSA at the plaque site divided by EEM CSA at the reference "nondiseased" vessel. *Positive remodeling* (index >1.0) occurs when there is an outward increase in EEM. *Negative remodeling* occurs with shrinkage of the vessel (ie, the EEM decreases in size, index <1).[38] Direct evidence of remodeling can only be demonstrated in serial studies showing changes in the EEM CSA over time because remodeling may also be encountered at the "normal-appearing" reference coronary segment.[38] IVUS is the optimal test for assessing remodeling—angiography images the lumen rather than the vessel wall, and OCT is limited by the limited penetration of light into tissue. Positive remodeling is linked to plaque vulnerability, increased inflammatory marker concentrations, larger lipid cores, a paucity of smooth muscle cells, and medial thinning, but not only positive remodeling, but also negative remodeling, predicts lesions that cause cardiovascular events at follow-up.[49]

Vulnerable Plaque and Thrombi

Approximately 60% to 80% of clinically evident plaque rupture originates within an inflamed TCFA.[50] Plaque ruptures occur at sites of significant plaque accumulation but are often not highly stenotic by coronary angiography because of positive vascular remodeling.[51] Although plaque characteristics do not yet influence current therapeutic guidelines, IVUS and OCT have

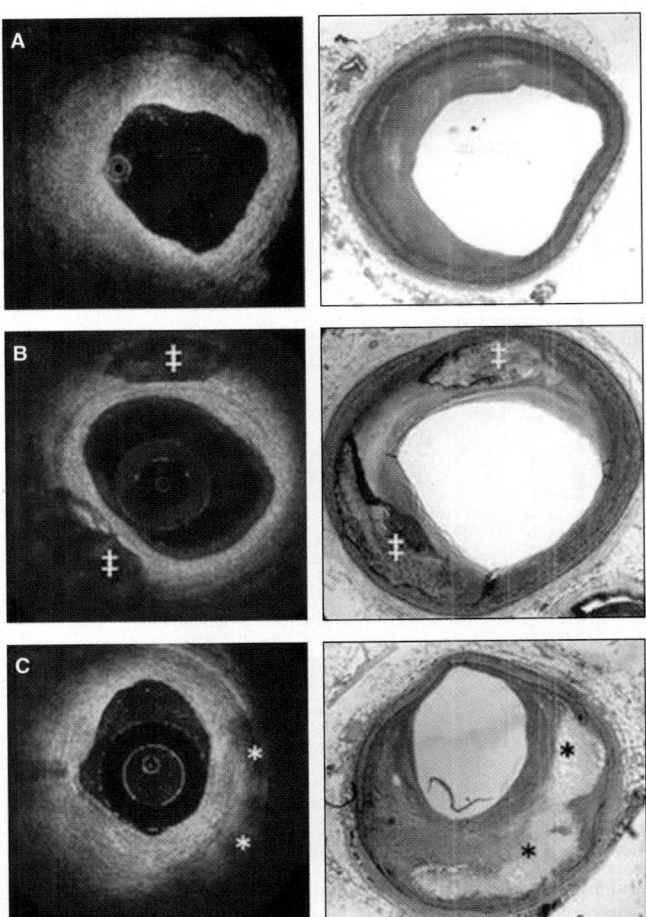

Figure 3–17. Correlation between optical coherence tomography (left) and histology (right). (A) Fibrotic plaque: characterized by high signal (high backscattering) and low attenuation (deep penetration). **(B)** Predominantly calcified plaque: calcified regions have a sharp border, low signal, and low attenuation, permitting deeper penetration. **(C)** Lipid-rich plaque: the lipid core has a diffuse border. Light attenuation results in poor tissue penetration (in contrast to calcified regions). The overlying fibrotic cap can be readily measured; in this case, a thick cap (>200 μm) is present. ‡Calcified region; *lipid core. Reproduced with permission from CY Xu and JM Schmitt, Light-Lab Imaging.

the ability to identify some of the aforementioned pathologic atheroma features (see Figs. 3–29 and 3–30). The clinical implications of plaque rupture appear to depend on the anatomical characteristics of the plaque. IVUS analysis demonstrated that the ruptured plaques causing events have smaller lumen area and increased plaque burden compared to the plaques having a silent rupture.

Thrombus, the ultimate pathologic feature leading to ACS, is usually recognized as an echolucent intraluminal mass, often with a layered or pedunculated appearance by IVUS.[38] As none of these IVUS features is a hallmark for thrombus, slow flow (fresh thrombus), air, stagnant contrast or black hole, an echolucent neointimal tissue observed after drug-eluting stents, and radiation therapy as differential diagnoses.[38] Overall, OCT possesses diagnostic advantages compared with both IVUS and angioscopy in the assessment of thrombus in culprit lesions.

Clinical Applications

The clinical applications of intravascular imaging are summarized in **Table 3–9**. Estimation of the severity and extent of atherosclerosis remains one of the main diagnostic clinical applications of intravascular imaging because angiography and noninvasive methods lack sufficient resolution for accurate disease assessment. The use of intravascular imaging to guide PCI is heterogeneously distributed across the world, varying from more than 60% of use in Japan to less than 20% in Europe and the United States. The explanation for such disparity is multifactorial but likely involves local reimbursement practices for the procedure, differences in clinical practice and training, and a relative lack of scientific evidence.

CARDIOVASCULAR COMPUTED TOMOGRAPHY

Technical Considerations

Advances in CT technology have made it possible to noninvasively image the beating heart. Multidetector computed tomography (MDCT) scanners produce images by rotating an x-ray tube around a circular gantry through which the patient advances on a moving table. Pitch is the speed of the table relative to the speed of the gantry rotation, which allows each cross-sectional level of the heart to be imaged during more than one cardiac cycle. The number of image slices acquired during each gantry rotation determines the overall duration of the MDCT scan. Improvements in gantry rotation speeds and the development dual source and large detector technologies have reduced effective temporal resolution to less than 100 milliseconds.

The temporal resolution of MDCT systems, may be further improved by selecting specific partial image sector data from different heartbeats and detector rings to reconstruct a complete data set. Cardiac CT is performed with electrocardiogram (ECG) gating in either prospective or retrospective mode. ECG gating synchronizes image acquisition with the cardiac cycle. The optimal phase or interval for image analysis is the period during which the heart is the least mobile (usually end-diastole) and therefore the least degraded by motion artifact. Prospective ECG gating entails scan initiation at a defined interval after the R wave, continues for a prespecified duration, and then stops until the same optimal period is reached in the subsequent cardiac cycle, at which time scanning resumes. Retrospective ECG gating uses continuous acquisition of images throughout the cardiac cycle. The images from multiple consecutive heartbeats are then reconstructed at various percentages of the R-R interval (eg, from 0% to 90% of an R-R cycle at 10% intervals). With retrospective gating, several thousand images can be acquired during a single cardiac study, allowing the interpreting physician to select the images with the least amount of motion-related distortion prior to final image reconstruction. However, the cost is radiation exposure that is an order of magnitude greater than prospective gating,[52] which has significantly reduced radiation exposure to potentially <1 mSv.[53] Gating is the most advantageous at relatively slower heart rates (<60 bpm, so careful preparation with β-blockade is

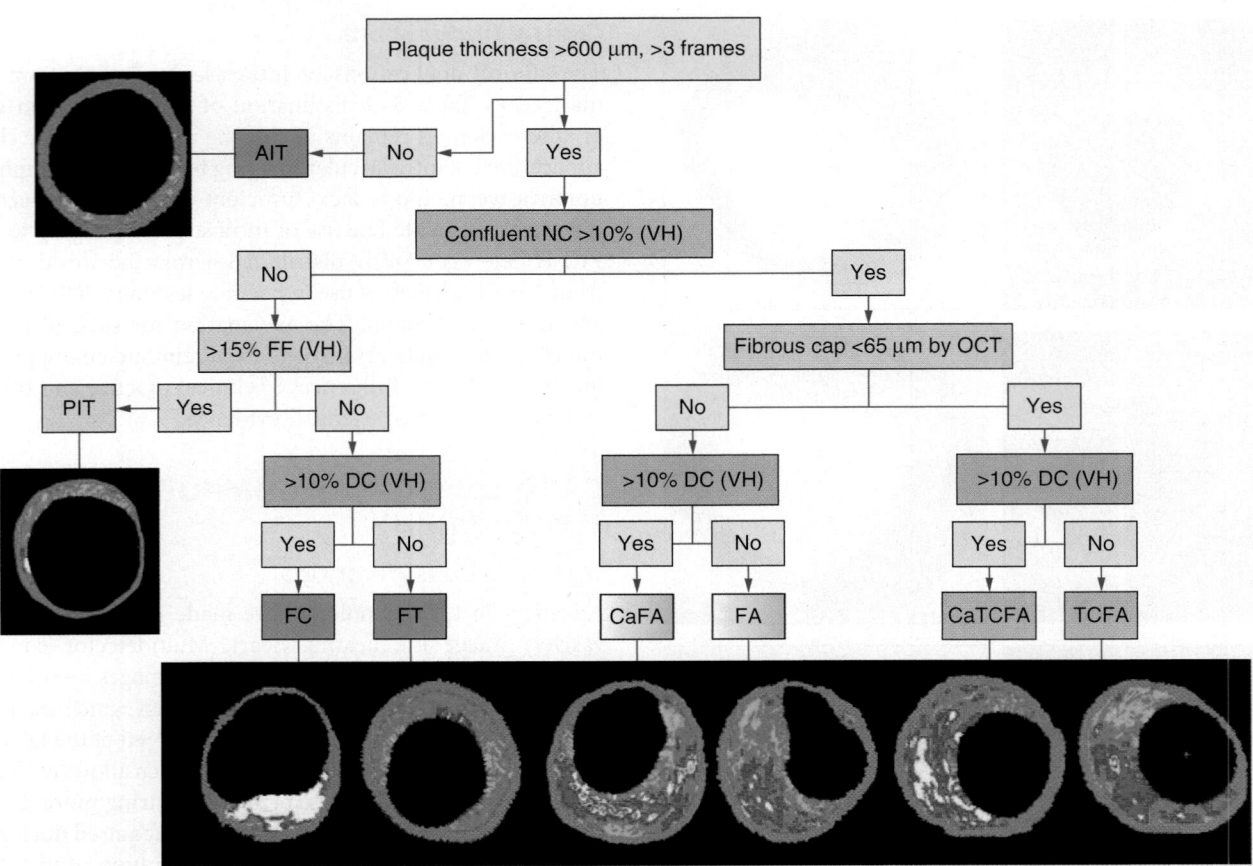

Figure 3–18. Plaque classification using optical coherence tomography (OCT) and intravascular ultrasound virtual histology (IVUS-VH). AIT, adaptive intimal thickening; CaFA, calcified fibroatheroma; CaTCFA, calcified thin cap fibroatheroma; DC, dense calcium; FA, fibroatheroma; FC, fibrocalcic (tissue); FF, fibrofatty (tissue); FT, fibrotic (tissue); NC, necrotic core; PIT, pathologic intimal thickening; TCFA, thin-cap fibroatheroma.

essential for high-quality coronary CT), where the R-R interval is more than 1000 milliseconds and the fastest imaging protocols may be used.

More recently, new iterative reconstruction algorithms have been introduced and validated for use in cardiac CT to allow for significant noise reduction, enabling an uncoupling of tube current and image noise and thereby allowing for significant tube current and dose reduction. New scan acquisition modes employing fast helical pitch technique afforded by dual source dual detector technology allows for rapid scan acquisition and significant dose reduction. Implementation of one or more of these strategies has been shown to consistently reduce radiation exposure to 1 to 3 mSv in suitable patients.

Evaluation of Cardiac Function

The combination of ECG gating and image postprocessing permits the reconstruction of multiple data sets at predetermined percentages of the R-R interval throughout the entire cardiac cycle (see Fig. 3–32). This multiphase image reconstruction can be displayed in cine mode as in echocardiography or cardiac magnetic resonance (CMR) imaging. Therefore, end-systolic and end-diastolic images can be obtained to assess ventricular volumes and function.

Both ventricles are well visualized by MDCT, allowing excellent spatial separation between the two structures. Delineation of the epicardial and endocardial surfaces allows accurate and reproducible measurement of LV and RV wall thickness and myocardial mass.[54] LVH can be quantified and serially assessed, and accurate and reproducible LV and RV end-diastolic and end-systolic volumes can be measured, with calculation of EF.[55] Cardiac CT is comparable to other tests for assessment of EF, albeit with minor differences in normal ranges.[56] CT can be used for assessment of regional LV thinning, morphology and function and LV thrombi.[57] RV volume and functional assessment by MDCT is feasible and has good correlation with other tests. LA imaging is feasible, and CT is a viable alternative to transesophageal echocardiography for the detection of intra-atrial thrombus.[58]

Evaluation of Coronary Artery Calcification

Coronary artery calcification (CAC) is more indicative of plaque burden than is angiographic stenosis severity.[59] A strong linear correlation exists between total coronary artery plaque area and the extent of CAC as found in individual hearts ($r = 0.93$, $P < 0.001$) and in individual coronary arteries ($r = 0.90$, $P < 0.001$). Calcification is an active, organized, and regulated

Diagnostic	Severity and extent of atherosclerosis	Quantification of luminal dimensions Assessment of atheroma burden
	Assessment of ambiguous anatomy on angiography Aneurysmal and large vessels Ostial and bifurcation disease Diffuse and cardiac allograft disease	
Interventional	Preintervention	Accurately determine vessel size, disease severity, character, extent, as well as location Guide therapeutic decision making in the cardiac catheterization laboratory
	Nonstent PCI PCI with stents Complications post-PCI	
Research	Drug effects on atherosclerosis Responses to device implantation	

TABLE 3–9. Indications for Intravascular Imaging

process occurring during atherosclerotic plaque development, and is found in the early stages of the disease. Although lack of calcification does not categorically exclude the presence of atherosclerotic plaque, calcification occurs exclusively in atherosclerotic arteries and is not found in normal coronary arteries.

Detection of Coronary Artery Calcification
MDCT imaging protocols vary among different camera systems and manufacturers. In general, images of 2.5- to 3-mm thickness, are acquired, and calcified lesions are defined one the basis of adjacent pixels exceeding a threshold density. Calcium scoring is usually based on the traditional Agatston method (ie, initial density of >130 HU). As with electron beam computed tomography (EBCT) scoring, the total coronary artery calcium score (CACS) is calculated as the sum of each calcified plaque over all the tomographic slices.

Prognostic Implications of Coronary Artery Calcification
Traditional risk factor assessment is routinely used to identify individuals who are at increased risk for developing cardiovascular disease based on standard clinical criteria.[60] However, symptomatic cardiovascular disease occurs almost exclusively in patients with atherosclerosis, and the likelihood of plaque rupture and the development of acute cardiovascular events is related to the total atherosclerotic plaque burden. CAC scoring is used in risk assessment on the basis that it directly characterizes the presence and severity of atherosclerotic burden. Although there is a clear relationship between the number of cardiac risk factors and the presence and

extent of CAC, 40% of men and 30% of women without risk factors in one series had CAC, whereas 26% of men and 36% of women with more than three traditional risk factors did not have any CAC.[61]

The prognostic implications of CAC scoring have been understood since the 1990s. A landmark study of 10,377 asymptomatic patients (4191 women and 6186 men) with a significant burden of cardiac risk factors (family history of CAD in 69%, hyperlipidemia in 62%, hypertension in 44%, and current cigarette smoking in 40%), followed for 5.0 ± 3.5 years, showed CACS was a strong independent predictor of mortality, with 43% additional predictive value contained within the CACS beyond risk factors alone.[62] A coronary calcium score of zero portends a very low risk over the subsequent decade.[63]

While there may be value in repeating a negative score to reassess risk after a significant interval, repetition of a positive score is probably not useful in patients on therapy. The use of high-intensity statin therapy promotes coronary calcification despite evidence of regression of overall coronary atheroma volume by IVUS, perhaps reflecting plaque stabilization.[64]

Coronary Computed Tomography Angiography
Assessment of Native Coronary Arteries
Coronary CT angiography (CCTA) has the ability to accurately detect luminal stenosis in the coronary arteries and characterize coronary artery plaques. Advances in MDCT technology have resulted in high spatial and temporal resolution capable of detecting coronary atherosclerosis approximating that seen with invasive catheter-based coronary angiography (ICA), but without the procedural risk (0.1%–0.2%) and procedural cost. Approximately up to 40% of patients who undergo coronary angiography have normal angiograms, and many patients with CAD do not require revascularization procedures.[65,66] CCTA has the potential to obviate the need for invasive procedures in select patients by demonstrating the absence of significant CAD, as well as improve prevention for patients with disease that does not require intervention.[67]

CCTA Acquisition
The coronary arteries move independently throughout the cardiac cycle and, even at relatively slower heart rates (ie, <70 bpm), exhibit significant translational motion of up to 60 mm/s for the RCA and 20 to 40 mm/s for the LAD and circumflex coronary arteries. The velocity of coronary artery motion increases significantly with increasing heart rates. Image acquisition of less than 50 milliseconds is required to completely avoid cardiac motion artifacts. Cardiac motion is minimized with the use of oral and/or intravenous β-blockers prior to scanning, thereby reducing the heart rate and prolonging the time during the cardiac cycle at which coronary artery velocity is low. For individuals without contraindication to β-blockade, these drugs are the medication of choice because they not only decrease the heart rate through the reduction of sympathetic tone, but may also reduce the number of premature atrial or ventricular beats, which adversely affect the overall quality of the images. Another crucial element for obtaining high-quality coronary images is to maximally dilate coronary vessels with

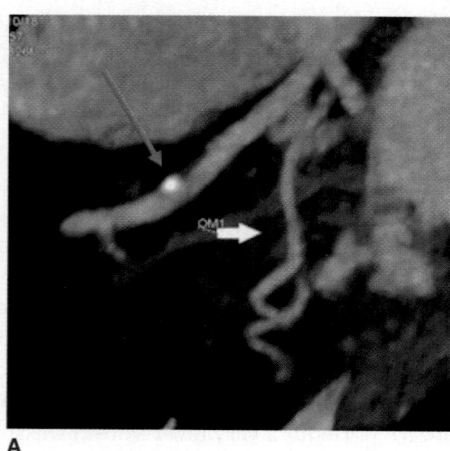 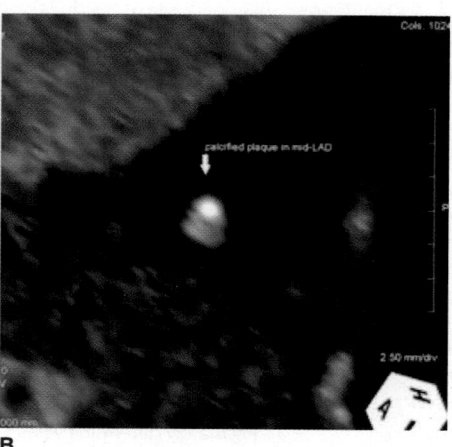

Figure 3–19. Evaluation of coronary atherosclerosis. (A) Longitudinal maximum-intensity projection view of the mid left anterior descending coronary artery showing a calcified plaque. **(B)** Axial multiplanar reconstruction view of the same nonobstructive plaque.

nitroglycerin through the use of sublingual tablets or spray. Respiratory motion is excluded by performing the scan during a breath-hold.

CCTA requires the intravenous administration of an iodinated contrast medium (usually 50–100 mL). The accurate timing of image acquisition relative to the contrast injection is a major determinant of overall image quality. A test bolus or bolus tracking technique is used to optimize this timing by determining the amount of time necessary to peak enhancement in the aorta. Advancements in MDCT technology have led to shorter scan times, reduced breath-hold duration, smaller intravenous contrast injections, and decreased motion-related artifacts, resulting in lower radiation exposure and improved diagnostic accuracy.

Image Interpretation

The coronary vasculature on CCTA is evaluated through axial images, multiplanar (coronal, sagittal, or oblique) reconstructions, and 3D data sets constructed from specific phases during the cardiac cycle (**Fig. 3–19**). Maximum-intensity projection images allow the evaluation of longer segments of the coronary vessels but can be limited by overlapping structures adjacent to the artery of interest. Curved multiplanar reformations are reconstructed on a plane to fit a curve and allow display of the entire vessel in a single image. 3D volume-rendered images are useful for selecting images with the least motion artifact and for assessing the relationships among different anatomic structures (**Fig. 3–20**).

The spatial resolution of the image depends on the size of the 3D pixels or volume elements (voxels) that constitute the image. Slice thickness affects the spatial resolution of CCTA. Temporal resolution is determined by the speed of rotation of the gantry around the patient. The reference standard for CT is invasive angiography, which has a spatial resolution of 0.2 mm and a temporal resolution of 5 to 20 milliseconds. A temporal resolution of 50 milliseconds or less is desirable for coronary artery imaging, and temporal and spatial resolution are an important potential cause of artifacts.[68]

Accuracy of CCTA

Acute Coronary Syndromes: In suspected ACS, a meta-analysis including nine studies totaling 566 patients using scanners with 64 or fewer detectors revealed a per-patient pooled sensitivity of 95% (95% confidence interval [CI], 90%–98%) and specificity of 90% (95% CI, 87%–93%) in comparison with ICA.[69] Another meta-analysis including 16 studies and 1119 patients found sensitivity and specificity of 96% (95% CI, 93%–98%) and 92% (95% CI, 89%–94%), respectively.[70] These findings demonstrate higher diagnostic accuracy for ACS with CCTA than with other previously studied modalities, including exercise treadmill, stress MRI, stress nuclear imaging, and stress echocardiography.

All trials demonstrated that absence of any coronary atherosclerosis by CCTA, which was observed in about half of the population, has an excellent negative predictive value (NPV) for presence of ACS. Indeed, the speed of CTCA and excellent NPV have led CT to be proposed for rapid assessment of acute chest pain in the emergency department. Three landmark trials—American College of Radiology Imaging Network–Pennsylvania Department of Health (ACRIN-PA) study, Coronary Computed Tomographic Angiography for Systematic Triage of Acute Chest Pain Patients to Treatment (CT-STAT), and the ROMICAT II—have shown that this is feasible and can lead to safe rapid discharge in about 50% by using a CCTA strategy, compared with 15% to 25% with standard care.[72-74]

However, presence of significant stenosis by CCTA is only moderately diagnostic for ACS. This is particularly problematic when combined with the low prevalence of ACS in the acute chest pain population in the emergency department (2%–8%). In order to improve the positive predictive value (PPV), assessment of stenosis severity may be supplemented by assessment of plaque morphology, identification of regional wall motion

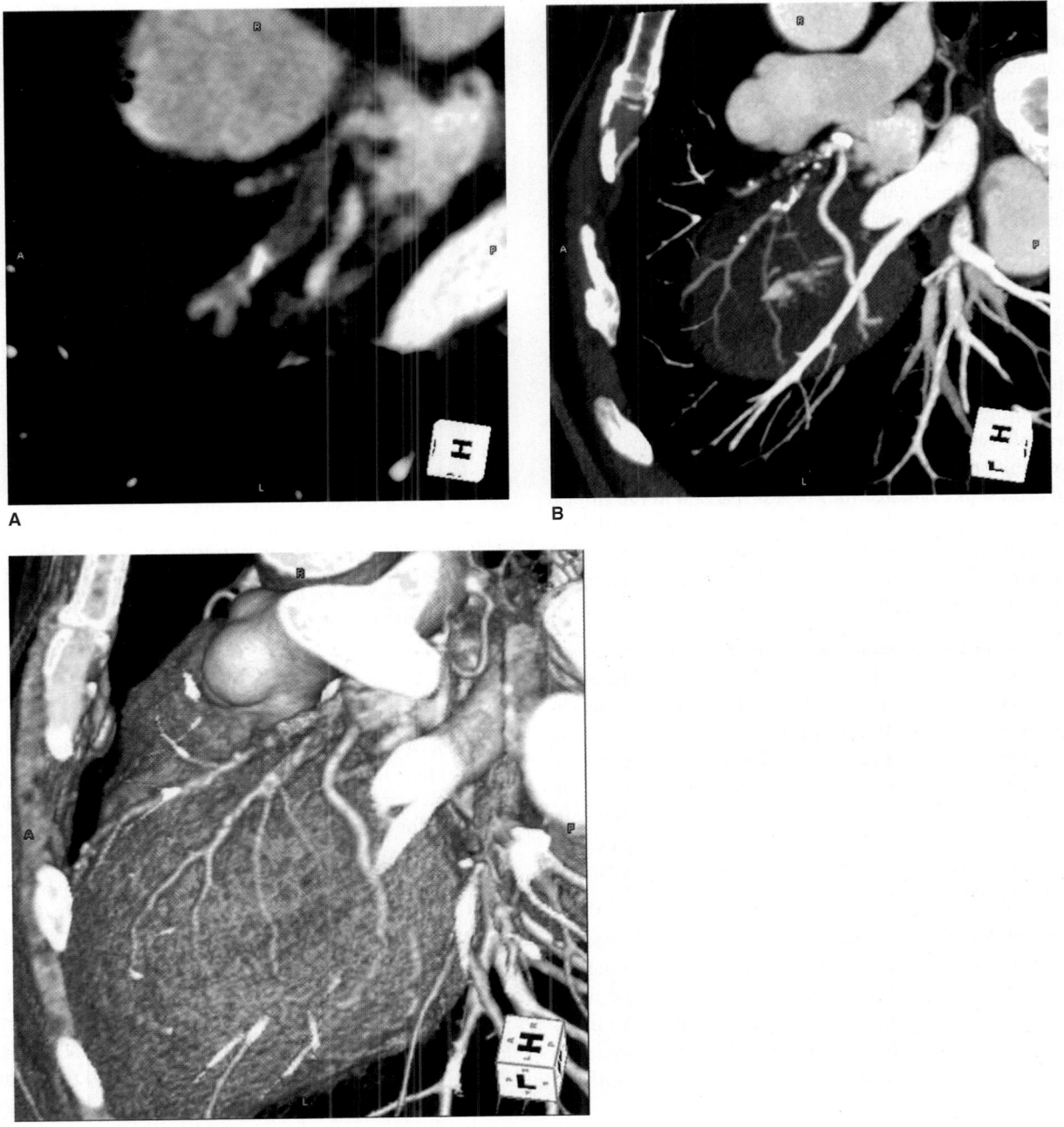

Figure 3–20. (A) Three-dimensional volume rendering image of severe proximal left anterior descending coronary artery (LAD) disease. (B) Maximum-intensity projection (15-mm thickness) of the same heart showing diffuse proximal LAD and diagonal branch stenoses. (C) Multiplanar reconstruction of the same heart focusing on the proximal LAD stenosis demonstrating total occlusion of the vessel segment with in situ thrombus (~20 HU).

abnormalities (albeit at the expense of higher radiation exposure), and physiologic assessment by CT perfusion (CTP) or CT FFR.

Stable Patients: In meta-analyses of diagnostic testing for the detection of obstructive CAD (>50% stenosis) in stable patients, 64-slice MDCT had a pooled sensitivity of 94% to 100%, a specificity of 89% to 100%, a positive predictive value (PPV) of 93% to 97%, and a negative predictive value (NPV) of 93% to 100%.[75–79]

These observational (mainly single-center) studies have been corroborated by two ensuing multicenter prospective clinical trials: Assessment by Coronary Computed Tomographic Angiography of Individuals Undergoing Invasive Coronary Angiography (ACCURACY)[80] and Coronary Artery Evaluation Using 64-Row Multidetector CT Angiography (CORE-64).[81] In the ACCURACY trial (230 patients with chest pain, undergoing both CCTA and ICA) the ability of CCTA to detect obstructive

CAD (>70% stenosis) had a sensitivity of 94%, specificity of 83%, PPV of 48%, and NPV of 99%. The high NPV of CCTA makes CCTA useful in the risk stratification of symptomatic patients and can reduce the need for invasive diagnostic coronary angiography in patients without obstructive CAD.

Assessment of Coronary Bypass Grafts: Because of their larger diameter and limited mobility, saphenous vein grafts are relatively easier to image with CCTA than native coronary arteries. CCTA has high diagnostic accuracy for evaluating arterial and venous bypass graft stenosis—sensitivity exceeds 97% and specificity exceeds 90%.[81] However, the assessment of bypass graft stenosis has several important limitations, namely the image artifacts caused by surgical clips and the presence of extensive coronary calcification in the native coronary arteries. These limitations can particularly hinder the evaluation in distal runoff vessels and nongrafted native coronary arteries. However, the percentage of segments of native coronary vessels that cannot be evaluated may be less relevant in the clinical decision-making process because the most extensively calcified vessels are often bypassed. In addition, in reoperation, CCTA may provide critically important information on the anatomic location of the bypass grafts.

Assessment of In-Stent Restenosis: The imaging artifacts caused by the metallic stents limits the overall visibility of the inner lumen of a deployed stent and can potentially reduce the diagnostic accuracy of CCTA for the noninvasive evaluation of in-stent restenosis. Stent location, heart rate, and stent diameter are also important determinants of accuracy and feasibility. The feasibility of stent visualization is approximately 95%, and a systematic review (including older CCTA methods) has reported moderate sensitivity (85%) and high specificity (97%) for the detection of coronary in-stent restenosis when compared with ICA.[82]

Evaluation of Coronary Anomalies: Anomalies of the coronary arteries are reported in 0.3% to 1% of the general population, and about 20% can be hemodynamically significant and manifest as arrhythmias, syncope, MI, or sudden death.[83] An interarterial course between the pulmonary artery and aorta is the anomaly most commonly associated with sudden cardiac death (**Fig. 3–21**).[129]

The diagnosis of coronary artery anomalies has previously required ICA; however, in up to 50% of patients, the coronary artery anomalies may be incorrectly classified during invasive angiography.[130] This misclassification may result from the difficulty in delineating the precise vessel path within a complex 3D geometry using a relatively restricted 2D view. CCTA has been shown to accurately depict the anomalous vessel origin, its subsequent course, and the relationship to the great vessels.[128] In contrast, although invasive angiography is able to detect most anomalous origins, it is inferior to CT in defining the anomalous coronary course.

CCTA versus Other Modalities: Three landmark randomized prospective studies have evaluated the role of CCTA compared to other commonly used noninvasive modalities for the evaluation of patients with stable CAD. In a multicenter European

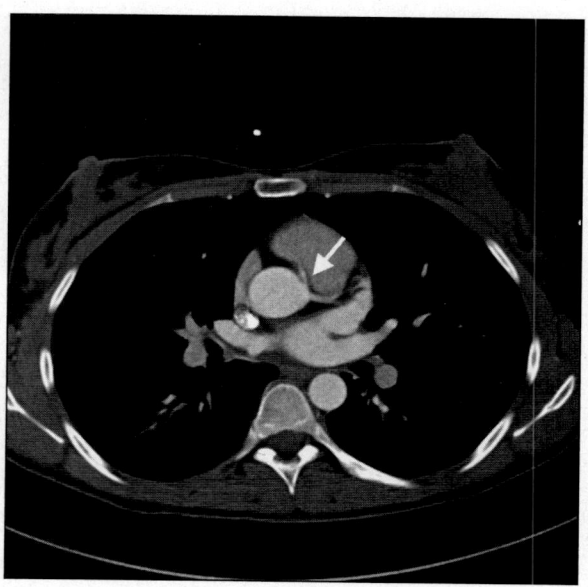

Figure 3–21. Anomalous right coronary artery. A 37-year-old woman with atypical chest pain who underwent coronary computed tomography angiography to exclude coronary artery disease. Note the right coronary artery (*arrowhead*) arising to the left of midline from the left sinus of Valsalva taking interarterial course.

study,[84] 475 patients with stable chest pain and low prevalence of CAD underwent CCTA and stress myocardial perfusion imaging (MPI) by single-photon emission computed tomography (SPECT) or positron emission tomography (PET), as well as ventricular wall motion imaging by stress echocardiography or CMR for detection of obstructive (>50%) CAD. CCTA had the highest diagnostic accuracy; the area under the receiver operating characteristics curve was 0.91 (95% CI, 0.88–0.94), with sensitivity of 91%, and specificity 92%. In the Scottish Computed Tomography of the Heart Trial (SCOT-HEART),[85] 4146 patients assessed for new-onset chest pain were randomized to standard care alone (documentation of angina and objective demonstration of exercise-induced myocardial ischemia through exercise stress testing) or CTA in addition to standard care. At 6 weeks, CTA reclassified the diagnosis of coronary heart disease in 27% of patients and the diagnosis of angina in 23%. Use of CTA increased the certainty of attributing the patient's symptoms to angina compared with usual care alone (relative risk [RR], 1.79; 95% CI, 1.62–1.96). The certainty of diagnosing CAD was also significantly improved (RR, 2.56; 95% CI, 2.33–2.79). Adding CTA changed planned investigations and treatment options and was associated with a reduction in MI, attributed to statin use in patients with plaque causing nonsignificant stenosis. Finally, The PROspective Multicenter Imaging Study for Evaluation of Chest Pain (PROMISE) trial[86] randomized a total of 10,003 patients and no prior diagnosis of CAD to a strategy of initial anatomical testing with CCTA or to functional testing (exercise electrocardiography, nuclear stress testing, or stress echocardiography). The study showed no difference in the primary endpoint, a composite rate of death, MI, major procedural complications or hospitalization for chest pain. However, select secondary endpoints, including level of radiation exposure and rate of subsequent procedures that did not reveal significant heart disease, favored CCTA.

Plaque Composition, and Noninvasive Identification of High-Risk Plaques

Although the visualization of the fibrous cap has required the spatial resolution of invasive studies, many aspects can be identified with noninvasive imaging—including CT and PET. In addition to characterizing the degree of narrowing of the coronary artery lumen, CCTA can assess the composition of the vessel wall, and assess coronary plaque extent, distribution, location, and composition. High-risk plaques are characterized by a large necrotic core, thin fibrous cap, positive remodeling (PR), spotty calcifications (SC), and perivascular inflammation.[87] The association of PR, low attenuation plaque (LAP) (<30 HU), and SC with plaque rupture and ACS has been recognized for over a decade.[88] A prospective study of 1059 patients followed for 27 months after the initial CCTA,[89] showed the copresence of LAP and PR was associated with a 22.5% chance of ACS, whereas absence of these features was associated with 0.5% event rates. There were no significant differences in the degree of stenosis between the plaques that led to ACS and those that did not. The long-term follow-up (10 years)

of this study[90] showed that ACS occurred in 23.0% of patients with two high-risk features, 10.7% of patients with one high-risk feature, 1.6% of patients with no such features, and 0.6% of patients without any plaque (log-rank P <0.0001).

The other CT finding suggestive of plaque vulnerability is the so-called "napkin ring" sign, characterized by napkin ring–like attenuation pattern and SC (**Fig. 3–22**).[91] The circumferential outer rim of noncalcified plaque has a higher CT attenuation in both the noncontrast and contrast-enhanced images as compared to the attenuation within the central part of the plaque, and are analogous to thin cap fibroatheroma. In a follow-up of 895 patients who had a CCTA and were followed for up to 5 years,[92] the "napkin ring" sign was predictive of events. Patients with plaques with no high-risk features had no events, whereas there was a 40% event rate for patients with lesions with the "napkin ring" sign, PR, and LAP.

The presence of high-risk plaque features is a strong predictor of ischemia independent of degree of luminal stenosis, and an important explanation of the inconsistency between anatomic and functional markers (often attributed to lesion length, entrance angle, exit angle, size of the reference vessel, and absolute flow relative to the territory supplied). Hence, FFR may indirectly identify stenotic plaques with large necrotic core.

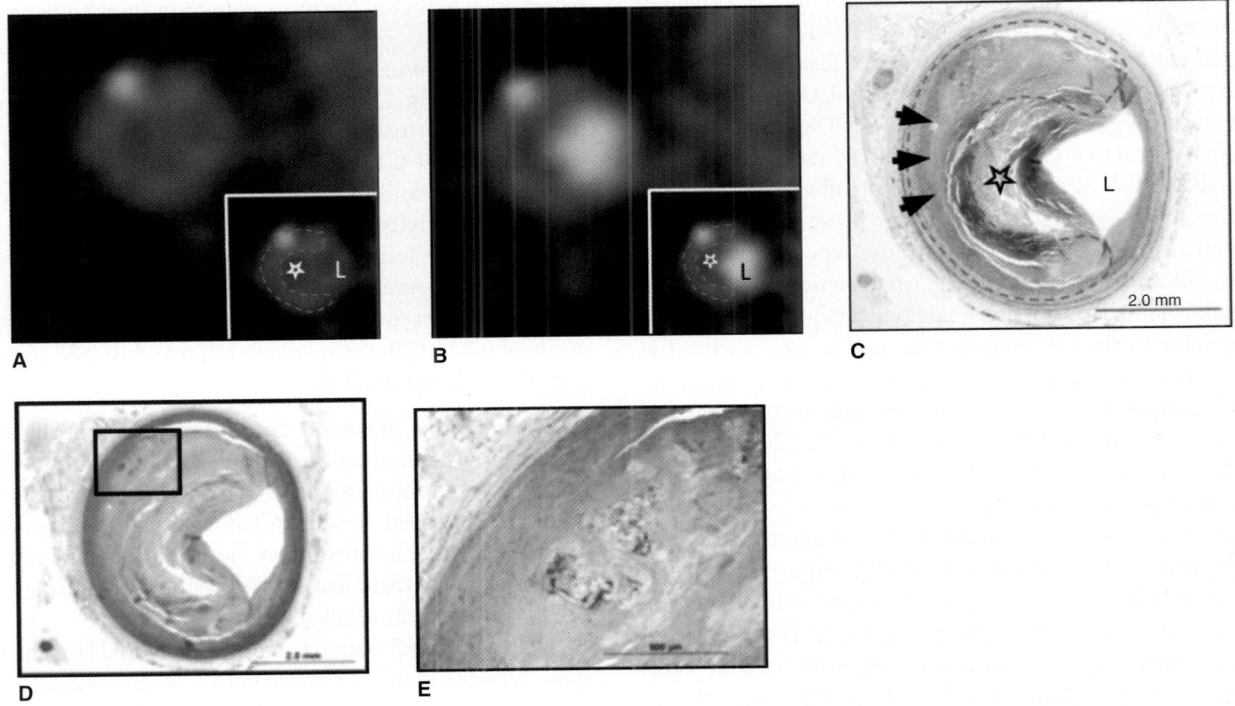

Figure 3–22. The cross-sectional computed tomography (CT) images show a coronary plaque with napkin ring–like attenuation pattern and spotty calcification. The circumferential outer rim (*red dashed line*) of the noncalcified plaque has a higher CT attenuation in both the noncontrast (**A**) and contrast-enhanced (**B**) images (44.0 ± 8.8 HU, range 23.0-61.0 HU vs 48.6 ± 5.8 HU, range 34.0–60.5 HU; respectively) as compared to the attenuation within the central part of the plaque (27.9 ± 4.2 HU, range 20.7–36.4 HU and 31.0 ± 6.6 HU, range 19.0–44.0 HU on noncontrast and contrast-enhanced images; respectively). The corresponding histological section (panels **C**, **D**, and **E**) revealed a late fibroatheroma, with spotty calcification (**E**). The lesion is characterized by a necrotic core (*star*), which is consistent with the low attenuation core of the plaque and a significant amount of fibrous plaque tissue, which is consistent with the high attenuation rim on the CT images (*red dashed line*). HU, Hounsfield units; L, lumen. Reproduced with permission from Maurovich-Horvat P, Hoffmann U, Vorpahl M, et al. The napkin-ring sign: CT signature of high-risk coronary plaques? *JACC Cardiovasc Imaging*. 2010 Apr;3(4):440-444.

Prognostic Value of CCTA

CCTA yields independent prognostic information in addition to clinical risk factors in patients with suspected or known CAD. The landmark study of 100 patients referred for cardiac evaluation, the cardiac event rate in the year following CCTA was 0% in patients without evidence of CAD, 8% in patients with nonobstructive CAD, and 63% when obstructive lesions were present.[92] A subsequent meta-analysis (11 studies, 7335 mostly symptomatic patients with suspected CAD followed for a median of 20 months), showed that the presence of any >50% stenosis at CCTA was associated with a 10-fold higher risk of cardiovascular events, and the finding of any CAD conferred a 4.5-fold risk, with each involved coronary segment increasing the risk of adverse outcomes by 23%.[93] The initial results from the Coronary CT Angiography Evaluation for Clinical Outcomes: An International Multicenter (CONFIRM) registry (27,125 patients with suspected obstructive CAD followed for a mean of 22.5 months), CAD severity provided information that was independent and incremental for predicting all-cause death over routine clinical predictors and left ventricular ejection fraction (LVEF).[94] A subsequent analysis of 17,793 CONFIRM registry patients with chest pain, followed over 2.3 years, showed that the number of proximal segments with mixed or calcified plaques and the number of proximal segments with ≥50% stenosis were the strongest CCTA predictive markers.[95]

The presence of any plaque increases the risk factor–adjusted mortality risk (hazard ratio [HR], 1.98), and risk is increased with multivessel nonobstructive disease (HR of 4.75 for three-vessel nonobstructive disease and HR of 5.12 when five or more segments were involved).[96] The increased risk from nonobstructive CAD is also seen in patients with low Framingham Risk Score (FRS), a patient subset that does not typically qualify for aggressive primary prevention. Mortality incrementally increases according to the type of nonobstructive disease; in the CONFIRM registry, patients with two or more noncalcified or partially calcified plaques had a prognosis similar to that of patients with one or two obstructive plaques. However, patients with up to seven calcified nonobstructive plaques had an excellent prognosis (<3% event rate in 2.3 years).[97] Annual MACE rates are 0.3%, 2.7%, and 6.0% in patients with normal CCTA, nonobstructive CAD, and obstructive CAD, respectively.[98]

In summary, the data available to date suggest that (1) the warranty period of a negative coronary CT angiogram appears to extend to at least 5 years, (2) the presence of any CAD and the burden of atherosclerotic changes at CCTA is strongly predictive for MACE and all-cause mortality in those with stable chest pain, and (3) plaque morphology by CT confers incremental prognostic information beyond that provided by percent stenosis alone.

Physiologic Assessment of CAD by CTA

Rationale: The association between coronary anatomy and ischemia is poor. An ideal diagnostic test would possess the technology that not only can give accurate assessment of the burden of atherosclerosis, location, and composition of each plaque, but also determine the physiological consequence of each lesion in the form of presence or absence of ischemia. Two such techniques are CTP and CT FFR.

Computed Tomography Myocardial Perfusion Imaging: In order to assess both coronary anatomy and myocardial ischemia using CTP, two separate CT acquisitions are required: one for vasodilator-induced stress MPI and one for rest MPI and coronary CTA.[99] Typically, a delay ranging from 10 to 30 minutes is currently employed between acquisitions to allow for CT contrast washout and/or reversal of the effects of the pharmacological vasodilator (adenosine, dipyridamole, or regadenoson).

The performance of CT MPI requires considerations specific to each CT platform—most importantly, the z-axis coverage. When images are acquired over multiple heartbeats, this technique results in nonhomogenous myocardial contrast enhancement resulting from the slight differences in acquisition time of each slab. Another important consideration is the estimated effective radiation dose delivered to the patient; estimated effective dose is significantly dependent on scanner technology and acquisition protocol. An axial acquisition with prospective ECG gating, as well as reduction in the tube voltage (kV) in nonobese patients and use of a single data set utilizing either a test bolus or bolus tracking are some of the techniques that could lead to reduction in effective radiation dose.

The multicenter, international study Coronary Artery Evaluation using 320-row multidetector CT angiography and myocardial perfusion (CORE 320) evaluated 381 patients who underwent CTP and CTA using the 320 MDCT, as well as SPECT MPI and invasive angiography. CTA ≥50% demonstrated a sensitivity of 94% and specificity of 64% for detecting obstructive lesions causing defects on MPI. There was a modest improvement in specificity with the addition of CTP to CTA.[100] The presence of stenosis by CTA had an area under the curve of 0.82 (0.78–0.85), which improved to 0.87 (0.84–0.89) with the addition of CTP.

Fractional Flow Reserve Computed Tomography: Recent advances in computational fluid dynamics and advanced imaging-based modeling have allowed for noninvasive calculation of FFR based on static CT images, without modification of image acquisition protocols, additional imaging or radiation, or need for vasodilators. The methods used in calculation of FFR CT are summarized in **Fig. 3–23**.[101]

Three landmark trials have shown that FFR CT technology is more accurate than CTA in predicting lesion-specific ischemia, as determined by invasive FFR. In 103 patients who underwent CTA and invasive FFR measurement in DISCOVER-FLOW (Diagnosis of ISChemia-Causing Stenoses Obtained Via Non-invasivE FRactional FLOW Reserve), FFR CT was superior to CTA as a predictor of lesion-specific ischemia with higher accuracy, specificity, PPV, and NPV in both per-patient and per-vessel analyses, with a significant improvement in accuracy

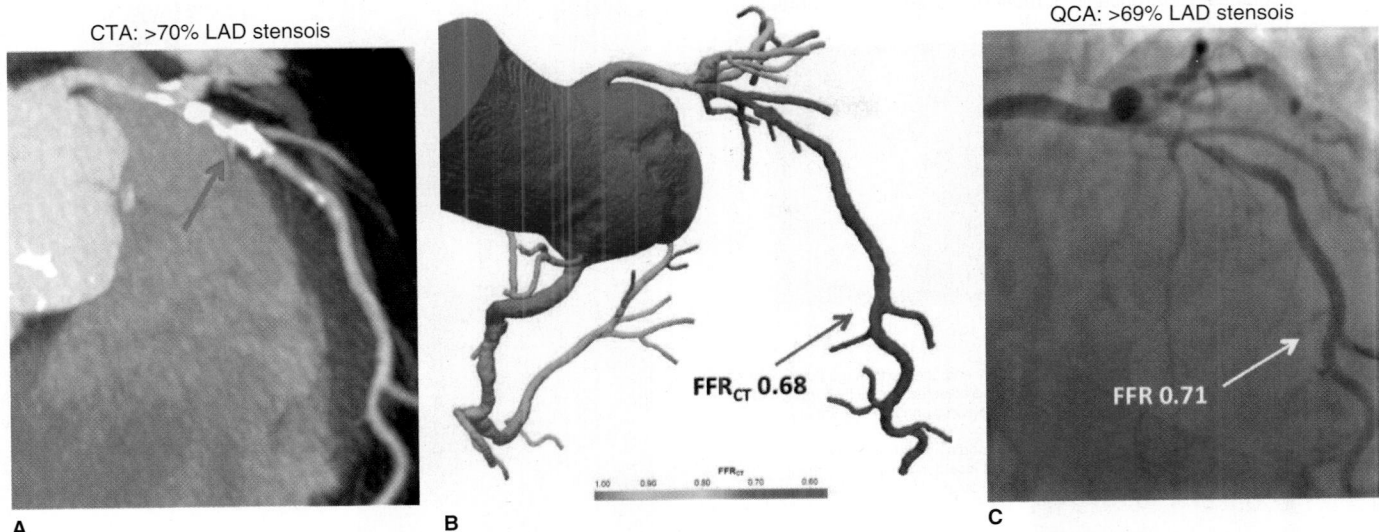

CTA: >70% LAD stensois

QCA: >69% LAD stensois

FFR$_{CT}$ 0.68

FFR 0.71

A   B   C

Figure 3–23. **Evaluation of a lesion by fractional flow reserve (FFR) computed tomography (CT). (A)** Cardiac computed tomography angiography (CTA) finding of heavily calcified left anterior descending coronary artery (LAD) lesion of >70% stenosis. **(B)** FFR CT of the same lesion demonstrating its clinical significance. **(C)** Invasive angiography and FFR of the same lesion, showing its clinical significance by quantitative coronary angiography (QCA).

of CCTA by FFR CT among the 50% to 69% stenosis group. In scans with motion artifact, calcium artifact or low signal-to-noise ratio, FFR CT performed significantly better than CTA.[102] Similarly, in 252 patients and 407 vessels were investigated by both FFR CT and invasive FFR in the DEFACTO trial (Determination of Fractional Flow Reserve from Anatomic Computed Tomographic Angiography) trial,[103] the per-patient diagnostic accuracy for FFR CT plus CT was 73% (95% CI, 67%–78%), which did not meet the prespecified primary end-point of the lower boundary of the confidence interval for diagnostic accuracy >70% (chosen to represent a 15% increase in accuracy over stress echocardiography or MPI). Nonetheless, DEFACTO confirmed the superiority of FFR CT over CT alone; the diagnostic accuracy of CTA alone was 64% (95% CI, 58%–70%), with FFR CT showing a 9% absolute improvement in accuracy—again, with a particular improvement in the evaluation of intermediate severity (30%–70%) stenosis. Finally, the NXT trial (Analysis of Coronary Blood Flow Using CT Angiography: Next Steps)[103] compared the FFR CT to ICA in predicting invasive FFR in 254 patients with CCTA stenosis of 30% to 90% before ICA. The area under the receiver-operating characteristic curve of FFR CT was 0.90 (95% CI, 0.87–0.94) versus 0.81 (95% CI, 0.76–0.87) for coronary CTA ($P = 0.0008$). The per-patient and per-vessel sensitivity, specificity, PPV, and NPV of FFR CT were superior to CTA and diameter stenosis by ICA for detecting lesion-specific ischemia.

The PLATFORM trial (Prospective LongitudinAl Trial of FFR CT: Outcome and Resource Impacts) compared the accuracy and clinical outcomes of a CCTA/FFR CT–guided approach to usual care in 584 patients at intermediate risk (20%–80%)

of obstructive CAD. Assessment of the primary endpoint confirmed that CTA/FFR CT was a potential gatekeeper to coronary angiography, as nonobstructive CAD was present in only 12% in the CCTA/FFR CT arm, compared with 73% in the standard-of-care invasive cohort ($P <0.0001$). In fact, 61% of CCTA/FFR CT patients had ICA canceled with no resultant adverse events over 90 days.[105] The CCTA/FFR approach was considerably less expensive than the usual care arm. The noninvasive group showed greater improvement in quality of life scores in the FFR CT group.[106]

CT in Aortic Valve Disease

MDCT is now the primary noninvasive imaging tool for the evaluation of patients prior to TAVR and includes annular sizing, aortic root assessment, provision of coplanar angles to guide implantation, evaluation of suitability of vascular access, and screening for procedural complications.[107]

Annulus and Root Assessment

MDCT has comparable spatial resolution in all reconstructed planes, and affords a robust platform to characterize the 3D complex anatomy of the aortic annulus in a granular and reproducible fashion[107] (see **Fig. 3–24**). The (virtual) basal ring, immediately below the hinge point of the aortic valve cusps, can be easily generated in its true short axis using standardized multiplanar reformatting (Fig. 3–24). Once generated, various measurements of the annulus can be performed that facilitate device sizing and selection. These include but are not limited to the short and long axes, the perimeter, and the area. It is import to consistently measure the annulus in systole. Given

For use with any imaging software that allows free manipulation of planes. Reference lines must be "locked" in 90° angles.

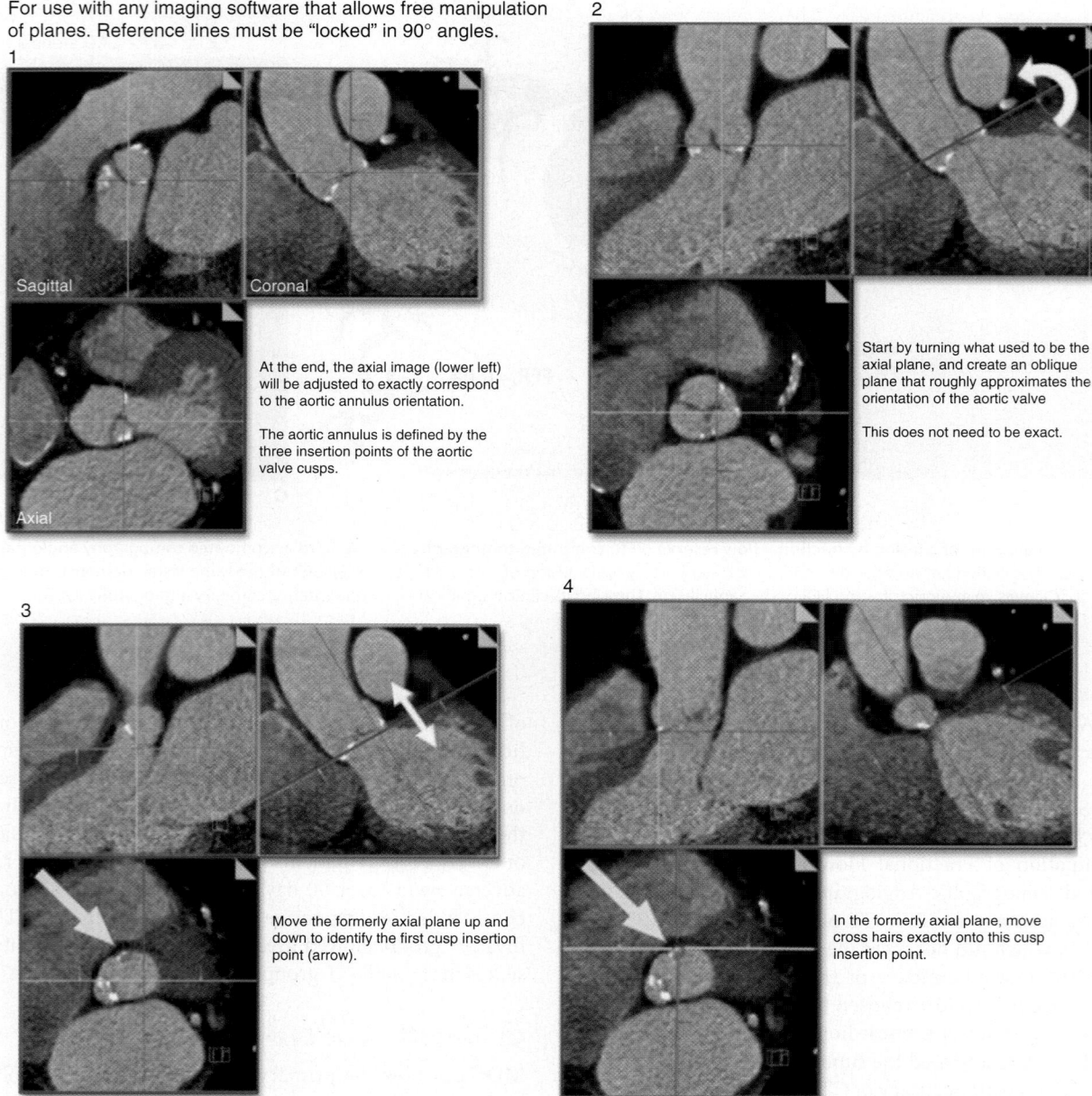

At the end, the axial image (lower left) will be adjusted to exactly correspond to the aortic annulus orientation.

The aortic annulus is defined by the three insertion points of the aortic valve cusps.

Start by turning what used to be the axial plane, and create an oblique plane that roughly approximates the orientation of the aortic valve

This does not need to be exact.

Move the formerly axial plane up and down to identify the first cusp insertion point (arrow).

In the formerly axial plane, move cross hairs exactly onto this cusp insertion point.

Figure 3–24. A method to create the aortic annulus plane in computed tomography. Reproduced with permission from Achenbach S, Schuhbäck A, Min JK, et al. Determination of the aortic annulus plane in CT imaging-a step-by-step approach. *JACC Cardiovasc Imaging.* 2013 Feb;6(2):275-278.

the dynamism of the annulus throughout the cardiac cycle, it is still recommended that retrospective ECG gating be performed with peak tube current in late systole. The goal of device selection is to place a transcatheter heart valve (THV) that is larger than the native annulus to help reduce the risk of nonapposition and paravalvular regurgitation

Subannular and extensive annular calcium is associated with increased frequency and severity of paravalvular regurgitation.[191] In addition, in a multicenter registry of patients who experienced annular rupture, Barbanti et al. showed that subannular calcification, particularly below the noncoronary cusp,[192]

is associated with an increased risk of annular rupture, particularly in conjunction with oversizing greater than 20% by area.[192,193] The identification and evaluation of the subannular zone is now routine and helps determine device sizing and often the type of THV used (**Fig. 3–25**).

MDCT is also extremely helpful in reducing the risk of coronary occlusion, caused by the native aortic valve leaflet being displaced up toward the coronary ostium. CT allows for accurate assessment of both the height of the coronaries as well as the size and capacity of the sinus of Valsalva. A left main height <12 mm, cusp to commissure diameter <30 mm and sinus of

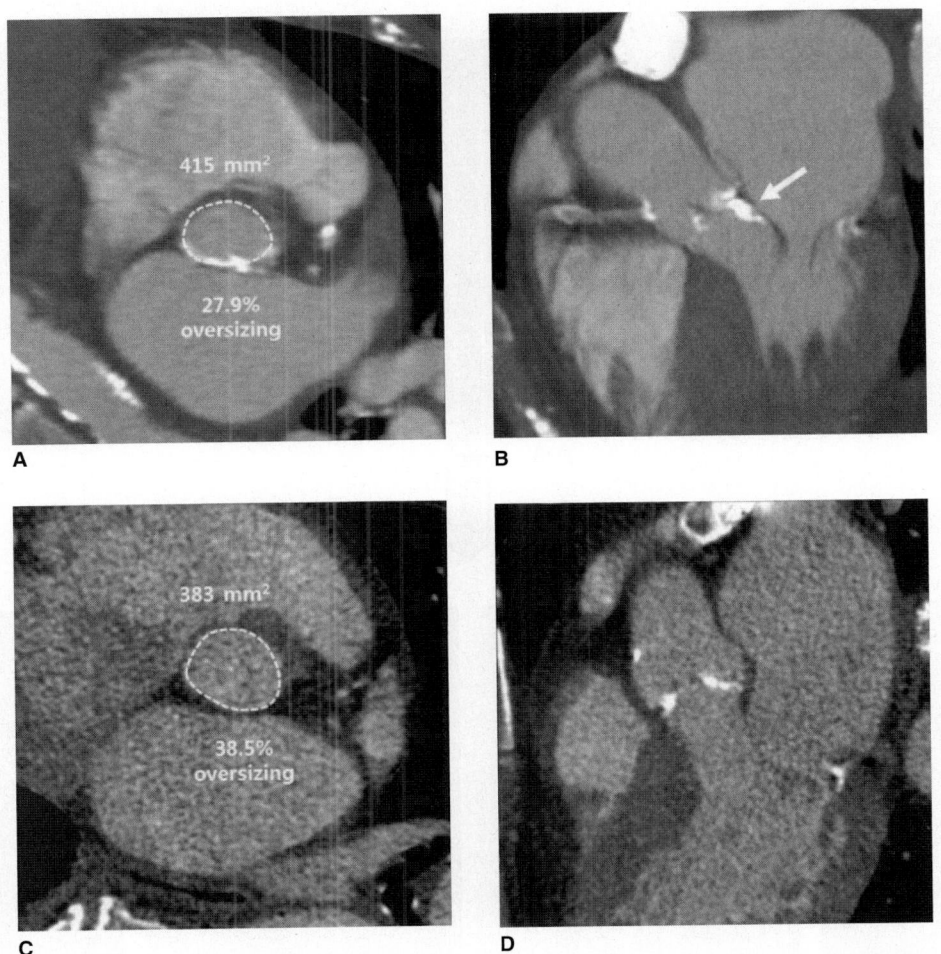

Figure 3–25. (**A**) Moderate annular calcium in an 89-year-old female patient. Annular measurement should traverse any annular calcium in order to maintain a "harmonic" elliptical configuration. (**B**) A large annular area measurement in an 85-year-old male patient reflecting noncircular geometry of the annulus. (**C**) An 84-year-old female patient with severe aortic stenosis and moderate annular calcium (*asterisk*). (**D**) Same patient with additional subannular (*asterisk*) and left ventricular outflow tract (LVOT) (#) calcification. AAo, ascending aorta; An, aortic annulus; LA, left atrium; LAA, left atrial appendage; LV, left ventricle; LVOT, left ventricular outflow tract; MPA, main pulmonary artery; RA; right atrium; RVOT, right ventricular outflow tract.

Valsalva–to–annular ratio <1.25 are associated with increased risk of coronary occlusion.

CT in Other Valve Lesions

The increasing use of transcatheter mitral valve interventions reflects the incidence of mitral regurgitation and the frequency that patients with functional mitral regurgitation in particular are not considered surgical candidates. Cardiac CT allows for a 3D and granular assessment of the saddle-shaped mitral annulus. In addition, using commercially available postprocessing, the annulus can be reconstructed in a highly reproducible fashion (**Fig. 3–26**). As in aortic interventions, CT facilitates procedural planning as well as procedural guidance. CT is helpful in determining the appropriateness of other anatomical parameters (such as nodular or extensive mitral annular calcification) that impact the feasibility of transcatheter mitral valve devices, or the risk of TMVR-related complications such as LVOT obstruction.

Other Uses of Cardiac CT

Pericardial Disease

CT scanning provides excellent visualization of the pericardium and associated lung and mediastinal structures. Even minimal (4–5 mm) pericardial thickening and calcification is easily detected,[109] and different processes within the pericardial space may be distinguished on the basis of density or attenuation. While caval distension and chamber compression can be recognized with CT, the detection of subtle filling changes due to early tamponade is more feasible with Doppler. Nonetheless, a pericardial thickness >4 mm in a patient with abnormal rapid early LV diastolic filling is diagnostic of pericardial constriction.[110]

Congenital Heart Disease

The often-complex anatomic relationships in patients with congenital heart disease may be clarified by both cardiac CT and MRI, because these modalities are readily rendered into

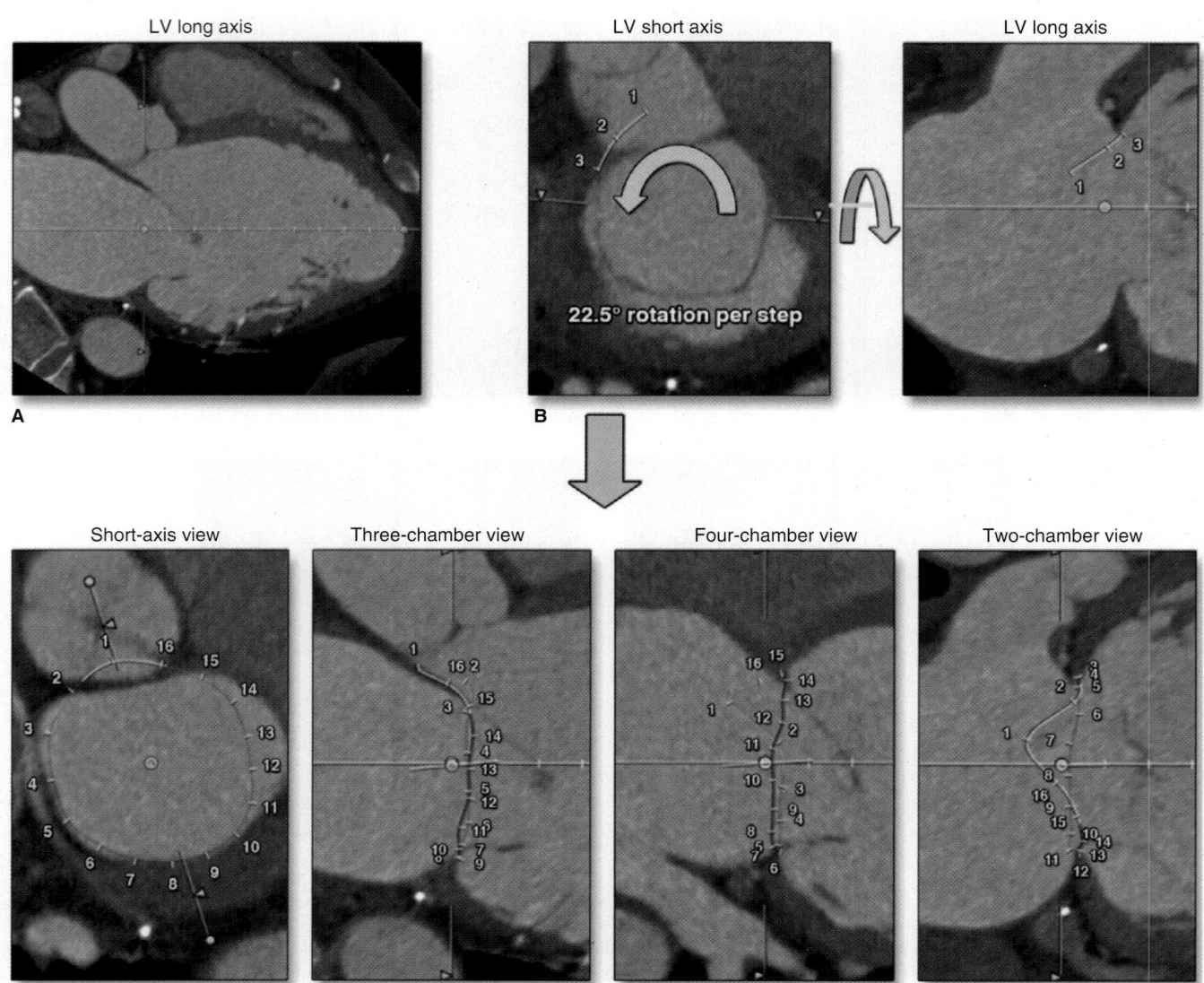

Figure 3–26. Mitral valve annulus evaluation. (A) The saddle-shaped mitral annulus is manually segmented by placing 16 seeding points along the insertion of the posterior mitral leaflet and along the contour of the fibrous continuity while rotating the long-axis view by 22.5° in a stepwise fashion. **(B)** (3mensio Structural Heart version 7.0, Pie Medical Imaging, Maastricht, the Netherlands). The *yellow line* denotes the orientation of the left ventricular (LV) long axis. **(C)** The fully segmented saddle-shaped annulus in standard views. The *blue line* on the short-axis view indicates the orientation of the long-axis view, the *red line* depicts the posterior aspect of the saddle-shaped annulus, and the *white line* indicates the anterior aspect of the saddle-shaped annulus.

3D images. MRI is preferred over MDCT in congenital heart disease because it does not involve ionizing radiation (important in the context of need for repeated imaging at young age) or nephrotoxic contrast agents and allows the precise quantification of flow with superior tissue characterization. However, advances in CT image quality, decreases in radiation dose, and the provision of accurate functional information have helped make CT a viable alternative, especially since fast CT study times may avoid the need for sedation and intubation.

Cardiac Tumors

Although echocardiography is usually the first diagnostic test, particularly in patients with tumor-related cardiac symptoms, such as tamponade, heart failure, or systemic emboli, CT has expanded the diagnostic capabilities of imaging beyond that of echocardiography. In the evaluation of cardiac tumors, MDCT can help differentiate benign from malignant masses and delineate metastatic tumor within the myocardial wall.[111] The precise anatomic information afforded by MDCT may facilitate presurgical assessment, including determining resectability and allowing planning for the reconstruction of cardiac chambers.

Imaging the Great Vessels

A complete study of the thoracic aorta can be completed using MDCT in only 10 to 15 seconds. After scan acquisition, 3D reconstructions are produced, which can be rotated and analyzed in multiple views. Aortic dissection is diagnosed with

>90% accuracy with MDCT, which can also diagnose atherosclerotic disease of the aorta, aortic intramural hematoma, penetrating aortic ulcer, sinus of Valsalva aneurysm, and coarctation of the aorta.[112] CTA is also used for monitoring of the expansion of thoracic aortic aneurysm over time.[112]

MDCT can diagnose acute and chronic pulmonary thromboembolism, and detailed assessment of thrombus location and burden is important for surgical planning. The triple rule-out (TRO) CTA can evaluate the coronary arteries, pulmonary arteries, aorta, and intrathoracic structures in select patients presenting with acute chest pain of unclear etiology.[113] When used in the emergency department in appropriately selected patients, TRO CTA can eliminate the need for further diagnostic testing in more than 75% of patients.[114]

Lastly, CTA can be used for the noninvasive evaluation of the coronary veins prior to lead placement for a biventricular pacemaker or to assess the pulmonary vein anatomy prior to pulmonary vein isolation with radiofrequency ablation for the treatment of atrial fibrillation.[113] CTA can also be used in the evaluation of the symptomatic patient after atrial fibrillation ablation to exclude the presence of pulmonary vein stenosis.

Summary

The clinical utility of cardiac CT has grown exponentially in conjunction with technological improvements. While coronary calcium scoring has seen an explosion in validation data, the diagnostic accuracy of coronary CTA is now well established and is considered the noninvasive gold standard for detection and exclusion of anatomical obstructive CAD. Recent multicenter randomized clinical trials have shown coronary CT to be a viable alternative to traditional stress testing in the setting of stable chest pain with higher diagnostic certainty. Evolving new applications for the adjudication of the hemodynamic significance of stenosis such as CT myocardial perfusion imaging and FFR-CT are now being used in clinical practice. Evaluation of plaque morphology and identification of high-risk plaque features and their prognosis is enhancing the understanding of mechanism of acute events in CAD and might prove very useful clinically in the near future. Finally, the field of structural heart disease interventions are now increasingly dependent on the spatial resolution and unparalleled anatomical evaluation noninvasively offered by cardiac CT.

NUCLEAR CARDIOLOGY

Background

Nuclear imaging has been used in cardiology since the development of the Anger scintillation camera in the late 1960s. Clinical MPI became feasible with the commercial availability of thallium-201 (^{201}Tl) in 1976, and the development of SPECT in the early 1980s, increased the ability to localize and quantify regional myocardial perfusion defects. The introduction of technetium-99m (^{99m}Tc) agents in the 1990s provided higher myocardial count rates and the development of gated SPECT. PET became available in the early 1980s, using ^{8}F-Fludeoxyglucose (FDG) for the assessment of myocardial viability, and ^{13}N-ammonia, ^{15}O-H$_2$O, and later, rubidium-82 (^{82}Rb) for MPI.

Nuclear Myocardial Perfusion Imaging

Basic Concepts

SPECT-MPI is performed using a scintillation camera and an intravenously injected radiopharmaceutical that distributes to the heart in proportion to regional myocardial perfusion. Various standardized SPECT-MPI protocols are used for imaging at rest and after exercise or pharmacologic stress. For SPECT, conventional scintillation camera detectors rotate to cover a 180-degree arc around the patient in a semicircular or elliptical fashion, collecting a series of planar *projection images* at regular angular intervals. The 3D distribution of radioactivity in the myocardium is then mathematically *reconstructed* from the 2D projections, and the resulting data are displayed in series of slices in the short-axis, vertical long-axis, and horizontal long-axis orientations. For gated SPECT, the feature that distinguishes it from nongated SPECT is that the projection images are acquired in 8 to 16 phases of the cardiac cycle based on ECG triggering (*gating*). Reconstruction of a summation of the frames is used to assess myocardial perfusion, and reconstruction of each of the separate phases is used to evaluate ventricular function. Recently, solid-state detector cameras with new acquisition geometries have been introduced that do not require detector rotation around the patient and offer the potential for reducing the time and the patient radiation dose associated with SPECT-MPI.[115]

Radiopharmaceuticals

The concept that CAD can be detected with MPI is based on the ability to detect a reduction in myocardial perfusion in a region supplied by a significantly stenosed vessel when compared with a normal region during hyperemia. The relationship between the quantitative degree of coronary artery narrowing and the maximal hyperemic response was first elucidated by Gould in 1974.[116] Resting myocardial perfusion is normal until the luminal diameter narrowing of a coronary artery exceeds 90% to 95%. With maximal coronary hyperemia produced by dipyridamole, Gould demonstrated a progressive decrease in the hyperemic response associated with increasing degrees of stenosis above a threshold of 50% diameter narrowing. As mentioned in the section Cardiovascular Computed Tomography, it has become widely recognized that factors beyond focal percent stenosis affect the degree of hyperemia achievable in diseased vessels—including stenosis length, myocardial mass distal to the stenosis, plaque composition, diffuse atherosclerosis, nonatherosclerotic microvascular disease, and endothelial dysfunction.[117] In general, a significant reduction in maximal hyperemia is usually present when stenosis severity exceeds 70%,[118] but only 35% of vessels visually assessed as having 50% to 70% stenosis manifest a decrease in maximal hyperemia by FFR.[119] Because moderate stenoses may produce a decrease in flow only at very high flow rates, net extraction is an important characteristic of perfusion tracers.

TABLE 3–10. Available Single-Photon Emission Computed Tomography Radiopharmaceuticals

Radiopharmaceutical	Isotope Half-Life (h)	Energy (keV)	Protocol	Injected Dose (mCi)	Radiation Dose (mSv)
^{99m}Tc-sestamibi OR	6	140	Stress only	5–12	1–3
^{99m}Tc-tetrofosmin			Stress/rest or rest/stress	5–12/15–36	5–13
^{201}Tl	73.1	69–83	Stress/redistribution (or rest/redistribution)	2.5–3.5	11–15

The radiopharmaceuticals share the characteristic that they are accumulated in viable myocardium in proportion to regional myocardial blood flow (**Table 3–10**).

Thallium-201 is avidly extracted from the blood by myocardial cells. Because of its relatively long half-life of 73 hours, the absorbed radiation dose per unit injected is much higher with ^{201}Tl than with ^{99m}Tc agents—for the same radiation dose to the patient, approximately one-tenth as much radioactivity can be injected with ^{201}Tl compared with ^{99m}Tc. This makes imaging times longer and generally providing lower information density ("counts") in the clinical images. ^{201}Tl has superior physiologic properties for MPI compared with the ^{99m}Tc agents, as the linear relationship between myocardial blood flow and ^{201}Tl uptake is better maintained during hyperemic stress up to high levels of flow (approximately >3 mL/min/g) before the previously noted roll-off in uptake occurs. ^{201}Tl is unbound within the myocardial cells, and redistributes over time[120]; its initial distribution is proportional to regional myocardial perfusion, and at equilibrium, the distribution of ^{201}Tl is proportional to the regional potassium pool, which represents viable myocardium.[121] By virtue of these properties, myocardial perfusion defect reversibility can be imaged at multiple times with a single injection of ^{201}Tl. The mechanisms of ^{201}Tl redistribution include differential washout rates between hypoperfused but viable myocardium and normal zones, and washin from the blood to initially hypoperfused zones. For practical purposes, the time it takes for ^{201}Tl to reach its ultimate distribution in viable myocardium varies, such that delayed redistribution imaging (at 24 hours rather than 3–4 hours) is commonly used to gain the greatest amount of information from thallium studies regarding defect reversibility and myocardial viability.

^{99m}Tc has a half-life of 6 hours, and provides better image quality than ^{201}Tl. From a practical standpoint, a main advantage of the ^{99m}Tc agents is flexibility. Unlike ^{201}Tl, ^{99m}Tc-sestamibi and ^{99m}Tc-tetrofosmin are quickly bound by mitochondria, and only a limited amount of myocardial washout (or washin) occurs. This means that imaging can commence as late as 2 hours after injection (more feasible than ^{201}Tl, which needs imaging as quickly as possible), and if artifact is a concern, image acquisition can simply be repeated (eg, in the prone position, **Fig. 3–27**). On the other hand, separate rest and stress injections are required to evaluate reversibility of perfusion defects. The gastrointestinal excretion of the ^{99m}Tc tracers results in high hepatic and gastrointestinal uptake which often interferes with inferior myocardial wall visualization, particularly after rest injection.

N-13 ammonia is a PET tracer with a small positron range (and therefore sharp images). Its longer half-life permits long acquisitions for 3D imaging, but limits the activity on first-pass bolus imaging. It requires an on-site or nearby cyclotron, close coordination of patient imaging with the cyclotron run, and slower patient throughput because of the longer half-life of N-13 (10 minutes) requiring decay time between rest and stress images.

Rb-82 has a short half-life permitting rapid serial rest-stress imaging or serial stress-stress images for research protocols, and a well-validated "simple" two-image acquisition protocol. However, the images are slightly less sharp than N-13 ammonia, although the small difference has no clinical consequences. The full dose

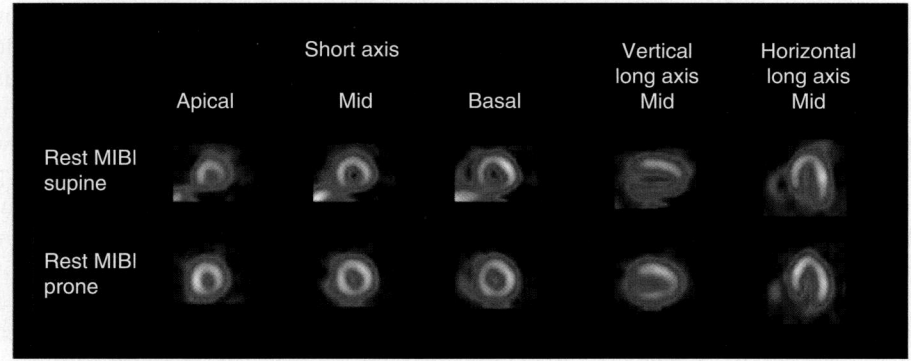

Figure 3–27. **Rest sestamibi (MIBI) single-photon emission computed tomography (SPECT) images in the supine position (*top row*) and prone position (*bottom row*) in a 55-year-old patient with a low likelihood of coronary artery disease.** Prone images are normal, demonstrating that the apparent inferior wall perfusion defect on the supine images is secondary to soft tissue attenuation. Normal wall motion was noted on gated SPECT-myocardial perfusion imaging (MPI). Gated resting MPI: end-diastolic volume 55 mL, end-systolic volume 35 mL, and ejection fraction 55%. Reproduced with permission from Germano G, Berman DS. *Clinical Gated Cardiac SPECT.* Armonk: Futura; 1999.

of 40 to 50 mCi of Rb-82 for the first-pass arterial input requires high scanner performance optimal with 2D imaging but not feasible with 3D scanners. The radiation dose for both radionuclides are similar at 1 to 2 mSV per image, compared to 3 times that dose from the CT attenuation scan of a PET-CT scanner.

Oxygen (O)-15 has a short half-life of 2 minutes and needs to be produced by an on-site cyclotron. Although 100% extracted by myocardium, myocardial uptake imaging is challenging because of its high concentration in the blood pool that requires subtraction of the blood-pool counts from the original image to visualize the myocardium. This subtraction requires acquiring a second set of images after a single inhalation of 40 to 50 mCi of O-15 carbon monoxide. Therefore, the imaging and processing protocol for the O-15 flow model is substantially more complex than the partially extracted tracers such as N-13 ammonia and Rb-82.

SPECT-MPI Stress Protocols

Patient Preparation

In general, for purposes of diagnosis or initial risk stratification, stress nuclear MPI is performed with the patient off antiischemic medications, because these medications may limit the detection of flow heterogeneity during the stress test.[122] This is true for both exercise and pharmacologic stress. Thus, in most cases, use of β-blockers or long-acting calcium channel blockers should be discontinued for 48 hours before stress imaging, and long-acting nitrates should be discontinued for 12 hours before stress imaging.

Methylxanthines, such as theophylline or caffeine, block adenosine binding and can reduce the coronary vasodilator effects of adenosine, regadenoson, or dipyridamole, leading to false-negative stress perfusion studies. Thus, patients should withhold compounds containing caffeine or theophylline for 24 hours prior to use of adenosine or dipyridamole, and 12 hours prior to use of regadenoson, prior to vasodilator stress testing.[123] In case there is a need for administration of pharmacologic stress, the recommendation that patients avoid caffeine for 24 hours is applied to all MPI studies. Dipyridamole-containing medications should be held for 48 hours prior to adenosine or regadenoson stress, because they can potentiate the effects of the vasodilator stress agents.

Exercise Stress Protocols

Exercise stress is preferred over pharmacologic stress for use with SPECT-MPI in patients who can exercise adequately because it allows assessment of exercise capacity, heart rate (HR), and blood pressure (BP) responses (including HR reserve and HR recovery); symptoms; and ST-segment response (although such ST-segment changes may occur with pharmacologic stress). This provides additional clinical information that can be useful in clinical decision-making.[122] For exercise SPECT-MPI, the tracer is injected at maximal stress. Exercise is continued for an additional 1 minute at peak workload to ensure that the myocardial tracer uptake reflects distribution of blood flow at the time of maximum flow achieved. Unless contraindicated, exercise stress testing should be maximal, terminated by symptoms, and not based on the HR achieved. If less than 85% of age-adjusted maximum predicted heart rate (MPHR; 220—age) is achieved, and unless there is clear clinical or ECG evidence of ischemia, the stress is considered inadequate, and switching to pharmacologic stress should be considered. When the exercise duration is less than 3 minutes on the Bruce protocol (or five or more metabolic equivalents [METs]), a normal SPECT is associated with a much greater event rate than in those with greater exercise capacity, similar to that seen in patients deemed unable to exercise. Postexercise stress imaging routinely commences 15 minutes after stress but, as already noted, with the ^{99m}Tc perfusion tracers, imaging can begin up to 2 hours after stress injection. Initiating image acquisition too early, before the patient has not fully recovered from stress, potentially introduces artifactual defects related to increased depth of respiration very early after stress, causing the heart to gradually move cephalad during the early portion of SPECT acquisition ("upward creep of the heart").[124]

Vasodilator Stress Protocols

For patients who cannot achieve an adequate level of exercise (at least 85% of MPHR), pharmacologic stress testing is the preferred approach to stress.[122] The preferred pharmacologic stress agents for SPECT-and PET-MPI are coronary vasodilators—adenosine, regadenoson, or dipyridamole—that provide a 3- to 5-fold increase in coronary flow (**Table 3-11**). As vasodilator stress is frequently associated with chest discomfort and shortness of breath, even in normal subjects, these symptoms are not considered to indicate the presence of ischemia. Vasodilator stress frequently causes an increase in HR, but unlike with exercise stress, the hemodynamic response is not critical to the vasodilator effect.

Dipyridamole is usually infused at 140 μg/kg/min for 4 minutes (total dose 0.56 mg/kg), and maximal hyperemia occurs

TABLE 3-11. Pharmaceutical Stress Agents				
Stress Agent	Half-Life	Dose	Infusion Protocol	Inhibitors/Antidote
Regadenoson	2–4 min[a]	0.4 mg	10 s	Methylxanthines
Adenosine	< 10 s	140 μg/kg/min	4–6 min	Methylxanthines
Dipyridamole	40 min	140 μg/kg/min	4 min	Methylxanthines
Dobutamine	2 min	5–40 μg/kg/min	Increase every 3 min up to 40 μg/kg/min, often with atropine	β-blockers

[a]Intermediate half-life 30 minutes; terminal half-life 120 minutes; methylxanthines are caffeine, theophylline, and aminophylline.

3 to 4 minutes after end of the infusion, and persists for 20 to 30 minutes. Chest pain, shortness of breath, dizziness, and flushing are common, but severe adverse effects are rare (1:10,000). Severe bronchospasm may occur, and dipyridamole is *contraindicated* in patients with asthma. Persistent side effects or significant adverse events after dipyridamole, adenosine, or regadenoson stress can usually be reversed by intravenous aminophylline (50–100 mg intravenous over 30–60 seconds).

Adenosine (140 µg/kg/min) is infused over 4 to 6 minutes, with radiopharmaceutical administration at 2 to 3 minutes of infusion. Side effects are frequent but transient (duration of action ~13 seconds), so reversal with aminophylline is rarely used. Adenosine is *contraindicated* for patients with second- or third-degree AV block, sick sinus syndrome, or bronchospasm.

Regadenoson is a selective A_{2A} receptor agonist, and therefore less likely than the other agents to provoke systemic adverse effects or bronchoconstriction. This has become the most commonly used vasodilator stress agent in the United States. It is injected over a 10-second period with a fixed dose (0.4 mg), without requiring an infusion pump. The radiopharmaceutical is injected over 10 to 20 seconds after intravenous injection of regadenoson.[123] The peak effect is seen approximately 1 minute after injection, and peak blood flow lasts for approximately 2 minutes. Regadenoson is considered *contraindicated* for patients with second- or third-degree AV block or sinus node dysfunction unless a functioning pacemaker is present.[123]

Combined Vasodilator Stress with Low-Level Exercise

It has become common to combine vasodilator stress with low-level exercise. Exercise, even at low levels, reduces splanchnic blood flow and, thereby, hepatic uptake of 99mTc-sestamibi or 99mTc-tetrofosmin, facilitating early postinfusion imaging with these tracers (10–15 minutes following injection) compared to the 1-hour delay required when adjunctive exercise is not performed. With dipyridamole, low-level exercise is begun after the end of dipyridamole infusion, and with adenosine, low-level exercise is performed during the infusion. With regadenoson, low-level exercise is started before injection, allowing the vasodilator and tracer to be injected during exercise, or the regadenoson can be added to inadequate exercise.

With exercise stress, patients with left bundle branch block (LBBB) frequently demonstrate reversible defects in the septal wall in the absence of CAD. Because of the relationship between the increase in HR and the presence of perfusion defects without CAD in LBBB and paced ventricular rhythms, vasodilator stress is preferred over exercise, and vasodilator stress protocols are performed without adjunctive low-level exercise.[122] With exercise SPECT-MPI, the perfusion defect associated with LBBB in the absence of LAD disease most commonly involves the interventricular septum with sparing of the LV apex (an uncommon pattern in LAD disease). Myocardial perfusion defects in the inferior and apical walls have also been reported in the absence of CAD in patients with prolonged RV pacing.

Dobutamine Stress

At present, dobutamine stress is usually reserved for patients with asthma, chronic obstructive pulmonary disease with bronchospasm, or patients who have ingested caffeine close to the time of testing. Dobutamine is not an ideal stressor because it results in a lower-rate pressure product than exercise and a lower peak coronary blood flow with vasodilator stress. Adverse effects, including ventricular ectopy, are more common than with vasodilator stress. The protocol used is the same as that used for dobutamine stress echocardiography, and is combined with atropine if the MPHR (>85%) is not achieved.

SPECT-MPI Imaging Protocols

Stress 99mTc-Sestamibi or 99mTc-Tetrofosmin

A variety of protocols can be used with these agents, including 2-day stress/rest, same-day rest/stress, same-day stress/rest, and dual-isotope. Because uptake and radiation dosimetry of these compounds are similar, the recommended acquisition protocols for these tracers are the same. After intravenous injection, the myocardial distribution of these agents does not change significantly over time. Therefore, in contrast to 201Tl, which redistributes into viable myocardium, separate rest and stress injections are needed with 99mTc-sestamibi or 99mtetrofosmin SPECT to assess reversibility of perfusion defects.

The most common 99mTc agent protocol is same-day low-dose rest/high-dose stress (see **Fig. 3–48A**),[43] which takes approximately 2 to 4 hours. Compared to a stress-first protocol, there is a reduction in stress-defect contrast, because approximately 15% of the radioactivity observed at the time of stress imaging comes from the preexisting resting injection. In patients with acute chest pain, the protocol has the advantage of allowing cancellation of stress if an unexpected perfusion defect is present. The same-day low-dose stress/high-dose rest sequence (see **Fig. 3–48B**) has the advantage of optimal perfusion defect contrast, with no contribution from a prior rest injection. An important advantage is that the sequence allows for cancellation of the rest portion of the test if the stress images are normal (see **Fig. 3–48C**). The resultant "stress-only" protocol reduces the overall radiation dose of the SPECT-MPI procedure by 75% and reduces the overall time of the study for the patient by a similar amount. The principal drawback of this approach is that the count rates associated with the low-dose stress images are low. In obese patients, in whom a low-dose injection may result in inadequate image quality, a 2-day stress/rest protocol may be preferred.

Stress 201Tl

Initial poststress image acquisition should be started promptly (within 15 minutes) because early 201Tl redistribution can decrease sensitivity for CAD if poststress imaging is delayed. Although the initially described stress/redistribution protocol is still commonly used, perfusion defect reversibility can be improved by reinjection with a small dose of 201Tl, use of a small dose of sublingual nitroglycerin prior to 201Tl reinjection, or additional 24-hour imaging.[125,126]

Dual-Isotope Protocols

A rest ^{201}Tl/stress ^{99m}Tc-sestamibi or ^{99m}Tc-tetrofosmin dual-isotope SPECT protocol takes advantage of the Anger camera's ability to collect data in different energy windows. Because of the increased radiation burden associated with the dual-isotope approach, its use is not recommended unless both ischemia and viability testing are needed.

Stress-Only Imaging

Stress-first protocols offer the opportunity to maximize the number of studies with stress-only imaging, resulting in several potential benefits. The rest study is not performed when stress imaging is not clearly normal; thus, there is reduced imaging time, lower radiation exposure, and lower cost.[127] Its limitations are that transient ischemic dilation (TID) and stunning cannot be assessed. The approach can also result in a higher false-positive rate than rest/stress imaging because failure of a minor defect to change between rest and stress can be used to identify artifact. The use of attenuation correction or two-position imaging is of greater importance for the stress-only protocol; they increase the percentage of normal stress images and thus reduce the percentage of patients who have to return for rest imaging.[127] The stress-only approach may be more appropriate for patients who can exercise, because patients undergoing pharmacologic stress are at higher risk. Stress-only imaging is not used in patients with known or expected resting perfusion defects.

SPECT Myocardial Viability Protocols

Rest/redistribution ^{201}Tl SPECT-MPI is the optimal SPECT approach for assessment of myocardial viability[14] (**Fig. 3–28**). Rest ^{99m}Tc-sestamibi and ^{99m}Tc-tetrofosmin can also be used for assessment of myocardial viability. However, they are not considered optimal because, unlike ^{201}Tl, they reflect only myocardial perfusion and do not redistribute into the potassium pool. These agents underestimate viability in the presence of myocardial hibernation with resting hypoperfusion. Administration of nitroglycerin prior to rest injection may improve the detection of hypoperfused but viable myocardium with these agents.

Technical and Radiation Dose Considerations

SPECT-MPI Instrumentation

Dramatic advances in cardiac SPECT instrumentation (gantry design, photon detectors, and collimators) and software reconstruction methods (incorporating resolution recovery and CT–based attenuation correction) have been introduced to clinical practice in recent years, allowing both a decrease in imaging time and a reduction in patient radiation dose. Compact cardiac scanners with cadmium-zinc-telluride (CZT) detectors, coupled with high-sensitivity collimation (multipinhole or high-sensitivity, parallel-hole—focusing on the myocardium) can achieve simultaneous improvement in sensitivity (5 to 8 times higher than with conventional MPI SPECT) and in image resolution (up to 2 times higher). To date, these new techniques have been utilized primarily to dramatically reduce the routine scan time. With faster imaging, patient comfort is markedly improved, and motion artifacts are reduced. However, these systems also allow low-dose (~4–6 mSv) stress/rest or rest/stress imaging at fast imaging times or ultra-low radiation dose (~1 mSv) stress-only scans at standard imaging times (10–12 minutes).[128,129]

Two-Position Imaging

One of the most difficult problems in interpretation of SPECT-MPI is the differentiation of artifactual from true perfusion defects. Soft-tissue attenuation and patient motion are the two major sources of artifact. Imaging the patient in two different positions decreases both types of artifacts. Regarding soft-tissue attenuation, shifting of attenuating organs occurs between supine and prone positions, particularly involving the breast and the diaphragm, the latter determining the position of sub-diaphragmatic structures. However, as prone imaging alone may create artifactual anteroseptal defects (caused by the more pronounced sternal attenuation in this position) combined prone and supine imaging (two-position imaging) has been described. With two-position SPECT, perfusion defects are considered present only when they are seen on the images in both positions.

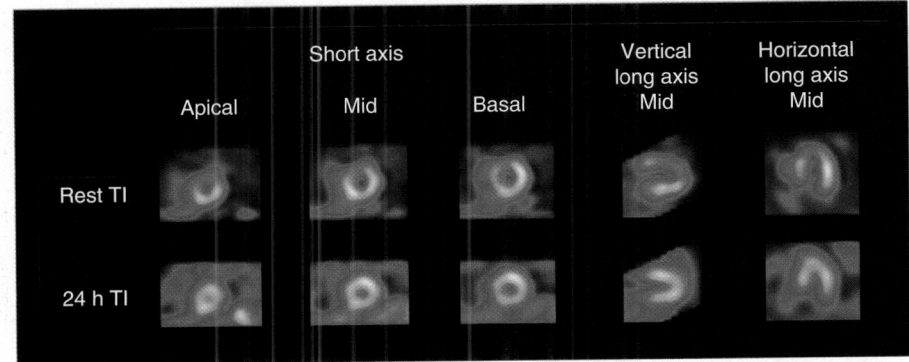

Figure 3–28. Rest and 24-hour redistribution thallium-201 (^{201}Tl) single-photon emission computed tomography (SPECT) myocardial perfusion imaging (MPI) of a 75-year-old man with atypical angina showing a large amount of resting ischemia in the left anterior descending coronary artery (LAD). Coronary angiography subsequently revealed a 95% proximal LAD stenosis. Of note, the left ventricle was larger at rest than at the time of redistribution imaging. The stress SPECT-MPI study was canceled in this patient because of the unexpected perfusion defect.

TABLE 3–12. Minimizing Radiation Dosimetry/Best Practices

Use stress/rest protocols instead of rest/stress protocols. Use stress-only protocols if stress normal.

Use weight-based dosing.

Use recommended radiopharmaceutical doses.

Avoid ^{201}Tl protocols (^{99m}Tc-based protocols are preferred).

Avoid dual-isotope (rest ^{201}Tl/stress ^{99m}Tc) protocols.

Use positron emission tomography when available.

Use newer high-efficiency solid-state single-photon emission computed tomography cameras with high-sensitivity crystal material.

Use advanced reconstruction software.

Attenuation Correction

Attenuation correction is mandatory for PET-MPI because of pronounced attenuation effects in positron emission. For SPECT, studies have demonstrated improved specificity with attenuation correction, with no change in overall sensitivity by both visual and automated computer analysis.[130,131] Hybrid SPECT/CT (and PET/CT) systems have minimized the risk of misregistration artifacts, as well as providing the capability to assess CAC and myocardial perfusion in a single examination.

Minimizing Radiation Dosimetry

The As Low As Reasonably Achievable (ALARA) principle highlights the goal to minimize radiation dosimetry in all patients while maintaining high-quality imaging. **Table 3–12** lists best practices that can help achieve this goal and/or minimize each patient's effective radiation dose.[132] Stress/rest protocols are preferred because they allow the potential for performance of stress-only SPECT if stress studies are normal. Ultra-low

radiation dose (~1 mSv) stress-only scans at standard imaging times (10–12 minutes) can now be achieved with CZT detector systems. ^{99m}Tc-based protocols are preferred over ^{201}Tl protocols due to more favorable radiation dosimetry. Because of the very short half-life of each of the PET-MPI tracers, rest/stress PET-MPI is associated with a very low radiation dose.

Interpretation of SPECT and PET-MPI

The interpretation of SPECT- and PET-MPI is performed by visual or computer-based quantitative methods. Perfusion defects are characterized by their type as well as their extent and severity. The various defect types are illustrated in **Fig. 3–29** for stress and rest SPECT-MPI and in **Fig. 3–30** for rest SPECT-MPI viability patterns. These perfusion defect patterns also apply to PET-MPI. The distribution of SPECT abnormalities provides information regarding the location of coronary artery stenoses. Representative examples of SPECT defect locations associated with individual coronary artery stenoses are illustrated in **Figs. 3–31** and **3–32**.

Semiquantitative Segmental Scoring

These scoring systems standardize the visual interpretation of scans and provide global indices for overall assessment of extent and severity of perfusion abnormality. They are more systematic and reproducible than simple qualitative evaluation. The 17-segment scoring system was adopted by the American Heart Association (AHA) in 2002 (**Fig. 3–33**).[133] Segmental assignment is based on three short-axis slices (four distal [apical], six middle, and six basal) representing the entire LV, with the apical segments visualized in a midventricular long-axis image. Each of the 17 segments has a distinct descriptor and is scored for defect severity using a five-point system (0 = normal;

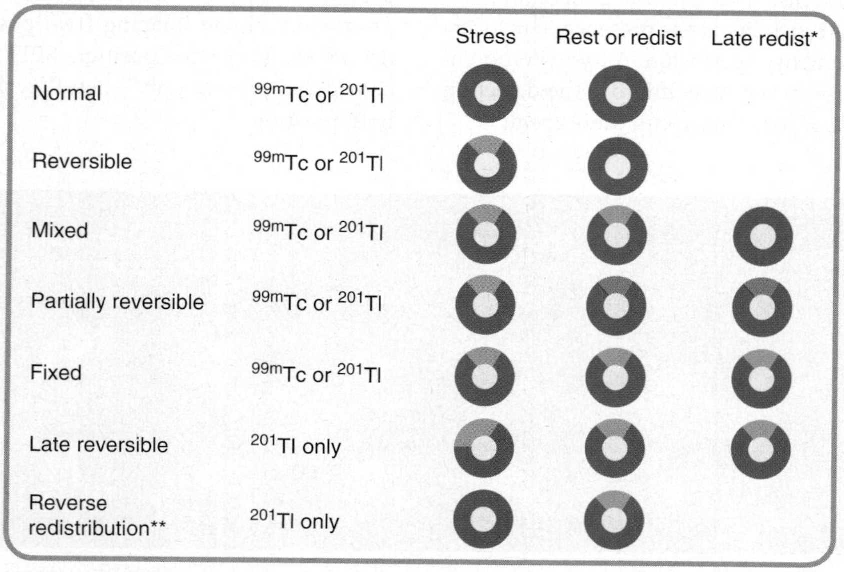

Figure 3–29. Patterns of stress/rest or redistribution (redist) single-photon emission computed tomography (SPECT) myocardial perfusion imaging (MPI) defects. Red represents normal tracer update; pink represents a definite perfusion defect; green represents less severe but still definite perfusion defect (seen in the partially reversible defect example). *Single asterisk* indicates redistribution or reinjection image. *Double asterisk* indicates stress/redist or rest/redist. ^{99m}Tc, technetium-99m–sestamibi or –tetrofosmin; ^{201}Tl, thallium-201.

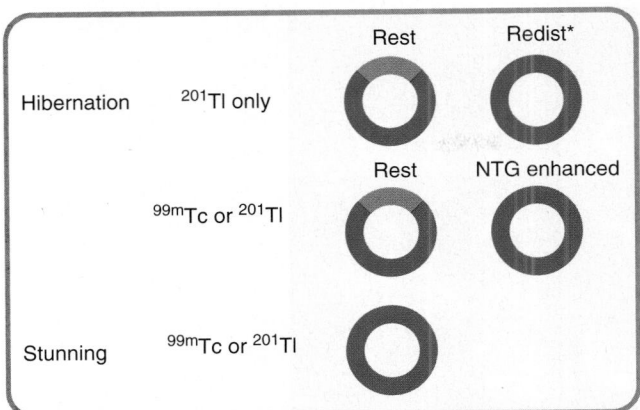

Figure 3–30. Single-photon emission computed tomography (SPECT) patterns of perfusion defects associated with myocardial viability and resting regional contractile abnormality. *Green* represents perfusion defect. The *asterisk* indicates 4- or 24-hours redistribution (Redist). NTG, nitroglycerin; ^{99m}Tc, technetium-99m-sestamibi or -tetrofosmin; ^{201}Tl, thallium-201.

1 = mild [equivocal]; 2 = moderate; 3 = severe reduction of a radioisotope; and 4 = absence of detectable tracer uptake).

The overall extent and severity of perfusion defects is reflected by the summed stress score (SSS), the summed rest score (SRS), and the summed differences score (SDS), with the latter defined by SSS – SRS and measuring the degree of reversibility. Risk groups have been defined by applying SSS categories in observational studies (**Table 3–13**).[134]

Quantitative Perfusion Analysis
Commercial software packages provide a variety of quantitative measurements (**Table 3–14**). With respect to myocardial perfusion assessment, these computer approaches generally operate by automatic determination of the amount of radioactivity observed at rest and stress within each voxel or small zone of the myocardium, scaling this amount by the maximal amount of radioactivity in the myocardium (normalization), and then comparing this scaled amount to the lower limit of normal. The perfusion defect size (extent) represents the proportion of voxels below the normal limit, which would correlate best with the number of visually abnormal segments. The total perfusion deficit (TPD) assesses both the proportion of voxels below normal limits and the degree by which they are abnormal and would correlate best with the summed segmental scores. The change between rest and stress is also assessed, providing information about perfusion defect reversibility. It is possible to automatically register and subtract the rest images from the stress images or serial stress or rest studies from previous studies, resulting in a "change" image without requiring comparison to protocol specific normal limits. The results are most commonly displayed using polar maps (**Fig. 3–34**). Quantitative analysis packages provide an objective assessment of the presence and magnitude of perfusion defects, gives the reader a "second expert" opinion and is more reproducible than expert visual assessment of serial studies. Significant advances are being made into the use of artificial intelligence for SPECT and PET interpretation.[135]

The quantitative MPI discussed thus far assesses with relative quantitation SPECT- or PET-MPI (ie, the presence and magnitude of regional myocardial perfusion abnormalities by comparison with more normal zones). With PET, the high count rates allow quantitation of the first-pass arrival of the radiotracer, permitting assessment of absolute myocardial perfusion in mL/g/min at rest and stress as well as myocardial

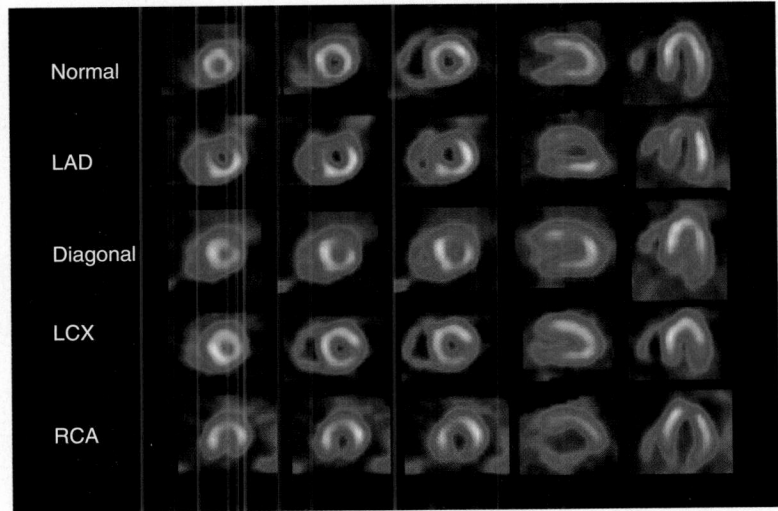

Figure 3–31. Examples of typical stress perfusion patterns corresponding to normal (*top row*) and various single-territory abnormalities. Coronary angiographic findings in these patients were as follows: left anterior descending coronary artery (LAD), proximal 95% stenosis; diagonal, occluded proximal first diagonal artery; left circumflex coronary artery (LCX), occluded first marginal artery branch; and right coronary artery (RCA), mid-95% stenosis. All patients had no evidence of myocardial infarction and normal single-photon emission computed tomography myocardial perfusion imaging at rest. From *left to right*, the images represent apical short axis, mid short axis, basal short axis, mid vertical long axis, and mid horizontal long axis. These patients show the typical distributions of perfusion defects associated with the specific coronary arteries involved.

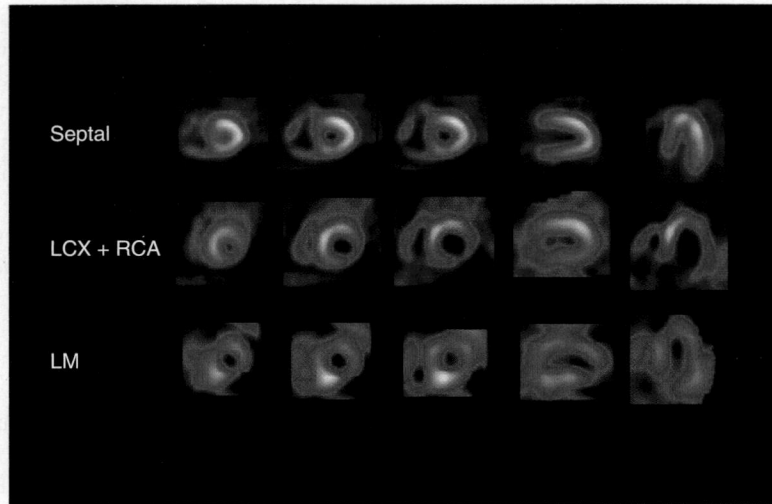

Figure 3–32. **Stress single-photon emission computed tomography myocardial perfusion imaging images demonstrating more complex patterns associated with known coronary lesions in patients with normal resting perfusion images and no history of prior myocardial infarction.** Septal refers to trapped septal perforator coronary artery (septal) in a patient with critical left anterior descending coronary artery (LAD) stenoses proximal and distal to the septal perforator takeoff and patent LAD internal mammary graft. Left circumflex coronary artery (LCX) plus right coronary artery (RCA) refers to occlusion of proximal LCX and proximal RCA. Left main (LM) refers to subtotal LM coronary artery stenosis.

flow reserve (**Figs. 3–35** and **3–36**), comparing rest and stress perfusion. With this approach, each segment or region can be assessed on its own, avoiding the reliance on comparison to perfusion of a normal area.[135]

Overall Perfusion Assessment

The final scan interpretation should express whether perfusion scan is abnormal and the degree to which it is abnormal. Summed stress scores 0 to 1 are considered normal, 2 to 3 borderline/equivocal, 3 probably abnormal, and 4 or more definitely abnormal. For percent myocardium abnormal or TPD,

2% to 3% is considered equivocal, 4% probably abnormal, and 5% or greater definitely abnormal. There is general agreement that the category of "borderline" or "equivocal" is needed for circumstances in which the interpreting physician is uncertain whether mild perfusion defects are attributable to true perfusion abnormality or to imaging artifact.

Ventricular Function

ECG gating should be performed with all SPECT- and PET-MPI protocols, whether ^{201}Tl or ^{99m}Tc tracers are used. Automatic computer-based methods quantify global function

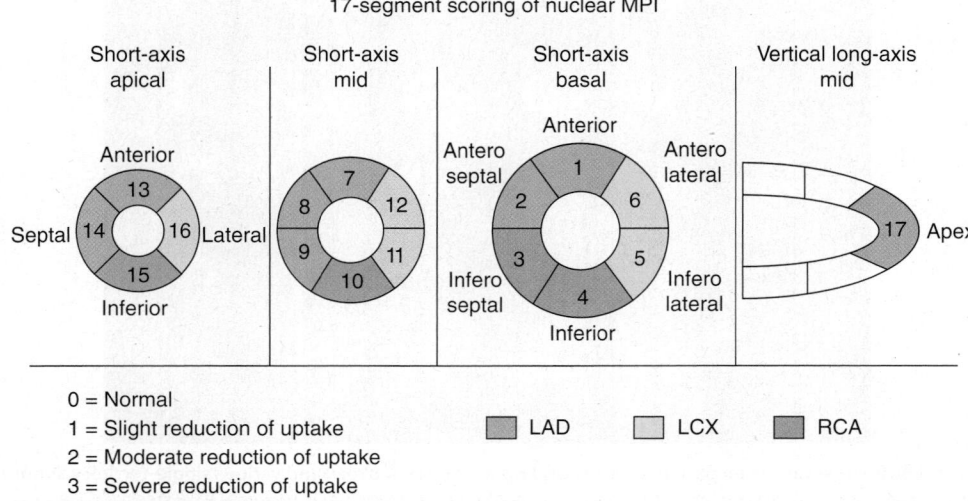

Figure 3–33. **Nuclear myocardial perfusion imaging (MPI) 17-segment scoring (diagrammatic representation of segmental division of the tomography slices and assignment of the segments to the individual coronary arteries using the 17-segment model).** LAD, left anterior descending coronary artery; LCX, left circumflex coronary artery; RCA, right coronary artery. Reproduced with permission from Imaging guidelines for nuclear cardiology procedures, part 2. American Society of Nuclear Cardiology. *J Nucl Cardiol.* 1999 Mar-Apr;6(2):G47-G84.

TABLE 3–13. Definitions of Summed Perfusion Scores and Percent Myocardium Hypoperfused

Perfusion Parameter	Derivation of Parameter	Clinical Relevance
Summed stress score (SSS)[a]	Sum of the segmental scores at stress	Amount of infarcted, ischemic, or jeopardized myocardium
Summed rest score (SRS)[a]	Sum of the segmental scores at rest	Amount of infarcted or hibernating myocardium
Summed difference score[a] (SDS)	SSS–SRS	Amount of ischemic or jeopardized myocardium
	20-Segment	**17-Segment**
Percent total	= SSS × 100/80	= SSS × 100/68
Percent ischemic	= SDS × 100/80	= SDS ×100/68
Percent fixed	= SRS × 100/80	= SRS × 100/68

[a]Reflects the extent and severity of perfusion abnormality/ischemia.
Data from Hachamovitch R, Hayes SW, Friedman JD, et al. Comparison of the short-term survival benefit associated with revascularization compared with medical therapy in patients with no prior coronary artery disease undergoing stress myocardial perfusion single photon emission computed tomography. *Circulation*. 2003 Jun 17;107(23):2900-2907.

parameters, including LVEF, end-diastolic volume, end-systolic volume, and diastolic function. Regional wall motion or thickening is most commonly assessed by semiquantitative visual analysis, using the same segmental system used for perfusion defect assessment, but wall motion and thickening can also be quantified from rest gated-MPI images. Regional function can be used to identify ischemia and stunning, distinction of perfusion defects from attenuation artifacts, and assessment of LV dyssynchrony.

Transient LV Ischemic Dilation

Several nonperfusion abnormalities can be observed with nuclear MPI, including size and shape of the LV, TID, RV myocardial uptake, RV size, and abnormalities of lung uptake or other abnormal extracardiac activity. TID is considered present when the LV cavity appears to be significantly larger in the poststress images than at rest. When accompanied by a perfusion defect, TID is considered to represent severe and extensive ischemia and has been shown to be highly specific for critical stenosis (>90% narrowing) in vessels supplying a large portion of the myocardium (ie, proximal left anterior descending or multivessel 90% lesions).[136] TID may represent true changes in LV size or may actually be an apparent cavity dilation secondary to diffuse subendocardial ischemia (obscuring the endocardial border). The latter would explain why TID may be seen for several hours following stress, when true cavity dilation would most likely no longer be present. The correlation between LV TID and lung uptake is weak, suggesting that there may be different pathophysiologic mechanisms for each, and their measurements may be complementary in assessing the extent and severity of CAD for risk stratification. Dipyridamole or adenosine-induced TID has similar implications as those associated with exercise.[129]

TABLE 3–14. Quantitative Measurements Possible with Gated Myocardial Perfusion Single-Photon Emission Computed Tomography

Type	Parameter	Comment
Perfusion	Perfusion defect extent	Expressed as percent of LV myocardium
	Perfusion defect severity	Related to the degree of hypoperfusion in the defect area
	Total perfusion deficit	Takes into account defect extent and severity; expressed as percent of LV myocardial perfusion deficit
	Segmental scores and summed scores (poststress, rest, reversibility)	Summed scores depend on specific myocardial model chosen; usually 0–4 with 17-segment model
	Change	Accounts for difference between two image sets (eg, stress/rest; study 1 vs study 2); expressed as percent of the myocardium
Function (global)	LV ejection fraction	
	LV end-systolic and end-diastolic volumes	
	PFR; time to PFR	LV diastolic function
Function (regional)	Wall motion and wall thickening	
Other	LV contraction histogram	LV contraction phase/dyssynchrony
	Lung:heart ratio	Ratio of uptake in lung and LV
	Transient ischemic dilation ratio	Ratio of LV cavity volume poststress vs at rest
	LV myocardial mass	Estimates of LV shape (global or regional)
	LV eccentricity, shape index	

Abbreviations: LV, left ventricular; PFR, peak filling rate.
Data from Sandler MP. *Diagnostic Nuclear Medicine*, 4th ed. Philadelphia, PA: Lippincott Williams & Wilkins; 2003.

Increased Lung Uptake

Increased lung uptake of tracer reflects increased pulmonary capillary wedge pressure. Nonischemic causes of increased pulmonary capillary wedge pressure, such as mitral regurgitation and mitral stenosis, are also associated with increased pulmonary uptake. Increased lung uptake after exercise has been shown to have incremental prognostic information over myocardial perfusion defect assessment.[137]

Markers of High Risk on Nuclear MPI

A number of patient characteristics, clinical and ECG stress test findings, and stress MPI findings have been found to be associated with increased patient risk of adverse events (**Table 3–15**). Clinical high-risk markers tend to be related to patient age,

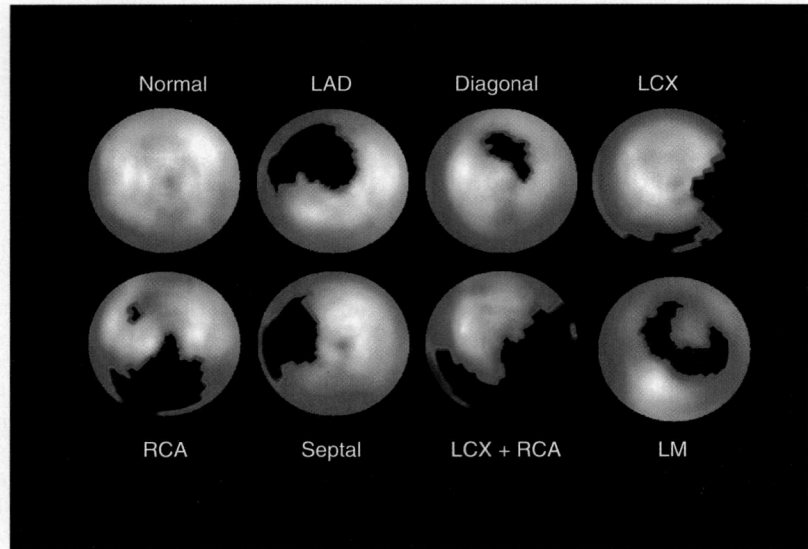

Figure 3–34. Quantitative stress polar maps of stress myocardial perfusion imaging in Figs. 3–32 and 3–33, demonstrating typical vascular perfusion pattern. *Black* represents regions of quantitative perfusion defect when compared to normal limit files. LAD, left anterior descending coronary artery; LCX, left circumflex coronary artery; LM, left main; RCA, right coronary artery.

rest ECG abnormalities, diabetes mellitus, presenting symptoms, functional capacity, and prior CAD. Stress test markers of risk include ability to perform exercise, exercise duration, stress-related BP and HR responses, ECG changes, and clinical response in terms of symptoms. MPI high-risk markers include the presence of extensive reversible or fixed defects and direct evidence of the presence of significant LV dysfunction. Hence, for any MPI result, the estimated risk of the patient is increased in proportion to the degree to which other higher risk markers are present. Consideration of markers beyond those provided by assessment of perfusion defects is particularly important in the case in patients found to have normal stress perfusion and

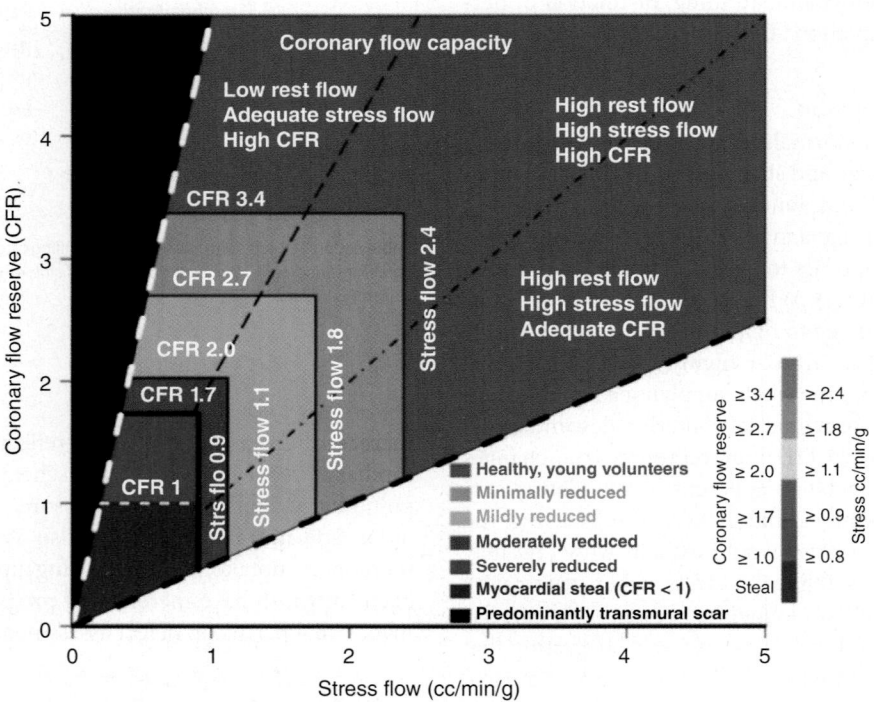

Figure 3–35. Ranges of stress flow and coronary flow reserve (CFR) for color-coding of the coronary flow capacity map. The color bar on the right of the map shows the thresholds of stress flow and CFR at each color transition (not combined stress flow–CFR values for pixels in the images). Adapted with permission from Johnson NP, Gould KL. Integrating noninvasive absolute flow, coronary flow reserve, and ischemic thresholds into a comprehensive map of physiological severity. *JACC Cardiovasc Imaging.* 2012 Apr;5(4):430-440.

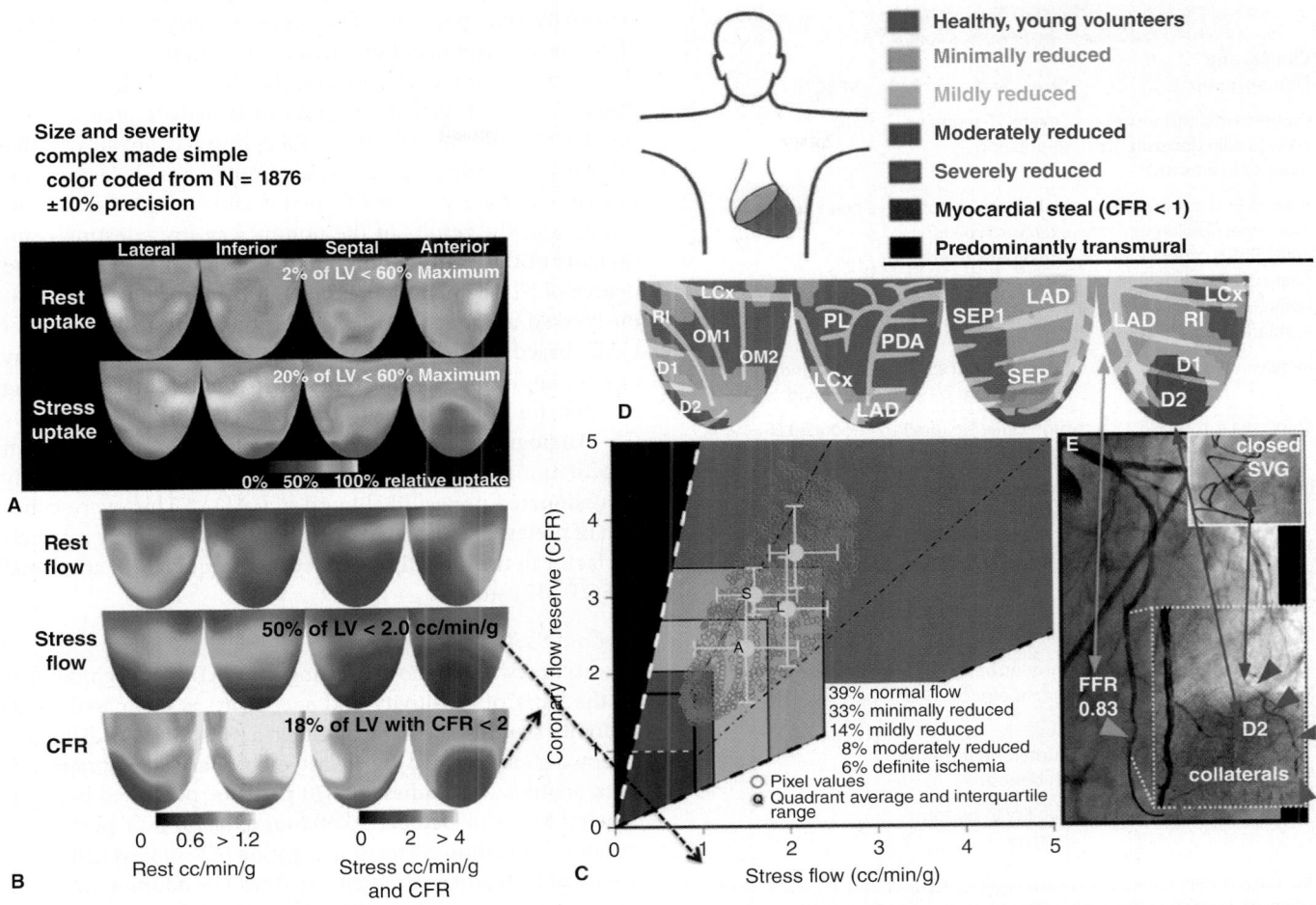

Figure 3–36. Integration of quantitative PET perfusion images. (**A**) Rest-stress relative images. (**B**) rest-stress perfusion in cc/min/g and coronary flow reserve (CFR). (**C**) Pixel plot of stress perfusion and CFR for color coding each pixel (**D**) Coronary flow capacity map made by projecting each color-coded pixel back to its original position in the topographic image. The percent of left ventricle (LV) in each of the color-coded groups are printed out on the pixel plot. The angiogram inset has arrows relating the angiogram to corresponding locations on the coronary flow capacity map. D, diagonal branch; FFR, fractional flow reserve; LAD, left anterior descending coronary artery; LCx, left circumflex coronary artery; OM, obtuse marginal branch; PDA, posterior descending artery; PL, posterior left ventricular branch; RI, ramus intermedius; SEP, septal perforator; SVG, saphenous vein graft. Reproduced with permission from Johnson NP, Gould KL. Integrating noninvasive absolute flow, coronary flow reserve, and ischemic thresholds into a comprehensive map of physiological severity. *JACC Cardiovasc Imaging.* 2012 Apr;5(4):430-440.

function, but with TID, LV enlargement, or severe ST-segment changes.

Sources of Artifact

As with any diagnostic test, quality control is critical to effective clinical application of nuclear-MPI. Artifactual perfusion defects have a variety of causes, the most common of which are patient motion, breast and diaphragmatic attenuation, reconstruction artifacts caused by adjacent or superimposed extracardiac radioactivity, and poor count statistics. With both SPECT- and PET-MPI, several technical artifacts can affect the accuracy of LVEF measurement. LVEFs can be overestimated in analyzing images of small hearts, because of the limitations of spatial resolution. In patients with LVH, LVEF may be underestimated because of failure to accurately determine the endocardial border in the presence of the large muscle mass. Marked arrhythmia results in a falsely low LVEF measurement.

SPECT two-view imaging—in supine/prone or upright/supine positions—reduces both attenuation and motion artifacts. With hybrid SPECT/CT or PET/CT systems, misregistration of perfusion and attenuation correction images is a major source of artifact.

Assessment of Myocardial Viability

Viability is considered present if the degree of uptake at rest, redistribution, or following nitrate-augmented rest injection is normal or nearly normal within segments showing contractile dysfunction. The presence of normal or near-normal tracer uptake in an abnormally contracting segment predicts improvement in ventricular function with successful revascularization. A dysfunctional segment or region with severely reduced or absent uptake of radioactivity on a viability study is considered to be nonviable. Areas with moderate reduction of counts in these conditions are usually partially viable,

TABLE 3–15. Markers of High Risk

Clinical and Demographic	Stress Test	SPECT
Diabetes mellitus (especially insulin dependence, more so in women)	Severe ST-segment depression	TID
Resting ECG abnormalities: atrial fibrillation, LBBB, RBBB, other block (first-or second-degree, hemiblocks), LVH with repolarization, PVCs	Inability to perform exercise/Type of stress performed	Lung uptake
Increasing age	Exercise-induced hypotension	Stress-induced stunning
Increased resting HR	High Duke Treadmill Score	Reduced EF
Dyspnea as presenting symptom	Stress-induced ventricular dysrhythmias	Severe and/or extensive defects
Typical angina Functional capacity	Tachycardic response to stress	Increased RV tracer uptake
Presentation with unstable angina	Exercise duration	Akinetic-dyskinetic LV segments
History of prior CAD (especially prior myocardial infarction)	Chronotropic incompetence	LV enlargement
	Blunted HR response to adenosine	
	Inability to perform exercise	

Abbreviations: CAD, coronary artery disease; ECG, electrocardiogram; EF, ejection fraction; HR, heart rate; LBBB, left bundle branch block; LV, left ventricular; LVH, left ventricular hypertrophy; PVC, premature ventricular contraction; RBBB, right bundle branch block; RV, right ventricular; SPECT, single-photon emission computed tomography; TID, transient ischemic dilation.

and patients in this group have a variable response in terms of improvement after revascularization. In a substudy involving about half of the 1212 patients with CAD suitable for coronary artery bypass graft (CABG) and an LVEF of <35% randomized in the STICH trial who underwent a baseline assessment of myocardial viability, 81% had viable myocardium. Patients with viable myocardium did not have a different mortality to the remainder, and viability did not influence the treatment effect of CABG.[138] These results have led to less interest in viability testing, but they may simply reflect that viability is but one aspect of decision-making regarding revascularization.

Clinical Applications of Nuclear Myocardial Perfusion Imaging

The most common applications are identifying inducible ischemia in patients with suspected disease, assessing the likelihood that a patient with known CAD has ischemia, evaluating patients prior to noncardiac interventions, and assessing the magnitude of ischemia for prognostic purposes.

Appropriate Patient Selection

For a given test result, the posttest likelihood is a function of three variables: patient pretest likelihood of disease and the test sensitivity and specificity. The degree to which the test result alters the posttest likelihood is directly affected by the pretest likelihood of disease. The greatest shift in posttest likelihood of disease occurs in patients with an intermediate pretest likelihood of CAD. Pretest likelihood takes into account all available information, including age, sex, symptoms, risk factors, the degree of coronary atherosclerosis if known (eg, from a CAC score), and the results of the nonnuclear stress testing components of the examination (eg, the duration of exercise and degree of ST-segment depression). It is important that previously-used approaches to assessing the pretest likelihood of CAD, based on the work of Diamond and Forrester,[139] may not be applicable in the types of patients currently being referred for noninvasive testing. In CONFIRM (COronary CT Angiography EvaluatioN For Clinical Outcomes: An InteRnational Multicenter registry), these criteria markedly overestimated pretest likelihood of CAD.[140] This overestimation of pretest likelihood of obstructive CAD is likely a principal factor in the recently observed low frequency of abnormal SPECT-MPI studies.

Diagnostic Accuracy of SPECT

The accuracy of diagnostic testing for CAD has been defined on the basis of sensitivity and specificity as compared to an anatomic stenosis standard of either a 50% or 70% diameter-narrowing determined by invasive coronary angiography. A meta-analysis (86 studies, 10,870 patients, published between January 2002 and October 2009) found that SPECT performed without attenuation correction or gating (63 studies) had a sensitivity of 87% and a specificity of 70%. The addition of gating information increased specificity to 78% (19 studies), and the use of attenuation correction further increased specificity to 81% (12 studies).[141]

In a meta-analyses comparing the sensitivity and specificity of 8 attenuation corrected and gated SPECT (1344 patients) versus 15 PET-MPI studies (1755 patients), McArdle et al. reported a pooled sensitivity of 90% (95% confidence interval [95% CI], 0.88–0.92) and specificity of 88% (95% CI, 0.85–0.91) for PET and a sensitivity of 85% (95% CI, 0.82–0.87) and specificity of 85% (95% CI, 0.82–0.87) for SPECT.[142] Pooling PET and SPECT studies, the areas under the summary receiver–operating characteristic curves were 0.95 and 0.90 for PET and SPECT (P <0.0001), respectively. As part of a comparison of multiple modalities (SPECT, PET, stress echocardiography, CT, or magnetic resonance [MR]) to invasive FFR, 37 studies were identified (n = 2048 patients).[143] This greater diagnostic accuracy of PET versus SPECT results from better resolution and attenuation correction of PET. Using FFR as a gold standard, PET had a lower negative likelihood ratio compared to SPECT (PET 0.14 [95% CI, 0.02–0.87]; SPECT 0.39 [95% CI, 0.27–0.55]) with a greater positive likelihood ratio (PET 7.43 [95% CI, 5.03–10.99]; SPECT 3.76 [95% CI, 2.74–5.16]). PET, MR, and CT perfusion performed similarly in excluding abnormal FFR, whereas MR and PET had similar positive likelihood ratios that were greater than that of CT. SPECT and stress echocardiography were inferior to the three other modalities with respect to both metrics.[143]

A major limitation in assessing the diagnostic accuracy of nuclear MPI to detect CAD is that the decision to perform the gold standard test—catheter-based coronary angiography—after nuclear testing is strongly influenced by the MPI result, thereby biasing the population available for the analysis of test accuracy. This is referred to as past test referral bias or verification bias. The referral to invasive angiography is largely driven by the presence of ischemia, particularly the extent and severity of perfusion abnormalities, as well as anginal symptoms, ECG changes, and other clinical factors. This referral pattern results in an overestimation of test sensitivity and a reduction in test specificity, because only a small proportion of patients with normal or low-risk MPI findings proceed to invasive coronary angiography, resulting in more variability in specificity measures than in sensitivity with the most dramatic change occurring in specificity.[144]

The normalcy rate has been suggested as surrogate for assessing test *specificity* without requiring the angiographic standard; thus, it is not being affected by the marked posttest referral bias associated with assessment of specificity based on invasive coronary angiographic stenosis.[144] The normalcy rate is defined as the percentage of patients with normal test results in a population with a low (<10%) pretest risk of CAD. Unfortunately, this measure is imperfect—it does not reflect the individuals being tested, and they may be less likely to show artifacts (eg, due to less frequent obesity, less likely to move during the study, more likely to have higher-quality images).

Risk Assessment with SPECT

The assessment of prognostic accuracy overcomes many of the limitations of diagnostic accuracy of stress MPI that have been previously discussed. Both the number and the severity of perfusion defects are related to adverse cardiac outcomes in an exponential fashion, with extent and severity of ischemia as independent predictors of outcome. Measurements of myocardial flow with PET-MPI add incremental information over perfusion defects. The incremental prognostic value of SPECT- and PET-MPI has since been documented extensively, including a broad spectrum of patient subsets.

In the resulting *risk-based approach* for to use of MPI in patients with known or suspected CAD with stable symptoms, the focus is not on predicting the presence of CAD but on identifying patients at risk for specific, potentially preventable adverse events. Subsequent management then focuses on reducing the risk of these outcomes—for example, by adherence and intensification of guideline-directed medical therapy or intervention.[145] Although this approach has been extensively evaluated using registry data for both SPECT- and PET-MPI, the recent ISCHEMIA randomized trial showed no benefit from an invasive strategy in those with moderate to severe ischemia.[66]

Risk evaluation seems to be most helpful when patients are identified as having low risk. A normal scan is generally associated with a less than 1% annual risk of cardiac death or MI, but all-cause mortality rates following a normal MPI are expectedly higher than that of cardiac-specific end points.[146] In higher risk cohorts, cardiovascular mortality risk can be about 2% per year

or higher. However, there are subsets of patients with a normal scan in whom the absolute risk is not low: those needing pharmacologic stress, known CAD, diabetes mellitus (especially in women), and advanced age. Patients with reduced EF, those presenting with dyspnea or showing reduced exercise duration, or with risk factors (hypertension, smoking, diabetes) all have a worse outcome.[147] In addition, a dynamic temporal component of risk is present, and it is possible to designate a *warranty* period for specific patient groups.

Risk Assessment with PET-MPI

As recently summarized,[148] a large number of studies have evaluated the prognostic value of stress PET-MPI. As described for SPECT-MPI, the risk of a normal stress PET is very low, with risk increasing as a function of the extent and severity of perfusion defects, as well as disturbances of absolute flow and CFR.[149]

Cost-Effectiveness and Comparative Effectiveness

A number of investigators have examined the relationship between SPECT-MPI and subsequent patient management. The extent and severity of reversible defects shown by the SPECT-MPI result are the dominant factors driving subsequent resource utilization.[134] A strategy of SPECT-MPI with selective subsequent catheterization produced a substantial reduction (31% to 50%) in costs for all levels of pretest clinical risk compared with a direct catheterization approach with essentially identical outcomes as assessed by cardiac death and MI rates. Importantly, in the SPECT-MPI strategy, rates of revascularization, rates of cardiac catheterization after normal SPECT-MPI, and the frequency of normal coronary angiographic findings were significantly reduced.[150]

However, proof of cost-effectiveness in imaging requires appropriate downstream decisions to embark on appropriate therapy. In many instances, this does not occur—for example, in SPARC (Study of Myocardial Perfusion and Coronary Anatomy Imaging Roles in Coronary Artery Disease), 38% to 61% of patients with the most abnormal SPECT, PET, and CCTA test results were not referred to catheterization.[151]

PROMISE (Prospective Multicenter Imaging Study for Evaluation of Chest Pain) randomized 10,003 symptomatic patients to an initial strategy of CCTA versus functional testing (67% nuclear MPI, 23% stress echocardiography, and 10% exercise ECG).[152] The primary endpoint (death, ACS, or major procedural complication) occurred in approximately 3% of randomized patients at 2 years of follow-up, and was similar by randomization strategy. The result emphasizes that, to provide value, MPI must be applied in a population with at least intermediate risk or likelihood of CAD. Notably, the PROMISE trial provided evidence that the pretest likelihood of obstructive CAD and of risk is overestimated by current clinical algorithms.

Appropriate Use Criteria

The appropriate use criteria (AUC) documents were developed to guide healthcare coverage decisions and are now mandated by many payers in the United States. A recent multimodality

AUC document has replaced prior modality-specific AUC papers on detection and risk-assessment of stable IHD,[153] and focuses on suspected stable ischemic heart disease, known stable ischemic heart disease, and preoperative cardiac assessment. The multimodality AUC categorizes indications for cardiac imaging as appropriate (usually ~70%), *maybe appropriate* (15%), or rarely appropriate (15%).[154] Moreover, the term *maybe appropriate* also indicates that some of the patients within a given indication will be candidates for MPI. Further, the term *appropriate* does not mandate testing but supports that a large proportion of patients within a given indication will be candidates for nuclear MPI. Importantly, the term *rarely appropriate* does not prohibit testing but implies that only a limited number of patients within a given indication will be candidates for nuclear MPI.

Radionuclide Angiography

Radionuclide angiography (RNA) can be performed by either equilibrium or first-pass methods, with assessments of LVEF, RV EF, LV regional wall motion, and LV volumes and LV diastolic function. Equilibrium RNA uses ECG-gated acquisition, in which each frame corresponds to a specific portion (interval or gate) of the cardiac cycle, identified relative to the R wave on the patient's ECG—the source of the term MUGA scan (multiple gated acquisition). Methods for automatically assessing LVEF from gated blood-pool SPECT have been developed and validated.[155] Because the SPECT approach avoids the overlap of cardiac chambers inherent in planar imaging, it enhances assessment of regional function and may well become the method of choice for RNA.

Myocardial Metabolic and Viability Imaging

Just as acutely reduced coronary blood flow causes ACSs, chronically reduced coronary blood flow causes "chronic coronary syndromes"—hibernating myocardium, stunned myocardium, or ischemic cardiomyopathy. These chronic coronary syndromes are usually caused by chronic total coronary occlusion with collateral perfusion or chronic subtotal occlusion with low forward coronary flow.

Clinical Myocardial Metabolism

With adequate oxygenated coronary blood flow, the myocardium preferentially metabolizes fatty acids aerobically as its primary source of energy for contraction. Following a high-sugar or a high-carbohydrate meal, the myocardium adapts by switching a substantial portion of its energy requirements for contraction to aerobic glucose metabolism. Ischemia resulting from low blood flow or hypoxia interrupts aerobic metabolism of either fatty acids or glucose. The myocardium then switches to anaerobic metabolism of glucose with production of lactic acid because complete metabolism to carbon dioxide requires an adequate supply of oxygenated coronary blood flow.

Under conditions of reduced coronary flow or hypoxia, the myocardial shift to anaerobic metabolism of glucose can provide only limited energy for contraction as a result of the accumulation of lactic acid, impeding further anaerobic metabolism of glucose and impeding LV contraction. Although this low-level fuel source from anaerobic metabolism of glucose at low coronary perfusion may inhibit regional contraction, it provides sufficient metabolism to maintain noncontracting myocardial cell integrity for prolonged periods. The dysfunctional myocardium recovers aerobic metabolism and contractile function on restoration of adequate oxygenated blood flow, hence the term *hibernating myocardium*.

The noninvasive study of the myocardium substrate's metabolism with PET extends beyond coronary perfusion and delivery of products necessary for metabolism. Energy-generating substrate oxidation relates to external cardiac work, myocardial efficiency, myocardial changes in energy needs, and substrate availability by shifting its metabolism among substrates in normal healthy myocardium. A wide spectrum of radionuclide probes is available for imaging these metabolic shifts, ranging from radiolabeled myocardial fatty acid, glucose, lactate, and amino acid metabolism to neuronal control and activity. The radioligand ^{18}F-FDG is the most important and widely used for clinical applications. As a glucose analog, it tracks the initial transport of glucose from blood into cells and its phosphorylation to glucose-6-phosphate as the initial metabolic step of transformation of exogenously derived glucose. Because phosphorylated ^{18}F-FDG cannot be metabolized further, it is metabolically trapped in the cell and accumulates in tissue in proportion to rates of exogenous glucose utilization.

Hibernating and Stunned Myocardium

The term *viable* is rather broad because, by definition, it also applies to normally contracting myocardium with adequate perfusion as well as ischemic myocardium with normal resting contraction without scar. By common use, *myocardial viability imaging* implies poorly contracting myocardium caused by chronic or transient low myocardial perfusion that recovers contractile function with restoration of normal perfusion. Improved segmental contractile function following revascularization serves as a measure of *myocardial viability*.

Myocardial hibernation is a response to chronically reduced resting myocardial blood flow, where the myocardium downregulates its energy expenditures for contractile work so that the diminished energy demand matches the diminished energy supply. Associated with this downregulation, the myocardium switches substrate selection from fatty acid to glucose as a more oxygen-efficient substrate to accommodate the reduced supply of coronary perfusion that is available. In hibernating myocardium, importantly, energy-producing cellular processes are maintained, although at a lower level, with high-energy phosphates expended mostly for the maintenance of transmembrane ion concentration gradients and for facilitation of basic cell maintenance rather than active contraction.[156]

Myocardial stunning is the myocardial response to a transient ischemic episode caused by a severe, but transient, decline in coronary flow or an increase in cardiac work without adequate flow increase (demand-induced ischemia). Following the ischemic episode, blood flow promptly recovers, but contractile dysfunction of the postischemic myocardium initially persists (ie, "stunning") and recovers only gradually over subsequent hours, weeks, or months.[157] In this scenario, repeated ischemic episodes interrupt the recovery of contractile function, leading to chronic impairment of contractile function despite normal resting coronary blood flow. A distinct feature of "repetitive" or "chronic stunning" is, therefore, the relatively well-preserved coronary flow at rest, which differs from the diminished resting coronary flow in "hibernating myocardium." Apart from hibernation, regional flow reductions may also reflect scar tissue and infarcted myocardium with irreversible loss or impairment of contractile function.

In patients, hibernation likely coexists with stunning in dysfunctional but viable myocardium. The delicate balance between supply and demand, although at a lower level, combined with the severe impairment in flow reserve renders "hibernating" myocardium susceptible to temporary increases in demand as, for example, related to physical and mental stress during daily life so that ischemia and stunning are superimposed on hibernation.[158] This possibly accounts for the "incomplete adaptation to ischemia" and for progressive loss of viable tissue.[159]

Imaging Myocardial Viability

Regional increases in myocardial glucose utilization are most reliably identified by comparing the myocardial ^{18}F-FDG uptake with myocardial perfusion. Resting myocardial perfusion is typically acquired first followed by assessment of ^{18}F-FDG uptake. ^{18}F-FDG is administered intravenously with image acquisition beginning 1 hour later. The F-18 glucose analog, ^{18}F-FDG, is taken up by viable myocardium in the LV regions of low resting perfusion, thereby imaged as a perfusion-FDG mismatch.[160] This perfusion-FDG "abnormal mismatch" pattern of high ^{18}F-FDG uptake in regions of low resting relative perfusion is the hallmark of hibernating myocardium.

Stress MPI after the rest perfusion image before ^{18}F-FDG imaging may add clinically useful diagnostic information. Although not essential for the assessment of viability, rest-stress perfusion imaging can delineate the extent and severity of epicardial CAD and provide explanations for increases in myocardial ^{18}F-FDG uptake in normally perfused but dysfunctional regions of myocardium. A stress-induced perfusion defect reflects a regional impairment in myocardial flow reserve and identifies the dysfunctional myocardium as chronically stunned. Furthermore, stress perfusion images aid in identifying possible reasons for impairments in LV function. Different from ischemic cardiomyopathies with regional stress-induced perfusion defects, myocardial perfusion in nonischemic idiopathic dilated cardiomyopathy is characteristically homogeneous both at rest and during vasodilator stress.

There are four basic clinical perfusion-FDG image patterns (**Fig. 3–37**):

- Normal perfusion and normal FDG or "normal match" of healthy subjects or patients with low LVEF caused by nonischemic cardiomyopathy (A)
- Abnormal perfusion and abnormal FDG or "abnormal match" of myocardial scar (B)

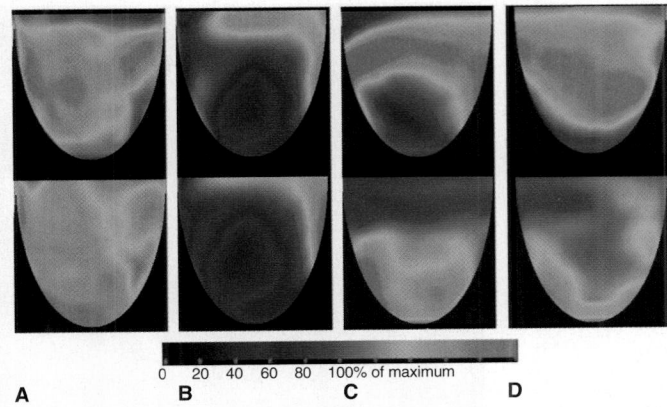

Figure 3–37. Single topographic views of left ventricle with patterns of relative perfusion and ^{18}F-FDG images. The color bar scales the relative activity with red being 100% of relative maximum activity. (**A**) Normal perfusion and normal ^{18}F-FDG or "normal match." (**B**) Abnormal perfusion and abnormal ^{18}F-FDG or "abnormal match" of myocardial scar. (**C**) Abnormal perfusion and normal ^{18}F-FDG or "abnormal mismatch" of hibernating myocardium. (**D**) Normal perfusion and low ^{18}F-FDG uptake or "reverse mismatch" of adequately perfused myocardium metabolizing fatty acids rather than glucose.

- Abnormal perfusion and normal ^{18}F-FDG or "abnormal mismatch" of hibernating myocardium in the distal half of the LV (C)
- Normal perfusion and low FDG uptake or "reverse mismatch" of adequately perfused myocardium metabolizing fatty acids rather than glucose (D)

Transaxially acquired perfusion and metabolism images are reoriented into short-axis and vertical and horizontal long-axis slices, using the same reorientation parameters for both (**Fig. 3–38**). Visual assessment of myocardial radiotracer concentrations employs the standard 17-segment model and grades segmental radiotracer activity concentrations separately for the perfusion and ^{18}F-FDG images on a four-point scale, where 1 is normal; 2, mildly reduced; 3, moderately reduced; and 4, severely reduced or absent radiotracer activity.[161] Differences in segmental radiotracer uptake between perfusion and metabolism images of at least one grade are considered "segmental metabolism perfusion-mismatches." The sum of segments with mismatch scores represents the extent of potentially reversible dysfunctional myocardium. The sum of all segmental mismatch scores serves as a measure of the combined extent and severity of the "mismatch myocardial region" or the amount of viable myocardium.

Semiquantitative information on regionally increased ^{18}F-FDG uptake relative to blood flow is available through polar or topographic map analysis of the PET ^{18}F-FDG and perfusion images as in **Fig. 3–39**. The analysis approach defines myocardial regions with the highest relative flow-tracer uptake as "normal" as the reference for normalizing the ^{18}F-FDG polar maps. "Mismatches" between metabolism and perfusion are identified by subtracting the perfusion from the normalized metabolism polar maps (regional differences) (Fig. 3–39). Regional count differences are compared to a database of normal values and predetermined thresholds defined as "mismatches" of ^{18}F-FDG

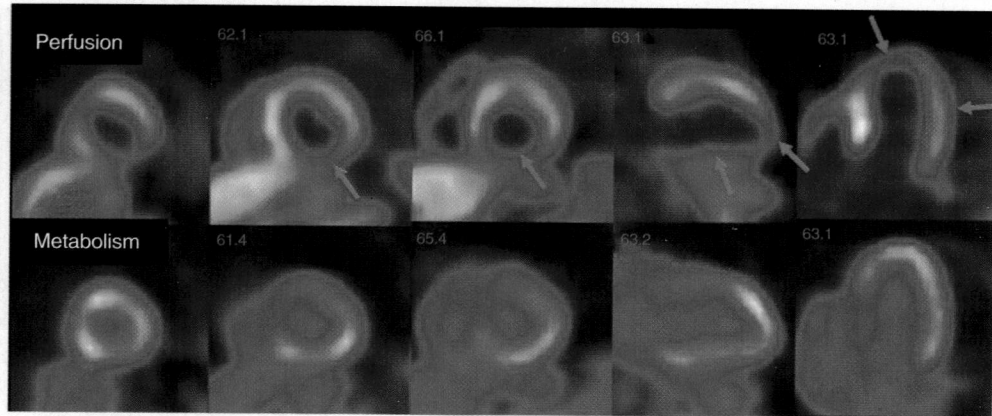

Figure 3–38. Myocardial viability with positron emission tomography myocardial perfusion and ¹⁸F-FDG imaging. The short-axis and vertical and horizontal long-axis images reveal an extensive moderate to severe perfusion defect in the distal anterior wall, the apex, and the inferior and inferolateral walls. Metabolic activity as shown on the ¹⁸F-FDG images is preserved throughout the hypoperfused myocardium, consistent with a large perfusion metabolism mismatch and thus myocardial viability. Note the low ¹⁸F-FDG uptake in apparently normally perfused myocardium, related to the patient's fasting prior to the study, leading to suppression of ¹⁸F-FDG uptake in normal myocardium.

uptake relative to perfusion. Accordingly, the quantitative image analysis approach generates a map of the geographic distribution and the total amount of viable (perfusion defect metabolism mismatch), nonviable (perfusion defect metabolism match), and normal myocardium (no perfusion defect normal metabolism match). Based on postrevascularization outcomes in regional wall motion, differences of more than two SDs from the normal indicate potential reversibility of wall motion impairment.[161] Importantly, the approach identifies those myocardial regions with increased extraction of ¹⁸F-FDG and thus of glucose relative to blood flow as an indication of persisting energy-producing metabolic processes that are essential for cell survival and identification of myocardial viability likely to benefit from improved coronary blood flow.

Some laboratories employ ¹⁸F-FDG imaging only for the assessment of reversible contractile dysfunction. Myocardial segments with normal or only mildly reduced (ie, <50%) ¹⁸F-FDG uptake are considered reversibly dysfunctional, whereas segments with more severe reductions in ¹⁸F-FDG uptake (usually >50%) are considered to be irreversibly dysfunctional.[163] Acquisition of gated ¹⁸F-FDG images affords assessments of regional myocardial systolic thickening as an

additional parameter of viability. However, ¹⁸F-FDG only may be diagnostically limited. Dysfunctional myocardial regions with only mild matched perfusion and metabolism defects that do not recover function following revascularization are identified as viable by ¹⁸F-FDG imaging only. Conversely, in regions with more severe reductions in ¹⁸F-FDG uptake, defined by the ¹⁸F-FDG–only approach as "nonviable," the ¹⁸F-FDG uptake may substantially exceed regional flow and, thus, reflect the presence of viable myocardium. Moreover, the variability of ¹⁸F-FDG uptake in normal myocardium (ie, low or no uptake because of fasting, fatty food, or diabetes), frequently limits accurate identification of "viable myocardium" without characterization of perfusion.

Patient Preparation

In view of these complex adaptive metabolic pathways, the preparation in the 24 hours before and at the time of the ¹⁸F-FDG PET scan is essential for clinically reliable results. This pre-PET preparation is largely due to the myocardium's ability to shift its energy needs among several fuel substrates including free fatty acid, glucose, and lactate. High carbohydrate meals in the 24 hours before the ¹⁸F-FDG PET are necessary to precondition

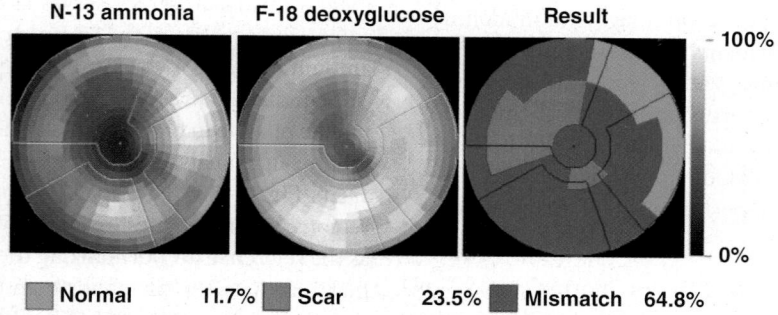

Figure 3–39. Polar map analysis of perfusion (N-13 ammonia) and glucose uptake (¹⁸F-FDG) images. Note the extensive perfusion defect in the interventricular septum and anterior wall associated with reduced ¹⁸F-FDG uptake. The "results" polar map delineates an extensive perfusion metabolism mismatch (*segments in blue*), a perfusion metabolism match (shown in *red*, reflecting scar tissue) with well-preserved ¹⁸F-FDG uptake and perfusion in the lateral and inferior wall, consistent with normal myocardium shown in *green*. Images derived with "Munich Heart" software package.

myocardium toward glucose metabolism and inhibit fatty acid metabolism. For resting perfusion-FDG imaging without stress, high-carbohydrate food can be eaten up to 2 hours before the scan. For combined vasodilator stress imaging with ^{18}F-FDG after the stress perfusion image, patients should fast for 4 hours before the study. Several standardization protocols are available:

1. Oral glucose loading. After an approximate 5-hour fasting period, oral glucose (50–100 g) is administered orally about 1 hour prior to the ^{18}F-FDG injection. Besides suppressing circulating free fatty acid levels, glucose loading raises plasma glucose concentrations and stimulates insulin secretion.

2. Administration of the antilipolytic agent acipimox. Acipimox diminishes lipolysis and, therefore, also circulating free fatty acid levels. It also increases glucose levels caused by prior carbohydrate ingestion.

3. Euglycemic-hyperinsulinemic clamping.[164] This entails continuous infusion of insulin with coinfusion of glucose at rates to maintain the plasma glucose concentrations within the range of normal. Among the standardization approaches, glucose clamping most consistently produces high-quality diagnostic ^{18}F-FDG images. However, it is so labor intensive that its use has remained confined to investigational settings.

4. Hybrid approach. After high-carbohydrate foods during the preceding 24 hours, a modified relatively simple insulin semiclamp can be easily applied. Just prior to the PET ^{18}F-FDG study, measure fingerstick blood sugar to determine the need for intravenous glucose and insulin to enhance myocardial uptake of ^{18}F-FDG for optimally differentiating viable myocardium from scar. The loading dose of intravenous glucose and addition of regular insulin intravenously depends on the baseline blood glucose. The aim is a controlled intravenous glucose load followed by a decreasing blood glucose indicating adequate response to native or exogenous injected insulin, thereby ensuring myocardial uptake of FDG.

Summary

The options for imaging in known or suspected CAD include echocardiography, CMR, MDCT, and PET as alternative or complementary modalities to stress SPECT-MPI. Each modality is likely to play an important clinical role for the foreseeable future. In many patients, these tests will be used in combination to most effectively guide patient management decisions. The ability of myocardial perfusion SPECT to provide standardized procedures that are not highly technologist dependent and provide objective quantization assessments of myocardial perfusion and function with equipment of only moderate expense offers a strength likely to sustain this approach for many years. Robust quantification will facilitate the application of artificial intelligence to image processing and interpretation.[165] Over a longer time frame, echocardiography, CT, and CMR may increasingly be used for many of the applications for which SPECT is commonly used today. During this time, however, opportunities for growth of molecular imaging methods both in SPECT and in PET are likely to be developed as growth areas for the field of nuclear cardiology. Although the basic SPECT camera has had little fundamental change over several decades, entirely new SPECT approaches have been introduced recently, offering the potential to increase both sensitivity (reducing imaging time or radiation dose) and resolution.

The current explosion of information in cell biology has led to initial formulations of numerous imaging agents with specific molecular targets. Perhaps the greatest future potential of the discipline of nuclear cardiology lies in molecular imaging because of the ability of the radiotracer technique to assess minute tracer concentrations in vivo. SPECT and PET methods are thousands of times more sensitive than ultrasound, MRI, or CT methods.[166] Although most work has occurred with PET in this regard, molecular SPECT tracers have also been developed.

ECHOCARDIOGRAPHY

The term *echocardiography* refers to the evaluation of cardiac structure and function with images and recordings produced by ultrasound. Currently, echocardiography (echo) provides essential (and sometimes unexpected) clinical information and is among the most frequently performed diagnostic procedures. The history of this technique has been closely linked with advances in computer processing, storage, and miniaturization. In the current era, handheld echographs that can be carried in a lab coat, use of 3D visualization, and the assessment of myocardial mechanics in the echo lab should be routine, and therapeutic ultrasound, artificial intelligence, and robotics are under development.

Physics and Instrumentation

Sound is an energy form that travels as a series of alternating compressions and rarefactions, typically characterized by wavelength and frequency (customarily expressed as cycles per second, or Hertz [Hz]). The velocity of sound is the product of wavelength and frequency; there is an inverse relationship between these two characteristics. Ultrasound is sonic energy with a frequency more than the audible range of the human ear (>20,000 Hz) and is useful for diagnostic imaging because it can be directed as a beam that obeys the laws of reflection and refraction. Thus, an ultrasound beam travels in a straight line through a homogeneous medium. If the beam meets an interface of different acoustic impedance, part of the energy reflects, and the remaining attenuated signal is transmitted. The reflected energy, or echo, is used to construct an image.

The transducer, which is responsible for both transmitting and receiving the ultrasound signal, consists of electrodes and a piezoelectric crystal, whose ionic structure results in deformation of shape when exposed to an electric current. *Harmonic imaging*, in which ultrasound energy is transmitted at a baseline (fundamental) frequency but then received at a higher multiple (harmonic) of that frequency (usually the first harmonic), has been implemented to enhance the signal-to-noise ratio. This allows capturing the change in the ultrasound frequency of a transmitted wave induced by the interaction with a reflecting target. Because structures close to the transducer do not generate much harmonic signal, harmonic imaging minimizes near-field and reverberation artifacts. Harmonic imaging has also been very useful in conjunction with echocardiographic contrast agents (subsequently discussed), the cyclic expansion and constriction of which produces a large amount of harmonic energy, exceeding that of myocardial tissue.[167] The net effect of harmonic imaging with echocardiographic contrast is a marked enhancement of the signal from the LV cavity and/or the coronary microcirculation compared with that of the myocardium.

Ultrasound presents several unique technical difficulties. Sound energy is poorly transmitted through air and bone, and the ability to record adequate images depends on a thoracic window that gives the interrogating beam adequate access to cardiac structures. The degree to which ultrasonic energy is reflected depends on how perpendicular the interrogating beam is to the interface. When the ultrasound beam is directed parallel to the interface, little or no sound energy reflects to the transducer. Therefore, poor signal transmission, a nonorthogonal orientation of the ultrasound beam to the surface, and energy attenuation can cause failure to record signals from cardiac structures—a phenomenon referred to as *echo dropout*.[168] Conversely, some structures may be such strong ultrasonic reflectors, being extremely dense and usually perpendicular to the beam, that sufficient energy returns to the transducer to reflect and again transmit into the field. This phenomenon can lead to *reverberations*, or the reproduction of the echoes of anatomic structures at multiple locations within the image.[169] Finally, very dense targets lying on the periphery of a 2D-sector ultrasound beam may be recorded and displayed as if they were located along the central scan line. This problem may be accentuated in the setting of strong reflectors that result in the formation of *side lobes*.[170]

The construction of a cardiac image from ultrasound signals is based on computation of the distance between an anatomic structure and the transducer. An ultrasound beam is produced by a handheld transducer positioned on the thorax and directed into the heart. This beam travels in a straight line until it reaches an interface between structures of different acoustic impedance, such as blood and myocardium. At this point, some ultrasonic energy reflects, some scatters, and some continues forward. The amplitude of the propagating signal is attenuated because of the reduction in energy at the interface. Circuitry within the echograph measures the time interval required for the transit of the ultrasound beam from the transducer to the interface and back again. Because the velocity of sound in soft tissue is constant (~1540 m/s), the instrument can calculate the total distance traveled to and from the reflecting surface as the product of transit time and velocity of sound. Interface location is derived as one-half of the total transit distance, and a signal is depicted on an oscilloscope or video monitor at that point. The amplitude of ultrasonic energy reflected from each target interface is represented by the brightness of the signal that is displayed.

In the most basic forms of echocardiography, a single scan line produced by a piezoelectric crystal is passed through the heart. At each structural interface, ultrasonic energy is reflected back and displayed at the appropriate distance as a signal, the amplitude of which represents the acoustic impedance or density of the material encountered. These signals are subsequently displayed as dots, the brightness of which is proportional to the amplitude of reflected ultrasonic energy. Accordingly, if repetitive B-mode scan lines are produced and swept across the screen over time, the movement of the heart can be obtained as a time-motion (or M-mode) recording, providing dynamic cardiac images. Because it transmits ultrasound signals at 1000 pulses/second, M-mode echocardiography provides very high temporal resolution and is excellent for timing cardiac events or recording high-velocity motion. 2D echocardiography acquires multiple B-mode scan lines that are aligned in the appropriate anatomic location to form a wedge-shaped sector image that provides additional spatial information in either superoinferior or mediolateral directions. High-quality images require optimal resolution—that is, the ability to distinguish two individual objects separated in space. Short wavelengths yield excellent resolution in echo imaging, because the shorter the cycle length, the smaller the object that will reflect the signal and be detected by the echo scanner. Because wavelength is inversely related to frequency, transducers that emit a high-frequency signal (≥ 3.5–7.0 MHz) yield high-resolution images. Because ultrasonic beams diverge as they propagate away from the transducer, the width of the beam can become sufficiently great to encompass multiple targets and decrease resolution. The degree of beam divergence is also less with high-frequency sonic energy than with low-frequency signals. The smaller wavelengths associated with high-frequency signals, however, are subject to greater reflection and scattering, with substantially higher attenuation as the beam propagates through tissue. The resultant attenuation is greater and leads to decreased sensitivity. Therefore, in clinical practice, echocardiographic examinations are performed using the highest-frequency transducer capable of sufficient penetration to obtain signals from all potential targets within the ultrasound field.

M-Mode Echocardiography

Despite the availability of 2D imaging, M-mode echocardiography remains a useful part of the ultrasound examination because of high temporal and spatial resolution. Measurements of the LV cavity dimension and wall thickness can be readily derived from M-mode recordings (**Fig. 3–40**) and are usually made according to the recommendations of the American Society of Echocardiography (ASE) at end diastole (the onset of the QRS complex) and end systole (the point of maximum upward motion of the LV posterior wall endocardium).[171] They are accurate if the beam is orthogonal to the long axis of the ventricle. Although M-mode LV cavity dimensions are still used in guidelines,[172] their use to measure LV volumes and EF) are based on several assumptions regarding LV geometry and should be discouraged. Normal M-mode measurements are summarized in **Table 3–16**.

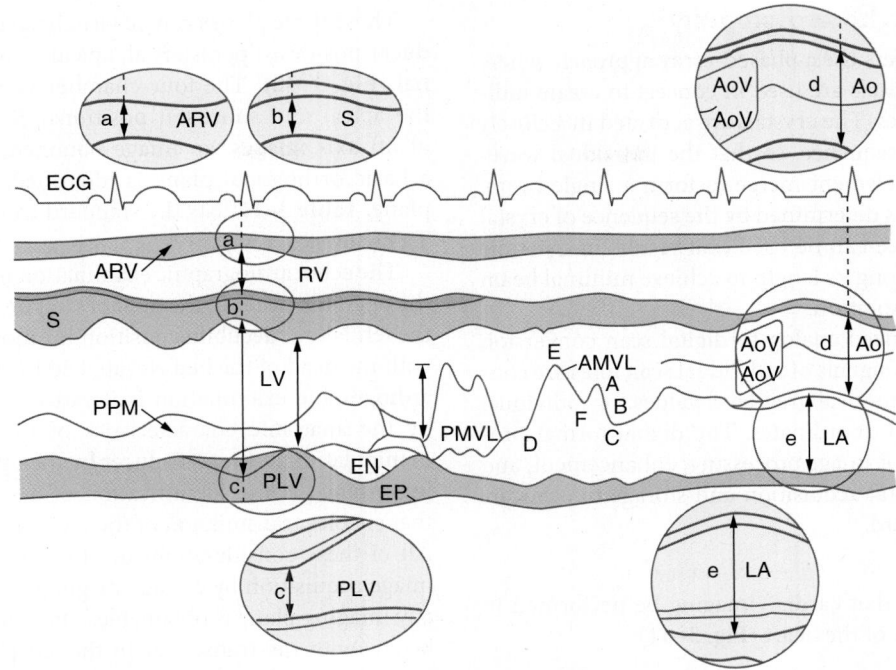

Figure 3–40. Recommended criteria for M-mode measurement of cardiac dimensions (see text for details). The figure and the elliptical inserts (a, b, c, d, and e) illustrate the leading-edge method. AMVL, anterior mitral valve leaflet; Ao, aorta; AoV, aortic valve; ARV, anterior right ventricular wall; ECG, electrocardiogram; EN, endocardium; EP, epicardium; LA, left atrium; LV, left ventricle; PLV, posterior left ventricular (wall); PPM, papillary muscle; PMVL, posterior mitral valve leaflet; RV, right ventricle; S, septum. Reproduced with permission from Sahn DJ, DeMaria A, Kisslo J, et al. Recommendations regarding quantitation in M-mode echocardiography: results of a survey of echocardiographic measurements. *Circulation.* 1978 Dec;58(6):1072-1083.

TABLE 3–16. Normal M-Mode Values of Cardiac Structure

	Mean ± Standard Deviation	Range	Mean ± Standard Deviation	Range
Number of patients	25	—	50	—
Age, years	10 ± 3	4–18	24 ± 0.6	1.10–2.53
BSA, m²	1.33 ± 0.38	0.72–2.04	1.81 ± 0.34	1.10–2.53
LVID$_d$, mm	44 ± 6	32–50	50 ± 3	42–60
LVID$_s$, mm	28 ± 7	32–50	50 ± 3	22–43
FSLV	34 ± 4	25–42	33 ± 3	28–37
IVS thickness, mm	8 ± 2	5–10	9 ± 1	7–12
IVS excursion, mm	7 ± 1	5–9	9 ± 1	7–12
PW$_d$ thickness, mm	7 ± 2	4–9	9 ± 1	7–12
PW$_s$ thickness, mm	12 ± 3	8–17	16 ± 2	13–20
α thickening PW	0.70 ± 0.25	0.41–0.95	0.50 ± 0.19	0.32–0.69
PW excursion, mm	9 ± 2	7–14	11 ± 2	9–17
RVD$_d$ supine, mm	—	—	15 ± 6	7–22
RVD$_d$ left lateral, mm	—	—	20 ± 8	10–37
Aorta$_d$ mm	23 ± 4	15–27	28 ± 5	26–36
LAD$_s$ mm	25 ± 5	20–31	27 ± 6	12–35

Abbreviations: BSA, body surface area; FSLV, fractional shortening of left ventricle; IVS, interventricular septum; LAD, left atrial dimension; LVID$_d$, left ventricular internal diameter, end diastole; LVID$_s$, left ventricular internal diameter, end systole; PW, posterior wall; RVD, right ventricular dimension.
Data from Felner JM, Schlant RC. *Echocardiography: A Teaching Atlas.* New York, NY: Grune & Stratton; 1976.

Two-Dimensional Echocardiography

Most current 2D scanners use a phased-array approach, where multiple ultrasonic crystals are used in concert to create individual B-mode scan lines. The crystals are activated in a closely coordinated temporal sequence, so that the individual wavelets produced by each element merge to form a single beam, the direction of which is determined by the sequence of crystal firing. A firing sequence can be used that results in dynamic focusing of the beam along its length to achieve minimal beam width and increased resolution.

Currently, computerized analog-to-digital scan conversion is standard, so the polar signals of individual scan lines are converted to a series of numerical gray-level values for individual pixels aligned along *x-y* coordinates. The digital format provides the opportunity for image processing, enhancement, and quantitation. Fully digital acquisition and storage of echocardiograms is now standard.

The Standard Two-Dimensional Examination

The ASE recommends that cardiac imaging be performed in three orthogonal planes of the heart (**Fig. 3–41**):

1. Long-axis (from aorta to the apex), including parasternal and apical two- and three-chamber views
2. Short-axis (perpendicular to long axis)
3. Four-chamber (traversing both ventricles and atria through the mitral and tricuspid valves)[173]

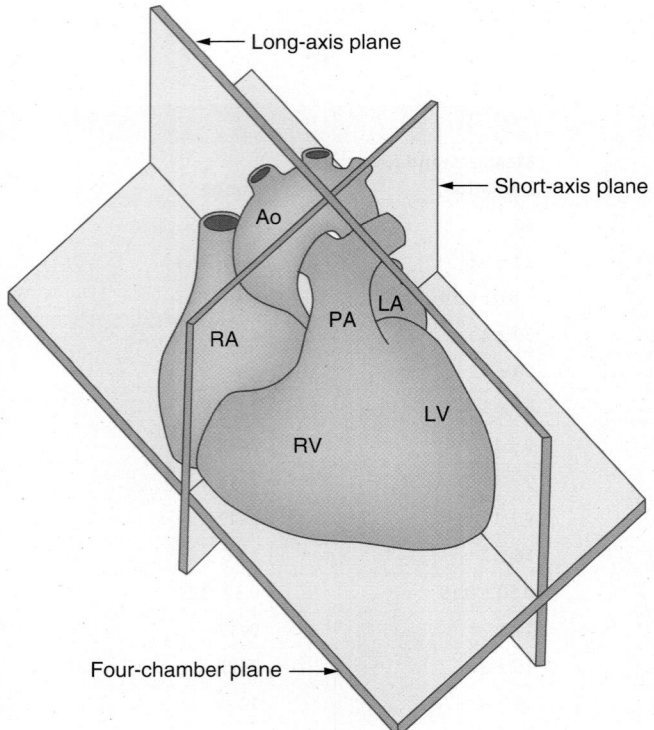

Figure 3–41. The three basic tomographic imaging planes used in echocardiography: long axis, short axis, and four chamber. Ao, aorta; LA, left atrium; LV, left ventricle; PA, pulmonary artery; RA, right atrium; RV, right ventricle. Reproduced with permission from Hagan AD, DeMaria AN. *Clinical Applications of Two-Dimensional Echocardiography and Cardiac Doppler,* 2nd ed. Boston, MA: Little, Brown; 1989.

These three planes can be visualized using four basic transducer positions: parasternal, apical, subcostal, and suprasternal (**Fig. 3–42**). The four-chamber views are obtained from the apical and subcostal positions. To permit classification of off-axis images, an image obtained within 45 degrees of a basic orthogonal plane is identified with that orthogonal plane. **Table 3–17** lists the standard transducer positions and TTE views.

The echocardiographic examination may be performed with the operator either to the patient's left or right. The patient is in the left lateral decubitus position for most of the examination, with the head of the bed elevated 20 to 30 degrees. The echocardiographic examination is iterative and largely determined by the anatomic characteristics of the patient and manual manipulation of the transducer by the operator. Of paramount importance is the identification of a thoracic site (window) that enables transmission of the ultrasound signal to the heart. All of these considerations are fundamentally different from image acquisition by cardiac magnetic resonance, from which any imaging plane is obtainable. The examination customarily begins with the transducer in the left parasternal position in the long-axis view (**Fig. 3–43**). This provides excellent images of the LV, aorta, LA, and the mitral valves (MVs) and aortic valves (AoVs). By angling the beam slightly rightward and inferiorly (RV inflow view), the RA, RV, and tricuspid valve (TV) are visualized (Fig. 3–43).

A 90-degree clockwise turn of the transducer produces the parasternal short-axis view. Slight axial angulation of the transducer enables visualization of the LV at various levels of the short axis, including the papillary muscle, mitral leaflets, and AoV (Fig. 3–43). With angulation toward the base, the LA, right heart structures, main pulmonary artery (PA), and occasionally the LA appendage are also recorded. The apical views are best acquired with the patient in a steep left lateral decubitus position and the transducer at the point of the apical impulse. The four-chamber view is obtained by turning the transducer so that both ventricles, atrioventricular valves, and atria are visualized (Fig. 3–43). In this view, the septal, apical, and lateral walls of the LV are visualized. Slight superior angulation of the transducer will add the AoV and proximal ascending aorta to the echocardiographic image (apical five-chamber view). From the four-chamber view, 90 degrees of counterclockwise transducer rotation produces the apical two-chamber view (Fig. 3–43). This imaging plane demonstrates the LA and the inferior, apical, and anterior wall segments of the LV (the right heart structures are absent). If the transducer is rotated slightly further, a three-chamber view similar to the parasternal long-axis view is produced (Fig. 3–43) and provides images of the posterior, apical, and anteroseptal LV wall segments, as well as the LA, aorta, and MVs and AoVs.

To facilitate subcostal imaging, the patient is moved into a supine position. The subcostal four-chamber view is much like the apical four-chamber view (Fig. 3–43), but because the ultrasound beam is now more perpendicular to the interventricular and interatrial septa, subcostal imaging is often helpful in the examination of these structures. A 90-degree rotation of the transducer will record a subcostal short-axis view. The transducer

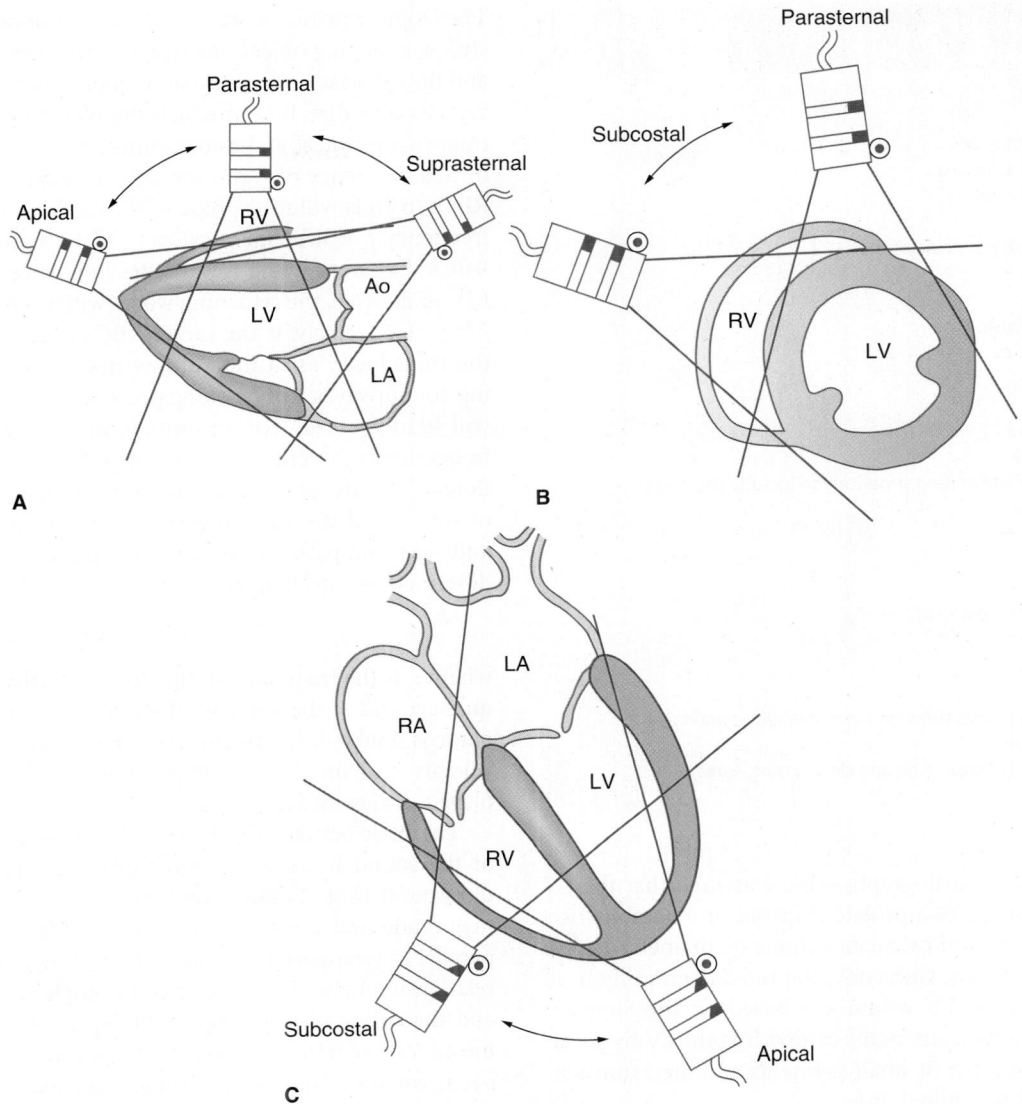

Figure 3–42. Visualization of the heart's basic tomographic imaging planes by various transducer positions. The long-axis plane (**A**) can be imaged in the parasternal, suprasternal, and apical positions; the short-axis plane (**B**) in the parasternal and subcostal positions; and the four-chamber plane (**C**) in the apical and subcostal positions. Ao, aorta; LA, left atrium; LV, left ventricle; RA, right atrium; RV, right ventricle. Reproduced with permission from Henry WL, DeMaria A, Gramiak R, et al. Report of the American Society of Echocardiography: nomenclature and standards in two-dimensional echocardiography. *Circulation.* 1980 Aug;62(2):212-217.

can also be angled to image the RV outflow tract (RVOT) and PA as well as the IVC (see Fig. 3–43).

The long-axis suprasternal imaging plane is shown in **Fig. 3–44B**. In adults, the LV is usually not visualized satisfactorily from the suprasternal position, but these imaging planes are well suited for examination of the thoracic aorta, PA, and great vessels. Normal values for 2D echocardiographic measurements are shown in **Table 3–18**.

Three-Dimensional Echocardiography

Using a transducer with a matrix array of crystals, a pyramid-shaped ultrasound beam can be produced that can often encompass the entire heart from one transducer location and acquire an entire data set in a single cardiac cycle. Advances in processing have improved surface rendering and endocardial border definition (**Fig. 3–44C**). Three-dimensional images

can be valuable in exact quantification of cardiac volumes and EF, assessing congenital heart disease (CHD), and evaluating structures of complex geometry such as the RV. Recent studies have shown an excellent correlation between real-time 3D echo and MRI in the measurement of regional and global LV volume and time-wall motion curves.[174] Real-time 3D transesophageal echocardiography (TEE) can provide rendered images that provide exquisite detail about native, repaired, and prosthetic valves (**Figs. 3–44D and 3–44F**).[175]

Assessment of Systolic Function by Echocardiography

Two-dimensional echocardiography is the standard clinical approach for measuring cardiac chamber volumes and EF.[172] Numerous algorithms have been applied to calculate

TABLE 3–17. Standard Two-Dimensional Echocardiographic Transducer Positions

Parasternal position
Long axis
    Left ventricular long axis
    Right ventricular long axis
    Right ventricular outflow
Short axis
    Short axis through the plane of the
        Cardiac base
        Mitral valve
        Chordae tendineae
        Papillary muscles
        Apex
Apical position
Four-chamber plane
Five-chamber plane
    (Four-chamber plane angled superiorly to include the aorta)
Two-chamber plane
Three-chamber plane
Subcostal position
Four-chamber plane
Short axis through the plane of the
    Mitral valve
    Papillary muscles
    Cardiac base
Posteriorly directed planes through the venae cavae and atria
Suprasternal position
Long axis (through the ascending and descending aorta)
Short axis

LV volumes by echocardiography—most assume that the LV conforms to the shape of a prolate ellipsoid or a combination of geometric shapes, and calculate volume by diameter-length or area-length formulas. Currently, the most commonly used algorithm to calculate LV volumes is based on the Simpson rule, which derives measurements by dividing the LV by parallel planes into a number of small segments and then summating the area of the individual disks.

Accurate calculations of LV volumes by echocardiography are critically dependent on high-quality images to delineate the endocardium and image the entire LV perimeter. LV opacification should be used when images are suboptimal.[176] Because of the 3D nature of the heart, 2D cut-planes are inevitably different between studies. Thus, the test-retest reproducibility of 2D echocardiography between individual studies is limited, with variations >10%, compared with 6% with 3D echocardiography.[177]

The assessment of regional function remains difficult. In addition to subjective assessment, recent approaches to quantitation of regional function have included tissue Doppler or tracking of speckle patterns. A variety of displays have been used to show the magnitude and time-course of contraction (**Fig. 3–45**).

Doppler Echocardiography

The Doppler Principle

Ultrasound can be used to determine the velocity and direction of blood flow by measuring the change in frequency produced when sound waves are reflected from red blood cells (RBCs).

The Doppler principle states that when a sound (or light) signal strikes a moving object, the frequency of that signal is altered, and the increase or decrease in frequency is proportional to the velocity and direction at which the object is moving. If a stationary transducer at the apex emits a sound wave with a transmitted frequency of f_o and the wave is reflected by nonmoving RBCs in an isovolumic phase of the cardiac cycle, the received frequency f_r will be identical to f_o. If the signal is reflected by RBCs that are moving toward the transducer, as through the MV in diastole, the returning waves will be compressed so that $f_r > f_o$. Conversely, if the target RBCs are moving away from the transducer, as in the outflow tract in systole, the returning sound waves will be elongated and the received frequency will be decreased. The magnitude of change in the received frequency is directly related to the velocity at which blood is flowing toward or away from the transducer.[178] If the velocity of sound and the angle θ between the direction of RBC flow and the beam path are known, then the velocity of the RBCs is described by the Doppler equation:

$$V = f_d \,(c)/2f_o \,(\cos\theta)$$

where f_d is the frequency shift recorded; f_o, the transmitted frequency; and c, the velocity of sound. Note that the denominator is doubled. By measuring Doppler shift frequencies, the velocity and direction of blood flow can be calculated, displayed, and recorded.

The angle between the direction of blood flow and the course of the sound beam is the most important factor in Doppler ultrasound (**Fig. 3–46A**). Velocity is a vectorial entity, having magnitude and direction, and Doppler best detects velocities parallel or near parallel to the interrogating signal. Because the relationship between velocity and the angle is a cosine function and the cosine of angles up to 20 degrees is 0.9, little error is introduced within this range.[178] However, considerable errors occur when the angle between the direction of blood flow and the course of the sound beam exceeds 20 degrees. Moreover, the angle of incidence in 3D space usually cannot be determined with certainty from 2D echocardiographic images. Therefore, it is crucial to position and direct the transducer so that the beam is as parallel to flow as possible. In clinical use, the frequency of transmitted ultrasound is in the range of 2 to 7 MHz, the velocity of sound in tissue is approximately 1540 m/s, and the Doppler shift frequency is relatively small (~1–4 kHz) as compared with the transmitted frequency. Because the Doppler shift frequencies are in the audible range, a speaker integrated into the Doppler echocardiography system can present them as an audible signal. Normal signals are tonal or musical.

Figure 3–46B shows the typical graphic pulsed Doppler pattern of normal systolic blood flow through the RVOT into the PA, with flow velocity on the y-axis and time on the x-axis. The location and size of the area from which Doppler recordings are derived is determined by positioning a sample volume on the echo image. The absence of flow is represented by the zero or no-flow line, termed the *baseline*. By convention, flow toward the transducer is displayed above the baseline and flow away from the transducer is displayed below the baseline. The velocities above and below baseline represent flow toward

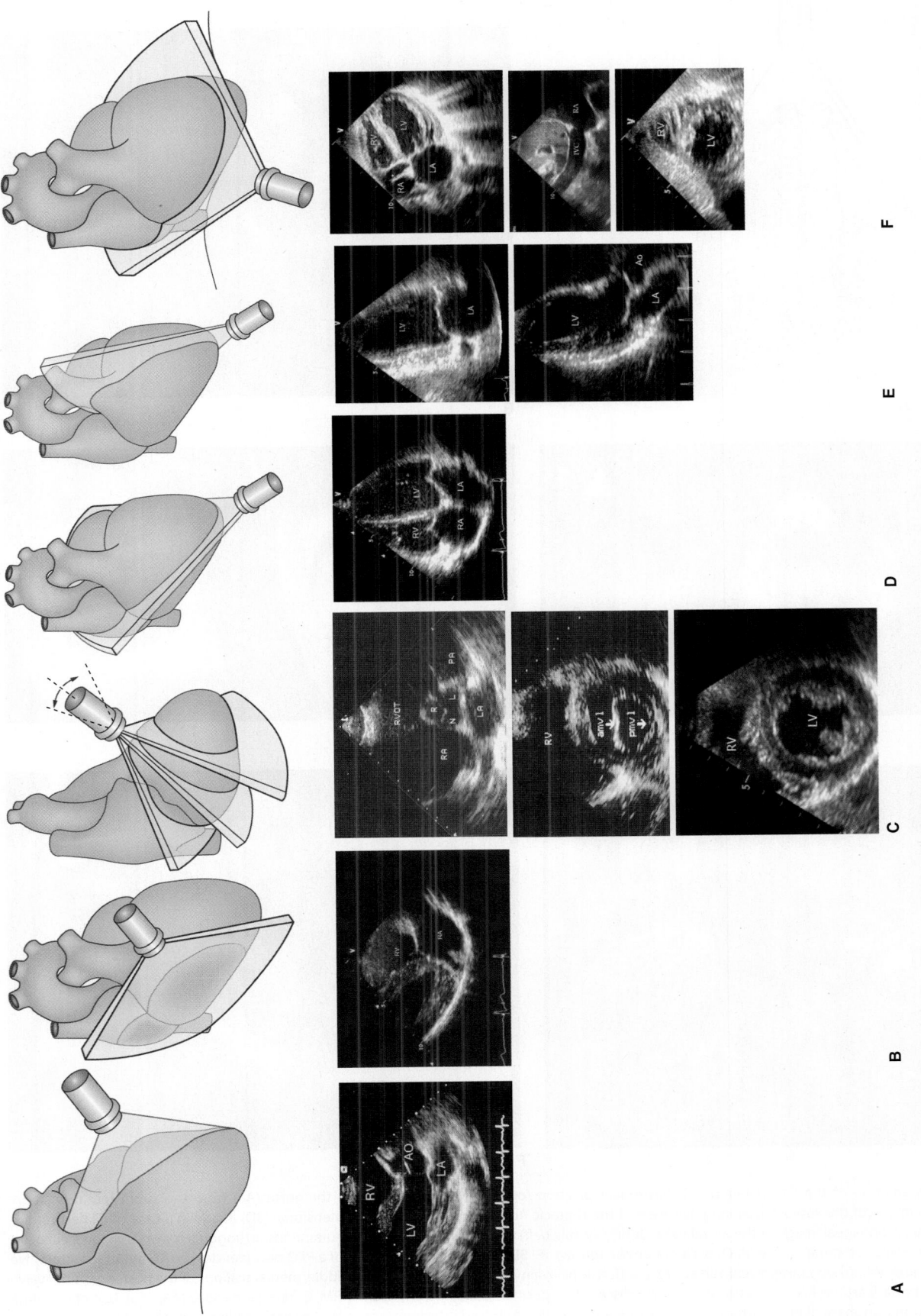

Figure 3–43. Orientation of the sector beam and transducer position and resulting 2D image for (**A**) the parasternal long-axis plane; (**B**) the parasternal RV inflow plan; (**C**) various short-axis sector planes obtained by angling the transducer in the parasternal position, including the base of the heart, level of the mitral valve leaflets, papillary muscle level; (**D**) apical four–chamber plane; (**E**) apical two- and three-chamber planes; and (**F**) subcostal four-chamber plane showing the subcostal four-chamber, RA and IVC, and subcostal short-axis views. AMVL, anterior mitral valve leaflet; Ao, aorta; *Asterisk*, a prominent eustachian valve; inferior vena cava (IVC); LA, left atrium; LV, left ventricle; N, noncoronary cusp of the aortic valve, PA, pulmonary artery; pmvl, posterior mitral valve leaflet; R, right cusp of the aortic valve; RA, right atrium; RV, right ventricle; RVOT, right ventricular outflow tract. Line drawings reproduced with permission from Hagan AD, DeMaria AN. *Clinical Applications of Two-Dimensional Echocardiography and Cardiac Doppler*, 2nd ed. Boston, MA: Little, Brown; 1989.

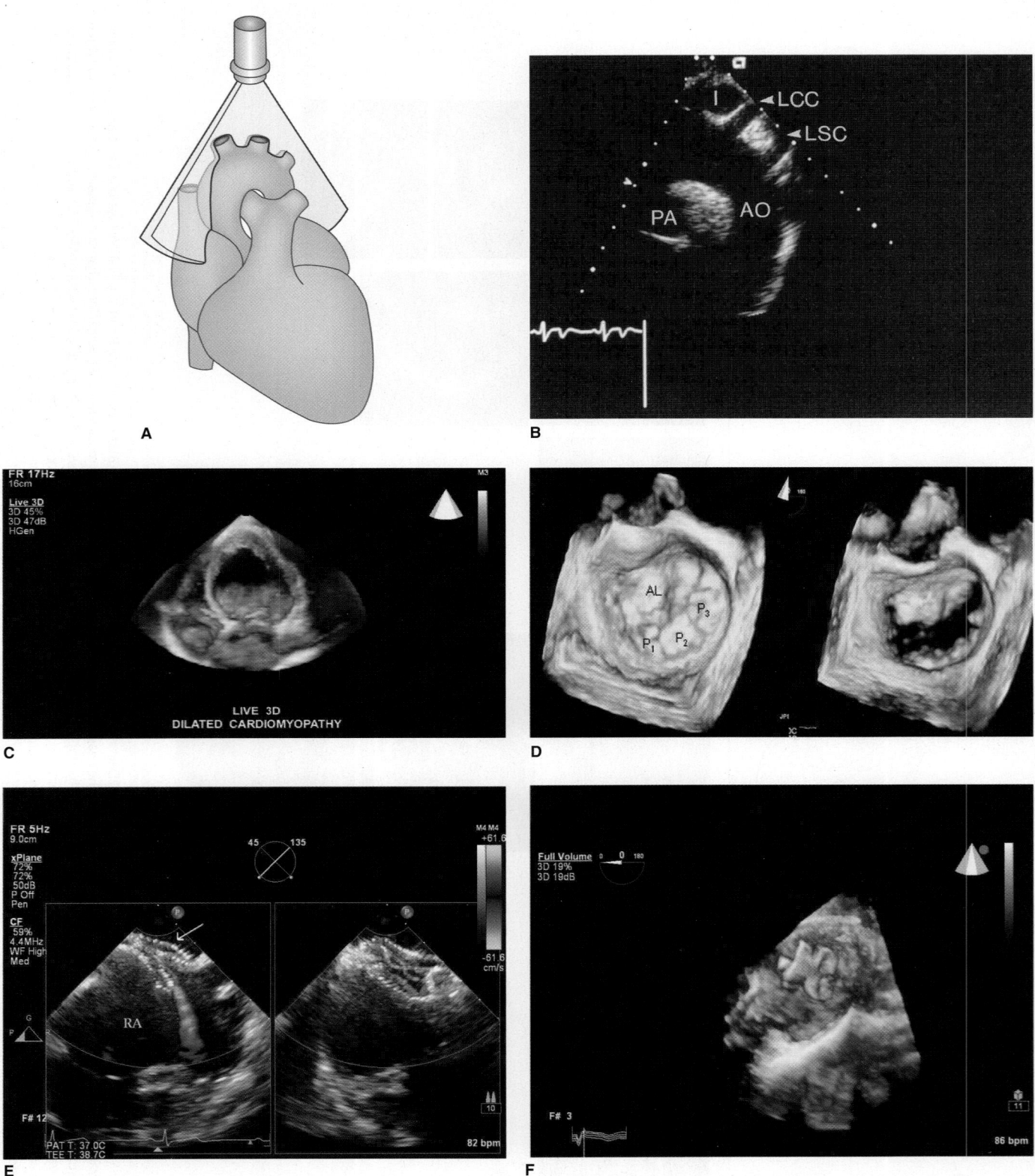

Figure 3–44. (**A**) Orientation of the sector beam and transducer position for long-axis plane through the aorta (Ao) from the suprasternal position. (**B**) Two-dimensional image of the suprasternal long-axis view of the thoracic Ao. (**C**) Example of three-dimensional (3D) image in a case of dilated cardiomyopathy. (**D**) 3D transesophageal image of the mitral valve during systole (*left*) and diastole (*right*). (**E**) Simultaneous orthogonal transesophageal echocardiography images of a patent foramen ovale (PFO) occluder device (*arrow*). (**F**) 3D transesophageal image of a PFO occluder device. AL, anterior mitral valve leaflet; I, innominate artery; LCC, left common carotid artery; LSC, left subclavian artery; P1/P2/P3, lateral/middle/medial scallops of the posterior mitral valve leaflet; PA, right pulmonary artery; RA, right atrium. (**D**) Reproduced with permission from Perk G, Lang RM, Garcia-Fernandez MA, et al. Use of real time three-dimensional transesophageal echocardiography in intracardiac catheter based interventions. *J Am Soc Echocardiogr.* 2009 Aug;22(8):865-882.

TABLE 3–18. Cardiac Dimensions by Two-Dimensional Echocardiography

Cardiac Feature	Range	Mean	Index (cm/m²)
Apical four-chamber view			
LV$_d$ major	6.9–10.3 cm	8.6 cm	4.1–5.7
LV$_d$ minor	3.3–6.1 cm	4.7 cm	2.2–3.1
LV$_s$ minor	1.9–3.7 cm	2.8 cm	1.3–2.0
LV$_d$ area	21.2–40.2 cm²	31.2 cm²	—
LV$_s$ area	8.0–21.1 cm²	14.2 cm²	—
RV major	6.5–9.5 cm²	8.0 cm	3.8–5.3
RV minor	2.2–4.4 cm²	3.3–3.5 cm	1.0–2.8
RV$_d$ area	12.0–22.2 cm²	18.6–2.1 cm²	—
RV$_s$ area	5.4–14.6 cm²	9.9 cm²	—
LA major	4.1–6.1 cm	5.1 cm	2.3–3.5
LA minor	2.8–4.3 cm	3.5 cm	1.6–2.4
LA area	10.2–17.8 cm²	14.7 cm²	—
RA major (inf-sup)	3.5–5.5 cm	4.3–4.5 cm	2.0–3.1
RA minor	2.5–4.9 cm	3.7 cm	1.7–2.5
RA area	11.3–16.7 cm²	13.8–14 cm²	—
Apical two-chamber view			
LV$_d$ major	6.8–9.4 cm	8.0 cm	—
LV$_d$ minor	3.8–5.7 cm	4.6 cm	—
LV$_d$ area	19.4–48.0 cm²	35.6 cm²	—
LV$_s$	8.9–27.0 cm	14.3 cm	—
Parasternal long-axis view			
LV$_d$	3.5–6.0 cm	4.8 cm	2.3–3.1
LV$_s$	2.1–4.0 cm	3.1 cm	1.4–2.1
RV	1.9–3.8 cm	2.8 cm	1.2–2.0
LA (A-P)	2.7–4.5 cm	3.6 cm	1.6–2.4
LA (S-I)	3.1–5.5 cm	4.4 cm	—
LA area	9.0–19.3 cm²	13.8 cm²	—
Ao	2.2–3.6 cm	2.9 cm	1.4–2.0
Parasternal short-axis view			
Ao	2.3–3.7 cm	3.0–2.3 cm	1.6–2.4
RVOT	1.9–2.2 cm	2.7 cm	—
RA	1.5–2.5 cm	1.9–2.2 cm	—
LA	2.6–4.5 cm	3.6 cm	1.6–2.4
LA area	7.2–13.0 cm²	10.8 cm²	—
LV$_d$ (PM level)	3.5–5.8 cm	4.7 cm	2.2–3.1
LV$_s$ (PM level)	2.2–4.0 cm	3.1 cm	1.4–2.2
LV$_d$ area (PM level)	16.0–31.2 cm²	22.2 cm²	—
LV$_s$ area (PM level)	5.2–13.4 cm²	8.5 cm²	—
LV$_d$ (Ch. level)	3.5–6.2	4.8 cm	2.3–3.2
LV$_s$ (Ch. level)	2.3–4.0	3.2 cm	1.5–2.2
LV$_d$ area (Ch. level)	16.4–32.3 cm²	22.5 cm²	—
LV$_s$ area (Ch. level)	6.1–16.8 cm²	10.7 cm²	—
Subcostal view			
IVC diameter		1.8 cm	—

Abbreviations: Ao, aorta; Ch., chordal; IVC, inferior vena cava; LA, left atrium; LV, left ventricle; LV$_d$, left ventricle, end diastole; LV$_s$, left ventricle, end systole; PM, papillary muscle; RA, right atrium; RV, right ventricle; RV$_d$, right ventricle, end diastole; RVOT, right ventricular outflow tract; RV$_s$, right ventricle, end systole.
Data from Schnittinger I, Gordon EP, Fitzgerald PJ, et al. Standardized intracardiac measurements of two-dimensional echocardiography. *J Am Coll Cardiol.* 1983;5:934. Weyman A. *Echocardiography.* Philadelphia, PA: Lea & Febiger; 1982. Hagan AD, DiSessa TG, Bloor CM, et al. *Two-Dimensional Echocardiography: Clinical-Pathological Corrections in Adult and Congenital Heart Disease.* Boston, MA: Little, Brown; 1983.

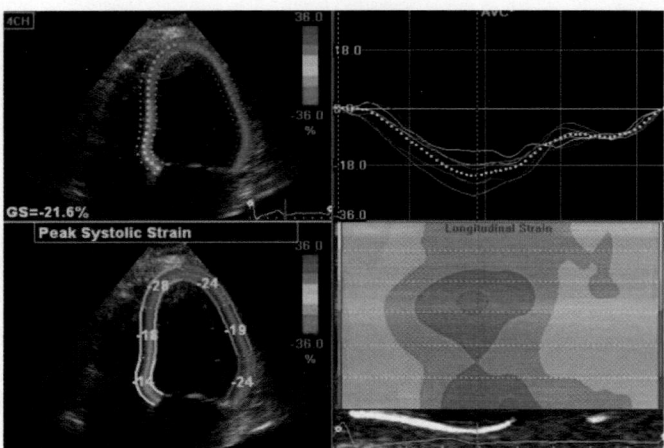

Figure 3–45. Speckle strain approach to the assessment of the magnitude and timing of strain in multiple segments, as well as averaging the longitudinal strain.

or away from the transducer, not forward or backward in the circulation. The sample volume almost invariably includes RBCs flowing at slightly different velocities. Even normal laminar blood flow in the great vessels varies in velocity across the lumen, because RBCs in the center of the vessel move at higher velocity than those exposed to viscous friction at the wall. Therefore, any returning Doppler-shifted signal contains a spectrum of velocities, each of which can be displayed by means of fast Fourier transform analysis. The graphic output of the Doppler signal displays the range of velocities within the sample volume site at any time in grayscale and the number of RBCs moving at any velocity as relative intensity. Normal laminar flow is characterized by a uniformity of velocity and direction of individual RBCs, and therefore a narrowly dispersed signal, whereas disturbed or turbulent flow is manifest by marked variability in velocity and direction and therefore a broad signal.

Continuous- and Pulsed-Wave Doppler

Time-velocity spectral recordings of blood flow are generally obtained with two types of Doppler interrogation: continuous and pulsed wave (**Fig. 3–47**).[178] In the continuous-wave (CW) mode, sound waves are both transmitted and received continuously. This requires two piezoelectric crystals in each transducer, one for transmitting and one for receiving. Because all flow velocities along the beam are recorded, CW Doppler cannot define individual signals at specific distances from the transducer—a problem referred to as *range ambiguity*. CW Doppler can accurately measure the direction and velocity of overall flow but cannot discern the precise site of origin of individual components within the signal.

The problem of range ambiguity can be overcome by pulsed-wave Doppler (PWD). Short bursts of signal are transmitted from the transducer at a given pulse repetition frequency (PRF). The instrument then receives the signal for only a brief period: an interval that corresponds to the time required for sound energy to travel and return from a specific site along the beam path. The operator selects the location at which flow is to be examined by positioning a sample volume,

and the instrument determines the period during which to receive the incoming reflected frequencies. With PWD only a single piezoelectric crystal is needed, and flow can be recorded in one small area within the heart or vasculature. Unfortunately, PWD techniques use intermittent sampling and are therefore susceptible to the problem of *aliasing*—the erroneous representation of flow in the direction opposite to that in which it is actually occurring. To correctly record the velocity of blood flow by PWD, the PRF must be at least double the Doppler shift frequency, a value known as the *Nyquist limit*. If the blood flow examined is of very high velocity or far from the transducer (requiring a long transit time), it may necessitate an unobtainably high PRF. In such cases, aliasing will occur as Doppler signals that depict flow at high velocity in ambiguous or opposite directions compared with actual flow (Fig. 3–47). An intermediate-mode, high-PRF Doppler is also available. This mode enables higher velocity recordings to be obtained at a compromise of depicting several sample sites simultaneously.

Tissue Doppler

Tissue Doppler has provided the opportunity to measure low-velocity, high-amplitude Doppler signals produced by moving tissue, as well as those of RBCs. This provides an evaluation of contraction and relaxation, and has become a cornerstone of the assessment of diastolic function. Doppler tissue provided the first opportunity to measure regional myocardial strain measurements, because differences in velocity of adjacent segments was a marker of deformation. More recently, the technique of tracking of the individual myocardial speckles of grayscale images has provided accurate measurements of strain independent of the orientation of the interrogating beam.

Color-Flow Doppler

The major limitation of PWD and CW Doppler (*spectral Doppler*) is that no spatial information regarding the size, shape, and 2D direction of flow is provided. An extension of PWD techniques, color-flow Doppler (CFD), provides real-time M-mode or 2D imaging of blood flow by presenting the velocity and direction of RBC movement, using a parametric display where colors representing velocities are superimposed on gray-level 2D tissue structure. In CFD, rapid pulsed-wave interrogations are performed at multiple sites for multiple scan lines to create a spatially correct and dynamic display of moving blood within the heart and vasculature (**Fig. 3–48**). Doppler signals are presented as colors assigned to individual sites (**Fig. 3–48**). Blood flow moving toward the transducer is displayed in red, flow away from the transducer is displayed in blue, and increasing velocity is depicted in brighter shades of each color. The variance within each signal is calculated as a statistical marker of turbulence and is presented by adding green to the image, so turbulent flow jets appear as a mosaic mix of colors. CFD can also be superimposed onto M-mode tracings often termed *color M-mode imaging*, and is helpful in clarifying the timing of flow phenomena.

Normal and Abnormal Flow Dynamics

Normal flow is laminar, with all RBCs exhibiting the same velocity and direction of flow. Most pathologic conditions,

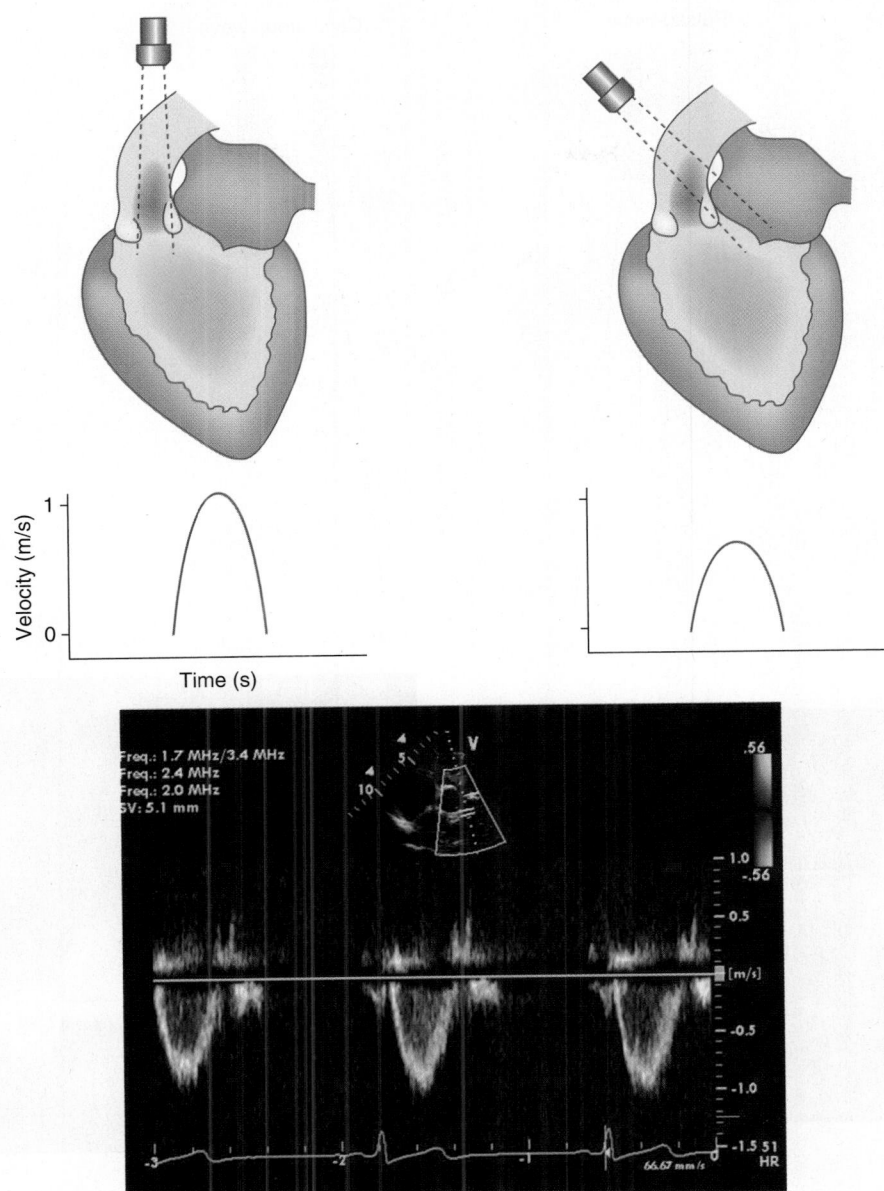

Figure 3–46. Basic principles of Doppler. (A) Effect of the angle of incidence on the velocity recorded with Doppler analysis. The true velocity is underestimated when the ultrasound beam is not parallel to the direction of blood flow. **(B)** Doppler spectral envelope of normal blood flow through the right ventricular outflow tract during systole. The transducer is in the parasternal position and the sample volume is placed just proximal to the pulmonic valve. **(A)** Reproduced with permission from Hagan AD, DeMaria AN. *Clinical Applications of Two-Dimensional Echocardiography and Cardiac Doppler*, 2nd ed. Boston, MA: Little, Brown; 1989.

with the exception of ASDs, involve disturbed or turbulent flow and share a common hydrodynamic basis for the resultant flow dynamics. Specifically, nearly all circulatory disturbances (stenosis, regurgitation, shunt) involve blood flow from a high-pressure chamber to a lower pressure chamber through a restricted orifice. In each case, the pressure gradient results in a high-velocity jet coursing through a restricted orifice, reaching its maximal velocity at a site just distal to the orifice, designated the vena contracta, at which time shear forces produce vortices resulting in flow of varying direction and velocity. In each case, the velocity of the jet is related to the pressure gradient across the orifice. On pulsed Doppler recordings, these hemodynamic abnormalities cause broadening of the spectral signal and aliasing. On CW recordings, high velocity represents the primary abnormality. By color-flow imaging, the disturbance is manifest by the increased variance and higher velocities in the signal.

The Standard Doppler Examination

Echocardiographic examinations include screening for flow disturbances by CFD. Because Doppler signals are best recorded with the ultrasound beam parallel to flow, screening is typically performed in long-axis or apical views. Any

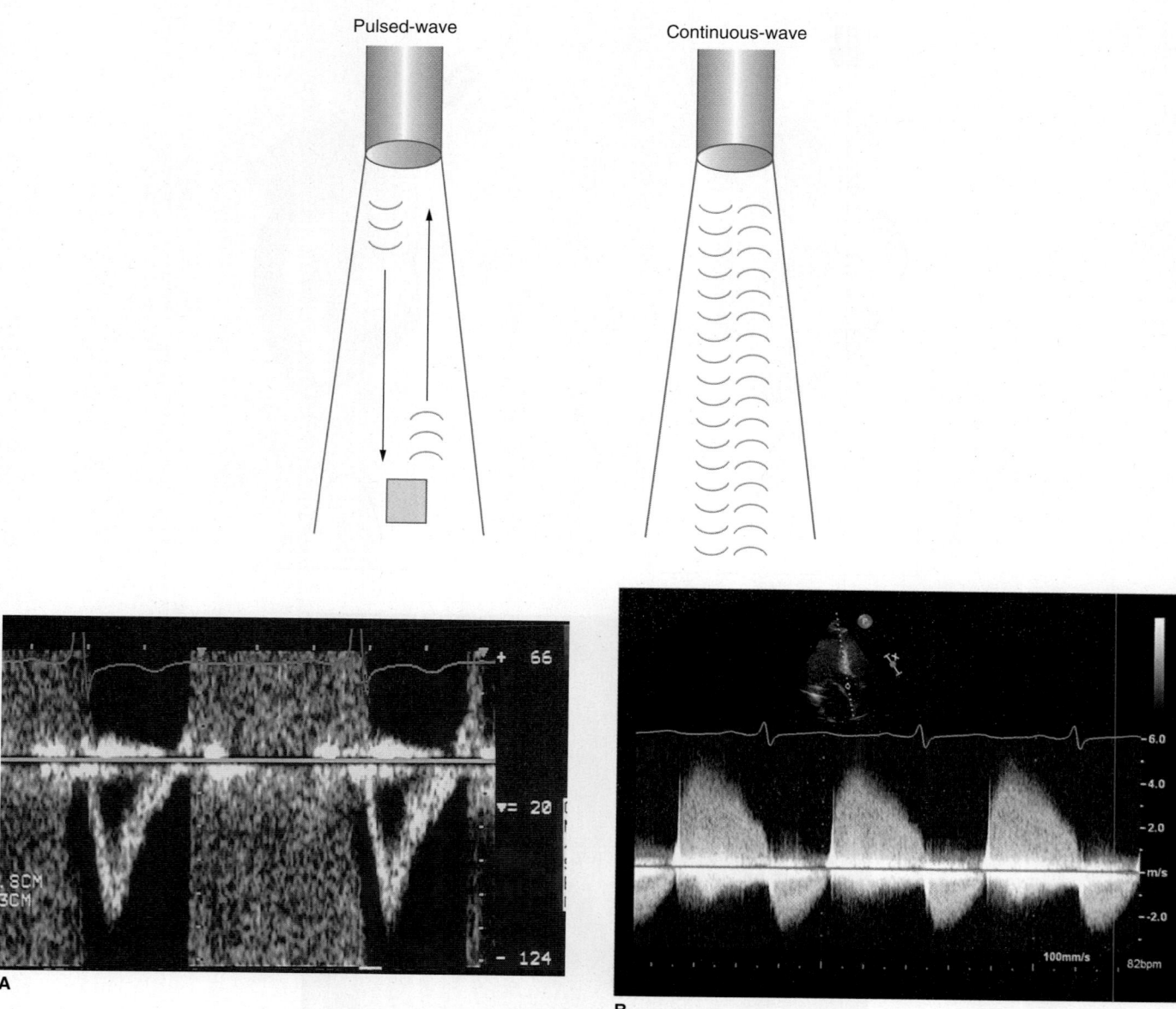

Figure 3–47. Pulsed-wave and continuous-wave Doppler. (A) Basic principles: with pulsed wave, a single pulse of ultrasound energy is emitted, and its reflection from a sample volume is received before the following pulse is transmitted. With continuous wave, there is continuous transmission and reception of ultrasound energy. **(B)** Pulsed-wave Doppler tracing from a patient with aortic regurgitation. The transducer is in the apical position and the sample volume is in the left ventricular outflow tract. A laminar envelope is seen during systole, whereas aliased flow is present during diastole because of high-velocity flow. **(C)** Continuous-wave Doppler tracing through the left ventricular outflow tract (with transducer in the apical position). The maximal velocity of the aortic regurgitation is now measurable, but all other velocities along the Doppler beam are recorded as well.

flow disturbances visualized are subsequently examined by CW spectral recordings and, in most laboratories, by PWD. Although CW examination is typically reserved for flow disturbances, PWD may also be of value in quantifying flow dynamics in the setting of laminar flow. In this regard, PWD recordings obtained at the mitral, tricuspid, and aortic valvular orifices, PA, and pulmonary veins constitute part of a standard echocardiogram (**Fig. 3–49**). Finally, the usual Doppler examination will include tissue Doppler recordings from a region of interest placed in the septal and lateral mitral annulus in the apical four-chamber view. Normal values for forward

flow velocity are given in **Table 3–19**—generally, blood moves through the heart at ~1m/s.

Assessment of Diastolic Function

Transmitral flow, annular tissue Doppler, LA volume, and PA pressure are the cornerstones of the evaluation of diastolic function and LV filling pressure.[179] Effective assessment is technically demanding—malposition of the Doppler sample volume away from the tip of the MV orifice and mitral annulus, off-axis views of the LA, and challenges with measurement of tricuspid regurgitation (TR) velocity are all

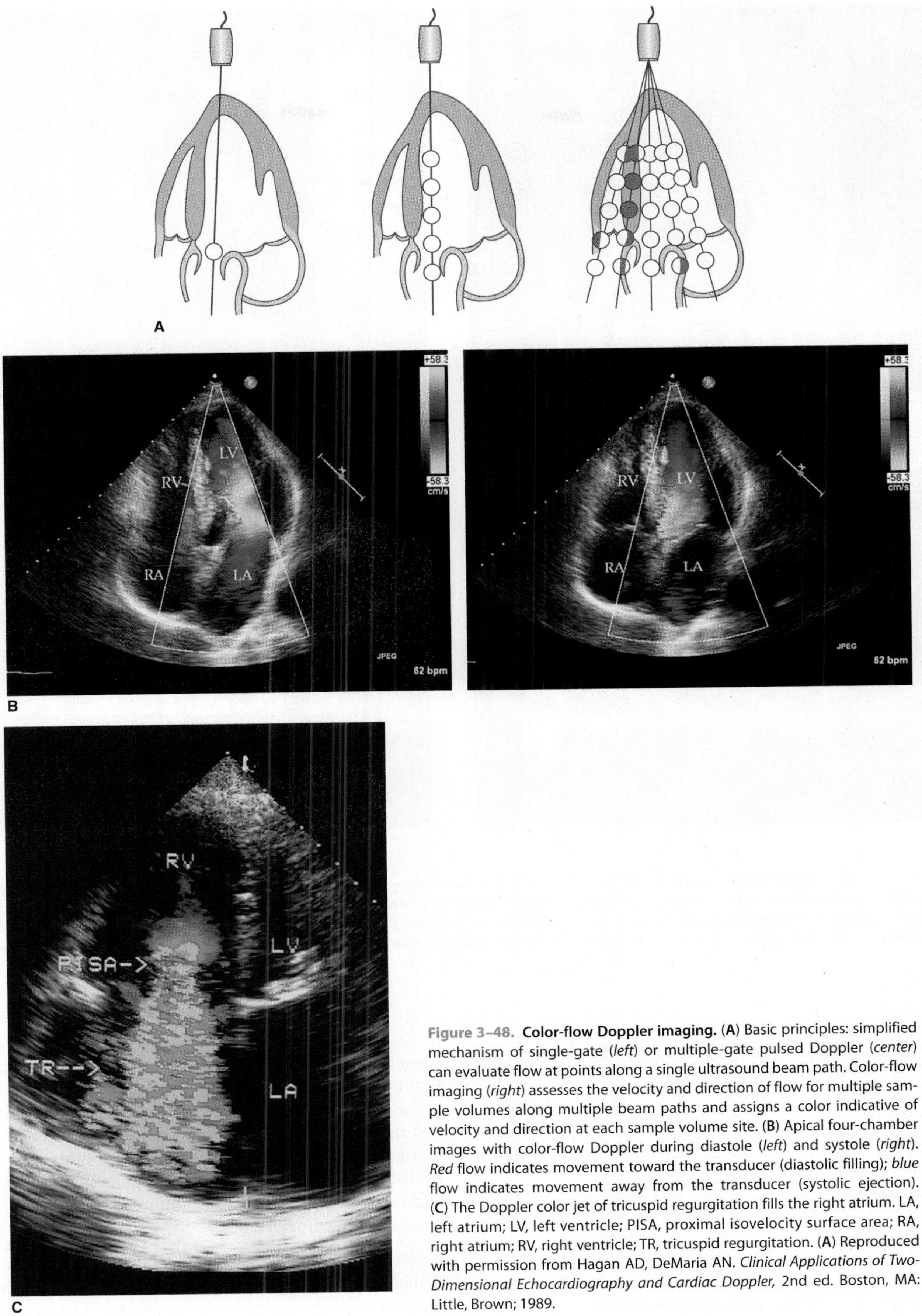

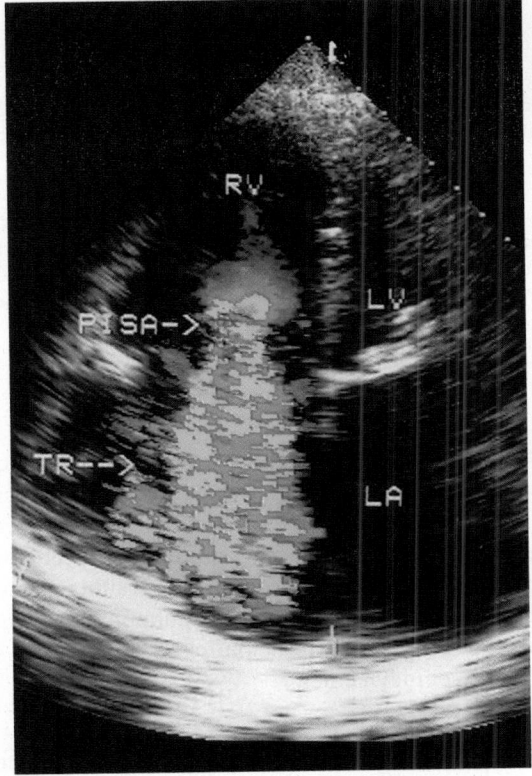

Figure 3–48. Color-flow Doppler imaging. (A) Basic principles: simplified mechanism of single-gate (*left*) or multiple-gate pulsed Doppler (*center*) can evaluate flow at points along a single ultrasound beam path. Color-flow imaging (*right*) assesses the velocity and direction of flow for multiple sample volumes along multiple beam paths and assigns a color indicative of velocity and direction at each sample volume site. **(B)** Apical four-chamber images with color-flow Doppler during diastole (*left*) and systole (*right*). *Red* flow indicates movement toward the transducer (diastolic filling); *blue* flow indicates movement away from the transducer (systolic ejection). **(C)** The Doppler color jet of tricuspid regurgitation fills the right atrium. LA, left atrium; LV, left ventricle; PISA, proximal isovelocity surface area; RA, right atrium; RV, right ventricle; TR, tricuspid regurgitation. **(A)** Reproduced with permission from Hagan AD, DeMaria AN. *Clinical Applications of Two-Dimensional Echocardiography and Cardiac Doppler,* 2nd ed. Boston, MA: Little, Brown; 1989.

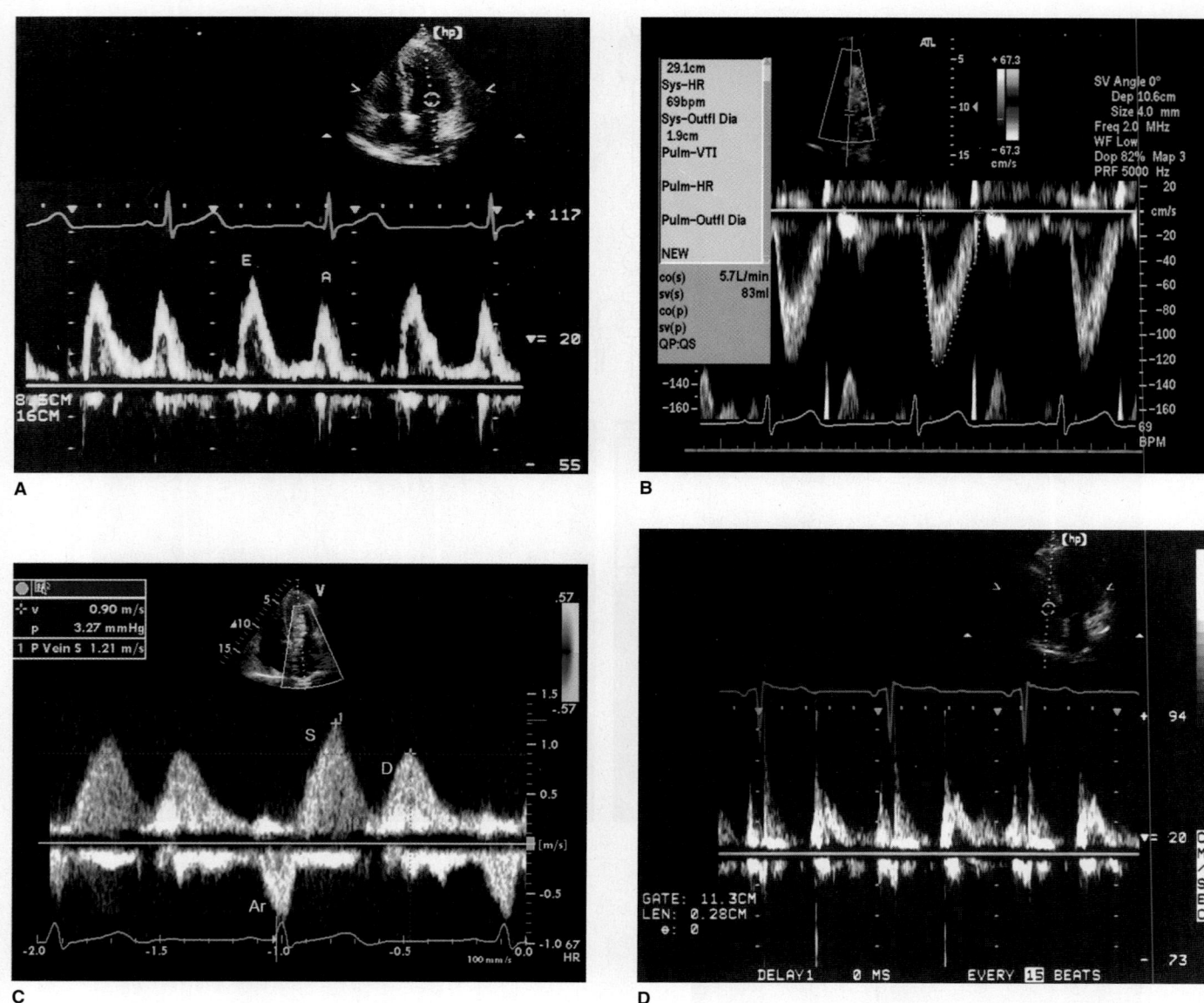

Figure 3–49. Normal pulsed-wave Doppler tracing from (**A**) the left ventricular inflow tract, displaying the early rapid filling (E) and atrial contraction (A) phases of diastolic flow. The transducer is in the apical position and the sample volume is at the mitral leaflet tips. (**B**) The left ventricular outflow tract (apical transducer position). (**C**) The right upper pulmonary vein (recorded from the apical transducer position). Flow toward the heart is biphasic, with peaks in systole (S) and diastole (D). A small amount of reversed flow is seen during atrial contraction (A$_r$). (**D**) The right ventricle inflow tract (apical transducer position).

TABLE 3–19. Normal Intracardiac Doppler Velocities	
	Velocity (m/s)
Right ventricle	
Tricuspid flow	0.3–0.7
Pulmonary artery	0.6–0.9
Left ventricle	
Mitral flow	0.6–1.3
Aorta	1.0–1.7

Data from Hatle L, Angelsen B. *Doppler Ultrasound in Cardiology: Physical Principles and Clinical Applications,* 2nd ed. Philadelphia, PA: Lea & Febiger; 1984.

potential problems. Several variables other than diastolic function are capable of influencing transmitral filling velocities—including patient age, changes in heart rate, respiration, mitral regurgitation (MR), and loading conditions. Inconsistencies between these parameters are common, and although less supported by guidelines than in the past, pulmonary venous flow and Valsalva response may be helpful, as may LA and LV strain, and exercise hemodynamics.

Assessment of Systolic Function and Cardiac Output

Doppler interrogation provides a unique and complementary noninvasive assessment of systolic function. Thus, LV systolic dysfunction often results in decreased aortic velocity and acceleration time. In the presence of MR, the acceleration of the MR jet (dP/dt) can provide information regarding contractile function.[180]

The Doppler-based calculation of the stroke volume[181] is important in hemodynamic assessment and fundamental to the continuity equation. The volume of flow through any orifice or tube can be calculated as the product of the CSA (measured from echocardiographic images) through which flow occurs and the velocity of that flow (determined by Doppler) (**Fig. 3–50A**).

Important sources of error are the LVOT measurement (which is squared) and off-axis Doppler. Recent advances may overcome some of the assumptions of the traditional calculation of stroke volume by this method. Multiple direct measurements of outflow tract area using 3D may avoid inaccuracies that arise from the assumption that the orifice is circular and constant in size. The assumption of uniform flow velocity throughout the CSA may be avoided by techniques using CFD. This calculation of stroke volume should be consistent with volumetric calculations from 2D or 3D echocardiography.

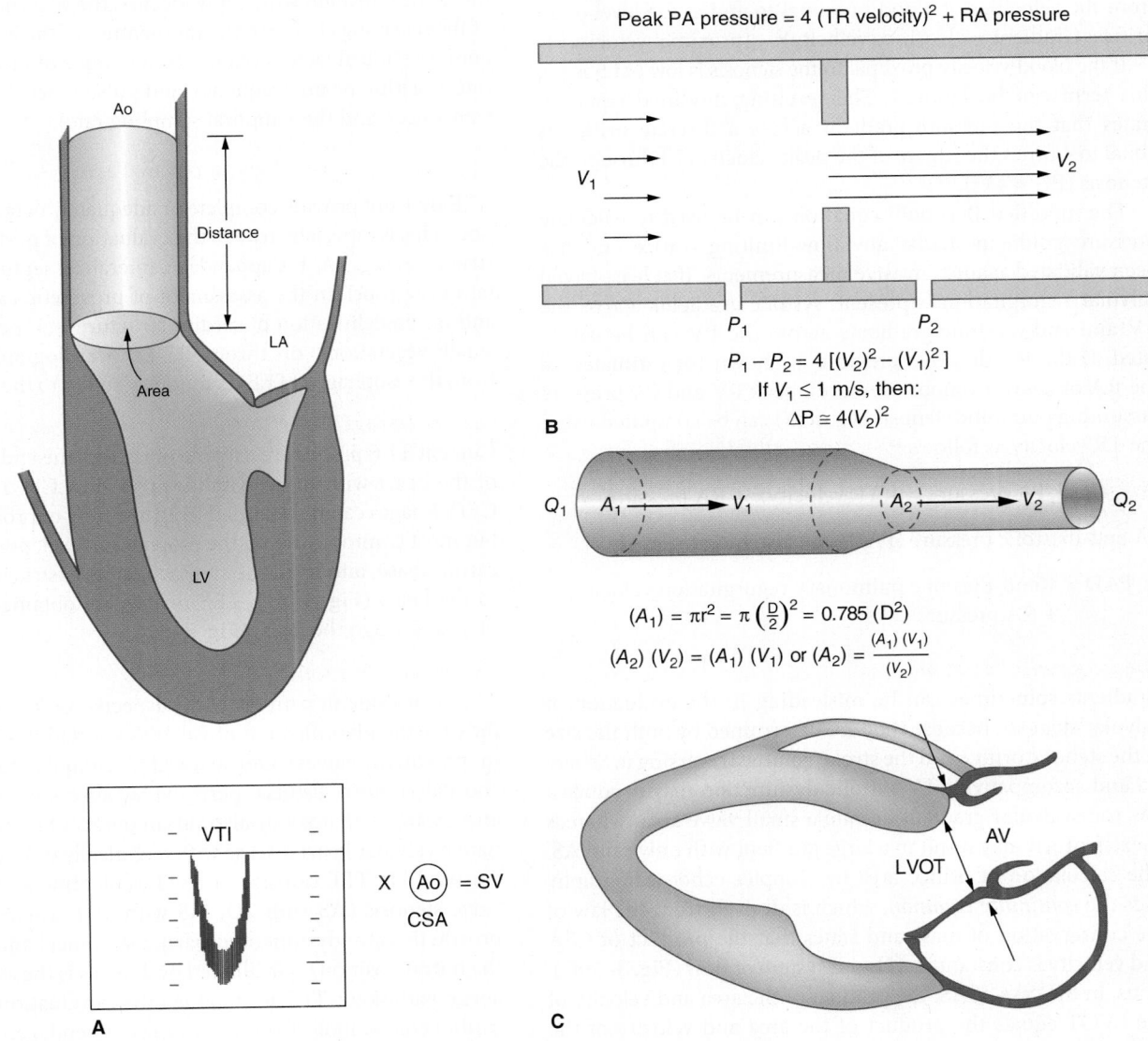

Figure 3–50. Basic Doppler calculations. (A) Stroke volume. Multiplying the cross-sectional area (CSA) of the blood column in the ascending aorta (Ao) by the distance the column moves during a single cardiac contraction yields the stroke volume (SV). The velocity-time integral (VTI), expressed in units of length, represents the *stroke distance*. **(B)** Modified Bernoulli equation. Pressure drop across a small orifice can be estimated as 4 times the square of the peak velocity (if the proximal velocity is <1 m/s). V_1 and P_1, proximal velocity and pressure; V_2 and P_2, distal velocity and pressure. **(C)** Continuity equation. In a closed system (*top*) with constant flow, $Q_1 = Q_2$. Therefore, $A_1 \times V_1$ must equal $A_2 \times V_2$. Determination of any three of the variables allows calculation of the fourth. Clinically (*bottom*), the area of the left ventricular outflow tract (LVOT) can be estimated and used to determine aortic valve (AV) area. V is usually incorporated as time-velocity integral, but mean or peak velocity have also been used. LA, left atrium; LV, left ventricle; PA, pulmonary arterial; RA, right atrial; TR, tricuspid regurgitation. A & B, Modified with permission from Schlant RC, Alexander RW. *The Heart, Arteries, and Veins*, 8th ed. New York, NY: McGraw Hill; 1994. C, Reproduced with permission from Hagan AD, DeMaria AN. *Clinical Applications of Two-Dimensional Echocardiography and Cardiac Doppler*, 2nd ed. Boston, MA: Little, Brown; 1989.

The Bernoulli Equation

An important application of Doppler echocardiography is the calculation of pressure gradients within the cardiovascular system using a modification of the Bernoulli equation.[182] This theorem states that the pressure drop across a discrete stenosis in the heart or vasculature occurs because of energy loss caused by three processes: (1) acceleration of blood through the orifice (*convective acceleration*), (2) inertial forces (*flow acceleration*), and (3) resistance to flow at the interfaces between blood and the orifice (*viscous friction*). Therefore, the pressure drop across any orifice can be calculated as the sum of these three variables (**Fig. 3–50B**). The pressure gradient can be calculated from the velocities of blood proximal to and at the level of an orifice: Gradient = $4[(\text{orifice velocity})^2 - (\text{proximal velocity})^2]$

If the blood velocity proximal to the stenosis is low (<1.5 m/s), this term can be ignored. The resulting modified equation states that the pressure gradient across a discrete orifice is equal to 4 times the square of the peak velocity (V) through the stenosis ($PG = 4V^2$).[182]

The modified Bernoulli equation can be used to calculate pressure gradients across any flow-limiting orifice and has been validated against invasive measurements. If at least trivial valvular regurgitation is present, systolic gradients across the TV and end-diastolic gradients across the PV can be calculated. If the RV diastolic pressure is known (or estimated as the RA or central venous pressure), peak RV and PA pressure (assuming pulmonic stenosis is absent) can be computed using the TR velocity as follows:[183]

$$\text{Peak PA pressure} = 4(\text{TR velocity})^2 + \text{RA pressure}$$

PA end-diastolic pressure (PAD) can also be calculated:

$$\text{PAD} = 4(\text{end-diastolic pulmonary regurgitation velocity})^2 + \text{RA pressure}$$

The Continuity Equation

Gradients sometimes can be misleading in the evaluation of valvular stenosis, because they are determined by both the size of the stenotic orifice and the stroke volume traversing it. Severe AS and accompanying LV systolic dysfunction may produce a low transvalvular gradient despite a small valve area, whereas coexistent AR may result in a large gradient with only mild AS. The calculation of orifice area by Doppler echocardiography uses the *continuity equation*, which is derived from the law of the conservation of mass and states that the product of CSA and velocity is constant in a closed system of flow (**Fig. 3–50C**). Thus, in the case of AS, the product of the area and velocity of the LVOT equals the product of the area and velocity of the AoV orifice. Measurements of annular diameter and integrated velocity are derived by the standard volumetric approach, and the velocity across the stenotic orifice is derived by CW Doppler. The equation is then solved for the valve area.[62]

The two most common pitfalls of the continuity equation are inaccurate estimation of the CSA proximal to the stenosis, and failure to measure blood velocity proximal to the stenosis outside the area of flow acceleration. Although the continuity equation actually solves for the area of the vena contracta, which is usually just distal to the stenotic orifice, this generally correlates well with the aortic valve area.

Regurgitation and the Size of Flow Disturbances

Quantitative measurement of valvular regurgitation is possible using the proximal isovelocity surface area (PISA).[184] If the area of flow acceleration and body of the jet are visualized, measurement of the vena contracta using 2D or 3D CFD provides a marker of effective orifice area.[184] However, other CFD parameters are primarily qualitative, especially the area of turbulence recorded by CFD. This has multiple determinants,[185] including the orifice through which flow occurs, the size and compliance of the receiving chamber, the momentum of the jet, and a number of technical factors (gain settings, angle of incidence of the interrogating beam, frequency and pulse repetition rate of the transducer, and the temporal sampling rate).

Transesophageal Echocardiography

TTE may not provide complete or adequately detailed information. This is especially true in the evaluation of posterior cardiac structures (eg, LA, LA appendage, interatrial septum, aorta distal to the root), in the assessment of prosthetic cardiac valves, and in the delineation of cardiac structures <3 mm in size (eg, small vegetations or thrombi). Echocardiographic imaging from the esophagus (TEE) is uniquely suited to these situations.

Technique and Views

Current TEE probes are capable of multiplane and 3D imaging of the heart with full capabilities of PWD, CW Doppler, and CFD. Images can be recorded from a variety of probe positions, but most commonly from the esophageal level, posterior to the cardiac base, and from the stomach (transgastric level), caudal to the heart (**Fig. 3–51**). TEE images are obtained in various planes through the heart (**Fig. 3–52**).

Clinical Applications

TEE is of value in patients with suspected or known endocarditis for the identification of valvular vegetations (particularly in prosthetic valves) and associated complications, such as chordal rupture, fistulas, perivalvular abscesses, and mycotic aneurysms. TEE imaging also aids in the accurate assessment of native valvular heart disease with technically difficult or inconclusive TTE. TEE can also be used to planimeter valve area in valve stenosis (AS with 2D; MS with 3D). The evaluation of prosthetic valve dysfunction (particularly mechanical valves in the mitral position) is facilitated by TEE, as is the assessment of aortic pathology. TEE is of value in the evaluation of possible cardiogenic emboli (from LA and LA appendage, ASD, patent foramen ovale (PFO), and aorta). Finally, TEE has become an important tool to assist structural heart disease specialists and surgeons in various cardiac interventions—especially with 3D imaging.

Handheld Echocardiography

Recent technical advances have led to the production of small, lightweight echocardiography units. These handheld devices

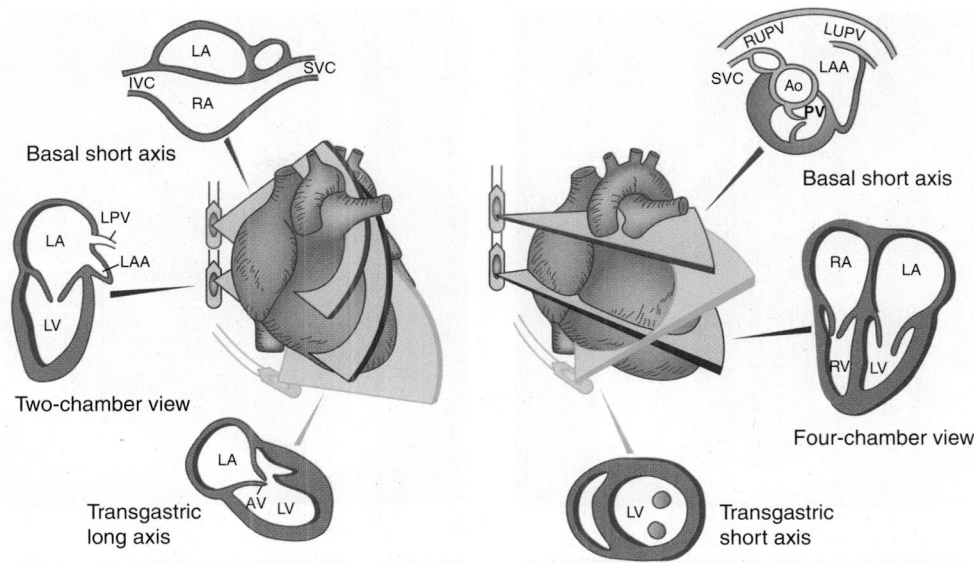

Figure 3–51. **Standard transesophageal echocardiography imaging planes in transverse and longitudinal axes.** Ao, aorta; AV, aortic valve; IVC, inferior vena cava; LA, left atrium; LAA, left atrial appendage; LPV, left pulmonary vein; LV, left ventricle, LUPV, left upper pulmonary vein; PV, pulmonary valve; RA, right atrium; RUPV, right upper pulmonary vein; RV, right ventricle; SVC, superior vena cava. Reproduced with permission from Fisher EA, Stahl JA, Budd JH, et al. Transesophageal echocardiography: procedures and clinical application. *J Am Coll Cardiol.* 1991 Nov 1;18(5):1333-1348.

can facilitate bedside, point-of-care echo evaluation. However, the sonographic and interpretive skills of the person performing the study are critical; however, it has been demonstrated that simple skills to evaluate overall cardiac function or pericardial effusion can be learned over a short period. Issues exist about the quality of the studies, technical skills required, potential misdiagnosis or omission, added time commitment during clinic visits, and overall quality control.[186] The recent development of an artificial intelligence–based process to assist nonexperts obtain on-axis images[187] may more effectively improve image quality than the recommendation that individuals performing handheld scanning have level 2 training in echocardiography.[188]

Contrast Echocardiography

Because few room-air microbubbles with the diameter of pulmonary capillaries persist intact in blood for longer than 1 second before dissolving, agitated agents injected intravenously rarely cross the lungs. Thus, the presence of echocardiographic contrast entering left heart chambers after intravenous injection of an agitated liquid indicates the presence of a right-to-left shunt, either intracardiac or through a pulmonary arteriovenous fistula—the two being distinguished by the absence or presence of a delay of 5-6 cardiac cycles before left heart opacification. Thus, the detection of a PFO remains a frequent indication for contrast echocardiography using simple agitated normal saline solution. As the passage of contrast across the interatrial septum requires right atrial to exceed left atrial pressure (at least transiently) a Valsalva maneuver or cough is performed in patients who do not readily show crossing of microbubbles across the septum. TEE (for assessing

the size and location of a PFO) is an adjunct to transthoracic echocardiogram (TTE), but the latter is more sensitive because Valsalva is more feasible without sedation.

The development of small (~3 micron), persistent bubbles has enabled successful crossing of the pulmonary capillaries and echocardiographic opacification of the LV cavity and myocardium after intravenous administration.[176] This has been accomplished by using a shell- or surface-modifying agent that inhibits the leakage of gas across the microbubble surface (eg, albumin or liposomes) and a dense, high-molecular-weight gas (eg, fluorocarbon) with a reduced capacity to diffuse across the bubble shell. These microbubbles permit LV opacification and myocardial imaging after intravenous injection.[176] Specific indications include improving the accuracy and reproducibility of LV volume measurements, improving endocardial border definition at rest and during stress echocardiography, and evaluation of possible LV thrombi.[176] Contrast can also enhance Doppler signal, thus improving spectral recordings of TR and AS jets if suboptimal, facilitating the quantitation of valvular lesions and PH.[176]

Stress Echocardiography

The combination of stress testing and echocardiography (stress echocardiography) has assumed an important role in the diagnosis of CAD. Its growth has been assisted by a number of technical advances, including side-by-side review of rest and stress images together in a cine-loop format, harmonic imaging, and LV opacification with intravenous echocardiographic contrast. The application of stress echocardiography is based on the concept that a stress-induced imbalance in the myocardial supply-to-demand ratio will produce regional ischemia and

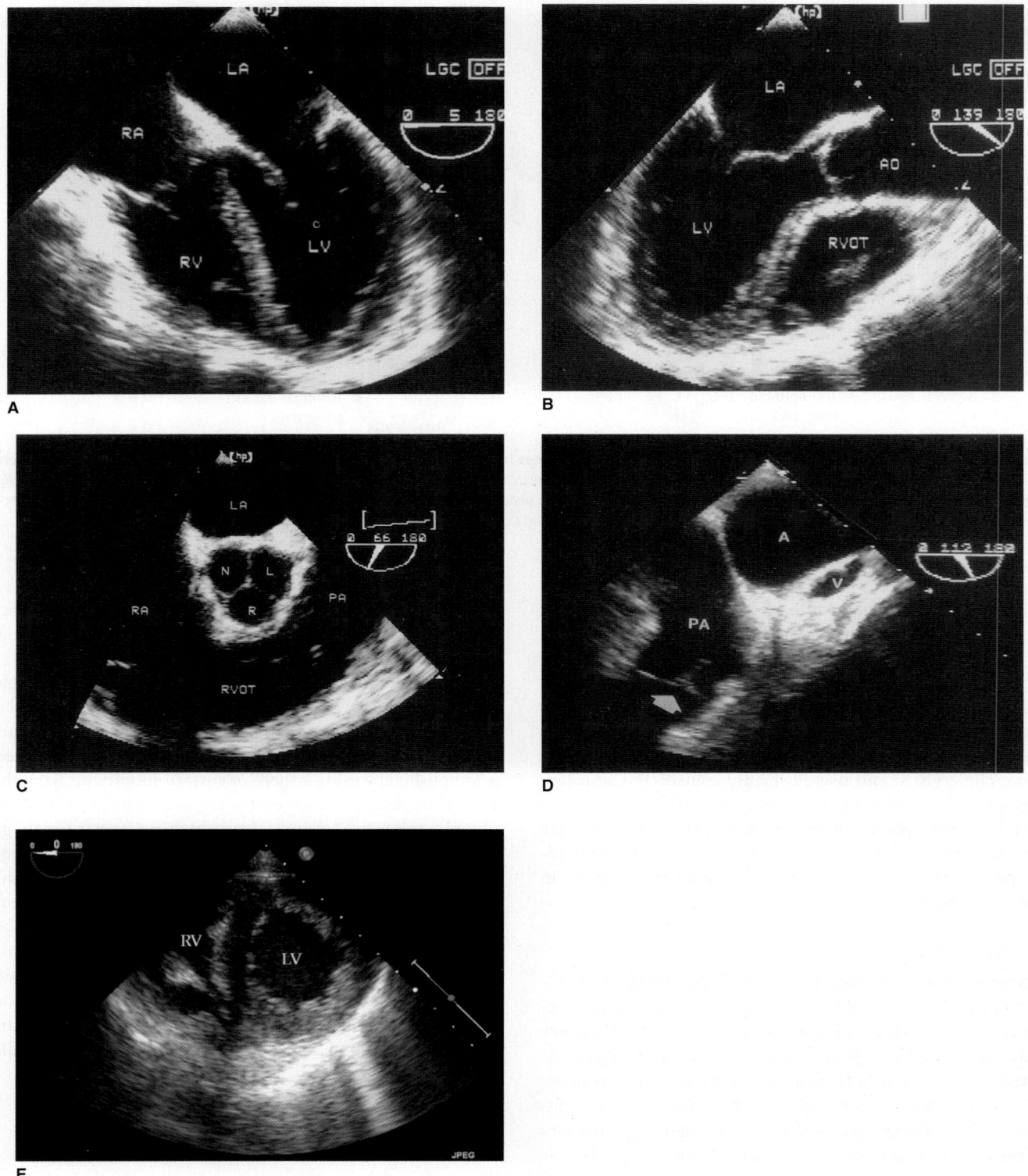

Figure 3–52. Transesophageal echocardiography views. (A) Transverse four-chamber. **(B)** Modified longitudinal (with transducer rotated to approximately 150 degrees), demonstrating a TEE apical three-chamber view. **(C)** Modified short-axis through the level of the aortic valve, demonstrating the left (*L*), right (*R*), and noncoronary (*N*) valvular cusps. **(D)** Longitudinal image at level of the aortic arch, demonstrating the transverse aorta (*A*), the brachiocephalic vein (*V*), and the main pulmonary artery (*PA*). The pulmonic valve is visible as well (*arrow*). **(E)** Short-axis transesophageal echocardiography plane through the left ventricle (LV) from transgastric position. The inferior wall is closest to the transducer, the anterior wall farthest. The interventricular septum is to the reader's left, the lateral wall to the right. Ao, ascending aorta; LA, left atrium; LV, left ventricle; PA, pulmonary artery; RA, right atrium; RV, right ventricle; RVOT, right ventricular outflow tract. **(D)** reproduced with permission from Blanchard DG, Kimura BJ, Dittrich HC, et al. Transesophageal echocardiography of the aorta, *JAMA.* 1994;272(7):546-551.

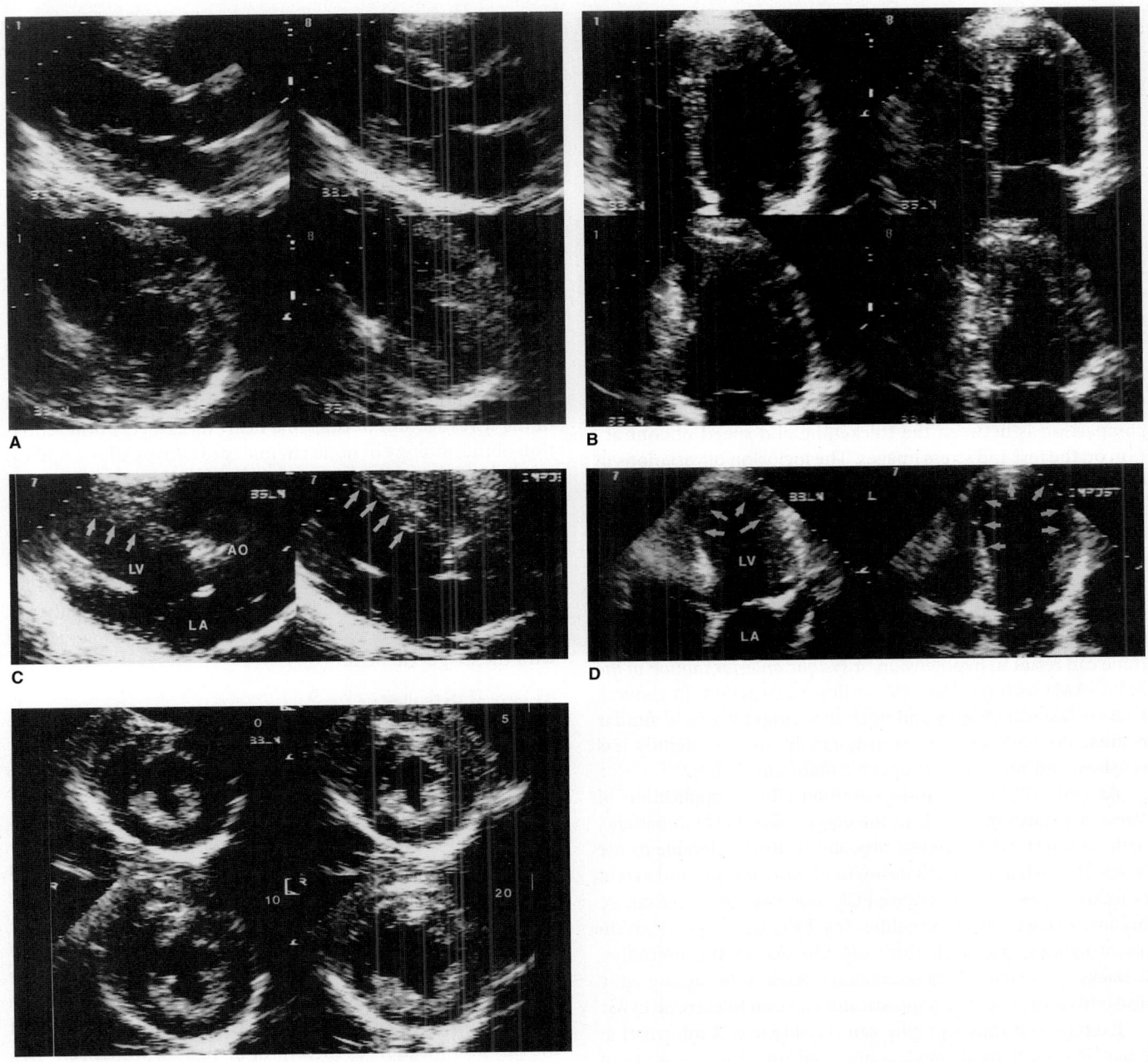

Figure 3–53. (**A**) Parasternal views during diastole (*left*) and systole (*right*) from a normal individual. *Upper panels*: long-axis plane; *lower panels*: short-axis plane. (**B**) Apical views during diastole (*left*) and systole (*right*) from a normal individual. *Upper panels*: four-chamber plane; *lower panels*: two-chamber plane. (**C**) Parasternal long-axis views at peak systole before (*left*) and immediately after exercise (*right*). The anteroseptal wall moves normally at rest (*arrows*) but becomes dyskinetic with exercise. (**D**) Apical four-chamber views at peak systole before (*left*) and immediately after exercise (*right*). The apical septal, apical, and apical lateral walls become dyskinetic with exercise, suggesting inducible ischemia in the left anterior descending coronary artery territory. (**E**) Parasternal short-axis views (all recorded at peak systole) during dobutamine echocardiography in a patient with three-vessel coronary artery disease. At baseline (*upper left panel*) the left ventricular systolic function is normal. With low-dose dobutamine (5 µg/kg/min; *upper right panel*), function improves. With 10 µg/kg/min, however (*lower left panel*), function is similar to that at baseline. At 20 µg/kg/min (*lower right panel*), systolic function deteriorates and the left ventricle (LV) dilates. This response suggests global ischemia induced by dobutamine infusion. Ao, aorta; LA, left atrium.

resultant abnormalities of regional contraction, which can be readily identified by echocardiography (**Fig. 3–53**). The location of wall motion abnormalities may be used to predict the stenosed coronary vessel(s), whereas the ratio of dyssynergic-to-normal myocardium can provide a quantitative assessment of LV ischemia.[189]

The types of stress used fall into two basic groups: exercise and pharmacologic. Exercise testing can be performed either on a treadmill or a stationary bicycle (either upright or supine). Echo imaging usually can be accomplished only before and after treadmill exercise, whereas bicycle exertion facilitates the acquisition of images during the exercise protocol. In the

United States, Australia, and the United Kingdom, a treadmill has been the preferred exercise modality, with bicycle exercise more widely used in Europe. All postexertional images should be obtained within a 1-minute window after exercise to avoid missing inducible wall motion abnormalities provoked by stress.

Pharmacologic stress has the advantages of reducing the motion artifact of exercise, enabling continuous imaging throughout the protocol and assessing myocardial viability. As with SPECT, pharmacologic stress echocardiography can use vasodilator agents such as dipyridamole or adenosine, which induce a heterogeneity of myocardial perfusion in ischemic heart disease, or inotropic agents such as dobutamine, which increase myocardial oxygen demand and directly produce ischemia. The diagnostic criteria include induction of regional wall motion abnormalities and LV dilatation. Although the normal response to exercise is hyperkinesis, the most important comparison is between the thickening and speed of contraction on the rest and stress images. The inclusion of variations in the degree of hyperkinesis as an ischemia signal may augment sensitivity at the cost of specificity. Myocardial viability can be assessed with dobutamine stress echocardiography.[190]

The safety and accuracy of stress echocardiography for the diagnosis of myocardial ischemia has been examined in several studies.[191] Both exercise and pharmacologic stress carry an extremely low risk of arrhythmia or infarction, but dobutamine can result in hypotension or *systolic anterior motion of the MV* (SAM) with resultant LV outflow obstruction. In general, stress echocardiography and nuclear scintigraphy yield similar results, although stress echocardiography may be slightly less sensitive and slightly more specific than scintigraphy.[192]

As with SPECT, the most common clinical application of stress echocardiography is in the diagnosis of CAD in patients with an intermediate pretest probability. It is preferable to the stress ECG when there is a desire to identify the site and extent of ischemia, and when exercise ECG alone would be inaccurate because of baseline abnormalities (eg, LVH with repolarization abnormalities, paced rhythm, digoxin use in the preceding 2 weeks or ventricular preexcitation). Stress echocardiography also adds independent prognostic information to exercise ECG.

Exercise echocardiography can provide useful information regarding the hemodynamic status and functional severity of valvular heart disease.[193] Specifically, stress echocardiography has been used to assess the degree of obstruction in patients with MS and AS, and contractile reserve. In MS, the critical findings of exercise echocardiography pertain not so much to gradient (which is related to the heart rate), but to the development of PH with exercise. In AS, exercise testing can uncover hitherto inapparent symptoms in asymptomatic patients and dobutamine echo can distinguish true AS from pseudo-AS in patients with low-flow, low-gradient AS with low EF.

Fetal Echocardiography

The average risk for significant heart disease in the fetus is approximately 0.4% to 0.8%. Fetal echocardiography has evolved over the last 20 years into a sophisticated method for intrauterine detection of cardiac abnormalities. The technique has been advocated for the preterm diagnosis of CHD, especially in higher risk cases. Fetal echocardiography has successfully identified a variety of congenital lesions.[194] Prenatal detection of these lesions may improve prognosis and guide therapy.

CARDIAC MAGNETIC RESONANCE

Over the last 30 years, CMR imaging has evolved from a technique used to acquire static images of the heart and chest into a versatile imaging modality for assessing many physiologic variables pertinent to the evaluation of patients with CVD. CMR-based methods accurately measure LV and RV volumes, mass, and function and are able to characterize the presence and extent of MI and viability. Hence, they now serve as "gold standard techniques" for assessing these metrics. Increasingly, CMR enables (1) assessments of myocardial perfusion in the investigation of ischemic heart disease; (2) differentiation of the etiology of nonischemic cardiomyopathies; and (3) characterization of congenital heart syndromes, pericardial disease, and cardiac masses. The advantages of this test are lack of ionizing radiation, ability to image in multiple tomographic planes, high spatial, temporal and contrast resolution, and reproducibility.[195] The disadvantages are access, need for special training, contraindications (claustrophobic patients, implanted ferrous devices), and potential hazards associated with the magnetic field.

Physical Principles

For the most CMR studies, image formulation relies on signals detected from hydrogen nuclei. In a strong magnetic field, these hydrogen nuclei (or protons) align and "precess" (spin) about the *z*-axis of the field (along the bore of the scanner). Pulse sequences or small magnetic field pulses alter this precession by delivering nonionizing electromagnetic radiation that transfers energy to ("excites") protons and tilts them into the *x-y* plane to a degree determined by the flip angle. The subsequent relaxation of the protons to their original orientation within the magnetic field creates a signal that is detected by a radiofrequency receiver (or coil). Spatial variations in the magnetic field (magnetic gradients) enable identification of the physical location of these proton signals, which can then be processed into an image of their spatial distribution (**Fig. 3–54**). After excitation, relaxation of protons within the magnetic field is governed by the field strength and the T1 and T2 magnetic times, which are intrinsic properties of the tissue. T2* time refers to T2 after accounting for inhomogeneity of the magnetic field. Quantification ("mapping") of these times can be performed with appropriate sequences.

Most CMR studies are performed on scanners with field strengths of 1.5 Tesla (T) or 3T. In addition to the room housing the magnet, there is a control room located just outside the scanner room housing the computer consoles to direct the scan acquisition as well as a small equipment room housing electrical and other scanner-related equipment. For CMR studies, additional equipment is required, including that for monitoring HR and BP, injecting intravenous contrast, and delivering intravenous medications. As images are obtained, they are

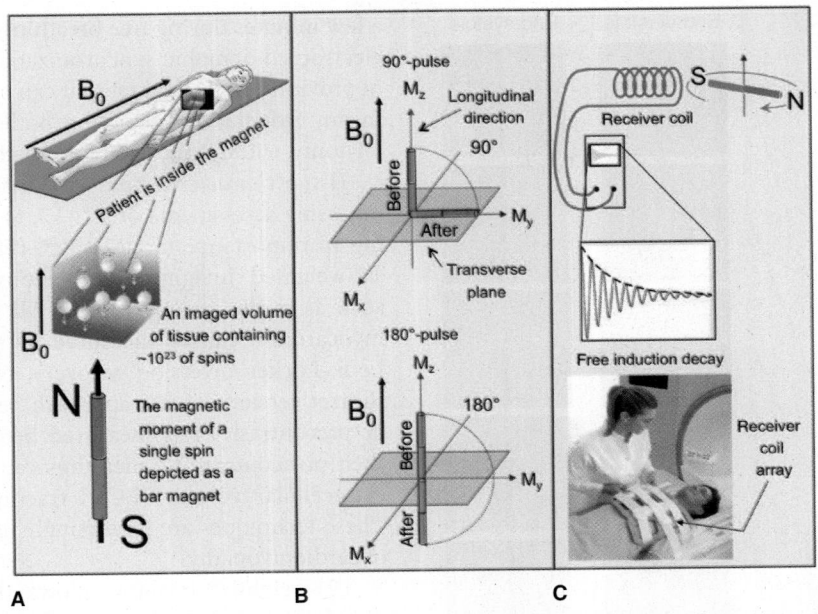

Figure 3–54. Basic operations of the magnetic resonance imaging scanner. (A) The protons align parallel or antiparallel to the static magnetic field (Bo), creating a small net magnetization vector. While aligned to the magnetic field, the protons precess at a frequency proportional to the strength of the magnetic field (the Larmor frequency). **(B)** Transmission of radiofrequency (RF) energy. Energy is transmitted to the rotating protons by an RF pulse at the Larmor frequency. RF pulses that result in a flip angle of 90 and 180 degrees are shown (*top* and *bottom*, respectively). The figures are presented in the rotating frame of reference, where the *x-y* axes are rotating at the Larmor frequency and thus appear stationary. **(C)** Generation of the magnetic resonance (MR) signal. Rotation of the net magnetization vector into the transverse plane results in the creation of a time-varying magnetic field, which in turn induces an alternating current in the receiver coil array; this is the MR signal.

typically transferred to additional computer workstations for independent image analysis and interpretation.

Recommendations for acquisition, reporting, and analysis of CMR images have been recently published to guide imagers on appropriate application of these techniques.[196–198]

Techniques

Steady-state free precession (SSFP) cine "bright-blood" imaging forms the foundation and primary acquisition strategy for most CMR examinations.[199] This mode of acquisition provides high contrast-to-noise between the dark myocardium and bright-blood pool and allows for the visualization of cardiac anatomy as well as atrial and ventricular contraction/relaxation. Multiple studies have demonstrated the accuracy and reproducibility of cine CMR bright-blood imaging for measuring LV volumes, LVEF, and LV regional systolic function.[195] To measure LV volumes, LV mass, and LVEF, short-axis images spanning the apex to the base of the heart are acquired throughout the cardiac cycle with slice thicknesses between 6 and 8 mm, with or without 2- to 4-mm gaps, and with temporal resolution ≤45 milliseconds[196] **(Fig. 3–55)**. Analysis is performed with computer software that uses semiautomated techniques for tracing endocardial and epicardial contours at end diastole and end systole and the summation of disks methods for adding volumes together from all of the short-axis slices. Measurements made with this 3D data set do not require geometric assumptions and are, therefore, less prone to error than 2D methods such as 2D echocardiography, especially in ventricles deformed by MI or cardiomyopathies. Interobserver and

interscan reproducibility is high, allowing for reduced sample sizes in clinical trials in heart failure.[200] Similarly, CMR is a highly reproducible technique for measurement of RV volumes because of its 3D analysis.[201] The RV can be measured using short-axis views or stacked axial scans; the latter improves identification of the tricuspid valve plane and correlates better with pulmonary flow measures.

Typically, long-axis images are also obtained in standard two-, three-, and four-chamber views. Most commonly, SSFP sequences are utilized; however, gradient-echo bright-blood images may also be acquired because these images are more sensitive to detect turbulent flow in the setting of valvular obstruction or regurgitation. Stress testing can be performed with SSFP cine in multiple planes at different stages of dobutamine ± atropine infusion. These cine bright-blood images may be acquired with high spatial and temporal resolution during 6- to 10-second breath-holds (known as a *segmented* acquisition), or at a slightly reduced spatial and temporal resolution in "real time" that does not require electrocardiographic gating or breath-holding. This latter technique is often used in those with arrhythmia or limited breath-holding ability.

Additional CMR methods are available for quantifying abnormalities of regional LV systolic function that may not be evident on visual inspection of the images.[202] "Tissue tagging" applies radiofrequency and gradient pulses to null the myocardium at end diastole, resulting in the placement of "tissue tags" that can be tracked through the cardiac cycle to enable assessment of myocardial deformation and measurement of

End-diastole   End-systole

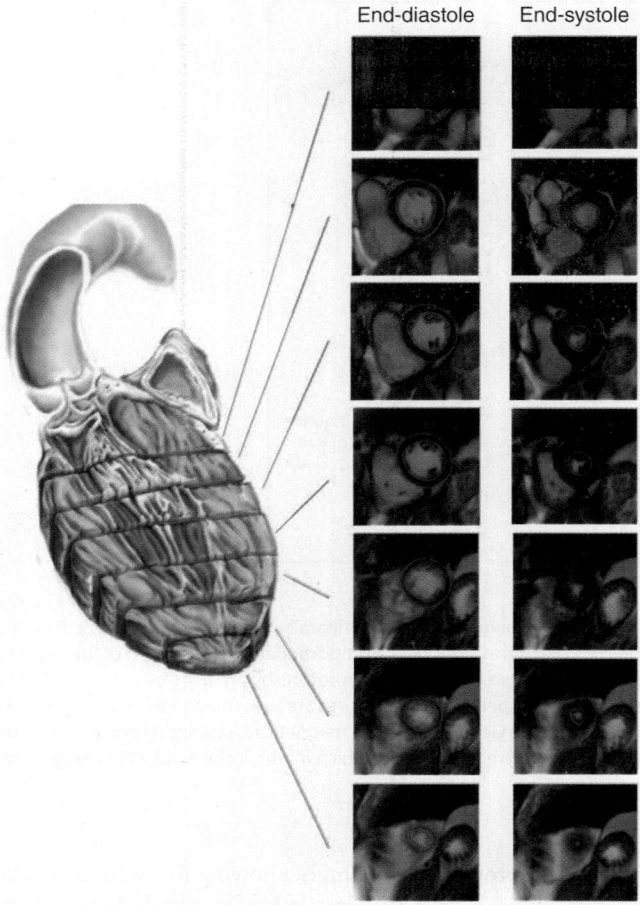

Figure 3–55. Cardiovascular magnetic resonance method to quantify left ventricular (LV) volumes, ejection fraction, and mass. The LV myocardium, cavity, mitral valve apparatus, and ascending thoracic aorta are depicted in the *left column*. As shown in the *right column*, a series of cine white blood images are acquired in short-axis planes positioned perpendicular to the long axis of the left ventricle. For each slice position, an end-diastolic frame and an end-systolic frame of the cine loop are displayed. On these images, the LV myocardial blood pool appears white and the myocardium gray. To calculate LV volumes, the area of the LV myocardial blood pool (red contour along the endocardial surface) is obtained. The LV volume is determined by summing the volume of all the slice positions (calculated for each slice by multiplying the area of each slice by the slice's thickness) spanning the cardiac base to the myocardial apex. The LV ejection fraction is calculated by subtracting the end-systolic volume from the end-diastolic volume and then dividing by the end-diastolic volume. Measurement of myocardial mass can be obtained by assessing the difference in the area bounded by the LV epicardial surface (*green line*) and endocardial surface (*red line*) and then summing myocardial volumes across the slices (and then multiplying by 1.05 g/cm³ the assumed density of the LV myocardium). Reproduced with permission from AE Hundley.

myocardial strain.[203] However, strain measurements are now more feasible using feature-tracking.

In spin echo black-blood images, the MRI signal of the spins from flowing blood is inverted, leaving the blood pool dark within the LV cavity. Once a staple of most CMR examinations, black-blood imaging has been largely replaced by SSFP cine imaging because of its utility for assessing cardiac structure and function during the same acquisition. It is important to note that stationary SSFP images may be acquired in 3D view over

a few minutes during free breathing with both respiratory and electrocardiographic synchronization. This has the advantage of providing a 3D data set that can be manipulated and viewed in any orientation, depicting both cardiac and extracardiac anatomy, without the need for breath-holding or contrast.

Tissue characterization with mapping or weighted imaging using assessments of T1, T2, or T2* relaxation is increasing in importance in CMR[204,205] (**Fig. 3–56**). High signal on T2-weighted imaging can demonstrate myocardial edema, such as in the setting of acute MI or myocarditis. T1 of the myocardium can be measured by mapping with a modified Look-Locker inversion recovery, or MOLLI, sequence[206] or shorter versions of this approach, termed shMOLLI.[207] Native or precontrast T1 is measured before contrast infusion and then postcontrast T1 measures can be used to calculate the extracellular volume (ECV) fraction of the myocardium.[208] These techniques are increasingly used to differentiate causes of cardiomyopathy.

T2*-weighted imaging allows the measurement of cardiac iron deposition because there is an inverse relationship between T2* and iron concentration. T2*-weighted imaging is sensitive to iron in the heart and can identify iron overload conditions and myocardial hemorrhage in the setting of acute MI. This mode of imaging has become quite important in iron overload states such as hemochromatosis and β-thalassemia major.[209] A T2* <10 milliseconds is an important predictor of clinical heart failure[209] (Fig. 3–56). This application has been carefully validated and performed in a large number of international sites. Clinical trials of chelation therapies have used T2* imaging to track reductions in cardiac iron and concomitant improvements in LVEF.

Phase contrast (PC) imaging (also known as velocity-encoded cine, velocity mapping, or flow imaging) is used to display and quantify velocities and flow. It relies on the principle that precession frequency of protons is directly proportional to the velocity of a particle moving across a magnetic field gradient. If a magnetic gradient is created along the direction of blood flow, protons moving faster will be subjected to a stronger or weaker magnetic field and experience a proportional shift in their precession. Measurement of this shift, therefore, allows for the quantification of blood velocity along the direction of the gradient. This is typically achieved by prescribing the acquisition perpendicular ("through-plane") to the expected direction of flow (ie, to the ascending aorta or pulmonary artery for quantification of systemic [aortic] or pulmonary forward cardiac outputs). PC sequences typically provide two reconstructions of the acquired data: a magnitude (or anatomic) image and a phase-difference reconstruction (velocity map) where the signal intensity of each voxel is rendered proportional to its velocity (**Fig. 3–57**). Accuracy is highest if the limit of measurable velocities is set close to, but below, the true velocity of blood. Using these sequences, flow is calculated by integrating changes in area and velocity throughout the cardiac cycle, and has been validated both in vitro and in vivo. Newer 3D sequences (also known as 4D PC or 4D flow imaging) have been developed that enable the quantification of velocities in all directions.[210]

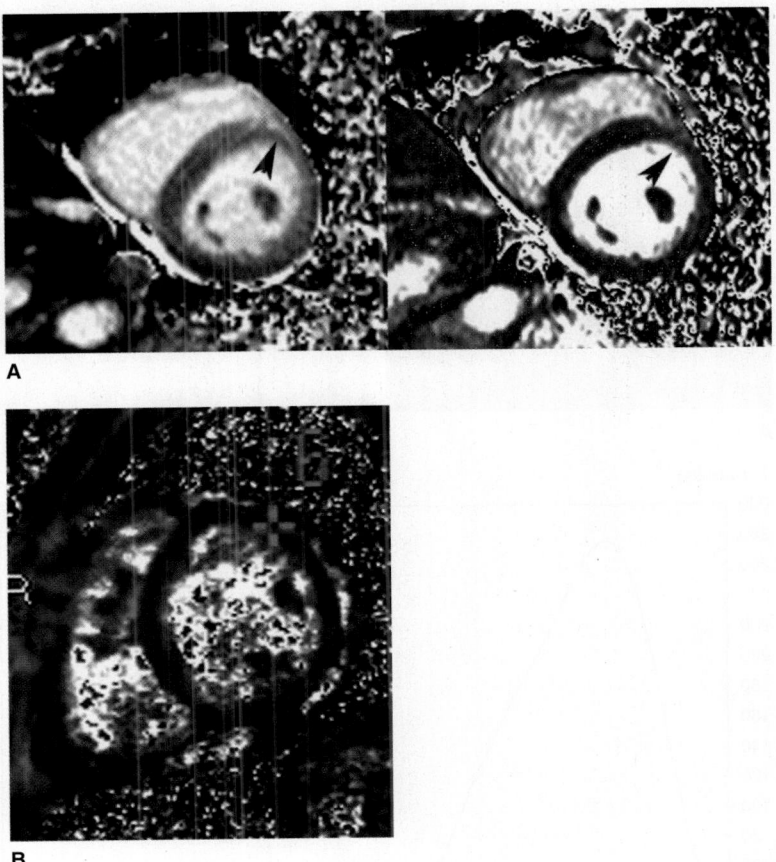

Figure 3–56. Myocardial tissue characterization with magnetic resonance imaging. (A) Short-axis T1 map in a patient with chest pain, troponin elevation, and normal coronary arteries with a recent viral infection and clinical diagnosis of myocarditis (*left*). There is higher T1 signal (brighter) in the anterior wall, which is also somewhat thinner. Short-axis T2 map in the same patient demonstrating bright signal (elevated T2) in the same region (*right*). **(B)** Basal short-axis T2* map in a patient with a history of multiple transfusions and systolic heart failure. The T2* is 6 milliseconds, which corresponds to the low ejection fraction noted on cine imaging in this patient.

Perfusion imaging has evolved significantly and is now a routine investigation.[211] In general, this is achieved by imaging the first-pass of a gadolinium-based contrast agent (GBCA) through the myocardium. It can be performed at rest (eg, to identify "tumor blush") and, for the purposes of stress testing, during vasodilator challenge to identify hypoperfusion associated with flow-limiting epicardial coronary artery stenoses.[212] Typically, images in three to five short-axis slices are acquired over 50 to 60 heartbeats. Images are assessed qualitatively for regions of low signal intensity consistent with hypoperfusion that encompass at least the subendocardial one-third of the myocardial wall of at least five frames or heartbeats in duration (**Fig. 3–58**). Comparing rest and stress imaging with late gadolinium-enhanced (LGE) imaging can differentiate perfusion defects caused by ischemia from those cause by artifacts or MI.

LGE refers to regions of scar and/or necrosis discriminated from normal tissue by prolonged retention of gadolinium-based contrast agents as visualized on T1-weighted imaging.[213] An inversion recovery-based pulse sequence is used to optimize the differentiation of normal dark myocardial tissue from bright areas of fibrosis or scar.[214] These fibrotic areas appear bright as a result of retention of gadolinium, in turn because of increased volume of distribution as well as delayed washout of the contrast agent. LGE is considered the gold standard technique for detecting and sizing MI (**Fig. 3–59**). However, LGE is not unique to infarct scar and can signify any cause of fibrosis or interstitial infiltration in cardiomyopathies, many of which have a unique pattern of LGE.[215]

Safety

Metallic and Electronic Devices

Although a relatively safe imaging modality, CMR does possess potential for serious and even lethal events. The magnetic field of clinical CMR scanners is 25,000 to 50,000 times stronger than that of the earth, and ferromagnetic metallic objects that come into close proximity with the field can be drawn toward the magnet in a projectile fashion. It is important to realize that the magnetic field is always "on," even when the scanner is not being used; therefore, all personnel involved in CMR operations need to be appropriately trained, and access

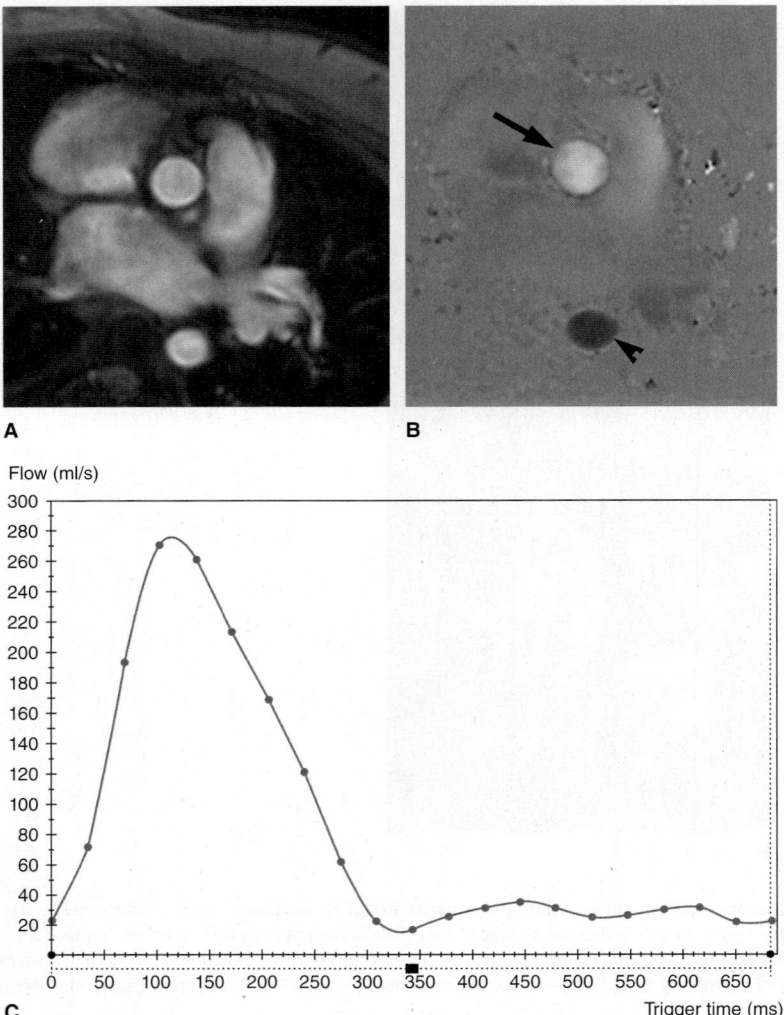

Figure 3–57. Magnitude image (A) and velocity map (B) of the ascending aorta as obtained with phase contrast. In (B), note that flow moving in one direction through the plane is encoded in *white* (ascending aorta; *arrow*) whereas flow in the opposite direction is encoded in *black* (descending aorta, *arrowhead*). Integration of velocities and cross-sectional area allows for the quantification of flow (**C**).

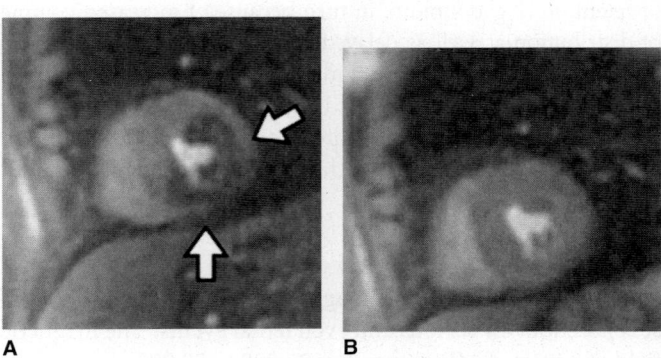

Figure 3–58. Hybrid gradient echo/echo planar first-pass contrast-enhanced perfusion images during vasodilator stress (A) and rest (B). At stress, there is a large perfusion defect in the anterolateral and inferolateral walls (*arrows*), whereas perfusion is normal at rest. This patient had two-vessel coronary artery disease (right and left circumflex) at subsequent cardiac catheterization.

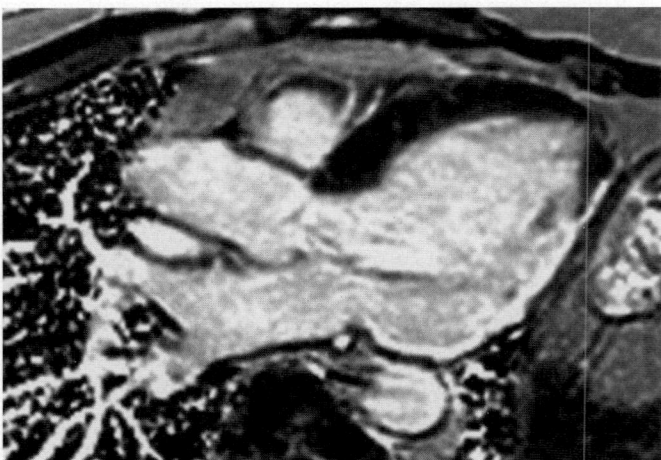

Figure 3–59. Three-chamber long-axis phase-sensitive inversion recovery late gadolinium-enhanced (LGE) image in a patient with a chronic inferolateral infarction. Note the wall thinning and near transmural LGE in that region.

to the CMR room and its vicinity must be severely restricted and adequately demarcated. Only MRI-compatible devices and materials (such as injections pumps or stretchers) may enter the magnet room, and individuals need to be appropriately screened.[216]

A CMR scanner may also pose danger to patients or personnel with implanted ferromagnetic or electronic devices. Aside from the potential for torque or pull by the magnetic field, the rapidly switching magnetic gradients can induce voltages in conducting materials, which in turn may heat surrounding tissues. In addition, depending on the sequence used, the magnetic field strength, and the specific device, changes in programming and functioning of implanted electronic devices may occur. Thus, the decision needs to be individualized for each patient to determine (1) whether the specific device is MRI-compatible and (2) at what field strength it is compatible. As a general rule, objects located in soft tissues that can be easily harmed are the greatest concern; these include the orbits and the brain (typically aneurysm clips, of which most modern ones are MRI-compatible). The vast majority of orthopedic implants are safe. Regarding devices frequently encountered in cardiac patients, safety recommendations[217] are summarized in **Table 3–20**. All current coronary stents and prosthetic valves are safe and can be imaged immediately after implantation. Many other cardiac or vascular implants are nonferromagnetic and can also be scanned at any time, or are weakly ferromagnetic and a delay of 6 weeks before MRI is recommended to allow for endothelialization. Swan-Ganz catheters contain metal and are considered unsafe. Similarly, some medication patches contain metallic foil and may need to be removed before the procedure.

Although pacemakers and ICDs have been traditionally considered absolute contraindications for CMR, an increasing body of literature indicates that it is feasible to safely scan select patients with select devices, as long as strict protocols and monitoring are followed. In the absence of such protocols, MRI with pacemakers and ICDs should still be considered unsafe. MRI-compatible pacemakers and ICD are available.

Nephrogenic Systemic Fibrosis

The administration of GBCAs in patients with renal failure risks the development of nephrogenic systemic fibrosis (a fibrosing disease primarily involving the skin and subcutaneous tissues, which can also affect internal organs). Symptoms typically include skin thickening and/or pruritus, with potential for contractures and joint immobility, and rarely, death through visceral fibrosis. The estimated incidence is 1% to 7% in those with an estimated glomerular filtration rate (eGFR) <30 mL/min/m^2, and it is more common in patients on dialysis and with specific GBCAs.[218] GBCAs should be avoided in patients with eGFR <30 mL/min/m^2 and in those with acute renal failure (where eGFR may be less accurate). Caution is recommended for those with eGFR between 30 and 40 mL/min/m^2 because of daily fluctuations in eGFR. For those patients on dialysis, prompt (within 2 hours) hemodialysis after the test should be considered to enhance elimination, although the benefit of this approach is unproven. Peritoneal dialysis is not considered effective.

Pregnancy and Lactation

There is no conclusive evidence that CMR can induce harm to the fetus, but there are also no solid safety data. Therefore, CMR is not recommended, although it can be performed after physician–patient discussion if the benefits are deemed to outweigh potential risks. The stage of the pregnancy plays no role in the decision.[216] The same applies to the use of GBCAs, which are known to cross the placental barrier and might be harmful to the fetus.[218] A very small amount of GBCA is excreted in the milk and it is considered safe to continue breastfeeding, although 12- to 24-hour interruption is occasionally recommended.[218]

Other

Magnetic gradients can cause peripheral stimulation that may be perceived as tingling. They also cause loud noises, so ear protection is systematically provided. The incidence of claustrophobia precluding CMR is approximately 4%; around half of these patients will be able to undergo the test with mild sedation.

CMR Stress Testing

Appreciation of LV myocardial ischemia has traditionally depended on identifying abnormalities of LV myocardial perfusion, wall motion, metabolism, or epicardial coronary artery blood flow after experiencing some form of stress. CMR is unique in that with a single imaging modality one can identify abnormalities of LV myocardial perfusion or wall motion in a single test with a relatively high spatial resolution and without administration of any form of ionizing radiation. Based on multimodality appropriate use criteria, stress CMR is considered appropriate for patients with high pretest probability for CAD or intermediate pretest probability of CAD with an uninterpretable ECG or inability to exercise.[153] It is also appropriate

TABLE 3–20. Safety of Common Metallic Implants and Electronic Devices Commonly Found in Patients Undergoing Cardiovascular Magnetic Resonance at ≤3 Tesla

Safe at Any Time	Safe at any Time or after 6 Weeks[a]	Unsafe
Valve prostheses/rings	Cardiac occluder devices	Pacemakers[b]
Coronary stents	Embolization coils	Defibrillators[b]
Retained epicardial leads	Peripheral stents	Retained intravenous leads
Sternotomy wires	Inferior vena cava filters	Swan-Ganz catheters
		Transdermal patches

[a]For weakly ferromagnetic devices, it is reasonable to wait 6 weeks after implantation; other devices can be scanned immediately after implantation.
[b]See text.

for patients with an abnormal ECG who are intermediate-to-high risk as well as those with an abnormal or uncertain exercise ECG or those with obstructive CAD of uncertain significance noted on CT or invasive coronary angiography.

Imaging Suite and Environment

Similar to stress testing environments used with other modalities, staff familiar with CV stress testing, including nursing personnel and physicians, should be present during and immediately after testing. In regard to safety, medication carts and defibrillators should be secured outside of, but in close proximity to, the CMR scanning room, and if defibrillation during testing should be required, patients should be removed from the CMR room to deliver cardioversions. Specialized MRI-compatible equipment for assessing BP, HR, oxygen saturation, and respiratory rate should be present in the MRI scanning room. Because the magnetic field alters the appearance of ST segments and T waves on the ECG once the patient enters the scanner, ECG tracings are used to monitor patients' rhythm and not to detect ST-segment changes associated with inducible ischemia. Consequently, many stress CMR facilities utilize near real-time image review to appreciate inducible ischemia. Major events during CMR stress testing are usually associated with continued infusions of pharmacologic stress agents in the setting of concurrent myocardial ischemia. A high level of attention is suggested so that termination of the stress procedure can occur once evidence of ischemia is present.

Dobutamine Stress

For dobutamine stress testing, baseline images are acquired in three standard long-axis and short-axis views at rest. The dobutamine-atropine protocol is similar to that used for echocardiography, and the process of wall motion scoring is similar. Myocardial ischemia is identified when a deterioration of ≥1 in a segment score occurs during the stress test.

The sensitivity and specificity of dobutamine stress CMR for detecting greater than 50% coronary arterial stenoses with wall motion analyses alone ranges from 78% to 96%.[219] Dobutamine wall motion analyses alone may underappreciate the presence of inducible ischemia and functionally important CAD, especially in those with resting LV segmental wall motion abnormalities, prior MI and scar, LVH or concentric remodeling, and in people exhibiting a hyperdynamic response with a decline in systolic blood pressure during testing. Several investigators have advocated for the incorporation of first-pass contrast-enhanced stress perfusion at peak heart rate response during intravenous dobutamine, and the acquisition of LGE images in the recovery phase. The simultaneous identification of LV wall motion and myocardial perfusion abnormalities was associated with an increase in the hazard ratio for future CV events.[220] The results of myocardial perfusion stress testing were most helpful in those with resting LV wall motion abnormalities or underlying LVH. As with echo contrast perfusion imaging, many individuals with perfusion defects indicative of myocardial ischemia exhibit no inducible wall motion abnormalities—especially those with reduced LV end-diastolic volume index (LV preload) or concentric LV remodeling.

Although LGE techniques identify myocardial scar and thus infer viability, LV myocardial contractile reserve is still important for assessing myocardial segments that have the potential to recover systolic function after successful revascularization.[221] Improvement in regional wall motion or radial thickening with low-dose dobutamine stress CMR may be superior to the assessments of LGE, particularly in individuals who have intermediate levels of LGE.[221]

Vasodilator Stress

CMR perfusion imaging in general is accomplished after the administration of contrast agents that help to demonstrate discrepancies in LV myocardial perfusion between adjacent myocardial segments as well as absolute perfusion within a particular segment.[222] As with nuclear perfusion studies, intravenous adenosine, dipyridamole and regadenoson are the agents of choice. Similar to nuclear perfusion, CMR perfusion may be assessed qualitatively (visual inspection), semiquantitatively, or by fully quantitative methods. Importantly, both quantitative as well as qualitative perfusion assessments by CMR have demonstrated very high correlations with fractional flow reserve measures using cutoff values of <0.75.[223] Studies using qualitative assessments may require larger amounts of gadolinium contrast (in the 0.1 mmol/kg range), whereas quantitative analysis may be achieved with much lower doses (0.05 mmol/kg). Although quantitative and qualitative analyses have similar accuracy on a per-patient basis, quantitative analysis of perfusion reserve identifies the extent of myocardial ischemia more accurately.[224]

The stress perfusion protocol includes a stress perfusion assessment, followed by evaluation of LV wall motion, rest perfusion, and LGE identification of myocardial injury/fibrosis. Utilizing this methodology, the sensitivities and specificities for identifying flow-limiting coronary arterial stenoses when compared to contrast coronary angiography have both exceeded 90%.[225] Several comparative study results have suggested that CMR perfusion imaging could realistically be used as an alternative (with superior results) to SPECT imaging. This was most convincingly demonstrated in the recent single-center Clinical Evaluation of Magnetic Resonance Imaging in Coronary Heart Disease (CE-MARC) study that directly compared CMR stress perfusion and LGE with SPECT.[226] In this study, CMR was found to have higher sensitivity and similar specificity to SPECT, using angiography stenosis severity as a study endpoint. The high spatial resolution of this technology enables identification of subendocardial infarcts that can be distinguished from small areas of subendocardial hypoperfusion related to reduced myocardial microcirculatory blood flow (**Fig. 3–60**) resulting from flow-limiting epicardial coronary arterial stenoses. In addition, this particular technique is useful for identifying inducible ischemia in those individuals with preexisting concentric LVH or remodeling, reduced LVEF, or female gender (when body habitus can impede acquisition with other methodologies).

Prognosis

Beyond the identification of flow-limiting coronary stenoses or inducible ischemia, both CMR myocardial perfusion as well as

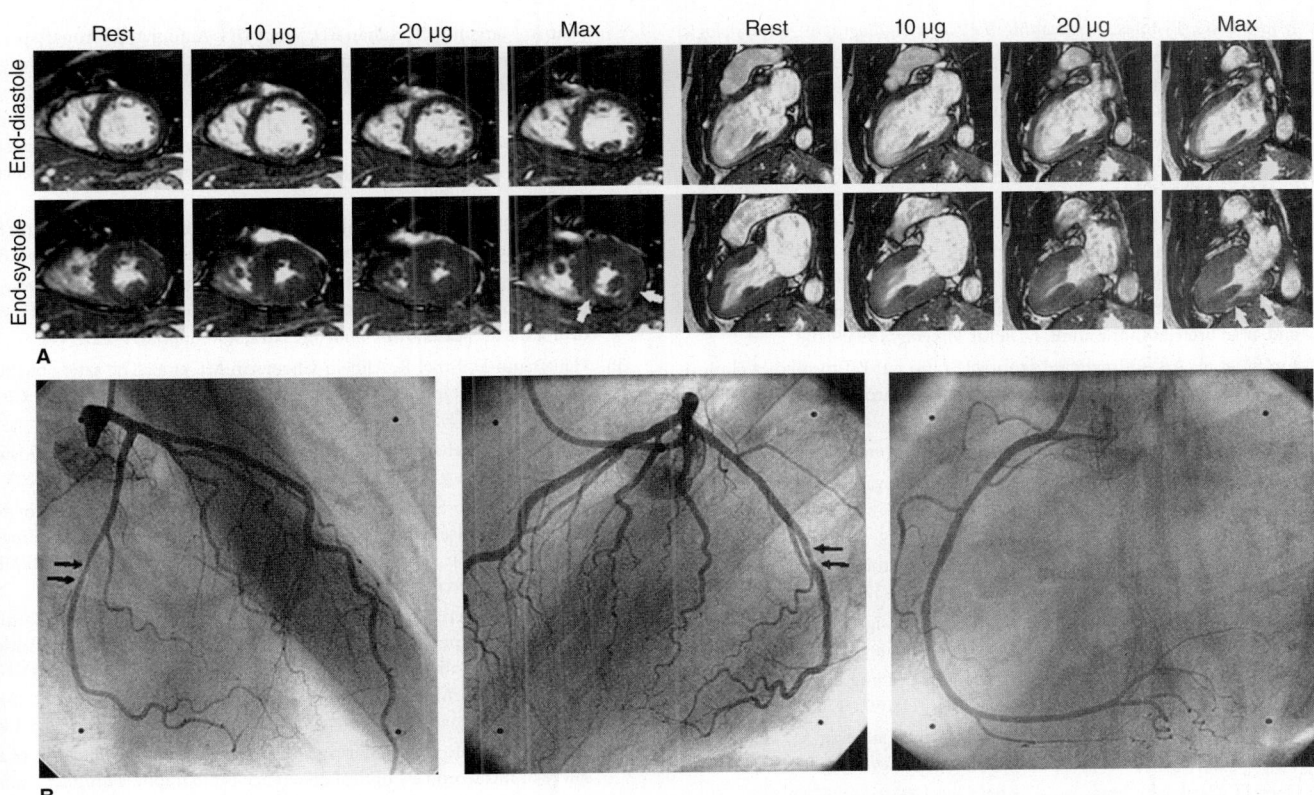

Figure 3–60. Positive dobutamine cardiac magnetic resonance (DCMR). DCMR cine images (short-axis and two-chamber view) of a patient with chest pain and suspected coronary artery disease (**A**). At rest and under increasing dobutamine, there is normal regional function. However, at maximum stress, an inferolateral wall motion abnormality is elicited. X-ray coronary angiography images demonstrating single-vessel left circumflex coronary artery disease (**B**, *black arrows*). Reproduced with permission from Paetsch I, Jahnke C, Fleck E, et al. Current clinical applications of stress wall motion analysis with cardiac magnetic resonance imaging. *Eur J Echocardiogr.* 2005 Oct;6(5):317-326.

CMR dobutamine wall motion stress are useful to determine cardiac prognosis.[227] A particular advantage for utilizing stress CMR for assessing myocardial perfusion or LV wall motion relates to the prognostic utility in women.[228] Stress CMR exhibits very high spatial resolution and fewer artifacts for imaging women relative to radioisotope techniques and, importantly, CMR stress does not involve ionizing radiation exposure to breast tissue.

Healthcare Expenditure

Participants managed through CMR-guided chest pain pathways experienced on average a reduction in the cost of the initial visit of $588 and reduction of $1641 over the ensuing year.[229] This decreased utilization and costs associated with managing the patients using CMR results was related to fewer return visits to the emergency department, cardiac catheterizations, and percutaneous coronary artery revascularization procedures, with no difference in the 30-day or 1-year occurrence of MI or cardiac death.

ACKNOWLEDGMENTS

We would like to thank Drs. Geoffrey D. Rubin, Morton J. Kern, Arnold H. Seto, Christos V. Bourantas, Yoshinobu Onuma, Renu Virmani, Jagat Narula, Patrick W. Serruys, Amir Ahmadi, Jonathon Leipsic, Daniel S. Berman, Rory Hachamovitch, Leslee J. Shaw, Sean W. Hayes, Piotr J. Slomka, Guido Germano, K. Lance Gould, Heinrich Schelbert, Anthony N. DeMaria, Daniel G. Blanchard, William A. Zoghbi, W. Gregory Hundley, Christopher M. Kramer, and Javier Sanz, who contributed the imaging chapters to the recent editions of this book.

REFERENCES

1. Chen, JT. The plain radiograph in the diagnosis of cardiovascular disease. *Radiolog Clin North Am.* 1983;4:609-621.

2. O'Rourke RA, Gilkeson RC. Cardiac radiography. In: Durkman D, Vander Belt. *Classic Teachings in Clinical Cardiology.* Washington, DC: Laennec Publishing; 1996:241-258.

3. Elliott E, Jue J, Amplatz K. A roentgen classification of cardiac malpositions. *Invest Radiol.* 1966:17-28.

4. Deleon D, Perloff P, Twigg T. Straight back syndrome. *Circulation.* 1965:193-203.

5. Aguilera AL, Volokhina YV, Fisher KL. Radiography of cardiac conduction devices: a comprehensive review. *Radiographics.* 2011;31: 1669-1682.

6. Mohamed I, et al: Building a bridge to save a failing ventricle: radiologic evaluation of short- and long-term cardiac assist devices. *Radiographics.* 2015;35:327-356.

7. Chen JT, Behar VS. Correlation of roentgen findings with hemodynamic data in pure mitral stenosis. *Am J Roentgenol.* 1968;102:280-292.

8. Milne ENC, Pistolesi M. *Reading the Chest Radiograph: A Physiologic Approach*. Mosby; 1993:164-241, 343-369.

9. Woolley K, Stark P. Pulmonary parenchymal manifestations of mitral valve disease. *Radiographics*. 1999;19:965-972.

10. Woodring JH. Pulmonary artery-bronchus ratios in patients with normal lungs, pulmonary vascular plethora, and congestive heart failure. *Radiology*. 1991;179:115-122.

11. Chen JT, Capp MP, Johnsrude IS, Goodrich JK, Lester RG. Roentgen appearance of pulmonary vascularity in the diagnosis of heart disease. *Am J Roentgenol Radium Ther Nucl Med*. 1971;112:559-570.

12. Boxt LM, Reagan K, Katz J. Normal plain film examination of the heart and great arteries in the adult. *J Thorac Imaging*. 1994;9:208.

13. Jun SJ, et al. An optimal cardiothoracic ratio cut-off to predict clinical outcomes in patients with acute myocardial infarction. *Int J Cardiovasc Imaging*. 2013;29:1889-1897.

14. Baron MG. The cardiac silhouette. *J Thorac Imaging*. 2000;15;230.

15. Koza Y. Mitral annular calcification and cardiovascular diseases: does correlation imply causation? *Angiology*. 2016;67(6):505-506.

16. Eleid MF, Foley TA, Said SM, Pislaru SV, Rihal CS. Severe mitral annular calcification multimodality imaging for therapeutic strategies and interventions. *JACC Cardiovasc Imaging*. 2016;9:1318-37.

17. Margolis JR, et al: The diagnostic and prognostic significance of coronary artery calcification. A report of 800 cases. *Radiology*. 1980;137:609-616.

18. Picano E, Scali MC, Ciampi Q, Lichtenstein D. Lung ultrasound for the cardiologist. *JACC Cardiovasc Imaging*. 2018;11:1692-1705.

19. Mondillo S, Giannotti G, Innelli P, Ballo PC, Galderisi M. Hand-held echocardiography: its use and usefulness. *Int J Cardiol*. 2006;111:1-5.

20. Chen JT. Cardiac fluoroscopy. *Cardiol Clin*. 1983;1:565-573.

21. Swischuck S. *Plain Film Interpretation in Congenital Heart Disease*. Baltimore, MD: Williams & Wilkins; 1979.

22. Kern MJ, Lim MJ, Sorajja P, eds. *The Cardiac Catheterization Handbook*. 6th ed., Philadelphia, PA: Elsevier; 2015.

23. Klein L, Sheldon MW, Brinker J, et al. The use of radiographic contrast media during PCI: a focused review: a position statement of the Society of Cardiovascular Angiography and Interventions. *Catheter Cardiovasc Interv*. 2009;74:728-746.

24. Levine GN, Bates ER, Blankenship JC, et al. American College of Cardiology Foundation; American Heart Association Task Force on Practice Guidelines; Society for Cardiovascular Angiography and Interventions. 2011 ACCF/AHA/SCAI Guideline for Percutaneous Coronary Intervention. A report of the American College of Cardiology Foundation/American Heart Association Task Force on Practice Guidelines and the Society for Cardiovascular Angiography and Interventions. *J Am Coll Cardiol*. 2011;58(24):e44–e122.

25. Gibson CM, Cannon CP, Daley WL, et al. TIMI frame count: a quantitative method of assessing coronary artery flow. *Circulation*. 1996;93:879-888.

26. Gould KL, Kirkeeide RL, Buchi M. Coronary flow reserve as a physiologic measure of stenosis severity. *J Am Coll Cardiol*. 1990;15:459-474.

27. Kern MJ, Lerman A, Bech JW, et al. Physiological assessment of coronary artery disease in the cardiac catheterization laboratory: a scientific statement from the American Heart Association Committee on Diagnostic and Interventional Cardiac Catheterization. *Circulation*. 2006;114:1321-1341.

28. Pijls NHJ, de Bruyne B, Peels K, et al. Measurement of fractional flow reserve to assess the functional severity of coronary-artery stenoses. *N Engl J Med*. 1996;334:1703-1708.

29. de Bruyne B, Bartunek J, Sys SU, et al. Simultaneous coronary pressure and flow velocity measurements in humans: feasibility, reproducibility and hemodynamic dependence of coronary flow velocity reserve, hyperemic flow versus pressure slope index and fractional flow reserve. *Circulation*. 1996;94:1842-1849.

30. Kern MJ, Bach RG, Mechem C, et al. Variations in normal coronary vasodilatory reserve stratified by artery, gender, heart transplantation and coronary artery disease. *J Am Coll Cardiol*. 1996;28:1154-1160.

31. Nair A, Margolis MP, Kuban BD, Vince DG. Automated coronary plaque characterisation with intravascular ultrasound backscatter: ex vivo validation. *EuroIntervention*. 2007;3(1):113-120.

32. Raber L, Taniwaki M, Zaugg S, et al. Effect of high-intensity statin therapy on atherosclerosis in non-infarct-related coronary arteries (IBIS-4): a serial intravascular ultrasonography study. *Eur Heart J*. 2015;36(8):490-500.

33. Schaar JA, De Korte CL, Mastik F, et al. Characterizing vulnerable plaque features with intravascular elastography. *Circulation*. 2003;108(21):2636-2641.

34. Brugaletta S, Garcia-Garcia HM, Serruys PW, et al. Relationship between palpography and virtual histology in patients with acute coronary syndromes. *JACC Cardiovasc Imaging*. 2012;5(3 Suppl):S19-S27.

35. Hausmann D, Erbel R, Alibelli-Chemarin MJ, et al. The safety of intracoronary ultrasound. A multicenter survey of 2207 examinations. *Circulation*. 1995;91(3):623-630.

36. Stone GW, Maehara A, Lansky AJ, et al. A prospective natural-history study of coronary atherosclerosis. *N Engl J Med*. 2011;364(3):226-235.

37. Stone PH, Saito S, Takahashi S, et al. Prediction of progression of coronary artery disease and clinical outcomes using vascular profiling of endothelial shear stress and arterial plaque characteristics: the PREDICTION Study. *Circulation*. 2012;126(2):172-181.

38. Mintz GS, Nissen SE, Anderson WD, et al. American College of Cardiology Clinical Expert Consensus Document on Standards for Acquisition, Measurement and Reporting of Intravascular Ultrasound Studies (IVUS). A report of the American College of Cardiology Task Force on Clinical Expert Consensus Documents. *J Am Coll Cardiol*. 2001;37(5):1478-1492.

39. Barlis P, Gonzalo N, Di Mario C, et al. A multicentre evaluation of the safety of intracoronary optical coherence tomography. *EuroIntervention*. 2009;5(1):90-95.

40. Tearney GJ, Regar E, Akasaka T, et al. Consensus standards for acquisition, measurement, and reporting of intravascular optical coherence tomography studies: a report from the International Working Group for Intravascular Optical Coherence Tomography Standardization and Validation. *J Am Coll Cardiol*. 2012;59(12):1058-1072.

41. Virmani R, Kolodgie FD, Burke AP, Farb A, Schwartz SM. Lessons from sudden coronary death: a comprehensive morphological classification scheme for atherosclerotic lesions. *Arterioscler Thromb Vasc Biol*. 2000;20(5):1262-1275.

42. Burke AP, Farb A, Malcom GT, Liang YH, Smialek J, Virmani R. Coronary risk factors and plaque morphology in men with coronary disease who died suddenly. *N Engl J Med*. 1997;336(18):1276-1282

43. Garcia-Garcia HM, Mintz GS, Lerman A, et al. Tissue characterisation using intravascular radiofrequency data analysis: recommendations for acquisition, analysis, interpretation and reporting. *EuroIntervention*. 2009;5(2):177-189.

44. Wang JC, Normand SL, Mauri L, Kuntz RE. Coronary artery spatial distribution of acute myocardial infarction occlusions. *Circulation*. 2004;110(3):278-284.

45. Virmani R, Burke AP, Kolodgie FD, Farb A. Vulnerable plaque: the pathology of unstable coronary lesions. *J Interv Cardiol*. 2002;15(6):439-446.

46. Fujii K, Hao H, Shibuya M, et al. Accuracy of OCT, grayscale IVUS, and their combination for the diagnosis of coronary TCFA: an ex vivo validation study. *JACC Cardiovasc Imaging*. 2015;8(4):451-460.

47. Manfrini O, Mont E, Leone O, et al. Sources of error and interpretation of plaque morphology by optical coherence tomography. *Am J Cardiol*. 2006;98(2):156-159.

48. Yabushita H, Bouma BE, Houser SL, et al. Characterization of human atherosclerosis by optical coherence tomography. *Circulation*. 2002;106(13):1640-1645.

49. Inaba S, Mintz GS, Farhat NZ, et al. Impact of positive and negative lesion site remodeling on clinical outcomes: insights from PROSPECT. *JACC Cardiovasc Imaging*. 2014;7(1):70-78.

50. Bourantas CV, Garcia-Garcia HM, Diletti R, Muramatsu T, Serruys PW. Early detection and invasive passivation of future culprit lesions:

a future potential or an unrealistic pursuit of chimeras? *Am Heart J.* 2013;165(6):869-881. e864.

51. Ambrose JA, Tannenbaum MA, Alexopoulos D, et al. Angiographic progression of coronary artery disease and the development of myocardial infarction. *J Am Coll Cardiol.* 1988;12(1):56-62.

52. Gopal A, Mao SS, Karlsberg D, et al. Radiation reduction with prospective ECG-triggering acquisition using 64-multidetector computed tomographic angiography. *Int J Cardiovasc Imaging.* 2009;25:405-416.

53. Carrascosa P, Leipsic JA, Capunay C, et al. Monochromatic image reconstruction by dual energy imaging allows half iodine load computed tomography coronary angiography. *Eur J Radiol.* 2015;84:1915-1920.

54. Orakzai SH, Orakzai RH, Nasir K, Budoff MJ. Assessment of cardiac function using multidetector row computed tomography. *J Comput Assist Tomogr.* 2006;30:555-563.

55. Budoff MJ, Gillespie R, Georgiou D, et al. Comparison of exercise electron beam computed tomography and sestamibi in the evaluation of coronary artery disease. *Am J Cardiol.* 1998;81:682-687.

56. Comparison of multiple modalities - ?Gerber/JLVO or JAMA-card

57. Henneman MM, Bax JJ, Schuijf JD, et al. Global and regional left ventricular function: a comparison between gated SPECT, 2D echocardiography and multi-slice computed tomography. *Eur J Nucl Med Mol Imaging.* 2006;33:1452-1460.

58. Pathan F, Hecht H, Narula J, Marwick TH. Roles of transesophageal echocardiography and cardiac computed tomography for evaluation of left atrial thrombus and associated pathology: a review and critical analysis. *JACC Cardiovasc Imaging.* 2018;11:616–627.

59. Sangiorgi G, Rumberger JA, Severson A, et al. Arterial calcification and not lumen stenosis is highly correlated with atherosclerotic plaque burden in humans: a histologic study of 723 coronary artery segments using nondecalcifying methodology. *J Am Coll Cardiol.* 1998;31:126-133.

60. Arnett DK, Blumenthal RS, Albert MA, et al. 2019 ACC/AHA guideline on the primary prevention of cardiovascular disease: a report of the American College of Cardiology/American Heart Association task force on clinical practice guidelines. *Circulation.* 2019;140(11):e596-e646.

61. Newman AB, Naydeck BL, Sutton-Tyrrell K, Feldman A, Edmundowicz D, Kuller LH. Coronary artery calcification in older adults to age 99: prevalence and risk factors. *Circulation.* 2001;104:2679-2684.

62. Shaw LJ, Raggi P, Schisterman E, Berman DS, Callister TQ. Prognostic value of cardiac risk factors and coronary artery calcium screening for all-cause mortality. *Radiology.* 2003;228:826-833.

63. Valenti V, ó Hartaigh B, Heo R, et al. A 15-year warranty period for asymptomatic individuals without coronary artery calcium: a prospective follow-up of 9,715 individuals. *J Am Coll Cardiol.* 2015;8:900-909.

64. Puri R, Nicholls SJ, Shao M, et al. Impact of statins on serial coronary calcification during atheroma progression and regression. *J Am Coll Cardiol.* 2015;65:1273-1282.

65. Boden WE, O'Rourke RA, Teo KK et al. Optimal medical therapy with or without PCI for stable coronary disease. *N Engl J Med.* 2007;356:1503-1516

66. Maron DJ, Hochman JS, Reynolds HR et al. Initial invasive or conservative strategy for stable coronary disease. *N Engl J Med.* 2020;382:1395-1407.

67. SCOT-HEART Investigators. Coronary CT angiography and 5-year risk of myocardial infarction. *N Engl J Med.* 2018;379:924-933.

68. Ghekiere O, Salgado R, Buls N, et al. Image quality in coronary CT angiography: challenges and technical solutions. *Br J Radiol.* 2017;90(1072):20160567.

69. Vanhoenacker PK, Decramer I, Bladt O, Sarno G, Bevernage C, Wijns W. Detection of non-ST-elevation myocardial infarction and unstable angina in the acute setting: meta-analysis of diagnostic performance of multi-detector computed tomographic angiography. *BMC Cardiovasc Disord.* 2007;7:39.

70. Athappan G, Habib M, Ponniah T, Jeyaseelan L. Multi-detector computerized tomography angiography for evaluation of acute chest pain—a meta analysis and systematic review of literature. *Int J Cardiol.* 2010;141:132-140.

71. Schlett CL, Hoffmann U, Geisler T, Nikolaou K, Bamberg F. Cardiac computed tomography for the evaluation of the acute chest pain syndrome: state of the art. *Radiol Clin North Am.* 2015;53:297-305.

72. Litt HI, Gatsonis C, Snyder B, et al. CT angiography for safe discharge of patients with possible acute coronary syndromes. *N Engl J Med.* 2012;366:1393-1403.

73. Goldstein JA, Chinnaiyan KM, Abidov A, et al. The CT-STAT (Coronary Computed Tomographic Angiography for Systematic Triage of Acute Chest Pain Patients to Treatment) trial. *J Am Coll Cardiol.* 2011;58:1414-1422.

74. Hoffmann U, Truong QA, Schoenfeld DA, et al. Coronary CT angiography versus standard evaluation in acute chest pain. *N Engl J Med.* 2012;367:299-308.

75. Mowatt G, Cook JA, Hillis GS, et al. 64-Slice computed tomography angiography in the diagnosis and assessment of coronary artery disease: systematic review and meta-analysis. *Heart.* 2008;94:1386-1393.

76. Schuijf JD, Bax JJ, Shaw LJ, et al. Meta-analysis of comparative diagnostic performance of magnetic resonance imaging and multislice computed tomography for noninvasive coronary angiography. *Am Heart J.* 2006;151:404-411.

77. Sun Z, Jiang W. Diagnostic value of multislice computed tomography angiography in coronary artery disease: a meta-analysis. *Eur J Radiol.* 2006;60:279-286.

78. Janne d' Othee B, Siebert U, Cury R, Jadvar H, Dunn EJ, Hoffmann U. A systematic review on diagnostic accuracy of CT-based detection of significant coronary artery disease. *Eur J Radiol.* 2008;65:449-461.

79. Budoff MJ, Dowe D, Jollis JG, et al. Diagnostic performance of 64-multidetector row coronary computed tomographic angiography for evaluation of coronary artery stenosis in individuals without known coronary artery disease: results from the prospective multicenter ACCURACY (Assessment by Coronary Computed Tomographic Angiography of Individuals Undergoing Invasive Coronary Angiography) trial. *J Am Coll Cardiol.* 2008;52:1724-1732.

80. Miller JM, Dewey M, Vavere AL, et al. Coronary CT angiography using 64 detector rows: methods and design of the multi-centre trial CORE-64. *Eur Radiol.* 2009;19:816-828.

81. Weustink AC, Nieman K, Pugliese F, et al. Diagnostic accuracy of computed tomography angiography in patients after bypass grafting: comparison with invasive coronary angiography. *JACC Cardiovasc Imaging.* 2009;2:816-824.

82. Sun Z, Davidson R, Lin CH. Multi-detector row CT angiography in the assessment of coronary in-stent restenosis: a systematic review. *Eur J Radiol.* 2009;69:489-495.

83. Budoff MJ, Ahmed V, Gul KM, Mao SS, Gopal A. Coronary anomalies by cardiac computed tomographic angiography. *Clin Cardiol.* 2006;29:489-493.

84. Neglia D, Rovai D, Caselli C, et al. Detection of significant coronary artery disease by noninvasive anatomical and functional imaging. *Circ Cardiovasc Imaging.* 2015;8.

85. SCOT-HEART Investigators. CT coronary angiography in patients with suspected angina due to coronary heart disease (SCOT-HEART): an open-label, parallel-group, multicentre trial. *Lancet.* 2015;385:2383-2391.

86. Douglas PS, Hoffmann U, Patel MR, et al. Outcomes of anatomical versus functional testing for coronary artery disease. *N Engl J Med.* 2015;372:1291-1300.

87. Kolodgie FD, Virmani R, Burke AP, et al. Pathologic assessment of the vulnerable human coronary plaque. *Heart.* 2004;90:1385-1391.

88. Motoyama S, Kondo T, Sarai M, et al. Multislice computed tomographic characteristics of coronary lesions in acute coronary syndromes. *J Am Coll Cardiol.* 2007;50:319-326.

89. Maurovich-Horvat P, Hoffmann U, Vorpahl M, Nakano M, Virmani R, Alkadhi H. The napkin-ring sign: CT signature of high-risk coronary plaques? *JACC Cardiovasc Imaging.* 2010;3:440-444.

90. Motoyama S, Ito H, Sarai M, et al. Plaque Characterization by coronary computed tomography angiography and the likelihood of acute coronary events in mid-term follow-up. *J Am Coll Cardiol.* 2015;66:337-346.

91. Maurovich-Horvat P, Hoffmann U, Vorpahl M, Nakano M, Virmani R, Alkhadi H. The napkin-ring sign: CT signature of high-risk coronary plaques? *JACC Cardiovasc Imaging*. 2010;3:440-444.

92. Pundziute G, Schuijf JD, Jukema JW, et al. Prognostic value of multislice computed tomography coronary angiography in patients with known or suspected coronary artery disease. *J Am Coll Cardiol*. 2007;49:62-70.

93. Bamberg F, Sommer WH, Hoffmann V, et al. Meta-analysis and systematic review of the long-term predictive value of assessment of coronary atherosclerosis by contrast-enhanced coronary computed tomography angiography. *J Am Coll Cardiol*. 2011;57:2426-2436.

94. Chow BJ, Small G, Yam Y, et al. Incremental prognostic value of cardiac computed tomography in coronary artery disease using CONFIRM: COroNary computed tomography angiography evaluation for clinical outcomes: an InteRnational Multicenter registry. *Circ Cardiovasc Imaging*. 2011;4:463-472.

95. Hadamitzky M, Achenbach S, Al-Mallah M, et al. Optimized prognostic score for coronary computed tomographic angiography: results from the CONFIRM registry (COronary CT Angiography EvaluatioN For Clinical Outcomes: An InteRnational Multicenter Registry). *J Am Coll Cardiol*. 2013;62:468-476.

96. Lin FY, Shaw LJ, Dunning AM, et al. Mortality risk in symptomatic patients with nonobstructive coronary artery disease: a prospective 2-center study of 2,583 patients undergoing 64-detector row coronary computed tomographic angiography. *J Am Coll Cardiol*. 2011;58:510-519.

97. Ahmadi A, Leipsic J, Blankstein R, et al. Do plaques rapidly progress prior to myocardial infarction? The interplay between plaque vulnerability and progression. *Circ Res*. 2015;117:99-104.

98. Dougoud S, Fuchs TA, Stehli J, et al. Prognostic value of coronary CT angiography on long-term follow-up of 6.9 years. *Int J Cardiovasc Imaging*. 2014;30:969-976.

99. Hulten E, Ahmadi A, Blankstein R. CT Assessment of Myocardial Perfusion and Fractional Flow Reserve. *Prog Cardiovasc Dis*. 2015;57:623-631.

100. Rochitte CE, George RT, Chen MY, et al. Computed tomography angiography and perfusion to assess coronary artery stenosis causing perfusion defects by single photon emission computed tomography: the CORE320 study. *Eur Heart J*. 2014;35:1120-1130.

101. Grunau GL, Min JK, Leipsic J. Modeling of fractional flow reserve based on coronary CT angiography. *Curr Cardiol Rep*. 2013;15:336.

102. Koo BK, Erglis A, Doh JH, et al. Diagnosis of ischemia-causing coronary stenoses by noninvasive fractional flow reserve computed from coronary computed tomographic angiograms. Results from the prospective multicenter DISCOVER-FLOW (Diagnosis of Ischemia-Causing Stenoses Obtained Via Noninvasive Fractional Flow Reserve) study. *J Am Coll Cardiol*. 2011;58:1989-1997.

103. Min JK, Leipsic J, Pencina MJ, et al. Diagnostic accuracy of fractional flow reserve from anatomic CT angiography. *JAMA*. 2012;308:1237-1245.

104. Norgaard BL, Leipsic J, Gaur S, et al. Diagnostic performance of noninvasive fractional flow reserve derived from coronary computed tomography angiography in suspected coronary artery disease: the NXT trial (Analysis of Coronary Blood Flow Using CT Angiography: Next Steps). *J Am Coll Cardiol*. 2014;63:1145-1155.

105. Douglas PS, Pontone G, Hlatky MA, et al. Clinical outcomes of FFRct guided diagnostic strategies vs usual care in patients with suspected coronary artery disease the prospective longitudinal trial of FFRct: outcome and resource impacts study. *Eur Heart J*. 2015:1-9.

106. Hlatky MA, De Bruyne B, Pontone G, et al. Quality of life and economic outcomes of assessing fractional flow reserve with computed tomography angiography: the PLATFORM study. *J Am Coll Cardiol*. 2015:1-9.

107. Achenbach S, Delgado V, Hausleiter J, Schoenhagen P, Min JK, Leipsic JA. SCCT expert consensus document on computed tomography imaging before transcatheter aortic valve implantation (TAVI)/transcatheter aortic valve replacement (TAVR). *J Cardiovasc Comput Tomogr*. 2012;6:366-380.

108. Khalique OK, Hahn RT, Gada H, et al. Quantity and location of aortic valve complex calcification predicts severity and location of paravalvular regurgitation and frequency of post-dilation after balloon-expandable transcatheter aortic valve replacement. *JACC Cardiovasc Interv*. 2014;7:885-894.

109. Oyama N, Oyama N, Komuro K, Nambu T, Manning WJ, Miyasaka K. Computed tomography and magnetic resonance imaging of the pericardium: anatomy and pathology. *Magn Reson Med Sci*. 2004;3:145-152.

110. Wang ZJ, Reddy GP, Gotway MB, Yeh BM, Hetts SW, Higgins CB. CT and MR imaging of pericardial disease. *Radiographics*. 2003;23 Spec No:S167-S180.

111. Kim EY, Choe YH, Sung K, Park SW, Kim JH, Ko YH. Multidetector CT and MR imaging of cardiac tumors. *Korean J Radiol*. 2009;10:164-175.

112. Litmanovich D, Bankier AA, Cantin L, Raptopoulos V, Boiselle PM. CT and MRI in diseases of the aorta. *AJR Am J Roentgenol*. 2009;193:928-940.

113. Taylor AJ, Cerqueira M, Hodgson JM, et al. ACCF/SCCT/ACR/AHA/ASE/ASNC/ NASCI/SCAI/SCMR 2010 appropriate use criteria for cardiac computed tomography. *J Am Coll Cardiol*. 2010;56:1864-1894.

114. Halpern EJ. Triple-rule-out CT angiography for evaluation of acute chest pain and possible acute coronary syndrome. *Radiology*. 2009;252:332-345.

115. Sharir T, et al. Multicenter trial of high-speed versus conventional single-photon emission computed tomography imaging: quantitative results of myocardial perfusion and left ventricular function. *J Am Coll Cardiol*. 2010;55(18):1965-1974.

116. Gould KL, Lipscomb K, Hamilton GW. Physiologic basis for assessing critical coronary stenosis. Instantaneous flow response and regional distribution during coronary hyperemia as measures of coronary flow reserve. *Am J Cardiol*. 1974;33(1):87-94.

117. Park HB, et al. Atherosclerotic plaque characteristics by CT angiography identify coronary lesions that cause ischemia: a direct comparison to fractional flow reserve. *JACC Cardiovasc Imaging*. 2015;8(1):1-10.

118. Ragosta M, et al. Comparison between angiography and fractional flow reserve versus single-photon emission computed tomographic myocardial perfusion imaging for determining lesion significance in patients with multivessel coronary disease. *Am J Cardiol*. 2007;99(7):896-902.

119. Tonino PA, et al. Angiographic versus functional severity of coronary artery stenoses in the FAME study fractional flow reserve versus angiography in multivessel evaluation. *J Am Coll Cardiol*. 2010;55(25):2816-2821

120. Beller GA, Smith TW. Radionuclide techniques in the assessment of myocardial ischemia and infarction. *Circulation*. 1976;53(3 Suppl):I123-I125.

121. Gewirtz H, et al. Transient defects of resting thallium scans in patients with coronary artery disease. *Circulation*. 1979;59(4):707-713.

122. Klocke FJ, et al. ACC/AHA/ASNC Guidelines for the clinical use of cardiac radionuclide imaging: A report of the American 1995 guidelines for the clinical use of radionuclide imaging. *Circulation*. 2003;108:1404-1418.

123. Henzlova MJ, et al. Stress protocols and tracers. *ASNC Imaging Guidelines for Nuclear Cardiology Procedures*; 2009.

124. Friedman J, et al. "Upward creep" of the heart: a frequent source of false-positive reversible defects during thallium-201 stress-redistribution SPECT. *J Nucl Med*. 1989;30(10):1718-1722.

125. Dilsizian V, et al. Enhanced detection of ischemic but viable myocardium by the reinjection of thallium after stress-redistribution imaging. *N Engl J Med*. 1990;323(3):141-146.

126. Kiat H, et al. Frequency of late reversibility in stress-redistribution thallium-201 SPECT using an early reinjection protocol. *Am Heart J*. 1991;122(3 Pt 1):613-619.

127. Des Prez RD, et al. Stress-only myocardial perfusion imaging. *J Nucl Cardiol*. 2009;16:329.

128. Duvall WL, et al. Reduced isotope dose and imaging time with a high-efficiency CZT SPECT camera. *J Nucl Cardiol*. 2011;18(5):847-857.

129. Einstein AJ, et al. Comparison of image quality, myocardial perfusion, and left ventricular function between standard imaging and single-injection ultra-low-dose imaging using a high-efficiency SPECT camera: the MILLISIEVERT study. *J Nucl Med*. 2014;55(9):1430-1437.

130. Heller GV, et al. American Society of Nuclear Cardiology and Society of Nuclear Medicine joint position statement: attenuation

correction of myocardial perfusion SPECT scintigraphy. *J Nucl Cardiol.* 2004;11(2):229-230.

131. Arsanjani R, et al. Comparison of fully automated computer analysis and visual scoring for detection of coronary artery disease from myocardial perfusion SPECT in a large population. *J Nucl Med.* 2013;54(2):221-228.

132. Cerqueira MD, et al. Recommendations for reducing radiation exposure in myocardial perfusion imaging. *J Nucl Cardiol.* 2010;17(4):709-718.

133. Cerqueira MD, et al. Standardized myocardial segmentation and nomenclature for tomographic imaging of the heart: a statement for healthcare professionals from the Cardiac Imaging Committee of the Council on Clinical Cardiology of the American Heart Association. *Circulation.* 2002;105(4):539-542.

134. Hachamovitch R, et al. Comparison of the short-term survival benefit associated with revascularization compared with medical therapy in patients with no prior coronary artery disease undergoing stress myocardial perfusion single photon emission computed tomography. *Circulation.* 2003;107(23):2900-2907.

135. Johnson NP, Gould KL. Integrating noninvasive absolute flow, coronary flow reserve, and ischemic thresholds into a comprehensive map of physiological severity. *JACC Cardiovasc Imaging.* 2012 Apr;5(4):430-440

136. Mazzanti M, et al. Identification of severe and extensive coronary artery disease by automatic measurement of transient ischemic dilation of the left ventricle in dual-isotope myocardial perfusion SPECT. *J Am Coll Cardiol.* 1996;27(7):1612-1620.

137. Leslie WD, et al. Prognostic value of lung sestamibi uptake in myocardial perfusion imaging of patients with known or suspected coronary artery disease. *J Am Coll Cardiol.* 2005;45(10):1676-1682.

138. Panza JA, Ellis AM, Al-Khalidi HR, et al. Myocardial viability and long-term outcomes in ischemic cardiomyopathy. *N Engl J Med.* 2019;381:739-748.

139. Diamond GA, Forrester JS. Analysis of probability as an aid in the clinical diagnosis of coronary-artery disease. *N Engl J Med.* 1979;300(24):1350-1358.

140. Cheng VY, et al. Performance of the traditional age, sex, and angina typicality-based approach for estimating pretest probability of angiographically significant coronary artery disease in patients undergoing coronary computed tomographic angiography: results from the multinational coronary CT angiography evaluation for clinical outcomes: an international multicenter registry (CONFIRM). *Circulation.* 2011;124(22):2423-2432, 1-8.

141. Anon. Single photon emission computed tomography for the diagnosis of coronary artery disease: an evidence-based analysis. *Ont Health Technol Assess Ser.* 2010;10(8):1-64.

142. Mc Ardle BA, et al. Does rubidium-82 PET have superior accuracy to SPECT perfusion imaging for the diagnosis of obstructive coronary disease? A systematic review and meta-analysis. *J Am Coll Cardiol.* 2012;60(18):1828-1837.

143. Takx RA, et al. Diagnostic accuracy of stress myocardial perfusion imaging compared to invasive coronary angiography with fractional flow reserve meta-analysis. *Circ Cardiovasc Imaging.* 2015;8(1).

144. Hachamovitch R, Di Carli MF. Methods and limitations of assessing new noninvasive tests: part I: Anatomy-based validation of noninvasive testing. *Circulation.* 2008;117(20):2684-2690.

145. Fihn SD, et al. 2012 ACCF/AHA/ACP/AATS/PCNA/SCAI/STS Guideline for the diagnosis and management of patients with stable ischemic heart disease. *J Am Coll Cardiol.* 2012;60(24):e44-e164.

146. Hachamovitch R, Di Carli MF. Methods and limitations of assessing new noninvasive tests: Part II: Outcomes-based validation and reliability assessment of noninvasive testing. *Circulation.* 2008;117(21):2793-2801.

147. Hachamovitch R, et al. Determinants of risk and its temporal variation in patients with normal stress myocardial perfusion scans: what is the warranty period of a normal scan? *J Am Coll Cardiol.* 2003;41:1329-1340.

148. Dorbala S, Di Carli MF. Cardiac PET perfusion: prognosis, risk stratification, and clinical management. *Semin Nucl Med.* 2014;44(5):344-357.

149. Murthy VL, et al. Improved cardiac risk assessment with noninvasive measures of coronary flow reserve. *Circulation.* 2011;124(20):2215-2224.

150. Shaw LJ, et al. The economic consequences of available diagnostic and prognostic strategies for the evaluation of stable angina patients: an observational assessment of the value of precatheterization ischemia. Economics of Noninvasive Diagnosis (END) Multicenter Study Group. *J Am Coll Cardiol.* 1999;33(3):661-669.

151. Hachamovitch R, et al. Patient management after noninvasive cardiac imaging results from SPARC (Study of myocardial perfusion and coronary anatomy imaging roles in coronary artery disease). *J Am Coll Cardiol.* 2012;59:462-474.

152. Douglas PS, et al. Outcomes of anatomical versus functional testing for coronary artery disease. *N Engl J Med.* 2015;372:1291-1300.

153. Wolk MJ, et al. ACCF/AHA/ASE/ASNC/HFSA/HRS/SCAI/SCCT/SCMR/STS 2013 multimodality appropriate use criteria for the detection and risk assessment of stable ischemic heart disease. *J Am Coll Cardiol.* 2014;63(4):380-406.

154. Hendel RC, et al. Multicenter assessment of the utilization of SPECT myocardial perfusion imaging using the ACCF appropriateness criteria. *J Am Coll Cardiol.* 2010;55:156-162.

155. Van Kriekinge SD, Berman DS, Germano G. Automatic quantification of left ventricular ejection fraction from gated blood pool SPECT. *J Nucl Cardiol.* 1999.6(5):498-506.

156. Rahimtoola SH. The hibernating myocardium. *Am Heart J.* 1989;117:211-221.

157. Vanoverschelde JL, Wijns W, Depre C, et al. Mechanisms of chronic regional postischemic dysfunction in humans. New insights from the study of noninfarcted collateral- dependent myocardium. *Circulation.* 1993;87:1513-1523.

158. Sun KT, Czernin J, Krivokapich J, et al. Effects of dobutamine stimulation on myocardial blood flow, glucose metabolism, and wall motion in normal and dysfunctional myocardium. *Circulation.* 1996;94:3146-3154.

159. Elsasser A, Schlepper M, Klovekorn WP, et al. Hibernating myocardium: an incomplete adaptation to ischemia. *Circulation.* 1997;96:2920-2931.

160. Tillisch J, Brunken R, Marshall R, et al. Reversibility of cardiac wall-motion abnormalities predicted by positron tomography. *N Engl J Med.* 1986; 314:884-888.

161. Schelbert HR, Beanlands R, Bengel F, et al. PET myocardial perfusion and glucose metabolism imaging: Part 2-Guidelines for interpretation and reporting. *J Nucl. Cardiol.* 2003;10:557-571.

162. Porenta G, Kuhle W, Czernin J, et al. Semiquantitative assessment of myocardial blood flow and viability using polar map displays of cardiac PET images. *J Nucl Med.* 1992;33:1628-1636.

163. Slart RH, Bax JJ, van Veldhuisen DJ et al. Prediction of functional recovery after revascularization in patients with coronary artery disease and left ventricular dysfunction by gated FDG-PET. *J Nucl Cardiol.* 2006;13:210-219.

164. Canty JM Jr, Fallavollita JA. Hibernating myocardium. *J Nucl Cardiol.* 2005;12:104-119.

165. Litjens G, Ciompi F, Wolterink JM, et al. State-of-the-Art Deep learning in cardiovascular image analysis. *JACC Cardiovasc Imaging.* 2019;12:1549-1565.

166. Dobrucki LW, Sinusas AJ. Cardiovascular molecular imaging. *Semin Nucl Med.* 2005;35(1):73-81.

167. Main ML, Asher CR, Rubin DN, et al: Comparison of tissue harmonic imaging with contrast (sonicated albumin echocardiography and Doppler myocardial imaging for enhancing endocardial border resolution. *Am J Cardiol.* 1999;83:218-222.

168. Kremkau FW, Taylor KJ. Artifacts in ultrasound imaging. *J Ultrasound Med.* 1986;5:227-237.

169. Yeh EL. Reverberations in echocardiograms. *J Clin Ultrasound.* 1977;5:84-86.

170. Weyman AE. Physical principles of ultrasound. In Weyman AE. *Principles and Practice of Echocardiography.* 2nd ed. Philadelphia, PA: Lea & Febiger; 1994:3-28.

171. Sahn DJ, Demaria A, Kisslo J, Weyman A. Recommendations regarding quantitation in M-mode echocardiography—results of a survey of echocardiographic measurements. *Circulation.* 1978;58:1072-1083.

172. Lang RM, Badano LP, Mor-Avi V, et al: Recommendations for cardiac chamber quantification by echocardiography in adults: an update from the American Society of Echocardiography and the European Association of Cardiovascular Imaging. *J Am Soc Echocardiogr.* 2015;28:1-39. e14.

173. Henry WL, DeMaria A, Gramiak R, et al: Report of the American Society of Echocardiography Committee on Nomenclature and Standards in Two-dimensional Echocardiography. *Circulation.* 1980;62:212-217.

174. Corsi C, Lang RM, Veronesi F, et al: Volumetric quantification of global and regional left ventricular function from real-time three-dimensional echocardiographic images. *Circulation.* 2005;112:1161-1170.

175. Salcedo EE, Quaife RA, Seres T, Carroll JD. A framework for systematic characterization of the mitral valve by real-time three-dimensional transesophageal echocardiography. *J Am Soc Echocardiogr.* 2009;22: 1087-1099.

176. Mulvagh SL, Rakowski H, Vannan MA, et al. American Society of Echocardiography Consensus Statement on the Clinical Applications of Ultrasonic Contrast Agents in Echocardiography. *J Am Soc Echocardiogr* 2008;21:1179-201.

177. Thavendiranathan P, Grant AD, Negishi T, Plana JC, Popović ZB, Marwick TH. Reproducibility of echocardiographic techniques for sequential assessment of left ventricular ejection fraction and volumes: application to patients undergoing cancer chemotherapy. *J Am Coll Cardiol.* 2013;61:77-84.

178. Hatle L, Angelsen B. *Doppler Ultrasound in Cardiology: Physical Principles and Clinical Applications.* Philadelphia, PA: Lea and Febiger; 1984.

179. Nagueh SF, Smiseth OA, Appleton CP, et al. Recommendations for the evaluation of left ventricular diastolic function by echocardiography. *J Am Soc Echocardiogr.* 2016;29:277-314

180. Chen C, Rodriguez L, Guerrero JL, Marshall S, et al: Noninvasive estimation of the instantaneous first derivative of left ventricular pressure using continuous-wave Doppler echocardiography. *Circulation.* 1991;83:2101-2110.

181. William GA, Labovitz AJ. Doppler estimation of cardiac output: principles and pitfalls. *Echocardiography.* 1987;4:355-374.

182. Currie PJ, Seward JB, Reeder GS, et al: Continuous-wave Doppler echocardiographic assessment of severity of calcific aortic stenosis: a simultaneous Doppler-catheter correlative study in 100 adult patients. *Circulation.* 1985;71:1162-1169.

183. Yock PG, Popp RL. Noninvasive estimation of right ventricular systolic pressure by Doppler ultrasound in patients with tricuspid regurgitation. *Circulation.* 1984;70:657-662.

184. Zoghbi WA, Enriquez-Sarano M, Foster E, et al: Recommendations for evaluation of the severity of native valvular regurgitation with two-dimensional and Doppler echocardiography. *J Am Soc Echocardiogr.* 2003;16:777-802.

185. Simpson IA, Sahn DJ, Valdescruz LM, Chung KJ, Sherman FS, Swensson RE. Color Doppler flow mapping in patients with coarctation of the aorta - new observations and improved evaluation with color flow diameter and proximal acceleration as predictors of severity. *Circulation.* 1988;77:736-744.

186. Schiller NB. Hand-held echocardiography: revolution or hassle? *J Am Coll Cardiol.* 2001;37:2023-2024.

187. Schneider M, Bartko P, Geller W, et al. A machine learning algorithm supports ultrasound-naïve novices in the acquisition of diagnostic echocardiography loops and provides accurate estimation of LVEF. *Int J Cardiovasc Imaging.* 2020. doi: 10.1007/s10554-020-02046-6.

188. Seward JB, Douglas PS, Erbel R, et al: Hand-carried cardiac ultrasound (HCU) device: recommendations regarding new technology. A report from the Echocardiography Task Force on New Technology of the Nomenclature and Standards Committee of the American Society of Echocardiography. *J Am Soc Echocardiogr.* 2002;15:369-373.

189. Sicari R, Nihoyannopoulos P, Evangelista A, et al, European Association of Echocardiography. Stress echocardiography expert consensus statement: European Association of Echocardiography (EAE) (a registered branch of the ESC). *Eur J Echocardiogr.* 2008;9:415-437.

190. Afridi I, Grayburn PA, Panza JA, Oh JK, Zoghbi WA, Marwick TH. Myocardial viability during dobutamine echocardiography predicts survival in patients with coronary artery disease and severe left ventricular systolic dysfunction. *J Am Coll Cardiol.* 1998;32:921-926.

191. Secknus MA, Marwick TH. Evolution of dobutamine echocardiography protocols and indications: safety and side effects in 3,011 studies over 5 years. *J Am Coll Cardiol.* 1997;29:1234-1240.

192. Marwick T, Willemart B, D'Hondt AM, et al: Selection of the optimal nonexercise stress for the evaluation of ischemic regional myocardial dysfunction and malperfusion. Comparison of dobutamine and adenosine using echocardiography and 99mTc-MIBI single photon emission computed tomography. *Circulation.* 1993;87:345-354.

193. Picano E, Pibarot P, Lancellotti P, Monin JL, Bonow RO. The emerging role of exercise testing and stress echocardiography in valvular heart disease. *J Am Coll Cardiol.* 2009;54:2251-2260.

194. Donofrio MT, Moon-Grady AJ, Hornberger LK, et al, American Heart Association Adults with Congenital Heart Disease Joint Committee of the Council on Cardiovascular Disease in the Young, Council on Clinical Cardiology Council on Cardiovascular Surgery and Anesthesia, Council on Cardiovascular and Stroke Nursing. Diagnosis and treatment of fetal cardiac disease: a scientific statement from the American Heart Association. *Circulation.* 2014;129:2183-2242.

195. Hundley WG, Bluemke DA, Finn JP, et al. ACCF/ACR/AHA/NASCI/ SCMR 2010 Expert Consensus Document on Cardiovascular Magnetic Resonance: a report of the American College of Cardiology Foundation Task Force on Expert Consensus Documents. *J Am Coll Cardiol.* 2010;55(23):2614-2662.

196. Kramer C, Barkhausen J, Flamm S, et al. Standardized cardiovascular magnetic resonance (CMR) protocols 2013 update. *J Cardiovasc Magn Reson.* 2013;15(1):91.

197. Hundley WG, Bluemke D, Bogaert JG, et al. Society for Cardiovascular Magnetic Resonance guidelines for reporting cardiovascular magnetic resonance examinations. *J Cardiovasc Magn Reson.* 2009;11:5.

198. Schulz-Menger J, Bluemke DA, Bremerich J, et al. Standardized image interpretation and post processing in cardiovascular magnetic resonance: Society for Cardiovascular Magnetic Resonance (SCMR) board of trustees task force on standardized post processing. *J Cardiovasc Magn Reson.* 2013;15:35.

199. Kramer CM. Role of cardiac MR imaging in cardiomyopathies. *J Nucl Med.* 2015;56(Suppl 4):39S-45S.

200. Grothues F, Smith GC, Moon JC, et al. Comparison of interstudy reproducibility of cardiovascular magnetic resonance with two-dimensional echocardiography in normal subjects and in patients with heart failure or left ventricular hypertrophy. *Am J Cardiol.* 2002;90(1):29-34.

201. Grothues F, Moon JC, Bellenger NG, Smith GS, Klein HU, Pennell DJ. Interstudy reproducibility of right ventricular volumes, function, and mass with cardiovascular magnetic resonance. *Am Heart J.* 2004;147(2):218-223.

202. Lorca MC, Haraldsson H, Ordovas KG. Ventricular mechanics: techniques and applications. *Magn Reson Imaging Clin North Am.* 2015;23(1): 7-13.

203. Kraitchman DL, Sampath S, Castillo E, et al. Quantitative ischemia detection during cardiac magnetic resonance stress testing by use of FastHARP. *Circulation.* 2003;107(15):2025-2030.

204. Ferreira VM, Piechnik SK, Robson MD, Neubauer S, Karamitsos TD. Myocardial tissue characterization by magnetic resonance imaging: novel applications of T1 and T2 mapping. *J Thorac Imaging.* 2014;29(3).

205. Salerno M, Kramer CM. Advances in parametric mapping with CMR imaging. *JACC Cardiovasc Imaging.* 2013;6(7):806-822.

206. Messroghli DR, Radjenovic A, Kozerke S, Higgins DM, Sivananthan MU, Ridgway JP. Modified Look-Locker inversion recovery (MOLLI) for high-resolution T1 mapping of the heart. *Magn Reson Med.* 2004;52(1):141-146.

207. Piechnik S, Ferreira V, Dall'Armellina E, et al. Shortened Modified Look-Locker inversion recovery (ShMOLLI) for clinical myocardial T1-mapping at 1.5 and 3 T within a 9 heartbeat breathhold. *J Cardiovasc Magn Reson.* 2010;12(1):69.

208. Moon J, Messroghli D, Kellman P, et al. Myocardial T1 mapping and extracellular volume quantification: a Society for Cardiovascular Magnetic Resonance (SCMR) and CMR Working Group of the European Society of Cardiology consensus statement. *J Cardiovasc Magn Reson.* 2013;15(1):92.

209. Pennell DJ, Udelson JE, Arai AE, et al. Cardiovascular function and treatment in beta-thalassemia major: a consensus statement from the American Heart Association. *Circulation.* 2013;128(3):281-308.

210. Lotz J, Meier C, Leppert A, Galanski M. Cardiovascular flow measurement with phase-contrast MR imaging: basic facts and implementation. *Radiographics.* 2002;22(3):651-671.

211. Stankovic Z, Allen BD, Garcia J, Jarvis KB, Markl M. 4D flow imaging with MRI. *Cardiovasc Diagn Ther.* 2014;4:173-192.

212. Coelho-Filho OR, Rickers C, Kwong RY, Jerosch-Herold M. MR myocardial perfusion imaging. *Radiology.* 2013;266(3):701-715.

213. Manka R, Wissmann L, Gebker R, et al. Multicenter evaluation of dynamic three-dimensional magnetic resonance myocardial perfusion imaging for the detection of coronary artery disease defined by fractional flow reserve. *Circ Cardiovasc Imaging.* 2015;8(5):pii. e003061.

214. Ambale-Venkatesh B, Lima JAC. Cardiac MRI: a central prognostic tool in myocardial fibrosis. *Nat Rev Cardiol.* 2015;12(1):18-29.

215. Simonetti OP, Kim RJ, Fieno DS, et al. An improved MR imaging technique for the visualization of myocardial infarction. *Radiology.* 2001;218(1):215-223.

216. Mahrholdt H, Goedecke C, Wagner A, et al. Cardiovascular magnetic resonance assessment of human myocarditis: a comparison to histology and molecular pathology. *Circulation.* 2004;109(10):1250-1258.

217. Expert Panel on MR Safety, Kanal E, Barkovich AJ, Bell C, et al. ACR guidance document on MR safe practices: 2013. *J Magn Reson Imaging.* 2013;37(3):501-530.

218. Levine GN, Gomes AS, Arai AE, et al. Safety of magnetic resonance imaging in patients with cardiovascular devices: an American Heart Association scientific statement from the Committee on Diagnostic and Interventional Cardiac Catheterization, Council on Clinical Cardiology, and the Council on Cardiovascular Radiology and Intervention: endorsed by the American College of Cardiology Foundation, the North American Society for Cardiac Imaging, and the Society for Cardiovascular Magnetic Resonance. *Circulation.* 2007;116(24):2878-2891.

219. American College of Radiology (ACR) Committee on Drugs and Contrast Media. *Manual on Contrast Media v10.1.* American College of Radiology; 2015.

220. Charoenpanichkit C, Hundley W. The 20 year evolution of dobutamine stress cardiovascular magnetic resonance. *J Cardiovasc Magn Reson.* 2010;12(1):59.

221. Gebker R, Jahnke C, Manka R, et al. Additional value of myocardial perfusion imaging during dobutamine stress magnetic resonance for the assessment of coronary artery disease. *Circ Cardiovasc Imaging.* 2008;1(2):122-130.

222. Wellnhofer E. Magnetic resonance low-dose dobutamine test is superior to scar quantification for the prediction of functional recovery. *Circulation.* 2004;109(18):2172-2174.

223. Klocke FJ, Simonetti OP, Judd RM, et al. Limits of detection of regional differences in vasodilated flow in viable myocardium by first-pass magnetic resonance perfusion imaging. *Circulation.* 2001;104(20):2412-2416.

224. Watkins S, McGeoch R, Lyne J, et al. Validation of magnetic resonance myocardial perfusion imaging with fractional flow reserve for the detection of significant coronary heart disease. *Circulation.* 2009;120(22):2207-2213.

225. Hamon M, Fau G, Née G, Ehtisham J, Morello R, Hamon M. Meta-analysis of the diagnostic performance of stress perfusion cardiovascular magnetic resonance for detection of coronary artery disease. *J Cardiovasc Magn Reson.* 2010;12(1):29.

226. de Jong MC, Genders TSS, van Geuns R-J, Moelker A, Hunink MGM. Diagnostic performance of stress myocardial perfusion imaging for coronary artery disease: a systematic review and meta-analysis. *Eur Radiol.* 2012;22(9):1881-1895.

227. Greenwood JP, Maredia N, Younger JF, et al. Cardiovascular magnetic resonance and single-photon emission computed tomography for diagnosis of coronary heart disease (CE-MARC): a prospective trial. *Lancet.* 2012;379(9814):453-460.

228. Gargiulo P, Dellegrottaglie S, Bruzzese D, et al. The prognostic value of normal stress cardiac magnetic resonance in patients with known or suspected coronary artery disease: a meta-analysis. *Circ Cardiovasc Imaging.* 2013;6(4):574-582.

229. Wallace EL, Morgan TM, Walsh TF, et al. Dobutamine cardiac magnetic resonance results predict cardiac prognosis in women with known or suspected ischemic heart disease. *JACC Cardiovasc Imaging.* 2009;2(3):299-307.

230. Miller CD, Case LD, Little WC, et al. Stress CMR reduces revascularization, hospital readmission, and recurrent cardiac testing in intermediate-risk patients with acute chest pain. *JACC Cardiovasc Imaging.* 2013;6(7):785-794.

4

Genomics and Epigenomics of Heart Diseases

June-Wha Rhee and Joseph C. Wu

CHAPTER OUTLINE

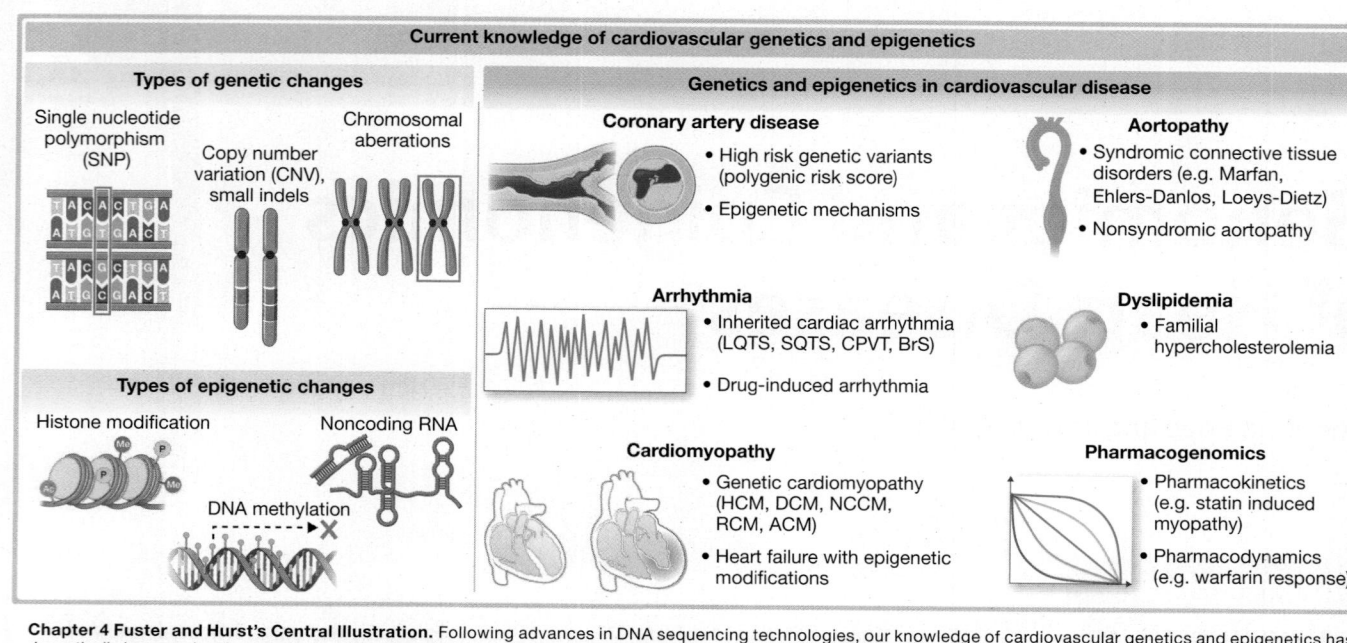

Chapter 4 Fuster and Hurst's Central Illustration. Following advances in DNA sequencing technologies, our knowledge of cardiovascular genetics and epigenetics has dramatically increased and we now appreciate integral roles of noncoding genes, polygenic mechanisms, and epigenetics in mediating heart diseases. Genetic variation can also influence drug response by altering pharmacokinetics (pertaining to drug bioavailability and metabolism) or pharmacodynamics (pertaining to either on- or off-target drug actions). ACM, arrhythmogenic cardiomyopathy; BrS, Brugada syndrome; CPVT, catecholaminergic polymorphic ventricular tachycardia; DCM, dilated cardiomyopathy; HCM, hypertrophic cardiomyopathy; LQTS, long QT syndrome; NCCM, noncompaction cardiomyopathy; RCM, restrictive cardiomyopathy; SQTS, short QT syndrome.

CHAPTER SUMMARY

This chapter discusses the genetics and epigenetics of cardiovascular disease (CVD) (see Fuster and Hurst's Central Illustration). Following the advances in deoxyribonucleic acid (DNA) sequencing technologies, our knowledge of cardiovascular genetics and epigenetics has dramatically increased. While we previously understood the genetics of heart disease mainly in the context of syndromic diseases, caused by chromosomal abnormalities, and Mendelian diseases, caused by single-gene defects, we now appreciate the integral roles of noncoding genes, polygenic mechanisms, and epigenetics in mediating heart disease. Herein, we first review conventional genetic mechanisms of heart disease, including chromosomal anomaly-related congenital heart defects and monogenic diseases such as genetic cardiomyopathy, inherited cardiac arrhythmia, and familial hypercholesterolemia. We then discuss the evolving evidence of polygenic mechanisms in heart disease, presenting an example of coronary artery disease and how polygenic risk score is used in its risk stratification. Next, we review epigenetic regulation of gene expression and discuss its role in CVD pathogenesis. Finally, we conclude by discussing a number of emerging technologies, including genome editing technologies, human-induced pluripotent stem cells, and advanced sequencing and bioinformatics technologies, which can further advance our knowledge of genetics and epigenetics of heart disease.

BRIEF CASE DESCRIPTION

A 57-year-old previously healthy man comes to the clinic for newly diagnosed nonischemic cardiomyopathy. He had been found to have severely reduced left ventricular systolic function and began guideline-directed medical therapy. He has no identifiable conventional cardiovascular risk factors. His family history is remarkable for multiple sudden cardiac deaths, premature atrial fibrillation, and heart failure, prompting a clinical genetic screening. His genetic panel identifies a pathogenic variant in Lamin A/C. How does this genetic information affect the management of his condition now and in the future?

INTRODUCTION

Over the past decade, our knowledge of genetics has exponentially increased as a result of advances in DNA sequencing technologies.[1] Whereas human genome sequencing initially took more than a decade and billions of dollars to accomplish, the whole human genome can now be sequenced in hours at a remarkably low cost. The advent of next-generation sequencing technology has accelerated genetic research in an unprecedented way,[2] allowing the genetic architecture of heart diseases to be gradually unveiled. Previously, the genetics of heart diseases was primarily understood in the context of syndromic diseases from large structural anomalies (eg, trisomy 21) or Mendelian diseases from single nucleotide variations in protein-coding genes. Accumulating research highlights critical roles of noncoding genes in regulating gene expression[3] and thereby contributing to disease mechanisms. Additionally, epigenetics, the reversible genetic modifications that regulate gene expression without altering the DNA sequence, has been implicated in various disease processes.[4] Here, we first review the basics and select examples of genetic mechanisms of heart diseases. We then discuss the role of epigenetics in the heart and heart diseases. Finally, we introduce emerging technologies, including genome editing tools and human-induced pluripotent stem cells, and describe how they can further our knowledge and offer therapeutic opportunities.

THE HUMAN GENOME

The human genome consists of approximately 3.3 billion DNA base pairs that are tightly packaged into 46 chromosomes. There are about 20,000 to 25,000 protein-coding genes comprising approximately 1.5% of the human genome (**Fig. 4–1**). The rest of the human genome contains introns, regulatory DNA sequences, DNA repeats, transposable elements (mobile genetic elements), and others. The exact amount and precise roles of the noncoding DNA are yet to be understood but may represent genomic diversity.[5] Available data thus far suggest that significant genetic variations exist among individuals, which can be classified into four major types (**Fig. 4–2A**): (1) large structural variants (eg, chromosomal aberrations such as trisomies, monosomies, and translocations), (2) copy number variants (duplications or deletions of intermediate-scale genetic contents at the cytogenetic-level resolution, typically on the

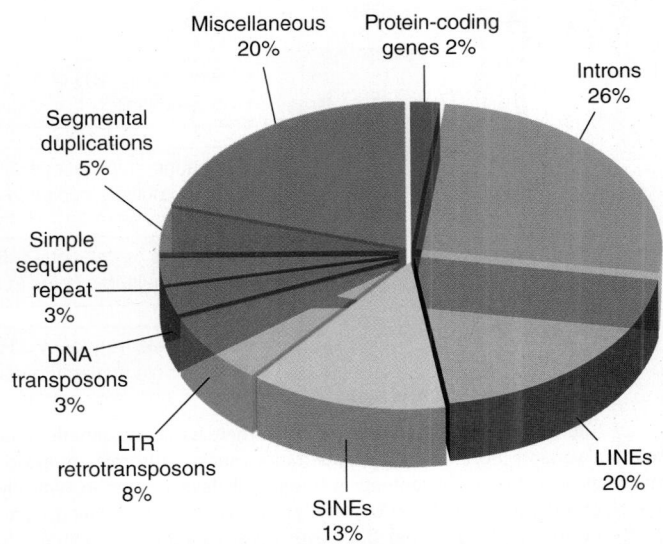

Figure 4–1. The human genome composition. The human genome consists of approximately 3.3 billion DNA base pairs tightly packaged into 46 chromosomes. There are about 20,000 to 25,000 protein-coding genes (exons, 1.5% of the human genome) interspersed by introns (26%). The vast majority of the rest are transposable elements (eg, DNA transposons, long terminal repeat [LTR] retrotransposons, long interspersed nuclear elements [LINEs], short interspersed nuclear elements [SINEs]).

order of kilobases to megabases), (3) small indels (insertions or deletions of nucleotides in genomic DNA, typically less than 50 bases in length), and (4) single nucleotide variants (variation of a single nucleotide base at a specific position in the genome).[2] Large structural variants are rare and typically present as syndromic diseases often associated with multiorgan defects. Other genetic variants can be found rather commonly without significant or definitive disease associations. For example, an average person's genome contains approximately 150 copy number variants, approximately 500,000 indels, and approximately 4 million single nucleotide polymorphisms (**Fig. 4–2B**). Therefore, understanding how these variants relate to clinical phenotypes and identifying disease-causing or disease-associated variants have been active areas of research.

DNA Sequencing Technology

The discovery of the aforementioned marked genetic diversity has been possible through the invention of next-generation sequencing (NGS) technology (**Fig. 4–3A**). Prior to NGS, DNA was primarily sequenced using the Sanger method, which uses a short primer binding to the genomic region of interest and forming DNA replication strands of various lengths that are terminated with fluorescent dideoxynucleotides.[6] Because this method can only sequence a single DNA fragment up to 100 base pairs at a time, it is rather laborious and time consuming. By contrast, NGS employs massively parallel, high-throughput sequencing of DNA, allowing billions of small DNA reads known as *short reads* to be simultaneously sequenced, aligned, and mapped against a reference genome.[1] NGS has revolutionized sequencing technology, dramatically speeding up the

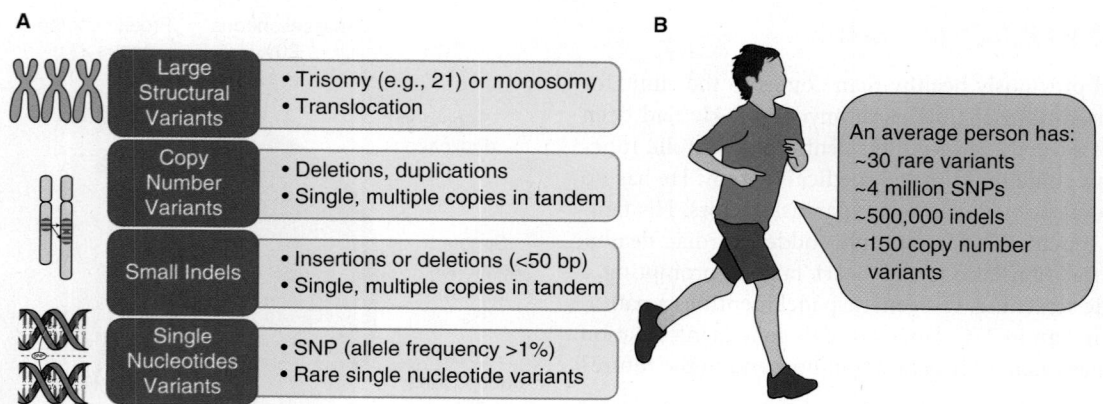

Figure 4–2. Variation of the human genome. There is marked genetic variation in the human genome. **A.** Four major types of the variation include (1) large structural variants (eg, chromosomal aberrations such as trisomies, monosomies, and translocations), (2) copy number variants (duplications or deletions of intermediate-scale genetic contents at cytogenetic-level resolution, typically in the order of kilobases to megabases), (3) small indels (insertions or deletions of nucleotides into genomic DNA, typically <50 base pairs [bp] in length), and finally (4) single nucleotide variants (variation of a single nucleotide base at a specific position in the genome). **B.** On average, a single person's genome contains approximately 150 copy number variants, approximately 500,000 indels, and approximately 4 million single nucleotide polymorphisms (SNPs).

sequencing process while reducing its cost.[7] It can now be used in clinics to sequence a single gene or a panel of genes, a whole exome, or a whole genome from a patient (**Fig. 4–3B**).

GENETIC MECHANISMS OF HEART DISEASE

Heart diseases or defects can arise from the following: (1) large structural variants involving a whole chromosome or a part of a chromosome (eg, trisomy 21–related congenital heart defects); (2) a single-gene defect, or monogenic disorder, which typically follows a Mendelian inheritance pattern (eg, hypertrophic cardiomyopathy); (3) a polygenic condition from the combined action of more than one gene (eg, hypertension or coronary artery disease); and (4) genetic disorders involving mitochondrial DNA. These genetic mechanisms of heart disease, along with examples, are discussed in the following sections.

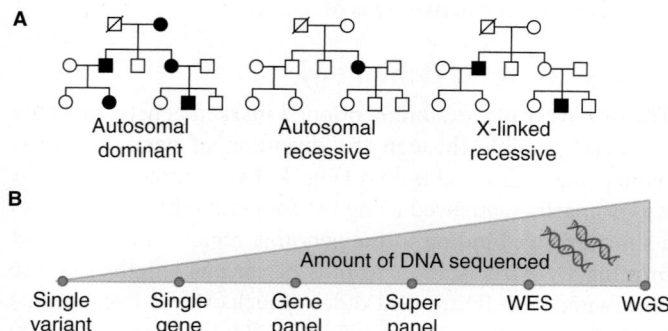

Figure 4–3. Genetic sequencing in clinical practice. A. Next-generation sequencing employs massively parallel, high-throughput sequencing of DNA, allowing billions of DNA fragments, called *short reads*, to be simultaneously sequenced, aligned, and mapped against a reference genome to create a final assembled sequence. **B.** Depending on clinical questions, DNA can be sequenced anywhere from a single variant to a whole genome. WES, whole exome sequencing; WGS, whole genome sequencing.

Chromosomal Disorders and Congenital Heart Defects

Large structural variations, or chromosomal disorders, occur when there is a gain or loss of a whole or a part of a chromosome. They often manifest clinically as syndromes with multiorgan involvement and distinct phenotypes. Several chromosomal abnormalities are associated with congenital heart defects (CHDs), including the following:

1. Trisomy 21 (T21) is the most common chromosomal defect, afflicting 1 in 500 live births worldwide. Up to 50% of T21 patients suffer from CHD, making it the leading genetic cause of CHD.[8] The most common cardiac anomalies associated with T21 include atrial septal defects, ventricular septal defects, and atrioventricular septal defects.

2. Turner syndrome is caused by a missing or partially missing X chromosome in female patients and often manifests with a bicuspid aortic valve, aortic coarctation, and aortic aneurysm.[9]

3. DiGeorge syndrome, also known as 22q11 deletion syndrome, is caused by the deletion of a small segment of chromosome 22. Up to 75% of patients with DiGeorge syndrome suffer from various forms of CHD, including tetralogy of Fallot, pulmonary atresia with ventricular septal defect, truncus arteriosus, and interrupted aortic arch.

Presently, CHDs caused by chromosomal disorders are thought to arise from errors during heart development, but the exact mechanisms of how these chromosomal aberrations lead to such a high rate of CHD remain incompletely understood.[10,11]

Monogenic Cardiovascular Diseases

Monogenic disease is caused by a single pathogenic variant in a single gene. Monogenic cardiovascular diseases typically follow a Mendelian inheritance pattern except in cases of de novo somatic mutations or mosaicism. These diseases include, but are not limited to, genetic cardiomyopathy (eg, hypertrophic or dilated cardiomyopathy),[11] familial hypercholesterolemia,[12] long QT syndrome,[13] and aortopathy.[14] Based on their inheritance pattern, these diseases can be further categorized into autosomal dominant (AD), autosomal recessive (AR), or X-linked (XL) diseases (**Fig. 4–4A**). The majority of genetic cardiovascular diseases are inherited as AD in which one mutated allele is sufficient for disease manifestation.[15] However, significant variabilities in disease expressivity and penetrance exist, especially in cases of familial cardiomyopathy, making it challenging to diagnose. AR inheritance, in which disease manifestation requires mutations in both alleles, is far less common than AD inheritance in cardiovascular disease. Examples of AR heart diseases include AR lysosomal storage diseases with cardiac involvement[16]; genetic cardiomyopathies caused by rare variants in *TNNC*, *PLN*, *NPPA*, or *MYL*[17]; and sick sinus syndrome caused by mutations in *SCN5A*.[18] Increased rates of AR diseases may be seen in cases of consanguinity or in the context of geographically isolated populations. Finally, XL diseases are caused by variants in the X chromosome, with examples such as Fabry-related hypertrophic cardiomyopathy (HCM) caused by mutations in *GLA* and dilated cardiomyopathies (DCMs) due to defects in dystrophin.[19] Clinical genetic testing, which typically sequences a single gene or panels of genes commonly linked to a particular disease, has a variable yield in identifying causative variants, ranging from approximately 80% to 85% in long QT syndrome to as low as 20% to 40% in DCM. Increasingly, with advances in sequencing technologies, whole exome sequencing and whole genome sequencing are being used in cases where causative variants are not identified.[7,20]

Determining Pathogenicity

Based on the level of evidence for the variant pathogenicity, variants can be categorized from benign to pathogenic (**Fig. 4–4B**).[21]

Traditionally, variant analysis is conducted among well-phenotyped family members to see whether particular variants would segregate among affected family members to determine pathogenicity. Applying genotyping or whole genome sequencing tools, genome-wide linkage analysis in families can also be employed to identify novel variants when a disease follows Mendelian inheritance. Additionally, to further investigate variant pathogenicity, variants should be comprehensively evaluated by comparing to previous reports of disease association, assessing rarity in the healthy population, and correlating with any available biological/experimental data and/or in silico computational prediction models.

Due to the subjectivity in annotating variant pathogenicity, there can be some level of disagreement in classifying variants among expert reviewers, national databases (eg, ClinVar), and various commercial clinical sequencing providers. Additionally, thus far, many variants have been classified as variants of uncertain significance (VUS), making it challenging to use genetic information in predictive testing and diagnosis.[22] Variants are more likely to be pathogenic if the variants are rare (<0.05%) or change protein structure or function. The variants are called *synonymous* if they do not alter the amino acid sequence of proteins and *nonsynonymous* if the variants are protein altering (**Fig. 4–4C**). Identifying pathogenic variants has many clinical implications, including but not limited to (1) establishing a diagnosis, (2) prognostication, (3) guiding management, (4) screening and identifying family members at risk, and (5) assisting in reproductive decision-making.[23]

Inherited Cardiomyopathy

As clinical genetic testing becomes widely available at a lower cost, more cardiomyopathies are being linked to genetic causes.[24] Genetic cardiomyopathies are typically caused by a

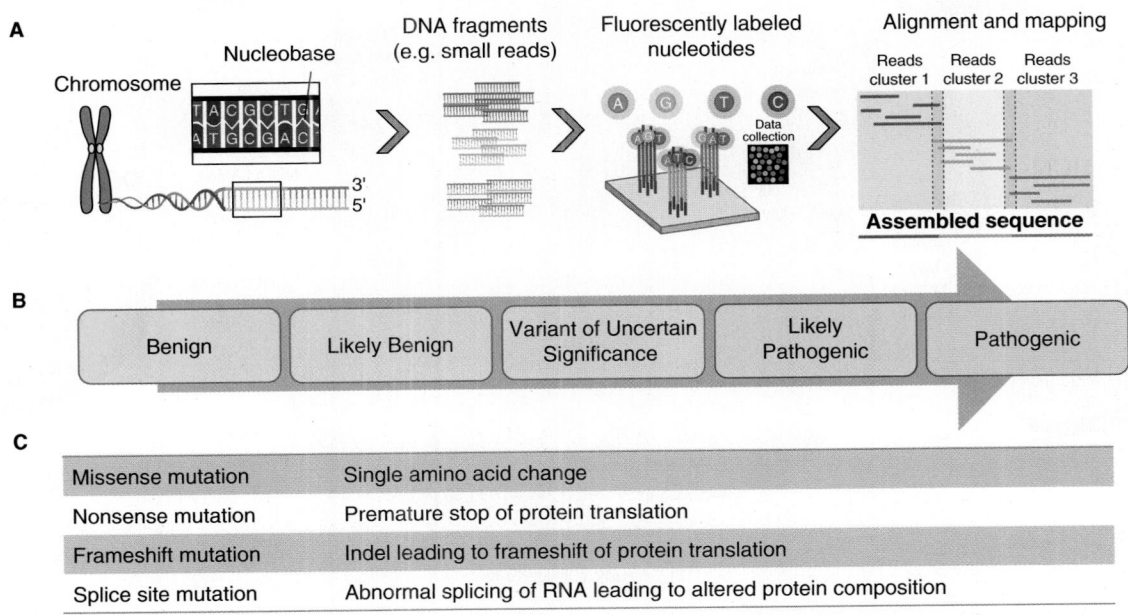

Figure 4–4. Monogenic disease: inheritance pattern and variant classification. A. Monogenic diseases follow the Mendelian inheritance pattern, which includes autosomal dominant, autosomal recessive, and X-linked. **B.** Based on the level of evidence for the variant pathogenicity, genetic variants can be categorized to be benign, likely benign, variant of uncertain significance (VUS), likely pathogenic, and pathogenic. **C.** Variants are more likely to be pathogenic if they are protein altering, termed *nonsynonymous*. Nonsynonymous variants include missense, nonsense, frameshift, and splice site mutations.

single-gene disorder (monogenic) and inherited in a pattern of AD or incomplete dominant depending on the disease penetrance and/or expressivity. Based on their clinical features and morphologic phenotypes, genetic cardiomyopathies can be categorized into several major types, including HCM, DCM, arrhythmogenic cardiomyopathy (ARM), restrictive cardiomyopathy (RCM), and noncompaction cardiomyopathy (NCCM). HCM is the most common genetic cardiomyopathy, affecting approximately 1 in 500 people worldwide.[25,26] It is the leading cause of sudden cardiac death in the young. Familial DCM is characterized by ventricular chamber dilatation and systolic dysfunction and is a leading indication for heart transplantation.[27,28] Its reported prevalence is 1 in 2500, although the true prevalence is thought to be higher. ACM,[29] RCM,[30] and NCCM[31] are rarer, with the prevalence for each estimated to be lower than 1 in 2000.

Significant progress has been made in defining genetic causes of cardiomyopathies. Thousands of mutations, or pathogenic variants, spanning many genes have been identified as causing genetic cardiomyopathies. These genes are of varying biological processes beyond the sarcomere, a basic contractile unit responsible for muscle contraction, suggesting diverse mechanisms underlying cardiomyopathies. Clinical expression of these variants can be widely heterogeneous; the same pathogenic variant can cause disease in some people but not in

others (incomplete/reduced penetrance) or manifest with different disease severities or phenotypes (variable expressivity).[32] For example, a pathogenic variant in *TNNT2* may be associated with cases of severe heart failure necessitating heart transplantation, mild cardiac dysfunction, or no apparent disease. This marked clinical heterogeneity may be due in part to the inherent wide spectrum of disease phenotypes (in fact, the normal hearts themselves have a broad range of sizes, functions, and anatomic features), the effects of modifier genes or genetic backgrounds, or the influence of nongenetic or environmental factors, among other causes. These complexities pose significant challenges for clinicians in determining how to translate genetic information in the clinic.

Further dissecting the genetic architecture of inherited cardiomyopathies, the genetics of cardiomyopathies is marked by significant genetic heterogeneity (mutations in many genes leading to the same disease phenotype) and allelic variation (same mutation in genetic loci causing different disease severity or phenotypes). For example, mutations in *MYBPC*, *TPM1*, and *MYH7* can all result in HCM (genetic heterogeneity). Additionally, the same mutation in *MYH7* can cause HCM, DCM, or RCM (allelic variation). Available data suggest that many genes are implicated in each genetic cardiomyopathy with frequent overlap with each other (**Fig. 4–5**). More information on clinical phenotypes and diagnostic and

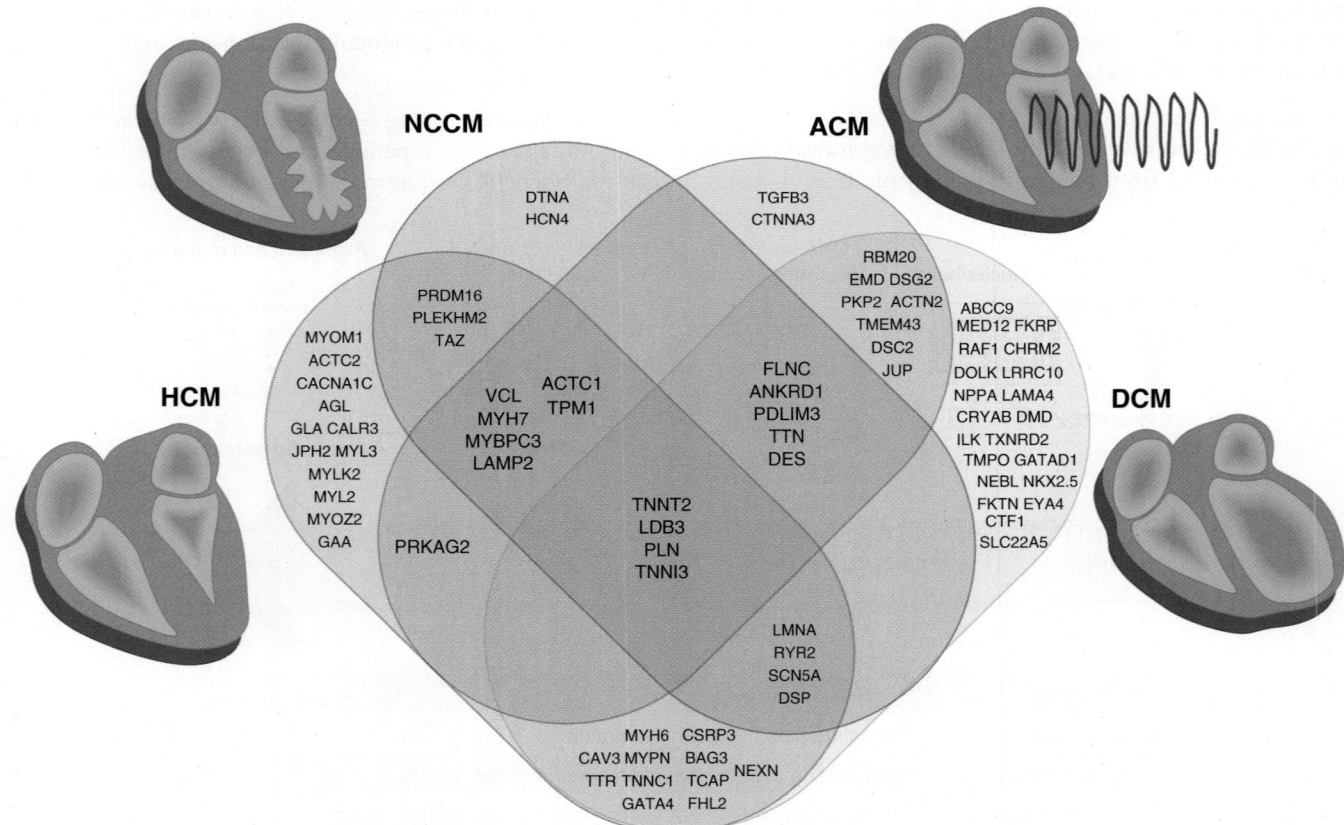

Figure 4–5. Common genes implicated in genetic cardiomyopathies. Based on their clinical features and morphologic phenotypes, genetic cardiomyopathies can be categorized into several major types including hypertrophic cardiomyopathy (HCM), dilated cardiomyopathy (DCM), arrhythmogenic cardiomyopathy (ARM), restrictive cardiomyopathy (RCM), and noncompaction cardiomyopathy (NCCM). Available data suggest that many genes are implicated in each genetic cardiomyopathy with frequent overlap with each other (genes on RCM not shown).

Inherited Cardiac Arrhythmia

Inherited cardiac arrhythmia is relatively rare and can cause life-threatening arrhythmia.[33] Given its association with defects in genes encoding or regulating activities of cardiac ion channels, the condition is often referred to as cardiac channelopathy. The main types include long QT syndrome (LQTS), short QT syndrome (SQTS), catecholaminergic polymorphic ventricular tachycardia (CPVT), Brugada syndrome (BrS), and hereditary atrial fibrillation. The diagnosis is based on clinical presentations, electrocardiography (ECG) characteristics at rest and/or during exercise, findings from electrophysiologic studies, and genetic analyses. LQTS is characterized by ECG findings of prolonged QT and T-wave abnormalities and is associated with potentially fatal tachyarrhythmias, namely the ventricular tachycardia torsade de pointes. It is relatively rare (1 in 2500 people) and inherited primarily as AD. There are three different types based on ECG characteristics and clinical manifestations. The genetics of LQTS is better defined than that of genetic cardiomyopathies, with approximately 80% genetic test yield among patients with definitive clinical diagnosis of LQTS identifying disease-causing mutations.[13] Most of these mutations are single nucleotide variants or small indels, and 90% of them lie in three LQTS susceptibility genes, namely *KCNQ1* (30%–35%, type 1), *KCNH2* (25%–40%, type 2), and *SNC5A* (5%–10%, type 3). About 5% to 10% of patients with LQTS have multiple mutations in LQTS genes, and these patients tend to have more severe phenotypes compared to those with a single mutation.[34]

Familial Hypercholesterolemia

Familial hypercholesterolemia (FH) is thus far the most common inherited cardiovascular disorder, affecting 1 in 300 patients, and is characterized by markedly elevated serum low-density lipoprotein cholesterol (LDL-C) levels from birth. Most cases (60%–80%) are caused by AD mutations in the LDL receptor, but other genes involved in cholesterol metabolism, such as *APOB* and *PCSK9*, have also been implicated, albeit more rarely. Thousands of rare mutations in the LDL receptor have been linked with FH, including small indels (~15%–20%), missense mutations altering a single amino acid (40%–50%), nonsense mutations (12%–15%), and mutations in noncoding regions (8%–10%). Because elevated LDL-C is the hallmark of the condition that leads to increased cardiovascular risk, the currently available diagnostic criteria do not require genetic testing to establish the diagnosis.[35,36]

Aortopathy

Thoracic aortic disease (TAD; aneurysm or dissection) can cause life-threatening vascular complications.[37] Several syndromic connective tissue disorders have been linked to TAD including Marfan, Loeys-Dietz, and Ehlers-Danlos syndromes.[38] Overall, about 20% of TAD cases are thought to be genetically mediated and generally follow an AD inheritance pattern.[14] A recent study by the ClinGen Aortopathy Working Group identified 11 susceptibility genes with mutations conferring significantly increased risk of TAD.[39] These genes encode proteins that are involved in vascular smooth muscle structure and function, extracellular matrix, and the transforming growth factor-β (TGF-β) pathway, including but not limited to FBN1/2 (commonly linked to Marfan), TGF-β receptor type I/II (linked to Loeys-Dietz), and α-1 procollagen type III (linked to vascular Ehlers-Danlos). Nevertheless, up to 70% of cases of familial aortopathy without syndromic features do not have identifiable genetic causes, suggesting that the genetic architecture of inherited aortopathy is not well understood.

Polygenic Cardiovascular Diseases

Common cardiovascular diseases such as coronary artery disease or atrial fibrillation often cluster in families ("disease running in a family") but may not follow Mendelian inheritance patterns as seen in the monogenic disorders. This is because the diseases are rarely caused by a single genetic variant but rather by complicated effects of multiple genes (polygenic) combined with lifestyle and environmental factors. Therefore, these common diseases are considered to be multifactorial in origin, and the familial clustering pattern is often referred to as *complex*, highlighting shared genetic background and environmental exposure among family members.

Genome-Wide Association Study

In monogenic diseases following Mendelian inheritance patterns, linkage analysis is primarily used among affected families to identify genetic causes of the diseases. In polygenic or common diseases, however, variants typically have small effects, and therefore, large-scale, population-based association studies are required to discover genetic variants associated with certain diseases or phenotypes of interest (either in the form of case-control or cross-sectional cohorts).[40] Previously, the association studies for a disease were undertaken by focusing on a single gene or a set of candidate genes believed to be linked to the disease. Assessing the whole genome in an unbiased fashion may discover novel genes implicated in a given disease. Genome-wide association studies (GWASs) conventionally use genotyping of approximately 300,000 to 1 million individual variants, also known as single nucleotide polymorphisms (SNPs), distributed across the whole genome (<0.03% of the whole genome) to identify any variants significantly associated with the disease of interest (**Fig. 4–6**). This approach exploits linkage disequilibrium of variants, the nonrandom association of alleles at two or more loci, to infer missing genetic information outside of the genotyped variants—a process called *imputation*. Therefore, when a variant is found through GWAS to alter disease susceptibility, it can be imputed to further determine genes or genetic loci associated with the disease susceptibility. As whole genome sequencing (WGS) is becoming more accessible, feasible, and affordable, it is also possible to employ WGS data in GWAS for novel gene discovery. However, thus far, this is largely limited by challenges in data processing and bioinformatics analysis.

Coronary artery disease (CAD) is the most common heart disease and a leading cause of death worldwide. It exhibits a complex inheritance pattern and is considered to be polygenic

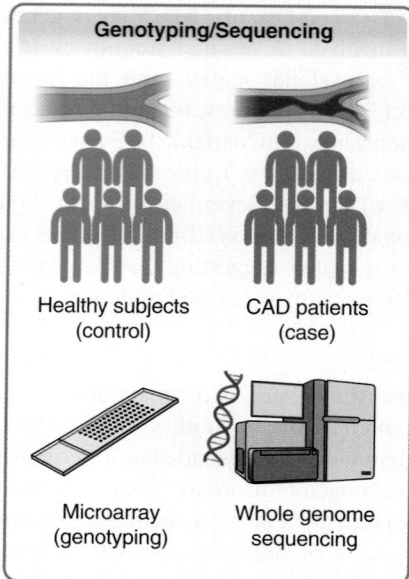

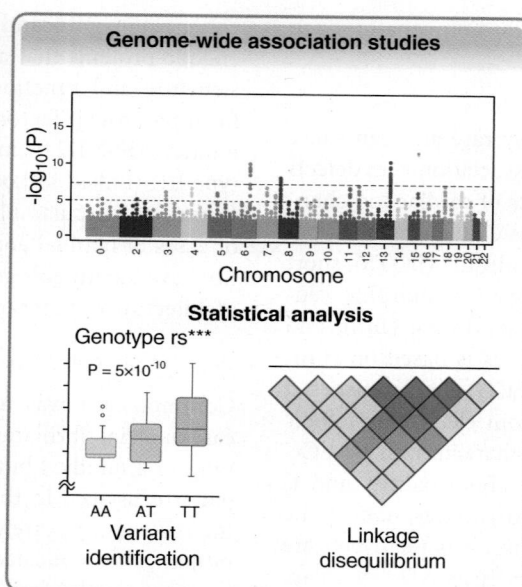

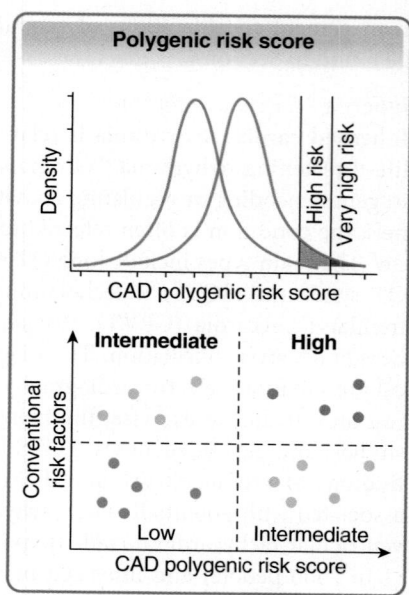

Figure 4–6. The applications of genome-wide association studies (GWASs). GWASs use genotyping of approximately 300,000 to 1 million individual variants, also known as single nucleotide polymorphisms (SNPs), distributed across the whole genome (<0.03% of the whole genome) to identify variants significantly associated with cases versus control subjects. The approach exploits linkage disequilibrium of variants to infer missing genetic information outside of the genotyped variants to further identify genes or genetic loci associated with the disease susceptibility. The information from GWAS can be used to compute a polygenic risk score to predict risk for disease and identify those at risk. CAD, coronary artery disease.

in nature. The first GWAS on CAD was jointly conducted by the Wellcome Trust Case Control Consortium and the Cardiogenics Consortium, using two respective cohorts of patients with premature CAD and family history of CAD.[41] The study identified several genetic loci significantly associated with CAD, including 9p21.3 (rs1333049), which had the strongest and most significant association with CAD in both cohorts. Since then, there have been multiple GWASs on CAD, with the largest cohort involving more than 100,000 subjects and identifying more than 150 genetic loci significantly linked to CAD.[42] Through linkage disequilibrium analysis, several candidate causal variants and associated genes have been inferred, although in the case of the 9p21.3 locus, no causal or pathogenic gene has been identified thus far. Although GWAS does not establish causality or functional implications of these variants, the studies nevertheless have opened doors for current and future mechanistic and confirmatory investigations on CAD.

Polygenic Risk Score

Even when causal variants and related mechanisms are not established, findings from GWASs can be useful in predicting risk for disease and identifying those at risk. Significant research has focused on identifying, prioritizing, and weighing SNPs from GWASs to compute polygenic risk scores to predict risk for complex cardiovascular diseases (see Fig. 4–6).[43] Polygenic risk scoring is well established in CAD; accumulating evidence suggests that those who have a high polygenic risk score for CAD are at significantly elevated risk for CAD, equivalent to the risk among those with unfavorable lifestyle (eg, smoking, obesity, and sedentary lifestyle).[44] Many studies are underway to develop, refine, and clinically apply polygenic

risk scores for complex cardiovascular diseases such as atrial fibrillation and diabetes.

Mitochondrial Disease

The mitochondrion is a key energy-producing organelle, and its function is critical for myocardial health. Mitochondria contain their own compact genomes separate from the nuclear genome. Mitochondrial proteins are encoded by both mitochondrial and nuclear DNA whose mutations can cause mitochondrial genetic disorders. The mitochondrial genome is thought to be exclusively inherited from the mother, although this notion has been challenged by a recent report suggesting biparental inheritance of mitochondrial DNA (mtDNA).[45] While mitochondrial disorders caused by nuclear DNA mutations follow Mendelian inheritance patterns, the ones caused by mtDNA mutations follow maternal inheritance (XL). Because there are mixed copies of both normal and diseased/mutant mitochondria in a myocyte (heteroplasmy), disease phenotypes tend to manifest when the amount of mutant mitochondria reaches a certain threshold.[46] Depending on the mutant mtDNA contents, family members may exhibit different disease types and severity. Mitochondria are more enriched in tissues with high energy demand, including the heart, brain, skeletal muscle, and endocrine system,[47] making them inherently more vulnerable to mitochondrial defects. Mitochondrial disorders typically manifest in the heart as mitochondrial cardiomyopathies, with clinical manifestations similar to those of HCM, DCM, and NCCM.[48]

Barth Syndrome

First described in 1983, Barth syndrome is an XL mitochondrial disease caused by mutations in *TAZ*, which encodes tafazzin, an essential regulator of mitochondrial structure and function.[49] It is associated with cardiac anomalies, skeletal myopathy, and growth retardation that affect approximately 1 in 300,000 to 400,000 live births. The disease typically manifests within the first year of life with failure to thrive and cardiac dysfunction. More than 90% of cases involve the heart, with manifestations that include DCM, endocardial fibroelastosis, NCCM, conduction abnormalities, and tachyarrhythmias. Presently, there is no curative treatment available, but early detection and management of heart failure can improve the disease course. Overall, more than 10% of patients will eventually require cardiac transplantation.

Pharmacogenomics

Patients have different responses to drugs; in some patients, a drug effectively treats their conditions, whereas in others, the same drug causes profound side effects without desirable effectiveness. Pharmacogenomics is the study of how genetic variants mediate beneficial versus adverse drug effects. Genetic variation can influence drug response by altering pharmacokinetics (pertaining to drug bioavailability and metabolism) or pharmacodynamics (pertaining to either on- or off-target drug actions).[50] For example, a subset of patients taking statins experience muscle symptoms such as muscle pain and weakness. A GWAS on those with and without statin-induced myopathy identified a variant in *SCLO1B1* that encodes the organic anion-transporting polypeptide OATP1B1, a dug transporter regulating the hepatic uptake of statins (pharmacokinetics).[51] In another example, patients have variable anticoagulation responses to warfarin, which inhibits an enzyme, vitamin K epoxide reductase (VKOR), and blocks synthesis of important clotting factors.[52,53] Studies have identified a genetic polymorphism of *VKORC1*, the gene encoding VKOR, which plays an important role in determining VKOR availability and predicting warfarin response (pharmacodynamics). As such, genetic polymorphisms can significantly affect the way patients respond to certain drugs. However, such potentially useful information mostly has not been incorporated into clinical practice due in part to the rather small effect size of the identified variants as well as lack of clinical benefits reported thus far. By combining accumulating genetic knowledge with clinical drug response data, pharmacogenetics may help guide clinicians in identifying the best drugs of choice for a given condition, determining optimal doses, and predicting risk of side effects.

Clonal Hematopoiesis of Indeterminate Potential

In a normal life span, somatic cells acquire random mutations, most of which are thought to be inconsequential. In some cases, however, these mutations can cause clonal expansion of hematopoietic stem cells in otherwise healthy patients. Termed *clonal hematopoiesis of indeterminate potential* (CHIP), these cells can become cancerous if there are any additional mutations acquired.[54] Moreover, emerging data suggest there is an increased risk of cardiovascular disease and mortality among patients with CHIP. About 10% to 15% of patients older than 65 years and approximately 30% older than 80 years may develop CHIP, shedding light on the link between aging and increased cardiovascular disease risk. To date, studies have identified several major genes (*TET2, JAK2, DNMT3A*) linked to CHIP, and active research is currently underway to further explore this important link.

EPIGENOMICS AND EPIGENETICS OF HEART DISEASE

Gene expression can be regulated by reversible modifications of the genes without changing their DNA sequences. For example, while all cell types of a person share the same genome, cell phenotypes can widely vary depending on which genes are turned on and off. As such, epigenomics is the study of how these reversible genetic modifications lead to changes in gene expression. Accumulating data suggest that environmental exposure (eg, nicotine),[55] different behaviors (eg, diet and exercise),[56] and aging[57] can alter the epigenome and thereby play important roles in the pathogenesis of cardiovascular diseases.[4,58,59]

There are three major mechanisms of how epigenetic regulation occurs in cells (**Fig. 4–7**); accumulating evidence indicates diverse epigenetic mechanisms in this process, which are beyond the scope of this chapter and have been comprehensively reviewed elsewhere. First, the accessibility and structure of chromatin, a complex of DNA and proteins that forms chromosomes, can be altered by DNA methylation.[60] When chromatin is tightly coiled, forming what is called heterochromatin, the genes are inaccessible for transcription and considered inactive. When chromatin is uncoiled (or loosely packed), the region of the chromosome can be transcriptionally active. Second, chromatin accessibility can be regulated by histone modification. Third, cells can also express noncoding RNAs such as microRNA (miRNA) and long noncoding RNA (lncRNA), which may directly interact with genes and their transcripts to modulate their expression.[61] Along with NGS, epigenetic technologies[62] have rapidly evolved, including technologies to sequence accessible chromatin regions (eg, ChIP-seq, ATAC-seq, DNase-seq), to interrogate methylation sites across the genome (methyl-seq), and to profile transcriptomes of noncoding RNAs.[63] Through these technologies, comprehensive epigenetic information at a single-cell level can now be obtained with only miniscule amounts of genomics samples. Additionally, large efforts are underway to establish reference human epigenomes, including ENCODE,[64] the Epigenome Roadmap, and BLUEPRINT.

Epigenetic Mechanism 1: DNA Methylation

DNA methylation is typically associated with gene silencing by decreasing chromatin accessibility and thereby inhibiting binding of transcription factors for gene transcription.[65] Among the four DNA nucleotides (A, C, T, and G), cytosines followed by guanine (so-called CpG sites) are most commonly (~60%–80%) methylated and best studied. Several enzymes have been identified to modify DNA methylations. Methylases such as

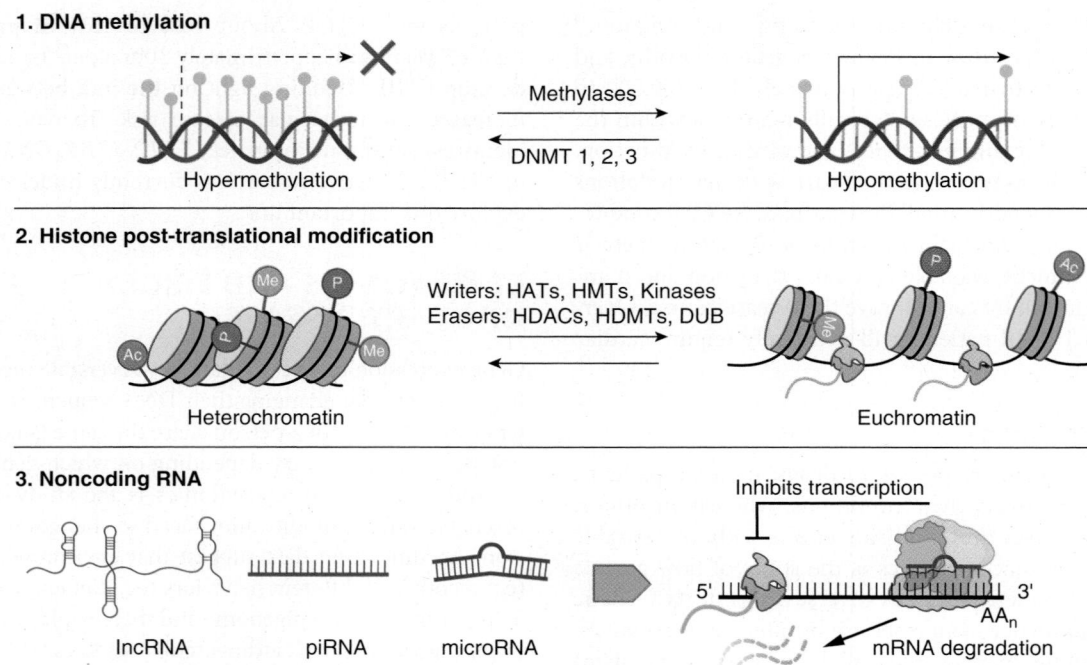

1. DNA methylation

Methylases →
← DNMT 1, 2, 3

Hypermethylation   Hypomethylation

2. Histone post-translational modification

Writers: HATs, HMTs, Kinases
Erasers: HDACs, HDMTs, DUB

Heterochromatin   Euchromatin

3. Noncoding RNA

Inhibits transcription

lncRNA   piRNA   microRNA

5'   3'
AA$_n$
mRNA degradation

Figure 4–7. Epigenetic mechanisms. There are three major ways of how epigenetic regulation occurs in cells. (1) DNA methylation and (2) histone posttranslational modification can change the accessibility and structure of chromatin for gene expression. When chromatin is tightly coiled, called heterochromatin, the genes are not accessible for transcription and considered inactive. When chromatin is loosely coiled, called euchromatin, the region of the chromosome can be transcriptionally active. (3) Noncoding RNAs, such as microRNA (miRNA), piwi-interacting RNA (piRNA), and long noncoding RNA (lncRNA), can also directly interact with genes and their transcripts to modulate their expression. DNMT, deoxyribonucleic acid methyltransferases; DUB, deubiquinating enzymes; HATs, histone acetylases; HDACs, histone deacetylases; HDMTs, histone demethylases; HMTs, histone methyltransferases.

deoxyribonucleic acid methyltransferases (DNMTs) add methyl groups to CpG sites, whereas demethylases remove the methyl groups. Both DNA hypomethylation and hypermethylation have been linked to various cardiovascular diseases, suggesting a complex interplay among DNA methylation, transcriptional regulation, and disease phenotypes. Advances in technologies now allow genome-wide interrogation of DNA methylation that may further advance the field. However, the epigenomic profiling of heart diseases thus far has been hampered by difficulties in obtaining myocardial or vascular tissues.

Heart Failure
Several studies have examined the relationship between DNA methylation and heart failure, identifying several epigenetic risk loci as well as patterns of methylation changes associated with heart failure. Meder et al.[66] performed epigenome-wide DNA methylation association studies using cardiac biopsies from 41 DCM patients and 31 controls. They reported 27 epigenetic loci that are significantly associated with DCM and correlated with transcriptomic changes, highlighting the importance of epigenetic changes in heart failure. Whether these changes are just bystander effects of the disease process or they have any causal relationships is currently under active investigation.

Cardiovascular Aging
DNA methylation changes with chronological age and the methylation status of these CpG sites have been used as an epigenetic clock correlating with aging or "biological age." Several

studies have examined DNA methylation with cardiovascular aging and found significant correlations between cardiovascular disease and aging-related epigenetic changes. Lind et al.[67] calculated biological age based on epigenetic profiles and found a 4% increased risk of future cardiovascular disease for each year of increased biological age. Evolving research suggests a potential role of age-associated mutations in *TET2*, a master epigenetic regulator of key cardiovascular genes as well as a main gene implicated in CHIP, in cardiovascular aging and diseases, but this potential link needs further exploration.

Epigenetic Mechanism 2: Posttranslational Histone Modifications

In a nucleosome, a basic structural unit of DNA packaging, four different histone proteins (H2A, H2B, H3, and H4) are organized as octamers with DNA wrapping around the protein complex. Given the close interaction between histone complex and DNA, the histone structure and organization are critical in how tightly DNA is packaged around the protein complex to be accessible for transcription (heterochromatin versus euchromatin). Emerging research suggests that posttranslational histone modifications such as phosphorylation, methylation, and acetylation of amino acid residues play key roles in altering DNA and histone complex interplay, thereby altering chromatin accessibility. These modifications can be done by "writer" enzymes such as histone acetyltransferases (HATs; adding an acetylation group) or "eraser" enzymes such as histone deacetylases (HDACs; removing an acetylation group). To describe specific histone modifications, a dedicated nomenclature has been developed that involves (1) the specific histone protein, (2) the location of the modification (eg, amino acid residue), and (3) the type of modification (eg, H3 acetylation at lysine 27 can be denoted as H3K27ac). Although some of these modifications last only minutes to hours, others last much longer and persist during cell division and differentiation to contribute to epigenetic memory.

Congenital Heart Disease

Thus far, the roles played by posttranslational modification of histones have been most extensively studied in cardiac development, and dysregulated epigenetics has been linked to an increased risk of congenital heart disease. A recent study[68] found that fetal hyperglycemia from maternal diabetes may decrease chromatin accessibility at the endothelial nitric oxide (NO) synthase (*NOS3*) locus, resulting in reduced NO synthesis. Subsequent upregulation of *JARID2*, a regulator of histone methyltransferase complexes, then leads to downregulation of Notch1, which is important in normal heart development, potentially resulting in CHDs. In another study[69] comparing incidence of de novo mutations in 362 severe congenital heart disease cases and 264 controls, a marked excess of de novo mutations in genes involved in H3K4 methylation (activating) and H3K27 methylation (inactivating) was found to be highly enriched in CHD patients. Further studies are warranted to better understand epigenetic mechanisms of congenital heart disease in the context of maternal-fetal exposure as well as de novo mutations.

Epigenetic Mechanism 3: Noncoding RNAs

Noncoding RNAs (ncRNAs) are highly expressed in the human heart and play diverse epigenetic roles in the cells, which include interfering with translation of target messenger RNA, remodeling chromatin, and modulating protein-protein scaffolding.[70] ncRNAs can be subcategorized based on their length as short ncRNAs (<200 nucleotides; eg, miRNAs,[71] piwi-interacting RNAs[72]) and lncRNA (>200 nucleotides),[73] among which miRNAs (~17–22 nucleotides) have been the most widely studied and implicated in cardiogenesis as well as a wide spectrum of cardiovascular diseases. Thus far, more than 1500 human miRNAs have been annotated in the miRBase database (http://www.mirbase.org). miRNAs primarily function to decrease gene expression by altering transcript stability or interfering with translation of messenger RNA.[71] Because miRNAs are stable and easily measured in serum, both diagnostic and therapeutic applications of miRNA have been explored in diverse cardiovascular diseases, including heart failure, coronary heart disease, limb ischemia, and angiogenesis. Other ncRNAs have not been as well studied due in part to poor conservation across species and the wide variety of regulatory mechanisms.

Myocardial Infarction

Acute myocardial infarction can result in myocardial injury and adverse cardiac remodeling with subsequent heart failure. Several studies have suggested important roles of miRNAs in mediating these processes.[74] Acute myocardial injury and subsequent inflammation can induce changes in miRNA expression in the heart, which in turn can modulate cardiomyocyte cell death and survival and also regulate postischemic neovascularization. For example, the expression of the miR-15 family was found to be increased after myocardial ischemia, which could induce myocardial cell death by targeting the apoptosis regulator Bcl-2. The inhibition of miR-15 family members reduced infarct size after ischemia-reperfusion injury in vivo.[75] As such, clinical applications of miRNA both as diagnostics and therapeutics are being actively explored. In contrast, few ncRNA candidates have thus far been validated across studies for their clinical utility, due in part to differences in isolation and measurement techniques.[76] Using rapidly advancing technologies to isolate, sequence, and quantify ncRNA, endeavors to harmonize and validate the measurement of ncRNAs would be critical for clinical applications.

EMERGING TECHNOLOGIES

GENOME EDITING

Over the past decade, genome editing tools have revolutionized biomedical research and become indispensable in genomic manipulation in cells and animal models.[77] These tools leverage the endogenous repair of DNA double-strand breaks generated by DNA site-specific nucleases such as zinc finger nucleases (ZFNs), transcription activator-like effector nucleases (TALENs), and clustered regularly interspaced short palindromic repeats (CRISPR)/CRISPR-associated 9 (Cas9).[78] In particular, the CRISPR/Cas9 system has been widely used due to its simplicity, efficiency, and ability to precisely change genomic sequences.[79] There are many comprehensive reviews on genome editing tools published previously, so we focus on cardiovascular applications of the CRISPR/Cas9 system.

Cardiovascular Applications of the CRISPR/Cas9 System

Originally identified as a mechanism of bacterial adaptive immunity, the CRISPR/Cas9 system uses guide RNAs (~100-nucleotide RNA to target Cas9 protein to a specific genomic site) and Cas9 protein to cleave the genome at specific sites. The first approximately 20 nucleotides of the guide RNA, termed the *protospacer*, are designed to specifically bind to the DNA site of interest and recruit Cas9. The DNA region of interest must include a protospacer-adjacent motif (PAM) for Cas9 to recognize and create a blunt-end double-strand DNA break adjacent to the PAM. When a double-strand DNA break is created, cells then activate their endogenous DNA repair pathways, during which desired genome editing can be achieved to fit experimental needs. In the cardiovascular field, CRISPR/Cas9 genome editing tools are primarily used to better define genetic mechanisms of diseases such as cardiomyopathy, arrhythmia, and dyslipidemia. Additionally, they are being actively investigated as therapeutic agents[80] primarily targeting the liver to modulate cholesterol levels. As such, genome editing tools have enormous potential for research, diagnostic, and therapeutic applications.[81]

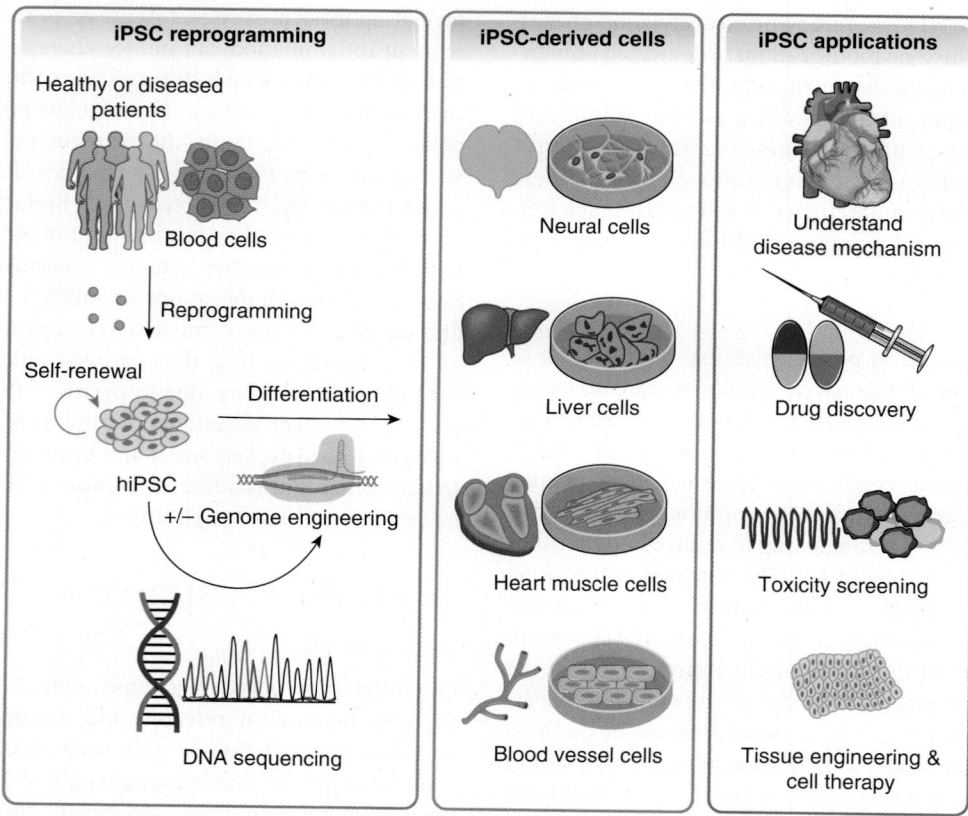

Figure 4–8. Applications of induced pluripotent stem cells (iPSCs) in medicine. Patients' somatic cells (eg, peripheral blood mononuclear cells) can be reprogrammed to iPSCs and their genetic sequences can be manipulated by genome editing technologies. Patient-specific human iPSCs can be differentiated into multiple disease-relevant cell types such as neural cells, liver cells, heart muscle cells, and blood vessel cells, which can then be used to better understand disease mechanisms, discover novel therapeutics, screen for toxicity, and apply in tissue engineering.

Human Induced Pluripotent Stem Cells

Recent advances in induced pluripotent stem cell (iPSC) biology provide an unprecedented opportunity to study cardiovascular diseases.[82] Since their first discovery by Dr. Shinya Yamanaka, who later received the Nobel Prize in 2012, remarkable progress has been made to differentiate human iPSCs into multiple cell types, including disease-relevant cardiovascular cell types such as cardiomyocytes, endothelial cells, and fibroblasts (**Fig. 4–8**).[83] Differentiated cells can then be used to better understand disease mechanisms, discover novel therapeutics, screen for toxicity, and apply in tissue engineering.[84] Notably, human cardiomyocytes (CMs) were previously nearly impossible to culture because the cells are difficult to obtain due to a significant procedural risk of endomyocardial biopsies and do not proliferate. With iPSCs, nearly limitless human iPSC-CMs can now be differentiated and cultured in a dish. Human iPSC-CMs represent a more physiologically relevant system compared to animal cell lines, with more similar biochemical, electrophysiologic, genomic, and mechanical properties as those of primary human CMs. Additionally, the ability to generate patient-specific iPSCs that retain patient-specific genetic information, combined with the use of CRISPR genome editing, now enables researchers to dissect the associations between genetic background and cardiovascular disease susceptibility. Examples include the use of iPSCs to model DCM,[28,85]

HCM,[26,86–88] NCCM,[89] LQTS,[90,91] BrS,[92] and LMNA-associated cardiomyopathy[93] and vasculopathy.[94]

Back To The Case: Combining Genome Editing and iPSC Technologies

The patient who was presented at the beginning of the chapter was found to carry a frameshift mutation in Lamin A/C (*LMNA*) that leads to the early termination of translation (348-349insG; K117fs). *LMNA* is one of the most frequently mutated genes associated with DCM with a high prevalence of early arrhythmia. Using iPSCs derived from the patient as well as several members of his family, our group recently modeled the LMNA-related DCM in vitro (**Fig. 4–9**).[93] We generated multiple iPSCs lines from the family members carrying this mutation as well as their genome-corrected isogenic lines. We also generated iPSC lines from the control members with type LMNA and their genome-edited isogenic lines to carry this specific mutation. We found that the LMNA-mutant iPSC-CMs (derived from both diseased and genome-edited lines) exhibited abnormal calcium handling, electrophysiologic disturbances, and proarrhythmic activities. These abnormalities were not present in both control and genome-corrected iPSC-CMs, establishing the pathogenic role of the LMNA variant. Further mechanistic investigations identified disturbed chromatin organization leading to an abnormally activated

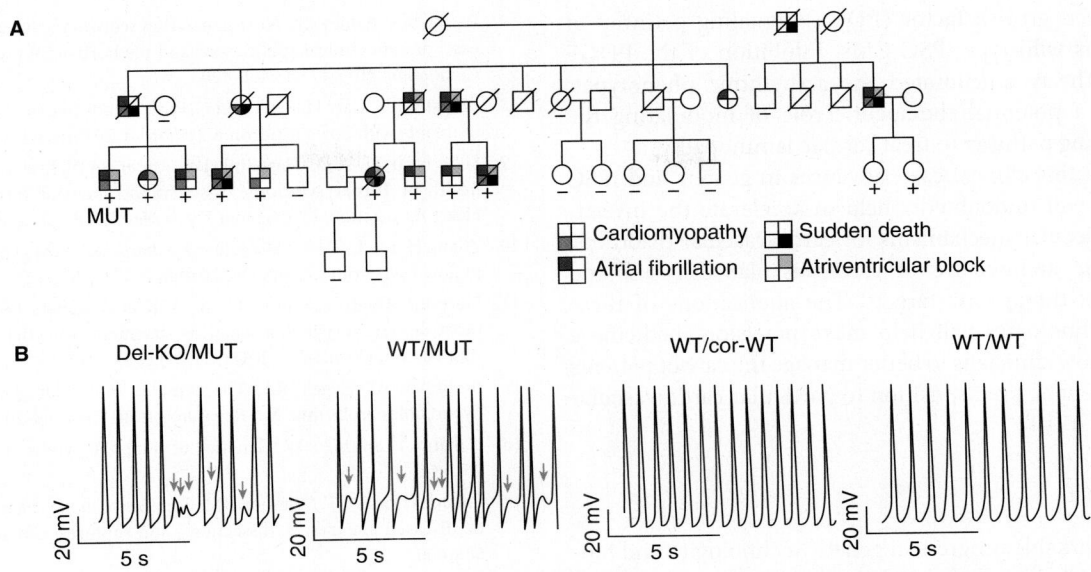

Figure 4–9. The case of cardiac laminopathy. A 57-year-old man was newly diagnosed with severely reduced left ventricular systolic function. **A.** His family history is remarkable for multiple sudden cardiac deaths, premature atrial fibrillation, and heart failure, prompting clinical genetic screening. His genetic panel identifies a pathogenic variant in Lamin A/C, which leads to the early termination of translation (348-349insG; K117fs). **B.** Multiple induced pluripotent stem cell (iPSC) lines were generated from family members with wild-type *LMNA* (WT/WT) as well as with this mutation (WT/MUT) and also their genome-edited/corrected isogenic lines (Del-KO/MUT to delete wild-type *LMNA* on the other allele while keeping the mutant *LMNA*, WT/cor-WT to genome correct mutant *LMNA*).

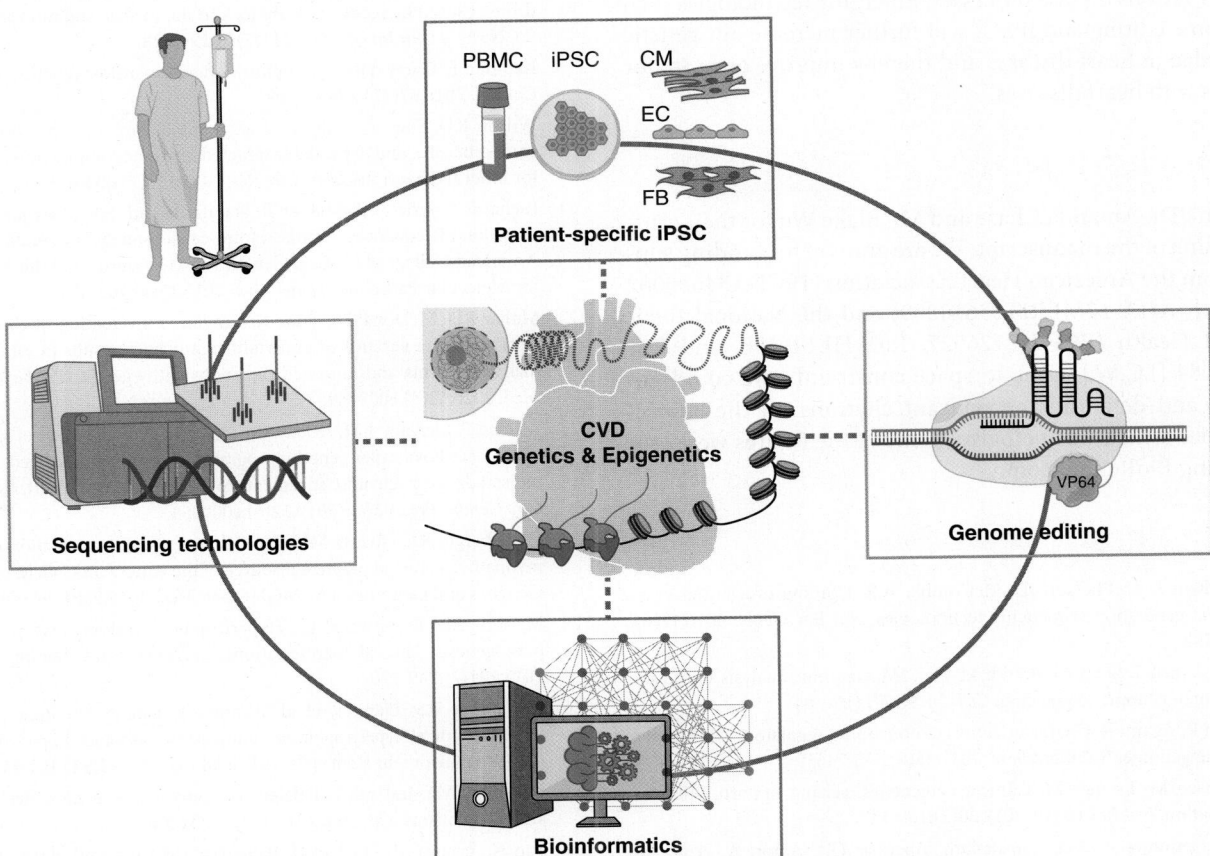

Figure 4–10. Emerging technologies for cardiovascular genetics and epigenomics. Advances in genetics, bioinformatics, and induced pluripotent stem cell (iPSC) technologies will accelerate the investigation of cardiovascular diseases (CVDs), define complex genetic architectures that exist among patients, and identify novel therapeutic targets, making precision medicine a reality. CM, cardiomyocyte; EC, endothelial cell; FB, fibroblast; PBMC, peripheral blood mononuclear cell.

platelet-derived growth factor (PDGF) signaling pathway in mutant versus wild-type iPSC-CMs. Inhibition of the PDGF signaling pathway ameliorated the arrhythmic phenotypes, highlighting a potential therapeutic role of modulating the PDGF signaling pathway to treat cardiac laminopathy.

As seen in this clinical case, advances in genetic and iPSC technologies will undoubtedly help to accelerate the investigation of molecular mechanisms for cardiovascular disorders, define genetic architecture of cardiovascular diseases, and identify novel therapeutic targets. The applications of these emerging technologies will help make precision medicine a reality and allow clinicians to better manage the care of patients who have a genetic predisposition to particular cardiovascular diseases (**Fig. 4–10**).

SUMMARY

With the remarkable progress in genetic technologies and bioinformatics tools in recent decades, we are starting to understand in ever greater detail the genetic architecture of heart diseases. Beyond conventional monogenic diseases following Mendelian inheritance, accumulating research highlights critical roles of polygenic mechanisms, somatic mutations (eg, CHIP), and noncoding genes in cardiovascular disease pathogenesis. Additionally, epigenetics is being increasingly implicated in various disease processes. Emerging technologies such as genome editing and iPSCs will further increase our genetic knowledge in heart diseases and thereby improve our care for patients with heart diseases.

ACKNOWLEDGMENTS

We thank Dr. Amanda Chase and Mr. Blake Wu for their critical reading of the manuscript. We are grateful for funding support from the American Heart Association (19CDA34680002 [J.-W.R.], AHA 17MERIT33610009) and the National Institutes of Health (R01 HL126527, R01 HL146690, and P01 HL141084 [J.C.W.]). Due to space constraints, we could not include and detail all the relevant citations on the subject matter, for which we apologize. Some of the figures were created using BioRender.com.

REFERENCES

1. Goodwin S, McPherson JD, McCombie WR. Coming of age: ten years of next-generation sequencing technologies. *Nat Rev Genet.* 2016;17(6): 333-351.

2. Lappalainen T, Scott AJ, Brandt M, Hall IM. Genomic analysis in the age of human genome sequencing. *Cell.* 2019;177(1):70-84.

3. Elkon R, Agami R. Characterization of noncoding regulatory DNA in the human genome. *Nat Biotechnol.* 2017;35(8):732-746.

4. Berdasco M, Esteller M. Clinical epigenetics: seizing opportunities for translation. *Nat Rev Genet.* 2019;20(2):109-127.

5. 1000 Genomes Project Consortium, Abecasis GR, Auton A, et al. An integrated map of genetic variation from 1,092 human genomes. *Nature.* 2012;491(7422):56-65.

6. Lander ES, Linton LM, Birren B, et al. Initial sequencing and analysis of the human genome. *Nature.* 2001;409(6822):860-921.

7. Parikh VN, Ashley EA. Next-generation sequencing in cardiovascular disease: present clinical applications and the horizon of precision medicine. *Circulation.* 2017;135(5):406-409.

8. Bergström S, Carr H, Petersson G, et al. Trends in congenital heart defects in infants with down syndrome. *Pediatrics.* 2016;138(1):e20160123.

9. Silberbach M, Roos-Hesselink JW, Andersen NH, et al. Cardiovascular health in Turner syndrome: a scientific statement from the American Heart Association. *Circ Genom Precis Med.* 2018;11(10):e000048.

10. Zhang H, Liu L, Tian J. Molecular mechanisms of congenital heart disease in down syndrome. *Genes Dis.* 2019;6(4):372-377.

11. Pierpont ME, Brueckner M, Chung WK, et al. Genetic basis for congenital heart disease: revisited: a scientific statement from the American Heart Association. *Circulation.* 2018;138(21):e653-e711.

12. Berberich AJ, Hegele RA. The complex molecular genetics of familial hypercholesterolaemia. *Nat Rev Cardiol.* 2019;16(1):9-20.

13. Nakano Y, Shimizu W. Genetics of long-QT syndrome. *J Hum Genet.* 2016;61(1):51-55.

14. Pinard A, Jones GT, Milewicz DM. Genetics of thoracic and abdominal aortic diseases: aneurysms, dissections, and ruptures. *Circ Res.* 2019;124(4): 588-606.

15. Kathiresan S, Srivastava D. Genetics of human cardiovascular disease. *Cell.* 2012;148(6):1242-1257.

16. Nagueh SF. Anderson-Fabry disease and other lysosomal storage disorders. *Circulation.* 2014;130(13):1081-1090.

17. Olson TM, Karst ML, Whitby FG, Driscoll DJ. Myosin light chain mutation causes autosomal recessive cardiomyopathy with mid-cavitary hypertrophy and restrictive physiology. *Circulation.* 2002;105(20):2337-2340.

18. Benson DW, Wang DW, Dyment M, et al. Congenital sick sinus syndrome caused by recessive mutations in the cardiac sodium channel gene (SCN5A). *J Clin Invest.* 2003;112(7):1019-1028.

19. Kamdar F, Garry DJ. Dystrophin-deficient cardiomyopathy. *J Am Coll Cardiol.* 2016;67(21):2533-2546.

20. Wilson KD, Shen P, Fung E, et al. A rapid, high-quality, cost-effective, comprehensive and expandable targeted next-generation sequencing assay for inherited heart diseases. *Circ Res.* 2015;117(7):603-611.

21. Richards S, Aziz N, Bale S, et al. Standards and guidelines for the interpretation of sequence variants: a joint consensus recommendation of the American College of Medical Genetics and Genomics and the Association for Molecular Pathology. *Genet Med.* 2015;17(5):405-424.

22. Muller RD, McDonald T, Pope K, Cragun D. Evaluation of clinical practices related to variants of uncertain significance results in inherited cardiac arrhythmia and inherited cardiomyopathy genes. *Circ Genom Precis Med.* 2020;13(4):e002789.

23. Ahmad F, McNally EM, Ackerman MJ, et al. Establishment of specialized clinical cardiovascular genetics programs: recognizing the need and meeting standards: a scientific statement from the American Heart Association. *Circ Genom Precis Med.* 2019;12(6):e000054.

24. Hershberger RE, Givertz MM, Ho CY, et al. Genetic evaluation of cardiomyopathy: a clinical practice resource of the American College of Medical Genetics and Genomics (ACMG). *Genet Med.* 2018;20(9):899-909.

25. Marian AJ, Braunwald E. Hypertrophic cardiomyopathy: genetics, pathogenesis, clinical manifestations, diagnosis, and therapy. *Circ Res.* 2017;121(7):749-770.

26. Lan F, Lee AS, Liang P, et al. Abnormal calcium handling properties underlie familial hypertrophic cardiomyopathy pathology in patient-specific induced pluripotent stem cells. *Cell Stem Cell.* 2013;12(1):101-113.

27. McNally EM, Mestroni L. Dilated cardiomyopathy: genetic determinants and mechanisms. *Circ Res.* 2017;121(7):731-748.

28. Sun N, Yazawa M, Liu J, et al. Patient-specific induced pluripotent stem cells as a model for familial dilated cardiomyopathy. *Sci Transl Med.* 2012;4(130):130ra47.

29. Corrado D, Basso C, Judge DP. Arrhythmogenic cardiomyopathy. *Circ Res.* 2017;121(7):784-802.

30. Muchtar E, Blauwet LA, Gertz MA. Restrictive cardiomyopathy: genetics, pathogenesis, clinical manifestations, diagnosis, and therapy. *Circ Res.* 2017;121(7):819-837.

31. van Waning JI, Caliskan K, Michels M, et al. Cardiac phenotypes, genetics, and risks in familial noncompaction cardiomyopathy. *J Am Coll Cardiol.* 2019;73(13):1601-1611.

32. Deacon DC, Happe CL, Chen C, et al. Combinatorial interactions of genetic variants in human cardiomyopathy. *Nat Biomed Eng.* 2019;3(2):147-157.

33. Schwartz PJ, Ackerman MJ, Antzelevitch C, et al. Inherited cardiac arrhythmias. *Nat Rev Dis Primers.* 2020;6(1):58.

34. Wu JC, Garg P, Yoshida Y, et al. Towards precision medicine with human iPSCs for cardiac channelopathies. *Circ Res.* 2019;125(6):653-658.

35. Sturm AC, Knowles JW, Gidding SS, et al. Clinical genetic testing for familial hypercholesterolemia: JACC scientific expert panel. *J Am Coll Cardiol.* 2018;72(6):662-680.

36. Knowles JW, Rader DJ, Khoury MJ. Cascade screening for familial hypercholesterolemia and the use of genetic testing. *JAMA.* 2017;318(4):381-382.

37. Kuijpers JM, Mulder BJ. Aortopathies in adult congenital heart disease and genetic aortopathy syndromes: management strategies and indications for surgery. *Heart.* 2017;103(12):952-966.

38. Rigelsky CM, Moran RT. Genetics of syndromic and nonsyndromic aortopathies. *Curr Opin Pediatr.* 2019;31(6):694-701.

39. Renard M, Francis C, Ghosh R, et al. Clinical validity of genes for heritable thoracic aortic aneurysm and dissection. *J Am Coll Cardiol.* 2018;72(6):605-615.

40. Musunuru K, Kathiresan S. Genetics of common, complex coronary artery disease. *Cell.* 2019;177(1):132-145.

41. Myocardial Infarction Genetics Consortium, Kathiresan S, Voight BF, et al. Genome-wide association of early-onset myocardial infarction with single nucleotide polymorphisms and copy number variants. *Nat Genet.* 2009;41(3):334-341.

42. Khera AV, Kathiresan S. Genetics of coronary artery disease: discovery, biology and clinical translation. *Nat Rev Genet.* 2017;18(6):331-344.

43. Khera AV, Chaffin M, Aragam KG, et al. Genome-wide polygenic scores for common diseases identify individuals with risk equivalent to monogenic mutations. *Nat Genet.* 2018;50(9):1219-1224.

44. Khera AV, Emdin CA, Drake I, et al. Genetic risk, adherence to a healthy lifestyle, and coronary disease. *N Engl J Med.* 2016;375(24):2349-2358.

45. Luo S, Valencia CA, Zhang J, et al. Biparental inheritance of mitochondrial DNA in humans. *Proc Natl Acad Sci USA.* 2018;115(51):13039-13044.

46. Stewart JB, Chinnery PF. The dynamics of mitochondrial DNA heteroplasmy: implications for human health and disease. *Nat Rev Genet.* 2015;16(9):530-542.

47. Duran J, Martinez A, Adler E. Cardiovascular manifestations of mitochondrial disease. *Biology.* 2019;8(2):34.

48. El-Hattab AW, Scaglia F. Mitochondrial cardiomyopathies. *Front Cardiovasc Med.* 2016;3:25.

49. Dudek J, Maack C. Barth syndrome cardiomyopathy. *Cardiovasc Res.* 2017;113(4):399-410.

50. Roden DM, Van Driest SL, Wells QS, Mosley JD, Denny JC, Peterson JF. Opportunities and challenges in cardiovascular pharmacogenomics: from discovery to implementation. *Circ Res.* 2018;122(9):1176-1190.

51. SEARCH Collaborative Group, Link E, Parish S, et al. SLCO1B1 variants and statin-induced myopathy: a genomewide study. *N Engl J Med.* 2008;359(8):789-799.

52. International Warfarin Pharmacogenetics Consortium, Klein TE, Altman RB, et al. Estimation of the warfarin dose with clinical and pharmacogenetic data. *N Engl J Med.* 2009;360(8):753-764.

53. Johnson JA, Cavallari LH. Warfarin pharmacogenetics. *Trends Cardiovasc Med.* 2015;25(1):33-41.

54. Jaiswal S, Natarajan P, Silver AJ, et al. Clonal hematopoiesis and risk of atherosclerotic cardiovascular disease. *N Engl J Med.* 2017;377(2):111-121.

55. Breitling LP. Current genetics and epigenetics of smoking/tobacco-related cardiovascular disease. *Arterioscler Thromb Vasc Biol.* 2013;33(7):1468-1472.

56. Barrès R, Zierath JR. The role of diet and exercise in the transgenerational epigenetic landscape of T2DM. *Nat Rev Endocrinol.* 2016;12(8):441-451.

57. Zhang W, Song M, Qu J, Liu G-H. Epigenetic modifications in cardiovascular aging and diseases. *Circ Res.* 2018;123(7):773-786.

58. van der Harst P, de Windt LJ, Chambers JC. Translational perspective on epigenetics in cardiovascular disease. *J Am Coll Cardiol.* 2017;70(5):590-606.

59. Liu C-F, Tang WHW. Epigenetics in cardiac hypertrophy and heart failure. *JACC Basic Transl Sci.* 2019;4(8):976-993.

60. Klemm SL, Shipony Z, Greenleaf WJ. Chromatin accessibility and the regulatory epigenome. *Nat Rev Genet.* 2019;20(4):207-220.

61. Holoch D, Moazed D. RNA-mediated epigenetic regulation of gene expression. *Nat Rev Genet.* 2015;16(2):71-84.

62. Wang KC, Chang HY. Epigenomics: technologies and applications. *Circ Res.* 2018;122(9):1191-1199.

63. Lau E, Paik DT, Wu JC. Systems-wide approaches in induced pluripotent stem cell models. *Annu Rev Pathol.* 2019;14:395-419.

64. Davis CA, Hitz BC, Sloan CA, et al. The Encyclopedia of DNA Elements (ENCODE): data portal update. *Nucleic Acids Res.* 2018;46(D1):D794-D801.

65. Greenberg MVC, Bourc'his D. The diverse roles of DNA methylation in mammalian development and disease. *Nat Rev Mol Cell Biol.* 2019;20(10):590-607.

66. Meder B, Haas J, Sedaghat-Hamedani F, et al. Epigenome-wide association study identifies cardiac gene patterning and a novel class of biomarkers for heart failure. *Circulation.* 2017;136(16):1528-1544.

67. Lind L, Ingelsson E, Sundström J. Methylation-based estimated biological age and cardiovascular disease. *Eur J Clin Invest.* 2018;48(2). doi: 10.1111/eci.12872.

68. Basu M, Zhu J-Y, LaHaye S, et al. Epigenetic mechanisms underlying maternal diabetes-associated risk of congenital heart disease. *JCI Insight.* 2017;2(20):e95085.

69. Zaidi S, Choi M, Wakimoto H, et al. De novo mutations in histone-modifying genes in congenital heart disease. *Nature.* 2013;498(7453):220-223.

70. Das Saumya, Shah Ravi, Dimmeler Stefanie, et al. Noncoding RNAs in cardiovascular disease: current knowledge, tools and technologies for investigation, and future directions: a scientific statement from the American Heart Association. *Circ Genom Precis Med.* 2020;13(4):e000062.

71. Jonas S, Izaurralde E. Towards a molecular understanding of microRNA-mediated gene silencing. *Nat Rev Genet.* 2015;16(7):421-433.

72. Ozata DM, Gainetdinov I, Zoch A, O'Carroll D, Zamore PD. PIWI-interacting RNAs: small RNAs with big functions. *Nat Rev Genet.* 2019;20(2):89-108.

73. Quinn JJ, Chang HY. Unique features of long non-coding RNA biogenesis and function. *Nat Rev Genet.* 2016;17(1):47-62.

74. Boon RA, Dimmeler S. MicroRNAs in myocardial infarction. *Nat Rev Cardiol.* 2015;12(3):135-142.

75. Hullinger TG, Montgomery RL, Seto AG, et al. Inhibition of miR-15 protects against cardiac ischemic injury. *Circ Res.* 2012;110(1):71-81.

76. Wright K, de Silva K, Purdie AC, Plain KM. Comparison of methods for miRNA isolation and quantification from ovine plasma. *Sci Rep.* 2020;10(1):825.

77. Musunuru K. Genome editing: the recent history and perspective in cardiovascular diseases. *J Am Coll Cardiol.* 2017;70(22):2808-2821.

78. Doudna JA, Charpentier E. The new frontier of genome engineering with CRISPR-Cas9. *Science.* 2014;346(6213):1258096.

79. Anzalone AV, Koblan LW, Liu DR. Genome editing with CRISPR-Cas nucleases, base editors, transposases and prime editors. *Nat Biotechnol.* 2020;38(7):824-844.

80. Nishiga M, Qi LS, Wu JC. Therapeutic genome editing in cardiovascular diseases. *Adv Drug Deliv Rev.* 2021;168:147-157.

81. Seeger T, Porteus M, Wu JC. Genome editing in cardiovascular biology. *Circ Res.* 2017;120(5):778-780.

82. Musunuru K, Sheikh F, Gupta RM, et al. Induced pluripotent stem cells for cardiovascular disease modeling and precision medicine: a scientific statement from the American Heart Association. *Circ Genom Precis Med.* 2018;11(1):e000043.

83. Shi Y, Inoue H, Wu JC, Yamanaka S. Induced pluripotent stem cell technology: a decade of progress. *Nat Rev Drug Discov.* 2017;16(2):115-130.

84. Liu C, Oikonomopoulos A, Sayed N, Wu JC. Modeling human diseases with induced pluripotent stem cells: from 2D to 3D and beyond. *Development.* 2018;145(5):dev156166.

85. Wu H, Lee J, Vincent LG, et al. Epigenetic regulation of phosphodiesterases 2A and 3A underlies compromised β-adrenergic signaling in an iPSC model of dilated cardiomyopathy. *Cell Stem Cell.* 2015;17(1):89-100.

86. Wu H, Yang H, Rhee J-W, et al. Modelling diastolic dysfunction in induced pluripotent stem cell-derived cardiomyocytes from hypertrophic cardiomyopathy patients. *Eur Heart J.* 2019;40(45):3685-3695.

87. Seeger T, Shrestha R, Lam CK, et al. A premature termination codon mutation in MYBPC3 causes hypertrophic cardiomyopathy via chronic activation of nonsense-mediated decay. *Circulation.* 2019;139(6):799-811.

88. Ma N, Zhang JZ, Itzhaki I, et al. Determining the pathogenicity of a genomic variant of uncertain significance using CRISPR/Cas9 and human-induced pluripotent stem cells. *Circulation.* 2018;138(23):2666-2681.

89. Kodo K, Ong S-G, Jahanbani F, et al. iPSC-derived cardiomyocytes reveal abnormal TGF-β signalling in left ventricular non-compaction cardiomyopathy. *Nat Cell Biol.* 2016;18(10):1031-1042.

90. Wang Y, Liang P, Lan F, et al. Genome editing of isogenic human induced pluripotent stem cells recapitulates long QT phenotype for drug testing. *J Am Coll Cardiol.* 2014;64(5):451-459.

91. Garg P, Oikonomopoulos A, Chen H, et al. Genome editing of induced pluripotent stem cells to decipher cardiac channelopathy variant. *J Am Coll Cardiol.* 2018;72(1):62-75.

92. Liang P, Sallam K, Wu H, et al. Patient-specific and genome-edited induced pluripotent stem cell–derived cardiomyocytes elucidate single-cell phenotype of Brugada syndrome. *J Am Coll Cardiol.* 2016;68(19):2086-2096.

93. Lee J, Termglinchan V, Diecke S, et al. Activation of PDGF pathway links LMNA mutation to dilated cardiomyopathy. *Nature.* 2019;572(7769):335-340.

94. Sayed N, Liu C, Ameen M, et al. Clinical trial in a dish using iPSCs shows lovastatin improves endothelial dysfunction and cellular cross-talk in LMNA cardiomyopathy. *Sci Transl Med.* 2020;12(554):eaax9276.

SECTION II

RISK FACTORS FOR CARDIOVASCULAR DISEASE

Epidemiology, Pathophysiology, and Treatment of Hypertension

Michael E. Hall, John E. Hall, and Paul K. Whelton

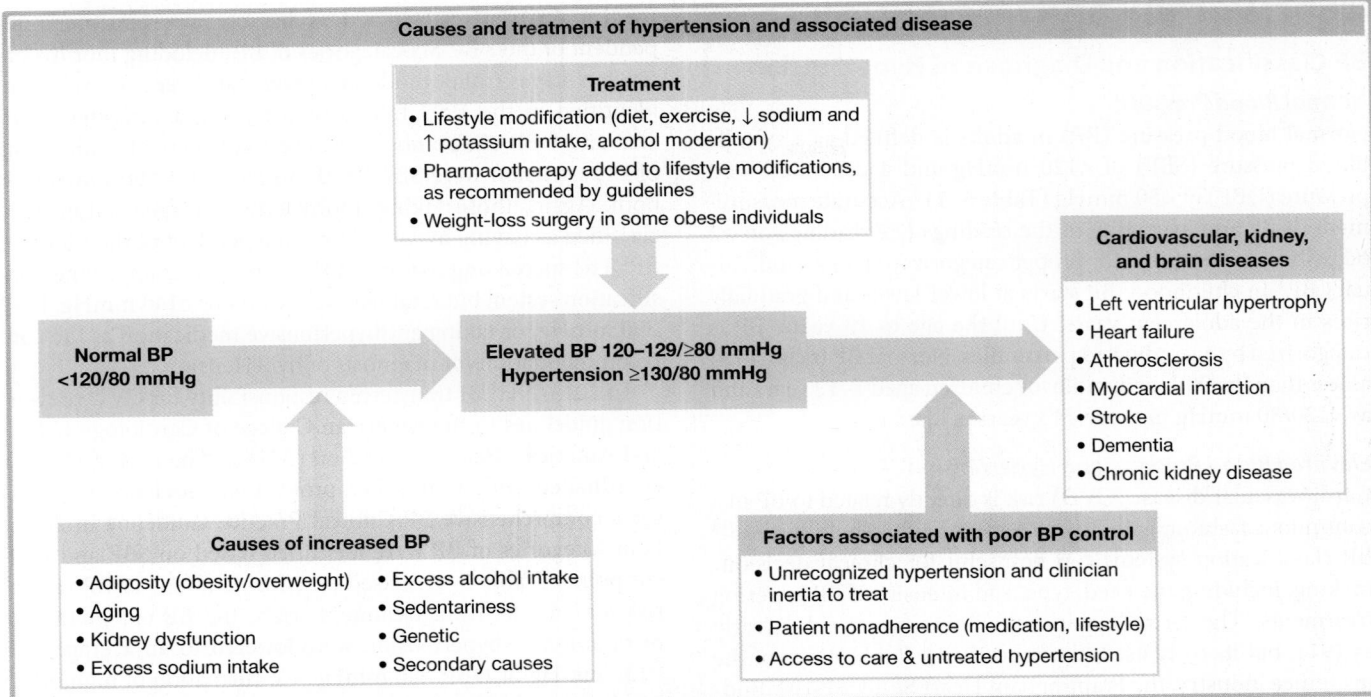

Chapter 5 Fuster and Hurst's Central Illustration. Hypertension is one of the strongest risk factors for cardiovascular, kidney and brain diseases, and overall mortality. Causes and treatment are shown. Lifestyle modifications are the cornerstone for treatment and prevention of hypertension but medications are often required to adequately control blood pressure (BP).

CHAPTER SUMMARY

This chapter reviews the epidemiology, pathophysiology, diagnosis, and treatment of hypertension. The worldwide prevalence of hypertension is increasing with an aging population and increased prevalence of overweight and obesity. Hypertension is one of the strongest risk factors for cardiovascular diseases (myocardial infarction, heart failure, atrial fibrillation, and stroke), kidney disease, dementia, and overall mortality. Modifiable risk factors for hypertension include poor diet, excessive sodium intake, reduced physical activity, excessive weight gain, and alcohol intake (see Fuster and Hurst's Central Illustration). Strategies focused on lifestyle modifications provide the cornerstone for the treatment and prevention of hypertension, although medications are often required to control blood pressure adequately. Effective control of blood pressure clearly reduces the risk for cardiovascular, kidney and brain disease, and death. Despite the availability of effective and inexpensive medications to control blood pressure, worldwide hypertension control continues to be unsatisfactory, with control rates in the United States <50% and as low as 8% to 14% in low- and middle-income countries. Unrecognized hypertension, patient nonadherence, and clinician inertia perpetuate this problem. Recent clinical trials indicate that blood pressure targets should be even lower than recommended in previous hypertension guidelines for more effective reduction of cardiovascular disease risk. Patient engagement in the treatment plan, home blood pressure monitoring (HBPM), and telehealth strategies may help improve hypertension control rates.

EPIDEMIOLOGY OF HYPERTENSION

BP Classification and Diagnosis of Hypertension

Normal Blood Pressure

Normal blood pressure (BP) in adults is defined as a systolic blood pressure (SBP) of <120 mmHg and a diastolic blood pressure (DBP) of <80 mmHg (**Table 5–1**).[1] Accurate measurement of BP and averaging of the readings (≥2 readings on ≥2 occasions) are essential for proper categorization of an individual's BP.[1] In childhood, BP starts at lower levels and gradually rises in the adolescent years. Until the age of 13 years, BP is categorized by age-adjusted percentiles. Normal BP is classified as less than the 90th percentile for children aged 1–12 years and as <120/80 mmHg in those ≥13 years of age.[2]

Elevated Blood Pressure and Hypertension

Cardiovascular disease (CVD) risk is directly related to BP in a continuous fashion, with no evidence for a threshold in risk.[3–5] BP classification systems can be useful for clinical decision-making, including the need, type, and intensity of BP-lowering treatments. The term "hypertension" was employed as early as 1911, but its early use lacked specificity. Publications of the insurance industry, the Framingham Heart Study BP-risk findings, and documentation of BP-lowering benefits in the 1967 and 1970 Veterans Administration Cooperative Study Group trials led to the creation of a National Heart, Lung, and Blood Institute (NHLBI) task force in 1973 and to the first BP clinical practice guideline (JNC 1) in 1977.[6]

The earliest detailed system of BP classification was introduced in the JNC 4 in 1988.[7] With the exception of an *isolated systolic hypertension* category, the JNC 4 BP classification of hypertension was based on DBP and characterized as *mild* (90–104 mmHg), *moderate* (105–114 mmHg), and *severe* (≥115 mmHg) hypertension. Those taking antihypertensive

medication were categorized as having hypertension, independent of their BP. Six categories of BP, including four hypertension stages (mild, moderate, severe, and very severe), were identified in the 1993 JNC 5 report using a combination of SBP and DBP cut points. The lowest cut points for diagnosis of hypertension were SBP ≥140 mmHg, DBP ≥90 mmHg, or both. Again, those taking antihypertensive medication were classified as having hypertension, independent of their level of BP.[8] The succeeding JNC 6 and JNC 7 reports changed the classification system but retained the use of SBP ≥140 mmHg, DBP ≥90 mmHg, or taking antihypertensive medication as the core recommendation for diagnosis of hypertension.

In 2013, NHLBI transferred responsibility for CVD prevention guidelines to the American College of Cardiology (ACC) and American Heart Association (AHA).[9] The ACC and AHA coordinated with nine other professional societies to sponsor a comprehensive BP Clinical Practice Guideline in 2017.[1] Four categories of BP were identified based on SBP and DBP cut points (**Table 5–1**). Based on considerations of BP-related risk and results from treatment trials, the BP cut points for recognition of hypertension were lowered to an average SBP ≥130 mmHg or DBP ≥80 mmHg. Confirmation of high office BPs by out-of-office measurements (home BPs or ambulatory BP measurements) was recommended before accepting a diagnosis of hypertension.

In an analysis of the National Health and Nutrition Examination Survey (NHANES; 2011–2014), approximately 24% of US adults reported taking antihypertensive medication, and approximately 46% met the criteria for diagnosis of hypertension.[10] This was about 12% higher than the corresponding prevalence using the JNC 7 criteria. The discrepancy in hypertension prevalence using the two sets of criteria was greatest at younger ages and least at older ages. Because NHANES estimates are based on office BPs measured on a single occasion rather than on the ACC/AHA recommendation to use an average of two or more office BPs on two or more occasions and confirmation of office hypertension using out-of-office measurements, the true general population prevalence of ACC/AHA-diagnosed hypertension is less than 46%.

It is worth noting that BP is a continuous variable and that even though a person's BP may not identify the presence of hypertension, there may be changes in cardiovascular risk associated with increases or decreases in BP. Distributions in BP likely vary based on factors such as body weight, physical activity, and sodium intake. For example, if a normal weight individual with a BP of 105/65 mmHg gains 25 pounds, leading to a BP of 119/79 mmHg, this would still be considered normal range BP. However, the increase in BP may be elevated for that person, although the quantitative effects of these changes and subsequent risk are unclear. An example of differences in BP distribution was described by Lowenstein in a study of two Amazonian tribes that had similar backgrounds and cultures but different levels of sodium intake.[11] The Mundurucus incorporated salt into their diet to preserve and season their food, but the Carajas consumed almost no salt. Although both tribes had similar average BP levels (~110/60 mmHg) in the teen years (16–20 years), by age 51–60 years, the mean BP in Mundurucus

TABLE 5–1. Guideline Recommendations for BP Classification in Adults and Children

Adults* and Children ≥ 13 years†			
	SBP		DBP
Normal	<120 mmHg	and	<80 mmHg
Elevated	120–129 mmHg	and	<80 mmHg
Hypertension			
Stage I	130–139 mmHg	or	80–89 mmHg
Stage II	≥140 mmHg	or	≥90 mmHg
Children 1–12 years (percentile based)†			
Normal	<90th percentile		
Elevated	≥90th percentile or ≥120/80 mmHg to <95th percentile		
Hypertension			
Stage I	≥95th percentile to <95th percentile + 12 mmHg or 130/80 to 139/89		
Stage II	≥95th percentile + 12 mmHg or 140/90 mmHg		

*Based on 2017 American College of Cardiology/American Heart Association BP Guidelines[1]
†Based on 2017 American Academy of Pediatrics Clinical Practice Guidelines for screening and management of high blood pressure in children and adolescents[2]

men was 133/77 mmHg; however, average BP did not increase with aging in Carajas men (109/70 mmHg at 51–60 years of age). Even though variations in "normal" distributions in BP exist, on a population level, elevated and hypertensive range BPs are associated with subsequent CVD.[12]

Comparison of ACC/AHA and European Society of Cardiology/European Society of Hypertension BP Classifications

In general, there are many similarities between the 2018 European Society of Cardiology (ESC)/European Society of Hypertension (ESH) guidelines[13] and the ACC/AHA BP guidelines; however, there are some notable differences in BP thresholds. The ESC/ESH defines hypertension as SBP ≥140 mmHg or DBP ≥90 mmHg. Further, ESC/ESH normal BP ranges include optimal BP being defined as <120/80 mmHg, normal as 120–129/80–84 mmHg, and high normal as 130–139/85–89 mmHg. The ESC/ESH guidelines also have three stages of hypertension: (1) Grade I: 140–159/90–99 mmHg, (2) Grade 2: 160–179/100–109 mmHg, and (3) Grade 3: ≥180/110 mmHg. While the ESC/ESH guidelines did not lower the hypertension threshold, they denote the "high normal BP" range as 130–139/80–89 mmHg.

BP Screening

The 2017 Clinical Practice Guidelines for the Diagnosis, Evaluation, and Treatment of High Blood Pressure in Children and Adolescents published by the American Academy of Pediatrics in 2017 recommends screening for high BP in children ≥3 years old at annual preventative visits. The United States Preventive Services Task Force (USPSTF) recommends annual screening for adults aged >40 years or for those with increased risk for high BP, including those with an elevated BP, those who are overweight or obese, and those who are Black. Recognizing differences in normal BP cut points defined by the 2017 ACC/AHA BP Guidelines, the USPSTF recommends rescreening adults with normal BP (defined by USPSTF as <130/85 mmHg) without risk factors every 3–5 years. Screening should be performed with properly measured office BPs, and if elevated, should be confirmed with out-of-office BP measurements, including ambulatory BP monitoring (ABPM) or home BP monitoring (HBPM). ABPM is the preferred form of out-of-office BP measurement, but HBPM is a reasonable and more practical substitute, provided that the patient is trained to measure BP accurately. The requirements for accurate home BP measurements are identical to those previously outlined for office measurements. Longer-term use of HBPM provides an excellent way to engage patients in their own care. Obtaining readings in the morning, prior to taking BP medications, helps to determine whether the regimen is providing sufficient duration of action. A repeated sequence of morning and evening BPs on three successive days can provide a good appraisal of the extent to which BP is being controlled and whether there is a need to escalate drug dosage or add an additional agent.

Proper BP Measurement

Although measuring BP is a relatively simple technique, errors are common. The 2017 ACC/AHA BP Guidelines recommend a checklist of technical considerations including proper preparation of the patient, proper BP measurement techniques, and proper measurement recording and documentation. These recommendations include taking an average of two or more readings obtained on two or more occasions. The basic requirements for an accurate BP are a period of quiet rest (5 minutes is optimal), no talking prior to or during the measurement, correct patient positioning (sitting in a chair, with back support, and feet flat on the floor), arm comfortably supported on a flat surface such that the midbrachial area is at heart level, choice of a valid instrument (several validation web sites provide guidance, including STRIDE BP web site), use of the correct cuff position (normally, midbrachial) and size (with 80% of the bladder encircling the arm). Oscillometric devices are generally considered the preferred measurement devices because they eliminate the need for auscultation, avoid the requirement for frequent calibration that is essential with aneroid devices, and preclude the toxicity risks of mercury manometers. Out-of-office BP measurements, including ABPM and HBPM, are recommended to confirm the diagnosis of hypertension. Many BP measurement training and certification courses are available, including several recent modules on the AHA/American Medical Association Target:BP web site (https://targetbp.org/tools-downloads/?sort=topic&) and an excellent certification course sponsored by the Pan American Health Organization, World Hypertension League, Lancet Commission on Hypertension Group, Hypertension Canada, and Resolve to Save Lives (https://www.whleague.org/index.php/j-stuff/awareness-and-screening/new-online-bp-certification-course).

White Coat and Masked Hypertension

White coat hypertension is defined as having an elevated BP in the clinical setting but normal BP when measured in the normal environment (ie, home) with either HBPM or ABPM. Conversely, *masked hypertension* is defined by normal BP in the clinical setting but consistently higher than normal BP measured by HBPM or ABPM.

White coat hypertension, also called *isolated clinic hypertension*, is not uncommon, affecting 15% to 30% of some hypertensive populations.[14] The *white-coat effect* is the term used when describing this phenomenon in treated patients. This effect is more common in women, older adults, and patients with newly diagnosed hypertension and a limited number of office BP measurements. White coat hypertension has been associated with target organ damage and cardiovascular mortality in some studies; however, the evidence has been inconsistent and dependent on the risk profiles of included participants. The definition of white coat hypertension also affects the interpretation of these relationships. In the International Database of Home Blood Pressure in Relation to Cardiovascular Outcome (IDACO) study, Asayama and colleagues demonstrated consistent associations of white coat hypertension and cardiovascular risk when using daytime or nighttime BPs Hazard ratio (HRs) both 1.3, p < 0.05). However, when using 24-hour ABPM alone or in combination with daytime or nighttime BP measures, these relationships were no longer significant.[15] There are currently no randomized controlled trials demonstrating reductions in CVD outcomes by treating patients with white coat hypertension with antihypertensive medications. White coat hypertension can convert to sustained hypertension in up to 5% of individuals each year, so close monitoring, particularly with HBPM or ABPM, may be warranted to determine whether antihypertensive therapies are indicated. Since white coat hypertension has typically been associated with minimal to only slightly increased risk of CVD and all-cause mortality, expert opinion suggests that it can be managed using nondrug lifestyle interventions and careful monitoring to recognize progression to established hypertension.

Unlike white coat hypertension, masked hypertension is associated with increased CVD and all-cause mortality risk. The prevalence of masked hypertension was estimated to be 13% to 19% of participants in the IDACO study.[15] Since the cardiovascular risk implications of masked uncontrolled hypertension appear to be similar to masked hypertension, further monitoring by HBPM or ABPM may be indicated in those under suspicion of having that condition. Patients with an average BP close to the cut point for diagnosis of hypertension and/or target organ damage (ie, left ventricular hypertrophy) or other cardiovascular risk factors may benefit from HBPM or ABPM to screen for masked hypertension. The 2017 ACC/ACC BP Guidelines recommended (Class IIa) continuation of lifestyle modification and initiation of antihypertensive drug therapy for patients suspected of masked hypertension and confirmed by ABPM or HBPM. Other characteristics associated with masked hypertension include older age, male sex, smoking, or patients with elevated body mass index (BMI), diabetes, or dyslipidemia.[14]

Resistant, Pseudoresistant, and Refractory Hypertension

Resistant hypertension is defined as high BP despite the use of at least three antihypertensive medications including (typically) a long-acting calcium channel blocker, a renin-angiotensin-aldosterone system (RAAS) blocker, and a diuretic (usually thiazide-like) at maximal or maximally tolerated doses.[16] Among nearly 24,000 patients on three or more antihypertensive medications for at least 1 month, the prevalence of resistant hypertension was 16%. Patients with resistant hypertension were more likely to be men, White, older, and diabetic compared to patients with nonresistant hypertension. Patients with resistant hypertension were also 50% more likely to experience a cardiovascular event over a median follow-up of 3.8 years compared to those without resistant hypertension.[17] Other comorbid conditions, including chronic kidney disease (CKD), obesity, and ischemic heart disease, are associated with resistant hypertension. It is important to note that healthy lifestyle factors, including normal waist circumference, diet, low sodium intake, physical activity, and nonsmoking, are associated with significantly lower risk for cardiovascular events in individuals with apparent treatment-resistant hypertension.[18]

The term *apparent treatment-resistant hypertension* is used when medication dose, adherence, or out-of-office BP is not documented or accounted for, and pseudoresistance cannot be excluded in a patient on three or more antihypertensive medications. In a recently published analysis of apparent treatment-resistant hypertension in Black participants from the Jackson Heart Study and the Reasons for Geographic and Racial Differences in Stroke (REGARDS) study, 28% of participants had apparent treatment-resistant hypertension. Among these, only 6% reported taking a thiazide-like diuretic and only 10% reported taking a mineralocorticoid receptor antagonist—therapies that are recommended in the 2018 AHA Scientific Statement on Resistant Hypertension.[19]

Pseudoresistance describes falsely elevated BPs in patients on three or more antihypertensive medications due to factors such as improper BP measurement techniques, white coat hypertension, medication nonadherance, or clinician undertreatment.[16] Among factors leading to pseudoresistant hypertension, medication nonadherence, undertreatment, and clinician inertia are the most common and most troubling. In an analysis of >200 community-based outpatient clinics including over 468,000 patients with hypertension, 44,644 were identified with apparent treatment-resistant hypertension.[20] Of these, only 15% had been prescribed optimal antihypertensive therapies, thus highlighting the role of clinician inertia in pseudoresistance.

Refractory hypertension is the term used to describe antihypertensive treatment failure in which BP remains uncontrolled on maximal or near-maximal therapy, typically with the use of five or more antihypertensive agents of different classes, including a thiazide-like diuretic and a mineralocorticoid antagonist.[16] From limited reported data, <5% to nearly 18% of patients with apparent treatment-resistant hypertension have refractory hypertension. Compared to patients with resistant hypertension, those with refractory hypertension are younger, more likely men, and have more target organ damage.[21]

Resistant and refractory hypertension are uncommon in randomized controlled trials, even in trials with low BP targets. In the Systolic Blood Pressure Intervention Trial (SPRINT), an average SBP of 121.5 mmHg was achieved in the intensive treatment group based on the use of an average of three medications.[22] A high percentage of patients have also met BP targets in health-care systems that employ a structured team-based treatment approach with careful monitoring of BP levels.[23,24]

Hypertensive Crises

Although most patients with severely elevated BPs (>180/120 mmHg) are asymptomatic, these patients may present with evidence of target organ damage or failure. When asymptomatic, these episodes are called *hypertensive urgencies*. In the setting of symptoms of acute or worsening target organ damage, these episodes are referred to as *hypertensive emergencies*. Target organ damage that can manifest during a hypertensive emergency includes acute myocardial ischemia or infarction, intracranial hemorrhage, pulmonary edema or heart failure, acute kidney injury, acute hypertensive encephalopathy, ischemic stroke, and aortic dissection. Fortunately, hypertensive emergencies are rare, with about 0.6% of adult emergency department visits carrying a diagnosis of hypertension.[25]

Hypertensive emergencies can be triggered by sympathetic overactivity, including (1) withdrawal of antihypertensive medications such as clonidine, (2) pain, (3) sympathomimetic agents including amphetamines or cocaine, (4) pheochromocytoma with adrenergic storm, and (5) severe autonomic dysfunction. In women, hypertensive emergencies can occur in preeclampsia or eclampsia.

Prevalence of Hypertension

According to data from 135 population-based studies of nearly 1 million adults from 90 countries, 31.1% of the world's adults (1.39 billion people) had hypertension (defined as SBP ≥140 mmHg, DBP ≥90 mmHg, or the use of antihypertensive medication) in 2010.[26] According to the 2017 ACC/AHA BP Guideline BP thresholds, the prevalence of hypertension, based on data from the 2011 to 2014 NHANES Survey, was 46% (>103 million) in US adults, and antihypertensive therapy was recommended for 36%.[1,27] This compares to BP thresholds from the Joint National Committee on Prevention, Detection, Evaluation, and Treatment of High Blood Pressure (JNC 7) guidelines, where the prevalence of hypertension was estimated to be 32% and 34% of US adults were recommended antihypertensive therapy. Implementation of the 2017 ACC/AHA BP Guidelines was therefore associated with an increased prevalence of hypertension due to the lower BP thresholds.[1] The most current NHANES estimate of hypertension prevalence (108 million adults) and trends using the 130/80 or antihypertensive medications definition was based on 2017–2018 data. They reported a decline in prevalence from 47% in 1999–2000 to 42% in 2013–2014, followed by an increase to 45% in 2017–2018.[27] Most contemporary population surveys like NHANES rely on BP measurements obtained at a single visit, which probably results in an overestimate of hypertension prevalence compared with what would be found by using an average of two or more readings taken on two or more visits as recommended by BP guidelines and out-of-office confirmation of office hypertension.

Lifetime Risk for Hypertension

Data were pooled from three large, contemporary cohort studies, the Coronary Artery Risk Development in Young Adults (CARDIA) study, the Atherosclerosis Risk in Communities (ARIC) study, and the Framingham Offspring Study, in order to determine the cumulative lifetime risk for hypertension from ages 20 through 85 years. Using the 2017 ACC/AHA BP Guideline definitions, the cumulative lifetime risks for hypertension were 86% for Black men and 84% for White men. The cumulative lifetime risks for Black and White women were 86% and 69%, respectively. These data are consistent with those published from the Framingham Heart Study, demonstrating a residual lifetime risk for hypertension for middle-aged and older adults around 90%.[28]

Hypertension and Race/Ethnicity

There are significant differences in hypertension prevalence and BP control rates based on race and ethnicity. The pathophysiologic mechanisms behind these racial/ethnic differences are not completely understood. Some explanations proposed for these differences in hypertension prevalence and responses to antihypertensive therapies include higher burden of adiposity, variability in sodium intake and retention, and socioeconomic

factors, such as access to health care and poverty, which may contribute to stress. These factors may interact with genetic and other environmental factors, leading to observed variations in BP across racial/ethnic populations. A subanalysis of incident myocardial infarction, acute coronary syndrome, stroke, decompensated heart failure, or CVD death in SPRINT demonstrated similar benefits and risks among non-Hispanic Whites, non-Hispanic Blacks, and Hispanics targeting an SBP goal of ≤120 mmHg compared to ≤140 mmHg (HRs 0.70, 0.71, 0.62, respectively, p-interaction = 0.85). It is important to note that in this study, Black participants required an average of ~0.3 more medications to control BP.[29]

Black Americans have a higher prevalence of hypertension than other racial/ethnic groups. Based on 2017–2018 data from NHANES, the age-adjusted prevalence was higher in non-Hispanic Black (57%) compared to non-Hispanic White (44%) and Hispanic (44%) adults in the United States (**Figure 5–1**). While the age-adjusted prevalence of hypertension is highest among Black men (57%) compared to White (50%) and Hispanic (50%) adult men, Black women also have a disproportionately higher prevalence of hypertension (57%) than White (37%) and Hispanic (37%) adult women.[27,30] In the United States, Black individuals develop hypertension at an earlier age compared to Whites, and they have higher average BP. They are also more likely to have resistant hypertension compared with other racial/ethnic groups.[31] Black adults are also more likely to develop left ventricular hypertrophy and heart failure compared with Whites. Compared to White adults, Black adults have higher rates of incident CVD and worse outcomes from stroke and end-stage kidney disease as well.

Many investigations have examined potential genetic and environmental etiologies for racial/ethnic differences in BPs. Although genetic polymorphisms affecting sodium and potassium exchange have been implicated to play a minor role,[32] research has failed to yield gene variants that explain racial/ethnic differences in BP. However, apolipoprotein L1 (APOL1) variants have been linked to worse outcomes, including advanced kidney disease,[33] in patients with hypertension. Environmental factors appear to play a much larger role in BP

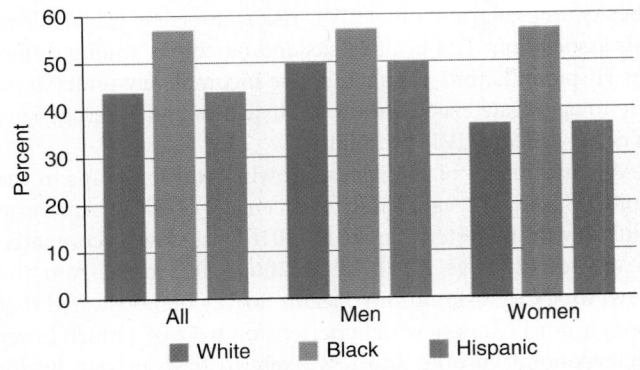

Figure 5–1. Hypertension prevalence (age-adjusted) in adults in the United States based on sex and race. Data from National Center for Health Statistics. National Health and Nutrition Examination Survey, 2017–2018.

disparities. This was highlighted in a study of members of the Luo tribe who migrated from rural western Kenya to an urban environment in Nairobi. Poulter and colleagues observed significantly higher mean SBPs and a right-shifted distribution of BPs in migrants compared to controls who stayed in the rural environment. Significantly higher BPs were observed within 1 month of urbanization. This was accompanied by rapid increases in body weight and urinary sodium:potassium ratio, suggesting that diet had played a major role in the BP increase.[34] This is consistent with results from a mediation analysis of a large prospective cohort of 30,239 participants in the United States demonstrating that key factors mediating the racial differences in incident hypertension rates were the Southern diet (high in fats, fried foods, processed meats, and sugar-sweetened beverages), dietary sodium:potassium ratio, and education.[35] Psychosocial factors are also associated with hypertension. Investigators from the Jackson Heart Study, a large community-based cohort of Black adults in Jackson, Mississippi, found that perceived stress was associated with incident hypertension[36] and lower perceived support was associated with reduced nocturnal BP dipping.[37]

The Hispanic American population, currently about 57 million, is the fastest-growing ethnic minority population in the United States and expected to double within the next four decades. Based on recent estimates, the prevalence of hypertension is similar in Hispanic and White adults in the United States.[38] However, there is significant heterogeneity in cultural, socioeconomic, and genetic factors that likely influence the prevalence of hypertension among the Hispanic/Latino populations. For example, the 6-year probability of developing hypertension was higher in Hispanic men of Dominican (28%) and Cuban (27%) ancestry compared with Mexican American men (18%) of the Hispanic Community Health Study/Study of Latinos. Among Hispanic/Latino women, the probability was higher among women of Cuban (23%), Dominican (23%), and Puerto Rican (28%) descent, compared with Mexican American women (16%).[39] Similar to other racial/ethnic populations, hypertension and CVD are a major cause of mortality in Hispanic populations. However, in 2018, Hispanics were 10% less likely to have coronary heart disease compared to Whites[40] and in 2017 were 30% less likely to die from heart disease,[41] leading to what has been termed the "Hispanic paradox." Lower rates of obesity, smoking, and other CVD risk factors may play a role in this association. The health risks and outcomes among different Hispanic/Latino populations are incompletely understood due to aggregate classification of Hispanics and heterogeneity in cause-specific CVD mortality.[42]

Asians are one of the fastest-growing ethnic groups in the United States. The age-adjusted percentage of Asian American adults with hypertension 2013–2016 was lower compared to Whites (27% vs 29%).[43] The 2009–2013 data from the New York City Community Health Survey demonstrated that foreign-born Chinese with hypertension were of a much lower socioeconomic profile and less likely to have private health insurance than were Whites. South Asians with hypertension were younger than Whites and had poorer diets. Chinese

and South Asian adults with hypertension had lower BMI than Whites (25 and 26 vs 29 kg/m², p < 0.001).[44] Aggregation of Asian/Pacific Islander subgroups has made it difficult to accurately assess outcomes for Asian American subgroups. Although standardized mortality rates for all CVD are lower in Asian Americans compared to Whites, there is greater proportionate mortality from hypertensive heart disease and cerebrovascular disease in every Asian American subgroup (Asian Indian, Filipino, Japanese, Chinese, Korean, and Vietnamese). Also, Asian Indians and Filipinos exhibited proportionately greater mortality from ischemic heart disease.[45]

Risk Factors for Hypertension

Elevated BP and hypertension have numerous causes, including many modifiable risk factors (**Table 5–2**). Only a small percentage of patients with hypertension have nonmodifiable genetic etiologies. The pathophysiology of hypertension will be discussed in more detail later in this chapter. One of the strongest nonmodifiable predictors of hypertension is age. Age-related increases in BP have been observed in almost every population studied. However, in certain populations, such as hunter-gatherers, age-related increases in BP are minimal, suggesting that lifestyle factors including diet, physical activity, and consumption of alcohol play important roles in the development of hypertension. For example, in the Tsimane forager-farmers, a longitudinal study of BP in adults for over 8 years demonstrated very low prevalence of hypertension in women and men (4% and 5%, respectively).[46] They observed SBP increases of only 2.86 mmHg per decade of life in women and 0.91 mmHg in men. Of note, the Tsimane are lean and very active. Obesity is rare among Tsimane people, but the effect of BMI on BP is similar for Tsimane and Americans, although the Tsimane display lower median BPs than expected based on comparative BMIs of other populations.

Increased weight and adiposity are strong predictors of elevated BP and hypertension. It is estimated that overweight and obesity may account for up to 75% of human essential hypertension, and systolic and diastolic BPs increased linearly with BMI.[47] Based on NHANES data, abdominal obesity (waist circumference ≥102 cm for men and ≥88 cm for women) was independently associated with hypertension (odds ratio 1.51, 95% confidence interval 1.27–1.81), even after adjusting for

TABLE 5–2. Modifiable and Nonmodifiable Risk Factors for Hypertension

Nonmodifiable Risk Factors	Modifiable Risk Factors
Older age	Obesity/adiposity
Male sex	Sedentariness/physical inactivity
Race	Sleep-disordered breathing
Genetic variants (rare)	Diabetes
Psychosocial stress	Smoking
Low socioeconomic status	Excessive alcohol intake
	High sodium intake
	Low potassium intake

BMI. Other important risk factors for hypertension include diabetes, CKD, obstructive sleep apnea, poor diet, reduced physical activity, sedentariness, and smoking. Of note, many of these risk factors, except perhaps smoking, occur in people who are overweight or obese.

Many patients with hypertension have other risk factors for CVD. For example, in the Action to Control Cardiovascular Risk in Diabetes Study Group (ACCORD) trial of 10,251 diabetic patients (mean age 62 years) designed to assess whether intensive glucose control would reduce CVD events, 85% of the participants were on antihypertensive therapy.[48] Further, the Centers for Disease Control and Prevention (CDC) reports that 68% of adults with diabetes in the United States from 2013–2016 with diabetes-related complications either had a BP ≥140/90 mmHg or were taking antihypertensive medication.[49] Given the collinearity of the prevalence of hypertension and diabetes, it is difficult to assess temporal relationships between the two commonly occurring comorbid conditions to determine cause and effect. In observational studies, type 2 diabetes has been associated with an increased risk of hypertension and vice versa. Sun and colleagues[50] examined the bidirectional relationships of type 2 diabetes with hypertension in 318,664 participants from the United Kingdom Biobank using Mendelian randomization analysis, and their results suggest type 2 diabetes was associated with increased hypertension risk; however, the converse (hypertension increasing risk for type 2 diabetes) was not observed. It is important to note that in many studies such as this one, it is difficult to fully assess these relationships, particularly due to the confounding of adiposity. As discussed previously, most people with type 2 diabetes are overweight or obese, and increased adiposity is a major cause of essential hypertension. Further, most studies assessing these relationships use BMI to assess adiposity, which has limitations for assessing body composition (distinguishing between muscle, bone, and adipose tissue).

There is an inverse relationship between physical activity and incident hypertension. A systematic review and meta-analysis of 29 studies demonstrated the risk of hypertension was also dose-dependently reduced by 6% with each 10 metabolic equivalents of task/hours per week of leisure-time physical activity.[51] Among treatment resistant hypertensive adults, 42% are physically inactive. At all levels of BP, physical activity levels are dose-dependently associated with lower mortality.[52] The 2018 Physical Activity Guidelines Advisory Committee reported strong evidence demonstrating that (1) there is an inverse dose-response relationship between physical activity and incident hypertension in adults with normal BP; (2) physical activity reduces the risk of CVD;[53] (3) physical activity reduces BP in adults with normal BP, prehypertension, and hypertension; and (4) the magnitude of the BP response to physical activity varies by resting BP, with greater benefits in adults with prehypertension than with normal BP.

Dietary factors such as excess sodium intake and inadequate potassium intake are also associated with hypertension. The International Study on Macro/Micronutrients and Blood Pressure (INTERMAP) data demonstrated higher dietary sodium and higher sodium-to-potassium intake ratio is associated with higher BP, and that multiple other macronutrients and micronutrients have minimal effects on the sodium-BP relationship, underscoring the need to reduce sodium intake to prevent and treat hypertension.[54] A systematic review of 24 trials including 23,858 participants demonstrated modest BP effects (−3.07/1.81 mmHg) from different dietary interventions, including the Dietary Approaches to Stop Hypertension (DASH) diet, low-calorie, low-sodium, and Mediterranean diets.[55] In the DASH-Sodium trial, the combination of the DASH diet (rich in fruits, vegetables, whole grains, nuts, legumes, lean protein, and low-fat dairy products, and low in refined sugars) and reduced sodium intake lowered SBP throughout the range of prehypertension and stage I hypertension with progressively greater reductions at higher levels of baseline SBP. Further, there were profound reductions (−20.8 mmHg) in SBP in adults with SBP ≥ 150 mmHg randomized to the low-sodium DASH diet compared to controls.[56] While these feeding trials probably demonstrate close to maximal potential for dietary change (with or without sodium reduction) to lower BP; in real-world practice settings where we have to rely on behavior change, the BP effect is (unfortunately) much less.

Social determinants of health are also risk factors for hypertension. These include socioeconomic factors such as income, education, employment, and access to health care, among others. These social determinants play a role in disparities of CVD prevalence and outcomes, particularly in minority populations. For example, hypertension is more prevalent in Blacks than Whites, and Blacks experience worse health outcomes, including increased risk for stroke, heart failure, and CKD.[57,58]

Blood Pressure and Cardiovascular Risk

Although the term "benign essential hypertension" has been used to refer to the most common form of hypertension, this is clearly a misnomer, as hypertension is neither benign nor essential. Data from numerous observational studies, including the Framingham Heart Study, have demonstrated that higher levels of BP are associated with increased risk for CVD.[59] The Prospective Studies Collaboration meta-analysis of 61 cohorts, including participants ages 40–89 years recruited between 1950 and 1990, reported log-linear associations of SBP and DBP with death from ischemic heart disease and stroke, with no apparent threshold below which no further risk reduction is observed, down to a BP of 115/75 mmHg (**Figure 5–2**).[3] Other large meta-analyses have shown similar findings, even studies of younger participants and those with a wider range of BP. In one of these analyses, the lifetime risk of total CVD at 30 years of age was estimated at 63% in people with hypertension (defined as ≥140/90 mmHg or taking antihypertensive medications) and 46% in those with normal BP <140/90 mmHg). They also observed that in each age group, the lowest risk for CVD was in people with an SBP 90–114 mmHg and a DBP 60–74 mmHg, with no evidence of a J-shaped increase at lower BPs.[4] In an analysis of participants from the Multi-Ethnic Study of Atherosclerosis without dyslipidemia, diabetes, or current tobacco use, and with an SBP level between 90 and 129 mmHg,

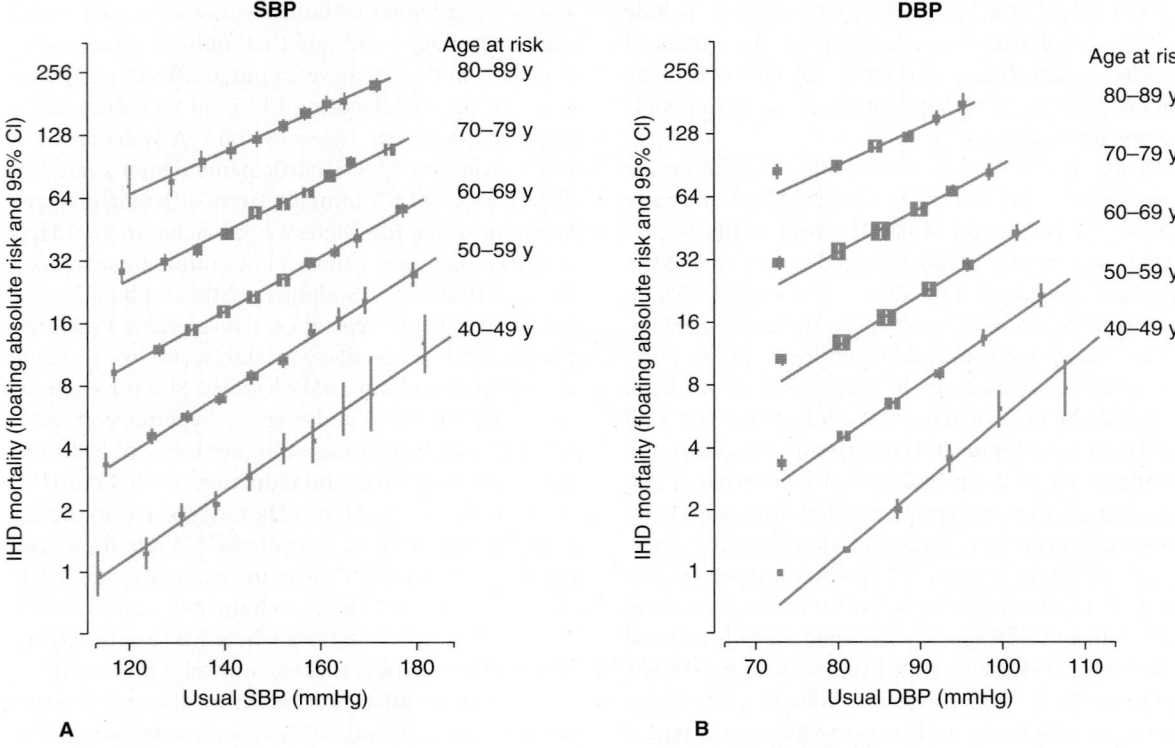

Figure 5–2. Risk of death from ischemic heart disease and stroke increases in a log-linear manner with both systolic and diastolic blood pressure. Reproduced with permission from Lewington S, Clarke R, Qizilbash N, et al. Age-specific relevance of usual blood pressure to vascular mortality: a meta-analysis of individual data for one million adults in 61 prospective studies. *Lancet.* 2002 Dec 14;360(9349):1903-1913.

Whelton and colleagues observed a stepwise increase in the presence of coronary artery calcium with increasing SBP and a 53% increased risk for incident atherosclerotic CVD for every 10 mmHg increase in SBP level. These results highlight the importance of primordial prevention for increases in SBP even in the lower end of the BP distribution, with BP values traditionally considered to be normal.[5]

Hypertension is a modifiable risk factor for CVD, including myocardial infarction, stroke, and heart failure. Most CVD can be attributed to several common modifiable risk factors, including hypertension. In the multinational, prospective cohort study Prospective Urban Rural Epidemiology (PURE), including 155,722 participants from 21 different countries, Yusuf and colleagues examined associations for modifiable risk factors with mortality and CVD. Metabolic factors including hypertension, diabetes, cholesterol, BMI, and waist-to-hip ratio were the predominant risk factors for CVD, with a population attributable fraction of 41%.[60,61] Among these metabolic factors, hypertension had the largest impact on CVD risk, accounting for 22% of the population attributable fraction (**Figure 5-3**).[61] In comparison, high cholesterol had a population attributable fraction of 8%, tobacco use 6%, and diabetes 5%. The Global Burden of Disease, Injuries, and Risk Factors Study (GBD) 2017 showed that high SBP was the leading risk factor (among 84 behavioral, environmental and occupational, and metabolic risks) accounting for 10.4 million deaths and 218 million disability-adjusted life-years.[60]

The risk for coronary heart disease increases in a log-linear manner with increases in BP above 115/75 mmHg in age

groups from 40 to 89 years. For each 20/10 mmHg increase in SBP/DBP, there is a doubling of mortality due to coronary heart disease.[3] This increase in risk has been primarily described in relation to associations with SBP. Strong relationships with

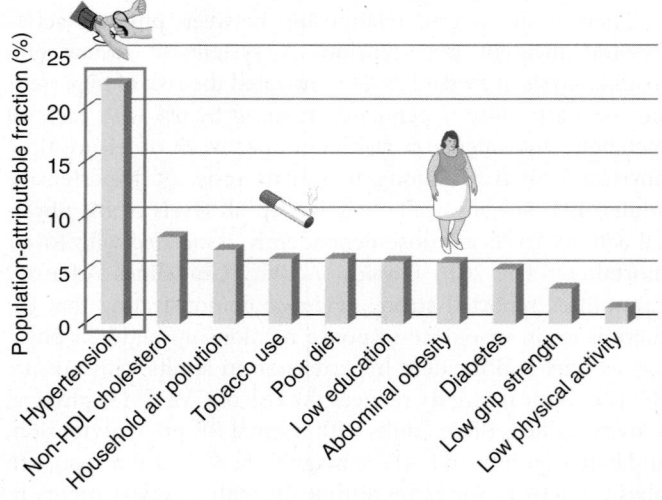

Figure 5–3. Population-attributable fraction (percentages) for 14 potentially modifiable risk factors for CVD (cardiovascular death, myocardial infarction, stroke, and heart failure) and mortality from 155,722 participants from the PURE prospective cohort study. Data from Yusuf S, Joseph P, Rangarajan S, et al. Modifiable risk factors, cardiovascular disease, and mortality in 155 722 individuals from 21 high-income, middle-income, and low-income countries (PURE): a prospective cohort study. *Lancet.* 2020 Mar 7;395(10226):795-808.

elevated DBP and CVD have been established; however, there has been some controversy over whether low DBP in patients with prevalent coronary heart disease is associated with increased mortality. Some hypothesize that a DBP below certain levels (70 mmHg) may be detrimental due to a reduction in coronary artery perfusion pressure that occurs during diastole. Paradoxical increases in mortality with "excessive" reductions in DBP, often called a "J-curve," were reported in the International Verapamil-Trandolapril Study (INVEST) trial,[62] and the CLARIFY registry observed a 50% higher risk for cardiovascular death or myocardial infarction in patients with DBP <70 mmHg.[63] However, evidence from other large analyses, such as the CALIBER (CArdiovascular research using LInked Bespoke studies and Electronic health Records) program including 1.25 million patients, demonstrated the lowest CVD risk in people with DBP of 60–74 mmHg with no evidence of a J-shaped increased risk at lower BPs.[4] SPRINT investigators did identify a U-shaped association with baseline DBP and CVD risk in nonrandomized analyses; however, participants randomized to intensive BP treatment had better CVD outcomes and lower all-cause mortality across the spectrum of baseline DBP, even among those in the lowest quintile of DBP at baseline.[64] Thus, low levels of DBP (within the range examined in SPRINT) probably should not be an impediment to treating hypertension to recommended goals.

Hypertension is a well-known major risk factor for development of heart failure. In the original Framingham Heart Study and the Framingham Offspring Study, Levy and colleagues observed that 91% of new cases of heart failure were preceded by a diagnosis of hypertension. The adjusted hazard ratio for incident heart failure in participants with hypertension (compared to men with normal BP) was twofold higher in men and threefold higher in women.[65] A similar association has been observed in other populations, including Black participants of the Jackson Heart Study where every 10 mmHg increase in SBP was associated with a 7% increase in risk for heart failure hospitalization.[66] Incident heart failure is much more common (20 times higher) in Black adults than White adults before the age of 50 years. This higher incidence is predicted by the presence of hypertension, obesity, and CKD prior to a heart failure diagnosis.[67] Higher SBP in mid- to late life was associated with worse late-life left ventricular structure and diastolic function and higher incident heart failure in the ARIC study. Teramato and colleagues also found that time-averaged cumulative SBP was more robustly associated with risk of incident heart failure than a single-time-point SBP.[68] These findings suggest that the risk of heart failure depends on the magnitude *and* duration of exposure to hypertension.

In patients with hypertension and left ventricular hypertrophy,[69] losartan-based treatment of BP reduced left ventricular mass in the LIFE trial,[70] and intensive BP lowering with an angiotensin receptor blocker and calcium channel blocker improved left ventricular diastolic function in patients with uncontrolled hypertension.[71] Although effective treatments for heart failure with preserved ejection fraction (HFpEF) have been elusive, data from a subanalysis of the Antihypertensive and Lipid-Lowering Treatment to Prevent Heart Attack Trial (ALLHAT) demonstrated a 50% reduction in incident HFpEF with chlorthalidone treatment. In the Prevention of Hypertension in Patients with Prehypertension (PREVER-Prevention) Trial, treatment of patients with prehypertension with chlorthalidone and amiloride prevented incident hypertension by nearly 50% and reduced left ventricular mass.[69] Taken together, these findings highlight the importance of prevention and control of hypertension, rather than specific antihypertensive medications, to prevent left ventricular structural and functional abnormalities and subsequent heart failure later in life.

Hypertension is more prevalent in Black adults in the United States compared to other racial/ethnic groups and therefore may be an even greater risk factor in Black adults. Clark and colleagues examined the attributable risk of hypertension using the 2017 ACC/AHA BP Guidelines on incident CVD in the Jackson Heart Study and Black participants in the REGARDS study. They observed a twofold higher risk for incident CVD over >14 years of follow-up in Black participants with hypertension compared to those with normal BP. The estimated population attributable risk for hypertension associated with incident CVD in Black participants was 33%. In addition, hypertension was associated with a substantial percentage of coronary heart disease (43%), heart failure (22%), and stroke (39%) events in this population.[72]

Pulse Pressure and Cardiovascular Risk

Systolic BP increases steadily with age, but DBP tends to fall after 50 years of age. *Pulse pressure*, which is the difference between systolic and diastolic BP and a measure of vascular stiffness, has been used to predict CVD risk in older adults. Factors associated with lower DBP and wide pulse pressure include older age, female sex, and diabetes.[73] In middle-aged and older adults (age 50–79 years) from the Framingham Heart Study, the risk for coronary heart disease increased with lower DBP at any level of SBP ≥120 mmHg, suggesting that higher pulse pressure was an important component of risk. They observed that neither SBP nor DBP was superior to pulse pressure in predicting coronary heart disease risk in this population.[74] However, investigators from the Chicago Heart Association Detection Project in Industry Study evaluated 25-year mortality rates for coronary heart disease in adults of different age groups and found that the relations of pulse pressure were weaker than were those of SBP for all end points in all age/sex groups. They found a stronger association between SBP and death compared with DBP, except for middle-aged men and for CVD in women. After controlling for SBP, DBP showed significant positive associations with death in middle-aged participants. They concluded that the long-term risk of hypertension should be assessed mainly on the basis of SBP or of SBP and DBP together, not on the basis of pulse pressure, in apparently healthy adults.[75] Other observational studies such as the REGARDS study demonstrated that pulse pressure was independently associated with incident coronary heart disease, even after adjustment for SBP, and there were no significant racial or regional differences in this association.[76]

Isolated Diastolic Hypertension

Based on the 2017 ACC/AHA BP Guidelines, isolated diastolic hypertension is defined as a DBP ≥80 mmHg with SBP <130 mmHg, which yields a prevalence of 1.3% to 6.5% in the United States.[77] Results from some large epidemiologic studies have demonstrated increased risk for ischemic heart disease and cerebrovascular disease with higher SBP and DBP (namely, DBP >75 mmHg).[3] Results from the ARIC study examined associations between isolated diastolic hypertension (using both the 2017 ACC/AHA BP Guidelines and the 2003 JNC7 definitions) and subclinical CVD or incident atherosclerotic CVD,[77] heart failure, or CKD. The ARIC investigators did not observe any significant associations with these outcomes or all-cause and cardiovascular mortality in ARIC and two other large external validation cohorts (NHANES and the CLUE II cohort study).

These findings do not suggest that elevated DBP is harmless, but rather that DBPs between 80 and 90 mmHg have no adverse prognostic significance when SBP is well controlled.[77] Comparing the 2017 ACC/AHA BP Guidelines with the 2018 ESC and the 2019 National Institute for Health Care Excellence (NICE) guidelines which uses a ≥140/90 mmHg BP threshold in participants of the United Kingdom Biobank, McGrath and colleagues observed a much higher prevalence of isolated diastolic hypertension with the 2017 ACC/AHA BP Guidelines compared to the latter (25% vs 6%, respectively). In this study, isolated diastolic hypertension using the 2017 AHA/ACC Guidelines was not associated with increased CVD risk compared to normal BP; however, it was associated with a modest increase in CVD (HR 1.15, 95% confidence interval 1.04–1.29) using the ESC/NICE definition.[78] The excess risk for the ESC/NICE definition of isolated diastolic hypertension was most evident in women and participants not on antihypertensive medications at baseline. While the 2017 ACC/AHA BP Guidelines recommend targets for both SBP and DBP, typically more attention is given to SBP, particularly for people over the age of 50. Incorporating average SBP and DBP marginally outperforms SBP in some populations; however, focusing on SBP is less complicated and easier to implement on a wide scale in clinical practice.

Nondipping Blood Pressure Increases Cardiovascular Risk

The 24-hour ABPM reading provides important information related to BP variation throughout the day and night. BP is variable in most individuals throughout the day and night, with higher levels observed in the day and a 10% to 20% fall in BP during sleep, often referred to as *nocturnal dipping*. Several large prospective studies have demonstrated increased risk of higher nighttime BP and a nondipping pattern with all-CVD, stroke, and cardiovascular mortality.[79–81] A large meta-analysis of 17,312 hypertensive patients in the Ambulatory Blood Pressure Collaboration in Patients with Hypertension (ABC-H) study demonstrated that nocturnal BP decline was an independent predictor of stroke, cardiovascular mortality, and total mortality even after adjustment for 24-hour SBP. Relative to participants with a normal dipping pattern, reverse dippers (ie, those with BP increases at night) had the worst prognosis for all outcomes, and reduced dippers had a 27% excess risk for total

cardiovascular events.[82] The pathophysiologic mechanisms associated with a blunted nocturnal BP fall include autonomic imbalance/sympathetic overactivity, altered baroreflex sensitivity, obesity, sleep-disordered breathing, endothelial dysfunction, and chronic inflammation, among others. Increased salt sensitivity and renal dysfunction may also play a role due to increased nocturnal volume overload requiring higher BPs to sustain natriuresis.[83]

Hypertension Control

Despite wide recognition that hypertension is a major risk factor for CVD, overall BP control rates remain suboptimal. Targeted strategies for controlling hypertension involve interventions to increase awareness, treatment, and control in individuals, and population-based strategies are designed to achieve small reductions in BP in the entire population. Limited access to health care, adherence, and therapeutic or clinician inertia are factors associated with suboptimal BP control.[84] Multilevel approaches and partnerships with all constituents (patient, provider, and health-care system) are required to optimize the prevention, recognition, and control of hypertension.

Awareness of having hypertension and insight into the risk associated with hypertension are both important factors that influence BP control in individuals. A recent study of a series of NHANES surveys (10 cycles conducted from 1999–2000 through 2017–2018) demonstrated that among adults with hypertension, the proportion who reported that they were aware they had hypertension initially increased from 70% in 1999–2000 to 85% in 2013–2014 and then declined to 77% in 2017–2018.[85] Hypertension awareness was more likely in participants with a usual health-care facility and in participants who had a health-care visit within the past year suggesting access to care is an important factor. Paulose-Ram and colleagues reported no significant differences in hypertension awareness between non-Hispanic Blacks and Whites (86 vs 85%, respectively); however, it was lower in Hispanics (80%) and Asian Americans (75%).[86]

Among all adults with hypertension, the number who had their BP controlled to <140/90 mmHg increased from 32% in 1999–2000 to 54% in 2013–2014. However, in 2017–2018, the control rate declined to 44%.[85] Among adults taking antihypertensive medication, the proportion with controlled BP increased from 53% in 1999–2000 to 72% 2013–2014, and then declined to 65% in 2017–2018. Younger adults with hypertension aged 18–44 years were less likely to have BP controlled compared to those aged 45–64 years. Controlled BP was less likely among Black adults compared to White adults (42% vs 48%, respectively) and ~50% more likely among those with private insurance or government insurance compared to no insurance.

The finding that younger adults are less likely to take antihypertensive medication highlights the need for increased efforts to ensure BP screening in younger adults. As Muntner and colleagues discuss, underuse of antihypertensive medications may be related to low perceived CVD risk, lack of access to health care, not having a usual source of care, or treatment discontinuation.[85] Given the high lifetime risk for CVD in young adults with hypertension[87] coupled with the higher likelihood of discontinuing antihypertensive medications,[88] greater focus should be placed on initiation of and adherence to antihypertensive medications in this group.

Low adherence is a major factor for uncontrolled hypertension. Among the 23.8 million US adults with hypertension who filled prescriptions for antihypertensive medications in 2015, the nonadherence rate was 31%, which was greater in women compared to men, greater in younger individuals, and differed by insurance plan type. Other factors associated with low adherence to antihypertensive medications include behavioral factors and depression, complex medication regimens and multiple pills, and issues with potential side effects from medications used to treat an asymptomatic disease.[84] Medication costs have been reported as presenting a barrier to antihypertensive medication adherence.[89] Fortunately, the costs of these medications have largely decreased, and many effective medications are now generic.

Although multiple patient-level factors affect BP control, there are also contributory physician- and health care–level factors (**Figure 5–4**). Therapeutic inertia or clinician inertia is a major barrier to achieving guideline-recommended BP control. In one large study of 7253 patients with hypertension, antihypertensive therapy was not intensified in 87% of visits when BP was ≥140/90 mmHg.[90] In another nationally representative ambulatory survey including 41.7 million primary care visits among US adults with hypertension with a BP ≥140/90 mmHg, only 17% (approximately 1 out of 6 visits) experienced

intensification with new medication.[91] There are several reasons that may contribute to clinicians not initiating or optimizing antihypertensive therapies, including time constraints (taking care of complex patients with many comorbidities), uncertainty about accuracy of BP measures (office BP vs HBPM by patients), inadequate knowledge of contemporary guidelines and BP targets, and concern about medication interactions or side effects.

In addition to initiation and optimization of antihypertensive medications for BP control, lifestyle modification is indicated in most individuals with hypertension. Lopez and colleagues reported that 84% of adult participants with hypertension receive recommendations for lifestyle modification, and among those receiving counseling, 88% reported adherence to the recommendations.[89] The most common advice that these participants reported was dietary sodium reduction (82%), exercise (79%), and weight loss (66%). However, recent evidence from Black participants in the Jackson Heart Study and REGARDS study with apparent treatment-resistant hypertension demonstrated low levels of ideal lifestyle factors, including physical activity (18%) or ideal BMI levels (10%). Only a fraction of Black adults with apparent treatment-resistant hypertension received appropriate antihypertensive therapies, including a thiazide-like diuretic (6%) or a mineralocorticoid receptor antagonist (10%).[92]

Control of BP requires multilevel (patient, provider, and health-care system) interactions to overcome these barriers to reduce long-term CVD risk. Primary care physicians are increasingly overwhelmed, and chronic disease guidelines appropriately call for greater recognition of risk and more

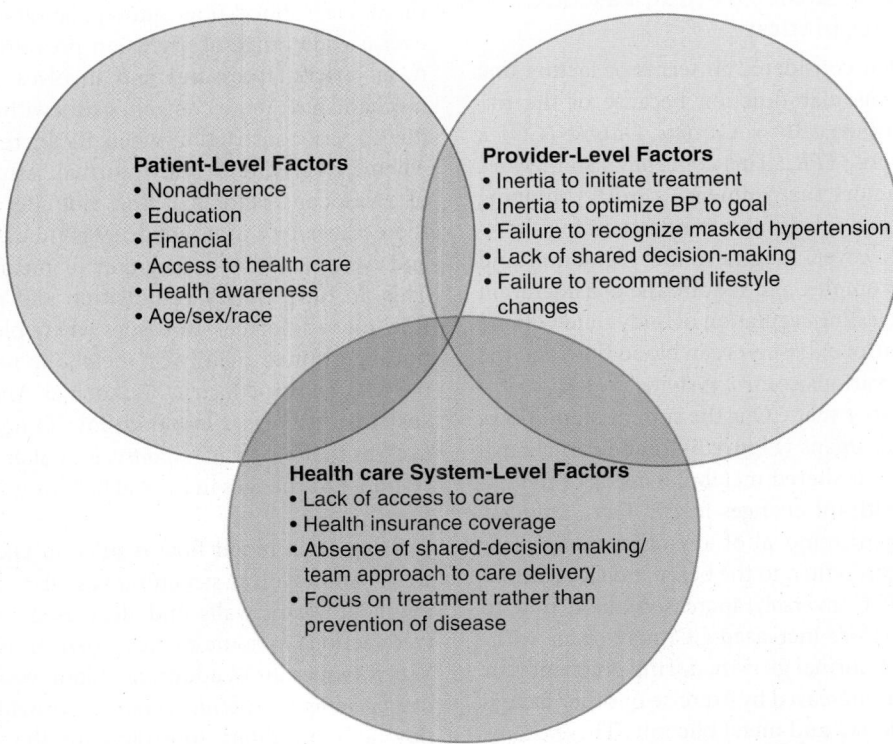

Figure 5–4. Many factors affect BP control. These include patient level (blue sphere), provider level (green sphere), and health-care system level factors (orange sphere), which intersect and overlap.

treatment to prevent CVD. The fundamental issue is that such a high percentage of the population is at increased risk for CVD, and clinical trials are progressively demonstrating the value of treating individuals at lower levels of risk factors (BP and lipids) and documenting the value of more intensive treatment. Strategies focused on increased shared decision-making, empowering patients to be their own primary caregivers, and collaborative team-based care may help address some of these barriers.[57,93,94] Other care delivery models, besides the classic in-person physician-patient model, may provide opportunities for optimal BP control on a wider population level. Incorporation of remote patient monitoring and telehealth delivery of care for BP control are obvious examples. Team-based care with multilevel implementation strategies has the biggest impact on improving BP treatment outcomes.[93] A community-based randomized controlled trial (HOPE-4) involving individuals with new or poorly controlled hypertension compared standard care and a comprehensive model of care led by nonphysician health workers that involved primary care physicians and families. This comprehensive model was associated with an absolute 11.5 mmHg additional reduction in SBP and an 11.2% reduction in the Framingham Risk Score in the group who received this comprehensive model, with no safety issues. Pragmatic strategies such as these models and the Chronic Care Model,[84] which include increased use of nonphysician health-care workers, have the potential to more effectively control BP and reduce CVD than current strategies that are typically physician based.[95]

PATHOPHYSIOLOGY OF HYPERTENSION

Basic Relationships of Cardiac Output, Vascular Resistance, and BP Regulation

Regulation of BP is often considered in terms of factors that influence cardiac and vascular function because of the following well-known formula: *BP = Cardiac Output (CO) x Total Peripheral Resistance (TPR)*. This conceptual framework focuses attention on factors that influence cardiac pumping and vascular resistance and is helpful for understanding short-term BP regulation. However, long-term BP regulation and hypertension are more complex and require the consideration of additional factors, including regulation of body fluid volume by the kidneys, local control of tissue/organ blood flow, and the time dependency of the various control systems for BP.

It is helpful to remember that CO is the sum of blood flows to the body's tissues and organs (**Figure 5–5**) and can change dramatically in response to altered metabolic needs of the tissues, often without significant changes in BP. Thus, amputation of an arm or a leg, or removal of any other tissue from the body, decreases venous return to the heart and CO without significantly altering BP. Conversely, increased blood flow to various tissues, and therefore increased CO, may occur without changes in BP during normal growth, during pregnancy, or when tissue blood flow is increased by exercise or other factors that increase tissue workload and metabolic rate. These examples illustrate that CO is determined not only by the pumping ability of the heart but also by the peripheral circulation.

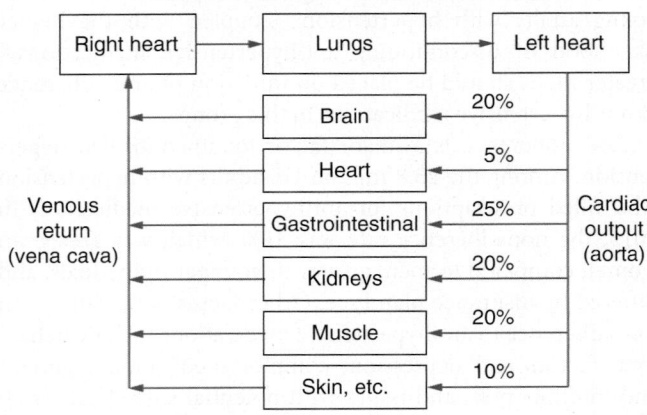

Figure 5–5. Relationship between cardiac output, peripheral blood flow regulation, and venous return.

Except when the heart is severely weakened and unable to adequately pump the venous return, CO and TPR are determined mainly by the metabolic needs and other special requirements of the body's tissues and organs. This conceptual framework helps to explain why CO and tissue blood flows are usually normal and TPR is elevated in chronic hypertension unless metabolic demands of the tissues are altered. With chronic hypertension, increases in TPR often occur secondary to increased BP, as a means of maintaining appropriate tissue blood flow rather than as a primary driver of hypertension.

One of the most fundamental principles of circulatory function is the ability of each tissue to *autoregulate* its own blood flow according to the metabolic needs and other functions of the tissue.[96] Blood flow autoregulation occurs in many tissues over a wide range of perfusion pressures (eg, 75–150 mmHg mean arterial pressure) and involves short- and long-term mechanisms. Acute control occurs within seconds or minutes due to vasoconstriction when BP increases or vasodilatation when BP is reduced below normal. Also, after administration of a vasoconstrictor that does not alter tissue metabolic rate, there is usually a transient decrease in tissue supply of nutrients and oxygen and accumulation of metabolic waste products. This, in turn, causes vasodilation and return of tissue blood flow toward normal. In tissues where blood flow regulation is not determined mainly by metabolic needs, such as the kidneys, some vasoconstrictors, such as Ang II, may cause small, sustained decreases in blood flow. Other short-term controls, such as the *myogenic response*, also alter vascular resistance in response to changes in BP and help to autoregulate tissue blood flow.[97]

Long-term blood flow regulation takes place over days or weeks and involves structural vascular changes, such as thickening of vessel walls and decreased numbers of capillaries (rarefaction) in some tissues when BP is chronically elevated. When tissues grow, additional blood vessels are generated (via *angiogenesis* or *vasculogenesis*) to provide the required blood flow and metabolic substrates for the tissues. Together, the short- and long-term mechanisms maintain the required levels of blood flow in each tissue to ensure normal function.

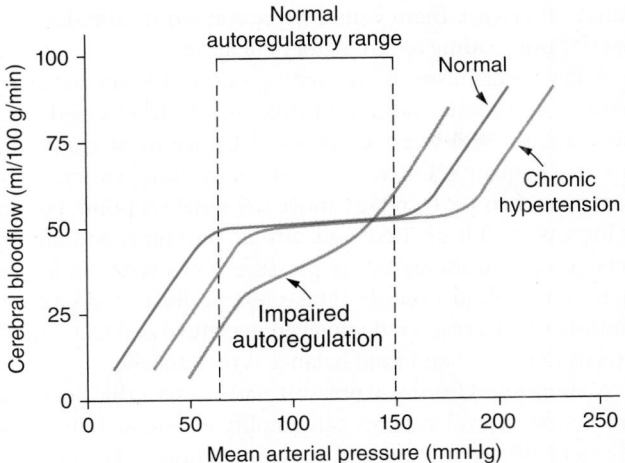

Figure 5–6. Autoregulation of blood flow during acute changes in mean arterial pressure in people with normal BP (blue curve), with chronic hypertension (red curve), and with impaired ability to autoregulate blood flow (black curve). The dashed vertical lines indicate the approximate normal range of autoregulation in many tissues.

In conditions such as heart failure, or when large increases in CO are needed to meet the metabolic demands of the body's tissues, such as exercise, various factors that alter cardiac pumping also play a major role in regulating CO.

Blood Flow Regulation in Hypertension

One characteristic of many, but not all, patients with hypertension is that they have increased TPR. This has led to the widely held belief that hypertension is usually caused by vasoconstriction. Yet, despite increased TPR in hypertension, tissue blood flows are approximately the same as in normotension and are regulated at a level that is adequate for the tissue needs. In many patients with hypertension, increased TPR appears to be an autoregulatory response that maintains normal tissue blood flow despite increased BP rather than a primary cause of hypertension. Thus, the hemodynamic pattern often observed in nonobese subjects with primary hypertension is normal blood flow, normal CO, and elevated vascular resistance.

Another important feature of blood flow regulation in hypertension is that the range of autoregulation is often shifted to higher BPs (**Figure 5–6**). This resetting is due partly to hypertrophic vascular remodeling as a compensation for chronic increases in BP. This adaptation helps prevent vascular wall stress as well as overperfusion and injury in organs such as the brain. With chronic antihypertensive therapy, the range of autoregulation gradually shifts back toward lower BP as regression of vascular hypertrophy occurs. However, rapid lowering of BP with overzealous antihypertensive therapy in patients with severe hypertension or in patients with impaired autoregulation due to endothelial/vascular injury (eg, atherosclerosis) may impair perfusion of some tissues, including the brain.

In the kidneys, autoregulation is determined by factors other than the metabolic needs and blood flow may be increased, normal, or decreased in primary hypertension. These seemingly disparate observations relate to the special mechanisms that balance glomerular filtration rate (GFR) with tubular reabsorption rate. For example, increased dietary protein, obesity, diabetes, and primary aldosteronism are all associated with increases in renal blood flow and GFR prior to nephron injury. In these cases, increases in renal blood flow and GFR serve as compensatory responses that offset elevated sodium reabsorption, helping to restore sodium balance. With prolonged, uncontrolled hypertension, obesity, and diabetes, there is often progressive nephron injury that leads to reductions in renal blood flow and GFR. Excessive renal vasoconstriction and decreased GFR may also initiate hypertension in some individuals.

Short-Term and Long-Term BP Regulation

BP varies throughout the day depending on activity of the body, environmental influences, and responses of multiple BP control systems. Although hypertension is usually considered to be a disorder of the average level at which BP is regulated during resting conditions, there is considerable interest in other measures of BP, including peak arterial pressure, lability of BP, nighttime and daytime BP, responses of BP to stress, and so forth when assessing cardiovascular risk.[98]

Feedback Control Systems for Blood Pressure Are Time Dependent

The quantitative importance of various BP controllers is highly time dependent, with some acting rapidly for moment-to-moment BP regulation while others are reacting slowly but powerfully for long-term control of BP. **Figure 5–7** shows the maximum feedback gains of some of the major control systems after a sudden change in BP, as might occur with rapid blood loss. Three neural control systems begin to function powerfully within seconds: (1) arterial baroreceptors, which

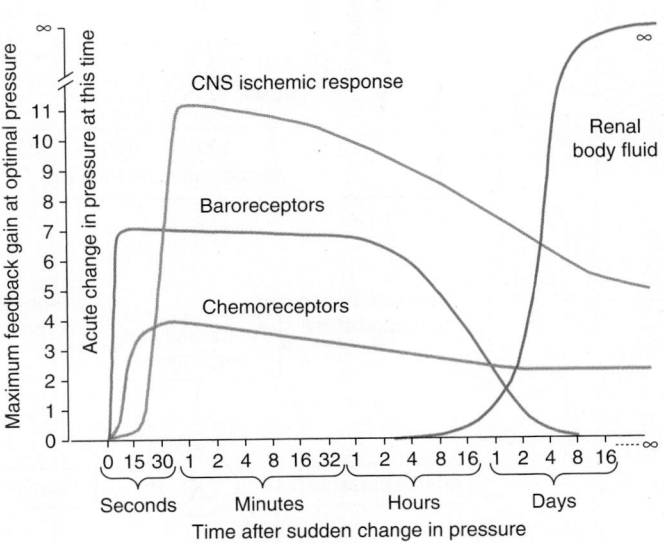

Figure 5–7. Time dependency of BP control mechanisms. Approximate maximum feedback gains of various BP control mechanisms at different time intervals after the onset of a disturbance to BP. Reproduced with permission from Hall JE, Hall ME. *Guyton and Hall Textbook of Medical Physiology,* 14th ed. Philadelphia, PA: Elsevier; 2021.

detect changes in BP and send appropriate autonomic reflex signals back to the heart and blood vessels to return the BP toward normal; (2) chemoreceptors, which detect changes in oxygen or carbon dioxide in the blood and initiate autonomic feedback responses that influence BP; and (3) the central nervous system (CNS), which responds within a few seconds to ischemia of the vasomotor centers in the medulla, especially when BP falls below about 50 mmHg. Each of these nervous mechanisms works rapidly and powerfully, but the feedback gains of these systems decrease with time if a BP disturbance is maintained.

Within a few minutes or hours after a BP disturbance, additional controls react, including (1) a shift of fluid from the interstitial spaces into the blood in response to decreased BP (or a shift of fluid out of the blood into the interstitial spaces in response to increased BP); (2) the RAAS, which is activated when BP falls too low and suppressed when BP increases above normal; and (3) multiple vasodilators systems (not shown in Figure 5–7) that are suppressed when BP decreases and stimulated when BP increases above normal.

Renal–Body Fluid Feedback for Long-Term BP Regulation

Figure 5–8 shows the conceptual framework for understanding a major long-term controller of BP and body fluid volume—the *renal–body fluid feedback*. Extracellular fluid volume is determined by the balance between intake and excretion of salt and water by the kidneys. Even temporary imbalances between intake and output can lead to changes in extracellular volume, and potentially changes in BP. During steady-state conditions, there must be a balance between intake and output of salt and water; otherwise, there would be continued accumulation or loss of fluid, leading to circulatory collapse.

A key mechanism for regulating salt and water balance is *pressure natriuresis* and *diuresis*, the effect of increased BP to raise sodium and water excretion.[99] Under most conditions, this mechanism stabilizes BP and body fluid volumes. For example, when BP increases above the renal set point, because of increased TPR or increased cardiac pumping, sodium and water excretion increases via pressure natriuresis. So long as excretion of fluid exceeds intake, extracellular fluid volume continues to decrease, reducing venous return and CO until BP returns to normal and fluid balance is reestablished.

An important feature of pressure natriuresis is that hormonal and neural control systems can amplify or attenuate the basic effects of BP on sodium and water excretion.[100] For example, during increases in sodium intake for several days, only small changes in BP occur in most people. One reason for this insensitivity of BP to changes in salt intake is decreased formation of Ang II and aldosterone, which enhances effectiveness of pressure natriuresis and allows sodium balance to be maintained with minimal increase in BP. On the other hand, overactivation of these antinatriuretic systems can reduce the effectiveness of pressure natriuresis, thereby necessitating greater increases in BP to maintain sodium balance.[100]

Another important feature of pressure natriuresis is that it continues to operate until BP returns to nearly the original set point. In other words, it acts as part of a near-infinite gain feedback control system.[101] It is the only known feedback system for BP regulation that displays near-infinite feedback gain, and this property makes it a dominant long-term BP controller.

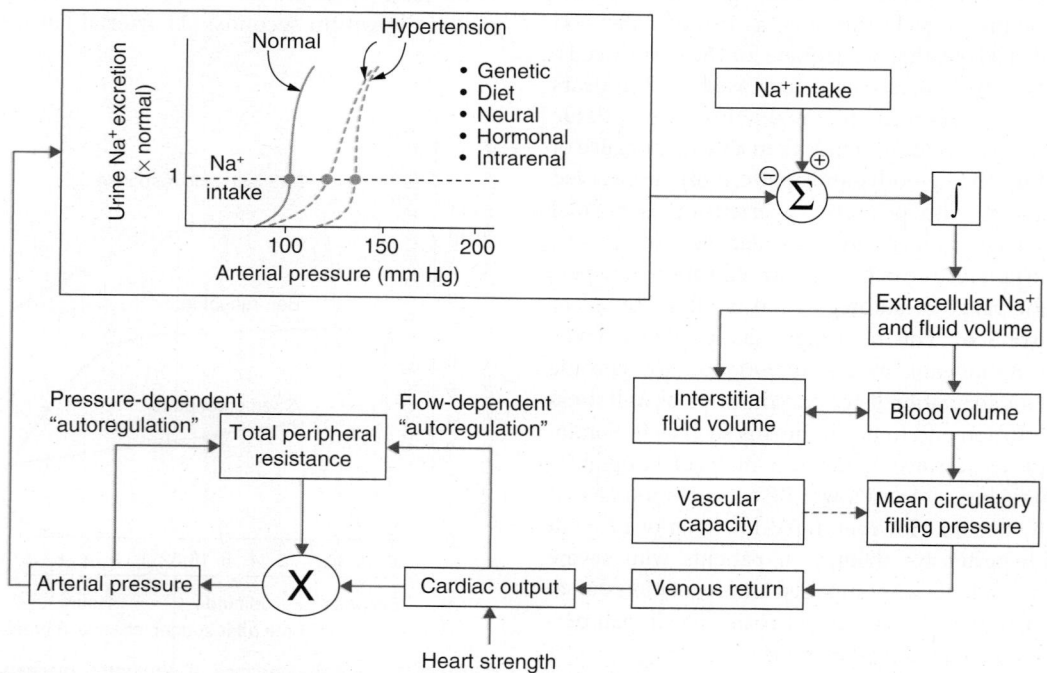

Figure 5–8. Basic elements of renal-body fluid feedback mechanism for long-term regulation of BP. A key component of this feedback is the effect of arterial pressure on urine sodium excretion, called *pressure natriuresis/diuresis*. The red dashed lines show altered pressure natriuresis in salt-sensitive and salt-resistant hypertension. Increased arterial pressure may cause secondary increases in total peripheral resistance via pressure-dependent or flow-dependent autoregulation in various tissues. Increased vascular capacity tends to reduce mean circulatory filling pressure.

In all types of human or experimental hypertension studied thus far, there is a shift of pressure natriuresis that sustains hypertension. In some cases, abnormal pressure natriuresis is caused by intrarenal disturbances that alter renal hemodynamics or tubular reabsorption. In other cases, altered kidney function is caused by extrarenal factors, such as increased sympathetic nervous system (SNS) activity or excessive formation of antinatriuretic hormones that reduce the kidney's ability to excrete sodium and water and eventually increase BP. Consequently, effective treatment of patients with hypertension requires interventions that reset pressure natriuresis toward normal BP, either by directly increasing renal excretory capability (eg, with diuretics) or by reducing antinatriuretic influences (eg, with RAAS blockers) on the kidneys.

Renal Mechanisms of Hypertension and Salt Sensitivity

Severe kidney disease is widely recognized as a cause and a consequence of hypertension. However, the importance of more subtle renal dysfunction in the pathogenesis of essential hypertension is not as well appreciated, partly because there are no obvious renal defects in many patients with primary hypertension. Measurements commonly used to evaluate kidney function, such as GFR, serum creatinine, and sodium excretion, are often within the normal range in the early stages of hypertension before kidney damage occurs. On the other hand, TPR is often increased in hypertensive subjects, leading many to conclude that vasoconstriction is the cause of increased BP. However, as discussed previously, increased TPR may be an autoregulatory response to increased BP in many hypertensive subjects.

Most experimental models of hypertension and monogenic forms of human hypertension are caused by obvious insults to the kidneys that alter renal hemodynamics or tubular reabsorption. For example, constriction of the renal arteries (eg, Goldblatt hypertension), compression of the kidneys (eg, perinephritic hypertension), and administration of sodium-retaining hormones (eg, mineralocorticoids or Ang II) are all associated with initial reductions in GFR or increases in renal tubular reabsorption prior to the development of hypertension. Likewise, in monogenic human hypertension, the common pathways to hypertension are (1) increased renal sodium reabsorption, caused by mutations that directly increase renal electrolyte transport or synthesis/activity of antinatriuretic hormones and (2) increased renal vascular resistance. As BP increases, the initial renal changes are obscured by compensations that restore kidney function toward normal. Increased BP then initiates a cascade of cardiovascular changes that may be more striking than the initial disturbance of kidney function. However, one aspect of kidney function that is abnormal in all types of experimental and clinical hypertension is renal pressure natriuresis.[100,101]

The general types of renal abnormalities that can alter pressure natriuresis and cause chronic hypertension include increased preglomerular resistance, decreased glomerular capillary filtration coefficient, reduced numbers of functional nephrons, and increased tubular reabsorption (**Table 5–3**). Some of these kidney abnormalities increase salt sensitivity of BP, whereas others cause salt-insensitive hypertension.[99,102]

Increased Preglomerular Resistance

Generalized Increases in Preglomerular Resistance Cause Salt-Insensitive Hypertension: Examples of generalized increases in preglomerular resistance are those caused by suprarenal aortic coarctation or constriction of one of the renal arteries and removal of the contralateral kidney (eg, one-kidney, one-clip Goldblatt hypertension). Immediately after constriction of the renal artery or aortic coarctation, renal blood flow decreases, renin secretion increases, and sodium excretion transiently decrease. Within a few days, sodium excretion returns to normal and sodium balance is reestablished (**Figure 5–9**). If sodium intake is normal, renin secretion also returns to normal in the established phase of hypertension. At this point, most indices of renal function are nearly normal, including BP distal to the stenosis, if the constriction is not too severe.[100]

How do these experimental models relate to human hypertension, other than the obvious conditions of aortic coarctation or renal artery stenosis? Presumably, functional or pathologic

TABLE 5–3. Renal Causes and Characteristics of Salt-Sensitive and Salt-Insensitive Hypertension[a]

Causes	BP	Pressure Natriuresis	Renal Blood Flow	GFR	Plasma Renin Activity	Glomerular Injury[b]
Salt-Sensitive Hypertension						
Decreased kidney mass	↑, ↔	Decreased slope	↓	↓	↓	Yes
Decreased glomerular capillary filtration coefficient (K_f)	↑	Decreased slope	↑	↓, ↔	↑, ↔	Yes
Increased distal and collecting tubule reabsorption	↑	Decreased slope	↑	↑	↓	Yes
Salt-Insensitive Hypertension						
Increased preglomerular resistance	↑	Parallel shift	↓, ↔	↓, ↔	↑, ↔	No[c]

[a]The changes shown in the table are those predicted to initially occur after the initial disturbances (causes). With chronic changes in arterial pressure and glomerular hydrostatic pressure, injury to the kidney may lead to secondary reductions in GFR and renal blood flow.

[b]Glomerular injury is predicted to occur secondary to hypertensive stimuli that cause chronic increases in glomerular hydrostatic pressure or hyperfiltration of surviving nephrons.

[c]Increased preglomerular resistance attenuates transmission of increased blood pressure to the glomerulus and protects against hypertension-induced glomerular injury. Severe increases in preglomerular resistance, however, can cause nephron ischemia and glomerular injury.

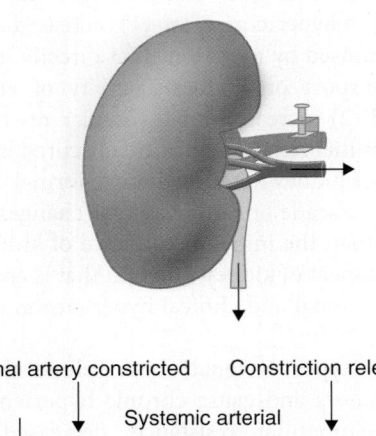

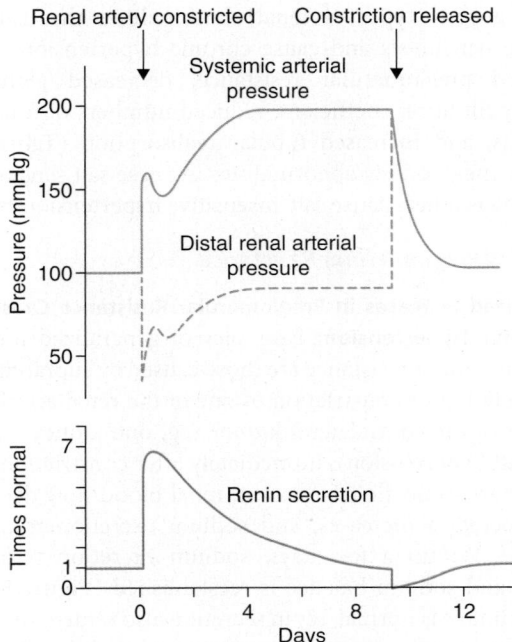

Figure 5–9. Effects of constriction of the renal artery of a sole remaining kidney. Renal artery pressure distal to the constriction, renin secretion, and sodium excretion rate return to nearly normal after a few days. Reproduced with permission from Hall JE, Hall ME. *Guyton and Hall Textbook of Medical Physiology,* 14th ed. Philadelphia, PA: Elsevier; 2021.

increases in preglomerular resistance at other sites besides the main renal arteries, such as the interlobular arteries or afferent arterioles, can increase BP through the same mechanisms as activated by clipping the renal artery. For example, widespread structural increases in afferent arteriolar resistance (eg, nephrosclerosis) or functional increases in resistance caused by excessive activation of the SNS or high levels of catecholamines (eg, pheochromocytoma) would also cause hypertension through the same mechanisms as constriction of the main renal artery.

Thus, hypertension in some patients may be caused by functional or pathologic increases in preglomerular resistance. This is almost certainly the case in patients who have severe atherosclerotic lesions in the renal blood vessels.

Patchy Increases in Preglomerular Resistance Cause Salt-Sensitive Hypertension: In the two-kidney, one-clip Goldblatt model of

hypertension, and in patients with stenosis in only one renal artery, there is a nonhomogeneous increase in preglomerular resistance with ischemia occurring in nephrons of the clipped or stenotic kidney; nephrons in the contralateral nonstenotic kidney have normal or increased single-nephron blood flow and GFR. Whereas the underperfused clipped kidney secretes large amounts of renin, the nonstenotic kidney secretes very little renin.[100]

An important distinction between a generalized increase in preglomerular resistance and patchy, nonhomogeneous increases in preglomerular resistance is the evolution of renal injury associated with hypertension. With homogeneous increases in preglomerular resistance, the glomeruli are protected from the damaging effects of increased BP. In the two-kidney, one-clip model, however, the glomeruli of the untouched kidney are subjected to the effects of increased BP, as well as the antinatriuretic effects of Ang II formed from increased secretion of renin by the clipped kidney. With prolonged hypertension, pathologic changes in the untouched kidney add to the impairment of overall renal excretory capability.

The relevance of experimental models of nonhomogeneous increases in preglomerular resistance to human hypertension is obvious when there is stenosis of only one renal artery, with the contralateral kidney being initially unaffected. Also, some patients with primary hypertension may have patchy nephrosclerosis within each kidney. In these instances, ischemic nephrons secrete large amounts of renin, and nonischemic nephrons may initially have increased single-nephron GFR. The combined effects of hypertension and hyperfiltration, however, may eventually damage the nephrons that were not initially ischemic, leading to progressive nephron loss.

Decreased Glomerular Capillary Filtration Coefficient

Reducing the glomerular capillary filtration coefficient (K_f) initially lowers GFR and sodium excretion while stimulating renin release and dilating afferent arterioles via macula densa feedback.[99,100] The sodium retention and increased Ang II formation increase BP, which then helps to restore GFR and renin secretion toward normal. After these compensations, the main persistent abnormalities of kidney function include reduced filtration fraction, increased glomerular hydrostatic pressure, and increased renal blood flow. BP is often salt sensitive when reductions in K_f are severe.

Compensatory increases in BP and glomerular hydrostatic pressure, which offset a decrease in K_f and restore sodium excretion to normal, may also lead to additional renal dysfunction over a period of years by causing further glomerular injury; the gradual injury and loss of glomeruli further reduce K_f and elicit additional increases in BP to maintain normal water and electrolyte balances. Such a sequence may initiate progressive kidney damage, worsening of hypertension, and greater salt sensitivity of BP. The clinical counterparts of this sequence may be found in hypertension caused by glomerulonephritis or by other conditions that cause thickening and damage to the glomerular capillary membranes, such as chronic diabetes mellitus.[100]

Nephron Loss

Complete loss of nephrons (eg, surgical reduction of kidney mass or unilateral nephrectomy), in the absence of other abnormalities, may not lead to significant hypertension so long as sodium intake is not excessive.[99,100] With surgical nephron loss, glomerular filtration and tubular reabsorption capability are proportionally reduced so that balance between filtration and reabsorption can be maintained without major adaptive changes in BP. In contrast, nephron loss because of ischemia or infarction of renal tissue usually induces hypertension that is initially caused by increased renin secretion and Ang II formation, and then is eventually mediated by additional abnormalities, such as immunologic and renal injury, in the established phase of the hypertension.[100]

Regardless of whether nephron loss initially causes hypertension, the kidneys become susceptible to additional insults that impair their function, or to additional challenges of sodium homeostasis. Thus, hypertension associated with excess mineralocorticoids is much more severe after nephron loss. Likewise, the kidney's response to the additional challenge of high sodium intake is accompanied by larger increases in BP when kidney mass is reduced.[99,100] Nephron loss may also initiate compensatory changes that damage surviving nephrons. For example, over long periods of time, renal vasodilation and increased single-nephron GFR may lead to glomerulosclerosis and reductions in K_f. These pathologic changes, in addition to the nephron loss, may eventually impair pressure natriuresis sufficiently to cause substantial hypertension.

With normal aging, especially after age 40 to 50 years, there is gradual nephron loss that is accelerated by renal disease such as glomerulonephritis, diabetes mellitus, or long-standing hypertension. Thus, even though hypertension may not begin with nephron loss, chronic elevations in glomerular pressure, metabolic abnormalities, and inflammation associated with hypertension may eventually cause progressive nephron loss that amplifies the hypertension and makes BP more salt sensitive.[99,103]

Increased Renal Tubular Sodium Reabsorption

Factors that increase renal sodium reabsorption, such as excessive levels of mineralocorticoids or Ang II, can also cause hypertension. The severity of hypertension depends on the degree to which tubular reabsorption is stimulated, as well as on other factors, such as the functional kidney mass and sodium intake.[99,100] With nephron loss or high sodium intake, the hypertensive potency of mineralocorticoids or Ang II is greatly enhanced.

Excessive distal and collecting tubule reabsorption causes salt-sensitive hypertension: Hypertension caused by increased distal or collecting tubular reabsorption is salt sensitive, with increased sodium intake exacerbating the hypertension.[104] Increased reabsorption at sites beyond the macula densa, such as the distal tubules and collecting tubules, causes chronic increased sodium chloride delivery to the macula densa, which, in turn, suppresses renin secretion.[99,100] Reduction of renin secretion to very low levels, characteristic of disorders associated with excessive distal or collecting tubular reabsorption,

prevents further suppression of Ang II formation during high sodium intake, making BP salt sensitive.

Another feature of hypertension caused by increased tubular reabsorption (eg, due to excess aldosterone secretion) is that it is often associated with moderate extracellular volume expansion. However, the initial volume expansion and increased CO usually subside because of pressure natriuresis, and TPR increases because of the vascular autoregulatory mechanisms discussed previously. When increased tubular reabsorption is also associated with marked peripheral vasoconstriction, as occurs with very high levels of Ang II, the degree of volume expansion depends on the relative vasoconstriction of peripheral blood vessels and the kidneys.[99,100] With severe vasoconstriction and marked reduction in vascular capacitance, there is a relative overfilling of the circulation but total blood volume may actually be reduced, despite impaired kidney function.

Reduced Responsiveness of the RAAS System Increases the Salt Sensitivity of Blood Pressure: Figure 5–10 shows the importance of appropriate changes in Ang II formation in keeping BP relatively constant over a wide range of sodium intakes.[105,106] When the RAAS was fully functional, only small increases in BP were associated with a 100-fold range of sodium intakes. However, when Ang II was infused at a low level that initially had little effect on BP but prevented Ang II from being suppressed as sodium intake was raised, BP became highly salt sensitive. After blockade of Ang II formation, BP was also salt sensitive but was maintained at a much lower level, especially when sodium intake was low.[106] Thus, a major function of the RAAS is to permit wide variations in intake and excretion of sodium without large fluctuations in BP that would otherwise be needed to maintain sodium balance.

Focal nephrosclerosis or patchy preglomerular vasoconstriction leads to increased renin secretion in ischemic nephrons and low levels of renin release by overperfused nephrons.[100] Thus, in ischemic as well as overperfused nephrons, the ability to adequately suppress renin secretion during high salt intake is impaired.

As discussed previously, reduced responsiveness of the RAAS also occurs with mineralocorticoid excess or mutations that increase distal and collecting tubule reabsorption (eg, Liddle syndrome). In these conditions, excess sodium retention causes nearly complete suppression of renin secretion and inability to further decrease renin release during high sodium intake. Consequently, BP becomes very salt sensitive.

Significance of Salt Sensitivity

There is considerable heterogeneity of BP responses to changes in sodium intake in normotensive and hypertensive individuals.[99] Clinical observations indicate that older individuals are usually more salt sensitive than young people, and Blacks are often more salt sensitive than Whites; however, there are many exceptions to these generalizations.

Genetic factors independent of ethnicity are also linked to BP salt sensitivity, especially monogenic disorders that increase distal and collecting tubule sodium reabsorption or that cause excess secretion of sodium-retaining hormones

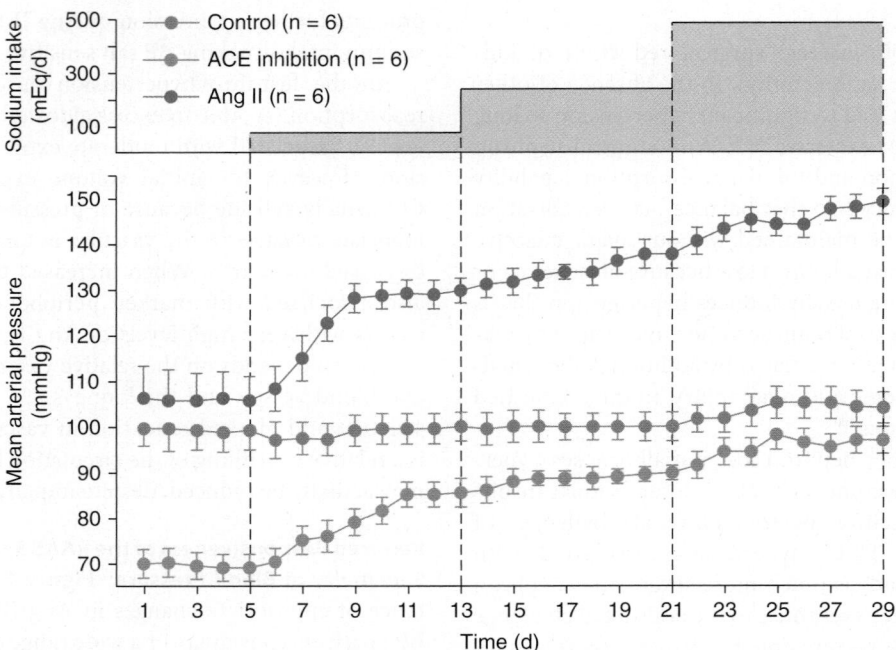

Figure 5–10. Changes in mean arterial pressure during chronic changes in sodium intake in normal control dogs, after ACE inhibition, or after Ang II infusion (5 ng/kg/min) to prevent Ang II from being suppressed when sodium intake was raised. Reproduced with permission from Hall JE, Guyton AC, Smith MJ, et al. Blood pressure and renal function during chronic changes in sodium intake: role of angiotensin. *Am J Physiol.* 1980 Sep;239(3):F271-F280.

(eg, mineralocorticoids).[99] Also, diabetes mellitus, renal diseases that cause nephron loss, and abnormalities of the RAAS are all associated with increased BP salt sensitivity.[99] Many of these examples may share two common pathways to salt sensitivity of BP: loss of functional nephrons or reduced responsiveness of the RAAS.

Salt sensitivity and target organ injury: Some studies suggest that salt sensitivity predicts greater risk for hypertensive target organ injury. Salt-sensitive hypertension is often associated with glomerular hyperfiltration and increased glomerular hydrostatic pressure (**Table 5–3**); together, the hypertension and renal hyperfiltration promote glomerular injury and may eventually cause loss of nephron function.

There is also evidence that salt-sensitive subjects die earlier than salt-resistant individuals. Weinberger et al.[107] followed patients for more than 20 years and found that normotensive individuals with increased salt sensitivity died almost at the same rate as people with hypertension and much faster than salt-resistant individuals who were normotensive. It is not clear whether chronic high salt intake, lasting over many years, may cause a person who is initially "salt insensitive" to become "salt sensitive" as a consequence of gradual renal injury.

Neurohumoral and Immune Mechanisms of Hypertension

Inappropriate activation of multiple antinatriuretic hormone systems, such as Ang II and aldosterone, that normally regulate sodium excretion, or deficiency of natriuretic influences on the kidneys, such as atrial natriuretic peptide (ANP) and nitric oxide (NO), can impair pressure natriuresis and cause chronic hypertension. Likewise, excessive SNS activation plays a major role in elevating BP in many hypertensive patients. The following sections discuss some of the neural, hormonal, and autacoid mechanisms that contribute to long-term BP regulation, their actions on the kidneys, and their potential roles in hypertension.

The Sympathetic Nervous System

Sympathetic vasoconstrictor fibers are distributed to almost all regions of the vasculature, the heart, and the kidneys, and SNS activation can raise BP within a few seconds by causing vasoconstriction, increased cardiac pumping capability, and increased heart rate. Conversely, sudden inhibition of SNS activity can decrease BP to as low as half of normal in less than 1 minute. Therefore, changes in SNS activity caused by various reflex mechanisms, CNS ischemia, or activation of higher centers in the brain provide powerful, rapid, and moment-to-moment regulation of BP.

The SNS also plays an important role in long-term BP regulation and in the pathogenesis of hypertension, in large part by activation of renal sympathetic nerves.[100,108–110] There is extensive innervation of the renal blood vessels, juxtaglomerular apparatus, and renal tubules, and excessive activation of these nerves promotes sodium retention, increased renin secretion, and impaired renal-pressure natriuresis. Except for extreme circumstances, such as severe hemorrhage or other conditions associated with marked circulatory depression, activation of the renal sympathetic nerves is usually not great enough to cause major reductions in renal blood flow or GFR. However, even mild increases in renal sympathetic activity stimulate renin secretion and sodium reabsorption in multiple segments of the nephron, including the proximal tubule, the loop of Henle, and distal segments.[100,108] Thus, the renal nerves provide a mechanism by which various reflex mechanisms and higher CNS centers may contribute to long-term BP regulation.

Evidence for a role of the renal nerves in hypertension comes from multiple studies showing that renal denervation (RDN) reduces BP in some models of experimental hypertension, including spontaneously hypertensive rats and obese, hypertensive dogs.[108,111] RDN may delay or attenuate increased BP in other forms of experimental hypertension, although some studies have not found an important role for the renal nerves in several forms of secondary hypertension. In Ang II hypertension, for example, renal sympathetic activity is reduced secondary to the activation of arterial baroreceptors.[112]

Human primary hypertension is often associated with increased renal sympathetic activity. In obese humans with resistant hypertension, catheter-based radiofrequency RDN lowered office BP for up to 36 months.[113] However, in many of the clinical trials, patients were already on at least three antihypertensive medications, including blockers of the RAAS, which may mediate at least part of the effect of the renal nerves on BP, and the extent of RDN was not verified.

The clinical trials conducted thus far likely underestimate the BP effects of RDN since catheter-based RDN typically causes <50% renal nerve ablation.[111] Some of the renal nerves bypass the main renal artery in route to the kidneys, making them inaccessible to catheter-based RDN. However, increased efficacy of RDN (up to 75% ablation of the renal nerves) can be achieved if the radiofrequency ablation procedure is performed in the branches of the main renal artery close to the kidneys.[114] In addition to the challenge of ensuring adequate RDN,[115] longer periods of follow-up will be needed to determine if the renal nerves eventually regrow and reinitiate increases in BP, as has been observed in experimental animal models of RDN.[111]

Whether RDN will prove to be an effective therapy for patients who are resistant to the usual pharmacological treatments remains to be determined. Although the mechanisms that activate the SNS in primary hypertension or in most experimental models are still unclear, we now briefly discuss three that have attracted the interest of many researchers.

Role of Baroreceptor Reflexes in Hypertension: The importance of the arterial baroreceptors in buffering moment-to-moment changes in BP is clearly evident in baroreceptor-denervated animals, in which there is extreme BP variability during normal daily activities. After baroreceptor denervation, BP oscillates between high and low levels with normal daily activities, although the average 24-hour mean arterial pressure is not markedly altered.

Although the arterial baroreceptors clearly provide a powerful means for acute BP regulation, their role in long-term BP regulation is controversial. Some studies suggest that the baroreceptors reset within a few days to higher BP in chronic hypertension. To the extent that baroreceptors reset, their potency as long-term controllers of BP would diminish.

Some experimental studies, however, suggest that the baroreceptors do not completely reset and with prolonged increases in BP may contribute to reductions in renal sympathetic activity, promoting sodium excretion and attenuating the increase in BP.[111] Thus, impaired baroreflexes may increase the lability of BP in hypertension and may fail to attenuate the increase in BP caused by other disturbances. However, there is currently little evidence that primary disturbances of baroreceptor function play a major role in causing chronic hypertension.

Chronic activation of the baroreceptors by electrical stimulation of the carotid sinus reduces BP in some forms of experimental hypertension, especially obesity-induced hypertension.[111] In humans with hypertension that were resistant to drug treatment, electrical stimulation of baroreceptors also significantly reduced BP for up to 6 years.[116] However, further randomized, controlled clinical trials will be required to test the feasibility, safety, efficacy, and long-term outcomes of baroreflex activation and other device-based therapies for treatment of resistant hypertension.

Does Chronic Stress Cause Hypertension by SNS Activation? Acute physiologic stresses, including pain, exercise, exposure to cold, and mental stress, can all lead to increased SNS activity and transient hypertension. It is also widely believed that unremitting psychosocial stress may lead to long-term increases in BP. Support for this concept comes largely from epidemiologic studies showing that people who are believed to lead stressful lives, such as those with chronic sleep disruption, some ethnic and economically disadvantaged groups, and people who experience posttraumatic stress disorder (PTSD) may have increased prevalence of hypertension.[117,118] Persistent emotional and mental stress following a traumatic event is associated with increased risk for developing hypertension and CVD.[119]

Although the factors that link PTSD with hypertension are uncertain, patients with PTSD and animal models of PTSD have increased SNS activity, decreased cardiac vagal control, and baroreflex dysfunction.[119] However, direct cause-and-effect relationships between psychosocial stress and mechanisms for chronic hypertension in humans have been challenging to elucidate.

Obesity Causes SNS Activation: Excess weight gain appears to be a major cause of human primary hypertension. The mechanisms responsible for obesity hypertension are closely linked to increased renal SNS activity.[100,120] People who are obese have elevated SNS activity in various tissues, including the kidneys and skeletal muscle, as assessed by microneurography, tissue catecholamine spillover, and other methods. Studies in experimental animals and humans indicate that combined α- and β-adrenergic blockade markedly attenuates hypertension associated with obesity.[109,120] Moreover, bilateral renal denervation greatly attenuates sodium retention and hypertension in obese dogs and obese patients with primary hypertension.[111] Thus, obesity increases renal sodium reabsorption, impairs pressure natriuresis, and causes hypertension partly by increasing renal SNS activity, as discussed in more detail later in this chapter.

The Renin-Angiotensin-Aldosterone System

The RAAS is perhaps the most powerful hormone system for regulating sodium balance and BP, as evidenced by the effectiveness of various RAAS blockers in reducing BP in normotensive and hypertensive subjects. Although the RAAS has many components, its most important effects on BP regulation are exerted by Ang II and aldosterone.

Ang II is a powerful vasoconstrictor that helps maintain BP in conditions associated with acute volume depletion (eg, hemorrhage), sodium depletion, or circulatory depression (eg, heart failure). The long-term effects of Ang II on BP, however, are closely intertwined with sodium and volume homeostasis through direct and indirect effects on the kidneys.[105,121,122]

When the RAAS is fully functional, sodium balance can be maintained over a wide range of intakes with minimal changes in BP (**Figure 5–10**). Blockade of the RAAS, with Ang II–receptor blockers (ARBs) or angiotensin-converting enzyme (ACE) inhibitors, increases renal excretory capability so that sodium balance can be maintained at reduced BP.[106] However, blockade of the RAAS also makes BP salt sensitive. Thus, the effectiveness of RAAS blockers in lowering BP is greatly diminished by high salt intake. Conversely, reducing sodium intake or addition of a diuretic improves the effectiveness of RAAS blockers in reducing BP.

Inappropriately high levels of Ang II reduce renal excretory capability and impair pressure natriuresis, thereby necessitating increased BP to maintain sodium balance. The mechanisms that mediate the potent antinatriuretic effects of Ang II include direct and indirect effects to increase tubular reabsorption, as well as renal hemodynamic effects.[105,106]

Ang II Stimulates Renal Sodium Reabsorption: Physiologic activation of the RAAS usually occurs as a compensation for conditions that cause volume depletion or underperfusion of the kidneys, such as sodium depletion, hemorrhage, or heart failure. Increased Ang II formation helps restore renal perfusion by increasing renal sodium reabsorption through stimulation of aldosterone secretion, direct effects on epithelial transport, and hemodynamic effects. The direct effects of Ang II on the renal tubules occur at low concentrations and are mediated by actions on the luminal and basolateral membranes of the proximal tubules, loops of Henle, and distal nephron segments.[100,105,109]

The renal hemodynamic effects of Ang II occur mainly by constriction of efferent arterioles, which reduces renal blood flow and peritubular capillary hydrostatic pressure and increases peritubular colloid osmotic pressure as a result of increased filtration fraction.[105] These changes in turn increase the driving force for fluid reabsorption across tubular epithelial cells.

Ang II Helps Prevent Excessive Decreases in Glomerular Filtration Rate When Renal Perfusion Is Threatened: In addition to its effect to enhance tubular reabsorption, efferent arteriolar constriction by Ang II acts in concert with other autoregulatory mechanisms, such as tubuloglomerular feedback and myogenic activity, to prevent excessive reductions in GFR when kidney perfusion is reduced, such as during sodium depletion, renal artery stenosis, or heart failure.[105] In these cases, administration of ARBs or ACE inhibitors may actually reduce GFR further, even though renal blood flow is preserved. Decreased GFR after RAAS blockade in these conditions is also caused in part by reductions in BP, as well as efferent arteriolar dilation.

The weak constrictor action of Ang II on preglomerular vessels during pathophysiological conditions that activate the RAAS, such as sodium depletion or renal artery stenosis, is due mainly to selective protection of these vessels by autacoid mechanisms such as prostaglandins or endothelial-derived NO.[105] When the ability of the kidneys to produce these autacoids is impaired by treatment with nonsteroidal anti-inflammatory drugs (NSAIDs) or by chronic vascular disease (eg, atherosclerosis), increased Ang II may reduce GFR by constricting afferent arterioles.

Blockade of Ang II Attenuates Glomerular Injury in Overperfused Kidneys: RAAS blockade is often beneficial when nephrons are hyperfiltering, especially if Ang II is not appropriately suppressed. For example, in diabetes mellitus and certain forms of hypertension associated with glomerulosclerosis and nephron loss, Ang II blockade decreases BP, dilates efferent arterioles, and attenuates glomerular hyperfiltration and kidney injury.[121]

Aldosterone and Mineralocorticoid Receptor Blockade in Hypertension: Aldosterone, the primary mineralocorticoid in humans, is a powerful sodium-retaining hormone and has important effects on renal pressure natriuresis and BP regulation. The primary sites of actions of aldosterone on sodium reabsorption are the principal and intercalated cells of the distal tubules, cortical collecting tubules, and collecting ducts where aldosterone stimulates sodium reabsorption, as well as secretion of potassium and hydrogen ions.[123,124] Aldosterone binds to intracellular mineralocorticoid receptors (MRs) and activates transcription by target genes, which, in turn, stimulate synthesis or activation of the Na^+-K^+-ATPase pump on the basolateral epithelial membrane and activation of amiloride-sensitive sodium channels on the luminal side of the epithelial membrane.[124]

The overall effects of aldosterone on pressure natriuresis are similar to those observed for Ang II. With low sodium intake, increased aldosterone helps prevent sodium loss and reductions in BP. Conversely, during high sodium intake, suppression of aldosterone helps prevent excessive sodium retention and attenuates increased BP.

Some investigators suggest that hyperaldosteronism and excess activation of MRs may be more common than previously believed, especially in patients with hypertension who are resistant to treatment with the usual antihypertensive medications.[125] Many of these patients, however, are overweight or obese, and MR antagonism may provide an important therapeutic tool for preventing target organ injury and reducing BP.[16]

The Endothelin System

Endothelin-1 (ET-1), the predominant effector of the endothelin system,[126] is the most powerful vasoconstrictor produced in humans, and tissue levels may be increased in some forms of hypertension.[127] However, in essential hypertension and most forms of experimental hypertension circulating ET-1 is not substantially elevated unless renal failure, endothelial damage,

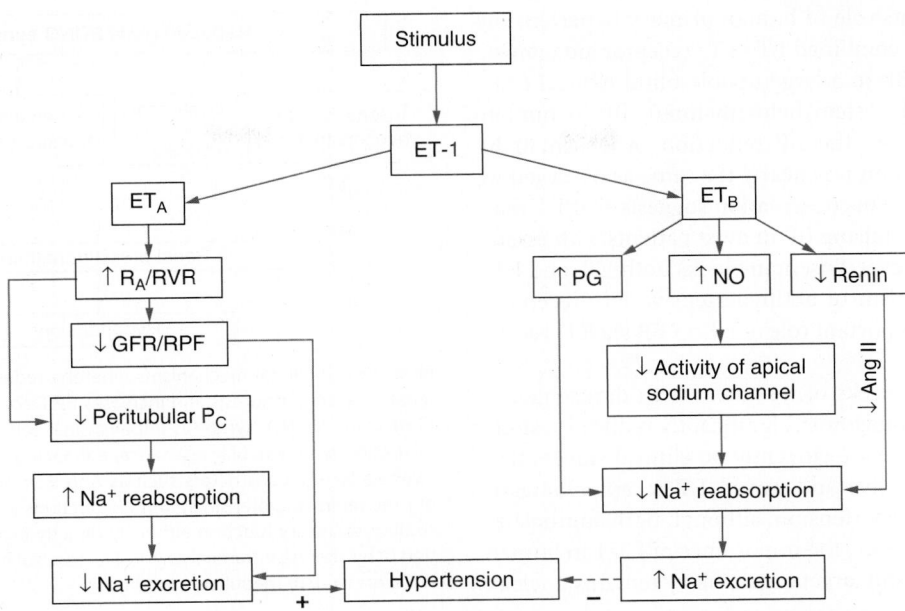

Figure 5–11. Summary of the prohypertensive and antihypertensive actions of ET-1. The ability of ET-1 to influence BP regulation and renal pressure natriuresis is highly dependent on where ET-1 is produced and which renal ET receptor type is activated. ET-1 elicits a prohypertensive antinatriuretic effect by activating ETA receptors in the kidneys. Activation of renal ETA receptors increases renal vascular resistance (RVR), which decreases renal plasma flow (RPF) and GFR, and enhances sodium reabsorption by decreasing peritubular capillary hydrostatic pressure (Pc). The net effect of renal ETA receptor activation is decreased sodium excretion and increased BP. Conversely, ET-1 can elicit an antihypertensive natriuretic effect via ETB receptor activation. Activation of the renal ETB receptor leads to enhanced synthesis of NO and prostaglandin E2 and suppression of the renin–angiotensin system. The net effect of renal ETB receptor activation is increased sodium excretion and decreased BP.

or atherosclerosis is present.[127] Circulating ET-1 levels, however, may not reflect local vascular production of the peptide and ET-1 acts in a paracrine fashion, regulating nearby vascular smooth muscle cells.

ET-1 Receptor Subtypes and Physiological Actions: ET-1 can either elicit hypertensive effects by activating ET type A (ET_A) receptors in the kidneys or antihypertensive effects via ET type B (ET_B) receptor activation. Thus, the ability of ET-1 to influence BP regulation is highly dependent on where ET-1 is produced and which ET receptors are activated (**Figure 5–11**).

ET-1, via ET_A receptor activation, exerts multiple actions within the kidney that, if sustained chronically, could contribute to hypertension and renal injury. ET-1 causes renal vasoconstriction and decreased GFR. Long-term effects of ET-1 on the kidney also include stimulation of mesangial cell proliferation and extracellular matrix deposition, as well as vascular smooth muscle hypertrophy in renal resistance vessels.[127–129]

Expression of ET-1 is greatly enhanced in several animal models of severe hypertension with renal vascular hypertrophy and in models of progressive renal injury. In addition, treatment with ET receptor antagonists attenuated hypertension and improved kidney function in several models of CKD.[126,130]

ET_B receptors are located on multiple cell types throughout the body, including endothelial cells and renal epithelial cells. ET_B activation causes vasodilation, enhances pressure natriuresis, and decreases BP. The most compelling evidence for a role of ET_B receptors in regulating BP comes from reports that transgenic mice deficient in ET_B receptors develop severe

salt-sensitive hypertension and that pharmacologic antagonism of ET_B receptors produces significant hypertension in rats.[131] Mice with selective deletion of ET_B in the renal collecting ducts were hypertensive even on a normal sodium diet and a high-sodium diet worsened the hypertension.[132] These findings suggest that ET_B receptor activation on the collecting ducts is an important physiologic regulator that increases renal sodium excretion and reduces BP.

ET-1 and Salt-Sensitive Hypertension: ET-1 may contribute to some forms of salt-sensitive hypertension. Chronic blockade of ET_A receptors attenuated hypertension and proteinuria and ameliorated glomerular and tubular damage associated with high salt intake in Dahl salt-sensitive (DS) rats.[133] Whether the beneficial effect of ET_A receptor blockade in reducing renal injury is mediated through lower BP or through direct renal mechanisms is unclear.

Renal ET-1 synthesis is also enhanced in other animal models of chronic hypertension including Ang II hypertension, deoxycorticosterone acetate (DOCA) hypertension, and placental ischemic-induced hypertension. Hypertension in these models is markedly attenuated or abolished by ET_A receptor antagonists.[126,127,129]

Role of Endothelin in Human Hypertension: Several selective and mixed endothelin receptor antagonists have been developed and utilized in clinical trials for renal disease, systemic and pulmonary arterial hypertension, and heart failure.[126,129,130] Although ET-1 clearly plays a significant role in the pathogenesis of some forms of experimental hypertension, especially salt-sensitive models, its role in human primary hypertension is unclear. Bosentan, a combined ET_A-ET_B receptor antagonist, significantly lowered BP in a large double-blind clinical trial, indicating that the ET system helps maintain BP in human hypertension.[134] However, the BP reduction by bosentan in patients with hypertension was nearly the same as observed in normotensive humans. This observation suggests that ET may not play a major role in raising BP in most patients with essential hypertension. However, bosentan blocks both ET_A and ET_B receptors, and antagonism of antihypertensive ET_B receptors may have masked an important role of ET on BP via ET_A receptor activation.

In another study, 6 weeks of treatment with darusentan, a selective ET_A receptor antagonist, significantly reduced systolic and diastolic BP.[135] There are currently no clinical studies that directly compared selective and mixed ET receptor antagonism for treatment of hypertension, although both approaches clearly reduce BP. Therefore, the importance of ET-1 in human essential hypertension and target organ injury remains unclear.

Nitric Oxide

Vascular NO is mainly produced from L-arginine by endothelial NO synthase (eNOS). Three distinct genes encode NOS isozymes that catalyze production of NO from L-arginine.[136] These include neuronal NOS (nNOS or NOS-1), cytokine-inducible NOS (iNOS or NOS-2), and endothelial NOS (eNOS or NOS-3). Production of NO from L-arginine by NOS also requires the various cofactors, including tetrahydrobiopterin (BH_4), flavin adenine dinucleotide, flavin mononucleotide, calmodulin, and iron protoporphyrin IX. Tonic release of eNOS-derived NO by the vascular endothelium plays a major role in regulating vascular function, and nNOS and NOS-derived NO from renal epithelial cells regulate sodium transport and renal hemodynamics.[136,137] Long-term inhibition of NOS causes sustained hypertension associated with impaired renal pressure natriuresis. The BP responses to NO inhibition depend on sodium intake, indicating salt sensitivity of BP.

Deficiency of Nitric Oxide Impairs Renal Pressure Natriuresis: Deficiency of NO synthesis impairs pressure natriuresis by several mechanisms, including hemodynamic and tubular effects, which may be modulated by processes that are intrinsic or extrinsic to the kidneys (**Figure 5–12**). For example, reductions in NO synthesis may decrease kidney function by increasing renal vascular resistance directly or by enhancing renal vascular responsiveness to vasoconstrictors such as Ang II or norepinephrine.[136–138] Reductions in NO synthesis also increase renal tubular sodium reabsorption via direct effects on tubular transport and through changes in intrarenal physical factors, such as renal interstitial hydrostatic pressure (RIHP) and medullary blood flow.

Evidence suggests that NO synthesis is impaired in some vascular beds in human primary hypertension, especially when associated with aging, atherosclerosis, obesity, diabetes, and other factors that cause endothelial injury.[136,137] However, whether impaired NO synthesis and release in blood vessels and kidneys are secondary to increased BP or reflect

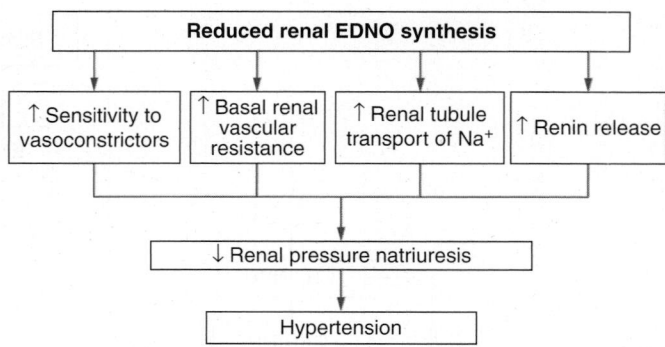

Figure 5–12. Renal mechanisms whereby reduced NO synthesis impairs renal pressure natriuresis and increases BP. Decreased endothelial-derived nitric oxide (EDNO) synthesis impairs renal sodium excretory function by increasing renal vascular resistance, enhancing the renal vascular responsiveness to vasoconstrictors such as Ang II or norepinephrine, or activating the renin–angiotensin system. Reductions in NO synthesis also impair sodium excretory function either by directly increasing tubular reabsorption or by altering intrarenal physical factors, such as renal interstitial hydrostatic pressure or medullary blood flow.

important mechanisms for the pathogenesis of hypertension remain unclear.

Oxidative Stress

Considerable evidence supports a role for increased reactive oxygen species (ROS) in animal models of hypertension.[139–142] DS rats, for example, have increased vascular and renal superoxide production and increased levels of H_2O_2. Renal expression of superoxide dismutase is decreased in kidneys of DS rats, and long-term administration of Tempol, a superoxide dismutase mimetic, significantly decreases BP and attenuates renal damage. Another salt-sensitive model, the stroke-prone, spontaneously hypertensive rat, has elevated levels of superoxide and decreased total plasma antioxidant capacity. Superoxide production is also increased in DOCA-salt hypertensive rats, and treatment with apocynin, a nicotinamide adenine dinucleotide phosphate (NADPH) oxidase inhibitor, decreases BP. Chronic administration of Tempol significantly decreases the BP response to Ang II, suggesting that ROS also may play an important role in Ang II-mediated hypertension.[141,142]

Despite evidence supporting a role for ROS in experimental hypertension, clinical studies on chronic antioxidant therapy have failed to confirm these findings. An imbalance between total oxidant production and the antioxidant capacity in human primary hypertension has been reported in some (but not all) studies. Equivocal findings in human studies are partly caused by the difficulty of assessing oxidative stress. Measurement of ROS in tissues is a challenge because of their low levels and relatively short half-lives.[143] Most human studies have found that chronic antioxidant therapy with vitamin E and C supplements has little or no effect on BP.[144]

Atrial Natriuretic Peptide

ANP is a 28-amino-acid peptide synthesized and released from atrial cardiomyocytes in response to stretch. It enhances sodium excretion through extrarenal and intrarenal mechanisms.[145–147] ANP increases GFR, but an increase in GFR is not a prerequisite for it to enhance sodium excretion. ANP may also directly inhibit renal tubular sodium reabsorption, or it may do so indirectly via alterations in medullary blood flow, peritubular capillary physical factors, and decreasing antinatriuretic hormones such as Ang II and aldosterone.[145,148]

Atrial Natriuretic Peptide Enhances Pressure Natriuresis and Lowers Blood Pressure: Plasma levels of ANP are elevated in physiologic and pathophysiological conditions associated with volume expansion.[145,148] Infusions of exogenous ANP at rates that increase plasma concentrations, comparable to those observed during volume expansion, elicit significant natriuresis, especially in the presence of high renal perfusion pressure. Long-term physiologic elevations in plasma ANP also enhance renal pressure natriuresis and reduce BP.

Blockade of the ANP System Produces Salt-Sensitive Hypertension: Genetic mouse models with altered expression of ANP or its receptors (eg, NPR-A, NPR-C) have provided compelling evidence for a role of ANP in chronic regulation of BP.[149] Whereas transgenic mice overexpressing ANP are hypotensive relative to their control litter mates, mice harboring functional disruptions of the ANP or NPR-A genes are hypertensive. ANP gene knockout mice develop BP salt-sensitivity associated with failure to adequately suppress the RAAS.

Obese hypertensive men have lower plasma pro-ANP levels, even though they have higher sodium intake and larger left atria than normotensive, lean men.[150] The ANP responses to volume loading are also impaired in obese subjects. Increased adipocyte-derived neprilysin, an endopeptidase that degrades ANP, may also contribute to a relative ANP deficiency in obesity. Although these studies suggest a potential role for ANP deficiency in hypertension, the significance of abnormal secretion and clearance of ANP in hypertension is still uncertain.[151] Novel ANP analogs that are resistant to degradation by neprilysin and activate guanylyl cyclase A receptors have been developed and are entering clinical trials for hypertension therapy.[152]

Innate and Adaptive Immunity

Immune and inflammatory cells interact with other cells to defend against pathogens and injury. However, if inflammatory responses are excessive or sustained too long, they may damage tissues, including the kidneys and blood vessels, leading to hypertension. Thus, in patients with and experimental models of systemic lupus erythematosus (SLE), rheumatoid arthritis, and psoriasis, immunosuppressive drugs attenuate hypertension.[153–155]

There is also an association between innate or adaptive immune system activation and renal inflammation, reduced pressure natriuresis, and increased BP in several experimental models of hypertension, including Ang II, aldosterone, salt-sensitive, and spontaneously hypertensive rats.[103,154,155] An important characteristic commonly observed in these models is increased infiltrating immune cells, including macrophage and T lymphocytes, in the kidneys. In support of a role for T cells in the pathogenesis of hypertension are studies demonstrating that treatment with mycophenolate mofetil attenuates

hypertension in association with reduced renal cortical T-cell infiltration in DS rats.[103]

Harrison and colleagues[155] reported that mice lacking recombination activating gene 1 (Rag1$^{-/-}$ mice), required for maturation and development of T and B cells, are protected from vascular dysfunction and hypertension during chronic infusion of Ang II, norepinephrine, or DOCA-salt. However, Seniuk et al.[156] have challenged the concept that T and B lymphocytes are critically involved in hypertension, reporting that Ang II-induced hypertension and target organ injury were not attenuated in Rag1$^{-/-}$ mice.

Despite these apparent inconsistencies, there is a large body of evidence that immune-inflammatory mechanisms contribute to, or exacerbate, increased BP and cardiorenal injury in several forms of experimental hypertension.[154,155,157] In some cases, activation of immune/inflammatory pathways may occur secondary to hypertension and pressure-induced tissue damage. For example, in DS rats, kidney infiltration of macrophages and monocytes and tissue damage were greatly attenuated when renal perfusion pressure was servocontrolled and prevented from increasing during development of hypertension induced by feeding the animals a high-salt diet.[103]

The mechanisms by which infiltrating immune cells in the kidneys exacerbate hypertension are not fully understood. Several effects of cytokines and ROS released by immune cells have been reported, including increased tubular sodium reabsorption, increased vascular resistance, reduced GFR, and ultimately loss of nephrons due to tissue injury.[103,154,157]

Although experimental studies in a variety of animal models suggest an important role for the immune system in the pathogenesis of hypertension, comparable studies in humans are limited. Low-grade inflammation occurs in many forms of human hypertension, but anti-inflammatory therapies have not yet proved to be effective for reducing BP in primary hypertension. Some anti-inflammatory therapies (such as NSAIDs) and some immunosuppressive therapies actually raise BP and exacerbate cardiorenal injury. However, the effect of immune modulators and anti-inflammatory drugs on BP and target organ injury may depend on when the drugs are administered during the evolution of hypertension and tissue injury.[158,159] Thus, the overall importance of the immune system and inflammatory cytokines in the pathogenesis of primary and secondary human hypertension remains an important area for further investigation to determine whether more specific, targeted approaches may be useful in treating hypertension or associated target organ injury.

Secondary Causes of Hypertension

In <10% of patients with hypertension, the clinical features, history, and physical examination point to a specific cause of increased BP, and the hypertension is therefore said to be *secondary*. Some types of secondary hypertension have a definite genetic basis, and others are associated with specific neurohormonal or kidney disorders. In some instances, hypertension is caused by drugs or treatments that the patient receives.

TABLE 5–4. Some Secondary Causes of Hypertension

A. Renal parenchymal disease:
 Acute and chronic glomerulonephritis
 Chronic nephritis (eg, pyelonephritis, radiation)
 Polycystic disease
 Diabetic nephropathy
 Hydronephrosis
 Neoplasms
B. Renovascular:
 Renal artery stenosis or compression
 Intrarenal vasculitis
 Suprarenal aortic coarctation
C. Renoprival (renal failure, loss of kidney tissue)
D. Endocrine disorders:
 Renin-producing tumors
 Cushing syndrome
 Primary aldosteronism
 Pheochromocytoma (adrenal or extraadrenal chromaffin tumors)
 Acromegaly
E. Pregnancy-induced hypertension
F. Sleep apnea
G. Increased intracranial pressure (brain tumors, encephalitis)
H. Exogenous hormones and drugs (partial list):
 Glucocorticoids
 Mineralocorticoids
 Sympathomimetics
 Tyramine-containing foods and monoamine oxidase inhibitors
 Apparent mineralocorticoid excess (eg, licorice)
 NSAIDs
 Cyclosporine
 Excess alcohol use
 Drug abuse (eg, amphetamines, cocaine)

Table 5–4 lists some of the more frequently diagnosed causes of secondary hypertension, including those caused by drugs that either themselves increase BP or exacerbate underlying disorders that contribute to hypertension. These drugs include NSAIDs, oral contraceptives, glucocorticoids, and sympathomimetics.

Appropriate treatment of various forms of secondary hypertension can often control the underlying condition as well as elevated BP, although discovering the causes of various forms of secondary hypertension may be challenging and require evaluation by clinicians with special expertise. Extensive testing is not warranted in all patients with elevated BP because of low occurrence of secondary hypertension, the potential for false-positive results, and the cost. However, more extensive evaluation may be recommended for patients who demonstrate some general clinical clues that suggest secondary hypertension: (1) severe or resistant/refractory hypertension, (2) an acute rise in BP compared to a previously stable value, (3) proven onset of hypertension before puberty, (4) nonobese patients with hypertension who are younger than 30 years, and (5) hypertension associated with electrolyte disorders such as hypokalemia and metabolic alkalosis.

The ACC/AHA guidelines indicate that "if an adult with sustained hypertension screens positive for a form of secondary hypertension, referral to a physician with expertise in that form of hypertension may be reasonable for diagnostic confirmation and treatment."[1] More detailed criteria for diagnosing and treating various forms of secondary hypertension have been reviewed by previous studies.[1,160–162]

Renovascular Hypertension

Renovascular hypertension, although accounting for only ~5% of all hypertension, is one of the most common causes of secondary hypertension. The pathophysiology of renovascular hypertension is related to reductions in renal perfusion resulting from stenosis of the main renal artery or one of its branches, or stenosis/injury of other smaller preglomerular blood vessels and glomeruli. The majority of renal vascular lesions reflect either fibromuscular dysplasia or atherosclerosis.[163,164] The predominant lesion found in the main renal artery or its branches in patients >50 years of age is atherosclerotic disease. More subtle functional (constriction) or structural changes in smaller blood vessels (eg, afferent arterioles, glomeruli), however, are difficult to detect clinically and can increase BP.

Renovascular hypertension may be unilateral or bilateral and due to homogeneous or nonhomogeneous ischemia of nephrons. As discussed previously, there are important differences in the pathophysiology of homogeneous compared with that of nonhomogeneous renal ischemia. In patients with nonhomogeneous increases in preglomerular resistance caused by patchy nephron ischemia or by stenosis of a single kidney, the pathophysiology of hypertension is complicated by some nephrons being underperfused and others having normal or increased blood flow. Ischemic nephrons (or the entire underperfused kidney, in the case of a unilateral renal artery stenosis) are exposed to reduced perfusion pressure, secrete more renin, and excrete less sodium and water than kidneys with normal blood flow. In contrast, the nonischemic nephrons (or the nonstenotic kidney) are exposed to increased renal perfusion pressure, decreased renin secretion, and increased sodium excretion. However, even with increased perfusion pressure, the function of the nonischemic nephrons is impaired because of increased circulating Ang II, which exerts an antinatriuretic effect and helps sustain hypertension. The higher BP experienced by the nonstenotic kidney may eventually damage its nephrons, sustaining increased BP even after correction of the stenosis in the other kidney.

Administration of ACE inhibitors or ARBs as a treatment for renovascular hypertension may improve the structure and function of the nonstenotic kidney, but in some cases, they may also produce shrinkage of the stenotic kidney, resulting in fibrosis and deterioration of its function. This is partly a result of decreased BP, which may reduce renal perfusion pressure distal to the lesion to a level below the range of autoregulation. Blockade of the RAAS also dilates efferent arterioles, which contributes to a decline in GFR in the stenotic kidney. In some patients with severe renal vascular lesions, administration of ACE inhibitors or ARBs may cause severe decreases in renal function, especially when there is also volume depletion because of concomitant use of diuretics. Therefore, renal function should be monitored frequently after administration of RAAS inhibitors in patients suspected of having renovascular hypertension. Fortunately, these effects appear to be reversible upon cessation of ACE inhibition or ARB, and in many patients, the beneficial BP-lowering effects of RAAS blockade can be achieved without precipitating further loss of kidney function.

Currently, atherosclerotic renal artery stenosis, the most common cause of renovascular hypertension in older patients, is often managed by medical therapy since three large, multicentric randomized trials [Cardiovascular Outcomes in Renal Atherosclerotic Lesions, (CORAL), Angioplasty and Stenting for Renal Artery Lesions (ASTRAL), and Stent Placement in Patients with Atherosclerotic Renal Artery Stenosis and Impaired Renal Function (STAR)] failed to prove the superiority of percutaneous transluminal renal-artery stenting (PTRAS). However, severe and sustained renal vascular stenosis can produce microvascular rarefaction and loss of function of the poststenotic kidney, sometimes with irreversible parenchymal injury. Therefore, identifying patients in whom revascularization is possible, as well as effective in slowing or preventing further kidney injury, remains challenging.[161,164]

Adrenal Cortex Hypertension

Aldosterone normally exerts nearly 90% of the mineralocorticoid activity of adrenocortical secretions. However, cortisol, the major glucocorticoid secreted by the adrenal cortex, can also provide significant mineralocorticoid activity in some conditions. Cortisol has a much higher plasma concentration than aldosterone and a high affinity for the MR, but the renal MR is normally protected from cortisol activation by the enzyme 11 β-hydroxysteroid dehydrogenase 2 (11β-HSD2), which converts active cortisol into inactive cortisone. However, when 11β-HSD2 activity is reduced or when cortisol levels are very high, the MR may be activated by cortisol.

Primary Aldosteronism (Conn Syndrome): *Primary aldosteronism*, also called *Conn syndrome*, results from hypersecretion of aldosterone in the absence of a known stimulus. The excess aldosterone secretion almost always comes from the adrenal cortex and is usually associated with a solitary adenoma or bilateral hyperplasia of the adrenal cortex. *Secondary aldosteronism* refers to increased aldosterone secretion resulting from a known stimulus, such as increased Ang II. This is the most common form of aldosteronism seen in clinical practice and occurs in various conditions associated with increased renin secretion, such as congestive heart failure, sodium depletion, or renal artery stenosis.

Primary aldosteronism may occur as a result of an aldosterone-producing adenoma (APA) or unilateral or bilateral adrenal hyperplasia (BAH).[125,160,165-167] The effects of excess aldosterone were discussed earlier, but the most important actions for BP regulation are increased sodium reabsorption and increased potassium secretion by the principal cells of the renal collecting tubules, and increased hydrogen ion secretion by the intercalated cells of the renal tubules. These effects cause expansion of extracellular fluid volume, hypertension, suppression of renin secretion, hypokalemia, and metabolic alkalosis—hallmarks of primary aldosteronism. Most of these effects are highly salt sensitive, and low sodium intake greatly attenuates the hypertension and hypokalemia associated with primary aldosteronism.

Diagnosis of primary aldosteronism is made by a multistep process that ends with adrenal venous sampling.[168] APA and BAH together account for more than 95% of primary aldosteronism. Patients with APA are often treated by surgical removal of the adenoma, whereas those with BAH are treated pharmacologically with MR antagonists.[165] With wider screening for primary aldosteronism, approximately 70% of cases appear to be caused by BAH, with APA comprising most of the remainder.[165]

In most studies of unselected patients, the classic form of primary aldosteronism was found in less than 1% of hypertensive patients. Some adrenal glands in patients with primary aldosteronism may have varying degrees of hyperplasticity, and the term *idiopathic hyperaldosteronism (IHA)* was coined to describe this condition. Clinically, APA and IHA are difficult to distinguish, although patients with APA often have more severe hypertension and hypokalemia than those with IHA.

Measurements of the aldosterone-renin ratio have been used to define more subtle cases of primary aldosteronism. This approach has led to the suggestion that excess aldosterone secretion may account for as much as 5% of essential hypertension. However, there is considerable debate about whether patients with increased aldosterone-renin ratios truly have primary aldosteronism. In many of these patients, the major reason for the increased aldosterone–renin ratio is the low level of renin rather than excess aldosterone secretion.

Sustained Hypokalemia and Metabolic Alkalosis with Hyperaldosteronism: Excess aldosterone not only increases the secretion of potassium ions by the renal tubules but also stimulates the transport of potassium from the extracellular fluid into most cells of the body. This shift of potassium from extracellular to intracellular fluid accounts for a significant part of the hypokalemia in hyperaldosteronism.

Increased aldosterone secretion also stimulates the secretion of hydrogen ions in exchange for sodium and bicarbonate reabsorption in the intercalated cells of the renal collecting tubules and collecting ducts. This decreases hydrogen ion concentration in the extracellular fluid, causing metabolic alkalosis.

Patients with IHA often have a milder form of aldosteronism than those with APA, although there may be an overlap in severity of the clinical features of these two groups. In patients with APA, plasma aldosterone concentration is not usually increased in response to an upright posture because of marked suppression of renin secretion and insensitivity of the aldosterone-secreting adenoma to Ang II. In contrast, patients with IHA usually have a significant increase in aldosterone concentration during an upright posture, suggesting that adrenal sensitivity to Ang II is maintained. These differences between IHA and APA in adrenal responsiveness to RAAS activation have been used to discriminate between these two forms of primary aldosteronism.

Cushing Syndrome (Glucocorticoid Excess): Cushing syndrome is characterized by excess secretion of glucocorticoids. Hypertension occurs in approximately 80% of patients with Cushing syndrome and is difficult to control.[169] The morbidity associated with cortisol excess is substantial, and risk of death is largely due to excess cardiovascular events, including heart attack and stroke.

Cushing syndrome may be caused by administration of excess cortisol (eg, for treatment of various inflammatory disorders) or by excess endogenous cortisol secretion. The most common cause of endogenous cortisol excess is overproduction of adrenocorticotropic hormone (ACTH) from a pituitary adenoma, a condition referred to as *Cushing disease*. Increased ACTH causes adrenal hyperplasia and stimulates cortisol secretion. Cushing disease may also occur as a result of ectopic secretion of ACTH by tumors outside the pituitary, such as an abdominal carcinoma.

ACTH-independent hypercortisolism may also be caused by adenomas of the adrenal cortex. Primary overproduction of cortisol by the adrenal glands, independent of ACTH, accounts for approximately 20% to 25% of cases of Cushing syndrome and is usually associated with suppressed ACTH levels caused by cortisol-induced feedback inhibition of ACTH secretion from the anterior pituitary gland. Administration of large doses of dexamethasone, a synthetic glucocorticoid, can be used to distinguish between ACTH-dependent and ACTH-independent Cushing syndrome. In patients with overproduction of cortisol because of an ACTH-secreting pituitary adenoma or hypothalamic-pituitary dysfunction, even large doses of dexamethasone usually do not suppress ACTH secretion. In contrast, patients with primary adrenal overproduction of cortisol (ACTH independent) usually have low or undetectable levels of ACTH. However, the dexamethasone test may occasionally give an incorrect diagnosis because some ACTH-secreting pituitary tumors respond to dexamethasone with suppression of ACTH secretion.

Other Forms of Adrenocortical Hypertension: There are several other rare forms of adrenocortical hypertension, as discussed in the section on genetic causes of hypertension later in this chapter. The clinical characteristics of these conditions are similar to those observed with primary increases in aldosterone secretion.

Pheochromocytoma

Although rare, occurring in only 0.05% of hypertensive patients, pheochromocytoma can provoke fatal hypertensive crises if unrecognized and untreated.[162] Pheochromocytoma can arise from neuroectodermal chromaffin cells, which are part of the sympathoadrenal system. The chromaffin cells have the capacity to synthesize and store catecholamines and are normally found mainly in the adrenal medulla. Although most chromaffin cell tumors are found in the adrenal medulla, as many as 15% to 30% may be extraadrenal, located along the sympathetic chain or, rarely, in other sites.

The symptoms and severity of hypertension associated with pheochromocytoma are highly variable, depending on the secretory pattern and amount of catecholamines released. With tumors that continuously release large amounts of catecholamines, there may be sustained hypertension with few paroxysms or sudden bursts of very high BP. Tumors that are less active may have cyclical release of catecholamines that induce paroxysms of hypertension.

The clinical presentation also depends on whether the predominant catecholamine secreted is norepinephrine or epinephrine. Whereas norepinephrine produces α-adrenergically mediated vasoconstriction with diastolic hypertension, epinephrine produces β-adrenergically mediated cardiac stimulation with mainly systolic hypertension and tachycardia, along with sweating, tremors, and flushing. Patients with predominantly epinephrine-secreting tumors sometimes have hypertension alternating with hypotension, and ~5% of patients with pheochromocytoma remain normotensive.

Although a high level of circulating catecholamine is the ultimate cause of hypertension in pheochromocytoma, BP is often only modestly correlated with plasma catecholamine levels. However, periodic bursts of catecholamine release may cause moderate to severe bouts of hypertension that lead to target organ injury. Consequently, diagnosis and effective treatment of pheochromocytoma are essential.

Preeclampsia

Preeclampsia is a complex maternal syndrome characterized by multiple disorders, including proteinuria, thrombocytopenia, renal insufficiency, impaired liver function, pulmonary edema, and cerebral or visual symptoms; however, preeclampsia is most identifiable by new-onset hypertension (SBP ≥140 mmHg/DBP ≥90 mmHg) after the 20th week of gestation.[170,171] Progression of the disease may lead to eclampsia, in which seizures develop in association with a high risk of fetal and maternal mortality. Despite being a leading cause of maternal death and a major contributor to maternal and perinatal morbidity, the pathophysiological mechanisms of preeclampsia have not been fully elucidated. Hypertension associated with preeclampsia remits after delivery, implicating the placenta as a central culprit in the disease.[170]

Although numerous factors, including genetic, immunologic, behavioral, and environmental mechanisms, have been implicated in the pathogenesis of preeclampsia, reduced uteroplacental perfusion as a result of abnormal cytotrophoblast invasion of spiral arterioles appears to play a key role.[172] Placental ischemia is thought to cause widespread dysfunction of the maternal vascular endothelium, which results in enhanced formation of ET-1, thromboxane, and superoxide; increased vascular sensitivity to Ang II; and decreased formation of vasodilators such as NO and prostacyclin. These endothelial abnormalities, in turn, cause hypertension by impairing renal function while increasing TPR.

One of the most intensely studied pathways in preeclampsia is that related to vascular endothelial growth factor (VEGF) signaling.[170,172] This signaling pathway came to prominence with the discovery of elevated circulating and placental levels of the soluble form of the VEGF receptor, fms-related tyrosine kinases (sFlt)-1 in preeclampsia.[170,172,173] Here, sFlt-1 is a circulating soluble receptor for VEGF and placental growth factor (PlGF), and when increased in maternal plasma, it leads to less circulating free VEGF and free PlGF, blocking their ability to stimulate angiogenesis and maintain endothelial integrity. In the kidney, inactivation of free VEGF may cause endotheliosis and proteinuria.

Animal studies have shown that a myriad of experimental models of preeclampsia (placental ischemia, sFlt-1 infusion, TNF-α infusion, and AT1-AA infusion) are associated with elevated tissue levels of ET-1. The fact that hypertension in pregnant rats, induced by placental ischemia or chronic infusion of sFlt-1, TNF-α, or AT1-AA can be attenuated by ET$_A$ receptor antagonism, strongly suggests that ET-1 may be a final common pathway linking factors produced during placental ischemia to elevations in BP.[174]

Unfortunately, effective treatments for patients with preeclampsia remain elusive. In light of the recent developments in our understanding of the pathophysiology of preeclampsia, treatment strategies aimed at improving endothelial dysfunction, safely lowering BP, and reducing maternal and perinatal morbidity are warranted.

Genetic Causes of Hypertension

Gene Variants and Human Primary Hypertension

With the development of superb tools for genetic studies and sequencing of the human genome, there has been great enthusiasm for the possibility that genetic causes of primary hypertension can be identified.[175–177] However, despite great effort, there has been limited success in identifying genes that contribute to human primary hypertension. Success thus far has been limited mainly to the identification of rare monogenic forms of hypertension. A detailed discussion of this topic is beyond the scope of this chapter, but other sources have discussed some reasons why the "geneticism of hypertension" approach has had limited success.[178]

When one considers the complexity of the multiple neural, hormonal, renal, and vascular mechanisms that contribute to short- and long-term BP regulation, perhaps it is not surprising that finding a few variant genes (alleles) to account for a substantial portion of BP variation has been challenging. The complexity of the problem is further amplified by the fact that genetic components of BP variation are likely to be mediated not only by single-gene variations but also by polymorphic genetic differences, complex interactions among several genes, and interactions among genetic and environmental factors. The observation that hypertension does not occur with significant frequency in multiple populations living in nonindustrialized regions of the world suggests that environmental influences play a major role in common forms of hypertension.

Although the hypertension research literature is replete with studies showing associations of gene polymorphisms and BP, the genetic alterations that contribute to primary hypertension remain unknown. All the polymorphisms studied thus far show weak, if any association with BP, and many of the early studies showing statistically significant associations have not been confirmed. Large-scale, genomewide association studies,

in which hundreds of thousands of common genetic variants are genotyped and analyzed for BP association, have shown limited success in identifying genes that contribute to hypertension.[179] The gene variations discovered thus far explain only a tiny part of the BP variation found in humans.

Epigenetic modification of gene expression may help to explain some of the "missing heritability" of human BP variation.[180–182] *Epigenetics* is the study of heritable changes in gene expression caused by factors that orchestrate changes in the expression of deoxyribonucleic acid (DNA) without altering the underlying DNA sequence.[180–182] Nucleic acid methylation, histone modification, nucleosome positioning, transcriptional control with DNA-binding proteins and noncoding ribonucleic acid (RNA), and translation control with microRNA and RNA-binding proteins could potentially contribute to epigenetic changes in gene expression. Evidence from rodent studies suggests that some epigenetically influenced phenotypes (eg, obesity, insulin resistance) may even be passed to more than one generation of offspring.[183] However, the importance of epigenetic changes in contributing to human primary hypertension is still unclear and is an emerging area of investigation.

Monogenic Disorders That Cause Hypertension

Table 5–5 shows some of the monogenic disorders associated with hypertension. An interesting feature of these genetic disorders is that all but one of them increase either electrolyte transport in the renal tubules or the synthesis/activity of mineralocorticoid hormones. The final common pathway to hypertension in most of these disorders appears to be increased renal sodium reabsorption;[184] hypertension in these disorders is salt sensitive, and treatment with diuretics reduces BP. One form of monogenic hypertension associated with increased vascular resistance is due to gain-of-function mutations in the gene encoding phosphodiesterase 3A (PDE3A).[185] Monogenic hypertension, however, is rare, and all the known forms together account for less than 1% of human hypertension.

Pathophysiology of Primary (Essential) Hypertension

Primary (essential) hypertension, which accounts for >90% of all cases of hypertension, has been traditionally defined as high BP for which an obvious secondary cause (eg, renovascular disease, aldosteronism, pheochromocytoma, or gene mutations) cannot be determined. Although primary hypertension is heterogeneous, some of the main causes of high BP are known. For example, overweight and obesity account for 65% to 75% of the risk for primary hypertension. Sedentary lifestyle, excess intake of sodium chloride or alcohol, and low potassium intake also contribute to increased BP in some patients. Thus, identifiable causes can often be found in patients classified as having primary hypertension.[100,120]

Overweight/Obesity: A Major Cause of Primary Hypertension

Current estimates indicate that more than 1.9 billion people in the world are overweight or obese as of 2016.[186] In the United States, >70% of adults are overweight, and >42% obese, with BMIs

TABLE 5–5. Some Known Genetic Causes of Hypertension

Genetic Disorder	Age of Onset	Pattern of Inheritance	Aldosterone Level	Serum Potassium Level	Treatment[a]
AME2[b,c]	Childhood	Autosomal recessive	Low	Low to normal	Dexamethasone, MR antagonist, amiloride
Liddle syndrome[d]	Third decade of life	Autosomal dominant	Low	Low to normal	Amiloride, triamterene
Gordon syndrome[e]	Second or third decade of life	Autosomal dominant	Low	High	Thiazide diuretic, low-sodium diet
FH-I (GRA)[f]	Second or third decade of life	Autosomal dominant	High	Decreased in most cases; marked decrease achieved with thiazides	Glucocorticoids, MR antagonist, amiloride
FH-II[b]	Middle age	Autosomal dominant	High	Low to normal	MR antagonist
DOC oversecretion caused by CAHb[g]	Childhood	Autosomal recessive	Low	Low to normal	Glucocorticoids, MR antagonist
Activating MR mutation exacerbated by pregnancy[h]	Second or third decade of life	Unknown	Low	Low to normal	Delivery of fetus, amiloride, triamterene
Brachydactly and hypertension[i]	Childhood	Autosomal dominant	Normal	Normal	Milrinone

[a]Treatment for underlying mechanisms and different antihypertensive medications that may be used to control blood pressure
[b]Excess production of nonaldosterone mineralocorticoids
[c]Apparent mineralocorticoid excess caused by either licorice ingestion or ectopic ACTH secretion
[d]Increased activity of sodium channels
[e]Increased activity of NaCl cotransporter in the distal tubule
[f]Familial hyperaldosteronism
[g]CAH-, DOC-producing tumors
[h]Increased activity of MRs
[i]Gain of function mutations of PDE3A
Abbreviations: ACTH, adrenocorticotropic hormone; AME, apparent mineralocorticoid excess; CAH, congenital adrenal hyperplasia; DOC, deoxycorticosterone; FH-I, familial hyperaldosteronism type I; FH-II, familial hyperaldosteronism type II; GRA, glucocorticoid-remediable aldosteronism; MR, mineralocorticoid receptor; PDE3A, phosphodiesterase 3A

above 30. Population studies show that excess weight gain predicts the development of hypertension, and the relationship between BMI and systolic and diastolic BP is nearly linear in diverse populations throughout the world.[109,120] Risk estimates from the Framingham Heart Study, for example, suggest that approximately 78% of primary hypertension in men and 65% in women can be ascribed to excess weight gain.[187] Clinical studies indicate that maintenance of a BMI <25 kg/m² is effective in primary prevention of hypertension and that weight loss reduces BP in most hypertensive subjects.[188]

One question often raised is why, if obesity is a major cause of increased BP, some persons who are overweight or obese are not hypertensive. Perhaps this is not surprising if one considers that BP is normally distributed and that excess weight gain shifts the frequency distribution of BP toward higher levels (**Figure 5–13**). However, even obese individuals who are considered normotensive have higher BP than they would at a lower body weight, and weight loss lowers BP in normotensive and hypertensive obese subjects.[109]

Distribution of adipose tissue is also important. Most population studies that have investigated the relationship between obesity and BP have measured BMI rather than visceral or retroperitoneal fat, which appear to be better predictors of increased BP than subcutaneous fat.[189]

Although the importance of obesity, especially excess visceral fat, is well established as a major risk factor for primary hypertension, the pathophysiologic mechanisms involved have

not been fully elucidated. **Table 5–6** summarizes some of the changes in hemodynamics, neurohumoral systems, and renal function that occur with excess weight gain in humans and experimental animals.

Mechanisms of Impaired Renal Pressure Natriuresis in Obesity Hypertension: Three mechanisms appear to be especially important in increasing sodium reabsorption and initiating

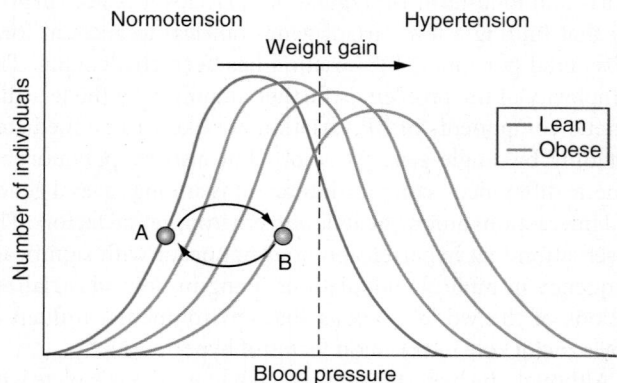

Figure 5–13. Obesity shifts the frequency distribution of BP. Not all individuals who are obese have BPs in the hypertensive range; however, obesity raises BP above the baseline level for an individual. (eg, from point A to B). Conversely, weight loss lowers BP in individuals who are obese but considered to be normotensive (eg, from point B to A), as well as in those who are obese and hypertensive. Increasing duration of obesity exacerbates the obesity-induced shift of the BP frequency distribution to higher levels of BP.

TABLE 5–6. Hemodynamic, Neurohumoral, and Renal Changes in Experimental Obesity Caused by a High-Fat Diet, as Well as in Human Obesity

Model	Arterial Pressure	Heart Rate	Cardiac Output	Renal Sympathetic Activity	Plasma Renin Activity	Na+ Balance	Renal Tubular Reabsorption	GFR[a]	Insulin Resistance
Obese rodents (high-fat diet)	↑→	↑→	↑	↑	↑→	↑→	↑→	↑→	↑
Obese rabbits (high-fat diet)	↑	↑	↑	↑	↑	↑	↑	↑	↑
Obese dogs (high-fat diet)	↑	↑	↑	↑	↑	↑	↑	↑	↑
Obese humans	↑	↑	↑	↑	↑	↑	↑	↑	↑

[a]GFR changes refer to the early phases of obesity, before major loss of nephron function has occurred.

obesity hypertension: (1) increased SNS activity, (2) activation of the RAAS, and (3) physical compression of the kidneys by fat accumulation within and around the kidneys, as well as by increased abdominal pressure (**Figure 5–14**). Also, chronic kidney injury, caused by interactions of increased BP, metabolic disorders, and inflammation, may gradually exacerbate obesity-associated hypertension, making it more difficult to control and less easily reversed by weight loss.[190]

SNS Activation in Obesity Hypertension: The following observations in experimental animals and in humans indicate that increased SNS activity contributes to obesity hypertension:[120,191] (1) SNS activation, especially renal sympathetic activity, is increased in obese subjects; (2) pharmacologic blockade of adrenergic activity lowers BP to a greater extent in obese than in lean individuals; and (3) RDN markedly attenuates the sodium retention and hypertension associated with obesity.

Increased SNS activity appears to be highly differentiated in obesity. For example, cardiac sympathetic activity may not be substantially elevated, but SNS activity is usually increased in kidneys and skeletal muscles of obese subjects. Obesity-induced SNS activation is usually not sufficient to cause vasoconstriction in most tissues, such as the kidneys or skeletal muscle, but it does increase renin secretion and renal tubular sodium reabsorption.[109,120]

Current evidence indicates that the chronic BP effects of SNS activation in obesity are mediated mainly by renal nerves. Bilateral RDN greatly attenuated sodium retention and

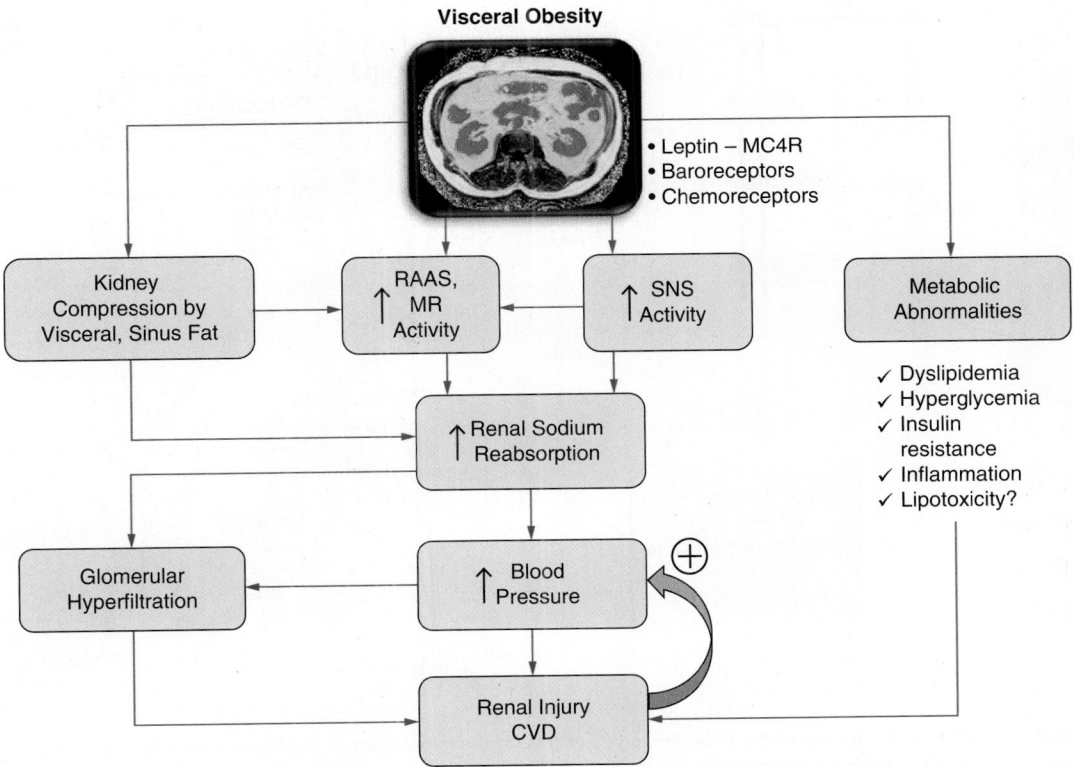

Figure 5–14. Summary of mechanisms by which obesity causes hypertension and renal injury. Visceral obesity increases BP by activation of the SNS and the RAAS, as well as by physical compression of the kidneys from fat surrounding them. These effects increase renal sodium reabsorption and impair pressure natriuresis. SNS activation may be caused by, in large part, the effects of leptin, which acts on POMC neurons in the hypothalamus and brain stem. Obesity-induced hypertension and glomerular hyperfiltration may cause renal injury, especially when combined with dyslipidemia, hyperglycemia, and other metabolic disorders. Renal injury then exacerbates the hypertension and makes it more difficult to control. MR, mineralocorticoid receptor.

hypertension in obese dogs.[111,192] Similar results were observed in obese humans with resistant hypertension in which catheter-based radiofrequency RDN lowered BP for up to 3 years, although not to the same extent as in experimental obesity hypertension.[113] However, in most of these clinical trials, the extent of RDN was not determined, and catheter-based RDN typically causes <50% renal nerve ablation unless nerves in renal segmental arteries are ablated.[111]

Potential mediators of SNS activation in obesity include (1) hyperinsulinemia; (2) Ang II; (3) increased levels of free fatty acids; (4) impaired baroreceptor reflexes; (5) activation of chemoreceptor-mediated reflexes associated with sleep apnea and intermittent hypoxia; and (6) cytokines released from adipocytes (ie, adipokines) such as leptin, TNF-α, and IL-6. Although the importance of most of these factors is still uncertain, leptin and the CNS proopiomelanocortin (POMC) pathway may contribute to obesity-induced SNS activation and hypertension (**Figure 5–15**).

Leptin is released from adipocytes and acts on the hypothalamus and other regions of the brain to reduce appetite and increase SNS activity.[109,120] In rodents, increasing plasma leptin concentration to levels comparable to those found in severe obesity increases SNS activity and BP.[109,120] Moreover, the hypertensive effects of leptin are enhanced when NO synthesis is inhibited,[109,120] as often occurs in obese subjects with endothelial dysfunction.

Another observation that points toward leptin as a potential mechanism of obesity hypertension is the finding that leptin-deficient, obese mice usually have little or no increase in BP compared with lean control subjects.[120,193] Similar results have been found in obese children with leptin gene mutations who have early-onset morbid obesity but normal BP despite having other characteristics of metabolic syndrome, including severe insulin resistance, hyperinsulinemia, and hyperlipidemia.[194] These observations suggest that the functional effects of leptin may be important in linking obesity with SNS activation and hypertension.

Leptin's stimulatory effect on SNS activity appears to be mediated by activation of POMC neurons in the hypothalamus and brain stem; these neurons release α-melanocyte

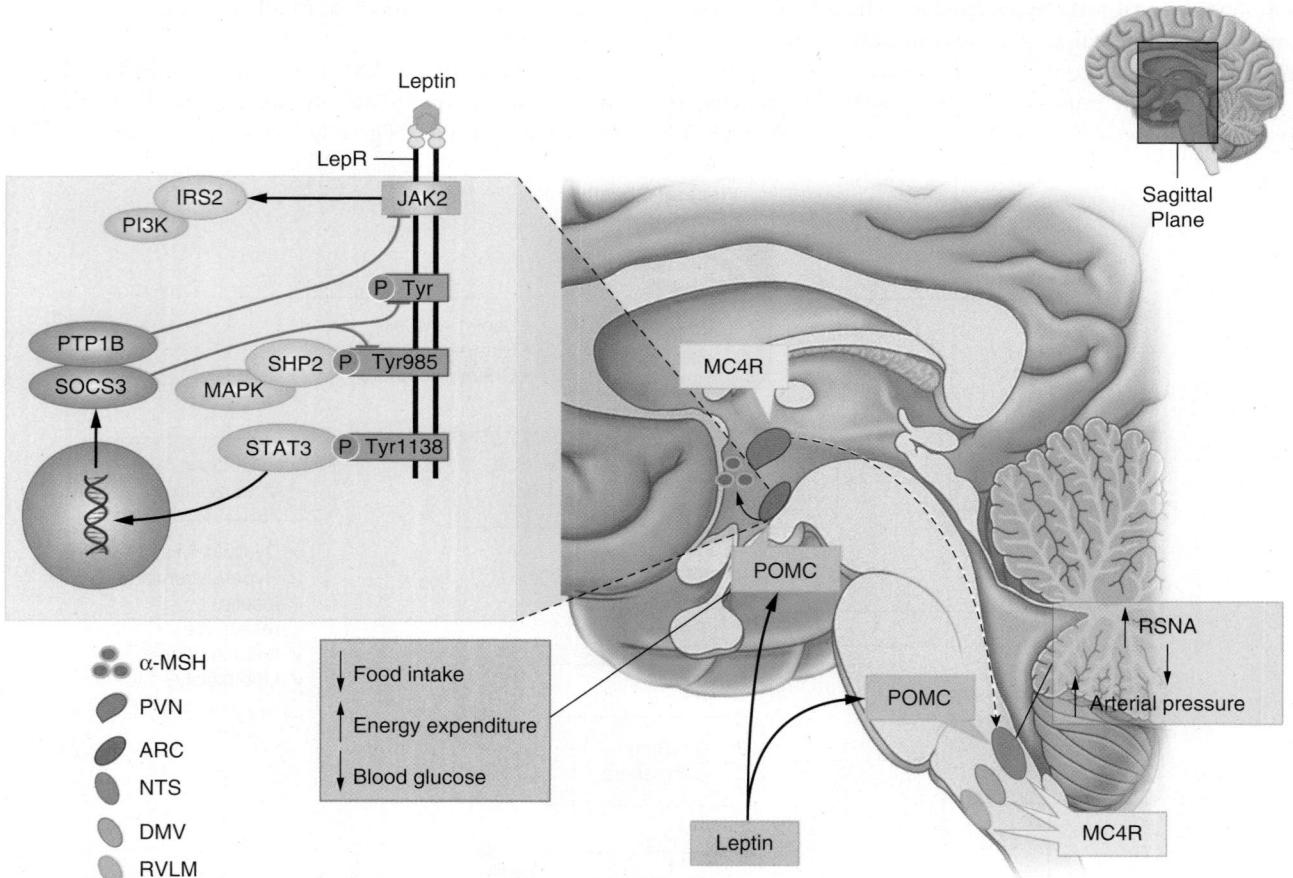

Figure 5–15. Possible link of increases in adiposity with leptin and its effects on the hypothalamus to initiate sympathetic activation and hypertension. Within the hypothalamus, one of the key pathways of leptin's action on food intake, energy expenditure, renal sympathetic nervous system activity (RSNA), and arterial pressure is stimulation of the POMC neurons in the arcuate nucleus (ARC). These neurons send projections to the paraventricular nucleus (PVN) and lateral hypothalamus, releasing α-melanocyte–stimulating hormone (α-MSH), which then acts as an agonist for MC4Rs. These neurons then send projections to the nucleus of the solitary tract (NTS) to effect changes in appetite, RSNA, and BP. Leptin may also stimulate POMC neurons in the NTS. MC4R activation in the dorsal motor nucleus of the vagus (DMV), rostral ventrolateral medulla (RVLM), and the spinal cord intermediolateral nucleus may also contribute to obesity-induced increases in RSNA and arterial pressure. LepR, leptin receptor.

stimulating hormone, which then activates melanocortin 4 receptors (MC4Rs) in second-order neurons in the hypothalamus and brain stem. Deletion of leptin receptors specifically in POMC neurons abolished the hypertensive effects of leptin.[195] Also, pharmacological antagonism or genetic deletion of MC4R completely abolished leptin's chronic BP effects. These findings indicate that activation of POMC neurons and subsequent stimulation of the MC4R mediate most of the effects of leptin to activate SNS activity and raise BP.[109,120,195] Studies in humans also suggest that MC4R activation may contribute to obesity-induced hypertension. The prevalence of hypertension is lower in MC4R-deficient humans than in control subjects, despite severe obesity and associated metabolic disorders.[196] Moreover, subcutaneous administration of an MC4R agonist for 7 days caused significant increases in BP that are similar to those observed in rodents. Thus, in humans and rodents, chronic activation of the MC4R increases BP, and the presence of a functional MC4R system appears to be necessary for obesity to increase SNS activity and BP.

RAAS Activation in Obesity: Obese subjects, especially those with visceral obesity, often have mild-to-moderate increases in plasma renin activity, angiotensinogen, ACE activity, Ang II, and aldosterone levels.[109,120] Activation of the RAAS in obese subjects occurs despite sodium retention, volume expansion, and hypertension, all of which would normally tend to suppress renin secretion and Ang II formation.

An important role for Ang II in stimulating renal sodium reabsorption and in mediating obesity hypertension is supported by experimental and clinical studies demonstrating that Ang II receptor blockade or ACE inhibition blunts sodium retention, volume expansion, increased BP, and target organ injury in obesity hypertension.[109,120] While major hypertension clinical trials have generally included RAAS blockers, randomized trials comparing the effectiveness of RAAS blockers with other antihypertensive agents in lean and obese patients have not been conducted.

Antagonism of MRs also provides an important therapeutic tool for reducing sodium retention, BP, and target organ injury in obesity hypertension.[109,120] Compared to other antihypertensive drugs, the MR antagonist spironolactone was superior for treating obese patients with resistant hypertension who were already on three or more antihypertensive medications, usually including an ARB or ACE inhibitor.[197] The antihypertensive benefit of an MR blockade appears to come mainly from reduced renal sodium reabsorption and the resulting natriuresis and diuresis.[197,198] The observation that MR antagonism reduces BP and protects against end-organ injury in obesity-hypertension, despite normal or even reduced plasma aldosterone after Ang II blockade, suggests that other factors, in addition to aldosterone, may activate MR.[109,120]

Kidney Compression Caused by Visceral Obesity: Increased visceral, retroperitoneal, and renal sinus fat obesity can compress the kidneys, causing increased intrarenal pressure, impaired renal pressure natriuresis, and increased BP.[109,120] Intra-abdominal pressure increases in proportion to abdominal diameter, reaching levels as high as 35 to 40 mmHg in some individuals.[109,120] In addition, retroperitoneal adipose tissue often encapsulates the kidneys and penetrates the renal hilum into the renal medullary sinuses, causing additional compression and increased intrarenal pressure.[190] Renal sinus fat was highly correlated with the number of BP medications and with stage II hypertension, as well as increased risk for CKD after adjusting for BMI, visceral adiposity, and other risk factors.[190] Although visceral adiposity and accumulation of renal sinus and retroperitoneal fat cannot account for the initial increase in BP that occurs with rapid weight gain, they may help to explain why visceral obesity is much more closely associated with hypertension than subcutaneous obesity.

Glomerular Injury and Nephron Loss in Obesity Hypertension: Obese patients often develop proteinuria, frequently in the nephrotic range, followed by progressive loss of kidney function.[190,199] The most common types of lesions observed in renal biopsies of obese subjects are focal and segmental glomerular sclerosis and glomerulomegaly.[199]

Animals placed on a high-fat diet for only a few weeks have significant structural changes in the kidneys, including enlargement of the Bowman space, glomerular cell proliferation, increased mesangial matrix, and increased expression of glomerular transforming growth factor (TGF)-β. These early changes, which occur with only modest hypertension, no evidence of diabetes, and only mild metabolic abnormalities, may be the precursors of more severe renal injury as obesity is sustained.

The impact of obesity on CKD is especially apparent when considering that type 2 diabetes and hypertension, which are driven largely by obesity, account for at least 70% to 75% of end-stage renal disease. However, obesity increases the risk for CKD even after adjustment for hypertension, diabetes, or preexisting renal disease.[199,200] Obesity also exacerbates the deleterious effects of other kidney insults, including unilateral nephrectomy, kidney transplantation, unilateral renal agenesis, and immunoglobulin A nephropathy.[190] Thus, obesity amplifies the loss of kidney function in patients with preexisting glomerulopathies, and weight loss may lessen the impact of renal injury from other causes.

Gradual loss of kidney function, as well as hypertension and diabetes that commonly coexist with obesity, may lead to progressive impairment of kidney function, increases in salt sensitivity, and progressive increases in BP. Thus, renal injury in obese subjects not only makes the hypertension more severe, but also more difficult to control with antihypertensive drugs. Early control of hypertension and effective weight management are crucial in preventing injury to the kidneys in obese patients.

What Is the Role of Insulin Resistance and Hyperinsulinemia in Primary Hypertension?

Dyslipidemia, hyperinsulinemia, and hyperglycemia often occur concurrently with hypertension, leading to the proposal of a unique pathophysiologic condition that is often called *metabolic syndrome*. Definitions of metabolic syndrome generally include disordered glucose homeostasis or measures of insulin resistance, dyslipidemia, hypertension, and obesity.[201]

Some researchers suggest that a defect in insulin action (ie, insulin resistance) is the main cause of all the CVD risk factors that constitute the different versions of the metabolic syndrome. Other analyses of metabolic syndrome, however, have questioned whether insulin resistance and hyperinsulinemia are the underlying causes of hypertension in this complex cluster of cardiovascular risk factors.[202–204]

Hyperinsulinemia Does Not Cause Hypertension in Humans: Evidence supporting a role for hyperinsulinemia in hypertension comes mainly from epidemiologic studies showing correlations between insulin resistance, hyperinsulinemia, and BP and from short-term studies indicating that insulin has sympathetic effects that, if sustained, could theoretically increase BP. However, chronic hyperinsulinemia, in the absence of obesity, does not raise BP in dogs or humans.[203,204] For example, chronic insulin infusions in dogs did not increase BP even when there was preexisting impairment of renal function caused by a 70% reduction of kidney mass and did not enhance the hypertensive effects of norepinephrine or Ang II.[203–205] Multiple studies in humans have also shown that chronic insulin treatment does not raise BP, and patients with severe hyperinsulinemia as a result of insulinoma are not hypertensive.[204,205] These observations suggest that hyperinsulinemia per se is insufficient to cause chronic hypertension.

Does Insulin Resistance Cause Hypertension Independent of Hyperinsulinemia? Insulin resistance has also been suggested to cause hypertension through mechanisms that are independent of hyperinsulinemia. However, experimental animals with obesity caused by mutations of the leptin gene or the leptin receptor, or by mutations of MC4Rs, have severe insulin resistance and many of the characteristics of the metabolic syndrome but do not have increased BP compared to control subjects.[120,204] Likewise, humans with leptin gene or MC4R mutations have severe insulin resistance, but no indication of SNS activation or hypertension.[194,196,204]

Although a direct causal relationship between insulin resistance and hypertension has not been established, abnormalities of glucose and lipid metabolism associated with insulin resistance may, over many years, lead to vascular and renal injury and contribute indirectly to increased BP, or at least exacerbate hypertension caused by obesity and its associated neurohormonal and renal changes.

Until more effective prevention and treatment strategies are developed, the impact of obesity on hypertension and related cardiovascular, renal, and metabolic disorders is likely to become even more important as the prevalence of obesity continues to increase. In the meantime, effective BP control is essential in treating patients with metabolic syndrome and preventing CVD. Weight reduction is an essential first step in the effective management of most patients with metabolic syndrome and hypertension, and more emphasis should be placed on lifestyle modifications that help patients to maintain a healthier weight and prevent CVD.

DIAGNOSIS AND TREATMENT OF HYPERTENSION

Initial Office Evaluation

The initial evaluation should include obtaining a personal history detailing lifestyle choices, record of health care, and use of medications, tobacco products, alcohol, or other forms of substance abuse. In addition, a patient's family history should be obtained to recognize occurrence of premature high BP and/or CVD. The physical examination should include measurement of sitting BP in both arms, with subsequent use of the arm with the higher reading. It is essential that BP is measured accurately, and that an average of two or more readings taken on two or more occasions is used to estimate usual office BP. This will ensure accurate BP classification and facilitate the practice of evidence-based medicine.

Basic laboratory testing enables CVD risk profiling, provides a baseline prior to the use of medication, and facilitates the recognition of secondary causes of hypertension. Minimally, it should include obtaining fasting blood glucose, serum sodium and potassium, serum creatinine, and estimation of glomerular filtration rate (eGFR), lipid profile, serum calcium, thyroid-stimulating hormone (TSH), complete blood count, urinalysis, and a 12-lead electrocardiogram. Blood uric acid and urinary albumin-to-creatinine ratio readings may be warranted in the context of specific medication choices, and echocardiography can be used as a complement to or in place of electrocardiography as a sensitive method for assessing left ventricular hypertrophy and function.

CVD Risk Assessment

CVD risk estimation is used as a complement to the level of BP for treatment decisions and is particularly valuable in adults with less severe forms of high BP, such as stage 1 hypertension. The concept is that CVD risk estimation will identify those who are most likely to experience a CVD clinical complication during a specified period (often 10 years), and this should be a consideration in the decision to recommend antihypertensive drug therapy.[206] Promoting a healthy lifestyle is in the best interest of all adults. Benefit-to-risk considerations make the addition of antihypertensive drug therapy increasingly justified at progressively higher levels of risk for CVD complications during the period specified. In addition, the landmark clinical trials that have proven the efficacy of antihypertensive drugs have all been conducted in patient populations at high risk for CVD.

Individuals who have already had a CVD event are at high risk for recurrent CVD complications. In others, it is often feasible to estimate CVD or atherosclerotic cardiovascular disease (ASCVD) risk based on the presence or absence of risk factors. Typically, CVD/ASCVD risk calculators have been validated in specific populations, and the use of a calculator in others is likely to provide a less accurate estimate.[207] In US adults aged 40–79 years who do not have a history of CVD, ASCVD risk should be estimated using the ACC/AHA Pooled Cohort Equations (PCE) risk calculator. This is available on many web sites, including those for the ACC and AHA. It is based on age; levels of SBP and DBP; total, high-density, and low-density cholesterol; history of diabetes mellitus; current cigarette smoking; and treatment with antihypertensive drugs, statins, and/or aspirin. The PCE calculator has been validated in both US White and Black adults.[208] For hypertension treatment decisions, those with a history of overt CVD or a PCE 10-year risk of ASCVD ≥10% should be considered as being at high CVD risk.

CVD risk estimation is recommended in all 40- to 79-year-old adults with hypertension who do not have a history of CVD complications. However, most adults with hypertension and either diabetes mellitus, CKD, or age ≥65 years are at high risk for ASCVD, and it is reasonable to assume high CVD risk in each of these settings. The role of ASCVD risk estimation in treatment decision-making is most important for adults with stage 1 hypertension. In adults <40 years, estimation of lifetime CVD risk can be helpful for treatment decision-making. Use of the Systematic Coronary Risk Evaluation (SCORE) calculator, which has been validated in Europe, is recommended in the 2018 ESC/ESH hypertension guidelines,[13] and other guidelines tend to employ locally validated CVD risk calculators.[209]

Nonpharmacological Treatments to Lower Blood Pressure

Nonpharmacological treatments to lower BP include pill supplementation and a variety of device therapies, but behavioral lifestyle change interventions represent the core of guideline recommendations. Promoting optimal health through healthy lifestyle choices is applicable across the entire spectrum of BP (**Figure 5–16**). However, the intensity of interventions to improve lifestyle should be matched to the needs to lower BP. The interventions best proved to be effective for prevention and treatment of hypertension are weight loss in those who are overweight or obese, changing to a healthier diet, reduction in sodium intake, enhanced potassium intake through diet, physical activity, and abstinence or moderation in alcohol consumption.[1]

Table 5–7 provides a summary of the intervention goals and expected BP lowering for each of these six interventions. Choice of interventions and intensity of treatment should be based on the clinician's assessment of a patient's greatest need and opportunity for benefit, as well as the patient's preference and commitment to achieve and maintain specific lifestyle changes. Combinations such as weight loss and sodium reduction in the context of a heart-healthy diet and moderation in alcohol consumption in combination with weight loss or sodium reduction are commonly required and can result in SBP reductions of ≥10 mmHg, especially in those with hypertension.

Sodium reduction and potassium supplementation are especially effective in Black adults with hypertension. A social compact between the clinician and patient is essential for success and should include written, time-specific, and achievable

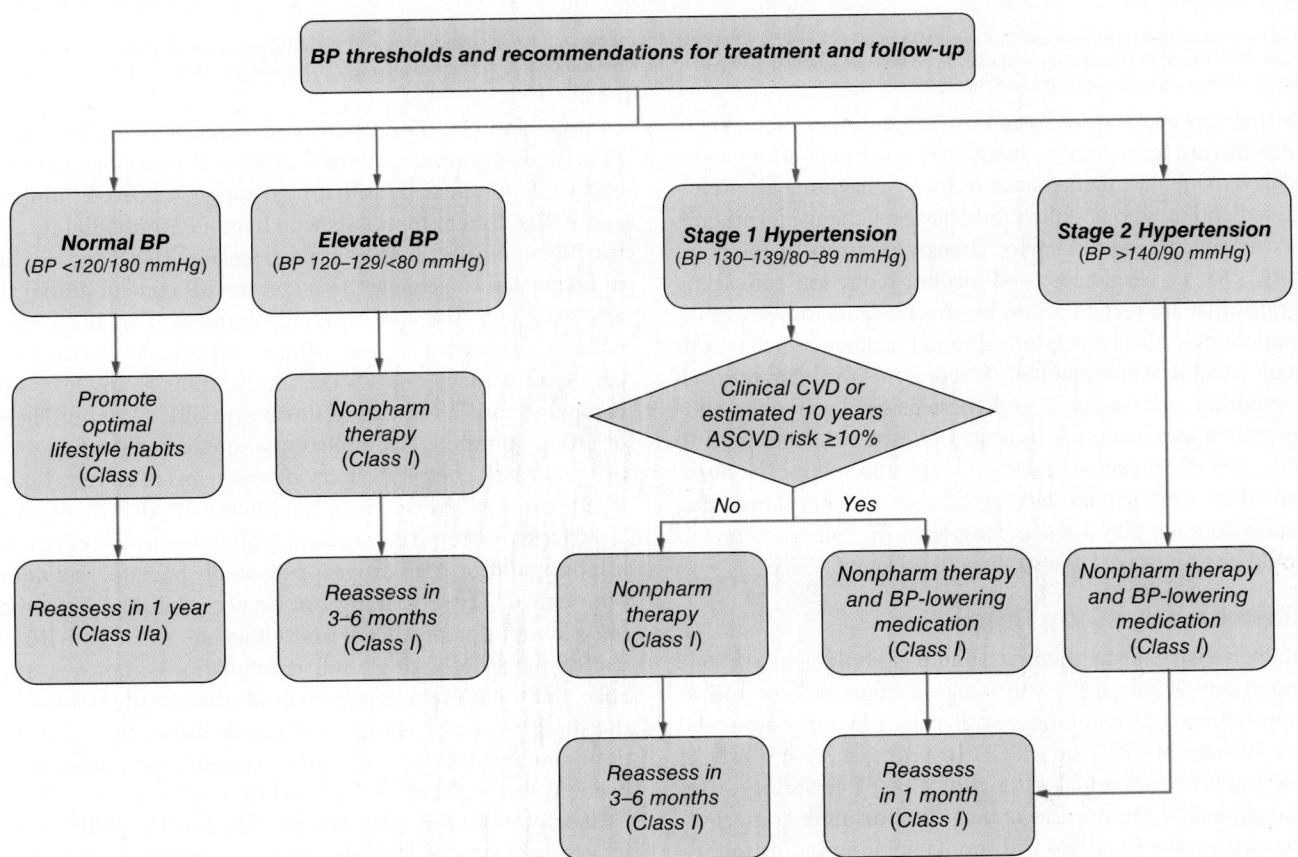

Figure 5–16. Management by BP category and ASCVD. ASCVD risk estimated using the PCE calculator. Adults with hypertension and either diabetes mellitus, CKD, or age ≥65 years can be assumed to be at high risk for CVD.

TABLE 5–7. Recommended Lifestyle Changes for Prevention and Treatment of Hypertension in Adults

Intervention	Goal	Expected SBP lowering	
		Hypertension	Nonhypertensive
Weight loss (in overweight or obese adults)	The optimal goal is achievement of ideal body weight, but any reduction in weight is helpful. Expect a reduction of approximately 1 mmHg for every 1 Kg reduction in body weight. Weight loss interventions employ a combination of reduced calorie consumption and physical activity.	−5 mmHg	−2/3 mmHg
Healthy diet	The DASH diet is preferred because it represents a healthy diet that has been customized to lower BP. BP lowering can also be achieved using the Mediterranean and other heart-healthy diets.	−11 mmHg in feeding studies but −4/5 mm Hg with behavioral change	−2/3 mmHg
Dietary sodium reduction	The optimal goal is a sodium intake of <1500 mg/d, but aim for a reduction of at least 1000 mg/d. A reduction of about 25% in sodium intake has been common in behavioral intervention trials, representing >1000 mg in most adults. Strategies to reduce sodium intake include choice of fresh rather than processed foods, use of food nutrition data and "no added sodium" labels to make informed purchasing decisions, avoidance or minimal addition of sodium during cooking and at the table, judicious use of condiments and high-sodium foods/snacks, control of portion size, and careful ordering when eating in fast-food and other restaurants.	−5/6 mmHg	−2/3 mmHg
Enhanced dietary potassium intake	Aim to exceed adequate intake of potassium (3400 mg/d) by consumption of additional fruits, vegetables, and other dietary sources.	−4/5 mmHg	−2 mmHg
Physical activity	Aerobic exercise such as brisk walking/running, swimming, and dancing is proved to be the best form of exercise for lowering BP, but dynamic and isometric resistance exercise also seems to be effective. Aerobic exercise several times per week, for a total of 90–150 min/week is recommended, as is achievement of 65% to 75% of heart rate reserve.	−5/7 mmHg	−2/3 mmHg
Abstinence or moderation in alcohol intake	In adults who drink alcohol, consumption of ≤2 standard drinks/d by men and ≤1 drink/d by women is recommended. A standard drink is about 12 ounces of beer, 5 ounces of wine, and 1.5 ounces of distilled spirits.	−4 mmHg	−3 mmHg

Modified with permission from Whelton PK, Carey RM, Aronow WS, et al. 2017 ACC/AHA/AAPA/ABC/ACPM/AGS/APhA/ASH/ASPC/NMA/PCNA Guideline for the Prevention, Detection, Evaluation, and Management of High Blood Pressure in Adults: A Report of the American College of Cardiology/American Heart Association Task Force on Clinical Practice Guidelines. *Hypertension.* 2018 Jun;71(6):e13-e115.

goals that can be measured and monitored. Other members of the health-care team may be better equipped to assist a patient in achievement and maintenance of their behavior goals. Referral to a dietitian who is skilled in behavioral change techniques or taking advantage of behavior change resources in the community, such as weight loss and alcohol reduction counseling programs that are recognized to be effective and convenient for the patient may also be helpful. Although change in behavior is difficult to achieve and maintain, it represents the best approach to prevention and treatment of hypertension. Even when antihypertensive medication is indicated, lifestyle changes tend to enhance the effectiveness of drug therapy and reduce the number and dosage of the pharmacological agents required. Smoking cessation does not play a role in long-term BP management, but it should be encouraged as a strategy to prevent CVD.

Antihypertensive Drug Therapy

Antihypertensive drug therapy should complement lifestyle interventions in all adults with stage 2 hypertension and in the approximately 30% of those with stage 1 hypertension who have a history of CVD or a PCE 10-year risk of ASCVD of ≥10%. In some individuals, the choice of BP-lowering drugs is determined by the need to manage one or more comorbidities concurrently. In adults with no compelling indication for choice of an antihypertensive agent, the following four drug classes have been shown to be effective for prevention of CVD

compared to placebo: (1) diuretics (especially the long-acting, thiazide-like diuretic chlorthalidone); calcium channel blockers (CCBs), especially dihydropyridine CCB; ACE inhibitors; and ARBs. Except for adults who have a BP only slightly above the BP cut points for stage 1 hypertension, two drugs are likely to be needed to achieve the target for BP control. Initial therapy with two drugs is especially important in Black people with hypertension, who are disproportionately at risk for target organ damage and CVD complications at any level of BP compared to Whites, and in those with SBP ≥150 mmHg and/or DBP ≥90 mmHg. Combinations should be based on the use of agents with complementary mechanisms of action. Taking a diuretic or CCB with an ACE inibitor or ARB represents an effective two-drug combination. Simultaneous use of two ACE inhibitor and/or ARB drugs is potentially harmful and not recommended. Triple therapy can be accomplished by combining a diuretic with a CCB and either an ACEI or ARB. The use of fixed-dose, single-pill combinations improves adherence, but the diuretic component of most combination pills is the shorter-acting hydrochlorothiazide rather than chlorthalidone, and the dosage employed is frequently less than what has been proven to prevent CVD in clinical trials.

If triple therapy does not provide sufficient BP lowering to achieve the desired BP target, substitution of a longer-acting diuretic in place of a shorter-acting agent or addition of spironolactone, an alpha-receptor blocker, or a β-blocker may prove to be effective. Lack of BP control with use of three or more antihypertensive agents at full doses merits a diagnosis of apparent resistant hypertension.

If there is no obvious explanation for the failure to control BP, such as use of inaccurate BP measurement methods, white coat hypertension, treatment nonadherence, use of agents that raise BP, or poor lifestyle decisions such as excessive consumption of alcohol, referral to a specialist in hypertension is warranted to confirm the diagnosis and search for an underlying cause. Individuals who present with a very high BP, such as SBP >180 mmHg or DBP >120 mmHg, need immediate careful evaluation. If there is a history of a rapid recent rise in BP, and/or there is evidence of new or worsening target organ damage, such as papilledema, overt renal disease, or heart failure, admission to an intensive care unit for parenteral therapy aimed at carefully supervised rapid reduction in BP is warranted. When the high BP is unaccompanied by signs or symptoms of acute target organ damage, oral outpatient therapy should be initiated with the initial goal of reducing SBP/DBP to <160/100 mmHg over several hours, with subsequent efforts to achieve target BP. Many of these patients have discontinued or are poorly adherent to a prior BP treatment regimen. Understanding and rectifying the underlying causes for nonadherence should be a high priority for the care team.

BP Target During Antihypertensive Therapy

Evidence from intensive therapy clinical trials and from meta-analyses has led to guideline recommendations for use of lower BP treatment targets compared to the BP-lowering goals that were previously advised.[1,13,210,211] The ACC/AHA guideline recommends an SBP/DBP treatment target of <130/80 mmHg, with the exception that SBP <130 mmHg is recommended for noninstitutionalized, ambulatory, community-dwelling adults ≥65 years old. In older adults with a high burden of comorbidity and limited life expectancy, the BP target should be based on clinical judgment, patient preference, and a team-based approach estimating the balance of benefit and risk. The general goal of SBP/DBP <130/80 mmHg should be the target in those with comorbidities, including a history of stroke, heart disease, CKD, and diabetes mellitus, provided that the treatment is well tolerated. The ESC/ESH guideline recommends an initial SBP/DBP goal of <140/90 mmHg, followed by an SBP/DBP target of 130/80 mmHg or lower in most patients, if tolerated, but SBP should not be targeted to <120 mmHg).[13] A lower SBP target of <120 mmHg, if tolerated, is supported by experience in recent trials[212,213] and meta-analyses,[214] and is recommended by the Canadian and Australian national guidelines.[210,211] An outlier recommendation from the American College of Physicians/American Academy of Family Physicians advises an SBP target of <150 mmHg in adults ≥60 years, with consideration of <140 mmHg in those with a history of a stroke or transient ischemic attack.[215]

Special Patient Groups and Considerations

Hypertension in Older Adults

Adults with hypertension who are older, have comorbidities such as heart disease, a history of stroke or transient ischemic

attacks, CKD, have diabetes mellitus, or are current cigarette smokers are at high risk for CVD and require special attention to manage their high BP and other CVD risk factors. The benefits of antihypertensive therapy in older adults are well established. It is often sensible to initiate antihypertensive treatment with lower doses of antihypertensive medication compared to those used in younger patients and intensify the treatment more gradually. Older adults tend to have isolated elevations of SBP, with DBPs that are often <70 mmHg. This has raised concerns that treatment to lower their SBP might inadvertently result in pathologically low DBPs and hypoperfusion, especially in the coronary arteries. Reports of J- or U-shaped curves, with an uptick in CVD risk at lower levels of BP, in nonrandomized analyses of several clinical trials have further fueled this concern. However, it is not possible to determine whether the excess risk is a consequence or cause of the lower levels of BP.

Randomized comparisons in the SPRINT and the Action to Control Cardiovascular Risk in Diabetes Blood Pressure trial (ACCORD BP) provide strong evidence that more intensive BP reduction is beneficial compared to less intensive treatment, even in those with low DBP prior to initiating the therapy.[64,216] In SPRINT, hypotension was less common in those randomized to intensive compared to standard antihypertensive drug therapy.[212] Care in the initiation of BP-lowering therapy and judicious monitoring for tolerance and treatment side effects is mandatory but concerns regarding the potential for adverse effects should not be a reason for therapeutic inertia and failure to reduce the high risk, resulting in elevated levels of BP in older adults. The ESC/ESH BP target recommendation in older adults is SBP/DBP of <140/80 mmHg, but not below an SBP of 130 mmHg.[13]

Hypertension in Adults with Diabetes Mellitus

Adults with diabetes mellitus are at high risk for CVD, with cohort studies suggesting that diabetes confers a risk equivalent to that associated with a myocardial infarction.[217] The combination of hypertension and diabetes mellitus in adults results in a CVD risk almost double that seen with either risk factor on its own.[218] Diabetes mellitus usually results from an unhealthy diet and physical inactivity, which in combination result in overweight/obesity and abdominal adiposity. As with hypertension, lifestyle change is a core management approach in the management of diabetes. However, in most patients with diabetes and hypertension, antihypertensive therapy provides the most effective and reliable means to reduce CVD risk. Increasing evidence suggests that intensive antihypertensive therapy is warranted, provided that standard approaches to glycemic control are utilized.[213] Intensive antihypertensive therapy has also been shown to confer great benefit with prediabetic patients with hypertension.[219] The ESC/ESH SBP target recommendation in adults <65 years with diabetes and hypertension is <130 mmHg, but SBP/DBP should not be lowered to <120/80 mmHg. In adults ≥65 years, an SBP target range of 130–140 mmHg is recommended.

Hypertension in Adults with Comorbid Clinical Complications

In general, lowering BP to SBP/DBP <130/80 mmHg is desirable, if tolerated, in adults with hypertension and stable ischemic heart disease, compensated heart failure, a history of a stroke or transient ischemic attacks, or CKD. Often, antihypertensive drug selection is influenced by the use of agents that are central to management of the comorbidity, but also lower BP. For example, β-blockers and ACE inhibitors or ARBs are typically the drugs of choice for management for those who have previously had a myocardial infarction or have stable angina. Likewise, the use of first-line antihypertensive agents may be undesirable in the context of specific comorbidities. For example, nondihydropyridine CCBs are not recommended in the treatment of patients with heart failure and a reduced ejection fraction. The ESC/ESH guideline recommends an SBP target of 130 mmHg in most adults with hypertension and a comorbidity, except for those with CKD, where SBP of 130–140 mmHg is recommended.[13]

Race, Ethnicity, Sex, and Treatment of Hypertension

Lifestyle modification is highly desirable but often difficult to achieve in race/ethnic minorities, including Black adults, Hispanics, Native Americans, and Pacific Islanders. The general approach to antihypertensive drug therapy is as outlined earlier in this chapter. Black people have a disproportionately high risk for CVD at any level of BP compared to Whites and should always be managed with combination antihypertensive drug therapy. Thiazide-like diuretics and CCBs are particularly effective for lowering BP in Black people, and one or both agents should be part of any antihypertensive drug combination used in treatment. Except during pregnancy, there is no evidence for a different approach to initiating or managing hypertension in women compared to men. ACE inhibitors, ARBs, and direct renin inhibitors should not be prescribed in women who are pregnant or likely to become pregnant because they are fetotoxic. It is beyond the scope of this chapter to address the management of high BP during pregnancy in detail. However, in general, methyldopa, nifedipine, and labetalol seem to be safe drugs for management of hypertension during pregnancy.

Follow-Up After Initiation of Treatment

The rapidity of BP reduction following initiation of lifestyle counseling varies, depending on the interventions selected and degree of success in implementation, but effects are usually seen within 1–4 weeks of treatment. Antihypertensive drugs tend to have more a rapid effect, but the full potential for BP reduction may take up to a month. Most adults should be evaluated at monthly intervals after initiation of BP-lowering therapy until control is achieved. In addition to measuring sitting BP, the initial follow-up evaluation should include obtaining a standing BP to recognize orthostatic hypotension, questioning to recognize potential adverse effects of the therapy, an assessment of adherence to the treatment, and laboratory testing in those taking medication (especially diuretics, ACE inhibitors, or ARBs) to monitor electrolyte level and renal function.

Follow-up visits can also be used to implement additional strategies that facilitate the achievement and maintenance of BP control, such as reinforcement of lifestyle change interventions, HBPM, and other approaches that empower patients to assume greater responsibility for their own care, greater utilization of a team-based care approach, and telehealth strategies. In patients with well-controlled chronic stable hypertension, the interval between visits can be lengthened to 3–6 months, with the understanding that a patient can request an earlier visit should circumstances change.

Plan of Care for Hypertension

Every adult with hypertension should have a clear, detailed, evidence-based plan of care that not only addresses the antihypertensive treatment plan, but empowers patient self-management, manages other CVD risk factors and comorbid conditions, and ensures timely follow-up with the health-care team. Clear and open communication between the patient and health-care team is essential. Use of language that is commensurate with a patient's level of literacy is important. In addition to verbal communication, a written visit summary that outlines the BP readings obtained at the visit, goals and specific patient actions, medication type and dosage, and contact instructions should be given to the patient. Lifestyle change is best achieved using a written contract that outlines plans and specific achievable goals.

When possible, it is highly desirable to have a patient measure BP at home. It is important that the patient be trained to obtain accurate BP measurements, and it is preferable to either transmit the readings to the health-care team electronically or use a memory function to store them until the patient's next clinic visit. A variety of technology options can be helpful, ranging from something as simple as use of the recording option on a patient's mobile phone to more advanced telehealth methods for monitoring BP. Use of a health-care team approach has been repeatedly demonstrated to improve BP control. Engaging spouses, family members, or friends in ways that support and encourage patients can be helpful. Likewise, taking advantage of resources in the community and understanding social and financial services that might apply can be very helpful. With care and attention to detail, target BP can be achieved in most patients.

SUMMARY

Definition and Epidemiology

- Normal BP in adults is defined as SBP <120 mmHg and DBP <80 mmHg.
- Nearly one-third of the world's adults have hypertension.
- Hypertension is one of the strongest modifiable risk factors for CVD, including myocardial infarction, heart failure, and stroke, as well as overall mortality.

Pathophysiology

- Most hypertension can be attributed to nongenetic etiologies, including sedentary lifestyle, excessive weight gain, visceral adiposity, and other modifiable risk factors such as high intake of sodium.
- Nongenetic causes of secondary hypertension, including excessive secretion of aldosterone and renal artery stenosis, may account for as much as 10% to 15% of hypertension and may warrant treatment by a hypertension specialist.

Management

- Based on outcomes in relatively recent clinical trials such as SPRINT, lower BP targets have been incorporated into some BP guidelines to reduce the risk of CVD.

- Although patient nonadherence is a factor in suboptimal BP control, other factors, including access to care and clinician inertia, play major roles.

- Telehealth strategies, empowered patient self-management, clear communication between patients and provider teams, and incorporation of lifestyle changes are critical to achieving optimal BP goals.

ACKNOWLEDGMENTS

The authors thank Stephanie Lucas for assistance with the manuscript preparation. The authors received support from National Institutes of Health (NIH) grants National Institutes of General Medical Sciences 5U54GM115428, P20GM104357, and the National Institute of Diabetes and Digestive and Kidney Diseases (R01 DK121411 and R01 DK121748).

REFERENCES

1. Whelton PK, Carey RM, Aronow WS, et al. ACC/AHA/AAPA/ABC/ACPM/AGS/APhA/ASH/ASPC/ NMA/PCNA Guideline for the prevention, detection, evaluation, and management of high blood pressure in adults: a report of the American College of Cardiology/American Heart Association Task Force on Clinical Practice Guidelines. *Hypertension.* 2018;71:e13-e115.

2. Flynn JT, Kaelber DC, Baker-Smith CM, et al. Clinical practice guideline for screening and management of high blood pressure in children and adolescents. *Pediatrics.* 2017;140.

3. Lewington S, Clarke R, Qizilbash N, Peto R, Collins R. Age-specific relevance of usual blood pressure to vascular mortality: a meta-analysis of individual data for one million adults in 61 prospective studies. *Lancet.* 2002;360:1903-1913.

4. Rapsomaniki E, Timmis A, George J, et al. Blood pressure and incidence of twelve cardiovascular diseases: lifetime risks, healthy life-years lost, and age-specific associations in 1.25 million people. *Lancet.* 2014;383:1899-1911.

5. Whelton SP, McEvoy JW, Shaw L, et al. Association of normal systolic blood pressure level with cardiovascular disease in the absence of risk factors. *JAMA Cardiol.* 2020;5:1011-1018.

6. Whelton PK. Evolution of blood pressure clinical practice guidelines: a personal perspective. *Can J Cardiol.* 2019;35:570-581.

7. The 1988 report of the Joint National Committee on Detection, Evaluation, and Treatment of High Blood Pressure. *Arch Intern Med.* 1988;148: 1023-1038.

8. The fifth report of the Joint National Committee on Detection, Evaluation, and Treatment of High Blood Pressure (JNC V). *Arch Intern Med.* 1993;153:154-183.

9. Gibbons GH, Harold JG, Jessup M, Robertson RM, Oetgen WJ. The next steps in developing clinical practice guidelines for prevention. *J Am Coll Cardiol.* 2013;62:1399-1400.

10. Muntner P, Carey RM, Gidding S, et al. Potential U.S. Population Impact of the 2017 ACC/AHA High Blood Pressure Guideline. *J Am Coll Cardiol.* 2018;71:109-118.

11. Fuchs FD, Whelton PK. High blood pressure and cardiovascular disease. *Hypertension.* 2020;75:285-292.

12. Lowenstein F. Blood-pressure in relation to age and sex in tropics and subtropics—a review of literature and an investigation in 2 tribes of Brazil Indians. *Lancet.* 1961;1:389-392.

13. Williams B, Mancia G, Spiering W, et al. 2018 ESC/ESH guidelines for the management of arterial hypertension. *Eur Heart J.* 2018;39:3021-3104.

14. Kario K, Thijs L, Staessen JA. Blood pressure measurement and treatment decisions. *Circ Res.* 2019;124:990-1008.

15. Asayama K, Thijs L, Li Y, et al. Setting thresholds to varying blood pressure monitoring intervals differentially affects risk estimates associated with white-coat and masked hypertension in the population. *Hypertension.* 2014;64:935-942.

16. Acelajado MC, Hughes ZH, Oparil S, Calhoun DA. Treatment of resistant and refractory hypertension. *Circ Res.* 2019;124:1061-1070.

17. Daugherty SL, Powers JD, Magid DJ, et al. Incidence and prognosis of resistant hypertension in hypertensive patients. *Circulation.* 2012;125: 1635-1642.

18. Diaz KM, Booth JN, 3rd, Calhoun DA, et al. Healthy lifestyle factors and risk of cardiovascular events and mortality in treatment-resistant hypertension: the Reasons for Geographic and Racial Differences in Stroke study. *Hypertension.* 2014;64:465-471.

19. Carey RM, Calhoun DA, Bakris GL, et al. Resistant hypertension: detection, evaluation, and management: a scientific statement from the American Heart Association. *Hypertension.* 2018;72:e53-e90.

20. Egan BM, Zhao Y, Li J, et al. Prevalence of optimal treatment regimens in patients with apparent treatment-resistant hypertension based on office blood pressure in a community-based practice network. *Hypertension.* 2013;62:691-697.

21. Armario P, Calhoun DA, Oliveras A, et al. Prevalence and clinical characteristics of refractory hypertension. *J Am Heart Assoc.* 2017;6.

22. Group SR, Wright JT, Jr., Williamson JD, et al. A randomized trial of intensive versus standard blood-pressure control. *N Engl J Med.* 2015;373: 2103-2116.

23. Jaffe MG, Lee GA, Young JD, Sidney S, Go AS. Improved blood pressure control associated with a large-scale hypertension program. *JAMA.* 2013;310:699-705.

24. Jaffe MG, Young JD. The Kaiser Permanente Northern California story: improving hypertension control from 44% to 90% in 13 years (2000 to 2013). *J Clin Hypertens (Greenwich).* 2016;18:260-261.

25. Janke AT, McNaughton CD, Brody AM, Welch RD, Levy PD. Trends in the incidence of hypertensive emergencies in US emergency departments from 2006 to 2013. *J Am Heart Assoc.* 2016;5.

26. Mills KT, Bundy JD, Kelly TN, et al. Global disparities of hypertension prevalence and control: a systematic analysis of population-based studies from 90 countries. *Circulation.* 2016;134:441-450.

27. Ostchega Y, Fryar CD, Nwankwo T, Nguyen DT. Hypertension prevalence among adults aged 18 and over: United States, 2017-2018. *NCHS Data Brief.* 2020:1-8.

28. Vasan RS, Beiser A, Seshadri S, et al. Residual lifetime risk for developing hypertension in middle-aged women and men: the Framingham Heart Study. *JAMA.* 2002;287:1003-1010.

29. Still CH, Rodriguez CJ, Wright JT, Jr., et al. Clinical outcomes by race and ethnicity in the Systolic Blood Pressure Intervention Trial (SPRINT): a randomized clinical trial. *Am J Hypertens.* 2017;31:97-107.

30. Centers for Disease Control and Prevention. Hypertension prevalence among adults aged 18 and over: United States, 2017-2018. https://www.cdc.gov/nchs/products/databriefs/db364.htm#section_2. Accessed May 11, 2021.

31. Maraboto C, Ferdinand KC. Update on hypertension in African-Americans. *Prog Cardiovasc Dis.* 2020;63:33-39.

32. Adeyemo A, Gerry N, Chen G, et al. A genome-wide association study of hypertension and blood pressure in African Americans. *PLoS Genet.* 2009;5:e1000564.

33. Parsa A, Kao WH, Xie D, et al. APOL1 risk variants, race, and progression of chronic kidney disease. *N Engl J Med.* 2013;369:2183-2196.

34. Poulter NR, Khaw KT, Hopwood BE, et al. The Kenyan Luo migration study: observations on the initiation of a rise in blood pressure. *BMJ.* 1990;300:967-972.

35. Howard G, Cushman M, Moy CS, et al. Association of clinical and social factors with excess hypertension risk in Black compared with white US adults. *JAMA*. 2018;320:1338-1348.

36. Spruill TM, Butler MJ, Thomas SJ, et al. Association between high perceived stress over time and incident hypertension in Black adults: findings from the Jackson Heart Study. *J Am Heart Assoc*. 2019; 8:e012139.

37. Ford CD, Sims M, Higginbotham JC, et al. Psychosocial factors are associated with blood pressure progression among African Americans in the Jackson Heart Study. *Am J Hypertens*. 2016;29:913-924.

38. Thomas IC, Allison MA. Hypertension in Hispanics/Latinos: epidemiology and considerations for management. *Curr Hypertens Rep*. 2019; 21:43.

39. Elfassy T, Zeki Al Hazzouri A, et al. Incidence of hypertension among US Hispanics/Latinos: the Hispanic Community Health Study/Study of Latinos, 2008 to 2017. *J Am Heart Assoc*. 2020;9:e015031.

40. Centers for Disease Control and Prevention. Summary of health statistics: National Health Interiew Survey: 2018, Table A-1a. https://www.cdc.gov/nchs/nhis/shs/tables.htm. Assessed October 16, 2020.

41. Centers for Disease Control and Prevention. National vital statistics report, vol. 68, no. 9. Table 10. https://www.cdc.gov/nchs/products/nvsr.htm. Accessed October 16, 2020.

42. Rodriguez F, Hastings KG, Boothroyd DB, et al. Disaggregation of cause-specific cardiovascular disease mortality among Hispanic subgroups. *JAMA Cardiol*. 2017;2:240-247.

43. Centers for Disease Control and Prevention. Health, United States, 2018, Table 22. https://www.cdc.gov/nchs/data/hus/hus18.pdf. Accessed October 16, 2020.

44. Yi SS, Thorpe LE, Zanowiak JM, Trinh-Shevrin C, Islam NS. Clinical characteristics and lifestyle behaviors in a population-based sample of Chinese and South Asian immigrants with hypertension. *Am J Hypertens*. 2016;29:941-947.

45. Jose PO, Frank AT, Kapphahn KI, et al. Cardiovascular disease mortality in Asian Americans. *J Am Coll Cardiol*. 2014;64:2486-2494.

46. Gurven M, Blackwell AD, Rodriguez DE, Stieglitz J, Kaplan H. Does blood pressure inevitably rise with age? Longitudinal evidence among forager-horticulturalists. *Hypertension*. 2012;60:25-33.

47. Jones DW, Kim JS, Andrew ME, Kim SJ, Hong YP. Body mass index and blood pressure in Korean men and women: the Korean National Blood Pressure Survey. *J Hypertens*. 1994;12:1433-1437.

48. Action to Control Cardiovascular Risk in Diabetes Study Group, Gerstein HC, Miller ME, et al. Effects of intensive glucose lowering in type 2 diabetes. *N Engl J Med*. 2008;358:2545-2559.

49. Centers for Disease Control and Prevention. National diabetes statistics report 2020: estimates of diabetes and its burden in the United States. https://www.cdc.gov/diabetes/pdfs/data/statistics/national-diabetes-statistics-report.pdf. Accessed October 16, 2020.

50. Sun D, Zhou T, Heianza Y, et al. Type 2 diabetes and hypertension. *Circ Res*. 2019;124:930-937.

51. Liu X, Zhang D, Liu Y, et al. Dose-response association between physical activity and incident hypertension: a systematic review and meta-analysis of cohort studies. *Hypertension*. 2017;69:813-820.

52. Joseph G, Marott JL, Torp-Pedersen C, et al. Dose-response association between level of physical activity and mortality in normal, elevated, and high blood pressure. *Hypertension*. 2019;74:1307-1315.

53. Pescatello LS, Buchner DM, Jakicic JM, et al. Physical activity to prevent and treat hypertension: a systematic review. *Med Sci Sports Exerc*. 2019;51:1314-1323.

54. Stamler J, Chan Q, Daviglus ML, et al. Relation of dietary sodium (salt) to blood pressure and its possible modulation by other dietary factors: The INTERMAP study. *Hypertension*. 2018;71:631-637.

55. Gay HC, Rao SG, Vaccarino V, Ali MK. Effects of different dietary interventions on blood pressure: systematic review and meta-analysis of randomized controlled trials. *Hypertension*. 2016;67:733-739.

56. Juraschek SP, Miller ER, 3rd, Weaver CM, Appel LJ. Effects of sodium reduction and the DASH diet in relation to baseline blood pressure. *J Am Coll Cardiol*. 2017;70:2841-2848.

57. Carey RM, Muntner P, Bosworth HB, Whelton PK. Prevention and control of hypertension: JACC Health Promotion Series. *J Am Coll Cardiol*. 2018;72:1278-1293.

58. Havranek EP, Mujahid MS, Barr DA, et al. Social determinants of risk and outcomes for cardiovascular disease: a scientific statement from the American Heart Association. *Circulation*. 2015;132:873-898.

59. Kannel WB. Elevated systolic blood pressure as a cardiovascular risk factor. *Am J Cardiol*. 2000;85:251-255.

60. Collaborators GBDRF. Global, regional, and national comparative risk assessment of 84 behavioural, environmental and occupational, and metabolic risks or clusters of risks for 195 countries and territories, 1990-2017: a systematic analysis for the Global Burden of Disease Study 2017. *Lancet*. 2018;392:1923-1994.

61. Yusuf S, Joseph P, Rangarajan S, et al. Modifiable risk factors, cardiovascular disease, and mortality in 155 722 individuals from 21 high-income, middle-income, and low-income countries (PURE): a prospective cohort study. *Lancet*. 2020;395:795-808.

62. Messerli FH, Mancia G, Conti CR, et al. Dogma disputed: can aggressively lowering blood pressure in hypertensive patients with coronary artery disease be dangerous? *Ann Intern Med*. 2006;144:884-893.

63. Vidal-Petiot E, Ford I, Greenlaw N, et al. CLARIFY Investigators. Cardiovascular event rates and mortality according to achieved systolic and diastolic blood pressure in patients with stable coronary artery disease: an international cohort study. *Lancet*. 2016; 388:2142-2152.

64. Beddhu S, Chertow GM, Cheung AK, et al. Influence of baseline diastolic blood pressure on effects of intensive compared with standard blood pressure control. *Circulation*. 2018;137:134-143.

65. Levy D, Larson MG, Vasan RS, Kannel WB, Ho KK. The progression from hypertension to congestive heart failure. *JAMA*. 1996;275:1557-1562.

66. Randolph TC, Greiner MA, Egwim C, et al. Associations between blood pressure and outcomes among Blacks in the Jackson Heart Study. *J Am Heart Assoc*. 2016;5.

67. Bibbins-Domingo K, Pletcher MJ, Lin F, et al. Racial differences in incident heart failure among young adults. *N Engl J Med*. 2009;360:1179-1190.

68. Teramoto K, Nadruz Jr. W, Matsushita K, et al. Mid- to late-life time-averaged cumulative blood pressure and late-life cardiac structure, function, and heart failure. *Hypertension*. 2020;76:808-818.

69. Fuchs SC, Poli-de-Figueiredo CE, Figueiredo Neto JA, et al. Effectiveness of chlorthalidone plus amiloride for the prevention of hypertension: the PREVER-Prevention randomized clinical trial. *J Am Heart Assoc*. 2016;5.

70. Devereux RB, Dahlof B, Gerdts E, et al. Regression of hypertensive left ventricular hypertrophy by losartan compared with atenolol: the Losartan Intervention for Endpoint Reduction in Hypertension (LIFE) trial. *Circulation*. 2004;110:1456-1462.

71. Solomon SD, Verma A, Desai A, et al. Effect of intensive versus standard blood pressure lowering on diastolic function in patients with uncontrolled hypertension and diastolic dysfunction. *Hypertension*. 2010;55:241-248.

72. Clark D, 3rd, Colantonio LD, Min YI, et al. Population-attributable risk for cardiovascular disease associated with hypertension in Black adults. *JAMA Cardiol*. 2019;4:1194-1202.

73. Franklin SS, Chow VH, Mori AD, Wong ND. The significance of low DBP in US adults with isolated systolic hypertension. *J Hypertens*. 2011;29:1101-1108.

74. Franklin SS, Khan SA, Wong ND, Larson MG, Levy D. Is pulse pressure useful in predicting risk for coronary heart disease? the Framingham Heart Study. *Circulation*. 1999;100:354-360.

75. Miura K, Dyer AR, Greenland P, et al. Pulse pressure compared with other blood pressure indexes in the prediction of 25-year cardiovascular and all-cause mortality rates: the Chicago Heart Association Detection Project in Industry Study. *Hypertension*. 2001;38:232-237.

76. Glasser SP, Halberg DL, Sands C, Gamboa CM, Muntner P, Safford M. Is pulse pressure an independent risk factor for incident acute coronary heart disease events? The REGARDS study. *Am J Hypertens.* 2014;27:555-563.

77. McEvoy JW, Daya N, Rahman F, et al. Association of isolated diastolic hypertension as defined by the 2017 ACC/AHA Blood Pressure Guideline with incident cardiovascular outcomes. *JAMA.* 2020;323:329-338.

78. McGrath BP, Kundu P, Daya N, et al. Isolated diastolic hypertension in the UK Biobank: comparison of ACC/AHA and ESC/NICE Guideline definitions. *Hypertension.* 2020;76:699-706.

79. Boggia J, Li Y, Thijs L, et al. Prognostic accuracy of day versus night ambulatory blood pressure: a cohort study. *Lancet.* 2007;370:1219-1229.

80. O'Brien E, Sheridan J, O'Malley K. Dippers and non-dippers. *Lancet.* 1988;2:397.

81. Muxfeldt ES, Cardoso CR, Salles GF. Prognostic value of nocturnal blood pressure reduction in resistant hypertension. *Arch Intern Med.* 2009;169:874-880.

82. Salles GF, Reboldi G, Fagard RH, et al. Prognostic effect of the nocturnal blood pressure fall in hypertensive patients: the Ambulatory Blood Pressure Collaboration in Patients with Hypertension (ABC-H) meta-analysis. *Hypertension.* 2016;67:693-700.

83. Sachdeva A, Weder AB. Nocturnal sodium excretion, blood pressure dipping, and sodium sensitivity. *Hypertension.* 2006;48:527-533.

84. Carey RM, Muntner P, Bosworth HB, Whelton PK. Reprint of: Prevention and Control of Hypertension: JACC Health Promotion Series. *J Am Coll Cardiol.* 2018;72:2996-3011.

85. Muntner P, Hardy ST, Fine LJ, et al. Trends in blood pressure control among US adults with hypertension, 1999-2000 to 2017-2018. *JAMA.* 2020;324:1190-1200.

86. Paulose-Ram R, Gu Q, Kit B. Characteristics of U.S. Adults with hypertension who are unaware of their hypertension, 2011-2014. *NCHS Data Brief.* 2017:1-8.

87. Pencina MJ, D'Agostino RB, Sr., Larson MG, Massaro JM, Vasan RS. Predicting the 30-year risk of cardiovascular disease: the Framingham Heart Study. *Circulation.* 2009;119:3078-3084.

88. Tajeu GS, Kent ST, Huang L, et al. Antihypertensive medication nonpersistence and low adherence for adults <65 years initiating treatment in 2007-2014. *Hypertension.* 2019;74:35-46.

89. Lopez L, Cook EF, Horng MS, Hicks LS. Lifestyle modification counseling for hypertensive patients: results from the National Health and Nutrition Examination Survey 1999-2004. *Am J Hypertens.* 2009;22:325-331.

90. Okonofua EC, Simpson KN, Jesri A, Rehman SU, Durkalski VL, Egan BM. Therapeutic inertia is an impediment to achieving the Healthy People 2010 blood pressure control goals. *Hypertension.* 2006;47:345-351.

91. Mu L, Mukamal KJ. Treatment intensification for hypertension in US ambulatory medical care. *J Am Heart Assoc.* 2016;5.

92. Langford AT, Akinyelure OP, Moore TL, Jr., et al. Underutilization of treatment for Black adults with apparent treatment-resistant hypertension: JHS and the REGARDS study. *Hypertension.* 2020;76:1600-1607.

93. Mills KT, Obst KM, Shen W, et al. Comparative effectiveness of implementation strategies for blood pressure control in hypertensive patients: a systematic review and meta-analysis. *Ann Intern Med.* 2018;168:110-120.

94. He J, Irazola V, Mills KT, et al. Effect of a community health worker–led multicomponent intervention on blood pressure control in low-income patients in Argentina: a randomized clinical trial. *JAMA.* 2017;318:1016-1025.

95. Schwalm JD, McCready T, Lopez-Jaramillo P, et al. A community-based comprehensive intervention to reduce cardiovascular risk in hypertension (HOPE 4): a cluster-randomised controlled trial. *Lancet.* 2019;394:1231-1242.

96. Hall JE. *Guyton and Hall Textbook of Medical Physiology.* 14th ed. Philadelphia, PA: Elsevier, 2021.

97. Carlstrom M, Wilcox CS, Arendshorst WJ. Renal autoregulation in health and disease. *Physiol Rev.* 2015;95:405-511.

98. Mancia G, Verdecchia P. Clinical value of ambulatory blood pressure: evidence and limits. *Circ Res.* 2015;116:1034-1045.

99. Hall JE. Renal dysfunction, rather than nonrenal vascular dysfunction, mediates salt-induced hypertension. *Circulation.* 2016;133:894-906.

100. Hall JE, Granger JP, do Carmo JM, et al. Hypertension: physiology and pathophysiology. *Compr Physiol.* 2012;2:2393-2442.

101. Guyton AC. The surprising kidney-fluid mechanism for pressure control—its infinite gain! *Hypertension.* 1990;16:725-730.

102. Clemmer JS, Pruett WA, Coleman TG, Hall JE, Hester RL. Mechanisms of blood pressure salt sensitivity: new insights from mathematical modeling. *Am J Physiol Regul Integr Comp Physiol.* 2017;312:R451-R466.

103. Mattson DL. Immune mechanisms of salt-sensitive hypertension and renal end-organ damage. *Nat Rev Nephrol.* 2019;15:290-300.

104. Bovee DM, Cuevas CA, Zietse R, Danser AHJ, Mirabito Colafella KM, Hoorn EJ. Salt-sensitive hypertension in chronic kidney disease: distal tubular mechanisms. *Am J Physiol Renal Physiol.* 2020;319:F729-F745.

105. Hall JE. Control of sodium excretion by angiotensin II: intrarenal mechanisms and blood pressure regulation. *Am J Physiol.* 1986;250:R960-R972.

106. Hall JE, Guyton AC, Smith MJ, Jr., Coleman TG. Blood pressure and renal function during chronic changes in sodium intake: role of angiotensin. *Am J Physiol.* 1980;239:F271-F280.

107. Weinberger MH, Fineberg NS, Fineberg SE, Weinberger M. Salt sensitivity, pulse pressure, and death in normal and hypertensive humans. *Hypertension.* 2001;37:429-432.

108. DiBona GF. Sympathetic nervous system and hypertension. *Hypertension.* 2013;61:556-560.

109. Hall JE, do Carmo JM, da Silva AA, Wang Z, Hall ME. Obesity, kidney dysfunction and hypertension: mechanistic links. *Nat Rev Nephrol.* 2019;15:367-385.

110. Kiuchi MG, Esler MD, Fink GD, et al. Renal denervation update from the international sympathetic nervous system summit: JACC state-of-the-art review. *J Am Coll Cardiol.* 2019;73:3006-3017.

111. Lohmeier TE, Hall JE. Device-based neuromodulation for resistant hypertension therapy. *Circ Res.* 2019;124:1071-1093.

112. Iliescu R, Lohmeier TE, Tudorancea I, Laffin L, Bakris GL. Renal denervation for the treatment of resistant hypertension: review and clinical perspective. *Am J Physiol Renal Physiol.* 2015;309:F583-F594.

113. Mahfoud F, Bohm M, Schmieder R, et al. Effects of renal denervation on kidney function and long-term outcomes: 3-year follow-up from the Global SYMPLICITY Registry. *Eur Heart J.* 2019;40:3474-3482.

114. Henegar JR, Zhang Y, Hata C, Narciso I, Hall ME, Hall JE. Catheter-based radiofrequency renal denervation: location effects on renal norepinephrine. *Am J Hypertens.* 2015;28:909-914.

115. Garcia-Touchard A, Maranillo E, Mompeo B, Sanudo JR. Microdissection of the human renal nervous system: implications for performing renal denervation procedures. *Hypertension.* 2020;76:1240-1246.

116. de Leeuw PW, Bisognano JD, Bakris GL, et al. Sustained reduction of blood pressure with baroreceptor activation therapy: results of the 6-year open follow-up. *Hypertension.* 2017;69:836-843.

117. Valenzuela PL, Carrera-Bastos P, Galvez BG, et al. Lifestyle interventions for the prevention and treatment of hypertension. *Nat Rev Cardiol.* 2021;18:251-275.

118. Hill LK, Thayer JF. The autonomic nervous system and hypertension: ethnic differences and psychosocial factors. *Curr Cardiol Rep.* 2019;21:15.

119. Johnson AK, Xue B. Central nervous system neuroplasticity and the sensitization of hypertension. *Nat Rev Nephrol.* 2018;14:750-766.

120. Hall JE, do Carmo JM, da Silva AA, Wang Z, Hall ME. Obesity-induced hypertension: interaction of neurohumoral and renal mechanisms. *Circ Res.* 2015;116:991-1006.

121. Hall JE, Brands MW, Henegar JR. Angiotensin II and long-term arterial pressure regulation: the overriding dominance of the kidney. *J Am Soc Nephrol.* 1999;10 (Suppl 12):S258-S265.

122. Crowley SD, Coffman TM. The inextricable role of the kidney in hypertension. *J Clin Invest.* 2014;124:2341-2347.

123. Wall SM, Verlander JW, Romero CA. The renal physiology of pendrin-positive intercalated cells. *Physiol Rev.* 2020;100:1119-1147.

124. Rossier BC, Baker ME, Studer RA. Epithelial sodium transport and its control by aldosterone: the story of our internal environment revisited. *Physiol Rev.* 2015;95:297-340.

125. Rossi GP. Primary aldosteronism: JACC state-of-the-art review. *J Am Coll Cardiol.* 2019;74:2799-2811.

126. Barton M, Yanagisawa M. Endothelin: 30 years from discovery to therapy. *Hypertension.* 2019;74:1232-1265.

127. Davenport AP, Hyndman KA, Dhaun N, et al. Endothelin. *Pharmacol Rev.* 2016;68:357-418.

128. Kohan DE. The renal medullary endothelin system in control of sodium and water excretion and systemic blood pressure. *Curr Opin Nephrol Hypertens.* 2006;15:34-40.

129. Dhaun N, Webb DJ. Endothelins in cardiovascular biology and therapeutics. *Nat Rev Cardiol.* 2019;16:491-502.

130. Benigni A, Buelli S, Kohan DE. Endothelin-targeted new treatments for proteinuric and inflammatory glomerular diseases: focus on the added value to anti-renin-angiotensin system inhibition. *Pediatr Nephrol.* 2021;36:763-775.

131. Gariepy CE, Ohuchi T, Williams SC, Richardson JA, Yanagisawa M. Salt-sensitive hypertension in endothelin-B receptor-deficient rats. *J Clin Invest.* 2000;105:925-933.

132. Ge Y, Bagnall A, Stricklett PK, et al. Collecting duct-specific knockout of the endothelin B receptor causes hypertension and sodium retention. *Am J Physiol Renal Physiol.* 2006;291:F1274-F1280.

133. Kassab S, Miller MT, Novak J, Reckelhoff J, Clower B, Granger JP. Endothelin-A receptor antagonism attenuates the hypertension and renal injury in Dahl salt-sensitive rats. *Hypertension.* 1998;31:397-402.

134. Krum H, Viskoper RJ, Lacourciere Y, Budde M, Charlon V. The effect of an endothelin-receptor antagonist, bosentan, on blood pressure in patients with essential hypertension. Bosentan Hypertension Investigators. *N Engl J Med.* 1998;338:784-790.

135. Nakov R, Pfarr E, Eberle S. Darusentan: an effective endothelin$_A$ receptor antagonist for treatment of hypertension. *Am J Hypertens.* 2002;15:583-589.

136. Vanhoutte PM, Zhao Y, Xu A, Leung SW. Thirty years of saying NO: sources, fate, actions, and misfortunes of the endothelium-derived vasodilator mediator. *Circ Res.* 2016;119:375-396.

137. Forstermann U, Xia N, Li H. Roles of vascular oxidative stress and nitric oxide in the pathogenesis of atherosclerosis. *Circ Res.* 2017;120:713-735.

138. Lu Y, Wei J, Stec DE, et al. Macula densa nitric oxide synthase 1beta protects against salt-sensitive hypertension. *J Am Soc Nephrol.* 2015;8:2346-2356.

139. Gimenez M, Schickling BM, Lopes LR, Miller FJ, Jr. Nox1 in cardiovascular diseases: regulation and pathophysiology. *Clin Sci (Lond).* 2016;130:151-165.

140. Brown DI, Griendling KK. Regulation of signal transduction by reactive oxygen species in the cardiovascular system. *Circ Res.* 2015;116:531-549.

141. Cowley AW, Jr., Abe M, Mori T, O'Connor PM, Ohsaki Y, Zheleznova NN. Reactive oxygen species as important determinants of medullary flow, sodium excretion, and hypertension. *Am J Physiol Renal Physiol.* 2015;308:F179-F197.

142. Touyz RM, Rios FJ, Alves-Lopes R, Neves KB, Camargo LL, Montezano AC. Oxidative stress: a unifying paradigm in hypertension. *Can J Cardiol.* 2020;36:659-670.

143. Griendling KK, Touyz RM, Zweier JL, et al. Measurement of reactive oxygen species, reactive nitrogen species, and redox-dependent signaling in the cardiovascular system: a scientific statement from the American Heart Association. *Circ Res.* 2016;119:e39-e75.

144. Forrester SJ, Kikuchi DS, Hernandes MS, Xu Q, Griendling KK. Reactive oxygen species in metabolic and inflammatory signaling. *Circ Res.* 2018;122:877-902.

145. Goetze JP, Bruneau BG, Ramos HR, Ogawa T, de Bold MK, de Bold AJ. Cardiac natriuretic peptides. *Nat Rev Cardiol.* 2020;17:698-717.

146. Burnett JC, Jr. Atrial natriuretic peptide, heart failure and the heart as an endocrine organ. *Clin Chem.* 2019;65:1602-1603.

147. Pandey KN. Molecular and genetic aspects of guanylyl cyclase natriuretic peptide receptor-A in regulation of blood pressure and renal function. *Physiol Genomics.* 2018;50:913-928.

148. Theilig F, Wu Q. ANP-induced signaling cascade and its implications in renal pathophysiology. *Am J Physiol Renal Physiol.* 2015;308:F1047-F1055.

149. Melo LG, Steinhelper ME, Pang SC, Tse Y, Ackermann U. ANP in regulation of arterial pressure and fluid-electrolyte balance: lessons from genetic mouse models. *Physiol Genomics.* 2000;3:45-58.

150. Asferg CL, Andersen UB, Linneberg A, Goetze JP, Jeppesen JL. Obese hypertensive men have lower circulating proatrial natriuretic peptide concentrations despite greater left atrial size. *Am J Hypertens.* 2018;31:645-650.

151. Jordan J, Birkenfeld AL, Melander O, Moro C. Natriuretic peptides in cardiovascular and metabolic crosstalk: implications for hypertension management. *Hypertension.* 2018;72:270-276.

152. Chen Y, Schaefer JJ, Iyer SR, et al. Long-term blood pressure lowering and cGMP-activating actions of the novel ANP analog MANP. *Am J Physiol Regul Integr Comp Physiol.* 2020;318:R669-R676.

153. Taylor EB, Wolf VL, Dent E, Ryan MJ. Mechanisms of hypertension in autoimmune rheumatic diseases. *Br J Pharmacol.* 2019;176:1897-1913.

154. Drummond GR, Vinh A, Guzik TJ, Sobey CG. Immune mechanisms of hypertension. *Nat Rev Immunol.* 2019;19:517-532.

155. Madhur MS, Kirabo A, Guzik TJ, Harrison DG. From rags to riches: moving beyond RAG1 in studies of hypertension. *Hypertension.* 2020;75:930-934.

156. Seniuk A, Thiele JL, Stubbe A, et al. B6.Rag1 knockout mice generated at the Jackson Laboratory in 2009 show a robust wild-type hypertensive phenotype in response to Ang II (angiotensin II). *Hypertension.* 2020;75: 1110-1116.

157. Norlander AE, Madhur MS, Harrison DG. The immunology of hypertension. *J Exp Med.* 2018;215:21-33.

158. Wu H, Ballantyne CM. Metabolic inflammation and insulin resistance in obesity. *Circ Res.* 2020;126:1549-1564.

159. Donath MY, Dinarello CA, Mandrup-Poulsen T. Targeting innate immune mediators in type 1 and type 2 diabetes. *Nat Rev Immunol.* 2019;19:734-746.

160. Zennaro MC, Boulkroun S, Fernandes-Rosa FL. Pathogenesis and treatment of primary aldosteronism. *Nat Rev Endocrinol.* 2020;16:578-589.

161. Herrmann SM, Textor SC. Renovascular hypertension. *Endocrinol Metab Clin N Am.* 2019;48:765-778.

162. Tevosian SG, Ghayee HK. Pheochromocytomas and paragangliomas. *Endocrinol Metab Clin N Am.* 2019;48:727-750.

163. Lerman LO, Textor SC. Gained in translation: protective paradigms for the poststenotic kidney. *Hypertension.* 2015;65:976-982.

164. Eirin A, Textor SC, Lerman LO. Novel therapeutic strategies for renovascular disease. *Curr Opin Nephrol Hypertens.* 2019;28:383-389.

165. Williams TA, Mulatero P, Bidlingmaier M, Beuschlein F, Reincke M. Genetic and potential autoimmune triggers of primary aldosteronism. *Hypertension.* 2015;66:248-253.

166. Fernandes-Rosa FL, Boulkroun S, Zennaro MC. Genetic and genomic mechanisms of primary aldosteronism. *Trends Mol Med.* 2020;26:819-832.

167. Stowasser M, Gordon RD. Primary aldosteronism: changing definitions and new concepts of physiology and pathophysiology both inside and outside the kidney. *Physiol Rev.* 2016;96:1327-1384.

168. Funder JW. Primary aldosteronism. *Hypertension.* 2019;74:458-466.

169. Pimenta E, Wolley M, Stowasser M. Adverse cardiovascular outcomes of corticosteroid excess. *Endocrinology.* 2012;153:5137-5142.

170. Rana S, Lemoine E, Granger JP, Karumanchi SA. Preeclampsia: pathophysiology, challenges, and perspectives. *Circ Res.* 2019;124:1094-1112.

171. Battarbee AN, Sinkey RG, Harper LM, Oparil S, Tita ATN. Chronic hypertension in pregnancy. *Am J Obstet Gynecol.* 2020;222:532-541.

172. Phipps EA, Thadhani R, Benzing T, Karumanchi SA. Pre-eclampsia: pathogenesis, novel diagnostics and therapies. *Nat Rev Nephrol.* 2019;15:275-289.

173. Ives CW, Sinkey R, Rajapreyar I, Tita ATN, Oparil S. Preeclampsia-pathophysiology and clinical presentations: JACC state-of-the-art review. *J Am Coll Cardiol.* 2020;76:1690-1702.

174. Granger JP, Spradley FT, Bakrania BA. The endothelin system: a critical player in the pathophysiology of preeclampsia. *Curr Hypertens Rep.* 2018;20:32.

175. Padmanabhan S, Caulfield M, Dominiczak AF. Genetic and molecular aspects of hypertension. *Circ Res.* 2015;116:937-959.

176. Manosroi W, Williams GH. Genetics of human primary hypertension: focus on hormonal mechanisms. *Endocr Rev.* 2019;40:825-856.

177. Padmanabhan S, Joe B. Towards precision medicine for hypertension: a review of genomic, epigenomic, and microbiomic effects on blood pressure in experimental rat models and humans. *Physiol Rev.* 2017;97:1469-1528.

178. Luft FC. What have we learned from the genetics of hypertension? *Med Clin N Am.* 2017;101:195-206.

179. Ehret GB, Caulfield MJ. Genes for blood pressure: an opportunity to understand hypertension. *Eur Heart J.* 2013;34:951-961.

180. Arnett DK, Claas SA. Omics of blood pressure and hypertension. *Circ Res.* 2018;122:1409-1419.

181. Arif M, Sadayappan S, Becker RC, Martin LJ, Urbina EM. Epigenetic modification: a regulatory mechanism in essential hypertension. *Hypertens Res.* 2019;42:1099-1113.

182. Liang M. Epigenetic mechanisms and hypertension. *Hypertension.* 2018;72:1244-1254.

183. King SE, Skinner MK. Epigenetic transgenerational inheritance of obesity susceptibility. *Trends Endocrinol Metab.* 2020;31:478-494.

184. Ceccato F, Mantero F. Monogenic forms of hypertension. *Endocrinol Metab Clin N Am.* 2019;48:795-810.

185. Ercu M, Marko L, Schachterle C, et al. Phosphodiesterase 3A and arterial hypertension. *Circulation.* 2020;142:133-149.

186. World Health Organization. Obesity and overweight—key facts. https://www.who.int/news-room/fact-sheets/detail/obesity-and-overweight. Accessed September 30, 2020.

187. Garrison RJ, Kannel WB, Stokes J, III, Castelli WP. Incidence and precursors of hypertension in young adults: the Framingham Offspring Study. *Prev Med.* 1987;16:235-251.

188. Stevens VJ, Obarzanek E, Cook NR, et al. Long-term weight loss and changes in blood pressure: results of the Trials of Hypertension Prevention, phase II. *Ann Intern Med.* 2001;134:1-11.

189. Piche ME, Tchernof A, Despres JP. Obesity phenotypes, diabetes, and cardiovascular diseases. *Circ Res.* 2020;126:1477-1500.

190. Hall ME, do Carmo JM, da Silva AA, Juncos LA, Wang Z, Hall JE. Obesity, hypertension, and chronic kidney disease. *Int J Nephrol Renovasc Dis.* 2014;7:75-88.

191. Grassi G, Biffi A, Seravalle G, et al. Sympathetic neural overdrive in the obese and overweight state. *Hypertension.* 2019;74:349-358.

192. Henegar JR, Zhang Y, Rama RD, Hata C, Hall ME, Hall JE. Catheter-based radiorefrequency renal denervation lowers blood pressure in obese hypertensive dogs. *Am J Hypertens.* 2014;27:1285-1292.

193. do Carmo JM, da Silva AA, Gava FN, Moak SP, Dai X, Hall JE. Impact of leptin deficiency compared with neuronal-specific leptin receptor deletion on cardiometabolic regulation. *Am J Physiol Regul Integr Comp Physiol.* 2019;317:R552-R562.

194. Ozata M, Ozdemir IC, Licinio J. Human leptin deficiency caused by a missense mutation: multiple endocrine defects, decreased sympathetic tone, and immune system dysfunction indicate new targets for leptin action, greater central than peripheral resistance to the effects of leptin, and spontaneous correction of leptin-mediated defects. *J Clin Endocrinol Metab.* 1999;84:3686-3695.

195. da Silva AA, do Carmo JM, Wang Z, Hall JE. Melanocortin-4 receptors and sympathetic nervous system activation in hypertension. *Curr Hypertens Rep.* 2019;21:46.

196. Greenfield JR, Miller JW, Keogh JM, et al. Modulation of blood pressure by central melanocortinergic pathways. *N Engl J Med.* 2009;360:44-52.

197. Williams B, MacDonald TM, Morant S, et al. Spironolactone versus placebo, bisoprolol, and doxazosin to determine the optimal treatment for drug-resistant hypertension (PATHWAY-2): a randomised, double-blind, crossover trial. *Lancet.* 2015;386:2059-2068.

198. Calhoun DA. Fluid retention, aldosterone excess, and treatment of resistant hypertension. *Lancet Diabetes Endocrinol.* 2018;6:431-433.

199. Denic A, Glassock RJ. Obesity-related glomerulopathy and single-nephron GFR. *Kidney Int Rep.* 2020;5:1126-1128.

200. Hsu CY, McCulloch CE, Iribarren C, Darbinian J, Go AS. Body mass index and risk for end-stage renal disease. *Ann Intern Med.* 2006;144:21-28.

201. Eckel RH, Alberti KG, Grundy SM, Zimmet PZ. The metabolic syndrome. *Lancet.* 2010;375:181-183.

202. Grundy SM. Metabolic syndrome update. *Trends Cardiovasc Med.* 2016;26:364-373.

203. Hall JE. Hyperinsulinemia: a link between obesity and hypertension? *Kidney Int.* 1993;43:1402-1417.

204. da Silva AA, do Carmo JM, Li X, Wang Z, Mouton AJ, Hall JE. Role of hyperinsulinemia and insulin resistance in hypertension: metabolic syndrome revisited. *Can J Cardiol.* 2020;36:671-682.

205. Hall JE, Brands MW, Zappe DH, Alonso GM. Insulin resistance, hyperinsulinemia, and hypertension: causes, consequences, or merely correlations? *Proc Soc Exp Biol Med.* 1995;208:317-329.

206. Muntner P, Whelton PK. Using predicted cardiovascular disease risk in conjunction with blood pressure to guide antihypertensive medication treatment. *J Am Coll Cardiol.* 2017;69:2446-2456.

207. Whelton PK, Campbell NRC, Lackland DT, et al. Strategies for prevention of cardiovascular disease in adults with hypertension. *J Clin Hypertens (Greenwich).* 2020;22:132-134.

208. Goff DC, Jr., Lloyd-Jones DM, Bennett G, et al. 2013 ACC/AHA guideline on the assessment of cardiovascular risk: a report of the American College of Cardiology/American Heart Association Task Force on Practice Guidelines. *J Am Coll Cardiol.* 2014;63:2935-2959.

209. Pylypchuk R, Wells S, Kerr A, et al. Cardiovascular disease risk prediction equations in 400 000 primary care patients in New Zealand: a derivation and validation study. *Lancet.* 2018;391:1897-1907.

210. Nerenberg KA, Zarnke KB, Leung AA, et al. Hypertension Canada's 2018 guidelines for diagnosis, risk assessment, prevention, and treatment of hypertension in adults and children. *Can J Cardiol.* 2018;34:506-525.

211. National Heart Foundation of Australia. *Guideline for the Diagnosis and Management of Hypertension in Adults—2016.* Melbourne: National Heart Foundation of Australia, 2016.

212. Wright JT, Jr., Williamson JD, Whelton PK, et al. A randomized trial of intensive versus standard blood-pressure control. *N Engl J Med.* 2015;373:2103-2116.

213. Beddhu S, Chertow GM, Greene T, et al. Effects of intensive systolic blood pressure lowering on cardiovascular events and mortality in patients with type 2 diabetes mellitus on standard glycemic control and in those without diabetes mellitus: reconciling results from ACCORD BP and SPRINT. *J Am Heart Assoc.* 2018;7:e009326.

214. Bundy JD, Li C, Stuchlik P, et al. Systolic blood pressure reduction and risk of cardiovascular disease and mortality: a systematic review and network meta-analysis. *JAMA Cardiol.* 2017;2:775-781.

215. Qaseem A, Wilt TJ, Rich R, et al. Pharmacologic treatment of hypertension in adults aged 60 years or older to higher versus lower blood pressure targets: a clinical practice guideline from the American College of Physicians and the American Academy of Family Physicians. *Ann Intern Med.* 2017;166:430-437.

216. Ilkun OL, Greene T, Cheung AK, et al. The influence of baseline diastolic blood pressure on the effects of intensive blood pressure lowering on cardiovascular outcomes and all-cause mortality in type 2 diabetes. *Diabetes Care.* 2020;43:1878-1884.

217. Haffner SM, Lehto S, Ronnemaa T, Pyorala K, Laakso M. Mortality from coronary heart disease in subjects with type 2 diabetes and in nondiabetic subjects with and without prior myocardial infarction. *N Engl J Med.* 1998;339:229-234.

218. Zafari N, Asgari S, Lotfaliany M, Hadaegh A, Azizi F, Hadaegh F. Impact of hypertension versus diabetes on cardiovascular and all-cause mortality in Iranian older adults: results of 14 years of follow-up. *Sci Rep.* 2017;7:14220.

219. Bress AP, King JB, Kreider KE, et al. Effect of intensive versus standard blood pressure treatment according to baseline prediabetes status: a post hoc analysis of a randomized trial. *Diabetes Care.* 2017;40(10):1401-1408.

Cardiometabolic Disease: Insulin Resistance, Obesity, and the Metabolic Syndrome

6

W. Timothy Garvey and Jeffrey I. Mechanick

CHAPTER OUTLINE

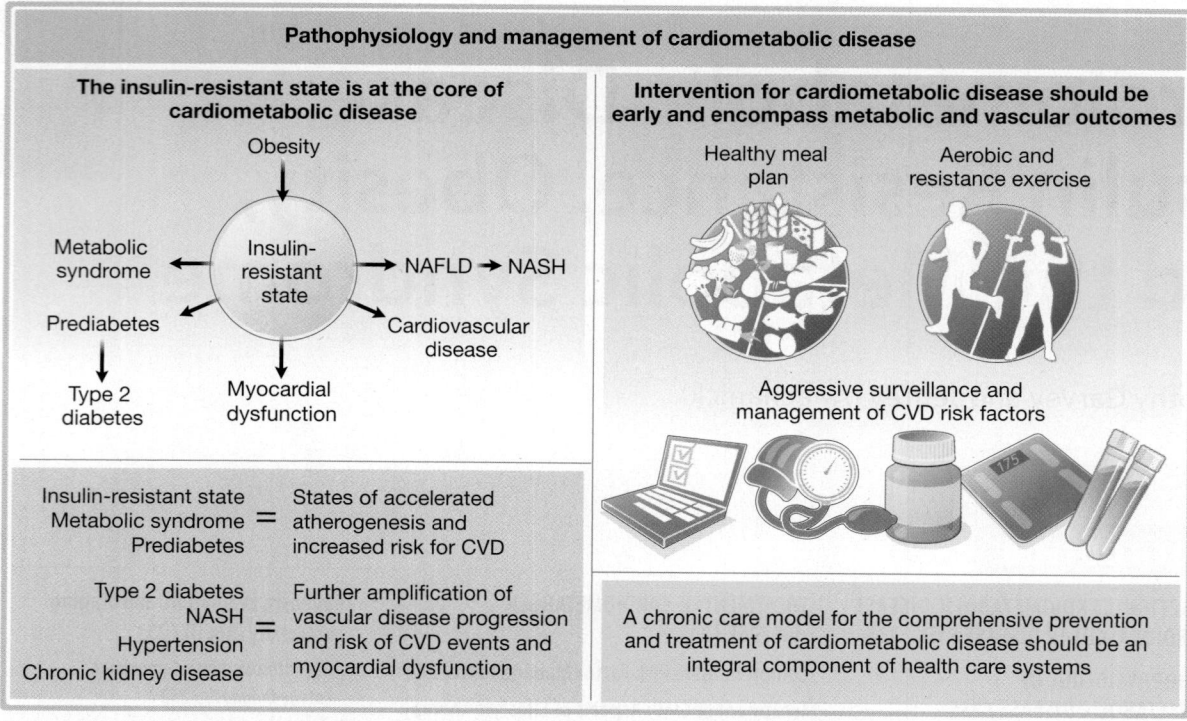

Chapter 6 Fuster and Hurst's Central Illustration. Cardiometabolic disease pathophysiology has the insulin-resistant state at its core. Obesity can exacerbate insulin resistance and promote cardiometabolic disease progression but can also exist independent of cardiometabolic disease. Early intervention is important and should involve a healthy meal plan, aerobic and resistance exercise, and aggressive surveillance and management of CVD risk factors. CVD, cardiovascular disease; NAFLD, non-alcoholic fatty liver disease; NASH, non-alcoholic steatohepatitis.

CHAPTER SUMMARY

This chapter discusses the pathophysiology and treatment of cardiometabolic disease and obesity. Insulin resistance is at the core of the pathophysiology of cardiometabolic disease and can give rise to metabolic syndrome, prediabetes, and non-alcoholic fatty liver disease (NAFLD) (see Fuster and Hurst's Central Illustration). Patients with insulin resistance, metabolic syndrome, and/or prediabetes have accelerated atherogenesis and increased risk for cardiovascular disease (CVD). Prediabetes and NAFLD can progress to type 2 diabetes and non-alcoholic steatohepatitis (NASH), respectively; these conditions further amplify the progression of vascular disease and risk of CVD events. Obesity can exacerbate insulin resistance and promote cardiometabolic disease progression, but it can also exist independent of cardiometabolic disease. In the prevention and treatment of cardiometabolic disease, intervention should be early and encompass metabolic and vascular outcomes. Healthy meal plans, aerobic and resistance exercise, and aggressive surveillance and management of CVD risk factors are all warranted. A chronic care model for cardiometabolic disease should be an integral component of health-care systems.

INTRODUCTION: CARDIOMETABOLIC DISEASE AND CARDIOVASCULAR DISEASE RISK

The term *cardiometabolic disease (CMD)* indicates that there is a common pathophysiological process that results in both metabolic and cardiovascular disease. This chapter will provide the clinical and mechanistic justifications for the term and contextualize cardiovascular disease (CVD) as an end-stage manifestation of this chronic disease process, thus providing opportunities for primordial, primary, secondary, and tertiary prevention and treatment. At the core of CMD is the insulin-resistant state that gives rise to clinically identifiable conditions at high risk for future CVD events—namely, metabolic syndrome (MetS), prediabetes, and non-alcoholic fatty liver disease (NAFLD). Obesity can exacerbate insulin resistance and impel this disease progression. Thus, insulin resistance, prediabetes, and MetS all represent states of accelerated atherogenesis and mark patients at higher risk for CVD.[1-3] Furthermore, once metabolic disease becomes overt, with the development of type 2 diabetes (T2D) and/or non-alcoholic steatohepatitis (NASH), there is further amplification of vascular disease progression and risk of CVD events. Within the context of CMD, treatment and prevention must concomitantly encompass both metabolic and vascular outcomes. Given the increasing burden of patient suffering and social costs exacted by this nexus of diseases interrelated via CMD pathophysiology, it becomes imperative to intervene early to halt CMD progression.

The acceleration of atherosclerosis by the insulin-resistant state is analogous to the impact of elevated low-density lipoprotein cholesterol (LDL-C) or cigarette smoking, which are emphasized as major targets for the primary prevention of CVD using a variety of dietary, behavioral, and pharmacological interventions. There is, perhaps, less of a concerted effort for prevention focused on the insulin-resistant state. The lowering of LDL-C levels in statin cardiovascular outcome trials results in an average risk reduction of approximately 30%, leaving a preponderant degree of "residual" risk.[4] Insulin resistance may account for the bulk of this residual risk and may be responsible for a greater degree of overall CVD risk than that ascribed to LDL-C. Using an Archimedes model and simulated trials involving NHANES data, investigators have estimated that insulin resistance accounts for 42% of overall CVD risk.[5] A comprehensive approach to the prevention and treatment of CVD must entail diligent efforts to address residual risk and impede the progression of CMD.

This chapter will address operative properties of the insulin-resistant state and the role of obesity in the pathophysiology of CMD. The clear majority of patients with CMD will be overweight or obese. In these patients, weight loss becomes the most effective way to prevent CMD progression, and the treatment of obesity will be given due emphasis in this chapter. Whether patients are lean or obese, healthy meal plan, physical activity, and aggressive surveillance and management of CVD risk factors are warranted in patients with CMD.

THE PATHOPHYSIOLOGY OF CARDIOMETABOLIC DISEASE

Overview

CVD, obesity, and T2D are epidemiologically linked and often present as comorbidities in single patients. Indeed, obesity increases the risk for T2D, and both are established risk factors for CVD events. The cooccurrence of these diseases is predictable since they represent at an advanced stage of CMD progression—the culmination of a chronic disease process that began early in life. As these diseases become overt, certain developments signal the need for therapeutic intervention: (i) for CVD, this often begins with the occurrence of events (eg, MI, stroke); (ii) for obesity, once the body mass index (BMI) is ≥30 kg/m²; and (iii) in T2D with the detection of hyperglycemia. The perspective of CVD, obesity, and T2D as end-stage developments of a chronic progressive disease assimilates the framework for designing rational preventive strategies. This will require an understanding of CMD pathogenesis as the scientific basis for designing effective interventions.

By way of overview, the spectrum of CMD and the pathophysiology driving its progression are illustrated in **Fig. 6–1**. Briefly stated, the abnormality central to pathogenesis is insulin resistance. Insulin resistance is a complex trait that not only involves defects in insulin-mediated glucose homeostasis but also multiple molecular abnormalities involving cell signaling, gene expression, oxidative stress, mitochondrial dysfunction, and inflammation. These molecular defects have systemic consequences producing vascular stiffness, abnormal glucose tolerance, elevated blood pressure, abnormal substrate metabolism, and ectopic lipid accumulation within muscle and liver cells. In aggregate, these abnormalities are referred to as the "insulin resistance state," which is subclinical early in CMD progression. As the disease progresses, clinical manifestations become apparent and signal the presence of CMD (Fig. 6–1), including dyslipidemia, abdominal obesity, MetS, prediabetes, and NAFLD. These clinical manifestations indicate the need to halt further progression to incident CVD and T2D. High LDL-C and smoking also worsen CVD risk, but independent of CMD. Progression to T2D involves insulin resistance combined with pancreatic beta cell defects, to the degree that insulin secretion can no longer compensate for ambient insulin resistance. With ongoing accumulation of intrahepatocellular lipid, some patients with NAFLD develop NASH as another metabolic end-stage manifestation of CMD. The presence of diabetes and/or NASH further worsens the risk of CVD events and myocardial dysfunction.

Obesity is a disease of positive energy balance that involves abnormalities in the mass, distribution, and/or function of adipose tissue.[6] Obesity can exist independent of CMD; indeed, not all patients with obesity are insulin resistant at increased risk of T2D or CVD, and lean individuals can also have CMD. However, obesity can exacerbate insulin resistance and promote CMD progression. The majority of patients with CMD will be overweight or obese, and, in this instance, weight loss is the most effective and comprehensive approach for treating CMD.

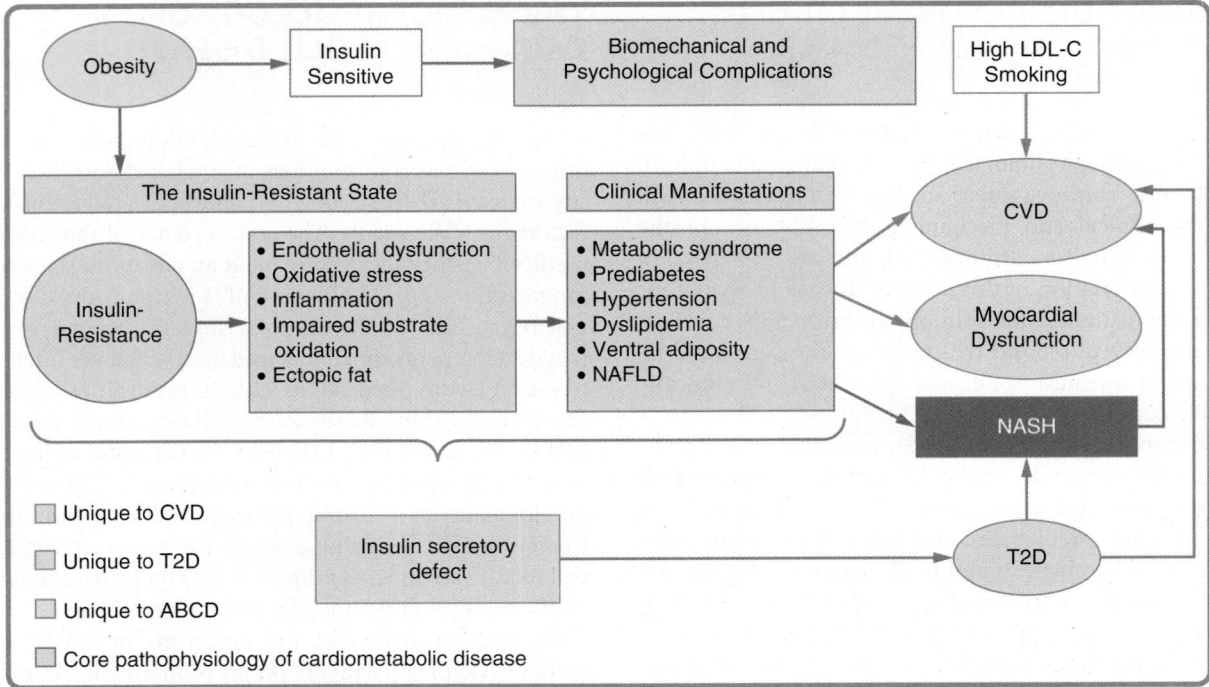

Figure 6-1. The spectrum of cardiometabolic disease. Pathophysiological properties of the insulin-resistant state (in gray) produce clinical manifestations that mark patients at increased risk of both metabolic disease, including T2D (in green) and nonalcoholic steatohepatitis (in blue), and vascular disease, including both atherosclerotic CVD and myocardial dysfunction (in red). Obesity can exacerbate insulin resistance and drive the progression of cardiometabolic disease to the end-stage developments of T2D and CVD. High LDL-C and smoking independently affect CVD risk, while CMD and the underlying insulin-resistant state account for the majority of residual risk.

Patients with obesity who remain insulin sensitive (ie, the metabolically healthy obese) are still at risk of biomechanical complications of the disease, such as obstructive sleep apnea, osteoarthritis, and impaired mobility.

Insulin Resistance and the Insulin-Resistant State

Insulin resistance constitutes the core pathophysiological abnormality in CMD and is integral to the pathogenesis of CVD and T2D.[4–10] The Insulin Resistance Atherosclerosis Study[7,8] and the Bezafibrate Infarction Prevention Trial[9] demonstrated that insulin resistance was independently associated with the development of CVD events and increased carotid wall thickness. Gast et al.[10] conducted a meta-analysis of 65 studies and found that the HOMA index of insulin sensitivity (based on fasting glucose and insulin) significantly increased the relative risk for incident CVD events. The term "insulin resistance" can be variably employed to describe different biological processes, and, within the context of CMD, it is important to provide a precise definition. The classic cardinal manifestations of insulin resistance include normoglycemia or hyperglycemia in the face of hyperinsulinemia. Using various in vivo metabolic techniques, investigators have shown that these manifestations of insulin resistance arise from impaired insulin action in muscle to promote glucose uptake and in liver to suppress glucose production. While classically conceptualized in relationship to insulin's glucoregulatory actions, insulin resistance also affects a broad range of insulin actions involving gene expression, vascular biology, and protein and lipid metabolism. Furthermore, insulin resistance is associated with multiple pathophysiological processes that exert adverse effects on both metabolism and the vasculature, including (1) defects in substrate oxidation and mitochondrial function, (2) increased inflammation and oxidative stress, (3) alterations in lipids and lipoproteins contributing to CVD risk, (4) impaired lipid storage in adipocytes via defects in both lipolysis and triacylglycerol synthesis, (5) accumulation of ectopic lipid within muscle and liver cells, and (6) abnormalities in vasoregulation due to a reduction in endothelial nitric oxide synthase activity and nitric oxide production. Thus, insulin resistance defined by abnormalities in glucose regulation due to insulin action defects is fundamentally linked with systemic inflammation, oxidative stress, impaired substrate metabolism, and dysfunctional adipose tissue. It is not clear whether the glucoregulatory defect precedes the development of these latter processes or vice versa. For this reason, in the context of what initiates and promulgates CMD, the combination of pathophysiological processes with defects in glucoregulation is referred to as the "insulin-resistant state." These processes constitute the mechanistic link between insulin resistance and CVD.

The insulin-resistant state is a complex trait that develops early in life and may develop in utero. Epigenetic factors can contribute; for example, epigenetic modifications arising in utero under conditions of maternal gestational diabetes can confer an insulin resistance phenotype in offspring that persists into adulthood.[11] These offspring are at increased risk for T2D, obesity, and CVD as adults. Genome-wide association studies have identified multiple chromosomal regions associated with various measures of insulin resistance reflecting abnormal glucose regulation, implicating a number of potentially causal genes, including *PPARG*, *IRS1*, *NAT2*, *IGF1*, *BCL2*, and *FAM19A2*.[12] Individually, these genes confer only a small relative risk for insulin resistance. The heritability scores (h^2) for insulin resistance are generally modest, usually in the range of ~30%,[13] indicating that factors such as physical inactivity and diet are responsible for a substantial amount of individual variation in insulin sensitivity.[14]

The interaction of genetic, epigenetic, environmental, and behavioral factors produces a wide range of individual variability in systemic insulin sensitivity. Among those at the more insulin-resistant range of the spectrum, there is preferential accumulation of fat in the intra-abdominal compartment, which contains an increased number of resident macrophages predominantly involving classically activated M1 and a lesser proportion of alternatively activated M2 macrophages.[15] These resident macrophages secrete cytokines and other factors that cross-talk with adipocytes and alter the systemic release of adipocytokines from adipose tissue. Altered release of adipose tissue factors such as adiponectin, resistin, free fatty acids, leptin, angiotensinogen, plasminogen activator inhibitor-1, and increased production of inflammatory cytokines, including interleukin (IL)-6 and IL-1, and tumor necrosis factor (TNF)–α alter metabolism in multiple organs. Adipocytes residing in the inflamed adipose tissue environment are dysfunctional and reach a limit where they are unable to store further calories as fat. Serum levels of free fatty acids become elevated and ectopic lipid accumulates within liver and muscle cells, leading to NAFLD and worsening insulin resistance.

Elevated levels of lipids (lipotoxicity) and glucose (glucose toxicity) coupled with mitochondrial dysfunction augment the production of reactive oxygen species (ROS) and oxidative stress. The systemic inflammation and oxidative stress activate nuclear factor (NF)–κB, further propagating inflammatory pathways and the production of cytokines. Intracellular levels of diacylglycerols and ceramides also increase and activate serine/threonine kinases that desensitize insulin action via the phosphorylation of signaling molecules (ie, insulin receptor substrate-1 and insulin receptor). These molecular events exacerbate insulin action defects in muscle and liver and worsen systemic inflammation and metabolism.

The Metabolic Syndrome and Prediabetes

The insulin-resistant state gives rise to clinically identifiable high-risk phenotypes in the form of MetS and prediabetes. The ATPIII criteria for MetS are widely used, and patients must exceed thresholds for abnormal values corresponding to any three out of five risk parameters for a diagnosis: waist circumference, blood pressure, triglycerides, high-density lipoprotein cholesterol (HDL-C), and fasting glucose.[16] However, additional sets of diagnostic criteria have been proposed (**Table 6–1**). The World Health Organization requires patients to have impaired fasting glucose or impaired glucose tolerance,

TABLE 6–1. Criteria for Metabolic Syndrome

RISK FACTOR	ATPIII	WHO	IDF
	3 out of 5	**IFG/IGT[a] + 2**	**Waist + 2**
I. Waist			
Men	>102 cm (40 in)	W/H > 0.90 BMI > 30 kg/m²	≥ 94 cm[b]
Women	>88 cm (35 in)	W/H > 0.85 BMI > 30 kg/m²	≥ 80 cm[b]
II. Triglycerides	≥150 mg/dL (1.7 mmol/L) or Tx	≥150 mg/dl (1.7 mmol/L)	≥150 mg/dL (1.7 mmol/L) or Rx
III. HDL cholesterol		and/or	
Men	<40 mg/dL (1.0 mmol/L) or Rx	<0.9 mmol/L (35 mg/dl)	<40 mg/dL (1.0 mmol/L) or Rx
Women	<50 mg/dL (1.3 mmol/L) or Rx	<1.0 mmol/L (39 mg/dl)	<50 mg/dL (1.3 mmol/L) or Rx
IV. Blood pressure	>130/>85 mmHg or Rx	≥140/90 mmHg	>130/>85 mmHg or Rx
IV. Fasting glucose	≥100 mg/dL (5.6 mmol/L) or Rx	IFG and/or IGT[d]	≥100 mg/dL (5.6 mmol/L)
V. Microalbuminuria		≥ 20 µg/min (≥30 mg/g creatinine)	

Abbreviations: IGF, impaired fasting glucose; IGT, impaired glucose tolerance; ATP, Advanced Treatment Panel; WHO, World Health Organization; IDF, International Diabetes Federation; HDL, high-density lipoprotein; W/H, waist-to-hip ratio; BMI, body mass index; Rx, pharmacologic treatment

a. IFG = fasting glucose ≥ 100 mg/dl (5.6 mmol/L); IGT = glucose ≥ 140 mg/dl (7.8 mmol/L) after a 75 oral gram glucose tolerance test.

b. Values apply to waist circumference applicable to Europeans. Criteria vary based on regional epidemiology.

plus any two additional risk factors, and therefore places greater emphasis on the dysglycemic component of the syndrome.[17]

Alternatively, the International Diabetes Federation (IDF) requires an elevated waist circumference plus any two additional risk factors, placing greater emphasis on this measure of abdominal adipose tissue accumulation.[18] In addition, the IDF advocates different waist circumference cut-points for indicating CMD risk based on geographical and ethnic variation as established by regional epidemiological studies. These studies, for example, have supported lower threshold values in South Asian, Southeast Asian, and East Asian adults in whom waist circumferences ≥90 cm in men and ≥80 cm in women more accurately identify those at greater CMD risk. MetS confers increased risk for T2D and CVD and has proved to be a useful clinical construct for identifying patients requiring more aggressive risk management. However, it is important to realize that in patients who present with one or two risk factors and fall short of the three criteria needed for the diagnosis, there remains elevated risk for CVD and T2D compared to individuals who lack any MetS traits (19; Fig. 10).

The diagnostic criteria for prediabetes are based upon fasting glucose values, the glucose level at 2 hours during a 75-gram oral glucose tolerance test (OGTT), and hemoglobin A1c (HbA1c) (**Table 6–2**). The clinical diagnosis requires three salient considerations. First, the categories of normoglycemia, prediabetes, and mild diabetes based on fasting or 2-hour OGTT glucose values can vary in individual patients over time, and it is reasonable to confirm the status by repeated testing on a separate day. Second, HbA1c has high specificity but relatively low sensitivity for diagnosing prediabetes or mild diabetes,[20] and clinicians should consider confirming glycemic status using fasting and/or 2-hour OGTT glucose rather than reliance on HbA1c alone. Third, with advancing age above 50 years old, an increasing majority of patients will have prediabetes on the basis of elevated 2-hour OGTT alone,[21] and the diagnosis will be missed unless an OGTT is performed.

In patient care, there is no accepted practical method of directly measuring insulin resistance, and research procedures used to identify and quantify insulin sensitivity are not feasible for clinical application. Even so, the presence of insulin resistance can be denoted in the clinic by the presence of MetS traits and prediabetes.[19] MetS traits represent the sequelae of processes integral to the insulin-resistant state, including dysfunctional inflamed adipose tissue, abnormal secretion of adipocytokines, endothelial dysfunction, and dyslipidemia.

Mechanisms Linking the Insulin-Resistant State to CVD

Dyslipidemia

The dyslipidemia associated with insulin resistance is characterized by (1) excessive and prolonged postprandial chylomicronemia, (2) high levels of plasma triglycerides, (3) low levels of HDL-C, and (4) increase in small, dense LDL particle concentration not necessarily accompanied by a rise in LDL-C levels. There is an increase in circulating large, triglyceride-containing, very low density lipoprotein (VLDL) molecules due to greater hepatic production driven by increased fatty acid flux to the liver and reduced clearance due to a decrease in lipoprotein lipase. The high levels of VLDL, together with the actions of cholesteryl ester transfer protein (CETP) and hepatic lipase, participate in the generation of small, dense LDL. CETP facilitates the exchange of cholesteryl esters and triglycerides between lipoproteins, resulting in a net loss of cholesterol esters and a gain of triacylglycerols by HDL and LDL, as well as a reciprocal net gain of cholesterol esters and loss of triacylglycerols by chylomicrons and VLDL. The resulting triglyceride-rich LDL becomes a substrate for the lipolytic action of hepatic lipase, resulting in the formation of small, dense LDL. Hepatic lipase also acts on triglyceride-rich HDL to produce small, dense HDL, which results in a decrease in HDL-C since small, dense HDL is susceptible to increased catabolism.

An increase in small, dense LDL particle concentration is a risk factor for CVD, independent of overall LDL-C levels. The Atherosclerosis Risk in Communities (ARIC) study, for example, prospectively demonstrated that the plasma levels of small, dense LDL were independently predictive of incident coronary heart disease.[22] Mechanistically, small, dense LDL particles are more susceptible to atherogenic modifications such as oxidation, and more readily enter the vascular wall where they induce endothelial adhesion molecules [ie, intercellular adhesion molecule (ICAM)-1 and vascular cell adhesion molecule (VCAM)-1 and monocyte chemoattractant protein-1]. Upon entering the vascular wall, macrophages preferentially take up modified LDL particles leading to cholesterol accumulation and foam cell formation together with induction of inflammation via toll-like receptor-4 and the NF-κB pathway. Thus, changes in lipids and lipoproteins that occur solely as a function of insulin resistance are atherogenic, and they act to accelerate atherosclerosis independent of overall LDL-C levels.

TABLE 6–2. Diagnostic Criteria for Diabetes and Prediabetes

Glycemic Status	Fasting Glucose	2-Hour OGTT Glucose	HbA1c
Normoglycemia	<100 mg/dl (<5.6 mmol/L)	<140 mg/dl (<7.8 mmol/L)	<5.7% (<39 mmol/mol)
Prediabetes	100–125 mg/dl (5.6–6.9 mmol/L)	140–199 mg/dl (7.8–11.0 mmol/L)	5.7%–6.4% (39-47 mmol/mol
Diabetes	≥126 mg/dl (≥7.0 mmol/L)	≥200 mg/dl (≥11.1 mmol/L)	≥6.5% (≥48 mmol/mol)

Data from American Diabetes Association. 2. Classification and Diagnosis of Diabetes: *Standards of Medical Care in Diabetes-2020*, Diabetes Care. 2020 Jan;43(Suppl 1):S14-S31.

Endothelial Dysfunction and Elevated Blood Pressure

Insulin signaling through phosphoinositide-3 kinase/Akt in endothelium regulates endothelial nitric oxide synthase (eNOS) activity and production of the vasodilator NO. In insulin resistance, this pathway is inhibited, while signaling through insulin's mitogenic ras/raf The mitogen-activated protein kinase (MAPK) pathway is unimpeded and, in fact, hyperactive due to hyperinsulinemia. MAPK signaling increases production of the vasoconstrictor endothelin-1, such that the net effect of imbalance between insulin's metabolic and mitogenic pathways is vasoconstriction. The mitogenic pathway also promotes vascular smooth muscle cell proliferation and expression of the vascular cell adhesion molecules VCAM-1 and E-selectin. In addition, insulin resistance is associated with increased activity of the sympathetic nervous system and the renin–angiotensin–aldosterone system (RAAS).[23] Augmented signaling through the mineralocorticoid receptor further increases the production of ROS, impairs vascular relaxation, and induces cell adhesion molecules. The endothelium is subject to increased inflammation and oxidative stress, as are other tissues in the metabolic milieu of the insulin-resistant state. The combination of these processes affecting the vascular wall enhances vasoreactivity and explains the relationship between insulin resistance, elevated blood pressure, development of hypertension, and progression over time to CVD events. In cross-sectional studies, ~50% of hypertensive subjects have hyperinsulinemia or glucose intolerance, and ~80% of patients with T2D have hypertension (23). The coexistence of hypertension and diabetes substantially enhances the risk of CVD. In addition, the insulin-resistant state is characterized by a clotting diathesis[24] due to endothelial dysfunction, insulin resistance, and decreased NO production, which increases platelet adhesiveness, combined with increased circulating fibrinogen and PAI-1 production by adipose tissue.

PROPERTIES OF THE INSULIN-RESISTANT STATE THAT PRODUCE CARDIOVASCULAR DISEASE

- Inflammation
- Oxidative stress
- Dyslipidemia
- Endothelial dysfunction
- Elevated blood pressure
- Impaired metabolism
- Hyperglycemia
- Clotting diathesis
- Myocardial dysfunction

Inflammation

A sine qua non of insulin resistance is inflamed dysfunctional adipose tissue that results in increased release of proinflammatory cytokines into the blood. These cytokines and other circulating factors such as oxidized and triglyceride-rich lipoproteins augment vascular wall inflammation, increase the expression of cell adhesion molecules promoting the margination and uptake of monocytes, and promote foam cell formation, as macrophages avidly accumulate cholesterol, particularly in the form of modified LDL. With insulin resistance, small, dense LDL particles are prone to modification by oxidation, acetylation, and glycation. These modifications render the lipoprotein particles proinflammatory and induce an immune response that leads to the formation of circulating LDL-Containing immune complexes that compound their atherogenicity. Foam cell formation due to the ready uptake of modified LDL particles leads to fatty streaks and plaque development.

Macrophages play an essential role at all stages of atherosclerotic lesion progression. Proinflammatory M1 macrophages differentiate in response to toll-like receptor (TLR) and interferon-γ signaling and are activated by lipopolysaccharides and lipoproteins. These cells secrete proinflammatory factors, such as TNFα, IL-1β, and various chemokines [C-X-C motif chemokine ligand (CXCL) 9, CXCL10, and CXCL11], and produce high levels of ROS. In contrast, M2 macrophages secrete anti-inflammatory factors, such as IL-1 receptor agonist and IL-10. With insulin resistance, resident M1 macrophages are increased in both the vascular wall and adipose tissue. While both macrophage phenotypes are detected in atherosclerotic lesions, proinflammatory M1 macrophages are enriched in progressing plaques, where they play a critical role in atherogenesis, and M2 macrophages are present in regressing plaques.[25] Insulin resistance favors the more inflammatory M1 macrophage phenotype residing in adipose tissue and the vascular wall.

Hyperglycemia

While patients with insulin resistance who maintain normal glucose levels have accelerated atherosclerosis, those who develop overt diabetes are at even greater risk of both CVD and myocardial dysfunction. Indeed, the United Kingdom Prospective Diabetes Study (UKPDS) was among the first to establish an epidemiological link between hyperglycemia and CVD by showing there was a linear relationship between HbA1c and CVD events including myocardial infarction.[26] The mechanisms by which hyperglycemia is associated with atherogenesis are not fully elucidated; however, it is clear that there are complex links between hyperglycemia, lipoprotein abnormalities, and systemic and vessel wall inflammation. High glucose itself worsens insulin resistance (ie, glucose toxicity). Glucose-induced insulin resistance is due at least in part to insulin action defects associated with the induction of tribbles homolog 3 (TRIB3), which binds Akt and blocks its phosphorylation in the insulin-signaling cascade.[27]

High glucose per se can also directly augment oxidative stress and activate inflammatory pathways, such as NFκB, in endothelial cells, monocyte-macrophages, and vascular smooth muscle cells. Hyperglycemia and mitochondrial dysfunction conspire to increase production of ROS and oxidative stress. Advanced glycation end-products (AGEs) can be formed as a result of prolonged exposure of proteins and lipids to high concentration of glucose. The ligation of AGEs to specific cell surface receptors contributes to increased expression of adhesion molecules that mediate margination and uptake of monocytes into the vascular wall. Lipoproteins are structurally modified by both AGEs and oxidation, and then are readily taken up by macrophages via surface scavenger receptors, thereby facilitating foam cell formation. In short, many of the properties of the insulin-resistant state and mechanisms responsible for accelerated atherosclerosis are intensified by hyperglycemia.

THE INSULIN-RESISTANT STATE AND PROGRESSION TO T2D AND NAFLD

Insulin resistance in muscle and liver increases the demand for insulin secretion from pancreatic beta cells to maintain glucose homeostasis. So long as robust insulin secretory responses are sustained, patients remain normoglycemic. Some individuals eventually exhibit elevations in postprandial glucose levels when early phase insulin secretion becomes insufficient to maintain normal postprandial glycemic excursions. Over time, insulin secretory capacity declines, further causing a rise in fasting glucose levels, and eventually patients satisfy the glycemic criteria for prediabetes, followed by progression to overt T2D. The development of abnormal glucose tolerance indicates that the chronic metabolic stress of insulin resistance has led to a reduction in insulin secretion to below the level needed to fully compensate for insulin resistance.

Thus, progression from the insulin-resistant state to T2D requires the predisposition to pancreatic beta cell exhaustion under conditions of the prolonged metabolic stress of insulin resistance. As was the case for CVD, processes associated with the insulin-resistant state create the conditions leading to beta cell injury, including inflammation, oxidative stress, glycotoxicity, and lipotoxicity. Reduced capacity for insulin secretion is due to a decrease in beta cell mass, as well as a defect in sensing glucose as a secretagogue. Beta cell failure under conditions of chronic metabolic stress appears to be a genetically determined trait that segregates independent of insulin resistance, consistent with the "two-hit" hypothesis for developing T2D. The majority of susceptibility genes found to be associated with diabetes in genome wide association study (GWAS) studies affect beta cell function, such as *TCF7L2, C2CD4A, ABCC8, KCNJ11, and SLC30A8*,[28] and the heritability factor for the insulin secretory defect is estimated as high as 70%.

It is well established that there is a higher incidence of acute myocardial infarction (AMI) in patients with T2D, and that patients with diabetes have greater mortality and re-infarction rates following AMI than patients without diabetes. In addition to T2D, NAFLD may also compound CVD risk. Increased accumulation of lipid in hepatocytes occurs as a function of the insulin-resistant state, and many patients with CMD have hepatic steatosis. In some patients, steatosis leads to inflammation and fibrosis and can progress to cirrhosis and hepatic failure. The entire spectrum of this disease is termed NAFLD, and can be categorized histologically as non-alcoholic fatty liver (NAFL), with the presence of ≥5% hepatocellular lipid content without evidence of hepatocellular injury, or NASH in the presence of ≥5% lipid content with inflammation and hepatocyte ballooning with or without fibrosis (29). NAFLD regularly coexists with T2D, obesity, and CVD, and the presence of T2D aggravates NAFLD to more severe forms of steatohepatitis.

It is also well established that NAFLD is associated with an increased risk of CVD events.[30] Some studies indicate that NAFLD increases CVD risk, independent of other risk factors, and that this risk becomes greater as NAFL progresses to more severe forms of NASH.[31,32] A Framingham Heart study of 3,529 patients undergoing computed tomography (CT) showed that NAFLD was associated with the presence of subclinical markers of atherosclerosis, such as calcium deposits in coronary arteries, even after adjustment for other metabolic risk factors.[33] On the other hand, a large, matched cohort study from Europe demonstrated that NAFLD was not associated with increased risk of AMI after controlling for other CVD risk factors.[34] While further studies are needed, NAFLD is an additional metabolic end-stage manifestation of CMD, and surveillance is required in patients with the clinical manifestations of CMD (Fig. 6–1), obesity, T2D, and CVD.

Role of Obesity

Obesity is a chronic disease of energy balance driven by dysregulated interactions involving satiety factors and the central nervous system (CNS), resulting in increased caloric intake and an excess in adipose tissue mass. The increase in adiposity causes chronic complications that confer increased morbidity and mortality. An abnormality in adipose tissue mass predisposes to biomechanical complications such as obstructive sleep apnea and osteoarthritis, while abnormalities in the mass, distribution, and function of adipose tissue contribute to cardiometabolic disease complications. In this context, adiposity-based chronic disease (discussed later in this chapter) is a precise clinical and diagnostic term referring to obesity.[6]

Obesity is a major risk factor for the development of MetS and prediabetes, as well as for progression to overt T2D, NASH, and CVD. However, many individuals with CMD who progress to T2D and/or CVD are lean. In addition, a certain proportion of patients with BMIs in the overweight or obesity range are insulin sensitive, do not develop MetS traits, and are not at increased risk of T2D and CVD.[3,35] These patients are referred to as the "metabolically healthy obese." When metabolic health is defined as the absence of any MetS traits, metabolically healthy obese individuals comprise ~15% to 20% of US adults with overweight or obesity in the NHANES cohort.[36] As shown in Fig. 6–1, insulin-sensitive individuals with obesity may develop the biomechanical complications of obesity, such as osteoarthritis or obstructive sleep apnea, but they may not be at increased risk of T2D or CVD. Weight gain in these patients occurs on an insulin-sensitive background, and adipose tissue is not inflamed and does not preferentially expand in the intra-abdominal compartment. Therefore, obesity as assessed by BMI is neither sufficient nor necessary as a pathogenic factor in the development of insulin resistance, MetS, and prediabetes.

The relationship between body weight gain and CMD is complex. The correlation between generalized adiposity and insulin sensitivity indicates that only ~11% of individual variability in insulin sensitivity can be explained by BMI.[14] However, if weight gain occurs on an insulin-resistant background, there is an asymmetrical accumulation of fat favoring the intra-abdominal depot and dysregulated secretion of adipocytokines due to adipose tissue inflammation and influx of macrophages. Weight gain can worsen insulin resistance and intensify processes such as inflammation, oxidative stress, and glucose intolerance that are components of the insulin-resistant state. In the setting of excessive caloric intake, insulin-resistant adipocytes cannot accommodate the need for increased fuel storage; consequently, free fatty acid (FFA) levels rise, and ectopic lipid accumulates in muscle and liver cells. Thus, there is an interaction between excess adiposity and insulin resistance that worsens pathophysiological processes associated with the insulin-resistant state and to promote progression toward end-stage developments in CMD. Clinically, the critical point is that in those patients with elevated BMI and insulin resistance, weight loss becomes a highly effective therapeutic modality to prevent and treat CMD.

Weight gain will increase the risk of overt T2D by worsening insulin resistance, thereby placing more metabolic stress on beta cells in those individuals predisposed to beta cell fatigue. Patients with insulin resistance who sustain robust insulin secretory responses to avoid T2D remain in a state of accelerated atherosclerosis and high risk of CVD events.

Adiponectin and the Macrophage: Paradigm for a Single Mechanism Common to Both Metabolic and Vascular Disease

A fundamental principle is that the insulin-resistant state constitutes a common pathophysiological mechanism leading to CVD and T2D. The role of adiponectin illustrates this paradigm, as an adipocyte-derived hormone involved in the pathogenesis of both metabolic and vascular disease.[37,38] As described previously, the expansion of visceral adipose tissue mass is associated with altered secretion of multiple adipocytokines from fat tissue into the circulation, and these factors alter metabolism in multiple organs, helping to produce the MetS trait complex. Adiponectin is one such adipokine. Epidemiological data clearly indicate that high adiponectin levels are associated with cardiometabolic wellness. Low levels, on the other hand, are associated with insulin resistance, high waist circumference, obesity, MetS and related traits, T2D, and CVD. Adiponectin circulates in high (duodecamers) and low (hexamers) molecular weight (MW) multimeric forms, and hyperinsulinemic euglycemic clamp studies have demonstrated that decrements in the high-MW form are more closely linked to insulin resistance than with the low-MW form.[38] Circulating adiponectin concentrations are also related to lipid metabolism, as evidenced by negative correlations with triglycerides and LDL-C, and positive correlations with whole-body fat oxidation and HDL-C levels. Finally, low adiponectin has been associated with endothelial dysfunction in coronary vessels, as well as the extent of coronary artery disease.[39]

Fig. 6–2 illustrates the mechanisms by which adiponectin can mediate both vascular and metabolic disease via its direct ability to influence macrophage biology. These effects on resident macrophages in the vascular wall can inhibit (high levels) or promote (low levels) foam cell formation

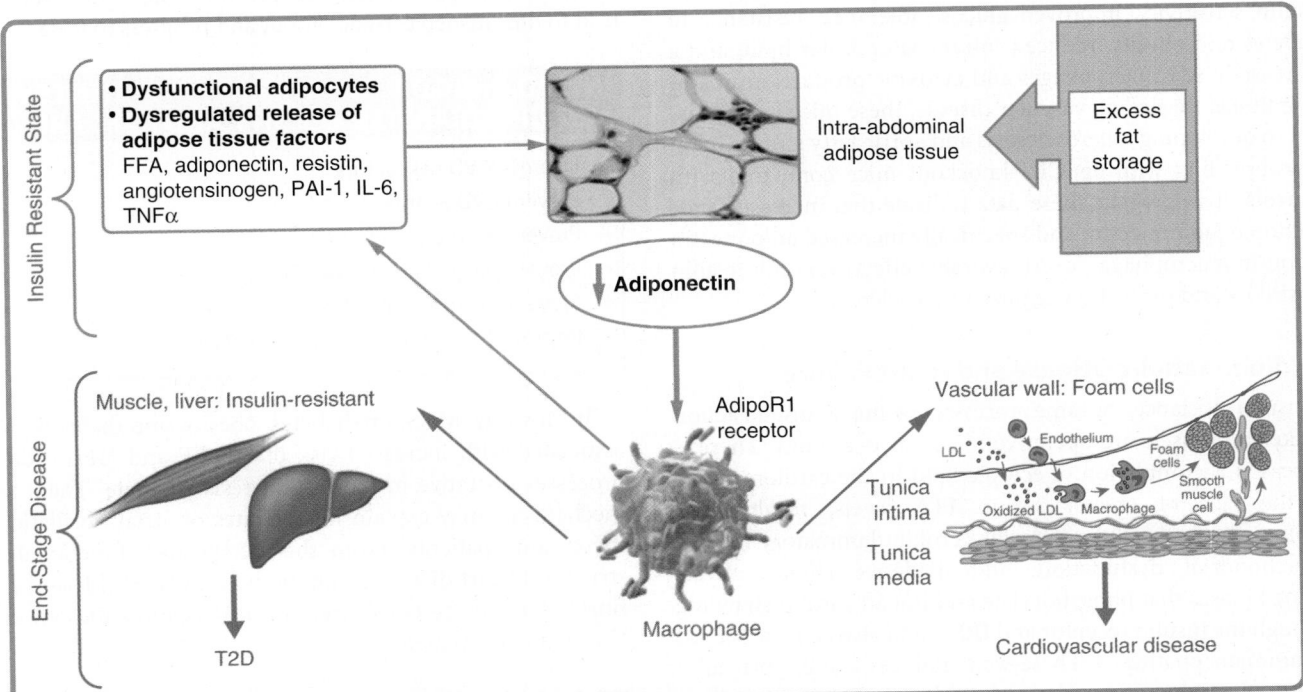

Figure 6–2. Adiponectin as a paradigm for common mechanism responsible for both metabolic and vascular disease. With increased fat storage in the intra-abdominal adipose tissue, adipocytes secrete less adiponectin. The reduction in adiponectin acts as an autocrine/paracrine factor that worsens insulin sensitivity and inflammation in adipose tissue. This factor leads to dysregulated secretion of adipocytokines and exacerbates peripheral insulin resistance. At the same time, decreased adiponectin augments the inflammatory posture of macrophages, which infiltrates adipose tissue and leads to further deterioration in adipose tissue function. Diminished adiponectin facilitates (1) increased monocyte entry into the vascular wall, (2) conversion to inflammatory macrophages, (3) cholesterol accumulation due to enhanced uptake of modified LDL and reduced HDL-mediated efflux, and (4) foam cell formation and initiation of fatty streaks.

and atherogenesis.[37] Mediated by changes in gene expression, adiponectin acts to impede foam cell formation in response to oxidized LDL inhibiting oxLDL uptake, as well as to enhance HDL-mediated cholesterol efflux.[40,41] Furthermore, adiponectin suppresses the migration of monocytes/macrophages and their uptake into the vascular wall.[37,41] Regarding effects in adipose tissue, adiponectin decreases macrophage content and promotes development of moderate-sized, well-functioning adipocytes that exhibit increased insulin-stimulated glucose transport, reduced release of inflammatory cytokines, and augmented capacity for lipid uptake and storage.[42] These actions underlie the systemic effects of adiponectin to augment insulin sensitivity and lipid oxidation in skeletal muscle, lower hepatic glucose production in liver, and reduce intracellular lipid in muscle and liver. Low levels of adiponectin have the opposite effect of impairing adipocyte function and promoting systemic insulin resistance. It is of interest that adiponectin may mediate the beneficial effects of insulin-sensitizing thiazolidinediones used to treat T2D; thiazolidinediones increase adiponectin production and expand well-functioning adipocytes in the subcutaneous fat depot, while decreasing intra-abdominal fat and ectopic lipid in muscle and fat cells.

Observations in transgenic mice corroborate the contention that adiponectin's ability to affect both metabolic and vascular disease in vivo is due to hormone action at the level of the macrophage. Transgenic mice that overexpress the adiponectin receptor (ie, adipoR1) solely in macrophages augment the effects of circulating adiponectin on only this cell type.[43] Regarding the metabolic impact, these mice exhibited increased insulin sensitivity, improved glucose tolerance, resistance to diabetes and obesity, reduced intrahepatocellular lipid, and a decrease in M1 macrophages and cytokine production in adipose tissue. Regarding vascular disease, these mice were resistant to developing atherosclerosis and aortic fatty streaks upon cross-breeding with apoCIII knockout mice compared with controls. In aggregate, these data indicate that increased production of adiponectin, and specifically increased adiponectin action in macrophages, exert favorable effects on both insulin sensitivity and protection against atherosclerosis.

Cardiometabolic Disease and Heart Failure

In insulin resistance, the same processes that impair insulin action in skeletal muscle are operative in the myocardium. There is increased accumulation of ectopic lipid in the cardiomyocyte in the face of greater serum FFA levels, resulting in lipotoxicity. Intracellular diacylglycerol, inflammatory factors, mitochondrial dysfunction, and oxidative stress activate serine kinases that phosphorylate and impair insulin signaling through the insulin receptor and IRS-1 and also activate NF-κB inflammatory pathways. These events reduce the ability of insulin to stimulate glucose uptake and oxidation. The myocardium uses fatty acids as its preferred fuel choice except in the presence of pacing or ischemia when the heart relies on glucose for fuel. Due to defects in insulin action and mitochondrial function, the flexibility to convert to glucose metabolism is diminished. The metabolic alterations in substrate utilization combined

with inappropriate activation of the renin–angiotensin–aldosterone system, endothelial dysfunction, sympathetic nervous system activation, oxidative stress, and inflammation produce structural abnormalities in the heart.[44] Cellular injury and abnormalities in contractile proteins promote cardiac tissue interstitial fibrosis, and cardiac stiffness impairs diastole relaxation and filling of the ventricle prior to systole. The result is heart failure with preserved ejection fraction (HFpEF), accompanied by increased left atrial size, left ventricular mass, and alterations in transmitral velocity.[45] Diastolic dysfunction can progress to systolic dysfunction and congestive heart failure with reduced ejection fraction (HFrEF).

Diabetes further worsens myocardial dysfunction, with greater risk of heart failure and atrial fibrillation at an earlier age.[46] Hyperglycemia and the diabetes milieu exacerbate pathophysiological processes due to insulin resistance including defective insulin signaling, impaired glucose utilization, inflammation, oxidative stress, and endothelial dysfunction. There is more fibrosis and myocardial stiffness due to AGE formation and collagen cross-linking.[47] Mitochondrial dysfunction results in greater ROS production through uncoupled respiration, and ROS signaling contributes to maladaptive hypertrophy, contractile dysfunction, damage to mitochondrial DNA, reduced adenosine triphosphate (ATP) generation, and apoptosis. As cardiac output diminishes, the RAAS becomes more active, increasing systemic blood pressure, endothelial injury, and oxidative stress in cardiomyocytes.[48] These changes in myocardial metabolism and structure impair diastole relaxation and filling of the ventricle prior to systole, and eventually lead to diminished cardiac output and progress to CHF.

> ### IN CMD, THE GOALS OF THERAPY IN PATIENTS WITH METS, PREDIABETES, OBESITY, AND NAFL ARE:
>
> - Improve CVD risk factors
> - Prevent CVD events
> - Prevent progression to T2D
> - Prevent progression to NASH
> - Prevent microvascular disease
> - Improve functionality and quality of life

In this way, MetS, prediabetes, obesity, and diabetes are all associated with increased risk of HFpEF and HFrEF due to processes operative in the insulin-resistant state. These same mechanisms may explain higher rates of atrial fibrillation in these same patients. From this perspective, functional and structural heart disease resulting in HFpEF, HFrEF, and atrial fibrillation can be considered as end-stage manifestations of CMD in many patients.

TREATMENT OF CARDIOMETABOLIC DISEASE

Comprehensive Risk Factor Management

Within the framework of CMD, the goals of therapy in patients with MetS, prediabetes, obesity, and/or NAFLD are the following: (1) prevent progression to CVD events, T2D, and NASH; (2) since hyperglycemia at the level of prediabetes is sufficient to cause background retinopathy and neuropathy in some patients, an additional goal is to prevent microvascular disease; and (3) improve the functionality and quality of life, particularly in sedentary individuals and patients with obesity. Since all these outcomes are the result of pathophysiological processes integral to the insulin-resistant state, the same interventions that effectively achieve any one of the treatment goals address many of the other goals as well. As described later in this chapter, weight loss in patients with overweight or obesity is highly effective in achieving treatment goals for CMD. In essence, treatment entails aggressive and comprehensive risk factor management.

Traditional risk factors epidemiologically linked to CVD are family history of premature disease (men age <55 years; women age <65 years), age (men age ≥45 years; women age ≥55 years), male sex, hypertension, elevated LDL-C, smoking, and diabetes.[49] Within the context of CMD, new risk factors include insulin resistance, in utero stress due to maternal obesity and/or gestational diabetes, abdominal obesity, MetS, prediabetes, NAFLD, biomarkers such as low adiponectin, inflammatory cytokines and other markers of systemic inflammation, and dyslipidemia characterized by high triglycerides, low HDL-C, and small, dense LDL particles.

Obesity is also a risk factor; however, obesity alone is not a prerequisite for CMD since lean individuals can be insulin-resistant and obese individuals can be insulin sensitive with no manifestations of MetS.[3,35] The association between BMI and CVD is largely explained by its association with other risk factors, such that independent risk conferred by BMI is usually minimized in multivariate analyses. For example, when adjusted for waist circumference, BMI is no longer a significant independent risk factor for CVD or becomes a much weaker predictor. Adjustment for MetS status similarly eliminates any independent effect of BMI on CVD risk.[35] Regarding the risk of developing T2D, the impact of high BMI is detrimental in patients with MetS and much less of a contributing factor in insulin-sensitive metabolically healthy individuals. In the ARIC study, lean individuals with MetS displayed a more than twofold increase in cumulative diabetes compared with obese metabolically healthy individuals.[35] Thus, weight gain against an insulin-sensitive background (ie, metabolically healthy) exerts a relatively small effect on increasing diabetes risk. This is consistent with the pathophysiological role of obesity to drive progression of CMD to CVD and T2D by exacerbating the insulin resistance state (Fig. 6–1).

To address comprehensive risk factor reduction in patients with MetS, prediabetes, obesity, and/or NAFLD, several key professional societies have made evidence-based recommendations for prevention of CVD or T2D (**Table 6–3**). A lifestyle characterized by a "healthy eating" plan and a program of aerobic and resistance exercise is consistently recommended. Management of blood pressure to a level of 130/80 mmHg or less (but not below 120/70 mmHg) is recommended for most patients, although a target of <140/90 mmHg is recommended by ACC/AHA and ADA if the 10-year

risk of ASCVD is <10% to 15%.[50] Recommended treatment to achieve blood pressure targets involves regular exercise, salt restriction, and sufficient potassium ingestion.[51] The drug of choice when needed to lower blood pressure is an angiotensin-converting enzyme inhibitor (ACEI) or an angiotensin receptor blocker (ARB). Many patients require dual therapy and the recommended second-line drug to be used with an ACEI or ARB is a calcium channel blocker or a diuretic. Regarding prediabetes, in addition to lifestyle therapy, both AACE and the ADA recommend the use of metformin in patients who are defined to be at a particularly high risk of T2D.[52-54]

Aggressive management of LDL-C and smoking cessation are critical components of CVD risk reduction in all patients, and exist outside of risk conferred by CMD. However, the dyslipidemia of insulin resistance does represent an important modifiable risk factor and, importantly, the recommended targets for LDL-C management should take into account the presence of small, dense LDL particles in CMD[55] (Table 6–3). In patients with prediabetes or MetS, the ACC/AHA and the ADA recommend treatment with statins based on the 10-year risk of ASCVD, and patients with diabetes should be prescribed a statin.[50,56] AACE recommends that LDL-C in patients with prediabetes be managed as if they had diabetes, and the recommendation is a target of LDL-C <100 mg/dl, <70 mg/dl, or <55 mg/dl depending on the presence of CVD, chronic kidney disease, and other risk factors.[55] The European Society of Cardiology/ European Society of Cardiology/European Association for the Study of Diabetes (ESC/EASD) recommend LDL-C lowering in patients with diabetes to <100 mg/dl, to <70 mg/dl if the patient with diabetes is at high risk of CVD, and to <55 mg/dl if at very high risk of CVD.[57] Thus, the AACE position in prediabetes and diabetes is similar to that of ESC/EASD in diabetes.

The contention that patients with prediabetes and/or MetS should be treated as aggressively as if they had diabetes is supported by the fact that the atherogenic processes inherent in the insulin-resistant state are ongoing in both groups of patients. Evidence to support aggressive management of LDL-C includes the results of the JUPITER trial in patients without diabetes but with elevated C-reactive protein (CRP). Ridker et al. demonstrated that LDL-C lowering by rosuvastatin from 108 mg/dl at baseline to 55 mg/dl by the end of the study substantially reduced CVD events compared with placebo, including patients with MetS at baseline.[58] In addition to LDL-C-lowering drugs, the REDUCE-IT trial[59,60] assessed the CVD benefits of a triglyceride-lowering drug, icosapent ethyl, in statin-treated patients with elevated triglycerides who had either established CVD disease (71%) or diabetes (29%) and included patients with MetS. Patients randomized to icosapent ethyl experienced reductions in first, subsequent, and total ischemic CVD events compared with placebo control subjects.

Treatment of CMD: Aspects of Lifestyle Therapy in Patients with and Without Obesity

Lifestyle therapy is the cornerstone of comprehensive risk management in all patients with CMD, while weight loss is critically important in those patients that are overweight or obese (ie, ABCD).

Healthy Meal Plan

Recommendations for a healthy meal plan generally include (1) limitations on fat intake; (2) emphasis on polyunsaturated/monounsaturated fats over saturated fats; (3) no trans fats; (4) avoidance of added sugar and sugar-sweetened beverages; (5) complex over simple carbohydrates; (6) whole grains; (7) fruits and vegetables; (8) dietary fiber, (9) limited sodium intake; (10) moderation in alcohol; and (11) reduced consumption of processed food[51] (**Table 6–3**). These recommendations are largely supported by epidemiological data and long-term controlled clinical trials assessing CVD events and progression to T2D as end-points are lacking. If there is lack of data addressing long-term outcomes, what evidence can be used to guide the dietary prescription? In CMD, dietary changes that enhance insulin sensitivity would predictably be effective in preventing or slowing disease progression.

Fortunately, there is a large body of data indicating that isocaloric substitution of specific macronutrients can influence insulin sensitivity and CVD risk factors.[14] Isocaloric enrichments or substitutions of macronutrients have been demonstrated to increase (favorable) or decrease (unfavorable) insulin sensitivity in studies employing gold-standard glucose clamps for measurement of insulin sensitivity (**Table 6–4**). It is clear that the recommendations concerning healthy meal plan align with macronutrients that enhance insulin sensitivity.

TABLE 6–3. Guidelines/Recommendations for Prevention of CVD or T2D in Patients with Prediabetes or Metabolic Syndrome

	ACC/AHA	AACE	ADA	ESC/EASD
References	87,88	89–92	93–95	96
Goals of intervention	• Prevent CVD events	• Prevent diabetes • Lower CVD risk • Prevent macrovascular/microvascular complications	• Prevent diabetes • Lower CVD risk • Prevent microvascular complications	• Prevent CVD events
Lifestyle	Structured lifestyle intervention	Structured lifestyle intervention	Structured lifestyle intervention	Structured lifestyle intervention
Diet	Healthy meal plan*; Replace SFAs with PUFAs	Healthy meal plan*	Healthy meal plan*	Mediterranean diet
Physical activity	• ≥150 min/week moderate exercise • Aerobic and resistance exercise • Limit sedentary activity	• ≥150 min/week moderate exercise • Aerobic and resistance exercise	• ≥150 min/week moderate exercise • Aerobic and resistance exercise	• ≥150 min/week moderate exercise • Aerobic and resistance exercise
Weight loss in patients with overweight/obesity	Weight loss; Clinically significant is >5%	5%–10%; 10% for diabetes prevention	5% or more	Reduce excessive weight
Obesity medications		As needed to achieve 10% weight loss	As needed to achieve >5% weight loss	
Diabetes medications if high risk		Metformin, acarbose with high risk of T2D	Metformin with high risk of T2D	
Definition of high T2D risk		Any 2 of IFG, IGT, or MetSyn; Worsening glycemia; CVD; NAFLD; GDM, PCOS	HbA1c 6.2%–6.4%, BMI≥35, age <60, GDM	
Blood pressure	Individualize based on 10-yr risk of ASCVD: <130/80 if risk ≥10%; <140/90 if risk <10%	<130/80 in most patients	Individualize based on 10-yr risk of ASCVD: <130/80 if risk ≥15%; <140/90 if risk <15%	Individualize but <130/80 if well tolerated; systolic 130–139 if >65 yrs
LDL-C (mg/dl)	Use statin based on 10-yr risk of CVD	Treat as T2D: LDL-C <100 or lower; <70 or <55 depending on CVD, diabetes, other risk factors	Use statin based on CVD risk; use statin in diabetes	<100; <55 in diabetes with high CVD risk
Tobacco use	Abstinence	Abstinence	Abstinence	Abstinence
Aspirin 75–100 mg/day	Not for primary prevention in most patients, but consider if high CVD risk	Not for primary prevention; use in diabetes or prediabetes with CVD or high CVD risk	Not for primary prevention; use in diabetes with CVD or high CVD risk	Not for primary prevention; use in diabetes with high CVD risk

*Healthy meals generally emphasize limitations on fat intake, emphasis on polyunsaturated/monounsaturated fats over saturated fats; no trans fats; avoidance of added sugar and sugar-sweetened beverages; complex over simple carbohydrates; whole grains; fruits and vegetables; dietary fiber, limited sodium intake; moderation in alcohol; limit processed food.

Abbreviations: ACC, American College of Cardiology; AHA, American Heart Association; AACE, American Association of Clinical Endocrinologists; ADA, American Diabetes Association; ESC, European Society of Cardiology; EASD, European Association for the Study of Diabetes; SFAs, saturated fatty acids; PUFAs, poly unsaturated fatty acids; IFG, impaired fasting glucose; IGT, impaired glucose tolerance; MetSyn, metabolic syndrome; NAFLD, non-alcoholic fatty liver disease; GDM, gestational diabetes mellitus; PCOS, polycystic ovary syndrome; ASCVD, atherosclerotic cardiovascular disease.

TABLE 6–4. Isocaloric Dietary Substitution on Enrichment: Impact on Insulin Sensitivity*

FAVORABLE	UNFAVORABLE
MUFAs	Saturated fat
PUFAs	Trans fat
Whole grains	Refined grains
High fiber	Low fiber
Low glycemic index	High glycemic index
Mediterranean diet	Western diet

*[27]

These observations can provide increased confidence in the dietary prescription consistent with the pathophysiology of CMD.

How can these recommendations for healthy macronutrients be integrated into real-world meal plans, and are there clinical trials demonstrating the ability of meal plans to prevent CVD and T2D independent of weight loss? Since the meal plan is intended over the lifetime of individuals, one consideration is that the diet should accommodate personal and cultural preferences, resulting in greater rates of compliance. Therefore, personal and cultural food preferences should be discussed with each patient to guide an optimal and more personalized healthy meal plan for a durable effect. The goal is to provide for a healthy macronutrient composition, and at the same time, identify foods that match personal and cultural preferences to assure adequate intake of required nutrients.

Clinical trial data addressing long-term outcomes exist for two meal plans that incorporate the macronutrient recommendations in large measure. The Mediterranean diet is characterized by a reliance on olive oil as a fat source, which contains the monounsaturated fatty acid (MUFA) oleic acid as ~75% of fatty acids. This diet is comprised largely of unprocessed foods and is rich in fiber, antioxidant polyphenols, vitamins and minerals, and phytochemicals. There are variations in the Mediterranean diet as it is followed in various regions and countries; however, there are commonalities relevant to cardiometabolic risk reduction. In addition to olive oil, these diets consistently feature high intake of vegetables, legumes, nuts, and fruits; a low intake of saturated fat; low to moderate consumption of dairy products; low intake of meat and poultry and relatively high intake of seafood; and regular consumption of red wine at meals (in most Mediterranean cultures). Epidemiologically, Mediterranean diets have been known to be associated with reduced CVD and mortality when compared with diets consumed in northern European countries.

The Predimed primary prevention trial demonstrated that over 4.8 years, a Mediterranean diet enriched in extra-virgin olive oil or nuts reduced the composite primary end-point of myocardial infarction, stroke, or cardiovascular death compared to a low-fat diet in individuals at risk for CVD.[61] The Lyon Diet Heart Study assessed the efficacy of Mediterranean diets for the secondary prevention of CVD events.[62] Patients who have had a previous myocardial infarction were randomized to a Mediterranean diet or a diet typically consumed in northern European countries, and after 4 years, the Mediterranean diet group had reduced rates of re-infarction and mortality. Adherence with this eating pattern is associated with decreased risk for MetS, reduced inflammation and hepatic steatosis, and improved renal function. Mediterranean diets have also been shown to reduce rates of progression to T2D independent of weight loss, and therefore can be recommended in lean patients with MetS or prediabetes.[63] In an umbrella evaluation of meta-analyses, Galbete et al.[64] affirmed that a higher adherence with a Mediterranean eating pattern was associated with lower incidence of mortality from T2D and CVD. Thus, Mediterranean diets are a highly rational choice as the dietary component of long-term lifestyle therapy in patients with cardiometabolic risk.

The second meal plan, the Dietary Approaches to Stop Hypertension (DASH) diet, has been shown to reduce blood pressure and is particularly effective in individuals who were hypertensive at baseline and/or self-identified as an African American.[65] This diet is rich in fruits, vegetables, and low-fat dairy foods, while being low in fat content (saturated fat, total fat, and cholesterol), red meat, sweets, and sugar-containing beverages. Improvements in blood pressure can occur without change in weight or sodium reduction. The DASH meal plan can also be combined with a reduced sodium intake, resulting in greater blood pressure reduction; in the DASH Sodium trial, combining the DASH dietary plan with 2400 mg sodium intake resulted in a blood pressure reduction of 7/4 mm Hg.[66] Sufficient potassium intake up to the level recommended in the US Food and Drug Administration (FDA) dietary guidelines for Americans (120 mmol/d; 4700 mg) can reduce blood pressure when dietary consumption falls below that level.[67] Finally, alcohol has a known pressor effect, and men should be counseled to consume ≤2 drinks per day and women ≤1 drink per day to avoid any adverse effect on blood pressure.

Physical Activity

Increased physical activity is an important component of lifestyle therapy. Regular exercise, by itself or as part of a comprehensive lifestyle plan, can prevent progression to T2D in high-risk individuals and improve CVD risk factors such as lipids and blood pressure. Structured exercise improves fitness, muscle strength, and insulin sensitivity. Studies have demonstrated the beneficial effects of both aerobic and resistance exercise, as well as additive benefits when both forms of exercise are combined.[68] For cardiometabolic conditioning, the guidelines proposed by the ACC/AHA, AACE, ADA, ESC/EASD, and the American College of Sports Medicine (ACSM) are well aligned (Table 6–3). The recommended targets for physical activity cannot always be achieved, and patients should be encouraged to engage in physical activity even if the level is suboptimal. For example, studies have consistently shown that a walking program is associated with a reduction in diabetes incidence. Reductions in sedentary behavior can also be helpful (eg, duration of sedentary periods lasting less than 90 min and interrupted by periods of activity) and are emphasized by the ACC/AHA[50,51] The health-care professional and the patient should together establish the physical activity prescription, with the goal for long-term adherence. Screening for coronary artery disease should also be performed in patients at risk.

Benefits of Weight Loss in Treating Patients with CMD and Overweight or Obesity

For patients with obesity and CMD (ie, with MetS, prediabetes, or NAFLD), there is an additional, all-important therapeutic prerogative to achieve treatment goals—namely, weight loss.[69] Approximately 90% of adults with MetS in the US NHANES survey are overweight or obese,[70] and weight loss is the most effective single intervention in these individuals. Weight loss, whether due to lifestyle therapy, obesity medications, or bariatric procedures, has been shown to (1) enhance insulin sensitivity; (2) prevent or delay progression to T2D, particularly in high-risk patients with prediabetes or MetS; (3) improve hepatic steatosis; (4) lower blood pressure; (5) improve dyslipidemia; and (6) ameliorate biomarkers of CVD risk, including CRP, IL-6, and other markers of inflammation, fibrinogen levels, and serum adiponectin concentrations. Thus, weight loss is perhaps the most effective therapeutic approach for treating and preventing the progression of CMD. By enhancing insulin sensitivity, weight loss mitigates the pathophysiological processes operative in the insulin-resistant state that confer a risk of future T2D and CVD events (Fig. 6–1). The specific benefits of weight-loss therapy in CMD are discussed later in this chapter.

Prevention of T2D

In patients who are overweight or obese, three major randomized clinical trials, the Diabetes Prevention Program, the Finnish Diabetes Study, and the Da Qing Study, all demonstrated that lifestyle/behavioral therapy featuring a reduced calorie diet (eg, caloric deficits of 500–1000 calories/day) is highly effective in preventing T2D.[2] These lifestyle interventions also improved other aspects of CMD, including improvements in insulin sensitivity and CVD risk factors, such as blood pressure, lipids, and markers of inflammation. The Diabetes Prevention Program study randomized subjects with impaired glucose tolerance to ordinary care, metformin, and lifestyle intervention, and after 4 years, lifestyle modification reduced progression to T2D by 58% and metformin by 31%, compared with placebo.[71] Subjects achieved approximately 6% mean weight loss at 2 years and 4% weight loss at 4 years in the lifestyle intervention arm, and there was a progressive 16% reduction in T2D risk with every kilogram of weight loss. With observational follow-up after termination of the study, there was still a significant reduction in the cumulative incidence of T2D in the lifestyle treatment group at 10 years, despite the fact that BMI levels had equalized among the three treatment arms.[72] In addition to T2D prevention, long-term follow-up of patients in the Da Qing Study revealed that CVD events and mortality were reduced when comparing the combined subgroups treated with diet and exercise with the controls.[73]

It is important to consider the degree of weight loss that is optimal for diabetes prevention. In the Diabetes Prevention Program, maximal prevention of diabetes over 4 years was observed at about 7% to 10% weight loss.[74] This is consistent with the study employing phentermine/topiramate extended-release (ER), where weight loss of 10% reduced incident diabetes by 79% over 2 years and any further weight loss to ≥15% did not lead to additional prevention.[75] Bariatric surgery produces greater weight loss than what is observed following lifestyle and pharmacotherapy interventions; and yet in two studies, there was a maximum of 76% to 80% reduction in diabetes rates.[76,77] similar to that observed with phentermine/topiramate ER and liraglutide 3 mg[75,78] despite less weight loss than achieved following bariatric surgery. These combined data suggest that 7% to 10% weight loss will reduce the risk of future T2D by ~80% and represents a threshold above which further weight loss may not result in additional preventive benefits. For this reason, 7% to 10% weight loss is the appropriate goal in treating patients with prediabetes,[69,79] whether as a component of a structured lifestyle intervention program or in conjunction with obesity medications.

Treatment of T2D

Weight-loss therapy in T2D has an outstanding therapeutic profile; it produces substantial reduction in HbA1c with less need for diabetes medications, can lead to diabetes remission, lowers blood pressure, improves triglycerides and HDL-C, improves NAFLD, is renal protective, improves sleep apnea, enhances mobility and decreases pain, and improves quality of life. These benefits were demonstrated in the Look AHEAD trial[80] and phase 3 clinical trials involving obesity medicines.[69] The Look AHEAD (Action for Health in Diabetes) trial randomized 5145 patients with T2D to an intensive lifestyle intervention, including caloric restriction, prespecified caloric intake of fats and protein, meal replacements, and 175 min/week of moderate-intensity physical activity or to usual care with diabetes support and education.[80] Despite weight loss of nearly 9% in the intervention group and greater improvements in HbA1c and CVD risk factors, the trial was stopped early for futility to reduce CVD events.

The DiRECT (Primary Care-Led Weight Management for Remission of Type 2 Diabetes) trial randomized patients with T2D followed in primary care clinics in the United Kingdom to a very-low-calorie diet versus standard care.[81,82] At 1 year, the very-low-calorie-diet group lost 10 kg and experienced a diabetes remission rate of 46%, compared to 1 kg of weight loss and a 4% remission rate in the control group. Remission of T2D was related to the amount of weight lost[81] with the remission rate rising to 86% in those patients losing 15 kg or more. Regarding pharmacotherapy, the efficacy and safety for all obesity medications in patients with T2D have been demonstrated in clinical trials.[69] Consistently, there are reductions in HbA1c despite the need for reduced use of diabetes drugs, as well as improvements in insulin sensitivity and CVD risk factors, in patients randomized to obesity medications compared with placebo. These data attest to the powerful benefits of weight loss, which should be considered as a primary treatment objective in patients with T2D and obesity.

Blood Pressure and Lipids

Additional benefits of weight loss are reductions in blood pressure and improvements in dyslipidemia. A meta-analysis of eight studies involving more than 2100 participants who were randomized to either a weight-reducing diet or a control intervention demonstrated that weight loss led to decrements in blood pressure of 4.5/3.2 mm Hg together with a 4.0 kg decrease in body weight, compared with the control groups after follow-up of 6 to 36 months.[83] The results of this meta-analysis are consistent with analyses suggesting that blood pressure decreases by 1.2/1.0 mm Hg for every kilogram of weight lost. Regarding dyslipidemia, weight loss decreases triglycerides, raises HDL-C, and lowers LDL-C in some studies; in addition, it amplifies the benefits of changes in dietary macronutrient composition. Meta-analyses have reported that for every kilogram of weight loss, triglyceride levels decrease about 1.9%.[84] Furthermore, there are beneficial effects of weight loss on LDL subclasses, characterized by reductions in small, dense LDL particle concentrations coupled with an increase in mean LDL particle size.[85]

NAFLD

The therapeutic imperative for patients with NAFLD is to delay or abrogate disease progression from hepatic steatosis (NAFL) to NASH to cirrhosis and liver failure. A 4% to 10% weight loss is sufficient to reduce hepatic steatosis; however, weight loss as high as 10% to 40% is required to decrease hepatic inflammation, hepatocellular injury, and fibrosis in NASH.[69] Liver biopsies obtained before and after weight loss produced by lifestyle modifications or bariatric surgery have exhibited histological improvements pertaining to NASH activity scores, hepatocellular fat, lobular inflammation, hepatocellular ballooning, and fibrosis. Mummadi et al.[86] conducted a meta-analysis of 15 interventional studies that included 766 paired liver biopsies in patients undergoing bariatric surgery. With the reductions in BMI after surgery, the pooled proportions of patients with improvement or resolution of steatosis, steatohepatitis, and fibrosis were 91.6%, 81.3%, and 65.5%, respectively, and a complete resolution of NASH was observed in 69.5% of patients.

Obstructive Sleep Apnea

Weight-loss therapy prevents or treats a wide variety of additional complications and comorbidities of obesity.[69] Obesity markedly augments the risk of obstructive sleep apnea, which interrupts normal sleep with periods of hypoxia and is highly prevalent among patients with CMD. By way of illustration, the Sleep AHEAD study found that 87% of patients with obesity and T2D had sleep apnea regardless of symptoms.[87] Obstructive sleep apnea adversely affects psychological health, causing fatigue and depression, metabolic health by predisposing to MetS and T2D, and cardiovascular health as an independent risk factor for refractory hypertension, stroke, and CVD. Severity of sleep apnea is quantified by the apnea-hypopnea index (AHI), which reflects the average number of apneic/hypopneic episodes per hour during a polysomnography study. The therapeutic options for obstructive sleep apnea include continuous positive airway pressure therapy and weight loss. Weight loss, whether achieved by lifestyle therapy[87] or obesity medications,[88] can dramatically improve both AHI scores and symptomatology, and therapeutic benefits are most predictably achieved with at least 10% weight loss.[69]

Cardiovascular Disease and Mortality

It is difficult to assess an independent effect of weight loss on CVD events and CVD mortality for several reasons: (1) the confounding effect of treatment targeted to risk factors can affect mortality (eg, statins and angiotensin-converting enzyme inhibitors); (2) the need to include only intentional weight loss in cohort studies and exclude unintentional weight loss; (3) studies that largely do not differentiate between patients with obesity with and without CVD risk factors, which could be the basis of heterogeneity in the response to weight loss; and (4) the need for long-term interventions and follow-up. While weight loss produces improvements in CVD risk factors, additional studies are needed to determine whether these effects translate into reductions in CVD events and mortality.

There are few, if any, long-term randomized clinical trials (RCTs) assessing the effects of weight loss on CVD events or mortality as a predetermined primary outcome measure. Most RCTs involve short-term lifestyle interventions and are not sufficient to demonstrate significant reductions in mortality when compared with control groups. However, meta-analyses of relevant RCTs have demonstrated that both lifestyle-induced and medication-assisted weight loss were associated with decreased mortality and CVD outcomes.[89,90] Large cohort studies have shown that intentional weight loss is associated with reduced mortality, particularly in subjects with weight-related complications such as T2D.[73,91]

The most convincing studies involve weight loss following bariatric surgery. In case-control cohort studies such as the Swedish Obese Subjects study[92] and a study involving Veterans Affairs Medical Centers,[93] data suggest that weight loss of more than 15% to 20% body weight is more likely to be associated with efficacy in this regard. Cardiovascular outcome trials assessing weight-loss medications approved by the FDA since 2012 are ongoing or planned. Two glucagon-like peptide 1 (GLP-1) receptor agonists, liraglutide 3 mg/day approved for obesity and semaglutide 2.4 mg/week under development for an obesity indication, have been found to be cardioprotective when used at lower doses in the treatment of T2D. Specifically, the LEADER (Liraglutide Effect and Action in Diabetes: Evaluation of Cardiovascular Outcome Results) study using liraglutide 1.8 mg/day[94] and SUSTAIN-6 study (Trial to Evaluate Cardiovascular and Other Long-Term Outcomes With Semaglutide in Subjects with Type 2 Diabetes) using semaglutide 1 mg/week[95] demonstrated superiority of the GLP-1 receptor agonist (GLP1ra) for the composite three-point MACE outcome in patients with T2D.

OBESITY AND OBESITY MEDICINE

Given the far-reaching clinical benefits produced by weight loss in patients with CMD, clinicians treating patients with CMD should ideally be competent in the comprehensive management of obesity or refer patents for this care.

The Pathophysiology of Obesity

Obesity is a disease of energy balance that produces excess adiposity sufficient to impair health. Like other chronic diseases, the

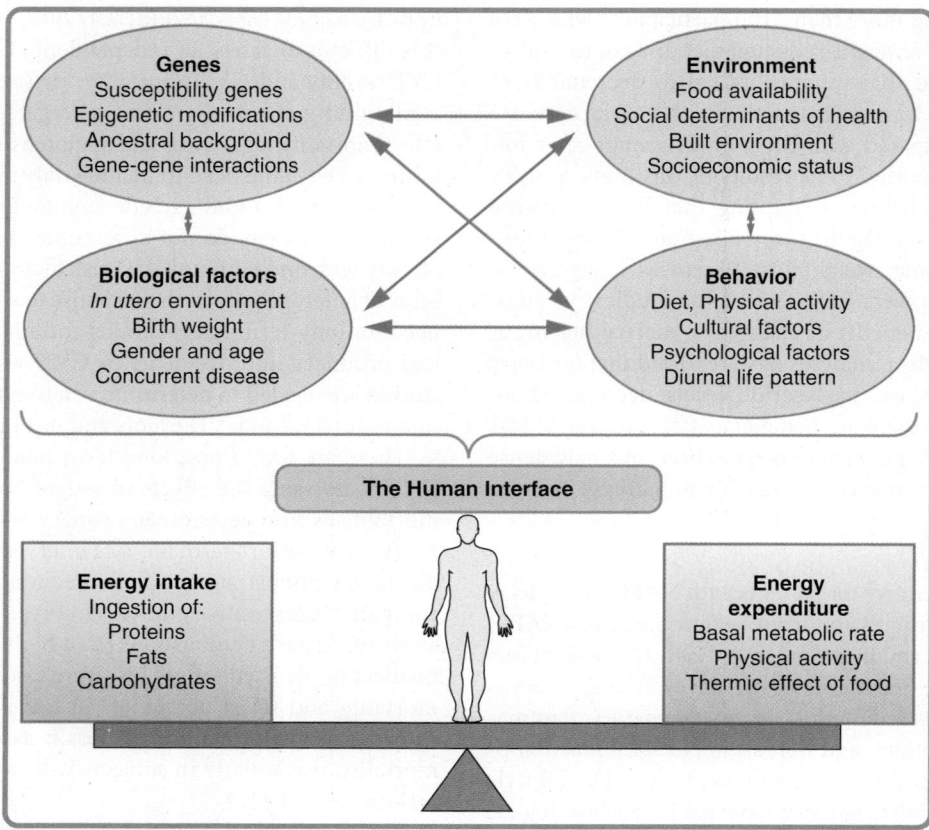

Figure 6–3. Pathophysiology of obesity. Obesity is a complex disease, with interactions involving genetic, environmental, biological, and behavioral factors that favor a positive energy balance.

pathophysiology of obesity is complex involving interactions among genes, biological factors, the environment, and behavior (**Fig. 6–3**). Genetic factors constitute a substantial component of disease risk that can explain 50% to 60% of individual variation in body weight in monozygotic/dizygotic twin studies. Monogenic forms of the disease are rare, such as in families with leptin or leptin receptor mutations or deletion of the *SNORD116* gene cluster in patients with Prader-Willi syndrome.

Susceptibility to obesity in the majority of individuals results from the inheritance of multiple genes, with each individual allele conferring a very small relative risk for the disease. Genome-wide association studies have identified more than 100 susceptibility loci for obesity.[96] Those individuals who inherit larger subsets of susceptibility genes will tend to be more overweight in any given environment. Progressive weight gain is not a lifestyle choice and cannot be viewed in terms of a simple thermodynamic equation of greater energy in than energy out. Rather, gene-environment interactions generate a human biological and behavioral interface unique to each individual that not only determines body weight but also explains individual variation in the net effect on body weight for any given amount of food intake or physical activity. To this point, among monozygotic twin pairs, the intratwin changes in body weight are highly correlated in response to overfeeding and underfeeding of the same number of calories, such that if one member of the twin pair lost a greater or lesser amount of weight, so did the corresponding twin. Thus, the genetic background determines differences in the amount of weight

gained or lost in response to an identical degree of caloric excess or deficit.

In obesity, a major consequence of gene-environment interactions is an alteration in caloric intake, as regulated by homeostatic satiety factors acting on CNS feeding centers (**Fig. 6–4**). Satiety hormones produced by peripheral organs register fuel availability and are released into the bloodstream to act on two cell types in the arcuate nucleus of the hypothalamus. Ghrelin from the stomach binds its receptor on neurons that release neuropeptide Y (NPY) as a neurotransmitter. This sends signals to higher cortical centers and activates the orexigenic pathway to increase hunger. Leptin from fat tissue and hormones from the gastrointestinal tract (including GLP-1, peptide YY, and amylin) activate proopiomelanocortin synthesizing cells to release alpha melanocyte-stimulating hormone (αMSH) as a neurotransmitter. This signals to higher centers to activate the anorexigenic pathway that decreases appetite. This system is altered in obesity to promote a higher set point for body weight regulation, wherein energy intake is relatively high compared with energy expenditure to generate and sustain an increase in adipose tissue mass.[97]

The pathophysiology of obesity is further operational in response to a weight-loss intervention. Weight loss activates multiple maladaptive responses that act to increase energy intake and decrease energy expenditure, thus driving weight regain back to the previous high level of body weight (**Fig. 6–5**). The combination of decrements in levels of anorexigenic hormones below baseline levels, as well as an increase in the

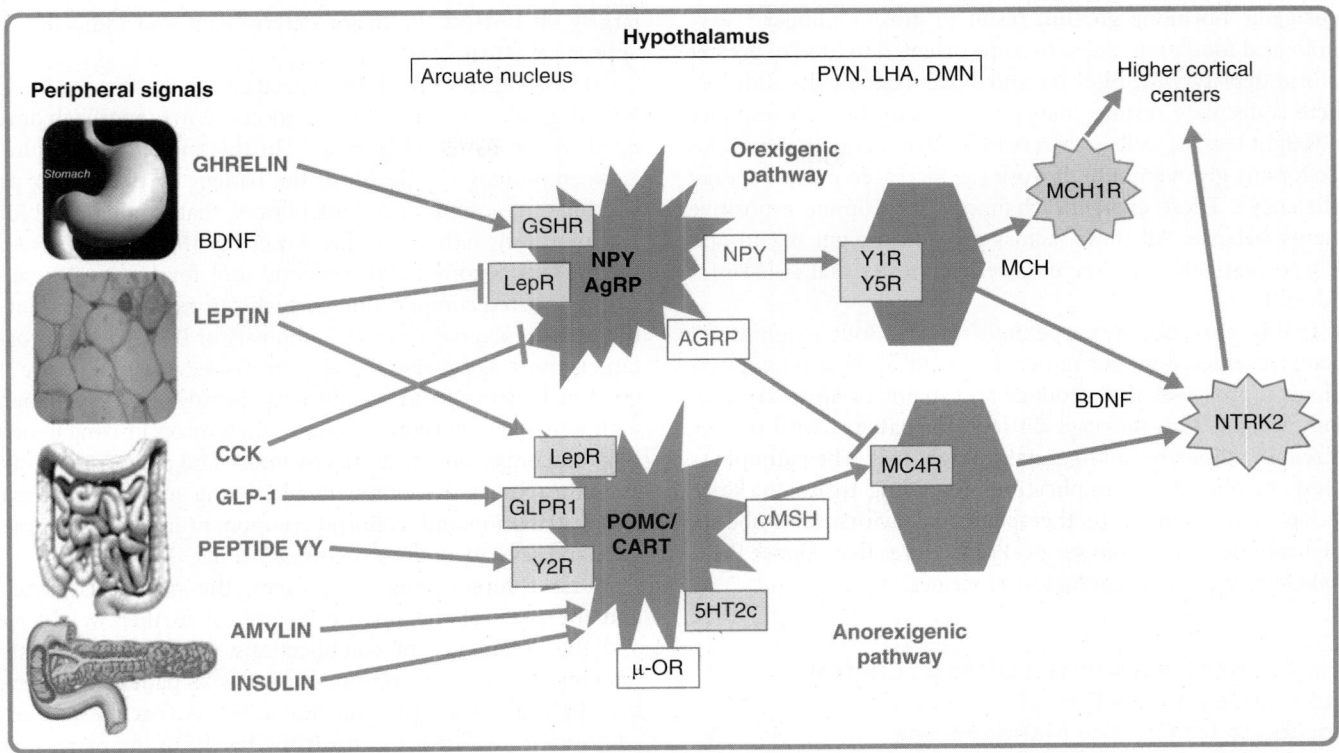

Figure 6–4. Regulation of caloric intake by satiety hormones and hypothalamic feeding centers. Satiety hormones are released from peripheral tissues and act on cells in the arcuate nucleus of the hypothalamus. The orexigenic hormone (ghrelin from the stomach) acts on cells releasing NPY as a neurotransmitter. Anorexigenic hormones (leptin from fat and CCK, GLP-1, peptide YY, and amylin from the gastrointestinal tract) act on cells producing the neurotransmitter αMSH. Both cell types signal to higher cortical centers to regulate hunger and satiety. CCK, cholecystokinin; GLP-1, glucagon-like peptide 1; NPY, neuropeptide Y; AgRP, agouti-related peptide; POMC, proopiomelanocortin; CART, cocaine and amphetamine-regulated transcript; αMSH, alpha melanocyte-stimulating hormone; PVN, paraventricular nucleus; LH, lateral hypothalamus; DMN, dorsomedial nucleus; GSHR, growth hormone secretagogue receptor.

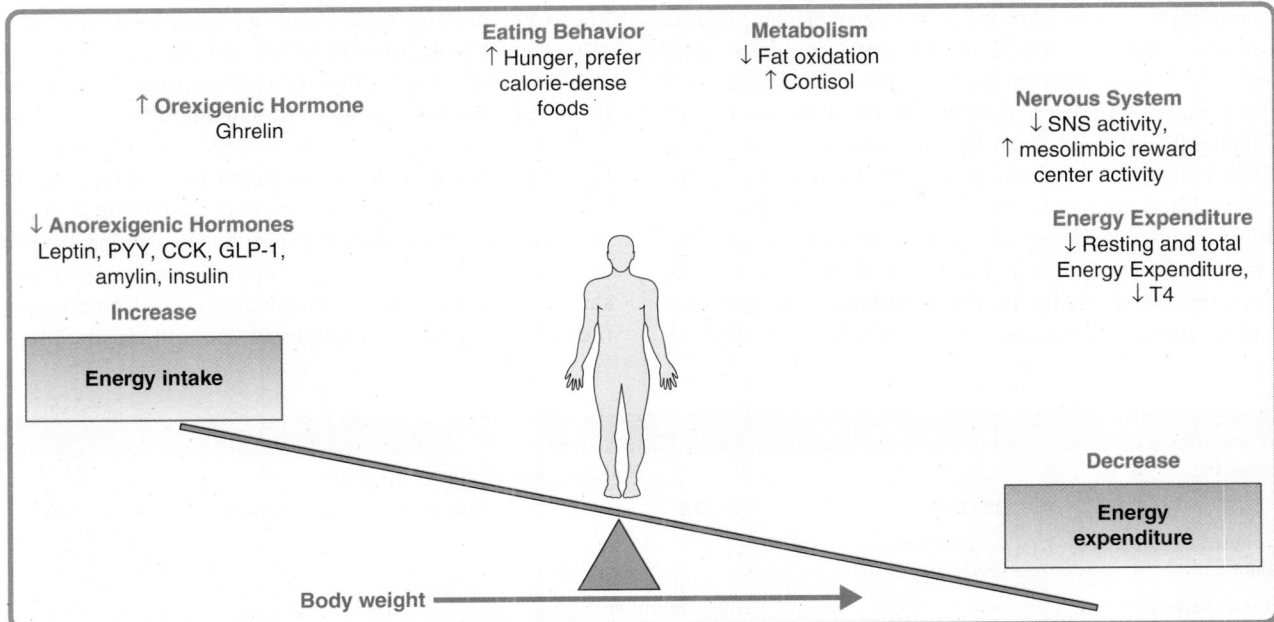

Figure 6–5. Maladaptive responses to weight loss in patients with the disease of obesity. Following a weight-loss intervention, multiple pathophysiological processes act to increase energy intake and decrease energy expenditure, and to drive weight regain and return to the previous high level of body weight. Anorexigenic hormones decrease and the orexigenic hormone ghrelin increases, resulting in greater hunger. Other mechanisms reduce the resting energy expenditure, further promoting a positive energy balance. PYY, peptide YY; CCK, cholecystokinin; GLP-1, glucagon-like peptide 1; SNS, sympathetic nervous system; T4, thyroxine.

orexigenic hormone ghrelin, result in greater hunger.[97] Psychological food preferences become oriented to food of greater caloric density with high fat and sugar content. In addition, there is decrease resting energy expenditure rates in response to weight loss, as well as a decrease in the energy that muscles use for any given amount of work (ie, increased muscle energy efficiency). These energetic changes also promote a positive energy balance. All these factors promote weight regain and help to maintain a degree of excess adiposity that is harmful to health.

In this sense, obesity perpetuates obesity. Body weight is not a cognitive decision, but rather the result of these pathophysiological processes that produce and maintain an increase in body weight. This makes it difficult for patients with obesity to reduce adiposity and to sustain weight loss. The pathophysiology of obesity has implications regarding treatment since patients must adhere to therapeutic behaviors, take obesity medications, or undergo surgical procedures that oppose these maladaptive pathophysiological processes.

Treatment of Obesity as a Disease: Clinical Guidelines and the Complications-Centric Approach for Obesity Management

Within the past decade, there have been improvements in all three therapeutic modalities for obesity treatment: evidence-based lifestyle interventions, new obesity medications, and more refined bariatric surgical and nonsurgical procedures. This has prompted the development of formal guidelines to achieve the best outcomes while balancing efficacy, safety, and costs. While emphasizing the health benefits of weight loss, these guidelines can be viewed as falling along a continuum from a more BMI-centric approach, with a goal of losing a given amount of weight, to a complications-centric model focused on preventing and treating obesity-related complications.[98] The BMI-centric approach is best illustrated by the obesity treatment guidelines set forth by the National Heart, Lung, and Blood Institute (NHLBI) in 1998[99] (**Table 6–5**). Under these guidelines, appropriate treatment was defined in terms of patients' initial BMI, with lifestyle interventions, pharmacotherapy, and surgery being added in a stepwise manner for those with progressively higher BMIs. Although this approach does make some allowances for comorbidities, it depends

largely on BMI as the major determinant and indication for appropriate treatment.

At the other end of the spectrum from the traditional NHLBI guidelines is the complications-centric approach developed by the AACE (**Fig. 6–6**).[69] In this model, the emphasis is on improving the health of the patient by treating or preventing the complications of obesity that confer morbidity and mortality, rather than just lowering BMI. In other words, weight loss becomes a therapeutic tool for the treatment of obesity-related complications, which can exist independent of the patients' degree of general adiposity or BMI. This approach targets more aggressive therapies to those who will derive the greatest benefits from weight-loss therapy—namely patients with weight-related complications, thereby optimizing benefit/risk, outcomes, and cost effectiveness. The diagnosis involves an anthropometric component addressing adipose tissue mass and distribution and a clinical component involving the presence and severity of obesity complications.

If no complications are present, the patient is stage 0, and the goals of therapy are to prevent further weight gain and the emergence of complications. A structured lifestyle intervention may be appropriate in these patients. However, if complications are present, this indicates that the degree of adiposity is sufficient to impair the health of the patient, and more aggressive weight-loss therapy is needed to ameliorate the complications and prevent further disease deterioration. The patient is stage 1 if the complications are mild-to-moderate, and the clinician should consider adding an obesity medication to the lifestyle intervention. If one or more complications are serious, the patient is stage 2, and treatment with both lifestyle and medications is likely appropriate and bariatric surgery should be considered for selected individuals. As targets for improvements in complications are monitored, intensification of treatment modalities (lifestyle, medication, and procedures) is implemented, together with direct treatment of complications if needed, to achieve the desired outcomes.

The evidence-based ACC/AHA/The Obesity Society (TOS) practice guidelines, published in 2014, update the earlier NHLBI guidelines and generally advocate a sequential approach, recommending that individuals who have never participated in a comprehensive lifestyle management program should be encouraged to do so before considering weight-loss medications or bariatric surgery.[100] By comparison, the AACE

TABLE 6–5. NHLBI Obesity Treatment Guidelines

Treatment	BMI Category (all values in kg/m²)				
	25–26.9	27–29.9	30–34.9	35–39.9	≥40
Diet, physical activity, and behavior	Appropriate NHLBI guidelines	+	+	+	+
Pharmacotherapy	No	With comorbidities	+	+	+
Surgery[a]	No	No	No[a]	With comorbidities	+

[a]US FDA-approved lap band surgery for patients with BMI of at least 30 kg/m² and one weight-related medical condition (February 2011).
Abbreviations: +, clinically indicated for consideration; **No,** not indicated.
Data from Clinical Guidelines on the Identification, Evaluation, and Treatment of Overweight and Obesity in Adults, National Institutes of Health/National Heart Lung and Blood Institute. September, 1998. http://www.nhlbi.nih.gov/guidelines/obesity/ob_gdlns.pdf.

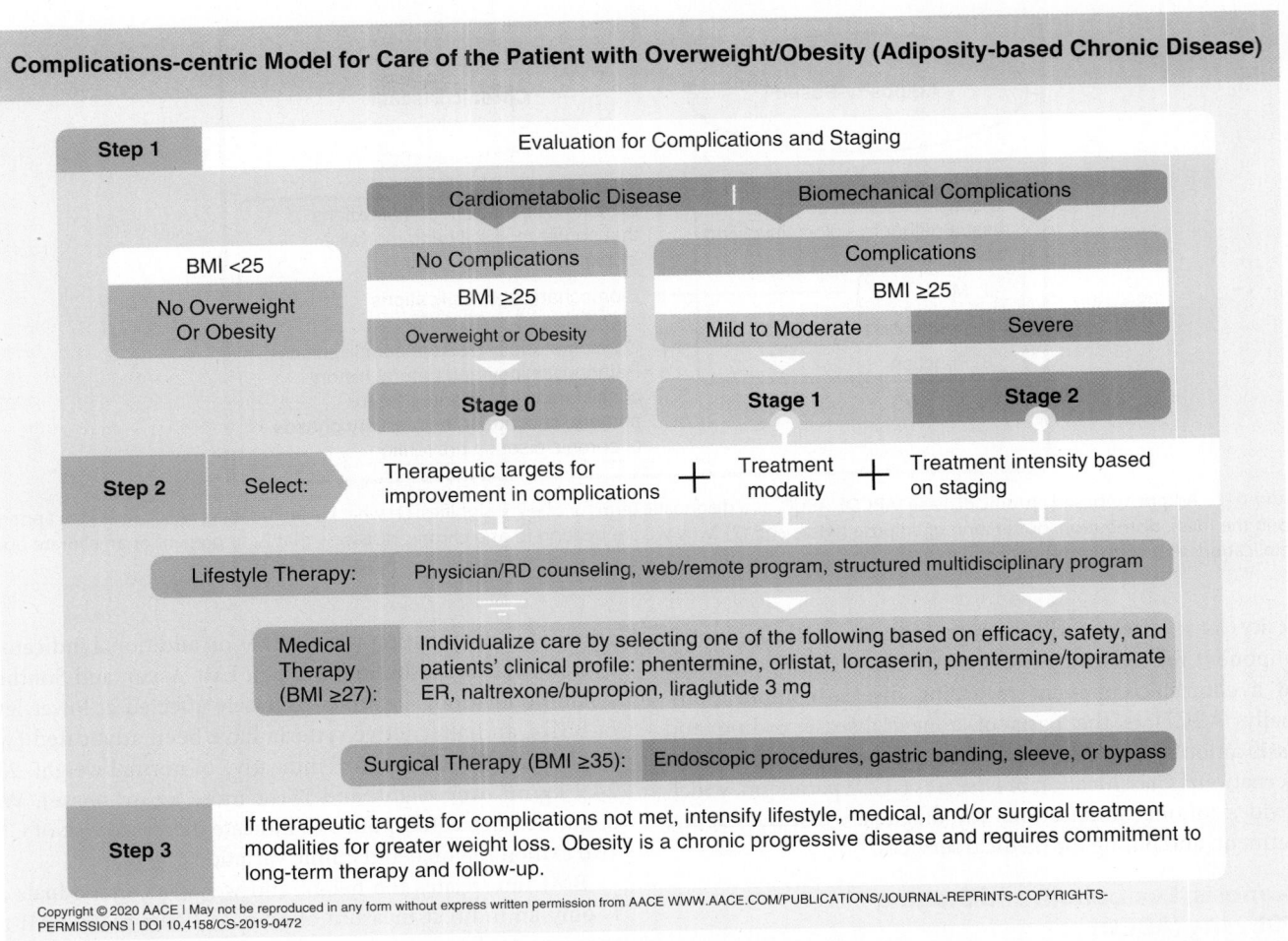

Complications-centric Model for Care of the Patient with Overweight/Obesity (Adiposity-based Chronic Disease)

Figure 6–6. The AACE Clinical Practice Guidelines for the Care of Patients with Obesity: an algorithm for complication-centric management. Modified with permission from Garber AJ, Handelsman Y, Grunberger G, et al: Consensus Statement by the American Association of Clinical Endocrinologists and American College of Endocrinology on the Comprehensive Type 2 Diabetes Management Algorithm–2020 Executive Summary, *Endocr Pract.* 2020 Jan;26(1):107-139.

algorithm stipulates that the aggressiveness of initial therapy (including lifestyle modification combined with an obesity medication) should be determined by the presence and severity of weight-related complications and their adverse impact on the health of the patient.

Adiposity-Based Chronic Disease

A new term, adiposity-based chronic disease (ABCD), has been proposed for medical diagnosis and disease coding, which is informative regarding pathophysiology and treatment goals in obesity. The diagnosis of obesity based only on BMI has led to confusion among the lay public and health-care professionals regarding the significance of obesity and the appreciation of obesity as a chronic disease.[6] This is primarily because BMI, which interrelates height and weight, conveys little information about how excess adiposity adversely affects health. Furthermore, the term "obesity" engenders stigma driven by negative perceptions concerning the personal character of patients, generating guilt, depression, and shame.[101] This bias, together with uncertainty regarding health implications, help perpetuate factors that limit access of patients to effective therapy.

ABCD has been proposed as a diagnostic term that conceptualizes obesity as a chronic disease associated with complications, considers the pathophysiological basis of the disease, and avoids the stigmata, ambiguity, differential use, and multiple meanings of the term "obesity"[6,102] (**Fig. 6–7**). This term alludes to what we are treating and why we are treating it. The phrase "adiposity-based" is used because the disease is primarily due to abnormalities in the mass, distribution, and/or function of adipose tissue. The phrase "chronic disease" is apropos because the disease is lifelong, is associated with complications that confer morbidity and mortality, and has a natural history that offers opportunities for primary, secondary, and tertiary prevention. Abnormalities in adipose tissue mass predispose to biomechanical complications, and defects in the function and distribution of adipose tissue lead to CMD complications, as well as other health problems.

This new diagnostic term provides a conceptual basis that can help inform and structure the evaluation and diagnosis of patients with obesity, as well as identifying high-risk patients suffering from disease complications. The term "ABCD" underscores the principle that the diagnostic evaluation of

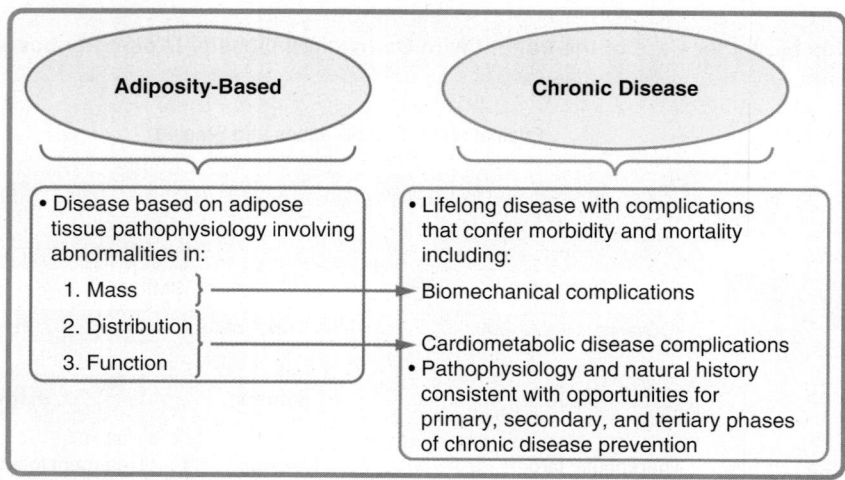

Figure 6–7. Adiposity-based chronic disease (ABCD). ABCD, as a diagnostic term for obesity, signifies: (1) what we are treating, which relates to abnormalities in the mass, distribution, or function of adipose tissue; and (2) "why we are treating it" as a chronic disease—that is, to prevent or ameliorate obesity complications that confer morbidity and mortality and impair the quality of life.

obesity as a disease will require both an anthropometric component related to mass and distribution of adipose tissue and a clinical component regarding disease complications. Finally, ABCD is the basis of a new disease coding and classification system proposed as an alternative to the current International Classification of Diseases (ICD) paradigm, which provides rational implications for diagnosis, disease staging, treatment, and billing for medical services.[103]

Diagnosis, Evaluation, and Staging of Obesity (ABCD)

The Anthropometric Component of the Diagnosis

The anthropometric component is largely satisfied by BMI, which is widely used in the screening, diagnoses, and classification of patients, as established by the World Health Organization in 1998 (**Table 6–6**). BMI values 18.5 to 24.9 kg/m^2 are indicative of lean individuals, BMIs 25 to 29.9 kg/m^2 overweight, and BMIs of 30 kg/m^2 or more represent obesity categorized as obese class I (BMI 30–34.9), class II (BMI 35–39.9), or class III (BMI ≥40). Waist circumference measurements provide additional information regarding fat distribution and CMD risk and

are used in conjunction with BMI as an additional indicator of overall health risk. In South Asian, East Asian, and Southeast Asian populations, health is adversely affected at lower levels of BMIs, and alternative criteria have been advocated (with BMIs of 18.5 to 22.9 kg/m^2 indicative of normal weight, 23 to 24.9 kg/m^2 overweight, and 25 or more kg/m^2 obese). Waist circumference cutoff points to indicate increased risk of CMD also exhibit regional and ethnic variations.

BMI interrelates the height and weight of individuals and is only an indirect measure of adipose tissue mass. BMI also incorporates lean mass, bone mass, and fluid status, all of which can vary independent of fat mass. BMI will overestimate adiposity in athletes with high muscle mass and in patients with edema, and it will underestimate adiposity in elderly patients with sarcopenia. For this reason, patients with elevated BMI measurements must be clinically evaluated to confirm excess adiposity.

The Clinical Component of the Diagnosis

Another limitation of BMI is that it does not indicate the impact of excess adiposity on the health of individual patients,

Classification	BMI		Waist	
	Measurement (kg/m²)	Comorbidity Risk	Waist Circumference and Comorbidity Risk	
			Men: ≤ 40 in Women: ≤ 35 in	Men: > 40 in Women: > 35 in
Underweight	<18.5	Low, but other problems		
Normal weight	18.5–24.9	Average		
Overweight	25–29.9	Increased	Increased	High
Obese class I	30–34.9	Moderate	High	Very high
Obese class II	35–39.9	Severe	Very high	Very high
Obese class III	≥40	Very severe	Extremely high	Extremely high

TABLE 6–6. Classification of Overweight and Obesity by BMI and Waist Circumference

Data from Obesity: preventing and managing the global epidemic. Report of a WHO consultation, World Health Organ Tech Rep Ser. 2000;894:i-xii, 1-253.

Cardiometabolic Complications   **Biomechanical Complications**

✓ = *Known to Respond to Weight Loss*

- Diabetes risk ✓ Prediabetes' ✓
  Metabolic syndrome ✓
- T2D ✓
- Hypertension ✓
- Dyslipidemia ✓
- Cardiovascular disease
- Nonalcoholic fatty liver disease ✓
- Polycystic ovary disease ✓
- Female infertility ✓
- Male hypogonadism ✓

- Obstructive sleep apnea ✓
- Osteoarthritis (knee, hip) ✓
- Urinary stress incontinence ✓
- Gastroesophageal reflux ✓
- Venous stasis ✓
- Immobility/disability ✓
- Obesity-hypoventilation syndrome ✓
- Poor quality of life ✓

Additional Important Factors in the Evaluation of Patients with Obesity

Other diseases:	Cholelithiasis, cancer risk
Psychological status:	Depression, binge-eating syndrome, stigmatization, anxiety, self-esteem, motivation
Iatrogenic medications:	Tricyclic antidepressants, antipsychotics, glucocorticoids, insulin and sulfonylureas, certain depot or oral contraceptives, certain anticonvulsants, certain β-blockers
Social and environmental determinants of health:	Certain cultural factors or practices, built environment, Access to healthy food, physical activity resources, work-related, time management, sleep hygiene, stress, socioeconomic

Figure 6–8. The clinical evaluation of patients with obesity. The clinical component of the-diagnosis of obesity includes an evaluation to identify obesity cardiometabolic and biomechanical complications, particularly those that respond to weight loss therapy. There are additional factors that should be ascertained that will need to be considered in formulating an individualized care plan.

as determined by the risk and presence of weight-related complications. Although the likelihood of complications generally increases as a function of progressive obesity, their development varies markedly among patients at any given BMI level. Patients with obesity need not have weight-related complications and can be free of disease-related morbidity and mortality. Therefore, individuals who meet the anthropometric criterion for overweight or obesity must then undergo a clinical evaluation for the presence and severity of obesity complications and other factors, such as iatrogenic medications, psychological factors, and social and environmental determinants of health, that place the patient at risk for poor outcomes.[103] These aspects of the clinical evaluation should be taken into account in formulating the treatment plan (**Fig. 6–8**).

The identification of complications and their severity are important for two reasons. First, complications or relevant risk factors determine disease staging and indicate the need for more aggressive therapy to improve the health of individual patients. Second, because these complications can be improved or reversed by weight loss, the evaluation establishes therapeutic targets based on the response of complications to weight-loss therapy. From this perspective, the goals of therapy are to improve the health of patients by treating and preventing weight-related complications, consistent with the complications-centric approach to obesity management advocated by the AACE obesity guidelines.[69]

The identification of complications does not involve an extensive or extraordinary degree of testing, but it can be ascertained in the course of an initial patient evaluation consisting of medical history, review of systems, physical examination, and laboratory studies (**Table 6–7**). The clinician will need to pay particular attention to aspects of the history and

examination relevant to obesity and conduct an obesity-focused review of systems that assesses the potential symptomatology of weight-related complications. In many cases, the information gathered in the initial examination is sufficient for the diagnosis of certain weight-related complications. For other complications, the initial information augments the degree of suspicion, and additional testing consistent with standards of care is then necessary to confirm the diagnosis and for staging the severity of the complication. Depending on the expertise of the clinician, referral may be indicated for further evaluation and treatment of specific complications.

Disease Staging

The presence and severity of obesity complications is the basis for staging disease severity. This information enables clinicians to target patients with advanced disease for more aggressive interventions to optimize the benefit/risk ratio. While several staging systems have been proposed, two have emerged as particularly useful for assessing overall disease severity.

The AACE obesity guidelines advocate a simple and clinically useful paradigm[69] (**Fig. 6–9**). Each complication is evaluated for severity and impact on the patient's health and used to designate obesity as Stage 0 (no complication is present), Stage 1 (any and all complications are mild-moderate), or Stage 2 (at least one complication is severe). The adjudication of a complication as mild-moderate versus severe is based on criteria unique to each complication, and in many instances will depend upon clinical judgment, together with objective findings and quantitative measures. In addition to severity determined by physical findings or objective laboratory measures, an important question is the degree to which the complication affects symptoms, patient-reported

TABLE 6–7. Screening and Diagnoses of Weight-Related Complications in Patients with Overweight/Obesity—the Clinical Component of the Diagnosis

Weight-Related Complication Checklist	Clinical Evaluation	Clinical Data	Diagnosis
☑ Prediabetes	Laboratory	Fasting glucose; HbA1c; OGTT	Fasting glucose 100–125 mg/dL; 2-hour OGTT glucose 140–199 mg/dL; HbA1c 5.7%–6.4%
☑ MetS	Examination	Waist circumference, blood pressure,	Waist circumference ≥40 inches in men and ≥3 5 inches in women; BP ≥130/85 mm Hg; fasting glucose ≥100 mg/dL; triglycerides ≥150 mg/dL; HDL-c ≤40 mg/dL in men and 50 mg/dL in women
	Laboratory	Fasting glucose, triglycerides, HDL-c	
☑ T2D	ROS	Symptoms of hyperglycemia	Overtly elevated glucose (≥200 mg/dL); repeat fasting glucose ≥126 mg/dL; 2-hour OGTT glucose ≥200 mg/dL; HbA1c ≥6.5%
	Laboratory	Fasting glucose; HbA1c; OGTT	
☑ Hypertension	Examination	Elevated BP	Repeated measurements of ≥140/90 mmHg, ambulatory monitoring
☑ Dyslipidemia	Laboratory	Lipid panel (total cholesterol, HDL-c, triglycerides, LDL-C, non-HDL-c)	Triglycerides ≥150 mg/dL; HDL-C ≤40 mg/dL in men and 50 mg/dL in women; LDL-C ≥100 or 130 mg/dL; lipoprotein subclasses, Lp(a), apolipoprotein B-100 may further define risk
☑ Nonalcoholic fatty liver disease	Examination	Firm or enlarged liver	Elevated hepatic transaminases; abnormal imaging (eg, ultrasound, magnetic resonance imaging, elastography); liver biopsy
	Laboratory	Liver function tests (see MetS)	
☑ Polycystic ovary syndrome	Examination	Hirsutism, ovarian cysts	Elevated androgen levels; oligo- or chronic anovulation; polycystic ovaries
	ROS	Hirsutism, menstrual irregularities, infertility	
	Laboratory	Androgen levels, LH/FSH (see MetS)	
☑ Obstructive sleep apnea	Examination	Neck circumference	Polysomnography needed to complete diagnosis
	ROS	Positive symptoms	
☑ Osteoarthritis	Examination	Joint tenderness, crepitance, structural changes	Radiographic imaging may be needed to complete diagnosis
	ROS	Joint pain, decreased function	
☑ Urinary stress incontinence	ROS	Urge or stress incontinence	Urine culture, urodynamic testing may be needed to complete diagnosis
☑ Gastroesophageal reflux disease	ROS	Esophagitis symptoms	Endoscopy, esophageal motility study may be needed to complete diagnosis
☑ Disability	Examination	Decreased mobility	Functional testing may be helpful
	ROS	Impaired function daily activities	
☑ Depression/ stigmatization	ROS	Symptoms of depression, binge eating disorder	Psychological testing and evaluation may be needed to complete diagnosis
☑ Obesity secondary to hormonal disorder	Examination	Signs of hyperthyroid/hypothyroid; Signs of hypercortisolism	Thyroid-stimulating hormone for suspected hypothyroidism; saliva/serum/urine cortisol for hypercortisolism; pituitary testing; magnetic resonance imaging (hypothalamus)
	ROS	Symptoms of hyperthyroid/hypothyroidism, hypercortisolism	
	Laboratory	Hormonal testing	
☑ Iatrogenic obesity (eg, secondary to medications)	History	Review current medications and medication history	Follow-up after withdrawal of offending medication and/or substitution with a weight-neutral alternative
☑ Monogenic or syndromic obesity	Examination	Signs of hypogonadism; short stature; dysmorphic features; visual or olfactory impairment; organ system defects	Genetic testing needed to complete diagnosis; intelligence testing
	ROS	Onset in childhood, strong family hx; infertility; delayed puberty; behavior problems; intellectual disability	

Abbreviations: BP, blood pressure; FSH, follicle-stimulating hormone; Hb, hemoglobin; HDL-c, high-density lipoprotein cholesterol; LDL-C, low-density lipoprotein cholesterol; LH, luteinizing hormone; OGTT, oral glucose tolerate test; ROS, review of symptoms.

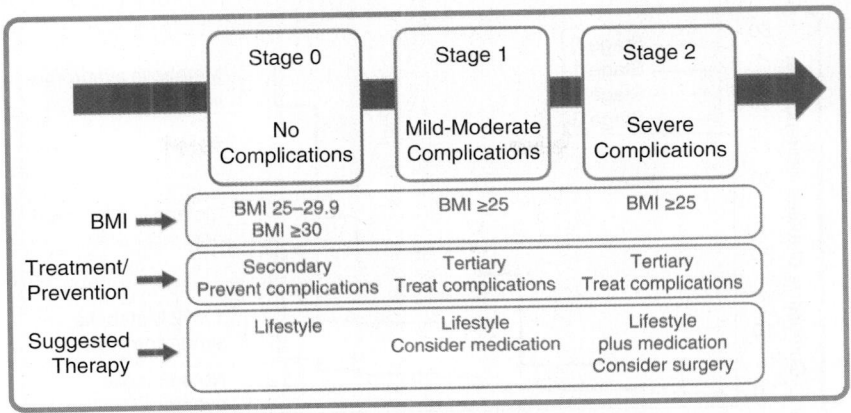

Figure 6–9. Staging the severity of obesity using the complications-centric AACE Clinical Practice Guidelines.

outcomes, impaired function, and adverse impact on quality of life. Patients with severe disease based on clinical findings and/or symptomatology can be treated more aggressively with weight-loss therapies to improve health.

The Edmonton obesity staging system is another useful staging approach that evaluates the medical, psychological, and functional impact of obesity in aggregate, and proposes five stages ranging from no limitations to severe impairment.[104] Stage 0 reflects no disease complications, psychological symptoms, or functional limitations. Stage 1 indicates subclinical factors and mild physical and psychological impairments that do not require medical intervention for obesity, and these patients should be managed using other preventative options. Stage 1 includes patients with prehypertension, prediabetes, MetS, and elevated liver enzymes, and the AACE guidelines would argue that these patients require active treatment of obesity to improve CVD risk factors and prevent progression to T2D and NASH. In Stage 2, patients have established obesity complications, such as T2D, obstructive sleep apnea, or osteoarthritis, together with moderate psychological or functional limitations; such patients require medical intervention. Stage 3 indicates significant end-organ damage (eg, CVD events or diabetes complications), significant psychological symptoms (eg, major depression or suicidality), and impairment of well-being. Stage 4 represents disabling and end-stage disease.

Special consideration must be given to staging patients with CMD before they develop the end-stage manifestations of T2D, CVD, and NASH. The at-risk population with prediabetes, MetS, and hepatic steatosis is quite large; for example, over two-thirds of the adult US population is overweight or obese[105] and 34.5% have prediabetes.[106] It is not feasible or safe to treat all at-risk patients aggressively using the tools of obesity medicine. However, the risk for developing the end-stage manifestations of T2D, CVD, and NASH varies greatly, and this presents opportunities for identifying and targeting patients at higher risk for more aggressive interventions.

One simple and accurate approach for staging patients for risk of future diabetes is referred to as Cardiometabolic Disease Staging (CMDS).[3,107] This framework uses quantitative MetS traits readily available to the clinician (namely, values for waist circumference, blood pressure, fasting glucose, triglycerides, and HDL-C) and can stratify risk of progression to

T2D over 40-fold among patients with overweight/obesity (**Fig. 6–10**). CMDS defines five stages of risk based on epidemiological observations and has been validated in large cohort studies. The lowest risk stratum consists of patients with overweight/obesity who have no MetS traits and represent metabolically healthy obesity. However, having one or two traits, or meeting the criteria for MetS or prediabetes but not both, confers progressively higher risk for future diabetes. The next risk stratum includes those patients who meet the criteria for both prediabetes and MetS. For these higher-risk patients, weight loss effectively prevents progression to diabetes with a lower "number-needed-to-treat" and a superior benefit/risk ratio.[108] The highest-risk stratum is comprised of patients who have the end-stage CMD manifestations of T2D and CVD.

Given the rising personal and social cost of diabetes, clinicians and health care systems can use this strategy to identify patients at high risk for diabetes and employ more aggressive interventions in those patients who will most benefit. Additional tools for predicting CVD risk include the American College of Cardiology (ACC)/American Heart Association (AHA) Omnibus risk estimator (109), Framingham Coronary Heart Disease Risk Score,[110] and the Reynolds Risk Score.[111]

Treatment

Treatment of patients with obesity incorporates three therapeutic modalities: lifestyle therapy, pharmacotherapy, and bariatric procedures, described next.

Lifestyle Therapy

Lifestyle therapy is the cornerstone of therapy for patients with obesity. It can constitute the sole approach to treatment, but it must also accompany treatment using weight-loss medications or bariatric surgery. The components of lifestyle therapy include a reduced-calorie, healthy meal plan, physical activity, and a package of behavioral interventions that are designed to promote adherence with the meal plan and physical activity prescription. Lifestyle therapy is most effective for weight loss when delivered as a structured program with the flexibility to accommodate the personal and cultural preferences of patients. The components of a structured lifestyle intervention can be delivered by a multidisciplinary team consisting of primary or specialty medical care professionals, health educators,

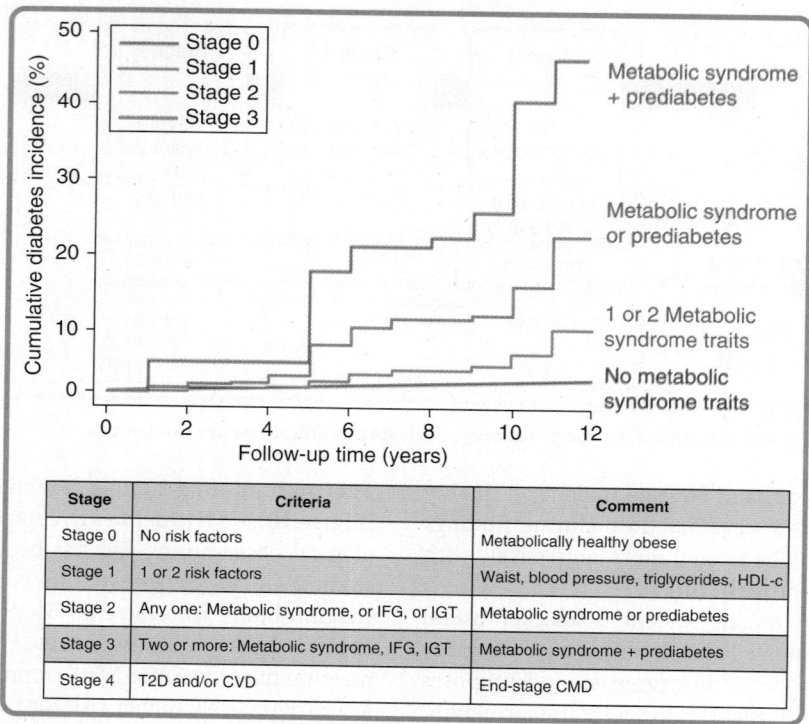

Stage	Criteria	Comment
Stage 0	No risk factors	Metabolically healthy obese
Stage 1	1 or 2 risk factors	Waist, blood pressure, triglycerides, HDL-c
Stage 2	Any one: Metabolic syndrome, or IFG, or IGT	Metabolic syndrome or prediabetes
Stage 3	Two or more: Metabolic syndrome, IFG, IGT	Metabolic syndrome + prediabetes
Stage 4	T2D and/or CVD	End-stage CMD

Figure 6–10. **Validation of CMDS using data from the Coronary Artery Risk Development in Young Adults study.** The data show cumulative diabetes incidence as a function of baseline CMDS risk category over 12 years beginning in 1995. Modified with permission from Guo F, Moellering DR, Garvey WT. The progression of cardiometabolic disease: validation of a new cardiometabolic disease staging system applicable to obesity, *Obesity* 2014 Jan;22(1):110-8.

dietitians, nurses, exercise trainers, and psychologists, and it may take place in a variety of venues in the clinic and in the community. Commercial programs featuring meal substitutes or delivered meals and interventions using remote technologies (telephone, text, Internet) have also been shown to be effective.

Reduced Calorie Healthy Meal Plan: The most important aspect of lifestyle therapy is a reduction in caloric intake, amounting to a 500- to 1000-kcal/d deficit in most instances. This can be achieved in the format of a healthy meal plan that provides all needed micronutrients and avoids processed foods. Examples of healthy meal plans for weight loss include low carbohydrate, low fat, low glycemic index, DASH, Mediterranean, and vegetarian. The macronutrient composition is less important than the patient's ability to adhere with the diet. Therefore, the meal plan should be individualized and selected to be compatible with the personal and cultural preferences of the patient. The use of meal substitutes in the form of shakes and bars add structure to the diet and have been shown to be effective. The patient should also be instructed in approaches to portion control and stimulus control.

Increased Physical Activity: A physical activity prescription can modestly increase caloric expenditure and is particularly helpful for maintaining lean body mass during weight loss and in helping sustain weight loss over a longer interval. The physical activity program optimally includes aerobic exercise, which should begin at a low level, allowing the patient to increase the intensity and duration of the exercise over time. Ideally, the patient will achieve at least 150 minutes per week of moderately

intense aerobic exercise accomplished in three to five sessions.[51] The combination of aerobic and resistance exercise provides better outcomes than either form of exercise alone.[68] Therefore, a resistance exercise program should be added and should consist of single-set repetitions targeting the major muscle groups two to three times per week. A final component of a physical activity program is to reduce sedentary behavior and increase active leisure activity. The physical activity prescription should be compatible with patient preferences and take into account any health-related or physical limitations.

Behavioral Therapy: Clinical trials have not only demonstrated the efficacy of lifestyle therapy programs that include behavioral interventions but also have underscored particular practices that are most likely to be associated with success.[71] For example, patients who self-monitor and record weight, food intake, and physical activity are more likely to achieve weight-loss goals. Patient education is also advantageous pertaining to obesity, obesity complications, nutrition, and physical activity, which can be delivered face-to-face, in group meetings, or using remote technologies (telephone, texting, and Internet). The program should also be able to provide for clear and reasonable goal setting, strategies for stimulus control, and systematic approaches for problem solving and stress reduction. Other components can include cognitive restructuring (ie, cognitive behavioral therapy), motivational interviewing, behavioral contracting, and mobilization of social support structures. Obesity can often be associated with depression, disordered eating (eg, binge eating disorder), anxiety, and other psychiatric disorders, which can impair the effectiveness of lifestyle

TABLE 6–8. Pharmacotherapy for Weight Loss in Patients with Obesity

Weight-Loss Medication	Dose	Mechanism	Side Effects	Warnings and Contraindications
Approved for Short-Term Therapy (≤3 Months)				
Phentermine (Adipex-P, Suprenza)	30 mg/d by mouth	Sympathomimetic amine	Restlessness, insomnia, dry mouth	Pregnancy; cardiovascular disease; hyperthyroidism; glaucoma; agitated states; abuse potential
Approved for Chronic Management of Obesity				
Orlistat (Xenical)	120 mg tid by mouth with meals	Gastrointestinal lipase inhibitor	Fat malabsorption, flatulence, fecal urgency, oily stools	Pregnancy; fat-soluble vitamin deficiency; malabsorption, renal oxalate stones; cholestasis
Phentermine/ topiramate ER (Qsymia)	Escalate to 7.5 mg/46 mg once a day by mouth; maximum dose 15 mg/92 mg	Sympathomimetic amine/ anticonvulsant, carbonic anhydrase inhibitor, gabaminergic	Dry mouth, insomnia/ Paresthesia, dysgeusia, mental clouding	Pregnancy; glaucoma; hyperthyroidism; fetal toxicity; suicidality; cognitive impairment; metabolic acidosis; urolithiasis
Naltrexone ER/ bupropion ER (Contrave)	Escalate to 8 mg/90 mg two pills twice a day by mouth	Opioid receptor antagonist/ dopamine-norepinephrine reuptake inhibitor	Nausea, headache, fatigue	Pregnancy; seizure risk; uncontrolled hypertension; chronic opioid use; suicidality
Liraglutide 3 mg (Saxenda)	Escalate to 3 mg/d subcutaneous injection	Glucagon-like peptide-1 receptor agonist	Nausea, vomiting, diarrhea, constipation,	Pregnancy; medullary thyroid cancer; MEN type II; increased pulse; acute pancreatitis; suicidality; acute gallbladder disease

Abbreviations: MEN, multiple endocrine neoplasia; ER, extended release.

interventions. For this reason, psychological counseling and psychiatric care may be necessary. The behavior intervention package is effectively accomplished by a multidisciplinary team that can include combinations of dietitians, nurses, health educators, physical activity trainers or coaches, and clinical psychologists. As with the meal plan and physical activity components, behavioral lifestyle interventions should be tailored to a patient's ethnic, cultural, socioeconomic, and educational background.

Pharmacotherapy

Since 2012, four weight-loss medications have been approved by the FDA for the chronic treatment of obesity (Table 6–8). Orlistat (120 mg) was the only preexisting medication for long-term pharmacotherapy approved in 1999, and it is the one most widely available worldwide. Phentermine as a single agent was approved over six decades ago, but only for short-term administration, generally regarded as three months or less, due to the lack of safety data with more chronic use. The newer medications include lorcaserin, phentermine/topiramate ER, naltrexone ER/bupropion ER, and high-dose liraglutide (3 mg). Lorcaserin was withdrawn in 2020 because the CAMELLIA-TIMI 61 cardiovascular outcomes trial, while demonstrated cardiovascular safety, found that more patients in the treatment group developed cancer than in the placebo group.[112]

Nevertheless, the availability of these new obesity medications has greatly expanded treatment options for patients with obesity and has led to more robust approaches to patient management. These weight-loss medications are approved by the FDA as adjuncts to lifestyle modification in patients with BMIs of 27 to 29.9 kg/m^2 (overweight) and having at least one weight-related comorbidity (generally taken to be

diabetes, hypertension, or dyslipidemia), or patients with BMI ≥30 kg/m^2 (obese) whether or not comorbidities are present. In adolescents with obesity, orlistat is approved for chronic administration beginning at age 12 years, and liraglutide 3 mg beginning at age 16. Regarding mechanism, orlistat acts as a lipase inhibitor in the gut to impair digestion and absorption of ingested lipids. The other approved weight-loss medications act on the mechanisms regulating appetite and satiety, helping to combat the pathophysiological adaptations that drive and sustain weight gain. In clinical trials, the addition of pharmacotherapy to lifestyle promotes greater weight loss and sustains weight loss for a greater period of time than that attributable to lifestyle interventions alone.

Long-term studies (ie, more than 2–3 years) using the recently approved weight-loss medications have not yet been conducted; however, it is important to consider that obesity is a lifelong disease that requires long-term management. Clinical experience needs to be developed in using medications, alone and in combination, to sustain weight loss and to prevent or treat obesity complications over a patient's lifetime. Postmarketing cardiovascular outcome trials are planned or ongoing for these weight-loss medications, and these studies should provide information pertinent to longer durations of therapy.

Bariatric Procedures

Bariatric surgery is the most effective method for treating class II and III obesity. It can be considered in patients with (1) BMI of 35 kg/m^2 or more and associated comorbidities or (2) BMI of ≥40 kg/m^2 whether accompanied by comorbidities or not, particularly after failure of lifestyle modification and medical therapies.[113] Bariatric surgery can provide substantial weight loss (15% to more than 40% of baseline body weight), but this varies by procedure. The most commonly performed procedures are Roux-en-Y gastric bypass (RYGB), sleeve gastrectomy, adjustable gastric banding, and biliopancreatic diversion, with or without duodenal switching. Many patients achieve long-term weight loss; however, it is not uncommon for patients to gradually regain weight over time.[114] Sustained weight loss also depends on ongoing lifestyle therapy, patient reeducation and recommitment to active lifestyle changes, and long-term medical follow-up. Nonsurgical endoscopic procedures have also been developed, including (1) placement of mucosal barriers preventing food absorption, (2) space-occupying intragastric balloons, (3) gastric remodeling using endoscopic suturing/plication devices (eg, endoscopic sleeve gastroplasty), and (4) aspiration of stomach contents via percutaneous gastrostomy.[113] Finally, oral hydrogel capsules have been approved as a device that absorbs water and expands in the stomach to promote satiety.[115]

A few key studies help highlight the clinical outcomes of bariatric surgery. Adams et al.[116] examined the impact of RYGB surgery on weight loss, T2D, and other health risks 6 years after surgery. Weight-loss maintenance was superior in patients undergoing RYGB compared with nonsurgical controls, with 76% of patients maintaining at least a 20% weight loss, higher rates of diabetes remission, and lower CVD risk. The Swedish Obese Subjects (SOS) study involved patients receiving any one of several bariatric procedures and matched conventionally treated obese controls.[117] The mean reported body weight changes after 2, 10, 15, and 20 years were –23%, –17%, –16%, and –18% in the surgery group, respectively, and little or no weight loss in the conventionally treated care group. Compared with standard care, bariatric surgery reduced overall mortality and decreased the incidence of diabetes, CVD events, and cancer. These studies suggest that sustained weight loss of ~20% can be demonstrated to reduce CVD events and mortality with sufficient duration of follow-up.

Obesity Pharmacotherapy and Surgery to Prevent and Treat T2D and Improve CVD Risk Factors

Since lifestyle interventions often do not achieve sustained weight loss, pharmacotherapy or surgery should be considered as an adjunct to lifestyle therapy in patients with CMD. Specifically, obesity medications have been shown to be highly effective in preventing or delaying progression to T2D and improving CVD risk factors. When used in combination with lifestyle therapy to achieve the recommended 7% to 10% weight loss,[69,79] phentermine/topiramate ER,[75] and liraglutide 3 mg[78] reduced rates of diabetes by up to 80% when compared with lifestyle plus placebo. Rates of incident diabetes were also dramatically reduced in patients treated with a variety of bariatric surgical procedures.[76,77] Since the at-risk pool is large and diabetes risk is highly variable among patients with obesity, CMDS can be used to target patients at greatest risk for future T2D and CVD, who will receive the greatest benefit[3,107] (Fig. 6–10). For example, the number-needed-to-treat to prevent one case of T2D using phentermine/topiramate ER is markedly reduced among high-risk patients compared with low-risk

patients using CMDS.[108] Bariatric surgery has also been shown to reduce rates of incident diabetes by up to 80%.[76,77]

Clinical trials have assessed the efficacy and safety of all obesity medications in patients with T2D.[118–120] The design of these studies was consistent, in that all T2D patients were treated with a lifestyle intervention and then randomized to placebo versus weight-loss medication. Obesity medications consistently resulted in (1) greater weight loss, (2) lower HbA1c values despite less need for diabetes medications in actively managed patients, (3) reductions in blood pressure, (4) lower triglycerides and higher HDL-C, (5) decreased levels of hepatic transaminases, and (6) improvements in biomarkers such as CRP, fibrinogen, and adiponectin when compared with patients treated with lifestyle plus placebo. Bariatric surgery also leads to substantial weight loss and improved diabetes control. While intensive lifestyle intervention can result in diabetes remission,[82] the additional weight loss that accompanies bariatric surgery results in higher remission rates and greater reductions in HbA1c.[121] The combined data do not point to a threshold of weight loss for maximal clinical benefits in T2D; rather, the more weight loss occurs, the better. Weight loss targeted at ≥15% is associated with superior outcomes in T2D[122] when this can feasibly and safely be accomplished.

CHRONIC DISEASE CARE MODEL FOR THE PREVENTION AND TREATMENT OF CARDIOMETABOLIC DISEASE

The conceptualization of CMD as a chronic disease process responsible for both metabolic and vascular disease outcomes enables opportunities for primary, secondary, and tertiary prevention of disease progression[1,2] (Fig. 6–11). Primordial prevention of CMD as a prevalent condition is relevant to the general population and includes better messaging about public health, creating a healthy environment, advocating healthy lifestyles, offering ready access to preventive care, and recognizing the importance of maternal-fetal health.

Primary prevention pertains to those at increased risk prior to any disease manifestations as a result of genetic predisposition and social and environmental determinants of health. These individuals require more targeted preventive measures regarding personalized prescriptions for healthy lifestyles and maintenance of healthy weight. Once it is clear that individuals are afflicted by the insulin-resistant state and can be identified as high risk by having MetS or prediabetes, secondary prevention strategies are warranted. Individuals that are lean or overweight/obese will need a meal plan featuring a macronutrient composition that enhances insulin sensitivity and a physical activity prescription. Patients with overweight/obesity also require weight loss to prevent progression to T2D and NASH and to ameliorate CVD risk factors.

Aggressive and comprehensive management of CVD risk factors, including elevated blood pressure, dyslipidemia, elevated LDL-C cholesterol, and hyperglycemia as delineated in Table 6–3, is warranted. Once the end-stage manifestations of CMD become evident, they should be managed aggressively

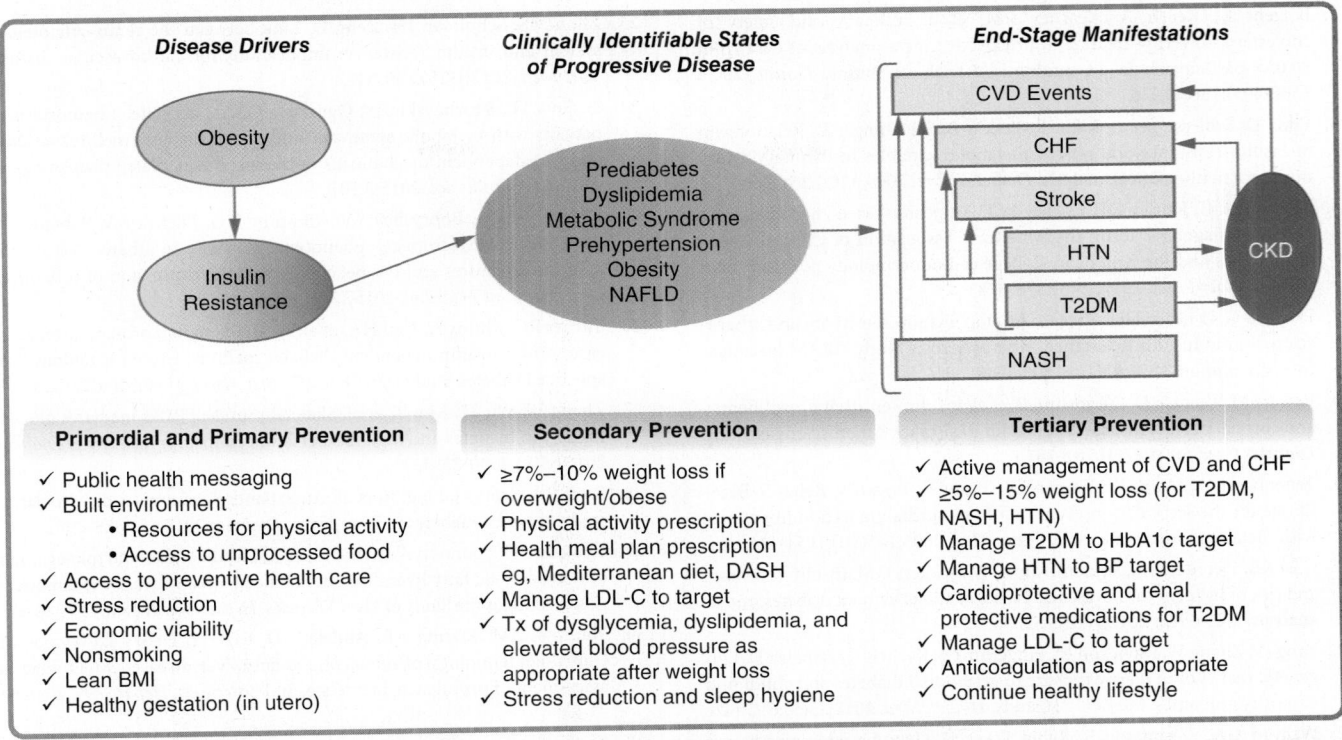

Figure 6–11. The chronic care model for the prevention and treatment of cardiometabolic disease and potential interventions that may be considered during the primordial/primary, secondary, and tertiary phases of disease progression.

in a tertiary prevention mode. In patients with T2D and obesity, weight-loss therapy should achieve 5% to 15% weight loss or more. Glucose-lowering agents should maintain HbA1c targets with a preference for those drugs such as sodium-glucose cotransporter-2 inhibitors and GLP-1 receptor agonists, which have been shown to prevent CVD events, hospitalizations for CHF, and progressive declines in renal function.[2] In addition, active management of T2D, CVD, and NASH should achieve targets for control of blood pressure and lipids.

The full force of our medical chronic care model should be brought to bear on the prevention and treatment of CMD, a disease nexus that presents this huge burden of social costs and patient suffering. It is not enough to begin treatment only at the time that end-stage manifestations appear as T2D, CVD, and NASH. Primary and secondary prevention strategies need to become commonplace in medical practice, particularly those involving weight loss. As the scientific understanding of obesity has progressed, it has become clear that obesity is not a lifestyle choice, and its treatment is not a merely cosmetic enterprise. The perspective of obesity as a disease mandates that the full force of our medical care model be implemented for prevention and treatment. This can be achieved only through activated and prepared health-care systems, activated and empowered patients, as well as regulatory and legislative measures that assure access of patients to therapies of proven benefit. Therefore, a chronic care model for CMD must become operational as an integral component of health-care systems and embraced by the larger society if it is to optimally benefit patients in particular and public health in general.

ACKNOWLEDGMENTS

The authors acknowledge support from the UAB Diabetes Research Center (P30 DK079626); the American Heart Association Strategically Focused Obesity Research Network center at the University of Alabama at Birmingham (17SFRN33610070); and the Merit Review program of the Department of Veterans Affairs (I01CX000432). The funders had no input regarding any aspect of this manuscript.

DISCLOSURES

W.T.G has served on ad hoc advisory boards for Sanofi, Novo Nordisk, Gilead, Boehringer-Ingelheim, Jazz Pharmaceuticals, BOYDSense, and the American Medical Group Association, and he has conducted research sponsored by the University of Alabama at Birmingham funded by Sanofi, Merck/Pfizer, and Novo Nordisk. J.I.M has received honoraria from Abbott Nutrition International and is on the advisory board of GoodSugar™.

REFERENCES

1. Mechanick JI, Farkouh ME, Newman JD, Garvey WT. Cardiometabolic-based chronic disease, adiposity and dysglycemia drivers: JACC state-of-the-art review. *J Am Coll Cardiol.* 2020;75(5):525-538.
2. Mechanick JI, Farkouh ME, Newman JD, Garvey WT. Cardiometabolic-based chronic disease, addressing knowledge and clinical practice gaps: JACC state-of-the-art review. *J Am Coll Cardiol.* 2020;75(5):539-555.
3. Guo F, Moellering DR, Garvey WT. The progression of cardiometabolic disease: validation of a new cardiometabolic disease staging system applicable to obesity. *Obesity.* 2014;22:110-118.

4. Baigent C, Keech A, Kearney PM, et al. Efficacy and safety of cholesterol-lowering treatment: prospective meta-analysis of data from 90,056 participants in 14 randomised trials of statins. *Lancet.* 2005; 366(9493):1267-1278.

5. Eddy D, Schlessinger L, Kahn R, Peskin B, Schiebinger R. Relationship of insulin resistance and related metabolic variables to coronary artery disease: a mathematical analysis. *Diabetes Care.* 2009;32(2):361-366.

6. Mechanick JI, Hurley DL, Garvey WT. Adiposity-based chronic disease as a new diagnostic term: the American Association of Clinical Endocrinologists and the American College of Endocrinology position statement. *Endocr Pract.* 2017;23(3):372-378.

7. Howard G, O'Leary DH, Zaccaro D, et al. Insulin sensitivity and atherosclerosis: the Insulin Resistance Atherosclerosis Study (IRAS) investigators. *Circulation.* 1996;93(10):1809-1817.

8. Rewers M, Zaccaro D, D'Agostino R, et al. Insulin sensitivity, insulinemia, and coronary artery disease: the Insulin Resistance Atherosclerosis Study. *Diabetes Care.* 2004;27(3):781-787.

9. Tenenbaum A, Motro M, Fisman EZ, Tanne D, Boyko V, Behar S. Bezafibrate for the secondary prevention of myocardial infarction in patients with metabolic syndrome. *Arch Intern Med.* 2005;165(10):1154-1160.

10. Gast KB, Tjeerdema N, Stijnen T, Smit JW, Dekkers OM. Insulin resistance and risk of incident cardiovascular events in adults without diabetes: meta-analysis. *PloS ONE.* 2012;7(12):e52036.

11. Yang IV, Zhang W, Davidson EJ, Fingerlin TE, Kechris K, Dabelea D. Epigenetic marks of *in utero* exposure to gestational diabetes and childhood adiposity outcomes: the EPOCH study. *Diabet. Med.* 2018;35(5):612-620.

12. Walford GA, Gustafsson S, Rybin D, et al. Genome-wide association study of the modified Stumvoll Insulin Sensitivity Index identifies BCL2 and FAM19A2 as novel insulin sensitivity loci. *Diabetes* 2016;65(10): 3200-3211.

13. Almgren P, Lehtovirta M, Isomaa B, et al. Heritability and familiality of type 2 diabetes and related quantitative traits in the Botnia Study. *Diabetologia.* 2011;54(11):2811-2819.

14. Garvey WT, Lara-Castro C. Diet, insulin resistance, and obesity: zoning in on data for Atkins dieters living in South Beach. *J Clin Endocrinol Metab.* 2004;89:4197-4205.

15. Olefsky JM, Glass CK. Macrophages, inflammation, and insulin resistance. *Annu Rev Physiol.* 2010;72:219-246.

16. Grundy SM, Cleeman JI, Daniels SR, et al. Diagnosis and management of the metabolic syndrome: an American Heart Association/National Heart, Lung and Blood Institute scientific statement. *Circulation.* 2005;112: 2735-2752.

17. Alberti KG, Zimmet PZ. Definition, diagnosis and classification of diabetes mellitus and its complications. Part 1: diagnosis and classification of diabetes mellitus provisional report of a WHO consultation. *Diabet Med.* 1998;15:539-553.

18. Zimmet P, Magliano D, Matsuzawa Y, Alberti G, Shaw J. The metabolic syndrome: a global public health problem and a new definition. *J Atheroscler Thromb.* 2005;12:295-300.

19. Liao Y, Kwon S, Shaughnessy S, et al. Critical evaluation of adult treatment panel III criteria in identifying insulin resistance with dyslipidemia. *Diabetes Care.* 2004;27(4):978-983.

20. Guo F, Moellering DR, Garvey WT. Use of HbA1c for diagnoses of diabetes and prediabetes: comparison with diagnoses based on fasting and 2-hr glucose values and effects of gender, race, and age. *Metab Syndr Relat Disord.* 2014;12(5):258-268.

21. Consequences of the new diagnostic criteria for diabetes in older men and women. DECODE Study (Diabetes epidemiology: Collaborative Analysis of Diagnostic Criteria in Europe). *Diabetes Care.* 1999;22(10): 1667-1671.

22. Hoogeveen RC, Gaubatz JW, Sun W, et al. Small dense low-density lipoprotein-cholesterol concentrations predict risk for coronary heart disease: the Atherosclerosis Risk in Communities (ARIC) study. *Arterioscler Thromb Vasc Biol.* 2014;34(5):1069-1077.

23. Zhou MS, Schulman IH, Zeng Q. Link between the renin–angiotensin system and insulin resistance: implications for cardiovascular disease. *Vasc Med.* 2012;17(5):330-341.

24. Suslova TE, Sitozhevskii AV, Ogurkova ON, et al. Platelet hemostasis in patients with metabolic syndrome and type 2 diabetes mellitus: cGMP- and NO-dependent mechanisms in the insulin-mediated platelet aggregation. *Front Physiol.* 2015;5:501.

25. Chistiakov DA, Bobryshev YV, Nikiforov NG, Elizova NV, Sobenin IA, Orekhov AN. Macrophage phenotypic plasticity in atherosclerosis: the associated features and the peculiarities of the expression of inflammatory genes. *Int J Cardiol.* 2015;184(1):436-445.

26. Turner RC, Millns H, Neil HA, et al. Risk factors for coronary artery disease in non-insulin dependent diabetes mellitus: United Kingdom Prospective Diabetes Study (UKPDS: 23). *Brit Med J.* 1998;316:823-828.

27. Zhang W, Wu M, Kim T, et al. Skeletal muscle TRIB3 mediates glucose toxicity in diabetes and high fat diet-induced insulin resistance. *Diabetes* 2016;65(8):2380-2391.

28. Scott RA, Scott LJ, Mägi R, et al. An expanded genome-wide association study of type 2 diabetes in Europeans. *Diabetes* 2017;66:2888-2902.

29. Chalasani N, Younossi Z, Lavine JE, et al. The diagnosis and management of nonalcoholic fatty liver disease: Practice guidance from the American Association for the Study of Liver Diseases. *Hepatology.* 2018;67(1): 328-357.

30. Younossi ZM, Koenig AB, Abdelatif D, Fazel Y, Henry L, Wymer M. Global epidemiology of nonalcoholic fatty liver disease—Meta-analytic assessment of prevalence, incidence, and outcomes. *Hepatology.* 2016;64: 73-84.

31. Targher G, Byrne CD, Lonardo A, Zoppini G, Barbui C. Non-alcoholic fatty liver disease and risk of incident cardiovascular disease: a meta-analysis. *J Hepatol.* 2016;65:589-600.

32. Yoshihisa A, Sato Y, Yokokawa T, et al. Liver fibrosis score predicts mortality in heart failure patients with preserved ejection fraction. *ESC Heart Fail.* 2018;5:262-270.

33. Mellinger JL, Pencina KM, Massaro JM, et al. Hepatic steatosis and cardiovascular disease outcomes: an analysis of the Framingham Heart Study. *J Hepatol.* 2015;63:470-476.

34. Alexander M, Loomis AK, van der Lei J, et al. Non-alcoholic fatty liver disease and risk of incident acute myocardial infarction and stroke: findings from matched cohort study of 18 million European adults. *Brit Med J.* 2019;367:l5367.

35. Guo F, Garvey WT. Cardiometabolic disease risk in metabolically healthy and unhealthy obesity: stability of metabolic health status in adults. *Obesity (Silver Spring).* 2016;24(2):516-525.

36. Guo F, Garvey WT. Trends in cardiovascular health metrics in obese adults: National Health and Nutrition Examination Survey (NHANES), 1988-2014. *J Am Heart Assoc.* 2016;5(7):e003619.

37. Lara-Castro C, Fu Y, Chung BH, Garvey WT. Adiponectin and the metabolic syndrome: mechanisms mediating the risk of metabolic and cardiovascular disease. *Curr Opin Lipidol.* 2007;18:263-270.

38. Lara-Castro C, Luo N, Wallace P, Klein RL, Garvey WT. Adiponectin multimeric complexes and the metabolic syndrome trait cluster. *Diabetes* 2006;55(1):249-259.

39. von Eynatten M, Schneider JG, Humpert PM, et al. Serum adiponectin levels are an independent predictor of the extent of coronary artery disease in men. *J Am Coll Cardiol.* 2006;47:2124-2126.

40. Tian L, Luo N, Klein RL, Chung BH, Garvey WT, Fu Y. Adiponectin reduces lipid accumulation in macrophage foam cells. *Atherosclerosis.* 2009;202(1):152-161.

41. Ouchi N, Kihara S, Arita Y, et al. Adipocyte-derived plasma protein, adiponectin, suppresses lipid accumulation and class A scavenger receptor expression in human monocyte-derived macrophages. *Circulation.* 2001;103:1057-1063.

42. Luo N, Liu J, Chung BH, et al. Macrophage adiponectin expression improves insulin sensitivity and protects against inflammation and atherosclerosis. *Diabetes* 2010;59:791-799.

43. Luo N, Chung BH, Wang X, et al. Enhanced adiponectin actions by over-expression of adiponectin receptor 1 in macrophages. *Atherosclerosis.* 2013;228:124-135.

44. Williams LJ, Nye BG, Wende AR. Diabetes-related cardiac dysfunction. *Endocrinol Metab (Seoul).* 2017;32(2):171-179.

45. Banerjee D, Biggs ML, Mercer L, et al. Insulin resistance and risk of incident heart failure: Cardiovascular Health Study. *Circ Heart Fail.* 2013;6:364-370.

46. Shah AD, Langenberg C, Rapsomaniki E, et al. Type 2 diabetes and incidence of cardiovascular diseases: a cohort study in 1.9 million people. *Lancet Diabetes Endocrinol.* 2015;3:105-113.

47. Bugger H, Abel ED. Molecular mechanisms of diabetic cardiomyopathy. *Diabetologia.* 2014;57:660-671.

48. Bernardi S, Michelli A, Zuolo G, Candido R, Fabris B. Update on RAAS modulation for the treatment of diabetic cardiovascular disease. *J Diabetes Res.* 2016;2016:8917578.

49. Khambhati J, Allard-Ratick M, Dhindsa D, et al. The art of cardiovascular risk assessment. *Clin Cardiol.* 2018;41(8):677-684.

50. Arnett DK, Blumenthal RS, Albert MA, et al. 2019 ACC/AHA guideline on the primary prevention of cardiovascular disease. *J Am Coll Cardiol.* 2019;74(10):e177-e232.

51. Eckel RH, Jakicic JM, Ard JD, et al. 2013 AHA/ACC guideline on lifestyle management to reduce cardiovascular risk: a report of the American College of Cardiology/American Heart Association Task Force on Practice Guidelines. *J. Am Coll Cardiol.* 2014;63(25 Pt B):2960-2984.

52. Garber AJ, Handelsman Y, Grunberger G, et al. Consensus statement by the American Association of Clinical Endocrinologists and American College of Endocrinology on the Comprehensive Type 2 Diabetes Management Algorithm—2020 executive summary. *Endocr Pract.* 2020;26(1): 107-139.

53. Garber AJ, Handelsman Y, Einhorn D, et al. Diagnosis and management of prediabetes in the continuum of hyperglycemia: when do the risks of diabetes begin? A consensus statement from the American College of Endocrinology and the American Association of Clinical Endocrinologists. *Endocr Pract.* 2008;14:933-946.

54. American Diabetes Association. 3. Prevention or delay of type 2 diabetes: Standards of Medical Care in Diabetes—2020. *Diabetes Care.* 2020;43(Suppl. 1):S32-S36.

55. Jellinger PS, Handelsman Y, Rosenblit PD, et al. 2017 American Association of Clinical Endocrinologists and American College of Endocrinology Guidelines for Management of Dyslipidemia and Prevention of Cardiovascular Disease. *Endocr Pract.* 2017;23(Suppl 2):1-87.

56. American Diabetes Association. 10. Cardiovascular disease and risk management: Standards of Medical Care in Diabetes—2020. *Diabetes Care.* 2020;43(Suppl.1):S111-S134.

57. Cosentino F, Grant PJ, Aboyans V, et al. 2019 Guidelines on diabetes, pre-diabetes and cardiovascular diseases developed in collaboration with the EASD. *Eur Heart J.* 2020;41(2):255-323.

58. Ridker PM, Danielson E, Fonseca FA, et al. Rosuvastatin to prevent vascular events in men and women with elevated C-reactive protein. *N Engl J Med.* 2008;359(21):2195-2207.

59. Bhatt DL, Steg PG, Miller M, et al. Cardiovascular risk reduction with icosapent ethyl for hypertriglyceridemia. *N Engl J Med.* 2019;380: 11-22.

60. Bhatt DL, Steg PG, Miller M, et al. Effects of icosapent ethyl on total ischemic events: from REDUCE-IT. *J Am Coll Cardiol.* 2019;73:2791-2802.

61. Estruch R, Ros E, Salas-Salvadó J, et al. Retraction and republication: primary prevention of cardiovascular disease with a Mediterranean diet. *N Engl J Med.* 2013;368:1279-90. *N Engl J Med.* 2018;378(25):2441-2442.

62. de Lorgeril M, Salen P, Martin JL, Monjaud I, Delaye J, Mamelle N. Mediterranean diet, traditional risk factors, and the rate of cardiovascular complications after myocardial infarction: final report of the Lyon Diet Heart Study. *Circulation.* 1999;99(6):779-785.

63. Salas-Salvadó J, Bulló M, Babio N, et al. Reduction in the incidence of type 2 diabetes with the Mediterranean diet: results of the PREDIMED-Reus nutrition intervention randomized trial. *Diabetes Care.* 2011;34:14-19.

64. Galbete C, Schwingshackl L, Schwedhelm C, Boeing H, Schulze MB. Evaluating Mediterranean diet and risk of chronic disease in cohort studies: an umbrella re- view of meta-analyses. *Eur J Epidemiol.* 2018;33: 909-931.

65. Svetkey LP, Simons-Morton D, Vollmer WM, et al. Effects of dietary patterns on blood pressure: subgroup analysis of the Dietary Approaches to Stop Hypertension (DASH) randomized clinical trial. *Arch Intern Med.* 1999;159(3):285-293.

66. Sacks FM, Svetkey LP, Vollmer WM, et al. Effects on blood pressure of reduced dietary sodium and the Dietary Approaches to Stop Hypertension (DASH) diet. DASH-Sodium Collaborative Research Group. *N Engl J Med.* 2001;344(1):3-10.

67. Aburto NJ, Hanson S, Gutierrez H, Hooper L, Elliott P, Cappuccio FP. Effect of increased potassium intake on cardiovascular risk factors and disease: systematic review and meta-analyses. *Brit Med J.* 2013;346:f1378.

68. Johannsen NM, Swift DL, Lavie CJ, Earnest CP, Blair SN, Church TS. Categorical analysis of the impact of aerobic and resistance exercise training, alone and in combination, on cardiorespiratory fitness levels in patients with type 2 diabetes: results from the HART-D study. *Diabetes Care.* 2013;36(10):3305-3312.

69. Garvey WT, Mechanick JI, Brett EM, et al. American Association of Clinical Endocrinologists and American College of Endocrinology clinical practice guidelines for comprehensive medical care of patients with obesity. *Endocr Pract.* 2016;22(Suppl 3):1-203.

70. Shi TH, Wang B, Natarajan S. The influence of metabolic syndrome in predicting mortality risk among US adults: importance of metabolic syndrome even in adults with normal weight. *Prev Chronic Dis.* 2020;17:E36.

71. Knowler WC, Barrett-Connor E, Fowler SE, et al. Reduction in the incidence of type 2 diabetes with lifestyle intervention or metformin. *N Engl J Med.* 2002;346(6):393-403.

72. Diabetes Prevention Program Research Group, Knowler WC, Fowler SE, et al. 10-year follow- up of diabetes incidence and weight loss in the Diabetes Prevention Program Outcomes Study. *Lancet.* 2009;374(9702): 1677-1686.

73. Li G, Zhang P, Wang J, et al. Cardiovascular mortality, all-cause mortality, and diabetes incidence after lifestyle intervention for people with impaired glucose tolerance in the Da Qing Diabetes Prevention Study: a 23-year follow-up study. *Lancet Diabetes Endocrinol.* 2014;2(6):474-480.

74. Hamman RF, Wing RR, Edelstein SL, et al. Effect of weight loss with lifestyle intervention on risk of diabetes. *Diabetes Care.* 2006;29(9):2102-2107.

75. Garvey WT, Ryan DH, Henry R, et al. Prevention of type 2 diabetes in subjects with prediabetes and metabolic syndrome treated with phentermine and topiramate extended release. *Diabetes Care.* 2014;37(4):912-921.

76. Carlsson LM, Peltonen M, Ahlin S, et al. Bariatric surgery and prevention of type 2 diabetes in Swedish obese subjects. *N Engl J Med.* 2012;367(8):695-704.

77. Booth H, Khan O, Prevost T, et al. Incidence of type 2 diabetes after bariatric surgery: population-based matched cohort study. *Lancet Diabetes Endocrinol.* 2014;2(12):963-968.

78. Le Roux CW, Astrup A, Fujioka K, et al. 3 years of liraglutide versus placebo for type 2 diabetes risk reduction and weight management in individuals with prediabetes: a randomised, double-blind trial. *Lancet.* 2017;389(10077): 1399-1409.

79. Evert AB, Dennison M, Gardner CD, et al. Nutrition Therapy for Adults With Diabetes or Prediabetes: A Consensus Report. *Diabetes Care.* 2019;42(5):731-754.

80. Wing RR, Lang W, Wadden TA, et al. Benefits of modest weight loss in improving cardiovascular risk factors in overweight and obese individuals with type 2 diabetes. *Diabetes Care.* 2011;34(7):1481-1486.

81. Lean MEJ, Leslie WS, Barnes AC, et al. Primary care-led weight management for remission of type 2 diabetes (DiRECT): an open-label, cluster-randomized trial. *Lancet.* 2018;391:541-551.

82. Lean MEJ, Leslie WS, Barnes AC, et al. Durability of a primary care-led weight-management intervention for remission of type 2 diabetes: 2-year

results of the DiRECT open-label, cluster-randomized trial. *Lancet Diabetes Endocrinol.* 2019;7:344-355.

83. Siebenhofer A, Jeitler K, Berghold A, et al. Long-term effects of weight-reducing diets in hypertensive patients. *Cochrane Database Syst Rev.* 2011;(9):CD008274.

84. Nordmann AJ, Nordmann A, Briel M, et al. Effects of low-carbohydrate vs low-fat diets on weight loss and cardiovascular risk factors: a meta-analysis of randomized controlled trials. *JAMA Intern Med.* 2006;166(3):285-293. Erratum in: *JAMA Intern Med.* 2006;166(8):932.

85. Varady KA, Bhutani S, Klempel MC, Kroeger CM. Comparison of effects of diet versus exercise weight loss regimens on LDL and HDL particle size in obese adults. *Lipids Health Dis.* 2011;10:119.

86. Mummadi RR, Kasturi KS, Chennareddygari S, Sood GK. Effect of bariatric surgery on nonalcoholic fatty liver disease: systematic review and meta-analysis. *Clin Gastroenterol Hepatol.* 2008;6(12):1396-1402.

87. Kuna ST, Reboussin DM, Borradaile KE, et al. Long-term effect of weight loss on obstructive sleeps apnea severity in obese patients with type 2 diabetes. *Sleep.* 2013;36(5):641-649.

88. Winslow DH, Bowden CH, DiDonato KP, McCullough PA. A randomized, double-blind, placebo-controlled study of an oral, extended-release formulation of phentermine/topiramate for the treatment of obstructive sleep apnea in obese adults. *Sleep.* 2012;35(11):1529-1539.

89. Kritchevsky SB, Beavers KM, Miller ME, et al. Intentional weight loss and all-cause mortality: a meta-analysis of randomized clinical trials. *PloS ONE.* 2015;10(3):e0121993.

90. Kane JA, Mehmood T, Munir I, et al. Cardiovascular risk reduction associated with pharmacological weight loss: a meta-analysis. *Int J Clin Res Trials.* 2019;4(1):131.

91. Williamson DF, Thompson TJ, Thun M, Flanders D, Pamuk E, Byers T. Intentional weight loss and mortality among overweight individuals with diabetes. *Diabetes Care.* 2000;23(10):1499-1504.

92. Sjostrom L, Lindroos AK, Peltonen M, et al. Lifestyle, diabetes, and cardiovascular risk factors 10 years after bariatric surgery. *N Engl J Med.* 2004;351:2683-2693.

93. Arterburn DE, Olsen MK, Smith VA, et al. Association between bariatric surgery and long-term survival. *J Am Med Assoc.* 2015;313(1):62-70.

94. Marso SP, Daniels GH, Brown-Frandsen K, et al. Liraglutide and cardiovascular outcomes in type 2 diabetes. *N Engl J Med.* 2016;375:311-322.

95. Marso SP, Bain SC, Consoli A, et al. Semaglutide and cardiovascular outcomes in patients with type 2 diabetes. *N Engl J Med.* 2016;375:1834-1844.

96. Haqq S, Ganna A, van der Laan SW, et al. Gene-based meta-analysis of genome-wide association studies implicates new loci involved in obesity. *Hum Mol Genet.* 2015;24(23):6849-6860.

97. Sumithran P, Proietto J. The defence of body weight: a physiological basis for weight regain after weight loss. *Clin Sci (Lond).* 2013;124:231-241.

98. Garvey WT. New tools for weight-loss therapy enable a more robust medical model for obesity treatment: rationale for a complications-centric approach. *Endocr Pract.* 2013;19(5):864-874.

99. National Heart, Lung, and Blood Institute. *Clinical Guidelines on the Identification, Evaluation, and Treatment of Overweight and Obesity in Adults: The Evidence Report.* Bethesda, MD: National Institutes of Health; 1998. Accessed at www.nhlbi.nih.gov/guidelines/obesity/ob_gdlns.pdf.

100. Jensen MD, Ryan DH, Apovian CM, et al. 2013 AHA/ACC/TOS guideline for the management of overweight and obesity in adults: a report of the American College of Cardiology/American Heart Association Task Force on Practice Guidelines and The Obesity Society. *J Am Coll Cardiol.* 2014;63:2985-3023.

101. Rubino F, Puhl RM, Cummings DE, et al. Joint international consensus statement for ending stigma of obesity. *Nat Med.* 2020;26(4):485-497.

102. Fruhbeck G, Busetto L, Dicker D, et al. The ABCD of obesity: an EASO position statement on a diagnostic term with clinical and scientific implications. *Obesity Facts.* 2019;12(2):131-136.

103. Garvey WT, Mechanick JI. Proposal for a scientifically correct and medically actionable disease classification system (ICD) for obesity. *Obesity (Silver Spring).* 2020;28(3):484-492.

104. Sharma AM, Kushner RF. A proposed clinical staging system for obesity. *Int J Obes (Lond).* 2009;33(3):289-295.

105. Hales CM, Carroll MD, Fryar CD, Ogden CL. *Prevalence of Obesity and Severe Obesity Among Adults: United States, 2017-2018.* NCHS Data Brief, no 360. Hyattsville, MD: National Center for Health Statistics. 2020.

106. Aguilar M, Bhuket T, Torres S, Liu B, Wong RJ. Prevalence of the metabolic syndrome in the United States, 2003-2012. *J Am Med Assoc.* 2015;313(19):1973-1974.

107. Wilkinson L, Yi N, Mehta T, Judd S, Garvey WT. Development and validation of a model for predicting incident type 2 diabetes using quantitative clinical data and a Bayesian logistic model: a nationwide cohort and modeling study. *PLoS Med.* 2020 Aug 7;17(8):e1003232.

108. Garvey WT, Guo F. Cardiometabolic disease staging predicts effectiveness of weight-loss therapy to prevent type 2 diabetes: pooled results from phase III clinical trials assessing phentermine/topiramate extended release. *Diabetes Care.* 2017;40(7):856-862.

109. Goff DC Jr, Lloyd-Jones DM, Bennett G, et al. 2013 ACC/AHA guideline on the assessment of cardiovascular risk: a report of the American College of Cardiology/American Heart Association Task Force on Practice Guidelines. *J Am Coll Cardiol.* 2014;63:2935-2959.

110. Kannel WB, McGee D, Gordon T. A general cardiovascular risk profile: the Framingham Study. *Am J Cardiol.* 1976;38(1):46-51.

111. Ridker PM, Buring JE, Rifai N, Cook NR. Development and validation of improved algorithms for the assessment of global cardiovascular risk in women: the Reynolds Risk Score. *J Am Med Assoc.* 2007;297(6):611-619.

112. Bohula EA, Wiviott SD, McGuire DK, et al. cardiovascular safety of lorcaserin in overweight or obese patients. *N Engl J Med.* 2018;379(12):1107-1117.

113. Mechanick JI, Apovian C, Brethauer S, et al. Clinical practice guidelines for the perioperative nutrition, metabolic, and non-surgical support of patients undergoing bariatric procedures—2019 update: co-sponsored by AACE/ACE, ASMBS OMA, and ASA. *Endocr Pract.* 2019;25(12):1346-1359.

114. Cooper TC, Simmons EB, Webb K, Burns JL, Kushner RF. Trends in weight regain following Roux-en-Y Gastric Bypass (RYGB) bariatric surgery. *Obes Surg.* 2015;25(8):1474-1481.

115. Greenway FL, Aronne LJ, Raben A, et al. A randomized, double-blind, placebo-controlled study of Gelesis100: a novel nonsystemic oral hydrogel for weight loss. *Obesity (Silver Spring).* 2019;27(2):205-216.

116. Adams TD, Davidson LE, Litwin SE, et al. Health benefits of gastric bypass surgery after 6 years. *J Am Med Assoc.* 2012;308:1122-1131.

117. Sjostrom L. Review of the key results from the Swedish Obese Subjects (SOS) trial—a prospective controlled intervention study of bariatric surgery. *J Intern Med.* 2013;273:219-234.

118. Garvey WT, Ryan DH, Bohannon NJ, et al. Weight loss therapy in type 2 diabetes: effects of phentermine and topiramate extended release. *Diabetes Care.* 2014;37(12):3309-3316.

119. Hollander P, Gupta AK, Plodkowski R, et al. Effects of naltrexone sustained release/bupropion sustained-release combination therapy on body weight and glycemic parameters in overweight and obese patients with type 2 diabetes. *Diabetes Care.* 2013;36(12):4022-4029.

120. Davies MJ, Bergenstal R, Bode B, et al. Efficacy of liraglutide for weight loss among patients with type 2 diabetes: the SCALE diabetes randomized clinical trial. *J Am Med Assoc.* 2015;314(7):687-699.

121. Schauer PR, Bhatt DL, Kirwan JP, et al. Bariatric surgery versus intensive medical therapy for diabetes--3-year outcomes. *N Engl J Med.* 2014;370(21):2002-2013.

122. Wing RR, Lang W, Wadden TA, et al. Benefits of modest weight loss in improving cardiovascular risk factors in overweight and obese individuals with type 2 diabetes. *Diabetes Care.* 2011;34(7):1481-1486.

Diabetes and Cardiovascular Disease

Jeffrey I. Mechanick and Michael E. Farkouh

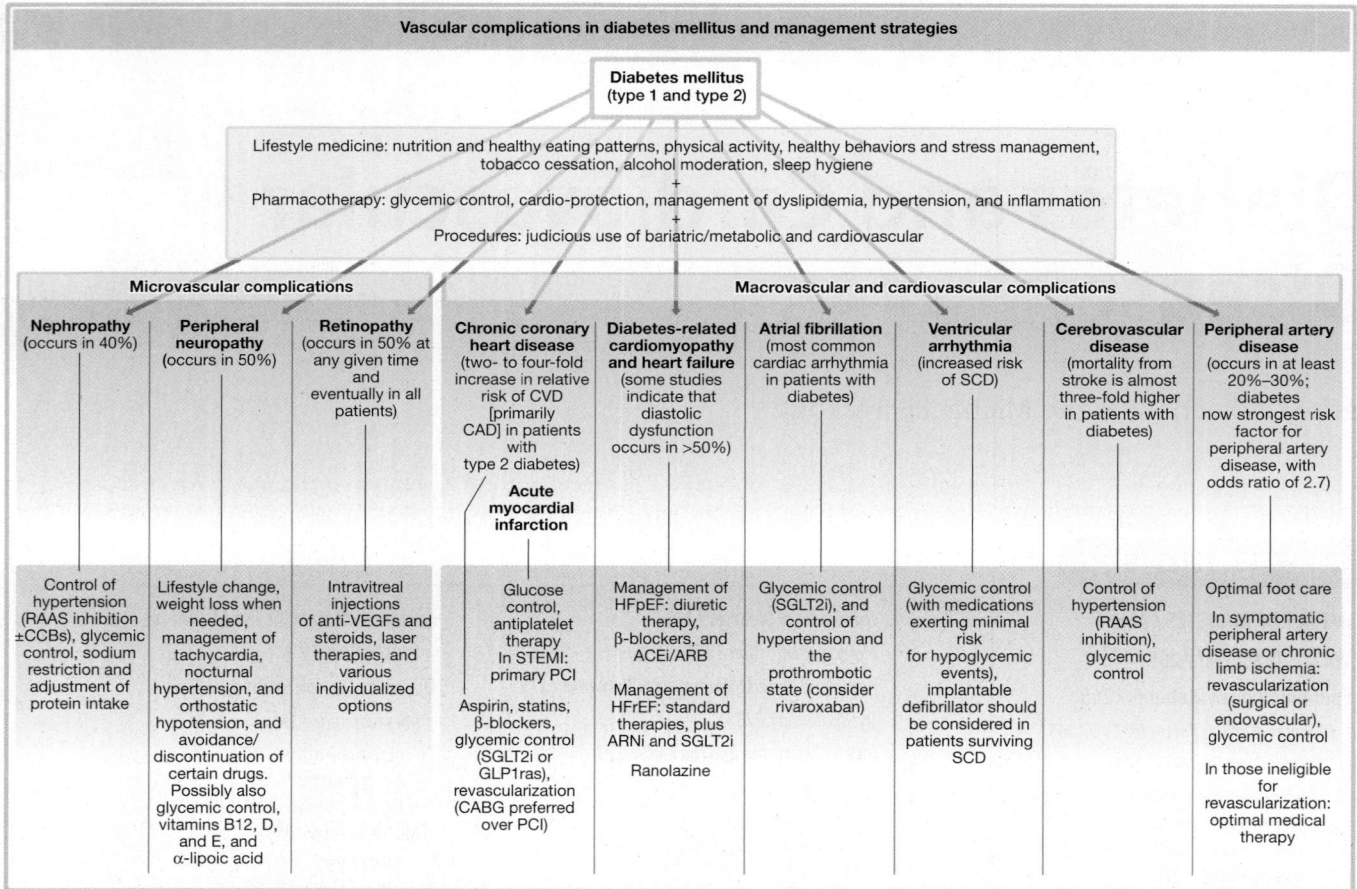

Chapter 7 Fuster and Hurst's Central Illustration. Microvascular and macrovascular complications of type 1 and type 2 diabetes mellitus. Cardiovascular disease is the most prevalent cause of mortality and morbidity in patients with diabetes. Major microvascular complications of diabetes include nephropathy, neuropathy, and retinopathy. Diabetes also significantly increases the risks of coronary heart disease and acute myocardial infarction, diabetes-related cardiomyopathy and heart failure, atrial fibrillation, ventricular arrhythmia, cerebrovascular disease, and peripheral artery disease. Preventative strategies are shown in green. Management strategies are shown in orange. ACEi, angiotensin-converting enzyme inhibitors; ARNi, dual angiotensin receptor-neprilysin inhibitor; CAD, coronary artery disease; CCBs, calcium channel blockers; CVD, cardiovascular disease; GLP1ras, glucagon-like peptide 1 receptor agonists; HFpEF, heart failure with preserved ejection fraction; HFrEF, heart failure with reduced ejection fraction; RAAS, renin-angiotensin-aldosterone system; SCD, sudden cardiac death; SGLT2i, sodium glucose transport protein 2 inhibitors.

CHAPTER SUMMARY

This chapter discusses the development, prevention, and management of cardiovascular disease in patients with diabetes mellitus. The number of patients with diabetes is rapidly increasing, and the condition is a major risk factor for the development of cardiovascular disease (see Fuster and Hurst's Central Illustration). Microvascular complications of diabetes include nephropathy, neuropathy, and retinopathy. Macrovascular and cardiovascular complications of diabetes include coronary heart disease—the leading cause of death in patients with type 2 diabetes (T2D)—diabetes-related cardiomyopathy and heart failure, atrial fibrillation, ventricular arrhythmia, cerebrovascular disease, and peripheral artery disease. Mechanisms of development of cardiovascular disease in patients with diabetes and insulin resistance include β-cell dysfunction and hyperglycemia, dyslipidemia, M1 macrophage activation, inflammation, endothelial dysfunction, and atherosclerosis. A major focus in the management of patients with type 1 or T2D is the prevention of cardiovascular disease. Strategies known to reduce cardiovascular events in patients with diabetes include diet and lifestyle modification, targeted glycemic and weight control, cardio-protective glucose-lowering medications, and effective management of dyslipidemia and hypertension.

IMPACT OF DIABETES

What Is Diabetes?

Diabetes mellitus refers to a group of diseases, with different etiologies and pathophysiological mechanisms, which result in blood glucose (BG) levels that are sufficiently high to cause specific clinical complications. Historically, diabetes was first an uncommon condition exclusively found in children, in whom there was a defect in insulin production, tendency toward diabetic ketoacidosis (DKA), and rapid natural progression of a catabolic state with classic symptoms of polyuria, polydipsia, polyphagia, weight loss, dehydration, and then death. Prior to the discovery and ability to harness insulin as a therapy in 1921, patients with diabetes could have their life extended with semi-starvation, although at the expense of severe cachexia and malnutrition. However, with insulin, patients with diabetes lived longer, though diabetes-related complications were still inevitable. It was only with the description of another form of hyperglycemia, referred to as type 2 diabetes (T2D) that the previously regarded form was referred to as type 1 diabetes (T1D), and the two types were distinguished separately in 1936. Classically, T2D was characterized by a tendency toward adult onset, overweight/obesity, insulin resistance, and elevated insulin levels, with treatment with insulin or, once available, oral agents or noninsulin injectable agents. Over the years, the prevalence rate of T2D far exceeded that of T1D.

Glycemic status can be described as normo-, dys-, hypo-, and hyperglycemia, which are defined by statistical-based classifiers correlating clinical metrics to stipulated risk levels for prediabetes, diabetes, and/or diabetes-related complications **(Table 7–1)**.[1] The salient differences among T1D, T2D, and atypical types with distinct management approaches are provided in **Table 7–2**.[2,3]

There are many reasons for the clinical cardiologist to be not only knowledgeable about diabetes but also aware of the subtleties of management that are swayed by a constant exposure to new clinical trial evidence. This chapter will explore these advances in adults with or at risk for diabetes in the context of cardiovascular disease (CVD), with an in-depth presentation of current scientific evidence and preventive/therapeutic approaches. From a broad standpoint, this chapter will provide the essential information for management of diabetes, and the use of diabetes medication, in the management of CVD. However, a more narrow question is posed: "How should acute and chronic coronary heart disease (CHD) be managed in patients with diabetes, and what is the nature of cardiac microvascular disease (MVD) in this decision-making?" Answers will follow a logical flow from establishing epidemiological/statistical associations that merit further interrogation, to relevant pathophysiological and mechanistic explanations to improve comprehension, to evidence-based management strategies, comments on education/training, and proposals on next steps to advance the field.

Epidemiology of Diabetes

Diabetes as a Risk Factor for CVD

The prevalence of diabetes is higher in developed countries than in developing countries, but the developing world will be hit the hardest by the diabetes epidemic in the future. Increased urbanization, westernization, and economic growth in developing countries have already contributed to a substantial rise in diabetes by promoting overweight/obesity and a sedentary lifestyle. Although diabetes is most common among the elderly in many populations, prevalence rates are rising among young populations in the developing world.

CVD continues to be a major cause of morbidity and mortality with diabetes and is expected to exponentially increase over the next 30 years. The global burden of CVD has emerged not only in the developed world, but also in low and middle-income countries. As a result, the major focus in patients with T1D and T2D is the prevention of the development of CVD. As the prevalence of diabetes increases, it is estimated that about 640 million adults ages 20–79 will have diabetes in 2014 with China, India, and the United States leading the way.[4] The risk profile for CVD in T1D differs from T2D in that inflammation and possibly cardiac autoimmunity may play a role in the former.[5] This concept is emphasized when considering that poor glycemic control (25%–30% of patients) with T1D increases the CVD mortality rate by about 10-fold, compared to the general population.[6] T2D accounts for 90% to 95% of all diabetes cases. Patients with T2D have a 6-fold increased risk for CVD death compared to those without diabetes.[7] More than one-half of deaths in T2D are due to a CVD cause. The age-adjusted odds ratio of developing heart failure (HF) is 2.8 for those with, compared to those without, diabetes. There is a greater than 2-fold increase in overall stroke risk with diabetes and a significant increase in the risk of both ischemic and hemorrhagic stroke subtypes. Patients with diabetes have a 2- to 4-fold increase in the prevalence of peripheral artery disease (PAD).[8] Although older evidence has suggested that diabetes is a CHD equivalent, recent data from the National Health and Nutrition Examination Survey show the mean Framingham and United Kingdom Prospective Diabetes Study (UKPDS) 10-year risk for CHD do not reach the thresholds as a CHD risk equivalent,[9,10] Nevertheless, evidence suggests that diabetes is a stronger risk factor in women (hazard ratio [HR]: 14.7; 95% confidence interval [CI]: 6.2–35.3) compared with men (HR: 3.8; 95% CI: 2.5–5.7).[11]

Diabetes Complications

Microvascular

Nephropathy: Nephropathy occurs in approximately 40% of patients with diabetes, especially those with poor glycemic control, hypertension (HTN), and certain ethnicities (Blacks, Latino/Hispanic, and Native Americans [eg, Pima Indians]).[12-14] Glomerular hyperfiltration is the hallmark of early renal hemodynamic disturbance and is an independent predictor of the development and progression of diabetic nephropathy in hypertensive T2D when only microalbuminuria is present. The earliest clinical finding of diabetic kidney disease is microalbuminuria, which may occur at a time when renal histology is essentially normal. The Diabetes Control and Complications Trial (DCCT) and the UKPDS both showed that the development and progression of microalbuminuria could be prevented through strict glycemic control.

TABLE 7–1. Clinical Terms Related to Glycemic Status[a]

Glycemic Status	Meaning	Biochemical Criteria
Normoglycemia	Normal glucose metabolism	FPG <100 mg/dl (IFG)
	Normal glucose levels	2hPG <140 mg/dl (IGT)
	Normal risk for diabetes	A1C <5.7%
	Normal risk for complications	Normal HOMA CGM: 97% time in 70–140 mg/dl range
Dysglycemia	Abnormal glucose metabolism	DBCD-1: Insulin resistance
	Normal or abnormal glucose levels	DBCD-2: Prediabetes
	Increased risk for diabetes	DBCD-3: Hyperglycemia
	Increased risk for vascular complications	DBCD-4: Vascular complications
Hyperglycemia	Abnormal glucose metabolism	FPG ≥100 mg/dl
	Abnormally high glucose levels	2hPG ≥140 mg/dl
	Diabetes or increased risk for diabetes	A1C ≥6.5%
	Increased risk for vascular complications	CGM: increased time >140–180 mg/dl range
Hypoglycemia	Abnormal glucose metabolism	any glucose <60 mg/dl
	Abnormally low glucose levels	CGM: increased time <70 mg/dl range
	May occur with dysglycemia	
	May be iatrogenic or secondary to disease	
	Increased risk for CVD events	
Insulin Resistance	Abnormal glucose metabolism	Abnormal HOMA
	Decreased insulin sensitivity	Normoglycemia
	β-cells can compensate	
	DBCD-1	
	Increased risk for prediabetes and T2D	
	Increased risk for macrovascular complications	
Prediabetes	Abnormal glucose metabolism	Abnormal HOMA
	Insulin Resistance + β-cell defect	FPG 100–125 mg/dl
	Predisease state (includes GDM, PCOS)	2hPG 140–199 mg/dl
	Mild hyperglycemia	A1C 5.7%–6.4%
	Increased risk for macrovascular complications	
	Increased risk for microvascular complications	
Diabetes	Abnormal glucose metabolism	Normal (T1D) or Abnormal (T2D) HOMA
	T1D: β-cell failure	FPG ≥126 mg/dl
	T2D: Insulin Resistance + β-cell defect	2hPG ≥200 mg/dl
	Disease state	A1C ≥6.5% on two separate occasions
	Moderate to severe hyperglycemia	Any glucose ≥200 mg/dl with classic symptoms (but without stress)
	Increased risk for macrovascular complications	CGM: controlled = >90% in 70–180 mg/dl target range
	Higher risk for microvascular complications	

[a]No consensus yet for "normal" CGM readings.

Abbreviations: 2hPG, two hour post-challenge glucose; A1C, hemoglobin A1c; CGM, continuous glucose monitoring; CVD, cardiovascular disease; DBCD-1,-2,-3,or -4, dysglycemia-based chronic disease stage 1,2,3, or 4; FPG, fasting plasma glucose; GDM, gestational diabetes; HOMA, homeostatic model assessment; IGT, impaired glucose tolerance; PCOS, polycystic ovary syndrome; T1D, type 1 diabetes; T2D, type 2 diabetes.

TABLE 7–2. The Different Types of Diabetes[b]

Type	Pathogenesis	Clinical Presentation	Management
T1D	Autoimmune β-cell destruction	Range from DKA, to polyuria, polydipsia,	Insulin
	Near absolute insulin deficiency	polyphagia, to severe hyperglycemia	Lifestyle change
	Polygenic, class II HLA	Dependent on insulin for life	Complication-specific
		Young age	
		Nonobese ("double diabetes" if ↑adiposity/IR)	
T2D	Impaired β-cell function	Hyperglycemia	Weight loss, healthy lifestyle
	Insulin resistance	Variable age	Noninsulin medication first
	Polygenic, environmental influence	Usually obese	Complication-specific
			Cardiovascular focus
			Insulin when needed
Gestational	Diabetes developing during pregnancy	Hyperglycemia in second or third trimester	Dietary change
		Routine screening <24–28 weeks gravid	Insulin
		No overt diabetes prior to pregnancy	Prevention of T2D
LADA	T1D spectrum, ↑β-cell antibodies	Usually as T1D	Insulin independence >6 months, then
	Polygenic, environmental influence	Adult and incomplete penetrance	insulin dependence
	May have insulin resistance	Usually nonobese	Lifestyle change
Ketosis-Prone	T1D-associated HLA alleles	Variable age, usually adulthood	Insulin with acute presentation
	Polygenic	Usually obese	60% require insulin by 10 years
	Lower titers of β-cell antibodies	Family history phenotypic T2D	Lifestyle change
	Insulin resistance		
Pancreatogenic	Postpancreatectomy	Consistent history and clinical diagnosis	Insulin
	Pancreatitis	Hyperglycemia	Lifestyle change
	Cystic fibrosis	↑ Risk hypoglycemia due to ↓ Glucagon	↑ Hypoglycemia precautions
	Tumor		
	Trauma		
	Fibrocalculous pancreatopathy		
	Hereditary hemochromatosis		
Monogenic	MODY (HNF1α/4α most common)	Young age	Lifestyle change
	Can affect mitochondrial function	High penetrance	Low-dose sulfonylurea in some forms
		Nonobese	Insulin in some forms
		↑ risk hypoglycemia	Meglitinides, GLP1ra, SGLT2i can be tried
		Postprandial hyperglycemia	
		Progresses to β-cell failure	
Mitochondrial	Nuclear and mitochondrial mutations	T1D and T2D phenotypes	Lifestyle
	Wide range of clinical syndromes	Child, young adult	Certain dietary supplements
		Multiorgan involvement	Insulin and noninsulin medications

[b]Abbreviations: DKA, diabetic ketoacidosis; HLA, human leukocyte antigen; HNF, hepatocyte nuclear factor; LADA, latent autoimmune diabetes in adults; MODY, maturity-onset diabetes of the young; T1D, type 1 diabetes; T2D, type 2 diabetes. See references. 2,3

Neuropathy: Diabetic peripheral neuropathy afflicts about 50% of patients with diabetes, with a risk of foot ulcer of about 25%, and is a leading causal factor for lower limb amputation and morbidity.[15,16] This risk is amplified by chronic hyperglycemia, as well as incretin impairment, insulinopenia, dyslipidemia, tobacco use, HTN, overweight/obesity, and involvement of other microvascular beds.[17–19] Autonomic neuropathy in patients with diabetes is strongly associated with CVD, including myocardial dysfunction and arrhythmia, and leads to increased mortality.[20]

Retinopathy: Diabetic retinopathy is the most prevalent microvascular complication, affecting nearly 50% of the diabetic population at a given time and eventually occurring in all patients with diabetes.[15] The main risk factors are genetic heritability, disease duration, poor glycemic control, glycemic variability, and HTN.[21] Significantly, diabetic retinopathy is an independent predictor of CVD, nephropathy and micro-/macroalbuminuria, peripheral and cardiovascular (CV) autonomic neuropathy, and stroke and cognitive impairment.[21]

Macrovascular and CV

CHD: Coronary artery disease (CAD) in patients with diabetes can be attributed to accelerated atherogenesis and atherothrombosis, as well as MVD.[22] Atherogenesis and macrovascular disease are linked to risk for atherosclerotic plaque and a pro-thrombotic state highlighted by increased platelet reactivity. MVD can lead to chronic coronary ischemia even when coronary lesions are revascularized.

CHD is strongly associated with T2D and is the leading cause of death regardless of the duration of disease. There is a 2- to 4-fold increase in the relative risk of CVD (primarily CAD) in T2D compared to the general population. This increase is particularly disproportionate in women with diabetes compared with men with diabetes. Evidently, the protection that premenopausal women have against CHD is not seen if they suffer from diabetes. The degree and duration of hyperglycemia are strong risk factors for the development of microvascular and macrovascular complications. Patients with acute coronary syndrome (ACS) and diabetes represent a high-risk group for developing and surviving acute myocardial infarction (MI). In particular, patients with T1D have a worse outcome than do patients with T2D, and women with diabetes have almost twice the risk of mortality of men with diabetes.

In chronic CHD with diabetes, there are epidemiological relationships with cardiomyopathy, represented by structural remodeling and MVD, with and without associations with atherosclerotic CAD. There is also an association with electrical remodeling, and resultant atrial fibrillation (AF) and ventricular arrhythmias (VAs). In diabetes, CHD is the most common CVD, while AF is the most common cardiac arrhythmia. The association of diabetes and AF is based on multiple covariates, including HTN, obesity, inflammation, and the concomitant alterations to the left atrium leading to dilatation and electrical abnormalities.[23] Of note, diabetes is a variable in the CHADS-VASC (*C*ongestive heart failure; *H*ypertension; *A*ge; [*D*iabetes]; prior *S*troke, transient ischemic attack, or thromboembolism;

*V*ascular disease; [*Age* again]; and *S*ex category) scoring system that estimates the risk of stroke in patients with nonrheumatic AF.

HF: Diabetes-related cardiomyopathy is a term used by clinicians to encompass the multifactorial etiologies of diabetes-related left ventricular (LV) failure characterized by both systolic and diastolic dysfunction. The Framingham Heart Study showed that men with diabetes who have congestive HF were twice as common as their nondiabetic counterpart, and that females with diabetes had a 5-fold increase, in the rate of congestive HF.[24] The spectrum of HF ranges from asymptomatic to overt systolic failure. Diabetes complicated by HTN represents a particularly high-risk group for the development of congestive HF. Diastolic dysfunction is exceedingly common (>50% prevalence in some studies) and may be linked to diabetes without the presence of concomitant HTN. Increases in N-terminal B-type natriuretic peptide over 6 months in patients with T2D have been found to be associated with a higher risk for the development of HF, hospitalization for HF, and CVD mortality.[25] In a recent report, Zareini et al.[26] found that the development of HF in patients with T2D, compared with any other CVD or renal diagnosis, was associated with the highest 5-year absolute and relative risk of death.

AF: There is a strong association between AF and diabetes. This association is based on multiple covariates including HTN, obesity, inflammation, and the concomitant alterations to the left atrium leading to dilatation and electrical abnormalities. Recently, studies of weight loss have demonstrated reductions in the burden of AF, suggesting that this association can be remedied.[27] Rhythm control is an important consideration in patients with diabetes. There remains a higher risk of AF recurrence after catheter ablation. Improved glycemic control appears to be a good predictor of reduced rates of recurrent AF.

VA: The Framingham Study showed that patients with diabetes are at higher risk of sudden cardiac death (SCD).[28] Diabetes was a greater predictor of SCD than obesity or HTN in the Nurse's Health Study.[29] However, diabetes was not associated with increased fatal MI despite the increased risk of SCD in the Paris Prospective Study.[30] In patients with a history of MI or HF, diabetes increases the risk of SCD.[31]

Cerebrovascular Disease: Compared to patients without diabetes, the mortality from stroke in patients with diabetes is almost 3-fold higher.[32] This is mainly due to increased cerebral lacunar infarction with relatively lower rates of cerebral hemorrhage. Risk factors in both T1D and T2D include advancing age, HTN, number of metabolic syndrome (MetS) traits, PAD and CAD, AF, and diabetic nephropathy. Though not a risk factor, uncontrolled hyperglycemia is associated with poorer outcomes. Carotid artery stenosis is a feature of cerebrovascular disease and also correlates with PAD. Cerebrovascular disease, or alterations of glucose homeostasis, can cause vascular cognitive impairment in patients with diabetes.

PAD: The presence of PAD in patients with T2D confers an increased risk for all-cause mortality and lower-extremity amputation.[33] With rates of cigarette smoking declining worldwide, diabetes is now the strongest risk factor for the development of PAD, with an odds ratio of 2.7.[34] The most conservative estimate is that 20% to 30% of patients with PAD have diabetes, with the association strongest in patients with diabetes and advanced age, increased duration of diabetes, and with peripheral neuropathy.[35] It has been documented that for every 1% increase in hemoglobin A1c (A1C), there was a 28% increase in the incidence of PAD with higher rates of major amputation.[36,37] The prevalence of chronic limb ischemia (CLI) is very high in diabetes, with a worse prognosis when compared to those without diabetes.

Key Statistical Associations for the Clinical Cardiologist

The rates of T1D and T2D are growing. T2D contributes disproportionately to these rising prevalence rates globally, compared to T1D. Diabetes (both T1D and T2D) is a strong risk factor for microvascular (nephropathy, neuropathy [especially CV autonomic], and retinopathy) and macrovascular (especially CAD] with consequent chronic CHD, HF, AF, and VA; but also cerebrovascular disease and PAD). CVD is the most prevalent cause of mortality and morbidity in patients with diabetes. Primarily due to the increased risk of MI and stroke, CVD death rates in the United States are 1.7 times higher in adults with diabetes than those without diabetes.[7] In diabetes, compared to no diabetes, the RR for CVD morbidity and mortality ranges from 1 to 3 in men and from 2 to 5 in women.[38] This increased risk for CVD is due to both the high rates of CVD risk factors and the direct biological effects of diabetes on the CV system. These strong epidemiological associations should prompt diligent attention to both diabetes and CVD when one of these components appears.

DISEASE MECHANISMS IN DIABETES

T1D

Etiology and Pathogenesis

T1D is caused by autoimmune destruction of the pancreatic β-cells, which normally produce insulin. This process can be represented by three stages: demonstrable autoimmunity/autoantibodies without dysglycemia or symptoms; with dysglycemia; and with frank hyperglycemia and symptoms.[39] Testing for autoantibodies (eg, anti-glutamic acid decarboxylase [GAD], islet-cell cytoplasmic, insulin, protein tyrosine phosphatase, and zinc transporter 8) may be considered in asymptomatic first-degree relatives, and those with severe, nonstress-related, insulin-requiring hyperglycemia. Further testing for other autoimmune disease, such as Hashimoto's thyroiditis (anti-thyroid peroxidase), and celiac disease (eg, antitransglutaminase) should be considered, particularly if an autoimmune polyglandular syndrome is suspected.

The sequelae of insulinopenia in patients with T1D are related to (1) profound decreases in physiological actions of insulin due to absent to near-absent production of insulin and (2) consequent organ dysfunction considered as diabetes-related complications. The net effect of near-absent insulin levels is a pathophysiological state resembling, in many ways,

carbohydrate starvation, except that there is a hyperglycemic ketoacidosis, and many times, hypertriglyceridemia.

"Double Diabetes" is a peculiar term first described in 1991[40] and applied to patients with features of both T1D and T2D. Specifically, double diabetes relates to children/adolescents with both autoimmune (but with generally lower autoantibody titers) and metabolic (generally with HTN, weight gain, low low-density lipoprotein [LDL]-cholesterol [LDL-C], and higher insulin dosing) loads. In fact, among patients with T1D over age 18 years, insulin resistance was demonstrated in about a third, and was related to adiposity, smoking, and diabetes duration.[41] Double diabetes is differentiated from late-stage, ketosis-prone T2D that exhibit features of T1D due to markedly reduced β-cell reserve. Conceptually, patients with double diabetes have T1D, but over time, generally due to an unhealthy lifestyle, overeating, and over-insulinization, they develop significantly increased adiposity, insulin resistance, and MetS traits. The prevalence of double diabetes among patients with T1D is 30% to 51%, depending on whether the definition includes MetS and/or nephropathy.[42] The association of CV risk, CVD, and mortality is higher in patients with double diabetes, compared to cohorts with T1D alone without MetS, and this increased risk is believed to be due to the proinflammatory, pro-thrombotic effects of insulin resistance.[42]

Complications

The indirect effects of hyperglycemia, or sustained organ dysfunction from near-absent insulin levels, within the context of networked relationships among multiple organs that are compromised, lead to a host of T1D-related complications.[15,43] Complications related to T1D are primarily microvascular, related to the adverse effects of hyperglycemia, but are also macrovascular, related to insidious metabolic derangements. CV complications with T1D are significant in terms of symptom burden, morbidity, and mortality, and therefore require early intervention.

T2D

Etiology and Pathogenesis

One of the most impactful approaches to the care of patients with T2D is expanding the chronic care model beyond a glucocentric approach (focusing primarily on achieving glycemic targets) to a comprehensive, complications-centric approach (focusing on optimal health, improved quality of life, and decreased complications). This paradigm shift is justified by the consistent demonstration of residual micro- and macrovascular risk after intensive vs. standard glycemic control.[44] With vascular events representing the most prevalent T2D-related complications, a novel framework has been constructed to consider pathogenic mechanisms of insulin resistance (euglycemia), prediabetes and T2D (β-cell enfeeblement leading to hyperglycemia), and vascular complications (micro- and macro-), as one all-encompassing chronic disease. Since abnormal regulation of BG is the principal driver of this encompassing chronic disease, the term *dysglycemia-based chronic disease* (DBCD) is applied and is composed of four distinct stages **(Table 7–3)**.[45]

TABLE 7–3. Primary and Metabolic Drivers for Dysglycemia-Based Chronic Disease Stages[a]

Category	Insulin Resistance	Prediabetes	Type 2 Diabetes	Complications
Primary drivers (Interact)	Genetics, Environment, Behavior	Genetics, Environment, Behavior	Genetics, Environment, Behavior	Genetics, Environment, Behavior
Metabolic drivers (Interact)	ABCD	Insulin Resistance β-Cell Defect	Insulin Resistance β-Cell Defect Medications Secondary Causes	ABCD Insulin Resistance Hyperglycemia MetS Traits
Phenotype	Euglycemia	Mild Hyperglycemia	Moderate-Severe Hyperglycemia	Macrovascular (CAD, CHD, CVA, PAD)
	ABCD PCOS	GDM ABCD PCOS	Diabetes Complications ABCD PCOS	Microvascular (Retinopathy, Neuropathy, Nephropathy) Structural Remodeling (HFpEF, HFrEF) Electrical Remodeling (AF/AFL, Ventricular Arrhythmias)

*The DBCD Framework unites insulin resistance, prediabetes, T2D, and vascular complications into one all-encompassing chronic disease to facilitate early and sustainable targeting and preventive care.

Abbreviations: ABCD, adiposity-based chronic disease; AF/FL, atrial fibrillation/flutter; CAD, coronary artery disease; CHD, coronary heart disease; CVA, cerebrovascular accident; GDM, gestational diabetes; HFpEF, heart failure with preserved ejection fraction; HFrEF, heart failure with reduced ejection fraction; PAD, peripheral arterial disease; PCOS, polycystic ovary syndrome. See reference.[45]

Insulin resistance, or Stage 1 DBCD, generally refers to patients with a molecular defect in insulin receptor signal transduction, where abnormally high, compensatory levels of insulin are required to inhibit ketogenesis, glycogenolysis, and gluconeogenesis, and glucose uptake. Insulin resistance can result from abnormal adiposity, particularly visceral and ectopic fat.[46] However, the relationship of abnormal adiposity with CVD risk in patients with T2D is not clear, especially in patients with overweight or mild (class I) obesity who due to an epidemiological artifact may have less CVD risk than their normal or underweight counterparts.[47] Insulin resistance is the predominant defect in more than 90% of patients with T2D, often preceding a diagnosis of T2D by 10 to 15 years corresponding to increased atherogenic exposure.[48,49] Not surprisingly, insulin resistance is a major pathological mechanism that underlies susceptibility to premature CVD. Relevant insulin resistance-related pathways include β-cell dysfunction and hyperglycemia; dyslipidemia; M1 macrophage activation; inflammation; endothelial dysfunction; and atherosclerosis; coronary artery spasm; cardiac dysmetabolism and structural remodeling; and CV events. In fact, insulin resistance is an independent risk factor when adjusted for lipid profile, HTN, and family history. Studies of multiple ethnic groups show increased carotid intima-medial thickness (a reliable marker for CHD) in subjects with insulin resistance. The gold standard for detecting and measuring insulin resistance is the euglycemic-insulin clamp, but simpler formulas are used in practice, such as the Homeostatic Model Assessment of Insulin Resistance (HOMA IR = [serum insulin × serum glucose] / 22.5).[48] The HOMA IR is predictive of CVD, with a one-unit increase associated with a 5.4% increased risk among patients with T2D.[48]

Prediabetes, or Stage 2 DBCD, is a term that describes a predisease state, in which patients with insulin resistance develop a β-cell defect that compromises the increase in insulin secretion needed to compensate for decreased insulin action. The controversy surrounding the need to diagnose and manage a distinct predisease state can be settled, not by considering prediabetes in isolation, but rather as a part of the fluid, holistic DBCD framework. Using this approach, CVD can be regarded in terms of early primary and metabolic drivers that are potential targets for preventive care.[50,51] Testing for prediabetes in patients with abnormal adiposity or acanthosis nigricans (especially post-puberal [or over 10 years of age] children), women desiring pregnancy, first-degree relative with prediabetes or T2D, certain ethnicities (eg, African-American, Latino/Hispanic, Asian American, Native American, and Pacific Islander), macrovascular disease (including CVD), polycystic ovary syndrome (PCOS), or other high-risk lifestyles (eg, physical inactivity and unhealthy eating patterns) is reasonable. Testing consists of a fasting BG, A1C level, or 2-hour post-challenge [75 gm oral glucose] plasma glucose [PG]), in whom a positive result would prompt prevention, such as structured lifestyle change, or pharmacotherapy.

T2D, or Stage 3 DBCD, is frank disease with increased risk for MVD from moderate-to-severe hyperglycemia, as well as macrovascular disease from the insulin resistance. Advancing age, abnormal adiposity, insulin resistance, and prediabetes, increase the risk for T2D. Testing for T2D should be risk-based, started no later than 45 years of age, and conducted at least annually.[52]

Complications

T2D with vascular complications, or Stage 4 DBCD, is composed of macrovascular disease and MVD and is therefore responsible for an array of adverse events in the natural history of T2D.[15,43] Microvascular complications are primarily related to nephropathy, neuropathy, and retinopathy. In patients with T2D and recent ACS, the presence of retinopathy and/or neuropathy increases the risk for recurrent CVD events.[53] Macrovascular complications are primarily related to accelerated atherosclerosis in various arterial beds: coronary, brain, carotid, peripheral, and great vessel. When primary

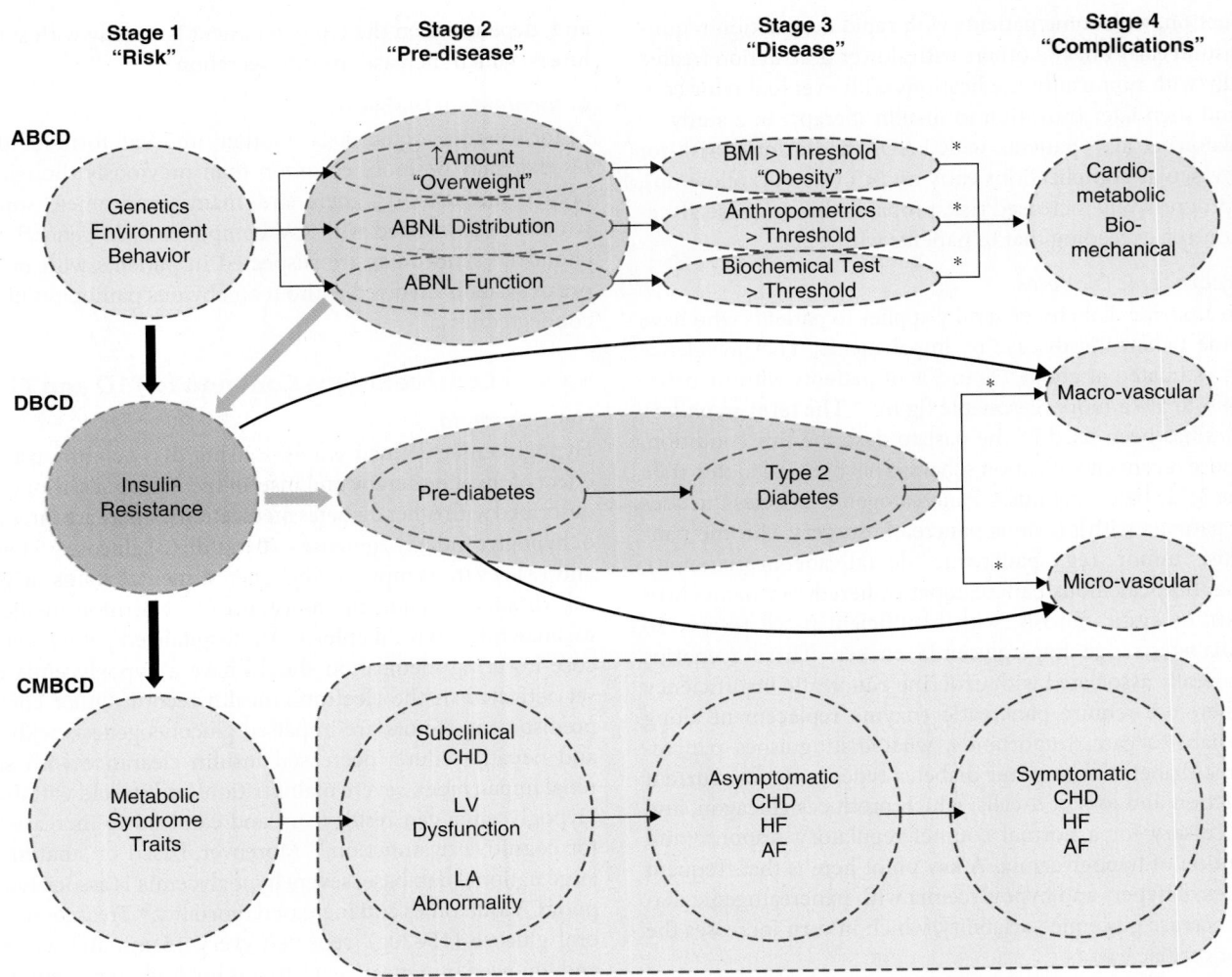

Figure 7–1. Cardiometabolic-Based Chronic Disease. Reproduced with permission from Mechanick JI, Farkouh ME, Newman JD, et al. Cardiometabolic-Based Chronic Disease, Addressing Knowledge and Clinical Practice Gaps: JACC State-of-the-Art Review. *J Am Coll Cardiol.* 2020 Feb 11;75(5):539-555.

and metabolic drivers of DBCD are considered together in a larger model of CVD, a *cardiometabolic-based chronic disease* (CMBCD) model emerges, which by design exposes actionable targets and thereby facilitates early and sustainable preventive care **(Fig. 7–1).**[50,51]

Gestational Diabetes

Gestational diabetes (GDM) increases the risk for spontaneous miscarriage, preeclampsia, fetal anomalies, macrosomia, and neonatal hypoglycemia, hyperbilirubinemia, and respiratory distress syndrome.[54] GDM is defined by abnormally high BG levels detected with testing during weeks 24–28 of pregnancy, though the upper limits of normal are lower than in the non-pregnant state. The A1C is also lower with pregnancy and usual targets are <6%, but if there is a problem with hypoglycemia, then 7%.[54] GDM is differentiated from diabetes complicating pregnancy, which occurs in women with preexisting dysglycemia, not unusual now with the increased prevalence rates of abnormal adiposity and T2D. In early pregnancy, there is increased insulin sensitivity (decreased insulin requirements)

but by 16 weeks, insulin resistance begins to increase. The significance of GDM to the cardiologist is that patients have an increased risk for T2D, which can lead to CVD.

Atypical Diabetes

The term *atypical* is used to describe biological features and clinical presentations of diabetes that are not typical for T1D, T2D, or GDM (Table 7–2).[3] The principal diagnostic challenge is determining, based on demonstrable pathophysiology and biochemistry, whether a significant β-cell defect is present that will require insulinization for the short and/ or longterm.

Latent Autoimmune Diabetes of Adults

Patients with Latent Autoimmune Diabetes of Adults (LADA) can present in a variety of ways, based on age at onset, presence/absence of DKA, specific ethnicity or environmental setting, insulin requirement, and comorbidities. Other names for this condition are type 1.5 diabetes mellitus, slowly progressive insulin-dependent T1D, and slowly evolving immune-related diabetes.[55] The etiology, pathophysiology, and clinical course of LADA is related to the autoantibody titers and rate of β-cell destruction, with some patients with rapid destruction requiring insulin early on, and others with slower destruction treated initially with noninsulin medications with eventual poor control and then later transition to insulin therapy. In a study by Maddaloni et al.,[56] patients with LADA had a lower risk for microvascular complications early on (<9 years of follow-up), with progressively increased risk, probably due to worse glycemic control, exceeding that in patients with T2D.

Pancreatogenic Diabetes

Pancreatogenic diabetes generally applies to patients who have exocrine pancreatic disease or impairments. The prevalence rate is estimated at about 1% to 9% of patients with diabetes, with 4% to 5% a more reasonable figure.[57] The term *secondary diabetes* has been used in the past to describe this condition, and more recent classification schemas have regarded this state as type 3c diabetes mellitus.[57] Pancreatogenic diabetes includes those patients with previous pancreatic surgery, chronic pancreatitis, tumor (eg, pancreatic ductal adenocarcinoma), trauma, fibrocalculous pancreatopathy, hereditary hemochromatosis, or cystic fibrosis, with insufficient β-cell reserve so that diabetes-range hyperglycemia ensues. These scenarios are generally associated with exocrine pancreatic insufficiency and therefore require pancreatic enzyme replacement along with diabetes care. Importantly, what distinguishes pancreatogenic diabetes from other diabetes types is the concurrent destruction and loss of α-cells, which produces glucagon, and are necessary for a normal counter-regulatory response and prevention of hypoglycemia. A key point here is that frequent episodes of hyper- and hypoglycemia with pancreatogenic diabetes increase glycemic variability, which in turn increases the risk for cardiac events.

Medications Causing Diabetes

Various medications cause hyperglycemia and a frank diabetes state. Chief among these are glucocorticoids, which lead to abnormal adiposity, insulin resistance, increased appetite, and impaired postprandial insulin secretion/action. In fact, an important finding in many, but not all, patients with steroid-associated diabetes is the postprandial > fasting hyperglycemia. Diabetes also occurs with the calcineurin inhibitors used in transplantation (usually accompanied by glucocorticoids early after transplantation and during episodes of rejection). New-onset diabetes after transplantation and posttransplantation diabetes mellitus are two terms describing this condition, which is not unusual after cardiac transplantation. Other medications that are associated with increased risk for development of T2D include thiazides, β-blockers, certain atypical antipsychotics (eg, olanzapine), anti-retrovirals, and statins.

Monogenic Diabetes

Maturity-onset diabetes of the young (MODY) and neonatal (<6 months age) diabetes are examples of monogenic diseases. Relatively uncommon (<5%), MODY is suspected in children or young adults with diabetes that is not clearly T1D or T2D (decreased insulin secretion, normal insulin action, no autoantibodies associated with T1D, and no obesity) with an autosomal dominant mode of inheritance. Genetic testing is required

and, depending on the type, treatment is usually with sulfonylureas, which increases insulin secretion.

Mitochondrial Diabetes

Mitochondrial diabetes is another unusual form of diabetes that may be more common than previously thought, but poorly understood. There are many syndromes, some of which are associated with CV components. In general, mitochondrial syndromes are suspected in patients with multiple organ systems involved without an obvious pathophysiological connectedness.

Special Considerations Common to T1D and T2D

Hypoglycemia

Hypoglycemia, defined as a BG <70 mg/dl is a common adverse effect of insulin therapy and insulin secretagogues, though also described with other diabetes medications. There are three levels of hypoglycemia: (1) glucose <70 mg/dl; (2) glucose <54 mg/dl; and (3) severe symptoms (eg, altered mental status or physical disability requiring assistance).[58] Nutrition-medication mismatch is a typical culprit. All hospitalized patients on glucose-lowering medication should have a hypoglycemia order set activated in the electronic health record. Other common predisposing factors are impaired gluconeogenesis with renal and hepatic failure, decreased insulin clearance with severe renal impairment, severe malnutrition, and steroid withdrawal. Hypoglycemia can result from and can lead to increased risk for cognitive dysfunction.[59] Moreover, based on analysis of a large national database, severe hypoglycemia is associated with poor CV outcomes and increased mortality.[60] Treatment is with oral glucose (15–20g), repeated every 15 minutes as needed and followed by a meal/snack that is not high in protein (which increases an endogenous insulin response in T2D), or in more severe cases, glucagon via auto-injector pen. Hypoglycemic unawareness results from repeated hypoglycemic episodes, autonomic dysfunction, chronic disease, and other conditions.

Glycemic Variability

The term *glycemic variability* refers to BG fluctuations over different time scales that are due to normal circadian rhythms, meals, and physical activity, as well as effects of stress, medications, and medical interventions. Patients can have different levels of glycemic variability despite similar levels of A1C or average glucose levels. Increased glycemic variability correlates with oxidative stress in T2D, but not T1D. This and other mechanistic relationships can lead to adverse events (many of which are related to the CV system) due to significant hypo- and hyperglycemia, as well as being statistically associated with adverse outcomes in the outpatient, general inpatient, and intensive care unit settings. In the Veterans Affairs Diabetes Trial (VADT), glycemic variability[61] and incident severe hypoglycemia[62] were independently associated with CVD complications. Glycemic variability can be gauged by simple daily ranges in glucose[63] or by sophisticated calculable metrics.[64]

Transcultural Diabetes

Many of the critical elements of diabetes etiology and pathophysiology are determined by primary drivers (genetics, environment, and behavior), each influenced by ethno-cultural variables.[13] In many instances, these culture-dependent phenotypes affect the CV system and should prompt modifications in the care plan. Examples of transcultural factors that should be routinely incorporated in patient encounters for diabetes and CVD include: dietary habits (eg, increased glutinous rice by Asians and Latino/Hispanics), attitudes toward clinicians (eg, decreased trust among many ethnic minority groups), appropriate anthropometric cutoffs for adiposity risk stratification (eg, body mass index [BMI] and waist circumference [WC]), interpretation of A1C (eg, South Asians have diminished β-cell reserve and more prone to postprandial hyperglycemia), and socioeconomics (eg, disparities in access to quality health care and affordability/availability of many diagnostic tests or therapeutic interventions).[13]

Molecular Nutrition

Dietary patterns are defined as the aggregated intake of foods over a certain period of time, such as a day. This concept distinguishes dietary patterns from strict "diets," which conform to scientific interventions or commercial product directions. Messaging dietary patterns can be more relevant for patients as they incorporate a real-world context and avoid classifying individual foods as "good" or "bad." Healthy dietary patterns are associated with specific proteomic/metabolomics signatures that characterize healthy cardiometabolic phenotypes with low risk for MetS and CVD.[65] The mechanisms by which healthy dietary patterns exert cardiometabolic benefit is understood at the molecular scale, through networking effects of nutrient molecules in a specific array of foods ("food-ome") with molecules participating in human metabolism ("metabolome").[66]

Adipokine-Based Inflammatory Networks

In the ABCD, DBCD, and CMBCD models, the effects of abnormal adiposity on insulin resistance, β-cell function, and the CV system, as well as insulin resistance and hyperglycemia on the CV system are mediated in part by complex interactions among various cytokines (eg, adipokines[67,68]) and physiological systems. The important adipokines are adiponectin, leptin, angiotensinogen/angiotensin II, tumor necrosis factor, and plasminogen activator inhibitor-1. These networks pose a unique intervention opportunity, which may prioritize lifestyle medicine (influencing many nodes in key sub-networks), over pharmacotherapy, (influencing only single or a few nodes in key sub-networks, even when there are proven pleiotropic drug effects [eg, statins and sodium glucose transport protein 2 inhibitors {SGLT2is}]), in a preventive care model (Fig. 7–2).[67,68] Examples of targetable adipokine-CVD sub-networks include: the response to hypoxia, lipopolysaccharides, glucocorticoids, and inflammation; positive regulation of cell migration, blood coagulation, and platelet activation; mitogen-activated protein kinase and tyrosine/serine/threonine phosphatase activity; peptidyl-tyrosine phosphorylation; and cachexia, appetite, and insulin receptor binding with insulin resistance.[67,68]

Viewed another way, the inflammatory, molecular mechanisms by which adipokines drive insulin resistance mediate development of macrovascular complications. This occurs via endothelial injury, vascular smooth muscle cell (VSMC) proliferation/migration, monocyte/macrophage adhesion and migration, and pro-atherogenesis. The normal endothelium regulates vasomotor tone and keeps the coagulation cascade in balance. With insulin resistance that is typically driven by adipokines, endothelial cell insulin receptor activation is decreased, resulting in endothelial dysfunction described by downregulated phosphoinositol-3 kinase and nitric oxide pathways, and consequently, impaired blood flow. In a parallel pathway, hyperglycemia triggers endothelial cell secretion of endothelin-1 and interleukin-6, inducing pro-atherogenic events, such as vasoconstriction, increased vascular permeability, and VSMC proliferation. Hyperglycemia stimulates proteoglycan synthesis on VSMCs. The insulin receptors on VSMCs are structurally and functionally similar to those in skeletal muscle and adipocytes, and stimulation by insulin is associated with cellular proliferation/migration. Insulin also acts synergistically with other atherogenic growth factors, such as platelet-derived growth factor, which promotes proliferation/migration of bovine aortic smooth muscle cells.

Circulating monocytes represent another feature in the adipokine-inflammatory network that characterizes insulin resistance. Insulin and insulin-like growth factor-1 receptors are present on circulating monocyte-macrophages, and defective insulin signaling contributes to macrophage foam cell formation. With insulin resistance, the protective effect of insulin to reduce macrophage apoptosis may be lost, which in the context of atherosclerotic plaques can lead to cytokine-mediated monocyte recruitment, accelerated development of the vascular lesion, and ultimately plaque rupture. Thus, through multiple concurrent and overlapping physiological mechanisms relating abnormal adiposity, adipokines, inflammation, and insulin resistance, CVD can evolve at varying paces, producing varying levels of severity.

Dyslipidemia

Dyslipidemia depends on glycemic status in patients with T1D or T2D. In uncontrolled T1D, LDL is moderately increased, triglycerides (TGs) are markedly increased, and high-density lipoprotein (HDL) is decreased. In uncontrolled T2D, the lipid abnormalities are related to both hyperglycemia and insulin resistance, and may be depicted by normal LDL levels despite high very-low-density lipoprotein (VLDL) and TG, as well as reduced HDL levels. On the other hand, even with controlled T1D or T2D, there is increased atherogenicity of the LDL particle. This occurs through glycosylation of apoprotein B and the phospholipid components of LDL, altering LDL clearance and oxidative modifications. These small, dense, and atherogenic LDLs are more avidly taken up by aortic intimal cells and macrophages, accelerating the formation of foam cells, and increasing the risk for CHD. Low HDL levels are also a strong risk factor for CHD in patients with diabetes, and result from decreased production (due to decreased lipoprotein lipase catabolism of VLDLs) and/or increased clearance (due to high TG content).

Insulin Resistance and the MetS

Insulin resistance is not only a key stage in DBCD, but also a mediator of the adipokine-inflammatory network,[67]

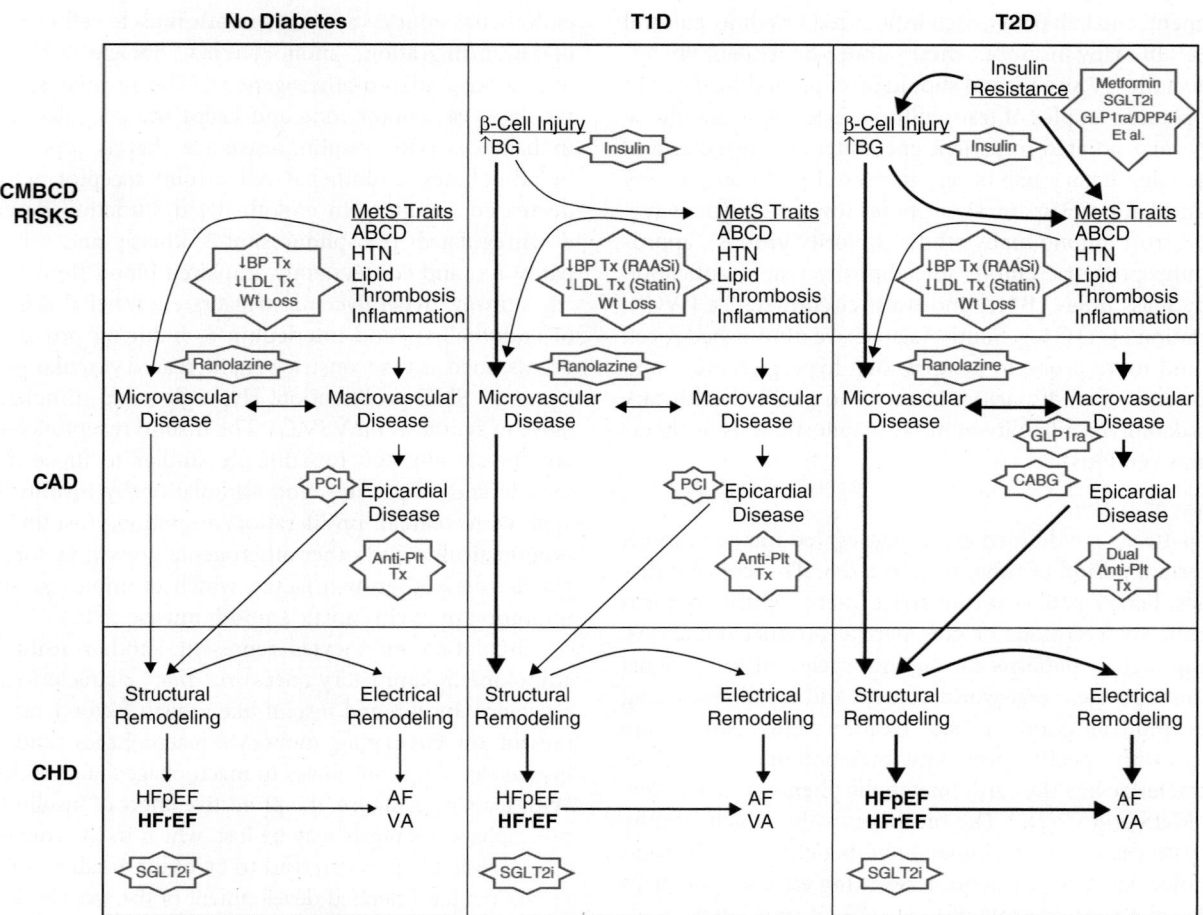

Figure 7–2. Coronary Heart Disease in Type 1 and Type 2 Diabetes. The progression from CMBCD risks to CAD and then CHD is depicted for patients with T1D and T2D and without diabetes. Important pathophysiological differences are indicated by thicker black arrows. Cardiometabolic interventions are provided in red and also with important evidence-based differences indicated by thicker stars and bolder fonts. In patients with T2D, compared with those with T1D or without diabetes, the cardiomyopathy that results from structural and electrical remodeling is driven by the combined impact of both microvascular and macrovascular complications. Abbreviations: ABCD, adiposity-based chronic disease; BP, blood pressure; CABG, coronary artery bypass grafting; CAD, coronary artery disease; CHD, coronary heart disease; CMBCD, cardiometabolic-based chronic disease; DPP4i, dipeptidyl-peptidase 4 inhibitor; GLP1ra, glucagon-like peptide 1 receptor agonist; HFpEF, heart failure with preserved ejection fraction; HFrEF, heart failure with reduced ejection fraction; HTN, hypertension; LDL, low-density lipoprotein; PCI, percutaneous coronary intervention; Plt, platelet; RAASi, renin-angiotensin-aldosterone system inhibition; SGLT2i, sodium glucose transport protein 2 inhibitors; T1D, type 1 diabetes; T2D, type 2 diabetes; Tx, treatment; Wt, weight.

feature of double diabetes, and hallmark of rare syndromes of extreme insulin resistance, as well as a critical aspect of MetS. Historically, MetS finds its roots in *Syndrome X* originally described by Reaven et al.,[69] and also referred to as *cardiometabolic syndrome*. Even though there are different definitions and diagnostic criteria for MetS, the principal components are the following cardiometabolic risk factors: insulin resistance, obesity, HTN, and hypertriglyceridemia; with residual risk factors including small LDL, vascular inflammation, coagulopathy, and pro-atherothrombosis.[70] In the San Antonio Heart Study, patients converting to overt diabetes had significantly higher blood pressure (BP), BMI, WC, TG levels, and lower HDL-cholesterol (HDL-c) levels at baseline compared to nonconverters.[71] The mechanisms underlying how diabetes increases CVD risk overlap with those pertaining to MetS and CVD risk, with insulin resistance as a common denominator.

CVD

There are multiple pathogenetic mechanisms linking CVD and diabetes. These mechanisms range from genetic factors and epigenetics to abnormal glucose regulation, insulin resistance, and increased oxidative stress. These mechanisms are common to both CVD and diabetes and contribute to the related co-morbidities. Atherosclerosis, microangiopathy, diabetic cardiomyopathy, and cardiac autonomic neuropathy, are caused by these pathogenetic mechanisms.

CHD: The development of CHD depends on the interplay of primary drivers (genetics and anatomical predisposition, environment, and behavior) to create a cardiometabolic risk profile for atherosclerosis. The mechanistic impact of diabetes on this process can be viewed in terms of networked effects of insulin resistance (T2D > T1D) and hyperglycemia (T1D and T2D) on other cardiometabolic risk factors (eg, HTN, dyslipidemia, inflammation, and thrombosis). From a pragmatic standpoint, early CHD is manifested by detectable cardiometabolic risk factors, acute CHD with ACS or other acute symptomatic presentations, and chronic CHD by angina, arrhythmia, or other chronic symptoms related to structural and/or electrical heart disease complications. Once CHD develops in the patient with diabetes, the LV systolic dysfunction (HF with preserved ejection fraction [HFpEF] and reduced ejection fraction [HFrEF]) that ensues responds to all the same therapies as in the population without diabetes.[72]

Chronic CHD: Chronic CHD, characterized by a mismatch in myocardial perfusion and metabolic demand, can arise from either atherosclerotic CAD leading to chronic ischemia and microvascular coronary disease. Atherosclerotic CAD results when lipid-rich lesions and smooth muscle cell proliferation lead to plaque formation and coronary obstruction, but how is this different in patients with diabetes?

In recent years, this problem has been clarified by understanding abnormalities in the coronary microcirculation, referred to as coronary MVD, in the context of diabetes. This centers on the effects of insulin resistance on reduced coronary flow reserve from abnormal endothelium-dependent and -independent vasomotor activity, and the effects of hyperglycemia on microvasculature and CV autonomic neuropathy. In aggregate, these processes are more complex than those resulting from just epicardial coronary artery stenosis in patients without diabetes.[73] A diagnosis of coronary MVD is the crux of the problem regarding the diabetic heart and is based on the following criteria: (1) symptoms of myocardial ischemia; (2) absence of obstructive epicardial CAD; (3) evidence of myocardial ischemia on noninvasive testing; and (4) evidence of impaired coronary flow reserve.

The pathogenesis of endothelial dysfunction in T2D is significant in chronic CHD and involves the confluence of multiple CV risk factors leading to increased oxidative stress. Insulin resistance in T2D leads to impaired insulin signaling, which leads to decreased production of endothelial nitric oxide synthase and nitric oxide. When this endothelial dysfunction accompanies CAD, the two combine to create progressive atherosclerosis and CHD.

HF: The etiology of impaired LV function may involve any of the following mechanisms: (1) coronary atherosclerotic disease, (2) HTN, (3) LV hypertrophy, (4) obesity, (5) endothelial dysfunction, (6) coronary MVD, (7) CV autonomic neuropathy, and (8) metabolic abnormalities. Commonly in diabetes, left HF is not characterized by systolic dysfunction. Right ventricular (RV) structural remodeling also occurs. In echocardiographic studies using strain techniques, independent of HTN, diabetes was associated with decreased RV diastolic and systolic dysfunction. Later work demonstrated that both RV and right atrial (RA) deformation and function were decreased in patients with diabetes compared to those without diabetes.[74] In multivariate regression analysis, RV global strain was correlated with A1C, underscoring the impact of dysglycemia on RV function.

HF with HFpEF is characterized by coronary microvascular endothelial dysfunction related to hyperglycemia, hyperinsulinemia, and lipotoxicity, leading to a restrictive picture.[75] Patients will have impaired diastolic dysfunction, so valvular, coronary, and hypertensive causes should always be excluded.

AF: The effects of diabetes on the heart can be attributed in part to structural and electrical remodeling of the left atrium (LA) independent of HTN and other MetS risk factors. Insulin resistance and subsequent impaired glucose regulation are linked to the following mechanisms: (1) LA enlargement seen in diabetes; (2) LV diastolic dysfunction linked to diabetes and leading to abnormal atrial function; (3) subendocardial fibrosis causing decreased atrial wall elasticity; (4) electrical remodeling of the LA; and (5) autonomic nervous system imbalance with enhanced sympathetic activation leading to an arrhythmogenic atrial substrate.[76]

The interaction of abnormal adiposity, particular ectopic, pericardial/epicardial fat, and insulin resistance affects the electrical function of the heart, increasing the risk for AF. The pathophysiological role of the autonomic nervous system in arrhythmogenesis is well established. Within minutes of myocardial ischemia there is a striking surge of sympathetic nerve activity, and with an increase in circulating catecholamines, an aggravation of myocardial ischemia occurs, establishing a vicious circle. As a result, the risk of developing supraventricular and ventricular tachyarrhythmias is increased.

VA: There are a number of mechanisms that underpin the electrical remodeling and substrate vulnerability in the ventricle, including: (1) cardiomyopathy (ischemic and nonischemic); (2) myocardial fibrosis; (3) coronary MVD, and (4) abnormalities in electrical repolarization and depolarization of the myocardium, including QTc interval prolongation.[77,78]

Cerebrovascular Disease

The small paramedial penetrating arteries are the most common sites of cerebrovascular disease. In addition, diabetes increases the likelihood of severe carotid atherosclerosis.[32] Patients with, compared to without, diabetes are more likely to suffer increased brain damage with carotid emboli that would result in a transient ischemic attack. Moreover, magnetic resonance imaging of patients with diabetes often uncovers asymptomatic lacunar infarctions in the basal ganglia and brain stem.[32]

PAD

The mechanisms leading to the development and progression of PAD are similar to the processes in other vascular beds.[79] They include derangements in the vessel wall through enhanced vascular inflammation and endothelial cell dysfunction. This is accompanied by abnormalities in smooth muscle cells and platelets, and an overall propensity to thrombosis.

Key Mechanistic Drivers That Are Actionable for Clinical Cardiologists

There are important mechanistic relationships among aspects of diabetes (insulin resistance and hyperglycemia), vascular complications of diabetes, and the CV system itself that expose opportunities for intervention early, during, and late in the natural history of CMBCD. These mechanisms are summarized below:

1. Critical role of abnormal adiposity, resulting from unhealthy lifestyles, on insulin resistance;

2. Interactions of MetS traits that increase risks for macrovascular disease;

3. Roles of chronic kidney disease (CKD), microalbuminuria, and CV autonomic neuropathy on the development and progression of CVD;

4. A pervasive role of inflammation on endothelial injury and vascular derangements;

5. An as yet unclear progression of atherosclerotic CAD and ACS to coronary MVD and structural/electrical remodeling, leading to HFpEF/HFrEF, AF, and VA; and

6. The atherothrombosis associated with diabetes is systemic and involves multiple vascular beds.

APPROACHES TO TREATMENT

Glucocentric and Complication-Centric

General Discussion

Historically, diabetes was approached with a primary focus on glycemic control and secondary focus on prevention or treatment of diabetes-related complications. Historically, there are many critical strong studies, not including the CV outcome trials (CVOTs) discussed below, correlating lifestyle, pharmacological, and surgical interventions with levels of glycemic control and development of complications **(Table 7–4)**.[80–119] A synthesis of these evidentiary findings can be summarized as follows:

- Intensive lifestyle intervention exerts primary and secondary prevention effects in patients with DBCD.

- Intensive glucose-lowering pharmacotherapy (with insulin or insulin secretagogues) in patients with T1D or T2D exerts beneficial effects primarily on microvascular complications (primarily driven by chronic hyperglycemia), with possible later secondary benefits on macrovascular complications (primarily driven by insulin resistance) but with an increased risk of hypoglycemia that can increase mortality.

- Statins are cardioprotective in prediabetes, T2D, and adult patients with T1D.

- Procedures involving the GI tract (eg, metabolic and bariatric) can exert significant benefit on glycemic control and CV risk in patients with abnormal adiposity, insulin resistance, prediabetes, and T2D.

- The stage is set for CVOTs in patients with T2D to demonstrate benefit of other diabetes medications on reduction of CV risk and events.

- An approach to whether or not to revascularize is linked to extent of CAD and degree of impairment of LV systolic function.

The most commonly used measurements of glycemic status are self-monitoring of blood glucose (SMBG; most patients perform intermittently and primarily fasting in the AM, but should be coordinated with meals and activity), the A1C (reflecting the average glucose level over about two to three months), and continuous glucose monitoring (CGM; recently much more popular due to lower cost, ease of use, and demonstrable benefits in glycemic control; requires SMBG for calibration, verification, and backup). All patients on diabetes medications should at least be taught SMBG. The A1C level should be checked at least twice a year with stable glycemic control and up to every three months with uncontrolled diabetes. Results are unreliable with anemia, certain hemoglobinopathies (eg, sickle cell), transfusion, end-stage kidney disease, and pregnancy. In general, glycemic targets for nonpregnant adults are 80–130 mg/dl preprandial and <180 mg/dl peak postprandial, with A1C <7%, though targets can be tighter (<6.5%) or looser (<8%) depending on individual variables: hypoglycemia risk, polypharmacy, age, comorbidities and complications, cognitive function, medical adherence, patient preference, resources, and overall goals of care.[120] Wih CGM, the time in range (70–180 mg/dl; target >70%) correlates with risk for microvascular complications; other CGM metrics are number of days worn (target 14 days), % time device is active (target 70%), glycemic variability (target ≤36%), and time in abnormal ranges above and below targets. In children and adults, with T1D or T2D, CGM improves glycemic control and reduces hypoglycemia risk.[121]

The majority of interventional studies in diabetes use stipulated glycemic targets and specific pharmacotherapies. However, more recent interventions have focused on structured lifestyle change, with the implicit context of using guideline-directed pharmacotherapy. Hypoglycemia risk should always be formally evaluated with special attention to minimizing/synchronizing insulin and secretagogues, liver and kidney impairments, frailty and cognitive impairments, dysautonomia and hypoglycemic unawareness, physical disabilities, alcohol and illicit drug use, and polypharmacy.[120] Moreover, there are many devices and procedures utilized for glycemic control, typically in the context of abnormal adiposity, but also with benefits on other cardiometabolic risks **(Fig. 7–3)**.[122]

Clinical practice algorithms have been constructed based on the most recent evidence at hand that integrates different treatment modalities to optimize glycemic status in diabetes **(Fig. 7–4)**.[123,124] Many of these algorithms comment on diabetes complication management, with directions for dental examinations, annual dilated eye exams, reproductive counseling for women and low testosterone assessment in men, evaluations for foot care, and consultations for nonalcoholic fatty liver disease/steatohepatitis, bone loss, hearing loss, neuropathy and cognitive dysfunction, sleep disorders, and mental health, as needed.[124] Guideline-directed routine vaccinations are also indicated for influenza, pneumococcal disease, and hepatitis B prophylaxis.[125]

An important feature of recent interventional approaches has been a shift away from purely glucocentric decision-making to more complex, comprehensive care plans. Indeed, the chronic care model figures prominently in diabetes management, including evidence-based guidelines based on biological and social determinants of health and disease, reliable

TABLE 7–4. Chronology of Key Randomized Controlled Trials in Patients with Prediabetes or Diabetes[a]

Year	Clinical Trial (Ref)	Intervention	Population (N)	Essential Findings
1993	DCCT (80)	P	T1D (1441)	Intensive therapy: delays microvascular disease; ↑hypoglycemia risk
1994	4S (89)	P	CHD (4444)	201 patients with diabetes; simvastatin 10–40 mg/d: 42% reduction in risk of CHD death over median 5.4 years
1997	DA QING (119)	L	PD (110,660)	Diet and exercise decreased incident T2D over 6 years
1998	CARE (90)	P	DM/PD (4159)	Pravastatin reduced recurrent MACE in patients with prediabetes and diabetes over 5 years
1998	UKPDS (109)	P	T2D (3867)	Intensive therapy: decreases microvascular but not macrovascular disease; ↑hypoglycemia risk
1998	HOT (104)	P	HTN (18,790)	In patients with T2D, 51% decreased CVD events with dBP <80 compared with <90 mmHg for up to 5 years
1999	EDIC (81,82)	P	T1D (1422)	DCCT cohort with durable ↓micro/macro-vascular disease (metabolic memory) after mean of 18 years
2000	HOPE (105)	P	DM+CVDr (3577)	Substudy: ramipril decreased MACE and overt nephropathy (81 [2.3%] with T1D)
2001	Tuomilehto (88)	L	PD (522)	ILI: 58% risk reduction for development of T2D after mean 3.2 years
2002	DPP (87)	L, P	PD (3234)	ILI: 58% risk reduction; metformin: 31% risk reduction for development of T2D after mean 2.8 years
2003	Steno-2 (85)	L, P	T2D/MA (80)	behavioral + intensive pharmacotherapy for CVDrf (e.g., A1C <6.5%): ↓microvascular/MACE by 50% after mean of 7.8 years
2004	HPS (91)	P	CVArf (20,536)	5963 with diabetes (615 [10.3%] with T1D); simvastatin 40 mg decreased coronary events and ischemic stroke
2004	CARDS (92)	P	T2D (2838)	Primary prevention study: atorvastatin 10 mg decreases risk 1st CVD or stroke event
2005	4D (93)	P	T2D+HD (1255)	No effect of atorvastatin 20 mg on CVD mortality, nonfatal MI, or stroke
2006	FIELD (100)	P	T2D (9795)	Fenofibrate (in patients not on statin) reduced total CVD events, albuminuria progression, and retinopathy requiring lased, but not coronary events over 5 years
2006	DREAM (114,115)	P	PD (5269)	Rosglitazone 8 mg/d x 3 years reduces incident T2D or death by 60% and ↑regression to normoglycemia by 70%–80%, with no effect on CVD outcomes; ramipril up to 15 mg/d x 3 years did not reduce incident T2D or death but had comparable ↑regression to normoglycemia as rosiglitazone
2008	ON-TARGET (106)	P	DM/VD (8596)	Ramipril and telmisartan equivalent in reducing MACE, but more adverse effects when used together
2008	ACCORD (110)	P	T2D (10,251)	Intensive therapy (A1C <6% vs. 7%–7.9%): increased mortality and hypoglycemia without CVD benefit
2008	ADVANCE (111)	P	T2D (11,140)	Intensive therapy (A1C 6.5% vs. 7.3%): ↓macro/microvascular (esp. renal) events; ↑hypoglycemia risk
2009	VADT (112)	P	T2D (1791)	Intensive therapy (>1.5% A1C reduction): no CVD, mortality, microvascular (except albuminuria) benefit; ↑hypoglycemia risk
2010	ACCORD lipid (101)	P	T2D (5518)	Fenofibrate added to simvastatin did not reduce MACE over mean of 4.7 years
2010	ACCORD BP (102)	P	T2D (4733)	Targeting sBP <120 compared with <140 mmHg did not ↓MACE over mean 4.7 years
2010	INVEST (103)	P	T2D+CAD (6400)	Subgroup analysis: targeting sBP <130 mmHg compared with usual control did not improve CVD outcomes
2010	NAVIGATOR (116,117)	P	PD+CVDr (9306)	Nateglinide 60 mg TID did not reduce incident T2D or MACE over median 5-6.5 years; ↑hypoglycemia risk; valsartan up to 160 mg/d reduced incident T2D by 14% but had no effect on MACE
2011	AIM-HIGH (98)	P	ASCVD (3414)	Niacin added to simvastatin+ezetimibe: no clinical benefit over 3 years (1158 [33.9%] with diabetes)
2012	MINGRONE (108)	S	T2D+Obesity (60)	Bariatric surgery resulted in more T2D remission & better glycemic control than medical therapy at 2 years
2013	Look AHEAD (83)	L	T2D (5145)	ILI and weight loss: no effect on MACE after median 9.6 years (↓A1C, fitness, CVD risks except LDL-c)
2014	HPS-2 THRIVE (99)	P	ASCVD (25,673)	Niacin-laropiprant added to statin: no effect on vascular events; ↑new diabetes/↓glycemic control; over median of 3.9 years (8,299 [32.3%] with diabetes)

(Continued)

TABLE 7–4. Chronology of Key Randomized Controlled Trials in Patients with Prediabetes or Diabetes[a] (Continued)

Year	Clinical Trial (Ref)	Intervention	Population (N)	Essential Findings
2015	TNT + IDEAL (94–96)	P	CVD (15,056)	Pooled study: atorvastin 80 mg cardioprotective for PreDM; ↑conversion rate to T2D compared with 10 mg dose
2015	IMPROVE-IT (97)	P	ACS (18,144)	Ezetimibe, when added to statin, lowers LDL-c and improves CVD outcomes (4.933 [27.2%] with diabetes)
2017	STAMPEDE (107)	S	T2D+OO (150)	Bariatric surgery, when added to intensive medical therapy, improves CVD risks, hyperglycemia, weight, and QOL at 5 years
2018	ASCEND (118)	P	DM (15,480)	Aspirin prevented serious events but counterbalanced by bleeding hazard over mean of 7.4 years (94.1% T2D)
2018	PREDIMED (84)	L	T2D/CVDrf (7447)	~50% T2D; Mediterranean Diet (energy-unrestricted; supplemented with EVOO/nuts): ↓MACE after mean
2019	DIRECT (86)	L	T2D (149)	ILI and stop DM meds: 36% diabetes remission (3% in controls) at 24 months and related to ↓wt (esp >10kg) of 4.8 years
2019	REDUCE-IT (113)	P	↑TG+[CVD or DM]	29% had T1D or T2D; IPE reduced burden of first, subsequent, and total ischemic events (8179)

[a]Not including Cardiovascular Outcome Trials (CVOT). Unless specifically clarified, studies denoting "diabetes" are presumed to include both T1D and T2D.

Abbreviations: A1C, hemoglobin A1c; ACS, acute coronary syndrome; ASCVD, atherosclerotic cardiovascular disease; CAD, coronary artery disease; CHD, coronary heart disease; CVAr, cerebrovascular accident risk(s); CVD, cardiovascular disease; CVDr, cardiovascular disease risk(s); dBP, diastolic blood pressure; DM, diabetes; EVOO, extra virgin olive oil; HD, hemodialysis; HTN, hypertension; ILI, intensive lifestyle intervention; LDL-c, low-density liproprotein cholesterol; MA, microalbuminuria; MACE, major adverse cardiac events; OO, overweight/obesity; PD, prediabetes; QOL, quality of life; sBP, systolic blood pressure; T1D, type 1 diabetes; T2D, type 2 diabetes; VD, vascular disease; S, strategy trials.

Surgical Procedure

Non-surgical Procedure

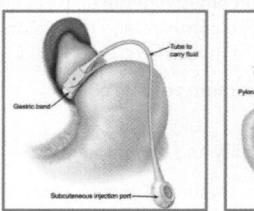
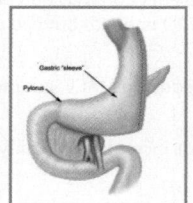
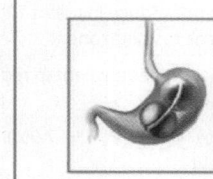
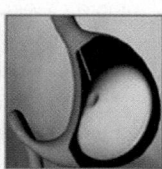
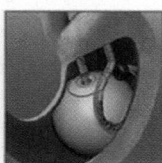
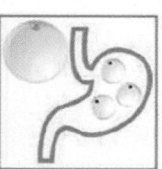
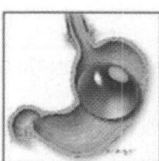

Adjustable Gastric Band   Sleeve Gastrectomy

ReShape Balloon   Ellipse Balloon   Spatz Balloon   Obalon Balloon   Orbera Balloon

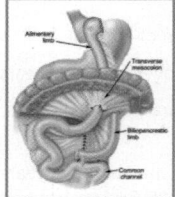
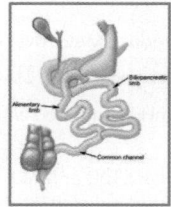
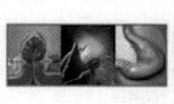
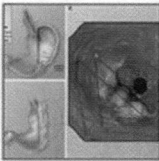
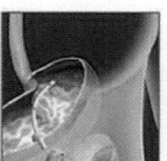
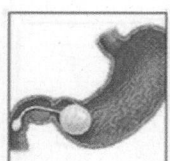
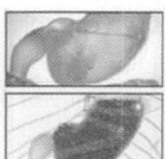

Roux-en-Y Gastric Bypass   Biliopancreatic Diversion with Duodenal Switch

POSE Procedure   Gastroplasty Apollo Device   Aspire Assist   Transpyloric Shuttle   Gelesis 100

Figure 7–3. Adjustable Gastric Band. Bariatric procedures with potential beneficial effects on glycemic control, diabetes remission, and cardiometabolic risk reduction. Left side sugical procedure: Adapted from Atlas of Metabolic and Weight Loss Surgery published by Cine-Med Publishing, Inc., 2010, www.cine-med.com. Right side non-surgical procedure: Reproduced with permission from Mechanick JI, Apovian C, Brethauer S, et al. Clinical Practice Guidelines for the Perioperative Nutrition, Metabolic, and Nonsurgical Support of Patients Undergoing Bariatric Procedures - 2019 Update: Cosponsored by American Association of Clinical Endocrinologists/American College of Endocrinology, The Obesity Society, American Society for Metabolic and Bariatric Surgery, Obesity Medicine Association, and American Society of Anesthesiologists. *Obesity.* 2020 Apr;28(4):O1-O58.

and current data metrics, collaborative teams and communication, community resources, and self-management strategies.

Lifestyle Medicine

Lifestyle medicine anchors preventive and therapeutic strategies for all types of diabetes, and is defined as the nonpharmacological and nonprocedural management of chronic disease.[125] Though nutrition and healthy eating patterns constitute the mainstay of lifestyle intervention, other modalities target physical inactivity, healthy behaviors and stress reduction, tobacco cessation (including e-cigarettes), alcohol moderation, and sleep hygiene (targeting 7 hours/night and referral to specialist for sleep apnea or other disturbances).[126–128] The complexity of lifestyle interventions, adipokines, and the CV system has been reviewed elsewhere.[67]

Nutrition: In patients with T1D, the major emphasis of lifestyle medicine is synchronizing carbohydrate consumption and physical activity with insulin administration to avoid hyperglycemia, hypoglycemia, and excessive glycemic variability. Carbohydrate counting should be taught to patients with T1D or other insulin-requiring states. Regular and consistent intake of healthy carbohydrates (fibers, nonstarchy plants, whole grains and pulses, and other low glycemic index foods, with minimal processing and added/refined sugars, especially sugar-sweetened beverages) at standard mealtimes, with predictable snacking, and with Registered Dietitian Nutritionist (RDN) oversight and counseling is advised. Formal medical nutrition therapy should be implemented for all patients, which is reimbursable in many instances. Foods with adequate protein and healthy fats are advised.

In patients with T2D the major emphasis of lifestyle medicine is on healthy eating and achieving a healthy body weight and composition. The nutritional guidelines above for healthy

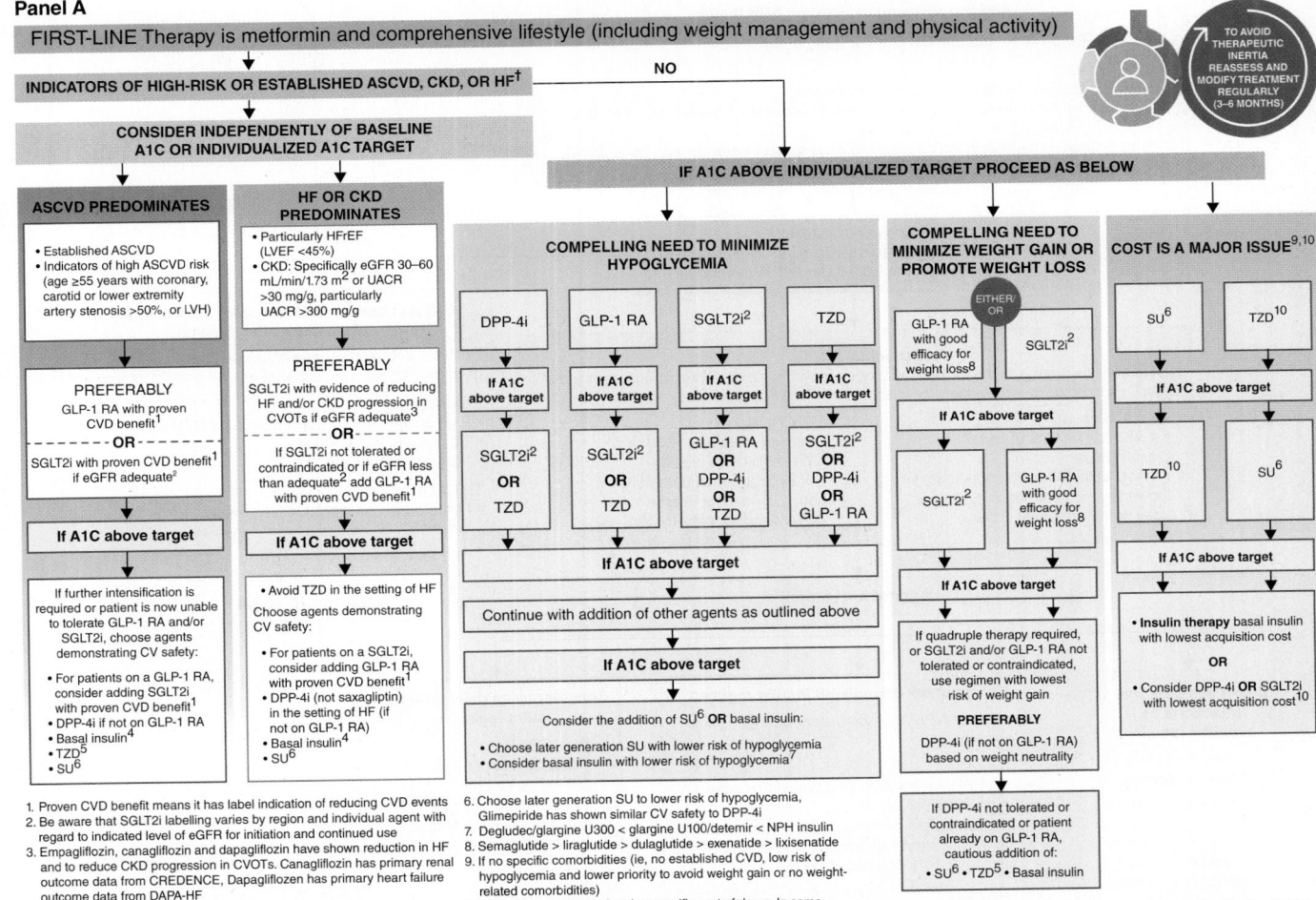

Figure 7–4. Clinical practice algorithms on diabetes management. Panel A—American Diabetes Association algorithm for glucose-lowering therapy in patients with T2D. Panel B—American Diabetes Association algorithm for injectable glucose-lowering therapies in patients with diabetes. Panel C—American Association of Clinical Endocrinologists algorithm for glycemic control in patients with T2D. Panel D—American Association of Clinical Endocrinologists algorithm for adding/intensifying insulin in patients with diabetes. Panel A & B, Modified with permission from American Diabetes Association.[9] Pharmacologic Approaches to Glycemic Treatment: Standards of Medical Care in Diabetes-2020, Diabetes Care. 2020 Jan;43(Suppl 1):S98-S110. Panel C–E, Modified with permission from Garber AJ, Handelsman Y, Grunberger G, et al. Consensus Statement by the American Association of Clinical Endocrinologists and American College of Endocrinology on the Comprehensive Type 2 Diabetes Management Algorithm - 2020 Executive Summary. *Endocr Pract.* 2020 Jan;26(1):107-139.

Panel B

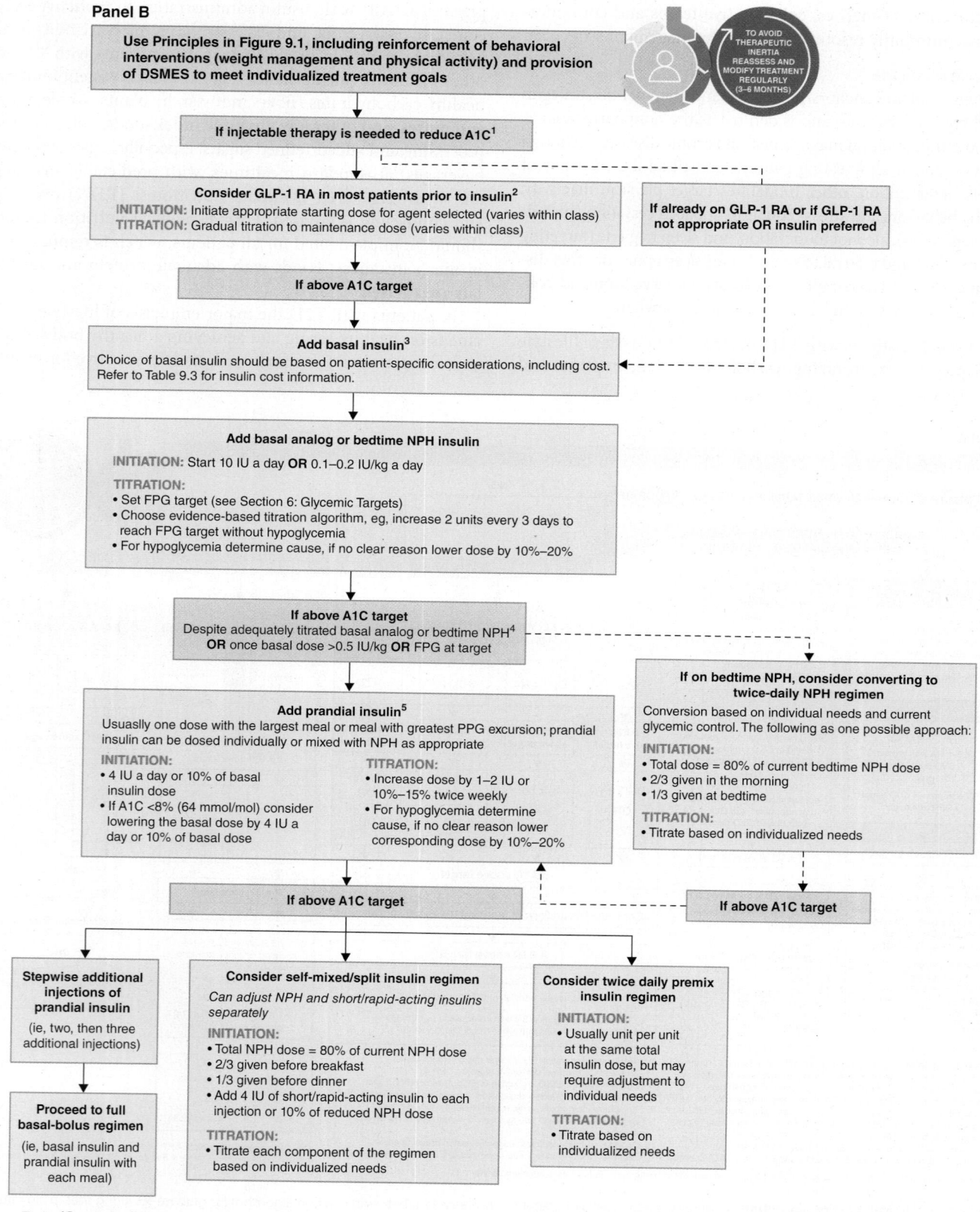

Use Principles in Figure 9.1, including reinforcement of behavioral interventions (weight management and physical activity) and provision of DSMES to meet individualized treatment goals

TO AVOID THERAPEUTIC INERTIA REASSESS AND MODIFY TREATMENT REGULARLY (3–6 MONTHS)

If injectable therapy is needed to reduce A1C[1]

Consider GLP-1 RA in most patients prior to insulin[2]
INITIATION: Initiate appropriate starting dose for agent selected (varies within class)
TITRATION: Gradual titration to maintenance dose (varies within class)

If already on GLP-1 RA or if GLP-1 RA not appropriate OR insulin preferred

If above A1C target

Add basal insulin[3]
Choice of basal insulin should be based on patient-specific considerations, including cost. Refer to Table 9.3 for insulin cost information.

Add basal analog or bedtime NPH insulin

INITIATION: Start 10 IU a day **OR** 0.1–0.2 IU/kg a day

TITRATION:
• Set FPG target (see Section 6: Glycemic Targets)
• Choose evidence-based titration algorithm, eg, increase 2 units every 3 days to reach FPG target without hypoglycemia
• For hypoglycemia determine cause, if no clear reason lower dose by 10%–20%

If above A1C target
Despite adequately titrated basal analog or bedtime NPH[4]
OR once basal dose >0.5 IU/kg **OR** FPG at target

If on bedtime NPH, consider converting to twice-daily NPH regimen
Conversion based on individual needs and current glycemic control. The following as one possible approach:

INITIATION:
• Total dose = 80% of current bedtime NPH dose
• 2/3 given in the morning
• 1/3 given at bedtime

TITRATION:
• Titrate based on individualized needs

Add prandial insulin[5]
Usuasly one dose with the largest meal or meal with greatest PPG excursion; prandial insulin can be dosed individually or mixed with NPH as appropriate

INITIATION:
• 4 IU a day or 10% of basal insulin dose
• If A1C <8% (64 mmol/mol) consider lowering the basal dose by 4 IU a day or 10% of basal dose

TITRATION:
• Increase dose by 1–2 IU or 10%–15% twice weekly
• For hypoglycemia determine cause, if no clear reason lower corresponding dose by 10%–20%

If above A1C target

If above A1C target

Stepwise additional injections of prandial insulin
(ie, two, then three additional injections)

Proceed to full basal-bolus regimen
(ie, basal insulin and prandial insulin with each meal)

Consider self-mixed/split insulin regimen
Can adjust NPH and short/rapid-acting insulins separately
INITIATION:
• Total NPH dose = 80% of current NPH dose
• 2/3 given before breakfast
• 1/3 given before dinner
• Add 4 IU of short/rapid-acting insulin to each injection or 10% of reduced NPH dose

TITRATION:
• Titrate each component of the regimen based on individualized needs

Consider twice daily premix insulin regimen
INITIATION:
• Usually unit per unit at the same total insulin dose, but may require adjustment to individual needs

TITRATION:
• Titrate based on individualized needs

Figure 7–4. (Continued)

Panel C

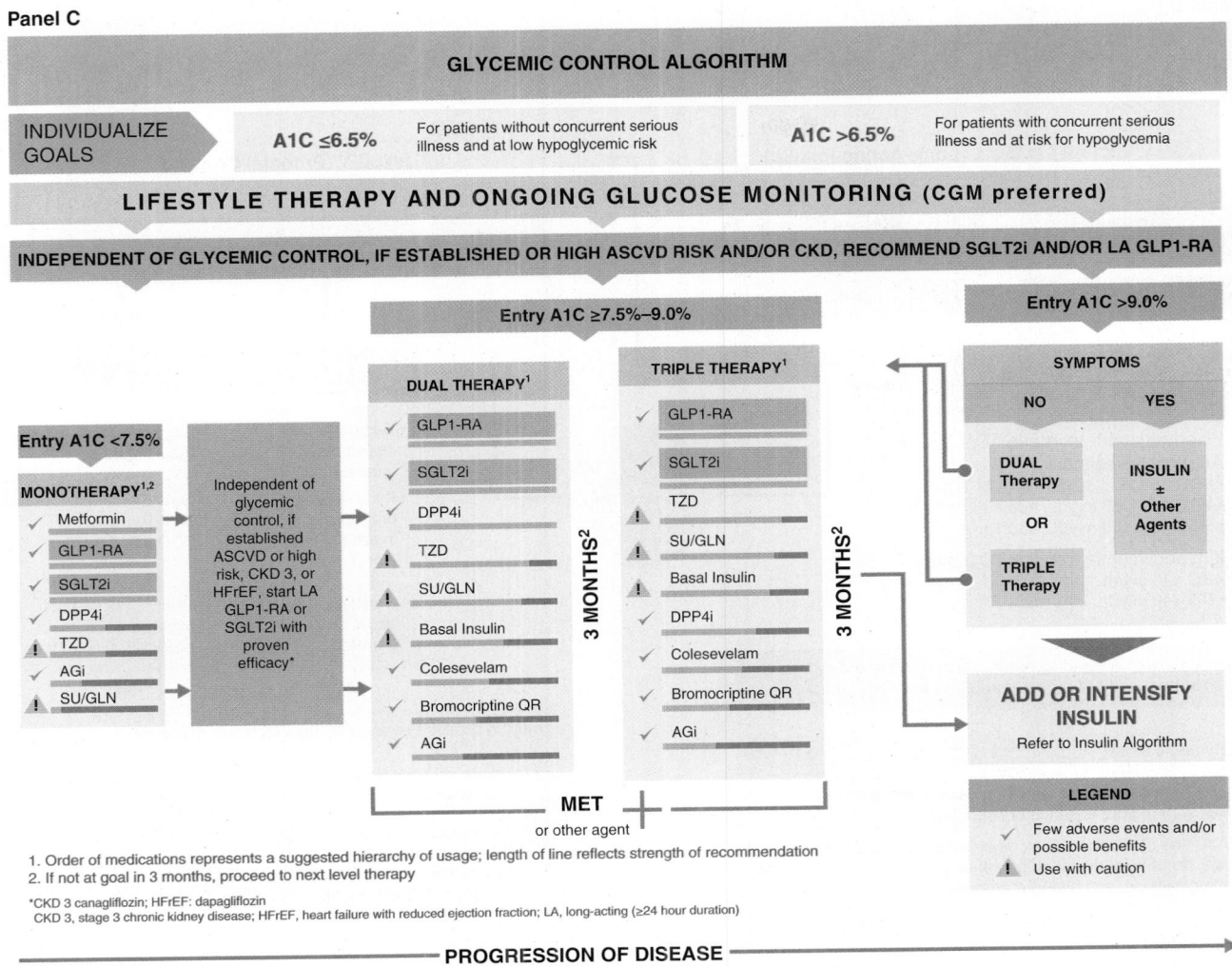

Figure 7–4. (Continued)

carbohydrates, protein, and fat also apply for patients with T2D. The management of abnormal adiposity within the CMBCD framework facilitates glycemic control and is complication-centric with respect to % weight loss needed for a desirable effect on a specific obesity-related complication. For instance, a weight loss of 5% to 7% is advised for patients with prediabetes and overweight/obesity to decrease the risk of T2D, 5% or more for those with T2D to reduce cardiometabolic risks, and >10% to 20% to address sleep apnea and nonalcoholic fatty liver disease or steatohepatitis.[129] In general, weight loss is achieved through a mild and consistent dietary energy deficit, such as 500–1000 kcal/d, corresponding in many patients to a loss of 1–2 pounds/week. This may be represented by a calorie controlled eating pattern of 1000–1200 kcal/d for women and 1200–1600 kcal/d for men. Failure to achieve weight loss targets should prompt consideration of weight loss medications or bariatric procedures. On the other hand, unintentional weight loss (not associated with beneficial lifestyle change) should trigger an evaluation for comorbidities and poor health.[130]

All patients should have height, weight, BMI calculations, and WC measurements, to assess cardiometabolic risk. There are many healthy eating patterns that can be individualized for glycemic control, overall health promotion, and weight loss/maintenance, though patient adherence is more important than the specific macronutrient composition.[131] One of the most evidence-based eating patterns for diabetes and cardioprotection, the Mediterranean Diet (MD; originally coined by Ansel Keys), is rich in fruits, vegetables, and olive oil, with the addition of chickpeas, bulgur, couscous, lentils, and fava beans. It is very limited in red meat and eggs. Emerging evidence has shown that adoption of the MD has positive effects on the progression of T2D and on CV outcomes. Shai et al.[132] first showed that the development and progression of T2D could be markedly reduced with the MD. After a revision to the original 2013 report of the landmark PREDIMED trial and acknowledging that not all of the patients may have been randomized, the final trial assigned 7447 patients at risk for, but without overt CVD, to three distinct diets: MD with extra-virgin olive oil,[84] MD with mixed nuts, or a reduced dietary fat control diet. For the

Panel D

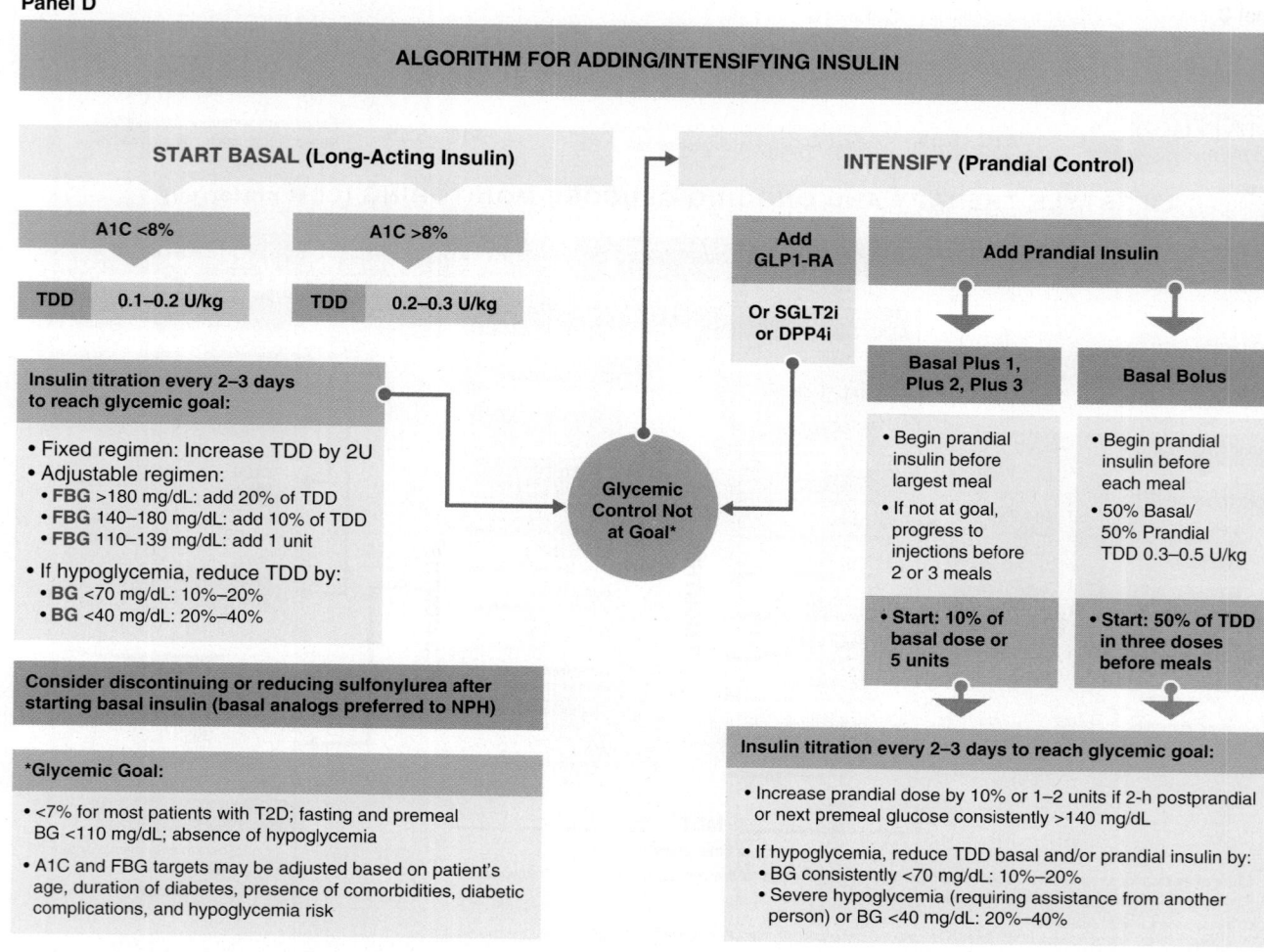

Figure 7–4. (Continued)

primary major adverse cardiac event (MACE) endpoint, and when compared to the control arm, the HR was 0.69 (95% CI, 0.53–0.91) for a MD with extra-virgin olive oil, and 0.72 (95% CI, 0.54–0.95) for a MD with nuts.

In the hospital, medical nutrition therapy should be provided to patients with diabetes, especially those managed with insulin. This consists of healthy eating patterns, adequate protein-energy, consistent carbohydrate meal plans, and a coordinated, safe transition to outpatient care.[133] Diabetes-specific nutritional formulas can be used as meal or snack replacements in patients with inconsistent intake (particularly with procedural interruptions where meals are held), and as tube feeds (particularly to control prandial glucose excursions with bolus feeding); in the ICU, this approach is associated with decreased mortality and cost savings.[134] An RDN should be consulted to implement and supervise medical nutrition therapy, as well as provide routine dietary counseling for all patients with diabetes.

There is insufficient evidence to support routine supplementation with micronutrients as dietary supplements or nutraceuticals in patients with diabetes, though the use of culinary herbs and spices with purported benefits on glucose

metabolism, diabetes complications and symptoms, and insulin receptor signaling may be safely incorporated into routine cooking practices and daily eating patterns.[135] Alcohol moderation is advised and though most guidelines advise <1 drink/day for women and <2 for men, a recent report on the global burden of disease supported complete avoidance of alcohol as part of a healthy diet.[136] Sodium intake should be <2300 mg/day for patients with prediabetes and diabetes. Nonnutritive sweeteners should be consumed in small amounts, if any, and the preferred beverage is simply water.

Physical Activity: Regular and predictable physical activity is associated with improvements in weight management, insulin sensitivity, glycemic control, and mitigation of other CVD risk factors (eg, HTN and dyslipidemia). Moderate-vigorous structured exercise should target at least 150 minutes/week (60 minutes/day in children and adolescents) and include safe, strength training, at least three to four times a week, after cardiac clearance, as needed. Greater activity levels of at least one hour per day of moderate (walking) or 30 minutes per day of vigorous (jogging) activity may be needed to achieve successful long-term weight

Panel E

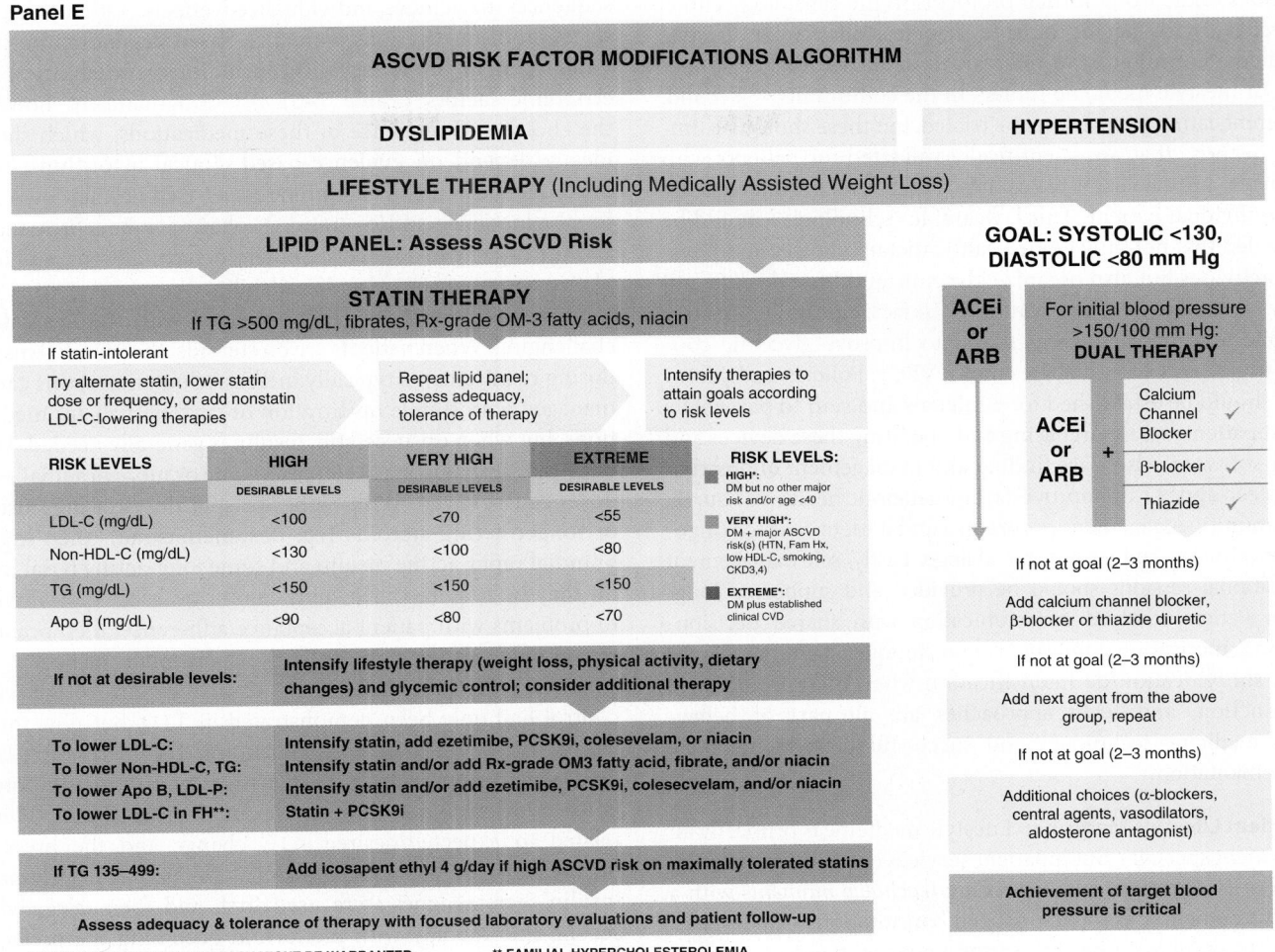

Figure 7–4. (Continued)

loss. High-intensity interval training was found to improve glycemic control, but not CV autonomic tone in patients with T2D.[137]

The American College of Sports Medicine now recommends that resistance training should be included in fitness programs for adults with T2D.[138] Resistance exercise improves insulin sensitivity to about the same extent as aerobic exercise. In older patients with diabetes, flexibility and mind-body activities (eg, yoga and tai chi) should be incorporated with aerobic and strength-training exercises.[127]

The NIH-sponsored Look-AHEAD trial of weight reduction and exercise in over 5000 patients with T2D sought to evaluate the role of modest weight loss and an exercise program on major CV events with at least 8 years of follow-up.[83] The trial was halted prematurely in 2012 due to futility bringing into question whether lifestyle provides adequate cardioprotection in T2D. The surrogate markers appeared favorable with a greater rate of modest weight loss in the intervention arm (4.7% vs 2.1% of initial weight was lost by year 8, p < 0.001) and with more than one-quarter of patients in the intervention group losing at least 10% of initial weight in the long-term. The real challenge in interpreting Look-AHEAD is that the control group was aggressively treated for CV risk through marked cointervention of evidence-based therapies.

Lifestyle Medicine Tactics: There are various lifestyle medicine tactics that can be employed to implement these strategies. First, large clinical trials demonstrating efficacy of intensive lifestyle intervention should be studied and adapted. These validated primary prevention programs can be scaled to a target population with appropriate reimbursement structures. In one pragmatic example, Diabetes Prevention Program (DPP)–like programs[139] reproduce study group interventions as closely as possible for weight management, glycemic control, and cardiometabolic risk reduction. Other programs demonstrating specific benefits of lifestyle interventions on prevention of T2D and related complications can also be emulated and include Look AHEAD,[183] Predimed,[84] Steno-2,[85] Da Qing,[119] and DiRECT.[186] Many lifestyle medicine primary and secondary prevention programs in diabetes incorporate a multidisciplinary and multi-modality (+pharmacotherapy/+procedures) approach.

Lifestyle medicine and other diabetes prevention programs can be leveraged in clinical practice in different ways. First, logistics range from: formal protocols in the cardiology clinic; to referrals to specific outside diabetes, obesity, or lifestyle medicine consultants; to referrals to dedicated diabetes, obesity, or lifestyle medicine centers in the community.[140] Second, different eating patterns can be trialed, but these should be limited to those that are scientifically validated for patients with diabetes, and also expected to have a high level of adherence by the individual patient. Third, wearable technologies should be provided that not only guide healthy dietary choices and physical activities but also organize glycemic and lifestyle data and provide "nudges" for motivation.[141] In fact, culturally sensitive mobile text messaging was found to improve glycemic control in patients with diabetes and CVD.[142] Policies and protocols should be established for clinicians and staff to personally assist patients with purchasing and operating these devices and their software. Also, case finding and management of obstructive sleep apnea can improve cardiometabolic health.[143] Fourth, community engagement programs can be identified for ongoing motivation and sustainable change. Lastly, self-management educational sessions should be provided and supported long-term. Patient-centered communication with shared decision-making, motivational interviewing techniques, cultural adaptation, simplification/de-intensification when there is cognitive dysfunction, and team approaches are all part of behavioral medicine techniques and successful lifestyle medicine implementation.

Inpatient Lifestyle Medicine: Lifestyle medicine is primarily an outpatient specialty, but inpatient services exist and are gaining popularity. Inpatient encounters are *teachable moments* with a captive audience, and personalized consultations can be fashioned to emphasize healthy eating patterns, types of physical activity, behavioral and mind-body techniques depending on cardiometabolic risk (eg, diabetes, obesity, HTN, and CVD), all within a chronic disease care model.[144] Evidence-based specialized programs can be implemented that involve art, music, imagery, massage, meditation, movement, and pet-assisted therapies.[144] Inpatient lifestyle medicine also promotes continuity of care for these therapeutic modalities and eases any fragmentation of chronic care that typically occurs with prolonged hospitalizations.[145]

Pharmacotherapy for Hyperglycemia

General: Various diabetes medications have exhibited primary prevention of T2D when given to patients with prediabetes in terms of various glycemic endpoints.[146] The primary prevention effects, expressed as risk reduction for T2D compared to controls, ranges from 49% to 89% for phentermine/topiramate (CONQUER/SEQUEL studies[147]); to 26% to 77% for metformin (DPP,[87] Chinese prevention study,[148] and Indian DPP[149]); to 55% to 70% for pioglitazone (ACT-NOW study[150]) and rosiglitazone (DREAM study[114]); to 45% for orlistat (XENDOS study[151]); to 25% for acarbose (STOP-NIDDM[152]). These and other medications constitute a larger portfolio of pharmacotherapies for the treatment, or secondary and tertiary prevention, of diabetes and its complications.[123,124] Many of these medications can be used in various combinations and

sequences to achieve individualized effects. Oftentimes, the selection of medications is nuance-based depending on individual patient preferences, comorbidities, availabilities, and economic factors (**Table 7–5**).[123,124] Pragmatically, however, the choice and sequence of these medications, which should ideally depend on evidence-based clinical algorithms, most often depends on clinician preference based on their own personal experience and/or training, pharmacy-benefit manager and third-party insurance formulary determinations, and local pharmacy supply chain and availability.

Glycemic control in patients treated with steroids can be challenging. When patients are on steroids, the prandial insulin dosing requirements typically increase. Sometimes, this can be managed with simple up-titration of current diabetes medications, but when unsuccessful, insulin is generally needed. With once-daily prednisone (4–6h peak), one or more prandial NPH doses can be given. With higher or split doses of prednisone, or longer-acting steroids (eg, dexamethasone), then higher prandial rapid-acting insulin and some long-acting basal insulin may be required. If insulin cannot be used, typically due to problems with patient acceptance/adherence, then prandial repaglinide or other noninsulin therapies can be trialed.

Historically, the benefit of intensification of glycemic control had only been demonstrated in T1D, but now this is commonplace in the management of T2D.[110–112,153–156] In a glucocentric approach to T2D management, the addition of glucose-lowering medications is primarily based on evidence related to expected/desired A1C change and the presence of any renal or hepatic impairment (Table 7–5). Originally, insulin secretagogues were used first, and then relegated to second-line therapy with metformin becoming the preferred first-line therapy.[157] Now, sulfonylureas are generally dissuaded based on adverse effects on appetite, weight (gain), hypoglycemia, and β-cell reserve (decreased). Incretin-based therapies (dipeptidyl-peptidase 4 inhibitors [DPP4is] and glucagon-like peptide 1 receptor agonists [GLP1ras]) and SGLT2is are currently viewed as the best add-ons, though this may change, as more evidence appears favoring GLP1ras and SGLT2is as potential first-line agents where cardiometabolic prevention is paramount. The use of insulin in patients with T2D is also dissuaded due to aggravation of weight gain, appetite stimulation, and hypoglycemia risk. However, insulin treatment in patients with T2D is appropriate to prevent significant hyperglycemia, hypertriglyceridemia, as well as DKA, not responding to noninsulin therapies, and usually in the setting of moderate-to-severe insulinopenia.

This management landscape changed beginning in 2008 when the US Food and Drug Administration (FDA) mandated that all anti-diabetic pharmacotherapies for T2D be subjected to evaluation in well-powered CVOTs (**Table 7–6**).[73,158–167] This was driven largely by a CV safety concern, but also afforded the opportunity to evaluate novel therapies for potential efficacy in reducing the burden of CV disease. Given the totality of the evidence, cardiologists are now well positioned to understand the clinical implications of these two new classes of agents. Guidelines have been modified internationally so that patients with CV disease are now considered for treatment with one or

TABLE 7–5. Diabetes Pharmacotherapy[a]

Class (ΔA1C)	Generic	Brand	Utility	Usual Dosing Strategy	Notes
Biguanides (−1.0–1.5)	Metformin	Glucophage Glucophage XR Riomet liquid Glumetza Fortamet	1st line T2D primary prevention T2D	500–850mg qPM to 2550mg/d	Dose po in middle of meal If GI side effects, consider XR) Avoid/limit alcohol use ↓ dose for eGFR 30–60 cc/min Hold for eGFR <30 cc/min
SGLT2i (−0.5–1.0)	Canagliflozin	Invokana	2nd line T2D 1st line T2D+CVD/HF/MA	100mg, then 300mg qAM	po; hold for eGFR <30 cc/min (except with MA >300 mg/day)
	Empagliflozin	Jardiance	2nd line T2D 1st line T2D+CVD/HF/MA	10mg, then 25mg qAM	po; hold for eGFR <30 cc/min (except with MA >300 mg/day)
	Dapagliflozin	Farxiga	2nd line T2D 1st line T2D+CVD/HF	5mg, then 10mg qAM	po; hold for eGFR <30 cc/min
	Ertugliflozin	Steglatro	2nd line T2D	5mg, then 15mg qAM	po; hold for eGFR <60 cc/min
GLP1ra (−1.0–1.5)	Exenatide	Byetta	2nd line T2D 1st line T2D+CVD/Ob/↑BG	5mg x 1mo, advance to 10 mg BID as needed	sq pen; ↓ dose for eGFR 30–60 cc/min hold for eGFR <30cc/min
		Bydureon	2nd line T2D 1st line T2D+CVD/Ob/↑BG	2mg q week	sq pen; hold for eGFR <45cc/min
	Liraglutide	Victoza	2nd line T2D 1st line T2D+CVD/Ob/↑BG	0.6mg x 7d, then 1.2mg advance to 1.8mg/d as needed	sq pen; no dose reduction for ↓eGFR
	Dulaglutide	Trulicity	2nd line T2D 1st line T2D+CVD/Ob/↑BG	0.75, then 1.5, then 3, then 4.5mg q wk advance q 4 week as needed	sq pen; no dose reduction for ↓eGFR
	Semaglutide	Ozempic	2nd line T2D 1st line T2D+CVD/Ob/↑BG	0.25mg, then 0.5mg, then 1.0mg q wk advance q 4 week as needed	sq pen; no dose reduction for ↓eGFR
		Rybelsus	2nd line T2D 1st line T2D+CVD/Ob/↑BG	3mg, then 7mg, then 14mg qD advance q 30d as needed	po; no dose reduction for ↓eGFR
DPP4i (−0.5–1.0)	Sitagliptin	Januvia	2nd line T2D	25/50/100mg qD	po; 50mg for eGFR 30–45 cc/min 25mg for eGFR <30 cc/min
	Linagliptin	Tradjenta	2nd line T2D	5mg qD	po; no dose reduction for ↓eGFR
	Saxagliptin	Onglyza	2nd line T2D	2.5–5mg qD	po; use 2.5mg for eGFR <45 cc/min consider avoiding with HF risk
	Alogliptin	Nesina	2nd line T2D	6.25/12.5/25mg qD	po; 12.5mg for eGFR 30–60cc/min 6.25mg for eGFR 15–30cc/min or HD
Amylin mimetic (−0.5–1.0)	Pramlintide	Symlin	2nd line T1D+postprandial ↑BG	15mcg, then 30/45/60mcg ac advance q 3d as needed	sq; no dose reduction for ↓eGFR reduce prandial insulin 50%
			3rd line T2D+postprandial ↑BG	60mcg, then 120mcg ac advance q 3–7d as needed	sq; no dose reduction for ↓eGFR reduce prandial insulin 50%
TZD (−1.0–1.5)	Pioglitazone	Actos	3rd line T2D	15–30mg qD ↑ monitoring with 45mg	po; avoid with HF/obesity/edema; √ALT no dose reduction for ↓eGFR
	Rosiglitazone	Avandia	3rd line T2D	4mg qd or 2mg BID after 8–12 weeks can double dose	po; avoid with HF/obesity/edema; √ALT no dose reduction for ↓eGFR

(Continued)

TABLE 7–5. Diabetes Pharmacotherapy[a] (Continued)

Class (ΔA1C)	Generic	Brand	Utility	Usual Dosing Strategy	Notes
SFU (−1.0–1.5)	Glimerpiride	Amaryl	3rd line T2D	1–2mg, ↑ by 1–2 mg q1–2 weeks Max 8mg qD or 4mg BID	po; start 1mg with ↓renal/liver monitor for ↓BG
	Glipizide	Glucotrol XL	3rd line T2D	5mg qD, then 10–20mg qD as needed Increase q 7d	po; start 2.5mg with ↓liver ↓50% with eGFR <50 cc/min monitor for ↓BG
	Glyburide	Diabeta	3rd line T2D	2.5–5mg qD, adjust to 1.25–20mg qD	po; ↓dose with eGFR <50 cc/min/↓liver monitor for ↓BG
		Micronase	3rd line T2D	2.5–5mg qD, adjust to 1.25–20mg qD	po; ↓dose with eGFR <50 cc/min/↓liver monitor for ↓BG
		Glynase PresTab	3rd line T2D	1.5–3mg qD, adjust to 1.5–12mg qD	po; ↓dose with eGFR <50 cc/min/↓liver monitor for ↓BG
Meglitinides (−0.5–1.0)	Repaglinide	Prandin	3rd line T2D	0.5 (A1C<8%)-1–2mg (A1C≥8%) ac Double q week to max 4mg ac tid	po; 0.5mg ac for eGFR 20–40cc/min hold for eGFR <20cc/min
	Nateglinide	Starlix	3rd line T2D	60 (near target)–120mg ac	po; caution with severe ↓renal/liver
AGI (−0.5–1.0)	Acarbose	Precose	3rd line T2D	25mg ac, then 50–100mg ac ↑4–8 weeks to 150mg/d (≤60kg) or 300mg/d (>60kg)	po; hold for eGFR <25 cc/min
	Miglitol	Glyset	3rd line T2D	25mg ac, then 50–100mg ac ↑ to target at 4–8 weeks	po; hold for eGFR <25 cc/min
Bile Acid Binding Resins (−0.5)	Colesevelam	Welchol	3rd line T2D	6 tab qD or 3 tab BID	po in water with meal hold with history bowel obstruction or TG >500mg/dl
Dopamine 2 Agonist (−0.1–0.6)	Bromocriptine QR	Cycloset	3rd line T2D	0.8mg qAM within 2h of waking ↑ by 0.8mg q week to 1.6–4.8mg/d	avoid with nursing, syncopal migraines, hypotension, and psychosis
Insulin (−1.5–3.5)			1st line T1D 1st line T2D + A1C > 9% 1st line GDM		
			2nd/3rd line T2D uncontrolled	Onset of Action	Time to Peak	Duration of Action
	Fast					
	Aspart	Fiasp		2.5 min	63 min	3–5 h
	Rapid					
	Lispro	Humalog		10–30 min	0.5–2 h	3–5 h
		Admelog		10–30 min	0.5–2 h	3–5 h
	Aspart	Novolog		10–30 min	1–2 h	3–5 h
	Glulisine	Apidra		5–15 min	1 h	4–5 h
	Inhaled	Afrezza		12 min	35–55 min	1.5–3 h
	Short					
	R	Humulin R		30–60 min	1–5 h	4–12 h
		Novolin R		30–60 min	1–5 h	4–12 h

(Continued)

TABLE 7–5. Diabetes Pharmacotherapy[a] (Continued)

Class (ΔA1C)	Generic	Brand	Utility	Usual Dosing Strategy		Notes
	Intermediate					
	NPH	Humulin N		1–2 h	4–8 h	12–24 h
		Novolin N		1–2 h	4–8 h	12–24 h
	Long					
	Detemir	Levemir U-100		1–2 h	6–12 h	12–24 h
	Glargine	Lantus U-100		1–4 h	no peak	~24 h
		Basaglar U-100		1–4 h	no peak	~24 h
		Tresiba U-100		1–9 h	no peak	>42 h
		Tresiba U-200		1–9 h	no peak	>42 h
		Toujeo U-300		1–6 h	no peak	24–36 h
	Premixed					
	NPH/lispro	Humalog-Mix75/25		5–15 min	2–4 h	14–24 h
		Humalog-Mix50/50		5–15 min	2–4 h	14–24 h
	NPH/aspart	Novolog-Mix70/30		5–15 min	2–4 h	14–24 h
	NPH/R	Humulin70/30		30–60 min	2–12 h	12–24 h
		Humulin50/50		30 min	2–5 h	24h
		Novolin70/30		30–60 min	2–12 h	12–24 h
	Degludec/aspart	Ryzodeg70/30		14 min	72 min	>42 h

[a]Diabetes medications are organized according to positioning in clinical practice algorithms. Second- and third-line agents are add-ons or to be considered if higher-level agents cannot be used. Utility is based on expected A1c change, cardiovascular effects, and side effect profiles. Pragmatically, medication selection should also be based on patient preferences and reimbursability. Combination tablets may be used once consistent dosing established to improve adherence: ActoPlus Met (pioglitazone + metformin); Avandamet (rosiglitazone + metformin); Avandaryl (rosiglitazone + glimeride); Duetact (pioglitazone + glimepiride); Glucovance (glyburide + metformin); Glyxambi (empagliflozin + linagliptin); Invokamet XR (canagliflozin + metformin); Janumet (metformin + sitagliptin); Jentadueto XR (linagliptin + metformin); Juvisync (simvastatin/sitagliptin); Kazano (alogliptin + metformin); Kombiglyze XR (metformin + saxagliptin); Metaglip (metformin + glipizide); Oseni (alogliptin + pioglitazone); Prandimet (metformin + repaglinide); Segluromet (ertugliflozin+metformin); Soliqua (insulin glargine + lixisenatide); Steglujan (ertugliflozin + sitagliptin); Synjardy XR (empagliflozin + metformin); Trijardy XR (empagliflozin + linagliptin + metformin); Xigduo XR (dapagliflozin + metformin); Xultophy (insulin degludec/liraglutide).

both of the SGLT2is or GLP1ras. First, CV specialists should be well prepared to prescribe these agents to the right patients. Patients with a history of HF should be considered for SGLT2i. For patients with a history of atherosclerotic CVD, both classes are appropriate. Meta-analysis demonstrated that the benefits of SGLT2i were observed in patients with established CVD (p for interaction = 0.05).[51] Similarly, the GLP1ras only definitively reduced three-point MACE in patients with established CVD.[51] The SGLT2is are favored for patients unable to self-inject the GLP1ras. The GLP1ras are favored for patients requiring more substantial weight loss to manage abnormal adiposity.

Metformin: For primary prevention of T2D in patients with prediabetes, intensive lifestyle interventions should be implemented first, with metformin specifically considered in patients with abnormal adiposity, other risk factors for T2D (eg, GDM or PCOS), or other MetS traits that increase risk for CVD. In addition, metformin can be considered in higher risk patients with prediabetes based on a fasting BG ≥110 mg/dl or A1C ≥6.0%.[45] For secondary and tertiary prevention in T2D, metformin offers the best combination of efficacy with safety

and relatively low cost meriting a "first-line" designation in algorithms. Metformin decreases hepatic glucose production by inhibiting glucose-6-dehydrogenase, stimulating insulin-mediated glucose uptake into skeletal muscle and adipocytes, and reducing intestinal glucose absorption. Metformin is used with caution in patients prone to hypoxia and/or lactic acidosis (eg, HF, pulmonary insufficiency, and CKD). Metformin dose reductions are warranted for eGFR <60 cc/min and should be avoided in patients with eGFR <30 cc/min. Metformin is typically continued until it is contra-indicated, replaced with full insulinization, or not tolerated. Other medications are typically added to metformin. Case finding for vitamin B12 insufficient/deficiency, preferably with a serum methylmalonic acid level, should be performed periodically, especially if there are neurological or even vague constitutional symptoms. All of the CVOTs reported herein were conducted on top of metformin. In a recent *post hoc* analysis of observations from the Saxagliptin Assessment of Vascular Outcomes Recorded in Patients with Diabetes Mellitus-Thrombolysis in Myocardial Infarction (SAVOR-TIMI) 53 Trial, metformin use was associated decreased all-cause mortality, but not decreased MACE.[168]

TABLE 7–6A. SGLT2i Cardiovascular Outcome Trials[a]

	EMPA-REG	CANVAS	DECLARE	CREDENCE	VERTIS
	Empagliflozin N = 7020	Canagliflozin N = 10,142	Dapagliflozin N = 17,160	Canagliflozin N = 4401	Ertugliflozin N = 8246
Median follow-up (years)	3.1	2.4	4.2	2.6	3.5
Mean age	63	63	64	63	64
Female (%)	29	36	37	34	30
BMI (kg/m2)	30.6	32.0	32.1	31.3	32.0
A1C (%)	8.1	8.3	8.3	8.3	8.3
Baseline eGFR	74	77	85	56	76
eGFR <60 ml/min (%)	26	20	7	59	22
Prior CVD (%)	99	66	41	50	100
Prior HF (%)	10	14	10	15	23
	HR (95% CI)	HR (95% CI)	HR (95% CI)	HR (95% CI)	HR (95%CI)
Three-point MACE	**0.86 (0.74–0.99)**	**0.86 (0.67–0.91)**	0.93 (0.84–1.03)	**0.80 (0.67–0.95)**	0.97 (0.85–1.11)
CV death or HHF	**0.66 (0.55–0.79)**	**0.78 (0.67–0.91)**	**0.83 (0.73–0.95)**	**0.69 (0.57–0.83)**	
CV death	**0.62 (0.49–0.77)**	0.87 (0.72–1.06)	0.98 (0.82–1.17)	**0.78 (0.61–1.00)**	
All-cause mortality	**0.68 (0.57–0.82)**	0.87 (0.74–1.01)	0.93 (0.82–1.04)	0.83 (0.68–1.02)	
MI	0.87 (0.70–1.09)	0.89 (0.73–1.09)	0.89 (0.77–1.01)	NR	
Nonfatal stroke	1.18 (0.89–1.56)	0.87 (0.69–1.09)	1.01 (0.84–1.21)	NR	
HHF	**0.65 (0.50–0.85)**	**0.67 (0.52–0.87)**	**0.73 (0.61–0.88)**	**0.61 (0.47–0.80)**	HR 0.70 (54–0.90)
Renal events[a]	**0.61 (0.53–0.70)**	**0.60 (0.47–0.77)**	**0.53 (0.43–0.66)**	**0.70 (0.59–0.82)**	

[a]Definition varied across trials for renal events. Figures in bold are statistically significant at p < 0.05.
Abbreviations: A1C, hemoglobin A1c; BMI, body mass index; CI, confidence interval; CV, cardiovascular; CVD, cardiovascular disease; eGFR, estimated glomerular filtration rate; HF, heart failure; HHF, hospitalization for heart failure; HR, hazard ratio; MACE, major adverse cardiac event; MI, myocardial infarction. Reproduced with permission from Mechanick JI, Farkouh ME, Newman JD, et al. Cardiometabolic-Based Chronic Disease, Addressing Knowledge and Clinical Practice Gaps: JACC State-of-the-Art Review. *J Am Coll Cardiol.* 2020 Feb 11;75(5):539-555.

Similar results were found by Charytan et al.,[169] in which metformin was associated with lower mortality and CVD event rates in patients with T2D and CKD Stage 3. The evidence for metformin and CV risk is currently sub-optimal, inconclusive, and largely based on the findings from the UKPDS trial in patients with obesity.[170] As with other medications, there have been various FDA alerts on potential adverse effects applicable to individual manufacturers of generic metformin, usually the extended-release formulations, and patients should be advised to check with their own pharmacists and prescribers with any concerns about these or future warnings.[171]

Sodium Glucose Transport Protein 2 Inhibitors: The SGLT2i class of diabetes medications block renal glucose resorption in the proximal tubule, thereby increasing urinary glucose excretion and eliminating significant kilocalories per day. Besides having significant therapeutic benefit in the management of hyperglycemia in patients with T2D, this class of drugs exhibits cardio-protection. To date four CVOTs have reported CV benefits for the three agents studied: empagliflozin (Empagliflozin Cardiovascular Outcome Event Trial in Type 2 diabetes Mellitus Patients [EMPA-REG OUTCOME]), canagliflozin (Canagliflozin Cardiovascular Assessment Study [CANVAS] and Canagliflozin and Renal Events in Diabetes with Established Nephropathy Clinical Evaluation

[CREDENCE]), and dapagliflozin (Dapagliflozin Effect on Cardiovascular Events—Thrombolysis in Myocardial Infarction [DECLARE TIMI] 58) (Table 7–6).[51,172-175] Independent of reductions in A1C between arms, the CV effects of SGLT2i were significant.[73] The four pivotal trials use the traditional three-point MACE atherothrombotic (CV death, nonfatal MI, and nonfatal stroke) and HF endpoints. EMPA-REG OUTCOME, CANVAS, and CREDENCE demonstrated reductions in a three-point MACE while in DECLARE TIMI 58 the three-point composite MACE was not met (HR 0.93, 95% CI 0.84–1.03; p-superiority = 0.17). For the HF endpoint and renal outcomes, all four trials demonstrated reductions in favor of a SGLT2i. Interestingly, empagliflozin was found to be associated with decreased LV mass indexed to body surface area, which may account for some of the observed benefit.[176] A fourth agent in this class, ertugliflozin, was evaluated in the Evaluation of Ertugliflozin Efficacy and Safety Cardiovascular Outcomes [VERTIS CV] trial and shown to be noninferior to placebo for reducing CV events in patients with T2D and established CVD, with a trend for beneficial effect on renal outcomes.[177] Meta-analysis demonstrated that the benefits of SGLT2is were observed in patients with established CVD (p for interaction = 0.05).[51,178] The SGLT2is were generally found to be safe and well tolerated. The most common adverse effect across the class was genital infection.

TABLE 7–6B. GLP1ra Cardiovascular Outcome Trials[a]

	ELIXA	LEADER	SUSTAIN-6	EXSCEL	HARMONY	REWIND	PIONEER-6
	Lixisenatide N = 6068	Liraglutide N = 9340	Semaglutide N = 3297	Exenatide QW N = 14,752	Albiglutide QW N = 9463	Dulaglutide QW N = 9901	Oral Semaglutide N = 3183
Median follow-up (y)	2.1	3.8	2.1	3.2	1.6	5.4	1.3
Mean age	60	64	54	62	64	66	66
Female (%)	30	36	39	38	31	46	32
BMI (kg/m2)	30.2	NR	NR	NR	32.3	32.3	32.3
A1C (%)	7.7	8.7	8.7	8.1	8.8	7.3	8.2
Baseline eGFR	76	75	75	76	79	75	74
eGFR <60 ml/min (%)	23	23	28.5	18	23	22	28
Prior CVD (%)	100	81	83	73	100	32	85
Prior HF (%)	22	18	24	16	20	9	N/A
	HR (95% CI)	HR (95% CI)	HR (95% CI)	HR (95% CI)	HR (95% CI)	HR (95% CI)	HR (95% CI)
Three-point MACE	1.02 (0.89–1.17)	**0.87 (0.78–0.97)**	**0.74 (0.58–0.95)**	0.91 (0.83–1.00)	**0.78 (0.68–0.90)**	**0.88 (0.79–0.99)**	0.79 (0.57–1.11)
CV death	0.98 (0.78–1.22)	**0.78 (0.66–0.93)**	0.98 (0.65–1.48)	0.88 (0.76–1.02)	0.93 (0.73–1.19)	0.91 (0.78–1.06)	**0.49 (0.27–0.92)**
All-cause mortality	0.94 (0.78–1.13)	**0.85 (0.74–0.97)**	1.05 (0.74–1.50)	0.86 (0.77–0.97)	0.95 (0.79–1.16)	0.90 (0.80–1.01)	**0.51 (0.31–0.84)**
MI	1.03 (0.87–1.22)	**0.86 (0.73–1.00)**	0.74 (0.51–1.08)	0.97 (0.85–1.10)	**0.75 (0.61–0.90)**	0.96 (0.79–1.16)	1.18 (0.73–1.90)
Nonfatal stroke	1.12 (0.79–1.58)	0.86 (0.71–1.06)	**0.61 (0.38–0.99)**	0.85 (0.70–1.03)	0.86 (0.66–1.14)	**0.76 (0.61–0.95)**	0.74 (0.35–1.57)
HHF	0.96 (0.75–1.23)	0.87 (0.73–1.05)	1.11 (0.77–1.61)	0.94 (0.78–1.13)	NR	0.93 (0.77–1.12)	0.86 (0.48–1.55)
Renal events[a]	0.81 (0.66–0.99)	**0.78 (0.67–0.92)**	**0.64 (0.46–0.88)**	0.85 (0.73–0.98)	NR	**0.85 (0.77–0.93)**	NR

[a]Definition varied across trials for renal events. Figures in bold are statistically significant at p<0.05.
Abbreviations: A1C, hemoglobin A1c; BMI, body mass index; CI, confidence interval; CV, cardiovascular; CVD, cardiovascular disease; eGFR, estimated glomerular filtration rate; HF, heart failure; HHF, hospitalization for heart failure; HR, hazard ratio; MACE, major adverse cardiac event; MI, myocardial infarction. Reproduced with permission from Mechanick JI, Farkouh ME, Newman JD, et al. Cardiometabolic-Based Chronic Disease, Addressing Knowledge and Clinical Practice Gaps: JACC State-of-the-Art Review. *J Am Coll Cardiol.* 2020 Feb 11;75(5):539-555.

In CANVAS there was a signal for an increased risk of lower extremity amputation and fractures with canagliflozin. This signal was not observed with the other agents and not replicated in posttrial registries.

Also, since only about 20% of patients with T1D are controlled, innovative adjuvant therapies using SGLT2is are being studied, but not yet recommended.[179] These medicines are available in pill form and for some patients, offer an advantage over injectables, such as the GLP1ras. Side effects are related to genital infections, primarily yeast, due to the glycosuria. Weight loss has been observed with SGLT2i use and in some patients, particularly older patients, unintentional weight loss can be severe enough to warrant down-titration or even discontinuation of the medication. Hypotension and dehydration can occur so patients should be advised to increase fluid intake. Euglycemic ketoacidosis has been observed in some patients warranting discontinuation of the medication.[180] Certain SGLT2i medications (eg, canagliflozin and empagliflozin) have also been shown to improve renal function in patients with diabetes and microalbuminuria, and though indicated for this reason in Stage 3 CKD, should be deferred in patients with Stages 4 or 5 CKD. In addition, recent studies have demonstrated benefit of dapagliflozin[181] or empagliflozin[182] in reducing hospitalization for HF in patients even without diabetes, further supporting a role for SGLT2is beyond glucose lowering.

Glucagon-Like Peptide 1 Receptor Agonists: The key incretins GLP-1 and glucose-dependent insulinotropic peptide (GIP) are secreted by the L and K cells in the small intestine, decreased in T2D, and when given pharmacologically, stimulate β-cell proliferation and delay the onset of diabetes. With respect to T2D, the GLP1ras increase insulin secretion in response to glucose, reduce glucagon secretion at nonfasting glucose levels, decrease gastric emptying leading to early satiety, and exert inhibitory effects on appetite, promoting weight loss and BP control.[183] These medications must be avoided in patients with a history of C-cell neoplasms of the thyroid. The risk for severe hypoglycemia is remarkably low. Liraglutide and semaglutide have been shown to have a potential increased risk of retinopathy and acute gallstones. Side effects are primarily related to nausea and other GI complaints. Concerns about associations with pancreatitis have not been sufficiently affirmed by clinical trials, though clinical monitoring should be performed. With the exception of oral semaglutide, these agents are self-injected daily or weekly. As with the SGLT2i class of drugs, the GLP1ra class has also exhibited superiority over placebo for cardio-protection, though subtle differences exist among individual chemical structures. Six of the agents have been evaluated in CVOTS with four of the injectables (liraglutide [Liraglutide Effect and Action in Diabetes trial; LEADER], semaglutide [Trial to Evaluate Cardiovascular and Other Long-term Outcomes with Semaglutide in Subjects With Type 2 Diabetes; SUSTAIN-6], albiglutide [Albiglutide and Cardiovascular Outcomes in Patients With Type 2 Diabetes and Cardiovascular Disease trial; HARMONY], and dulaglutide [Researching Cardiovascular Events with a Weekly Incretin in Diabetes trial; REWIND]) demonstrating superiority in reducing MACE compared to placebo (Table 7–6).[51,162-167] Exenatide and lixisenatide are derived from exogenous Gila monster venom and both agents have not met superiority in reducing MACE. Recently, a trial of oral semaglutide demonstrated noninferiority compared with placebo for CV outcomes.[184] Meta-analysis demonstrated that the GLP1ra class only definitively reduced three-point MACE in patients with established CVD, consistent with secondary prevention.[51,185] It is these salutary effects on CV health and weight loss that have repositioned GLP1ra drugs in a higher position in clinical algorithms. In addition, as with SGLT2i, the GLP1ra class of medications is also under investigation as an adjunct therapy in patients with T1D.[179]

Dipeptidyl-Peptidase 4 Inhibitors: The DPP4i class of diabetes medications exerts their action through inhibition of GLP-1 and GIP degradation, effectively raising the levels of these incretins. The DPP4is are available only in pill form, weight neutral, and without cardio-protection effects. The SAVOR TIMI-53, Examination of Cardiovascular Outcomes with Alogliptin versus Standard of Care in Patients with Type 2 Diabetes Mellitus and Acute Coronary Syndrome trial (EXAMINE), and Trial Evaluating Cardiovascular Outcomes with Sitagliptin (TECOS) trials evaluating saxagliptin, alogliptin and sitagliptin, respectively, showed HRs around 1.0 for the MACE rates when compared to usual care.[186-188] Recently, the Cardiovascular Safety and Renal Microvascular Outcome Study with Linagliptin (CARMELINA)[189] and Cardiovascular Outcome Study of Linagliptin versus Glimepiride in Patients with Type 2 Diabetes (CAROLINA)[190] investigators demonstrated the noninferiority of linagliptin, compared with placebo or glimepiride, respectively, on CV outcomes. Overall, the CV safety profile (noninferiority compared with placebo) has been seen as favorable to the diabetologists, but lack of any superiority over placebo rather disappointing for the CV community. Moreover, though the majority of DPP4is exhibited noninferiority compared with placebo, saxagliptin was actually inferior to placebo for hospitalization for HF.

Amylin Mimetic: Pramlintide activates amylin receptors, and similar to GLP1ras, decreases glucagon secretion, slows gastric emptying, and increases satiety. This drug is available as an injection to be dosed prior to a meal to decrease postprandial glucose excursions for use in patients with both T1D and T2D. Adverse effects include nausea, vomiting, headache, stomachache, fatigue, and excessive (unintentional) weight loss. In a pooled analysis of clinical trials, pramlintide was not associated with any CV adverse events.[191]

Thiazolidinediones: The TZDs induce peroxisome proliferator-activated receptor (PPAR)-γ binding to nuclear receptors in muscle and adipocytes, allowing insulin-stimulated glucose transport. There are demonstrable primary prevention benefits of TZDs for T2D incidence. However, the TZD class of agents has been scrutinized due to associations with edema and weight gain, precluding their use in patients with HF and relegating their position in clinical practice algorithms to third line. The pivotal outcome trial of pioglitazone—Prospective Pioglitazone Clinical Trial In Macrovascular Events (PROACTIVE)—was not definitive.[192] However, a comprehensive meta-analysis did confirm a favorable CV risk profile for pioglitazone.[193] On the other hand, the evidence for a cardio-protective effect of rosiglitazone is lacking. In fact, the meta-analysis by Nissen and Wolski[194] created a media firestorm by reporting a 43% excess in MI and a 60% excess for CV death for patients treated with rosiglitazone in clinical trials with an active comparator. Pioglitazone has greater beneficial effects on LDL particle concentration and size, TGs, and HDL-c, than rosiglitazone, which may explain the differences observed in clinical trials. Furthermore, in a pharmaco-epidemiological study by Mendes et al.,[195] CV risk was higher for rosiglitazone compared with pioglitazone. In short, pioglitazone confers benefit in terms of primary prevention, glycemic control, and lipid metabolism, but its role as an "add-on" agent needs to be weighed against the risks of edema and weight gain for a particular patient.

Sulfonylureas: This is the oldest class of oral medication for T2D. Sulfonylureas stimulate β-cell insulin secretion via (1) SFU receptor-mediated inhibition of the ATP-sensitive K^+ channel (K^+-ATP) causing membrane depolarization; then (2) voltage-dependent Ca^{++} channel opening allowing calcium entry into the cell; and then (3) insulin-containing secretory granule exocytosis. Commercially available second-generation SFUs have shorter half-lives than first-generation SFUs, decrease the A1C by 1% to 2%, and overall have a better safety profiles and are used more globally than first-generation SFUs, but are still associated with hypoglycemia, especially with skipped meals.[196] The SFUs have also been relegated to a lower position in guideline-directed diabetes management, not only due to the higher incident hypoglycemia rates, but also: increased association with higher CV risk; poorer outcomes; increased appetite and weight gain, thus exacerbating the insulin resistance and cardiometabolic risk; and accelerated decline in β-cell mass over time.

Meglitinides: These drugs act via β-cell membrane K_{ATP} channel closing and are therefore insulin secretagogues similar to the SFUs. They are short acting and are dosed prior to a meal to decrease postprandial glucose excursions. If the medication is taken but the meal is skipped, then the patient may experience hypoglycemia. However, with inconsistent meal timing, these drugs offer a distinct advantage since the medication can be synchronized for when the patient is actually eating. Based on the Long-term Study of Nateglinide+Valsartan to Prevent or Delay Type II Diabetes Mellitus and Cardiovascular Complications (NAVIGATOR) of 9306 patients with IGT and CV disease or risk factors, nateglinide use was not associated with reduced T2D incidence or adverse CV outcomes.[116]

Alpha-Glucosidase Inhibitors: This class of medications inhibits intestinal α-glucosidase resulting in slower carbohydrate digestion and absorption, and in effect, dampening post-prandial glucose excursions. There is no hypoglycemia associated with these medications, but patients can experience flatulence, upset stomach, diarrhea, and constipation. Among patients with IGT, the use of α-glucosidase inhibitors was associated with reduced incidence of T2D; among those with IGT or T2D, the impact on CV outcomes was neutral.[197] These agents may also have beneficial effects in patients with postprandial hypoglycemia due to accelerated gastric emptying.[198]

Bile Acid-Binding Resins: Colesevelam is a nonabsorbed, lipid-lowering polymer that binds bile acids in the small intestine. This depletes the bile acid pool, up-regulates hepatic cholesterol-7α-hydroxylase and hydroxymethylglutaryl (HMG)-CoA reductase, increasing hepatic LDL receptors and lowering serum LDL-C by 15% to 19%.[199] Colesevelam is also used for glycemic control in patients with T2D, in part due to increased GLP-1 secretion, splanchnic glucose utilization, bile acid induction of energy metabolism, and cholecystokinin secretion.[200] TG levels can increase with colesevelam and side effects include headache, myalgia, flatulence, constipation, nausea, vomiting, diarrhea, and abdominal discomfort. In a retrospective cohort study of 42,549 patients with T2D and hyperlipidemia newly starting colesevelam, increased adherence with the medication (by proportion of days covered by prescription claims) was associated with a lower risk for acute MI and hospitalization for stroke.[201]

Dopamine 2 Agonist: Bromocriptine activates dopamine type 2 receptors and modulates hypothalamic function to increase insulin sensitivity, possible by resetting circadian rhythmicity.[202] There is no hypoglycemia associated with this drug, but patients can experience dizziness, syncope, nausea, fatigue, and rhinitis. There was noninferiority compared with placebo for CV outcomes.[203]

Insulin: Insulin therapy is necessary in the management of patients with T1D and other forms of significantly insulinopenic or otherwise recalcitrant diabetes. For most patients with T1D, insulin dosing consists of (1) 50% of total daily dose (TDD) as rapid-acting insulin ("bolus" or "prandial" insulin) administered immediately before, during, or immediately after the meal based on the premeal glucose, carbohydrate content in the meal, anticipated activity level, and prior postprandial BG levels, and (2) 50% TDD as long-acting insulin ("basal") based on the fasting glucose levels. The TDD ranges from 0.4 to 1.0 units/kg/day (general rule of thumb = 0.5 units/kg/day) depending on the degree of insulin resistance (eg, increased with puberty, pregnancy, certain medications, and certain co-morbidities). In patients with T1D, glycemic control is associated with lower rates of microvascular complications as with

T2D, but also with lower rates of CVD events. Insulinization in patients is initialized along with lifestyle modification at the time of diagnosis and glycemic targets are based on risks of hypoglycemia, self-monitoring resources, age, frailty, or presence of multiple comorbidities.

Patients with T2D require insulin for glycemic control that cannot be accomplished with noninsulin modalities (lifestyle and other medications) alone. However, the weight of evidence from strong clinical studies on T2D supports dose-dependent associations of insulin with increased CV risk and mortality.[204] Potential mechanisms mediating this adverse effect include weight gain, increased hypoglycemia risk, and adverse effects of exogenous hyperinsulinemia on inflammation, atherosclerosis, MetS traits, and cardiac function.[204] As with patients with T1D, in patients with "insulin-requiring T2D," the type and regimen of subcutaneous (sq) insulin depends on synchronization with food (especially carbohydrate) intake. Subcutaneous insulins range in terms of rate of absorption and duration of action (Table 7–5). Currently used insulins are synthetic human or analogs of human insulin that are fast-, rapid-, short-, intermediate-, long-acting, or mixtures thereof.

There are three main insulin-delivering systems for chronic care as outpatients: syringe, needle, and insulin vial; insulin pen devices with attachable needles; and continuous subcutaneous insulin infusion or insulin pumps. U-100 (100 units/cc) formulations of insulin are typical. U-300 (300 units/cc) and U-500 (500 units/cc) formats for insulin as vials or pens are available for certain insulins, and particularly suitable when larger volumes are needed with significant insulin resistance, such as in patients with obesity. Insulin pump innovations, such as sensor-augmentation, are commercially available and associated with improved glycemic control metrics and outcomes.[121,205] Insulin pump settings are in terms of basal rates for different times of the day based on activity and circadian rhythms, boluses to be given with meals/snacks, and correction doses for hyperglycemia. The catheter is changed every 2 to 3 days, and abdominal infusion sites are most commonly used. Innovation with insulin pumps is ongoing, with many new features that, for example, adjust bolus morphology, closed-loop technology and algorithms, and programming to alert patients about impending hypoglycemia. Referral to a Certified Diabetes Educator (CDE) is recommended for patients on insulin pumps, as well as any patient with diabetes requiring additional support with diabetes technology, self-management logistics (eg, insulin injection, BG testing, and synchronization with diet), diabetes education, or individualization of diabetes care.

Inpatient diabetes management

All inpatients with diabetes, hyperglycemia, or risk for hyperglycemia should have an A1C within 3 months of hospital admission. The specific type of diabetes must be indicated, especially if T1D, in whom insulin must be on-board at all times. Insulin is the preferred glucose-lowering medication in the hospital for all diabetes types, though other agents may be used if available on the formulary and safely dosed in terms of patients' individual comorbidities. For inpatients, insulin may be delivered as sq injections, insulin pump infusions, IV boluses, dedicated IV continuous infusions for acute care, or IV in parenteral nutrition. Tight glycemic control is advocated for critically ill patients using intensive insulin therapy (via IV insulin drips), which vary by glycemic target (eg, 80–110 mg/dl, 100–140 mg/dl, or 140–180 mg/dl), duration (ICU days 0–2 or longer), and protocol (simple sliding scale; higher-order algorithms based on glucose, insulin rate, and changes; or proprietary software) according to institutional preferences, ICU culture, and physiological insult (eg, general, neurological, or cardiothoracic surgery; sepsis; and respiratory failure). Education for insulin administration may be provided by the physician, nurse, or CDE.

Perioperative glucose targets are usually 80–180 mg/dl.[133] Metformin and any other glucose-lowering medication should be held on the day of surgery, and only 60% to 80% of the usual long-acting basal dosing (sq or pump) the night before or morning of surgery. While fasting, glucose determinations should be performed every 3–6 hours depending on risk and corrected with rapid-acting insulin.

Patients with DKA require prompt insulinization with an IV insulin drip to lower the BG by approximately 100 mg/dl/hr until the 250 mg/dl range is reached, when dextrose can be added to the IV fluids to start rendering an anabolic state and avoid hypoglycemia. Patients also require aggressive volume with saline or a mixed solute infusion (chloride + bicarbonate/acetate) to help correct the acidosis, potassium, and other electrolytes, including phosphate with severe hypophosphatemia. Once the BG is at or below the 250 mg/dl range and patients are able to tolerate oral (or enteral) nutrition, then the IV insulin drip can be transitioned to sq insulin (with the first sq basal insulin dosed 2–4 hours before the drip stops). Patients with DKA typically have T1D, but they may also have late-stage, atypical, or otherwise insulinopenic T2D, pancreatogenic diabetes, or acute COVID-19 due to viral binding to type 2 ACE on β-cells.[206] Moreover, there can be elements of hyperosmolar hyperglycemia states that overlap with DKA, where fluid resuscitation takes on greater importance. Also, the SGT2i class of medications is associated with a euglycemic ketoacidosis state that resolves with discontinuation of the SGLT2i and hydration.[180]

Bariatric, Metabolic, and Diabetes Procedures

There are various surgical and nonsurgical procedures for diabetes management. Historically, bariatric surgical procedures have been recommended for weight loss in patients with severe obesity inadequately responsive to lifestyle and pharmacotherapy. However, this landscape has changed in recent years with respect to: novel surgical and nonsurgical procedures, clinical trials reporting improvements in glycemic control and CV outcomes, and guideline-directed protocols for these procedures to decrease cardiometabolic risk.[122] In fact, there have been at least 11 prospectives, randomized controlled studies demonstrating superiority of bariatric surgery over medical treatment on glycemic control and CV risk factors. Specifically, the Surgical Treatment and Medications Potentially Eradicate

Diabetes Efficiently (STAMPEDE)[107] and Mingrone et al.[108] trials demonstrated a significant remission or improvement in T2D glycemic parameters and other cardiometabolic metrics, with sustained reductions in BMI for both sleeve gastrectomy and Roux-en Y gastric bypass surgeries. Earlier observational studies of bariatric surgery cohorts have reported a lower risk of mortality and macrovascular and microvascular complications of T2D.[207] More recently, the Cleveland Clinic investigators published a landmark observational study on the long-term CV outcomes of patients undergoing bariatric surgery compared to matched patients with diabetes and obesity who were managed medically.[208] A six-point MACE outcome and all-cause mortality were reduced by about 40% during long-term follow-up. This study sets the stage for a definitive CVOT for metabolic surgery, which is currently under discussion. Evidence from Sweden and the Swedish national registries demonstrated reduced rates of HF, particularly in those undergoing Roux-en Y gastric bypass surgery.[209,210] The data for recurrence or severity of AF are divergent and warrant further study in CVOTs.[211,212] Taken together, the decision to proceed with a bariatric procedure to treat T2D, especially in the context of reducing CV risk, can be difficult but should take into account the following points:

1. Has the patient maximally benefitted from structured lifestyle and all available pharmacotherapy?

2. Is the patient at sufficiently high risk for significant morbidity that compromises quality of life and/or mortality due to uncontrolled hyperglycemia, abnormal adiposity, and cardiometabolic risk factors?

3. Did the patient have an adequate trial of optimal medical therapy (OMT) to reduce weight and cardiometabolic risk and were they adherent with the program?

4. Will the patient have access to an expert bariatric proceduralist, where the risks of the procedure are minimal (absolutely, and relative to the risks of not doing the procedure) and acceptable?

5. Is the patient agreeable to having a bariatric procedure and expected to adhere with postprocedure instructions and care?

Whole pancreas transplantation for labile T1D, refractory to medical therapy, is generally limited to those also undergoing kidney transplantation.[213] This procedure has been associated with restoration of insulin secretion with 1-year graft survival rates as high as 78% to 83%. Additionally, recipients experience reversal of glomerular and tubular basement membrane thickening and increased mesangial volume. Also, motor, sensory, and autonomic neuropathies reverse within 12 to 24 months after transplantation. Immunosuppression, viral and fungal infections, and increased risk of malignancy post-transplant are the main complications. Alternatively, islet cell transplantation can be considered but is experimental, involving the infusion of islet cells into the portal vein. At present, patients can achieve independence of exogenous insulin and improvement of hypoglycemic unawareness for up to 5 years after transplantation.[214] Obstacles still include donor availability and selection, engraftment, and adverse effects of immunosuppression.[214] Other procedures that are expected to gain in popularity with successful clinical trials include mechanical closed-loop sensors, closed-loop artificial pancreas, one of which delivers both insulin and glucagon,[215] gene therapy targeting auto-reactive T-cells,[216] stem cells,[217] and regenerative factors, such as harmine,[218] to restore deficient β-cell mass.

Diabetes Complications

Diabetes-specific complications need to be addressed in a protocol-driven manner, preferably with the assistance of a checklist or algorithm to avoid omissions and delays in detection and action.[123,124]

Microvascular

Nephropathy: Renal dysfunction is evaluated with annual 24-hour urine collections for creatinine clearance and spot urinary microalbumin-to-creatinine ratios, preferably in the morning. Values >30 mg/g creatinine (microalbuminuria) merit consideration of renin-angiotensin-aldosterone system (RAAS) antagonist therapy (along with glycemic control, sodium restriction, and adjustment of protein intake) to mitigate progression of renal disease. Analysis of the extant evidence on RAAS inhibition is confounded by pooled patient populations that have different pathophysiological mechanisms (eg, primary glomerular nephropathy with T1D, but multifactorial causes in T2D) and challenged by conflation of different endpoints: presence or absence of HTN, primary vs. secondary prevention, and cardio- vs reno-prevention. Angiotensin-converting enzyme (ACE) inhibitors (ACEi) were found to reduce: proteinuria; risk of CKD progression to end-stage renal disease; mortality in T1D; and microalbuminuria in patients with T2D, HTN, and normoalbuminuria. These effects are best observed with early CKD.[219] Even though there is insufficient evidence to recommend ACEi in patients who are normotensive and without microalbuminuria, physicians should still recommend case finding in patients with diabetes on at least a yearly basis. This is because the risk-to-benefit ratio of diagnosing microalbuminuria justifies treatment with an ACEi, if not for renal disease alone, but also for reducing the incidence of MI. While ACEi are reno-protective and cardio-protective in patients with T1D and T2D, the role of angiotensin II receptor blockers (ARBs; eg, irbesartan and losartan) is more narrow. Based on the weight of the evidence, ARBs may be favored in patients with T2D, HTN, macroalbuminuria (>300 mg/day), and renal insufficiency.[220] Since BP control is an essential part of reno-protection, and HTN generally requires more than one medication in most patients with diabetes, there are clear indications to add antihypertensive medications, namely calcium-channel blockers as second-line therapy. The use of certain SGLT2is (eg, canagliflozin and empagliflozin) has been advocated in patients with renal hyperfiltration (an early stage of diabetic nephropathy) to retard progress of microalbuminuria to frank albuminuria.[221,222]

Dietary protein restriction in patients who have progressive renal insufficiency will reduce accumulation of nitrogen-containing waste products and can have a beneficial influence on progression of renal insufficiency. In addition, the DCCT and UKPDS showed that the development and progression of microalbuminuria could be prevented through strict glycemic control.

Values over 300 mg/g creatinine are consistent with macroalbuminuria, are generally not reversible with RAAS antagonists, and along with patients with values >3 g/d consistent with nephrotic syndrome, merit referral to a nephrologist. A nephrology consult should also be considered for patients with a rising creatinine from 1.4 to >2.0 mg/dl, symptoms of uremia, microalbuminuria not responding to RAAS antagonism, and urinanalysis with red cells, pyuria, or casts. It is strongly recommended that renal arteriography be avoided in patients with diabetic nephropathy.

Neuropathy: All patients with diabetes should be evaluated for neuropathy, and those with neuropathy, evaluated for CVD. There are plenty of likely drivers for CV autonomic neuropathy, each representing a potential therapeutic target and ultimately contributing to the diabetes heart phenotype. Broadly speaking, glycemic control is the prime target in T1D, and management of cardiometabolic risk factors for T2D. Specifically, each of these pathways converges on vagal depression and sympathetic predominance, aggravating CVD as well as other diabetes complications.[271] A comprehensive therapeutic approach consists of: case finding and risk stratification; lifestyle change; weight loss when needed; management of tachycardia (eg, β-blockers), nocturnal HTN (eg, olmesartan and enalapril), and orthostatic hypotension (eg, midodrine, droxidopa, fludrocortisone, salt, pyridostigmine, acarbose, octreotide, desmopressin, and erythropoietin); avoidance/discontinuation of drugs with a negative impact; and addressing clinical inertia and patient adherence problems.[223] There are also emerging data showing benefits on CV autonomic neuropathy with SGLT2i and GLP1ra use, as well as vitamins B12, D, and E, and α-lipoic acid use.[223]

Retinopathy: Diabetes remains the leading cause of visual loss in adults, usually as a result of proliferative retinopathy or macular edema. Tight glycemic control reduces risks associated with diabetic retinopathy in patients with T1D (DCCT[80]) and T2D (UKPDS[224]). Protocol-based therapies have been reviewed by the UK Consensus Working Group[225] and include case finding programs, use of optical coherence tomography and wide-field imaging, home monitoring, intravitreal injections of anti-VEGFs and steroids, laser therapies, and various individualization options.

Macrovascular

CHD

Screening Asymptomatic Patients with Diabetes: The DIAD (Detection of Ischemia in Asymptomatic Diabetics[226]) trial publication answered an important question in the diabetes and CAD field: namely, what is the role of routine screening for myocardial ischemia in asymptomatic patients with diabetes? For many years, the American Heart Association had advocated for optimal management of coronary risk factors as frontline therapy. Colleagues from the American Diabetes Association (ADA) argued strongly for routine stress testing in these patients. Over 1000 asymptomatic patients were randomized to undergo myocardial perfusion imaging or no screening. After 5 years, there was no difference in the rates of nonfatal MI or cardiac death between the two arms. The DIAD trial demonstrated a very low rate of significant ischemia in the screening arm (about 6% with moderate to large perfusion defects) and a very high adherence to a robust medical risk factor modification program. In fact, the excellent medical therapy in DIAD is responsible for a very low 5-year primary event rate. The one question that remains is what is the best therapy for patients with moderate to large perfusion defects if they were to be treated aggressively in an adequately powered trial?

Stable Ischemic CHD: Patients with diabetes can present in an atypical fashion and patients are often unaware of myocardial ischemic pain, so silent ischemia and MI are markedly increased in this population. Therapeutic modalities in patients with diabetes and CHD revolve around standard therapy with aspirin, statins, β-blockers, calcium channel blockers, and nitrates. The outcomes of medical and revascularization management of obstructive CAD are often sub-optimal when compared to patients without diabetes. This is because in T2D, actual disease progression can outpace the detected extensiveness of disease, furthering the argument in favor of early prevention and comprehensive care. Clinical outcomes in CAD with T2D are poor despite improvement in medications and intervention devices.

Coronary Revascularization vs OMT: The management of patients with diabetes with CHD entails both pharmacological and revascularization strategies. Advances in the OMT of the patient with diabetes and CHD are based on emerging data on aspirin, β-blockers, statins, and ACEi use. These agents may provide clinical benefit not only by treating ischemia but also by stabilizing atherosclerotic plaque and inhibiting endovascular thrombosis, thereby preventing acute coronary events. In addition, the SGLT2i and GLP1ra agents have changed the landscape for OMT. Coronary revascularization procedures are a mainstay of therapy for CHD patients, providing both symptomatic relief and mortality reduction in certain anatomic subsets. Several studies have attempted to rationalize the use of different revascularization techniques by comparing them to OMT and to each other in various clinical settings, such as with vs without diabetes.

About one-third of the patients randomized in the Clinical Outcomes Utilizing Revascularization and Aggressive Drug Evaluation (COURAGE) trial had diabetes.[227] The trial demonstrated no difference in the 5-year MACE rate. Nevertheless, this required further confirmation. The Bypass Angioplasty Revascularization Investigation 2 Diabetes (BARI 2D) trial was a multicenter, National Heart, Lung, and Blood Institute–sponsored study.[228] The principal research question was whether patients with diabetes and relatively mild or no

symptoms could be treated with deferred (ie, receiving only OMT) compared with prompt revascularization (plus OMT). The important feature was that patients were randomized post-catheterization with anatomy defined and requiring at least one lesion to be amenable for revascularization. It is critical to emphasize that the decision to undertake PCI or CABG was left to the discretion of the investigators with the caveat that patients with multivessel and more extensive disease were more likely to undergo CABG. In BARI 2D, survival did not differ significantly between the revascularization group (88.3%) and the OMT group (87.8%, P = 0.97). Moreover, MACE rates did not differ between the two arms, but in the CABG stratum, the MACE rate was significantly lower in the revascularization group (22.4%), compared with the OMT group (30.5%, P = 0.01; P = 0.002 for interaction). These results suggested that OMT up front is a viable option in patients able to defer a revascularization strategy. The BARI 2D trial was an important contribution based on two key conclusions. First, patients with diabetes who are asymptomatic or have mild symptoms can be first treated with OMT alone. By 5 years, 40% of these patients will require a deferred revascularization procedure. Second, when OMT is applied, the A1C target of 7% can be achieved by an individualized approach.

More Aggressive CAD: Percutaneous Coronary Intervention vs Coronary Artery Bypass Grafting: The evaluation of coronary revascularization in patients with diabetes comparing PCI with CABG was enriched by a number of important trials: Coronary Artery Risk Development in Young Adults (CARDIA),[229] Coronary Artery Revascularization in Diabetes (VA-CARDS),[230] Synergy between Percutaneous Coronary Intervention with Taxus and Cardiac Surgery (SYNTAX),[231] and Future Revascularization Evaluation in Patients with Diabetes Mellitus: Optimal Management of Multivessel Disease (FREEDOM).[232] The SYNTAX program[231] consisted of a randomized trial of patients with three-vessel or left main disease comparing PCI with paclitaxel-eluting stents vs CABG, as well as two parallel registries of patients ineligible for PCI or CABG respectively. In the SYNTAX trial, about 28% or 452 of the 1800 patients had diabetes. At 12 months of follow-up, the only difference between PCI and CABG for patients with diabetes was the excess of repeat revascularization in the PCI arm (20.3% vs 6.4%, p < 0.001).[231] As expected, when compared to patients without diabetes, the 12-month rate of death, MI, or stroke was higher for the diabetes cohort (10.2% vs 6.8%).[231] Interestingly, when moving across the spectrum of nondiabetes to MetS to insulin-treated diabetes, the 12-month major adverse cardiovascular and cerebrovascular event (MACCE) rate for CABG was consistent between 12% and 14%, whereas, the MACCE rates for PCI progressed from 15% in nondiabetes to 30% in insulin-treated diabetes.[231] The SYNTAX program followed patients out to 10 years and the results confirmed the effectiveness of CABG over PCI in patients with diabetes.[231]

The CARDIA trial[229] evaluated patients with diabetes and multivessel disease exclusively to either drug-eluting stent (DES)-PCI or CABG. This 500-patient trial was underpowered to detect important clinical differences in death, MI, or stroke at 12 months.[229] In a noninferiority analysis, the primary event rate was greater in the PCI arm (11.6 vs. 10.2%, p = NS) but this failed to meet statistical significance.[229] PCI was not proven to be noninferior to CABG due to wide 95% CIs.[229] As in SYNTAX, there was excess repeat revascularization in the PCI arm.[229] CARDIA set the stage for the FREEDOM trial, which had 1900 subjects with a mean follow-up of 3.8 years.[232] The primary outcome (composite of all-cause mortality, nonfatal MI, and nonfatal stroke) was more likely to occur at 5 years in the PCI group as opposed to the CABG group (26.6% vs. 18.7%, respectively; p = 0.005). The %-year rates of nonfatal MI and all-cause mortality were greater in the PCI arm (13.9% vs 6.0%, p < 0.001 for nonfatal MI and 16.3% vs 10.9%, p = 0.049 for all-cause mortality), while the rate of nonfatal stroke was significantly lower in the PCI-DES arm (2.4% vs 5.2%, p = 0.03). Given the findings from COURAGE[227] and from BARI 2D,[228] FREEDOM[232] had strict medical management targets for both strategies. FREEDOM led to a Class 1 indication for CABG in patients with diabetes with multivessel CAD when using the heart team approach. In 2019, the long-term mortality benefit of CABG was shown in the FREEDOM Follow On trial.[233]

Another important aspect of the SYNTAX program was the derivation and evaluation of the SYNTAX scoring system for grading the complexity of CAD. Simply put, the SYNTAX score is the summation of the points assigned for each individual lesion in the coronary tree (divided into 16 segments). Esper et al.[234] from FREEDOM have shown that the SYNTAX score does not discriminate who will benefit from CABG, since MACE reduction is realized across all tertiles of the SYNTAX score.

Evidence suggests that later generation stents have closed the gap between CABG and PCI in patients with diabetes in terms of short-term CV outcomes. The Taxus Element versus Xience Prime in a Diabetic Population (TUXEDO) trial and meta-analysis that included patients from 68 randomized controlled trials showed that cobalt-chromium everolimus-eluting stents may be promising.[235] From BARI to the Arterial Revascularization Trial (ART) to FREEDOM, the point estimate for mortality remains unchanged so that it would be a mistake to continue to test the CABG vs PCI hypothesis without first demonstrating that systemic therapy with OMT can be improved to the point where nontarget lesions are no longer an issue **(Table 7–7)**.[236]

A large database of 190,000 patients 65 years or older from the American College of Cardiology Foundation, the Society of Thoracic Surgeons, Medicare, and Medicaid databases confirmed reduced 4-year mortality in CABG patients vs PCI.[237] This benefit persisted across subgroups, including patients with diabetes treated with insulin (risk ratio [RR]: 0.72; 95% CI: 0.66–0.78) or not (RR: 0.78; 95% CI: 0.72–0.83). This was confirmed in a population-based study from Ontario, Canada in 2020.[238] Head et al.[239] published an individual patient-level meta-analysis (N = 11,518 patients) demonstrating that when compared to CABG, PCI exhibited a higher likelihood of 5-year all-cause mortality in the subgroup with diabetes (N = 3266 patients; HR: 1.48; 95% CI: 1.19–1.84; p = 0.0004). As observed in FREEDOM alone, PCI was associated with significantly

TABLE 7–7. Coronary Revascularization Strategies in Patients with Diabetes and Coronary Artery Disease[a]

PCI can be Considered	CABG Recommended
Single-vessel CAD not involving the left anterior descending artery	Multi-vessel CAD
Frailty	Robust
Porcelain aorta	DAPT contraindications
Complications of thoracic radiotherapy	Previous PCI complications (eg, recurrent restenosis)
Limited life expectancy	Reduced left ventricular function
Multiple morbidities	Mild to moderate chronic kidney disease
	Need for combined surgery (valvular or aortic)
	Anatomy not feasible for PCI intervention

[a]Features to be considered in the clinical decision-making process of revascularization strategies in patients with CAD and diabetes. Abbreviations: CABG, coronary artery bypass grafting; CAD, coronary artery disease; DAPT, dual anti-platelet therapy; PCI, percutaneous coronary intervention. Data from Neumann FJ, Sousa-Uva M, Ahlsson A, et al. 2018 ESC/EACTS Guidelines on myocardial revascularization. *Eur Heart J.* 2019 Jan 7;40(2):87-165.

lower 5-year stroke rates in patients with diabetes (HR: 0.52; 95%CI: 0.37–0.75; p < 0.001; p for interaction = 0.004).[240] The increased risk of stroke appears to be most pronounced in the first 30 post-operative days. In a landmark analysis, stroke rates from the 31st day to 5 years were comparable between PCI and CABG.

Arterial conduits have been shown to have better long-term patency when compared to venous grafts, but concerns of sternal wound infections have remained.[241] In ART, there was no difference in the 10-year mortality rate comparing the use of bilateral internal mammary artery grafting with single internal mammary artery grafting, including the subgroup with diabetes.[242]

ACS: In ACS, diabetes is associated with more severe CAD; whereas ST-elevation MI (STEMI) is optimally managed by primary PCI, the revascularization strategy for non-STEMI (NSTEMI) is more controversial.[243]

The use of insulin and glucose infusion for at least 24 hours after admission followed by intensive long-term insulin was compared with usual care in the Diabetes and Insulin-Glucose infusion in Acute Myocardial Infarction (DIGAMI) trial.[244] A total of 620 patients with diabetes were randomized, and the trial demonstrated a 30% reduction in mortality at 12 months for the group treated under the intensive program.[244] However, the follow-up DIGAMI-2 trial (N = 1253), which compared three strategies—intensive insulin infusion followed by long-term insulin therapy, intensive insulin infusion followed by long-term standard glucose control, and regular metabolic control, was unable to show a difference in short- and long-term mortality and morbidity among any of the arms. DIGAMI-2 concluded that intensive glucose control was of great importance in the peri-ischemic period irrespective of the strategy used to achieve it.[245]

HF: Over time in patients with diabetes and CAD, microvascular dysfunction develops as a result of chronic ischemia, insulin resistance, and hyperglycemia, and coupled with the adverse metabolic effects of other MetS traits, can lead to diabetic cardiomyopathy. In many cases, both atherosclerotic disease and microvascular dysfunction coexist. Novel therapies have been tested to address the increased ischemic burden experienced by patients with diabetes and CAD. Ranolazine reduces the late inward sodium current and intracellular calcium, as well as beneficial effects on β-cell function and glucose-dependent insulin secretion.[246] Ranolazine lowers the weekly angina frequency when compared to placebo (3.8 vs 4.3 episodes per week, p = 0.008), as well as the use of sublingual nitroglycerin in the Type 2 Diabetes Evaluation of Ranolazine in Subjects with Chronic Stable Angina (TERISA) trial.[247] Ranolazine has been evaluated in microvascular CHD and works by favoring myocardial relaxation and diastolic microvascular perfusion. Four trials have demonstrated the potential effectiveness of ranolazine in coronary MVD: patients with reduced coronary flow reserve and exercise-induced myocardial ischemia without coronary obstructive disease.[248–251] In a secondary analysis of the Ranolazine in Patients with Incomplete Revascularization after Percutaneous Coronary Intervention (RIVER-PCI) trial, ranolazine was found to reduce angina in patients more when the A1C was ≥7.5%, compared with <7.5%.[252] However, in an analysis from the CARISA trial, ranolazine produced similar improvements in angina frequency, exercise parameters, and nitroglycerin use in the diabetes and no diabetes groups.[253]

Ranolazine can be considered as chronic therapy in diabetes as there are definite A1C lowering effects when used in patients with diabetes and CAD. In patients with diabetes, the potential benefits in diastolic dysfunction positions ranolazine a therapeutic option. In patients without diabetes it can also be used on a chronic basis in selected patients.[254]

Coronary MVD is now strongly linked to HFpEF. Indeed, HFpEF is characterized by the absence of a relevant reduction of LV ejection fraction. The management of HFpEF is typically diuretic therapy and usually includes β-blockers and ACEi, but evidence for this is sparse. No therapeutic intervention has been shown to consistently improve patient outcomes; consequently, the treatment for both coronary MVD and HFpEF is mainly empirical. By tackling the underlying impairment in coronary flow reserve and treating traditional and novel risk factors in patients with diabetes, progress is likely to be realized.[255]

Recently, a number of novel therapies for patients with HFrEF have emerged. A dual angiotensin receptor-neprilysin inhibitor (ARNi; sacubitril-valsartan) combination improved insulin sensitivity and glucose control in T2D in the Prospective comparison of ARNI with ACEI to Determine Impact on Global Mortality and morbidity in Heart Failure (PARADIGM-HF) trial.[256] The findings of the PARADIGM-HF trial demonstrated that the sacubitril-valsartan combination was superior to enalapril in reducing the combination of mortality and hospitalization for HF, but the Prospective Comparison of ARNI with ARB Global Outcomes in HF With Preserved Ejection Fraction (PARAGON-HF) trial failed to show that sacubitril-valsartan reduced adverse events among patients with HFpEF.[257] The Dapagliflozin and Prevention of Adverse Outcomes in Heart Failure (DAPA-HF) trial evaluating the SGLT2i, dapagliflozin, showed an impressive reduction in worsening HF and death in patients HFrEF, with and without diabetes.[181] Beyond mortality and hospitalization for HF, quality of life metrics also deserve consideration. The Change the Management of Patients with Heart Failure (CHAMP-HF) registry evaluated the longitudinal clinical features of HFrEF diagnosis and management across the United States over 18 months.[258] Across major classes of HF drugs, patients with diabetes are often underdosed. Unfortunately, the current mainstays of T2D therapy are still metformin, SFUs, and insulin with poor uptake of the cardio-protective SGLT2i and GLP1ra agents. Of particular significance, SFUs and insulin are associated with higher incident hypoglycemia rates, which in turn, are also associated with increased risk for hospitalization for HF.[259]

AF: The early treatment of tachyarrhythmias is important since increased ventricular rates and loss of atrial systole result in more cardiac ischemia and lead to a reduction in cardiac output. Among patients with diabetes and AF, treatment focuses on control of hyperglycemia, HTN, and the pro-thrombotic state. Drivers of CVD in diabetes contribute to many complications, and in the case of AF, the key pathophysiological steps that may be targetable are increased sympathetic activity, with resultant atrial fibrosis and electrical remodeling. With abnormal adiposity, there is also inflammation and peri/epi-cardial fat accumulation, which contributes to the increased AF risk.[50] Weight loss with structured lifestyle change[260,261] with/without bariatric surgery[211] can reduce AF risk.

Diabetes medications that lower insulin resistance (eg, TZDs[262]) may also decrease AF risk, whereas diabetes medications that can cause hypoglycemia (eg, insulin and SFUs[263]) increase AF risk. In the DECLARE-TIMI 58 trial of patients with T2D and ASCVD or multiple ASCVD risk factors randomized to dapagliflozin or placebo, there was a 19% reduction in the risk of AF or atrial flutter (AFL) with dapagliflozin, regardless of prior history of AF, ASCVD, or HF.[264] In a recent meta-analysis of GLP1ra clinical trials >1 year treatment duration in patients with T2D, there was no increased risk for AF.[265] The DPP4i appear to have a neutral effect on AF risk.

There are also special considerations regarding anticoagulant therapy for patients with diabetes as well. In patients with diabetes, the newer agents are more effective and safer than warfarin.[266] Dabigatran is a direct thrombin inhibitor, but is associated with more bleeding in patients with diabetes, compared to those without diabetes.[267] More bleeding is also associated with apixaban—a direct factor Xa inhibitor—in patients with diabetes.[268] On the other hand, diabetes was not associated with excess bleeding risk in patients treated with rivaroxaban, also a direct factor Xa inhibitor.[269]

VAs: As in patients without diabetes, premature ventricular beats and nonsustained ventricular tachycardia are common in patients with diabetes who exhibit cardiomyopathy or ischemic heart disease. It is critical to rule out cardiomyopathy and/or ischemia in these patients. Similarly, the prognosis with sustained ventricular tachycardia or resuscitated SCD is no different in those with or without diabetes.

The key message regarding initial VA and diabetes care is that hypoglycemia is a distinct risk factor.[270] In a nationwide cohort study of patients with T2D, hypoglycemic episodes were associated with VA and sudden cardiac arrest events, with insulin exposure further increasing this risk.[271] Hyperglycemia also increases the risk for ventricular tachycardia after MI, arguing for diligent attention to glycemic control in this population, but with medications exerting minimal risk for hypoglycemic events.[272] This poses a problem in hospitals with limited formularies for patients with severe hyperglycemia, where insulin and SFUs are frequently used and newer agents (eg, SGLT2i and GLP1ra) are not available.

The management of VAs is similar for patients with and without diabetes. Patients surviving SCD are candidates for an implantable defibrillator as are patients with a LV ejection fraction less than 30% to 35%. There are no clear data distinguishing prognosis or management between T1D and T2D.

Cerebrovascular Disease: Management should concentrate on OMT with evidence that glycemic control and BP treatment are the cornerstones. The evidence suggests that HTN is the most important single risk factor increasing the risk of stroke by 30% to 40%.[273] The RAAS antagonists—ACEis and ARBs—have demonstrated the greatest efficacy in the prevention of stroke.

PAD: The management of PAD is based on optimization of medical therapy. Poor glycemic control is linked to a greater prevalence of PAD, need for revascularization, and amputation.[274] Revascularization, either a surgical or endovascular approach is reserved for treatment of symptomatic PAD and/or in those with CLI. Primary graft patency is improved with glycemic control at the time of a procedure.[274]

Overall, survival in patients with diabetes who are free of amputation is comparable for endovascular and surgical approaches.[275] Guidelines recommend that arterial revascularization should be considered in those with CLI who have a predicted 1-year amputation-free survival of around 75%.[275] Furthermore, in CLI, immediate revascularization is superior to delayed revascularization. Optimal medical treatment of those ineligible for revascularization reduces amputation rates.[276] The presence of a diabetic foot ulcer is associated with a greater incidence of impaired wound healing and amputation. Optimal foot care is the most important preventive measure for limb preservation.

Cardiometabolic Risk Factor Mitigation

Abnormal Adiposity and Obesity

Abnormal adiposity is not only a driver of dysglycemia but can also result from certain diabetes medications (eg, SFUs and insulin). Therefore, weight loss medications should be considered in patients with T2D (an obesity-related comorbidity) and BMI ≥27 kg/m^2 (or ≥30 kg/m^2 without an obesity-related comorbidity) who are not responding to lifestyle interventions alone. Weight-loss medications currently approved for long-term use include orlistat, phentermine/topiramate extended release, naltrexone-buproprion, and high-dose liraglutide.

Bariatric procedures should be considered for higher risk patients with obesity, in which lifestyle and pharmacotherapy interventions are not successful for inducing sufficient weight loss or glycemic control.[122]

Dyslipidemia

Among high-risk patients with T2D and CVD in the TECOS study, only about a third achieved an LDL-C <70 mg/dl and a sixth <55 mg/dl, with each 10 mg/dl higher LDL-C conferring a 5% and 6% increased 5-year incidence of MACE and CVD mortality, respectively.[277] Management of dyslipidemia in patients with diabetes consists of case finding initially at age 40 years, then every 1 to 2 years, with institution of a plant-based diet containing viscous fibers and sterols, and weight loss as needed. Statins are the mainstay of treatment to reduce LDL-C[89–94] with ongoing monitoring to assess adherence with therapy.

Statins are the frontline therapy in lowering LDL-c levels in patients with diabetes, without having a significantly adverse effect on glycemic control. The goal for LDL-C is <100 mg/dL for all those with diabetes regardless of CHD. The Scandinavian Simvastatin Survival Study (4S) study enrolled 202 patients with diabetes and a prior history of CHD.[89] Although this study was under-powered, the comparison of simvastatin with a placebo showed almost a 50% reduction in coronary events in favor of simvastatin (45% vs 23%; p = NS). Similar trends were observed in the Cholesterol and Recurrent Events (CARE) Trial, which compared pravastatin with a placebo in secondary prevention.[90] In the CARE trial, the baseline mean LDL-C in patients with diabetes was 136 mg/dL. LDL cholesterol was reduced by 27% in the group receiving pravastatin, which translated into a 25% reduction in coronary events over 5 years, compared with that of the control group. The Heart Protection Study (HPS), with a subgroup of 5963 patients with diabetes, showed a 28% reduction in total CHD (nonfatal MI and CHD death), nonfatal and fatal strokes, coronary and noncoronary revascularizations, and major vascular events (total CHD, total stroke, or revascularizations) with simvastatin therapy.[91] In aggregate, trials of statin therapy in patients with hyperlipidemia demonstrate a relative benefit similar between patients with and without diabetes. The Collaborative Atorvastatin Diabetes Study (CARDS) trial showed that among 2838 diabetic subjects with at least one heart disease risk factor, but without elevated cholesterol levels, randomized to atorvastatin vs placebo and followed up for 3.9 years, statin therapy was associated with a 37% reduction in the primary composite endpoint of CHD death, fatal MI, hospitalized unstable angina, resuscitated cardiac arrest, coronary revascularization, and stroke.[92] In contrast, The Deutsche Diabetes Dialysis Study (4D), investigated 1255 patients with diabetes on maintenance hemodialysis, but was unable to show a significant reduction in CHD death, fatal MI, or stroke with atorvastatin compared with placebo.[93]

The current 2020 ADA recommendations for lipid lowering are presented in terms of primary and secondary prevention.[55] For primary prevention, moderate-intensity statin therapy is recommended in addition to lifestyle therapy for patients with diabetes aged 40–75 years without atherosclerotic CVD. For secondary prevention in patients with diabetes and atherosclerotic CVD, a high-intensity statin therapy should be added to lifestyle therapy; and if LDL cholesterol is ≥70 mg/dl on maximally tolerated statin dose, the addition of ezetimibe or a proprotein convertase subtilisin/kexin type 9 inhibitor (PCSK9i) is recommended (ezetimibe may be preferred on the basis of cost).[43]

Ezetimibe decreases MACE in patients with ACS and can be considered as an add-on in high-risk patients.[97] In the Improved Reduction of Outcomes: Vytorin Efficacy International Trial (IMPROVE-IT) trial,[97,278] there were 4933 patients with diabetes enrolled out of the over 18,000 total sample size randomized to receive simvastatin with or without ezetimide. The prespecified subgroup of patients with diabetes enjoyed greater benefit in CV reduction (5.5% absolute difference; HR: 0.86; 95% CI: 0.78–0.94), compared to patients without diabetes (0.7% absolute difference; HR: 0.98; 95% CI: 0.92–1.04; p-interaction = 0.02).

The PCSK9is alirocumab and evolocumab can lower LDL-C by 60% and are indicated in patients (with/without diabetes) unable to reach LDL-C targets with statins alone (due to suboptimal LDL effects or statin intolerance).[279,280] The PCSK9is bind to LDL receptors, leading to their degradation and reduction in LDL levels. At present, there are no specific differences in the efficacy and safety of these compounds between patients with or without diabetes. The Further Cardiovascular Outcomes Research with PCSK9 Inhibition in Subjects with Elevated Risk (FOURIER) trial was the first to report and enroll patients with prior atherosclerotic CVD with enrichment with a high risk feature where LDL-C remained ≥70 mg/dL on maximum tolerated statin therapy.[281] Patients with diabetes comprised 40% of the trial and were treated with evolocumab (either 140 mg every 2 weeks or 420 mg every month) or placebo.[282] For the primary endpoint of MACE, including hospitalization for angina and coronary revascularization, the HRs were 0.83 (95% CI 0·75–0·93; p = 0.0008) for patients with diabetes and 0·87 (0.79–0.96; p = 0.0052) for patients without diabetes ($i_{interaction}$ = 0.60). For MACE (triple endpoint), the HRs were 0.82 (0.72–0.93; p = 0.0021) for those with diabetes and 0.78 (0.69–0.89; p = 0.0002) for those without diabetes ($p_{interaction}$ = 0.65). Importantly, PCSK9 inhibition with evolocumab did not increase the incidence of new onset diabetes or worsen glycemic control. The Evaluation of Cardiovascular Outcomes After an Acute Coronary Syndrome During Treatment With Alirocumab (ODYSSEY OUTCOMES) trial evaluated alirocumab in patients with ACS.[283] For the primary endpoint of MACE plus hospitalization, the relative risk reductions for alirocumab were consistent across glycemic categories, with a greater absolute reduction in patients with diabetes (2.3%, 95% CI: 0.4–4.2) than in those with prediabetes (1.2%, 0.0–2.4) or normoglycaemia (1.2%, −0.3–2.7; absolute risk reduction $p_{interaction}$ = 0.0019).[98] Unfortunately, the cost for PCSK9i therapy may be prohibitive for the majority of eligible patients. In a study by Arbel et al.,[284] ezetimibe was a cost-effective medication compared with evolocumab as an add-on strategy with statins for secondary prevention of CVD events in patients with T2D.

In patients with diabetes and hypertriglyceridemia, fibric acid derivatives can lower TG levels, may raise LDL-C levels, and have not been shown to have a cardio-protective effect.[100,101,285] The addition of niacin and fibrates to statin has not been shown to provide any additional CV benefit.[98,101] Niacin can raise HDL-c levels in patients with diabetes.[98,99] The Reduction of Cardiovascular Events with Icosapent Ethyl–Intervention Trial (REDUCE-IT) randomized patients with atherosclerotic CVD or diabetes and one additional risk factor and moderately elevated TG (135–499 mg/d, median baseline of 216 mg/dL) to icosapent ethyl (IPE) 4 g/day (2 g twice daily with food) vs. placebo.[113] In this CVOT, there was a significant benefit in favor of IPE in both the primary expanded MACE endpoint and in the reduction in CV death, nonfatal MI, and nonfatal stroke (relative risk reduction 26%. P < 0.001). These benefits were found to be independent of TG strata. In the diabetes sub-group of a real-world study of patients with diabetes and ACS, one-sixth of patients met the REDUCE-IT eligibility criteria and would merit IPE therapy.[286] As a result, the 2020 ADA guidelines recommend that in the setting of well-controlled LDL-C levels, patients with diabetes and elevated TG should be considered for IPE therapy.[43]

HTN

The presence of HTN in patients with diabetes significantly increases their risk of micro- and macrovascular complications. Current guidelines distinguish the target BP based on the 10-year ASVD risk of 15%.[26] For patients below the 15% threshold, the target BP is <140/90. For those at higher risk, the recommendation is for a target BP <130/80, if it can be safely achieved. These targets are based both on observational studies and randomized trial evidence.[102,103] As with all other cardiometabolic risk factors, lifestyle change is the first-line therapy for HTN, including increased physical activity and a plant-based, Dietary Approaches to Stop Hypertension (DASH) diet. Pharmacotherapy begins with RAAS inhibition using an ACEi or ARB, with at least one medicine dosed at night.[287] The Hypertension Optimal Treatment (HOT) study showed that the risk of MACE in patients with diabetes was halved if they had a target diastolic BP ≤80 mmHg, compared with those with a diastolic BP ≤90 mmHg (p for trend = 0.005).[104] There was a lower but still significant decrease in the risk of silent MI and approximately a 30% risk reduction in the rate of stroke in the ≤80 mmHg group compared with the ≤90 mmHg group. The HOPE trial evaluated over 9000 high-risk patients with evidence of vascular disease or diabetes in a randomized trial comparing ramipril with placebo over a 5-year period.[105] A total of 3578 of these patients had diabetes. This study demonstrated a 22% reduction in primary CV endpoints of death, MI, and stroke in favor of ramipril. The beneficial effect of ramipril was observed over all predefined subgroups. Interestingly, there was a 30% reduction in a new diagnosis of diabetes in the ramipril-treated arm. The data from more recent evidence has still created controversy around the optimal BP target in a patient with diabetes. The NIH- sponsored Action to Control Cardiovascular Risk in Diabetes Blood Pressure (ACCORD BP) trial compared intensive BP control (systolic <120 mmHg) with standard BP control (target systolic blood pressure <140 mmHg), and showed that intensive BP control did not reduce MACE. However, intensive BP control did reduce the risk of stroke, but with increased adverse events. After ACCORD BP, meta-analyses demonstrate that antihypertensive treatment appears to be beneficial when mean baseline blood pressure is ≥140/90 mmHg or mean attained intensive blood pressure is ≥130/80 mmHg.[288–290] When lower targets are achieved, there is evidence that antihypertensive treatment reduces the risk of albuminuria, stroke, retinopathy, but not MACE.

β-blocker use in diabetes has come under great scrutiny in recent years. These medications are recommended for the treatment of prior MI, active angina, or HF, but have not been shown to reduce mortality when used for isolated HTN.[291] Furthermore, the use of nonselective β-blockade in patients using insulin or SFUs has been associated with prolonged hypoglycemia. However, in a large study of over 13,000 elderly patients there was no increased risk of hypoglycemia for β-blockers in patients with vs without diabetes.[292] Moreover, in a subgroup, observational analysis of patients enrolled in the TECOS study, baseline β-blocker use was not associated with severe hypoglycemia or CVD risk reduction over 3 years of follow-up.[293] Overall, the use of cardio-selective β-blockers, such as bisoprolol, is favored.

Atherothrombosis

In general, aspirin therapy at 81 mg/day is recommended with statin-based primary prevention for patients with diabetes over age 50 years (men) or 60 years (women) with at least one other cardiometabolic risk factor.[43] The effects of aspirin in patients with diabetes are still being clarified. For instance, there is a reduced immediate effect of aspirin on endothelium-dependent vasodilation in patients with diabetes, compared to controls without diabetes.[294]

The use of antiplatelet therapy is the mainstay of management of ACS in patients with diabetes (**Table 7–8**).[295] With the advent of newer antiplatelet drugs, there have been recommendations for greater utilization of prasugrel and ticagrelor. The evidence suggests that there is no heterogeneity in the response to newer agents and strategies based on diabetes status.[295–301] What is clear is that consideration of renal insufficiency plays a major role in the outcomes using these agents after ACS.[302] In a study by Franchi et al.,[303] the ischemic benefit of ticagrelor over clopidogrel was greatest in patients with both diabetes and CKD. In 2019, the Effect of Ticagrelor on Health Outcomes in Diabetes Mellitus Patients Intervention Study (THEMIS) investigators published the long-awaited results of a dual antiplatelet strategy with aspirin and ticagrelor compared to aspirin alone in patients with stable ischemic heart disease without a prior

TABLE 7–8. Anti-platelet Therapy in Patients with Acute Coronary Syndrome, With or Without Diabetes[a]

Study	Primary endpoint	n	Standard treatment: % of events	Active treatment: % of events	HR (95% CI)	P-value for interaction
CURE (placebo vs clopidogrel)	1-year CV death, nonfatal MI or stroke	No DM:9722 DM:2840	9.9% 16.7%	7.9% 14.2%	0.78 (0.71–0.86) 0.83 (0.71–0.96)	0.31
PCI CLARITY (placebo vs clopidogrel in STEMI)	30-day CV death, recurrent MI or stroke	No DM:1555 DM:282	5.3% 10.1%	2.9% 6.0%	0.51 (0.30–0.87) 0.61 (0.24–1.53)	0.93
CURRENT-OASIS 7 (standard-dose clopidogrel vs double-dose clopidogrel; low-dose aspirin vs highdose aspirin)	30-day CV death, MI or stroke	No DM:19,203 DM:5880 No DM:19,203 DM:5880	Standard-dose clopidogrel: 3.9% 6.1% Low-dose aspirin: 4.0% 5.6%	Double-dose clopidogrel: 3.9% 5.2% High-dose aspirin: 3.8% 5.7%	0.98 (0.81–1.20) 0.86 (0.68–1.13) 0.95 (0.76–1.10) 1.01 (0.76–1.25)	0.32 0.62
CURRENT-OASIS 7 PCI subgroup (standard-dose clopidogrel vs double-dose clopidogrel; low-dose aspirin vs highdose aspirin)	30-day CV death, MI or stroke	No DM:13,418 DM:3844 No DM:13,418 DM:3844	Standard-dose clopidogrel: 4.2% 5.6% Low-dose aspirin: 4.0% 5.0%	Double-dose clopidogrel: 3.5% 4.9% High-dose aspirin: 3.7% 5.6%	0.84 (0.71–1.00) 0.89 (0.68–1.18) 0.92 (0.77–1.10) 1.12 (0.85–1.48)	0.87 0.22
TRITON-TIMI 38 (clopidogrel vs prasugrel)	15-month CV death, nonfatal MI or nonfatal stroke	No DM:10,462 DM:3146	10.6% 17.0%	9.2% 12.2%	0.86 (0.76–0.98) 0.70 (0.58–0.85)	0.09
PLATO (clopidogrel vs ticagrelor)	1-year CV death, MI or stroke	No DM:13,951 DM:4662	10.2% 16.2%	8.4% 14.1%	0.83 (0.74–0.93) 0.88 (0.76–1.03)	0.49

Abbreviations: CI, confidence interval; CV, cardiovascular; DM, diabetes mellitus; MI, myocardial infarction; STEMI, ST-segment elevation MI.
[a]These data show consistent benefit in MACE reduction for oral anti-P2Y$_{12}$ agents in patients with and without diabetes and acute coronary syndromes. There is a consistent treatment benefit regardless of diabetes status. See reference 295.

MI or stroke.[304] There was modest 10% reduction in ischemic CV events that was offset by a doubling of TIMI major bleeding. Nevertheless, the dual antiplatelet approach is particularly beneficial in patients with prior PCI at low bleeding risk.[305] Notably, ticagrelor therapy does not modify the excess risk for composite MACE in patients with T2D who also have PAD.[306]

The use of dual antiplatelet therapy post-PCI is recommended for up to 12 months in those with and without diabetes and stable CAD. Newer stent platforms have allowed for shorter duration of dual antiplatelet therapy, but there is no clear evidence that patients with diabetes should be treated differently. The evidence post-CABG, non-ACS, and diabetes supports an aspirin-only approach.

Key Treatment Strategies for Diabetes for Clinical Cardiologists

Many of the management strategies for diabetes in the context of CVD are derived from recent clinical practice guidelines in cardiology **(Table 7–9)**.[236,307–311] In addition, the following listing summarizes key clinical actions for cardiologists managing patients with diabetes.

1. Diligently avoid therapies that increase the risk for hypoglycemia.
2. Implement case finding strategies for diabetes in the clinic and hospital settings with particular attention to patients with recent ACS or HF admission.
3. Adopt a strategy of OMT in the primary and secondary care setting.
4. Treat to target for major cardiovascular risk factors: A1C 7.0%; LDL-C <70 mg/dL and in high risk patients <50 mg/dL; and systolic BP <130/80 mmHg. Statin therapy for all patients over age 40 years, regardless of CVD status.
5. Adopt adjunctive therapies: aspirin as secondary prevention, and in selected high-risk patients, as primary prevention; IPE in high-risk patients.
6. Perform coronary artery calcium scoring to stratify risk.

TABLE 7–9. Management Strategies for Diabetes and Cardiovascular Disease from Current Clinical Practice Guidelines in Cardiology[a]

Topic	Recommendation	Guidelines (reference)
• CV Risk Assessment	• Resting ECG is recommended in patients with diabetes with HTN or suspected CVD • Carotid or femoral ultrasound should be considered for plaque detection as a CV risk modifier • CAC scoring may be considered as a risk modifier • ABI may be considered a risk modifier • Carotid ultrasound intima-media thickness for CV risk is not recommended	• 2020 ESC guidelines for the management of acute coronary syndromes in patients presenting without persistent ST-segment elevation (307) • 2019 ESC/EASD guidelines on diabetes, prediabetes, and cardiovascular diseases (308)
• Lifestyle Medicine	• For all adults with T2D, a tailored nutrition plan focusing on a heart-healthy dietary pattern is recommended to improve glycemic control, achieve weight loss if needed, and improve other ASCVD risk factors • Adults with T2D should perform at least 150 minutes per week of moderate-intensity or 75 minutes per week of vigorous-intensity physical activity to improve glycemic control, achieve weight loss if needed, and improve other ASCVD risk factors	• 2019 ACC/AHA guideline on the primary prevention of cardiovascular disease (309)
• Glycemic Control	• Empagliflozin, canagliflozin, or dapagliflozin are recommended in patients with T2D and CVD, or at very high/high CV risk, to reduce CV events • Empagliflozin is recommended in patients with T2D and CVD to reduce the risk of death • Liraglutide is recommended in patients with T2D and CVD, or at very high/high CV risk, to reduce the risk of Death • Saxagliptin is not recommended in patients with T2D and a high risk of HF	• 2019 ESC/EASD guidelines on diabetes, prediabetes, and cardiovascular diseases (308)
• Revascularization	• PCI ------------: 1- or 2-vessel CAD, no proximal LAD • PCI or CABG: 1- or 2-vessel CAD, proximal LAD • -------- CABG: 3-vessel CAD, low complexity • PCI or CABG: Left main CAD, low complexity • -------- CABG: 3-vessel CAD, intermediate or high complexity • -------- CABG: Left main CAD, intermediate complexity • -------- CABG: High complexity	• 2018 ESC/EACTS guidelines on myocardial revascularization (286)
• Acute Coronary Syndrome	• Glucose-lowering therapy should be considered when BG >180 mg/dl (target adapted to comorbidities), while episodes of hypoglycemia should be avoided • A multifactorial approach to diabetes management with treatment targets should be considered in patients with diabetes and CVD • Less stringent glucose control should be considered, both in the acute phase and at follow-up, in patients with more advanced CVD, older age, longer diabetes duration, and more comorbidities	• 2020 ESC guidelines for the management of acute coronary syndromes in patients presenting without persistent ST-segment elevation (307)

(Continued)

TABLE 7–9. Management Strategies for Diabetes and Cardiovascular Disease from Current Clinical Practice Guidelines in Cardiology[a] (Continued)

Topic	Recommendation	Guidelines (reference)
• Heart Failure	• Device therapy with an ICD, CRT, or CRT-D is recommended • Sacubitril/valsartan instead of ACEIs is recommended in patients with HFrEF and diabetes who remain symptomatic despite treatment with ACEIs, β-blockers, and MRAs • CABG is recommended in HFrEF and diabetes and 2- or 3-vessel CAD • Ivabradine should be considered in patients with HF and diabetes in sinus rhythm, and with a resting heart rate ≥70 bpm, if symptomatic despite full HF treatment • Aliskiren is not recommended for patients with HFrEF and diabetes • SGLT2is are recommended to lower risk of HF hospitalization • Metformin should be considered in patients with diabetes and HF if eGFR >30ml/min/1.73m • Saxagliptin is not recommended in HF • Thiazolidinediones are not recommended in HF	• 2019 ESC/EASD guidelines on diabetes, prediabetes, and cardiovascular diseases (308)
• Arrythmia	• Oral anticoagulation in AF (paroxysmal or persistent) is preferably accomplished with the NOACs (dabigatran, rivaroxaban, apixaban, or edoxaban) • attempts to diagnose structural heart disease should be considered in patients with diabetes with frequent premature ventricular contractions • Hypoglycemia should be avoided as it can trigger arrhythmias	• 2019 ESC/EASD guidelines on diabetes, prediabetes, and cardiovascular diseases (308)
• Peripheral Arterial Disease and Chronic Kidney Disease	• Low-dose rivaroxaban 2.5 mg BID plus aspirin 100 mg/day may be considered in patients with diabetes and symptomatic lower extremity arterial disease • SGLT2is are recommended to reduce progression of diabetic kidney disease	• 2019 ESC/EASD guidelines on diabetes, prediabetes, and cardiovascular diseases (308)
• Dyslipidemia	• In patients with T2D at moderate CV risk, an LDL-c target of <100 mg/dl is recommended • In patients with T2D at high CVD risk, an LDL-c target of <70 mg/dl and LDL-c reduction ≥50% is recommended • In patients with T2D at very high CVD risk, and LDL-c target of <55 mg/dl and LDL-c reduction ≥50% is recommended • In adults 40 to 75 years of age with diabetes, regardless of 10-year ASCVD risk, moderate-intensity statin therapy is indicated • In patients at very high risk, with persistent high LDL-c despite treatment with maximum tolerated statin dose in combination with ezetimibe, or in patients with intolerance to statins, a PCSK9i is recommended • Statins are not recommended in women of childbearing potential	• 2019 ESC/EASD guidelines on diabetes, prediabetes, and cardiovascular diseases (308) • 2018 AHA/ACC/AACVPR/AAPA/ABC/ACPM/ADA/AGS/AphA/ASPC/NLA/PCNA guidelines on the management of blood cholesterol (310)
• Hypertension	• In diabetes and HTN, antihypertensive drug treatment should be initiated at a BP ≥130/80 mmHg with a treatment goal of <130/80 mmHg • All first-line classes of antihypertensive agents are useful and effective • ACEIs and ARBs should be considered in the presence of albuminuria	• 2019 ESC/EASD guidelines on diabetes, prediabetes, and cardiovascular diseases (308) • 2017 ACC/AHA/AAPA/ABC/ACPM/AGS/APhA/ASH/ASPC/NMA/PCNA guideline for the prevention, detection, evaluation, and management of high blood pressure in adults (311)
• Atherothrombosis	• Aspirin <100 mg/d for primary prevention in diabetes and high CV risk if bleeding risk is low • DAPT for 3 years in patients at high risk for CVD who have tolerated DAPT in the short-term • PPIs in patients at high GI bleeding risk	• 2019 ESC/EASD guidelines on diabetes, pre-diabetes, and cardiovascular diseases (308) • 2019 ACC/AHA guideline on the primary prevention of cardiovascular disease (309)

[a]Abbreviations: AACVPR, American Association of Cardiovascular and Pulmonary Rehabilitation; AAPA, Association of Physician Assistants in Cardiology; ABC, Association of Black Cardiologists; ABI, ankle-brachial index; ACC, American College of Cardiology; ACEI, angiotensin converting enzyme inhibitor; ACPM, American College of Preventive Medicine; ADA, American Diabetes Association; AF, atrial fibrillation; AGS, American Geriatrics Society; AHA, American Heart Association; APhA, American Pharmacists Association; ARB, angiotensin II receptor blocker; ASCVD, atherosclerotic cardiovascular disease; ASPC, American Society for Preventive Cardiology; BG, blood glucose; CABG, coronary artery bypass grafting; CAC, coronary artery calcium; CAD, coronary artery disease; CRT, cardiac resynchronization therapy; CRT-D, cardiac resynchronization therapy with defibrillation; CV, cardiovascular; CVD, cardiovascular disease; DAPT, dual anti-platelet therapy; EACTS, European Association for Cardio-Thoracic Surgery; EASD, European Association for the Study of Diabetes; eGFR, estimated glomerular filtration rate; ESC, European Society of Cardiology; GI, gastrointestinal; HF, heart failure; HFrEF, heart failure with reduced ejection fraction; HTN, hypertension; ICD, implantable cardioverter defibrillator; LDL-c, low-density lipoprotein cholesterol; MRA, mineral corticoid receptor antagonist; NLA, National Lipid Association; NOAC, novel oral anticoagulants; PCI, percutaneous coronary intervention; PCNA, Preventive Cardiovascular Nurses Association; PCSK9i, Proprotein convertase subtilisin/kexin type 9 inhibitor; PPI, proton pump inhibitor; SGLT2i, sodium-glucose cotransporter-2 inhibitor; T2D, type 2 diabetes.

7. Prescribe the SGLT2is and GLP-1RAs in patients with established or at high-risk for CVD. The SGLT2is are preferred in those with HFpEF.

8. No definite role for case finding for myocardial ischemia in asymptomatic patients with diabetes.

9. Coronary revascularization approaches should always include a heart team approach with consideration of CABG in patients with advanced CAD and/or reduced ejection fraction.

TRAINING AND EDUCATION

Core Concepts for Diabetes Training

In a 2010 report by Chan et al.[312] from a registry of US patients, only 13% of those with CAD evaluated by cardiologists had diabetes screening. Currently, general training in diabetes care occurs in conventional undergraduate and graduate medical education, across all specialties and subspecialties due to the relatively high prevalence rates for this disease. Specialized training in diabetes typically occurs in endocrine fellowship programs, although there is a recent interest in extending this to primary care medicine. Other programs that formally include diabetes training do so within the context of how diabetes-related complications overlap with a particular field. Examples include pediatrics with T1D, obstetrics/gynecology with GDM, critical illness and stress hyperglycemia, bariatric surgery with T2D, and cardiology with CMBCD. Core concepts can be envisioned as basic and advanced depending on the program.

Basic concepts in diabetes training need to be covered for all educational programs for clinicians and include:

1. Epidemiology of diabetes with a focus on complications and differences in phenotypic expressions of disease;

2. Pathophysiology of T1D and T2D, including etiology, mechanistic drivers, and complications;

3. The role of lifestyle medicine, especially nutrition, in prevention of disease progression; and

4. Mechanism of action and dosing principles of insulin and noninsulin therapeutics.

Advanced concepts in diabetes training should be tailored to the particular medical/surgical specialty/subspecialty and may include one or more of the following:

1. In-depth pathophysiology, including molecular mechanisms;

2. Practical training in structured lifestyle medicine, including behavioral medicine, clinical dietetics and nutrition, and exercise physiology;

3. Nuance-based clinical decision-making using all available pharmacotherapies, devices (eg, CGMs, pumps, other wearables, and cloud-based software), and gastrointestinal procedures (ie, metabolic and bariatric).

Diabetes Training for CVD Specialists

Recently, the American College of Cardiology Solution Set Oversight Committee 2020 Expert Consensus Decision Pathway on Novel Therapies for Cardiovascular Risk Reduction in Patients with Type 2 Diabetes published their recommendations.[313] Comprehensive evidence for CV risk reduction in patients with T2D now requires CV practitioners to champion and advocate for optimization of patient care. This includes a full knowledge of the prescription of anti-diabetes therapies. To quote the panel, "CV specialists now need to incorporate these agents into their care of patients with T2D, and coordinate care with the primary diabetes care providers, to optimize clinical outcomes in patients with diabetes." To make this actionable, new approaches to training are required. The CV community needs to advocate for at least 2 months of core training in diabetes in their outpatient cardiology clinic. This will require a team approach with prevention cardiologists and diabetologists. Endocrinology training will also benefit from time in the prevention cardiology clinics.

Key Training Recommendations

The training of CV specialists should incorporate a rotation in the diabetes clinic to better understand the link with diabetes and CVD and to better understand the multidisciplinary approach to the patient with diabetes. This affords the opportunity to learn how to prescribe SGLT2is and GLP-1RAs as the CV specialist will be needed to roll these therapies out to patients at increased CV risk. The American Board of Internal Medicine and other specialty boards in CV medicine should adopt a core competency for this diabetes-CVD link. Cardiovascular specialists should demonstrate practical, clinical proficiency with cardiometabolic care with specific attention to diabetes. There should be a demonstrated competency of cardiometabolic disorders for maintenance of certification by licensing authorities with a set number of hours in ongoing education in cardiometabolic disorders.

FUTURE DIRECTIONS

Diabetes care has experienced an inflection point with a dramatic impact on CV health. This is supported by epidemiological, mechanistic, and strong clinical trial data. Research gaps represent unanswered scientific questions, knowledge gaps represent the nonuniform distribution of scientific information, and practice gaps represent this scientific information, which has not been implemented. For diabetes and CVD, each of these gaps need to be closed; potential actions are given below:

- To further demonstrate a class effect of SGLT2is on cardio-protection independent of glucose lowering, with extension to other medication classes (eg, GLP1ras), other CVD scenarios/endpoints (eg, HFpEF, MACE, AF, and CVA), and other prevention modalities (eg, primary).

- To evaluate the role of tight glycemic control vs. standard control with incorporation of SGLT2is and GLP-1RAs in the patient at risk for, or with established CVD.

- To investigate the role of β-blockers and aspirin in primary prevention of diabetes in the context of personalized medicine strategies.

- To evaluate the role of minimally invasive CABG and hybridized PCI approaches.

- To design and perform a CVOT on metabolic surgery vs OMT.
- To understand and address the clinical inertia and barriers to prescribe and adopt the newer T2D agents into CV practice with a focus on education and training.
- To consider the establishment of a stand-alone cardiometabolic subspecialty and its potential impact on health care delivery.
- To evaluate the role of multidisciplinary clinics with combined diabetes/ cardiology/nephrology experts working with allied medical experts to provide a holistic approach to CMBCD.

ACKNOWLEDGMENT

The authors would like to acknowledge Elliot J. Rayfield and Valentin Fuster who wrote the chapter on "Diabetes and Cardiovascular Disease" in the previous edition.

DISCLOSURES

Dr. Mechanick reports that he received honoraria from Abbott Nutrition for lectures and program development and is on the Advisory Board of GoodSugar™.

Dr. Farkouh reports that he received grant support from Amgen, Novartis, and Novo Nordisk.

REFERENCES

1. Rodriguez-Segade S, Rodriguez J, Camiña F, et al. Continuous glucose monitoring is more sensitive than HbA1c and fasting glucose in detecting dysglycaemia in a Spanish population without diabetes. *Diabetes Res Clin Pract.* 2018;142:100-109.

2. Urbanova J, Brunerova L, Broz J. Hypoglycemia and antihyperglycemic treatment in adult MODY patients—a systematic review of literature. *Diabetes Res Clin Pract.* 2019;158:107914.

3. Steenkamp DW, Alexanian SM, Sternthal E. Approach to the patient with atypical diabetes. *CMAJ.* 2014;186(9):678-684.

4. WHO. Global report on diabetes. Geneva: World Health Organization; 2016.

5. Sousa GR, Pober D, Galderisi A, et al. Glycemic control, cardiac autoimmunity, and long-term risk of cardiovascular disease in type 1 diabetes: a DCCT/EDIC cohort-based study. *Circulation.* 2019;139(6):730-743.

6. Lind M, Svensson AM, Kosiborod M, et al. Glycemic control and excess mortality in type 1 diabetes. *N Engl J Med.* 2014;371:1972-1982.

7. Centers for Disease Control and Prevention. National diabetes statistics report: estimates of diabetes and its burden in the United States. Atlanta, GA: US Department of Health and Human Services; 2014.

8. Newman AB, Siscovick DS, Manolio TA, et al. Ankle-arm index as a marker of atherosclerosis in the Cardiovascular Health Study. Cardiovascular Heart Study (CHS) Collaborative Research Group. *Circulation.* 1993;88:837-845.

9. Ford ES. Trends in the risk for coronary heart disease among adults with diagnosed diabetes in the US Findings from the National health and nutrition examination survey, 1999–2008. *Diabetes Care.* 2011;34:1337-1343.

10. Fan W. Epidemiology in diabetes mellitus and cardiovascular disease. *Cardiovasc Endocrinol.* 2017;6(1):8-16.

11. Manson JE, Colditz GA, Stampfer MJ, et al. A prospective study of maturity-onset diabetes mellitus and risk of coronary heart disease and stroke in women. *Arch Intern Med* 1991;151:1141-1147.

12. Menke A, Casagrande S, Geiss L, Cowie CC. Prevalence of and trends in diabetes among adults in the United States, 1988–2012. *JAMA.* 2015;314(10):1021-1029.

13. Mechanick JI, Davidson JA, Fergus IV, et al. Transcultural diabetes care in the United States—a position statement by the American Association of Clinical Endocrinologists. *Endocr Pract.* 2019;25(7):729-765.

14. Narres M, Claessen H, Droste S, et al. The incidence of end-stage renal disease in the diabetic (compared to the non-diabetic) population: a systematic review. *PLoS One.* 2016;11(1):e0147329.

15. American Diabetes Association. Microvascular complications and foot care: standards of medical care in diabetes—2020. *Diabetes Care.* 2020;43(Suppl 1):S135-S151.

16. Hicks CW, Selvin E. Epidemiology of peripheral neuropathy and lower extremity disease in diabetes. *Curr Diab Rep.* 2019;19(10):86. doi: 10.1007/s11892-019-1212-8.

17. Behroozian A, Beckman JA. Microvascular disease increases amputation in patients with peripheral artery disease. *Arterioscler Thromb Vasc Biol.* 2020;40(3):534-540.

18. Lee KA, Park TS, Jin HY. Non-glucose risk factors in the pathogenesis of diabetic peripheral neuropathy. *Endocrine.* 2020;70(3):465-478. doi: 10.1007/s12020-020-02473-4.

19. Hicks CW, Selvin E. Epidemiology of peripheral neuropathy and lower extremity disease in diabetes. *Curr Diab Rep.* 2019;19(10):86.

20. Ang L, Dillon B, Mizokami-Stout K, et al. Cardiovascular autonomic neuropathy: a silent killer with long reach. *Auton Neurosci.* 2020;225:102646.

21. Simo-Servat O, Hernandez C, Simo R. Diabetic retinopathy in the context of patients with diabetes. *Ophthalmic Res.* 2019;62:211-217.

22. Brownrigg JR, Hughes CO, Burleigh D, et al. Microvascular disease and risk of cardiovascular events among individuals with type 2 diabetes: a population level cohort study. *Lancet Diabetes Endocrinol.* 2016;4:588-597.

23. Wang A, Green JB, Halperin JL, Piccini JP, Sr. Atrial fibrillation and diabetes mellitus: JACC review topic of the week. *J Am Coll Cardiol.* 2019;74(8):1107-1115.

24. Palmieri V, Bella JN, Arnett DK, et al. Effect of type 2 diabetes mellitus on left ventricular geometry and systolic function in hypertensive subjects. *Circulation.* 2001;103:102-107.

25. Jarolim P, White WB, Cannon CP, et al. Serial measurement of natriuretic peptides and cardiovascular outcomes in patients with type 2 diabetes in the EXAMINE Trial. *Diabetes Care.* 2018;41:1510-1515.

26. Zareini B, Blanche P, D'Souza M, et al. Type 2 diabetes mellitus and impact of heart failure on prognosis compared to other cardiovascular diseases. *Circ Cardiovasc Qual Outcomes.* 2020;13:e006260.

27. Pathak RK, Middeldorp ME, Meredith M, et al. Long-Term effect of goal-directed weight management in an atrial fibrillation cohort: a long-term follow-up study (LEGACY). *J Am Coll Cardiol.* 2015;65(20):2159-2169.

28. Kannel WB, Thomas HE Jr. Sudden coronary death: the Framingham Study. *Ann N Y Acad Sci.* 1982;382:3-21.

29. Albert CM, Chae CU, Grodstein F, et al. Prospective study of sudden cardiac death among women in the United States. *Circulation.* 2003;107:2096-2101.

30. Jouven X, Lemaitre RN, Rea TD, et al. Diabetes, glucose level, and risk of sudden cardiac death. *Eur Heart J.* 2005;26:2142-2147.

31. MacDonald MR, Petrie MC, Varyani F, et al. CHARM Investigators. Impact of diabetes on outcomes in patients with low and preserved ejection fraction heart failure: an analysis of the Candesartan in Heart failure: Assessment of Reduction in Mortality and morbidity (CHARM) programme. *Eur Heart J.* 2008;29:1377-1385.

32. Umemura T, Kawamura T, Hotta N. Pathogenesis and neuroimaging of cerebral large and small vessel disease in type 2 diabetes: a possible link between cerebral and retinal microvascular abnormalities. *J Diabetes Investig.* 2017;8(2):134-148.

33. Badjatiya A, Merrill P, Buse JB, et al. Clinical outcomes in patients with type 2 diabetes mellitus and peripheral artery disease. Results from the EXSCEL Trial. *Circ Cardiovasc Interv.* 2019;13:e009018.

34. Fowkes FG, Rudan D, Rudan I, et al. Comparison of global estimates of prevalence and risk factors for peripheral artery disease in 2000 and 2010: a systematic review and analysis. *Lancet.* 2013;382:1329-1340.

35. Marso SP, Hiatt WR. Peripheral arterial disease in patients with diabetes. *J Am Coll Cardiol.* 2006;47:921-929.

36. Selvin E, Marinopoulos S, Berkenblit G, et al. Meta-analysis: glycosylated hemoglobin and cardiovascular disease in diabetes mellitus. *Ann Intern Med.* 2004;141:421-431.

37. Jude EB, Oyibo SO, Chalmers N, et al. Peripheral arterial disease in diabetic and nondiabetic patients: a comparison of severity and outcome. *Diabetes Care.* 2001;24:1433-1437.

38. Rivellese AA, Riccardi G, Vaccaro O. Cardiovascular risk in women with diabetes. *Nutr Metab Cardiovasc Dis.* 2010;20:474-480.

39. American Diabetes Association. Classification and diagnosis of diabetes: standards of medical care in diabetes—2020. *Diabetes Care.* 2020;43(Suppl 1):S14-S31.

40. Teupe B, Bergis K. Epidemiological evidence for "double diabetes." *Lancet.* 1991;337:361-362.

41. Simonlene D, Platukiene A, Prakapiene E, et al. Insulin resistance in type 1 diabetes mellitus and its association with patient's micro- and macrovascular complications, sex hormones, and other clinical data. *Diabetes Ther.* 2020;11:161-174.

42. Kietsiriroje N, Pearson S, Campbell M, et al. Double diabetes: a distinct high-risk group? *Diabetes Obes Metab.* 2019;21(12):2609-2618.

43. American Diabetes Association. Cardiovascular disease and risk management: standards of medical care in diabetes—2020. *Diabetes Care* 2020;43(Suppl 1):S111-S134.

44. Giugliano D, Mariorino MI, Bellastella G, et al. Glycemic control in type 2 diabetes: from medication nonadherence to residual vascular risk. *Endocrine.* 2018;61:23-27.

45. Mechanick JI, Garber AJ, Grunberger G, et al. Dysglycemia-based chronic disease: An American Association of Clinical Endocrinologists position statement. *Endocr Pract.* 2018;24:995-1011.

46. Lee JJ, Pedley A, Hoffmann U, et al. Visceral and intrahepatic fat are associated with cardiometabolic risk factors above other ectopic fat depots: the Framingham Heart Study. *Am J Med.* 2018;131:684-692.e12.

47. Pagidipati NJ, Zheng Y, Green JB, et al. Association of obesity with cardiovascular outcomes in patients with type 2 diabetes and cardiovascular disease: insights from TECOS. *Am Heart J.* 2020;219:47-57.

48. Hanley AJ, Williams K, Stern MP, et al. Homeostasis model assessment of insulin resistance in relation to the incidence of cardiovascular disease: the San Antonio Heart Study. *Diabetes Care.* 2002;25(7):1177-1184.

49. Forst T, Lubben G, Hohberg C, et al. Influence of glucose control and improvement of insulin resistance on microvascular blood flow and endothelial function in patients with diabetes mellitus type 2. *Microcirculation.* 2005;12:543-550.

50. Mechanick JI, Farkouh ME, Newman JD, et al. Cardiometabolic-based chronic disease—adiposity and dysglycemia drivers. *J Am Coll Cardiol.* 2020;75:525-538.

51. Mechanick JI, Farkouh ME, Newman JD, et al. Cardiometabolic-based chronic disease—addressing knowledge and clinical practice gaps in the preventive care plan. *J Am Coll Cardiol.* 2020;75:539-555.

52. American Diabetes Association. Prevention of delay of type 2 diabetes: standards of medical care in diabetes—2020. *Diabetes Care.* 2020;43(Suppl 1):S32-S36.

53. Seferovic JP, Bentley-Lewis R, Claggett B, et al. Retinopathy, neuropathy, and subsequent cardiovascular events in patients with type 2 diabetes and acute coronary syndrome in the ELIXA: the importance of disease duration. *J Diabetes Res.* 2018;1631263. doi: 10.1155/2018/1631263.

54. American Diabetes Association. Management of diabetes in pregnancy: standards of medical care in diabetes—2020. *Diabetes Care* 2020;43(Suppl 1):S183-S192.

55. Rajkumar V, Levine SN. Latent autoimmune diabetes. StatPearls [Internet]. Treasure Island (FL): StatPearls Publishing; 2020 Jan. 2020 Jun 25.

56. Maddaloni E, Coleman RL, Agbaje O, et al. Time-varying risk of microvascular complications in latent autoimmune diabetes of adulthood compared with type 2 diabetes in adults: a post-hoc analysis of the UK Prospective Diabetes Study 30-year follow-up data (UKPDS 86). *Lancet Diabetes Endocrinol.* 2020;8:206-215.

57. Hart PA, Bellin MD, Andersen DK, et al. Type 3c (pancreatogenic) diabetes mellitus secondary to chronic pancreatitis and pancreatic cancer. Lancet Gastroenterol Hepatol. 2016;1(3):226-237.

58. American Diabetes Association. Glycemic targets: standards of medical care in diabetes—2020. *Diabetes Care* 2020;43(Suppl 1):S66-S76.

59. Mattishent K, Loke YK. Bi-directional interaction between hypoglycaemia and cognitive impairment in elderly patients treated with glucose-lowering agents: a systematic review and meta-analysis. *Diabetes Obes Metab.* 2016;18(2):135-141.

60. Choi SY, Ko SH. Severe hypoglycemia as a preventable risk factor for cardiovascular disease in patients with type 2 diabetes mellitus. *Korean J Intern Med.* 2021;36(2):263-370. doi: 10.3904/kjim.2020.327.

61. Davis SN, Duckworth W, Emanuele N, et al. Effects of severe hypoglycemia on cardiovascular outcomes and death in the Veterans Affairs Diabetes Trial. *Diabetes Care.* 2019;42:157-163.

62. Zhou JJ, Schwenke DC, Bahn G, et al. Glycemic variation and cardiovascular risk in the Veterans Affairs Diabetes Trial. *Diabetes Care.* 2018;41:2187-2194.

63. Schulman RC, Moshier EL, Rho L, et al. Intravenous pamidronate is associated with reduced mortality in patients with chronic critical illness. *Endocr Pract.* 2016;22(7):799-808.

64. Kovatchev B. Glycemic variability: risk factors, assessment, and control. *J Diabetes Sci Technol.* 2019;13(4):627-635.

65. Walker ME, Song RJ, Xu Xiang, et al. Proteomic and metabolomics correlates of healthy dietary patterns: the Framingham Heart Study. *Nutrients.* 2020;12(5):1476. doi: 10.3390/nu12051476.

66. Zhao S, Mechanick JI. Targeting foodome-metabolome interactions: a combined modeling approach. In, Mechanick JI, Via MA, Zhou S (eds.). *Molecular Nutrition: The Practical Guide.* Endocrine Press, Washington, DC, 2015, pp. 182-205.

67. Mechanick JI, Zhao S, Garvey WT. The adipokine-cardiovascular-lifestyle network. *J Am Coll Cardiol.* 2016;68:1785-1803.

68. Mechanick JI, Zhao S, Garvey WT. Leptin, an adipokine with central importance in the global obesity problem. *Global Heart.* 2018;13:113-127.

69. Reaven GM. Syndrome X. *Blood Press Suppl.* 1992;4:13-16.

70. Sperling LS, Mechanick JI, Neeland IJ, et al. The CardioMetabolic Health Alliance: working toward a new care model for the metabolic syndrome. *J Am Coll Cardiol.* 2015;66(9):1050-1067.

71. Haffner SM, Mykanen L, Festa A, et al. Insulin-resistant pre-diabetic subjects have more atherogenic risk factors than insulin-sensitive pre-diabetic subjects: implications for preventing coronary heart disease during the pre-diastolic state. *Circulation.* 2000;101:975-980.

72. Ghosh-Swaby OR, Goodman SG, Leiter LA, et al. Glucose-lowering drugs or strategies, atherosclerotic cardiovascular events, and heart failure in people with or at risk of type 2 diabetes: an updated systematic review and meta-analysis of randomised cardiovascular outcome trials. *Lancet Diabetes Endocrinol.* 2020;8(5):418-435.

73. Kibel A, Selthofer-Relatic K, Drenjancevic I, et al. Coronary microvascular dysfunction in diabetes mellitus. *J Int Med Res.* 2017;45(6):1901-1929.

74. Tadic M, Celic V, Cuspidi C, et al. Right heart mechanics in untreated normotensive patients with prediabetes and type 2 diabetes mellitus: a two- and three-dimensional echocardiographic study. *J Am Soc Echocardiogr.* 2015;28(3):317-327.

75. McHugh K, DeVore AD, Wu J, Matsouaka RA, et al. Heart Failure With Preserved Ejection Fraction and Diabetes: JACC State-of-the-Art Review. *J Am Coll Cardiol.* 2019;73(5):602-611.

76. Tadic M, Cuspidi C. The influence of type 2 diabetes on left atrial remodeling. *Clin Cardiol.* 2015;38(1):48-55.

77. O'Brien IA, McFadden JP, Corrall RJ. The influence of autonomic neuropathy on mortality in insulin-dependent diabetes. *Q J Med.* 1991;79:495-502.

78. Forsen A, Kangro M, Sterner G, et al. A 14-year prospective study of autonomic nerve function in type 1 diabetic patients: association with nephropathy. *Diabet Med.* 2004;21:852-858.

79. MacGregor AS, Price JF, Hau CM, et al. Role of systolic blood pressure and plasma triglycerides in diabetic peripheral arterial disease. The Edinburgh Artery Study. *Diabetes Care.* 1999;22:453-458.

80. The Diabetes Control and Complications Trial Research Group. The effect of intensive treatment of diabetes on the development and progression of long-term complications in insulin-dependent diabetes mellitus. *N Engl J Med.* 1993;329:977-986.

81. Epidemiology of Diabetes Interventions and Complications (EDIC) Research Group. Epidemiology of Diabetes Interventions and Complications (EDIC): Design and implementation of a long-term follow-up of the Diabetes Control and Complications Trial cohort. *Diabetes Care.* 1999;22:99-111.

82. Nathan DM and for the DCCT/EDIC Research Group. The diabetes control and complications trial/epidemiology of diabetes interventions and complications study at 30 years: overview. *Diabetes Care.* 2014;37(1):9-16.

83. The Look AHEAD Research Group. Cardiovascular effects of intensive lifestyle intervention in type 2 diabetes. *N Engl J Med.* 2013;369(2):145-154.

84. Estruch R, Ros E, Salas-Salvadó J, et al. Primary prevention of cardiovascular disease with a mediterranean diet supplemented with extra-virgin olive oil or nuts. *N Engl J Med.* 2018;378(25):e34.

85. Gæde P, Vedel P, Larsen N, et al. Multifactorial intervention and cardiovascular disease in patients with type 2 diabetes. *N Engl J Med.* 2003;348:383–393.

86. Lean MEJ, Leslie WS, Barnes AC, et al. Durability of a primary care-led weight-management intervention for remission of type 2 diabetes: 2-year results of the DiRECT open-label, cluster-randomised trial. *Lancet Diabetes Endocrinol.* 2019;7(5):344-355.

87. Knowler WC, Barrett-Connor E, Fowler SE, et al.; Diabetes Prevention Program Research Group. Reduction in the incidence of type 2 diabetes with lifestyle intervention or metformin. *N Engl J Med.* 2002; 346(6):393-403.

88. Tuomilehto J, Lindstrom J, Eriksson JG, et al. Prevention of type 2 diabetes mellitus by changes in lifestyle among subjects with impaired glucose tolerance. *N Engl J Med.* 2001;344:1343-1350.

89. Scandinavian Simvastatin Survival Study Group. Randomized trial of cholesterol lowering in 4444 patients with coronary heart disease: Scandinavian Simvastatin Survival Study (4S). *Lancet.* 1994;344:1383-1389.

90. Goldberg RB, Mellies MJ, Sacks FM, et al. Cardiovascular events and their reduction with pravastatin in diabetic and glucose-intolerant myocardial infarction survivors with average cholesterol levels: subgroup analyses in the cholesterol and recurrent events (CARE) trial: the Care investigators. *Circulation.* 1998;98:2513-2519.

91. Collins R, Armitage J, Parish S, et al. Heart Protection Study Collaborative Group. Effects of cholesterol-lowering with simvastatin on stroke and other major vascular events in 20536 people with cerebrovascular disease or other high-risk conditions. *Lancet.* 2004;363(9411):757-767.

92. Colhoun HM, Betteridge DJ, Durrington PN, et al. CARDS investigators. Primary prevention of cardiovascular disease with atorvastatin in type 2 diabetes in the Collaborative Atorvastatin Diabetes Study (CARDS): Multicentre randomised placebo-controlled trial. *Lancet.* 2004;364(9435):685-696.

93. Wanner C, Krane V, Marz W, et al. German Diabetes and Dialysis Study Investigators. Atorvastatin in patients with type 2 diabetes mellitus undergoing hemodialysis. *N Engl J Med.* 2005;353(3):238-248.

94. Kohli P, Waters DD, Nemr R, et al. Risk of new-onset diabetes and cardiovascular risk reduction from high-dose statin therapy in pre-diabetes and non-pre-diabetics: an analysis from TNT and IDEAL. *J Am Coll Cardiol.* 2015;65(4):402-404.

95. LaRosa JC, Grundy SM, Waters DD, et al. Intensive lipid lowering with atorvastatin in patients with stable coronary disease. *N Engl J Med.* 2005;352:1425-1435.

96. Pedersen TR, Faergeman O, Kastelein JJ, et al. High-dose atorvastatin vsusual-dose simvastatin for secondary prevention after myocardial infarction: the IDEAL study: a randomized controlled trial. *JAMA.* 2005;294:2437-2445.

97. Cannon CP, Blazing MA, Giugliano RP, et al. Ezetimibe added to statin therapy after acute coronary syndromes. *N Engl J Med.* 2015;372:2387-2397.

98. Boden WE, Probstfield JL, Anderson T, et al.; AIM-HIGH Investigators. Niacin in patients with low HDL cholesterol levels receiving intensive statin therapy. *N Engl J Med.* 2011;365:2255-2267.

99. Landray MJ, Haynes R, Hopewell JC, et al.; HPS2-THRIVE Collaborative Group. Effects of extended-release niacin with laropiprant in high-risk patients. *New Engl J Med.* 2014;371(3):203-212.

100. Keech A, Simes RJ, Barter P, et al.; FIELD Study Investigators. Effects of long-term fenofibrate therapy on cardiovascular events in 9795 people with type 2 diabetes mellitus (the FIELD study): randomized controlled trial. *Lancet.* 2005;366(9500):1849-1861.

101. Ginsberg HN, Elam MB, Lovato LC, et al.; ACCORD Study Group. Effects of combination lipid therapy in type 2 diabetes mellitus. *N Engl J Med.* 2010;362:1563-1574.

102. Cushman WC, Evans GW, Byington RP, et al.; ACCORD Study Group. Effects of intensive blood pressure control in type 2 diabetes. *N Engl J Med.* 2010;362(17):1575-1585.

103. Cooper-DeHoff RM, Gong Y, Handberg EM, et al. Tight blood pressure control and cardiovascular outcomes among hypertensive patients with diabetes and coronary artery disease. *JAMA.* 2010;304(1):61-68.

104. Hansson L, Zanchetti A, Carruthers SG, et al. Effects of intensive blood-pressure lowering and low-dose aspirin in patients with hypertension: principal results of Hypertension Optimal Treatment (HOT) randomized trial. *Lancet.* 1998;351:1755-1762.

105. Heart Outcomes Prevention Evaluation Study Investigators. Effects of ramipril on cardiovascular and microvascular outcomes in people with diabetes mellitus: results of the HOPE study and MICRO-HOPE substudy. *Lancet.* 2000;355:253-259.

106. ONTARGET Invesitgators. Telmisartan, ramipril, or both in patients at high risk for vascular events. *N Engl J Med.* 2008;358:1547-1559.

107. Schauer PR, Bhatt DL, Kirwan JP, et al. Bariatric surgery versus intensive medical therapy for diabetes—5-Year Outcomes. *N Engl J Med.* 2017;376(7):641-651.

108. Mingrone G, Panunzi S, De Gaetano A, et al. Bariatric surgery versus conventional medical therapy for type 2 diabetes. *N Engl J Med.* 2012;366(17):1577-1585.

109. UK Prospective Diabetes Study (UKPDS) Group. Intensive blood-glucose control with sulphonylureas or insulin compared with conventional treatment and risk of complications in patients with type 2 diabetes (UKPDS 33). *Lancet.* 1998;352(9131):837-853.

110. Action to Control Cardiovascular Risk in Diabetes Study Group, et al. Effects of intensive glucose lowering in type 2 diabetes. *N Engl J Med.* 2008;358(24):2545-2559.

111. ADVANCE Collaborative Group, et al. Intensive blood glucose control and vascular outcomes in patients with type 2 diabetes. *N Engl J Med.* 2008;358(24):2560-2572.

112. Duckworth W, Abraira C, Moritz T, et al. Glucose control and vascular complications in veterans with type 2 diabetes. *N Engl J Med.* 2009;360(2):129-139.

113. Bhatt DL, Steg PG, Miller M, et al; REDUCE-IT Investigators. Effects of icosapent ethyl on total ischemic events: from REDUCE-IT. *J Am Coll Cardiol.* 2019;73(22):2791–2802.

114. The DREAM (Diabetes Reduction Assessment with ramipril and rosiglitazone Medication) Trial Investigators. Effect of rosiglitazone on the frequency of diabetes in patients with impaired glucose tolerance

or impaired fasting glucose: a randomised controlled trial. *Lancet.* 2006;368(9541):1096-1105.

115. The DREAM Trial Investigators. Effect of ramipril on the incidence of diabetes. *N Engl J Med.* 2006;355:1551-1562.

116. Holman RR, Haffner SM, McMurray JJ, Bethel MA, Holzhauer B, Hua TA, et al. Effect of nateglinide on the incidence of diabetes and cardiovascular events. *N Engl J Med.* 2010;362:1463-1476.

117. NAVIGATOR Study Group; McMurray JJ, Holman RR, Haffner SM, et al. Effect of valsartan on the incidence of diabetes and cardiovascular events. *N Engl J Med.* 2010;362:1477-1490.

118. Bowman L, Mafham M, Stevens W, et al.; ASCEND Study Collaborative Group. ASCEND: a study of cardiovascular events in diabetes: characteristics of a randomized trial of aspirin and of omega-3 fatty acid supplementation in 15,480 people with diabetes. *Am Heart J.* 2018;198:135–144.

119. Pan XR, Li GW, Hu YH, et al. Effects of diet and exercise in preventing NIDDM in people with impaired glucose tolerance: the Da Qing IGT and Diabetes study. *Diabetes Care.* 1997;20:537-544.

120. American Diabetes Association. Glycemic targets: standards of medical care in diabetes—2020. *Diabetes Care.* 2020;43(Suppl 1):S66-S76.

121. American Diabetes Association. Diabetes technology: standards of medical care in diabetes—2020. *Diabetes Care* 2020;43(Suppl 1):S77-S88.

122. Mechanick JI, Apovian C, Brethauer S, et al. Clinical practice guidelines for the perioperative nutrition, metabolic, and nonsurgical support of patients undergoing bariatric procedures—2019 update: cosponsored by American Association of Clinical Endocrinologists/American College of Endocrinology, The Obesity Society, American Society for Metabolic & Bariatric Surgery, Obesity Medicine Association, and American Society of Anesthesiologists. *Obesity.* 2020;28:1-58.

123. Garber AJ, Handelsman Y, Grunberger G, et al. Consensus statement by the American Association of Clinical Endocrinologists and American College of Endocrinology on the comprehensive type 2 diabetes management algorithm—2020 executive summary. *Endocr Pract.* 2020;26(1):107-139.

124. American Diabetes Association. Pharmacologic approaches to glycemic treatment: standards of medical care in diabetes—2020. *Diabetes Care.* 2020;43(Suppl 1):S98-S110.

125. American Diabetes Association. Comprehensive medical evaluation and assessment of comorbidities: standards of medical care in diabetes—2020. *Diabetes Care.* 2020;43(Suppl 1):S37-S47.

126. Mechanick JI, Kushner RF. Why lifestyle medicine? In: Mechanick JI, Kushner RF (eds.). Lifestyle Medicine—A Manual for Clinical Practice; 2016, Springer, New York, pp. 1-8.

127. American Diabetes Association. Improving care and promoting health in populations: standards of medical care in diabetes—2020. *Diabetes Care* 2020;43(Suppl 1):S7-S13.

128. American Diabetes Association. Facilitating behavior change and well-being to improve health outcomes: standards of medical care in diabetes—2020. *Diabetes Care* 2020;43(Suppl 1):S48-S65.

129. Garvey WT, Mechanick JI, Brett EM, et al. American Association of Clinical Endocrinologists and American College of Endocrinology comprehensive clinical practice guidelines for medical care of patients with obesity—executive Summary. *Endocr Pract.* 2016;22(7):842-884.

130. Lee AK, Woodward M, Wang D, et al. The risks of cardiovascular disease and mortality following weight change in adults with diabetes: results from ADVANCE. *J Clin Endocrinol Metab.* 2020;105(1):152-162.

131. Dansinger ML, Augustin Gleason J, Griffith JL, et al. Comparison of the Atkins, Ornish, Weight Watchers, and Zone diets for weight loss and heart disease risk reduction: a randomized trial. *JAMA.* 2005;293(1):43-53.

132. Shai I, Schwarzfuchs D, Henkin Y, et al. Dietary Intervention Randomized Controlled Trial (DIRECT) Group. Weight loss with a low-carbohydrate, mediterranean, or low-fat diet. *N Engl J Med.* 2008;359(3):229-241.

133. American Diabetes Association. Diabetes care in the hospital: standards of medical care in diabetes—2020. *Diabetes Care* 2020;43(Suppl 1):S193-S202.

134. Han YY, Lai SR, Partridge JS, et al. The clinical and economic impact of the use of diabetes-specific enteral formula on ICU patients with type 2 diabetes. *Clin Nutr.* 2017;36(6):1567-1572.

135. Mechanick JI, Brett EM, Chausmer AB, et al. American Association of Clinical Endocrinologists medical guidelines for the clinical use of dietary supplements and nutraceuticals. *Endocr Pract.* 2003;9(5):417-470.

136. Global Burden of Disease 2016 Alcohol Collaborators. Alcohol use and burden for 195 countries and territories, 1990–2016: a systematic analysis for the Global Burden of Disease Study 2016. *Lancet.* 2018;392(10152):1015-1035.

137. Cassidy S, Vaidya V, Houghton D, et al. Unsupervised high-intensity interval training improves glycaemic control but not cardiovascular autonomic function in type 2 diabetes patients: a randomised controlled trial. *Diabetes Vasc Dis Res.* 2019;16(1):69-76.

138. Kemps H, Kränkel N, Dörr M, et al. Exercise training for patients with type 2 diabetes and cardiovascular disease: what to pursue and how to do it. A Position Paper of the European Association of Preventive Cardiology (EAPC). *Eur J Prev Cardiol.* 2019;26(7):709-727.

139. Sheinfeld Gorin S, Davis C. Implementing behavioral medicine in a lifestyle medicine practice. In: Mechanick JI, Kushner RF (eds.). Creating a Lifestyle Medicine Center, Springer Nature, Switzerland AG, 2020, pp. 161-179.

140. Mechanick JI, Kushner RF. Synthesis: deriving a core set of recommendations for planning, building, and operating a lifestyle medicine center. In: Mechanick JI, Kushner RF (eds.). Creating a Lifestyle Medicine Center, Springer Nature, Switzerland AG, 2020, pp. 355-361.

141. Mechanick JI, Zhao S. Wearable technologies. In: Mechanick JI, Kushner RF (eds.). Creating a Lifestyle Medicine Center, Springer Nature, Switzerland AG, 2020, pp. 133-143.

142. Huo X, Bai X, Spatz ES, et al. Effects of mobile text messaging on glycemic control in patients with coronary heart disease and diabetes mellitus. *Circ Cardiovas Qual Outcomes.* 2019;12:e005805.

143. Reutrakul S, Mokhlesi B. Obstructive sleep apnea and diabetes: A state of the art review. *Chest.* 2017;152(5):1070-1086.

144. Mechanick JI. The inpatient lifestyle medicine consultation service. In: Mechanick JI, Kushner RF (eds.). Creating a Lifestyle Medicine Center, Springer Nature, Switzerland AG, 2020, pp. 215-231.

145. Perish E, Meltzer D, McDonald E. Models for caring for patients with complex lifestyle, medical, and social needs. In: Mechanick JI, Kushner RF (eds.). Creating a Lifestyle Medicine Center, Springer Nature, Switzerland AG, 2020, pp. 37-45.

146. Samson SL, Garber AJ. Prevention of type 2 diabetes mellitus: potential of pharmacological agents. *Best Pract Res Clin Endocrinol Metab.* 2016;30(3):357-371.

147. Garvey WT, Ryan DH, Look M, et al. Two-year sustained weight loss and metabolic benefits with controlled-release phentermine/topiramate in obese and overweight adults (SEQUEL): a randomized, placebo-controlled, phase 3 extension study. *Am J Clin Nutr.* 2012;95:297e308.

148. Yang W, Lin L, Qi J, et al. The preventive effect of acarbose and metformin on the progression to diabetes mellitus in the IGT population: a 3-year multicenter prospective study. *Chin J Endocrinol Metab* 2001;17:131e6.

149. Ramachandran A, Snehalatha C, Mary S, et al. The Indian Diabetes Prevention Programme shows that lifestyle modification and metformin prevent type 2 diabetes in Asian Indian subjects with impaired glucose tolerance (IDPP-1). *Diabetologia.* 2006;49:289e97.

150. DeFronzo RA, Tripathy D, Schwenke DC, et al. Pioglitazone for diabetes prevention in impaired glucose tolerance. *N Engl J Med.* 2011;364:1104e15.

151. Torgerson JS, Hauptman J, Boldrin MN, et al. XENical in the prevention of diabetes in obese subjects (XENDOS) study: a randomized study of orlistat as an adjunct to lifestyle changes for the prevention of type 2 diabetes in obese patients. *Diabetes Care.* 2004;27:155e61.

152. Chiasson JL, Josse RG, Gomis R, et al. Acarbose for prevention of type 2 diabetes mellitus: the STOP-NIDDM randomised trial. *Lancet.* 2002;359:2072e7.

153. Macisaac RJ, Jerums G. Intensive glucose control and cardiovascular outcomes in type 2 diabetes. *Heart Lung Circ.* 2011;20(10):647-654.

154. Fullerton B, Jeitler K, Seitz M, Horvath K, Berghold A, Siebenhofer A. Intensive glucose control versus conventional glucose control for type 1 diabetes mellitus. *Cochrane Database Syst Rev.* 2014;2:CD009122.

155. Holman RR, Paul SK, Bethel MA, Matthews DR, Neil HA. 10-year follow-up of intensive glucose control in type 2 diabetes. *N Engl J Med.* 2008;359(15):1577-1589.

156. Kähler P, Grevstad B, Almdal T, Gluud C, Wetterslev J, Lund SS, Vaag A, Hemmingsen B. Targeting intensive versus conventional glycaemic control for type 1 diabetes mellitus: a systematic review with meta-analyses and trial sequential analyses of randomised clinical trials. *BMJ Open.* 2014;4(8).

157. Insulins for type 2 diabetes. *Med Lett Drugs Ther.* 2019;61:65-68.

158. Zinman B, Wanner C, Lachin JM, et al. Empagliflozin, cardiovascular outcomes, and mortality in type 2 diabetes. *N Engl J Med.* 2015;373:2117-2128.

159. Neal B, Perkovic V, Mahaffey KW, et al. Canagliflozin and cardiovascular and renal events in type 2 diabetes. *N Engl J Med.* 2017;377:644–657.

160. Percovic V, Jardine MJ, Neal B, et al.; CREDENCE Trial Investigators. Canagliflozin and renal outcomes in type 2 diabetes and nephropathy. *N Engl J Med.* 2019;380(24):2295-2306.

161. Wiviott SD, Raz I, Bonaca MP, et al. Dapagliflozin and cardiovascular outcomes in type 2 diabetes. *N Engl J Med.* 2019;380:347-357.

162. Pfeffer MA, Claggett B, Diaz R, et al. Lixisenatide in patients with type 2 diabetes and acute coronary syndrome. *New Engl J Med.* 2015;373:2247-2257.

163. Marso SP, Daniels GH, Brown-Frandsen K, et al. Liraglutide and cardiovascular outcomes in type 2 diabetes. *N Engl J Med.* 2016;375:311-322.

164. Marso SP, Bain SC, Consoli A, et al.; SUSTAIN-6 Investigators. Semaglutide and cardiovascular outcomes in patients with type 2 diabetes. *New Engl J Med.* 2016;375:1834-1844.

165. Holman RR, Bethel MA, Mentz RJ, et al. Effects of once-weekly exenatide on cardiovascular outcomes in type 2 diabetes. *New Engl J Med.* 2017;377:1228-1239.

166. Hernandez AF, Green JB, Janmohamed S, et al. Albiglutide and cardiovascular outcomes in patients with type 2 diabetes and cardiovascular disease (Harmony Outcomes): a double-blind, randomised placebo-controlled trial. *Lancet.* 2018;392:1519-1529.

167. Gerstein HC, Colhoun HM, Dagenais GR, et al. Dulaglutide and cardiovascular outcomes in type 2 diabetes (REWIND): a double-blind, randomized placebo-controlled trial. *Lancet.* 2019;13:121-130.

168. Bergmark BA, Bhatt DL, McGuire DK, et al. Metformin use and clinical outcomes among patients with diabetes mellitus with or without heart failure or kidney dysfunction. *Circulation.* 2019;140:1004-1014.

169. Charytan DM, Solomon SD, Ivanovich P, et al. Metformin use and cardiovascular events in patients with type 2 diabetes and chronic kidney disease. *Diabetes Obes Metab.* 2019;21:1199-1208.

170. Griffin SJ, Leaver JK, Irving GJ. Impact of metformin on cardiovascular disease: a meta-analysis of randomised trials among people with type 2 diabetes. *Diabetologia.* 2017;60(9):1620-1629.

171. U.S. Food and Drug Administration. Search list of recalled metformin products. https://www.fda.gov/drugs/drug-safety-and-availability/search-list-recalled-metformin-products (accessed on October 11, 2020).

172. Zinman B, Wanner C, Lachin JM, et al. Empagliflozin, cardiovascular outcomes, and mortality in type 2 diabetes. *N Engl J Med.* 2015;373:2117-2128.

173. Neal B, Perkovic V, Mahaffey KW, et al. Canagliflozin and cardiovascular and renal events in type 2 diabetes. *N Engl J Med.* 2017;377:644–657.

174. Percovic V, Jardine MJ, Neal B, et al.; CREDENCE Trial Investigators. Canagliflozin and renal outcomes in type 2 diabetes and nephropathy. *N Engl J Med.* 2019;380(24):2295-2306.

175. Wiviott SD, Raz I, Bonaca MP, et al. Dapagliflozin and cardiovascular outcomes in type 2 diabetes. *N Engl J Med.* 2019;380:347–357.

176. Verma S, Mazer CD, Yan AT, et al. Effect of empagliflozin on left ventricular mass in patients with type 2 diabetes mellitus and coronary artery disease. The EMPA-HEART CardioLink-6 Randomized Clinical Trial. *Circulation.* 2019;140:1693-1702.

177. Cannon CP, Pratley R, Dagogo-Jack S, et al. Cardiovascular outcomes with ertugliflozin in type 2 diabetes. *N Engl J Med.* 2020;383:1425-1435. doi: 10.1056/NEJMoa2004967.

178. Zelniker TA, Wiviott SD, Raz I, et al. SGLT2 inhibitors for primary and secondary prevention of cardiovascular and renal outcomes in type 2 diabetes: a systematic review and meta-analysis of cardiovascular outcome trials. *Lancet.* 2019;393:31-39.

179. Goyal I, Sattar A, Johnson M, et al. Adjunct therapies in treatment of type 1 diabetes. *J Diabetes.* 2020;12(10):742-753. doi: 10.1111/1753-0407.13078.

180. Blau JE, Tella SH, Taylor SI, et al. Ketoacidosis associated with SGLT2 inhibitor treatment: analysis of FAERS data. *Diabetes Metab Res Rev.* 2017;33:10.

181. McMurray JJV, Solomon SD, Inzucchi SE, et al. Dapagliflozin in patients with heart failure and reduced ejection fraction. *N Engl J Med.* 2019;381(21):1995-2008.

182. Packer M, Anker SD, Butler J, et al. Cardiovascular and renal outcomes with empagliflozin in heart failure. *N Engl J Med.* 2020;383:1413-1424. doi: 10.1056/NEJMoa2022190.

183. Müller TD, Finan B, Bloom SR, et al. Glucagon-like peptide 1 (GLP-1). *Mol Metab.* 2019;30:72-130.

184. Husain M, Birkenfeld AL, Donsmark M, et al. Oral semaglutide and cardiovascular outcomes in patients with type 2 diabetes. *N Engl J Med.* 2019;381:841-851.

185. Jia X, Alam M, Ye Y, Bajaj M, Birnbaum Y. GLP-1 receptor agonists and cardiovascular disease: a meta-analysis of recent cardiac outcome trials. *Cardiovasc Drugs Ther.* 2018;32(1):65-72.

186. Scirica BM, Bhatt DL, Braunwald E, et al.; Committee S-TS, Investigators. Saxagliptin and cardiovascular outcomes in patients with type 2 diabetes mellitus. *N Engl J Med.* 2013;369:1317-1326.

187. White WB, Cannon CP, Heller SR, et al.; Investigators E. Alogliptin after acute coronary syndrome in patients with type 2 diabetes. *N Engl J Med.* 2013;369:1327-1335.

188. Green JB, Bethel MA, Armstrong PW, et al.; Group TS. Effect of sitagliptin on cardiovascular outcomes in type 2 diabetes. *N Engl J Med.* 2015;373:232-242.

189. Rosenstock J, Perkovic V, Johansen OE, et al. Effect of linagliptin vs placebo on major cardiovascular events in adults with type 2 diabetes and high cardiovascular and renal risk: The CARMELINA Randomized Clinical Trial. *JAMA.* 2019;321(1):69-79.

190. Rosenstock J, Kahn SE, Erik Johansen O, et al. Effect of linagliptin vs glimepiride on major adverse cardiovascular outcomes in patients with type 2 diabetes: The CAROLINA Randomized Clinical Trial. *JAMA.* 2019;322(12):1155-1166.

191. Herrmann K, Zhou M, Wang A, et al. Cardiovascular safety assessment of pramlintide in type 2 diabetes: results from a pooled analysis of five clinical trials. *Clin Diabetes Endocrinol.* 2016;2:12. doi: 10.1186/s40842-016-0030-z. eCollection 2016.

192. Dormandy JA, Charbonnel B, Eckland DJA, et al.; PROactive Investigators. Secondary prevention of macrovascular events in patients with type 2 diabetes in the PROactive Study (PROspective pioglitAzone Clinical Trial In macroVascular Events): a randomised controlled trial. *Lancet.* 2005;366:1279-1289.

193. Erdmann E, Harding S, Lam H, Perez A. Ten-year observational follow-up of PROactive: a randomized cardiovascular outcomes trial evaluating pioglitazone in type 2 diabetes [published correction appears in *Diabetes Obes Metab.* 2017;19(6):912]. *Diabetes Obes Metab.* 2016;18(3):266-273.

194. Nissen SE, Wolski K. Effect of rosiglitazone on the risk of myocardial infarction and death from cardiovascular causes. *N Engl J Med.* 2007;356:2457–2471.

195. Mendes D, Alves C, Batel-Marques F. Number needed to harm in the post-marketing safety evaluation: results for rosiglitazone and pioglitazone. *Pharmacoepidemiol Drug Saf.* 2015;24:1259-1270.

196. Scheen AJ. Cardiovascular safety of DPP-4 inhibitors compared with sulphonylureas: Results of randomized controlled trials and observational studies. *Diabetes Metab.* 2018;44(5):386-392.

197. Coleman RL, Scott CAB, Lang Z, et al. Meta-analysis of the impact of alpha-glucosidase inhibitors on incident diabetes and cardiovascular outcomes. *Cardiovasc Diabetol.* 2019;18(1):135. doi: 10.1186/s12933-019-0933-y.

198. Playford RJ, Pither C, Gao R, et al. Use of the alpha glucosidase inhibitor acarbose in patients with 'Middleton syndrome': normal gastric anatomy but with accelerated gastric emptying causing postprandial reactive hypoglycemia and diarrhea. *Can J Gastroenterol.* 2013;27(7):403-404.

199. Insull W, Toth P, Mullican W, et al. Effectiveness of colesevelam hydrochloride in decreasing LDL cholesterol in patients with primary hypercholesterolemia: a 24-week randomized controlled trial. *Mayo Clin Proc.* 2001;76:971-982.

200. Holst Nerild H, Christensen B, Krag Knop F, et al. Preclinical discovery and development of colesevelam for the treatment of type 2 diabetes. *Exp Opin Drug Discovery.* 2018;12:1161-1167.

201. Ye X, Qian C, Liu J, et al. Lower risk of major cardiovascular events associated with adherence to colesevelam HCl. *Pharmacotherapy.* 2013;33(10):1062-1070.

202. Kerr JL, Timpe EM, Petkewicz KA. Bromocriptine mesylate for glycemic management in type 2 diabetes mellitus. *Ann Pharmacother.* 2010;44:1777-1785.

203. Gaziano JM, Cincotta AH, O'Connor CM, et al. Randomized clinical trial of quick-release bromocriptine among patients with type 2 diabetes on overall safety and cardiovascular outcomes. *Diabetes Care.* 2010;33(7):1503-1508.

204. Herman ME, O'Keefe JH, Bell DSH, et al. Insulin therapy increases cardiovascular risk in type 2 diabetes. *Prog Cardiovasc Dis.* 2017;60(3):422-434.

205. Bailey TS, Grunberger G, Bode BW, et al. American Association of Clinical Endocrinologists and American College of Endocrinology 2016 outpatient glucose monitoring consensus statement. *Endocr Pract.* 2016;22(2):231-261.

206. Mechanick JI, Rosenson RS, Pinney SP, et al. Coronavirus and cardiometabolic syndrome. *J Am Coll Cardiol.* 2020;76(17):2024-2035.

207. Sjöström L, Peltonen M, Jacobson P, et al. Bariatric surgery and long-term cardiovascular events. *JAMA.* 2012;307(1):56-65.

208. Aminian A, Zajichek A, Arterburn DE, et al. Association of Metabolic Surgery with Major Adverse Cardiovascular Outcomes in Patients with Type 2 Diabetes and Obesity [published online ahead of print, 2019 Sep 2]. *JAMA.* 2019;322(13):1271-1282.

209. Jamaly S, Carlsson L, Peltonen M, et al. Surgical obesity treatment and the risk of heart failure. *Eur Heart J.* 2019;40(26):2131-2138.

210. Sundstrom J, Bruze G, Ottosson J, et al. Weight loss and heart failure. *Circulation.* 2017;135:1577-1585.

211. Jamaly S, Carlsson L, Peltonen M, et al. Bariatric surgery and the risk of new-onset atrial fibrillation in Swedish obese subjects. *J Am Coll Cardiol.* 2016;68:2497-2504.

212. Lynch KT, Mehaffey JH, Hawkins RB, et al. Bariatric surgery reduces incidence of atrial fibrillation: a propensity score-matched analysis. *Surg Obes Rel Dis.* 2019;15:279-287.

213. Gruessner AC, Sutherland DE. Pancreas transplant outcomes for the United States (US) and non-US cases as reported to the United Network for Organ Sharing (UNOS) and the International Pancreas Transplant Registry (IPTR) as of June 2004. *Clin Transplant.* 2005;19(4):433-455.

214. Qi M, Kinzer K, Danielson KK, et al. Five-year follow-up of patients with type 1 diabetes transplanted with allogeneic islets: the UIC experience. *Acta Diabetol.* 2014;51:833-843.

215. Russell SJ, El-Khatib SH, Sinha M, et al. Outpatient glycemic control with a bionic pancreas in type 1 diabetes. *N Engl J Med.* 2014;311:313-325.

216. Tian C, Bagley J, Cretin N, et al. Prevention of type 1 diabetes by gene therapy. *J Clin Invest.* 2004;114(7):969-978.

217. Zulewski H, Abraham EJ, Gerlach MJ, et al. Multipotential nestling-positive stem cells isolated from adult pancreatic islets differentiate ex vivo into pancreatic endocrine, exocrine and hepatic phenotypes. *Diabetes.* 2001;50(3):521-533.

218. Kumar K, Wang P, Swartz EA, et al. Structure-activity relationships and biological evaluation of 7-substituted harmine analogs for human β-cell proliferation. *Molecules.* 2020;25:1983. doi: 10.3390/molecules25081983.

219. Nistor I, De Sutter J, Drechsler C, et al. Effect of renin–angiotensin–aldosterone system blockade in adults with diabetes mellitus and advanced chronic kidney disease not on dialysis: a systematic review and meta-analysis. *Nephrol Dial Transplant.* 2018;33:12-22.

220. Brenner BM, Cooper ME, de Zeeuw D, et al. Effects of losartan on renal and cardiovascular outcomes in patients with type 2 diabetes and nephropathy. *N Engl J Med.* 2001;345:861–869.

221. Barnett AH, Mithal A, Manassie J, et al.; EMPA-REG RENAL Trial Investigators. Efficacy and safety of empagliflozin added to existing antidiabetes treatment in patients with type 2 diabetes and chronic kidney disease: a randomised, double-blind, placebo-controlled trial. *Lancet Diabetes Endocrinol.* 2014;2:369-384.

222. Mudaliar S, Polidori D, Zambrowicz B, et al. Sodium-glucose cotransporter inhibitors: effects on renal and intestinal glucose transport: from bench to bedside. *Diabetes Care.* 2015;38(12):2344-2353.

223. Spallone V. Update on the impact, diagnosis and management of cardiovascular Autonomic neuropathy in diabetes: what is defined, what is new, and what is unmet. *Diabetes Metab J.* 2019;43:3-30.

224. UK Prospective Diabetes Study Group. Tight blood pressure control and risk of macrovascular and microvascular complications in type 2 diabetes: UKPDS 38. *BMJ.* 1998;317(7160):703–713.

225. Amoaku WM, Ghanchi F, Bailey C, et al. Diabetic retinopathy and diabetic macular oedema pathways and management: UK Consensus Working Group. *Eye.* 2020;34:1-51.

226. Young LH, Wackers FJ, Chyun DA, et al.; DIAD Investigators. Cardiac outcomes after screening for asymptomatic coronary artery disease in patients with type 2 diabetes: the DIAD study: a randomized controlled trial. *JAMA.* 2009;301(15):1547-1555.

227. Boden WE, O'Rourke RA, Teo KK, et al. Optimal medical therapy with or without PCI for stable coronary disease. *N Engl J Med.* 2007;356(15):1503-1516.

228. BARI 2D Study Group; Frye RL, August P, Brooks MM, et al. A randomized trial of therapies for type 2 diabetes and coronary artery disease. *N Engl J Med.* 2009;360(24):2503-2515.

229. Kapur A, Hall RJ, Malik IS, et al. Randomized comparison of percutaneous coronary intervention with coronary artery bypass grafting in diabetic patients. 1-year results of the CARDia (Coronary Artery Revascularization in Diabetes) trial. *J Am Coll Cardiol.* 2010;55(5):432-440.

230. Kamalesh M, Sharp TG, Tang XC, et al. Percutaneous coronary intervention versus coronary bypass surgery in United States veterans with diabetes. *J Am Coll Cardiol.* 2013;61(8):808-816.

231. Kappetein AP, Head SJ, Morice MC, et al. Treatment of complex coronary artery disease in patients with diabetes: 5-year results comparing outcomes of bypass surgery and percutaneous coronary intervention in the SYNTAX trial. *Eur J Cardiothoracic Surg.* 2013;43(5):1006-1013.

232. Farkouh ME, Domanski M, Sleeper LA, et al. Strategies for multivessel revascularization in patients with diabetes. *N Engl J Med.* 2012;367(25):2375-2384.

233. Farkouh ME, Domanski M, Dangas GD, et al. Long-term survival following multivessel revascularization in patients with diabetes: the FREEDOM follow-on study. *J Am Coll Cardiol.* 2019;73(6):629-638.

234. Esper RB, Farkouh ME, Ribeiro EE, et al. SYNTAX Score in patients with diabetes undergoing coronary revascularization in the FREEDOM trial. *J Am Coll Cardiol.* 2018;72(23 Pt A):2826-2837.

235. Kaul U, Bangalore S, Seth A, et al.; TUXEDO–India Investigators. Paclitaxel-eluting versus everolimus-eluting coronary stents in diabetes. *N Engl J Med.* 2015;373(18):1709-1719.

236. Neumann FJ, Sousa-Uva M, Ahlsson A, et al. 2018 ESC/EACTS Guidelines on myocardial revascularization. *Eur Heart J.* 2019;40:87-165.

237. Weintraub WS, Grau-Sepulveda MV, Weiss JM, et al. Comparative effectiveness of revascularization strategies. *N Engl J Med.* 2012;366:1467-1476.

238. Tam DY, Dharma C, Rocha R, et al. Long-term survival after surgical or percutaneous revascularization in patients with diabetes and multivessel coronary disease. *J Am Coll Cardiol.* 2020;76(10):1153-1164.

239. Head SJ, Milojevic M, Daemen J, et al. Mortality after coronary artery bypass grafting versus percutaneous coronary intervention with stenting for coronary artery disease: a pooled analysis of individual patient data. *Lancet.* 2018;391:939-948.

240. Head SJ, Milojevic M, Daemen J, et al. Stroke rates following surgical versus percutaneous coronary revascularization. *J Am Coll Cardiol.* 2018;72:386-398.

241. Dorman MJ, Kurlansky PA, Traad EA, et al. Bilateral internal mammary artery grafting enhances survival in diabetic patients: a 30-year follow-up of propensity score-matched cohorts. *Circulation.* 2012;126:2935-2942.

242. Taggart DP, Benedetto U, Gerry S, et al. Bilateral versus single internal-thoracic-artery grafts at 10 years. *N Engl J Med.* 2019;380:437-446.

243. Ramanathan K, Abel JG, Park JE, et al. Surgical versus percutaneous coronary revascularization in patients with diabetes and acute coronary syndromes. *J Am Coll Cardiol.* 2017;70(24):2995-3006.

244. Malmberg K, for the DIGAMI Study Group. Prospective randomised study of intensive insulin treatment on long-term survival after acute myocardial infarction in patients with diabetes mellitus. *BMJ.* 1997;314:1512-1515.

245. Malmberg K, Ryden L, Wedel H, et al.; DIGAMI 2 Investigators. Intense metabolic control by means of insulin in patients with diabetes mellitus and acute myocardial infarction (DIGAMI 2): effects on mortality and morbidity. *Eur Heart J.* 2005;26(7):650-661.

246. Lisi D, Andrews E, Parry C, et al. The effect of ranolazine on glycemic control: a narrative review to define the target population. *Cardiovasc Drugs Ther.* 2019;33(6):755-761.

247. Kosiborod M, Arnold SV, Spertus JA, et al. Evaluation of ranolazine in patients with type 2 diabetes mellitus and chronic stable angina: results from the TERISA randomized clinical trial (Type 2 diabetes evaluation of ranolazine in subjects with chronic stable angina). *J Am Coll Cardiol.* 2013;61(20):2038-2045.

248. Mehta PK, Goykhman P, Thomson LE, et al. Ranolazine improves angina in women with evidence of myocardial ischemia but no obstructive coronary artery disease. *JACC Cardiovasc Imaging.* 2011;4(5):514-522.

249. Tagliamonte E, Rigo F, Cirillo T, et al. Effects of ranolazine on noninvasive coronary flow reserve in patients with myocardial ischemia but without obstructive coronary artery disease. *Echocardiography.* 2015;32(3):516-521.

250. Villano A, Di Franco A, Nerla R, et al. Effects of ivabradine and ranolazine in patients with microvascular angina pectoris. *Am J Cardiol.* 2013;112(1):8-13.

251. Bairey Merz CN, Handberg EM, Shufelt CL, et al. A randomized, placebo-controlled trial of late Na current inhibition (ranolazine) in coronary microvascular dysfunction (CMD): impact on angina and myocardial perfusion reserve. *Eur Heart J.* 2016;37(19):1504-1513.

252. Fanaroff AC, James SK, Weisz G, et al. Ranolazine after incomplete percutaneous coronary revascularization in patients with versus without diabetes mellitus: RIVER-PCI trial. *J Am Coll Cardiol.* 2017;69(18):2304-2313.

253. Timmis AD, Chaitman BR, Crager M. Effects of ranolazine on exercise tolerance and HbA1c in patients with chronic angina and diabetes. *Eur Heart J.* 2006;27(1):42-48.

254. Banerjee K, Ghosh RK, Kamatam S, et al. Role of Ranolazine in cardiovascular disease and diabetes: exploring beyond angina. *Int J Cardiol.* 2017;227:556-564.

255. Filippo Crea, C. Noel Bairey Merz, John F. Beltrame, et al.; On behalf of the Coronary Vasomotion Disorders International Study Group (COVADIS). The parallel tales of microvascular angina and heart failure with preserved ejection fraction: a paradigm shift. *Eur Heart J.* 2017;38:473-477.

256. McMurray JJ, Packer M, Desai AS, et al. Angiotensin-neprilysin inhibition versus enalapril in heart failure. *N Engl J Med.* 2014;371(11):993-1004.

257. Solomon SD, McMurray JJV, Anand IS, et al. Angiotensin-neprilysin inhibition in heart failure with preserved ejection fraction. *N Engl J Med.* 2019;381(17):1609-1620.

258. Vaduganathan M, Fonarow GC, Greene SJ, et al. Contemporary treatment patterns and clinical outcomes of comorbid diabetes mellitus and HFrEF: The CHAMP-HF Registry. *JACC Heart Fail.* 2020;8(6):469-480.

259. Pratley RE, Husain M, Lingvay I, et al. Heart failure with insulin degludec versus glargine U100 in patients with type 2 diabetes at high risk of cardiovascular disease: DEVOTE 14. *Cardiovasc Diabetol.* 2019;18:156.

260. Pathak RK, Middeldorp ME, Meredith M, et al. Long-term effect of goal-directed weight management in an atrial fibrillation cohort: a Long-Term Follow-Up Study (LEGACY). *J Am Coll Cardiol.* 2015;65:2159-2169.

261. Abed HS, Wittert GA, Leong DP, et al. Effect of weight reduction and cardiometabolic risk factor management on symptom burden and severity in patients with atrial fibrillation: a randomized clinical trial. *JAMA.* 2013;310:2050-2060.

262. Pallisgaard JL, Lindhardt TB, Staerk L, et al. Thiazolidinediones are associated with a decreased risk of atrial fibrillation compared with other antidiabetic treatment: a nationwide cohort study. *Eur Heart J Cardiovasc Pharmacother.* 2017;3:140-146.

263. Chen HY, Yang FY, Jong GP, Liou YS. Antihyperglycemic drugs use and new-onset atrial fibrillation in elderly patients. *Eur J Clin Invest.* 2017;47:388-393.

264. Zelniker TA, Bonaca MP, Furtado RHM, et al. Effect of dapagliflozin on atrial fibrillation in patients with type 2 diabetes mellitus. *Circulation.* 2020;141:1227-1234.

265. Nreu B, Dicembrini I, Tinti F, et al. Major cardiovascular events, heart failure, and atrial fibrillation in patients treated with glucagon-like peptide-1 receptor agonists: an updated meta-analysis of randomized controlled trials. *Nutr Metab Cardiovasc Dis.* 2020;30(7):1106-1114.

266. Lega JC, Bertoletti L, Gremillet C, et al. Consistency of safety and efficacy of new oral anticoagulants across subgroups of patients with atrial fibrillation. *PLoS One.* 2014;9:e91398.

267. Reilly PA, Lehr T, Haertter S, et al. The effect of dabigatran plasma concentrations and patient characteristics on the frequency of ischemic stroke and major bleeding in atrial fibrillation patients: the RE-LY Trial (Randomized Evaluation of Long-Term Anticoagulation Therapy). *J Am Coll Cardiol,* 2014;63:321-328.

268. Hylek EM, Held C, Alexander JH, et al. Major bleeding in patients with atrial fibrillation receiving apixaban or warfarin: The ARISTOTLE Trial (apixaban for reduction in stroke and other thromboembolic events in atrial fibrillation): predictors, characteristics, and clinical outcomes. *J Am Coll Cardiol,* 2014;63:2141-2147.

269. Goodman SG, Wojdyla DM, Piccini JP, et al. Factors associated with major bleeding events: insights from the ROCKET AF trial (rivaroxaban once-daily oral direct factor Xa inhibition compared with vitamin K antagonism for prevention of stroke and embolism trial in atrial fibrillation). *J Am Coll Cardiol.* 2014;63:891-900.

270. Clark AL, Best CJ, Fisher SJ. Even silent hypoglycemia induces cardiac arrhythmias. *Diabetes.* 2014;63(5):1457-1459.

271. Hsieh YC, Liao YC, Li CH, et al. Hypoglycaemic episodes increase the risk of ventricular arrhythmia and sudden cardiac arrest in patients with type 2 diabetes—A nationwide cohort study. *Diabetes Metab Res Rev.* 2020;36:e3226.

272. Tran HV, Gore JM, Darling CE, et al. Hyperglycemia and risk of ventricular tachycardia among patients hospitalized with acute myocardial infarction. *Cardiovasc Diabetol.* 2018;17(1):136.

273. Petznick AM, Shubrook JH. Treatment of specific macrovascular beds in patients with diabetes mellitus. *Osteopath Med Prim Care.* 2010;4:5. doi: 10.1186/1750-4732-4-5 .

274. Singh S, Armstrong EJ, Sherif W, et al. Association of elevated fasting glucose with lower patency and increased major adverse limb events among patients with diabetes undergoing infrapopliteal balloon angioplasty. *Vasc Med.* 2014;19:307-314.

275. Dick F, Diehm N, Galimanis A, et al. Surgical or endovascular revascularization in patients with critical limb ischemia: influence of diabetes mellitus on clinical outcome. *J Vasc Surg.* 2007;45:751-761.

276. Forsythe RO, Jones KG, Hinchliffe RJ. Distal bypasses in patients with diabetes and infrapopliteal disease: technical considerations to achieve success. *Int J Low Extrem Wounds.* 2014;13:347-362.

277. De Ferrari GM, Stevens SR, Ambrosio G, et al. Low-density lipoprotein cholesterol treatment and outcomes in patients with type 2 diabetes and established cardiovascular disease: insights from TECAS. *Am Heart J.* 2020;220:82-88.

278. Giugliano RP, Cannon CP, Blazing MA, et al. Benefit of adding ezetimibe to statin therapy on cardiovascular outcomes and safety in patients with versus without diabetes mellitus: results from IMPROVE-IT (Improved Reduction of Outcomes: Vytorin Efficacy International Trial). *Circulation.* 2018;137(15):1571-1582.

279. Blom DJ, Hala T, Bolognese M, et al. A 52-week placebo-controlled trial of evolocumab in hyperlipidemia. *N Engl J Med.* 2014;370:1809-1819.

280. Stein EA, Mellis S, Yancopoulos GD, et al. Effects of a monoclonal antibody to PCSK9 on LDL cholesterol. *N Engl J Med.* 2012;366:1108-1118.

281. Sabatine MS, Giugliano RP, Keech AC, et al.; FOURIER Steering Committee and Investigators. Evolocumab and clinical outcomes in patients with cardiovascular disease. *N Engl J Med.* 2017;376:1713-1722.

282. Sabatine MS, Leiter LA, Wiviott SD, et al. Cardiovascular safety and efficacy of the PCSK9 inhibitor evolocumab in patients with and without diabetes and the effect of evolocumab on glycaemia and risk of new-onset diabetes: a prespecified analysis of the FOURIER randomised controlled trial. *Lancet Diabetes Endocrinol.* 2017;5:941-950.

283. Ray KK, Colhoun HM, Szarek M, et al.; ODYSSEY OUTCOMES Committees and Investigators. Effects of alirocumab on cardiovascular and metabolic outcomes after acute coronary syndrome in patients with or without diabetes: a prespecified analysis of the ODYSSEY OUTCOMES randomised controlled trial. *Lancet Diabetes Endocrinol.* 2019;7(8):618-628.

284. Arbel R, Hammerman A, Azuri J. Usefulness of ezetimibe versus evolocumab as add-on therapy for secondary prevention of cardiovascular events in patients with type 2 diabetes mellitus. *Am J Cardiol.* 2019;123:1273-1276.

285. Reyes-Suffer G, Ngai CI, Lovato L, et al. Effect of combination therapy with fenofibrate and simvastatin on postprandial lipemia in the ACCORD lipid trial. *Diabetes Care.* 2013;36:422-428.

286. Lan NSR, Fegan PG, Yeap BB, et al. Icosapent ethyl for dyslipidaemia in patients with diabetes and coronary artery disease: Act now to reduce it. *Diabetes Obes Metab.* 2019;21(7):1734-1736.

287. Boer-Martins L, Figueiredo VN, Demacq C, et al. Relationship of autonomic imbalance and circadian disruption with obesity and type 2 diabetes in resistant hypertensive patients. *Cardiovasc Diabetol.* 2011; 10:24.

288. Emdin CA, Rahimi K, Neal B, et al. Blood pressure lowering in type 2 diabetes: a systematic review and meta-analysis. *JAMA.* 2015;313:603–615.

289. Brunström M, Carlberg B. Effect of antihypertensive treatment at different blood pressure levels in patients with diabetes mellitus: systematic review and meta-analyses. *BMJ.* 2016;352:i717.

290. Thomopoulos C, Parati G, Zanchetti A. Effects of blood-pressure-lowering treatment on outcome incidence in hypertension: 10—should blood pressure management differ in hypertensive patients with and without diabetes mellitus? Overview and meta-analyses of randomized trials. *J Hypertens.* 2017;35:922-944.

291. Ettehad D, Emdin CA, Kiran A, et al. Blood pressure lowering for prevention of cardiovascular disease and death: a systematic review and meta-analysis. *Lancet.* 2016;387:957-967.

292. Shorr RI, Ray WA, Daugherty JR, et al. Antihypertensives and the risk of serious hypoglycemia in older persons using insulin or sulfonylureas. *JAMA.* 1997;278(1):40-43.

293. Shavadia JS, Zheng Y, Green JB, et al. Associations between β-blocker therapy and cardiovascular outcomes in patients with diabetes and established cardiovascular disease. *Am Heart J.* 2019;218:92-99.

294. Vernstrom L, Laugesen E, Graove EL, et al. Differential vascular effects of aspirin in people with type 2 diabetes without cardiovascular disease and matched controls without diabetes. *Diabet Med.* 2019;36:1141-1148.

295. Patti G, Proscia C, Di Sciascio G. Antiplatelet therapy in patients with diabetes mellitus and acute coronary syndrome. *Circ J.* 2014;78(1):33-41.

296. CURRENT-OASIS 7 Investigators, Mehta SR, Bassand JP, Chrolavicius S, et al. Dose comparisons of clopidogrel and aspirin in acute coronary syndromes. *N Engl J Med.* 2010;363:930-942.

297. James S, Angiolillo DJ, Cornel JH, et al. Ticagrelor versus. clopidogrel in patients with acute coronary syndromes and diabetes: a substudy from the PLATelet inhibition and patient Outcomes (PLATO) trial. *Eur Heart J.* 2010;31:3006-3016.

298. Ferreiro JL, Ueno M, Tello-Montoliu A, et al. Effects of cangrelor in coronary artery disease patients with and without diabetes mellitus: an in vitro pharmacodynamics investigation. *J Thromb Thrombolysis.* 2013;35:155-164.

299. Angiolillo DJ, Capranzano P, Ferreiro JL, et al. Impact of adjunctive cilostazol therapy on platelet function profiles in patients with and without diabetes mellitus on aspirin and clopidogrel therapy. *Thromb Haemost.* 2011;106:253-262.

300. Angiolillo DJ, Badimon JJ, Saucedo JF, et al. A pharmacodynamic comparison of prasugrel versus high-dose clopidogrel in patients with type 2 diabetes mellitus and coronary artery disease: Results of the OPTIMUS-3 trial. *Eur Heart J.* 2011;32:838-846.

301. Wiviott SD, Braunwald E, Angiolillo DJ, et al.; TRITON-TIMI 38 Investigators. Greater clinical benefit of more intensive oral antiplatelet therapy with prasugrel in patients with diabetes mellitus in the trial to assess improvement in therapeutic outcomes by optimizing platelet inhibition with prasugrel-Thrombolysis in Myocardial Infarction 38. *Circulation.* 2008;118(16):1626-1636.

302. Morel O, Muller C, Jesel L, et al. Impaired platelet P2Y12 inhibition by thienopyridines in chronic kidney disease: mechanisms, clinical relevance and pharmacological options. *Nephrol Dial Transplant.* 2013;28(8):1994-2002.

303. Franchi F, James SK, Ghukasyan T, et al. Impact of diabetes mellitus and chronic kidney disease on cardiovascular outcomes and platelet P2Y$_{12}$ receptor antagonist effects in patients with acute coronary syndromes: insights from the PLATO Trial. *J Am Heart Assoc.* 2019;8:e011139.

304. Steg PG, Bhatt DL, Simon T, et al.; THEMIS Steering Committee and Investigators. Ticagrelor in patients with stable coronary disease and diabetes. *N Engl J Med.* 2019;381(14):1309-1320.

305. Bhatt DL, Steg PG, Mehta SR, et al.; THEMIS Steering Committee and Investigators. Ticagrelor in patients with diabetes and stable coronary artery disease with a history of previous percutaneous coronary intervention (THEMIS-PCI): a phase 3, placebo-controlled, randomised trial. *Lancet.* 2019;394(10204):1169-1180.

306. Low Wang CC, Blomster JI, Heizer G, et al. Cardiovascular and limb outcomes in patients with diabetes and peripheral artery disease. The Euclid Trial. *J Am Coll Cardiol.* 2018;72:3274-3284.

307. Collet JP, Thiele H, Barbato E, et al.; the ESC Scientific Document Group. 2020 ESC Guidelines for the management of acute coronary syndromes in patients presenting without persistent ST-segment elevation. *Eur Heart J.* 2020;42(14):1289-1367. doi: 10.1093/eurheartj/ehaa575.

308. Cosentino F, Grant PJ, Aboyans V, et al.; the ESC Scientific Document Group. 2019 ESC Guidelines on diabetes, pre-diabetes, and

cardiovascular diseases developed in collaboration with the EASD. *Eur Heart J.* 2020;41(2):255-323.

309. Arnett DK, Blumenthal RS, Albert MA, et al. 2019 ACC/AHA guidelines on the primary prevention of cardiovascular disease: executive summary: a report of the American College of Cardiology/American Heart Association Task Force on Clinical Practice Guidelines. *Circulation.* 2019;140(11):e563-e595.

310. Grundy SM, Stone NJ, Bailey AL, et al. AHA/ACC/AACVPR/AAPA/ABC/ACPM/ADA/AGS/AphA/ASPC/NLA/PCNA guideline on the management of blood cholesterol: a report of the American College of Cardiology/American Heart Association Task Force on Clinical Practice Guidelines. *Circulation.* 2019;139(25):e1082-e1143.

311. Whelton PK, Carey RM, Aronow WS, et al. 2017 ACC/AHA/AAPA/ABC/ACPM/AGS/AphA/ASH/ASPC/NMA/PCNA guideline for the prevention, detection, evaluation, and management of high blood pressure in adults: a report of the American College of Cardiology/American Heart Association Task Force on Clinical Practice Guidelines. *Circulation.* 2018;138(17):e426-e483.

312. Chan PS, Oetgen WJ, Buchanan D, et al. Cardiac performance measure compliance in outpatients: the American College of Cardiology and National Cardiovascular Data Registry's PINNACLE (Practice Innovation And Clinical Excellence) program. *J Am Coll Cardiol.* 2010;56:8-14.

313. Das SR, Everett BM, Birtcher KK, et al. 2020 ACC expert consensus decision pathway on novel therapies for cardiovascular risk reduction in patients with type 2 diabetes and atherosclerotic cardiovascular disease: a report of the American College of Cardiology Solution Set Oversight Committee. *J Am Coll Cardiol.* 2020;76. doi: 10.1016/j.jacc.2020.05.037.

8

Tobacco-Related Cardiovascular Disease

Nancy A. Rigotti, Sara Kalkhoran, and Neal L. Benowitz

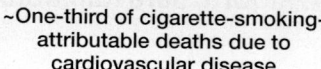

Effects of cigarette smoking on cardiovascular disease and events

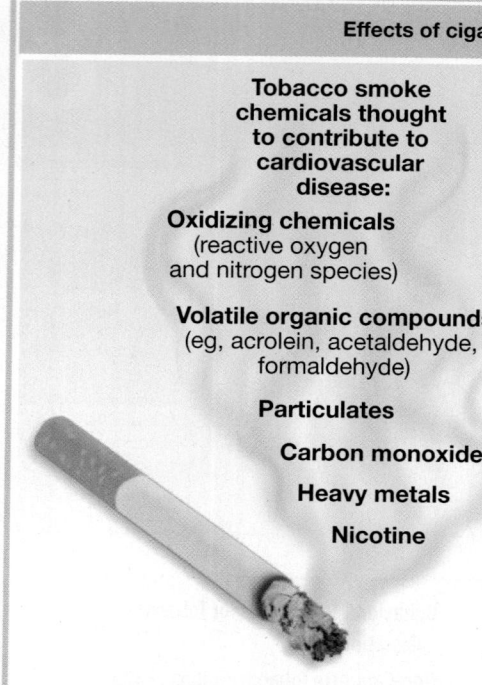

Tobacco smoke chemicals thought to contribute to cardiovascular disease:

Oxidizing chemicals (reactive oxygen and nitrogen species)

Volatile organic compounds (eg, acrolein, acetaldehyde, formaldehyde)

Particulates

Carbon monoxide

Heavy metals

Nicotine

- Oxidative injury
- Endothelial damage and dysfunction
- Enhanced plaque rupture and thrombosis
- Chronic inflammation
- Hemodynamic stress
- Adverse effects on blood lipids
- Insulin resistance and diabetes mellitus
- Reduced oxygen delivery by red blood cells
- Arrhythmogenesis

Cardiovascular disease and events
including

myocardial infarction, stroke, peripheral arterial disease, abdominal aortic aneurysm, sudden cardiac death, left ventricular hypertrophy and diastolic dysfunction, cardiac arrhythmias (atrial fibrillation and ventricular arrhythmias), higher risk of restenosis after coronary revascularization

---

~One-third of cigarette-smoking-attributable deaths due to cardiovascular disease

~20% of annual cardiovascular deaths are attributable to cigarette smoking

Smokers have double the risk of cardiovascular death as never smokers

Excess cardiovascular risk caused by cigarette smoking is rapidly reversible after smoking cessation

Chapter 8 Fuster and Hurst's Central Illustration. Cigarette smoking is associated with excess risk of cardiac events. Pathophysiological mechanisms of tobacco-related cardiovascular disease are shown. Smoking cessation results in an immediate reduction in risk of cardiac events, which continues to decline rapidly.

CHAPTER SUMMARY

This chapter discusses the epidemiology and pathophysiology of tobacco-related cardiovascular disease (CVD), as well as the cardiovascular benefits of and effective strategies for cessation of tobacco use (see Fuster and Hurst's Central Illustration). Around 20% of annual cardiovascular deaths are attributed to cigarette smoking. The oxidizing chemicals (reactive oxygen and nitrogen species), volatile organic compounds (such as acrolein, acetaldehyde, and formaldehyde), particulates, carbon monoxide, heavy metals, and nicotine found in tobacco smoke are all thought to contribute to CVD. Smoking has been associated with the development of multiple cardiovascular conditions and events, and smoking cessation results in an immediate reduction in the risk of cardiac events, which continues to decline rapidly. Behavioral support and pharmacotherapy are effective strategies for smoking cessation, and combining these strategies produces the best results. Approved pharmacotherapies include nicotine-replacement therapy (available in the form of patches, gum, lozenges, oral inhalers, and nasal sprays), varenicline, and bupropion. The long-term health effects of electronic cigarettes (e-cigarettes) are not well established and clinicians should thus recommend the use of smoking cessation treatments approved by the US Food and Drug Administration (FDA) first.

PREVALENCE AND IMPACT OF TOBACCO USE

Tobacco use causes over 8 million annual deaths worldwide through both active tobacco use and secondhand smoke exposure.[1] In the United States, over 480,000 deaths per year are attributable to cigarette smoking,[2] and approximately one-third of these smoking-attributable deaths are due to cardiovascular disease (CVD),[2] the leading cause of death.[3] CVD causes approximately 800,000 deaths a year.[4] Approximately 160,000 deaths (20% of annual cardiovascular deaths) are attributable to cigarette smoking, which is also responsible for over 113,000 deaths from respiratory diseases and over 163,000 deaths from cancers.[5] The life expectancy of a lifelong smoker is reduced by at least 10 years compared to that of a nonsmoker,[6] and smokers have double the risk of cardiovascular mortality as never smokers.[7] Therefore, treating tobacco use is a critical component of overall preventive care and cardiovascular risk reduction.

Trends in Prevalence of Tobacco Use

Over 1 billion people use tobacco globally, and over 80% of tobacco users live in low- and middle-income countries.[8] The majority of smokers worldwide are men. In 2015, the prevalence of daily smoking was 25% among men and 5.4% among women.[9]

In the United States, cigarette consumption has been declining since the 1960s when over 40% of Americans smoked (**Fig. 8–1**). The 1964 Surgeon General's report highlighted the negative health effects associated with cigarette smoking, laying the foundation for several tobacco control policies and increased public awareness of the risks of smoking. These policies came several years after aggressive and deceptive advertising and marketing campaigns by the tobacco industry to increase the popularity of cigarette smoking, as well as conflicts of interests and fostering a rhetoric of scientific uncertainty about the evidence surrounding the harms associated with tobacco use.

Despite these advances, 34-million US adults (approximately 14% of the adult population) reported smoking cigarettes in 2018.[10] There are significant disparities in smoking prevalence among US adults, with higher rates of use among adults with less education; lower income; lesbian, gay, or bisexual sexual orientation; and serious psychological distress.[10] Cigarette smoking among youth in the United States continues to decrease, with only 5.8% of high school students and 2.3% of middle school students reporting current use in 2019.[11]

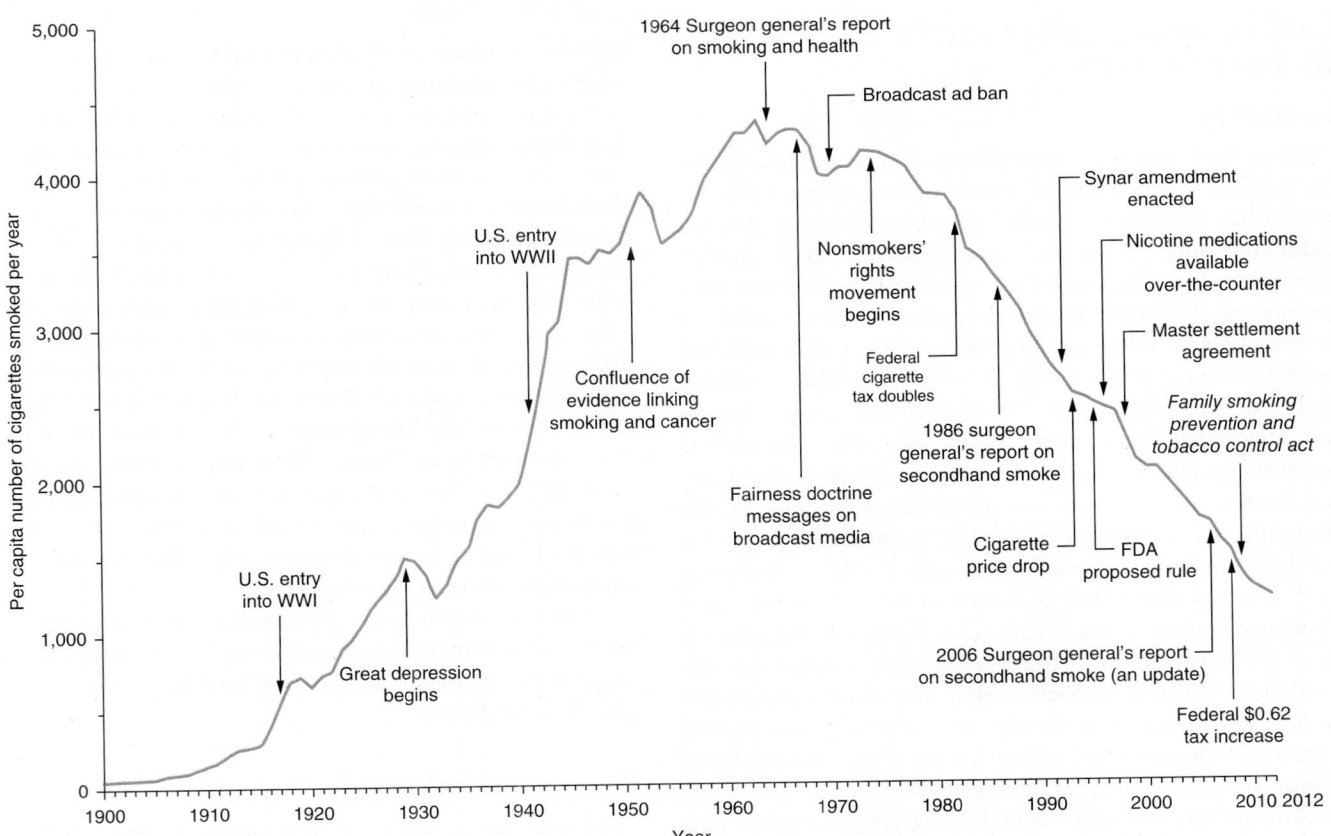

Adults ≥18 years of age as reported annually by the Census Bureau.

Figure 8–1. Trends in per capita cigarette consumption among the US adult population. Reproduced with permission from US Department of Health and Human Services. *The Health Consequences of Smoking: 50 Years of Progress. A Report of the Surgeon General*. Atlanta, GA: US Department of Health and Human Services, Centers for Disease Control and Prevention, National Center for Chronic Disease Prevention and Health Promotion, Office on Smoking and Health, 2014.

Types of Tobacco Products

While cigarette smoking is most prevalent, millions of US adults and youth use non-cigarette nicotine and tobacco products.[10,11] In 2017, an estimated 19% of adult tobacco users used multiple tobacco products, and in 2019,[12] 11% of high school students reported use of two or more tobacco products over the past 30 days.[11] Non-cigarette nicotine and tobacco products come in many forms that can be organized into two categories: smoked (or combustible) and smokeless (or noncombustible). Combustible products are those that burn tobacco, producing smoke that is inhaled. These products include cigars, cigarillos, pipes, and waterpipes (also called hookah, narghile, or shisha). Noncombustible products include smokeless tobacco, which is chewed, sniffed, or placed between the gum and cheek, and two newer alternative tobacco products: electronic cigarettes (e-cigarettes), which heat a solution containing nicotine to create an aerosol that is inhaled, and heated tobacco products, which heat tobacco without burning it, also producing an inhaled aerosol. The distinction between combustible and noncombustible tobacco products is made because while both categories carry health risks, the large majority of tobacco-related cardiovascular risks are due to the chemicals produced when tobacco leaf is burned and the smoke inhaled by users of combustible tobacco products.[13]

CARDIOVASCULAR EFFECTS OF TOBACCO USE

Cigarettes

Cigarette smoking is associated with accelerated atherosclerosis, acute plaque rupture, and all cardiovascular events, including myocardial infarction, stroke, peripheral arterial disease, abdominal aortic aneurysm, and sudden cardiac death.[13] Smoking is also associated with a higher risk of restenosis after coronary revascularization, including after coronary angioplasty or thrombolysis. While smoking increases the risk of ischemic heart disease and stroke 2-fold, it increases the risk of sudden cardiac death 3-fold and the risk of peripheral arterial disease and abdominal aortic aneurysm 5-fold.[5] The relationship between cigarettes smoked per day and coronary heart disease is nonlinear, such that the risk associated with smoking five cigarettes per day is more than 50% that of smoking 20 cigarettes per day.[14] Smoking is also associated with cardiac arrhythmias such as atrial fibrillation and ventricular arrhythmias, and smoking cessation results in clinical improvement and reduced mortality in patients with heart failure with reduced ejection fraction.[15–17] Cigarette smokers demonstrate a higher prevalence of left ventricular hypertrophy and diastolic dysfunction compared to nonsmokers, independently from coronary heart disease or alcohol use.[18] Other adverse vascular effects of smoking include impaired wound healing, erectile dysfunction, and macular degeneration.[5] Smoking acts synergistically with hypertension, diabetes, and hyperlipidemia to increase cardiovascular risk.[5] While the absolute risk of myocardial infarction is greatest in elderly smokers, the relative risk is much higher in younger smokers.[5]

Secondhand Tobacco Smoke Exposure

Exposure to secondhand smoke has been reported in many studies to be associated with an increase in coronary heart disease and stroke risk in nonsmokers, with meta-analyses indicating a 25% to 30% increased risk.[19,20] A higher coronary calcium score has been reported among never smokers who are exposed to secondhand smoke.[21] Exposure to cigarette smoke from parental smoking during childhood was associated with a higher risk of developing carotid atherosclerotic plaques and higher carotid intima-media thickness during adulthood, even 25 years after last exposure among Cardiovascular Risk in Young Finns Study participants.[22,23]

In addition to long-term effects, secondhand smoke exposure acutely causes endothelial dysfunction and platelet activation, which can trigger acute ischemic events in vulnerable people.[24] Reduced hospital admissions for myocardial infarction are seen soon after communities implement smoke-free laws.[25] A decrease in cardiovascular morbidity and mortality has been reported immediately following workplace bans of cigarette smoking, even among people who have never smoked.[26] These studies provide a compelling rationale for cardiologists to ask all patients about their exposure to secondhand smoke and provide clear advice to avoid such exposures.

Cigars and Pipes

Cigars are products in which shredded tobacco is wrapped with a tobacco-containing substance or tobacco leaf. Cigars come in various types, including little cigars, cigarillos, and large (premium) cigars. In the United States, 3.9% of adults reported current use of cigars/cigarillos in 2018,[10] and 7.6% of high school students and 2.3% of middle school students reported a past-30-day use of cigars in 2019.[11] Cigar smoke contains the same toxins as cigarette smoke. Cigar use has been associated with coronary heart disease among men, with greater cigar consumption associated with greater risk.[27] Exclusive cigar smokers have also been shown to have increased all-cause mortality compared to never tobacco users.[28] One study found that men 75 years old or younger who smoke cigars to be at higher risk of death from coronary heart disease.[29] However, in general, the risk of coronary heart disease is lower in cigar smokers because they smoke less frequently and/or do not inhale the smoke. Of note, former cigarette smokers are more likely to inhale cigar smoke compared to primary cigar smokers.

Smoking tobacco from a pipe also exposes users to many of the toxins that are also in cigarette smoke, and some evidence suggests that pipe smoking can increase risk of cardiovascular[30] and all-cause mortality.[31]

Waterpipe (Hookah)

Waterpipe users inhale tobacco smoke through a mouthpiece connected to a hose that transports smoke from tobacco burned in a bowl through a base containing water. Waterpipe tobacco is often a combination of dried fruit and tobacco. Worldwide, waterpipe use prevalence is highest in the Middle East and Europe and is higher among youths than adults.[32,33]

In the United States, 3.4% of high school students, 1.6% of middle school students, and 1% of adults report current waterpipe use.[10,11]

Similar to cigarette smoke, waterpipe tobacco smoke contains combustion-derived toxins,[34] but with higher levels of carbon monoxide from the burning charcoal. There is wide variability in how waterpipes are used, which in turn will impact a user's exposure. The health effects of waterpipe tobacco use likely depend on the length of waterpipe tobacco use sessions and how frequently waterpipe tobacco is smoked. Studies have raised concerns about both acute and long-term effects of waterpipe tobacco use on CVD.[35]

Smokeless Tobacco Products

While smokeless tobacco does not expose users to the products of tobacco combustion, users are exposed to nicotine, carcinogens, and other toxins.[36,37] Smokeless tobacco comes in several different forms, including chewing tobacco, moist snuff, and snus. The prevalence of current smokeless tobacco use is 2.4% among US adults[10] and 3.5% among US middle and high school students.[11] Most studies on the cardiovascular risk of smokeless tobacco have focused on snus, a product that is widely used in Sweden, where it is subject to government regulation, and which contains fewer toxins than other smokeless tobacco products such as those sold in the United States. Epidemiological studies in Sweden have generally found no increased risk of nonfatal CVD among smokeless tobacco users,[36] but some report a higher risk of fatal myocardial infarction and

stroke.[38] Additionally, among snus users who have suffered acute myocardial infarction, those who continue using snus have a higher subsequent cardiovascular mortality than those who quit.[39] International studies of smokeless tobacco use and coronary heart disease report wide regional differences, presumably related to different composition of smokeless products, as well as differences in other cardiac risk factors among users compared to nonusers.[40] Concern that use of both cigarettes and chewing tobacco increases the odds of acute myocardial infarction compared to use of either product alone has also been raised.[40]

MECHANISM OF CARDIOVASCULAR EFFECTS OF TOBACCO USE

Cigarette smoke is a mixture of more than 7000 chemicals[41] and generates 10^{15} to 10^{17} free radicals per puff.[42,43] The main tobacco smoke chemicals thought to contribute to CVD include oxidizing chemicals (reactive oxygen and nitrogen species), volatile organic compounds (such as acrolein, acetaldehyde, formaldehyde), particulates, carbon monoxide, heavy metals, and nicotine.[44]

Cigarette smoke acts to promote CVD through several pathophysiological mechanisms.[45-50] These mechanisms include oxidative injury, endothelial damage and dysfunction, enhanced thrombosis, chronic inflammation, hemodynamic stress adverse effects on blood lipids, insulin resistance and diabetes mellitus, reduced oxygen delivery by red blood cells, and arrhythmogenesis (**Fig. 8–2**).

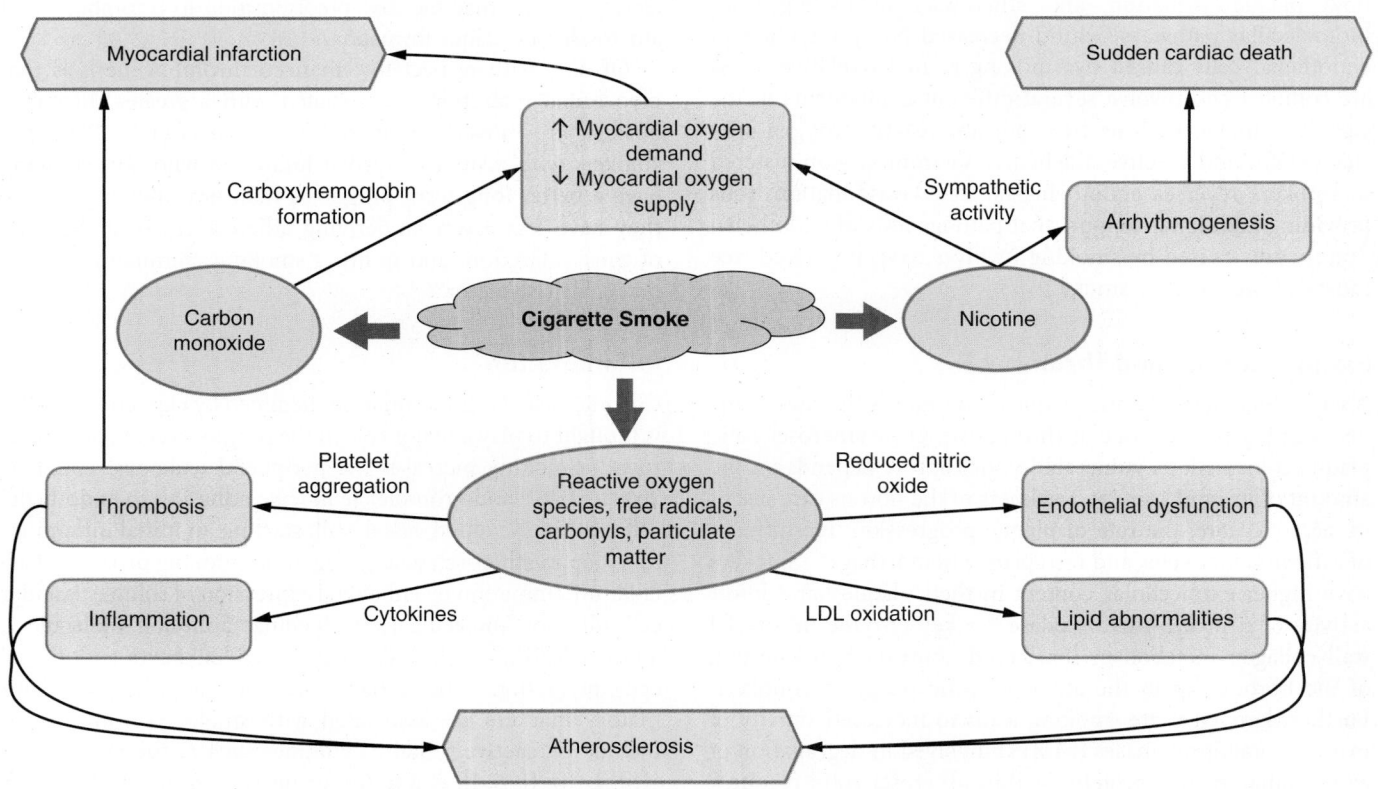

Figure 8–2. Pathophysiology of smoking-related cardiovascular disease.

Oxidative Stress

The most important mechanism in the cigarette smoking–related cardiovascular pathogenesis is oxidative stress. Most of the molecular changes associated with cigarette smoking are triggered by high concentration of oxidizing chemicals inhaled by smokers with the cigarette smoke. These changes include reducing the bioavailability of nitric oxide (NO), depletion of endogenous antioxidants, inflammation and generation of atherogenic oxidized low-density lipoprotein (LDL), effects that are the main contributors to atherogenesis, and thrombogenesis.[51,52]

Endothelial Dysfunction

Cigarette smoking–induced endothelial dysfunction is an important factor in coronary hemodynamic disturbances and the progression of atherosclerosis. The endothelium is an active regulator of the vascular tone through the release of NO, prostacyclin, tissue plasminogen activator (tPA), and plasminogen activator inhibitor-1.[53] Endothelium-dependent vasodilation in coronary and peripheral vessels is diminished in smokers when compared to nonsmokers. The primary mechanism by which smoking leads to vascular and endothelial dysfunction is thought to be suppression of endothelial nitric oxide synthase (eNOS) expression and decreased bioavailability of NO caused by oxidant chemicals from cigarette smoke.[54] The main roles of endothelial NO are vasodilation, inhibition of platelet aggregation and adhesion, inhibition of leukocyte adhesion, and reduction of smooth muscle proliferation.[47] Therefore, deficiency of NO can contribute to reduced coronary blood flow, plaque formation, and atherosclerosis pathogenesis. Biomolecular pathways behind decreased NO production in endothelial cells caused by smoking-related oxidative stress are complex and involve several different components of the cigarette smoke, such as free radicals, reactive oxygen species (ROS), and reactive aldehydes. Vitamin C administered to smokers reverses endothelial-mediated vasodilation, thus providing additional support that pathogenesis of endothelial dysfunction caused by smoking involves oxygen-derived free radicals from cigarette smoke.[55]

Plaque Rupture and Thrombosis

A ruptured atherosclerotic plaque is commonly the site of coronary or peripheral vascular thrombosis. Once atherosclerotic plaque is formed, its vulnerability for rupture depends on the amount of its lipid content, thickness of the fibrous cap, size of its necrotic core, the rate of plaque progression, recruitment of inflammatory cells, and intraplaque hemorrhage.[57] Smokers have higher extracellular content in their plaque[58] and lower activity of n-prolyl-4-hydroxylase,[59] a key enzyme in arterial wall collagen metabolism that could contribute to thinning of the fibrous cap in the atherosclerotic plaque of smokers. Furthermore, cigarette smoking leads to increased activity of matrix metalloproteinases (MMPs) involved in degradation of extracellular matrix proteins within atherosclerotic plaque.[60] Taken together, most of pathologic changes associated with

highly vulnerable plaque and plaque rupture and coronary thrombosis[56] are potentiated by smoking.[57]

Cigarette smoking promotes a prothrombotic state through several mechanisms. These mechanisms include increased platelet aggregation as well as alterations in antithrombotic and prothrombotic factors, including fibrinolytic factors and platelet-mediated pathways.[61,62]

Platelets isolated from smokers exhibit an increased spontaneous and stimulated aggregation compared to nonsmokers.[63] Not only does smoking decrease endothelial NO production, but it also leads to diminished bioavailability of platelet-derived NO and decreased platelet sensitivity to NO.[49,50,64] Both mechanisms promote platelet activation and adhesion, making smokers' platelets more thrombogenic. In addition to impaired NO release from platelets, cigarette smoke also triggers the release of thromboxane A_2, a potent vasoconstrictor, and inhibits coronary endothelial release of prostacyclin, a potent vasodilator and inhibitor of platelet aggregation.[45] An increased level of circulating von Willebrand factor, an important ligand of platelet binding, is seen in smokers compared to nonsmokers.[65,66] Furthermore, cigarette smoking is associated with increased concentration of fibrinogen;[67,68] increased expression of tissue factor that contributes to thrombosis after plaque rupture;[69] and reduced basal production of tPA,[54] which is an essential regulator of plasminogen-plasmin transformation. A lower level of activated plasmin leads to diminished lysis of fibrin and propagation of thrombus. As previously mentioned, carbon monoxide from cigarette smoke causes relative hypoxemia, which compensatorily leads to an increase in the number (and mass) of erythrocytes in the circulation, which increases blood viscosity.[70] Increased blood viscosity may increase predisposition to thrombosis and atherosclerotic plaque formation.

Of note with respect to enhanced thrombogenesis is that myocardial infarction is associated with a greater thrombus burden in smokers compared to nonsmokers.[71] Relatedly, smokers with acute myocardial infarction who quit smoking have a better long-term prognosis than nonsmokers because they have less severe underlying atherosclerosis at the time of their infarction, and quitting smoking eliminates a major reversible risk factor.[72]

Inflammation

Chronic vascular inflammation mediated by cigarette smoking is thought to play a major role in the progression of atherosclerosis.[73] Smoking increases the peripheral leukocyte count by 20% to 25%[74] and promotes leukocyte adhesion to endothelial cells within the blood vessel wall, starting an initial inflammatory step in atherosclerosis.[75] Cigarette smoking promotes vascular inflammation by enhanced expression of soluble vascular cell adhesion molecule-1, intercellular adhesion molecule-1, and E-selectin, which leads to increased leukocyte-endothelial cell interaction.[76] Increased levels of multiple proinflammatory markers are associated with smoke exposure; these include C-reactive protein, cytokines such as the interleukins (IL) IL-1β, IL-6, IL-8, and tumor necrosis factor-α (TNF-α).[48] Cigarette smoking induces release of proinflammatory cytokines in macrophages[77] and lymphocytes by activation of NF-κB and posttranslational modification of histone deacetylase.[73]

Hemodynamic Effects

Nicotine is responsible for most hemodynamic changes caused by cigarette smoking. Nicotine is a sympathomimetic drug that stimulates release of catecholamines from the adrenal medulla and sympathetic neurons.[46] Via sympathetic stimulation, nicotine leads to an increase in cardiac contractility, acute and sustained increase in heart rate up to 7 to 10 beats per minute,[46] and elevation in systolic blood pressure up to 5 to 10 mm Hg compared to a nonsmoking baseline.[53] Consistent with activation of the sympathetic nervous system, cigarette smoking results in reduced heart rate variability, which is a risk factor for future cardiovascular events. While smoking significantly and acutely increases blood pressure, it is not associated with hypertension per se. However, smoking does increase the risk of vascular and renal complications of hypertension. A large study using Mendelian randomization selecting genes associated with smoking heaviness to overcome the observational nature of studies did not find any relationship with hypertension.[78]

The net result of increased cardiac contraction and heart rate is increased myocardial oxygen demand that, in the presence of reduced coronary blood flow, can result in myocardial ischemia. In smokers with coronary artery disease, cigarette smoking causes coronary vasoconstriction and reduced coronary flow reserve. Smoking-induced coronary vasoconstriction can be prevented with the α-adrenergic blocker phentolamine, indicating that the α-adrenergic pathway is the mechanism of reduced coronary blood flow.[45]

Lipid Metabolism

Cigarette smoking promotes an atherogenic lipid profile that may contribute to CVD. Cigarette smoking has its major effect in lowering serum high-density lipoprotein (HDL), but it also increases triglycerides, cholesterol, and LDL.[79] Importantly, smokers have higher levels of oxidized LDL, which is involved in pathogenesis of atherosclerosis.[80] Exposure of human plasma to cigarette smoke causes oxidative modification of plasma LDL that is actively taken up by the macrophages and forms foam cells in the culture.[80] In addition to this, smoking increases hepatic lipase activity, which leads to production of small dense LDL cholesterol (sdLDL-c) and sdHDL-c. LDL-c has toxic effects on endothelium and promotes release of even more ROS. HDL-c has no protective antiatherogenic effects, which are normally attributed to HDL.[81] A nicotine-induced increase in circulating catecholamines induces lipolysis and release of plasma-free fatty acids.[53,82]

Insulin Resistance

Cigarette smoking increases the risk of development of diabetes mellitus type 2.[83] Data from the Cancer Prevention Study shows that there is a 45% higher diabetes rate among smokers than among men who had never smoked. Smoking increases requirements for insulin and causes insulin resistance in nondiabetics.[84] Microvascular complications of diabetes such as diabetic neuropathy and faster progression of renal disease are more common in smokers.[85] The pathogenesis of smoking and glucose metabolism is not fully understood, but nicotine appears to have a central role in this process.[43,86] Nicotine stimulates catecholamine release from the adrenal medulla and sympathetic nervous system, which may lead to insulin resistance. It also increases the release of corticosteroids, which are known hyperglycemic hormones.[53]

Cardiac Remodeling

Smoking has been associated with left ventricular hypertrophy and left atrial enlargement in animal models.[87,88] Smokers exhibit higher level of activation of MMPs that degrade elastin and collagen in the extracellular matrix. Within myocardium, increased MMP activity leads to breakdown of the supporting fibrillary collagen and ventricular wall thinning.[89] Smoke-related ROS stimulate fibroblasts to proliferate and induce myocardial cell apoptosis, leading to cardiac fibrosis and remodeling.[90] Cigarette smoking–induced cardiac remodeling has also been linked to increased activation of mitogen-activated protein kinases by either norepinephrine, which is increased in smokers, serum, or directly by free radicals from cigarette smoke.[89] Within the heart, norepinephrine can lead to myocyte hypertrophy by binding to α_1-adrenergic receptors or apoptosis by binding to β_1-adrenergic receptors.[91]

Impaired Oxygen Delivery

Cigarette smoke delivers high levels of carbon monoxide, which binds tightly to hemoglobin, producing a functional anemia. Reduced oxygen delivery can aggravate angina pectoris, congestive heart failure, intermittent claudication, and chronic obstructive lung disease, and can lower the ventricular fibrillation threshold. Chronic carbon monoxide exposure also produces erythrocytosis, which increases blood viscosity and contributes to thrombogenesis.

Arrhythmogenesis

Cigarette smoking is associated with a higher incidence of sudden cardiac death, which is likely related to ventricular arrhytmias.[92] Catecholamines released by nicotine may facilitate arrhythmogenesis, and carbon monoxide reduces the ventricular fibrillation threshold. Smokers with implanted cardiac defibrillators have a higher incidence of inappropriate shocks compared to nonsmokers.[93,94] Cigarette smoking increases the risk of atrial fibrillation, thought to be a consequence of atrial fibrosis and remodeling and systemic catecholamine release.[17]

TOBACCO CESSATION

Health Benefits of Smoking Cessation

The risk of overall mortality is substantially reduced among patients who quit smoking.[95,96] Smoking cessation before the age of 40 years eliminates nearly all of the risk of premature death from smoking-related disease, and even those who quit at older ages, including over the age of 65 years, gain years of life compared to those who continue to smoke.[97–99] This highlights the importance of encouraging smokers of all ages to quit.

Within hours of stopping smoking, heart rate and levels of carbon monoxide in the blood decrease,[100] and within days of stopping smoking, platelet activation is reduced.[101] The risk of cardiac events declines rapidly after quitting, such that half of the excess risk of coronary heart disease is eliminated after 1 year of cessation.[102] Smokers who quit cigarettes nearly eliminate all excess risk of stroke after 5 to 15 years.[100] The excess lung cancer risk among former smokers is slower to decline than the cardiovascular risks,[103] and former smokers who quit many years ago still carry increased risk compared to never smokers.[100]

Smokers with heart disease also greatly reduce their cardiovascular risk after smoking cessation, highlighting the importance of smoking cessation in secondary prevention. Among patients with coronary heart disease, a systematic review of 20 studies found an overall 36% reduction in risk of all-cause mortality among those who quit smoking compared to those who continued to smoke.[104] Smoking cessation after myocardial infarction has been associated with a decrease in mortality by 15% to 61%[105] and improvements in both health-related quality of life and anginal symptoms.[106] One study found that the risk of repeat coronary events in patients who quit smoking after their first myocardial infarction decreased to that of nonsmokers 3 years after cessation.[107] In patients with a previous myocardial infarction or stable angina followed for a mean of 8 years, risk of sudden cardiac death was significantly increased in current smokers compared to those who had never smoked, while there was no significant difference between former smokers and never smokers.[108] In patients with left ventricular dysfunction, quitting smoking was associated with decreased morbidity and mortality within 2 years.[109]

In addition to reducing CVD risks, smoking cessation improves the excess risks of other smoking-related diseases. Smokers with chronic obstructive pulmonary disease (COPD) who quit smoking have slower decline in lung function,[110] fewer symptoms,[111] fewer exacerbations,[112] and lower mortality.[113] Smokers with lung cancer who quit can reduce the risk of recurrence, development of other cancers, and mortality.[114]

Because of the nonlinear epidemiologic relationship between the amount of cigarette smoking and the degree of cardiovascular risk, even low levels of cigarette smoking are associated with an increased risk of CVD.[115] Smokers who reduce their cigarette consumption by over 50% have a similar risk of death from any cause, cardiovascular death, or smoking-related cancers compared to those who continue to smoke more heavily.[116] Smoking reduction has been associated with improvements in blood pressure and heart rate,[117] but a randomized controlled trial of smoking reduction found no difference in angina, quality of life, or adverse events in smokers assigned to the reduction group.[118] A study in Denmark found a decreased risk of myocardial infarction among individuals who had stopped smoking (hazard ratio [HR] 0.71, 95% confidence interval [CI] 0.59–0.85), but not among individuals who reduced cigarette consumption by at least 50% (HR 1.15, 95% CI 0.94–1.40).[119] Thus, there are unlikely to be major health benefits to smoking

reduction without eventual cessation,[120] and all smokers should be encouraged to have the goal of abstinence from all cigarette use.

Tobacco Use Behavior and Nicotine Dependence

Cigarette smoking is a behavior that almost always begins in childhood or adolescence,[121] but once established persists for decades. Tobacco use is tenacious because it is both a physical dependence on nicotine and a deeply ingrained learned behavior.[5,122] Nicotine binds to nicotinic acetylcholine receptors in the brain, leading to the release of neurotransmitters with rewarding and reinforcing effects. Repeated use leads to the upregulation of nicotine receptors, tolerance, and physical dependence.[5] The rewarding aspects of nicotine dependence become associated with specific triggers that prompt craving to smoke and contribute to repeated use. Triggers can include smoking in specific contexts such as the end of a meal, drinking coffee or alcohol, seeing other smokers, or even seeing cigarette advertisements. Many smokers report smoking in response to stress or other negative emotional states, and quitting smoking is particularly difficult for such smokers. This behavior is likely due both to the positive effects of nicotine and to the fact that smoking reverses the dysphoria and cognitive impairment induced by nicotine withdrawal in addicted smokers.

Smoking cessation triggers symptoms of nicotine withdrawal, which include the specific symptom of cigarette craving and also a range of nonspecific symptoms that are often not recognized as withdrawal symptoms; these include irritability, anxiety, restlessness, dysphoria, impaired concentration, and hunger.[123] The intensity and duration of nicotine withdrawal symptoms vary among smokers, generally lasting 2 weeks to 1 month, although some experience cigarette cravings for 6 months or more.[124]

Because tobacco use is a chronic relapsing disorder, most smokers make numerous attempts to quit before they achieve success, passing through cycles of making a quit attempt leading to a period of abstinence followed by relapse to smoking. Over half of smokers attempt to quit each year, but only 7.5% of them achieve long-term tobacco abstinence following an attempt.[10] However, most smokers who continue to try eventually succeed. In the United States, 62% of all living adults who have ever smoked have now quit smoking.[10] A major reason for the low success rate of individual quit attempts is that only one-third of smokers who make a quit attempt use any effective treatment.[125]

The degree of a smoker's nicotine dependence is a major predictor of success in quitting. Stronger nicotine dependence is associated with smoking more cigarettes per day and with smoking the day's first cigarette within 30 minutes of awakening.[126] Other factors are associated with greater difficulty stopping smoking include initiation of smoking at an early age, the degree of a smoker's nicotine dependence, an individual's degree of motivation to stop smoking, confidence in the ability to stop smoking, presence of a comorbid psychiatric disorder (eg, depression and anxiety), other substance use, especially heavy alcohol use, and having a smoker in the household. These factors can be used to tailor the intensity of cessation treatment recommended.

TREATMENT OF TOBACCO USE

Behavioral support and pharmacotherapy are the treatment modalities with the strongest evidence of effectiveness for smoking cessation.[127-129] While each modality is effective when used alone, combining them produces the best success.[127,130] Pharmacotherapy addresses the nicotine withdrawal symptoms that arise from a smoker's physical addiction to nicotine, while behavioral treatment addresses the conditioned behavior of smoking. Nicotine withdrawal symptoms consist of craving for a cigarette and a group of nonspecific symptoms that are often not recognized by smokers as representing nicotine withdrawal (see previous section). Withdrawal symptoms have a variable time course but largely resolve over 1 month, although cravings can persist much longer.[124,131]

Pharmacologic Treatment for Tobacco Cessation

Pharmacotherapy should be offered to virtually every smoker. The US Food and Drug Administration (FDA) has approved seven medications as cessation aids, including bupropion, varenicline, and five nicotine replacement therapy (NRT) products. Meta-analyses and a recent large randomized controlled trial indicate that each of these medications is more effective than placebo in promoting smoking cessation for 6 months or more and that each is safe for use in patients with CVD.[132,133] **Table 8–1** summarizes dosing, precautions, and adverse effects of the FDA-approved smoking cessation medications. They are all first-line treatments for smoking cessation and the choice of medication should consider patient preference, medical comorbidities, and potential drug interactions. The American College of Cardiology (ACC) Expert Consensus Decision Pathway on Tobacco Cessation Treatment's[133] guidance for selection of pharmacotherapy in patients with CVDs is presented in **Table 8–2**. Nearly all clinical trials that have demonstrated the efficacy of these medications also provided behavioral support, highlighting the importance of providing behavioral support along with a pharmacotherapy prescription.

Nicotine Replacement Therapy

The nicotine in tobacco products produces a physical dependence that sustains smoking and generates symptoms of nicotine withdrawal when smoking stops abruptly. NRT aids smoking cessation by delivering nicotine in a noninhaled form to reduce withdrawal symptoms. The efficacy of NRT for smoking cessation is well-established in both the general population and in patients with stable CVD.[134] Regarding safety, controlled trials, longitudinal studies, and case-control studies of NRT in patients with CVD report no increase in adverse cardiovascular events compared with those treated with placebo.[135-138] A meta-analysis of NRT studies found no increase in major cardiovascular events (death, myocardial infarction, stroke),[139] indicating that the risks associated with NRT are much lower than the risks of continued smoking even in patients with CVD.

Five forms of NRT are sold in the United States. Patches, gum, and lozenges are available without prescription, while the nasal spray and oral inhaler are sold only by prescription. Each NRT product has roughly comparable efficacy in clinical trials. Use of NRT in any form increases smoking abstinence by 55% compared to placebo (risk ratio [RR] 1.55, 95% CI 1.49–1.61) in a meta-analysis.[140] Consequently, the choice of NRT product can reflect a patient's preference. Nicotine patches deliver nicotine in a sustained manner throughout the day and are the most convenient delivery system for reducing withdrawal symptoms. More rapidly absorbed forms of NRT (gum, lozenges, inhaler, and spray) relieve withdrawal symptoms more quickly than the patch, although not as rapidly as cigarette smoking. They require more frequent use to suppress withdrawal symptoms because their effect has a shorter duration. The patch is generally used as the primary product because the convenience of the once-daily dose produces the best compliance and sustained suppression of withdrawal symptoms.

Combining the nicotine patch with a more rapidly absorbed form of NRT (combination NRT) is more effective than using a single product, with a risk ratio of 1.25 compared with use of a single product in a meta-analysis.[141] Combination NRT is now the standard of care for using NRT and should be recommended as initial therapy when NRT is chosen.[129] Combination NRT is one of the two first-line pharmacotherapy choices recommended by the ACC for smokers with CVD[133] (Table 8–2). Individual NRT products are second-line choices in that algorithm.

Nicotine patches are marketed for 8 to 12 weeks of use, but a randomized trial of longer durations of nicotine patch treatment found higher rates of smoking abstinence at 24 weeks, supporting a longer treatment duration,[142] and many smoking cessation experts treat smokers for longer periods until the patient is confident that they will not return to smoking. No harm from long-term NRT use has been reported.[142] There is some evidence that starting nicotine patches prior to a patient's quit date is associated with increased smoking cessation compared to starting after the quit date.[130] Thus, it is not necessary to wait until the quit date to initiate treatment with nicotine patches.

The nicotine in nicotine gum, lozenge, and inhaler (a cigarette-like plastic device) is absorbed through the oral mucosa, while nicotine in the spray is absorbed through the nasal mucosa. Peak nicotine levels for these products are reached less rapidly than by inhaling cigarette smoke but much more rapidly than they occur with a skin patch. Oral NRT products produce relatively low blood nicotine levels and require frequent use (once every 1–2 hours) to relieve withdrawal symptoms. Smokers tend not to use the product frequently enough unless carefully instructed.

Varenicline

Varenicline is a partial agonist at the α4β2 nicotinic cholinergic receptor that generates brain dopamine release and is believed to be the primary mediator of nicotine addiction.[143] As a partial agonist, varenicline activates the nicotine receptor to a limited extent, thereby reducing nicotine withdrawal symptoms. At the same time, varenicline binding to the nicotine receptor prevents the nicotine in any cigarettes subsequently smoked from binding to the receptor, reducing the rewarding effects of smoking.

TABLE 8-1. FDA-Approved Smoking Cessation Medications

1st line Medications for Tobacco Cessation Treatment[a]						
Drug (Available Doses)	How Sold (US)	Dosing Instructions[b]	Administration	Common Side Effects	Advantages	Disadvantages
Nicotine patch - 21 mg - 14 mg - 7 mg	OTC or Rx	Starting dose: 21 mg for ≥10 cigarettes per day 14 mg for <10 cigarettes per day Use >3 months After 6 weeks, continue original dose or taper to lower doses (either option acceptable.)	Apply a new patch each morning to dry skin Rotate application site to avoid skin irritation May start patch before or on quit date Keep using even if a slip occurs	Skin irritation Trouble sleeping Vivid dreams (Remove patch at bedtime to manage insomnia or vivid dreams.)	Easiest nicotine product to use Provides a steady nicotine level Combination NRT therapy is recommended: add gum, lozenge, inhaler, or nasal spray as needed to patch to cover situational cravings	User cannot alter dose if cravings occur during the day. Combination of patch + gum, lozenge, inhaler, or spray is used to manage situational cravings
Nicotine lozenge - 4 mg - 2 mg	OTC or Rx	If 1st cigarette is ≤30 min of waking: 4 mg If 1st cigarette is >30 minutes of waking: 2 mg Use >3 months	Place between gum and cheek, let it melt slowly Use 1 piece every 1–2 hours as needed (Max: 20/day)	Mouth irritation Hiccups Heartburn Nausea	User controls nicotine dose Oral substitute for cigarettes May be added to patch to cover situational cravings Easier to use than gum for those with dental work or dentures	No food or drink 15 minutes prior to use and during use
Nicotine gum - 4 mg - 2 mg	OTC or Rx	If 1st cigarette is ≤ 30 min of waking: 4 mg If 1st cigarette is >30 minutes of waking: 2 mg Use >3 months	Chew briefly until mouth tingles, then "park" gum inside cheek until tingle fades Repeat chew-and-park each time tingle fades Discard gum after 30 minutes of use Use ~1 piece per hour as needed (Max: 24/day) No food or drink 15 minutes prior to use and during use	Mouth irritation Jaw soreness Heartburn Hiccups Nausea	User controls nicotine dose Oral substitute for cigarettes May be added to patch to cover situational cravings	Not chewed in same way as regular gum; requires careful instruction Can damage dental work and be difficult to use with dentures
Nicotine inhaler - 10 mg cartridge	Rx only	10 mg/cartridge Each cartridge has ~80 puffs Use >3 months	Puff into mouth/throat until cravings subside Do not inhale into lungs Change cartridge when nicotine taste disappears Use 1 cartridge every 1–2 hours as needed (Max: 16/day)	Mouth and throat irritation Coughing if inhaled too deeply	User controls nicotine dose Mimics hand-to-mouth ritual of smoking cigarettes May be added to patch to cover situational cravings	Frequent puffing required to achieve adequate nicotine delivery
Nicotine nasal spray - 10 mg/ml (10 ml bottle)	Rx only	10 mg/ml 0.5 mg per spray Each bottle has ~200 sprays Use >3 months	Use 1 spray to each nostril Use spray every 1–2 hours as needed (Max: 80/day)	Nasal and throat irritation Rhinitis Sneezing Coughing Tearing	User controls nicotine dose Most rapid delivery of nicotine among all NRT products May be added to patch to cover situational cravings	Has the most side effects of all NRT products Some users cannot tolerate local irritation to nasal mucosa

(Continued)

TABLE 8–1. FDA-Approved Smoking Cessation Medications (Continued)

1st line Medications for Tobacco Cessation Treatment[a]

Drug (Available Doses)	How Sold (US)	Dosing Instructions[b]	Administration	Common Side Effects	Advantages	Disadvantages
Varenicline (tablet) - 0.5 mg - 1.0 mg	Rx only	Days 1–3: 0.5 mg/day Days 4–7: 0.5 mg twice a day Day 8+: 1 mg twice a day. Use 3–6 months	Start 1–4 weeks before quit date Alternative is gradual smoking reduction: reduce smoking to 50% by week 4, to 25% by week 8, quit by week 12 Take with food and a tall glass of water to minimize nausea	Nausea Insomnia Vivid dreams Headache (Skip PM dose or take it earlier to manage vivid dreams or insomnia.)	Quit date can be flexible, from 1 week to 3 months after starting drug Dual action: relieves nicotine withdrawal and blocks reward of smoking Oral agent (pill)	Because of previous FDA boxed warning (now removed), many patients fear psychiatric adverse events, even though they are no more common than with other cessation medications
Bupropion sustained release (SR) (tablet) - 150 mg	Rx only	150 mg/day for 3 days, then 150 mg twice a day Use 3–6 months	Start 1–2 weeks before quit date	Insomnia Agitation Dry mouth Headache (Lower dose to 150 mg qAM for insomnia or agitation)	May lessen post-cessation weight gain while drug is being taken Oral agent (pill)	Increases seizure risk: not for use if seizure disorder or binge drinking

Abbreviations: OTC, over the counter (no prescription required); Rx, prescription required.
[a]All are FDA approved as smoking cessation aids and listed as a 1st line medication by US Clinical Practice Guidelines (Fiore, 2008).
[b]Recommended duration of use for medications is at least 3 months but extending to 6 months is frequently done to prevent relapse to tobacco use. Patch dosing differs slightly from FDA labeling.
Reproduced with permissions from Barua RS, Rigotti NA, Benowitz NL, et al: 2018 ACC Expert Consensus Decision Pathway on Tobacco Cessation Treatment: A Report of the American College of Cardiology Task Force on Clinical Expert Consensus Documents, J Am Coll Cardiol. 2018 Dec 25;72(25):3332-3365.

TABLE 8–2. Recommended Pharmacotherapy for Smoking Cessation in Patients With Cardiovascular Disease, American College of Cardiology Consensus Decision Pathway

	Outpatient with Stable CVD	Inpatient with ACS
1st line	Varenicline OR combination NRT[a]	*In-hospital to relieve nicotine withdrawal:* nicotine patch OR combination NRT[a] *At discharge:* combination NRT or varenicline[b]
2nd line	Bupropion OR single NRT product	*At discharge:* single NRT product
3rd line	Nortriptyline[c]	Bupropion[d]
If single agent is insufficient to achieve abstinence	Combine categories of FDA-approved drugs: Varenicline + NRT (single agent) Varenicline + bupropion Bupropion + NRT (single agent)	n/a

[a]Combination NRT comprises a nicotine patch plus the patient's choice of nicotine gum or lozenge or inhaler or spray.
[b]Some committee members planning to use varenicline would start it in hospital; others would not start until discharge. Regardless, continue nicotine patch or short-acting form for 1 week to manage nicotine withdrawal symptoms during up-titration of varenicline dose.
[c]Nortriptyline is not FDA-approved for smoking cessation indication and there are few data on use in patients with CVD.
[d]Bupropion is listed as 3rd line because of no evidence of efficacy when started during hospitalization for acute ACS or acute MI. However, there are no special safety concerns for bupropion in this setting.
Reproduced with permissions from Barua RS, Rigotti NA, Benowitz NL, et al: 2018 ACC Expert Consensus Decision Pathway on Tobacco Cessation Treatment: A Report of the American College of Cardiology Task Force on Clinical Expert Consensus Documents, J Am Coll Cardiol. 2018 Dec 25;72(25):3332-3365.

Randomized clinical trials have found that varenicline more than doubles quit rates compared to placebo (RR 2.24, 95% CI 2.06–2.43) and that it is more effective for smoking cessation than placebo, single-product NRT, or bupropion.[144] The largest randomized clinical trial for smoking, the EAGLES trial (Evaluating Adverse Events in a Global Smoking Cessation Study), enrolled more than 8000 smokers and compared varenicline, bupropion, nicotine patch, and placebo given for 12 weeks.[132] Continuous quit rates from weeks 9 to 24 were: varenicline (21.8%); bupropion (16.2%); nicotine patch (15.7%); and placebo (9.4%). Varenicline has also been shown to be more effective than placebo in smokers with stable CVD (odds ratio [OR] 3.14, 95% 1.94–5.11) and acute coronary syndrome (ACS).[145,146] No clinical trials have directly compared the efficacy of varenicline to combination NRT. In the absence of clinical trial data, many experts consider them to be roughly comparable first-line pharmacotherapies for smoking cessation,[147] and they are recommended as such in the ACC Consensus Decision Pathway on Tobacco Cessation Treatment for patients with CVD (Table 8–2).[133]

Concerns about potential adverse neuropsychiatric and cardiovascular effects of varenicline limited its use for several years but proved to be largely unfounded. Case reports submitted to the FDA after varenicline entered the US market in 2006 raised concerns about possible neuropsychiatric effects, including depression, psychosis and suicidal ideation, and behavior.[148] In 2009, the FDA required varenicline to be marketed with a warning about such events, leading many physicians and patients reluctant to use varenicline. These concerns were not confirmed in the landmark EAGLES trial,[132] which enrolled over 8000 smokers, half of whom had stable mild to moderate psychiatric symptoms. Neuropsychiatric side effects were no more frequent with varenicline than with NRT, bupropion, or placebo.[132] For all medications in the trial, adverse neuropsychiatric effects were more frequent among smokers with a history of psychiatric disease than among those without. This evidence led the FDA to remove the warning on varenicline in 2016.

Because varenicline has nicotine-like properties, concern about its potential for adverse cardiovascular effects has been raised, but this is not supported by the majority of evidence. A large clinical trial of varenicline in smokers with stable CVD found low cardiovascular event rates and no significant differences from placebo.[145] Similar results were found in a clinical trial of varenicline in smokers with ACS,[146] in several meta-analyses[139,149] and in a study that analyzed data from the large EAGLES trial. It found no evidence of increased cardiovascular events with varenicline compared to bupropion, nicotine patch, or placebo.[150]

In clinical practice, varenicline is started at least 1 week before a smoker's quit date and continued for 12 weeks. Among those who quit at the end of a 12-week course, extending varenicline for 6 months to prevent relapse is effective.[151] The most common side effect is nausea, which can generally be managed by administering the drug with food and a large glass of water.

Bupropion

Bupropion is FDA-approved as both an antidepressant and a smoking cessation aid. It acts primarily by blocking the neuronal uptake of dopamine, thereby simulating some of nicotine's effects on the brain and relieving nicotine withdrawal symptoms.[152]

Sustained-release bupropion increases quit rates at 6-month follow-up with a relative risk of 1.55 (95% CI 1.49–1.61) in a systematic review.[153] It is similar in efficacy to NRT and is effective in smokers with and without depression.[132] Bupropion is efficacious in smokers with stable CVD,[154] but has not shown efficacy when started in hospitalized patients with acute coronary syndrome, likely because hospitalization is often too brief to allow bupropion to achieve therapeutic drug levels before discharge.[155] No significant increase in cardiovascular events was observed in either a meta-analysis or in very large clinical trial that compared patients treated with bupropion versus placebo.[139,150] Clinical trials of bupropion in patients with CVD have found no increase in cardiovascular events compared with placebo.[154] A prior potential concern about neuropsychiatric adverse events similar to those potentially associated with varenicline was laid to rest by the EAGLES trial[132]. Bupropion is recommended as a second-line agent in the ACC's treatment algorithm[133] (Table 8–2).

Bupropion is started 1 week before a smoker's quit date and approved for 12 weeks' use; however, extended treatment for 1 year reduced the relapse rate after initial cessation in one clinical trial.[156]

Combination Pharmacotherapy

Combining long-acting (patch) and short-acting (gum, lozenge, inhaler, spray) NRT products increases smoking cessation rates compared to using a single type of NRT and is now the recommended way to use NRT.[129,141] A small number of trials have tested the efficacy and tolerability of combining various pairings of NRT, bupropion, and varenicline. In one trial adding NRT to varenicline produced higher tobacco abstinence for 6 months than varenicline alone,[157] but another trial did not.[158] Another randomized controlled trial found that adding bupropion to varenicline produced more smoking cessation than treatment with varenicline alone for up to 26 weeks, but not at 1-year follow-up.[159] In a meta-analysis, combinations of bupropion and nicotine patch were more effective than either drug alone.[134] While more evidence is needed, experts generally recommend considering combinations of drug classes when single agents have been partially helpful but have failed to produce complete tobacco abstinence. This is recommended by the ACC algorithm.[133]

Gradual Reduction Prior to Quitting

Pharmacotherapy has traditionally not been used in smokers who are not ready to plan a quit attempt. Newer evidence suggests that for these smokers, the alternative strategy of pharmacotherapy-assisted gradual reduction in the number of cigarettes smoked daily for weeks to a few months before a planned quit date can be effective in producing abstinence. In a randomized controlled trial that enrolled smokers who were not ready to quit in the next 30 days, varenicline produced higher abstinence rates than placebo when used for gradual reduction in smoking over 3 months before the quit date.[160] A meta-analysis of gradual reduction versus abrupt quitting found similar quit rates,[161] although a subsequent randomized trial that compared abrupt quitting versus reducing cigarette smoking for 2 weeks before quitting found that abruptly quitting cigarette was more effective. However, in that trial, a substantial number of those in the gradual reduction group were also successful in quitting.

Other Smoking Cessation Medications

Other medications have some evidence for smoking cessation efficacy but are not FDA-approved for smoking cessation in the United States. Nortriptyline, a tricyclic antidepressant, has been associated with increased smoking cessation compared to placebo.[153] However, it should be avoided in patients with underlying heart disease because of the association between tricyclic antidepressants and cardiac disease. Clonidine has some clinical trial evidence of efficacy for smoking cessation, but it is rarely used due to the limitations of these trials and its substantial side effects.[162] Cytisine, a nicotine receptor partial agonist, has been associated with increased smoking cessation compared to placebo in several randomized trials and is marketed in some Eastern European countries but is not approved for smoking cessation in the United States.[163,164]

Behavioral Treatments for Tobacco Cessation

Effective nonpharmacologic treatments for tobacco dependence include cognitive-behavioral skills training and motivational interviewing strategies.[127,130,133,165] Smoking cessation counseling programs often combine these techniques. In contrast, acupuncture and hypnotherapy have not shown a consistent benefit for smoking cessation.[166,167]

TABLE 8–3. Community-Based Behavioral Support Resources to Help Smokers Quit[133]

Resource	Services Provided
Telephone Quitline 1-800-QUIT-NOW (1-800-784-8669)	• Counseling by telephone from a trained tobacco coach who offers support via a series of scheduled telephone calls before and after a smoker's quit date • Many quitlines also offer text messaging and web coaching support • Many quitlines also offer a free sample of non-prescription nicotine replacement products • Providers can directly refer to Quitlines using fax or web enrollments. Quitline then contacts smoker directly to offer services
Smokefree.gov (National Cancer Institute website)	• SmokefreeTXT (text messaging program) • QuitGuide (mobile phone app) • Web-based information about quitting resources
Becomeanex.org (Truth Initiative)	• Web-based support program that includes support from experts and an online community to help smokers quit

The principles of behavioral and cognitive psychology are combined in cognitive-behavioral treatments that aim to help smokers increase their ability to control their tobacco use. Cognitive treatments help smokers to change unhelpful thoughts, beliefs, and attitudes. Behavioral treatments provide structure to change smoking behavior using techniques such as goal setting (eg, setting a quit date), self-monitoring (eg, recording when and where each cigarette is smoked), and skills training to help smokers learn, practice, and implement behaviors that help them resist urges to smoke. Motivational interviewing is a patient-centered counseling style that attempts to help smokers change behavior by exploring and resolving ambivalence about making changes in their behavior.

Counseling strategies can be provided to smokers in a variety of ways. They are effective when provided at in-person individual or group sessions, by telephone call, text messages, or web-based programs.[129,168–171] Clinicians can refer smokers to programs located in their healthcare system if such a program is available. Alternately, clinicians can refer to free resources that are available nationally (**Table 8–3**).[173]

Non-Cigarette Tobacco Products

The evidence base for treating non-cigarette tobacco use is far more limited than it is for cigarette smoking. For smokeless tobacco users, varenicline, nicotine lozenges, and behavioral interventions have evidence of effectiveness for cessation in randomized clinical trials.[172] Behavioral interventions and bupropion have limited evidence of effectiveness to aid cessation in a few studies of waterpipe users.[173]

TREATING TOBACCO USE IN CLINICAL PRACTICE

Tobacco cessation treatment is a key element of both primary and secondary CVD prevention because cessation reduces the excess risk of CVD attributable to cigarette smoking, even when cessation occurs after the onset of clinical cardiovascular events.[102,103] A strong evidence base supports the effectiveness of even brief clinical interventions done routinely in cardiovascular practice. Advice to quit smoking from a physician or nurse is associated with increased smoking cessation rates compared to no advice or usual care, and brief office-based counseling is even more effective than advice alone.[174,175] Furthermore, a new diagnosis of CVD, a cardiovascular procedure, and hospital admission for acute myocardial infarction or acute coronary syndrome all serve as teachable moments that can motivate a smoker to attempt cessation. This evidence provides a strong rationale for the routine delivery of tobacco cessation treatment as a standard component of all cardiovascular care. According to national surveys, most smokers want to quit but only a minority of them use evidence-based treatments when making a quit attempt, contributing to modest success rates.[125] Clinicians who care for patients with CVD are well positioned to narrow this treatment gap by routinely screening for tobacco use and not only providing advice to quit but also ensuring that current smokers access and use evidence-based tobacco cessation treatment.

Tobacco Treatment in Outpatient Practice

Treating tobacco use resembles the management of other chronic disorders such as hypertension or diabetes, for which a routine offer of treatment is the standard of care. The delivery of tobacco treatment is a task that can be distributed across the care team rather than being the responsibility of a single individual. A framework for brief office-based tobacco treatment was initially outlined by the US Public Health Service's Clinical Practice Guideline for Tobacco Dependence Treatment.[127] This 5A's model consists of five steps: *Ask* about tobacco use, *Advise* tobacco users to quit, *Assess users'* readiness to quit, *Assist* tobacco users to quit by providing medications or brief counseling for those ready to set a quit date and motivational interventions for those not yet ready to quit, and *Arrange* follow-up care by referring tobacco users to counseling resources outside the office and by monitoring a patient's progress at subsequent clinical visits.

The 5A's model has been condensed into several three-step models that are now commonly used. Each reflects the understanding of tobacco use as a chronic relapsing disorder for which treatment is likely to be needed repeatedly and should be offered proactively. Rather than assessing whether a smoker is ready to quit, these newer models offer tobacco cessation treatment to every smoker, recognizing that some may refuse treatment (ie, opt out).[176] **Figure 8–3** outlines a simplified workflow that consists of these three steps: *Ask* about tobacco use, *Advise* tobacco users to make a quit attempt and offer treatment, and *Connect* them to appropriate treatment resources.

Ask: Every patient is routinely screened for tobacco use and secondhand tobacco smoke exposure, a task that might be done by a medical assistant. Tobacco use is best assessed with a broad question such as "Do you ever use/smoke any tobacco product?" because the use of multiple types of tobacco products is increasing.[10] Furthermore, one-quarter of cigarette smokers

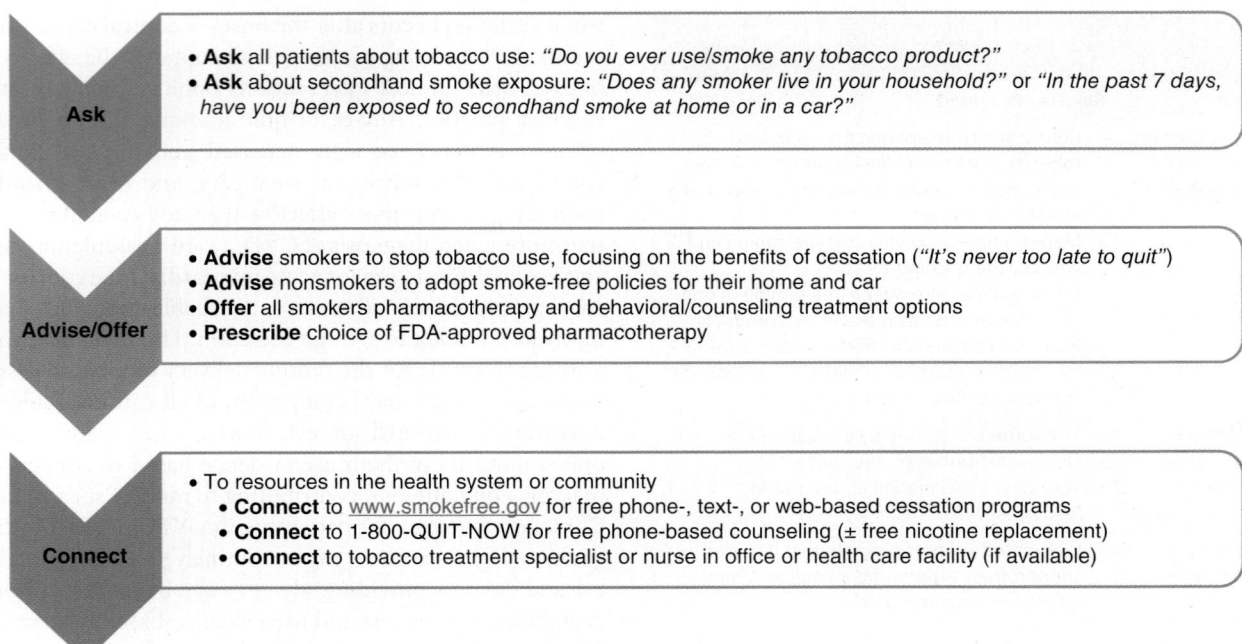

Ask
- **Ask** all patients about tobacco use: *"Do you ever use/smoke any tobacco product?"*
- **Ask** about secondhand smoke exposure: *"Does any smoker live in your household?"* or *"In the past 7 days, have you been exposed to secondhand smoke at home or in a car?"*

Advise/Offer
- **Advise** smokers to stop tobacco use, focusing on the benefits of cessation (*"It's never too late to quit"*)
- **Advise** nonsmokers to adopt smoke-free policies for their home and car
- **Offer** all smokers pharmacotherapy and behavioral/counseling treatment options
- **Prescribe** choice of FDA-approved pharmacotherapy

Connect
- To resources in the health system or community
  - **Connect** to www.smokefree.gov for free phone-, text-, or web-based cessation programs
  - **Connect** to 1-800-QUIT-NOW for free phone-based counseling (± free nicotine replacement)
  - **Connect** to tobacco treatment specialist or nurse in office or health care facility (if available)

Figure 8–3. Tobacco treatment model for outpatient practice.

do not smoke every day, and some of them may not identify themselves as smokers.[10] Nonsmokers should be screened for secondhand tobacco smoke exposure by a question such as, "Does any smoker live in your household?" or "In the past 7 days, have you been exposed to secondhand smoke at home or in a car?"[177]

Advise/Offer: A key role for the cardiology clinician is to provide firm advice to stop all forms of tobacco use as soon as possible. The advice should focus on the benefits of cessation even after cardiovascular events have occurred ("It's never too late to quit") and be followed by an offer to help the tobacco user make a plan to quit. The treatment offered should incorporate both pharmacological and behavioral components. The primary role in treatment delivery is to prescribe the cessation medication(s) selected after the options are reviewed with the patient and the patient's preferences considered. Table 8–2 provides an algorithm for medication selection for cardiology patients that is endorsed by the ACC. The clinician should also emphasize the critical role of behavioral support for quitting smoking. Additionally, clinicians can help nonsmokers avoid the health risks of secondhand tobacco smoke exposure on CVD through routine screening of all nonsmokers and giving advice to adopt strict smoke-free policies for their home and car.

Connect: The clinician or office staff review behavioral treatment options available in the health-care system or in the community (outlined in Table 8–3) and help the patient to make a choice. The key step is to make a specific referral to the selected resource. These can include referral to a tobacco treatment specialist or nurse in the office or hospital, or to free community-based resources. Telephone quitlines, available in all US states by calling 1-800-QUIT-NOW, provide free telephone counseling and often offer free samples of NRT to callers.

The website www.smokefree.gov[178] provides easy access to the National Cancer Institute's SmokefreeTXT program and web-based resources (Table 8–3). The smoker should leave the office with a tobacco cessation pharmacotherapy prescription, an explicit plan for connection to a behavioral support resource, and the understanding that the clinician will monitor progress at future visits.

Tobacco Treatment in Inpatient Care

Hospitalization, especially for a CVD, provides an opportunity to promote smoking cessation and initiate treatment.[179] The onset or worsening of a tobacco-related disease makes the risks of tobacco use personally salient, while admission to a hospital's smoke-free environment requires a smoker to abstain temporarily from tobacco use and provides an opportunity to start a quit attempt, initiate a cessation medication, and connect the smoker to treatment resources after discharge. Among smokers hospitalized for CVD, providing a smoking cessation intervention in the hospital and sustaining it for at least 1 month after discharge increases smoking cessation rates by 42%.[179]

A national hospital quality measure developed by the Joint Commission calls for hospitals to (1) assess and document the tobacco use status of all admitted patients, (2) provide tobacco cessation treatment, including pharmacotherapy and counseling, to all current smokers during the hospitalization, and (3) offer tobacco cessation treatment at hospital discharge.[180] Most hospitals screen for tobacco use by building a question about tobacco use in the past 30 days into the electronic health record admission template routinely completed by clinical staff.

To minimize the discomfort of nicotine withdrawal following abrupt tobacco abstinence, virtually all smokers should be offered NRT at admission, whether or not the patient plans to quit after discharge. The nicotine patch is the most often used product because of its ability to sustain nicotine levels over a 24-hour period but is best supplemented by short-acting nicotine products (lozenges, gum, or an inhaler) on an as-needed basis to manage acute cravings in the hospital. Using nicotine replacement in hospital also increases the odds that a smoker will use the medication after discharge.[181] Physicians and nurses should advise all admitted smokers to quit, emphasizing that it is not too late to benefit from cessation. Nursing staff or a hospital-based tobacco treatment counselor can provide a brief intervention in the hospital and make referrals for postdischarge treatment (Table 8–3). A prescription for a smoking cessation medication should be included on the discharge medication list, using the algorithm endorsed by the ACC (Table 8–2).[133]

Sustaining tobacco cessation counseling and pharmacotherapy begun in the hospital during the transition to outpatient care has been shown to increase cessation rates for 6 months after discharge.[182,183] One model that provided cessation medications in hand at discharge and proactive telephone calls for 3 months after discharge for behavioral support and cessation medication management increased cessation rates at 6 months by 71% (26% vs 15%, P = .009).[182] Another model that has demonstrated effectiveness in combining inpatient-to-outpatient treatment is the Ottawa Model.[183]

Reducing Secondhand Tobacco Smoke Exposure

The population-level studies showing a reduction in hospital admissions for acute myocardial infarction following the adoption of comprehensive smoke-free laws[25] provide a compelling rationale for clinicians to take action to reduce the secondhand smoke exposure of all patients. In the United States, laws and policies ban smoking in most indoor public places and workplaces, in many restaurants and bars, and increasingly extending to outdoor areas such as beaches and outdoor eating areas. As a result, homes and cars are the sites of most secondhand smoke exposure.[184] These private areas are less amenable to governmental action, but clinicians can and should provide strong advice to all patients to adopt a strict smoke-free

policy for their homes and cars. The ACC recommends that clinicians take these actions to reduce secondhand tobacco smoke (SHS) exposure: (1) regularly ask all patients (especially nonsmokers) about their SHS exposure; (2) educate patients that SHS exposure increases the risk of cardiovascular events in nonsmokers; (3) advise all patients (especially nonsmokers) to adopt a smoke-free policy for their home and car and avoid other sites of SHS exposure; and (4) actively support smoke-free policies for worksites, including health-care centers, and promote smoke-free legislation in their communities.[133]

ALTERNATIVE TOBACCO PRODUCTS

Electronic Cigarettes

Electronic cigarettes (e-cigarettes) are devices that use battery power to heat a solution consisting of a humectant (vegetable glycerin and/or propylene glycol), usually nicotine, and flavorings (**Fig. 8–4**) to create an aerosol that the user inhales, a process referred to as vaping. Electronic cigarette devices have widely varying designs that continue to evolve (**Fig. 8–5**). Devices vary in power and in the temperature at which the liquid is heated, as well as the nature of the heating coil and the wick material that holds the liquid while it is heated. Pod devices have become increasingly popular in the United States.[185] These rechargeable devices have replaceable cartridges that contain nicotine in the form of nicotine salts, in which nicotine is combined with an acid.[186] The e-cigarettes containing nicotine salts are less irritating to the throat,[186] and therefore can deliver higher nicotine concentrations compared to e-cigarettes containing freebase nicotine. The high levels of nicotine delivery raise concerns about the potential for creating and/or sustaining nicotine dependence among users.

E-cigarettes are nicotine-delivery devices but because they do not burn tobacco to create smoke, they expose users to fewer toxins than are found in cigarette smoke, giving them the potential to be harm-reduction products.[187] Smokers who use e-cigarettes to quit smoking combustible tobacco products should reduce their tobacco-related health risks, even if they continue to use e-cigarettes after smoking stops. This potential

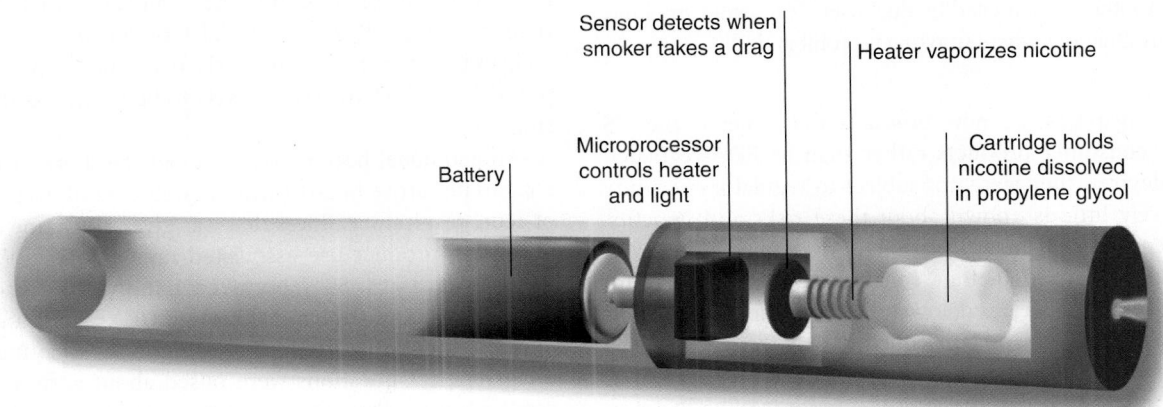

Figure 8–4. Basic design of an electronic cigarette.

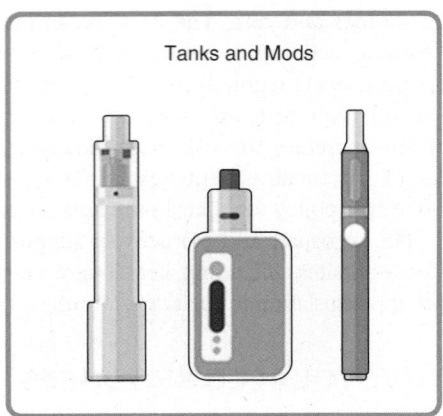
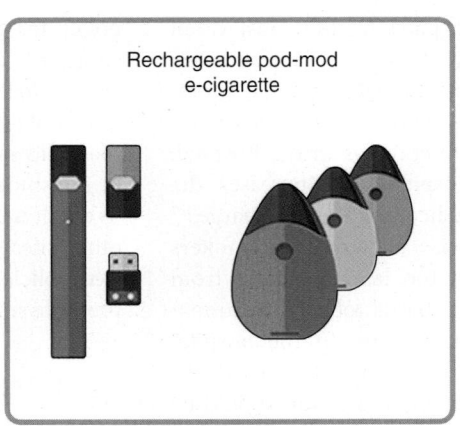
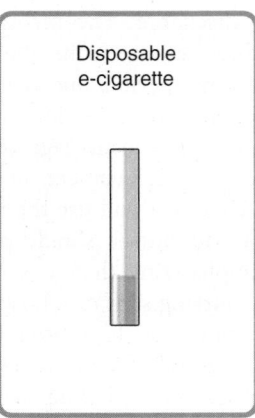

Tanks and Mods

Rechargeable pod-mod
e-cigarette

Disposable
e-cigarette

Figure 8–5. Different types of electronic cigarette devices. Reproduced with permission from About Electronic Cigarettes (E-Cigarettes). Office on Smoking and Health, National Center for Chronic Disease Prevention and Health Promotion, 2021. https://www.cdc.gov/tobacco/basic_information/e-cigarettes/about-e-cigarettes.Html

benefit of e-cigarettes must be balanced against any health risks for users of the devices themselves. From a public health perspective, the potential benefit must also be balanced against the risk that nonsmokers who would not otherwise be exposed to nicotine will use them.[188] In practice, the devices have generally not been taken up by adult nonsmokers but have proven to be attractive to adolescents and young adults.

Prevalence and Patterns of Use

Electronic cigarette use has increased dramatically among adolescents and young adults in the United States. In 2019, approximately 27.5% of high school students and 10.5% of middle school students reported current e-cigarette use,[11] defined as use in the past 30 days. This was an increase from 20.8% of high school students to 4.9% of middle school students in 2018.[189] However, in 2020, the rising prevalence of e-cigarette use among adolescents reversed; the prevalence of current e-cigarette use decreased to 19.6% among high school students and 4.7% among middle school students.[190]

Among US adults, prevalence of e-cigarette use was approximately 3.2% in 2018.[10] Most adult e-cigarette users are current or former cigarette smokers.[192] Most e-cigarette users also continue to smoke cigarettes, a practice known as dual use. Most smokers report that they use e-cigarettes to help them to quit or reduce their cigarette smoking. Another reason cited by dual users is to avoid smoking, especially in situations where smoking is prohibited.[193]

Health Effects

Because e-cigarettes are new products that entered the US market as consumer products rather than as FDA-regulated drugs or devices, they were not subject to regulatory scrutiny and relatively little is known about these risks and benefits. A 2018 report from the US National Academies of Science, Engineering, and Medicine concluded that e-cigarettes exposed users to fewer and lower levels of toxins than did combustible cigarettes and consequently they were likely to be far less harmful than continuing to smoke cigarettes. However, the report also noted that the long-term effects of e-cigarettes are not yet known, although there was no clinical evidence of cardiovascular harms.[188]

The potential cardiovascular risk of e-cigarettes compared to tobacco cigarettes is a key question under investigation. Because CVD takes many years to develop and e-cigarettes have been used for relatively few years, and because most vapers are current or former smokers, there are no reliable empirical data on the long-term cardiovascular risk from vaping. Thus, to assess the risk to current smokers who might switch to e-cigarettes, the risk assessment at present must be based on data from toxicity of constituents, levels of exposure, potential mechanisms of harm, and studies in experimental models, with comparison to cigarette smoke. Toxic constituents, with the exception of nicotine and particulates, are present in much lower levels in e-cigarette aerosol compared to cigarette smoke.[188,194] The particulates from e-cigarette aerosol are liquid and evaporate quickly, as opposed to the carbonaceous particles of cigarette smoke, and the toxicity of e-cigarette particles is as yet unknown. Most of the cardiovascular effects of e-cigarette use are related to nicotine and are similar to cigarette smoking. However, exposure to oxidative chemicals and other combustion products such as carbon monoxide and acrolein that are thought to mediate most cardiovascular risks of smoking is much lower with e-cigarette use.[194] In people, e-cigarette use acutely impairs endothelial function,[195] as indicated by flow-mediated dilation, but when smokers switch from cigarettes to e-cigarettes, endothelial function improves.[196] While e-cigarettes may pose some risk, particularly in people with preexisting CVD, the risk is likely to be much less than that of smoking.

An additional health concern about the short-term safety of e-cigarettes arose in 2019 with an outbreak of over 2000 cases of acute respiratory illness that was given the name e-cigarette or vaping product use associated lung injury (EVALI). The majority of cases (>80%) occurred in individuals who reported vaping of tetrahydrocannabinol (THC).[197] Although some affected individuals reported using only nicotine in their e-cigarettes,[198] questions were raised about accuracy of these reports given that recreational cannabis use is illegal in many states. Subsequently, the EVALI outbreak was strongly associated with exposure to Vitamin E acetate contaminating illicit THC-containing vaping devices.[199] Very little evidence was found to associate commercially produced e-cigarettes containing only nicotine with the EVALI cases.

Efficacy for Smoking Cessation

Currently, evidence from two clinical trials demonstrates the benefit of e-cigarettes to aid smoking cessation. One trial performed in smoking cessation clinics in the United Kingdom found that compared to nicotine replacement therapy, e-cigarettes nearly doubled quit rates at 1 year (18.0% vs 9.9%).[200] More than 80% of quitters in the e-cigarette group continued to vape, consistent with the idea of nicotine harm reduction. Another trial, conducted in New Zealand, compared the nicotine patch alone with patch plus nicotine e-cigarettes and patch plus non-nicotine e-cigarettes. Smokers treated with the nicotine patch and nicotine e-cigarette combination had significantly higher quit rates at 6 months compared to the patch alone (7% vs 2%).[201] The Cochrane systematic review of the effectiveness and safety of e-cigarettes for smoking cessation was updated in 2020.[202] It concluded that "moderate certainty evidence" supports the effectiveness of nicotine-containing e-cigarettes to aid cessation for 6 months when compared to NRT (RR = 1.69, 95% CI = 1.25–2.27) or to non-nicotine e-cigarettes (RR = 1.71, 95% CI = 1.00–2.92). The evidence also suggests a benefit of e-cigarettes over counseling only or no treatment (RR = 2.50, 95% CI = 1.24–5.04), although confidence in this last comparison is lower due to the quality of the trials identified. Epidemiological studies also indicate that e-cigarettes substantially increase quit rates, particularly when the intent of vaping is to quit smoking, and e-cigarettes are used daily.[203]

Role for Clinicians

While many uncertainties still exist with respect to the health effects of e-cigarettes and their efficacy for smoking cessation, smokers are using these products and asking their clinicians for guidance about their use. Because of the limited evidence about the health consequences of e-cigarette use, guidelines from the ACC and other health organizations recommend that clinicians advise smokers who are attempting to quit to use FDA-approved smoking cessation treatments first, rather than e-cigarettes. However, clinicians should be prepared to discuss the health risks and benefits of e-cigarette use. Smokers who choose to use e-cigarettes should be encouraged to switch completely to e-cigarettes and stop all cigarette use due to the lack of evidence that dual use of these products has meaningful benefits. Because of uncertainty about the safety of long-term e-cigarette use, smokers who stop smoking combustible cigarettes by switching to e-cigarettes should be encouraged to have the eventual goal of stopping e-cigarette use as well. There is no reason for nonsmokers to use e-cigarettes, and to minimize the risk of EVALI, smokers who use e-cigarettes should be advised not to purchase e-cigarettes illegally or to alter commercial e-cigarettes in any way.

Evidence on how to quit e-cigarette use is currently very limited. In the interim, a reasonable approach is to adapt the strategies used to help cigarette smokers to stop, including both behavioral resources (Table 8–3) and consideration of FDA-approved smoking cessation aids.

Heated Tobacco Products

Heated tobacco products (also called heat-not-burn tobacco products) are newer devices that heat tobacco leaf without burning it to create an aerosol. Heated tobacco products are marketed in several countries and have become quite popular in Japan and South Korea, where the sale of e-cigarettes is not allowed.[204] In 2020, one heated tobacco product (IQOS) was authorized for marketing in the United States as a modified-risk tobacco product.[205] The long-term health effects of heated tobacco product use are not yet known. Based on chemical analysis of emissions, the risk is likely to be intermediate in toxicity between an e-cigarette and a tobacco cigarette.[204]

SUMMARY

Tobacco use, especially cigarette smoking, is a major risk factor for CVD morbidity and mortality. Cigarette smoking increases virtually all clinical manifestations of atherosclerotic CVD, and cigarette smoke promotes CVD through multiple pathophysiological mechanisms. Fortunately, the excess cardiovascular risk caused by cigarette smoking is rapidly reversible after smoking cessation, even when that occurs at an advanced age or following an acute cardiovascular event. The reversible relationship between cigarette smoking and CVD mortality provides a strong rationale for healthcare providers to make the routine delivery of tobacco cessation treatment a standard component of cardiovascular care. There is firm evidence that FDA-approved cessation pharmacotherapies and psychosocial interventions each promote smoking cessation but are most effective when provided together. A framework for delivering tobacco cessation treatment in both outpatient and inpatient clinical settings has been outlined in the Expert Consensus Decision Pathway developed by the ACC.[133]

REFERENCES

1. World Health Organization. *Fact Sheets: Tobacco.* https://www.who.int/news-room/fact-sheets/detail/tobacco. Accessed August 14, 2020.
2. Centers for Disease Control and Prevention (CDC). Smoking-attributable mortality, years of potential life lost, and productivity losses—United States, 2000-2004. *MMWR.* 2008;57(45):1226.
3. Xu J, Murphy SL, Kockanek KD, Arias E. Mortality in the United States, 2018. *NCHS Data Brief.* 2020;355:1-8.
4. Benjamin EJ, Virani SS, Callaway CW, et al. Heart disease and stroke statistics-2018 update: a report from the American Heart Association. *Circulation.* 2018;137(12):e67-e492. doi:10.1161/CIR.0000000000000558
5. U.S. Department of Health and Human Services. *The Health Consequences of Smoking: 50 Years of Progress. A Report of the Surgeon General.* Atlanta, GA: U.S. Department of Health and Human Services, Centers for Disease Control and Prevention, National Center for Chronic Disease Prevention and Health Promotion, Office on Smoking and Health, 2014. Printed with corrections, January 2014.
6. Jha P, Ramasundarahettige C, Landsman V, et al. 21st-century hazards of smoking and benefits of cessation in the United States. *N Engl J Med.* 2013;368(4):341-350.
7. Mons U, Müezzinler A, Gellert C, et al. Impact of smoking and smoking cessation on cardiovascular events and mortality among older adults: meta-analysis of individual participant data from prospective cohort studies of the CHANCES consortium. *BMJ.* 2015;350:h1551. doi:10.1136/bmj.h1551

8. World Health Organization. *WHO Report on the Global Tobacco Epidemic, 2019*. Geneva: World Health Organization; 2019. Licence: CC BY-NC-SA 3.0 IGO.

9. Smoking prevalence and attributable disease burden in 195 countries and territories, 1990-2015: a systematic analysis from the Global Burden of Disease Study 2015. *Lancet*. 2017;389(10082):1885-1906. doi:10.1016/S0140-6736(17)30819-X

10. Creamer MR, Wang TW, Babb S, et al. Tobacco product use and cessation indicators among adults—United States, 2018. *MMWR*. 2019;68(45):1013-1019. doi:10.15585/mmwr.mm6845a2

11. Wang TW, Gentzke AS, Creamer MR, et al. Tobacco product use and associated factors among middle and high school students—United States, 2019. *MMWR Surveill Summ*. 2019;68(12):1-22. doi:10.15585/mmwr.ss6812a1

12. Wang TW. Tobacco product use among adults—United States, 2017. *MMWR*. 2018;67. doi:10.15585/mmwr.mm6744a2

13. Fiore MC, Schroeder SA, Baker TB. Smoke, the chief killer—strategies for targeting combustible tobacco use. *N Engl J Med*. 2014;370(4):297-299. doi:10.1056/NEJMp1314942

14. Law MR, Wald NJ. Environmental tobacco smoke and ischemic heart disease. *Prog Cardiovasc Dis*. 2003;46(1):31-38. doi:10.1016/s0033-0620(03)00078-1

15. Shah AM, Pfeffer MA, Hartley LH, et al. Risk of all-cause mortality, recurrent myocardial infarction, and heart failure hospitalization associated with smoking status following myocardial infarction with left ventricular dysfunction. *Am J Cardiol*. 2010;106(7):911-916. doi:10.1016/j.amjcard.2010.05.021

16. Evangelista LS, Doering LV, Dracup K. Usefulness of a history of tobacco and alcohol use in predicting multiple heart failure readmissions among veterans. *Am J Cardiol*. 2000;86(12):1339-1342. doi:10.1016/s0002-9149(00)01238-8

17. Zhu W, Yuan P, Shen Y, Wan R, Hong K. Association of smoking with the risk of incident atrial fibrillation: a meta-analysis of prospective studies. *Int J Cardiol*. 2016;218:259-266. doi:10.1016/j.ijcard.2016.05.013

18. Nadruz WJ, Claggett B, Gonçalves A, et al. Smoking and cardiac structure and function in the elderly: the ARIC Study (Atherosclerosis Risk in Communities). *Circ Cardiovasc Imaging*. 2016;9(9):e004950. doi:10.1161/CIRCIMAGING.116.004950

19. Barnoya J, Glantz SA. Cardiovascular effects of secondhand smoke: nearly as large as smoking. *Circulation*. 2005;111(20):2684-2698. doi:10.1161/CIRCULATIONAHA.104.492215

20. Oono IP, Mackay DF, Pell JP. Meta-analysis of the association between secondhand smoke exposure and stroke. *J Public Health (Oxf)*. 2011;33(4):496-502. doi:10.1093/pubmed/fdr025

21. Yankelevitz DF, Henschke CI, Yip R, et al. Second-hand tobacco smoke in never smokers is a significant risk factor for coronary artery calcification. *JACC Cardiovasc Imaging*. 2013;6(6):651-657. doi:10.1016/j.jcmg.2013.02.004

22. West HW, Juonala M, Gall SL, et al. Exposure to parental smoking in childhood is associated with increased risk of carotid atherosclerotic plaque in adulthood: the Cardiovascular Risk in Young Finns Study. *Circulation*. 2015;131(14):1239-1246. doi:10.1161/CIRCULATIONAHA.114.013485

23. Gall S, Huynh QL, Magnussen CG, et al. Exposure to parental smoking in childhood or adolescence is associated with increased carotid intima-media thickness in young adults: evidence from the Cardiovascular Risk in Young Finns study and the Childhood Determinants of Adult Health Study. *Eur Heart J*. 2014;35(36):2484-2491. doi:10.1093/eurheartj/ehu049

24. Heiss C, Amabile N, Lee AC, et al. Brief secondhand smoke exposure depresses endothelial progenitor cells activity and endothelial function: sustained vascular injury and blunted nitric oxide production. *J Am Coll Cardiol*. 2008;51(18):1760-1771. doi:10.1016/j.jacc.2008.01.040

25. Tan CE, Glantz SA. Association between smoke-free legislation and hospitalizations for cardiac, cerebrovascular, and respiratory diseases: a meta-analysis. *Circulation*. 2012;126(18):2177-2183. doi:10.1161/CIRCULATIONAHA.112.121301

26. CDCTobaccoFree. *Smokefree Policies Improve Health*. Centers for Disease Control and Prevention. Published December 1, 2016. https://www.cdc.gov/tobacco/data_statistics/fact_sheets/secondhand_smoke/protection/improve_health/index.htm. Accessed September 10, 2020.

27. Iribarren C, Tekawa IS, Sidney S, Friedman GD. Effect of cigar smoking on the risk of cardiovascular disease, chronic obstructive pulmonary disease, and cancer in men. *N Engl J Med*. 1999;340(23):1773-1780. doi:10.1056/NEJM199906103402301

28. Christensen CH, Rostron B, Cosgrove C, et al. Association of cigarette, cigar, and pipe use with mortality risk in the US population. *JAMA Intern Med*. 2018;178(4):469-476. doi:10.1001/jamainternmed.2017.8625

29. Jacobs EJ, Thun MJ, Apicella LF. Cigar smoking and death from coronary heart disease in a prospective study of US men. *Arch Intern Med*. 1999;159(20):2413-2418. doi:10.1001/archinte.159.20.2413

30. Henley SJ, Thun MJ, Chao A, Calle EE. Association between exclusive pipe smoking and mortality from cancer and other diseases. *J Natl Cancer Inst*. 2004;96(11):853-861. doi:10.1093/jnci/djh144

31. Tverdal A, Bjartveit K. Health consequences of pipe versus cigarette smoking. *Tob Control*. 2011;20(2):123-130. doi:10.1136/tc.2010.036780

32. Jawad M, Charide R, Waziry R, Darzi A, Ballout RA, Akl EA. The prevalence and trends of waterpipe tobacco smoking: a systematic review. *PLoS One*. 2018;13(2):e0192191. doi:10.1371/journal.pone.0192191

33. Maziak W, Taleb ZB, Bahelah R, et al. The global epidemiology of waterpipe smoking. *Tob Control*. 2015;24(Suppl 1):i3. doi:10.1136/tobaccocontrol-2014-051903

34. Cobb C, Ward KD, Maziak W, Shihadeh AL, Eissenberg T. Waterpipe tobacco smoking: an emerging health crisis in the United States. *Am J Health Behav*. 2010;34(3):275-285. doi:10.5993/ajhb.34.3.3

35. Bhatnagar A, Maziak W, Eissenberg T, et al. Water pipe (hookah) smoking and cardiovascular disease risk: a scientific statement from the American Heart Association. *Circulation*. 2019;139(19):e917-e936. doi:10.1161/CIR.0000000000000671

36. Piano MR, Benowitz NL, Fitzgerald GA, et al. Impact of smokeless tobacco products on cardiovascular disease: implications for policy, prevention, and treatment: a policy statement from the American Heart Association. *Circulation*. 2010;122(15):1520-1544. doi:10.1161/CIR.0b013e3181f432c3

37. National Cancer Institute and Centers for Disease Control and Prevention. *Smokeless Tobacco and Public Health: A Global Perspective*. Bethesda, MD: U.S. Department of Health and Human Services, Centers for Disease Control and Prevention and National Institutes of Health, National Cancer Institute. NIH Publication No. 14-7983; 2014.

38. Boffetta P, Straif K. Use of smokeless tobacco and risk of myocardial infarction and stroke: systematic review with meta-analysis. *BMJ*. 2009;339:b3060. doi:10.1136/bmj.b3060

39. Arefalk G, Hambraeus K, Lind L, Michaëlsson K, Lindahl B, Sundström J. Discontinuation of smokeless tobacco and mortality risk after myocardial infarction. *Circulation*. 2014;130(4):325-332. doi:10.1161/CIRCULATIONAHA.113.007252

40. Teo KK, Ounpuu S, Hawken S, et al. Tobacco use and risk of myocardial infarction in 52 countries in the INTERHEART study: a case-control study. *Lancet*. 2006;368(9536):647-658. doi:10.1016/S0140-6736(06)69249-0

41. Borgerding M, Klus H. Analysis of complex mixtures—cigarette smoke. *Exp Toxicol Pathol*. 2005;57 (Suppl 1):43-73. doi:10.1016/j.etp.2005.05.010

42. Rafacho BPM, Azevedo PS, Polegato BF, et al. Tobacco smoke induces ventricular remodeling associated with an increase in NADPH oxidase activity. *Cell Physiol Biochem*. 2011;27(3-4):305-312. doi:10.1159/000327957

43. Kitami M, Ali MK. Tobacco, Metabolic and inflammatory pathways, and CVD Risk. *Glob Heart*. 2012;7(2):121-128. doi:10.1016/j.gheart.2012.06.004

44. U.S. Department of Health and Human Services. *How Tobacco Smoke Causes Disease: The Biology and Behavioral Basis for Smoking-Attributable Disease: A Report of the Surgeon General*. U.S. Department of Health and Human Services, Centers for Disease Control and Prevention, National Center for Chronic Disease Prevention and Health Promotion, Office on Smoking and Health; 2010.

45. Winniford MD, Wheelan KR, Kremers MS, et al. Smoking-induced coronary vasoconstriction in patients with atherosclerotic coronary artery disease: evidence for adrenergically mediated alterations in coronary artery tone. *Circulation*. 1986;73(4):662-667. doi:10.1161/01.cir.73.4.662

46. Benowitz NL, Kuyt F, Jacob P. Influence of nicotine on cardiovascular and hormonal effects of cigarette smoking. *Clin Pharmacol Ther*. 1984;36(1):74-81. doi:10.1038/clpt.1984.142

47. Toda N, Toda H. Nitric oxide-mediated blood flow regulation as affected by smoking and nicotine. *Eur J Pharmacol*. 2010;649(1-3):1-13. doi:10.1016/j.ejphar.2010.09.042

48. Barbieri SS, Zacchi E, Amadio P, et al. Cytokines present in smokers' serum interact with smoke components to enhance endothelial dysfunction. *Cardiovasc Res*. 2011;90(3):475-483. doi:10.1093/cvr/cvr032

49. Ichiki K, Ikeda H, Haramaki N, Ueno T, Imaizumi T. Long-term smoking impairs platelet-derived nitric oxide release. *Circulation*. 1996;94(12):3109-3114. doi:10.1161/01.cir.94.12.3109

50. Takajo Y, Ikeda H, Haramaki N, Murohara T, Imaizumi T. Augmented oxidative stress of platelets in chronic smokers. Mechanisms of impaired platelet-derived nitric oxide bioactivity and augmented platelet aggregability. *J Am Coll Cardiol*. 2001;38(5):1320-1327. doi:10.1016/s0735-1097(01)01583-2

51. Niemann B, Rohrbach S, Miller MR, Newby DE, Fuster V, Kovacic JC. Oxidative stress and cardiovascular risk: obesity, diabetes, smoking, and pollution: part 3 of a 3-part series. *J Am Coll Cardiol*. 2017;70(2):230-251. doi:10.1016/j.jacc.2017.05.043

52. Csordas A, Bernhard D. The biology behind the atherothrombotic effects of cigarette smoke. *Nat Rev Cardiol*. 2013;10(4):219-230. doi:10.1038/nrcardio.2013.8

53. Benowitz NL. Cigarette smoking and cardiovascular disease: pathophysiology and implications for treatment. *Prog Cardiovasc Dis*. 2003;46(1):91-111. doi:10.1016/s0033-0620(03)00087-2

54. Barua RS, Ambrose JA, Srivastava S, DeVoe MC, Eales-Reynolds L-J. Reactive oxygen species are involved in smoking-induced dysfunction of nitric oxide biosynthesis and upregulation of endothelial nitric oxide synthase: an in vitro demonstration in human coronary artery endothelial cells. *Circulation*. 2003;107(18):2342-2347. doi:10.1161/01.CIR.0000066691.52789.BE

55. Heitzer T, Just H, Münzel T. Antioxidant vitamin C improves endothelial dysfunction in chronic smokers. *Circulation*. 1996;94(1):6-9. doi:10.1161/01.cir.94.1.6

56. Ahmadi A, Leipsic J, Blankstein R, et al. Do plaques rapidly progress prior to myocardial infarction? *Circ Res*. 2015;117(1):99-104. doi:10.1161/CIRCRESAHA.117.305637

57. Barua RS, Sy F, Srikanth S, et al. Effects of cigarette smoke exposure on clot dynamics and fibrin structure: an ex vivo investigation. *Arterioscler Thromb Vas Biol*. 2010;30(1):75-79.

58. Wissler RW. New insights into the pathogenesis of atherosclerosis as revealed by PDAY. *Atherosclerosis*. 1994;108:S3-S20.

59. Raveendran M, Senthil D, Utama B, et al. Cigarette suppresses the expression of P4Hα and vascular collagen production. *Biochem Bioph Res Co*. 2004;323(2):592-598.

60. Perlstein TS, Lee RT. Smoking, metalloproteinases, and vascular disease. *Arterioscler Thromb Vasc Biol*. 2006;26(2):250-256.

61. Ambrose JA, Barua RS. The pathophysiology of cigarette smoking and cardiovascular disease: an update. *J Am Col Cardiol*. 2004;43(10):1731-1737.

62. Salahuddin S, Prabhakaran D, Roy A. Pathophysiological mechanisms of tobacco-related CVD. *Global Heart*. 2012;7(2):113-120. doi:10.1016/j.gheart.2012.05.003

63. Fusegawa Y, Goto S, Handa S, Kawada T, Ando Y. Platelet spontaneous aggregation in platelet-rich plasma is increased in habitual smokers. *Thromb Res*. 1999;93(6):271-278. doi:10.1016/S0049-3848(98)00184-4

64. Sawada M, Kishi Y, Numano F, Isobe M. Smokers lack morning increase in platelet sensitivity to nitric oxide. *J. Cardiovasc Pharmacol*. 2002;40(4):571-576.

65. Price J, Mowbray PI, Lee AJ, Rumley A, Lowe GDO, Fowkes FGR. Relationship between smoking and cardiovascular risk factors in the development of peripheral arterial disease and coronary artery disease; Edinburgh Artery Study: Edinburgh Artery Study. *Eur Heart J*. 1999;20(5):344-353.

66. Smith FB, Lowe GDO, Fowkes FGR, et al. Smoking, haemostatic factors and lipid peroxides in a population case control study of peripheral arterial disease. *Atherosclerosis*. 1993;102(2):155-162. doi:10.1016/0021-9150(93)90157-P

67. Ogston D, Bennett NB, Ogston CM. The influence of cigarette smoking on the plasma fibrinogen concentration. *Atherosclerosis*. 1970;11(2):349-352.

68. Dotevall A, Johansson S, Wilhelmsen L. Association between fibrinogen and other risk factors for cardiovascular disease in men and women results from the Göteborg MONICA Survey 1985. *Ann Epidemiol*. 1994;4(5):369-374.

69. Matetzky S, Tani S, Kangavari S, et al. Smoking increases tissue factor expression in atherosclerotic plaques: implications for plaque thrombogenicity. *Circulation*. 2000;102(6):602-604.

70. Czernin J, Waldherr C. Cigarette smoking and coronary blood flow. *Prog Cardiovasc Dis*. 2003;45(5):395-404.

71. Burke AP, Farb A, Malcom GT, Liang YH, Smialek J, Virmani R. Coronary risk factors and plaque morphology in men with coronary disease who died suddenly. *N Engl J Med*. 1997;336(18):1276-1282. doi:10.1056/NEJM199705013361802

72. Metz L, Waters DD. Implications of cigarette smoking for the management of patients with acute coronary syndromes. *Prog Cardiovasc Dis*. 2003;46(1):1-9. doi:10.1016/s0033-0620(03)00075-6

73. Hasnis E, Bar-Shai M, Burbea Z, Reznick AZ. Cigarette smoke-induced NF-kappaB activation in human lymphocytes: the effect of low and high exposure to gas phase of cigarette smoke. *J Physiol Pharmacol*. 2007;58 Suppl 5(Pt 1):263-274.

74. Smith CJ, Fischer TH. Particulate and vapor phase constituents of cigarette mainstream smoke and risk of myocardial infarction. *Atherosclerosis*. 2001;158(2):257-267. doi:10.1016/s0021-9150(01)00570-6

75. Lehr HA, Frei B, Arfors KE. Vitamin C prevents cigarette smoke-induced leukocyte aggregation and adhesion to endothelium in vivo. *Proc Natl Acad Sci USA*. 1994;91(16):7688-7692. doi:10.1073/pnas.91.16.7688

76. Mazzone A. Leukocytes-endothelial interaction in vascular pathology: from host defence mechanism to promoter of vascular injury. *Minerva Cardioangiol*. 2001;49(6):417-420.

77. Yang S-R, Chida AS, Bauter MR, et al. Cigarette smoke induces proinflammatory cytokine release by activation of NF-κB and posttranslational modifications of histone deacetylase in macrophages. *Am J Physiol-Lung Cellul Molecul Physiol*. 2006;291(1):L46-L57.

78. Linneberg A, Jacobsen RK, Skaaby T, et al. Effect of smoking on blood pressure and resting heart rate: a Mendelian randomization meta-analysis in the CARTA consortium. *Circ Cardiovasc Gene*. 2015;8(6):832-841.

79. Craig WY, Palomaki GE, Haddow JE. Cigarette smoking and serum lipid and lipoprotein concentrations: an analysis of published data. *BMJ*. 1989;298(6676):784-788. doi:10.1136/bmj.298.6676.784

80. Yokode M, Kita T, Arai H, Kawai C, Narumiya S, Fujiwara M. Cholesteryl ester accumulation in macrophages incubated with low density lipoprotein pretreated with cigarette smoke extract. *Proc Natl Acad Sci USA*. 1988;85(7):2344-2348. doi:10.1073/pnas.85.7.2344

81. Kong C, Nimmo L, Elatrozy T, et al. Smoking is associated with increased hepatic lipase activity, insulin resistance, dyslipidaemia and early atherosclerosis in Type 2 diabetes. *Atherosclerosis*. 2001;156(2):373-378. doi:10.1016/s0021-9150(00)00664-x

82. Hellerstein MK, Benowitz NL, Neese RA, et al. Effects of cigarette smoking and its cessation on lipid metabolism and energy expenditure in heavy smokers. *J Clin Invest*. 1994;93(1):265-272. doi:10.1172/JCI116955

83. Eliasson B. Cigarette smoking and diabetes. *Prog Cardiovasc Dis*. 2003;45(5):405-413. doi:10.1053/pcad.2003.00103

84. Zhu Y, Zhang M, Hou X, et al. Cigarette smoking increases risk for incident metabolic syndrome in Chinese men-Shanghai diabetes study. *Biomed Environ Sci*. 2011;24(5):475-482. doi:10.3967/0895-3988.2011.05.004

85. Chuahirun T, Khanna A, Kimball K, Wesson DE. Cigarette smoking and increased urine albumin excretion are interrelated predictors of nephropathy progression in type 2 diabetes. *Am J Kidney Dis*. 2003;41(1):13-21. doi:10.1053/ajkd.2003.50009

86. Axelsson T, Jansson PA, Smith U, Eliasson B. Nicotine infusion acutely impairs insulin sensitivity in type 2 diabetic patients but not in healthy subjects. *J Intern Med.* 2001;249(6):539-544. doi:10.1046/j.1365-2796.2001.00840.x

87. Meurrens K, Ruf S, Ross G, Schleef R, von Holt K, Schlüter K-D. Smoking accelerates the progression of hypertension-induced myocardial hypertrophy to heart failure in spontaneously hypertensive rats. *Cardiovasc Res.* 2007;76(2):311-322.

88. Talukder MH, Johnson WM, Varadharaj S, et al. Chronic cigarette smoking causes hypertension, increased oxidative stress, impaired NO bioavailability, endothelial dysfunction, and cardiac remodeling in mice. *Am J Physiol-Heart Circ Physiol.* 2011;300(1):H388-H396.

89. Gu L, Pandey V, Geenen DL, Chowdhury SA, Piano MR. Cigarette smoke-induced left ventricular remodelling is associated with activation of mitogen-activated protein kinases. *Eur J Heart Fail.* 2008;10(11):1057-1064.

90. Varela Carver A, Parker H, Kleinert C, Rimoldi O. Adverse effects of cigarette smoke and induction of oxidative stress in cardiomyocytes and vascular endothelium. *Curr Pharm Des.* 2010;16(23):2551-2558.

91. Singh K, Xiao L, Remondino A, Sawyer DB, Colucci WS. Adrenergic regulation of cardiac myocyte apoptosis. *J Cell Physiol.* 2001;189(3):257-265.

92. Plank B, Kutyifa V, Moss AJ, et al. Smoking is associated with an increased risk of first and recurrent ventricular tachyarrhythmias in ischemic and nonischemic patients with mild heart failure: a MADIT-CRT substudy. *Heart Rhythm.* 2014;11(5):822-827. doi:10.1016/j.hrthm.2014.02.007

93. Desai H, Aronow WS, Ahn C, et al. Risk factors for appropriate cardioverter-defibrillator shocks, inappropriate cardioverter-defibrillator shocks, and time to mortality in 549 patients with heart failure. *Am J Cardiol.* 2010;105(9):1336-1338. doi:10.1016/j.amjcard.2009.12.057

94. Goldenberg I, Moss AJ, McNitt S, et al. Cigarette smoking and the risk of supraventricular and ventricular tachyarrhythmias in high-risk cardiac patients with implantable cardioverter defibrillators. *J Cardiovasc Electrophysiol.* 2006;17(9):931-936. doi:10.1111/j.1540-8167.2006.00526.x

95. Jha P, Peto R. Global effects of smoking, of quitting, and of taxing tobacco. *N Engl J Med.* 2014;370(1):60-68.

96. Proctor RN. The cigarette catastrophe continues. *Lancet.* 2015;385(9972):938-939.

97. Yang G, Wang Y, Wu Y, Yang J, Wan X. The road to effective tobacco control in China. *Lancet.* 2015;385(9972):1019-1028.

98. Ezzati M, Henley SJ, Thun MJ, Lopez AD. Role of smoking in global and regional cardiovascular mortality. *Circulation.* 2005;112(4):489-497.

99. Nash SH, Liao LM, Harris TB, Freedman ND. Cigarette smoking and mortality in adults aged 70 years and older: results from the NIH-AARP cohort. *Am J Prevent Med.* 2017;52(3):276-283.

100. US Department of Health and Human Services. *The Health Consequences of Smoking: A Report of the Surgeon General.* Vol 62. U.S. Department of Health and Human Services, Centers for Disease Control and Prevention, National Center for Chronic Disease Prevention and Health Promotion, Office on Smoking and Health; 2004.

101. Benowitz NL, Fitzgerald GA, Wilson M, Zhang QI. Nicotine effects on eicosanoid formation and hemostatic function: comparison of transdermal nicotine and cigarette smoking. *J Am Col Cardiol.* 1993;22(4):1159-1167.

102. Pujades-Rodriguez M, George J, Shah AD, et al. Heterogeneous associations between smoking and a wide range of initial presentations of cardiovascular disease in 1 937 360 people in England: lifetime risks and implications for risk prediction. *Int J Epidemiol.* 2015;44(1):129-141.

103. Peto R, Darby S, Deo H, Silcocks P, Whitley E, Doll R. Smoking, smoking cessation, and lung cancer in the UK since 1950: combination of national statistics with two case-control studies. *BMJ.* 2000;321(7257):323-329.

104. Critchley JA, Capewell S. Mortality risk reduction associated with smoking cessation in patients with coronary heart disease: a systematic review. *JAMA.* 2003;290(1):86-97.

105. Wilson K, Gibson N, Willan A, Cook D. Effect of smoking cessation on mortality after myocardial infarction: meta-analysis of cohort studies. *Arch Intern Med.* 2000;160(7):939-944.

106. Buchanan DM, Arnold SV, Gosch KL, et al. Association of smoking status with angina and health-related quality of life after acute myocardial infarction. *Circulation: Cardiovasc Qual Outcomes.* 2015;8(5):493-500.

107. Rea TD, Heckbert SR, Kaplan RC, Smith NL, Lemaitre RN, Psaty BM. Smoking status and risk for recurrent coronary events after myocardial infarction. *Ann Intern Med.* 2002;137(6):494-500.

108. Goldenberg I, Jonas M, Tenenbaum A, et al. Current smoking, smoking cessation, and the risk of sudden cardiac death in patients with coronary artery disease. *Arch Intern Med.* 2003;163(19):2301-2305.

109. Suskin N, Sheth T, Negassa A, Yusuf S. Relationship of current and past smoking to mortality and morbidity in patients with left ventricular dysfunction. *J Am Col Cardiol.* 2001;37(6):1677-1682.

110. Anthonisen NR, Connett JE, Kiley JP, et al. Effects of smoking intervention and the use of an inhaled anticholinergic bronchodilator on the rate of decline of FEV1: the Lung Health Study. *JAMA.* 1994;272(19):1497-1505.

111. Kanner RE, Connett JE, Williams DE, Buist AS, Group LHSR. Effects of randomized assignment to a smoking cessation intervention and changes in smoking habits on respiratory symptoms in smokers with early chronic obstructive pulmonary disease: the Lung Health Study. *Am J Med.* 1999;106(4):410-416.

112. Au DH, Bryson CL, Chien JW, et al. The effects of smoking cessation on the risk of chronic obstructive pulmonary disease exacerbations. *J Gen Intern Med.* 2009;24(4):457-463.

113. Anthonisen NR, Skeans MA, Wise RA, Manfreda J, Kanner RE, Connett JE. The effects of a smoking cessation intervention on 14.5-year mortality: a randomized clinical trial. *Ann Intern Med.* 2005;142(4):233-239.

114. Parsons A, Daley A, Begh R, Aveyard P. Influence of smoking cessation after diagnosis of early stage lung cancer on prognosis: systematic review of observational studies with meta-analysis. *BMJ.* 2010;340:b5569.

115. Hackshaw A, Morris JK, Boniface S, Tang J-L, Milenković D. Low cigarette consumption and risk of coronary heart disease and stroke: meta-analysis of 141 cohort studies in 55 study reports. *BMJ.* 2018;360.

116. Tverdal A, Bjartveit K. Health consequences of reduced daily cigarette consumption. *Tob Control.* 2006;15(6):472-480.

117. Hatsukami DK, Kotlyar M, Allen S, et al. Effects of cigarette reduction on cardiovascular risk factors and subjective measures. *Chest.* 2005;128(4):2528-2537.

118. Joseph AM, Hecht SS, Murphy SE, et al. Smoking reduction fails to improve clinical and biological markers of cardiac disease: a randomized controlled trial. *Nicotine Tob Res.* 2008;10(3):471-481.

119. Godtfredsen NS, Osler M, Vestbo J, Andersen I, Prescott E. Smoking reduction, smoking cessation, and incidence of fatal and non-fatal myocardial infarction in Denmark 1976-1998: a pooled cohort study. *J Epidemiol Comm Heal.* 2003;57(6):412-416.

120. Begh R, Lindson-Hawley N, Aveyard P. Does reduced smoking if you can't stop make any difference? *BMC Med.* 2015;13(1):1-5.

121. U.S. Department of Health and Human Services,. *Preventing Tobacco Use among Youth and Young Adults: A Report of the Surgeon General.* U.S. Department of Health and Human Services, Centers for Disease Control and Prevention, National Center for Chronic Disease Prevention and Health Promotion, Office on Smoking and Health; 2012.

122. Prochaska JJ, Benowitz NL. Current advances in research in treatment and recovery: Nicotine addiction. *Sci Adv.* 2019;5(10):eaay9763. doi:10.1126/sciadv.aay9763

123. Hughes JR, Hatsukami D. Signs and symptoms of tobacco withdrawal. *Arch Gen Psychiat.* 1986;43(3):289-294.

124. Herd N, Borland R. The natural history of quitting smoking: findings from the International Tobacco Control (ITC) Four Country Survey. *Addiction.* 2009;104(12):2075-2087.

125. Babb S. Quitting smoking among adults—United States, 2000-2015. *MMWR.* 2017;65.

126. Borland R, Yong H-H, O'Connor RJ, Hyland A, Thompson ME. The reliability and predictive validity of the Heaviness of Smoking Index and its two components: findings from the International Tobacco Control Four Country study. *Nicotine Tob Res.* 2010;12(suppl_1):S45-S50.

127. Fiore MC, Jaén CR, Baker TB, et al. *Treating Tobacco Use and Dependence: 2008 Update*. Rockville, MD: US Department of Health and Human Services. Published online 2008.

128. Siu AL. Behavioral and pharmacotherapy interventions for tobacco smoking cessation in adults, including pregnant women: US Preventive Services Task Force recommendation statement. *Ann Intern Med*. 2015;163(8):622-634.

129. U.S. Department of Health and Human Services. *Smoking Cessation. A Report of the Surgeon General*. U.S. Department of Health and Human Services, Centers for Disease Control and Prevention, National Center for Chronic Disease Prevention and Health Promotion, Office on Smoking and Health; 2020. Accessed September 10, 2020, https://www.ncbi.nlm.nih.gov/books/NBK555591

130. Stead LF, Koilpillai P, Fanshawe TR, Lancaster T. Combined pharmacotherapy and behavioural interventions for smoking cessation. *Cochrane Database Syst Rev*. 2016;3.

131. Piper ME. Withdrawal: expanding a key addiction construct. *Nicotine Tob Res*. 2015;17(12):1405-1415.

132. Anthenelli RM, Benowitz NL, West R, et al. Neuropsychiatric safety and efficacy of varenicline, bupropion, and nicotine patch in smokers with and without psychiatric disorders (EAGLES): a double-blind, randomised, placebo-controlled clinical trial. *Lancet*. 2016;387(10037):2507-2520.

133. Barua RS, Rigotti NA, Benowitz NL, et al. 2018 ACC expert consensus decision pathway on tobacco cessation treatment: a report of the American College of Cardiology Task Force on Clinical Expert Consensus Documents. *J Am Col Cardiol*. 2018;72(25):3332-3365.

134. Suissa K, Larivière J, Eisenberg MJ, et al. Efficacy and safety of smoking cessation interventions in patients with cardiovascular disease: a network meta-analysis of randomized controlled trials. *Circ Cardiovasc Qual Outcomes*. 2017;10(1). doi:10.1161/CIRCOUTCOMES.115.002458

135. Joseph AM, Norman SM, Ferry LH, et al. The safety of transdermal nicotine as an aid to smoking cessation in patients with cardiac disease. *N Engl J Med*. 1996;335(24):1792-1798. doi:10.1056/NEJM199612123352402

136. Murray RP, Bailey WC, Daniels K, et al. Safety of nicotine polacrilex gum used by 3,094 participants in the Lung Health Study. Lung Health Study Research Group. *Chest*. 1996;109(2):438-445. doi:10.1378/chest.109.2.438

137. Meine TJ, Patel MR, Washam JB, Pappas PA, Jollis JG. Safety and effectiveness of transdermal nicotine patch in smokers admitted with acute coronary syndromes. *Am J Cardiol*. 2005;95(8):976-978. doi:10.1016/j.amjcard.2004.12.039

138. Pack QR, Priya A, Lagu TC, et al. Short-term safety of nicotine replacement in smokers hospitalized with coronary heart disease. *J Am Heart Assoc*. 2018;7(18):e009424. doi:10.1161/JAHA.118.009424

139. Mills EJ, Thorlund K, Eapen S, Wu P, Prochaska JJ. Cardiovascular events associated with smoking cessation pharmacotherapies: a network meta-analysis. *Circulation*. 2014;129(1):28-41. doi:10.1161/CIRCULATIONAHA.113.003961

140. Hartmann-Boyce J, Chepkin SC, Ye W, Bullen C, Lancaster T. Nicotine replacement therapy versus control for smoking cessation. *Cochrane Database Syst Rev*. 2018;5:CD000146. doi:10.1002/14651858.CD000146.pub5

141. Lindson N, Chepkin SC, Ye W, Fanshawe TR, Bullen C, Hartmann-Boyce J. Different doses, durations and modes of delivery of nicotine replacement therapy for smoking cessation. *Cochrane Database Syst Rev*. 2019;4:CD013308. doi:10.1002/14651858.CD013308

142. Schnoll RA, Goelz PM, Veluz-Wilkins A, et al. Long-term nicotine replacement therapy: a randomized clinical trial. *JAMA Intern Med*. 2015;175(4):504-511.

143. Rollema H, Chambers LK, Coe JW, et al. Pharmacological profile of the α4β2 nicotinic acetylcholine receptor partial agonist varenicline, an effective smoking cessation aid. *Neuropharmacology*. 2007;52(3):985-994.

144. Cahill K, Lindson-Hawley N, Thomas KH, Fanshawe TR, Lancaster T. Nicotine receptor partial agonists for smoking cessation. *Cochrane Database Syst Rev*. 2016;(5):CD006103. doi:10.1002/14651858.CD006103.pub7

145. Rigotti NA, Pipe AL, Benowitz NL, Arteaga C, Garza D, Tonstad S. Efficacy and safety of varenicline for smoking cessation in patients with cardiovascular disease: a randomized trial. *Circulation*. 2010;121(2):221-229. doi:10.1161/CIRCULATIONAHA.109.869008

146. Eisenberg MJ, Windle SB, Roy N, et al. Varenicline for smoking cessation in hospitalized patients with acute coronary syndrome. *Circulation*. 2016;133(1):21-30.

147. Fiore MC, Jaén CR. A clinical blueprint to accelerate the elimination of tobacco use. *JAMA*. 2008;299(17):2083-2085.

148. US Food and Drug Administration. *Drug Approval Package: Chantix (Varenicline) NDA #021928*. Accessed September 10, 2020, https://www.accessdata.fda.gov/drugsatfda_docs/nda/2006/021928_s000_chantixtoc.cfm

149. Sterling LH, Windle SB, Filion KB, Touma L, Eisenberg MJ. Varenicline and adverse cardiovascular events: a systematic review and meta-analysis of randomized controlled trials. *J Am Heart Ass*. 2016;5(2):e002849.

150. Benowitz NL, Pipe A, West R, et al. Cardiovascular safety of varenicline, bupropion, and nicotine patch in smokers: a randomized clinical trial. *JAMA Intern Med*. 2018;178(5):622-631.

151. Tonstad S, Tønnesen P, Hajek P, et al. Effect of maintenance therapy with varenicline on smoking cessation: a randomized controlled trial. *JAMA*. 2006;296(1):64-71.

152. Slemmer JE, Martin BR, Damaj MI. Bupropion is a nicotinic antagonist. *J Pharmacol Exp Ther*. 2000;295(1):321-327.

153. Howes S, Hartmann-Boyce J, Livingstone-Banks J, Hong B, Lindson N. Antidepressants for smoking cessation. *Cochrane Database Syst Rev*. 2020;4:CD000031. doi:10.1002/14651858.CD000031.pub5

154. Tonstad S, Farsang C, Klaene G, et al. Bupropion SR for smoking cessation in smokers with cardiovascular disease: a multicentre, randomised study. *Eur Heart J*. 2003;24(10):946-955.

155. Eisenberg MJ, Grandi SM, Gervais A, et al. Bupropion for smoking cessation in patients hospitalized with acute myocardial infarction: a randomized, placebo-controlled trial. *J Am Col Cardiol*. 2013;61(5):524-532.

156. Hays JT, Hurt RD, Rigotti NA, et al. Sustained-release bupropion for pharmacologic relapse prevention after smoking cessation: a randomized, controlled trial. *Ann Intern Med*. 2001;135(6):423-433.

157. Koegelenberg CF, Noor F, Bateman ED, et al. Efficacy of varenicline combined with nicotine replacement therapy vs varenicline alone for smoking cessation: a randomized clinical trial. *JAMA*. 2014;312(2):155-161.

158. Hajek P, Smith KM, Dhanji A-R, McRobbie H. Is a combination of varenicline and nicotine patch more effective in helping smokers quit than varenicline alone? A randomised controlled trial. *BMC Med*. 2013;11(1):1-7.

159. Ebbert JO, Hatsukami DK, Croghan IT, et al. Combination varenicline and bupropion SR for tobacco-dependence treatment in cigarette smokers: a randomized trial. *JAMA*. 2014;311(2):155-163.

160. Ebbert JO, Hughes JR, West RJ, et al. Effect of varenicline on smoking cessation through smoking reduction: a randomized clinical trial. *JAMA*. 2015;313(7):687-694.

161. Lindson N, Klemperer E, Hong B, Ordóñez-Mena JM, Aveyard P. Smoking reduction interventions for smoking cessation. *Cochrane Database Syst Rev*. 2019;9.

162. Gourlay SG, Stead LF, Benowitz NL. Clonidine for smoking cessation. *Cochrane Database Syst Rev*. 2004;3:CD000058. doi:10.1002/14651858.CD000058.pub2

163. Walker N, Howe C, Glover M, et al. Cytisine versus nicotine for smoking cessation. *N Engl J Med*. 2014;371(25):2353-2362.

164. West R, Zatonski W, Cedzynska M, et al. Placebo-controlled trial of cytisine for smoking cessation. *N Engl J Med*. 2011;365(13):1193-1200.

165. Lindson N, Thompson TP, Ferrey A, Lambert JD, Aveyard P. Motivational interviewing for smoking cessation. *Cochrane Database Syst Rev*. 2019;7:CD006936. doi:10.1002/14651858.CD006936.pub4

166. White AR, Rampes H, Liu JP, Stead LF, Campbell J. Acupuncture and related interventions for smoking cessation. *Cochrane Database Syst Rev*. 2014;1:CD000009. doi:10.1002/14651858.CD000009.pub4

167. Barnes J, McRobbie H, Dong CY, Walker N, Hartmann-Boyce J. Hypno-therapy for smoking cessation. *Cochrane Database Syst Rev.* 2019;6.

168. Lancaster T, Stead LF. Individual behavioural counselling for smoking cessation. *Cochrane Database Syst Rev.* 2017;3.

169. Stead LF, Carroll AJ, Lancaster T. Group behaviour therapy programmes for smoking cessation. *Cochrane Database Syst Rev.* 2017;3.

170. Matkin W, Ordóñez-Mena JM, Hartmann-Boyce J. Telephone counselling for smoking cessation. *Cochrane Database Syst Rev.* 2019;5.

171. Whittaker R, McRobbie H, Bullen C, Rodgers A, Gu Y. Mobile phone-based interventions for smoking cessation. *Cochrane Database Syst Rev.* 2016;4.

172. Ebbert JO, Elrashidi MY, Stead LF. Interventions for smokeless tobacco use cessation. *Cochrane Database Syst Rev.* 2015;10.

173. Maziak W, Jawad M, Jawad S, Ward KD, Eissenberg T, Asfar T. Interventions for waterpipe smoking cessation. *Cochrane Database Syst Rev.* 2015;7.

174. Stead LF, Buitrago D, Preciado N, Sanchez G, Hartmann-Boyce J, Lancaster T. Physician advice for smoking cessation. *Cochrane Database Syst Rev.* 2013;5:CD000165. doi:10.1002/14651858.CD000165.pub4

175. Rice VH, Heath L, Livingstone-Banks J, Hartmann-Boyce J. Nursing interventions for smoking cessation. *Cochrane Database Syst Rev.* 2017;12:CD001188. doi:10.1002/14651858.CD001188.pub5

176. Richter KP, Ellerbeck EF. It's time to change the default for tobacco treatment. *Addiction.* 2015;110(3):381-386. doi:10.1111/add.12734

177. Prochaska JJ, Grossman W, Young-Wolff KC, Benowitz NL. Validity of self-reported adult secondhand smoke exposure. *Tob Control.* 2015;24(1):48-53. doi:10.1136/tobaccocontrol-2013-051174

178. Home | Smokefree. Accessed September 10, 2020, https://smokefree.gov

179. Rigotti NA, Clair C, Munafò MR, Stead LF. Interventions for smoking cessation in hospitalised patients. *Cochrane Database Syst Rev.* 2012;5:CD001837. doi:10.1002/14651858.CD001837.pub3

180. Fiore MC, Goplerud E, Schroeder SA. The Joint Commission's new tobacco-cessation measures—will hospitals do the right thing? *N Engl J Med.* 2012;366(13):1172-1174. doi:10.1056/NEJMp1115176

181. Regan S, Reyen M, Richards AE, Lockhart AC, Liebman AK, Rigotti NA. Nicotine replacement therapy use at home after use during a hospitalization. *Nicotine Tob Res.* 2012;14(7):885-889. doi:10.1093/ntr/ntr244

182. Rigotti NA, Regan S, Levy DE, et al. Sustained care intervention and postdischarge smoking cessation among hospitalized adults: a randomized clinical trial. *JAMA.* 2014;312(7):719-728. doi:10.1001/jama.2014.9237

183. Reid RD, Mullen K-A, Slovinec D'Angelo ME, et al. Smoking cessation for hospitalized smokers: an evaluation of the "Ottawa Model." *Nicotine Tob Res.* 2010;12(1):11-18. doi:10.1093/ntr/ntp165

184. CDCTobaccoFree. *Secondhand Smoke (SHS) Facts.* Centers for Disease Control and Prevention. Published February 21, 2017. Accessed September 10, 2020, https://www.cdc.gov/tobacco/data_statistics/fact_sheets/secondhand_smoke/general_facts/index.htm

185. Barrington-Trimis JL, Leventhal AM. Adolescents' use of "pod mod" e-cigarettes—urgent concerns. *N Engl J Med.* 2018;379(12):1099-1102. doi:10.1056/NEJMp1805758

186. Harvanko AM, Havel CM, Jacob P, Benowitz NL. Characterization of nicotine salts in 23 electronic cigarette refill liquids. *Nicotine Tob Res.* 2020;22(7):1239-1243. doi:10.1093/ntr/ntz232

187. Rigotti NA. Balancing the benefits and harms of e-cigarettes: a National Academies of Science, Engineering, and Medicine report. *Ann Intern Med.* 2018;168(9):666-667. doi:10.7326/M18-0251

188. National Academies of Sciences, Engineering, and Medicine, Health and Medicine Division, Board on Population Health and Public Health Practice, Committee on the Review of the Health Effects of Electronic Nicotine Delivery Systems. *Public Health Consequences of E-Cigarettes.* (Eaton DL, Kwan LY, Stratton K, eds.). National Academies Press (US); 2018. Accessed September 10, 2020, http://www.ncbi.nlm.nih.gov/books/NBK507171

189. Cullen KA, Ambrose BK, Gentzke AS, Apelberg BJ, Jamal A, King BA. Notes from the field: use of electronic cigarettes and any tobacco product among middle and high school students—United States, 2011-2018. *MMWR.* 2018;67(45):1276-1277. doi:10.15585/mmwr.mm6745a5

190. Wang TW. E-cigarette use among middle and high school students—United States, 2020. *MMWR.* 2020;69. doi:10.15585/mmwr.mm6937e1

191. Cullen KA, Gentzke AS, Sawdey MD, et al. E-cigarette use among youth in the United States, 2019. *JAMA.* 2019;322(21):2095-2103. doi:10.1001/jama.2019.18387

192. Bao W, Liu B, Du Y, Snetselaar LG, Wallace RB. Electronic cigarette use among young, middle-aged, and older adults in the United States in 2017 and 2018. *JAMA Intern Med.* 2020;180(2):313-314. doi:10.1001/jamainternmed.2019.4957

193. Patel D, Davis KC, Cox S, et al. Reasons for current E-cigarette use among U.S. adults. *Prev Med.* 2016;93:14-20. doi:10.1016/j.ypmed.2016.09.011

194. Benowitz NL, Fraiman JB. Cardiovascular effects of electronic cigarettes. *Nat Rev Cardiol.* 2017;14(8):447-456. doi:10.1038/nrcardio.2017.36

195. Carnevale R, Sciarretta S, Violi F, et al. Acute impact of tobacco vs electronic cigarette smoking on oxidative stress and vascular function. *Chest.* 2016;150(3):606-612. doi:10.1016/j.chest.2016.04.012

196. George J, Hussain M, Vadiveloo T, et al. Cardiovascular effects of switching from tobacco cigarettes to electronic cigarettes. *J Am Coll Cardiol.* 2019;74(25):3112-3120. doi:10.1016/j.jacc.2019.09.067

197. Krishnasamy VP, Hallowell BD, Ko JY, et al. Update: characteristics of a nationwide outbreak of e-cigarette, or vaping, product use-associated lung injury—United States, August 2019-January 2020. *MMWR.* 2020;69(3):90-94. doi:10.15585/mmwr.mm6903e2

198. Ghinai I, Navon L, Gunn JKL, et al. Characteristics of persons who report using only nicotine-containing products among interviewed patients with e-cigarette, or vaping, product use-associated lung injury—Illinois, August-December 2019. *MMWR.* 2020;69(3):84-89. doi:10.15585/mmwr.mm6903e1

199. Blount BC, Karwowski MP, Shields PG, et al. Vitamin E acetate in bronchoalveolar-lavage fluid associated with EVALI. *N Engl J Med.* 2020;382(8):697-705. doi:10.1056/NEJMoa1916433

200. Hajek P, Phillips-Waller A, Przulj D, et al. A randomized trial of e-cigarettes versus nicotine-replacement therapy. *N Engl J Med.* 2019;380(7):629-637. doi:10.1056/NEJMoa1808779

201. Walker N, Parag V, Verbiest M, Laking G, Laugesen M, Bullen C. Nicotine patches used in combination with e-cigarettes (with and without nicotine) for smoking cessation: a pragmatic, randomised trial. *Lancet Respir Med.* 2020;8(1):54-64. doi:10.1016/S2213-2600(19)30269-3

202. Hartmann-Boyce J, McRobbie H, Lindson N, et al. Electronic cigarettes for smoking cessation. *Cochrane Database Syst Rev.* 2020;(10):CD010216. doi:10.1002/14651858.CD010216.pub4

203. Kalkhoran S, Chang Y, Rigotti NA. Electronic cigarette use and cigarette abstinence over 2 years among U.S. smokers in the population assessment of tobacco and health study. *Nicotine Tob Res.* 2020;22(5):728-733. doi:10.1093/ntr/ntz114

204. Ratajczak A, Jankowski P, Strus P, Feleszko W. Heat not burn tobacco product—a new global trend: impact of heat-not-burn tobacco products on public health, a systematic review. *Int J Environ Res Public Health.* 2020;17(2):409. doi:10.3390/ijerph17020409

205. Office of the Commisioner. *FDA Authorizes Marketing of IQOS Tobacco Heating System with 'Reduced Exposure' Information.* FDA. Published July 7, 2020. Accessed September 10, 2020, https://www.fda.gov/news-events/press-announcements/fda-authorizes-marketing-iqos-tobacco-heating-system-reduced-exposure-information

Air Pollution and Cardiovascular Disease

Michael B. Hadley and Sanjay Rajagopalan

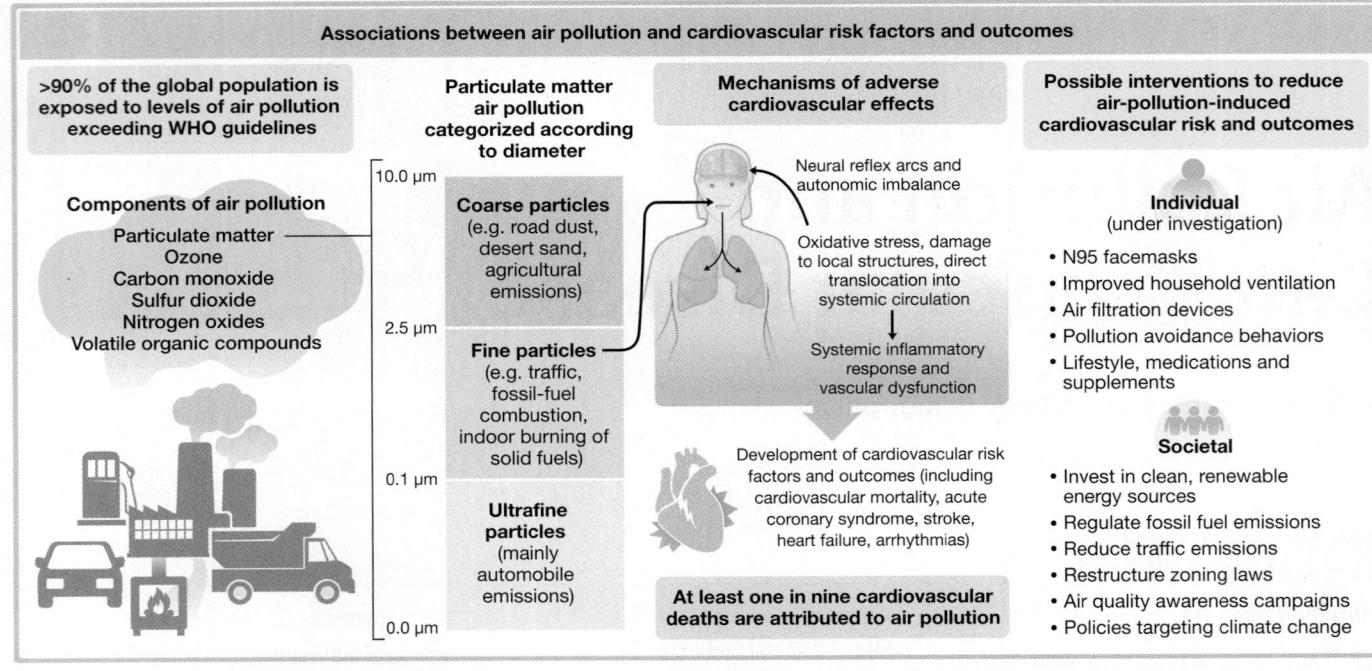

Chapter 9 Fuster and Hurst's Central Illustration. At least one in nine cardiovascular deaths are attributed to air pollution. Fine particulate matter (<2.5 μm in diameter) is the component of air pollution most linked to adverse cardiovascular effects. Inhaled fine particulate matter triggers multiple interdependent initiating mechanisms. Subsequent effector pathways—including a systemic inflammatory response, prothrombotic pathways, acute vascular dysfunction, neurohormonal dysregulation, and epigenomic changes—lead to the development and exacerbation of cardiovascular risk factors and outcomes.

CHAPTER SUMMARY

This chapter discusses the effects of air pollution on cardiovascular risk factors and outcomes. The vast majority (>90%) of the world's population is exposed to ambient fine particulate matter air pollution that exceeds World Health Organization guidelines. Almost 5 million deaths (8.7% of global mortality) were attributed to air pollution in 2017, and >50% of air pollution deaths are due to cardiovascular disease. Indeed, at least one in nine cardiovascular deaths are attributed to air pollution. Fine particulate matter is the component of air pollution most linked to adverse cardiovascular effects; the particles have diameter <2.5 μm and are largely derived from fossil-fuel combustion from power generation, industrial emissions, motorized vehicles, and household burning of solid fuel. Inhaled fine particulate matter triggers multiple interdependent initiating mechanisms (see Fuster and Hurst's Central Illustration), with subsequent effector pathways leading to development and exacerbation of cardiovascular risk factors such as elevated blood pressure, elevated blood glucose, atherosclerosis, and myocardial remodeling. A large body of evidence links air pollution exposure with cardiovascular mortality, acute coronary syndrome, stroke, heart failure, and arrhythmias. Cardiovascular risk from air pollution is modifiable at the individual and population levels. Various strategies for mitigating the harmful effects of air pollution are discussed.

INTRODUCTION

Air pollution is responsible for one in nine cardiovascular deaths globally, with attributable mortality expected to double by 2050.[1-4] The American Heart Association and other medical societies now list air pollution as a key modifiable risk factor for cardiovascular morbidity and mortality.[5-7] Importantly, reductions in air pollution exposures are estimated to avert cardiovascular (CV) events, increase population life expectancy, and reduce health care expenses.[6-9] Health care providers and policymakers therefore have an opportunity and a responsibility to mitigate pollution exposures and improve CV health.[10] In this chapter, we discuss the burden of air pollution-attributable cardiovascular disease (CVD), the complex pathophysiology of air pollution CV effects, and strategies to assess and intervene on air pollution exposure mediated CV events.

GLOBAL BURDEN OF DISEASE ATTRIBUTABLE TO AIR POLLUTION

Air pollution is the leading environmental cause of reversible premature morbidity and mortality worldwide.[1,11] In 2017 alone, 4.9 million deaths were attributed to air pollution (8.7% of global mortality).[1] Air pollution is responsible for more deaths than obesity, renal disease, alcohol use, malnutrition, physical inactivity, or HIV/AIDS, malaria, and tuberculosis combined[1] (**Fig. 9–1**). The large global impact of air pollution exposure is on account of its ubiquitous exposure. Over 90% of the global population is exposed to levels of ambient fine particulate matter air pollution exceeding World Health Organization (WHO) guidelines (<10 μg/m³ annually and <25 μg/m³ daily).[12] In densely populated regions of Asia and Africa, virtually the entire population is exposed to hazardous levels of ambient air pollution.[2] Similarly, nearly 3 billion people are exposed to hazardous levels of household air pollution from cooking and heating.[13,14] Although the relative risk of CV outcomes attributable to air pollution may be low for a single individual, near-universal exposures result in a significant burden of disease.[9] The burden of disease is higher in regions with more air pollution. In India, for example, one in five CV deaths is attributed to air pollution.[1] By comparison, one in 14 CV deaths is attributable to air pollution in the United States and the European Union, where exposure levels are lower.[1] **Figure 9–2** illustrates the number of people exposed to different levels of fine particulate matter air pollution across different countries.

More than 50% of air pollution deaths are due to CV disease.[2,11] According to the Global Burden of Disease project, most deaths are due to ischemic heart disease (1.39 million) and stroke (0.68 million).[1] Globally, at least one in nine CV

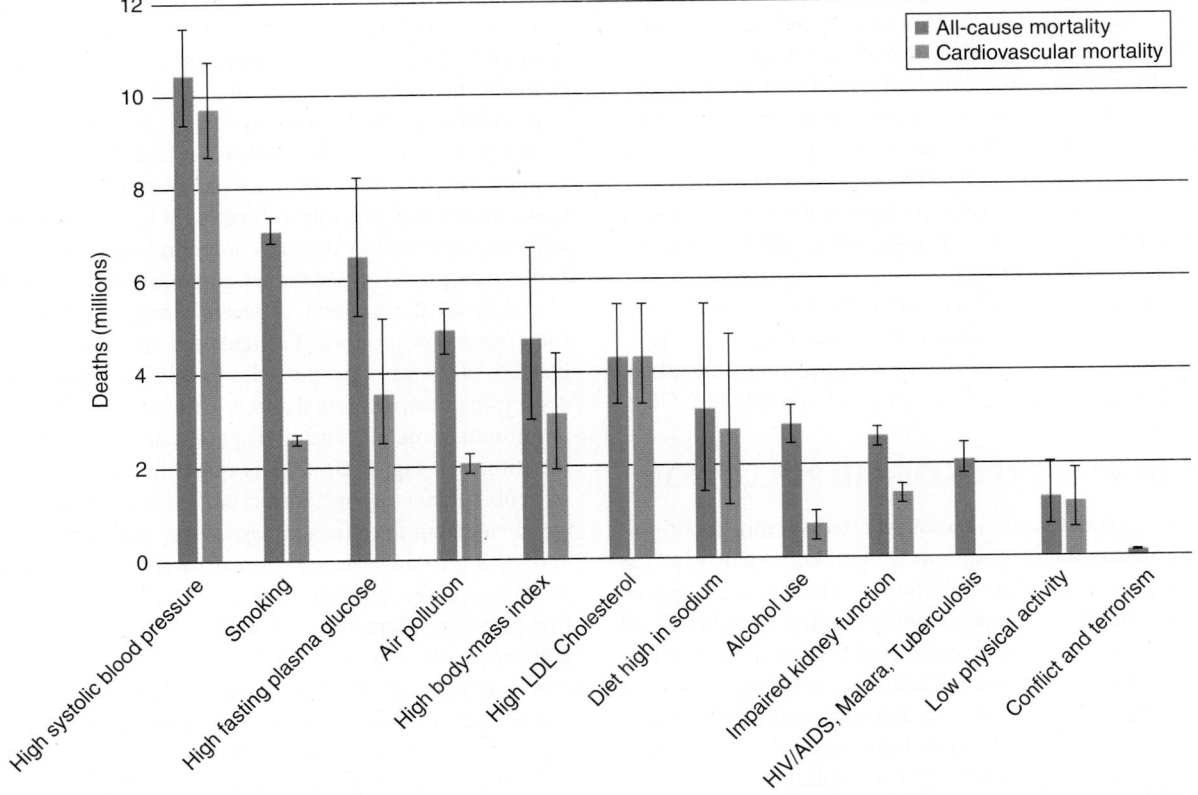

Figure 9–1. **Global All-Cause and Cardiovascular Mortality Attributed to Various Risk Factors** (with 95% Confidence Intervals) All-cause mortality attributed to air pollution is similar to traditional risk factors, including high fasting plasma glucose, high body-mass index, and high LDL cholesterol. Data from *Institute for Health Metrics & Evaluation: Global Health Data Exchange* (*2020*).

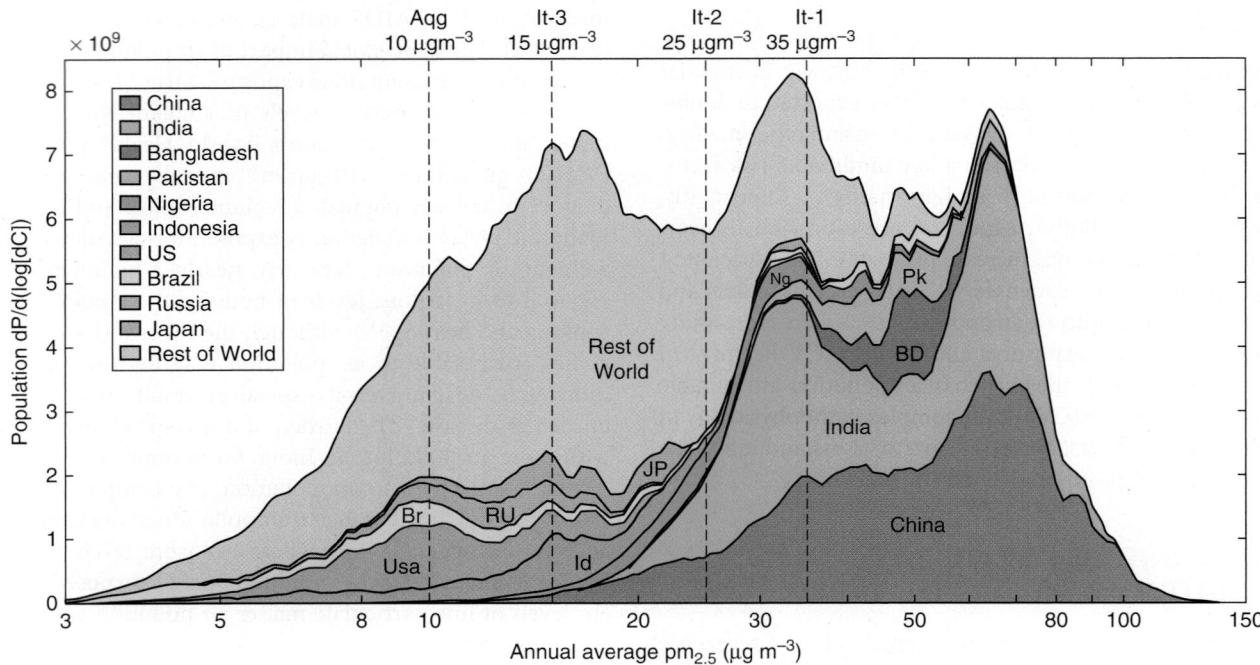

Figure 9–2. **Distribution of the Global Population According to Exposures to Fine Particulate Matter Air Pollution (PM$_{2.5}$)** The world's 10 most populous countries are shown. Pollution exposures are shown on a logarithmic scale, with population adjusted to ensure equal-sized plotted areas reflect equal populations. World Health Organization recommendations for average annual exposures are shown as: AQG = air quality guideline; IT = interim targets. Reproduced with permission from *Brauer M, Freedman G, Frostad J, et al*: Ambient Air Pollution Exposure Estimation for the Global Burden of Disease 2013, *Environ Sci Technol 2016 Jan 5;50(1):79-88.*

deaths (2.1 million) is due to air pollution.[1] This approximates the risk of other traditional risk factors, including high body-mass index, low physical activity, and diet high in sodium[1] (Fig. 9–1). In more recent estimates using the global exposure mortality model (GEMM) relying on ambient air pollution exposure risk estimates, this mortality appears to be much higher.[15] The GEMM mortality estimates may be more realistic, given that air pollution is partly responsible for the burden of other CV risk factors (e.g., hypertension), which themselves are implicated in CV mortality.[9]

Global exposures to ambient air pollution are rising due to increasing urbanization and industrialization.[3,8] As rising exposures affect an aging global demographic, mortality attributable to outdoor air pollution is expected to double by 2050.[2–4]

SOURCES AND TYPES OF AIR POLLUTION

Air pollution exposures often are categorized as ambient air pollution and household air pollution (HAP), consistent with the rather distinct sources of air pollution for these two categories. Ambient air pollution is predominantly emitted from fossil fuel combustion (e.g., motorized road traffic, power generation, industrial emissions, residential heating), smelting ores, and brake and tire wear.[7,8] Agricultural burning, wildfires, volcanic eruptions, and resuspended soil and dust may play a dominant role in specific environments.[6,7] HAP is typically emitted from indoor cooking and heating, typically with the burning of solid fuels and oils in inefficient cookstoves and furnaces.[13,14] In many urban environments in Africa and Asia, indoor penetration

of ambient air pollution is highly prevalent. In certain environments, solid fuel burning resulting in HAP may co-mingle with high ambient air pollution penetration. No clear line exists between these exposures, as ambient pollution infiltrates buildings and household pollution is vented outdoors.

Air pollution is a heterogeneous mixture of gaseous and particulate components.[6–9] Primary gaseous pollutants include carbon monoxide (CO), sulfur dioxide (SO$_2$), nitrogen oxides (NO and NO$_2$), and volatile organic compounds (e.g., benzene). Ozone is the most prevalent secondary gaseous pollutant, formed from photochemical reactions between nitrogen oxides and volatile organic compounds. Particulate matter air pollution (PM) consists of microscopic particles of solid or liquid matter, often combining dust, elemental and organic carbon, sulfates, nitrates, ammonium, metals, and a disparate array of other chemical constituents (**Fig. 9–3**). PM is quantified by particulate mass per cubic meter (μg/m^3) and classified into three size fractions which segment specific sources: coarse particles (diameter <10 and ≥2.5 μm) are derived from natural (e.g., road dust, desert sand) and anthropogenic sources (e.g., agricultural emissions); fine particles (diameter <2.5 μm) are principally derived from anthropogenic sources including traffic and fossil fuel based power emissions; ultrafine particles (diameter <0.1 μm) are almost exclusively derived from automobile emissions. The fine particulate fraction, "PM$_{2.5}$," is the component with the largest body of evidence implicating adverse CV effects.[6,7,9]

The Environmental Protection Agency (EPA) is responsible for establishing and maintaining national ambient air quality standards (NAAQS) for six of the most common air

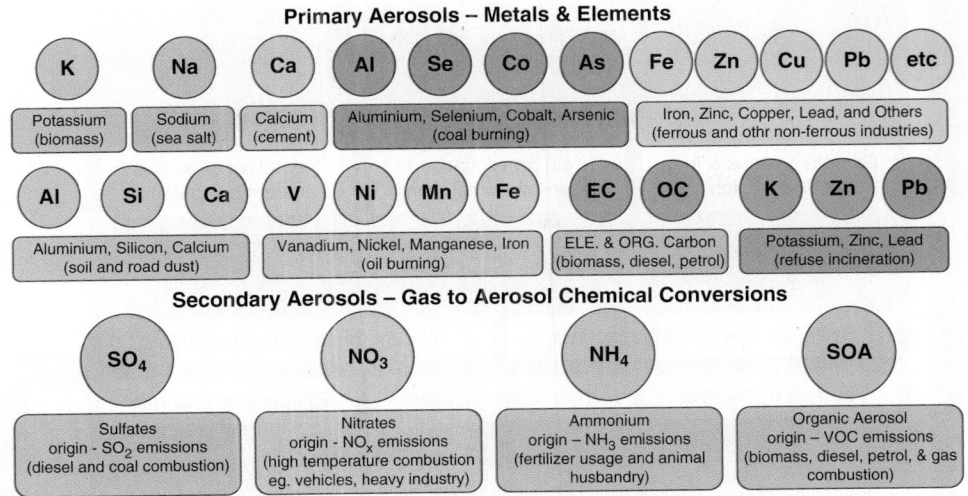

Figure 9–3. Composition of Particulate Matter (PM) The components and health effects of particulate matter vary according to source. Primary aerosols include metals and other elements resulting from fuel combustion and other aerosolizing processes. Secondary aerosols typically result from oxidation and condensation of primary gaseous emissions. Reproduced with permission from *Guttikunda, S. Primer on pollution source apportionment. Urban Emissions (2020) http://www.urbanemissions.info/publications/primer-on-pollution-source-apportionment/*

pollutants—carbon monoxide, lead, ground-level ozone, particulate matter, nitrogen dioxide, and sulfur dioxide (also known as "criteria" air pollutants). The primary NAAQS standards are set to protect public health while secondary NAAQS are meant to protect the public from adverse effects including protection against visual impairment, damage to crops, vegetation, or buildings. Understanding the specific health effects of PM components can help regulate the sources.[8]

Cohort studies and a recent systematic review have identified sulfates, nitrates, and organic carbons as components of PM strongly associated with CV mortality.[16,17] PM containing these components is derived primarily from the combustion of fossil fuels in industry and motorized vehicles (Fig. 9–3). Fittingly, fossil fuel combustion has been identified as a source of particularly hazardous PM exposures.[8,18] For example, an analysis of a large cohort from the American Cancer Society demonstrated that the attributable risk of ischemic heart disease mortality was five times higher for $PM_{2.5}$ derived from coal combustion compared to overall $PM_{2.5}$ exposure.[18] Similarly, the National Particle Component Toxicity Initiative demonstrated that PM from oil combustion was closely associated with short-term health effects, whereas PM from coal combustion was closely associated with long-term health effects.[19] These relationships between specific PM sources, components, and health outcomes is an area of active research. Meanwhile, general PM exposures continue to be used as a convenient though imperfect surrogate marker for a variety of chemical species hazardous to CV health.

PATHOPHYSIOLOGY OF POLLUTION-ATTRIBUTABLE CARDIOVASCULAR DISEASE

Our understanding of the complex pathophysiology of air pollution exposure continues to evolve. Broadly, air pollution exposures trigger initiating pathways, leading to the development of CV risk factors and ultimately to adverse CV outcomes (**Fig. 9–4**). Here, we focus primarily on the health effects of fine particulate matter ($PM_{2.5}$), responsible for most pollution-attributable CVD. These pathways have been extensively reviewed elsewhere.[5–9,20–22]

Initiating Mechanisms

Inhaled $PM_{2.5}$ is deposited in the alveoli where it triggers a cascade of interdependent physiologic events.[6–8] In the lungs, $PM_{2.5}$ damages local structures (e.g., cell membranes, surfactant lipids) and activates resident macrophages and dendritic cells. Activated cellular enzyme systems, as well as metallic and organic components of $PM_{2.5}$, generate reactive oxygen species (ROS) and reactive nitrogen species, resulting in *oxidative stress*, inflammation, and the recruitment of monocytes from the bone marrow.[21,23] Additional proinflammatory pathways may be triggered by the long-term accumulation of particles in macrophages, resulting in frustrated phagocytosis.[24] Recent studies have demonstrated that upregulation of the pulmonary antioxidant barrier reduces the adverse effects of air pollution exposure, illustrating the critical role of oxidative stress in disease pathophysiology.[8]

At the biochemical level, this process appears to be mediated by families of membrane-associated receptors (e.g., Toll-like receptors TLR2 and TLR4, chemokine receptors CCR2 and CXCR3, Nod-like receptors) and ion channels (e.g., transient receptor potential channels TRPA1, TRPV1), that together sense particulate pollutants, ROS, and other secondary mediators.[8] A deficiency in TLR4, for example, has been shown to attenuate the effect of $PM_{2.5}$ on increasing ROS generation and monocyte infiltration.[23] Other initiating mechanisms include the *direct translocation* of particles and gaseous co-pollutants into the systemic circulation, resulting in

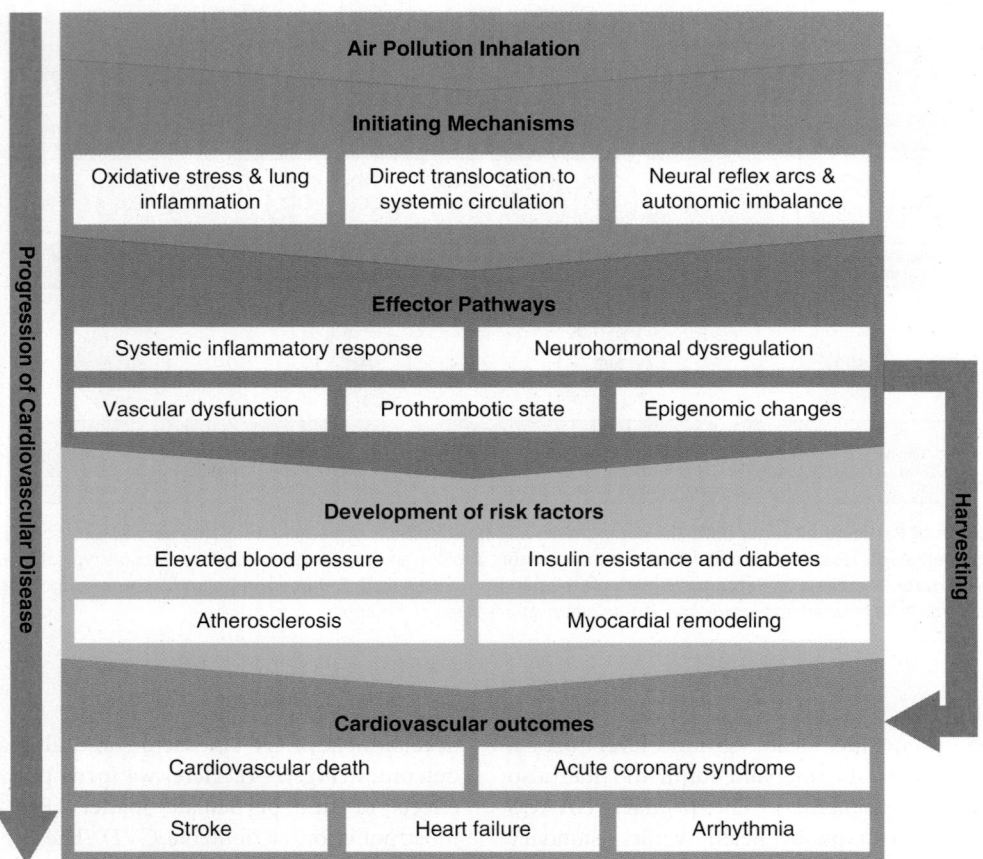

Figure 9–4. Pathophysiology of Pollution-Attributable Cardiovascular Disease Inhalation of air pollution triggers *initiating mechanisms*, including oxidative stress, neural reflex arcs, and direct translocation of pollutants to the systemic circulation. These mechanisms activate *effector pathways*, such as systemic inflammation, neurohormonal dysregulation, vascular dysfunction, prothrombotic pathways, and neurohormonal dysregulation. With *acute* exposures to air pollution, the effector pathways may lead directly to CV events in individuals with preexisting atherosclerotic disease (the so-called "harvesting hypothesis"). With *chronic* exposures to air pollution, the effector pathways lead to the development of CV risk factors, including hypertension, diabetes, atherosclerosis, and myocardial remodeling. These risk factors increase susceptibility to CV outcomes, particularly CV death, acute coronary syndromes, stroke, arrhythmias, and decompensated heart failure.

direct effects at remote sites.[9,25] Ultrafine particles have been shown to penetrate the systemic circulation where they could potentially mediate inflammatory effects. In an important translational study, inhaled gold nanoparticles in both humans and rodents demonstrated facile translocation within hours, deposition in atherosclerotic plaque, and excretion in the urine for weeks following inhalation.[26] Ultrafine particles may also disrupt the blood-brain barrier and perturb ***neural reflex arcs*** resulting in autonomic imbalance, central nervous system inflammation, and cause hypertension and dysregulated metabolism in experimental models.[9] In animal models, rapid activation of ion channels (TRPA1, TRPV1, P2X) in the lungs and nasal passages activate afferent C-fiber signaling, resulting in increased blood pressure and decreased heart rate variability.[8] Gaseous pollutants also trigger various initiating pathways. Ozone inactivates native antioxidant and surfactant defenses, which may potentiate oxidative stress from concomitant $PM_{2.5}$ exposure.[9] Sulfur dioxide reacts with water to create acid and sulfites, which cause inflammation. Nitrogen dioxide reacts with antioxidants and lipids, resulting

in reactive species causing inflammation. These initiating mechanisms remain an area of active research.

Effector Pathways

Several pathways amplify the initiating mechanisms. Oxidative stress in the respiratory tract produces secondary mediators that trigger a broader ***systemic inflammatory response***.[8,25] Oxidized phospholipids, for example, activate cytokine pathways and recruit inflammatory cells in the vasculature.[8,23] Similarly, oxidized cholesterol derivatives may prompt endothelial dysfunction, thrombosis, and atherosclerosis.[8,27] Receptor signaling (e.g., TLR4, CCR2, CXCR3) also promotes the migration of monocytes from the bone marrow to the vasculature, adipose tissue, and other sites.[21,23] Both PM_{10} and $PM_{2.5}$, and likely UFP, stimulate migration of monocyte populations from the bone marrow and spleen into atherosclerotic lesions.[28] The transmission of inflammatory signals from lung to circulation and ultimately to atherosclerotic plaques likely involves oxidative stress pathways and the generation of oxidized intermediates, such as oxidation products of phospholipids and cholesterol.

Air pollution exposure may induce acute *vascular dysfunction*, including increased arterial stiffness and impaired vasodilation.[7,21,22] The mechanisms appear to involve generation of ROS (e.g., superoxide) and depletion of nitric oxide, which may potentiate vasoconstrictor responses.[9] Similarly, depletion of endothelial progenitor cells has been associated with $PM_{2.5}$ and traffic proximity in human studies suggesting that this could potentially represent another mechanism by which endothelial dysfunction could occur. In experimental models, air pollution exposure has been associated with impaired release of endothelial progenitor cells.[23] In human studies, for example, acute $PM_{2.5}$ exposure results in brief reversible endothelial dysfunction as measured by a reduction in vasodilatory responses.[29] Long-term exposures to low levels of $PM_{2.5}$ in prospective cohort studies also have been linked to endothelial dysfunction.[30]

Exposure to air pollution activates *prothrombotic pathways*. Studies in animals and humans demonstrate that pulmonary inflammation may lead to platelet activation, imbalance of tissue plasminogen activator, and increased systemic thrombosis.[31] For example, double-blind, controlled studies in humans have demonstrated that exposure to diesel exhaust increases the thrombotic area of platelet-leukocyte aggregates[32] and reduces release of tissue plasminogen activator in response to bradykinin.[31] At least in experimental murine models, the pathway to heightened thrombosis involves mitochondrial electron transport ROS, opening of calcium release-activated channels, and release of IL-6.[33]

Air pollution exposures act in a variety of ways to precipitate *neurohormonal dysregulation*. Exposure to $PM_{2.5}$ has been linked to disruption of blood-brain barrier integrity and resulting hypothalamic inflammation.[8,9] This is associated with metabolic reprogramming, including insulin resistance and adipose dysfunction.[21,34,35] Pollution exposures may also activate the adrenal axis and increase glucocorticoid levels.[36]

Finally, air pollution exposures result in *epigenomic changes*. Preliminary studies have demonstrated correlations between pollution exposures and altered blood DNA methylation profiles.[37] Given the importance of epigenomic pathways in the regulation of transcriptional programming, these changes could play an important role as a buffer in response to environmental stimuli. In a recent paper, chronic exposure to $PM_{2.5}$ in mice was associated with metabolic reprogramming as evidenced by insulin resistance, altered metabolism, and increased hepatic steatosis.[38] Importantly, widespread epigenomic reprogramming was noted in multiple circadian genes. Cessation of air pollution exposure resulted in reversal of many of these changes, including epigenomic changes. Prenatal exposure to air pollution has been associated with persistent metabolic changes and alterations in intima thickness and DNA methylation.[39] Epigenomic changes may in turn be transmitted for multiple generations and carry forward the harmful effects of ancestors' exposures.[6]

Development of Cardiovascular Risk Factors

Air pollution exposures lead to the development and exacerbation of multiple CV risk factors, including elevated blood pressure and elevated blood glucose, which in turn may exacerbate atherosclerosis.[6,7,9]

Elevated Blood Pressure

Air pollution exposures trigger elevated blood pressure via increased vascular tone, endothelial dysfunction, and autonomic imbalance.[9,29,30,40,41] Carefully performed controlled-exposure studies routinely demonstrate a linear relationship between $PM_{2.5}$ exposure and elevations in blood pressure.[8,9,21,22,29,40–42] This relationship persists both at low levels of ambient pollution exposure (e.g., Canada and the United States) and at high levels of exposure (e.g., China), and appears to be stronger among men and Asian individuals,[8,42,43] Additionally, individuals with underlying endothelial dysfunction may exhibit exaggerated hemodynamic responses to air pollution exposure.[31] Recent meta-analyses find that an acute increase in $PM_{2.5}$ exposure by 10 µg/m³ is consistently associated with an increase of 1–3 mmHg in systolic and diastolic blood pressure.[43,44] Chronic air pollution exposure also is linked to chronic elevations in blood pressure and the incidence of hypertension.[44] Importantly, interventions to decrease personal air pollution exposures result in reductions in blood pressure.[8,21]

Insulin Resistance and Diabetes

Air pollution exposures result in insulin resistance and diabetes, likely via systemic inflammation, neurohormonal dysregulation, and epigenomic changes.[21,22,35] A recent meta-analysis of 2.3 million individuals and 21,095 incident cases of type 2 diabetes found that each 10 µg/m³ increase in $PM_{2.5}$ exposure was associated with a 10% relative increase in incident diabetes.[45] A prior meta-analysis suggested that each 10 µg/m³ increase in $PM_{2.5}$ exposure increased the risk for diabetes by 39% and the risk of diabetes-related mortality by 49%.[46] The relationship appears to be stronger in women and those with underlying risk factors including diet and inflammatory disorders.[34,35,45] Globally, over 3 million incident cases of diabetes and over 0.2 million diabetes deaths are attributed to ambient $PM_{2.5}$ exposure.[47]

Atherosclerosis

Air pollution exposures potentiate atherosclerosis via vascular inflammation, accumulation of oxidized lipids, and macrophage infiltration.[7,8,27,48] Cohort studies and cross-sectional analyses have demonstrated an increase in carotid intima-media thickness, carotid plaques, and coronary artery calcium associated with air pollution exposures.[9,21,48–50] For example, a cohort study of 6795 individuals across six regions in the United States demonstrated that a 5 µg/m³ increase in long-term exposure to $PM_{2.5}$ was associated with progression of coronary artery calcification.[49] A meta-analysis of eight cross-sectional and three prospective studies found that $PM_{2.5}$ exposures significantly increase carotid intima-media thickness.[51] Importantly, $PM_{2.5}$ exposure is also associated with the transition to more vulnerable, high-risk atherosclerotic lesions.[23,48]

Myocardial Remodeling

Air pollution exposure is associated with myocardial remodeling, likely via systemic inflammation, elevated blood pressure, hyperglycemia, and the upregulation of profibrotic genes.[8,9,52] This leads to left ventricular hypertrophy, diastolic dysfunction, and myocardial fibrosis discernible on cardiac imaging and pathology.[8,52] In animal models air pollution exposure has been associated with incipient heart failure and abnormal calcium cycling (i.e., downregulation of SERCA2a).[52]

Fatal and Nonfatal Cardiovascular Outcomes

A large body of evidence supports associations between air pollution exposures and CV mortality, acute coronary syndrome, stroke, heart failure, and arrhythmias.[6–8,19,53,54] The American Heart Association released a comprehensive review of this literature in 2010, concluding that there is a *causal* and *modifiable* relationship between $PM_{2.5}$ exposure and CV morbidity and mortality.[7] The European Society of Cardiology released a similar statement, writing that air pollution should be viewed as one of several major modifiable risk factors in the prevention and management of CVD.[6]

Cardiovascular Mortality

Mortality has the strongest supporting evidence as a pollution-attributable outcome.[6,7,9] The Harvard Six-Cities Study was the first large prospective cohort study to demonstrate a clear relationship between CV mortality and acute $PM_{2.5}$ exposure in six large U.S. cities.[55,56] This finding has been corroborated by numerous large cohort studies.[57,58] For example, the American Cancer Society Study cohort of 1.2 million individuals across 172 metropolitan areas found a 15% relative increase in ischemic heart disease (IHD) mortality per 10 $\mu g/m^3$ increase in $PM_{2.5}$ exposure, after controlling for 44 other variables.[59] Most pollution-attributable CV deaths are due to ischemic heart disease and stroke (see below).[1,6,7,9]

The association between pollution exposure and CV mortality is seen with both short- and long-term exposures.[7,8] Across major cohorts, short-term exposures are associated with increased relative risk in CV mortality typically ranging from 0.3% to 1.0% per 10 $\mu g/m^3$ increase in ambient $PM_{2.5}$ exposure, with substantial regional variation.[7,8,60,61] Long-term exposures are linked to larger increases in mortality.[7,9,62] Across major cohorts, long-term exposures are associated with an increased relative risk in CV mortality typically ranging from 7% to 11% per 10 $\mu g/m^3$ increase in ambient $PM_{2.5}$ exposure.[57,62] These relationships persist across both high exposures (e.g., China) and low exposures (e.g., Europe and the United States). Additionally, mortality is attributable to both ambient and household $PM_{2.5}$ exposure. A large prospective study in China demonstrated that burning of household solid fuel, compared with clean energy, was associated with increased all-cause and CV mortality.[63]

Gaseous pollutants have been associated with increased mortality, although these relationships require further study. Ozone exposure appears to potentiate the risk of cardiopulmonary mortality, even at exposure levels below national standards (<70 ppb).[8,64] Similarly, nitrogen dioxide has been associated with CV and all-cause mortality, in a relationship independent of $PM_{2.5}$ exposure.[65]

Acute Coronary Syndrome

Numerous controlled studies have identified associations between air pollution exposure and incident fatal or non-fatal myocardial infarction.[6,7,9,18,58,66–68] The strongest associations are for ST-elevation myocardial infarction in patients with underlying coronary artery disease.[9,66]

ACS is associated with both short- and long-term $PM_{2.5}$ exposures at both ends of the exposure spectrum, such as at very high levels (e.g., China) and also at levels well below current NAAQS limits (e.g., Canada).[8,15,58,67,69] A meta-analysis of 17 times-series studies and 17 case-crossover studies found that short-term exposure (<24 hours) was associated with a 2.5% relative increase in the risk of MI with each 10 $\mu g/m^3$ increase in $PM_{2.5}$ exposure.[69] Similarly, in the ESCAPE cohort of more than 100,000 participants across Europe, long-term exposures were associated with a 13% relative increase in nonfatal MI per 10 $\mu g/m^3$ increase in $PM_{2.5}$.[67] Long-term survival after ACS is also worse among individuals with higher $PM_{2.5}$ exposures.[70] Evidence is building to support associations between myocardial infarction and exposure to ultrafine PM,[54] nitrogen dioxide, sulfur dioxide, and carbon monoxide.[71]

Stroke

Cohort studies and time series have identified associations between air pollution exposures and both ischemic and hemorrhagic stroke.[8,20,68] The association persists for both high- and low-level exposures.[8,20]

Recent meta-analyses combining over 100 studies of various designs (case-crossover, cohort, time-series, cross-sectional, and case-control) have identified significant associations between $PM_{2.5}$ exposures and both stroke and stroke mortality.[72,73] Short-term exposures increased the relative risk of stroke mortality by 1% to 2% per 10 $\mu g/m^3$ increase in $PM_{2.5}$.[72,73] Long-term exposures were associated with a 14% relative increase in the risk of stroke mortality per 10 $\mu g/m^3$ increase in $PM_{2.5}$.[73] Of note, some carefully performed cohort studies have demonstrated a more profound association.[20,68] The Women's Health Initiative study, for example, identified a 35% and 83% relative increase in stroke and stroke mortality, respectively, per 10 $\mu g/m^3$ increase in $PM_{2.5}$.[68] Growing evidence supports the association between stroke and exposure to PM_{10} and nitrogen dioxide.[74]

Heart Failure

Several mechanisms lead to heart failure in patients exposed to air pollution.[6] Systemic and pulmonary vasoconstriction result in increased cardiac afterload; ventricular remodeling leads to decrease cardiac output and increased diastolic pressures; and new arrhythmias may lead to deteriorating cardiac function. Indeed, the risk of decompensated heart failure attributed to air pollution exposures is higher in those with preexisting heart failure, hypertension, or arrhythmias.[75]

In a systematic review and meta-analysis of 35 studies, short-term pollution exposures were associated with a 2.1% increase in the relative risk of heart failure hospitalization or death, per 10 $\mu g/m^3$ increase in $PM_{2.5}$.[75] This association has also been observed with coarse and ultrafine PM, as well as with nitrogen dioxide, sulfur dioxide, and carbon monoxide.[54,75] Additional research is needed to determine the association between decompensated heart failure and long-term exposures to $PM_{2.5}$, as well as whether the relationship varies between ischemic versus non-ischemic cardiomyopathies.

Air pollution also affects heart transplant recipients. A recent retrospective study of 21,800 heart transplant patients demonstrated an association between $PM_{2.5}$ exposure and mortality.[76] After adjusting for individual and neighborhood variables, the mortality hazard ratio was 1.26 per 10 µg/m³ increase in annual $PM_{2.5}$ exposure. Further research is needed to determine the mechanisms of disease, which may include heart transplant rejection due to systemic inflammation and immune activation.

Arrhythmia

Air pollution is associated with both atrial and ventricular arrhythmias, likely via autonomic imbalance, decreased heart-rate variability, systemic inflammation, and myocardial ischemia and remodeling. A recent meta-analysis of four observational studies combining 461,441 participants demonstrated a 0.89% increase in the relative risk of atrial fibrillation per 10 µg/m³ short-term increase in $PM_{2.5}$ exposures.[77] Other studies have demonstrated an association between air pollution exposures and ventricular tachycardia or ventricular fibrillation, particularly in individuals with prior MI and left ventricular dysfunction.[21,77–79] Similarly, case-crossover studies have identified associations between out-of-hospital cardiac arrest and exposure to PM and ozone pollution.[80] However, not all investigations have demonstrated an association, so confirmation is needed from larger prospective studies.[6]

Other Emerging Cardiovascular Outcomes

It is plausible that *venous thromboembolism* could result from systemic inflammation, vascular dysfunction, and hypercoagulability due to air pollution exposure.[6] However, studies have revealed mixed results.[8,81,82] One study of 605,242 individuals identified an increased risk of venous thromboses associated with a 10 µg/m³ increase in $PM_{2.5}$ exposure.[83] Specifically, there was an increased risk of deep vein thrombosis of 0.63% for short-term exposure and 6.98% for long-term exposure, and an increased risk of pulmonary embolism of 0.38% for short-term exposure and 2.67% for long-term exposure.[83] Further studies are needed to corroborate these associations.

Several other adverse outcomes have been linked to air pollution exposures, including peripheral arterial disease,[84] pregnancy-related blood pressure complications,[85] and diseases related to the cardiometabolic syndrome, including obesity,[86] chronic kidney disease,[87] and sleep apnea.[88] These associations require additional investigation.

Although this chapter focuses on CVD, it is important to recognize that air pollution exposures are associated with a variety of other health outcomes, including preterm birth, low birth weight, lower respiratory infection, asthma exacerbation, chronic obstructive pulmonary disease, lung cancer, and neurodevelopmental and neurodegenerative disorders.[3,9,11]

Time Frames of Exposure

Chronic air pollution exposures lead to the development of CV risk factors, including hypertension, diabetes, myocardial remodeling, and atherosclerosis.[6–9] These disease states exponentially increase the risk of future CV events, which may be triggered by acute air pollution exposures.[7,9,50] Acute exposures trigger CV events via inflammation, destabilization of atherosclerotic plaques, prothrombotic pathways, vascular dysfunction, autonomic imbalance, pulmonary and systemic vasoconstriction, and increased myocardial oxygen demand. Many individuals experience both of these processes, as acute exposures often occur in the setting of chronic exposures over a lifetime.

The "harvesting hypothesis" describes a key mechanism by which *acute* exposures may lead to CV events[8,9,89] (Fig. 9–4). Here, acute $PM_{2.5}$ exposures destabilize (or "harvest") vulnerable atherosclerotic plaques, leading to acute coronary syndromes and ischemic stroke.[8,9,89] Harvesting may trigger CV events in individuals with known atherosclerotic disease, or in previously asymptomatic individuals with subclinical atherosclerosis. Conversely, because harvesting requires both an exposure and an underlying vulnerability, individuals with *no* atherosclerosis are unlikely to experience ACS or ischemic stroke from acute pollution exposures.

Long-term exposures are associated with larger CV risks than short-term exposures.[7,9,21,22,50,68] This supports the theory that chronic air pollution exposures lead to the development of a vulnerable state more prone to CV events. In vulnerable individuals, CV events are more likely to occur with acute exposures (e.g., within hours to months), with progressively smaller increases in risk at longer time intervals (e.g., years), consistent with the harvesting hypothesis.[9]

EXPOSURE-RESPONSE RELATIONSHIP

Air pollution exposures vary worldwide (**Fig. 9–5**). WHO air quality guidelines recommend that average annual exposures not exceed 10 µg/m³ and daily exposures not exceed <25 µg/m³. Most of the global population is exposed to average annual levels above this guideline, including 99% of the population of Asia.[9] Across China, for example, the average annual population-weighted ambient $PM_{2.5}$ exposure is 59 µg/m³.[90] In the United States, by comparison, population-weighted ambient exposure is 12 µg/m³.[90] Daily ambient exposures may reach as high as 500–1000 µg/m³ in industrializing urban centers.[9,91,92] Household pollution exposures from low-efficiency combustion of biomass fuels typically range from 200–2000 µg/m³, and may reach as high as 30,000 µg/m³.[91] The WHO provides data on mean $PM_{2.5}$ levels for specific cities and countries.[12]

The *exposure-response relationship* defines CV risk attributable to different levels of air pollution exposure. Several approaches have been used to develop models describing this relationship for long-term exposures. These curves may underestimate the true relationship, due to measurement error and bias toward the null.[71] Additionally, these models provide estimates of *relative* risk, rather than *absolute* risk. That is, for an

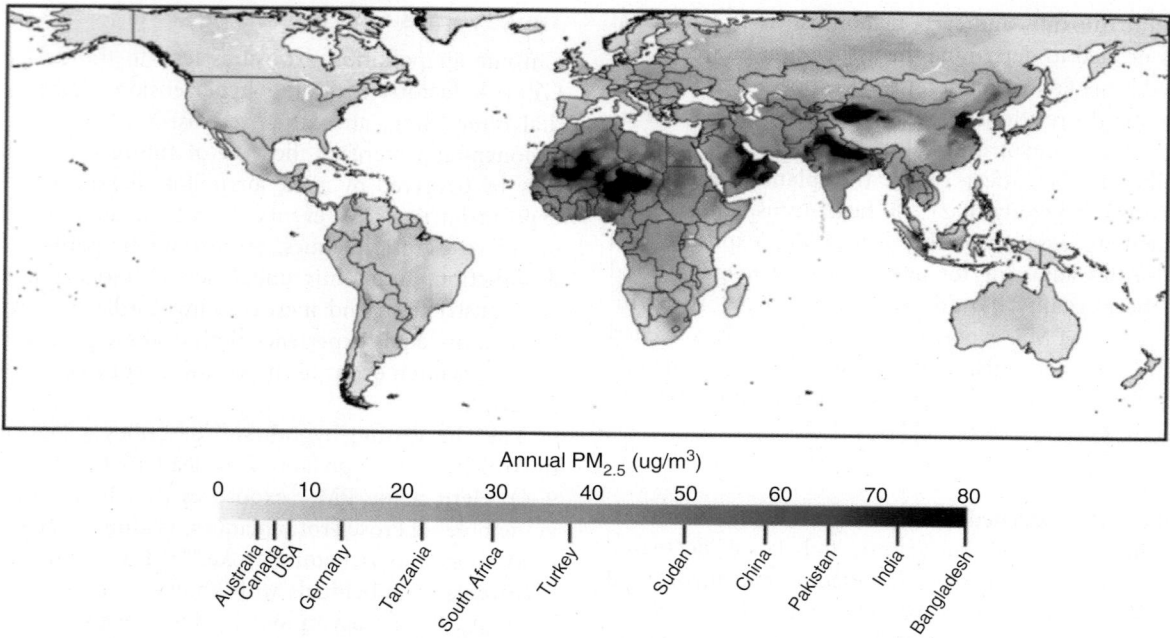

Figure 9–5. Global Distribution of Average Ambient PM₂.₅ The highest concentrations are observed in populous areas, particularly across Asia, as well as in desert regions. WHO guidelines recommend average annual exposures <10 μg/m³. Reproduced with permission from *Rajagopalan S, Al-Kindi SG, Brook RD. Air Pollution and Cardiovascular Disease: JACC State-of-the-Art Review, J Am Coll Cardiol. 2018 Oct 23;72(17):2054-2070.*

individual with low baseline cardiac risk, exposure to air pollution may increase relative risk significantly, while the absolute risk of a cardiac event remains low.

The most widely cited exposure-response relationship is the Integrated Exposure-Response (IER) model.[93] The IER arrives at dose-response relationships for a wide range of air pollution exposures by integrating information from cohort studies of ambient air pollution, household air pollution, active smoking, and second-hand smoke. For each cohort study, the total mass of inhaled particles is converted to an equivalent concentration of ambient PM₂.₅ pollution. A single dose-response curve is then fitted to outcome data for a range of PM₂.₅ concentrations. Curves are available for specific age groups and countries. Studies of chronic air pollution exposures appear to confirm the IER relationship, particularly at lower levels of exposure.[8,94] **Figure 9–6** illustrates IER curves developed for the outcomes of ischemic heart disease mortality and stroke mortality. The shape of these exposure-response relationships leads to several conclusions. First, there appears to be no lower concentration of exposure that can be considered safe.[9] Indeed, studies from Europe and North America have demonstrated that even concentrations below the WHO AQG target (average annual PM₂.₅ <10 μg/m³) pose elevated CV risk.[20,57,58,64] Second, the IER curve flattens out at higher levels of exposure, such as those seen with household air pollution. This suggests that the largest health benefits will accrue from interventions that reduce exposures to low levels.[95] For example, an intervention that reduces PM₂.₅ exposure from 300 to 100 μg/m³ may have a smaller benefit than one that reduces PM₂.₅ exposure from 100 to 30 μg/m³.[10] An important limitation of the IER model is the assumption that pollutants from different sources have equivalent composition and toxicity.[8,93,94]

The Global Exposure Mortality Model (GEMM) incorporates data only from studies of ambient air pollution (41 cohorts from 16 countries).[8,15] As shown in Fig. 9–6, this model has a steeper, linear dose-response relationship. Using the GEMM, there were an estimated 8.9 million deaths attributable to ambient air pollution exposures in 2015, which is twice the number of deaths calculated using the IER model for the global burden of disease study.[1,15] Ongoing cohort studies in regions with high levels of ambient pollution will help to define the shape of the GEMM curve for even higher doses of PM₂.₅.[94]

Other air pollutants may also have a predictable dose-response relationship. Di et al., for example, have defined the relationship between acute ozone exposure and mortality.[64] Likewise, Weichenthal et al., demonstrated that ozone exposure modifies the effect of PM₂.₅ on CV mortality,[96] perhaps by inactivating native antioxidant defenses.[9]

RISK ASSESSMENT

Individuals at the highest risk from air pollution exposures may be more *susceptible*, more *vulnerable*, or both. A recent review article examined different approaches to identifying such individuals.[10] *Susceptible* individuals are those at higher risk of CV events for any given level of exposure. Following data from cohort studies, these groups include children under 5 and adults over age 60, socioeconomically disadvantaged groups and minorities, and individuals patients with hypertension, diabetes, obesity, and atherosclerotic CVD.[3,6,7,9,57,97] Clinicians and policymakers should be sensitive to air pollution exposures in these susceptible groups.[10]

Vulnerable individuals are those exposed to higher levels of air pollution. The key predictor of *household* pollution

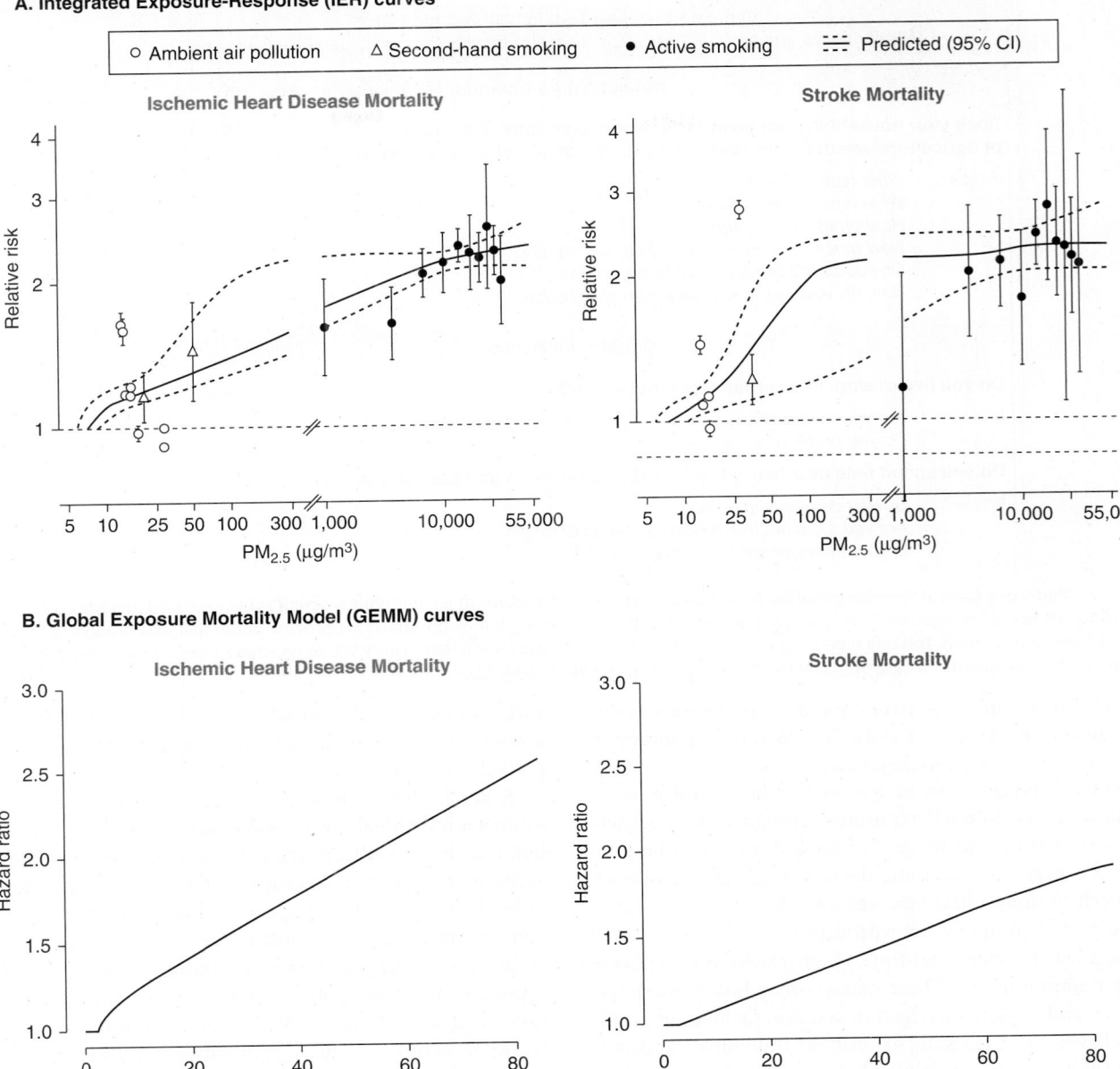

Figure 9–6. **Exposure-Response Relationships for Air Pollution and Cardiovascular Outcomes** (Ischemic Heart Disease Mortality and Stroke Mortality) **A.** Integrated exposure-response (IER) curves combine information from cohort studies of air pollution, second-hand smoking, and active smoking. **B.** Global Exposure Mortality Model (GEMM) curves fit data from cohorts studying only ambient air pollution across a narrower range of exposures. **A,** Reproduced with permission from *Burnett RT, Pope CA 3rd, Ezzati M, et al*: An integrated risk function for estimating the global burden of disease attributable to ambient fine particulate matter exposure, *Environ Health Perspect.* 2014 Apr;122(4):397-403. **B,** Modified with permission from *Burnett R, Chen H, Szyszkowicz M, et al*: Global estimates of mortality associated with long-term exposure to outdoor fine particulate matter, *Proc Natl Acad Sci USA* 2018 Sep 18;115(38):9592-9597.

exposure is the frequent indoor burning of solid fuels (e.g., wood, coal, charcoal, dung, agricultural residues) for cooking or heating.[13,98,99] Other predictors include female gender, low socioeconomic status, rural household, cold weather climates, and poor household ventilation (e.g., windows, chimneys, hoods, filtration systems).[13,14,98,99] Key predictors of *ambient* pollution exposures include proximity to an urban industrial center (e.g., Beijing), heavy traffic, wildfires, seasonal agricultural burning, and local wind and weather patterns.[6,7,10] Ambient $PM_{2.5}$ can travel large distances (i.e., >100 km),

creating high background concentrations around polluted cities.[6] Additionally, ambient $PM_{2.5}$ may infiltrate buildings, so individuals need not be outdoors to be exposed.[100]

A clinical screening tool has been proposed to identify these exposures, but requires validation[10] (**Fig. 9–7**). Screening for exposures may identify possible targets for intervention. Additionally, open-ended questions about pollution sources in the community may identify sources.[10] Clinicians may ask these questions along with other social screening questions about exercise or tobacco use. Of note, screening may provide

Clinical Screening Tool for Air Pollution Risk
An affirmative answer to any question is associated with increased cardiovascular risk

Household Air Pollution

Does your household burn solid fuels (wood, coal, charcoal, dung, or agricultural residues) for cooking, heating, lighting or other purposes?   Yes   No

If "yes":   *What type of fuel do you use?*
What type of stove do you use?
How often do you burn solid fuel?
How much time do you spend around the fire?
Do you burn solid fuels inside the home?
How do you ventilate smoke from your house?

Outdoor Air Pollution

Do you live or work in an urban industrial center?   Yes   No

If "yes":   *Are you aware of any sources of pollution near your home?*
Do you perform physical exertion outdoors?

Do you spend time near heavy traffic (e.g., multi-lane, high-speed roads)   Yes   No

If "yes":   *Do you commute in traffic?*
Are you exposed to the open air when driving?
Is your home located near major roads?

Figure 9–7. Model of a Clinical Screening Tool for Air Pollution Risk This tool contains three questions covering evidence-based predictors of household and outdoor air pollution exposure. For questions answered in the affirmative, follow-up questions provide additional information to help guide patient-tailored interventions. This tool is pending validation. Reproduced with permission from *Hadley MB, Baumgartner J, Vedanthan R*. Developing a Clinical Approach to Air Pollution and Cardiovascular Health, *Circulation. 2018 Feb 13;137(7):725-742.*

no benefit in regions with virtually universal exposures (e.g., urban industrial centers in Asia, low-income communities without access to clean cooking fuels).[10,13]

Personal exposures can be assessed using *wearable monitors*, allowing one to track exposures through various activity patterns over time and space.[101,102] Such devices can be integrated into personal electronic devices (e.g., cellular phones, wristwatches) and collect relevant data for patients and clinicians.[8,21,101,102] Similarly, crowdsourced data from personal devices may provide real-time, high-resolution exposure maps for communities.[8] These datasets may link to alert systems may and personal navigation systems, facilitating avoidance behaviors and reducing exposures.[8] Individual exposures might also be quantified via biomarkers in blood, urine, saliva, or exhaled air, but such tests require further development and validation.[8-10]

Meanwhile, *exposure modeling* remains the primary method to quantify ambient pollution exposures for specific geographic locations. Exposure models are generated using data from over 10,000 ground-level air-monitoring stations in over 1000 cities around the world.[8,10,103] Regression analysis ("spatial estimation") can be used to predict pollution levels for any location between these measured points.[10] In areas with limited ground-based monitoring, exposure estimates can be generated with satellite measurements of aerosol optical depth, which may be integrated with chemical transport models and available ground-level monitor data.[8,104] This technique is used to estimate the global burden of disease attributable to ambient air pollution.[104] Other methods of exposure mapping include: modeling emissions from known pollution sources; land-use regression models using pollution-related predictor

variables (e.g., nearby traffic, population density); and mixed models combining multiple methodologies.[10] Many models are publicly available.[8,10,12,103]

A key limitation of ambient exposure modeling is that it estimates individual exposures based on specific locations (e.g., home address) with insufficient spatiotemporal resolution to account for the local microenvironment and movements of individuals over time and space.[8,105] Indeed, some studies have demonstrated that only moderate correlation exists between ambient estimates and personal exposures, leading to possible exposure misclassification error.[8,105] Modeling *household* exposures also remains difficult, since exposures covary with types of cookstove, fuels, ventilation, weather, geography, individual time-activity patterns, and penetration of ambient pollution into the home.[10,95,98] Regression models based on these covariates have been developed to estimate household pollution exposures around the world, with modest success.[98]

Quantified exposures can be translated into estimates of CV risk via the exposure-response relationships described above.[10,93] In the United States, for example, the average population-weighed ambient annual exposure is about 12 µg/m³, corresponding on the IER to a relative risk of approximately 1.1 for IHD mortality.[10,90,93] Likewise in China, average exposures are approximately 59 µg/m³, corresponding to a relative risk of approximately 1.4 mortality.[10,90,93]

Exposures and associated risks can be mapped for regions of interest.[10] For example, **Fig. 9–8** illustrates the risk of ischemic heart disease mortality associated with chronic pollution exposures across New York City.[10] Similar maps can be developed for other pollutants or for short-term exposures.[10] Health care providers and policymakers can use such maps to estimate

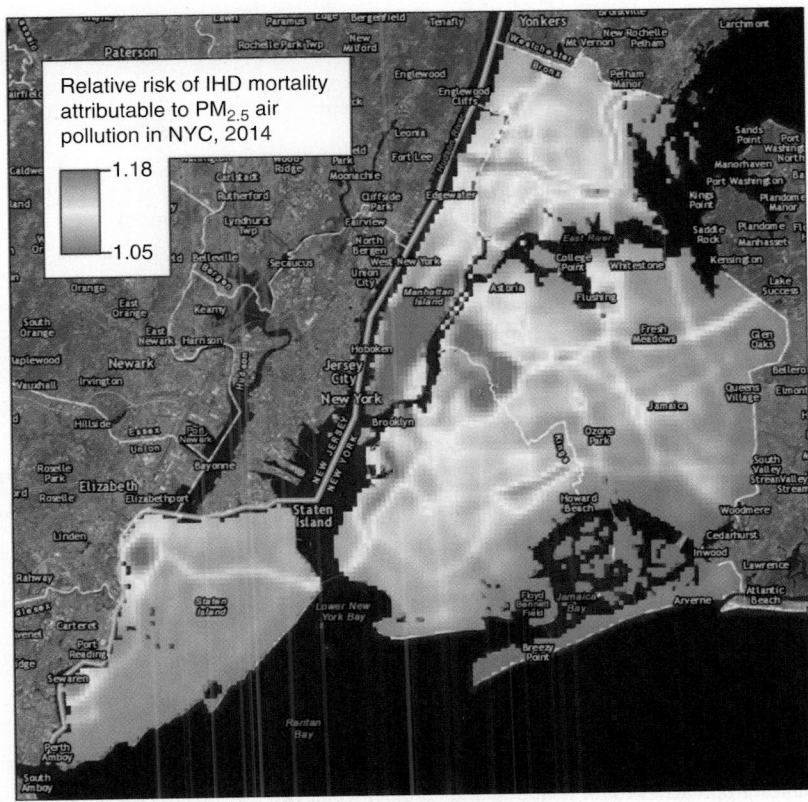

Figure 9–8. Risk Map Prototype This map depicts the estimated risk of ischemic heart disease mortality attributable to fine particular matter exposures in New York City in 2014. The map combines a frequently cited exposure-response curve[93] with annual average $PM_{2.5}$ concentration estimates based on a land-use regression model.[149] Risk estimates apply to populations and may not be predictive of individual risk. Exposure estimates used with permission from The New York City Department of Health and Mental Hygiene, Queens College Center for the Biology of Natural Systems, and Zev Ross Spatial Analysis. Reproduced with permission from *Hadley MB, Baumgartner J, Vedanthan R*. Developing a Clinical Approach to Air Pollution and Cardiovascular Health, *Circulation. 2018 Feb 13;137(7):725-742.*

the burden of pollution-attributable CVD in their communities and identify hot spots for intervention.[10] Of note, since the exposure-response relationship varies with individual characteristics, these risk estimates should be applied to populations and are not necessarily predictive of individual risk.[10]

At present, there is no accepted consensus on approaches to communicate air pollution levels or associated risks to individuals and communities. A recent AHA document details current approaches and provides practical recommendations.[106] Indices such as the United States Environmental Protection Agency (EPA)'s Air Quality Index (AQI) and the Air Quality Health Index (AQHI) in Canada are focused on the population health impact of short-term exposures and are most applicable to bouts of high air pollution episodes. While only a small proportion of individuals follow the accompanying behavioral recommendations, those who do can reduce their exposure. Evidence indicating that such communications and/or recommendations reduce health impact amongst the general, more susceptible, or even compliant populations is still limited, particularly for CV outcomes. Tools to communicate long-term exposure are needed to more accurately convey the health risk due to air pollution. Such tools could be used by health care providers to prioritize the use of personal preventive measures (e.g., indoor air cleaners) and target treatment and/or

prevention strategies, or by public health officials to highlight areas in greatest need for air quality management. The increased access and availability of air pollution monitoring data from low-cost sensors and portable monitors at high spatial and temporal resolution has generated a need for interpretation of the impact of short term personal exposures on CV health.[107] To avoid confusion, messaging must be uniform, consistent, and aligned with established approaches from regulatory monitors.[107] Open-source platform technologies, harmonization of values/reporting, and recommendations that are consistent and valid are needed before use in messaging. Not addressing these issues has the potential for creating mass anxiety and misinterpretation, and potentially unnecessary modification of behavior and activity.

INTERVENTIONS

Cardiovascular risk from air pollution is modifiable at the individual and population levels.[1,6,7,21,22,93,102] Observational studies demonstrate that reducing exposures decreases the risk of CV mortality, ACS, stroke, heart failure, arrhythmias, and progression of atherosclerosis.[6,8,10,108,109] A modeling study demonstrated that elimination of all fossil fuel emissions could reduce global mortality by 3.6 million annual deaths.[110] Across the

---

Clinical approaches to air pollution and cardiovascular disease

Risk assessment

Susceptible groups
- Age: children under age 5, adults over age 60
- Socioeconomically disadvantaged groups and minorities
- Preexisting cardiovascular risk factors (e.g., hypertension, atherosclerosis)

Vulnerable groups
- Exposed to hazardous levels of ambient or household air pollution
- Can assess via screening tools, wearable monitors, or exposure modeling

Interventions

Policy interventions
- Invest in clean, renewable energy sources (e.g., wind, tidal, solar, geothermal)
- Regulate fossil fuel emissions using taxes, penalties, and emissions trading programs
- Reduce traffic emissions (e.g., low-emission vehicles, particle traps, catalytic converters)
- Restructure zoning laws to separate residential districts from traffic and industry
- Empower civil society with air quality alert networks and awareness campaigns
- Seek co-benefits with policies targeting climate change

Individual interventions
- Facemasks
- Clean stove-fuel combinations and improved household ventilation
- Air filtration devices (e.g. central air, high efficiency particulate arrestance air filters)
- Avoidance behaviors (e.g., avoid rush hour, keep windows closed)
- Medications and supplements (e.g., antioxidants, omega-3 fatty acids)
- Preventive medicine (e.g., reduce risk factors for atherosclerosis)

Figure 9–9. Summary of Key Clinical Approaches to Air Pollution and Cardiovascular Disease. Health care providers can perform a risk assessment to identify individuals who are susceptible and/or vulnerable to air pollution exposures. Policy interventions can mitigate air pollution exposures across populations. Individual interventions can help reduce personal air exposures for susceptible individuals. Interventions must be tailored to local sociocultural structures and economic resources. The interventions listed here show promise in early studies but require confirmation by larger randomized trials looking at CV events.

United States, a reduction in long-term exposure of 10 μg/m³ was estimated to increase average life expectancy by more than 7 months. Similarly in Europe, compliance with WHO guidelines (average annual exposure <10 μg/m³) is estimated to increase life expectancy by 22 months or more, and save tens of billions of dollars in health care expenses.[111,112] Health care providers and policymakers have an opportunity and responsibility to act. In what follows, we review strategies for mitigating the harmful effects of air pollution (summarized in **Fig. 9–9**).

Policy Interventions

Policies to reduce air pollution exposures are critical to reducing the attributable burden of disease.[8] Such policies have a proven track record of improving public health.[8,11] The Clean Air Act, for example, is estimated to have prevented 130,000 myocardial infarctions in 2010.[113] Policies may also save resources. In 2013, the European Commission estimated that an annual investment of €3.4 billion to reduce pollution exposures would result in savings of at least €40 billion per year from decreased health care expenditures and increased productivity.[6]

There are several key policy interventions. These should be directed toward the most vulnerable communities and tailored to local economic and sociocultural structures.[10] First, emissions must be regulated to reduce the burning of fossil fuels and encourage the transition to clean energy sources (e.g., wind, solar, tidal, and geothermal power).[8] Regulations should

target sources of pollution with the strongest associations with CV events (e.g., coal burning, traffic).[18,53] Second, zoning laws should separate residential areas from emitters[6,8] and support the development of green areas that may attenuate pollution exposures and CV risk.[114,115] Third, building codes can require indoor air filtration and minimize the indoor penetration of outdoor pollution.[8] Fourth, air quality monitoring systems are needed to identify vulnerable populations and evaluate the efficacy of policies targeting pollution. These monitoring systems should be linked to alert networks providing real-time warnings of hazardous exposures.[8]

Enforcing these policies requires a system of taxes, penalties, incentives, and offsetting programs.[8–11] Resulting tax revenues can be directed toward clean energy projects, urban landscape reform, air quality monitoring systems, and media campaigns to improve public awareness of pollution.[9] The *Lancet* Commission stressed the need for strong leadership, planning, and legally enforced targets and timetables.[11] Similarly, strong partnership is needed between health care providers, patient organizations, insurers, and governmental and nongovernmental organizations to share exposure data, enforce quality standards, and subsidize technologies to reduce patient exposures.[10] Unfortunately, leadership, partnership, and enforcement sometimes are lacking in the nations where reductions in pollution are most needed.[8,9]

Policies to reduce emissions should look for co-benefits in mitigating climate change.[8,9,11] Climate change is the single greatest threat confronting global public health and has a complex relationship with air pollution.[8,116] Toxic pollutants and greenhouse gases are emitted largely from the same sources (e.g., burning of fossil fuels).[6,8] Moreover, climate change increases air pollution exposures via extreme weather conditions, dust storms, wildfires, and elevated ground-level ozone concentrations.[8,116] A recent systematic review found that strategies to reduce greenhouse gas emissions had substantial public health benefits.[117]

Individual Interventions

Dramatic reductions in air pollution are unlikely in the short-term across much of the world.[8] Therefore, personal measures are critical to mitigate exposures.

Current approaches to mitigate air pollution and their impact have been reviewed in a recently published AHA Scientific Statement[118] and can be broadly classified into: (1) Active personal exposure mitigation with personal masks and home air filtration; (2) Modification of human behavior to reduce passive exposures; and (3) Pharmacologic approaches (**Fig. 9–10**).

Early trials have shown promising results for several interventions, including air filtration devices, clean stoves, facemasks, and avoidance behaviors (discussed in detail below).[6-8,21,22] However, these remain primarily hypothesis-generating investigations. Large randomized trials are needed to evaluate the efficacy of these interventions on CV events over various timeframes of exposure.[8,9] We now turn to a review of promising interventions to reduce individual risk from air pollution exposures.

Personal Masks

Inexpensive facemasks made of cloth, cotton, or gauze can reduce the inhalation of PM, but are not uniformly effective because of a poor seal around the face.[8] In a small study in Beijing, simple facemasks were associated with a reduction in blood pressure.[119] Alternatively, N95 respirators provide a better seal and block 95% of particles larger than 0.3μm in size, including the majority of $PM_{2.5}$ inhalation. In small studies of acute pollution exposures, N95 respirators have demonstrated reductions in blood pressure, increased heart rate variability, and prevention of ST-depression.[22,92,119,120] A randomized case-crossover trial enrolled 98 patients with known coronary artery disease who wore a respirator while ambulating in Beijing, then went through a brief washout period, then walked the same route without a mask. The use of a mask was associated with small but significant increases in heart rate variability, as well as reductions in blood pressure and maximal ST-segment depression.[121] In another small crossover trial, 26 patients with known heart failure were willingly exposed to diesel exhaust while wearing and while *not* wearing a filtration mask.[122] The use of the mask significantly reduced a reactive hyperemia index and brain natriuretic peptide levels in the presence of diesel exhaust. Larger, randomized trials are needed to test the efficacy of facemasks on reducing CV events.

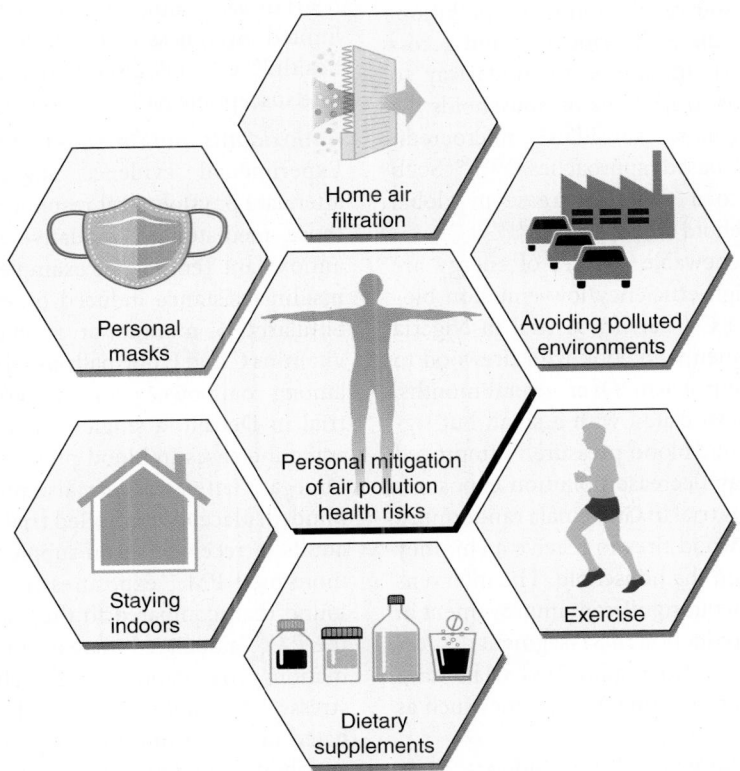

Figure 9–10. Summary of Personal Measures to Reduce Air Pollution Exposure.[150]

Air Filters

Indoor air pollution may result both from the indoor burning of unclean fuels or from the infiltration of outdoor pollution indoors. Indeed, up to 65% of the exposure to outdoor air particles is from inhalation while indoors.[123] High-efficiency particulate arrestance (HEPA) filters can reduce indoor $PM_{2.5}$ levels by >50% when windows are closed and are less intrusive than face masks.[6,8,9,124,125] HEPA filters can be added to heating, ventilation, and air-conditioning systems, or used independently in portable air cleaners.[8] Analysis of cohort data has demonstrated that central air may reduce the risk of CV hospitalizations.[126] Small trials have demonstrated that air filters can improve several surrogate endpoints, including blood pressure, insulin sensitivity, microvascular function, stress hormones, and inflammatory biomarkers.[8,9,124,125,127,128] For example, a crossover trial randomized 35 college students to functional versus sham air purifiers, then monitored difference in blood pressure and 14 circulating biomarkers following a 2-week washout period. The study found a significant decrease in blood pressure and inflammatory biomarkers among individuals with the functional air purifier.[124] In a crossover study in Canada, 45 adults that use wood fires indoors were randomized to portable air filters and monitored for biomarkers and endothelial function as measured by tonometry.[125] The investigators found that use of air filtration improved endothelial function and significantly decreased levels of C-reactive protein. No randomized trials have yet studied the impact of air filtration on CV outcomes.

Clean Stoves

Household burning of fossil fuels (e.g., oil, coal) and biomass (e.g., wood, dung) is a key source of indoor air pollution. Key interventions therefore include electrification and access to clean-burning gas.[129] Global initiatives are underway to provide cleaner-burning stoves to millions of households via government-sponsored programs, subsidies, microcredit programs, and other market-based approaches.[10,129,130] Such programs have contributed to a steady decrease in global mortality attributable to household air pollution.[3,9,10]

In regions where clean, renewable sources of energy are unavailable, provision of a high-efficiency/low-emission biomass stove may provide some CV benefit. A trial in Nigeria randomized 324 pregnant women who cook with firewood to either an ethanol stove or a control arm. Over several months, use of the ethanol stove was associated with a small but significant improvement in diastolic blood pressure.[131] Improved household ventilation also may decrease pollution exposures and provide some CV benefit. A trial in Guatemala randomized 534 households using indoor wood fires to receive a chimney with a hood to vent smoke from the household. The intervention was associated with a small but significant improvement in diastolic blood pressure and a reduction in ST-segment depression on electrocardiograms.[132,133] No randomized trials have yet studied the impact of clean stoves on CV outcomes such as stroke, MI, or mortality.

For households burning solid or fossil fuels indoors, clinicians can recommend clean stove-fuel sources and improved household ventilation.[129] Provider organizations can partner with governmental organizations and charities to assist in the provision of clean stoves.[10] The International Organization for Standardization offers frameworks for identifying safe, low-emission stoves.[134] These interventions appear to be cost-effective; costing as little as U.S. $50–100 per disability-adjusted life year averted.[91]

Avoidance Behaviors

Behavioral modifications can significantly reduce air pollution exposures and may provide some CV benefit. Susceptible individuals can connect to local air quality alert networks (e.g., EPA AirNow[135]) to receive warnings and strategies to minimize time outdoors.[6,7] Similarly, exposure to vehicular emissions can be reduced by avoiding peak morning and evening rush hours,[6,53,136] closing vehicle windows, and using car air conditioning/purifiers.[6–10]

It remains unclear whether the CV benefits of outdoor exercise outweigh the CV risks of pollution exposure. Animal studies have suggested that exercise may attenuate the adverse effects of air pollution.[137] Quasi-experimental and modeling studies have suggested that there may be a threshold of exposure, beyond which additional inhalation of pollutants with exercise, due to increased respiratory rate and tidal volumes (and hence exposure) may outweigh any protective benefits.[8,9,138] As a general rule, high-intensity exercise under heavy pollution should be avoided, particularly for susceptible individuals.[6–8]

Studies have found that awareness of air quality indices and media alerts along with advice from a health professional can increase pollution-avoiding behaviors.[139] Still, individuals with heart disease, compared to those with respiratory disease, have limited awareness of the harmful effects of air pollution on health.[140] Cardiologists therefore have an opportunity to educate susceptible patients about an important risk factor.[10]

Antioxidants and Omega-3 Fatty Acids

Experimental evidence suggests that antioxidants may attenuate physiological responses to air pollution, particularly those mediated by oxidative stress.[141] Treatment with the antioxidant Tempol, for example, prevented inflammation and insulin resistance induced by exposure to $PM_{2.5}$ exposure.[142] Similarly, 6 months of supplementation with antioxidant vitamins C and E normalized serum markers of oxidative stress among coal power plant workers in Brazil.[143] In a randomized trial in Detroit, a single dose of vitamin C did not mitigate acute increases in blood pressure from acute PM exposures.[29] Omega-3 fatty acids may also provide some benefit. A double-blinded, placebo-controlled trial randomized 65 healthy young adults to receive fish-oil supplementation versus placebo and monitored $PM_{2.5}$ exposures in real time.[144] The investigators found that, compared to the control group, fish-oil mitigated the $PM_{2.5}$-associated increase in serum biomarkers of inflammation, coagulation, endothelial function, and oxidative stress.[144] A smaller randomized trial found that olive oil attenuated the effect of acute air pollution exposures on heart rate variability, but found no benefit to fish oil.[145] A prospective cohort of 548,845 individuals followed for 17 years across the

United States demonstrated that a Mediterranean diet reduced CVD mortality risk related to long-term exposure to air pollutants in a large prospective US cohort.[146] Future prospective randomized studies are needed to examine the impact of therapeutic interventions in heavily polluted environments.

Clinicians

A recent review article described how clinicians can play a central role in mitigating risk to individuals.[10] Since susceptibility to air pollution depends on traditional risk factors (e.g., atherosclerosis), clinical management of these risk factors by Cardiologists and Internists is critical to protect patients from air pollution.[7,8] Additionally, clinicians can use the aforementioned methods to assess individual exposures, estimate risk, and provide tailored interventions. Some interventions require patient education (e.g., avoidance behaviors) while others require the provision of equipment (e.g., air filters). These interventions may be reimbursed as the health benefits of clean air become increasingly clear, and as personal exposure monitors and alert networks accelerate the incorporation of air pollution into clinical conversations.[10] To empower clinicians accordingly, medical education and training should now include the pathophysiology and management of pollution-attributable diseases, including cardiovascular, pulmonary, and neurologic consequences of air pollution exposure.[8-10]

FUTURE RESEARCH

Further research is needed to improve our understanding and management of pollution-attributable CVD. First, randomized, controlled trials are needed to evaluate the efficacy of interventions on hard CV outcomes.[92] Key interventions to be tested include: facemasks, air filtration systems, clean stove-fuel combinations, and cardioprotective medications. Well-designed prospective observational studies and case-crossover studies may be required to answer questions when trials are too expensive or logistically difficult. Trials should quantify exposures with personal monitoring devices, test for effect modification by traditional CV risk factors, and collect data on cost-effectiveness to guide policy decisions.[134]

Second, studies are needed to better characterize exposure-response relationships. Specifically, cohort studies are needed to define the effect of specific *sources* (e.g., coal burning, traffic) and *types* of air pollution (e.g., NO_2, ultrafine PM) on specific *outcomes* (e.g., heart failure, non-fatal MI) in specific patient populations (e.g., diabetics).[10,62,95] Special attention is needed to characterize the risk of occupational exposures (e.g., mining, manufacturing, constructions), which may contribute over 1 million premature deaths, but remain poorly understood.[10] Improved understanding of exposure-response relationships will facilitate the development of screening tools, clinical guidelines, and government policies to target hazardous pollutants in at-risk populations.[6,8] Ultimately, the goal would be to provide custom estimates of the *absolute* risk of CV events for individual exposures. These developments, along with increasingly available personal exposure monitors, will lead to personalized medicine where air pollution exposures

can be integrated as potentially modifiable components into the framework of other well-known risk factors.[8]

Finally, investigations are needed to delineate the effects of other environmental risk factors. These include climate, temperature, soil and water contamination, noise exposure, psychosocial stress, socioeconomic environment, nighttime light, agricultural methods, proximity to health services, and climate change.[9,11] These risk factors may covary with air pollution and potentiate CV risk.[8]

SUMMARY

Air pollution is an important modifiable risk factor for CV morbidity and mortality.[5-7] Here, we have described the burden of disease attributable to air pollution, various sources and types of air pollution, and the complex pathophysiology of pollution-attributable CVD. We have shared approaches to assess risk among individuals and communities, as well as summarized potential interventions to mitigate risk and improve CV health. The field of air pollution mediated health effects and that of environmental risk factors as mediators of CVD continues to offer promise as an avenue for sustainable global health.

REFERENCES

1. Institute for Health Metrics and Evaluation (2020). Global Health Data Exchange. Available at: ghdx.healthdata.org. Accessed June 8, 2020.
2. Collaborators GRF. Global, regional, and national comparative risk assessment of 84 behavioural, environmental and occupational, and metabolic risks or clusters of risks for 195 countries and territories, 1990–2017: a systematic analysis for the Global Burden of Disease Study 2017. *Lancet (London, England)*. 2018;392:1923.
3. Cohen AJ, Brauer M, Burnett R, et al. Estimates and 25-year trends of the global burden of disease attributable to ambient air pollution: an analysis of data from the Global Burden of Diseases Study 2015. *Lancet*. 2017;389:1907-1918.
4. Lelieveld J, Evans JS, Fnais M, Giannadaki D, and Pozzer A. The contribution of outdoor air pollution sources to premature mortality on a global scale. *Nature*. 2015;525:367-371.
5. World Health Organization (2016). Ambient air pollution: A global assessment of exposure and burden of disease. Available at: http://www.who.int/phe/publications/air-pollution-global-assessment/en/. Accessed December 10, 2019.
6. Newby DE, Mannucci PM, Tell GS, et al., Esc Working Group on Thrombosis EAfCP, Rehabilitation and Association ESCHF. Expert position paper on air pollution and cardiovascular disease. *Eur Heart J*. 2015;36:83-93b.
7. Brook RD, Rajagopalan S, Pope CA, 3rd, et al., American Heart Association Council on E, Prevention CotKiCD, Council on Nutrition PA and Metabolism. Particulate matter air pollution and cardiovascular disease: An update to the scientific statement from the American Heart Association. *Circulation*. 2010;121:2331-2378.
8. Al-Kindi SG, Brook RD, Biswal S, and Rajagopalan S. Environmental determinants of cardiovascular disease: lessons learned from air pollution. *Nature Reviews Cardiology*. 2020:1-17.
9. Rajagopalan S, Al-Kindi SG, and Brook RD. Air pollution and cardiovascular disease: JACC state-of-the-art review. *Journal of the American College of Cardiology*. 2018;72:2054-2070.
10. Hadley MB, Baumgartner J, and Vedanthan R. Developing a Clinical Approach to Air Pollution and Cardiovascular Health. *Circulation*. 2018;137:725-742.
11. Landrigan PJ, Fuller R, Acosta NJR, et al. The Lancet Commission on pollution and health. *Lancet*. 2017.

12. World Health Organization. Global Health Observatory (GHO) data. Available at: https://www.who.int/gho/en. Accessed December 10, 2019.

13. Martin WJ, 2nd. On the Global Epidemic of CVD and Why Household Air Pollution Matters. *Glob Heart*. 2012;7:201-206.

14. Smith KR, Bruce N, Balakrishnan K, et al. Millions dead: how do we know and what does it mean? Methods used in the comparative risk assessment of household air pollution. *Annu Rev Public Health*. 2014;35:185-206.

15. Burnett R, Chen H, Szyszkowicz M, et al. Global estimates of mortality associated with long-term exposure to outdoor fine particulate matter. *Proceedings of the National Academy of Sciences*. 2018;115:9592-9597.

16. Atkinson RW, Mills IC, Walton HA, and Anderson HR. Fine particle components and health—a systematic review and meta-analysis of epidemiological time series studies of daily mortality and hospital admissions. *Journal of Exposure Science & Environmental Epidemiology*. 2015;25:208-214.

17. Ostro B, Hu J, Goldberg D, Reynolds P, et al. Associations of mortality with long-term exposures to fine and ultrafine particles, species and sources: results from the California Teachers Study Cohort. *Environmental Health Perspectives*. 2015;123:549-556.

18. Thurston GD, Burnett RT, Turner MC, et al. Ischemic heart disease mortality and long-term exposure to source-related components of US fine particle air pollution. *Environmental Health Perspectives*. 2016;124:785-794.

19. Lippmann M, Chen LC, Gordon T, Ito K, and Thurston GD. National Particle Component Toxicity (NPACT) Initiative: integrated epidemiologic and toxicologic studies of the health effects of particulate matter components. *Res Rep Health Eff Inst*. 2013:5-13.

20. Stafoggia M, Cesaroni G, Peters A, et al. Long-term exposure to ambient air pollution and incidence of cerebrovascular events: results from 11 European cohorts within the ESCAPE project. *Environmental Health Perspectives*. 2014;122:919-925.

21. Munzel T, Sorensen M, Gori T, et al. Environmental stressors and cardio-metabolic disease: part II-mechanistic insights. *Eur Heart J*. 2017;38:557-564.

22. Munzel T, Sorensen M, Gori T, et al. Environmental stressors and cardio-metabolic disease: part I-epidemiologic evidence supporting a role for noise and air pollution and effects of mitigation strategies. *Eur Heart J*. 2017;38:550-556.

23. Kampfrath T, Maiseyeu A, Ying Z, et al. Chronic fine particulate matter exposure induces systemic vascular dysfunction via NADPH oxidase and TLR4 pathways. *Circulation Research*. 2011;108:716-726.

24. O'Neill LA. How frustration leads to inflammation. *Science*. 2008;320:619-620.

25. Rao X, Zhong J, Brook RD, and Rajagopalan S. Effect of particulate matter air pollution on cardiovascular oxidative stress pathways. *Antioxidants & redox signaling*. 2018;28:797-818.

26. Miller MR, Raftis JB, Langrish JP, et al. Inhaled nanoparticles accumulate at sites of vascular disease. *ACS Nano*. 2017;11:4542-4552.

27. Rao X, Zhong J, Maiseyeu A, et al. CD36-dependent 7-ketocholesterol accumulation in macrophages mediates progression of atherosclerosis in response to chronic air pollution exposure. *Circulation Research*. 2014;115:770-780.

28. Suwa T, Hogg JC, Quinlan KB, et al. Particulate air pollution induces progression of atherosclerosis. *Journal of the American College of Cardiology*. 2002;39:935-942.

29. Brook RD, Urch B, Dvonch JT, et al. Insights into the mechanisms and mediators of the effects of air pollution exposure on blood pressure and vascular function in healthy humans. *Hypertension*. 2009;54:659-667.

30. Krishnan RM, Adar SD, Szpiro AA, et al. Vascular responses to long-and short-term exposure to fine particulate matter: MESA Air (Multi-Ethnic Study of Atherosclerosis and Air Pollution). *Journal of the American College of Cardiology*. 2012;60:2158-2166.

31. Mills NL, Törnqvist H, Gonzalez MC, et al. Ischemic and thrombotic effects of dilute diesel-exhaust inhalation in men with coronary heart disease. *New England Journal of Medicine*. 2007;357:1075-1082.

32. Lucking AJ, Lundback M, Mills NL, et al. Diesel exhaust inhalation increases thrombus formation in man. *European Heart Journal*. 2008;29:3043-3051.

33. Soberanes S, Misharin AV, Jairaman A, et al. Metformin targets mitochondrial electron transport to reduce air-pollution-induced thrombosis. *Cell Metabolism*. 2019;29:335-347.e5.

34. Rao X, Montresor-Lopez J, Puett R, Rajagopalan S, and Brook RD. Ambient air pollution: an emerging risk factor for diabetes mellitus. *Current Diabetes Reports*. 2015;15:1-11.

35. Rajagopalan S and Brook RD. Air pollution and type 2 diabetes: mechanistic insights. *Diabetes*. 2012;61:3037-3045.

36. Miller DB, Ghio AJ, Karoly ED, et al. Ozone exposure increases circulating stress hormones and lipid metabolites in humans. *American Journal of Respiratory and Critical Care Medicine*. 2016;193:1382-1391.

37. Sayols-Baixeras S, Fernández-Sanlés A, Prats-Uribe A, et al. Association between long-term air pollution exposure and DNA methylation: the REGICOR study. *Environmental Research*. 2019;176:108550.

38. Rajagopalan S, Park B, Palanivel R, et al. Metabolic effects of air pollution exposure and reversibility. *The Journal of Clinical Investigation*. 2020.

39. Breton CV, Yao J, Millstein J, et al. Prenatal air pollution exposures, DNA methyl transferase genotypes, and associations with newborn LINE1 and Alu methylation and childhood blood pressure and carotid intima-media thickness in the Children's Health Study. *Environmental Health Perspectives*. 2016;124:1905-1912.

40. Byrd JB, Morishita M, Bard RL, et al. Acute increase in blood pressure during inhalation of coarse particulate matter air pollution from an urban location. *Journal of the American Society of Hypertension*. 2016;10:133-139.e4.

41. Cosselman KE, M. Krishnan R, Oron AP, et al. Blood pressure response to controlled diesel exhaust exposure in human subjects. *Hypertension*. 2012;59:943-948.

42. Zhao X, Sun Z, Ruan Y, et al. Personal black carbon exposure influences ambulatory blood pressure: air pollution and cardiometabolic disease (AIRCMD-China) study. *Hypertension*. 2014;63:871-877.

43. Yang B-Y, Qian Z, Howard SW, et al. Global association between ambient air pollution and blood pressure: a systematic review and meta-analysis. *Environmental Pollution*. 2018;235:576-588.

44. Cai Y, Zhang B, Ke W, et al. Associations of short-term and long-term exposure to ambient air pollutants with hypertension: a systematic review and meta-analysis. *Hypertension*. 2016;68:62-70.

45. Eze IC, Hemkens LG, Bucher HC, et al. Association between ambient air pollution and diabetes mellitus in Europe and North America: systematic review and meta-analysis. *Environmental Health Perspectives*. 2015;123:381-389.

46. Wang B, Xu D, Jing Z, Liu D, Yan S, and Wang Y. Effect of long-term exposure to air pollution on type 2 diabetes mellitus risk: a systemic review and meta-analysis of cohort studies. *Eur J Endocrinol*. 2014;171:R173-82.

47. Bowe B, Xie Y, Li T, Yan Y, Xian H, and Al-Aly Z. The 2016 global and national burden of diabetes mellitus attributable to PM2· 5 air pollution. *The Lancet Planetary Health*. 2018;2:e301-e312.

48. Sun Q, Wang A, Jin X, et al. Long-term air pollution exposure and acceleration of atherosclerosis and vascular inflammation in an animal model. *JAMA*. 2005;294:3003-3010.

49. Kaufman JD, Adar SD, Barr RG, et al. Association between air pollution and coronary artery calcification within six metropolitan areas in the USA (the Multi-Ethnic Study of Atherosclerosis and Air Pollution): a longitudinal cohort study. *Lancet*. 2016;388:696-704.

50. Brook RD and Rajagopalan S. Particulate matter air pollution and atherosclerosis. *Curr Atheroscler Rep*. 2010;12:291-300.

51. Provost EB, Madhloum N, Panis LI, De Boever P, and Nawrot TS. Carotid intima-media thickness, a marker of subclinical atherosclerosis, and particulate air pollution exposure: the meta-analytical evidence. *PloS one*. 2015;10:e0127014.

52. Wold LE, Ying Z, Hutchinson KR, et al. Cardiovascular remodeling in response to long-term exposure to fine particulate matter air pollution. *Circulation: Heart Failure*. 2012;5:452-461.

53. Krzyzanowski M and Cohen A. Update of WHO air quality guidelines. *Air Quality, Atmosphere & Health.* 2008;1:7-13.

54. Downward GS, van Nunen EJ, Kerckhoffs J, et al. Long-term exposure to ultrafine particles and incidence of cardiovascular and cerebrovascular disease in a prospective study of a Dutch cohort. *Environmental Health Perspectives.* 2018;126:127007.

55. Dockery DW, Pope CA, 3rd, Xu X, et al. An association between air pollution and mortality in six U.S. cities. *N Engl J Med.* 1993;329:1753-1759.

56. Lepeule J, Laden F, Dockery D, and Schwartz J. Chronic exposure to fine particles and mortality: an extended follow-up of the Harvard Six Cities study from 1974 to 2009. *Environmental Health Perspectives.* 2012;120:965-970.

57. Di Q, Wang Y, Zanobetti A, et al. Air Pollution and Mortality in the Medicare Population. *N Engl J Med.* 2017;376:2513-2522.

58. Crouse DL, Peters PA, van Donkelaar A, et al. Risk of nonaccidental and cardiovascular mortality in relation to long-term exposure to low concentrations of fine particulate matter: a Canadian national-level cohort study. *Environmental Health Perspectives.* 2012;120:708-714.

59. Krewski D, Jerrett M, Burnett RT, et al. Extended follow-up and spatial analysis of the American Cancer Society study linking particulate air pollution and mortality. *Res Rep Health Eff Inst.* 2009:5-114; discussion 115-136.

60. Lu F, Xu D, Cheng Y, Dong S, Guo C, Jiang X, and Zheng X. Systematic review and meta-analysis of the adverse health effects of ambient PM2. 5 and PM10 pollution in the Chinese population. *Environmental Research.* 2015;136:196-204.

61. Atkinson RW, Kang S, Anderson HR, Mills IC, and Walton HA. Epidemiological time series studies of PM2.5 and daily mortality and hospital admissions: a systematic review and meta-analysis. *Thorax.* 2014;69:660-665.

62. Hoek G, Krishnan RM, Beelen R, et al. Long-term air pollution exposure and cardio- respiratory mortality: a review. *Environ Health.* 2013;12:43.

63. Yu K, Qiu G, Chan K-H, et al. Association of solid fuel use with risk of cardiovascular and all-cause mortality in rural China. *JAMA* 2018;319:1351-1361.

64. Di Q, Dai L, Wang Y, et al. Association of short-term exposure to air pollution with mortality in older adults. *JAMA.* 2017;318:2446-2456.

65. Faustini A, Rapp R, and Forastiere F. Nitrogen dioxide and mortality: review and meta-analysis of long-term studies. *European Respiratory Journal.* 2014;44:744-753.

66. Pope III CA, Muhlestein JB, Anderson JL, et al. Short-term exposure to fine particulate matter air pollution is preferentially associated with the risk of ST-segment elevation acute coronary events. *Journal of the American Heart Association.* 2015;4:e002506.

67. Cesaroni G, Forastiere F, Stafoggia M, et al. Long term exposure to ambient air pollution and incidence of acute coronary events: prospective cohort study and meta-analysis in 11 European cohorts from the ESCAPE Project. *BMJ.* 2014;348:f7412.

68. Miller KA, Siscovick DS, Sheppard L, et al. Long-term exposure to air pollution and incidence of cardiovascular events in women. *New England Journal of Medicine.* 2007;356:447-458.

69. Mustafic H, Jabre P, Caussin C, et al. Main air pollutants and myocardial infarction: a systematic review and meta-analysis. *JAMA.* 2012;307:713-21.

70. Chen H, Burnett RT, Copes R, et al. Ambient fine particulate matter and mortality among survivors of myocardial infarction: population-based cohort study. *Environmental Health Perspectives.* 2016;124:1421-1428.

71. Mustafić H, Jabre P, Caussin C, et al. Main air pollutants and myocardial infarction: a systematic review and meta-analysis. *JAMA.* 2012;307:713-721.

72. Shah AS, Lee KK, McAllister DA, et al. Short term exposure to air pollution and stroke: systematic review and meta-analysis. *BMJ.* 2015;350:h1295.

73. Fu P, Guo X, Cheung FMH, and Yung KKL. The association between PM2. 5 exposure and neurological disorders: a systematic review and meta-analysis. *Science of the Total Environment.* 2019;655:1240-1248.

74. Zhang P, Dong G, Sun B, et al. Long-term exposure to ambient air pollution and mortality due to cardiovascular disease and cerebrovascular disease in Shenyang, China. *PloS One.* 2011;6:e20827.

75. Shah AS, Langrish JP, Nair H, et al. Global association of air pollution and heart failure: a systematic review and meta-analysis. *Lancet.* 2013;382:1039-1048.

76. Al-Kindi SG, Sarode A, Zullo M, et al. Ambient air pollution and mortality after cardiac transplantation. *Journal of the American College of Cardiology.* 2019;74:3026-3035.

77. Shao Q, Liu T, Korantzopoulos P, Zhang Z, Zhao J, and Li G. Association between air pollution and development of atrial fibrillation: a meta-analysis of observational studies. *Heart & Lung.* 2016;45:557-562.

78. Peralta AA, Link MS, Schwartz J, et al. Exposure to Air Pollution and Particle Radioactivity with the Risk of Ventricular Arrhythmias. *Circulation.* 2020.

79. Folino F, Buja G, Zanotto G, et al. Association between air pollution and ventricular arrhythmias in high-risk patients (ARIA study): a multicentre longitudinal study. *The Lancet Planetary health.* 2017;1:e58-e64.

80. Raza A, Bellander T, Bero-Bedada G, et al. Short-term effects of air pollution on out-of-hospital cardiac arrest in Stockholm. *European Heart Journal.* 2014;35:861-868.

81. Baccarelli A, Martinelli I, Pegoraro V, et al. Living near major traffic roads and risk of deep vein thrombosis. *Circulation.* 2009;119:3118.

82. Shih RA, Griffin BA, Salkowski N, et al. Ambient particulate matter air pollution and venous thromboembolism in the Women's Health Initiative Hormone Therapy trials. *Environmental Health Perspectives.* 2011;119:326-331.

83. Kloog I, Zanobetti A, Nordio F, Coull BA, Baccarelli AA, and Schwartz J. Effects of airborne fine particles (PM 2.5) on deep vein thrombosis admissions in the northeastern United States. *Journal of Thrombosis and Haemostasis.* 2015;13:768-774.

84. Kloog I. Fine particulate matter (PM2. 5) association with peripheral artery disease admissions in northeastern United States. *International Journal of Environmental Health Research.* 2016;26:572-577.

85. van den Hooven EH, de Kluizenaar Y, Pierik FH, et al. Air pollution, blood pressure, and the risk of hypertensive complications during pregnancy: the generation R study. *Hypertension.* 2011;57(3):406-412.

86. Li W, Dorans KS, Wilker EH, et al. Residential proximity to major roadways, fine particulate matter, and adiposity: the Framingham Heart Study. *Obesity.* 2016;24:2593-2599.

87. Mehta AJ, Zanobetti A, Bind M-AC, et al. Long-term exposure to ambient fine particulate matter and renal function in older men: the veterans administration normative aging study. *Environmental Health Perspectives.* 2016;124:1353-1360.

88. Zanobetti A, Redline S, Schwartz J, et al. Associations of PM10 with sleep and sleep-disordered breathing in adults from seven US urban areas. *American Journal of Respiratory and Critical Care Medicine.* 2010;182:819-825.

89. Schwartz J. Harvesting and long term exposure effects in the relation between air pollution and mortality. *American Journal of Epidemiology.* 2000;151:440-448.

90. Apte JS, Marshall JD, Cohen AJ, and Brauer M. Addressing Global Mortality from Ambient PM2.5. *Environ Sci Technol.* 2015;49:8057-66.

91. Rajagopalan S and Brook RD. The Indoor-Outdoor Air-Pollution Continuum and the Burden of Cardiovascular Disease: An Opportunity for Improving Global Health. *Glob Heart.* 2012;7:207-213.

92. Brook RD, Newby DE, and Rajagopalan S. The Global Threat of Outdoor Ambient Air Pollution to Cardiovascular Health: Time for Intervention. *JAMA Cardiol.* 2017;2:353-354.

93. Burnett RT, Pope CA, 3rd, Ezzati M, et al. An integrated risk function for estimating the global burden of disease attributable to ambient fine particulate matter exposure. *Environ Health Perspect.* 2014;122:397-403.

94. Pope III CA, Cohen AJ, and Burnett RT. Cardiovascular disease and fine particulate matter: lessons and limitations of an integrated exposure–response approach. *Circulation research.* 2018;122:1645-1647.

95. Clark ML, Peel JL, Balakrishnan K, et al. Health and household air pollution from solid fuel use: the need for improved exposure assessment. *Environ Health Perspect.* 2013;121:1120-1128.

96. Weichenthal S, Pinault LL, and Burnett RT. Impact of oxidant gases on the relationship between outdoor fine particulate air pollution and nonaccidental, cardiovascular, and respiratory mortality. *Scientific Reports.* 2017;7:1-10.

97. Bell ML, Zanobetti A, and Dominici F. Evidence on vulnerability and susceptibility to health risks associated with short-term exposure to particulate matter: a systematic review and meta-analysis. *American Journal of Epidemiology.* 2013;178:865-876.

98. Balakrishnan K, Ghosh S, Ganguli B, et al. State and national household concentrations of PM2.5 from solid cookfuel use: results from measurements and modeling in India for estimation of the global burden of disease. *Environ Health.* 2013;12:77.

99. Baumgartner J, Schauer JJ, Ezzati M, et al. Patterns and predictors of personal exposure to indoor air pollution from biomass combustion among women and children in rural China. *Indoor Air.* 2011;21:479-488.

100. Chen C and Zhao B. Review of relationship between indoor and outdoor particles: I/O ratio, infiltration factor and penetration factor. *Atmospheric Environment.* 2011;45:275-288.

101. McKercher GR, Salmond JA, and Vanos JK. Characteristics and applications of small, portable gaseous air pollution monitors. *Environmental Pollution.* 2017;223:102-110.

102. Steinle S, Reis S, and Sabel CE. Quantifying human exposure to air pollution—moving from static monitoring to spatio-temporally resolved personal exposure assessment. *Sci Total Environ.* 2013;443:184-93.

103. Environmental Protection Agency. Air Pollution in World: Real-time Air Quality Index Visual Map. 2016. Available at: http://aqicn.org/map/world/. Accessed December 15, 2016.

104. Brauer M, Amann M, Burnett RT, et al. Exposure assessment for estimation of the global burden of disease attributable to outdoor air pollution. *Environ Sci Technol.* 2012;46:652-660.

105. Holliday KM, Avery CL, Poole C, et al. Estimating personal exposures from ambient air-pollution measures: Using meta-analysis to assess measurement error. *Epidemiology (Cambridge, Mass).* 2014;25:35.

106. Rajagopalan S, Brauer M, Bhatnagar A, et al. Personal-Level Protective Actions Against Particulate Matter Air Pollution Exposure. A Scientific Statement from the American Heart Association. *Circulation.* 2020 (In press).

107. Cromar KR, Duncan BN, Bartonova A, et al. Air Pollution Monitoring for Health Research and Patient Care. An Official American Thoracic Society Workshop Report. *Ann Am Thorac Soc.* 2019;16:1207-1214.

108. Laden F, Schwartz J, Speizer FE, and Dockery DW. Reduction in fine particulate air pollution and mortality: Extended follow-up of the Harvard Six Cities study. *Am J Respir Crit Care Med.* 2006;173:667-672.

109. Pope CA, 3rd, Ezzati M, and Dockery DW. Fine-particulate air pollution and life expectancy in the United States. *N Engl J Med.* 2009;360:376-86.

110. Lelieveld J, Klingmüller K, Pozzer A, Burnett R, Haines A, and Ramanathan V. Effects of fossil fuel and total anthropogenic emission removal on public health and climate. *Proceedings of the National Academy of Sciences.* 2019;116:7192-7197.

111. Pascal M, Corso M, Chanel O, et al. Assessing the public health impacts of urban air pollution in 25 European cities: results of the Aphekom project. *Science of the Total Environment.* 2013;449:390-400.

112. Beelen R, Raaschou-Nielsen O, Stafoggia M, et al. Effects of long-term exposure to air pollution on natural-cause mortality: an analysis of 22 European cohorts within the multicentre ESCAPE project. *The Lancet.* 2014;383:785-795.

113. Environmental Protection Agency Office of Air and Radiation. The benefits and costs of the clean air act from 1990 to 2020, Final Report, Rev A. Available at: https://www.epa.gov/sites/production/files/2015-07/documents/fullreport_rev_a.pdf (2011). Accessed December 10, 2019.

114. James P, Kioumourtzoglou M-A, Hart JE, Banay RF, Kloog I, and Laden F. Interrelationships between walkability, air pollution, greenness, and body mass index. *Epidemiology (Cambridge, Mass).* 2017;28:780.

115. Nowak DJ, Hirabayashi S, Bodine A, and Greenfield E. Tree and forest effects on air quality and human health in the United States. *Environmental pollution.* 2014;193:119-129.

116. Kim EJ. The impacts of climate change on human health in the United States: A scientific assessment, by us global change research program. *Journal of the American Planning Association.* 2016;82:418-419.

117. Gao J, Kovats S, Vardoulakis S, et al. Public health co-benefits of greenhouse gas emissions reduction: a systematic review. *Science of the Total Environment.* 2018;627:388-402.

118. Rajagopalan S, Brauer M, Bhatnagar A, et al. Personal-Level Protective Actions Against Particulate Matter Air Pollution Exposure. A Scientific Statement from the American Heart Association; on behalf of the American Heart Association Council on Lifestyle and Cardiometabolic Health, Council on Arteriosclerosis, Trombosis and Vascular Biology, Council on Clinical Cardiology, Council on Cardiovascular and Stroke Nursing, Stroke Council. *Circulation.* 2020 (in press).

119. Langrish JP, Mills NL, Chan JK, et al. Beneficial cardiovascular effects of reducing exposure to particulate air pollution with a simple facemask. *Particle and Fibre Toxicology.* 2009;6:8.

120. Shi J, Lin Z, Chen R, et al. Cardiovascular benefits of wearing particulate-filtering respirators: a randomized crossover trial. *Environmental Health Perspectives.* 2017;125:175-180.

121. Langrish JP, Li X, Wang S, et al. Reducing personal exposure to particulate air pollution improves cardiovascular health in patients with coronary heart disease. *Environmental Health Perspectives.* 2012;120:367-372.

122. Vieira JL, Guimaraes GV, de Andre PA, Cruz FD, Saldiva PHN, and Bocchi EA. Respiratory filter reduces the cardiovascular effects associated with diesel exhaust exposure: a randomized, prospective, double-blind, controlled study of heart failure: the FILTER-HF trial. *JACC: Heart Failure.* 2016;4:55-64.

123. Fisk WJ and Chan WR. Effectiveness and cost of reducing particle-related mortality with particle filtration. *Indoor Air.* 2017;27:909-920.

124. Chen R, Zhao A, Chen H, et al. Cardiopulmonary benefits of reducing indoor particles of outdoor origin: a randomized, double-blind crossover trial of air purifiers. *Journal of the American College of Cardiology.* 2015;65:2279-2287.

125. Allen RW, Carlsten C, Karlen B, et al. An air filter intervention study of endothelial function among healthy adults in a woodsmoke-impacted community. *American Journal of Respiratory and Critical Care Medicine.* 2011;183:1222-1230.

126. Bell ML, Ebisu K, Peng RD, and Dominici F. Adverse health effects of particulate air pollution: modification by air conditioning. *Epidemiology.* 2009;20:682-6.

127. Morishita M, Adar SD, D'Souza J, et al. Effect of portable air filtration systems on personal exposure to fine particulate matter and blood pressure among residents in a low-income senior facility: a randomized clinical trial. *JAMA Internal Medicine.* 2018;178:1350-1357.

128. Li H, Cai J, Chen R, et al. Particulate matter exposure and stress hormone levels: a randomized, double-blind, crossover trial of air purification. *Circulation.* 2017;136:618-627.

129. Baumgartner J, Smith KR, and Chockalingam A. Reducing CVD Through Improvements in Household Energy: Implications for Policy-Relevant Research. *Glob Heart.* 2012;7:243-7.

130. Sagar A, Balakrishnan K, Guttikunda S, Roychowdhury A, and Smith KR. India Leads the Way: A Health-Centered Strategy for Air Pollution. *Environ Health Perspect.* 2016;124:A116-A117.

131. Olopade CO, Frank E, Bartlett E, et al. Effect of a clean stove intervention on inflammatory biomarkers in pregnant women in Ibadan, Nigeria: a randomized controlled study. *Environ Int.* 2017;98:181-190.

132. McCracken JP, Smith KR, Diaz A, Mittleman MA, and Schwartz J. Chimney stove intervention to reduce long-term wood smoke exposure lowers blood pressure among Guatemalan women. *Environ Health Perspect.* 2007;115:996-1001.

133. McCracken J, Smith KR, Stone P, Diaz A, Arana B, and Schwartz J. Intervention to lower household wood smoke exposure in Guatemala reduces

ST-segment depression on electrocardiograms. *Environ Health Perspect.* 2011;119:1562-1568.

134. International Organization for Standardization. Guidelines for evaluating cookstove performance. 2012. Available at: https://www.iso.org/obp/ui/#iso:std:iso:iwa:11:ed-1:v1:en. Accessed October 17, 2016.

135. Environmental Protection Agency. AirNow. 2016. Available at: https://www.airnow.gov. Accessed December 16, 2016.

136. Zuurbier M, Hoek G, Oldenwening M, et al. Commuters' exposure to particulate matter air pollution is affected by mode of transport, fuel type, and route. *Environ Health Perspect.* 2010;118:783-789.

137. Vieira RdP, Toledo AC, Silva LB, et al. Anti-inflammatory effects of aerobic exercise in mice exposed to air pollution. *Medicine & Science in Sports & Exercise.* 2012;44:1227-1234.

138. Tainio M, de Nazelle AJ, Götschi T, et al. Can air pollution negate the health benefits of cycling and walking? *Preventive Medicine.* 2016;87:233-236.

139. Wen XJ, Balluz L, and Mokdad A. Association between media alerts of air quality index and change of outdoor activity among adult asthma in six states, BRFSS, 2005. *J Community Health.* 2009;34:40-46.

140. Mirabelli MC, Boehmer TK, Damon SA, et al. Air quality awareness among US adults with respiratory and heart disease. *American Journal of Preventive Medicine.* 2018;54:679-687.

141. Romieu I, Castro-Giner F, Kunzli N, and Sunyer J. Air pollution, oxidative stress and dietary supplementation: a review. *Eur Respir J.* 2008;31:179-197.

142. Haberzettl P, O'Toole TE, Bhatnagar A, and Conklin DJ. Exposure to fine particulate air pollution causes vascular insulin resistance by inducing pulmonary oxidative stress. *Environmental health perspectives.* 2016;124:1830-1839.

143. Possamai FP, Júnior SÁ, Parisotto EB, et al. Antioxidant intervention compensates oxidative stress in blood of subjects exposed to emissions from a coal electric-power plant in South Brazil. *Environmental Toxicology and Pharmacology.* 2010;30:175-180.

144. Lin Z, Chen R, Jiang Y, et al. Cardiovascular benefits of fish-oil supplementation against fine particulate air pollution in China. *Journal of the American College of Cardiology.* 2019;73:2076-2085.

145. Tong H, Rappold AG, Diaz-Sanchez D, et al. Omega-3 fatty acid supplementation appears to attenuate particulate air pollution-induced cardiac effects and lipid changes in healthy middle-aged adults. *Environ Health Perspect.* 2012;120:952-957.

146. Lim CC, Hayes RB, Ahn J, et al. Mediterranean diet and the association between air pollution and cardiovascular disease mortality risk. *Circulation.* 2019;139:1766-1775.

147. Brauer M, Freedman G, Frostad J, et al. Ambient air pollution exposure estimation for the global burden of disease 2013. *Environmental Science & Technology.* 2016;50:79-88.

148. Guttikunda, S. Primer on pollution source apportionment. 2020. Available at: http://www.urbanemissions.info/publications/primer-on-pollution-source-apportionment. Accessed June 1, 2020.

149. Matte TD, Ross Z, Kheirbek I, Eisl H, et al. Monitoring intraurban spatial patterns of multiple combustion air pollutants in New York City: design and implementation. *J Expo Sci Environ Epidemiol.* 2013;23:223-231.

150. Munzel T, Rajagopalan S, et al. Reduction of environmental pollutants for prevention of cardiovascular disease: it's time to act. *European Heart Journal.* 2020;41(41), p.3989.

Hypercholesterolemia, Hyperlipoproteinemia(a), Hypertriglyceridemia, and Low HDL

10

Robert S. Rosenson, Marlys L. Koschinsky, Børge G. Nordestgaard, and Robert A. Hegele

Lipoproteins and atherosclerotic cardiovascular disease

Risk assessment

- History of clinical cardiovascular events and subclinical CVD
- Assessment and evaluation of cardiovascular risk factors
- Family history
  - First-degree and multigenerational family trees including CVD history, age of onset of first and recurrent events, untreated lipid and lipoprotein levels, genetic analysis

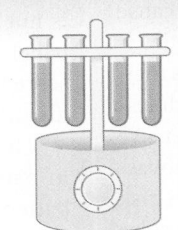

Laboratory assessment

- Lipid panel (total cholesterol, LDL cholesterol, HDL cholesterol, non-HDL cholesterol, triglycerides)
- Apolipoprotein B (or LDL particle number)
- Lp(a)
- TGRL/remnant cholesterol
- Screen for secondary causes of dyslipidemia
  - Obesity, poor diet, diabetes, hypothyroidism, renal disease, liver disease, autoimmune disease

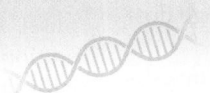

Genetic assessment

- Major genes in monogenic dyslipidemias
- Polygenic risk

Interventions to reduce lipoprotein CVD risk

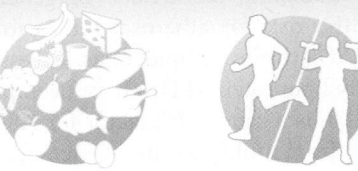

Healthy diet

Aerobic and resistance exercise

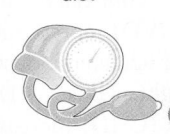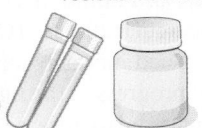

Aggressive surveillance and management of CVD risk factors

Aggressive reduction in LDL cholesterol based on underlying risk, adhering to treatment targets

Once LDL cholesterol targets are achieved:

TGRL-lowering therapies

Lp(a)-lowering therapies

Chapter 10 Fuster and Hurst's Central Illustration. Lipoprotein abnormalities are interpreted in the context of the history of clinical cardiovascular events or subclinical cardiovascular disease (CVD). This evaluation requires a complete assessment of other major cardiovascular risk factors and detailed multigenerational family trees. The evaluation of hyperlipidemia must include assessment of secondary causes of dyslipidemia. Confirmation of underlying lipoprotein disorders may include genetic assessment. The implementation of a strategy to reduce cardiovascular risk involves lifestyle interventions, aggressive surveillance and management of cardiovascular risk factors with therapies supported by clinical outcomes, and aggressive treatment of low-density lipoprotein (LDL) cholesterol. After LDL cholesterol targets are achieved, evaluation of strategies to lower triglyceride-rich lipoprotein (TGRL) and lipoprotein(a) (Lp(a)) may be considered.

CHAPTER SUMMARY

This chapter discusses the prevalence, genetics, pathophysiology, and management of lipoprotein abnormalities, which are interpreted in the context of the history of clinical cardiovascular events or subclinical cardiovascular disease (CVD) (see Fuster and Hurst's Central Illustration). Evaluation requires a complete assessment of other major cardiovascular risk factors and detailed, multigenerational family trees that include cardiovascular history, age of onset of the first and recurrent events, untreated lipid and lipoprotein levels, and genetic analysis. Laboratory assessment begins with the standard lipid panel and may extend to measures of atherogenic lipoprotein concentrations (apolipoprotein B [apoB], and low-density lipoprotein [LDL] particle number), lipoprotein(a) (Lp[a]), and triglyceride-rich lipoproteins/remnant cholesterol. The evaluation must include assessment of secondary causes of dyslipidemia, such as obesity, poor diet, diabetes, hypothyroidism, renal disease (chronic kidney disease and nephrotic syndrome), liver disease (hepatosteatosis and primary biliary cirrhosis), and autoimmune conditions. Confirmation of underlying lipoprotein disorders may include genetic assessment of major genes in monogenic dyslipidemias and polygenic factors. A strategy to reduce cardiovascular risk involves implementation of lifestyle interventions (healthy diet, and aerobic and resistance exercise), aggressive surveillance and management of cardiovascular risk factors with therapies supported by clinical outcomes, and aggressive treatment of LDL cholesterol (LDL-C). Once LDL-C targets are achieved, strategies to lower triglyceride-rich lipoproteins and Lp(a) may be considered.

HYPERLIPIDEMIA

The term hyperlipidemia comprises multiple disorders of high levels of circulating blood fats. In general, hyperlipidemia increases the risk for atherosclerotic cardiovascular disease (ASCVD). Of the hyperlipidemias, excess concentrations of low-density lipoprotein (LDL) have been the most extensively studied. LDL is a causal risk factor for ASCVD that has been established from multiple sources encompassing natural selection studies (Mendelian randomization), prospective population studies, and randomized, controlled clinical trials.[1]

Cardiovascular disease (CVD) represents the leading cause of morbidity and mortality for adults in industrialized societies.[2,3] Decades of progress in the fight against CVD is eroding as incident coronary heart disease (CHD) increases among adolescents and young adults.[4] Lifestyle changes and comprehensive medical therapy has reduced the risk of recurrent cardiovascular events and mortality in high-risk and very high-risk patients.[1,5-7] However, the risk of recurrent cardiovascular events after hospitalization for a myocardial infarction (MI) remains high even among many patients treated with high dosages of high-intensity statins.[8-10]

Despite multiple advances in LDL therapeutics, investigations are needed to improve understanding of lipoprotein associated risk beyond aggressive lowering of LDL cholesterol (LDL-C). Other hyperlipidemias characterized as disorders of cholesterol metabolism include lipoprotein(a) (Lp[a]) excess, while disorders of triglyceride metabolism contribute to increased cardiovascular risk through accumulation of remnant lipoproteins. Although high-density lipoprotein cholesterol (HDL-C), an inadequate surrogate for HDL, is inversely associated with cardiovascular risk, the causal association between the concentration, composition, and functional properties of HDL particles and atherosclerosis is far more complex.

This chapter reviews the prevalence, mechanism, genetics, and approaches to treatment for categories of hyperlipidemias categorized under as disorders of LDL, Lp(a) excess, and triglyceride-rich lipoproteins. Low HDL levels are considered pathologic under most circumstances and will be addressed separately. Lipoproteins are contextualized by the contribution to ASCVD and other noncardiovascular diseases. Thus, risk assessment is an essential embarkment for this discussion.

ASSESSMENT OF ATHEROSCLEROTIC CARDIOVASCULAR RISK

CVD risk assessment represents the initial process in the evaluation of the patient with hyperlipidemia. The underlying risk of the patient provides context for the healthcare professional–patient dialogue and guides evaluation and treatment of the hyperlipidemia. The term hyperlipidemia is more accurately described by the concentration(s) of abnormal lipoproteins or conditions known as dyslipoproteinemias.

As clinicians, we evaluate patients with abnormal risk factors that fall in the category of primary prevention of CVD and risk assessment in patients with established ASCVD that falls under the umbrella of secondary prevention of CVD. The use of risk assessment tools in the at-risk patient provides an integrated measure of near-term and lifetime risk for a cardiovascular event using widely evaluable major risk factors. Several risk assessment tools have been evaluated and validated in various populations.[11-15]

Noninvasive measures of atherosclerosis may assist with identification of high-risk patients in whom a specific lipoprotein abnormality is less well established or studied, and as a tool to guide investigation into lipoprotein associated risk that is not adequately identified by the conventional plasma lipid panel. Of the noninvasive measures, coronary artery calcium score identifies patients with either a higher or lower risk than identified by risk equations.[16,17]

The simplicity of commonly used risk assessment tools in patients with hyperlipidemia diminishes the accuracy in patients for whom cardiovascular risk is not accurately captured by the total cholesterol and HDL-C level. Other major limitations include the absence of family history for early onset ASCVD events and more detailed sex-specific generational approaches to encapsulating the risks associated with family history of CVD. As an example, family history of MI in first-degree relatives, and the number of relatives and age of onset of MI was associated with an increased risk of acute MI after adjustment for several major CHD risk factors in the Gruppo Italiano per lo Studio della Sopravvivenza nell'Inferno Miocardio (GISSI-2) trial.[18] Specifically, when compared with individuals without a family history of MI in first-degree relatives, the relative risk for MI in was 2.0 (95% confidence interval [CI]: 1.6–2.5) in patients with one affected relative with an MI <55 years and 3.0 (95% CI: 2.0–4.4) in those with two or more affected relatives. The risk of acute MI was higher when there was a family history of MI <55 years (relative risk [RR] 20.0; 95% CI: 3.3–121.2) versus later onset of MI (≤65 years). This more expansive family history is a useful construct in the assessment of risk in patients with dyslipoproteinemias that are not adequately captured by the serum cholesterol or other major CHD risk factors. Optimization of cardiovascular risk assessment in the encounter with the patient will be enhanced by the availability of untreated lipid and Lp(a) concentrations, identification of major risk factors and behaviors, and age of onset of atherosclerotic cardiovascular events and interventional procedures used in the treatment of ischemic CVD.

Among patients with clinical ASCVD, risk assessment is based on categorizing patients into high-risk and very-high risk strata[6,7] (**Table 10–1**). Evidence from large insurance claims data identifies individuals who remain at extremely high risk despite optimal risk of evidence-based secondary preventive therapies. In a study of 67,412 patients who underwent percutaneous coronary intervention while hospitalized for MI who received intensive medical management (dual anti-platelet therapy, beta adrenergic blocker, angiotensin converting enzyme inhibitor (ACE-I) or angiotensin receptor blocker (ARB), and high-intensity statin therapy) within 30 days after hospital discharge, certain characteristics were associated with

TABLE 10–1. Definition of Major Atherosclerotic Cardiovascular Disease Events and High-Risk Conditions in the 2018 AHA/ACC Blood Cholesterol Guideline

Major atherosclerotic cardiovascular disease events

1. Recent acute coronary syndrome within the last 12 months
2. History of myocardial infarction other than a recent acute coronary syndrome event
3. History of ischemic stroke
4. Symptomatic peripheral arterial disease

High-risk conditions

1. Age ≥65 years
2. Heterozygous familial hypercholesterolemia
3. History of prior coronary artery bypass surgery or percutaneous coronary intervention outside of the major atherosclerotic cardiovascular disease event(s)
4. Diabetes mellitus
5. Hypertension
6. Chronic kidney disease defined by an estimated glomerular filtration rate between 15 and 59 mL/min/1.73 m²
7. Current smoking
8. Persistently elevated LDL-C defined by LDL-C ≥100 mg/dL (2.6 mmol/L) despite maximally tolerated statin therapy and ezetimibe
9. History of congestive heart failure

Very high-risk conditions

1. Recent acute coronary syndrome within the last 12 months
2. History of MI (other than recent ACS event listed above)
3. History of ischemic stroke
4. Symptomatic peripheral arterial disease (history of claudication with ABI <0.85, or previous revascularization or amputation)

Extremely high-risk conditions

1. Two major cardiovascular events in preceding 2 years.
2. Myocardial infarction with prior CKD and diabetes, particularly insulin-requiring diabetes

LDL-C, low-density lipoprotein cholesterol Symptomatic peripheral arterial disease includes a history of claudication with ankle-brachial index <0.85, or previous revascularization or amputation.

an extremely high risk of recurrent MI, CHD hospitalization, and all-cause mortality beginning 30 days after hospital discharge.[8] As compared with MI survivors without a diagnosis of CHD, diabetes, or chronic kidney disease (CKD) prior to the hospitalization, a 2-fold higher event rate was observed in patients with prior CHD, diabetes, and CKD (**Fig. 10–1**). The presence of cardiovascular events increases with the number of ASCVD events and the number of vascular territories involved. A study of 15,366 US adults aged <65 years of age with health insurance evaluated cardiovascular events in patients with ASCVD who met the definition of very high risk versus high risk by the American Heart Association/American College of Cardiology (AHA/ACC) cholesterol guidelines.[9] Among patients with ≥2 major ASCVD events and with 1 event and ≥2 high-risk conditions, the age- and sex-adjusted hazard ratios versus those without very high risk were 2.98 (95% CI: 2.6–33.37), 4.89 (95% CI: 4.22–5.66), and 2.33 (95% CI: 2.04–2.66), respectively (**Fig. 10–2**).[9] A retrospective cohort study of 943,232 adults age ≥19 years who had a history of CHD, cerebrovascular disease, or peripheral arterial disease (PAD) compared the risk for ASCVD events among patients with

ASCVD in different vascular distributions and multiple vascular distributions or polyvascular disease.[19] The ASCVD event rate among patients with CHD only, cerebrovascular disease only, and PAD only was 42.2 (95% CI: 41.5–42.8), 38.9 (95% CI: 37.6–40.1), and 34.7 (95% CI: 33.2–36.2), respectively. The age-standardized ASCVD event rate per 1000 person-years for those with a history of 1, 2, and 3 conditions including CHD, cerebrovascular disease, and PAD was 40.8 (95% CI: 40.3–41.3), 68.9 (95% CI: 67.9–70.0), and 119.5 (95% CI: 117.0–122.0), respectively (**Fig. 10–3**).

HYPERCHOLESTEROLEMIA

Overview

Hypercholesterolemia is a common lipid disorder that is strongly associated with premature ASCVD.[20] If the 95th percentile of age- and sex-adjusted plasma cholesterol level is taken as the diagnostic threshold, then 1 in 20 people have hypercholesterolemia.[21] Because most cholesterol is carried within LDL particles, isolated hypercholesterolemia most often results from elevated LDL-C.[22] Causes of isolated LDL-C elevation are classified as primary, which encompasses genetic etiologies, and secondary, which includes numerous nongenetic factors.[22,23] Genetic etiologies can be broken down into either single gene causes, such as heterozygous or homozygous familial hypercholesterolemia (FH), or complex polygenic hypercholesterolemia.[24] Secondary nongenetic causes must be ruled out before pursuing a genetic diagnosis. While clinical criteria can establish a diagnosis of heterozygous FH, strategically applied deoxyribonucleic acid (DNA) testing allows for a definitive diagnosis in many patients and families.[24]

Irrespective of the precise cause of hypercholesterolemia, the primary goal of treatment is to reduce LDL-C levels in order to reduce ASCVD risk. In addition to diet and lifestyle modification, drug treatments include statins, ezetimibe, and monoclonal antibody inhibitors of proprotein convertase subtilisin kexin type 9 (PCSK9) and angiopoietin like 3 (ANGPTL3).[25] Some treatment-resistant cases of hypercholesterolemia may benefit from older therapies such as bile acid sequestrants,[25] while in children and young adults with homozygous FH, lipoprotein apheresis is the standard of care.[26] Emerging therapies include inclisiran, bempedoic acid, and evinacumab.[25]

Approach to the Patient with Hypercholesterolemia

Hypercholesterolemia is typically asymptomatic and is usually discovered through biochemical screening (**Table 10–2**). Mild-to-moderate hypercholesterolemia often results from a combination of a polygenic susceptibility component (**Table 10–3**) aggravated by one or more secondary factors (**Table 10–4**). Secondary causes, including lifestyle and diet, some medical conditions, and certain medications can be identified through careful medical history taking and physical examination, focusing on a review of diet, lifestyle, and medications. For instance, physical inactivity and a diet high in saturated and/or trans fatty acids are associated with increased LDL-C.

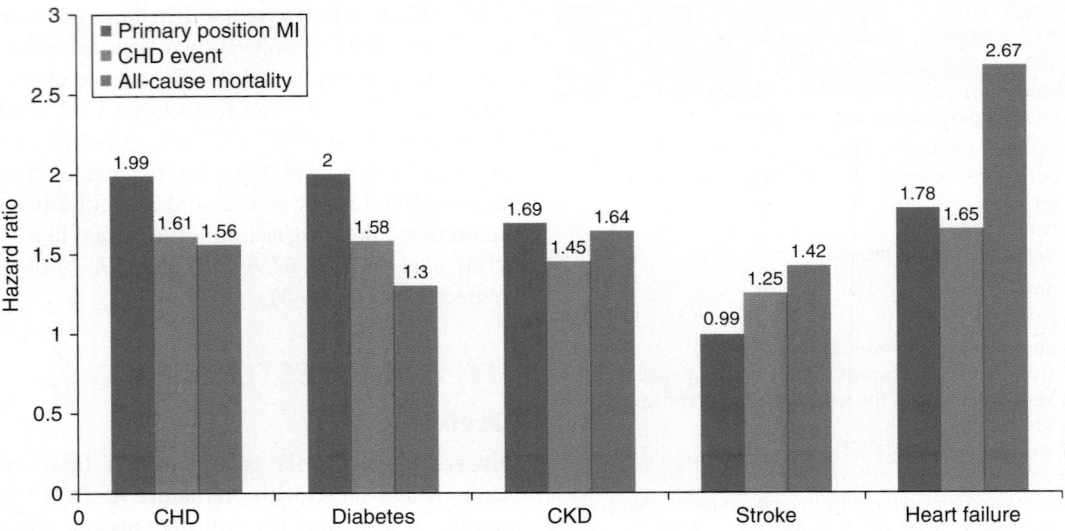

Figure 10–1. Cardiovascular risk among subgroups of survivors of MI undergoing in hospital percutaneous coronary intervention who are treated with intensive medical therapy. Data from Brown TM, Bittner V, Colantonio LD, et al. Residual risk for coronary heart disease events and mortality despite intensive medical management after myocardial infarction. *J Clin Lipidol.* 2020 Mar-Apr;14(2):260-270.

Also, increased LDL-C is seen in patients with hypothyroidism, nephrotic syndrome, obstructive liver disease, and anorexia nervosa (Table 10–4). Furthermore, several drugs, including cyclosporine, amiodarone, thiazide diuretics, and rosiglitazone can cause hypercholesterolemia (**Table 10–5**). A detailed mechanistic description of how these various secondary factors cause hypercholesterolemia is beyond the scope of this chapter, but impaired catabolism of LDL particles via cellular LDL receptors is often implicated. Irrespective of specific mechanisms, secondary causes of hypercholesterolemia must always be ruled out, both clinically and through targeted laboratory investigations (**Table 10–6**).

If a secondary cause for hypercholesterolemia is found, treatment should target the underlying cause before progressing to a lipid-modifying drug. Hypercholesterolemia associated with a secondary factor often resolves, at least partially, with treatment or elimination of the secondary factor. If residual hypercholesterolemia remains, it suggests an underlying endogenous susceptibility and indicates that further specific lipid-modifying drug treatment is needed.

When hypercholesterolemia is severe, a monogenic or single gene cause, such as FH, is likely (**Table 10–7**). Once a monogenic condition is suspected, certain characteristic clinical features should be searched for. For instance, cholesterol

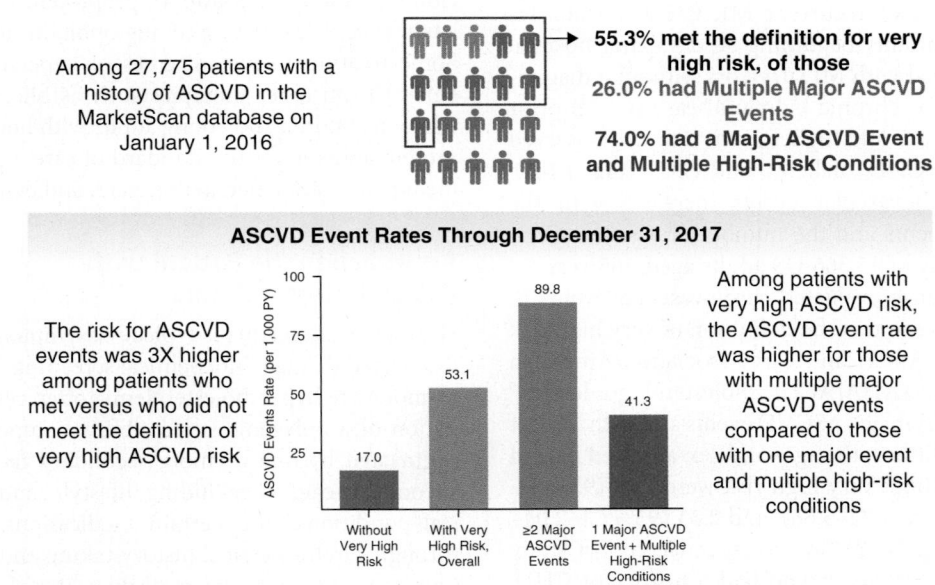

Figure 10–2. Cardiovascular events among very high-risk patients with ASCVD based on the number of events. Reproduced with permission from Colantonio LD, Shannon ED, Orroth KK, et al. Ischemic Event Rates in Very-High-Risk Adults. *J Am Coll Cardiol.* 2019 Nov 19;74(20):2496-2507.

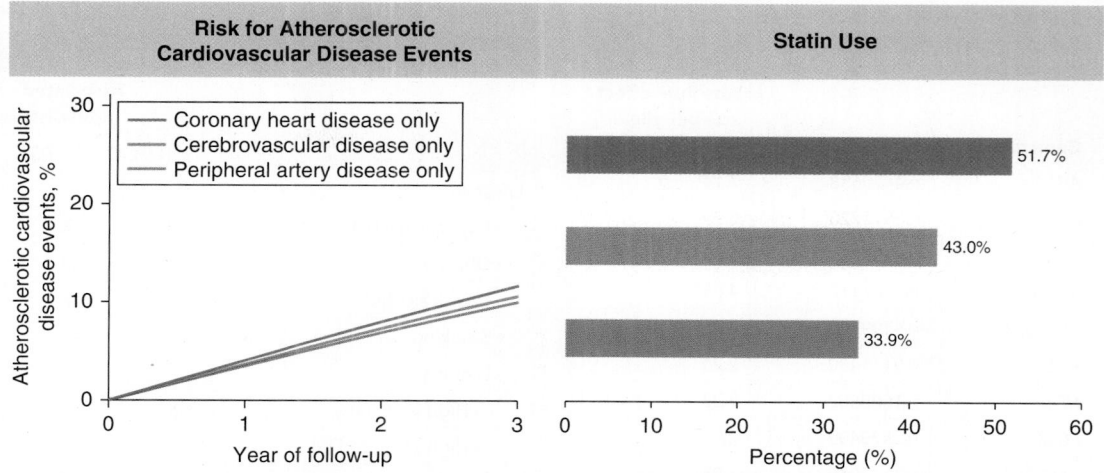

Figure 10–3. Cardiovascular events in high-risk patients with different vascular conditions. Reproduced with permission from Colantonio LD, Hubbard D, Monda KL, et al. Atherosclerotic Risk and Statin Use Among Patients With Peripheral Artery Disease. *J Am Coll Cardiol.* 2020 Jul 21;76(3):251-264.

deposits in the eyelids are called "xanthelasmas."[26] Cholesterol deposits in connective tissues within and surrounding extensor tendons, especially of the hands and Achilles tendons are called "xanthomas."[26] Deposits along the corneal margin are called "arcus cornealis" or "corneal arcus."[26] The most life-threatening deposits are within arteries, leading to premature CHD, occlusive stroke, and peripheral vascular disease.[26] Heterozygous FH is a potent risk factor for early ASCVD and death if undetected and untreated. However, in many cases, a discrete monogenic cause cannot be found and hypercholesterolemia has instead resulted from polygenic susceptibility that has further been aggravated by secondary factors. Targeted genetic analysis may clinically help with the diagnosis of monogenic hypercholesterolemia.[26,27]

Prevalence of Hypercholesterolemia

As mentioned, isolated hypercholesterolemia is seen in about 1 in 20 individuals.[21] Given the importance of distinguishing between primary and secondary causes of hypercholesterolemia,

a longstanding goal has been to enable clinicians to impute a genetic cause. Practically, this simplifies to a diagnosis of heterozygous FH, the most common single gene cause of severe hypercholesterolemia, with prevalence estimated at 1 in 250 to 300 according to epidemiologic and genetic studies.[28] A positive DNA test is considered the gold standard for a definitive diagnosis of heterozygous FH, but this may not always be the case, as discussed next.

In the 1990s, when DNA testing was available only in research laboratories, algorithms were developed to help clinicians diagnose heterozygous FH using a combination of LDL-C levels, physical findings, and personal and family history. Such scoring algorithms include the Simon Broome Register (SBR) criteria and Dutch Lipid Clinic Network (DLCN) score, both of which are still widely used to help clinicians diagnose a patient as having heterozygous FH with confidence levels ranging from "possible" to "definite."[29] These and other diagnostic systems are shown in **Table 10–8**.[29-31] Generally, these scoring schemes provide predictive surrogates for the presence of a pathogenic DNA variant. Some also allow for inclusion of genetic testing

TABLE 10–2. Biochemical Levels for Dyslipidemia			
	LDL-C	**TG**	**HDL-C**
Mild-to-moderate deviation			
- levels	130 to 189 mg/dL	200 to 999 mg/dL	25 to 35 mg/dL
	3.4 to 4.9 mmol/L	2.3 to 11.1 mmol/L	0.7 to 0.9 mmol/L
- etiology	polygenic predisposition (see Table 10–3) plus secondary factors (see Tables 10–4 and 10–5)		
Severe deviation			
- levels	≥190 mg/dL	≥1000 mg/dL	<25 mg/dL
	≥4.9 mmol/L	≥11.1 mmol/L	<0.7 mmol/L
- etiology	monogenic disorders (see Table 10–7) and/or marked polygenic predisposition (see Table 2) plus secondary factors (see Tables 10–4 and 10–5)		

Abbreviations: LDL-C, low-density lipoprotein cholesterol; TG, triglyceride; HDL-C, high-density lipoprotein cholesterol.

TABLE 10–3. Top Ten Common Polygenic Determinants (DNA Polymorphisms) for Major Plasma Lipids

Lipid trait	Gene name	Associated SNP	Absolute effect size per allele in mg/dL
LDL-C	APOE	rs4420638	7.14
	LDLR	rs6511720	6.99
	SORT1	rs629301	5.65
	APOB	rs1367117	4.05
	ABCG5/8	rs4299376	2.75
	ABO	rs9411489	2.24
	HFE	rs1800562	2.22
	PCSK9	rs2479409	2.01
	ST3GAL4	rs11220462	1.95
	MYLIP	rs3757354	1.43
TG	APOA5	rs964184	17.0
	LPL	rs12678919	13.6
	MLXIPL	rs17145738	9.32
	GCKR	rs1260326	8.76
	TYW1B	rs13238203	7.91
	APOB	rs1042034	5.99
	TRIB1	rs2954029	5.64
	APOE	rs439401	5.50
	FRMD5	rs2929282	5.13
	ANGPTL3	rs2131925	4.94
HDL-C	CETP	rs3764261	3.39
	HNF4A	rs1800961	1.88
	LIPC	rs1532085	1.45
	LIPG	rs7241918	1.31
	LCAT	rs16942887	1.27
	PPP1R3B	rs9987289	1.21
	ABCA1	rs1883025	0.94
	PLTP	rs6065906	0.93
	SLC39A8	rs13107325	0.84
	LILRA3	rs386000	0.83

Abbreviations: SNP, single nucleotide polymorphism; LDL-C, low-density lipoprotein cholesterol; TG, triglyceride; HDL-C, high-density lipoprotein cholesterol; APOE, apolipoprotein E; LDLR, low density lipoprotein receptor; SORT1, sortilin 1; APOB, apolipoprotein B; ABCG5/8, ATP-binding cassette sub-family G member 5 and 8; ABO, ABO blood group transferase A, alpha 1-3-N-acetylgalactosaminyltransferase transferase B, alpha 1-3-galactosyltransferase; HFE, hemochromatosis; PCSK9, proprotein convertase subtilisin/kexin type 9; ST3GAL4, ST3 beta-galactoside alpha-2,3-sialyltransferase 4; MYLIP, myosin regulatory light chain interacting protein; APOA5, apolipoprotein A-V; LPL, lipoprotein lipase; MLXIPL, MLX interacting protein-like; GCKR, glucokinase (hexokinase 4) regulator; TYW1B, tRNA-yW synthesizing protein 1 homolog B (S. cerevisiae); TRIB1, tribbles homolog 1 (Drosophila); FRMD5, FERM domain containing 5; ANGPTL3, angiopoietin-like 3; CETP, cholesteryl ester transfer protein, plasma; HNF4A, hepatocyte nuclear factor 4, alpha; LIPC, hepatic lipase; LIPG, endothelial lipase; LCAT, lecithin-cholesterol acyltransferase; protein phosphatase 1; PPP1R3B, regulatory subunit 3B; ABCA1, ATP-binding cassette, sub-family A (ABC1), member 1; PLTP, phospholipid transfer protein; SLC39A8, solute carrier family 39 (zinc transporter), member 8; LILRA3, leukocyte immunoglobulin-like receptor, subfamily A (without TM domain), member 3. Data from Rosenson RS, Hegele RA, Fazio S, Cannon CP. The Evolving Future of PCSK9 Inhibitors. *J Am Coll Cardiol.* 2018 Jul 17;72(3):314-329.

TABLE 10–4. Secondary Lifestyle Factors and Medical Conditions Associated with Dyslipidemia

	Associated primary lipid disturbance		
	↑LDL-C	↑TG	↓HDL-C
Lifestyle			
- Physical inactivity	X	X	
- Obesity		X	X
- Excess alcohol		X	
- Smoking			X
- Dietary			
• High trans-fat	X		
• High saturated fat	X		
• High carbohydrate		X	X
Medical conditions			
- Obstructive liver disease	X		
- Hypothyroidism	X		
- Nephrotic syndrome	X		
- Anorexia	X		
- Metabolic syndrome		X	X
- Insulin resistance		X	X
- Diabetes mellitus		X	X
- Non-alcoholic fatty liver disease		X	X
- Chronic renal failure		X	X
- Cushing syndrome		X	X
- HIV infection		X	X
- Systemic lupus erythematosus		X	X

Abbreviations: LDL-C, low-density lipoprotein cholesterol; TG, triglyceride; HDL-C, high-density lipoprotein cholesterol. Data from Rosenson RS, Hegele RA, Fazio S, et al: The Evolving Future of PCSK9 Inhibitors, *J Am Coll Cardiol.* 2018 Jul 17;72(3):314-329.

results when available. For instance, a positive DNA test alone yields a "definite" diagnosis of heterozygous FH in both SBR and DLCN scoring systems.

All schemes concur suspicion of heterozygous FH is raised by: (1) elevated plasma total or LDL-C found incidentally; (2) a positive family history for premature onset of symptomatic ASCVD in a first-degree male relative <55 years and/or first degree female relative <65 years and/or possibly very high total and/or LDL-C; and (3) suggestive physical findings. Furthermore, patients who develop ASCVD endpoints at young ages should be carefully evaluated for heterozygous FH.

More recently, high throughput genomic analysis in large populations shows that most individuals who meet clinical criteria for "probable" or "definite" FH do not have an identifiable FH mutation. For instance, among individuals ascertained on the basis of an LDL-C >190 mg/dL (>4.9 mmol/L), a pathogenic FH variant was found in <5% of them.[32] By contrast, among patients assessed at a tertiary referral lipid clinic with a diagnosis of at least "probable" FH and LDL-C ≥194 mg/dL

TABLE 10–5. Medications Associated with Dyslipidemia

	Associated primary lipid disturbance		
	↑ LDL-C	↑ TG	↓ HDL-C
Cyclosporine	X		
Amiodarone	X		
High-dose chlorthalidone	X		
Hydrochlorothiazide	X		
Rosiglitazone	X		
Fibrates	X		
Oral estrogens		X	
Tamoxifen		X	
Corticosteroids		X	X
β-blockers		X	X
Retinoids		X	X
Protease inhibitors (especially ritonavir)		X	X
Bile acid binding resins		X	X
Sirolimus		X	X
L-asparaginase		X	X
Atypical antipsychotic agents		X	X

Abbreviations: LDL-C, low-density lipoprotein cholesterol; TG, triglyceride; HDL-C, high-density lipoprotein cholesterol. Data from Rosenson RS, Hegele RA, Fazio S, et al: The Evolving Future of PCSK9 Inhibitors, *J Am Coll Cardiol*. 2018 Jul 17;72(3):314-329.

TABLE 10–6. Investigations for Secondary Causes of Dyslipidemia

Secondary cause	Investigations
Chronic renal failure	Creatinine Urea
Diabetes and insulin resistance	Fasting glucose Hemoglobin A1c Consider serum insulin or C-peptide
Hypothyroidism	Thyroid stimulating hormone (TSH)
Nephrotic syndrome	Urinalysis, 24 hour urine for albumin
Obstructive liver disease	Aspartate aminotransferase (AST) Alanine aminotransferase (ALT) Total bilirubin Alkaline phosphatase (ALP)

assessment suggests a clinical suspicion of FH and also in proportion to the degree of LDL-C elevation.

Classification of Hypercholesterolemia

Table 10–9 shows a classification system[21] for hypercholesterolemia based on two key parameters: (1) presence of absence of severe hypercholesterolemia, defined as LDL-C ≥190 mg/dL (≥4.9 mmol/L); and (2) presence or absence of a pathogenic DNA variant in an FH-associated gene (*LDLR*, *APOB*, or *PCSK9*). In this system, there are four classes of individuals: (1) hypercholesterolemia positive and mutation positive (ie, heterozygous FH); (2) hypercholesterolemia positive and mutation negative (ie, severe hypercholesterolemia); (3) hypercholesterolemia negative and mutation positive (ie, patient at risk for hypercholesterolemia); and (4) neither hypercholesterolemia

(≥5 mmol/L), ~50% had a pathogenic FH-related DNA variant. For those with LDL-C ≥310 mg/dL (≥8 mmol/L), this prevalence rose to >90%.[33] Thus, the prevalence of pathogenic variants among patients referred to lipid clinic increases if medical

TABLE 10–7. Severe Monogenic Dyslipidemias

Primary lipid disturbance	Disease name	Inheritance	Causative gene/location	OMIM numbers
↑ LDL-C	Hypercholesterolemia	Codominant	*LDLR* / 19p13.3	143890, 606945
	Hypercholesterolemia	Codominant	*APOB* / 2p24-p23	144010
	Hypercholesterolemia	Codominant	*PSCK9* / 1p32.3	603776, 607786
	Hypercholesterolemia	Recessive	*LDLRAP1* / 1p36-p35	603813, 605747
↑ TG	Familial chylomicronemia	Recessive	*LPL* / 8p22	609708, 238600
			APOC2 / 19q13.2	608083, 207750
			APOA5 / 11q23	606368
			LMF1 / 16p13.3	611761, 246650
			GPIHBP1 / 8q24.3	612757
	Transient infantile HTG	Recessive	*GPD1* / 12q12	138420, 614480
	Dysbetalipoproteinemia	Dominant	*APOE* / 19q13	107741
		Recessive	*APOE* / 19q13	107741
↓HDL-C	Tangier disease	Recessive	*ABCA1* / 9q31	600046, 205400
	LCAT deficiency	Recessive	*LCAT* / 16q22	606967, 245900
	Hypoalphalipoproteinemia	Codominant	*APOA1* / 11q23	107680, 604091

Abbreviations: LDL-C, low-density lipoprotein cholesterol; TG, triglyceride; HDL-C, high-density lipoprotein cholesterol; OMIM, Online Inheritance in Man. Data from Rosenson RS, Hegele RA, Fazio S, et al: The Evolving Future of PCSK9 Inhibitors, *J Am Coll Cardiol*. 2018 Jul 17;72(3):314-329.

TABLE 10–8. Comparison of Clinical Scoring Systems for Familial Hypercholesterolemia (FH)

Criteria	Simon Broome Register	Dutch Lipid Clinic Network	MED-PED	ICD-10	Canadian Criteria
Lipids					
Total cholesterol (mmol/l)	>7.5 (adult) (a) >6.7 (child) (a)	NA	NA	NA	NA
LDL cholesterol (mmol/l)	>4.9 (adult) (a) >4.0 (child) (a)	>8.5 (8) 6.5–8.4 (5) 5.0–6.4 (3) 4.0–4.9 (1)	5.7–9.3[b]	>5.0 (adult) (a) >4.0 (child) (a)	>4.0 (child) (a) >4.5 (18–39 years) (a) >5.0 (>40 years) (a) >8.5 (b)
Physical stigmata					
Personal	Tendon xanthoma (b)	Tendon xanthoma (6) Arcus cornealis[c] (4)	NA	NA	Tendon xanthoma (c)
Family	Tendon xanthoma in one relative (b)	Tendon xanthoma or arcus cornealis (2)	NA	NA	NA
Family history					
CAD	MI aged <50 years in two relatives or aged <60 years in one relative (d)	Premature CAD[d] (2) Premature CVD or PVD[d]	NA	Premature CAD in one relative (b)	Premature CAD in one relative[d] (d)
LDL cholesterol (mmol/l)	>7.5 in one or two relatives (e)	Child with LDL-cholesterol >95th percentile (2)	NA	One affected relative (c)	One relative with high LDL-cholesterol level (d)
Genetics	NA	NA	Known FH in family member	NA	FH mutation in one family member (c)
Genetics					
Genetic mutations	*APOB, LDLR,* or *PCSK9* gene mutation (c)	*APOB, LDLR,* or *PCSK9* gene mutation (8)	NA	*APOB, LDLR,* or *PCSK9* gene mutation (d)	*APOB, LDLR,* or *PCSK9* gene mutation (c)
Diagnosis					
Diagnosis of FH	Definite: a + b or c Probable: a + d OR a + e	Definite: >8 Probable: 6–8 Possible: 3–5	Meets adjusted LDL-cholesterol cut-off point	a + (b or c) OR d	Definite: (a + c) OR b Probable: a + d

[a]Requires a diagnosis of FH in a family member. [b]Cut-off based on year and degree of separation from affected relative. [c]Arcus cornealis when aged <45 years. [d]Aged <55 years in men and aged <60 years in women.
Abbreviations: CAD, coronary artery disease; CVD, cerebrovascular disease; FH, familial hypercholesterolaemia; ICD, International Classification of Diseases; MED-PED, Make Early Diagnosis – Prevent Early Death; MI, myocardial infarction; NA, not applicable; PVD, peripheral vascular disease. Data from Wang J, Dron JS, Ban MR, et al. Polygenic Versus Monogenic Causes of Hypercholesterolemia Ascertained Clinically. *Arterioscler Thromb Vasc Biol.* 2016 Dec;36(12):2439-2445.

TABLE 10–9. Classification of Hypercholesterolemia

	Familial hypercholesterolemia	Severe hypercholesterolemia	Genetic risk factor for hypercholesterolemia	Neither variant nor severe hypercholesterolemia
LDL cholesterol ≥190 mg/dL (>4.9 mmol/L)	yes	yes	no	no
pathogenic FH variant	yes	no (either untested or undetected)	yes	no
population prevalence	~1:300 to 500	1:20	~1:500 to 1000	>90%
inheritance	autosomal dominant	some are polygenic	incomplete penetrance	not applicable
physical exam findings (xanthomas, arcus cornealis)	up to 50%	very low to absent	absent	absent
causative genes	heterozygous variants in *LDLR, APOB, PCSK9*	not applicable	heterozygous variants in *LDLR, APOB, PCSK9*	not applicable
ASCVD risk	>20-fold increase	>5-fold increase	>2-fold increase	reference
genetic cascade screening warranted	yes	no	yes	no
biochemical cascade screening warranted	yes	yes	yes	no

Abbreviations: FH, familial hypercholesterolemia; ASCVD, Atherosclerotic Cardiovascular Disease. Reproduced with permission from Khera AV, Hegele RA. What Is Familial Hypercholesterolemia, and Why Does It Matter? *Circulation.* 2020 Jun 2;141(22):1760-1763.

nor mutation (ie, general or normal population). Clinical features of these groups are described as follows:

1. Familial hypercholesterolemia: Pathogenic FH variant and severe hypercholesterolemia. These patients fit our classical concept of heterozygous FH, with prevalence of about 1 in 300.[34] Some have physical findings—corneal arcus, xanthelasma, and xanthomas—and are susceptible to early ASCVD, with >20-fold increased risk compared to those with normal LDL-C and no mutation (ie, group 4 in this list).[32] The presence of a pathogenic mutation should prompt cascade screening of relatives. Furthermore, knowledge of genotype may improve compliance with lipid management.

2. Severe hypercholesterolemia: No pathogenic variant, but severe hypercholesterolemia. These individuals are quite prevalent in the population (ie, 1 in 20). Genetic testing when performed in these patients is reported as "negative" for various

reasons. For example, the patient carries a rare DNA variant that does not meet standard criteria for pathogenicity, or carries a variant in an undiscovered gene, or has a polygenic inherited basis for their dyslipidemia (see Genetics section). Patients in this large subgroup are still very susceptible to premature ASCVD, with >5-fold increased risk compared to those with normal LDL-C and no mutation (ie, group 4 in this list).[32] They should be treated assertively with lipid-lowering according to treatment guidelines (**Table 10–10**). Furthermore, about one-third of relatives of these patients also have hypercholesterolemia. Thus, biochemical screening of family members of patients with severe hypercholesterolemia but no mutation is recommended.

3. Pathogenic variant, but no hypercholesterolemia. Such individuals are rare in the population, with prevalence of 1 in 500 to 1000.[34] Normal LDL-C may be explained by a

TABLE 10–10. Key Recommendations for Primary and Secondary ASCVD Prevention

	AHA/ACC	ESC/EAS
Primary prevention		
Risk assessment	*PCE:* - Measures 10-year risk fatal and non-fatal MI and stroke - Incorporates age, race, gender, TC, HDL-C, SBP, DM2, HTN treatment, smoking - Risk groups: high (≥ 20%), intermediate (≥ 7.5 to < 20%), borderline (≥ 5 to < 7.5%), low (< 5%) *Risk-enhancing factors:* FHx premature ASCVD, LDL-C 160–189 mg/dL, metabolic syndrome, CKD, chronic inflammation, premature menopause, preeclampsia ethnicity, ↑ hsCRP, ↑ Lp(a), ↑ apoB, ABI < 0.9 *CAC (class IIa):* Used in intermediate PCE risk. If 0 → defer statin (except FHx premature ASCVD, DM2, smoking)	*SCORE:* - Measures 10-year risk of first fatal atherosclerotic event (2 charts for high- and low-risk countries) - Incorporates age, gender, TC, HDL-C, SBP, smoking - Risk groups: Very high (≥ 10%), high (≥ 5 to < 10%), moderate (≥ 1 to < 5%), low (< 1%) *Risk-modifying factors:* social deprivation, obesity, physical inactivity, psychosocial stress, FHx premature ASCVD, chronic inflammation, atrial fibrillation, LVH, CKD, OSA, NAFLD, major psychiatric disorders, treatment for HIV infection *CAC (class IIb):* Used in low-moderate risk.
Treatment	*Statin (class I):* LDL-C ≥ 190 mg/dL (> 4.9 mmol/L) (high intensity), DM2 and age 40–75 years (moderate), intermediate PCE risk (moderate); high PCE risk (high) *Non-statin:* Only in FH (class IIa/IIb)	*LDL-C treatment goals:* ≥ 50% reduction and LDL-C < 70 mg/dL (high total risk*) or < 55 mg/dL (very high total risk†). Using statin + non-statin.
Secondary prevention		
Risk groups	Very high ASCVD risk: Multiple ASCVD events OR 1 ASCVD event + multiple high-risk conditions. All others are not very high risk.	All are considered very high total risk†.
LDL-C goal	LDL-C < 70 mg/dL (< 1.8 mmol/L) (very high risk)	LDL-C < 55 mg/dL (< 1.4 mmol/L) and ≥ 50% reduction from baseline
Non-statins		
Ezetimibe	Primarily for secondary prevention (class IIa). Add to statin to reach LDL-C goal if not already met.	For primary and secondary prevention (class I). Add to high-intensity statin to reach LDL-C goal if not already met.
PCSK-9	Primarily for secondary prevention (class IIa). Add to statin + ezetimibe to reach LDL-C goal if not already met.	For primary (class I-FH, IIb-other) and secondary (class I) prevention. Add to statin + ezetimibe to reach LDL-C goal if not already met.
Icosapent ethyl	Not included.	For high or very high total risk when TG 135–499 mg/dL despite statin (class IIa)

Abbreviations: ASCVD, atherosclerotic cardiovascular disease; AHA/ACC, American Heart Association/American College of Cardiology; ESC/EAS European Society of Cardiology/ European Atherosclerosis Society; PCE pooled cohort equations; MI, myocardial infarction; TC, total cholesterol; HDL-C, high-density lipoprotein cholesterol; SBP, systolic blood pressure; DM2, type 2 diabetes mellitus; HTN. hypertension; FHx, family history; LDL-C, low-density lipoprotein cholesterol; CKD, chronic kidney disease; hsCRP, high-sensitivity C-reactive protein; Lp(a), lipoprotein(a), apo B, apolipoprotein B; ABI, ankle brachial index; CAC, coronary artery calcium; SCORE. Systematic Coronary Risk Estimation; LVH, left ventricular hypertrophy; OSA, obstructive sleep apnea; NAFLD, non-alcoholic fatty liver disease; PCSK9, proprotein convertase subtilisin/kexin type 9; FH, familial hypercholesterolemia.

*High total ASCVD risk (ESC/EAS): SCORE ≥5 to <10%, TC >310 mg/dL, LDL-C >190 mg/dL (> 4.9 mmol/L) or BP ≥ 180/110 mmHg; FH without risk factors, moderate CKD, DM without target organ damage with DM duration ≥10 years or other additional risk factors

†Very high total ASCVD risk (ESC/EAS): ASCVD (clinical/imaging), SCORE ≥10%, FH with ASCVD, severe CKD, DM2 with target organ damage. Reproduced with permission from Raygor V, Khera A. New Recommendations and Revised Concepts in Recent Guidelines on the Management of Dyslipidemias to Prevent Cardiovascular Disease: the 2018 ACC/AHA and 2019 ESC/EAS Guidelines. *Curr Cardiol Rep.* 2020 Jul 9;22(9):87.

milder or variably penetrant DNA variant, offsetting beneficial DNA variants, or positive influences from nongenetic factors. These patients still have ~2-fold increased risk of ASCVD compared to those with normal LDL-C and no mutation (ie, group 4 in this list).[34] LDL-C levels may be elevated at various times outside of laboratory testing, which might explain increased ASCVD risk. Periodic monitoring of the LDL-C level is recommended, and lipid lowering therapy should be considered if an elevated level is subsequently observed. Treatment in primary prevention of ASCVD for such patients might be lower than in those without a pathogenic variant. Because the DNA variant has variable impact on LDL-C levels, biochemical screening of family members is warranted. More research is needed on long-term outcomes and interventions for this patient subgroup.

4. Neither pathogenic variant nor severe hypercholesterolemia. About 90% of the adult population would fit into this category. Recommendations for lipid screening and treatment for these individuals would follow the appropriate national guidelines, which in the absence of severe hypercholesterolemia, typically recommend LDL-lowering treatment for individuals with established ASCVD or for primary prevention in those at high risk of ASCVD due to other risk factors (Table 10–10).

Mechanism of Hypercholesterolemia

LDL particles transport the majority of circulating cholesterol from the liver to the periphery.[29] After a lifespan of about 3 days, LDL particles return to and are catabolized by the liver. Apolipoprotein B-100 (apoB-100) on the LDL particle surface binds to the LDL receptor; the LDL particle is degraded and the LDL receptor is recycled to the cell surface. Increased LDL-C levels in FH results from impaired LDL-receptor activity, which is often caused by different classes of mutations that directly affect the receptor.[29] Because of the central role of the LDL receptor in FH, its life cycle is briefly summarized in **Fig. 10–4** and its legend, including the roles of several interacting proteins.

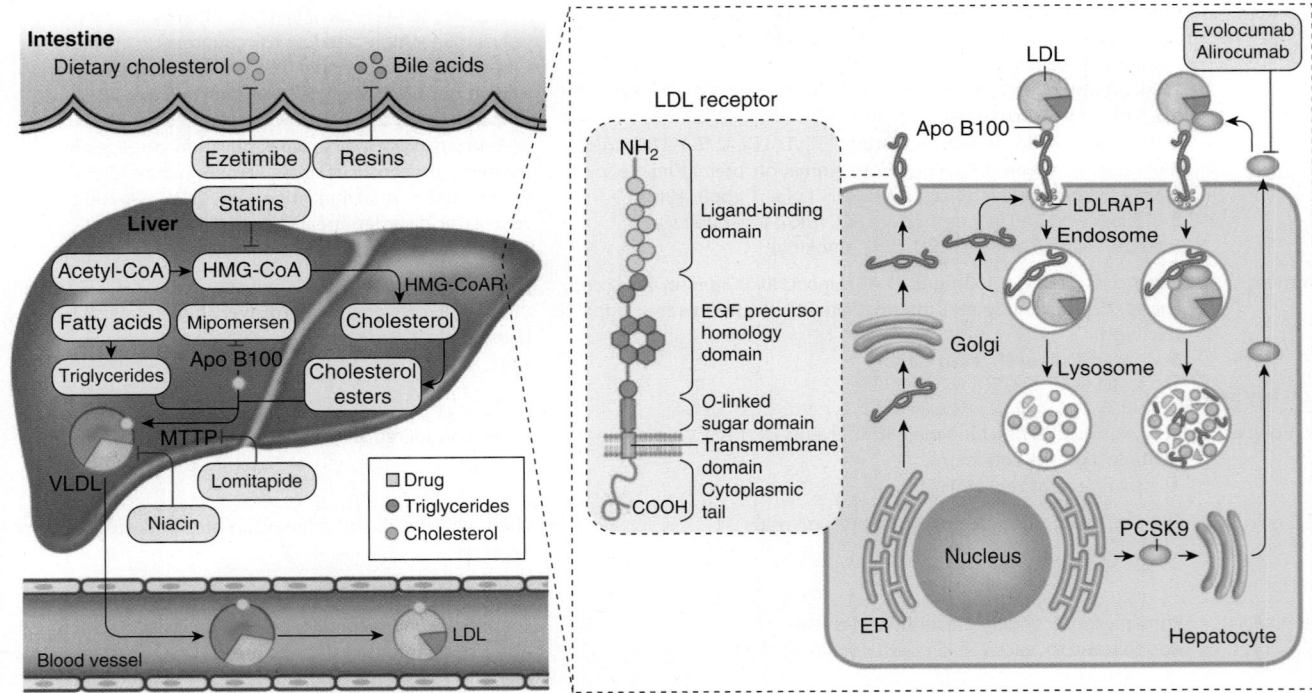

Figure 10–4. Basic pathways in LDL synthesis and LDLR-mediated uptake. Dietary cholesterol and bile acids enter the circulation through the upper and lower small intestine, respectively. These uptake pathways are disrupted by the cholesterol absorption inhibitor ezetimibe and bile acid sequestrants (resins), which both reduce the intrahepatic cholesterol pool. Cholesterol is synthesized within the liver by a multistep process that begins with acetyl coenzyme A (CoA). 3-hydroxy-3-methyl-glutaryl (HMG) CoA reductase (HMGCoAR) is the rate-limiting enzyme, whose activity is inhibited by statin drugs. Triglycerides are synthesized by esterification of fatty acids on a 3-carbon glycerol backbone. Microsomal triglyceride transfer protein (MTTP) assembles triglycerides and esterified cholesterol into nascent very low density lipoprotein (VLDL) particles, with apoB-100 on their surface. In the circulation, endovascular lipases process VLDL to LDL. LDL is catabolized by the LDL receptor mainly on hepatocytes. After synthesis and secretion from endoplasmic reticulum (ER), LDLRs are processed in the Golgi where sugars are added and finally transported to the plasma membrane, where they cluster within clathrin coated pits. The exposed ligand-binding domain binds to the apoB-100 moiety on LDL and the LDL-LDLR complex undergoes endocytosis, which is assisted by LDL receptor associated protein 1 (LDLRAP1). Within the cell, LDL components are targeted for lysosomal degradation, whereas the LDLR is recycled to the cell surface. Intracellular cholesterol upregulates the expression of proprotein convertase subtilisin kexin type 9 (PCSK9), which undergoes autocatalytic processing in the ER, is secreted and circulates briefly in plasma. In the presence of PCSK9, all components of the endocytosed complex are degraded, thereby short circuiting normal LDLR recycling and reducing the overall capacity for LDL catabolism. EGF, epidermal growth factor. Reproduced with permission from Defesche JC, Gidding SS, Harada-Shiba M, et al. Familial hypercholesterolaemia. *Nat Rev Dis Primers.* 2017 Dec 7;3:17093.

Elevated Low-Density Lipoprotein Cholesterol and Atherogenesis

Chronically excessive levels of LDL-C in FH are directly causal for ASCVD.[35,36] LDL has manifold deleterious effects on vascular function, which have been comprehensively documented, including attenuated arterial endothelial dilation, which is an early manifestation of vascular dysfunction.[35] LDL that does not undergo regulated receptor-mediated uptake is taken up in an unregulated manner by scavenger receptors on arterial wall macrophages. Entrapped LDL lipids can become oxidized, generating toxic intermediates that induce cytokine production and chemotaxis of inflammatory cells. Arterial wall macrophages can become engorged with cholesterol from LDL, creating foam cells, which are a key component of atherogenic plaques. Lipids engulfed by macrophages become oxidized, generating toxic intermediates, which induce cytokine production and inflammatory cell chemotaxis. Occlusive plaques, often the result of rupture compounded by thrombosis, result in ASCVD, such as CHD or stroke. Because ASCVD risk is increased in hypercholesterolemia, it is essential to clinically evaluate the cardiovascular system. Risk factors that can accelerate onset of ASCVD in patients with hypercholesterolemia include advanced age, elevated body mass index, type 2 diabetes mellitus, hypertension, and poor lifestyle habits, such as an unhealthy diet and smoking.[36]

Genetics of Familial Hypercholesterolemia

Research on FH has strongly impacted on basic science, cardiology, and public health. Michael Brown and Joseph Goldstein's Nobel Prize–winning research on the LDL receptor in FH patients provided the first model of receptor-mediated endocytosis of cellular ligands.[29] Clinical observations in FH patients have contributed to our understanding of LDL-C's causal role in ASCVD.[29] The US Center for Disease Control and Prevention recognizes FH as a "Tier 1" genomic condition in which genetic testing to identify carriers of a pathogenic variant is clinically valuable.[37]

Although previously regarded as a monogenic disorder whose inheritance followed Mendelian rules of inheritance, FH is more accurately envisioned as a group of conditions with variable inheritance patterns, molecular etiologies, and clinical presentations (Table 10–7).[29] Three main FH-causing genes are the *LDLR* gene on chromosome 19p13.3, the *APOB* gene on chromosome 2p24-p23, and the *PCSK9* gene on chromosome 1p32.3.[29] FH results from deficiency or defective function of the LDL receptor, either directly because of molecular defects in the receptor itself, or indirectly because of aberrantly functioning interacting proteins such as binding defective apoB-100 or abnormally overactive PCSK9. For the three main FH genes, one copy of a pathogenic variant acts dominantly to produce the disease phenotype (ie, the conventional model of heterozygous FH). Furthermore, many patients who inherit two pathogenic variants or alleles have a more severe phenotype, consistent with homozygous FH.[29]

The observed inheritance of FH is thus more complicated than implied by a simple autosomal dominant or recessive model. FH is more precisely viewed as an autosomal codominant condition, given that both variant alleles from each affected parent contribute to the much worse clinical phenotype in a homozygote (eg, by additively acting to raise the LDL-C level). The result is a very severe phenotype in homozygotes, and a dramatic but less severe phenotype in heterozygotes. The two forms are often considered separately because heterozygous FH is relatively common, comprising a substantial proportion of adult lipid clinic patients with twice-normal LDL-C levels who can be managed with pharmacological treatment.[29] In contrast, homozygous FH primarily affects children and young adults with four- to six-times normal LDL-C levels; patients often require periodic lifelong extracorporeal plasma exchange or apheresis to offload the excess LDL particles.[29] Most cardiologists will never encounter a case of homozygous FH over their entire career.

LDLR Gene Mutations in Familial Hypercholesterolemia

At least 80% of genetically defined cases of FH are caused by *LDLR* variants, with >2000 such rare variants reported in the literature, and >3000 deposited in the international ClinVar database of genetic variants.[38] Several types of DNA variant can cause FH, including: (1) large-scale DNA copy number variations (~10% of all mutations); (2) null alleles that prevent secretion of receptor; (3) small insertions or deletions in or near the coding sequence; (4) nonsense mutations within the coding region; (5) splicing mutations, typically noncoding and occurring at intron-exon boundaries; and (6) missense mutations typically altering a single amino acid residue anywhere in the protein.[29]

LDLR mutations affect function at all stages of receptor-mediated endocytosis (Fig. 10–4).[29] Six mutation classes correlate with malfunctions in cell biology: class 1: absent receptor synthesis; class 2: impaired receptor release from the endoplasmic reticulum; class 3: abnormal binding to apoB; class 4: defective clustering in clathrin pits or internalization; class 5: defective recycling; and class 6: failed targeting to the basolateral membrane. These six classes can be reduced to two broad categories of *LDLR* mutations: (1) those resulting in synthesis of either no protein or a completely nonfunctional receptor (ie, receptor-negative or receptor-null mutations); and (2) those resulting in synthesis of an ineffective receptor (ie, receptor-defective mutations).

Only ~10% of *LDLR* variants that have been deemed pathogenic have actually been studied functionally in cell biology experiments in vitro.[38] Such experiments provide the highest level of biological proof of pathogenicity. For other mutations, indirect approaches are used to infer their pathogenicity and possible clinical relevance. Some mutations that were initially reported as pathogenic based on computer predictions were later reclassified after family studies showed the variant failed to cosegregate with FH status or functional studies showed normal function of the protein expressed from the variant allele. Predictions of a variant's pathogenicity by computer programs can show up to 50% discordance with gold standard laboratory experiments.[38] The clinical consequences of reporting either false-positive or false-negative genetic diagnoses of FH to patients are obvious, and range from labeling and stigmatization in the case of the former to a false sense of security in the case of the latter.[24,27] The American College of Medical Genetics and Genomics has developed criteria for reporting variant pathogenicity in genetic disorders, including FH in order to reduce the risk of misdiagnosis.[39]

Variations in lipid profile among individuals with the identical pathogenic mutation might be the result of interacting genetic effects, either large-effect variants, polygenic effects, gene–environment interactions (including the effects of diet and lifestyle), or non-Mendelian mechanisms.[29] The non-Mendelian mechanisms include environmentally induced epigenetic effects, mitochondrial influences, or somatically acquired DNA variation in the liver or other tissues.

Other Genes Causing Familial Hypercholesterolemia

In addition to pathogenic variants in *LDLR*, rare mutations within the LDL receptor binding domain of the *APOB* gene cause a dominantly segregating FH-like phenotype called "familial defective apoB."[26,29] Between 5% and 10% of patients clinically diagnosed with heterozygous FH have such *APOB* mutations and not *LDLR* mutations.[23,29] In addition, rare gain-of-function mutations in *PCSK9* were found to underlie a few cases of dominantly segregating FH, such that <1% of patients clinically diagnosed with heterozygous FH have *PCSK9* gain-of-function mutations.[40] Attributing causality to potential FH-causing variants in *APOB* and *PCSK9* is even more complicated than for *LDLR*, because both genes are very polymorphic and in vitro functional studies are more difficult to perform compared with studies on the LDL receptor.[38] Finally, next-generation DNA sequencing efforts in FH families negative for *LDLR*, *APOB*, and *PCSK9* variants have found that in certain rare variants in *APOE*, encoding apoE can rarely cause a dominantly segregating FH-like phenotype.[29]

Other reported causal genes for FH (eg, *LDLRAP1*, *LIPA*, *ABCG5*, and *ABCG8*) should be included in genetic testing, but these together explain <1% of all FH cases.[29] For these "minor genes," two mutant alleles act recessively, sometimes resulting in a relatively severe phenotype consistent with homozygous FH. Some of the "minor genes" for FH were already known to cause well-known non-FH dyslipidemia syndromes: for example, sitosterolemia in the case of *ABCG5* and *ABCG8*, dysbetalipoproteinemia in the case of *APOE*, and cholesterol ester storage disease (lysosomal acid lipase deficiency) in the case of *LIPA*.[41] The reason that FH is clinically expressed in such patients is unexplained. Comprehensive exome-wide and genome-wide sequencing efforts have not identified other FH-related genes.

Homozygous Familial Hypercholesterolemia

Homozygous FH can be treated as a distinct entity from heterozygous FH.[29] Homozygous FH is an ultrarare but significant pediatric disorder usually caused by loss-of-function variants on both *LDLR* alleles. In the era before statins and lipoprotein apheresis, patients with homozygous FH sometimes died from ASCVD end points aged ≤25 years. Patients can be simple homozygotes (same mutation in both alleles of the same gene)

or compound heterozygotes (different mutations in each allele of the same gene) or, rarely, double heterozygotes (mutations in two different genes). Archetypally, patients with homozygous FH have two mutant *LDLR* alleles, with both parents affected by heterozygous FH but, less commonly, patients with mutations on both alleles of *APOB*, *LDLRAP1*, and *PCSK9* genes can express homozygous FH, with codominant inheritance seen with *APOB* and *PCSK9*, and a recessive pattern with *LDLRAP1*. Untreated LDL-C levels vary across genotypes: levels are highest with two *LDLR* null alleles, lower with two *LDLR* defective alleles or two mutant PCSK9 alleles, and lowest with two mutant *APOB* alleles and in double heterozygotes.[29] However, wide variations in LDL-C levels are seen among homozygous FH patients with identical genotypes. Classic pediatric homozygous FH with xanthomatosis, severe hypercholesterolemia, bi-allelic mutations, and plasmapheresis eligibility is, therefore, a severe subgroup of a heterogeneous spectrum of patients with homozygous FH. Management is primarily determined by LDL-C levels.[26]

Screening to Find Familial Hypercholesterolemia Patients

What is the best screening method to find new cases of FH: universal screening or cascade screening? Universal population-wide screening has been proposed in the adult, adolescent, child, or infant populations, using lipid values, DNA testing, or both. A pilot screening project obtained capillary blood samples from 10,095 children aged 1 to 2 years during routine immunization visits and tested for both cholesterol levels and known genetic mutations; family members of positive cases were then also screened.[42] This program had an overall case-finding rate of eight FH cases identified for every 1000 children screened (four children and four parents), allowing for early monitoring and intervention. Other childhood universal screening programs using lipid levels and prediction scores have shown success. Universal screening programs minimize missed cases, but can be costly especially if genetic testing is included. However, preventing morbidity and mortality makes universal screening potentially cost-effective, especially with declining costs for DNA analysis.

By contrast, cascade screening tests all first-degree relatives of patients identified with FH, followed by all first-degree relatives of further identified cases, and so on.[41] The target population is enriched for positive cases because first-degree, second-degree, and third-degree relatives will have a 50%, 25%, and 12.5% likelihood, respectively, of carrying the causative mutation, which maximizes cost-effectiveness.[29] Both lipid-only and genetic-only screening of relatives has been proposed, as has a combination approach, whereby relatives are screened with lipid levels followed by genetic testing when values exceed diagnostic thresholds. Cascade screening might fail to ascertain some cases, since it depends on acceptance by family members[43] and requires the starting point of an identified FH case.

Polygenic Influences

Between 20% and 40% of patients with severe hypercholesterolemia and no FH mutation have polygenic hypercholesterolemia.[29] In this situation, patients inherit numerous small-effect alleles of common single nucleotide polymorphisms (SNPs) from across the genome. Each SNP genotype is associated in genome-wide association studies with subtle but reproducible and significant increases in LDL-C level.[44] Out of the thousands of genomic loci have been associated with increased LDL-C levels, the top ten are shown in Table 10–3.[45] Cumulatively, these raise LDL-C into the range seen in patients with mutation-positive FH. Some of the top small-effect loci associated with LDL-C level overlap with large-effect loci causing heterozygous FH, such as *APOB*, *LDLR*, and *PCSK9*, whereas others have no connection to lipid metabolism. In the general population, most individuals carry a balance of LDL-C–raising and –lowering alleles. But individuals at the high extreme of this distribution have unfortunately inherited a preponderance of LDL-C–raising alleles at most of these loci.

At present, there is no clinical standard for the precise loci and alleles that should be included in a future clinical polygenic risk score for LDL-C; some research based scores have incorporated literally millions of SNPs.[46] Although inheritance of polygenic hypercholesterolemia does not follow not simple Mendelian rules, the LDL-C–raising alleles cluster in families. Also, a high polygenic score can worsen the biochemical phenotype when a heterozygous large-effect FH variant is present. Patients with FH owing to polygenic risk appear to have less severe preclinical atherosclerosis compared with individuals with large effect FH-causing mutations.[44]

Combined Hyperlipidemia

Combined hyperlipidemia (CHL, formerly hyperlipoproteinemia type 2B) is characterized by concurrently elevated total and LDL-C and triglyceride (TG) (all >90th percentile for age and sex) in probands and affected relatives.[47] The elevated TG in this phenotype is due to liver derived VLDL and not intestinally-derived chylomicrons. ASCVD risk in CHL is related to the degree of LDL-C and TG elevation, which is integrated by the number of apoB-containing particles, a laboratory measurement that is discussed elsewhere. Some clinicians still believe that CHL is a monogenic disorder, like FH. However, after almost 40 years of careful searching, no single gene has yet been identified. Instead, evidence shows CHL is a complex trait that results from the accumulation of numerous small-effect common alleles from many different chromosomes and genetic loci.[47] In addition, there are important contributions from secondary nongenetic metabolic factors. There is no consensus about the best approach to genetic testing for this condition, either with polygenic scoring or next-generation sequencing, or both. The diagnosis is mainly based on clinical and biochemical criteria.

There are no recent published guidelines or best practice statements for management of patients with the CHL profile. Because elevated LDL-C is a core biochemical feature of this phenotype, it is reasonable to follow treatment principles from management of heterozygous FH patients who have an equivalent degree of LDL-C elevation.[22,23] This would include statin treatment if LDL-C is sufficiently elevated, and especially with a positive family history of premature ASCVD and the presence of other risk factors including elevated LDL-C. In addition, the associated hypertriglyceridemia in CHL may exacerbate the risk of the elevated LDL-C. Treatment of the TG component would center on nonpharmacologic approaches such as weight reduction through a prudent diet with reduced intake of saturated and trans fats and of high glycemic index foods. With the exception of the omega-3 preparation icosapent ethyl, the role of adjunctive pharmacologic agents for TG-reduction on top of statins to reduce ASCVD risk is not proven.

Other Genetic Dyslipidemias

Other dyslipidemias can be present in cohorts of patients with hypercholesterolemia. For instance, a Danish study observed that LDL-C levels in 25% of patients with hypercholesterolemia were raised due to elevated Lp(a) cholesterol levels.[48] In addition, hyperlipoprotein(a) levels increased ASCVD risk in patients with heterozygous FH.[49] Furthermore, a large US study showed that ~4% of individuals with LDL-C levels ≥190 mg/dL (≥ 4.9 mmol/L) had plasma β sitosterol levels >99th percentile, and ~0.3% had levels consistent with sitosterolemia, in turn consistent with genetic studies showing that some patients with FH have pathogenic mutations in sitosterolemia-related genes.[50] Finally, in a cohort of 750 individuals from Portugal with suspected FH, about 0.5% had lysosomal acid lipase deficiency owing to *LIPA* gene variants.[51] Therefore, other genetic dyslipidemias, including elevated Lp(a), sitosterolemia, or lysosomal acid lipase deficiency, are sometimes found in individuals with suspected FH.

Treatment of Hypercholesterolemia

Numerous agencies recommend LDL-C as the primary target of therapy to reduce ASCVD risk (Table 10–10). These guidelines are directly relevant for patients with hypercholesterolemia, irrespective of the underlying cause.[22,23] LDL-C goals are recommended for patients who are stratified into particular risk categories, as determined using risk algorithms such as the Framingham risk score.[52] For instance, subjects at very high ASCVD risk should aim for optimal LDL-C <1.4 mmol/L (< 70 mg/dL) according to recent European and North American treatment guidelines (Table 10–10). Treatment of patients at lower ASCVD risk follows along a graded algorithm of intensity of treatment based on LDL-C target levels.[52] Treatment includes lifestyle interventions and drug therapy.

Lifestyle Interventions

Lifestyle modification is the foundation of treatment in most individuals with hypercholesterolemia. Patients with hypercholesterolemia are encouraged to attain and maintain a desirable body weight through appropriate dietary modification and exercise. Of critical importance in these patients is modification of major ASCVD risk factors, including smoking cessation and control of glycemia and blood pressure.

Dietary interventions for the patient with hypercholesterolemia include: (1) overall reduction in intake and reduced portion sizes; (2) redistribution of relative quantities of sources of calories (eg, replace high glycemic index foods with complex carbohydrates, and replace trans and saturated fats with monounsaturated and polyunsaturated fats); (3) addition or enhancement of specific foods that may have functional effects on the lipid profile (eg, add soluble fiber or consider plant sterols if sitosterolemia has been ruled out); and (4) elimination of specific components that perturb the lipid profile (eg, eliminate alcohol in patients with concurrently elevated triglyceride).

The recommended cardioprotective diet for patients with hypercholesterolemia is thus low in saturated fat, relatively high in polyunsaturated fat, all within a framework of a beneficial healthy heart diet, such as the Mediterranean diet or Dietary Approaches to Stop Hypertension (DASH) diet. Dietary advice should be culturally appropriate. A specialized dietician can be helpful in these circumstances.

Pharmacological Therapy

Drug therapy may be started concurrently with lifestyle interventions in high-risk patients (**Fig. 10–5**). Pharmacotherapy is very frequently required in patients with severe hypercholesterolemia, particularly those with heterozygous FH, because LDL-C targets usually cannot be reached with diet and lifestyle changes alone. Available agents for dyslipidemia treatment are shown in **Table 10–11**.

The patient's levels of ASCVD risk and of LDL-C guide the timing of treatment initiation and the intensity of the treatment. Moderate- or low-risk patients may be started on medication after a trial period of lifestyle interventions. The main priority of drug therapy is to achieve the LDL-C target level. Therefore, once drug therapy has been decided upon for a general patient with high ASCVD risk and mild-to-moderate complex dyslipidemia, an LDL-lowering drug is almost always the first step.

Response to drug therapy should be checked in about 8 weeks. If the LDL-C target is not achieved, options include upward titration, switching to a more potent member of the same drug class, or addition of a second-line agent. If the patient develops a drug-related adverse event, alternatives include a trial period off the medication to confirm a temporal relationship, empirically switching with the same class in the event that the side effect is agent-specific rather than class-specific, or switching to a second-line drug, such as ezetimibe or a PCSK9 inhibitor.

Statins: 3-hydroxy-3-methylglutaryl coenzyme A (HMG-CoA) reductase inhibitors (statins) block the rate-limiting step in de novo cholesterol biosynthesis, which depletes intracellular cholesterol and upregulates the LDL receptor, thus increasing catabolism of LDL particles and reducing LDL-C levels.[53] Statins also appear to have a minor effect on reducing secretion

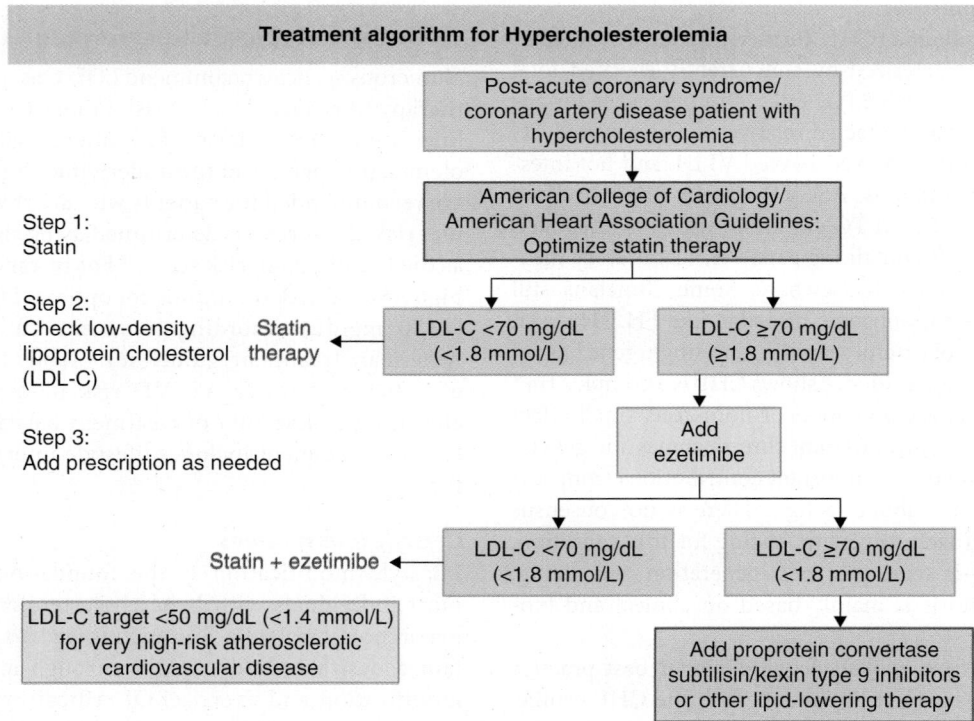

Figure 10–5. Clinical algorithm for managing LDL-C. Managing LDL-C begins with therapeutic lifestyle changes. Statin therapy (Step 1) is recommended in the four statin benefit groups, which include patients with ASCVD, LDL-C >190 mg/dL (>4.9 mmol/L), or diabetes mellitus, as well as primary prevention patients with an ASCVD risk score of >7.5%. Response to statin therapy is evaluated (Step 2). If the LDL-C target is not reached, ezetimibe is added (Step 3), and if the LDL-C target is not attained, PCSK9 inhibitor is added. Data from Rosenson RS, Hegele RA, Fazio S, et al: The Evolving Future of PCSK9 Inhibitors, *J Am Coll Cardiol*. 2018 Jul 17;72(3):314-329.

TABLE 10–11. Dosing and Efficacy of Currently Available Drugs for the Treatment of Dyslipidemia

Drug	Class	Mechanism	Dosing	Approximate LDL cholesterol reduction
Atorvastatin	Statin	HMG-CoA inhibition	10–80 mg/day	35%–50%
Fluvastatin	Statin	HMG-CoA inhibition	20–80 mg/day	24%–38%
Lovastatin	Statin	HMG-CoA inhibition	20–80 mg/day	26%–38%
Pitavastatin	Statin	HMG-CoA inhibition	1–4 mg/day	22%–39%
Pravastatin	Statin	HMG-CoA inhibition	10–40 mg/day	25%–40%
Rosuvastatin	Statin	HMG-CoA inhibition	20–80 mg/day	37%–52%
Simvastatin	Statin	HMG-CoA inhibition	5–80 mg/day	32%–46%
Ezetimibe	Cholesterol absorption inhibitor	Blocks NPC1L1 transporter	10 mg/day	18%–25%
Cholestyramine	Bile acid sequestrant	depletes liver cholesterol	4–8 g/1–2 times daily	18%–20%
Colesevelam	Bile acid sequestrant	depletes liver cholesterol	625 mg 2–3 times daily	7%–18%
Evolocumab	PCSK9 inhibitor	prevents LDLR degradation	140 mg sc biweekly or 420 mg sc monthly	50%–70%
Alirocumab	PCSK9 inhibitor	prevents LDLR degradation	75 -150 mg sc every two weeks	50%–70%

Abbreviations: PCSK9, proprotein convertase subtilisin kexin 9; LDL, HMG-CoA; 3-hydroxy-3-methylglutaryl-coenzyme A; NPC1L1, Niemann Pick C like transporter; sc, subcutaneously

of apoB-containing lipoproteins. In subjects with heterozygous FH who have one normal *LDLR* allele to upregulate, plasma LDL-C reductions of ~50% can be achieved with high dose intensive statin monotherapy. Heterozygous FH patients generally require more than one medication to reach guideline LDL-C targets because their baseline levels of LDL-C are so elevated.

The evidence that ASCVD endpoints and mortality are reduced by statins is overwhelming.[53] Considering their very widespread use in cardioprotection, statins are generally well tolerated and only rarely cause myopathy. Hepatic toxicity is no longer considered to be a relevant concern. The place of statins as front-line drug therapy in patients with hypercholesterolemia is incontrovertible. Available statins include lovastatin, pravastatin, simvastatin, fluvastatin, atorvastatin, rosuvastatin, and pitavastatin (Table 10–11).

Ezetimibe: There is one clinically available cholesterol absorption inhibitor, namely ezetimibe.[25] This agent works preferentially at luminal brush border of enterocytes in the upper intestine, reducing cholesterol content of nascent lipoproteins while maintaining absorption of lipid-soluble vitamins or steroid hormones. Ezetimibe lowers plasma LDL-C by upregulating activity of hepatic LDL receptors. Ezetimibe is available at a single dose of 10 mg daily and lowers LDL-C levels by 18-25%, with no effect on other components of the lipid profile. Ezetimibe is considered as a second-line drug added to statin therapy when LDL-C targets have not been reached or when statins cannot be tolerated as first-line therapy.[25]

PCSK9 Inhibitors: Two monoclonal antibodies against PCSK9 are currently available for clinical use, namely evolocumab and alirocumab.[54] These agents lower LDL-C by >50% when given on top of background statin therapy, plus or minus ezetimibe, and by >60% when given as monotherapy. They are administered subcutaneously biweekly or monthly. Both agents reduce ASCVD events when used in combination with a statin. Evolocumab has also been shown to induce

regression of coronary arterial plaques. Current indications for these agents include patients with FH and patients with ASCVD who are not at target LDL-C levels despite statin with or without ezetimibe therapy. Both agents are very well tolerated, with only occasional mild injection site reactions. These agents are also worth considering in individuals at high ASCVD risk who cannot tolerate a statin. Due to cost, many treatment algorithms suggest that current PCSK9 inhibitors are reserved for the second or third-line in LDL-C management after statins and ezetimibe. A promising long-acting RNA-based interference therapy that targets PCSK9 message, namely inclisiran, is being approved in certain jurisdictions.[55] Other approaches to target PCSK9 include new monoclonal antibodies, adnectins, vaccines, and gene editing.[56]

Bile Acid Sequestrants: Bile acid sequestrants, such as cholestyramine, cholestipol, and colesevelam, are basic anion-exchange resins that bind bile acids in the intestine, interrupting the enterohepatic bile acid recirculation, depleting intrahepatic cholesterol stores, with resulting upregulation of the LDL receptor and reduction of LDL-C levels.[29] Despite evidence for ASCVD benefit and a long track record of safety, compliance with bile acid sequestrants is poor due to adverse gastrointestinal effects. These agents also tend to raise serum TG, so they should be avoided in persons with hypertriglyceridemia (>400 mg/dL or >5 mmol/L). They are third-line agents to be added to maximally-tolerated statin plus or minus ezetimibe and also might be considered in people who develop statin-related adverse effects.[25]

Nicotinic Acid: Nicotinic acid (niacin) is now rarely used because of definitive clinical trials that showed no incremental benefit when used in combination with a statin in the preventing ASCVD outcomes.[57] Niacin may have a role when other therapies are poorly tolerated or inaccessible.

Microsomal Triglyceride Transfer Protein (MTP) Inhibition: The cardioprotective biochemical phenotype in ABL due to

TABLE 10–12. Novel Therapeutics for Hypercholesterolemia

Indication	Name	Mechanism of action	Stage
severe hypercholesterolemia	bempedoic acid	oral ACL inhibitor	approved in US, Europe
homozygous FH	lomitapide	oral MTP inhibitor	approved in North America, Europe, Latin America and Asia
homozygous FH	mipomersen	anti-*APOB* antisense	withdrawn in 2019
severe hypercholesterolemia	inclisiran	anti-*PCSK9* antisense	approved in UK, Canada
severe hypercholesterolemia	gemcabene	oral acetyl-CoA carboxylase inhibitor	phase 2-3
homozygous FH	AAV8.TBG.hLDLR (RGX-501)	*LDLR* gene therapy	phase 1-2
homozygous FH; severe hypercholesterolemia	evinacumab	anti-*ANGPTL3* antibody	approved in US, Europe
homozygous FH; severe hypercholesterolemia	vupanorsen	anti-*ANGPTL3* antisense	phase 2

Abbreviations: ACL, ATP citrate lyase; ANGPTL3, angiopoietin like protein 3; APOA1, apolipoprotein A-I; APOB, apolipoprotein B; APOC3, apolipoprotein C-III; HDL, high density lipoprotein; HoFH, homozygous familial hypercholesterolaemia; HDL-C, high-density lipoprotein cholesterol (HDL-C); LAL, lysosomal acid lipase; LCAT, lecithin cholesterol acyl transferase; LDLR, low density lipoprotein receptor; LPL, lipoprotein lipase; MTP, microsomal triglyceride transfer protein

mutations in *MTTP*—such as extremely low levels of chylomicrons, VLDL, and LDL—inspired the development of an orally administered inhibitor of MTP, namely lomitapide (**Table 10–12**).[25] In homozygous FH patients, lomitapide significantly reduced plasma total and LDL-C and apoB by up to 40%. However, ~25% of patients in short term studies developed transaminase elevations and accumulation of hepatic fat, although this became less severe with prolonged treatment. Fat-soluble vitamin supplements should also be given. Lomitapide is reserved for treatment of homozygous FH.

Interference with Apolipoprotein B Synthesis: The cardioprotective biochemical phenotype in HBL due to mutations in *APOB*—such as extremely low levels of VLDL and LDL—inspired the development of parenteral antisense RNA therapies. Antisense RNA therapy refers to agents that have a range of mechanisms that result in specific targeting and degradation of mRNA. Instead of pharmacological targeting, these newer methods, including antisense oligonucleotides (ASOs) and ribonucleic acid (RNA) interference (RNAi), reduce translation by selectively degrading mRNAs. The first antisense RNA for the treatment of dyslipidemia was mipomersen, an ASO administered subcutaneously week.[58] Mipomersen reduced both apoB and LDL-C levels by up to 50% in homozygous FH. Adverse effects include skin site reactions and to a lesser extent fatty liver.[58] The manufacturer discontinued market availability of mipomersen in 2019.

Bempedoic Acid: Bempedoic acid is a new oral agent whose dominant mechanism of action in humans is probably competitive inhibition of ATP citrate lyase (Table 10–12). In early phase clinical trials, LDL-C was reduced by 15% to 20% as monotherapy and up to 48% when given together with ezetimibe.[59] Headaches were commonly reported, while muscle and liver adverse effects were uncommon. Bempedoic acid was approved in the United States in 2020 as monotherapy and in combination with ezetimibe for LDL-C reduction, although there are no ASCVD outcomes data yet.

Apheresis for Homozygous Familial Hypercholesterolemia and Severe Refractory Hypercholesterolemia

The current standard of care for patients with homozygous FH is LDL-apheresis (or less preferably plasmapheresis); extracorporeal removal of LDL particles prolongs endpoint free survival. LDL-apheresis has the advantages of reduced exposure to blood products, no significant changes in HDL-C levels, and smaller extracellular fluid volume shifts compared to nonspecific plasma exchange.[26] Concurrent intensive statin therapy plus or minus ezetimibe may enhance LDL clearance by upregulating expression of partially functional LDL receptors, but most homozygous FH patients have only a marginal response to these oral therapies.[26] Apheresis may also be considered for patients with severe hypercholesterolemia but without homozygous FH.[60] PCSK9 monoclonal antibody inhibitors reduce LDL-C in homozygous FH patients who have at least one receptor-defective allele with at least some incremental residual function.[61] Nevertheless, all patients with homozygous FH should undergo an empirical therapeutic trial with PCSK9 inhibition irrespective of their genotype.

Other Therapies

Other targets and strategies for lowering LDL-C include inhibition of acetyl-CoA carboxylase with gemcabene (Table 10–12).[62] A recombinant liver-tropic adeno-associated virus 8 (AAV8) vector carrying an *LDLR* transgene is in development, namely AAV8.TBG.hLDLR and may prove to be valuable for homozygous FH patients who have bi-allelic loss of function mutations of the *LDLR* gene.[29] Other promising agents for treatment of homozygous FH and heterozygous FH include inhibitors of angiopoietin like-protein 3 (ANGPTL3) with or example, using the monoclonal antibody evinacumab,[63,64] or anti-RNA strategies such as vupanorsen.[65] The LDL-C lowering effect of monoclonal antibodies has been consistently greater than anti-RNA approaches suggesting differences in mechanism of action on endothelial lipase-mediated VLDL production and clearance. Finally, lowering of elevated Lp(a) levels in FH is likely to be an important adjunct for ASCVD risk reduction, as discussed in the section on Lp(a).

Children and Adolescents with Hypercholesterolemia

What is the appropriate management of children or adolescents with heterozygous FH for ASCVD prevention?[66] Dietary and lifestyle advice form the therapeutic cornerstone. Statin treatment of pediatric heterozygous FH is an evolving field because there are still few long-term data. Some advocate for initiation of statin treatment at a very young age and maintaining treatment over a patient's lifetime. Bile acid sequestrants have the advantage of not being systemically absorbed, but they are poorly tolerated. Ezetimibe has theoretical advantages but there is limited evidence for its use in children or adolescents. Evolocumab effectively reduces LDL-C in children and adolescents with heterozygous FH, although long term use in these patients has not been reported.[67] The exact age to initiate treatment and the applicability of adult targets in children has not been definitively settled. Referral for specialist opinion is appropriate for young patients with heterozygous FH.[66]

Training and Education

Training and education[68] issues related to hypercholesterolemia are targeted to both patients and healthcare providers. For FH patients, the heritable nature of the condition should be reinforced together with the option for cascade screening of close relatives to identify new cases. The cost-effectiveness of cascade screening is similar to that of other widely implemented screening programs (eg, for breast cancer). It is also important to emphasize the need to comply with dietary and drug management of hypercholesterolemia. Finally, as part of the global risk management in patients with hypercholesterolemia, the presence of other modifiable risk factors should be assessed, and their cumulative effect on ASCVD risk should be explained. If appropriate, the healthcare provider should offer assistance with smoking cessation, initiation of an exercise and weight reduction regimen, and controlling glycemia and blood pressure in those with coexisting diabetes and hypertension, respectively.

The second immediate educational challenge is to maximize awareness of FH among healthcare providers and patients to promote early diagnosis and treatment. There is a critical need among providers to improve awareness of the diagnosis and appropriate management of patients with hypercholesterolemia. This should begin with dedicated education of allied care providers who work in general practice, cardiology, pediatrics, genetics, imaging, and transfusion medicine. These various specialties must increase their awareness of diagnosis and treatment of hypercholesterolemia. They must together collegially develop cooperative norms of interacting with patients and families.

At present, there is considerable room for improvement of care models for hypercholesterolemia, which need to optimize diagnosis, prediction and prevention of complications, and delivery of high-quality personalized treatment.[68] The design of optimal models of care must also take into account local practices, expectations from patients, and available resources.

Medical and related services for patients with hypercholesterolemia should integrate a broad continuum of care and deliver a whole-life healthcare plan. A team approach would engage frontline primary care physicians, nurses and nurse practitioners, pharmacy practice members, nutritionists, dieticians, social workers, and genetic counsellors. Each team member would require updating of their knowledge of hypercholesterolemia and FH. For all integrated care visions, education, skills training, and research capacity building is central in designing an effective care plan.

Furthermore, patient support groups and networks can facilitate for advocacy of value-based health care for patients with hypercholesterolemia. A successful example is the US patient driven Familial Hypercholesterolemia Foundation.[69] Since healthcare and government policies vary widely across the globe, approaches should be appropriate to the particular jurisdiction. Sharing experiences between patients and stakeholder via networking platforms is essential. Awareness can be raised through social media, general education, and counselling opportunities. Tangible successful examples include government-run screening programs, national clinical registries, and the development of specific ASCVD risk prediction algorithms. Clinical registries on FH capture "real-world" clinical practice data and are important not only to raise overall awareness of FH but also to garner information for clinical trials and for health service research, as a means to improve the quality of patient care and outcomes. Finally, a new International Statistical Classification of Diseases and Related Health Problems 10th revision (ICD-10) code for FH has been established, and this has helped with access to new treatments.

Conclusions

Hypercholesterolemia is common—1 in 20 people—and greatly increases risk of ASCVD. In evaluating a patient with hypercholesterolemia, secondary causes must be ruled out and possible genetic etiologies of primary isolated hypercholesterolemia, in particular FH should be considered. FH has surprising genetic complexity. DNA testing to find the precise monogenic defect can reduce diagnostic uncertainty and may have implications for family members, since there is a greater likelihood that additional cases can be identified by cascade screening. Furthermore, hypercholesterolemic mutation positive patients have remarkably elevated risk of ASCVD. But even mutation negative patients with severe hypercholesterolemia have greatly increased ASCVD risk. Thus, irrespective of the cause of hypercholesterolemia, the main goal of treatment is to reduce LDL-C levels in order to reduce ASCVD risk. Treatment begins with diet and lifestyle modification, frequently supplemented by drugs to help attain guideline recommended target levels of LDL-C. First-line drug treatment is statins with second-line therapies being ezetimibe and PCSK9 inhibitors. Until the value of genotyping is formally proven scientifically, therapeutic decisions can be safely based on the degree of LDL-C elevation with adjustments based empirically on the response to treatment. Thus, irrespective of the precise genetic basis, individuals diagnosed with severe hypercholesterolemia require intensive therapy for their condition, including possible consideration of future therapies, based on their high ASCVD risk.

LIPOPROTEIN(a)

Overview

Lp(a) was first described in 1963 as an antigenic variant of LDL. However, more than 50 years later, there remain many unanswered questions about Lp(a), ranging from gaps in fundamental biological and pathophysiological knowledge to understanding of its contribution to cardiovascular risk and how it can be used in the clinic for risk stratification.

Lp(a) is a unique lipoprotein class that contains a LDL-like moiety in which the distinguishing protein apolipoprotein(a) (apoB-100) is covalently linked to apoB-100 (**Fig. 10–6**). Hepatocytes are the source of plasma Lp(a): these cells synthesize and secrete both apo(a) and apoB-100, the latter of which requires assembly of a lipoprotein particle to be secreted. In terms of particle density, Lp(a) is primarily found in the lower

end of the LDL density range, with variability attributable to the presence of differently sized apo(a) molecules. Although overall highly similar to LDL in lipid composition, lipidomic analyses to discern differences in the lipid content of Lp(a)-derived LDL have not yet been reported.

Kringles are structural protein motifs containing three invariant disulfide bonds and are characterized by their ability to bind a variety of substrates. Kringles are present in several proteins associated with the thrombotic and fibrinolytic cascades. The apo(a) component of Lp(a) bears striking sequence similarity to the serine protease zymogen plasminogen:[70] apo(a) contains multiply repeated copies of a plasminogen kringle IV (KIV)-like sequence, followed by a single plasminogen kringle V (KV)-like domain (**Figs. 10–6** and **10–7**).[70] At its carboxyl-terminus, apo(a) has a protease domain that is highly similar to that of plasminogen, although the apo(a) protease-like domain contains amino acid substitutions/deletion that render it catalytically inactive.[70] The KIV domains in apo(a) are organized into 10 types (KIV_{1-10}) based on amino acid sequence (Fig. 10–7)[71] Each domain contains 114 amino acids, with a

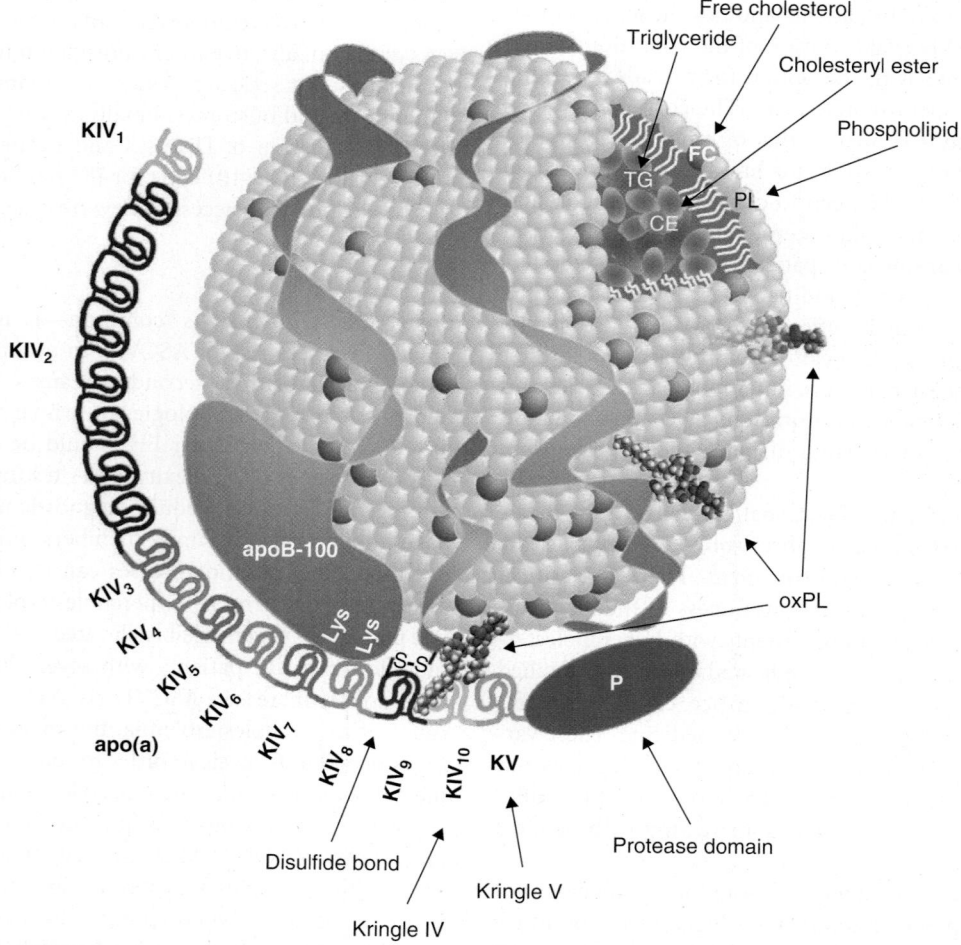

Figure 10–6. Structure of Lp(a). Lp(a) consists of an LDL-like moiety covalently linked by a single disulfide bond to apo(a). The LDL-like moiety contains a single molecule of apoB-100, an outer shell of phospholipids and unesterified cholesterol, and a neutral lipid core consisting of cholesteryl esters (primarily) and triglycerides. Apo(a) consists of multiple plasminogen-like kringles and an inactive protease-like domain. Also shown are the oxPL that are predominantly covalently bonded to apo(a) but are also found covalently linked to apoB-100 and free in the lipid moiety.

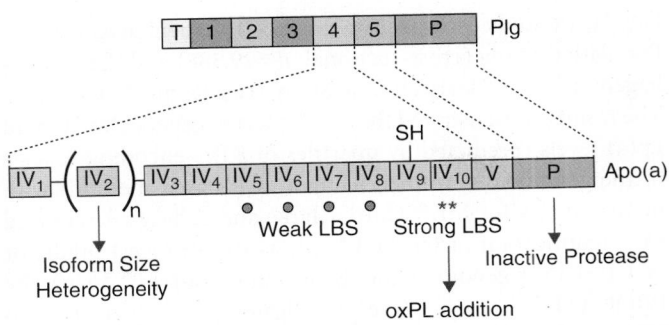

Figure 10–7. Apo(a) kringle organization and relationship to plasminogen. Apo(a) consists of multiply repeated copies of 10 different domains homologous to plasminogen (Plg) kringle 4, followed by kringle 5-like and protease-like domains. There are two different types of apo(a) KIV, of which KIV_2 is present in different numbers of copies in different apo(a) isoforms while the remainder are present in single copy. Specific functionalities have been ascribed to specific KIV types, as indicated. T, tail domain; P, protease domain; LBS, lysine binding site; SH, free thiol in KIV_9; oxPL, oxidized phospholipids.

36 amino acid-long flexible linker sequence separating each of the kringle IV domains (28 between KIV_6 and KIV_7).[70] Apo(a) KIV domains have variable functions ascribed to them including: (1) mediating assembly of Lp(a) particles via noncovalent and covalent linkages to apoB-100 (see below); (2) binding to substrates in a lysine-dependent manner; and (3) harboring the covalent attachment of an oxidized phospholipid moiety (Fig. 10–6).[72] The most distinct feature of apo(a) is the presence of a variable number of identically-repeated KIV_2 sequences (ranging from 3 to greater than 40 copies) in different alleles of *LPA*, the gene encoding apo(a).[73] This copy number variation gives rise to the many differently sized Lp(a) isoforms observed in the population.

Unlike plasminogen, apo(a) is highly glycosylated—approximately 28% carbohydrate by weight. Each KIV domain contains at least one site for *N*-linked glycan addition, with up to 6 sites for *O*-linked modification present within each inter-kringle sequence. As such, the apparent molecular weight of the apo(a) moiety can range from approximately 200 kDa to greater than 1000 kDa depending on the apo(a) isoform size. The significance of the extensive glycosylation in apo(a)/Lp(a) function remains unclear.

Plasma Lp(a) levels vary remarkably in the population, ranging from undetectable (< 1 mg/dL) to greater than 500 mg/dL.[74] Lp(a) levels are stable by 1 or 2 years of age and remain relatively unchanged throughout life.[75] While a large component of this variability is determined at the level of the *LPA* gene itself (see below), many gaps persist in our knowledge of the production and catabolism of Lp(a). It has been shown using in vivo tracer labeling studies that plasma Lp(a) levels are predominantly determined at the level of production of the particle rather than its catabolism.[76] There are several possible regulatory steps in apo(a)/Lp(a) production, many of which remain unstudied (**Fig. 10–8**). We do know that the efficiency of apo(a) movement through the initial phases of the secretory pathway is determined by its size: different apo(a) isoforms all fold at the same rate but larger isoforms are retained longer

in the endoplasmic reticulum (ER).[77] They are thus subject to proteasome-mediated degradation leading to less efficient secretion compared to smaller apo(a) species. Another possible point of regulation of Lp(a) production is the efficiency of assembly of Lp(a) particles from apo(a) and apoB-100 (Fig. 10–8). Their assembly to form plasma Lp(a) occurs through a two-step process. In the first step, apo(a) interacts noncovalently with apoB-100, involving weak lysine binding sites located in each of apo(a) KIV_7 and KIV_8 with lysine residues in the globular domain of apoB-100.[78] The second step involves the formation of a covalent bond between apo(a) and apoB-100 to form circulating Lp(a) particles (Figs. 10–6 and 10–8).[79] The location of each of the two steps remains controversial, with in vivo human kinetics studies suggesting intracellular and/or extracellular sites as possible locations for Lp(a) assembly.[80] The origin of the apoB-100 component of Lp(a) also remains unclear. There are kinetic data to suggest that a separate pool of hepatocyte apoB-100 is involved in Lp(a) assembly,[80] although direct evidence for this is lacking at present.

Relatively little is known about how Lp(a) is removed from the circulation. Several candidate hepatic receptors have been

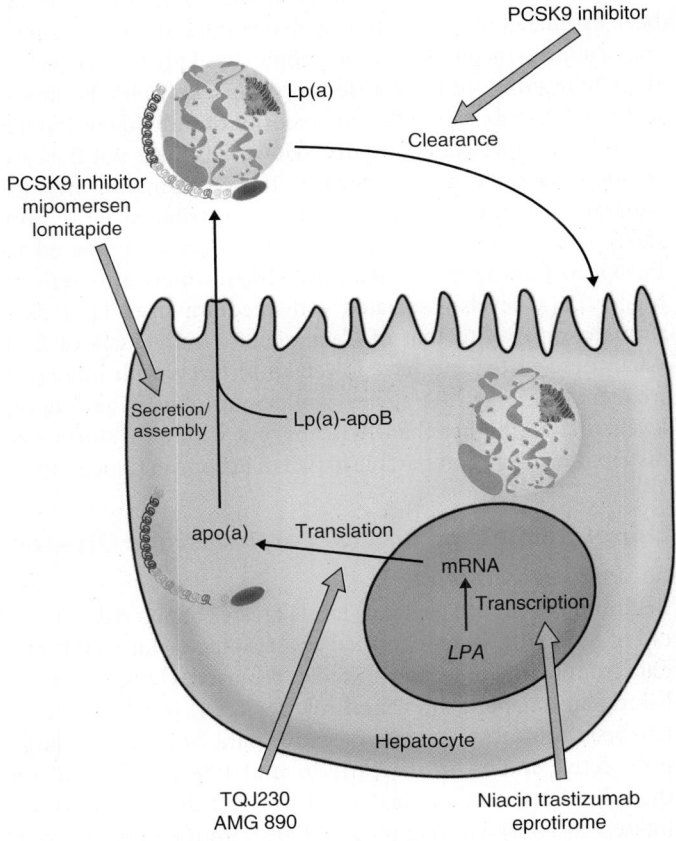

Figure 10–8. Control of Lp(a) biosynthesis and catabolism. Lp(a) plasma levels are primarily controlled at the level of production of the lipoprotein in the hepatocyte. Apo(a) production is regulated at the levels of transcription in the nucleus, protein folding and processing in the endoplasmic reticulum, and possibly other compartments of the secretory pathway. Lp(a) assembly may occur intracellularly or on the cell surface, and may use a cholesterol-rich apoB-100-containing particle produced within the hepatocyte. Lp(a) may be cleared by several different hepatic receptors. Drugs that affect he respective metabolic events are indicated with the *blue arrows*.

suggested to play a role in Lp(a) catabolism (**Fig. 10–8**). Conflicting results addressing the role of the LDL receptor (LDL-R) in Lp(a) catabolism have been generated using both in vitro and in vivo approaches.[81,82] A number of additional candidate receptors have been suggested to play a role including LDL receptor-related proteins 1 and 8, scavenger receptor B1[82] and, most recently, the plasminogen receptor Plg-R$_{KT}$.[83] It is reasonable to assume that there are multiple receptors operating in vivo, the relative contributions of which may vary under certain physiological or pathophysiological conditions. For example, it has been argued that Lp(a) may be catabolized by the LDL-R under conditions in which LDL levels are very low, and both LDL-R and Lp(a) levels are elevated;[84] this can be seen both in vitro[81,85] and in vivo with the use of PCSK9 inhibitors and statin therapy.[86]

Prevalence of Elevated Lipoprotein(a)

A large meta-analysis demonstrated that Lp(a) risk for CHD and ischemic stroke increases with increasing Lp(a) concentrations,[87] with risk for CHD becoming significant over 30 mg/dL. Other studies have shown the presence of significant risk for CVD events associated with Lp(a) levels above 50 mg/dL.[88,89] It has been estimated that 20% of the global population (corresponding to approximately 1.4 billion people) has Lp(a) levels greater than 50 mg/dL.[90] In most ancestry groups, Lp(a) levels exhibit a skewed distribution with the majority of individuals having Lp(a) levels less than 20 mg/dL.[88] However, this is not the case in some ancestry groups, such as those originating in sub-Saharan Africa, where Lp(a) levels are distributed more normally and are in fact relatively higher overall compared to European Caucasian populations.[88] Interestingly, this reflects higher Lp(a) levels associated with medium-sized Lp(a) isoforms compared to that of Caucasians.[91] Individuals of East Asian descent tend to have lower Lp(a) levels with increased frequency of large *LPA* alleles, while South Asians have Lp(a) levels that are higher than Africans, but with an isoform size distribution more comparable to that of European Caucasians.[88]

Lipoprotein(a) and Risk for Cardiovascular Disease

Coronary Heart Disease

Beginning in the 1970s, Lp(a) levels greater than a risk threshold of 30 mg/dL were identified as a risk factor for CHD with data from many case-control studies reported. However, establishing an independent, causal role for Lp(a) in CHD disease has been more challenging. Negative data from several large prospective studies in the early to mid-1990s cast doubt on the role of Lp(a) as a casual agent in CHD disease. However, interest in Lp(a) was reignited in 2009 with the publication of three seminal studies. First, a large meta-analysis performed by Erqou and colleagues (analysis of 126,634 subjects corresponding to 36 studies from 1970 to 2009) reported that Lp(a) is an "independent" risk factor for CHD and ischemic stroke, with a continuous relationship to risk corresponding to Lp(a) levels greater than ~30 mg/dL.[87] Second, Kamstrup and colleagues reported the results of a seminal Mendelian randomization study in 2009, using individuals from the Copenhagen

City Heart Study (prospective; $n = 8637$), Copenhagen General Population Study (cross-sectional; $n = 29,388$) and the Copenhagen Ischemic Heart Disease Study (case/control; $n = 2461$). The results demonstrated the association of genetically elevated Lp(a) levels (predicted by quartiles of KIV$_2$-encoding repeats in the genome determined using a PCR-based method) with increased risk for MI.[92] Third, Clarke and colleagues reported the identification of the *LPA* locus as the strongest predictor of CHD in a genome-wide association analysis.[93] Using the PROCARDIS cohort, these investigators also identified two *LPA* single nucleotide polymorphisms (SNPs) (rs10455872 and rs3798220) that each predicted elevated Lp(a) levels and increased CHD risk in an additive fashion.[93] Although these landmark studies are frequently cited, there are many additional publications that support an independent, causal role for Lp(a) in CHD risk.[94]

Most studies of Lp(a) as a CHD risk factor have been conducted in European Caucasian subjects. Because Lp(a) concentration distribution and the *LPA* genetic architecture differs substantially between ethnic groups, it has been of interest to assess if Lp(a)-attributable risk similarly varies. A recent study in a multiethnic population found that Lp(a)-attributable risk for MI is highest in South Asians, Southeast Asians, and Latin Americans, but is absent in Arabs and Africans.[88] However, the power to detect an association between Lp(a) and MI was low for both Arabs and Africans in this study; indeed, previous studies showed a similar association between Lp(a) levels and CVD events in Whites and Blacks.[95] A recent report from the Multi-Ethnic Study of Atherosclerosis (MESA) found that Lp(a) levels greater than 30 mg/dL significantly predicted risk for Blacks but a higher cutoff of 50 mg/dL was required for Whites and Hispanics.[96]

Few studies have considered the role of sex as a factor in the determination of Lp(a) risk. Data from an early prospective study (the Stanford Five-City Project[97]) suggested that women with elevated Lp(a) were not at risk for MI or cardiac death compared to men. On the other hand, results from the Women's Health Study found that Lp(a) in the highest quintile increased risk for CHD in women, particularly those with elevated LDL-C.[98] In addition, the large meta-analysis by Erqou and colleagues found a similar impact of elevated Lp(a) on CHD risk in men and women.[87] In a recent publication by Cook and colleagues, analysis of three different cohorts of women indicated that elevated Lp(a) does not increase CHD risk in the absence of elevated total cholesterol.[99] This is clearly an important area that requires further study.

The extent to which isoform sizes per se contribute to risk is not clear. A meta-analysis of 58,000 subjects across 40 studies showed that having a small apo(a) isoform (≤22 KIV repeats) doubled the risk for CHD, although whether or not this was independent of the impact of apo(a) isoform on Lp(a) levels was not explored.[100] In the INTERHEART study, isoform size did not predict risk independently of Lp(a) levels in a study of six ethnic groups.[88] On the other hand, a recent study has shown that small isoform sizes contribute to risk independently of Lp(a) levels in the PROMIS cohort.[101] Moreover, a SNP (rs2457564) associated with isoform size but not Lp(a) levels was used in Mendelian randomization to show that smaller isoform size alone could predict CHD in subjects from the CARDIoGRAMplusC4D consortium.[101]

Calcific Aortic Valve Disease

While the majority of studies involving genome-wide association study (GWAS) and Mendelian randomization approaches have focused on the role of Lp(a) as a risk factor for CHD, similar approaches have identified a causal role for Lp(a) in calcific aortic valve disease (CAVD) risk.[102,103] Studies over the last 10 years have established elevated Lp(a) as an important inherited risk factor for CAVD and its clinical manifestation as aortic stenosis (AS). Although CAVD is recognized as a distinct pathophysiological process from atherosclerosis, it does share some features and risk factors.[104] The Cohorts for Heart and Aging Research in Genomic Epidemiology (CHARGE) Consortium was the first to show a link between genetically-elevated Lp(a) and CAVD: a SNP in the *LPA* gene associated with elevated plasma Lp(a) levels (rs10455872) was the only one of 2.5 million SNPs considered that was associated with CAVD and the need for aortic valve replacement in multiple cohorts.[102] Subsequent studies showed that elevated Lp(a) is a causal risk factor for AS[105] and that elevated Lp(a) levels predict the progression of CAVD.[106] Recently, using data from the Aortic Stenosis Progression Observation: Measuring Effects of Rosuvastatin (ASTRONOMER) Trial, it was shown that elevated Lp(a)-apoCIII complexes in conjunction with high levels of Lp(a)-associated oxidized phospholipids (oxPL) predict accelerated CAVD progression.[107]

Heart Failure

Using a Mendelian randomization approach with data from both the Copenhagen City Heart Study ($n = 10,855$) and the Copenhagen General Population Study ($n = 87,242$), Kamstrup and colleagues demonstrated that genetically-elevated Lp(a) levels are causally associated with increased risk for heart failure.[108] The authors postulate that this may result from the ability of elevated Lp(a) to increase arterial stiffness including aortic noncompliance. Recently, using 6,089 participants from the MESA, Steffen and colleagues reported that over a median 13 year follow-up, the relationship between Lp(a) and heart failure was restricted to Caucasians, with no significant relationships observed in Black, Hispanic, or Chinese participants.[109]

Other Diseases of the Vasculature

It has been demonstrated using Mendelian randomization approaches that Lp(a) is also a causal risk factor for peripheral arterial disease (PAD).[110,111] Most recently, GWAS of 32 million sequence variants from the Million Veteran Program reported that the *LPA* locus is associated with disease in the peripheral vasculature as well as the coronary and cerebral beds.[112]

While Lp(a) is well-recognized risk factor for ischemic stroke in children,[113] the role of Lp(a) in adult stroke is less clear. Although the meta-analysis of Erqou and colleagues did identify Lp(a) as a risk factor for stroke,[87] the evidence base is not as compelling as for Lp(a) and CHD. This likely reflects the variable etiology for stroke (eg, ischemic versus hemorrhagic stroke; different ischemic stroke subtypes) and the frequent lack of reporting of the underlying cause of the event. Data have been provided to suggest that Lp(a) is an independent risk factor for stroke, particularly in younger study populations[114] and that elevated Lp(a) levels may increase risk of early stroke recurrence after an initial stroke event.[115] Interestingly, compelling evidence from the Copenhagen General Population Study and Copenhagen City Heart Study data indicate that Lp(a) can contribute to ischemic stroke in patients over 70 years of age; this was not related to elevated LDL as is often observed in younger stroke patients.[87,116,117] However, findings from other studies point to either a modest or nonsignificant role for Lp(a) in stroke risk.[111,117-119] Interestingly, it has been reported that elevated Lp(a) may pose a differential risk for stroke in women, although the data are inconsistent and further research is required.[114]

Lipoprotein(a) in Familial Hypercholesterolemia

Elevated Lp(a) levels are more prevalent in heterozygous FH patients compared to the general population,[120] putting heterozygous FH patients with hyperlipoprotein(a) at even greater CVD risk. Results from the Spanish Familial Hypercholesterolemia Cohort Study (SAFEHEART) using data from 1960 patients with FH and 957 relatives without reported that median Lp(a) was significantly higher in FH 23.6 mg/dL (intraquartile range [IQR] 9.6–59.2) versus 21.0 mg/dL (IQR 7–47.2) and that Lp(a) levels ≥50 mg/dL were more common in FH (29.3% versus 22.2%).[120] There is also strong evidence that elevated Lp(a) levels contribute to atherothrombotic CVD events in patients with genetic FH. In family members from 755 index FH cases enrolled in SAFEHEART who were tested for elevated Lp(a) (>50 mg/dL) and genetic FH it was found that over a 5 year period, FH and elevated Lp(a) each contributed to ASCVD and risk for death (hazard ratio [HR] 2.47; $P = 0.036$, and 3.17; $P = 0.024$ respectively); the greatest risk was observed in relatives with both FH and elevated Lp(a) (HR 4.40; $P < 0.001$).[121] Lp(a) levels are consistently elevated in FH patients with deleterious LDL receptor mutations, strongly suggesting a role for the LDL receptor in Lp(a) catabolism under these conditions.[84]

Subsequently, it has been reported in several studies that Lp(a) levels are elevated in a large proportion of patients with FH and that clinical presentation of FH in these individuals can be attributed to Lp(a) cholesterol.[122,123] In this sense, it is debatable as to whether elevated Lp(a) is a genetic cause of FH, or results in the misclassification of FH.[124]

Lipoprotein(a) in Secondary Prevention

Although the risk for Lp(a) in primary prevention settings is well established, the role of Lp(a) in secondary prevention remains controversial.[125] A related question is whether Lp(a) can confer residual risk even after aggressive LDL-lowering. It has been reported that elevated Lp(a) persists as a risk factor in the context of low (<70 mg/dL) LDL.[126] Most recently, there is evidence of residual risk for clinically elevated Lp(a) even in the context of dramatic LDL lowering such as can be obtained using PCSK9 inhibitors together with statins. Outcomes data from the FOURIER trial suggest that Lp(a) levels in the highest quartile (>165 nmol/L) predict risk for a composite endpoint of

CHD death, MI, or urgent revascularization.[127] Moreover, those with the lowest achieved levels of both Lp(a) and LDL-C had the lowest risk.[127] As this large study enrolled patients only with preexisting CHD, it is strong evidence that Lp(a) is an important risk factor in secondary as well as primary prevention. Most recently, the role of alirocumab in Lp(a) in residual risk was demonstrated in a prespecified analysis of the ODYSSEY OUTCOMES trial of patients with recent acute coronary syndrome.[128] Although the patients with elevated Lp(a) levels were not specifically enrolled and treated (median Lp[a] was 21.2 mg/dL; IQR 6.7–59.6 mg/dL) and Lp(a) lowering was modest overall (5 mg/dL versus 51.5 mg/dL for LDL-C), the study was able to show that reduction of Lp(a) with alirocumab treatment lowered risk of events independently of LDL-lowering and after adjustment for baseline Lp(a) and LDL-C. It was reported that a 1 mg/dL reduction in Lp(a) with alirocumab was associated with a HR of 0.994 (95% CI: 0.990–0.999; $P = 0.0081$). Taken together, these findings underscore that lowering Lp(a) represents a potentially important target to reduce risk of recurrent CHD events.

In a large meta-analysis by Willeit and colleagues, data from seven randomized, placebo-controlled, statin outcomes trials were harmonized to calculate HRs for cardiovascular events, defined as fatal or nonfatal CHD, stroke, or revascularization procedures.[89] Initiation of statin therapy reduced LDL-C (mean change −39%; 95% CI: −43 to −35]) without a significant change in Lp(a).[89] Associations of baseline and on-statin treatment Lp(a) with CVD risk were approximately linear, with increased risk at Lp(a) values of ≥30 mg/dL for baseline Lp(a) and ≥50 mg/dL for on-statin Lp(a). This study underscores the important contribution of elevated Lp(a) to residual risk in the context of LDL-C lowering with statins. Importantly, Lp(a) was a significant risk factor at all levels of LDL-C, and thus lowering LDL-C on its own cannot mitigate the risk attributable to elevated Lp(a). This underscores the importance of developing specific Lp(a)-lowering strategies to reduce residual risk including in secondary prevention settings.[125]

Genetics of Lipoprotein(a)

Lp(a) is the most common monogenic cause of inherited CHD. The *LPA* gene is located in a cluster of homologous genes on chromosome 6q27.[129] *LPA* arose from duplication of the *PLG* (plasminogen) gene which is also located in this cluster. A third *LPA*-like gene (*LPAL2*) that is also present in this cluster does not appear to correspond to a functional protein. Interestingly, it appears that the gene duplication event that gave rise to *LPA* occurred after the divergence of New World and Old World monkeys (ie, less than 6 million years ago) since only humans, apes, and Old World monkeys have the *LPA* gene.

Plasma Lp(a) concentrations are primarily determined at the level of the gene with some estimates of heritability of Lp(a) concentrations greater than 90%.[129] The vast majority of the variability in Lp(a) levels is attributable to the *LPA* gene itself;[130] most of the contribution of *LPA* is in turn conferred by differences in *LPA* size where smaller alleles are strongly associated with higher plasma Lp(a) levels, although the strength of this association differs between ancestry groups.[131] As aforementioned, larger apo(a) isoforms are secreted more slowly from hepatic cells and this has been shown to correspond to differences in apo(a) production rates between isoform sizes in in vivo stable isotope kinetics studies in humans.[76] Plasma Lp(a) concentrations reflect a codominant inheritance pattern where Lp(a) levels correspond to the sum of the contribution of each allele. Owing to the strong contribution of the *LPA* gene to plasma Lp(a) concentrations, levels are relatively resistant to lowering through alterations in diet and lifestyle or most lipid-lowering therapies.[132]

Many SNPs within *LPA* have been identified that are associated with plasma Lp(a) concentrations.[130] Clarke and colleagues screened ~50,000 SNPs in 2100 candidate genes to identify loci associated with CHD in individuals of European Caucasian descent.[93] From this study, two SNPs were identified in *LPA*: rs10455872 (intronic) and rs3798220 (causes an Ile to Met substitution in the protease domain). Both SNPs were associated with smaller apo(a) isoform size, increased Lp(a) levels, and increased risk for CHD; the CHD risk associated with these SNPs disappears with adjustment for Lp(a) levels, indicating that the presence of small isoforms per se does not increase CHD risk.[93] The Ile/Met substitution does not result in increased secretion of apo(a), suggesting that the impact of this mutation is through its linkage to smaller *LPA* alleles.[133] However, it has been shown that apo(a) bearing this mutation does have a greater effect on inhibition of clot lysis through effects of fibrin clot structure.[133]

Haplotype studies in different ethnic groups by Hegele and colleagues showed that both *LPA* SNPs and KIV$_2$ copy number are genomic determinants of plasma Lp(a) concentration, but that these relationships differ across ethnic groups.[134] SNPs that have been identified in *LPA* haplotypes are linked to both levels and KIV$_2$ copy number in Caucasian, East Asian, and South Asian populations. Interestingly, however, the KIV$_2$ copy number explains a larger proportion of variability in plasma Lp(a) levels in European Caucasians, compared to that observed in the East Asian and South Asian populations.[134] This may reflect the rs10455872 SNP, which is only found in European Caucasians, and which is significantly associated with both KIV$_2$ copy number and Lp(a) levels. This highlights the importance of performing Mendelian randomization studies in different ethnic groups to confirm the causal role of Lp(a) in non-European Caucasian populations. Additionally, SNPs identified that contribute to Lp(a) levels independently of the size of the KIV$_2$ domain should be investigated as this may shed new light on the regulation of Lp(a) production.

Several mutations resulting in "null" *LPA* alleles have been identified, and these can take the form of nonsense codons or splice-site mutations.[135,136] Importantly, such null alleles are strong predicters of both lower Lp(a) levels and lower risk for CHD.[135] Ultradeep sequencing of the KIV$_2$ repeat region of *LPA* revealed a large number of missense mutations as well as a substantial number of loss-of-function and splice-site mutations.[137] Importantly, many of these mutations were common in some ancestry groups and absent in others, indicating that they may play a role in the different relationships between *LPA* allele size and

Lp(a) levels in these groups. The KIV$_2$ repeat region has been comparatively impenetrable to discovery of mutations because of its highly repetitive nature, and advances in next-generation sequencing have allowed these recent insights into the mutation burden in this region. A strong implication of the findings is that *LPA* has the characteristics of an expressed pseudogene. This calls into question whether there is truly a physiological role played by Lp(a) apart from its pathological effects.

GWAS has revealed only one locus (*APOE*) outside the *LPA*-containing gene cluster on chromosome 6 that is significantly associated with Lp(a) levels.[130] Interestingly, *APOE* genotype appears to play a role in determining Lp(a) levels, with a 65% increase in Lp(a) mass associated with individuals with ε4/ε4 genotype compared to ε2/ε2.[138] The ε2/ε2 genotype is associated with elevated triglycerides as *APOE2* has impaired association with the LDL-R; the mechanism underlying the association of *APOE* genotype with Lp(a) may reflect enhanced LDL-R–mediated clearance of Lp(a) compared to *APOE2*-containing lipoproteins, or an effect on apoB availability for Lp(a) assembly.

There are clearly factors underlying variation in Lp(a) levels that are not attributable to genetics. Regulation of *LPA* transcription has been reported: for example, proinflammatory cytokines such as IL-6 increase *LPA* transcription through binding to response elements in the promoter.[139] Subjects with FH appear to have higher Lp(a) levels, through an as-yet unknown mechanism.[120] A weak to moderate inverse correlation between triglycerides and Lp(a) has been reported;[138] a causal relationship between metabolism of Lp(a) and VLDL is suggested by Mendelian randomization studies indicating that *LPA* genetic signatures of elevated Lp(a) causally reduce VLDL size and density.[140] Lp(a) levels are inversely related to risk of incident and prevalent type 2 diabetes mellitus.[141] While it has been suggested that hyperinsulinemia decreases *LPA* transcription in vitro, a recent genetic studies using SNPs associated with either Lp(a) levels or number of KIV$_2$ repeats shown that KIV$_2$ repeat number, rather than low Lp(a) concentrations, are associated with increased risk for type 2 diabetes mellitus.[142]

Mechanism of Action of Lipoprotein(a) in Cardiovascular Disease

The strong genetic control of Lp(a) levels facilitated the design of Mendelian randomization studies demonstrating that elevated Lp(a) is a causal risk factor for both ASCVD and CAVD. However, the mechanisms underlying causal role of elevated Lp(a) in vascular diseases remain to be precisely defined (**Fig. 10–9**).

When the complementary DNA (cDNA) sequence of apo(a) was published by McLean and colleagues in 1987, a striking similarity between apo(a) and the proteolytic precursor plasminogen was observed.[70] Upon plasminogen activation to plasmin by either tissue plasminogen activator (tPA) or urokinase plasminogen activator (uPA) action, the resulting enzyme then cleaves many substrates including fibrin; this results in dissolution of thrombi through the process of fibrinolysis. Owing to its homology with plasminogen, it was hypothesized that apo(a) and Lp(a) could counteract this process, which

spawned tremendous excitement in the field as it suggested a link between the processes of atherosclerosis and thrombotic events. However, the data supporting a role for Lp(a) in fibrinolysis in vivo have been disappointing.[113] Indeed, Mendelian randomization studies suggested against a causal role of elevated Lp(a) in venous thromboembolism.[143] It has recently been demonstrated that Lp(a) does not inhibit fibrinolysis in human plasma (although apo(a) alone does).[144] However, this does not rule out a potential role for Lp(a) in the promotion of thrombus formation in the vasculature. For example, Lp(a) may modulate platelet reactivity and/or stimulate the pathways that result in thrombus formation and/or stabilization.[113] These mechanisms would be independent of the similarity between apo(a) and plasminogen.

The key observation that Lp(a), and not LDL, is the preferential carrier of oxidized phospholipids (oxPL) in plasma has provided a different lens through which to consider the basis of Lp(a) pathogenicity (Fig. 10–9). Indeed, apo(a) contains a covalently-linked oxPL moiety within the KIV$_{10}$ domain, the addition of which requires the strong lysine binding site present in this kringle.[145] The basis for this observation is unclear, as is the location of the oxPL addition (intracellular versus extracellular). Lp(a) accumulates at and is retained in the site of developing atherosclerotic lesions to greater extent than LDL; the extent of accumulation is directly proportional to the plasma Lp(a) concentration. The retention of Lp(a) in lesions is likely facilitated by its ability to bind to several extracellular matrix proteins including collagen, fibrinogen, and fibronectin. This, in turn, provides a route by which Lp(a) can deliver OxPL to arterial lesions.[146] The oxPL present on apo(a) has been linked to a number of proinflammatory effects of Lp(a) including increased expression of inflammatory mediators in cultured cells as well as in human PBMCs.[147,148] Interestingly, the oxPL moiety in apo(a) has also been shown to play a role in the development of CAVD through its ability to stimulate osteogenic differentiation in isolated valve interstitial cells.[149,150] As such, it has been hypothesized that the oxPL on Lp(a) provides a link between ASCVD and CAVD by virtue of its proinflammatory properties.[72]

The oxPL on Lp(a) has also been implicated in alteration of vascular endothelial cell phenotype through activation of glycolysis, promoting adhesion and transmigration of monocytes (Fig. 10–9).[151] This is in keeping with previous studies that have demonstrated a role for Lp(a) in endothelial cell signaling pathways that result in cellular contraction and disruption of cell-cell adhesion molecules.[152]

Taken together, the role of Lp(a) in the progression of ASCVD and CAVD is likely dependent in large part on its intrinsic proinflammatory properties (Fig. 10–9). This also helps to explain the independent nature of the risk associated with Lp(a) and vascular diseases.

Clinical Management of Elevated Lipoprotein(a)
Approach to Treatment

Although accounting for Lp(a) levels aids in risk prediction,[153] treatment options for patients with elevated Lp(a) are currently

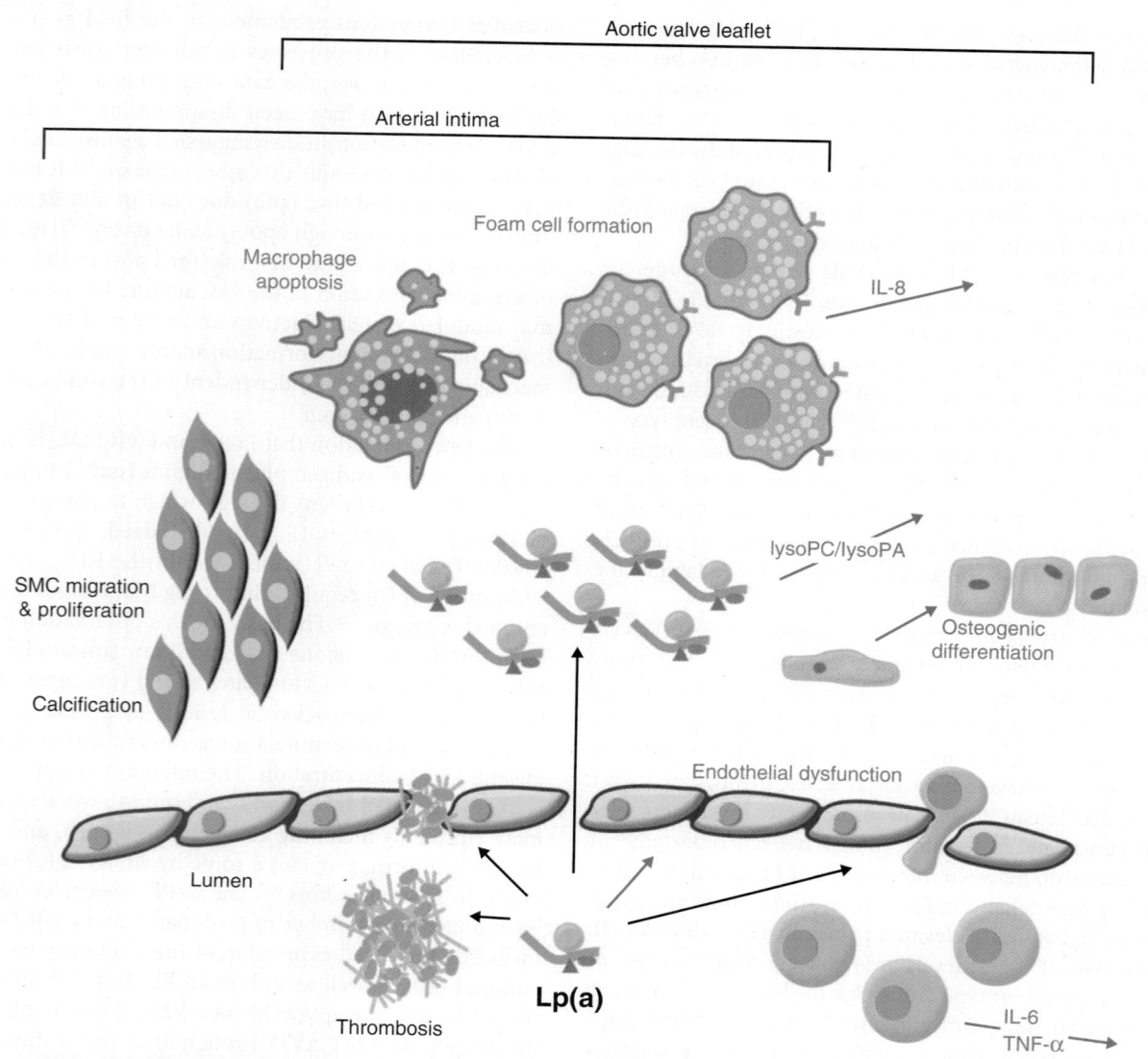

Figure 10–9. Pathological effects of Lp(a) and Lp(a)-associated oxPL. Lp(a) promotes endothelial damage by causing mural thrombosis and endothelial dysfunction; the latter includes decreased barrier function and a proinflammatory phenotype. Lp(a) can also activate monocytes in the circulation. The roles of Lp(a) in the arterial intima in atherosclerosis and in the valve interstitium in the aortic leaflet are overlapping and involve promotion of lipid deposition, inflammation, and calcification. The activities in red have been shown to be mediated by oxPLs on apo(a)/Lp(a). IL, interleukin; lysoPC, lysophosphatidyl choline; LysinePA, lysophosphatidic acid; SMC, smooth muscle cell; TNF, tumor necrosis factor.

limited. Owing to the large genetic component in the determination of Lp(a) levels, lifestyle interventions to lower Lp(a) are relatively ineffective. Despite the similarity between Lp(a) and LDL as already discussed, Lp(a) is resistant to lowering by statin therapy—in fact, statins may result in a small increase in Lp(a) levels.[154] However, several compounds that lower LDL also do lower Lp(a), albeit to a lesser extent (see **Table 10–13**). This includes PCSK9 inhibitors that lower Lp(a) by approximately 15% to 30%[127,128] and may lower risk for CHD events through Lp(a)-lowering independently;[128] it must be noted that these drugs are not approved for use in Lp(a) lowering at this time. A very effective way to lower Lp(a) levels is through lipoprotein apheresis.[155] However, this is an expensive and highly invasive approach that in North America is reserved for extreme cases. In Germany and the United Kingdom, however, lipoprotein apheresis has been approved by the government for patients

with Lp(a) levels in excess of 60 mg/dL and existing CVD, even if LDL-C is well-controlled.[156,157]

Other agents have also been identified that modestly lower Lp(a); these include niacin and lomitapide (Table 10–13), as well as aspirin, the thyroid hormone mimetic eprotirome, and estrogen.[158] However, clinical data on the effectiveness of these agents in Lp(a) lowering is not always robust and there are safety issues and/or lack of proven efficacy with each. Interestingly, analysis of the HPS2-THRIVE data shows, not unexpectedly, that the absolute Lp(a) lowering effect of niacin is proportionally dependent on Lp(a) isoform size: a greater absolute reduction was observed with smaller apo(a) isoform sizes which correspond to higher Lp(a) levels.[159] Given that the mean proportional lowering of Lp(a) even in the highest quintile was only 18%, this is likely insufficient to reduce Lp(a) risk that may require treatments that result in at least 40% lowering.[159]

TABLE 10-13. Established and Experimental Therapies to Lower Plasma Lp(a)

Agent	Class	% Lp(a) ↓	Specific for Lp(a)?[a]	Mechanism of action	Status	Ref.
Antibodies						
Evolocumab	mAb	30	N	Inhibition of PCSK9; ↑ LDL receptors; ↓ apo(a) secretion	Established	(85)
Alirocumab	mAb[b]	30	N	Inhibition of PCSK9; ↑ LDL receptors; ↓ apo(a) secretion	Established	(85)
Tocilizumab	mAb	30	N	IL-6 receptor blockade; ↓ transcription of *LPA* mRNA	Established	(358,359)
E06	mAb	?	N	Blockade of pro-inflammatory oxPL on Lp(a)	Experimental	(360)
Nucleic acid-based						
Mipomersen	Antisense oligonucleotide	21 – 39	N	↓ *APOB* mRNA	Established	(361)
IONIS-APO(a)$_{Rx}$	Antisense oligonucleotide	70	Y	↓ *LPA* mRNA	Experimental	(362,363)
AKCEA-APO(a)-L$_{Rx}$	Antisense oligonucleotide	90	Y	↓ *LPA* mRNA	Experimental	(362,363)
Inclisiran	RNAi[c]	14-25	N	↓ translation of *PCSK9* mRNA	Experimental	(364,365)
AMG 890	RNAi[c]	85-90[d]	Y	↓ translation of *LPA* mRNA	Experimental	(366)
Small molecule						
Niacin	Small molecule	25	N	Unknown (Transcription of *LPA*?)	Established	(367)
Lomitapide	Small molecule	15-20	N	MTP inhibitor; ↓ secretion of apoB-containing lipoproteins	Established	(368)
Other						
Lipoprotein-apheresis	Not applicable	70 (acute) 25-40 (sustained)	N	ApoB- or apo(a) affinity-based extracorporeal removal of lipoproteins from plasma	Established	(369-372)

[a]Refers to lipid profile
[b]Monoclonal antibody
[c]RNA interference
[d]Observed in nonhuman primates

Blockade of *LPA* mRNA translation has been the target of several exciting molecules in development which can dramatically lower Lp(a) levels (Fig. 10-8). One of these is a small interfering ribonucleic acid (siRNA), which is in early stages of clinical study (https://clinicaltrials.gov/ct2/show/NCT04270760). The other is an antisense oligonucleotide, which has shown very promising results in both Phase I and Phase II clinical trials.[160,161] Recruitment is ongoing for the Phase III outcome trial (https://clinicaltrials.gov/ct2/show/NCT04023552) studying major adverse cardiovascular events (cardiovascular death, nonfatal MI, nonfatal stroke, and urgent coronary revascularization requiring hospitalization) in subjects with hyperlipoprotein(a) (≥ 70 mg/dL or ≥90 mg/dL) and established ASCVD. This study will allow, for the first time, direct assessment of whether lowering of Lp(a) decreases risk for CVD events in a secondary prevention setting.

Training and Education

Lp(a) remains poorly understood from the clinical perspective as a possible tool for cardiovascular risk management.

Efforts are ongoing to increase both physician and patient awareness of elevated Lp(a) as an ASCVD and CAVD risk factor, particularly its importance in contributing to residual risk. There are a number of questions regarding Lp(a) that are frequently asked by clinicians. These are summarized here, with responses based on recent lipid statements,[132,157,162-165] and can serve as a guideline for managing patients with elevated Lp(a).

1. **In whom should Lp(a) be measured?** The most recent EAS/ESC guidelines recommend the measurement of Lp(a) in every individual at least once.[165] This is based on the relative stability of Lp(a) levels through an individual's lifetime.[166] It is important to measure Lp(a) in clinical practice as part of an individual's risk profile such that management of modifiable risk factors can be maximized.[132,163] Other recent lipid guidelines suggest that Lp(a) measurement should be performed in individuals with the following: a strong family history of premature CVD (<55 years old for men; <65 years old for women) in first degree relatives, and/or moderate to high CVD risk.[132,157,162-165] It has also been suggested that Lp(a) should be measured in all individuals with hypercholesterolemia (LDL ≥190 mg/dL) or confirmed/suspected FH.[124,132]

For individuals with high very ASCVD risk, Lp(a) measurement can be considered to identify individuals in whom PCSK9 inhibitor therapy may be considered.[132]

Although specific recommendations for measurement of Lp(a) in youth are lacking, there is growing interest in measuring Lp(a) in individuals less than/equal to 20 years old who have had ischemic or hemorrhagic stroke, and/or family history of premature CVD and/or if one or both biological parents have diagnosed hypercholesterolemia and/or elevated Lp(a).[75]

2. **How should Lp(a) be measured?** Although Lp(a) has been historically measured in mass concentration units (ie, mg/dL), the variation in Lp(a) isoform size necessitates the use of a particle concentration (ie, nmol/L) for accurate measurement. In the latter case, the risk threshold for Lp(a) in Caucasian populations has been identified as greater than 100 nmol/L (~ 50 mg/dL). Additionally, assays must be carefully chosen to minimize apo(a) isoform size bias by using a 5-point calibrator, and to use calibrators traceable to the IFCC secondary reference material. Proper measurement of Lp(a) is essential for standardization and harmonization of assays.[167]

3. **How to manage patients with elevated Lp(a) levels:** At the present time, the recommendation is to optimize control of modifiable risk factors in these individuals and ensure adherence to a healthy lifestyle including diet and exercise.[132] This approach has been proven effective to manage risk in patients with elevated Lp(a) in the absence of an Lp(a)-specific treatment.[168] The use of Lp(a)-lowering agents that have been identified to date including PCSK9 inhibitors are considered as off-label treatments since their effectiveness in lowering risk associated with elevated Lp(a) has not been proven. The ongoing trials with the *LPA* antisense drug which specifically and significantly lowers Lp(a) will address this question. The use of hormone replacement therapy to manage Lp(a) risk in postmenopausal women is not recommended at this time.[132]

4. **Awareness of Lp(a) risk:** Lp(a) is generally poorly understood from the clinical perspective. Enhanced communication is ongoing to increase both physician and patient awareness of elevated Lp(a) through the efforts of several national and international groups. There is a particular focus on increasing understanding of the role of Lp(a) in determining residual risk for ASCVD.

Concluding Remarks

While many unanswered questions remain concerning the biology, genetics, epidemiology, and clinical management of Lp(a), a new era where elevated Lp(a) is a legitimate treatment target is within sight. It is now crucial to define as precisely as possible the at-risk populations who might benefit from Lp(a)-lowering therapy. Moreover, a better understanding of the pathophysiology of Lp(a) could also pave the way to the development of drugs to specifically lower Lp(a) and/or to interfere with the harmful effects of this lipoprotein in the vasculature.

HYPERTRIGLYCERIDEMIA

Residual Atherosclerotic Cardiovascular Disease Risk

Despite aggressive LDL-C lowering for prevention of ASCVD, considerable lipid-related residual risk exists. Most important is the role of elevated triglyceride-rich lipoproteins at mild-to-moderate hypertriglyceridemia (150–1000 mg/dL; 1.7–11.4 mmol/L). This can be referred to as hypertriglyceridemia or combined hyperlipidemia, that is, elevation of both plasma triglycerides and plasma cholesterol. Clinically, either of these will typically be identified through elevated plasma triglycerides, or elevated non-HDL-C or apoB in the absence of elevated LDL-C.

It is most likely the cholesterol and not the triglyceride content of triglyceride-rich lipoproteins that lead to atherosclerosis, MI, and ASCVD[169] (**Fig. 10–10**). This is referred to as elevated remnant cholesterol (remnant-C), elevated very low-density lipoprotein cholesterol (VLDL-C), or elevated triglyceride-rich lipoprotein cholesterol (TRL-C). For simplicity, this chapter mainly uses the term remnant-C.

Numerous studies of patients on statin therapy have documented that part of residual ASCVD and all-cause mortality risk is due to elevated triglyceride-rich lipoproteins and remnant-C.[170-173] Of these studies, some examined elevated plasma triglycerides while others examined elevated remnant-C or elevated VLDL-C as explanations for the residual ASCVD risk. Despite these different study designs, all studies came to the same conclusion: triglyceride-rich lipoproteins explain residual ASCVD morbidity and mortality risk beyond statin therapy, independent of LDL-C and HDL-C levels.

Historical Development

In the 1970s and 1980s, clinicians treating lipid disorders focused on patients at high risk of ASCVD due to either FH with elevated LDL-C or to remnant hyperlipidemia with combined hyperlipidemia, elevated remnant-C, and elevated triglyceride-rich lipoproteins (see next subsection). These were the typical two types of patients followed in lipid clinics, together with the rare genetic form of the familial chylomicronemia syndrome with severe hypertriglyceridemia (subsequently discussed).

Later on, focus centered on elevated LDL-C clinically, partly due to understanding of the genetic cause of FH as mutations in the LDL-receptor; this pioneering work by Michael S. Brown and Joseph L. Goldstein lead to the Nobel Prize in 1985. The LDL-C focus clinically was further supported by statin trials convincingly showing reduced ASCVD morbidity as well as reduced cardiovascular and all-cause mortality.[174] For easy communication statins were marketed as LDL-C lowering drug, as statins work via upregulation of the LDL-receptor on hepatocytes and as LDL-C in consequence is lowered; however, statins also reduce triglyceride-rich lipoproteins[175] and remnant-C, a fact that was partly ignored by most drug companies during marketing of statins. Therefore, even today, this important added value of statins remains unrecognized by many clinicians prescribing statins.

Explained Risk From ApoB-containing Lipoproteins to Myocardial Infarction

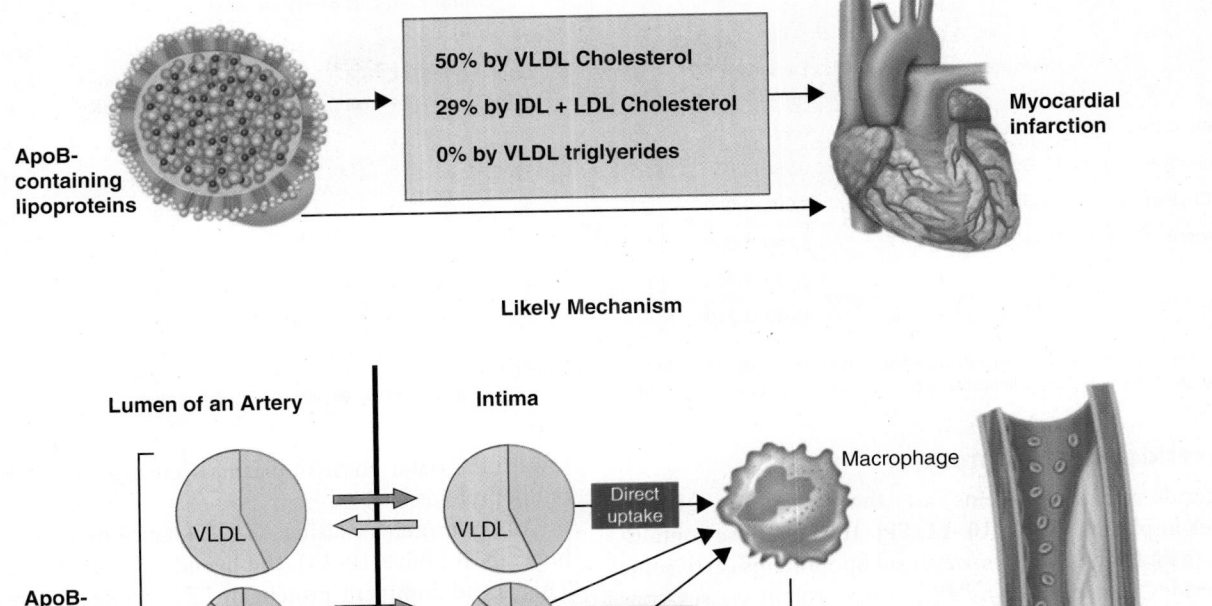

Likely Mechanism

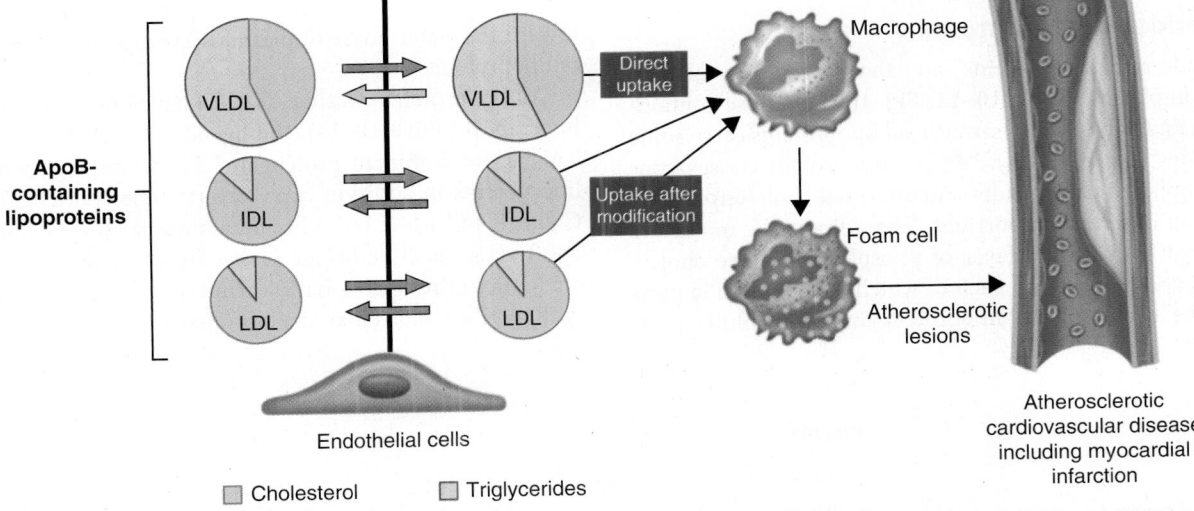

Figure 10–10. Fractions of risk explained and likely mechanism from apoB-containing triglyceride-rich remnants or VLDL to ASCVD including MI. VLDL cholesterol explained 50% of the risk from apoB-containing lipoproteins to MI. ApoB, apolipoprotein B; IDL, intermediate-density lipoprotein; LDL, low-density lipoprotein; VLDL, very low-density lipoprotein. Reproduced with permission from Balling M, Afzal S, Varbo A, et al. VLDL Cholesterol Accounts for One-Half of the Risk of Myocardial Infarction Associated With apoB-Containing Lipoproteins. *J Am Coll Cardiol.* 2020 Dec 8;76(23):2725-2735.

Thereafter came a period of scientific (and partly clinical) focus on low HDL-C starting in the 1990s due to very strong epidemiological evidence that low HDL-C is associated with high risk of ASCVD, shown in numerous studies including in meta-analyses.[176] It was believed by many that raising HDL-C would reduce ASCVD events, like through lowering of LDL-C, and many drug companies developed HDL-C increasing drugs. However, starting around year 2000, genetic studies questioned high HDL-C as cardioprotective because such studies could not confirm a causal relationship between low HDL-C and increased risk of ASCVD, or vice versa.[177-179] The hypothesis that HDL-C could be cardioprotective was largely abandoned when none of the HDL-C–raising trials led to cardiovascular benefit through HDL-C increases,[180-182] with one trial even increasing cardiovascular morbidity and mortality.[180] Looking back, it appears that scientists and drug companies were misled by confounding, that is, the fact that individuals with low HDL-C often have high levels of remnant-C and triglyceride-rich lipoproteins—the real cause of high ASCVD risk in those with low HDL-C.[177,183]

Renewed interest in elevated plasma triglycerides, remnant-C, and triglyceride-rich lipoproteins surfaced in 2007, with special focus on the nonfasting state to better capture the risk associated with these lipoproteins;[184,185] these studies build on the original 1979 hypothesis by Donald B. Zilversmit stating that "atherogenesis is a postprandial phenomenon." The 2007 renewed interest in elevated triglyceride-rich lipoproteins as a risk factor for ASCVD and all-cause mortality was followed by numerous genetic Mendelian randomization studies documenting causality from elevated remnant-C and triglyceride-rich lipoproteins to increased risk of ASCVD and all-cause mortality.[177-179,186-200] Finally, three large-scale triglyceride-lowering trials in patients with elevated triglyceride-rich lipoproteins despite statin therapy were initiated.[201-203]

TABLE 10–14. Size, Density and Core, and Surface Components of Different Lipoprotein Classes

| | Diameter (nm) | Molecular weight X10⁶ (daltons) | Density (g/mL) | Components (% of dry weight) | | | | | Main apolipo-proteins |
| | | | | Core | | Surface | | | |
				Trigly-cerides	Cholesterol ester	Chole-sterol	Phospho-lipid	Apolipo-proteins	
Chylomicrons	75–1200	50–1000	0.93	86	3	2	7	2	A, B-48, C, E
VLDL (+ChylRem*)	30–80	10–80	0.93–1.006	55	12	7	18	8	B-100, C, E
IDL (+ChylRem*)	25–35	5–10	1.006–1.019	23	29	9	19	19	B-100, C, E
Lipoprotein(a)	25–30	4–5	1.040–1.090	8	30	8	25	29	B-100, a
LDL	18–25	2.3	1.019–1.063	6	42	8	22	22	B-100
HDL	5–12	0.2—0.4	1.063–1.210	4	15	5	34	42	A, C, E

*Chylomicron remnants will be present in these fractions in nonfasting plasma in the postprandial phase.
Abbreviations: HDL, high-density lipoprotein; LDL, low-density lipoprotein; IDL, intermediate-density lipoprotein; VLDL, very low-density lipoprotein.

Triglyceride-Rich Lipoproteins

Triglyceride-rich lipoproteins are the largest fat-carrying particles in plasma (**Table 10–14, Fig. 10–11**), those containing the most triglycerides; however, all lipoproteins carry some triglycerides (Table 10–14).[204,205] All lipoprotein classes contain hydrophobic triglycerides and esterified cholesterol in the core, but in different proportions. These lipophilic molecules are covered by a surface layer of phospholipids, free cholesterol, and apolipoproteins, each of which have lipophilic parts toward the center of the lipoprotein and hydrophilic parts toward the water phase in plasma securing the spherical form of lipoproteins.

All lipoproteins causing ASCVD have one molecule of the huge apoB (Table 10–14), the ligand for the LDL-receptor.[206] This is the dominant protein in LDL, while triglyceride-rich lipoproteins in addition carry several other proteins like apo C and E and while Lp(a) has an additional apo(a) attached to apoB via a disulfide bridge (Table 10–14). Chylomicrons and chylomicron remnants have a truncated form of apoB (B-48) with 48% the molecular size of full-size apoB (B-100) present

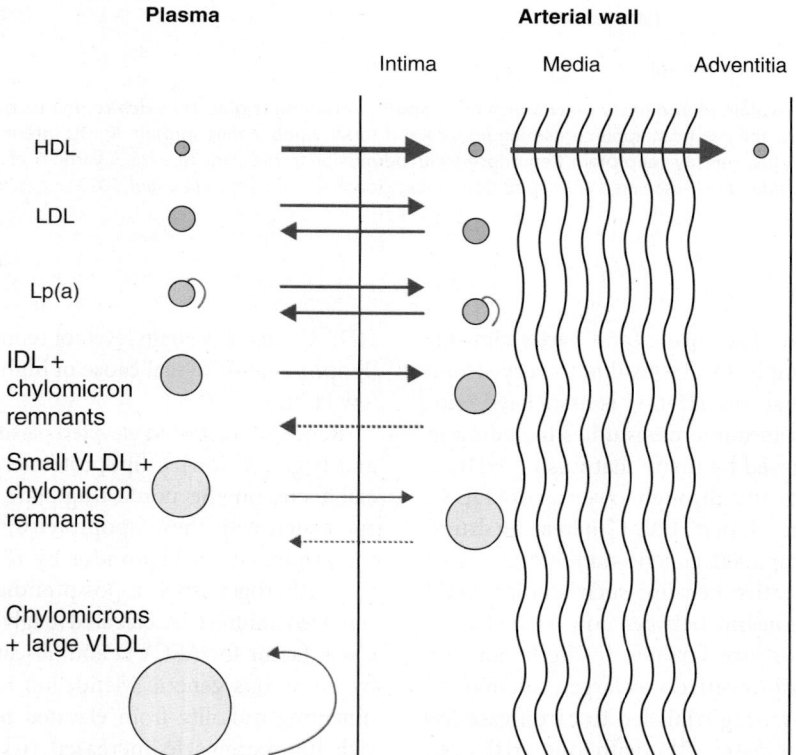

Figure 10–11. Transport of plasma lipoproteins in and out of the arterial intima. HDL, high-density lipoprotein; IDL, intermediate-density lipoprotein; LDL, low-density lipoprotein; Lp(a), lipoprotein(a); VLDL, very low-density lipoprotein. Reproduced with permission from Nordestgaard BG. A Test in Context: Lipid Profile, Fasting Versus Nonfasting. *J Am Coll Cardiol.* 2017 Sep 26;70(13):1637-1646.

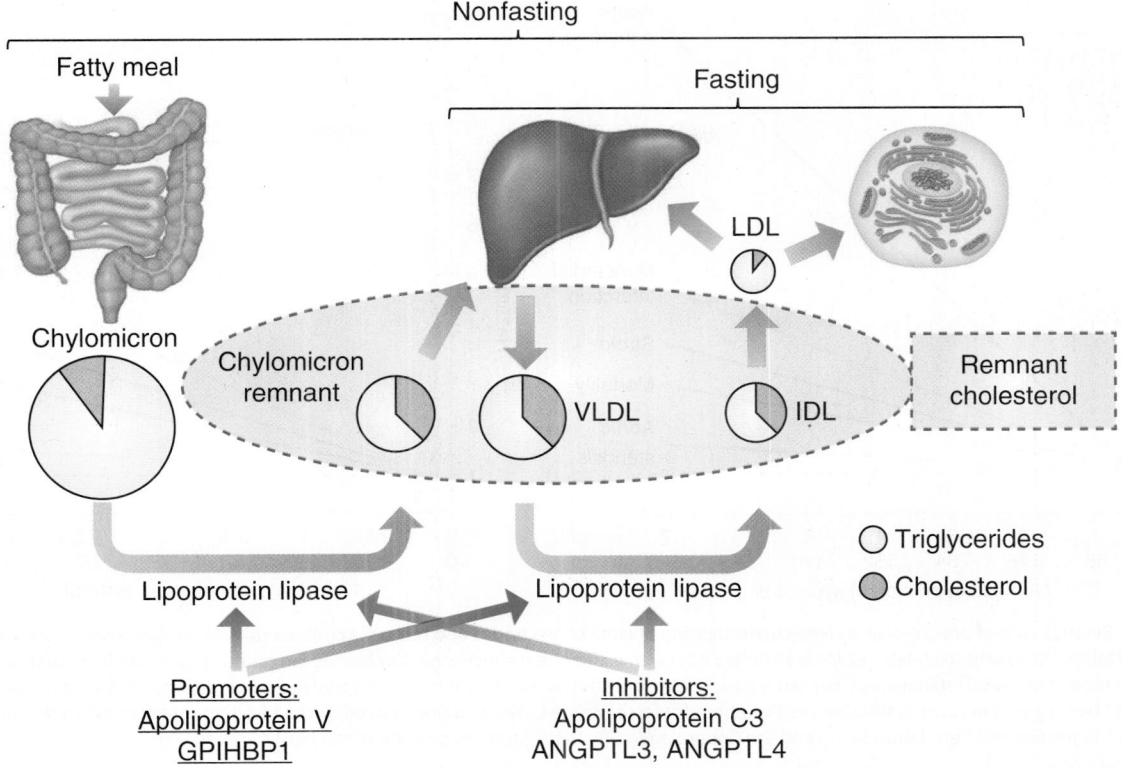

Figure 10–12. Metabolism of apolipopprotein B containing lipoproteins. These particles are immediately being acted upon by lipoprotein lipase, leading to triglyceride hydrolysis and reduction in lipoprotein size. These lipoproteins with some triglyceride hydrolysis (VLDL, chylomicron remnants, and IDL) can collectively be called remnants and the cholesterol content remnant cholesterol. The triglyceride degradation in plasma by lipoprotein lipase is promoted and inhibited by different proteins. IDL, intermediate-density lipoprotein; LDL, low-density lipoprotein; VLDL, very low-density lipoprotein; GPIHBP1, glycosylphosphatidylinositol anchored high-density lipoprotein binding protein 1; ANGPTL3, angiopoietin-like 3; ANGPTL4, angiopoietin-like 4. Reproduced with permission from Professor Børge G. Nordestgaard.

in LDL, Lp(a), intermediate-density lipoprotein (IDL), and VLDL.

After intake of a fatty meal, triglyceride-rich lipoproteins in the form of chylomicrons are transported from the intestine via lymph to the blood stream[207] (**Fig. 10–12**); lipoprotein lipase then immediately start triglyceride hydrolysis rapidly converting chylomicrons to cholesterol-enriched chylomicron remnants to be taken up by liver cells.[208] Liver cells resecrete triglycerides together with esterified cholesterol in VLDL particles into the blood stream; during lipoprotein lipase-mediated triglyceride hydrolysis in plasma VLDL particles are converted first into IDL and then further into LDL, representing a continuous process where lipoproteins decrease in size and increasingly are depleted of triglycerides. This process also includes cholesterol ester transfer protein (CETP)–mediated cholesterol ester enrichment of VLDL, IDL, and LDL in exchange for triglycerides from other lipoproteins. Understanding lipoprotein metabolism may seem complicated for many clinicians; however, it is not essential to understand the details when it comes to clinical relevance.

For clinical use, all triglyceride-rich lipoproteins can be lumped into one group, to differentiate this class from LDL, Lp(a), and HDL.[206,208] For simplicity, triglyceride-rich lipoproteins can collectively be referred as remnants.[209] This is because a remnant means a breakdown product, and because all

chylomicrons and VLDL are immediately partly broken down due to triglyceride hydrolysis by lipoprotein lipase after entering the plasma space (Fig. 10–12); in hypertriglyceridemia and combined hyperlipidemia in nonfasting conditions, elevated levels of triglyceride-rich lipoproteins usually represent a mixture of intestine-derived chylomicron remnants and liver-derived VLDL remnants.[210] The only exception is in familial chylomicronemia syndrome (seen in 1 in 1 million), characterized by a total lack of lipoprotein lipase activity and therefore no triglyceride hydrolysis.

For LDL in clinical use, we measure the cholesterol content; this is also pathologically meaningful because after degradation of triglycerides, proteins, and phospholipids, the remainder undegradable cholesterol is what is deposited in the arterial intima to cause atherosclerosis. In analogy, for clinical use, one should examine remnant-C (= VLDL-C = TRL-C).[204,208,209] Elevated plasma triglycerides represent a less precise marker of elevated triglyceride-rich lipoproteins as plasma triglycerides include triglycerides in all lipoproteins combined (Table 10–14).

Risk of Atherosclerotic Cardiovascular Disease

Progressively higher levels of triglyceride-rich lipoproteins measured either as plasma triglycerides or remnant-C are associated with progressively higher risk of MI, ischemic stroke, ASCVD, aortic valve stenosis, and all-cause mortality

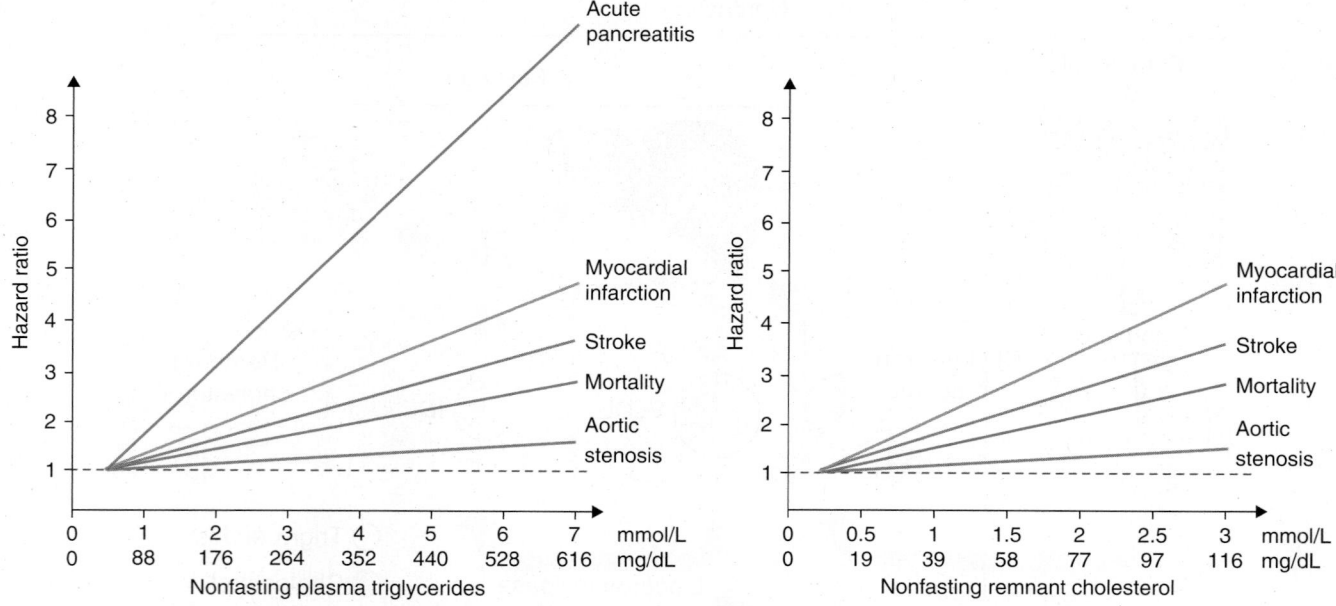

Figure 10–13. **Relationship of progressive increase in nonfasting plasma triglycerides and remnant cholesterol with progressive increase in risk of morbidity and mortality.** Observational relationships are shown; however, using genetic instrument in Mendelian randomization analysis such associations are all confirmed to represent causal relationships. For acute pancreatitis, only the relationship with plasma triglycerides is depicted because remnant cholesterol is not thought of being a part in causing this disease. Data from Professor Børge G. Nordestgaard based on data from roughly 100,000 individuals participating in the Copenhagen General Population Study and the Copenhagen City Heart Study as published previously.

(**Fig. 10–13**)[191,211-215] When plasma triglycerides are above 440 mg/dL (5 mmol/L) versus below 88 mg/dL (1 mmol/L) or remnant-C is above 89 mg/dL (2.3 mmol/L) versus below 19 mg/dL (0.5 mmol/L), risk is approximately 5-fold for MI, 3-fold for ischemic stroke, 2-fold for all-cause mortality, 1.5-fold for aortic stenosis, and 10-fold for acute pancreatitis; in other words, with the same increase in plasma triglycerides the relative risk of acute pancreatitis is double that of MI (Fig. 10–13);[216] however, roughly 10 times as many MIs compared to acute pancreatitis events developed during 7 years of follow-up. Fig. 10–13 only shows risk of acute pancreatitis as a function of elevated plasma triglycerides, because this is the likely causal factor for acute pancreatitis through triglyceride hydrolysis and inflammation,[217] while elevated remnant-C is more likely the cause of ASCVD.[212]

Measurement

A standard lipid profile includes plasma cholesterol, LDL-C, HDL-C, and plasma triglycerides (**Fig. 10–14**).[204] These four values will not accurately determine the amount of triglyceride-rich lipoproteins in plasma, as plasma triglycerides is a composite marker of triglycerides in all lipoproteins (Table 10–14). Ideally, laboratories should measure or calculate remnant-C to direct focus toward the cholesterol content on triglyceride-rich lipoproteins.[208,218,219] As cholesterol, and not triglycerides, accumulates in the atherosclerotic plaque, clinicians and patients need to understand that the cholesterol in these particles likely are equally important to LDL-C in leading to atherosclerosis and ASCVD (Fig. 10–10).

Remnant-C can be calculated from a standard lipid profile as total cholesterol minus HDL-C minus LDL-C; LDL-C can be calculated or measured directly. Either nonfasting or fasting blood samples can be used; nonfasting values have the advantage of capturing the average levels seen during a 24-hour cycle.[204,218] Remnant-C levels are typically 8 mg/dL (0.2 mmol/L) higher 3 to 4 hours after a normal meal compared with in the fasting state; for plasma triglycerides, the corresponding value is 26 mg/dL (0.3 mmol/L) higher levels. The calculated version of remnant-C comes at no additional cost; however, remnant-C (= TRL-C) can also be measured directly using a newly developed homogenous assay for auto-analyzers from Denka Seiken,[220,221] ultracentrifugation, or nuclear magnetic resonance (NMR) technology.[222]

United States,[223] European,[224] and Canadian[225] cholesterol guidelines advise to also examine non-HDL-C and plasma apoB levels, because these indirectly identify elevated triglyceride-rich lipoproteins, that is, if LDL-C is low (Fig. 10–14). Because the cholesterol content of Lp(a) is normally included in the LDL-C value, the difference between non-HDL-C and LDL-C solely represents remnant-C.

Prevalence

According to the US National Health and Nutrition Examination Survey (NHANES), the prevalence during 2007 to 2014 of plasma triglycerides of <150 mg/dL (1.7 mmol/L) was 75%, of 150–199 mg/dL (1.7–2.3 mmol/L) 13%, and of ≥200 mg/dL (2.3 mmol/L) was 12% in adults not taking statins; among statin users corresponding values were 68%, 16%, and 15%,

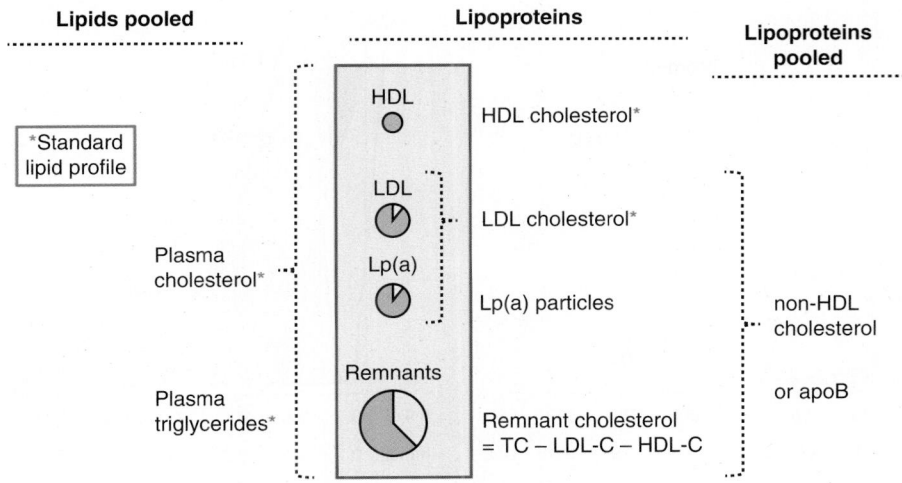

Figure 10–14. Lipids and lipoproteins as part of standard and expanded lipid profiles. Standard lipid profiles consist of plasma cholesterol, LDL-C, HDL-C, and plasma triglycerides; however, a standard lipid profile could also report calculated remnant cholesterol and calculated non-HDL-C because these come at no additional cost. Calculated remnant cholesterol is nonfasting total cholesterol minus LDL-C minus HDL-C. Calculated non-HDL-C is total cholesterol minus HDL-C. Lipoprotein(a) should be measured at least once in every individual screened for cardiovascular risk in order to detect potentially high concentrations of this genetic risk factor. Finally, apoB can be used as an alternative to non-HDL-C, which comes at an extra cost.

respectively.[226] In other words, one-fourth of US adults overall, including nearly one-third of those on statin therapy, have suboptimal plasma triglyceride levels.[226] Plasma triglycerides in US populations appear to be highest in Hispanics, lowest in African Americans, and in between in South Asian American, Whites, and Chinese American.[227]

The population distribution of remnant-C and plasma triglycerides are skewed with a tail toward elevated levels (**Fig. 10–15**).[212] In a typical affluent country exemplified by Denmark, 26% of women and 45% of men have remnant-C of 30-100 mg/dL (0.8-2.6 mmol/) while 0.2% of women and 0.7% of men have even higher levels. Likewise, 27% of women and 45% of men have triglycerides of 150–500 mg/dL (1.7-5.7 mmol/) while 0.5% of women and 1.9% of men have triglycerides above 500 mg/dL (5.7 mmol/L). Newborns on average have triglycerides of 20 mg/dL (0.3 mmol/L) while levels in children and adolescent are double those values, unless overweight or obesity are present in the child when values are even higher (see below). In men including those with overweight or obesity, levels of both triglycerides and remnant-C increase from age 20 onward, while a similar increase is only observed in women after age 40.

Overweight and obesity are the most common causes of elevated remnant-C and plasma triglycerides.[212] Indeed, body mass index (BMI) explains 12% of all variation in remnant-C in individuals in the population at large.[220] In individuals in affluent countries, average remnant-C levels are 15 mg/dL (0.4 mmol/L) in underweight individuals, 19 mg/dL (0.5 mmol/L) in normal weight individuals, 27 mg/dL (0.7 mmol/L) in overweight individuals, 32 mg/dL (0.8 mmol/L) in obese individuals, 34 mg/dL (0.9 mmol/L) in severe obese individuals, and 34 mg/dL (0.9 mmol/L) in extreme obese individuals.[220] Corresponding values are 30 mg/dL (0.8 mmol/L) and 24 mg/dL (0.6 mmol/L) in those with and without diabetes mellitus,

partly explained by the higher BMI in those with diabetes versus without diabetes.

Genetics, fat intake, carbohydrate intake, alcohol intake, and exercise will also influence remnant-C and plasma triglyceride levels. Numerous genetic variants in many different genes influence levels of remnant-C and plasma triglycerides, genetic variants that together with lifestyle and BMI determine the concentrations in plasma in the individual.[228] Therefore, within each BMI category there will be a remnant-C and plasma triglyceride distributions like those shown in Fig. 10–15, such that some individuals will have lower and some individuals will have higher levels than those observed in the average person.[220] Nevertheless, because BMI is the strongest determinant of remnant-C and plasma triglyceride levels, the simplest possible explanation is as follows: when energy intake in the form of fat, carbohydrates, and alcohol surpasses that used to exercise, triglycerides are deposited in fat and liver tissue with overflow of increasingly higher levels of triglyceride-rich lipoproteins and remnant-C in plasma as BMI increases.[220]

Nonfasting versus Fasting

The postprandial or nonfasting state predominates during most of a 24-hour cycle.[206,229] In contrast, fasting for more than 8 hours, as previously used before lipid profile testing, in most people only occurs just before breakfast. Therefore, and because plasma only contains triglyceride-rich lipoproteins of hepatic origin in the fasting state but additionally those of intestinal origin in the nonfasting state (Fig. 10–12), the nonfasting state optimally evaluate the total amount of triglyceride-rich lipoproteins in plasma averaging over a 24-hour period. Also, using fasting lipid profiles may disguise the real residual risk in a patient due to elevated triglyceride-rich lipoproteins.[229]

Further and likewise important, nonfasting lipid profiles represent a simplification for patients, laboratories, and clinicians

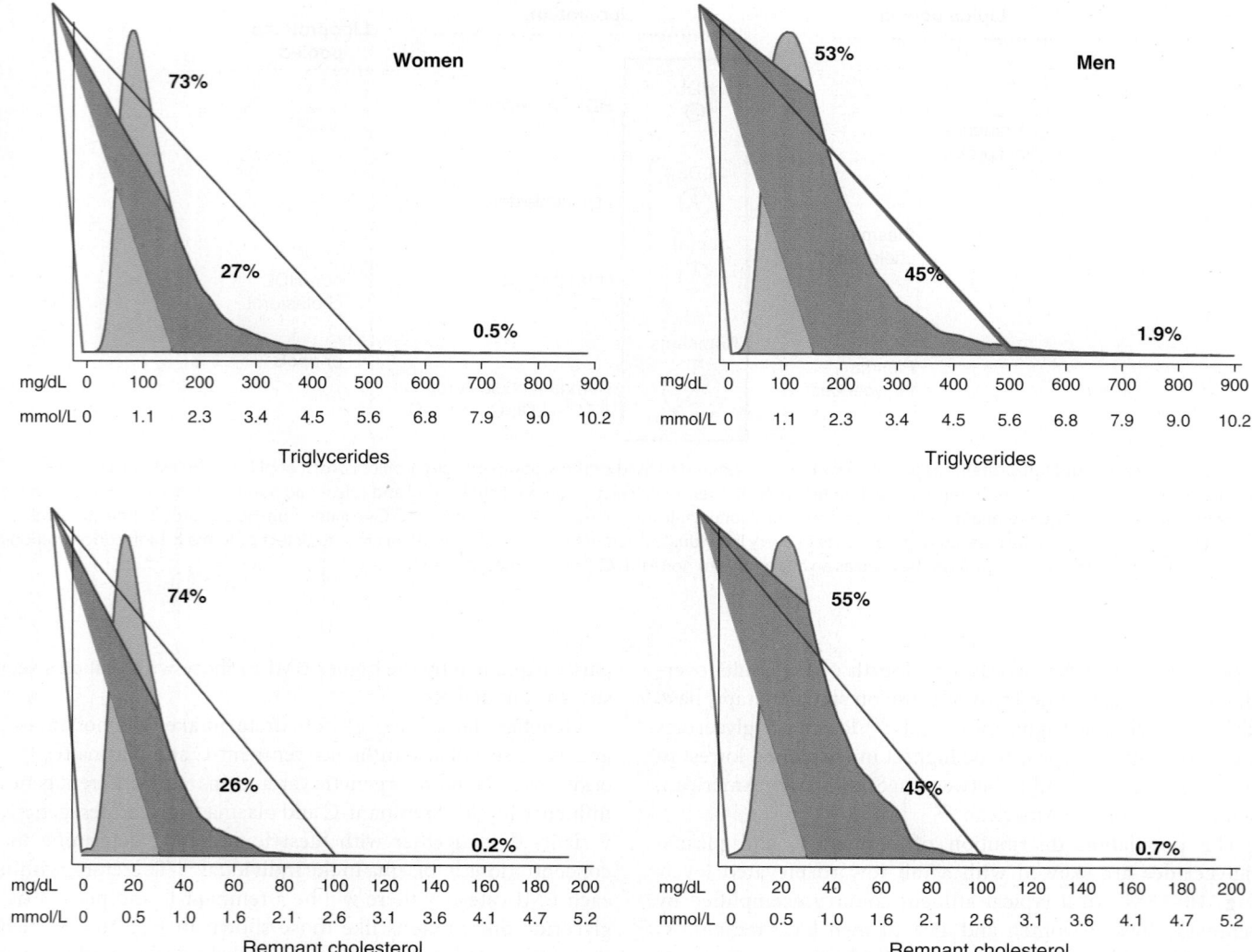

Figure 10–15. Distributions of plasma triglycerides and remnant cholesterol in 60,000 women and 50,000 men from the Copenhagen General Population Study, representing a typical affluent society. Green indicates normal levels, orange high levels, and red very high levels. Reproduced with permission from Professor Børge G. Nordestgaard.

alike without negative implications for prognostic, diagnostic, and therapeutic options for CVD prevention.[206,208,229,230] In accordance, United States and European guidelines on prevention of ASCVD now endorse widespread use of nonfasting lipid profiles,[223,224] as do guidelines in several other countries.[204]

Mechanism

The most likely scenario from elevated triglyceride-rich lipoproteins to atherosclerosis and ASCVD is simple and straightforward.[211,212] At elevated levels in plasma and irrespective of intestinal or hepatic origin, triglyceride-rich lipoproteins smaller than chylomicrons penetrate from plasma into the arterial intima where they, due to being a larger size than LDL and HDL, get trapped selectively (Fig. 10–11). Triglyceride hydrolysis in the intima lead to liberation of tissue-toxic free fatty acids and consequent local inflammation,[207] while the entire triglyceride-rich lipoprotein particle is taken up directly

by macrophages to produce foam cells and atherosclerosis (**Fig. 10–16**).

Vulnerable atherosclerotic plaques, possibly due to inflammation from liberated free fatty acids during triglyceride hydrolysis, then lead to plaque rupture and subsequent MI or ischemic stroke (Figs. 10–10 and 10–16). Supporting this idea, elevated plasma triglycerides and remnant-C are observationally and causally through human genetics related to increased whole-body low-grade inflammation, while elevated LDL-C is not.[189,217]

Genetics

Mendelian Randomization Studies to Document Causality
Numerous studies document that genetically elevated triglyceride-rich lipoproteins, measured as elevated plasma triglycerides or remnant-C, are causally related to increased risk of ASCVD or even all-cause mortality irrespective of levels of LDL-C and

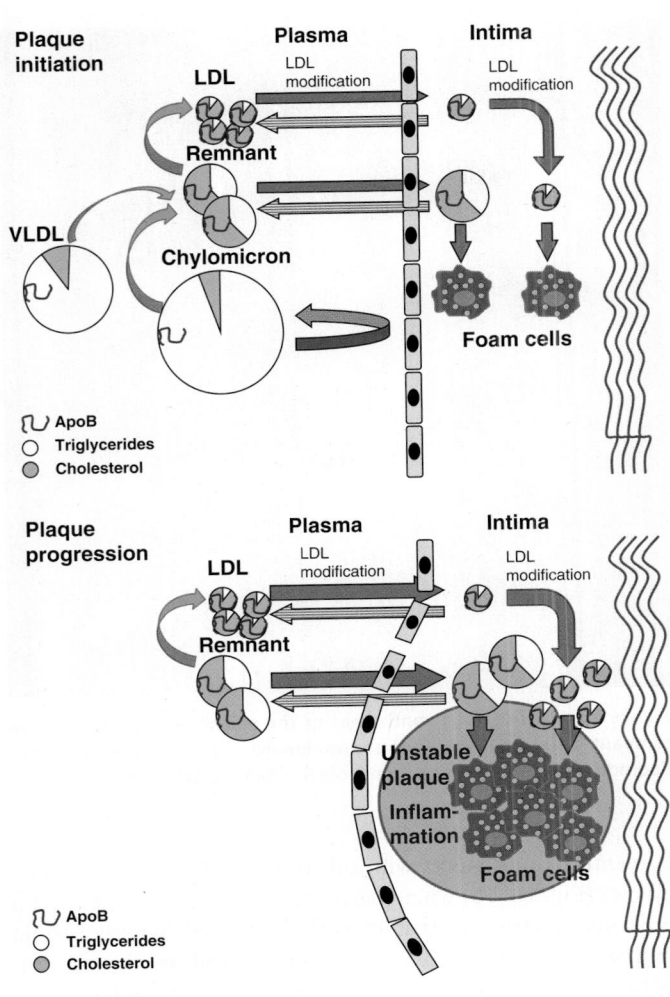

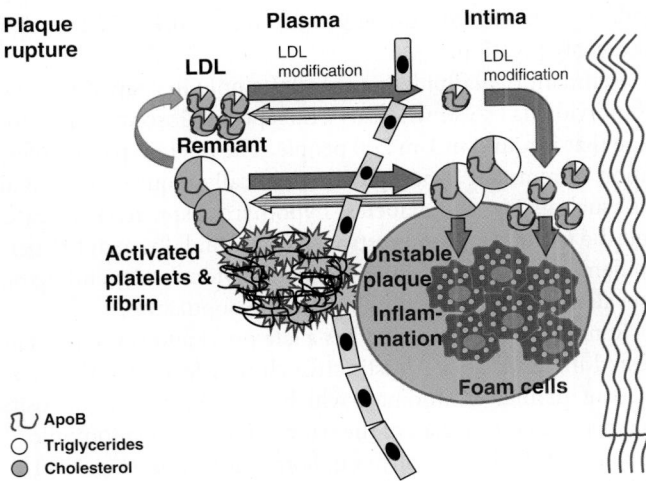

Figure 10–16. From elevated triglyceride-rich lipoproteins to atherosclerotic plaque initiation, plaque progression, and finally plaque rupture causing MI or ischemic stroke. This mechanistic cartoon depicts the situation in the nonfasting or postprandial state with lipoproteins in plasma both of intestinal (chylomicrons and chylomicron remnants) and hepatic origin (very low-density lipoproteins [VLDL], VLDL remnants [= intermediate-density lipoproteins, IDL] and low-density lipoproteins [LDL]). Reproduced with permission from Parhofer KG, Chapman MJ, Nordestgaard BG. Efficacy and safety of icosapent ethyl in hypertriglyceridaemia: a recap. *Eur Heart J Suppl.* 2020 Oct 6;22(Suppl J):J21-J33.

HDL-C.[177-179,186-200,207,211,212] These studies take advantage of the Mendelian randomization design where genetic variants generally are unconfounded and where reverse causation is not an issue, because genotypes are present from birth and therefore always precede ASCVD development.[231]

Genetic variants leading to lifelong high or low levels of triglyceride-rich lipoproteins and corresponding high and low risk of ASCVD are observed in many single genes of direct importance for triglyceride metabolism:[186,187,190,193-200] the proteins apolipoprotein AV and glycosylphosphatidylinositol anchored high density lipoprotein binding protein 1 (GPI-HBP1) promote the action of lipoprotein lipase and thus lower remnant-C and plasma triglyceride levels, while the lipoprotein lipase inhibitors apolipoprotein C3, angiopoietin-like 3 (ANGPTL3), and ANGPTL4 increase remnant-C and plasma triglyceride levels (Fig. 10–12).

Monogenic Disorders in Clinical Practice

Familial Chylomicronemia Syndrome (Type I Hyperlipidemia; OMIM 238600): Clinically, this syndrome is identified when plasma triglycerides are severely elevated above 1000 mg/dL (11.4 mmol/L) or when eruptive xanthomas are present (**Fig. 10–17**), but should also be suspected when other blood test cannot be measured due to lipid interference; if you receive such information from the laboratory, a plasma triglyceride test should be ordered. Severe hypertriglyceridemia found in 1 in 1000 is most often due to obesity, dysregulated diabetes, or reduced kidney function,[232] each of which should be excluded before considering the familial form of the chylomicronemia syndrome; in a few women, third trimester pregnancy may also cause the chylomicronemia syndrome due to very high plasma estrogen levels (subsequently discussed). The familial form is found in 1 in 1 million, or maybe slightly more common.

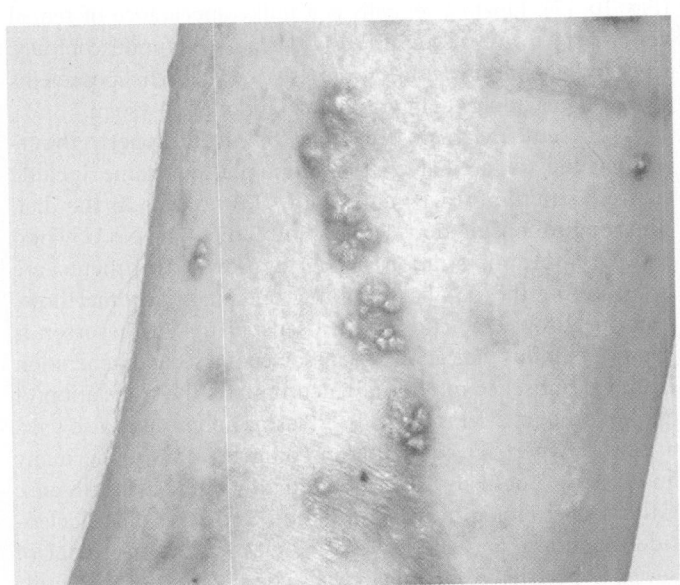

Figure 10–17. Eruptive xanthomas on the torso, elbows, or buttocks as typically seen in the familial chylomicronemia syndrome with severe hypertriglyceridemia (type I hyperlipidemia). Reproduced with permission from Professor Børge G. Nordestgaard.

Familial chylomicronemia syndrome is due to homozygosity or compound heterozygosity for large-effect loss-of-function mutations in genes that regulate catabolism of triglyceride-rich lipoproteins: lipoprotein lipase (*LPL*), apoC-II (*APOC2*), glucosylphosphatidylinositol-anchored high-density lipoprotein-binding protein 1 (*GPIHBP1*), lipase maturation factor 1 (*LMF1*), apoA-V (*APOA5*), or glycerol-3-phosphate dehydrogenase (*GPD1*).[228]

The typical onset of familial chylomicronemia syndrome is in childhood to adolescent due to episodes of acute pancreatitis, but onset has also been described in infants as well as in older adults; however, the clinical diagnosis of familial chylomicronemia syndrome is often delayed and is often only considered after recurrent episodes of abdominal pain due to acute pancreatitis. Acute pancreatitis is the most serious manifestation and the main morbidity of familial chylomicronemia syndrome, which can be fatal. Risk of acute pancreatitis increases already at mild-to-moderate hypertriglyceridemia (Fig. 10–13);[216,217,233] however, at these levels, the absolute risk of ASCVD surpasses by many folds the risk of acute pancreatitis.

When triglycerides are constantly elevated above 2000 to 5000 mg/dL (23-57 mmol/L; exact levels are not known), atherosclerosis does not appear to develop,[228] simply because chylomicrons and very large VLDL are too large to enter into the arterial intima (Fig. 10–11).[234] However, at triglycerides below these levels, triglyceride-rich lipoproteins are able to enter the intima of arteries (Fig. 10–11) and thus are highly atherogenic leading to premature ASCVD.

Other clinical manifestations include eruptive xanthomas (Figure 10-17), lipemia retinalis, and hepatosplenomegaly. Eruptive xanthomas are dermatological features of severe hypertriglyceridemia: localized or wide-spread small yellowish papules with erythematous bases of 3 to 5 mm due to triglyceride accumulation in subcutaneous macrophages on the torso, elbows, or buttocks (Fig. 10–17). Lipemia retinalis is a milky appearance of retinal vessels loaded with viscous lipemic plasma, seen funduscopically. Hepatosplenomegaly results from triglyceride-rich lipoproteins uptake by macrophages in the reticulo-endothelial system.

At present, the main treatment of severe hypertriglyceridemia due to familial chylomicronemia syndrome include severe restriction of fat intake with <15% of fats in the diet. This require consultations with a clinical dietitian. No US Food and Drug Administration (FDA)–approved treatments are available for the familial chylomicronemia syndrome; however, in Europe, the apo-CIII antisense drug Volanesorsen is approved for this indication: Volanesorsen is a second-generation chimeric antisense inhibitor, which impairs the translation of apolipoprotein C-III mRNA.[235,236] Plasma apheresis is also used at severe hypertriglyceridemia in countries such as Germany and Austria, but likely used less frequently in the United States. Other novel biologics using antibody, antisense oligonucleotide inhibition, and siRNA technologies for the treatment of severe hypertriglyceridemia may also be effective for the familial chylomicronemia syndrome in the future.[237]

Remnant Hyperlipidemia (Dysbetalipoproteinemia; Type III Hyperlipidemia; OMIM 617347) : Clinically, this condition

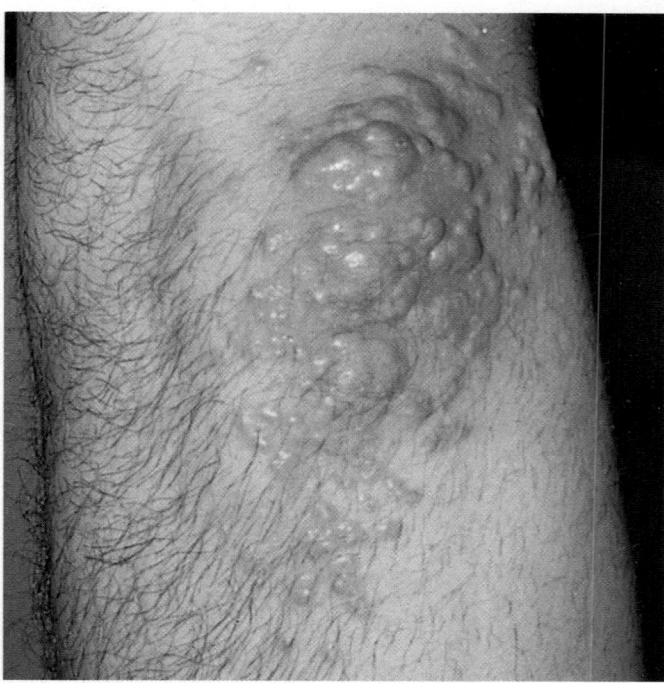

Figure 10–18. Tuberous xanthomas at the elbow as typically seen in remnant hyperlipidemia (dyslipoproteinemia; type III hyperlipidemia). Reproduced with permission from Professor Børge G. Nordestgaard.

is identified in patients with tuberous xanthomas at knees or elbows (**Fig. 10–18**) when plasma triglycerides and cholesterol are equally elevated, that is, with combined hyperlipidemia and elevated remnant-C.[238] Lacking typical xanthomas but with combined hyperlipidemia, remnant hyperlipidemia can be diagnosed either due to apoE-2/2 isoform (or genotype) and/or a cholesterol-to-triglyceride ratio >0.4 i VLDL after ultracentrifugation.

Remnant hyperlipidemia manifests only in a small portion of individuals (<5%) who carry the apoE-2/2 isoform, a genotype that is found in 1 in 200 people. The phenotypic manifestation of remnant hyperlipidemia typically requires a "second hit" such as obesity, diabetes, hypothyroidism, renal disease, and the use of exogenous estrogen or alcohol. Remnant hyperlipidemia is found in 1 to 5 in 1000 individuals, depending on prevalence of these "second hits" in the population.

Remnant hyperlipidemia has a late onset and is rarely manifested in childhood. A distinctive clinical feature is the presence of palmar xanthomas, which describe yellow deposits that occur in the creases of the palms and is pathognomonic.[238] Tuberous and tuberoeruptive xanthomas also occur (**Fig. 10–18**), but they are not unique to this condition. Premature ASCVD develops in up to half of these patients, as least as common as that seen for FH. Remnant hyperlipidemia is often missed due to lack of awareness and infrequent use of definitive diagnostic tests, such as genetic testing or detailed lipoprotein diagnostics. Once diagnosed, remnant hyperlipidemia is relatively easy to treat using lifestyle changes (low-fat diet and weight loss) combined with cholesterol and triglyceride-lowering drugs, as described in the next subsection.

TABLE 10–15. Main Targets and Goals for Reduction in Lipid Values in Adults Aged 40 to 75 using Statins or Similar Drugs According to UK, Canadian, European, and US Atherosclerotic Cardiovascular Disease (ASCVD) Prevention Guidelines

Target	UK 2016 NICE	Canada 2016 CCS	Europe 2019 ESC/EAS	US 2018 ACC/AHA
Secondary prevention: ASCVD				
LDL cholesterol	≥50%	>50% or <77 mg/dL <2.0 mmol/L	≥50% & <55 mg/dL <1.4 mmol/L	≥50% & <70 mg/dL <1.8 mmol/L
Non-HDL cholesterol		<100 mg/dL <2.6 mmol/L	<85 mg/dL <2.2 mmol/L	<100 mg/dL <2.6 mmol/L
Apolipoprotein B		<80 mg/dL	<65 mg/dL	
Primary prevention: Familial hypercholesterolemia				
LDL cholesterol	≥50%	>50%	≥50% & <55 or <70 mg/dL <1.4 or <1.8 mmol/L	≥50%
Primary prevention: Absolute 10-year risk based, diabetes or chronic kidney disease				
LDL cholesterol	≥40% ≥50% if ↑nonHDL-C	>50% or <77 mg/dL <2.0 mmol/L	≥50% & <55, <70 or (<100 mg/dL) <1.4, <1.8 or (<2.6 mmol/L)	≥30% or ≥50%
Non-HDL cholesterol		<100 mg/dL <2.6 mmol/L	<85 mg/dL <2.2 mmol/L	
Apolipoprotein B		<80 mg/dL	<65 mg/dL	

Abbreviations: LDL, low-density lipoprotein; HDL, high-density lipoprotein cholesterol; ASCVD, atherosclerotic cardiovascular disease; ACC, American College of Cardiology; AHA, American Heart Association; CCS, Canadian Cardiovascular Society; NICE, National Institute for Health and Care Excellence; ESC, European Society of Cardiology; EAS, European Atherosclerosis Society.

Approaches to Treatment

According to guidelines on prevention of ASCVD in the United States, Canada, the UK and Europe, the primary lipid target and goal is reduction of LDL-C (**Table 10–15**).[223-225,239] This is true for secondary prevention in patients already diagnosed with ASCVD and in primary prevention in people with FH, diabetes, CKD, or otherwise with elevated risk of ASCVD, that is, if LDL-C is above certain thresholds. However, a secondary target and goal for reduction in United States, Canadian, and European guidelines include elevated non-HDL-C, while Canadian and European guidelines also mention elevated apoB as a secondary target and goal for reduction. The difference in non-HDL-C and LDL-C is remnant-C, while correspondingly elevated apoB when LDL is low is due to elevated triglyceride-rich lipoproteins.

As outlined elsewhere in this chapter, elevated triglyceride-rich lipoproteins like elevated LDL and elevated Lp(a) are causally linked to increased ASCVD risk,[211,212,240-243] all of which carry one apoB molecule. Therefore, it is not surprising that LDL-lowering (and thus non-HDL-C and apoB lowering) approaches can also decrease ASCVD morbidity and mortality in subjects with hypertriglyceridemia or combined hyperlipidemia.[244] Indeed, LDL-C reduction remains the primary therapeutic approach in patients with elevated triglyceride-rich lipoproteins, with LDL-C goals dependent on the overall risk for ASCVD in any given individual (Table 10–15).[223-225,239]

If LDL-C is at the guideline-recommended goal but not at the goal for apoB and/or non-HDL-cholesterol, then the latter goals can be achieved by either further LDL-C reduction or by reduction of remnant-C levels. While LDL-C reduction has been shown to reduce ASCVD events, data on reduction of remnant-C (ie, reduction of triglyceride-rich lipoprotein concentrations) are more ambiguous because most studies did not recruit patients specifically with elevated plasma triglycerides and elevated remnant-C; however, reduction of triglyceride-rich lipoproteins in the subgroup of participants with elevated triglyceride-rich lipoproteins at study entry reduced ASCVD events in all individual studies.[211,215] Based on these observations, a number of algorithms have been developed to treat patients with elevated plasma triglycerides and remnant-C, that is, hypertriglyceridemia or combined hyperlipidemia.[245] The following subsections describe the approach for reduction of elevated triglyceride-rich lipoproteins at mild-to-moderate hypertriglyceridemia (150–1000 mg/dL; 1.7–11.4 mmol/L); for the treatment of chylomicronemia syndrome with severe hypertriglyceridemia (>1000 mg/dL; 11.4 mmol/L), see the pervious subsection on familial chylomicronemia syndrome.

Secondary Hypertriglyceridemia

Mild-to-moderate hypertriglyceridemia (150–1000 mg/dL; 1.7–11.4 mmol/L) can be due to lifestyle and genetics (primary hypertriglyceridemia), other drug treatment and other diseases (secondary hypertriglyceridemia), or combinations hereof. Therefore, other drug treatment and other diseases as explanation for all or part of an observed hypertriglyceridemia needs to be excluded, and potentially corrected if possible, before other efforts are directed toward triglyceride and remnant-C reduction (**Table 10–16**).

In the case of diabetes, diabetes control needs to be optimized (Table 10–16). Nephrotic syndrome and CKD also need to be dealt with if present. The same is true for high alcohol intake and suspected alcoholism, with the aim of reducing alcohol intake. Finally, use of triglyceride-increasing drugs like

TABLE 10–16. Approaches to Treatment at Elevated Plasma Triglycerides and Remnant Cholesterol at Mild-to-Moderate Hypertriglyceridemia (150–1000 mg/dL; 1.7–11.4 mmol/L)

Correct secondary hypertriglyceridemia if possible

  Optimize diabetes control

  Chronic kidney disease treatment

  Reduce alcohol intake if alcoholism is suspected

  Consider stopping triglyceride-increasing drugs

  At third trimester pregnancy, monitor triglycerides closely until delivery (estrogen effect)

Lifestyle changes

Weight loss

  Increase physical activity

  Reduce food intake

  Reduce soft drink and alcohol intake

Drug treatment

LDL cholesterol reduction

  Statin

  Ezetimibe

  PCSK9-inhibitor

Plasma triglyceride and remnant cholesterol reduction

  High-intensity statin

  Fibrates

  Icosapent ethyl

high-dose thiazide, some betablockers, steroids given systemically, estrogens in contraceptive pills or hormone replacement therapy, isotretinoin, protease inhibitors, and yet other drugs may need to be stopped to bring down elevated plasma triglycerides. Naturally, this is only possible if alternative drugs are available or if the patient can do without the drug.

At third trimester pregnancy, high plasma levels of estrogen may in some women induce severe hypertriglyceridemia and the chylomicronemia syndrome. Because this is a very serious condition potentially leading to acute pancreatitis and death of the pregnant woman and the child, close monitoring of plasma triglycerides is necessary. At plasma triglycerides above 1000 mg/dL (11.4 mmol/L), advise from a dietician on how to minimize any fat intake is needed to keep plasma triglycerides as low as possible until delivery. Immediately after delivery, plasma estrogen and triglycerides rapidly decrease and the dangerous situation dissolves itself. There is no medication approved to lower plasma triglycerides during pregnancy. Plasma apheresis to remove triglyceride-rich lipoproteins can also be used in this situation.

Lifestyle

In patients with elevated plasma triglycerides and remnant-C, weight reduction through increase in physical activity and reduction in intake of food, soft drinks, and alcohol can improve the lipid profile (Table 10–16).[245] Concerning diet, reduction in the consumption of refined carbohydrate-rich foods and drinks, as well as sucrose and fructose, is important. Similarly, reduction of alcohol intake and the replacement of saturated fat with mono- or polyunsaturated fats translate into triglyceride reduction. However, randomized, placebo-controlled trial evidence for these nutritional recommendations is lacking. If insufficient lowering of LDL-C, remnant-C, non-HDL-C, and apoB is achieved through lifestyle changes, drug treatment is advised as described in Table 10–16 and the next subsection.

Statins and Other Drugs for Low-Density Lipoprotein Cholesterol Reduction

LDL-C reduction is the primary lipid approach for ASCVD risk reduction, independent of the underlying hyperlipidemia (Tables 10–15 and 10–16; except at severe hypertriglyceridemia and the chylomicron syndrome; see previous section). LDL-C treatment goals depend on the overall ASCVD risk and should be achieved with lifestyle modification initially and with drugs if required. Statins, frequently in combination with ezetimibe and sometimes with PCSK9 inhibitors, should be used as the primary pharmacological approach (Table 10–16).[223,224] Although these agents (except high-intensity statins[175]) have little effect on plasma triglyceride levels, this strategy is also successful in reducing ASCVD morbidity and mortality in patients with elevated triglyceride-rich lipoproteins, that is, hypertriglyceridemia and combined hyperlipidemia.

High-Intensity Statins

If mild-to-moderate hypertriglyceridemia (150–1000 mg/dL; 1.7–11.4 mmol/L) persists despite pharmacological LDL-C reduction, the first drug of choice is high-intensity statins (IB recommendation).[224] This entail atorvastatin 40 to 80 mg daily or rosuvastatin 20 to 40 mg daily,[223] because these doses will reduce plasma triglycerides typically by 30%.[175] Further, use of statins to reduced ASCVD is proven beyond doubt.[174,240]

Fibrates

In primary prevention patients who are at LDL-C goal but with hypertriglyceridemia, fenofibrate or bezafibrate may be considered in combination with statins (IIb recommendation).[224] The same is true for patients at high risk of ASCVD (IIb recommendation).

Fibrates can reduce plasma triglyceride levels by up to 70% with considerable inter-individual variation.[246] In monotherapy, fibrates have been shown to reduce ASCVD risk, but no additional benefit was observed when used in combination with statins in individuals without elevated triglycerides. It remains unclear as to whether the lack of additional benefit relates to methodological issues (study design, enrolment criteria), or true failure. This question is of some importance as post hoc subgroup analyses indicate that patients with hypertriglyceridemia associated with low HDL-C may benefit from statin-fibrate combination therapy.[211,247] The results of an ongoing outcome trial (PROMINENT) using a new selective PPA-Ralpha modulator (pemafibrate), an improved novel type of fibrate, will probably clarify the value of fibrate therapy in high-risk patients recruited to have hypertriglyceridemia together with low HDL-C.[203,248]

Omega-3 Fatty Acids and Icosapent Ethyl

In high-risk (or above) patients with plasma triglyceride levels of 135 to 499 mg/dL (1.5–5.6 mmol/L) despite statin treatment, icosapent ethyl 2×2 g/day should be considered in combination with a statin (IIaB recommendation).[224]

A number of studies have evaluated the effect of low-dose omega-3-fatty acids (1 g/day) on cardiovascular events. With the exception of one early Italian study, none of the trials (and especially those involving adequate background therapy including statins, aspirin, and beta-blockers), showed any benefit with respect to ASCVD risk reduction.[249,250] Therefore, low-dose omega-3 fatty acids should not be used for cardiovascular risk reduction.

A higher dose of the omega-3-fatty acid icosapent ethyl (4 g/day), a precursor of eicosapentaenoic acid (EPA), was used in the REDUCE-IT trial.[201] In that trial, icosapent ethyl versus mineral oil produced 20% lower plasma triglycerides, 40% lower C-reactive proteins, and over a 5-year period 25% fewer ASCVD events. However, part of this effect could be due to deleterious effect of mineral oil that by itself increased LDL-C by 10% and CRP by 30%. The STRENGTH trial also used high-dose omega-3-fatty acid (4 g/day, consisting of 75% EPA and 25% docosahexaenoic acid (DHA). In that study versus corn oil, plasma triglycerides was lowered by 18% and C-reactive protein by 11%; however, over a 3.5-year period there was no effect on ASCVD events.[251]

Training and Education

The key problem leading to elevated plasma triglycerides and remnant-C is overweight and obesity, the only cardiovascular risk factor that has increased substantially over the last couple of decades. Primordial prevention, primary prevention, and secondary prevention to reduce ASCVD in individuals and societies are all theoretical possible;[252] however, reversing the worldwide pandemic of overweight and obesity is a huge task that needs to involve the individual, local community, and society at large.

Individuals need to understand the ideal of keeping within the normal weight range, or in case of overweight or obesity, the need for losing weight. Naturally, this can only occur if the intake of calories from food, sugar-sweetened soft drinks, and alcohol does not exceed the calories used through basal metabolism and exercise.

At the community level, education of children and adults about getting the right balance between intake of calories and calories burnt through exercise in order to keep normal body weight is essential. Communities can also facilitate exercise as part of normal life by building bicycle and walking trails allowing people to use this form of transport to and from school, university, or workplace lifelong, rather than using cars or public transport; this is already done in many countries in Europe, such as the Netherlands and Denmark. Access to healthy low-calorie meals at schools, universities, and workplaces will also help prevent overweight and obesity, particularly if unhealthy high-calorie items cannot be purchased at the school, university, or workplace.

At society levels, politicians and governments can through reduced taxation promote higher intake of low-calorie food items including vegetables and fruits, and conversely though higher taxation discourage intake of high-calorie processed food items, sugar-sweetened soft drinks, and alcohol. Laws preventing large servings of high-calorie items like sugar-sweetened soft drinks, cakes, and fast food will likely also reduce calorie intake in many individuals in a society.

HIGH-DENSITY LIPOPROTEIN DISORDERS

HDLs represent heterogeneous subpopulations of discrete particles (**Fig. 10–19**) that differ quantitatively and qualitatively in composition of surface proteins and lipids and core lipids (**Table 10–17**).[253-255] Historically, HDLs have been characterized by their cholesterol content for analytical simplicity. However, the cholesterol content is neither causally associated with cardiovascular risk nor an effective target for pharmacological intervention.[256,257] Analytical methods commonly used in the isolation and quantification of HDLs are based on particle size (**Table 10–18**).[254] In 2011, a unifying nomenclature for various HDL methods was

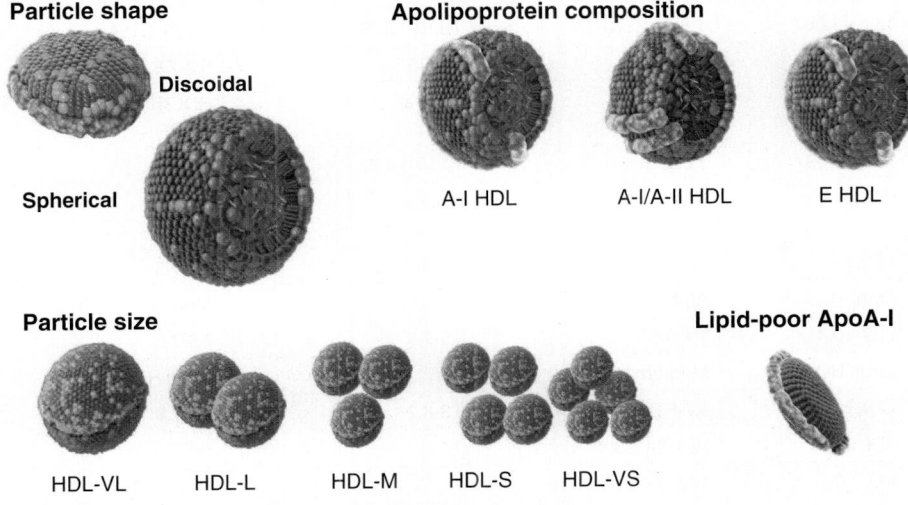

Figure 10–19. HDLs represent discrete subpopulations of particles that differ in composition.

TABLE 10–17. Composition of High-Density Lipoprotein Acceptors

| | HDL-VL (HDL$_{2b}$) | HDL-L (HDL$_{2a}$) | HDL-M (HDL$_{3a}$) | HDL-S (HDL$_{3b}$) | HDL-VS | | Free Apolipoprotein (ApoA-I) |
					HDL$_{3c}$	Pre-β–HDL	
Density, g/mL	1063–1090	1090–1120	1120–1150	1150–1180	1180–1210	x	x
Composition, %							
TG	4	4	3	2	1	0	0
FC	4	3	2	1	0.1	0.1	0
CE	29	27	25	23	17	0	0
PL	30	33	29	24	16	16	0
Proteins	33	34	41	50	66	84	100
Apolipoproteins							
ApoA-I, mol/mol HDL	3.6	4.1	4.4	3.7	3	1	1
ApoA-II, mol/mol HDL	0.8	1.1	1.4	1	0.4	0	0
Other	ApoC, apoD, apoE			ApoC, apoD		x	ApoE

Abbreviations: HDL, high-density lipoprotein; HDL-VL, very large HDL; HDL-L, large HDL; HDL-M, medium HDL; HDL-S, small HDL; apo, apolipoprotein; TG, triglycerides; FC, free cholesterol; CE, cholesteryl ester; and PL, phospholipid. HDL nomenclature.
Reproduced with permission from Rosenson RS, Brewer HB Jr, Davidson WS, et al. Cholesterol efflux and atheroprotection: advancing the concept of reverse cholesterol transport. *Circulation*. 2012 Apr 17;125(15):1905-1919.

proposed. HDL particle size increases with the cholesterol content of the particle, and early prospective studies suggested that large HDL particle size and its major protein constituent apoA-I were associated with lower cardiovascular risk.[258,259]

The GENES study investigated the associations of multiple HDL measures in long-term prospective study of 214 men with angiographically determined stable coronary artery disease.[260] In this study, HDL-C and all-cause mortality (0.71 [0.55–0.92], $P = 0.01$) and cardiovascular mortality (0.72 [0.53–0.99], $P = 0.05$). ApoA-I was inversely associated with all-cause mortality (0.68 [0.52–0.89], $P = 0.005$) and cardiovascular mortality (0.69 [0.51–0.84]; $P = 0.02$). Serum NMR-measured total HDL particle concentration (HDL-P) and small HDL-P were inversely associated with cardiovascular and all-cause

mortality in multivariate analysis that adjusted for cardiovascular risk factors and bio-clinical variables. Hazard ratios per 1 standard deviation higher for all-cause mortality and cardiovascular mortality was strongest for HDL-P (0.60 [0.49–0.79, $P = 0.001$) and 0.63 [0.46–0.86], $P = 0.001$) respectively, and small HDL-P (0.63 [0.46–0.84], $P = 0.002$) and (0.64 [0.45–0.90], $P = 0.01$, respectively. Inverse associations were observed between. However, none of these multivariate models were adjusted for apoB.

Since HDL particle size is inversely associated with apoB-containing lipoproteins,[261] it was subsequently reported from classical epidemiology studies that large HDL particle size is a biomarker of lower concentrations of atherogenic lipoproteins[262,263] (**Fig. 10–20**). However, in studies that adjust for the

TABLE 10–18. Classification of HDL by Physical Properties

Proposed term	Very large HDL (HDL-VL)	Large HDL-V (HDL-L)	Medium HDL (HDL-M)	Small HDL (HDL-S)	Very small HDL (VS-HDL)
Density range, g/mL	1.063-1.087	1.088-1.110	1.110-1.129	1.129-1.154	1.154-1.25
Size range, nm	12.9-9.7	9.7-8.8	8.8-8.2	8.2-7.8	7.8-7.2
Density gradient ultracentrifugation	HDL2b	HDL2a	HDL3a	HDL3b	HDL3c
Density range, g/mL	1.063-1.087	1.088-1.110	1.110-1.129	1.129-1.154	1.154-1.170
Gradient gel electrophoresis	HDL2b	HDL2a	HDL3a	HDL3b	HDL3c
Size range, nm	12.9-9.7	9.7-8.8	8.8-8.2	8.2-7.8	7.8-7.2
2D gel electrophoresis	Alpha-1	Alpha-2	Alpha-3	Alpha-4	Preβ-1 HDL
Size range, nm	11.2-10.8	9.4-9.0	8.5-7.5	7.5-7.0	6.0-5.0
NMR	Large HDL-P	Medium HDL-P		Small HDL-P	
Size range, nm	12.9-9.7	9.7-8.8	8.8-8.2	8.2-7.8	7.8-7.2
Ion mobility	HDL 2b	HDL 2a + 3			
Size range, nm	14.5-10.5	10.5-7.65			

Reproduced with permission from Rosenson RS, Brewer HB Jr, Chapman MJ, et al. HDL measures, particle heterogeneity, proposed nomenclature, and relation to atherosclerotic cardiovascular events. *Clin Chem*. 2011 Mar;57(3):392-410.

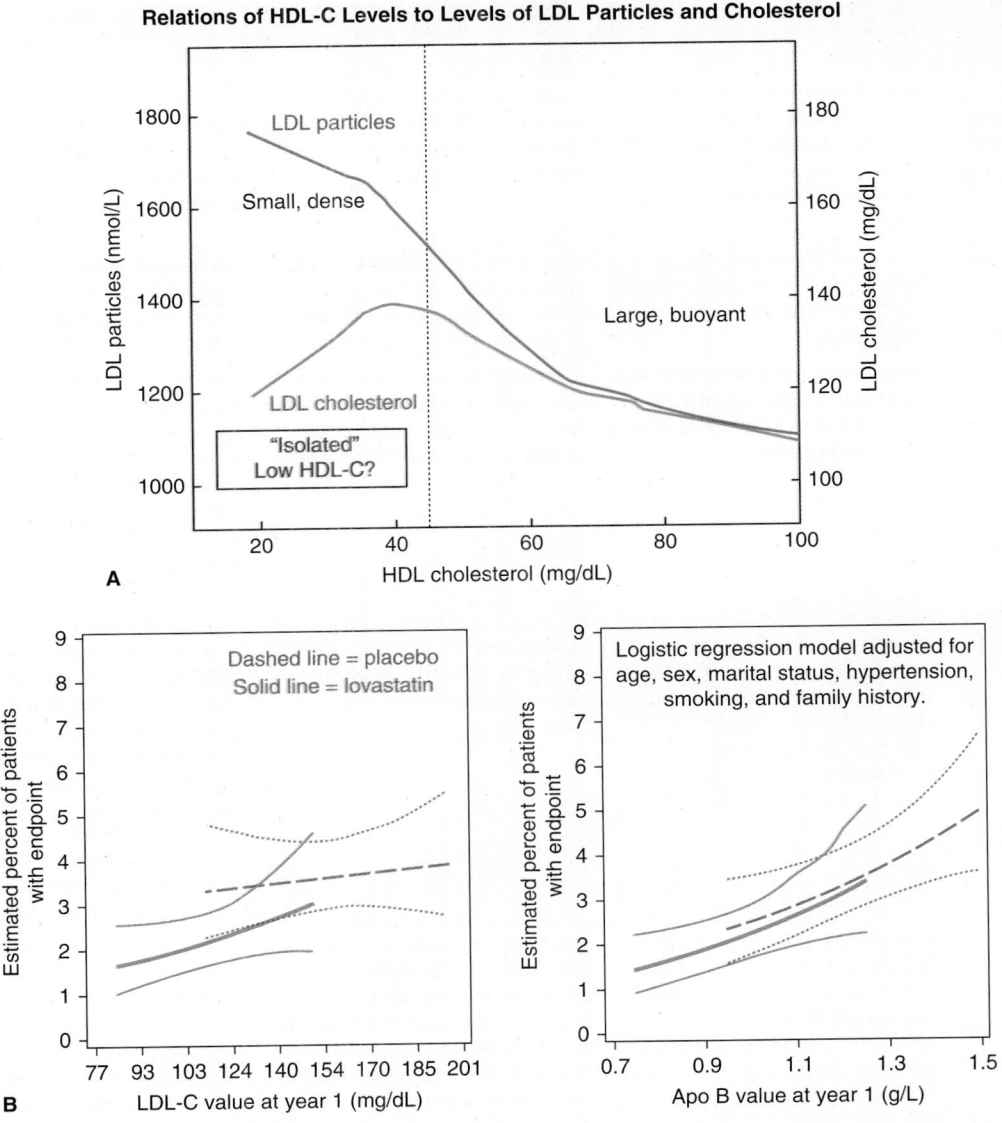

Figure 10–20. Disconnect between LDL-C and LDL particles/apoB in persons with low HDL-C. A. Low HDL-C is inversely associated with high concentrations of small and total LDL particles. Thus, the residual risk assocaited with low HDL-C is partly accounted for higher concentrations of small and total LDL particles. **B.** In a primary prevention trial with lovastatin, the Airforce/Texas Coronary Atherosclerosis Prevention Study, cardiovascular risk was more highly associated with high baseline and on-trial concentrations of apolipoprotein B than LDL-C.

concentration of apoB (or LDL particle concentration [LDL-P]), the associations between large HDL particle size was not associated with reduced cardiovascular risk.[264] In an analysis of the United Kingdom Biobank (UKBB), CHD risk was inversely associated with a 1-standard deviation higher HDL-C (odds ratio [OR] 0.80 [95% CI: 0.75–0.86) and apoA-I (OR 0.83; 95% CI: 0.77–0.89). These risk estimates were nullified after accounting for apoB.[264]

HDL-P is a more robust measure of cardiovascular risk than other static HDL measures. Numerous prospective population studies and subgroup analyses of clinical trials that adjust for LDL-P have shown that atheroprotective properties of HDL are associated with total HDL-P and small HDL-P[265-275] (**Table 10–19**). In a nested case-control study of the JUPITER trial (Justification for the Use of Statins in Prevention: An Intervention Trial Evaluating Rosuvastatin), baseline HDL-P

(adjusted odds ratio per standard deviation [SD] increment [OR/SD] 0.69; 95% CI: 0.56–0.86; *P* <0.001) was more inversely correlated with incident cardiovascular events, whereas no significant associations was observed for HDL-C (OR/SD, 0.82; 95% CI; 0.66–1.02; *P* = 0.08) or apoA-I (OR/SD, 0.83; 95% CI; 0.67–1.03; *P* = 0.08).[269] On treatment with high-intensity statin therapy (eg, rosuvastatin 20 mg daily), HDL-P increased by 5.2% and this HDL biomarker most strongly associated with incident cardiovascular events (OR/SD, 0.51; 95% CI, 0.33–0.77; *P* <0.001). The association between HDL-P and a biomarker of inflammation was investigated in the Dallas Heart Study.[270] In this multiethnic cohort of 2,643 adults followed for an average 12.4 years, levels of GlycA, an integrated glycosylation NMR-derived marker of five acute phase reactants, was associated with higher HDL-P.[270] Increasing quartiles of GlycA were associated with ASCVD events in models that adjusted

TABLE 10–19. Prospective Clinical studies Showing HDL Particle number (HDL-P) and Incident Cardiovascular Disease (CVD) Events

Study name	Population	Study outcome	Significant study findings
Veterans Affairs High-Density Lipoprotein Intervention Trial (VA-HIT)[1]	Nested case-control study of 364 men with a new CHD event (nonfatal myocardial infarction or cardiac death) during a median 5.1-year follow-up and 697 age-matched controls.	Associations of baseline levels of lipids and each of the lipoprotein classes and subclasses by NMR with incident CVD events	HDL particles achieved with gemfibrozil were significant, independent predictors of new CHD events. For total HDL particles, odds ratios predicting CHD benefit was 0.71 (95% CI: 0.61 to 0.81).
Women's Health Study (WHS)[2]	27,673 healthy women; 26,658 without a CVD event and 1015 with a CVD event after an 11-year follow-up period	Associations of baseline levels of lipids, apoB, apoA-I and each of the lipoprotein classes and subclasses by NMR with incident CVD events	CVD risk prediction associated with lipoprotein profiles evaluated by NMR, including HDL-P was comparable but not superior to that of standard lipids, apoB-100 or apoA-I
Heart Protection Study (HPS)[3]	Randomized trial of simvastatin versus placebo (>5000 vascular events during 5.3 years of follow-up among 20,000 participants)	Associations of baseline levels of lipids, apoB, apoA-I and each of the lipoprotein classes and subclasses by NMR with incident CVD events	After adjustment for LDL-P, the hazard ratios for major occlusive coronary event per 1-SD-higher level were 0.91 (95% CI: 0.86–0.96) for HDL-C and 0.89 (95% CI: 0.85– 0.93) for HDL-P. Other cardiac events were inversely associated with total HDL-P (HR, 0.84; 95% CI: 0.79–0.90) and small (0.82; 95% CI: 0.76–0.89) HDL-P but only very weakly associated with HDL-C (0.94; 95% CI: 0.88–1.00).
Justification for the Use of statins in Prevention: an Intervention Trial Evaluating Rosuvastatin (JUPITER)[4]	Randomized trial of 17,802 individuals; women ≥60 years and men ≥50 years without a previous history of CVD or diabetes mellitus who had LDL-C <130 mg/dL, hsCRP ≥2.0 mg/L, and triglycerides <500 mg/dL.	HDL size and HDL-P were measured by NMR, and HDL-C and apoA-I were chemically assayed in 10,886 participants before and after treatment	Among rosuvastatin-allocated individuals, on-treatment HDL-P remained significant (0.72, 0.53–0.97, P = 0.03) even after additionally adjusting for HDL-C. Therefore, in the setting of potent statin therapy, HDL-P may be a better marker of residual risk than HDL-C or apoA-I. Note: Khera et al[5] showed that for both baseline and on-statin analyses, HDL-P was the strongest of four HDL-related biomarkers (including HDL-C, apoA-I and cholesterol efflux capacity) as an inverse predictor of incident events and biomarker of residual risk.
Dallas Heart Study (DHS)[6]	A multiethnic population study of Dallas County residents, with deliberate oversampling of black participants. From 2000 to 2002, 2971 participants were enrolled. For this study the population comprised 1977 participants.	HDL-C was measured by chemistry assay and HDL-P by NMR; Participants were followed for a median of 9.3 years for incident CHD events which was defined as the composite of first MI, stroke, coronary revascularization, or CVD death.	HDL-P, adjusted for risk factors and HDL-C, was inversely associated with incident CHD overall (adjusted HR per 1 SD 0.73, 95% CI: 0.62 to 0.86), with no interaction by Black race/ethnicity (P interaction [0.57]). In contrast to HDL-C, the inverse relation between HDL-P and incident CHD events is consistent across ethnicities.
Atherothrombosis Intervention in Metabolic Syndrome with Low HDL/High Triglycerides and Impact on Global Health Outcomes trial (AIM-HIGH)[7]	AIM-HIGH participants (n = 3,414) included men and women who were ≥45 years old and had established stable atherosclerotic disease with low HDL-C (<40 mg/dL for men and <50 mg/dL for women), high TG (150–400 mg/dL), and LDL-C <180 mg/d.; 1387 were treated with a statin plus placebo and 1367 were treated with a statin and extended release niacin (ERN)	Associations of baseline levels of lipids, apoB, apoA-I, GlycA and each of the lipoprotein classes and subclasses by NMR (at baseline and 1-year treatment) with incident CVD events.	None of the lipoprotein particle classes or subclasses was associated with incident CVD in this trial.
Meta-analysis of the Multi-Ethnic Study of Atherosclerosis (MESA), Dallas Heart Study (DHS), Atherosclerosis Risk in Communities (ARIC) and Prevention of Renal and Vascular Endstage Disease (PREVEND studies[8]	Pooled cohort of four large population studies without baseline CVD: DHS (n = 2535), ARIC (n = 1595), MESA (n = 6632), and PREVEND (n = 5022) for a total of 15,784 subjects.	HDL-C measured chemically and HDL-P measured by NMR; combined outcome of MI and ischemic stroke	HDL-P was inversely associated with the CVD outcome even when adjusted for cardiometabolic risk factors (HR for quartile 4 [Q4] versus quartile 1 [Q1], 0.64 [95% CI: 0.52–0.78]), as was HDL-C (HR for Q4 versus Q1, 0.76 [95% CI: 0.61–0.94]). Adjustment for HDL-C did not attenuate the inverse relationship between HDL-P and CVD disease, whereas adjustment for HDL-P attenuated all associations between HDL-C and CVD events.

Prospective population studies and subgroup analyses of clinical trials that adjust for LDL-P have shown that atheroprotective properties of HDL are associated with total HDL-P and small HDL-P.[266,268,269,273-277]

TABLE 10–20. Genetic Causes of Severe HDL Deficiency

Mutation	Variants	Prevalence	ASCVD Prevalence rates
ABCA1	rs9282541/p.R230C rs111292742/c.-279C>G	26.9%	37.0%
LCAT	rs4986970/p.S232T	12.4%	4.0%
APOA1	c.718C>T (p.Q240)	5.0%	40.0%
LPL	rs268/p.N318S	4.5%	11.1%
None		52.2%	6.4%

Data from Geller AS, Polisecki EY, Diffenderfer MR, et al. Genetic and secondary causes of severe HDL deficiency and cardiovascular disease. *J Lipid Res*. 2018 Dec;59(12):2421-2435.

for HDL-P (HR for GlycA, upper quartile vs. lowest quartile, 3.46 [95% CI: 2.06–5.84]).

Prevalence

Low levels of HDL-C have been defined in gender specific terms as less than 40 mg/dL in men and less than 50 mg/dL in women.[276] Often, low HDL-C levels are associated with high triglyceride levels representing a pattern of insulin resistance.[277-279] Since low levels of HDL-C are associated with unhealthy behaviors and characteristics (overweight, insulin resistance, sedentary lifestyle, and cigarette smoking), the utility of this measure in describing disorders of HDL metabolism is severely limited. Furthermore, the cholesterol content transported by HDL particles is not causally related to CHD risk. Most genetic disorders of HDL metabolism that are causally related to early-onset CVD are rare[280] (**Table 10–20**).

Mechanism

HDLs encompass a constellation of particles with multifarious functions involving cellular transport, immunoregulation, inflammation and hemostasis that modulate atherosclerois[281] (**Fig. 10–21**).[282] Thus, the nomenclature for HDLs has evolved into structure–function relationships that incorporates composition with mechanism (**Fig. 10–22**).

Reverse cholesterol transport is the process used to define elimination of excess cholesterol from tissues to its ultimate elimination in the feces. The process involves multiple components (**Table 10–21**). Macrophage cholesterol efflux, the initial step in the reverse cholesterol transport process, has been considered the primary atheroprotective mechanism associated with HDLs[255,281,283,284] (**Fig. 10–23**). The initiation of cholesterol mobilization from the macrophage involves interaction of either a cholesterol deficient and phospholipid depleted ApoA-I or apoE complex with the ABCA1 transporter (**Fig. 10–24**). This interaction activates Acyl-CoA cholesterol acyltransferase (ACAT), which elaborates cholesteryl esters from the foam cell as unesterified cholesterol. The mobilization of unesterified cholesterol from the membrane onto the nascent HDL particle and consequent esterification of cholesterol by lecithin–cholesteryl acyltransferase (LCAT) transforms the nascent HDL into a very small spherical particle (HDL-VS). Spherical HDL particles interact with different receptors than nascent HDL acquire cholesterol via interactions with *ABCG1* and *SRB1*. Passive diffusion of unesterified cholesterol from the plasma membrane is another mechanism for cholesterol disposition from the arterial wall. Ongoing cholesterol accumulation in the HDL particle results in a

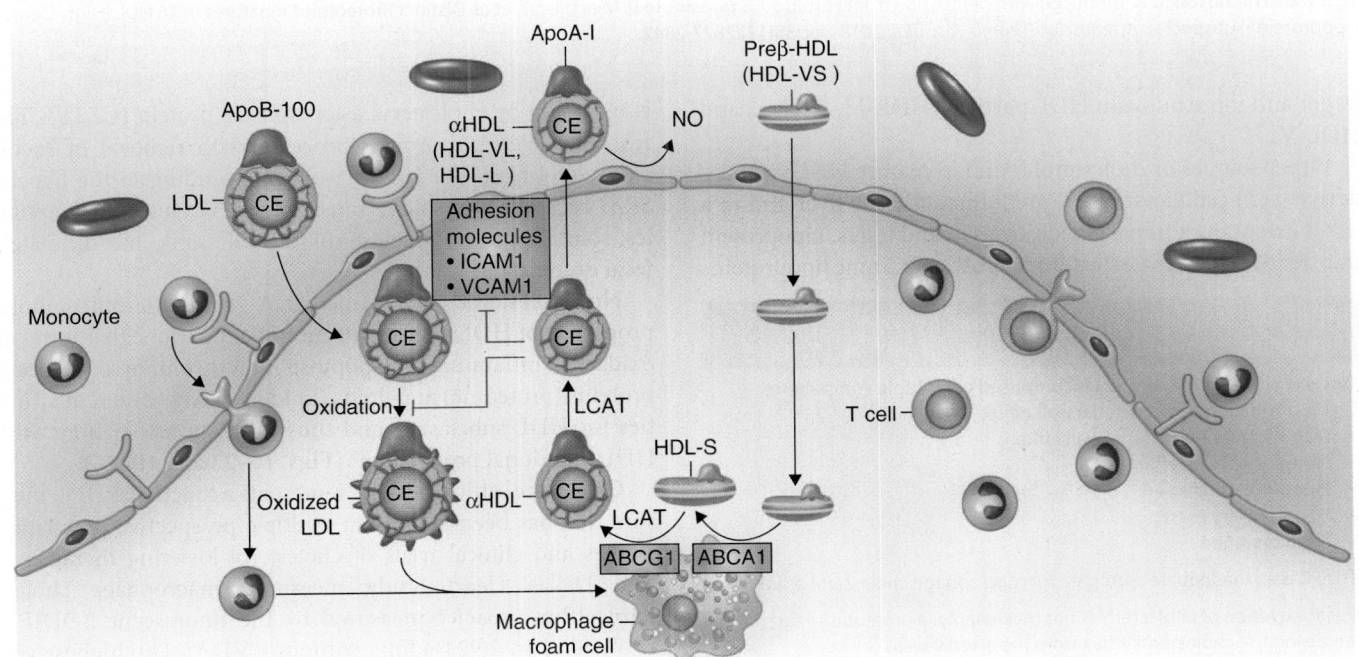

Figure 10–21. HDL modulation of atherosclerosis. Reproduced with permission from Rosenson RS, Brewer HB, Ansell BJ, et al. Dysfunctional HDL and atherosclerotic cardiovascular disease. *Nat Rev Cardiol*. 2016 Jan;13(1):48-60.

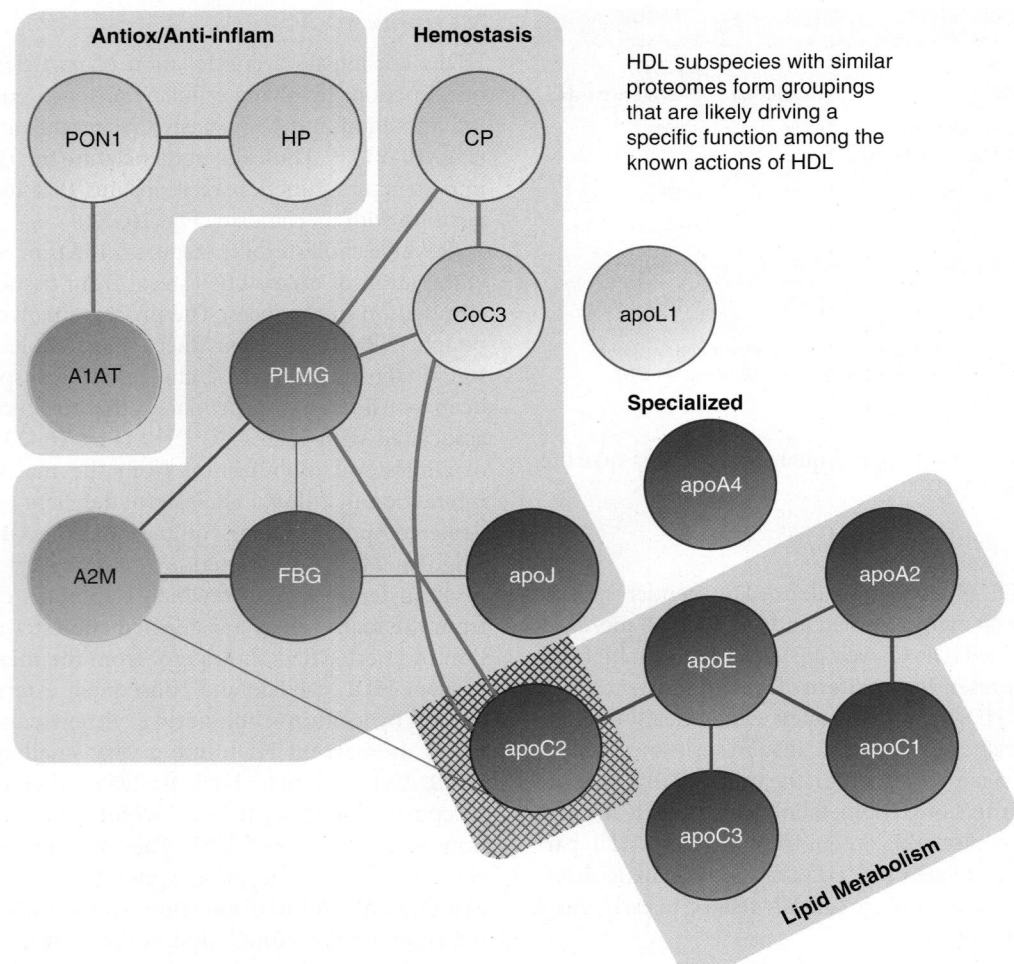

Figure 10–22. **Distinct HDL subspecies participate in diverse HDL functions encompassing lipid metabolism, antioxidant and anti-inflammatory properties, and hemostasis.** Reproduced with permission from Furtado JD, Yamamoto R, Melchior JT, et al. Distinct Proteomic Signatures in 16 HDL (High-Density Lipoprotein) Subspecies. *Arterioscler Thromb Vasc Biol.* 2018 Dec;38(12):2827-2842.

larger and more buoyant HDL particle (HDL-M, HDL-L, and HDL-VL).

Other sources of cholesterol found in mature HDL particles derive from cellular sources, predominantly the liver and to a lesser extent the adrenal glands, ovaries, and testes. Lipoprotein transfer of cholesterol esters from apoB-containing lipoproteins is mediated by cholesteryl ester transfer protein (CETP). The reverse cholesterol process proceeds with removal of excess cholesterol from the HDL particle via binding to the hepatic *SRB1* receptor, sinusoidal transport of HDL into the lymphatics, solubilization of cholesterol into bile salts, and ultimately fecal excretion.

Noncholesterol efflux-mediated anti-atherothrombotic properties of HDL encompass multiple functions that mitigate oxidation, inflammation, apoptosis, and thrombosis.[283] Surface proteins (proteome) and lipids (lipidome) have different affinities for HDL subclasses, and thus different associations with HDL functional properties[285] (**Figs. 10–22** and **10–25**).

Cholesterol efflux capacity represents a functional HDL measure that has been studied in multiple prospective population studies and clinical trials of cholesterol lowering therapies.[255] The Dallas Heart Study measured macrophage cholesterol efflux capacity measured by the fluorescent BODIPY-cholesterol in 2,924 adults without CVD.[284] The highest versus lowest quartile of cholesterol efflux capacity was associated with a 67% reduction in CVD risk in a fully adjusted model that included traditional risk factors that included

TABLE 10–21. Multiple Components in Reverse Cholesterol Transport

Reverse cholesterol transport is comprised of multiple components
- Macrophage-specific arterial wall efflux
- Non-macrophage arterial wall efflux
- Non-arterial wall efflux
- Lipoprotein transport
- Hepatobiliary excretion
- Fecal excretion

HDL-C is an inadequate surrogate for macrophage cholesterol efflux

Fecal excretion of cholesterol is not (necessarily) a prerequisite for assessing the cholesterol efflux from the arterial wall

Reproduced with permission from Rosenson RS, Brewer HB Jr, Davidson WS, et al. Cholesterol efflux and atheroprotection: advancing the concept of reverse cholesterol transport. *Circulation.* 2012 Apr 17;125(15):1905-1919.

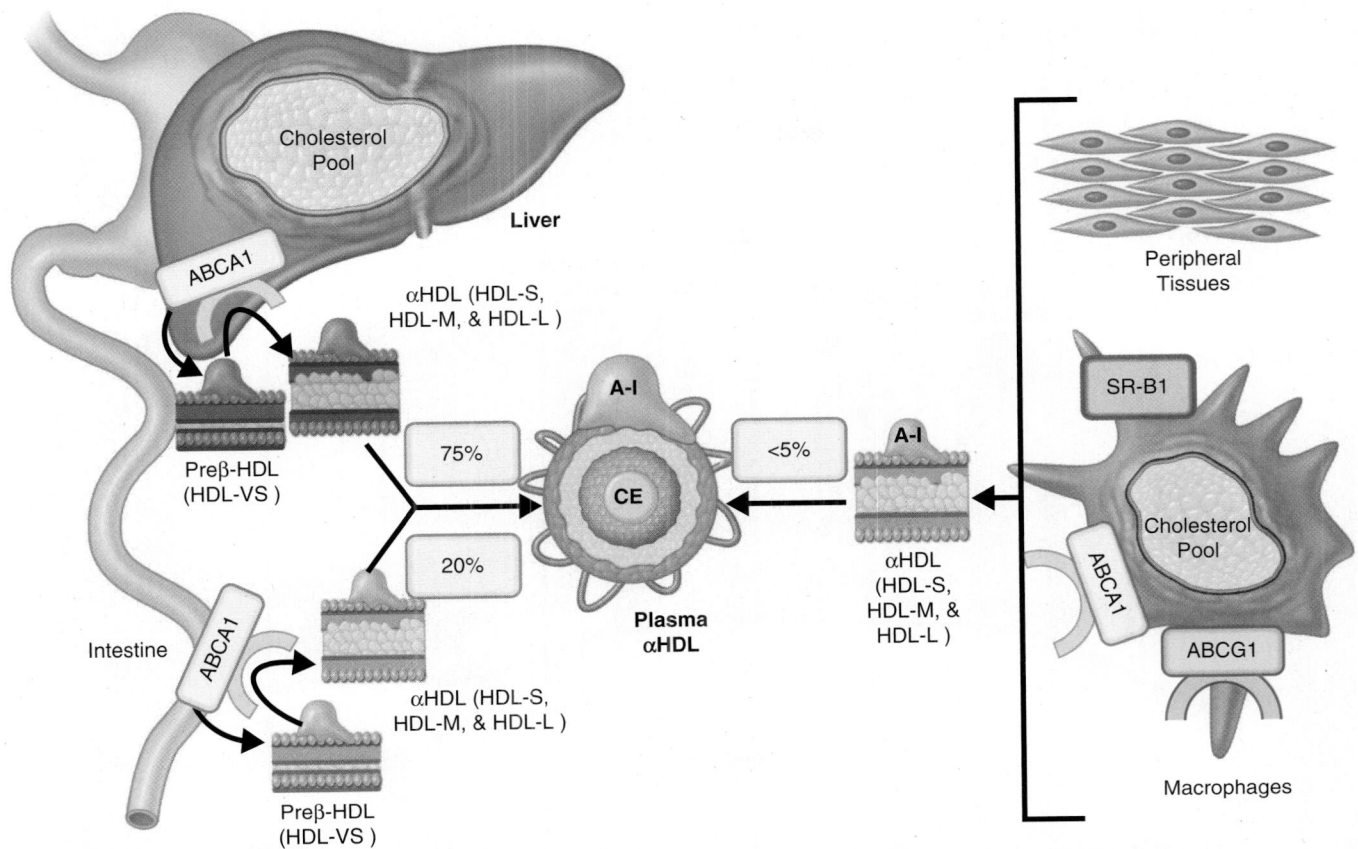

Figure 10–23. Reverse cholesterol transport. Sources of cholesterol in HDL are derived from the liver, intestine, and peripheral cells.

HDL-C and HDL-P. The EPIC Norfolk Study measured macrophage cholesterol efflux capacity using radiolabeled cholesterol in 1,745 of 25,639 participants.[281] After multivariable adjustment that included HDL-C and apoA-I, the risk of incident CHD was 0.80 (95% CI: 0.70–0.90) for a per-SD change in cholesterol efflux capacity. In JUPITER, baseline cholesterol efflux capacity was not significantly associated with cardiovascular events (OR/SD, 0.89; 95% CI: 0.72–1.10; P = 0.28), but in participants randomized to high-intensity statin therapy, cholesterol efflux capacity measured at 12 months was inversely associated with incident CVD (OR/SD, 0.62; 95% CI: 0.42–0.92; P = 0.02).[269] In a study of 1609 MI patients undergoing primary angioplasty, cholesterol efflux capacity was inversely associated with all-cause mortality at an average follow-up of 1.9 years.[286] Similar findings were reported from the HPFS (Health Professionals Follow-Up Study) that included a generally healthy primary-prevention population of 701 cases and 696 controls followed for more than 16 years.[287] The risk of CHD per standard deviation of cholesterol efflux capacity (using J774 cells) was 0.82 (0.71–0.96), but this association was attenuated when HDL-C was included in the model (1.08 [0.85–1.37]). This study suggests that cholesterol efflux capacity may not be associated with risk independent of HDL-C in a cohort of predominantly Caucasian men. In summary, these studies support that cholesterol efflux capacity provides

incremental data on the risk of a first cardiovascular event in persons with multiple risk factors and treated with high intensity statin therapy for the primary prevention of CVD.[288,289]

Efforts to quantify multiple steps in the reverse cholesterol transport process have used multicompartment modeling with radiolabeled cholesterol nanoparticles.[290] This method provides estimates of the fractional transfer rate of free cholesterol from the reticuloendothelial system compartment to HDL (macrophage cholesterol efflux and availability of the acceptor), the fractional transfer rate of the tracer from free cholesterol to cholesteryl ester (CE) (LCAT-dependent pathway), and fractional transfer rate of the HDL-CE into non-HDL particles (cholesteryl ester transfer protein activity). After the administration of the cholesterol nanoparticles, the radiolabeled tracer is excreted and measured in stool.

HDL transports nearly 100 proteins that include apoA-I as the major protein[291,292] (Fig. 10–25). Proteomic analyses have identified distinct HDL subspecies with unique proteomes involved in specific functions including lipid metabolism, antioxidant and anti-inflammatory properties and hemostasis.

HDL structure and function is perturbed after an MI resulting in a dysfunctional HDL particle.[282] During the first several days after MI, plasma cholesterol declines and then increases gradually after many weeks.[293] The reduction in HDL-C results from fewer HDL particles and a decrease in LCAT activity that

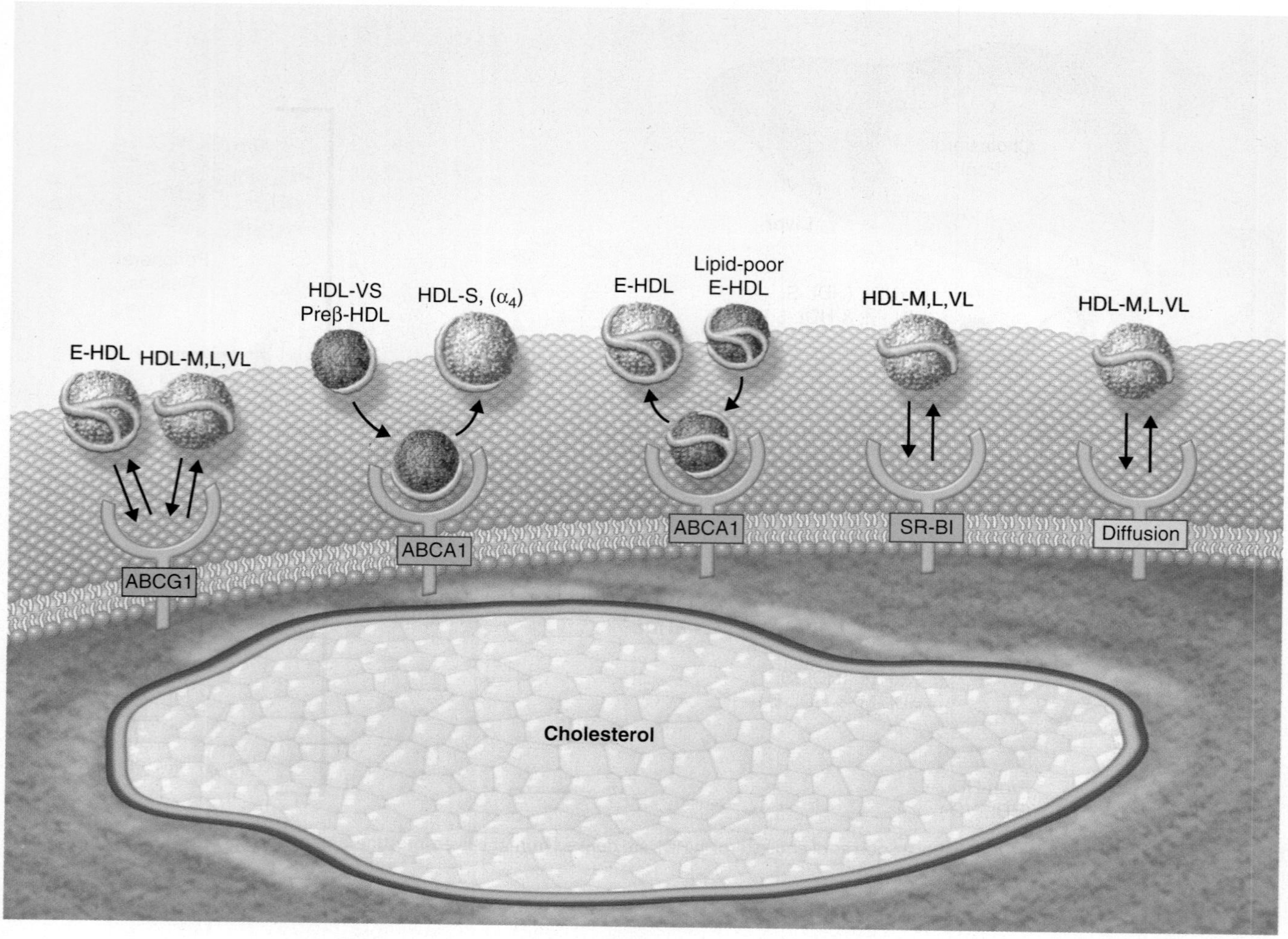

E-HDL HDL-M,L,VL   HDL-VS Preβ-HDL   HDL-S, (α₄)   E-HDL   Lipid-poor E-HDL   HDL-M,L,VL   HDL-M,L,VL

ABCG1   ABCA1   ABCA1   SR-BI   Diffusion

Cholesterol

Figure 10–24. HDL particle subclasses and cholesterol efflux from cholesterol loaded cells.

reduces the cholesteryl content of HDL more than the unesterified fraction.[282,283] Initial studies on HDL compositional perturbations in the acute phase demonstrated that serum amyloid A (SAA)[394] in the bloodstream increases inflammation through activation of NF-kB (nuclear factor-kB) in endothelial cells.[295]

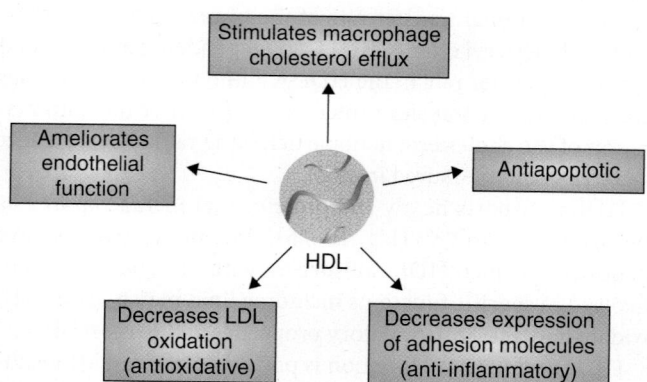

Figure 10–25. **Diverse antiatherosclerotic influences of HDL particles and/or its major protein constituent apoA-I.** Reproduced with permission from Rosenson RS, Brewer HB, Ansell BJ, et al. Dysfunctional HDL and atherosclerotic cardiovascular disease. *Nat Rev Cardiol.* 2016 Jan;13(1):48-60.

In addition, SAA binds to HDL and displaces apoA-I creating a very large HDL dysfunctional particle with reduced antioxidant anti-inflammatory capacity.[283,293]

After an MI, an imbalance in anti-apoptotic and proapoptotic HDL proteins increase abnormal myocardial remodeling, particularly in the peri-infarct zone.[289] ApoJ (clusterin), an HDL protein involved in the inhibition of cellular death pathways, is decreased in MI patients. On contrast, enrichment of HDL with apoC-III increases proapoptotic signaling by stimulating phosphorylation of p38-MAPK (mitogen-activated protein kinase) and upregulates endothelial expression of Bid (BH3-interacting domain death agonist), which is a member of the proapoptosis regulator proteins.

In addition to SAA enrichment, proinflammatory conditions increase the content of LBP (lipopolysaccharide binding protein) and complement proteins in HDL[296] In an analysis of the HDL proteome, the Heinecke laboratory identified that complement components C3 and C4, and a complement regulatory protein vitronectin and several distinct serpins with serine-type endopeptidase inhibitor activity were higher in patients with CVD than controls (**Fig. 10–26**).[297] These observations reveal that HDL particles that include protein families

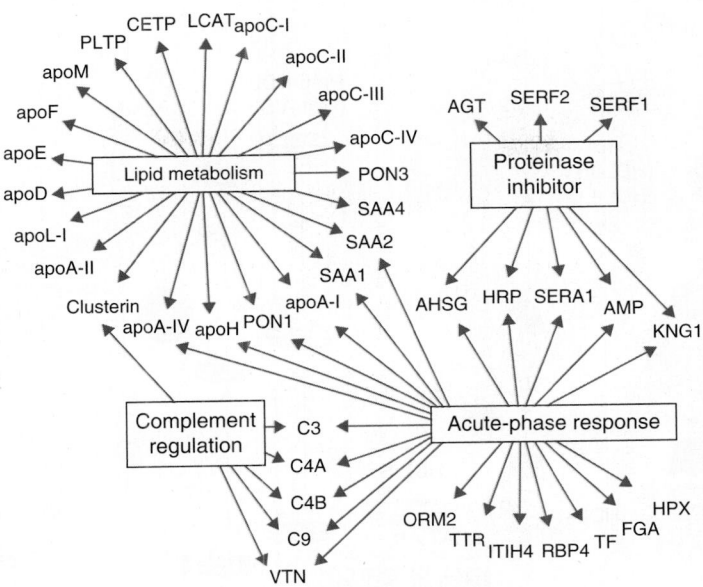

Quantification of HDL proteins by MS/MS analysis. Pioneering MS/MS studies from the Heinecke laboratory identified 48 proteins in HDL. This study showed that HDL carries multiple complement-regulatory proteins and a diverse array of distinct serpins with serine-type endopeptidase inhibitor activity. Many acute-phase response proteins were also detected, strongly supporting the proposal that HDL is of central importance in inflammation.

Figure 10–26. Shotgun proteomics identified multiple proteins involved in inflammation and tissue injury. Reproduced with permission from Vaisar T, Pennathur S, Green PS, et al. Shotgun proteomics implicates protease inhibition and complement activation in the antiinflammatory properties of HDL. *J Clin Invest.* 2007 Mar;117(3):746-756.

involved in regulating complement and proteolysis, both of which have been implicated in inflammation, immune function, and infection.

In human atherosclerotic tissue, monocytes, macrophages, and neutrophils express myeloperoxidase (MPO), a heme protein expressed in high concentrations by inflammatory macrophages in human atherosclerotic tissue.[298,299] Oxidation of apoA-I by the myeloperoxidase-H_2O_2-Cl^- system occurs mainly within the subendothelial compartment,[300] resulting in increased oxidation of multiple residues that have been detected by proteomic analysis.[285,286] Oxidation of Try72 on apoA-I is a site-specific target for MPO-dependent oxidation that results in the formation of oxindolyl alanine (2-hydroxyl L-tryptophan, or 2-OH –Trp) moiety that was detected in 20% of apoA-I recovered from human atherosclerotic lesions.[301] Methionine oxidation and site-specific chlorination of Tyr192 of apoA-I impairs *ABCA1*-dependent cholesterol efflux.[302] Lipid-poor apoA-I in atheroma is cross-linked and oxidized resulting in impaired *ABCA1* interaction that impairs *ABCA1*-mediated macrophage cholesterol efflux, promoting human atherosclerosis and atherosclerotic coronary events[298,299,301] (**Fig. 10–27**). As compared with apoA-I, ox-apoA-I is nonfunctional in reducing inflammatory M1 and increasing anti-inflammatory M2 macrophage markers in atherosclerotic plaques. OxTrp72-apoA-I has dysfunctional properties that increase inflammatory responses through its effects on promoting endothelial cell NF-kB activation and nuclear localization, and consequently increases in surface vascular cell adhesion molecule (VCAM-1) protein content.[301]

In human studies, levels of protein-bound 3-chlorotyrosine, an MPO-mediated product, are markedly higher in circulating HDL from patients with established CHD compared to circulating HDL from healthy subjects.[299] When HDL was isolated from coronary atherosclerotic lesions, concentrations of 3-chlorotyrosine and 3-nitrotyrosine were higher than in plasma HDL. Stable CAD patients and ACS patients have higher levels of chlorinated tyrosine-192 and oxidized methionine-148 than control subjects, and levels of both chlorinated tyrosine-192 and oxidized methionine-148 were associated with reduced ABCA1-mediated macrophage cholesterol efflux and CAD status.[303] In addition to its effects on ABCA1-medicated macrophage cholesterol efflux, oxidation of methionine in apoA-I inhibits LCAT activity, a key enzyme involved in HDL maturation.[303]

Lipid-poor apoA-I diffuses into the circulation and the 2-Ox-Trp72 apoA-I moiety accounts for 0.007% of apoA-I in plasma. In a cohort of 627 individuals, high levels of circulating oxTrp72-apoA-I were associated within increased CVD risk in both unadjusted and multivariate-adjusted models.[301] An imprecise measure of MPO-mediated modification of apoA-I is the serum MPO/HDL particle ratio. In the Dallas Heart Study, the highest versus lowest quartile of MPO/HDL-P was associated with a 74% increase in incident ASCVD events in fully adjusted models.[304]

The combined effects of multiple HDL antioxidant proteins contribute to oxidative modification of HDL proteins. The reduction in PON1 (paraoxonase/arylesterase 1) activity post MI is inversely associated with the risk of recurrent coronary

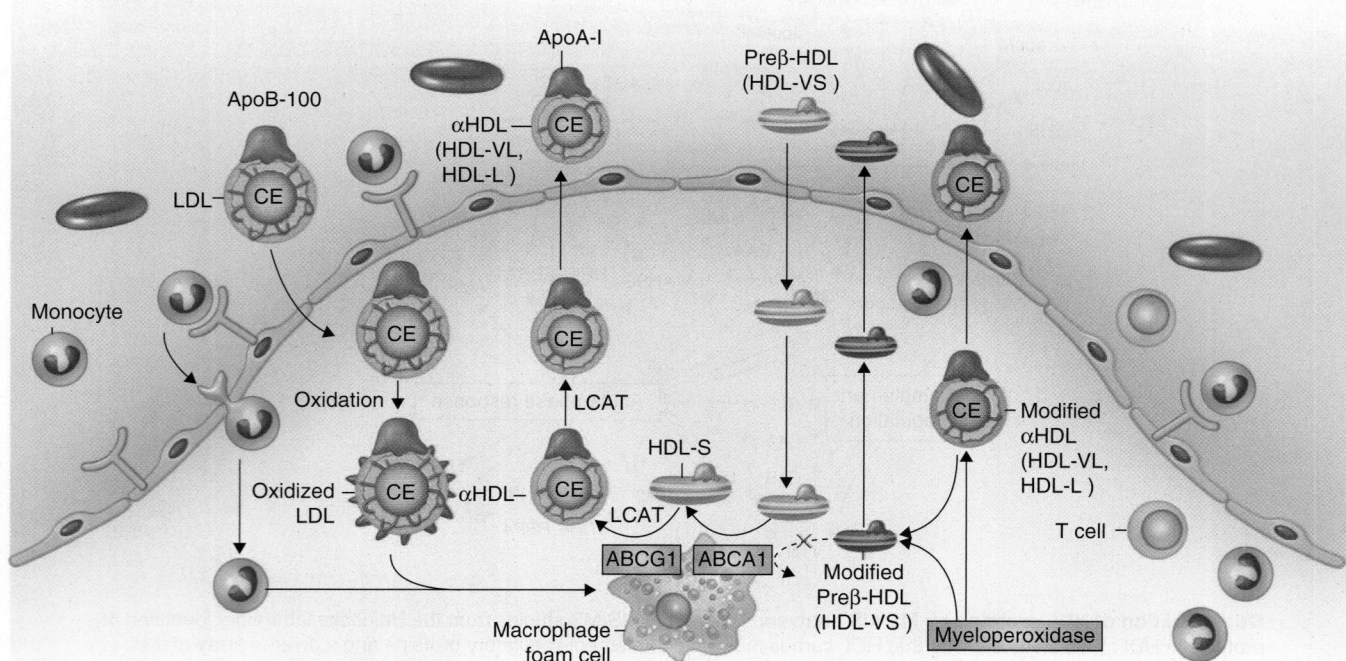

Figure 10–27. Myeloperoxidase-mediated modification of apoA-I and sterol efflux. Reproduced with permission from Rosenson RS, Brewer HB, Ansell BJ, et al. Dysfunctional HDL and atherosclerotic cardiovascular disease. *Nat Rev Cardiol.* 2016 Jan;13(1):48-60.

events[304,305] in MI patients predict a worse outcome. S1P (sphingosine-1 phosphate) is predominantly bound to HDL and limits vascular inflammation by two major mechanisms. S1P inhibits phosphorylation of the p65 NF-kB subunit in endothelial cells decreasing leukocyte adhesion to the endothelium by suppressing TNF (tumor necrosis factor) alpha-mediated VCAM-1 (vascular adhesion molecule 1) and ICAM-1 (intercellular adhesion molecule 1) release. HDL-S1P also limits endothelial inflammation by increasing PI3K (phosphatidylinositol-4,5-bisphosphate 3 kinase)/AKT (serine/threonine kinase 1/eNOS) signaling, which enhances the endothelial barrier, reduces apoptosis and counteracts TNF signaling.[306,307] In addition, HDL/S1P inhibits macrophage apoptosis that may improve myocardial tissue repair after infarction.[308]

Glycosylation of HDL (glycomes) is highly diverse and impacts on the efficacy of cholesterol efflux. The N-glycans in HDL include sialylation with one or two sialic acid residues with the most common a complex type biantennary N-glycan with one sialic acid (A2G2S1). The efficiency of cholesterol efflux from THP-1 cells was greater in native HDL versus desialysated HDL[309]

In human studies, the antioxidant and anti-inflammatory properties have been measured with cell-based and cell-free assays.[282,283] An HDL inflammatory index was defined as the relative ability of the "test" HDL to inhibit monocyte chemotaxis induced by oxidized LDL.[310] The monocyte chemotaxis assay (MCA) involves adding standardized LDL added to a co-culture of human vascular endothelial and smooth muscle cells and quantifying monocyte entry into the co-culture. The impact of test HDL on the MCA is compared to this reference measurement, and the resulting "inflammatory index" contrasts HDL that reduces MCA (anti-inflammatory, index <1.0)

from HDL or one that enhances MCA ("proinflammatory," index >1.0).[310] The MCA has been able to distinguish cases of CHD from control patients without vascular disease with greater accuracy than HDL-C levels.[310] A study of 26 patients with CHD with normal HDL-C levels (57 ± 12 mg/dL) showed an inflammatory index of 1.38 ± 0.91, compared to 0.38 ± 0.14 (*P* <0.001) for 26 age and sex-matched controls free of the disease who had comparable HDL-C levels (63.5 ± 6.1 mg/dL, *P* = 0.008).

A cell-free, fluorometric, high-throughput assay that measures HDL lipid peroxidation fluorometrically has been used assess HDL function. In the presence of horseradish peroxidase, the conversion of fluorochrome Amplex Red to highly fluorescent resorufin is used to quantify the endogenous lipid hydroperoxides present in the captured HDL-C sample. This cell-free assay correlated modestly with the current cell-based assay (Pearson's correlation coefficient [r] = 0.47, *p* <0.001) and cell-free assays (r = 0.46, p <0.001).[311,312] In the MASHAD cohort that included 330 participants followed for a median 7 years, increased serum HDL peroxidation (HDLox) was associated with a 1.62-fold (95% CI: 1.41–1.86) higher risk for cardiovascular events in multivariable models that included HDL-C.[313] Larger studies with a difference population of statin-treated patients will be required to further advance this concept. These studies will require adjustment of HDLox per HDL particle concentration and corroboration with support from HDL proteomics and lipidomics.[256]

Genetics

Studies of human genetics do not support a causal role for HDL-C in ASCVD.[314] However, certain components of HDL and the functional attributes of HDL particles may include genetically determined atheroprotective effects. A GWAS analysis conducted in 441,016 participants from the United Kingdom Biobank (UKBB) identified many new SNPs associated with plasma lipid traits (HDL-C and apoA-I), but in multivariate Mendelian randomization analysis, the risk of CHD was attenuated after accounting for apoB.[264] In a human genetics study of five population-based Finnish cohorts ($n = 20,270$ individuals) combined with a large-scale genomic-wide data ($n = 122,733$ CAD cases), apoA-I was associated with a lower risk of CHD in observational studies (HR 081: 95% CI: 0.75, 0.88 per 1-SD higher apoA-I), but the *rs12225230* variant associated with apoA-I concentration was not in Mendelian randomization studies (OR 1.12; 95% CI: 0.98–1.30 per 1-SD higher apoA-I).[315]

Over the last four decades, monogenic disorders that impair HDL biogenesis, maturation, macrophage cholesterol efflux, and hepatic clearance have been associated with increased cardiovascular risk.[280] Genes implicated in monogenic low HDL-C states include *APOA1* encoding apoA-I, *LCAT* encoding lecithin cholesterol acyl transferase, and *ABCA1* encoding the ATP binding cassette subfamily A member 1 transporter, and *LPL* encoding lipoprotein lipase. Expression of the extreme phenotype requires mutations on both alleles (either simple homozygosity or compound heterozygosity), and in some cases, simple heterozygotes have HDL-C levels that are intermediate between homozygotes and normolipidemic individuals.[280] In an analysis of 258,252 subjects with severe HDL deficiency (HDL-C <20 mg/dL), genetic causes included 0.33% of men and 0.0999% of women (Table 10–20).[280] The racial distribution of the participants undergoing genetic analysis included 85.6% Caucasian, 5.0% Hispanic, 5.0% African American, and 1.5% Asian. Mutations and select loci were found in the following gene loci: *APOA1* (5.0%), *ABCA1* (26.9%), *LCAT* (12.4%), and *LPL* (4.5%).

Monogenic Disorders Associated with Low High-Density Lipoprotein Cholesterol

APOA-I Deficiency: ApoA-I is the key structural and defining protein of the HDL particle. Selective deficiency of apoA-I, the 243 amino acid–defining structural protein of HDL, has been reported in several human kindreds.[316] Human apoA-I deficiency is characterized by undetectable levels of plasma apoA-I, normal triglycerides and apoB-containing lipoproteins, and premature atherosclerosis. In a small series of five cases of familial apoA-1 deficiency (FAID) and 5 age-matched normolipidemic Caucasian controls, perturbations in the HDL lipidome that includes increased concentrations of lysophosphatidylcholine, ceramides and phosphatidylserine, phosphatidic acid and phosphatidylglycerol, and reduced concentrations of phosphatidylethanolamine species.[317] The content of specific phospholipid and sphingolipid species is associated with impaired antiatherogenic properties of HDL in FAID.

The first human deficiencies of apoA-I involved large scale rearrangements involving permutations of the contiguous *APOA1*, *APOC3*, and *APOA4* genes on chromosome 11q23.[318] Probands for both the *APOA1-C3* and *APOA1-C3-A4* deletions had reduced HDL-C, reduced plasma triglycerides consistent with apoC-III deficiency, normal LDL-C, and severe premature atherosclerosis. In addition, *APOA1-C3-A4* deficiency was associated with mild malabsorption of fat and fat-soluble vitamins, consistent with apoA-IV deficiency.

Since then, additional reported *APOA1* mutations in HDL-C deficiency include small insertions and deletions, splicing variants, and numerous nonsense or missense variants.[319,320] Most of these probands are heterozygous for the *APOA1* mutation and have either normal or reduced plasma apoA-I and HDL-C levels. Mutations that result in premature truncation of apoA-I generally have negligible or no circulating protein, with increased catabolism of apoA-I and impaired lipid binding.[321]

Physical findings including planar, as well as tuberoeruptive xanthomas and moderate cornea opacification. These individuals exhibit a wide spectrum of clinical manifestations ranging from significant premature CHD to a normal prevalence of CHD.[322] In one large cohort, ASCVD was present in 40% of subjects with *APOA1* mutations.[280]

ABCA1 Deficiency–Tangier Disease: ABCA1 governs the efflux of esterified cholesterol from peripheral tissues and is a central component of reverse cholesterol transport. The genetic defect in Tangier disease is a mutation in the ABCA1 transporter and the subsequent identification of preβ-HDL as the primary ligand for the ABCA1 transporter provided a major advance in the understanding of the function of HDL in cellular cholesterol efflux and the reverse cholesterol transport pathway.[322]

The role of rare *ABCA1* variants in the development of premature atherosclerosis has proven to be controversial. Although there are several well documented cases of increased premature atherosclerosis in Tangier disease homozygotes, this is not universally observed.

Observational studies in Tangier disease heterozygotes with rare variants in *ABCA1* associated with reduced cholesterol efflux reported increased carotid wall thickness.[323] However, Mendelian randomization experiments in the Combined Copenhagen Heart Study revealed that lower plasma HDL-C levels due to heterozygosity for rare loss-of-function mutations in *ABCA1* were not associated with increased risk of CVD end points.[324] One possible factor contributing to the variable relationship between homozygous *ABCA1* loss of function variants and CVD risk is the associated low plasma LDL-C. In the cohort assembled by Geller and colleagues, the prevalence of atherosclerotic CVD in participants with *ABCA1* mutations was 37% (Table 10–20).[280]

Lecithin–Cholesterol Acyltransferase Deficiency: Lecithin–cholesterol acyltransferase (LCAT) converts cholesterol and phosphatidylcholines to cholesteryl esters and lysophosphatidylcholines on the surface of HDL, a key step in reverse cholesterol transport.[255] In humans, two separate clinical phenotypes, classic homozygous LCAT deficiency[325] and fish eye disease (FED),[326] have been reported in individuals with rare loss-of-function variants affecting both *LCAT* alleles. Classic homozygous LCAT deficiency is characterized by the absence of plasma LCAT activity, increased plasma free cholesterol, marked reduction in HDL-C and apoA-I, decreased LDL-C, and formation of lipoprotein-X. Clinically, these individuals exhibit corneal opacification, anemia, and renal disease, but not premature CVD.[280] The lack of association with CVD risk has been attributed to the concomitantly low plasma LDL-C levels observed in many LCAT deficient homozygotes. However, development of progressive renal disease may indirectly increase CVD risk in some patients.

Probands with the FED phenotype also have two *LCAT* alleles harboring rare variants and low but detectable levels of LCAT activity. However, the LCAT enzyme is located on the apoB-containing lipoproteins rather than HDL and thus termed α LCAT deficiency.[327,328] FED probands have decreased HDL-C and apoA-I, normal to increased LDL-C, and significant corneal opacification and increased CVD risk. It has been proposed that the small residual LCAT activity prevents the development of anemia, lipoprotein-X, and renal disease.[329]

Genetic variants of HDL function have been investigated from studies of genomic, transcriptomic, and lipidomics in individuals with extremely low HDL-C.[330] Low HDL-C subjects were selected based on HDL-C <10th age-and sex-specific population percentile and high HDL-C was >90th percentile selected from a large Finnish cohort study ($n = 11,211$). Genes involved in inflammatory response-related pathways were overexpressed in subjects with low versus high HDL-C status. A biological link between genomics and transcriptomics was supported by gene expression analysis of subcutaneous adipose tissue showing an upregulation in inflammatory pathways involving mitochondrial dysfunction and oxidative phosphorylation. The proinflammatory status in subjects with low HDL-C was supported by mass spectrometry analysis of the HDL particle lipidome. In these studies, low HDL-C subjects had lower content of the ether bond containing phosphatidylethanolamines (plasmalogens) with antioxidant properties and lysophsphatidylcholines involved in cellular cholesterol efflux, and higher content of proinflammatory ceramides than subjects with high HDL-C. This combined inflammatory pathway was associated with *cis*-expression quantitative trait loci (*cis*-eQTL) variants in the *HLA* region with the most significant reported eQTL SNPs *HLA-DRA* rs3135338 and *HLA-DRB1* rs9272143. These data support the concept that HDL particles are regulated by inflammatory signals, which is consistent with mechanistic data that the macrophages from subjects with low HDL-C have a proinflammatory gene expression pattern,[330] and a dysfunctional HDL particle with reduced macrophage cholesterol efflux.[331,332]

Lipoprotein Lipase Deficiency: LPL deficiency is associated with elevated triglycerides and low HDL-C. In the analysis of Geller and colleagues, LPL traits in participants with extremely low HDL-C levels were associated with a low prevalence of ASCVD (Table 10–20).[280]

Approaches to Treatment

Lifestyle factors contribute to the variation observed in HDL-C levels. Higher HDL-C levels are observed in physically fit men and women without prediabetes or diabetes who do not smoke or are exposed to passive smoking and consume moderate amounts of alcohol. Thus, HDL-C is a biomarker of a healthy lifestyle. Efforts to mitigate HDL-associated cardiovascular risk require ongoing efforts at improving healthy behaviors.

Physical activity is associated with higher levels of HDL-C in several epidemiological studies.[333,334] The most compelling data supporting an improvement in total HDL particle concentration and atheroprotective properties derives from the studies of high-impact and high-intensity aerobic exercise.[334] STRRIDE (Studies of Targeted Risk Reduction Interventions through Defined Exercise) was a randomized clinical study that investigated the effects of exercise amount and intensity on serum lipoproteins in overweight and obese men and women with mild to moderate dyslipidemia. Study participants were randomized to a control group of one of three exercise groups that included high-amount high-intensity exercise defined as the equivalent of jogging 20 miles per week at 65% to 80% of peak oxygen consumption; low-amount high-intensity exercise defined as the equivalent of jogging 12 miles at 65% to 80% of peak oxygen consumption; and low-amount of moderate exercise defined as the equivalent of walking 12 miles per week at 40% to 55% of peak oxygen consumption. After 8 months, the high-amount, high-intensity exercise group had higher levels of HDL-C and large HDL particle concentration than the control group or other exercise regimens. These data support recommendations to increase HDL require high amounts of high intensity exercise performed over many months.[334] The STRRIDE-PD (Studies of Target Risk Reduction Interventions through Defined Exercise, in individuals with Pre-Diabetes) trial investigated the effects of exercise on HDL-C efflux in 106 volunteers with prediabetes.[335] High amounts of high-intensity exercise increased global radiolabeled efflux capacity by 6.2% when compared with the other STRIDDE-PD groups. However, exercise had no effect on BODIPY-labeled cholesterol efflux.

The variable effects of exercise on HDL-C is partly impacted by certain HDL regulating polymorphisms. In a prospective cohort study of 22,939 apparently healthy US women of European ancestry, a genome-wide association examined the effect modification of physical activity with HDL-C levels.[336] Per-minor-allele increases in HDL-C among active versus inactive women were observed in carriers of rs1800588 in *LIPC*, rs1532624 in *CETP*, and rs10096633 at *LPL* among active than inactive women. A reduced risk of MI was associated with minor-allele carrier status at the *LPL* SNP (HR, 0.51; 95% CI: 0.30–0.86) but not among inactive women (HR 1.13; 95% CI: 0.79–1.61; *P*-interaction = 0.007). No associations between carrier status in *LIPC* and *CETP* SNPs and MI risk was noted. Protection from MI associated with higher plasma levels of HDL-C may depend both on variation in the genetic determinants of those levels and healthy behaviors.

Statin therapy is first line treatment for the prevention of cardiovascular events in patients with low levels of HDL-C. In addition to the anti-atherosclerotic and anti-inflammatory effects of statins, low HDL-C is often inversely associated with high levels of apoB/LDL-P,[2262,263] which is an established target of statin therapy. Statins differ with respect to HDL effects. In the COMETS (Comparative Study with Rosuvastatin in Subjects with Metabolic Syndrome) trial, rosuvastatin was more effective than atorvastatin in elevating HDL-C and HDL-P.[337]

However, the clinical relevance of these differences in patients with low HDL-C levels remains unknown.

Pharmacotherapy directed at increasing HDL-C has no impact on cardiovascular events.[256] These interventions have involved niacin and CETP inhibitors. Niacin has been investigated in two clinical trials of patients with well controlled LDL-C levels (<70 mg/dL) on statin therapy. The Atherosclerosis Intervention in Metabolic syndrome with Low HDL/HIGH Triglycerides: impact on Global Health Outcomes (AIM-HIGH) trial was designed to investigate the effects of HDL-C–raising therapy with niacin versus placebo in statin-treated patients with ASCVD and LDL-C levels less than 70 mg/dL.[338] The trial randomized 3314 patients to either niacin ($n = 1718$) or placebo ($n = 1696$). The initial primary outcome measure included a composite of CHD death, nonfatal MI, ischemic stroke, or hospitalization for high-risk acute coronary syndrome, but due to the lower than expected event rate the expanded composite endpoint included symptom-driven revascularization procedure for coronary or cerebral revascularization At 2 years, the niacin group had an increase in HDL-C by 25%, while the placebo group had an increase in HDL-C of 9.8%. LDL-C levels were reduced by 12.0% in the niacin group and by 5.5% in the placebo group. The primary endpoint occurred in 16.4% of the niacin group and 16.2% of the placebo group (HR 1.02; 95% CI: 0.87–1.21; $P = 0.79$ by the log-rank test. Due to futility at this interim analysis, the data and safety monitoring board recommended early termination of the trial.

The Heart Protection Study-2-THRIVE trial (A Randomized Trial of the Long-term Clinical Effects of Raising HDL Cholesterol With Extended Release Niacin/Laropiprant) was designed to investigate the effect increasing HDL-C with extended release niacin (ERN) 2 g plus laropiprant (LRPT) 40 mg daily versus placebo on the time to the first major vascular event (composite of nonfatal MI, CHD death, stroke, or arterial revascularization) in patients with a history of occlusive arterial disease (MI, ischemic stroke or transient ischemic attack, peripheral arterial disease, or diabetes with other CHD) who were receiving simvastatin 40 mg daily as background therapy.[339] A total of 25,673 participants were randomized to receive ERN/LRPT or placebo. The mean (SD) baseline total cholesterol was 128 (22) mg/dL, direct LDL-C was 63 (17) mg/dL, HDL-C was 44 (11) mg/Dl, and triglycerides were 125 (74) mg/dL. On trial, ERN/LRPT treatment reduced LDL-C by an average 10 mg/dL (0.25 mmol/L), and increased HDL-C by 6 mg/dL. After a median of 3.9 years, the primary endpoint was no different among participants allocated to ERN/LRPT or placebo (14.5% vs. 15.0%, RR 0.96 [95% CI: 0.90–103], logrank $P = 0.29$). At the end of the study, 25.4% of participants allocated to ERN/LRPT and 16.6% of placebo-treated participants discontinued the therapy. Leading serious adverse events included a 1.55-fold excess risk for diabetes complications ($P <0.0001$); 1.4% excess infections ($P <0.0001$), 1.28-fold more gastrointestinal events ($P <0.0001$) that were attributed to 0.2% more gastrointestinal bleeds, 0.5% more peptic ulcer/upper gastrointestinal complaints, and 0.2% more lower gastrointestinal complaints; and 1.26-fold excess risk for musculoskeletal events (0.0008)

that included 0.5% more myopathy and 0.1% more gout. In addition to these adverse events that have been associated with niacin therapy, there was a 1.22-fold excess risk for infections that were primarily due to 0.6% increased lower respiratory tract infections. This large, multinational trial demonstrated that ERN/LRPT had no impact on the major vascular events when added to effective simvastatin-induced LDL-C lowering treatment. Treatment with ERN/LRPT was accompanied by more serious adverse events of both niacin-related side effects and side effects not previously reported with niacin.

Therapies involving HDL infusions have shown promise in small studies with imaging endpoints. The initial human study involved infusions of the mutant apoA-I Milano protein.[340] The metabolism of apoA-I Milano differs from normal apoA-I due to increased catabolism and reduced activation of LCAT, which reduces the conversion of HDL unesterified cholesterol to esterified cholesterol.[120] In the MILANO-PILOT, a reformulated apoA-I formulation of the mutant apoA-I Milano, was administered to ACS patients in 5 weekly infusions, reduced coronary intravascular ultrasound percent atheroma volume by 0.21% and 0.73% in the placebo group ($P = 0.07$).[341] This mutant dimeric form of apoA-I did not activate LCAT resulting in hypercatabolism of endogenous apoA-I,[342] and does not result in lipid-poor apoA-I during remodeling.[343]

Synthetic HDL mimetics have been studies in ACS patients. CER-001 is a recombinant apoA-I complex containing sphingomyelin and phospholipid enriched with dipalmityl phosphoglycerol. Sphingomyelin interferes with lipid poor A-I release from HDL-impairing ABCA1 interactions,[344] and additionally inhibits LCAT, the second step in cholesterol efflux.[345] In the CARAT (CER-001 Atherosclerosis Regression Acute Coronary Syndrome) trial, investigated the effect of 10 weekly intravenous infusions of CER-001 (3 mg/kg) versus placebo on coronary atherosclerosis progression in statin-treated patients with acute coronary syndrome.[346] The primary efficacy measure, percent atheroma volume, decreased by 0.41% with placebo ($P = 0.005$ compared with baseline), but no change with CER-001 (–0.09%; $P = 0.67$ compared with baseline; between group differences, 0.32%; $P = 0.15$).

Subsequently, a modified human apoA-I complex with reduced phospholipid content was formulated as CSL 112.[346] Although these synthetics discs are poor substrates for ABCA1, they interact with spherical HDL particles generating a lipid-poor A-I that is effectively mediates cholesterol efflux from RAW264.7 cells.[347] The AEGIS-I trial (Apo-I Event Reducing in Ischemic Syndromes I) was a multicenter, randomized, double-blind, placebo-controlled, dose-ranging phase 2b trial. This phase 2b clinical trial randomized 1258 patients with a recent acute MI to CSL112 (2 g apoA-I per dose) and high-dose CSL112 (6 g apoA-I per dose), or placebo for four consecutive weekly infusions. Infusion of CSL112 caused a dose-dependent elevation of both apoA-I and cholesterol efflux capacity. For the 2-g dose elevated total cholesterol efflux capacity by 1.87-fold, whereas the 6-g dose elevated total cholesterol efflux capacity by 2.45-fold. The elevation of ABCA1-dependent cholesterol efflux capacity increased by 3.67-fold for the 2-g dose, and by 4.30-fold for the 6-g dose.

Currently, the results of AEGIS-II (Study to Investigate CSL112 in Subjects With Acute Coronary Syndrome) trial are ongoing with results anticipated in 2022[347] (ClinicalTrials.gov Identifier: NCT03473223). This trial is investigating the effects of 7 weekly infusions of CSL112 versus an albumin comparator on the time to first occurrence of any component of composite MACE (cardiovascular death, MI, or stroke) through 90 days in 17,400 participants with acute coronary syndrome.

Other synthetic HDL mimetics include L-4F and D-4F. In experimental models, both L-4F and D-4F are trapped in the small intestine and transported into the intestinal lumen.[348] Transintestinal cholesterol efflux is one of the major mechanisms for removal of cholesterol from the body. L-4F is a peptide mimetic of apoA-I comprised of L-amino acids with a structure based on tandem repeating amphipathic helical domains. In experimental studies, L-4F exhibits antioxidant, anti-inflammatory and anti-atherogenic properties.[349] L-4F inhibits proinflammatory and glycolytic gene expression in macrophages,[350] changes immune cell profiles by promoting differentiation of M2 monocyte differentiated macrophages, and inhibits endothelial adhesion and migration.[351] In a murine model of MI reperfusion injury, L-4F inhibits inflammation after MI, improves post-MI LV remodeling and diminishes progression to heart failure.[352] Infusions of L-4F in patients with CVD has no effect on the HDL inflammatory index.[352] D-4F is a peptide comprising 18 amino acids with a tertiary structure resembling apoA-I, but without sequence homology.[353] In a first-in-human multiple-dose trial, CHD treated patients treated with statins were randomized to double-blind treatment with oral D-4F or placebo, and treatment with D-4F reduced the HDL inflammatory index.

Selective HDL delipidation techniques generate nascent HDL particles that have similar composition and metabolism to native nascent HDL particles.[354] In a proof-of-concept study of 28 patients with acute coronary syndromes who were randomized to 7 weeks of treatment with autologous delipidate nascent HDL or placebo, pre-beta HDL increased from 5.6% to 79.1% while coronary intravascular ultrasound volume was reduced by -12.18 mm^3 in the treatment group versus an increase of $+2.80$ mm^3 in the control group ($P = 0.238$).[355] In a subsequent study of six patients with homozygous FH, seven weekly infusions of autologous delipidated HDL reduced CT angiography total atheroma area by 18% and noncalcified plaque by 20% including reductions in low-density ("soft") plaque (-38%) and the necrotic core (-33%).[356]

Clinical trials in patients with low HDL levels have focused on increasing the cholesterol content of HDL; however, cholesterol loading of HDL may diminish the antioxidant and anti-inflammatory capacity of HDL.[256] Subsequently, HDL-directed therapies have emphasized increasing the availability of ApoA-I complexes through direct intravenous infusions or delipidation of HDL. The initial studies demonstrate reductions in atherosclerosis with infusions of phospholipid-deficient and cholesterol absent ApoA-I complexes and generation of these complexes achieved by HDL delipidation. Currently, the efficacy of increasing ABCA1-mediated cholesterol efflux on the risk of cardiovascular events remains unproven.

Training and Education

Nearly 60 years ago, Glomset identified HDL in the reverse cholesterol transport process.[357] This pathway centered on the LCAT pathway that allowed for more efficient cholesterol

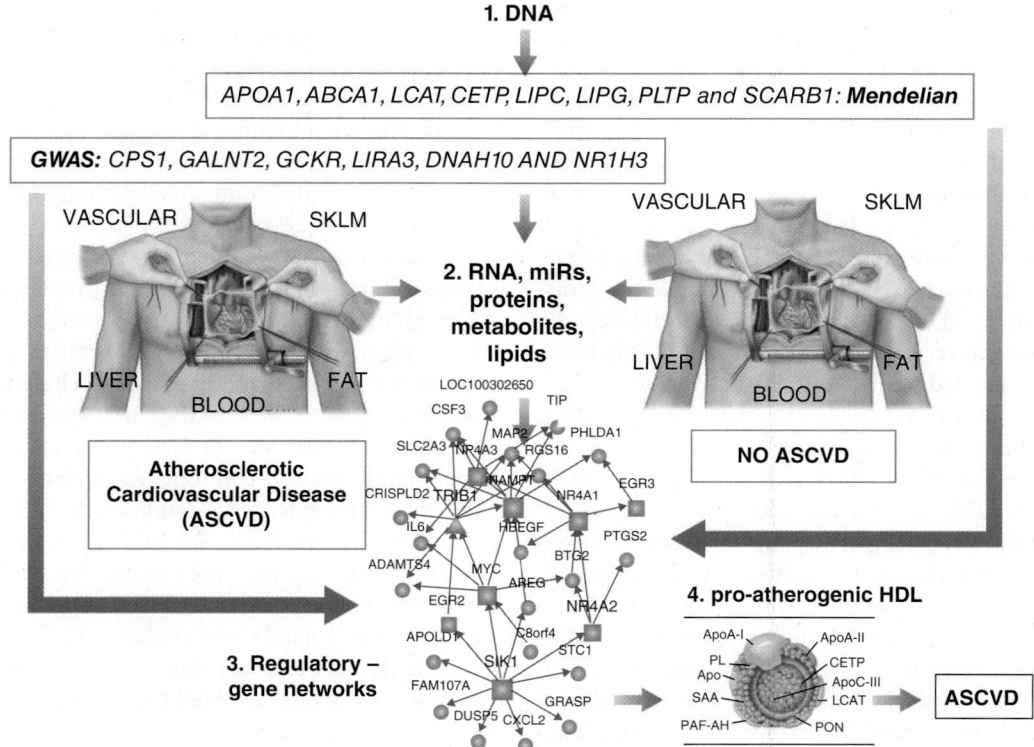

Figure 10–28. A systems-based approach to understanding the dynamic processes involved in HDL metabolism and contribution to atherosclerosis.

accumulation by HDL particles. This concept led to decades of investigations and clinical trials designed to increase the cholesterol carrying capacity of HDL. After a multitude of failures with multiple classes of HDL-C raising therapies, the field of HDL requires a resurrection with novel strategies that integrate HDL structure–function relationships. These approaches must consider the dynamic aspects of HDL within the circulation, and by multiple cells and tissues[314] (**Fig. 10–28**). This systems-based approach is complex, but it provides the most comprehensive approach to advancing improved understanding in the field.

SUMMARY

Hypercholesterolemia

Pathogenesis

- Hypercholesterolemia is most often due to elevated LDL-C, which is an established causal agent for atherosclerosis.

Genetics

- The most common single gene disorder characterized by elevated LDL-C is heterozygous FH, which is typically due to a single copy of a loss-of-function mutated allele of the *LDLR* gene.
- Many cases of elevated LDL-C are polygenic in nature.

Diagnosis

- A combination of clinical features, including family history, elevated LDL-C, and positive DNA testing can help with definitive diagnosis of FH.

Treatment

- Even if a single gene cause is not detected, elevated LDL-C should still be treated according to clinical practice guidelines using diet and lifestyle and, if necessary, statins in combination with ezetimibe and a PCSK9 inhibitor.
- Newer agents that reduce LDL-C are in development.

Lipoprotein(a)

Pathogenesis

- Strong evidence indicates that elevated Lp(a) levels are a causal and independent risk factor for ASCVD and CAVD.
- The mechanism of action of Lp(a) in ASCVD and CAVD likely involves a proinflammatory role mediated by apo(a)-associated oxPL, although a prothrombotic role for Lp(a) in the former cannot be ruled out.

Genetics

- Lp(a) levels are strongly heritable, with 60 to >90% of the variation determined at the level of the LPA gene itself.
- Copy number variants in LPA result in alleles carrying a variable number of KIV type 2-encoding sequences (from 3 to greater than 40). This results in a wide range of plasma Lp(a) isoform sizes.
- A general inverse correlation exists between apo(a) isoform size and plasma Lp(a) levels, which is the major driver of plasma Lp(a) concentrations.

- There is little evidence for contributions of other genes to Lp(a) levels with the exception of *APOE*.

Diagnosis

- Elevated Lp(a) levels are defined as greater than 30 to 50 mg/dL, or greater than 100 nmol/L.
- Assays should be carefully selected where possible to avoid isoform size bias with values reported in particle concentration rather than mass units.
- Measurement of Lp(a) levels is reasonable to consider in several circumstances, including:
- a strong family history of premature CVD in first degree relatives, and/or moderate to high CVD risk.
- hypercholesterolemia (LDL>190 mg/dL) or confirmed/suspected FH.
- in individuals ≤20 years old who have had ischemic or hemorrhagic stroke or with family histories of premature CVD, hypercholesterolemia, or elevated Lp(a).

Treatment

- There is currently no specific therapy to lower Lp(a) levels. An LPA antisense oligonucleotide that lowers plasma Lp(a) up to 80% is currently in Phase III trials. This will conclusively demonstrate that significant specific lowering of Lp(a) has clinical benefit.
- At this time, the recommendation to manage elevated Lp(a) is to aggressively treat modifiable risk factors.

Hypertriglyceridemia

Pathogenesis

- Mild-to-moderate hypertriglyceridemia (150–1000 mg/dL; 1.7–11.4 mmol/L) is due to elevated triglyceride-rich lipoproteins and their remnants, which are established causal agents for atherosclerosis.
- Severe hypertriglyceridemia (>1000 mg/dL; >11.4 mmol/L) is due to elevated chylomicrons and/or very large VLDL, both of which can lead to acute pancreatitis.

Genetics

- The most common cause of hypertriglyceridemia is obesity in individuals with polygenic predisposition.
- Remnant hyperlipidemia is found in individuals with the apoE-2/2 isoform together with some other predisposing factor, and is characterized by combined hypertriglyceridemia and hypercholesterolemia.
- Chylomicronemia syndrome occurs in a rare familial form and in a slightly more common form.

Diagnosis

- Hypertriglyceridemia is diagnosed as elevated plasma triglycerides while elevated remnant cholesterol (cholesterol in triglyceride-rich lipoproteins) assess risk of CVD.

Treatment

- Mild-to-moderate hypertriglyceridemia is best approached with weight loss supplemented with high-intensity statin.

- In certain circumstances, fibrates or icosapent ethyl can be added to high-intensity statin.
- Newer agents that reduce severe hypertriglyceridemia (>1000 mg/dL; >11.4 mmol/L) are in development.

Low High-Density Lipoprotein Cholesterol

Pathogenesis

- HDL has multiple atheroprotective properties that are inadequately expressed by the cholesterol carrying capacity of HDL particles.
- The mechansims whereby HDLs protects against atherosclerotic vascular disease include the quintessential macrophage cholesterol efflux pathway, but other properties may be equally or more important including antioxidant, anti-inflammatory, and anti-apoptotic effects mediated by the HDL proteins and lipids.

Genetics

- Genetically low HDL-C levels have variable associations with early onset ASCVD.
- Future studies are required to improve understanding of genetic susceptibilities associated specific HDL proteins and pathways.

Diagnosis

- A low HDL-C level is often associated with unhealthy behaviors and hence a marker of disease.
- A more precise measure of HDL associated cardiovascular risk is the HDL particle concentration.

Treatment

- The treatment of HDL associated risk is an evolving area.
- Ongoing clinical trials emphasize therapies that increase the concentrations of cholesterol depleted and phospholipid deficient apoA-1 moieties either through infusions or regeneration via delipidation.

REFERENCES

1. Ference BA, Ginsberg HN, Graham I, et al. Low-density lipoproteins cause atherosclerotic cardiovascular disease. 1. Evidence from genetic, epidemiologic, and clinical studies. A consensus statement from the European Atherosclerosis Society Consensus Panel. *Eur Heart J.* 2017;38: 2459–2472.
2. Benjamin EJ, Muntner P, Alonso A, et al. Heart disease and stroke statistics-2019 update: a report From the American Heart Association. *Circulation* 2019;139:e56–e528.
3. World Health Organization. *Global Status Report on Noncommunicable Diseases.* 2014. https://www.who.int/nmh/publications/ncd-status-report-2014/en/
4. Kavey RE, Allada V, Daniels SR, et al. Cardiovascular risk reduction in high-risk pediatric patients: a scientific statement from the American Heart Association Expert Panel on Population and Prevention Science; the Councils on Cardiovascular Disease in the Young, Epidemiology and Prevention, Nutrition, Physical Activity and Metabolism, High Blood Pressure Research, Cardiovascular Nursing, and the Kidney in Heart Disease; and the Interdisciplinary Working Group on Quality of Care and Outcomes Research. *J Cardiovasc Nurs.* 2007;22:218–253.
5. Cholesterol Treatment Trialists C. Efficacy and safety of statin therapy in older people: a meta-analysis of individual participant data from 28 randomised controlled trials. *Lancet* 2019;393:407–415.
6. Grundy SM, Stone NJ, Bailey AL, et al. 2018 AHA/ACC/AACVPR/AAPA/ABC/ACPM/ADA/AGS/APhA/ASPC/NLA/PCNA guideline on the management of blood cholesterol: executive summary: a report of the American College of Cardiology/American Heart Association Task Force on Clinical Practice Guidelines. *J Am Coll Cardiol.* 2019;73:3168–3209.
7. Mach F, Baigent C, Catapano AL, et al. 2019 ESC/EAS Guidelines for the management of dyslipidaemias: lipid modification to reduce cardiovascular risk. *Eur Heart J.* 2020;41:111–188.
8. Brown TM, Bittner V, Colantonio LD, et al. Residual risk for coronary heart disease events and mortality despite intensive medical management after myocardial infarction. *J Clin Lipidol.* 2020;14:260–270.
9. Colantonio LD, Shannon ED, Orroth KK, et al. Ischemic Event Rates in Very-High-Risk Adults. *J Am Coll Cardiol.* 2019;74:2496–2507.
10. Rosenson RS, Farkouh ME, Mefford M, et al. Trends in use of high-intensity statin therapy after myocardial infarction, 2011 to 2014. *J Am Coll Cardiol.* 2017;69:2696–2706.
11. Goff DC, Jr., Lloyd-Jones DM, Bennett G, et al. 2013 ACC/AHA guideline on the assessment of cardiovascular risk: a report of the American College of Cardiology/American Heart Association Task Force on Practice Guidelines. *J Am Coll Cardiol.* 2014;63:2935–2959.
12. Muntner P, Colantonio LD, Cushman M, et al. Validation of the atherosclerotic cardiovascular disease Pooled Cohort risk equations. *JAMA.* 2014;311:1406–1415.
13. Ridker PM, Buring JE, Rifai N, Cook NR. Development and validation of improved algorithms for the assessment of global cardiovascular risk in women: the Reynolds Risk Score. *JAMA.* 2007;297:611–619.
14. National Institute for Health and Care Excellence (NICE) clinical guideline CG181: lipid modification, cardiovascular risk assessment and the modification of blood lipids for the primary and secondary prevention of cardiovascular disease. 2019. https://www.nice.org.uk/guidance/cg181.
15. Cooney MT, Selmer R, Lindman A, et al. Cardiovascular risk estimation in older persons: SCORE O.P. *Eur J Prev Cardiol.* 2016;23:1093–1103.
16. Greenland P, Blaha MJ, Budoff MJ, Erbel R, Watson KE. Coronary calcium score and cardiovascular risk. *J Am Coll Cardiol.* 2018;72:434–447.
17. Blaha MJ, Whelton SP, Al Rifai M, et al. Comparing risk scores in the prediction of coronary and cardiovascular deaths: Coronary Artery Calcium Consortium. *JACC Cardiovasc Imaging* 2020.
18. Roncaglioni MC, Santoro L, D'Avanzo B, et al. Role of family history in patients with myocardial infarction. An Italian case-control study. GISSI-EFRIM Investigators. *Circulation* 1992;85:2065–2072.
19. Colantonio LD, Hubbard D, Monda KL, et al. Atherosclerotic risk and statin use among patients with peripheral artery disease. *J Am Coll Cardiol.* 2020;76:251–264.
20. Garg A, Garg V, Hegele RA, Lewis GF. Practical definitions of severe versus familial hypercholesterolaemia and hypertriglyceridaemia for adult clinical practice. *Lancet Diabetes Endocrinol.* 2019; 7:880–886.
21. Khera AV, Hegele RA. What is familial hypercholesterolemia, and why does it matter? *Circulation.* 2020; 141:1760–1763.
22. Grundy SM, Stone NJ, Bailey AL, et al. 2018 AHA/ACC/AACVPR/AAPA/ABC/ACPM/ADA/AGS/APhA/ASPC/NLA/PCNA guideline on the management of blood cholesterol: executive summary: a report of the American College of Cardiology/American Heart Association Task Force on Clinical Practice Guidelines. *Circulation.* 2019; 139:e1046–e1081.
23. Mach F, Baigent C, Catapano A, et al. 2019 ESC/EAS Guidelines for the management of dyslipidaemias: lipid modification to reduce cardiovascular risk. *Eur Heart J.* 2020; 41:111–188.
24. Sturm AC, Knowles JW, Gidding SS, et al. Clinical genetic testing for familial hypercholesterolemia: JACC Scientific Expert Panel. *J Am Coll Cardiol.* 2018; 72:662–680.
25. Robert SR. Existing and emerging therapies for the treatment of familial hypercholesterolemia. *J. Lipid. Res.* 2021;62:100060.

26. Defesche JC, Gidding SS, Harada-Shiba M, Hegele RA, Santos RD, Wierzbicki AS. Familial hypercholesterolaemia. *Nat Rev Dis Primers.* 2017; 3:17093.

27. Brown EE, Sturm AC, Cuchel M, et al. Genetic testing in dyslipidemia: A scientific statement from the National Lipid Association. *J Clin Lipidol.* 2020; 14:398–413.

28. Hu P, Dharmayat KI, Stevens CAT, et al. Prevalence of familial hypercholesterolemia among the general population and patients with atherosclerotic cardiovascular disease: a systematic review and meta-analysis. *Circulation.* 2020; 141:1742–1759.

29. Berberich AJ, Hegele RA. The complex molecular genetics of familial hypercholesterolaemia. *Nat Rev Cardiol.* 2019; 16:9–20.

30. Gidding SS, Champagne MA, de Ferranti SD, et al. The agenda for familial hypercholesterolemia: a scientific statement from the American Heart Association. *Circulation.* 2015; 132:2167–2192.

31. Brunham LR, Ruel I, Aljenedil S, et al. Canadian Cardiovascular Society position statement on familial hypercholesterolemia: update 2018. *Can J Cardiol.* 2018; 34:1553–1563.

32. Khera AV, Won HH, Peloso GM, et al. Diagnostic yield and clinical utility of sequencing familial hypercholesterolemia genes in patients with severe hypercholesterolemia. *J Am Coll Cardiol.* 2016; 67:2578–2589.

33. Wang J, Dron JS, Ban MR, et al. Polygenic versus monogenic causes of hypercholesterolemia ascertained clinically. *Arterioscler Thromb Vasc Biol.* 2016; 36:2439–2445.

34. Abul-Husn NS, Manickam K, Jones LK, et al. Genetic identification of familial hypercholesterolemia within a single U.S. health care system. Science 2016; 354(6319). pii: aaf7000. doi: 10.1126/science.aaf7000.

35. Ference BA, Ginsberg HN, Graham I, et al. Low-density lipoproteins cause atherosclerotic cardiovascular disease. 1. Evidence from genetic, epidemiologic, and clinical studies. A consensus statement from the European Atherosclerosis Society Consensus Panel. *Eur Heart J.* 2017; 38: 2459–2472.

36. Borén J, Chapman MJ, Krauss RM, et al. Low-density lipoproteins cause atherosclerotic cardiovascular disease: pathophysiological, genetic, and therapeutic insights: a consensus statement from the European Atherosclerosis Society Consensus Panel. *Eur Heart J.* 2020; 41:2313–2330.

37. George R, Kovak K, Cox SL. Aligning policy to promote cascade genetic screening for prevention and early diagnosis of heritable diseases. *J Genet Couns.* 2015; 24:388–399.

38. Iacocca MA, Chora JR, Carrié A, et al. ClinVar database of global familial hypercholesterolemia-associated DNA variants. *Hum Mutat* 2018; 39:1631–1640.

39. Richards S, Aziz N, Bale S, et al. Standards and guidelines for the interpretation of sequence variants: a joint consensus recommendation of the American College of Medical Genetics and Genomics and the Association for Molecular Pathology. *Genet Med.* 2015; 17:405–424.

40. Dron JS, Hegele RA. Complexity of mechanisms among human proprotein convertase subtilisin-kexin type 9 variants. *Curr Opin Lipidol.* 2017; 28:161–169.

41. Hegele RA, Borén J, Ginsberg HN, et al. Rare dyslipidaemias, from phenotype to genotype to management: a European Atherosclerosis Society task force consensus statement. *Lancet Diabetes Endocrinol.* 2020; 8:50–67.

42. Wald DS, Bestwick JP, Morris JK, Whyte K, Jenkins L, Wald NJ. Child-parent familial hypercholesterolemia screening in primary care. *N Engl J Med.* 2016; 375:1628–1637.

43. Gidding SS, Sheldon A, Neben CL, et al. Patient acceptance of genetic testing for familial hypercholesterolemia in the CASCADE FH Registry. *J Clin Lipidol.* 2020; 14:218–223.

44. Sharifi M, Futema M, Nair D, Humphries SE. Polygenic hypercholesterolemia and cardiovascular disease risk. *Curr Cardiol Rep.* 2019; 21:43.

45. Hegele RA, Ban MR, Cao H, McIntyre AD, Robinson JF, Wang J. Targeted next-generation sequencing in monogenic dyslipidemias. *Curr Opin Lipidol.* 2015; 26:103–113.

46. Khera AV, Chaffin M, Aragam KG, et al. Genome-wide polygenic scores for common diseases identify individuals with risk equivalent to monogenic mutations. *Nat Genet.* 2018; 50:1219–1224.

47. Brahm AJ, Hegele RA. Combined hyperlipidemia: familial but not (usually) monogenic. *Curr Opin Lipidol.* 2016; 27:131–140.

48. Langsted A, Kamstrup PR, Benn M, Tybjærg-Hansen A, Nordestgaard BG. High lipoprotein(a) as a possible cause of clinical familial hypercholesterolaemia: a prospective cohort study. *Lancet Diabetes Endocrinol.* 2016; 4:577–587.

49. Watanabe J, Hamasaki M, Kotani K. Risk of cardiovascular disease with lipoprotein(a) in familial hypercholesterolemia: a review. *Arch Med Sci Atheroscler Dis.* 2020; 5:e148–e152.

50. Brinton EA, Hopkins PN, Hegele RA, et al. The association between hypercholesterolemia and sitosterolemia, and report of a sitosterolemia kindred. *J Clin Lipidol.* 2018; 12:152–161.

51. Chora JR, Alves AC, Medeiros AM, et al. Lysosomal acid lipase deficiency: a hidden disease among cohorts of familial hypercholesterolemia? *J Clin Lipidol.* 2017; 11:477–484.

52. Raygor V, Khera A. New recommendations and revised concepts in recent guidelines on the management of dyslipidemias to prevent cardiovascular disease: the 2018 ACC/AHA and 2019 ESC/EAS guidelines. *Curr Cardiol Rep.* 2020; 22: 87 doi: 10.1007/s11886-020-01331-z.

53. Rached F, Santos RD. The role of statins in current guidelines. *Curr Atheroscler Rep.* 2020; 22:50.

54. Rosenson RS, Hegele RA, Fazio S, Cannon CP. The evolving future of PCSK9 inhibitors. *J Am Coll Cardiol.* 2018; 72:314–329.

55. Ray KK, Wright RS, Kallend D, et al. Two Phase 3 trials of inclisiran in patients with elevated LDL cholesterol. *N Engl J Med.* 2020; 382:1507–1519.

56. Catapano AL, Pirillo A, Norata GD. New pharmacological approaches to target PCSK9. *Curr Atheroscler Rep.* 2020; 22:24.

57. D'Andrea E, Hey SP, Ramirez CL, Kesselheim AS. Assessment of the role of niacin in managing cardiovascular disease outcomes: a systematic review and meta-analysis. *JAMA Netw Open.* 2019; 2:e192224.

58. Parham JS, Goldberg AC. Mipomersen and its use in familial hypercholesterolemia. *Expert Opin Pharmacother.* 2019; 20:127–131.

59. Marrs JC, Anderson SL. Bempedoic acid for the treatment of dyslipidemia. *Drugs Context.* 2020; 9:2020-6-5.

60. Santos RD, Gidding SS, Hegele RA, et al. Defining severe familial hypercholesterolaemia and the implications for clinical management: a consensus statement from the International Atherosclerosis Society Severe Familial Hypercholesterolemia Panel. *Lancet Diabetes Endocrinol.* 2016; 4:850–861.

61. Raal FJ, Hovingh GK, Blom D, et al. Long-term treatment with evolocumab added to conventional drug therapy, with or without apheresis, in patients with homozygous familial hypercholesterolaemia: an interim subset analysis of the open-label TAUSSIG study. *Lancet Diabetes Endocrinol.* 2017; 5:280–290.

62. Gaudet D, Durst R, Lepor N, et al. Usefulness of gemcabene in homozygous familial hypercholesterolemia (from COBALT-1). *Am J Cardiol.* 2019; 124:1876–1880.

63. Raal FJ, Rosenson RS, Reeskamp LF, et al. Evinacumab for homozygous familial hypercholesterolemia. *N Engl J Med.* 2020; 383:711–720.

64. Gaudet D, Karwatowska-Prokopczuk E, Baum SJ, et al. Vupanorsen, an N-acetyl galactosamine-conjugated antisense drug to ANGPTL3 mRNA, lowers triglycerides and atherogenic lipoproteins in patients with diabetes, hepatic steatosis, and hypertriglyceridaemia. *Eur Heart J.* 2020 Aug 29: ehaa689.

65. Rosenson RS, Burgess LJ, Ebenbichler CF, et al. Evinacumab in patients with refractory hypercholesterolemia. *N Engl J Med.* 2020;383(24): 2307–2319. doi: 10.1056/NEJMoa2031049.

66. Wiegman A, Gidding SS, Watts GF, et al. Familial hypercholesterolaemia in children and adolescents: gaining decades of life by optimizing detection and treatment. *Eur Heart J* 2015; 36:2425–2437.

67. Santos RD, Ruzza A, Hovingh GK, et al. Evolocumab in pediatric heterozygous familial hypercholesterolemia. *N Engl J Med.* 2020; 383:1317–1327.

68. Watts GF, Gidding SS, Mata P, et al. Familial hypercholesterolaemia: evolving knowledge for designing adaptive models of care. *Nat Rev Cardiol.* 2020; 17:360–377.

69. Sturm AC, Knowles JW, Gidding SS, et al. Clinical genetic testing for familial hypercholesterolemia: JACC Scientific Expert Panel. *J Am Coll Cardiol.* 2018; 72:662–680.

70. McLean JW, Tomlinson JE, Kuang WJ, et al. cDNA sequence of human apolipoprotein(a) is homologous to plasminogen. *Nature.* 1987;330(6144):132–137.

71. van der Hoek YY, Wittekoek ME, Beisiegel U, Kastelein JJ, Koschinsky ML. The apolipoprotein(a) kringle IV repeats which differ from the major repeat kringle are present in variably-sized isoforms. *Hum Mol Genet.* 1993;2(4):361–366.

72. Boffa MB, Koschinsky ML. Oxidized phospholipids as a unifying theory for lipoprotein(a) and cardiovascular disease. *Nat Rev Cardiol.* 2019;16(5):305–318.

73. Lackner C, Cohen JC, Hobbs HH. Molecular definition of the extreme size polymorphism in apolipoprotein(a). *Hum Mol Genet.* 1993;2(7):933–940.

74. Varvel S, McConnell JP, Tsimikas S. Prevalence of Elevated Lp(a) mass levels and patient thresholds in 532 359 patients in the United States. *Arterioscler Thromb Vasc Biol.* 2016;36(11):2239–2245.

75. McNeal CJ, Peterson AL. Lipoprotein (a) in youth. In: Feingold KR, Anawalt B, Boyce A, Chrousos G, de Herder WW, Dungan K, et al., eds. *Endotext.* South Dartmouth, MA; 2000.

76. Chan DC, Watts GF, Coll B, Wasserman SM, Marcovina SM, Barrett PHR. Lipoprotein(a) particle production as a determinant of plasma lipoprotein(a) concentration across varying apolipoprotein(a) isoform sizes and background cholesterol-lowering therapy. *J Am Heart Assoc.* 2019;8(7): e011781.

77. White AL, Hixson JE, Rainwater DL, Lanford RE. Molecular basis for "null" lipoprotein(a) phenotypes and the influence of apolipoprotein(a) size on plasma lipoprotein(a) level in the baboon. *J Biol Chem.* 1994;269(12):9060–9066.

78. Becker L, Cook PM, Wright TG, Koschinsky ML. Quantitative evaluation of the contribution of weak lysine-binding sites present within apolipoprotein(a) kringle IV types 6-8 to lipoprotein(a) assembly. *J Biol Chem.* 2004;279(4):2679–2688.

79. Becker L, Nesheim ME, Koschinsky ML. Catalysis of covalent Lp(a) assembly: evidence for an extracellular enzyme activity that enhances disulfide bond formation. *Biochemistry.* 2006;45(32):9919–9928.

80. Reyes-Soffer G, Ginsberg HN, Ramakrishnan R. The metabolism of lipoprotein (a): an ever-evolving story. *J Lipid Res.* 2017;58(9):1756–1764.

81. Romagnuolo R, Scipione CA, Boffa MB, Marcovina SM, Seidah NG, Koschinsky ML. Lipoprotein(a) catabolism is regulated by proprotein convertase subtilisin/kexin type 9 through the low density lipoprotein receptor. *J Biol Chem.* 2015;290(18):11649–11662.

82. Yang X.-P. et al. Scavenger receptor-BI is a receptor for lipoprotein(a). *J. Lipid Res.* 2013; 54(9): 2450–2457.

83. Sharma M, Redpath GM, Williams MJ, McCormick SP. Recycling of apolipoprotein(a) after plgrkt-mediated endocytosis of lipoprotein(a). *Circ Res.* 2017;120(7):1091–1102.

84. Vuorio A, Watts GF, Schneider WJ, Tsimikas S, Kovanen PT. Familial hypercholesterolemia and elevated lipoprotein(a): double heritable risk and new therapeutic opportunities. *J Intern Med.* 2020;287(1):2–18.

85. Raal FJ, Giugliano RP, Sabatine MS, et al. PCSK9 inhibition-mediated reduction in Lp(a) with evolocumab: an analysis of 10 clinical trials and the LDL receptor's role. *J Lipid Res.* 2016;57(6):1086–1096.

86. Watts GF, Chan DC, Somaratne R, et al. Controlled study of the effect of proprotein convertase subtilisin-kexin type 9 inhibition with evolocumab on lipoprotein(a) particle kinetics. *Eur Heart J.* 2018;39(27):2577–2585.

87. Emerging Risk Factors Collaboration, Erqou S, Kaptoge S, et al. Lipoprotein(a) concentration and the risk of coronary heart disease, stroke, and nonvascular mortality. *JAMA.* 2009;302(4):412–423.

88. Pare G, Caku A, McQueen M, et al. Lipoprotein(a) Levels and the risk of myocardial infarction among 7 ethnic groups. *Circulation.* 2019;139(12):1472–1482.

89. Willeit P, Ridker PM, Nestel PJ, et al. Baseline and on-statin treatment lipoprotein(a) levels for prediction of cardiovascular events: individual patient-data meta-analysis of statin outcome trials. *Lancet.* 2018;392(10155):1311–1320.

90. Tsimikas S, Fazio S, Ferdinand KC, et al. NHLBI working group recommendations to reduce lipoprotein(a)-mediated risk of cardiovascular disease and aortic stenosis. *J Am Coll Cardiol.* 2018;71(2):177–192.

91. Marcovina SM, Albers JJ, Wijsman E, Zhang Z, Chapman NH, Kennedy H. Differences in Lp[a] concentrations and apo[a] polymorphs between black and white Americans. *J Lipid Res.* 1996;37(12):2569–2585.

92. Kamstrup PR, Tybjaerg-Hansen A, Steffensen R, Nordestgaard BG. Genetically elevated lipoprotein(a) and increased risk of myocardial infarction. *JAMA.* 2009;301(22):2331–2339.

93. Clarke R, Peden JF, Hopewell JC, et al. Genetic variants associated with Lp(a) lipoprotein level and coronary disease. *N Engl J Med.* 2009;361(26):2518–2528.

94. Forbes CA, Quek RG, Deshpande S, et al. The relationship between Lp(a) and CVD outcomes: a systematic review. *Lipids Health Dis.* 2016;15:95.

95. Virani SS, Brautbar A, Davis BC, et al. Associations between lipoprotein(a) levels and cardiovascular outcomes in black and white subjects: the Atherosclerosis Risk in Communities (ARIC) Study. *Circulation.* 2012;125(2):241–249.

96. Guan W, Cao J, Steffen BT, et al. Race is a key variable in assigning lipoprotein(a) cutoff values for coronary heart disease risk assessment: the Multi-Ethnic Study of Atherosclerosis. *Arterioscler Thromb Vasc Biol.* 2015;35(4):996–1001.

97. Wild SH, Fortmann SP, Marcovina SM. A prospective case-control study of lipoprotein(a) levels and apo(a) size and risk of coronary heart disease in Stanford Five-City Project participants. *Arterioscler Thromb Vasc Biol.* 1997;17(2):239–245.

98. Suk Danik J, et al. Lipoprotein(a), measured with an assay independent of apolipoprotein(a) isoform size, and risk of future cardiovascular events among initially healthy women. *JAMA.* 2006 Sep 20;296(11):1363–1370.

99. Cook NR, Mora S, Ridker PM. Lipoprotein(a) and Cardiovascular risk prediction among women. *J Am Coll Cardiol.* 2018;72(3):287–296.

100. Erqou S, Thompson A, Di Angelantonio E, et al. Apolipoprotein(a) isoforms and the risk of vascular disease: systematic review of 40 studies involving 58,000 participants. *J Am Coll Cardiol.* 2010;55(19):2160–2167.

101. Saleheen D, Haycock PC, Zhao W, et al. Apolipoprotein(a) isoform size, lipoprotein(a) concentration, and coronary artery disease: a mendelian randomisation analysis. *Lancet Diabetes Endocrinol.* 2017;5(7):524–533.

102. Thanassoulis G, Campbell CY, Owens DS, et al. Genetic associations with valvular calcification and aortic stenosis. *N Engl J Med.* 2013;368(6):503–512.

103. Kamstrup PR, Tybjaerg-Hansen A, Nordestgaard BG. Elevated lipoprotein(a) and risk of aortic valve stenosis in the general population. *J Am Coll Cardiol.* 2014;63(5):470–477.

104. Mathieu P, Arsenault BJ, Boulanger MC, Bosse Y, Koschinsky ML. Pathobiology of Lp(a) in calcific aortic valve disease. *Expert Rev Cardiovasc Ther.* 2017;15(10):797–807.

105. Tsimikas S. Potential causality and emerging medical therapies for lipoprotein(a) and its associated oxidized phospholipids in calcific aortic valve stenosis. *Circ Res.* 2019;124(3):405–415.

106. Capoulade R, Chan KL, Yeang C, et al. Oxidized phospholipids, lipoprotein(a), and progression of calcific aortic valve stenosis. *J Am Coll Cardiol.* 2015;66(11):1236–1246.

107. Capoulade R, Torzewski M, Mayr M, et al. ApoCIII-Lp(a) complexes in conjunction with Lp(a)-OxPL predict rapid progression of aortic stenosis. *Heart.* 2020;106(10):738–745.

108. Kamstrup PR, Nordestgaard BG. Elevated lipoprotein(a) levels, lpa risk genotypes, and increased risk of heart failure in the general population. *JACC Heart Fail.* 2016;4(1):78–87.

109. Steffen BT, Duprez D, Bertoni AG, Guan W, Tsai MY. Lp(a) [Lipoprotein(a)]-related risk of heart failure is evident in whites but not in other racial/ethnic groups. *Arterioscler Thromb Vasc Biol.* 2018;38(10):2498–2504.

110. Laschkolnig A, Kollerits B, Lamina C, et al. Lipoprotein (a) concentrations, apolipoprotein (a) phenotypes, and peripheral arterial disease in three independent cohorts. *Cardiovasc Res.* 2014;103(1):28–36.

111. Emdin CA, Khera AV, Natarajan P, et al. Phenotypic characterization of genetically lowered human lipoprotein(a) levels. *J Am Coll Cardiol.* 2016;68(25):2761–2772.

112. Klarin D, Lynch J, Aragam K, et al. Genome-wide association study of peripheral artery disease in the Million Veteran Program. *Nat Med.* 2019;25(8):1274–1279.

113. Boffa MB, Koschinsky ML. Lipoprotein (a): truly a direct prothrombotic factor in cardiovascular disease? *J Lipid Res.* 2016;57(5):745–757.

114. Nave AH, Lange KS, Leonards CO, et al. Lipoprotein (a) as a risk factor for ischemic stroke: a meta-analysis. *Atherosclerosis.* 2015;242(2):496–503.

115. Hong XW, Wu DM, Lu J, Zheng YL, Tu WJ, Yan J. Lipoprotein (a) as a predictor of early stroke recurrence in acute ischemic stroke. *Mol Neurobiol.* 2018;55(1):718–726.

116. Langsted A, Nordestgaard BG, Kamstrup PR. Elevated lipoprotein(a) and risk of ischemic stroke. *J Am Coll Cardiol.* 2019;74(1):54–66.

117. Arora P, Kalra R, Callas PW, et al. Lipoprotein(a) and risk of ischemic stroke in the REGARDS study. *Arterioscler Thromb Vasc Biol.* 2019;39(4):810–818.

118. Gurdasani D, Sjouke B, Tsimikas S, et al. Lipoprotein(a) and risk of coronary, cerebrovascular, and peripheral artery disease: the EPIC-Norfolk prospective population study. *Arterioscler Thromb Vasc Biol.* 2012;32(12):3058–3065.

119. Brandt EJ, Mani A, Spatz ES, Desai NR, Nasir K. Lipoprotein(a) levels and association with myocardial infarction and stroke in a nationally representative cross-sectional US cohort. *J Clin Lipidol.* 2020;14(5):695–706.

120. Alonso R, Andres E, Mata N, et al. Lipoprotein(a) levels in familial hypercholesterolemia: an important predictor of cardiovascular disease independent of the type of LDL receptor mutation. *J Am Coll Cardiol.* 2014;63(19):1982–1989.

121. Ellis KL, Pérez de Isla L, Alonso R, Fuentes F, Watts GF, Mata P. Value of measuring lipoprotein(a) during cascade testing for familial hypercholesterolemia. *J Am Coll Cardiol.* 2019;73(9):1029–1039.

122. Langsted A, Kamstrup PR, Benn M, Tybjaerg-Hansen A, Nordestgaard BG. High lipoprotein(a) as a possible cause of clinical familial hypercholesterolaemia: a prospective cohort study. *Lancet Diabetes Endocrinol.* 2016;4(7):577–587.

123. Chan DC, Pang J, Hooper AJ, Bell DA, Burnett JR, Watts GF. Effect of lipoprotein(a) on the diagnosis of familial hypercholesterolemia: does it make a difference in the clinic? *Clin Chem.* 2019;65(10):1258–1266.

124. Langsted A, Nordestgaard BG. Lipoprotein(a) should be measured in all individuals suspected of having familial hypercholesterolemia. *Clin Chem.* 2019;65(10):1190–1192.

125. Boffa MB, Stranges S, Klar N, Moriarty PM, Watts GF, Koschinsky ML. Lipoprotein(a) and secondary prevention of atherothrombotic events: A critical appraisal. *J Clin Lipidol.* 2018;12(6):1358–1366.

126. Khera AV, Everett BM, Caulfield MP, et al. Lipoprotein(a) concentrations, rosuvastatin therapy, and residual vascular risk: an analysis from the JUPITER Trial (Justification for the Use of Statins in Prevention: an Intervention Trial Evaluating Rosuvastatin). *Circulation.* 2014;129(6):635–642.

127. O'Donoghue ML, Fazio S, Giugliano RP, et al. Lipoprotein(a), PCSK9 inhibition, and cardiovascular risk. *Circulation.* 2019;139(12):1483–1492.

128. Bittner VA, Szarek M, Aylward PE, et al. Effect of Alirocumab on lipoprotein(a) and cardiovascular risk after acute coronary syndrome. *J Am Coll Cardiol.* 2020;75(2):133–144.

129. Schmidt K, Noureen A, Kronenberg F, Utermann G. Structure, function, and genetics of lipoprotein (a). *J Lipid Res.* 2016;57(8):1339–1359.

130. Mack S, Coassin S, Rueedi R, et al. A genome-wide association meta-analysis on lipoprotein (a) concentrations adjusted for apolipoprotein (a) isoforms. *J Lipid Res.* 2017;58(9):1834–1844.

131. Enkhmaa B, Anuurad E, Zhang W, Tran T, Berglund L. Lipoprotein(a): genotype-phenotype relationship and impact on atherogenic risk. *Metab Syndr Relat Disord.* 2011;9(6):411–418.

132. Wilson DP, Jacobson TA, Jones PH, et al. Use of Lipoprotein(a) in clinical practice: a biomarker whose time has come. A scientific statement from the National Lipid Association. *J Clin Lipidol.* 2019;13(3):374–392.

133. Scipione CA, McAiney JT, Simard DJ, et al. Characterization of the I4399M variant of apolipoprotein(a): implications for altered prothrombotic properties of lipoprotein(a). *J Thromb Haemost.* 2017;15(9):1834–1844.

134. Lanktree MB, Anand SS, Yusuf S, Hegele RA, Investigators S. Comprehensive analysis of genomic variation in the LPA locus and its relationship to plasma lipoprotein(a) in South Asians, Chinese, and European Caucasians. *Circ Cardiovasc Genet.* 2010;3(1):39–46.

135. Coassin S, Erhart G, Weissensteiner H, et al. A novel but frequent variant in LPA KIV-2 is associated with a pronounced Lp(a) and cardiovascular risk reduction. *Eur Heart J.* 2017;38(23):1823–1831.

136. Di Maio S, Gruneis R, Streiter G, et al. Investigation of a nonsense mutation located in the complex KIV-2 copy number variation region of apolipoprotein(a) in 10,910 individuals. *Genome Med.* 2020;12(1):74.

137. Coassin S, Schonherr S, Weissensteiner H, et al. A comprehensive map of single-base polymorphisms in the hypervariable LPA kringle IV type 2 copy number variation region. *J Lipid Res.* 2019;60(1):186–199.

138. Moriarty PM, Varvel SA, Gordts PL, McConnell JP, Tsimikas S. Lipoprotein(a) mass levels increase significantly according to apoe genotype: an analysis of 431 239 patients. *Arterioscler Thromb Vasc Biol.* 2017;37(3):580–588.

139. Muller N, Schulte DM, Turk K, et al. IL-6 blockade by monoclonal antibodies inhibits apolipoprotein (a) expression and lipoprotein (a) synthesis in humans. *J Lipid Res.* 2015;56(5):1034–1042.

140. Kettunen J, Demirkan A, Wurtz P, et al. Genome-wide study for circulating metabolites identifies 62 loci and reveals novel systemic effects of LPA. *Nat Commun.* 2016;7:11122.

141. Tsimikas S. In search of a physiological function of lipoprotein(a): causality of elevated Lp(a) levels and reduced incidence of type 2 diabetes. *J Lipid Res.* 2018;59(5):741–744.

142. Tolbus A, Mortensen MB, Nielsen SF, Kamstrup PR, Bojesen SE, Nordestgaard BG. kringle IV Type 2, Not low lipoprotein(a), as a cause of diabetes: a novel genetic approach using SNPs associated selectively with lipoprotein(a) concentrations or with kringle IV Type 2 repeats. *Clin Chem.* 2017;63(12):1866–1876.

143. Kamstrup PR, Tybjaerg-Hansen A, Nordestgaard BG. Genetic evidence that lipoprotein(a) associates with atherosclerotic stenosis rather than venous thrombosis. *Arterioscler Thromb Vasc Biol.* 2012;32(7):1732_1741.

144. Boffa MB, Marar TT, Yeang C, , et al. Potent reduction of plasma lipoprotein (a) with an antisense oligonucleotide in human subjects does not affect ex vivo fibrinolysis. *J Lipid Res.* 2019;60(12):2082–2089.

145. Leibundgut G, Scipione C, Yin H, et al. Determinants of binding of oxidized phospholipids on apolipoprotein (a) and lipoprotein (a). *J Lipid Res.* 2013;54(10):2815–2830.

146. van Dijk RA, Kolodgie F, Ravandi A, et al. Differential expression of oxidation-specific epitopes and apolipoprotein(a) in progressing and ruptured human coronary and carotid atherosclerotic lesions. *J Lipid Res.* 2012;53(12):2773–2790.

147. Scipione CA, Sayegh SE, Romagnuolo R, et al. Mechanistic insights into Lp(a)-induced IL-8 expression: a role for oxidized phospholipid modification of apo(a). *J Lipid Res.* 2015;56(12):2273–2285.

148. van der Valk FM, Bekkering S, Kroon J, et al. Oxidized phospholipids on lipoprotein(a) elicit arterial wall inflammation and an inflammatory monocyte response in humans. *Circulation.* 2016;134(8):611–624.

149. Bouchareb R, Mahmut A, Nsaibia MJ, et al. Autotaxin derived from lipoprotein(a) and valve interstitial cells promotes inflammation and mineralization of the aortic valve. *Circulation.* 2015;132(8):677–690.

150. Zheng KH, Tsimikas S, Pawade T, et al. Lipoprotein(a) and oxidized phospholipids promote valve calcification in patients with aortic stenosis. *J Am Coll Cardiol.* 2019;73(17):2150–2162.

151. Schnitzler JG, Hoogeveen RM, Ali L, et al. Atherogenic lipoprotein(a) increases vascular glycolysis, thereby facilitating inflammation and leukocyte extravasation. *Circ Res.* 2020;126(10):1346–1359.

152. Cho T, Romagnuolo R, Scipione C, Boffa MB, Koschinsky ML. Apolipoprotein(a) stimulates nuclear translocation of β-catenin: a novel pathogenic mechanism for lipoprotein(a). *Mol Biol Cell.* 2013;24(3):210–221.

153. Willeit P, Kiechl S, Kronenberg F, et al. Discrimination and net reclassification of cardiovascular risk with lipoprotein(a): prospective 15-year outcomes in the Bruneck Study. *J Am Coll Cardiol.* 2014;64(9):851–860.

154. Tsimikas S, Gordts P, Nora C, Yeang C, Witztum JL. Statin therapy increases lipoprotein(a) levels. *Eur Heart J.* 2020;41(24):2275–2284.

155. Waldmann E, Parhofer KG. Lipoprotein apheresis to treat elevated lipoprotein(a). *J Lipid Res.* 2016;57(10):1751–1757.

156. Roeseler E, Julius U, Heigl F, et al. Lipoprotein apheresis for lipoprotein(a)-associated cardiovascular disease: prospective 5 years of follow-up and apo(a) characterization. *Arterioscler Thromb Vasc Biol.* 2016;36(9):2019–2027.

157. Cegla J, Neely RDG, France M, et al. HEART UK consensus statement on Lipoprotein(a): a call to action. *Atherosclerosis.* 2019;291:62–70.

158. Borrelli MJ, Youssef A, Boffa MB, Koschinsky ML. New frontiers in Lp(a)-targeted therapies. *Trends Pharmacol Sci.* 2019;40(3):212–225.

159. Parish, S. et al. HPS2-THRIVE Collaborative Group. Impact of apolipoprotein(a) isoform size on lipoprotein(a) lowering in the HPS2-THRIVE study. *Circ Genom Precis Med.* 2018;11(2):e001696.

160. Viney NJ, van Capelleveen JC, Geary RS, et al. Antisense oligonucleotides targeting apolipoprotein(a) in people with raised lipoprotein(a): two randomised, double-blind, placebo-controlled, dose-ranging trials. *Lancet.* 2016;388(10057):2239–2253.

161. Tsimikas S, Karwatowska-Prokopczuk E, Gouni-Berthold I, et al. Lipoprotein(a) reduction in persons with cardiovascular disease. *N Engl J Med.* 2020;382(3):244–255.

162. Catapano AL, Graham I, De Backer G, et al. 2016 ESC/EAS guidelines for the management of dyslipidaemias. *Eur Heart J.* 2016;37(39):2999–3058.

163. Grundy SM, Stone NJ, Bailey AL, et al. 2018 AHA/ACC/AACVPR/AAPA/ABC/ACPM/ADA/AGS/APhA/ASPC/NLA/PCNA guideline on the management of blood cholesterol: a report of the American College of Cardiology/American Heart Association Task Force on clinical practice guidelines. *Circulation.* 2019;139(25):e1082–e143.

164. Anderson TJ, Gregoire J, Pearson GJ, et al. 2016 Canadian Cardiovascular Society guidelines for the management of dyslipidemia for the prevention of cardiovascular disease in the adult. *Can J Cardiol.* 2016;32(11):1263–1282.

165. Mach F, Baigent C, Catapano AL, et al. 2019 ESC/EAS Guidelines for the management of dyslipidaemias: lipid modification to reduce cardiovascular risk. *Eur Heart J.* 2020;41(1):111–188.

166. Tsimikas S. A *test in context: lipoprotein(a): diagnosis, prognosis, controversies, and emerging therapies. J Am Coll Cardiol.* 2017;69(6):692–711.

167. Marcovina SM, Albers JJ. Lipoprotein (a) measurements for clinical application. *J Lipid Res.* 2016;57(4):526–537.

168. Perrot N, Verbeek R, Sandhu M, et al. Ideal cardiovascular health influences cardiovascular disease risk associated with high lipoprotein(a) levels and genotype: The EPIC-Norfolk prospective population study. *Atherosclerosis.* 2017;256:47–52.

169. Balling M, Afzal S, Varbo A, et al. VLDL cholesterol accounts for one-half the risk of myocardial infarction associated with apoB-containing lipoproteins. *J Am Coll Cardiol.* 2020; 76:2725–2735.

170. Jepsen AM, Langsted A, Varbo A, et al. Increased remnant cholesterol explains part of residual risk of all-cause mortality in 5414 patients with ischemic heart disease. *Clin Chem.* 2016;62(4):593–604.

171. Klempfner R, Erez A, Sagit BZ, et al. Elevated triglyceride level is independently associated with increased all-cause mortality in patients with established coronary heart disease: twenty-two-year follow-up of the bezafibrate infarction prevention study and registry. *Circ Cardiovasc Qual Outcomes.* 2016;9(2):100–108.

172. Lawler PR, Akinkuolie AO, Harada P, et al. Residual risk of atherosclerotic cardiovascular events in relation to reductions in very-low-density lipoproteins. *J Am Heart Assoc.* 2017;6(12).

173. Vallejo-Vaz AJ, Fayyad R, Boekholdt SM, et al. Triglyceride-*Rich Lipoprotein Cholesterol and Risk of Cardiovascular Events Among Patients Receiving Statin Therapy in the* TNT trial. *Circulation.* 2018;138(8):770–781.

174. Baigent C, Blackwell L, Emberson J, et al. Efficacy and safety of more intensive lowering of LDL cholesterol: a meta-analysis of data from 170,000 participants in 26 randomised trials. *Lancet.* 2010;376(9753):1670–1681.

175. Karlson BW, Palmer MK, Nicholls SJ, Lundman P, Barter PJ. A VOYAGER meta-analysis of the impact of statin therapy on low-density lipoprotein cholesterol and triglyceride levels in patients with hypertriglyceridemia. *Am J Cardiol.* 2016;117(9):1444–1448.

176. The Emerging Risk Factors Collaboration. Major lipids, apolipoproteins, and risk of vascular disease. *JAMA.* 2009;302(18):1993–2000.

177. Varbo A, Benn M, Tybjaerg-Hansen A, Jorgensen AB, Frikke-Schmidt R, Nordestgaard BG. Remnant cholesterol as a causal risk factor for ischemic heart disease. *J Am Coll Cardiol.* 2013;61(4):427–436.

178. Do R, Willer CJ, Schmidt EM, Sengupta S, et al. Common variants associated with plasma triglycerides and risk for coronary artery disease. *Nat Genet.* 2013;45(11):1345–1352.

179. Helgadottir A, Gretarsdottir S, Thorleifsson G, et al. Variants with large effects on blood lipids and the role of cholesterol and triglycerides in coronary disease. *Nat Genet.* 2016;48(6):634–639.

180. Barter PJ, Caulfield M, Eriksson M, et al. Effects of torcetrapib in patients at high risk for coronary events. *N Engl J Med.* 2007;357(21):2109–2122.

181. Lincoff AM, Nicholls SJ, Riesmeyer JS, et al. Evacetrapib and cardiovascular outcomes in high-risk vascular disease. *N Engl J Med.* 2017;376(20):1933–1942.

182. Bowman L, Hopewell JC, Chen F, , et al. Effects of anacetrapib in patients with atherosclerotic vascular disease. *N Engl J Med.* 2017;377(13):1217–1227.

183. Langsted A, Jensen AMR, Varbo A, Nordestgaard BG. Low high-density lipoprotein cholesterol to monitor long-term average increased triglycerides. *J Clin Endocrinol Metab.* 2020;105(4).

184. Nordestgaard BG, Benn M, Schnohr P, Tybjaerg-Hansen A. Nonfasting triglycerides and risk of myocardial infarction, ischemic heart disease, and death in men and women. *JAMA.* 2007;298(3):299–308.

185. Bansal S, Buring JE, Rifai N, Mora S, Sacks FM, Ridker PM. Fasting compared with nonfasting triglycerides and risk of cardiovascular events in women. *JAMA.* 2007;298(3):309–16.

186. Nordestgaard BG, Abildgaard S, Wittrup HH, Steffensen R, Jensen G, Tybjaerg-Hansen A. Heterozygous lipoprotein lipase deficiency: frequency in the general population, effect on plasma lipid levels, and risk of ischemic heart disease. *Circulation.* 1997;96(6):1737–1744.

187. Wittrup HH, Tybjaerg-Hansen A, Nordestgaard BG. Lipoprotein lipase mutations, plasma lipids and lipoproteins, and risk of ischemic heart disease. A meta-analysis. *Circulation.* 1999;99(22):2901–2907.

188. Sarwar N, Sandhu MS, Ricketts SL, et al. Triglyceride-mediated pathways and coronary disease: collaborative analysis of 101 studies. *Lancet.* 2010;375(9726):1634–1639.

189. Varbo A, Benn M, Tybjaerg-Hansen A, Nordestgaard BG. Elevated remnant cholesterol causes both low-grade inflammation and ischemic heart disease, whereas elevated low-density lipoprotein cholesterol causes ischemic heart disease without inflammation. *Circulation.* 2013;128(12):1298–1309.

190. Jorgensen AB, Frikke-Schmidt R, West AS, Grande P, Nordestgaard BG, Tybjaerg-Hansen A. Genetically elevated non-fasting triglycerides and calculated remnant cholesterol as causal risk factors for myocardial infarction. *Eur Heart J.* 2013;34(24):1826–1833.

191. Thomsen M, Varbo A, Tybjaerg-Hansen A, Nordestgaard BG. Low nonfasting triglycerides and reduced all-cause mortality: a mendelian randomization study. *Clin Chem.* 2014;60(5):737–746.

192. Varbo A, Benn M, Smith GD, Timpson NJ, Tybjaerg-Hansen A, Nordestgaard BG. Remnant cholesterol, low-density lipoprotein cholesterol, and blood pressure as mediators from obesity to ischemic heart disease. *Circ Res.* 2015;116(4):665–673.

193. Jorgensen AB, Frikke-Schmidt R, Nordestgaard BG, Tybjaerg-Hansen A. Loss-of-function mutations in APOC3 and risk of ischemic vascular disease. *N Engl J Med.* 2014;371(1):32–41.

194. Crosby J, Peloso GM, Auer PL, et al. Loss-of-function mutations in APOC3, triglycerides, and coronary disease. *N Engl J Med.* 2014;371(1):22–31.

195. Dewey FE, Gusarova V, O'Dushlaine C, et al. Inactivating Variants in ANGPTL4 and Risk of Coronary Artery Disease. *N Engl J Med.* 2016;374(12):1123–1133.

196. Stitziel NO, Stirrups KE, Masca NG, et al. Coding variation in ANGPTL4, LPL, and SVEP1 and the risk of coronary disease. *N Engl J Med.* 2016;374(12):1134–1144.

197. Stitziel NO, Khera AV, Wang X, et al. ANGPTL3 deficiency and protection against coronary artery disease. *J Am Coll Cardiol.* 2017;69(16):2054–2063.

198. Dewey FE, Gusarova V, Dunbar RL, et al. Genetic and pharmacologic inactivation of ANGPTL3 and cardiovascular disease. *N Engl J Med.* 2017;377(3):211–221.

199. Khera AV, Won HH, Peloso GM, et al. Association of rare and common variation in the lipoprotein lipase gene with coronary artery disease. *JAMA.* 2017;317(9):937–946.

200. Ference BA, Kastelein JJP, Ray KK, Ginsberg HN, et al. Association of triglyceride-lowering lpl variants and ldl-c-lowering LDLR variants with risk of coronary heart disease. *JAMA.* 2019;321(4):364–373.

201. Bhatt DL, Steg PG, Miller M, et al. Cardiovascular risk reduction with icosapent ethyl for hypertriglyceridemia. *N Engl J Med.* 2019;380(1):11–22.

202. Nicholls SJ, Lincoff AM, Bash D, et al. Assessment of omega-3 carboxylic acids in statin-treated patients with high levels of triglycerides and low levels of high-density lipoprotein cholesterol: rationale and design of the STRENGTH trial. *Clin Cardiol.* 2018;41(10):1281–1288.

203. Pradhan AD, Paynter NP, Everett BM, et al. Rationale and design of the Pemafibrate to Reduce Cardiovascular Outcomes by Reducing Triglycerides in Patients with Diabetes (PROMINENT) study. *Am Heart J.* 2018;206:80–93.

204. Nordestgaard BG. A test in context: lipid profile, fasting versus nonfasting. *J Am Coll Cardiol.* 2017;70(13):1637–1646.

205. Balling M, Langsted A, Afzal S, Varbo A, Davey Smith G, Nordestgaard BG. A third of nonfasting plasma cholesterol is in remnant lipoproteins: lipoprotein subclass profiling in 9293 individuals. *Atherosclerosis.* 2019;286:97–104.

206. Nordestgaard BG, Langsted A, Mora S, et al. Fasting is not routinely required for determination of a lipid profile: clinical and laboratory implications including flagging at desirable concentration cut-points-a joint consensus statement from the European Atherosclerosis Society and European Federation of Clinical Chemistry and Laboratory Medicine. *Eur Heart J.* 2016;37(25):1944–1958.

207. Rosenson RS, Davidson MH, Hirsh BJ, Kathiresan S, Gaudet D. Genetics and causality of triglyceride-rich lipoproteins in atherosclerotic cardiovascular disease. *J Am Coll Cardiol.* 2014;64(23):2525–2540.

208. Langlois MR, Chapman MJ, Cobbaert C, et al. Quantifying Atherogenic lipoproteins: current and future challenges in the era of personalized medicine and very low concentrations of LDL cholesterol. A consensus statement from EAS and EFLM. *Clin Chem.* 2018;64(7):1006–1033.

209. Varbo A, Langsted A, Nordestgaard BG. Commentary: Nonfasting remnant cholesterol simplifies triglyceride-rich lipoproteins for clinical use, and metabolomic phenotyping ignites scientific curiosity. *Int J Epidemiol.* 2016;45(5):1379–1385.

210. Salinas CAA, Chapman MJ. Remnant lipoproteins: are they equal to or more atherogenic than LDL? *Curr Opin Lipidol.* 2020;31(3):132–139.

211. Nordestgaard BG, Varbo A. Triglycerides and cardiovascular disease. *Lancet.* 2014;384(9943):626–635.

212. Nordestgaard BG. Triglyceride-rich lipoproteins and atherosclerotic cardiovascular disease: new insights from epidemiology, genetics, and biology. *Circ Res.* 2016;118(4):547–563.

213. Varbo A, Nordestgaard BG. Remnant cholesterol and risk of ischemic stroke in 112,512 individuals from the general population. *Ann Neurol.* 2019;85(4):550–559.

214. Kaltoft M, Langsted A, Nordestgaard BG. Triglycerides and remnant cholesterol associated with risk of aortic valve stenosis: Mendelian randomization in the Copenhagen General Population Study. *Eur Heart J.* 2020; 21;41(24):2288–2299.

215. Parhofer KG, Chapman MJ, Nordestgaard BG. Efficacy and safety of icosapent ethyl in hypertriglyceridaemia: a recap. *Eur Heart J Suppl.* 2020;22(Suppl J):J21–j33.

216. Pedersen SB, Langsted A, Nordestgaard BG. Nonfasting mild-to-moderate hypertriglyceridemia and risk of acute pancreatitis. *JAMA Intern Med.* 2016;176(12):1834–42.

217. Hansen SEJ, Madsen CM, Varbo A, Nordestgaard BG. Low-grade inflammation in the association between mild-to-moderate hypertriglyceridemia and risk of acute pancreatitis: a study of more than 115000 individuals from the general population. *Clin Chem.* 2019;65(2):321–332.

218. Nordestgaard BG, Langsted A, Mora S, et al. Fasting Is Not routinely required for determination of a lipid profile: clinical and laboratory implications including flagging at desirable concentration cutpoints-a joint consensus statement from the European Atherosclerosis Society and European Federation of Clinical Chemistry and Laboratory Medicine. *Clin Chem.* 2016;62(7):930–946.

219. Langlois MR, Nordestgaard BG, Langsted A, et al. Quantifying atherogenic lipoproteins for lipid-lowering strategies: consensus-based recommendations from EAS and EFLM. *Clin Chem Lab Med.* 2020;58(4):496–517.

220. Varbo A, Freiberg JJ, Nordestgaard BG. Remnant cholesterol and myocardial infarction in normal weight, overweight, and obese individuals from the Copenhagen General Population Study. *Clin Chem.* 2018;64(1):219–230.

221. Duran EK, Aday AW, Cook NR, Buring JE, Ridker PM, Pradhan AD. Triglyceride-rich lipoprotein cholesterol, small dense ldl cholesterol, and incident cardiovascular disease. *J Am Coll Cardiol.* 2020;75(17):2122–2135.

222. Wurtz P, Wang Q, Soininen P, et al. Metabolomic profiling of statin use and genetic inhibition of HMG-CoA reductase. *J Am Coll Cardiol.* 2016;67(10):1200–1210.

223. Grundy SM, Stone NJ, Bailey AL, et al. 2018 AHA/ACC/AACVPR/AAPA/ABC/ACPM/ADA/AGS/APhA/ASPC/NLA/PCNA guideline on the management of blood cholesterol: a report of the American College of Cardiology/American Heart Association Task Force on Clinical Practice Guidelines. *Circulation.* 2019;139(25):e1082–e143.

224. Mach F, Baigent C, Catapano AL, et al. 2019 ESC/EAS guidelines for the management of dyslipidaemias: lipid modification to reduce cardiovascular risk. *Eur Heart J.* 2020;41(1):111–188.

225. Anderson TJ, Gregoire J, Pearson GJ, et al. 2016 Canadian Cardiovascular Society guidelines for the management of dyslipidemia for the prevention of cardiovascular disease in the adult. *Can J Cardiol.* 2016;32(11):1263–1282.

226. Fan W, Philip S, Granowitz C, Toth PP, Wong ND. Hypertriglyceridemia in statin-treated US adults: the National Health and Nutrition Examination Survey. *J Clin Lipidol.* 2019;13(1):100–108.

227. Flowers E, Lin F, Kandula NR, et al. Body composition and diabetes risk in south asians: findings from the MASALA and MESA studies. *Diabetes Care.* 2019;42(5):946–953.

228. Hegele RA, Ginsberg HN, Chapman MJ, et al. The polygenic nature of hypertriglyceridaemia: implications for definition, diagnosis, and management. *Lancet Diabetes Endocrinol.* 2014;2(8):655–666.

229. Nordestgaard BG. A test in context: lipid profile, fasting versus nonfasting. *J Am Coll Cardiol.* 2017;70(13):1637–1646.

230. Mora S. Nonfasting for routine lipid testing: from evidence to action. *JAMA Intern Med.* 2016;176(7):1005–1006.

231. Benn M, Nordestgaard BG. From genome-wide association studies to Mendelian randomization: novel opportunities for understanding cardiovascular disease causality, pathogenesis, prevention, and treatment. *Cardiovasc Res.* 2018;114(9):1192—1208.

232. Pedersen SB, Varbo A, Langsted A, Nordestgaard BG. Chylomicronemia risk factors ranked by importance for the individual and community in 108 711 women and men. J *Intern Med.* 2018;283(4):392–404.

233. Hansen SEJ, Madsen CM, Varbo A, Tybjærg-Hansen A, Nordestgaard BG. Genetic variants associated with increased plasma levels of triglycerides, via effects on the lipoprotein lipase pathway, increase risk of acute pancreatitis. *Clin Gastroenterol Hepatol.* 2020;S1542–3565(20)31125–31123.

234. Nordestgaard BG, Stender S, Kjeldsen K. Reduced atherogenesis in cholesterol-fed diabetic rabbits. Giant lipoproteins do not enter the arterial wall. *Arteriosclerosis.* 1988;8(4):421–428.

235. Gaudet D, Alexander VJ, Baker BF, et al. Antisense inhibition of apolipoprotein C-III in patients with hypertriglyceridemia. *N Engl J Med.* 2015;373(5):438–447.

236. Witztum JL, Gaudet D, Freedman SD, et al. Volanesorsen and triglyceride levels in familial chylomicronemia syndrome. *N Engl J Med.* 2019;381(6):531–542.

237. Nordestgaard BG, Nicholls SJ, Langsted A, Ray KK, Tybjaerg-Hansen A. Advances in lipid-lowering therapy through gene-silencing technologies. *Nat Rev Cardiol.* 2018;15(5):261–272.

238. Mahley RW, Rall SC. Type III hyperlipoproteinemia (dysbetalipoproteinemia): the role of apolipoprotein E in normal and abnormal lipoprotein metabolism. In: Scriver CR, Beaudet AL, Sly WS, Valle D, eds. *The Metabolic & Molecular Bases of Inherited Disease.* 8th ed. McGraw-Hill; 2001: 2835–2862.

239. Guidance N. Cardiovascular disease: risk assessment and reduction, including lipid modification. 2016. https://www nice org uk/guidance/cg181. (accessed June 17, 2017).

240. Ference BA, Ginsberg HN, Graham I, et al. Low-density lipoproteins cause atherosclerotic cardiovascular disease. 1. Evidence from genetic, epidemiologic, and clinical studies. A consensus statement from the European Atherosclerosis Society Consensus Panel. *Eur Heart J.* 2017;38(32):2459–2472.

241. Borén J, Chapman MJ, Krauss RM, et al. Low-density lipoproteins cause atherosclerotic cardiovascular disease: pathophysiological, genetic, and therapeutic insights: a consensus statement from the European Atherosclerosis Society Consensus Panel. *Eur Heart J.* 2020;41(24):2313–2330.

242. Nordestgaard BG, Chapman MJ, Ray K, et al. Lipoprotein(a) as a cardiovascular risk factor: current status. *Eur Heart J.* 2010;31(23):2844–2853.

243. Nordestgaard BG, Langsted A. Lipoprotein (a) as a cause of cardiovascular disease: insights from epidemiology, genetics, and biology. *J Lipid Res.* 2016;57(11):195–175.

244. Collins R, Reith C, Emberson J, et al. Interpretation of the evidence for the efficacy and safety of statin therapy. *Lancet.* 2016;388(10059):2532–2561.

245. Laufs U, Parhofer KG, Ginsberg HN, Hegele RA. Clinical review on triglycerides. *Eur Heart J.* 2020;41(1):99–109c.

246. Katsiki N, Nikolic D, Montalto G, Banach M, Mikhailidis DP, Rizzo M. The role of fibrate treatment in dyslipidemia: an overview. *Curr Pharm Des.* 2013;19(17):3124–3131.

247. Jun M, Foote C, Lv J, et al. Effects of fibrates on cardiovascular outcomes: a systematic review and meta-analysis. *Lancet.* 2010;375(9729):1875–1884.

248. Araki E, Yamashita S, Arai H, et al. Effects of pemafibrate, a novel selective PPARalpha modulator, on lipid and glucose metabolism in patients with type 2 diabetes and hypertriglyceridemia: a randomized, double-blind, placebo-controlled, phase 3 trial. *Diabetes Care.* 2018;41(3):538–546.

249. Aung T, Halsey J, Kromhout D, et al. Associations of omega-3 fatty acid supplement use with cardiovascular disease risks: meta-analysis of 10 trials involving 77917 individuals. *JAMA Cardiol.* 2018;3(3):225–234.

250. Manson JE, Cook NR, Lee IM, et al. Vitamin D supplements and prevention of cancer and cardiovascular disease. *N Engl J Med.* 2019;380(1):33–44.

251. Nicholls, S. J. et al. Effect of high-dose omega-3 fatty acids vs corn oil on major adverse cardiovascular events in patients at high cardiovascular risk: the STRENGTH randomized clinical trial. *JAMA.* 2020;324(22): 2268–2280. doi: 10.1001/jama.2020.22258.

252. Turco JV, Inal-Veith A, Fuster V. Cardiovascular health promotion: an issue that can no longer wait. *J Am Coll Cardiol.* 2018;72(8):908–913.

253. Barter PJ. Hugh sinclair lecture: the regulation and remodelling of HDL by plasma factors. *Atheroscler Suppl.* 2002;3:39–47.

254. Rosenson RS, Brewer HB, Jr., Chapman MJ, et al. HDL measures, particle heterogeneity, proposed nomenclature, and relation to atherosclerotic cardiovascular events. *Clim Chem.* 2011;57:392–410.

255. Rosenson RS, Brewer HB, Jr., Davidson WS, et al. Cholesterol efflux and atheroprotection: advancing the concept of reverse cholesterol transport. *Circulation* 2012;125:1905–1919.

256. Rosenson RS. The high-density lipoprotein puzzle: why classic epidemiology, genetic epidemiology, and clinical trials conflict? *Arterioscler Thromb Vasc Biol.* 2016;36:777–782.

257. Voight BF, Peloso GM, Orho-Melander M, et al. Plasma HDL cholesterol and risk of myocardial infarction: a mendelian randomisation study. *Lancet* 2012;380:572–580.

258. Freedman DS, Otvos JD, Jeyarajah EJ, et al. Sex and age differences in lipoprotein subclasses measured by nuclear magnetic resonance spectroscopy: the Framingham Study. *Clin Chem.* 2004;50:1189–200.

259. Asztalos BF, Collins D, Horvath KV, Bloomfield HE, Robins SJ, Schaefer EJ. Relation of gemfibrozil treatment and high-density lipoprotein subpopulation profile with cardiovascular events in the Veterans Affairs High-Density Lipoprotein Intervention Trial. *Metabolism* 2008;57:77–83.

260. Duparc T, Ruidavets JB, Genoux A, et al. Serum level of HDL particles are independently associated with long-term prognosis in patients with coronary artery disease: The GENES study. *Sci Rep.* 2020;10:8138.

261. Austin MA, King MC, Vranizan KM, Krauss RM. Atherogenic lipoprotein phenotype. A proposed genetic marker for coronary heart disease risk. *Circulation* 1990;82:495–506.

262. Otvos JD, Jeyarajah EJ, Cromwell WC. Measurement issues related to lipoprotein heterogeneity. *Am J Cardiol.* 2002;90:22i-9i.

263. Gotto AM, Jr., Whitney E, Stein EA, et al. Relation between baseline and on-treatment lipid parameters and first acute major coronary events in the Air Force/Texas Coronary Atherosclerosis Prevention Study (AFCAPS/TexCAPS). *Circulation* 2000;101:477–484.

264. Richardson TG, Sanderson E, Palmer TM, et al. Evaluating the relationship between circulating lipoprotein lipids and apolipoproteins with risk of coronary heart disease: a multivariable Mendelian randomisation analysis. *PLoS Med.* 2020;17:e1003062.

265. Mackey RH, Greenland P, Goff DC, Jr., Lloyd-Jones D, Sibley CT, Mora S. High-density lipoprotein cholesterol and particle concentrations, carotid atherosclerosis, and coronary events: MESA (multi-ethnic study of atherosclerosis). *J Am Coll Cardiol.* 2012;60:508–516.

266. Otvos JD, Collins D, Freedman DS, et al. Low-density lipoprotein and high-density lipoprotein particle subclasses predict coronary events and are favorably changed by gemfibrozil therapy in the Veterans Affairs High-Density Lipoprotein Intervention Trial. *Circulation* 2006;113:1556–1563.

267. McGarrah RW, Craig DM, Haynes C, Dowdy ZE, Shah SH, Kraus WE. High-density lipoprotein subclass measurements improve mortality risk prediction, discrimination and reclassification in a cardiac catheterization cohort. *Atherosclerosis* 2016;246:229–235.

268. Mora S, Glynn RJ, Ridker PM. High-density lipoprotein cholesterol, size, particle number, and residual vascular risk after potent statin therapy. *Circulation* 2013;128:1189–1197.

269. Khera AV, Demler OV, Adelman SJ, et al. Cholesterol efflux capacity, high-density lipoprotein particle number, and incident cardiovascular

events: an analysis from the JUPITER Trial (Justification for the Use of Statins in Prevention: An Intervention Trial Evaluating Rosuvastatin). *Circulation* 2017;135:2494–2504.

270. Riggs KA, Joshi PH, Khera A, et al. Impaired HDL metabolism links GlycA, a novel inflammatory marker, with incident cardiovascular events. *J Clin Med.* 2019;8.

271. Mora S, Otvos JD, Rifai N, Rosenson RS, Buring JE, Ridker PM. Lipoprotein particle profiles by nuclear magnetic resonance compared with standard lipids and apolipoproteins in predicting incident cardiovascular disease in women. *Circulation* 2009;119:931–939.

272. Parish S, Offer A, Clarke R, et al. Lipids and lipoproteins and risk of different vascular events in the MRC/BHF Heart Protection Study. *Circulation* 2012;125:2469–2478.

273. Chandra A, Neeland IJ, Das SR, et al. Relation of black race between high density lipoprotein cholesterol content, high density lipoprotein particles and coronary events (from the Dallas Heart Study). Am J Cardiol. 2015;115:890–894.

274. Otvos JD, Guyton JR, Connelly MA, et al. Relations of GlycA and lipoprotein particle subspecies with cardiovascular events and mortality: a post hoc analysis of the AIM-HIGH trial. *J Clin Lipid.* 2018;12:348–355 e2.

275. Singh K, Chandra A, Sperry T, et al. Associations Between high-density lipoprotein particles and ischemic events by vascular domain, sex, and ethnicity: a pooled cohort analysis. *Circulation* 2020;142:657–669.

276. Wilson PW, D'Agostino RB, Levy D, Belanger AM, Silbershatz H, Kannel WB. Prediction of coronary heart disease using risk factor categories. *Circulation* 1998;97:1837–1847.

277. Reaven GM, Chen YD, Jeppesen J, Maheux P, Krauss RM. Insulin resistance and hyperinsulinemia in individuals with small, dense low density lipoprotein particles. *J Clin Invest.* 1993;92:141–146.

278. Lamarche B, Tchernof A, Mauriege P, et al. Fasting insulin and apolipoprotein B levels and low-density lipoprotein particle size as risk factors for ischemic heart disease. *JAMA.* 1998;279:1955–1961.

279. Garvey WT, Kwon S, Zheng D, et al. Effects of insulin resistance and type 2 diabetes on lipoprotein subclass particle size and concentration determined by nuclear magnetic resonance. *Diabetes* 2003;52:453–462.

280. Geller AS, Polisecki EY, Diffenderfer MR, et al. Genetic and secondary causes of severe HDL deficiency and cardiovascular disease. *J Lipid Res.* 2018;59:2421–2435.

281. Saleheen D SR, Javad S, Zhao W, et al. HDL cholesterol efflux capacity is inversely associated with incident CHD events independent of HDL-C and APO-I concentrations. Abstract Oral Session: Novel Biomarkers and Cardiovascular Disease Risk Prediction-American Heart Association; 2014.

282. Rosenson RS, Brewer HB, Jr., Ansell BJ, et al. Dysfunctional HDL and atherosclerotic cardiovascular disease. *Nature Rev Cardiol.* 2016;13:48–60.

283. Rosenson RS, Brewer HB, Jr., Ansell B, et al. Translation of high-density lipoprotein function into clinical practice: current prospects and future challenges. *Circulation* 2013;128:1256–1267.

284. Rohatgi A, Khera A, Berry JD, et al. HDL cholesterol efflux capacity and incident cardiovascular events. *New Engl J Med.* 2014;371:2383–2393.

285. Cukier AMO, Therond P, Didichenko SA, et al. Structure-function relationships in reconstituted HDL: Focus on antioxidative activity and cholesterol efflux capacity. *Biochim Biophys Acta Mol Cell Biol Lipids* 2017;1862:890–900.

286. Guerin M, Silvain J, Gall J, et al. Association of serum cholesterol efflux capacity with mortality in patients with ST-segment elevation myocardial infarction. *J Am Coll Cardiol.* 2018;72:3259–3269.

287. Cahill LE, Sacks FM, Rimm EB, Jensen MK. Cholesterol efflux capacity, HDL cholesterol, and risk of coronary heart disease: a nested case-control study in men. *J Lipid Res.* 2019;60:1457–1464.

288. Distelmaier K, Schrutka L, Seidl V, et al. Pro-oxidant HDL predicts poor outcome in patients with ST-elevation acute coronary syndrome. *Thromb Haemostas.* 2015;114:133–138.

289. Riwanto M, Rohrer L, Roschitzki B, et al. Altered activation of endothelial anti- and proapoptotic pathways by high-density lipoprotein

from patients with coronary artery disease: role of high-density lipoprotein-proteome remodeling. *Circulation* 2013;127:891–904.

290. Cuchel M, Raper AC, Conlon DM, et al. A novel approach to measuring macrophage-specific reverse cholesterol transport in vivo in humans. *J Lipid Res.* 2017;58:752–262.

291. Furtado JD, Yamamoto R, Melchior JT, et al. Distinct Proteomic Signatures in 16 HDL (High-Density Lipoprotein) Subspecies. *Arterioscler Thromb Vasc Biol.* 2018;38:2827–2842.

292. Vaisar T, Pennathur S, Green PS, et al. Shotgun proteomics implicates protease inhibition and complement activation in the antiinflammatory properties of HDL. *J Clin Invest.* 2007;117:746–756.

293. Rosenson RS, Brewer HB, Rader DJ. Lipoproteins as biomarkers and therapeutic targets in the setting of acute coronary syndrome. *Circulation Res.* 2014;114:1880–1889.

294. Cabana VG, Lukens JR, Rice KS, Hawkins TJ, Getz GS. HDL content and composition in acute phase response in three species: triglyceride enrichment of HDL a factor in its decrease. *J Lipid Res.* 1996;37:2662–2674.

295. Chami B, Barrie N, Cai X, et al. Serum amyloid A receptor blockade and incorporation into high-density lipoprotein modulates its pro-inflammatory and pro-thrombotic activities on vascular endothelial cells. *Int J Mol Sci.* 2015;16:11101–11124.

296. Sposito AC, de Lima-Junior JC, Moura FA, et al. Reciprocal multifaceted interaction between hdl (high-density lipoprotein) and myocardial infarction. *Arterioscler Thromb Vasc Biol.* 2019;39:1550–1564.

297. Sankaranarayanan S, de la Llera-Moya M, Drazul-Schrader D, Asztalos BF, Weibel GL, Rothblat GH. Importance of macrophage cholesterol content on the flux of cholesterol mass. *J Lipid Res.* 2010;51:3243–3249.

298. Zheng L, Nukuna B, Brennan ML, et al. Apolipoprotein A-I is a selective target for myeloperoxidase-catalyzed oxidation and functional impairment in subjects with cardiovascular disease. *J Clin Invest.* 2004;114:529–541.

299. Bergt C, Pennathur S, Fu X, et al. The myeloperoxidase product hypochlorous acid oxidizes HDL in the human artery wall and impairs ABCA1-dependent cholesterol transport. Proc. National Academy of Sciences 2004;101:13032–13037.

300. Baldus S, Eiserich JP, Brennan ML, Jackson RM, Alexander CB, Freeman BA. Spatial mapping of pulmonary and vascular nitrotyrosine reveals the pivotal role of myeloperoxidase as a catalyst for tyrosine nitration in inflammatory diseases. *Free Radic Biol Med.* 2002;33:1010.

301. Huang Y, DiDonato JA, Levison BS, et al. An abundant dysfunctional apolipoprotein A1 in human atheroma. *Nature Med.* 2014;20:193–203.

302. Shao B, Cavigiolio G, Brot N, Oda MN, Heinecke JW. Methionine oxidation impairs reverse cholesterol transport by apolipoprotein A-I. Proc. National Academy of Sciences 2008;105:12224–12229.

303. Shao B, Tang C, Sinha A, et al. Humans with atherosclerosis have impaired ABCA1 cholesterol efflux and enhanced high-density lipoprotein oxidation by myeloperoxidase. *Circulation Res.* 2014;114:1733–1742.

304. Besler C, Heinrich K, Rohrer L, et al. Mechanisms underlying adverse effects of HDL on eNOS-activating pathways in patients with coronary artery disease. *J. Clin Invest.* 2011;121:2693–2708.

305. Mackness B, Durrington P, McElduff P, et al. Low paraoxonase activity predicts coronary events in the Caerphilly Prospective Study. *Circulation* 2003;107:2775–2779.

306. Wilkerson BA, Grass GD, Wing SB, Argraves WS, Argraves KM. Sphingosine 1-phosphate (S1P) carrier-dependent regulation of endothelial barrier: high density lipoprotein (HDL)-S1P prolongs endothelial barrier enhancement as compared with albumin-S1P via effects on levels, trafficking, and signaling of S1P1. *J Bio Chem.* 2012;287:44645–44653.

307. Ruiz M, Frej C, Holmer A, Guo LJ, Tran S, Dahlback B. High-density lipoprotein-associated apolipoprotein M limits endothelial inflammation by delivering sphingosine-1-phosphate to the sphingosine-1-phosphate receptor 1. *Arterioscler Thromb Vasc Biol.* 2017;37:118–129.

308. Feuerborn R, Becker S, Poti F, et al. High density lipoprotein (HDL)-associated sphingosine 1-phosphate (S1P) inhibits macrophage apoptosis

by stimulating STAT3 activity and survivin expression. *Atherosclerosis* 2017; 257:29–37.

309. Sukhorukov V, Gudelj I, Pucic-Bakovic M, et al. Glycosylation of human plasma lipoproteins reveals a high level of diversity, which directly impacts their functional properties. *Biochim Biophys Acta Mol Cell Biol Lipids* 2019;1864:643–653.

310. Ansell BJ, Navab M, Hama S, et al. Inflammatory/antiinflammatory properties of high-density lipoprotein distinguish patients from control subjects better than high-density lipoprotein cholesterol levels and are favorably affected by simvastatin treatment. *Circulation* 2003;108:2751–2756.

311. Kelesidis T, Roberts CK, Huynh D, et al. A high throughput biochemical fluorometric method for measuring lipid peroxidation in HDL. *PloS One* 2014;9:e111716.

312. Sen Roy S, Nguyen HCX, Angelovich TA, et al. Cell-free biochemical fluorometric enzymatic assay for high-throughput measurement of lipid peroxidation in high density lipoprotein. *J Vis Exp.* 2017;128:56325.

313. Samadi S, Mehramiz M, Kelesidis T, et al. High-density lipoprotein lipid peroxidation as a molecular signature of the risk for developing cardiovascular disease: Results from MASHAD cohort. *J Cell Physiol.* 2019. doi: 10.1002/jcp.28276.

314. Rosenson RS, Brewer HB, Jr., Barter PJ, et al. HDL and atherosclerotic cardiovascular disease: genetic insights into complex biology. *Nature Rev Cardiol.* 2018;15:9–19.

315. Karjalainen MK, Holmes MV, Wang Q, et al. Apolipoprotein A-I concentrations and risk of coronary artery disease: A Mendelian randomization study. *Atherosclerosis* 2020;299:56–63.

316. Norum RA, Lakier JB, Goldstein S, et al. Familial deficiency of apolipoproteins A-I and C-III and precocious coronary-artery disease. *New Engl J Med.* 1982;306:1513–1519.

317. Zakiev E, Rached F, Lhomme M, et al. Distinct phospholipid and sphingolipid species are linked to altered HDL function in apolipoprotein A-I deficiency. *J Clin Lipid.* 2019;13:468–80 e8.

318. Ordovas JM, Cassidy DK, Civeira F, Bisgaier CL, Schaefer EJ. Familial apolipoprotein A-I, C-III, and A-IV deficiency and premature atherosclerosis due to deletion of a gene complex on chromosome 11. *J Bio Chem.* 1989;264:16339–16342.

319. von Eckardstein A, Funke H, Walter M, Altland K, Benninghoven A, Assmann G. Structural analysis of human apolipoprotein A-I variants. Amino acid substitutions are nonrandomly distributed throughout the apolipoprotein A-I primary structure. *J Bio Chem.* 1990;265:8610–8617.

320. Lee EY, Klementowicz PT, Hegele RA, Asztalos BF, Schaefer EJ. HDL deficiency due to a new insertion mutation (ApoA-INashua) and review of the literature. *J Clin Lipid.* 2013;7:1697–1693.

321. Schmidt HH, Remaley AT, Stonik JA, et al. Carboxyl-terminal domain truncation alters apolipoprotein A-I in vivo catabolism. *J Bio Chem.* 1995;270:5469–5475.

322. Hooper AJ, Hegele RA, Burnett JR. Tangier disease: update for 2020. *Curr Op Lipid.* 2020;31:80–84.

323. Baldassarre D, Amato M, Pustina L, et al. Increased carotid artery intima-media thickness in subjects with primary hypoalphalipoproteinemia. *Arterioscler Thromb Vasc Biol.* 2002;22:317–322.

324. Frikke-Schmidt R, Nordestgaard BG, Stene MC, et al. Association of loss-of-function mutations in the ABCA1 gene with high-density lipoprotein cholesterol levels and risk of ischemic heart disease. *JAMA.* 2008;299:2524–2532.

325. Roshan B, Ganda OP, Desilva R, et al. Homozygous lecithin:cholesterol acyltransferase (LCAT) deficiency due to a new loss of function mutation and review of the literature. *J Clin Lipid.* 2011;5:493–499.

326. Saeedi R, Li M, Frohlich J. A review on lecithin:cholesterol acyltransferase deficiency. *Clin Biochem.* 2015;48:472–475.

327. Klein HG, Lohse P, Duverger N, et al. Two different allelic mutations in the lecithin:cholesterol acyltransferase (LCAT) gene resulting in classic LCAT deficiency: LCAT (tyr83-->stop) and LCAT (tyr156-->asn). *J Lipid Res.* 1993;34:49–58.

328. McNeish J, Aiello RJ, Guyot D, et al. High density lipoprotein deficiency and foam cell accumulation in mice with targeted disruption of ATP-binding cassette transporter-1. Proc. National Academy of Sciences. 2000;97:4245–4250.

329. Klein HG, Lohse P, Pritchard PH, Bojanovski D, Schmidt H, Brewer HB, Jr. Two different allelic mutations in the lecithin-cholesterol acyltransferase gene associated with the fish eye syndrome. Lecithin-cholesterol acyltransferase (Thr123----Ile) and lecithin-cholesterol acyltransferase (Thr347----Met). *J Clin Invest.* 1992;89:499–506.

330. Laurila PP, Surakka I, Sarin AP, et al. Genomic, transcriptomic, and lipidomic profiling highlights the role of inflammation in individuals with low high-density lipoprotein cholesterol. *Arterioscler Thromb Vasc Biol.* 2013;33:847–857.

331. de la Llera Moya M, McGillicuddy FC, Hinkle CC, et al. Inflammation modulates human HDL composition and function in vivo. Atherosclerosis 2012;222:390–394.

332. McGillicuddy FC, de la Llera Moya M, Hinkle CC, et al. Inflammation impairs reverse cholesterol transport in vivo. *Circulation* 2009;119:1135–1145.

333. Mora S, Cook N, Buring JE, Ridker PM, Lee IM. Physical activity and reduced risk of cardiovascular events: potential mediating mechanisms. *Circulation* 2007;116:2110–2118.

334. Kraus WE, Houmard JA, Duscha BD, et al. Effects of the amount and intensity of exercise on plasma lipoproteins. *New Engl J Med.* 2002;347: 1483–1492.

335. Sarzynski MA, Ruiz-Ramie JJ, Barber JL, et al. Effects of increasing exercise intensity and dose on multiple measures of hdl (high-density lipoprotein) function. *Arterioscler Thromb Vasc Biol.* 2018;38:943–952.

336. Ahmad T, Chasman DI, Buring JE, Lee IM, Ridker PM, Everett BM. Physical activity modifies the effect of LPL, LIPC, and CETP polymorphisms on HDL-C levels and the risk of myocardial infarction in women of European ancestry. *Circ Cardiovasc Genet.* 2011;4:74–80.

337. Rosenson RS, Otvos JD, Hsia J. Effects of rosuvastatin and atorvastatin on LDL and HDL particle concentrations in patients with metabolic syndrome: a randomized, double-blind, controlled study. *Diabetes Care* 2009;32:1087–1091.

338. Investigators A-H, Boden WE, Probstfield JL, et al. Niacin in patients with low HDL cholesterol levels receiving intensive statin therapy. *New Engl J Med.* 2011;365:2255–2267.

339. Group HTC, Landray MJ, Haynes R, et al. Effects of extended-release niacin with laropiprant in high-risk patients. *New Engl J Med.* 2014;371:203–212.

340. Nissen SE, Tsunoda T, Tuzcu EM, et al. Effect of recombinant ApoA-I Milano on coronary atherosclerosis in patients with acute coronary syndromes: a randomized controlled trial. *JAMA.* 2003;290:2292–300.

341. Nicholls SJ, Puri R, Ballantyne CM, et al. Effect of infusion of high-density lipoprotein mimetic containing recombinant apolipoprotein A-I Milano on coronary disease in patients with an acute coronary syndrome in the MILANO-PILOT trial: a randomized clinical trial. *JAMA Cardiol.* 2018;3:806–814.

342. Roma P, Gregg RE, Meng MS, et al. In vivo metabolism of a mutant form of apolipoprotein A-I, apo A-IMilano, associated with familial hypoalphalipoproteinemia. J Clin Invest. 1993;91:1445–1452.

343. Kempen HJ, Schranz DB, Asztalos BF, et al. Incubation of MDCO-216 (ApoA-IMilano/POPC) with human serum potentiates ABCA1-mediated cholesterol efflux capacity, generates new prebeta-1 HDL, and causes an increase in HDL size. *J Lipids* 2014;2014:923903.

344. Navdaev AV, Sborgi L, Wright SD, Didichenko SA. Nascent HDL (High-density lipoprotein) discs carry cholesterol to HDL Spheres: effects of HDL particle remodeling on cholesterol efflux. *Arterioscler Thromb Vasc Biol.* 2020;40:1182–1194.

345. Bolin DJ, Jonas A. Sphingomyelin inhibits the lecithin-cholesterol acyltransferase reaction with reconstituted high density lipoproteins by decreasing enzyme binding. *J Biol Chem.* 1996;271:19152–19158.

346. Nicholls SJ, Andrews J, Kastelein JJP, et al. Effect of serial infusions of CER-001, a pre-beta high-density lipoprotein mimetic, on coronary

atherosclerosis in patients following acute coronary syndromes in the CER-001 atherosclerosis regression acute coronary syndrome trial: a randomized clinical trial. *JAMA Cardiol.* 2018;3:815–822.

347. *Study to Investigate CSL112 in Subjects With Acute Coronary Syndrome (AEGIS-II).* 2018. https://clinicaltrials.gov/ct2/show/NCT03473223?term=NCT03473223&draw=2&rank=1. (Accessed 08/21/2020)

348. Navab M, Reddy ST, Anantharamaiah GM, et al. Intestine may be a major site of action for the apoA-I mimetic peptide 4F whether administered subcutaneously or orally. *J Lipid Res.* 2011;52:1200–1210.

349. Van Lenten BJ, Wagner AC, Jung CL, et al. Anti-inflammatory apoA-I-mimetic peptides bind oxidized lipids with much higher affinity than human apoA-I. *J Lipid Res.* 2008;49:2302–2311.

350. Hamid T, Ismahil MA, Bansal SS, et al. The apolipoprotein A-I mimetic L-4F attenuates monocyte activation and adverse cardiac remodeling after myocardial infarction. *Int J Mol Sci.* 2020;21.

351. Smythies LE, White CR, Maheshwari A, et al. Apolipoprotein A-I mimetic 4F alters the function of human monocyte-derived macrophages. *Am J Physiol Cell Physiol.* 2010;298:C1538–C1548.

352. Watson CE, Weissbach N, Kjems L, et al. Treatment of patients with cardiovascular disease with L-4F, an apo-A1 mimetic, did not improve select biomarkers of HDL function. *J Lipid Res.* 2011;52:361–373.

353. Navab M, Anantharamaiah GM, Hama S, et al. Oral administration of an Apo A-I mimetic Peptide synthesized from D-amino acids dramatically reduces atherosclerosis in mice independent of plasma cholesterol. *Circulation* 2002;105:290–292.

354. Sacks FM, Rudel LL, Conner A, et al. Selective delipidation of plasma HDL enhances reverse cholesterol transport in vivo. *J Lipid Res.* 2009;50:894–907.

355. Waksman R, Torguson R, Kent KM, et al. A first-in-man, randomized, placebo-controlled study to evaluate the safety and feasibility of autologous delipidated high-density lipoprotein plasma infusions in patients with acute coronary syndrome. *J Am Coll Cardiol.* 2010;55:2727–2735.

356. Ghoshhajra, B. B. et al. Coronary atheroma regression from infusions of autologous selectively delipidated Preβ-HDL-enriched plasma in homozygous familial hypercholesterolemia. *J Am Coll Cardiol.* 2020;76(25):3062–3064. doi: 10.1016/j.jacc.2020.10.038.

357. Glomset JA. The plasma lecithins:cholesterol acyltransferase reaction. *J Lipid Res.* 1968;9:155–167.

358. McInnes IB, Thompson L, Giles JT, et al. Effect of interleukin-6 receptor blockade on surrogates of vascular risk in rheumatoid arthritis: MEASURE, a randomised, placebo-controlled study. *Ann Rheum Dis.* 2015;74(4):694–702.

359. Garcia-Gomez C, Martin-Martinez MA, Castaneda S, et al. Lipoprotein(a) concentrations in rheumatoid arthritis on biologic therapy: results from the CARdiovascular in rheuMAtology study project. *J Clin Lipidol.* 2017;11(3):749–56 e3.

360. Que X, Hung MY, Yeang C, Gonen A, Prohaska TA, Sun X, et al. Oxidized phospholipids are proinflammatory and proatherogenic in hypercholesterolaemic mice. *Nature.* 2018;558(7709):301–306.

361. Nandakumar R, Matveyenko A, Thomas T, et al. Effects of Mipomersen, an apoB100 antisense, on Lp(a) metabolism in healthy subjects. *J Lipid Res.* 2018.

362. Tsimikas S, Viney NJ, Hughes SG, Singleton W, Graham MJ, Baker BF, et al. Antisense therapy targeting apolipoprotein(a): a randomised, double-blind, placebo-controlled phase 1 study. *Lancet.* 2015;386(10002):1472–1483.

363. Graham MJ, Viney N, Crooke RM, Tsimikas S. Antisense inhibition of apolipoprotein (a) to lower plasma lipoprotein (a) levels in humans. *J Lipid Res.* 2016;57(3):340–351.

364. Ray KK, Landmesser U, Leiter LA, et al. Inclisiran in patients at high cardiovascular risk with elevated LDL cholesterol. *N Engl J Med.* 2017;376(15): 1430–1440.

365. Ray KK, Stoekenbroek RM, Kallend D, et al. Effect of an siRNA therapeutic targeting PCSK9 on atherogenic lipoproteins: pre-specified secondary end points in ORION 1. *Circulation.* 2018.

366. Melquist S, Wakefield D, Hamilton H, et al. Targeting apolipoprotein(a) with a novel RNAi delivery platform as a prophylactic treatment to reduce risk of cardiovascular events in individuals with elevated lipoprotein (a) [Abstract]. *Circulation*: 2018;134:Suppl.1.

367. Albers JJ, Slee A, O'Brien KD, Robinson JG, et al. Relationship of apolipoproteins A-1 and B, and lipoprotein(a) to cardiovascular outcomes: the AIM-HIGH trial (Atherothrombosis Intervention in Metabolic Syndrome with Low HDL/High Triglyceride and Impact on Global Health Outcomes). *J Am Coll Cardiol.* 2013;62(17):1575–1579.

368. Samaha FF, McKenney J, Bloedon LT, Sasiela WJ, Rader DJ. Inhibition of microsomal triglyceride transfer protein alone or with ezetimibe in patients with moderate hypercholesterolemia. *Nat Clin Pract Cardiovasc Med.* 2008;5(8):497–505.

369. Waldmann E, Parhofer KG. Lipoprotein apheresis to treat elevated lipoprotein (a). *J Lipid Res.* 2016;57(10):1751–1757.

370. Roeseler E, Julius U, Heigl F, et al. Lipoprotein apheresis for lipoprotein(a)-associated cardiovascular disease: prospective 5 years of follow-up and apolipoprotein(a) characterization. *Arterioscler Thromb Vasc Biol.* 2016;36(9):2019–2027.

371. Rosada A, Kassner U, Vogt A, Willhauck M, Parhofer K, Steinhagen-Thiessen E. Does regular lipid apheresis in patients with isolated elevated lipoprotein(a) levels reduce the incidence of cardiovascular events? *Artif Organs.* 2014;38(2):135–141.

372. Jaeger BR, Richter Y, Nagel D, et al. Longitudinal cohort study on the effectiveness of lipid apheresis treatment to reduce high lipoprotein(a) levels and prevent major adverse coronary events. *Nat Clin Pract Cardiovasc Med.* 2009;6(3):229–239.

Psychological Factors in Cardiovascular Health and Disease

Darwin R. Labarthe and Rosalba Hernandez

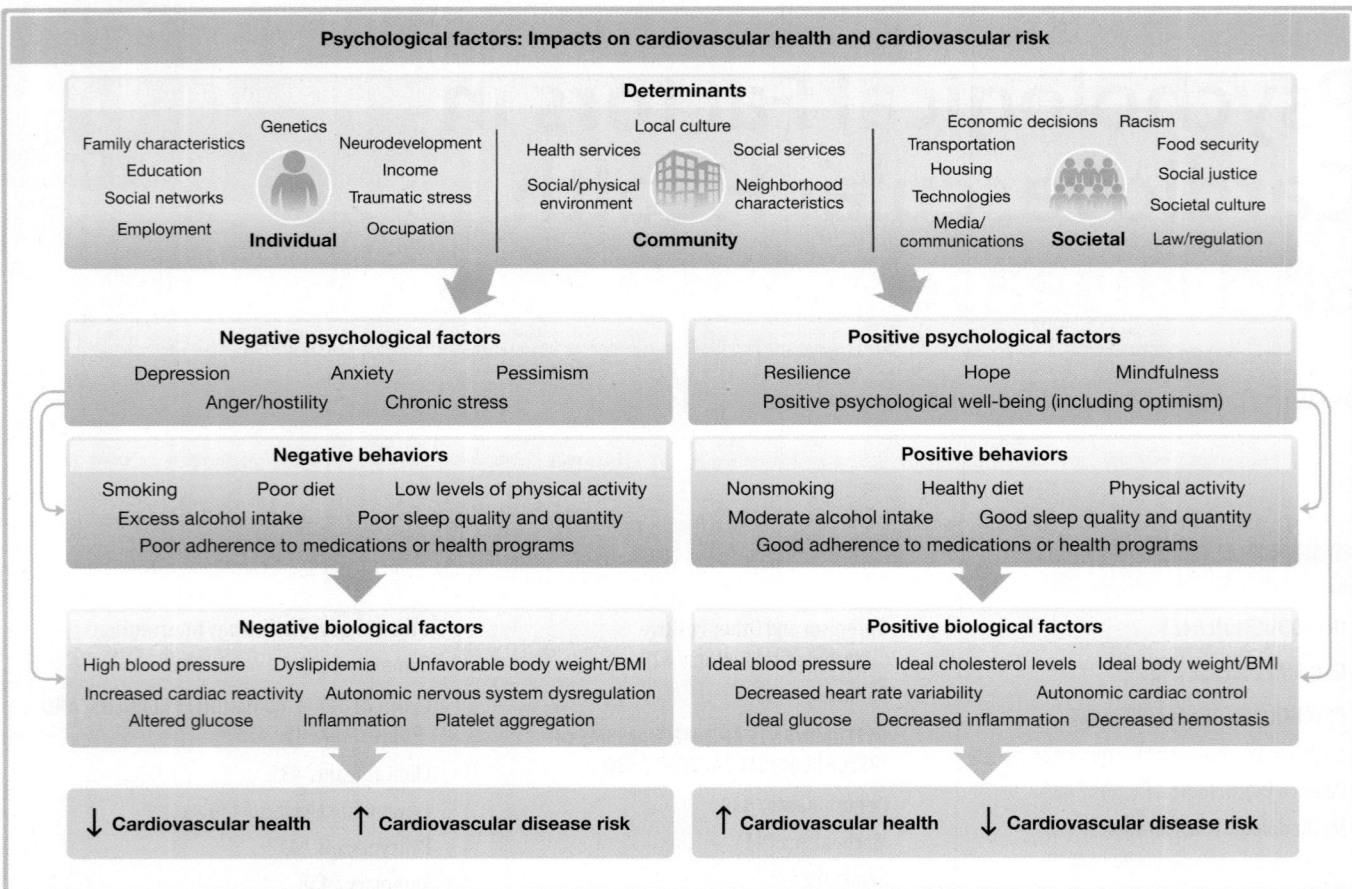

Chapter 11 Fuster and Hurst's Central Illustration. Individual, community, and societal determinants of psychological factors known to impact cardiovascular health and cardiovascular disease risk are shown. Various negative psychological factors result in reduced cardiovascular health and increased risk of cardiovascular disease. Conversely, positive psychological factors are associated with improved cardiovascular health and reduced risk of cardiovascular disease.

CHAPTER SUMMARY

This chapter discusses the impact that psychology can have on cardiovascular health (CVH) and cardiovascular disease (CVD); the individual, community, and societal determinants of various psychological factors that impact CVH and CVD risk; and interventions that could be used to reduce/enhance the influence of negative/positive psychological factors. Negative psychological factors such as depression, chronic stress, anxiety, anger/hostility, and pessimism have been shown to affect multiple behaviors and biological factors to result in reduced CVH and increased risk of CVD (see Fuster and Hurst's Central Illustration). Conversely, positive psychological factors such as positive psychological well-being (including optimism), mindfulness, resilience, and hope are associated with several favorable health behaviors and biological factors to result in improved CVH and reduced risk of CVD. Individual-level interventions that can improve psychological health include stress management, mindfulness, meditation, and other mind-body techniques, as well as other positive psychology approaches. The clinical team, community leaders, and policymakers can also all impact the psychological factors that influence CVH and CVD. While the evidence base on psychological factors in CVH and CVD is still expected to grow, sufficient evidence currently exists to guide the care of patients to promote CVH and prevent CVD.

INTRODUCTION

The role of psychological factors is an important part of our understanding of cardiovascular (CV) health and disease, with respect to both its origins and its potential prevention and treatment. A new CV perspective broadens the long-standing focus on cardiovascular disease (CVD) events and outcomes to include the earlier life course of cardiovascular health (CVH). This concept adds to CVD prevention (primary, secondary, and tertiary) the potential for CVH promotion (primordial prevention), to avert CVD in the first place.

Psychological factors related to CVH and CVD may be negative (eg, depression) or positive (eg, optimism) and include a wide array of factors with varying degrees of research to date. Evidence for their relations to CV conditions is reviewed. Translation of this evidence into practice by cardiologists and others at individual, community, and societal levels has potential to improve both patient and population health. More widespread training and increased resources are required at each level. Implementation research and other studies will be needed to answer several specific questions, including how best to utilize emerging technologies to improve psychological health.

CVH AND DISEASE

Cardiovascular and cerebrovascular diseases (CVD) and CV risk have long been considered consequences of adverse psychological factors, such as depression, stress, or any of several other negative conditions. A substantial body of research addresses links between these factors and CVD events.[1-3] Recommendations have been published for intervention with patients to reduce risk of a first CV event, a fatal outcome, or—for survivors—a recurrent event or impaired quality of life. The field of behavioral cardiology has evolved to foster such interventions in clinical practice.[4]

Since 2010, discussion of "CV risk" has taken a new, positive direction. In the context of *cardiovascular health (CVH)*, in contrast to CVD, "risk factors" have become "health factors" and "risk behaviors," or "health behaviors."[5] The concept of CVH, in persons remaining free of CVD, is anchored in the most favorable measures of each of seven metrics: diet, physical activity, smoking exposure, body weight/body mass index (BMI), blood pressure (BP), cholesterol, and blood glucose (BG). Ideal CVH is defined by an optimal composite score across the seven metrics. It can be measured at the individual level in terms of its status or its longitudinal developmental trajectory. CVH can also be measured at the population level, in terms of its prevalence, distribution, disparities, and trends.[6] Ideal CVH and its metrics represent important CV outcomes in themselves.

In addition, while CVD in terms of events is largely a phenomenon of adulthood, CVH is lifelong.[7] A life course perspective embraces both CVH and CVD (**Fig. 11–1**). CVH typically declines, as shown, from ideal to intermediate to poor from childhood through adolescence and adulthood, as unfavorable changes develop and persist in its defining behavioral and health factors. In consequence of poor CVH, CVD events occur with survival or death as the immediate outcomes and, for survivors, recurrence risk and impaired quality of life to be mitigated through long-term management. The strategy to prevent this progression from ideal CVH to CVD death, proposed by Strasser in 1978, is "primordial prevention," aimed to avert CV risk in the first place.[8] This concept has been reinforced recently in a JACC Focus Seminar on CV Health Promotion.[9]

This perspective identifies four phases in which intervention could in principle promote CVH, prevent CVD, and ameliorate adverse consequences when events do occur: (1) promoting healthy gestation, development, and aging to prevent unfavorable behaviors and factors in the first place (primordial prevention); (2) reversing adverse behaviors and factors to improve CVH and thereby prevent incident CV events (primary prevention); (3) delivering effective acute and long-term case management and rehabilitation to increase survival and quality

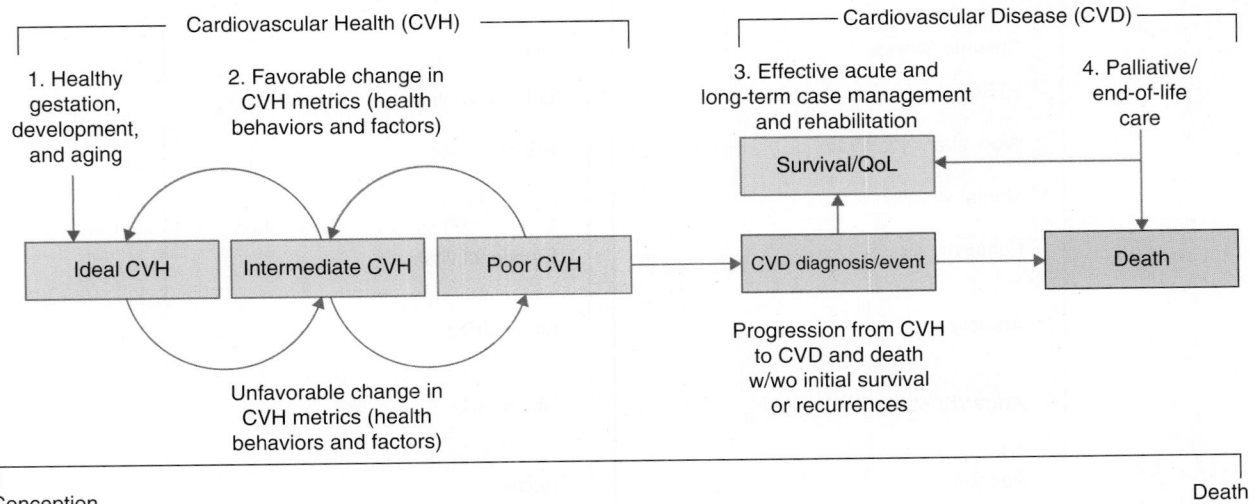

Figure 11–1. The life course of CVH and CVD: Four opportunities for positive psychology intervention. Reproduced with permission from Labarthe DR, Kubzansky LD, Boehm JK, et al. Positive Cardiovascular Health: A Timely Convergence. *J Am Coll Cardiol.* 2016 Aug 23;68(8):860-867.

of life and reduce recurrence risk (secondary and tertiary prevention); and (4) palliative and end-of-life care.[7]

Interest in understanding the role of psychological factors in etiology and prevention of CVD events and their consequences is a familiar concept. Attention is now called as well to opportunities for promotion of CVH throughout the life course to improve patient and population CVH in the first place, averting development of CVD altogether.

PSYCHOLOGICAL FACTORS

The term "psychological factors" embraces a wide array of characteristics, much as "biologic factors" or "behavioral factors" do in their own domains. Interest in psychological factors has previously focused on those potentially associated with high CV risk and occurrence of CVD events. Several examples are noted in **Fig. 11–2**. Two broad categories of these and related factors can readily be distinguished as negative or positive. Depression and optimism, respectively, are leading examples and serve as illustrations.

Depression is a well-established such factor, preceding and following CV events, and can range in severity from a mild condition to major depressive disorder (MDD).[10] "Stress" is a multifaceted concept regarding its acuteness or chronicity, sources in objective external social circumstances, and effects whether perceived or "buffered" by other factors. "Chronic stress" is often represented by post traumatic stress disorder (PTSD), a term once used chiefly in relation to military combat exposures but now applied more widely to exposures to traumatic events or threats to personal safety, such as adverse

childhood experiences (ACEs). It also includes such conditions as work stress or "job strain," marital stress, and others.

Anxiety, anger and hostility, and pessimism are distinct conditions that may be either momentary or chronic, as "states" or "traits," with their own CV consequences.

However, especially since the development of positive psychology and the concept of positive CVH, factors associated with low CVD risk, or better outcomes of CV events, have also been studied.[11-13] Several of these factors are subsumed under the term "positive psychological well-being (PPWB)." Commonly measured components of PPWB, as described by Boehm and Kubzansky, broadly include three categories.[13]

The first category is "fulfilling one's potential and identifying meaningful life pursuits," or "evaluations of functioning in life" ("eudaimonic well-being"). It is measured by purpose in life, personal growth, self-acceptance, environmental mastery, autonomy, and *ikigai* ("a sense that life is worth living"). The second category, "evaluations of feelings about life" ("hedonic well-being"), which is focused more on affective domains, includes happiness, satisfaction with life, and positive affect. The third is optimism and other measures of well-being, including hope and vitality. Also notable are mindfulness and resilience. Mindfulness has been described by Levine and others as "a present, moment-by-moment, non-judgmental awareness of one's thoughts, emotions, and actions."[14] Resilience has been characterized as a set of those intrapersonal skills and protective factors that defend against the effects of cumulative stress.[15] "Coping" and "buffering" share some features of this concept.

Another composite construct, developed by Seligman, combines Positive emotion, Engagement, Relationships, Meaning,

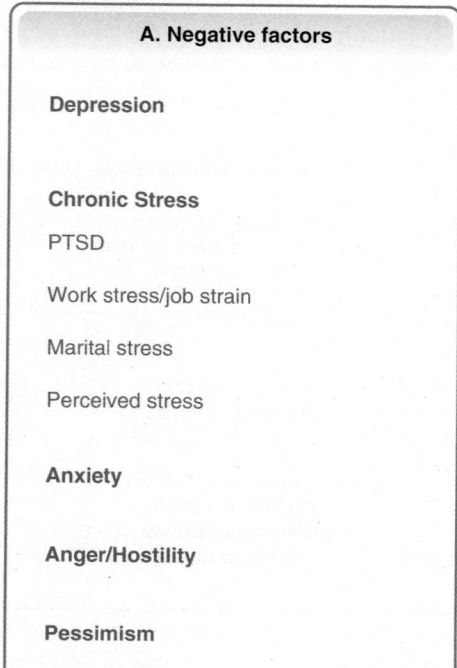

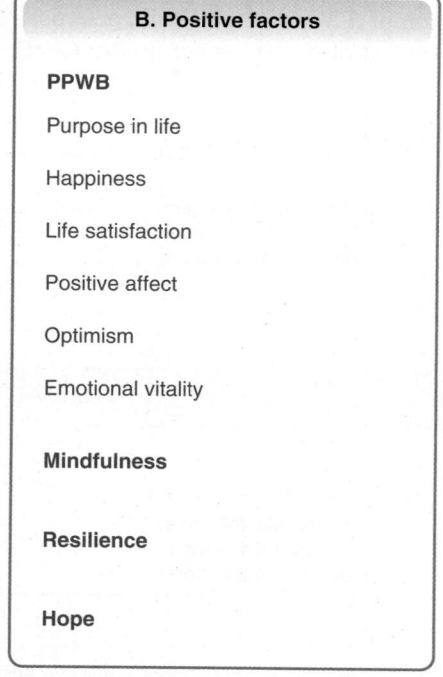

Figure 11–2. Examples of psychological factors in CVH and CVD—negative and positive factors.

and Accomplishment (PERMA) to provide metrics and an integrated score for happiness. PERMA has generated an online assessment tool and a multicomponent curriculum.[16]

Negative Psychological Factors

Depression can be assessed in many ways, reviewed recently in the *Handbook of Depression*.[17] They are distinguished broadly as clinician ratings and self-report inventories. The former are generally used by health professionals trained in their use and may conform closely to elements of the Diagnostic and Statistical Manual of Mental Disorders (DSM) of the American Psychiatric Association, as revised in 2000.[18] The latter are more commonly utilized in population studies and as screening tools in primary care and similar clinical settings. A simple self-report questionnaire can be used in clinical practice to screen for depression and rate its severity and has been recommended in a 2008 American Heart Association (AHA) Science Advisory on management of depression in coronary heart disease (CHD) (**Box 11-1**).[2]

Evaluation of instruments to assess depression in research and practice has shown important variation in their correspondence to specific psychological constructs and their sensitivity and specificity in relation to more definitive diagnostic assessments.[17] For example, the Cardiac Depression Scale is specifically intended to identify MDD in patients with cardiac

---

BOX 11-1. SCREENING QUESTIONS FOR DEPRESSION[2]

Over the past 2 weeks, how often have you been bothered by any of the following problems?

(1) Little interest or pleasure in doing things.

(2) Feeling down, depressed, or hopeless.

"Yes" to either question is an indication for either referral to a qualified health professional or administration of the following:
   Over the past 2 weeks, how often have you been bothered by any of the following problems?

(1) Little or no interest or pleasure in doing things.

(2) Feeling down, depressed, or hopeless.

(3) Trouble falling asleep, staying asleep, or sleeping too much.

(4) Feeling tired or having little energy.

(5) Poor appetite or overeating.

(6) Feeling bad about yourself, feeling that you are a failure, or feeling that you have let yourself or family down.

(7) Trouble concentrating on things such as reading the newspaper or watching television.

(8) Moving or speaking so slowly that other people could have noticed. Or being so fidgety or restless that you have been moving around a lot more than usual.

(9) Thinking that you would be better off dead or that you want to hurt yourself in some way.

Each question is answered categorically, as none = 0, several days = 1, more than half the days = 2, and nearly every day = 3. The 9 scores are summed to find the overall depression severity score.

BOX 11-2. SCREENING QUESTIONNAIRE FOR OPTIMISM AND PESSIMISM[25]

Please be as honest and accurate as you can throughout. Try not to let your response to one statement influence your responses to other statements. There are no "correct" or "incorrect" answers. Answer according to your own feelings, rather than how you think "most people" would answer.

   A = I agree a lot B = I agree a little C = I neither agree nor disagree D = I disagree a little E = I disagree a lot

1. In uncertain times, I usually expect the best.
2. It's easy for me to relax.
3. If something can go wrong for me, it will. (R)
4. I'm always optimistic about my future.
5. I enjoy my friends a lot.
6. It's important for me to keep busy.
7. I hardly ever expect things to go my way. (R)
8. I don't get upset too easily.
9. I rarely count on good things happening to me. (R)
10. Overall, I expect more good things to happen to me than bad.

Scoring:
Items 3, 7, and 9 are reverse scored (or scored separately as a pessimism measure). Items 2, 5, 6, and 8 are fillers and should not be scored. Scoring is kept continuous—there is no benchmark for being an optimist/pessimist.

---

disease, where depression is especially common, with a 26-item questionnaire. There remains need for further development of methods with respect to definitions of depression, validation of their use across diverse cultures, and appropriate utilization of computerized assessments and other emerging technologies. Such research is needed with respect to the other negative measures as well.

Positive Psychological Factors

Optimism has been considered the most consistent component of PPWB in being associated with decreased CV events both in patients and in healthy populations (and as the leading candidate among positive psychological factors for further research).[14,19-24] Optimism is often assessed by one or another variation of the Life Orientation Test—Revised (LOT-R) (**Box 11-2**).[25]

Assessment of optimism is sometimes reduced to item 10 (Box 11-2), "Overall, I expect more good things to happen to me than bad." Boehm and Kubzanski noted that optimism can be viewed not only in terms of future expectations but as a personal explanatory style regarding causality of past events.[14] They also called attention to the need for assessments of PPWB (presumably including optimism) in life course studies to identify critical periods most influential for subsequent CV events. Finally, a more recent measurement tool for optimism was created to tap into more momentary emotional states influenced by time, context, and situational events versus the less mutable personality trait.[26]

Methodologic Considerations

Study of each of the conventional CV risk factors has encountered and, to varying degrees, overcome a variety of methodologic challenges. The same is true in the area of psychological factors. Noting these challenges and solutions offers an appreciation of both the strengths and the remaining limitations of the science to date.[13,25]

Definition and Measurement

Terms used to characterize psychological attributes can be difficult to define precisely, and discerning their overlap or distinctness one from another is sometimes difficult. As one consequence, methods of assessment—whether by structured interviews or questionnaires, or others—often lack standardization. This poses challenges for communication, replication, and synthesis of study findings. In some cases, however, tools developed to standardize definitions and ascertainment—for example, in depression and optimism—have become widely adopted and have greatly strengthened research and practice. Approaches to measurement must take into account whether the factors of interest are regarded as only momentary responses to immediate circumstances (states) or enduring characteristics (traits). In some cases, surrogate measures may sufficiently represent the factors of interest but be ascertained indirectly rather than by self-report.

Multiplicity of Psychological Factors

Where one factor is specified as the "exposure" of interest and studied in isolation from others, questions may arise whether the resulting observations reflect other psychological factors that are unmeasured, or may not capture well the influential aspect of a complex attribute. Recent studies have more often assessed more than a single psychological factor in order to evaluate their separate effects, for example, whether optimism protects against CVD independent of absence of depression or perceived stress.

Relation to Behavioral and Biological Factors

In CV studies, dominant interest in established risk factors, especially biological ones, has tended to limit investment in research on psychological factors. Studies of traditional risk factors have paid little attention to psychological factors, and conversely. As a result, joint or independent contributions of these multiple factors on CVD and CVH are difficult to evaluate. Where studied together, it has been possible to demonstrate contributions of certain psychological factors independent of biological ones.

Study Design

Studies of psychological factors in CVD and CVH have often been cross-sectional in design and small in size—unlike the large body of long-term cohort studies on predominantly biological factors. However, the major CV cohort studies often include one-time psychological assessments that then become available subsequently for analysis. In some cases, data collection in their more recent follow-up examination cycles has included a more extensive psychological component. Approaches to small study sizes have been to conduct larger-scale studies and meta-analyses to assess effects over multiple studies. Recent publications of both kinds have provided important contributions.[14] Finally, to permit rigorous interpretation of potential intervention effects, randomized controlled trials are necessary—but relatively few such studies have been reported to date.

Interpretation

For the foregoing reasons, interpretation of observed associations between psychological attributes and CVH or CVD status may be quite limited. Questions may remain, for example, as to the direction of association: Is a particular psychological attribute a cause or a consequence of other factors, or of CVH or CVD status? Or is the association bi directional, indicating a reciprocal relationship? Further, how are other considerations about causal interpretation met, such as temporal relationships, independence from other factors, and consistency with other evidence? The most robust observational studies in these respects are longitudinal/prospective follow-up studies with multiple assessments not only of the factor of primary interest but of co variables and potentially confounding factors.

Summary

Many psychological factors, both negative and positive, are potentially important to more fully understanding CVH and CVD. Increasing rigor of research in this area is strengthening the evidence for these relationships.

In the discussion that follows, emphasis is placed on those psychological factors that have been studied most extensively and rigorously are addressed in recent reviews and are of greatest potential interest for cardiologists and other health professionals concerned with CVH promotion and CVD prevention.

A simple scheme represents: (1) a direct relationship from their underlying determinants to psychological factors; (2) the links from these factors to CV outcomes; (3) mechanisms through which (a) the determinants affect psychological factors and (b) the factors in turn lead to their CV effects; and (4) targets for intervention—(a) the determinants, (b) the mechanisms of the determinants, (c) the psychological factors themselves, (d) mechanisms of the factors, and (e) the CV outcomes (**Fig. 11–3**).

Following review of associations between psychological factors and CVH and CVD, this scheme provides a framework for discussion of determinants, mechanisms, and interventions to improve CVH and outcomes of CVD.

PSYCHOLOGICAL FACTORS ASSOCIATED WITH CVH AND CVD

Depression and other Negative Psychological Factors

A substantial body of research provides good evidence on the CV impact of depression.[2,27–31] To consider first the relation of negative psychological factors to CVH, **Table 11–1A** represents several negative psychological factors and indicates (X) where, according to these recent reviews, studies have found them associated with any or all of the seven CVH metrics.

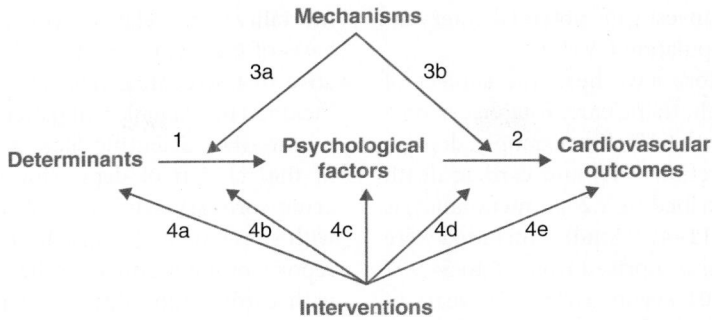

Figure 11–3. Psychological factors in CVH and CVD: Determinants, mechanisms, CV outcomes, and interventions.

Depression, for example, is associated with smoking and unfavorable body weight/BMI, BP, cholesterol, and glucose. For PTSD and anxiety, findings have been similar. For anger and hostility, only BP has been found associated, while for pessimism each of the CVH metrics appears associated.

The many studies represented here have mainly been cross-sectional surveys, leaving unclear whether these psychological characteristics precede or follow the behavioral or biological ones. Complicating interpretation of these associations with

respect to possible causal direction is whether they may be bidirectional, such that each influences the other in a reciprocal way—smoking, for example, resulting in part from depression and persisting or increasing partly in consequence of smoking. A further consideration is the limited number and quality of studies in this area. Empty cells in Table 11–1 reflect lack of sufficient data and not absence of associations. Clarification of relationships between negative psychological factors and CVH will require more and better studies. This can help to

TABLE 11–1. Associations of Psychological Factors with CVH and CVD

A. Negative Factors	Association with CVH Metrics						
	Less favorable:						
	smoking	diet	physical act	body weight	BP	Chol	Glucose
DEPRESSION	X	X	X	X	X	X	X
PTSD	X	X	X	X	X	X	X
ANXIETY	X	X	X	X	X	X	X
ANGER/HOSTILITY					X		
PESSIMISM	X	X	X	X	X	X	X
	Association with CVD Indicators						
	Increases in:						
DEPRESSION	Incident and recurrent CVD events in clinical and community populations						
CHRONIC STRESS	Incident CVD events						
PTSD	CHD and other events; abnormal myocardial perfusion imaging						
ANXIETY	Incident CVD events and case fatality						
ANGER/HOSTILITY	Multiple CVD events: MI/ACS, ventricular arrythmias, stroke, heart failure						
PESSIMISM	Stroke and other CVD events						
B. Positive Factors	Association with CVH Metrics						
	More favorable:						
	smoking	diet	physical act	body weight	BP	Chol	Glucose
OPTIMISM	X	X	X	X	X	X	X
MINDFULNESS	X	X	X	X	X	X	X
	Association with CVD Indicators						
	Decreases in:						
PPWB	CDV risk, brain infarcts, dementia						
OPTIMISM	CDV events, stroke, heart failure, hospital readmission						

determine where and how to investigate potential interventions to improve patient and population CVH.

Negative psychological factors have been the subject of more and better quality research, that clearly establishes prospective associations of some with CVD. For example, depression predicts myocardial infarction (MI) and cardiac death in community cohorts, as described in a 2006 meta-analysis by Nicholson and others (**Fig. 11–4**).[30] Studies included were reported from 1993 to 2003 and comprised from 76 to 54,997 participants and from 7 to 1401 events, over 2–29 years of followup. Eleven of these studies reported adjusted relative risks ranging from 0.7 (95% confidence interval [CI] 0.4–1.5) to 5.7 (95% CI 2.6–12.8), with the overall risk estimate 1.9 (95% CI 1.5–2.4).

This finding is consistent with other systematic reviews and meta-analyses, beginning as early as the late 1990s, including studies of both clinical and community populations. Three reports from the AHA, in 2008, 2014, and 2021 assessed the evidence for association between depression and CV outcomes.[2,14,27] The first of these, an AHA Science Advisory, noted that more than 100 narrative reviews and many meta-analyses on the role of depression in CV morbidity and mortality were "relatively consistent" in their findings.[2] On the basis of this evidence, the writing group considered it imperative that screening, referral, and treatment of depression be included in evaluation of patients with CHD.

An AHA Scientific Statement in 2014 reviewed evidence of the relation of depression to prognosis in patients with acute coronary syndrome (ACS).[27] Association of depression with subsequent all-cause mortality was summarized from 32 reports of longitudinal studies, published from 1992 to 2009; with cardiac mortality in 12 reports of longitudinal studies published from 1993 to 2011; and with all-cause and cardiac mortality as well as nonfatal cardiac events in 22 reports of longitudinal studies published from 1990 to 2010. The great majority of study cohorts were in the United States, some in Canada and the UK, and a few in Europe as well as Japan, Australia, and Iran. Women were included in all but two of these studies. While methodologic variation was noted, such as differences in definition and ascertainment of depression, associations were judged to be consistent among the better-designed studies. The statement concluded that the AHA should elevate depression to be regarded as a risk factor for adverse outcomes in patients with ACS.

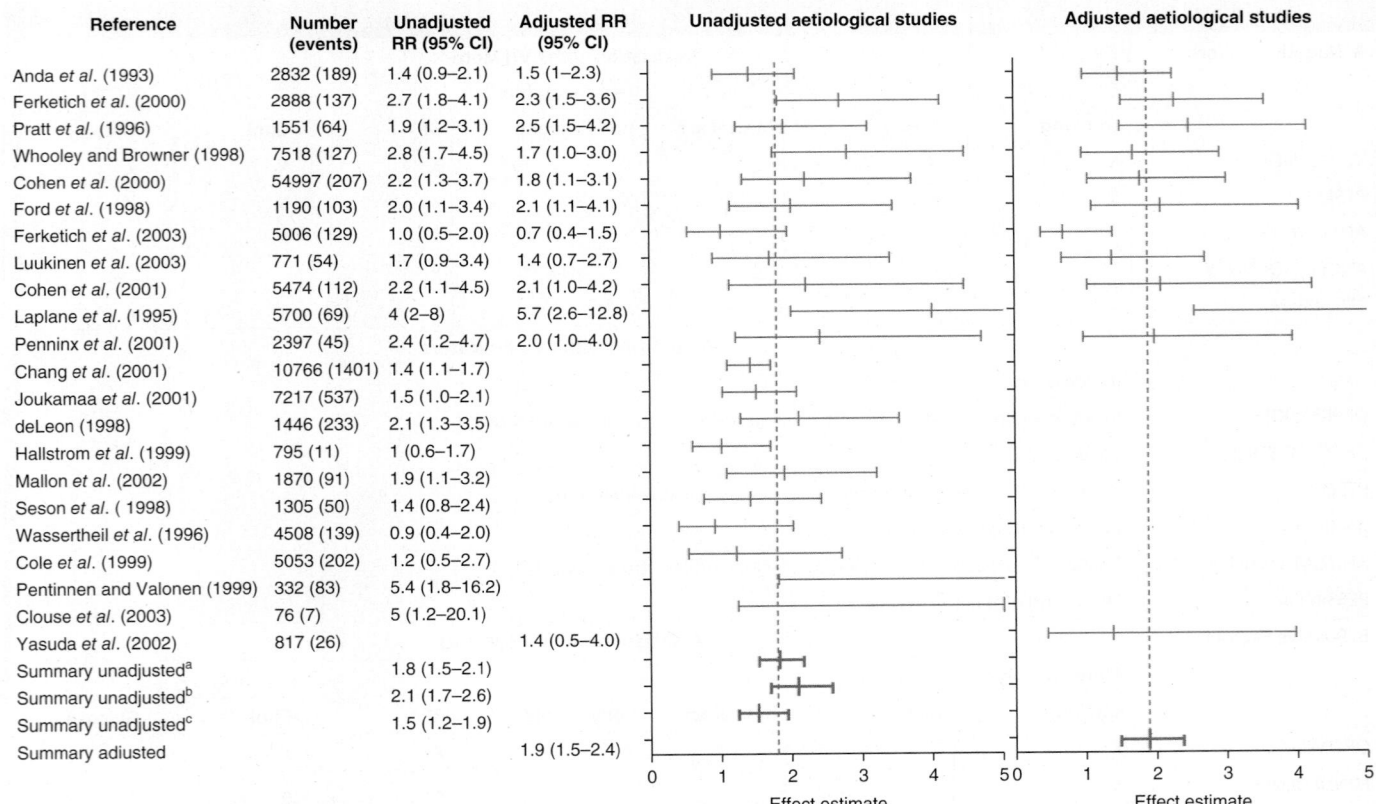

Aetiological studies: Forrest plot of the effect of depression on the incidence of CHD

Reference	Number (events)	Unadjusted RR (95% CI)	Adjusted RR (95% CI)	Unadjusted aetiological studies	Adjusted aetiological studies
Anda et al. (1993)	2832 (189)	1.4 (0.9–2.1)	1.5 (1–2.3)		
Ferketich et al. (2000)	2888 (137)	2.7 (1.8–4.1)	2.3 (1.5–3.6)		
Pratt et al. (1996)	1551 (64)	1.9 (1.2–3.1)	2.5 (1.5–4.2)		
Whooley and Browner (1998)	7518 (127)	2.8 (1.7–4.5)	1.7 (1.0–3.0)		
Cohen et al. (2000)	54997 (207)	2.2 (1.3–3.7)	1.8 (1.1–3.1)		
Ford et al. (1998)	1190 (103)	2.0 (1.1–3.4)	2.1 (1.1–4.1)		
Ferketich et al. (2003)	5006 (129)	1.0 (0.5–2.0)	0.7 (0.4–1.5)		
Luukinen et al. (2003)	771 (54)	1.7 (0.9–3.4)	1.4 (0.7–2.7)		
Cohen et al. (2001)	5474 (112)	2.2 (1.1–4.5)	2.1 (1.0–4.2)		
Laplane et al. (1995)	5700 (69)	4 (2–8)	5.7 (2.6–12.8)		
Penninx et al. (2001)	2397 (45)	2.4 (1.2–4.7)	2.0 (1.0–4.0)		
Chang et al. (2001)	10766 (1401)	1.4 (1.1–1.7)			
Joukamaa et al. (2001)	7217 (537)	1.5 (1.0–2.1)			
deLeon (1998)	1446 (233)	2.1 (1.3–3.5)			
Hallstrom et al. (1999)	795 (11)	1 (0.6–1.7)			
Mallon et al. (2002)	1870 (91)	1.9 (1.1–3.2)			
Seson et al. (1998)	1305 (50)	1.4 (0.8–2.4)			
Wassertheil et al. (1996)	4508 (139)	0.9 (0.4–2.0)			
Cole et al. (1999)	5053 (202)	1.2 (0.5–2.7)			
Pentinnen and Valonen (1999)	332 (83)	5.4 (1.8–16.2)			
Clouse et al. (2003)	76 (7)	5 (1.2–20.1)			
Yasuda et al. (2002)	817 (26)		1.4 (0.5–4.0)		
Summary unadjusted[a]		1.8 (1.5–2.1)			
Summary unadjusted[b]		2.1 (1.7–2.6)			
Summary unadjusted[c]		1.5 (1.2–1.9)			
Summary adjusted			1.9 (1.5–2.4)		

[a]Studies reporting an unadjusted effect estimate.
[b]Studies reporting an unadjusted effect estimate that also reported an adjusted effect estimate.
[c]Studies reporting an unadjusted effect estimate that do not reported an adjusted effect estimate.

Figure 11–4. Aetiological studies: Forrest plot of the effect of depression on the incidence of CHD. Reproduced with permission from Nicholson A, Kuper H, Hemingway H. Depression as an aetiologic and prognostic factor in coronary heart disease: a meta-analysis of 6362 events among 146 538 participants in 54 observational studies. *Eur Heart J.* 2006 Dec;27(23):2763-2774.

Overall, from decades of research, generally consistent associations have been found between depression and not only these outcomes, but also poor adherence to medications, decreased participation in cardiac rehabilitation programs, and reduced responsiveness to interventions to modify other risk factors, as well as increased health care costs and lower quality of life. All of these findings result from research including many longitudinal cohort studies. Depression is exceptional among negative psychological factors in the extent of research interest and investment it has received with respect to CVD risk.

Other negative psychological characteristics, including those described above, have also been found associated with several CVD outcomes, such as incident and recurrent coronary events and case fatality, heart failure (HF), stroke, and other manifestations: PTSD, chronic stress, adverse childhood events, anxiety, anger/hostility, and pessimism.[14]

Optimism and Other Positive Psychological Factors

Overall PPWB as well as both optimism and mindfulness has been found associated with more favorable levels of each of the seven CVH metrics—including diet and physical activity—or with an aggregated CVH score (**Table 11–1B**). Data are too limited for the other positive factors in Table 11–1 to draw firm conclusions. Regarding overall PPWB, associations have been found not only with CVD risk, but with brain infarcts and dementia and with both onset and progression of CVD.

In addition to the separate positive factors, the composite measure of PPWB warrants further evaluation as an entity in relation to CVH and CVD. There were generally mixed findings for specific factors and behaviors—associations being found between optimism and moderate intake, and reduced problem drinking; some components of PPWB, including optimism, associated with sleep quality and quantity; and both optimism and PPWB associated with food patterns. These observations were largely reported in cross-sectional studies, with limitations to their interpretation.

The association of optimism with CV events and all-cause mortality was examined recently through a systematic review and meta-analysis by Rozanski and others (**Fig. 11–5**).[32] This appears to be the first such review regarding optimism. For CV events (fatal CV events and nonfatal MI, stroke, and new-onset angina), 10 longitudinal community cohort studies were included in the meta-analysis. These studies were published between 2001 and 2016 and ranged from 545 to 97,253 participants with from 2 to 15 years of follow-up. They were conducted primarily in the United States but also in Europe.

The relative risk of CV events ranged across these studies from 0.94 (95% CI 0.86–1.02) to 0.23 (95% CI 0–0.46), overall 0.65 (95% CI 0.51–0.78). The decreased risk of CV events was reflected in results for all-cause mortality which, though less strong, were also significant (relative risk [RR] 0.86, 95% CI 0.80–0.92). Those studies in which pessimism was also assessed demonstrated independence of optimism as a predictor of outcomes; adjustments for other risk factors showed optimism to be independent of these as well. Reference to previous studies noted consistency of findings with other favorable outcomes in HF, cognitive dysfunction, carotid atherosclerosis, respiratory disease, infection, and cancer. Rozanski earlier found optimism to be associated with improved recovery from MI and cardiac procedures.[4]

The authors concluded that these findings are potentially important for behavioral cardiology. At the same time, several limitations of the evidence to date call for further research on the role of optimism with respect to CVD: improvement in methods of assessment; clearer conception of whether it represents a momentary state or an enduring personality trait; better

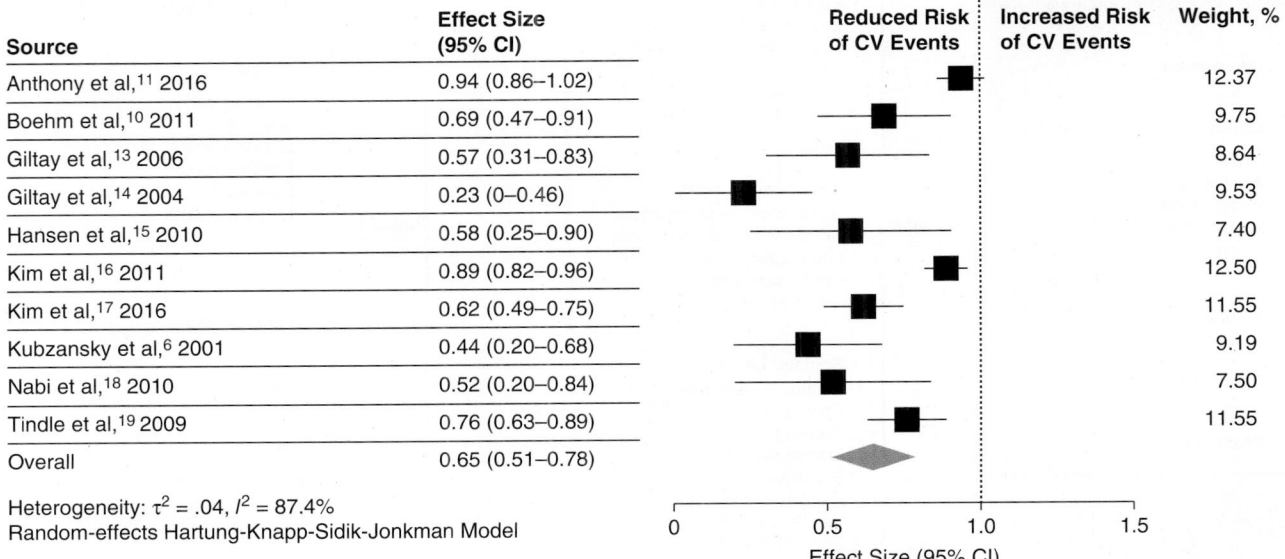

Source	Effect Size (95% CI)		Weight, %
Anthony et al,[11] 2016	0.94 (0.86–1.02)		12.37
Boehm et al,[10] 2011	0.69 (0.47–0.91)		9.75
Giltay et al,[13] 2006	0.57 (0.31–0.83)		8.64
Giltay et al,[14] 2004	0.23 (0–0.46)		9.53
Hansen et al,[15] 2010	0.58 (0.25–0.90)		7.40
Kim et al,[16] 2011	0.89 (0.82–0.96)		12.50
Kim et al,[17] 2016	0.62 (0.49–0.75)		11.55
Kubzansky et al,[6] 2001	0.44 (0.20–0.68)		9.19
Nabi et al,[18] 2010	0.52 (0.20–0.84)		7.50
Tindle et al,[19] 2009	0.76 (0.63–0.89)		11.55
Overall	0.65 (0.51–0.78)		

Heterogeneity: $\tau^2 = .04$, $I^2 = 87.4\%$
Random-effects Hartung-Knapp-Sidik-Jonkman Model

Reduced Risk of CV Events | Increased Risk of CV Events

Effect Size (95% CI) — 0, 0.5, 1.0, 1.5

Figure 11–5. Association of optimism with CV events and all-cause mortality: A systematic review and meta-analysis. Reproduced with permission from Rozanski A, Bavishi C, Kubzansky LD, et al. Association of Optimism With Cardiovascular Events and All-Cause Mortality: A Systematic Review and Meta-analysis. *JAMA Netw Open.* 2019 Sep 4;2(9):e1912200.

understanding of mechanisms; and development of intervention methods to both increase optimism and decrease pessimism.

Summary

Reviews of the growing body of evidence present many identified associations of both negative and positive psychological factors separately with CVH and CVD. For CVH, these studies have typically addressed only one or a few of the seven defining metrics, rarely all. Especially infrequent are data regarding diet and physical activity. Most common are findings regarding smoking and the clinical factors—body weight, BP, cholesterol, and glucose. In all instances, the negative psychological factors are associated with unfavorable health and positive factors with favorable levels of CVH.

For CVD, the principal negative psychological factors, including depression, are associated with excess incidence and recurrence of clinical events, chiefly in patient populations but also in community-based studies. These include both cardiac events (ACS, MI, HF) and stroke. Conversely, the positive psychological factors, including optimism, predict lower rates of these events.

Interpretation of these findings, as well as those for the other negative and positive psychological factors, requires caution for the reasons summarized above. To enable fuller understanding of these relationships, both determinants of psychological factors and their possible mechanisms of action have been investigated.

DETERMINANTS AND MECHANISMS OF PSYCHOLOGICAL FACTORS

Determinants

In principle, understanding what determines psychological factors in CVH and CVD is important for promoting and preserving positive psychological factors as well as preventing or ameliorating negative ones. Many aspects of life can be considered as such determinants. Clinical interest centers primarily on the individual, while a public health perspective calls for attention to the community and societal levels as well. A combined perspective is shown in **Fig. 11–6**, in which both the negative and positive psychological factors discussed above are shown in relation to potential determinants at all three levels.

The center panel of Fig. 11–6 illustrates, though not exhaustively, the types of influences on psychological factors that could be considered at each level. It is intuitively plausible that any of these could have psychological effects. But the evidence is less clear where a specific relationship may obtain between a particular determinant and psychological factor. Further, the preponderance of evidence appears to relate to adverse life circumstances—such as low household income, unemployment, or inadequate social networks—and negative psychological factors—such as depression or chronic stress (left panel). But if a determinant is seen as on a continuous scale, from unfavorable to favorable, then positive effects on psychological factors as well as negative ones can be considered (right panel).

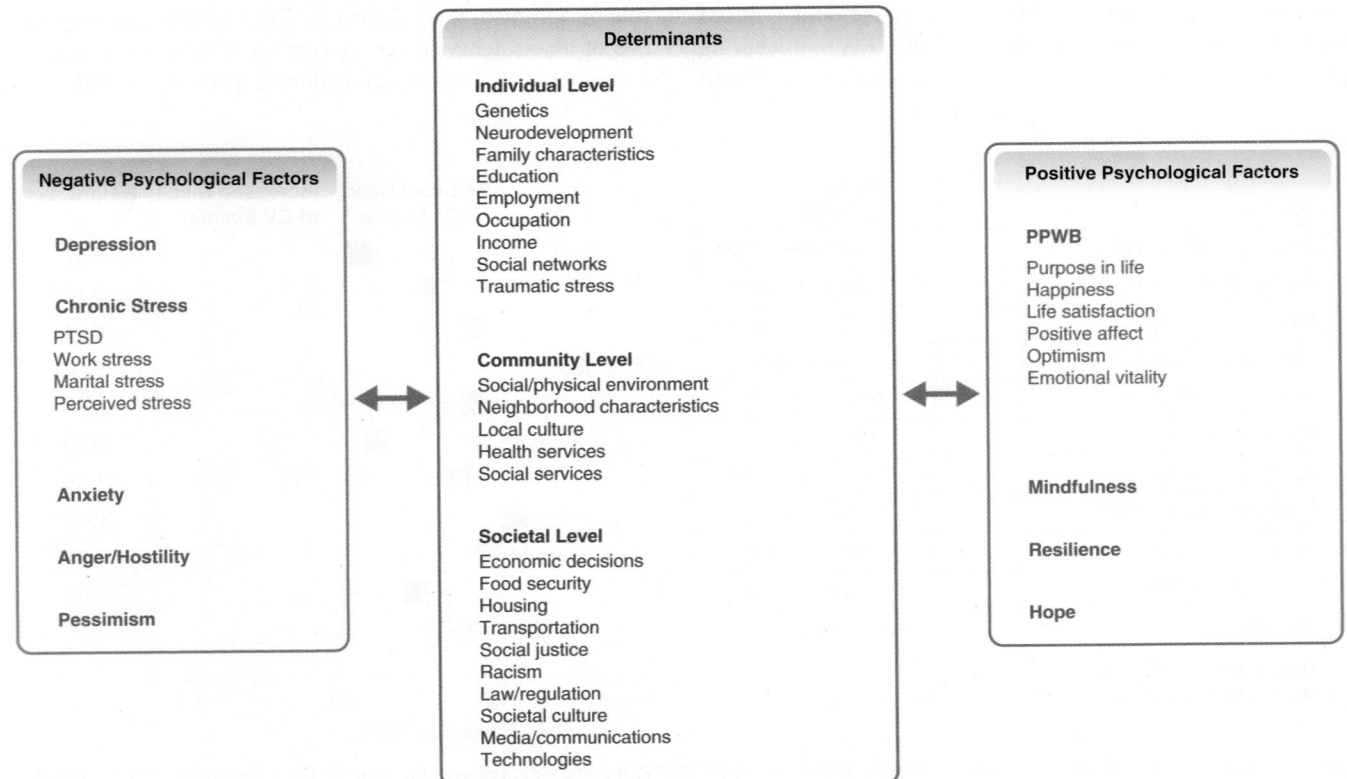

Figure 11–6. Determinants of psychological factors in CVH and CVD.

A core concept in this context is that of social determinants of health. Impetus to this concept was provided by the 2008 report of the WHO Commission.[33] Its thesis was that health equity across populations could be achieved by global action on these determinants, subsequently defined as including "… early years' experiences, education, economic status, employment and decent work, housing and environment, and effective systems of preventing and treating ill health."[33]

Various expressions of this concept have been published over ensuing years, as in the decennial publication of *Healthy People*.[34] Most relevant to the immediate discussion is an AHA Scientific Statement, *Social Determinants of Risk and Outcomes for Cardiovascular Disease*.[35] That report defines social determinants of health broadly as socioeconomic position (SEP); race, ethnicity; social support; culture and language; access to care; and residential environment. Further elements are specified for some of these—for example, eight conditions are listed as markers of SEP. The central panel of Fig. 11–6 represents these and other related terms as they might be considered at individual, community, and societal levels.

The AHA Statement reviews evidence on how the social determinants act on psychological factors, together with behavioral and biological ones, as mechanisms for causing CVD.[35] The present focus is on how the determinants affect the psychological factors in themselves, rather than as mechanisms for further consequences. Depression, in particular, was judged to result from several social conditions: socioeconomic disadvantage; economic stressors; job stress; being nonwhite; having low social capital, trust and cohesion; racial and other forms of discrimination; limited social support or social networks; poor built environments; crime and low personal safety; deprived and densely populated neighborhoods; social disorganization; poor-quality built environments; and living in adverse environments.

Conversely one favorable determinant, higher levels of green space in low-income neighborhoods, was associated with lower levels of perceived stress. This last example points to the idea that any of the determinants, if seen as positive, could be considered fruitfully as a means for promoting positive psychological factors—"social determinants of healthy." Further, relationships between factors (negative or positive) and the determinants may be reciprocal, as indicated in Fig. 11–6— for example, depression or optimism leading to restriction or enrichment, respectively, of social networks.

Finally, beyond their contributions to psychological factors, these determinants often contribute to CV outcomes in other ways, in part through behavioral and biological factors and their mutual interactions with psychological ones. The AHA Statement concludes that the traditional view of CVD as caused by physiological, lifestyle, and genetic risk factors must now include the social determinants of health as well. The additional consideration of CVH, defined in terms of seven behavioral and biological factors, as a CV outcome in itself presents another perspective on their relationships with psychological factors. These relationships are considered further below.

Mechanisms

Evidence regarding mechanisms of action by which the determinants affect psychological factors which in turn affect CV outcomes (Fig. 11–3, arrows 3a and 3b) is important to understand associations and identify causal relations, and thereby to recognize potential points of intervention to counter negative and promote positive psychological factors. **Figure 11–7** presents a framework for considering such mechanisms.

Broadly, the negative/positive duality between categories of psychological factors, determinants, and outcomes remains a useful, though simple, distinction. In general, negative determinants result in negative psychological factors, shown in Fig. 11–7 as leading to two kinds of effects—negative behaviors and negative biological factors that together cause reduced CVH and increased CVD. The corresponding relationships of positive determinants and factors promote positive behaviors,

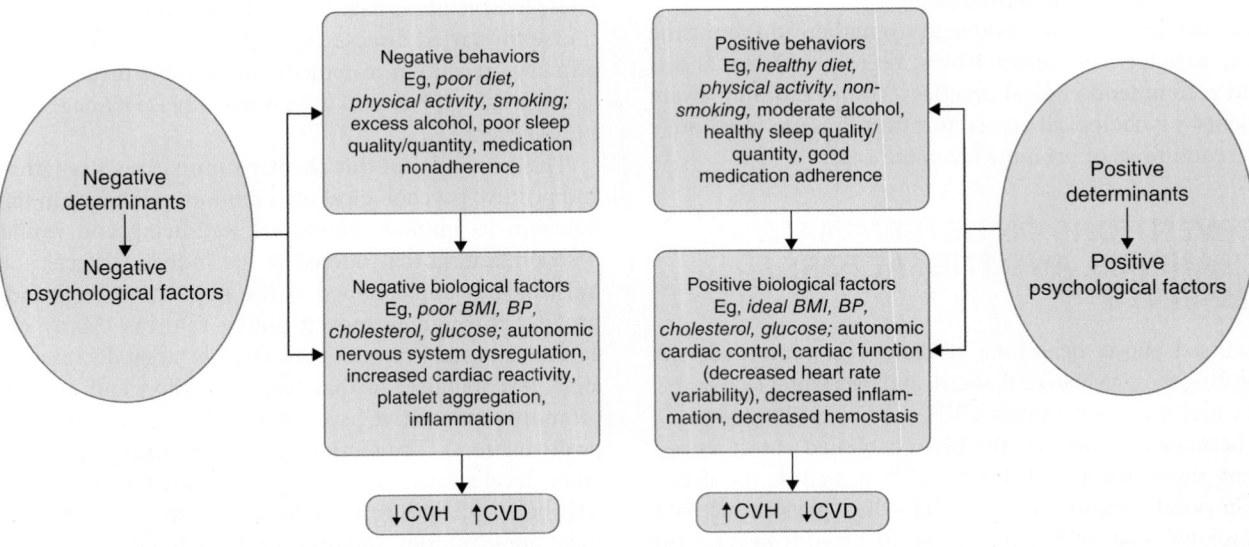

Figure 11–7. Mechanisms of action—determinants and psychological factors.

biological factors, and greater CVH and less CVD. Specific behaviors and biological factors for which evidence is sufficient to comment are illustrated in their respective panels in Fig. 11–7. In each panel, the first entries, in italics, identify the behavioral or biological metrics that define CVH. The additional items are noted in recent reviews as being associated with negative or positive psychological factors.

Overall, each of the indicated relationships has scientific support, albeit often mixed. Study results are in some cases inconsistent in magnitude or even direction of effect measures, due in part to the methodological issues discussed above. Variation in findings might be expected, as well, given the mixed representation of healthy populations versus CV patients; groups of differing age, sex, race, culture, and geography; and study of acute versus chronic psychological states. Though studies of negative factors strongly predominate, the lists of mechanisms with the most meaningful overall evidence are essentially the same, between negative and positive, and opposite in their effects.

Among the most consistent findings, both negative and positive, are those with respect to the CVH metrics—whether considered separately, as behavioral or biological mechanisms, or collectively, as the CVH outcome. Depression, PTSD, and anxiety are associated with poor behavioral and biological mechanisms while, conversely, optimism and PPWB are associated with favorable mechanisms.

One conceptual model of these relationships posits a contrast between "deteriorative" and "restorative" processes, with positive psychological factors both countering the deteriorative and enhancing the restorative ones. Stress, as an external exposure, may be modified directly, or its deteriorative effects buffered, by PPWB.[36] However, Boehm and Kubzansky have noted that distinction between these roles of PPWB has received little study.[13]

Summary

Negative psychological factors have been shown to affect multiple pathophysiological pathways, while positive ones are associated with several favorable biological processes as well as health behaviors and overall well-being.[4,7,13]

Much work remains to be done to strengthen and refine the evidence base for these relationships. Yet it is sufficient at this stage to recommend clinical practices, from becoming aware of patients' psychological status, to intervening to ameliorate adverse conditions or promote favorable ones.

INTERVENTIONS ON DETERMINANTS, MECHANISMS, AND THE FACTORS THEMSELVES

As discussed above, behavioral cardiology is concerned with investigating the psychological, social, and behavioral factors that directly, and indirectly, impact CVH, CVD, and longevity.[4] Of these, behavioral factors are the best-established antecedents—including sleep quality and duration,[37,38] as well as the defining behavioral components of CVH—diet, physical activity, and smoking. The field is increasing in breadth beyond the detrimental effects of negative psychological factors such as depression alone and now also includes investigation of positive psychological assets such as optimism.

The preceding discussion suggests that interventions could potentially apply at multiple points along the course of development of CVH and CVD (Fig. 11–3, points 4a–e): They could address determinants, their mechanisms of action, the psychological factors themselves, the mechanisms of their effects of CVH and CVD, or CVH and CVD as outcomes to be promoted or prevented. They could be intended to counter negative or support positive psychological factors that may result from determinants operating at individual, community, or societal levels (Fig. 11–6). And they could act on either negative or positive behaviors and biological factors as remedial or primordial interventions, respectively, in order to reduce adverse or promote favorable CV status (Fig. 11–7). Accordingly, the types of interventions that are available or could be developed are wide-ranging in their approaches, strength of evidence for their effectiveness, and current extent of implementation. The following discussion illustrates some of the types of interventions presently available and where they fit along this array.

Figure 11–8 presents a framework detailing the multiple levels in which intervention are delivered, at the individual level or to a broader segment of the population, and across different domains of influence, and targeting behavioral factors (eg, healthy eating), the physical or built environment, or entire health care systems. In an effort to promote CVH, a multipronged approach is necessary and can involve health professionals delivering individual counseling to their patients or advocating for changes to the health care system to modify treatment access and delivery. It also can involve other key players including community-based organizations, policymakers, and governmental agencies.

Some behavioral interventions have been designed to boost psychological health and promote factors of resilience as a means to promote healthy longevity.[36] To date, multiple trials have tested the impact of strengths-based behavioral interventions on psychological well-being and indicators of CVH. These interventions have targeted improvements across the life course for varied disease states—for instance, for purposes of primary prevention to remedy unfavorable measures of CVH or secondary prevention to improve disease management after a CVD event.

The remainder of this chapter summarizes strengths-based and positive psychological interventions published in the field, that aim to improve emotional well-being and resilience—first, presenting that offered at the individual-level, followed by strategies implemented at the population level and more broadly through proposed policy reforms. Many of these evidence-based strategies concurrently target decreases in negative psychological factors (eg, depression and anxiety) and promotion of positive psychological factors (eg, optimism and positive affect). The section ends with identification of population-level strategies targeting determinants of psychological well-being, including such factors as social capital, employment opportunities, and overt or implicit policies and practices based on racial and ethnic differences.

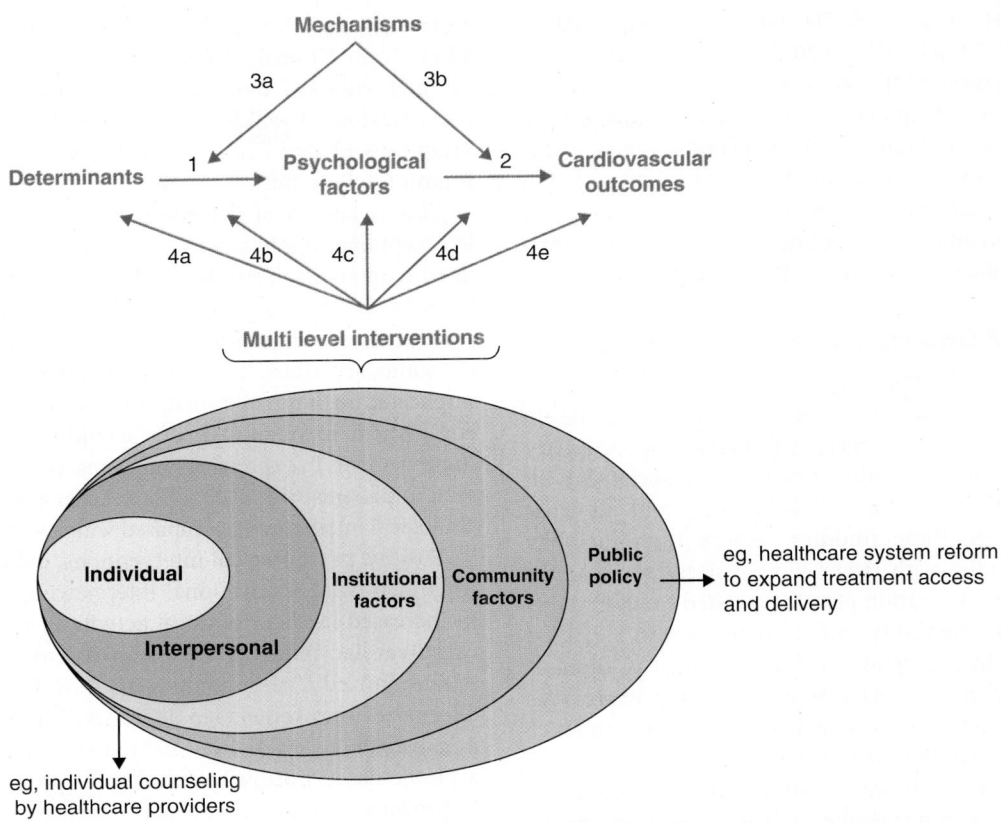

Figure 11–8. Ecological Levels of Intervention Implementation to Improve Psychological Health. Expanding on the framework linking determinants with psychological factors and downstream CVH outcomes, we now illustrate the multiple levels for delivery of strengths-based interventions. Specifically, interventions can be deployed at the individual level or more broadly though targeting of entire communities or larger ecological systems (eg, state-level policies). These multipronged strategies can effect change directly on determinants, psychological factors, and CVH outcomes, or they can indirectly act as modifiers that change the impact that each exerts.

Stress Management

Reductions in anxiety and stress have been targets of multiple intervention programs. These programs, not typically designed to directly heighten psychological health but instead focused more on alleviating psychiatric syndromes (eg, generalized anxiety), nonetheless present collateral benefits by augmenting levels of psychological well-being. Three randomized trials test the efficacy of psychotherapy as a form of stress reduction to improve health outcomes in patients with diagnosed heart disease. Gulliksson et al. (2011) compared group-based cognitive behavioral therapy (CBT) with treatment-as-usual, in a trial that included patients hospitalized in the past 12 months for a CHD event (ie, MI, percutaneous coronary intervention, or coronary artery bypass grafting [CABG]).[39] Patients who participated in the yearlong CBT arm experienced a 41% lower rate of fatal and nonfatal first recurrent CVD events (hazard ratio [HR], 0.59, 95% CI 0.42–0.83, $p = 0.002$) when compared to those receiving standard care, after adjusting for possible confounders.[39] In contrast, after approximately 12 months of follow-up, no differences in psychological well-being or cardiac health were observed when comparing treatment-as-usual to programs implementing stepped-care psychotherapy, psychiatric screening paired with a home-based nursing intervention, and a nurse-delivered stepped depression intervention.[40–43]

Mindfulness

Evidence is also accumulating on the benefits of mindfulness-based interventions.[44,45] Mindfulness is a practice focused on paying attention to the present moment, while exploring one's thoughts and feelings both calmly and with curiosity, nonjudgmentally. In relatively healthy adults, those with no preexisting cardiac conditions, engagement in mindfulness practice is associated with reductions in anxiety, stress, and symptoms of depression, improved quality of life and physical functioning, higher rates of smoking cessation, and greater engagement in healthful behaviors (eg, exercise, healthy dietary adherence).[46–48] Mindfulness is also associated with increased energy, eagerness, intrinsic motivation, healthier immune and cognitive function, neuroplasticity, and social connectedness.[49–51]

In primary prevention, in adults with preexisting CVD risk factors, mindfulness is associated with improved weight loss,[52] BP[53] and glucose control,[54,55] greater engagement in self-management practices,[54,55] and use of more healthful coping strategies.[53] Mindfulness for secondary prevention has also been tested. A meta-analysis pooling data across eight randomized trials and inclusive of 578 patients with vascular disease (including heart disease) found that mindfulness-based interventions, when compared to control conditions, were associated with greater reductions in stress (standard mean difference ([SMD]: −0.36; 95% CI: −0.67 to −0.09; p = 0.01), anxiety (SMD: −0.50; 95% CI: −0.70 to −0.29; p < 0.001), and symptoms of depression (SMD: −0.35; 95% CI: −0.53 to −0.16; p = 0.003), with effects largely evident at the 8-week follow-up.[56] Triangulating these findings, a 2019 systematic review summarizing data across 16 trials found that mindfulness-based interventions resulted in greater improvements in a variety of mental health outcomes (eg, anxiety, depression, and stress) and significant reductions in systolic BP in adults with CVD.[57]

Meditation and Other Mind-Body Techniques

Meditation, often a component of mindfulness-based interventions, also has recorded cardio protective effects. Modestly sized single-center studies targeting primary and secondary prevention find that meditation practice is associated with significant reductions in nonfatal MI, CVD- and all-cause mortality; although, these findings require reproducibility in multicenter studies with larger sample sizes.[58-61] In adults with hypertension, meditation practice resulted in lower overall rates of all-cause mortality; and, in patients with HF, it led to improvements in depression and management of disease-related symptoms.[62] A recent AHA Scientific Statement provides a comprehensive review of the benefits of meditation practice and associated interventions for cardiac risk reduction.[61]

Though findings remain somewhat mixed, when results are pooled across single-center studies and meta-analyses, meditation practice is generally associated with reductions in anxiety, negative affect, perceived stress, higher rates of smoking cessation, and moderate reductions in systolic and diastolic BP values. Conclusions of AHA identify meditation as a promising adjunct therapy to existing risk reduction methods for CVD, particularly given low risk and associated cost effectiveness. They do recommend, however, implementation of larger multicenter studies with more rigorous methodologies to improve overall quality and to deter potential risk of bias in data collection.

Other related mind-body techniques that have undergone clinical testing include activities such as yoga, tai chi, deep breathing exercises, and guided imagery, among other, which also show evidence for improvements in psychological health.[63-66] In HF patients, tai chi and yoga have resulted in improvements across multiple cardiac outcomes, and, in other CVD-related groups, improvements in BP and exercise capacity have been recorded.

Other Positive Psychology Interventions

Positive psychological interventions systematically target boosting of well-being indicators (eg, happiness, optimism, positive affect) through teaching of multiple evidence-based skills. These include not only mindfulness and meditation, but also identification of positive events in daily life, positive reappraisal of negative events, engagement in acts of kindness, and use of personal intrinsic strengths. Sustained positive effects on psychological health are consistently documented for positive psychological interventions when delivered in healthy adults, with evidence summarized in systematic reviews and meta-analyses.[67,68] A 2013 meta-analysis pooling data of 6139 adults from 39 distinct trials found that positive psychological interventions led to positive sustained effects across multiple indicators of well-being (SMD: 0.34; p = 0.001), including symptoms of depression (SMD: 0.23; p < 0.001), at 3- and 6-month follow-up.[67]

Less is known of the effects of positive psychology-based interventions in adults with CVD or those at risk for cardiac disease. In adults at risk for CVD (eg, patients with type 2 diabetes [T2D] mellitus), positive psychological interventions are associated with improvements in psychological health,[69-71] and on some occasions, these strengths-based interventions are implicated in improved medication adherence[69-72] and greater engagement in other self-care activities. Significantly greater improvements in depressive symptoms (β = −0.21; p = 0.05) were seen in patients with T2D who received a 5-week positive psychological intervention, compared with a waitlist control arm.[70]

Positive psychological interventions, delivered occasionally in tandem with motivational interviewing, have also resulted in increased levels of physical activity in patients with preexisting cardiac illness when compared to control conditions. A randomized trial in adults with ACS documented medium effect size improvements in depressive symptoms, anxiety, and positive affect (SMD: 0.47-0.71) after patients participated in a phone-based positive psychological program for 8 weeks.[73] Improvements in functional performance are also seen in clinical samples.

However, such strengths-based interventions present mixed findings when targeting cardiac biomarkers. Some trials find positive psychology-based interventions to be associated with positive changes in heart rate variability (HRV) and markers of inflammation in HF patients (ie, CRP, TNF-α, IL-6, and sTNFr1),[74] modest improvements in glycosylated hemoglobin in patients with diabetes, and minimal effects across other relevant biomarkers.[75] More recently, in a randomized trial where patients with coronary artery disease received optimism training, significant improvements were seen across multiple biological markers, including high-sensitivity C-reactive protein, fibrinogen, and irisin, compared to an active control condition.[76] However, two large single-center trials illustrate inconsistency of findings. After implementing a positive psychology-based intervention targeting improvements in BP control over a 1-year period, investigators reported no differences in systolic and diastolic values when compared to an active control condition.[71,77]

The studies described thus far focus on delivery of strengths-based interventions at an individual level or within the context of a small group setting. Less is known about higher-level interventions targeting entire communities at the societal level. Larger benefits can be derived by targeting improvements in psychological health at the community-level by partnering with workplace settings, churches, or other neighborhood-based organizations. Thus far, positive psychological interventions have been used in the school setting with adolescents[78,79] and in older adults through partnership with senior centers.[80]

These community-based interventions have resulted in improvements in quality of life and emotional well-being, with reductions in symptoms of depression and physical complaints.[79,80] Two randomized, controlled trials (RCTs) testing interventions aimed at cultivating gratitude and enhanced engagement in acts of kindness, in university students, resulted in greater levels of positive affect and academic engagement.[81] A church-based intervention in Hispanic/Latinos adults at risk for CVD found improvements in subjective happiness, emotional vitality, and engagement in happiness-inducing behavior (eg, meditation).[82]

The richest developments in strengths-based interventions have occurred in the context of work-site-based programs. This is particularly relevant in the United States where a majority of adults are employed and often identify work as a significant stressor. And, the literature suggests that work-related stress and long work hours are associated with greater risk of developing CVD.[83] In the UK, a 5-week online positive psychological intervention made available through the workplace, resulted in significant improvements in positive affect and flourishing, when compared to a waitlist control group.[84] In 2018, the AHA published the *Workplace Health Playbook* focused on fostering resilience in the workplace.[85] Rooted in theories of positive psychology, these resiliency-based interventions have resulted in small but significant improvements in psychological and physical health, accompanied by enhancements in work-based performance.[85,86]

Finally, although individual-level concepts of positive psychological interventions have yet to be applied explicitly across entire communities, there are concerted efforts targeting improvements in CVH in specific community settings.[87] For example, Chicago and San Diego are engaged in community-wide efforts to improve population health through their signature programs, the *Healthy Chicago/Healthy Hearts Action Plan*[88] and *Be There San Diego*,[89] both aiming to reduce incidence of CVD and stroke. San Diego County aspires to become "heart healthy and stroke free" and is one of some 30 sentinel communities in the Robert Wood Johnson Foundation *Culture of Health Initiative*.[90] This Initiative seeks to "make health a shared value, fostering cross-sector collaboration to improve well-being, creating healthier, more equitable communities, and strengthening integration of health services and systems."

Summary

Several examples of individual-level interventions to improve psychological health illustrate potential clinical practices, including stress management, mindfulness, meditation, and other mind-body techniques, and further positive psychology approaches. Evidence syntheses support the concept that such interventions can result in sustained positive changes in healthy populations. Less is known about their specific effects in patients with CVD, or in promoting and preserving ideal CVH. However, strength-based interventions have been shown in some, but not all, studies to be associated with such biomarkers as HRV and inflammatory markers, mechanisms that connect both psychological and behavioral factors with CVH and CVD.

Community-level intervention programs designed to improve population CVH and prevent CVD include worksite wellness programs and school health activities, among others. They offer opportunities for more explicit and fully developed application of principles and concepts of positive psychology. Insofar as these become well developed and adequately evaluated, they may be implemented in public health practice and policy as well as in clinical settings.

CLINICAL TEAM, COMMUNITY LEADERS, AND POLICYMAKERS

Clinical Team

Clinic encounters with patients in the hospital or outpatient medical setting provide ample opportunity for cardiologists and front-line staff (eg, medical assistants, nurses) to assess and intervene on indicators of psychological well-being—which, as the literature suggests, can lead to positive upstream CV effects. Multiple systematic approaches are available to assess psychological health during a cardiology encounter to identify mild to major depression or optimism and psychological well-being as discussed above.[2,25] Brief validated instruments are available to measure whether a patient is experiencing elevated symptoms of depression or anxiety; these include the two-item measures known as the Patient Health Questionnaire-2[91] and the Generalized Anxiety-Disorder questionnaire-2,[92] among others. Screening tools facilitate initial assessment as to whether a cardiac patient or patient at risk for CVD is experiencing emotional distress, which may elicit a discussion on symptomatology and the perceived consequences to overall health and functioning—or, it may trigger the need for immediate follow-up or a referral to a mental health specialist.

In certain patient populations, such as hemodialysis patients (who are at increased risk for CVD), screening for depression is federally mandated and often prompts development of a treatment plan and next steps for follow-up. When this is not the case, however, front-line staff can use clinical encounters to probe patients on feelings of optimism, positive emotion, and happiness, and their overall intrinsic motivation, and how these might impact engagement in important self-care activities (eg, healthy eating, physical activity). Potential screening items have been previously published and include questions such as, "How do you think things will go with your health in the future," "How often do you experience pleasure or happiness in your life."[36]

Clinical cardiologists may not always feel equipped to initiate a detailed discussion on mental health with their patients. However, after screening positive for a possible psychiatric syndrome, brief targeted discussions delivered by front-line staff are perceived as valuable and highly effective by patients. **Table 11–2** presents possible probes or points of discussion when addressing mental health with patients during a clinical encounter.[36] A dialogue focused on health-related optimism and gratitude may flow seamlessly within the typical conversation of a clinical encounter—and it is precisely these well-being indicators that are consistently linked to superior cardiac recovery after a CVD event.

After determining whether a referral to a mental health specialist is warranted, clinicians can complement these services

TABLE 11–2. Brief Clinician Questions and Statements to Address and Promote Psychological Well-being during Clinical Encounters

Characteristic or Asset	Questions and Sample Statements
Optimism	Questions: • "Do you expect that good things will happen for you in the future?" • "How do you think things will go with your health in the future?" Sample statements to support positive psychological well-being: *I have managed many patients with this health problem before, and I have seen many of them do very well. I think you can, too.*
Positive affect or life satisfaction	Questions: • "How often do you experience pleasure or happiness in your life?" • "Are you satisfied with how your life has gone and how you have lived it?" Sample statements to support positive psychological well-being: *There is a lot of research finding connections between feeling happy and satisfied with your life, and your heart health. So I want to really support you in taking time for yourself and engaging in [healthy hobbies or meaningful activities].*
Gratitude	Questions: • "What, if anything, do you have to feel grateful for in your life?" • "Do you ever feel grateful about your health? Tell me about that." Sample statements to support positive psychological well-being: *We were lucky to catch this problem when we did, and I think that means that there is a good chance that your health can remain strong if we work together.*
Leveraging personal strengths	Questions: • "What are your greatest strengths and skills?" • "When have you applied your best skills to improving your health?" Sample statements to support positive psychological well-being: *I have been so impressed with how you have succeeded in your life when [life situation]. You can use those same skills to be successful in taking care of your heart health.*

Reproduced with permission from Kubzansky LD, Huffman JC, Boehm JK, et al. Positive Psychological Well-Being and Cardiovascular Disease: JACC Health Promotion Series. *J Am Coll Cardiol*. 2018 Sep 18;72(12):1382-1396.

with "prescriptions" for patients to engage in activities known to boost psychological and cardiac health, such as exercise, mindfulness meditation, or other self-care activities; recommendations can be annotated on prescription-pad-style paper to heighten credibility and stimulate positive change. The Chicago-based *Food Rx* program[93] provides coupons and community resources tailored on nutritional recommendations of the attending physician. Exercise prescription can be individually tailored based on age and underlying medical conditions and can offer evidence-based details on type, dosage, and frequency of exercise activities. For example, in Vermont and South Dakota physicians are writing prescriptions recommending that patients go hiking and that they spend time outdoors to enjoy nature. These discussions can be time consuming in a setting with tight time constraints. But they are well worth the investment if they help identify substantial psychosocial barriers leading to poor adherence and risky behaviors. This can translate into reduced morbidity and cost savings through better adherence, enhanced quality of life, and improved CV outcomes.

Technology has a major role to play in supplementing efforts of clinicians. Known as behavioral health technologies (BITs),[94,95] behavioral medicine is advancing the science that leverages state-of-the-art technology to deliver mental health services to improve psychological and physical health. BITs include systems such as telehealth, mobile health apps, and Internet sites, all meant to digitally dispense intervention strategies to improve physical and emotional well-being in healthy and clinical samples. Technological interventions have shown efficacy comparable to traditional face-to-face therapy and offer the ability to "scale up" proven interventions to much larger numbers of end users without comparable increases in cost. Because many of these interventions are self-paced and incorporate practices into daily life, they can transcend geographical space and time.[94] BITs have proven a useful tool to improve human wellness. In **Box 11–3**, we present a case study in which a 5-week positive psychological intervention was delivered chairside using Apple iPads in hemodialysis patients during maintenance treatment. This pilot trial documents significant improvements in depressive symptoms from baseline to immediately post intervention at 5 weeks.[96]

Community Leaders

Less is known about the role that community organizations and governmental policies play in promoting psychological health. Only recently are governments across the world systematically including well-being measures in their national polls—asking, for instance, "*All things considered, how satisfied are you with your life as a whole these days*?" In the last decade, questions probing life satisfaction, social cohesion, and positive/negative affect, among others, were incorporated into national measures deployed in Italy, Israel, Canada,

BOX 11–3. CASE STUDY: INTERNET-BASED POSITIVE PSYCHOLOGICAL INTERVENTION IN HEMODIALYSIS PATIENTS[96]

Depression is the most pervasive psychological issue experienced in hemodialysis (HD) patients and it serves as a significant added burden with one-third of HD patients in the United States reporting compromised psychological health. Comorbid depression considerably exacerbates disease progression and is associated with lower rates of adherence to dialysis prescriptions, increased markers of systemic inflammation, compromised cellular immunity, greater risk of hospitalization, and decreased survival.

A positive psychological intervention delivered remotely using investigator-purchased tablet computers may serve as a low-resource intensive strategy to reduce symptoms of depression and enhance associated psychological assets in HD patients. Accordingly, HD patients (n = 14) with elevated symptoms of depression were enrolled in a single-arm pre-post trial with clinical assessments at baseline and immediately post intervention. Chairside during regularly scheduled HD treatment, patients utilized a web browser to complete online modules promoting skills for increasing positive emotion over a 5-week period using Apple iPads. Targeted skills included noting of daily positive events, gratitude, positive reappraisal, acts of kindness, and mindfulness/meditation.

Twelve of 14 patients completed the program for an 85.7% retention rate. Participants felt satisfied with each session and offered consistently positive feedback. On average, participants visited the website 3.5 times per week. Significant improvements were evident for depressive symptoms (15.3 vs 10.9; $p = 0.04$), as per the Center for Epidemiological Studies Depression Scale. This case highlights important concerns when delivering services in the clinical setting to patients with, or at risk for, CVD: (1) use of technology may be an inexpensive option to deliver mental health programming, (2) opportunities should be explored during clinic encounters or treatment sessions when patients have downtime and are receptive to educational programming, and (3) more counter intuitive technology should be explored that minimizes need to consume textual content and that requires little tech savviness—this includes use of fully immersive virtual reality requiring a head-mounted display.

and the UK. And, there are instances where findings have informed policy. For instance, survey results of the UK found low levels of social connectedness in their older adult population. As a result, the "Silver Line" hotline, was created, which resulted in 70% of older adult callers indicating improvements in their social life and levels of happiness; after which, the first UK Minister of Loneliness was appointed in 2018.[97] As such, at the population level, systematic monitoring is an important first step in informing policy change aimed at improving well-being profiles.

Growing awareness of the importance and impact of community leadership in determining the health status of populations is reflected in the initiatives discussed previously—in Chicago, San Diego, and the Robert Wood Johnson Foundation Sentinel Communities. When communities of multiple kinds are considered—not only localities such as neighborhoods or political units, but also schools, worksites, regional or national organizations, and health systems—the potential roles of community leaders can be more fully appreciated. As CVH promotion assumes greater prominence as a clinical, community, and societal priority, community leadership can be expected to contribute significantly.

Policymakers

First launched in Australia, Europe, and Canada, the *Health in All Policies* (HiAP) approach is now being considered and adopted across US local and state governments.[98] The HiAP advocates for consideration of social determinants of health and associated disease outcomes across all policymaking sectors regardless of their jurisdiction or area of oversight.[99] HiAP recognizes that multiplex factors contribute to societal health, and as such, overall responsibility extends well beyond the health care system. In this way, HiAP represents an approach to societal issues that could be considered more explicitly as a high-level strategy to improve population CVH, as well as other social priorities.

A coordinated approach is necessary where all public sectors are charged with advocating for policies that enhance population health, thus removing sole onus on the public health sector. Parks and recreation and the housing authority have responsibility for enacting policies that are geared toward health promotion, for example ensuring access to greenspace, affordable housing in neighborhoods with low disorder and violence.[98] Cross-sector communication and systems of evaluation can lead to synergistic efforts, which for instance, simultaneously target building of better transportation infrastructures (eg, safe paths for walking and biking) and that sponsor reductions in carbon emissions and air pollutants. These cross-sector efforts can more efficiently give rise to environments that by default promote psychological health, which can lead to positive downstream effects on health behaviors and CVD risk factors (eg, reductions in obesity and sedentarism).

Under this new paradigm, all governmental agencies collaborate to ensure that residents have access to safe outdoor space, local fresh produce, and affordable health care access, among others. Finally, HiAP efforts at the municipal and state levels may further benefit by deploying evidence-based skillsets identified in well-being science though implementation of low-cost and brief resiliency-based interventions at the community or neighborhood level. Indeed, concerted cross-sector policies can translate to great synergistic gains at the population level.

Another area for focused governmental policy is targeting of antecedents or upstream social determinants that directly impact psychological health—in other words, intervening on factors that negatively impact psychological well-being. The literature consistently finds that low socioeconomic status as measured by education and income, unemployment, and limited social capital are all associated with lower levels of psychological health.[36,100–102] For instance, the gross domestic product

(GDP) in both developed and developing countries shows a positive correlation with levels of happiness and life satisfaction. Policies that promote affordable access to higher education and that provide job training in growing industrial sectors (eg, renewable energy jobs), particularly in vulnerable or underserved populations, have the potential to promote financial stability and mobility, which can lead to improvements in psychological health.[98]

A prime example of national policy is the 1972 Equal Employment Opportunity Act, which safeguards against discrimination in hiring practices based on factors of race/ethnicity, gender, and sexual orientation.[103] Anti-discrimination policies that are strictly enforced can continue to be useful tools to ensure equitable job opportunities for the US populace and to promote equal distribution of gains in well-being. Another example illustrates state-level policy, whereby lawmakers in Hawaii sought to allow physicians to prescribe 6 months of subsidized housing for homeless patients.

Finally, policies regarding reimbursement for mental health treatment could remove a barrier to receiving psychotherapy or other mental health services. A value-based payment approach takes a holistic view of medicine where lifestyle counseling and programs to enhance psychological health are viewed as essential components for positive health outcomes and as effectual targets for long-term cost savings—and, some large health systems are embracing this approach, including Kaiser Permanente Medical Group and the Benson-Henry Institute for Mind Body Medicine at the Massachusetts General Hospital.

Summary

The clinical team, community leaders, and policymakers all have potential to impact the psychological factors influential in CVH and CVD in multiple complementary ways. Through the work of Rozanski in championing behavioral cardiology and of others engaged in evaluation of positive psychological interventions, approaches to this aspect of patient care have become more widely recognized. The provider team, which may include other health professionals experienced in assessment of psychological factors and social circumstances, can collectively determine patients' assets and liabilities as a basis for their management. Applying available tools in practice and learning from the experience can be expected to lead to more effective care.

Community leaders and influential policymakers can make essential contributions to improving population CVH by adapting principles and concepts of behavioral cardiology and positive psychology to community and societal levels of action. Examples of such developments offer promise of wider implementation of these concepts in the future.

FUTURE RESEARCH AND PRACTICE

Research

There is need and opportunity for further research to deepen understanding of the relation between psychological factors and CV outcome—both CVH and CVD, including stroke. A 2012 review called for studies to address methodologic challenges in measurement and conceptualization of psychological factors, greater use of longitudinal rather than cross-sectional designs, and specific emphasis on the CV role of optimism, among other issues.[13] These remain important considerations in setting research priorities.

The science informing how psychological well-being is measured is in need of further development, along with consideration and inclusion of non-Western constructs and viewpoints. The field needs to come to consensus on terminology, how psychological well-being is conceptualized, what domains should be included, and identification of the best survey instruments. Psychological well-being is largely captured using self-report surveys. Technology should be mined to explore more objective indicators of emotional well-being, such as facial recognition, voice frequency or vibration, or skin conductance, among other possible techniques.

Regardless of methods in measuring psychological well-being, cultural differences should be at the forefront, especially given the US diversity in race/ethnicity. Race/ethnicity may dictate how psychological health is expressed and interpreted as informed by social norms, historical events, and cultural systems—and measures traditionally used in those of European ancestry may not perform well in minority populations. Indeed, instrument malfunctioning can result from biases related to social desirability, flawed translation, or problematic wording of items that constrain understanding, dissimilar interpretation and responses across positively and negatively worded items, that is, differential item functioning, and imperfect Likert-based response options or problematic formatting, among others.

The field is expanding to be more inclusive of non-Western cultural experiences when conceptualizing indicators of psychological health. This is especially important in the United States, which has great racial/ethnic diversity and where Eastern philosophies inform beliefs of numerous racial/ethnic groups (eg, Hispanics/Latinos, Asian-Pacific Islanders); in fact, according to the Eastern worldview, more low arousal emotional states such as tranquility and balance are valued and communal well-being of family and friends is favored over individualistic parameters.[104] Recently, the Gallup World Poll (GWP) and Well-Being for Planet Earth Foundation teamed up to design a more inclusive global measure of well-being where culturally relevant questions are identified and included in their international polls to ensure a global well-being perspective.[105] The new GWP expands items to include the following indicators of psychological health: (1) low-arousal emotion (eg, calm), (2) feelings of balance or harmony, (3) communal well-being and connectivity to family and friends, and (4) metrics of meaning and purpose in life.[105] A more global and cross-cultural perspective is also important when designing positive psychological interventions in the United States, particularly when targeting racial/ethnic minority groups. As an example, the Spanish-language "¡*Alégrate!*" ["*Be Happy!*"] positive psychological intervention targeting Hispanic/Latino adults with hypertension, was adapted from previously published and empirically validated curricula, with additional content informed by formative qualitative work identifying the cultural importance of infusing curricular activities with aspects of religiosity and familialism (ie, the ideology of putting family first).[82,106]

A research agenda outlined in 2016 included six lines of investigation: methodologic studies, population studies, mechanistic studies, intervention studies, modeling studies, and policy studies. Each area would require specific hypotheses, multidisciplinary collaborations bridging preventive cardiology and positive psychology, and appropriate laboratory, clinical, and population settings.[7] A more fully developed agenda will specify research questions in detail and seek the funding needed to make substantial progress in the near future.

Particular emphasis has been placed on the importance of well-designed and executed intervention trials. Clearly these are needed to further inform clinical practice and establish the optimum approaches to both ameliorating negative psychological factors and strengthening positive ones. The several points of intervention indicated in Fig. 11–3 offer opportunities for investigation, with targets among the determinants, the factors themselves, states of CVH or CVD, and the mechanisms linking them. Correspondingly, several levels of outcomes are suggested, not only CVD events and their sequelae. It is important to know more about interventions to promote, preserve, and improve psychological health and well-being, as well as their impact on intervening behavioral and biological factors and both CVH and CVD as ultimate outcomes. Implementation and dissemination research will contribute significantly to putting effective practices into widespread use.

An innovative technology with potential utility in intervention is fully immersive virtual reality (VR), where end users wear a head-mounted display that uses tracking systems and physical motion to navigate digitally created artificial worlds. This is another potential tool to deliver evidence-based programming in the cardiology setting. VR technology is most frequently used in video gaming and for simulation training with clinicians and military personnel.[107–109] More recently, VR technology has been included in treatment plans for pain management (eg, burn victims), physical rehabilitation, and in treatment of psychological phobias (eg, acrophobia or fear of heights), with evident improvements in emotional well-being and lessening of physical complaints.[110–114] VR merits evaluation in intervention research given its potential for application in the clinical cardiology setting.

At the community level, programs such as school health, worksite wellness, and others require rigorous evaluation including assessment of their feasibility, acceptability, costs, and impact on indicators of community health. How closely they can be replicated in varied social, cultural, and economic settings, and the extent to which they must be adapted to be impactful in such different circumstances, are all questions for investigation if promising programs are to be disseminated effectively.

At the still broader societal level, attention has been urged for research on social determinants of health in relation to CVH and CVD.[35] Specific topics to be addressed include previously under-recognized institutionalized racism, intergenerational transmission of social disadvantage, interactions among social factors, and others. Resulting knowledge is expected to inform policies that will have broad societal impact. In the US context of 2020 and beyond, the fundamental importance of these issues in enabling effective community- and patient-level programs and practices is clearer than ever before.

Finally, as a framework for undertaking all of the proposed research, there is a need for further epidemiologic research on distributions and disparities in occurrence of the psychological factors of interest. In contrast to depression and other negative psychological factors,[10] epidemiology of optimism and other components of PPWB has received less attention.[115] Further standardization of definitions and methods for measurement of these factors will greatly facilitate this work.

Practice

Future growth of the evidence base on psychological factors in CVH and CVD is anticipated from research in the areas outlined above. But evidence is sufficient now to guide practice by cardiologists and other health professionals in caring for patients to promote CVH and prevent CVD. For example, Rozanski has championed the development of behavioral cardiology, citing evidence on both negative and positive social and psychological factors and their relationship with CVD. He proposes a "tiered behavioral care delivery system" to further develop this field. His system includes health counseling/coaching, emotional/cognitive counseling, stress management, goal setting, and social support.[4] He calls for action to increase recognition of the importance of these factors, to overcome challenges to bringing about change in cardiology practice especially in the contemporary context of rapid social change.

To realize this development in practice may depend not only on pursuit of the research agenda outlined above but on initiative taken in practice to implement and evaluate direct practitioner experience. Green argued in 2008 for the concept of "practice-based evidence" to complement, and perhaps exceed, the impact the traditional view that "pushing information to the practitioner" would suffice to bring about progress.[116] Relevant at all three levels considered here—individual, community, and societal—is the following perspective:

What practitioners in clinical, community, and policy making roles crave, it appears, is more evidence from practices or populations like their own, more evidence-based in real time, real jurisdictions, typical patients, without all the screening and control, and staff like their own. The ideal setting in which to conduct such studies would be their own … [p. i23]

Given current evidence, practitioners can take the lead in adopting strengths-based strategies into procedural practice. In this way, practitioners use clinical encounters to introduce the concept of psychological well-being to their patients, with discussion of its importance to cardiac health, and subsequent recommendation of activities to boost emotional well-being. However, clinicians will need to determine best ways to disseminate the information. That is, is it best done before, during, or after the clinical encounter and what co-provider might best deliver the message on benefits of psychological well-being, for example nurse practitioner, physician, or medical assistant? Or, is it best introduced during a "teachable moment," perhaps in the context a new medical diagnosis when patients are most susceptible to medical advice and strategies to lessen disease impact? And, how might technology be used to deliver the message? After implementing these strategies, practitioners can scan their clinical data, viewed using electronic medical systems (if possible), to see if trends are evident where positive gains are seen across metrics of CVH, both behavioral (if diet, physical activity, and smoking are appropriately documented) and biological (BMI, BP, cholesterol, and BG). In this way, providers generate practice-based solutions to promote CVH, prevent CVD, and extend healthy longevity.

Summary

Research on psychological factors in CVH and CVD has grown in scale and quality, sufficient to increase understanding and point to candidate approaches to intervention affecting the impact of these factors in patient and population health. The methodologic considerations discussed above continue to be addressed, and a substantial research agenda remains to be fulfilled. Among the several aspects identified, well-designed and executed trials of candidate interventions have been emphasized in recent reviews of the field. Additional areas needing special attention are social determinants of health—favorable and unfavorable; cultural differences in psychological health, its contribution to CVH and CVD, and efficacy of interventions; and utility of new technologies, such as VR, in improvement in psychological well-being.

Application of current knowledge, and insights to be gained through expanded research, can be expected to grow at all levels of practice—patient care, community programs, and policy development. However, the long-recognized lag between scientific progress and translation into practice should be overcome for this progress to have meaningful impact in the near future. The concept of "practice-based evidence" is complementary to the suggested research priority of intervention trials. More generally, implementation and evaluation of practices for assessment and improvement of psychological factors can both accelerate the research and foster more timely adoption of its findings.

It can be hoped that through these developments the value of understanding the role of psychological factors in CVH and CVD will be translated soon into greatly improved patient and population CVH, with corresponding reduction in deaths, disabilities, and disparities attributable to the global CV problem of today.

REFERENCES

1. Rozanski A, Blumenthal JA, Kaplan J. Impact of psychological factors on the pathogenesis of cardiovascular disease and implications for therapy. *Circulation*. 1999;99(16):2192-2217.

2. Lichtman JH, Bigger Jr JT, Blumenthal JA, et al. Depression and coronary heart disease: recommendations for screening, referral, and treatment: a science advisory from the American Heart Association

Prevention Committee of the Council on Cardiovascular Nursing, Council on Clinical Cardiology, Council on Epidemiology and Prevention, and Interdisciplinary Council on Quality of Care and Outcomes Research: endorsed by the American Psychiatric Association. *Circulation*. 2008;118(17):1768-1775.

3. Steptoe A, Kivimäki M. Stress and cardiovascular disease: an update on current knowledge. *Annu Rev Public Health*. 2013;34:337-354.

4. Rozanski A. Behavioral cardiology: current advances and future directions. *J Am Coll Cardiol*. 2014;64(1):100-110.

5. Lloyd-Jones DM, Hong Y, Labarthe D, et al. Defining and setting national goals for cardiovascular health promotion and disease reduction: the American Heart Association's strategic Impact Goal through 2020 and beyond. *Circulation*. 2010;121(4):586-613.

6. Virani SS, Alonso A, Benjamin EJ, et al. Heart disease and stroke statistics—2020 update: a report from the American Heart Association. *Circulation*. 2020:E139-E596.

7. Labarthe DR, Kubzansky LD, Boehm JK, Lloyd-Jones DM, Berry JD, Seligman ME. Positive cardiovascular health: a timely convergence. *J Am Coll Cardiol*. 2016;68(8):860-867.

8. Strasser T. Reflections on cardiovascular diseases. *Interdiscipl Sci Rev*. 1978;3(3):225-230.

9. Turco JV, Inal-Veith A, Fuster V. Cardiovascular health promotion: an issue that can no longer wait. *J Am Coll Cardiol*. 2018.

10. Kessler RC, de Jonge P, Shahly V, van Loo HM, Wang PS-E, Wilcox MA. Epidemiology of depression. 2014.

11. Lloyd-Jones DM, Leip EP, Larson MG, et al. Prediction of lifetime risk for cardiovascular disease by risk factor burden at 50 years of age. *Circulation*. 2006;113(6):791-798.

12. Allen NB, Zhao L, Liu L, et al. Favorable cardiovascular health, compression of morbidity, and healthcare costs: forty-year follow-up of the CHA Study (Chicago Heart Association Detection Project in Industry). *Circulation*. 2017;135(18):1693-1701.

13. Boehm JK, Kubzansky LD. The heart's content: the association between positive psychological well-being and cardiovascular health. *Psychol Bull*. 2012;138(4):655.

14. Levine GN, Cohen BE, Commodore-Mensah Y, et al. Psychological health, well-being, and the mind-heart-body connection: a scientific statement from the American Heart Association. *Circulation*. Under Review.

15. Burton NW, Pakenham KI, Brown WJ. Evaluating the effectiveness of psychosocial resilience training for heart health, and the added value of promoting physical activity: a cluster randomized trial of the READY program. *BMC Public Health*. 2009;9(1):427.

16. Seligman M. The PERMA Model: Your scientific theory of happiness. 2017.

17. Nezu AM, Nezu CM, Lee M, Stern JB. Assessment of depression. 2014.

18. Association AP. Diagnostic and Statistical Manual of Mental Disorders (4th ed.) Washington, DC: American Psychiatric Association. *Developmental Considerations in Treatment*. 1994;35.

19. Kubzansky LD, Sparrow D, Vokonas P, Kawachi I. Is the glass half empty or half full? A prospective study of optimism and coronary heart disease in the normative aging study. *Psychosom Med*. 2001;63(6):910-916.

20. Giltay EJ, Geleijnse JM, Zitman FG, Hoekstra T, Schouten EG. Dispositional optimism and all-cause and cardiovascular mortality ina prospective cohort of elderly Dutch men and women. *Arch Gen Psychiatry*. 2004;61(11):1126-1135.

21. Kim ES, Smith J, Kubzansky LD. Prospective study of the association between dispositional optimism and incident heart failure. *Circ Heart Fail*. 2014;7(3):394-400.

22. Tindle HA, Chang Y, Kuller LH, et al. Optimism, Hostility and Incident Coronary Heart Disease and Mortality in the Women's Health Initiative. Am Heart Assoc; 2008.

23. Vaillant GE. *Aging Well: Surprising Guideposts to a Happier Life from the Landmark Study of Adult Development*. UK: Hachette; 2008.

24. Hernandez R, Kershaw KN, Siddique J, et al. Optimism and cardiovascular health: multi-ethnic study of atherosclerosis (MESA). *Health Behav Policy Rev.* 2015;2(1):62-73.

25. Scheier MF, Carver CS, Bridges MW. Distinguishing optimism from neuroticism (and trait anxiety, self-mastery, and self-esteem): a reevaluation of the Life Orientation Test. *J Pers Soc Psychol.* 1994;67(6):1063.

26. Millstein RA, Chung W-J, Hoeppner BB, et al. Development of the State Optimism Measure. *Gen Hosp psychiatry.* 2019;58:83-93.

27. Lichtman JH, Froelicher ES, Blumenthal JA, et al. Depression as a risk factor for poor prognosis among patients with acute coronary syndrome: systematic review and recommendations: a scientific statement from the American Heart Association. *Circulation.* 2014;129(12):1350-1369.

28. Gan Y, Gong Y, Tong X, et al. Depression and the risk of coronary heart disease: a meta-analysis of prospective cohort studies. *BMC Psychiatry.* 2014;14(1):1-11.

29. Van der Kooy K, van Hout H, Marwijk H, Marten H, Stehouwer C, Beekman A. Depression and the risk for cardiovascular diseases: systematic review and meta analysis. *Int J Geriatr Psychiatry.* 2007;22(7):613-626.

30. Nicholson A, Kuper H, Hemingway H. Depression as an aetiologic and prognostic factor in coronary heart disease: a meta-analysis of 6362 events among 146 538 participants in 54 observational studies. *Eur Heart Journal.* 2006;27(23):2763-2774.

31. Serlachius A, Pulkki-Råback L, Elovainio M, et al. Is dispositional optimism or dispositional pessimism predictive of ideal cardiovascular health? The Young Finns Study. *Psychol Health.* 2015;30(10):1221-1239.

32. Rozanski A, Bavishi C, Kubzansky LD, Cohen R. Association of optimism with cardiovascular events and all-cause mortality: a systematic review and meta-analysis. *JAMA Netw Open.* 2019;2(9):e1912200.

33. Organization WH. Rio political declaration on social determinants of health. Paper presented at: World Conference on Social Determinants of Health, 2011.

34. Prevention OoD, Promotion H. Healthy people 2020 framework. *HealthyPeople gov.* 2018.

35. Havranek E, Mujahid M, Barr D, et al. American Heart Association Council on quality of care and outcomes research, council on epidemiology and prevention, council on cardiovascular and stroke nursing, council on lifestyle and Cardiometabolic health, and stroke council. Social determinants of risk and outcomes for cardiovascular disease: a scientific statement from the American Heart Association. *Circulation.* 2015;132(9):873-898.

36. Kubzansky LD, Huffman JC, Boehm JK, et al. Positive psychological well-being and cardiovascular disease: JACC health promotion series. *J Am Coll Cardiol.* 2018;72(12):1382-1396.

37. Sofi F, Cesari F, Casini A, Macchi C, Abbate R, Gensini GF. Insomnia and risk of cardiovascular disease: a meta-analysis. *Eur J Prev Cardiol.* 2014;21(1):57-64.

38. Cappuccio FP, Cooper D, D'Elia L, Strazzullo P, Miller MA. Sleep duration predicts cardiovascular outcomes: a systematic review and meta-analysis of prospective studies. *Eur Heart J.* 2011;32(12):1484-1492.

39. Gulliksson M, Burell G, Vessby B, Lundin L, Toss H, Svärdsudd K. Randomized controlled trial of cognitive behavioral therapy vs standard treatment to prevent recurrent cardiovascular events in patients with coronary heart disease: Secondary Prevention in Uppsala Primary Health Care project (SUPRIM). *Arch Intern Med.* 2011;171(2):134-140.

40. Frasure-Smith N, Lespérance F, Prince RH, et al. Randomised trial of home-based psychosocial nursing intervention for patients recovering from myocardial infarction. *Lancet.* 1997;350(9076):473-479.

41. Herrmann-Lingen C, Beutel ME, Bosbach A, et al. A stepwise psychotherapy intervention for reducing risk in coronary artery disease (SPIRR-CAD): results of an observer-blinded, multicenter, randomized trial in depressed patients with coronary artery disease. *Psychosom Med.* 2016;78(6):704-715.

42. Pols AD, Adriaanse MC, van Tulder MW, et al. Two-year effectiveness of a stepped-care depression prevention intervention and predictors of incident depression in primary care patients with diabetes type 2 and/or coronary heart disease and subthreshold depression: data from the Step-Dep cluster randomised controlled trial. *BMJ open.* 2018;8(10):e020412.

43. Pols AD, Van Dijk SE, Bosmans JE, et al. Effectiveness of a stepped-care intervention to prevent major depression in patients with type 2 diabetes mellitus and/or coronary heart disease and subthreshold depression: a pragmatic cluster randomized controlled trial. *PloS One.* 2017;12(8):e0181023.

44. Kabat-Zin J. *Full Catastrophe Living: Using the Wisdom of Your Body and Mind to Face Stress, Pain and Illness.* New York: Random House Publishing Group; 1990.

45. Teasdale JD, Segal ZV, Williams JMG, Ridgeway VA, Soulsby JM, Lau MA. Prevention of relapse/recurrence in major depression by mindfulness-based cognitive therapy. *J Consult Clin Psychol.* 2000;68(4):615.

46. Ruffault A, Czernichow S, Hagger MS, et al. The effects of mindfulness training on weight-loss and health-related behaviours in adults with overweight and obesity: a systematic review and meta-analysis. *Obes Res Clin Pract.* 2017;11(5):90-111.

47. Gotink RA, Chu P, Busschbach JJ, Benson H, Fricchione GL, Hunink MM. Standardised mindfulness-based interventions in healthcare: an overview of systematic reviews and meta-analyses of RCTs. *PloS One.* 2015;10(4):e0124344.

48. Oikonomou MT, Arvanitis M, Sokolove RL. Mindfulness training for smoking cessation: a meta-analysis of randomized-controlled trials. *J Health Psychol.* 2017;22(14):1841-1850.

49. Buchholz L. Exploring the promise of mindfulness as medicine. *JAMA.* 2015;314(13):1327-1329.

50. Catalino LI, Fredrickson BL. A Tuesday in the life of a flourisher: the role of positive emotional reactivity in optimal mental health. *Emotion.* 2011;11(4):938.

51. Fredrickson BL, Cohn MA, Coffey KA, Pek J, Finkel SM. Open hearts build lives: positive emotions, induced through loving-kindness meditation, build consequential personal resources. *J Pers Soc Psychol.* 2008;95(5):1045.

52. Olson KL, Emery CF. Mindfulness and weight loss: a systematic review. *Psychosom Med.* 2015;77(1):59-67.

53. Nejati S, Zahiroddin A, Afrookhteh G, Rahmani S, Hoveida S. Effect of group mindfulness-based stress-reduction program and conscious yoga on lifestyle, coping strategies, and systolic and diastolic blood pressures in patients with hypertension. *J Tehran Univ Heart Cent.* 2015;10(3):140.

54. Gregg JA, Callaghan GM, Hayes SC, Glenn-Lawson JL. Improving diabetes self-management through acceptance, mindfulness, and values: a randomized controlled trial. *J Consult Clin Psychol.* 2007;75(2):336.

55. Youngwanichsetha S, Phumdoung S, Ingkathawornwong T. The effects of mindfulness eating and yoga exercise on blood sugar levels of pregnant women with gestational diabetes mellitus. *Appl Nurs Res.* 2014;27(4):227-230.

56. Abbott RA, Whear R, Rodgers LR, et al. Effectiveness of mindfulness-based stress reduction and mindfulness based cognitive therapy in vascular disease: a systematic review and meta-analysis of randomised controlled trials. *J Psychosom Res.* 2014;76(5):341-351.

57. Scott-Sheldon LA, Gathright EC, Donahue ML, et al. Mindfulness-based interventions for adults with cardiovascular disease: a systematic review and meta-analysis. *Ann Behav Med.* 2020;54(1):67-73.

58. Schneider RH, Grim CE, Rainforth MV, et al. Stress reduction in the secondary prevention of cardiovascular disease: randomized, controlled trial of transcendental meditation and health education in Blacks. *Circ Cardiovasc Qual Outcomes.* 2012;5(6):750-758.

59. Schneider RH, Alexander CN, Staggers F, et al. Long-term effects of stress reduction on mortality in persons≥ 55 years of age with systemic hypertension. *Am J Cardiol.* 2005;95(9):1060-1064.

60. Barnes VA, Schneider RH, Alexander CN, Rainforth M. Impact of the transcendental meditation program on mortality in older African

Americans with hypertension-eight-year follow-up. *J Soc Behav Pers.* 2005;17(1):201.

61. Levine GN, Lange RA, Bairey-Merz CN, et al. Meditation and cardiovascular risk reduction: a scientific statement from the American Heart Association. *J Am Heart Assoc.* 2017;6(10):e002218.

62. Viveiros J, Chamberlain B, O'Hare A, Sethares KA. Meditation interventions among heart failure patients: An integrative review. *Eur J Cardiovasc Nurs.* 2019;18(8):720-728.

63. Howie-Esquivel J, Lee J, Collier G, Mehling W, Fleischmann K. Yoga in heart failure patients: a pilot study. *J Card Fail.* 2010;16(9):742-749.

64. Yeh GY, Chan CW, Wayne PM, Conboy L. The impact of tai chi exercise on self-efficacy, social support, and empowerment in heart failure: insights from a qualitative sub-study from a randomized controlled trial. *PLoS One.* 2016;11(5):e0154678.

65. Yeh GY, McCarthy EP, Wayne PM, et al. Tai chi exercise in patients with chronic heart failure: a randomized clinical trial. *Arch Intern Med.* 2011;171(8):750-757.

66. Yeh GY, Wang C, Wayne PM, Phillips R. Tai chi exercise for patients with cardiovascular conditions and risk factors: a systematic review. *J Cardiopulm Rehabil Prev.* 2009;29(3):152.

67. Bolier L, Haverman M, Westerhof GJ, Riper H, Smit F, Bohlmeijer E. Positive psychology interventions: a meta-analysis of randomized controlled studies. *BMC Public Health.* 2013;13(1):119.

68. Malouff JM, Schutte NS. Can psychological interventions increase optimism? A meta-analysis. *J Posit Psychol.* 2017;12(6):594-604.

69. DuBois CM, Millstein RA, Celano CM, Wexler DJ, Huffman JC. Feasibility and acceptability of a positive psychological intervention for patients with type 2 diabetes. *Prim Care Companion CNS Disord.* 2016;18(3).

70. Cohn MA, Pietrucha ME, Saslow LR, Hult JR, Moskowitz JT. An online positive affect skills intervention reduces depression in adults with type 2 diabetes. *J Posit Psychol.* 2014;9(6):523-534.

71. Boutin-Foster C, Offidani E, Kanna B, et al. Results from the trial using motivational interviewing, positive affect, and self-affirmation in African Americans with hypertension (TRIUMPH). *Ethn Dis.* 2016; 26(1):51.

72. Kahler CW, Spillane NS, Day AM, et al. Positive psychotherapy for smoking cessation: a pilot randomized controlled trial. *Nicotine Tob Res.* 2015;17(11):1385-1392.

73. Huffman JC, Millstein RA, Mastromauro CA, et al. A positive psychology intervention for patients with an acute coronary syndrome: treatment development and proof-of-concept trial. *J Happiness Stud.* 2016;17(5):1985-2006.

74. Redwine LS, Henry BL, Pung MA, et al. Pilot randomized study of a gratitude journaling intervention on heart rate variability and inflammatory biomarkers in patients with stage B heart failure. *Psychosom Med.* 2016;78(6):667-676.

75. Nikrahan GR, Laferton JA, Asgari K, et al. Effects of positive psychology interventions on risk biomarkers in coronary patients: a randomized, wait-list controlled pilot trial. *Psychosomatics.* 2016;57(4):359-368.

76. Mohammadi N, Aghayousefi A, Nikrahan GR, et al. The impact of an optimism training intervention on biological measures associated with cardiovascular health: data from a randomized controlled trial. *Psychosom Med.* 2020;82(7):634-640.

77. Ogedegbe GO, Boutin-Foster C, Wells MT, et al. A randomized controlled trial of positive-affect intervention and medication adherence in hypertensive African Americans. *Arch Intern Med.* 2012;172(4):322-326.

78. Seligman ME, Ernst RM, Gillham J, Reivich K, Linkins M. Positive education: Positive psychology and classroom interventions. *Oxf Rev Educ.* 2009;35(3):293-311.

79. Ruini C, Ottolini F, Tomba E, et al. School intervention for promoting psychological well-being in adolescence. *J Behav Ther Exp Psychiatry.* 2009;40(4):522-532.

80. Friedman EM, Ruini C, Foy R, Jaros L, Sampson H, Ryff CD. Lighten UP! A community-based group intervention to promote psychological well-being in older adults. *Aging Ment Health.* 2017;21(2):199-205.

81. Ouweneel E, Le Blanc PM, Schaufeli WB. On being grateful and kind: Results of two randomized controlled trials on study-related emotions and academic engagement. *J Psychol.* 2014;148(1):37-60.

82. Hernandez R, Cheung E, Carnethon M, et al. Feasibility of a culturally adapted positive psychological intervention for Hispanics/Latinos with elevated risk for cardiovascular disease. *Transl Behav Med.* 2018;8(6):887-897.

83. Kivimäki M, Kawachi I. Work stress as a risk factor for cardiovascular disease. *Curr Cardiol Rep.* 2015;17(9):74.

84. Oliver JJ, MacLeod AK. Working adults' well-being: an online self-help goal-based intervention. *J Occup Organ Psychol.* 2018;91(3):665-680.

85. *Workplace Health Playbook: Strategies for a Healthier Workforce.* Dallas, TX: American Heart Association.

86. Vie LL, Griffith KN, Scheier LM, Lester PB, Seligman ME. The Person-Event Data Environment: leveraging big data for studies of psychological strengths in soldiers. *Front Psychol.* 2013;4:934.

87. Pearson TA, Palaniappan LP, Artinian NT, et al. American Heart Association Guide for Improving Cardiovascular Health at the Community Level, 2013 update: a scientific statement for public health practitioners, healthcare providers, and health policy makers. *Circulation.* 2013;127(16):1730-1753.

88. Chicago Department of Public Health. *Healthy Chicago, healthy hearts: a local response to the national forum updated public health action plan to prevent heart disease and stroke.* Chicago DPH: Chicago, IL. Available at: https://www.chicago.gov/content/dam/city/depts/cdph/CDPH/CDPH_CardiovascularHealthBrochure_v4.pdf. Accessed October 1, 2020.

89. Be There San Diego. *Organizational approach to hypertension management using team-based care.* Be There San Diego; San Diego, CA. Available at: http://betheresandiego.org/. Accessed October 4, 2020.

90. Robert Wood Johnson Foundation. *Building a Culture of Health.* Princeton, NJ: RWJF. Available at: https://www.rwjf.org/en/how-we-work/building-a-culture-of-health.html. Accessed October 4, 2020.

91. Kroenke K, Spitzer RL, Williams JB. The Patient Health Questionnaire-2: validity of a two-item depression screener. *Med Care.* 2003:1284-1292.

92. Kroenke K, Spitzer RL, Williams JB, Monahan PO, Löwe B. Anxiety disorders in primary care: prevalence, impairment, comorbidity, and detection. *Ann Intern Med.* 2007;146(5):317-325.

93. Goddu AP, Roberson TS, Raffel KE, Chin MH, Peek ME. Food Rx: a community–university partnership to prescribe healthy eating on the South Side of Chicago. *J Prev Interv Community.* 2015;43(2):148-162.

94. Schueller SM, Muñoz RF, Mohr DC. Realizing the potential of behavioral intervention technologies. *Curr Dir Psychol Sci.* 2013;22(6):478-483.

95. Schueller SM, Hunter JF, Figueroa C, Aguilera A. Use of digital mental health for marginalized and underserved populations. *Current Treatment Options in Psychiatry.* 2019:1-13.

96. Hernandez R, Burrows B, Wilund K, Cohn M, Xu S, Moskowitz JT. Feasibility of an Internet-based positive psychological intervention for hemodialysis patients with symptoms of depression. *Soc Work Health Care.* 2018;57(10):864-879.

97. *The Silver Line: helpline for older people.* Annual report and financial statements. Calico Row: Trade Tower; 2018.

98. The World Health Organization. Adelaide statement health in all policies. Adelaide: Government of South Australia; 2010.

99. Baum F, Lawless A, Delany T, et al. Evaluation of health in all policies: concept, theory and application. *Health Promot Int.* 2014;29(suppl_1):i130-i142.

100. Steptoe A. Happiness and health. *Ann Rev Public Health.* 2019;40:339-359.

101. Kobau R, Seligman ME, Peterson C, et al. Mental health promotion in public health: Perspectives and strategies from positive psychology. *Am J Public Health.* 2011;101(8):e1-e9.

102. Patel V, Saxena S, Lund C, et al. The Lancet Commission on global mental health and sustainable development. *Lancet.* 2018;392(10157):1553-1598.

103. Hahn RA, Truman BI, Williams DR. Civil rights as determinants of public health and racial and ethnic health equity: health care, education,

employment, and housing in the United States. *SSM-Popul Health.* 2018;4:17-24.

104. Joshanloo M. Eastern conceptualizations of happiness: fundamental differences with western views. *J Happiness Stud.* 2014;15(2):475-493.

105. Lambert L, Lomas T, van de Weijer MP, et al. Towards a greater global understanding of wellbeing: a proposal for a more inclusive measure. *Int J Wellbeing.* 2020;10(2).

106. Hernandez R, Daviglus ML, Martinez L, et al. "¡Alegrate!"—A culturally adapted positive psychological intervention for Hispanics/Latinos with hypertension: Rationale, design, and methods. *Contemp Clin trials Commun.* 2019;14:100348.

107. Ghanbarzadeh R, Ghapanchi AH, Blumenstein M, Talaei-Khoei A. A decade of research on the use of three-dimensional virtual worlds in health care: a systematic literature review. *J Med Internet Res.* 2014;16(2):e47.

108. Lindner P, Miloff A, Zetterlund E, Reuterskiöld L, Andersson G, Carlbring P. Attitudes toward and familiarity with virtual reality therapy among practicing cognitive behavior therapists: a cross-sectional survey study in the era of consumer VR platforms. *Front Psychol.* 2019;10:176.

109. Motraghi TE, Seim RW, Meyer EC, Morissette SB. Virtual reality exposure therapy for the treatment of posttraumatic stress disorder: a methodological review using CONSORT guidelines. *J Clin Psychol.* 2014;70(3):197-208.

110. Indovina P, Barone D, Gallo L, Chirico A, De Pietro G, Giordano A. Virtual reality as a distraction intervention to relieve pain and distress during medical procedures. *Clin J Pain.* 2018;34(9):858-877.

111. Jerdan SW, Grindle M, van Woerden HC, Boulos MNK. Head-mounted virtual reality and mental health: critical review of current research. *JMIR Serious Games.* 2018;6(3):e14.

112. Mishkind MC, Norr AM, Katz AC, Reger GM. Review of virtual reality treatment in psychiatry: evidence versus current diffusion and use. *Curr Psychiatry Rep.* 2017;19(11):80.

113. Dascal J, Reid M, IsHak WW, et al. Virtual reality and medical inpatients: a systematic review of randomized, controlled trials. *Innov Clin Neurosci.* 2017;14(1-2):14.

114. Malloy KM, Milling LS. The effectiveness of virtual reality distraction for pain reduction: a systematic review. *Clin Psychol Rev.* 2010;30(8):1011-1018.

115. Boehm JK, Chen Y, Williams DR, Ryff C, Kubzansky LD. Unequally distributed psychological assets: are there social disparities in optimism, life satisfaction, and positive affect? *PloS One.* 2015;10(2):e0118066.

116. Green LW. Making research relevant: if it is an evidence-based practice, where's the practice-based evidence? *Fam Pract.* 2008;25(suppl_1):i20-i24.

12

Sedentary Lifestyle and Role of Exercise in Cardiovascular Diseases

Ambarish Pandey, Nitin Kondamudi, and Carl J. Lavie

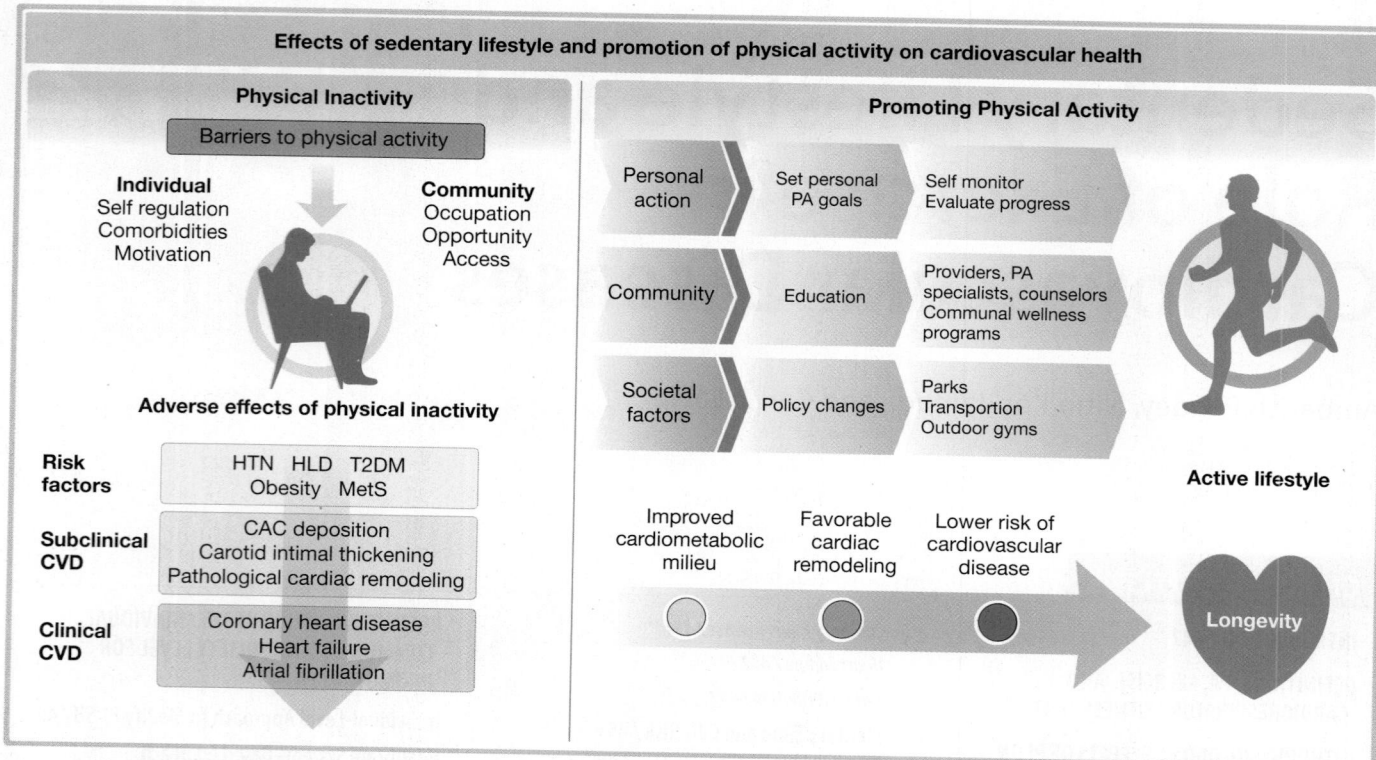

Chapter 12 Fuster and Hurst's Central Illustration. Sedentary lifestyle contributes to the cardiovascular disease (CVD) risk through excess burden of CVD risk factors and development of intermediate at-risk phenotypes. Identification of barriers to physical activity (PA) may help inform strategies for PA promotion at an individual, community, and societal level, and thus improve cardiovascular health. CAC, coronary artery calcium; HLD, hyperlipidemia; HTN, hypertension; MetS, metabolic syndrome; T2DM, type 2 diabetes mellitus.

CHAPTER SUMMARY

This chapter discusses the effects of sedentary lifestyle and physical activity (PA) on cardiovascular disease (CVD) and cardiovascular health. PA and cardiorespiratory fitness (CRF) are risk factors for CVD and have garnered attention as targets for primary and secondary prevention of CVD. Low PA and CRF are independently associated with atherosclerotic CVD as well as heart failure (HF). Sedentary lifestyle contributes to CVD risk through excess burden of CVD risk factors and development of intermediate at-risk phenotypes (see Fuster and Hurst's Central Illustration). Among individuals with prevalent CVD, low PA and CRF levels portend higher risk of adverse outcomes. However, adoption of healthy exercise behavior and adherence to guideline-recommended levels of PA are low in the general population due to individual, interpersonal, and societal barriers. Identification of these barriers to PA may help inform strategies for PA promotion at an individual, community, and societal level. By increasing healthcare provider awareness of the salutary effects of PA, equipping providers with the training and resources needed to optimize PA adherence, and leveraging a multidisciplinary approach to PA promotion, society can move closer toward realizing the cardiovascular benefits of an active lifestyle.

INTRODUCTION

Cardiovascular disease (CVD) is the leading cause of death in the United States, and accounts for ~32% of deaths globally.[1] Since 1992, the age-standardized mortality rate for CVD has decreased in most countries.[2] However, in 2017, CVD was responsible for 17.8 million deaths worldwide, reflecting a 21% increase in annual CVD deaths since 2007.[1] In addition, the prevalence of CVD has been increasing globally. In 2017, the prevalence of CVD was 486 million cases, reflecting a 29% increase in CVD prevalence since 2007.[1] These trends may in part reflect an increase in the prevalence of CVD risk factors such as hypertension (HTN), diabetes mellitus (DM), obesity, dyslipidemia, and physical inactivity (PI).[1]

A concerning trend among CVD risk factors is the recent increase in sedentary behavior (SB) and PI. In 2008, the US Department of Health and Human Services published federal guidelines for physical activity (PA),[3] which was updated in 2018.[4] The purpose of this guideline was to prescribe PA and specify the type, dose, and duration most likely to improve cardiovascular (CV) health based on available evidence. The guidelines recommend participation in at least 150 minutes a week of moderate-intensity or 75 minutes a week of vigorous-intensity aerobic PA. Despite these recommendations, data suggests that adherence to these PA levels in the United States and worldwide has not improved in the last decade; rather, time spent in SB has significantly increased.[5] Furthermore, a significant proportion of individuals in the United States and worldwide lead a lifestyle marked by PI.[6–9] This is particularly concerning in light of the favorable pleiotropic effects of PA. Exercise and PA have salutary effects on a wide variety of disease processes, including DM, osteoporosis, depression, HTN, dyslipidemia, and mental health. Specifically, the CV benefits of PA and exercise have been demonstrated in several population-based epidemiological studies, physiological experiments, and randomized controlled clinical trials (RCTs). Thus, there is a global need to promote a physically active lifestyle to reduce CVD burden and mitigate downstream risk of adverse outcomes.[10–13] In this chapter, we will discuss the biological effects of SB that lead to the development of CVD risk factors, pathological intermediate phenotypes, and clinical CVD, including coronary heart disease (CHD), heart failure (HF), and atrial fibrillation (AF). We will highlight the potential role of exercise as primary and secondary prevention, discuss the personal, communal, and societal determinants of PI, the role of PA promotion at the personal, communal, and societal level, and provide pragmatic guidance for caregivers of health promotion.

DEFINITIONS: PA, EXERCISE, AND CARDIORESPIRATORY FITNESS

PA reflects energy utilized beyond basal energy expenditure using skeletal muscle. PA typically encompasses activities of daily life, including lawn care, occupation-related work, transportation (ie, walking, cycling), and housekeeping. Exercise is distinct from PA, in that exercise is a form of PA that is planned, repetitive, and structured. Energy expended with PA is expressed as kilocalories. A metabolic equivalent (MET) unit refers to the amount of energy consumed at rest, with more METs consumed depending on the type and intensity of PA. Alternatively, PA can be quantified by classifying activity counts over a specific duration of time. In contrast to PA and exercise, SB refers to any waking behavior that consumes ≤1.5 METs, while in a sitting, reclining, or lying posture.[14]

Methods of capturing PA and SB vary with regard to their precision, their simplicity, and the information that they provide. Historically, self-reporting assessments using questionnaires have been used to ascertain PA because they are cost-effective, offer minimal work to the respondent, and are generally accepted by research and medical communities.[15] Some studies have shown that self-reported PA is valid and reproducible.[16,17] Furthermore, investigators have linked PA type, intensity, duration, and frequency with significant morbidity and mortality. Self-reported PA can be obtained from global questionnaires, quantitative history recall questionnaires, short-term recall questionnaires, PA logs, and PA diaries. The sensitivity of self-reported measures of PA range from 20% to 70% and the specificity ranges from 70% to 94%.[18] Despite the advantages of using questionnaires to quantify PA, there are several limitations of self-reported PA that warrant mention. Self-reporting inherently introduces bias into PA data, which may lead to over or underestimation of PA and SB. Consistently, multiple studies have shown that self-reported PA may be inaccurate, especially in young individuals.[19] Alternatives to self-reported PA include more objective measures of PA assessment, including accelerometers, pedometers, and wearable heart monitors. These PA assessment tools can improve estimates of exercise volume and intensity and have been shown to validate subjective reporting. While self-reported PA can provide info regarding PA intensity and duration over specific time blocks, direct measures of activity can quantify PA volume, duration, intensity, distance traveled, and energy expended.[15] These direct data points more reliably relate PA to cardiometabolic risk factors, morbidity, and mortality.[20]

Accelerometers are wearable devices that can measure the acceleration of a particular body segment. Of the commercially available brands of accelerometers, ActiGraph accelerometers are used most frequently in research studies. Accelerometers are appealing because they are precise, minimally invasive, and can provide PA intensity, pattern, duration, and frequency over days, weeks, or months.[19] Although calibrations studies have shown a wide range of correlations (Pearson's correlation coefficient [r] = 0.45–0.93), these observations are likely related to variation in study protocols rather than imprecision of the device itself. The recent emergence of SB as an independent predictor of CVD morbidity and mortality has made the accelerometer an attractive method to capture sedentary time and body posture to assess SB. Studies have shown that accelerometers can detect postural transitions, such as sitting to standing, making them a useful tool to ascertain SB.[21,22] Along these lines, accelerometers used in the context of mobile health (mHealth) predicted 5-year all-cause mortality incremental to known risk

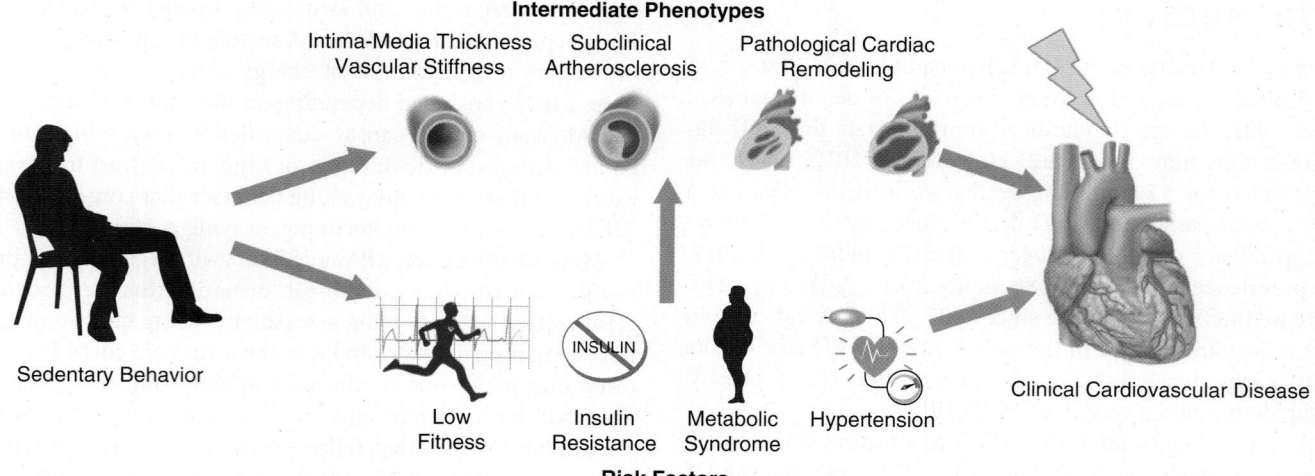

Figure 12–1. Progression from sedentary behavior to cardiovascular risk factors to intermediate phenotypes to clinical cardiovascular disease.

factors such as age, cigarette smoking, and various comorbidities.[22] In light of the precision, feasibility, and predictive utility of accelerometers, there has been an uptick in the use of accelerometers for the evaluation and implementation of PA.[22–25]

In contrast to PA, cardiorespiratory fitness (CRF) is a measurement of maximal exercise oxygen uptake, and reflects the cardiorespiratory system's efficiency in meeting the metabolic needs of the body during exercise. CRF can be estimated by peak work rate during exercise on a cycle ergometer or treadmill, or directly measured during peak exercise as maximal oxygen consumption based on the Fick equation. Oxygen consumption during cardiopulmonary exercise testing is expressed as VO_2, and CRF is usually expressed as maximal oxygen consumption (VO_{2max}) or as peak oxygen consumption (VO_{2peak}).[26] VO_2 can be expressed as liters of oxygen consumed per minute (L/min) or relatively as milliliters of oxygen consumed per kilogram of body weight per minute (mL/kg/min).[27,28] Given the technical challenges of direct CRF measurement, CRF can be predicted from highest attained work rate during graded, maximal, or submaximal exercise protocols. This method of CRF estimation is most frequently used to compute fitness in large-scale studies.[27] Both methods of CRF assessment have been validated in epidemiological studies.[27]

CRF represents the functional reserve of an individual and is determined by interconnected physiological processes related to right and left ventricular function, ventriculo-arterial coupling, vascular health, peripheral muscle metabolism, and lung ventilation/diffusion.[27] Consistently, data suggests that age-related decline in exercise capacity is mediated through cardiac mechanisms, such as reduced inotropic and chronotropic reserve.[29] Notably, CRF is an independent predictor of death and CVD death in both healthy and diseased populations,[30–33] making it a meaningful prognostic indicator.

Taken together, assessments of PA, SB, and CRF are all data points that are influenced by PA, and each has far-reaching pleiotropic effects on CV health. PI, SB, and low CRF can initiate a plethora of physiological pathways that hasten the

development of CVD at each stage: development of risk factors, progression of subclinical abnormalities in vascular health and cardiac structure and function, and manifestation of clinical CVD (**Fig. 12–1**). Once CVD is diagnosed, these exercise parameters continue to impact functional status, and remain prognostic for morbidity and mortality. Thus, promotion of PA and exercise behavior represents the most efficient, comprehensive, and holistic approach to advancing CV health and mitigating the downstream adverse effects of PI and SB. In this section of the chapter, we will discuss the effects of exercise behavior on each of these stages in the progression from at-risk to clinical CVD.

PATHOPHYSIOLOGICAL EFFECTS OF PI ON CVD RISK FACTORS, INTERMEDIATE CV PHENOTYPES, AND CLINICAL CVD

Effect of PA, Exercise, and CRF on CVD Risk Factor Burden

Numerous epidemiological studies have linked low levels of PA with higher prevalence of CVD risk factors, including DM, HTN, obesity, dyslipidemia, and metabolic syndrome (MetS).[10,34–36] Consistently, higher levels of PA and CRF have been associated with reduced burden of CVD risk factors.[10,37] In a multiethnic cohort of individuals with abnormal glucose tolerance, vigorous and nonvigorous PA, assessed by self-report, were associated with improved glucose sensitivity. Furthermore, an analysis of over 12,000 participants of the Hispanic Community Health Study/Study of Latinos cohort demonstrated that SB measured by accelerometer was associated with increased insulin resistance and higher glycosylated hemoglobin independent of PA.[38] These data are supported by a study that demonstrated that more than 3 hours a week of moderate to vigorous leisure time PA reduced the risk of developing MetS by 50%, even after adjustment for potential confounders. In the same study, high CRF was protective against the development of MetS. Another prospective observational study of over 5000 healthy men showed that self-reported PA, categorized as regular walking or cycling, recreational activity, and sporting (vigorous), is associated with improvement in blood pressure (BP) and cardiometabolic parameters, including triglycerides (TGs), high-density lipoprotein cholesterol (HDL-C), and insulin levels. Furthermore, prospective cohort studies from the Nurses' Health Study II, Aerobic Center Longitudinal Study (ACLS), and Coronary Artery Risk Development in Young Adults (CARDIA) have shown that self-reported PA is inversely associated with risk of incident HTN.[39-41] Likewise, these observational studies have demonstrated the inverse association between CRF and the development of HTN. It is noteworthy that SB assessed by questionnaire was associated with HTN independent of PA.[42] Interactive SBs, such as driving and computer use, were associated with incident HTN, but not behaviors such as television viewing and sleeping. These data highlight the independent contribution of specific SBs to incident HTN. Taken together, numerous studies have established the epidemiological link between SB, PI, and the development of CVD risk factors.

These epidemiological observations are supported by physiological data showing the direct pathophysiological effects of SB. Available evidence from animal models offer insight into the mechanisms by which an inactive lifestyle can promote the development of CVD risk factors. Recent animal studies suggest that aerobic exercise may prevent HTN via beneficial alterations in autonomic nervous system and vasoconstriction regulation.[43,44] In a rat model emulating human SB, a day of SB resulted in lower TG uptake into skeletal muscle,

lipoprotein lipase activity (reducing hydrolysis of triglyceride rich lipoproteins), and HDL-C concentrations. An analysis of mice with impaired glucose tolerance showed that exercise was associated with increased insulin stimulated phosphorylated protein kinase B (Akt) expression in adipose tissue, and improved glucose homeostasis.[45] Another study that relegated mice to an active lifestyle versus a sedentary lifestyle for 9 weeks found that SB resulted in reduced citrate synthase activity, lower expression of endothelial nitric oxide synthase, and impaired endothelial relaxation.[46] Consistently, a recent study observed that PI in mice was not only associated with endothelial dysfunction, but also with accelerated atherosclerosis.[47] In sum, SB may directly promote derangements in the CV system's cardiometabolic milieu by causing abnormalities in lipid metabolism, mitochondrial dysfunction, insulin insensitivity, increased oxidative stress, and endothelial dysfunction, predisposing individuals to the development of CVD risk factors (**Fig. 12–2**).

Similar mechanisms relating PA, SB, and CRF to CVD risk factors have been described in human studies. Abnormalities in mitochondrial regulation and function have been observed among sedentary individuals due to lower expression of proliferator-activated receptor γ coactivator 1-α,[48] which may contribute to enhanced oxidative stress. Furthermore, evidence suggests that sedentary individuals have higher postprandial glucose and insulin levels compared to more active individuals.[49] SB also has adverse effects on vascular health. In an analysis of healthy volunteers who reduced their PA from more than 10,000 steps a day to less than 5000 steps a day, PI reduced

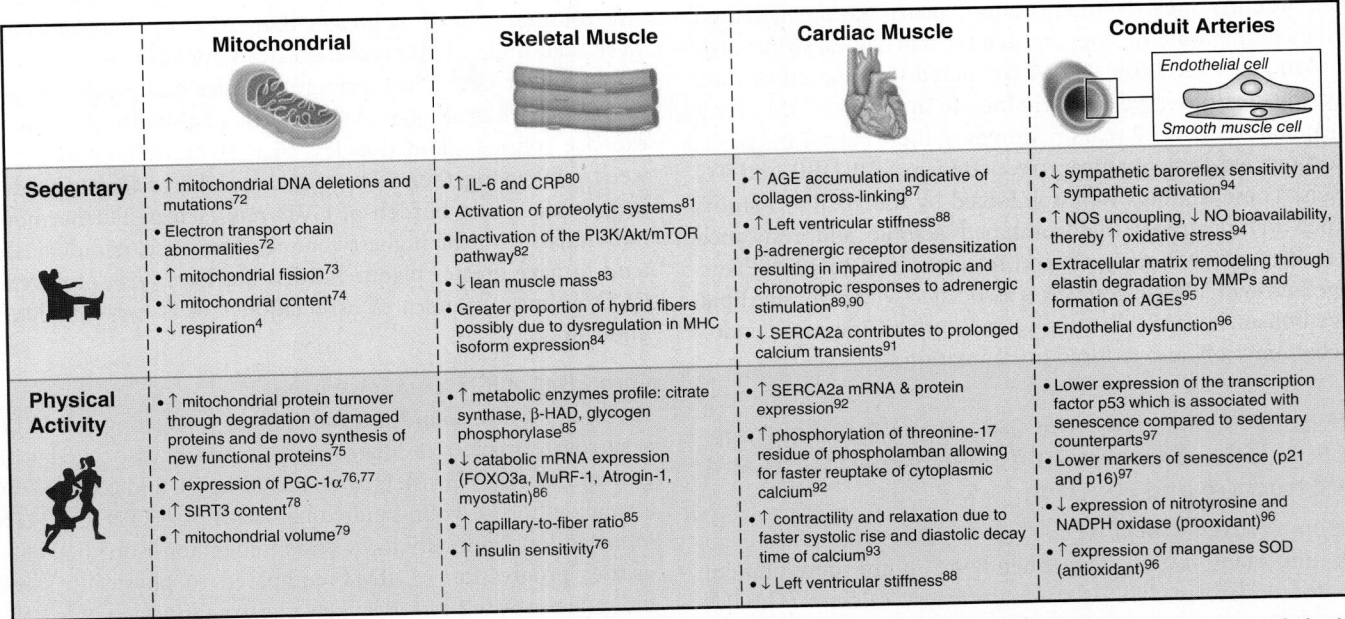

	Mitochondrial	Skeletal Muscle	Cardiac Muscle	Conduit Arteries
Sedentary	• ↑ mitochondrial DNA deletions and mutations[72] • Electron transport chain abnormalities[72] • ↑ mitochondrial fission[73] • ↓ mitochondrial content[74] • ↓ respiration[4]	• ↑ IL-6 and CRP[80] • Activation of proteolytic systems[81] • Inactivation of the PI3K/Akt/mTOR pathway[82] • ↓ lean muscle mass[83] • Greater proportion of hybrid fibers possibly due to dysregulation in MHC isoform expression[84]	• ↑ AGE accumulation indicative of collagen cross-linking[87] • ↑ Left ventricular stiffness[88] • β-adrenergic receptor desensitization resulting in impaired inotropic and chronotropic responses to adrenergic stimulation[89,90] • ↓ SERCA2a contributes to prolonged calcium transients[91]	• ↓ sympathetic baroreflex sensitivity and ↑ sympathetic activation[94] • ↑ NOS uncoupling, ↓ NO bioavailability, thereby ↑ oxidative stress[94] • Extracellular matrix remodeling through elastin degradation by MMPs and formation of AGEs[95] • Endothelial dysfunction[96]
Physical Activity	• ↑ mitochondrial protein turnover through degradation of damaged proteins and de novo synthesis of new functional proteins[75] • ↑ expression of PGC-1α[76,77] • ↑ SIRT3 content[78] • ↑ mitochondrial volume[79]	• ↑ metabolic enzymes profile: citrate synthase, β-HAD, glycogen phosphorylase[85] • ↓ catabolic mRNA expression (FOXO3a, MuRF-1, Atrogin-1, myostatin)[86] • ↑ capillary-to-fiber ratio[85] • ↑ insulin sensitivity[76]	• ↑ SERCA2a mRNA & protein expression[92] • ↑ phosphorylation of threonine-17 residue of phospholamban allowing for faster reuptake of cytoplasmic calcium[92] • ↑ contractility and relaxation due to faster systolic rise and diastolic decay time of calcium[93] • ↓ Left ventricular stiffness[88]	• Lower expression of the transcription factor p53 which is associated with senescence compared to sedentary counterparts[97] • Lower markers of senescence (p21 and p16)[97] • ↓ expression of nitrotyrosine and NADPH oxidase (prooxidant)[96] • ↑ expression of manganese SOD (antioxidant)[96]

Figure 12-2. The multidimensional mechanisms associated with the deleterious effects of sedentary behavior and the beneficial effects of physical activity that occur within the mitochondria, skeletal muscle, myocardium, and conduit arteries. β-HAD, β-hydroxyacyl CoA dehydrogenase; AGE, advanced glycation end products; Akt, protein kinase B; CRP, C-reactive protein; FOXO3a, forkhead box O3;IL-6, interleukin-6; MHC, myosin heavy chain; MMP, matrix metalloproteinase; mTOR, mammalian target of rapamycin; MuRF-1, muscle RING-finger protein-1; NADPH, nicotinamide adenine dinucleotide phosphate; NO, nitric oxide; NOS, nitric oxide synthase; PGC-1α, peroxisome proliferator-activated receptor γ coactivator 1-α; PI3K, phosphoinositide 3-kinase; SERCA2a, sarcoplasmic reticulum calcium adenosine triphosphatase; and SIRT3; nicotinamide adenine dinucleotide-dependent deacetylase sirtuin-3 SOD. Reproduced with permission from Lavie CJ, Ozemek C, Carbone S, et al. Sedentary Behavior, Exercise, and Cardiovascular Health. *Circ Res.* 2019 Mar;124(5):799-815.

endothelial cell activation, decreased popliteal flow-mediated dilation, and enhanced endothelial cell apoptosis.[50] Conversely, frequent, light intensity activity has been associated with upregulation of antioxidant and anti-inflammatory pathway modulators such as nicotinamide N-methyltransferase.[51] Consistently, the pathophysiological consequences of prolonged bedrest in humans are impaired lipid trafficking, heightened insulin resistance, abnormal shifts in muscle fiber type, and ectopic fat storage.[52] These cardiometabolic and vascular disturbances accelerate the development of CVD risk factors and CVD. Consistently, regular exercise has numerous positive pleiotropic effects that mitigate the biological consequences of SB. Exercise training increases insulin stimulated glycogen synthesis, promotes fatty acid oxidation from free fatty acids and triglycerides, and increases translocation of muscle glucose transporter-4(GLUT-4), all of which improve the cardiometabolic milieu of the body.[53]

The degree to which exercise modifies risk factor burden is less established. In the seminal Dose Response to Exercise (DREW) study, hypertensive, postmenopausal women randomized to graded levels of exercise exposure did not experience improvement in BP compared to controls, despite an observed improvement in CRF.[54] In contrast, Kokkinos et al. reported a significant reduction in diastolic BP (DBP) in response to exercise training among African American men with severe HTN.[55] Furthermore, a pooled analysis of studies evaluating the effect of aerobic exercise and resistance training (RT) on BP reported a net reduction in systolic BP (SBP) and DBP of 4.3 mm Hg and 1.7 mm Hg, respectively, due to exercise.[56] Given the data relating exercise to improved glycemic control, the Finnish Diabetes Prevention Study Group examined whether lifestyle modification incorporating increased PA, including walking, jogging, aerobic ball games, swimming, or skiing, reduced risk of DM compared to standard of care. Investigators observed a 58% reduction in incident DM over a mean follow up of 3.2 years.[57] Moreover, these behavioral modifications led to a significant reduction in SBP, DBP, and TG levels. These findings were reinforced by the HART D study, which demonstrated that combined aerobic and resistance exercise improves glycemic control compared to PI.[58] Taken together, evidence suggests PA is associated with favorable lipid metabolism, lower BP, better glycemic control, improved endothelial function, and reduced inflammation.[59]

Effect of PA, Exercise, and CRF on the Development of Subclinical Abnormalities in Atherosclerosis and CV Structure and Function

Coronary Artery Calcium

An important intermediate phenotype in the development of atherosclerotic CHD is coronary artery calcium (CAC).[60] Recent studies have established the predictive utility of CAC score for incident CHD incremental to current risk assessment tools.[61-65] However, the longitudinal association between PA and CAC is not clear. In an analysis of over 3000 participants from the CARDIA study, investigators did not observe an association between PA levels and incident CAC on 25 years of

follow up after adjustment for traditional CVD risk factors.[66] In contrast, an analysis of the Multi-Ethnic of Atherosclerosis (MESA) cohort showed that self-reported vigorous PA was inversely associated with incident CAC and CAC progression after 3 years of follow up.[67]

CRF has a more consistent, inverse association with the development of CAC. In a study of over 2300 participants from the CARDIA study, high sex-specific CRF in young adulthood, measured using the Balke treadmill protocol, was independently and inversely associated with incident CAC after 15 years of follow up.[68] Similarly, in an analysis of over 5000 healthy women from the Cooper Center Longitudinal Study (CCLS), high CRF levels, estimated from maximal treadmill exercise testing using the Balke protocol, were associated with lower prevalence of CAC. However, this association was attenuated and no longer significant after adjustment for CVD risk factors.[69] The analysis was repeated in men from the same cohort, and in the unadjusted analysis, high CRF was inversely associated with CAC score.[70]

Moreover, some studies have demonstrated a more J-shaped relationship between PA, CRF, and CAC burden. In an analysis of over 21,000 men from the CCLS, investigators showed that men with over 3000 MET-min/week of PA had a higher prevalence of CAC score ≥100 as compared to those who were less active. It is noteworthy that CAC score remained predictive of all-cause and CVD death across all strata of PA. Mortality risk among those with PA levels greater than 3000 MET-min/week and CAC score ≥100 was comparable to those with PA less than 1500 MET-min/week.[71] Similarly, another study evaluating subclinical coronary atherosclerosis and its determinants among athletes showed that individuals with high lifelong exercise volume, defined as greater than 2000 MET-minutes per week, had higher CAC score, greater CAC area, and nearly a 3-fold higher CAC. Furthermore, athletes had greater plaque prevalence when compared with participants with low lifelong exercise volume, defined as less than 1000 MET-minutes per week.[72] Taken together, SB may mediate atherosclerotic burden in part via excess burden of CVD risk factors. Furthermore, individuals with the highest volume of exercise, paradoxically tend to have greater plaque burden but lower risk of adverse CVD events, a pattern of association that is not completely understood.

Carotid Intimal Thickening

Assessed by ultrasound, carotid intimal thickening (cIMT) is a surrogate marker of atherosclerosis and is associated with greater risk of CVD risk factors, including PI, and CVD.[73-75] In a small cohort of young individuals with pre-HTN and HTN followed longitudinally for 6 years, sedentary individuals had greater progression of cIMT compared to physically active individuals (by self-report), likely due to a more favorable CVD risk factor profile among individuals with higher PA.[76] In an analysis of German firefighters and sedentary clerks, investigators examined the effect of the physical work environment on cIMT. CRF and PA were inversely associated with cIMT in firefighters compared to sedentary clerks.[75] A similar pattern of association has been observed between PA and cIMT among individuals with CHD. However, the cross-sectional association between PA and cIMT is less consistent.[77,78] In a cross-sectional analysis from the MESA cohort, PA was not associated with cIMT in men or women. Walking pace was associated with cIMT, but this association was attenuated by CVD risk factors. Consistently, in a cohort of children with obesity and dyslipidemia, PA was not significantly associated with greater cIMT in multivariable analysis.[78] Taken together, SB is linked to cIMT via excess burden of cardiometabolic risk factors. Furthermore, high PA and CRF may impede the progression of cIMT.

Cardiac Structure and Function

Abnormal cardiac remodeling patterns characterized by impaired left ventricular (LV) systolic and diastolic dysfunction, increased LV mass, LV concentricity, LV stiffness, and left atrial (LA) enlargement are epidemiologically linked with greater risk of mortality, incident HF, and incident AF. These stages in cardiac remodeling represent intermediate phenotypes in the progression to HF and AF.[79-83] Several cross-sectional studies have highlighted the association between PA, CRF, and abnormalities in cardiac structure and function. In a cohort of participants from the CCLS, CRF was strongly associated with higher LV filling pressure and impairment in diastolic filling, but not reduced systolic dysfunction as measured by ejection fraction (EF).[84] However, in a cross-sectional analysis of the Dallas Heart Study, there was an inverse, independent association between CRF and peak systolic circumferential strain.[85] Furthermore, a longitudinal analysis of the CARDIA study spanning ~20 years, demonstrated that low CRF at a young age was independently associated with greater risk of impaired diastolic LV filling.[84-86] These findings are reinforced by data demonstrating the relationship between SB and LV stiffness. In a small study comparing sedentary seniors to young adult controls, SB was associated with decreased LV compliance and impaired diastolic performance.[87] Consistently, cross-sectional and prospective observational data have shown that individuals with higher PA and CRF have reduced arterial stiffness compared to sedentary individuals.[88-89]

LV stiffness and diastolic LV dysfunction are associated with LA enlargement (LAE).[90-91] Despite the overwhelming evidence linking SB to reduced LV compliance and worse LV diastolic dysfunction, there is scarce evidence linking SB to LA size. Rather, LAE is more often observed in master athletes, and is considered an adaption to extreme doses of exercise.[92-93] Furthermore, endurance training is associated with LAE in a graded fashion, such that greater lifetime exposure to endurance training leads to LAE,[94-95] although short duration intensive exercise training can also induce changes in LA volume and function.[96,97] Consistently, in an analysis of the CCLS, individuals with higher CRF levels tended to have higher LA volumes.[84] Most recently, investigators demonstrated that LA volume index is independently, positively associated with CRF in a healthy cohort.[98] In general, athletes tend to have larger LV end diastolic diameters, greater LV wall thickness (≥13 mm), and marked LV hypertrophy. Despite these well described CV adaptions to prolonged endurance training, the clinical implications of these cardiac remodeling patterns in athletes are not completely clear.

The consequences of SB on subclinical atherosclerosis, vascular stiffness, and pathological cardiac remodeling suggest that these intermediate phenotypes may be modifiable with exercise training. In a small study of patients with DM and CHD, 12 months of combined aerobic and RT was associated with reduced cIMT progression among individuals with carotid plaques. Exercise training did not reduce cIMT progression in patients with carotid plaques.[99] These results are consistent with prior work showing that exercise training for higher risk individuals may have a limited impact on cIMT progression incremental medical therapy. For example, patients with HTN or CHD requiring statin therapy do not experience a reduction in cIMT progression in response to exercise. In contrast, a mild-to-modest benefit in halting cIMT progression can be observed with exercise training among lower-risk patients, suggesting lifestyle interventions may be beneficial if initiated earlier in the natural history of disease.

A similar pattern of association is observed in parameters of LV structure and function. In nine sedentary seniors at least 65 years old, 1 year of endurance training did not improve LV compliance, despite an observed increase in arterial elastance and exercise capacity.[100] Similarly, in a larger study of 62 health sedentary aged adults, aerobic exercise training for 1 year had little impact on LV stiffness.[101] In contrast, 2 years of exercise training in middle-aged adults (45–64 years old) improved exercise capacity and reduced LV stiffness, suggesting that exercise may modify LV compliance associated with sedentary aging, if initiated in middle age. Exercise training has beneficial effects on LV parameters beyond LV compliance. In a cohort of African American men with severe HTN, 32 weeks of exercise reduced LV mass, interventricular septum thickness, and LV mass index.[55] Furthermore, in a pooled analysis of randomized control trials examining the effect of exercise on LV parameters of structure and function in patients with DM, exercise was associated with improvement in early diastolic velocity and global longitudinal strain as compared with control groups.[102] The effects of exercise training on vascular compliance have yielded mixed results, but pooled data suggests there is benefit. In a meta-analysis of 14 trials comprising 472 pre-HTN patients, aerobic exercise did not reduce arterial stiffness, except among individuals who concomitantly experienced a reduction in BP.[103] Consistently, a more recent meta-analysis of 14 trials consisting of 642 HTN patients demonstrated that aerobic, combined, or isometric exercise improved arterial compliance.[104]

Effect of PA, Exercise, and CRF on Incidence of CVD

Coronary Heart Disease

Individuals with CVD risk factors and pathological intermediate at-risk phenotypes are at heightened risk for CHD, HF, and AF. The epidemiological link between PA and CRF and incident CHD is well established. Obeservational studies have consistently shown that higher PA levels are independently associated with lower risk of CHD.[105-110] The association between PA and CHD risk appears to be dose-dependent in a curvilinear fashion, such that the highest risk reduction afforded by PA occurs early in the dose-response curve. This pattern of association was observed in a meta-analysis showing that moderate intensity PA levels at 150 and 300 minutes per week (min/week) were associated with a 14% and 20% lower risk of CHD, respectively, as compared to SB.[111] Reduction in CHD risk from PA levels greater than 300 min/week were only modest. Observational studies have demonstrated a similar relationship between CRF and CHD risk.[112-117] High CRF is independently associated with lower risk of CHD, independent of traditional CVD risk factors.[118] Furthermore, there is a 10% higher risk of myocardial infarction later in life for every 1-metabolic equivalent (MET) decline in CRF.[112]

Heart Failure

In contrast to risk associated with CHD, there is a more distinct and robust association between PA, CRF, and incident HF. High PA is independently associated with lower risk of HF in a graded fashion. However, PA levels beyond guideline recommended PA doses for CHD risk reduction continue to afford significant reduction in risk of HF[112,119,120] (**Fig. 12–3**).

It is noteworthy that HF risk associated with low PA predominantly manifests as HF with preserved EF (HFpEF), consistent with the cardiometabolic risk and cardiac remodeling patterns previously discussed. Along these lines, a pooled analysis showed that lower leisure-time PA was associated with higher risk of HFpEF in a dose-dependent fashion, but not HF with reduced EF (HFrEF).[121] Similarly, CRF is inversely associated with HF risk, independent of traditional CVD risk factors. Low CRF at midlife has a more robust association with risk of HF compared to risk of CHD.[112,122-126] Furthermore, a secondary analysis of the Look AHEAD trial showed that higher CRF at baseline was associated with lower risk of HFpEF but not HFrEF after adjustment for CVD risk factors.[127] Taken together, SB and low CRF may render individuals more susceptible to HF (HFpEF in particular) compared to other CV conditions. This is relevant, because limited therapeutic options are available for HFpEF, which is projected to be the predominant subtype of HF.[128-131]

Atrial Fibrillation

Unlike CHD, and HF, PA has a more U-shaped association with AF risk.[132-140] The beneficial effects of PA doses appear to

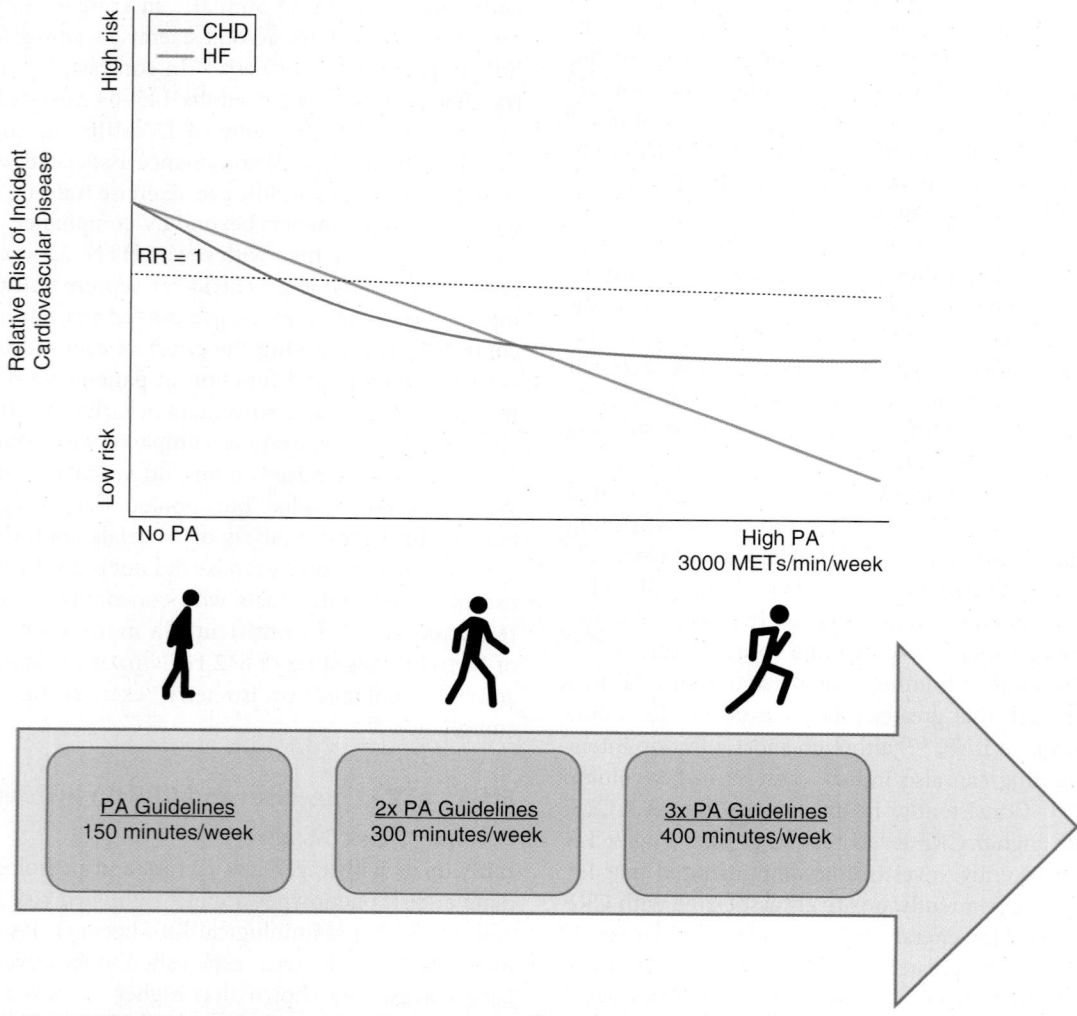

Figure 12–3. Dose-response relationship between physical activity and cardiovascular disease. PA, physical activity.

plateau around 1200 MET-min/week.[141,142] However, studies report a trend toward increased AF risk at extreme doses of PA.[140] These observations in community dwelling individuals are reinforced by data showing that elite athletes are at greater risk of AF compared to the general population.[143] Athletes with high lifetime exposure to high-intensity PA, such as skiers, are particularly susceptible to risk of AF later in life.[134,144-148] Thus, PA levels ranging from mild to moderate doses are most protective against the development of AF compared to PA levels at either extremes.

Studies examining the association between CRF and AF have yielded conflicting results. In a cohort of 1.1 million Swedish men, investigators observed a U-shaped relationship between CRF and risk of AF, such that higher levels CRF conferred excess risk of AF.[149] Consistently, in a cohort of Finnish middle-aged men, Khan et al. reported a nonlinear association between CRF and AF.[150] In the adjusted analysis, fitness levels between 6 and 9 METs resulted in the greatest AF risk reduction; however, at 10 to 12 METs, there was increased risk for AF.[150] In contrast, studies in the United States suggest a more linear association between higher CRF and lower risk of AF.[150-153] The heterogeneity in study findings may be related to differences in populations across study cohorts in US and European studies. More investigation is needed to clarify how CRF modifies AF risk.

Sedentary Time and CVD Risk

Sedentary time refers to the time spent performing activities of low energy expenditure (1.0–1.5 METs), such as watching television, driving, or sitting. Compared to older generations, more time is being spent in environments that promote SB. This is important because epidemiological evidence suggests that the deleterious health consequences of sedentary time are distinct from those associated with PI. As previously mentioned in this chapter, the advent of the accelerometer enabled researchers to capture time spent in SB, which has improved measurement of sedentary time beyond self-reported data.[154] Such innovations have allowed investigators to shed light on the time spent in SB in the United States. Accelerometer data captured over 7 days from ~1700 individuals from the US National Health and Nutrition demonstrated that Americans spend a majority of their time performing SB (58%) or light intensity activity (39%).[155] These findings are striking and are particularly concerning given epidemiological data linking sedentary time with cardiometabolic risk and incident CVD.

Numerous studies have documented the association between sedentary time and central obesity, insulin resistance, and increased triglyceride levels. Importantly, breaks in sedentary time are favorably associated with BMI, waist circumference, insulin resistance, and triglyceride levels, independent of total sedentary time and exercise time. Consistently, several epidemiological studies have demonstrated the association between sedentary time and incident CVD.[156-158] Moreover, the relationship between sedentary time and CVD risk is nonlinear, such that only sedentary duration greater than 10 hours confers excess risk of CVD.[159] This association is consistent across subtypes of CVD, including CHD,[160,161] HF,[162] and AF,[163]

and is independent of PA and traditional CVD risk factors. These data highlight the potential additive benefits of exercise on CV health via reduction in sedentary time and improvement in PA and CRF.

Exercise for Primary Prevention of CVD

Observational studies have suggested that improvement in PA and CRF may reduce downstream risk of CVD.[164,165] However, clinical trials have not yet decisively shown that exercise reduces risk of incident CVD. In the seminal Look AHEAD trial, over 5000 individuals with DM were randomized to intensive lifestyle changes, involving unsupervised exercise training, versus usual care to assess the effect of lifestyle behavioral modification on CVD risk.[166] The primary outcome was a composite of death from CVD causes, nonfatal myocardial infarction (MI), and nonfatal stroke. Due to a low event rate, investigators extended the follow up period from 11.5 years to 13.5 years and added hospitalization for angina as part of the primary composite outcome. HF hospitalization was included as a secondary outcome. Trial results did not show a significant difference between treatment arms for the risk of the primary composite outcome or the secondary outcome of HF hospitalization. These null findings were attributed to several factors, including the difficulty with monitoring unsupervised exercise, the low number of primary and secondary outcome events, and the regression of weight loss and fitness gain initially achieved in the trial. Given the low number of HF events (218) and the preponderance of observational data suggesting a link between SB and HFpEF, investigators adjudicated more HF events into HF subtypes in the Look AHEAD trial cohort and extended follow up until 2015. In this analysis, which included 257 HF events, lifestyle interventions were not associated with reduced risk of HF or its subtypes. Importantly, sustained improvement in CRF and body mass index (BMI) was associated with lower risk of HF, suggesting lifestyle interventions that lead to sustained changes to relevant cardiometabolic parameters may modify risk of HF.[127] Although AF was not adjudicated in the initial Look AHEAD trial, a secondary analysis was performed to examine the effect of lifestyle intervention on incident AF.[167] However, investigators did not observe reduced risk of AF in the lifestyle intervention arm. Taken together, evidence irrefutably supports the salutary effects of exercise on a variety of cardiometabolic parameters. It is less established to what degree exercise can modify intermediate phenotypes of CVD such as subclinical atherosclerosis and abnormalities in cardiac structure and function. Although trial data have yet to establish a direct link between lifestyle interventions and primary prevention of CHD, HF, and AF, it is plausible that interventions resulting in sustained improvement in cardiometabolic parameters can mitigate the risk of developing CVD.

Exercise as Secondary Prevention

Once individuals are diagnosed with CVD, PA and exercise remain staples for the prevention of recurrent CVD events and death. In a cohort of patients predominantly with CHD, CRF was an independent prognostic factor for mortality, such that each 1-MET increase in CRF conferred a 12% improvement in survival.[168] Consistently, CRF has been established as an important, independent predictor of mortality in HF and AF.[169] Not surprisingly, interventions aimed at improving CRF, such as cardiac rehabilitation (CR) and exercise training, have been shown to improve outcomes among individuals with CVD. In a pooled analysis of 48 trials including ~9000 patients with CHD, CR was associated with reduction in all-cause mortality and CVD mortality. In addition, CR was associated with lower smoking rates and reduction in BP, total cholesterol, and TG levels. Even light-to-moderate PA can lower risk of death compared to SB in patients with CHD. These benefits are most realized in individuals with CHD; however, in recent decades, evidence has emerged showing the utility of exercise in other CV conditions, including HF and AF.[59,170–173]

The seminal HF-ACTION trial examined whether supervised exercise training modified risk of adverse outcomes among patients with HFrEF. The initial benefits in the first 3 months of supervised exercise training were somewhat offset by lack of adherence following supervised training. Nevertheless, trial results demonstrated that exercise training significantly reduces risk of HF hospitalization, increases CRF, and improves quality of life (QoL)[174]; findings that have been reproduced in multiple studies.[175] Less data is available regarding the beneficial effects of lifestyle intervention in HFpEF patients. However, a pooled analysis of exercise intervention trials showed that exercise improves CRF and QoL in HFpEF patients,[175] suggesting exercise training may be a useful adjunctive therapy in the management of HFpEF, which is particularly relevant given the dearth of effective therapies available for this condition.

Exercise training in patients with AF has consistently been shown to reduce AF burden and symptoms. In a small cohort of 51 AF patients referred for ablation, investigators found that aerobic interval training significantly reduced AF burden compared to no exercise.[176] In the exercise group, ~40% of patients experienced a decline in arrhythmia burden. In another study of over 300 symptomatic, overweight, obese patients with AF, 1-MET improvement in CRF corresponded to 9% reduction in AF recurrence over 4 years of follow up,[177] suggesting improvement in CRF may in part mediate the beneficial effects of exercise on AF burden. These data are in keeping with prior work demonstrating the favorable impact of lifestyle interventions on AF. In the landmark LEGACY trial, lifestyle interventions aimed at weight loss via diet and exercise resulted in reduced AF burden, fewer symptoms, and longer arrhythmia-free survival.[178] More recently, Kato et al.[179] demonstrated the efficacy and safety of CR in patients with AF. Among patients with AF treated with catheter ablation, those who underwent CR experienced improvement in exercise capacity without excess risk of AF recurrence.[179] Ongoing clinical trials, including Exercise-AF and the OPPORTUNITY study will provide further insight into the potential benefits of exercise training in patients with AF. Taken together, multiple lines of evidence demonstrate the benefits of exercise and CR for secondary prevention of CVD.

Muscular Strength and CVD Risk

Muscular strength (MusS) is another marker of exercise health and is associated with excess risk of developing cardiometabolic risk factors[180] and CVD. MusS can be captured reliably, accurately, and safely by measuring handgrip strength (HGS) using a dynamometer. Measuring HGS involves maximal isometric contraction of the forearm, in the sitting or standing positions without elbow support. Individuals are asked to squeeze the dynamometer three times for 3 to 5 seconds; the highest measurement of the three attempts is recorded. HGS is correlated with measures of MusS obtained from other muscle groups including the legs, trunk, and arms, suggesting that HGS is a pragmatic, accurate assessment of total body MusS.

Numerous studies have linked MusS with CVD risk factors including DM, HTN, MetS, and obesity. In an analysis of the Health, Aging, and Body Composition cohort, investigators found that both men and women with DM tended to have lower MusS. Moreover, poor glycemic control (A1c >8%) and longer duration of DM were associated with lower MusS. Notably, physiologic decline of MusS with aging is accelerated among individuals with DM compared to individuals without DM. The independent contribution of MusS to HTN risk is less established. In an analysis of over 4000 men, low MusS was associated with excess risk of incident HTN in men with pre-HTN. MusS was not associated with risk of developing HTN among normotensive individuals.[181] It is noteworthy that association between MusS and incident HTN among individuals with pre-HTN was attenuated and no longer significant after adjustment for CRF.[181] However, a pooled analysis of five RCTs including ~200 participants, showed that RT was significantly associated with reduction in SBD and DBP in both prehypertensive and hypertensive patients.[182] In an analysis of data from the National Health and Nutrition Examination Survey, investigators found that high HGS was associated with lower DBP in both men and women. However, high HGS was associated with a 34% lower risk of incident HTN in men but not women.[183] A clearer relationship exists between MusS and MetS. In a study of over 8000 healthy men, MusS was associated with MetS, such that the highest quartile of MusS afforded a 24% risk reduction for the development of MetS, an observation that has been replicated in other studies.[184–186] Few studies have evaluated the relationship between MusS and obesity. In an analysis of ~600 individuals from the Physical Activity Longitudinal Study, investigators observed that lower MusS was associated with 70% greater risk of ≥10-kg weight gain over a 20-year follow up period. Notably, both weight and height were self-reported in this analysis. Another study using objective measures of body weight, investigators reported similar findings in men, such that the highest quintile of MusS was associated with a 70% reduction in bodyfat.[187]

There is extensive evidence supporting the association between MusS and CVD risk. In an analysis of ~40,000 men, investigators observed that dynapenia in childhood is associated with greater risk of incident CVD.[188] In this study, MusS was evaluated in youth using a composite score of three different strength assessments including knee extension, elbow extension, and HGS. Individuals with greater MusS had a 12% lower risk of developing CVD as adults, independent of CRF.[188] Furthermore, data supports an association between MusS and CVD subtypes including CHD, HF, and AF. A study of over 1 million healthy adults showed that greater MusS at baseline was associated with lower risk of downstream CHD and cerebrovascular disease at 25 years follow up.[189] A study of ~500,000 participants using UK Biobank data demonstrated that lower HGS is significantly associated with greater risk of HF even after adjustment for confounders including age, sex, ethnicity, and CVD risk factors.[190] These findings have been replicated in study populations with greater prevalence of cardiometabolic risk factors. One study demonstrated that higher MusS is significantly associated with lower risk of MI and HF in men and women with prediabetes and diabetes.[191] It is noteworthy that this analysis did not adjust for fitness. Limited data is available relating MusS with risk of AF. In an analysis of over 1.1 million young Swedish men, MusS assessed by HGS was not associated with risk of AF but was associated with lower risk of bradyarrhythmia and sudden cardiac death.[149] However, in an analysis of UK Biobank data, HGS was significantly associated with lower risk of AF, even with adjustment for potential confounders including PA.[115]

In light of the epidemiological data supporting the relationship between MusS, cardiometabolic risk factors, and CVD, emerging data suggests that improvement in MusS can modify risk of CVD. RT is a validated method of improving MusS in both older and younger adults.[180,192,193] Moreover, data suggests that RT can optimize cardiometabolic risk factors and improve CRF, mitigating downstream risk of CVD. A study of over ~7000 individuals showed that individuals who met the requirement for RT in the PA guidelines had a 17% lower risk of developing MetS.[194] Notably, RT beyond guideline-recommended doses did not afford greater risk reduction for MetS. Consistently, individuals who met the PA guideline recommendation for RT have a 13% lower risk of developing hyperlipidemia. Similar studies have linked RT to improved glycemic control and lower blood pressure.[195] In analysis of over 12,000 patients from the ACLS, <1 hour/week of RT was associated with lower risk of CVD, independent of aerobic exercise time.[196] The salutatory effects of RT were in part mediated by weight loss. These findings were replicated in an analysis of the Women's Health Study. RT was associated with lower risk of CVD; however, the risk reduction afforded by RT plateaued at RT >150 min/week.[197] In sum, observational data suggests that RT can improve cardiometabolic parameters and modify risk of CVD.

While observational data supports the primary prevention of CVD with RT, RCTs have not demonstrably shown that RT reduces risk of CVD. The HART D study was an RCT evaluating whether exercise training improved glycemic control in patients with diabetes. About 260 patients with an HbA1c ≥6.5% were randomized to four study groups: the nonexercise control group, the aerobic exercise group (12 kcal/kg per week), the RT group (3 days of RT per week), and the combined aerobic and RT exercise group.[58] RT alone was not associated with reduction in HgbA1c. However, patients in the combined aerobic and RT exercise group experienced a significant improvement in glycemic control.[58] In contrast to the RT only exercise group, the combined exercise group experienced significant weight loss and improvement in CRF. In a recent randomized

crossover trial evaluating the effect of exercise on ambulatory BP among patients with HTN, investigators showed that aerobic exercise reduced BP during awake periods, while RT reduced BP more significantly during the nighttime periods among patients with resistant hypertension. Combined aerobic and RT exercise significantly reduced BP during both awake and nighttime periods. Among patients without resistant hypertension, aerobic exercise resulted in more sustained postexercise decline in BP compared to RT.[198] In another small RCT, both aerobic exercise and RT were associated with reduction in 24-hour systolic BP; however, only aerobic exercise was associated with a reduction in inflammatory markers.[199] Whether RT alone reduces cardiometabolic parameters is less clear. In a small RCT of obese individuals with MetS, combined aerobic exercise and RT was associated with greater improvement in cardiometabolic parameters, included waist circumference, TGs, LDL, and VLDL, compared to diet alone.[200] In a recent RCT evaluating the effect of RT on cardiometabolic parameters among adolescents, a 12-week RT program was associated with reduction in TGs, LDL, serum glucose, and systolic BP. However, a meta-analysis of RCTs assessing the effect of RT on CV risk factors showed that RT did not reduce waist circumference, improve glycemic control, or improve lipid parameters.[201] These findings were replicated in a larger meta-analysis of 28 RCTs evaluating the effect of resistance training on CVD risk factors.[202] Taken together, RT may confer favorable effects on CVD risk factors. More investigation is needed to evaluate the role of RT for primary prevention of CVD.

DETERMINANTS OF PA AND SB

To modify SB in individuals, it is crucial to understand the drivers of PI (**Table 12–1**). Several factors ranging from individual, interpersonal, environmental, to social influences likely play an important role in determining SB and are discussed in detail in this section.

Individual-Level Factors That Influence PA Behavior

Individual factors related to PA include demographic, genetic, psychological, behavioral, and biological variables.[203] Among demographic factors, the male sex is strongly associated with PA in children aged 4 to 9 years old, and only modestly associated with PA in older age groups up until adolescence.[203] It is less clear whether sex influences PA in adulthood, with only some reviews observing an inverse association between the female sex and PA from adolescence into adulthood.[203,204] White ethnicity has been reported as a determinant of PA in adolescents, but this has not been consistently observed.[205,206] Age is an important determinant of PA, such that young age is associated with higher PA[203,204] and SB is consistently reported among the elderly.[207] In a multiethnic nationally represented cohort, individuals reported lower PA in adulthood compared to childhood, consistent with prior literature reporting decline in PA in old age. Several factors may account for the observed temporal decline in PA with aging. The transition from adolescence to adulthood is marked by significant social transitions related to work, marriage status, and other major life events

TABLE 12-1. Barriers to Physical Activity and Preventive Strategies to Reduce Sedentary Behavior

	Barriers	**Solution**	**Implementation**
Intrapersonal	Lack of self-efficacy	Individual Behavioral Change	Education on goal setting, monitoring progress, problem solving, focus on preventing relapse into sedentary behavior
	Lack of education	Healthcare-based intervention	Didactic and behavioral counseling by healthcare professionals (provider, dietician, nursing, exercise physiologist)
Interpersonal	Minimal social support	Nonfamily social support	Expanding and maintaining social network, such as buddy system and walking groups
Community	Lack of education	School-based intervention	Increase amount of time spent in moderate or vigorous PA during PE class, inclusion of PA education in school curriculum
		Work-based intervention	Improve PA among employees by providing educational sessions on PA, coordinating supervised exercise, and reducing gym memberships
	Minimal social support	Community-wide campaigns	Providing health education and social support via community sectors
	Suboptimal infrastructure for promoting PA	Environment interventions	Motivational signs around base of elevators or stairwell, creating walking trails, building exercise facilities, urban changes to reduce distance from homes to schools, work, and recreational areas

Abbreviations: PA, physical activity; PE, physical education

known to decrease PA. Furthermore, comorbidities such as obesity, DM, and chronic degenerative disease are being diagnosed at a younger age, which may deter participation in PA, resulting in PA decline during the transition from adolescence to adulthood. Consistently, SB in the elderly is mediated to a great degree by excess burden of chronic medical conditions.[208]

Genetics contribute a significant proportion of influence over the tendency for SB. Genome-wide association studies suggest that genes determine an individual's inclination to participate in exercise in tandem with external factors. The degree to which genetics affect PA is known as heritability, formally defined as the percent influence of genetics on the variance observed among individuals with a given phenotype. The estimated heritability of PA has varied across different studies. In the Quebec Family Study, 3-day activity surveys from 300 families were analyzed to compare the degree of PA variation between families versus within families. Investigators reported a heritability of 20% to 29% for PA, a range that is in agreement with prior familial aggregation studies using self-reported PA. Twin study designs leverage comparisons between monozygotic twins and dizygotic twins to disentangle the contribution of genetic versus external factors to SB. In a study of ~13,500 monozygotic twins and ~23,000 dizygotic twins, from seven different countries, investigators observed a median heritability of 62% for self-reported leisure time PA/exercise. Heritability ranged from 27% among men in Norway to 71% among women in the United Kingdom, with higher genetic correlation observed in monozygotic versus dizygotic twins. Multiple cohort studies of adult Finnish twins have reported heritability ranging from 35% to 50% for self-reported sedentary work and self-reported sitting time.[209] It is noteworthy that these estimates were derived from self-reported measures of SB and PA. Limited data is available on the heritability of PA based on more objective assessments. In a recent analysis of twins from the Netherlands, investigators computed a heritability of 56% for sedentary time based on objective measurements

via accelerometer.[210] Although the magnitude of genetic influence over SB is fairly well characterized in the literature, few studies have identified specific genes and pathways involved in determining SB. In the Framingham Heart study, investigators reported an association between the fat mass and obesity-associated gene and prolonged sitting time.[211] Moreover, Simonen et al. found an association between a variant of the melanocortin-4 receptor and PI.[212] Current data suggests that genes involved in the heritability of PA are related to pathways responsible for neurotransmitter trafficking, glucose metabolism, and myelination regulation.[213] More genome-wide association studies are needed to identify specific genes and metabolic pathways that are implicated in PA.

An important psychological factor influencing PA is the mindset of "self-efficacy," confidence in the ability to carry out a specific action. Self-efficacy appears to be strongly associated with PA in adolescents, but less so in younger children. In adults, self-efficacy and health status are consistently associated with PA, with some reports identifying both as determinants.[203] Additionally, the perception of having family support for PA and close friendships are positively associated with PA. In contrast, positive attitudes toward using a computer and watching television, less positive attitudes toward exercise, and stress are all associated with greater likelihood of PI.[214-216] Among behavioral factors affecting PA, history of PA and exercise are consistently positively associated with PA across age groups.[203] Furthermore, pet ownership is a positive behavioral determinant of PA; data suggests that owning a dog may increase daily walking by ~20 minutes.[217] In contrast, external biological factors seem to have a more limited effect on PI. Weight and BMI are not associated with PI across age groups due to insufficient evidence.[203,204] Family history of obesity and CVD have been periodically linked to PI in children; however the strength of evidence is weak.[204] In contrast, physical health concerns, particularly among individuals with CHD and musculoskeletal disorders, have been reported as barriers to PA.[218]

Interpersonal Factors That Influence PA Behavior

Interpersonal factors play a significant role in determining PA in adolescents and young adults. In an analysis of ~28,000 young adults from Europe, occupational status was a significant determinant of SB. Moreover, social details such as marital status, number of children, and household size were all linked to SB.[219] Indeed, studies report greater PA correlation between spouses compared to same-sex siblings, potentially due to shared life experiences and prolonged cohabitation among partners. Consistently, social support for PA from family is strongly associated with PA across age groups.[203] In contrast, environmental variables seem to affect PA in older adults to a greater degree compared to interpersonal/social variables. For example, data suggests that SB later in life is associated with the availability of recreational facilities, social clubs, outdoor activities, urbanization, and perceived support from municipal authorities in promoting active living.[219] Consistently, studies have identified walkability (areas designed such that residents can walk to nearby destinations from their residence), and street connectivity (grid-like pattern of streets) as factors strongly associated with PA in older adults.[203] Other studies have linked leisure time PA to factors related to transportation, such as availability of walking pavement and safe crossings.[203] These data highlight the differential contribution of PA determinants to specific age groups.

Societal Factors That Influence PA Behavior

There are multiple factors at the societal level that may influence PA. Evidence suggests that policies focusing on cycling infrastructure, park upgrades, and biking trails improved PA among citizens of Germany, Denmark, and the Netherlands.[220] However, the relationship between legislation and PA is not consistent, because studies evaluating the effect of policies on PA participation in schools have not yielded consistent results. In addition to policy and legislation, major crises at the societal level such as civil unrest, economic depression, and natural disasters can all influence PA. For example, data suggests that economic crises can increase transportation-related PA but reduce leisure-time PA.[221]

The mechanisms driving PA in the US population are not necessarily homogeneous across different geographical and cultural contexts. Within the United States, PI is particularly prevalent in rural areas compared to urban areas, due to unique challenges related to lack of indoor recreation facilities, poor infrastructure for transportation, lack of PA programs, and limited social support.[222] In China and East Asian nations, PA increases with age as adults retire, in contrast to the United States, where age tends to be inversely correlated with PA.[223] In urban sub-Saharan Africa, determinants of PI are related to lack of education regarding the benefits of PA, long working hours, prioritization of family needs, preference for SB, and specific cultural understandings of PA, such as the idea that walking is considered a sign of idleness.[224] Furthermore, the sub-Saharan Africa cultural tradition that women should not engage in outdoor PA and the negative perception of exercise attire negatively influences incentive for PA among women.[224] Similar cultural influences affect PA in the United States. For example, African American women report hair maintenance as a barrier to PA.[218]

Determinants of Response to Exercise Behavior

The determinants of PA highlight the complex interplay of internal and external influences over exercise behavior. Moreover, exercise alone does not necessarily guarantee improvement in CRF and other cardiometabolic parameters. In fact, there is significant heterogeneity in the magnitude of CRF change in response to exercise training. In early exercise training studies, changes in peak oxygen uptake in response to aerobic exercise ranged from 0% (no improvement) to 100% improvement. Sisson et al. observed comparable variation in CRF in response to exercise training in the DREW trial.[225] Variables that modify CRF response to exercise training are not well-established. Physiological factors are important determinants of CRF response. For example, cardiac output accounts for 70% to 85% of the variance of peak oxygen uptake, and chronotropic incompetence is inversely related to CRF change after exercise.[226] Factors related to cardiac structure and function such as cardiac size and myocardial strain influence CRF response to exercise.[227] Details of exercise training, including exercise volume and intensity, have also been identified as determinants of CRF response.[54,228] At the individual level, factors such as age, body habitus, and genetics have all been posited as determinants of CRF response to exercise. Taken together, there is substantial variation in CRF change in response to exercise. Moreover, the factors that drive CRF heterogeneity are not well characterized. These data highlight the importance of personalized, targeted exercise training regimens, to maximize improvement in fitness with exercise training.

PREVENTIVE ACTION AT THE INDIVIDUAL, COMMUNITY, AND SOCIETY LEVEL FOR PROMOTING PA

Despite compelling evidence demonstrating the salutary effects of PA and the detailed recommendations of the PA guidelines,[3] a sizeable proportion of the US population does not participate in PA at guideline-recommended doses. In fact, involvement in PA has historically been low, with only 50% of individuals reporting compliance with the PA guidelines for aerobic exercise, and only 20% engaging with both aerobic and muscle strengthening. In recent years, a favorable trend in PA guideline compliance has been observed (**Fig. 12–4**). It is therefore incumbent on medical practitioners to help address modifiable personal, communal, and societal barriers to PA to maximize adherence to the PA guidelines (**Fig. 12–5**).

Individual-Level Approach to Modify PI/SB

Modifiable personal barriers to PA previously discussed in this chapter include, but are not limited to, lack of self-efficacy, misconceptions of the types/doses of PA, disinterest in PA, lack of companionship, lack of social support, and concerns about safety.[229] The presence of one or more of these barriers poses a challenge to adopting an active lifestyle in accordance with

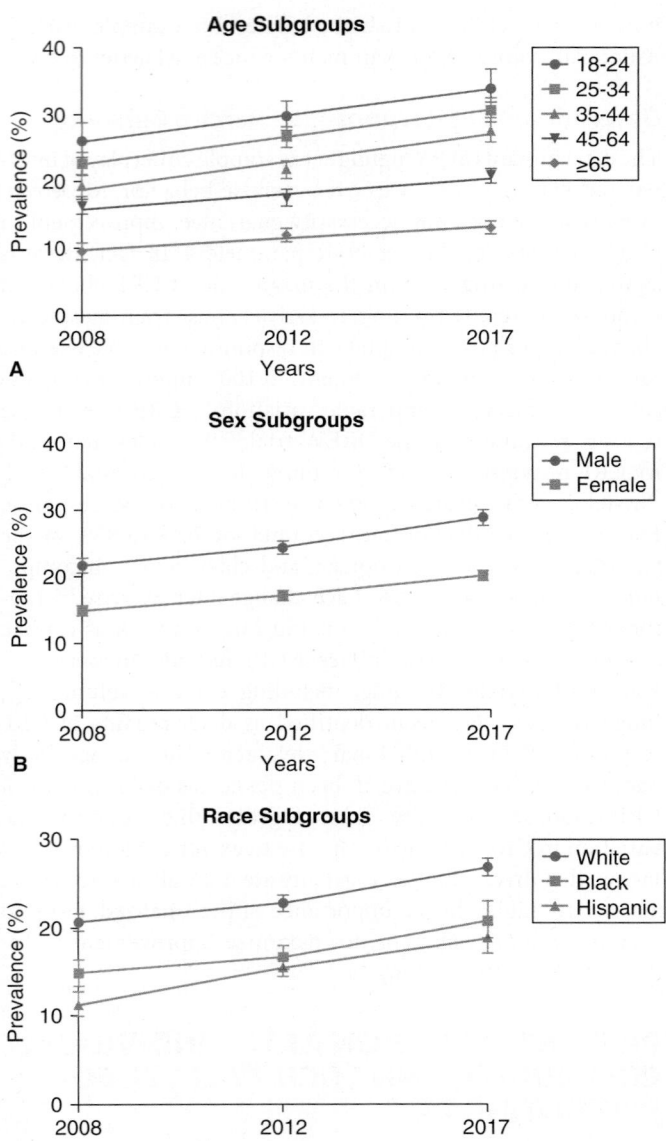

Figure 12–4. Prevalence trend of individuals meeting physical activity guideline recommendations for aerobic exercise and resistance training. A, age subgroups; B, sex subgroups; C, race subgroups. Prevalence age adjusted, except age-specific estimates. Data from Whitfield GP, Carlson SA, Ussery EN, et al. Trends in Meeting Physical Activity Guidelines Among Urban and Rural Dwelling Adults-United States, 2008-2017. *MMWR Morb Mortal Wkly Rep*. 2019 Jun 14;68(23):513-518.

the recommendations laid out in the PA guidelines. An important strategy in mitigating the effects of these barriers involves the development of self-regulatory skills, which can lead to sustained exercise behaviors. Fostering self-regulation for an individual requires: identification of a goal the individual aims to accomplish, capability to self-monitor behavior and establish a link to the goal, access to information regarding progress toward that goal, a mechanism for self-evaluating progress, and the opportunity to correct behavior to be more in line with their goal. This strategy relies on self-monitoring of PA. Technological advances have created a market for commercial devices such

as Fitbit, Apple, Garmin, Samsung Gear, TomTom, Misfit, and Lumo, which allow individuals to be more involved in monitoring their own PA.[230] Data suggests that individual utilization of self-monitoring devices can lead to sustained improvements in PA. In a pooled analysis of ~700 individuals, self-monitoring PA using commercial technology led to a 2,500 daily step increase.[43] Moreover, commercial self-monitoring can be leveraged with mHealth for a more streamlined approach to self-monitoring. Merging commercial self-monitoring devices and smartphone applications has proven effective in improving PA.[232] However, limitations of such strategies warrant mention. There is modest heterogeneity in the precision of these devices. For example, wrist and forearm devices tend to underestimate heart rate. Furthermore, step count tends to be underestimated at slow walking speeds and more accurate at faster walking speeds. Errors such as these may provide incorrect information regarding PA to the user. Consistently, in a recent large-scale trial, individuals who followed an evidence-based weight-loss program with a wearable PA device experienced less weight loss compared to individuals who followed the weight-loss program alone,[233] presumably due to false reassurance of PA due to inaccuracies in the wearable device measurements. Recent iterations of wearable self-monitoring devices incorporate advanced algorithms to accurately determine time spent in moderate to vigorous heart rate ranges.[234] As technology advances, wearable self-monitoring devices with mHealth smartphone applications may become a staple of PA promotion via self-regulation.

Healthcare System–Based Approach to Modify PI/SB

Individual motivation and behavioral modification are not enough to improve adherence to the PA guidelines at a population level. The 2008 PA guidelines are the product of landmark interventional trials and observational studies highlighting the impact of PA on CV health.[3] Yet, only 36% of adults in the United States have heard of these guidelines. Even more sobering, 1% of the population is aware of the optimal guideline recommended doses of PA.[235] Thus, there is urgent need to more directly improve awareness and education regarding the health benefits of PA at the community level. One such avenue is through endorsement of PA by outpatient healthcare providers. In a large healthcare system, adopting the concept of treating PA as a vital sign wherein 80% to 96% of physicians addressed PA during outpatient visits, patients experienced improvements in PA and reduction in CVD risk factor burden.[236–238] Another study reviewing data from five meta-analyses, three systematic reviews, and two literature reviews published over the last decade demonstrated that PA counseling by primary care providers (PCPs) had a significant effect on increasing PA levels.[239] Accordingly, the US Preventive Services Task Force recommends that healthcare providers provide lifestyle counseling regarding PA and dietary habits for individuals with CVD risk factors.[240] Dependence solely on healthcare providers for PA education may be challenging, because providers are often inundated with clinical responsibilities, with little time to discuss PA and assess patient adherence PA.[241] Thus, a

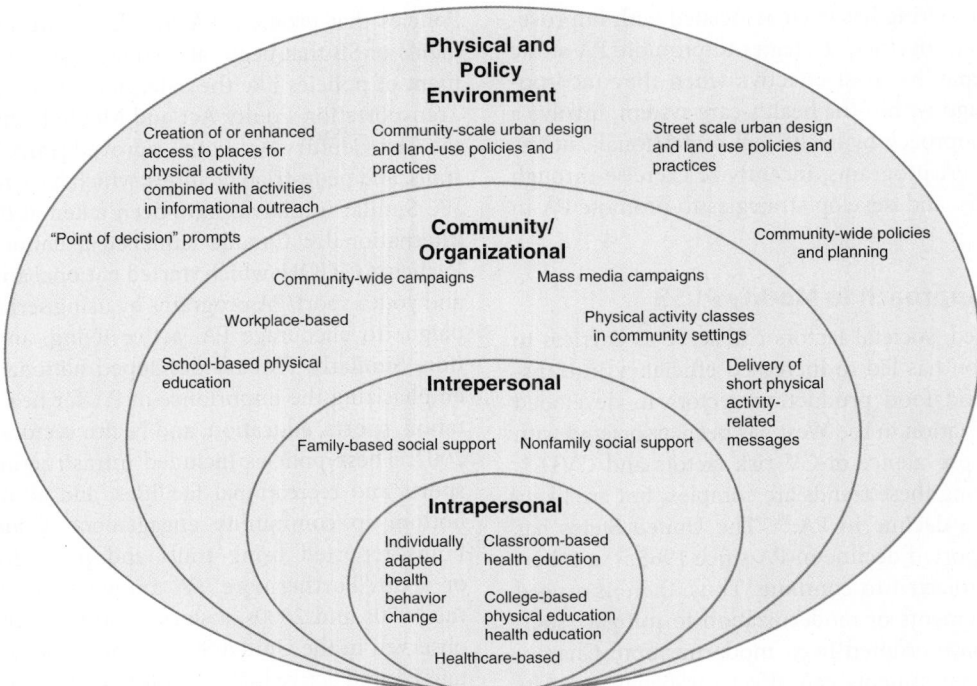

Figure 12–5. Mapping physical activity intervention strategies on the socio-ecological model. Reproduced with permission from Pratt M, Perez LG, Goenka S, et al. Can population levels of physical activity be increased? Global evidence and experience. *Prog Cardiovasc Dis.* 2015 Jan-Feb;57(4):356-367.

multidisciplinary approach involving ancillary staff such as nursing, exercise physiologists, and behavioral counselors may more effectively promote PA within the health-care system.[242-243] It is important to highlight that data from these intervention trials do not necessarily capture the experience of patients receiving health care outside the context of a clinical trial. Patients in the community do not have as frequent contact with their healthcare providers. Therefore, involvement of community PA programs may help reinforce exercise behaviors that were promoted and developed within the healthcare system. Accordingly, studies have shown that increasing referrals to community-based PA programs result in modest improvement in PA.[244]

Outside of the healthcare system, there are other methods of incentivizing PA at the community level. For example, multiple models exist that make provisions for insurance compensation for PA/exercise. The Silver Sneakers program for Medicare-eligible individuals includes a fitness benefit at almost no cost, and provides access to a fitness center, personal trainer, and exercise classes. Collaboration among the YMCA, selected health insurance entities, and healthcare providers has led to the implementation of the Diabetes Prevention Program,[245] which links physicians and health insurance providers to community-based health promotion specialists, including fitness professionals. These mechanisms allow coordination between the healthcare system, insurance programs, and fitness professions to enhance engagement with PA in the community.

Workplace-Based Approach to Modify PI/SB

An integral aspect of life in the community is the workplace. Unfortunately, the workplace is the single most contributor to daily sitting time. The percentage of industrial work that entails SB is increasing, highlighting the need for workplace-based interventions to reduce the burden of sedentary time.[246] Even modest changes to workplace exercise behavior can be beneficial. Observational studies have demonstrated that time spent standing is associated with lower risk of death in a dose-dependent fashion.[247] Such a simple intervention has proven pragmatic and efficacious in the workplace. Recent workplace intervention trials have shown that ~42-minute reduction in workplace sitting resulted in an equivalent increase in standing.[248,249] Furthermore, this small change led to improvement in cardiometabolic risk scores at 12 months.[250] Such strategies are not only beneficial for workers, but also cost-effective for healthcare systems.[251] In addition to workplace interventions targeting reduction in SB, exercise behavior can be modified via promotion of PA in the workplace. Most individuals spend a significant proportion of their time in the workplace, making the occupational setting an ideal place to promote PA.[252,253] A number of PA promotion strategies in the workplace have been effective in improving PA. One such strategy is designating goals for individuals, allowing them to follow their own progress, and providing feedback as they move toward completion of their goal in a stepwise fashion. Consistently, incorporating self-monitoring of PA with goal setting, feedback, and progression toward goal completion has been shown to be effective in promoting PA. In addition to goal setting, providing tangible educational resources is a valid method of promoting PA in the occupational setting. For example, studies have shown that making printed material about PA readily available in the workplace increases PA of workers. Furthermore, offering pedometers in the occupational setting has been associated with improvement in PA.[254] Taken together, strategies to promote PA at the community level may be most effective when they incorporate PA as a vital sign within the health-care system, involve a multidisciplinary approach by healthcare professionals, utilize community-based PA programs, incentivize exercise through insurance programs, and develop strategies to promote PA in the workplace.

Societal-Level Approach to Modify PI/SB

As already discussed, societal factors can serve as barriers to PA. Industrialization has led to increased efficiency in transportation, labor, and food production sectors in developed countries. Modernization in the West has been associated with an increase in the prevalence of CV risk factors and CVD.[255] The factors mediating these trends are complex, but are likely in part driven by a decline in PA.[256] The United States has observed a 32% reported decline in PA since 1965,[256] a sobering trend that is projected to continue. Thus, there is a need to leverage advancements of modernization to mitigate societal barriers that have erupted from modernization. Characteristics of built environments can affect the behavior of its members.[257] Areas that have advanced transportation infrastructure, positive perceived walkability, and easy access to parks tend to have active individuals.[258] Consistently, an analysis in the MESA cohort demonstrated that improvements in built environment characterized by increased access to destinations and improved street connectivity are associated with increases in self-reported PA.[259] These findings are reinforced by data showing that cycling to work is associated with lower prevalence of cardiometabolic risk factors compared to driving.[260] These built infrastructures are more prevalent in safe neighborhoods of higher socioeconomic status. Compared to affluent neighborhoods, underserved communities tend to have poorer transportation infrastructure, less sidewalks, and reduced perception of safety from crime, characteristics that are associated with lower walk time and higher vehicle time.[261] In sum, health-care providers must be mindful of the environmental context of their patient as they discuss and promote PA.

Health Policy–Based Approach to Modify PI/SB

The societal make up of a community is in large part determined by the policies put in place by governance. Consequently, legislation and policy are important platforms on which reforms can be made to create a society that emphasizes and fosters PA. Unlike individual and communal interventions, policy changes tend to impact a broader group of people and have the potential to make changes more sustainable over time.[262] Historically, there have been numerous policies enacted by the United States that have encouraged PA in many domains. In 1895, New York City put in place a law that states "No school house shall be considered in the city of New York without an open-air playground attached,"[262] a law that encourages kids to play outside in school. More recently, Michelle Obama led the "Let's Move!" initiative, which encouraged schools to incorporate strategies to ensure adequate moderate-to-vigorous PA for 60 minutes.[263]

Policies that promote PA in schools are necessary to reverse habits of SB that begin at a young age.[264] Furthermore, enactment of policies like the Safe, Accountable, Flexible, Efficient Transportation Equity Act and Moving Ahead for Progress in the 21st Century Act both improved transit systems, bicycling trails, and pedestrian facilities, which have indirectly promoted PA. Similar initiatives have been taken at the population level internationally. Canada launched a national initiative called ParticipACTION, which started national and regional worksite and youth sport/PA programs by using serial mass media campaigns to encourage PA, active living, and sports participation. Similarly, Finland developed national policy statements emphasizing the importance of PA for health in the transportation, sports, education, and health sectors between 1970 and 2002. These policies included infrastructure for trails, parks, sports and recreational facilities, and additional funding for bottom-up community engagement. Consequently, 90% of Finns reported using trails and paths for recreation and/or sport. Furthermore, PA among Finns increased between the 1970s and 2000s, a stark contrast to the historical trends observed in the United States. Thus, policy changes can facilitate PA and active living to a broad population through a variety of mechanisms (**Table 12–2**).

Guidance for Caregivers of Health Promotion

Altogether, poor lifestyle choices are at the center of the observed trends involving SB and PI. The deleterious ramifications of these choices with regard to CV health are firmly established, and the salutary, pleiotropic effects of PA and high CRF in reducing CVD risk are indisputable. Awareness of potential barriers to PA, and the implementation of strategies at the individual, communal, and societal level are paramount to improving the adherence to PA for the betterment of CV health worldwide. A key facet of PA promotion within the healthcare system that warrants further discussion is provider awareness. Without proper training, practicing physicians are less likely to devote the appropriate time to discuss PA. In one study, obese patients reported that their outpatient providers discussed PA ~20% of the time.[263] Moreover, a recent survey of physicians showed that <10% of physicians provided exercise prescriptions prior to receiving training in lifestyle counseling.[266] Addressing this lack of awareness is a critical step to ensuring lifestyle counseling is a cornerstone of the primary care outpatient visit.

Insufficient preparation for lifestyle counseling with regard to PA and SB among physicians is likely rooted in the lack of education during medical school. A minority of medical schools emphasize the importance of PA, regular exercise, and CRF into the curriculum.[267,268] This deficiency in PA education may lead to the perception among medical students that this subject is unimportant, which in turn can hinder integration of lifestyle counseling into clinical practice. Along these lines, medical training that integrates lifestyle counseling meaningfully into curricula results in greater likelihood of physicians incorporating these concepts into clinical practice.[269] Accordingly, many healthcare societies, such as the American

TABLE 12–2. National Initiatives to Promote Physical Activity at the Population Level

Country	National Initiative	Implementation
Canada	ParticipACTION	- Mass media campaigns encouraging PA, sports participation, active living - Development of national and regional worksite, youth sport, and activity programs
Finland	National PA promotion programs	- Funding allocated to improving infrastructure for trails, parks, sports, community centers, and recreational facilities - Mass media campaigns
Brazil	Academia da Cidade	- Free daily classes in the mornings and afternoons taught by trained physical educators - Restructuring parks and plazas in poor, less safe neighborhoods
Columbia	National Development Plan	- PA promotion through sports, recreation, public health, and physical education - Focus on training PA and public health professionals - Free PA classes in parks, plazas, and community centers
Portugal	National Strategy for Promotion of Physical Activity	- Enhanced training of healthcare workers on the importance of PA - Computer-based tools to assist providers with assessing PA and counseling - Collective participation in PA by doctors and the community—Walk with a Doc
United States	Let's Move!	- Schools encouraged to implement strategies to ensure 60 minutes of moderate to vigorous PA in school-aged children
United States	Move Your Way	- Promote PA by providing education regarding PA benefits, offering interactive online tools to learn ways to participate in PA, and displaying motivational videos
International	Walk with a Doc	- Grassroots, community level promotion of PA, with physicians and community individuals participating in physician led walks across the world
United States	GirlTrek	- Nonprofit organization that encourages African American women and girls to walk in their neighborhoods to promote health, advocacy, and civil liberties
United States	Mall Walking	- Program that promotes walking in malls when neighborhood infrastructure is not conducive to PA
United States	Promoting Airport Walking	- Program that promotes walking in airports rather than using available amenities
United States	Active People, Healthy Nation	- Initiative to implement programs to promote PA at national, state, and community levels - Disseminate knowledge regarding the benefits of an active lifestyle, through education and mass media campaign - Train state and community leaders on how to promote and support PA

Abbreviation: PA, physical activity.

College of Cardiology (ACC), the American Heart Association (AHA), the Institute of Medicine, and the American College of Physicians, have supported incorporation of medical education that teaches students how to recognize detrimental SB and PI patterns and effectively provide counseling to modify patient PA/exercise behavior.[267,270,271] Furthermore, educating practicing physicians on the importance of PA and exercise can augment integration of these principles into their management plans.[266,272,273] The Centers for Disease Control and Prevention developed an initiative to improve PA levels in the United States called Active People, Healthy Nation. A key component of this initiative is to train practitioners how to create and promote walkable communities. Furthermore, practitioners are taught how to concentrate efforts across sectors, (ie, public health, elected official, transportation, planning) to develop a plan to create walkable communities through policy, systems, and environmental approaches.[8]

Education of these concepts need not be limited to physicians. A multidisciplinary approach to lifestyle counseling by ancillary staff including nursing, dieticians, physical and occupational therapists, and exercise physiologists, increases the likelihood of improving PA in patients. Indeed, physicians are somewhat limited by the time constraints imposed by modern day medicine,[241] necessitating more involvement of ancillary staff in lifestyle counseling as previously discussed in this chapter. However, insufficient education regarding the nuance of lifestyle counseling is still problematic in education among ancillary staff, perhaps with the exception of exercise physiologists. Curricular of other healthcare professionals often do not allocate the required time needed to meaningfully provide education regarding exercise and PA assessment and counseling.[274,275] Fortunately, there are new models for education in this area that are being incorporated into the curriculum for other healthcare professsionals.[268,276]

A component of PA intervention that physicians may struggle with is the incorporation of pragmatic PA recommendations and exercise prescriptions into clinical practice. As previously stated in this chapter, the relationship between PA and reduced risk of CVD is curvilinear, with minimal gains in risk reduction above a specific PA threshold. Physicians should be aware that these thresholds vary among subtypes of CVD, such as CHD, HF, and AF, with higher thresholds affording greater reduction in HF compared to CHD, and extreme doses possibly enhancing risk of AF. Similarly, the PA formula most effective for the secondary prevention of CVD is not established. Some studies even suggest a U- or J-shaped relationship between PA and mortality among individuals with CVD, such that extreme doses of exercise confer excess risk of mortality.[277-281] Despite these nuances in PA, there is consensus that even modest PA can have numerous benefits on CV health. The PA guidelines recommend 150 min/week of moderate or 75 min/week of vigorous PA/aerobic exercise with muscle strengthening.[3] However, weekend warriors who only engage in just 75 minutes of exercise one to two times a week have lower risk of death and CVD mortality compared to sedentary individuals.[6,282] Furthermore, several types of light exercise have been shown to reduce CVD and mortality, such as brisk walking for more than 30 minutes a day, running for 1 hour or more a week, rowing for 1 hour or more a week, or lifting weights for 30 minutes or more a week.[7,283,284] Moreover, a large study of over 50,000 individuals showed that runners have 45% and 30% lower risk of CVD death and all-cause mortality respectively, compared to nonrunners. Consistently, even those who participated in running for 5 to 10 minutes a day at slow speeds had significantly lower risk of CVD death and all-cause mortality.[283] These data highlight the many benefits of even modest PA, which physicians must keep in mind as they prescribe exercise doses to their patients.

A final consideration for physicians aiming to promote PA to patients is the importance of exemplifying role model behavior when it comes to PA and exercise. Modeling a healthy lifestyle for patients can help motivate them to adhere to ideal exercise behavior. This is particularly challenging among physicians, since life as a student, trainee, and clinical practitioner are all marked by stress and SB if conscious efforts are not made to be more active.[285,286] The importance of the physical and mental benefits that come with exercise must be understood and internalized, for physicians to maintain a healthy, active lifestyle themselves. The significance of physician role modeling cannot be overstated, because patients who perceive their doctors as self-consistent are more likely to be self-motivated to make major lifestyle changes themselves.[287]

In conclusion, the far-reaching benefits of living an active lifestyle are irrefutable and the levels of PA needed to optimize CV health are clearly established. Promotion of PA at personal, communal, and societal levels is essential for the population to engage in PA and reap the benefits of an active lifestyle. Importantly, healthcare providers are in a prime position to promote PA, not just with the tools and mechanisms available, but also by modeling a healthy lifestyle.

Guidelines for the Primary Prevention of CVD

The importance of regular exercise and active living in the primary prevention of CVD cannot be overstated. As such, these data have been incorporated into the 2019 AHA/ACC and 2016 European Society of Cardiology (ESC) CVD prevention guidelines. The 2019 AHA/ACC CVD prevention guidelines recommend individuals should receive routine counseling of PA during their healthcare visits and should participate in at least 75 minutes of vigorous aerobic PA per week or at least 150 minutes of moderate aerobic PA per week to reduce CVD risk, class of recommendation (COR) I[288] (**Table 12–3**). The 2019 AHA/ACC CVD prevention guidelines encourage individuals to participate in some PA rather than none, if they are unable to achieve the aforementioned recommended PA thresholds, COR IIa. Finally, the 2019 AHA/ACC CVD prevention guidelines recommend reducing SB to mitigate CVD risk, COR IIb[288] (Table 12–3).

TABLE 12–3. The 2019 ACC/AHA and 2016 ESC Cardiovascular Disease Prevention Guidelines for Physical Activity

Organization	Recommendation	Class of Recommendation	Level of Evidence
ACC/AHA	Adults should routinely be counseled in health-care visits to optimize a physically active lifestyle	I	B-R
	Adults should engage in at least 150 minutes of moderate aerobic PA per week or at least 75 minutes of vigorous aerobic PA per week to reduce CVD risk	I	B-NR
	For adults unable to meet the minimum PA recommendations, engaging in some moderate or vigorous PA can be beneficial to reduce CVD risk	IIa	B-NR
	Decreasing sedentary behavior in adults may be reasonable to reduce CVD risk	IIb	C-LD
ESC	It is recommended for healthy adults of all ages to perform at least 150 minutes a week of moderate intensity or at least 75 minutes a week of vigorous intensity aerobic PA or an equivalent combination thereof	I	A
	For additional benefits in healthy adults, a gradual increase in aerobic PA to 300 minutes per week of moderate intensity or 150 minutes per week of vigorous intensity aerobic PA, or an equivalent thereof is recommended	I	B
	Regular assessment and counseling of PA are recommended to promote the engagement, and if necessary, to support an increase in PA volume over time.	I	C
	Multiple sessions of PA should be considered, each lasting ≥10 minutes and evenly spread out throughout the week	IIa	B
	Clinical evaluation including exercise testing should be considered for sedentary people with CV risk factors who intend to engage in vigorous PAs or sports	IIa	C

Abbreviations: AHA, American Heart Association; ACC, American College of Cardiology; ESC, European Society of Cardiology; PA, physical activity; CVD, cardiovascular disease; CV, cardiovascular.

Similarly, the 2016 ESC CVD prevention guidelines recommend participation in at least 75 minutes of vigorous aerobic PA per week or at least 150 minutes of moderate aerobic PA per week, COR I[289] (Table 12–3). In contrast, the ESC guidelines also recommend doubling the thresholds for vigorous and moderate aerobic PA to at least 150 and 300 minutes per week respectively, when able, COR I. Furthermore, PA is recommended in low risk individuals without additional workup, and regular assessment and counseling on PA are expected in the healthcare system, COR I (Table 12–3). ESC encourages multiple PA sessions a week lasting at last 10 minutes, COR IIa. Finally, the 2016 ES CVD prevention guidelines recommend clinically evaluating sedentary individuals at high risk for CVD who intend on playing sports COR IIa. Taken together, both CVD prevention guidelines recommend PA doses at thresholds established in the PA guidelines and also recommend regular PA counseling in the healthcare setting. The AHA/ACC guidelines endorse participation in some PA (even at doses below guideline recommended thresholds) compared to complete PI to achieve modest CVD risk reduction, while the ESC guidelines take into account the potential salutary effects of PA doses above guideline-recommended thresholds. Both guidelines incontrovertibly support the notion that participation in PA and reduction in SB are key components of CVD primary prevention.

REFERENCES

1. Virani SS, Alonso A, Benjamin EJ et al. Heart disease and stroke statistics-2020 update: a report from the American Heart Association. *Circulation.* 2020;141:e139-e596.
2. Collaborators GBDCoD. Global, regional, and national age-sex-specific mortality for 282 causes of death in 195 countries and territories, 1980-2017: a systematic analysis for the Global Burden of Disease Study 2017. *Lancet.* 2018;392:1736-1788.
3. Physical activity guidelines for Americans. *Okla Nurse.* 2008;53:25.
4. Piercy KL, Troiano RP. Physical activity guidelines for Americans from the US Department of Health and Human Services. *Circ Cardiovasc Qual Outcomes.* 2018;11:e005263.
5. Du Y, Liu B, Sun Y, Snetselaar LG, Wallace RB, Bao W. Trends in adherence to the physical activity guidelines for Americans for aerobic activity and time spent on sedentary behavior among US adults, 2007 to 2016. *JAMA Netw Open.* 2019;2:e197597.
6. Fletcher GF, Ades PA, Kligfield P, et al. Exercise standards for testing and training: a scientific statement from the American Heart Association. *Circulation.* 2013;128:873-934.
7. Lavie CJ, Arena R, Swift DL, et al. Exercise and the cardiovascular system: clinical science and cardiovascular outcomes. *Circ Res.* 2015;117:207-219.
8. Katzmarzyk PT, Lee IM, Martin CK, Blair SN. Epidemiology of physical activity and exercise training in the United States. *Prog Cardiovasc Dis.* 2017;60:3-10.
9. Dumith SC, Hallal PC, Reis RS, Kohl HW 3rd. Worldwide prevalence of physical inactivity and its association with human development index in 76 countries. *Prev Med.* 2011;53:24-28.
10. Wisloff U, Lavie CJ. Taking physical activity, exercise, and fitness to a higher level. *Prog Cardiovasc Dis.* 2017;60:1-2.
11. Vuori IM, Lavie CJ, Blair SN. Physical activity promotion in the health care system. *Mayo Clin Proc.* 2013;88:1446-1461.
12. Harber MP, Kaminsky LA, Arena R, et al. Impact of cardiorespiratory fitness on all-cause and disease-specific mortality: advances since 2009. *Prog Cardiovasc Dis.* 2017;60:11-20.
13. Nauman J, Tauschek LC, Kaminsky LA, Nes BM, Wisloff U. Global fitness levels: findings from a web-based surveillance report. *Prog Cardiovasc Dis.* 2017;60:78-88.
14. Tremblay MS, Aubert S, Barnes JD, et al. Sedentary Behavior Research Network (SBRN)—Terminology Consensus Project process and outcome. *Int J Behav Nutr Phys Act.* 2017;14:75.
15. Strath SJ, Kaminsky LA, Ainsworth BE, et al. Guide to the assessment of physical activity: clinical and research applications: a scientific statement from the American Heart Association. *Circulation.* 2013;128:2259-2279.
16. Silsbury Z, Goldsmith R, Rushton A. Systematic review of the measurement properties of self-report physical activity questionnaires in healthy adult populations. *BMJ Open.* 2015;5:e008430.
17. Ball TJ, Joy EA, Gren LH, Shaw JM. Concurrent validity of a self-reported physical activity "vital sign" questionnaire with adult primary care patients. *Prev Chronic Dis.* 2016;13:E16.
18. Steene-Johannessen J, Anderssen SA, van der Ploeg HP et al. Are self-report measures able to define individuals as physically active or inactive? *Med Sci Sports Exerc.* 2016;48:235-244.
19. Ainsworth B, Cahalin L, Buman M, Ross R. The current state of physical activity assessment tools. *Prog Cardiovasc Dis.* 2015;57:387-395.
20. Celis-Morales CA, Perez-Bravo F, Ibanez L, Salas C, Bailey ME, Gill JM. Objective vs. self-reported physical activity and sedentary time: effects of measurement method on relationships with risk biomarkers. *PLoS One.* 2012;7:e36345.
21. Owen N, Healy GN, Matthews CE, Dunstan DW. Too much sitting: the population health science of sedentary behavior. *Exerc Sport Sci Rev.* 2010;38:105-113.
22. Kozey-Keadle S, Libertine A, Lyden K, Staudenmayer J, Freedson PS. Validation of wearable monitors for assessing sedentary behavior. *Med Sci Sports Exerc.* 2011;43:1561-1567.
23. Adam Noah J, Spierer DK, Gu J, Bronner S. Comparison of steps and energy expenditure assessment in adults of Fitbit Tracker and Ultra to the Actical and indirect calorimetry. *J Med Eng Technol.* 2013;37:456-462.
24. Bonn SE, Lof M, Ostenson CG, Trolle Lagerros Y. App-technology to improve lifestyle behaviors among working adults—the Health Integrator study, a randomized controlled trial. *BMC Public Health.* 2019;19:273.
25. Tanaka C, Tanaka M, Tanaka S. Objectively evaluated physical activity and sedentary time in primary school children by gender, grade and types of physical education lessons. *BMC Public Health.* 2018;18:948.
26. Guazzi M, Adams V, Conraads V, et al. EACPR/AHA Scientific Statement. Clinical recommendations for cardiopulmonary exercise testing data assessment in specific patient populations. *Circulation.* 2012;126:2261-2274.
27. Ross R, Blair SN, Arena R, et al. Importance of assessing cardiorespiratory fitness in clinical practice: a case for fitness as a clinical vital sign: a scientific statement from the American Heart Association. *Circulation.* 2016;134:e653-e699.
28. Fleg JL, Pina IL, Balady GJ, et al. Assessment of functional capacity in clinical and research applications: an advisory from the Committee on Exercise, Rehabilitation, and Prevention, Council on Clinical Cardiology, American Heart Association. *Circulation.* 2000;102:1591-1597.
29. Pandey A, Kraus WE, Brubaker PH, Kitzman DW. Healthy aging and cardiovascular function: invasive hemodynamics during rest and exercise in 104 healthy volunteers. *JACC Heart Fail.* 2020;8:111-121.
30. Myers J, McAuley P, Lavie CJ, Despres JP, Arena R, Kokkinos P. Physical activity and cardiorespiratory fitness as major markers of cardiovascular risk: their independent and interwoven importance to health status. *Prog Cardiovasc Dis.* 2015;57:306-314.
31. Kokkinos P, Myers J. Exercise and physical activity: clinical outcomes and applications. *Circulation.* 2010;122:1637-1648.
32. Swift DL, Lavie CJ, Johannsen NM, et al. Physical activity, cardiorespiratory fitness, and exercise training in primary and secondary coronary prevention. *Circ J.* 2013;77:281-292.

33. Fogelholm M. Physical activity, fitness and fatness: relations to mortality, morbidity and disease risk factors. A systematic review. *Obes Rev.* 2010;11:202-221.

34. Ekelund U, Steene-Johannessen J, Brown WJ, et al. Does physical activity attenuate, or even eliminate, the detrimental association of sitting time with mortality? A harmonised meta-analysis of data from more than 1 million men and women. *Lancet.* 2016;388:1302-1310.

35. Lee DC, Pate RR, Lavie CJ, Sui X, Church TS, Blair SN. Leisure-time running reduces all-cause and cardiovascular mortality risk. *J Am Coll Cardiol.* 2014;64:472-481.

36. Lee IM, Shiroma EJ, Lobelo F, et al. Effect of physical inactivity on major non-communicable diseases worldwide: an analysis of burden of disease and life expectancy. *Lancet.* 2012;380:219-229.

37. Moreau KL, Ozemek C. Vascular adaptations to habitual exercise in older adults: time for the sex talk. *Exerc Sport Sci Rev.* 2017;45:116-123.

38. Diaz KM, Goldsmith J, Greenlee H, et al. Prolonged, uninterrupted sedentary behavior and glycemic biomarkers among US Hispanic/Latino adults: The HCHS/SOL (Hispanic Community Health Study/Study of Latinos). *Circulation.* 2017;136:1362-1373.

39. Carnethon MR, Evans NS, Church TS, et al. Joint associations of physical activity and aerobic fitness on the development of incident hypertension: coronary artery risk development in young adults. *Hypertension.* 2010;56:49-55.

40. Forman JP, Stampfer MJ, Curhan GC. Diet and lifestyle risk factors associated with incident hypertension in women. *JAMA.* 2009;302:401-411.

41. Asferg C, Mogelvang R, Flyvbjerg A, et al. Interaction between leptin and leisure-time physical activity and development of hypertension. *Blood Press.* 2011;20:362-369.

42. Beunza JJ, Martinez-Gonzalez MA, Ebrahim S, et al. Sedentary behaviors and the risk of incident hypertension: the SUN Cohort. *Am J Hypertens.* 2007;20:1156-1162.

43. Moraes-Silva IC, Mostarda C, Moreira ED, et al. Preventive role of exercise training in autonomic, hemodynamic, and metabolic parameters in rats under high risk of metabolic syndrome development. *J Appl Physiol.* (1985) 2013;114:786-791.

44. Araujo AJ, Santos AC, Souza Kdos S, et al. Resistance training controls arterial blood pressure in rats with L-NAME- induced hypertension. *Arq Bras Cardiol.* 2013;100:339-346.

45. Carter LG, Ngo Tenlep SY, Woollett LA, Pearson KJ. Exercise improves glucose disposal and insulin signaling in pregnant mice fed a high fat diet. *J Diabetes Metab.* 2015;6.

46. Suvorava T, Lauer N, Kojda G. Physical inactivity causes endothelial dysfunction in healthy young mice. *J Am Coll Cardiol.* 2004;44:1320-1327.

47. Laufs U, Wassmann S, Czech T, et al. Physical inactivity increases oxidative stress, endothelial dysfunction, and atherosclerosis. *Arterioscler Thromb Vasc Biol.* 2005;25(4):809-814.

48. Joseph AM, Adhihetty PJ, Buford TW, et al. The impact of aging on mitochondrial function and biogenesis pathways in skeletal muscle of sedentary high- and low-functioning elderly individuals. *Aging Cell.* 2012;11:801-809.

49. Pulsford RM, Blackwell J, Hillsdon M, Kos K. Intermittent walking, but not standing, improves postprandial insulin and glucose relative to sustained sitting: a randomised cross-over study in inactive middle-aged men. *J Sci Med Sport.* 2017;20:278-283.

50. Boyle LJ, Credeur DP, Jenkins NT, et al. Impact of reduced daily physical activity on conduit artery flow-mediated dilation and circulating endothelial microparticles. *J Appl Physiol.* (1985) 2013;115:1519-1525.

51. Latouche C, Jowett JB, Carey AL, et al. Effects of breaking up prolonged sitting on skeletal muscle gene expression. *J Appl Physiol.* (1985) 2013;114:453-460.

52. Bergouignan A, Rudwill F, Simon C, Blanc S. Physical inactivity as the culprit of metabolic inflexibility: evidence from bed-rest studies. *J Appl Physiol.* (1985) 2011;111:1201-1210.

53. Pinckard K, Baskin KK, Stanford KI. Effects of exercise to improve cardiovascular health. *Front Cardiovasc Med.* 2019;6:69.

54. Church TS, Earnest CP, Skinner JS, Blair SN. Effects of different doses of physical activity on cardiorespiratory fitness among sedentary, overweight or obese postmenopausal women with elevated blood pressure: a randomized controlled trial. *JAMA.* 2007;297:2081-2091.

55. Kokkinos PF, Narayan P, Colleran JA, et al. Effects of regular exercise on blood pressure and left ventricular hypertrophy in African-American men with severe hypertension. *N Engl J Med.* 1995;333:1462-1467.

56. Cornelissen VA, Buys R, Smart NA. Endurance exercise beneficially affects ambulatory blood pressure: a systematic review and meta-analysis. *J Hypertens.* 2013;31:639-648.

57. Tuomilehto J, Lindstrom J, Eriksson JG, et al. Prevention of type 2 diabetes mellitus by changes in lifestyle among subjects with impaired glucose tolerance. *N Engl J Med.* 2001;344:1343-1350.

58. Church TS, Blair SN, Cocreham S, et al. Effects of aerobic and resistance training on hemoglobin A1c levels in patients with type 2 diabetes: a randomized controlled trial. *JAMA.* 2010;304:2253-2262.

59. Kachur S, Chongthammakun V, Lavie CJ, et al. Impact of cardiac rehabilitation and exercise training programs in coronary heart disease. *Prog Cardiovasc Dis.* 2017;60:103-114.

60. Greenland P, Blaha MJ, Budoff MJ, Erbel R, Watson KE. Coronary calcium score and cardiovascular risk. *J Am Coll Cardiol.* 2018;72:434-447.

61. Polonsky TS, McClelland RL, Jorgensen NW, et al. Coronary artery calcium score and risk classification for coronary heart disease prediction. *JAMA.* 2010;303:1610-1616.

62. Elias-Smale SE, Proenca RV, Koller MT, et al. Coronary calcium score improves classification of coronary heart disease risk in the elderly: the Rotterdam study. *J Am Coll Cardiol.* 2010;56:1407-1414.

63. Erbel R, Mohlenkamp S, Moebus S, et al. Coronary risk stratification, discrimination, and reclassification improvement based on quantification of subclinical coronary atherosclerosis: the Heinz Nixdorf Recall study. *J Am Coll Cardiol.* 2010;56:1397-1406.

64. Paixao AR, Ayers CR, El Sabbagh A, et al. Coronary artery calcium improves risk classification in younger populations. *JACC Cardiovasc Imaging.* 2015;8:1285-1293.

65. Hoffmann U, Massaro JM, D'Agostino RB Sr., Kathiresan S, Fox CS, O'Donnell CJ. Cardiovascular event prediction and risk reclassification by coronary, aortic, and valvular calcification in the framingham heart study. *J Am Heart Assoc.* 2016;5.

66. Laddu DR, Rana JS, Murillo R, et al. 25-year physical activity trajectories and development of subclinical coronary artery disease as measured by coronary artery calcium: the Coronary Artery Risk Development in Young Adults (CARDIA) study. *Mayo Clin Proc.* 2017;92:1660-1670.

67. Delaney JAC, Jensky NE, Criqui MH, Whitt-Glover MC, Lima JAC, Allison MA. The association between physical activity and both incident coronary artery calcification and ankle brachial index progression: the Multi-Ethnic Study of Atherosclerosis. *Atherosclerosis.* 2013;230:278-283.

68. Lee CD, Jacobs DR, Jr., 68. Hankinson A, Iribarren C, Sidney S. Cardiorespiratory fitness and coronary artery calcification in young adults: The CARDIA Study. *Atherosclerosis.* 2009;203(1):263-268.

69. DeFina L, Radford N, Leonard D, Gibbons L, Khera A. Cardiorespiratory fitness and coronary artery calcification in women. *Atherosclerosis.* 2014;233:648-653.

70. Radford NB, DeFina LF, Leonard D, et al. Cardiorespiratory fitness, coronary artery calcium, and cardiovascular disease events in a cohort of generally healthy middle-age men: results from the Cooper Center Longitudinal Study. *Circulation.* 2018;137:1888-1895.

71. DeFina LF, Radford NB, Barlow CE, et al. Association of all-cause and cardiovascular mortality with high levels of physical activity and concurrent coronary artery calcification. *JAMA Cardiol.* 2019;4:174-181.

72. Aengevaeren VL, Mosterd A, Braber TL, et al. Relationship between lifelong exercise volume and coronary atherosclerosis in athletes. *Circulation.* 2017;136:138-148.

73. Polak JF, Pencina MJ, Pencina KM, O'Donnell CJ, Wolf PA, D'Agostino RB Sr. Carotid-wall intima-media thickness and cardiovascular events. *N Engl J Med.* 2011;365:213-221.

74. O'Leary DH, Polak JF, Kronmal RA, Manolio TA, Burke GL, Wolfson SK Jr. Carotid-artery intima and media thickness as a risk factor for myocardial infarction and stroke in older adults. Cardiovascular Health Study Collaborative Research Group. *N Engl J Med.* 1999;340:14-22.

75. Leischik R, Foshag P, Strauss M, et al. Physical activity, cardiorespiratory fitness and carotid intima thickness: sedentary occupation as risk factor for atherosclerosis and obesity. *Eur Rev Med Pharmacol Sci.* 2015;19:3157-3168.

76. Palatini P, Puato M, Rattazzi M, Pauletto P. Effect of regular physical activity on carotid intima-media thickness. Results from a 6-year prospective study in the early stage of hypertension. *Blood Press.* 2011;20:37-44.

77. Baldassarre D, Nyyssonen K, Rauramaa R, et al. Cross-sectional analysis of baseline data to identify the major determinants of carotid intima-media thickness in a European population: the IMPROVE study. *Eur Heart J.* 2010;31:614-622.

78. Morrison KM, Dyal L, Conner W, et al. Cardiovascular risk factors and non-invasive assessment of subclinical atherosclerosis in youth. *Atherosclerosis.* 2010;208:501-505.

79. Jain A, McClelland RL, Polak JF, et al. Cardiovascular imaging for assessing cardiovascular risk in asymptomatic men versus women: the multi-ethnic study of atherosclerosis (MESA). *Circ Cardiovasc Imaging.* 2011;4:8-15.

80. Kane GC, Karon BL, Mahoney DW, et al. Progression of left ventricular diastolic dysfunction and risk of heart failure. *JAMA.* 2011;306:856-863.

81. Sardana M, Konda P, Hashmath Z, et al. Usefulness of left ventricular strain by cardiac magnetic resonance feature-tracking to predict cardiovascular events in patients with and without heart failure. *Am J Cardiol.* 2019;123:1301-1308.

82. Redfield MM, Jacobsen SJ, Burnett JC, Mahoney DW, Bailey KR, Rodeheffer RJ. Burden of systolic and diastolic ventricular dysfunction in the community—appreciating the scope of the heart failure epidemic. *JAMA.* 2003;289:194-202.

83. Lam CS, Lyass A, Kraigher-Krainer E, et al. Cardiac dysfunction and noncardiac dysfunction as precursors of heart failure with reduced and preserved ejection fraction in the community. *Circulation.* 2011;124:24-30.

84. Brinker SK, Pandey A, Ayers CR, et al. Association of cardiorespiratory fitness with left ventricular remodeling and diastolic function: the Cooper Center Longitudinal Study. *JACC Heart Fail.* 2014;2:238-246.

85. Pandey A, Park B, Martens S, et al. Relationship of cardiorespiratory fitness and adiposity with left ventricular strain in middle-age adults (from the Dallas Heart Study). *Am J Cardiol.* 2017;120:1405-1409.

86. Pandey A, Allen NB, Ayers C, et al. Fitness in young adulthood and long-term cardiac structure and function: the CARDIA Study. *JACC Heart Fail.* 2017;5:347-355.

87. Arbab-Zadeh A, Dijk E, Prasad A, et al. Effect of aging and physical activity on left ventricular compliance. *Circulation.* 2004;110:1799-1805.

88. Boreham CA, Ferreira I, Twisk JW, Gallagher AM, Savage MJ, Murray LJ. Cardiorespiratory fitness, physical activity, and arterial stiffness: the Northern Ireland Young Hearts Project. *Hypertension.* 2004;44:721-726.

89. Ferreira I, Twisk JW, Van Mechelen W, et al. Current and adolescent levels of cardiopulmonary fitness are related to large artery properties at age 36: the Amsterdam Growth and Health Longitudinal Study. *Eur J Clin Invest.* 2002;32:723-731.

90. Tsang TS, Barnes ME, Gersh BJ, Bailey KR, Seward JB. Left atrial volume as a morphophysiologic expression of left ventricular diastolic dysfunction and relation to cardiovascular risk burden. *Am J Cardiol.* 2002;90:1284-1289.

91. Abhayaratna WP, Seward JB, Appleton CP, et al. Left atrial size: physiologic determinants and clinical applications. *J Am Coll Cardiol.* 2006;47:2357-2363.

92. Schillaci MA, Jones-Engel L, Engel GA, et al. Prevalence of enzootic simian viruses among urban performance monkeys in Indonesia. *Trop Med Int Health.* 2005;10:1305-1314.

93. Iskandar A, Mujtaba MT, Thompson PD. Left atrium size in elite athletes. *JACC Cardiovasc Imaging.* 2015;8:753-762.

94. Elliott AD, Mahajan R, Linz D, et al. Atrial remodeling and ectopic burden in recreational athletes: implications for risk of atrial fibrillation. *Clin Cardiol.* 2018;41:843-848.

95. Pelliccia A, Maron BJ, Di Paolo FM, et al. Prevalence and clinical significance of left atrial remodeling in competitive athletes. *J Am Coll Cardiol.* 2005;46:690-696.

96. Opondo MA, Aiad N, Cain MA, et al. Does high-intensity endurance training increase the risk of atrial fibrillation? A longitudinal study of left atrial structure and function. *Circ Arrhythm Electrophysiol.* 2018;11:e005598.

97. McNamara DA, Aiad N, Howden E, et al. Left atrial electromechanical remodeling following 2 years of high-intensity exercise training in sedentary middle-aged adults. *Circulation.* 2019;139:1507-1516.

98. Letnes JM, Nes B, Vaardal-Lunde K, et al. Left atrial volume, cardiorespiratory fitness, and diastolic function in healthy individuals: the HUNT study, Norway. *J Am Heart Assoc.* 2020;9:e014682.

99. Byrkjeland R, Stensaeth KH, Anderssen S, et al. Effects of exercise training on carotid intima-media thickness in patients with type 2 diabetes and coronary artery disease. Influence of carotid plaques. *Cardiovasc Diabetol.* 2016;15:13.

100. Fujimoto N, Prasad A, Hastings JL, et al. Cardiovascular effects of 1 year of progressive and vigorous exercise training in previously sedentary individuals older than 65 years of age. *Circulation.* 2010;122:1797-1805.

101. Fujimoto N, Hastings JL, Carrick-Ranson G, et al. Cardiovascular effects of 1 year of alagebrium and endurance exercise training in healthy older individuals. *Circ Heart Fail.* 2013;6:1155-1164.

102. Anand V, Garg S, Garg J, Bano S, Pritzker M. Impact of exercise training on cardiac function among patients with type 2 diabetes: a systematic review and meta-analysis. *J Cardiopulm Rehabil Prev.* 2018;38:358-365.

103. Montero D, Roche E, Martinez-Rodriguez A. The impact of aerobic exercise training on arterial stiffness in pre- and hypertensive subjects: a systematic review and meta-analysis. *Int J Cardiol.* 2014;173:361-368.

104. Lopes S, Afreixo V, Teixeira M, et al. Exercise training reduces arterial stiffness in adults with hypertension: a systematic review and meta-analysis. *J Hypertens.* 2020.

105. Wahid A, Manek N, Nichols M, et al. Quantifying the association between physical activity and cardiovascular disease and diabetes: a systematic review and meta-analysis. *J Am Heart Assoc.* 2016;5.

106. Renninger M, Lochen ML, Ekelund U, et al. The independent and joint associations of physical activity and body mass index with myocardial infarction: the Tromso Study. *Prev Med.* 2018;116:94-98.

107. Barengo NC, Antikainen R, Borodulin K, Harald K, Jousilahti P. Leisure-time physical activity reduces total and cardiovascular mortality and cardiovascular disease incidence in older adults. *J Am Geriatr Soc.* 2017;65:504-510.

108. Kubota Y, Iso H, Yamagishi K, Sawada N, Tsugane S, Group JS. Daily total physical activity and incident cardiovascular disease in Japanese men and women: Japan Public Health Center-based prospective study. *Circulation.* 2017;135:1471-1473.

109. Lear SA, Hu W, Rangarajan S, et al. The effect of physical activity on mortality and cardiovascular disease in 130 000 people from 17 high-income, middle-income, and low-income countries: the PURE study. *Lancet.* 2017;390:2643-2654.

110. Chomistek AK, Cook NR, Rimm EB, Ridker PM, Buring JE, Lee IM. Physical activity and incident cardiovascular disease in women: is the relation modified by level of global cardiovascular risk? *J Am Heart Assoc.* 2018;7.

111. Sattelmair J, Pertman J, Ding EL, Kohl HW 3rd, Haskell W, Lee IM. Dose response between physical activity and risk of coronary heart disease: a meta-analysis. *Circulation.* 2011;124:789-795.

112. Berry JD, Pandey A, Gao A, et al. Physical fitness and risk for heart failure and coronary artery disease. *Circ Heart Fail*. 2013;6:627-634.

113. Gander JC, Sui XM, Hebert JR, et al. Association of cardiorespiratory fitness with coronary heart disease in asymptomatic men. *Mayo Clin Proc*. 2015;90:1372-1379.

114. Khan H, Jaffar N, Rauramaa R, Kurl S, Savonen K, Laukkanen JA. Cardiorespiratory fitness and nonfatalcardiovascular events: a population-based follow-up study. *Am Heart J*. 2017;184.

115. Tikkanen E, Gustafsson S, Ingelsson E. Associations of fitness, physical activity, strength, and genetic risk with cardiovascular disease longitudinal analyses in the UK Biobank study. *Circulation*. 2018;137:2583-2591.

116. Letnes JM, Dalen H, Vesterbekkmo EK, Wisloff U, Nes BM. Peak oxygen uptake and incident coronary heart disease in a healthy population: the HUNT Fitness Study. *Eur Heart J*. 2019;40:1633-1639.

117. Al-Mallah MH, Sakr S, Al-Qunaibet A. Cardiorespiratory fitness and cardiovascular disease prevention: an update. *Curr Atheroscler Rep*. 2018;20:1.

118. Lakka TA, Venalainen JM, Rauramaa R, et al. Relation of leisure-time physical activity and cardiorespiratory fitness to the risk of acute myocardial infarction. *N Engl J Med*. 1994;330:1549-1554.

119. Andersen K, Mariosa D, Adami HO, et al. Dose-response relationship of total and leisure time physical activity to risk of heart failure: a prospective cohort study. *Circ Heart Fail*. 2014;7:701-708.

120. Pandey A, Garg S, Khunger M, et al. Dose-response relationship between physical activity and risk of heart failure: a meta-analysis. *Circulation*. 2015;132:1786-1794.

121. Pandey A, LaMonte M, Klein L, et al. Relationship between physical activity, body mass index, and risk of heart failure. *J Am Coll Cardiol*. 2017;69:1129-1142.

122. Kupsky DF, Ahmed AM, Sakr S, et al. Cardiorespiratory fitness and incident heart failure: the Henry Ford ExercIse Testing (FIT) Project. *Am Heart J*. 2017;185:35-42.

123. Lindgren M, Aberg M, Schaufelberger M, Aberg D, Schioler L, Toren K, Rosengren A. Cardiorespiratory fitness and muscle strength in late adolescence and long-term risk of early heart failure in Swedish men. *Eur J Prev Cardiol*. 2017;24:876-884.

124. Myers J, Kokkinos P, Chan K, et al. Cardiorespiratory fitness and reclassification of risk for incidence of heart failure: the veterans exercise testing study. *Circ Heart Fail*. 2017;10.

125. Khan H, Kunutsor S, Rauramaa R, et al. Cardiorespiratory fitness and risk of heart failure: a population-based follow-up study. *Eur J Heart Fail*. 2014;16:180-188.

126. Kokkinos P, Faselis C, Franklin B, et al. Cardiorespiratory fitness, body mass index and heart failure incidence. *Eur J Heart Fail*. 2019;21:436-444.

127. Pandey A, Patel KV, Bahnson JL, et al. Association of intensive lifestyle intervention, fitness, and body mass index with risk of heart failure in overweight or obese adults with type 2 diabetes mellitus: an analysis from the look AHEAD trial. *Circulation*. 2020;141:1295-1306.

128. Horwich TB, Fonarow GC, Clark AL. Obesity and the obesity paradox in heart failure. *Prog Cardiovasc Dis*. 2018;61:151-156.

129. Lavie CJ, Laddu D, Arena R, Ortega FB, Alpert MA, Kushner RF. Healthy weight and obesity prevention: JACC Health Promotion Series. *J Am Coll Cardiol*. 2018;72:1506-1531.

130. Pandey A, Patel KV, Vaduganathan M, et al. Physical activity, fitness, and obesity in heart failure with preserved ejection fraction. *JACC Heart Fail*. 2018;6:975-982.

131. Oktay AA, Rich JD, Shah SJ. The emerging epidemic of heart failure with preserved ejection fraction. *Curr Heart Fail Rep*. 2013;10:401-410.

132. Azarbal F, Stefanick ML, Salmoirago-Blotcher E, et al. Obesity, physical activity, and their interaction in incident atrial fibrillation in postmenopausal women. *J Am Heart Assoc*. 2014;3.

133. Bapat A, Zhang Y, Post WS, et al. Relation of physical activity and incident atrial fibrillation (from the Multi-Ethnic Study of Atherosclerosis). *Am J Cardiol*. 2015;116:883-888.

134. Calvo N, Ramos P, Montserrat S, et al. Emerging risk factors and the dose-response relationship between physical activity and lone atrial fibrillation: a prospective case-control study. *Europace*. 2016;18:57-63.

135. Diouf I, Magliano DJ, Carrington MJ, Stewart S, Shaw JE. Prevalence, incidence, risk factors and treatment of atrial fibrillation in Australia: The Australian Diabetes, Obesity and Lifestyle (AusDiab) longitudinal, population cohort study. *Int J Cardiol*. 2016;205:127-132.

136. Drca N, Wolk A, Jensen-Urstad M, Larsson SC. Atrial fibrillation is associated with different levels of physical activity levels at different ages in men. *Heart*. 2014;100:1037-1042.

137. Drca N, Wolk A, Jensen-Urstad M, Larsson SC. Physical activity is associated with a reduced risk of atrial fibrillation in middle-aged and elderly women. *Heart*. 2015;101:1627-1630.

138. Everett BM, Conen D, Buring JE, Moorthy MV, Lee IM, Albert CM. Physical activity and the risk of incident atrial fibrillation in women. *Circ Cardiovasc Qual Outcomes*. 2011;4:321-327.

139. Huxley RR, Misialek JR, Agarwal SK, et al. Physical activity, obesity, weight change, and risk of atrial fibrillation: the Atherosclerosis Risk in Communities study. *Circ Arrhythm Electrophysiol*. 2014;7:620-625.

140. Morseth B, Graff-Iversen S, Jacobsen BK, et al. Physical activity, resting heart rate, and atrial fibrillation: the Tromso Study. *Eur Heart J*. 2016;37:2307-2313.

141. Ricci C, Gervasi F, Gaeta M, Smuts CM, Schutte AE, Leitzmann MF. Physical activity volume in relation to risk of atrial fibrillation. A nonlinear meta-regression analysis. *Eur J Prev Cardiol*. 2018;25:857-866.

142. Elliott AD, Maatman B, Emery MS, Sanders P. The role of exercise in atrial fibrillation prevention and promotion: Finding optimal ranges for health. *Heart Rhythm*. 2017;14:1713-1720.

143. Li X, Cui S, Xuan D, Xuan C, Xu D. Atrial fibrillation in athletes and general population: a systematic review and meta-analysis. *Medicine (Baltimore)*. 2018;97:e13405.

144. Myrstad M, Nystad W, Graff-Iversen S, et al. Effect of years of endurance exercise on risk of atrial fibrillation and atrial flutter. *Am J Cardiol*. 2014;114:1229-1233.

145. Myrstad M, Lochen ML, Graff-Iversen S, et al. Increased risk of atrial fibrillation among elderly Norwegian men with a history of long-term endurance sport practice. *Scand J Med Sci Sports*. 2014;24:e238-e244.

146. Myrstad M, Aaronaes M, Graff-Iversen S, Nystad W, Ranhoff AH. Does endurance exercise cause atrial fibrillation in women? *Int J Cardiol*. 2015;184:431-432.

147. Andersen K, Farahmand B, Ahlbom A, et al. Risk of arrhythmias in 52 755 long-distance cross-country skiers: a cohort study. *Eur Heart J*. 2013;34:3624-3631.

148. Svedberg N, Sundstrom J, James S, Hallmarker U, Hambraeus K, Andersen K. Long-term incidence of atrial fibrillation and stroke among cross-country skiers. *Circulation*. 2019;140:910-920.

149. Andersen K, Rasmussen F, Held C, Neovius M, Tynelius P, Sundstrom J. Exercise capacity and muscle strength and risk of vascular disease and arrhythmia in 1.1 million young Swedish men: cohort study. *BMJ*. 2015;351:h4543.

150. Khan H, Kella D, Rauramaa R, Savonen K, Lloyd MS, Laukkanen JA. Cardiorespiratory fitness and atrial fibrillation: a population-based follow-up study. *Heart Rhythm*. 2015;12:1424-1430.

151. Qureshi WT, Alirhayim Z, Blaha MJ, et al. Cardiorespiratory fitness and risk of incident atrial fibrillation: results from the Henry Ford Exercise Testing (FIT) project. *Circulation*. 2015;131:1827-1834.

152. Faselis C, Kokkinos P, Tsimploulis A, et al. Exercise capacity and atrial fibrillation risk in veterans: a cohort study. *Mayo Clin Proc*. 2016;91:558-566.

153. Hussain N, Gersh BJ, Gonzalez Carta K, et al. Impact of cardiorespiratory fitness on frequency of atrial fibrillation, stroke, and all-cause mortality. *Am J Cardiol*. 2018;121:41-49.

154. Matthews CE, Hagstromer M, Pober DM, Bowles HR. Best practices for using physical activity monitors in population-based research. *Med Sci Sports Exerc*. 2012;44:S68-S76.

155. National Health and Nutrition Examination Survey Data 2003-2004, 2005-2006, Centers for Disease Control and Prevention (CDC), National Center for Health Statistics (NCHS), Atlanta, GA (2009-2010) [article online], Available from http://www.cdc.gov/nchs/nhanes.htm.

156. Borodulin K, Kärki A, Laatikainen T, Peltonen M, Luoto R. Daily sedentary time and risk of cardiovascular disease: the national FINRISK 2002 study. *J Physic Activ Health.* 2015;12:904-908.

157. Biswas A, Oh PI, Faulkner GE, et al. Sedentary time and its association with risk for disease incidence, mortality, and hospitalization in adults: a systematic review and meta-analysis. *Ann Intern Med.* 2015;162:123-132.

158. Chomistek AK, Manson JE, Stefanick ML, et al. Relationship of sedentary behavior and physical activity to incident cardiovascular disease: results from the Women's Health Initiative. *J Am Coll Cardiol.* 2013;61:2346-2354.

159. Pandey A, Salahuddin U, Garg S, A. Continuous dose-response association between sedentary time and risk for cardiovascular disease: a meta-analysis. *JAMA Cardiol.* 2016;1:575-583.

160. Bellettiere J, LaMonte MJ, Evenson KR, et al. Sedentary behavior and cardiovascular disease in older women: the Objective Physical Activity and Cardiovascular Health (OPACH) Study. *Circulation.* 2019;139:1036-1046.

161. Bjørk Petersen C, Bauman A, Grønbæk M, Wulff Helge J, Thygesen LC, Tolstrup JS. Total sitting time and risk of myocardial infarction, coronary heart disease and all-cause mortality in a prospective cohort of Danish adults. *Int J Behav Nutr Phys Act.* 2014;11:13.

162. Rariden BS, Boltz AJ, Brawner CA, et al. Sedentary time and cumulative risk of preserved and reduced ejection fraction heart failure: from the Multi-Ethnic Study of Atherosclerosis. *J Cardiac Fail.* 2019;25:418-424.

163. Kubota Y, Alonso A, Shah AM, Chen LY, Folsom AR. Television watching as sedentary behavior and atrial fibrillation: the Atherosclerosis Risk in Communities study. *J Physic Activ Health.* 2018;15:895-899.

164. Kraigher-Krainer E, Lyass A, Massaro JM, et al. Association of physical activity and heart failure with preserved vs. reduced ejection fraction in the elderly: the Framingham Heart Study. *Eur J Heart Fail.* 2013;15:742-746.

165. Florido R, Kwak L, Lazo M, et al. Six-year changes in physical activity and the risk of incident heart failure: ARIC study. *Circulation.* 2018;137:2142-2151.

166. Look ARG, Wing RR, Bolin P, et al. Cardiovascular effects of intensive lifestyle intervention in type 2 diabetes. *N Engl J Med.* 2013;369:145-154.

167. Alonso A, Bahnson JL, Gaussoin SA, et al. Effect of an intensive lifestyle intervention on atrial fibrillation risk in individuals with type 2 diabetes: the Look AHEAD randomized trial. *Am Heart J.* 2015;170:770-777, e775.

168. Myers J, Prakash M, Froelicher V, Do D, Partington S, Atwood JE. Exercise capacity and mortality among men referred for exercise testing. *N Engl J Med.* 2002;346:793-801.

169. Garnvik LE, Malmo V, Janszky I, et al. Physical activity, cardiorespiratory fitness, and cardiovascular outcomes in individuals with atrial fibrillation: the HUNT study. *Eur Heart J.* 2020;41:1467-1475.

170. Lavie CJ, Menezes AR, De Schutter A, Milani RV, Blumenthal JA. Impact of cardiac rehabilitation and exercise training on psychological risk factors and subsequent prognosis in patients with cardiovascular disease. *Can J Cardiol.* 2016;32:S365-S373.

171. Anderson L, Oldridge N, Thompson DR, et al. Exercise-based cardiac rehabilitation for coronary heart disease: Cochrane Systematic Review and Meta-Analysis. *J Am Coll Cardiol.* 2016;67:1-12.

172. Lavie CJ, Arena R, Franklin BA. Cardiac rehabilitation and healthy lifestyle interventions: rectifying program deficiencies to improve patient outcomes. *J Am Coll Cardiol.* 2016;67:13-15.

173. Lavie CJ, Kachur S, Milani RV. Making cardiac rehabilitation more available and affordable. *Heart.* 2019;105:94-95.

174. O'Connor CM, Whellan DJ, Lee KL, et al. Efficacy and safety of exercise training in patients with chronic heart failure: HF-ACTION randomized controlled trial. *JAMA.* 2009;301:1439-1450.

175. Davies EJ, Moxham T, Rees K, et al. Exercise training for systolic heart failure: Cochrane Systematic Review and Meta-Analysis. *Eur J Heart Fail.* 2010;12:706-715.

176. Malmo V, Nes BM, Amundsen BH, et al. Aerobic interval training reduces the burden of atrial fibrillation in the short term: a randomized trial. *Circulation.* 2016;133:466-473.

177. Pathak RK, Elliott A, Middeldorp ME, et al. Impact of CARDIOrespiratory FITness on arrhythmia recurrence in obese individuals with atrial fibrillation: the CARDIO-FIT study. *J Am Coll Cardiol.* 2015;66:985-996.

178. Pathak RK, Middeldorp ME, Meredith M, et al. Long-term effect of goal-directed weight management in an atrial fibrillation cohort: a long-term follow-up study (LEGACY). *J Am Coll Cardiol.* 2015;65:2159-2169.

179. Kato M, Ogano M, Mori Y, et al. Exercise-based cardiac rehabilitation for patients with catheter ablation for persistent atrial fibrillation: a randomized controlled clinical trial. *Eur J Prev Cardiol.* 2019;26:1931-1940.

180. Artero EG, Lee DC, Lavie CJ, et al. Effects of muscular strength on cardiovascular risk factors and prognosis. *J Cardiopulm Rehabil Prev.* 2012;32:351-358.

181. Maslow AL, Sui X, Colabianchi N, Hussey J, Blair SN. Muscular strength and incident hypertension in normotensive and prehypertensive men. *Med Sci Sports Exerc.* 2010;42:288-295.

182. de Sousa EC, Abrahin O, Ferreira ALL, Rodrigues RP, Alves EAC, Vieira RP. Resistance training alone reduces systolic and diastolic blood pressure in prehypertensive and hypertensive individuals: meta-analysis. *Hypertens Res.* 2017;40:927-931.

183. Ji C, Zheng L, Zhang R, Wu Q, Zhao Y. Handgrip strength is positively related to blood pressure and hypertension risk: results from the National Health and nutrition examination survey. *Lipids Health Dis.* 2018;17:86.

184. Rodrigues de Lima T, Gonzalez-Chica DA, Santos Silva DA. Clusters of cardiovascular risk factors and its association with muscle strength in adults. *J Sports Med Phys Fitness.* 2020;60:479-485.

185. Ko KJ, Kang SJ, Lee KS. Association between cardiorespiratory, muscular fitness and metabolic syndrome in Korean men. *Diabetes Metab Syndr.* 2019;13:536-541.

186. Hong S. Association of relative handgrip strength and metabolic syndrome in Korean older adults: Korea national health and nutrition examination survey VII-1. *J Obes Metab Syndr.* 2019;28:53-60.

187. Jackson AW, Lee DC, Sui X, et al. Muscular strength is inversely related to prevalence and incidence of obesity in adult men. *Obesity (Silver Spring).* 2010;18:1988-1995.

188. Timpka S, Petersson IF, Zhou C, Englund M. Muscle strength in adolescent men and risk of cardiovascular disease events and mortality in middle age: a prospective cohort study. *BMC Med.* 2014;12:62.

189. Silventoinen K, Magnusson PK, Tynelius P, Batty GD, Rasmussen F. Association of body size and muscle strength with incidence of coronary heart disease and cerebrovascular diseases: a population-based cohort study of one million Swedish men. *Int J Epidemiol.* 2009;38:110-118.

190. Sillars A, Celis-Morales CA, Ho FK, et al. Association of fitness and grip strength with heart failure: findings from the UK Biobank population-based study. *Mayo Clin Proc.* 2019;94:2230-2240.

191. Lopez-Jaramillo P, Cohen DD, Gómez-Arbeláez D, et al. Association of handgrip strength to cardiovascular mortality in pre-diabetic and diabetic patients: a subanalysis of the ORIGIN trial. *Int J Cardiol.* 2014;174:458-461.

192. Csapo R, Alegre LM. Effects of resistance training with moderate vs heavy loads on muscle mass and strength in the elderly: a meta-analysis. *Scand J Med Sci Sports.* 2016;26:995-1006.

193. Franco CMC, Carneiro MAS, de Sousa JFR, Gomes GK, Orsatti FL. Influence of high- and low-frequency resistance training on lean body mass and muscle strength gains in untrained men. *J Strength Cond Res.* 2019.

194. Bakker EA, Lee DC, Sui X, et al. Association of resistance exercise, independent of and combined with aerobic exercise, with the incidence of metabolic syndrome. *Mayo Clin Proc.* 2017;92:1214-1222.

195. Sigal RJ, Kenny GP, Boulé NG, et al. Effects of aerobic training, resistance training, or both on glycemic control in type 2 diabetes: a randomized trial. *Ann Intern Med.* 2007;147:357-369.

196. Liu Y, Lee DC, Li Y, et al. Associations of resistance exercise with cardiovascular disease morbidity and mortality. *Med Sci Sports Exerc.* 2019;51:499-508.

197. Kamada M, Shiroma EJ, Buring JE, Miyachi M, Lee IM. Strength training and all-cause, cardiovascular disease, and cancer mortality in older women: a cohort study. *J Am Heart Assoc.* 2017;6.

198. Pires NF, Coelho-Júnior HJ, Gambassi BB, et al. Combined aerobic and resistance exercises evokes longer reductions on ambulatory blood pressure in resistant hypertension: a randomized crossover trial. *Cardiovasc therapeut.* 2020;8157858.

199. Boeno FP, Ramis TR, Munhoz SV, et al. Effect of aerobic and resistance exercise training on inflammation, endothelial function and ambulatory blood pressure in middle-aged hypertensive patients. *J Hypertens.* 2020.

200. Said MA, Abdelmoneem M, Alibrahim MC, Elsebee MA, Kotb AAH. Effects of diet versus diet plus aerobic and resistance exercise on metabolic syndrome in obese young men. *J Exer Sci Fitness.* 2020;18:101-108.

201. Lemes IR, Ferreira PH, Linares SN, et al. Resistance training reduces systolic blood pressure in metabolic syndrome: a systematic review and meta-analysis of randomised controlled trials. *Br J Sports Med.* 2016;50:1438-1442.

202. Cornelissen VA, Fagard RH, Coeckelberghs E, Vanhees L. Impact of resistance training on blood pressure and other cardiovascular risk factors: a meta-analysis of randomized, controlled trials. *Hypertension.* 2011;58:950-958.

203. Bauman AE, Reis RS, Sallis JF, et al. Correlates of physical activity: why are some people physically active and others not? *Lancet.* 2012;380:258-271.

204. Aleksovska K, Puggina A, Giraldi L, et al. Biological determinants of physical activity across the life course: a "Determinants of Diet and Physical Activity" (DEDIPAC) umbrella systematic literature review. *Sports Med Open.* 2019;5:2.

205. Craggs C, Corder K, van Sluijs EM, Griffin SJ. Determinants of change in physical activity in children and adolescents: a systematic review. *Am J Prev Med.* 2011;40:645-658.

206. Uijtdewilligen L, Nauta J, Singh AS, et al. Determinants of physical activity and sedentary behaviour in young people: a review and quality synthesis of prospective studies. *Br J Sports Med.* 2011;45:896-905.

207. Schlaff RA, Baruth M, Boggs A, Hutto B. Patterns of sedentary behavior in older adults. *Am J Health Behav.* 2017;41:411-418.

208. Ward BW, Schiller JS. Prevalence of multiple chronic conditions among US adults: estimates from the National Health Interview Survey, 2010. *Prev Chronic Dis.* 2013;10:E65.

209. Piirtola M, Kaprio J, Ropponen A. A study of sedentary behaviour in the older Finnish twin cohort: a cross sectional analysis. *Biomed Res Int.* 2014;2014:209140.

210. Schutte NM, Huppertz C, Doornweerd S, Bartels M, de Geus EJC, van der Ploeg HP. Heritability of objectively assessed and self-reported sedentary behavior. *Scand J Med Sci Sports.* 2020;30:1237-1247.

211. Klimentidis YC, Arora A, Chougule A, Zhou J, Raichlen DA. FTO association and interaction with time spent sitting. *Int J Obes (Lond).* 2016;40:411-416.

212. Simonen RL, Rankinen T, Perusse L, et al. A dopamine D2 receptor gene polymorphism and physical activity in two family studies. *Physiol Behav.* 2003;78(4-5):751-757.

213. Lin X, Chan KK, Huang YT, et al. Genetic determinants for leisure-time physical activity. *Med Sci Sports Exerc.* 2018;50:1620-1628.

214. Rollo S, Gaston A, Prapavessis H. Cognitive and motivational factors associated with sedentary behavior: a systematic review. *AIMS Public Health.* 2016;3:956-984.

215. Koeneman MA, Verheijden MW, Chinapaw MJ, Hopman-Rock M. Determinants of physical activity and exercise in healthy older adults: a systematic review. *Int J Behav Nutr Phys Act.* 2011;8:142.

216. van Stralen MM, Lechner L, Mudde AN, de Vries H, Bolman C. Determinants of awareness, initiation and maintenance of physical activity among the over-fifties: a Delphi study. *Health Educ Res.* 2010;25:233-247.

217. Dall PM, Ellis SLH, Ellis BM, et al. The influence of dog ownership on objective measures of free-living physical activity and sedentary behaviour in community-dwelling older adults: a longitudinal case-controlled study. *BMC Public Health.* 2017;17:496.

218. Siddiqi Z, Tiro JA, Shuval K. Understanding impediments and enablers to physical activity among African American adults: a systematic review of qualitative studies. *Health Educ Res.* 2011;26:1010-1024.

219. Buck C, Loyen A, Foraita R, et al. Factors influencing sedentary behaviour: a system based analysis using Bayesian networks within DEDIPAC. *PLoS One.* 2019;14:e0211546.

220. McCormack GR, Shiell A. In search of causality: a systematic review of the relationship between the built environment and physical activity among adults. *Int J Behav Nutr Phys Act.* 2011;8:125.

221. Hou N, Popkin BM, Jacobs DR Jr., et al. Longitudinal trends in gasoline price and physical activity: the CARDIA study. *Prev Med.* 2011;52:365-369.

222. Lo BK, Morgan EH, Folta SC, et al. Environmental influences on physical activity among rural adults in Montana, United States: views from built environment audits, resident focus groups, and key informant interviews. *Int J Environ Res Public Health.* 2017;14.

223. Bauman A, Ma G, Cuevas F, et al. Cross-national comparisons of socio-economic differences in the prevalence of leisure-time and occupational physical activity, and active commuting in six Asia-Pacific countries. *J Epidemiol Community Health.* 2011;65:35-43.

224. Yiga P, Seghers J, Ogwok P, Matthys C. Determinants of dietary and physical activity behaviours among women of reproductive age in urban sub-Saharan Africa: a systematic review. *Br J Nutr.* 2020;124:761-772.

225. Sisson SB, Katzmarzyk PT, Earnest CP, Bouchard C, Blair SN, Church TS. Volume of exercise and fitness nonresponse in sedentary, postmenopausal women. *Med Sci Sports Exerc.* 2009;41(3):539-545.

226. Schmid JP, Zurek M, Saner H. Chronotropic incompetence predicts impaired response to exercise training in heart failure patients with sinus rhythm. *Eur J Prev Cardiol.* 2013;20:585-592.

227. La Gerche A, Burns AT, Taylor AJ, Macisaac AI, Heidbuchel H, Prior DL. Maximal oxygen consumption is best predicted by measures of cardiac size rather than function in healthy adults. *Eur J Appl Physiol.* 2012;112:2139-2147.

228. Slentz CA, Duscha BD, Johnson JL, et al. Effects of the amount of exercise on body weight, body composition, and measures of central obesity: STRRIDE—a randomized controlled study. *Arch Intern Med.* 2004;164:31-39.

229. Lee C, Ory MG, Yoon J, Forjuoh SN. Neighborhood walking among overweight and obese adults: age variations in barriers and motivators. *J Community Health.* 2013;38:12-22.

230. Bunn JA, Navalta JW, Fountaine CJ, Reece JD. Current state of commercial wearable technology in physical activity monitoring 2015-2017. *Int J Exerc Sci.* 2018;11:503-515.

231. Kanejima Y, Kitamura M, Izawa KP. Self-monitoring to increase physical activity in patients with cardiovascular disease: a systematic review and meta-analysis. *Aging Clin Exp Res.* 2019;31:163-173.

232. Feldman DI, Theodore Robison W, Pacor JM, et al. Harnessing mHealth technologies to increase physical activity and prevent cardiovascular disease. *Clin Cardiol.* 2018;41:985-991.

233. Jakicic JM, Davis KK, Rogers RJ, et al. Effect of wearable technology combined with a lifestyle intervention on long-term weight loss: the IDEA randomized clinical trial. *JAMA.* 2016;316:1161-1171.

234. Zisko N, Skjerve KN, Tari AR, et al. Personal Activity Intelligence (PAI), sedentary behavior and cardiovascular risk factor clustering—the HUNT Study. *Prog Cardiovasc Dis.* 2017;60:89-95.

235. Kay MC, Carroll DD, Carlson SA, Fulton JE. Awareness and knowledge of the 2008 Physical Activity Guidelines for Americans. *J Phys Act Health.* 2014;11:693-698.

236. Lobelo F, Rohm Young D, Sallis R, et al. Routine assessment and promotion of physical activity in healthcare settings: a scientific statement from the American Heart Association. *Circulation*. 2018;137:e495-e522.

237. Sallis R, Franklin B, Joy L, Ross R, Sabgir D, Stone J. Strategies for promoting physical activity in clinical practice. *Prog Cardiovasc Dis*. 2015;57:375-386.

238. Grant RW, Schmittdiel JA, Neugebauer RS, Uratsu CS, Sternfeld B. Exercise as a vital sign: a quasi-experimental analysis of a health system intervention to collect patient-reported exercise levels. *J Gen Intern Med*. 2014;29:341-348.

239. Sanchez A, Bully P, Martinez C, Grandes G. Effectiveness of physical activity promotion interventions in primary care: a review of reviews. *Prev Med*. 2015;76 (Suppl):S56-S67.

240. LeFevre ML, Force USPST. Behavioral counseling to promote a healthful diet and physical activity for cardiovascular disease prevention in adults with cardiovascular risk factors: U.S. Preventive Services Task Force Recommendation Statement. *Ann Intern Med*. 2014;161:587-593.

241. Albert FA, Crowe MJ, Malau-Aduli AEO, Malau-Aduli BS. Physical activity promotion: a systematic review of the perceptions of healthcare professionals. *Int J Environ Res Public Health*. 2020;17.

242. Arena R, Lavie CJ. The healthy lifestyle team is central to the success of accountable care organizations. *Mayo Clin Proc*. 2015;90:572-576.

243. Arena R, Guazzi M, Lianov L, et al. Healthy lifestyle interventions to combat noncommunicable disease-a novel nonhierarchical connectivity model for key stakeholders: a policy statement from the American Heart Association, European Society of Cardiology, European Association for Cardiovascular Prevention and Rehabilitation, and American College of Preventive Medicine. *Mayo Clin Proc*. 2015;90:1082-1103.

244. Pavey TG, Taylor AH, Fox KR, et al. Effect of exercise referral schemes in primary care on physical activity and improving health outcomes: systematic review and meta-analysis. *BMJ*. 2011;343:d6462.

245. Ely EK, Gruss SM, Luman ET, et al. A national effort to prevent type 2 diabetes: participant-level evaluation of CDC's national diabetes prevention program. *Diabetes Care*. 2017;40:1331-1341.

246. Neuhaus M, Healy GN, Fjeldsoe BS, et al. Iterative development of Stand Up Australia: a multi-component intervention to reduce workplace sitting. *Int J Behav Nutr Phys Act*. 2014;11:21.

247. van der Ploeg HP, Chey T, Ding D, Chau JY, Stamatakis E, Bauman AE. Standing time and all-cause mortality in a large cohort of Australian adults. *Prev Med*. 2014;69:187-191.

248. Healy GN, Eakin EG, Owen N, et al. A cluster randomized controlled trial to reduce office workers' sitting time: effect on activity outcomes. *Med Sci Sports Exerc*. 2016;48:1787-1797.

249. Edwardson CL, Yates T, Biddle SJH, et al. Effectiveness of the Stand More AT (SMArT) Work intervention: cluster randomised controlled trial. *BMJ*. 2018;363:k3870.

250. Healy GN, Winkler EAH, Eakin EG, et al. A cluster RCT to reduce workers' sitting time: impact on cardiometabolic biomarkers. *Med Sci Sports Exerc*. 2017;49:2032-2039.

251. Gao L, Nguyen P, Dunstan D, Moodie M. Are office-based workplace interventions designed to reduce sitting time cost-effective primary prevention measures for cardiovascular disease? A systematic review and modelled economic evaluation. *Int J Environ Res Public Health*. 2019;16.

252. Aittasalo M, Rinne M, Pasanen M, Kukkonen-Harjula K, Vasankari T. Promoting walking among office employees—evaluation of a randomized controlled intervention with pedometers and e-mail messages. *BMC Public Health*. 2012;12:403.

253. McEachan RR, Lawton RJ, Jackson C, Conner M, Meads DM, West RM. Testing a workplace physical activity intervention: a cluster randomized controlled trial. *Int J Behav Nutr Phys Act*. 2011;8:29.

254. Tudor-Locke C, Craig CL, Aoyagi Y, et al. How many steps/day are enough? For older adults and special populations. *Int J Behav Nutr Phys Act*. 2011;8:80.

255. Mortality GBD, Causes of Death C. Global, regional, and national age-sex specific all-cause and cause-specific mortality for 240 causes of death, 1990-2013: a systematic analysis for the Global Burden of Disease Study 2013. *Lancet*. 2015;385:117-171.

256. Ng SW, Popkin BM. Time use and physical activity: a shift away from movement across the globe. *Obes Rev*. 2012;13:659-680.

257. Sallis JF, Cerin E, Conway TL, et al. Physical activity in relation to urban environments in 14 cities worldwide: a cross-sectional study. *Lancet*. 2016;387:2207-2217.

258. Smith M, Hosking J, Woodward A, et al. Systematic literature review of built environment effects on physical activity and active transport—an update and new findings on health equity. *Int J Behav Nutr Phys Act*. 2017;14:158.

259. Hirsch JA, Moore KA, Clarke PJ, et al. Changes in the built environment and changes in the amount of walking over time: longitudinal results from the multi-ethnic study of atherosclerosis. *Am J Epidemiol*. 2014;180:799-809.

260. Berger AT, Qian XL, Pereira MA. Associations between bicycling for transportation and cardiometabolic risk factors among Minneapolis-Saint Paul area commuters: a cross-sectional study in working-age adults. *Am J Health Promot*. 2018;32:631-637.

261. Serrano N, Perez LG, Carlson J, et al. Sub-population differences in the relationship between the neighborhood environment and Latinas' daily walking and vehicle time. *J Transp Health*. 2018;8:210-219.

262. In *Physical Activity: Moving toward Obesity Solutions: Workshop Summary*. Washington, DC; 2015.

263. Let's move!. [article online], 2012. Available from https://web.archive.org/web/20120423172843/, http://www.letsmove.gov/active-schools

264. Kohl HW III, Cook HD, eds. *Educating the Student Body: Taking Physical Activity and Physical Education to School*. Washington, DC: The National Academies Press; 2013.

265. Jensen MD, Ryan DH, Apovian CM, et al. 2013 AHA/ACC/TOS guideline for the management of overweight and obesity in adults: a report of the American College of Cardiology/American Heart Association Task Force on Practice Guidelines and The Obesity Society. *J Am Coll Cardiol*. 2014;63:2985-3023.

266. O'Brien MW, Shields CA, Oh PI, Fowles JR. Health care provider confidence and exercise prescription practices of exercise is medicine Canada workshop attendees. *Appl Physiol Nutr Metab*. 2017;42:384-390.

267. Hivert MF, Arena R, Forman DE, et al. Medical training to achieve competency in lifestyle counseling: an essential foundation for prevention and treatment of cardiovascular diseases and other chronic medical conditions: a scientific statement from the American Heart Association. *Circulation*. 2016;134:e308-e327.

268. Hivert MF, McNeil A, Lavie CJ, Arena R. Training health professionals to deliver healthy living medicine. *Prog Cardiovasc Dis*. 2017;59:471-478.

269. Luckman S, Xiao C, McLennan E, Anderson AS, Mutrie N, Moug SJ. An investigation into UK medical students' knowledge of lifestyle factors on cancer. *Scott Med J*. 2017;62:110-114.

270. Bairey Merz CN, Alberts MJ, Balady GJ, et al. ACCF/AHA/ACP 2009 competence and training statement: a curriculum on prevention of cardiovascular disease: a report of the American College of Cardiology Foundation/American Heart Association/American College of Physicians Task Force on Competence and Training (Writing Committee to Develop a Competence and Training Statement on Prevention of Cardiovascular Disease): developed in collaboration with the American Academy of Neurology; American Association of Cardiovascular and Pulmonary Rehabilitation; American College of Preventive Medicine; American College of Sports Medicine; American Diabetes Association; American Society of Hypertension; Association of Black Cardiologists; Centers for Disease Control and Prevention; National Heart, Lung, and Blood Institute; National Lipid Association; and Preventive Cardiovascular Nurses Association. *J Am Coll Cardiol*. 2009;54:1336-1363.

271. Cuff PA, Vanselow NA, eds. *Improving Medical Education: Enhancing the Behavioral and Social Science Content of Medical School Curricula*. Washington, DC: The National Academies Press; 2004.

272. Windt J, Windt A, Davis J, Petrella R, Khan K. Can a 3-hour educational workshop and the provision of practical tools encourage family physicians to prescribe physical activity as medicine? A pre-post study. *BMJ Open.* 2015;5:e007920.

273. Fowles JR, O'Brien MW, Solmundson K, Oh PI, Shields CA. Exercise is medicine Canada physical activity counselling and exercise prescription training improves counselling, prescription, and referral practices among physicians across Canada. *Appl Physiol Nutr Metab.* 2018;43:535-539.

274. Lang J, James C, Ashby S, et al. The provision of weight management advice: an investigation into occupational therapy practice. *Aust Occup Ther J.* 2013;60:387-394.

275. Curran AE, Caplan DJ, Lee JY, et al. Dentists' attitudes about their role in addressing obesity in patients: a national survey. *J Am Dent Assoc.* 2010;141:1307-1316.

276. Arena R, Lavie CJ, Hivert MF, Williams MA, Briggs PD, Guazzi M. Who will deliver comprehensive healthy lifestyle interventions to combat non-communicable disease? Introducing the healthy lifestyle practitioner discipline. *Expert Rev Cardiovasc Ther.* 2016;14:15-22.

277. Schnohr P, O'Keefe JH, Marott JL, Lange P, Jensen GB. Dose of jogging and long-term mortality: the Copenhagen City Heart Study. *J Am Coll Cardiol.* 2015;65:411-419.

278. Williams PT, Thompson PD. Increased cardiovascular disease mortality associated with excessive exercise in heart attack survivors. *Mayo Clin Proc.* 2014;89:1187-1194.

279. Mons U, Hahmann H, Brenner H. A reverse J-shaped association of leisure time physical activity with prognosis in patients with stable coronary heart disease: evidence from a large cohort with repeated measurements. *Heart.* 2014;100:1043.

280. Lavie CJ, O'Keefe JH, Sallis RE. Exercise and the heart-the harm of too little and too much. *Curr Sports Med Rep.* 2015;14:104-109.

281. Lee D-c, Lavie CJ, Vedanthan R. Optimal dose of running for longevity: is more better or worse? *J Am Coll Cardiol.* 2015;65:420-422.

282. Zubin Maslov P, Schulman A, Lavie CJ, Narula J. Personalized exercise dose prescription. *Eur Heart J.* 2018;39:2346-2355.

283. Lee D-c, Pate RR, Lavie CJ, Sui X, Church TS, Blair SN. Leisure-time running reduces all-cause and cardiovascular mortality risk. *J Am Coll Cardiol.* 2014;64:472-481.

284. Lee D-c, Brellenthin AG, Thompson PD, Sui X, Lee IM, Lavie CJ. Running as a key lifestyle medicine for longevity. *Progress Cardiovasc Dis.* 2017;60:45-55.

285. Banday AH, Want FA, Alris FF, Alrayes MF, Alenzi MJ. A cross-sectional study on the prevalence of physical activity among primary health care physicians in Aljouf Region of Saudi Arabia. *Mater Sociomed.* 2015;27:263-266.

286. Biernat E, Poznanska A, Gajewski AK. Is physical activity of medical personnel a role model for their patients. *Ann Agric Environ Med.* 2012;19:707-710.

287. Morishita Y, Miki A, Okada M, Tsuboi S, Ishibashi K, Ando Y, Kusano E. Association of primary care physicians' exercise habits and their age, specialty, and workplace. *J Multidiscip Healthc.* 2013;6:409-414.

288. Arnett DK, Blumenthal RS, Albert MA, et al. 2019 ACC/AHA guideline on the primary prevention of cardiovascular disease: executive summary: a report of the American College of Cardiology/American Heart Association Task Force on Clinical Practice Guidelines. *J Am Coll Cardiol.* 2019;74:1376-1414.

289. Piepoli MF, Hoes AW, Agewall S, et al. 2016 European Guidelines on cardiovascular disease prevention in clinical practice: The Sixth Joint Task Force of the European Society of Cardiology and Other Societies on Cardiovascular Disease Prevention in Clinical Practice (constituted by representatives of 10 societies and by invited experts). Developed with the special contribution of the European Association for Cardiovascular Prevention & Rehabilitation (EACPR). *Eur Heart J.* 2016;37:2315-2381.

13

Nutrition, Diet, and Alcohol in Health and Cardiovascular Disease

Marta Guasch-Ferré and Frank Hu

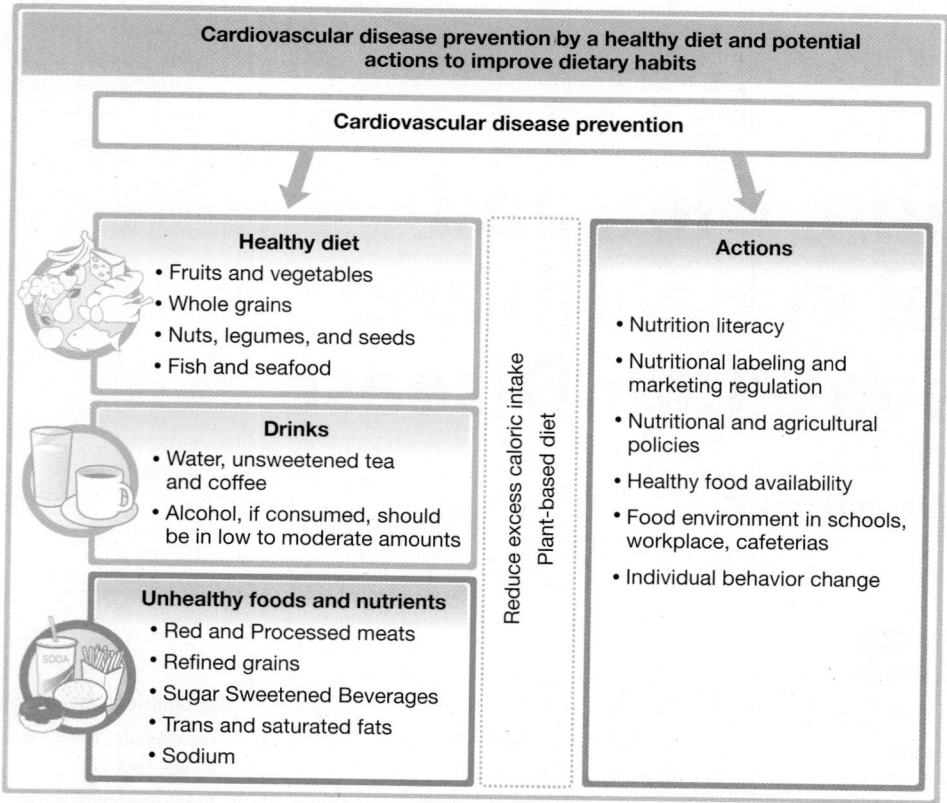

Chapter 13 Fuster and Hurst's Central Illustration. A healthy diet that reduces excess caloric intake and is plant-based should be emphasized for cardiovascular disease prevention. In green, healthy food that have been associated with lower risk of CVD, and in red, unhealthy food that has been associated with higher risk of CVD. Actions to reduce CVD burden need to address personal and clinical strategies, education and community, and societal/authoritative actions.

CHAPTER SUMMARY

This chapter discusses the state of knowledge for several food groups, nutrients, and dietary patterns, and their relation with cardiovascular health. The chapter also discusses factors influencing food choices, the public health impact of diet on cardiovascular disease (CVD), and recommendations for achieving better cardiovascular health (see Fuster and Hurst's Central Illustration). Cardiovascular health can be improved through lifestyle changes such as not smoking, increasing physical activity, and adhering to a healthy diet. Current evidence gathered from decades of nutritional research emphasizes avoidance of excess caloric intake, greater consumption of vegetables, fruits, nuts and legumes, whole grains, and fish; moderate consumption of low-fat dairy products, and coffee; and lower intake of processed meats and unprocessed red meats, refined grains, sodium, and sugar-sweetened beverages (SSBs). Alcohol, if consumed, should be consumed in low-to-moderate amounts. Preventive efforts by healthcare providers, dietitians, and governments should be focused on promoting better overall eating habits and diet quality. The strategies to improve the diet of the population should include addressing nutrition literacy of the general population, the availability of healthy affordable foods, the food environment including restaurants and school cafeterias, social and cultural norms regarding eating habits, and limiting marketing of unhealthy products.

INTRODUCTION

Importance of Nutrition and Diet for Health

Cardiovascular diseases (CVD), specifically coronary heart disease (CHD) and stroke, are the leading causes of death and disability-adjusted life-years worldwide.[1] However, CVD and its related risk factors are largely preventable by primary prevention. Hence, effective approaches for the prevention of CVD, including changes in lifestyle and diet, are key to reduce disease burden and improve overall population health.

Among the many established risk factors for CVD, diet is one of the primary modifiable risk factors.[2] In the last several decades, numerous studies have enhanced our understanding of the relationship between diet and cardiovascular health. Understanding the relationship between individual dietary factors and patterns with cardiometabolic disease is crucial to identify priorities, guide public health policies, and inform strategies to improve dietary habits and health. Indeed, suboptimal diet was responsible for an estimated 1 in 5 premature deaths globally from 1990 to 2016.[2] In the United States, suboptimal diets were associated with more deaths than any other risk factors. In 2016, they were responsible for an estimated 529,300 deaths, of which 84% were due to CVD.[3] Among individual dietary components, the largest estimated mortality was associated with suboptimal sodium intake (9.5%), followed by nuts and seeds, seafood omega-3 fatty acids, vegetables, fruits, sugar-sweetened beverages (SSBs), and whole grains (each between 5.9% and 8.5%) and, finally, polyunsaturated fats (2.3%) and unprocessed red meats (0.4%).[4]

A growing body of evidence highlights the importance of diet in reducing the risk of CVD and death and, consequently, the burden that this causes in health systems and economic growth around the globe. Therefore, effective dietary interventions aimed at improving population health and reducing the risk of chronic diseases should be at the forefront of public health initiatives.

Current Dietary Guidelines and CVD Prevention

Randomized controlled clinical trials (RCTs) are the gold standard for determining causation between an exposure and outcome. Similar to what is required for new drugs and medical devices, it would be ideal to use RCTs to evaluate the effects of diet on cardiovascular health. However, it is often not feasible to use RCT designs for many nutrients and foods. For cardiovascular events, in particular, the intervention would need to last for several years and a large sample size is required to have sufficient statistical power.[5] Another potential caveat is the difficulty to maintain a high adherence to diets for long periods of time. The use of RCTs on surrogate markers of CVD that require shorter intervention periods can also provide insights into the relationships of dietary factors and cardiovascular health.

Due to the constraints of RCTs, prospective cohort studies are the strongest observational study design to examine the association between diet and CVD[6] (**Fig. 13–1**). Nevertheless, these studies are not immune from limitations including random and systematic measurement errors due to the self-reported data and potential problems with generalizability and confounding.[6] Finally, dietary biomarkers in biofluids, mainly blood and urine, can be complementary to other self-reported measurements of diet and estimate objective intake for nutrients that are not available using only self-reported nutritional assessment methods. While there are few biomarkers established for some nutrients (ie, protein intake by urinary nitrogen, salt intake by urinary sodium/potassium, etc.), for most of the individual foods and dietary patterns, there are no specific biomarkers. In addition, short-term measurements may not adequately represent long-term dietary exposures. Thus, current dietary recommendations and dietary guidelines are largely based on a combination of human observational and intervention trial evidence coupled with findings from mechanistic studies.[7]

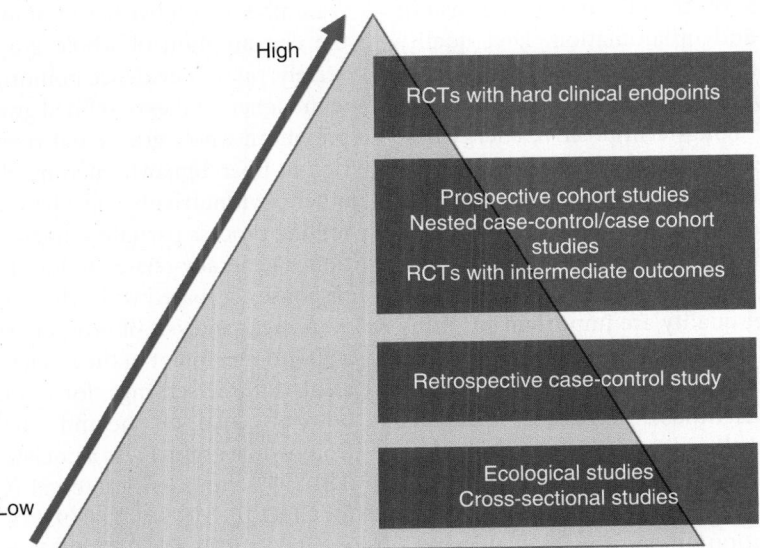

Figure 13–1. Hierarchy of study designs based on causality inference. RCTs, randomized controlled trials.

Current Dietary Guidelines for Americans 2015–2020 recommend several healthy eating patterns that incorporate a variety of nutrient-dense foods and healthy beverages, mainly water, coffee, or tea. The main recommendation is to include a variety of vegetables from all subgroups, fruits, whole grains, fat-free and low-fat dairy products, plant-based oils, and a variety of protein foods including seafood, lean meats and poultry, eggs, legumes, nuts and seeds, and soy products. The dietary guidelines also recommend reducing consumption of sodium, saturated fats, trans fats, added sugars (especially SSBs), and refined grains. If alcohol is consumed, it should be in moderation, up to one drink per day for women, and the 2020 Dietary Guidelines Advisory Committee report has redefined moderate alcohol consumption as up to one drink per day for men as well.[8] Finally, balance calories with physical activity to maintain a healthy weight and reduce the risk of chronic diseases is another key recommendation. Of note, most of these recommendations are consistent with many other dietary guidelines from several countries and other dietary recommendations from major health organizations.

In the present chapter, we summarize the current state of knowledge for several food groups, nutrients, and dietary patterns, and their relation with cardiovascular health. In addition, we explore factors influencing food choices, the public health impact of diet on CVD, strategies to facilitate behavioral change, and recommendations for achieving better cardiovascular health.

PATHOPHYSIOLOGICAL EFFECTS OF DIETARY COMPONENTS AND BENEFITS FOR CARDIOVASCULAR HEALTH

Dietary components can influence a number of cardiometabolic risk factors, including blood pressure, blood lipids, inflammation, endothelial function, glucose-insulin homeostasis, visceral adiposity, adipocyte metabolism, and weight regulation, among others. Maintaining caloric balance is key for cardiometabolic benefits, specifically, improving insulin sensitivity, blood glucose, and inflammation. Diet quality can affect several pathways related to weight homeostasis, including satiety hunger, brain reward, adipocyte function, and metabolic expenditure.[9] Long-term positive energy balance is the main cause of overweight and obesity, which are strong risk factors of CVD. However, not all calories are created equal and specific foods and overall diet patterns, rather than single isolated nutrients, are most relevant to cardiometabolic health. Emerging evidence suggests that dietary composition and overall diet quality are important for minimizing overconsumption, and that low-carbohydrate and Mediterranean diets are superior to low-fat high carbohydrate diets in maintaining weight loss.[10] **Figure 13–2** depicts the prevention of CVD and disease risk factors through a healthy eating pattern.[11] The impact of dietary composition is important for primary and secondary prevention of CVD, including secondary prevention among myocardial infarction survivors.

Foods and Food Groups

Figure 13–3 shows the summary estimates from various meta-analyses of key individual foods and food groups, beverages, and dietary patterns with CVD.

Fruits and Vegetables

Fruits and vegetables provide high amounts of vitamins and minerals (beta-carotene, folate, vitamin C, potassium, among others), dietary fiber, and also phytosterols and polyphenols (mainly flavonoids). Increased consumption of fruits and vegetables has been widely recommended for the prevention of chronic diseases and it is a common recommendation in most, if not all, healthy diets. Most dietary guidelines and health organizations recommend the intake of at least five servings per day of a variety of fruits and vegetables.[7] The protective constituents of fruits and vegetables act through a variety of mechanisms, such as reducing antioxidant stress, improving lipoprotein profiles, lowering blood pressure, and increasing satiety and insulin sensitivity. These observed long-term benefits are supported by RCTs of surrogate cardiovascular markers and large observational studies.[12]

In general, observational epidemiological studies report inverse associations between fruit and vegetable consumption and CHD incidence. In a meta-analysis including 24 observational studies, increasing fruit intake by 200 g/d (grams per day) was associated with a 10% lower risk of total CVD. For vegetables, the respective risk reduction was 16%. Findings from this meta-analysis showed consistent results of risk reductions in CHD and stroke incidence, and all-cause death.[12] Conversely, the benefits of fruit and vegetable subgroups have not been studied to the same degree, and may vary considerably. Potatoes, and especially French fries, have been associated with an increased risk of weight gain, hypertension, type 2 diabetes, and CHD in several studies.[13-15] The potential mechanism may be explained by the fact that potatoes have high starch content, which is rapidly digested and can increase glucose response, thus affecting the risk of diabetes.[15]

Whole Grains

A number of studies have found inverse associations between the consumption of whole grains and risk of CVD.[16] Conversely, there is evidence pointing to an increased risk of CVD with higher intakes of refined grains. The bran and germ layers, present in whole grains, but removed from refined grains, are rich in fiber, lignans, micronutrients, fatty acids, protein, and other phytonutrients.[17] Depletion of these nutrients during the milling process partially explains why refined grain consumption is generally related to lower satiety and a higher glycemic response compared with whole grains.[18]

A meta-analysis of prospective cohort studies suggests that a 90-g/d increment in the intake of whole grains (90 g is equivalent to three servings, for example: two slices of bread, one bowl of cereal, or one-and-a-half pieces of pita bread made from whole grains) was associated with a hazard ratio (HR) of 0.81 (95% confidence interval (CI), 0.75–0.87; n = 7 studies) for CHD, the HR was 0.88 (95% CI, 0.75–1.03; n = 6) for stroke, and 0.78 (95% CI, 0.73–0.85; n = 10) for total CVD.[19] The intake of specific types of whole grains including whole grain

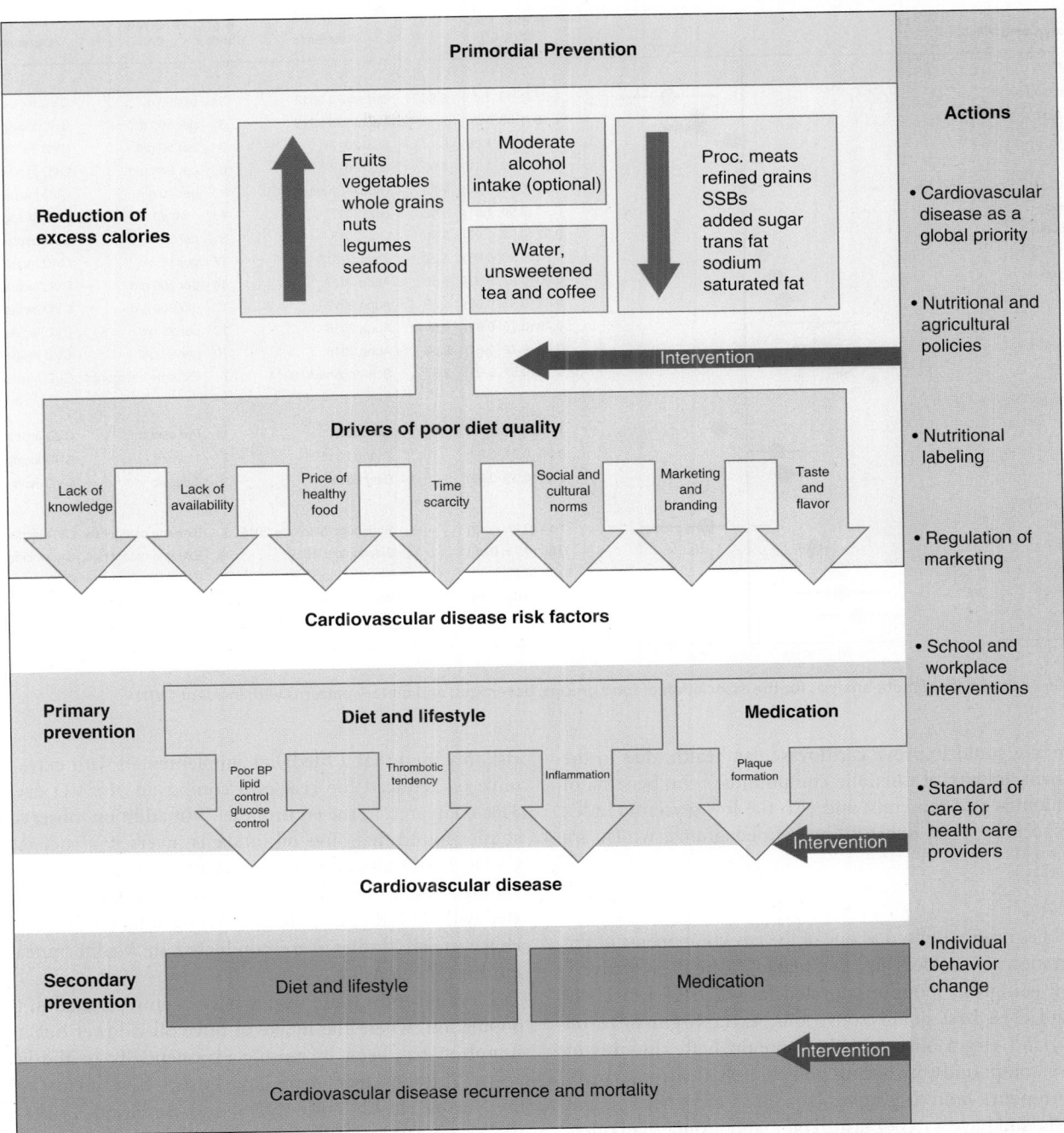

Figure 13–2. Flow diagram of the development of CVD and possible prevention by a healthy diet. Avoiding excess calories is an integral part of halting the development of CVD risk factors (ie, primordial prevention). Unfavorable eating patterns are driven by a variety of biological, social, economic, and psychological factors, and a robust intervention from all levels of society may steer populations toward a healthier diet and prevent disease progression. Diet and other lifestyle changes remain crucial steps in primary and secondary prevention of CVD, although the relative importance of medication and clinical procedures increases over time with disease progression. CVD, cardiovascular disease; SSB, sugar-sweetened beverage. Reproduced with permission from Yu E, Malik VS, Hu FB. Cardiovascular Disease Prevention by Diet Modification: JACC Health Promotion Series. *J Am Coll Cardiol.* 2018 Aug 21;72(8):914-926.

bread, whole grain breakfast cereals, and added bran, as well as total bread and total breakfast cereals, were also associated with reduced risks of CVD and all-cause mortality, but there was little evidence of an association with these outcomes for refined grains, white rice, total rice, or total grains.[19] Similarly, a prospective cohort study including 158,259 women and 36,525 men followed for up to 30 years, revealed that after adjusting

for lifestyle and dietary factors for diabetes, participants in the highest category for total whole grain consumption had a 29% (95% CI, 26%–33%) lower risk of type 2 diabetes. In addition, higher consumption of several commonly eaten whole grain foods, including whole grain cold breakfast cereal, dark bread, oatmeal, brown rice, added bran, and wheat germ, was significantly associated with a lower risk of type 2 diabetes.[20] Whole

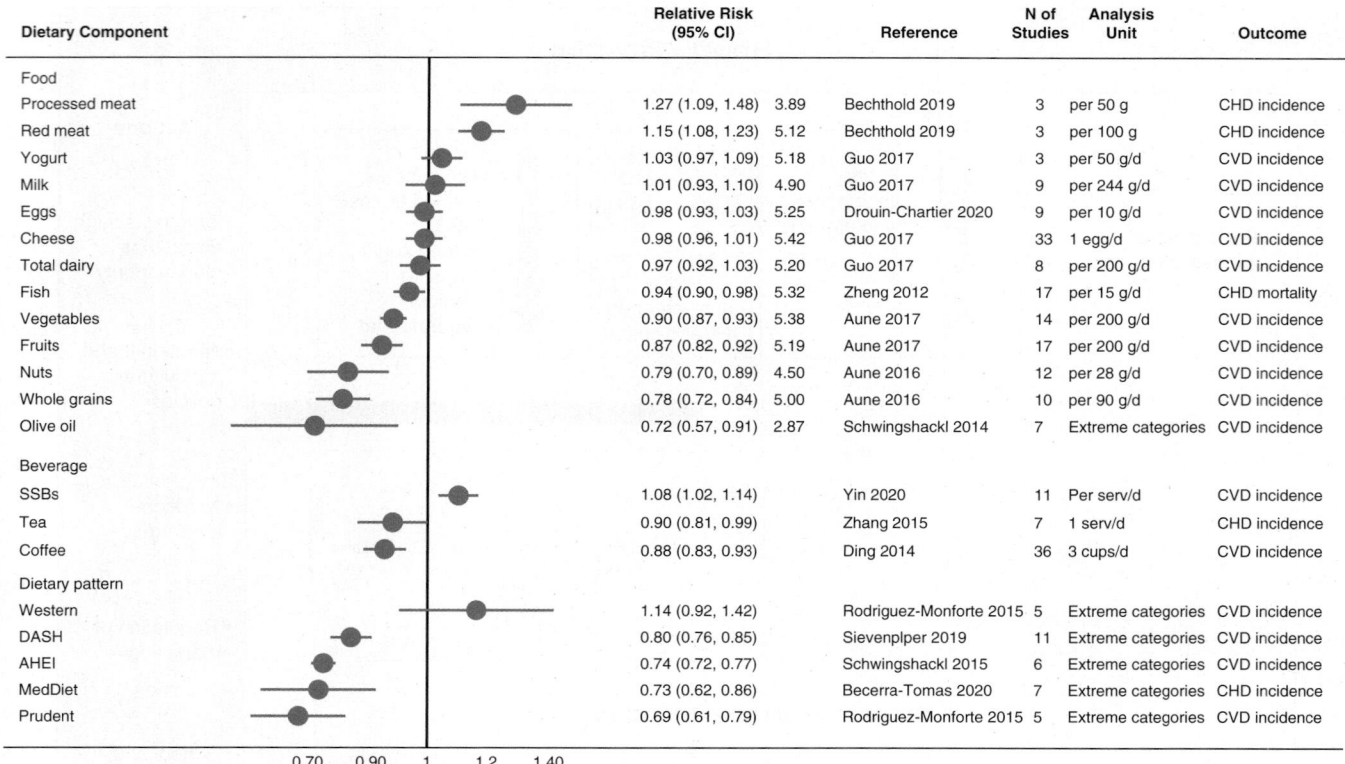

Dietary Component	Relative Risk (95% CI)		Reference	N of Studies	Analysis Unit	Outcome
Food						
Processed meat	1.27 (1.09, 1.48)	3.89	Bechthold 2019	3	per 50 g	CHD incidence
Red meat	1.15 (1.08, 1.23)	5.12	Bechthold 2019	3	per 100 g	CHD incidence
Yogurt	1.03 (0.97, 1.09)	5.18	Guo 2017	3	per 50 g/d	CVD incidence
Milk	1.01 (0.93, 1.10)	4.90	Guo 2017	9	per 244 g/d	CVD incidence
Eggs	0.98 (0.93, 1.03)	5.25	Drouin-Chartier 2020	9	per 10 g/d	CVD incidence
Cheese	0.98 (0.96, 1.01)	5.42	Guo 2017	33	1 egg/d	CVD incidence
Total dairy	0.97 (0.92, 1.03)	5.20	Guo 2017	8	per 200 g/d	CVD incidence
Fish	0.94 (0.90, 0.98)	5.32	Zheng 2012	17	per 15 g/d	CHD mortality
Vegetables	0.90 (0.87, 0.93)	5.38	Aune 2017	14	per 200 g/d	CVD incidence
Fruits	0.87 (0.82, 0.92)	5.19	Aune 2017	17	per 200 g/d	CVD incidence
Nuts	0.79 (0.70, 0.89)	4.50	Aune 2016	12	per 28 g/d	CVD incidence
Whole grains	0.78 (0.72, 0.84)	5.00	Aune 2016	10	per 90 g/d	CVD incidence
Olive oil	0.72 (0.57, 0.91)	2.87	Schwingshackl 2014	7	Extreme categories	CVD incidence
Beverage						
SSBs	1.08 (1.02, 1.14)		Yin 2020	11	Per serv/d	CVD incidence
Tea	0.90 (0.81, 0.99)		Zhang 2015	7	1 serv/d	CHD incidence
Coffee	0.88 (0.83, 0.93)		Ding 2014	36	3 cups/d	CVD incidence
Dietary pattern						
Western	1.14 (0.92, 1.42)		Rodriguez-Monforte 2015	5	Extreme categories	CVD incidence
DASH	0.80 (0.76, 0.85)		Sievenpiper 2019	11	Extreme categories	CVD incidence
AHEI	0.74 (0.72, 0.77)		Schwingshackl 2015	6	Extreme categories	CVD incidence
MedDiet	0.73 (0.62, 0.86)		Becerra-Tomas 2020	7	Extreme categories	CHD incidence
Prudent	0.69 (0.61, 0.79)		Rodriguez-Monforte 2015	5	Extreme categories	CVD incidence

0.70 0.90 1 1.2 1.40

Figure 13–3. Summary of meta-analysis for the association of food groups, beverages, and dietary patterns with incident CVD.

grain intake could improve cardiovascular health, due to the antioxidant activity of phenolic compounds,[21] the benefits of fiber, vitamins and minerals, and also the low glycemic index (GI), especially when substituting refined grains, which are high in GI.[22]

Olive Oil

Olive oil has been proposed as one of the key components of the Mediterranean Diet (MedDiet) that makes it cardio-protective.[23] Olive oil is high in monounsaturated fat (MUFA), especially oleic acid. The best quality olive oils, extra-virgin olive oil (EVOO) and virgin olive varieties, contain high amounts of bioactive compounds, including polyphenols (hydroxytyrosol and oleuropein), lipid derivatives (squalene, tocopherols), and vitamin E, and have a richer taste, color, and aroma than other common varieties.[24] Olive oil has been traditionally used as the main culinary and dressing fat in Mediterranean regions, and recently, it has become more popular worldwide.

Early ecological studies observed inverse associations between average country-level consumption of olive oil and the risk of CVD.[25] Experimental studies and clinical trials have shown that olive oil, especially virgin olive oil, due to its antioxidant capacity, is beneficial for the prevention of CHD and reducing its risk factors.[26] A MedDiet supplemented with olive oil has been observed to improve the lipid profile, and have beneficial effects on endothelial dysfunction, hypertension, inflammation, insulin sensitivity, and diabetes.[26–30] Results from the landmark PREDIMED trial, a primary prevention trial that included 7,447 participants at high cardiovascular

risk, revealed that a MedDiet supplemented with extra-virgin olive oil reduced the risk of a composite of CVD events by 31% compared to the control diet.[31] In addition, observational studies found that olive oil intake is inversely associated with CVD[32–34] and all-cause death.[33] A meta-analysis of six observational studies found that higher olive oil intake was associated with an HR of 0.72 (0.57–0.91) for total CVD incidence.[35] However, all studies were conducted in Mediterranean and European regions.

More recently, these results have been replicated in the US population, where the intake of olive oil is lower but its consumption has been increasing exponentially in the last few years. Findings from two large prospective cohort studies, the Nurses' Health Study (NHS) and the Health Professionals Follow-up Study (HPFS), showed that in a study including 61,181 women and 31,797 men, who were followed for up to 24 years, higher intake of olive oil (>0.5 tablespoons/day) was associated with a 14% lower risk of CVD (HR, 0.86; 95% CI, 0.79–0.94), and an 18% lower risk of CHD (HR, 0.82; 95% CI, 0.73–0.91). Of note, replacing 5 g/d of margarine, butter, mayonnaise, or dairy fat with the equivalent amount of olive oil was associated with a 5% to 7% lower risk of total CVD and CHD. No significant associations were observed when olive oil was compared with other plant oils combined. Thus, suggesting that replacing fat-based salad dressings and other fats with olive oil or other plant oils should be considered to reduce cardiometabolic risk.[36] Olive oil can also be used to replace tropical oils such as coconut and palm oil to improve blood lipids and other CVD risk factors.

Nuts and Legumes

Nuts and legumes are a good source of unsaturated fatty acids, rich in vegetable fat and fiber, minerals (potassium, calcium, and magnesium), vitamins (folate, vitamins C and E), and other bioactive compounds (phytosterols and polyphenols). There is strong evidence demonstrating that a higher intake of nuts confers multiple benefits for cardiovascular health, and such an effect can be attributed to their unique nutritional composition.[37]

Frequent nut consumption has been associated with reduced cardiovascular risk factors including dyslipidemia, type 2 diabetes, and metabolic syndrome, as well as with a lower risk of CHD.[38–40] Small intervention studies have reported lower total cholesterol, low-density lipoprotein cholesterol, apolipoprotein B, and triglycerides among those randomized to consuming tree nuts compared with the control arms.[38] Furthermore, findings from the large PREDIMED trial demonstrated that participants randomized to a MedDiet supplemented with mixed nuts—hazelnuts, almonds, and walnuts—had a 28% reduction in the incidence of major cardiovascular events after 5 years of follow-up.[31]

Along these lines, similar results have been observed in large observational studies. Findings from the NHS and the HPFS, including 92,946 participants and 14,136 incident CVD cases during up to 32 years of follow-up, have provided further evidence that the intake of total nuts is inversely associated with CVD risk in the US general population. The pooled multivariable HR for CVD and CHD among participants who consumed one serving of nuts (28 g) five or more times per week, compared with to those who never or almost never consumed nuts, was 0.86 (95% CI, 0.79–0.93) and 0.80 (95% CI, 0.72–0.89), respectively.[41] Of note, the results were consistent when peanuts, tree nuts, and walnuts were analyzed separately. Several meta-analyses on the topic have been published. A meta-analysis of 25 observational studies found that four servings per week of nut intake was associated with an HR of 0.76 (95% CI, 0.69–0.84) for fatal CHD and an HR of 0.78 (95% CI, 0.67–0.92) for nonfatal CHD.[42]

Fish and Seafood

Fish and seafood are rich in protein of high biologic value and are a major source of poly-unsaturated fatty acids (PUFA), namely, omega-3 and omega-6 fatty acids. Long-chain omega-3 fatty acids present in marine fish have been shown to reduce arrhythmias, thrombosis, inflammation, blood pressure, as well as favorably modify the lipid profile, thus reducing the risk of CVD.[43]

Consistent findings from observational studies have shown inverse associations between higher fish (~2+ servings/week) consumption and lower risk of CHD.[44] A meta-analysis of observational studies has found that higher fish consumption versus little to no fish consumption was associated with a reduced relative risk of fatal and nonfatal CHD. Specifically, a 15-g/d increment in fish intake was associated with an HR of 0.96 (95% CI, 0.90–0.98) for CHD mortality.[44] The benefits of long-chain omega-3 fatty acids have been studied for decades. A recent meta-analysis including study-level data from 13 trials,

suggests that daily marine omega-3 supplementation had a modest benefit in lowering the risk for coronary heart disease and most other cardiovascular endpoints, including myocardial infarction, CHD death, total CVD, and cardiovascular death. However, no benefits were observed for stroke.[45] While methylmercury consumed from fish does not appear to have detectable adverse effects on hypertension, diabetes, and cardiovascular events in adults,[46,47] the Food and Drug Administration (FDA) recommends that children and pregnant women limit the intake of fish high in mercury (tuna, swordfish, king mackerel, etc.) and consume a variety of fish lower in mercury about two to three servings per week.

Dairy Products

Dairy products are good sources of vitamins (retinol, riboflavin, and vitamin D) and minerals (particularly calcium and magnesium). The lactic acid bacteria found in fermented dairy products (eg, yogurt and cheese) contribute to gut microbial balance, which may reduce the risk of cardiometabolic diseases.[48] Dairy products also contain a myriad of fatty acids, including high amounts of saturated fat. The association between specific dairy fatty acids and risk of cardiometabolic diseases has been controversial. In general, long, even-chain saturated fatty acids have been associated with higher risk, whereas medium- and odd-chain saturated fatty acids are associated with lower risk of cardiometabolic diseases.[49,50] There is conflicting evidence on the health benefits of dairy products, mainly because dairy products represent a heterogeneous group of food with potential differing effects on health outcomes. Nevertheless, the moderate intake of dairy products, especially yogurt, is recommended in many dietary guidelines.

Based on the evidence from observational studies, the consumption of milk and dairy products has shown null results or has been weakly inversely related to the incidence of CVD. In a recent meta-analysis including a total of 29 cohort studies, with 938,465 participants and 93,158 deaths, 28,419 CHD, and 25,416 CVD cases, no associations were found for total (high-fat/low-fat) dairy, and milk with several health outcomes including CHD, CVD, and mortality. Inverse associations were found between total fermented dairy (including sour milk products, cheese, or yogurt; per 20 g/d) with mortality (relative risk [RR] 0.98; 95% CI, 0.97–0.99) and CVD risk (RR 0.98; 95% CI, 0.97–0.99).[51] In a recent analysis of three large prospective cohorts, moderate dairy consumption of one to two servings per day was associated with lower total and CVD mortality, but higher consumption was associated with increased cancer mortality. Of note, the effects of dairy may depend on substitution foods. Consumption of nuts, legumes, or whole grains instead of dairy foods was associated with lower mortality, whereas consumption of red and processed meat instead of dairy foods was associated with higher mortality.[52]

It has been suggested that dairy products could ameliorate characteristics of the metabolic syndrome, a cluster of risk factors that increase the risk of diabetes and CVD.[53] Dairy products, such as cheese, do not exert the negative effects on blood lipids, as predicted solely due to the content of saturated fat. Calcium and other bioactive components may modify the effects on low-density lipprotein cholesterol (LDL-C) and triglycerides. However, cheese consumption still increases LDL-C levels compared to vegetable oils, although it has smaller cholesterol-raising effects than butter.[54] Yogurt may also contribute to beneficial probiotic effects.[53] The consumption of yogurt, and other dairy products, in observational studies, has been associated with loss of body weight in the context of energy restriction.[53] These findings are, in part, supported by small randomized trials.[55] It has been observed that when cheese consumption is consumed with refined carbohydrates, it could lead to more weight gain, whereas if it replaces carbohydrates, it is associated with less weight gain and even weight loss.[56]

Red and Processed Meat

A large body of evidence has shown that higher consumption of red meat, especially processed red meat (hamburgers, hot dogs, and deli meats), is associated with a higher risk of developing type 2 diabetes, CVD, and certain cancers.[57,58] Dietary iron and heme iron, which are found primarily in red meat, have been associated with risk of myocardial infarction and CHD.[59] Excess heme iron may impose oxidative injury, which is associated with several cardiovascular risk factors, including dyslipidemia, insulin resistance, and inflammation, and may contribute to the development of atherosclerosis.[60] Meat is also high in phosphatidylcholine, choline, and carnitine, which are dietary precursors of trimethylamine N-oxide (TMAO) produced by intestinal microbes. Higher TMAO in mice and humans has been associated with an increased risk of atherosclerosis and CVD.[61] In addition, processed meats have higher amounts of sodium, which are linked to increases in blood pressure, one of the main cardiovascular risk factors.[62]

Findings from RCTs and meta-analyses assessing the effect of red meat intake on CVD risk factors have shown inconsistent results.[63,64] However, most of the meta-analyses did not consider the substitution source for red meat. In a recent meta-analysis totaling 1898 participants from 37 RCTs, relative to all comparison diets combined, red meat consumption had no differential effect on total cholesterol, LDL-C, high-density lipoprotein cholesterol (HDL-C), apolipoproteins A1 and B, or blood pressure but triglyceride concentrations were higher in the red meat groups. In analyses stratified by type of comparison diet, substituting red meat with high-quality plant foods (ie, soy, nuts, and legumes) led to more favorable changes in total cholesterol and LDL-C concentrations. These results suggest improvements in some lipid parameters when red meat was consumed versus combined animal protein, usual diet, or carbohydrates; and mixed effects compared to fish or poultry. In addition, these findings underscore the importance of considering the comparison diet interventions as a determinant of the relative effects of red meat on CVD risk factors.[64]

Systematic reviews and meta-analyses of prospective cohort studies have indicated an adverse association of consumption of red meat, in particular processed meat, with CVD and mortality.[65,66] For example, a meta-analysis found that comparing the highest to the lowest categories of red meat consumption, a positive association between red meat and risk of CHD (RR, 1.16; 95% CI, 1.08–1.24) and stroke (RR, 1.16; 95% CI,

1.08–1.25) was observed. In the dose-response meta-analysis, each additional daily 100 g of red meat increase were positively associated with risk of CHD and stroke. Similar associations and even stronger associations were observed for processed meat.[65] Likewise, a meta-analysis including 17 prospective cohorts suggested that total red meat consumption was significantly associated with increased risk of total death, cardiovascular and cancer death, and the increased risk was more pronounced for processed meat than for unprocessed red meat.[67]

Eggs

Whether eggs can be a part of a healthy diet has been a topic of intense debate in previous decades. Eggs are a major source of dietary cholesterol and it was previously recommended to limit the intake of dietary cholesterol to 300 mg/d to prevent CVD. However, because there is no appreciable association between dietary cholesterol and blood cholesterol, the current Dietary Guidelines for Americans does not include this recommendation.[7] Besides the high cholesterol content, eggs are a good source of high-quality protein, unsaturated fatty acids, vitamins, phospholipids, and carotenoids.

The evidence regarding egg consumption and CVD has been inconsistent. However, a recent study including results from three large US cohorts and from an updated meta-analysis including 27 prospective cohort studies showed that moderate egg consumption (up to one egg per day) is not associated with CVD risk (the relative risk for CVD for one egg per day increase was 0.98 [95% CI, 0.93–1.03]), and similar results were observed for CHD and stroke. Egg consumption was associated with potentially lower CVD risk in Asian populations. Finally, when the meta-analysis was restricted to people with type 2 diabetes only, higher egg consumption was associated with an increased risk of CVD, but considerable heterogeneity between studies was observed.[68] Overall, moderate egg consumption appears to be relatively neutral for cardiometabolic health for generally healthy people and it can be considered an alternative to less healthy foods such as processed meats or refined grains, but not as healthy as other foods with established health benefits such as vegetables, nuts, or legumes.

Beverages

Sugar-Sweetened Beverages

The term sugar-sweetened beverages (SSBs) refers to any beverage with added sugar or other sweeteners and includes carbonated and noncarbonated soft drinks, fruit punch, fruit juice concentrates, sweetened powdered drinks, and energy drinks. SSBs contain 140 to 150 kcal and 35 to 37.5 g of sugar per 12-oz (0.35 L) serving, and they are the largest source of added sugars in the US diet.

There is compelling evidence that higher intakes of SSBs are associated with a wide range of health consequences including tooth decay, weight gain, type 2 diabetes, fatty liver disease, and CVD.[69] The associations between SSBs, type 2 diabetes, and CVD are partially mediated by an increase in body weight. Independent of weight change, intake of SSBs increases postprandial blood glucose and insulin concentrations through a high glycemic load, as well as confer adverse effects on fat deposition, lipid metabolism, blood pressure, insulin sensitivity, and lipogenesis.[70]

A meta-analysis of 17 prospective cohort studies evaluating SSB consumption and risk of type 2 diabetes found that a one-serving-per-day increment in SSB was associated with an 18% higher risk of type 2 diabetes (95% CI, 9%–28%) among studies that did not adjust for adiposity.[71] Among studies that adjusted for adiposity, the estimate was attenuated to 13% (6%–21%), suggesting a partial mediating role of adiposity in this association. A meta-analysis of four prospective cohort studies also found a 16% higher risk of CHD (95% CI, 6%–27%) comparing extreme SSB intake categories and a 16% higher risk of CHD per one-serving-per-day increment (10%–24%).[72]

Another meta-analysis suggested that similar to studies of type 2 diabetes, when estimates that did not adjust for BMI or energy intake were included, the magnitude of the association increased (RR: 1.26; 95% CI, 1.16–1.37), suggesting these factors as partial mediators of the association.[73] A recent study conducted in the HPFS and NHS showed that comparing extreme categories of SSBs intake, the relative risk of cardiovascular mortality was 31% (95% CI, 15%–49%) higher in participants consuming more than two servings per day of SSBs after adjusting for major diet and lifestyle factors, including BMI.[74] These results are consistent with a meta-analysis including 11 prospective cohort studies evaluating the consumption of SSBs, that found that one serving per day increment of SSBs was associated with an 8% (RR: 1.08; 95% CI, 1.02, 1.14, I2 = 43.0%) higher risk of CVD incidence and an 8% (RR: 1.08; 95% CI, 1.04, 1.13, I2 = 40.6%) higher risk of CVD mortality.[75]

Conversely, the evidence for artificially sweetened beverages (ASB) is less clear; however, there is some evidence suggesting that higher consumption of ASBs is also associated with a higher risk of cardiometabolic diseases. Some research has suggested that ASBs may increase body weight and contribute to cardiometabolic risk despite containing few to no calories. It has been suggested that the intense sweetness of artificial sweeteners may habituate toward a preference for sweets or stimulate a cephalic insulin response and was more recently linked to insulin resistance through alterations in gut microflora.[74] However, these mechanisms are not well understood, and reverse causation and residual confounding may partly explain the positive associations observed with cardiometabolic outcomes in some cohort studies. Short-term trials that assessed ASBs as a replacement for SSBs reported modest benefits on body weight and metabolic risk factors. Consumption of ASBs in place of SSBs could be a helpful strategy to reduce cardiometabolic risk among regular SSB consumers with the ultimate goal of switching to water or other healthy beverages. However, a recent meta-analysis showed that a one serving per day increment in low-calorie sweetened beverages was associated with a 7% (RR, 1.07; 95% CI, 1.05, 1.10, I2 = 0.0%) higher risk of CVD incidence.[75]

The evidence for fruit juices and health outcomes is much less abundant and consistent. Findings from the European Prospective Investigation into Cancer and Nutrition-Netherlands study showed that the moderate consumption of pure fruit juice (100% fruit juice) up to seven glasses/week (one glass = 5 oz), but not eight or more glasses per week, was associated with a 17% (95% CI, 5%–27%) lower risk of CVD and a 24% (95% CI, 6%–39%) lower risk of stroke.[76] The potential underlying mechanisms for the observed inverse associations may be related to the high content in antioxidants and bioactive substances (including vitamins, minerals, and polyphenols) in some 100% fruit juices. The same polyphenols can also be obtained from whole fruits, which have higher amounts of dietary fiber and more satiating effects, thus, consumption of whole fruit is preferable because the evidence of their health benefits is strong.[77]

The deleterious effects of SSBs are well-established and thus, individual efforts and policy solutions are needed to reduce its consumption. Although fruit juices and ASBs are not as deleterious as SSBs, their consumption should be moderated in both children and adults, especially for individuals who attempt to control their body weight.

Coffee and Tea

Several beverages have been suggested as alternatives to SSBs. Among them, water is the optimal calorie-free beverage for most people with access to safe drinking water. Other beverages that have been shown to be healthy when no sugar or creams are added include coffee and tea, which are among the most popular beverages consumed worldwide.

Evidence from prospective cohort studies has shown that regular consumption of coffee is associated with lower risk of CVD. A meta-analysis including more than 1 million participants from 36 prospective studies showed a nonlinear relationship of coffee with CVD risk. The greatest risk reduction occurred at around three to five cups per day conferring an 11% lower risk. Similar results were observed when CHD and stroke were analyzed separately.[78] Coffee contains high amounts of polyphenols and other antioxidants, including chlorogenic acid, lignans, phytochemicals, modest amounts of magnesium, potassium, and vitamin B[3], that may in part explain the biological mechanisms through which regular consumption of coffee is associated with lower risk of cardiometabolic diseases.[79] These compounds found in coffee may also reduce oxidative stress, improve the gut microbiome, and modulate glucose and fat metabolism.[79] A large body of evidence suggests that consumption of caffeinated coffee does not increase the risk of CVDs and cancer, and regular consumption of coffee has been consistently associated with lower risk of chronic diseases including CVDs, several cancers, type 2 diabetes, Parkinson disease, and premature death.[79]

Likewise, tea has been reported to be inversely associated with CVD incidence. Evidence from a meta-analysis of prospective studies has shown that an increase in tea consumption by three cups per day was associated with a reduced risk of CHD (RR, 0.73; 95% CI, 0.53–0.99), cardiac death (RR, 0.74; 95% CI, 0.63–0.86), stroke (RR, 0.82; 95% CI, 0.7–0.92), and total mortality (RR, 0.76; 95% CI, 0.63–0.91).[80] Tea flavonoids, specifically flavonols, have received considerable attention and are themselves independently associated with reduced CVD risk.[81]

Alcohol and Alcoholic Beverages

Habitual heavy alcohol consumption is clearly associated with detrimental effects for health and is also an important cause of traffic accidents, domestic violence, homicides, and suicides. Heavy alcohol consumption is associated with a higher risk of cardiomyopathy, atrial fibrillation, several cancers, and liver disease. In addition, it is associated with higher long-term weight gain.[82]

Nevertheless, epidemiological evidence has shown that alcohol is associated with CVD risk in a U-shaped relationship. Compared to nondrinkers, regular moderate consumption (1 to 2 drinks per day for men and ~1 to 1.5 drinks per day for women) was associated with lower incidence of several cardiovascular outcomes including CVD mortality, CHD incidence and mortality.[83] A dose-response analysis revealed that the lowest risk of CHD mortality occurred with one to two drinks a day. The associations were nonsignificant for stroke. Alcohol use has also been shown to exhibit a "J-shape" with all-cause mortality, with lowest risk observed between one drink per week and one drink per day and higher risk thereafter.[83] These findings may have been masked by the fact that never drinkers could include individuals who avoid alcohol use due to underlying health causes or other confounding factors. Of note, the risk differs widely according to age, sex, ethnicity, and baseline disease.

The pattern of alcohol consumption is also an important determinant in these associations. It is likely not the same to consume a moderate amount of red wine within meals, such as in the traditional MedDiet pattern, than consuming high levels of alcohol or binge drinking during the weekend.

Several controlled trials have suggested that moderate alcohol intake may increase HDL cholesterol, adiponectin, and decrease fibrinogen levels.[84] In addition, these effects have not only been observed for red wine but also for white wine, beer, and some spirits, suggesting that the potential benefits could be related to alcohol itself but also the phenolic compounds and other bioactive compounds present in wine and beer.

Based on current recommendations, adults who already drink alcohol should be advised to follow guidance to consume moderate-to-low levels of alcohol, and alcohol should not be recommended as a means to reduce the risk of cardiometabolic diseases because it has been clearly demonstrated that it can increase the risk of a number of cancers. Of note, recent guidelines have lowered the cutoff of moderate alcohol consumption from two drinks per day to one drink per day in men, which is the same cutoff for women.[8]

Dietary Patterns and Diet Quality

Dietary patterns represent the overall combination of food habitually consumed, allowing us to assess the cumulative and synergistic effects of all the nutrients and compounds in different foods. Dietary patterns can be assessed by diet quality indices based on a priori scoring, such as the Alternative Mediterranean diet score, Alternative Healthy Eating Index (AHEI), and DASH (Dietary Approaches to Stop Hypertension) diet score, as well as exploratory methods including principal component analysis and cluster analysis. Certain types of dietary patterns are considered beneficial for health such as "Mediterranean" and "prudent" patterns, but others are considered disruptive for health, such as "Western" patterns, and have been associated with higher risk for chronic diseases[85] (Fig. 13–3). In general, beneficial dietary patterns share several key characteristics including the intake of minimally processed foods such as vegetables, fruits, nuts and seeds, legumes, yogurt, whole grains, and vegetable oils; and fewer intake of red and processed meats, refined grains, starches, desserts/pastry, and other added sugars. Healthy dietary patterns can influence cardiovascular health by modifying risk factors such as obesity, dyslipidemia, and hypertension, as well as factors involved in systemic inflammation, insulin sensitivity, glucose-insulin homeostasis, hepatic function, oxidative stress, endothelial function, and thrombosis (Fig. 13–2).

Prudent and Western Dietary Patterns

Principal component and factor analyses have generally identified two dietary patterns that explain most of the variation in population-level eating habits: Prudent and Western. Prudent diets are rich in fruits, vegetables, legumes, whole grains, fish, and poultry, whereas Western diets include high amounts of processed meat, French fries, desserts, SSBs, red meat, and high-fat dairy. A meta-analysis of 22 cohort studies found that those in the highest category of adherence to a prudent diet had a 31% lower risk of CVD compared with those with the lowest adherence,[86] whereas a Western dietary pattern was associated with a 14% increase in risk.[86] In general, the definition of these dietary patterns is consistent with the recommendations of major current dietary guidelines emphasizing higher intake of plant-based food, healthy protein sources such as legumes, and healthy dietary fats while discouraging high intake of animal fat, saturated fat, sugars, and sodium. Other indices such as the Alternative Mediterranean diet score (aMED) and Alternative Healthy Eating (AHEI) have also been strongly associated with better cardiovascular outcomes and reduced risk of mortality.[87,88]

Plant-Based Diets

The term "plant-based diet" encompasses a wide variety of dietary patterns that contain lower amounts of animal-source foods, such as dairy and meat, and higher amounts of plant-source foods. Due to the large diversity in plant-based diets, conceptual and statistical definitions of these dietary patterns differ greatly between studies. Although plant-based diets do not exclude any food groups, they are sometimes defined as vegetarian (excluding meat) or vegan (excluding all animal products).[89] Several meta-analyses of RCTs have shown that vegetarian diets seem to exert benefits on cardiovascular risk factors including blood pressure, blood lipids, as well as greater weight loss. Similarly, meta-analyses of prospective cohort studies have demonstrated that vegetarians (defined as not eating meat or fish) have lower risk of mortality from ischemic heart disease compared to nonvegetarians.[89]

To fully understand the health benefits of plant-based diets, it is crucial to consider the quality of the plant foods included as well as to account for dietary patterns that contain animal products. A vegetarian diet per se is not necessarily a healthy diet if unhealthy plant foods, such as soda, French fries, and refined grains, are included. To address these issues, Satija et al. used a graded approach, positively scoring plant foods and negatively scoring animal foods, to create an overall plant-based diet index (PDI), a healthy plant-based diet index (hPDI), and an unhealthy plant-based diet index (uPDI).[90] The hPDI positively weighs high-quality plant foods associated with health benefits (whole grains, fruits, vegetables, nuts, legumes, vegetable oils, tea, and coffee) and negatively weighs animal and low-quality plant foods. The uPDI positively scores low-quality plant foods associated with higher chronic disease risk (fruit juices, refined grains, potatoes, sugar-sweetened beverages, and sweets/desserts) and negatively weighs animal and high-quality plant foods. In multivariable adjusted analyses including over 200,000 participants followed for up to 28 years in the NHS, NHS II, and HPFS, the overall PDI was modestly associated with a decreased CHD risk (HR per 10-U PDI increase 0.93; 95% CI, 0.90–0.97; P trend = 0.003). The hPDI was more strongly associated with a decreased CHD risk (HR per 10-U hPDI increase 0.88; 95% CI, 0.85–0.91; P trend <0.001). However, the uPDI was associated with an increased CHD risk (HR per 10-U uPDI increase 1.10; 95% CI, 1.06–1.14; P trend <0.001).[90]

The Mediterranean Diet

The much appreciated MedDiet is characterized by high intake of fruits, vegetables, legumes, fish, whole grains, nuts, and olive oil; moderate consumption of dairy products and wine, and low intake of red and processed meat and foods that contain high levels of added sugar.[91] The relatively high intake of nuts, olive oil, and moderate intake of wine, particularly red wine during meals, makes the MedDiet unique and different from the other healthy diet patterns, but it can be considered a plant-based diet. The traditional MedDiet has been allied with a reduced risk of cardiovascular risk factors, CVD, and mortality.[92]

The first scientific evidence indicating the health benefits of the MedDiet probably came from a study in which patterns of food consumption in seven different countries were compared. The ecological study, which was conducted several decades ago[93] in the Mediterranean region, revealed that the dietary habits and the type of fat consumed had healthy compounds that reduced mortality from CVDs.[93]

Over the years, a number of significant prospective cohort studies and intervention trials have been conducted. The foremost findings of such prospective cohort studies demonstrated associations between MedDiet pattern and a reduced risk of CHD and mortality.[92] For instance, in the NHS, a greater adherence to the MedDiet, as reflected by a higher Alternate MedDiet Score, was found to be associated with a 29% (RR: 0.71; 95% CI, 0.62–0.82) lower risk of CHD incidence and a 27% (RR:0.87; 95% CI, 0.73–1.02) lower risk of stroke in women.[94] In the EPIC-Spain cohort study, the MedDiet was associated with a 27% (RR: 0.73; 95% CI, 0.57–0.94) lower risk of CHD.[95] EPIC also showed that a 2-point increase in a Med-Diet score was related to a 25% and 8% reduced risk of all-cause

mortality in a Greek population[91] and in elderly subjects,[96] respectively. Moreover, a meta-analysis of prospective cohort studies showed inverse associations with total CVD mortality (RR: 0.79; 95% CI, 0.77–0.82, n = 21), CHD incidence (RR: 0.73; 95% CI, 0.62–0.86, n = 7), and stroke incidence (RR: 0.80; 95% CI, 0.71–0.90, n = 5) when comparing the highest versus lowest categories of MedDiet adherence.[97]

Intervention studies have also helped to confirm causality on the protective role of the MedDiet on cardiovascular health. The Lyon Diet Heart Study was an RCT of secondary prevention and evaluated the effect of the MedDiet on the risk of suffering from a second myocardial infarction after 3.8 years of follow-up.[98] It was observed that the individuals who were randomized to the MedDiet group had a 47% reduced risk of myocardial infarction and cardiovascular death, as compared to the control group.[98] The PREDIMED trial is the largest intervention study designed to evaluate the effects of the MedDiet on primary cardiovascular prevention.[31] The main results of the trial demonstrated that among persons who are at high risk of CVD, an energy-unrestricted MedDiet supplemented with extra-virgin olive oil led to a reduced risk of the primary endpoint (a composite of myocardial infarction, stroke, and cardiovascular death) by 30% (RR: 0.70; 95% CI, 0.54–0.92) and by 28% when the MedDiet was supplemented with nuts (RR: 0.72; 95% CI, 0.54–0.96) compared to the control diet (recommendations to reduce all types of dietary fat) after a median of 4.8 years of follow-up.[31] A recent meta-analysis including RCTs further confirmed these associations, showing that total CVD incidence was reduced by 38% after adhering to a MedDiet pattern (RR: 0.62; 95% CI, 0.50–0.78, n = 2).[97]

The DASH Diet

The Dietary Approaches to Stop Hypertension (DASH) has emerged as a healthy eating guideline. The diet consists of a set of recommendations including increased consumption of whole grains, fruits and vegetables, low-fat dairy products, and nuts, and reduced consumption of sweets, sodium, and red and processed meats. Published systematic reviews have shown that the better compliance with the DASH dietary pattern could reduce systolic and diastolic blood pressure, total cholesterol, LDL, body weight, and fat, and also improve glycemic control and serum inflammatory markers; thus, it might significantly protect against CVD, stroke, diabetes, and cancers, which are associated with a lower life expectancy rate.[99] In a recent umbrella systematic review and meta-analysis, findings from 11 prospective cohort studies showed that the DASH dietary pattern was associated with a decreased risk of incident CVD (RR: 0.80 [0.76–0.85]), CHD (RR: 0.79 [0.71–0.88]), and stroke (RR: 0.81 [0.72–0.92]).[100]

The NORDIC Diet

The Nordic diet highlights the local, seasonal, and nutritious foods from Denmark, Finland, Iceland, Norway, and Sweden. It's quite similar to the MedDiet in that it emphasizes whole grains such as barley, rye and oats, berries, vegetables, legumes, rapeseed oil, fatty fish, shellfish, seaweed, and low-fat dairy, and it is low in sweets and red meat. The Nordic dietary pattern reduced body weight, insulin resistance, and improved blood lipids in RCTs of individuals with obesity or metabolic syndrome.[101,102] A recent meta-analysis of prospective cohort studies showed beneficial associations between the Nordic dietary pattern and reduced risk of CVD (RR: 0.93; 95% CI, 0.88–0.99) and stroke incidence (RR: 0.87; 95% CI, 0.77–0.97).[102]

Other Healthy Diets

A wide range of other dietary patterns, mainly prioritizing fruits and vegetables, whole grains, legumes, healthy dietary fats, and moderate intakes of healthy proteins, have also been identified for being protective against cardiometabolic risk factors and cardiovascular events. For example, the Portfolio dietary pattern, which includes four individual components that have shown to improve LDL-C including plant sterols/stanols, viscous fibers, plant proteins, and nuts, improved cardiometabolic risk factors and reduced estimated 10-year CHD risk by 13% (−1.34%; 95% CI, −2.19 to −0.49).[102]

Other popular diets such as the "low-carb diet" and the "paleo diet" have been a matter of recent interest in the community. One of the potential benefits of these diets is the reduced intake of refined grains, added sugars, and other ultra-processed foods. However, paleo diets allow ad libitum intakes of red meat and other animal products, which have shown detrimental effects on cardiovascular health, and low-carb diets may limit the intake of healthy carbohydrates such as legumes, whole grains, or fruits.

Macronutrients and Micronutrients

Traditionally, the evaluation of the relationship between the intake of macronutrients (carbohydrates, protein, and fat) and the risk of CVD has been focused on the total consumption rather than their quality. However, several studies conducted during recent years have highlighted the relevance of the differential effects of types of carbohydrates, proteins, and fats, and the replacement of one macronutrient by another on cardiovascular health, along with the evaluation of the effects of total macronutrients.[103]

Carbohydrate Quality

The scientific evidence relating carbohydrates to CVD remains inconsistent, probably because total carbohydrate consumption is less important than the quality of carbohydrates consumed. Even though some evidence suggests that low-carbohydrate diets are associated with improvement in certain risk factors (such as serum triglycerides, HDL-levels, glycemia, and weight loss),[104] data from two cohort prospective studies have reported that a low-carbohydrate diet based on animal sources was associated with a 23% higher risk of all-cause mortality (RR = 1.23; 95% CI, 1.01–1.24, comparing extreme deciles) in both men and women. On the contrary, a vegetable-based low-carbohydrate diet was found to be associated with about a 20% lower risk of all-cause and CVD mortality rates,[105] thus highlighting the importance of the quality of carbohydrates. A cohort study conducted in Europe, comprising more than 40,000 participants who were followed-up for 15 years, found that a 2-unit increase in the low carbohydrate-high protein

score was significantly associated with a 5% higher incidence of CVD.[106] In addition, a meta-analysis of more than 272,216 individuals revealed that the risk of all-cause mortality, among the individuals who had higher low-carbohydrate scores, was significantly increased: the pooled RR (95% CI) was 1.31 (1.07–1.59). The risks of CVD incidence and mortality were not statistically significant, but showed a trend toward a higher risk.[107]

The source and the type of carbohydrates consumed and the amount of fiber they contain are more important than the total intake of carbohydrates. High intake of dietary fiber is known to be associated with low risk of CVD as shown in several meta-analyses.[108] In a meta-analysis of 22 cohorts, a 7-g/d increase in fiber intake was associated with a 9% decrease in CHD incidence.[108] Intake of fiber, particularly cereal fiber, has also been shown to reduce all-cause mortality among myocardial infarction survivors, with a 27% (HR: 0.73; 95% CI, 0.58–0.91) reduction in risk of death in the highest compared with the lowest quintile of cereal fiber intake.[109]

Other factors that have been widely studied in relation to the carbohydrates of the diet are the glycemic index (GI) and the glycemic load (GL). GI has been defined as the incremental area under the blood glucose response curve of a 50-g carbohydrate portion of a test food, and is expressed as a percent of the response to the same amount of carbohydrate from a standard food taken by the same subject.[110] A low-GI and energy-restricted diet containing moderate amounts of carbohydrates may be more effective than a high-GI and a low-fat diet in reducing body weight and controlling the metabolic risk factors.[111] There is evidence from epidemiological cohort studies that suggests that high dietary GI and GL increase the risk of CHD.[112] A report from the NHS found that after adjustment for potential confounders, dietary GL was directly associated with the risk of CHD (HR: 1.98; 95% CI, 1.41–2.77, for the highest quintile of GL compared to the reference quintile).[113] The results from the *ARIC* study indicated that every 30-units increase in GL was associated with 14% (HR: 1.14; 95% CI, 1.02–1.26) increased risk of incident CHD in White nondiabetic individuals.[114] Among the Dutch and the Italian women who consumed modest GL diets, high dietary GL and GI increase the risk of CVD, particularly in overweight women.[115,116] On the contrary, in a large prospective cohort study (*EPIC-MORGEN*), it was observed that the high dietary GL and carbohydrate intake from high-GI foods increases the overall risk of CVD in men but not in women.[117] Two meta-analyses concluded that the high dietary GL and GI significantly increase the risk of CHD in women but not in men, the unfavorable effects being more pronounced in overweight or obese participants.[112–118] Results from another meta-analysis indicated that there is a linear dose-response relationship between the GL and CHD risk.[119] Despite the findings that the dietary GI is slightly associated with the risk of CHD, the results of the meta-analysis were nonsignificant for stroke and stroke-related death.[119]

Protein

The data relating to the effects of protein consumption on health outcomes has been controversial.[120] The intake of protein has increased in recent decades, and high-protein diets have been linked to improvements in cardiometabolic biomarkers, including blood glucose and blood pressure levels, as well as potential benefits for weight loss. While the association between total protein and CVD has been inconsistent across studies, in general, the intake of plant proteins is associated with decreased risk of CVD and total mortality, and the intake of animal protein is associated with higher risk.[121] Results from the *PREDIMED* Study demonstrated a U-shape relationship between protein consumption and both body weight and mortality.[122] In particular, total protein intake was found to be associated with a significant increase in risk of all-cause mortality in a Mediterranean population, which is at high cardiovascular risk. These data are in line with the earlier studies, which indicated that a high protein intake leads to increased risk of CVD and mortality.[105,123] However, the evidence is still inconclusive because some of the studies have found no associations[124,125] or suggested protection due to high protein intake.[106,126,127] Dietary recommendations should focus on the type of proteins consumed, giving preference to the plant proteins and restricting the animal proteins.[105,120] As described above, replacing processed and unprocessed red meat with other sources of protein such as fish, poultry, and nuts was associated with lower incidence of CHD.[128] Moreover, substituting red meat with high-quality plant foods (ie, soy, nuts, and legumes) leads to improvements in blood lipids.[64] Findings from a meta-analysis of 31 prospective cohort studies including 715,128 participants, showed that the intake of total protein was associated with a lower risk of all-cause mortality, and the intake of plant protein was significantly associated with a lower risk of all-cause and CVD mortality, but not with cancer mortality. On the other hand, intake of total and animal protein was not significantly associated with risk of CVD and cancer mortality.[121]

Dietary Fat

Dietary fatty acids play significant roles in the cause and prevention of cardiometabolic diseases. In brief, the type of fat, rather than the total, or the ratio or balance between the saturated and certain unsaturated fats, may be more important than total amount of fat. CVD risk could be reduced by decreasing the intake of saturated fatty acids and replacing them with a combination of PUFA and MUFA. The trans-fatty acids, from partially hydrogenated vegetable oils, are known for their adverse effects on CVD and should be significantly decreased. Indeed, they have been banned in the United States and other countries in recent years. Regarding the intake of the trans-fatty acids, there is strong evidence from meta-analyses supporting a highly significant association between the consumption of trans fat and CVD morbidity and mortality.[129-131] This may be explained by the adverse effects of the trans fat on HDL-C and LDL-C levels, particularly the industrial hydrogenated trans fat.[132,133]

Substantial evidence from meta-analyses of prospective cohort studies and RCTs indicates that the effects of consumption of saturated fatty acids on CVD risk vary depending upon the replaced macronutrient. In general, no consistent associations for risk reduction have been observed when saturated

fatty acids are substituted for refined carbohydrates, but lower risk of CVD has been observed when saturated fatty acids are substituted for PUFA and/or MUFA.[134,135] Recently, the research in the field has questioned if there are actually significant positive associations between saturated fat intake and CVD, as traditionally speculated. Most of the meta-analyses failed to show associations between the intake of saturated fat and risk of CHD, stroke, or mortality. However, the studies were unable to consider the effects of replacing nutrients alone and bias in self-reporting the intake of saturated fat in dietary questionnaires should be considered.[129,130,136,137] There is clear evidence demonstrating that PUFA in place of saturated fat is associated with reduced risk of CHD and death. A pooled analysis of eight RCTs concluded that the CHD risk is reduced by 10% for every 5% intake of energy from PUFA replacing saturated fatty acid.[138] The long-chain PUFA, most often, includes n-6 PUFA (linolenic and arachidonic acid) and n-3 PUFA (alpha-linolenic acid [ALA], eicosapentaenoic, and docosahexanoic acid). It has been suggested that PUFA improves blood lipids, blood pressure, inflammation, and vascular function. The American Heart Association concluded that consumption of at least 5% to 10% energy intake from n-6 PUFA reduces the risk of CHD as compared to its lower intake.[139] In addition, for every 5% energy substitution of mainly n-6 PUFA, in place of saturated fat, a reduction of 10% in the CHD risk was observed.[138] The n-6 PUFA has also been inversely associated with sudden cardiac death.[140]

A meta-analysis of 20 RCTs suggested that the n-3 PUFA supplementation protected against cardiovascular death, but had no significant effect on CVD and total mortality.[141] Another meta-analysis among individuals with high CVD risk from 21 clinical trials reported a 10% decrease in risk of cardiac death and a 9% reduction in risk of CVD events and a trend toward low total mortality.[142] Two RCTs did not observe any significant association for major cardiovascular events, cardiovascular death, and death from any cause.[143,144] Thus, the evidence on n-3 PUFA is still inconclusive, but it seems that the protective effect of fish on CVD could be attributed to its n-3 PUFA content.[134] Moreover, ALA exposure was found to be associated with moderately low risk of CVD in healthy adults.[145]

Even though MUFA (oleic acid is the major dietary MUFA) is reported to have various benefits against cardiovascular risk factors (eg, high HDL-C, low blood pressure, and improved inflammatory status), there is no clear evidence available which indicates a reduction in the risk of CVD and mortality by MUFA consumption.[134] In a pooled analysis of 11 prospective cohort studies, no association with CVD was observed when saturated fats were replaced with MUFA.[146] The associations between MUFA and cardiometabolic health are complex. One possible reason is that dietary MUFAs come from both plant and animal sources with divergent dietary components that may potentially obscure the associations for MUFAs and health outcomes. In recent analyses, findings from large cohort prospective studies have shown that MUFAs from plant-based foods were associated with a lower risk of CHD and mortality,[147,148] whereas the opposite was observed for MUFAs from animal products, suggesting that food sources may play an important role in the relation between MUFAs and human health.

In summary, replacing saturated fats, refined carbohydrates, and trans fats with unsaturated fatty acids, including PUFA and MUFA mainly from plant-sources, is a good strategy to reduce the risk of cardiometabolic risk factors and CVD incidence.

PERSONAL AND SOCIAL FACTORS INFLUENCING FOOD CHOICE

Eating habits are sculpted over a lifetime and are influenced by a large number of personal and social triggering factors including biological, economic, physical, psychological, and sociocultural determinants that lead individuals and communities to eat one way or the other. Other societal and environmental influences may have additional effects, including education, income, race/ethnicity, industry marketing, food availability, and pricing (Fig. 13–2).

Although strong scientific evidence and nutritional knowledge of the population are important factors influencing food choice, other factors such as lack of availability of healthy food, price, and other social behaviors have been recognized as potential drivers of unhealthy eating, especially in low-income populations. The simultaneous availability of cheap, low-quality food and expensive, or lack of availability of high-quality food can drive individuals to choose unhealthy eating options.[149,150]

Another important determinant of excess obesity and adiposity (which may lead to cardiometabolic diseases) is eating out, which can be a predictor of overconsumption and lower micronutrient intake. Indeed, in the last few decades, the American society switched from a society that cooked at home to one that buys nearly half its meals prepared or consumed elsewhere, in part, due to the successful marketing of the US food industry. The availability of cheap, low-quality food coupled with the marketing strategies creates an obesogenic environment that can lead to excess adiposity and consequently cardiometabolic disease.[151] Branding and marketing have been identified as factors that can influence food choices. Regulations on food branding and restriction of advertising to children have also been proposed as ways to improve diet quality and reduce obesity.[152]

More recently, a growing interest in understanding the determinants of inter-individual variation in responses to diet and food choices has emerged. Epidemiological data suggest that certain individuals are more likely to be susceptible than others to unhealthy choices and are at increased risk of obesity and type 2 diabetes.[153-155] For example, preliminary data has shown that some genetic variations alter carbohydrate and sugar intake,[156-158] and affects body-fat distribution.[158] Other data has suggested that some individuals may be more biologically driven to prefer food high in fat, while others prefer food higher in sugar or salt. However, this is only preliminary evidence and taste preferences are highly complex and are influenced by a wide range of factors including appearance, color, texture, and aroma, as well as other cultural determinants. Advertising has also been known to affect taste preferences, possibly by linking positive sensory thoughts with the target product.

In sum, although some biological factors may influence food choices, tackling the environmental and sociocultural determinants is crucial to develop helpful strategies to reduce the burden of obesogenic environments and the subsequent risk of cardiometabolic disease in the population.

STRATEGIES TO FACILITATE BEHAVIORAL CHANGE

A wide range of factors may affect dietary habits. From the individual level, many factors can influence the dietary choices of individuals besides personal preferences including education, income, nutritional and cooking knowledge, as well as health status. Motivation, ethical values, and religion are other relevant psychological factors that affect attitudes toward food and health.[149,150] Several lifestyle factors also appear to interact with diet and can play a role in the development of CVD. These include TV watching, physical activity, sleep duration, smoking, and possibly maternal–fetal influences.[159]

To influence behavior change, and specifically to improve the dietary habits of the population, several actions need to be addressed namely personal and clinical strategies, education/community, and societal/authoritative. These approaches range from clinical counseling, food and menu labeling, to dietary guidelines and food tax regulations.

Societal/Authoritative

Broader drivers of food choice and availability include agricultural production and policies, food industry marketing, trade agreements, availability, convenience, price, and taxation. All these factors have a huge impact on how consumers perceive nutrition and health. While policies to reduce smoking have been quite effective; addressing cigarette smoking requires only a single change in behavior: Don't smoke. But because people must eat to survive, advice about dietary improvements is much more complicated. The dietary recommendations often conflict directly with the food industry that demands that people eat more of their products.

Two good examples of effective policies for improving public health include banning trans fat from food systems and the taxation of SSBs. First, following evidence-based recommendations demonstrating that trans fats have harmful effects on health, and cardiovascular health in particular, the United States legislated in 2018 that industrially produced trans fat needed to be removed from the food supply. This action is expected to reduce at least 20,000 coronary events and 7,000 cardiovascular deaths.[160] Second, taxing SSBs, which are clearly detrimental for health, has been considered by some governments as a means to improve the choice of consumers and also generate revenue. A study in Mexico has shown that taxing SSBs has resulted in an average reduction in sales of 7.6% of taxed beverages 2 years after implementation; on the contrary, purchases of untaxed beverages increased by 2.1%. During this time, families with lower socioeconomic status had the largest decreases in purchases of taxed beverages.[161] Recently, a microsimulation study estimated incremental changes in diabetes mellitus and CVD, quality-adjusted life-years, costs, and cost-effectiveness of different SSBs tax designs in the United States. This study demonstrated that all SSBs tax designs would generate substantial health gains and savings. More research is needed to quantify the effect that these policies have made, but they are an excellent first step in improving public health.[162]

Education/Community

In addition, other policies that can be implemented to improve diets in the population, and in turn the risk of cardiometabolic diseases, include regulation of school lunch programs by the government or other health authorities, as well as providing healthy snack options in vending machines at educational centers.[163] Regulations for labeling calorie and nutrient content of foods and displaying calorie information in menus at restaurants are also good strategies to help the consumers in making healthy and informed dietary choices, as demonstrated in several studies conducted around the globe.[164] Worksite-based interventions and improving the accessibility to healthy food choices in the workplace can also be excellent strategies to enhance healthy dietary habits in the general population. A systematic review of 17 studies in Europe focusing on promoting a healthy diet in the workplace found limited to moderate evidence of effectiveness for the prevention of obesity and obesity-related conditions.[165] Another systematic review of 16 studies, mostly in Europe and North America, found that diet-based worksite interventions of moderate methodological quality led to positive changes in fruit, vegetable, and total fat intake.[166]

Personal Strategies

While multiple complex factors influence dietary choice, ultimately dietary habits are an individual choice. Providing simple and meaningful nutrition information, reducing nutrition misinformation, and providing clear public health messages, as well as providing options to access healthy food and regulating food marketing, could help individuals make better food choices.[167] In the clinical setting, dietitians need to work with patients to set specific achievable goals, strategies for self-monitoring, follow-up visits, provide regular feedback, use motivational interviewing, as well as promote family and peer support, and ideally combine several strategies adapted to each patient.[9]

The role and education of clinicians are key to improving lifestyle factors. Although physicians may have several barriers in health systems that may preclude their ability to implement effective behavior change strategies such as limited time for patient visits, strategies such as monitoring the body weight of patients and providing lifestyle counseling, including dietary recommendations, can help in decreasing obesity rates and consequently cardiometabolic diseases. A good strategy could be to refer patients to registered dietitians and nutrition services when needed.

The use of novel technology may also facilitate dietary behavioral changes through the use of web-based methods to assess diet and health apps that encourage improving lifestyle behaviors, including diet.

Overall, each of these factors are powerful and can influence the selection of healthier foods. Of note, education and information alone, without additional economic or environmental changes, has limited influence on behavior, and to improve diet quality and overall health, integrated, multicomponent approaches should be implemented.

SUMMARY AND FUTURE DIRECTIONS

CVD remains by far the leading cause of morbidity and death globally; however, it is largely preventable by implementing prevention strategies for uncontrolled risk factors, including obesity, high blood pressure, diabetes, and hypercholesterolemia, but also by improving cardiovascular health through lifestyle changes such as not smoking, increasing physical activity, and adhering to a healthy diet.

Current evidence gathered from decades of nutritional research emphasizes avoidance of excess caloric intake, a greater consumption of vegetables, fruits, nuts and legumes, whole grains, and fish; moderate consumption of low-fat dairy, especially yogurt, and coffee; and lower intake of processed meats, refined grains, sodium, and SSBs. Alcohol, if consumed, should be consumed in moderation. Preventive efforts by physicians, dietitians, healthcare providers, and governments, should be focused on promoting better overall eating habits and diet quality.

The roadmap for the present and future to improve the diet of the population should address several factors including improving nutrition literacy of the consumers, improving the quality of the products and the availability of healthy affordable foods, the environment including restaurants and school cafeterias, cultural unhealthy eating habits, and reducing marketing of unhealthy products.

REFERENCES

1. Roth GA, Abate D, Abate KH, et al. Global, regional, and national age-sex-specific mortality for 282 causes of death in 195 countries and territories, 1980–2017: a systematic analysis for the Global Burden of Disease Study 2017. *Lancet.* 2018;392:1736-1788.
2. Gakidou E, Afshin A, Abajobir AA, et al. Global, regional, and national comparative risk assessment of 84 behavioural, environmental and occupational, and metabolic risks or clusters of risks, 1990–2016: a systematic analysis for the Global Burden of Disease Study 2016. *Lancet.* 2017;390:1345-1422.
3. Murray CJL, Mokdad AH, Ballestros K, et al. The state of US health, 1990–2016: burden of diseases, injuries, and risk factors among US states. *JAMA.* 2018;319:1444-1472.
4. Micha R, Peñalvo JL, Cudhea F, Imamura F, Rehm CD, Mozaffarian D. Association between dietary factors and mortality from heart disease, stroke, and type 2 diabetes in the United States. *JAMA.* 2017;317:912-924.
5. Pan A, Lin X, Hemler E, Hu FB. Diet and cardiovascular disease: advances and challenges in population-based studies. *Cell Metab.* 2018;27:489-496.
6. Satija A, Yu E, Willett WC, Hu FB. Understanding nutritional epidemiology and its role in policy. *Adv Nutr.* 2015;6:5-18.
7. U.S. Department of Agriculture and U.S. Department of Health and Human Services. Scientific Report of the 2015 Dietary Guidelines Advisory Committee. Washington, DC: U.S. Departments of Agriculture and Health and Human Services, 2015.
8. U.S. Department of Agriculture and U.S. Department of Health and Human Services. Scientific Report of the 2015 Dietary Guidelines

Advisory Committee. Washington, DC: U.S. Departments of Agriculture and Health and Human Services, 2020.

9. Mozaffarian D. Dietary and policy priorities for cardiovascular disease, diabetes, and obesity: a comprehensive review. *Circulation.* 2016; 133(2):187-225.

10. Shai I, Schwarzfuchs D, Henkin Y, et al. Weight loss with a low-carbohydrate, Mediterranean, or low-fat diet. *N Engl J Med.* 2008;359:229-241.

11. Yu E, Malik VS, Hu FB. Cardiovascular disease prevention by diet modification: jacc health promotion series. *J Am Coll Cardiol.* 2018;72:914-926.

12. Aune D, Giovannucci E, Boffetta P, et al. Fruit and vegetable intake and the risk of cardiovascular disease, total cancer and all-cause mortality-a systematic review and dose-response meta-analysis of prospective studies. *Int J Epidemiol.* 2017;46(3):1029-1056.

13. Borch D, Juul-Hindsgaul N, Veller M, Astrup A, Jaskolowski J, Raben A. Potatoes and risk of obesity, type 2 diabetes, and cardiovascular disease in apparently healthy adults: a systematic review of clinical intervention and observational studies. *Am J Clin Nutr.* 2016;104:489-498.

14. Lea B, Eric B, Walter C, John PF. Potato intake and incidence of hypertension: results from three prospective US cohort studies. *BMJ.* 2016 353:i2351.

15. Muraki I, Rimm EB, Willett WC, Manson JE, Hu FB, Sun Q. Potato consumption and risk of type 2 diabetes: results from three prospective cohort studies. *Diabetes Care.* 2016;39:376-384.

16. Hu FB. Plant-based foods and prevention of cardiovascular disease: an overview. *Am J Clin Nutr.* 2003;78:544S-551S.

17. Okarter N, Liu RH. Health benefits of whole grain phytochemicals. *Crit Rev Food Sci Nutr.* 2010;50:193-208.

18. Holt SHA, Brand-Miller JC, Stitt PA. The effects of equal-energy portions of different breads on blood glucose levels, feelings of fullness and subsequent food intake. *J Am Diet Assoc.* 2001;101:767-773.

19. Aune D, Keum N, Giovannucci E, et al. Whole grain consumption and risk of cardiovascular disease, cancer, and all cause and cause specific mortality: systematic review and dose-response meta-analysis of prospective studies. BMJ. 2016;353; i2716.

20. Hu Y, Ding M, Sampson L, et al. Intake of whole grain foods and risk of type 2 diabetes: results from three prospective cohort studies. *BMJ.* 2020;370:i2716.

21. Flight I, Clifton P. Cereal grains and legumes in the prevention of coronary heart disease and stroke: a review of the literature. *Eur J Clin Nutr.* 2006;60:1145-1159.

22. Salas-Salvado J, Bullo M, Perez-Heras A, Ros E. Dietary fibre, nuts and cardiovascular diseases. *Br J Nutr.* 2006;96(Suppl 2):S46-S51.

23. Gaforio JJ, Visioli F, Alarcón-de-la-Lastra C, et al. Virgin olive oil and health: summary of the III International Conference on Virgin Olive Oil and Health consensus report, JAEN (Spain) 2018. *Nutrients* 2019;11:2039.

24. Ros E. Olive oil and CVD: accruing evidence of a protective effect. *Br J Nutr.* 2012;108:1931-1933.

25. Keys A. Olive oil and coronary heart disease. *Lancet* 1987;329:983-984.

26. López-Miranda J, Pérez-Jiménez F, Ros E, et al. Olive oil and health: summary of the II International Conference on Olive Oil and Health consensus report, Jaén and Córdoba (Spain) 2008. *Nutr Metab Cardiovasc Dis.* 2010;20:284-294.

27. Estruch R, Martínez-González MA, Corella D, et al. Effects of a Mediterranean-style diet on cardiovascular risk factors: a randomized trial. *Ann Intern Med.* 2006;145:1-11.

28. Salas-Salvado J, Fernandez-Ballart J, Ros E, et al. Effect of a Mediterranean diet supplemented with nuts on metabolic syndrome status: one-year results of the PREDIMED randomized trial. *Arch Intern Med.* 2008;168:2449-2458.

29. Salas-Salvadó J, Garcia-Arellano A, Estruch R, et al. Components of the Mediterranean-type food pattern and serum inflammatory markers among patients at high risk for cardiovascular disease. *Eur J Clin Nutr.* 2008;62:651-659.

30. Salas-Salvadó J, Bulló M, Estruch R, et al. Prevention of diabetes with Mediterranean diets: a subgroup analysis of a randomized trial. *Ann Intern Med.* 2014;160:1-10.

31. Estruch R, Ros E, Salas-Salvadó J, et al. Primary prevention of cardiovascular disease with a Mediterranean diet supplemented with extra-virgin olive oil or nuts. *N Engl J Med.* 2018;378:e34.

32. Bendinelli B, Masala G, Saieva C, et al. Fruit, vegetables, and olive oil and risk of coronary heart disease in Italian women: the EPICOR Study. *Am J Clin Nutr.* 2011;93:275-283.

33. Buckland G, Travier N, Barricarte A, et al. Olive oil intake and CHD in the European Prospective Investigation into Cancer and Nutrition Spanish cohort. *Br J Nutr.* 2012:1-8.

34. Guasch-Ferré M, Hu FB, Martínez-González MA, et al. Olive oil intake and risk of cardiovascular disease and mortality in the PREDIMED Study. *BMC Med.* 2014;12:78.

35. Schwingshackl L, Hoffmann G. Monounsaturated fatty acids, olive oil and health status: a systematic review and meta-analysis of cohort studies. *Lipids Health Dis.* 2014;13:154.

36. Guasch-Ferré M, Liu G, Li Y, et al. Olive oil consumption and cardiovascular risk in U.S. Adults. *J Am Coll Cardiol.* 2020;75:1729-1739.

37. Ros E. Health benefits of nut consumption. *Nutrients.* 2010;2:652-682.

38. Sabaté J, Oda K, Ros E. Nut consumption and blood lipid levels: a pooled analysis of 25 intervention trials. *Arch Intern Med.* 2010;170:821-827.

39. Kendall CW, Josse AR, Esfahani A, Jenkins DJ. Nuts, metabolic syndrome and diabetes. *Br J Nutr.* 2010;104:465-473.

40. Luo C, Zhang Y, Ding Y, et al. Nut consumption and risk of type 2 diabetes, cardiovascular disease, and all-cause mortality: a systematic review and meta-analysis. *Am J Clin Nutr.* 2014;100:256-269.

41. Guasch-Ferré M, Liu X, Malik VS, et al. Nut consumption and risk of cardiovascular disease. *J Am Coll Cardiol.* 2017;70:2519-2532.

42. Aune D, Keum N, Giovannucci E, et al. Nut consumption and risk of cardiovascular disease, total cancer, all-cause and cause-specific mortality: a systematic review and dose-response meta-analysis of prospective studies. *BMC Med.* 2016;14:207.

43. Galli C, Risé P. Fish consumption, omega 3 fatty acids and cardiovascular disease. The science and the clinical trials. *Nutr Health.* 2009;20: 11-20.

44. Zheng J, Huang T, Yu Y, Hu X, Yang B, Li D. Fish consumption and CHD mortality: an updated meta-analysis of seventeen cohort studies. *Public Health Nutr.* 2012;15:725-737.

45. Hu Y, Hu FB, Manson JAE. Marine omega-3 supplementation and cardiovascular disease: an updated meta-analysis of 13 randomized controlled trials involving 127 477 participants. *J Am Heart Assoc.* 2019; 8(19):e013543.

46. Mozaffarian D, Shi P, Morris JS, et al. Mercury exposure and risk of hypertension in US men and women in 2 prospective cohorts. *Hypertension* 2012;60:645-652.

47. Mozaffarian D, Shi P, Morris JS, et al. Methylmercury exposure and incident diabetes in U.S. men and women in two prospective cohorts. *Diabetes Care* 2013;36:3578-3584.

48. Fernandez MA, Panahi S, Daniel N, Tremblay A, Marette A. Yogurt and cardiometabolic diseases: a critical review of potential mechanisms. *Adv Nutr.* 2017;8:812-829.

49. Yakoob MY, Shi P, Willett WC, et al. Circulating biomarkers of dairy fat and risk of incident diabetes mellitus among US men and women in two large prospective cohorts. *Circulation.* 2016:133(17):1645-1654.

50. de Oliveira Otto MC, Nettleton JA, Lemaitre RN, et al. Biomarkers of dairy fatty acids and risk of cardiovascular disease in the Multi-ethnic Study of Atherosclerosis. *J Am Heart Assoc.* 2013;2(4):e000092.

51. Guo J, Astrup A, Lovegrove JA, Gijsbers L, Givens DI, Soedamah-Muthu SS. Milk and dairy consumption and risk of cardiovascular diseases and all-cause mortality: dose–response meta-analysis of prospective cohort studies. *Eur J Epidemiol.* 2017;32:269-287.

52. Ding M, Li J, Qi L, et al. Associations of dairy intake with risk of mortality in women and men: three prospective cohort studies. *BMJ.* 2019;367:l6204.

53. Astrup A. Yogurt and dairy product consumption to prevent cardiometabolic diseases: epidemiologic and experimental studies. *Am J Clin Nutr.* 2014;99:1235S-1242S.

54. Lordan R, Tsoupras A, Mitra B, Zabetakis I. Dairy fats and cardiovascular disease: Do we really need to be concerned? *Foods.* 2018;7(3):29.

55. Chen M, Pan A, Malik VS, Hu FB. Effects of dairy intake on body weight and fat: a meta-analysis of randomized controlled trials. *Am J Clin Nutr.* 2012;96:735-747.

56. Mozaffarian D, Hao T, Rimm EB, Willett WC, Hu FB. Changes in diet and lifestyle and long-term weight gain in women and men. *N Engl J Med.* 2011;364:2392-2404.

57. Micha R, Wallace SK, Mozaffarian D. Red and processed meat consumption and risk of incident coronary heart disease, stroke, and diabetes mellitus: a systematic review and meta-analysis. *Circulation* 2010;121:2271-2283.

58. Wu J, Zeng R, Huang J, et al. Dietary protein sources and incidence of breast cancer: a dose-response meta-analysis of prospective studies. *Nutrients.* 2016;8:730.

59. Qi L, van Dam RM, Rexrode K, Hu FB. Heme iron from diet as a risk factor for coronary heart disease in women with type 2 diabetes. *Diabetes Care.* 2007;30:101-106.

60. Yuan XM, Anders WL, Olsson AG, Brunk UT. Iron in human atheroma and LDL oxidation by macrophages following erythrophagocytosis. *Atherosclerosis.* 1996;124:61-73.

61. Tang WHW, Wang Z, Levison BS, et al. Intestinal microbial metabolism of phosphatidylcholine and cardiovascular risk. *N Engl J Med.* 2013;368:1575-1584.

62. Bibbins-Domingo K, Chertow GM, Coxson PG, et al. Projected effect of dietary salt reductions on future cardiovascular disease. *N Engl J Med.* 2010;362:590-599.

63. O'Connor LE, Kim JE, Campbell WW. Total red meat intake of ≥0.5 servings/d does not negatively influence cardiovascular disease risk factors: a systemically searched meta-analysis of randomized controlled trials. *Am J Clin Nutr.* 2017;105:57-69.

64. Guasch-Ferré M, Satija A, Blondin SA, et al. Meta-analysis of randomized controlled trials of red meat consumption in comparison with various comparison diets on cardiovascular risk factors. *Circulation* 2019;139:1828-1845.

65. Bechthold A, Boeing H, Schwedhelm C, et al. Food groups and risk of coronary heart disease, stroke and heart failure: a systematic review and dose-response meta-analysis of prospective studies. *Crit Rev Food Sci Nutr.* 2019;59:1071-1090.

66. Zheng Y, Li Y, Satija A, et al. Association of changes in red meat consumption with total and cause specific mortality among US women and men: two prospective cohort studies. *BMJ* 2019;365:l2110.

67. Wang X, Lin X, Ouyang YY, et al. Red and processed meat consumption and mortality: dose-response meta-analysis of prospective cohort studies. *Public Health Nutr.* 2016;19:893-905.

68. Drouin-Chartier JP, Chen S, Li Y, et al. Egg consumption and risk of cardiovascular disease: three large prospective US cohort studies, systematic review, and updated meta-analysis. *BMJ.* 2020;368:m513.

69. Malik VS. Sugar sweetened beverages and cardiometabolic health. *Curr Opin Cardiol.* 2017;32:572-579.

70. Malik VS, Popkin BM, Bray GA, Després JP, Hu FB. Sugar-sweetened beverages, obesity, type 2 diabetes mellitus, and cardiovascular disease risk. *Circulation* 2010;121:1356-1364.

71. Imamura F, O'Connor L, Ye Z, et al. Consumption of sugar sweetened beverages, artificially sweetened beverages, and fruit juice and incidence of type 2 diabetes: systematic review, meta-analysis, and estimation of population attributable fraction. *BMJ.* 2015;351:h3576.

72. Xi B, Huang Y, Reilly KH, et al. Sugar-sweetened beverages and risk of hypertension and CVD: a dose–response meta-analysis. *Br J Nutr.* 2015;113:709-717.

73. Huang C, Huang J, Tian Y, Yang X, Gu D. Sugar sweetened beverages consumption and risk of coronary heart disease: a meta-analysis of prospective studies. *Atherosclerosis* 2014;234:11-16.

74. Malik VS, Li Y, Pan A, de Koning L, Schernhammer E, Willett WC. Long-term consumption of sugar-sweetened and artificially sweetened beverages and risk of mortality in US adults. *Circulation.* 2019;139(18):2113-2125.

75. Yin J, Zhu Y, Malik V, et al. Intake of sugar-sweetened and low-calorie sweetened beverages and risk of cardiovascular disease: a meta-analysis and systematic review. *Adv Nutr.* 2021;1;12(1):89-101.

76. Scheffers FR, Boer JMA, Verschuren WMM, et al. Pure fruit juice and fruit consumption and the risk of CVD: the European Prospective Investigation into Cancer and Nutrition-Netherlands (EPIC-NL) study. *Br J Nutr.* 2019;121:351-359.

77. Muraki I, Imamura F, Manson JE, et al. Fruit consumption and risk of type 2 diabetes: results from three prospective longitudinal cohort studies. *BMJ.* 2013;347:f5001.

78. Ding M, Bhupathiraju SN, Satija A, van Dam RM, Hu FB. Long-term coffee consumption and risk of cardiovascular disease. *Circulation* 2014;129:643-659.

79. van Dam RM, Hu FB, Willett WC. Coffee, Caffeine, and Health. *N Engl J Med.* 2020;383:369-378.

80. Zhang C, Qin YY, Wei X, Yu FF, Zhou YH, He J. Tea consumption and risk of cardiovascular outcomes and total mortality: a systematic review and meta-analysis of prospective observational studies. *Eur J Epidemiol.* 2015;30:103-113.

81. Wang X, Ouyang YY, Liu J, Zhao G. Flavonoid intake and risk of CVD: a systematic review and meta-analysis of prospective cohort studies. *Br J Nutr.* 2014;111:1-11.

82. Shield KD, Parry C, Rehm J. Chronic diseases and conditions related to alcohol use. *Alcohol Res Curr Rev.* 2013;35:155-171.

83. Ronksley PE, Brien SE, Turner BJ, Mukamal KJ, Ghali WA. Association of alcohol consumption with selected cardiovascular disease outcomes: a systematic review and meta-analysis. *BMJ.* 2011;342:479.

84. Brien SE, Ronksley PE, Turner BJ, Mukamal KJ, Ghali WA. Effect of alcohol consumption on biological markers associated with risk of coronary heart disease: systematic review and meta-analysis of interventional studies. *BMJ.* 2011;342:d636.

85. Jacobs DR, Tapsell LC. Food synergy: the key to a healthy diet. *Proc Nutr Soc.* 2013;72:200-206.

86. Rodríguez-Monforte M, Flores-Mateo G, Sánchez E. Dietary patterns and CVD: a systematic review and meta-analysis of observational studies. *Br J Nutr.* 2013;114:1341-1359.

87. Sotos-Prieto M, Bhupathiraju SN, Mattei J, et al. Changes in diet quality scores and risk of cardiovascular disease among US men and women. *Circulation.* 2015;132:2212-2219.

88. Sotos-Prieto M, Bhupathiraju SN, Mattei J, et al. Association of changes in diet quality with total and cause-specific mortality. *N Engl J Med.* 2017;377:143-153.

89. Hemler EC, Hu FB. Plant-based diets for cardiovascular disease prevention: all plant foods are not created equal. *Curr Atheroscler Rep.* 2019;21(5):18.

90. Satija A, Bhupathiraju SN, Spiegelman D, et al. Healthful and unhealthful plant-based diets and the risk of coronary heart disease in U.S. adults. *J Am Coll Cardiol.* 2017;70:411-422.

91. Trichopoulou A, Costacou T, Bamia C, Trichopoulos D. Adherence to a Mediterranean diet and survival in a Greek population. *N Engl J Med.* 2003;348:2599-2608.

92. Sofi F, Abbate R, Gensini GF, Casini A. Accruing evidence on benefits of adherence to the Mediterranean diet on health: an updated systematic review and meta-analysis. *Am J Clin Nutr.* 2010;92:1189-1196.

93. Keys A, Menotti A, Karvonen MJ, et al. The diet and 15-year death rate in the seven countries study. *Am J Epidemiol.* 1986;124:903-915.

94. Fung TT, Rexrode KM, Mantzoros CS, Manson JE, Willett WC, Hu FB. Mediterranean diet and incidence of and mortality from coronary heart disease and stroke in women. *Circulation* 2009;119:1093-100.

95. Guallar-Castillón P, Rodríguez-Artalejo F, Tormo MJ, et al. Major dietary patterns and risk of coronary heart disease in middle-aged persons from a Mediterranean country: the EPIC-Spain cohort study. *Nutr Metab Cardiovasc Dis.* 2012;22:192-199.

96. Trichopoulou A, Bamia C, Norat T, et al. Modified Mediterranean diet and survival after myocardial infarction: the EPIC-Elderly study. *Eur J Epidemiol.* 2007;22:871-881.

97. Becerra-Tomás N, Blanco Mejía S, Viguiliouk E, et al. Mediterranean diet, cardiovascular disease and mortality in diabetes: a systematic review and meta-analysis of prospective cohort studies and randomized clinical trials. *Crit Rev Food Sci Nutr.* 2020;60:1207-1227.

98. de Lorgeril M, Salen P, Martin JL, Monjaud I, Delaye J, Mamelle N. Mediterranean diet, traditional risk factors, and the rate of cardiovascular complications after myocardial infarction: final report of the Lyon Diet Heart Study. *Circulation* 1999;99:779-785.

99. Schwingshackl L, Hoffmann G. Diet quality as assessed by the Healthy Eating Index, the Alternate Healthy Eating Index, the Dietary Approaches to Stop Hypertension score, and health outcomes: a systematic review and meta-analysis of cohort studies. *J Acad Nutr Diet.* 2015;115:780-800.e5.

100. Chiavaroli L, Viguiliouk E, Nishi SK, et al. DASH dietary pattern and cardiometabolic outcomes: an umbrella review of systematic reviews and meta-analyses. *Nutrients.* 2019;11(2):338.

101. Adamsson V, Reumark A, Fredriksson IB, et al. Effects of a healthy Nordic diet on cardiovascular risk factors in hypercholesterolaemic subjects: a randomized controlled trial (NORDIET). *J Intern Med.* 2011;269:150-159.

102. Kahleova H, Salas-Salvadó J, Rahelić D, Kendall CWC, Rembert E, Sievenpiper JL. Dietary patterns and cardiometabolic outcomes in diabetes: a summary of systematic reviews and meta-analyses. *Nutrients* 2019;11(9):2209.

103. Siri-Tarino PW, Sun Q, Hu FB, Krauss RM. Saturated fat, carbohydrate, and cardiovascular disease. *Am J Clin Nutr.* 2010;91:502-509.

104. Zarraga IGE, Schwarz ER. Impact of dietary patterns and interventions on cardiovascular health. *Circulation.* 2006;114:961-973.

105. Fung TT, van Dam RM, Hankinson SE, Stampfer M, Willett WC, Hu FB. Low-carbohydrate diets and all-cause and cause-specific mortality: two cohort studies. *Ann Intern Med.* 2010;153:289-298.

106. Lagiou P, Sandin S, Lof M, Trichopoulos D, Adami H-O, Weiderpass E. Low carbohydrate-high protein diet and incidence of cardiovascular diseases in Swedish women: prospective cohort study. *BMJ.* 2012;344:e4026.

107. Noto H, Goto A, Tsujimoto T, Noda M. Low-carbohydrate diets and all-cause mortality: a systematic review and meta-analysis of observational studies. *PLoS One.* 2013;8:e55030.

108. Threapleton DE, Greenwood DC, Evans CEL, et al. Dietary fibre intake and risk of cardiovascular disease: systematic review and meta-analysis. *BMJ.* 2013;347:f6879.

109. Li S, Flint A, Pai JK, et al. Dietary fiber intake and mortality among survivors of myocardial infarction: prospective cohort study. *BMJ.* 2014;348:g2659.

110. Jenkins DJ, Wolever TM, Buckley G, et al. Low-glycemic-index starchy foods in the diabetic diet. *Am J Clin Nutr.* 1988;48:248-254.

111. Juanola-Falgarona M, Salas-Salvadó J, Ibarrola-Jurado N, et al. Effect of the glycemic index of the diet on weight loss, modulation of satiety, inflammation, and other metabolic risk factors: a randomized controlled trial. *Am J Clin Nutr.* 2014;100(1):27-35.

112. Dong J-Y, Zhang Y-H, Wang P, Qin L-Q. Meta-analysis of dietary glycemic load and glycemic index in relation to risk of coronary heart disease. *Am J Cardiol.* 2012;109:1608-1613.

113. Liu S, Willett WC, Stampfer MJ, et al. A prospective study of dietary glycemic load, carbohydrate intake, and risk of coronary heart disease in US women. *Am J Clin Nutr.* 2000;71:1455-1461.

114. Hardy DS, Hoelscher DM, Aragaki C, et al. Association of glycemic index and glycemic load with risk of incident coronary heart disease among Whites and African Americans with and without type 2 diabetes: the Atherosclerosis Risk in Communities study. *Ann Epidemiol.* 2010;20:610-616.

115. Beulens JWJ, de Bruijne LM, Stolk RP, et al. High dietary glycemic load and glycemic index increase risk of cardiovascular disease among middle-aged women: a population-based follow-up study. *J Am Coll Cardiol.* 2007;50:14-21.

116. Sieri S, Krogh V, Berrino F, et al. Dietary glycemic load and index and risk of coronary heart disease in a large italian cohort: the EPICOR study. *Arch Intern Med.* 2010;170:640-647.

117. Burger KNJ, Beulens JWJ, Boer JMA, Spijkerman AMW, van der A DL. Dietary glycemic load and glycemic index and risk of coronary heart disease and stroke in Dutch men and women: the EPIC-MORGEN study. *PLoS One.* 2011;6:e25955.

118. Mirrahimi A, de Souza RJ, Chiavaroli L, et al. Associations of glycemic index and load with coronary heart disease events: a systematic review and meta-analysis of prospective cohorts. *J Am Heart Assoc.* 2012;1:e000752.

119. Fan J, Song Y, Wang Y, Hui R, Zhang W. Dietary glycemic index, glycemic load, and risk of coronary heart disease, stroke, and stroke mortality: a systematic review with meta-analysis. *PLoS One.* 2012;7:e52182.

120. Clifton PM. Protein and coronary heart disease: the role of different protein sources. *Curr Atheroscler Rep.* 2011;13:493-498.

121. Naghshi S, Sadeghi O, Willett WC, Esmaillzadeh A. Dietary intake of total, animal, and plant proteins and risk of all cause, cardiovascular, and cancer mortality: systematic review and dose-response meta-analysis of prospective cohort studies. *BMJ.* 2020;370:m2412.

122. Hernández-Alonso P, Salas-Salvadó J, Ruiz-Canela M, et al. High dietary protein intake is associated with an increased body weight and total death risk. *Clin Nutr.* 2016;35:496-506.

123. Halbesma N, Bakker SJL, Jansen DF, et al. High protein intake associates with cardiovascular events but not with loss of renal function. *J Am Soc Nephrol.* 2009;20:1797-804.

124. Preis SR, Stampfer MJ, Spiegelman D, Willett WC, Rimm EB. Dietary protein and risk of ischemic heart disease in middle-aged men. *Am J Clin Nutr.* 2010;92:1265-1272.

125. Preis SR, Stampfer MJ, Spiegelman D, Willett WC, Rimm EB. Lack of association between dietary protein intake and risk of stroke among middle-aged men. *Am J Clin Nutr.* 2010;91:39-45.

126. Hu FB, Stampfer MJ, Manson JE, et al. Dietary protein and risk of ischemic heart disease in women. *Am J Clin Nutr.* 1999;70:221-227.

127. Bates CJ, Mansoor MA, Pentieva KD, Hamer M, Mishra GD. Biochemical risk indices, including plasma homocysteine, that prospectively predict mortality in older British people: the National Diet and Nutrition Survey of People Aged 65 Years and Over. *Br J Nutr.* 2010;104:893-899.

128. Bernstein AM, Sun Q, Hu FB, Stampfer MJ, Manson JE, Willett WC. Major dietary protein sources and risk of coronary heart disease in women. *Circulation.* 2010;122:876-883.

129. Skeaff CM, Miller J. Dietary fat and coronary heart disease: summary of evidence from prospective cohort and randomised controlled trials. *Ann Nutr Metab.* 2009;55:173-201.

130. Mente A, de Koning L, Shannon HS, Anand SS. A systematic review of the evidence supporting a causal link between dietary factors and coronary heart disease. *Arch Intern Med.* 2009;169:659-669.

131. Mozaffarian D, Clarke R. Quantitative effects on cardiovascular risk factors and coronary heart disease risk of replacing partially hydrogenated vegetable oils with other fats and oils. *Eur J Clin Nutr.* 2009;63(Suppl 2):S22-S33.

132. Brouwer IA, Wanders AJ, Katan MB. Effect of animal and industrial trans fatty acids on HDL and LDL cholesterol levels in humans–a quantitative review. *PLoS One.* 2010;5:e9434.

133. Bendsen NT, Christensen R, Bartels EM, Astrup A. Consumption of industrial and ruminant trans fatty acids and risk of coronary heart

disease: a systematic review and meta-analysis of cohort studies. *Eur J Clin Nutr.* 2011;65:773-783.

134. Michas G, Micha R, Zampelas A. Dietary fats and cardiovascular disease: putting together the pieces of a complicated puzzle. *Atherosclerosis* 2014;234:320-328.

135. Wang DD, Li Y, Chiuve SE, et al. Association of specific dietary fats with total and cause-specific mortality. *JAMA Intern Med.* 2016;176:1134.

136. Siri-Tarino PW, Sun Q, Hu FB, Krauss RM. Meta-analysis of prospective cohort studies evaluating the association of saturated fat with cardiovascular disease. *Am J Clin Nutr.* 2010;91:535-546.

137. Chowdhury R, Warnakula S, Kunutsor S, et al. Association of dietary, circulating, and supplement fatty acids with coronary risk: a systematic review and meta-analysis. *Ann Intern Med.* 2014;160:398-406.

138. Mozaffarian D, Micha R, Wallace S. Effects on coronary heart disease of increasing polyunsaturated fat in place of saturated fat: a systematic review and meta-analysis of randomized controlled trials. *PLoS Med.* 2010;7:e1000252.

139. Harris WS, Mozaffarian D, Rimm E, et al. Omega-6 fatty acids and risk for cardiovascular disease: a science advisory from the American Heart Association Nutrition Subcommittee of the Council on Nutrition, Physical Activity, and Metabolism; Council on Cardiovascular Nursing; and Council on Epidem. *Circulation.* 2009;119:902-907.

140. Chiuve SE, Rimm EB, Sandhu RK, et al. Dietary fat quality and risk of sudden cardiac death in women. *Am J Clin Nutr.* 2012;96:498-507.

141. Kotwal S, Jun M, Sullivan D, Perkovic V, Neal B. Omega 3 Fatty acids and cardiovascular outcomes: systematic review and meta-analysis. *Circ Cardiovasc Qual Outcomes.* 2012;5:808-818.

142. Delgado-Lista J, Perez-Martinez P, Lopez-Miranda J, Perez-Jimenez F. Long chain omega-3 fatty acids and cardiovascular disease: a systematic review. *Br J Nutr.* 2012;107(Suppl 2):S201-S213.

143. Bosch J, Gerstein HC, Dagenais GR, et al. n-3 fatty acids and cardiovascular outcomes in patients with dysglycemia. *N Engl J Med.* 2012;367:309-318.

144. Roncaglioni MC, Tombesi M, Avanzini F, et al. n-3 fatty acids in patients with multiple cardiovascular risk factors. *N Engl J Med.* 2013;368:1800-1808.

145. Pan A, Chen M, Chowdhury R, et al. α-Linolenic acid and risk of cardiovascular disease: a systematic review and meta-analysis. *Am J Clin Nutr.* 2012;96:1262-1273.

146. Jakobsen MU, O'Reilly EJ, Heitmann BL, et al. Major types of dietary fat and risk of coronary heart disease: a pooled analysis of 11 cohort studies. *Am J Clin Nutr.* 2009;89:1425-1432.

147. Zong G, Li Y, Sampson L, et al. Monounsaturated fats from plant and animal sources in relation to risk of coronary heart disease among US men and women. *Am J Clin Nutr.* 2018;107:445-453.

148. Guasch-Ferré M, Zong G, Willett WC, et al. Associations of monounsaturated fatty acids from plant and animal sources with total and cause-specific mortality in two US prospective cohort studies. *Circ Res.* 2019;124:1266-1275.

149. Nestle M, Wing R, Birch L, et al. Behavioral and social influences on food choice. In: *Nutrition Reviews. Vol 56.* Blackwell Publishing Inc., 1998: 50-64.

150. Brug J, Kremers SP, Lenthe F Van, Ball K, Crawford D. Environmental determinants of healthy eating: in need of theory and evidence. *Proc Nutrition Soc.* 2008;67:307-316.

151. Lake A, Townshend T. Obesogenic environments: exploring the built and food environments. *J R Soc Promot Health.* 2006;126:262-267.

152. Kelly B, Halford JCG, Boyland EJ, et al. Television food advertising to children: a global perspective. *Am J Public Health.* 2010;100:1730-1736.

153. Hare TA, Camerer CF, Rangel A. Self-control in decision-making involves modulation of the vmPFC valuation system. *Science.* 2009;324:646-648.

154. Christine PJ, Auchincloss AH, Bertoni AG, et al. Longitudinal associations between neighborhood physical and social environments and incident type 2 diabetes mellitus. *JAMA Intern Med.* 2015;175:1311.

155. Siegel KR, Bullard KM, Imperatore G, et al. Prevalence of major behavioral risk factors for type 2 diabetes. *Diabetes Care.* 2018:dc171775.

156. Chu AY, Workalemahu T, Paynter NP, et al. Novel locus including FGF21 is associated with dietary macronutrient intake. *Hum Mol Genet.* 2013;22:1895-1902.

157. Merino J, Dashti HS, Li SX, et al. Genome-wide meta-analysis of macronutrient intake of 91,114 European ancestry participants from the cohorts for heart and aging research in genomic epidemiology consortium. *Mol Psychiatry.* 2018;24(12):1920-1932.

158. Frayling TM, Beaumont RN, Jones SE, et al. A common allele in FGF21 associated with sugar intake is associated with body shape, lower total body-fat percentage, and higher blood pressure. *Cell Rep.* 2018;23:327-336.

159. Gonnissen HKJ, Hulshof T, Westerterp-Plantenga MS. Chronobiology, endocrinology, and energy- and food-reward homeostasis. *Obes Rev.* 2013;14:405-416.

160. Dietz WH, Scanlon KS. Eliminating the use of partially hydrogenated oil in food production and preparation. *JAMA.* 2012;308:143-144.

161. Arantxa Cochero M, Rivera-Dommarco J, Popkin BM, Ng SW. In Mexico, evidence of sustained consumer response two years after implementing a sugar-sweetened beverage tax. *Health Aff.* 2017;36:564-571.

162. Lee Y, Mozaffarian D, Sy S, et al. Health impact and cost-effectiveness of volume, tiered, and absolute sugar content sugarsweetened beverage tax policies in the United States: a microsimulation study. *Circulation* 2020;142(6):523-534.

163. Condon EM, Crepinsek MK, Fox MK. School meals: types of foods offered to and consumed by children at lunch and breakfast. *J Am Diet Assoc.* 2009;109:S67-S78.

164. Long MW, Tobias DK, Cradock AL, Batchelder H, Gortmaker SL. Systematic review and meta-analysis of the impact of restaurant menu calorie labeling. *Am J Public Health.* 2015;105:e11-e24.

165. Maes L, Van Cauwenberghe E, Van Lippevelde W, et al. Effectiveness of workplace interventions in Europe promoting healthy eating: a systematic review. *Eur J Public Health.* 2012;22(5):677-683.

166. Ni Mhurchu C, Aston LM, Jebb SA. Effects of worksite health promotion interventions on employee diets: a systematic review. *BMC Public Health.* 2010;10.

167. Roberto CA, Kawachi I. Use of psychology and behavioral economics to promote healthy eating. *Am J Prev Med.* 2014;47:832-837.

14

Inflammation and Atherosclerosis

Hasan K. Siddiqi and Paul M. Ridker

CHAPTER OUTLINE

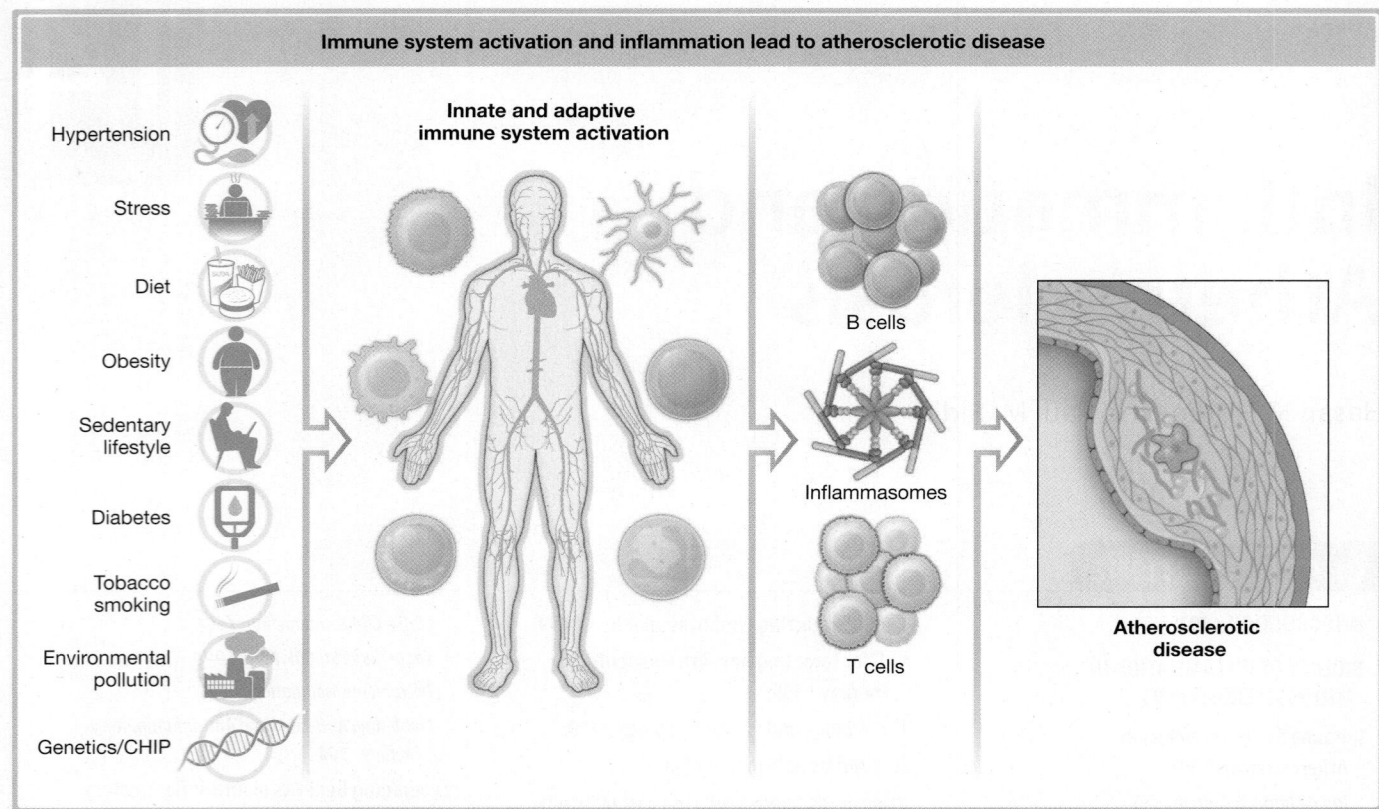

Chapter 14 Fuster and Hurst's Central Illustration. Activation of the immune system by medical comorbidities and environmental inputs leads to enhanced inflammation in the body. Multiple pathways in the immune system converge to establish and accelerate atherosclerotic disease.

CHAPTER SUMMARY

This chapter discusses the role of inflammation in the development of atherosclerotic disease, with lessons from basic science and clinical studies informing future strategies for prevention and treatment. Historically considered a disease driven by dyslipidemia, the central role of inflammation in atherosclerosis has been elucidated in recent years with the concept of residual inflammatory risk as an important contributor to atherosclerotic disease. Various stimuli and insults converge on the immune system leading to activation of multiple immune effectors, including the innate and adaptive immune system, that have key roles in the development of atherosclerosis (see Fuster and Hurst's Central Illustration). The use of biomarkers and inflammatory intermediaries including C-reactive protein (CRP), interleukin (IL)-1, and IL-6 for risk stratification and mechanistic elucidation is of key interest. Recent therapies targeting inflammatory pathways, including the NLRP3 inflammasome and IL-1 pathway, have shown promise in reducing this residual inflammatory risk for atherosclerosis in high-risk populations, with positive results seen in multiple large clinical trials. In addition, public health efforts to improve nutrition, reduce obesity, and combat environmental pollution will play a role in reducing the inflammatory contribution to atherosclerosis.

INTRODUCTION

The critical role of inflammation in the development and progression of atherosclerotic plaque has opened multiple new avenues for the diagnosis, treatment, and prevention of atherosclerotic cardiovascular disease (ASCVD). Early concepts of ASCVD focused on the critical role of cholesterol deposition in the arterial wall as the main driver of atherosclerosis.[1] Cell biology studies then focused on the processes of endothelial dysfunction, smooth muscle cell (SMC) hyperplasia, and SMC proliferation in the arterial intima with subsequent formation of an atherosclerotic plaque.[2] The widespread use of statins led to a major leap forward in the prevention and treatment of ASCVD. Yet despite effective anti-lipid therapies, "residual inflammatory risk" has only recently become a target for treatment. As described in this chapter, recent preclinical and clinical trial data have established the key role of inflammation in atherosclerotic disease, ushering in a new paradigm of atherosclerosis.

BIOLOGY OF INFLAMMATION IN ATHEROSCLEROSIS

Immune System Effectors in Atherosclerosis

Pathological examination of atherosclerotic plaques provides insight into the role of the immune system and inflammation in atherosclerosis. Experimental studies in the 1980s revealed that human atherosclerotic plaques contained vascular endothelial cells, smooth muscle cells, lipids, extracellular matrix and lipid-rich debris, and importantly, inflammatory and immune cells including macrophages and T cells.[3] Initially, atherosclerotic plaques present as thickening in the intimal layer of the arterial wall. Depending on factors that promote or counteract atherosclerotic disease (such as diet, environmental exposures such as pollution and smoking, blood pressure, lipids, and physical activity), these early atherosclerotic lesions may progress or regress. Mature plaques (atheromas) continue to evolve and have more complex immunological features than these early fatty streaks. Both the innate and acquired immune systems have central roles in modulating vascular inflammation.

Innate Immune System

The innate immune system is the evolutionarily older component of the intrinsic immune system and has an important role in surveying the host's internal environment for threats that can be rapidly addressed. Cells of the innate immune system that play a role in inflammation and atherosclerosis are outlined in **Fig. 14–1**.[4]

Monocytes: Monocytes and cells derived from them (macrophages) are the most prominent in atherosclerotic plaques. Human monocytes are divided into two main types: CD14+/CD16- classic (Mon1 [similar to mouse Ly6C/GR-1 high cells]) and CD14+/CD16++ nonclassic (Mon3 [similar to mouse Ly6C/GR-1 low cells]). Mon1 cells are highly proinflammatory, and express several important receptors and ligands including CCR2, CD62L, CD64, and CD115. These cells, when activated, induce an inflammatory milieu by releasing reactive oxygen species, interleukin 1 (IL-1), and tumor necrosis factors (TNFs), along with other proinflammatory cytokines. Release of these cytokines leads to further immune activation and propagation of inflammation. On the other hand, Mon3 cells express CXCR1 and elaborate factors that promote metabolic tissue repair, including transforming growth factor (TGF)-β, CD36, CD163, and vascular endothelial growth factor (VEGF). A recently described subtype of monocytes, Mon2, is characterized by CD14++/CD16+ expression, and is thought to have a more inflammatory effect. Additional cells from the innate immune system include dendritic cells that are antigen-presenting cells using human leukocyte antigen (HLA) molecules that interact with other immune cells to regulate and potentiate inflammatory responses.[5]

Mast Cells: While the population of mast cells (MCs) in atheromas is fairly small, experimental data show that these cells also play an important role in the atherosclerotic process. Committed progenitor cells of MCs are found in the circulation after being produced from pluripotent hematopoietic progenitors. Various chemokines are responsible for the migration of MC progenitors into specific tissues, with the most prominent known as stem cell factor (SCF). SCF is secreted by vascular SMCs and endothelial cells (ECs), therefore attracting MC progenitors to the vascular site of injury from atherosclerosis.[6] Once MC progenitors enter the arterial wall, SCF further acts as a growth factor to induce the maturation of MCs. The specific inflammatory milieu in tissue further informs the specific phenotype of the MC. Stored within MCs are several cytokines including tumor necrosis factor (TNF), basic fibroblast growth factor (bFGF or FGF-2), and TGF-β, which can be rapidly released via degranulation.[7] MCs also secrete soluble heparin proteoglycans that form complexes with low-density lipoprotein (LDL) in the intimal layer that are then phagocytosed by macrophages through scavenger-receptors, helping transform macrophages into foam cells.[8]

Histamine, one of the major products released by MCs, increases vascular permeability and has been hypothesized to lead to increased EC permeability that allows LDL to enter the intima of the vessel wall, one of the inciting and propagating steps in atherogenesis. Additionally, MCs inhibit cholesterol efflux mediated by high-density lipoproteins (HDL), which leads to greater subendothelial accumulation of cholesterol products.[9] Studies on the distribution of MCs in atheromas have shown that these cells are found in much higher concentrations in the shoulder region of the plaque where they preferentially demonstrate degranulation, further leading to a localized proinflammatory milieu.[10] MCs also play a role in the process of plaque erosion and rupture. Serine proteases and other enzymes released by MCs lead to activation of matrix metalloproteinases (MMP) in the fibrous cap of atheromas, leading to degradation of collagen and other structural proteins that stabilize this layer of the atheroma and protect its contents from vascular exposure.[11]

Platelets: While not officially classified as part of the immune system, platelets teleologically are an important part of the

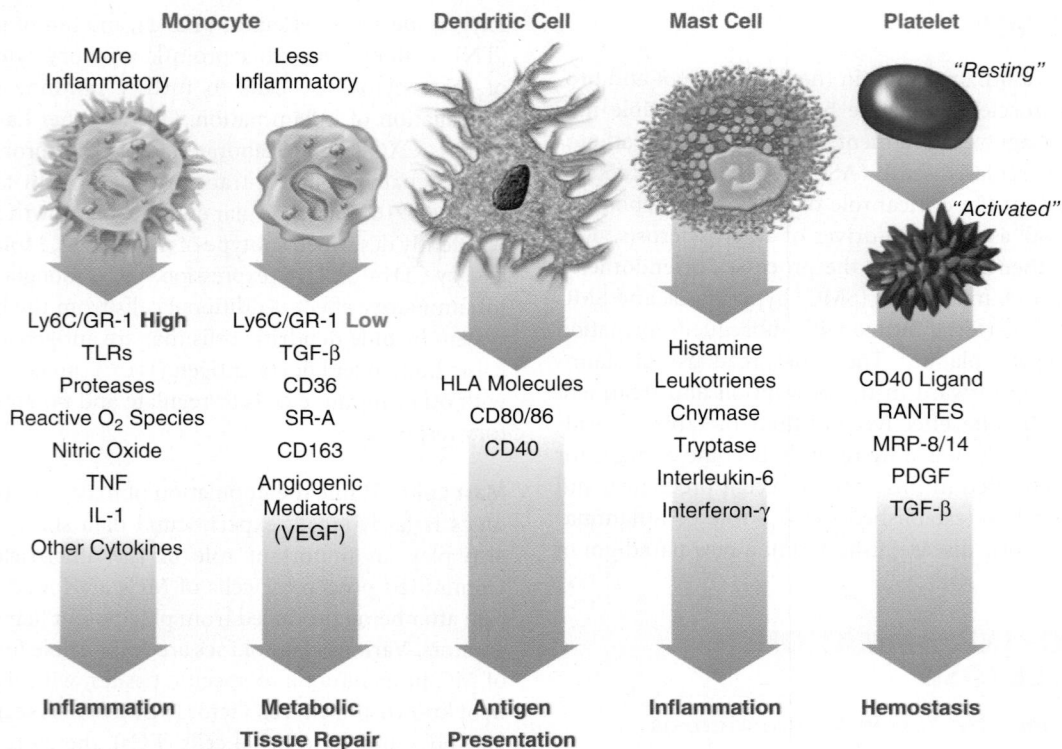

Figure 14–1. Several key participants in the innate cellular immunity pathway in atherosclerosis. This figure illustrates several of the key participants in the innate cellular immunity pathway in atherosclerosis. The effects of each of these participants are shown in detail. Activation of Ly6C/GR-1-expressing monocytes leads to an inflammatory milieu, whereas those monocytes with low Ly6C/GR-1 expression are associated with mediators of metabolic tissue repair. Dendritic cells are associated with antigen presentation to T cells, forming a bridge between the innate and adaptive immune systems. Mast cells harbor many mediators of inflammation that are also thought to play an important role in atherosclerosis. Finally, platelets also have an important role in immune activation when exposed to stimulatory signals. TLR, toll-like receptor; TNF, tumor necrosis factor; IL, interleukin; TGF, transforming growth factor; SR-A, scavenger receptor A; VEGF, vascular endothelial growth factor; RANTES, regulated and T-cell expressed secreted; MRP, myeloid related protein; PDGF, platelet-derived growth factor. Reproduced with permission from Libby P, Ridker PM, Hansson GK. Leducq Transatlantic Network on Atherothrombosis. Inflammation in atherosclerosis: from pathophysiology to practice. *J Am Coll Cardiol.* 2009 Dec 1;54(23):2129-2138.

inflammatory process for host protection.[12] In atherosclerosis, platelets are well known to play a key role in the late stage of disease, particularly in promoting plaque rupture and atherothrombosis. However, there is newfound appreciation of the proinflammatory role that platelets play in atherosclerotic disease. Activated ECs express P-selectin, E-selectin, and integrins on their luminal surface, which facilitate platelet rolling and adhesion.[13] Platelet activation during adhesion to the EC surface releases many powerful inflammatory mediators from platelets, further altering the EC phenotype to a proinflammatory and activated one. Platelets can release proinflammatory cytokines and chemokines such as IL-1β, CD40 ligand (CD40L), Regulated upon Activation Normal T Cell Expressed and Presumably Secreted cytokine (RANTES), and platelet factor 4 (PF4).[12] Each of these agents has important and overlapping roles in the activation of ECs, chemoattraction and recruitment of leukocytes, triggering of further inflammatory cascades, and resulting remodeling of the atheroma.

Adaptive Immune System

The adaptive immune system is the evolutionarily newer part of the immune system, and also plays an important role in atherosclerosis.[14,15] The two arms of the adaptive immune system include those that enact cellular responses and those involved in humoral responses. Complex mechanisms are involved in the interaction between the adaptive immune system and developing atherosclerotic plaque.[4] Dendritic cells (part of the innate immune system) within atherosclerotic plaque present antigens to B and T cells. While the antigens that stimulate these cells in atherosclerotic disease are not clear, candidates include heat shock proteins, plasma lipoprotein, and possibly microbial signatures as well. Stimulation of T cells leads to proliferation of the specific clone that recognizes the antigen, with resulting initiation of cellular immune responses. B cells activate humoral immunity with antibody production and trigger proinflammatory cytokine production. Cells of the adaptive immune system that play a role in inflammation and atherosclerosis are outlined in **Fig. 14–2.**

T Cells: Several subclasses of T cells are involved in the immune response in atherosclerosis. The major classification system for T cells distinguishes between CD4+ and CD8+ T cells. Among CD4+ T cells, T helper cells (Th) have multiple subtypes, each of which have different roles in the inflammatory process in atherosclerosis.[15] Th1 cells are the most prominent T cell subtype in plaques and promote atherosclerosis.[16] Th1 cells secrete TNF and IFNγ, which further activate nearby macrophages and other T cells to accelerate the inflammatory response. Th2

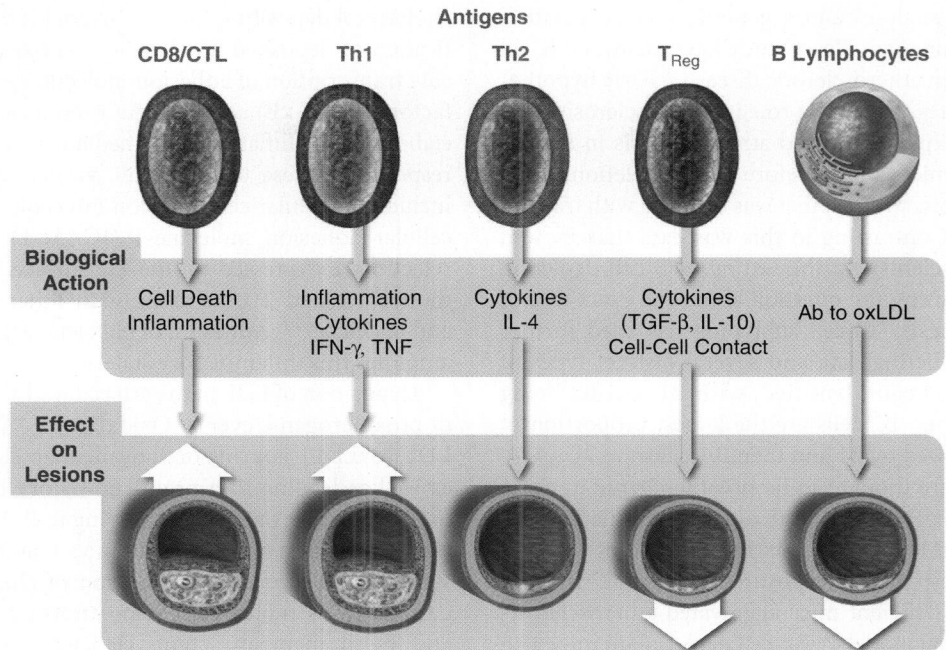

Figure 14–2. The various cells involved in adaptive immunity. B cells elaborate antibodies to various antigens including oxidized LDL, leading to a reduction in atherosclerotic plaque burden. T cells have a variety of different effects depending on subtype as shown in the figure. The effect of each type of response on atherosclerotic lesions is shown in the bottom row, with *upward arrows* indicating increased plaque formation and *downward arrows* indicating reduced plaque formation, realizing that this diagram may simplify the complex biology at play in these processes. CTL, cytolytic T lymphocytes; IFN, interferon; hsp, heat shock protein; Th, T helper cells; T_{Reg}, regulatory T cells. Reproduced with permission from Libby P, Ridker PM, Hansson GK. Leducq Transatlantic Network on Atherothrombosis. Inflammation in atherosclerosis: from pathophysiology to practice. *J Am Coll Cardiol.* 2009 Dec 1;54(23):2129-2138.

cells are the second-largest population of T cells and may have anti-inflammatory and stabilizing effects in atheroma. Key cytokines associated with Th2 cells include IL-4, IL-5, IL-10, and IL-13. Data thus far show that patients with higher numbers of Th2 cells in their peripheral blood mononuclear cell fraction tend to have decreased carotid intimal media thickening, a proxy for atherosclerotic plaque burden.[17] In vitro data points to decreased atherosclerosis in models with IL-4 release, a cytokine associated with Th2 cells.[17] However, various other experimental models have conflicting data on the role of IL-4 in atherosclerosis.[18]

Atherosclerotic plaques also contain Th17 cells that primarily secrete IL-17 and exhibit variable inflammatory effects in different settings. Th17 cells induce secretion of proinflammatory and proatherogenic cytokines including IL-6, granulocyte colony-stimulating factor (G-CSF), and granulocyte-macrophage colony-stimulating factor (GM-CSF) when found in endothelial and immune cell settings.[19] However, a subset of Th17 cells also produce atheroprotective IL-10.[19]

An additional population of CD4+ T cells that may have an important role in atherosclerosis is that of regulatory T (T_{reg}) cells.[20] These cells secrete the anti-inflammatory cytokine IL-10, and both T_{reg} numbers and IL-10 concentration are lower in patients with myocardial infarction (MI) compared to those without coronary disease.[21] Cohort studies have shown mixed clinical effects of T_{reg} numbers and prevalence of atherosclerotic disease. Overall, T_{reg} cells are believed to have an atheroprotective effect mainly through IL-10 and TGFβ secretion.[22]

In contrast to CD4+ T cells, CD8+ T cells can mature into cytotoxic T cells and target specific cells (such as cancer cells or virus-infected cells) for cytotoxic destruction. The antigens responsible for this activation and transformation to cytotoxic T cells in atherosclerosis are unknown. CD8+ T cells are found in higher concentrations in the blood of patients with coronary artery disease (CAD) and in atherosclerotic plaque.[23] Pathologic analyses of atherosclerotic plaques show large populations of CD8+ cells, often concentrated in the fibrous cap of the plaque, and advanced atheromas have a larger proportion of CD8+ cells than CD4+ cells.[24] The damage inflicted by these cells on vascular SMCs and other stabilizing cell types in plaque may lead to destabilization and acceleration of atherosclerosis. In atherogenic mouse models, targeting of cytotoxic T cells by antibodies led to reduced atherosclerotic burden, suggesting a proatherogenic role for cytotoxic T cells.[25] Furthermore, CD8+ T cells may promote maturation and development of monocytes by an IFNγ mediated pathway, although this axis is not clearly defined.[25] While these data appear to implicate CD8+ T cells in accelerating atherosclerosis, studies about the regulatory nature of these cells indicate that they may have a tempering effect on the atherosclerotic disease process as well.[26] Therefore, while CD8+ cytotoxic T cells are thought to have deleterious consequences in atherosclerotic disease, more studies are needed to define the true and multifaceted role of these cells in atherosclerosis.

B Cells: Humoral immunity and the role of B lymphocytes in atherosclerosis have recently received attention.[27] Recent large-scale network analyses and a genome-wide association study from the Framingham Heart Study have identified B cell activity as causative in atherosclerotic disease.[28] Early hypotheses that B lymphocytes may play a role in atherosclerosis were based on data showing exaggerated atherosclerosis in apoE[-/-] mice with splenectomies (and therefore B-cell depletion) compared to sham controls, an effect that was reversed with transfer of splenic B cells.[29] Contrasting to this was data that showed reduction of atherosclerosis in the setting of B-cell depleting therapies in mice, raising the question about the exact role of B cells in atherogenesis.[30] B-cell subtyping has shed further light into these conflicting data and several distinct types of B lymphocytes have been identified, with B1 and B2 being the predominant types. B2 cells are the largest proportion of B lymphocytes, followed by B1 and then B$_{reg}$ cells.

B2 lymphocytes are thought to be proatherogenic in mice. B2 cells interact with T cells through antigen stimulation and produce adaptive IgM, IgG, IgA, or IgE antibodies through class-switching in response to exposure to antigens. Transfer of B2 cells in B-cell deficient mice aggravated atherosclerosis in two different animal models.[31] B2-cell depletion in mice also led to reduction in plaque formation, further supporting the atherogenic role of B2 cells.[32]

B1 cells, in contrast to B2 cells, are generally considered to be protective against atherosclerosis in mice. B1 cells primarily secrete germline-encoded IgM and IgA antibodies that arise without immunization or prior infection. These cells are found on mucosal surfaces and provide rapid immunologic protection. Current theories about the protective mechanism of B1 cells are related to the action of IgM antibodies against inflammatory epitopes in atherosclerosis.

CURRENT MODEL OF ATHEROGENESIS

The concept of atherosclerosis as an inflammatory state has a long history. In 1856, Rudolf Virchow termed atherosclerosis as "entzündung" (inflammation) in a seminal publication.[33] In subsequent years, the role of cholesterol in atherosclerosis took center stage. In 1913, experimental models showed that feeding high cholesterol diets to rabbits induced atherosclerosis, with Nikolai Anitschkow declaring that "without cholesterol, there is no atherosclerosis."[34] Pathologic and mechanistic studies in the last few decades have helped develop the sophisticated current model of atherosclerosis as a lipid-driven inflammatory disease, with contributions from all arms of the immune system (**Fig. 14–3**).[35]

Today, investigators recognize that cholesterol accumulation and an activated immune system augment each other and are not competing hypotheses.[4,14,36,37] ECs lining the arterial lumen do not actively recruit immune cells when in a resting state. Two important and contemporaneous events lead to the inciting lesions in early atherosclerosis. First, exposure of ECs to irritating stimuli such as shear stress, hypertension, dyslipidemia, or proinflammatory mediators leads to EC activation with resulting expression of selective leukocyte adhesion molecules. The second inciting event for atherosclerosis is when a state of hyperlipidemia leads to LDL and its accompanying cholesterol depositing into the arterial intimal layer.[35,38] Modification of deposited lipoproteins via oxidative pathways activate transcription of adhesion molecule genes through nuclear factor-κB (NF-κB) activity.[39] As a result of these processes and elaboration of inflammatory mediators in the vascular wall in response to these toxic stimuli, various adhesion molecules, including vascular cell adhesion molecule-1 (VCAM-1), intercellular adhesion molecule-1 (ICAM-1), E-selectin, and P-selectin are expressed on the EC surface with recruitment of monocytes and T cells along with other immune mediators and platelets.[40-43] Adhesion of platelets to activated ECs further amplifies this inflammatory state.

Deposition of LDL in the arterial wall also triggers a cascade of proatherogenic events. Oxidation of LDL to yield oxidized LDL (oxLDL) is a major intermediate step in atherogenesis as well as leading to a proinflammatory cascade. Circulating oxLDL promotes monocyte binding to ECs independent of the classic adhesion molecules VCAM-1 and ICAM-1.[44] In this stage of atherogenesis, production of chemoattractant molecules such as monocyte chemoattractant protein-1 (MCP-1) and T-cell chemoattractants lead to transmigration of these cells into the intima.[45] The entry of monocytes and leukocytes (predominantly T cells) into the arterial intima establishes and propagates atherosclerosis. Modified LDLs (such as oxLDL) interact and activate monocytes and macrophages in the tunica intima, potentially acting as pathogen-associated molecular patterns (PAMPs) and damage-associated molecular patterns (DAMPs) to activate specific pattern recognition receptors (PRRs) including toll-like receptors (TLR) and scavenger receptor-A (SR-A) that are found on a various immune cells.[46,47] Other ligands of TLRs that are present in the plaque (such as heat shock protein and viral glycoproteins, among others) may also play a role in this activation.

Immune cells (predominated by monocytes and T cells) in the early atherosclerotic plaque undergo various transformations in response to local and systemic signals. Monocytes convert to specific inflammatory macrophage subtypes (such as Mon1) and foam cells, induced by exposure to oxLDL and M-CSF.[48] Expression of scavenger receptors on macrophages leads to ingestion of oxLDL and the formation of foam cells that reside in the arterial wall.[49] Human ECs and SMCs themselves produce cytokines that potentiate these immune cell changes in the vessel wall.[43]

Along with cellular immunity, important effects of the humoral immune system are also emerging. In the setting of activated ECs, the endothelial layer becomes more porous to immunoglobulin entry into the plaque. In addition, B cells and plasma cells take up residence in the adventitial layer of the arterial wall, and organize as an artery tertiary lymphoid organ.[50] Here, they produce a myriad of immunoglobulins, which have variable effects on atherosclerosis. IgM antibodies appear to target oxLDL and clear apoptotic/necrotic debris in the plaque, therefore playing an atheroprotective role.[51] Meanwhile, IgG antibodies complex with oxLDL to form immune complexes that interact with macrophages and other immune cells, ultimately activating the inflammasome, promoting phagocytosis and antigen presentation, and cytokine

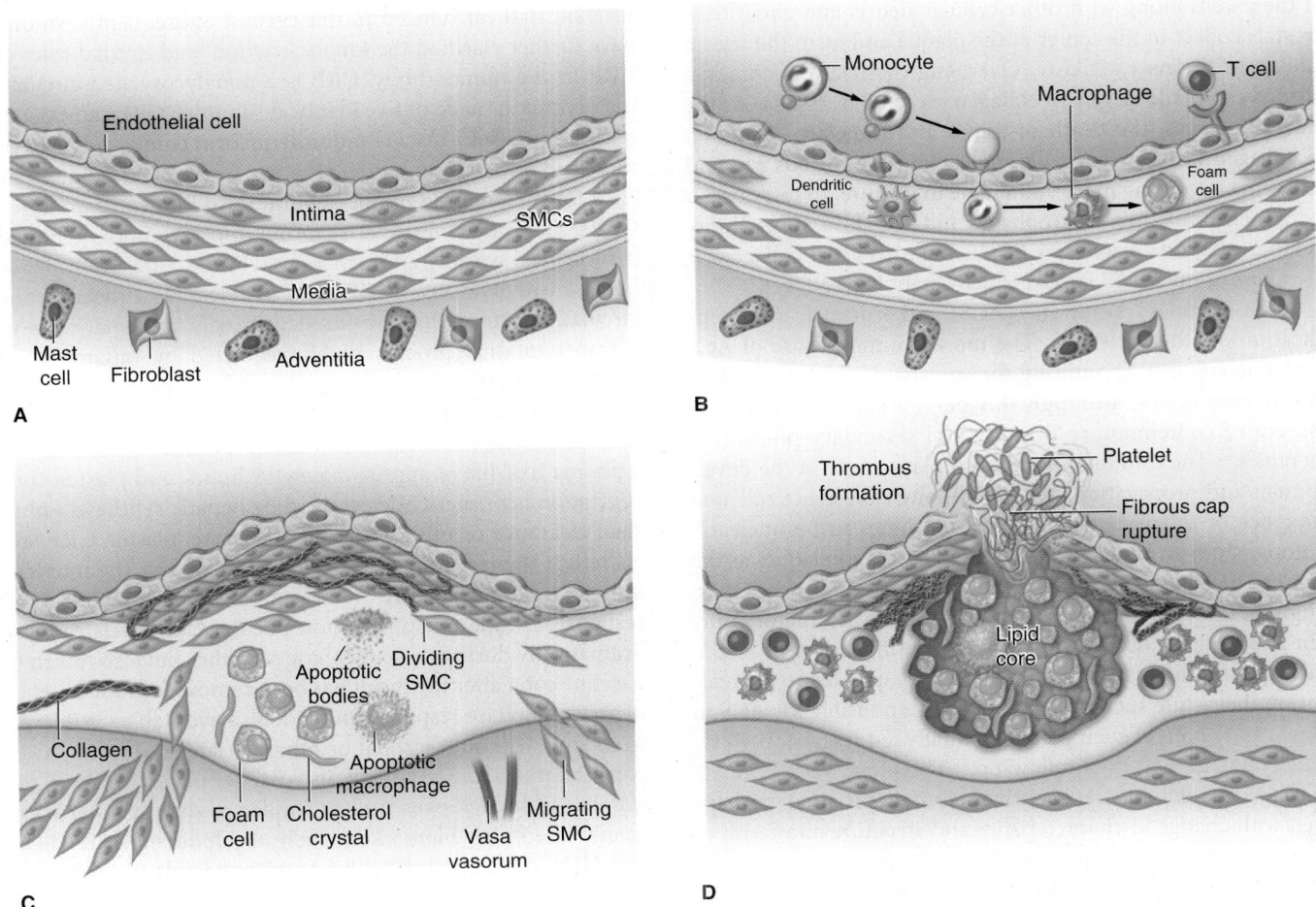

Figure 14–3. A schematic of the proposed pathway in formation of atherosclerotic plaque. (A) The normal resting artery has three layers, with the inner layer lined by endothelial cells. The intimal and medial layers of the human artery contain smooth muscle cells (SMCs). The outer layer of the artery, the adventitia, contains fibroblasts, mast cells, nerve endings, and small blood vessels. (B) Early steps in atherosclerosis include adhesion of leukocytes to the endothelial cells with transmigration into the intimal layer, along with maturation of monocytes into macrophages that take up lipid particles to transform into foam cells. (C) Atherosclerotic plaque growth involves proliferation of intimal SMCs along with migration of SMCs from the media to the intimal layer, as well as production of extracellular matrix components including proteoglycans and collagen. Cellular components including macrophages and SMCs undergo cell death, with debris and extracellular lipid components collecting in a necrotic core. (D) Through various mechanisms, some of which are not understood, the fibrotic cap overlying the necrotic core can rupture, exposing prothrombotic components in the core to circulating factors that promote acute thrombosis, the most feared complication of atherosclerosis. Reproduced with permission from Libby P, Ridker PM, Hansson GK. Progress and challenges in translating the biology of atherosclerosis. *Nature.* 2011 May 19;473(7347):317-325.

production.[52] IgE also appears to have a proatherogenic role in the plaque primarily through activation of macrophages and mast cells in the plaque.[53] Besides antibody production, B cells themselves produce cytokines (including the proatherogenic TNFα and antiatherogenic IL-10) and thus may modulate the inflammatory milieu in atheromas directly.

Another key inflammatory pathway in atherosclerosis centers around inflammasomes, which are protein and enzyme complexes that lead to inflammatory activation and cytokine production. Cholesterol, particularly oxLDL, leads to activation of inflammasome immune complexes through various mechanisms, including recognition by TLRs, intracellular stress, and cytokine receptors.[54] The NLRP3 inflammasome, a specific inflammasome complex, leads to activation of caspase-1 (also known as IL-1β-converting enzyme), which converts pro-IL-1β to the inflammatory cytokine IL-1β, and

pro-IL-18 to IL-18.[55] Activation of the IL-1 receptor family by IL-1β leads to potentiation of local and systemic inflammation. IL-1 type 1 receptor activity is carefully balanced between activation by IL-1α and IL-1β and inhibition through IL-1 receptor antagonist (IL-1Ra). Both IL-1β and IL-1Ra are found in atherosclerotic plaques and the balance of these two opposing forces participates in determining the trajectory of atherosclerosis.[56] In vitro and in vivo data have established IL-1β as a significant proatherogenic cytokine.[57] IL-1β also leads to expression of adhesion molecules on SMCs and ECs, further attracting immunocytes to the inflamed plaque.[58] IL-1 is also one of the most potent inducers of IL-6 production, an axis that has considerable import in the etiology of cardiovascular disease (CVD).[59]

As atherosclerotic plaques mature, foam cells and SMCs undergo programmed cell death, or apoptosis. The remains of these cells along with other cellular debris and cholesterol crystals collect in the center of the plaque and form the region known as the necrotic core. Overlying the necrotic core is a fibrous cap made largely of collagen secreted by SMCs. As the plaque matures, the death of SMCs and therefore reduction in collagen integrity and volume leads to the fibrous cap and atheroma becoming more vulnerable to rupture. In response to cytokine stimulation, macrophages and MCs lead to instability in atherosclerotic plaques by producing interstitial collagenase members of the MMP family, which catabolize collagen.[60]

Acute coronary syndrome (ACS) is the most feared complication of atherosclerosis. The most common cause of ACS is plaque rupture, accounting for approximately 70% of ACS in one case series, although this percentage is dropping in the era of contemporary primary and secondary prevention therapies.[61] The immune system also plays a role in the development and propagation of ACS, although the exact role and sequence of inflammation in ACS continues to be unclear.[62] Autopsy studies in the 1980s identified ruptured plaques as the cause of most fatal ACS, a finding that informed the early paradigm of the vulnerable plaque with a high inflammatory burden and thinned fibrous cap as the initiating lesion in ACS.[63] Subsequent studies to characterize these plaques led to the realization that while such plaques may be responsible for ACS in some cases, <5% of such plaques actually led to clinically evident events in 3 years of follow-up.[64] Therefore, such "vulnerable" plaques demonstrate relative stability over time, perhaps even with change in characteristics and structure as a result of primary and secondary prevention efforts. Nonetheless, a subset of ACS cases is likely driven by inflammatory stimuli, as evidenced by studies assessing inflammatory biomarkers such as C-reactive protein (CRP).[65] Macrophage and T-cell populations in ACS-related plaque appear to shift toward a catabolic and inflammatory phenotype compared to reparative and stable characteristics.

TRANSLATING INFLAMMATION BIOLOGY TO BIOMARKERS AND TARGETS FOR THERAPY IN ATHEROSCLEROTIC DISEASE

Translating the understanding of the role of inflammation in atherosclerosis to clinical relevance requires detection of biomarkers that reflect the unique inflammatory state and risk for each individual. Prospective epidemiological studies have evaluated several serum markers to understand their relationship with systemic inflammation and CVD.[66] Some candidates that have been examined for this role include myeloperoxidase,[67] adhesion molecules (such as ICAM-1 and P-selectin),[41,68,69] Lp-PLA2,[70] IL-6,[71,72] IL-1β,[73] MMP9[74], and CRP[65,75–77] (contemporarily measured as high-sensitivity CRP). Of these, CRP has emerged as the most widely used clinical biomarker for the assessment of inflammatory activation and risk of future CVD.[78]

CRP Biology

CRP was first described in the 1930s in the context of pneumococcal infection, with the concept of CRP as an acute phase reactant first introduced in the 1940s.[79] Subsequently, studies have further clarified the kinetics, action, and myriad roles of CRP in the human body. CRP is a nonglycosylated circulating pentraxin made of five identical subunits. CRP can exist in one of three isoforms: (1) multimeric form composed of 10 or more subunits, (2) pentameric (native) form, or (3) monomeric CRP form composed of one subunit (also known as modified CRP).[80] The pentameric native form is most commonly studied in biological systems, and is measured by the clinically available high-sensitivity assay, hsCRP. CRP is released in the systemic circulation after being produced primarily in hepatocytes in a transcriptional process highly regulated by inflammatory cytokines, particularly IL-1 and IL-6. While extrahepatic sites of CRP production have been identified, they do not produce enough protein to substantively change plasma levels. CRP has a plasma half-life of approximately 19 hours, and plasma concentration is primarily determined by hepatic synthesis rather than clearance or other factors.[81] Therefore, plasma CRP levels reflect the inflammatory drive as encoded by the interleukins that determine CRP transcription, and as a result, CRP response to inflammation is nonspecific. CRP levels can rise dramatically during an acute phase stimulus, but also return to baseline soon after the insult has been removed. In the absence of an acute phase response, individuals have stable CRP levels over time, without seasonal or other variation, although CRP concentration does gradually increase with age.[82] Indeed, the stability of hsCRP over time is similar to that of other commonly used risk biomarkers such as blood pressure, LDL, and HDL cholesterol. CRP binds to its ligands in a calcium-dependent process, and can bind to lipids including LDL and lipoprotein(a).[83]

CRP Physiology

As will be subsequently described, hsCRP is a powerful clinical predictor of residual inflammatory risk for atherosclerotic events. Whether CRP itself is more than a biomarker and plays a direct role in atherothrombosis remains controversial. Physiologic studies of CRP have found it to have pleiotropic effects in the human body. Ligand-bound CRP acts as an opsonin to activate the classical complement pathway through interaction with C1q and also activates phagocytic cells through immunoglobulin receptors, thereby promoting an immune response.[84] However, CRP may also have anti-inflammatory properties, and has been found to induce IL1-Ra expression in humans, while also increasing secretion of IL-10 in mice.[85] CRP also interacts with neutrophils in both activating and inhibitory fashion.[86] In addition to its effects on immune cells, CRP has direct effects on the endothelial and vascular system. CRP induces expression of adhesion molecules (such as ICAM-1, VCAM-1, and E-selectin) on ECs and amplifies monocyte adhesion to the endothelium.[87] CRP also opsonizes LDL particles, thereby mediating LDL uptake by macrophages in an essential step of atherogenesis.[88] In additional effects on the vascular system, CRP reduces nitric oxide release in ECs through reducing nitric oxide synthase activity and expression.[89] CRP has also been noted to induce EC apoptosis and endothelial inflammatory cytokine production, with resulting potential deleterious vascular effects.[90] On the other hand, Mendelian randomization studies have suggested that CRP may simply be a biomarker of risk with upstream activation of IL-1 and IL-6 as causal agents and, therefore, targets for intervention.

CRP in Predicting Cardiovascular Risk

Case reports in the 1940s and 1950s indicated that CRP concentrations were elevated in patients after acute MI, first linking CVD and CRP. In the 1980s and 1990s, several studies demonstrated CRP elevations in the setting of ACS, although such studies could not address whether ischemia was a cause or a result of an activated inflammatory process.[91] Multiple prospective cohort studies were subsequently conducted to better understand the relationship of CRP with future incident cardiovascular (CV) events. In one of these, the Multiple Risk Factor Intervention Study (MRFIT) investigators looked at the risk of CV events in a case-control study of male subjects with risk factors for CVD but without clinical ASCVD, and found a significant relationship between baseline CRP and risk of coronary heart disease (CHD) death in smokers.[92] Given these findings in smokers only and with knowledge that smoking itself increases CRP, the question of the independent risk prediction of CRP for CVD remained uncertain.

The Physicians' Health Study (PHS) was the pivotal investigation that answered this question and established the modern paradigm of risk assessment with CRP. The PHS investigators measured baseline CRP levels in healthy men and followed them in a prospective cohort study. The key findings in this study showed that baseline CRP levels were significantly higher in those who had a subsequent MI or stroke, and that this relationship was not modified by smoking status or controlling for lipid and nonlipid-related risk factors.[75] Further investigations in this cohort showed that CRP added incremental prognostic information to that of total and HDL cholesterol in a lipid and nonlipid risk factor independent manner, and that CRP was predictive of incident peripheral arterial disease as well as sudden death.[75,76,93] The results of PHS were replicated in healthy women enrolled in the Women's Health Study.[77] With the development of a commercial and accurate hsCRP assay, the ability of CRP to independently predict future CV events was replicated in more than 50 diverse cohorts. In 2010, a comprehensive meta-analysis of these studies by the Emerging Risk Factor Consortium included >160,000 individuals with 1.3 million person-years of follow-up and showed that each standard deviation increase in log-normalized hsCRP associated with a multivariate adjusted relative increase in risk of 1.37 (95% confidence interval [CI], 1.27–1.48) for future CHD and 1.55 (95% CI, 1.37–1.76) for future CV mortality.[94] These effects were similar in magnitude to that of other traditional risk factors such as total cholesterol, HDL, and blood pressure. Given the significant predictive power of hsCRP, the Reynold's Risk Score (www.reynoldsriskscore.org) was developed to incorporate hsCRP and family history in CV risk prediction.[95,96] This score has been shown to appropriately reclassify 20% to 30% of individuals in intermediate risk categories to either higher or lower risk. The use of hsCRP was also subsequently affirmed in the Framingham Risk Score.[97]

CRP for Targeting Anti-Atherosclerotic Therapy

Another important aspect of PHS was the critical evidence it provided that CRP might help identify a population that may benefit the most from targeted interventions. In PHS, participants were randomized to receive aspirin (ASA) 325 mg every other day or matching placebo. As an antiplatelet and anti-inflammatory agent, ASA was an attractive therapy to explore CVD risk reduction. While ASA resulted in a 44% reduction in vascular events in the whole cohort, the attributable risk reduction from ASA was greatest in those with the highest baseline CRP. The next major step in translating the emerging understanding of inflammation in atherosclerosis was taken when the Cholesterol and Recurrent Events (CARE) trial showed that the reduction in CVD events in pravastatin treated patients was greatest in those with elevated CRP, and that pravastatin reduced CRP concentrations in an LDL-independent manner.[98] These data provided early clinical proof that statin therapy was both lipid lowering and anti-inflammatory. Subsequent trials replicated these findings for other statins as well. The next important step in the use of CRP for targeting therapy most effectively came from data in the Air Force/Texas Coronary Atherosclerosis Prevention Study (AFCAPS/TexCAPS), which showed that statin therapy reduced CVD events amongst those with low LDL concentrations but with an elevated CRP.[99] In contrast, subjects in this study who had low CRP and low LDL did not derive any significant benefit from statin therapy. This finding identified an important group of individuals who did not meet statin therapy requirements by lipid guidelines, but were shown to have elevated CVD risk. However, since these were not the primary analyses but rather post hoc observations, a dedicated trial to test this hypothesis in patients with low LDL but high CRP was necessary.

The Justification for the Use of Statins in Prevention: an Intervention Trial Evaluating Rosuvastatin (JUPITER) was published in 2008 after being stopped early by its data safety monitoring board due to the finding that there was a significant benefit of rosuvastatin in healthy participants with low LDL cholesterol (<130 mg/dL) but elevated hsCRP (>2 mg/L).[100] The trial showed a highly statistically significant 54% reduction in MI, 48% reduction in stroke, 47% reduction in coronary revascularization procedures, and a 20% reduction in all-cause mortality for subjects on rosuvastatin when compared to placebo. These effects persisted amongst several subgroups, including women and those with LDL <100 mg/dL. In addition, the beneficial effect of rosuvastatin in patients with high hsCRP but low LDL was apparent within a few months of therapy. With a number-needed-to-treat of 25 to prevent one event in 5 years, this trial established the role of targeted CV therapies based on inflammatory risk as measured by hsCRP, regardless of lipid level.

The question of whether lipid lowering and concomitant CRP reduction in ACS would yield benefit was addressed in two pivotal trials—the Pravastatin or Atorvastatin Evaluation and Infection Therapy: Thrombolysis in Myocardial Infarction 22 (PROVE IT–TIMI 22) trial and the Aggrastat to Zocor (A to Z) trial—both of which demonstrated that the best clinical outcomes with statin therapy in ACS were observed in those with reduction of LDL <70 mg/dL and hsCRP <2 mg/L.[101,102] This data was further supported by findings from the Reversing Atherosclerosis with Aggressive Lipid Lowering (REVERSAL) trial that used intravascular ultrasound (IVUS) to demonstrate that atherosclerotic plaque regression was observed only amongst those with reductions in both hsCRP and LDL after initiating statin therapy.[103]

IL-6 Biology and Pathophysiology

While the evidence presented demonstrates the ability of CRP to both predict CVD risk and identify those most likely to benefit from statin therapy, biological and genetic studies to date have not established a clear causal link between CRP and CVD. Contemporary Mendelian randomization studies have consistently shown neutral results for the relationship between CRP and CVD.[104] In an attempt to better understand the pathways through which CRP associates with CVD, the upstream regulator of CRP, IL-6 has been studied rigorously and emerged as an important candidate as a causal link between inflammation and atherosclerosis.

Similar to studies for CRP, 1L-6 predicts vascular risk in healthy men and women, a finding that has been robustly replicated in multiple large diverse cohorts.[72,77] A meta-analysis of inflammatory markers in CVD showed a 26% increased risk of vascular events for each standard deviation increase in log IL-6 levels, data that was similar to the CRP meta-analysis described previously.[105] Biologically, IL-6 correlates with evidence of vascular dysfunction as measured by arterial stiffness, endothelial dysfunction, and degree of subclinical atherosclerosis.[106,107] Clinical studies have shown IL-6 to be associated with microvascular dysfunction, atherosclerotic plaque initiation, and destabilization, along with worse outcomes in acute ischemia.[108,109] A phenome-wide association study showed that IL-6 receptor single nucleotide polymorphisms led to a lower risk of aortic aneurysms and CHD.[110] In an interesting experiment, sampling of coronary blood in the setting of coronary occlusion and resulting ischemia showed elevations in IL-6 with concomitant CRP reduction.[111] In contradistinction to CRP, Mendelian randomization studies of IL-6 polymorphisms have shown a concordantly low level of hsCRP and lower lifetime risk of vascular disease.[71,112] Therefore, IL-6 appears to be a unifying mediator of the association between hsCRP level and CV risk, and appears to lie on the causal pathway to ASCVD. These findings have led to considerable interest in targeting IL-6 for the prevention of ASCVD.

IL-1 and Its Role in CVD

As research continues to understand the specific pathways involved in the inflammatory contribution to ASCVD, attention has turned to IL-1 as a potential powerful mediator of this relationship.[113] IL-1 is one of the key proinflammatory cytokines in the human body, and lies directly upstream of IL-6 in the inflammatory cascade. The NLRP3 inflammasome converts pro-IL-1β to active IL-1β, which then exerts its effects on downstream targets.[114] IL-1β has been implicated in several autoinflammatory diseases with dysfunctional involvement of monocyte–macrophage interactions leading to pathologic inflammation, a process similar to atherogenesis.[115] Treatment of these disorders with IL-1β targeted therapies such as canakinumab (anti-IL-1β antibody), anakinra (a synthetic IL-1Ra), and rilonocept (IL-1 trap) has led to improvement in symptoms, thereby providing an open armamentarium of targeting this cytokine in atherosclerosis.

Due to challenges in accurately and reliably measuring IL-1β, large epidemiological studies relating IL-1β levels and CVD risk are not available. Recent data shows that IL-1β measured on admission to the hospital for ST-segment elevation MI (STEMI) was associated with risk of mortality and major adverse CV events, independent of hsCRP and clinical risk factors.[73] Those who had the highest levels of IL-1β and hsCRP on admission were at the highest risk for adverse events.[73] IL-1 has direct effects on the arterial wall by inducing procoagulant activity and leukocyte adhesion in ECs while also inducing release of growth-inhibitory prostanoids in SMCs.[116,117] Deficiency of IL-1β leads to reduced atherosclerotic plaque formation in mouse models, possibly as a result of reduced immune cell recruitment and adhesion.[118] With modulation of IL1-Ra activity, atherosclerosis burden was noted to be increased in states of IL1-Ra depletion and reduced in states of IL1-Ra overexpression, further implicating the IL-1 pathway in ASCVD.[119,120] In human studies, genetic polymorphisms of the IL-1Ra gene have effects on coronary plaque and restenosis rates, implicating the effect of IL-1 in the atherosclerotic process.[121]

THERAPIES TARGETING INFLAMMATION IN ATHEROSCLEROTIC DISEASE

Targeting IL-1β in CVD

Integrating all the epidemiological and experimental data already presented, the next logical step in reducing ASCVD burden was to test the hypothesis that intervention in the central IL-1 to IL-6 to CRP signaling pathway would lead to clinical improvement in patients with atherosclerosis, regardless of baseline lipid levels or lipid lowering (**Fig. 14–4**).[59] The agent canakinumab, a fully human monoclonal antibody targeting IL-1β, was chosen to help answer this question by specifically interrupting the IL-1β pathway. A phase IIb trial of canakinumab in diabetic patients with high vascular risk showed >50% reductions in IL-6 and CRP, without significant effect on HDL or LDL, thus providing important data supporting the use of this drug to test the hypothesis of IL-1β inhibition in ASCVD.[122] The Canakinumab Anti-Inflammatory Thrombosis Outcomes Study (CANTOS) was designed to test this specific hypothesis as a proof-of-principle trial.[123] In CANTOS, the investigators randomly allocated 10,061 patients with prior MI and hsCRP ≥2 mg/L to either placebo or one of three canakinumab doses (given subcutaneously every 3 months).

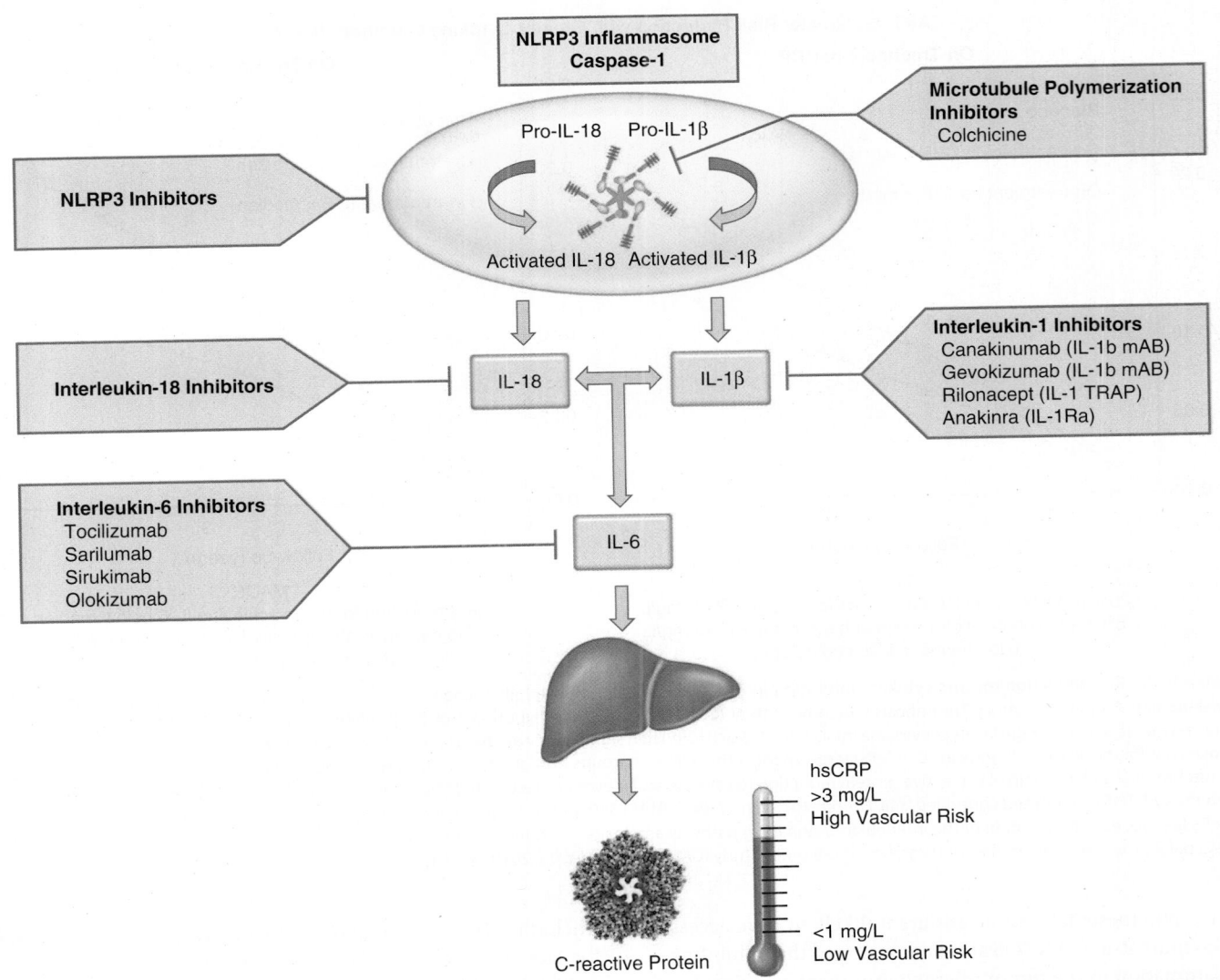

Figure 14–4. Schematic of NLRP3 inflammasome activation and possible targets of therapy. Inflammatory stimuli (including cholesterol crystals) lead to stimulation of the NLRP3 inflammasome, with subsequent conversion of pro–IL-18 and pro–IL-1β into activated IL-18 and IL-1β by the proteinase caspase-1, with downstream production of IL-6. These important mediators have significant vascular effects, with IL-6 also promoting hepatic CRP production. The *yellow boxes* in this diagram indicate targets of the signaling pathway and, where available, approved agents that potentially could be repurposed as vascular therapeutics. IL-1β, interleukin-1β; IL-1βmAB, interleukin-1β monoclonal antibody; IL-1Ra, interleukin-1 receptor antagonist; IL-1 TRAP, dimeric fusion protein of an interleukin-1 receptor component and an IL-1 receptor accessory protein; IL-6, interleukin-6; IL-18, interleukin-18; NLRP3 inflammasome, NOD-like receptor family pyrin domain containing 3 inflammasome. Reproduced with permission from Ridker PM. From CANTOS to CIRT to COLCOT to Clinic: Will All Atherosclerosis Patients Soon Be Treated With Combination Lipid-Lowering and Inflammation-Inhibiting Agents? *Circulation.* 2020 Mar 10;141(10):787-789.

After 48 months of therapy, CANTOS participants allocated to the higher doses of canakinumab had a 35% to 40% reduction in IL-6 and hsCRP compared to placebo participants.[124] Concomitant with this, actively treated participants in CANTOS experienced a 15% reduction in nonfatal MI, any nonfatal stroke, or CV death (MACE hazard ratio [HR], 0.85; 95% CI, 0.76–0.96; $P = 0.007$ for the pooled 150 mg and 300 mg canakinumab doses) and a 17% reduction in MACE plus the additional end point of hospitalization for unstable angina requiring urgent revascularization (MACE+; HR, 0.83; 95% CI, 0.74–0.92; $P = 0.0006$ for the pooled 150 mg and 300 mg canakinumab doses). Interestingly, the lower dose of canakinumab was associated with lesser reductions in IL-6 and hsCRP, with a

nonsignificant reduction in MACE and MACE+.[124] In line with this, CANTOS participants who achieved greater than average levels of cytokine inhibition (IL-6 or hsCRP) had significantly greater clinical benefit compared to those with lower than average cytokine inhibition (**Fig. 14–5**).[125,126] The results of this pivotal trial established the role of targeted anti-inflammatory therapy in the reduction of CV events in patients with established ASCVD, and ushered in a fundamentally new era in the treatment and prevention of CVD. Indeed, CANTOS provided the first hard evidence in over 40 years that a therapy not directly related to lipid lowering, blood pressure, glucose modulation, or thrombosis could in fact substantially reduce CV event rates.

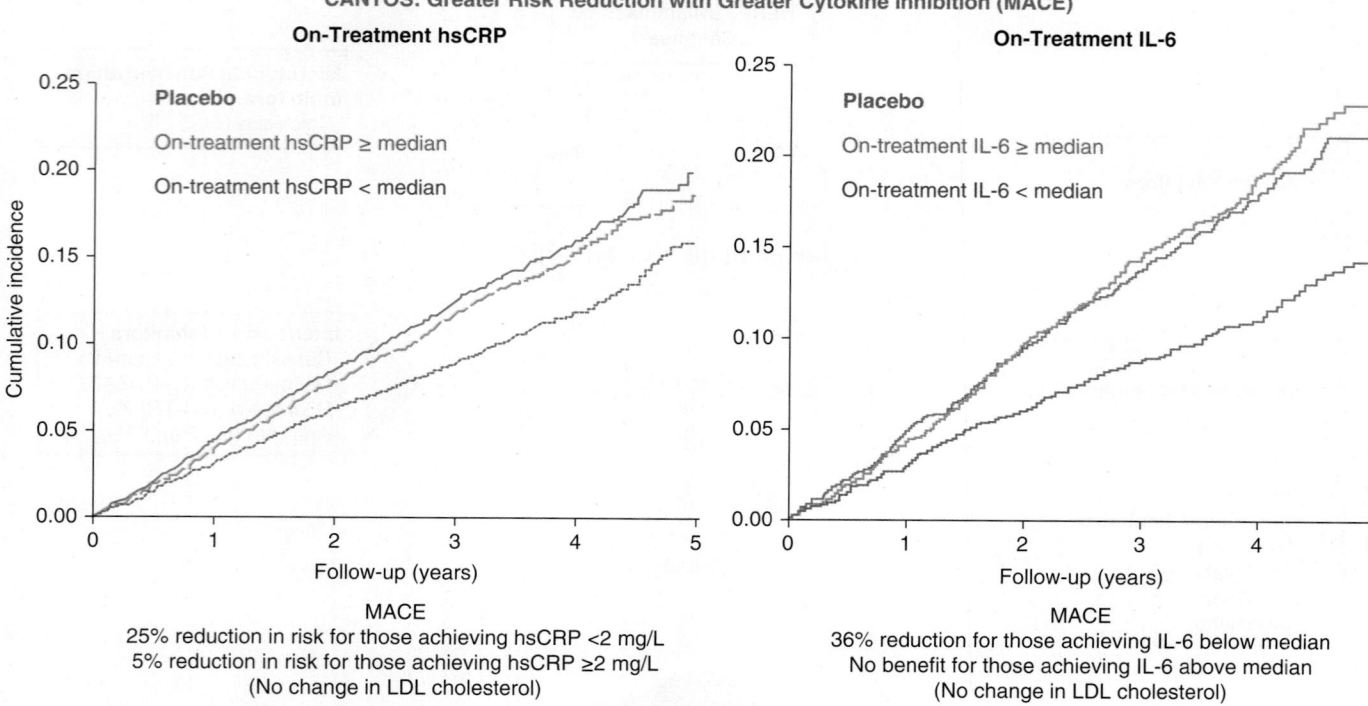

Figure 14–5. Risk reduction mirrors cytokine inhibition in CANTOS. Canakinumab, a fully human monoclonal antibody targeting IL-1β was used in the Canakinumab Anti-Inflammatory Thrombosis Outcomes Study (CANTOS) to test the hypothesis of IL-1β inhibition in ASCVD. CANTOS participants who achieved greater than average levels of cytokine inhibition (IL-6 or hsCRP) had significantly greater clinical benefit compared to those with lower than average cytokine inhibition, with no change in LDL cholesterol amongst the different groups. Left graph, reproduced with permission from Ridker PM, MacFadyen JG, Everett BM, et al. Relationship of C-reactive protein reduction to cardiovascular event reduction following treatment with canakinumab: a secondary analysis from the CANTOS randomised controlled trial. *Lancet.* 2018 Jan 27;391(10118):319-328 and right graph reproduced with permission from Ridker PM, Libby P, MacFadyen JG, et al. Modulation of the interleukin-6 signalling pathway and incidence rates of atherosclerotic events and all-cause mortality: analyses from the Canakinumab Anti-Inflammatory Thrombosis Outcomes Study (CANTOS). *Eur Heart J.* 2018 Oct 7;39(38):3499-3507.

Despite these data, clinicians are unlikely to have access to canakinumab as CANTOS also demonstrated that inhibition of inflammation in the tumor microenvironment associated with IL-1β inhibition lowers mortality from lung cancer by 50% to 60% in a dose-dependent manner.[127] For this reason, canakinumab is currently under intense investigation as adjunctive therapy in several oncologic settings. Data from CANTOS has also shown marked reductions in gout, anemia, and the need for total hip or total knee replacement all benefits secondary to inhibition of low-grade systemic inflammation.[128–130]

Methotrexate for Secondary Prevention of CVD

Where CANTOS studied the effect of narrowly targeted IL-1β inhibition on CVD, the Cardiovascular Inflammation Reduction Trial (CIRT) was designed to study the role of broader immunomodulation in reducing vascular events. Low dose methotrexate (LDM, 15–20 mg weekly) has been safely and successfully used for treatment of autoimmune disorders and is first-line therapy for rheumatoid arthritis. In observational data, the use of LDM appears to have lowered CV events.[131] Given this rationale, CIRT enrolled 4786 patients with known ASCVD and either diabetes or metabolic syndrome who were assigned to either LDM or placebo, on a background of aggressive standard of care therapy. In ≤5 years of follow-up, LDM did not reduce cytokine or biomarker concentrations

(including IL-1β, IL-6, and hsCRP). CIRT was stopped early for lack of benefit for the primary endpoint of nonfatal MI, nonfatal stroke, unstable angina requiring unplanned coronary revascularization, or CV death, with an HR for incident MI, stroke, or CV death of 1.04 (95% CI, 0.83–1.30).[132]

While several explanations are possible for the difference in results between CANTOS and CIRT, the combined interpretation of these two contemporary trials is highly informative. First, CANTOS specifically tested treatment of residual inflammatory risk in patients with ASCVD by enrolling patients with elevated hsCRP at baseline. On the other hand, CIRT enrolled patients without any baseline hsCRP screening criteria. This difference emphasizes the concept of residual inflammatory risk, a principle that stresses the independent effect of inflammation on ASCVD, beyond lipid and other risk factors. Furthermore, the two trials tested very different biological therapies. Whereas canakinumab specifically targeted the IL-1 to IL-6 to CRP axis, LDM did not affect the IL-1 pathway. The neutral results of CIRT therefore points toward modulation of the IL-1 to IL-6 axis as being most likely to yield benefits in CVD. This conclusion is further supported by null results from trials of anti-inflammatory therapies that, like methotrexate, also do not target the IL-1 pathway. For example, trials of losmapimod (an oral selective inhibitor of the Lp-PLA2 enzyme) and darapladib (a p38 Mitogen-activated protein kinase inhibitor) did not show benefit in CV events in patients with atherosclerotic disease.[133,134]

Colchicine as Anti-Inflammatory Therapy for Secondary Prevention of CVD

One attractive anti-inflammatory agent that has recently been tested in large CV trials is the antimitotic agent colchicine. Colchicine has pleiotropic effects on inflammation, where it exerts its primary effect through inhibition of tubulin polymerization and subsequent microtubule formation. However, colchicine is also known to have other effects on the immune system, including inhibition of neutrophil chemotaxis, adhesion and mobilization, superoxide production, as well as NLRP3 inflammasome inhibition and reduction in IL-1β processing and release (Fig. 14–4).[135]

The Low-Dose Colchicine (LoDoCo) open-label trial randomized 532 secondary prevention patients with stable CAD to either standard therapy or standard therapy and colchicine 0.5 mg daily.[136] In this Australian study with a median follow-up of 3 years, there was a 67% reduction in primary endpoint that was a composite of ACS, out-of-hospital cardiac arrest, and noncardioembolic ischemic stroke (95% CI, 0.18–0.59; $P < 0.001$).[136] Despite the limitations of this small trial in a relatively homogenous population without blinding or placebo, these outcomes were suggestive and encouraging, leaving the door open for more powerful studies to be conducted.

The Colchicine Cardiovascular Outcomes Trial (COLCOT) enrolled 4745 patients after MI and randomized them in a one-to-one fashion to either colchicine 0.5 mg daily or placebo.[137] The primary results of this trial showed a significant 23% relative reduction in the primary trial outcome including MI, stroke, resuscitated cardiac arrest, urgent hospitalization for angina requiring revascularization, and CV death (95% CI, 0.61–0.96; $P = 0.02$). While only the coronary revascularization and stroke components of the primary outcome were significantly lower in the treatment group, all other outcomes were directionally similarly reduced. There was a significantly increased risk of pneumonia with this therapy (0.9% in the colchicine group versus 0.4% in the placebo group [$P = 0.03$]) but no change in all-cause mortality.[137]

The LoDoCo2 (the second Low-Dose Colchicine) randomized, controlled, double-blind, event-driven trial tested the hypothesis whether colchicine 0.5 mg once daily could safely reduce the composite primary endpoint of CV death, MI, ischemic stroke, or ischemia-driven coronary revascularization in 5522 patients with stable CAD in Australia and the Netherlands.[138] Over a median follow-up of 28.6 months, there was a significant 31% reduction in the composite primary endpoint amongst treated patients compared to placebo (95% CI, 0.57–0.83; $P < 0.001$). This effect was also seen for the key composite secondary outcome of CV death, MI, or ischemic stroke. There was, however, a statistically nonsignificant increase in non-CV mortality in the colchicine group compared to the placebo group (HR 1.51; 95% CI, 0.99–2.31), without an increase in hospitalization for infection or pneumonia.[138]

While COLCOT and LoDoCo2 gave positive results for colchicine in secondary prevention of CV events, the smaller contemporaneous Colchicine in Patients with Acute Coronary Syndrome (COPS) randomized, double-blind, placebo-controlled trial of 795 patients with ACS did not show a benefit of colchicine for the primary outcome (a composite of all-cause mortality, ACS, ischemia-driven unplanned urgent revascularization and noncardioembolic ischemic stroke) over 12 months of follow-up (HR 0.65, 95% CI, 0.38–1.09, $P = 0.10$).[139]

The release of this group of trials further strengthens the role of anti-inflammatory therapies in secondary prevention of CVD and highlights colchicine as an inexpensive and potentially effective intervention.

Future Therapies Targeting Inflammatory Pathways for CVD

Multiple additional anti-inflammatory strategies are now being tested in preclinical settings and clinical trials (Fig. 14–4). Results from these trials will add invaluable information in piecing together the role and clinical benefit of targeting inflammation to treat and prevent ASCVD. Additional therapies may target IL-1Ra, the NLRP3 inflammasome, IL-6, CD40-CD40L, autonomic inflammatory reflexes, and the microbiome. By contrast, trials targeting TNF, adhesion molecules, leukotrienes, secretory phospholipases, and inflammation-associated antioxidants have not been effective.[140,141]

IL-1 Receptor Antagonists

In addition to direct IL-1 inhibition, there is also interest in leveraging IL-1Ra to modulate the inflammatory response (Fig. 14–4). Anakinra is a recombinant IL-1Ra that is approved for use in autoimmune diseases such as rheumatoid arthritis. The Virginia Commonwealth University Anakinra Remodeling Trials (VCUART) phase 2 clinical trial program included three studies in which patients with STEMI were given 14 days of anakinra. The primary outcome of the trials, the area under the curve (AUC) for hsCRP, was significantly reduced in treated patients compared to placebo controls.[142-144] In addition, incidence of heart failure and heart failure hospitalizations were also significantly reduced in the anakinra group.

NLRP3 Inflammasome Inhibition

Moving one step upstream of IL-1β inhibition, several efforts are underway to develop small-molecule inhibitors of the NLRP3 inflammasome.[145] In a mouse model, use of MCC950, a selective NLRP3 inhibitor, showed reduction in atherosclerotic lesion development, and reduced VCAM and ICAM mRNA expression.[146] Meanwhile, in pig experiments, MCC950 led to reduction in infarct size and preservation of myocardial function.[147] Another direct NLRP3 inhibitor, CY-09, showed improvements in metabolic parameters and hepatic steatosis in diabetic mice with treatment in an NLRP3 dependent manner.[148] These early studies provide optimism for the development of future direct NLRP3 modulators for human trials.

IL-6 Inhibition

Moving downstream from IL-1β inhibition in CANTOS, attention has also shifted to the possibility of IL-6 inhibition for ASCVD (Fig. 14–4). As seen in CANTOS, IL-6 was an important mediator of the protective effect of canakinumab, and therefore targeting IL-6 could be expected to yield salutary effects.[125] Two strategies for IL-6 specific therapies include blocking IL-6 binding to its receptor (as seen with the anti-IL-6-receptor humanized monoclonal antibody tocilizumab or anti-IL-6-receptor human monoclonal antibody sarilumab) or altering IL-6 receptor activity. A small randomized trial of tocilizumab in patients with non-STEMI showed reduced AUC for hsCRP and troponin in patients given tocilizumab, suggesting a smaller infarct size with therapy without an increase in adverse events.[149] This promising result is now being tested in a larger phase 2 trial (ASSAIL, ClinicalTrials.gov Identifier: NCT03004703) of patients arriving at three Norwegian hospitals with a STEMI.[150] One large-scale trial of ziltivekimab, a novel IL-6 inhibitor, will focus on patients with chronic kidney disease, a group with high residual inflammatory risk where lipid lowering is known to be less effective (ClinicalTrials.gov Identifier: NCT03926117).

CD40–CD40L Interactions

In looking at other inflammatory pathways relevant to atherothrombosis, the role of the costimulatory CD40–CD40L receptor–ligand signaling dyad appears to be prominent.[151] Inhibition of CD40 leads to a reduction in atherosclerosis in mice.[152] CD40–CD40L binding recruits TNF receptor-associated factor 6 (TRAF6), and inhibition of CD40-TRAF6 by small molecule inhibitors appears to reduce atherosclerosis and slow plaque progression in mice without adverse immune effects.[152–154] Development of novel therapies to target this interaction may help address the residual inflammatory risk in ASCVD.

Vagal Nerve Stimulation

Vagal nerve stimulation (VNS) is employed in several disorders including epilepsy, depression, and eating disorders to modulate the autonomic immune system. Data suggests that the vagus nerve mediates autonomic anti-inflammatory processes in a pathway known as the cholinergic anti-inflammatory pathway (CAP). While the mechanism of CAP is not completely delineated, it appears that inflammatory stimuli and tissue damage lead to afferent vagal signaling to the brain, and that efferent vagal signaling leads to adrenocorticotropic hormone production with resulting inhibition of cytokine production.[155] VNS has been shown to suppress inflammation in multiple ways, including lowering TNF synthesis, with vagotomy producing the opposite effect.[156,157] An interesting question is whether VNS can produce sustainable and substantial effects to leverage this relationship to translate into clinical benefit for ASCVD.

Microbiome Modulation

The role of the microbiome in human biology is the subject of much focus currently and may be implicated in the relationship between inflammation and CVD.[158] A low gene count of gut microbiota has been associated with elevated CRP levels, along with decreased presence of specific gut microbes associated with a similar response.[159] Modulation of PRRs by the gut microbiome and subsequent altered recognition of PAMPs leading to immune responses is also a putative pathway linking the effect of diet, inflammation, and atherogenesis. As a result, deeper mechanistic and epidemiologic studies examining these relationships are important, and may offer interventions to alter the immune and inflammatory response.

Combining Anti-Lipid and Anti-Inflammatory Therapy

Now recognized as a disease with important influences from both lipid disorder and inflammation, the use of combined therapies in preventing atherosclerosis and CVD is a new frontier. With recent groundbreaking advances in lipid lowering with the development of proprotein convertase subtilisin/kexin type 9 inhibitors (PCSK9i), the time is ripe for consideration of concurrent targeting of both cholesterol metabolism and immune responses. Trials with PCSK9i show that these novel agents do not have significant effects on hsCRP or other inflammatory markers, indicating that their primary mechanism of efficacy is through cholesterol metabolism. The magnitude of effect seen with intensive lipid lowering with PCSK9i is virtually identical to that seen with anti-inflammatory therapy in CANTOS.[160,161] Several lines of evidence lead to the conclusion that combination therapy with a PCSK9i and a targeted anti-inflammatory agent would yield at least additive effects. Extensive evidence with statins shows that there is no significant relationship between on-treatment hsCRP and on-treatment LDL, indicating the independence of these two pathways.[101] Furthermore, the beneficial effects of hsCRP reduction are apparent regardless of LDL level.[101,126] And finally, in both individual anti-lipid and anti-inflammatory trials, significant residual risk remains from the untreated parallel mechanism. That is, in patients with low LDL on PCSK9i therapy, significant residual risk was observed in those with elevated hsCRP; conversely, in CANTOS, those patients with low hsCRP but high LDL continued to have higher CVD residual risk.[162,163] A strategy targeting both lipid and inflammatory risk may yield dividends in reducing the CVD in high-risk patients, and may be most effectively tested using a thoughtful 2×2 factorial clinical trial design that would greatly move the field forward.

Leveraging Genetics in Anti-Inflammatory Therapy

Clonal Hematopoiesis of Indeterminate Potential

Clonal hematopoiesis of indeterminate potential (CHIP) may lead to novel approaches in anti-atherogenic therapy and interventions. CHIP is a primarily age-related phenomenon in which bone marrow stem cells acquire somatic mutations through human aging, with some mutations leading to expansion of monoclonal leukocyte populations detectable in peripheral blood.[164] This condition has been associated with MI, stroke, and ischemic heart failure, and has higher mortality compared to those without CHIP.[164,165] The two most common mutations in CHIP, *TET2 and DNMT3A*, encode enzymes that regulate DNA methylation, and thus mutations in these genes likely lead to epigenetic alterations in transcriptional activity.[166] Introduction of a *TET2* CHIP mutation in mice accelerates atherosclerosis development.[167] Interestingly, CHIP mutations are not strongly correlated with hsCRP, and leukocytes from mice with the CHIP *TET2* mutation show higher IL-1β and IL-6 levels.[141] These findings raise the question of the exact mechanism by which CHIP leads to exaggerated ASCVD, although the involvement of the immune system and inflammation is highly likely. In one example of how CHIP status and anti-inflammatory therapy could intersect, a specific CHIP mutation in Janus kinase 2 (JAK2) promotes thrombosis by promoting the formation of neutrophil extracellular traps by granulocytes, which leads to larger lipid cores in atheromas and induction of the NLRP3 inflammasome/IL-1β axis.[168] Given the availability of JAK2 inhibitors, identifying patients who harbor this mutation and have a resulting higher ASCVD risk could lead to targeted precision therapy to neutralize the inflammatory risk for ASCVD.[141]

Gene Editing Using CRISPR/Cas9 Techniques

The advent of clustered, regularly interspaced, short palindromic repeat (CRISPR) and CRISPR-associated protein 9 (Cas9) technology also holds promise in modulating inflammatory pathways.[169] CRISPR/Cas9 techniques allow for targeted genetic alterations that can alter the expression and activity of various proteins, including those involved in inflammatory pathways. Already, experiments show effective targeting of genes to disrupt NLRP3 in mouse macrophages, with inhibition of NLRP3 activation both in vitro and in vivo associated with a reduction in lipopolysaccharide-induced septic shock in mice. Interestingly, this reduction in NLRP3 activity also improved glucose tolerance and insulin sensitivity in diabetic mice models. Furthermore, IL-1β, IL-18, TNF-α, and MCP-1 levels were reduced in mice who underwent this treatment. With this technique in hand, future treatment strategies could identify patients at high inflammatory residual risk, and then delivery gene-specific therapy to ameliorate the drivers of this risk.

SOCIAL, BEHAVIORAL, AND PREVENTIVE MEASURES TO REDUCE INFLAMMATORY RISK FOR ATHEROSCLEROSIS

The pharmacologic interventions described have proven that inflammation inhibition can lower vascular event rates. Yet, multiple environmental, social, and behavioral interventions also have anti-inflammatory effects. Key risk factors that may play a role in inflammatory risk for atherogenesis include exposure to air pollution, and the role of nutrition and the obesity epidemic.

Pollution

Epidemiological and environmental studies have established environmental pollution as the most significant cause of premature and reversible morbidity and mortality globally. With continuing climate change, deforestation, and rapid industrialization leading to acceleration in pollution, it is necessary to address its public health effects. The 2015 Global Burden of Disease study estimated that approximately 9 million deaths annually were directly due to environmental pollution, of which

7 million were due to air pollution.[170] Fine particles defined as those <2.5 μm ($PM_{2.5}$) are thought to be the air pollutant with the greatest threat to the global population. Per the World Health Organization, more than 90% of the world's population is exposed to air quality levels that are below acceptable global standards.[171] Multiple studies have shown that even short-term exposure to $PM_{2.5}$ resulted in significant increases in risk of ACS and CV mortality.[172] In addition, survival post-ACS was reduced with long-term $PM_{2.5}$ exposure.[173] A meta-analysis of 59 studies examining the association of air pollution to CV mortality showed an absolute 0.63% increase in CV mortality for every 10 mg/m³ increase in $PM_{2.5}$ across a wide range of concentrations.[174] Furthermore, other studies indicate that this risk may not be linear, and further exaggerated at higher levels of exposure.

Mechanisms for the elevated risk of CVD in the setting of air pollution remain to be clearly delineated, but several possibilities include (1) endothelial barrier dysfunction/disruption; (2) inflammation, involving both innate and adaptive immune components; (3) prothrombotic pathways; (4) autonomic imbalance favoring sympathetic tone via afferent pathways; (5) central nervous system effects on metabolism and hypothalamic-pituitary adrenal axis activation; and (6) epigenomic changes, with interactions between these pathways.[175] Particulate matter inhaled and ingested in the body can activate the immune system through various receptors including PAMPs and DAMPs to trigger the immune cascade resulting in cytokine production and activation of immune cells.[176] NLRP3 inflammasome activation by various environmental pollutants including $PM_{2.5}$ has also been shown in mice, perhaps pointing to an important mechanism linking pollution to CVD.[177] Pollutant facilitated oxidation of cholesterol and other products in the body that translocate within LDL and lead to atherosclerosis is another pathway of inflammatory atherogenesis in relationship to pollution.[178] Long-term exposure to $PM_{2.5}$ has been shown to increase efflux of Mon1 monocytes from the bone marrow to vascular cells, increasing inflammatory burden in these sites.[179] Environmental exposure to fine particulate matter may also lead to epigenetic and genetic changes that could potentiate the effect of CHIP in exposed populations and lead to increased CV burden.

Nutrition and Obesity

Whereas malnourishment and starvation were previously the most prevalent nutritional disorders globally, the disease burden has now shifted toward obesity and weight excess. There are myriad causes of obesity including easier access to high-fat, high-carbohydrate, processed foods, and reduction in physical activity on a regular basis. The increase in adiposity, a central feature of obesity, has important immunomodulatory effects that may link it to CVD and atherogenesis.[180] Adipose tissue is responsive to several cytokines, and switches to a proinflammatory phenotype with exposure to IL-1β and IL-6, leading to production of further inflammatory cytokines and modulators.[181] Adipokines elaborated from adipose tissue may also impact inflammation and CVD risk. Levels of leptin have been correlated with increased CVD, although these results are not consistent across studies.[182] Adiponectin is another adipokine that has been shown to have mixed associations with CVD, with some studies showing a protective effect while others showing a pathogenic effect in CVD.[183,184] Resistin is an adipokine that may have proinflammatory and proatherogenic effects, and is related to adiposity.[185] Furthermore, resident macrophages in adipose tissue also directly modulate inflammation.[186] Production of free fatty acids in adipose tissue lead to activation of TLRs, with subsequent cytokine production including TNF-α.[187] Directly connecting obesity to inflammation, subjects with elevated levels of total and visceral obesity have the highest CRP levels and are associated with the greatest prevalence of metabolic syndrome for any given body mass index.[188] Furthermore, the increased incidence of diabetes in obese individuals and its resulting cardiometabolic effects plays an important role connecting obesity to ASCVD.

Given the ever-increasing burden of obesity and adiposity in the global population, the inflammatory, metabolic, and proatherogenic effects of obesity will become a bigger contributor to the burden of ASCVD. Targeted interventions at all levels, from the personal to community to national to global strategies are of utmost importance in reducing this epidemic. Availability of nutritious and well-balanced food, particularly in the most vulnerable populations that are exposed to food deserts and only have suboptimal quality nutrition available, is a key intervention that must be stressed. In addition, campaigns and systems encouraging physical activity starting in youth and continuing in the elderly population would also reduce the burden of this disease and induce the positive effects known to associate with physical activity.

SUMMARY

The modern era in understanding the pathobiology of atherosclerosis has led to a novel paradigm that encapsulates two parallel risk pathways: lipid-related risk and inflammation-related risk. While traditional therapies have targeted lipid lowering with resulting improvement in the burden of ASCVD, there continues to be a prominent residual inflammatory risk as a driver of disease. Recent clinical trials have shown efficacy in secondary prevention using targeted anti-inflammatory therapy, opening a new chapter in cardioprotective therapy. In addition, understanding unique drivers and contributors to the inflammatory risk will provide new targets for intervention with the ultimate goal of further reducing the burden of CVD globally.

REFERENCES

1. Goldstein JL, Brown MS. A century of cholesterol and coronaries: from plaques to genes to statins. *Cell*. 2015;161:161-172.
2. Ross R, Glomset JA. The pathogenesis of atherosclerosis. *N Engl J Med*. 1976;295:369-377.
3. Jonasson L, Holm J, Skalli O, Bondjers G, Hansson GK. Regional accumulations of T cells macrophages and smooth muscle cells in the human atherosclerotic plaque. *Arteriosclerosis*. 1986;6:131-138.
4. Libby P, Ridker PM, Hansson GK. Inflammation in atherosclerosis. *J Am Coll Cardiol*. 2009;54:2129-2138.
5. Libby P, Nahrendorf M, Swirski FK. Leukocytes link local and systemic inflammation in ischemic cardiovascular disease. *J Am Coll Cardiol*. 2016;67:1091-1103.
6. Miyamoto T, et al. Expression of stem cell factor in human aortic endothelial and smooth muscle cells. *Atherosclerosis*. 1997;129:207-213.
7. Galli SJ, et al. Mast cells as "tunable" effector and immunoregulatory cells: recent advances. *Annu Rev Immunol*. 2005;23:749-786.
8. Lindstedt KA, Kokkonen JO, Kovanen PT. Soluble heparin proteoglycans released from stimulated mast cells induce uptake of low density lipoproteins by macrophages via scavenger receptor-mediated phagocytosis. *J Lipid Res*. 1992;33:65-75.
9. Kovanen PT. Mast cells: multipotent local effector cells in atherothrombosis. *Immunol Rev*. 2007;217:105-122.
10. Kaartinen M, Penttilä A, Kovanen PT. Accumulation of activated mast cells in the shoulder region of human coronary atheroma the predilection site of atheromatous rupture. *Circulation*. 1994;90:1669-1678.
11. Saarinen J, Kalkkinen N, Welgus HG, Kovanen PT. Activation of human interstitial procollagenase through direct cleavage of the Leu83-Thr84 bond by mast cell chymase. *J Biol Chem*. 1994;269:18134-18140.
12. Gawaz M, Langer H, May AE. Platelets in inflammation and atherogenesis. *J Clin Invest*. 2005;115:3378-3384.
13. Frenette PS, et al. P-Selectin glycoprotein ligand 1 (PSGL-1) is expressed on platelets and can mediate platelet-endothelial interactions in vivo. *J Exp Med*. 2000;191:1413-1422.
14. Hansson GK, Libby P. The immune response in atherosclerosis: a double-edged sword. *Nat Rev Immunol*. 2006;6:508-519.
15. Saigusa R, Winkels H, Ley K. T cell subsets and functions in atherosclerosis. *Nat Rev Cardiol*. 2020;17:387-401.
16. Frostegård J, et al. Cytokine expression in advanced human atherosclerotic plaques: dominance of pro-inflammatory (Th1) and macrophage-stimulating cytokines. *Atherosclerosis*. 1999;145:33-43.
17. Engelbertsen D, et al. T-Helper 2 Immunity is associated with reduced risk of myocardial infarction and stroke. *Arterioscler Thromb Vasc Biol*. 2013;33:637-644.
18. Davenport P, Tipping PG. The role of interleukin-4 and interleukin-12 in the progression of atherosclerosis in apolipoprotein E-deficient mice. *Am J Pathol*. 2003;163:1117-1125.
19. McGeachy MJ, Cua DJ, Gaffen SL. The IL-17 family of cytokines in health and disease. *Immunity*. 2019;50:892-906.
20. Ait-Oufella H, et al. Natural regulatory T cells control the development of atherosclerosis in mice. *Nat Med*. 2006;12:178-180.
21. George J, et al. Regulatory T cells and IL-10 levels are reduced in patients with vulnerable coronary plaques. *Atherosclerosis*. 2012;222:519-523.
22. Foks AC, Lichtman AH, Kuiper J. Treating atherosclerosis with regulatory T cells. *Arterioscler Thromb Vasc Biol*. 2015;35:280-287.
23. Hwang Y, et al. Expansion of CD8+ T cells lacking the IL-6 receptor α chain in patients with coronary artery diseases (CAD). *Atherosclerosis*. 2016;249:44-51.
24. Fernandez DM, et al. Single-cell immune landscape of human atherosclerotic plaques. *Nat Med*. 2019;25:1576-1588.
25. Kyaw T, et al. Cytotoxic and proinflammatory CD8+ T lymphocytes promote development of vulnerable atherosclerotic plaques in apoE-deficient mice. *Circulation*. 2013;127:1028-1039.
26. van Duijn J, et al. CD8+ T-cells contribute to lesion stabilization in advanced atherosclerosis by limiting macrophage content and CD4+ T-cell responses. *Cardiovasc Res*. 2019;115:729-738.
27. Tsiantoulas D, Diehl CJ, Witztum JL, Binder CJ. B Cells and humoral immunity in atherosclerosis. *Circ Res*. 2014;114:1743-1756.
28. Huan T, et al. a systems biology framework identifies molecular underpinnings of coronary heart disease. *Arterioscler Thromb Vasc Biol*. 2013;33:1427-1434.
29. Caligiuri G, Nicoletti A, Poirier B, Hansson GK. Protective immunity against atherosclerosis carried by B cells of hypercholesterolemic mice. *J Clin Invest*. 2002;109:745-753.

30. Kyaw T, et al. Conventional B2 B Cell depletion ameliorates whereas its adoptive transfer aggravates atherosclerosis. *J Immunniol.* 2010;185:4410-4419.

31. Ait-Oufella H, et al. B cell depletion reduces the development of atherosclerosis in mice. *J Experiment Med.* 2010;207:1579-1587.

32. Kyaw T, et al. Depletion of B2 but not B1a B Cells in BAFF receptor-deficient apoE$^{-/-}$ mice attenuates atherosclerosis by potently ameliorating arterial inflammation. *PLoS ONE.* 2012;7:e29371.

33. Virchow R. *Gesammelte Abhandlungen zur Wissenschaftlichen Medicin.* Meidinger Sohn Corp; 1856.

34. Anitschkoff N. Über Veränderungen der Kaninchen-Aorta bei experimentelle Cholesterolinsteatose. *Beitr Path Anat.* 1913;379-391.

35. Hansson GK. Inflammation atherosclerosis and coronary artery disease. *N Engl J Med.* 2005;11.

36. Libby P, Ridker PM, Hansson GK. Progress and challenges in translating the biology of atherosclerosis. *Nature.* 2011;473:317-325.

37. Gisterå A, Hansson GK. The immunology of atherosclerosis. *Nat Rev Nephrol.* 2017;13:368-380.

38. Libby P, Ridker PM, Maseri A. Inflammation and atherosclerosis. *Circulation.* 2002;105:1135-1143.

39. Collins T, Cybulsky MI. NF-κB: pivotal mediator or innocent bystander in atherogenesis? *J Clin Invest.* 2001;107:255-264.

40. Nakashima Y, Raines EW, Plump AS, Breslow JL, Ross R. Upregulation of VCAM-1 and ICAM-1 at Atherosclerosis-prone sites on the endothelium in the apoE-deficient mouse. *Arterioscler Thromb Vasc Biol.* 1998;18:842-851.

41. Dong ZM, et al. The combined role of P- and E-selectins in atherosclerosis. *J Clin Invest.* 1998;102:145-152.

42. Lipton BA, et al. Components of the protein fraction of oxidized low density lipoprotein stimulate interleukin-1 alpha production by rabbit arterial macrophage-derived foam cells. *J Lipid Res.* 1995;36:2232-2242.

43. Libby P, et al. Endotoxin and tumor necrosis factor induce interleukin-1 gene expression in adult human vascular endothelial cells. *Am J Pathol.* 1986;124:179-185.

44. Dwivedi A, Änggård EE, Carrier MJ. Oxidized LDL-mediated monocyte adhesion to endothelial cells does not involve NFκB. *Biochem Biophys Res Comm.* 2001;284:239-244.

45. Boring L, Gosling J, Cleary M, Charo IF. Decreased lesion formation in CCR2$^{-/-}$ mice reveals a role for chemokines in the initiation of atherosclerosis. *Nature.* 1998;394:894-897.

46. Miller YI, et al. Minimally modified LDL binds to CD14 induces macrophage spreading via TLR4/MD-2 and inhibits phagocytosis of apoptotic cells. *J Biol Chem.* 2003;278:1561-1568.

47. West XZ, et al. Oxidative stress induces angiogenesis by activating TLR2 with novel endogenous ligands. *Nature.* 2010;467:972-976.

48. Quinn MT, Parthasarathy S, Fong LG, Steinberg D. Oxidatively modified low density lipoproteins: a potential role in recruitment and retention of monocyte/macrophages during atherogenesis. *Proc Nat Acad Sci.* 1987;84:2995-2998.

49. Kunjathoor VV, et al. Scavenger receptors Class A-I/II and CD36 are the principal receptors responsible for the uptake of modified low density lipoprotein leading to lipid loading in macrophages. *J Biol Chem.* 2002;277:49982-49988.

50. Srikakulapu P, et al. Artery tertiary lymphoid organs control multilayered territorialized atherosclerosis B-cell responses in aged apoE$^{-/-}$ mice. *Arterioscler Thromb Vasc Biol.* 2016;36:1174-1185.

51. Chou MY, et al. Oxidation-specific epitopes are dominant targets of innate natural antibodies in mice and humans. *J Clin Invest.* 2009;119:1335-1349.

52. Rhoads JP, et al. Oxidized low-density lipoprotein immune complex priming of the Nlrp3 inflammasome involves TLR and FcγR cooperation and is dependent on CARD9. *J Immuniol.* 2017;198:2105-2114.

53. Sage AP, Tsiantoulas D, Binder CJ, Mallat Z. The role of B cells in atherosclerosis. *Nat Rev Cardiol.* 2019;16:180-196.

54. Duewell P, et al. NLRP3 inflammasomes are required for atherogenesis and activated by cholesterol crystals. *Nature.* 2010;464:1357-1361.

55. Strowig T, Henao-Mejia J, Elinav E, Flavell R. Inflammasomes in health and disease. *Nature.* 2012;481:278-286.

56. Dewberry R, Holden H, Crossman D, Francis S. Interleukin-1 receptor antagonist expression in human endothelial cells and atherosclerosis. *Arterioscler Thromb Vasc Biol.* 2000;20:2394-2400.

57. Galea J, et al. Interleukin-1 beta in coronary arteries of patients with ischemic heart disease. *Arterioscler Thromb Vasc Biol.* 1996;16:1000-1006.

58. Wang X, Feuerstein GZ, Gu JL, Lysko PG, Yue TL. Interleukin-1 beta induces expression of adhesion molecules in human vascular smooth muscle cells and enhances adhesion of leukocytes to smooth muscle cells. *Atherosclerosis.* 1995;115:89-98.

59. Ridker PM. From C-reactive protein to interleukin-6 to interleukin-1: moving upstream to identify novel targets for atheroprotection. *Circulation Res.* 2016;118:145-156.

60. Sukhova GK, et al. Evidence for increased collagenolysis by interstitial collagenases-1 and -3 in vulnerable human atheromatous plaques. *Circulation.* 1999;99:2503-2509.

61. Kubo T, et al. Assessment of culprit lesion morphology in acute myocardial infarction: ability of optical coherence tomography compared with intravascular ultrasound and coronary angioscopy. *J Am Coll Cardiol.* 2007;50:933-939.

62. Crea F, Libby P. Acute coronary syndromes: the way forward from mechanisms to precision treatment. *Circulation.* 2017;136:1155-1166.

63. Finn AV, Nakano M, Narula J, Kolodgie FD, Virmani R. Concept of vulnerable/unstable plaque. *Arterioscler Thromb Vasc Biol.* 2010;30:1282-1292.

64. Stone PH, et al. Role of Low endothelial shear stress and plaque characteristics in the prediction of nonculprit major adverse cardiac events: the PROSPECT study. *JACC Cardiovasc Imaging.* 2018;11:462-471.

65. Ridker PM. Morrow DAC-reactive protein inflammation and coronary risk. *Cardiol Clin.* 2003;21:315-325.

66. Vasan RS. Biomarkers of cardiovascular disease: molecular basis and practical considerations. *Circulation.* 2006;113:2335-2362.

67. Brennan M.-L, et al. Prognostic value of myeloperoxidase in patients with chest pain. *N Engl J Med.* 2003;349:1595-1604.

68. de Lemos JA, Hennekens CH, Ridker PM. Plasma concentration of soluble vascular cell adhesion molecule-1 and subsequent cardiovascular risk. *J Am Coll Cardiol.* 2000;36:423-426.

69. Scialla JJ, et al. Soluble P-selectin levels are associated with cardiovascular mortality and sudden cardiac death in male dialysis patients. *Am J Nephrol.* 2011;33:224-230.

70. Rosenson RS, Hurt-Camejo E. Phospholipase A2 enzymes and the risk of atherosclerosis. *Eur Heart J.* 2012;33:2899-2909.

71. IL6R Genetics Consortium, Emerging Risk Factors Collaboration, et al. Interleukin-6 receptor pathways in coronary heart disease: a collaborative meta-analysis of 82 studies. *Lancet.* 2012;379:1205-1213.

72. Ridker PM, Rifai N, Stampfer MJ, Hennekens CH. Plasma concentration of interleukin-6 and the risk of future myocardial infarction among apparently healthy men. *Circulation.* 2000;101:1767-1772.

73. Silvain J, et al. Interleukin-1. Beta and risk of premature death in patients with myocardial infarction. *J Am Coll Cardiol.* 2020;S0735109720363233. doi:10.1016/j.jacc.2020.08.026.

74. Hlatky MA, et al. Matrix metalloproteinase circulating levels genetic polymorphisms and susceptibility to acute myocardial infarction among patients with coronary artery disease. *Am Heart J.* 2007;154:1043-1051.

75. Ridker PM, Hennekens CH. Inflammation aspirin and the risk of cardiovascular disease in apparently healthy men. *N Engl J Med.* 1997;7.

76. Ridker PM, Glynn RJ, Hennekens CH. C-reactive protein adds to the predictive value of total and HDL cholesterol in determining risk of first myocardial infarction. *Circulation.* 1998;97:2007-2011.

77. Ridker PM. C-reactive protein and other markers of inflammation in the prediction of cardiovascular disease in women. *N Engl J Med.* 2000;8.

78. Ridker PM. C-reactive protein: eighty years from discovery to emergence as a major risk marker for cardiovascular disease. *Clin Chem.* 2009;55:209-215.

79. Macleod CM, Avery OT. The occurrence during acute infections of a protein not normally present in the blood: isolation and properties of the reactive protein. *J Exp Med.* 1941;73:183-190.

80. Boncler M, Wu Y, Watala C. The multiple faces of c-reactive protein-physiological and pathophysiological implications in cardiovascular disease. *Molecules.* 2019;24.

81. Hutchinson WL, Noble GE, Hawkins PN, Pepys MB. The pentraxins C-reactive protein and serum amyloid P component are cleared and catabolized by hepatocytes in vivo. *J Clin Invest.* 1994;94:1390-1396.

82. Tang Y, Fung E, Xu A, Lan H-Y. C-reactive protein and ageing. *Clin Exp Pharmacol Physiol.* 2017;44 Suppl 1:9-14.

83. Pepys MB, Rowe IF, Baltz ML. C-reactive protein: binding to lipids and lipoproteins. *Int Rev Exp Pathol.* 1985;27:83-111.

84. Lu J, Mold C, Du Clos TW, Sun PD. Pentraxins and Fc receptor-mediated immune responses. *Front Immunol.* 2018;9:2607.

85. Sproston NR, Ashworth JJ. Role of C-reactive protein at sites of inflammation and infection. *Front Immunol.* 2018;9:754.

86. Heuertz RM, Ahmed N, Webster RO. Peptides derived from C-reactive protein inhibit neutrophil alveolitis. *J Immunol.* 1996;156:3412-3417.

87. Pasceri V, Cheng JS, Willerson JT, Yeh ET, Chang J. Modulation of C-reactive protein-mediated monocyte chemoattractant protein-1 induction in human endothelial cells by anti-atherosclerosis drugs. *Circulation.* 2001;103:2531-2534.

88. Zwaka TP, Hombach V, Torzewski J. C-reactive protein-mediated low density lipoprotein uptake by macrophages: implications for atherosclerosis. *Circulation.* 2001;103:1194-1197.

89. Venugopal SK, Devaraj S, Yuhanna I, Shaul P, Jialal I. Demonstration that C-reactive protein decreases eNOS expression and bioactivity in human aortic endothelial cells. *Circulation.* 2002;106:1439-1441.

90. Nabata A, et al. C-reactive protein induces endothelial cell apoptosis and matrix metalloproteinase-9 production in human mononuclear cells: Implications for the destabilization of atherosclerotic plaque. *Atherosclerosis.* 2008;196:129-135.

91. Haverkate F, Thompson SG, Pyke SD, Gallimore JR, Pepys MB. Production of C-reactive protein and risk of coronary events in stable and unstable angina. European Concerted Action on Thrombosis and Disabilities Angina Pectoris Study Group. *Lancet.* 1997;349:462-466.

92. Kuller LH, Tracy RP, Shaten J, Meilahn EN. Relation of C-reactive protein and coronary heart disease in the MRFIT nested case-control study. Multiple Risk Factor Intervention Trial. *Am J Epidemiol.* 1996;144:537-547.

93. Albert CM, Ma J, Rifai N, Stampfer MJ, Ridker PM. Prospective study of C-reactive protein homocysteine and plasma lipid levels as predictors of sudden cardiac death. *Circulation.* 2002;105:2595-2599.

94. Emerging Risk Factors Collaboration, et al. C-reactive protein concentration and risk of coronary heart disease stroke and mortality: an individual participant meta-analysis. *Lancet.* 2010;375:132-140.

95. Ridker PM, Buring JE, Rifai N, Cook NR. Development and validation of improved algorithms for the assessment of global cardiovascular risk in women: the Reynolds Risk Score. *JAMA.* 2007;297:611-619.

96. Ridker PM, Paynter NP, Rifai N, Gaziano JM, Cook NR. C-reactive protein and parental history improve global cardiovascular risk prediction: the Reynolds Risk Score for men. *Circulation.* 2008;118:2243-2251.

97. Wilson PWF, et al. C-reactive protein and reclassification of cardiovascular risk in the Framingham Heart Study. *Circ Cardiovasc Qual Outcomes.* 2008;1:92-97.

98. Ridker PM, Rifai N, Pfeffer MA, Sacks F, Braunwald E. Long-term effects of pravastatin on plasma concentration of C-reactive protein. The Cholesterol and Recurrent Events (CARE) Investigators. *Circulation.* 1999;100:230-235.

99. Ridker PM, et al. Measurement of C-reactive protein for the targeting of statin therapy in the primary prevention of acute coronary events. *N Engl J Med.* 2001;344:1959-1965.

100. Ridker PM, et al. Rosuvastatin to prevent vascular events in men and women with elevated C-reactive protein. *N Engl J Med.* 2008;359:2195-2207.

101. Ridker PM, et al. C-reactive protein levels and outcomes after statin therapy. *N Engl J Med.* 2005;352:20-28.

102. Morrow DA, et al. Clinical relevance of C-reactive protein during follow-up of patients with acute coronary syndromes in the Aggrastat-to-Zocor Trial. *Circulation.* 2006;114:281-288.

103. Nissen SE, et al. Statin therapy LDL cholesterol C-reactive protein and coronary artery disease. *N Engl J Med.* 2005;352:29-38.

104. C Reactive Protein Coronary Heart Disease Genetics Collaboration (CCGC), et al. Association between C reactive protein and coronary heart disease: mendelian randomisation analysis based on individual participant data. *BMJ.* 2011;342:d548.

105. Kaptoge S, et al. Inflammatory cytokines and risk of coronary heart disease: new prospective study and updated meta-analysis. *Eur Heart J.* 2014;35:578-589.

106. Esteve E, et al. Serum interleukin-6 correlates with endothelial dysfunction in healthy men independently of insulin sensitivity. *Diabetes Care.* 2007;30:939-945.

107. Mahmud A, Feely J. Arterial stiffness is related to systemic inflammation in essential hypertension. *Hypertension.* 2005;46:1118-1122.

108. Schieffer B, et al. Impact of interleukin-6 on plaque development and morphology in experimental atherosclerosis. *Circulation.* 2004;110:3493-3500.

109. Guo F, et al. Association between local interleukin-6 levels and slow flow/microvascular dysfunction. *J Thromb Thrombolysis.* 2014;37:475-482.

110. Cai T, et al. Association of Interleukin 6 receptor variant with cardiovascular disease effects of interleukin 6 receptor blocking therapy: a phenome-wide association study. *JAMA Cardiol.* 2018;3:849-857.

111. Maier W, et al. Inflammatory markers at the site of ruptured plaque in acute myocardial infarction: locally increased interleukin-6 and serum amyloid A but decreased C-reactive protein. *Circulation.* 2005;111:1355-1361.

112. Interleukin-6 Receptor Mendelian Randomisation Analysis (IL6R MR) Consortium, et al. The interleukin-6 receptor as a target for prevention of coronary heart disease: a mendelian randomisation analysis. *Lancet.* 2012;379:1214-1224.

113. Van Tassell BW, Toldo S, Mezzaroma E, Abbate A. Targeting interleukin-1 in heart disease. *Circulation.* 2013;128:1910-1923.

114. Agostini L, et al. NALP3 forms an IL-1beta-processing inflammasome with increased activity in Muckle-Wells autoinflammatory disorder. *Immunity.* 2004;20:319-325.

115. Dinarello CA, Simon A, van der Meer JWM. Treating inflammation by blocking interleukin-1 in a broad spectrum of diseases. *Nat Rev Drug Discov.* 2012;11:633-652.

116. Bevilacqua MP, Pober JS, Wheeler ME, Cotran RS, Gimbrone MA. Interleukin 1 acts on cultured human vascular endothelium to increase the adhesion of polymorphonuclear leukocytes monocytes and related leukocyte cell lines. *J Clin Invest.* 1985;76:2003-2011.

117. Libby P, Warner SJ, Friedman GB. Interleukin 1: a mitogen for human vascular smooth muscle cells that induces the release of growth-inhibitory prostanoids. *J Clin Invest.* 1988;81:487-498.

118. Kirii H, et al. Lack of interleukin-1β decreases the severity of atherosclerosis in apoE-deficient mice. *ATVB.* 2003;23:656-660.

119. Isoda K, et al. Lack of interleukin-1 receptor antagonist modulates plaque composition in apolipoprotein E-deficient mice. *Arterioscler Thromb Vasc Biol.* 2004;24:1068-1073.

120. Merhi-Soussi F, et al. Interleukin-1 plays a major role in vascular inflammation and atherosclerosis in male apolipoprotein E-knockout mice. *Cardiovasc Res.* 2005;66:583-593.

121. Kastrati A, et al. Protective role against restenosis from an interleukin-1 receptor antagonist gene polymorphism in patients treated with coronary stenting. *J Am Coll Cardiol.* 2000;36:2168-2173.

122. Ridker PM, et al. Effects of interleukin-1β inhibition with canakinumab on hemoglobin A1c lipids C-reactive protein interleukin-6 and

fibrinogen: a phase IIb randomized placebo-controlled trial. *Circulation.* 2012;126:2739-2748.

123. Ridker PM, Thuren T, Zalewski A, Libby P. Interleukin-1β inhibition and the prevention of recurrent cardiovascular events: rationale and design of the Canakinumab Anti-inflammatory Thrombosis Outcomes Study (CANTOS). *Am Heart J.* 2011;162:597-605.

124. Ridker PM, et al. Antiinflammatory Therapy with Canakinumab for Atherosclerotic Disease. *N Engl J Med.* 2017;377:1119-1131.

125. Ridker PM, et al. Modulation of the interleukin-6 signalling pathway and incidence rates of atherosclerotic events and all-cause mortality: analyses from the Canakinumab Anti-Inflammatory Thrombosis Outcomes Study (CANTOS). *Eur Heart J.* 2018;39:3499-3507.

126. Ridker PM, et al. Relationship of C-reactive protein reduction to cardiovascular event reduction following treatment with canakinumab: a secondary analysis from the CANTOS randomised controlled trial. *Lancet.* 2018;391:319-328.

127. Ridker PM, et al. Effect of interleukin-1β inhibition with canakinumab on incident lung cancer in patients with atherosclerosis: exploratory results from a randomised double-blind placebo-controlled trial. *Lancet.* 2017;390:1833-1842.

128. Schieker M, et al. Effects of interleukin-1β inhibition on incident hip and knee replacement: exploratory analyses from a randomized double-blind placebo-controlled trial. *Ann Intern Med.* 2020;173:509-515.

129. Solomon DH, et al. Relationship of interleukin-1β blockade with incident gout and serum uric acid levels: exploratory analysis of a randomized controlled trial. *Ann Intern Med.* 2018;169:535.

130. Vallurupalli M, et al. Effects of interleukin-1β inhibition on incident anemia: exploratory analyses from a randomized trial. *Ann Intern Med.* 2020;172:523.

131. Micha R, et al. Systematic review and meta-analysis of methotrexate use and risk of cardiovascular disease. *Am J Cardiol.* 2011;108:1362-1370.

132. Ridker PM, et al. Low-dose methotrexate for the prevention of atherosclerotic events. *N Engl J Med.* 2019;380:752-762.

133. O'Donoghue ML, et al. Effect of darapladib on major coronary events after an acute coronary syndrome: the SOLID-TIMI 52 randomized clinical trial. *JAMA.* 2014;312:1006-1015.

134. O'Donoghue ML, et al. Effect of losmapimod on cardiovascular outcomes in patients hospitalized with acute myocardial infarction: a randomized clinical trial. *JAMA.* 2016;315:1591-1599.

135. Leung YY, Hui LLY, Kraus VB. Colchicine—update on mechanisms of action and therapeutic uses. *Semin Arthritis Rheum.* 2015;45:341-350.

136. Nidorf SM, Eikelboom JW, Budgeon CA, Thompson PL. Low-dose colchicine for secondary prevention of cardiovascular disease. *J Am Coll Cardiol.* 2013;61:404-410.

137. Tardif J.-C, et al. Efficacy and safety of low-dose colchicine after myocardial infarction. *N Engl J Med.* 2019;381:2497-2505.

138. Nidorf SM, et al. Colchicine in patients with chronic coronary disease. *N Engl J Med.* 2020. doi:10.1056/NEJMoa2021372

139. Tong DC, et al. Colchicine in patients with acute coronary syndrome: the Australian COPS randomized clinical trial. *Circulation.* 2020. doi:10.1161/CIRCULATIONAHA.120.050771

140. Ridker PM. Anticytokine agents: targeting interleukin signaling pathways for the treatment of atherothrombosis. *Circ Re.* 2019;124:437-450.

141. Libby P, Everett BM. Novel antiatherosclerotic therapies. *ATVB.* 2019;39:538-545.

142. Abbate A, et al. Interleukin-1 blockade with anakinra to prevent adverse cardiac remodeling after acute myocardial infarction (Virginia Commonwealth University Anakinra Remodeling Trial [VCU-ART] Pilot study). *Am J Cardiol.* 2010;105:1371-1377.e1.

143. Abbate A, et al. Interleukin-1 blockade inhibits the acute inflammatory response in patients with ST-segment–elevation myocardial infarction. *JAHA.* 2020;9.

144. Abbate A, et al. Effects of interleukin-1 blockade with anakinra on adverse cardiac remodeling and heart failure after acute myocardial infarction

[from the Virginia Commonwealth University-Anakinra Remodeling Trial (2) (VCU-ART2) pilot study]. *Am J Cardiol.* 2013;111:1394-1400.

145. Mangan MSJ, et al. Targeting the NLRP3 inflammasome in inflammatory diseases. *Nat Rev Drug Discov.* 2018;17:688.

146. van der Heijden T, et al. NLRP3 inflammasome inhibition by MCC950 reduces atherosclerotic lesion development in apolipoprotein E-deficient mice-brief report. *Arterioscler Thromb Vasc Biol.* 2017;37:1457-1461.

147. van Hout GPJ, et al. The selective NLRP3-inflammasome inhibitor MCC950 reduces infarct size and preserves cardiac function in a pig model of myocardial infarction. *Eur Heart J.* 2017;38:828-836.

148. Jiang H, et al. Identification of a selective and direct NLRP3 inhibitor to treat inflammatory disorders. *J Exp Med.* 2017;214:3219-3238.

149. Kleveland O, et al. Effect of a single dose of the interleukin-6 receptor antagonist tocilizumab on inflammation and troponin T release in patients with non-ST-elevation myocardial infarction: a double-blind randomized placebo-controlled phase 2 trial. *Eur Heart J.* 2016;37:2406-2413.

150. Anstensrud AK, et al. Rationale for the ASSAIL-MI-trial: a randomised controlled trial designed to assess the effect of tocilizumab on myocardial salvage in patients with acute ST-elevation myocardial infarction (STEMI). *Open Heart.* 2019;6:e001108.

151. Bosmans LA, Bosch L, Kusters PJH, Lutgens E, Seijkens TTP. The CD40-CD40L dyad as immunotherapeutic target in cardiovascular disease. *J Cardiovasc Transl Res.* 2020. doi:10.1007/s12265-020-09994-3.

152. Mach F, Schönbeck U, Sukhova GK, Atkinson E, Libby P. Reduction of atherosclerosis in mice by inhibition of CD40 signalling. *Nature.* 1998;394:200-203.

153. Lutgens E, et al. Deficient CD40-TRAF6 signaling in leukocytes prevents atherosclerosis by skewing the immune response toward an antiinflammatory profile. *J Exp Med.* 2010;207:391-404.

154. Seijkens TTP, et al. Targeting CD40-induced TRAF6 signaling in macrophages reduces atherosclerosis. *J Am Coll Cardiol.* 2018;71:527-542.

155. Pavlov VA, Tracey KJ. Neural regulation of immunity: molecular mechanisms and clinical translation. *Nat Neurosci.* 2017;20:156-166.

156. Tracey KJ. The inflammatory reflex. *Nature.* 2002;420:853-859.

157. Borovikova LV, et al. Vagus nerve stimulation attenuates the systemic inflammatory response to endotoxin. *Nature.* 2000;405:458-462.

158. van den Munckhof ICL, et al. Role of gut microbiota in chronic low-grade inflammation as potential driver for atherosclerotic cardiovascular disease: a systematic review of human studies. *Obes Rev.* 2018;19:1719-1734.

159. Le Chatelier E, et al. Richness of human gut microbiome correlates with metabolic markers. *Nature.* 2013;500:541-546.

160. Sabatine MS, et al. Evolocumab and clinical outcomes in patients with cardiovascular disease. *N Engl J Med.* 2017;376:1713-1722.

161. Ridker PM, et al. Cardiovascular efficacy and safety of bococizumab in high-risk patients. *N Engl J Med.* 2017;376:1527-1539.

162. Bohula EA, et al. Inflammatory and cholesterol risk in the FOURIER trial. *Circulation.* 2018;138:131-140.

163. Pradhan AD, Aday AW, Rose LM, Ridker PM. Residual inflammatory risk on treatment with PCSK9 inhibition and statin therapy. *Circulation.* 2018;138:141-149.

164. Jaiswal S, et al. Clonal hematopoiesis and risk of atherosclerotic cardiovascular disease. *N Engl J Med.* 2017;377:111-121.

165. Dorsheimer L, et al. Association of mutations contributing to clonal hematopoiesis with prognosis in chronic ischemic heart failure. *JAMA Cardiol.* 2019;4:25-33.

166. Costantino S, et al. Epigenetics and precision medicine in cardiovascular patients: from basic concepts to the clinical arena. *Eur Heart J.* 2018;39:4150-4158.

167. Fuster JJ, et al. Clonal hematopoiesis associated with TET2 deficiency accelerates atherosclerosis development in mice. *Science.* 2017;355:842-847.

168. Wolach O, et al. Increased neutrophil extracellular trap formation promotes thrombosis in myeloproliferative neoplasms. *Sci Transl Med.* 2018;10.

169. Sander JD. Joung JK. CRISPR-Cas systems for editing regulating and targeting genomes. *Nature Biotechnol.* 2014;32:347-355.

170. Cohen AJ, et al. Estimates and 25-year trends of the global burden of disease attributable to ambient air pollution: an analysis of data from the Global Burden of Diseases Study 2015. *Lancet.* 2017;389:1907-1918.

171. World Health Organization. *Ambient air pollution: a global assessment of exposure and burden of disease.* 2016. https://apps.who.int/iris/handle/10665/250141.

172. Pope CA, et al. Short-term exposure to fine particulate matter air pollution is preferentially associated with the risk of ST-segment elevation acute coronary events. *J Am Heart Assoc.* 2015;4.

173. Chen H, et al. Ambient fine particulate matter and mortality among survivors of myocardial infarction: population-based cohort study. *Environ Health Perspect.* 2016;124:1421-1428.

174. Lu F, et al. Systematic review and meta-analysis of the adverse health effects of ambient PM2.5 and PM10 pollution in the Chinese population. *Environ Res.* 2015;136:196-204.

175. Rajagopalan S, Al-Kindi SG, Brook RD. Air pollution and cardiovascular disease. *J Am Coll Cardiol.* 2018;72:2054-2070.

176. Miyata R, van Eeden SF. The innate and adaptive immune response induced by alveolar macrophages exposed to ambient particulate matter. *Toxicol Appl Pharmacol.* 2011:257:209-226.

177. Du X, et al. Air pollution is associated with the development of atherosclerosis via the cooperation of CD36 and NLRP3 inflammasome in ApoE−/− mice. *Toxicol Lett.* 2018;290:123-132.

178. Rao X, et al. CD36-dependent 7-ketocholesterol accumulation in macrophages mediates progression of atherosclerosis in response to chronic air pollution exposure. *Circ Res.* 2014;115:770-780.

179. Münzel T, et al. Environmental stressors and cardio-metabolic disease: part II-mechanistic insights. *Eur Heart J.* 2017;38:557-564.

180. Mathieu P, Lemieux I, Després J-P. Obesity Inflammation and cardiovascular risk. *Clinic Pharmacol Therapeut.* 2019;87:407-416.

181. Blackburn P, et al. Postprandial variations of plasma inflammatory markers in abdominally obese men. *Obesity (Silver Spring).* 2006;14:1747-1754.

182. Wallace AM, et al. Plasma leptin and the risk of cardiovascular disease in the west of Scotland coronary prevention study (WOSCOPS). *Circulation.* 2001;104:3052-3056.

183. Ouchi N, et al. Novel modulator for endothelial adhesion molecules: adipocyte-derived plasma protein adiponectin. *Circulation.* 1999;100:2473-2476.

184. Schnabel R, et al. Association of adiponectin with adverse outcome in coronary artery disease patients: results from the AtheroGene study. *Eur Heart J.* 2008;29:649-657.

185. Reilly MP, et al. Resistin is an inflammatory marker of atherosclerosis in humans. *Circulation.* 2005;111:932-939.

186. Spalding KL, et al. Dynamics of fat cell turnover in humans. *Nature.* 2008;453:783-787.

187. Nguyen MTA, et al. A subpopulation of macrophages infiltrates hypertrophic adipose tissue and is activated by free fatty acids via Toll-like receptors 2 and 4 and JNK-dependent pathways. *J Biol Chem.* 2007;282:35279-35292.

188. Arsenault BJ, Pibarot P, Després J-P. The quest for the optimal assessment of global cardiovascular risk: are traditional risk factors and metabolic syndrome partners in crime? *Cardiology.* 2009;113:35-49.

189. Zheng G, et al. Effect of aerobic exercise on inflammatory markers in healthy middle-aged and older adults: a systematic review and meta-analysis of randomized controlled trials. *Front Aging Neurosci.* 2019;11:98.

190. Nimmo MA, Leggate M, Viana JL, King JA. The effect of physical activity on mediators of inflammation. *Diabetes Obes Metab.* 2013;15:51-60.

15

Location and Level of Care, Education, Availability of Medicines, and Cardiovascular Mortality

Rajeev Gupta, Philip Joseph, Annika Rosengren, and Salim Yusuf

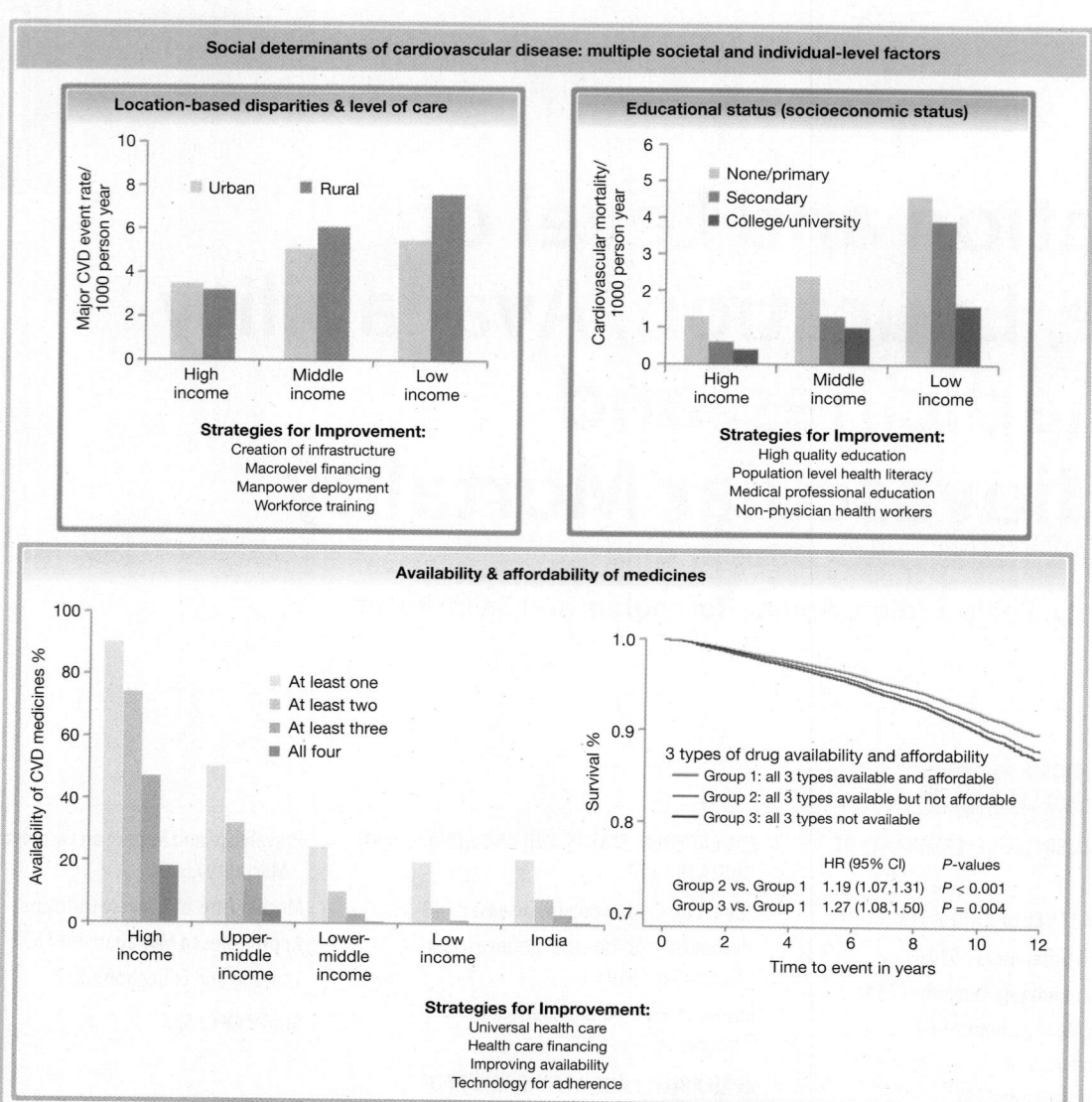

Chapter 15 Fuster and Hurst's Central Illustration. Social determinants of cardiovascular disease include location-based disparities in health care, educational status, and availability and affordability of medicines. Policy-level interventions are needed to improve cardiovascular health in deprived communities. Data from Yusuf S, et al. Cardiovascular risk and events in 17 low, middle-and high-income countries. *N Engl J Med*. 2014;371:818-827; Rosengren A, et al. Socioeconomic status and risk of cardiovascular disease in 20 low-income, middle-income and high income countries: the Prospective Urban Rural Epidemiology (PURE) study. *Lancet Glob Health*. 2019; 7:e748-e760; Khatib R, et al. Availability and affordability of cardiovascular disease medicines and their effect on use in high-income, middle-income, and low-income countries: an analysis of the PURE study data. *Lancet*. 2016; 387:61-69. Survival curves (lower right) reproduced from Chow CK, et al. Availability and affordability of medicines and cardiovascular outcomes in high-income, middle-income and low-income countries: an analysis of the PURE study data. *BMJ Glob Health*. 2020; 5:e002640.

CHAPTER SUMMARY

This chapter discusses societal and individual-level social determinants of cardiovascular health. Understanding these social determinants of cardiovascular health is important for improving the outcomes among individuals and the community through better prevention and treatments for ischemic heart disease (IHD). Epidemiological studies have reported that populations in rural and underserved urban locations have greater cardiovascular events and mortality than urbanites in developed and developing countries. This risk is mediated through location-based disparities in health care, lower educational status (a marker of lower socioeconomic status), and lower availability and affordability of medicines (see Fuster and Hurst's Central Illustration). Policy-level interventions that focus on each of these three factors are needed to improve quality of health systems and health care in these underserved locations. Essential to this improvement is the requirement for novel health financing mechanisms to provide comprehensive universal primary and secondary health care, especially in developing countries. High-quality and free universal health care are crucial for improving access and use of proven medicines and other interventions, and promotion of lifelong adherence can lead to substantially better cardiovascular health.

INTRODUCTION: SOCIAL DETERMINANTS OF HEALTH

Healthy lifestyles are crucial in the prevention of cardiovascular disease (CVD) and mortality. Pharmacological measures are also needed among those with cardiovascular risk factors and established disease. Healthy lifestyle in individuals and populations, type of health care, and access to medications are, however, determined by social and economic factors that are in turn influenced by multiple social, economic, and cultural circumstances. These factors, collectively known as social determinants of health, are increasingly being identified as important in health and also in causation and treatment of CVDs.[1,2] Physicians have known for centuries that social factors such as poor living conditions and poverty are associated with poor health and higher all-cause mortality.[3] It is also well known that cardiovascular conditions such as rheumatic heart disease and other infection-related conditions (tubercular pericarditis, Chagas disease) and nutritional deficiency cardiomyopathies are more common among the poor and those living in crowded conditions.[4] Until the middle of the 20th century, diseases such as ischemic heart disease (IHD) and stroke and their risk factors—hypertension, diabetes, hypercholesterolemia, and unhealthy lifestyles—were more prevalent among richer individuals in developed countries. This has changed and poor individuals in these countries currently have higher incidence and mortality from IHD and stroke.[5,6] Similar trends are emerging in developing countries.[6]

The World Health Organization (WHO) has defined social determinants of health as the conditions in which people are born, grow, live, work, and age.[7] These circumstances are shaped by the distribution of money, power, and resources at global, national, and local levels. Key concepts that influence the social determinants of health include globalization, urbanization, early child development, employment conditions, social exclusion and isolation, women and gender equity, health systems, and public health programs. Marmot and Wilkinson have suggested that social gradients, social exclusion, social support, work, unemployment, stress, addiction, food, and transport in early life are also relevant and exert their influences throughout the lifecourse.[1] Research over the last 100 years has identified several social determinants of CVD and a summary list is provided in **Table 15–1**. Both macrolevel social factors as well as individual-level risk factors are important.[8–10] Social determinants and social factors contribute to the pathophysiology of CVD, especially IHD, via multiple pathways (**Table 15–2**).[11] Some of the pathways involved are direct consequences of upstream political and social determinants such as location-based economic and social factors, housing characteristics, social discrimination, economic deprivation, employment status, parental education and values, and family structure.[11]

Low socioeconomic status is also associated with poor health literacy and harmful health behaviors.[2] Studies from developed as well as developing countries have shown greater prevalence of smoking and tobacco use and alcohol abuse (both among men), consumption of unhealthy foods, and sedentary lifestyle,

TABLE 15–1. Important Socioeconomic Factors for Cardiovascular Diseases	
Macrolevel factors	– Community and residence (urban, rural, slums, etc.) – Personal safety, freedom from crime, and conflicts – Social and human development – Social isolation, social capital, and support systems – Reduced Income inequality – Health systems and access to health care – Policies that affect health, such as tobacco taxation and advertisement, food security, and access and affordability of healthy foods – Environmental pollution
Microlevel individual factors	– Individual-level social and income gradient – Social class throughout life – Social exclusion – Stress – Adverse early life events – Employment status – Working conditions – Social support – Addiction including tobacco and alcohol – Healthy food availability and affordability – Availability of transport – Education – Adoption of healthy lifestyles and other treatments – Control of major cardiovascular risk factors – Smoking, abnormal lipid levels, hypertension, diabetes, obesity – Availability and affordability of secondary/tertiary prevention and treatments – Factors affecting adherence to medications and healthy behaviors

and exposure to ambient and indoor pollution, along with low awareness and treatment of major proximate cardiovascular risk factors such as hypertension, diabetes, and hypercholesterolemia among individuals of lower socioeconomic status.[9,10] Risk factor control and other preventive care is also poor among lower socioeconomic status individuals. This is due, in part, because of their low access and relative unaffordability. Multiple studies, in both the developing countries of Asia, Africa, and South America, as well as in the developed countries of Europe and North America, have shown lower quality of acute cardiovascular care among the poor.[9] In the present review, we will describe the impact of three of the more important social determinants of IHD: (1) location and level of care; (2) educational status; and (3) availability and affordability of cardiovascular medicines.

LOCATION AND LEVEL OF CARE

Location-based disparities and level of health care are interrelated. Living or working in poor and deprived locations in rural and urban areas is associated with higher all-cause mortality.[3] In the early 20th century, it was reported that cardiovascular risk factors including smoking, unhealthy diet, hypertension, hypercholesterolemia, and diabetes were more prevalent in the rich compared to the poor and that cardiovascular mortality was higher among individuals living in more affluent locations.[5,8] However, this has now changed and cardiovascular mortality is now higher in less affluent and poor locations

TABLE 15–2. Pathways Leading to Adverse Cardiovascular Consequences of Social Determinants

Pathways	Cardiovascular consequences
Psychobiological pathways	• Deprivation, discrimination, and chronic stress • Abnormal sympathetic-parasympathetic functions • Neuroendocrine axes: hypothalamic-pituitary influence • Allostasis and the metabolic syndrome • Disturbance of coagulation • Endothelial function • Influence on inflammation and Immunity

Cardiovascular risk factors	• Low educational status and poor preventative health literacy
	• Adverse health behaviors
	  • Greater prevalence of tobacco use, smoking, and alcohol
	  • Consumption of unhealthy foods: low-quality carbohydrates, trans fats, comfort foods, prepackaged ultra-processed food
	  • Poor intake of healthy foods: fruits, green vegetables, nuts, legumes, whole grain cereals
	  • Sedentary lifestyle
	• Low awareness, treatment, and control of major risk factors such as hypertension, diabetes, hypercholesterolemia

Access to preventive care and affordability	• Variations in universal health care: type of services, populations covered, and extent of coverage • Financial coverage and copayments • Access to lifelong preventative care • Availability and affordability of medicines and health economic issues
Access to acute cardiovascular care	• Universal availability and access to high quality of secondary and tertiary cardiovascular care • Affordability and lack of financial protection systems

in most countries. The transition of risk factors from rich to poor individuals and from affluent to poor urban and rural populations was initially reported in the mid-20th century in developed countries but is now becoming a global phenomenon.[5] Greater all-cause as well as cardiovascular mortality in deprived urban and rural as compared to richer urban locations has also been observed in the United States.[12] Three factors have likely influenced this epidemiologic transition: changes in social determinants (Table 15–1), health delivery systems, and individual level risk factors.[13]

Location-Based Differences

Studies from several developed countries have reported higher prevalence and incidence of CVDs (stroke and myocardial infarction) among deprived populations in rural and urban locations.[8,9,13] Data from the US National Center for Health Statistics reported that between 1999 and 2009, IHD death rates declined in both urban and rural locations; however from 2007 onward, deaths in rural areas have been higher than in urban locations.[14] Analysis of the CDC-WONDER database reported age-adjusted differences in cardiovascular mortality

in large, medium, and small metropolitan and rural locations in the United States.[15] Rural locations reported consistently higher age-adjusted mortality rates per 100,000 population per year. Rural mortality in 1999 was 371.6 per 100,000 and decreased in 2017 to 251.4 per 100,000. In medium/small metropolitan areas, it declined from 343.7 to 221.8 per 100,000, and in large metropolitan locations it declined from 347.6 to 208.6 per 100,000.[15] Higher cardiovascular mortality has also been reported among homeless adults in the United States.[16] Such differences in cardiovascular mortality in urban compared to rural areas are larger in low- and middle-income countries.

The Prospective Urban Rural Epidemiology (PURE) study systematically evaluated the importance of location-based measures (urban vs rural residence) on incidence and mortality from CVDs in high-, middle-, and low-income countries.[17] In this study, baseline data were recorded between 2003 and 2008 on cardiovascular risk factors in urban and rural locations in 17 countries among 150,000 participants. Prevalence of cumulative cardiovascular risk, estimated as the INTERHEART risk score, was the highest in high-income countries. After a mean of 5 years of follow-up, it was reported that despite the INTERHEART risk score being the highest in high-income countries, paradoxically, the incidence of major cardiovascular events as well as cardiovascular mortality were highest in low-income countries. Case-fatality rates were highest in rural areas in low-income countries (**Fig. 15–1**). In China, IHD mortality increased from 2004 to 2010, mainly in rural areas.[18] In India, a nationwide study involving an analysis of more than 112,000 CVD deaths from 2001 to 2013 reported higher IHD death rates in rural versus urban individuals aged 30 to 69 years in men (255 vs 234/100,000), with lesser differences in women (127 vs 123/100,000).[19] These findings confirm evidence of greater cardiovascular mortality in rural and deprived urban locations globally.

Level of Care and Adverse Outcomes

In rural locations, as well as in deprived urban communities, the quality of primary and secondary preventive care, and care for acute CVD is significantly inferior.[9,13] For example, in the United Kingdom primary care system, significant gaps in risk assessment, communication, surveillance, and management were reported as barriers to risk prevention.[20] In the United States, it has been reported that rural populations are younger than urban populations and have different health issues such as occupational respiratory diseases, suicides, accidents, and unintentional injuries compared to urban populations.[21] They also have higher mortalities from a number of noncommunicable diseases including IHD.[21] The Behavioral Risk Factor Surveillance System survey (2013) reported that nonmetropolitan counties in the United States, compared to metropolitan, had lower prevalence of health-promoting behaviors (avoidance of smoking, maintaining normal body weight, and increasing aerobic leisure-time physical activity).[22] Higher prevalence of unhealthy behaviors in rural and nonmetropolitan counties were associated with enhanced rates of IHD. Similar data have been reported from Europe[23] and other regions of the world.[24–27]

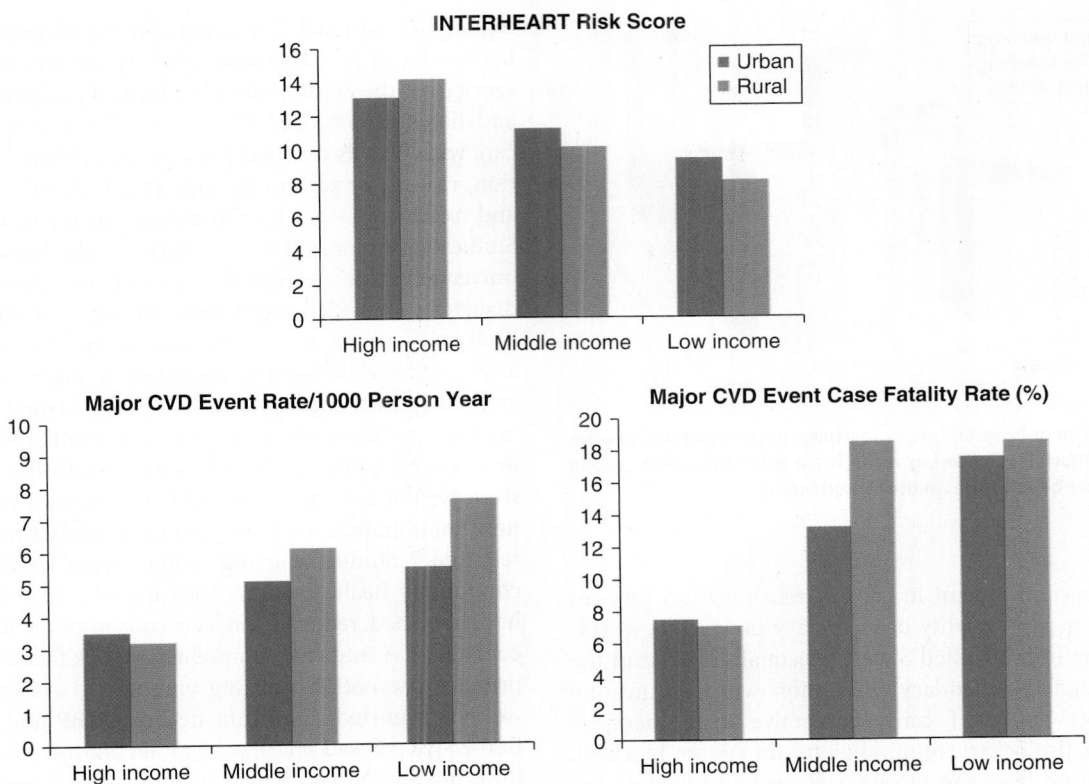

Figure 15–1. The Prospective Urban Rural Epidemiology (PURE) Study: higher major cardiovascular disease event rate and case fatality in rural areas in middle- and low-income countries despite having lower burden of cardiovascular risk. Reproduced with permission from Yusuf S, Rangarajan S, Teo K, et al. Cardiovascular risk and events in 17 low-, middle-, and high-income countries. *N Engl J Med*. 2014 Aug 28;371(9):818-827.

Primary and secondary prevention is also less well developed in rural areas in the United States,[13] as well as in low- and middle-income countries.[27,28] There is high prevalence and poor control of most lifestyle-related IHD risk factors—tobacco use, alcohol, unhealthy diet (high carbohydrates, low fruits and vegetables, high trans fats, and food pollutants), and indoor and ambient air pollution.[10] Awareness, treatment and control of these risk factors is low in rural locations in developed as well as developing countries.[28] Hypertension awareness, treatment, and control is a marker of overall cardiovascular risk management. In the United States, hypertension awareness, treatment, and control are significantly lower in rural and inner city deprived populations.[29] In another study in 44 low- and middle-income countries with data of 1.1 million participants, hypertension was reported in 17.6%. In those with hypertension, 73.6% had had their blood pressure (BP) measured, 39.2% were aware of the diagnosis, 29.9% received treatment, and 10.3% had it under control.[30] This was much lower than in the high-income countries of Europe and North America; although even in these countries, hypertension control rates varied from 40% to 70%.[31] Low rates of diabetes control have also been reported from rural primary care in developed as well as developing countries.[32,33] Use of statins to control hypercholesterolemia is low globally.[34] Achievement of target cholesterol levels (in primary prevention) is low among the insured in the United States (21.4%), and lower among the uninsured (10.5%).[35] It is also low in primary care.[36]

Disparities by location also exist in secondary-level health care in management of acute coronary syndromes.[28] In the United States, it has been reported that outcomes following an acute coronary syndrome are inferior in county-level hospitals compared to teaching hospitals. In a study of relationship of teaching status of hospitals with quality of care and mortality for Medicare patients with acute myocardial infarction, a gradient of increasing mortality was observed from major teaching hospitals to minor teaching hospitals and nonteaching hospitals (**Fig. 15–2**).[37] This was attenuated after adjustment for patient characteristics and receipt of therapies. Among major teaching, minor teaching, and nonteaching hospitals, respectively, administration rates for aspirin were 91.2%, 86.4%, and 81.4% (*P* < 0.001); for angiotensin-converting enzyme inhibitors, 63.7%, 60.0%, and 58.0% (*P* < 0.001); for β-blockers, 48.8%, 40.3%, and 36.4% (*P* < 0.001); and for reperfusion therapy, 55.5%, 58.9%, and 55.2% (*P* = 0.29).[37] It has also been reported that myocardial infarction mortality was lower among patients who were treated by cardiologists versus generalists.[38] Cardiovascular specialists are not available in large parts of the world including in the United States[13] In the United States, although rural hospitals provide 40% of acute care they only have 20% of beds and have inferior management capabilities.[13] They are smaller in size and volumes and have less capacity to provide critical care.[13] District hospitals, the most important location for management of acute coronary syndrome, function poorly in large parts of the world.[39]

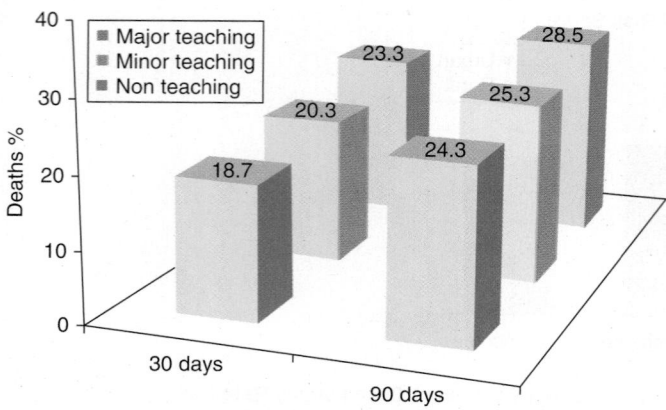

Figure 15–2. Type of hospital (major teaching, minor teaching, or non-teaching) and mortality following acute myocardial infarction among 114,411 Medicare beneficiaries in the United States.

There is low enrollment in cardiac rehabilitation services and there are gaps in quality of secondary prevention worldwide including in the United States.[40] Inequalities exist in the use of high-quality secondary prevention with significantly lower rates of intake of cardio-protective drug therapies (anti-platelets, β-blockers, renin-angiotensin system blockers, and statins) in primary and secondary care.[38,41] In Europe, the EUROASPIRE-3 study reported that less than half of patients after discharge from coronary care units were formally enrolled in cardiac rehabilitation and intake of secondary prevention medications was low.[42] The status of secondary prevention therapies is even poorer in primary and secondary care in developing countries. In the PURE study, extremely low use of such medications in patients with known CVDs was observed in low- and lower-middle income countries compared to high middle- and high-income countries.[43] Prescription audits in China and India have reported lower secondary prevention therapies in primary care clinics, compared to IHD patients in secondary and tertiary care.[44,45] There are multiple reasons for compromised quality of long-term care in primary and secondary health care globally.[28,46,47] Barriers exist at healthcare-system level (availability, access, and affordability), healthcare-provider level (quality of medical education, physician shortage, physician inertia, and lack of task-sharing with nonphysician health workers), and at the patient level (health illiteracy, poverty, and drug-costs).

Approaches to Management

Primary Prevention

Improving cardiovascular prevention in resource-limited settings require strategies to increase health and disease awareness, capacity building of healthcare workers, and improving access.[10] Political and policy initiatives are important. Health-promotion policies implemented at population level have similar benefits in both high- and low-resource communities. For example, taxation of tobacco products has proven successful in reducing tobacco use across different types of communities, and

regional or national restrictions on use of trans fats in food have reduced its consumption.[10,47] Strong primary healthcare services in the community with focus on control of BP, lipids, and diabetes are needed. Universal and efficient primary health care with a focus on CVD primary prevention—health education, risk factor screening, appropriate lifestyle interventions, and treatments—can lead to changes in the health behaviors. Studies have reported that countries in the highest quintile of universal health coverage have lower rates of smoking, BP, and diabetes—all evidence of better risk factor control.[48] A major limiting factor in risk factor control in rural areas in many low- and middle-income countries is dearth of physicians and other health professionals trained in prevention. Sharing tasks between physicians and community health workers or other nonphysician health workers with the help of novel strategies for risk factor control (eg, information and communication initiatives, empowerment, and mobile technology) are required.[28] Studies utilizing nonphysician health workers or community health workers for cardiovascular risk reduction have reported reduced tobacco consumption and better BP control.[49,50] A study for comprehensive risk factor reduction for primary prevention utilizing empowered community health workers reported significant decline in BP and cholesterol.[51] Barber-shop based pharmacist's intervention led to greater BP lowering among Black men in the United States.[52] Enhanced and better education of physicians, nurses, and health workers for prevention of CVDs via risk factor control should be strengthened.[28,53,54]

Acute Coronary Syndrome

Better management of acute coronary syndromes at primary and secondary levels are important in low-resource settings. Combined with preventive medical therapies, this accounts for a third of the decline in IHD mortality in developed countries.[55,56] Acute coronary syndrome management has improved significantly in developed countries due to pharmacological and technological innovations.[57] The Royal Colleges in the United Kingdom,[58] Canadian Society of Cardiology,[59] American Heart Association (AHA) and American College of Cardiology,[60] and European Society of Cardiology[61] have described optimum organizational structure, staffing, resources, and educational initiatives. These include dedicated (closed) intensive care units, leadership of intensivists, high-intensity staffing, advanced training of cardiologists in general intensive care, and balancing training with critical care needs.[62] In deprived locations in developed countries, there has been a focus on rapid transfer to coronary intervention capable centers, home or ambulance-based thrombolysis, and pharmaco-invasive approaches.[60–62] Implementation of guideline-based management of acute coronary syndrome using validated protocols could be useful for better management in low- and middle-income countries.[64,64] There have been a number of policy initiatives to provide rapid access to high-quality acute coronary syndrome care in many countries.[47] There is focus on provision of 24-hour free ambulance services, creation of systems for central telediagnosis, telemonitoring, and rapid transfer of patients to facilities with capabilities for pharmacological reperfusion therapies or coronary interventions.[64] These approaches are being evaluated in low- and middle-income countries such as the ST elevation myocardial infarction (STEMI)-India model in South India,[65] and the LATIN Telemedicine project in South America.[66] Both are focused on early coronary interventions utilizing pharmaco-invasive approaches to improving acute coronary syndrome care in low- and middle-income countries. However, high-quality randomized clinical trials and economic evaluation of technology-supported interventions are needed. In addition, improving health literacy among the general population and heart-literacy among primary care nurses and physicians are important for early symptom identification and to ensure rapid transport of patients to hospitals for acute management. This involves efforts to improve health literacy and access to care along with task-shifting simple but proven key tasks from physicians to trained nonphysicians (eg, for risk identification, risk management, and early diagnosis).

Secondary Prevention

A number of strategies to improve quality of care have been evaluated for better secondary prevention. Referral to formal cardiac rehabilitation units is useful, but limited availability of such units in developed countries and nonavailability in developing countries is a barrier.[67] Task-shifting alone with involvement of healthcare workers to promote adherence has been evaluated with some short-term success,[49,68] although it can be a key component of a more comprehensive strategy and lead to a larger impact as in the HOPE-4 study.[51] Telehealth strategies including telemedicine-enabled diagnosis, algorithm-based management, and discharge check lists have been evaluated with limited success in both developed and developing countries.[69] The American College of Cardiology Task Force recommends confluence of advances in digital health, big data, and precision health approaches through research and sharing of resources with stakeholder engagement and partnerships to improve quality of care.[70] With respect to medications, use of combination therapy with a polypill (aspirin, a statin, and two BP-lowering drugs) has been shown to reduce CVD events by about one-third.[71,72] Publicly funded insurance schemes and free medicine supply schemes have also been implemented.[73] However, results of most of these initiatives have been equivocal and no study has reported clear reductions in clinical outcomes, perhaps because the changes in individual processes were modest. In the HOPE-4 study, with nonphysician health workers–based systematic door-to-door screening, free combination drugs when needed, and use of family members or friends as treatment supporters, there was a large reduction in risk (by 50%) as assessed by the Framingham and INTERHEART risk scores in individuals who had hypertension. This trial was not designed to demonstrate a lower incidence of cardiovascular events but the changes in risk factors were substantial and sustained and should be considered a viable strategy to reduce cardiovascular risk in the community to a significant degree.[51]

Training and Education

Training healthcare professionals in cardiovascular prevention and management at primary and secondary level is important.[10] The World Health Organization (WHO) has suggested that physicians should be adequately trained to have proficiency to meet demands of the health needs of people while maintaining the systems needed to provide medical care to sick.[74] The AHA has recognized that there are gaps in physician knowledge regarding cardiovascular preventive medicine.[75] Suggested educational strategies to reorient undergraduate and postgraduate education are: focus on healthy lifestyles and related domains, prehospital management of acute cardiovascular events, and the importance of lifelong medical treatment. This could be performed using multidimensional curricula, pedagogies, technologies, and competency-based assessments. It has been argued that better physician education and enhancing collaborative care delivery can reduce the health and economic burdens from CVDs to a degree not previously realized.[76]

An important adjunct to change in physician education is training of nurses and allied professionals in general cardiovascular and preventive medicine, especially for primary and secondary prevention. Education of community health workers and nurses for prevention is important.[28,47,77] In low- and middle-income countries, where the burden of coronary disease is substantial and physician shortage is common, task-sharing with other health workers is important.[49] Public health education (starting from schools) for adoption for healthy lifestyles and education regarding CVD risk factors is crucial for prevention.

Management of acute coronary syndromes can be improved by training healthcare workers, nurses, and emergency room physicians, especially at the secondary care level, such as those working in district and rural hospitals.[13,78] Coronary intensive care units can be improved by better organizational structure, staffing, and continuing education.[13] An AHA scientific statement suggests transformation of cardiac intensive care units from basic to advanced evidence-based staffing models that are adaptable to a variety of clinical settings.[79] It also recommends procedural competencies including through training in noninvasive and invasive cardiology, advanced cardiac life support, airway management and ventilator training, and proficiency in use of ultrasound and interventional pulmonary procedures.[79]

EDUCATIONAL STATUS AND CARDIOVASCULAR DISEASE

A variety of approaches to conceptualization and measurement of socioeconomic status have been used. These reflect different theoretical orientations and exigencies in conducting research.[80] Four measures have been consistently associated with greater cardiovascular risk in developed countries: low education, low income, lower employment status, and neighborhood socioeconomic factors.[81]

Low education or socioeconomic status has been recognized as a leading modifiable risk factor for CVD and overall mortality.[5-9] Educational status has been used as marker of

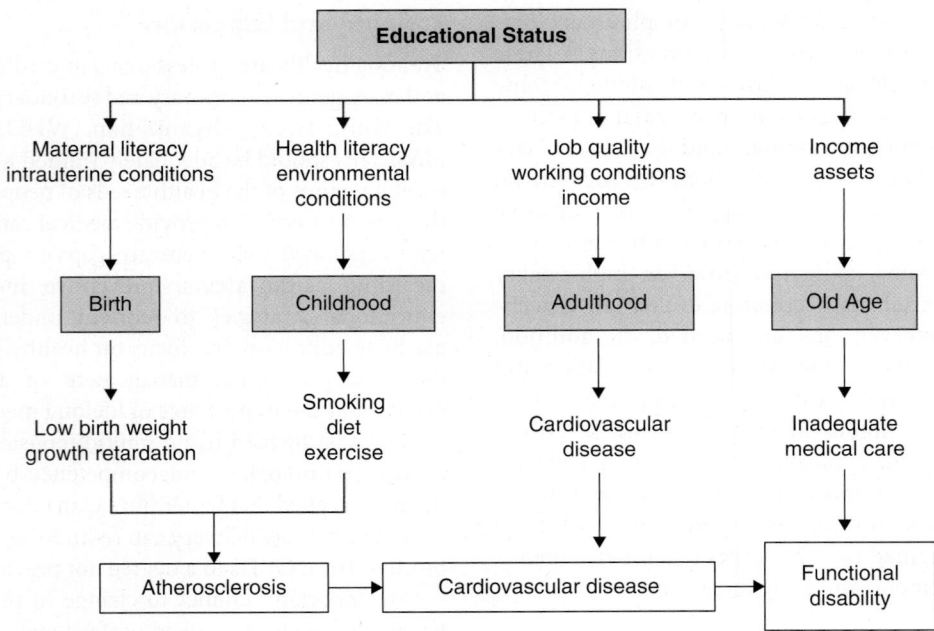

Figure 15–3. Education and cardiovascular disease from a life-course perspective.

socioeconomic position and is the most frequent method of assessment of socioeconomic status in cardiovascular epidemiological studies.[8] In addition, it is a marker of social networks and support, discrimination, work demands and control, and is important for developmental and life-course perspective.[9] Educational status may be a more important marker in developing countries where prevalence of illiteracy and low educational status is high and where public and health resources are more limited.[81] Education is one of the most important modifiable social determinant of CVD and mortality as reported in the PURE study.[82] It has been argued that education shapes lives and is key to lifting people out of poverty and reducing socioeconomic and political inequalities.[83] Educational status is used as a measure of social class mainly because it is simple to measure, changes infrequently after young adulthood, and is less prone to reverse causality.[8] Low educational status means less ability to determine one's own destiny, deprivation of material resources, and having limited opportunities. Educational status influences cardiovascular risk across the life-course (**Fig. 15–3**).

Impact on Cardiovascular Disease

Low educational status as marker of increased risk cardiovascular risk has been extensively studied in developed countries and hundreds of studies have consistently reported greater incidence and prevalence of cardiovascular risk factors (smoking, unhealthy diets, physical inactivity, hypertension, lipid abnormalities, and diabetes) and greater CVD incidence as well as cardiovascular mortality among the less literate.[8,80] Emerging data from lower-middle income countries also highlight the importance of low socioeconomic status (educational status) in adverse cardiovascular outcomes.[84] In a prospective study of >90,000 persons, the Asia Pacific Cohort Studies Collaboration from Australasia and Eastern Asia reported greater

cardiovascular risk, mortality, and all-cause mortality in those with low or no education as compared to those with tertiary education.[85] Greater cardiovascular mortality among the less literate has also been reported in a large prospective study in India.[86]

The INTERHEART case-control study of risk factors for acute myocardial infarction in individuals from 52 countries reported low educational status as a risk factor (odds ratio [OR] 1.31; 95% confidence interval [CI] 1.20–1.44). The relative risk (RR), comparing low to high educational status, was greater in high-income countries (RR 1.6; CI, 1.33–1.94) than in middle and lower income countries (RR 1.25; CI, 1.14–1.37).[87] The importance of educational status, as marker of socioeconomic status and wealth among 154,000 participants from 20 countries has been prospectively evaluated in the PURE study.[88] After a mean follow-up of 7.5 years, all-cause mortality and major cardiovascular events were more common in low-income countries and among low educational status participants as compared to high (**Fig. 15–4**). While the INTERHEART study reported a steeper gradient by education in high-income compared to low-income and middle-income countries, the reverse was observed in PURE study. The hazard ratio (HR) for low versus high level of education in high-income countries was 1.23 (CI, 0.96–1.58), middle-income countries 1.59 (CI, 1.42–1.78), and low-income countries 2.23 (CI, 1.79–2.77). In another report from the PURE study, a low educational status was identified as one of the six leading cardiovascular risk factors, the others being hypertension, high non-high-density lipoprotein cholesterol, household air pollution, tobacco use, and poor diet.[82] It was considered the leading risk factor for mortality with a greater importance in low- and middle-income countries.[82] These studies clearly highlight the importance of the independent effects of living in poorer countries and low educational

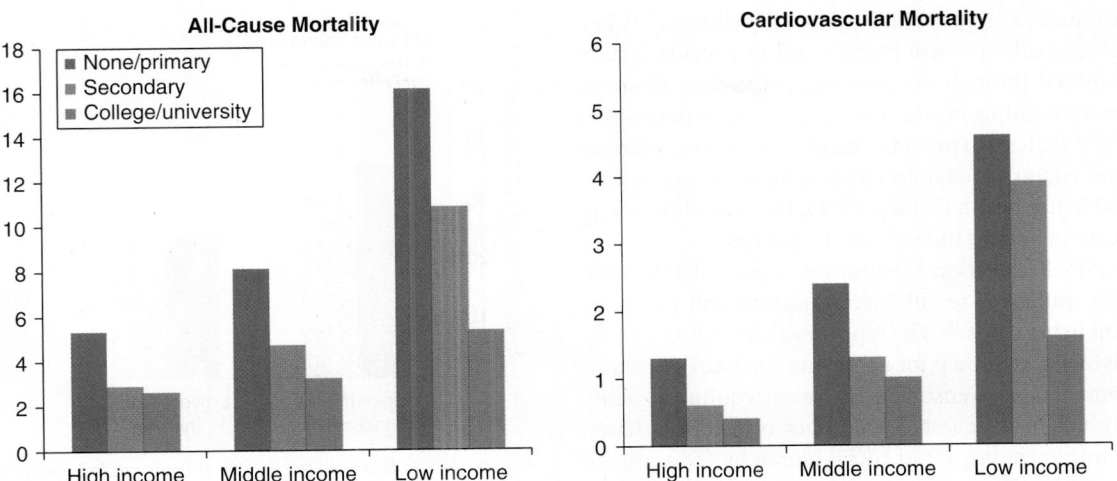

Figure 15–4. Educational status and age- and sex-standardized all-cause and cardiovascular mortality in high-, middle-, and low-income countries in the PURE study. Data from Rosengren A, Smyth A, Rangarajan S, et al. Socioeconomic status and risk of cardiovascular disease in 20 low-income, middle-income, and high-income countries: the Prospective Urban Rural Epidemiologic (PURE) study. *Lancet Glob Health*. 2019 Jun;7(6):e748-e760.

status as an important risk factor for CVDs and mortality. Educational and social status are now recognized as a mainstream cardiovascular risk factor, in addition to standard behavioral and cardiometabolic factors.[81]

Mechanisms of Adverse Cardiovascular Outcomes

The mechanisms by which low educational status affect CVD and outcomes are poorly understood. Initial studies were focused on individual psychosocial and personality patterns and highlighted the importance of chronic stress.[8,11] Recent studies have emphasized the importance of environmental factors—physical, social, occupational, psychological, etc.[80,89] Adverse consequences of low educational status evolve over the life-course and are important determinants of CVDs (Fig. 15–3). Low maternal education is associated with maternal poverty and poor-quality nutrition. These factors lead to fetal undernutrition, growth retardation, and birth of small-for-age babies. In adulthood, this is associated with multiple cardiovascular risk factors (hypertension, diabetes, lipid abnormalities, reduced pulmonary, and kidney function) and premature CHD.[90] Low educational status in childhood could also be due to low parental education and socioeconomic influences. It has been reported that important cardiovascular risk factors such as tobacco use, poor-quality diet, childhood obesity, BP, blood cholesterol and triglycerides, and metabolic syndrome start in early childhood and adolescence and track through adulthood.[91] Early-age elevations of these risk factors are known to be associated with premature CVDs in low-income countries.[92] Greater prevalence of cardiovascular risk factors—tobacco, unhealthy diet, hypertension, and hypercholesterolemia—has been consistently reported among low educational status and low socioeconomic status populations in several studies.[93] In developed countries, the prevalence of obesity, metabolic syndrome, and diabetes is also higher among less educated groups.[80] An emerging area of interest is the presence of coronary risk enhancers (chronic kidney disease, premature menopause, inflammatory diseases, and raised inflammatory biomarkers) in individuals with low educational status.[94]

Studies have reported an increased incidence of acute coronary events in persons of low educational status related to not only greater presence of major risk factors but also due to more risk enhancers.[9,94]

Lower educational status also predicts worse short-term (<30 days) as well as long term (>1 year) outcomes following an acute event.[9,95] Low-educational-status patients have more comorbidities, receive lesser number of expensive medications (thrombolysis, high dose statins, etc.), and fewer interventions, especially in low-income countries.[95] They are less likely to be referred to tertiary prevention programs, including cardiac rehabilitation.[96] Quality of secondary prevention and adherence to therapies are also lower among low-educational-status patients.[96-98] A strong contributor to greater cardiovascular risk in low-educational-status individuals is low health literacy (Fig. 15–3). Individuals with poor health literacy are more likely to be noncompliant with their medications, have poorer control of the risk factors, experience a higher incidence of cardiovascular events, and have greater all-cause and cardiovascular mortality.[99] The absolute effect of health literacy on cardiovascular risk and the influence of interventions require further studies.

Approaches to Management and Interventions

Given the importance of education as a major risk factor for CVD and mortality, there is a need to prioritize it as a modifiable risk factor from a health policy perspective. The United Nations (UN) has promulgated 17 Sustainable Development Goals for countries to address key social and health issues.[100] Each goal has the potential to promote cardiovascular health. Especially important are goals to eliminate poverty; to provide good health and well-being; to provide quality education, affordable and clean energy, decent working conditions, and economic growth; to develop industry, innovation, and infrastructure; and to forge action for a healthy climate.[10] A key goal is to substantially increase literacy and to provide quality education achieved through improved access, greater financial support, capacity building of educators, and focus on developing relevant skills.[100] Policies to provide universal basic education are present in most countries but unless there is focus on high-quality education and better health literacy, the higher mortality among the low-educational-status individuals shall persist.

The UN Global Education Monitoring Report 2020 focused on supporting initiatives to enhance education and to ensure that education never stops.[101] The report evaluated global progress and provided a roadmap for achieving the fourth Sustainable Development Goal to ensure inclusive and equitable quality education. Tobias has suggested a number of evidence-based strategies to minimize impact of social hierarchy (educational status) on health.[81] These strategies focus on investment in children, getting the welfare mix right, provision of safety nets, implementation of active labor policies, strengthening of local communities, provision of wrap-around services for the disadvantaged, promotion of healthy lifestyles, and ensuring universal access to high-quality education and primary health care. Ensuring universal access to high-quality secondary and tertiary health care should be an important component. Social prescribing (obtaining detailed social history at each healthcare visit and efforts to modify them) and transforming relationships between physicians and their patients to improve health literacy among patients and medical literacy among physicians also are crucial interventions.[102]

AVAILABILITY AND AFFORDABILITY OF MEDICINES

Health economics is the study of allocation of scarce resources among alternative uses for care of sickness and for promotion, maintenance, and improvement of health, including the study of how health care and health-related services, their costs and benefits, and health itself are distributed among individuals and groups in society.[103] It is important at both the macro or policy level as well as micro or individual level of health care. Availability and affordability of cardiovascular health care are crucial to prevent premature deaths across the globe.[104,105] One of the important consequences of low medication availability and affordability is nonadherence, a major problem in CVDs. In the United States, it has been estimated that medication nonadherence leads to 125,000 preventable annual deaths.[106] Medicines are essential "building blocks" of a well-functioning health system and involve a substantial portion of health expenditure. Five aspects of medicine supply are important: availability, affordability, accessibility, acceptability, and quality.[105] In the context of CVDs, both availability and affordability of medicines are important because medicines are to be consumed lifelong and because availability and affordability are driven both by national and local policies as well as individual practices.[107]

Prevalence and Impact on Cardiovascular Mortality

Availability is defined as the relationship between type and/or quality of medicine required and type and/or quality of

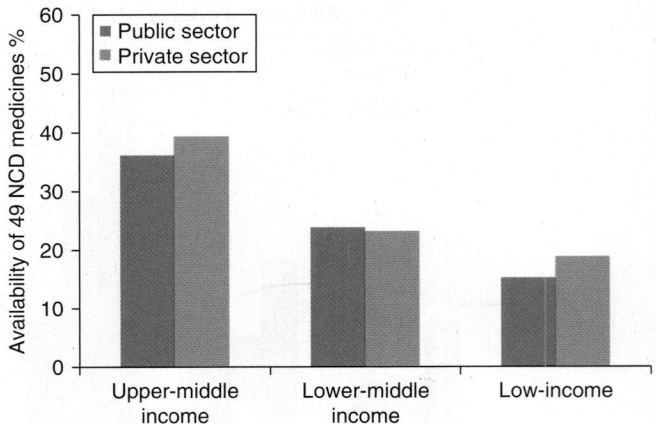

Figure 15–5. Availability of 49 recommended medicines for noncommunicable disease (NCD) in public and private sectors in upper-middle, lower-middle, and low-income countries. Data from Wirtz VJ, Kaplan WA, Kwan GF, et al. Access to Medications for Cardiovascular Diseases in Low- and Middle-Income Countries. *Circulation.* 2016 May 24;133(21):2076-2085.

medicine delivered.[105] Availability of cardiovascular medicines varies widely across the globe. In a review of surveys in low- and middle-income countries during 2008 to 2015 using the WHO target of availability of 80% of recommended 49 medicines, Ewen et al. reported significant variations in availability of these medicines in low-, lower-middle and upper-middle income countries.[108] Availability was lower in low-income countries in both private and public outlets, compared to lower-middle and upper-middle income countries (**Fig. 15–5**).[108] In the PURE study, it was reported that cardiovascular medicines for secondary prevention were more commonly available in high- and middle-income countries compared to low-income countries (**Fig. 15–6**).[109] Antihypertensive medications were also more often available in high- and middle-income countries compared to low-income countries in a study published in 2017.[110] More recent data (2020), however, report better availability of these medicines in low- and lower-middle income countries (54%) as well as upper-middle and high-income countries (60%) with generic brands being more available than branded medicines (61% vs 41%).[111] Availability is an important issue, especially in public health systems, where delays related to policies, procurement, financing, and logistics are common.[112]

Affordability of the medicines is also important, especially in developing countries.[104] Medicines account for 20% to 60% of healthcare costs in low- and lower-middle income countries compared to high-income countries where they constitute 18% of such costs.[111] Affordability of medicines is influenced by patent status of the medicine, market authorization requirements, and pricing and reimbursement policies.[105] Epidemiologic studies have reported low affordability of cardiovascular medicines in many low- and middle-income countries.[105] In a systematic study in 36 developing countries, it was reported that despite better availability of medications in the public sector, the affordability of even generic medicines was low. In almost half of these countries studied, the procurement prices for generics were 1.11 times the corresponding international

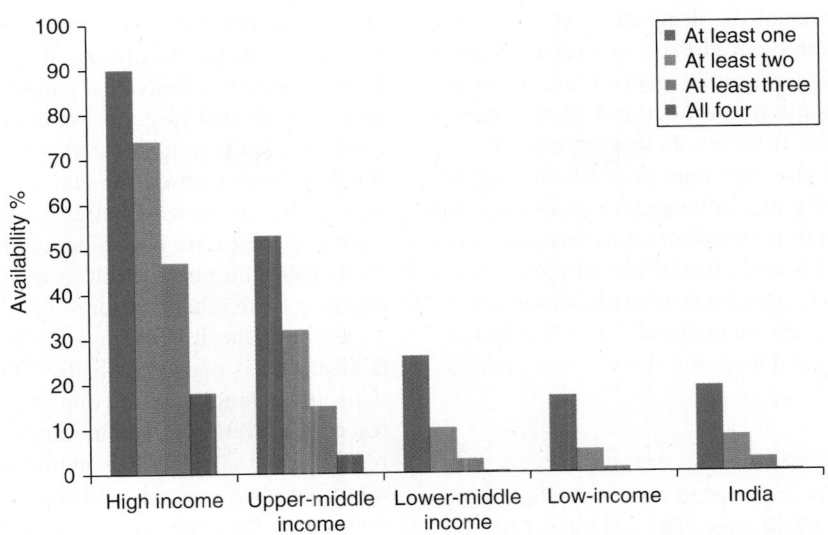

Figure 15–6. Availability of medicines for cardiovascular secondary prevention in high-, middle-, and low-income countries and India. Data from Khatib R, McKee M, Shannon H, et al. Availability and affordability of cardiovascular disease medicines and their effect on use in high-income, middle-income, and low-income countries: an analysis of the PURE study data. *Lancet.* 2016 Jan 2;387(10013):61-69.

reference prices (calculated as wholesale price of these drugs adjusted to purchasing power parity) and purchasing efficiency (ratio of wholesale procurement cost to international references price) varied from 0.1 to 5.4 times the base price.[112] Lower costs than international reference cost in some countries is due to government subsidies. In the PURE study, it was reported that while secondary prevention medicines were unaffordable to less than 1% in high-income countries and 5% in upper middle-income countries, they were not affordable to 21% of patients in lower-middle income countries and to 45% in low-income countries.[109]

Low availability and affordability of cardiovascular care and medicines are associated with less use of these medications (nonadherence) and greater incidence of adverse cardiovascular outcomes.[106] Residing in deprived locations, poverty, illiteracy, and other social factors that are associated with greater poverty (Table 15–1) are associated with reduced availability and affordability of medicines.[104,106] These differences are present not only in developing and less developed countries but also among the deprived communities in developed countries.[13,106] Studies have reported that in the United States, availability and affordability of cardiovascular care as well as cardiovascular medicines are lower in rural populations,[13] as well as selected ethnic groups such as African Americans, Latin Americans, and Pacific Islanders.[113] Although these ethnic and socioeconomic status–related differences have been known for decades, they still persist.[114] Individuals with low socioeconomic status as well as low educational status, with poor affordability of medicines and health care have high risk of all-cause mortality, cardiovascular mortality, and incident CVD.[88] In the PURE study, a systematic evaluation of the relationship of availability and affordability of essential cardiovascular medicines (anti-platelet, BP-lowering, and statins) with cardiovascular outcomes among 93,000 high-risk participants was performed.[115] Compared to participants to whom all medicines were available and

affordable, major adverse cardiovascular events (MACE) as well as deaths (adjusted HR, 95% CI) were significantly greater in participants when medicines were either not affordable (HR MACE 1.19, CI, 1.07–1.31; HR death 1.20, CI, 1.08–1.33) or not available (HR MACE 1.25, CI, 1.08–1.50; HR death 1.25, CI, 1.04–1.50). The increases in hazards were significantly greater in low-income countries compared to others.[115]

Mechanisms of Adverse Outcomes

Availability and affordability of medicines depend on type of health systems. Traditionally, they are classified based on their type of financing into: (1) predominantly tax funded (eg, British National Health Service) or publicly funded regional systems; (2) statutory social health insurance (eg, in Germany, France, and the Netherlands); (3) various hybrid arrangements as in the United States and former Soviet countries; and (4) predominantly self-funded or out-of-pocket expenditures as in most developing countries.[116] Pharmaceutical expenditures as a proportion of total health expenditures vary widely across types of health system. Such data are readily available in developed countries and show that 10% to 30% of total health expenditures arise from pharmaceuticals.[117]

Developing countries with more public- and insurance-funded schemes display a lower proportion of health expenditures from pharmaceuticals while those that rely on out-of-pocket expenditures have greater spending on pharmaceuticals.[118] In the PURE study, it was reported that consumption of medicines varied with availability as well as affordability of medicines and monthly household capacity to pay.[109] When fewer than four categories of secondary prevention medicines (anti-platelets, β-blockers, renin-angiotensin blockers, statins) were available, compared with all four drug categories being available, their use was 84% lower (95% CI, 43%–96%). Similarly, use of these medications was 84% (45%–96%) lower when the drugs were not affordable.[109] Low socioeconomic status was associated with lower intake of the drugs in all the 20 countries studied in the PURE study.[118] The strongest predictors for socioeconomic differences were public expenditure on health as proportion of gross domestic product and gross national income. Clearly, macrolevel social factors, related to health system financing (Table 15–1) are important determinants of poor availability and affordability of cardiovascular medicines. An important mechanism leading to greater cardiovascular mortality due to non-availability and affordability of medicines is low medication compliance. Adherence to medicines is a complex issue and multiple factors are involved.[98] The factors vary from policy level to individual level and this has regulatory as well as clinical relevance.[106]

Approaches to Management

Major health-care reforms are needed to provide adequate, accessible, and affordable health care. The AHA has prepared a blueprint that focuses on the following principles: (1) universal and affordable health coverage; (2) high-quality patient-centered health care; (3) evidence-based preventive services, (4) elimination of socioeconomic disparities; (5) growth of a healthcare workforce; and (6) support of biomedical and health research.[117] The targets are: expanding access to affordable health care and coverage; enhancing the availability of evidence-based preventive services; eliminating disparities that limit the availability and equitable delivery of health care; strengthening the public health infrastructure to respond to social determinants of health; prioritizing and accelerating investments in biomedical research; and growing a diverse, culturally competent health and healthcare workforce prepared to meet the challenges of delivering high value health care. Similar principles would be appropriate for large developing countries with fractured and unstable health systems (India, Brazil, Indonesia, Pakistan, Bangladesh, etc.) who experience more than two-thirds of the global CVD burden.[119]

Interventions are possible at health-care-system level to promote availability, affordability, and consumption of medicines.[28] Improving access and affordability of health care, revised health insurance policies with inclusion of outpatient services and elimination of copayments for primary and secondary preventive services, policies for greater involvement of nonphysician health professionals, and better medical education can yield dividends. At the health-care-provider level, interventions suggested are simplification of medication regimens and use of combination pharmacotherapy (eg, the polypill, etc.). A review has identified that in the United States, patient access to drugs is controlled by complex interaction between government and third-party payers, pharmacy benefit managers, distributers, manufacturers, health systems, pharmacies, and patients. Creation of a shared standardized and transparent process for coverage decisions that minimizes administrative barriers has been suggested.[107]

Training and Education

Education of politicians and health bureaucrats in policy development and in critical evaluation of interventions is important.[120] Elimination of poverty and creation of stable healthcare systems are crucial to improving cardiovascular health.[121] Universally applicable healthcare financing mechanisms need to be developed and individual nations should develop their own interventions that are contextually appropriate. The COVID-19 pandemic has highlighted deficiencies in health systems across the globe and focused the attention of politicians and policy makers for creation of better health infrastructure.[113] Short-term and long term consequences of CVDs can be prevented by focusing on public health measures, better intensive care, and long-term rehabilitation.

Universal health coverage for high-quality preventive and clinical care is needed globally.[121] Physicians have to improve their understanding of the importance of evidence-based clinical care, preventive medicine, and cost-effective care. Waste of resources is a worldwide phenomenon, but its effects are greatest in diverting scarce health resources in low and lower-middle income countries. This can be curtailed by better education of health providers and patients and audits of clinical practices with feedback. More than one-third of the adult global population has elevated cardiovascular risk factors or CVD. To reach this large population, which is about 1.5 billion individuals, simple, safe, and effective aspects of health care have to be delegated to nonphysician health workers not just in developing countries but also in developed countries. Suitable training of such professionals for improving prescriptions and promoting adherence to health recommendations and medications in patients is needed.[123] Health-care technology can be used to bring low-cost solutions for promoting affordability, availability, and adherence.[124] Finally, it is important to teach and train health professionals and community health workers, nurses, and pharmacists to promote adherence to proven cardiovascular medicines. Patient education and counseling are also important to promote adherence using motivation, technology, and behavioral support. Assurance of continuity of care is crucial. Family support in social and financial domains is important in less educated, elderly, and marginalized populations.

SUMMARY

Knowledge and understanding of social determinants of cardiovascular health and disease is crucial for better patient management. A large number of social and economic factors have been implicated in CVDs, especially IHD (Table 15–1). In this chapter, we have highlighted three of the more important factors: location and level of care, educational status, and availability and affordability of medicines. Each has high impact on cardiovascular mortality and are amenable to interventions. Focus on the three is important to reduce cardiovascular mortality, the most important cause of death globally.[125] Cardiovascular risk factors and IHD can be better managed when high-quality preventive and emergency services are available at all types of locations (rural, underserved urban, and urban). High-quality health systems for acute cardiovascular care that are available, accessible, and affordable are crucial. Novel health financing mechanisms should be developed to provide comprehensive universal health care globally. Strategies to improve care include better training of physicians and task-sharing for routine preventive care with nonphysician health workers. Low educational status influences cardiovascular risk over the life-course, from womb to tomb. Better quality of general education is crucial to prevent cardiovascular risk factors and diseases. And finally, high-quality universal primary health care, free at the point of delivery, is crucial to promote availability and affordability of medicines and promote lifelong adherence.

REFERENCES

1. Marmot M, Wilkinson RG. *Social Determinants of Heath*. Oxford: Oxford University Press; 1999.

2. Berkman L, Kawachi I. *Social Epidemiology*. New York: Oxford University Press; 2000:13-35.

3. Leon D, Walt G. *Poverty, Inequality and Health: an International Perspective*. Oxford: Oxford University Press; 2001.

4. Gaziano TA, Prabhakaran D, Gaziano JM. Global burden of cardiovascular disease. In: Zipes D, Libby P, Bonow RO, Mann DL, Tomaselli GF, Eds. *Braunwald's Heart Disease: a Textbook of Cardiovascular Medicine*. 11th Ed. New York: Elsevier; 2019:1-18.

5. Marmot M, Bartley M. Social class and coronary heart disease. In: Stansfeld S, Marmot M, Eds. *Stress and the Heart*. London: BMJ Books; 2002:5-19.

6. Braveman P, Egerter S, Williams DR. The social determinants of health: coming of age. *Annu Rev Public Health*. 2011;32:381-398.

7. World Health Organization. Social determinants of health. Accessed July 12, 2020. www.who.int/social_determinants/sdh_definition/en/

8. Kaplan GA, Keil JE. Socioeconomic factors and cardiovascular disease: a review of the literature. *Circulation*. 1993;88:1973-1998.

9. Havranek EP, Mujahid MS, Barr DA, et al. American Heart Association Council on Quality of Care and Outcomes Research, Council on Epidemiology and Prevention, Council on Cardiovascular and Stroke Nursing, Council on Lifestyle and Cardiometabolic Health, and Stroke Council. Social determinants of risk and outcomes for cardiovascular disease: a scientific statement from the American Heart Association. *Circulation*. 2015;132:873-898.

10. Gupta R, Wood DA. Primary prevention of ischemic heart disease: populations, individuals and healthcare professionals. *Lancet*. 2019;394:685-696.

11. Brunner EJ. Social factors and cardiovascular morbidity. *Neurosci Biobehavioral Rev*. 2017;74B:260-268.

12. Cosby AG, McDoom-Echebiri MM, James W, et al. Growth and persistence of place-based mortality in the United States: the rural mortality penalty. *Am J Public Health*. 2019;109:155-162.

13. Harrington RA, Califf RM, Balamurugan A, et al. Call to action: rural health: a Presidential Advisory from the American Heart Association and American Stroke Association. *Circulation*. 2020;141:e615-e644.

14. Kulshreshtha A, Goyal A, Dabhadkar K, et al. Urban-rural differences in coronary heart disease mortality in the United States: 1999-2009. *Pub Health Rep*. 2014;129:19-29.

15. Cross SH, Mehra MR, Bhatt DL, et al. Rural-urban differences in cardiovascular mortality in the US. *JAMA*. 2020;323:1852-1854.

16. Wadhera RK, Khatana SAM, Choi E, et al. Disparities in care and mortality among homeless adults hospitalised for cardiovascular conditions. *JAMA Intern Med*. 2019;180:357-366.

17. Yusuf S, Rangarajan S, Teo K, et al. Cardiovascular risk and events in 17 low-, middle- and high-income countries. *N Engl J Med*. 2014;371:818-827.

18. Zhang X, Khan AA, Haq EU, et al. Increasing mortality from ischemic heart disease in China from 2004 to 2010: disproportionate rise in rural areas and elderly subjects, 438 million person-years follow-up. *Eur Heart J Qual Care Clin Outcomes*. 2017;3:47-52.

19. Ke C, Gupta R, Xavier D, et al. Divergent trends in ischemic heart disease and stroke mortality in India from 2000 to 2015: a nationally representative mortality survey. *Lancet Glob. Health*. 2018;6:e914-e923.

20. Chauhan U. Cardiovascular disease prevention in primary care. *Br Med Bull*. 2007;81:65-79.

21. Deligiannidis KE. Primary care issues in rural populations. *Prim Care*. 2017;44:11-19.

22. Matthews KA, Croft JB, Liu Y, et al. Health related behaviours by urban-rural county classification—United States, 2013. *MMWR Surveill Summ*. 2017;66:1-8.

23. Piepoli MF, Hoes AW, Agewall S, et al. 2016 European Guidelines on cardiovascular disease primary prevention in clinical practice. *Eur Heart J*. 2016;37:2315-2381.

24. Yusuf S, Reddy KS, Ounpuu S, et al. Global burden of cardiovascular diseases: part 1: general considerations, the epidemiological transition, risk factors and impact of urbanization. *Circulation*. 2001;104:2746-2753.

25. Kreatsoulas C, Anand SS. The impact of social determinants on cardiovascular disease. *Can J Cardiol*. 2010; 26(Suppl C):8C-13C.

26. Gupta R, Khedar RS, Gaur K, et al. Low quality cardiovascular care is important coronary risk factor in India. *Indian Heart J*. 2018;70(Suppl 3):s419-s430.

27. Neissen LW, Mohan D, Akuoko JK, et al. Tackling socioeconomic inequalities and non-communicable diseases in low-income and middle-income countries under the Sustainable Development agenda. *Lancet*. 2018;391:2036-2046.

28. Gupta R, Yusuf S. Challenges in ischemic heart disease management and prevention in low socioeconomic status people in low and lower-middle income countries. *BMC Med*. 2019;17:e209.

29. Samanic CM, Barbour KE, Liu Y, et al. Prevalence of self-reported hypertension and antihypertensive medication use by county and rural-urban classification-United States 2017. *MMWR Morb Mortal Wkly Rep*. 2020;69:533-539.

30. Geldsetzer P, Manne-Goehler J, Marcus M-E, et al. The state of hypertension care in 44 low-income and middle-income countries: a cross sectional study of nationally representative individual-level data from 1.1 million adults. *Lancet*. 2019;393:652-662.

31. NCD Risk Factor Collaboration. Long term and recent trends in hypertension awareness, treatment and control in 12 high-income countries: an analysis of 123 nationally representative surveys. *Lancet*. 2019;394:639-651.

32. Kelley AT, Nocon RS, O'Brien MJ. Diabetes management in community health centers: a review of policies and programs. *Curr Diab Rep*. 2020;20:e8.

33. Shivashankar R, Kirk K, Kim WC, et al. Quality of diabetes care in low- and middle-income Asian and Middle Eastern countries (1993-2012): 20-year systematic review. *Diabetes Res Clin Pract*. 2015;107:203-223.

34. Murphy A, Fario-Neto JR, Al-Rasadi K, et al. World Heart Federation cholesterol roadmap. *Glob Heart*. 2017;12:179-197.

35. Egan MBM, Li J, Sarasua SM, et al. Cholesterol control among uninsured adults did not improve from 2001-2004 to 2009-2012 as disparities with both publicly and privately insured adults doubled. *J Am Heart Assoc*. 2017;6:e0006.

36. Goff DC, Bertoni AG, Kramer H, et al. Dyslipidemia prevalence, treatment and control in the Multi-Ethnic Study of Atherosclerosis(MESA): Gender, ethnicity and coronary artery calcium. *Circulation*. 2006;113:647-656.

37. Allison JJ, Kiefe CI, Weissman NW, et al. Relationship of hospital teaching status with quality of care and mortality for Medicare patients with acute MI. *JAMA*. 2000;284:1256-1262.

38. Hartz A, James PA. A systematic review of studies comparing myocardial infarction mortality for generalists and specialists: lessons for research and health policy. *J Am Board Fam Med*. 2006;19:291-302.

39. Rajbhandari R, McMahon DE, Rhatigan JJ, et al. The neglected hospital-the district hospital's central role in global health care delivery. *N Engl J Med*. 2020;382:397-400.

40. Smith SC, Benjamin EJ, Bonow RO, et al. AHA/ACCF secondary prevention and risk reduction therapy for patients with coronary and other vascular disease: 2011 update. *J Am Coll Cardiol*. 2011;58:2432-2446.

41. Virani SS, Alonso A, Benjamin EJ, et al. Heart disease and stroke statistics-2020 update: a report from the American Heart Association. *Circulation*. 2020;141:e139-596.

42. Kotseva K, De Baquer D, Jennings C, et al. Time trends in lifestyle, risk factor control and use of evidence based medications in patients with coronary heart disease in Europe: Results from 3 EUROASPIRE surveys, 1999-2013. *Glob Heart*. 2017;12:315-322.

43. Yusuf S, Islam S, Chow CK, et al. Low use of secondary prevention medications for cardiovascular disease in the community in 17 high, middle and low income countries (The PURE Study). *Lancet*. 2011;378:1231-1243.

44. Niu S, Zhao D, Zhu J, et al. The association between socioeconomic status of high-risk patients with coronary heart disease secondary prevention in China: Results from the Bridging the Gap on CHD Secondary Prevention in China (BRIG) Project. *Am Heart J*. 2009;157:709-715.

45. Sharma KK, Gupta R, Agrawal A, et al. Low use of statins and other coronary secondary prevention therapies in primary and secondary care in India. *Vasc Health Risk Manag*. 2009;5:1007-1014.

46. Bansilal S, Castalleno JM, Fuster V. Global burden of CVD: focus on secondary prevention of cardiovascular disease. *Int J Cardiol*. 2015;201 (Suppl 1):S1-S7.

47. Yusuf S, Wood D, Ralston J, et al. The World Heart Federation's vision for worldwide cardiovascular disease prevention. *Lancet*. 2015;386:399-402.

48. Kruk ME, Gage AD, Joseph NT, et al. Mortality due to low-quality health systems in the universal health coverage era: a systematic analysis of amenable deaths in 137 countries. *Lancet*. 2018;392:2203-2212.

49. Joshi R, Thrift AG, Smith C, et al. Task-shifting for cardiovascular risk factor management: lessons from the Global Alliance for Chronic Diseases. *BMJ Glob Health*. 2018;3:e001092.

50. Joshi R, Agarwal T, Fathima F, et al. Evaluation of community health worker led intervention in control of cardiovascular risk factors in rural populations in India: a cluster randomized trial. *Am Heart J*. 2019;216:9-19.

51. Schwalm JD, McCready T, Lopez-Jaramillo P, et al. a community based comprehensive intervention to reduce cardiovascular risk in hypertension (HOPE-4): a cluster randomized controlled trial. *Lancet*. 2019;394:1231-1242.

52. Victor RG, Lynch K, Li N, et al. A cluster randomized trial of blood pressure reduction in black barbershops. *N Engl J Med*. 2018;378:1291-1301.

53. Nugent R, Bertram MY, Jan S, et al. Investing in non-communicable disease prevention and management to advance the Sustainable Development Goals. *Lancet*. 2018;391:2029-2035.

54. Pahigiannis K, Thompson-Paul AM, Barfield W, et al. Progress towards improved cardiovascular health in the United States. *Circulation*. 2019;139:1957-1973.

55. Unal B, Critchley JA, Capewell S. Explaining the decline in coronary heart disease mortality in England and Wales between 1981 and 2000. *Circulation*. 2004;109:1101-1107.

56. Ford ES, Ajani UA, Croft JB, et al. Explaining the decrease in US deaths from coronary disease, 1980-2000. *N Engl J Med*. 2007;356:2388-2398.

57. Szummer K, Wallentin L, Lindhagen L, et al. Relations between implementation of new treatments and improved outcomes in patients with non-ST elevation myocardial infarction during the last 20 years: experience from SWEDEHEART registry 1995 to 2014. *Eur Heart J*. 2018;39:3766-3776.

58. British Cardiac Society, Royal College of Physicians London, Royal College of Physicians Edinburgh, Royal College of Physicians and Surgeons Glasgow. The changing interface between district hospital cardiology and major cardiac centres. *Heart*. 1997;78:519-523.

59. Le May M, van Diepen S, Liszkowski M, et al. From coronary care units to cardiac intensive care units: recommendations for organizational, staffing and educational transformation. *Can J Cardiol*. 2016;32:1204-1213.

60. Jneid H, Addison D, Bhatt DL, et al. 2017 AHA/ACC clinical performance and quality measures for adults with ST-elevation and non-ST-elevation myocardial infarction: a report for the American College of Cardiology/American Heart Association Taskforce on performance measures. *J Am Coll Cardiol*. 2017;70:2048-2090.

61. Ibanez B, James S, Agewall S, et al. 2017 ESC guidelines for the management of patients of acute myocardial infarction in patients presenting with ST-segment elevation: the Task Force for the management of acute myocardial infarction in patients presenting with ST-segment elevation of the European Society of Cardiology. *Eur Heart J*. 2018;39:119-177.

62. Van Diepen S, Fordyce CBV, Wegerman ZK, et al. Organizational structure, staffing, resources, and educational initiatives in cardiac intensive care units in the United States. *Circ Cardiovasc Qual Outcomes*. 2017;10:e003864.

63. Lodi-Junqueira L, Ribeiro AL. Tackling acute coronary syndrome in low-income and middle-income countries. *Heart*. 2018;104:1390-1391.

64. Nascimento BR, Brant LCC, Marino BCA, et al. Implementing myocardial infarction systems of care in low/middle income countries. *Heart*. 2019;105:20-26.

65. Alexander T, Mullasari AS, Joseph G, et al. A system of care for patients with ST-segment elevation myocardial infarction in India: The Tamilnadu ST-segment elevation myocardial infarction program. *JAMA Cardiol*. 2017;2:498-505.

66. Mehta S, Botelho R, Cade J, et al. Global challenges and solutions: role of telemedicine in ST-elevation myocardial infarction interventions. *Interv Cardiol Clin*. 2016;5:569-581.

67. Corra U. Cardiac rehabilitation and exercise training. In: Camm AJ, Luscher TF, Maurer G, Serruys PW, Eds. *ESC Textbook of Cardiovascular Medicine*. 3rd Ed. Oxford: Oxford University Press; 2019:882-892.

68. Xavier D, Gupta R, Sigamani A, et al. Community health worker based intervention for adherence to medications and lifestyle modifications after acute coronary syndrome: a randomized controlled trial. *Lancet Diab Endocrinol*. 2016;4:244-253.

69. Huang K, Liu W, He D, et al. Telehealth interventions versus center-based cardiac rehabilitation of coronary artery disease: a systematic review and meta-analysis. *Eur J Prev Cardiol*. 2015;22:959-971.

70. Bhavnani SP, Parakh K, Atreja A, et al. 2017 Roadmap for innovation-ACC health policy statement on healthcare transformation in the era of digital, big data and precision health: a report of the American College of Cardiology task force on health policy statements and systems of care. *J Am Coll Cardiol*. 2017;70:2696-2718.

71. Castellano JM, Sanz G, Penalvo JL, et al. A polypill strategy to improve adherence: results from the FOCUS project. *J Am Coll Cardiol*. 2014;64:2071-2082.

72. Roshandel G, Khoshina M, Poustchi H, et al. Effectiveness of polypill for primary and secondary prevention of cardiovascular diseases (PolyIran): a pragmatic, cluster-randomised trial. *Lancet*. 2019;394:672-683.

73. Choudhry NK. Randomized controlled trials in health insurance systems. *N Engl J Med*. 2017;377:957-964.

74. World Health Organization. *Teaching of public health in medical schools: report of the regional meeting, Bangkok, Thailand*. New Delhi: South East Asia Regional Office; 2010.

75. Aspry KE, Van Horn L, Carson JAS, et al. American Heart Association Nutrition Committee of the Council on Lifestyle and Cardiometabolic Health; Council on Cardiovascular and Stroke Nursing; Council on Cardiovascular Radiology and Intervention; and Stroke Council. Medical nutrition education, training and competencies to advance guideline-based diet counselling by physicians: a science advisory from the American Heart Association. *Circulation*. 2018;137:e821-e841.

76. Lianov L, Johnson M. Physician competencies for prescribing lifestyle medicine. *JAMA*. 2010;304:202-203.

77. Connolly SB, Kotseva K, Jennings C, et al. Outcomes of an integrated community based nurse-led cardiovascular prevention programme. *Heart*. 2017;103:840-847.

78. Gupta R. Health systems in post-covid-19 era: strengthening primary care and district hospitals. *RUHS J Health Sciences*. 2020;5:61-65.

79. Morrow DA, Fang JC, Fintel DJ, et al. Evolution of critical care cardiology: transformation of the cardiovascular intensive care unit and the emerging need for new medical staffing and training modules: a scientific statement from the American Heart Association. *Circulation.* 2012;126:1408-1428.

80. Schultz WM, Kelli HM, Lisko JC, et al. Socioeconomic status and cardiovascular outcomes: Challenges and interventions. *Circulation.* 2018;137: 2166-2178.

81. Tobias M. Social rank: a risk factor whose time has come? *Lancet.* 2017;389:1172-1174.

82. Yusuf S, Joseph P, Rangarajan S, et al. Modifiable risk factors, cardiovascular disease, and mortality in 155,722 individuals from 21 high-income, middle-income, and low-income countries (PURE): a prospective cohort study. *Lancet.* 2020;395:795-808.

83. Editorial. Education: a neglected social determinant of health. *Lancet Public Health.* 2020;5:e361.

84. Prabhakaran D, Jeemon P, Roy A. Cardiovascular diseases in India: current epidemiology and future directions. *Circulation.* 2016;133:1605-1620.

85. Woodward M, Peters SA, Batty GD, et al. Asia Pacific Cohort Studies Collaboration. *BMJ Open.* 2015;5:e006408.

86. Pednekar M, Gupta R, Gupta PC. Illiteracy, low educational status and cardiovascular mortality in India. *BMC Public Health.* 2011;11:e568.

87. Rosengren A, Subramanian SV, Islam S, et al. Education and risk of acute myocardial infarction in 52 high, middle and low-income countries: INTERHEART case-control study. *Heart.* 2009;95:2014-2022.

88. Rosengren A, Smyth A, Rangarajan S, et al. Socioeconomic status and risk of cardiovascular disease in 20 low-income, middle-income and high income countries: the Prospective Urban Rural Epidemiology (PURE) study. *Lancet Glob Health.* 2019;7:e748-e760.

89. Rozanski A, Blumenthal JA, Davidson KW, et al. The epidemiology, pathophysiology and management of psychosocial risk factors in cardiac practice: the emerging field of behavioral cardiology. *J Am Coll Cardiol.* 2005;45:637-651.

90. Lindblom R, Ververis K, Tortorella SM, et al. The early life origin theory in the development of cardiovascular disease and type 2 diabetes. *Mol Biol Rep.* 2015;42:791-797.

91. O'Keefe LM, Simkin AJ, Tilling K, et al. Data on trajectories of measures of cardiovascular health in the Avon Longitudinal Study of Parents and Children (ALSPAC). *Data Brief.* 2019;23:103687.

92. Joshi P, Islam S, Pais P, et al. Risk factors for early myocardial infarction in South Asians compared with individuals in other countries. *JAMA* 2007;297:286-294.

93. Allen L, Williams J, Townsend N, et al. Socioeconomic status and non-communicable disease behavioral risk factors in low-income and lower-middle income countries. *Lancet Glob Health.* 2017;5:e277-e289.

94. Arnett DK, Blumenthal RS, Albert MA, et al. 2019 ACC/AHA guidelines on the primary prevention of cardiovascular disease: a report of the American College of Cardiology/American Heart Association Task Force on Clinical Practice guidelines. *J Am Coll Cardiol.* 2019;74: e177-e232.

95. Xavier D, Pais P, Devereaux PJ, et al. Treatment and outcomes of acute coronary syndromes in India (CREATE): a prospective analysis of registry data. *Lancet.* 2008;371:1435-1442.

96. Alter DA, Iron K, Austin PC, et al. Socioeconomic status, service patterns, and perceptions of care among survivors of acute myocardial infarction in Canada, *JAMA.* 2004;291:1100-1107.

97. Ades PA. Cardiac rehabilitation and secondary prevention of coronary heart disease. *N Engl J Med.* 2001;345:892-902.

98. Oserberg L, Blaschke T. Adherence to medication. *N Engl J Med.* 2005;353:487-497.

99. Zhang NJ, Terry A, McHorney CA. Impact of health literacy on medication adherence: a systematic review and meta-analysis. *Ann Pharmacother.* 2014;48:741-751.

100. United Nations. Sustainable development goals. Accessed Aug 3, 2020. https://www.un.org/sustainabledevelopment/sustainable-development-goals/

101. Global Education Monitoring Report Team. 2020 global education monitoring report: all means all. Accessed August 3, 2020. https://unesdoc.unesco.org/ark:/48223/pf0000373718

102. Roland M, Everington S, Marshall M. Social prescribing—transforming the relationship between physicians and their patients. *N Engl J Med.* 2020;383:97-99.

103. National Information Center on Healthcare Resources and Healthcare Technology. Health economics information resource. Accessed August 3, 2020. https://www.nlm.nih.gov/nichsr/edu/healthecon/glossary.html

104. Joshi R, Jan S, Wu Y, et al. Global inequalities in access to cardiovascular health care: our greatest challenge. *J Am Coll Cardiol.* 2008;52:1817-1825.

105. Wirt VJ, Kaplan WA, Kwan GF, et al. Access to medications for cardiovascular diseases in low- and middle-income countries. *Circulation.* 2016;133:2076-2085.

106. Ferdinand KC, Senatore FF, Clayton-Jeter H, et al. Improving medical adherence in cardiometabolic disease: practical and regulatory implications. *J Am Coll Cardiol.* 2017;69:437-445.

107. Psotka MA, Fiuzat M, Solomon SD, et al. Challenges and potential improvements to patient access to pharmaceuticals. *Circulation.* 2020;142:790-798.

108. Ewen M, Zwekhorst M, Reeger B, et al. Baseline assessment of WHO's target for both availability and affordability of essential medicines to treat non-communicable diseases. *PLoS One.* 2017;12:e0171284.

109. Khatib R, McKee M, Shannon H, et al. Availability and affordability of cardiovascular disease medicines and their impact on use: comparison across high, middle, and low-income countries. *Lancet.* 2016;387:61-69.

110. Attaei MW, Khatib R, McKee M, et al. Availability and affordability of blood pressure-lowering medicines and the effect on blood pressure control in high-income, middle-income, and low-income countries: an analysis of the PURE study data. *Lancet Public Health.* 2017;2:e411-e419.

111. Husain MJ, Datta BK, Kostova D, et al. Access to cardiovascular disease and hypertension medicines in developing countries: an analysis of essential medicine price lists, price, availability and affordability. *J Am Heart Assoc.* 2020;9:e015302.

112. Cameron A, Ewen M, Ross-Degnan D, et al. Medicine prices, availability and affordability in 36 developing and middle-income countries: a secondary analysis. *Lancet.* 2009;373:240-249.

113. Schneider EC. Healthcare as an ongoing policy project. *N Engl J Med.* 2020;383:405-408.

114. Evans MK. Covid's color line: infectious disease, inequity and racial justice. *N Engl J Med.* 2020;383:408-410.

115. Chow CK, Nguyen T, Marschner S, et al. Availability and affordability of medicines and cardiovascular outcomes in high-income, middle-income and low-income countries: an analysis of the PURE study data. *BMJ Glob Health.* 2020. doi: 10.1136/bmjgh-2020-002640.

116. Saltman RB. Health care systems in developed countries. In: Jameson JL, Kasper DL, Longo DL, Fauci AS, Hauser SL, Loscalzo J, Eds. *Harrison's Principles of Internal Medicine.* 20th Ed. New York: McGraw Hill; 2018: 27-33.

117. Warner JJ, Benjamin IJ, Churchwell K, et al. Advancing healthcare reform: the American Heart Association's 2020 statement of principles for adequate, accessible and affordable health care. *Circulation.* 2020;141:e1-e14.

118. Murphy A, Palafox B, O'Donnell O, et al. Inequalities in the use of secondary prevention of cardiovascular disease by socioeconomic status: evidence from the PURE observational study. *Lancet Glob Health.* 2018;6:e292-e301.

119. Gaur K, Mohan I, Kaur M, et al. Escalating ischemic heart disease burden among women in India: Insights from GBD, NCDRisC and NFHS reports. *Am J Prev Cardiol.* 2020;2:100035.

120. Marmot M, Allen J, Boyce T, et al. *Health Equity in England: the Marmot Review Ten Years on.* London: Institute of Health Equity; 2020.

121. Neissen LW, Mohan D, Akuoko JK, et al. Tackling socioeconomic inequalities and non-communicable diseases in low-income and middle-income countries under the Sustainable Development agenda. *Lancet.* 2018;391:2036-2046.

122. Blumenthal D, Fowler EJ, Abrams M, et al. Covid-19: implications for the healthcare system. *N Engl J Med.* 2020. doi: 10.1056/NEJMsb2021088.

123. Seidman G, Atun R. Does task shifting yield cost savings and improve efficiency for health systems? A systematic review of evidence from low-income and middle-income countries. *Hum Resources Health.* 2017;15:29.

124. Widmer RJ, Collins NM, Collins CS, et al. Digital health interventions for the prevention of cardiovascular disease: a systematic review and meta-analysis. *Mayo Clin Proc.* 2015;90:469-480.

125. Global Burden of Disease Study 2019 Diseases and Injuries Collaborators. Global burden of 369 diseases and injuries in 204 countries and territories, 1990-2019: a systematic analysis for the Global Burden of Disease Study 2019. *Lancet.* 2020;396:1204-1222.

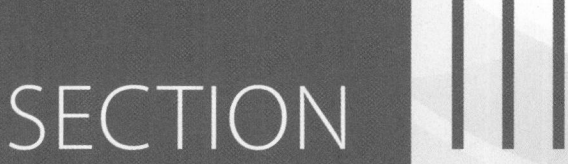

SECTION III

ATHEROSCLEROSIS AND CORONARY HEART DISEASE

Pathological Basis of Atherosclerotic Coronary Artery Disease

Jagat Narula, Renu Virmani, Navneet Narula, Borja Ibanez, and Valentin Fuster

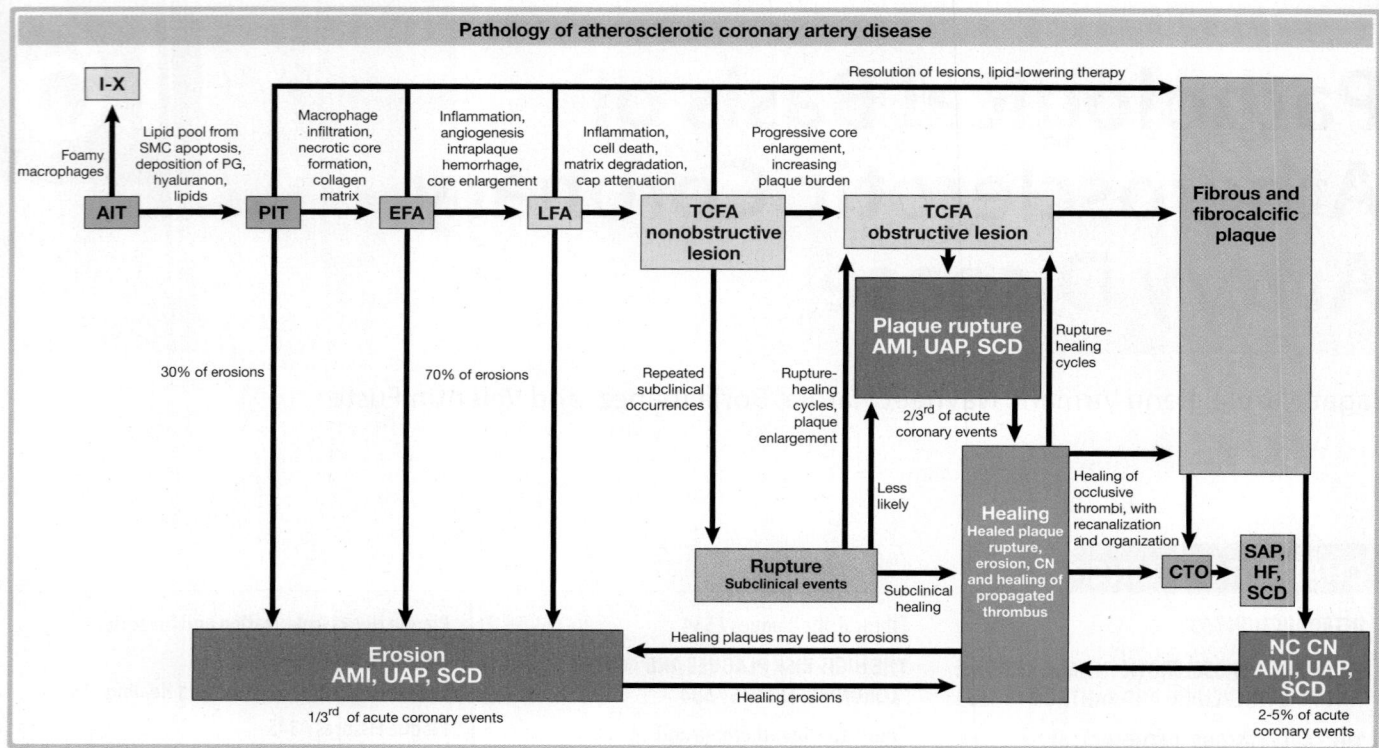

Chapter 16 Fuster and Hurst's Central Illustration. The red boxes (plaque rupture, erosion or calcified nodules) represent the pathologic basis of acute coronary syndromes. Plaque rupture is thought to be responsible for at least two-thirds of cases of coronary thrombosis and subsequent acute coronary events; plaque erosion accounts for most of the remaining cases, and calcified nodules contribute to less than 5% of adverse outcomes. I-X, intimal xanthoma; AIT, adaptive intimal thickening; PIT, pathological intimal thickening; EFA, early fibroatheroma; LFA, late fibroatheroma; TCFA, thin-cap fibroatheraoma; AMI, acute myocardial infarction; UAP, unstable angina pectoris; SCD, sudden cardiac death; CTO, chronic total occlusion; SAP, stable angina pectoris; HF, heart failure; NC, nodular calcification; CN, calcified nodules.

CHAPTER SUMMARY

This chapter describes plaque characteristics contributing to coronary thrombosis, provides mechanistic insights into lesion progression, and summarizes diagnostic imaging. At least half of both physiologically and anatomically significant lesions do not fair worse with modern medical therapy than with revascularization, and it is likely that the plaques of event-free patients are stable or have low wall shear stress. Recognition of high-risk plaques is prudent, and it is thus important for clinicians to understand the pathology of atherosclerotic disease of coronary arteries (see Fuster and Hurst's Central Illustration). Plaque rupture is thought to be responsible for at least two-thirds of cases of coronary thrombosis and subsequent acute coronary events, including sudden death; plaque erosion accounts for most of the remaining cases of thrombosis, and calcified nodules contribute to less than 5% of adverse outcomes. The importance of progressively increasing necrotic core burden covered by thin and inflamed fibrous caps is highlighted. The rapid enlargement of plaques is attributed to repeated subclinical plaque rupture–thrombosis–healing cycles. On the other hand, fibroatheromatous, fibrous or fibrocalcific plaques in the absence of overlying thrombosis, and the presence of significant luminal obstruction form the basis of stable chest pain syndromes. Native coronary atherosclerosis develops over decades to result in clinical events and differs from clinical events associated with accelerated vein graft atherosclerosis or in-stent neoatherosclerosis.

INTRODUCTION

More than 50 years ago, when the risk factors for coronary artery disease had become established, injury to the arterial wall from the risk factors was proposed to be the basis of phenotypic alteration and proliferation of medial smooth muscle cell (SMC) resulting in their subendothelial migration and development of neointimal atherosclerotic lesions.[1,2] Although SMC migration remains a major player in the pathogenesis of atherosclerosis, inflammatory cells and consequent local cytokine milieu were later found to be the *primum movens* for disease initiation, maturation, progression, and plaque rupture or even erosion.[3–5] With the increasing understanding of pathogenesis of atherosclerosis, a pathological classification was developed to describe the evolution of disease.[6–8] The classification captured pathological manifestations of early neointimal lesions and advanced plaques, and recognized that deep plaque fissures and ulcerations were responsible for development of luminal thrombosis and clinical manifestations of acute coronary syndrome. The lesions were classified by the American Heart Association (AHA) as (I) intimal thickening, (II) fatty streak formation, (III) pre-atheroma, (IV) atheroma with well-defined intimal cap, (V) fibroatheroma or atheroma with overlaid new fibrous connective tissue, and (VI) complicated lesions with surface defects, hemorrhage, thrombosis, calcification, or a combination of these characteristics.[8] An appropriate emphasis on the recognition of precursor lesions that potentially gave rise to clinical events was subsequently incorporated in the clinicopathological correlative classification.[9] Identification of important structural plaque characteristics conceivably leading to coronary thrombosis was expected to provide mechanistic insights into lesion progression, and develop diagnostic imaging.[9] Whereas plaque rupture was suggested to be responsible for 65% to 75% cases of coronary thrombosis and hence acute events including sudden death; plaque erosion accounted for 25% to 30% of thrombosis, and the less frequent eruptive calcified nodules occurred in up to 5% of victims of sudden death. In the modified scheme,[9] AHA lesion types I to IV were replaced by descriptive terms including adaptive intimal thickening, intimal xanthoma, pathological intimal thickening (PIT), and (early and late) fibroatheroma (see Fuster and Hurst's Central Illustration).[10] Early and late fibroatheromas could evolve as fibrous and fibrocalcific plaques or thin-cap fibroatheroma (TCFA). AHA categories V and VI were modified to assign pathological substrate to three major complications: rupture, erosion, and calcified nodule associated with overlying luminal thrombosis. Whereas the precursor lesion to plaque rupture (high-risk or vulnerable plaque) was descriptively included as TCFA, erosion was expected to emanate from PIT, and calcified nodules could result from fibrocalcific plaques.[9] The plaque fissures and ulcers, described in the mid-1980s as communication between the lumen and necrotic core,[11] were considered nuanced terms for disruption of surface continuity and could fall under the broader category of plaque rupture. The sudden enlargement of plaques was attributed to repeated subclinical plaque rupture–thrombosis–healing cycles, referred to as healed plaque rupture (HPR).[9] The HPR or even healed erosions could lend to luminal narrowing and chronic total occlusion (CTO). The modified classification attributed plaque stability to fibroatheromatous, fibrous or fibrocalcific plaques in the absence of overlying thrombosis; such plaques in presence of significant luminal obstruction formed the basis of stable chest pain syndromes. The native coronary atherosclerosis develops over decades to result in clinical events and differs from clinical events associated with accelerated vein graft atherosclerosis or in-stent neoatherosclerosis that evolve within months to a few years.

THE NONATHEROSCLEROTIC INTIMAL LESIONS: INTIMAL THICKENING AND XANTHOMAS

The diffuse intimal thickening is observed in medium and large arteries including coronary arteries, which are prone to develop atherosclerosis.[12] It is an adaptive response of the vasculature in postnatal physiology. The adaptive thickening progressively worsens at the branch point where more-advanced lesions are expected to develop in adults.[13,14] The regions of intimal thickening contain widely spaced SMC accumulation with proteoglycan-rich extracellular matrix (ECM) but without inflammation. Intimal xanthomas or fatty streaks, on the other hand, represent early subendothelial foam cells that are predominantly macrophages and few SMC.[15,16] These lesions do not progress to advanced atherosclerosis and are more likely to regress[17–19] (**Fig. 16–1**).

Imaging data addressing the occurrence and fate of intimal thickening and xanthoma are scant. Correlative pathological and optical coherence tomography (OCT) imaging studies have respectively demonstrated intimal thickening with a signal-rich high backscatter appearance, and presence of foamy macrophages as focal signal-rich regions close to the luminal surface.

THE EARLY LESIONS: PATHOLOGICAL INTIMAL THICKENING WITH OR WITHOUT INFLAMMATION

PIT (**Fig. 16–2**) is the first atherosclerotic lesion that progresses and could evolve into more mature lesions over time or even lend itself to an erosive thrombotic complication. The ECM is rich in proteoglycans which could define evolving characteristics of the lesions. For instance, Decorin is not observed in SMC-rich healthy intima,[20] but has been reported in zones with reduced staining for SMC α-actin,[21] which facilitates the retention of apoB-100 in early PIT.[22] In addition to direct insudation from plasma low-density lipoprotein (LDL),[23] small cholesterol pools in PIT might also be derived from membranes of dead SMC.[24] On the other hand, ECM rich in versican promotes monocyte adhesion,[25–27] and might be one of the initial amplification steps contributing to inflammation in atherosclerosis, wherein macrophages are attracted to the lipid pools, evolve into foam cells, and eventually undergo necrosis.[28] The inflammatory cells are observed more superficially in these lesions, and the extracellular lipid is observed under layers of macrophage-derived foam cells close to the medial wall,[9,29] often

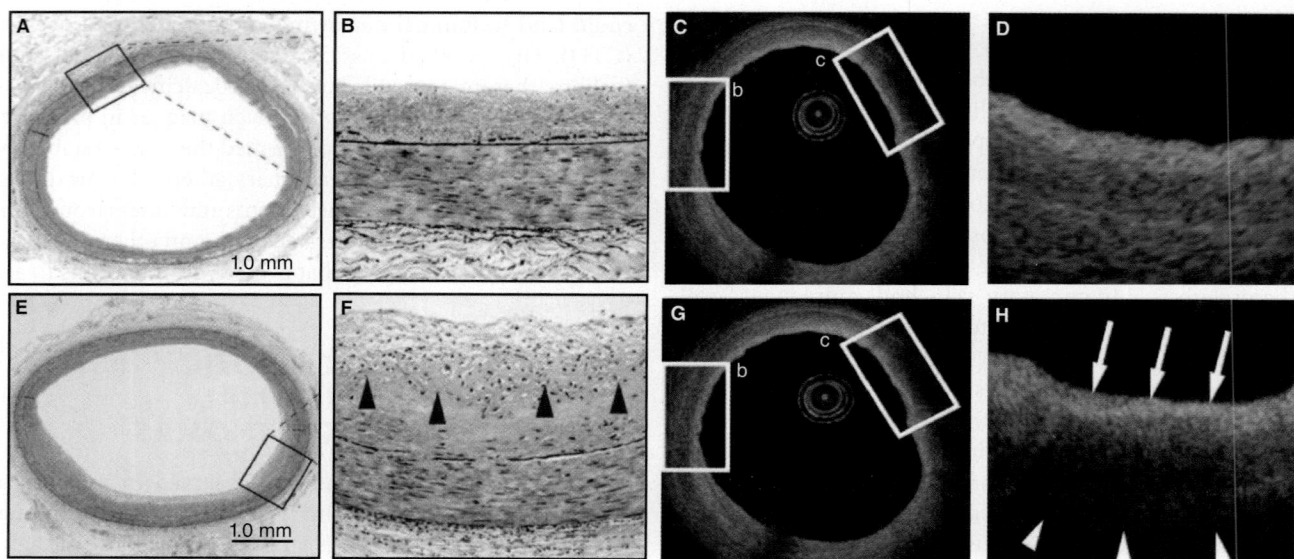

Figure 16–1. Nonatherosclerotic intimal lesions. Histological and OCT images are shown for intimal thickening (**A–D**), and intimal xanthoma (**E–H**). Intimal thickening is characterized by proteoglycan-rich ECM with widely spaced SMC accumulation but no inflammation or lipid accumulation. Intimal xanthomas represent early subendothelial foam cells that are predominantly macrophages and few lipid-laden SMC. Adaptive intimal thickening progresses at branch points where advanced atherosclerotic lesions develop in adults. Xanthomas usually regress. The correlative OCT imaging studies ex vivo have demonstrated signal-rich high backscatter appearance in AIT, and presence of foamy macrophages in xanthomas is seen as focal signal-rich regions close to the luminal surface (arrowheads). A, B, E, F, Reproduced with permission from Abdelrahman KM, Chen MY, Dey AK, et al. Coronary Computed Tomography Angiography From Clinical Uses to Emerging Technologies: JACC State-of-the-Art Review. *J Am Coll Cardiol.* 2020 Sep 8;76(10):1226-1243. C, D, G, H, Reproduced with permission from Otsuka F, Joner M, Prati F, et al. Clinical classification of plaque morphology in coronary disease. *Nat Rev Cardiol.* 2014 Jul;11(7):379-389.

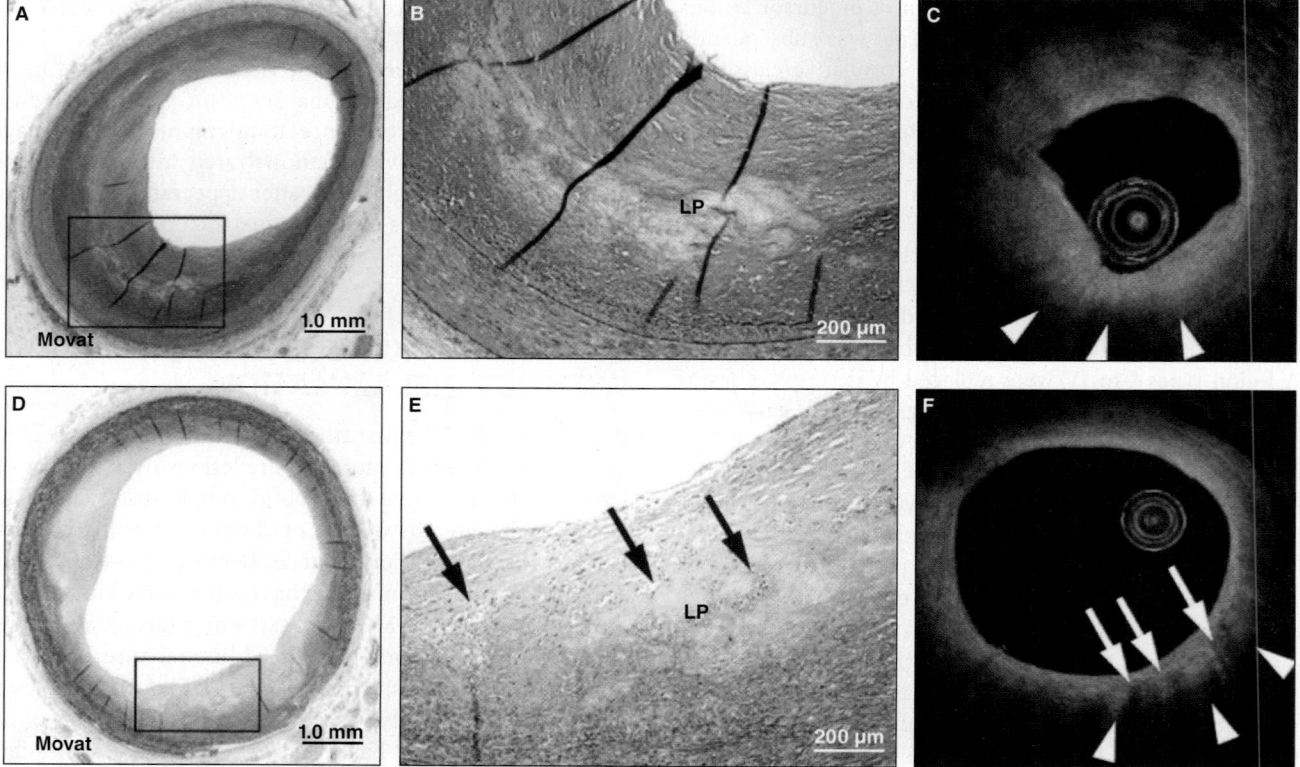

Figure 16–2. The early lesions: pathological intimal thickening. The histological and OCT images are shown for PIT without (**A–C**) and with (**D–F**) inflammation. As illustrated, PIT is composed of ECM rich in proteoglycans, collagen type III, SMC remnants, and lipid pools. Decorin-rich proteoglycan in the intima loses SMC and facilitates retention of lipid predominantly from the plasma LDL as well as small pools may be derived from membranes of dead SMC. ECM that is rich in versican promotes monocyte accumulation (**E**). Hyaluranon-rich ECM is characteristically seen in erosive complications of PIT. The earliest signs of calcification (not shown here) could be seen associated with lipid pool. OCT imaging, in the absence of macrophages demonstrates focal thickening of the intimal layer with high backscattering signal (**C**), with or without modest attenuation of the light beam from a lipid pool deeper in the intimal layers (**F**). Reproduced with permission from Otsuka F, Joner M, Prati F, et al. Clinical classification of plaque morphology in coronary disease. *Nat Rev Cardiol.* 2014 Jul; 11(7):379-389.

near branch points.[30] The earliest signs of calcification can be observed within the lipid pool in PIT as a stippled von Kossa staining that likely originates from dying SMC.[31]

By OCT imaging, PIT in the absence of macrophages typically demonstrates focal thickening of the intimal layer with high backscattering signal, and moderate attenuation of the light beam from lipid pool deeper in the intimal layers. Distinct or confluent punctate signal-rich areas with shadowing of the underlying tissue is seen when macrophages are present in the superficial intima.[32,33] Rapid attenuation of the penetrating light beam is an important component of macrophage-rich lesions and explains the difficulty to distinguish the lipid pool of PIT from the necrotic core of fibroatheroma and TCFA.

THE MATURE LESIONS: DEVELOPMENT AND RESOLUTION OF ATHEROMATOUS CORES

Maturation of PIT leads to the development of fibroatheromatous lesions, and is associated with increasing inflammation, changing cytokine milieu, altered ground substance composition, differentiation of necrotic cores, and distinct evolution of a fibrous cap. The loss of scavenging inflammatory cells is associated with progressive calcification. Spontaneous and pharmacological resolution results in healing by fibrous and fibrocalcific elements.

Early and Late Fibroatheromas

Fibroatheromas consist of clearly demarcated lipid-rich necrotic core encapsulated by surrounding fibrous tissue[8,9] (Fig. 16–3). Macrophage proliferation into the extracellular lipid pool, foam cell formation, and cell death lead to the development of characteristic acellular necrotic core. The release of peptidases of *a disintegrin and metalloproteinase with thrombospondin motifs family* (ADAMTS) and active metalloproteinases (MMP) lead to a reduction in the proteoglycan and collagen ground substance with growing necrotic cores.[9,34] Formation of the necrotic core and shrinking ECM creates an overlying fibrous cap.[35–37] Two temporally distinct phases of the necrotic core formation have been described mostly on the basis of the extent of proteoglycans loss. Whereas in the early fibroatheroma, a transition from the lipid pool to the formation of the necrotic core begins, the late phase is associated with almost complete loss of proteoglycans, and the development of the necrotic core with debris, where the invading neoangiogenesis is associated with red blood cell (RBC) extravasation and intraplaque hemorrhage.[10,38,39] The fibrous cap in late fibroatheromas are typically thick, and composed of collagen type I and III and proteoglycans interspersed with SMC. However, enlarging necrotic core and diminishing ECM with cytokine excess leads to fibrous cap attenuation—hence, thin-cap fibroatheroma (TCFA), a forerunner of plaque rupture and

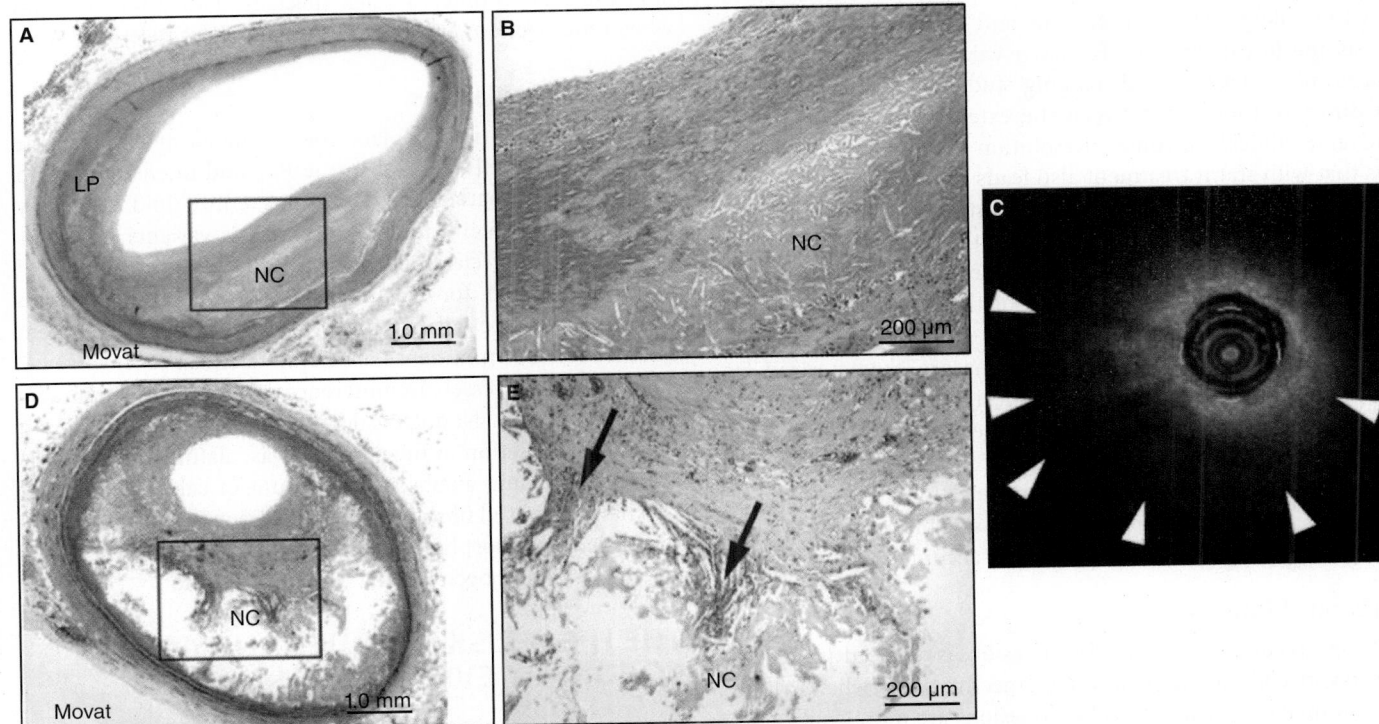

Figure 16–3. Early and late fibroatheromas. This mature lesion demonstrates formation of distinct necrotic core (NC) in presence of progressive inflammation and macrophage death, and overlying fibrous cap. The release of matrix-dissolving peptidases and metalloproteinases lead to a reduction in the proteoglycans and hyaluronan. With the initial proteoglycans loss and a transition of a lipid pool to a necrotic core first, the early fibroatheroma is established (A, B). The late fibroatheroma (D) is associated with complete loss of proteoglycans, with necrotic debris, associated with neoangiogenesis, erythrocytic leak, and intraplaque hemorrhage. RBC excess is associated with increased cholesterol clefts (*arrows*, E). The fibrous caps in late fibroatheromas are typically thick. Calcification (not shown here) occurs in the vicinity of dying cells in and around necrotic cores. OCT imaging (C) reveals superficial high backscattering bright signal and signal attenuation in the deeper plaque from necrotic core or intraplaque hemorrhage (C). Reproduced with permission from Otsuka F, Joner M, Prati F, et al. Clinical classification of plaque morphology in coronary disease. *Nat Rev Cardiol.* 2014 Jul;11(7):379-389.

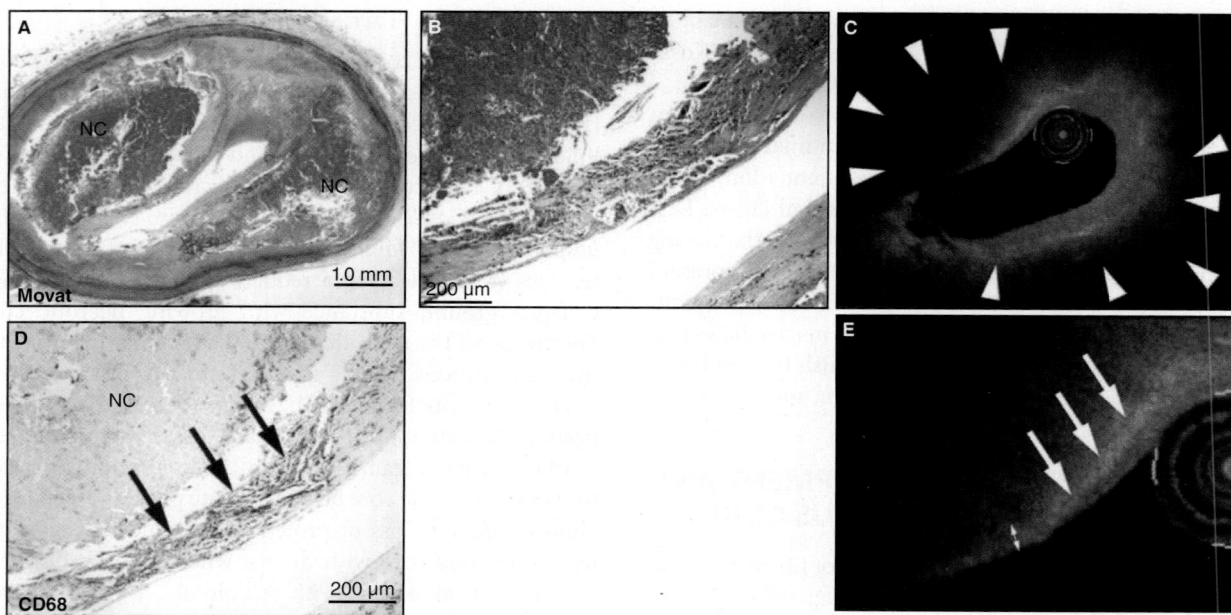

Figure 16–4. Thin-cap fibroatheroma. (A) A fibroatheromatous lesion in which the necrotic core (NC) is covered by a thin intact fibrous cap rendering the plaque vulnerable to rupture. The fibrous cap usually measures between 55 μm and 84 μm. These plaques are usually voluminous with a large NC burden and luminal stenosis. Whereas TCFA that are stenotic result in acute events, subclinical rupture of less occlusive lesions contributes to healing–rupture cycles, and plaque progression. The immunohistochemical staining (**D**) for macrophages (CD68) shows infiltration in the fibrous cap (*arrows*). OCT images demonstrate necrotic core (*arrowheads*, **C**) and the higher magnification of the OCT image (**E**) shows a high backscattering, signal-rich region that corresponds to the macrophages infiltration in thin fibrous cap. Reproduced with permission from Otsuka F, Joner M, Prati F, et al. Clinical classification of plaque morphology in coronary disease. *Nat Rev Cardiol.* 2014 Jul;11(7):379-389.

acute event (**Fig. 16–4**). The hydroxyapetite deposition occurs in the vicinity of dying cells in and around necrotic cores resulting in calcification. Excessive calcification could lead to fibrocalcific lesions, and imaging studies have demonstrated a direct relationship between the extent of calcification and adverse clinical outcomes. Resolution of necrotic cores such as that with statin treatment also leads to greater calcification. Rarely, nodular calcification grows nestled within the necrotic core and could serve as a precursor to the calcific nodule leading to acute plaque rupture regardless of the fibrous cap thickness. The restricted development of the necrotic core could lead to lipid-poor fibrous lesion.

Upon OCT imaging, fibroatheroma are characterized by superficial high backscattering bright signal, and there is a substantial signal attenuation of light in the deeper plaque regions, which could result from the necrotic core and hemorrhage. Since OCT only has limited tissue penetration, it does not lend to differentiation of necrotic core areas and intraplaque hemorrhage, and plaque areas also cannot be accurately measured.[40]

Fibrous Plaques

The intima or neointima in fibrous lesions is replaced and thickened with collagenous or fibrous connective tissue, wherein lipid is minimal or absent,[41,42] and such lesions are more commonly observed in arteries of the lower extremities.[43] Fibrotic lesions evolve from organization of thrombi, extension of the fibrous component of an adjacent fibroatheroma, or regression of lipid cores.[8] Increased wall shear stress associated with increased hydrostatic pressure in the lower extremities or hypertension as risk factor may play a role, but fibrogenic effects of cigarette smoking remain to be demonstrated. A restricted amount of

lipid can be encountered when specially stained for lipid and when serial sections are sought through the entire lesion.[8]

Fibrocalcific Plaques

Mineral deposits may replace the remnants of extracellular lipid and dead cells, earliest in the PIT and intensifying with evolution of fibroatheromatous lesions; entire lipid cores may be replaced by calcification.[8] Morphologic variants of calcification have been classified histologically according to size;[44] microcalcification for calcium particles ≥0.5 μm <15 μm diameter, punctate calcification >15 μm <1 mm, and fragment calcification ≥1 mm; dense sheets of calcification involve >1 quadrant of the vessel circumference or >3 mm in circumferential dimension. Nodular calcification is the least common form of calcification in the coronary vasculature. Fibrocalcific lesions containing a substantial amount of calcium generally also have increased fibrous connective tissue, and often there is the underlying morphology of fibroatheroma.[8] Elsewhere, the calcific lesion has been labeled the type VII lesion.[45–47]

THE HIGH-RISK PLAQUES AND ACUTE CORONARY EVENTS

Acute coronary events including myocardial infarction, sudden death, and unstable angina result from fibrous cap disruption of TCFA in two-thirds of patients. In the remaining one-third, surface erosion is responsible for the acute event; rarely, calcified nodules formed within the necrotic cores erupt through the fibroatheromatous lesion irrespective of the fibrous cap thickness.[48–50] Plaque rupture is more common in older men and women and is associated with traditional coronary risk factors.[51] The erosive lesions are observed in younger patients, more often women, and their lesions reveal less calcification and inflammation compared with plaque rupture; smoking is the commonest risk factor especially so in younger women.

Thin-Cap Fibroatheroma and Plaque Rupture

TCFA pathologically represent commonly used terms such as *vulnerable* or *high-risk* plaques.[9] They are a fibroatheromatous lesion where the distinct necrotic core is covered by a thin, well delineated, intact fibrous cap. The attenuated caps are prone to rupture and acute coronary events including myocardial infarction and sudden death. Histologically, TCFA has been described as the plaque that has all the characteristics of the disrupted plaques (below) except that they have an intact cap in the absence of luminal thrombus. An elegant histomorphological comparison of late fibroatheromas, TCFA, and disrupted plaques in a large number of victims of sudden death and heart attacks addressed the important discriminators of TCFA that may help identify lesions at risk of developing acute events. The most important characteristic of TCFA is the attenuated fibrous cap composed

predominantly of collagen type I, with few SMC, varying degrees of inflammation including cells of monocyte-macrophage lineage, and often spotty calcification.[52] The fibrous cap usually measures between 55 µm and 84 µm for TCFA, and is almost always <55 µm for ruptured plaques.[52] These plaques are usually voluminous with a large plaque area, necrotic core burden, and luminal stenosis (Fig. 16–4). Disrupted plaques in up to 75% of cases demonstrated >75% cross-sectional luminal area narrowing, and 50% to 75% narrowing in the remaining cases, and the necrotic core occupied 30% of the plaque area with abundant macrophage infiltration. Compared with plaque ruptures, TCFA showed lesser plaque burden, less luminal encroachment, smaller necrotic core, and fewer macrophages within the fibrous cap, underscoring that the plaques would need to evolve before they disrupt. Whereas those lesions that are sufficiently occlusive result in acute events, subclinical rupture of less occlusive lesions is also possible. The latter lesions may undergo multiple plaque rupture and healing cycles to contribute to plaque enlargement for subsequent major events or CTO.[52]

Disruption of the fibrous cap of TCFAs exposes the thrombogenic necrotic cores to luminal blood (**Figs. 16–5**

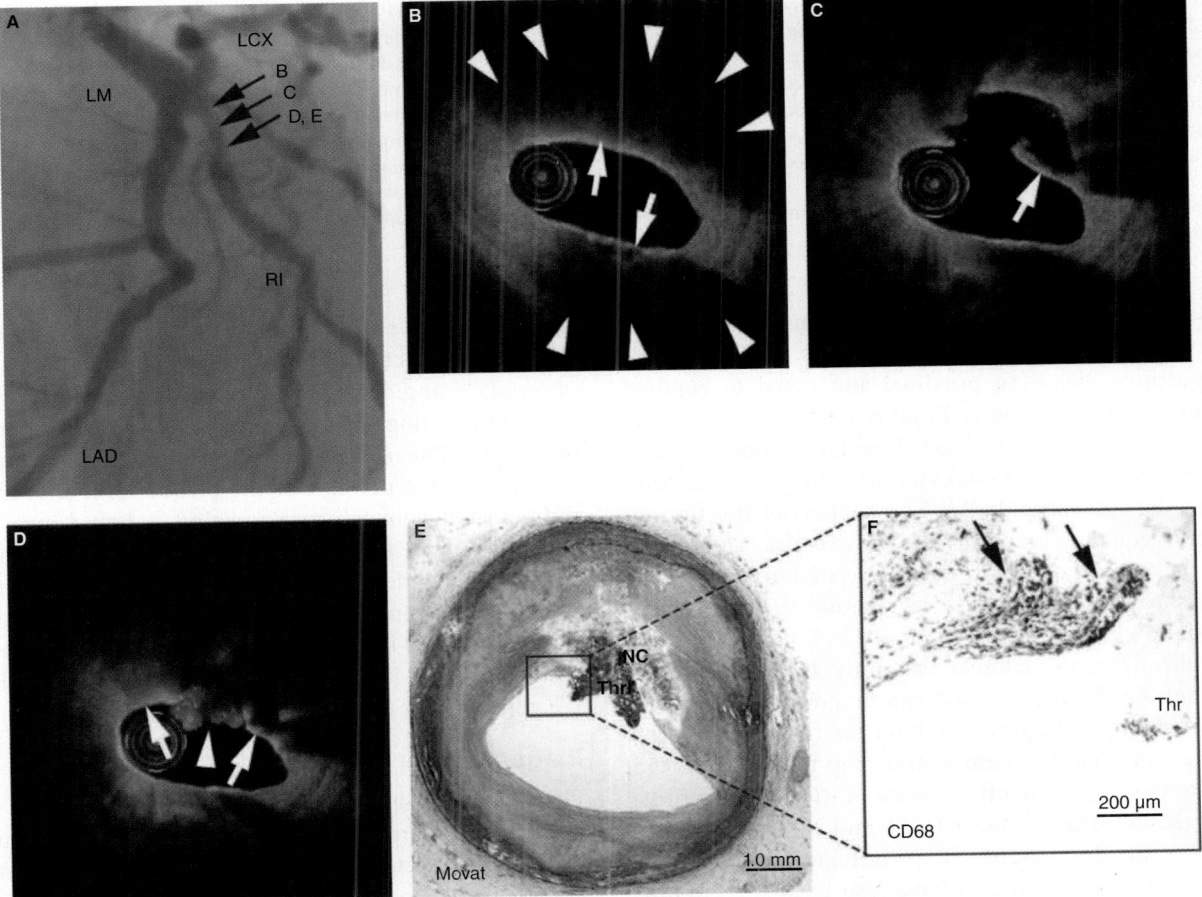

Figure 16–5. Plaque rupture and acute coronary syndrome. Disruption of the fibrous cap of thin-cap fibroatheromas exposes the thrombogenic necrotic cores to luminal blood and is considered the most common cause of acute coronary events. The OCT images from the ramus (**A**) demonstrate that the fibrous cap thickness is <55 µm at the site of plaque rupture (*arrows*, **C**); images of the proximal portion shows characteristics of TCFA (**B**) with thin cap (*arrows*) and large necrotic core (*arrowheads*) and the distal portion shows propagated thrombus (**D**, *arrowhead*). The overlying luminal thrombus (Thr) at the site of rupture (**E**, Movat pentachrome) is almost always a white thrombus, and the propagated portions including proximal and distal to rupture sites comprises red thrombus. The disrupted cap is inflamed with macrophages (**F**). Reproduced with permission from Otsuka F, Joner M, Prati F, et al. Clinical classification of plaque morphology in coronary disease. *Nat Rev Cardiol.* 2014 Jul;11(7):379-389.

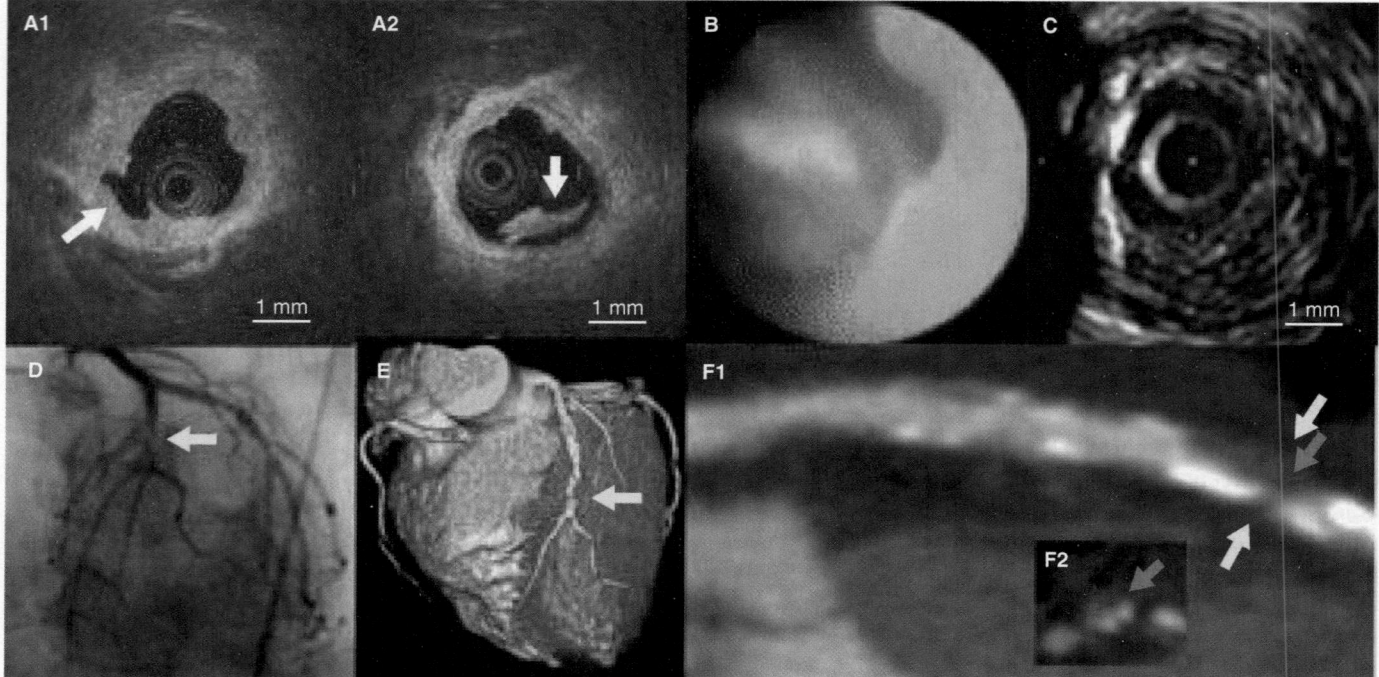

Figure 16–6. Intravascular imaging: acute coronary syndrome with ruptured fibrous cap. OCT (**A1** and **A2**), coronary angioscopy (**B**), IVUS (**C**), angiography (**D**), CT volume rendering (**E**), CT curved multiplanar reformation (**F1**), and the cross-sectional images (**F2**) were obtained in a culprit lesion with plaque rupture in a 67-year-old male presenting with acute coronary event. OCT images revealed fibrous cap disruption (*white arrow* in **A1**) and thrombus formation in adjacent slices (*white arrow* in **A2**). Coronary angioscopy (**B**) showed yellow plaque and red thrombus formation through the blue coronary angioscopy guide catheter. IVUS (**C**) indicates two focal calcium deposits <90°. Angiography (**D**) and volume-rendered CT images (**E**) disclose a significant stenosis in the middle segment of the left anterior descending coronary artery (*yellow arrows* in **D** and **E**). Curved multiplanar reformation CT images (**F1**) reveal positive remodeling associated with focal calcium deposits (*yellow arrows* in **F1**). Curved multiplanar reformation and the cross-sectional images (**F2**) display the presence of soft plaque with an attenuation of <30 HU (*red arrow* in **F1** and **F2**). Reproduced with permission from Ozaki Y, Okumura M, Ismail TF, et al. Coronary CT angiographic characteristics of culprit lesions in acute coronary syndromes not related to plaque rupture as defined by optical coherence tomography and angioscopy. *Eur Heart J*. 2011;32(22):2814-2823.

and **16–6**). The overlying luminal thrombus at the site of rupture is almost always a white thrombus, and the propagated portions including proximal and distal to rupture sites comprises red thrombus. Rupture of the fibrous cap, at rest, occurs mostly at the weakest shoulder regions, wherein the neointimal inflammation, cytokines and proteases contribute to the susceptibility.[53–55] The rupture of the fibrous caps occurs equally commonly during exercise,[56] but more likely at the summit of the fibrous cap related to high hemodynamic shear and local stress aggregation through spotty calcification.[57]

The fibrous cap thickness can only be measured in life through OCT imaging, and can be employed to identify TCFA using a <85 μm threshold for the thin cap; the eventful plaques usually demonstrate cap thickness of <55 μm.[52,58] Previously, a cut-off measure of <65 μm was proffered for the detection of both TCFA and ruptured plaques based on a smaller number of pathological specimens.[59] Intravascular imaging studies have also used the circumferential extent of the necrotic core exceeding 120° as a surrogate accomplice of TCFA.[32,60] Computed tomography (CT) angiographic evidence of the necrotic core and positive remodeling has been referred to as 2-feature positive plaques, suggestive of a 10-fold greater risk of developing

adverse cardiac events up to 10 years of follow-up of more than 3000 subjects[61–63] (**Fig. 16–7**). In the case of availability of serial CT angiographic examinations, plaque progression substantially improved the predictive value of unfavorable outcomes. The reliable assessment of inflammation has not yet become possible at the plaque level and, although radiolabeled deoxyglucose imaging is being investigated, measures of the systemic biomarkers provide the best circumstantial evidence of plaque inflammation (**Fig. 16–8**).[64] It has also been proposed that the pericoronary adipogenesis is minimized in the presence of vessel wall inflammation and could be measured as a fat attenuation index (FAI) on CT angiography (Fig. 16–8).[65]

Plaque Erosion

Plaque erosion is distinctly different from plaque rupture wherein the fibrous cap remains intact[49] and thrombi are directly in contact with a denuded intimal surface. There are no known morphological characteristics of *erosion-prone* lesions.

Plaque erosion has typically been associated with the composition of ground substance and may occur regardless of the maturity of the lesions; relatively immature lesion compared with ruptured plaques, such as PIT or early fibroatheromas served as substrate for plaque erosion in 16% and 50%

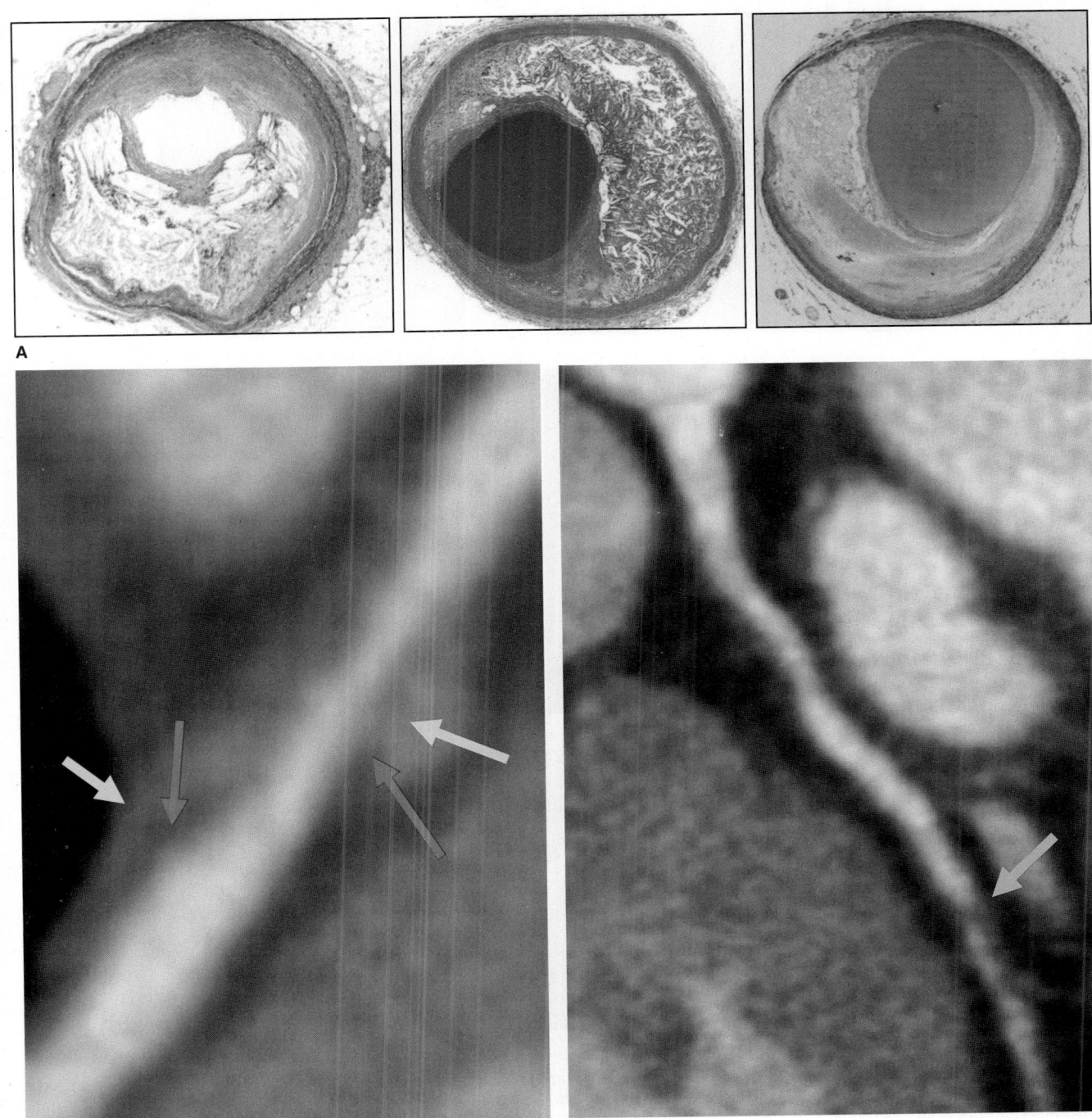

Figure 16–7. Noninvasive assessment of plaques vulnerable to rupture. (A) Histologically vulnerable plaques are referred to as thin-cap fibroatheroma that are characterized by large necrotic cores covered by attenuated and inflamed fibrous caps. The plaque burden is substantial but the extent of luminal obstruction is variable. The three TCFAs in **(A)** demonstrate significant, moderate, and minimal luminal stenosis. These plaques initially expand outward (positive remodeling) to accommodate large plaque burden. Accordingly, the right top TCFA shows significant plaque burden but minimal luminal stenosis due to positive remodeling. **(B)** Noninvasive assessment of vulnerable plaques by CT angiography has been based on presence or absence of two features: positive remodeling (*yellow arrows*) and large necrotic cores (*red arrows*); IVUS-verified necrotic cores in CT angiography are defined as low-attenuation plaque (LAP) of Hounsfield densities of less than 30 units. A, Reproduced with permission from Narula J, Nakano M, Virmani R, et al. Histopathologic characteristics of atherosclerotic coronary disease and implications of the findings for the invasive and noninvasive detection of vulnerable plaques. *J Am Coll Cardiol.* 2013 Mar 12; 61(10):1041-1051. B, Reproduced with permission from Motoyama S, Kondo T, Sarai M, et al. Multislice computed tomographic characteristics of coronary lesions in acute coronary syndromes. *J Am Coll Cardiol.* 2007 Jul 24;50(4):319-326.

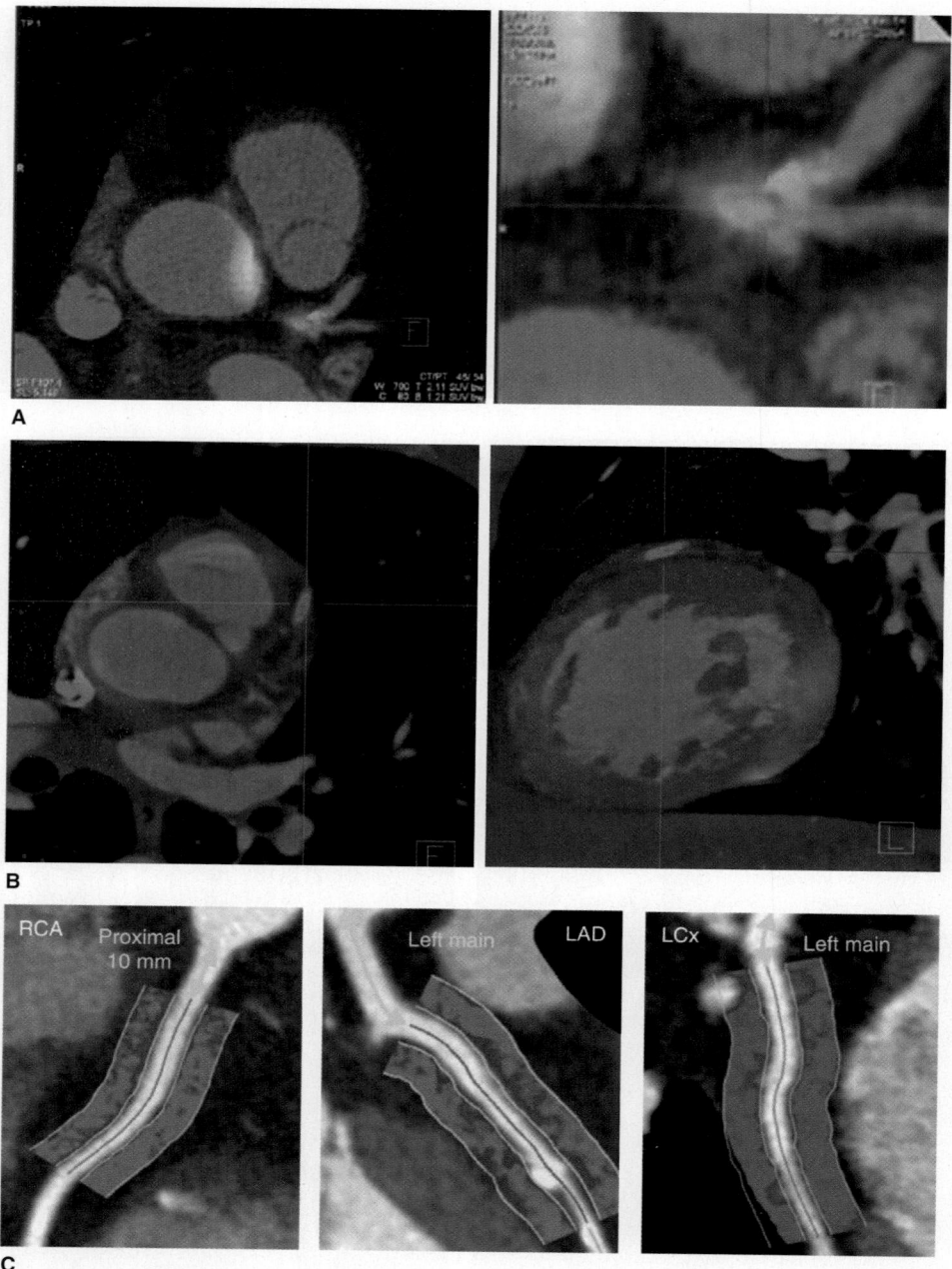

Figure 16–8. Noninvasive identification of vascular inflammation as a surrogate marker of plaque vulnerability. Inflammation can be detected either by simultaneous PET imaging with F-18 FDG (that targets macrophage infiltration) (**A,B**), or by fat attenuation index of perivascular fat (**C**). FDG uptake in the left main bifurcation and aortic root suggests inflammatory lesions (**A**); FDG uptake is not seen in stented plaque presenting with stable angina (**B**). The Fat Attenuation Index represents lower prevalence of adipocytes consequent to greater cytokines in neointima in high-risk plaques. A, B Reproduced with permission from Rogers IS, Nasir K, Figueroa AL, et al. Feasibility of FDG imaging of the coronary arteries: comparison between acute coronary syndrome and stable angina. *JACC Cardiovasc Imaging.* 2010 Apr;3(4):388-397. C, Reproduced with permission from Oikonomou EK, Marwan M, Desai MY, et al. Non-invasive detection of coronary inflammation using computed tomography and prediction of residual cardiovascular risk (the CRISP CT study): a post-hoc analysis of prospective outcome data. *Lancet.* 2018 Sep 15;392(10151):929-939.

of acute erosive events and the remaining 34% occurred over late fibroatheromas[66] (**Fig. 16–9**). The underlying lesions rarely carried large necrotic cores, or significant inflammation, calcification, and hemorrhage.[67] Abundant SMCs were observed embedded within a proteoglycan-rich matrix comprising hyaluronan and versican, and collagen-type III; the ground substance of fibrous caps in disrupted or stable plaques was richer in biglycan, decorin, and collagen type I[49,67] (**Fig. 16–10**). From a susceptibility perspective, erosions occurred more commonly at a younger age, and more frequently in women.[49,69] The risk of smoking significantly correlated with erosion;[67] whereas lipid profiles did not correlate with erosions.[51,69] Postmortem

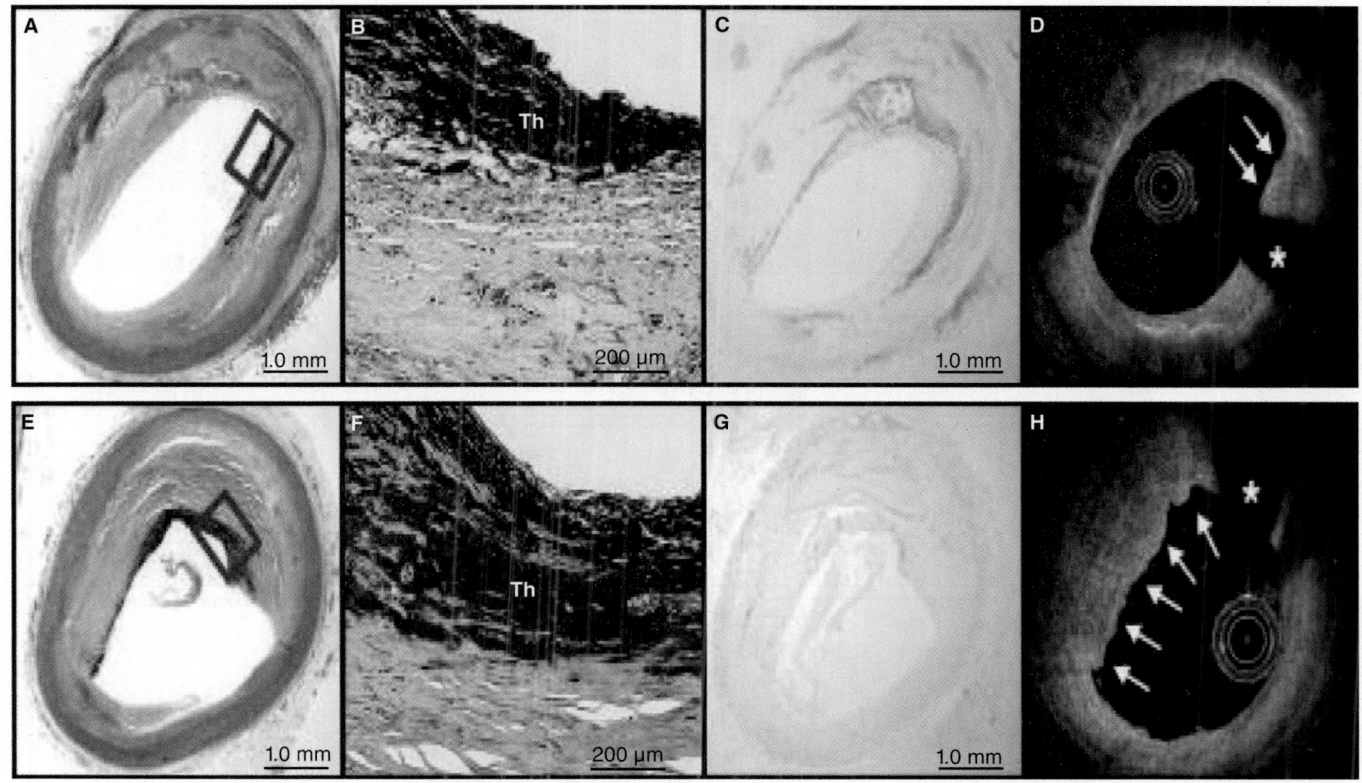

Figure 16–9. Plaque erosion and acute coronary event. Plaque erosion is the second most common cause of acute coronary event and differs from plaque rupture by having an intact fibrous cap. The underlying plaque in (**A–D**) is PIT and the underlying plaque in (**E–H**) is an early fibroatheromatous lesion. These lesions are present in different coronary arteries in the same victim who suffered an acute event. Reproduced with permission from Yahagi K, Zarpak R, Sakakura K, et al. Multiple simultaneous plaque erosion in 3 coronary arteries. *JACC Cardiovasc Imaging.* 2014 Nov;7(11):1172-1174.

data revealed more organized thrombi with eroded plaques,[70] and their fragments embolized downstream as intramyocardial microemboli.[71]

Clinical OCT studies[72,73] have suggested that in the setting of an acute coronary event, the presence of luminal thrombus over an intact fibrous cap is indicative of plaque erosion (**Fig. 16–11**). Substantial hurdles have limited the clinical utility of OCT in reliably distinguishing plaque erosion from other causes of coronary thrombosis; in particular, its limited axial resolution in detecting a disrupted endothelial monolayer. Additionally, the presence of luminal thrombus further amplifies the hindrance of light and sound into deeper tissue regions of the underlying plaque, making a reliable judgment of plaque morphology impossible. Although presumptive clinical documentation of plaque erosion is now available, demonstrating OCT characteristics of pathologically verified plaque erosion will be important.

Nodular Calcification and Calcified Nodules

Nodular calcification is the precursor lesion for eruptive calcified nodules, which is the least common pathogenetic mechanism of an acute coronary event. It is composed of areas of nodular calcification of varying size, nestled within the necrotic cores and often accompanied by intraplaque fibrin and an overlying thick, intact fibrous cap (**Fig. 16–12**). The calcified

nodules as the basis of adverse events is rare because a combination of multiple unusual features is needed, including the location of nodular calcification at the knee of a tortuous vessel within the large necrotic core flanked both proximally and distally by fibrocalcific, collagen-rich plaques and the systemic milieu of diabetes and chronic kidney disease.[74,75]

In the tortuous coronary segments, the changes in shear stress are produced by the loss of flow linearity especially when the direction of the flow abruptly changes[76,77] and could result in fragmentation of nodular calcification, squeezing dense calcific deposits out of relatively softer necrotic cores, and fibrous cap disruption. Such changes in shear stress further weaken and dilate aneurysmal vessels in monogenic autosomal recessive SLC2A10-related hereditary arterial tortuosity syndrome[78] The loose necrotic cores homing the nodular calcification compared with the circumferential sheet calcium and collagen-rich matrix of the flanking fibrocalcific plaques create substantial disparity in local tensile strength.[74,75]

The rupture of a fibrous cap is a mechanical event that could occur when the local stress levels within the cap exceed the local tissue strength. Biomechanical models based on histology of plaque rupture have suggested that plaque macrocalcification does not increase fibrous cap stress. In contrast, a soft core is associated with increased local stress[57,79] and microcalcific deposits embedded in the thin fibrous cap overlying necrotic cores act as stress concentrators facilitating plaque rupture.[57]

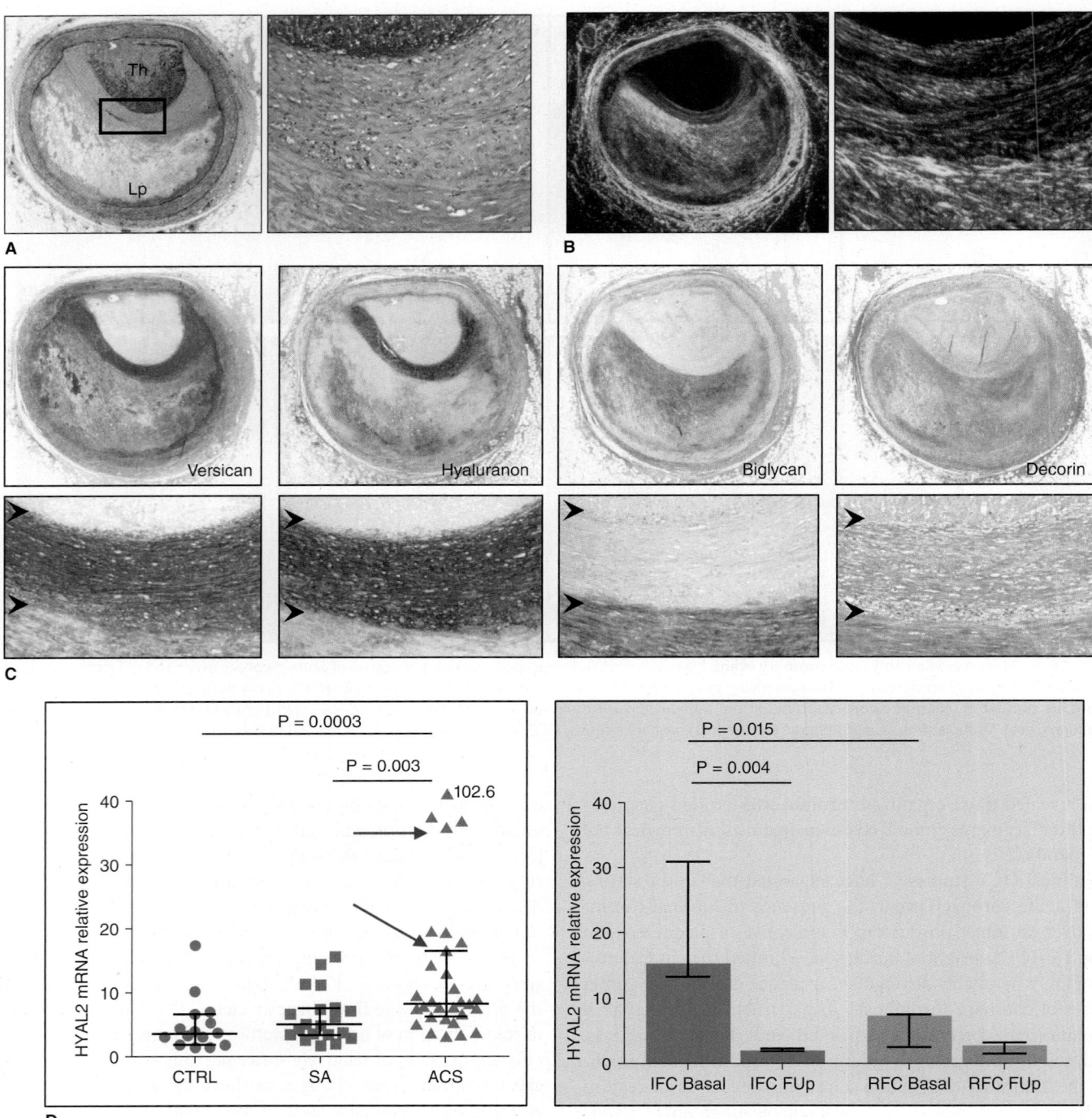

Figure 16–10. ECM characterization in plaque erosion picrosirius red staining and identification of proteoglycans. (A) Low-power (×20) and high-power (×200) micrographs of an eroded plaque (Movat pentachrome stain). *The black box* outlines a region at the plaque/thrombus interface. SMC- and proteoglycan-rich (*blue-green*) ECM is seen adjacent to the thrombus. **(B)** Corresponding picrosirius red staining showing a plaque surface rich in collagen type III. **(C)** Immunohistochemical staining for versican, hyaluronan, biglycan, and decorin, respectively. Note intense staining for versican and hyaluronan at the plaque/thrombus interface, whereas staining for decorin was weak, and that for biglycan is negative. Lp, lipid pool; Th, thrombus. **(D)** HYAL2 messenger RNA expression in peripheral mononuclear cells was evaluated in acute coronary syndromes. HYAL2 encodes for an enzyme that degrades Hyaluranon to a proinflammatory molecule. Increased expression of HYAL2 is seen in patients with plaque erosion and not plaque ruptures, there is a phasic rise in HYAL2 expression. A–C, Reproduced with permission from Kolodgie FD, Burke AP, Farb A, et al. Differential accumulation of proteoglycans and hyaluronan in culprit lesions: insights into plaque erosion. *Arterioscler Thromb Vasc Biol.* 2002 Oct 1;22(10):1642-1648. D, Reproduced with permission from Pedicino D, Vinci R, Giglio AF, et al. Alterations of Hyaluronan Metabolism in Acute Coronary Syndrome: Implications for Plaque Erosion. *J Am Coll Cardiol.* 2018 Sep 25;72(13):1490-1503.

Subsequent computational studies based on a higher resolution micro-CT showed that microcalcification oriented along the tensile axis in fibrous caps could increase the local stress levels more than 5-fold.[80] The possibility that a large necrotic core calcification can fragment into multiple pieces and pop through a thick fibrous cap is intriguing. Nodular calcification in highly tortuous coronary arteries flanked by stable fibrocalcific plaques represents a distinctively unique morphology and complex loading conditions. In addition to the circumferential stress, a tortuous artery experiences axial stress arising from

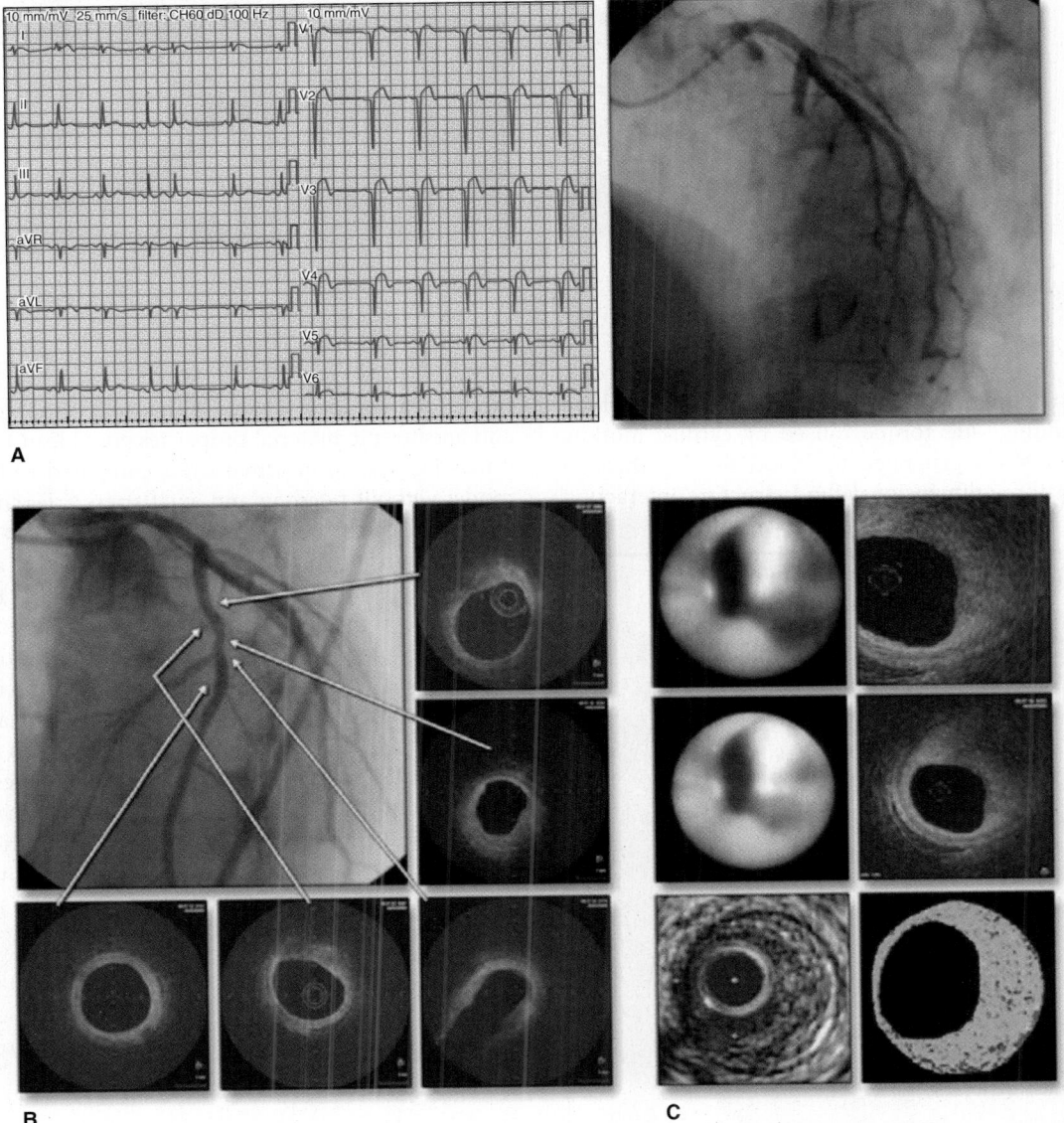

Figure 16–11. Acute coronary syndrome with an intact fibrous cap. Severe chest discomfort and shortness of breath developed in a 66-year-old man after 12 h of intermittent and stuttering retrosternal discomfort. He presented to a local hospital; his blood pressure was 96/57 mm Hg, his heart rate was 84 bpm, and an electrocardiogram revealed ST-segment elevation in precordial leads **(A)**. The coronary risk factors included dyslipidemia and a 46-pack-year smoking history. An emergent coronary angiography was performed 4 h after the onset of chest pain, which revealed total occlusion of the proximal segment of LAD coronary artery **(A)**. Then, intravenous administration of heparin (10,000 IU) and half-dose alteplase was started, and he was transferred to a tertiary cardiovascular care center for a percutaneous coronary intervention. Repeat coronary angiography (8 h after the onset of chest pain) demonstrated no thrombus or stenosis at the original site of total occlusion. OCT, angioscopy, grayscale IVUS, and integrated backscatter IVUS **(B, C)** were performed. On arrival, CK-MB was 399 (normal: 0.6 to 3.5) ng/mL, and TnI was 60.80 (normal: 0.00 to 0.06) ng/mL. Coronary angioscopy showed faint red thrombus formation through the blue coronary angioscopy guide catheter, whereas OCT did not show a typical red thrombus with a high backscattering protrusion mass with signal-free shadowing, but some signal reduction was observed from 12 to 3 o'clock positions **(C)**. Multiple slices of OCT images revealed an intact fibrous cap **(B)**. IVUS and integrated backscatter IVUS demonstrated predominantly a fibrous plaque (*green*) and negligible lipid-rich component (*blue*) **(C)**. No intervention was undertaken. Predischarge curved multiplanar reconstruction CT images confirmed the absence of positive remodeling and no significant stenosis at the site of the original occlusion **(D)** and mainly normal coronary arteries. Reproduced with permission from Prati F, Uemura S, Souteyrand G, et al. OCT-based diagnosis and management of STEMI associated with intact fibrous cap. *JACC Cardiovasc Imaging.* 2013 Mar;6(3):283-287.

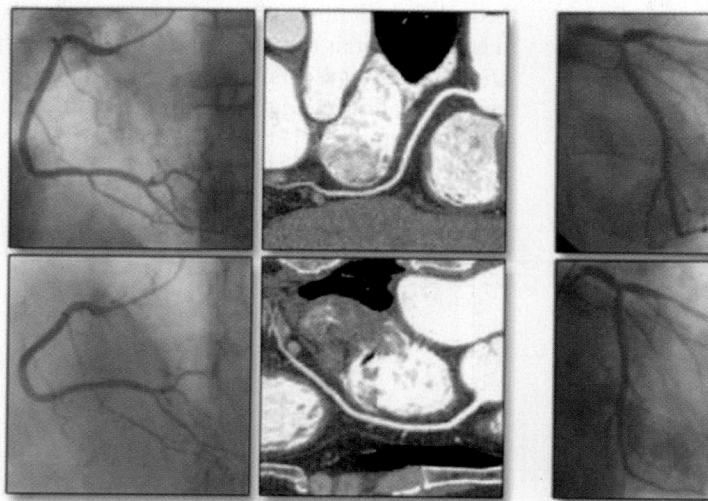
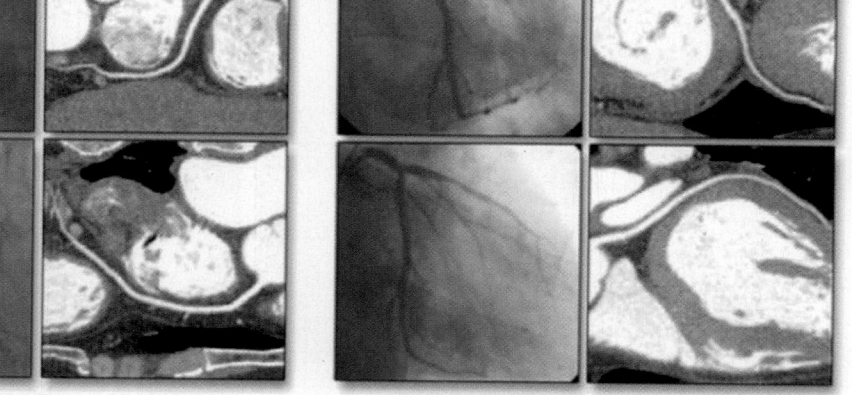

D

Figure 16–11. (Continued)

longitudinal stretching of vessels exposed to cyclical blood flow, cyclic bending, and torque caused by cardiac motion, as well as shear stress generated by blood flowing through the vessel. In a three-dimensional fluid structure interaction model of a coronary plaque with cyclic bending, axial stretch and anisotropic material properties could lead to more than a 4-fold increase in maximal stress compared with an isotropic model without bending and axial stress,[81] leading to rupture of the core calcification through even a thick cap (**Fig. 16–13**).

Although uncommon, calcified nodules are clinically recognizable by intracoronary imaging (**Fig. 16–14**),[82] and potentially associated with a worse prognosis compared with superficial plaque calcification.[83] Besides the role of micro-calcification and calcified nodules in acute coronary syndrome, the presence of coronary artery calcification remains a disease marker, and in patients treated with statins, large calcific plates are suggestive of stabilized plaques.[4] The mural thrombi and the calcific mass can be recognized by intravascular imaging,[83] but the assessment of nodular calcification and the fibrin distribution amongst calcific fragments cannot be identified by in vivo imaging. The in vivo characterization of tortuous coronary segments is feasible with imaging.[84]

THE DYNAMIC AND PROGRESSIVE LESIONS

Plaque progression happens to be the most important characteristic of high-risk plaques that are susceptible to plaque rupture. Plaque progression and increasing positive remodeling occur consequent to necrotic core expansion and is closely associated with plaque inflammation. Necrotic core expansion occurs with free cholesterol abundance that is unlikely to be derived from circulating LDL and macrophages, which deliver esterified form of cholesterol.[85] It has been reported that the RBC extravasation through the leaky neovascularization and intraplaque hemorrhage facilitate free cholesterol accumulation that is derived from the RBC membrane. Plaque fissures and subclinical ruptures also help incorporate red thrombus within

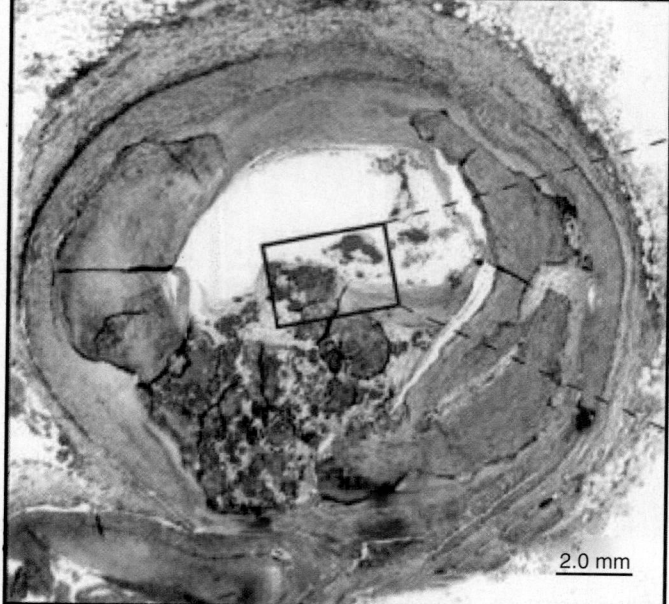

2.0 mm

Figure 16–12. **Histological images are shown for luminal thrombus associated with a calcified nodule.** This is the least-frequent cause of luminal thrombus. Calcific fragments disrupt through luminal surface (regardless of fibrous cap thickness). Calcific nodules are nestled in residual necrotic core and the nodule is usually situated at the significantly tortuous coronary arterial segments. Proximal and distal portions of this situation have significant fibrocalcific plaques. Although the precise nature of this lesion remains incompletely understood, fragmentation of calcified plates is believed to be the etiology of the nodular calcification. These lesions are generally more prevalent in older men, and in patients with diabetes mellitus, or chronic renal failure. Reproduced with permission from Falk E, Nakano M, Bentzon JF, et al. Update on acute coronary syndromes: the pathologists' view. *Eur Heart J*. 2013 Mar;34(10):719-728.

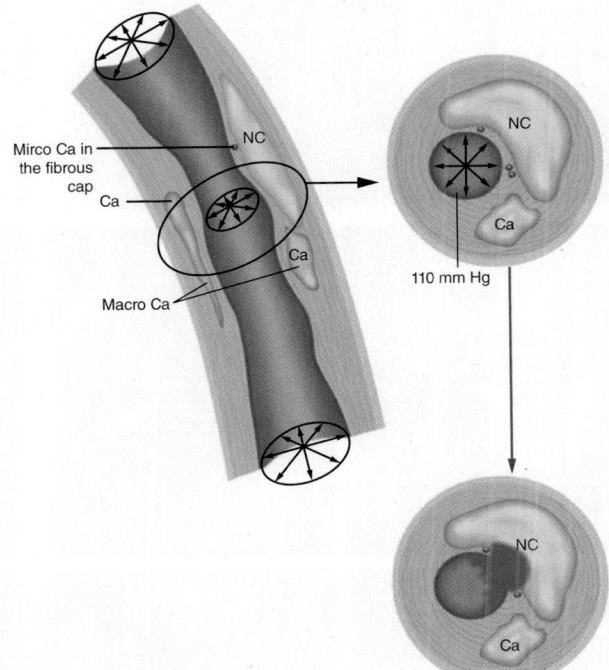

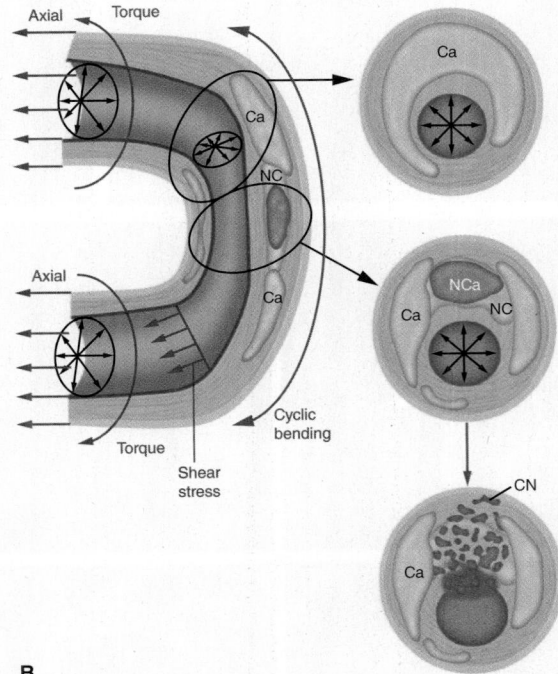

Figure 16–13. Fibrous cap microcalcification and necrotic core nodular calcification, and the mechanical modeling of plaque instability in linear versus tortuous coronary segments. (A) Two-dimensional finite-element model of plaque rupture due to local stress concentration around microcalcifications embedded in the fibrous cap. Plaque rupture occurs mainly in proximal segments with low tortuosity, when circumferential stress in the fibrous cap resulting from blood pressure exceeds the local tissue strength. **(B)** Advanced three-dimensional model of calcific nodule located in a tortuous vessel incorporates complex lesion morphology and loading conditions. In addition to circumferential stretch generated by blood pressure, axial stretch, torque, and cyclic bending may contribute to critical stress variations responsible for the fragmentation of necrotic core calcification and subsequent plaque disruption. Ca, calcification; CN, calcified nodule; NC, necrotic core. Reproduced with permission from Arbustini E, Vengrenyuk Y, Narula J. On the Shades of Coronary Calcium and Plaque Instability. *J Am Coll Cardiol.* 2021 Apr 6;77(13):1612-1615.

the healing plaque and contribute to increasing RBC mass and free cholesterol. CTO might also represent a logical consequence of expanding lesions, and plaque rupture and healing cycles.

Plaque Neovascularization and Necrotic Core Expansion

The concept of plaque enlargement by erythrocyte and fibrin accumulation within the necrotic core has been reported by autopsy and clinical magnetic resonance imaging (MRI) studies.[10,86,87] With evolving necrotic core, plaque neovascularization occurs as adventitial vasa vasorum penetrated through the vascular SMC medial layer into the neointima. The penetrating neoangiogenic vessels lose their own smooth muscle layers and the endothelium loses competent intercellular junctions and

exhibits intracytoplasmic vacuoles, and is detached from the basement membrane.[88] The fragile neoangiogenic sprouting is associated with an RBC leak and intraplaque hemorrhage.[89] The extent of neovascularization correlates with plaque burden and plaque inflammation, and vascular density is reduced in fibrous and calcified arteries. RBC membranes have a rich free cholesterol-to-phospholipid ratio and substantial amount of free cholesterol deposition could occur from neovascularization. Employing immunohistochemical staining for glycophorin A (an RBC membrane-specific marker) together with iron staining for hemoglobin, intraplaque hemorrhage was found to be common in ruptured plaques, TCFA, and late fibroatheromas, and their distribution directly correlated with the size of the necrotic core and the extent of inflammation.[88,89] **(Fig. 16–15).**

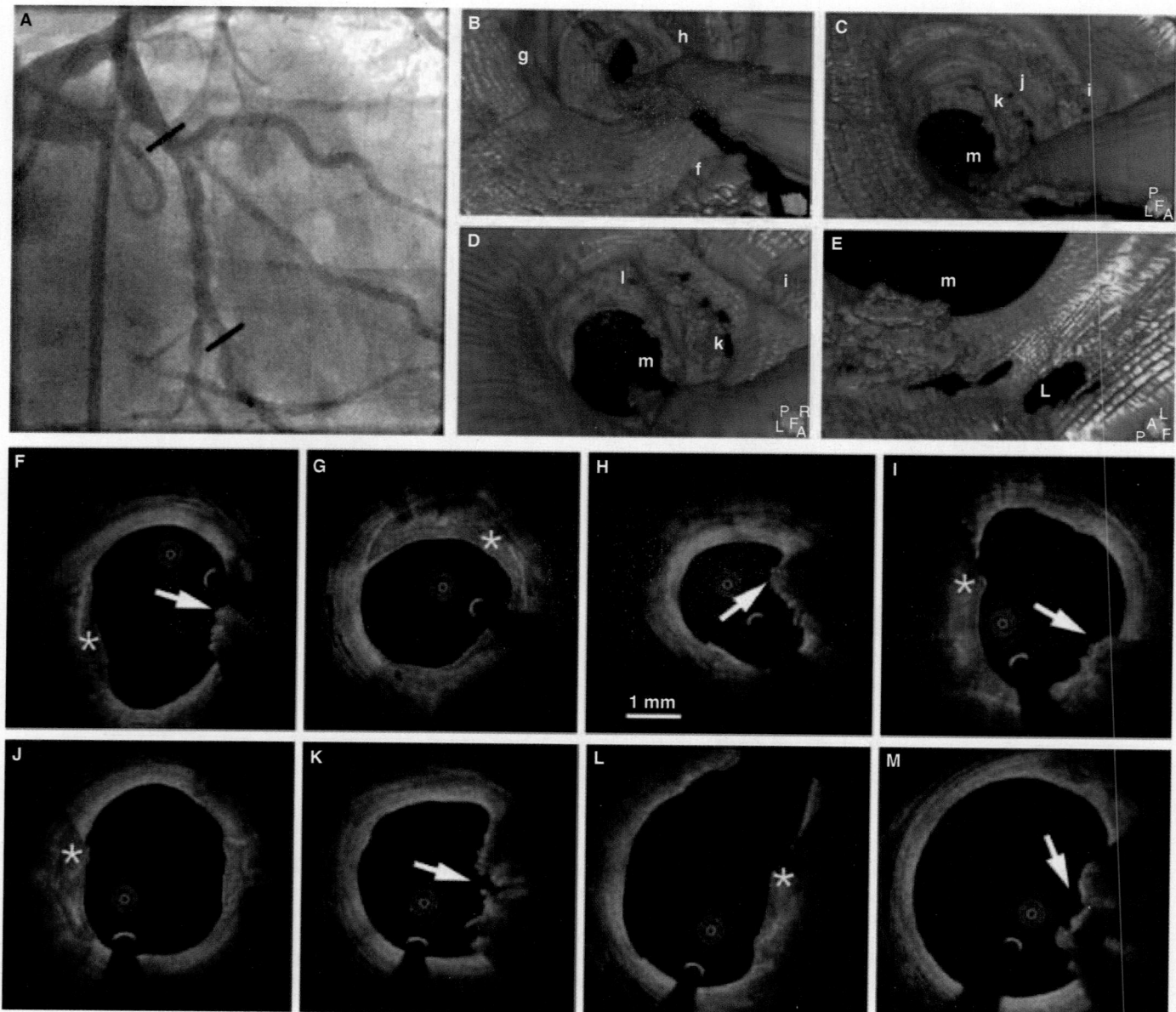

Figure 16-14. Calcified nodule and acute coronary event. A 57-year-old man underwent percutaneous coronary intervention in the LAD coronary artery for stable angina. The LCX coronary artery was evaluated for the presence of clinically significant lesions by OCT. (**A**) Coronary angiography of the left circumflex coronary artery. *Black lines* indicate the studied segment. (**B–E**) Upstream fly-through view (distal-to-proximal) of three-dimensional reconstruction of OCT images indicated the sites corresponding to (**F–M**). OCT shows presence of red thrombus (*white arrows*) in areas of fibrocalcific plaque (*asterisks*) in the absence of plaque rupture. Sharp protrusions of calcium into the lumen are seen in (**G, J, L**) (*asterisks*) with very thin, or absent overlying intimal layer. Reproduced with permission from Karanasos A, Ligthart JM, Witberg KT, et al. Calcified nodules: an underrated mechanism of coronary thrombosis? *JACC Cardiovasc Imaging.* 2012 Oct;5(10):1071-1072.

Subclinical Plaque Rupture and Healing

The concept of plaque progression through subclinical rupture and healing in coronary arteries has been well known from autopsy studies in victims of unstable angina and acute myocardial infarction.[88] Healed lesions are characterized by reparative process surrounding sites of previously disrupted fibrous cap and organizing thrombus,[90] wherein thrombi resolve with RBC-derived free cholesterol deposits, and the matrix comprising SMC, proteoglycans, and type III collagen. With complete healing, type III collagen matures to type I collagen, and the luminal surface is eventually endothelialized. Picrosirius red staining allows identification of high risk plaques represented by collagen layers of different ages. The earliest rupture site is always located in the deepest intima.[90] Healed ruptures could contribute to episodic increase in plaque burden and luminal narrowing (**Fig. 16–16**).

It is conceivable that high-risk plaques with subcritical stenosis are associated with subclinical rupture-healing cycles and lead to plaque progression. Healing with thin caps could

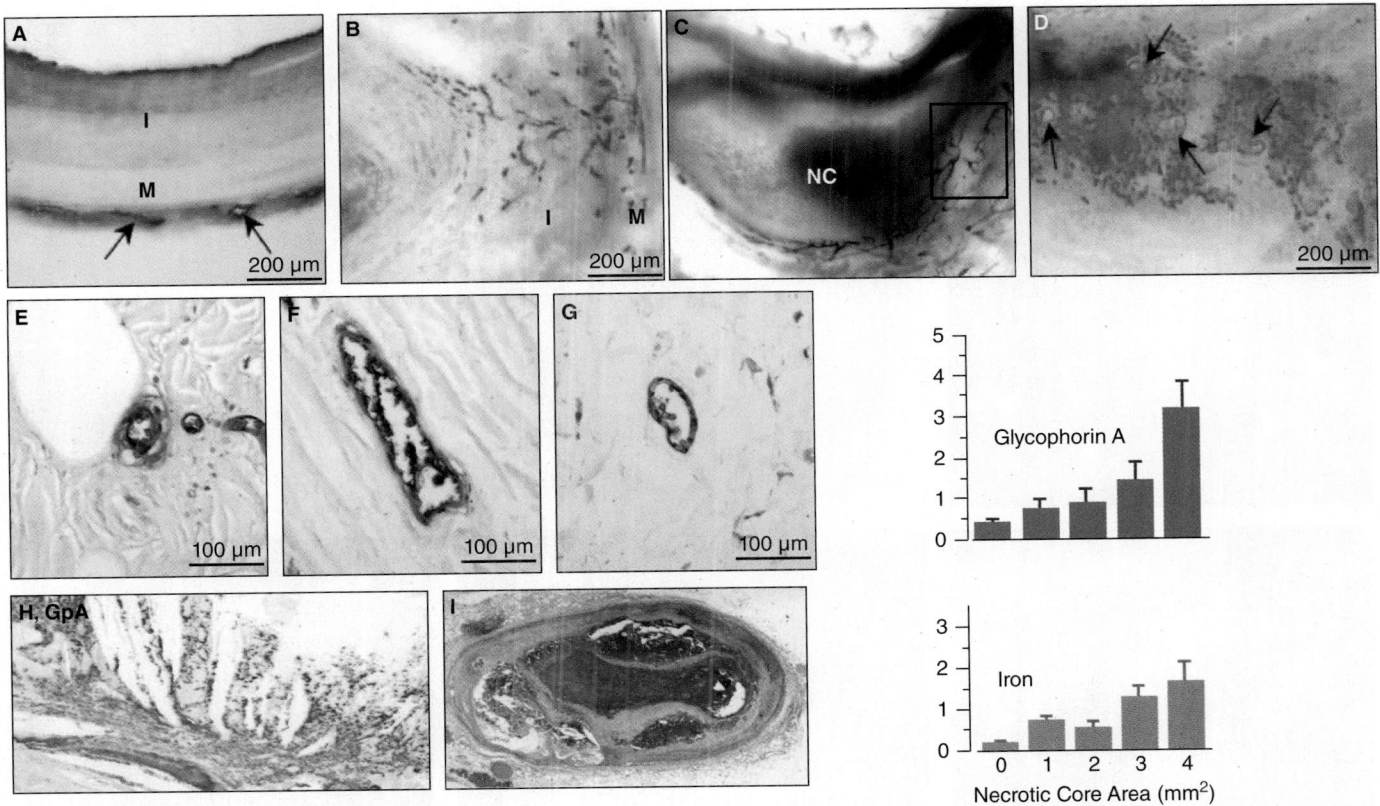

Figure 16–15. Plaque neoangiogenesis and necrotic core. Plaque expansion is associated with proliferation of adventitial vasa vasorum that penetrates to neointima through the medial layer. (Ulex, 150 mic) In the vicinity of necrotic core (NC), the vessels are leaky in the neo intima (**A–D**). The vessels are leaky because upon penetration from adventitia (**E**, 3-layer SMC) to media (**F**, single-layer SMC) vasa vasorum lose their SMC layer upon arrival in neointima (**G**). RBC extravasation contributes to deposition of free cholesterol (**H**) as confirmed by immunohistochemical staining for the RBC membrane-specific protein, glycophorin A. RBC deposition is exaggerated by intraplaque hemorrhage of the fragile neovasculature (**I**). (**J**) The more glycophorin A and iron load in the plaque, the greater is the plaque magnitude. (A,B,D) Reproduced with permission from Jain RK, Finn AV, Kolodgie FD, et al. Antiangiogenic therapy for normalization of atherosclerotic plaque vasculature: a potential strategy for plaque stabilization. *Nat Clin Pract Cardiovasc Med.* 2007 Sep;4(9):491-502. (C) Reproduced with permission from Virmani R, Kolodgie FD, Burke AP, et al. Atherosclerotic plaque progression and vulnerability to rupture: angiogenesis as a source of intraplaque hemorrhage. *Arterioscler Thromb Vasc Biol.* 2005 Oct;25(10):2054-2061. (H,J) Reproduced with permission from Kolodgie FD, Gold HK, Burke AP, et al. Intraplaque hemorrhage and progression of coronary atheroma. *N Engl J Med.* 2003 Dec 11;349(24):2316-2325.

lead to rupture again. Nonocclusive thrombi resulting from silent plaque ruptures or erosions, but not incorporated in plaque, could organize with granulation tissue and SMC proliferation with proteoglycan and collagen deposition;[91] thrombus could propagate proximally and distally to heal into a fibrous plaque. On the other hand, stenotic high-risk plaque ruptures should induce overt major clinical events. Silent luminal thrombi are usually nonocclusive, but could result in chronic total occlusion.

In data from three decades ago, a mean of 2.4 episodes of coronary thrombosis had occurred as subclinical nonocclusive thrombi, which had reendothelialized and seemed to have contributed to luminal narrowing.[92] The prevalence of silent ruptures is not known, but earlier studies have suggested less than 20% of silent plaque rupture in lesions with <50% diameter stenosis, and almost 75% of plaques with >50% diameter stenosis. The HPRs are most commonly seen in the most stenotic lesion in chronic coronary syndromes patients or culprit plaques in those dying of acute coronary event; less than 10% of erosive plaques demonstrate background of HPR.[91] Luminal stenosis is greater in plaques with multiple healed ruptures compared with virgin ruptures. Healed ruptured plaques can be detected by OCT as multiple tissue layers of different optical density overlying a large necrotic core in the presence or absence of calcification.[93] When healing of ruptured plaque is complete, and type III collagen has been replaced by type I collagen, a typical band of high backscattering signal occurs between individual tissue layers, probably because of the differential optical density of different types of collagen.

Plaque Fissures

The cracks or fissures on the luminal plaque surface have been described as contributing to fibrin deposition within the necrotic core.[94] The fissures and plaque ruptures have been described as distinct entities; the latter are always accompanied by luminal thrombus, whereas fissures usually have a confined intraintimal thrombus consisting of fibrin and platelets with scattered erythrocytes. When present, luminal thrombi associated with fissures are rather tiny. Therefore, unlike an overt disruption of the attenuated fibrous cap with overlying thrombus, a plaque fissure is characterized by a marginal tear in an eccentric plaque with a small underlying necrotic core; the separation plane of the fissure begins from the necrotic core and extends into the lumen and is lined by few macrophages, RBC, and fibrin.

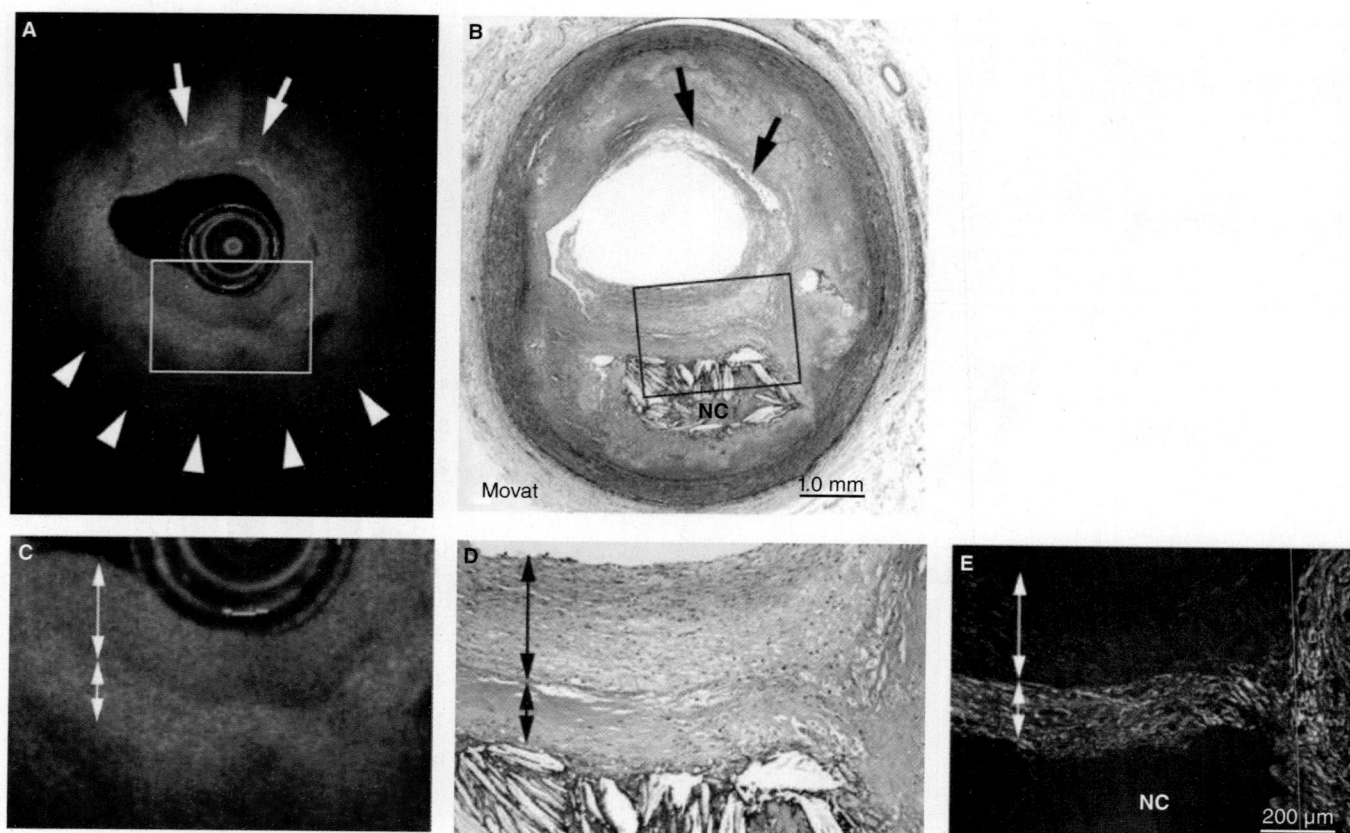

Figure 16–16. Healed plaques. An ex vivo OCT image shows a layered pattern of the signals and underlying signal-poor region with diffuse border (*white arrow heads*) and a focal signal-rich confluent punctate area with rapid attenuation (*white arrows*) (**A**). A corresponding histological section (**B**) of the human coronary plaque (stained with Movat pentachrome) shows healed plaque rupture and underlying NC with extensive hemorrhage and the presence of foamy macrophages close to the luminal surface (*black arrows*). The layered pattern of the OCT signals is highlighted in a high-power image (*white double arrows*, **C**), and the corresponding high-power histological section shows numerous SMCs within the newly formed proteoglycan-rich neointima (*black double arrows* close to the luminal surface), with clear demarcation from the underlying old collagen-rich fibrous cap. In a high-power image of a Sirius-red-stained section (under polarized light) corresponding with the image in (**D**), dense (type I) collagen forms a fibrous cap, seen as a reddish-yellow region, and is overlaid with newer (type III) collagen, detected as a greenish area, confirming collagen of different ages and healing (**E**). NC, necrotic core. Reproduced with permission from Otsuka F, Joner M, Prati F, et al. Clinical classification of plaque morphology in coronary disease. *Nat Rev Cardiol.* 2014 Jul;11(7):379-389.

Chronic Total Occlusion

Histological examination of angiographically verified CTO reveals the lumen area to be occupied by both mature atherosclerotic lesions and resolving thrombus.[92] The vessels with aged CTO usually show underlying fibrous plaque, rich in type I collagen with negative vascular remodeling; the thrombus is completely healed and no fibrin can be seen at any level.[92] CTO of short standing, on the other hand, have underlying plaques with necrotic core and positive vascular remodeling,[92] and organizing thrombus comprising inflammation, angiogenesis, and SMC infiltration with proteoglycan matrix and collagen type III[92] (**Figs. 16–17** and **16–18**). Macrophage infiltration is usually greater in younger occlusion,[95] and plays an active role in angiogenesis and recanalization.[96,97] Approximately half of the angiographically verified CTO show histological evidence of recanalization,[98] and the size of small microchannels is 160 μm to 230 μm.[99] Microchannel size is an important guide for development of guidewires and catheters aimed at crossing the occlusive lesions. CTO lesions with lesser microchannels of 20 μm to 40 μm are not amenable to crossing and might involve penetration of soft tissue. The relatively high failure rate of recanalization procedures of long-duration CTOs can be explained on the basis of extensive negative remodeling and is the likely source for failure of guidewire penetration.[46] In addition, the proximal lumen tapered pattern is strongly associated with successful guidewire penetration and antegrade revascularization of CTO, whereas the abrupt lumen pattern is associated with failure of successful wire passage.[45,47] Similarly, the distal lumen tapered pattern is conducive to the successful retrograde revascularization approach.[100,101]

VENOUS BYPASS GRAFTS AND IN-STENT ATHEROSCLEROSIS

Unlike the protracted process of atherogenesis in native coronary arteries spread over dozens of years, in-stent and vein graft neoatherosclerosis develop over several months to a few years. Similar to adaptive intimal thickening seen in native arteries, the neointimal hyperplasia evolves within the first year after

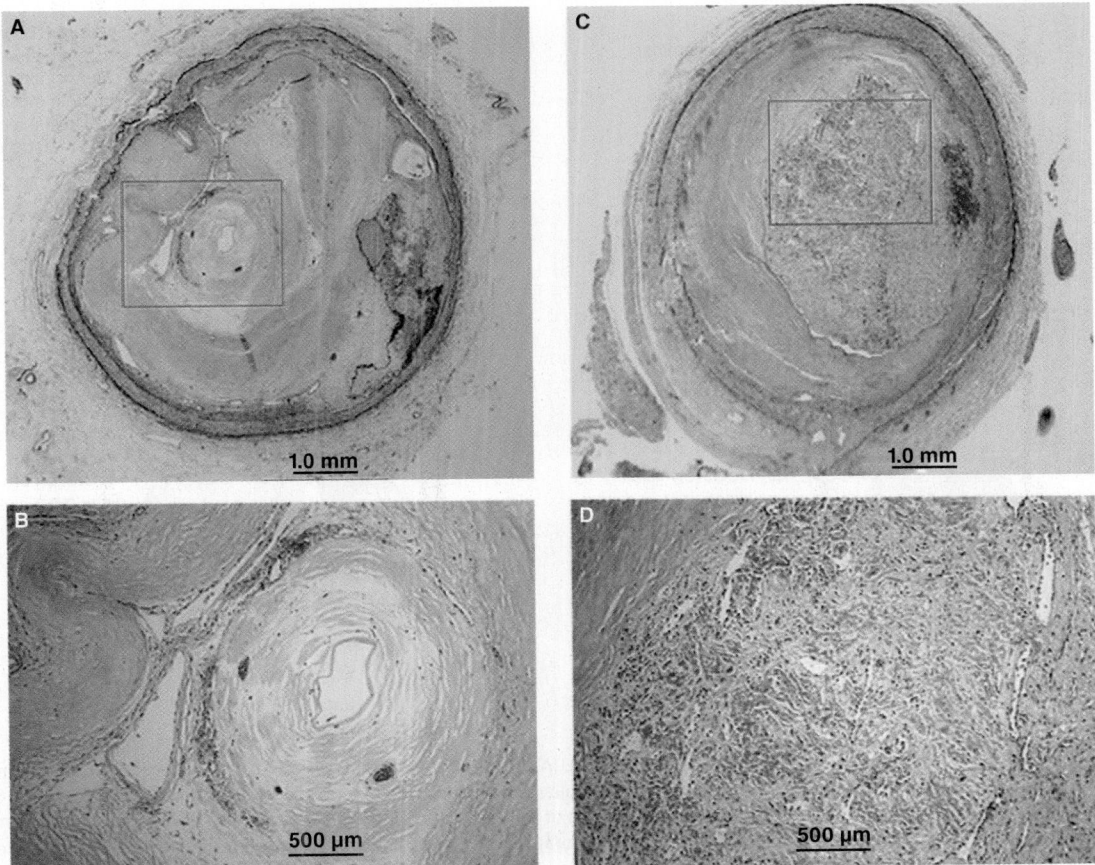

Figure 16–17. **Chronic total occlusion (CTO).** Low-power images of long-duration (**A** and **B**) and short-duration chronic total occlusion (**C** and **D**). (**B**) and (**D**) are high-power images of the boxed areas in (**A**) and (**C**), respectively. The matrix is predominantly made up of collagen type I in (**B**). In (**D**), the matrix predominantly consists of proteoglycan and fibrin. Underlying atherosclerotic plaques and propagated thrombus heals with CTO, and with aging thrombus it demonstrates recanalization. Reproduced with permission from Sakakura K, Nakano M, Otsuka F, et al. Comparison of pathology of chronic total occlusion with and without coronary artery bypass graft. *Eur Heart J.* 2014 Jul 1;35(25):1683-1693.

stent implantation, and also in vein grafts. Although macrophage infiltration in vein grafts and stents resembles intimal xanthomas of native arteries, the macrophages preferentially accumulate as surface clusters or in peri-strut regions. However, unlike native arteries where fatty streaks almost always are nonprogressive lesions,[9,19] the neointimal macrophage clusters in venous grafts or stents rapidly form necrotic cores through dying macrophages, and usually bypass the need to evolve through the necessary step of PIT in native coronary disease. The lipid pools and necrotic cores are located in the deep intimal layers in native disease but they are superficial in neoatherosclerotic lesions and appear as late fibroatheromas or TCFA based on the cap thickness. Although intraplaque hemorrhage is common in neoatherosclerosis similarly to native disease, it is driven from blood entering on the luminal side from fissure or rupture, and not from vasa vasorum and neoangiogenesis.

In vein graft or in-stent neoatherosclerosis, coronary thrombi are almost always associated with plaque rupture. Plaque erosions and eruptive calcified nodules are rarely seen in vein grafts or in stent lesions. Similarly, HPRs are also not seen in neoatherosclerosis. CTO could occur in vein grafts from organization of luminal thrombus.[91] CTO lesions within the stent might infrequently result from neoatherosclerotic plaque rupture or incomplete healing of the stent. Thrombus organization could be associated with microcalcification, calcified sheets, or calcified fragments.

INTRAVASCULAR IMAGING OF HIGH-RISK PLAQUES AND ACUTE EVENTS

The recursive partitioning analysis of 105 stable fibroatheromatous, 88 thin-capped fibroatheromatous, and 102 disrupted plaques from victims of sudden death was performed to determine the hierarchical discriminatory value of various pathological characteristics (**Fig. 16–19**). For this analysis, fibrous cap thickness, luminal stenosis, plaque area, necrotic core area, macrophage area, and calcification were included.[52] The most important discriminator, fibrous cap thickness, was found to be greater than 85 μm in thickness for stable plaques, and less than 55 μm in plaque ruptures; fibrous caps in most of the TCFA measured between 55 μm and 85 μm. The intact caps were less than 55 μm thick in a minority of the TCFA that were less occlusive than 75% cross-sectional area narrowing. In addition, the extent of inflammatory cell infiltration of monocyte-macrophage lineage and the magnitude of necrotic core size

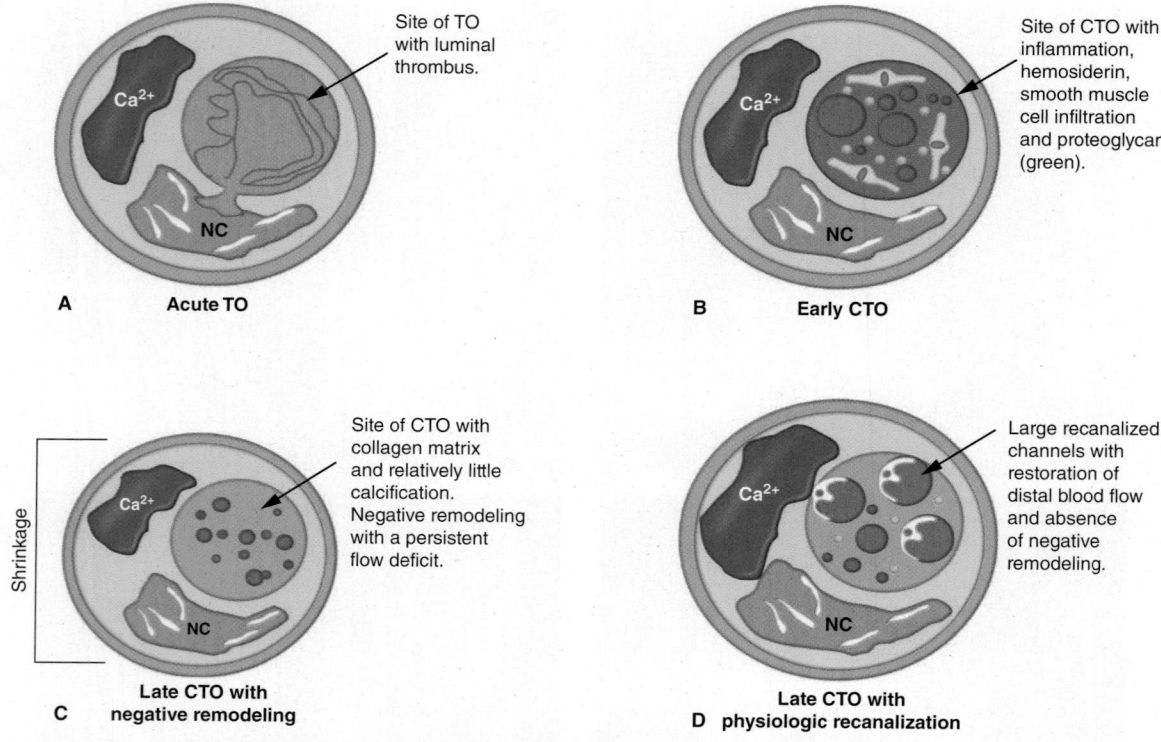

Figure 16–18. Schematic representation of chronic total occlusion (CTO). (A) Acute plaque rupture is shown, with luminal thrombus eventually resulting in CTO. **(B)** Inflammation with early thrombus organization and early recanalization accompanied by proteoglycan matrix (*green*) is seen in the area of total occlusion. **(C)** The late chronic phase of healed CTO is shown, with deposition of collagen type I where the cross-linking of collagen promotes negative remodeling of the vessel. **(D)** Physiological recanalization is accompanied by restoration of flow distally, thus preventing negative remodeling. Reproduced with permission from Finn AV, Kolodgie FD, Nakano M, et al. The differences between neovascularization of chronic total occlusion and intraplaque angiogenesis. *JACC Cardiovasc Imaging.* 2010 Aug;3(8):806-810.

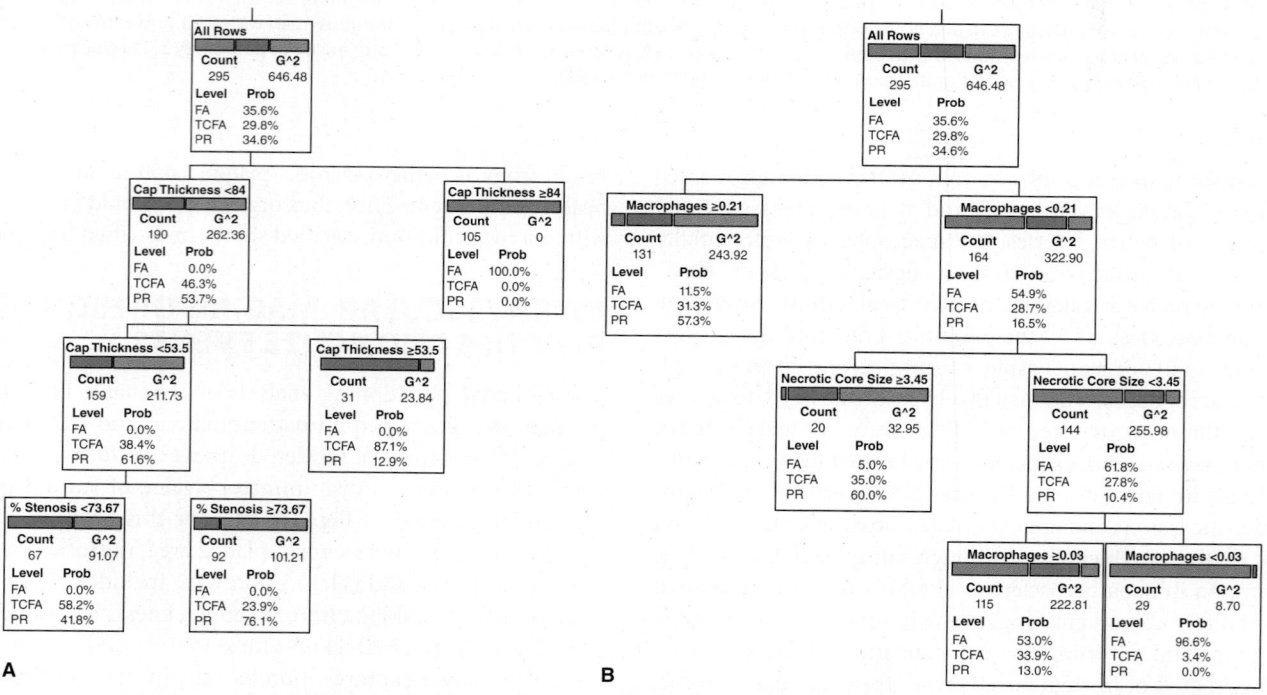

Figure 16–19. Hierarchical importance of morphological characteristics of plaque vulnerability by recursive partitioning analyses. Pathological characterization of nearly 300 stable (*green*), high-risk (*blue*), and disrupted (*red*) plaques revealed fibrous cap thickness (FCT) to be the most important determinant of plaque vulnerability (**A**); FCT was <85 μm in high-risk and <55 μm in disrupted plaques. Since FCT can only be assessed by an invasive procedure, reanalysis without including FCT suggested the extent of plaque inflammation and the magnitude of the necrotic core to be the best determinants (**B**). Both these characteristics can be measured to CT angiography. Reproduced with permission from Narula J, Nakano M, Virmani R, et al. Histopathologic characteristics of atherosclerotic coronary disease and implications of the findings for the invasive and noninvasive detection of vulnerable plaques. *J Am Coll Cardiol.* 2013 Mar 12;61(10):1041-1051.

were important determinants of plaque instability. This study[52] also reported disrupted plaques to be more occlusive than TCFA underscoring the importance of plaque progression. The angiographic and intravascular analysis[102] have also supported the concept of plaque progression as a prerequisite for plaque rupture. Therefore, the finding that the disrupted plaques are luminally significantly occlusive does not contradict the belief that the plaque responsible for acute coronary events is more likely to be mildly stenotic,[103] because even if less occlusive initially, it evolves to hemodynamic significance at the time of rupture.[104,105]

The pathologic findings of TCFA and plaque rupture were confirmed in a prospective 3-vessel intravascular ultrasound (IVUS) imaging PROSPECT study of nonculprit plaques in patients presenting with acute coronary events.[106] Of 697 patients followed for a period of 3.4 years, major adverse cardiovascular events occurred in 74 patients (cumulative rate 11.6%), wherein a 100% increase in angiographic diameter stenosis of the eventful lesions was observed.[106] The IVUS identified baseline plaque burden of greater than 70%, minimal luminal area of smaller than 4.0 mm^2, and the presence of TCFA (represented by necrotic core abutting the lumen) to be the strongest imaging characteristics predictive of eventful lesions. The ATHEROREMO IVUS study[107] similarly showed TCFA to be the independent predictor of composite end point of death or acute coronary event.

Because of the high resolution of OCT, the thickness of the fibrous cap can be measured (Fig. 16–6). The high-risk plaques demonstrated wide circumferential lipid arc and longitudinal lipid extent.[108,109] Numerous OCT studies have been reported in patients presenting with acute coronary events.[110,111] The median minimum thickness of the fibrous cap was 47 μm in patients presenting with myocardial infarction, 54 μm in unstable angina, and 103 μm in patients with chronic stable coronary syndrome,[110] confirming the pathological findings.[52,110] Similarly, another large OCT study of 103 lesions from patients with acute coronary syndrome and 163 lesions from patients with stable angina[60] showed the median minimum plaque cap thickness of 54 μm of ruptured plaques.[60] It has been proposed[112] that relatively thicker fibrous caps of vulnerable plaques could rupture during exercise. OCT studies have also demonstrated a significant increase in the fibrous cap thickness after statin therapy.[113,114] The standard deviation of the OCT signal intensity has been demonstrated to correlate well with histological measurements of fibrous cap macrophage density,[33] and a greater macrophage density was confirmed in the fibrous caps of culprit plaques in patients presenting with acute coronary events compared with the target lesions in the patients presenting with chronic coronary syndromes.[115] Even though an excellent agreement has been demonstrated between the plaque characteristics on postmortem OCT imaging and the histology, prospective outcomes studies similar to the PROSPECT trial are needed to evaluate the clinical utility of OCT imaging for the development of plaque level management algorithms for high-risk and/or culprit plaques.

It has been proposed that accurate identification of TCFA at an impending risk of rupture could be treated by preemptive self-expanding stent or bioabsorbable scaffold placement as a preventive measure (**Fig. 16–20**). A proof-of-principle feasibility and safety SECRITT trial[116] used a bare-metal self-expanding stent that allowed development of a thick fibrous cap similar to a stable plaque.[116] It has been further suggested that bioresorbable vascular scaffolds might prove superior to bare-metal stents because they are fully degraded within 4 years, leaving behind symmetric neointimal tissue exceeding 200 μm thickness similar to a stable fibroatheromatous plaque.[117] Although not with OCT, randomized prospective study designs have been reported for preemptive management employing IVUS and near-infrared spectroscopy (NIRS).

The PROSPECT II (Providing Regional Observations to Study Predictors of Events in the Coronary Tree II Combined with a Randomized, Controlled, Intervention Trial)[118] study quite like its predecessor recruited 898 patients after successful percutaneous coronary intervention (PCI) of all flow-limiting coronary lesions and performed 3-vessel imaging with a combination of IVUS and NIRS and followed them for 3.7 years. During follow-up, 84 events occurred attributed to 78 unique untreated nonculprit lesions in 66 (8.0%) patients. The mean baseline angiographic diameter stenosis of 46.9% progressed by the time of event to 68.4%. Event rate was substantially greater in nonculprit lesions with high-risk plaque characteristics including large lipid content (NIRS Max LCBI4mm = 325; adjusted odds ratio [aOR] 7.47), greater plaque burden (IVUS >70%; aOR 11.37), and lower minimum lumen area (<4 mm^2; aOR 4.99) compared with nonculprit lesions without high-risk character. A subset of patients with an angiographically nonobstructive stenosis not intended for PCI were randomized to preemptive treatment of the lesion with a bioresorbable vascular scaffold compared with guideline-directed medical therapy if IVUS-verified plaque burden was at least 65% (PROSPECT ABSORB). The primary (powered) effectiveness endpoint was the minimum lumen area (MLA), primary (nonpowered) safety endpoint target lesion failure defined as cardiac death, target vessel-related myocardial infarction, or revascularization, and secondary (nonpowered) clinical effectiveness endpoint lesion-related major adverse cardiovascular events including cardiac death, myocardial infarction, unstable angina, or progressive angina by 24 months. Of 182 randomized patients (median angiographic diameter stenosis 41.6%, median IVUS plaque burden 73.7%, median angiographic MLA 2.9 mm^2, median maximum lipid plaque content 33.4%), the median angiographic MLA in scaffold-treated lesions was substantially greater compared with medically treated lesions (OR 0.38). Even though 60% lower in the preemptively-treated patients due to a small number of events, the lesion-related major adverse cardiovascular events were statistically not significant, and there was no difference in target lesion failure.

The feasibility of differentiation of acute events associated with disrupted fibrous caps (plaque rupture) or intact fibrous caps (plaque erosion) by intravascular imaging,[73] could theoretically help improve management of the two distinct

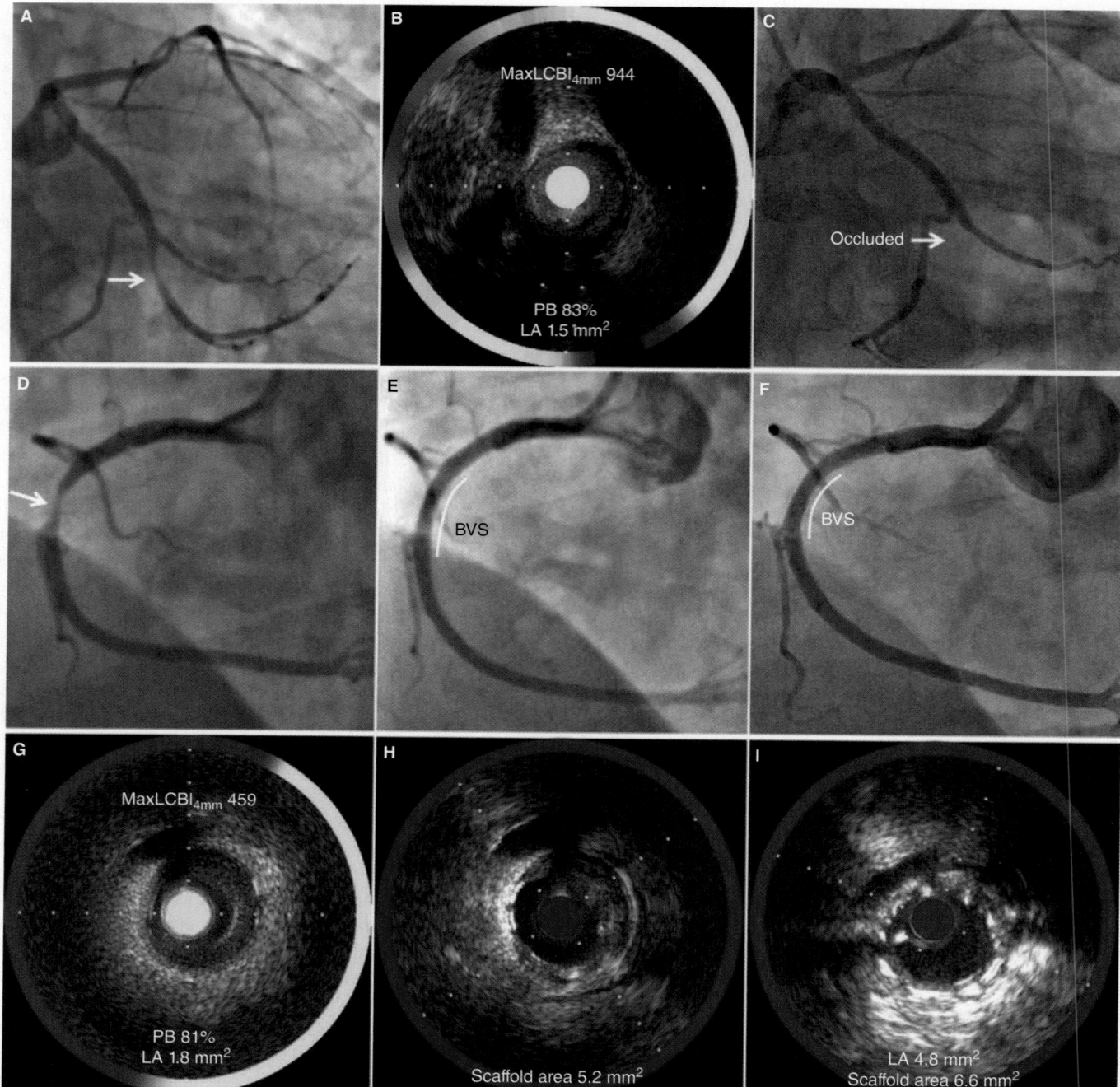

Figure 16–20. PROSPECT-II Absorb study. A 57-year-old man was admitted with a non-STEMI due to a high-grade stenosis of the LAD. After successful metallic stent implantation in the LAD, a 3-vessel imaging was performed. The operator considered two possible lesions for randomization to conservative treatment versus preemptive bioresorbable stent placement on the basis of a grayscale IVUS demonstrating a PB of >65% (*arrows* in **A, D**). Both lesions were angiographically moderately severe, but both were negative by FFR testing (FFR was 0.90 in both lesions). (**A**) The lesion in the obtuse marginal branch of the left circumflex artery had (**B**) a PB of 83%, an MLA of 1.5 mm², and a maxLCBI4mm of 944, consistent with 94% lipid at its most severe location. (**D**) The mid RCA lesion had (**G**) a PB of 81%, an MLA of 1.8 mm², and a maxLCBI4mm of 459, consistent with 46% lipid at its most severe location. The operator chose to randomize the RCA lesion, which was allocated to BVS plus GDMT. (**E**) The final result is shown. (**H**) Post–scaffold implant, the lumen had been enlarged to 5.2 mm². The patient was initially asymptomatic but presented 9 months later with severe progressive angina. (**C**) Repeat angiography demonstrated occluded OM branch of the LCX adjacent to the site of the original high-risk lesion; stented RCA was patent RCA (not shown). The operator chose to treat the LCX conservatively, and the patient remained stable with mild angina. At the 25-month protocol-driven routine follow-up, angiography and imaging were performed. (**F**) The LCX OM remained occluded (not shown), and (**I**) the RCA was widely patent, with a scaffold area of 6.6 mm² and a minimal luminal area of 4.8 mm², the difference representing neointimal hyperplasia, functionally, a thickened neocap covering the prior fibroatheroma. Reproduced with permission from Stone GW, Maehara A, Ali ZA, et al. Percutaneous Coronary Intervention for Vulnerable Coronary Atherosclerotic Plaque. *J Am Coll Cardiol.* 2020 Nov 17;76(20):2289-2301.

mechanisms of acute coronary events (Fig. 16–11). In erosive pathology, when stenosis of the arterial lumen is not clinically significant and the vessel wall not disrupted, aspiration of intraluminal thrombus could preclude the need for coronary stent placement.[73,119] In an observational report, standard-of-care stent placement in 60% of the patients was compared with the aspiration only in the remaining 40% of patients in the absence of a severely obstructive plaque. The latter patients were treated with aspirin, heparin, and a thienopyridine, with or without a glycoprotein IIb/IIIa inhibitor. The luminal stenosis was no different for the two groups, postprocedurally and after a 2-year follow-up; none of the thrombectomy-only patients required an additional revascularization. This approach seems attractive, but it would be necessary to determine in a randomized evaluation whether the benefit of adding OCT imaging to the diagnostic regimen would outweigh the detrimental effects of delay incurred in revascularization procedure.[119] The antithrombotic regimen needs to be perfected and the role of intracoronary plasmin would be explored. Owing to the limited resolution, other intravascular imaging modalities than OCT are not likely to be useful for clinically decision-making.

REFERENCES

1. Ross R. The pathogenesis of atherosclerosis–an update. *N Engl J Med.* 1986;314(8):488-500.

2. Ross R, Glomset JA. The pathogenesis of atherosclerosis (first of two parts). *N Engl J Med.* 1976;295(7):369-377.

3. Hansson GK. Inflammation, atherosclerosis, and coronary artery disease. *N Engl J Med.* 2005;352(16):1685-1695.

4. Hansson GK, Libby P, Schonbeck U, Yan ZQ. Innate and adaptive immunity in the pathogenesis of atherosclerosis. *Circ Res.* 2002;91(4):281-291.

5. Libby P. Inflammation in atherosclerosis. *Nature.* 2002;420(6917):868-874.

6. Fuster V. Lewis A. Conner Memorial Lecture. Mechanisms leading to myocardial infarction: insights from studies of vascular biology. *Circulation.* 1994;90(4):2126-2146.

7. Stary HC, Chandler AB, Dinsmore RE, et al. A definition of advanced types of atherosclerotic lesions and a histological classification of atherosclerosis. A report from the Committee on Vascular Lesions of the Council on Arteriosclerosis, American Heart Association. *Arterioscler Thromb Vasc Biol.* 1995;15(9):1512-1531.

8. Otsuka F, Joner M, Prati F, et al. Clinical classification of plaque morphology in coronary disease. *Nat Rev Cardiol.* 2014;11:379-389.

9. Virmani R, Kolodgie FD, Burke AP, Farb A, Schwartz SM. Lessons from sudden coronary death: a comprehensive morphological classification scheme for atherosclerotic lesions. *Arterioscler Thromb Vasc Biol.* 2000;20(5):1262-1275.

10. Kolodgie FD, Gold HK, Burke AP, et al. Intraplaque hemorrhage and progression of coronary atheroma. *N Engl J Med.* 2003;349(24):2316-2325.

11. Davies MJ, Thomas A. Thrombosis and acute coronary-artery lesions in sudden cardiac ischemic death. *N Engl J Med.* 1984;310(18):1137-1140.

12. Nakashima Y, Chen YX, Kinukawa N, Sueishi K. Distributions of diffuse intimal thickening in human arteries: preferential expression in atherosclerosis-prone arteries from an early age. *Virchows Arch.* 2002;441(3):279-288.

13. Ikari Y, McManus BM, Kenyon J, Schwartz SM. Neonatal intima formation in the human coronary artery. *Arterioscler Thromb Vasc Biol.* 1999;19(9):2036-2040.

14. McGill HC, Jr., McMahan CA, Tracy RE, et al. Relation of a postmortem renal index of hypertension to atherosclerosis and coronary artery size in young men and women. Pathobiological Determinants of Atherosclerosis in Youth (PDAY) Research Group. *Arterioscler Thromb Vasc Biol.* 1998;18(7):1108-1118.

15. Aikawa M, Rabkin E, Okada Y, et al. Lipid lowering by diet reduces matrix metalloproteinase activity and increases collagen content of rabbit atheroma: a potential mechanism of lesion stabilization. *Circulation.* 1998;97(24):2433-2444.

16. Fan J, Watanabe T. Inflammatory reactions in the pathogenesis of atherosclerosis. *J Atheroscler Thromb.* 2003;10(2):63-71.

17. McGill HC, Jr., McMahan CA, Herderick EE, et al. Effects of coronary heart disease risk factors on atherosclerosis of selected regions of the aorta and right coronary artery. PDAY Research Group. Pathobiological Determinants of Atherosclerosis in Youth. *Arterioscler Thromb Vasc Biol.* 2000;20(3):836-845.

18. Velican C. Relationship between regional aortic susceptibility to atherosclerosis and macromolecular structural stability. *J Atheroscler Res.* 1969;9(2):193-201.

19. Velican C. A dissecting view on the role of the fatty streak in the pathogenesis of human atherosclerosis: culprit or bystander? *Med Interne.* 1981;19(4):321-337.

20. Kockx MM, De Meyer GR, Bortier H, et al. Luminal foam cell accumulation is associated with smooth muscle cell death in the intimal thickening of human saphenous vein grafts. *Circulation.* 1996;94(6):1255-1262.

21. Radhakrishnamurthy B, Tracy RE, Dalferes ER, Jr., Berenson GS. Proteoglycans in human coronary arteriosclerotic lesions. *Exp Mol Pathol.* 1998;65(1):1-8.

22. Gustafsson M, Levin M, Skalen K, et al. Retention of low-density lipoprotein in atherosclerotic lesions of the mouse: evidence for a role of lipoprotein lipase. *Circ Res.* 2007;101(8):777-783.

23. Smith EB, Slater RS. The microdissection of large atherosclerotic plaques to give morphologically and topographically defined fractions for analysis. 1. The lipids in the isolated fractions. *Atherosclerosis.* 1972;15(1):37-56.

24. Tulenko TN, Chen M, Mason PE, Mason RP. Physical effects of cholesterol on arterial smooth muscle membranes: evidence of immiscible cholesterol domains and alterations in bilayer width during atherogenesis. *J Lipid Res.* 1998;39(5):947-956.

25. Otsuka F, Kramer MC, Woudstra P, et al. Natural progression of atherosclerosis from pathologic intimal thickening to late fibroatheroma in human coronary arteries: a pathology study. *Atherosclerosis.* 2015;241(2):772-782.

26. Wight TN, Kang I, Merrilees MJ. Versican and the control of inflammation. *Matrix Biol.* 2014;35:152-161.

27. Wight TN, Kinsella MG, Evanko SP, Potter-Perigo S, Merrilees MJ. Versican and the regulation of cell phenotype in disease. *Biochim Biophys Acta.* 2014;1840(8):2441-2451.

28. Bogels M, Braster R, Nijland PG, et al. Carcinoma origin dictates differential skewing of monocyte function. *Oncoimmunology.* 2012;1(6):798-809.

29. Stary HC, Chandler AB, Glagov S, et al. A definition of initial, fatty streak, and intermediate lesions of atherosclerosis. A report from the Committee on Vascular Lesions of the Council on Arteriosclerosis, American Heart Association. *Arterioscler Thromb.* 1994;14(5):840-856.

30. Nakashima Y, Fujii H, Sumiyoshi S, Wight TN, Sueishi K. Early human atherosclerosis: accumulation of lipid and proteoglycans in intimal thickenings followed by macrophage infiltration. *Arterioscler Thromb Vasc Biol.* 2007;27(5):1159-1165.

31. Kolodgie FD, Burke AP, Nakazawa G, Virmani R. Is pathologic intimal thickening the key to understanding early plaque progression in human atherosclerotic disease? *Arterioscler Thromb Vasc Biol.* 2007;27(5):986-989.

32. Tearney GJ, Regar E, Akasaka T, et al. Consensus standards for acquisition, measurement, and reporting of intravascular optical coherence tomography studies: a report from the International Working Group for Intravascular Optical Coherence Tomography Standardization and Validation. *J Am Coll Cardiol.* 2012;59(12):1058-1072.

33. Tearney GJ, Yabushita H, Houser SL, et al. Quantification of macrophage content in atherosclerotic plaques by optical coherence tomography. *Circulation.* 2003;107(1):113-119.

34. Stupka N, Kintakas C, White JD, et al. Versican processing by a disintegrin-like and metalloproteinase domain with thrombospondin-1 repeats proteinases-5 and -15 facilitates myoblast fusion. *J Biol Chem.* 2013;288(3):1907-1917.

35. Edsfeldt A, Goncalves I, Grufman H, et al. Impaired fibrous repair: a possible contributor to atherosclerotic plaque vulnerability in patients with type II diabetes. *Arterioscler Thromb Vasc Biol.* 2014;34(9):2143-2150.

36. Johnson JL, Jenkins NP, Huang WC, et al. Relationship of MMP-14 and TIMP-3 expression with macrophage activation and human atherosclerotic plaque vulnerability. *Mediators Inflamm.* 2014;2014:276457.

37. Lee CW, Hwang I, Park CS, et al. Comparison of ADAMTS-1, -4 and -5 expression in culprit plaques between acute myocardial infarction and stable angina. *J Clin Pathol.* 2011;64(5):399-404.

38. Sluimer JC, Kolodgie FD, Bijnens AP, et al. Thin-walled microvessels in human coronary atherosclerotic plaques show incomplete endothelial junctions relevance of compromised structural integrity for intraplaque microvascular leakage. *J Am Coll Cardiol.* 2009;53(17):1517-1527.

39. Virmani R, Joner M, Sakakura K. Recent highlights of ATVB: calcification. *Arterioscler Thromb Vasc Biol.* 2014;34(7):1329-1332.

40. Lowe HC, Narula J, Fujimoto JG, Jang IK. Intracoronary optical diagnostics current status, limitations, and potential. *JACC Cardiovasc Interv.* 2011;4(12):1257-1270.

41. Stary HC. Composition and classification of human atherosclerotic lesions. *Virchows Arch A Pathol Anat Histopathol.* 1992;421(4):277-290.

42. Stary HC. Changes in components and structure of atherosclerotic lesions developing from childhood to middle age in coronary arteries. *Basic Res Cardiol.* 1994;89 (Suppl 1):17-32.

43. Ross R, Wight TN, Strandness E, Thiele B. Human atherosclerosis. I. Cell constitution and characteristics of advanced lesions of the superficial femoral artery. *Am J Pathol.* 1984;114(1):79-93.

44. Torii S, Mustapha JA, Narula J, et al. Histopathologic characterization of peripheral arteries in subjects with abundant risk factors: correlating imaging with pathology. *JACC Cardiovasc Imaging.* 2019;12(8 Pt 1): 1501-1513.

45. Dong S, Smorgick Y, Nahir M, et al. Predictors for successful angioplasty of chronic totally occluded coronary arteries. *J Interv Cardiol.* 2005;18(1):1-7.

46. Ehara M, Terashima M, Kawai M, et al. Impact of multislice computed tomography to estimate difficulty in wire crossing in percutaneous coronary intervention for chronic total occlusion. *J Invasive Cardiol.* 2009;21(11):575-582.

47. Morino Y, Abe M, Morimoto T, et al. Predicting successful guidewire crossing through chronic total occlusion of native coronary lesions within 30 minutes: the J-CTO (Multicenter CTO Registry in Japan) score as a difficulty grading and time assessment tool. *JACC Cardiovasc Interv.* 2011;4(2):213-221.

48. van der Wal AC, Becker AE, van der Loos CM, Das PK. Site of intimal rupture or erosion of thrombosed coronary atherosclerotic plaques is characterized by an inflammatory process irrespective of the dominant plaque morphology. *Circulation.* 1994;89(1):36-44.

49. Farb A, Burke AP, Tang AL, et al. Coronary plaque erosion without rupture into a lipid core. A frequent cause of coronary thrombosis in sudden coronary death. *Circulation.* 1996;93(7):1354-1363.

50. Falk E, Nakano M, Bentzon JF, Finn AV, Virmani R. Update on acute coronary syndromes: the pathologists' view. *Eur Heart J.* 2013;34(10): 719-728.

51. Burke AP, Farb A, Malcom GT, Liang YH, Smialek J, Virmani R. Coronary risk factors and plaque morphology in men with coronary disease who died suddenly. *N Engl J Med.* 1997;336(18):1276-1282.

52. Narula J, Nakano M, Virmani R, et al. Histopathologic characteristics of atherosclerotic coronary disease and implications of the findings for the

invasive and noninvasive detection of vulnerable plaques. *J Am Coll Cardiol.* 2013;61(10):1041-1051.

53. Gijsen FJ, Wentzel JJ, Thury A, et al. Strain distribution over plaques in human coronary arteries relates to shear stress. *Am J Physiol Heart Circ Physiol.* 2008;295(4):H1608-H1614.

54. Sukhova GK, Schonbeck U, Rabkin E, et al. Evidence for increased collagenolysis by interstitial collagenases-1 and -3 in vulnerable human atheromatous plaques. *Circulation.* 1999;99(19):2503-2509.

55. Kolodgie FD, Narula J, Burke AP, et al. Localization of apoptotic macrophages at the site of plaque rupture in sudden coronary death. *Am J Pathol.* 2000;157(4):1259-1268.

56. Burke AP, Farb A, Malcom GT, Liang Y, Smialek JE, Virmani R. Plaque rupture and sudden death related to exertion in men with coronary artery disease. *JAMA.* 1999;281(10):921-926.

57. Vengrenyuk Y, Carlier S, Xanthos S, et al. A hypothesis for vulnerable plaque rupture due to stress-induced debonding around cellular microcalcifications in thin fibrous caps. *Proc Natl Acad Sci U S A.* 2006;103(40):14678-14683.

58. Yonetsu T, Kakuta T, Lee T, et al. In vivo critical fibrous cap thickness for rupture-prone coronary plaques assessed by optical coherence tomography. *Eur Heart J.* 2011;32(10):1251-1259.

59. Burke AP, Farb A, Malcolm GT, Liang YH, Smialek J, Virmani R. Coronary risk factors and plaque morphology in men with coronary disease who died suddenly. *N Engl J Med.* 1997;336:1276-82.

60. Prati F, Regar E, Mintz GS, et al. Expert review document on methodology, terminology, and clinical applications of optical coherence tomography: physical principles, methodology of image acquisition, and clinical application for assessment of coronary arteries and atherosclerosis. *Eur Heart J.* 2010;31(4):401-415.

61. Motoyama S, Kondo T, Sarai M, et al. Multislice computed tomographic characteristics of coronary lesions in acute coronary syndromes. *J Am Coll Cardiol.* 2007;50:319-326.

62. Motoyama S, Ito H, Sarai M, et al. Plaque characterization by coronary computed tomography angiography and the likelihood of acute coronary events in mid-term follow-up. *J Am Coll Cardiol.* 2015;66(4):337-346.

63. Motoyama S, Sarai M, Harigaya H, et al. Computed tomographic angiography characteristics of atherosclerotic plaques subsequently resulting in acute coronary syndrome. *J Am Coll Cardiol.* 2009;54(1):49-57.

64. Rogers IS, Nasir K, Figueroa AL, et al. Feasibility of imaging of coronary arteries: comparison between acute coronary syndromes. *JACC Cardiovasc Imaging.* 2010;3:388-97.

65. Oikonomou E, Marwan M, Desai MY, et al. Noninvasive detection of coronary inflammation using computed tomography and prediction of residual cardiovascular risk (CRISP-CT study). *Lancet.* 2018;392:929-39.

66. Yahagi K, Zarpak R, Sakakura K, et al. Multiple simultaneous plaque erosion in 3 coronary arteries. *JACC Cardiovasc Imaging.* 2014;7(11): 1172-1174.

67. Kolodgie FD, Burke AP, Farb A, et al. Differential accumulation of proteoglycans and hyaluronan in culprit lesions: insights into plaque erosion. *Arterioscler Thromb Vasc Biol.* 2002;22(10):1642-1648.

68. Pedicino D, Vinci R, Giglio AF, et al. Alterations of hyaluranon metabolism in acute coronary syndrome: implications for plaque erosion. *J Am Coll Cardiol.* 2018;72:1490-1503.

69. Burke AP, Farb A, Malcom GT, Liang Y, Smialek J, Virmani R. Effect of risk factors on the mechanism of acute thrombosis and sudden coronary death in women. *Circulation.* 1998;97(21):2110-2116.

70. Kramer MC, Rittersma SZ, de Winter RJ, et al. Relationship of thrombus healing to underlying plaque morphology in sudden coronary death. *J Am Coll Cardiol.* 2010;55(2):122-132.

71. Schwartz RS, Burke A, Farb A, et al. Microemboli and microvascular obstruction in acute coronary thrombosis and sudden coronary death: relation to epicardial plaque histopathology. *J Am Coll Cardiol.* 2009;54(23):2167-2173.

72. Ozaki Y, Okumura M, Ismail TF, et al. Coronary CT angiographic characteristics of culprit lesions in acute coronary syndromes not related to plaque rupture as defined by optical coherence tomography and angioscopy. *Eur Heart J.* 2011;32(22):2814-2823.

73. Prati F, Uemura S, Souteyrand G, et al. OCT-based diagnosis and management of STEMI associated with intact fibrous cap. *JACC Cardiovasc Imaging.* 2013;6:283-7.

74. Torii S, Sato Y, Otsuka F, et al. Eruptive calcified nodules as a potential mechanism of acute coronary thrombosis and sudden death. *J Am Coll Cardiol.* 2021;77(13):1599-1611.

75. Arbustini E, Vengrenyuk Y, Narula J. On the shades of coronary calcium and plaque instability. *J Am Coll Cardiol.* 2021;77(13):1612-1615.

76. Ciurica S, Lopez-Sublet M, Loeys BL, et al. Arterial tortuosity. *Hypertension.* 2019;73(5):951-960.

77. Kahe F, Sharfaei S, Pitliya A, et al. Coronary artery tortuosity: a narrative review. *Coron Artery Dis.* 2020;31(2):187-192.

78. Callewaert BL, Willaert A, Kerstjens-Frederikse WS, et al. Arterial tortuosity syndrome: clinical and molecular findings in 12 newly identified families. *Hum Mutat.* 2008;29(1):150-158.

79. Huang H, Virmani R, Younis H, Burke AP, Kamm RD, Lee RT. The impact of calcification on the biomechanical stability of atherosclerotic plaques. *Circulation.* 2001;103(8):1051-1056.

80. Kelly-Arnold A, Maldonado N, Laudier D, Aikawa E, Cardoso L, Weinbaum S. Revised microcalcification hypothesis for fibrous cap rupture in human coronary arteries. *Proc Natl Acad Sci U S A.* 2013;110(26):10741-10746.

81. Yang C, Bach RG, Zheng J, et al. In vivo IVUS-based 3-D fluid-structure interaction models with cyclic bending and anisotropic vessel properties for human atherosclerotic coronary plaque mechanical analysis. *IEEE Trans Biomed Eng.* 2009;56(10):2420-2428.

82. Karanosos A, Ligthart JM, Witberg KT, Regar E. Calcified nodules: an underrated mechanism of coronary thrombosis. *JACC Cardiovasc Imaging.* 2012;5:1071-72.

83. Prati F, Gatto L, Fabbiocchi F, et al. Clinical outcomes of calcified nodules detected by optical coherence tomography: a sub-analysis of the CLIMA study. *EuroIntervention.* 2020;16(5):380-386.

84. Sakamoto A, Virmani R, Finn AV, Gupta A. Calcified nodule as the cause of acute coronary syndrome: connecting bench observations to the bedside. *Cardiology.* 2018;139(2):101-104.

85. Tabas I. Consequences of cellular cholesterol accumulation: basic concepts and physiological implications. *J Clin Invest.* 2002;110(7):905-911.

86. Takaya N, Yuan C, Chu B, et al. Presence of intraplaque hemorrhage stimulates progression of carotid atherosclerotic plaques: a high-resolution magnetic resonance imaging study. *Circulation.* 2005;111(21):2768-2775.

87. Chistiakov DA, Orekhov AN, Bobryshev YV. Contribution of neovascularization and intraplaque haemorrhage to atherosclerotic plaque progression and instability. *Acta Physiol (Oxf).* 2015;213(3):539-553.

88. Virmani R, Kolodgie FD, Burke AP, et al. Atherosclerotic plaque progression and vulnerability to rupture: angiogenesis as a source of intraplaque hemorrhage. *Arterioscler Thromb Vasc Biol.* 2005;25(10):2054-2061.

89. Mulligan-Kehoe MJ, Simons M. Vasa vasorum in normal and diseased arteries. *Circulation.* 2014;129(24):2557-2566.

90. Burke AP, Kolodgie FD, Farb A, et al. Healed plaque ruptures and sudden coronary death: evidence that subclinical rupture has a role in plaque progression. *Circulation.* 2001;103(7):934-940.

91. Sakakura K, Nakano M, Otsuka F, et al. Comparison of pathology of chronic total occlusion with and without coronary artery bypass graft. *Eur Heart J.* 2014;35(25):1683-1693.

92. Mann J, Davies MJ. Mechanisms of progression in native coronary artery disease: role of healed plaque disruption. *Heart.* 1999;82(3):265-268.

93. Zadeh AA, Jang IK, Blumenthal R, Libby P, Fuster V. Atherosclerosis imaging for preventing acute coronary events. *J Am Coll Cardiol.* 2021;78:1257-66.

94. Constantindes P. Coronary thrombosis linked to fissure in atherosclerotic vessel wall. *JAMA.* 1964;188:SUPPL:35-37.

95. Finn AV, Kolodgie FD, Nakano M, Virmani R. The differences between neovascularization of chronic total occlusion and intraplaque angiogenesis. *JACC Cardiovasc Imaging.* 2010;3(8):806-810.

96. Blotnick S, Peoples GE, Freeman MR, Eberlein TJ, Klagsbrun M. T lymphocytes synthesize and export heparin-binding epidermal growth factor-like growth factor and basic fibroblast growth factor, mitogens for vascular cells and fibroblasts: differential production and release by CD4+ and CD8+ T cells. *Proc Natl Acad Sci U S A.* 1994;91(8):2890-2894.

97. Kumamoto M, Nakashima Y, Sueishi K. Intimal neovascularization in human coronary atherosclerosis: its origin and pathophysiological significance. *Hum Pathol.* 1995;26(4):450-456.

98. Srivatsa SS, Edwards WD, Boos CM, et al. Histologic correlates of angiographic chronic total coronary artery occlusions: influence of occlusion duration on neovascular channel patterns and intimal plaque composition. *J Am Coll Cardiol.* 1997;29(5):955-963.

99. Katsuragawa M, Fujiwara H, Miyamae M, Sasayama S. Histologic studies in percutaneous transluminal coronary angioplasty for chronic total occlusion: comparison of tapering and abrupt types of occlusion and short and long occluded segments. *J Am Coll Cardiol.* 1993;21(3):604-611.

100. Surmely JF, Katoh O, Tsuchikane E, Nasu K, Suzuki T. Coronary septal collaterals as an access for the retrograde approach in the percutaneous treatment of coronary chronic total occlusions. *Catheter Cardiovasc Interv.* 2007;69(6):826-832.

101. Rathore S, Katoh O, Tuschikane E, Oida A, Suzuki T, Takase S. A novel modification of the retrograde approach for the recanalization of chronic total occlusion of the coronary arteries intravascular ultrasound-guided reverse controlled antegrade and retrograde tracking. *JACC Cardiovasc Interv.* 2010;3(2):155-164.

102. Glaser R, Selzer F, Faxon DP, et al. Clinical progression of incidental, asymptomatic lesions discovered during culprit vessel coronary intervention. *Circulation.* 2005;111(2):143-149.

103. Moreno PR, Narula J. Thinking outside the lumen: fractional flow reserve versus intravascular imaging for major adverse cardiac event prediction. *J Am Coll Cardiol.* 2014;63(12):1141-1144.

104. Niccoli G, Stefanini GG, Capodanno D, Crea F, Ambrose JA, Berg R. Are the culprit lesions severely stenotic? *JACC Cardiovasc Imaging.* 2013;6(10):1108-1114.

105. Stone GW, Narula J. The myth of the mild vulnerable plaques. *JACC Cardiovasc Imaging.* 2013;6(10):1124-1126.

106. Stone GW, Maehara A, Lansky AJ, et al. A prospective natural-history study of coronary atherosclerosis. *N Engl J Med.* 2011;364(3):226-235.

107. Cheng JM, Garcia-Garcia HM, de Boer SP, et al. In vivo detection of high-risk coronary plaques by radiofrequency intravascular ultrasound and cardiovascular outcome: results of the ATHEROREMO-IVUS study. *Eur Heart J.* 2014;35(10):639-647.

108. Kato K, Yonetsu T, Kim SJ, et al. Nonculprit plaques in patients with acute coronary syndromes have more vulnerable features compared with those with non-acute coronary syndromes: a 3-vessel optical coherence tomography study. *Circ Cardiovasc Imaging.* 2012;5(4):433-440.

109. Kubo T, Imanishi T, Takarada S, et al. Assessment of culprit lesion morphology in acute myocardial infarction: ability of optical coherence tomography compared with intravascular ultrasound and coronary angioscopy. *J Am Coll Cardiol.* 2007;50(10):933-939.

110. Jang IK, Tearney GJ, MacNeill B, et al. In vivo characterization of coronary atherosclerotic plaque by use of optical coherence tomography. *Circulation.* 2005;111(12):1551-1555.

111. Kubo T, Imanishi T, Kashiwagi M, et al. Multiple coronary lesion instability in patients with acute myocardial infarction as determined by optical coherence tomography. *Am J Cardiol.* 2010;105(3):318-322.

112. Tanaka A, Imanishi T, Kitabata H, et al. Morphology of exertion-triggered plaque rupture in patients with acute coronary syndrome: an optical coherence tomography study. *Circulation.* 2008;118(23):2368-2373.

113. Hattori K, Ozaki Y, Ismail TF, et al. Impact of statin therapy on plaque characteristics as assessed by serial OCT, grayscale and integrated backscatter-IVUS. *JACC Cardiovasc Imaging.* 2012;5(2):169-177.

114. Takarada S, Imanishi T, Kubo T, et al. Effect of statin therapy on coronary fibrous-cap thickness in patients with acute coronary syndrome: assessment by optical coherence tomography study. *Atherosclerosis.* 2009;202(2):491-497.

115. MacNeill BD, Jang IK, Bouma BE, et al. Focal and multi-focal plaque macrophage distributions in patients with acute and stable presentations of coronary artery disease. *J Am Coll Cardiol.* 2004;44(5):972-979.

116. Wykrzykowska JJ, Diletti R, Gutierrez-Chico JL, et al. Plaque sealing and passivation with a mechanical self-expanding low outward force nitinol vShield device for the treatment of IVUS and OCT-derived thin cap fibroatheromas (TCFAs) in native coronary arteries: report of the pilot study vShield Evaluated at Cardiac hospital in Rotterdam for Investigation and Treatment of TCFA (SECRITT). *EuroIntervention.* 2012;8(8):945-954.

117. Onuma Y, Serruys PW, Perkins LE, et al. Intracoronary optical coherence tomography and histology at 1 month and 2, 3, and 4 years after implantation of everolimus-eluting bioresorbable vascular scaffolds in a porcine coronary artery model: an attempt to decipher the human optical coherence tomography images in the ABSORB trial. *Circulation.* 2010;122(22):2288-2300.

118. Stone GW, Maehara A, Ali ZA et al. Percutaneous coronary intervention for vulnerable coronary atherosclerotic plaque. *J Am Coll Cardiol.* 2020;76:2289-2301.

119. Braunwald E. Coronary plaque erosion: recognition and management. *JACC Cardiovasc Imaging.* 2013;6(3):288-289.

Pathogenesis of Coronary Thrombosis and Myocardial Infarction

Gemma Vilahur, Valentín Fuster, and Borja Ibanez

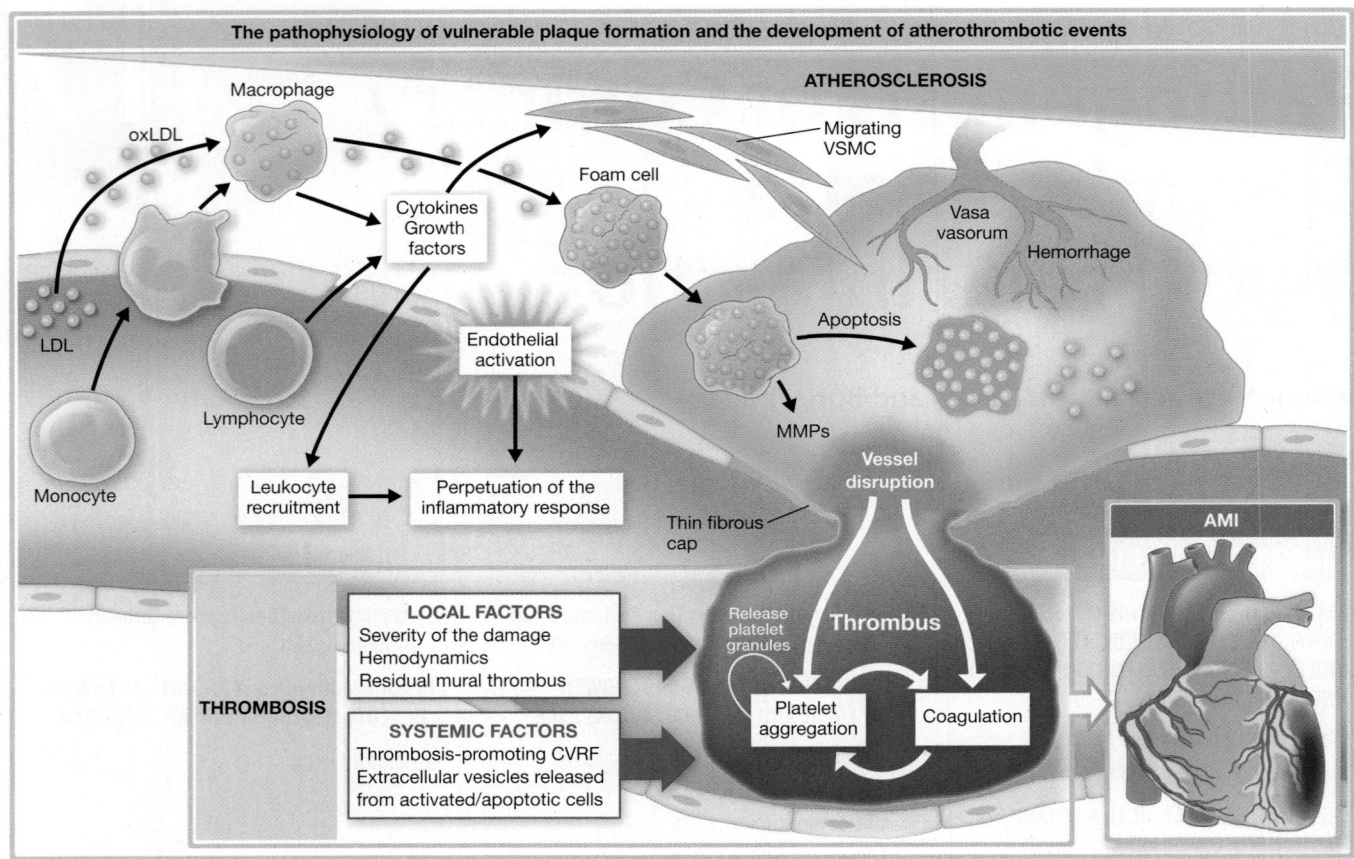

Chapter 17 Fuster and Hurst's Central Illustration. High-risk atherosclerotic plaques are characterized by a high inflammatory burden and the formation of leaky neovessels that penetrate from the adventitia, favoring intraplaque hemorrhage. Atherosclerotic plaque disruption (fibrous cap rupture or superficial erosion) exposes thrombogenic surfaces that trigger activation of platelets and the coagulation system, leading to thrombus formation and subsequent atherothrombotic events. CVRF, cardiovascular risk factors; LDL, low-density lipoprotein; MMPs, matrix metalloproteases; VSMC, vascular smooth muscle cell.

CHAPTER SUMMARY

This chapter discusses the most recent advances in the understanding of the pathophysiology of vulnerable plaque formation and provides new insights into the molecular mechanisms and sequence of events that drive thrombus formation at the culprit site (see Fuster and Hurst's Central Illustration). High-risk atherosclerotic plaques are characterized by a high inflammatory burden tightly intertwined with the formation of leaky neovessels that penetrate from the adventitia, favoring intra-plaque hemorrhage. Atherosclerotic plaque disruption (either fibrous cap rupture or superficial erosion) exposes thrombogenic surfaces that trigger a complex and coordinated activation of platelets and the coagulation system, leading to thrombus formation and the perpetuation of the inflammatory response. Recent large-scale clinical trials have verified the benefits of anti-inflammatory therapies in the reduction of cardiovascular events. Other factors are also known to affect or modulate thrombus growth either locally (eg, degree of stenosis and lesion injury, and fluid dynamics) or systemically (traditional and newly identified cardiovascular risk factors and extracellular vesicles). Further progress toward better characterization of rupture-prone atherosclerotic plaques and the higher susceptibility to thrombosis (the so-called vulnerable patient) will reduce the risk of atherothrombotic events, the leading cause of morbidity and mortality worldwide.

FEATURES OF THE HIGH-RISK ATHEROSCLEROTIC PLAQUE: THE KEY ROLE OF NEOVASCULARIZATION AND INFLAMMATION

Atherosclerosis is a systemic and nonresolving chronic inflammatory disease that occurs in the intima of large and medium-sized arteries (ie, aorta, carotids, coronaries, and peripheral arteries) and is characterized by intimal thickening caused by the accumulation of cells and lipids (**Fig. 17–1**).[1] Atherothrombosis mainly represents the clinical manifestation of this pathology in which atherosclerotic plaque rupture or erosion triggers the formation of an acute thrombus, obstructing coronary blood flow and reducing the oxygen supply to the myocardium, leading to the onset of acute coronary syndromes (ACS).[2,3] ACS represents a spectrum of ischemic myocardial events that share similar pathophysiology; these include unstable angina (UA)/non–ST-segment elevation myocardial infarction (UA/NSTEMI) and ST-segment elevation myocardial infarction (STEMI), which may lead to the occurrence of sudden cardiac death.

The early atherosclerotic lesions might progress without compromising the lumen, because of compensatory vascular enlargement (Glagovian remodeling) to preserve luminal dimensions and coronary flow reserve.[4] Importantly, the culprit lesions leading to ACS are usually nonobstructive and, therefore, barely detected by angiography.[5] It is well recognized that the culprit plaques contain vulnerable features, including a large lipid core; a low vascular smooth muscle cell content (VSMC); microcalcification; a thin fibrous cap (<65 μm thick); neovascularization; and a high density of inflammatory cells (particularly at the shoulder region where disruptions most often occur).[6] In fact, these plaque characteristics have become potentially important imaging targets to identify high-risk plaques (**Fig. 17–2**).[7-10] Implementation of "molecular and cellular imaging" has allowed a more specific, refined characterization of atherosclerotic lesions. As such, within recent years, multiple engineered molecular imaging probes have been developed to noninvasively characterize plaque components including foam cells, macrophages, matrix metalloproteinase (MMP)-2, vascular endothelial growth factor (VEGF), oxidized low-density lipoprotein (Ox-LDL), and vascular cell adhesion molecule (VCAM) as well as to identify the fibrin mesh.[11-14] Yet, whereas plaque burden seems to fairly predict the occurrence of thrombotic events (the more plaques a patient has, the more likely a rupture will occur), there is still a scarce direct predictive value between features of plaque vulnerability and clinical events.[9] Nevertheless, it certainly helps to identify vulnerable patients with a higher likelihood of plaque rupture and clinical events.[9] Studies from the Multi-Ethnic Study of Atherosclerosis (MESA) trial suggest that adding coronary artery calcium (CAC) to the American College of Cardiology (ACC)/American Heart Association (AHA) risk calculator may improve prediction of atherosclerotic cardiovascular disease (ASCVD) events[15] and may also guide more rationale aspirin allocation for primary prevention.[16] There is also an abundance of

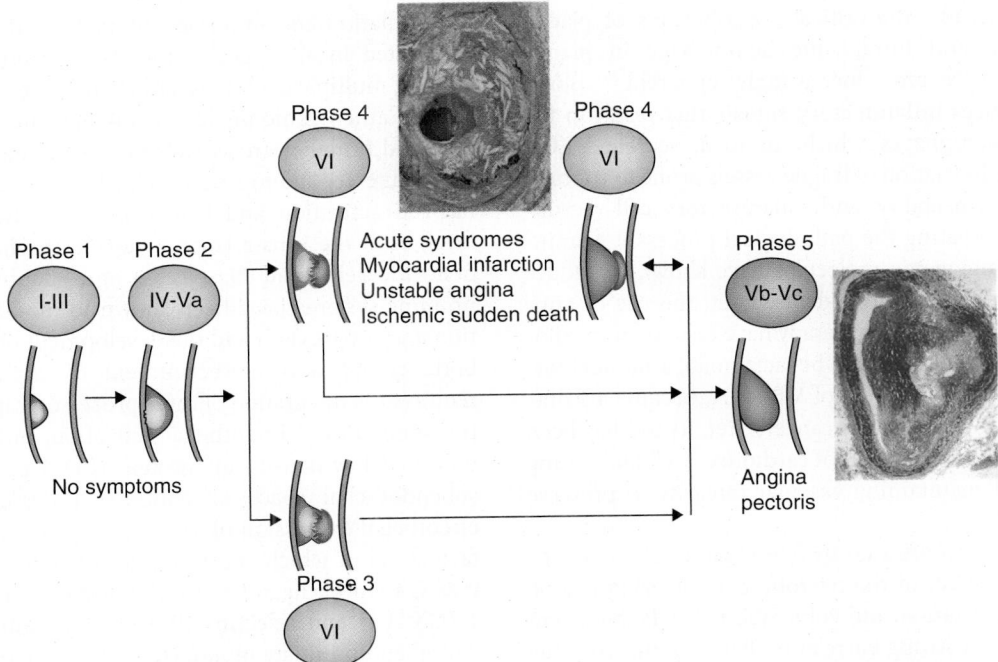

Figure 17–1. Simplified diagram of the evolution of coronary atherosclerosis. Phases and morphology of lesion progression. Roman numbers designate the sequence of atherosclerotic lesion progression according to histological classification being type I the initial lesion that contains scattered foam cells and type VI those plaque that have undergone fissure, hematoma, and thrombus superimposition. Type V lesions have been subclassified into those plaques that contain a rich lipid core and connective tissue (type Va lesion), those largely calcified (type Vb), or those rich in fibrous connective tissue and little or no accumulated lipid or calcium (type Vc).

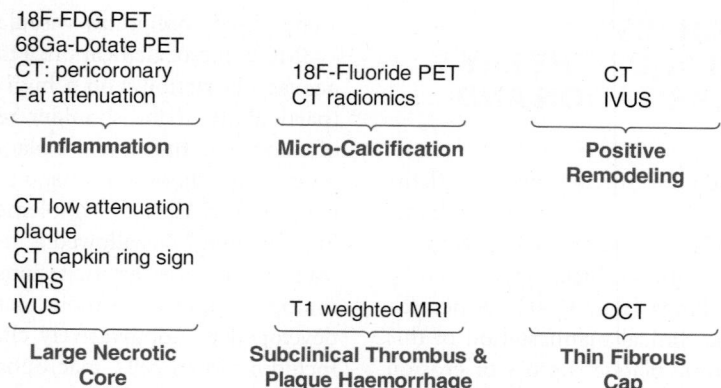

Figure 17–2. Invasive and noninvasive imaging techniques used to depict vulnerable plaque features. CT, computed tomography; IVUS, intravascular ultrasound; NIRS, near infrared spectroscopy; OCT, optical coherence tomography; PET, Positron emission tomography.

evidence, mostly from imaging studies, supporting an association between inflammation and calcium deposition, but whether inflammation precedes calcification or rather calcification triggers inflammation still needs to be determined.[17,18] Careful stratification of atherosclerotic plaque based on the stage of calcification, not alone but in combination with a full patient vulnerability profile or with the degree of coronary stenosis, has shown potential value in providing additional information as per the risk of suffering an event.[19] Randomized controlled trials are needed to determine the optimal imaging approach to identify culprit plaques and the clinical utility of plaque phenotyping.

Plaque Neovascularization

Within the last decade, the critical contributions of plaque neovascularization and intraplaque hemorrhage in plaque vulnerability have become increasingly apparent.[20] Blood extravasation induces inflammatory signals that result in the infiltration of macrophages which, in turn, secrete VEGF. VEGF induces the formation of fragile vessels prone to rupture, favors vascular permeability, and inflammatory cell recruitment further exacerbating the pathological process.[21] Administration of anti-angiogenic molecules have shown to reduce atherosclerotic progression in rodents.[22] Yet, the use of anti-angiogenic drugs in anticancer therapy have resulted in cardiovascular adverse effects. As such, bevacizumab, a monoclonal antibody that binds all isoforms of VEGF-A, became a front-line treatment option for several cancers. Yet, its use has been associated with the development of cardiotoxicity highlighting the importance of maintaining vascular integrity to preserve cardiac function.[23]

Erythrocytes, which are rich in free cholesterol, also contribute to the expansion of the necrotic core favoring plaque progression, destabilization, and vulnerability.[24-27] Postmortem studies have shown a strong correlation between macrophage infiltration and increased vasa vasorum in human atherosclerotic lesions. Preexisting vasa vasorum in the adventitia is thought to spread into the intima, prompting intimal neovascularization.[28] The use of optical coherence tomography (OCT) has associated vasa vasorum increase with fibrous plaque

volume and intraplaque neovessels with plaque vulnerability becoming a potential new biomarker for plaque vulnerability.[29] On the other hand, inhibition of plaque neovascularization has been regarded as a potential new therapeutic intervention to minimize plaque disruption.[30] A recent pilot clinical study in atherosclerotic patients has demonstrated that a short period of sonodynamic therapy (ie, the use of ultrasonography to stimulate the production of reactive oxygen species) reduces atherosclerotic plaque inflammation and neovascularization assessed in both the carotid and femoral arteries.[31] Interestingly, the benefits of this short-period intervention was equivalent to that detected after a 3-month intensive statin treatment.[31]

Plaque Inflammation

Inflammation and immune system activation are key factors implicated in all stages of the atherothrombotic process.[32,33] Among multiple cytokines and chemokines secreted throughout the atherogenic process, cytokines interleukin (IL)-1 and IL-6 and tumor necrosis factor (TNF)-α, have been shown to contribute to atherogenesis, largely by promoting endothelial cell activation and leukocyte recruitment. At a cellular level, both the innate (monocytes/macrophages, neutrophils, dendritic cells, and mast cells) and adaptive (lymphocytes) immune systems have been shown to modulate lesion initiation and progression and the development of potential thrombotic complications. Recruitment of circulating monocyte requires the integration of three processes; capture, rolling, and transmigration.[34] Endothelial activation, induced by retained modified low-density lipoprotein (LDL) particles within the subendothelial space or endothelial dysfunction, leads to endothelial expression of selectins, integrins, and chemotactic factors, all of which contribute to monocyte arrest. Chemokines C-C motif ligand 5 (CCL5) and CXC-chemokine ligand 1 (CXCL1) and selectins (P, E, and L) immobilized on the endothelium initiate monocyte capture, rolling, and tethering, whereas VCAM1 and intercellular adhesion molecule (ICAM) 1, as well as some of the integrins, mediate firm adhesion at the vascular surface. Monocyte transmigration is mainly mediated by platelet endothelial cell adhesion molecule (PECAM)-1 as well as locally produced chemokines CCL2, CX3CL1, and

CCL5.[34] Once internalized monocytes release inflammatory mediators that perpetuate monocyte recruitment favoring lesion progression. Monocytes are divided into three major types according to their expression of CD14 and CD16.[35] CD14+/CD16- monocytes, also known as "classical" or Mon1, are the most abundant subtype. They express CCR2 (receptor for MCP-1), CD62L, CD64, and CD115, but not CXCR1, and they perpetuate the inflammatory status by releasing reactive oxygen species (ROS), TNF-α, IL-1, and other inflammatory cytokines. A second subtype is the CD14+/CD16++ Mon3 cells, also called "nonclassical" or patrolling monocytes. These do not express CCR2 or CD64 but express CXCR1 (receptor for fractalkine). They release transforming growth factor-beta, CD36, CD163, and VEGF. They are less inflammatory and responsible for metabolic tissue repair. Finally, Mon2 consists of a subtype of CD14++/CD16+ monocytes, also called intermediate, that express high levels of CCR2, CX3CR1, and CDS115, but not CD62. Their role is still not well understood, although they may be proinflammatory.[36] High Mon2 levels have been associated with a poor outcome in patients with STEMI.[37]

Once in the intimal space, two cytokines, macrophage colony-stimulating factor (M-CSF; constitutively expressed in the circulation) and granulocyte-macrophage colony stimulating factor (GM-CSF; induced under inflammatory stimuli), facilitate monocyte proliferation and their phenotypic transformation into macrophages. Moreover, they also modulate macrophage polarization into proinflammatory (M1) and anti-inflammatory (M2) phenotypes.[38] More precisely, in vitro studies have suggested that M-CSF mostly promotes M2 polarization whereas GM-CSF induces the proinflammatory phenotype.[39] Within atherosclerotic lesions, macrophages have been described to present both phenotypes with a higher tendency toward M1 macrophages being more densely populated within the vulnerable shoulder region of a plaque.[35] The attenuation of the proatherogenic state, as occurs in conditions characterized by high-density lipoprotein (HDL)-raising or LDL-lowering by statins, seems to facilitate the efflux of the wall macrophages removing the excess of cholesterol deposited in the intima. Whether it is due to reduced levels of the retaining factors or systemic lipid-lowering is not clear yet.[36]

Macrophages also play a key role in plaque vulnerability. As such, in the developed plaque, proinflammatory macrophages secrete MMP (mainly MMP9) that degrade the extracellular matrix (ECM), providing physical strength to the fibrous cap and increasing its susceptibility to disruption.[40] In fact, an association between the activity of the leukocyte enzyme myeloperoxidase (MPO) and features of vulnerable plaque have been reported.[41] LDL has also been shown to downregulate the expression of lysyl-oxidase (LOX), an enzyme that contributes to the maturation of the elastin and collagen fibrils that compose the ECM. In addition to secreting proteases and increasing the likelihood of plaque rupture, lipid-rich intraplaque macrophages undergo apoptosis, expressing tissue factor (TF) and increasing the thrombogenic status of the vascular lesions.

Plaque vulnerability and thrombogenic status can be reduced by long-term treatment with lipid-lowering agents.[42] Whether the same holds for HDL-raising therapies remains to be proven. HDLs have long been considered to exert multiple cardiovascular benefits based on epidemiological and retrospective data in patients with no baseline cardiovascular disease and multiple experimental animal studies.[43–46] In this later regard, preclinical evidence and small human studies suggest that acute treatment with recombinant apo A-I Milano or other HDL-targeting interventions can induce acute plaque stabilization, representing a promising approach for high-risk patients.[47,48] Yet, lately, conflicting results have been reported in humans as to the beneficial effects afforded by the infusion of different HDL-related constructs, some reporting benefits, and others not.[49,50] Moreover, pharmacotherapy-based approaches for raising HDL-cholesterol in secondary prevention, including the use of fibrates, niacin, and CETP inhibitors, have not led to the expected favorable outcomes.[51–53] Moreover, Mendelian randomization studies have failed to confirm the causal relationship between HDL cholesterol levels and atherosclerosis. The apparent discordance has initiated an important discussion on the physiological value of the quality versus quantity of HDL.[54] In this regard, it has become increasingly evident that the presence of comorbidities including diabetes, metabolic syndrome, chronic inflammatory conditions, hypertriglyceridemia, or hypercholesterolemia impairs HDL-related protective effects.[48,55–57] Moreover, recent studies have linked the lack of HDL functionality with subclinical cardiovascular disorders.[58] Further research is needed to identify the components involved in the loss of HDL function to select those targets that will allow restoring or enhancing HDL cardiovascular beneficial effects.

Besides monocyte/macrophages, the *acquired or trained immune system* has also shown to play an important role in atherogenesis.[59] T lymphocytes constitute 10% of all cells in human lesions and enter the intima by binding to VCAM-1 where they become activated by interferon (IFN)-γ, recognize modified autoantigens (eg, OxLDL and heat shock protein [HSP]-60), and start releasing inflammatory cytokines. As occurs with monocytes, among the T lymphocytes, the T helper (Th) 1 and 17 lineages release IFN-γ and are proinflammatory while the Th2 subtype and regulatory T cells (Treg) are anti-inflammatory **(Fig. 17–3)**.

While the role of T cells in atherosclerosis has been studied extensively, the role of B cells has only recently begun to gain attention, probably because they accumulate in small numbers in atherosclerotic plaques. Among B-cell subsets, B1 has shown to be atheroprotective by secreting antibodies against modified LDL to favor oxLDL clearance, whilst B2 cells have been shown to exert both atherogenic (B2 cells formed in the follicular region of lymph nodes and spleen) and atheroprotective (B2 cells formed in the marginal zone of the spleen and lymph nodes) effects.[60] The possibility of modulating the adaptive immune system has been regarded as a novel therapeutic target to treat atherosclerosis.[61,62] Studies are ongoing into the development of vaccines that could effectively interfere with the proportion of pro- and anti-inflammatory cells in the lesions and the secretion of protective antibodies while affecting the general host defense. Multiple studies have also highlighted the contribution of dendritic cells (DCs), mast

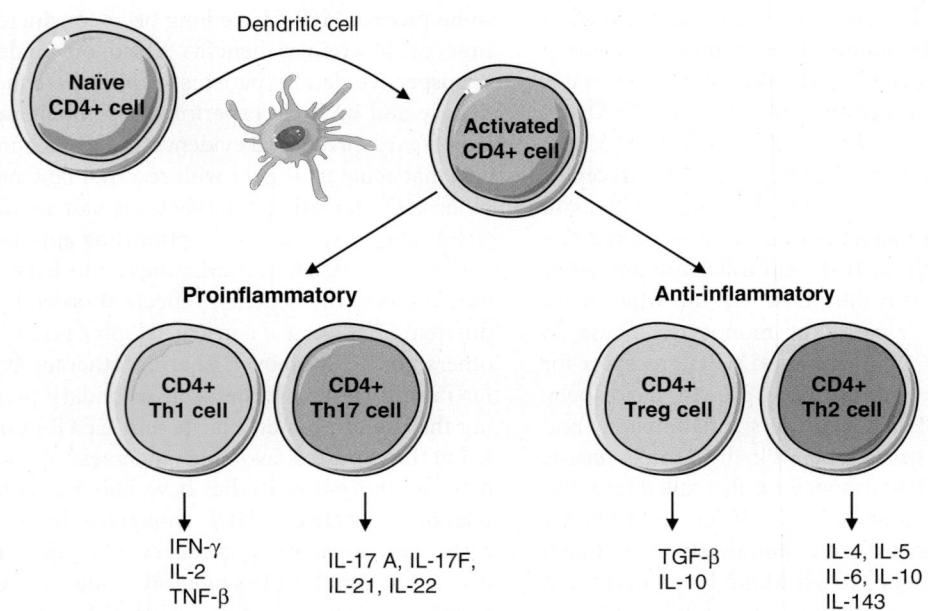

Figure 17–3. Types of CD4+ T cells involved in the pathogenesis of the atherosclerotic process.

cells, and neutrophils on atherosclerosis progression. Mast cells are inflammatory by releasing histamine, leukotrienes, IL-6, and IFN-γ.[36] Despite the contribution of DCs remaining poorly understood, they have been suggested to contain antigen to naive T cells promoting lymphocyte recruitment into the atherosclerotic lesion thereby modulating both cellular and humoral immunity.[63] Neutrophils are thought to be recruited to the atherosclerotic lesion partly via platelet CCL5, and further retained by the interaction with P- and E- selectins. Cholesterol crystals and oxLDL have shown to activate neutrophils with the consequent release of web-like filamentous structures of decondensed chromatin (so-called neutrophil extracellular traps [NETs]), which are composed of DNA, histones, and granular components (MPO, neutrophil elastase, and cathepsin G). NETs have been detected in human atherosclerotic plaques and have been demonstrated to contribute to atherosclerosis formation by priming macrophages for cytokine production, thus amplifying inflammatory cell recruitment.[64]

Platelet activation may be a further mechanism by which inflammation may be modulated in the context of atherosclerosis.[65] Although platelets were formerly suggested to be passive players because they are organelles lacking nuclei, we currently know that they are very active, being important not only in thrombosis itself but also in perpetuating the inflammatory environment. Platelets secrete various vasoactive chemokines and cytokines with autocrine and paracrine effects detailed in **Fig. 17–4.** Accordingly, it has been postulated the use of antiplatelet drugs in primary prevention as a potential approach to target platelet-mediated inflammation.[66] However, these anti-inflammatory properties are counteracted by the increased bleeding risk associated with available antiplatelet drugs. Novel therapeutic antiplatelet approaches able to limit platelet activation without affecting hemostasis are strongly needed. In this regard, nutraceuticals (nutritional supplements

or functional foods with health-promoting properties) with antiplatelet effects have rendered promising results.[67,68]

The role of inflammation as an important atherosclerotic factor is illustrated by the increased cardiovascular risk conferred by chronic inflammatory conditions such as rheumatoid arthritis, systemic lupus erythematosus, and psoriasis, as well as with infections such as periodontal disease and human immunodeficiency virus (HIV).[69] Despite a clear link between inflammation and atherothrombosis, clinical data demonstrating a direct benefit of targeting inflammation on patient outcomes has only recently emerged, as in the CANTOS (Canakinumab Antiinflammatory Thrombosis Outcomes Study).[70] The PROVE-IT-TIMI 22 (Pravastatin or Atorvastatin Evaluation and Infection Therapy Thrombolysis in Myocardial Infarction) and JUPITER (Justification for the Use of Statins in Prevention: an Intervention Trial Evaluating Rosuvastatin) trials evidenced a reduction of MACE associated with a reduction in high-sensitivity CRP, regardless of the decline in LDL-cholesterol concentration.[71] Yet, the recent CANTOS trial demonstrated the successful anti-inflammatory benefit of canakinumab, a monoclonal antibody targeting IL-1β, toward MACE reduction in patients with a previous history of MI.[72] MACE reduction was directly attributed to a reduction in IL-6 and high-sensitivity C-reactive protein (hsCRP) and was independent of lipid-lowering. IL-1β is involved in the downstream activation of the IL-6 receptor, which itself has been previously implicated as a target for atherothrombosis from Mendelian randomization studies.[73] While there was a reduction in MACE, the drawback with canakinumab was a significantly higher incidence of sepsis and fatal infection, compared to placebo. The recent CIRT (Cardiovascular Inflammation Reduction Trial) failed to show similar favorable cardiovascular effects through the use of low-dose methotrexate. Low-dose methotrexate was unable

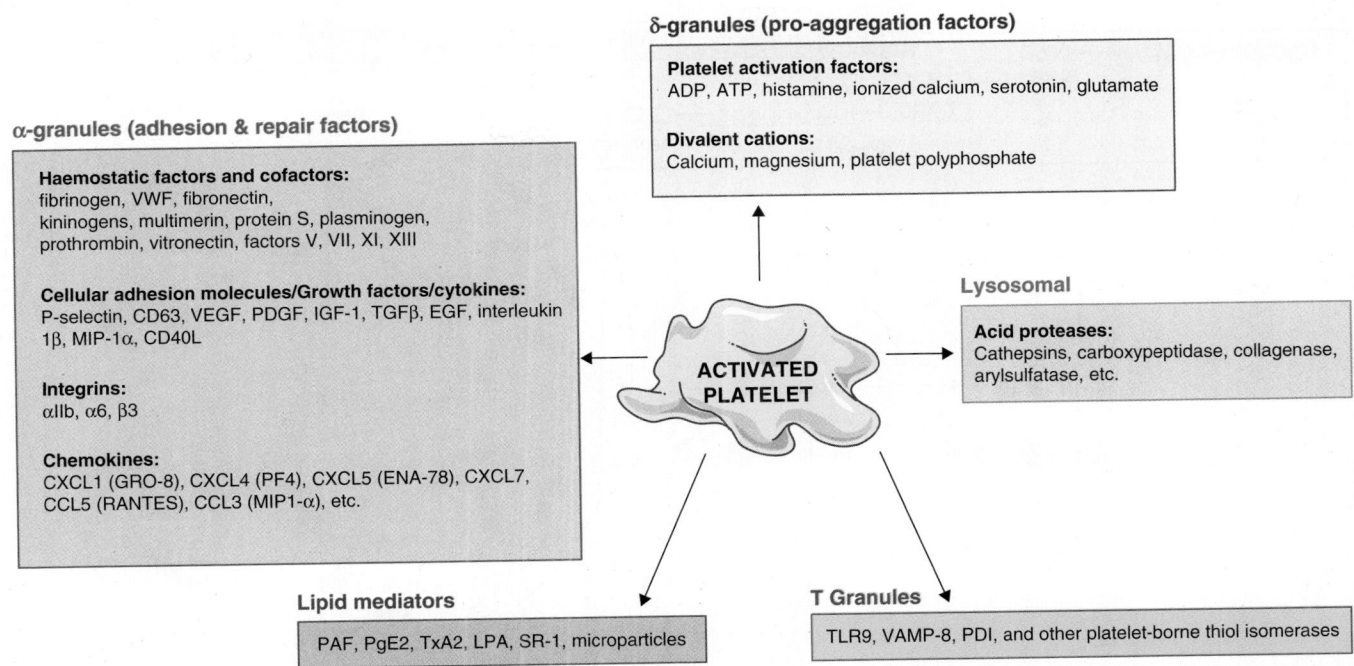

Figure 17–4. Platelet granule content secreted upon activation. ADP, adenosine diphosphate; ATP, adenosine triphosphate; vWF, von Willebrand factor; VEGF, vascular endothelial growth factor; PDGF, platelet-derived growth factor; IGF-1, insulin growth factor; TGF, tissue growth factor; EGF, epidermal growth factor; MIP, macrophage inflammatory protein; TLR9, toll-like receptor 9; VAMP-8, vesicle-associated membrane protein; PDI, protein disulfide isomerase; PAF, platelet activating factor; PgE2, prostaglandin-E2; TxA2, thromboxane A2; LPA, Lysophosphatidic acid; SR, scavenger receptor; CXCL, hemokine (C-X-C motif) ligand; CCL, chemokine ligand.

to reduce IL-1β, IL-6, or hsCRP in addition to MACE among patients with prior myocardial infarction (MI) or multivessel coronary artery disease (CAD) but with normal hsCRP levels.[74] Therefore, elucidation of therapeutic targets against the IL-1β pathway is currently of immense interest for treating atherothrombosis. Upstream and serving as an activator of IL-1β lies the nucleotide-binding oligomerization domain-like receptor protein 3 (NLRP3) inflammasome (a vital player in innate immunity and inflammation; **Fig. 17–5**). Several experimental studies have evidenced that NLRP3 is activated by cholesterol crystals or hypoxia, promoting cleavage and secretion of IL-1β and IL-18 (Fig. 17–5).[75,76] Given the direct implication of an atherogenic role to the NLRP3 inflammasome in generating these cytokines, NLRP3 inhibitors are of interest with the consideration to move upstream from the initial success of anti-IL-1β therapy.[77,78] Supporting this concept, preliminary data from CANTOS showed that plasma IL-18 levels remained a determinant of residual risk despite this targeted anti-IL-1β therapy, suggesting the need to explore NLRP3 inflammasome as a potential therapeutic target.[77,79,80] Finally, administration of colchicine, a potent anti-inflammatory drug that prevents microtubule assembly and thereby disrupts inflammasome activation, microtubule-based inflammatory cell chemotaxis, has also shown promising data in the cardiovascular arena. Both, the Low-Dose Colchicine 2 (LoDoCo2) trial (stable CAD patients)[81] and the Colchicine Cardiovascular Outcomes Trial (COLCOT) (recent MI patients)[82] showed improved cardiovascular outcomes among patients treated with low-dose colchicine as compared with placebo.

CELLULAR AND MOLECULAR MECHANISMS INVOLVED IN CORONARY THROMBUS FORMATION

Regulation of Platelet Adhesion, Activation, and Aggregation

Platelets are anucleated cells (2μm in diameter) originating from bone marrow megakaryocytes and have a life span of 7 to 10 days. In the presence of healthy endothelium, circulating platelets remain in a quiescent discoid state, with laminar blood flow close to the endothelium, nonadherent to each other and the endothelial surface because of the presence of electrostatic repulsive forces between platelets and the endothelial cells, and the antiplatelet, anticoagulant, and fibrinolytic properties of the healthy endothelium (**Fig. 17–6**).[3] It is worth mentioning the protective role of the ecto-nucleotidase CD39 expressed on the luminal surface of endothelial cells. CD39, in association with CD73, promotes the catabolism of adenosine triphosphate (ATP) and adenosine diphosphate (ADP) with the consequent generation of adenosine known to exert antiplatelet, anti-inflammatory, and vasodilatory effects.[83] Furthermore, CD39 has also shown to prevent endothelial cell and apoptosis[84] becoming a potential therapeutic target in the management of thromboinflammatory diseases.

Recent experimental studies have also revealed the existence of key checkpoints within the platelet molecular machinery by which platelets may control and limit their activation preventing undesired platelet adhesion to occur.[85] Platelets are devoid of genomic DNA but contain messenger RNA and ribosomes

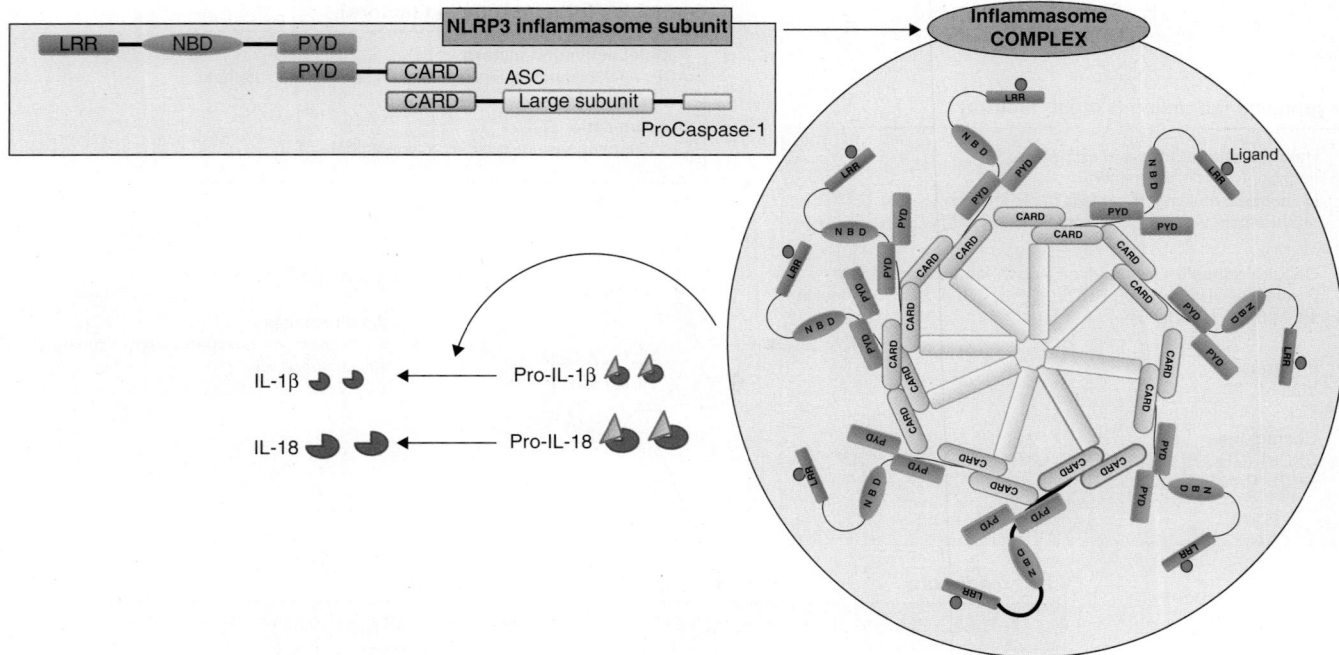

Figure 17–5. Inflammasome NLR3 complex. NLR3, NLR family pyrin domain containing 3 ; LRR, leucine-rich repeat; NBD, nucleotide-binding domain; PYD, pyrin domain; CARD, Caspase activation and recruitment domain; ASC, apoptosis-associated speck-like protein containing a CARD; IL, interleukin.

that enable them to synthesize a subset of proteins, a function that is enhanced upon platelet activation.[86,87] Upon plaque disruption, exposure of inner plaque components to the blood favors platelet–vascular interactions and consequent thrombus formation.[3] Most of the glycoproteins (GPs) on the platelet membrane surface are receptors for adhesive proteins. Many of these receptors have been identified, cloned, sequenced, and classified within large gene families that mediate a variety of cellular interactions (**Table 17–1**). The initial recognition of damaged vessel wall by platelets involves (1) adhesion, activation, and adherence to recognition sites on the thrombogenic substrate; (2) spreading of the platelet on the surface; and (3) aggregation of platelets to form a platelet plug or white thrombus. (3)

The initial tethering of platelets at sites of injured vessels is mainly driven by the interaction of the collagen-anchored A3 domain of vWF with the platelet GPIbα receptor (from the GPIb/IX/V platelet complex) binding site of vWF located in the A1 domain (**Fig. 17–7**).[88,89] Under pathological conditions and in response to changes in shear stress, vWF can be secreted from the storage organelles in platelets or endothelial cells, reinforcing the adhesion process. Although GPIb/IX–vWF interaction is enough to promote binding of platelets to subendothelium, this interaction is highly transient, resulting in rapid dislocation of platelets from the site of injury.[89] Recent studies have shown that the intracellular adaptor signaling molecule 14-3-3ζ, found associated with the GPIb subunit, regulates vWF binding to GPIb-IX-V and mediates

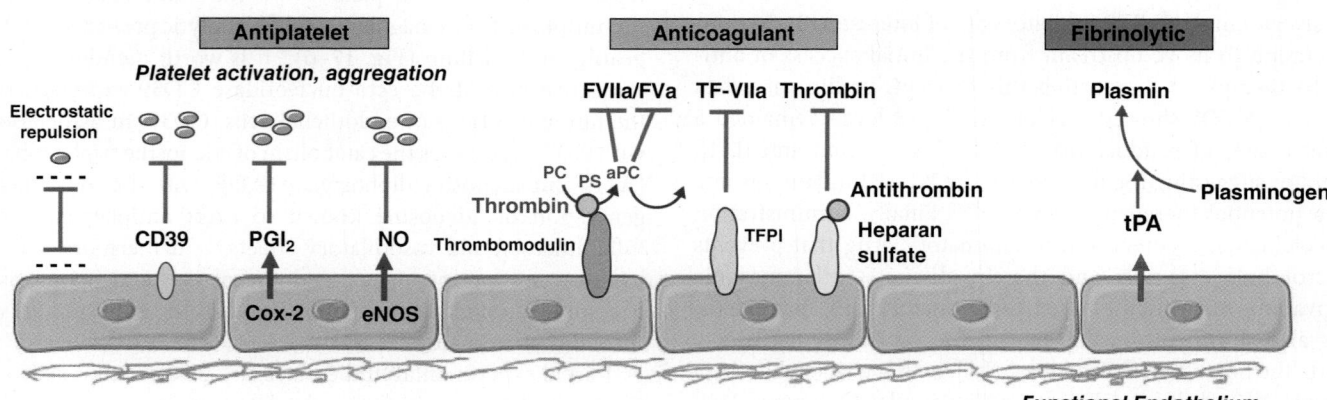

Figure 17–6. Antithrombotic and fibrinolytic properties of a healthy endothelium. CD39, cluster of differentiation 39; PGI2, prostacyclin; NO, nitric oxide; Cox2, cyclooxygenase-2; eNOS, endothelial nitric oxide synthase; PC, protein C; PS: protein S; aPC, activated PC; TFPI, tissue factor pathway inhibitor; tPA, tissue plasminogen activator.

TABLE 17–1. Platelet Receptors Involved in Platelet Adhesion and Aggregation

Receptor	Ligand	Action
INTEGRIN		
$\alpha_2\beta_1$ (glycoprotein Ia / IIa)	Collagen	Adhesion
$\alpha_5\beta_1$ (glycoprotein Ic / IIa)	Fibronectin	Adhesion
$\alpha_6\beta_1$	Laminin	Adhesion
$\alpha_V\beta_3$	Vitronectin Fibrinogen Fibronectin von Willebrand factor	Adhesion
$\alpha_{II}\beta_3$ (glycoprotein IIb / IIIa)	von Willebrand factor Fibrinogen Vitronectin Fibronectin	Adhesion Aggregation
NON-INTEGRIN		
Glycoprotein Ib-IX-V	von Willebrand factor	Adhesion
Glycoprotein VI-FcRϒ	Collagen	Adhesion
Glycoprotein IV	Thrombospondin	Adhesion

that involve phospholipase (PL)-C and protein kinase (PK)-G activation leading to the activation of integrins α2β1 (or GPI-a-IIa) and αIIbβ3 (GPIIb/IIIa) (Fig. 17–7).[91] Both integrins directly support firm platelet adhesion and further activation by binding to collagen (α2β1), or indirectly through fibrinogen and vWF interaction (αIIbβ3). Besides, fibronectin, vitronectin, and thrombospondin also contribute to platelet adhesion by binding to GPIc-IIa, vitronectin receptors, and to GPIV, respectively, although to a lesser extent. Of note, P-selectin, leukocyte integrin MAC-1, and Factor XII have also been shown to interact with GPIb-IX-V, suggesting the ability of this platelet receptor to modulate thrombin generation and inflammation beyond platelet activation.

Platelet adhesion and further activation modify platelet morphology and stimulate the release of its granule content-rich soluble agonists, adhesion molecules, and coagulation factors among others all of which amplify the thrombotic response (Fig. 17–4). Besides, platelet activation favors TXA$_2$ generation through cyclooxygenase-1 (Cox-1) dependent arachidonic acid metabolism and exposes phosphatidylserine on the outer leaflet of the platelet plasma membrane providing the surface to form the prothrombinase complex (Xa, Va, phospholipid, and Ca^{2+}). The prothrombinase complex catalyzes the conversion of prothrombin into thrombin through factor Xa and co-factor Va.[3] Yet, thrombin generation is mainly driven by TF-mediated activation of the extrinsic coagulation pathway through FVII/FVIIa interaction (subsequently detailed).

vWF/GPIb-IX-V–dependent signal transduction.[90] GPVI-Fc receptor gamma-chain complex (GPVI-FcRγ) interaction with vascular collagen has slower binding kinetics than does GP Ib/IX–vWF, but when initiated promotes firm adhesion of platelet to the vessel surface and triggers "inside-out" signals

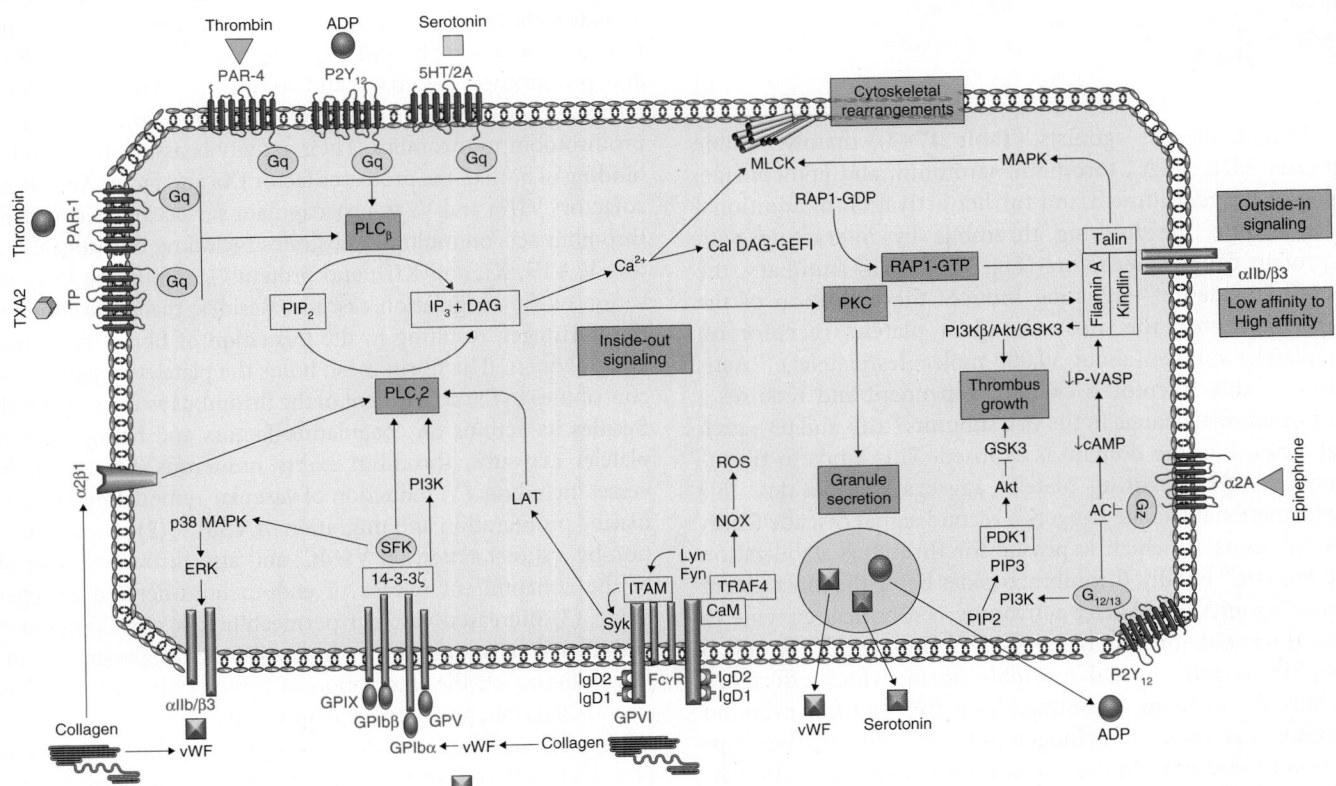

Figure 17–7. Platelet inside-out and out-side in signaling. Modified with permission from Vilahur G, Gutiérrez M, Arzanauskaite M, et al. Intracellular platelet signalling as a target for drug development. *Vascul Pharmacol.* 2018 Dec;111:22-25.

TABLE 17-2. Platelet Agonists and Their Receptors

Platelet Agonists	Platelet Receptors
ADP	$P2X_1$, $P2Y_1$, $P2Y_{12}$
Epinephrine	α_2A
Thrombin	PAR-1, PAR-4, GPIbα
Thromboxane A_2	TP
PAF and PAFLL	PAF-R
Collagen	$\alpha_2\beta_1$ (GPIa-IIa)
Fibronectin	$\alpha_5\beta_1$ (Fibronectin Receptor)
Laminin, collagen	GPVI
VWF	(GP Ib-IX-V Complex)
VWF, fibrinogen, fibronectin	$\alpha_{IIb}\beta_3$ (GP IIb / IIIa)
Laminin	$\alpha_6\beta_1$
Vitronectin, fibrinogen, VWF, osteoponin	$\alpha_V\beta_3$
Podoplanin	CLEC-2
PGE_2	PGE_2 receptor (EP3)
Lysophosphatidic acid	Lysophosphatidic acid receptor
Chemokines	Chemokine receptors
Vasopressin	$V1_a$ vasopressin receptor
Adenosine	$A2_a$ adenosine receptor
Serotonin (5-hydroxytryptamin)	Serotonin receptor
Dopamine	Dopamine receptor
TPO	c-mpl
Leptin	Leptin receptor
Insulin	Insulin receptor
PDGF	PDGF receptor

Multiple platelet agonists (**Table 17-2**), mainly soluble agonists ADP, TXA_2, thrombin, serotonin, and epinephrine, enhance the recruitment and further activation of additional platelets into the forming thrombus by interacting with G-protein coupled receptors (Fig. 17-7).[89] In summary, the overall "inside-out" signaling induces the activation of the αIIbβ3 receptor, the most abundant platelet receptor on the platelet surface (about 50,000 molecules/platelet).[92] Activation of this receptor is calcium-dependent and requires a conformational change in the two subunits (αIIb and β3), such that a new binding domain is exposed. This binds to fibrinogen and vWF-favoring platelet aggregation. Besides, this conformational change triggers a second signal cascade ("outside-in" signals), which is pivotal for thrombus stabilization and growth.[93] Finally, thrombin, besides being the most potent known agonist for platelet activation, is a critical enzyme in early thrombus formation, cleaving fibrinopeptides A and B from fibrinogen to yield insoluble fibrin, which effectively anchors the evolving thrombus. Both free and fibrin-bound thrombin can convert fibrinogen to fibrin, allowing the propagation of thrombus at the site of injury. Also, other circulating cells, including red blood cells and leucocytes, are trapped within the expanding thrombus, contributing to its growth.

The Coagulation System

During plaque rupture, flowing blood interacts with inner components of the lesions, TF among them. Exposure of the TF is considered the initial event triggering arterial thrombosis because it induces activation of the coagulation cascade and consequent formation of a fibrin monolayer covering the exposed surface onto which circulating platelets are further recruited.[3,94,95] TF is highly expressed in deep vascular layers and atherosclerotic plaque components (macrophages, foam cells, and VSMC). Yet, other potential sources of TF include NETs,[96,97] platelets,[98] monocytes, and microparticles,[99] which overall contribute to a high local TF concentration in the disrupted site. One issue yet to be clarified is the individual contribution of the TF from the plaque versus the contribution of systemic TF to thrombus formation.[100]

The blood coagulation system involves a sequence of reactions integrating zymogens (proteins susceptible to activation into enzymes via limited proteolysis) and cofactors (nonproteolytic enzyme activators) and involves two distinct, yet cross-talking pathways: the extrinsic, or TF-dependent pathway and the intrinsic or contact activation pathway[101] (**Fig. 17-8**). Both pathways converge on a final common pathway: activated Xa converts prothrombin into thrombin (Fig. 17-8). The complex that catalyzes the formation of thrombin consists of factors Xa and Va in a 1:1 complex, FII, and Calcium (the prothrombinase complex). The protrombinase complex activates prothrombin (FII) to form fragment 1.2 and thrombin (from fragment 2). The interaction of the four components of the prothrombinase complex enhances the efficiency of the reaction. In this regard, as stated above, activated platelets provide a procoagulant surface for the assembly and expression of both intrinsic Xase and prothrombinase enzymatic complexes.[3] These complexes respectively catalyze the activation of factor X to factor Xa and prothrombin to thrombin. Their activity is associated with the binding of both of the proteases factor IXa and factor Xa and the cofactors VIIIa and Va to procoagulant surfaces. Once formed, thrombin acts on multiple substrates including fibrinogen; factors V, VIII, XI, and XIII; and protein C, amplifying the activation of the coagulation cascade. Besides, thrombin binds to the fibrinogen resulting in the formation of fibrin monomers and polymers. The fibrin mesh holds the platelets together and contributes to the attachment of the thrombus to the vessel wall. Besides its actions on coagulation factors and being a potent platelet activator, thrombin exerts numerous effects on the vessel including: (1) induction of vascular remodeling by stimulating proliferation and migration of VSMC; (2) vasoconstriction by a direct action on VSMC, and also through regulation of the concomitant release of endothelium-derived nitrogen oxide; (3) increased vascular permeability; (4) proliferation of endothelial cells and thereby modulation of angiogenesis; and (5) influence on the interaction of tumor cells with platelets, endothelial cells, and extracellular matrix.

Finally, activated platelets have recently been shown to play a critical role in triggering the contact/intrinsic coagulation pathway. As such, activated platelets release inorganic polyphosphates from their dense granules, which trigger the

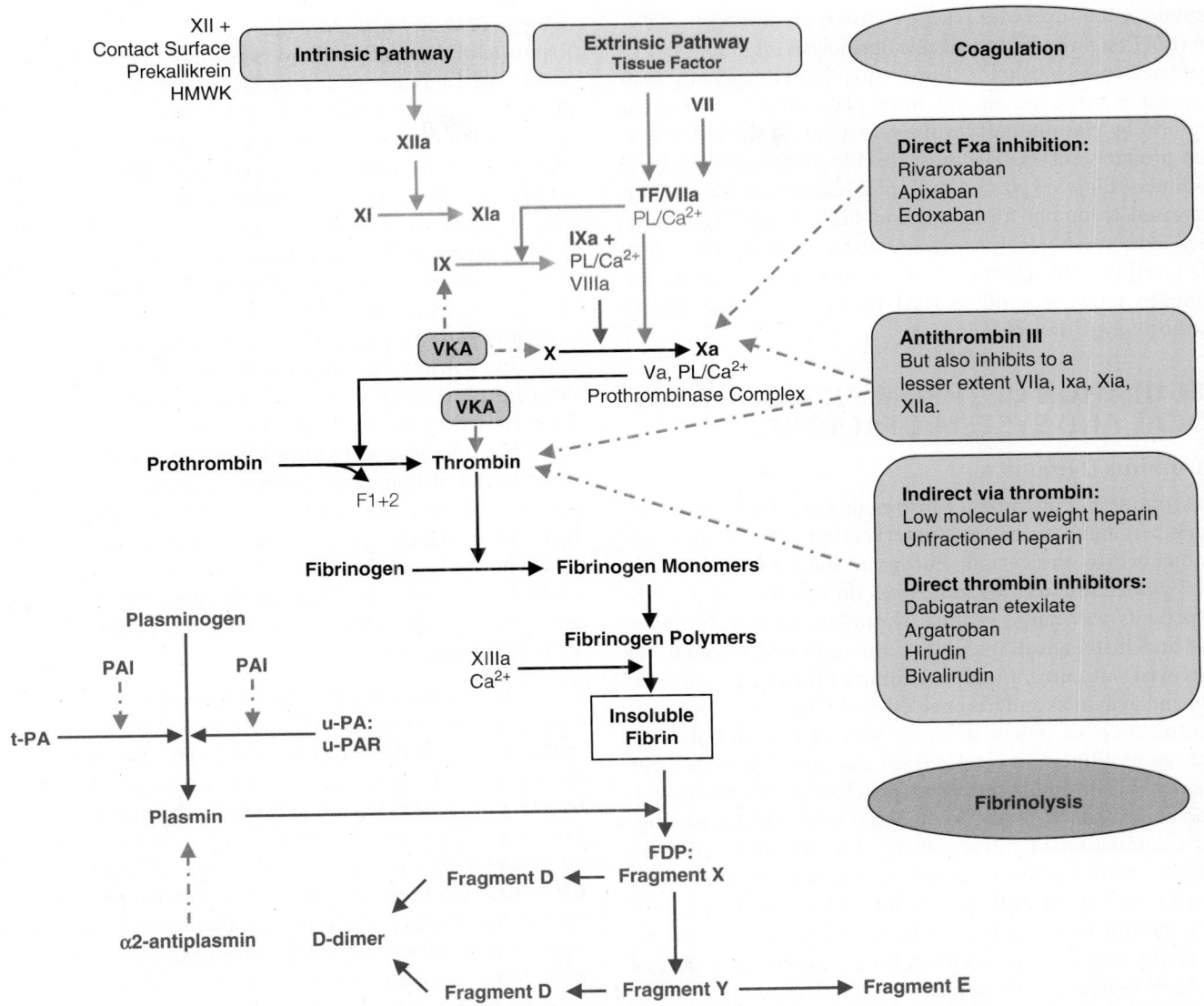

Figure 17–8. Coagulation and fibrinolytic pathways and anticoagulant and antifibrinolytic agents. PAI, plasminogen activator inhibitor; u-PA, urokinase plasminogen activator; t-PA, tissue plasminogen activator; VKA, vitamin K antagonists. FPD, fibrin derived products.

activation FXII/prekallikrein enhancing FXI-related thrombin activation (intrinsic coagulation pathway; Fig. 17–8).[102,103]

As to prevent and/or treat thrombosis-related complications, the progression in understanding the receptors and signaling pathways involved in platelet adhesion/activation/aggregation[89] as well as activation of the coagulation cascade has led to the development and widespread use of antiplatelet and anticoagulant agents[104,105] and has fostered the discovery of new antithrombotic compounds aimed to prevent thrombosis without the side effect of increased bleeding.[89,103,106]

Physiological Pathways That Regulate Blood Coagulation and Clot Dissolution

The control of the coagulation reactions occurs by diverse mechanisms, such as hemodilution and flow effects, proteolytic feedback by thrombin, inhibition by plasma proteins (eg, antithrombin III [ATIII]), endothelial cell–localized activation

of an inhibitory enzyme (protein C), and fibrinolysis. Although ATIII readily inactivates thrombin in solution, its catalytic site is inaccessible while bound to fibrin; it may still cleave fibrinopeptides even in the presence of heparin. Binding of thrombin with thrombomodulin, its specific receptor on the endothelial cell surface, triggers an anticoagulant response. The thrombin–thrombomodulin complex serves as a receptor for the vitamin K–dependent protein C, which is activated and released from the endothelial cell surface. Thrombin generated at the site of injury binds to thrombomodulin, initiating activation of protein C, which in turn (in the presence of protein S) inactivates factors Va and VIIIa and limits the effects of thrombin. The loss of Va decreases the role of thrombin formation to negligible levels. Thrombin not only plays a pivotal role in maintaining the complex balance of initial prothrombotic reparative events and subsequent endogenous anticoagulant but also promotes endogenous fibrinolysis. As such, thrombin stimulates the successive release of tissue plasminogen activator (tPA) via thrombin activatable fibrinolysis inhibitor (TAFI)-mediated mechanisms,[107] thus initiating endogenous lysis through plasmin generation from plasminogen. Proteolysis of fibrin by plasmin induces the generation of fibrin degradation products (FDP). The most specific of stabilized FDP are D-dimers. Elevated plasma levels of D-dimers are a marker for increased thrombin formation and fibrin degradation turnover. However, fibrinolysis is found to be limited in the culprit site given that the atheromatous core is a rich source of plasminogen activator inhibitor (PAI-1), a powerful endogenous antifibrinolytic molecule.[3]

REGULATION OF THROMBUS GROWTH BY LOCAL AND SYSTEMIC FACTORS

Thrombus Dynamics

The routine use of coronary thrombus aspiration before primary percutaneous catheter intervention (PCI) is not recommended by the current European Society of Cardiology 2017 guidelines. Yet, the guidelines do consider its practice in patients with large residual thrombus burden.[108] Molecular and histological analyses of the aspirated thrombi has improved our current understanding of thrombus composition and dynamics and has enabled, by proteomic approaches, identification of potential biomarkers of ischemic damage such as profiline-1, a cytoskeleton-associated protein likely released by thrombin-activated platelets at the atherosclerotic culprit site.[109,110] A study focused on the histopathological examination of intracoronary thrombi retrieved from 211 consecutive STEMI patients within 6 hours after onset of symptoms revealed that, in at least 50% of patients, coronary thrombi were days or weeks old suggesting that plaque instability may precede sudden coronary occlusion by days or weeks.[111] Besides, characterization of intracoronary thrombus from STEMI patients within the first hours after the onset-of-pain-to-PCI revealed a rapid (3 hours) recruitment of neutrophils and monocytes and a late appearance (6 hours) of T and B lymphocytes along with few undifferentiated cells.[109] Moreover, the content of fibrin increased over time contrary to the pattern observed for platelet content.[109] Recent studies have further revealed that the composition of intracoronary thrombi in STEMI patients does not differ from that seen on postmortem examination of those with sudden cardiac death; time from symptom onset to coronary reperfusion is the strongest factor influencing thrombus composition.[112]

Local Factors That Regulate Thrombus Growth

The cellular and molecular mechanisms of platelet deposition and thrombus formation after vascular damage are modulated by the severity of the injury, the local geometry at the site of damage (degree of stenosis), and local hemodynamic conditions.[113] Similarly, the major factors that determine the vulnerability of the fibrous cap include circumferential wall stress, or cap "fatigue"; lesion characteristics (location, size, and consistency); and blood flow characteristics.

Severity of Vessel Wall Damage

Exposure of deendothelialized vessel wall, native fibrillar collagen type I bundles with a rough surface, or atherosclerotic plaque components at similar blood shear rate conditions lead to increasing degrees of platelet deposition.[114,115] Overall, it is likely that when an injury to the vessel wall is mild, the thrombogenic stimulus is relatively limited, and the resulting thrombotic occlusion is transient, as occurs in UA. On the other hand, deep vessel injury secondary to plaque rupture or ulceration results in exposure of collagen, TF, and other elements of the vessel matrix, leading to relatively persistent thrombotic occlusion and MI. Likely, the nature of the substrate exposed after spontaneous or angioplasty-induced plaque rupture determines whether an unstable plaque proceeds rapidly to an occlusive thrombus or persists as a nonocclusive mural thrombus. The analysis of the relative contribution of different components of human atherosclerotic plaques (fatty streaks, sclerotic plaques, fibrolipid plaques, atheromatous plaques, hyperplasic cellular plaque, and normal intima) to acute thrombus formation has shown that the atheromatous core is up to 6-fold more active than are the other substrates in triggering thrombosis and the plaque TF content is directly related to its thrombogenicity.[113,115]

The Impact of Local Geometry and Hemodynamics

Platelet deposition is directly related to the degree of stenosis in the presence of the same degree of injury, indicating a shear-induced platelet activation.[116] Besides, analysis of the axial distribution of platelet deposition indicates that the apex, not the flow recirculation zone distal to the apex, is the segment of greatest platelet accumulation. These data suggest that the severity of the acute platelet response to plaque disruption partly depends on the sudden changes in geometry after rupture. Interestingly, hemodynamic effects play a role in the regulation of the thrombotic response in different arteries. In the absence of atherosclerotic lesions, dilatation of carotid and coronary arteries in normocholesterolemic pigs lead to significantly different levels of platelet deposition in the two arterial beds, with significantly more in the coronary circulation than in the carotids.[117]

Spontaneous lysis of thrombus does occur, not only in UA but also in acute MI. In these patients as well as in those undergoing thrombolysis for acute infarction, the presence of a residual mural thrombus predisposes to recurrent thrombotic vessel occlusion. In fact, residual thrombus, and a fragmented thrombus are the two main factors that contribute to rethrombosis.[116] Residual mural thrombus encroaching into the vessel lumen may result in an increased shear rate, facilitating deposition and activation of platelets on the lesion and a fragmented thrombus appears to present one of the most powerful thrombogenic surfaces. Hence, although a gradual increase in platelet deposition in the area of maximal stenosis may be followed by an abrupt decrease in platelet deposition, probably because of spontaneous embolization of the thrombus or platelet de-aggregation, this episode is likely to be immediately followed by a rapid increase in platelet deposition. In fact, platelet deposition is increased two to four times on residual thrombus compared with that on the deeply injured arterial wall.

TABLE 17–3. Factors Implicated in Thrombus Formation

	Plaque Disruption	Blood flow	Blood Thrombogenicity
Coronaries	+++	++	+
Carotids	++	+	++
Peripherals	+	++	+++

Systemic Factors That Regulate Coronary Thrombosis

When a plaque ruptures, in addition to the aforementioned local factors, systemic factors modulate, predispose, or lead to MI. Current knowledge supports the concept that the rupture of atherosclerotic plaques happens more frequently than initially thought. This disruption may occur in an asymptomatic fashion and may be clinically unnoticed. Postmortem evidence has demonstrated the existence of repeated and healed thrombotic episodes within the same lesion.[119] This plaque rupture without a superimposed thrombus suggests that, in addition to local factors implicated in coronary thrombosis, other circulating systemic factors modulate coronary thrombosis (**Table 17–3**). This knowledge led to the concept of vulnerable patients as a composite of vulnerable plaque plus vulnerable blood.[120] One-third of ACS cases, particularly those involving ischemic sudden cardiac death, develop without plaque disruption but instead superficial erosion of a markedly stenotic and fibrotic plaque. Under such conditions, thrombus formation seems to depend on the hyperthrombogenic state triggered by systemic factors (**Table 17–4**). Indeed, a wide range of factors has been identified in prospective epidemiological studies to have a systemic effect on blood thrombogenicity. There is increasing evidence of a close relationship between the traditional cardiovascular risk factors, such as diabetes mellitus, obesity, hypertension, or hyperlipidemia, and the increased thrombogenicity, which is characterized by hypercoagulability, hypofibrinolysis, and/

TABLE 17–4. Factors Modulating Thrombus Formation

Local Fluid Dynamics	Nature of the Exposed Substrate	Systemic Thrombogenic Factors
• Shear stress • Tensile stress	• Degree of injury (mild vs. severe arterial injury) • Composition of atherosclerotic plaque • Residual mural thrombus	• Hypercholesterolemia • Catecholamines (smoking, cocaine, stress, amphetamines) • Smoking • Diabetes and obesity • Pollution • Homocysteine • Lipoprotein (a) • Infections (*Chlamydia pneumoniae*, Helicobacter, cytomegalovirus, SARS-CoV-2, influenza) • Hypercoagulable state (fibrinogen, von Willebrand factor, tissue factor, FVII) • Defective fibrinolytic state

or increased platelet reactivity. Other cardiovascular risk factors such as lipoprotein(a), pollution, and infections have also been shown to directly increase the risk of thrombosis.[121,122] With regards to the latter, a significant association between respiratory infections, especially influenza, and acute MI has recently been reported.[123] Furthermore, although venous thrombosis is the predominant thrombotic complication, arterial thrombotic events including stroke, MI, and mesenteric artery occlusion have all been reported in COVID-19 patients.[124] Indeed, the enhanced inflammatory response induced by SARS-CoV-2 induces endothelial injury, NETosis, procoagulant disturbances, and impaired fibrinolysis overall favoring thrombus formation.[125]

Importantly, however, improvements in some of these cardiovascular risk factors have been associated with a lower prothrombotic tendency.[126] Blood thrombogenicity has been found increased in patients with hyperlipidemia or diabetes; most importantly, however, effective management of these risk factors has been shown to normalize thrombogenicity.[127] In fact, lifestyle changes and improved medical therapy over the last few years have led to less vulnerable lesions assessed by histological analyses.[128] Finally, local fluid dynamics also modulate thrombus progression. On the one hand, high shear stress (a force that acts parallel to the surface) favors a conformational change in ultra-large vWF from its globular to an elongated form, exposing the platelet GPIb binding site in the vWF A1 domain and resulting in platelet tethering to vWF.[129] On the other hand, tensile stress (a force that acts perpendicular to the surface) has shown to influence the localization of metalloproteinase ADAMTS13, a metalloproteinase known to regulate vWF activity by cleaving pro-thrombotic ultra-large vWF.[130] Extracellular vesicles (EVs) have also been considered to regulate thrombus growth beyond their key role in intracellular communication. EVs are released from vascular (endothelial cells, macrophages, and VSMC) and circulating cells (platelets, red blood cells, and leukocytes) upon their activation or apoptosis. EVs include apoptotic bodies (50–5000 nm in diameter), exosomes (30–150 nm in diameter), and microvesicles (0.1–1 micron in diameter; previously known as microparticles). During the last few years, multiple studies have reported that circulating EV levels increase in a wide range of cardiovascular diseases, including uncontrolled cardiovascular risk factors, atherosclerosis progression, heart failure, thrombosis, arrhythmias, and inflammatory vascular disease.[131] The cargo of EVs includes the proteins, lipids, and nucleic acids from their parent cell and have been shown to enhance endothelial cell activation, promote inflammation, induce VSMC migration, and favor thrombus formation (particularly platelet-derived microvesicles [MVs]) thereby regulating each stage of the atherothrombotic process.[132–134] EVs also support coagulation by the exposure of phosphatidylserine on their outer leaflet. As such, both circulating and platelet MVs have been shown to enhance thrombosis on atherosclerotic plaques.[135] Besides, the platelet MV surface presents an array of platelet-derived adhesion and chemokine receptors (eg, P-selectin, GPIIb/IIIa, GPIbα, and PF4 receptor) that induce monocyte and endothelium cytokine production and enhanced leukocyte aggregation.

Circulating, platelet- and monocyte/leukocyte-related MVs have been found increased in patients with complete coronary thrombotic occlusion (ie, STEMI patients) as compared to those with partial coronary thrombotic occlusion (ie, NSTEMI), thereby serving as a marker of thrombus burden.[136] Furthermore, erythrocyte-derived MPs, which are continuously released from evolving growing thrombi, have appeared as a potential biomarker of ongoing thrombosis.[137]

PLAQUE MORPHOLOGY AND SITE OF THROMBUS IN ACUTE MYOCARDIAL INFARCTION

It has been recognized that besides vulnerable plaque rupture, between 25% and 60% of the events are caused by plaque erosion, by calcified nodule, or by functional coronary alterations.[138] An OCT study conducted in 822 STEMI patients revealed that current smoking, absence of coronary risk factors, lack of multivessel disease, reduced lesion severity, larger vessel size, nearby bifurcation, and being under 50 years old were factors significantly associated with plaque erosion.[139] Gender differences have also been observed as per the prevalence of plaque erosion leading to acute MI being 37% in women and only 18% in men.[140] The thrombus age also varies; the majority of acute thrombi (<1 day) have been observed in plaque rupture, whereas in plaque erosion, thrombi are organizing (>1 day).[140] Autopsy data have revealed that most culprit lesions in patients dying of sudden cardiac death have angiographic lumen diameter stenoses of 40% to 69% (**Fig. 17–9**).[120] A possible explanation is that although individual severe stenosis is more likely to become occluded by a thrombus than a lesion with less severe stenosis, less severely narrowed plaques give rise to more occlusions because there are many more sites that are mild-to-moderately narrowed.[141] It has been described that the mean percent stenosis underlying coronary plaque erosion is 70% versus 80% at the site of plaque rupture; however, 82% of fatal plaque erosions result in total occlusions compared with only 57% of plaque ruptures.[142] The majority of thin cap

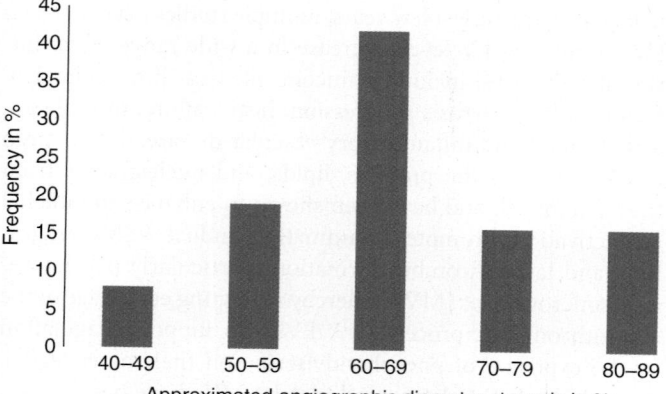

Figure 17–9. Estimates of angiographic stenosis of culprit coronary artery lesions in 50 consecutive patients experiencing sudden coronary death. Reproduced with permission from Arbab-Zadeh A, Fuster V. From Detecting the Vulnerable Plaque to Managing the Vulnerable Patient: JACC State-of-the-Art Review. *J Am Coll Cardiol.* 2019 Sep 24;74(12):1582-1593.

fibroatheromas, acute and healed ruptures, and lesions with fibroatheromas occur predominantly in the proximal portion of the three major coronary arteries, and about 50% arise in the midportion of these arteries. By far, the culprit coronary artery of infarction at autopsy is most frequently the proximal portion of the left anterior descending artery (~50%), followed by the right coronary artery (30%–45%) and then the left circumflex artery (15%–20%).[140]

SUMMARY

The formation of a thrombus within a coronary artery with obstruction of coronary blood flow and reduction in oxygen supply to the myocardium produces the several types of ACS. These thrombotic episodes largely occur in response to atherosclerotic lesions that have progressed to a high-risk inflammatory, prothrombotic stage by a process modulated by local and systemic factors. Although distinct from each other, these atherosclerotic and thrombotic processes appear to be closely related as the cause of ACS through a complex multifactorial process called atherothrombosis. The cellular and molecular mechanisms at play in the formation, growth, and stabilization of a coronary thrombus are being thoroughly investigated, and many of the activation pathways and receptor–ligand interactions have been identified. Inflammation has been revealed as a great player in the systemic and diffuse pattern of atherothrombotic disease. Strategies combining dietary, pharmacologic/medical, and interventional/surgical therapies have shown considerable success in the prevention and treatment of major cardiovascular events. These regimens focus on inhibiting the various pathways involved in thrombus generation. Novel strategies based on the knowledge of the biochemistry of platelet aggregation and the coagulation processes, as well as the geometric conditions encountered in the circulation, are presently in different stages of development and clinical trials. Advances in noninvasive imaging techniques will help to identify plaques at risk and reduce the clinical impact of atherothrombosis.

REFERENCES

1. Libby P, Buring JE, Badimon L et al. Atherosclerosis. *Nature Rev Dis Primers.* 2019;5:56.
2. Ahmadi A, Argulian E, Leipsic J, Newby DE, Narula J. From subclinical atherosclerosis to plaque progression and acute coronary events: JACC State-of-the-Art Review. *J Am Coll Cardiol.* 2019;74:1608-1617.
3. Badimon L, Vilahur G. Thrombosis formation on atherosclerotic lesions and plaque rupture. *J Intern Med.* 2014;276:618-632.
4. Davies MJ. Glagovian remodelling, plaque composition, and stenosis generation. *Heart.* 2000;84:461-462.
5. Narula J, Nakano M, Virmani R et al. Histopathologic characteristics of atherosclerotic coronary disease and implications of the findings for the invasive and noninvasive detection of vulnerable plaques. *J Am Coll Cardiol.* 2013;61:1041-1051.
6. Kolodgie FD, Virmani R, Burke AP et al. Pathologic assessment of the vulnerable human coronary plaque. *Heart.* 2004;90:1385-1391.
7. Ibanez B, Badimon JJ, Garcia MJ. Diagnosis of atherosclerosis by imaging. *Am J Med.* 2009;122:S15-25.
8. Koskinas KC, Ughi GJ, Windecker S, Tearney GJ, Raber L. Intracoronary imaging of coronary atherosclerosis: validation for diagnosis, prognosis and treatment. *Eur Heart J.* 2016;37:524-535a-c.

9. Dweck MR, Maurovich-Horvat P, Leiner T et al. Contemporary rationale for non-invasive imaging of adverse coronary plaque features to identify the vulnerable patient: a Position Paper from the European Society of Cardiology Working Group on Atherosclerosis and Vascular Biology and the European Association of Cardiovascular Imaging. *Eur Heart J Cardiovasc Imaging.* 2020.

10. Abdelrahman KM, Chen MY, Dey AK et al. Coronary computed tomography angiography from clinical uses to emerging technologies: JACC State-of-the-Art Review. *J Am Coll Cardiol.* 2020;76:1226-1243.

11. Keliher EJ, Ye YX, Wojtkiewicz GR et al. Polyglucose nanoparticles with renal elimination and macrophage avidity facilitate PET imaging in ischaemic heart disease. *Nature Comm.* 2017;8:14064.

12. Qin H, Zhao Y, Zhang J, Pan X, Yang S, Xing D. Inflammation-targeted gold nanorods for intravascular photoacoustic imaging detection of matrix metalloproteinase-2 (MMP2) in atherosclerotic plaques. *Nanomed: Nanotech Biol Med.* 2016;12:1765-1774.

13. Khamis RY, Woollard KJ, Hyde GD et al. Near infrared fluorescence (NIRF) molecular imaging of oxidized LDL with an autoantibody in experimental atherosclerosis. *Sci Rep.* 2016;6:21785.

14. Qiao R, Huang X, Qin Y et al. Recent advances in molecular imaging of atherosclerotic plaques and thrombosis. *Nanoscale.* 2020;12:8040-8064.

15. Nasir K, Bittencourt MS, Blaha MJ et al. Implications of coronary artery calcium testing among statin candidates according to American College of Cardiology/American Heart Association cholesterol management guidelines: MESA (Multi-Ethnic Study of Atherosclerosis). *J Am Coll Cardiol.* 2015;66:1657-1668.

16. Cainzos-Achirica M, Miedema MD, McEvoy JW et al. Coronary artery calcium for personalized allocation of aspirin in primary prevention of cardiovascular disease in 2019: The MESA Study (Multi-Ethnic Study of Atherosclerosis). *Circulation.* 2020;141:1541-1553.

17. Joshi FR, Rajani NK, Abt M et al. Does vascular calcification accelerate inflammation?: a substudy of the dal-PLAQUE trial. *J Am Coll Cardiol.* 2016;67:69-78.

18. Nakahara T, Narula J, Strauss HW. Calcification and inflammation in atherosclerosis: which is the chicken, and which is the egg? *J Am Coll Cardiol.* 2016;67:79-80.

19. Iwasaki K, Matsumoto T. Relationship between coronary calcium score and high-risk plaque/significant stenosis. *World J Cardiol.* 2016;8:481-487.

20. Chistiakov DA, Melnichenko AA, Myasoedova VA, Grechko AV, Orekhov AN. Role of lipids and intraplaque hypoxia in the formation of neovascularization in atherosclerosis. *Annals Med.* 2017;49:661-677.

21. Guo L, Harari E, Virmani R, Finn AV. Linking hemorrhage, angiogenesis, macrophages, and iron metabolism in atherosclerotic vascular diseases. *Arterioscler Thromb Vasc Biol.* 2017;37:e33-e39.

22. Winter PM, Neubauer AM, Caruthers SD et al. Endothelial alpha(v) beta3 integrin-targeted fumagillin nanoparticles inhibit angiogenesis in atherosclerosis. *Arterioscler Thromb Vasc Biol* 2006;26:2103-2109.

23. Touyz RM, Herrmann J. Cardiotoxicity with vascular endothelial growth factor inhibitor therapy. *NPJ Precis Oncol.* 2018;2:13.

24. Moulton KS, Vakili K, Zurakowski D et al. Inhibition of plaque neovascularization reduces macrophage accumulation and progression of advanced atherosclerosis. *Proc Natl Acad Sci.* 2003;100:4736-4741.

25. Ahmadi A, Leipsic J, Blankstein R et al. Do plaques rapidly progress prior to myocardial infarction? The interplay between plaque vulnerability and progression. *Circulation Res.* 2015;117:99-104.

26. Kolodgie FD, Gold HK, Burke AP et al. Intraplaque hemorrhage and progression of coronary atheroma. *N Engl J Med.* 2003;349:2316-25.

27. Moreno PR, Purushothaman KR, Fuster V et al. Plaque neovascularization is increased in ruptured atherosclerotic lesions of human aorta: implications for plaque vulnerability. *Circulation.* 2004;110:2032-2038.

28. Virmani R, Kolodgie FD, Burke AP et al. Atherosclerotic plaque progression and vulnerability to rupture: angiogenesis as a source of intraplaque hemorrhage. *Arterioscler Thromb Vasc Biol.* 2005;25:2054-2061.

29. Taruya A, Tanaka A, Nishiguchi T et al. Vasa vasorum restructuring in human atherosclerotic plaque vulnerability: a clinical optical coherence tomography study. *J Am Coll Cardiol.* 2015;65:2469-2477.

30. Badimon L, Pena E, Arderiu G et al. C-reactive protein in atherothrombosis and angiogenesis. *Frontiers Immunol.* 2018;9:430.

31. Yao J, Gao W, Wang Y et al. Sonodynamic therapy suppresses neovascularization in atherosclerotic plaques via macrophage apoptosis-induced endothelial cell apoptosis. *JACC Basic Translation Sci.* 2020;5:53-65.

32. Oikonomou E, Leopoulou M, Theofilis P et al. A link between inflammation and thrombosis in atherosclerotic cardiovascular diseases: clinical and therapeutic implications. *Atherosclerosis* 2020;309:16-26.

33. Libby P, Loscalzo J, Ridker PM et al. Inflammation, immunity, and infection in atherothrombosis: JACC review topic of the week. *J Am Coll Cardiol.* 2018;72:2071-2081.

34. Moore KJ, Koplev S, Fisher EA et al. Macrophage Trafficking, inflammatory resolution, and genomics in atherosclerosis: JACC macrophage in CVD series (part 2). *J Am Coll Cardiol.* 2018;72:2181-2197.

35. Biessen EAL, Wouters K. Macrophage complexity in human atherosclerosis: opportunities for treatment? *Curr Opinion Lipidol.* 2017;28:419-426.

36. Libby P, Nahrendorf M, Swirski FK. Leukocytes link local and systemic inflammation in ischemic cardiovascular disease: an expanded "cardiovascular continuum". *J Am Coll Cardiol.* 2016;67:1091-1103.

37. Shantsila E, Ghattas A, Griffiths HR, Lip GYH. Mon2 predicts poor outcome in ST-elevation myocardial infarction. *J Intern Med.* 2019;285:301-316.

38. Kuznetsova T, Prange KHM, Glass CK, de Winther MPJ. Transcriptional and epigenetic regulation of macrophages in atherosclerosis. *Nature Rev Cardiol.* 2020;17:216-228.

39. Trus E, Basta S, Gee K. Who's in charge here? Macrophage colony stimulating factor and granulocyte macrophage colony stimulating factor: Competing factors in macrophage polarization. *Cytokine.* 2020;127:154939.

40. Gough PJ, Gomez IG, Wille PT, Raines EW. Macrophage expression of active MMP-9 induces acute plaque disruption in apoE-deficient mice. *J Clin Invest.* 2006;116:59-69.

41. Teng N, Maghzal GJ, Talib J, Rashid I, Lau AK, Stocker R. The roles of myeloperoxidase in coronary artery disease and its potential implication in plaque rupture. *Redox Rep: Comm Free Radical Res.* 2017;22:51-73.

42. Hohensinner PJ, Baumgartner J, Ebenbauer B et al. Statin treatment reduces matrix degradation capacity of proinflammatory polarized macrophages. *Vasc Pharmacol.* 2018;110:49-54.

43. Ben-Aicha S, Badimon L, Vilahur G. Advances in HDL: Much more than lipid transporters. *Int J Mol Sci.* 2020;21.

44. Badimon L, Vilahur G. LDL-cholesterol versus HDL-cholesterol in the atherosclerotic plaque: inflammatory resolution versus thrombotic chaos. *Ann N Y Acad Sci.* 2012;1254:18-32.

45. Vilahur G. High-density lipoprotein benefits beyond the cardiovascular system: a potential key role for modulating acquired immunity through cholesterol efflux. *Cardiovascular Res.* 2017;113:e51-e53.

46. Vilahur G, Gutierrez M, Casani L et al. Hypercholesterolemia abolishes high-density lipoprotein-related cardioprotective effects in the setting of myocardial infarction. *J Am Coll Cardiol.* 2015;66:2469-2470.

47. Ibanez B, Vilahur G, Cimmino G et al. Rapid change in plaque size, composition, and molecular footprint after recombinant apolipoprotein A-I Milano (ETC-216) administration: magnetic resonance imaging study in an experimental model of atherosclerosis. *J Am Coll Cardiol.* 2008;51:1104-1109.

48. Ben-Aicha S, Casani L, Munoz-Garcia N et al. HDL (high-density lipoprotein) remodeling and magnetic resonance imaging-assessed atherosclerotic plaque burden: study in a preclinical experimental model. *Arterioscler Thromb Vasc Biol.* 2020:ATVBAHA120314956.

49. Nicholls SJ, Andrews J, Kastelein JJP et al. Effect of serial infusions of CER-001, a pre-beta high-density lipoprotein mimetic, on coronary atherosclerosis in patients following acute coronary syndromes in the CER-001

Atherosclerosis Regression Acute Coronary Syndrome Trial: a randomized clinical trial. *JAMA Cardiol.* 2018;3:815-822.

50. Nicholls SJ, Puri R, Ballantyne CM et al. Effect of infusion of high-density lipoprotein mimetic containing recombinant apolipoprotein A-I Milano on coronary disease in patients with an acute coronary syndrome in the MILANO-PILOT trial: a randomized clinical trial. *JAMA Cardiol.* 2018;3:806-814.

51. Bagdade J, Barter P, Quiroga C, Alaupovic P. Effects of torcetrapib and statin treatment on ApoC-III and apoprotein-defined lipoprotein subclasses (from the ILLUMINATE Trial). *Am J Cardiol.* 2017;119:1753-1756.

52. Lincoff AM, Nicholls SJ, Riesmeyer JS et al. Evacetrapib and cardiovascular outcomes in high-risk vascular disease. *N Engl J Med.* 2017;376:1933-1942.

53. Group HTRC, Bowman L, Hopewell JC et al. Effects of anacetrapib in patients with atherosclerotic vascular disease. *N Engl J Med.* 2017;377:1217-1227.

54. Badimon L, Vilahur G. HDL particles–more complex than we thought. *Thrombo Haemost.* 2014;112:857.

55. Ben-Aicha S, Escate R, Casani L et al. High-density lipoprotein remodelled in hypercholesterolaemic blood induce epigenetically driven down-regulation of endothelial HIF-1alpha expression in a preclinical animal model. *Cardiovasc Res.* 2020;116:1288-1299.

56. Padro T, Cubedo J, Camino S et al. Detrimental effect of hypercholesterolemia on high-density lipoprotein particle remodeling in pigs. *J Am Coll Cardiol.* 2017;70:165-178.

57. Cubedo J, Padro T, Garcia-Arguinzonis M et al. A novel truncated form of apolipoprotein A-I transported by dense LDL is increased in diabetic patients. *Journal Lipid Res.* 2015;56:1762-1773.

58. Fadaei R, Poustchi H, Meshkani R, Moradi N, Golmohammadi T, Merat S. Impaired HDL cholesterol efflux capacity in patients with non-alcoholic fatty liver disease is associated with subclinical atherosclerosis. *Sci Rep.* 2018;8:11691.

59. Tabas I, Lichtman AH. Monocyte-macrophages and T cells in atherosclerosis. *Immunity.* 2017;47:621-634.

60. Nus M, Sage AP, Lu Y et al. Marginal zone B cells control the response of follicular helper T cells to a high-cholesterol diet. *Nature Med.* 2017;23:601-610.

61. Pfeiler S, Gerdes N. Atherosclerosis: cell biology and lipoproteins—focus on anti-inflammatory therapies. *Curr Opinion Lipidol.* 2018;29:53-55.

62. Back M, Hansson GK. Anti-inflammatory therapies for atherosclerosis. *Nature Rev Cardiol.* 2015;12:199-211.

63. Cybulsky MI, Cheong C, Robbins CS. Macrophages and dendritic cells: partners in atherogenesis. *Circulation Res.* 2016;118:637-652.

64. Warnatsch A, Ioannou M, Wang Q, Papayannopoulos V. Inflammation. Neutrophil extracellular traps license macrophages for cytokine production in atherosclerosis. *Science.* 2015;349:316-320.

65. Nording H, Baron L, Langer HF. Platelets as therapeutic targets to prevent atherosclerosis. *Atherosclerosis.* 2020;307:97-108.

66. Lordan R, Tsoupras A, Zabetakis I. Platelet activation and prothrombotic mediators at the nexus of inflammation and atherosclerosis: potential role of antiplatelet agents. *Blood Rev.* 2020:100694.

67. O'Kennedy N, Raederstorff D, Duttaroy AK. Fruitflow((R)): the first European Food Safety Authority-approved natural cardio-protective functional ingredient. *Eur J Nutrition.* 2017;56:461-482.

68. Vilahur G, Badimon L. Antiplatelet properties of natural products. *Vascular Pharmacol.* 2013;59:67-75.

69. Ley K. 2015 Russell Ross memorial lecture in vascular biology: protective autoimmunity in atherosclerosis. *Arterioscler Thromb Vasc Biol.* 2016;36:429-438.

70. Ibanez B, Fuster V. CANTOS: A gigantic proof-of-concept trial. *Circulation Res.* 2017;121:1320-1322.

71. Ridker PM, Cannon CP, Morrow D et al. C-reactive protein levels and outcomes after statin therapy. *N Engl J Med.* 2005;352:20-28.

72. Ridker PM, Everett BM, Thuren T et al. Antiinflammatory therapy with canakinumab for atherosclerotic disease. *N Engl J Med.* 2017;377:1119-1131.

73. Collaboration IRGCERF, Sarwar N, Butterworth AS et al. Interleukin-6 receptor pathways in coronary heart disease: a collaborative meta-analysis of 82 studies. *Lancet.* 2012;379:1205-1213.

74. Ridker PM, Everett BM, Pradhan A et al. Low-dose methotrexate for the prevention of atherosclerotic events. *N Engl J Med.* 2019;380:752-762.

75. Tall AR, Marit W. Inflammasomes, neutrophil extracellular traps, and cholesterol. *J Lipid Res.* 2019 Apr; 60(4):721-727.

76. Grebe A, Hoss F. NLRP3 Inflammasome and the IL-1 Pathway in Atherosclerosis. *Circ Res.* 2018 Jun 8; 122(12):1722-1740.

77. Satish M, Agrawal DK. Atherothrombosis and the NLRP3 inflammasome - endogenous mechanisms of inhibition. *Translational Res: J Lab Clin Med.* 2020;215:75-85.

78. Wang Y, Liu X, Shi H et al. NLRP3 inflammasome, an immune-inflammatory target in pathogenesis and treatment of cardiovascular diseases. *Clin Translation Med.* 2020;10:91-106.

79. Ridker PM. Anticytokine agents: targeting interleukin signaling pathways for the treatment of atherothrombosis. *Circulation Res.* 2019;124:437-450.

80. Ridker PM. From C-reactive protein to interleukin-6 to interleukin-1: moving upstream to identify novel targets for atheroprotection. *Circulation Res.* 2016;118:145-156.

81. Nidorf SM, Fiolet ATL, Mosterd A et al. Colchicine in patients with chronic coronary disease. *N Engl J Med.* 2020;383:1838-1847.

82. Tardif JC, Kouz S, Waters DD et al. Efficacy and safety of low-dose colchicine after myocardial infarction. *N Engl J Med.* 2019;381:2497-2505.

83. Kanthi YM, Sutton NR, Pinsky DJ. CD39: Interface between vascular thrombosis and inflammation. *Curr Atheroscler Rep.* 2014;16:425.

84. Goepfert C, Imai M, Brouard S, Csizmadia E, Kaczmarek E, Robson SC. CD39 modulates endothelial cell activation and apoptosis. *Mol Med.* 2000;6:591-603.

85. Stefanini L, Bergmeier W. Negative regulators of platelet activation and adhesion. *J Thromb Haemost.* 2018;16:220-230.

86. Mills EW, Green R, Ingolia NT. Slowed decay of mRNAs enhances platelet specific translation. *Blood.* 2017;129:e38-e48.

87. Fountain JH, Lappin SL. *Physiology, platelet.* Treasure Island, FL: StatPearls; 2020.

88. Badimon L, Badimon JJ, Turitto VT, Fuster V. Role of von Willebrand factor in mediating platelet-vessel wall interaction at low shear rate; the importance of perfusion conditions. *Blood.* 1989;73:961-967.

89. Vilahur G, Gutierrez M, Arzanauskaite M, Mendieta G, Ben-Aicha S, Badimon L. Intracellular platelet signalling as a target for drug development. *Vascular Pharmacol.* 2018;111:22-25.

90. Chen Y, Ruggeri ZM, Du X. 14-3-3 proteins in platelet biology and glycoprotein Ib-IX signaling. *Blood.* 2018;131:2436-2448.

91. Manne BK, Badolia R, Dangelmaier C, et al. Distinct pathways regulate Syk protein activation downstream of immune tyrosine activation motif (ITAM) and hemITAM receptors in platelets. *J Biologic Chem.* 2015;290:11557-11568.

92. Stefanini L, Bergmeier W. RAP1-GTPase signaling and platelet function. *J Mol Med.* 2016;94:13-19.

93. Laurent PA, Severin S, Gratacap MP, Payrastre B. Class I PI 3-kinases signaling in platelet activation and thrombosis: PDK1/Akt/GSK3 axis and impact of PTEN and SHIP1. *Adv Biologic Regulat.* 2014;54:162-174.

94. Grover SP, Mackman N. Tissue factor in atherosclerosis and atherothrombosis. *Atherosclerosis.* 2020;307:80-86.

95. Camera M, Toschi V, Brambilla M et al. The role of tissue factor in atherothrombosis and coronary artery disease: insights into platelet tissue factor. *Seminars Thromb Hemostas.* 2015;41:737-746.

96. Badimon L, Vilahur G. Neutrophil extracellular traps: a new source of tissue factor in atherothrombosis. *Eur Heart J.* 2015;36:1364-1366.

97. Stakos DA, Kambas K, Konstantinidis T et al. Expression of functional tissue factor by neutrophil extracellular traps in culprit artery of acute myocardial infarction. *Eur Heart J.* 2015;36:1405-1414.

98. Muller I, Klocke A, Alex M et al. Intravascular tissue factor initiates coagulation via circulating microvesicles and platelets. *FASEB J.* 2003;17:476-478.

99. Rauch U, Bonderman D, Bohrmann B et al. Transfer of tissue factor from leukocytes to platelets is mediated by CD15 and tissue factor. *Blood.* 2000;96:170-175.

100. Fuster V, Moreno PR, Fayad ZA, Corti R, Badimon JJ. Atherothrombosis and high-risk plaque: part I: evolving concepts. *J Am Coll Cardiol.* 2005;46:937-954.

101. Chaudhry R, Usama SM, Babiker HM. *Physiology, Coagulation Pathways.* Treasure Island, FL: StatPearls; 2020.

102. Rai V, Balters MW, Agrawal DK. Factors IX, XI, and XII: potential therapeutic targets for anticoagulant therapy in atherothrombosis. *Rev Cardiovasc Med.* 2019;20:245-253.

103. Szekely O, Borgi M, Lip GYH. Factor XI inhibition fulfilling the optimal expectations for ideal anticoagulation. *Expert Opin Emerg Drugs.* 2019;24:55-61.

104. Chan NC, Weitz JI. Antithrombotic agents. *Circulation Res.* 2019;124:426-436.

105. Patrono C, Morais J, Baigent C et al. Antiplatelet agents for the treatment and prevention of coronary atherothrombosis. *J Am Coll Cardiol.* 2017;70:1760-1776.

106. McFadyen JD, Schaff M, Peter K. Current and future antiplatelet therapies: emphasis on preserving haemostasis. *Nature Rev Cardiol.* 2018;15:181-191.

107. Ni R, Neves MAD, Wu C et al. Activated thrombin-activatable fibrinolysis inhibitor (TAFIa) attenuates fibrin-dependent plasmin generation on thrombin-activated platelets. *J Thromb Haemost.* 2020.

108. Ibanez B, James S, Agewall S et al. 2017 ESC Guidelines for the management of acute myocardial infarction in patients presenting with ST-segment elevation: the Task Force for the management of acute myocardial infarction in patients presenting with ST-segment elevation of the European Society of Cardiology (ESC). *Eur Heart J.* 2018;39:119-177.

109. Ramaiola I, Padro T, Pena E et al. Changes in thrombus composition and profilin-1 release in acute myocardial infarction. *Eur Heart J.* 2015;36:965-975.

110. Helseth R, Seljeflot I, Opstad T et al. Genes expressed in coronary thrombi are associated with ischemic time in patients with acute myocardial infarction. *Thromb Res.* 2015;135:329-333.

111. Rittersma SZ, van der Wal AC, Koch KT et al. Plaque instability frequently occurs days or weeks before occlusive coronary thrombosis: a pathological thrombectomy study in primary percutaneous coronary intervention. *Circulation.* 2005;111:1160-1165.

112. Silvain J, Collet JP, Guedeney P et al. Thrombus composition in sudden cardiac death from acute myocardial infarction. *Resuscitation.* 2017;113:108-114.

113. Badimon L, Badimon JJ, Turitto VT, Vallbhajosula S, Fuster V. Platelet thrombus formation on collagen type I. A model of deep vessel injury. Influence of blood rheology, von Willebrand factor, and blood coagulation. *Circulation.* 1988;78:1431-1442.

114. Badimon L, Badimon JJ. Mechanisms of arterial thrombosis in nonparallel streamlines: platelet thrombi grow on the apex of stenotic severely injured vessel wall. Experimental study in the pig model. *J Clinic Invest.* 1989;84:1134-1144.

115. Fernandez-Ortiz A, Badimon JJ, Falk E et al. Characterization of the relative thrombogenicity of atherosclerotic plaque components: implications for consequences of plaque rupture. *J Am Coll Cardiol.* 1994;23:1562-1569.

116. Badimon JJ, Ortiz AF, Meyer B et al. Different response to balloon angioplasty of carotid and coronary arteries: effects on acute platelet deposition and intimal thickening. *Atherosclerosis.* 1998;140:307-314.

117. Pallares J, Senan O, Guimera R et al. A comprehensive study on different modelling approaches to predict platelet deposition rates in a perfusion chamber. *Sci Rep.* 2015;5:13606.

118. Meyer BJ, Badimon JJ, Mailhac A et al. Inhibition of growth of thrombus on fresh mural thrombus. Targeting optimal therapy. *Circulation.* 1994;90:2432-2438.

119. Ziada KM, Misumida N. In vivo identification of healed plaques in culprit lesions: is what we're seeing really there? *J Am Coll Cardiol.* 2019;73:2264-2266.

120. Arbab-Zadeh A, Fuster V. From detecting the vulnerable plaque to managing the vulnerable patient: JACC state-of-the-art review. *J Am Coll Cardiol.* 2019;74:1582-1593.

121. Boffa MB, Koschinsky ML. Lipoprotein (a): truly a direct prothrombotic factor in cardiovascular disease? *J Lipid Res.* 2016;57:745-757.

122. Lacey B, Herrington WG, Preiss D, Lewington S, Armitage J. The role of emerging risk factors in cardiovascular outcomes. *Curr Atheroscleros Rep.* 2017;19:28.

123. Kwong JC, Schwartz KL, Campitelli MA. Acute myocardial infarction after laboratory-confirmed influenza infection. *N Engl J Med.* 2018;378:2540-2541.

124. Shi S, Qin M, Shen B et al. Association of cardiac injury with mortality in hospitalized patients with COVID-19 in Wuhan, China. *JAMA Cardiol.* 2020;5:802-810.

125. Ali MAM, Spinler SA. COVID-19 and thrombosis: from bench to bedside. *Trends Cardiovasc Med.* 2020.

126. Osende JI, Badimon JJ, Fuster V et al. Blood thrombogenicity in type 2 diabetes mellitus patients is associated with glycemic control. *J Am Coll Cardiol.* 2001;38:1307-1312.

127. Sambola A, Osende J, Hathcock J et al. Role of risk factors in the modulation of tissue factor activity and blood thrombogenicity. *Circulation.* 2003;107:973-977.

128. Nilsson J. Atherosclerotic plaque vulnerability in the statin era. *Eur Heart J.* 2017;38:1638-1644.

129. Bryckaert M, Rosa JP, Denis CV, Lenting PJ. Of von Willebrand factor and platelets. *Cell Mol Life Sci.* 2015;72:307-26.

130. Shida Y, Swystun LL, Brown C et al. Shear stress and platelet-induced tensile forces regulate ADAMTS13-localization within the platelet thrombus. *Res Pract Thromb Haemost.* 2019;3:254-260.

131. Amabile N, Rautou PE, Tedgui A, Boulanger CM. Microparticles: key protagonists in cardiovascular disorders. *Seminars Thromb Hemost.* 2010;36:907-916.

132. Badimon L, Suades R, Arderiu G, Pena E, Chiva-Blanch G, Padro T. Microvesicles in atherosclerosis and angiogenesis: from bench to bedside and reverse. *Frontiers Cardiovasc Med.* 2017;4:77.

133. Badimon L, Suades R, Vilella-Figuerola A et al. Liquid biopsies: microsicles in cardiovascular disease. *Antioxidants Redox Signaling.* 2019.

134. Chiva-Blanch G, Badimon L. Cross-talk between lipoproteins and inflammation: the role of microvesicles. *J Clin Med.* 2019;8.

135. Suades R, Padro T, Vilahur G, Badimon L. Circulating and platelet-derived microparticles in human blood enhance thrombosis on atherosclerotic plaques. *Thromb Haemost.* 2012;108:1208-1219.

136. Chiva-Blanch G, Laake K, Myhre P et al. Platelet-, monocyte-derived and tissue factor-carrying circulating microparticles are related to acute myocardial infarction severity. *PloS One.* 2017;12:e0172558.

137. Suades R, Padro T, Vilahur G et al. Growing thrombi release increased levels of CD235a(+) microparticles and decreased levels of activated platelet-derived microparticles. Validation in ST-elevation myocardial infarction patients. *J Thromb Haemost.* 2015;13:1776-1786.

138. Tomaniak M, Katagiri Y, Modolo R et al. Vulnerable plaques and patients: state-of-the-art. *Eur Heart J.* 2020;41:2997-3004.

139. Dai J, Xing L, Jia H et al. In vivo predictors of plaque erosion in patients with ST-segment elevation myocardial infarction: a clinical, angiographical, and intravascular optical coherence tomography study. *Eur Heart J.* 2018;39:2077-2085.

140. Kramer MC, Rittersma SZ, de Winter RJ et al. Relationship of thrombus healing to underlying plaque morphology in sudden coronary death. *J Am Coll Cardiol.* 2010;55:122-132.

141. Falk E, Shah PK, Fuster V. Coronary plaque disruption. *Circulation.* 1995;92:657-671.

142. Farb A, Burke AP, Tang AL et al. Coronary plaque erosion without rupture into a lipid core. A frequent cause of coronary thrombosis in sudden coronary death. *Circulation.* 1996;93:1354-1363.

18

ST-Elevation Myocardial Infarction

Borja Ibanez, Manesh Patel, Inés García-Lunar, Usman Baber, Jonathan Halperin, and Valentin Fuster

CHAPTER OUTLINE

ST-segment elevation myocardial infarction

Epidemiology

- The incidence, acute and long-term mortality of STEMI are decreasing in the USA and Europe

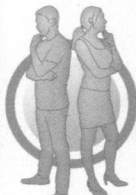

- Mortality associated with STEMI is still substantial: in-hospital death rate is 4-12%

- STEMI is relatively more common in younger than older people

- STEMI is relatively more common in men than in women, although the incidence in women increases after the menopause

  - Compared to men, women tend to present later and more frequently with atypical symptoms, and end to undergo fewer interventions despite receiving equal benefit from these therapies

Mechanisms of disease

- STEMI results from acute occlusion of an epicardial coronary artery

- Prolonged ischemia results in irreversible replacement of the myocardium with fibrotic non-contracting scar

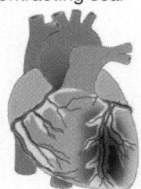

- Reperfusion itself may also induce damage to the formerly ischemic myocardium

- The final extent of necrosis (infarct size) is a major determinant of postinfarction mortality

Management

- Timely reperfusion (primary PCI vs. pharmacoinvasive strategy)

- Class I pharmacological agents (acute & chronic phases)
  - Dual antiplatelet therapy
  - Lipid-lowering therapies
  - RAAS inhibition and beta-blockers

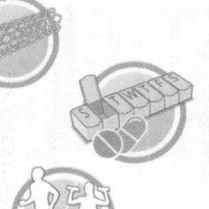

- Revascularization of non-culprit disease (not necessarily at the time of addressing the culprit lesion)

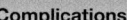

- Cardiac rehabilitation

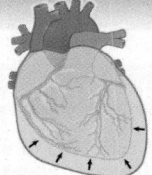

Complications

- The incidence of mechanical and pericardial complications after STEMI has fallen significantly in the primary PCI era

- Electrical complications (arrhythmias and conduction disturbances) are relatively common during the early hours of STEMI and are important prognostic factors

Chapter 18 Fuster and Hurst's Central Illustration. The epidemiology, mechanisms of disease, management and complications of ST-segment elevation myocardial infarction (STEMI). PCI, percutaneous coronary intervention; RAAS, renin-angiotensin-aldosterone system; STEMI, ST-segment elevation myocardial infarction.

CHAPTER SUMMARY

This chapter describes the epidemiology, mechanisms of disease, and management of ST-segment elevation myocardial infarction (STEMI; see Fuster and Hurst's Central Illustration). The incidence of STEMI is decreasing in the United States and Europe. However, while advances in treatment and secondary prevention strategies have led to a reduction of short-term and long-term mortality in patients with STEMI, mortality remains substantial. STEMI results from acute occlusion of an epicardial coronary artery. Depending on the size of the territory distal to the occlusion site, the global left ventricular function can be significantly impaired, resulting in postinfarction chronic heart failure. Electrical and mechanical complications may also complicate STEMI and are discussed. The final extent of necrosis (myocardial infarct size) is one of the major determinants of prognosis after STEMI and is mainly the result of two processes: ischemia and subsequent reperfusion. Timely reperfusion (by primary percutaneous coronary intervention [PCI] or a pharmaco-invasive strategy, i.e. fibrinolysis combined with early PCI) is the cornerstone of STEMI treatment. Antithrombotic therapy comprising both anticoagulants and platelet inhibitors is also central to the management of patients with STEMI, as is timing of revascularization of nonculprit multivessel disease. Since thrombotic potential diminishes over time after myocardial infarction, and ongoing exposure to dual antiplatelet therapy increases the risk of bleeding, the risk-benefit calculus favoring potent antithrombotic therapy gradually declines beyond the acute phase of STEMI. The benefits of lipid-lowering therapies, ß-blockers, renin-angiotensin-aldosterone system inhibitors, and other pharmacological and nonpharmacological interventions are additionally discussed.

EPIDEMIOLOGY OF STEMI: CHANGE IN TEMPORAL TRENDS IN PROGNOSIS

ST-elevation myocardial infarction (STEMI, **Fig. 18–1**), resulting from an abrupt coronary artery occlusion, is the most severe presentation of ischemic heart disease, the leading cause of death worldwide. Opposed to non-STEMI (NSTEMI), the relative incidence of STEMI is decreasing.[1,2] The adjusted incidence of STEMI in the United States has decreased from 133 per 100,000 in 1999 to 50 per 100,000 in 2008.[3] While there are regional differences, incidence rates of STEMI in Europe are similar, as shown by a Swedish registry in 2015, which was 58 per 100,000 per year.[4] STEMI is relatively more common in younger than older people and in men than in women; however, the incidence in women increases after the menopause.[4,5] Average age at first myocardial infarction (MI) is 65.6 years for males and 72.0 years for females.[6]

Mortality in STEMI patients is influenced by many factors, such as age, Killip class, time to reperfusion, presence of networks for STEMI care including the emergency medical system, reperfusion strategy, patient's risk profile, presence of multivessel disease, and left ventricular (LV) systolic function, among others. The widespread use of reperfusion therapy, adoption of primary percutaneous coronary intervention (pPCI), refinement in antithrombotic therapy, and improvement in secondary prevention strategies have resulted in a reduction of short- and long-term mortality in STEMI patients. Despite these advances, mortality associated with STEMI is still substantial: in-hospital death rate is between 4% and 12%,[7] increasing to 10% at 1 year according to registries.[6,7] A study of the MONICA population-based registries showed that although event rates, incidence, and mortality associated with MI all showed significant reductions between 2006 and 2014, these were seen primarily in the 65 to 74 year age group, and there were no substantial declines in younger people except for mortality in young women.

MI remains a leading cause of death in women even though the development of ischemic heart disease is delayed about one decade compared to that in males. The incidence of acute MI has declined in the last 20 years; however, declines in hospitalization for MI have slowed in women compared to those in men.[8] Women tend to present later and more frequently with atypical symptoms than men.[9] Outcomes may be poorer in women than in men with STEMI.[8-10] Women tend to undergo fewer interventions than do men and undergo coronary angiography and/or pPCI less frequently, even though both men and women receive equal benefit from these therapies.[9,11-13] When hospitalized, women tend to be older and have more comorbidities than do their male counterparts. In the Prospective Urban Rural Epidemiological (PURE) study, women less frequently received secondary prevention treatment, diagnostic tests, and coronary revascularization, but paradoxically they had lower 30-day mortality than men after an MI. Black males have a higher incidence of MI in all age groups. In the United States, 35% of MIs occur in patients 75 years and older and 11% occur in patients older than 85 years of age.[14]

MECHANISMS OF MYOCARDIAL INJURY DURING STEMI: ISCHEMIA/REPERFUSION INJURY

STEMI is the result of an acute occlusion of an epicardial coronary artery. The myocardium supplied by the occluded artery suffers severe ischemia. Prolonged ischemia, if there is no collateral circulation, results in irreversible myocardial damage, with replacement of the myocardium by fibrotic noncontracting scar. Depending on the size of the territory distal to the occlusion site, the global ventricular function can be significantly impaired resulting in postinfarction chronic heart failure (HF).[15] Classical studies performed in large animal models have demonstrated that restoration of blood flow (reperfusion) is able to efficiently limit the progression of myocardial injury.[16] Reperfusion was shown not only to limit the progression of myocardial death but also to change the pattern of myocardial tissue healing. This concept was rapidly introduced into practice, and a long series of successful trials demonstrated that early reperfusion was able to reduce the extent of myocardial injury and, more importantly, to reduce mortality. Since then, timely reperfusion has become the standard treatment

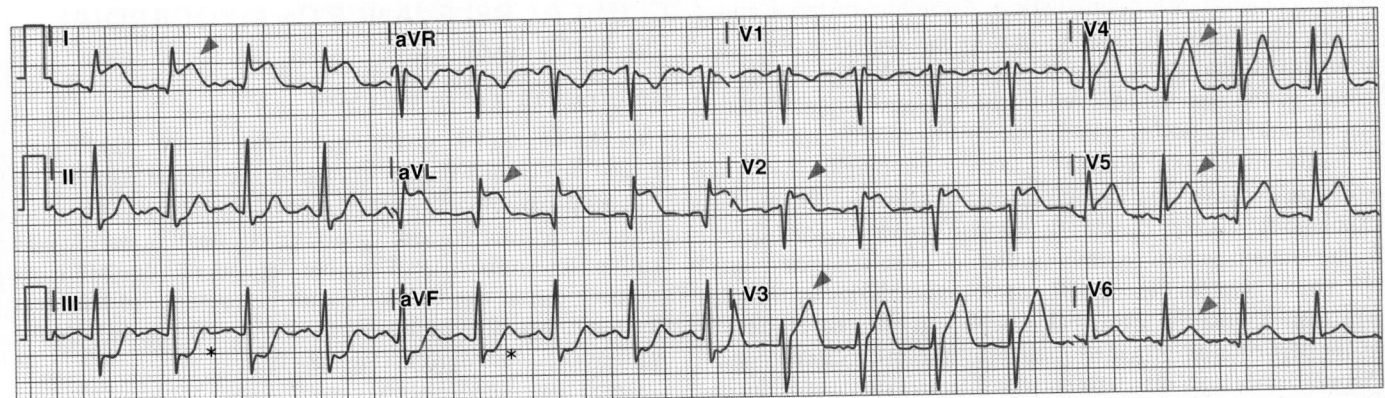

Figure 18–1. **Twelve-lead ECG tracing in a patient with an anterolateral acute STEMI.** *Red arrowheads* point the ST-segment elevation in anterior (V2–V4) and lateral leads (I-aVL; V5–V6). *Asterisks* mark ST-segment depression in inferior leads (reciprocal changes).

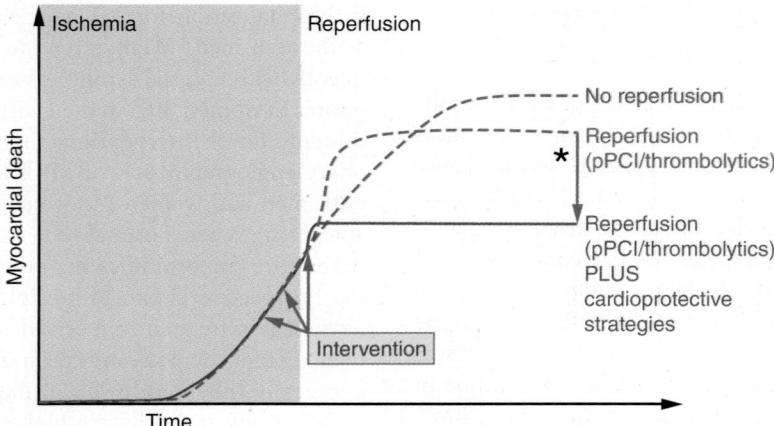

Figure 18–2. Impact of reperfusion injury on final infarct size. Myocardial death during coronary occlusion increases exponentially with time. Unrelieved ischemia (no reperfusion) results in death of the entire area at risk (*brown dashed line*). Reperfusion, either mechanical by primary angioplasty (primary pPCI) or pharmacological by thrombolytic agents results in myocardial salvage and reduction of infarct size compared to no reperfusion (*red dashed line*). Reperfusion injury adds to the injury developed during initial ischemia (note the progression of death [stepped slope of *red line*] immediately after reperfusion). If reperfusion-related damage is abrogated by cardioprotective strategies, infarct size does not progress after reperfusion (*blue line*). The difference between infarct size presented in *red and blue lines* is the contribution of reperfusion injury to final infarct size (represented by an *arrow*). The administration of a given therapy, *dashed arrows*, any time before reperfusion (including immediately before) can attenuate reperfusion injury. Adapted with permission from Garcia-Dorado D, Piper HM. Postconditioning: reperfusion of "reperfusion injury" after hibernation. *Cardiovasc Res.* 2006 Jan;69(1):1-3.

for patients suffering an acute MI. However, extensive pre- and clinical studies have shown that reperfusion itself may induce damage to the formerly ischemic myocardium (**Fig. 18–2**). Since reperfusion is the prerequisite for myocardial salvage, the damage inflicted on the myocardium during a STEMI is known as *ischemia/reperfusion injury* (IRI) (ie, the result of ischemia- and reperfusion-related damages). Myocardial IRI is a complex phenomenon involving many factors, all contributing to the final damage inflicted on the myocardium.[15] **Figure 18–3** summarizes the highly complex process of IRI and its multiple mechanisms. The first critical player is the epicardial artery (represented as 1 in Fig. 18–3). Atherosclerotic plaque rupture with superimposed thrombus formation results in abrupt cessation of oxygen and nutrient supply distal to the occlusion. Recanalization of the epicardial vessel by mechanical or pharmacological means, as well as the reduction in thrombus burden by adjuvant antiplatelet/anticoagulant therapies, is only the first step toward the salvage of myocardium. During the reperfusion process (either if it is mechanical by pPCI or pharmacological by thrombolytics), thrombus material and other plaque debris can be distally embolized, contributing to microvascular obstruction (MVO).[17] Circulating cells contribute to the damage inflicted to the myocardium: activated platelets and leukocytes in the bloodstream not only contribute to the thrombus generation but also can form plugins that can embolize distally into the microcirculation through the residual blood flow across the culprit lesion (a process independent from plaque debris microembolization). The microcirculation is a critical player in the fate of the myocardium during ischemia/reperfusion. Once the epicardial vessel flow is restored, efficient tissue perfusion is provided mainly by the microcirculation. Plaque debris and platelet/neutrophil aggregates can induce a mechanical obstruction of the microcirculation precluding efficient tissue perfusion despite the opening of the epicardial

artery (known as the no-reflow phenomenon). The generation of tissue edema following reperfusion can result in external compression of the microcirculation, reducing the perfusion capacity of the capillary network (*arrowheads* in Fig. 18–3). Finally, the microcirculation can be disintegrated due to previous damage and allow the circulating cells to leak the interstitial space (*dashed lines* in the capillary of Fig. 18–3). Hemorrhage is especially harmful due to the release of iron, contributing to subsequent inflammatory reactions. Cardiomyocytes that have survived the ischemic phase may suffer from several intracellular pathways activated during reperfusion. After the acute phase of the IRI insult has passed, the significant infiltration of myocardial tissue by inflammatory cells can induce additional damage to the myocardium. In this chapter, we summarize the cellular and molecular mechanisms involved in IRI; however, it is important to keep in mind that it is the combination of these different, interconnected mechanisms that leads to the progression of myocardial injury during reperfusion.

CLINICAL RELEVANCE OF MYOCARDIAL INFARCT SIZE

Determinants of Infarct Size

After the onset of a MI (ie, coronary occlusion), the hypoperfused myocardial region, known as the area at risk (AAR), is at jeopardy of developing irreversible injury. Unrelieved ischemia, in the absence of significant collateral flow, results in death of the entire AAR. The time-dependent slope of infarct size progression can be blunted in the presence of therapies ameliorating ischemic injury, such as ischemic preconditioning or intravenous metoprolol (**Fig. 18–4**).

Given that today's mainstay treatment for MI is reperfusion, part of the AAR remains free of necrosis: the so-called salvaged myocardium. The seminal studies by Ross and coworkers four

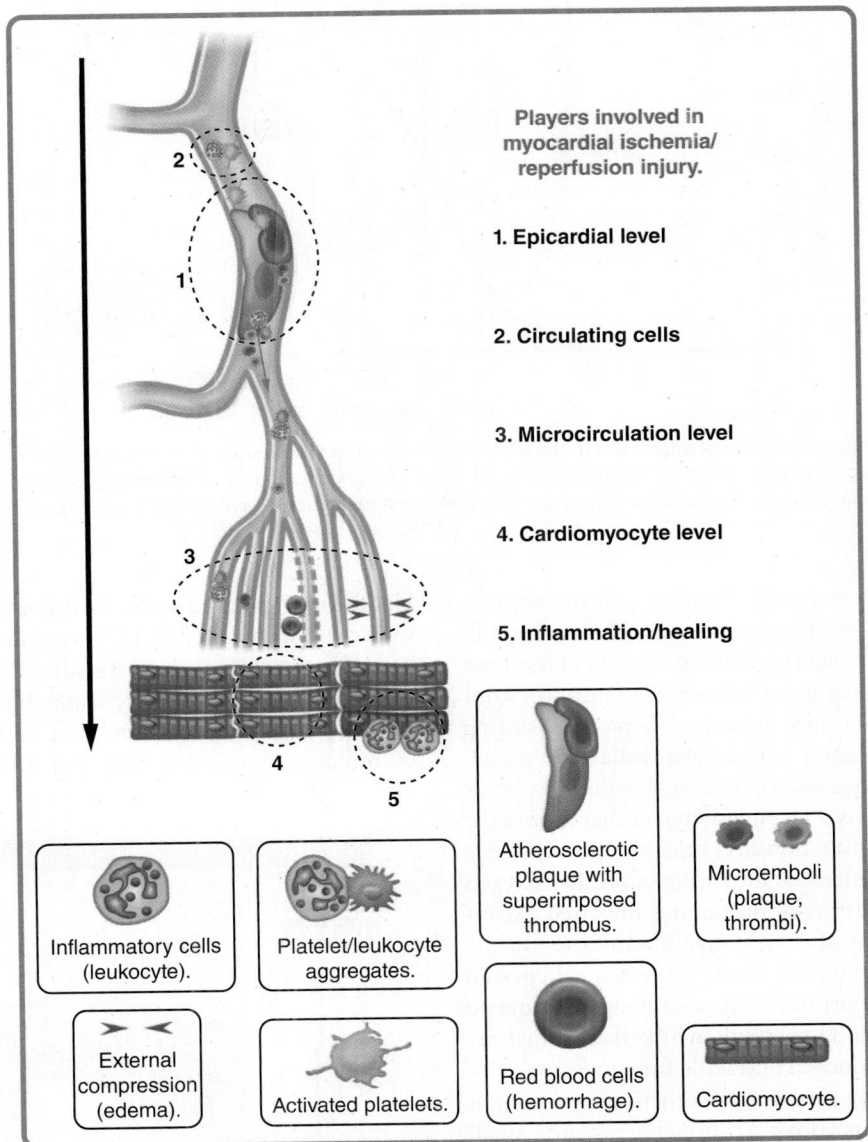

Players involved in
myocardial ischemia/
reperfusion injury.

1. Epicardial level

2. Circulating cells

3. Microcirculation level

4. Cardiomyocyte level

5. Inflammation/healing

Atherosclerotic plaque with superimposed thrombus.

Microemboli (plaque, thrombi).

Inflammatory cells (leukocyte).

Platelet/leukocyte aggregates.

External compression (edema).

Activated platelets.

Red blood cells (hemorrhage).

Cardiomyocyte.

Figure 18–3. Gradient of events during ischemia/reperfusion injury. *Arrow* in the left side of the figure illustrates the sequence of events (see text for details). To attain cardioprotection and salvage the jeopardized myocardium, a hierarchical chain of events must occur. The *arrow* in the left side of the figure represents the gradient of events contributing to final damage during ischemia/reperfusion injury (IRI). If any of these events is not managed, the chain of protection is broken and damage will continue (eg, if the microcirculation is severely damaged, no matter how well the cardiomyocyte mitochondrial transition pore is preserved, that cardiomyocyte will not survive the event due to poor tissue perfusion). According to this scheme, it is intuitive to understand that protective interventions targeting only these layers are unlikely to significantly protect the heart from damage. Therapies targeting multiple layers of this chain of damage or multiple therapies applied simultaneously will have higher chances of resulting in protection.

decades ago[16] first demonstrated that early restoration of blood flow (reperfusion) salvages myocardium from infarction. These landmark studies demonstrated that there is a temporal progression of myocardial death during ongoing coronary occlusion: the sooner the reperfusion, the smaller the proportion of AAR that becomes necrotic. These experimental studies primed the development of reperfusion strategies to limit the size of necrosis in patients suffering an acute MI.[15] Interventions applied at the end of the ischemic period (ie, coinciding with reperfusion) can reduce infarct size. It was already recognized in the mid-1980s that gentle reperfusion at low pressure resulted in significantly less edema and a smaller infarct

size than did standard abrupt reperfusion at normal pressure. This idea was later developed into ischemic postconditioning, a strategy to reduce infarct size by brief episodes of coronary re-occlusion/reflow at the time of reperfusion, a strategy called ischemic postconditioning.[15] Since these interventions are applied at the end of the ischemic period, they cannot reduce infarct size by reducing ischemic damage and thus must act through a reduction of reperfusion-related damage. From these observations it is clear not only that reperfusion injury contributes to infarct size, but also that all conditioning strategies that protect the myocardium and reduce infarct size act only in conjunction with eventual reperfusion.[15]

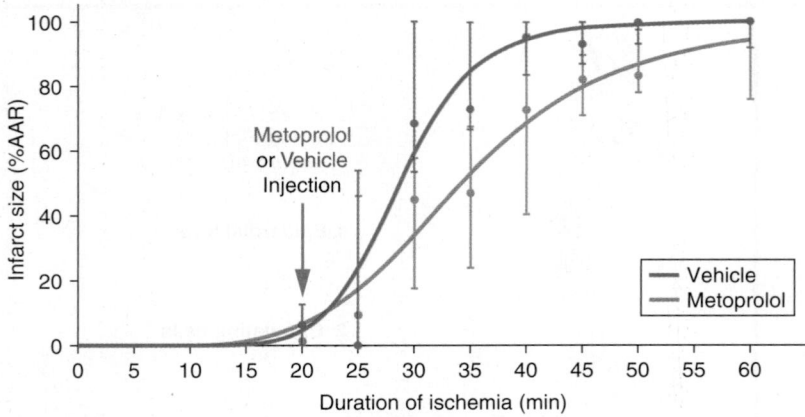

Figure 18–4. Time-dependent progression of infarct size in the presence or absence of metoprolol. Slope progression of infarct size (% AAR) with time of ischemia (minutes) in a pig model of ischemia/reperfusion injury. *Blue*, vehicle group; *orange*, metoprolol group. Reproduced with permission from Lobo-Gonzalez M, Galán-Arriola C, Rossello X, et al. Metoprolol blunts the time-dependent progression of infarct size. *Basic Res Cardiol*. 2020 Aug 3;115(5):55.

Within a given AAR, both the duration and the severity of coronary blood flow reduction determine the nature and amount of injury.[15] A complete coronary occlusion of less than 20 minutes duration results in only reversible injury (ie, contractile dysfunction with a slow, but complete recovery during reperfusion), a phenomenon called myocardial stunning.[18] This time-dependent progression of irreversible injury is influenced by several conditions. The underlying mechanisms of the prolonged contractile dysfunction after brief ischemic episodes (stunning) relate to the enhanced formation of reactive oxygen species (ROS) during early reperfusion and impaired excitation–contraction coupling after oxidative modification of the sarcoplasmic reticulum and the contractile proteins. Repeated coronary occlusions of short duration or prolonged moderate reduction in coronary blood flow result in hibernating myocardium, a viable state of reduced contractile function capable of eventual recovery after reperfusion.[18] Hibernating myocardium displays both signs of injury (loss of contractile proteins, small donut-like mitochondria, fibrosis) and of adaptation (short-term energetic recovery, altered expression of mitochondrial proteins, and expression of cardioprotective proteins).[19] When the reduction in coronary blood flow is severe and lasts longer than 20 to 40 minutes, infarction develops first in the inner subendocardial layers of the core of the AAR and then spreads in a "wavefront" to the outer subepicardial layers and the borders of the AAR. The wavefront of infarct development reflects the lateral and transmural distribution of coronary blood flow, which is less in the inner than the outer layers of the myocardium and less in the core than in the borders of the AAR. Recently, it has been demonstrated that while the predominant spatial progression of the wavefront is from endo- to epicardium, there is also a lateral progression of infarction (**Fig. 18–5**). The evolution of infarction varies with species and depends on the existence and extent of a collateral circulation. Dogs have a well-developed native collateral circulation, and infarction starts after 40 minutes of coronary occlusion and spreads to affect 70% of the AAR after 6 hours; in dogs, therefore, infarct size is best quantified as a fraction of the AAR and normalized to the residual

blood flow. Pigs have a negligible native collateral circulation, and infarction starts after 20 to 25 minutes of coronary occlusion and affects ≥80% of the AAR after 40 minutes (Fig. 18–4).[20] Primates have few innate collaterals but are relatively resistant to myocardial ischemia; there is no infarction after 40 to 60 minutes of coronary occlusion, and even after 90 minutes

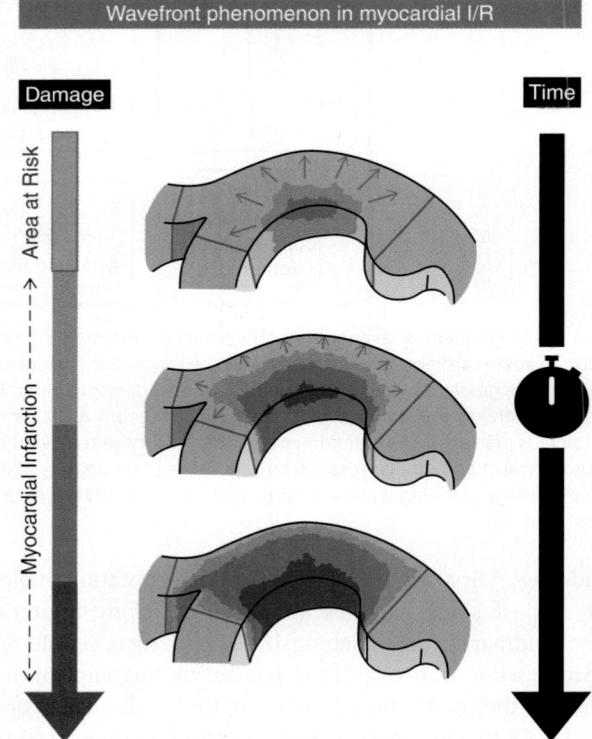

Figure 18–5. Wavefront phenomenon in myocardial infarction. According to cardiac MRI data generated in the METOCARD-CNIC trial, the wavefront progression of a myocardial infarct takes place not only in the transmural direction, but also laterally in the human heart. Reproduced with permission from Lorca R, Jiménez-Blanco M, García-Ruiz JM, et al. Coexistence of transmural and lateral wavefront progression of myocardial infarction in the human heart. *Rev Esp Cardiol (Engl Ed)*. 2021 Oct;74(10):870-877.

of coronary occlusion, infarct size is smaller than it is in pigs. Fortunately, infarct development in humans is slower than it is in these large mammals. Even after 4 to 6 hours of coronary occlusion, 30% to 50% of the AAR remains viable and thus salvageable, as one can estimate from magnetic resonance imaging (MRI) and from the amount of salvage by reperfusion.[21] Salvageable myocardium remains even after 12 hours from symptom onset (BRAVE-2 trial). To what extent the resistance of the diseased human heart is attributable to a developed collateral circulation at the time of infarction, as in the native dog heart, or reflects an inherently greater resistance to ischemic injury, such as in the primate heart, or is a result of preceding episodes of brief ischemia/ reperfusion, is unclear at present. In contrast to prior notions, hemodynamic changes have little impact on the development of MI, and, if they do exert an impact, it is largely through their effect on coronary blood flow and its spatial distribution. Heart rate determines infarct progression to some extent. Variations in coronary blood flow not only determine the nature and extent of myocardial injury, but paradoxically also protection from it. Repeated brief episodes of coronary occlusion preceding a prolonged coronary occlusion with reperfusion reduce infarct size, a phenomenon known as ischemic preconditioning. Likewise, repeated brief coronary occlusion during early reperfusion reduces infarct size, a phenomenon known as ischemic postconditioning.[15]

Therefore, there are several determinants of myocardial infarct size (**Table 18–1**).

Infarct Size Determines Postinfarction Mortality and Morbidity

The final extent of necrosis (infarct size) is a major determinant of postinfarction mortality.[22] Large infarctions are associated with an irreversible impairment of the contractile function of the heart and concomitant chronic HF. Beyond their impact on LV systolic function, large infarctions are associated with an increased risk of sudden death. The widespread implementation of reperfusion strategies has resulted in a very significant

reduction in the acute mortality associated with MI. In fact, in-hospital mortality has decreased from ~20% in the late-1980s to ~5% in the mid-2010s.[6,7] Paradoxically, this significant reduction of infarction-related acute mortality has resulted in an increase in the incidence of chronic HF. The obvious reason is that patients with a severely depressed cardiac function would not have survived the acute phase of infarction in the past, but with the advent of reperfusion, patients now survive the index episode and live with a significantly damaged heart. In fact, prior MI is still one of the main etiologies of chronic HF worldwide. Chronic HF treatment is one of the main contributors to healthcare expenditures and thus it is important to implement strategies to reduce its incidence. After acknowledging that infarct size is the main determinant of adverse postinfarction outcomes, including HF, therapies able to reduce infarct size are therefore urgently sought under the hypothesis that smaller infarctions will result in better long-term heart performance, and that this will translate into fewer adverse clinical events. The identification of therapies able to reduce infarct size, including through amelioration of IRI, is a major challenge to 21st-century society.[23]

MANAGEMENT OF STEMI

Reperfusion Strategies (PCI vs Fibrinolysis)

Timely reperfusion constitutes the most effective method to restore the balance between myocardial oxygen supply and demand in STEMI. Its widespread implementation in STEMI patients has resulted in a reduction of in-hospital mortality from 20% to 5% in three decades[25] and also in improved myocardial healing and remodeling, thus lowering the risk of post-STEMI arrhythmia and HF. Timely reperfusion by means of fibrinolysis or pPCI is therefore recommended in STEMI patients presenting within 12 hours of symptom onset.[24,25] Fibrinolysis has been a vital reperfusion strategy for decades and involves the administration of an intravenous agent to produce lysis of the thrombus associated with STEMI, restore anterograde coronary flow, and interrupt infarct formation. After publication of the first GISSI trial in 1986 in which intravenous streptokinase significantly reduced mortality in 11,000 STEMI patients within 6 hours of symptom onset, the use of fibrinolytic therapy for STEMI was established. The advent of pPCI provided an alternative and more effective method for the emergent recanalization of an occluded infarct artery. This technique has undergone remarkable progress over the last four decades with adjunctive pharmacological treatments, transradial access and new generation drug-eluting stents, significantly lowering the rates of complications and stent restenosis and thrombosis.

Early Phase of STEMI (<12 Hours from Symptom Onset)

In a large meta-analysis including 23 randomized clinical trials (RCTs), pPCI was better than thrombolytic therapy at reducing death, reinfarction, and stroke in STEMI patients.[26] Accordingly, clinical practice guidelines recommend pPCI over fibrinolysis in STEMI provided it can be performed timely and by an experienced team.[24,25] One of the running debates in this area is the definition of "timely" reperfusion. Since no single

TABLE 18–1. Determinants of Infarct Size

Determinant	Effect on infarct size	Refs
Area at risk (AAR) extent	The larger the AAR, the larger the extent of infarction	142
Duration of myocardial ischemia	The longer the duration of myocardial ischemia (coronary occlusion), the larger the extent of infarction	143
Collateral circulation	Poor collaterals are associated with larger infarctions	142, 143, 144
Temperature of the tissue during ischemia	The lower the temperature during coronary occlusion, the larger the extent of infarction	145
Ischemia/Reperfusion injury (IRI)	Damage driven by reperfusion increases the size of infarction	15

Major determinants of infarct size and some references as guide. The table shows those determinants with stronger evidence from experimental studies. There are other determinants that have been associated with the extent of infarct size but are less widely validated.

study has specifically addressed this issue, experts have agreed, based on information from relatively old registries and trials on a cut-off point of 120 minutes (time from STEMI diagnosis to PCI-mediated reperfusion, that is, wire crossing of the occluded artery) to choose pPCI over fibrinolysis.[24] Of note, most of the aforementioned trials treated postlytic patients conservatively, which is no longer the state-of-the-art. The efficacy and clinical benefit of fibrinolysis decrease as the time from symptom onset elapses.[24] One possible explanation is that coronary thrombi mature with the passage of time, making them harder to lyse. Besides, fibrinolysis is associated with increased odds of stroke, largely attributable to intracranial hemorrhage and several absolute and relative contraindications to its use should be evaluated prior to the bolus administration (**Table 18–2**). In the absence of contraindications, it is recommended that intravenous fibrinolytics (fibrin-specific agents are preferred) should be administered as soon as possible and with a maximum target delay of 10 minutes from STEMI diagnosis.[24] This also includes the lytic bolus administration at the prehospital setting whenever possible since this strategy has demonstrated to be feasible and safe and associated with a reduction in long-term mortality.[24]

However, in practice, it is very difficult to estimate time from STEMI diagnosis to wire crossing and multiple structural as well as unexpected additional delays may present.[27] For example, in a very recent French registry, more than one quarter of STEMI patients underwent pPCI later than recommended (>120 minutes).[28] Delays are even greater in patients that need to be transferred from a non-PCI center for pPCI.[29] Treatment delays also come with an increased rate of morbidity and mortality in STEMI patients. In a previous report, each 30-minute

---

TABLE 18–2. Contraindications of Fibrinolytic Therapy

Absolute
Previous intracranial hemorrhage or stroke of unknown origin at any time.
Ischemic stroke in the preceding 6 months.
Central nervous system damage, neoplasms, or arteriovenous malformation.
Recent major trauma/surgery/head injury (within the preceding month).
Gastrointestinal bleeding within the last month.
Aortic dissection.
Noncompressible punctures in the last 24 hours.
Relative
Transient ischemic attack in the preceding 6 months.
Oral anticoagulant therapy.
Pregnancy or within 1 week postpartum.
Refractory hypertension (SBP >180 mm Hg and/or DBP >110 mm Hg).
Advanced liver disease.
Infective endocarditis.
Active peptic ulcer.
Prolonged or traumatic resuscitation.

Reproduced with permission from Ibanez B, James S, Agewall S, et al. 2017 ESC Guidelines for the management of acute myocardial infarction in patients presenting with ST-segment elevation: The Task Force for the management of acute myocardial infarction in patients presenting with ST-segment elevation of the European Society of Cardiology (ESC). *Eur Heart J.* 2018 Jan 7;39(2):119-177.

---

delay in pPCI was associated with an 8% higher 1-year mortality risk.[30] In addition to the deleterious effect of time on myocardial salvage itself, pPCI is less capable to achieve microvascular reperfusion in evolved STEMI patients.[31] Accumulating contemporary evidence indicates that a mixed procedure, the so-called pharmaco-invasive strategy—fibrinolysis combined with rescue PCI (in case of failed reperfusion) or routine-early PCI (ideally 2–24 hours after fibrinolysis)— achieves clinical outcomes at least as good as pPCI in the first hours after symptom onset. Failed fibrinolysis is defined as <50% ST-segment resolution within 60 to 90 minutes of fibrinolytic administration. Rescue PCI is also recommended in the presence of hemodynamic or electrical instability, worsening ischemia, or persistent chest pain.[24] In the STREAM RCT, there were no differences in clinical events (death, shock, congestive HF, or reinfarction) acutely and mortality rates at 1-year follow-up[32] in early STEMI presenters (<3 hours) without the possibility of immediate PCI between a delayed PCI strategy or pharmaco-invasive strategy with Tenecteplase. A subanalysis of this trial suggested that the equipoise when the benefit of pPCI is lost in favor of pharmaco-invasive strategy is around 60 to 70 minutes, much earlier than the 120-minute universally accepted limit to choose pPCI.[33] It has been suggested that the clinical benefit associated with early pharmaco-invasive strategy may be secondary to reduced rates of cardiogenic shock and congestive HF,[34] although this hypothesis should be further tested in large RCTs. Further observational studies in Canada (Vital Heart) and Korea (KAMIR) have found that 1-year mortality and major adverse cardiovascular event (MACE) rates were similar between the pharmaco-invasive strategy and pPCI[35] or even lower for the pharmaco-invasive population.[36] In the French FAST-MI registry,[28] patients who underwent late pPCI (>120 minutes) had an increased risk of death and MACE 5 years after STEMI whereas prognosis for pharmaco-invasive or timely (<120 minutes) pPCI patients did not significantly differ. Importantly, in the STREAM trial, the dose of Tenecteplase was halved in patients ≥75 years by a protocol amendment after evidencing an excess of intracranial hemorrhage in that age group. This same strategy was replicated (using half-dose Alteplase) in the EARLY-MYO trial[37] for patients 18 to 75 years presenting ≤6 hours after symptom onset and with an expected PCI-related delay. Though not powered for clinical outcomes, infarct size and LV ejection fraction (LVEF) (assessed with cardiac MRI) were similar between pharmaco-invasive and pPCI strategies. The STREAM-2 trial (NCT02777580) is currently evaluating the effect of this reduced dose of Tenecteplase in a much larger population of STEMI patients ≥60 years.

Ultimately, the decision to choose one or another reperfusion strategy should evaluate, apart from the time required to initiate pPCI, the time elapsed since the onset of symptoms, the individual's ischemic versus bleeding risk, and the risk of complications related to STEMI (mechanical complications, shock, or severe HF). **Figure 18–6** shows factors that favor fibrinolysis or pPCI and **Fig. 18–7** summarizes the decision algorithm for reperfusion strategies in STEMI.

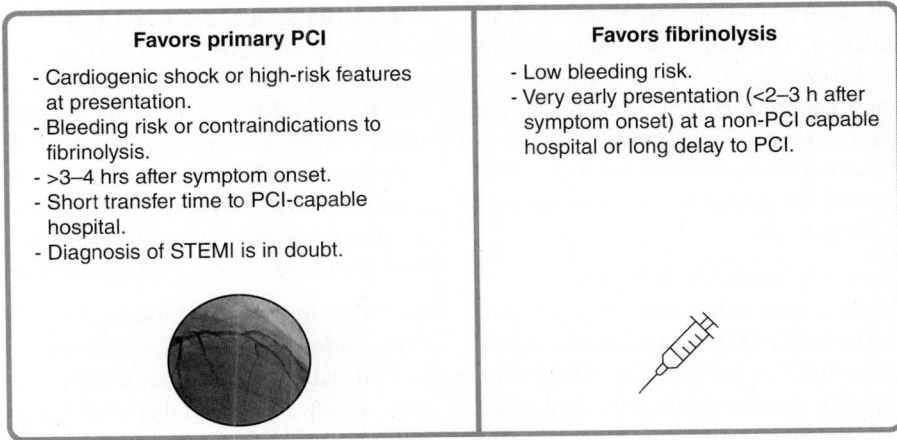

Favors primary PCI

- Cardiogenic shock or high-risk features at presentation.
- Bleeding risk or contraindications to fibrinolysis.
- >3–4 hrs after symptom onset.
- Short transfer time to PCI-capable hospital.
- Diagnosis of STEMI is in doubt.

Favors fibrinolysis

- Low bleeding risk.
- Very early presentation (<2–3 h after symptom onset) at a non-PCI capable hospital or long delay to PCI.

Figure 18–6. Factors to be considered when choosing a reperfusion strategy.

Evolved (12–48 Hours) or Recent (>48 Hours) STEMI

In patients presenting late after symptom onset (12–48 hours), a routine pPCI strategy should be considered.[24] However, in stable patients with persistent occlusion of the infarct related artery >48 hours after symptom onset, routine PCI is not indicated since it has shown no additional benefit compared with medical treatment alone (OAT trial)[38] (Fig. 18–7).

Finally, during the COVID-19 pandemic, some countries recommended to adopt a strategy of fibrinolysis for STEMI patients due to concerns of resource allocation, sufficient personal protective equipment (PPE), and challenges in transfer of patients to PCI-capable hospitals. Thus, in such regions (such as the Hubei province in China), the proportion of STEMI patients receiving pPCI decreased in favor of fibrinolysis during the outbreak.[39] Increases in time to reperfusion therapy have also been reported, together with higher odds of in-hospital mortality and HF. A dedicated consensus statement from scientific societies[40] has very recently emphasized that pPCI should remain the standard of care during the COVID-19 pandemic provided it can be delivered timely by an expert time outfitted with PPE in a dedicated laboratory.

Management of Multivessel Disease in STEMI Patients

Patients with STEMI often have obstructive coronary disease in one or more non–infarct-related artery (IRA). In a large

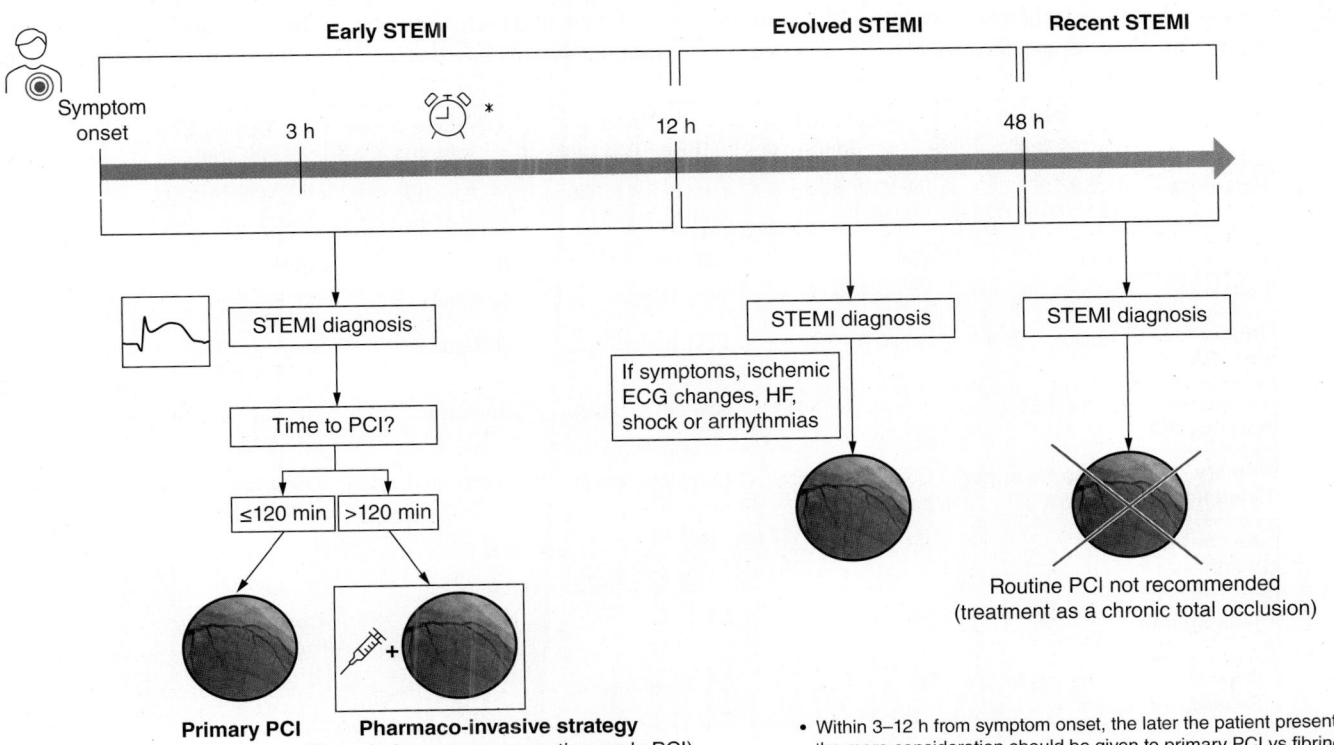

Figure 18–7. Selection of reperfusion strategy according to time from symptoms onset.

retrospective analysis of several randomized trials in AMI patients (over 68,765 patients), 52% had at least one non-IRA with obstructive disease and 18.8% with three vessel disease.[41] Given this prevalence and common clinical occurrence, the acute and subacute management of multivessel disease in patients with STEMI has been the subject of several recent clinical trials that have impacted the guideline recommendations for both stable and unstable patients.

Complete Revascularization in Stable STEMI Patients

In the early 2010s, complete revascularization (ie, perform non-IRA PCI) during the initial STEMI revascularization procedure or as a staged procedure was not recommended in the absence of clinical instability. Several trials published from 2013 completely changed the approach to multivessel disease in STEMI patients. The 2016 update of the American Heart Association/American College of Cardiology (AHA/ACC) STEMI guideline[42] proposed that PCI in a non-IRA (either during index procedure or staged during hospitalization) may be appropriate, while the 2017 European Society of Cardiology (ESC) document proposed that routine PCI of non-IRA severe stenoses should be considered before hospital discharge.[24] These major changes in the recommendation were motivated by several trials in the topic. **Figure 18–8** contains the characteristics of these studies.[43]

The largest and more recent trial in the topic is the COMPLETE trial, which randomized 4041 patients to culprit only PCI compared to complete revascularization at either the time of primary PCI or in a staged fashion. This trial enrolled at 140 centers in 31 countries and evaluated the primary endpoint of cardiovascular death and MI and a co-primary endpoint of cardiovascular death, MI, or ischemia driven revascularization. The trial found complete revascularization to be superior for

both cardiovascular death and MI (7.8% vs 10.5% at 3 years; hazard ratio [HR], 0.74; $P = 0.004$) and for the primary endpoint plus ischemia driven revascularization, (8.9% vs 16.7% at 3 years; HR, 0.51; $P <0.001$). The findings were consistent irrespective of the timing of the revascularization (P value for interaction $P = 0.62$ for initial intervention and $P = 0.27$ for staged intervention).[44] A meta-analysis of over 10 trials also confirmed a benefit for complete revascularization in patients with STEMI and multivessel disease without cardiogenic shock.[45]

Complete Revascularization in STEMI Patients Presenting with Cardiogenic Shock

STEMI patients presenting with shock are a special subgroup with a very high mortality risk. Until recently, the accepted rationale was when multivessel disease was present, and the patient remained in shock despite PCI of the culprit artery, non-IRA immediate PCI should improve perfusion and thus prognosis. However, the only trial performed to date demonstrated that this approach was not associated with improved outcomes. The CULPRIT-SHOCK trial randomized 706 patients with cardiogenic shock and acute MI to culprit only PCI versus multivessel revascularization. The primary endpoint of death or severe renal failure requiring renal replacement therapy was reported both at 30 days and 1 year. Over 60% of the randomized patients had STEMI. The 1-year findings showed that death or renal replacement was 52% in the culprit only group and 59.5% in the multivessel revascularization group (HR 0.87; confidence interval [CI], 0.76–0.99).[46,47] Based on this trial, the 2018 ESC myocardial revascularization guidelines recommended against routine non-IRA PCI in STEMI patients presenting in shock (class III, level of evidence [LOE] B).[48]

Taken together, the recent clinical trials provide a common evidenced based strategy for the numerous patients with

	PRAMI trial	CvLPRIT trial	DANAMI-3-PRIMULTI trial	Compare-Acute trial	COMPLETE trial
Reference	NEJM 2013; 369: 1115–1123	JACC 2015; 65: 963–972	Lancet 2015; 386: 665–671	NEJM 2017; 376: 1234–1244	NEJM 2019; 381: 1411–1421
N	465	296	627	885	4041
Follow-up	23 months	12 months	27 months	12 months	12 months
Trigger for non-IRA PCI	Angio (>50%)	Angio (>70%)	FFR-guided	FFR-guided	Angio (>70%) or FFR in 50-70%
Timing of non-IRA PCI	Immediate	Immediate (64%) or staged*	Staged* (2 days)	Immediate	Staged (1day (64%) 23 days (36%))
Primary outcome	Complete revasc superior	Complete revasc superior	Complete revasc superior	Complete revasc superior	Complete revasc superior
All cause death	NS	NS	NS	NS	NS
Reinfarction	Complete revasc superior	NS	NS	NS	Complete revasc superior
Repeat Revasc	Complete revasc superior	NS	Complete revasc superior	Complete revasc superior	Complete revasc superior

Figure 18–8. Major trials testing the clinical benefit of complete revascularization in STEMI patients with multivessel disease. Reproduced with permission from Ibanez B, Roque D, Price S. The year in cardiovascular medicine 2020: acute coronary syndromes and intensive cardiac care. *Eur Heart J.* 2021 Mar 1;42(9): 884-895.

multivessel disease and STEMI. In patients without cardiogenic shock, there is relatively strong evidence with several RCT that complete revascularization of the non-IRA coronary artery disease either at the time of pPCI or during a staged procedure is clinically beneficial in reducing cardiovascular death and MI. In patients with cardiogenic shock, CULPRIT-SHOCK RCT has shown that culprit artery only PCI reduced the rate of death and renal replacement therapy at 1 year.

Antithrombotic Therapy (Acute, subacute and chronic phases of STEMI)

Acute Phase: From Clinical Presentation Until Hospital Discharge

Coronary atherosclerotic plaque rupture is the most common pathologic substrate for STEMI. Components of disrupted plaque, including oxidized lipoproteins and tissue factor, activate the coagulation cascade, generate thrombin, and promote platelet aggregation. Thus, antithrombotic therapy comprising both anticoagulants and platelet inhibitors is central to the management of patients during the acute phase of STEMI, defined as the time from clinical presentation until hospital discharge. Coronary reperfusion may be achieved using either pharmaco-invasive (ie, fibrinolysis followed by routine angiography) or mechanical (ie, pPCI) strategies. Irrespective of reperfusion strategy, clinical guidelines recommend adjunctive use of antithrombotic drugs to maintain vessel patency and prevent recurrent thrombosis.[24,49] Compared with fibrinolytics, pPCI yields superior outcomes if performed by experienced personnel within a reasonable interval after symptom onset, which is generally within 120 minutes from diagnosis (ideally within 60 minutes if the patient presents to a PCI center or 90 minutes if they present elsewhere).[24] Here, we focus mainly on the use of antithrombotic therapy in the setting of pPCI, which is the preferred reperfusion strategy endorsed by current guidelines.

Anticoagulants: Unfractionated heparin (UFH) binds antithrombin III and enhances its capacity to inactivate thrombin and, to a lesser extent, factor Xa. Although there are no data from placebo-controlled randomized trials to guide UFH dosing in the setting of pPCI, current guidelines recommend an initial bolus of 70 to 100 U/kg in the absence of concomitant glycoprotein (GP) IIb/IIIa inhibition, based on studies involving patients undergoing balloon angioplasty. UFH is the most commonly used anticoagulant for management of patients with STEMI, resulting from long experience with this agent, relatively low cost, and widespread availability. Among the disadvantages of UFH are its variable anticoagulant effect, inability to bind clot-bound thrombin, and potential for causing heparin-induced thrombocytopenia. Alternatives to UFH include low-molecular-weight heparin (LMWH) and direct thrombin inhibitors. LMWHs have a more predictable anticoagulant effect, greater activity against factor Xa, and lower risk of thrombocytopenia than UFH. The largest randomized comparison of LMWH versus UFH in patients with STEMI undergoing pPCI is a 910-patient open-label trial.[50] The difference between groups in the 30-day primary composite endpoint of death, complication of MI, procedure failure, or major bleeding was not significant (28% vs 34%; $P = 0.06$), nor did

the individual components of the composite favor LMWH over UFH. In the per-protocol analysis of the ATOLL trial (87% of the study population), intravenous enoxaparin was superior to UFH in reducing ischemic and bleeding events.[51] In a meta-analysis of 23 PCI trials (30,966 patients, 33% pPCI), enoxaparin outperformed UFH in mortality endpoints, mainly in patients undergoing pPCI.[52] While the AHA/ACC guidelines do not recommend LMWH,[49] two ESC guidelines (STEMI and revascularization) recommend these agents as an alternative to UFH for patients undergoing pPCI (class IIa).[24,48] Fondaparinux is not recommended as the sole anticoagulant for patients with STEMI (class III: Harm) based on its association with excess catheter thrombosis in the OASIS-6 randomized trial.[49]

The direct thrombin inhibitor (DTI) bivalirudin, extensively studied in patients with STEMI, offers several advantages over UFH, including shorter half-life, binding of clot-bound thrombin, and consistent anticoagulant effect.[53] Five dedicated randomized controlled trials have compared bivalirudin with UFH with or without planned use of GP IIb/IIIa inhibitors in patients with STEMI (**Table 18–3**).[54-59] A meta-analysis of these trials showed no mortality advantage with bivalirudin and a reduction in the risk of major bleeding, but at the cost of an increased risk of acute in-stent thrombosis.[60] Less frequent use of GP IIb/IIIa inhibitors[61] and a lower dose of UFH[62] may reduce the benefit in lowering the bleeding risk with bivalirudin. The MATRIX study, including 7213 acute coronary syndrome (ACS) patients, showed that prolonging bivalirudin infusion after PCI did not improve the outcomes compared with bivalirudin infusion confined to the duration of PCI.[63] The more recent VALIDATE-SWEDEHEART trial (Bivalirudin versus Heparin in ST-segment and non-ST-segment myocardial infarction in Patients on Modern Antiplatelet Therapy in the Swedish Web System for Enhancement and Development of Evidence-based Care in Heart Disease Evaluated according to Recommended Therapies Registry Trial) enrolled 6006 MI patients (3005 with STEMI) undergoing PCI under potent P2Y$_{12}$ inhibitors without GP IIb/IIIa to bivalirudin or heparin during the index procedure. The rate of the combined endpoint of all cause death, MI or major bleeding was not different among groups.[64] Although bivalirudin may be considered as an alternative to UFH during primary PCI, its main indication during pPCI is for patients with heparin-induced thrombocytopenia.[65]

Antiplatelets: The evidence supporting platelet inhibitors in management of patients with STEMI is iterative, with the use of aspirin foundational. The historical Second International Study of Infarct Survival (ISIS-2) demonstrated that, compared with placebo, aspirin lowered vascular mortality by an absolute 2% in patients with STEMI. Clinical practice guidelines provide a class I recommendation for dosing aspirin, 150 to 325 mg orally or, in the European guidelines, 150 mg intravenously for those unable to swallow, for all patients with STEMI, irrespective of treatment strategy.[24] Aspirin exerts only a modest platelet inhibitory effect, however, through irreversible inhibition of the cyclooxygenase-1 enzyme, reducing production of thromboxane A$_2$. Concurrent administration of

TABLE 18–3. Selected Clinical Trials Comparing Heparin and Bivalirudin in Patients with Acute Coronary Syndrome

	HORIZONS	EUROMAX	HEAT	MATRIX	VALIDATE SWEDEHEART
Design	Multicenter (n = 3602)	Multicenter (n = 2198)	Single center (n = 1829)	Multicenter (n = 7213)	Multicenter, registry-based (n = 6006)
Comparators	Heparin + routine GPI vs bivalirudin	Upstream heparin + frequent GPI vs upstream bivalirudin	Heparin with infrequent GPI vs bivalirudin	Heparin vs bivalirudin	Heparin vs bivalirudin with bail-out GPI
Antiplatelet use	Aspirin + clopidogrel	Aspirin plus clopidogrel (50%); ticagrelor/prasugrel (50%)	Aspirin plus clopidogrel (11%) and ticagrelor/prasugrel 89%	Aspirin plus clopidogrel (47%)/ticagrelor (24%)/prasugrel (13%)	Aspirin plus ticagrelor (94.9%)/prasugrel (2.1%)
GP IIb/IIIa inhibitor use	Heparin arm–94.5% Bivalirudin arm–7.2%	Heparin arm–69% Bivalirudin arm–11%	Heparin arm–16% Bivalirudin arm–14%	Heparin arm–0.2% Bivalirudin arm–0.1%	Heparin arm–2.8% Bivalirudin arm–2.4%
Bivalirudin use	Bolus with infusion terminated at end of PCI	Bolus with low-dose infusion for 4 hours	Bolus with infusion terminated at end of PCI	Bolus with infusion terminated at end of PCI (50%); prolonged infusion (50%)	Bolus with infusion terminated at end of PCI (34.7%); prolonged infusion (65.3%)
30-day mortality	3.1% vs 2.1%; P = 0.05	3.1% vs 2.9%; P = 0.86	4.3% vs 5.1%; P = 0.43	2.3% vs 1.7%; P = 0.04	1.7% vs 1.9%; P = 0.63
Bleeding, %	8.3% vs 4.9%; P <0.001	6.0% vs 2.6%; P <0.001	3.1% vs 3.5%; P = 0.59	13.6% vs 11.4%; P = 0.001	5.6% vs 5.1%; P = 0.32
Stent thrombosis, %	0.3% vs 1.3%; P <0.001	0.2% vs 1.1%; P = 0.007	0.9% vs 2.9%; P = 0.007	0.6% vs 1.0%; P = 0.048	1.8% vs 1.7%; P = 0.77

Modified with permission from Dauerman HL. Anticoagulation strategies for primary percutaneous coronary intervention: current controversies and recommendations. *Circ Cardiovasc Interv.* 2015 May;8(5):e001947.

aspirin plus a platelet $P2Y_{12}$ receptor inhibitor—dual antiplatelet therapy (DAPT)—exerts more potent antiplatelet effects. The first generation thienopyridine, clopidogrel, is the most extensively studied $P2Y_{12}$ receptor inhibitor in the setting of STEMI. Compared with aspirin alone, aspirin plus clopidogrel significantly reduces recurrent ischemic events among patients with STEMI treated with fibrinolytics with or without PCI.[66,67] Among patients undergoing coronary intervention, a clopidogrel loading dose of 600 mg is recommended because this increases efficacy without apparent harm, compared with 300 mg.[68,69] Limitations of clopidogrel include relatively slow onset of action and substantial heterogeneity in pharmacodynamic responses.[70] This variation is largely attributable to demographic, clinical and genetic factors that modulate hepatic conversion of clopidogrel to its active metabolite. Compared with clopidogrel,[71,72] the second-generation thienopyridine, prasugrel, and the nonthienopyridine, ticagrelor, are characterized by more potent, durable and consistent platelet inhibitory effects. Experiences in clinical trials evaluating these agents are consistent with these pharmacodynamic observations and led to regulatory approval of prasugrel and ticagrelor. Because these trials excluded patients receiving fibrinolytics as the primary mode of reperfusion, clopidogrel remains the only oral $P2Y_{12}$ inhibitor recommended as part of the pharmaco-invasive strategy.

The TRITON-TIMI 38 trial compared prasugrel (60 mg loading dose followed by 10 mg daily) with clopidogrel (300 mg loading dose followed by 75 mg daily) in 13,608 moderate- to high-risk patients with acute coronary syndromes managed with an invasive strategy.[73] The primary endpoint of cardiovascular death, nonfatal MI, and non-fatal stroke was reduced by 19% with prasugrel, while major bleeding increased 32%.

Findings were qualitatively similar among trial participants with STEMI (n = 3534). Use of prasugrel was associated with a higher risk of ischemic events in patients with a history of stroke or transient cerebral ischemic attack (p_{int} = 0.02), so this agent is not recommended for such patients. Among patients at least 75 years of age or older, prasugrel is generally not recommended due to unclear benefit and propensity for increased bleeding. In addition, patients weighing less than 60 kg have increased exposure to the active metabolite of prasugrel and therefore a lower maintenance dose of 5 mg is recommended in such patients.

The Platelet Inhibition and Patient Outcomes (PLATO) trial compared ticagrelor (180 mg loading dose followed by 90 mg twice daily) to clopidogrel (300 or 600 mg loading dose and 75 mg daily thereafter) in 18,624 patients with ACS,[74] 38% of whom presented with STEMI. Approximately two-thirds of patients underwent PCI. Over 12 months follow-up, ticagrelor significantly reduced the composite outcome of vascular death, MI, or stroke by 16%, while the incidence of major bleeding unrelated to coronary bypass surgery was higher with ticagrelor (4.5% vs 3.8%; P = 0.03), as was fatal intracranial bleeding.

Despite the evidence supporting use of clopidogrel, prasugrel or ticagrelor in patients with STEMI undergoing pPCI, all are administered orally and thienopyridines require metabolic activation. These distinctions are clinically relevant as delayed gastric absorption and heightened platelet reactivity may alter the pharmacodynamic profiles of orally administered platelet inhibitors. In one study, more than 30% of patients undergoing pPCI for STEMI who were treated with a loading dose of either ticagrelor or prasugrel displayed high degrees of platelet reactivity for up to 2 hours after drug ingestion.[75] This delay in onset of full platelet inhibitory effect suggests that some patients with

STEMI remain vulnerable to recurrent thrombosis even after receiving potent $P2Y_{12}$ inhibitors. Therapeutic strategies to address this issue include prehospital administration, tablet crushing, and administration of intravenous platelet inhibitors.

The ATLANTIC (Administration of Ticagrelor in the Cath Lab or in the Ambulance for New ST Elevation Myocardial Infarction to Open the Coronary Artery) trial tested the hypothesis that prehospital administration of ticagrelor (in the ambulance or emergency department) is superior to in-hospital administration (in the catheterization laboratory) with respect to surrogate markers of coronary perfusion in STEMI patients undergoing PCI (n = 1862).[76] The median delay of 31 minutes in ticagrelor administration between groups did not translate into significant differences in electrocardiographic or angiographic markers of coronary perfusion, but the pre-specified secondary endpoint of definite stent thrombosis was reduced with prehospital administration (0.0% vs 0.8% in the first 24 hours). A nested pharmacodynamic substudy found that differences in platelet reactivity between treatment arms favoring prehospital administration appeared 1 to 3 hours after PCI and were negligible thereafter.[77] The MOJITO (Mashed Or Just Integral pill of TicagrelOr) study of ticagrelor administered as crushed versus intact tablets in 82 patients with STEMI undergoing pPCI[78] found significantly reduced platelet reactivity 1 hour after PCI and attenuated differences after administration of the crushed tablets, similar to findings in a randomized comparison of crushed versus intact prasugrel tablets.[79]

Intravenous platelet inhibitors offer an alternative for patients unable to ingest oral agents. Cangrelor is a reversible, direct-acting intravenous $P2Y_{12}$ inhibitor with a very short half-life that results in rapid, potent platelet inhibition and recovery of platelet function within 1 to 2 hours after discontinuation.[80] A series of randomized trials compared the safety and efficacy of cangrelor versus clopidogrel among patients undergoing PCI for a variety of clinical indications. In a pooled analysis (n = 24,910), cangrelor reduced the primary 48-hour efficacy endpoint of death, MI, ischemia-driven revascularization, and stent thrombosis by 19% (odds ratio [OR] 0.81; 95% CI, 0.71–0.91) with no difference in the overall incidence of severe or life-threatening bleeding (OR 1.22; 95% CI, 0.70–2.11).[81] Results were consistent among patients presenting with STEMI (n = 2884; P_{int} = 0.866). These data led to regulatory approval of cangrelor as an adjunct to lower periprocedural thrombotic events among patients undergoing PCI. Other studies focused on surrogate endpoints examined the use of cangrelor in patients with STEMI receiving more potent $P2Y_{12}$ inhibitors. The CANTIC (Cangrelor and Crushed Ticagrelor in STEMI Patients Undergoing Primary Percutaneous Coronary Intervention) trial compared cangrelor to placebo among 50 patients presenting with STEMI treated with crushed ticagrelor.[82] Cangrelor was associated with reductions in the primary outcome of $P2Y_{12}$ reaction units (PRU) within 30 minutes, and the difference was sustained throughout the 2-hour infusion, similar to findings in a small study of orally administered intact ticagrelor tablets.[83] An important limitation of these studies is the lack of comparison to a glycoprotein IIb/IIIa inhibitor. To address this evidence gap, a trial comparing tirofiban, cangrelor or prasugrel in 122 patients with STEMI undergoing PCI found 3-fold greater degree of platelet inhibition at 30 minutes with tirofiban than with cangrelor (95% vs 34%; P <0.001); both parenteral agents were superior to crushed or intact prasugrel tablets.[84] It remains unsettled, however, whether these findings should be incorporated in clinical practice.

Selatogrel is a new highly selective reversible $P2Y_{12}$ inhibitor with a fast onset of action. In a recent phase II trial, a single subcutaneous administration of selatogrel to MI patients reached maximum plasma concentration at approximately 1 hour (with profound platelet inhibition as early as 15 minutes), without major bleeding complications.[85]

Evidence supporting GP IIb/IIIa inhibitors derives largely from the era before widespread use of DAPT and availability of the more potent $P2Y_{12}$ inhibitors. Hence, GP IIb/IIIa inhibitors are recommended as "bail-out" therapy in the event of periprocedural complications, such as vessel closure or acute stent thrombosis.[48]

Subacute Phase: From Hospital Discharge to 1 Year

The primary goal of antithrombotic therapy during the subacute phase after STEMI (ie, during the first year following hospital discharge) is to prevent recurrent thrombosis with oral antiplatelet or anticoagulant drugs. Current practice guidelines recommend DAPT for 1 year for all survivors of STEMI, irrespective of original reperfusion strategy. Ongoing exposure to DAPT increases the risk of bleeding, and hemorrhagic events are associated with greater morbidity and mortality. Since thrombotic potential diminishes over time after MI, the risk-benefit calculus favoring potent antithrombotic therapy gradually declines beyond the acute phase of STEMI. Several studies have evaluated alternative therapeutic strategies, including shortening the duration of DAPT and de-escalation of therapy, in attempts to preserve anti-ischemic efficacy while lessening harm due to bleeding.

Shortening DAPT Duration: Implicit in the construct of DAPT is that addition of an oral $P2Y_{12}$ inhibitor to aspirin is superior to aspirin alone when administered for at least one year following STEMI. Shortening the duration of DAPT could be achieved by earlier discontinuation of either aspirin or the $P2Y_{12}$ inhibitor. At least 2 randomized trials compared a 6-month duration of DAPT followed by aspirin alone versus longer DAPT durations in patients with STEMI who underwent PCI. In the DAPT-STEMI trial, 870 patients who had completed 6 months of DAPT were randomized to continue aspirin alone or continue DAPT for another 6 months.[86] The incidence of the primary endpoint of all-cause death, MI, revascularization, stroke, or major bleeding was noninferior between groups at 18 months after randomization (4.8% vs 6.6%; HR, 0.73; 95% CI, 0.41–1.27; P_{ni} = 0.04). The claim of noninferiority in this trial must be interpreted with caution, however, because the observed event rate at 18 months was significantly lower than originally projected (15%), potentially leading to type I error. In a larger trial involving 2712 patients with ACS (38% with STEMI), 6 months of DAPT was associated with a higher risk of MI than was a longer duration of DAPT (1.8% vs 0.8%; P = 0.02).[87] Moreover, a landmark analysis at 6 months demonstrated a

69% higher incidence of major adverse cardiovascular events with the shorter DAPT duration. In aggregate, these studies do not support discontinuation of $P2Y_{12}$ inhibition earlier than 6 months post-STEMI as a safe or effective strategy.

Other studies have explored early discontinuation of aspirin while continuing $P2Y_{12}$ inhibition as an alternative approach to avoid bleeding while maintaining potent platelet inhibition. The pharmacodynamic basis for this strategy is supported by in vitro studies showing that aspirin exerts a minimal inhibitory effect when added to ticagrelor or prasugrel,[88] and aspirin does not modulate validated markers of thrombogenicity in patients receiving potent $P2Y_{12}$ inhibitors or target-specific oral anticoagulants.[89,90] Results from clinical trials are concordant with and extend these physiologic observations to the clinical setting.

The GLOBAL LEADERS trial was the first to examine $P2Y_{12}$ inhibitor monotherapy with ticagrelor versus DAPT in a large (n = 15,968) population of patients who underwent PCI.[91] The experimental strategy involved 1 month of DAPT with aspirin and ticagrelor followed by ticagrelor alone for an additional 23 months, while the comparator arm included a conventional 1-year DAPT duration followed by aspirin alone. Among participants with ACS, the study design mandated aspirin and ticagrelor for the first year in the conventional group. Although there was no difference in the rate of the primary endpoint of death or Q-wave MI, several subgroup analyses suggested a benefit among participants with ACS (n = 7487; 2092 with STEMI). Ticagrelor monotherapy reduced major bleeding by 48% between 31 and 365 days compared with ticagrelor plus aspirin,[92] while differences in death or Q-wave MI were not significant. The Ticagrelor Monotherapy After 3 Months in the Patients Treated With New Generation Sirolimus Stent for Acute Coronary Syndrome (TICO) trial formally addressed the safety and efficacy of ticagrelor monotherapy exclusively in patients with ACS.[93] The study included 3056 patients (36% with STEMI) randomized to ticagrelor alone versus continuation of ticagrelor-based DAPT after a 3-month course of DAPT. Major bleeding was significantly less frequent with ticagrelor monotherapy (1.7% vs 3.0%; HR, 0.56: 95% CI, 0.34–0.91) while the incidence of major ischemic events was comparable between groups (2.3% vs 3.4%; HR, 0.69; 95% CI, 0.45–1.06). Results were consistent in a prespecified subgroup analysis of the patients with STEMI (n = 1103).

De-Escalation of Therapy: De-escalation, defined as transition from a potent $P2Y_{12}$ inhibitor (prasugrel or ticagrelor) to clopidogrel during the course of DAPT often occurs as a result of drug-related side effects, economic considerations, or accumulation of bleeding-related risk factors. The putative advantage of adopting this approach a priori centers on calibrating the intensity of platelet inhibition to temporal variations in thrombotic and bleeding risks following ACS. In the single-center, open-label Timing of Platelet Inhibition after Acute Coronary Syndromes (TOPIC) trial (n = 646), patients treated with ticagrelor or prasugrel who remained event-free over the first month after ACS and PCI were randomized to either continue DAPT with a potent $P2Y_{12}$ inhibitor or transition

to clopidogrel-based DAPT.[94] Among the participants, 40% had presented with STEMI, and prasugrel was used more frequently than was ticagrelor (57% vs 43%). Over 1 year, DAPT adherence among switched participants was greater (86% vs 75%; P <0.001), and nonadherence among the group continuing the initially assigned DAPT regimen was due mainly to bleeding or medication side effects. The primary endpoint of minor or major bleeding and ischemic events favored de-escalation (13.4% vs 26.3%; HR, 0.48, 95% CI, 0.34–0.68), the benefit driven by bleeding, because there was no significant difference in ischemic events. Findings were uniform across clinical presentation with STEMI or NSTEMI (P_{int} = 0.85). Although intriguing, the single-center design and modest sample size precludes conclusive inferences about the efficacy of this strategy with respect to ischemic events.

Another de-escalation strategy through platelet function testing (PFT) was examined in the TROPICAL-ACS (Testing Responsiveness to Platelet Inhibition on Chronic Antiplatelet Treatment for Acute Coronary Syndromes) trial of 2610 patients with biomarker-positive ACS (55% STEMI) randomized to DAPT with prasugrel versus PFT-guided de-escalation.[95] Patients in the experimental arm received 1 week of prasugrel followed by 1 week of clopidogrel and platelet function testing. Patients demonstrating an adequate platelet inhibitory response continued clopidogrel, while poor responders (~40%) resumed prasugrel. The primary endpoint of cardiovascular death, MI, stroke, or clinically significant bleeding at 12 months (7.3% vs 9.0%; P = 0.12) fulfilled the prespecified criterion for noninferiority. The treatment effect varied by presentation, with accentuated benefit among survivors of STEMI (HR_{stemi}: 0.54% vs. HR_{nstemi}:1.10; P_{int} = 0.01). Although this approach introduces implementation challenges (ie, requirements for PFT and adjusting the antiplatelet regimen), the results of TROPICAL-ACS demonstrate the safety and feasibility of PFT-guided de-escalation, and guidelines suggest that this bleeding-reduction strategy for management of patients following ACS may be considered (class IIb, LOE A) in patients deemed unsuitable for potent $P2Y_{12}$ inhibitors.[96]

Ticagrelor versus Prasugrel: The ISAR-REACT 5 (Intracoronary Stenting and Antithrombotic Regimen: Rapid Early Action for Coronary Treatment) trial compared the safety and efficacy of ticagrelor versus prasugrel among patients with ACS (n = 4018; 41% with STEMI) undergoing an invasive strategy.[97] Patients allocated to ticagrelor received a 180 mg loading dose followed by 90 mg twice daily, and patients allocated to prasugrel received a loading dose of 60 mg followed by 10 mg daily (reduced to 5 mg for patients over 75 years of age or those with body weight less than 60 kg). Over 1 year, prasugrel significantly reduced the primary endpoint of death, MI, or stroke (6.9% vs 9.3%; P = 0.006), with the benefit driven mainly by reduction of MI (3.0% vs 4.8%). The incidence of major bleeding did not differ significantly between groups. These results were unexpected and against the original hypothesis of the investigators, since prior studies found the platelet inhibitory effect of ticagrelor comparable to or greater than that of prasugrel. In addition, the reduction in coronary thrombosis were not accompanied by excess bleeding, discordant with the experience in numerous large trials. One plausible interpretation of these findings is that ISAR-REACT 5 involved not only different drugs but also different therapeutic strategies that minimized the bleeding hazard previously observed with prasugrel pretreatment and in elderly or low body weight patients. In a prespecified subanalysis of the ISAR-REACT 5 trial STEMI population (41% of the sample), no significant differences in the primary endpoint (composite of 1-year death, MI, or stroke) were found between prasugrel and ticagrelor, albeit the latter was associated with a higher incidence of recurrent MI.[98] Conversely, a post hoc analysis of the trial undertaken in the NSTEMI population (59% of the sample), prasugrel was superior to ticagrelor in reducing the primary endpoint without increasing the risk of bleeding.[99]

In line with the ISAR-REACT 5 results, a small mechanistic study showed that, compared with ticagrelor and clopidogrel, pre-PCI administered prasugrel is associated with improved endothelial function, stronger platelet inhibition, and lower IL-6 levels, thus limiting stent-induced endothelial dysfunction and inflammation.[100] However, a recent meta-analysis of 12 trials found that of the three $P2Y_{12}$ receptor inhibitors, only ticagrelor was associated with decreased mortality.[101] A more recent large study of three databases including 31,290 ACS patients undergoing PCI found no differences in net adverse clinical events between patients taking ticagrelor or clopidogrel.[102]

Chronic Phase: Beyond the First Year

Among patients with STEMI undergoing PCI, the risk of recurrent MI may be attributed to the originally treated culprit coronary lesion or to other (non-IRA or nonculprit) lesions. In a prospective natural history study of coronary atherosclerosis involving patients with ACS (n = 697; 30% with STEMI), recurrent ischemic events were equally likely to derive from nonculprit or culprit lesions over 3 years follow-up.[103] In a large population-based cohort of patients with acute MI (n = 44,332), the risk of recurrent MI due to nonculprit versus culprit lesions was 2-fold higher over 8 years.[104] In addition, while coronary stenting is highly effective at stabilizing and recanalizing near-occlusive lesions, nonculprit lesions resulting in subsequent MI are usually either not flow-limiting or angiographically inapparent. In aggregate, these studies suggest that long-term antithrombotic therapy (ie, beyond 1 year following acute MI) may reduce the risk of recurrent ischemic events. Evolving approaches involve long-term DAPT or dual pathway inhibition (DPI), comprising the combination of antiplatelet and anticoagulant drugs.

DAPT: The PEGASUS-TIMI 54 (Prevention of Cardiovascular Events in Patients with Prior Heart Attack Using Ticagrelor Compared to Placebo on a Background of Aspirin–Thrombolysis in Myocardial Infarction 54) trial examined DAPT with aspirin plus ticagrelor at either a 90 or 60 mg twice daily dose versus aspirin alone in 21,162 patients with prior MI.[105] The median time from MI to enrollment was 1.7 years and in 53% of participants the qualifying event was STEMI. Over 3 years follow-up, DAPT with aspirin plus ticagrelor significantly reduced the primary endpoint of cardiovascular death, MI, or

stroke (absolute risk reduction ~1.2%) while increasing major bleeding to a comparable extent (~1.5%). Outcomes were similar with both doses of ticagrelor, but the incidence rates of bleeding and treatment discontinuation were lower with 60 mg twice daily than with 90 mg twice daily. Subgroup analyses of clinical trials involving patients with prior MI or PCI have shown consistent results with prolonged DAPT using aspirin and clopidogrel. A pooled analysis comprising 6 trials and 33,345 patients with prior MI found significant reductions in ischemic events with DAPT durations beyond 1 year and uniform benefit among those with STEMI or NSTEMI (P_{int} 0.29).[106] Current guidelines suggest that continuation of DAPT beyond 1 year may be reasonable for patients with STEMI managed medically without revascularization or who have undergone coronary stent implantation and who are not at high bleeding risk based, for example, on prior bleeding on DAPT, coagulopathy, or concurrent oral anticoagulant therapy.[107]

Dual Pathway Inhibition: The addition of target-specific oral anticoagulants (DOACs) to antiplatelet therapy—dual pathway inhibition (DPI)—following ACS has been examined in both phase II and III trials. As these trials enrolled patients in the acute or subacute phases of ACS, most patients were already receiving DAPT. In general, these have shown reductions in thrombotic events with DPI at the expense of major bleeding. In the ATLAS-2 study, two doses of rivaroxaban (2.5 or 5 mg) twice daily were compared to placebo among patients with recent ACS (~50% STEMI), the majority of whom were receiving DAPT.[108] While low-dose rivaroxaban reduced the primary endpoint of cardiovascular death, MI or stroke (8.9% vs 10.7%; $P = 0.008$), major bleeding not related to coronary artery bypass surgery was significantly increased (1.8% vs 0.6%; $P < 0.001$). The magnitude of incremental bleeding risk associated with rivaroxaban observed in this study is higher than that previously observed with prior comparisons of ticagrelor or prasugrel to clopidogrel.[73,74] Contemporary practice guidelines do not support use of DOACs or vitamin K antagonists in this setting unless there is another indication for anticoagulation, such as atrial fibrillation, venous thromboembolism, mechanical heart valve prostheses, or LV mural thrombus. A combination of rivaroxaban 2.5 mg twice daily plus DAPT was compared with rivaroxaban 15 mg once daily plus a $P2Y_{12}$ inhibitor or conventional therapy with a vitamin K antagonist plus DAPT for 1, 6, or 12 months in patients with atrial fibrillation undergoing PCI with stenting in the PIONEER AF/PCI trial.[109] Of the randomized cohort, 12.3% were enrolled following STEMI. In the primary analysis of the entire trial population (with or without STEMI), either low-dose rivaroxaban combination was associated with a lower rate of clinically significant bleeding than was the combination of DAPT with a vitamin K antagonist. Although efficacy against thrombotic events was similar across the three regimens, wide confidence bounds around the event rates preclude conclusions regarding efficacy.

The COMPASS (Cardiovascular Outcomes for People Using Anticoagulation Strategies) trial enrolled 27,395 patients with stable atherosclerotic cardiovascular disease to compare cardiovascular outcomes during treatment with the factor Xa inhibitor rivaroxaban, 2.5 mg twice daily with aspirin, rivaroxaban 5 mg without aspirin, or aspirin alone.[110] A key exclusion criterion was ongoing DAPT. Over a median follow-up of 23 months, the primary endpoint of cardiovascular death, MI, or stroke was significantly reduced with rivaroxaban plus aspirin compared with aspirin alone (absolute reduction 1.3%) while the absolute increase in major bleeding was 1.2%. The consistent results with respect to a common composite endpoint observed in both PEGASUS and COMPASS suggest that DAPT and DPI may be efficacious options for long-term secondary prevention in patients with prior MI. Key differences in study design, trial participants, and event distributions should be considered in selecting an optimal antithrombotic strategy for individual patients (**Fig. 18–9**). While all patients in PEGASUS had a history of MI, ischemic stroke was an exclusion and only 5% of patients had documented peripheral arterial disease (PAD). In contrast, PAD was present in 27% of COMPASS trial participants and prior stroke in 5%. These differences in case-mix may account for the variable effects observed for individual endpoints. Specifically, among aspirin-treated patients in PEGASUS the incidence of MI was 2.7-fold higher than stroke, whereas in COMPASS, the incidence of MI in patients randomized to aspirin monotherapy was only 38% higher than stroke. The absolute reduction in MI associated with DAPT in PEGASUS was much greater than that for stroke (0.9% vs 0.3%), while the opposite was observed with DPI in COMPASS (0.3% vs 0.7%). As the case-fatality rate of stroke is much higher than that associated with MI, the higher rate of stroke, coupled with the greater benefit associated with DPI for this endpoint, may account for the larger reduction in cardiovascular death observed in COMPASS versus PEGASUS. Patients at higher risk of coronary versus noncoronary events may benefit more from DAPT, while those with atherosclerosis involving more than one vascular bed (coronary, cerebral, or peripheral limb territories—polyvascular disease) or those more likely to sustain stroke, may derive greater benefit from DPI. This hypothesis remains speculative, however, and requires prospective confirmation.

Other Pharmacological Therapy (Acute, subacute and chronic phases of STEMI)

Figure 18–10 illustrates the recommended maintenance therapies for patients after STEMI.

β-Blockers

The effect of β-blockers in STEMI patients can be divided into immediate (early intravenous [IV] administration early in the course of MI) and mid- or long-term effect.

In patients undergoing fibrinolysis, the large COMMIT trial showed no benefit on mortality of pre reperfusion intravenous β-blocker administration and even potential for harm in patients with Killip class III at presentation. In patients undergoing pPCI, the METOCARD-CNIC RCT[21] showed that in stable patients with anterior STEMI, the pre-reperfusion administration of IV metoprolol (15 mg) was associated with a reduction in infarct size and MVO[111] measured by cardiac MRI at 5 to 7 days as well as higher LVEF at 6 month follow-up,[112] with no excess of adverse events during the first 24 hours after STEMI. These results were not confirmed in the EARLY-BAMI RCT, that included patients with different STEMI localizations randomized to pre-reperfusion IV metoprolol (10 mg) or placebo. In EARLY-BAMI, the incidence of adverse events was not different between the metoprolol and placebo groups, and there was a borderline significant reduction of ventricular arrhythmia in patients treated with IV metoprolol.[113] In both trials, all patients received oral metoprolol within the first 12 to 24 hours. It has been demonstrated that the timing of metoprolol administration in the course of STEMI has a clear impact on its cardioprotective abilities.[114] When metoprolol is injected long before reperfusion, it can delay the progression of irreversible injury and thus results in a significant effect on infarct size (Fig. 18–4).[20] However, if metoprolol is injected close to reperfusion (ie, in the cath lab), it has no cardioprotective effect.[114] The fact that in the EARLY-BAMI trial, metoprolol was injected close to reperfusion (and at low dose) and in the METOCARD-CNIC trial, it was injected long before reperfusion and at higher doses probably explains the differences in primary outcomes of the trials.

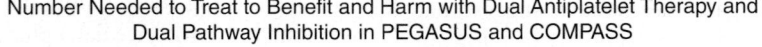

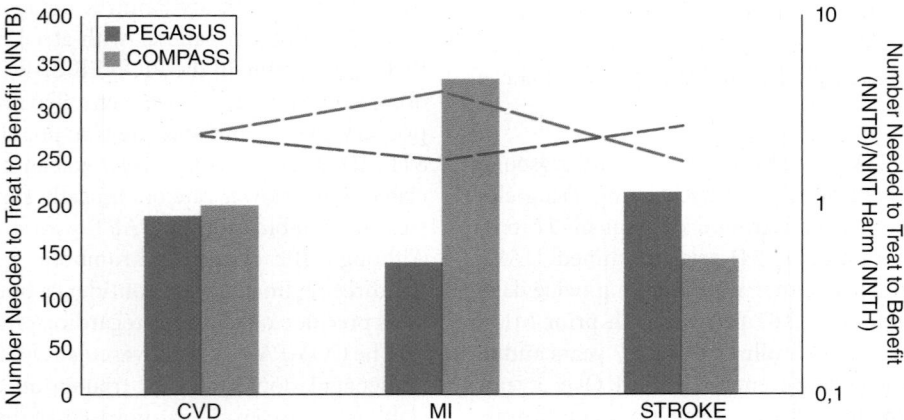

Figure 18–9. Trade-off between ischemic and bleeding events associated with very long-term ticagrelor and Rivaroxaban.

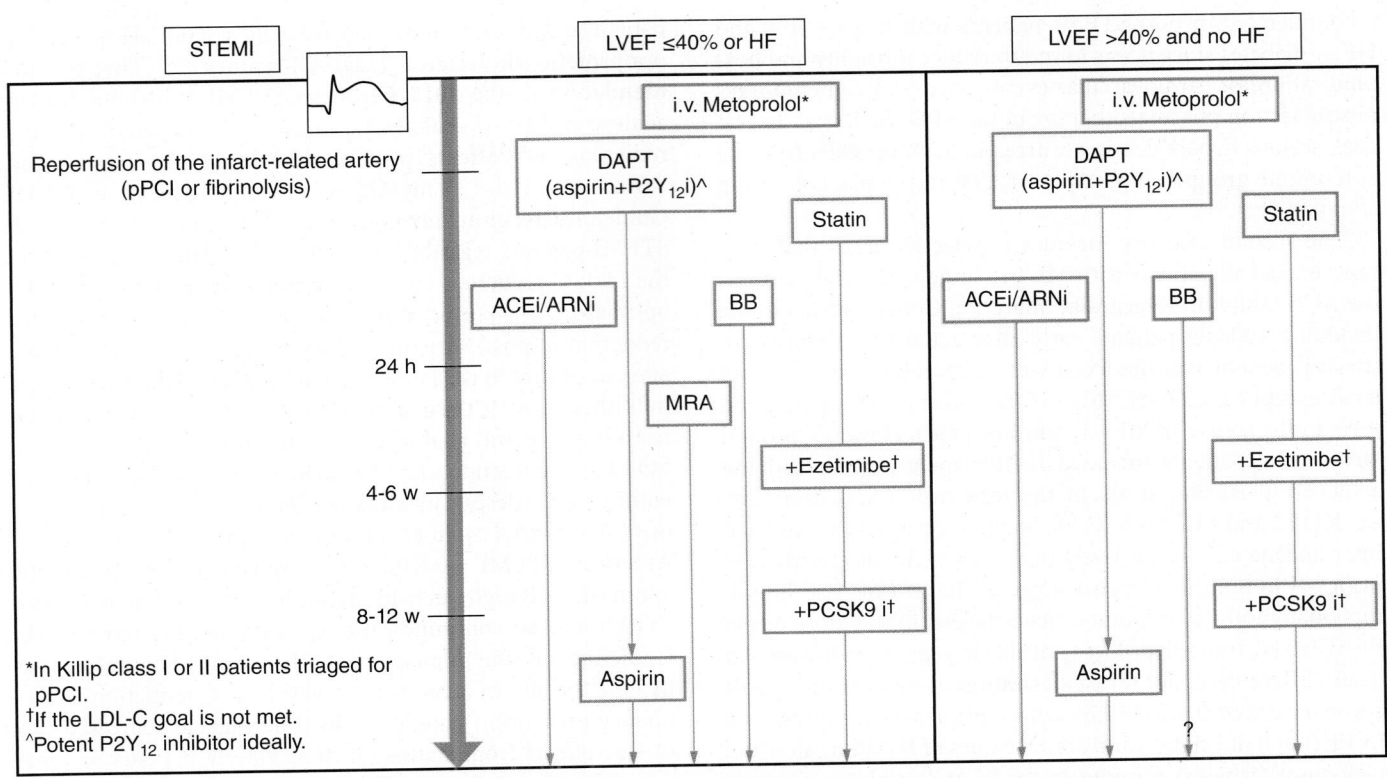

Figure 18–10. Evidence-based and timely delivery of other pharmacological treatment in patients with STEMI. *Green boxes* correspond to class I indication in the European STEMI guidelines (European Dyslipidemia guidelines for lipid-lowering therapy) and *yellow boxes* to class IIa indication. ACE-I, angiotensin-converting enzyme inhibitors; ARB, angiotensin II receptor blocker; BB, β-blocker; HF, heart failure; LVEF, left ventricular ejection fraction; MRA, mineralocorticoid receptor antagonist; PCI, primary percutaneous intervention, PCSK9 i, proprotein convertase subtilisin-kexin type 9 inhibitor.

Very recently, it has been demonstrated that not all IV β-blockers exert the same cardioprotective effect.[115] Metoprolol exerts a unique effect on the β-1 adrenergic receptor explaining its cardioprotective effects.[115] Therefore, the IV β-blocker of choice in the acute phase of STEMI is metoprolol, given immediately after diagnosis (Fig 18–10).

The benefit of long-term treatment with β-blockers on mortality, reinfarction, and cardiac arrest was well established in the pre-reperfusion era. The only large trial testing the effect of long-term β-blocker treatment on reperfused MI patients is the CAPRICORN trial, which randomized post-MI patients with a reduced LVEF (≤40%) to carvedilol or placebo and found that β-blocker treatment was associated with significantly reduced all-cause mortality over 2.5 years of follow-up.[116] Many observational studies and large registries have evaluated the effect of β-blockers in contemporary post-MI patients and have yielded conflicting results.[117-120] However, these trials are confounded by indication and statistical propensity score analyses have a number of additional limitations, thus making the results difficult to interpret.[121] The need for and duration of β-blocker therapy after MI in the absence of LV systolic dysfunction or HF are currently being investigated in four large European clinical trials (that will recruit in total 29,000 patients): REBOOT-CNIC (n = 8500, Spain and Italy, NCT03596385), REDUCE-SWEDEHEART (n = 7000, Sweden NCT03278509),

ABYSS (n = 3700, France, NCT03498066), and BETAMI (n = 10,000, Norway, NCT03646357).

Based on this evidence, according to European clinical practice guidelines, early administration of IV β-blockers (metoprolol) followed by oral treatment should be considered in hemodynamically stable patients undergoing primary PCI (class IIa, LOE A). Long-term treatment with β-blockers is indicated by both European[24] and US guidelines[25] for STEMI patients with a LVEF ≤40% or HF (class I, LOE A). For patients with LVEF >40% and no HF, treatment with β-blockers should be considered routinely (class IIa, LOE B recommendation in European guidelines vs. class I, LOE B in US guidelines for 3 years after STEMI and IIa, LOE B thereafter) (Fig 18–10).

Inhibition of the Renin-Angiotensin-Aldosterone System

Trials testing the effect of inhibition of the renin-angiotensin-aldosterone system (RAAS) in STEMI may be grouped in two categories: the first category includes patients with clinical HF or a reduced (≤40%) LVEF. In this scenario, treatment with different angiotensin-converting enzyme (ACE) inhibitors has shown to reduce all-cause mortality as well as reinfarction and HF hospitalizations (SAVE trial).[122,123] Patients who do not tolerate an ACE inhibitor should be given an angiotensin II receptor blocker (ARB) instead (VALIANT trial). Additionally, mineralocorticoid receptor antagonist (MRA) therapy is also recommended in post-STEMI patients with LVEF ≤40% and HF or diabetes since it was found to reduce mortality and hospitalization for cardiovascular events on top of contemporary postinfarction pharmacotherapy in the EPHESUS trial. In this trial, serious hyperkalemia occurred in 5.5% of patients in the eplerenone group compared with 3.9% in the placebo group ($P = 0.002$).

The second category includes unselective trials that have randomized all patients with MI. In a large meta-analysis from the ACE Inhibitor Myocardial Infarction Collaborative Group, including 100,000 patients early after acute MI, a consistent survival benefit was observed with ACE inhibitors across all trials except for CONSENSUS-II (in which an IV preparation early in the course of MI was administered). However, around 40% of the patients included in this meta-analysis did not achieve reperfusion at all. In the reperfusion era, data from the HOPE and EUROPA RCTs, including patients at high and intermediate risk, respectively (approximately two-thirds with prior MI in both trials), also suggest a benefit of ACE inhibitors on composite endpoints. Nevertheless, in the more recent PEACE trial, trandolapril was not able to reduce cardiovascular death, MI, or coronary revascularization in patients with stable coronary artery disease (55% with a prior MI) and preserved LVEF (but it did significantly reduce rates of HF admission and new onset diabetes). Of note, in the PEACE trial, there was an intensive management of risk factors including high percentages of statin use and complete revascularization, which may explain little left to be gained with RAAS inhibition. Treatment with MRAs has also been tried in STEMI patients without HF. The REMINDER trial found a significant reduction in the combined primary endpoint (mainly due to differences in B-type natriuretic peptide levels) in STEMI patients treated with eplerenone compared with placebo. However, in the ALBATROSS trial, no beneficial effect of early MRA use was found in post-MI patients. An individual participant pooled analysis including both trials showed that active treatment was associated with less mortality, although event rate was overall low.[124]

Considering the previous evidence, current guidelines recommend treatment with ACE inhibitors in STEMI patients with evidence of HF, LV systolic dysfunction, diabetes, or an anterior infarct (class I, LOE A indication). Demonstration of an early benefit (within the first 24 hours after STEMI) supports the prompt use of these agents in the absence of contraindications (mainly hypotension, known hypersensitivity and pregnancy).[123,125] ARBs (particularly Valsartan) are an alternative for those patients who are intolerant to ACE inhibitors. In post-MI patients with HF or low LVEF, MRAs are recommended on top of ACE-inhibitors and β-blockers, provided there is no renal failure or hyperkalemia. Additionally, in all patients, ACE inhibitors should be considered (class IIa, LOE A recommendation) in the absence of contraindications[24,25] (Fig. 18–10).

Lipid-Lowering Therapy

The clinical benefit of early and intensive treatment with statins has been widely demonstrated in post-MI patients.[24] Early and high-intensity statin therapy is indicated in all STEMI patients unless contraindicated, regardless of initial low-density lipoprotein cholesterol (LDL-C) values.[24,25] The recommendation in the 2017 European STEMI guidelines was to achieve an LDL-C goal of <1.8 mmol/L (70 mg/dL) or a ≥50% reduction for patients with baseline levels between 1.8 and 3.5 mmol/L (70–135 mg/dL), whereas the American STEMI Guidelines recommend high intensity statin therapy for all STEMI patients regardless of LDL level.[126] However, based on the LDL-C reduction observed in more recent RCTs,[127-129] the optimal LDL-C cut-off values for optimal cardiovascular risk reduction in post-MI patients have been (again) moved down and, according to the latest European Dyslipidemia guidelines published in 2019, the goal is to reach a ≥50% LDL-C reduction from baseline and goal levels <1.4 mmol/L (<55 mg/dL) (IIa, LOE C recommendation).[130] In patients with recurrent events within 2 years despite maximally tolerated statin therapy, a goal of <1.0 mmol/L (<40 mg/dL) for LDL-C should be considered. American STEMI guidelines recommend a more pragmatic approach with high intensity statin therapy for all patients with STEMI and no contraindications,[49] although the more recent Guideline on the Management of Blood Cholesterol does include the aim of achieving a ≥50% LDL-C reduction in secondary prevention patients.[126] In subgroups at increased risk of side effects from statins (such as elderly patients or those with hepatic or renal insufficiency, previous side effects, or a potential for interaction with essential concomitant therapy), the use of lower-intensity statin regimens should be weighed. In patients who are intolerant of any dose of statin, treatment with ezetimibe should be considered.[130] It is recommended to maintain statin treatment in the long term in post-MI patients.

To pursue these goals, a lipid profile should be obtained as early as possible after admission for STEMI (nonfasting values are admissible since LDL-C variation is only within 10%).[24] Lipids should be reevaluated 4 to 6 weeks after MI and treatment adjusted accordingly. In the IMPROVE-IT trial, patients with a recent acute coronary syndrome (29% STEMI) were randomized to Ezetimibe 10 mg/Simvastatin 40 mg or Simvastatin 40 mg alone.[127] Patients on the combined treatment arm presented a relative risk reduction of 6.4% ($P = 0.016$) in the composite primary endpoint at 7 years follow-up. The FOURIER trial randomized patients with atherosclerotic cardiovascular disease (81% prior MI) and LDL-C levels ≥70 mg/dL despite maximum tolerated statin dose to receive Evolocumab (a human monoclonal antibody that inhibits proprotein convertase subtilisin-kexin type 9 [PCSK9]) or placebo.[128] At 2.2 years follow-up, there was a significant 15% relative reduction in the composite primary endpoint (cardiovascular death, MI, stroke, hospitalization for unstable angina, or coronary revascularization). In terms of individual outcomes, neither cardiovascular mortality nor all-cause mortality were significantly reduced with evolocumab. Similarly, in the ODYSSEY trial,[129] patients with a prior (<1 year) ACS and suboptimal LDL-C levels (≥70 mg/dL) despite maximum tolerated statin dose were randomized to receive Alirocumab (a different PCSK9 inhibitor) or placebo. Allocation to Alirocumab was associated with a 15% relative risk reduction in the primary endpoint (composite of coronary heart disease death, non-fatal MI, ischemic stroke, or unstable angina requiring hospitalization) at 2.8 years follow-up. Although there was a significant reduction in all-cause mortality, this was an exploratory outcome and was not supported by a significant reduction of cardiovascular death.

In summary, if the LDL-C target is not reached within 4 to 6 weeks with the highest tolerable statin dose, it is recommended to add Ezetimibe as a first step (class I, LOE B recommendation) and a PCSK9 inhibitor as a second step (class I, LOE B recommendation).[130]

Other Pharmacological Therapy

The routine use of nitrates and calcium channel antagonists in the acute phase of STEMI has proven no benefit and these agents are therefore not recommended. Treatment with Verapamil may be considered in the chronic phase of MI for patients without HF or LV systolic dysfunction and contraindications to β-blockers.[24]

Colchicine is a drug with anti-inflammatory effects approved for the treatment of gout, familial Mediterranean fever, and pericarditis. Recently, there has been growing interest on colchicine as a potential therapy adjunct to the secondary prevention pharmacological armamentarium in post-MI patients (distinct to the use of colchicine as an adjuvant to aspirin/nonsteroidal anti-inflammatory drug therapy in post-STEMI pericarditis; see Pericarditis in section Complications Following STEMI). After several initial positive pilot trials using inflammation markers as the primary endpoint, the COLCOT trial randomized ≈4700 patients 30 days after acute MI (not specified whether STEMI or NSTEMI) to treatment with 0.5 mg of Colchicine daily versus placebo.[131] Patients received standard of care treatment before enrolling in the study including high percentages of aspirin, a second antiplatelet agent, statin, and β-blocker use as well as revascularization for the index MI (PCI in ≈93%). At 23 months follow-up, there was a significant reduction in the combined primary endpoint (5.5% vs 7.1%, P = 0.02) in patients receiving Colchicine, which was driven by significant reductions in stroke and angina leading to revascularization. In the very recent LoDoCo2 trial,[132] treatment with Colchicine (0.5 mg daily) compared with placebo in patients with chronic coronary disease (≈84% prior ACS) was associated with a reduced risk of major cardiovascular events but rates of death from any cause and noncardiovascular death were higher in the Colchicine arm.

Further specific anti-inflammatory treatment was tested in the CANTOS trial[133] that randomized patients with previous MI on optimal medical treatment and with chronic elevation of high-sensitivity C-reactive protein (hs-CRP) to treatment with Canakinumab (a monoclonal antibody targeting interleukin-1β) or placebo. At 3.7 years follow-up, there was a dose-dependent reduction in inflammatory markers together with significantly lower recurrent cardiovascular events in the Canakinumab arm. The risk of severe and fatal infections was also worrisomely higher in the treatment arm and the US Food and Drug Administration (FDA) did not approve Canakinumab for cardiovascular risk reduction. Despite this, CANTOS was considered as a gigantic proof-of-concept trial of the inflammatory hypothesis in atherotrombosis.[134]

Special Patient Subsets
Conservative Management of STEMI

Those patients who, for specific reasons, do not receive reperfusion therapy within the first 12 hours after STEMI should undergo clinical evaluation. In the case of signs or symptoms of ongoing ischemia, HF, or hemodynamic/arrhythmic instability, a pPCI strategy is recommended[24] (Fig 18–7). In stable asymptomatic patients, pPCI should be considered between 12 and 48 hours after symptom onset. After that (>48 hours), patients should be managed as those with a chronic total occlusion since routine coronary intervention has not shown any clinical benefit compared to medical management alone (OAT trial). Pharmacological treatment should include DAPT (clopidogrel preferred, COMMIT trial), anticoagulation (preferably with fondaparinux)[135] until hospital discharge or coronary revascularization as well as other guideline-directed medical therapy for secondary prevention.

STEMI with Cardiogenic Shock

Cardiogenic shock is defined as persistent hypotension (systolic blood pressure [SBP] <90 mm Hg or need for inotropes/mechanical support to maintain a SBP >90 mm Hg) with signs of hypoperfusion in the presence of adequate filling status.[24] It is present in up to 10% of patients with STEMI and it is associated with high mortality rates, approaching 50%. In STEMI patients presenting with cardiogenic shock, immediate reperfusion (pPCI preferred, Fig. 18–6) is mandatory. If multivessel disease is present, recent European myocardial revascularization guidelines recommend against routine non-IRA PCI after the results of the CULPRIT-SHOCK trial.[48] An urgent transthoracic Doppler echocardiogram is indicated in order to evaluate the biventricular and valvular function, loading status and to rule out mechanical complications. Besides immediate reperfusion, intravenous inotropic agents or vasopressors should be administered, if required, to maintain adequate organ perfusion. However, intra-aortic balloon pump (IABP) counterpulsation has not been found to improve outcomes in patients with STEMI and cardiogenic shock (IABP-SHOCK II trial) nor to significantly reduce infarct size in those with potentially large anterior MIs (CRISP AMI trial) and thus is not routinely recommended.[24] Some selected patients may benefit from IABP counterpulsation though (such as those with mechanical complications). Finally, short-term mechanical circulatory support with a mechanical left ventricular assist device (LVAD) has theoretical advantages over an IABP by unloading the LV and may be considered in the STEMI setting as a bridge to recovery, cardiac transplantation, or even to LVAD as destination therapy. Randomized controlled trials are needed to evaluate whether these devices could have a mortality benefit in patients with STEMI and cardiogenic shock.[136]

Complications Following STEMI
Pericarditis

The incidence of pericardial complications following STEMI (ie, early pericarditis, late pericarditis or Dressler syndrome, and pericardial effusion) has fallen significantly in the pPCI era. Early pericarditis should be considered in the differential diagnosis of recurrent chest pain after STEMI, particularly when the patient presents with pleuritic pain, accompanied by a pericardial rub and typical ECG changes.[49] In contrast, Dressler syndrome (presumed to be immune-mediated) typically occurs later (at least 1 to 2 weeks after STEMI). Both entities are treated with anti-inflammatory therapy (de-escalating doses of aspirin as the first choice, together with colchicine).[24] Pericardial effusion may be a consequence of post-MI pericarditis, but patients should be investigated to rule out a potential subacute rupture.

Mechanical Complications

Similar to post-STEMI pericarditis, the incidence of mechanical complications has been drastically reduced after the generalization of pPCI. These devastating complications of MI include free wall rupture, ventricular septal defect, and papillary muscle rupture and are associated with early mortality and need for surgical intervention. Clinical suspicion should rise in the presence of sudden hypotension, recurrent chest pain, systolic cardiac murmurs, pulmonary congestion, or jugular vein distension.[24] In a recent observational study including nearly 4 million hospitalizations for STEMI in the United States, mechanical complications occurred in 0.27% patients and the mortality rate was 42%.[137] There was no significant change over a contemporary 12-year period (2003 to 2015) in the mechanical complications prevalence or mortality rates, suggesting that these remain to be catastrophic sequelae of STEMI even today. During the COVID-19 pandemic, some groups have reported a higher incidence of mechanical complications presumed to be secondary to delayed presentation times,[138] although others have not.[139]

Electrical Complications

Arrythmias and conduction disturbances are relatively common during the early hours of STEMI and are also important prognostic factors. Among supraventricular arrhythmia, atrial fibrillation (AF) is by far the most frequent after STEMI with up to 21% of patients affected. Patients with AF are at higher risk for short and long-term complications, including reinfarction, stroke, and heart HF. Acute management includes β-blocker or amiodarone administration for rate/rhythm control as well as anticoagulation. Electrical cardioversion may be considered especially in the presence of hemodynamic or clinical instability but early AF recurrences are common.[24]

Ventricular arrhythmia (ventricular tachycardia [VT] or ventricular fibrillation [VF]) are encountered in 6% to 8% of patients with STEMI, often triggered by ischemia, hemodynamic and electrolyte abnormalities, reentry, and enhanced automaticity.[24,49] Treatment includes expeditious reperfusion, electrical cardioversion or defibrillation with advanced cardiac life support, and β-blockers and/or amiodarone if clinically indicated. In case of contraindications to amiodarone, IV lidocaine may be considered, although no studies comparing superiority of either drug in STEMI patients are available. VT or VF may also occur during coronary reperfusion. In general, patients with early VT/VF (within the first 48 hours of STEMI) are considered to be at low long-term arrhythmic risk. Conversely, VT or VF that develops 48 hours after the onset of

STEMI and in the absence of recurrent ischemia is associated with worse prognosis and warrants evaluation for implantable cardioverter-defibrillator (ICD) implantation for secondary prevention.[136]

Conduction abnormalities and bradyarrhythmia associated with acute STEMI are common, especially in the presence of an inferior MI. Early sinus bradycardia is often mediated through increased vagal tone and is usually self-limited. Various degrees of atrioventricular block may also occur, potentially requiring temporary pacing if hemodynamic instability is present. Atrioventricular block associated with inferior wall infarction is usually supra-Hisian and generally resolves after reperfusion. However, atrioventricular block associated with anterior infarction is mostly infra-Hisian and reflects a large extent of myocardial injury. The development of a new bundle branch or hemiblock also usually indicates an extensive anterior MI.[24]

Postdischarge Care

Key lifestyle interventions after STEMI include smoking cessation, blood pressure control, diet and weight management, as well as regular physical activity. All patients should participate in a cardiac rehabilitation program at hospital discharge[24] since systematic reviews have shown a significant reduction (13% to 25%) of global and cardiovascular mortality rates with this approach. Cardiac rehabilitation programs typically include risk factor control, education, exercise with individual programs, titration, and monitoring of secondary prevention medication and stress management/psychological support.[136]

REFERENCES

1. Sugiyama T, Hasegawa K, Kobayashi Y, Takahashi O, Fukui T, Tsugawa Y. Differential time trends of outcomes and costs of care for acute myocardial infarction hospitalizations by ST elevation and type of intervention in the United States, 2001-2011. *J Am Heart Assoc.* 2015;4(3):e001445.

2. McManus DD, Gore J, Yarzebski J, Spencer F, Lessard D, Goldberg RJ. Recent trends in the incidence, treatment, and outcomes of patients with STEMI and NSTEMI. *Am J Med.* 2011;124(1):40-47.

3. Mozaffarian D, Benjamin EJ, Go AS, et al. Heart disease and stroke statistics—2015 update: a report from the American Heart Association. *Circulation.* 2015;131(4):e29-e322.

4. Jernberg T. *Swedeheart Annual Report 2015.* Stockholm, Sweden: Karolinska University Hospital; 2016.

5. Khera S, Kolte D, Gupta T, et al. Temporal trends and sex differences in revascularization and outcomes of ST-segment elevation myocardial infarction in younger adults in the United States. *J Am Coll Cardiol.* 2015;66(18):1961-1972.

6. Pedersen F, Butrymovich V, Kelbaek H, et al. Short- and long-term cause of death in patients treated with primary PCI for STEMI. *J Am Coll Cardiol.* 2014;64(20):2101-2108.

7. Fokkema ML, James SK, Albertsson P, et al. Population trends in percutaneous coronary intervention: 20-year results from the SCAAR (Swedish Coronary Angiography and Angioplasty Registry). *J Am Coll Cardiol.* 2013;61(12):1222-1230.

8. Kang SH, Suh JW, Yoon CH, et al. Sex differences in management and mortality of patients with ST-elevation myocardial infarction (from the Korean Acute Myocardial Infarction National Registry). *Am J Cardiol.* 2012;109(6):787-793.

9. EUGenMed Cardiovascular Clinical Study Group, Regitz-Zagrosek V, Oertelt-Prigione S, et al. Gender in cardiovascular diseases: impact

on clinical manifestations, management, and outcomes. *Eur Heart J.* 2016;37(1):24-34.

10. Kyto V, Sipila J, Rautava P. Gender and in-hospital mortality of ST-segment elevation myocardial infarction (from a multihospital nation-wide registry study of 31,689 patients). *Am J Cardiol.* 2015;115(3):303-306.

11. Hvelplund A, Galatius S, Madsen M, et al. Women with acute coronary syndrome are less invasively examined and subsequently less treated than men. *Eur Heart J.* 2010;31(6):684-690.

12. Jackson AM, Zhang R, Findlay I, et al. Healthcare disparities for women hospitalized with myocardial infarction and angina. *Eur Heart J Qual Care Clin Outcomes.* 2020;6(2):156-165.

13. DeFilippis EM, Collins BL, Singh A, et al. Women who experience a myocardial infarction at a young age have worse outcomes compared with men: the Mass General Brigham YOUNG-MI registry. *Eur Heart J.* 2020;41(42):4127-4137.

14. Puymirat E, Aissaoui N, Cayla G, et al. Changes in one year mortality in elderly patients admitted with acute myocardial infarction in relation with early management. *Am J Med.* 2017;130:555-63.

15. Ibanez B, Heusch G, Ovize M, Van de Werf F. Evolving Therapies for Myocardial Ischemia/Reperfusion Injury. *J Am Coll Cardiol.* 2015;65(14):1454-1471.

16. Maroko PR, Libby P, Ginks WR, et al. Coronary artery reperfusion. I. Early effects on local myocardial function and the extent of myocardial necrosis. *J Clin Invest.* 1972;51:2710-2716.

17. Heusch G. Coronary microvascular obstruction: the new frontier in cardioprotection. *Basic Res Cardiol.* 2019;114(6):45.

18. Heusch G. Myocardial stunning and hibernation revisited. *Nat Rev Cardiol.* 2021.

19. Martinez-Milla J, Galan-Arriola C, Carnero M, et al. Translational large animal model of hibernating myocardium: characterization by serial multimodal imaging. *Basic Res Cardiol.* 2020;115(3):33.

20. Lobo-Gonzalez M, Galan-Arriola C, Rossello X, et al. Metoprolol blunts the time-dependent progression of infarct size. *Basic Res Cardiol.* 2020;115(5):55.

21. Ibanez B, Macaya C, Sanchez-Brunete V, Pizarro G, et al. Effect of Early Metoprolol on Infarct Size in ST-Segment-Elevation Myocardial Infarction Patients Undergoing Primary Percutaneous Coronary Intervention: The Effect of Metoprolol in Cardioprotection During an Acute Myocardial Infarction (METOCARD-CNIC) Trial. *Circulation.* 2013;128(14):1495-1503.

22. Ibanez B, Aletras AH, Arai AE, Arheden H, et al. Cardiac MRI Endpoints in Myocardial Infarction Experimental and Clinical Trials: JACC Scientific Expert Panel. *J Am Coll Cardiol.* 2019;74(2):238-256.

23. Heusch G. Cardioprotection: chances and challenges of its translation to the clinic. *Lancet.* 2013;381(9861):166-175.

24. Ibanez B, James S, Agewall S, et al. 2017 ESC Guidelines for the management of acute myocardial infarction in patients presenting with ST-segment elevation: the Task Force for the management of acute myocardial infarction in patients presenting with ST-segment elevation of the European Society of Cardiology (ESC). *Eur Heart J.* 2018;39(2):119-177.

25. O'Gara PT, Kushner FG, Ascheim DD, et al. 2013 ACCF/AHA guideline for the management of ST-elevation myocardial infarction: executive summary: a report of the American College of Cardiology Foundation/American Heart Association Task Force on Practice Guidelines. *J Am Coll Cardiol.* 2013;61(4):485-510.

26. Keeley EC, Boura JA, Grines CL. Primary angioplasty versus intravenous thrombolytic therapy for acute myocardial infarction: a quantitative review of 23 randomised trials. *Lancet.* 2003;361(9351):13-20.

27. Sinnaeve P, Van de Werf F. Primary PCI and the indistinct 120 min time limit. *Eur Heart J.* 2020;41(7):867-869.

28. Danchin N, Popovic B, Puymirat E, et al. Five-year outcomes following timely primary percutaneous intervention, late primary percutaneous intervention, or a pharmaco-invasive strategy in ST-segment elevation myocardial infarction: the FAST-MI programme. *Eur Heart J.* 2020;41(7):858-866.

29. Vora AN, Holmes DN, Rokos I, et al. Fibrinolysis use among patients requiring interhospital transfer for ST-segment elevation myocardial infarction care: a report from the US National Cardiovascular Data Registry. *JAMA Intern Med.* 2015;175(2):207-215.

30. De Luca G, Suryapranata H, Ottervanger JP, Antman EM. Time delay to treatment and mortality in primary angioplasty for acute myocardial infarction: every minute of delay counts. *Circulation.* 2004;109(10):1223-1225.

31. Prasad A, Gersh BJ, Mehran R, et al. Effect of ischemia duration and door-to-balloon time on myocardial perfusion in ST-segment elevation myocardial infarction: an analysis from HORIZONS-AMI Trial (Harmonizing Outcomes with Revascularization and Stents in Acute Myocardial Infarction). *JACC Cardiovasc Interv.* 2015;8(15):1966-1974.

32. Sinnaeve PR, Armstrong PW, Gershlick AH, et al. ST-segment-elevation myocardial infarction patients randomized to a pharmaco-invasive strategy or primary percutaneous coronary intervention: Strategic Reperfusion Early After Myocardial Infarction (STREAM) 1-year mortality follow-up. *Circulation.* 2014;130(14):1139-1145.

33. Gershlick AH, Westerhout CM, Armstrong PW, et al. Impact of a pharmacoinvasive strategy when delays to primary PCI are prolonged. *Heart.* 2015;101(9):692-698.

34. Vanhaverbeke M, Bogaerts K, Sinnaeve PR, Janssens L, Armstrong PW, Van de Werf F. Prevention of cardiogenic shock after acute myocardial infarction. *Circulation.* 2019;139(1):137-139.

35. Sim DS, Jeong MH, Ahn Y, et al. Pharmacoinvasive strategy versus primary percutaneous coronary intervention in patients with ST-segment-elevation myocardial infarction: a propensity score-matched analysis. *Circ Cardiovasc Interv.* 2016;9(9).

36. Bainey KR, Armstrong PW, Zheng Y, et al. Pharmacoinvasive strategy versus primary percutaneous coronary intervention in ST-elevation myocardial infarction in clinical practice: insights from the vital heart response registry. *Circ Cardiovasc Interv.* 2019;12(10):e008059.

37. Pu J, Ding S, Ge H, et al. Efficacy and safety of a pharmaco-invasive strategy with half-dose alteplase versus primary angioplasty in ST-segment-elevation myocardial infarction: EARLY-MYO trial (Early Routine Catheterization After Alteplase Fibrinolysis Versus Primary PCI in Acute ST-Segment-Elevation Myocardial Infarction). *Circulation.* 2017;136(16):1462-1473.

38. Hochman JS, Lamas GA, Buller CE, et al. Coronary intervention for persistent occlusion after myocardial infarction. *N Engl J Med.* 2006;355(23):2395-2407.

39. Xiang D, Xiang X, Zhang W, et al. Management and outcomes of patients with STEMI during the COVID-19 pandemic in China. *J Am Coll Cardiol.* 2020;76(11):1318-1324.

40. Mahmud E, Dauerman HL, Welt FGP, et al. Management of acute myocardial infarction during the COVID-19 pandemic: a position statement from the Society for Cardiovascular Angiography and Interventions (SCAI), the American College of Cardiology (ACC), and the American College of Emergency Physicians (ACEP). *J Am Coll Cardiol.* 2020;76(11):1375-1384.

41. Park DW, Clare RM, Schulte PJ, et al. Extent, location, and clinical significance of non-infarct-related coronary artery disease among patients with ST-elevation myocardial infarction. *JAMA.* 2014;312(19):2019-2027.

42. Patel MR, Calhoon JH, Dehmer GJ, et al. ACC/AATS/AHA/ASE/ASNC/SCAI/SCCT/STS 2016 appropriate use criteria for coronary revascularization in patients with acute coronary syndromes: a report of the American College of Cardiology Appropriate Use Criteria Task Force, American Association for Thoracic Surgery, American Heart Association, American Society of Echocardiography, American Society of Nuclear Cardiology, Society for Cardiovascular Angiography and Interventions, Society of Cardiovascular Computed Tomography, and the Society of Thoracic Surgeons. *J Am Coll Cardiol.* 2017;69(5):570-591.

43. Ibanez B, Roque D, Price S. The year in cardiovascular medicine 2020: acute coronary syndromes and intensive cardiac care. *Eur Heart J*. 2021; 42(9):884-895.

44. Mehta SR, Wood DA, Storey RF, et al. Complete revascularization with multivessel PCI for myocardial infarction. *N Engl J Med*. 2019; 381(15):1411-1421.

45. Atti V, Gwon Y, Narayanan MA, et al. Multivessel versus culprit-only revascularization in STEMI and multivessel coronary artery disease: meta-analysis of randomized trials. *JACC Cardiovasc Interv*. 2020;13(13): 1571-1582.

46. Thiele H, Akin I, Sandri M, et al. PCI strategies in patients with acute myocardial infarction and cardiogenic shock. *N Engl J Med*. 2017;377(25): 2419-2432.

47. Thiele H, Akin I, Sandri M, et al. One-year outcomes after PCI strategies in cardiogenic shock. *N Engl J Med*. 2018;379(18):1699-1710.

48. Neumann FJ, Sousa-Uva M, Ahlsson A, et al. 2018 ESC/EACTS guidelines on myocardial revascularization. *Eur Heart J*. 2018;40(2):87-165.

49. O'Gara PT, Kushner FG, Ascheim DD, et al. 2013 ACCF/AHA guideline for the management of ST-elevation myocardial infarction: a report of the American College of Cardiology Foundation/American Heart Association Task Force on Practice Guidelines. *Circulation*. 2013;127(4):e362-e425.

50. Montalescot G, Zeymer U, Silvain J, et al. Intravenous enoxaparin or unfractionated heparin in primary percutaneous coronary intervention for ST-elevation myocardial infarction: the international randomised open-label ATOLL trial. *Lancet*. 2011;378(9792):693-703.

51. Collet JP, Huber K, Cohen M, et al. A direct comparison of intravenous enoxaparin with unfractionated heparin in primary percutaneous coronary intervention (from the ATOLL trial). *Am J Cardiol*. 2013;112(9):1367-1372.

52. Silvain J, Beygui F, Barthelemy O, et al. Efficacy and safety of enoxaparin versus unfractionated heparin during percutaneous coronary intervention: systematic review and meta-analysis. *BMJ*. 2012;344:e553.

53. Dauerman HL. Anticoagulation strategies for primary percutaneous coronary intervention: current controversies and recommendations. *Circ Cardiovasc Interv*. 2015;8(5).

54. Stone GW, Witzenbichler B, Guagliumi G, et al. Bivalirudin during primary PCI in acute myocardial infarction. *N Engl J Med*. 2008;358(21): 2218-2230.

55. Steg PG, van 't Hof A, Hamm CW, et al. Bivalirudin started during emergency transport for primary PCI. *N Engl J Med*. 2013;369(23):2207-2217.

56. Schulz S, Richardt G, Laugwitz KL, et al. Prasugrel plus bivalirudin vs. clopidogrel plus heparin in patients with ST-segment elevation myocardial infarction. *Eur Heart J*. 2014;35(34):2285-2294.

57. Shahzad A, Kemp I, Mars C, et al. Unfractionated heparin versus bivalirudin in primary percutaneous coronary intervention (HEAT-PPCI): an open-label, single centre, randomised controlled trial. *Lancet*. 2014;384(9957):1849-1858.

58. Han Y, Guo J, Zheng Y, et al. Bivalirudin vs heparin with or without tirofiban during primary percutaneous coronary intervention in acute myocardial infarction: the BRIGHT randomized clinical trial. *JAMA*. 2015;313(13):1336-1346.

59. Zeymer U, van 't Hof A, Adgey J, et al. Bivalirudin is superior to heparins alone with bailout GP IIb/IIIa inhibitors in patients with ST-segment elevation myocardial infarction transported emergently for primary percutaneous coronary intervention: a pre-specified analysis from the EUROMAX trial. *Eur Heart J*. 2014;35(36):2460-2467.

60. Capodanno D, Gargiulo G, Capranzano P, Mehran R, Tamburino C, Stone GW. Bivalirudin versus heparin with or without glycoprotein IIb/IIIa inhibitors in patients with STEMI undergoing primary PCI: an updated meta-analysis of 10,350 patients from five randomized clinical trials. *Eur Heart J Acute Cardiovasc Care*. 2016;5(3):253-262.

61. Cavender MA, Sabatine MS. Bivalirudin versus heparin in patients planned for percutaneous coronary intervention: a meta-analysis of randomised controlled trials. *Lancet*. 2014;384(9943):599-606.

62. Bavry AA, Elgendy IY, Mahmoud A, Jadhav MP, Huo T. Critical appraisal of bivalirudin versus heparin for percutaneous coronary intervention: a meta-analysis of randomized trials. *PLoS One*. 2015;10(5):e0127832.

63. Valgimigli M, Frigoli E, Leonardi S, et al. Bivalirudin or unfractionated heparin in acute coronary syndromes. *N Engl J Med*. 2015;373(11): 997-1009.

64. Erlinge D, Omerovic E, Frobert O, et al. Bivalirudin versus heparin monotherapy in myocardial infarction. *N Engl J Med*. 2017;377(12):1132-1142.

65. Neumann FJ, Sousa-Uva M, Ahlsson A, et al. 2018 ESC/EACTS guidelines on myocardial revascularization. *Eur Heart J*. 2019;40(2):87-165.

66. Sabatine MS, Cannon CP, Gibson CM, et al. Addition of clopidogrel to aspirin and fibrinolytic therapy for myocardial infarction with ST-segment elevation. *N Engl J Med*. 2005;352(12):1179-1189.

67. Sabatine MS, Cannon CP, Gibson CM, et al. Effect of clopidogrel pretreatment before percutaneous coronary intervention in patients with ST-elevation myocardial infarction treated with fibrinolytics: the PCI-CLARITY study. *JAMA*. 2005;294(10):1224-1232.

68. Mehta SR, Tanguay JF, Eikelboom JW, et al. Double-dose versus standard-dose clopidogrel and high-dose versus low-dose aspirin in individuals undergoing percutaneous coronary intervention for acute coronary syndromes (CURRENT-OASIS 7): a randomised factorial trial. *Lancet*. 2010;376(9748):1233-1243.

69. Patti G, Colonna G, Pasceri V, Pepe LL, Montinaro A, Di Sciascio G. Randomized trial of high loading dose of clopidogrel for reduction of periprocedural myocardial infarction in patients undergoing coronary intervention: results from the ARMYDA-2 (Antiplatelet therapy for Reduction of MYocardial Damage during Angioplasty) study. *Circulation*. 2005;111(16):2099-2106.

70. Gurbel PA, Bliden KP, Hiatt BL, O'Connor CM. Clopidogrel for coronary stenting: response variability, drug resistance, and the effect of pretreatment platelet reactivity. *Circulation*. 2003;107(23):2908-2913.

71. Gurbel PA, Bliden KP, Butler K, et al. Randomized double-blind assessment of the ONSET and OFFSET of the antiplatelet effects of ticagrelor versus clopidogrel in patients with stable coronary artery disease: the ONSET/OFFSET study. *Circulation*. 2009;120(25):2577-2585.

72. Wiviott SD, Trenk D, Frelinger AL, et al. Prasugrel compared with high loading- and maintenance-dose clopidogrel in patients with planned percutaneous coronary intervention: the Prasugrel in Comparison to Clopidogrel for Inhibition of Platelet Activation and Aggregation-Thrombolysis in Myocardial Infarction 44 trial. *Circulation*. 2007;116(25):2923-2932.

73. Wiviott SD, Braunwald E, McCabe CH, et al. Prasugrel versus clopidogrel in patients with acute coronary syndromes. *N Engl J Med*. 2007;357(20): 2001-2015.

74. Wallentin L, Becker RC, Budaj A, et al. Ticagrelor versus clopidogrel in patients with acute coronary syndromes. *N Engl J Med*. 2009;361(11):1045-1057.

75. Alexopoulos D, Xanthopoulou I, Gkizas V, et al. Randomized assessment of ticagrelor versus prasugrel antiplatelet effects in patients with ST-segment-elevation myocardial infarction. *Circ Cardiovasc Interv*. 2012;5(6):797-804.

76. Montalescot G, Hof AW, Lapostolle F, et al. Prehospital ticagrelor in ST-segment elevation myocardial infarction. *N Eng J Med*. 2014;371(11): 1016-1027.

77. Silvain J, Storey RF, Cayla G, et al. P2Y12 receptor inhibition and effect of morphine in patients undergoing primary PCI for ST-segment elevation myocardial infarction. The PRIVATE-ATLANTIC study. *Thromb Haemost*. 2016;116(2):369-378.

78. Parodi G, Xanthopoulou I, Bellandi B, et al. Ticagrelor crushed tablets administration in STEMI patients: the MOJITO study. *J Am Coll Cardiol*. 2015;65(5):511-512.

79. Rollini F, Franchi F, Hu J, et al. Crushed prasugrel tablets in patients with STEMI undergoing primary percutaneous coronary intervention: the CRUSH study. *J Am Coll Cardiol*. 2016;67(17):1994-2004.

80. Akers WS, Oh JJ, Oestreich JH, Ferraris S, Wethington M, Steinhubl SR. Pharmacokinetics and pharmacodynamics of a bolus and infusion of

cangrelor: a direct, parenteral P2Y12 receptor antagonist. *J Clin Pharmacol.* 2010;50(1):27-35.

81. Steg PG, Bhatt DL, Hamm CW, et al. Effect of cangrelor on periprocedural outcomes in percutaneous coronary interventions: a pooled analysis of patient-level data. *Lancet.* 2013;382(9909):1981-1892.

82. Franchi F, Rollini F, Rivas A, et al. Platelet inhibition with cangrelor and crushed ticagrelor in patients with ST-segment-elevation myocardial infarction undergoing primary percutaneous coronary intervention. *Circulation.* 2019;139(14):1661-1670.

83. Alexopoulos D, Pappas C, Sfantou D, et al. Cangrelor in ticagrelor-loaded STEMI patients undergoing primary percutaneous coronary intervention. *J Am Coll Cardiol.* 2018;72(14):1750-1751.

84. Gargiulo G, Esposito G, Avvedimento M, et al. Cangrelor, tirofiban, and chewed or standard prasugrel regimens in patients with ST-segment-elevation myocardial infarction: primary results of the FABOLUS-FASTER Trial. *Circulation.* 2020;142(5):441-454.

85. Sinnaeve P, Fahrni G, Schelfaut D, et al. Subcutaneous selatogrel inhibits platelet aggregation in patients with acute myocardial infarction. *J Am Coll Cardiol.* 2020;75(20):2588-2597.

86. Kedhi E, Fabris E, van der Ent M, et al. Six months versus 12 months dual antiplatelet therapy after drug-eluting stent implantation in ST-elevation myocardial infarction (DAPT-STEMI): randomised, multicentre, non-inferiority trial. *BMJ.* 2018;363:k3793.

87. Hahn JY, Song YB, Oh JH, et al. 6-month versus 12-month or longer dual antiplatelet therapy after percutaneous coronary intervention in patients with acute coronary syndrome (SMART-DATE): a randomised, open-label, non-inferiority trial. *Lancet.* 2018;391(10127):1274-1284.

88. Leadbeater PD, Kirkby NS, Thomas S, et al. Aspirin has little additional anti-platelet effect in healthy volunteers receiving prasugrel. *J Thromb Haemost.* 2011;9(10):2050-2056.

89. Baber U, Zafar MU, Dangas G, et al. Ticagrelor with or without aspirin after PCI: the TWILIGHT platelet substudy. *J Am Coll Cardiol.* 2020;75(6):578-586.

90. Franchi F, Rollini F, Garcia E, et al. Effects of edoxaban on the cellular and protein phase of coagulation in patients with coronary artery disease on dual antiplatelet therapy with aspirin and clopidogrel: results of the EDOX-APT study. *Thromb Haemost.* 2020;120(1):83-93.

91. Vranckx P, Valgimigli M, Juni P, et al. Ticagrelor plus aspirin for 1 month, followed by ticagrelor monotherapy for 23 months vs aspirin plus clopidogrel or ticagrelor for 12 months, followed by aspirin monotherapy for 12 months after implantation of a drug-eluting stent: a multicentre, open-label, randomised superiority trial. *Lancet.* 2018;392(10151):940-949.

92. Tomaniak M, Chichareon P, Onuma Y, et al. Benefit and risks of aspirin in addition to ticagrelor in acute coronary syndromes: a post hoc analysis of the randomized GLOBAL LEADERS trial. *JAMA Cardiol.* 2019;4(11):1092-1101.

93. Kim BK, Hong SJ, Cho YH, et al. Effect of ticagrelor monotherapy vs ticagrelor with aspirin on major bleeding and cardiovascular events in patients with acute coronary syndrome: the TICO randomized clinical trial. *JAMA.* 2020;323(23):2407-2416.

94. Cuisset T, Deharo P, Quilici J, et al. Benefit of switching dual antiplatelet therapy after acute coronary syndrome: the TOPIC (timing of platelet inhibition after acute coronary syndrome) randomized study. *Eur Heart J.* 2017;38(41):3070-3078.

95. Sibbing D, Aradi D, Jacobshagen C, et al. Guided de-escalation of antiplatelet treatment in patients with acute coronary syndrome undergoing percutaneous coronary intervention (TROPICAL-ACS): a randomised, open-label, multicentre trial. *Lancet.* 2017;390(10104):1747-1757.

96. Collet JP, Thiele H, Barbato E, et al. 2020 ESC guidelines for the management of acute coronary syndromes in patients presenting without persistent ST-segment elevation. *Eur Heart J.* 2020;42(14):1289-1367.

97. Schupke S, Neumann FJ, Menichelli M, et al. Ticagrelor or prasugrel in patients with acute coronary syndromes. *N Engl J Med.* 2019;381(16):1524-1534.

98. Aytekin A, Ndrepepa G, Neumann FJ, et al. Ticagrelor or prasugrel in patients with ST-segment-elevation myocardial infarction undergoing primary percutaneous coronary intervention. *Circulation.* 2020;142(24):2329-2337.

99. Valina C, Neumann FJ, Menichelli M, et al. Ticagrelor or prasugrel in patients with non-ST-segment elevation acute coronary syndromes. *J Am Coll Cardiol.* 2020;76(21):2436-2446.

100. Schnorbus B, Daiber A, Jurk K, et al. Effects of clopidogrel vs. prasugrel vs. ticagrelor on endothelial function, inflammatory parameters, and platelet function in patients with acute coronary syndrome undergoing coronary artery stenting: a randomized, blinded, parallel study. *Eur Heart J.* 2020;41(33):3144-3152.

101. Navarese EP, Khan SU, Kolodziejczak M, et al. Comparative efficacy and safety of oral P2Y12 inhibitors in acute coronary syndrome: network meta-analysis of 52 816 patients from 12 randomized trials. *Circulation.* 2020;142(2):150-160.

102. You SC, Rho Y, Bikdeli B, et al. Association of ticagrelor vs clopidogrel with net adverse clinical events in patients with acute coronary syndrome undergoing percutaneous coronary intervention. *JAMA.* 2020;324(16):1640-1650.

103. Stone GW, Maehara A, Lansky AJ, et al. A prospective natural-history study of coronary atherosclerosis. *N Engl J Med.* 2011;364(3):226-235.

104. Varenhorst C, Hasvold P, Johansson S, et al. Culprit and nonculprit recurrent ischemic events in patients with myocardial infarction: data from SWEDEHEART (Swedish Web System for Enhancement and Development of Evidence-Based Care in Heart Disease Evaluated According to Recommended Therapies). *J Am Heart Assoc.* 2018;7(1):e007174.

105. Bonaca MP, Bhatt DL, Cohen M, et al. Long-term use of ticagrelor in patients with prior myocardial infarction. *N Engl J Med.* 2015;372(19):1791-1800.

106. Udell JA, Bonaca MP, Collet JP, et al. Long-term dual antiplatelet therapy for secondary prevention of cardiovascular events in the subgroup of patients with previous myocardial infarction: a collaborative meta-analysis of randomized trials. *Eur Heart J.* 2016;37(4):390-399.

107. Levine GN, Bates ER, Bittl JA, et al. 2016 ACC/AHA guideline focused update on duration of dual antiplatelet therapy in patients with coronary artery disease: a report of the American College of Cardiology/American Heart Association Task Force on Clinical Practice Guidelines: an update of the 2011 ACCF/AHA/SCAI Guideline for Percutaneous Coronary Intervention, 2011 ACCF/AHA Guideline for Coronary Artery Bypass Graft Surgery, 2012 ACC/AHA/ACP/AATS/PCNA/SCAI/STS Guideline for the Diagnosis and Management of Patients With Stable Ischemic Heart Disease, 2013 ACCF/AHA Guideline for the Management of ST-Elevation Myocardial Infarction, 2014 AHA/ACC Guideline for the Management of Patients With Non-ST-Elevation Acute Coronary Syndromes, and 2014 ACC/AHA Guideline on Perioperative Cardiovascular Evaluation and Management of Patients Undergoing Noncardiac Surgery. *Circulation.* 2016;134(10):e123-e155.

108. Mega JL, Braunwald E, Wiviott SD, et al. Rivaroxaban in patients with a recent acute coronary syndrome. *N Engl J Med.* 2012;366(1):9-19.

109. Gibson CM, Mehran R, Bode C, et al. Prevention of bleeding in patients with atrial fibrillation undergoing PCI. *N Engl J Med.* 2016;375(25):2423-2434.

110. Eikelboom JW, Connolly SJ, Bosch J, et al. Rivaroxaban with or without aspirin in stable cardiovascular disease. *N Engl J Med.* 2017;377(14):1319-1330.

111. Garcia-Prieto J, Villena-Gutierrez R, Gomez M, et al. Neutrophil stunning by metoprolol reduces infarct size. *Nat Commun.* 2017;8:14780.

112. Pizarro G, Fernandez-Friera L, Fuster V, et al. Long-term benefit of early pre-reperfusion metoprolol administration in patients with acute myocardial infarction: results from the METOCARD-CNIC Trial (Effect of Metoprolol in Cardioprotection During an Acute Myocardial Infarction). *J Am Coll Cardiol.* 2014;63(22):2356-2362.

113. Roolvink V, Ibanez B, Ottervanger JP, et al. Early intravenous beta-blockers in patients with ST-segment elevation myocardial infarction before primary

percutaneous coronary intervention. *J Am Coll Cardiol.* 2016;67(23): 2705-2715.

114. Garcia-Ruiz JM, Fernandez-Jimenez R, Garcia-Alvarez A, et al. Impact of the timing of metoprolol administration during STEMI on infarct size and ventricular function. *J Am Coll Cardiol.* 2016;67(18):2093-2104.

115. Clemente-Moragon A, Gomez M, Villena-Gutierrez R, et al. Metoprolol exerts a non-class effect against ischaemia-reperfusion injury by abrogating exacerbated inflammation. *Eur Heart J.* 2020;41(46):4425-4440.

116. Dargie HJ. Effect of carvedilol on outcome after myocardial infarction in patients with left-ventricular dysfunction: the CAPRICORN randomised trial. *Lancet.* 2001;357(9266):1385-1390.

117. Goldberger JJ, Bonow RO, Cuffe M, et al. Effect of beta-blocker dose on survival after acute myocardial infarction. *J Am Coll Cardiol.* 2015;66(13): 1431-1441.

118. Dondo TB, Hall M, West RM, et al. Beta-blockers and mortality after acute myocardial infarction in patients without heart failure or ventricular dysfunction. *J Am Coll Cardiol.* 2017;69(22):2710-2720.

119. Holt A, Blanche P, Zareini B, et al. Effect of long-term beta-blocker treatment following myocardial infarction among stable, optimally treated patients without heart failure in the reperfusion era: a Danish, nationwide cohort study. *Eur Heart J.* 2021;42(9):907-914.

120. Kim J, Kang D, Park H, et al. Long-term beta-blocker therapy and clinical outcomes after acute myocardial infarction in patients without heart failure: nationwide cohort study. *Eur Heart J.* 2020;41(37):3521-3529.

121. Ibanez B, Raposeiras-Roubin S, Garcia-Ruiz JM. The swing of beta-blockers: time for a system reboot. *J Am Coll Cardiol.* 2017;69(22):2721-2724.

122. Pfeffer MA, Braunwald E, Moye LA, et al. Effect of captopril on mortality and morbidity in patients with left ventricular dysfunction after myocardial infarction. Results of the survival and ventricular enlargement trial. The SAVE Investigators. *N Engl J Med.* 1992;327(10):669-677.

123. Flather MD, Yusuf S, Kober L, et al. Long-term ACE-inhibitor therapy in patients with heart failure or left-ventricular dysfunction: a systematic overview of data from individual patients. ACE-Inhibitor Myocardial Infarction Collaborative Group. *Lancet.* 2000;355(9215):1575-1581.

124. Beygui F, Van Belle E, Ecollan P, et al. Individual participant data analysis of two trials on aldosterone blockade in myocardial infarction. *Heart.* 2018;104(22):1843-1849.

125. Indications for ACE inhibitors in the early treatment of acute myocardial infarction: systematic overview of individual data from 100,000 patients in randomized trials. ACE Inhibitor Myocardial Infarction Collaborative Group. *Circulation.* 1998;97(22):2202-2212.

126. Grundy SM, Stone NJ, Bailey AL, et al. 2018 AHA/ACC/AACVPR/AAPA/ABC/ACPM/ADA/AGS/APhA/ASPC/NLA/PCNA guideline on the management of blood cholesterol: a report of the American College of Cardiology/American Heart Association Task Force on Clinical Practice Guidelines. *Circulation.* 2019;139(25):e1082-e1143.

127. Cannon CP, Blazing MA, Giugliano RP, et al. Ezetimibe added to statin therapy after acute coronary syndromes. *N Engl J Med.* 2015;372(25): 2387-2397.

128. Sabatine MS, Giugliano RP, Keech AC, et al. Evolocumab and clinical outcomes in patients with cardiovascular disease. *N Engl J Med.* 2017; 376(18):1713-1722.

129. Schwartz GG, Steg PG, Szarek M, et al. Alirocumab and cardiovascular outcomes after acute coronary syndrome. *N Engl J Med.* 2018;379(22): 2097-2107.

130. Mach F, Baigent C, Catapano AL, et al. 2019 ESC/EAS guidelines for the management of dyslipidaemias: lipid modification to reduce cardiovascular risk. *Eur Heart J.* 2020;41(1):111-188.

131. Tardif JC, Kouz S, Waters DD, et al. Efficacy and safety of low-dose colchicine after myocardial infarction. *N Engl J Med.* 2019;381(26):2497-2505.

132. Nidorf SM, Fiolet ATL, Mosterd A, et al. Colchicine in patients with chronic coronary disease. *N Engl J Med.* 2020;383(19):1838-1847.

133. Ridker PM, Everett BM, Thuren T, et al. Antiinflammatory therapy with canakinumab for atherosclerotic disease. *N Engl J Med.* 2017;377(12): 1119-1131.

134. Ibanez B, Fuster V. CANTOS: a gigantic proof-of-concept trial. *Circ Res.* 2017;121(12):1320-1322.

135. Yusuf S, Mehta SR, Chrolavicius S, et al. Effects of fondaparinux on mortality and reinfarction in patients with acute ST-segment elevation myocardial infarction: the OASIS-6 randomized trial. *JAMA.* 2006;295(13): 1519-1530.

136. Vogel B, Claessen BE, Arnold SV, et al. ST-segment elevation myocardial infarction. *Nat Rev Dis Primers.* 2019;5(1):39.

137. Elbadawi A, Elgendy IY, Mahmoud K, et al. Temporal trends and outcomes of mechanical complications in patients with acute myocardial infarction. *JACC Cardiovasc Interv.* 2019;12(18):1825-1836.

138. Kitahara S, Fujino M, Honda S, et al. COVID-19 pandemic is associated with mechanical complications in patients with ST-elevation myocardial infarction. *Open Heart.* 2021;8(1).

139. Rodriguez-Leor O, Cid-Alvarez B, Perez de Prado A, et al. Impact of COVID-19 on ST-segment elevation myocardial infarction care. The Spanish experience. *Rev Esp Cardiol.* 2020;73(12):994-1002.

140. Garcia-Dorado D, Piper HM. Postconditioning: reperfusion of "reperfusion injury" after hibernation. *Cardiovasc Res.* 2006;69(1):1-3.

141. Lorca R, Jimenez-Blanco M, Garcia-Ruiz JM, et al. Coexistence of transmural and lateral wavefront progression of myocardial infarction in the human heart. *Rev Esp Cardiol (Engl Ed).* 2020 Aug 24.

142. Miura T, Yellon DM, Hearse DJ, Downey JM. Determinants of infarct size during permanent occlusion of a coronary artery in the closed chest dog. *J American Col Card.* 1987;9(3):647-54.

143. Reimer KA, Lowe JE, Rasmussen MM, Jennings RB. The wavefront phenomenon of ischemic cell death. 1. Myocardial infarct size vs duration of coronary occlusion in dogs. *Circulation.* 1977;56(5):786-94.

144. Reimer KA, Jennings RB. The "wavefront phenomenon" of myocardial ischemic cell death. II. Transmural progression of necrosis within the framework of ischemic bed size (myocardium at risk) and collateral flow. *Lab Invest.* 1979;40(6):633-44.

145. Duncker DJ, Klassen CL, Ishibashi Y, Herrlinger SH, Pavek TJ, Bache RJ. Effect of temperature on myocardial infarction in swine. *The American J of phys.* 1996;270(4 Pt 2):H1189-99.

Evaluation and Management of Non–ST-Segment Elevation Acute Coronary Syndromes

19

Eric R. Bates, David J. Moliterno, and Manesh R. Patel

Pathophysiology, diagnosis, and treatment of non-ST-segment elevation acute coronary syndromes

Pathophysiology

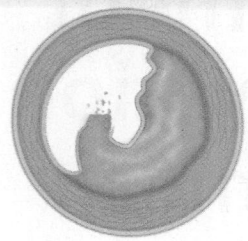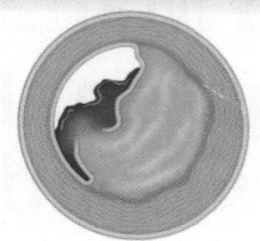

Platelet-rich thrombus formation usually does not completely occlude the coronary lumen

Plaque rupture is the most common cause of coronary thrombosis, but superficial plaque erosion is present in ~30% of patients

Diagnosis

- History
- Electrocardiography
- Biomarkers
- Cardiac catheterization

Unstable angina options:
- Stress testing
- Coronary CT angiography

Management

In-hospital treatment

- Anti-ischemic
  - Nitrate
  - Beta blocker
- ACEi/ARB
- High-intensity statin therapy
- Anticoagulant

- Antiplatelets
  - ASA
  - P2Y$_{12}$ inhibitor
- Revascularization
  - PCI
  - CABG

Outpatient management

- ASA*
- 12 months P2Y$_{12}$ inhibitor
- Beta blocker
- ACEi/ARB
- High-intensity statin therapy

- Lifestyle interventions (diet, weight control, exercise, smoking cessation)
- Risk factor control (diabetes, hypertension, hyperlipidemia)
- Cardiac rehabilitation participation

Chapter 19 Fuster and Hurst's Central Illustration. The most common etiology of non-ST-segment elevation acute coronary syndromes is disruption of an atherosclerotic coronary artery plaque with subsequent platelet-rich thrombus formation. The clearest separation between unstable angina and non–ST-segment elevation myocardial infarction is the absence or presence of abnormal concentrations of myocardial biomarkers; the clearest separation between non-ST-segment elevation acute coronary syndromes and ST-segment elevation myocardial infarction is made by the electrocardiogram. The aims of therapy are to relieve ischemia, control symptoms, and prevent complications. *May be discontinued in some patients from 3-12 months to decrease bleeding risk. ACEi, angiotensin-converting enzyme inhibitor; ARB, angiotensin receptor blocker; ASA, acetylsalicylic acid/aspirin; CABG, coronary artery bypass graft; CT, computed tomography; PCI, percutaneous coronary intervention.

CHAPTER SUMMARY

This chapter discusses the pathophysiology, epidemiology, diagnosis, and treatment of non–ST-segment elevation acute coronary syndromes (see Fuster and Hurst's Central Illustration). The most common etiology is disruption of an atherosclerotic coronary artery plaque with subsequent platelet-rich thrombus formation that may be flow limiting, but usually does not completely occlude the coronary lumen. Downstream microembolization of platelet aggregates and components of the disrupted plaque are likely responsible for the release of myocardial injury biomarkers. The clearest separation between unstable angina (UA) and non–ST-segment elevation myocardial infarction (NSTEMI) is the absence or presence of abnormal concentrations of myocardial biomarkers. The aims of therapy are to relieve ischemia, control symptoms, and prevent complications. Nitrates, β-blockers, and calcium channel blockers reduce the risk of recurrent ischemia. The risk of progression to myocardial infarction (MI), or recurrent MI, is diminished by antiplatelet and antithrombotic drugs and by revascularization of the culprit lesion, usually with percutaneous coronary intervention (PCI). Hospitalized patients should be treated with ASA, a platelet P2Y$_{12}$ receptor inhibitor, antithrombin therapy, a β-blocker, an angiotensin-converting enzyme (ACE) inhibitor, and a high-intensity statin. Outpatient therapy includes lifestyle interventions, risk factor control, and education about the importance of medication adherence. Discharge planning protocols and cardiac rehabilitation programs are the best way to achieve these goals.

INTRODUCTION

Acute coronary syndromes (ACSs) refer to a pattern of clinical symptoms that are consistent with acute myocardial ischemia.[1,2] The pathophysiology, findings, and treatment of ACS range along a clinical spectrum. This chapter discusses two closely related forms of non-ST-segment elevation ACS (NSTE-ACS), namely unstable angina (UA) and non–ST-segment elevation myocardial infarction (NSTEMI). Coronary angiographic and intravascular studies indicate that acute NSTE-ACS usually results from the disruption of an atherosclerotic plaque with subsequent platelet-rich thrombus formation that may be flow limiting, but usually does not completely occlude the epicardial lumen. Plaque rupture is the most common cause of coronary thrombosis, but superficial plaque erosion is increasingly recognized and is present in approximately 30% of patients (**Fig. 19–1**).[3] Downstream microembolization of platelet aggregates and components of the disrupted plaque are key components of NSTE-ACS and are likely responsible for the release of myocardial injury biomarkers that help distinguish NSTEMI from UA (**Fig. 19–2**). Factors that modulate the development of ACS are listed in **Table 19–1**.

EPIDEMIOLOGY AND NATURAL HISTORY

Atherosclerotic coronary artery disease (CAD) is the leading cause of morbidity and mortality in the world and is dramatically increasing in developing countries.[4] There are more than 1 million annual ACS hospital admissions in the United States. The mean patient age is 68 years and the male-to-female ratio is 3:2. In the United States, the prevalence of myocardial infarction (MI) is 4.0% and the prevalence of angina is 3.6%.[5] The estimated annual incidence of MI is 600,000 new events and 200,000 recurrent events. Of these, it is estimated that 170,000 are silent. In a meta-analysis of eight randomized trials comparing a routine versus a selective invasive diagnostic strategy in patients with NSTE-ACS, the risk of all-cause mortality at a mean of 10.3 years was 28% for both strategies.[6]

Prognosis in patients with NSTE-ACS depends on the combination of the morbidity or mortality expected from the extent of coronary stenosis and left ventricular (LV) dysfunction and the short-term risk associated with the culprit lesion and the unstable state of ACS. Risk is highest early after the onset of symptoms. Published reports are influenced by patient selection and treatment and can be misleading. The inclusion and

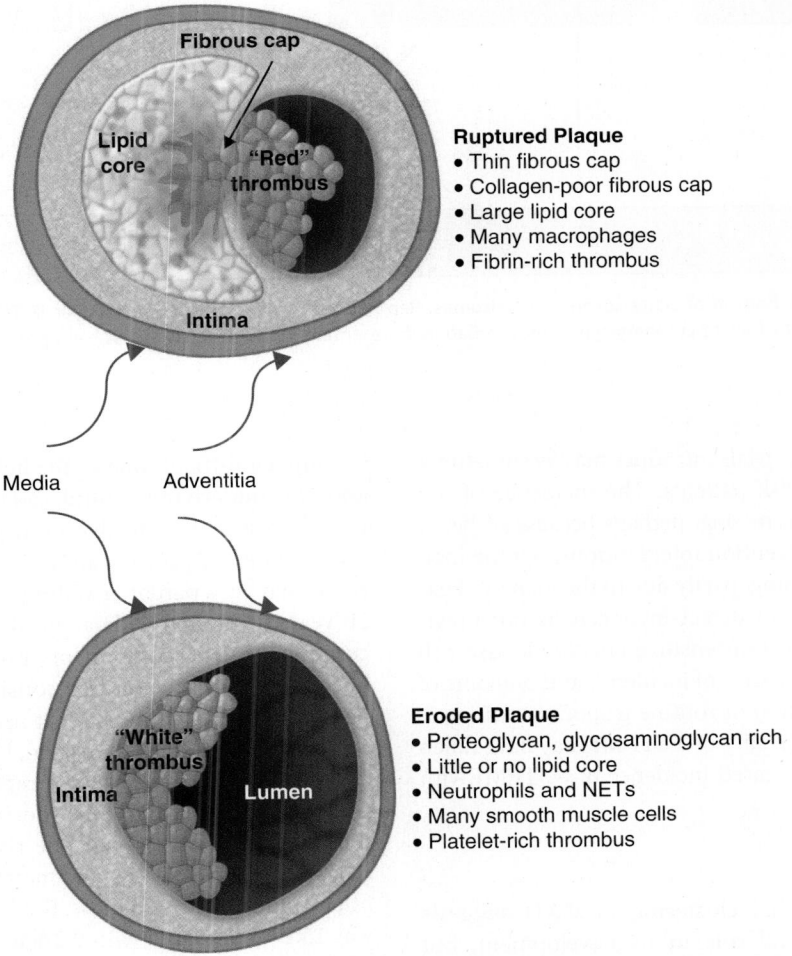

Figure 19–1. Comparisons of coronary atheroma complicated by thrombosis due to plaque rupture (top) or superficial erosion (bottom).

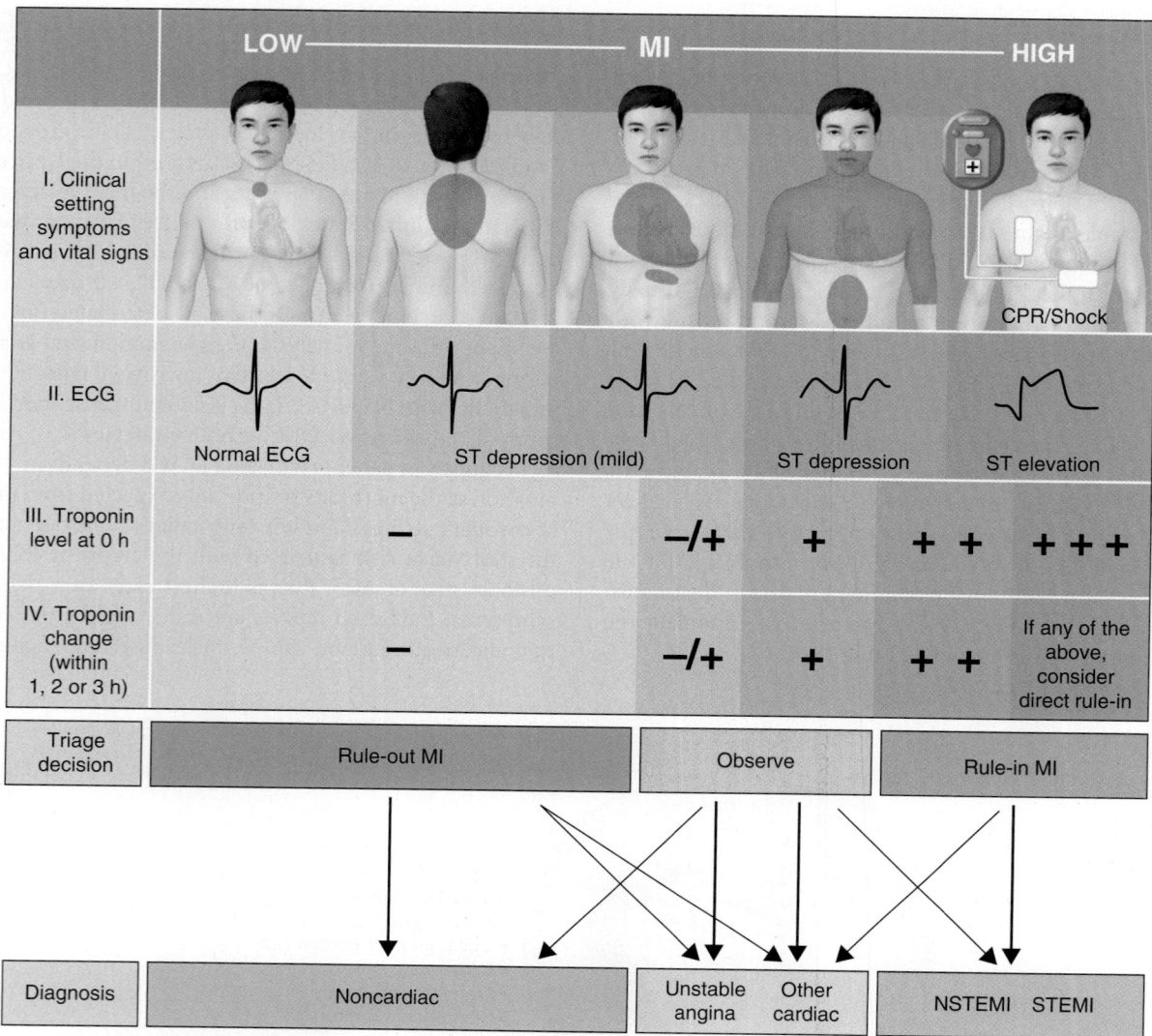

Figure 19–2. Framework for definition of acute coronary syndromes. Reproduced with permission from Collet JP, Thiele H, Barbato E, et al: 2020 ESC Guidelines for the management of acute coronary syndromes in patients presenting without persistent ST-segment elevation. *Eur Heart J.* 2021 Apr 7; 42(14):1289-1367.

exclusion criteria for clinical trials introduce bias by sometimes eliminating low- or high-risk patients. The incidence of ST-elevation MI (STEMI) is decreasing, perhaps because of better primary and secondary prevention interventions, but the incidence of NSTEMI is increasing, partly due to the increased use of troponin measurements to detect myonecrosis not previously recognized by the more insensitive creatine kinase MB band (CK-MB) test. Comparisons of incidence and outcome of NSTE-ACS since the adoption of routine troponin testing are problematic; the overall mortality of NSTEMI may have fallen as a consequence of the increased incidence of NSTEMI with troponin testing.

GENETICS

The long-recognized familial clustering of CAD suggests that genetics plays a central role in its development, but understanding the genetic architecture of CAD and ACS

has proven difficult due to the heterogeneity of clinical CAD and the underlying multidecade complex pathophysiological processes that involve both genetic and environmental interactions.[7] Approximately 12% of patients with CAD report having a parent or sibling with angina or MI before age 50 years.[8] Genome-wide association studies have implicated common genetic components in the development of CAD, but very few have identified consistent, replicated, and independent genetic variants. Most involve lipid metabolism, cell proliferation, and inflammation; but all have had small effect sizes.[9] The most consistently replicated genetic marker for CAD and MI in a European-derived population is on chromosome 9p21.3; 50% had one risk allele and 23% had two risk alleles.[10] In a 65-year-old man with two risk alleles and no other traditional risk factors, the 10-year risk for heart disease was 13.2% compared with 9.2% in a similar man with no risk alleles.

TABLE 19–1. Factors That Modulate the Development and Complications of Acute Coronary Syndromes

Inflammatory substrate
Endothelial function
Platelet aggregability and reactivity
Resistance to antiplatelet agents
Leukocyte activation
Thrombotic factors and intrinsic clotting activity
Level of fibrinolytic activity
Blood viscosity
Catecholamine levels (smoking, cocaine, stress)
Heart rate and blood pressure
Blood lipid levels
Extent of plaque rupture or erosion
Degree of coronary vasoconstriction
Microembolization and microvascular obstruction
Location of the culprit coronary lesion
Stenosis morphology and severity
Extent of collaterals
Medical comorbidities (eg, thyroid, renal, pulmonary disease)
Compliance with lifestyle and pharmacologic therapies

NONINVASIVE AND INVASIVE DIAGNOSTIC APPROACHES

Acute Coronary Syndrome Definition and Classification

The diagnosis of UA depends mostly on history and sometimes on electrocardiogram (ECG) or imaging abnormalities that suggest myocardial ischemia in the setting of normal troponin values. Patients with NSTE-ACS most commonly present with retrosternal chest discomfort occurring at rest or with minimal exertion and lasting at least 10 minutes. New onset angina, rest angina, nocturnal angina, prolonged angina, and progressive angina are some of the different presentations of UA. Ischemia lasting less than 20 minutes usually does not result in myocyte necrosis or elevated troponin, whereas longer durations of ischemia result in MI. The Fourth Universal Definition of MI separates patients with troponin elevations into three groups: Type I MI, Type II MI, and myocardial injury (**Fig. 19–3**).[11] Type I MI includes STEMI and NSTEMI caused by acute reductions in myocardial oxygen supply from a platelet-rich thrombus that develops after rupture or erosion of an atherosclerotic plaque. Type II MI is caused by supply and demand ischemia.[12] Coronary artery etiologies include severe fixed narrowing due to progressive atherosclerosis or restenosis after percutaneous coronary intervention (PCI), vasospasm, vasculitis, embolism, or spontaneous coronary artery dissection (SCAD).[13] Noncoronary cardiac and noncardiac causes of Type II MI are shown in Fig. 19–3. Importantly, NSTEMI is a Type I MI, not a Type II MI. The diagnosis of Type I or Type II MI requires both an elevated troponin value plus clinical evidence of ischemia (symptoms of ischemia, new EKG evidence of ischemia, new pathologic Q waves, new regional wall motion abnormalities on imaging, or coronary thrombosis on angiography or autopsy). Troponin elevation without clinical

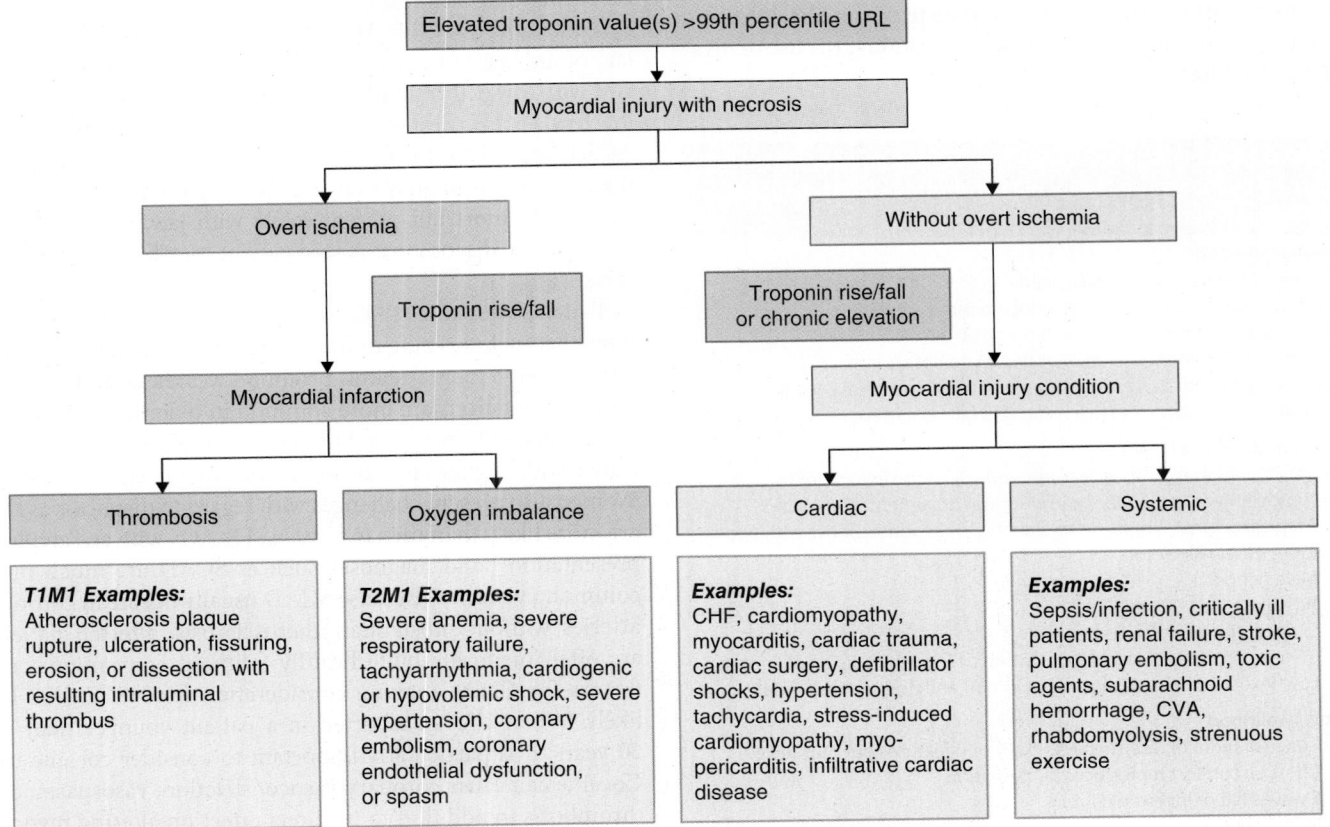

Figure 19–3. Fourth universal definition of myocardial infarction. Adapted with permission from Thygesen K, Alpert JS, Jaffe AS, et al: Fourth Universal Definition of Myocardial Infarction (2018), *J Am Coll Cardiol.* 2018 Oct 30;72(18):2231-2264.

myocardial ischemia is termed myocardial injury secondary to an underlying cause (eg, pulmonary embolism).

Initial Presentation

Initial patient evaluation includes rapid efforts to distinguish noncardiac chest pain from myocardial ischemia. The clearest separation between UA and NSTEMI is the absence or presence of abnormal concentrations of myocardial biomarkers, usually the troponins (which are structural proteins) but rarely CK-MB (which is a cardiac enzyme); the clearest separation between this end of the ACS spectrum and STEMI is made by the ECG.

A patient with symptoms consistent with ACS should have an ECG performed and interpreted within 10 minutes. The most important goal of the early ECG is to identify patients with STEMI who are candidates for immediate reperfusion therapy. Each patient should be given a provisional diagnosis of; (1) definite ACS, which should be classified as STEMI, NSTEMI, or UA; (2) possible ACS; (3) a non-ACS cardiac condition (eg, chronic stable angina or heart failure); or (4) a noncardiac diagnosis, which should be as specific as possible (**Table 19–2**). If a provisional diagnosis of ACS is assigned, risk assessment should be performed to determine the probability of major cardiac complications.[1,2] Such risk assessment is not only important among individuals with definite ACS; among patients with possible ACS, risk assessment should be used to determine the contingent probability of an adverse cardiac event if the diagnosis of ACS is ultimately confirmed, because this information will guide appropriate triage, medical therapy, and timing of subsequent evaluation, including the use of invasive procedures.

TABLE 19–2. Likelihood That Chest Symptoms Are Caused by Myocardial Ischemia Attributable to Obstructive Coronary Artery Disease

High likelihood
Known coronary disease (particularly recent PCI)
Typical angina reproducing prior documented angina
Hemodynamic or ECG changes during pain
Dynamic ST-segment elevation or depression of ≥1 mm
Marked symmetric T-wave inversion in multiple precordial leads
Elevated cardiac enzymes in a rising and falling pattern

Intermediate likelihood
Absence of high-likelihood features and any of the following:
  Typical angina in a patient without prior documented angina
  Atypical anginal symptoms in diabetics or in nondiabetics with two or more other risk factors
  Male gender
  Age older than 70 years
  Extracardiac vascular disease
  ST-segment depression of 0.5–1.0 mm or T-wave inversion of ≥1 mm
  Low-level troponin elevation that is "flat" and does not rise or fall

Low likelihood
Absence of high- or intermediate-likelihood features but may have:
  Chest discomfort reproduced by palpation
  T waves flat or inverted <1 mm
  Normal ECG

Abbreviations: ECG, electrocardiogram; PCI, percutaneous coronary intervention.

Patients with symptoms suggestive of ACS require rapid evaluation and expedient decision-making, with the intensity of monitoring and therapy determined both by the probability of ACS and the associated likelihood of a poor outcome if ACS is subsequently confirmed and/or managed without revascularization. Approximately 15% of patients evaluated in US emergency departments with symptoms suggestive of ACS ultimately have an ACS diagnosis confirmed; conversely, patients with unrecognized ACS have a substantially higher mortality risk. Thus, an organized, efficient, and systematic strategy is needed to avoid unnecessarily exposing patients to risk associated with diagnostic procedures and therapies, and unnecessary resource utilization, while simultaneously ensuring accuracy of diagnosis. Formal chest pain or ACS protocols, or critical pathways, are recommended strategies to provide a systematic approach to the evaluation of possible ACS and to provide greater adherence to guideline recommendations.[1,2]

History

Obtaining an accurate chest pain history to make a diagnosis of myocardial ischemia requires diligence. Onset, location, duration, intensity, character, radiation, exacerbating factors, alleviating factors, and associated symptoms are important variables. The pretest likelihood of a positive diagnosis is increased by older age and background cardiovascular risk factors including smoking, diabetes, hypertension, hyperlipidemia, obesity, family history of premature cardiovascular disease, and prior cardiovascular diagnoses.

Patients with NSTE-ACS often experience discomfort typical of angina, but such episodes are more severe, prolonged, and with lower threshold; they often occur at rest or with very low levels of exertion. Also, chest discomfort because of NSTE-ACS is less likely to be completely relieved by nitroglycerin than is pain from stable angina. Some patients may have no chest discomfort but present solely with jaw, neck, ear, arm, or epigastric discomfort. A rare patient may have Prinzmetal's variant angina.

Patients with NSTE-ACS may present with "atypical" symptoms that include acute dyspnea, indigestion, diaphoresis, agitation, altered mental status, profound weakness, and syncope. Such presentations are more common in older individuals and in patients with long-standing diabetes mellitus and are associated with higher risk for death and major complications.[13] Women also present challenges with regard to diagnosis as they are more likely than men to have NSTE-ACS with an "atypical" presentation[13] and diagnoses such as SCAD are much more common in women. Because SCAD usually occurs in coronary arteries without substantial atherosclerosis, affected patients are often medically quite healthy (without conventional risk factors for CAD), making consideration for NSTE-ACS less likely. When UA is suspected in a patient younger than age 50 years, it is particularly important to consider cocaine use. Cocaine can cause coronary vasoconstriction, vasospasm, and thrombosis in addition to its direct effect on altering myocardial oxygen demands through increases in heart rate and blood pressure.[14] In addition, NSTE-ACS may be present without evident clinical symptoms, particularly among patients in the perioperative state and those with comorbid medical conditions such as diabetes.

Electrocardiography

The ECG is too often overlooked as a powerful risk stratification tool in patients with NSTE-ACS. The diagnostic yield of the 12-lead ECG is enhanced greatly if it can be recorded during an episode of chest discomfort. Transient ST-segment depression of at least 0.5 mm that appears during chest discomfort and disappears after relief provides objective evidence of transient myocardial ischemia. When it is a constant finding with or without chest pain, it is less specific but even minor ST-segment depression is associated with increased mortality.[15] A common but nonspecific ECG pattern in patients with NSTE-ACS consists of transient or persistent negative T waves over the involved area. Deeply negative T waves across the precordial leads suggest a proximal, severe, left anterior descending coronary artery stenosis as the culprit lesion and is considered a marker of high risk. Although a completely normal ECG during chest pain does not rule out NSTE-ACS, it significantly reduces the probability and is a favorable prognostic sign.

ECG abnormalities may appear or progress in the absence of new symptoms or signs in patients with NSTE-ACS. Accordingly, it is appropriate and diagnostically useful to obtain serial ECGs during the initial observation period, during recurrent episodes of chest pain, and before hospital discharge.

Biochemical Cardiac Markers

Troponin measurements should be used in the risk stratification of patients with possible NSTE-ACS to supplement the assessment from clinical and electrocardiographic data, both for diagnosis of myocardial necrosis and for estimation of prognosis. Cardiac troponins are the preferred biomarkers for the diagnosis of MI, whereas CK-MB is a less preferred option and should only be used when troponin is not available.[11] Cardiac troponins T and I (cTnT and cTnI) are structural components of the cardiac contractile apparatus and are found in the sarcomere of the cardiomyocyte and in small concentrations within the cytosol. Both cTnT and cTnI are thought to be nearly entirely cardiac in origin; this confers very high cardiac specificity. Numerous studies have demonstrated that even minor troponin elevations are independently associated with adverse events in populations with NSTE-ACS.[16] Many of these patients will have normal levels of CK-MB. The association of troponin elevation with high-risk coronary lesion morphology provides mechanistic insight into studies demonstrating that patients with even minor elevations in cTnT or cTnI derive substantial benefit from an aggressive approach with antithrombotic therapies and an early invasive management strategy.[17] Coronary angiographic trials have demonstrated that in patients with NSTE-ACS, troponin elevation is associated with multivessel coronary disease, complex lesion morphology, and visible thrombus, as well as with impairment in microvascular function.[18] These findings explain the consistent association

between troponin concentration, even at low levels, and recurrent ischemic events in patients with NSTE-ACS.

As troponin assays have become more sensitive, the proportion of individuals with elevation has increased; with cTnI or cTnT assays, more than 30% of individuals with a presentation of NSTE-ACS have detectable levels, and with highly sensitive troponin (hsTn), the proportion is 2- to 3-fold higher. The main advantages of hsTn assays over conventional methods are superior sensitivity to detect minute quantities in TnT or TnI concentrations and increased analytical precision at these very low concentrations. In this regard, compared with conventional troponin methods, hsTnT and hsTnI are both more likely to be abnormal at first draw, to provide incremental prognostic information, and to reclassify the diagnosis from UA to NSTEMI in approximately 30% of patients.[19] The increased sensitivity of hsTn assays also allows for very rapid exclusion of myocardial injury when extremely low concentrations are noted at presentation[20]; such patients could still have UA, however. Lastly, the increased analytical precision (which allows for resolution of small changes in hsTn over short periods of time) facilitates strategies of accelerated diagnostic pathways to exclude NSTEMI in as little as 1 hour.[21]

Present recommendations support serial measurement of troponins in patients with suspected NSTE-ACS, seeking a rise and/or fall in troponin concentration and reserving the diagnosis of NSTEMI for patients with both elevated troponin levels and clinical evidence for myocardial ischemia.[11] Otherwise, caution is necessary. A reflex cardiac evaluation based solely on an elevated cardiac biomarker without considering whether the episode is indeed consistent with NSTE-ACS is inappropriate and may be harmful. In recent years, several different "rule-in" and "rule-out" protocols have been proposed.

Although troponins are highly specific for myocardial injury, they are not specific for the cause of myocardial injury. Multiple noncardiac diagnoses may cause cardiac injury and lead to troponin elevation (**Table 19–3**). Particular consideration should be given to the diagnosis of acute pulmonary embolism, which may present with nonspecific chest symptoms, tachycardia, and ST-segment and T-wave changes along with low-level elevation in cardiac troponins.[22] Moreover, among individuals with chronic cardiovascular conditions; such as heart failure or stable CAD, as well as individuals from the general population with diabetes, chronic kidney disease, or asymptomatic LV hypertrophy or LV dysfunction; chronic troponin elevation may be seen, even in the absence of signs and symptoms of ischemia.[23,24] Therefore, it is crucial to interpret troponin values in the context of the clinical presentation and available clinical information.

In most non-ACS conditions associated with cardiac injury, patients with detectable troponin are at increased risk for adverse cardiac outcomes.[25] However, it should be recognized that in patients with atypical presentations, elevation in troponin may be caused by a process other than NSTE-ACS. Interpreting troponins in patients with renal failure presents a unique challenge. Although persistent troponin elevation frequently occurs in patients on hemodialysis even in the absence of signs of NSTE-ACS, detectable cTnT or cTnI is still associated

TABLE 19–3. Causes of Troponin Elevation Other Than Acute Coronary Syndromes

Acute Disease

Cardiac and vascular
- Acute heart failure
- Acute aortic dissection
- Apical ballooning syndrome
- Endocarditis
- Myocarditis
- Pericarditis
- Cerebrovascular accident
  - Ischemic stroke
  - Intracerebral hemorrhage
  - Subarachnoid hemorrhage
- Kawasaki disease
- Critical illness
  - Hypotension
  - Gastrointestinal bleeding
  - Thrombotic thrombocytopenic purpura

Respiratory
- Acute pulmonary embolism
- Acute respiratory distress syndrome

Muscular damage
- Rhabdomyolysis

Infectious
- Sepsis
- Viral illness

Other acute causes of troponin elevation
- Toxic exposure
  - Carbon monoxide
  - Hydrogen sulfide
  - Colchicine

Chronic Disease
- Chronic heart failure
- Cardiac infiltrative disorders
  - Amyloidosis
  - Sarcoidosis
  - Hemochromatosis
  - Scleroderma
- Hypertension
- Diabetes
- Hypothyroidism
- End-stage renal disease

Myocardial Injury
- Cancer chemotherapy
- Envenomation
- Endurance athletics

with high cardiac event rates.[26] Knowledge of prior troponin values may help to assess whether a current troponin elevation is new or changing (ie, potentially caused by NSTE-ACS) or chronic. If NSTE-ACS is suspected, troponin elevation should be interpreted similarly in patients with and without chronic kidney disease. Measurement of CK-MB may also be helpful.

As troponin assays have become increasingly sensitive, elevations from causes other than NSTE-ACS are becoming more common and more frustrating for consultant cardiologists. Indeed, recent estimates suggest that as many as 50% of troponin elevations occurring in the hospital setting may be attributable to disease processes other than ACS, including heart failure.[27] Misdiagnosis of NSTE-ACS leads to over-testing and

over-treatment; and adversely impacts diagnostic coding, quality improvement efforts, reimbursement, and public reporting of outcomes.[28] In such patients, clinical decisioning and documentation should indicate the underlying mechanism of myocardial injury and establish that MI did not occur.

At present, few data are available to help clinicians distinguish NSTE-ACS causes of troponin elevation from other causes. Elevations caused by NSTE-ACS are usually of a greater magnitude and should demonstrate a dynamic pattern characterized by a transient increase and decrease in values. When a cause other than NSTE-ACS is suspected, treatment should focus on the underlying disease process. An echocardiogram should be considered, given the frequent association of chronic troponin elevation with cardiac structural abnormalities.

Plasma levels of B-type natriuretic peptide (BNP) and the N-terminal fragment of its prohormone (NT-proBNP) may increase in response to cardiac ischemia in proportion to the size and severity of the ischemic insult.[29] In patients with NSTE-ACS, higher levels of BNP or NT-proBNP measured at presentation or during hospitalization are associated with increased risk for subsequent death or heart failure. As such, measurement of BNP or NT-proBNP may provide information additive to that provided by troponin values. Because coronary ischemia in a patient with incident or prevalent heart failure is associated with substantially greater risk than in a patient without heart failure, and because coronary ischemia may lead to decompensation of heart failure itself, use of natriuretic peptide testing may be helpful to round out the diagnostic picture in such patients.

Although many other biomarkers have been proposed for measurement at various time points after NSTE-ACS, with the exception of troponin and BNP or NT-proBNP, few have demonstrated the level of robust evidence necessary for consideration of measurement in routine practice.[30] With increased use of hsTn, the bar will be even higher for newer biomarkers to show clinical utility.

Risk Stratification

Risk models and risk scores predict a probability for adverse outcomes based on combinations of clinical, ECG, and laboratory data available at presentation. It is increasingly recognized that risk assessment should be both integrative and dynamic. Tools that account for multiple risk predictors provide clear enhancement over evaluation of single variables. Moreover, the risk assessment should be updated during hospitalization.

Initial risk assessment of NSTE-ACS dictates the appropriate intensity of initial therapy. At the low end of the risk scale, a patient may be discharged home with ASA (acetylsalicylic acid commonly known as aspirin) and possibly an early outpatient stress test. By contrast, high-risk patients may be hospitalized in a coronary care unit, treated with multiple drugs, and undergo coronary angiography urgently as a prelude to revascularization. Guideline committees recommend using risk-stratification models, such as the Thrombolysis in Myocardial Infarction (TIMI) Risk Score[31] or the Global Registry of Acute Coronary Events (GRACE) Risk Model Nomogram[32] to assess prognosis. Web-based applications for TIMI (timi.org) and GRACE (gracescore.org) scores are available.

Features suggesting high risk include ongoing chest pain that lasts longer than 20 minutes, reversible ST-segment changes of at least 0.5 mm, elevated markers of myonecrosis, and signs of significant LV dysfunction. In addition to these features, the GRACE Risk Model Nomogram uses Killip class, vital signs, age, and creatinine in a stepwise scoring system and considers whether the patient had cardiac arrest at admission. Generally, lower risk patients are younger, have worsening angina without rest pain, have a normal or unchanged ECG without evidence of previous infarction, and have normal cardiac enzymes.

Whereas the TIMI and PURSUIT scores were derived from clinical trial databases, the GRACE score was derived from a large international registry.[13,31,32] Although all three methods discriminate patients at high versus low risk for short- and intermediate-term adverse outcomes, the GRACE model provides better calibration between predicted and observed rates of death.[33] The TIMI score does not include any measurement of heart failure. The GRACE model was developed in a less-selected patient population and includes renal insufficiency as a variable, which are two potential advantages over the other methods. The major advantage of the TIMI score is that it is a simple integer sum that can be calculated at the bedside without a calculator; PURSUIT and GRACE use weighted averages of multiple risk factors and may require a computer to calculate. None of the models incorporates information from biomarkers, such as troponin or BNP/NT-proBNP.

Chest Pain Units

The evaluation of patients with chest pain who may have a NSTE-ACS can be difficult and uncertain. Hospitalizing all such patients for an extensive workup is unwise and results in unnecessary tests with patient risk and expense. However, missing the diagnosis of MI is one of the leading causes of malpractice claims for emergency department physicians in the United States, and patients with missed MI have a higher mortality. The chest pain unit was developed as a strategy to provide systematic care, prevent missed MI diagnoses, and avoid unnecessary hospitalizations. However, the utilization of hsTn testing has led many hospitals to close their chest pain units. If cardiac biomarkers remain negative over a few hours, a symptom-limited stress test may be performed for diagnostic and prognostic purposes or the patient may be discharged and sent home with the option to perform the stress test as an outpatient, if indicated.

Noninvasive Stress Testing

Stress testing (**Table 19–4**) is commonly used for risk assessment in patients with NSTE-ACS who are managed with an initial selective invasive strategy (also called a conservative strategy or an ischemia-guided strategy). Low-risk and some intermediate-risk patients who stabilize with medical therapy are candidates for stress testing for risk stratification. Stress tests should be symptom limited rather than submaximal, and a stress ECG without adjunctive imaging is appropriate unless

TABLE 19–4. American College of Cardiology/American Heart Association Noninvasive Risk Stratification

High risk (>3% annual mortality)
1. Severe resting LV dysfunction (LVEF <0.35)
2. High-risk treadmill (score ≤11)
3. Severe exercise LV dysfunction (exercise LVEF <0.35)
4. Stress-induced large perfusion defect (particularly if anterior)
5. Stress-induced multiple perfusion defects of moderate size
6. Large, fixed perfusion defect with LV dilatation or increased lung uptake
7. Stress-induced moderate perfusion defect with LV dilatation or increased lung uptake (thallium-201)
8. Echocardiographic wall motion abnormality (involving >2 segments) developing at a low dose of dobutamine (≤10 mg/kg/min) or at a low heart rate (≤120 bpm)
9. Stress echocardiographic evidence of extensive ischemia

Intermediate risk (1%–3% annual mortality)
1. Mild to moderate resting LV dysfunction (LVEF 0.35–0.49)
2. Intermediate-risk treadmill score (score −11 to +5)
3. Stress-induced moderate perfusion defect without LV dilatation or increased lung intake
4. Limited stress echocardiographic ischemia with a wall motion abnormality only at higher doses or dobutamine involving ≤2 segments

Low risk (<1% annual mortality)
1. Low-risk treadmill (score ≥+5)
2. Normal or small myocardial perfusion defect at rest or with stress
3. Normal stress echocardiographic wall motion or no change of limited resting wall motion abnormalities during stress

Abbreviations: LV, left ventricular; LVEF, left ventricular ejection fraction.

baseline ECG abnormalities would preclude adequate interpretation. Those with high-risk findings, such as ST-segment depression at low exercise levels, or large, reversible perfusion defects should undergo coronary arteriography; those with negative or low-risk results can be treated medically. Low-risk patients without objective evidence of myocardial ischemia can safely undergo stress testing for diagnosis and prognostic purposes either immediately or as an outpatient.

In patients who are unable to exercise, pharmacologic testing with dipyridamole, adenosine, regadenoson, or dobutamine can be used as an alternative, and sestamibi imaging or echocardiography can be used as a method of assessment. Stress testing is not needed in patients whose clinical features already put them into a high-risk category; instead, they should undergo early coronary angiography.

Coronary Computed Tomography Angiography

Coronary computed tomography angiography (CCTA) is a potentially useful test among some patients undergoing a chest pain evaluation,[34] providing high-quality imaging of the coronary artery anatomy and high sensitivity for CAD (**Fig. 19–4**). The high sensitivity of CCTA for coronary plaque has been found to impart a high negative predictive value for NSTE-ACS among low- to intermediate-risk patients. Emerging techniques, such as identification of high-risk plaque, help to add to the evaluation of patients with CAD detected on CCTA.[35,36] Other advantages include visualization of other cardiac and

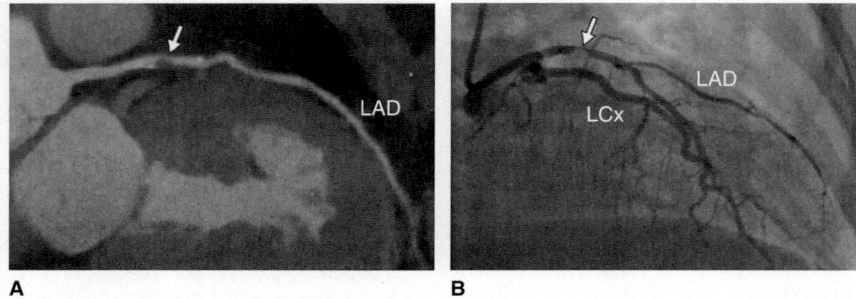

Figure 19–4. Side-by-side comparison of computed tomographic coronary angiography versus invasive angiography in a patient presenting with chest discomfort, ambiguous electrocardiography, and normal troponin concentrations. A severe stenosis of the left anterior descending artery (LAD) is identified using (**A**) coronary computed tomography angiography (CCTA) (*white arrow*) and confirmed at (**B**) invasive angiography (*white arrow*). LCx, left circumflex artery.

pulmonary structures (potentially allowing for detection of unsuspected pathology, such as pericardial effusion) and good sensitivity for detection of less common causes of NSTE-ACS, including SCAD.

In contrast to the high sensitivity of CCTA for plaque presence, specificity is a limitation because many lesions that appear obstructive by CCTA are nonobstructive with coronary angiography; this is most often a result of "positive remodeling" of the coronary vessel, such that large plaque burden may not project into the lumen of the artery. Because of this, the positive predictive value is only moderate for significant luminal obstruction. Ongoing studies are evaluating computationally derived fractional flow reserve to improve specificity (FFR-CT). Additional limitations of CCTA include difficulty in plaque severity quantification in the context of heavy coronary calcification, the requirement for intravenous contrast administration, and exposure to ionizing radiation; newer algorithms for CCTA performance now allow for substantial reduction in radiation exposure.

Randomized comparative effectiveness studies suggest that appropriate use of CCTA in patients at low-to-intermediate risk for NSTE-ACS may shorten time to disposition from the emergency department and reduce need for hospital admission.[37] In such studies, CCTA was highly sensitive to detect presence of CAD and thus provided high sensitivity for NSTE-ACS. Outcomes are largely the same in those evaluated with CCTA versus standard methods (such as myocardial perfusion imaging); however, downstream testing (such as invasive coronary angiography) may also be increased, presumably as a result of visualization of coronary anatomy.

In the balance, CCTA represents a potentially useful test when the probability of severe CAD is low to moderate, study quality may be optimized (heart rate can be reduced to 70 bpm or lower with a β-blocker, and nitrates may be provided), contrast medium exposure is not contraindicated, and anatomic rather than physiologic information is preferred.

Coronary Angiography

Among patients with stable CAD, risk is proportional to the number of vessels with greater than 50% diameter stenosis

and the presence and severity of LV dysfunction. However, the relative prognostic impact of the extent of CAD is probably less with NSTE-ACS because the risk of short-term events is dominated by features of the culprit lesion, such as whether it induces ST-segment depression or troponin release.

Among patients with NSTE-ACS who undergo coronary angiography, approximately 25% have one-vessel disease; 25% have two-vessel disease; and 25% have three-vessel disease. Ten percent have significant left main stenosis, and the other 15% will have coronary luminal narrowing of less than 50% or normal-appearing vessels on angiography. In patients with no significant angiographic lesions, noncardiac causes of chest pain should be considered. If the coronary arteries are angiographically normal, antithrombotic and antiplatelet drugs can often be discontinued and the need for antianginal medication reassessed. Importantly, symptomatic patients without significant obstructive CAD on angiography may have atherosclerosis detected by intravascular ultrasound (IVUS) caused by eccentric coronary artery remodeling that preserves the lumen size. Therefore, in selected patients, more invasive testing at the time of coronary arteriography, including use of IVUS, or measurement of coronary fractional flow reserve using adenosine as a vasodilating agent, or use of resting coronary physiology measurement, may be indicated to help better establish the cause of the acute chest pain.

Early Invasive versus Selective Invasive Strategies

The early invasive strategy of performing coronary angiography for diagnosis and prognosis has become routine for NSTEMI. In the selective invasive strategy, more common in patients with UA, angiography is deferred and reserved for patients with spontaneous recurrent ischemia, development of heart failure, or evidence of significant ischemia or LV dysfunction detected on a predischarge noninvasive evaluation.

The decision between early invasive and selective invasive strategies has been moved to a very proximal time point in the management algorithm of NSTE-ACS.[1] Although initial treatments for these strategies are very similar, patients who undergo an early invasive approach are separated into immediate (<2 hours), early (<24 hours), and delayed (1–3 days) groups according to the urgency of coronary angiography. Patients needing immediate angiography are those with refractory angina, sustained ventricular tachyarrhythmias, worsening heart failure or shock, or new or worsening mitral regurgitation. Early, but not immediate, angiography is performed for patients at increased risk, whereas a selective invasive approach can be considered for patients at intermediate or low risk.

Among high-risk patients, the benefits of an invasive approach are well established and include a reduction in early and late MI, a halving of refractory angina events, and cost effectiveness, but no change in long-term mortality.[38,39] Thus, in high-risk patients, a routine invasive strategy is generally preferred if there are no contraindications to coronary angiography and if the patient is a good candidate for prolonged dual antiplatelet therapy (DAPT). Among low-risk patients, no benefit exists for a routine early invasive approach.

CLINICAL AND THERAPEUTIC CHALLENGES

Treatment Overview

The aims of therapy for patients with NSTE-ACS are to relieve ischemia, control symptoms, and prevent complications. Complications may include recurrent episodes of myocardial ischemia or MI, heart failure, and death. Supplemental oxygen should only be administered for oxygen saturation <90% or respiratory distress. Sublingual or intravenous nitroglycerin should be administered for pain relief. Morphine sulfate can be added for unrelieved pain, but has been shown to delay absorption of oral medications, especially important antiplatelet drugs.[40] Nitrates, β-blockers, and calcium channel blockers reduce the risk of recurrent ischemia. The risk of progression to MI, or recurrent MI, is diminished by antiplatelet and antithrombotic drugs and by revascularization of the culprit lesion, usually with PCI. Hospitalized patients with NSTE-ACS should be treated with ASA, a platelet $P2Y_{12}$ inhibitor, antithrombin therapy, a β-blocker, an angiotensin converting enzyme (ACE) inhibitor, and a high intensity statin. Regardless of whether an early invasive strategy or a selective invasive strategy is used, an assessment of LV function should be performed because it helps guide therapy and carries prognostic information. Neurohormonal inhibition with β-blockers and renin-angiotensin-aldosterone system inhibitors improve long-term outcomes in patients with heart failure.

Anti-Ischemic Therapy

Nitrates

Nitroglycerin is an endothelium-independent vasodilator with venous, peripheral, and coronary vascular effects. Nitrates improve oxygen supply by dilating coronary and collateral arteries and reduce myocardial oxygen demand (MVO_2) by dilating the venous bed and reducing preload. Patients whose symptoms are not relieved with sublingual nitroglycerin may experience symptom relief from intravenous nitroglycerin, and such therapy is recommended in the absence of contraindications for patients with ongoing ischemia, hypertension,

or heart failure. Side effects include headache or hypotension. Nitrates are absolutely contraindicated with concomitant use of phosphodiesterase-5 inhibitors because concomitant therapy may lead to severe hypotension.

Clinical trial evidence does not support benefit of nitrates in reducing adverse cardiovascular outcomes beyond the first 48 hours of treatment.[41] Thus, nitrates should not be administered routinely or for extended periods in the absence of ongoing or recurrent chest pain or heart failure symptoms.

β-Blockers

β-blockers reduce heart rate, blood pressure, and contractility, thereby reducing MVO_2. Slowing of the heart rate with β-blockers also increases the duration of diastole, which improves coronary and collateral blood flow. These effects are mediated by competitive antagonism of β-1 receptors in cardiomyocytes. In contrast, antagonism of β-2 receptors in the peripheral circulation and the lungs may cause vasoconstriction and bronchoconstriction.

It is recommended that β-blockers be initiated orally within the first 24 hours after it has been determined that the patient is not in heart failure or at significant risk for cardiogenic shock and does not otherwise have contraindications, such as significant sinus bradycardia (heart rate <50 bpm), hypotension (systolic blood pressure <90 mm Hg), or evidence of significant heart failure (pulmonary congestion). If there are concerns about possible intolerance to β-blockers, initial selection should favor a short-acting β-1 specific drug such as metoprolol, or esmolol if a very short-acting agent is needed. Mild wheezing or a history of asthma or chronic obstructive pulmonary disease does not preclude use of a β-blocker, but initiating therapy with a low dose of a short-acting cardioselective agent is prudent. Intravenous β-blockers should be reserved for patients with a clear indication for parenteral therapy and absence of risk factors for cardiogenic shock or other contraindications.

Calcium Channel Blockers

These agents inhibit vascular smooth muscle cell function and have effects on sinus node and atrioventricular (AV) nodal function. All of these agents are coronary and peripheral vasodilators, but members of the drug class differ notably with regard to their effects on cardiac contractility and electrical conduction. Verapamil and diltiazem have broad effects, slowing heart rate and AV nodal conduction, reducing contractility, and causing peripheral vasodilation. In contrast, the dihydropyridines (amlodipine and nifedipine) have a vasodilatory effect but show minimal or no direct effects on sinus or AV nodal function.

Rate-limiting calcium antagonists should be considered second- or third-line agents to treat persistent or recurring ischemia in patients on full doses of β-blockers and nitrates or in whom these agents are contraindicated or poorly tolerated. Several randomized trials assessing the use of diltiazem or verapamil in patients with NSTE-ACS suggest that these agents relieve or prevent symptoms and ischemia, but should be avoided in patients with heart failure or known LV dysfunction, because they have been shown to increase mortality in this setting.[1]

Dihydropyridines do not play a primary role in the management of NSTE-ACS, but may be useful agents for blood pressure control when persistent hypertension is present after initiation of β-blockers and ACE inhibitors or angiotensin receptor blockers (ARBs). Only long-acting dihydropyridines, such as amlodipine, should be used for this purpose; short-acting preparations of nifedipine should be avoided in NSTE-ACS because they may cause adverse outcomes.

Antiplatelet Therapy

Antiplatelet and antithrombin agents are cornerstone therapies to help passivate the active vascular disease process and prevent thrombotic complications. Currently, a combination of ASA plus a $P2Y_{12}$ receptor inhibitor (clopidogrel, prasugrel, or ticagrelor), known as DAPT, antithrombin therapy (unfractionated heparin [UFH], low-molecular-weight heparin [LMWH]), and in certain instances, a platelet GP IIb/IIIa receptor inhibitor (eptifibatide, tirofiban) represent the antithrombotic treatment options. The intensity and duration of treatment are tailored to individual risk, although nearly all patients should receive DAPT and an antithrombin agent initially.[1]

ASA

ASA irreversibly acetylates and inhibits the cyclooxygenase-1 enzyme within platelets, preventing the formation of thromboxane A_2, which is a potent platelet activator and a vasoconstrictor. In patients with NSTE-ACS, ASA monotherapy reduced the probability of death or MI by 25% to 30% in older studies.[42] ASA should be initiated in patients with NSTE-ACS at a dose of 150 mg to 325 mg, with the first dose chewed to rapidly establish a high blood level.[1] Thereafter, daily doses of 75 mg to 100 mg are prescribed, continued indefinitely, and interrupted only if necessary and for the shortest possible time that is feasible.

$P2Y_{12}$ Receptor Inhibitors

Clopidogrel: Clopidogrel is a thienopyridine derivative that blocks binding of adenosine diphosphate (ADP) to the $P2Y_{12}$ receptor on the platelet surface, inhibiting ADP–mediated platelet activation and aggregation by approximately 50% to 60%. The Clopidogrel in Unstable Angina to Prevent Recurrent Ischemic Events (CURE) trial randomized 12,562 patients with NSTE-ACS to ASA monotherapy or DAPT with ASA and clopidogrel for 3 to 12 months (average of 9 months).[43] The composite end point of cardiovascular death, MI, or stroke occurred in 11.5% of patients assigned to ASA monotherapy versus 9.3% assigned to DAPT (relative risk [RR] 0.80; $P < 0.001$). Major bleeding was increased with DAPT (3.7% vs 2.7%; $P = 0.003$). Bleeding was notably increased in patients who underwent coronary artery bypass graft (CABG) surgery within the first 5 days of stopping clopidogrel. Thus, elective CABG (and other major surgery) should be delayed for at least 5 days after the last dose of clopidogrel. Some physicians prefer withholding oral $P2Y_{12}$ inhibitor therapy until the coronary anatomy is known to be certain that CABG will not be delayed if needed. The clopidogrel loading dose is 300 mg and the maintenance dose is 75 mg/d; a 600-mg loading dose is recommended before PCI.

Thienopyridines are prodrugs that require more than one step of metabolism before achieving their antiplatelet effects. Clopidogrel has complex pharmacokinetic and pharmacodynamic properties that result in widely variable levels of the circulating active metabolite. After absorption, clopidogrel requires a two-step oxidation by the hepatic cytochrome P450 (CYP) system to generate an active metabolite. Multiple CYP enzymes are involved (CYP3A4, CYP3A5, CYP2C9, CYP1A2, CYP2B6, and CYP2C19), several of which have important genetic variants and are affected by concomitant medications in pharmacodynamic studies, but no important clinical drug-drug interactions have been proven. First, many studies have defined "clopidogrel resistance" on the basis of a single measurement of platelet reactivity performed after clopidogrel; however, residual platelet aggregation to ADP is determined only in part by response to clopidogrel because patient-related factors such as diabetes, smoking, and proximity to the ACS event also contribute to platelet aggregation. Second, the limitations of currently available platelet function tests are noteworthy because the available tests correlate poorly with each other and capture neither the full functionality of the platelet nor the response to clopidogrel.

Prasugrel: Prasugrel is a thienopyridine that, similar to clopidogrel, requires conversion to an active metabolite to bind to the $P2Y_{12}$ receptor. Prasugrel requires only a one-step hepatic metabolism with CYP3A, CYP2B6, CYP2C9, and CYP2C19. This more favorable pharmacokinetic profile translates into better pharmacodynamics with faster onset of action, more potent and irreversible platelet inhibition, and lower interindividual variability compared with even high doses of clopidogrel. In the Trial to Assess Improvement in Therapeutic Outcomes by Optimizing Platelet Inhibition with Prasugrel–Thrombolysis in Myocardial Infarction (TRITON-TIMI) 38 trial,[44] which enrolled 13,608 patients with STEMI or high-risk NSTE-ACS who were scheduled to undergo PCI, prasugrel (60-mg load; then 10 mg/d) plus ASA was compared with clopidogrel (300-mg load; 75 mg/d) plus ASA. Both drugs were initiated at the time of PCI with no pretreatment administered in advance of PCI. The primary efficacy composite endpoint of cardiovascular death, MI, and stroke and was reduced from 12.1% with clopidogrel to 9.9% with prasugrel over a median 14.5 months of follow-up (hazard ratio [HR], 0.81; 95% confidence interval [CI], 0.73–0.90; $P < 0.001$). This benefit was mediated by a 24% reduction in nonfatal MI without a significant reduction in mortality or stroke rates. Two-thirds of the MI events were procedural MI detected by serial cardiac enzyme measurement rather than clinical recognition of symptoms and signs. Definite or probable stent thrombosis was reduced from 2.4% with clopidogrel to 1.1% with prasugrel ($P < 0.001$).

TIMI major bleeding rates were significantly increased with prasugrel (1.8% to 2.4%; HR 1.32; 95% CI, 1.03–1.68; $P = 0.03$) and life-threatening and fatal bleeding were increased. There was no net benefit in patients older than 75 years or with body weight below 60 kg. Net harm was seen in patients with prior stroke or transient ischemic attack, so prasugrel is contraindicated in these patients. Among individuals who underwent CABG after at least one dose of study drug, major bleeding rates were 13.4% with prasugrel and 3.2% with clopidogrel (*P* <0.0001), so CABG should be delayed 7 days after prasugrel administration. No benefit has been shown for prasugrel pretreatment before PCI in patients with NSTE-ACS.[45] Similarly, no benefit has been shown for prasugrel in place of clopidogrel in patients with NSTE-ACS not treated with revascularization.[46]

Ticagrelor: Ticagrelor, a nonthienopyridine, is a direct-acting and reversible $P2Y_{12}$ receptor inhibitor. It does not require conversion to an active metabolite and provides more rapid onset of action and a more potent and predictable antiplatelet response than clopidogrel.[47] In the Study of Platelet Inhibition and Patient Outcomes (PLATO) trial,[48] ticagrelor (180-mg loading dose; 90 mg twice daily) was compared with clopidogrel (300- to 600-mg loading dose; 75 mg/d) in 18,624 patients with STEMI or NSTE-ACS, including patients managed with and without PCI. At 12 months, the primary composite endpoint of cardiovascular death, MI, and stroke was reduced from 11.7% with clopidogrel to 9.8% with ticagrelor (HR, 0.84; 95% CI, 0.77–0.92; *P* <0.001). In addition to significant reductions in MI with ticagrelor, there was also a surprising reduction in total mortality (4.5% vs 5.9%; *P* <0.001), a finding that has not been reproduced in subsequent studies. Stent thrombosis was reduced, but there was an increase in non-CABG major bleeding with ticagrelor (4.5% vs 3.8%; *P* = 0.03); bleeding rates after CABG were lower than in other studies, likely because of the more rapid reversibility of the drug (3–5 days).

Several unique side effects have been observed with ticagrelor, which may be adenosine mediated, and contribute to a higher rate of discontinuation than seen with clopidogrel or prasugrel.[49] Dyspnea can occur early in 10% to 15% of patients, but is not associated with evidence of heart failure and usually lasts less than a week. Ventricular pauses can also occur, but decrease in frequency over time, are rarely symptomatic, and are not associated with clinically significant bradycardia.

Cangrelor: Cangrelor is an intravenous non-thienopyridine ATP analogue that blocks the platelet $P2Y_{12}$ receptor. Three Cangrelor versus Standard Therapy to Achieve Optimal Management of Platelet Inhibition (CHAMPION) trials enrolled patients with NSTE-ACS or stable angina undergoing PCI and randomized them to cangrelor or clopidogrel. The first two trials showed no benefit.[50,51] But in the third trial,[52] the definition for MI was modified, more patients with stable symptoms were enrolled, the threshold for detection of periprocedural MI was lowered, and the definition of stent thrombosis was expanded and added to the efficacy composite endpoint. Cangrelor was better than clopidogrel in this trial, but clopidogrel was not preloaded and not all patients received the recommended loading dose of 600 mg. Since most of the benefit with cangrelor was due to a reduction in periprocedural MI within 2 hours of randomization, it could be argued that maximal cangrelor effect was compared with minimal clopidogrel effect. Earlier clopidogrel treatment might have attenuated the benefit seen with cangrelor; the benefit of cangrelor has yet to be proven compared with prasugrel or ticagrelor. Cangrelor is approved as an adjunct to PCI in patients not pretreated with a $P2Y_{12}$ inhibitor or receiving a GP IIb/IIIa inhibitor.

Glycoprotein IIb/IIIa Receptor Inhibitors
When the platelet is activated, the GP IIb/IIIa receptors on the platelet surface increase in number and demonstrate improved binding affinity for fibrinogen. The binding of fibrinogen to receptors on different platelets results in platelet aggregation. The intravenous platelet GP IIb/IIIa receptor antagonists (eptifibatide, tirofiban) act by occupying the receptor sites, thus opposing fibrinogen and von Willebrand factor binding. The occupancy of 80% or more of the receptor sites and inhibition of platelet aggregation to ADP by 80% or more results in potent antiplatelet effects. Use has decreased significantly in recent years in patients undergoing PCI because of no pretreatment benefit and increased bleeding compared with provisional use,[53,54] and improved acute platelet inhibition with oral prasugrel and ticagrelor. They are most useful when recurrent ischemia develops despite oral antiplatelet therapy and intravenous antithrombin therapy, during emergency PCI when oral $P2Y_{12}$ receptor inhibitor therapy has not been initiated,[55] or with extensive intracoronary thrombus formation. Another PCI strategy is to use the bolus dosing alone and not give the prolonged infusion to decrease bleeding risk since the oral $P2Y_{12}$ inhibitors and newest generation coronary stents have mostly eliminated the occurrence of acute stent thrombosis.[56]

Anticoagulant Therapy

Anticoagulants available for parenteral use include UFH, LMWH, and direct thrombin inhibitors. UFH is a heterogenous mixture of polysaccharide chains of various lengths that accelerate the action of circulating antithrombin, a proteolytic enzyme that inactivates factor Xa, factor IXa, and factor IIa (thrombin). UFH prevents thrombus generation but is not active against clot-bound thrombin. LMWHs contain more short chain polysaccharides and are more potent inhibitors of upstream factor Xa than of downstream factor IIa. Compared with UFH, LMWHs have more specific binding, longer half-life, and more predictable anticoagulation, permitting once- or twice-daily subcutaneous administration. Use of LMWHs does not usually require laboratory monitoring, except during pregnancy and with changing renal function. Direct thrombin inhibitors act by binding directly to the anion binding and catalytic sites of thrombin to produce potent, predictable anticoagulation. Unlike UFH and LMWH, these agents are active against clot-bound thrombin.

Unfractionated Heparin
Pharmacokinetic limitations of UFH translate into poor bioavailability and marked variability in anticoagulant response. An initial weight-adjusted regimen is recommended, with a bolus of 60 U/kg (maximum, 5000 U) and an infusion of 12 U/kg/1h (maximum, 1000 U/h). Dosage adjustments should be made to achieve antifactor Xa levels of 0.3 to 0.7 U/mL, which correlate with aPTT values of 50 to 75 seconds. Therapy can be

discontinued after PCI or after 48 hours in patients not treated with PCI. Several trials have compared UFH with placebo. In an older meta-analysis of six trials with end-point assessment varying from 2 to 12 weeks, UFH reduced death or MI rates by 33% ($P = 0.06$).[57]

Serial platelet counts are necessary to monitor for heparin-induced thrombocytopenia for patients receiving more than 96 hours of therapy or who receive readministration following a recent prolonged UFH course. Thrombocytopenia from UFH takes two forms. One form involves a mild decrease in platelet counts (rarely <100,000/μL) that occurs early (1–4 days) after initiation of therapy, reverses quickly after UFH discontinuation, and is of little clinical consequence because it is not antibody mediated. The more severe form of thrombocytopenia is an immune-mediated thrombocytopenia that typically occurs more than 4 days from therapy, although it may occur earlier in patients who have received UFH within the previous several months. Heparin immune thrombocytopenia is caused by a heparin-dependent, antiplatelet antibody that can activate normal platelets. This syndrome can be associated with thrombosis that can produce severe morbidity and mortality. It should be treated with fondaparinux or a direct thrombin inhibitor initially, especially if thrombosis is present, and then with an oral anticoagulant after hospital discharge.

Low Molecular Weight Heparin

Several large randomized trials have directly compared LMWH with UFH. Important differences have emerged depending on the approach to revascularization used in the studies. Among the earlier trials, those studying enoxaparin versus UFH for medical therapy found a 15% to 20% reduction in death or MI at 4- to 6-week follow-up with a small excess in bleeding in the enoxaparin arms.[58,59] In contrast, a trial comparing enoxaparin with UFH among patients with a planned early-invasive strategy found no benefit with major bleeding rates increased in patients receiving enoxaparin.[60]

Direct Thrombin Inhibitors

Several direct thrombin inhibitors are commercially available (argatroban, lepirudin, and bivalirudin), although bivalirudin has been the most studied and widely used. Bivalirudin is a semisynthetic direct-acting antithrombin with a 25-minute half-life. Efficacy and safety appears to be similar between bivalirudin and UFH monotherapy. Compared with UFH plus a GP IIb/IIIa inhibitor, bivalirudin monotherapy has been associated with similar ischemic outcomes, with a small excess in early stent thrombosis, but lower bleeding risk.[61,62] In the current era with radial artery access, $P2Y_{12}$ receptor inhibitors, lower UFH doses, and newer generation stents, there are no major advantages with bivalirudin monotherapy instead of UFH.[63]

Long-Term Anticoagulation

Anticoagulants may be required for NSTE-ACS patients on DAPT who also have atrial fibrillation, mechanical prosthetic heart valves, or chronic venous thromboembolism. Evidence suggests that "triple therapy" (ASA, $P2Y_{12}$ inhibitor, and oral anticoagulant) is associated with substantially increased risks

for bleeding.[64] As such, it is recommended that attempts be made to minimize the duration of triple therapy. Additionally, the ASA dose should be reduced to 81 mg, prasugrel and ticagrelor should be avoided, the international normalized ratio should be maintained at the lower end of the therapeutic range, and gastrointestinal prophylaxis should be considered.

There have been several trials testing "double therapy" (non-vitamin K antagonist plus a $P2Y_{12}$ receptor inhibitor) versus triple antithrombotic therapy in patients with atrial fibrillation undergoing PCI, with or without ACS.[65] At follow-up, bleeding events including intracerebral hemorrhage were significantly less frequent in the double therapy group without an increase in ischemic events, although there was an insignificant trend toward more MI and stent thrombosis.

Inhibitors of the Renin-Angiotensin-Aldosterone System

ACE inhibitors inhibit neurohormonal pathways that contribute to adverse LV remodeling and heart failure after ACS. In patients with acute MI, particularly when complicated by LV systolic dysfunction, ACE inhibitors show long-term mortality benefits. Although data focusing specifically on populations with NSTE-ACS are sparse, ACE inhibitors have also demonstrated risk reduction among high-risk subsets with chronic CAD, including those with normal LV function. Accordingly, ACE inhibitors should be used in patients with NSTE-ACS complicated by heart failure or LV dysfunction, as well as in those with hypertension, diabetes, or stable chronic kidney disease. ARBs are effective alternatives to ACE inhibitors after MI, but should not routinely be used in combination with ACE inhibitors. Because of the larger evidence base for ACE inhibitors, ARBs should predominantly be used in place of ACE inhibitors in patients with ACE inhibitor intolerance.

Spironolactone or eplerenone are mineralocorticoid receptor antagonists that should be considered for high-risk NSTE-ACS patients with LV ejection fraction ≤40% and either symptomatic heart failure or diabetes mellitus, provided they are receiving adequate doses of ACE inhibitors and do not have significant renal dysfunction or hyperkalemia.[1]

Lipid Lowering Therapy

A series of large randomized controlled trials has evaluated the role of statin therapy in patients with ACS. In the Myocardial Ischemia Reduction with Aggressive Cholesterol Lowering (MIRACL) study, patients were randomized to atorvastatin 80 mg/d or placebo 24 to 96 hours after ACS. The primary 16-week end point of death, MI, resuscitated cardiac arrest, or recurrent myocardial ischemia was reduced with atorvastatin (14.8% vs 17.4%; $P = 0.048$).[66] The Zocor (Z) phase of the A to Z trial compared an early intensive simvastatin regimen (40 mg followed by 80 mg) with a delayed and less intensive regimen (placebo for 4 months followed by simvastatin 20 mg) for up to 24 months.[67] The primary end point of cardiovascular death, MI, readmission for ACS, or stroke favored the early intensive strategy (14.4% vs 16.7%; HR, 0.89; 95% CI, 0.76–1.04). Cardiovascular death was reduced by 25% in the early intensive group ($P = 0.05$). During the first 4 months, no difference was evident between treatment groups, but from 4 to 24 months, the primary end point was reduced in the intensive statin group. In the Pravastatin or Atorvastatin Evaluation and Infection Therapy (PROVE IT)-TIMI 22 trial, atorvastatin 80 mg was compared with pravastatin 40 mg/d.[68] The atorvastatin group achieved an average low-density lipoprotein (LDL) cholesterol of 62 mg/dL versus an average of 95 mg/dL in the pravastatin group. The primary end point of 30-day death, MI, UA, or revascularization was reduced by 16% with atorvastatin ($P <0.0001$). Thus, findings are generally consistent with a "lower is better" approach to LDL-cholesterol management after ACS.

A recent study supports additional LDL lowering by the addition of ezetimibe to maximally tolerated statin therapy as the second lipid-lowering agent.[69] If the LDL goal is not achieved, the addition of a proprotein convertase subtilisin/kexin type 9 (PCSK9) inhibitor is now possible.[70]

Coronary Revascularization

Coronary revascularization (PCI or CABG) is performed to relieve symptoms, prevent ischemic complications, improve functional capacity, and improve prognosis. The decision to proceed from diagnostic angiography to revascularization is influenced not only by the coronary anatomy but also by a number of additional factors including anticipated life expectancy, LV function, comorbidity, functional capacity, severity of symptoms, quantity of viable myocardium at risk, and patient preference.

In patients with NSTE-ACS, PCI of the culprit lesion is usually performed. Careful clinical judgment is required when deciding which nonculprit lesions to revascularize. Complete revascularization of all significant coronary stenoses may have prognostic benefit.[71] Data from both retrospective observational reports and randomized clinical trials indicate that PCI success rates are now very high in patients with NSTE-ACS. Procedural safety appears to be enhanced by the use of radial artery access. Patients with multivessel disease can now often undergo complete revascularization by PCI with the use of multiple stents. Although the timing of nonculprit lesion PCI at the time of culprit lesion PCI is under debate, increasing procedural safety and improving revascularization durability support more single-setting complete revascularization procedures compared with staged PCI. In general, the indications for CABG in NSTE-ACS are similar to those for stable angina.[1] Although the Synergy Between Percutaneous Coronary Intervention With Taxus and Cardiac Surgery (SYNTAX) study did not focus specifically on patients with ACS, the demonstration of CABG benefit over multivessel PCI among individuals with more diffuse and complex disease likely applies to the ACS population as well.[72] A multidisciplinary discussion of treatment options is recommended in patients with more complex anatomy before deciding on the elective revascularization option. Conversely, patients with cardiogenic shock should undergo emergency PCI of the culprit lesion; routine nonculprit PCI should not be performed. In these patients, CABG is recommended if the coronary anatomy is not amenable to PCI.

Hospital Discharge and Outpatient Care

The risk of progression to MI or the development of recurrent MI or death is highest during the first few months after the index ACS event. At 1 to 3 months after the acute phase, most patients resume a clinical course similar to that in patients with chronic stable CAD.

Preparing patients for resumption of normal activities after hospital discharge should include lifestyle interventions (diet, weight control, exercise, smoking cessation), risk factor control (diabetes, hypertension, hyperlipidemia), and education about the importance of medication adherence (DAPT, β-blockers, statins, and ACE inhibitors). Patients should also be advised to avoid nonsteroidal anti-inflammatory drugs (except for ASA). Discharge planning protocols and cardiac rehabilitation programs are the best way to achieve these goals. Monitoring for depression after hospital discharge is also recommended, as is an annual influenza vaccination.[1]

Special Patient Groups

Vasospastic angina

In 1959, Prinzmetal described a syndrome characterized by angina at rest with transient marked ST-segment elevation. The attacks can be cyclic in nature, often occurring at rest and in the early morning hours. Ventricular arrhythmias and AV block sometimes occur at the peak of an attack, and both MI and sudden death are potential consequences. Vasospastic angina is more common in heavy cigarette smokers; 25% have a history of migraine headaches and approximately 25% have symptoms of Raynaud phenomenon. Syncope that occurs during rest angina, likely caused by ischemia-induced ventricular arrhythmia or AV block, is a clue to the diagnosis. Coronary angiography has demonstrated coronary spasm as the etiology.

Nitroglycerin relieves angina attacks within minutes and should be used promptly. Calcium channel blockers are first-line therapy in preventing attacks; higher calcium channel blocker doses are frequently required. Long-acting nitrates are also effective when combined with calcium channel blockers, Statins, magnesium supplements, and alpha-receptor blockers may also be useful.

Spontaneous Coronary Artery Dissection

SCAD is an increasingly recognized cause of ACS, usually in women aged 30 to 50 years.[73] Many cases occur in situations such as uncontrolled hypertension, in the puerperium, in those with fibromuscular dysplasia, or as a complication of disorders of collagen integrity, such as Marfan syndrome. The diagnosis of SCAD should be entertained when symptoms and signs of acute coronary ischemia occur in the absence of other risk factors. Diagnostic studies should be similar to those without SCAD. The presence of coronary dissection may be challenging to recognize, so a high level of suspicion should be maintained during angiography.

Avoiding PCI is recommended if normal coronary flow is present and symptoms have resolved; spontaneous healing of the dissection is often seen at follow-up. If ischemia persists or flow is decreased, either PCI or CABG can restore myocardial perfusion. Given the high prevalence of unrecognized fibromuscular dysplasia in affected patients, some recommend screening other vascular beds for fibromuscular dysplasia or aneurysm formation.

Stress Cardiomyopathy

Widely recognized as an ACS "mimic," stress cardiomyopathy ("apical ballooning" syndrome or takotsubo cardiomyopathy), is now found in approximately 2% of patients presenting with NSTE-ACS symptoms, with 90% women.[74] Stress cardiomyopathy most often results from a severe acute emotional stress, such as the death of a loved one, and may appear indistinguishable from NSTE-ACS, with typical angina, a small rise and fall of troponin, and sometimes the onset of heart failure symptoms. Characteristic ECG changes of stress cardiomyopathy include development of T-wave inversion in many leads. At angiography, nonobstructed coronary arteries are the rule. LV akinesis does not follow a coronary artery distribution, there may be compensatory basal hyperkinesis, and the wall motion abnormalities are greater than would be suggested by the biomarker release.

Management of patients with stress cardiomyopathy is typically supportive; patients most often recover rapidly after presentation, although shock at presentation is possible. Use of vasodilating inotropic agents or intra-aortic balloon counterpulsation in those with shock may actually worsen hemodynamics by precipitating LV outflow tract obstruction in the context of basal hyperkinesis. β-blockers and ACE inhibitors or ARBs are often used during convalescent periods, but their value in stress cardiomyopathy is unknown.

Diabetes Mellitus

More than 30% of patients with NSTE-ACS have diabetes. They have higher risk profiles, longer treatment delays, and more renal insufficiency and heart failure. Patients less frequently undergo angiography and revascularization and have higher adverse outcome rates after NSTE-ACS. It is important to avoid hypoglycemia and to control hyperglycemia. Revascularization with CABG instead of PCI is more commonly considered.[75] Greater success in implementing guideline-directed medical therapy is needed in these patients.

Chronic Kidney Disease

Chronic kidney disease is associated with more comorbidities and worse outcomes with NSTE-ACS. Creatinine clearance should be estimated in every patient and doses of renally cleared medications should be adjusted accordingly. Patients undergoing angiography should be well hydrated and the contrast medium load should be minimized to avoid contrast-induced nephropathy. More evidence is needed to support the benefit of an invasive strategy in patients with more advanced kidney disease.

Perioperative Patients

Perioperative ACS may occur in as many as 5% of patients after noncardiac surgery, typically within 48 hours and often without obvious symptoms since the patients are less able to give a history. Frequency will depend on the intensity of monitoring troponin values and ECGs. Medical therapy with nitrates, β-blockers, and ACE inhibitors should be optimized. Antiplatelet, anticoagulant, and coronary angiography use need to be modified based on the limitations imposed by the surgical procedure.

Older Patients

Patients at least 75 years of age have the highest incidence, prevalence, and adverse outcomes of NSTE-ACS. They also benefit more from pharmacological and interventional therapies, but receive less guideline recommended therapy than do younger patients. They should generally be managed similarly to younger patients, but patient-centered decision-making is important and pharmacotherapy needs to be individualized, given more medical comorbidities and differences in renal function.[76]

Future Therapeutic Opportunities

The burden of recurrent cardiovascular ischemic events and mortality remains unacceptably high despite impressive advances in diagnosis and treatment. In the future, we may be able to better predict who is at risk for ACS through genetic profiling, artificial intelligence algorithms, or advanced imaging techniques. Inflammation is important in atherothrombosis and could be a new treatment target. Early trials of anti-inflammatory therapy with methotrexate, canakinumab, and colchicine have yielded mixed results, but this is an active area for investigation.[77-79] Advances are needed in personalizing antiplatelet therapy to improve efficacy and decrease bleeding risk by tailoring duration and intensity of therapy. Great progress is being make in cholesterol-lowering therapy. There is exciting potential for risk reduction in NSTE-ACS with PCSK9 inhibitors[70] and inclisiran,[80] a small interfering RNA agent that inhibits synthesis of PCSK9 and only requires twice-yearly dosing. Icosapent ethyl[81] and bempedoic acid[82] are additional agents that can be used for lipid lowering. Improved LV remodeling with angiotensin receptor neprilysin inhibitors (ARNI)[83] and the role for vericiguat,[84] sodium-glucose cotransporter (SGLT-2) inhibitors, and glucagon-like peptide-1 receptor (GLP-1) agonists in patients with NSTE-ACS and heart failure need more evaluation. Additionally, more precise selection of patients who might benefit from implantable cardioverter defibrillator devices is needed. There is a great therapeutic opportunity to improve hypertension control by home monitoring with wearable technology and telemedicine. Advances in utilization of structured registries and the organization of claims and electronic health record data are needed to more quickly test the clinical effectiveness of new treatments and to better use in quality improvement efforts. Greater uptake of guideline-directed care by providers and better treatment adherence by patients would maximize the benefit of the many treatment options available to patients with NSTE-ACS.

GUIDELINES

The most recent clinical practice guidelines for NSTE-ACS were released by the American College of Cardiology (ACC)/ American Heart Association (AHA) in 2014[1] and by the

European Society of Cardiology (ESC) in 2020.[2] In 2015, the AHA published an important document on pharmacotherapy in patients with chronic kidney disease and ACS,[85] and a scientific statement on acute MI in women.[86] Both committees harmonized recommendations for antiplatelet therapy across all of their guideline statements with guideline updates.[87,88]

ACC/AHA made 168 recommendations and ESC made 125 recommendations in their guideline documents (**Tables 19–5**

and **19–6**). Both recommend early evaluation, a clinical history, physical examination, ECG within 10 minutes of patient arrival, hsTn measurements, and risk scores to assess prognosis. ESC promotes a shortened algorithm for diagnosis with early repeat hsTn measurements, takes a stronger position on recommending noninvasive stress tests or CCTA to diagnose NSTE-ACS in patients without recurrent symptoms and with normal hsTn levels, and specifically recommends the radial

TABLE 19–5. Selected Key Class I Guideline Treatment Recommendations

ACC/AHA Guidelines[1,87]	ESC Guidelines[2]
Administer sublingual nitroglycerin every 5 minutes × 3 for continuing ischemic pain and then assess need for IV nitroglycerin.	Sublingual or IV nitrates are recommended in patients with ongoing ischemic symptoms and without contraindications.
IV nitroglycerin is indicated for patients for the treatment of persistent ischemia, HF, or hypertension.	IV nitrates are recommended in patients with uncontrolled hypertension or signs of HF.
Initiate oral β-blockers within the first 24 hours in the absence of HF, low-output state, risk for cardiogenic shock, or other contraindications to beta blockade.	Early initiation of β-blocker treatment and chronic β-blocker therapy is indicated unless the patient is in overt HF.
Non–enteric-coated, chewable ASA (162 mg to 325 mg) should be given to *all* patients without contraindications as soon as possible after presentation, and a maintenance dose of ASA (81 mg/d) should be continued indefinitely.	ASA is recommended for all patients without contraindications at an initial oral dose of 150 mg to 300 mg and at a maintenance dose of 75 mg to 100 mg daily for long-term treatment.
A P2Y$_{12}$ inhibitor therapy (clopidogrel, prasugrel, or ticagrelor) should be given for at least 12 months.	A P2Y$_{12}$ receptor inhibitor is recommended in addition to ASA, and maintained over 12 months unless there are contraindications or an excessive risk of bleeding.
Anticoagulation, in addition to antiplatelet therapy, is recommended for all patients irrespective of initial treatment strategy.	Parenteral anticoagulation is recommended for all patients, in addition to antiplatelet treatment, at the time of diagnosis and during revascularization procedures according to both ischemic and bleeding risks.
The duration of triple antithrombotic therapy with a vitamin K antagonist, ASA, and a P2Y$_{12}$ receptor inhibitor in patients with NSTE-ACS should be minimized to the extent possible to limit the risk of bleeding.	In patients with AF and CHA2DS2-VASc score ≥1 in men and ≥2 in women, after a short period of triple therapy (up to 1 week from the acute event), dual therapy is recommended as the default strategy using a NOAC at the recommended dose for stroke prevention and a single oral antiplatelet agent (preferably clopidogrel).
Initiate or continue high-intensity statin therapy in patients with no contraindications.	Statins are recommended in all patients. The aim is to reduce LDL-C by ≥50% from baseline and/or to achieve LDL <55 mg/dL.
	If the LDL-C goal is not achieved after 4 to 6 weeks with the maximally tolerated statin dose, combination with ezetimibe is recommended.
	If the LDL-C goal is not achieved after 4 to 6 weeks despite maximally tolerated statin therapy and ezetimibe, the addition of a PCSK9 inhibitor is recommended.
ACE inhibitors should be started and continued indefinitely in all patients with LVEF less than 0.40 and in those with hypertension, diabetes mellitus, or stable CKD, unless contraindicated.	ACE inhibitors are recommended in patients with HF with reduced LVEF (<40%), diabetes, or CKD unless contraindicated.
ARBs are recommended in patients with HF or MI with LVEF less than 0.40 who are ACE inhibitor intolerant.	ARBs are recommended in cases of intolerance to ACE inhibitors in patients with HF with reduced LVEF (<40%), diabetes, or CKD unless contraindicated.
Aldosterone blockade is recommended in patients post–MI without significant renal dysfunction (creatinine >2.5 mg/dL in men or >2.0 mg/dL in women) or hyperkalemia (K >5.0 mEq/L) who are receiving therapeutic doses of ACE inhibitor and β-blocker and have a LVEF 0.40 or less, diabetes mellitus, or HF.	MRAs are recommended in patients with HF with reduced LVEF (<40%) in order to reduce all-cause and cardiovascular mortality and cardiovascular morbidity.
Proton pump inhibitors should be prescribed in patients with a history of gastrointestinal bleeding who require triple antithrombotic therapy with a vitamin K antagonist, ASA, and a P2Y$_{12}$ receptor inhibitor.	Concomitant use of a proton pump inhibitor is recommended in patients who are at high risk of gastrointestinal bleeding in order to reduce the risk of gastric bleeds.
All eligible patients with NSTE-ACS should be referred to a comprehensive cardiovascular rehabilitation program either before hospital discharge or during the first outpatient visit.	Multidisciplinary exercise-based cardiac rehabilitation is recommended as an effective means for patients with CAD to achieve a healthy lifestyle and manage risk factors in order to reduce all-cause and cardiovascular mortality and morbidity, and improve health-related quality of life.

Abbreviations: ACE, angiotensin converting enzyme; AF, atrial fibrillation; ARB, angiotensin receptor blocker; CAD, coronary artery disease; CKD, chronic kidney disease; HF, heart failure; IV, intravenous; LDL-C, low-density lipoprotein cholesterol; LVEF, left ventricular ejection fraction; MI, myocardial infarction; MRA, mineralocorticoid receptor antagonist; NOAC, non–vitamin K anticoagulant.

TABLE 19–6. Selected Key Class III Guideline Treatment Recommendations

ACC/AHA Guidelines[1]	ESC Guidelines[2]
Nitrates should not be administered to patients who recently received a phosphodiesterase inhibitor.	
Nonsteroidal anti-inflammatory drugs (except ASA) should not be initiated and should be discontinued during hospitalization.	
Administration of intravenous β-blockers is potentially harmful in patients who have risk factors for shock.	
	Crossover of unfractionated heparin and low molecular weight heparin is not recommended.
	It is not recommended to administer routine pre-treatment with a P2Y$_{12}$ receptor inhibitor in patients in whom coronary anatomy is not known and an early invasive management is planned.
Prasugrel should not be administered to patients with a prior history of stroke or transient ischemic attack.	The use of ticagrelor or prasugrel as part of triple antithrombotic therapy is not recommended.
	Treatment with GP IIb/IIIa antagonists in patients in whom coronary anatomy is not known is not recommended.
An early invasive strategy is not recommended in patients with extensive comorbidities or low likelihood of acute coronary syndrome who are troponin-negative, especially women.	

approach for arterial access in coronary angiography. ESC also recommends a diagnostic algorithm, including cardiac myocardial resonance imaging, to evaluate MI with nonobstructive coronary arteries (MINOCA).

Supplemental oxygen is only recommended for hypoxia. Morphine sulfate is reasonable to treat persistent chest pain. Anti-ischemic agents are recommended to decrease myocardial oxygen demand. Nitrates are recommended for angina, heart failure, or hypertension. β-blockers are recommended in patients without contraindications to treat ischemia and improve prognosis in patients with LV dysfunction or heart failure. Calcium channel blockers are a supplemental strategy.

DAPT for 12 months is recommended by both with indefinite ASA for maintenance therapy and the option for longer or shorter DAPT duration. Ticagrelor and prasugrel are recommended over clopidogrel more strongly by ESC, with prasugrel limited to patients with a planned PCI. ACC/AHA recommends against genetic or platelet function testing, whereas ESC suggests testing may be considered to screen for clopidogrel resistance. ESC recommends against routine upstream GP IIb/IIIa receptor inhibitor administration whereas ACC/AHA states that it is reasonable in high-risk patients with planned early angiography if oral therapy has not been administered.

There are several recommendations for the use of UFH, LMWH, fondaparinux, and bivalirudin in the documents, but many are dated because of the rapid uptake in the use of radial access and the move toward lower-dose UFH as a routine anticoagulation strategy. Enoxaparin and fondaparinux are easier to administer at hospitals without PCI capability and bivalirudin may be useful in patients with high bleeding risk.

Both recommend an early invasive strategy for most patients. Interestingly, ACC/AHA states that women with low-risk should not undergo early invasive treatment because of

bleeding risk. Both recommend the heart team approach for revascularization decisions.

Discharge recommendations include use of ASA, P2Y$_{12}$ inhibitors, β-blockers, ACE inhibitors, statins, lifestyle counseling, control of risk factors, and referral to a cardiac rehabilitation program. Both recommend high-intensity statins, with ESC setting a target LDL < 55 mg/dl to be achieved by sequentially adding ezetimibe and a PCSK-9 inhibitor. Both recommend participation in quality improvement registries and continuous quality improvement programs.

SUMMARY

Pathogenesis

- NSTE-ACS usually results from the disruption of an atherosclerotic plaque with subsequent platelet-rich thrombus formation that may be flow limiting, but usually does not completely occlude the coronary lumen.

- Downstream microembolization of platelet aggregates and components of the disrupted plaque are key components of NSTE-ACS and are likely responsible for the release of myocardial injury biomarkers that help distinguish NSTEMI from UA.

Genetics

- Genome-wide association studies have implicated common genetic components in the development of CAD, but very few have identified consistent, replicated, and independent genetic variants. Most involve lipid metabolism, cell proliferation, and inflammation; but all have had small effect sizes.

Treatment and Management

- The aims of therapy for patients with NSTE-ACS are to relieve ischemia, control symptoms, and prevent complications.

- Sublingual or intravenous nitroglycerin should be administered for pain relief, with morphine sulfate limited to patients with unrelieved pain.
- Nitrates, β-blockers, and calcium channel blockers reduce the risk of recurrent ischemia.
- The risk of progression to MI, or recurrent MI, is diminished by antiplatelet and antithrombotic drugs and by revascularization of the culprit lesion, usually with PCI.
- Hospitalized patients should be treated with ASA, a platelet P2Y$_{12}$ inhibitor, antithrombin therapy, a β-blocker, an ACE inhibitor, and a high-intensity statin.

ACKNOWLEDGMENTS

We would like to thank Dr. James A de Lemos, Dr. Robert A O'Rourke, Dr. Robert A Harrington, and Dr. James L Januzzi, Jr. who substantially contributed to the previous versions of this chapter.

REFERENCES

1. Amsterdam EA, Wenger NK, Brindis RG, et al. 2014 AHA/ACC guideline for the management of patients with non-ST-elevation acute coronary syndromes: a report of the American College of Cardiology/American Heart Association Task Force on Practice Guidelines. *J Am Coll Cardiol.* 2014;64(24):e139-e228.

2. Collett JP, Thiele H, Barbato E, et al. 2020 ESC guidelines for the management of acute coronary syndromes in patients presenting without persistent ST-segment elevation: Task Force for the Management of Acute Coronary Syndromes in Patients Presenting without Persistent ST-Segment Elevation of the European Society of Cardiology (ESC). *Eur Heart J.* 2021;42(14):1289-1367.

3. Libby P, Pasterkamp G, Crea F, Jang IK. Reassessing the mechanisms of acute coronary syndromes. *Circ Res.* 2019;124(1):150-160.

4. Mensah GA, Roth GA, Fuster V. The global burden of cardiovascular diseases and risk factors: 2020 and beyond. *J Am Coll Cardiol.* 2019;74(20):2529-2532.

5. Virani SS, Alonso A, Benjamin EJ, et al. Heart disease and stroke statistics-2020 update: a report from the American Heart Association. *Circulation.* 2020;141(9):e139-e596.

6. Elgendy IY, Mahmoud AN, Wen X, Bavry AA. Meta-analysis of randomized trials of long-term all-cause mortality in patients with non-ST-elevation acute coronary syndrome managed with routine invasive versus selective invasive strategies. *Am J Cardiol.* 2017;119(4):560–564.

7. Dai X, Wiernek S, Evans JP, Runge MS. Genetics of coronary artery disease and myocardial infarction. *World J Cardiol.* 2016;8(1):1-23.

8. National Center for Health Statistics. National Health and Nutrition Examination Survey (NHANES) public use data files. *Centers for Disease Control and Prevention.* Accessed April 1, 2019. https://www.cdc.gov/nchs/nhanes

9. Franchini M. Genetics of the acute coronary syndrome. *Ann Transl Med.* 2016;4(10):192-197.

10. Helgadottir A, Thorleifsson G, Manolescu A, et al. A common variant on chromosome 9p21 affects the risk of myocardial infarction. *Science.* 2007;316(5830):1491-1493.

11. Thygesen K, Alpert JS, Jaffe AS, et al. Fourth universal definition of myocardial infarction. *J Am Coll Cardiol.* 2018;72(18):2231-2264.

12. Sandoval Y, Jaffe AS. Type 2 myocardial infarction: JACC review topic of the week. *J Am Coll Cardiol.* 2019;73(14):1846-1860.

13. Bastante T, Rivero F, Cuesta J, Benedicto A, Restrepo J, Alfonso F. Nonatherosclerotic causes of acute coronary syndrome: recognition and management. *Curr Cardiol Rep.* 2014;16(11):543.

14. Richards JR, Garber D, Laurin EG, et al. Treatment of cocaine cardiovascular toxicity: a systematic review. *Clin Toxicol (Phila).* 2016;54(5):345-364.

15. Boersma E, Pieper KS, Steyerberg EW, et al. Predictors of outcome in patients with acute coronary syndromes without persistent ST-segment elevation. Results from an international trial of 9461 patients. The PURSUIT Investigators. *Circulation.* 2000;101(22):2557-2567.

16. Segraves JM, Frishman WH. Highly sensitive cardiac troponin assays: a comprehensive review of their clinical utility. *Cardiol Rev.* 2015;23(6):282-289.

17. Morrow DA, Cannon CP, Rifai N, et al. Ability of minor elevations of troponins I and T to predict benefit from an early invasive strategy in patients with unstable angina and non-ST elevation myocardial infarction: results from a randomized trial. *JAMA.* 2001;286(19):2405-2412.

18. Wong GC, Morrow DA, Murphy S, et al. Elevations in troponin T and I are associated with abnormal tissue level perfusion: a TACTICS-TIMI 18 substudy. Treat Angina with Aggrastat and Determine Cost of Therapy with an Invasive or Conservative Strategy-Thrombolysis in Myocardial Infarction. *Circulation.* 2002;106(2):202-207.

19. Januzzi JL Jr, Bamberg F, Lee H, et al. High-sensitivity troponin T concentrations in acute chest pain patients evaluated with cardiac computed tomography. *Circulation.* 2010;121(10):1227-1234.

20. Body R, Carley S, McDowell G, et al. Rapid exclusion of acute myocardial infarction in patients with undetectable troponin using a high-sensitivity assay. *J Am Coll Cardiol.* 2011;58(13):1332-1339.

21. Reichlin T, Twerenbold R, Wildi K, et al. Prospective validation of a 1-hour algorithm to rule-out and rule-in acute myocardial infarction using a high-sensitivity cardiac troponin T assay. *CMAJ.* 2015;187(8):E243-E252.

22. Yalamanchili K, Sukhija R, Aronow WS, Sinha N, Fleisher AG, Lehrman SG. Prevalence of increased cardiac troponin I levels in patients with and without acute pulmonary embolism and relation of increased cardiac troponin I levels with in-hospital mortality in patients with acute pulmonary embolism. *Am J Cardiol.* 2004;93(2):263-264.

23. Eggers KM, Lagerqvist B, Venge P, Wallentin L, Lindahl B. Persistent cardiac troponin I elevation in stabilized patients after an episode of acute coronary syndrome predicts long-term mortality. *Circulation.* 2007;116(17):1907-1914.

24. Wallace TW, Abdullah SM, Drazner MH, et al. Prevalence and determinants of troponin T elevation in the general population. *Circulation.* 2006;113(16):1958-1965.

25. Ammann P, Maggiorini M, Bertel O, et al. Troponin as a risk factor for mortality in critically ill patients without acute coronary syndromes. *J Am Coll Cardiol.* 2003;41(11):2004-2009.

26. de Filippi C, Wasserman S, Rosanio S, et al. Cardiac troponin T and C-reactive protein for predicting prognosis, coronary atherosclerosis, and cardiomyopathy in patients undergoing long-term hemodialysis. *JAMA.* 2003;290(3):353-359.

27. Januzzi JL, Jr., Filippatos G, Nieminen M, Gheorghiade M. Troponin elevation in patients with heart failure: on behalf of the third Universal Definition of Myocardial Infarction Global Task Force: Heart Failure Section. *Eur Heart J.* 2012;33(18):2265-2271.

28. McCarthy C, Murphy S, Cohen JA, et al. Misclassification of myocardial injury as myocardial infarction: implications for assessing outcomes in value-based programs. *JAMA Cardiol.* 2019;4(5):460-464.

29. Sabatine MS, Morrow DA, de Lemos JA, et al. Acute changes in circulating natriuretic peptide levels in relation to myocardial ischemia. *J Am Coll Cardiol.* 2004;44(10):1988-1995.

30. Morrow DA, de Lemos JA. Benchmarks for the assessment of novel cardiovascular biomarkers. *Circulation.* 2007;115(8):949-952.

31. Antman EM, Cohen M, Bernink PJ, et al. The TIMI risk score for unstable angina/non-ST elevation MI: a method for prognostication and therapeutic decision making. *JAMA.* 2000;284(7):835-842.

32. Eagle KA, Lim MJ, Dabbous OH, et al. A validated prediction model for all forms of acute coronary syndrome: estimating the risk of

6-month postdischarge death in an international registry. *JAMA.* 2004;291(22):2727-2733.

33. de Araujo Goncalves P, Ferreira J, Aguiar C, Seabra-Gomes R. TIMI, PURSUIT, and GRACE risk scores: sustained prognostic value and interaction with revascularization in NSTE-ACS. *Eur Heart J.* 2005;26(9):865-872.

34. Samad Z, Hakeem A, Mahmood SS, et al. A meta-analysis and systematic review of computed tomography angiography as a diagnostic triage tool for patients with chest pain presenting to the emergency department. *J Nucl Cardiol.* 2012;19(2):364-376.

35. Bittner DO, Mayrhofer T, Puchner SB, et al. Coronary computed tomography angiography-specific definitions of high-risk plaque features improve detection of acute coronary syndrome. *Circ Cardiovasc Imaging.* 2018;11(8):e007657.

36. Lee JM, Choi G, Koo BK, et al. Identification of high-risk plaques destined to cause acute coronary syndrome using coronary computed tomographic angiography and computational fluid dynamics. *JACC Cardiovasc Imaging.* 2019;12(6):1032-1043.

37. Hoffmann U, Truong QA, Schoenfeld DA, et al. Coronary CT angiography versus standard evaluation in acute chest pain. *N Engl J Med.* 2012;367(4):299-308.

38. Hoenig MR, Aroney CN, Scott IA. Early invasive versus conservative strategies for unstable angina and non-ST elevation myocardial infarction in the stent era. *Cochrane Database Syst Rev.* 2010;3:CD004815.

39. Mahoney EM, Jurkovitz CT, Chu H, et al. Cost and cost-effectiveness of an early invasive vs conservative strategy for the treatment of unstable angina and non-ST-segment elevation myocardial infarction. *JAMA.* 2002;288(15):1851-1858.

40. Furtado RHM, Nicolau JC, Guo J, et al. Morphine and cardiovascular outcomes among patients with non-ST-segment elevation acute coronary syndromes undergoing coronary angiography. *J Am Coll Cardiol.* 2020;75(3):289-300.

41. Perez MI, Musini VM, Wright JM. Effect of early treatment with antihypertensive drugs on short and long-term mortality in patients with an acute cardiovascular event. *Cochrane Database Syst Rev.* 2009;4:CD006743.

42. Collaborative overview of randomised trials of antiplatelet therapy–I: Prevention of death, myocardial infarction, and stroke by prolonged antiplatelet therapy in various categories of patients. Antiplatelet Trialists' Collaboration. *BMJ.* 1994;308(6921):81-106.

43. Yusuf S, Zhao F, Mehta SR, et al. Effects of clopidogrel in addition to aspirin in patients with acute coronary syndromes without ST-segment elevation. *N Engl J Med.* 2001;345(7):494-502.

44. Wiviott SD, Braunwald E, McCabe CH, et al. Prasugrel versus clopidogrel in patients with acute coronary syndromes. *N Engl J Med.* 2007;357(20):2001-2015.

45. Montalescot G, Bolognese L, Dudek D, et al. Pretreatment with prasugrel in non-ST-segment elevation acute coronary syndromes. *N Engl J Med.* 2013;369(11):999-1010.

46. Roe MT, Armstrong PW, Fox KA, et al. Prasugrel versus clopidogrel for acute coronary syndromes without revascularization. *N Engl J Med.* 2012;367(14):1297-309.

47. Gurbel PA, Bliden KP, Butler K, et al. Randomized double-blind assessment of the ONSET and OFFSET of the antiplatelet effects of ticagrelor versus clopidogrel in patients with stable coronary artery disease: the ONSET/OFFSET study. *Circulation.* 2009;120(25):2577-2585.

48. Wallentin L, Becker RC, Budaj A, et al. Ticagrelor versus clopidogrel in patients with acute coronary syndromes. *N Engl J Med.* 2009;361(11):1045-1057.

49. Arora S, Shemisa K, Vaduganathan M, et al. Premature ticagrelor discontinuation in secondary prevention of atherosclerotic CVD: JACC Review Topic of the Week. *J Am Coll Cardiol.* 2019;73(19):2454-2464.

50. Bhatt DL, Lincoff AM, Gibson CM, et al. Intravenous platelet blockade with cangrelor during PCI. *N Engl J Med.* 2009;361:2330-2341.

51. Harrington RA, Stone GW, McNulty S, et al. Platelet inhibition with cangrelor in patients undergoing PCI. *N Engl J Med.* 2009;361:2318-2329.

52. Bhatt DL, Stone GW, Mahaffey KW, et al. Effect of platelet inhibition with cangrelor during PCI on ischemic events. *N Engl J Med.* 2013;368:1303-1313.

53. Stone GW, Bertrand ME, Moses JW, et al. Routine upstream initiation vs deferred selective use of glycoprotein IIb/IIIa inhibitors in acute coronary syndromes: the ACUITY Timing trial. *JAMA.* 2007;297(6):591-602.

54. Giugliano RP, White JA, Bode C, et al. Early versus delayed, provisional eptifibatide in acute coronary syndromes. *N Engl J Med.* 2009;360(21):2176-2190.

55. Kastrati A, Mehilli J, Neumann FJ, et al. Abciximab in patients with acute coronary syndromes undergoing percutaneous coronary intervention after clopidogrel pretreatment: the ISAR-REACT 2 randomized trial. *JAMA.* 2006;295(13):1531-1538.

56. Fung AY, Saw J, Starovoytov A, et al. Abbreviated infusion of eptifibatide after successful coronary intervention. The BRIEF-PCI (Brief Infusion of Eptifibatide Following Percutaneous Coronary Intervention) randomized trial. *J Am Coll Cardiol.* 2009;53:837-845.

57. Oler A, Whooley MA, Oler J, Grady D. Adding heparin to aspirin reduces the incidence of myocardial infarction and death in patients with unstable angina. A meta-analysis. *JAMA.* 1996;276(10):811-815.

58. Cohen M, Demers C, Gurfinkel EP, et al. A comparison of low-molecular-weight heparin with unfractionated heparin for unstable coronary artery disease. Efficacy and Safety of Subcutaneous Enoxaparin in Non-Q-Wave Coronary Events Study Group. *N Engl J Med.* 1997;337(7):447-452.

59. Antman EM, McCabe CH, Gurfinkel EP, et al. Enoxaparin prevents death and cardiac ischemic events in unstable angina/non-Q-wave myocardial infarction. Results of the thrombolysis in myocardial infarction (TIMI) 11B trial. *Circulation.* 1999;100(15):1593-1601.

60. Ferguson JJ, Califf RM, Antman EM, et al. Enoxaparin vs unfractionated heparin in high-risk patients with non-ST-segment elevation acute coronary syndromes managed with an intended early invasive strategy: primary results of the SYNERGY randomized trial. *JAMA.* 2004;292(1):45-54.

61. Stone GW, McLaurin BT, Cox DA, et al. Bivalirudin for patients with acute coronary syndromes. *N Engl J Med.* 2006;355(21):2203-2216.

62. Navarese EP, Schulze V, Andreotti F, et al. Comprehensive meta-analysis of safety and efficacy of bivalirudin versus heparin with or without routine glycoprotein IIb/IIIa inhibitors in patients with acute coronary syndrome. *JACC Cardiovasc Interv.* 2015;8(1 Pt B):201-213.

63. Valgimigli M, Frigoli E, Leonardi S, et al. Radial versus femoral access and bivalirudin versus unfractionated heparin in invasively managed patients with acute coronary syndrome (MATRIX): final 1-year results of a multicentre, randomised controlled trial. *Lancet.* 2018;392(10150):835-848.

64. Sorensen R, Hansen ML, Abildstrom SZ, et al. Risk of bleeding in patients with acute myocardial infarction treated with different combinations of aspirin, clopidogrel, and vitamin K antagonists in Denmark: a retrospective analysis of nationwide registry data. *Lancet.* 2009;374(9706):1967-1974.

65. Gargiulo G, Goette A, Tijssen J, et al. Safety and efficacy outcomes of double vs. triple antithrombotic therapy in patients with atrial fibrillation following percutaneous coronary intervention: a systematic review and meta-analysis of non-vitamin K antagonist oral anticoagulant-based randomized clinical trials. *Eur Heart J.* 2019;40:3757-3767.

66. Schwartz GG, Olsson AG, Ezekowitz MD, et al. Effects of atorvastatin on early recurrent ischemic events in acute coronary syndromes: the MIRACL study: a randomized controlled trial. *JAMA.* 2001;285(13):1711-1718.

67. de Lemos JA, Blazing MA, Wiviott SD, et al. Early intensive vs a delayed conservative simvastatin strategy in patients with acute coronary syndromes: phase Z of the A to Z trial. *JAMA.* 2004;292(11):1307-1316.

68. Cannon CP, Braunwald E, McCabe CH, et al. Intensive versus moderate lipid lowering with statins after acute coronary syndromes. *N Engl J Med.* 2004;350(15):1495-1504.

69. Cannon CP, Blazing MA, Giugliano RP, et al. Ezetimibe added to statin therapy after acute coronary syndromes. *N Engl J Med.* 2015;372(25): 2387-2397.

70. Schwartz GG, Steg PG, Szarek M, et al. Alirocumab and cardiovascular outcomes after acute coronary syndrome. *N Engl J Med.* 2018;379(22): 2097-2107.

71. Bainey KR, Alemayehu W, Armstrong PW, Westerhout CM, Kaul P, Welsh RC. Long-term outcomes of complete revascularization with percutaneous coronary intervention in acute coronary syndromes. *JACC Cardiovasc Interv.* 2020;13(13):1557-1567.

72. Serruys PW, Morice MC, Kappetein AP, et al. Percutaneous coronary intervention versus coronary artery bypass grafting for severe coronary artery disease. *N Engl J Med.* 2009;360(10):961-972.

73. Hayes SN, Tweet MS, Adlam D, et al. Spontaneous coronary artery dissection: JACC State-of-the-Art Review. *J Am Coll Cardiol.* 2020;76(8):961-984.

74. Ono R, Falcao LM. Takotsubo cardiomyopathy systematic review: pathophysiologic process, clinical presentation and diagnostic approach to Takotsubo cardiomyopathy. *Int J Cardiol.* 2016;209:196-205.

75. Farkouh ME, Domanski M, Sleeper LA, et al. Strategies for multivessel revascularization in patients with diabetes. *N Engl J Med.* 2012;367(25):2375-2384.

76. McCune C, McKavanagh P, Menown IB. A review of current diagnosis, investigation, and management of acute coronary syndromes in elderly patients. *Cardiol Ther.* 2015;4(2):95-116.

77. Ridker PM, Everett BM, Thuren T, et al. Antiinflammatory therapy with canakinumab for atherosclerotic disease. *N Engl J Med.* 2017;377(12): 1119-1131.

78. Ridker PM, Everett BM, Pradhan A, et al. Low-dose methotrexate for the prevention of atherosclerotic events. *N Engl J Med.* 2019;380(8):752-762.

79. Tardif JC, Kouz S, Waters DD, et al. Efficacy and safety of low-dose colchicine after myocardial infarction. *N Engl J Med.* 2019;381(26):2497-2505.

80. Ray KK, Wright RS, Kallend D, et al. Two phase 3 trials of inclisiran in patients with elevated LDL cholesterol. *N Engl J Med.* 2020;382(16): 1507-1519.

81. Bhatt DL, Steg PG, Miller M, et al. Cardiovascular risk reduction with icosapent ethyl for hypertriglyceridemia. *N Engl J Med.* 2019;380(1):11-22.

82. Ray KK, Bays HE, Catapano AL, et al. Safety and efficacy of bempedoic acid to reduce LDL cholesterol. *N Engl J Med.* 2019;380(11):1022-1032.

83. McMurray JJ, Packer M, Desai AS, et al. Angiotensin-neprilysin inhibition versus enalapril in heart failure. *N Engl J Med.* 2014;371(11):993-1004.

84. Armstrong PW, Pieske B, Anstrom KJ et al. Vericiguat in patients with heart failure and reduced ejection fraction. *N Engl J Med.* 2020;382(20):1883-1893.

85. Washam JB, Herzog CA, Beitelshees AL, et al. Pharmacotherapy in chronic kidney disease patients presenting with acute coronary syndrome: a scientific statement from the American Heart Association. *Circulation.* 2015;131(12):1123-1149.

86. Mehta LS, Beckie TM, DeVon HA, et al. Acute myocardial infarction in women: a scientific Statement from the American Heart Association. *Circulation.* 2016;133(9):916-947.

87. Levine GN, Bates ER, Bittl JA, et al. 2016 ACC/AHA guideline focused update on duration of dual antiplatelet therapy in patients with coronary artery disease: a report of the American College of Cardiology/American Heart Association Task Force on Clinical Practice Guidelines. *J Am Coll Cardiol.* 2016;68(10):1082-1115.

88. Valgimigli M, Bueno H, Byrne RA, et al. 2017 ESC focused update on dual antiplatelet therapy in coronary artery disease developed in collaboration with EACTS: The Task Force for dual antiplatelet therapy in coronary artery disease of the European Society of Cardiology (ESC) and of the European Association for Cardio-Thoracic Surgery (EACTS). *Eur Heart J.* 2018;39(3):213-260.

Mimickers of Atherosclerotic Myocardial Infarction

SCAD, Coronary Vasospasm, Myocarditis, and takotsubo Syndrome

Jacqueline Saw, Jaya Chandrasekhar, Sarah Zaman, and Harmony Reynolds

CHAPTER OUTLINE

INTRODUCTION / 621

SPONTANEOUS CORONARY ARTERY DISSECTION (SCAD) / 621

Epidemiology / 621

Pathophysiology (Predisposing and Precipitating Causes) / 621

Genetics / 622

Diagnosis / 622

Management / 623

Prognosis / 625

Guidelines and Knowledge Gaps / 625

CORONARY VASOSPASM / 625

Epidemiology / 626

Pathogenesis and Role of Genetics / 626

Presentation, Triggers, and ECG Changes / 627

Diagnosis / 628

Treatment / 629

Natural History and Prognosis / 631

Summary / 632

MYOCARDITIS / 632

Epidemiology / 632

Natural History / 633

Pathogenesis / 633

Viral Myocarditis / 633

Autoimmune Myocarditis / 635

Toxic Myocarditis / 635

Myocarditis as an ACS Mimicker / 635

Diagnostic Approaches / 636

Invasive Approaches / 636

Endomyocardial Biopsy / 637
Coronary Angiography / 637

Noninvasive Approaches / 637

Echocardiography / 637
Cardiac Magnetic Resonance Imaging / 637
Viral Serology / 638

Genetics / 639

Clinical Challenges / 639

Therapeutic Challenges / 639

Treatment / 639

Immunosuppression / 639

Immunomodulation / 640

Guidelines / 640

Summary / 640

TAKOTSUBO SYNDROME / 640

Definition / 640

Epidemiology / 640

Pathogenesis / 641

Presentation: Symptoms, Triggers, ECG Findings, and Laboratory Test Results / 643

Patterns of Cardiac Wall Motion Abnormalities / 643

Distinguishing TTS from Acute MI / 645

Suggested Diagnostic Approach / 645

Acute Complications / 645

Outcomes / 646

Summary / 646

CONGENITAL ANOMALIES AND KAWASAKI DISEASE / 646

Anomalous Coronary Arteries / 646

Kawasaki Disease / 647

SUMMARY / 648

ACKNOWLEDGMENT / 648

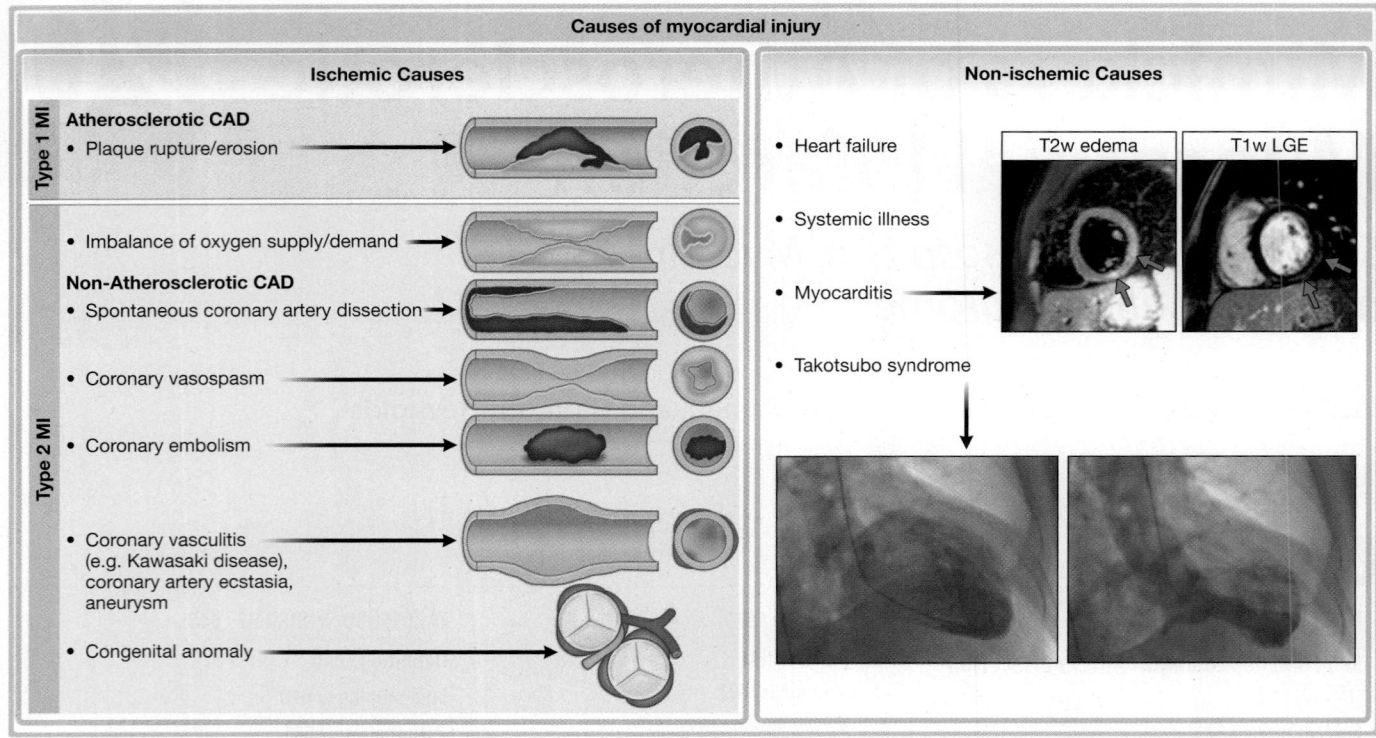

Chapter 20 Fuster and Hurst's Central Illustration. Causes of myocardial injury can be ischemic or non-ischemic. Both type 1 and type 2 MI may occur without obstructive disease (MINOCA). Differentiating the etiology of myocardial injury is important for prompt and appropriate management of acute coronary syndrome. Red arrows indicate patchy focal edema in the subepicardium of the inferolateral wall. CAD, coronary artery disease; LGE, late gadolinium enhancement; MI, myocardial infarction. Magnetic resonance images of myocarditis reproduced from Caforio et al. Current state of knowledge on aetiology, diagnosis, management and therapy of myocarditis: a position statement of the European Society of Cardiology Working Group on Myocardial and Pericardial Diseases. *Eur Heart J.* 2013;34:2636-2648.

CHAPTER SUMMARY

This chapter discusses important nonatherosclerotic etiologies of myocardial injury, which can be due to ischemic or non-ischemic causes (see Fuster and Hurst's Central Illustration). Differentiating the etiology of myocardial injury is critical because the management strategy differs for atherosclerotic versus nonatherosclerotic causes. Type 1 myocardial infarctions (MIs) are due to atherosclerotic plaque rupture/erosion with thrombus formation and typically require invasive management for restoration of coronary perfusion. Type 2 MIs can result from ischemia due to imbalance of oxygen supply and demand, or nonatherosclerotic causes such as spontaneous coronary artery dissection, coronary vasospasm, coronary embolism, coronary vasculitis, coronary ectasia, and anatomic coronary artery anomaly. Causes of nonischemic myocardial injury include myocarditis, takotsubo syndrome, and heart failure. The management of type 2 MIs and nonischemic causes of myocardial injury depends on the underlying etiology, and thus discerning these "mimickers" of non-type 1 MI is pertinent for prompt and appropriate management of acute coronary syndromes.

INTRODUCTION

Acute coronary syndrome (ACS) denotes the presence of myocardial ischemia that can result in a spectrum of clinical symptoms and presentations, including unstable angina, ST-elevation myocardial infarction (STEMI), and non-ST-elevation MI (NSTEMI). As per the Fourth Universal Definition of Myocardial Infarction,[1] the term myocardial infarction (MI) requires not only the presence of myocardial injury (acute rise and fall of troponin) but also acute myocardial ischemia as the underlying cause, together with symptoms and/or signs of ischemia/infarction. Myocardial injury has numerous causes (ischemic and nonischemic causes) and can easily be detected by modern highly sensitive assays for cardiac biomarkers. Differentiating the etiology of myocardial injury is critical as the management strategy differs for atherosclerotic versus nonatherosclerotic causes of cardiomyocyte deaths. Type 1 MIs are due to atherosclerotic plaque rupture/erosion with thrombus that typically requires invasive management with percutaneous coronary intervention (PCI), with the exception of MI with nonobstructive coronary arteries (MINOCA) whereby medical stabilization may suffice. Type 2 MIs result from ischemia due to imbalance of oxygen supply and demand, which may occur in the setting of atherosclerotic obstructive coronary disease, or nonatherosclerotic causes such as spontaneous coronary artery dissection (SCAD), coronary vasospasm, coronary embolism, hypotension/shock, arrhythmia, respiratory failure, and anemia. Myocardial injury can also result from nonischemic causes such as myocarditis, takotsubo syndrome (TTS), heart failure, cardiac procedures, and systemic illnesses. The management of type 2 MIs and nonischemic causes of myocardial injury obviously depends on the underlying etiology, and thus discerning these "mimickers" of non-type 1 MI is pertinent for prompt and appropriate management of ACS. It is important to keep in mind that SCAD and coronary vasospasm both cause true MI, which meets the universal definition of MI and can cause cardiac magnetic resonance imaging (MRI) evidence of scarring that is indistinguishable from that induced by type 1 MI. In this chapter, we review in-depth the "mimickers" that are important causes of ACS and MI, highlighting the differences in diagnosis, management, and investigations compared to atherosclerotic type 1 MI.

SPONTANEOUS CORONARY ARTERY DISSECTION (SCAD)

Epidemiology

SCAD is defined as a nontraumatic, noniatrogenic, and non-atherosclerotic separation of the coronary arterial wall by spontaneous rupture of the intima or vasa vasorum within the vessel wall.[2] This results in accumulation of intramural hematoma (IMH) within the false lumen that compresses the true lumen, causing myocardial ischemia or infarction. SCAD was first reported in 1931 and was initially thought to be rare. Subsequent early reports for several decades were limited by case reports and small case series. However, since 2010, publications on SCAD rapidly expanded due to increased recognition

from the use of high-resolution intracoronary imaging (especially optical coherence tomography [OCT]), which led to better angiographic recognition of SCAD. This is coupled with heightened awareness of cardiac disease in young women and increased rate of coronary angiography in women presenting with ACS. This recent increase in diagnosis led to the recognition that SCAD is much more common and is an important cause of MI in women. The true incidence and prevalence of SCAD remains unknown due to under and misdiagnosis of the condition. Among patients presenting with ACS, SCAD was reported to be the cause in 1% to 4% on coronary angiography,[3,4] and a rare cause of sudden cardiac death in 0.5% of autopsy cases.[5] These values are believed to be underestimated due to underrecognition. In recent series, SCAD was shown to be the cause of MI in 25% to 35% of women age <50, and in up to 25% of women age <60.[6-8] It is also the most common cause of pregnancy-associated MI (up to 43%), primarily occurring in the third trimester or postpartum stage.[9] SCAD predominantly affects women in >90% of cases, and ~60% of these women are post menopausal.[10-12] The mean age of SCAD patients ranges from 45 to 53 years, thus affecting mostly young-to-middle-aged women.[7,12-16] Most patients have few or no conventional cardiovascular risk factors. Instead, they have different risk profiles with high prevalence of migraine (~40%), depression (~25%), and anxiety (~15%).[15,17,18]

Pathophysiology (Predisposing and Precipitating Causes)

The etiology of SCAD appears to be multifactorial, usually with an underlying predisposing arteriopathy, and often precipitated by additional emotional or physical stressors (**Table 20–1**). Fibromuscular dysplasia (FMD) is the most commonly observed associated disease, reported in 50% to 86% of patients with SCAD.[10,15,19] Other less commonly associated diseases include inherited connective tissue disorders (~5%), systemic inflammatory diseases (5%–12%), hormonal therapy usage (eg, estrogen, progesterone, gonadotrophin, clomiphene, fertility treatment), and pregnancy-associated cases (eg, peripartum [<5%], multiple pregnancies).[17,20,21] These conditions are believed to weaken the coronary artery wall through various mechanisms, acutely, or chronically through repetitive insults.

FMD is a noninflammatory, nonatherosclerotic disorder of the arterial vasculature that can cause arterial stenosis, occlusion, aneurysm, and/or dissection. It can involve any small-to-medium-sized arterial beds, especially the renal, carotid, and iliac arteries. FMD affecting the coronary arteries have also been reported in several histopathological SCAD case reports. Coronary FMD can cause dysplasia, disorganization, and/or destruction of cells (eg, smooth muscle cells and fibroblasts) and connective tissue matrix (eg, collagen, elastic fibers, and proteoglycan) that can affect any of the three arterial layers and elastic laminas.[22] Clinically, coronary FMD can be challenging to diagnose since the angiographic appearance of tortuosity, stenosis (irregular or smooth), and segmental dilatation/ectasia are not unique to FMD.[22] Nevertheless, case series of coronary FMD observed on angiography in SCAD patients were reported.[23]

TABLE 20–1. Predisposing Arteriopathies and Precipitating Stressors for SCAD

Predisposing causes
Fibromuscular dysplasia
Pregnancy-related: antepartum, early postpartum, late postpartum, very late postpartum
Recurrent pregnancies: multiparity or multigravida
Connective tissue disorder: Marfan syndrome, Loeys-Dietz syndrome, Ehler-Danlos syndrome type 4, cystic medical necrosis, alpha-1 anti-trypsin deficiency, polycystic kidney disease
Systemic inflammatory disease: systemic lupus erythematosus, Crohn's disease, ulcerative colitis, polyarteritis nodosa, sarcoidosis, Churg-Strauss syndrome, Wegener's granulomatosis, rheumatoid arthritis, Kawasaki, giant cell arteritis, celiac disease
Hormonal therapy: oral contraceptive, estrogen, progesterone, beta-HCG, testosterone, corticosteroids
Coronary artery spasm
Idiopathic

Precipitating stressors
Intense exercises (isometric or aerobic activities)
Intense emotional stress
Labor and delivery
Intense Valsave-type activities (eg, retching, vomiting, bowel movement, coughing)
Recreational drugs (eg, cocaine, amphetamines, methamphetamines)
Intense hormonal therapy (eg, beta-HCG injections, corticosteroids injections)

Abbreviations: HCG, human chronic gonadotropin; SCAD, spontaneous coronary artery dissection.
Reproduced with permission from Saw J, Mancini GBJ, Humphries KH. Contemporary Review on Spontaneous Coronary Artery Dissection. *J Am Coll Cardiol*. 2016 Jul 19; 68(3):297-312.

Conditions that increase intracoronary shear stress, such as physical (increase thoraco-abdominal pressure) and emotional triggers may precipitate SCAD. Emotional stress was reported in ~50% of patients, and intense physical stress in 29%, with isometric activities lifting >50 pounds in 10% of SCAD cases.[24] The combination of these triggers in the setting of underlying arteriopathies set up the "perfect storm" inciting the dissection in many cases.

Genetics

Aside from infrequent monogenic vascular connective tissue diagnoses (eg, Marfan syndrome due to FBN1 and vascular Ehlers–Danlos syndrome due to COL3A1 pathogenic variation) observed in <5% of cases, familial studies of SCAD inheritance are lacking, although familial clustering had been reported.[25,26] A common variant on chromosome 6p24.1 in the *PHACTR1* gene (rs9349379-A) had been associated with both FMD (odds ratio [OR] = 1.4) and SCAD (OR = 1.7).[27,28] This allele has also been associated with cervical artery dissection and migraine. In a genome-wide association study of SCAD, a number of alleles were identified that associated with SCAD. Importantly, rs12740679 at chromosome 1q21.2 (OR = 1.8) influences ADAMTSL4 expression.[40] *ADAMTSL4* is a member of the ADAMTS (a disintegrin and metalloproteinase with thrombospondin motifs)-like gene family, which encodes an

extracellular matrix protein that binds to fibrillin-1 to promote the formation of microfibrils in the matrix.[29] In the study by Saw et al, histopathological data localized ADAMTSL4 protein and mRNA expression to the medial layer of the arterial wall and medial vascular smooth muscle cells, which was consistent with the arterial media as the site of dissection and IMH.[30] Other associations were chromosome 6p24.1 in PHACTR1, chromosome 12q13.3 in LRP1, and in females-only, at chromosome 21q22.11 near LINC00310.[31] The derived polygenic risk score for SCAD from this study was associated with higher risk of SCAD in FMD patients ($P = 0.021$, OR = 1.82) and lower risk of atherosclerotic coronary artery disease and MI. Thus, SCAD-related MI and atherosclerotic MI appear to exist at opposite ends of a genetic risk spectrum. These recent studies support a complex genetic basis of SCAD, and ongoing large meta-analysis efforts are anticipated to reveal further genomic insights.

Diagnosis

Most patients with SCAD present with chest pain and biomarker evidence of MI.[24,32] Coronary angiography remains the cornerstone for diagnosing SCAD, which can appear with characteristic dissection features or subtle findings that can mimic atherosclerosis. Intracoronary imaging with OCT or intravascular ultrasound (IVUS) can help with the diagnosis of SCAD; however, there are associated risks with propagation of dissection and iatrogenic catheter-induced dissection, and therefore usage should be limited to cases where the diagnosis is unclear. A novel angiographic SCAD classification stratifying angiographic variants of SCAD into three types have facilitated diagnosis and is increasingly adopted (**Fig. 20–1**).[13,17,24] Type 1 describes the presence of contrast within arterial wall exposing multiple radiolucent lumens. Type 2 depicts diffuse and smooth stenosis (usually >20 mm in length) due to IMH and can be of varying severity. Type 3 describes focal or tubular stenosis that mimics atherosclerosis and generally requires intracoronary imaging to confirm IMH or double-lumen.

In the largest angiographic SCAD series of 1002 dissected arteries evaluated by core laboratory in the Canadian SCAD Study, the most common angiographic appearance was Type 2 SCAD in 60.2% of cases, with Type 3 SCAD being least frequent in 10.8% of cases.[17,24] The classic Type 1 SCAD was observed in 29.0% of cases. In this series, 5.5% had OCT-confirmed SCAD, and 2.1% had IVUS-confirmed SCAD. Any coronary artery can be affected by SCAD, although the most commonly involved is the left anterior descending artery (LAD) in 52.1% of cases, followed by the circumflex artery (37.7%) and the right coronary artery (23.2%).[17] The mean length of dissection was 33.2 mm. The majority had only one artery (86.9%) and one segment (74.8%) affected. Multivessel noncontiguous dissections occur in ~15% of cases.[17,24] Four or more simultaneous noncontiguous dissected arteries in one SCAD presentation is rare but has been reported.[33]

Coronary computed tomography angiography (CCTA) is increasingly utilized to evaluate low and intermediate risk patients presenting with ACS; however, its role in SCAD has

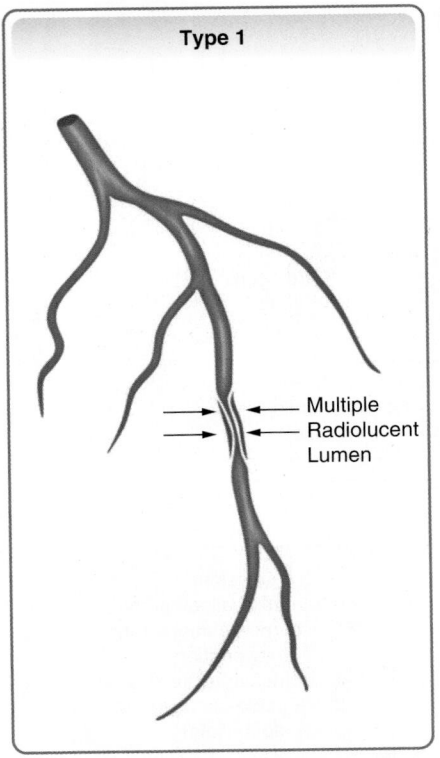
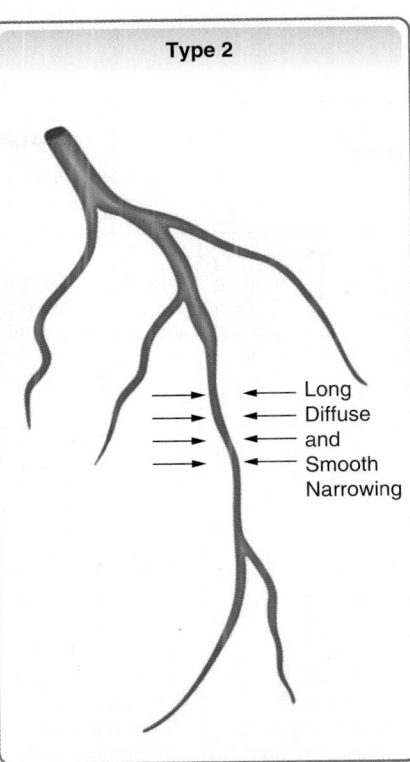
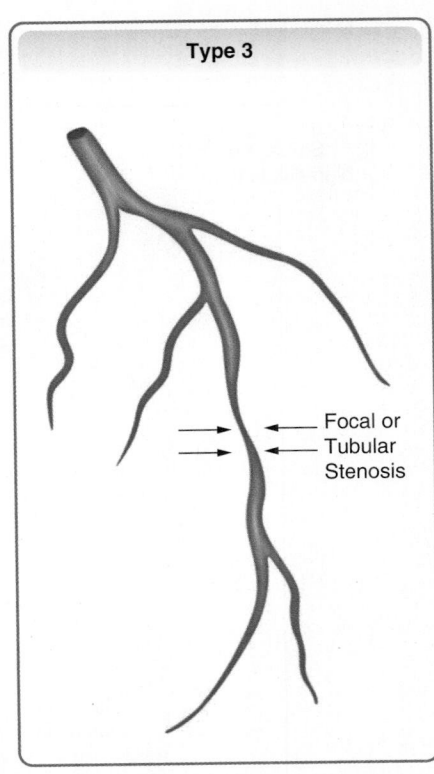

Figure 20–1. Angiographic subtypes of SCAD. Reproduced with permission from Saw J, Humphries K, Aymong E, et al. Spontaneous Coronary Artery Dissection: Clinical Outcomes and Risk of Recurrence. *J Am Coll Cardiol*. 2017 Aug 29;70(9):1148-1158.

not been established. CCTA is not recommended as the first-line imaging modality for suspected acute SCAD since it does not have sufficient sensitivity to exclude SCAD, due to its lower spatial and temporal resolution compared to invasive coronary angiography. IMH can mimic the appearance of cardiac motion artifact and further limits CCTA. In two small series, CCTA identified 2 out of 14 and 10 out of 14 SCAD cases, respectively, compared to angiography.[34,35] However, CCTA can be utilized to noninvasively monitor for resolution of SCAD in cases where proximal or large arteries are dissected, particularly given the risk of iatrogenic catheter-induced dissection with angiography. Indeed, the risk of iatrogenic dissection during angiography of SCAD patients was reported at 3.4% (2.0% with diagnostic catheterization, and 14.3% with ad hoc PCI), and therefore, careful meticulous techniques with angiography is necessary.[36]

Cardiac magnetic resonance imaging (CMR) may be helpful to differentiate SCAD versus other etiology (eg, nonobstructive atherosclerotic plaque rupture/erosion, myocarditis, or TTS) especially when SCAD diagnosis is elusive on coronary angiography. In acute SCAD cases, late gadolinium enhancement was observed in the majority of patients in small case series with varying degrees of severity (transmural, subendocardial, or patchy),[37,38] and large infarcts can have associated microvascular obstruction and intramyocardial hemorrhage.[39] CMR can help rule-out other/concurrent causes of MI-mimics (eg, myocarditis, TTS). The utility of CMR in the chronic phase to prognosticate post-SCAD is not established.

Management

The management recommendations for SCAD have been derived from observational studies and expert opinions since there is no randomized trial data available. Conservative therapy is the preferred management strategy for stable patients. Revascularization with PCI or coronary artery bypass graft (CABG) surgery is recommended only if high-risk features are present (ie, left main dissection, ongoing ischemia, hemodynamic instability, sustained ventricular arrhythmias). This is based on the observation that the majority of SCAD arteries heal spontaneously, and that revascularization is challenging and associated with high failure rates.[2] The recommended management algorithm is depicted in **Fig. 20–2.**[2] Patients managed conservatively should be monitored in-hospital for 3 to 5 days depending on symptoms and anatomic location of SCAD.[7] Peripartum SCAD (P-SCAD) patients should be admitted for longer duration given their higher complication rates in-hospital.[24]

For conservatively-managed patients, several small retrospective studies had shown that spontaneous angiographic healing occurred in 73% to 97% of cases on repeat angiography.[2] In the largest series from Vancouver of 156 patients with 182 SCAD lesions, 95% of lesions healed (improved stenosis severity, residual stenosis <50%, and TIMI-3 flow) when repeat angiograms were performed ≥30 days post-SCAD.[40] There was time-dependency for arterial healing to occur, with early resorption of IMH beginning within days as shown on OCT,[17]

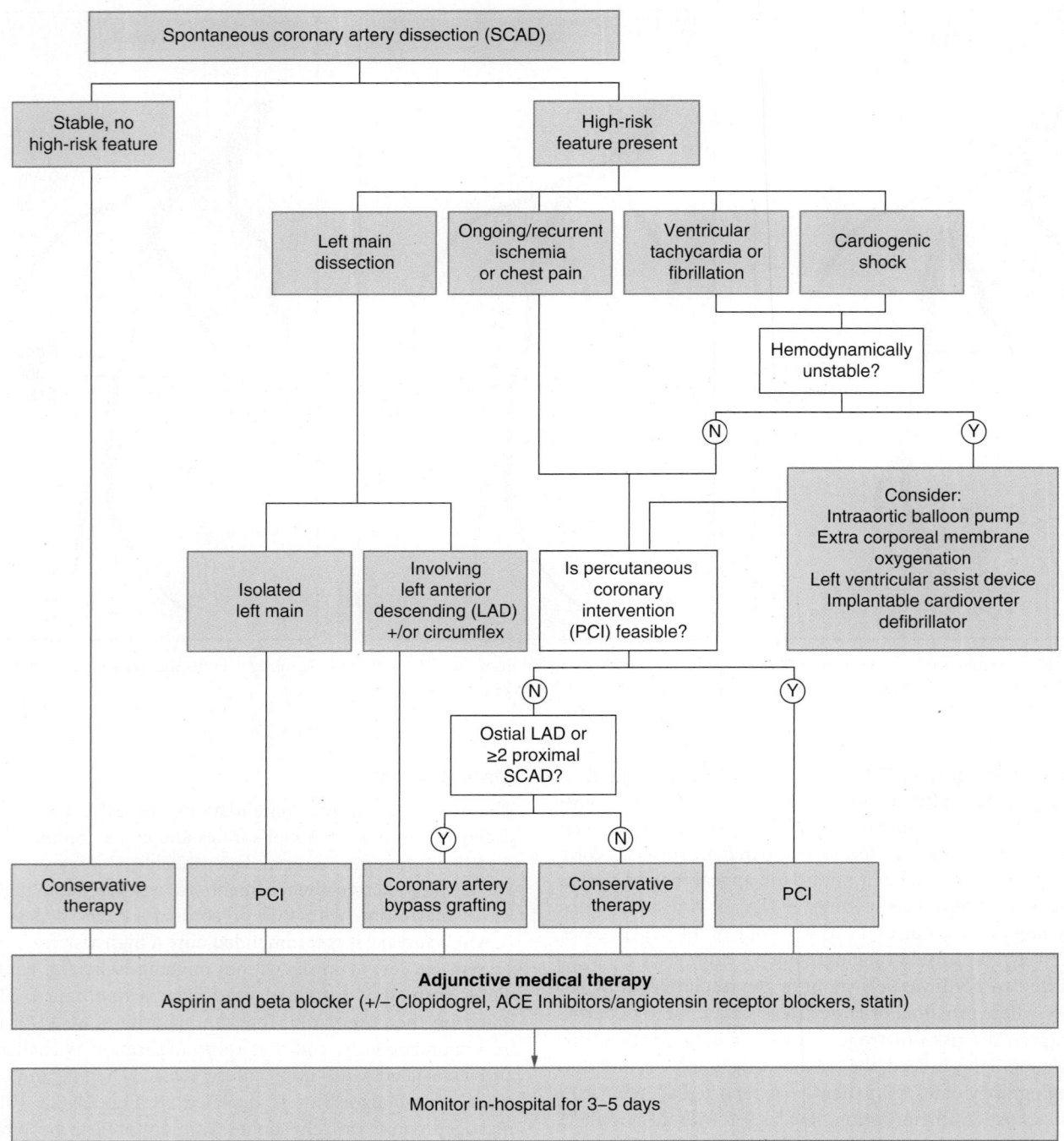

Figure 20–2. Management algorithm for SCAD. Reproduced with permission from Saw J, Mancini GBJ, Humphries KH. Contemporary Review on Spontaneous Coronary Artery Dissection. *J Am Coll Cardiol*. 2016 Jul 19;68(3):297-312.

and full resorption often requiring several weeks depending on IMH volume within the false lumen.

In cases where revascularization is necessary and if technically feasible, PCI is preferred over CABG, unless patients have left main dissection or failed PCI. However, PCI for SCAD can be technically challenging and associated with high complication and failure rates. Reported PCI success rates ranged from 47% to 91%.[2] The technical challenges include iatrogenic catheter-induced coronary artery dissection, difficulty wiring into the true lumen, and propagation of dissection or IMH with wiring, angioplasty, or stenting. If stenting is required, often multiple long stents are required due to extensive dissections, which increases the risk of restenosis and stent thrombosis. Late stent malapposition can also occur with natural resorption of IMH, potentially increasing the risk of late stent thrombosis.[41] PCI strategies include balloon angioplasty alone, cutting balloon angioplasty to fenestrate and decompress IMH, use of long stents to cover both edges of dissections by >5 mm, stenting the distal and proximal ends of the dissection with short stents before stenting the middle of the dissection, and use of bioabsorbable stents if available.

For medical management, SCAD patients are routinely administered aspirin and beta-blocker long-term. Short-term P2Y$_{12}$ receptor antagonist therapy (eg, clopidogrel) is often administered for 1 to 12 months post-SCAD; however, this agent is controversial in patients not receiving intracoronary stenting. Angiotensin-converting enzyme (ACE) inhibitor or angiotensin receptor blocker (ARB) is administered if there is left ventricular (LV) dysfunction, and statin is administered if there is underlying dyslipidemia. With the exception of beta-blocker, none of the other pharmaceutical agents have been demonstrated to be beneficial in SCAD. In a 327 SCAD series from Vancouver, beta-blocker use was associated with lower risk of recurrent SCAD (hazard ratio [HR] 0.36, $P = 0.004$).[17]

Following the acute SCAD event, cardiac rehabilitation is recommended, preferably with modified protocol avoiding heavy isometric and intense aerobic activities.[42] Weight restrictions to less than 30 lb for women and 50 lb for men (<14 kg and <23 kg, respectively) have been suggested.[42] Also, competitive and high-intensity aerobic sports should be curtailed. Other strategies to prevent recurrent SCAD include minimizing emotional triggers, avoiding hormonal therapy (ie, estrogen, progesterone, beta-HCG), and avoiding future pregnancies.[3]

Prognosis

In the Canadian SCAD Study, acute survival was excellent, with low in-hospital mortality of only 0.1%. However, other in-hospital and 30-day outcomes were not benign. Other important in-hospital major adverse events included recurrent MI (4.0%), severe ventricular arrhythmia (3.9%), cardiogenic shock (2.0%), stroke/TIA (0.8%), congestive heart failure (CHF) (0.3%), and unplanned revascularization in 2.5%. The majority of SCAD patients were treated conservatively (86.4%), only 11.9% underwent PCI and 0.3% underwent CABG.[24] Of those treated conservatively, only 2.0% subsequently required PCI and 0.3% required CABG. The median hospital stay was 4 days. The 30-day major adverse cardiovascular events (MACE) occurred in 8.8% of patients, including recurrent MI, unplanned revascularization, stroke/TIA, and CHF. P-SCAD and connective tissue disorder were independent predictors of 30-day MACE.[24] Therefore, these patients may require more aggressive management.

Following hospital discharge, early readmission rates in SCAD patients are high. Emergency room visit for cardiac reasons was 4.9% and admission for chest pain was 2.5% at 30 days in the Canadian SCAD Study.[24] Two recent analyses from the National Readmission Database also showed higher readmission rate at 30 days among SCAD patients (12.3% vs 9.9%, $P = 0.022$) compared to a propensity-matched non-SCAD cohort, and readmission rate of 22% at 90 days (median time to readmission 29 days) with 55.4% due to cardiac reasons.[43,44] At longer-term follow-up, 2-year MACE were reported in 10% to 30% of patients, which was primarily comprised of recurrent MI due to recurrent SCAD.[7,17,45] Overall long-term survival was

>95% despite relatively high MACE rates between 15% and 37% at 5 to 7 years.[14,15,45,46] MACE-rates at 10 years post-SCAD were estimated at 50%, with 30% due to recurrent SCAD.[14,15,46] The risks associated with recurrent SCAD are not clearly elucidated; however, presence of underlying hypertension and coronary tortuosity were associated with higher risk, and the use of beta-blockers was associated with lower risk of recurrent SCAD.[17,47] There is limited published data on the risk of recurrent SCAD with pregnancy post-SCAD. A recent series from the Mayo Clinic reported that 2 out of 23 women who had pregnancy post-SCAD had a recurrent SCAD event (out of 32 pregnancies with 20 live births).[48]

Guidelines and Knowledge Gaps

The American Heart Association (AHA) and the European Society of Cardiology (ESC) published their SCAD scientific statements in 2018.[3,49] And both documents have similar recommendations from expert consensus with regards to diagnosis, management, and investigation for associated diseases. Several knowledge gaps remain with SCAD, with regards to prevalence, etiology, management, and outcomes. This disease remains underdiagnosed and misdiagnosed, which results in inaccuracies in estimating the true prevalence. The underlying etiology for SCAD appears multifactorial, but the proportional contribution and importance of genetic, hormonal, and environment causes leading to predisposing arteriopathies, and the relative role of overlying triggers, remain unknown. Many uncertainties remain as to the best management strategy, and post-SCAD lifestyle changes and medical therapies to reduce recurrent SCAD and cardiac events. Real-world registries are instrumental since this being a relatively rare disease makes conducting large randomized trials challenging; thus, registries will continue to be the main data source to guide the management of SCAD patients.

CORONARY VASOSPASM

Myron Prinzmetal first referred to coronary vasospasm as variant angina in 1959.[50] He noted that his patients experienced diurnal symptoms of chest pain at rest with ST-segment elevation on electrocardiography (ECG). Such patients were subsequently found on coronary angiography to have nonobstructive coronary artery disease (CAD), with constrictions that could be localized, multifocal, or multivessel, suggestive of a supply rather than demand issue. Coronary vasospasm is currently a well-recognized cause for functional angina, usually starting in the fifth decade of life. Particularly common among Asian patients, the Japanese circulation society was among the first to have a dedicated guidance document on this condition, referred to as vasospastic angina, which has since been updated.[51] In recent years widespread reports have become available globally; nevertheless, vasospastic angina frequently remains a suspected rather than proven diagnosis in common clinical practice even after exclusion of obstructive disease, due to the limited uptake of provocation testing. Recent studies have amply demonstrated the morbidity associated with ischemia and nonobstructive coronary artery disease (INOCA), and have shown compelling evidence for the overlapping prevalence of coronary vasospasm and coronary microvascular dysfunction (CMD).[52-55] While vasospasm may be related to endothelial dysfunction, CMD is linked with endothelial independent processes. Most recently, the Coronary Vasomotion Disorders International Study Group (COVADIS) group has defined the criteria for vasospastic angina based on coronary reactivity testing,[56] which is commonly undertaken with acetylcholine or ergonovine to test for endothelial dysfunction. Adenosine is commonly used to test endothelial independent dysfunction under conditions of hyperemia to assess for coexisting CMD. The CorMicA trial is a recent landmark trial that reported the prevalence of vasospasm and CMD among INOCA patients, and in a randomized setting examined the effect of diagnostic accuracy on recurrent angina and quality of life after interventional diagnostic testing compared to usual care based on angiography alone.[57]

Epidemiology

Approximately 6% of patients with MI can have MI nonobstructive disease (MINOCA), which can include causes such as vasospasm; however, some have reported the prevalence of coronary vasospasm to be approximately 50% in ACS and all-comer patients.[54,58] Some experts consider microvascular coronary vasospasm, a component of microvascular angina to be encompassed in the diagnosis of vasospasm.[55] Microvascular spasm can cause MI. In a registry of 921 White patients with nonobstructive CAD, Ong et al. noted 33.4% with epicardial spasm and 24.2% with microvascular spasm.[59] In a sample of 80 MINOCA patients, Montone et al. observed 64.9% with epicardial spasm and 35.1% with microvascular spasm.[60]

Coronary vasospasm can affect both men and women, although there are conflicting reports on sex differences in prevalence.[61-64] In a European population of 1327 German and Danish patients, Aziz et al. noted that vasomotor dysfunction with acetylcholine testing was more common in women by a greater odds of 4.2 for epicardial or microvascular spasm, after multivariable adjustment.[61] The mean age of patients in this registry was 62 years. A pathological acetylcholine test was more common in women (70% vs 43%, $P < 0.001$) and was observed at lower doses of acetylcholine. Di Fiore et al. found that in an Australian population of 183 patients undergoing acetylcholine challenge in the absence of obstructive CAD, the mean age was 54.1 ± 11.1 years and nearly 78% of patients were women;[62] 82% were White, 10% Indigenous Australians, and 4% Asian. However, there were no differences in the proportion of women with or without evidence of spasm (75% vs 79%, $P = 0.51$) on acetylcholine testing in this study.

Conversely several groups have shown that variant angina was more common in men, who also had a higher prevalence of concurrent CAD and smoking.[63-65] Lee et al. reported on 986 patients undergoing ergonovine challenge, and 85% were men with high prevalence of smoking.[65] Women were younger with less CAD. Women required more ergonovine to induce spasm. While women had more spasm in the right coronary artery

(RCA), men had greater spasm in the left circumflex (LCx). On long-term follow-up to 11 years, major adverse cardiac events (MACE) was similar in both sexes. Coma-Conella et al. examined 162 patients, out of which 85 patients underwent ergonovine testing.[64] Of these, 47% had RCA spasm; 14% had left anterior descending (LAD) artery and RCA spasm; 7%, 6%, and 6%, respectively, had spasm in the LAD, LAD and LCx, and LCx respectively; and 18% had spasm in all arteries. Men had a higher proportion of positive ergonovine tests (61% vs 34%, $P = 0.001$). Functional stress testing did not correlate with ergonovine testing, rather it predicted spasm only in 55.2%.

Kobayashi et al. reported on sex differences in vasomotor testing from a prospective cohort of 117 women and 40 men with INOCA who underwent interventional procedures with coronary flow reserve (CFR) and index of maximum hyperemia (IMR) using thermodilution, fractional flow reserve (FFR), and quantitative coronary angiography (QCA) in the LAD.[66] CFR was assessed using the thermodilution method for obtaining mean coronary blood flow transit time at rest and hyperemia. By QCA, mean diameter stenosis was $23.2 \pm 12.3\%$. Women had slightly higher FFR (0.88 ± 0.04 vs 0.87 ± 0.04; $P = 0.04$), lower CFR (3.8 ± 1.6 vs 4.8 ± 1.9; $P = 0.004$) but similar IMR to men (20.7 ± 9.8 vs 19.1 ± 8.0; $P = 0.45$). This was due to greater resting coronary flow and thus shorter resting mean transit time in women, without differences in hyperemic transit time. Female sex was an independent predictor of lower CFR.

Coronary spasm can also occur in the setting of recreational drug usage, such as cocaine, cannabis, or amphetamines,[67] which is commonly seen in younger patients, and in response to cancer chemotherapeutics such as 5-fluorouracil, or its prodrug capecitabine, or triptan antimigraine agents.[68,69] The incidence of coronary spasm and possible thrombosis on 5-fluorouracil, or capecitabine, has been reported to vary from 1% to 68%.[68] In a study of 377 patients with 5-fluorouracil induced cardiotoxicity, over one-third had traditional cardiovascular risk factors, including smoking, which was the most common risk factor.[70] 5-fluorouracil treatment with an infusion rather than a bolus has been linked with greater likelihood of coronary events, and usually this resolves with cessation of treatment. Treatment with sumatriptan, a serotonin agonist, has been noted to cause coronary spasm in patients with variant angina, from a small study of nine patients.[69] Serotonin has previously been shown to be a strong trigger for coronary vasospasm.[71]

Pathogenesis and Role of Genetics

The pathogenesis of vasospasm is considered to be related to endothelial dysfunction and smooth muscle hyperreactivity in response to vasoconstrictor stimuli or postreceptor alterations and autonomic dysregulation.[72] Endothelial dysfunction hampers the normal vasodilatory response or promotes vasoconstriction in response to certain stimuli. Inflammation, oxidative stress, and genetics may also have a role. Inflammatory markers such as C-reactive protein, interleukin-6, soluble CD40 ligand, monocytes, and polymorphonuclear neutrophils have been linked with vasospasm.[73-75] Other biochemical molecules including endothelin-1, bradykinin, histamine, serotonin, thromboxane A2, vasopressin, and rho-kinase have also been implicated.[73,76]

Nitric oxide (NO) plays a crucial role in healthy endothelial function. NO synthase mutation and Glu298Asp and T786C polymorphisms have been shown to result in reduced production of NO and endothelial dysfunction. Polymorphisms in the paraoxonase-1 gene has been associated with greater oxidative stress and coronary spasm. Polymorphisms in the endothelin-1 gene have been shown to be associated with endothelial dysregulation and spasm in Koreans.[77]

Vasospasm has been described to a greater extent in Japanese patients than Caucasians.[78] Murase et al. noted that the NADH/NADPH oxidase *p22phox* gene was a susceptibility locus for coronary spasm in men, and the stromelysin-1 and interleukin-6 genes were susceptibility loci in women. Smoking was also noted to be an independent risk factor in this study.

In addition, hyperresponsiveness to smooth muscle contraction may result in spasm. The implicated molecules are rho-kinase and protein kinase C that affect calcium sensitization of the myosin light chain.[72] Recreational drug usage can enhance smooth muscle contraction, and contribute to coronary vasospasm via this mechanism.

Presentation, Triggers, and ECG Changes

Patients with coronary vasospasm can present with stable angina, rest pain, or ACS including cardiac arrest or aborted sudden cardiac death (ASCD). In the registry by Ong et al., 35% patients had chest pain at rest, 22% had exertional chest pain, 24% had mixed symptoms, and 4% presented with troponin-positive ACS.[59] Coma-Conella et al. studied chest pain characteristics among 162 enrolled patients. Of these, 36.4% had rest pain, 24.7% had effort pain, 9% had pain at night, 19.1% had mixed pain, and 11% had atypical pain.[64] Resting angina was a strong predictor of spasm in the study by Ong et al.,[59] but not in other studies.[61,64]

Patients with vasospasm, particularly males, may have a high prevalence of smoking, prior CAD, and dyslipidemia whereas other traditional cardiovascular risk factors including hypertension and diabetes tend to be low. Vasospastic angina may be associated with other vasospastic conditions such as migraine and Raynaud's disease.[53]

Some groups have noted that patients may demonstrate both epicardial vasospasm and microvascular angina.[55] The two have previously been considered to be distinct entities with vasospasm occurring at rest and microvascular angina with exercise. Vasospasm is frequently linked with mild CAD, whereas microvascular angina patients may have no disease on angiography. Typically, there are also diurnal changes with vasospasm with patients experiencing symptoms at night or early in the morning and on exposure to cold and with hyperventilation, usually at rest but also with effort; whereas in microvascular angina, symptoms are classically produced with effort. The circadian rhythm of variant angina has been described by other authors. Autonomic changes are implicated as a trigger, with either an increase in adrenergic surge or withdrawal of vagal stimulation.

Togashi et al. examined a small sample of patients with sudden cardiac arrest (n = 18) or syncope (n = 28) triggered by coronary spasm, compared to spasm patients with angina only (n = 52).[79] Cardiac arrest and syncope frequently occurred during daytime in 57% and 68% patients, respectively. Conversely, nocturnal angina occurred less frequently in these patients compared to angina-only patients (33% and 32% vs 83%, $P < 0.01$ for each). Spontaneous ST-segment changes during daytime were recorded in 50% and 39% respectively compared to 4% in angina-only patients ($P < 0.01$ for all). Severe multivessel spasm, daytime ST-segment changes, and younger age were significant predictors of sudden cardiac arrest, whereas daytime ST-segment changes and active smoking were related to syncope.

A strong association has been noted between anxiety, depression, and coronary spasm. Hung et al. describe the association of anxiety and depression with spasm in a large retrospective cohort study based on the Taiwanese National Health Insurance Research Database.[80] They examined three large propensity score matched groups for the period between 2000 and 2012 including 10,473 patients with spasm based on symptoms, ECG changes, and positive ergonovine test; 10,473 with obstructive CAD; and 10,325 controls with neither diagnosis. A diagnosis of anxiety and depression was identified retrospectively in the previous 3 years. Anxiety and depression diagnoses were more frequent in patients with new-onset spasm than in those with new-onset CAD and controls. Compared with CAD, risk of developing spasm was higher in patients with anxiety (OR = 2.29, 95% CI, 2.14–2.45, $P < 0.001$), and depression (OR 1.34, 95% CI, 1.08–1.66, $P = 0.007$). More significant associations for anxiety and depression were noted when comparing spasm patients to controls without spasm or CAD, (OR 5.20, 95% CI, 4.72–5.74, $P < 0.001$, and OR 1.98, 95% CI, 1.50–2.62, $P < 0.001$, respectively). This increased risk of spasm in individuals with prior anxiety and depression diagnoses showed no sex differences.

Sohn et al. found an association between alcohol intake and occurrence of spasm[81] from a sample of 5491 patients with typical or atypical chest pain who underwent an acetylcholine provocation test, and were stratified as current drinkers (n = 1792) or nondrinkers (n = 3699). After propensity score matched analysis, alcohol consumption was a strong risk factor for spasm. As compared with nondrinkers, current drinkers showed higher incidence of spasm on provocation (58% vs 62%, $P = 0.016$), spontaneous spasm (17% vs 22%, $P = 0.004$), multivessel spasm (31% vs 37%, $P = 0.009$), proximal epicardial spasm (39% vs 46%, $P = 0.002$), ischemic ECG changes (0.4% vs 1.2%, $P < 0.001$), and chest pain (42% vs 46%, $P = 0.047$) during the provocation test. However, the status and pattern of alcohol consumption had no influence on long-term clinical MACE or recurrent angina.

Coronary vasospasm can often present with ST-segment changes on ECG and cardiac biomarker rise. On occasion, it may also present with positive changes on functional stress testing. ECG changes can include ST-segment deviation, T-wave inversion, and negative U-wave changes coinciding with episodes of spasm. Onaka et al. published findings on 24-hour ECG analysis in patients with variant angina.[82] Thirty out of 122 patients were included, 22 of whom showed ST-segment changes on two channel Holter, including 138 ST-segment elevation episodes and 13 ST-segment depression episodes. About 19% of the episodes of ST-segment elevation were associated with arrhythmias: premature ventricular ectopics, ventricular bigeminy or complete atrioventricular block, and sinus bradycardia <45 beats per min. Nearly 45% of these patients had multivessel spasm, which was either migratory at different sites on different occasions; sequential in two different sites; or simultaneous in more than a single site. Patients with sequential and simultaneous spasm had longer durations of ST-segment elevation and higher frequency of arrhythmia.

Diagnosis

Diagnosis of vasospasm is frequently based on history and ECG changes with exclusion of obstructive CAD on angiography. However, if there is no ECG documented during an attack, the diagnosis may be elusive. Thus, the accuracy of diagnosis can be significantly improved with invasive testing using coronary reactivity testing or provocation testing in specialist centers. Given the overlap in vasospasm and CMD, assessment of endothelial dependent and endothelial independent hyperemia testing proves to be invaluable in the same setting. **Fig. 20–3** summarizes the presentation and diagnostic features of this condition.

Noninvasive testing for coronary vasospasm can be performed but may be challenging since intracoronary nitrate cannot be delivered during the test, and angiography cannot be conducted to confirm the findings. The sensitivity and specificity may be low, reported to be 41% and 57%, respectively.[53] Noninvasive methods for testing CMD have included positron emission tomography scan, single-photon emission computed tomography, Doppler echocardiography, contrast echocardiography with microbubbles, and cardiac MRI. Correlation between stress testing and provocation testing is low.

Invasive testing can be conducted with acetylcholine, ergonovine, or papaverine provocation testing, although the first two agents are more commonly used. Sueda et al. have described the differences between acetylcholine and ergonovine testing based on a comprehensive review of literature.[83] While definitions for vasospasm based on provocation testing have been varied, the COVADIS group have recently drafted the consensus criteria for diagnosis to include three key features: presence of nitrate responsive chest pain, ischemic ST-segment changes on ECG, and >=90% spasm of the artery on acetylcholine provocation testing.[56] The Class I indications for undertaking testing are classic symptoms with ACS or recurrent presentations in the absence of obstructive CAD, unexplained cardiac arrest or syncope, and recurrent angina following successful PCI. Class II indications include an existing diagnosis on noninvasive testing with ergonovine

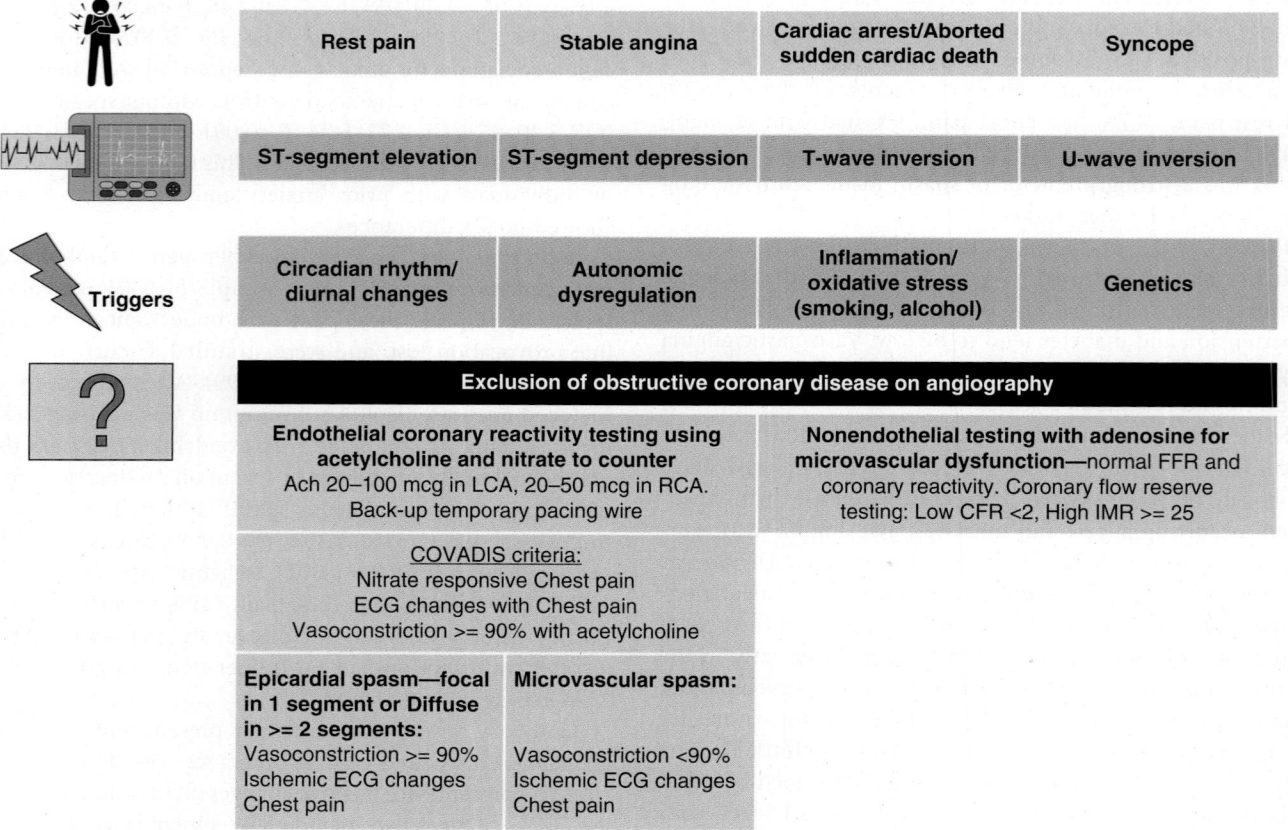

Figure 20–3. **Presentation and diagnostic features of coronary vasospasm.** CFR, coronary flow reserve; ECG, electrocardiography; LCA, left coronary artery; RCA, right coronary artery; RFF, fractional flow reserve.

stress test for purposes of confirmation, or for assessing improvement on medications. Invasive testing is not indicated in the presence of obstructive CAD (Class III).[56] Several testing algorithms have been put together, a common one prescribes the use of acetylcholine 20 mcg to 100 mcg in the left coronary artery (LCA), and 20 mcg to 50 mcg in the RCA followed by nitrate to counter the effect. Usually, acetylcholine results in vasodilation but in the presence of endothelial dysfunction, it can result in vasoconstriction. Microvascular spasm may be diagnosed in the presence of ECG changes and chest pain without sufficient vasoconstriction on provocation to meet the criteria for vasospastic angina.

Side effects of provocation testing include hypotension and bradycardia. A temporary pacing wire may be required prophylactically. With ergonovine testing, significant hypertension and ventricular tachyarrhythmia have been noted.[55] The overall rate of complications, however, is low with invasive testing and the safety and feasibility have been shown by several groups.[57,59,62,84] In the study by Ong et al., no irreversible fatal or nonfatal complications occurred. Minor complications occurred in nine patients (1%) including nonsustained ventricular tachycardia (n = 1), rapid paroxysmal atrial fibrillation (n = 1), symptomatic bradycardia (n = 6), and catheter-induced spasm (n = 1).[59] In the study by Di Fiore et al. using acetylcholine challenge, atrial fibrillation occurred in four patients and bradycardia in one patient due to loss of temporary pacemaker position.[62] Nevertheless, some data have shown that paroxysmal atrial fibrillation (AF) may be common after acetylcholine challenge. Saito et al. examined 377 patients without persistent AF who underwent an intracoronary acetylcholine provocation test.[85] A total of 31 patients (8%) developed paroxysmal AF during the test. Eleven patients (35%) required antiarrhythmic drugs; however, no patients required electrical cardioversion, and all patients reverted to sinus rhythm within 48 hours. Paroxysmal AF was more common during testing of the RCA versus the left coronary artery (90% vs 10%). On multivariate logistic regression analysis, predictors of AF during testing included history of paroxysmal AF (OR 4.38, 95% CI, 1.42–13.51, $P = 0.01$) and lower body mass index (OR 0.88, 95% CI, 0.78–0.99, $P = 0.03$). Saito et al. also studied the feasibility and safety of an acetylcholine provocation test in the outpatient services. A total of 323 patients were included, of which 201 patients (62%) were hospitalized inpatients and 122 (38%) were elective. The incidence of a positive acetylcholine provocation test was similar between the two groups (47% vs 54%, $P = 0.21$). The rate of complications was low, two cases (1.0%) in the hospitalization group, and one case (0.8%) in the elective group requiring hospitalization.

Sueda and others found acetylcholine to be more sensitive than ergonovine in both sexes for provocation testing.[86] They performed both acetylcholine and ergonovine challenge in 461 patients (294 males) of mean age 64.4 ± 11.3 years, over a 23-year period. Acetylcholine was administered in incremental doses of 20/50/(80) mcg into the RCA and 20/50/100/(200) mcg into the LCA over 20 seconds. Ergonovine was administered in a total dose of 40 mcg into the RCA and of 64 mcg into the LCA over 2 to 4 minutes. A positive test was defined as >99 % coronary narrowing with chest pain symptoms and/or ischemic ECG changes. In females, acetylcholine provoked spasm in almost all patients (59 patients, 96.7%), whereas ergonovine provoked spasm in only 32.8% of patients. In males, acetylcholine provoked spasm in 80.6% of patients, which was higher than with ergonovine, which provoked spasm in 60.6% of patients.

In a separate study, Sueda et al. compared acetylcholine and ergonovine in 1508 patients (873 acetylcholine tests) over 11 years.[87] Intracoronary acetylcholine provoked more spasms than ergonovine (36.0% vs 29.8%) overall. When stratified by presence of prior ischemic heart disease (IHD), there was no difference in the incidence of provoked spasms between acetylcholine (50.9%) and ergonovine tests (43.8%) in IHD patients. However, in patients without IHD, the incidence of provoked spasms with acetylcholine was significantly higher than with ergonovine (11.0% vs 6.4%, $P < 0.05$). Acetylcholine also provoked more spasms than did ergonovine in patients without fixed stenosis (36.2% compared with 25.5%, $P < 0.01$), and provoked multiple spasms (40.0% compared with 27.0%, $P < 0.01$). Major complications were observed in 1.4% of patients with acetylcholine and in 0.2% with ergonovine. Intracoronary nitrate to relieve spasm was more frequently required with acetylcholine tests (5.04% vs 1.49%, $P < 0.01$). There was a significant difference in sex, history of smoking, and hyperlipidemia between patients with and without spasms for both tests.

Treatment

Treatment of coronary vasospasm is largely conservative with medical therapy. Use of beta-blockers can often provoke more spasms, whereas calcium channel blockers can be useful for management of angina and hypertension. Other treatments include anti-anginal therapy with nitrates. Rho-kinase inhibitors are currently being studied in clinical trials. Attention toward risk factor optimization and weight loss is necessary. Recreational drug users may also often be smokers and have other modifiable cardiovascular risks including metabolic syndrome. Some specific studies examining individual treatment agents are subsequently described.

In a Korean study of 1586 patients with positive provocation tests, second-generation calcium channel blockers such as amlodipine and benidipine were equivalent to first-generation agents such as diltiazem and nifedipine with respect to incidence of the primary composite endpoint of death, arrhythmia or ACS (HR 0.54, 95% CI, 0.25–1.17, $P = 0.12$) during follow-up. However, second-generation drugs were associated with lower incidence of ACS (HR 0.22, 95% CI, 0.05–0.89, $P = 0.034$).[88] Benidipine was associated with better angina control compared to diltiazem at 3 years (HR 0.17, 95% CI, 0.07–1.32, $P < 0.001$). In a meta-analysis comparing MACE between four different calcium channel blockers, benidipine resulted in lower MACE than did diltiazem after adjusting for patient characteristics (HR 0.41, $P = 0.016$).[89]

In a cohort of 777 patients, Lim et al. noted that patients with vasospasm and atherosclerotic disease on low-dose aspirin had higher MACE (22.8% vs 12.1%, $P = 0.04$) and higher rate of rehospitalization (20.6% vs 11.2%; $P = 0.08$) but no difference in death.[90] After propensity matching, aspirin was associated with greater MACE (HR 1.54, 95% CI, 1.04–2.28). However, there was no impact of aspirin use on MACE in patients without atherosclerotic disease. Despite these findings, residual confounding from the observational nature of the study may have been an issue. Ishii et al. examined 640 patients with vasospasm and nonsignificant atherosclerotic disease to find no increased risk associated with low-dose aspirin on 5-year MACE (cardiac death, nonfatal MI, and unstable angina, 4.4% vs 3.6%, $P = 0.64$), concluding that low-dose aspirin may be safe to use.[91] Aspirin use had a neutral effect on 5-year MACE in univariable (HR 1.25, 95% CI, 0.50–3.14, $P = 0.64$) and multivariable statistical models (HR 1.5, 95% CI, 0.59–3.79, $P = 0.39$) in this study.

Ishii et al. also examined the effect of statins in this vasospastic angina cohort using propensity score matching.[92] Dyslipidemia was noted in 95.2% patients of the statin group compared to 26.5% of the nonstatin group. Of the 640 patients, 24 (3.8%) developed MACE. On multivariate Cox regression analysis, statin use was a significant negative predictor of MACE (HR, 0.11; 95% CI, 0.02–0.84; $P = 0.033$). In the propensity-score matched arms (n = 128 each), the 5-year MACE-free survival rate was higher among patients on statins (100% vs 91.7%, respectively; $P = 0.002$). Conversely, other groups have found a neutral effect of statins on MACE.[93,94]

Kim et al. examined 1154 vasospastic angina patients proven by ergonovine provocation, who were stratified by nitrate use (n = 676 on nitrate and n = 478 nonnitrate patients), including isosorbide mononitrate (ISMN) and nicorandil.[95] MACE was a composite of cardiac death, MI, any revascularization, or rehospitalization with recurrent angina. The nitrate group had higher MACE (22.9% vs 17.6%, HR 1.32, 95% CI, 1.01–1.73, $P = 0.043$) than did the nonnitrate group, which persisted after propensity score matching (HR 1.32, 95% CI, 1.01–1.73, $P = 0.049$). Patients receiving immediate-release ISMN (HR 1.80, 95% CI, 1.35–2.39, $P < 0.001$) and those receiving any form of ISMN other than at bedtime (HR 1.90, 95% CI, 1.41–2.57, $P < 0.001$) had higher risk of MACE than did non-nitrate patients. Nicorandil, however, had a neutral effect on MACE (HR 1.11, 95% CI, 0.73–1.69, $P = 0.62$).

The effect of nitrate use was also analyzed in another study of 1429 vasospastic angina patients of median age 66 years and including majority males (n = 1090).[96] Of these patients, 695 (49%) received nitrates, including nicorandil in 306 patients. Over 90% patients were also maintained on calcium channel blockers. Over a median follow-up of 32 months, 85 patients (5.9%) experienced a MACE event. Propensity score-matched analysis demonstrated that risk of 5-year MACE was similar in patients with and without nitrate use (11% vs 8%; HR 1.28, 95% CI, 0.72–2.28, $P = 0.40$). Nicorandil also had a neutral effect (HR 0.80, 95% CI, 0.28–2.27, $P = 0.67$) in propensity matched groups. However, in a multivariable Cox model concomitant use of conventional nitrates and nicorandil was found to be harmful (HR 2.14; 95% CI, 1.02–4.47; $P = 0.044$), particularly when conventional nitrate and nicorandil were simultaneously taken.

In another recent study, Suda et al. studied 187 patients of mean age 63.2 ± 12.3, including 60% males,[97] and undertook acetylcholine provocation and IMR testing in all patients, and additionally explored the therapeutic impact of rho-kinase inhibitor fasudil. Acetylcholine provocation identified 68% with vasospastic angina and cardiac adverse events occurred in 5.3% during follow-up. Multivariable regression analysis showed that IMR was an independent predictor of adverse outcomes (HR 1.05, 95% CI, 1.02–1.09, $P = 0.002$) with IMR of 18.0 shown to be the optimal cut-off value. Among four patient groups stratified based on IMR cut-off of 18.0 and the presence or absence of vasospastic angina on acetylcholine provocation, survival was significantly worse in the group with high IMR (≥18.0) and vasospasm compared with others (log rank $P = 0.002$). Treatment with intracoronary fasudil reduced IMR in this high-risk group ($P < 0.0001$); however, larger studies are necessary to confirm these findings.

With respect to interventional treatment, PCI is unsuitable due to high risk of stent failure due to ongoing vasospasm, and the risk of ongoing symptoms from spasm in another vessel or segment. Surgical management with CABG is not routinely recommended in patients with vasospasm, since spasm of vessels can occur beyond anastomosis, and grafts may become atretic in the absence of obstructive native coronary disease.

Implantable cardioverter defibrillator (ICD) implantation should be considered in case of patients with vasospasm and ventricular tachyarrhythmias, who have a greater risk of adverse outcomes.[98,99] Takagi et al. studied 1429 patients with vasospastic angina between September 2007 and December 2008 of which 35 patients survived out-of-hospital cardiac arrest (OHCA).[100] The OHCA survivors were younger with higher incidence of LAD spasm. Fourteen patients underwent ICD implantation. Five-year survival from MACE was significantly lower in the OHCA survivors (72% vs 92%, $P < 0.001$; HR 3.25, 95% CI, 1.39–7.61, $P < 0.01$).

In a study of 188 South Korean patients with variant angina and ASCD (mean age 52.8 ± 9.9 years) and 1844 patients with variant angina without ASCD (mean age 55.3 ± 9.5 years), Ahn et al. examined for differences in cardiac death on follow-up.[101] Predictors of ASCD included age (OR 0.98 by 1 year increase, 95% CI, 0.96–1.00, $P = 0.013$), hypertension (OR 0.51, 95% CI, 0.37–0.70, $P < 0.001$), hyperlipidemia (OR 0.38, 95% CI, 0.25–0.58, $P < 0.001$), family history of sudden cardiac death (OR 3.67, 95% CI, 1.27–10.6, $P = 0.016$), multivessel spasm (OR 2.06, 95% CI, 1.33–3.19, $P = 0.001$), and LAD spasm (OR 1.40, 95% CI, 1.02–1.92, $P = 0.04$). Over a median follow-up of 7.5 years, the risk of cardiac death was significantly higher in ASCD patients (HR 7.26, 95% CI, 4.21–12.5, $P < 0.001$). The incidence of recurrent ventricular tachyarrhythmia in ASCD patients was 32.4 per 1000 patient-years. A total of 24 out of 188 ASCD patients received ICDs. There was a trend for lower rate of cardiac death in patients with versus without ICDs (4.3% vs 19.3%, $P = 0.15$).

Aligned with this are findings from a nationwide Korean population-based database comparing outcomes between VSA patients presenting with and without ASCD.[102] Nearly 598 out of 6972 (8.6%) VSA patients presented with ASCD between

July 1, 2007, and May 31, 2015. On inverse probability of treatment weighting, ASCD patients had a significantly increased risk of the composite of cardiac arrest and acute MI (adjusted HR 2.52; 95% CI, 1.72–3.67; P <0.001) during the median follow-up duration of 4 years. ASCD patients treated with an ICD had a lower incidence of the composite of cardiac arrest and acute MI during follow-up (P = 0.009).

In a small study of 23 patients with vasospastic angina and VT, 5 patients had recurrent VT. No predictors were identified associated with recurrence of VT, including medications used, smoking, or angina status after ICD implantation.[103] Sueda et al. investigated the appropriateness of medications and ICD shocks in a systematic review of 137 patients with a history of ASCD due to coronary spasm.[98] Approximately 15.6% of the 96 patients with ICDs received aggressive medical therapy, including multiple calcium channel blockers. During a mean 41 months of follow-up, 24.1% of patients received ICD shocks which were appropriate. The remaining patients received no ICD shocks. The rate of appropriate ICD shocks was significantly higher in Western than Asian countries (42.9% vs 19.3%, P <0.01), whereas medications used did not significantly differ between the two regions; however, this analysis may be limited by the small sample size of the study. Appropriate ICD shocks successfully resuscitated 33 patients, but 3 patients died due to fatal arrhythmias. The authors concluded that medical therapy after ICD implantation in patients with ASCD remains crucial to optimize.

Natural History and Prognosis

In 1983, Bott-Silverman et al. published data on 5-year follow-up in 59 patients, 32 of who were women.[104] One-third of these patients had positive stress tests; 27% presented with syncope and angina, 10% required pacemaker insertion, and 19% had MI. With respect to ECG changes during angina episodes, 64% had ST-segment elevation; 19% had ST-segment depression; and 15% had no changes. Improvement with long-acting nitrate was seen in 31% and with calcium channel blockers in 83%. The natural history of these patients included frequent episodes of angina at rest, spontaneous remission for long periods, poor response to long-acting nitrates, but good response to calcium channel blockers. While MI and arrhythmia were not uncommon, mortality was rare on medical therapy.

Shin et al. studied the 2-year prognosis of patients with vasospasm.[105] Out of 2129 patients in the VA-KOREA registry, patients with ergonovine positive spasm had worse prognosis compared to intermediate or negative patients. Two-thirds of positive patients had diffuse spasm, 23% had focal spasm, and 10% had mixed spasm. Patients with spasm had a higher prevalence of smoking, elevated triglycerides, high C-reactive protein, and greater angina frequency. From the same registry, Han et al. described that patients with multivessel spasm (n = 104) had worse outcomes than did those with single vessel spasm (n = 163), or no spasm (n = 737).[106] Multivessel vasospastic angina was an independent predictor of the 3-year primary composite endpoint of death, ACS, or arrhythmia (HR 8.5, 95% CI, 2.6–27.2, P <0.0001). The rate of death or ACS was higher in

multi- versus single-vessel vasospasm or non-vasospasm patients (5.8% vs 1.2% vs 0.9%, P <0.05).

Conversely, out of 2797 patients undergoing acetylcholine provocation testing from 2004 to 2010 in a single Korean tertiary center, Park et al. noted that the 3-year incidence of death, MI, PCI, cerebrovascular accidents, and MACE were similar among patients with (n = 528) or without multivessel diffuse spasm (n = 1081) or no spasm (n = 1188).[107] However, recurrent angina occurred more frequently in the multivessel spasm group than those with no spasm (HR 1.96; 95% CI, 1.27–3.02, P = 0.002).

Sato et al. examined 873 out of 1673 patients with acetylcholine provoked spasm from 1991 to 2010, from a single center and reported 20-year outcomes.[63] They noted that in response to acetylcholine, women were more likely to demonstrate diffuse spasm in the absence of significant CAD, and these patients had better prognosis with respect to MACE and 5-year survival than the focal spasm subtype.

Moderate as well as severe spasm on acetylcholine testing was found to have adverse outcomes in vasospastic angina by Hoshino et al.[108] A total of 298 consecutive patients were divided into three groups according to the diameter reduction during the acetylcholine testing: severe spasm showing ≥75 % diameter reduction, moderate spasm showing ≥50 % reduction, and others with <50% reduction. Over median follow-up of 4.6 years, MACE rates was significantly greater in severe (11.1%, P = 0.009) and moderate (8.5%) spasm compared to controls (1.9%, P = 0.029). No differences in MACE were noted between severe and moderate spasm groups (P = 0.534). In adjusted analyses, moderate spasm was an independent predictor of MACE (HR 7.18, 95 % CI, 1.42–36.4, P = 0.017).

Nam et al. included 812 patients with myocardial bridge (MB) without significant CAD, who underwent an acetylcholine provocation test with spasm defined as ≥70% narrowing, and MB defined as phasic systolic compression of the coronary artery with a decrease of more than 30% in diameter on the angiogram after intracoronary nitroglycerin.[109] MACE was defined as recurrent angina requiring repeat coronary angiography at 5 years. MB was closely associated with a high incidence of spasm, ischemic ECG change, and chest pain during the provocation test. Severe MB was a strong risk factor of coronary spasm. MB patients with spasm were shown to have a higher rate of recurrent angina compared with MB patients without coronary spasm, up to a 5-year follow-up, without differences in MACE.

In a large study of 4644 consecutive patients with rest angina and nonobstructive CAD,[110] patients were categorized into four types based on vasomotor response to acetylcholine testing: normal vasomotion (no chest pain, ischemic ECG changes, or vasoconstriction); microvascular spasm (chest pain with <75% vasoconstriction and relief after nitrate); epicardial spasm (chest pain with ≥75% vasoconstriction); and inconclusive tests (vasoconstriction and/or electrocardiographic changes, but no chest pain). Angina requiring repeat angiography recurred in 7.9% of patients and was more frequent in patients with abnormal vasomotion (5.4%, 9.8%, 10.9%, and 8.2% in normal vasomotion, microvascular spasm, epicardial spasm, and inconclusive types, respectively, $P = 0.009$). Independent positive predictors for recurrent angina were male sex, obstructive CAD, and medications including calcium channel blockers, nitrates, and statins, whereas alcohol consumption (at least one alcoholic drink per week) at baseline was a negative predictor. The rate of MACE was low in 1.6%, and similar among the different vasomotor subtypes ($P = 0.42$).

In a multicenter registry from the Japanese Coronary Spasm Association, Takagi et al. analyzed 1429 patients of median age 66 years for median follow-up of 32 months.[111] The authors identified seven predictors of MACE (cardiac death, nonfatal MI, hospitalization with unstable angina or heart failure, appropriate ICD shocks) on a multivariable Cox regression model with an integer score assigned to each; history of out-of-hospital cardiac arrest (4 points), smoking status, rest angina, obstructive coronary disease, multivessel spasm (2 points each), ST-segment elevation with angina, and beta-blocker use (1 point each). Based on these predictors, three risk groups were defined: low (score 0 to 2, n = 598), intermediate (score 3 to 5, n = 639), and high (score 6 or more, n = 192). MACE during follow-up showed a stepwise increase from the low-, intermediate-, and high-risk patients at 2.5%, 7.0%, and 13.0% ($P <0.001$), respectively. The average prediction rates of the scoring system in the development and validation sets were 86.6% and 86.5%, respectively.

From the same registry database, Kawana et al. examined for sex differences in outcomes.[112] Females were older (median 69 vs 66 years), with lower prevalence of smoking (20% vs 72%) and obstructive CAD (9% vs 16%) ($P = 0.001$ for all). Predictors of MACE were different by sex; in women, age and electrical abnormalities were found to be independent predictors, whereas in men, structural abnormalities were found. A 5-year MACE-free survival was comparable by sex; however, the survival was significantly lower in young women <50 years (young 82%, middle-aged [50–64 years] 92%, elderly [≥65 years] 96%; $P <0.01$). There was also significant interaction between age and smoking, with a higher prevalence of smokers in young women. In contrast, the survival was similar among the three age groups in men.

In the recent CorMicA trial, authors grouped 391 patients as having obstructive CAD, vasospastic angina, or microvascular angina or normal coronary arteries. Further, they randomized 151 patients without obstructive CAD into treatment guided by interventional diagnostic procedure versus standard of care with angiography alone. At a median follow-up of 19 months, the group receiving interventional diagnostic procedures for an accurate diagnosis had improved Seattle angina scores and quality of life, without differences in MACE (12% vs 11%, $P = 0.80$).[113]

Summary

In summary, coronary vasospasm is a challenging diagnosis that can cause ACS, including MI. Coronary vasospasm frequently overlaps with microvascular angina in stable patients. The uptake of provocation testing in clinical practice is low at this time, increasing the risk of morbidity from wrong or missed diagnosis. Patients may experience high psychological distress, particularly in younger age groups, due to recurrent symptoms, lack of accurate diagnosis, and uncertainty in the direction of management. Accurate diagnosis and tailored therapy result in improved quality of life. Treatment is conservative mainly with the use of calcium channel blockers, although ICD implantation has a specific role in patients with ventricular tachyarrhythmias. Future studies focused on targeted therapy are warranted.

MYOCARDITIS

Myocarditis is an inflammatory disease of the myocardium defined as the histological presence of inflammatory infiltrate on endomyocardial biopsy (EMB).[114] Fulminant myocarditis is a less common form characterized by sudden and severe myocardial inflammation requiring inotropic or mechanical circulatory support.[115] As myocarditis often presents with chest pain, ECG changes and elevated cardiac biomarkers, it can mimic ACS. Important distinguishing characteristics between myocarditis and a coronary event are subsequently highlighted. Myocarditis is a highly heterogeneous condition, with a myriad of underlying causes, both infectious and noninfectious. The most common infectious etiologies are viral, with bacterial, fungal, protozoal, and helminths all causative. Noninfectious etiologies include drugs, toxins, or in association with autoimmune diseases such as systemic lupus erythematosus (SLE), scleroderma, sarcoidosis, and myositis. The natural history, diagnosis, and management of myocarditis is highly dependent on the clinical presentation and underlying etiology.

Epidemiology

The epidemiology of myocarditis has been difficult to describe due to its highly heterogeneous nature and frequent lack of biopsy-proven disease. However, with these limitations in mind, the incidence of myocarditis has been estimated to be 10 to 22 per 100,000 people, or 1.5 million global cases in a 2013 worldwide population.[116,117] Using global hospital discharge data, the burden of myocarditis as a percentage of heart failure cases ranged from 0.5% to 4%.[117] A Finnish study of >90,000 patients with acute MI found that myocarditis was the diagnosis in 2.3%, with this rate 11-fold higher than atherosclerotic MI in younger patients (age 18–29 years).[118] Prevalence of myocarditis described at autopsy has been highly variable, ranging from 0.11% to 0.53% of all-cause deaths and 2% to 42% of sudden cardiac deaths in young adults.[119,120] However, an important consideration when assessing rates of myocarditis at autopsy is that inflammatory infiltrates have been described in noncardiac deaths and healthy donor hearts. This suggests that inflammatory infiltrates on cardiac histopathology at the time of death, in the absence of clinical manifestations, do not equal a myocarditis diagnosis.

Viral myocarditis is the most common form of myocarditis. A cardiac viral pathogen is identified or implicated in a third of myocarditis cases and also a large proportion of dilated cardiomyopathies. Coxsackievirus myocarditis has been described in 3.5% to 5% of all infected patients while smallpox vaccination causes suspected myocarditis in 5 to 6 per 10,000 vaccinated individuals.[121] With the emergence of the COVID-19 pandemic, myocarditis has been thrust back into the spotlight. Infection with severe acute respiratory syndrome coronavirus 2 (SARS-CoV-2) results in acute cardiac injury in 12% to 33% of hospitalized patients and myocarditis has been postulated to be an underlying contributor.[122–126] Case reports have described acute and fulminant myocarditis diagnosed on multimodal imaging in the presence of SARS-CoV-2 infection without detection of cardiac SARS-CoV-2 genome.[127,128] Further studies are needed to confirm if viral myocarditis is a major contributor to SARS-CoV-2-related myocardial injury.

Natural History

The natural history and prognosis of myocarditis is as variable as its presentation and underlying etiologies. In general, most mild cases of myocarditis without significant LV dysfunction have excellent prognosis with complete recovery.[129] However, acute myocarditis has the potential to progress to dilated cardiomyopathy, heart failure, life-threatening arrhythmia, and sudden cardiac death.[129–133] Overall, approximately half of acute myocarditis cases completely recover, a quarter experience slow decline in LV function, and another quarter rapidly progress to severe LV dysfunction, need for cardiac transplantation, or death.[132,134] Independent predictors of poor prognosis include an initial presentation with biventricular failure, sustained ventricular arrhythmia, low cardiac output, and left ventricular ejection fraction (LVEF) <50%.[134,135] Fulminant myocarditis, despite its severe initial presentation, has a better chance of full recovery in adult patients.[115] Certain myocarditis subtypes, namely giant cell myocarditis (GCM) and necrotizing eosinophilic myocarditis (NEM), have markedly worse prognosis, frequently resulting in transplantation or death, and are subsequently discussed in further detail.

Pathogenesis

Infectious etiologies of myocarditis are viral (DNA and RNA), bacterial, fungal, protozoal, and helminths. Noninfectious etiologies include systemic autoimmune diseases, eosinophilic syndromes, and toxins (**Table 20–2**).

Viral Myocarditis

Viral myocarditis can be caused by a myriad of viruses, commonly enterovirus (such as coxsackievirus), adenovirus, parvovirus B-19, influenza virus, Epstein–Barr virus, human herpes virus 6, hepatitis C, and cytomegalovirus (CMV). This leads to lymphocytic myocarditis whereby the virus triggers or binds to receptors in the myocardium resulting in production of proinflammatory cytokines, which in turn recruit T cells (**Fig. 20–4a**). Viral pathogens can directly invade the myocardium leading to myocyte death rapidly followed by exposure of host proteins and immune system activation. In addition, in genetically susceptible individuals, viral myocarditis can lead to the production of anticardiac autoantibodies, propagating downstream myocardial inflammation, in the absence of ongoing viral infection (**Fig. 20–5**).

TABLE 20–2. Pathogenesis of Myocarditis

Infectious		Autoimmune/immune-mediated	Toxic
Viral (RNA):	**Bacterial:**	**Systemic:**	- Checkpoint inhibitors (atezolizumab, avelumab, cemiplimab, durvalumab, ipilimumab, nivolumab, pembrolizumab)
- Coxsackievirus A and B	- Staphylococcus	- Systemic lupus erythematous	
- Echovirus	- Streptococcus	- Rheumatoid arthritis	
- Coronavirus	- Pneumococcus	- Scleroderma	- Amphetamines
- Poliovirus	- Meningococcus	- Polymyositis	- Cocaine
- Influenza A/B	- Gonococcus	- Type 1 diabetes mellitus	- Heroin
- Respiratory syncytial virus	- Salmonella	- Kawasaki's disease	- Ethanol
- Mumps, measles, rubella viruses	- Corynebacterium diphtheria	- Wegener's granulomatosis	- Iron
- Chikungunya	- Hemophilus influenza	- Inflammatory bowel disease	- Copper
- Hepatitis C	- Mycobacterium tuberculosis	- Myasthenia Gravis	- Lead
- HIV	- Mycoplasma pneumoniae	- Thyrotoxicosis	- Arsenic
- Dengue, yellow fever, rabies virus	- Brucella	- Sarcoidosis	- Radiation
Viral (DNA)	**Fungal**	- Giant cell	- Electric shock
- Adenovirus	- Aspergillus	- Celiac	- Insect stings or bites
- Parvovirus B19	- Actinomyces	**Eosinophilic:**	
- Cytomegalovirus	- Candida	- Antibiotics (penicillin, cephalosporin, sulfonamides, isoniazid)	
- Human herpes virus-6	- Cryptococcus	- Smallpox vaccine	
- Epstein–Barr	- Blastomyces	- Dobutamine	
- Varicella-zoster	- Histoplasma	- Clozapine/olanzapine	
- Herpes simplex	**Parasitic**	- Diuretics	
Protozoal	- *Trichinella spiralis*	- Methyldopa	
- Malaria	- *Echinococcus granulosus*	- Tetanus	
- Trypanosoma (Chagas disease)	- *Taenia solium*	- Phenytoin, carbamazepine	
- Toxoplasma	**Rickettsial**	- Reactive: parasitic, Churg-Strauss, familial	
- Leishmania	- *Coxiella burnetti*	- Neoplastic	
	- *R. rickettsii*		
	- *R. tsutsugamuschi*		

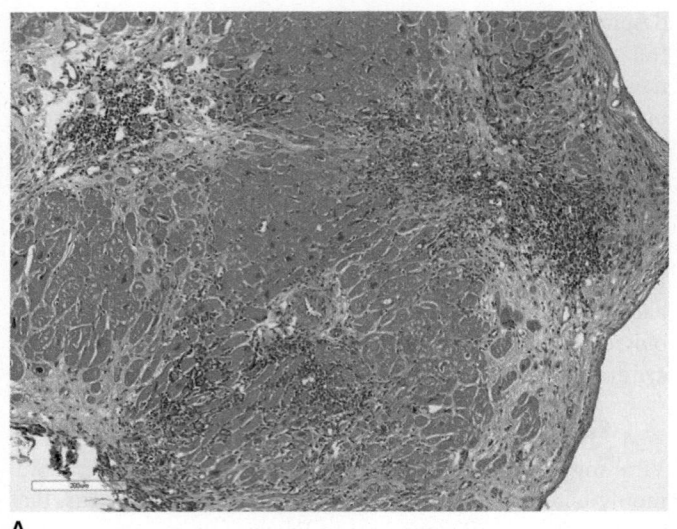

A

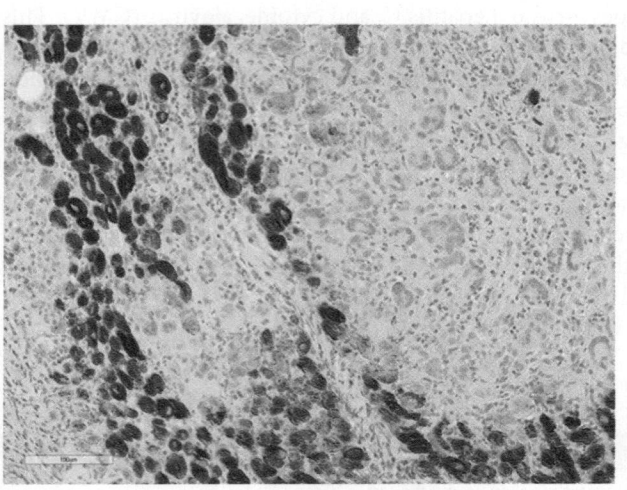

B

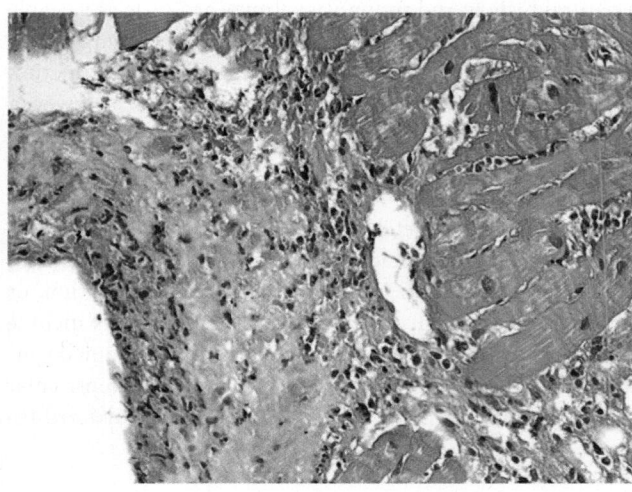

C

CD68

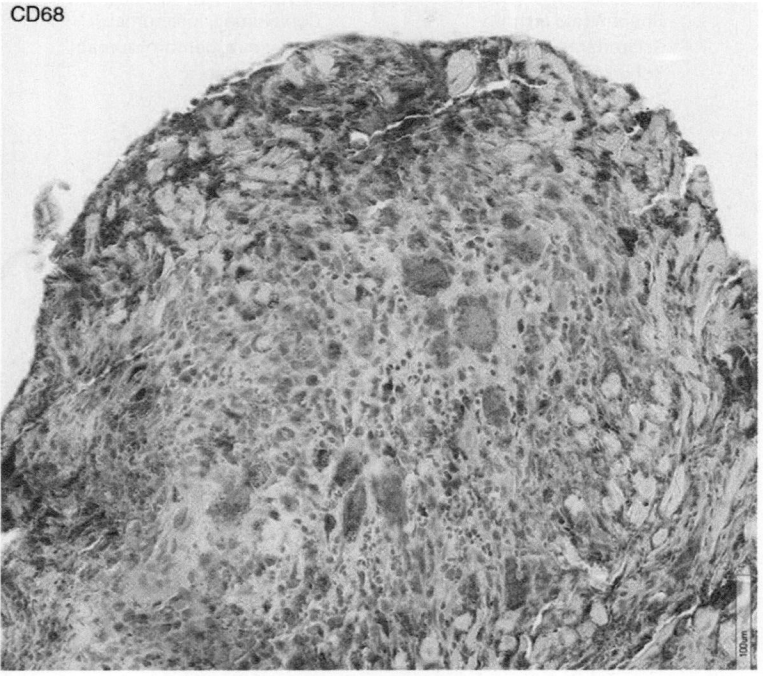

Figure 20–4. Endomyocardial biopsy. (A) Endomyocardial biopsy showing active inflammation and early granulation tissue in coxsackievirus B3-positive viral myocarditis. **(B)** Endomyocardial biopsy showing classical giant cells in giant cell myocarditis (left panel) and with positive immunostaining for anti-CD68 antibodies (right panel). **(C)** Endomyocardial biopsy showing interstitial inflammatory infiltrates, largely consisting of eosinophils. The patient had peripheral hypereosinophilia with an underlying neoplasm and a diagnosis of eosinophilic myocarditis.

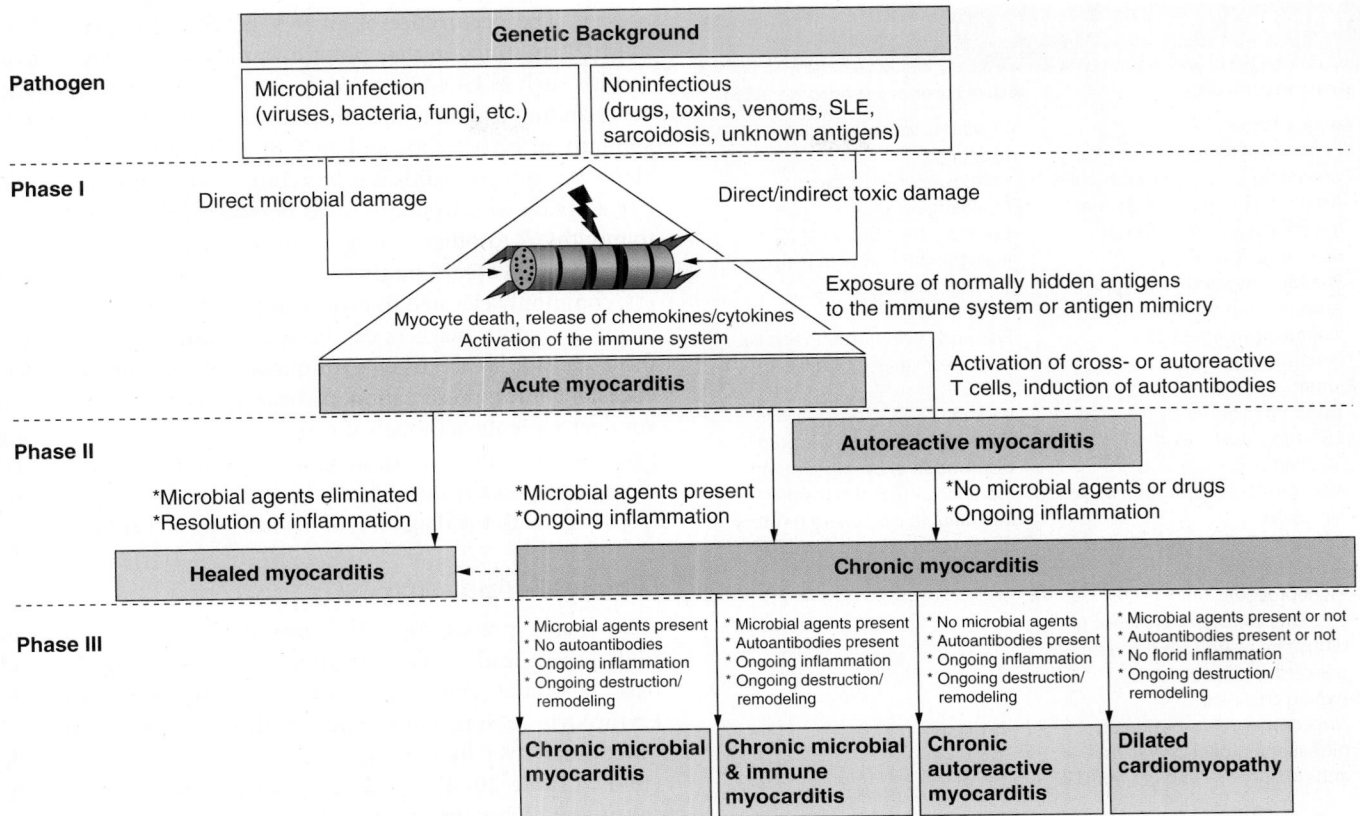

Figure 20-5. Pathogenetic mechanisms involved in myocarditis and progression to dilated cardiomyopathy. Reproduced with permission from Caforio AL, Pankuweit S, Arbustini E, et al. Current state of knowledge on aetiology, diagnosis, management, and therapy of myocarditis: a position statement of the European Society of Cardiology Working Group on Myocardial and Pericardial Diseases. *Eur Heart J.* 2013 Sep;34(33):2636-2648.

Autoimmune Myocarditis

Autoimmune myocarditis is often found in association with noncardiac autoimmune conditions, such as SLE, scleroderma, and myositis. Sarcoidosis (idiopathic granulomatous myocarditis) is an autoimmune condition with noncaseating granulomas with fibrosis, few eosinophils, and little to no necrosis. Cardiac sarcoidosis occurs in about a quarter of patients with systemic sarcoidosis and requires a negative stain for underlying infectious causes.[136,137] GCM is a rare autoimmune myocarditis characterized by giant cells (**Fig. 20-4b**) that often progresses rapidly to fulminant heart failure, death, or transplantation.[137,138] GCM is also commonly associated with several noncardiac autoimmune conditions such as thymoma and drug hypersensitivity. Hypersensitivity myocarditis is a form of eosinophilic autoimmune myocarditis (**Fig. 20-4c**), most often drug-related, characterized by rash, fever, and peripheral eosinophilia. Numerous drugs have been implicated including antibiotics, diuretics, antipsychotics and antiepileptics (Table 20-2). Eosinophilic myocarditis can also occur in the context of malignancy or parasitic infection. Acute NEM is a rare form of eosinophilic myocarditis that is usually a result of drug hypersensitivity (Table 20-2). NEM is characterized by diffuse inflammation with prominent myocyte necrosis and thrombosis. It also has a rapidly progressive course resulting in fulminant myocarditis with cardiogenic shock, death, or transplantation in half of patients.[115,139,140]

Toxic Myocarditis

Toxic myocarditis can be caused by heavy metals, illicit drugs, and insect stings or bites. An emerging cause of toxic myocarditis due to their increasing use as cancer therapies, are the immune checkpoint inhibitors. These are monoclonal antibodies (eg, ipilimumab, tremelimumab, and atezolizumab) that target the body's immune checkpoints to activate the immune system in order to fight off malignancies such as metastatic melanoma, non-small cell lung cancer, renal cell carcinoma, and many others. Since 2016, descriptions of fulminant and fatal myocarditis with T cell and macrophage infiltration of the myocardium have been reported.[141-144]

Myocarditis as an ACS Mimicker

Myocarditis has a broad range of clinical presentations ranging from very mild symptoms, to fulminant cardiogenic shock. Acute myocarditis is a common mimicker of ACS, presenting frequently with chest pain, ST-T wave changes on ECG, elevated cardiac biomarkers, and new LV dysfunction. Similar to a coronary event, acute myocarditis can be rapidly progressive, leading to heart failure, cardiogenic shock, ventricular tachyarrhythmias, and sudden cardiac death. However, several features may be used to clinically distinguish myocarditis from an acute coronary event (**Table 20-3**). On history, patients with viral myocarditis may describe a febrile or flu-like illness with cough, fever, and constitutional symptoms such as myalgia

TABLE 20–3. Features Supporting Acute Myocarditis versus an Acute Coronary Event*

Acute myocarditis	Acute coronary syndrome (ACS)
Medical History of: - Fever =>38 at presentation or preceding 30 days, malaise, chills - Respiratory or gastrointestinal infective symptoms (cough, vomiting, diarrhea) - Previous myocarditis diagnosis - Autoimmune conditions, allergic asthma, toxic agent use - Peripartum period Biomarkers: - Troponin persistently elevated - CRP and ESR elevated ECG changes: - Noncoronary distribution of ST elevation - Concave ST elevation without reciprocal changes - PR depression - Low QRS voltage in presence of diffuse myocardial oedema or pericardial effusion Imaging changes: - Noncoronary distribution of global or regional LV wall motion abnormality on echo or CMR-LGE	Medical History of: - Older age - Cardiovascular risk factors ECG changes: - Coronary distribution of ST elevation on ECG with reciprocal ST depression Biomarkers: - Rise and fall in troponin levels - Normal or small elevations in CRP, ESR Imaging: - Coronary territory implicated in distribution of LV impairment - Subendocardial or transmural infarction in a coronary territory distribution seen on CMR-LGE

*In patients with an acute coronary syndrome-like presentation, coronary angiography is still necessary to exclude obstructive coronary artery disease.

and fatigue. The viral illness, if present, precedes the cardiac manifestations. However, the absence of prodromal symptoms does not exclude myocarditis, given their variable penetrance. In myocarditis, ECG changes can include ST elevation or depression, nonspecific TW inversion or changes, conduction disturbances, and atrial or ventricular arrhythmias. Imaging can demonstrate global or regional LV wall motion abnormalities. However, unlike a coronary event, ECG and LV involvement in myocarditis is unlikely to follow a coronary artery territory distribution. ST-elevation in myocarditis is also more likely to be concave (rather than convex in coronary obstruction), without reciprocal changes. Pericarditis-type pattern with widespread ST elevation and PR depression may also be

present. The occurrence of an A-V block in the presence of mild LV dysfunction may point toward certain types of myocarditis such as GCM or sarcoidosis.[129,138,145] Cardiac biomarkers including troponin and creatinine kinase (CK) are elevated similarly in myocarditis and ACS to indicate myocyte injury. However, in myocarditis it is less common to see an ACS-type rise and fall, with troponin often persistently high over weeks to months.[129] Another distinguishing marker between myocarditis and ACS would be the presence of inflammatory markers, commonly elevated in myocarditis. While small elevations of inflammatory markers can be seen in atherosclerotic ACS, these elevations are usually minimal. In addition to differences in clinical presentation, myocarditis is more common in younger patients, although it can occur at any age.[118] Among patients with a provisional diagnosis of MINOCA, the finding of angiographically normal coronary arteries is independently associated with the diagnosis of myocarditis on cardiac MRI.

Diagnostic Approaches

All patients presenting with suspected myocarditis should undergo 12-lead ECG, transthoracic echocardiogram, and basic laboratory investigations including troponins, CK-MB, erythrocyte sedimentation rate (ESR), CRP blood count and differential, liver function tests, and brain natriuretic peptide (BNP) (**Table 20–4**). Cardiac troponins, particularly high-sensitivity troponins, are sensitive to myocardial injury, but not specific for myocarditis. When troponin levels are normal, myocarditis is not excluded. Similarly, brain natriuretic peptide (BNP) levels are commonly raised in myocarditis particularly in the presence of LV dysfunction and heart failure, but may also be normal.[129] Inflammatory markers are often, but not always, elevated in myocarditis.[115,129,146] In suspected hypersensitivity or drug-related myocarditis, peripheral blood eosinophilia is an important maker; however, similar to above, a normal result does not exclude the diagnosis.[140] All patients should then be considered for endomyocardial biopsy (EMB), invasive coronary angiography, cardiac magnetic resonance imaging (CMR), viral serology, and cardiac auto-antibody testing.

Invasive Approaches

According to the original World Health Organization (WHO) criteria, the diagnosis of myocarditis requires the presence of

TABLE 20–4. Diagnostic Approach to Suspected Myocarditis

Basic investigations	Invasive tests	Imaging tests	Serology and cardiac autoantibodies
- 12-lead ECG - Chest x-ray - Complete full blood count and differential: eosinophils - Metabolic panel - Liver function - ESR and CRP - Troponin T/I - BNP level - Lactate -Blood cultures (if febrile)	-Endomyocardial biopsy: consider if diagnosis unclear, fulminant myocarditis, suspected sarcoid, GCM or NEM - Coronary angiography to exclude CAD	- Trans-thoracic echocardiogram in all cases - Cardiac magnetic resonance imaging if available	- Serum viral serology if clinical suspicion for Hepatitis C, HIV, Lyme disease, and Rickettsia - Anticardiac autoantibodies if clinically available

inflammatory infiltrate on a histopathological specimen.[130] Without a histologically confirmed diagnosis, myocarditis is considered suspected, rather than proven.

Endomyocardial Biopsy: EMB is considered the gold standard for myocarditis diagnosis.[129–131] This can be performed through right heart catheterization, or opportunistically, at the time of implantation of circulatory support devices or heart transplantation. Conventional Dallas criteria for myocarditis diagnosis includes the presence of inflammatory infiltrate associated with myocyte degeneration and necrosis.[114] The histological findings on EMB are classified according to type of inflammatory cell infiltrate: lymphocytic, eosinophilic, polymorphic, giant cell, and sarcoidosis.[147] Immunohistochemistry can be combined with monoclonal and polyclonal antibodies to better identify the inflammatory infiltrate type: anti-CD3, T lymphocytes, anti-CD68, macrophages, and anti-Human Leukocyte Antigen (HLA)-DR. EMB is important to distinguish lymphocytic myocarditis from giant cell or necrotizing eosinophilic myocarditis, with the later conditions more likely to benefit from immunosuppression and have a poorer prognosis.

Since the original Dallas criteria were coined, immunohistochemistry has now been combined with molecular viral polymerase chain reaction (PCR). This includes viral DNA and RNA extraction with reverse transcriptase (RT)-PCR amplification of the viral genome. This enables the direct detection of viral genome in the myocardium with significant improvements in EMB sensitivity. As a result, additional histological diagnostic criteria to the Dallas criteria have been proposed, including viral myocarditis associated with positive viral PCR, autoimmune myocarditis with negative viral PCR with or without serum cardiac autoantibodies, and viral and immune myocarditis with both positive viral PCR and the presence of cardiac autoantibodies.[129] Of note, the findings on EMB in the context of viral myocarditis is dependent upon the stage of the disease in which it is taken. If taken early in the disease course, viral infection is often present, while a later biopsy may demonstrate viral-negative immune-mediated myocarditis, more likely to respond to immunosuppression.

While EMB has been held up as the gold standard for myocarditis diagnosis, the updated ESC guidelines acknowledge its significant limitations.[129] Utilizing Dallas criteria in clinical myocarditis, the sensitivity of EMB is low, ranging from 30% to 60%.[148,149] Sampling error plays a major role due to the often localized nature of the disease, with many samples required from the right or left ventricle to achieve a higher sensitivity.[131] Sensitivity may be improved by incorporating CMR to help identify the best site for biopsy. Even the detection of viral PCR in the heart can represent a false positive, in the presence of peripheral viral blood infection. A false negative for viral PCR can also occur in chronic viral myocarditis, where low amounts of viral RNA are common.[129] As a result of these limitations, in real-world studies, EMB is performed in the minority of suspected myocarditis cases.[135]

Coronary Angiography: The diagnosis of myocarditis requires exclusion of CAD, particularly in the case of ACS mimickers

(Table 20–4).[129] This can be achieved with invasive coronary angiography or, in the instance of a young and stable patient without cardiovascular risk factors, a computed tomography coronary angiogram.

Noninvasive Approaches

Due to the limitations associated with invasive EMB, the ESC working group on myocarditis has suggested alternate diagnostic criteria using a range of clinical and investigation features (**Table 20–5**).[129]

Echocardiography: Echocardiography is a requirement in the investigation of myocarditis. It can show the presence of focal or global LV dysfunction, right ventricular involvement, pericardial effusion with or without tamponade features, and cardiac thrombus. Myocardial inflammation can result in longitudinal and circumferential strain, with the degree of strain associated with prognosis.[150,151] Acute or fulminant myocarditis often manifests as a nondilated, LV thickened from interstitial edema. In addition, echocardiography is a requirement to exclude other causes of cardiac disease such as valvular or hypertensive heart disease. In the case of worsening hemodynamic status in myocarditis, echocardiography should be repeated to reassess LV function.

Cardiac Magnetic Resonance Imaging: CMR is incredibly useful in the diagnosis of myocarditis due to its ability to delineate tissue characteristics. It can demonstrate myocardial tissue edema through global myocardial signal intensity in T2-weighted images, and a nonischemic distribution of myocardial injury in late gadolinium enhancement (LGE).[152] T1 mapping techniques can also be used to show diffuse

---

TABLE 20–5. Diagnostic Criteria for Clinically Suspected Myocarditis

Clinically suspected myocarditis if =>1 clinical presentation and =>1 diagnostic criteria from each category, in the absence of coronary artery disease with stenosis =>50%, known preexisting cardiovascular disease or extra-cardiac causes that could explain the syndrome. Suspicion is higher with higher number of fulfilled criteria.

Clinical presentation:	*Diagnostic criteria:*
1. Acute chest pain, pericarditis or pseudoischemic	1. New ECG/Holter or stress test abnormalities of I-III degree AV block, bundle branch block, ST-TW changes, sinus arrest, VT or VF or asystole, AF, reduced R wave height, broad QRS, low voltage, frequent premature beats, SVT
2. New-onset (days-3 months) or worsening dyspnea, fatigue with or without left or right heart failure signs	
3. Subacute/chronic (>3 months) worsening dyspnea, fatigue with or without left or right heart failure signs	2. Elevated troponin T/I
	3. New, unexplained LV and/or RV regional or global function abnormality on echocardiogram, angiography or CMR
4. Palpitations and/or unexplained arrhythmia, syncope or sudden cardiac death	4. Myocardial edema and/or LGE on CMR
5. Unexplained cardiogenic shock	

Data from from Caforio AL, Pankuweit S, Arbustini E, et al. Current state of knowledge on aetiology, diagnosis, management, and therapy of myocarditis: a position statement of the European Society of Cardiology Working Group on Myocardial and Pericardial Diseases. *Eur Heart J.* 2013 Sep;34(33):2636-2648.

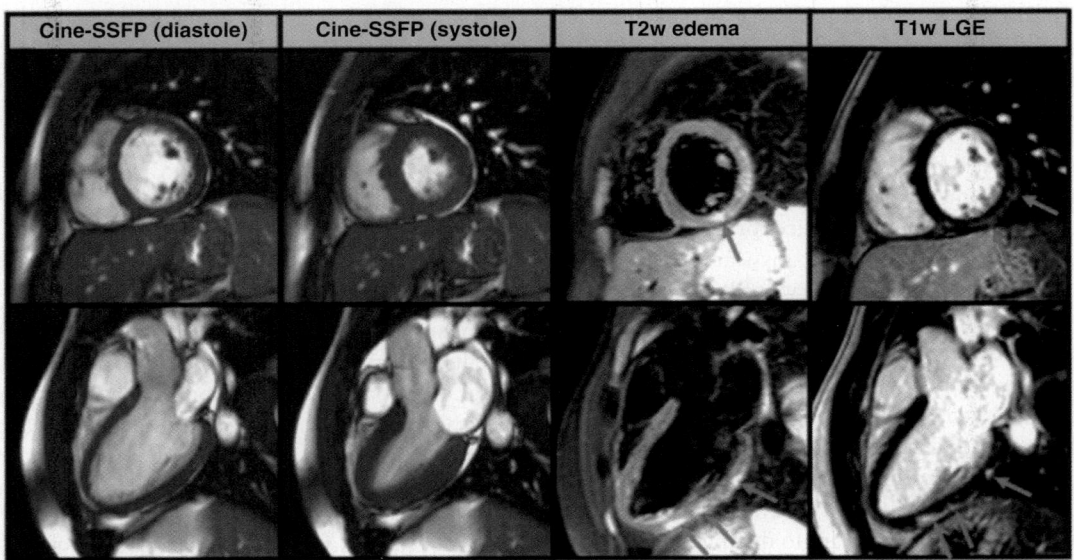

Figure 20–6. Cardiac magnetic resonance imaging of acute myocarditis. This figure shows cine images in diastole and systole without evidence of regional wall motion abnormality (columns 1 and 2), and with T2-weighted oedema images showing patchy focal oedema in the subepicardium of the inferolateral wall (*red arrows*, column 3) and on T1-weighted late gadolinium enhancement (LGE) (*red arrows*, Column 4). Reproduced with permission from Caforio AL, Pankuweit S, Arbustini E, et al. Current state of knowledge on aetiology, diagnosis, management, and therapy of myocarditis: a position statement of the European Society of Cardiology Working Group on Myocardial and Pericardial Diseases. *Eur Heart J.* 2013 Sep;34(33):2636-2648.

inflammatory processes (**Fig. 20–6**). The Lake Louise criteria (**Table 20–6**) proposes CMR diagnostic criteria for myocarditis.[153,154] The location of LGE on CMR has been associated with specific viral etiology, with parvovirus B19 causing lateral wall inflammation, and human herpesvirus associated with septal LGE. Of note, a repeat CMR study should be considered after 1 to 2 weeks if the initial CMR is normal but the onset of symptoms has been very recent and there is strong clinical suspicion for myocardial inflammation.[153]

Other imaging types, such as nuclear imaging, are not recommended in myocarditis diagnosis, due to low specificity.[129] The only exception would be in cardiac sarcoidosis where Thallium 201 and technetium 99m scintigraphy have been described to detect myocardial metabolism and inflammation.

Viral Serology: Viral serology can be performed for antibodies (IgM and IgG) to specific viruses known to cause myocarditis. However, their clinical utility is hindered by the fact that no

TABLE 20–6. Guideline Differences for Diagnosis and Management of Myocarditis		
	ACC/AHA guidelines[147, 115, 155]	ESC Guidelines[129, 250]
Endomyocardial biopsy	- Recommended in heart failure that is rapidly progressing with a high suspicion that the cause can only be confirmed on biopsy or in unexplained cardiomyopathy requiring inotropic or mechanical support, Mobitz type 2 or higher degree HB, ventricular tachycardia or failure to respond to medical management within 1-2 weeks	Should be considered in *all* patients with suspected myocarditis or in heart failure that is rapidly progressing with a high suspicion that the cause can only be confirmed on biopsy
EMB number of samples	5-10 samples each 1-2mm³ in size	At least 3 samples, each 1-2mm³ in size
Coronary angiography	Recommended in all patients	Recommended in all patients
Routine testing for viral serology	Do not recommend	Do not recommend
Testing for cardiac autoantibodies	Can test for if clinically available	Strongly recommend if clinically available
Consideration of ICD	- ICD implantation deferred until resolution of the acute episode if possible - ICD may be considered in GCM with ventricular fibrillation or unstable ventricular tachycardia, if survival >1 year expected	- ICD implantation deferred until resolution of the acute episode if possible - ICD may be considered earlier in GCM or sarcoidosis with hemodynamic unstable ventricular tachyarrhythmia or aborted sudden death if survival >1 year expected
Return to competitive or amateur sport	At 3-6 months after normal stress test, echocardiogram and Holter monitor	At =>6 months after resolution

correlation has been seen between positive viral serology and EMB findings.[147] This has led to both the ESC and the American Heart Association (AHA) recommending that routine viral serology should not be performed.[115,129] This is because it is very common to find IgG antibodies to cardiotropic viruses in the general population, in the absence of viral myocarditis. The caveat to this recommendation is serological testing for hepatitis C, HIV, and rickettsia or Lyme disease in suspected cases or endemic areas.

Genetics

Several autoimmune conditions are associated with immune-mediated myocarditis, hence the overlapping genetic predisposition for both. A vast array of cardiac autoantibodies (aabs) have been described both in autoimmune myocarditis and in familial dilated cardiomyopathy.[133] These are not yet used routinely in clinical practice, but include muscle-specific antisarcolemmal aab, antiheart aab, antiinterfibrillary aabs, organ-specific antiheart aabs, antitropomyosin aabs, anti-troponin I, T aabs, and others.[129,133] Detected by indirect immunofluorescence, they have been found to predict disease development in relatives of patients with dilated cardiomyopathy.[133] While the ESC guidelines recommend testing for these autoantibodies, they are not yet widely available for clinical use. In addition, the major histocompatibility complex (MHC) genes that predispose to autoimmune disease such as Type 1 diabetes mellitus (T1DM) also appear to predispose to myocarditis in animal models. However, apart from the context of associated autoimmune disease and as a predictor of disease progression, major genetic components to myocarditis are not well described.

Clinical Challenges

The diagnosis of myocarditis remains challenging due to its heterogeneous clinical presentation and multiple underlying etiologies. In addition, access to appropriate diagnostic tools may be limited depending on availability of resources. While EMB is the gold standard for myocarditis diagnosis, in real-world observational studies it is performed in the minority of suspected cases.[135,147] Due to sampling error and progression of the type of inflammatory infiltrate with time, repeat EMBs may be needed to achieve a diagnosis.[145] Even with the addition of molecular viral PCR, the EMB results must be interpreted with caution. This is because intercurrent or previous viral infection unrelated to the current myocarditis cannot be excluded. In addition, patients with positive cardiac viral PCR have been found in some cases to have a different viral pathogen identified on peripheral cultures.[134] CMR provides noninvasive tissue characterization, and is highly useful in myocarditis diagnosis. However, its availability and expertise may be limited, and performing CMR in clinically unstable patients is not always feasible. The other challenge is the management of fulminant myocarditis in centers that cannot undertake mechanical circulatory support. Patients with myocarditis who are hemodynamically unstable should be transferred to tertiary centers experienced in appropriate diagnostic and treatment options.[129]

Therapeutic Challenges

Myocarditis also presents a therapeutic challenge. The mainstay of treatment for all cases is supportive, following the usual principles of heart failure care.[155,156] In the instance of heart failure with reduced ejection fraction this includes diuretics, angiotensin-converting enzyme inhibitors or angiotensin receptor blockers and cardioselective beta-blockers. Aldosterone antagonists (ie, spironolactone) should also be introduced in those with ongoing heart failure symptoms. If there is hemodynamic instability, treatment can include ionotropic, vasopressor, and/or mechanical circulatory support. When pharmacological blood pressure support is needed, vasopressor therapy with noradrenaline has been associated with fewer arrhythmias than has dopamine in the acute MI setting. In the instance of rapid deterioration or incessant ventricular tachyarrhythmia, ventricular assist devices or extracorporeal membrane oxygenation (ECMO) may be required. These can provide a bridge to recovery or, less commonly, cardiac transplantation. ECMO therapy, in particular, has been shown to be effective in bridging patients with acute or fulminant myocarditis to recovery.[115] In the occurrence of fulminant myocarditis, recognition of the deteriorating patient is critical in order to institute circulatory support and prevent end-organ damage. Early warning signs of circulatory collapse may include sinus tachycardia, narrow arterial pulse pressure, cool/mottled extremities, or elevated lactate. Avoidance of rate control agents such as beta-blockers or calcium-channel blockers, particularly those with negative inotropic effects, are crucial in maintaining stroke volume and cardiac output. The ACC/AHA recommend that patients be transferred and treated in centers that have the capability for mechanical support procedures, endomyocardial biopsy, and advanced cardiac imaging, as this improves outcomes.[157]

In addition to treating the myocarditis-related heart failure, it is important to identify the cause and remove the trigger, where applicable. For instance, in the event of eosinophilic or toxic myocarditis identifying a medication or toxin and removing it. Anticoagulation should also be considered in the event of acute necrotizing eosinophilic myocarditis due to the association with microvascular thrombosis.[115] Of note, unlike for pericarditis, nonsteroidal anti-inflammatories (NSAIDs) are not indicated for myocarditis and have been found to be harmful in animal models.

Treatment

Immunosuppression

In regards to specific treatments for myocarditis, this is highly dependent on the underlying cause. Immunosuppressive therapy can be with steroids alone or in combination with cyclosporine A or azathioprine.[158-161] In the case of viral myocarditis or myocarditis of unknown cause, broad immunosuppressive therapy has not been shown to be beneficial.[162] Immunosuppression in autoimmune myocarditis (autoantibody positive or in association with systemic autoimmune disease), GCM, and cardiac sarcoidosis has been shown to improve LVEF and survival.[158-161] In the instance of autoimmune myocarditis, EMB is useful in guiding appropriate therapy with HLA-DR upregulation indicating a benefit for immunosuppression.[131] In the case of eosinophilic myocarditis, particularly acute NEM, high-dose corticosteroids have been found to be beneficial.[163,164] For toxic myocarditis related to checkpoint inhibitors, intravenous corticosteroids are also recommended to prevent progression to fulminant myocarditis.[115,165]

Immunomodulation

Antiviral medications have also been studied in viral myocarditis. This includes acyclovir, ganciclovir, and valacyclovir in herpes virus infection and antiretrovirals in HIV infection. However, while these have a benefit in clearing the peripheral virus, they have not been shown to improve myocardial function itself. Interferon-beta treatment has been studied in enteroviral and adenoviral infection where it has been associated with an improvement in LV function.[166] High-dose intravenous immunoglobulin has also been studied in all-cause myocarditis, where little benefit was seen in adults despite clinical utility in pediatric populations.[167] Despite the lack of prospective studies, in unstable patients not responding to steroids, IVIG can be considered.[115] Statin therapy has also been tested, in a small randomized trial with improvement in LVEF.[168]

Guidelines

Patients with myocarditis may have severely reduced LVEF that falls within primary prevention ICD guidelines.[157] However, implanting a primary prevention ICD in the setting of myocarditis is not recommended due to the likelihood for LVEF recovery. Use of a wearable defibrillator in patients deemed high risk based on impaired LVEF, or with ventricular tachyarrhythmia episodes, might bridge to recovery of LVEF, but there is little data to guide their use. ESC guidelines recommend that ICD implantation be deferred until resolution of the acute episode and then placed based on ESC device guidelines (Table 20–6).[129] ACC/AHA guidelines recommend that patients with GCM and VF/unstable VT or cardiac sarcoidosis with sustained VT, cardiac arrest, or LVEF<=35% can be considered for an ICD if life expectancy is greater than 1 year.[157] The ESC guidelines recommend that physical activity and competitive or amateur sports be avoided during acute myocarditis and for at least 6 months after resolution due to the risk of ventricular arrythmia.[129,164] This is based upon expert opinion with little clinical study data to guide this area. The ACC/AHA guidelines temper this recommendation slightly, advising that after 3 to 6 months, patients with a normal stress test, echocardiogram, and Holter monitor can resume sport activity.[115]

Summary

Myocarditis is a heterogeneous disease with the overarching finding of myocardial inflammation. Its clinical presentation with chest pain, ECG changes, and elevated cardiac biomarkers can masquerade as an acute MI. While classically diagnosed on invasive myocardial biopsy, it can now be diagnosed with the use of clinical and diagnostic criteria, ideally with incorporation of tissue characteristics on cardiac MRI. Management is largely supportive, including all guideline-directed heart failure therapy with immunosuppressive and immunomodulatory therapy reserved for certain myocarditis subtypes. Further study will help close the knowledge gap surrounding the true epidemiology, underlying genetic predispositions, and short- and long-term management of myocarditis.

TAKOTSUBO SYNDROME

Takotsubo syndrome (TTS) is an LV dysfunction syndrome that presents similarly to ACS, but has several characteristic features: (1) there is no coronary artery culprit stenosis; (2) TTS is often triggered by emotional or physical stress; and (3) there are extensive LV wall motion abnormalities that are transient in survivors. The extent of the wall motion abnormalities is larger than would be expected for the degree of troponin elevation. The name "takotsubo" derives from the resemblance between the LV dysfunction pattern in the apical form to a Japanese octopus trapping pot of the same name. Over the 30 years since the initial publication describing TTS by Sato in Japan in 1990,[169] nomenclature and definitions have evolved. Several alternate terms for the syndrome have largely been discarded because they describe features that are not universal, such as apical ballooning cardiomyopathy, stress cardiomyopathy, and broken heart syndrome. TTS should be diagnosed only after acute MI has been excluded, typically via invasive coronary angiography.

Definition

Several definitions have been proposed and those in most common use are the International takotsubo Registry (InterTAK) definition[170] and the revised Mayo Clinic criteria.[171] We prefer the InterTAK definition (**Table 20–7**), because it formally recognizes the possibility of coexisting coronary artery obstructive disease, which may be present but not part of the pathogenesis, and because it includes a broader array of ECG abnormalities than do the revised Mayo Clinic criteria. However, it must be recognized that the InterTAK definition is also imperfect in that many cases of MINOCA appear to fit the definition, and MINOCA is a distinct entity (ie, infarction due to vascular causes). Some patients with hypertrophic cardiomyopathy develop apical ballooning during their clinical course, and this is not termed TTS. Thus, as is often the case in medicine, clinical judgment must be exercised to apply diagnostic criteria for TTS appropriately.

Epidemiology

TTS is ultimately diagnosed in 0.5% to 3% of ACS cases[172,173] overall and in 5% to 6% of women presenting with ACS.[172,175] Approximately 90% of patients with TTS are female, and approximately 80% are aged 50 years or older, although people of any age can be affected (**Fig. 20–7**).[176–177] The mean age at presentation is between 65 and 70 years.[177,178] The incidence of TTS has increased over time, likely due to increased recognition (**Fig. 20–8**).[172,179,180] Incidence is somewhat higher in the summer and lower in winter months in the Northern Hemisphere.[181,182] The true incidence among people at risk,

TABLE 20-7. InterTAK Diagnostic Criteria for TTS[170]

1. Patients show transient[a] left ventricular dysfunction (hypokinesia, akinesia, or dyskinesia) presenting as apical ballooning or midventricular, basal, or focal wall motion abnormalities. Right ventricular involvement can be present. Besides these regional wall motion patterns, transitions between all types can exist. The regional wall motion abnormality usually extends beyond a single epicardial vascular distribution; however, rare cases can exist where the regional wall motion abnormality is present in the subtended myocardial territory of a single coronary artery (focal TTS).[b]
2. An emotional, physical, or combined trigger can precede the takotsubo syndrome event, but this is not obligatory.
3. Neurologic disorders (eg, subarachnoid hemorrhage, stroke/transient ischemic attack, or seizures) as well as pheochromocytoma may serve as triggers for takotsubo syndrome.
4. New ECG abnormalities are present (ST-segment elevation, ST-segment depression, T-wave inversion, and QTc prolongation); however, rare cases exist without any ECG changes.
5. Levels of cardiac biomarkers (troponin and creatine kinase) are moderately elevated in most cases; significant elevation of brain natriuretic peptide is common.
6. Significant coronary artery disease does not exclude takotsubo syndrome.
7. Patients have no evidence of infectious myocarditis.[b]
8. Postmenopausal women are predominantly affected.

[a]Wall motion abnormalities may remain for a prolonged period of time or documentation of recovery may not be possible. For example, death before evidence of recovery is captured.
[b]Cardiac magnetic resonance imaging is recommended to exclude infectious myocarditis and support the diagnosis of takotsubo syndrome.

including those who experience severe emotional or physical stressors, remains unknown. Risk factors for CAD are commonly present, such as hypertension in 54% to 65%, diabetes in 14% to 17%, dyslipidemia in 31% to 32%, and smoking in 20% to 22% of patients.[176,183] In addition, TTS patients are more

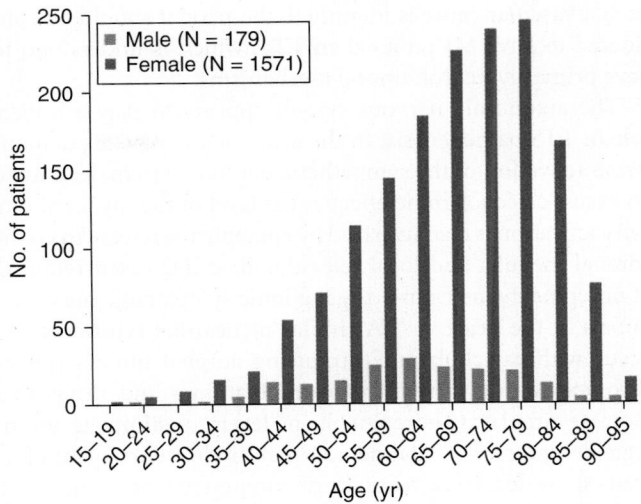

Figure 20–7. Age and sex distribution of 1,750 patients with takotsubo syndrome in the InterTAK registry. Reproduced with permission from Templin C, Ghadri JR, Diekmann J, et al. Clinical Features and Outcomes of Takotsubo (Stress) Cardiomyopathy. *N Engl J Med.* 2015 Sep 3;373(10):929-938.

likely to have history of mood or anxiety disorders than other ACS patients.[175]

Pathogenesis

LV dysfunction is induced via direct catecholamine toxicity, epinephrine-induced changes in adrenoceptor stimulus trafficking, and/or vascular effects (endothelial dysfunction and spasm).[184] Some TTS events represent plaque rupture in a large LAD coronary artery or left main coronary artery, or initially unrecognized coronary dissection.[185–187] Strictly speaking, once

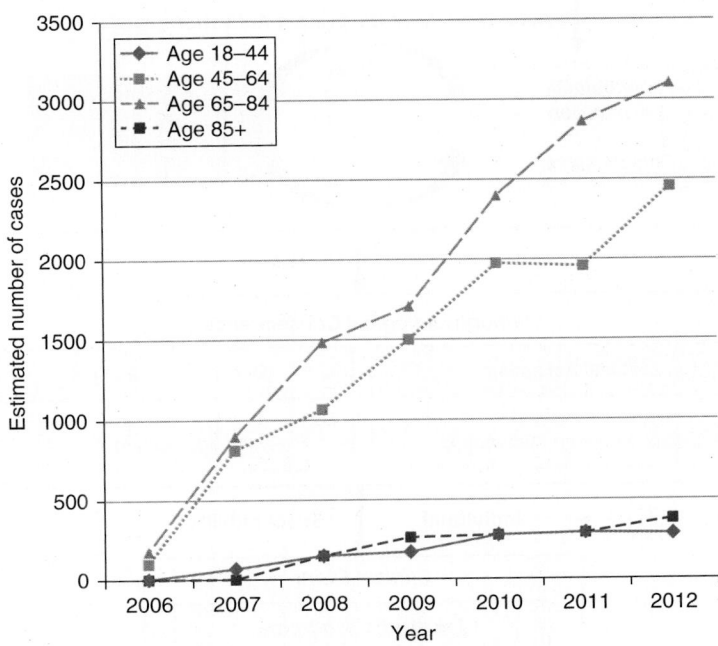

Figure 20–8. Estimated number of cases of TTS in the United States by age group from 2006 to 2012 in the National Inpatient Sample. Reproduced with permission from Minhas AS, Hughey AB, Kolias TJ. Nationwide Trends in Reported Incidence of Takotsubo Cardiomyopathy from 2006 to 2012. *Am J Cardiol.* 2015 Oct 1;116(7):1128-1131.

such a vascular cause is identified, the patient should be considered to have MI rather than TTS, which is understood to have primarily neurohumoral mechanisms.

The autonomic nervous system appears to play a critical role in TTS pathogenesis. In the acute phase, patients demonstrate activation of the sympathetic nervous system, leading to an excess catecholamine effect at the level of the myocardium. This activation is characterized by epinephrine release from the adrenal medulla and local release and/or decreased reuptake of norepinephrine from postganglionic sympathetic nerve terminals in the heart.[184,188] A similar myocardial syndrome can occur with catecholamine-producing adrenal tumors (pheochromocytoma), infusion of catecholamines and drugs that increase circulating norepinephrine levels, or stimulate adrenergic receptors.[189–191] Iodine-123 meta-iodo-benzyl-guanidine scans show decreased reuptake of norepinephrine in the heart, consistent with elevated coronary sinus catecholamine levels. In addition, there may be diminished parasympathetic influences on the heart in the acute phase and at follow-up (reduced heart rate variability [HRV]).[192] Some investigators have identified marked elevation of catecholamines in the acute phase, but this has not been consistent across studies.[193] The net effect of autonomic nervous system imbalance is the clinical event, with LV dysfunction. There may be more than one mechanism

by which LV dysfunction occurs (**Fig. 20–9**). There is evidence for direct toxic catecholamine effect, with histological analysis of myocardial biopsies confirming contraction bands without necrosis; these persist for months.[194] Myocardial stunning may be mediated by a switch from stimulatory to inhibitory G-protein coupling of myocardial beta-2 adrenoceptors induced by high levels of epinephrine. This switch was associated with reduced mortality in an animal model.

Large artery and/or microvascular endothelial dysfunction/spasm may also play a pathogenetic role, inducing transient ischemia and LV dysfunction, even present on provocative testing years after the event.

LV and mitral apparatus geometry may contribute to susceptibility to catecholamine stress and therefore TTS. Apical ballooning occurs in response to stress among patients with hypertrophic cardiomyopathy, and patients with a clinical diagnosis of TTS were more likely than controls to have morphologic features consistent with a mild form of hypertrophic cardiomyopathy (eg, longer anterior mitral leaflets and larger interventricular septal thickness).[195,196]

Hormonal and genetic factors are likely to have at least a partial role in susceptibility based on the strong predominance of postmenopausal females among patients with the disorder, and familial clustering in some cases. Adrenoceptor gene

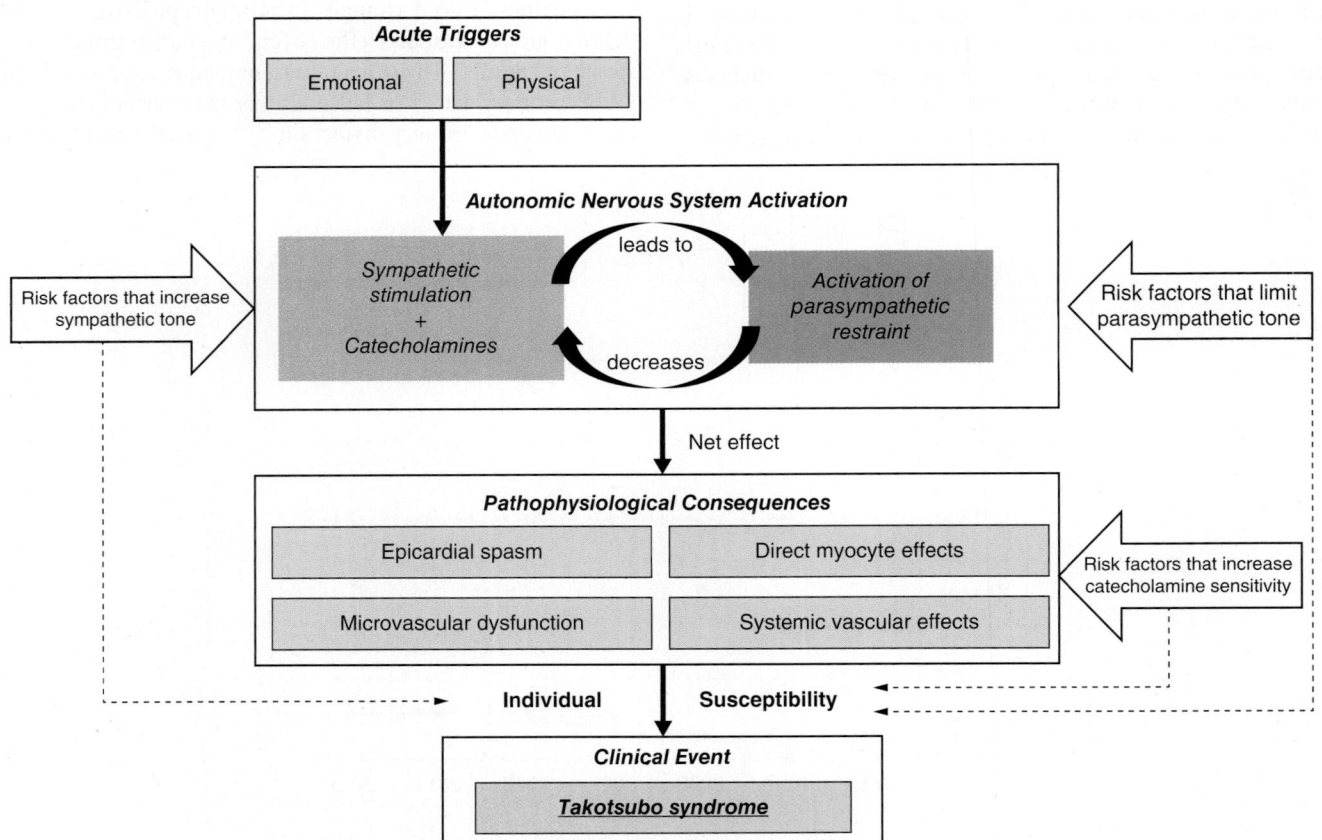

Figure 20–9. Interplay between the sympathetic and parasympathetic nervous systems in takotsubo syndrome, and risk factors that may mediate individual susceptibility.

polymorphisms have been implicated in some studies, but data are inconsistent.[191]

Presentation: Symptoms, Triggers, ECG Findings, and Laboratory Test Results

The most common presenting symptoms are chest discomfort (76%), shortness of breath (47%), and syncope (8%).[176] ECG changes may include ST-segment elevation (44%), T-wave inversion (41%), QTc-interval prolongation (48%), and less commonly, ST-segment depression (8%).[180] Numerous emotional and physical triggering events have been described (**Fig. 20–10**). However, a substantial minority of patients have no triggering event identified. Most emotional triggers involve unpleasant emotions, but some are pleasant ("happy heart syndrome"). Trigger events all have the potential to increase sympathetic outflow or catecholamine levels or action, thought to be central in TTS pathogenesis. Some find the term "broken heart syndrome" derogatory, because it minimizes the physical causes and effects of the syndrome and implies self-causation by the patient. TTS may develop in the midst of or just after triggering events, or days or weeks later. During clinical interviews, TTS patients often describe having been under high stress chronically, and state that a triggering event was simply "the straw that broke the camel's back."[197]

Cardiac troponin is elevated in nearly all patients, as is B-type natriuretic peptide. Troponin tends to be less markedly elevated and BNP more elevated in TTS than in MI.[176] A hallmark of TTS is the relatively modest nature of troponin elevation in relation to the extent of abnormal LV wall motion; for example, the median peak troponin was just 13 times the upper limit of normal in the InterTAK registry while the median LVEF was 40%.[176]

Patterns of Cardiac Wall Motion Abnormalities

The most common pattern of LV wall motion abnormalities observed in TTS is the apical pattern, which includes at least the apical segments of the left ventricle and also typically the mid segments, sparing the basal segments and extending beyond the usual territory of the LAD coronary artery (**Fig. 20–11**). Interestingly, a long, "wrap-around" LAD serving the inferior wall is no more common among apical type TTS patients than among consecutive sex-matched patients without TTS.[197] The midventricular wall motion pattern demonstrates preserved wall motion in the apex. The basal or inverted wall motion pattern is far less common, affecting the basal and mid segments of the left ventricle with preserved wall motion at the apex. Also infrequent is the focal pattern of wall motion abnormality, which affects one or more segments and does not meet the criteria for other wall motion patterns. The focal type may be confused with MINOCA of a vascular cause such as plaque rupture, erosion, or coronary spasm. The diagnosis of focal TTS, in particular, should be made only after excluding MI or myocarditis, such as via cardiac MRI. Right ventricular

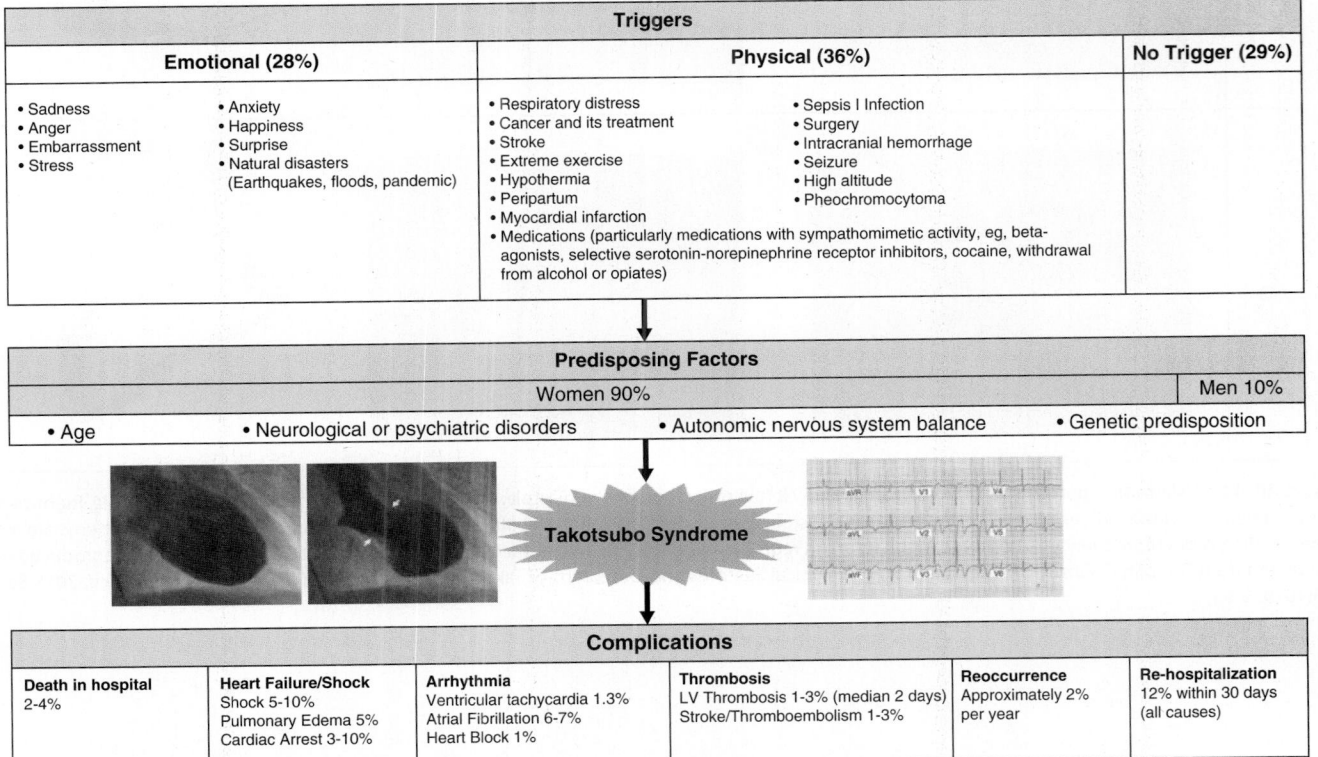

Figure 20–10. Triggers, predisposing factors, and complications of TTS. Note that an additional ~7% of patients have both an emotional and a physical trigger.

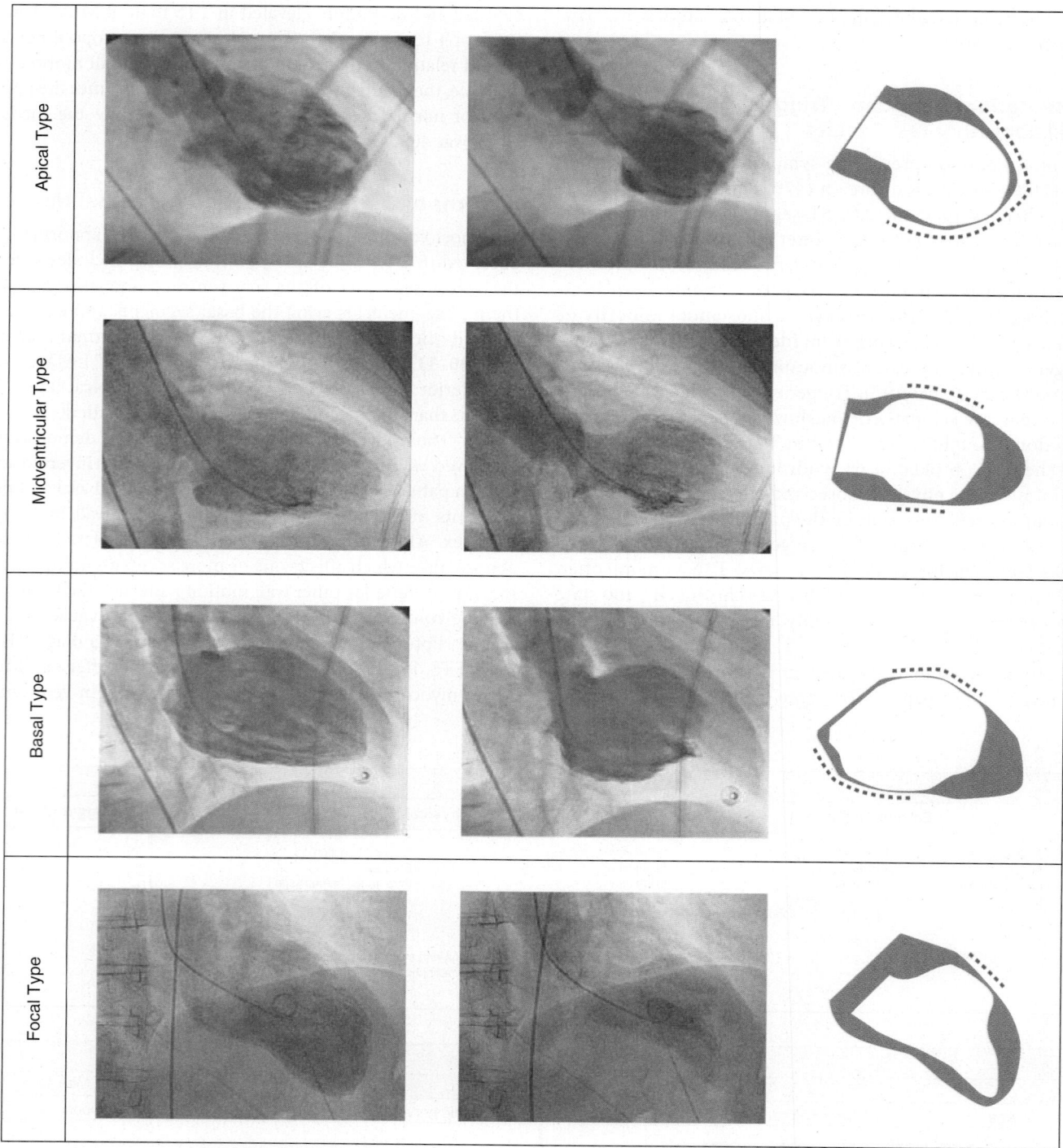

Figure 20–11. Wall motion patterns in TTS. Left panels show left ventriculography in diastole. Center panels, left ventriculography in systole. Right panels show a schematic of the left ventricle in diastole (red) and systole (white), demonstrating the affected areas with blue dots. The different patterns are listed in descending order of frequency as observed in the InterTAK registry: apical in 82%, midventricular in 15%, basal in 2%, and focal in 1.5%. Reproduced with permission from Templin C, Ghadri JR, Diekmann J, et al. Clinical Features and Outcomes of Takotsubo (Stress) Cardiomyopathy. *N Engl J Med.* 2015 Sep 3; 373(10):929-938.

hypokinesis may accompany LV dysfunction, most commonly with the apical type, or may occur alone.[199,200] In-hospital and long-term outcomes are no different based on the wall motion pattern, and the same patient may present with a different wall motion pattern if TTS recurs.[199,201,202]

Distinguishing TTS from Acute MI

Coronary angiography should not be deferred in a patient with suspected acute MI based solely on the ECG or wall motion pattern, even in a patient thought to be at high risk for TTS. Emotional and physical stress are well known to precipitate plaque rupture and acute MI. For example, the apical ballooning wall motion pattern in a postmenopausal woman who is under emotional stress may certainly be due to occlusion of the LAD coronary artery if the distribution of that artery is large, and the larger the myocardial territory affected, the greater the concern should treatable coronary occlusion be missed. On the other hand, not all patients with a clinical diagnosis of TTS who prove to have some obstructive CAD have MI. Some do not have sufficient culprit CAD to explain takotsubo-like wall motion abnormalities. These patients are considered to have bystander CAD that is unrelated to the pathogenesis, or may have TTS triggered by acute MI.[203]

The InterTAK investigators developed a score that may be useful in assessing the likelihood of TTS in a patient presenting with features of ACS.[204,205] Components of the score include female sex, emotional or physical trigger, ECG findings, and the presence of psychiatric or neurologic disease. The specificity of different constellations of ECG findings[206–209] and wall motion patterns[210,211] for TTS is imperfect, as it is for the InterTAK score. Noninvasive angiography should be reserved for patients with very high likelihood of TTS and without ST elevation or hemodynamic compromise, and should be performed promptly in case the diagnosis of TTS proves not to be correct.[212] Clinical judgment is necessary. As noted earlier, SCAD may be the cause of a TTS presentation if the LAD coronary artery is affected.[185,186] The diagnosis of SCAD may be missed, so careful angiographic review is necessary.

Suggested Diagnostic Approach

Patients who are ultimately diagnosed with TTS usually present with symptoms that could represent myocardial ischemia. Given that there is usually either ST-segment elevation on the ECG, extensive wall motion abnormality on echocardiography, or both, in association with troponin elevation, most patients will undergo invasive angiography in the acute setting to rule out coronary artery occlusion or severe stenosis. Such stenosis may be atherosclerotic in origin or due to coronary dissection or embolism. When there is no obstructive CAD, the differential diagnosis is MINOCA (ie, a vascular cause of infarction in the absence of significant CAD[213]), myocarditis, or TTS. This differential diagnosis may be resolved most definitively using cardiac MRI. MINOCA patients may have an area of subendocardial or transmural late gadolinium enhancement (LGE) indicative of MI or may have an area of myocardial edema on T1- or T2-weighted imaging in a coronary territory consistent with coronary ischemia, or normal MRI.[214] Myocarditis patients have nonischemic LGE with or without myocardial edema.[215] Those with TTS often have circumferential myocardial edema in the area of affected LV segments, without dense LGE.[216] Cardiac MRI is not necessary in all cases but may be strongly considered when the demographics or presentation of the patient are atypical for TTS (eg, young male, larger degrees of troponin elevation) and with the focal wall motion pattern.

Acute Complications

Cardiogenic shock complicates TTS in approximately 5% to 10% of patients (Fig. 20–10).[176–178,217–219] Pulmonary edema occurs in 5%.[177] Shock may be due to pump failure alone or in association with left ventricular outflow tract (LVOT) obstruction. LVOT obstruction occurs due to the combination of preserved contraction of basal LV segments, poor contractility of the mid and/or apical segments, and in some cases, predisposing mitral anatomy and LV geometry.[195]

The identification of LVOT obstruction in the TTS patient with shock is critical because it influences management. Patients with pump failure alone as the mechanism of shock may benefit from administration of vasoactive agents. Levosimendan may be preferred where available, given that excess catecholamines have been implicated in TTS pathogenesis; further study is needed.[212,220] In those who do have LVOT obstruction, inotropic agents should be avoided because they will worsen LVOT obstruction and therefore shock. Increasing preload via leg elevation or administration of fluids may be helpful, even with mild pulmonary congestion, since it may relieve obstruction and improve forward flow. Beta blockade is used in shock with LVOT obstruction, as a negative inotrope, to relieve obstruction. If vasopressor support is needed, a pure alpha agonist (eg, phenylephrine) is used in the setting of LVOT obstruction. Mechanical circulatory support may be considered when these measures fail.

Arrhythmia (atrial and ventricular) and cardiac arrest may complicate TTS, but ventricular rupture is rare (0.2%).[176,178,218,219,221,222]

LV thrombus is identified in 1% to 3% of patients with TTS and may embolize, causing stroke.[176,216,218] LV thrombus formation is associated with larger degrees of troponin elevation and with the apical wall motion pattern.[176]

In-hospital death occurs in 1% to 5% of patients, a rate intermediate between that of NSTEMI and STEMI.[176,177,178,179,217] Predictors of in-hospital death are shock, older age, male sex, non-White race, atrial fibrillation, ventricular arrhythmia, cardiac arrest, and comorbidity.[179,222,223] Echocardiographic predictors of in-hospital adverse events include lower LVEF, poorer diastolic parameters, and mitral regurgitation.[224]

Rehospitalization within 30 days occurs in 12%, and mortality associated with rehospitalization is 3.5% of patients.[178,179,225] Overall, rehospitalization is more likely to be due to noncardiac than cardiac causes, but the single most common readmission diagnosis is heart failure.[178] Readmission is associated with older age, history of heart failure, atrial fibrillation, malignancy,

SECTION III • Atherosclerosis and Coronary Heart Disease

chronic kidney disease, chronic lung disease, CAD risk factors, and depression, among other factors.[178,225]

Outcomes

Long-term unadjusted mortality is 2% to 6% per year, similar to MI patients in most comparative studies.[176,179,217,226–229] Unlike MI, noncardiovascular causes are more common than cardiovascular causes of death after TTS.[226,228] The presence of a physical trigger or absence of a trigger is associated with higher risk of mortality, as are male sex, older age, history of diabetes, lower LVEF, and shock.[219,226,227,229] Triggering by a neurologic disorder is associated with a particularly adverse prognosis.[229] A mortality prediction score has been derived from the Inter-TAK registry (**Fig. 20–12**).

Recurrent TTS occurs at a rate of approximately 2% per year in larger studies, and more than one recurrence is possible.[176,218] Predictors of recurrence remain unclear.[218]

Although cancer is associated with TTS, a case-control study demonstrated no increase in the incidence of cancer after a takotsubo event.[230] Strain imaging demonstrated persistent abnormalities in patients who recovered from TTS, including with normalization of EF.[231–232] An increase in the extracellular volume fraction has also been observed after normalization of global function, on cardiac MRI.[232]

Despite implication of the autonomic nervous system in the pathogenesis of TTS, beta-blockade has not been associated with reduced risk of recurrence or lower mortality.[176,219] The use of ACE inhibitors and/or angiotensin receptor blockers has been associated with reduced risk in multiple observational studies.[176,219] Further research is needed, but clinical trial execution is limited by the relatively low event rate.

Summary

TTS is a transient, reversible LV dysfunction syndrome that mimics MI in the acute phase. It occurs almost exclusively in postmenopausal women. Patients have similar symptoms, ECG changes, and cardiac biomarker release to typical MI and have extensive LV wall motion abnormalities, in the absence of culprit CAD. The syndrome is often preceded by an acute physical or emotional stressor, but may not have an obvious trigger. Risk of shock, in-hospital death, readmission, and long-term mortality are substantial. The recurrence rate is low. Treatment is unknown; ACE inhibition may be useful based on observational studies. Survivors have complete recovery of LV function on echocardiography, but emerging evidence demonstrates subtle abnormalities of the myocardium, even after recovery.

CONGENITAL ANOMALIES AND KAWASAKI DISEASE

Anomalous Coronary Arteries

Variation from the normal origin and course of the coronary arteries is observed in approximately 1% to 2% of the population. These patterns of variation include anomalous origin (coronary atresia, separate ostia for circumflex and anterior descending arteries, coronary arising from the wrong aortic cusp, and coronary arising from the pulmonary artery), anomalous course (interarterial, intraarterial, retroaortic), and anomalous branching (single coronary artery). The two most commonly observed patterns are right coronary artery arising from the left cusp coursing between the aorta and pulmonary artery, and the circumflex artery arising from the right sinus coursing retrograde around the aorta.[234] Single coronary artery is rare in the absence of other associated anomalies of the heart. Atresia of one of the two main coronary ostia may occur and may result in myocardial ischemia and infarction in infancy or childhood. The involved vessel becomes dependent on collateral coronary blood flow from the contralateral coronary artery. Anomalous left coronary artery arising from the pulmonary artery (ALCAPA; also known

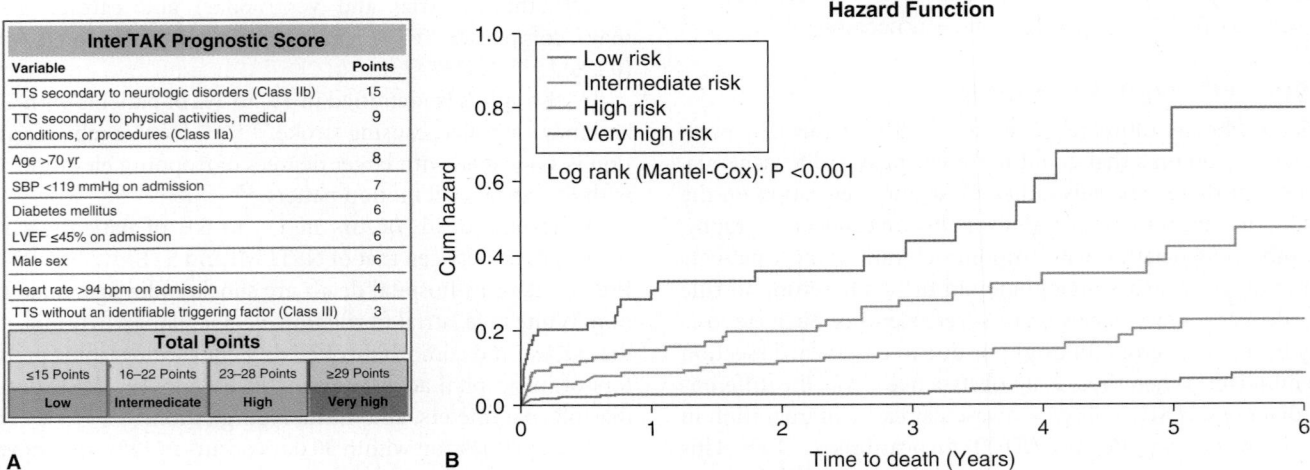

Figure 20–12. InterTAK prognostic score. Five-year overall survival in low risk, intermediate risk, high risk, and very-high risk groups rated as high as 93.5%, 79.9%, 65.6%, and 45.1%, respectively. Using the low-risk group as the reference group, the following HR with 95% CI were obtained: intermediate risk: HR 3.15, 95% CI, 1.74–5.72, *P* <0.001; high risk: HR 6.16, 95% CI, 3.46–10.98, *P* <0.001, and very-high risk: HR 11.82, 95% CI, 6.56–21.28, *P* <0.001. Reproduced with permission from Wischnewsky MB, Candreva A, Bacchi B, et al. Prediction of short- and long-term mortality in takotsubo syndrome: the InterTAK Prognostic Score. *Eur J Heart Fail.* 2019 Nov; 21(11):1469-1472.

as Bland-White-Garland syndrome) is frequently fatal during infancy. Those surviving into adulthood typically have developed a robust collateral system where the myocardium is supplied with oxygen from the right coronary alone, and flow is reversed in the left system into the pulmonary artery.[235] This causes a coronary steal phenomenon, LV dysfunction, and sometimes ischemia and even sudden death.

Some of these patterns may be associated with myocardial ischemia and raise concern for adverse events, including sudden death.[236] A multitude of causal mechanisms have been proposed, including hypoplasia of the artery, the acute angle of origin, a flaplike mechanism of the endothelium at the origin, and direct compression of the artery between the great arteries. The primary concern among these anomalies relates to arterial courses between the aorta and pulmonary artery. Normally, the coronary ostia are round to oval in shape, but in anomalous origin, the coronary artery has an acute angle of origin that makes the ostium slit-like in shape. Although the precise mechanism is unclear, what appears to occur is that with increased cardiac output, some combination of hemodynamic changes (eg, increase in systolic pressures, aortic dilation with stretching of the aortic wall) results in diminished flow down the coronary artery, leading to ischemia. Further investigation into the mechanisms of ischemia is underway.[237] Single coronary arteries do not commonly have the same acute take-off, but may have elevated risk of adverse cardiac events caused by excessive blood flow in the single artery (**Figs 20–13 and 20–14**).[238,239]

When compared to patients with coronary arteries that do not travel between the great arteries, patients with an interarterial/intraarterial course are more likely to undergo surgical revascularization and may be at higher risk for MI and/or sudden death.[234] Perhaps the most comprehensive understanding of risk associated with anomalous coronaries comes from Eckart, who reviewed sudden deaths in 6.3 million military recruits.[240] This selected population had gone through screening necessary for military service; 126 deaths were observed (64 caused by an identifiable cardiac abnormality) at a rate of 13 per 100,000 recruit years. Among them, anomalous coronary arteries were considered responsible for one-third of deaths (21 of 64), all of which were left coronary arteries arising from the right sinus with a course between the aorta and pulmonary artery.[241]

Less clear is the relationship between anomalous coronary arteries and clinical symptoms such as dyspnea, angina, and syncope, particularly among older patients. With cardiac computed tomography growing in popularity as an imaging modality to evaluate chest pain patients, anomalous coronary arteries are increasingly incidentally detected. When these anomalies are discovered in older patients, aggressive management becomes difficult to justify as these defects, present from birth, have not caused MI or death in the patients up to the time of their discovery. Surgical revascularization can be performed; often surgeons request evidence of myocardial ischemia before embarking on a repair. Surgical approach is individualized to the anatomy of the patient and could take the form of reimplantation, pulmonary artery relocation, surgical repair of the coronary ostium, bypass grafting, or unroofing.[242] Surgical management of anomalous coronary from the pulmonary artery is typically achieved with coronary reimplantation.[243,244]

Kawasaki Disease

Kawasaki disease, also known as mucocutaneous lymph node syndrome, is a common childhood vasculitis that can manifest with coronary abnormalities, and is rare in adults. Typical presentation includes erythema of mucous membranes (conjunctivitis, mucositis, and rash) and lymphadenopathy. Although an infectious agent is suspected, no causative agent has been identified.[245] Pathologically, necrotizing angiitis of the vaso vasorum damages the media and adventitia. Widespread

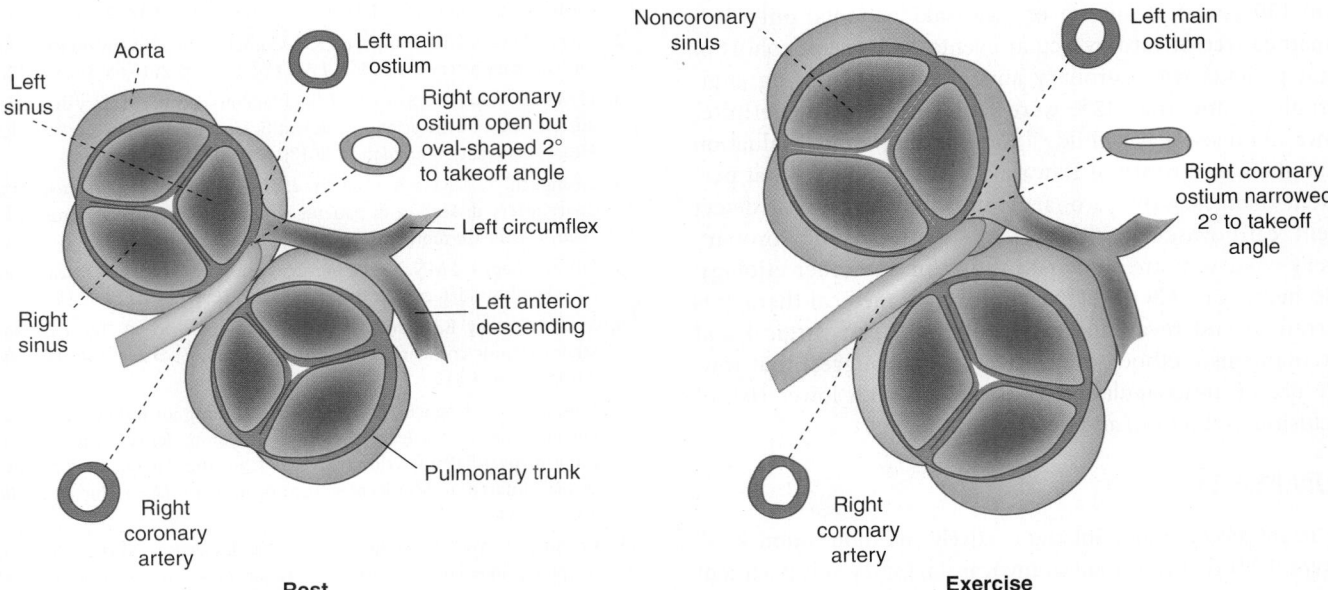

Figure 20–13. Diagram showing the proposed mechanism of myocardial ischemia produced by anomalous origin of the right coronary artery from the left sinus of Valsalva. With exercise, the aorta and pulmonary trunk dilate, thereby reducing the already narrowed coronary ostium of the anomalous right coronary.

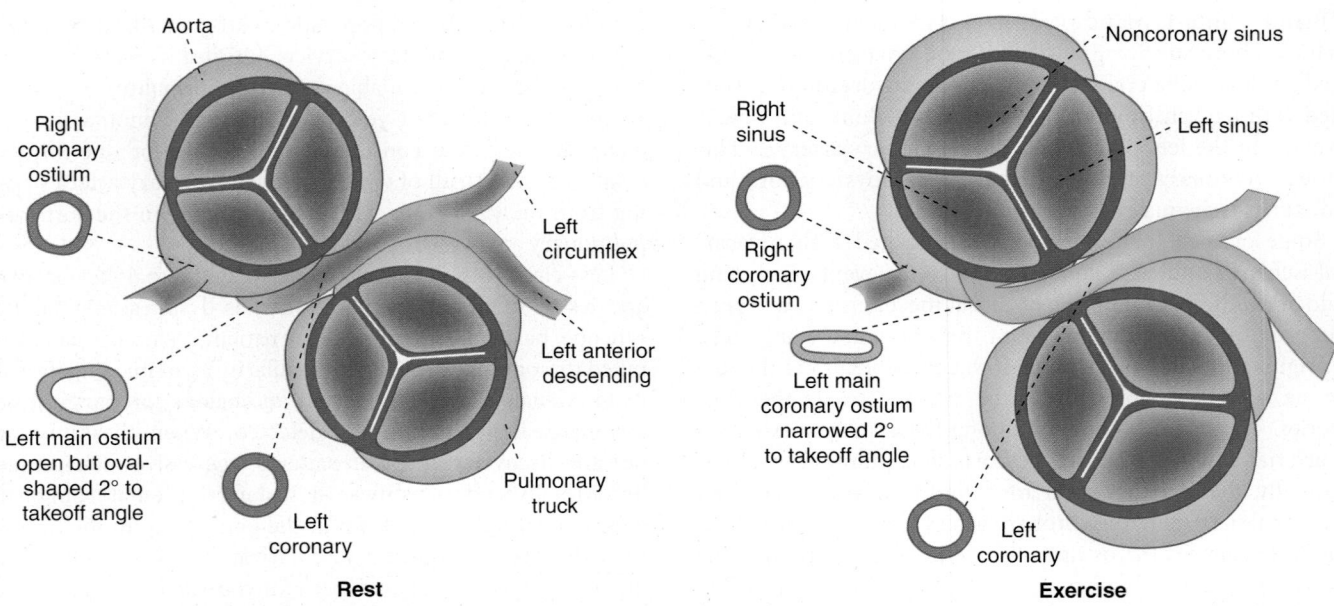

Figure 20–14. Diagram showing the proposed mechanism of myocardial ischemia produced by anomalous origin of the left coronary artery from the right sinus of Valsalva. With exercise, the aorta and pulmonary trunk dilate, thereby reducing the already narrowed coronary ostium of the anomalous left coronary.

inflammation of medium-sized arteries results in coronary artery aneurysms, typically developing between 4 days and 4 weeks of symptom onset in about 25% to 30% of patients who are not treated early. Widespread use of intravenous immunoglobulin has resulted in dramatic reductions in morbidity and mortality. Treatment with other immune modulating drugs is a current area of study.[246] Spontaneous regression of the aneurysm occurs in about half of vessels 1 to 2 years after illness, predominantly determined by the size of the initial aneurysm. Pericarditis, myocarditis, and arrhythmias can also occur. Noncoronary vascular symptoms include peripheral ischemia and, rarely, gangrene.

When Kawasaki disease goes undiagnosed in childhood, adults can suffer from late clinical manifestations. In long-term (30 years) follow-up of Kawasaki patients, only 36% remained free of cardiovascular events.[247] A recent cohort of adult patients with coronary aneurysm noted during angiography found that 22% were believed to have "definite" Kawasaki disease as a child.[248] Echocardiographic evaluation of adults with history of Kawasaki disease suggests that persistent changes in the coronary intima may be a way to detect latent cardiovascular risk.[249] Late treatments of coronary artery aneurysm are similar to those for any other etiology. If ischemia or ACS develops, appropriate medical therapy is warranted and revascularization options span surgical and percutaneous methods. Retrospective data suggest that routine use of anticoagulation is associated with lower risk of occlusion, infarction, and death.[250]

SUMMARY

There are several important and relatively common "mimickers" of type 1 MI that can result in myocardial injury. It is pertinent to differentiate these entities from atherosclerotic causes of MI since the management and outcomes can differ substantially as

described in this chapter. Clinicians need to comprehend the diagnostic criteria, investigations, and management strategies of these pathologically distinct conditions to optimally manage patients presenting with myocardial injury.

ACKNOWLEDGMENT

In the previous edition(s), some sections of this chapter were written by David E. Winchester and Carl J. Pepine, and this text has been retained.

REFERENCES

1. Thygesen K, Alpert JS, Jaffe AS, et al. Fourth universal definition of myocardial infarction (2018). *J Am Coll Cardiol.* 2018;72(18):2231-2264.
2. Saw J, Mancini GB, Humphries KH. Contemporary review on spontaneous coronary artery dissection. *J Am Coll Cardiol.* 2016;68(3):297-312.
3. Hayes SN, Kim ESH, Saw J, et al. Spontaneous coronary artery dissection: current state of the science: a scientific statement from the American Heart Association. *Circulation.* 2018;137(19):e523-e557.
4. Nishiguchi T, Tanaka A, Ozaki Y, et al. Prevalence of spontaneous coronary artery dissection in patients with acute coronary syndrome. *Eur Heart J Acute Cardiovasc Care.* 2016;5(3):263-270.
5. Hill SF, Sheppard MN. Non-atherosclerotic coronary artery disease associated with sudden cardiac death. *Heart.* 2010;96(14):1119-1125.
6. Saw J, Aymong E, Mancini J, Sedlak T, Starovoytov A, Ricci D. Non-atherosclerotic coronary artery disease in young women. *Can J Cardiol.* 2014;30(7):814-819.
7. Nakashima T, Noguchi T, Haruta S, et al. Prognostic impact of spontaneous coronary artery dissection in young female patients with acute myocardial infarction: a report from the Angina Pectoris-Myocardial Infarction Multicenter Investigators in Japan. *Int J Cardiol.* 2016;207:341-348.
8. Rashid HN, Wong DT, Wijesekera H, et al. Incidence and characterisation of spontaneous coronary artery dissection as a cause of acute coronary syndrome-a single-centre Australian experience. *Int J Cardiol.* 2016;202:336-338.

9. Elkayam U, Jalnapurkar S, Barakkat MN, et al. Pregnancy-associated acute myocardial infarction: a review of contemporary experience in 150 cases between 2006 and 2011. *Circulation*. 2014;129(16):1695-1702.

10. Saw J, Ricci D, Starovoytov A, Fox R, Buller CE. Spontaneous coronary artery dissection: prevalence of predisposing conditions including fibromuscular dysplasia in a tertiary center cohort. *JACC Cardiovasc Interv*. 2013;6(1):44-52.

11. Tweet MS, Eleid MF, Best PJ, et al. Spontaneous coronary artery dissection: revascularization versus conservative therapy. *Circ Cardiovasc Interv*. 2014;7(6):777-786.

12. Rogowski S, Maeder MT, Weilenmann D, et al. Spontaneous coronary artery dissection: angiographic follow-up and long-term clinical outcome in a predominantly medically treated population. *Catheter Cardiovasc Interv*. 2017;89(1):59-68.

13. Saw J. Coronary angiogram classification of spontaneous coronary artery dissection. *Catheter Cardiovasc Interv*. 2014;84(7):1115-1122.

14. Tweet MS, Hayes SN, Pitta SR, et al. Clinical features, management, and prognosis of spontaneous coronary artery dissection. *Circulation*. 2012;126(5):579-588.

15. Saw J, Aymong E, Sedlak T, et al. Spontaneous coronary artery dissection: association with predisposing arteriopathies and precipitating stressors and cardiovascular outcomes. *Circ Cardiovasc Interv*. 2014;7(5):645-655.

16. Godinho AR, Vasconcelos M, Araujo V, Maciel MJ. Spontaneous coronary artery dissection in acute coronary syndrome: report of a series of cases with 17 patients. *Arq Bras Cardiol*. 2016;107(5):491-494.

17. Saw J, Humphries K, Aymong E, et al. Spontaneous coronary artery dissection: clinical outcomes and risk of recurrence. *J Am Coll Cardiol*. 2017;70(9):1148-1158.

18. McGrath-Cadell L, McKenzie P, Emmanuel S, Muller DWM, Graham RM, Holloway CJ. Outcomes of patients with spontaneous coronary artery dissection. *Openheart*. 2016;3:e000491.

19. Prasad M, Tweet MS, Hayes SN, et al. Prevalence of extracoronary vascular abnormalities and fibromuscular dysplasia in patients with spontaneous coronary artery dissection. *Am J Cardiol*. 2015;115(12):1672-1677.

20. Tweet MS, Hayes SN, Codsi E, Gulati R, Rose CH, Best PJM. Spontaneous coronary artery dissection associated with pregnancy. *J Am Coll Cardiol*. 2017;70(4):426-435.

21. Henkin S, Negrotto SM, Tweet MS, et al. Spontaneous coronary artery dissection and its association with heritable connective tissue disorders. *Heart*. 2016;102(11):876–881.

22. Saw J, Bezerra H, Gornik HL, Machan L, Mancini GB. Coronary fibromuscular dysplasia angiographic manifestations. *Circulation*. 2015;132:A16282.

23. Moulson N, Kelly J, Iqbal MB, Saw J. Histopathology of coronary fibromuscular dysplasia causing spontaneous coronary artery dissection. *JACC Cardiovasc Interv*. 2018;11(9):909-910.

24. Saw J, Starovoytov A, Humphries K, et al. Canadian spontaneous coronary artery dissection cohort study: in-hospital and 30–day outcomes. *Eur Heart J*. 2019.

25. Goel K, Tweet M, Olson TM, Maleszewski JJ, Gulati R, Hayes SN. Familial spontaneous coronary artery dissection: evidence for genetic susceptibility. *JAMA Intern Med*. 2015;175(5):821-826.

26. Turley TN, Theis JL, Sundsbak RS, et al. Rare missense variants in TLN1 are associated with familial and sporadic spontaneous coronary artery dissection. *Circ Genom Precis Med*. 2019;12(4):e002437.

27. Adlam D, Olson TM, Combaret N, et al. Association of the PHACTR1/EDN1 genetic locus with spontaneous coronary artery dissection. *J Am Coll Cardiol*. 2019;73(1):58-66.

28. Kiando SR, Tucker NR, Castro-Vega LJ, et al. PHACTR1 is a genetic susceptibility locus for fibromuscular dysplasia supporting its complex genetic pattern of inheritance. *PLoS Genet*. 2016;12(10):e1006367.

29. Hubmacher D, Apte SS. ADAMTS proteins as modulators of microfibril formation and function. *Matrix Biol*. 2015;47:34-43.

30. Lie JT, Berg KK. Isolated fibromuscular dysplasia of the coronary arteries with spontaneous dissection and myocardial infarction. *Hum Pathol*. 1987;18(6):654-656.

31. Saw J, Yang M-L, Trinder M, et al. Chromosome 1q21.2 and additional loci influence risk of spontaneous coronary artery dissection and myocardial infarction. *Nature Comm*. 2020;11. doi: 10.1038/s41467-020-17558-x

32. Luong C, Starovoytov A, Heydari M, Aymong E, Saw J. Clinical presentation of patients with spontaneous coronary artery dissection. *Catheter Cardiovasc Interv*. 2016;89(7):1149-1154.

33. Lempereur M, Gin K, Saw J. Multivessel spontaneous coronary artery dissection mimicking atherosclerosis. *JACC Cardiovasc Interv*. 2014;7(7):e87-e88.

34. Pozo-Osinalde E, Garcia-Guimaraes M, Bastante T, et al. Characteristic findings of acute spontaneous coronary artery dissection by cardiac computed tomography. *Coron Artery Dis*. 2020;31(3):293-299.

35. Tweet MS, Akhtar NJ, Hayes SN, Best PJ, Gulati R, Araoz PA. Spontaneous coronary artery dissection: Acute findings on coronary computed tomography angiography. *Eur Heart J Acute Cardiovasc Care*. 2019;8(5):467-475.

36. Prakash R, Starovoytov A, Heydari M, Mancini GB, Saw J. Catheter-induced iatrogenic coronary artery dissection in patients with spontaneous coronary artery dissection. *JACC Cardiovasc Interv*. 2016;9(17):1851-1853.

37. Tan NY, Hayes SN, Young PM, Gulati R, Tweet MS. Usefulness of cardiac magnetic resonance imaging in patients with acute spontaneous coronary artery dissection. *Am J Cardiol*. 2018;122(10):1624-1629.

38. Chandrasekhar J, Thakkar J, Starovoytov A, Lee C, Mayo J, Saw J. Characteristics of cardiac magnetic resonance imaging in spontaneous coronary artery dissection. *PCRonline*. 2018:Euro18A-OP004.

39. Saw J. Is there a role for cardiac magnetic resonance imaging in patients with SCAD? *Eur Heart J*. 2020;41(23):2206-2208.

40. Hassan S, Prakash R, Starovoytov A, Saw J. Natural history of spontaneous coronary artery dissection with spontaneous angiographic healing. *JACC Cardiovasc Interv*. 2019;12(6):518-527.

41. Lempereur M, Fung A, Saw J. Stent mal-apposition with resorption of intramural hematoma with spontaneous coronary artery dissection. *Cardiovasc Diag Ther*. 2015;5(4):323-329.

42. Chou AY, Prakash R, Rajala J, et al. The first dedicated cardiac rehabilitation program for patients with spontaneous coronary artery dissection: description and initial results. *Can J Cardiol*. 2016;32(4):554-560.

43. Gad MM, Mahmoud AN, Saad AM, et al. Incidence, clinical presentation, and causes of 30–day readmission following hospitalization with spontaneous coronary artery dissection. *JACC Cardiovasc Interv*. 2020;13(8):921-932.

44. Virk HUH, Tripathi B, Kumar V, et al. Causes, trends, and predictors of 90–day readmissions after spontaneous coronary artery dissection (from a nationwide readmission database). *Am J Cardiol*. 2019;124(9):1333-1339.

45. Saw J, Mancini GBJ, Humphries KH. Contemporary review on spontaneous coronary artery dissection. *J Am Coll Cardiol*. 2016;68(3):297-312.

46. Lettieri C, Zavalloni D, Rossini R, et al. Management and long-term prognosis of spontaneous coronary artery dissection. *Am J Cardiol*. 2015;116(1):66-73.

47. Eleid MF, Guddeti RR, Tweet MS, et al. Coronary artery tortuosity in spontaneous coronary artery dissection: angiographic characteristics and clinical implications. *Circ Cardiovasc Interv*. 2014;7(5):656-662.

48. Tweet MS, Young KA, Best PJM, et al. Association of pregnancy with recurrence of spontaneous coronary artery dissection among women with prior coronary artery dissection. *JAMA Network Open*. 2020;3(9):e2018170-e2018170.

49. Adlam D, Alfonso F, Maas A, Vrints C, Writing C. European Society of Cardiology, acute cardiovascular care association, SCAD study group: a position paper on spontaneous coronary artery dissection. *Eur Heart J*. 2018;39(36):3353-3368.

50. Prinzmetal M, Ekmekci A, Kennamer R, Kwoczynski JK, Shubin H, Toyoshima H. Variant form of angina pectoris, previously undelineated syndrome. *JAMA*. 1960;174:1794-1800.

51. Group JCSJW. Guidelines for diagnosis and treatment of patients with vasospastic angina (Coronary Spastic Angina) (JCS 2013). *Circ J*. 2014;78(11):2779-2801.

52. Ford TJ, Rocchiccioli P, Good R, et al. Systemic microvascular dysfunction in microvascular and vasospastic angina. *Eur Heart J*. 2018;39(46):4086-4097.

53. Konst RE, Meeder JG, Wittekoek ME, et al. Ischaemia with no obstructive coronary arteries. *Neth Heart J*. 2020;28(Suppl 1):66-72.

54. Beijk MA, Vlastra WV, Delewi R, et al. Myocardial infarction with non-obstructive coronary arteries: a focus on vasospastic angina. *Neth Heart J*. 2019;27(5):237-245.

55. Song JK. Coronary Artery Vasospasm. *Korean Circ J*. 2018;48(9):767-777.

56. Beltrame JF, Crea F, Kaski JC, et al. International standardization of diagnostic criteria for vasospastic angina. *Eur Heart J*. 2017;38(33):2565-2568.

57. Ford TJ, Stanley B, Good R, et al. Stratified medical therapy using invasive coronary function testing in angina: the CorMicA trial. *J Am Coll Cardiol*. 2018;72(23 Pt A):2841-2855.

58. Smilowitz NR, Mahajan AM, Roe MT, et al. Mortality of myocardial infarction by sex, age, and obstructive coronary artery disease status in the ACTION registry-GWTG (Acute Coronary Treatment and Intervention Outcomes Network Registry-Get With the Guidelines). *Circ Cardiovasc Qual Outcomes*. 2017;10(12):e003443.

59. Ong P, Athanasiadis A, Borgulya G, et al. Clinical usefulness, angiographic characteristics, and safety evaluation of intracoronary acetylcholine provocation testing among 921 consecutive white patients with unobstructed coronary arteries. *Circulation*. 2014;129(17):1723-1730.

60. Montone RA, Niccoli G, Fracassi F, et al. Patients with acute myocardial infarction and non-obstructive coronary arteries: safety and prognostic relevance of invasive coronary provocative tests. *Eur Heart J*. 2018;39(2):91-98.

61. Aziz A, Hansen HS, Sechtem U, Prescott E, Ong P. Sex-related differences in vasomotor function in patients with angina and unobstructed coronary arteries. *J Am Coll Cardiol*. 2017;70(19):2349-2358.

62. Di Fiore DP, Zeitz CJ, Arstall MA, Rajendran S, Sheikh AR, Beltrame JF. Clinical determinants of acetylcholine-induced coronary artery spasm in Australian patients. *Int J Cardiol*. 2015;193:59-61.

63. Sato K, Kaikita K, Nakayama N, et al. Coronary vasomotor response to intracoronary acetylcholine injection, clinical features, and long-term prognosis in 873 consecutive patients with coronary spasm: analysis of a single-center study over 20 years. *J Am Heart Assoc*. 2013;2(4):e000227.

64. Coma-Canella I, Castano S, Macias A, Calabuig J, Artaiz M. Ergonovine test in angina with normal coronary arteries. Is it worth doing it? *Int J Cardiol*. 2006;107(2):200-206.

65. Lee DH, Park TK, Seong CS, et al. Gender differences in long-term clinical outcomes and prognostic factors in patients with vasospastic angina. *Int J Cardiol*. 2017;249:6-11.

66. Kobayashi Y, Fearon WF, Honda Y, et al. Effect of sex differences on invasive measures of coronary microvascular dysfunction in patients with angina in the absence of obstructive coronary artery disease. *JACC Cardiovasc Interv*. 2015;8(11):1433-1441.

67. Manninger M, Perl S, Brussee H, G GT. Sniff of coke breaks the heart: cocaine-induced coronary vasospasm aggravated by therapeutic hypothermia and vasopressors after aborted sudden cardiac death: a case report. *Eur Heart J Case Rep*. 2018;2(2):yty041.

68. Chong JH, Ghosh AK. Coronary artery vasospasm induced by 5-fluorouracil: proposed mechanisms, existing management options and future directions. *Interv Cardiol*. 2019;14(2):89-94.

69. Shimizu M, Hata K, Takaoka H, et al. Sumatriptan provokes coronary artery spasm in patients with variant angina: possible involvement of serotonin 1B receptor. *Int J Cardiol*. 2007;114(2):188-194.

70. Saif MW, Shah MM, Shah AR. Fluoropyrimidine-associated cardiotoxicity: revisited. *Expert Opin Drug Saf*. 2009;8(2):191-202.

71. Kanazawa K, Suematsu M, Ishida T, et al. Disparity between serotonin- and acetylcholine-provoked coronary artery spasm. *Clin Cardiol*. 1997;20(2):146-152.

72. Lanza GA, Careri G, Crea F. Mechanisms of coronary artery spasm. *Circulation*. 2011;124(16):1774-1782.

73. Li L, Jin YP, Xia SD, Feng C. The biochemical markers associated with the occurrence of coronary spasm. *Biomed Res Int*. 2019;2019:4834202.

74. Matta A, Bouisset F, Lhermusier T, et al. Coronary artery spasm: new insights. *J Interv Cardiol*. 2020;2020:5894586.

75. Ong P, Carro A, Athanasiadis A, et al. Acetylcholine-induced coronary spasm in patients with unobstructed coronary arteries is associated with elevated concentrations of soluble CD40 ligand and high-sensitivity C-reactive protein. *Coron Artery Dis*. 2015;26(2):126-132.

76. Ford TJ, Corcoran D, Padmanabhan S, et al. Genetic dysregulation of endothelin-1 is implicated in coronary microvascular dysfunction. *Eur Heart J*. 2020.

77. Lee J, Cheong SS, Kim J. Association of endothelin-1 gene polymorphisms with variant angina in Korean patients. *Clin Chem Lab Med*. 2008;46(11):1575-1580.

78. Murase Y, Yamada Y, Hirashiki A, et al. Genetic risk and gene-environment interaction in coronary artery spasm in Japanese men and women. *Eur Heart J*. 2004;25(11):970-977.

79. Togashi I, Sato T, Soejima K, et al. Sudden cardiac arrest and syncope triggered by coronary spasm. *Int J Cardiol*. 2013;163(1):56-60.

80. Hung MY, Mao CT, Hung MJ, et al. Coronary artery spasm as related to anxiety and depression: a nationwide population-based study. *Psychosom Med*. 2019;81(3):237-245.

81. Sohn SM, Choi BG, Choi SY, et al. Impact of alcohol drinking on acetylcholine-induced coronary artery spasm in Korean populations. *Atherosclerosis*. 2018;268:163-169.

82. Onaka H, Hirota Y, Shimada S, et al. Clinical observation of spontaneous anginal attacks and multivessel spasm in variant angina pectoris with normal coronary arteries: evaluation by 24-hour 12-lead electrocardiography with computer analysis. *J Am Coll Cardiol*. 1996;27(1):38-44.

83. Sueda S, Kohno H, Ochi T, Uraoka T, Tsunemitsu K. Overview of the pharmacological spasm provocation test: Comparisons between acetylcholine and ergonovine. *J Cardiol*. 2017;69(1):57-65.

84. Wei J, Mehta PK, Johnson BD, et al. Safety of coronary reactivity testing in women with no obstructive coronary artery disease: results from the NHLBI-sponsored WISE (Women's Ischemia Syndrome Evaluation) study. *JACC Cardiovasc Interv*. 2012;5(6):646-653.

85. Saito Y, Kitahara H, Shoji T, et al. Paroxysmal atrial fibrillation during intracoronary acetylcholine provocation test. *Heart Vessels*. 2017;32(7):902-908.

86. Sueda S, Miyoshi T, Sasaki Y, Sakaue T, Habara H, Kohno H. Gender differences in sensitivity of acetylcholine and ergonovine to coronary spasm provocation test. *Heart Vessels*. 2016;31(3):322-329.

87. Sueda S, Kohno H, Fukuda H, et al. Clinical impact of selective spasm provocation tests: comparisons between acetylcholine and ergonovine in 1508 examinations. *Coron Artery Dis*. 2004;15(8):491-497.

88. Kim SE, Jo SH, Han SH, et al. Comparison of calcium-channel blockers for long-term clinical outcomes in patients with vasospastic angina. *Korean J Intern Med*. 2020.

89. Nishigaki K, Inoue Y, Yamanouchi Y, et al. Prognostic effects of calcium channel blockers in patients with vasospastic angina—a meta-analysis. *Circ J*. 2010;74(9):1943-1950.

90. Lim AY, Park TK, Cho SW, et al. Clinical implications of low-dose aspirin on vasospastic angina patients without significant coronary artery stenosis; a propensity score-matched analysis. *Int J Cardiol*. 2016;221:161-166.

91. Ishii M, Kaikita K, Sato K, et al. Impact of aspirin on the prognosis in patients with coronary spasm without significant atherosclerotic stenosis. *Int J Cardiol*. 2016;220:328-332.

92. Ishii M, Kaikita K, Sato K, et al. Impact of statin therapy on clinical outcome in patients with coronary spasm. *J Am Heart Assoc*. 2016;5(5).

93. Park SJ, Park H, Kang D, et al. Association of statin therapy with clinical outcomes in patients with vasospastic angina: Data from Korean health insurance review and assessment service. *PLoS One*. 2019;14(1):e0210498.

94. Seo WW, Jo SH, Kim SE, et al. Clinical impact of statin therapy on vasospastic angina: data from a Korea nation-wide cohort study. *Heart Vessels*. 2020;35(8):1051-1059.

95. Kim CH, Park TK, Cho SW, et al. Impact of different nitrate therapies on long-term clinical outcomes of patients with vasospastic angina: A propensity score-matched analysis. *Int J Cardiol*. 2018;252:1-5.

96. Takahashi J, Nihei T, Takagi Y, et al. Prognostic impact of chronic nitrate therapy in patients with vasospastic angina: multicentre registry study of the Japanese coronary spasm association. *Eur Heart J*. 2015;36(4):228-237.

97. Suda A, Takahashi J, Hao K, et al. Coronary functional abnormalities in patients with angina and nonobstructive coronary artery disease. *J Am Coll Cardiol*. 2019;74(19):2350-2360.

98. Sueda S, Kohno H. Optimal medications and appropriate implantable cardioverter-defibrillator shocks in aborted sudden cardiac death due to coronary spasm. *Intern Med*. 2018;57(10):1361-1369.

99. Tan NS, Almehmadi F, Tang ASL. Coronary vasospasm-induced polymorphic ventricular tachycardia: a case report and literature review. *Eur Heart J Case Rep*. 2018;2(1):yty021.

100. Takagi Y, Yasuda S, Tsunoda R, et al. Clinical characteristics and long-term prognosis of vasospastic angina patients who survived out-of-hospital cardiac arrest: multicenter registry study of the Japanese Coronary Spasm Association. *Circ Arrhythm Electrophysiol*. 2011;4(3):295-302.

101. Ahn JM, Lee KH, Yoo SY, et al. Prognosis of variant angina manifesting as aborted sudden cardiac death. *J Am Coll Cardiol*. 2016;68(2):137-145.

102. Park TK, Gwag HB, Park SJ, et al. Differential prognosis of vasospastic angina according to presentation with sudden cardiac arrest or not: Analysis of the Korean Health Insurance Review and Assessment Service. *Int J Cardiol*. 2018;273:39-43.

103. Matsue Y, Suzuki M, Nishizaki M, Hojo R, Hashimoto Y, Sakurada H. Clinical implications of an implantable cardioverter-defibrillator in patients with vasospastic angina and lethal ventricular arrhythmia. *J Am Coll Cardiol*. 2012;60(10):908-913.

104. Bott-Silverman C, Heupler FA, Jr. Natural history of pure coronary artery spasm in patients treated medically. *J Am Coll Cardiol*. 1983;2(2):200-205.

105. Shin DI, Baek SH, Her SH, et al. The 24-month prognosis of patients with positive or intermediate results in the intracoronary ergonovine provocation test. *JACC Cardiovasc Interv*. 2015;8(7):914-923.

106. Han SH, Lee KY, Her SH, et al. Impact of multi-vessel vasospastic angina on cardiovascular outcome. *Atherosclerosis*. 2019;281:107-113.

107. Park SH, Choi BG, Rha SW, Kang TS. The multi-vessel and diffuse coronary spasm is a risk factor for persistent angina in patients received anti-angina medication. *Medicine (Baltimore)*. 2018;97(47):e13288.

108. Hoshino M, Yonetsu T, Mizukami A, et al. Moderate vasomotor response to acetylcholine provocation test as an indicator of long-term prognosis. *Heart Vessels*. 2016;31(12):1943-1949.

109. Nam P, Choi BG, Choi SY, et al. The impact of myocardial bridge on coronary artery spasm and long-term clinical outcomes in patients without significant atherosclerotic stenosis. *Atherosclerosis*. 2018;270:8-12.

110. Lee EM, Choi MH, Seo HS, et al. Impact of vasomotion type on prognosis of coronary artery spasm induced by acetylcholine provocation test of left coronary artery. *Atherosclerosis*. 2017;257:195-200.

111. Takagi Y, Takahashi J, Yasuda S, et al. Prognostic stratification of patients with vasospastic angina: a comprehensive clinical risk score developed by the Japanese Coronary Spasm Association. *J Am Coll Cardiol*. 2013;62(13):1144-1153.

112. Kawana A, Takahashi J, Takagi Y, et al. Gender differences in the clinical characteristics and outcomes of patients with vasospastic angina–a report from the Japanese Coronary Spasm Association. *Circ J*. 2013;77(5):1267-1274.

113. Ford TJ, Stanley B, Sidik N, et al. 1–year outcomes of angina management guided by invasive coronary function testing (CorMicA). *JACC Cardiovasc Interv*. 2020;13(1):33-45.

114. Aretz HT, Billingham ME, Edwards WD, et al. Myocarditis. A histopathologic definition and classification. *Am J Cardiovasc Pathol*. 1987;1(1):3-14.

115. Kociol RD, Cooper LT, Fang JC, et al. Recognition and initial management of fulminant myocarditis: a scientific statement from the American Heart Association. *Circulation*. 2020;141(6):e69-e92.

116. Collaborators GMaCoD. Global, regional, and national age-sex specific all-cause and cause-specific mortality for 240 causes of death, 1990–2013: a systematic analysis for the Global Burden of Disease Study 2013. *Lancet*. 2015;385(9963):117-171.

117. Cooper LT, Keren A, Sliwa K, Matsumori A, Mensah GA. The global burden of myocarditis: part 1: a systematic literature review for the Global Burden of Diseases, Injuries, and Risk Factors 2010 study. *Glob Heart*. 2014;9(1):121-129.

118. Kytö V, Sipilä J, Rautava P. Acute myocardial infarction or acute myocarditis? Discharge registry-based study of likelihood and associated features in hospitalised patients. *BMJ Open*. 2015;5(5):e007555.

119. Gore I, Saphir O. Myocarditis; a classification of 1402 cases. *Am Heart J*. 1947;34(6):827-830.

120. Basso C, Calabrese F, Corrado D, Thiene G. Postmortem diagnosis in sudden cardiac death victims: macroscopic, microscopic and molecular findings. *Cardiovasc Res*. 2001;50(2):290-300.

121. Casey CG, Iskander JK, Roper MH, et al. Adverse events associated with smallpox vaccination in the United States, January-October 2003. *JAMA*. 2005;294(21):2734-2743.

122. Huang C, Wang Y, Li X, et al. Clinical features of patients infected with 2019 novel coronavirus in Wuhan, China. *Lancet*. 2020;395(10223):497-506.

123. Arentz M, Yim E, Klaff L, et al. Characteristics and outcomes of 21 critically ill patients with COVID-19 in Washington State. *JAMA*. 2020;323(16):1612-1614.

124. Shi S, Qin M, Shen B, et al. Association of cardiac injury with mortality in hospitalized patients with COVID-19 in Wuhan, China. *JAMA Cardiol*. 2020;5(7):802-810.

125. Zhou F, Yu T, Du R, et al. Clinical course and risk factors for mortality of adult inpatients with COVID-19 in Wuhan, China: a retrospective cohort study. *Lancet*. 2020;395(10229):1054-1062.

126. Yang X, Yu Y, Xu J, et al. Clinical course and outcomes of critically ill patients with SARS-CoV-2 pneumonia in Wuhan, China: a single-centered, retrospective, observational study. *Lancet Respir Med*. 2020;8(5):475-481.

127. Yao XH, Li TY, He ZC, et al. A pathological report of three COVID-19 cases by minimal invasive autopsies. *Zhonghua Bing Li Xue Za Zhi*. 2020;49(5):411-417.

128. Xu Z, Shi L, Wang Y, et al. Pathological findings of COVID-19 associated with acute respiratory distress syndrome. *Lancet Respir Med*. 2020;8(4):420-422.

129. Caforio AL, Pankuweit S, Arbustini E, et al. Current state of knowledge on aetiology, diagnosis, management, and therapy of myocarditis: a position statement of the European Society of Cardiology Working Group on Myocardial and Pericardial Diseases. *Eur Heart J*. 2013;34(33):2636-2648, 2648a-2648d.

130. Richardson P, McKenna W, Bristow M, et al. Report of the 1995 World Health Organization/International Society and Federation of Cardiology Task Force on the definition and classification of cardiomyopathies. *Circulation*. 1996;93(5):841-842.

131. Leone O, Veinot JP, Angelini A, et al. 2011 consensus statement on endomyocardial biopsy from the Association for European Cardiovascular Pathology and the Society for Cardiovascular Pathology. *Cardiovasc Pathol*. 2012;21(4):245-274.

132. Felker GM, Hu W, Hare JM, Hruban RH, Baughman KL, Kasper EK. The spectrum of dilated cardiomyopathy. The Johns Hopkins experience with 1,278 patients. *Medicine (Baltimore)*. 1999;78(4):270-283.

133. Caforio AL, Mahon NG, Baig MK, et al. Prospective familial assessment in dilated cardiomyopathy: cardiac autoantibodies predict disease development in asymptomatic relatives. *Circulation.* 2007;115(1):76-83.

134. Caforio AL, Calabrese F, Angelini A, et al. A prospective study of biopsy-proven myocarditis: prognostic relevance of clinical and aetiopathogenetic features at diagnosis. *Eur Heart J.* 2007;28(11):1326-1333.

135. Ammirati E, Cipriani M, Moro C, et al. Clinical presentation and outcome in a contemporary cohort of patients with acute myocarditis: Multicenter Lombardy Registry. *Circulation.* 2018;138(11):1088-1099.

136. Silverman KJ, Hutchins GM, Bulkley BH. Cardiac sarcoid: a clinicopathologic study of 84 unselected patients with systemic sarcoidosis. *Circulation.* 1978;58(6):1204-1211.

137. Cooper LT. Myocarditis. *N Engl J Med.* 2009;360(15):1526-1538.

138. Blauwet LA, Cooper LT. Idiopathic giant cell myocarditis and cardiac sarcoidosis. *Heart Fail Rev.* 2013;18(6):733-746.

139. Al Ali AM, Straatman LP, Allard MF, Ignaszewski AP. Eosinophilic myocarditis: case series and review of literature. *Can J Cardiol.* 2006;22(14):1233-1237.

140. Janík M, Hejna P. Necrotizing eosinophilic myocarditis. *Forensic Sci Med Pathol.* 2017;13(2):255-258.

141. Johnson DB, Balko JM, Compton ML, et al. Fulminant myocarditis with combination immune checkpoint blockade. *N Engl J Med.* 2016;375(18):1749-1755.

142. Escudier M, Cautela J, Malissen N, et al. Clinical features, management, and outcomes of immune checkpoint inhibitor-related cardiotoxicity. *Circulation.* 2017;136(21):2085-2087.

143. Mahmood SS, Fradley MG, Cohen JV, et al. Myocarditis in patients treated with immune checkpoint inhibitors. *J Am Coll Cardiol.* 2018;71(16):1755-1764.

144. Moslehi JJ, Salem JE, Sosman JA, Lebrun-Vignes B, Johnson DB. Increased reporting of fatal immune checkpoint inhibitor-associated myocarditis. *Lancet.* 2018;391(10124):933.

145. Kandolin R, Lehtonen J, Salmenkivi K, Räisänen-Sokolowski A, Lommi J, Kupari M. Diagnosis, treatment, and outcome of giant-cell myocarditis in the era of combined immunosuppression. *Circ Heart Fail.* 2013;6(1):15-22.

146. Caforio AL, Marcolongo R, Basso C, Iliceto S. Clinical presentation and diagnosis of myocarditis. *Heart.* 2015;101(16):1332-1344.

147. Cooper LT, Baughman KL, Feldman AM, et al. The role of endomyocardial biopsy in the management of cardiovascular disease: a scientific statement from the American Heart Association, the American College of Cardiology, and the European Society of Cardiology. Endorsed by the Heart Failure Society of America and the Heart Failure Association of the European Society of Cardiology. *J Am Coll Cardiol.* 2007;50(19):1914-1931.

148. Wu LA, Lapeyre AC, Cooper LT. Current role of endomyocardial biopsy in the management of dilated cardiomyopathy and myocarditis. *Mayo Clin Proc.* 2001;76(10):1030-1038.

149. Hauck AJ, Kearney DL, Edwards WD. Evaluation of postmortem endomyocardial biopsy specimens from 38 patients with lymphocytic myocarditis: implications for role of sampling error. *Mayo Clin Proc.* 1989;64(10):1235-1245.

150. Escher F, Kasner M, Kühl U, et al. New echocardiographic findings correlate with intramyocardial inflammation in endomyocardial biopsies of patients with acute myocarditis and inflammatory cardiomyopathy. *Mediators Inflamm.* 2013;2013:875420.

151. Hsiao JF, Koshino Y, Bonnichsen CR, et al. Speckle tracking echocardiography in acute myocarditis. *Int J Cardiovasc Imaging.* 2013;29(2):275-284.

152. Ferreira VM, Schulz-Menger J, Holmvang G, et al. Cardiovascular magnetic resonance in nonischemic myocardial inflammation: expert recommendations. *J Am Coll Cardiol.* 2018;72(24):3158-3176.

153. Friedrich MG, Sechtem U, Schulz-Menger J, et al. Cardiovascular magnetic resonance in myocarditis: A JACC White Paper. *J Am Coll Cardiol.* 2009;53(17):1475-1487.

154. Lurz P, Eitel I, Adam J, et al. Diagnostic performance of CMR imaging compared with EMB in patients with suspected myocarditis. *JACC Cardiovasc Imaging.* 2012;5(5):513-524.

155. Yancy CW, Jessup M, Bozkurt B, et al. 2017 ACC/AHA/HFSA Focused update of the 2013 ACCF/AHA Guideline for the Management of Heart Failure: a report of the American College of Cardiology/American Heart Association Task Force On Clinical Practice Guidelines and the Heart Failure Society of America. *J Am Coll Cardiol.* 2017;70(6):776-803.

156. Ponikowski P, Voors AA, Anker SD, et al. 2016 ESC Guidelines for the diagnosis and treatment of acute and chronic heart failure: The Task Force for the diagnosis and treatment of acute and chronic heart failure of the European Society of Cardiology (ESC)Developed with the special contribution of the Heart Failure Association (HFA) of the ESC. *Eur Heart J.* 2016;37(27):2129-2200.

157. Al-Khatib SM, Stevenson WG, Ackerman MJ, et al. 2017 AHA/ACC/HRS Guideline for management of patients with ventricular arrhythmias and the prevention of sudden cardiac death: a report of the American College of Cardiology/American Heart Association Task Force on Clinical Practice Guidelines and the Heart Rhythm Society. *J Am Coll Cardiol.* 2018;72(14):e91-e220.

158. Cooper LT, Hare JM, Tazelaar HD, et al. Usefulness of immunosuppression for giant cell myocarditis. *Am J Cardiol.* 2008;102(11):1535-1539.

159. Frustaci A, Chimenti C, Calabrese F, Pieroni M, Thiene G, Maseri A. Immunosuppressive therapy for active lymphocytic myocarditis: virological and immunologic profile of responders versus nonresponders. *Circulation.* 2003;107(6):857-863.

160. Frustaci A, Russo MA, Chimenti C. Randomized study on the efficacy of immunosuppressive therapy in patients with virus-negative inflammatory cardiomyopathy: the TIMIC study. *Eur Heart J.* 2009;30(16):1995-2002.

161. Wojnicz R, Nowalany-Kozielska E, Wojciechowska C, et al. Randomized, placebo-controlled study for immunosuppressive treatment of inflammatory dilated cardiomyopathy: two-year follow-up results. *Circulation.* 2001;104(1):39-45.

162. Mason JW, O'Connell JB, Herskowitz A, et al. A clinical trial of immunosuppressive therapy for myocarditis. The Myocarditis Treatment Trial Investigators. *N Engl J Med.* 1995;333(5):269-275.

163. Allen SF, Godley RW, Evron JM, Heider A, Nicklas JM, Thomas MP. Acute necrotizing eosinophilic myocarditis in a patient taking Garcinia cambogia extract successfully treated with high-dose corticosteroids. *Can J Cardiol.* 2014;30(12):1732.e1713-e1735.

164. Yonenaga A, Hasumi E, Fujiu K, et al. Prognostic improvement of acute necrotizing eosinophilic myocarditis (ANEM) through a rapid pathological diagnosis and appropriate therapy. *Int Heart J.* 2018;59(3):641-646.

165. Wang DY, Okoye GD, Neilan TG, Johnson DB, Moslehi JJ. Cardiovascular toxicities associated with cancer immunotherapies. *Curr Cardiol Rep.* 2017;19(3):21.

166. Kühl U, Pauschinger M, Schwimmbeck PL, et al. Interferon-beta treatment eliminates cardiotropic viruses and improves left ventricular function in patients with myocardial persistence of viral genomes and left ventricular dysfunction. *Circulation.* 2003;107(22):2793-2798.

167. Amabile N, Fraisse A, Bouvenot J, Chetaille P, Ovaert C. Outcome of acute fulminant myocarditis in children. *Heart.* 2006;92(9):1269-1273.

168. Mishra PK. Variations in presentation and various options in management of variant angina. *Eur J Cardiothorac Surg.* 2006;29(5):748-759.

169. Sato H, Tateishi H, Uchida T, et al. Clinical aspect of myocardial injury: from ischemia to heart failure. 1990:55-64.

170. Ghadri J-R, Wittstein IS, Prasad A, et al. International expert consensus document on Takotsubo syndrome (part I): clinical characteristics, diagnostic criteria, and pathophysiology. *Eur Heart J.* 2018;39(22):2032-2046.

171. Prasad A, Lerman A, Rihal CS. Apical ballooning syndrome (Tako-Tsubo or stress cardiomyopathy): a mimic of acute myocardial infarction. *Am Heart J.* 2008;155(3):408-417.

172. Redfors B, Vedad R, Angerås O, et al. Mortality in Takotsubo syndrome is similar to mortality in myocardial infarction—A report from the SWEDEHEART registry. *Int J Cardiol.* 2015;185:282-289.

173. Prasad A, Dangas G, Srinivasan M, et al. Incidence and angiographic characteristics of patients with apical ballooning syndrome (Takotsubo/

stress cardiomyopathy) in the HORIZONS-AMI trial: an analysis from a multicenter, international study of ST-elevation myocardial infarction. *Catheter Cardiovasc Intervent.* 2014;83(3):343-348.

174. Sy F, Basraon J, Zheng H, Singh M, Richina J, Ambrose JA. Frequency of Takotsubo cardiomyopathy in postmenopausal women presenting with an acute coronary syndrome. *Am J Cardiol.* 2013;112(4):479-482.

175. Kurowski V, Kaiser A, von Hof K, Killermann DP, Mayer B, Hartmann F, Schunkert H and Radke PW. Apical and midventricular transient left ventricular dysfunction syndrome (tako-tsubo cardiomyopathy): frequency, mechanisms, and prognosis. *Chest.* 2007;132:809-16.

176. Templin C, Ghadri JR, Diekmann J, et al. Clinical features and outcomes of Takotsubo (stress) cardiomyopathy. *N Engl J Med.* 2015;373(10):929-938.

177. El-Battrawy I, Santoro F, Stiermaier T, et al. Incidence and clinical impact of recurrent Takotsubo syndrome: results from the GEIST registry. *J Am Heart Assoc.* 2019;8(9):e010753.

178. Smilowitz NR, Hausvater A, Reynolds HR. Hospital readmission following Takotsubo syndrome. *Eur Heart J: Qual Care Clinic Outcomes.* 2018;5(2):114-120.

179. Murugiah K, Wang Y, Desai NR, et al. Trends in short- and long-term outcomes for Takotsubo cardiomyopathy among Medicare fee-for-service beneficiaries, 2007 to 2012. 2016;4(3):197-205.

180. Minhas AS, Hughey AB, Kolias TJ. Nationwide trends in reported incidence of Takotsubo cardiomyopathy from 2006 to 2012. *Am J Cardiol.* 2015;116(7):1128-1131.

181. Deshmukh A, Kumar G, Pant S, Rihal C, Murugiah K, Mehta JL. Prevalence of Takotsubo cardiomyopathy in the United States. *Am Heart J.* 2012;164(1):66-71.e61.

182. Çatalkaya Demir S, Demir E, Çatalkaya S. Electrocardiographic and seasonal patterns allow accurate differentiation of Tako-tsubo cardiomyopathy from acute anterior myocardial infarction: results of a multicenter study and systematic overview of available studies. *Biomolecules.* 2019;9(2).

183. Pelliccia F, Parodi G, Greco C, et al. Comorbidities frequency in Takotsubo syndrome: an international collaborative systematic review including 1109 patients. *Am J Med.* 2015;128(6):654.e611-e659.

184. Wittstein IS. The sympathetic nervous system in the pathogenesis of Takotsubo syndrome. *Heart Failure Clinics.* 2016;12(4):485-498.

185. Hausvater A, Smilowitz NR, Saw J, et al. Spontaneous coronary artery dissection in patients with a provisional diagnosis of Takotsubo syndrome. *J Am Heart Assoc.* 2019;8(22):e013581.

186. Chou AY, Sedlak T, Aymong E, et al. Spontaneous coronary artery dissection misdiagnosed as Takotsubo cardiomyopathy: a case series. *Can J Cardiol.* 2015;31(8):1073.e1075-e1078.

187. Reynolds HR, Srichai MB, Iqbal SN, et al. Mechanisms of myocardial infarction in women without angiographically obstructive coronary artery disease. *Circulation.* 2011;124(13):1414-1425.

188. Y-Hassan S, Tornvall P. Epidemiology, pathogenesis, and management of Takotsubo syndrome. *Clinic Autonom Res.* 2017.

189. Nakagawa N, Fukawa N, Tsuji K, Nakano N, Kato A. Takotsubo cardiomyopathy induced by dopamine infusion after carotid artery stenting. *Int J Cardiol.* 2016;205:62-64.

190. Ramanath VS, Andrus BW, Szot CR, Kaplan AV, Robb JF. Takotsubo cardiomyopathy after midodrine therapy. *Texas Heart Instit J.* 2012;39(1):158-159.

191. Ghadri J-R, Wittstein IS, Prasad A, et al. International expert consensus document on Takotsubo syndrome (part I): clinical characteristics, diagnostic criteria, and pathophysiology. *Eur Heart J.* 2018;39(22):2032-2046.

192. Norcliffe-Kaufmann L, Kaufmann H, Martinez J, Katz SD, Tully L, Reynolds HR. Autonomic findings in Takotsubo cardiomyopathy. *Am J Cardiol.* 2016;117(2):206-213.

193. S YH, Henareh L. Plasma catecholamine levels in patients with Takotsubo syndrome: Implications for the pathogenesis of the disease. *Int J Cardiol.* 2015;181:35-38.

194. Pelliccia F, Kaski JC, Crea F, Camici PG. Pathophysiology of Takotsubo syndrome. *Circulation.* 2017;135(24):2426-2441.

195. Sherrid MV, Riedy K, Rosenzweig B, et al. Distinctive hypertrophic cardiomyopathy anatomy and obstructive physiology in patients admitted with Takotsubo syndrome. *The Am J Cardiol.* 2020;125(11):1700-1709.

196. Sherrid MV, Riedy K, Rosenzweig B, et al. Hypertrophic cardiomyopathy with dynamic obstruction and high left ventricular outflow gradients associated with paradoxical apical ballooning. *Echocardiography.* 2019;36(1): 47-60.

197. Wallström S, Ulin K, Määttä S, Omerovic E, Ekman I. Impact of long-term stress in Takotsubo syndrome: Experience of patients. *Eur J Cardiovasc Nurs.* 2016;15(7):522-528.

198. To AC, Kay P, Khan AA, Kerr AJ. Coronary artery anatomy and apical sparing in apical ballooning syndrome: implications for diagnosis and aetiology. *Heart Lung Circ.* 2010;19(4):219-224.

199. Becher T, El-Battrawy I, Baumann S, et al. Characteristics and long-term outcome of right ventricular involvement in Takotsubo cardiomyopathy. *Int J Cardiol.* 2016;220:371-375.

200. Kagiyama N, Okura H, Kume T, Hayashida A, Yoshida K. Isolated right ventricular Takotsubo cardiomyopathy. *Eur Heart J—Cardiovasc Imag.* 2014;16(3):285-285.

201. Ghadri JR, Cammann VL, Napp LC, et al. Differences in the clinical profile and outcomes of typical and atypical Takotsubo syndrome: data from the international Takotsubo registry. *JAMA Cardiology.* 2016;1(3):335-340.

202. Ghadri JR, Jaguszewski M, Corti R, Lüscher TF, Templin CJIjoc. Different wall motion patterns of three consecutive episodes of Takotsubo cardiomyopathy in the same patient. 2012;160(2):e25-e27.

203. Rendón ISH, Alcivar D, Rodriguez-Escudero JP, Silver KJTAjom. Acute myocardial infarction and stress cardiomyopathy are not mutually exclusive. 2018;131(2):202-205.

204. Samul-Jastrzębska J, Roik M, Wretowski D, et al. Evaluation of the Inter-TAK Diagnostic Score in differentiating Takotsubo syndrome from acute coronary syndrome. A single center experience. *Cardiol J.* 2019.

205. Ghadri JR, Cammann VL, Jurisic S, et al. A novel clinical score (Inter-TAK Diagnostic Score) to differentiate Takotsubo syndrome from acute coronary syndrome: results from the International Takotsubo Registry. *Eur J Heart Fail.* 2017;19(8):1036-1042.

206. Frangieh AH, Obeid S, Ghadri JR, et al. ECG criteria to differentiate between Takotsubo (stress) cardiomyopathy and myocardial infarction. *J Am Heart Assoc.* 2016;5(6).

207. Parkkonen O, Allonen J, Vaara S, Viitasalo M, Nieminen MS, Sinisalo J. Differences in ST-elevation and T-wave amplitudes do not reliably differentiate Takotsubo cardiomyopathy from acute anterior myocardial infarction. *J Electrocardiol.* 2014;47(5):692-699.

208. Vervaat FE, Christensen TE, Smeijers L, et al. Is it possible to differentiate between Takotsubo cardiomyopathy and acute anterior ST-elevation myocardial infarction? *J Electrocardiol.* 2015;48(4):512-519.

209. Johnson NP, Chavez JF, Mosley WJ, 2nd, Flaherty JD, Fox JM. Performance of electrocardiographic criteria to differentiate Takotsubo cardiomyopathy from acute anterior ST elevation myocardial infarction. *Int J Cardiol.* 2013;164(3):345-348.

210. Patel SM, Lennon RJ, Prasad A. Regional wall motion abnormality in apical ballooning syndrome (Takotsubo/stress cardiomyopathy): importance of biplane left ventriculography for differentiating from spontaneously aborted anterior myocardial infarction. *Int J Cardiovasc Imag.* 2012;28(4): 687-694.

211. Citro R, Rigo F, Ciampi Q, et al. Echocardiographic assessment of regional left ventricular wall motion abnormalities in patients with tako-tsubo cardiomyopathy: comparison with anterior myocardial infarction. *Eur J Echocardiogr.* 2011;12(7):542-549.

212. Ghadri JR, Wittstein IS, Prasad A, et al. International expert consensus document on Takotsubo syndrome (part ii): diagnostic workup, outcome, and management. *Eur Heart J.* 2018;39(22):2047-2062.

213. Tamis-Holland JE, Jneid H, Reynolds HR, et al. Contemporary diagnosis and management of patients with myocardial infarction in the absence of obstructive coronary artery disease: a scientific statement from the American Heart Association. *Circulation.* 2019;139(18):e891-e908.

214. Agewall S, Beltrame JF, Reynolds HR, et al. ESC working group position paper on myocardial infarction with non-obstructive coronary arteries. *Eur Heart J.* 2017;38(3):143-153.

215. Friedrich MG, Sechtem U, Schulz-Menger J, et al. Cardiovascular magnetic resonance in myocarditis: A JACC White Paper. *J Am Coll Cardiol.* 2009;53(17):1475-1487.

216. Eitel I, von Knobelsdorff-Brenkenhoff F, Bernhardt P, et al. Clinical characteristics and cardiovascular magnetic resonance findings in stress (Takotsubo) cardiomyopathy. *JAMA.* 2011;306(3).

217. Redfors B, Vedad R, Angerås O, et al. Mortality in Takotsubo syndrome is similar to mortality in myocardial infarction—A report from the SWE-DEHEART11Swedish web system for enhancement of evidence-based care in heart disease evaluated according to recommended therapies. registry. *Int J Cardiol.* 2015;185:282-289.

218. Ding KJ, Cammann VL, Szawan KA, et al. Intraventricular thrombus formation and embolism in Takotsubo syndrome. 2020;40(1):279-287.

219. Citro R, Radano I, Parodi G, et al. Long-term outcome in patients with Takotsubo syndrome presenting with severely reduced left ventricular ejection fraction. *Eur J Heart Fail.* 2019;21(6):781-789.

220. Guo Y, Zhou C, Yang X. Efficacy and safety of levosimendan in Chinese elderly patients with Takotsubo syndrome. *Ann Transl Med.* 2018;6(22):438-438.

221. Stiermaier T, Santoro F, Eitel C, et al. Prevalence and prognostic relevance of atrial fibrillation in patients with Takotsubo syndrome. *Int J Cardiol.* 2017;245:156-161.

222. Jesel L, Berthon C, Messas N, et al. Ventricular arrhythmias and sudden cardiac arrest in Takotsubo cardiomyopathy: Incidence, predictive factors, and clinical implications. *Heart Rhythm* 2018;15(8):1171-1178.

223. Sharkey SW, Windenburg DC, Lesser JR, et al. Natural history and expansive clinical profile of stress (tako-tsubo) cardiomyopathy. *J Am Coll Cardiol.* 2010;55(4):333-341.

224. Citro R, Rigo F, D'Andrea A, et al. Echocardiographic correlates of acute heart failure, cardiogenic shock, and in-hospital mortality in tako-tsubo cardiomyopathy. *JACC Cardiovasc Imag.* 2014;7(2):119-129.

225. Nayeri A, Bhatia N, Xu M, et al. Prognostic significance of early rehospitalization after Takotsubo cardiomyopathy. *Am J Cardiol.* 2017;119(10):1572-1575.

226. Uribarri A, Núñez-Gil IJ, Conty DA, et al. short- and long-term prognosis of patients with Takotsubo syndrome based on different triggers: importance of the physical nature. *J Am Heart Assoc.* 2019;8(24):e013701.

227. Stiermaier T, Moeller C, Oehler K, et al. Long-term excess mortality in Takotsubo cardiomyopathy: predictors, causes and clinical consequences. *Eur J Heart Fail.* 2016;18(6):650-656.

228. Tornvall P, Collste O, Ehrenborg E, Järnbert-Petterson H. A case-control study of risk markers and mortality in Takotsubo stress cardiomyopathy. *J Am Coll Cardiol.* 2016;67(16):1931-1936.

229. Ghadri JR, Kato K, Cammann VL, et al. Long-term prognosis of patients with Takotsubo syndrome. *J Am Coll Cardiol.* 2018;72(8):874-882.

230. Tornvall P, Collste O, Pettersson H. Prevalence and cumulative incidence of cancer, and mortality in patients with Takotsubo syndrome with focus on the index event. *QJM: Int J Med.* 2019;112(11):861-867.

231. Kim S-A, Jo S-H, Park K-H, Kim H-S, Han S-J, Park W-J. Functional recovery of regional myocardial deformation in patients with Takotsubo cardiomyopathy. *J Cardiol.* 2017;70(1):68-73.

232. Schwarz K, Ahearn T, Srinivasan J, et al. Alterations in cardiac deformation, timing of contraction and relaxation, and early myocardial fibrosis accompany the apparent recovery of acute stress-induced (Takotsubo) cardiomyopathy: an end to the concept of transience. *J Am Soc Echocardiogr.* 2017;30(8):745-755.

233. Nowak R, Fijalkowska M, Gilis-Malinowska N, et al. Left ventricular function after Takotsubo is not fully recovered in long-term follow-up: A speckle tracking echocardiography study. *Cardiol J.* 2017;24(1):57-64.

234. Ripley DP, Saha A, Teis A, et al. The distribution and prognosis of anomalous coronary arteries identified by cardiovascular magnetic resonance: 15 year experience from two tertiary centres. *J Cardiovasc Magn Reson.* 2014;16:34.

235. Wu WH, Sun JP, Ma L, Xie XY, Yang XS, Yu CM. Anomalous origin of the left coronary artery from the pulmonary trunk. *Int J Cardiol.* 2015;201:165-167.

236. Cheitlin MD, De Castro CM, McAllister HA. Sudden death as a complication of anomalous left coronary origin from the anterior sinus of Valsalva, a not-so-minor congenital anomaly. *Circulation.* 1974;50(4):780-787.

237. Angelini P. Novel imaging of coronary artery anomalies to assess their prevalence, the causes of clinical symptoms, and the risk of sudden cardiac death. *Circ Cardiovasc Imaging.* 2014;7(4):747-754.

238. Aldana-Sepulveda N, Restrepo CS, Kimura-Hayama E. Single coronary artery: spectrum of imaging findings with multidetector CT. *J Cardiovasc Comput Tomogr.* 2013;7(6):391-399.

239. Roberts WC, Siegel RJ, Zipes DP. Origin of the right coronary artery from the left sinus of Valsalva and its functional consequences: analysis of 10 necropsy patients. *Am J Cardiol.* 1982;49(4):863-868.

240. Eckart RE, Scoville SL, Campbell CL, et al. Sudden death in young adults: a 25–year review of autopsies in military recruits. *Ann Intern Med.* 2004;141(11):829-834.

241. Attili A, Hensley AK, Jones FD, Grabham J, DiSessa TG. Echocardiography and coronary CT angiography imaging of variations in coronary anatomy and coronary abnormalities in athletic children: detection of coronary abnormalities that create a risk for sudden death. *Echocardiography.* 2013;30(2):225-233.

242. Poynter JA, Bondarenko I, Austin EH, et al. Repair of anomalous aortic origin of a coronary artery in 113 patients: a Congenital Heart Surgeons' Society report. *World J Pediatr Congenit Heart Surg.* 2014;5(4):507-514.

243. Li D, Zhu Z, Zheng X, et al. Surgical treatment of anomalous left coronary artery from pulmonary artery in an adult. *Coron Artery Dis.* 2015;26(8):723-725.

244. Quah JX, Hofmeyr L, Haqqani H, et al. The management of the older adult patient with anomalous left coronary artery from the pulmonary artery syndrome: a presentation of two cases and review of the literature. *Congenit Heart Dis.* 2014;9(6):E185-E194.

245. Shulman ST, Rowley AH. Kawasaki disease: insights into pathogenesis and approaches to treatment. *Nat Rev Rheumatol.* 2015;11(8):475-482.

246. Tremoulet AH, Jain S, Jaggi P, et al. Infliximab for intensification of primary therapy for Kawasaki disease: a phase 3 randomised, double-blind, placebo-controlled trial. *Lancet.* 2014;383(9930):1731-1738.

247. Tsuda E, Hamaoka K, Suzuki H, et al. A survey of the 3–decade outcome for patients with giant aneurysms caused by Kawasaki disease. *Am Heart J.* 2014;167(2):249-258.

248. Rizk SR, El Said G, Daniels LB, et al. Acute myocardial ischemia in adults secondary to missed Kawasaki disease in childhood. *Am J Cardiol.* 2015;115(4):423-427.

249. Giacchi V, Sciacca P, Stella I, et al. Assessment of coronary artery intimal thickening in patients with a previous diagnosis of Kawasaki disease by using high resolution transthoracic echocardiography: our experience. *BMC Cardiovasc Disord.* 2014;14:106.

250. Su D, Wang K, Qin S, Pang Y. Safety and efficacy of warfarin plus aspirin combination therapy for giant coronary artery aneurysm secondary to Kawasaki disease: a meta-analysis. *Cardiology.* 2014;129(1):55-64.

251. Priori SG, Blomström-Lundqvist C, Mazzanti A, Blom N, Borggrefe M, Camm J, et al. 2015 ESC Guidelines for the management of patients with ventricular arrhythmias and the prevention of sudden cardiac death: The Task Force for the Management of Patients with Ventricular Arrhythmias and the Prevention of Sudden Cardiac Death of the European Society of Cardiology (ESC). Endorsed by: Association for European Paediatric and Congenital Cardiology (AEPC). *Eur Heart J.* 2015;36(41):2793-867.

21

Chronic Coronary Syndromes

Sripal Bangalore, Ziad Ali, Jagat Narula, John Puskas, and Gregg W. Stone

The natural history, diagnosis, and management of chronic coronary syndromes

Chronic coronary artery disease =

"Stable ischemic heart disease"
or
"Stable angina"
or
"Chronic coronary syndromes"

The ischemic cascade = progressive mismatch between coronary blood flow and myocardial oxygen demand

Increasingly severe coronary stenosis with impairment of myocardial perfusion

Regional diastolic dysfunction

Regional systolic dysfunction

Ischemic electrocardiographic changes

Angina pectoris

Diagnosis

Angina or anginal equivalents

Silent ischemia

Pretest probability
Duke risk score
Diamond–Forrester (updated) risk score
CORSCORE risk model

Noninvasive test
Anatomical:
• Coronary CT angiography with FFR$_{CT}$ as necessary
Functional:
• Exercise treadmill test
• Stress echocardiography
• SPECT/PET
• Cardiac MRI

Management

Guideline-directed medical therapy

Lifestyle measures (smoking cessation, exercise, and diet), antiplatelet therapy, lipid-lowering therapy, anti-ischemic treatment, hypertension management, and diabetes management

Revascularization

Relieves angina, improves survival in certain subsets (left main disease or left ventricular systolic dysfunction), reduces the risk of acute coronary syndromes

Chapter 21 Fuster and Hurst's Central Illustration. The Duke, updated Diamond–Forrester, and CORSCORE risk models are the most accurate in prediction of coronary artery disease. Diagnostic tests that rely on detection of perfusion defects (such as SPECT) are more sensitive than those that detect wall motion abnormalities (such as stress echocardiography) because perfusion defects occur earlier than wall motion abnormalities in the ischemic cascade. Patients with refractory symptoms despite goal-directed medical therapy, and/or elevated clinical or angiographic risk profiles and suitable coronary anatomy, may benefit from revascularization.

CHAPTER SUMMARY

This chapter reviews the epidemiology, diagnosis, and management of chronic coronary syndromes (see Fuster & Hurst's Central Illustration). Assessment of pretest probability of coronary artery disease (CAD) aids in appropriate risk stratification of patients with suspected chronic coronary syndromes. The Duke, updated Diamond–Forrester, and CORSCORE risk models are the most accurate in predicting CAD. The ischemic cascade is based on progressive mismatch between coronary blood flow and myocardial oxygen demand and, since perfusion defects occur earlier than do wall motion abnormalities, tests that rely on detection of perfusion defects (such as SPECT) are more sensitive than those that detect wall motion abnormalities (such as stress echocardiography), which are more specific for the detection of obstructive CAD. Detection of CAD by coronary computed tomography angiography is associated with a reduced incidence of myocardial infarction. Goal-directed medical therapy consists of intensive and comprehensive secondary prevention and includes lifestyle and pharmacological approaches. Patients with refractory symptoms despite goal-directed medical therapy, and/or elevated clinical or angiographic risk profiles and suitable coronary anatomy, may benefit from revascularization. Coronary artery anatomy, left ventricular systolic function, systemic factors (eg, diabetes), and patient values and preferences should be considered when choosing the revascularization strategy (ie, percutaneous coronary intervention versus coronary artery bypass graft surgery).

EPIDEMIOLOGY AND NATURAL HISTORY

Coronary artery disease (CAD) is a leading cause of death and disability nationally and internationally. In the United States, 18.2 million adults have coronary heart disease and 9.4 million have angina.[1] Although deaths from CAD have been steadily declining, it is still responsible for 1 in 7 deaths per year in the United States, which in 2017 totaled 365,914 fatalities.[1] Annually, it is estimated that 720,000 Americans are hospitalized or die from an initial myocardial infarction (MI), 335,000 suffer from recurrent MI, and an additional 170,000 individuals develop a clinically silent MI.[1]

Chronic CAD has been variously termed stable ischemic heart disease (SIHD) or stable angina by the American College of Cardiology/American Heart Association (ACC/AHA) guidelines or chronic coronary syndromes (CCS) by the European Society of Cardiology (ESC) guidelines. Atherosclerosis is a chronic, most often progressive process and the natural history varies based on the underlying comorbidity burden, degree of atherosclerosis, and primary and secondary preventative measures (**Fig. 21–1**). The condition can have long, stable periods but can also become unstable at any time, typically due to an acute atherothrombotic event caused by plaque rupture or erosion. This chapter reviews the epidemiology, natural history, etiology, and diagnostic, clinical, and therapeutic approaches of patients with CCS.

ETIOLOGY AND CLASSIFICATION

Myocardial ischemia is mediated by an imbalance between oxygen supply and demand at the cardiomyocyte cellular level. Supply-demand mismatch may be caused by cardiac and noncardiac causes (**Table 21–1**). Coronary atherosclerosis impairs coronary blood flow (CBF) via a variety of mechanisms and is the dominant cause of angina under conditions of elevated myocardial oxygen demand, such as exercise or emotional stress. However, CBF is impaired even in the absence of epicardial CAD in several other disease states, including severe aortic valve disease with left ventricular hypertrophy (LVH), systemic hypertension, idiopathic dilated cardiomyopathy, and hypertrophic cardiomyopathy. In patients with LVH, ischemia may result from a combination of inadequate capillary density, pathologic changes within small intramyocardial arteries and arterioles, reduced coronary flow reserve (CFR), systolic compressive forces, and markedly elevated diastolic pressures within the vulnerable subendocardium. Nonobstructive epicardial CAD may result in endothelial dysfunction and impaired CFR, which is a major mechanism underlying ischemia and no obstructive coronary artery disease (INOCA). A primary reduction in myocardial oxygen supply following intraluminal thrombus formation and/or epicardial constriction underlies the development of acute coronary syndromes (ACS) (Table 21–1). There are other, nonatherosclerotic causes

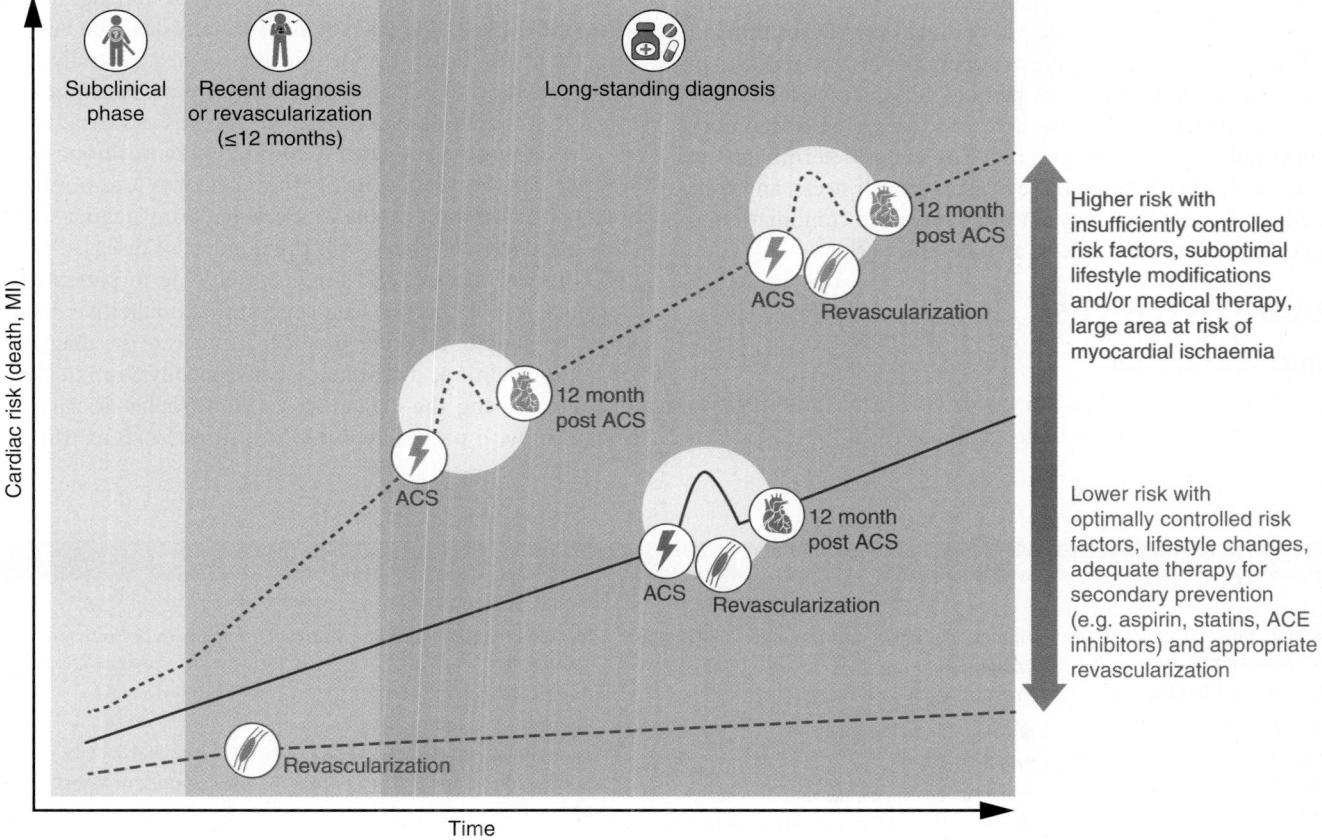

Figure 21–1. Natural history of chronic stable ischemic heart disease. Reproduced with permission from Knuuti J, Wijns W, Saraste A, et al. 2019 ESC Guidelines for the diagnosis and management of chronic coronary syndromes. *Eur Heart J.* 2020 Jan 14;41(3):407-477.

TABLE 21–1. Conditions Provoking or Exacerbating Ischemia

Increased Oxygen Demand	Decreased Oxygen Supply
Noncardiac	*Noncardiac*
Thyroid dysfunction	Anemia
Sympathomimetic toxicity (cocaine)	Hypoxemia: pneumonia, asthma, COPD, pulmonary hypertension, IPF, OSA
Hypertension	Sickle cell anemia
Anxiety	Hyperviscosity
Arteriovenous fistulae	Polycythemia
Cardiac	*Cardiac*
Hypertrophic cardiomyopathy	Aortic stenosis
Aortic stenosis	Hypertrophic cardiomyopathy
Dilated cardiomyopathy	High-grade coronary artery obstruction
Tachycardia	Microvascular circulatory disease

Abbreviations: COPD, chronic obstructive pulmonary disease; IPF, idiopathic pulmonary fibrosis; OSA, obstructive sleep apnea.
Reproduced with permission from Fihn SD, Gardin JM, Abrams J, et al. 2012 ACCF/AHA/ACP/AATS/PCNA/SCAI/STS Guideline for the diagnosis and management of patients with stable ischemic heart disease: a report of the American College of Cardiology Foundation/American Heart Association Task Force on Practice Guidelines, and the American College of Physicians, American Association for Thoracic Surgery, Preventive Cardiovascular Nurses Association, Society for Cardiovascular Angiography and Interventions, and Society of Thoracic Surgeons. *J Am Coll Cardiol.* 2012 Dec 18;60(24):e44-e164.

TABLE 21–2. Classification of Chest Pain

Chest Pain	Characteristics
Typical angina (definite)	1. Substernal chest discomfort with a characteristic quality and duration that is provoked by exertion or emotional stress and relieved by rest or nitroglycerin
Atypical angina (probable)	Meets 2 of the above characteristics
Noncardiac chest pain	Meets 1 or none of the typical anginal characteristics

Reproduced with permission from Fihn SD, Gardin JM, Abrams J, et al. 2012 ACCF/AHA/ACP/AATS/PCNA/SCAI/STS Guideline for the diagnosis and management of patients with stable ischemic heart disease: a report of the American College of Cardiology Foundation/American Heart Association Task Force on Practice Guidelines, and the American College of Physicians, American Association for Thoracic Surgery, Preventive Cardiovascular Nurses Association, Society for Cardiovascular Angiography and Interventions, and Society of Thoracic Surgeons. *J Am Coll Cardiol.* 2012 Dec 18;60(24):e44-e164.

of abrupt reductions in CBF, including spontaneous dissection and embolization. Chronic reductions in oxygen supply may also occur with severe, diffuse, and extensive CAD, resulting in myocardial hibernation. Oxygen supply can also be reduced in the setting of severe anemia or hemoglobinopathies, and under these circumstances, the threshold for developing ischemia or myocardial injury can be lowered. The major determinants of myocardial oxygen demand are heart rate, wall stress, and contractility. These factors may act singularly or in combination to trigger an ischemic cascade in a vulnerable patient.

DIAGNOSIS OF CCS

Clinical Evaluation

The spectrum of CCS may vary widely from asymptomatic to symptomatic phases with stable angina or ACS.

Angina or Anginal Equivalents

For over two centuries, it has been recognized that cardiac angina can be diagnosed effectively by a careful patient interview. William Heberden is credited with the initial description of angina in 1772 in his chapter entitled "Pectoris Dolor," in *Commentaries on the History and Cure of Diseases*.[2] Characteristics of chest pain including location, character, duration, and relationship to aggravating and relieving factors can be used to classify chest pain into typical, atypical, or nonanginal chest pain (**Table 21–2**). Typical angina is usually described as pressure, tightness, heaviness, or burning located centrally in the chest, radiating to left arm, jaw/neck or back, brought about by exertion or emotion and relieved with rest or nitroglycerine use. Symptoms are unrelated to respiration or position. Angina severity can be graded using the Canadian Cardiovascular Society classification (**Table 21–3**).[3] Increasing angina severity class positively correlates with the number of diseased epicardial coronary arteries and predicts outcome in patients with chronic CAD.[4] However, data suggest that qualitative descriptions of symptoms alone may be inaccurate in diagnosing CAD.[5] In addition, discordance between physician's estimate of angina (using the Canadian Cardiovascular Society classification) with patient-reported measures (such as using the

TABLE 21–3. The Canadian Cardiovascular Society Angina Scale

I	II	III	IV
Ordinary physical activity does not cause angina including: Walking and climbing stairs *Angina occurs:* Only with strenuous, rapid, or prolonged exertion at work or recreation	Slight limitation of ordinary activity including: Walking stairs rapidly Walking uphill Stair climbing after meals *Angina occurs:* A few hours after awakening Walking >2 city blocks (level ground) Walking 1 flight of ordinary stairs at a normal pace	Marked limitation of ordinary physical activity. *Angina occurs:* Walking ≤1 city block (level ground) Climbing one flight of stairs under normal conditions and at a normal pace	Inability to perform any physical activity without discomfort. *Angina occurs:* With minimal activity May be present at rest

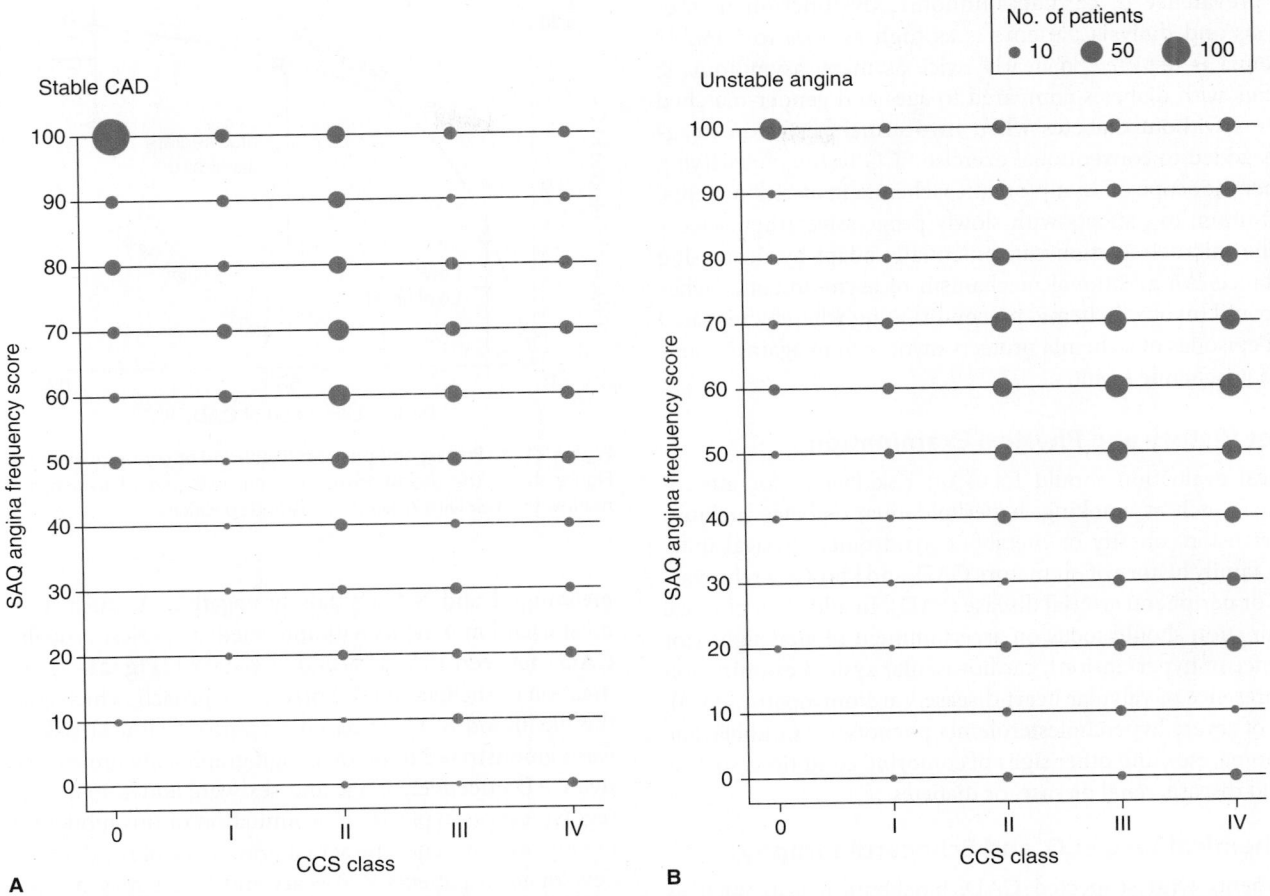

Figure 21–2. Comparison of physician-estimated Canadian Cardiovascular Society (CCS) Class versus Seattle Angina Questionnaire (SAQ) angina frequency scores in patients undergoing percutaneous coronary intervention for (A) stable ischemic heart disease and (B) unstable angina. Reproduced with permission from Saxon JT, Chan PS, Tran AT, et al. Comparison of Patient-Reported vs Physician-Estimated Angina in Patients Undergoing Elective and Urgent Percutaneous Coronary Intervention. *JAMA Netw Open*. 2020 Jun 1;3(6):e207406.

Seattle Angina Questionnaire) have been reported (**Fig. 21–2**).[6] Moreover, some patients do not report chest pain, but report jaw, neck, ear, arm, or epigastric discomfort. Among this constellation of cardiac angina equivalent symptoms, exertional dyspnea should be considered a potentially high-risk finding as a result of the association between this symptom and adverse outcome in patients with CAD.[7,8] In a series of 17,991 patients undergoing cardiac evaluation, dyspnea identified a subgroup of patients at increased risk for all-cause death and cardiovascular death even when compared with patients presenting with typical angina.[8] In addition, patients may present with fatigue. Traditionally it is believed that compared to men, women are less likely to present with typical angina symptoms, but more likely to present with throat, jaw, or neck pain, shortness of breath, fatigue, and non-chest discomfort.[9] However, more recent studies demonstrate the substantial overlap of shared symptoms between men and women with obstructive CAD.[10]

In patients presenting with angina, determination of stable from unstable angina should be made rapidly as the diagnosis and subsequent management differs. Among patients with unstable angina, low-risk unstable angina (age <70 years, exertional pain lasting <20 minutes, pain not rapidly accelerating,

normal or unchanged electrocardiogram [ECG], no elevation of cardiac biomarkers) may be managed similar to CCS.[11]

Asymptomatic Ischemia

Myocardial ischemia is characterized as asymptomatic, or *silent*, when it occurs in the absence of angina or an anginal equivalent.[12] When present, asymptomatic ischemia confers an unfavorable prognosis.[13] It is estimated that silent myocardial ischemia accounts for more than 75% of ischemic episodes during daily life as assessed by ECG monitoring in patients with known CAD and, as such, this is the most common manifestation of CCS.[13] The pathophysiology of asymptomatic ischemia remains controversial. Leading contemporary theories emphasize the presence of defective sensory afferent nerve function, which impairs normal sensory conduction from the atria and ventricles to the thoracic sympathetic ganglia and dorsal roots of the spinal cord. Asymptomatic ischemia is frequently observed among patients with diabetes, presumably due to the associated neuropathy and autonomic dysfunction. Other patient populations at risk for asymptomatic ischemia include those with a previous MI, the elderly, and those with chronic kidney disease (CKD) including those on dialysis.[14]

The prevalence of cardiac autonomic dysfunction in pre-dialysis and dialysis patients is as high as 40% to 90%.[14,15] Ischemia is detected in nearly twice as many asymptomatic patients with diabetes compared to age- and gender-matched patients without diabetes when myocardial perfusion imaging is added to conventional exercise ECG testing,[16] clarifying further the scope of asymptomatic ischemia in at-risk patients. In addition, in patients with slowly progressive atherosclerosis, the microcirculation can potentially adapt by decreasing resistance. An additional mechanism of asymptomatic ischemia could involve ischemic preconditioning whereby repeated short episodes of ischemia protects myocardium against a subsequent ischemic insult.

Other History and Physical Examination

Clinical evaluation should focus on risk factors for atherosclerosis such as smoking, hyperlipidemia, diabetes mellitus, hypertension, obesity or metabolic syndrome, physical inactivity, family history of premature CAD, and known cerebrovascular or peripheral arterial disease (PAD). In addition, physical examination should focus on ascertainment of vital signs (for presence of hypertension), cardiovascular system examination (for presence of valvular heart disease, cardiomyopathy, PAD), signs of severe hypercholesterolemia phenotype (xanthelasma, xanthoma, etc), and other signs of comorbid conditions such as thyroid disease, renal disease, or diabetes.

Biochemical Test, ECG, and Echocardiography

In patients with suspected CAD, biochemical tests such as complete blood count (to evaluate for anemia), basic metabolic panel (to evaluate for renal disease), fasting blood glucose, hemoglobin A1c, lipid panel, and cardiac biomarkers are recommended. Other tests such as a thyroid function test are recommended based on clinical suspicion. In patients without an obvious noncardiac cause of symptoms, resting ECG may provide useful information including presence of ischemic ST-segment depression, evidence of prior MI (Q waves), or conduction abnormalities (bundle branch block). It is often normal in patients with CCS. Similarly, a resting echocardiogram should be considered to exclude alternate cause of angina, for the identification of wall motion abnormalities suggestive of CAD, for the measurement of left ventricular ejection fraction (LVEF) for risk stratification, and for evaluation of diastolic function.

Pretest Probability of CAD

Assessment of pretest probability of CAD aids in appropriate risk stratification of patients with suspected CCS. Pretest probability estimates can guide whether or not further testing is needed. When the pretest probability is low (<10%–15%), a negative test result is merely confirmatory whereas a positive stress test results will not increase the posttest odds to an extent that is clinical meaningful and is likely falsely positive. In patients with a high pretest probability (>85%–90%), a positive test result is merely confirmatory whereas a negative stress test will not decrease the posttest odds sufficiently to be clinically

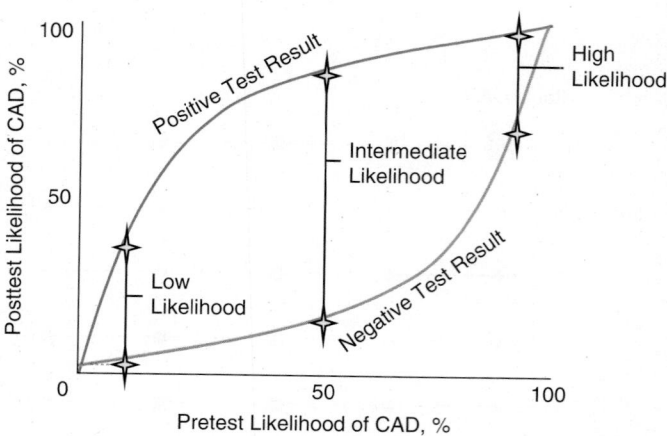

Figure 21–3. Pretest and posttest likelihood of coronary artery disease. Figure shows the use of Bayes' theorem with regard to a hypothetical noninvasive test with 70% sensitivity and specificity.

meaningful and is likely falsely negative. As such, testing is most useful in patients with intermediate pretest probability of CAD (between 10%–15% and 85%–90%) (**Fig. 21–3**). A modification of the Diamond–Forrester approach, which considers the likelihood of CAD based on various clinical risk factors, was demonstrated to predict angiographically proven obstructive CAD effectively if age and sex were added to angina type (eg, typical or atypical).[17,18] A limitation of this model is that it greatly overestimates the actual prevalence of the disease;[19] was developed in patients ≤70 years and hence may not perform well in older adults; and tends to perform less well in women since they have a lower prevalence of obstructive CAD.[20] Other models incorporating risk factors, ECG findings, and biochemical variables (such as high-density lipoprotein cholesterol [HDL-C] levels) have improved the identification of patients with obstructive CAD.[21,22] In a study that compared the performance of five risk models (Diamond–Forrester, the updated Diamond–Forrester, Morise, Duke, and COronary Risk SCORE [CORSCORE]) in predicting significant CAD in patients with chest pain suggestive of stable angina pectoris, the Duke, updated Diamond–Forrester, and CORSCORE risk models were most accurate in predicting CAD.[21]

Diagnostic Testing

In patients with suspected CAD, diagnostic testing with either a functional noninvasive test, an anatomic noninvasive test, or invasive coronary angiography for detection of obstructive CAD are potential options, with invasive coronary angiography limited to patients with high pretest probability of CAD.

The Ischemic Cascade

The ischemic cascade is based on progressive mismatch between coronary blood flow and myocardial oxygen demand with increasing severity of coronary stenosis. When the degree of stenosis is <50%, patients are typically asymptomatic and testing for the presence of atherosclerotic plaque is typically used to optimize medical therapy to prevent disease progression. Persistent symptoms in such patients may be an indicator

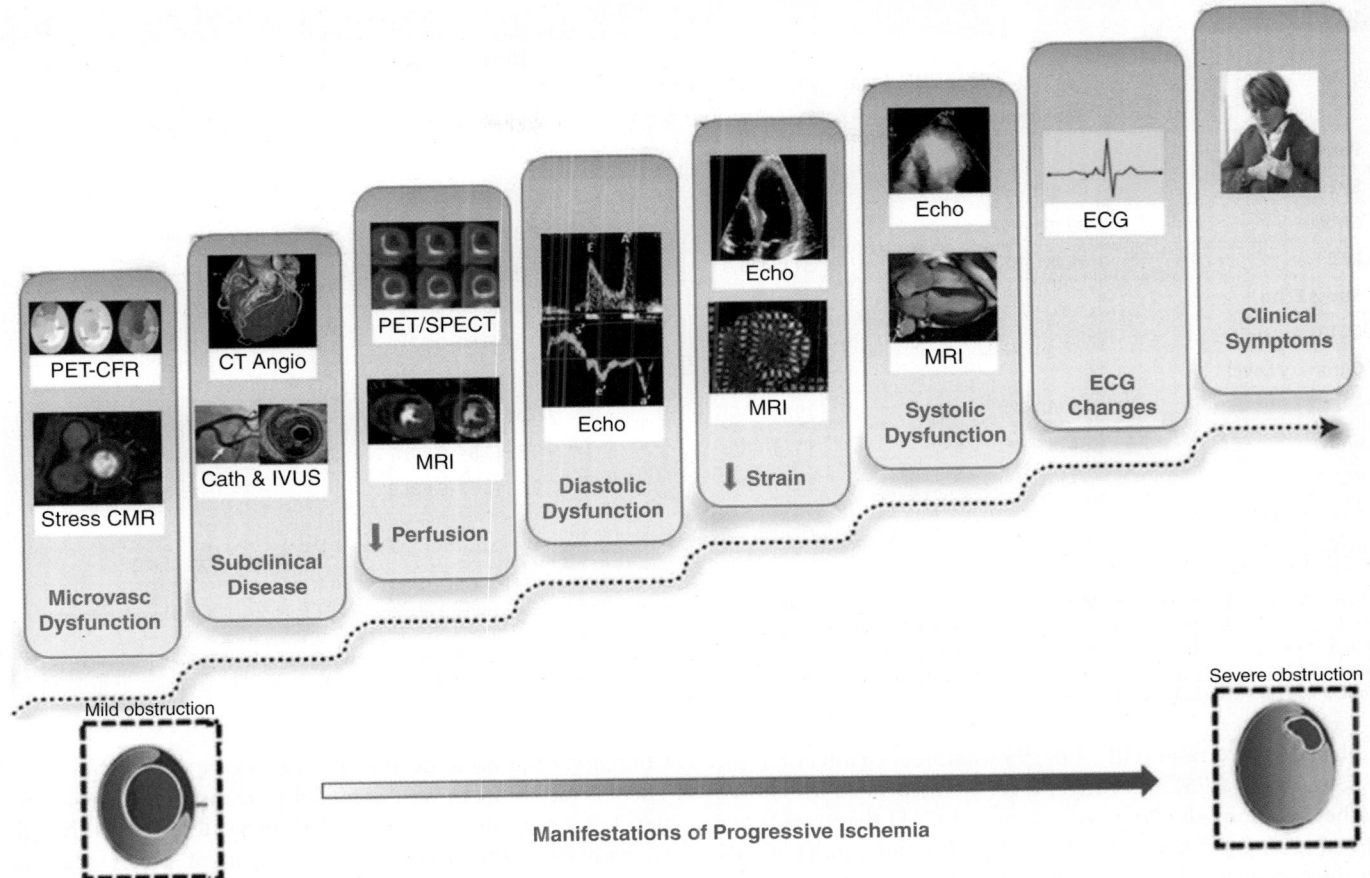

Figure 21–4. The ischemic cascade. Reproduced with permission from Aggarwal NR, Bond RM, Mieres JH. The role of imaging in women with ischemic heart disease. *Clin Cardiol.* 2018 Feb;41(2):194-202.

of microvascular disease and endothelial dysfunction. With stenosis severity ≥50%, reduction in blood flow leads to functional consequences in the myocardium characterized by impairment of myocardial perfusion, followed by regional diastolic dysfunction, regional systolic dysfunction, ischemic ECG changes, and finally angina pectoris. An array of cardiovascular testing is useful across the spectrum of the ischemic cascade from detection of microvascular dysfunction, subclinical disease, to detection of functional and ECG consequences (**Fig. 21–4**).

Diagnostic Accuracy

The diagnostic accuracy of noninvasive testing to detect obstructive disease has been compared in a number of studies with the gold standard of invasive coronary angiography. However, in the 1990s with the introduction of fractional flow reserve (FFR), detection of physiologically/hemodynamically significant disease has emerged to be of greater importance. The diagnostic accuracy of various functional tests when compared with either detection of visually obstructive disease on invasive coronary angiography or hemodynamically significant disease as characterized by FFR is outlined in **Table 21–4**. Since perfusion defects occur earlier than do wall motion abnormalities, tests that rely on detection of perfusion defects

(such as SPECT) are more sensitive than are those that detect wall motion abnormalities (such as stress echocardiography), which are more specific for the detection of obstructive CAD. In addition, test characteristics depend on the prevalence of CAD in the population under consideration (**Table 21–5**). Under conditions of lower prevalence of CAD, the positive predictive value decreases but the negative predictive value increases. In addition, diagnostic test accuracy is reduced in certain patient populations, such as the elderly, women, and those with CKD.

Functional versus Anatomic Noninvasive Testing

A number of clinical trials have tested the outcomes of functional versus anatomic noninvasive testing in patients with suspected CAD. The Prospective Multicenter Imaging Study for Evaluation of Chest Pain (PROMISE) study evaluated anatomic testing with coronary computed tomography angiography (CTA) versus functional testing (exercise electrocardiography, nuclear stress testing, or stress echocardiography) as an initial diagnostic strategy for symptomatic patients with suspected CAD (n = 10,003). Compared to functional testing, anatomic testing did not result in a reduction in the composite endpoint of death, MI, hospitalization for unstable angina, or major procedural complications at 25 months (3.3% vs 3.0%;

TABLE 21-4. Diagnostic Accuracy of Stress Testing for Detecting Significant CAD

	Diagnostic Accuracy for ≥50% on ICA[1]		Diagnostic Accuracy for Hemodynamically Significant Stenosis Based on FFR[2]	
	Sensitivity (95% CI)	Specificity (95% CI)	Sensitivity (95% CI)	Specificity (95% CI)
Patient Level				
SPECT	88 (88–89)	61 (59–62)	0.74 (0.67–0.79)	0.79 (0.74–0.83)
CMR	89 (88–91)	76 (73–78)	0.89 (0.86–0.92)	0.87 (0.83–0.90)
PET	84 (81–87)	81 (74–87)	0.84 (0.75–0.91)	0.87 (0.80–0.92)
Stress Echo			0.69 (0.56–0.79)	0.84 (0.75–0.90)
CCTA			0.88 (0.82–0.92)	0.80 (0.73–0.86)
Coronary Level				
SPECT	69 (68–70)	79 (78–80)	0.61 (0.56–0.66)	0.84 (0.81–0.87)
CMR	84 (81–86)	83 (81–86)	0.87 (0.84–0.90)	0.91 (0.89–0.92)
PET	77 (73–81)	88 (84–90)	0.83 (0.77–0.88)	0.89 (0.86–0.91)
Stress Echo				
CCTA			0.78 (0.72–0.82)	0.86 (0.83–0.88)

Abbreviations: CAD, coronary artery disease; CCTA, computed coronary tomographic angiography; CMR, cardiac magnetic resonance; FFR, fractional flow reserve; ICA, invasive coronary angiography; PET, positron emission tomography; SPECT, single photon emission tomography.
[1]Adapted with permission from Jaarsma C, Leiner T, Bekkers SC, et al. Diagnostic performance of noninvasive myocardial perfusion imaging using single-photon emission computed tomography, cardiac magnetic resonance, and positron emission tomography imaging for the detection of obstructive coronary artery disease: a meta-analysis. *J Am Coll Cardiol.* 2012 May 8;59(19):1719-1728.

adjusted hazard ratio [HR], 1.04; 95% confidence interval [CI], 0.83–1.29; $P = 0.75$).[23] Coronary CTA was associated with fewer catheterizations showing no obstructive CAD than was functional testing (3.4% vs 4.3%; $P = 0.02$), although more patients in the coronary CTA group underwent catheterization within 90 days after randomization (12.2% vs 8.1% [CI and P not reported]).[23] In contrast, in the Scottish Computed Tomography of the HEART (SCOT-HEART) trial, a significantly lower rate of the combined endpoint of cardiovascular death or nonfatal MI (2.3% vs 3.9%; HR, 0.59; 95% CI, 0.41–0.84; $P = 0.004$), driven by reduction in nonfatal MI (HR, 0.60; 95% CI, 0.41–0.87) was observed in patients in whom coronary CTA was performed in addition to routine testing, which consisted predominantly of exercise ECG.[24] Meta-analysis of randomized trials (13 trials, 20,092 participants) showed that coronary CTA is associated with a reduced incidence of MI driven by an increased incidence of invasive coronary angiography, revascularization, CAD diagnoses, and new prescriptions for aspirin and statins when compared with functional testing.[25]

Guideline Recommendations for the Choice of Testing

There is variability in various guideline recommendations as to the choice of testing in patients with suspected CAD, although all emphasize the need to consider patient preference and comorbidities. In patients with suspected CAD and no history of prior CAD, the 2016 UK National Institute for Health and Care Excellence (NICE) recommends 64-slice (or above) CT to be the first-line investigation for all patients with typical or atypical chest pain as well as those with nonanginal pain but with ECG changes.[26] The guidelines recommend noninvasive functional testing as second-line investigation if coronary CTA has shown CAD of uncertain functional significance or is nondiagnostic. NICE discourages the use of exercise ECG in such patients and recommends functional testing with imaging (with the choice of modality left to the locally available technology and expertise, and patient preference, and comorbidities).[26] The guidelines recommend invasive coronary angiography as the third-line investigation if the results of noninvasive functional imaging are inconclusive. In patients with known CAD, NICE

TABLE 21-5. Accuracy of Exercise Testing Depends on CAD Prevalence

Chest Pain Type	Gender	Prevalence of CAD	False Positive	False Negative
Typical angina	Male	89	4%	65%
Typical angina	Female	63	27%	23%
Atypical angina	Male	70	13%	44%
Atypical angina	Female	40	46%	22%
Nonanginal chest pain	Male	22	91%	14%
Nonanginal chest pain	Female	5	96%	5%

Abbreviation: CAD, coronary artery disease.
Data from Weiner DA, Ryan TJ, McCabe CH, et al. Exercise stress testing. Correlations among history of angina, ST-segment response and prevalence of coronary-artery disease in the Coronary Artery Surgery Study (CASS). *N Engl J Med.* 1979 Aug 2;301(5):230-235.

recommends noninvasive functional testing with exercise ECG as an alternative to stress testing with imaging provided the ECG is interpretable.[26] The 2019 ESC chronic coronary syndrome guidelines recommend use of either noninvasive functional imaging or noninvasive anatomical imaging as the initial test for diagnosing CAD (class I).[27] The use of exercise ECG was downgraded as an alternative test to when other noninvasive or invasive imaging methods are not available (class IIb). Invasive angiography is recommended as an alternative test to diagnose CAD in patients with a high clinical likelihood of disease and severe symptoms refractory to medical therapy, or typical angina at a low level of exercise, clinical evaluation that indicates high event risk, and in those where the noninvasive test is nondiagnostic.[27] The 2012 ACC/AHA SIHD guidelines recommend exercise ECG as the first-line in patients with intermediate pretest probability of CAD, and who are able to exercise and who have interpretable ECG.[11] In patients with intermediate or high pretest probability and inability to exercise, pharmacological stress with nuclear myocardial perfusion imaging (MPI) or echocardiography is recommended. Coronary CTA is recommended for patients with an intermediate pretest probability of SIHD who (1) have continued symptoms despite prior normal test findings, or (2) have inconclusive or discordant results from prior exercise or pharmacological stress testing, or (3) are unable to undergo stress with nuclear MPI or echocardiography.[11] Guideline updates for the ACC/AHA recommendations are awaited.

Coronary Artery Calcification Score
Calcium is a common component of atherosclerotic plaque and is easily detected by CT using low radiation and without the use of contrast. Coronary artery calcification observed on cardiac CT strongly correlates with the presence of established atherosclerosis, although it does not correlate with the degree

of luminal obstruction.[28] As such, quantification of coronary artery calcium should be reserved for asymptomatic patients who need further risk stratification or in those with low-to-intermediate pretest probability of obstructive CAD. The Agatston score is commonly used as an overall measure of calcium burden in the coronary arteries and is predictive of coronary heart disease events and survival.[29] In fact, it is estimated that measures of coronary calcium can be used as an estimate of an individual's "biological age."[30] Serial coronary artery calcification scoring to assess the rate of disease progression is not recommended.[31] In fact, studies have shown that lipid-lowering therapy promotes plaque regression but increases plaque calcification and hence the coronary artery calcification score, especially with statin.[32] The absence of coronary calcium (an Agatston score of zero) in asymptomatic patients is associated with an excellent prognosis with a negative predictive value for excluding severe stenosis (on coronary CTA) of 99.5%.[33] In addition, a zero calcium score was associated with a low prevalence of obstructive CAD (<5%), low risk of death or nonfatal MI (<1% annual risk), and identified a subset of patients less likely to benefit from statin therapy (**Fig. 21–5**).[34,35] Of note, noncalcified plaques (a majority of which are nonobstructive) can be seen in approximately 13% of individuals with a zero calcium score.[36]

Coronary Computed Tomographic Angiography
Coronary CTA provides an anatomic assessment of the epicardial coronary arteries. Because of its high spatial resolution and negative predictive value (97%–99%), coronary CTA is especially helpful to exclude important CAD in patients with a low pretest likelihood of disease. Coronary CTA is also well suited to visualize suspected congenital coronary artery anomalies and great vessel anatomy. More recently, anatomical

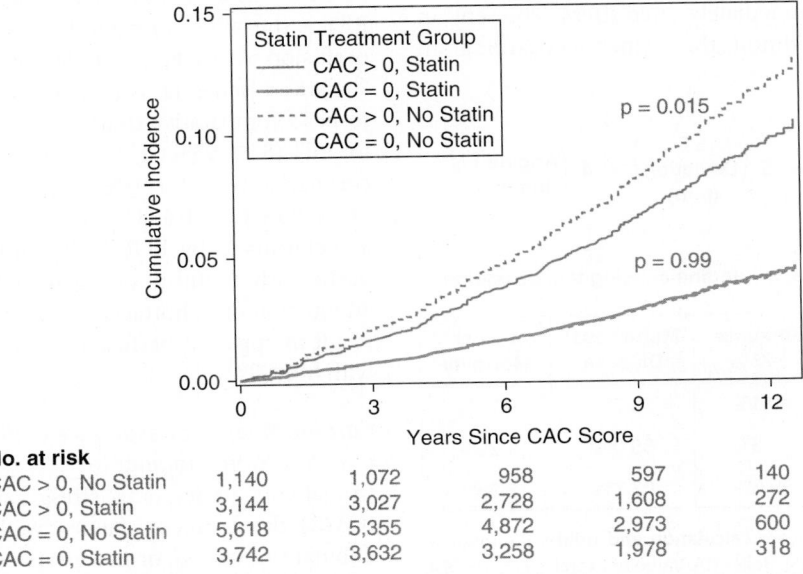

Figure 21–5. Cumulative incidence of MACE by statin treatment and CAC score. Reproduced with permission from Mitchell JD, Fergestrom N, Gage BF, et al. Impact of Statins on Cardiovascular Outcomes Following Coronary Artery Calcium Scoring. *J Am Coll Cardiol.* 2018 Dec 25;72(25):3233-3242.

assessment by coronary CTA has been combined with functional data using a postprocessing technique called FFR_{CT}. This uses computational fluid dynamics applied to a standard coronary CTA data set. The use of FFR_{CT} (pooled specificity of 0.78; 95% CI, 0.72–0.83) substantially improved identification of hemodynamically significant CAD in intermediate lesions when compared with CTA alone (pooled specificity of 0.61; 95% CI, 0.54–0.68) in a meta-analysis of 54 studies with 5330 patients.[37] Ongoing studies will determine whether FFR_{CT} will improve clinical outcomes.

Exercise ECG Stress Testing

In patients undergoing exercise ECG with interpretable baseline ECG (defined as a normal 12-lead ECG or one with minimal resting ST-T-wave abnormalities [<0.5 mm]), a ≥1-mm horizontal or down-sloping ST-segment depression (at 80 ms after the J point) at peak exercise or ST-segment elevation (in a non–Q-wave lead) during or after exercise are considered abnormal responses. A number of studies have validated the prognostic utility of ECG treadmill testing. However, the diagnostic sensitivity and specificity is low and ranges from 70% to 77% resulting in high rates of both false positive and false negative results. Diagnostic accuracy is improved with addition of non-ECG variables such as exercise duration, chronotropic competence, heart rate recovery, angina, ventricular arrhythmias, and hemodynamic response to exercise (ie, drop in systolic blood pressure).[38–40] The Duke Treadmill Score (DTS) is commonly used in clinical practice for predicting the probability of a future MI or cardiovascular death in patients with CAD. In this model, a numeric score is generated that reflects a patient's exercise time, extent of ST-segment depression, and presence of anginal symptoms (**Fig. 21–6**). The DTS correlates with future cardiovascular mortality.[41]

Stress Echocardiography

In patients undergoing stress echocardiography, new or worsening wall motion abnormalities and changes in global LV function during or immediately after stress represent an abnormal response. In addition, the resting echocardiogram provides information on left ventricular systolic function, diastolic function, and valvular abnormalities. Stress echocardiography is more sensitive (70% to 85% for exercise and 85% to 90% for pharmacological) and specific than exercise ECG for the detection of CAD (Table 21–4).[42,43] In addition, a number of studies have shown the utility of stress echocardiography in risk stratification and prognosis of patients with known or suspected CAD.[44–49] A normal stress echocardiography response in these studies portends a favorable prognosis with a cardiac death or MI rate of <1% per year.[44–49] High-risk markers include greater extent and severity of ischemia, transient ischemic dilatation, concomitant RV ischemia, left atrial size, and abnormal exercise parameters (as aforementioned).[44–50]

Myocardial Perfusion SPECT and PET Imaging

In patients undergoing myocardial MPI, decrease in myocardial perfusion with stress when compared to that with rest represents ischemia. In addition, gated SPECT can provide information on regional and global LV systolic function and ejection fraction. In general, perfusion imaging is more sensitive than is stress echocardiography. Diagnostic sensitivity ranged from 82% to 88% for exercise and 88% to 91% for pharmacological stress nuclear MPI (Table 21–4). In addition, a number of studies have shown the utility of SPECT in risk stratification and prognosis of patients with known or suspected CAD.[51–59] A normal SPECT in these studies portends a favorable prognosis with a cardiac death or MI rate of <1% per year.[51–59] High-risk markers include a markedly abnormal ECG, extensive stress-induced wall motion abnormalities or ischemia (≥10% of the myocardium), reduced poststress LVEF drop ≥5%, transient ischemic LV dilation, increased lung or right ventricular uptake, or abnormal coronary flow reserve with myocardial perfusion positron emission tomography (PET).[51–59]

Myocardial perfusion PET is characterized by high spatial resolution compared with SPECT and as such has the ability to better assess for endocardial ischemia. An added advantage of PET is the ability to quantify absolute blood flow or absolute perfusion. As such, the limitation of SPECT in demonstrating "balanced ischemia" is potentially avoided by PET. In a head-to-head comparative study of 208 adults, accuracy was highest for PET (85%; 95% CI, 80%–90%), when compared with that of coronary CTA (74%; 95% CI, 67%–79%; P = 0.003) and SPECT (77%; 95% CI, 71%–83%; P = 0.02) for the diagnosis of CAD as determined by FFR.[60] Myocardial perfusion PET may be particularly useful in the extremely obese where nonuniform attenuation of radiotracer counts by excess adipose tissue may result in apparent perfusion defects and false-positive studies with SPECT.[61]

Cardiac Magnetic Resonance Wall Motion and Perfusion Imaging

In patients undergoing stress cardiac magnetic resonance (CMR), development of a new wall motion abnormality (with dobutamine stress), or new perfusion abnormality (on vasodilator stress) defines the presence of ischemia. Stress CMR has a high sensitivity and specificity for the detection of obstructive

$$\text{Duke Treadmill Score} = \text{Exercise Duration (min)} - 5\left(\frac{\text{ST Deviation (mm)}}{}\right) - 4\left(\frac{\text{Angina Index}}{}\right)$$

Angina Index
0 – none, 1 – typical angina, 2 – angina causing test cessation

Score	Risk Group	Stenosis ≥ 75%	Multivessel Disease	1-Year Mortality
≥ 5	Low	40.1%	23.7%	0.25%
−10 to 4	Intermediate	67.3%	55.0%	1.25%
≤ −11	High	99.6%	93.7%	5.25%

Figure 21–6. Duke treadmill score calculation and utility. Reproduced with permission from Bourque JM, Beller GA. Value of Exercise ECG for Risk Stratification in Suspected or Known CAD in the Era of Advanced Imaging Technologies. *JACC Cardiovasc Imaging.* 2015 Nov;8(11):1309-1321.

CAD with a sensitivity and specificity of 83% and 86%, respectively, for dobutamine stress CMR and 91% and 81% respectively for vasodilator stress CMR (Table 21–4).[62] In addition, CMR can provide additional information on LV regional and global function, valvular abnormalities and the quantification of scar tissue and viability.

Invasive Coronary Angiography

Referral for invasive coronary angiography in patients with CCS is most often indicated for refractory symptoms or high-risk features on noninvasive testing and serves as a prelude to revascularization. In individuals with symptoms suggestive but not diagnostic of CAD, invasive angiography may be appropriate if their occupations constitute a risk to themselves or others (eg, airline pilots, firefighters, etc).[63] In certain patients for whom the diagnosis of CAD on clinical grounds may be elusive as a result of atypical chest pain characteristics, asymptomatic ischemia (eg, patients with diabetes), or suspicion for balanced ischemia on stress testing, a lower threshold for coronary angiography may be appropriate. As a result of atypical symptomatology and relatively lower diagnostic accuracy rates on conventional stress testing, women are more frequently considered for invasive angiography in the setting of an ambiguous presentation and/or inconsistent noninvasive data, but consideration of this approach should be weighed against the low, but finite, risks of the procedure. Moreover, findings from population studies suggest that in the United States, coronary angiography may be overused as an initial diagnostic test for CAD.[64] Additional indications for invasive angiography include the evaluation of CAD in patients with reduced EF (<0.40), patients surviving sudden cardiac death, or patients with ventricular arrhythmias and a high or intermediate likelihood of CAD.[63]

TREATMENT OF STABLE ISCHEMIC HEART DISEASE

Goal-directed therapy in the management of CCS is focused on (1) prevention of death and MI and (2) reduction of symptoms of myocardial ischemia. The intensity of treatment is dictated by the magnitude of risk and the severity of the ischemic burden. The decision to initiate medical, percutaneous, surgical, or hybrid treatment is developed in the context of a patient's specific clinical, coronary angiographic, and LV functional profiles. Patient values and preferences should be taken into account.

Goal-Directed Medical Therapy

Goal-directed medical therapy consists of intensive and comprehensive secondary prevention and includes lifestyle and pharmacological approaches.

Lifestyle Measures

Lifestyle measures include physical activity, weight management, implementation of a heart-healthy diet, and smoking cessation. Patients should be encouraged to do 30 to 60 minutes of moderate intensity aerobic activity (like brisk walking) 5 to 7 times a week. Cardiac rehabilitation and physician-directed home-based programs are recommended for high-risk individuals with CCS. In a meta-analysis of 63 randomized trials with 14,486 participants with median follow-up of 12 months, cardiac rehabilitation reduced cardiovascular mortality by 26% (risk ratio [RR], 0.74; 95% CI 0.64–0.86) and the risk of hospital admissions by 18% (RR, 0.82; 95% CI, 0.70–0.96) when compared with usual care.[65] In overweight or obese individuals, weight loss and weight maintenance should be encouraged by a combination of physical activity, structured exercise, reduction in caloric intake, and formal behavioral programs. Excessive weight fluctuations in patients with CAD have been shown to be harmful and should be avoided.[66] Dietary measures to reduce low-density lipoprotein cholesterol (LDL-C) include replacing saturated and trans fatty acids with unsaturated fatty acids, reducing dietary cholesterol, and adding plant stanols/sterols (2 g/day) and fiber (>10 g/day). Smoking cessation using non-pharmacological and pharmacological approaches should be encouraged to reduce the risk of future cardiovascular events. In addition, patients with CCS should be screened for depression and referred for treatment as needed. Patients with CCS are more likely to experience comorbid depressive symptoms which have been known to be strong predictors of adverse outcomes including mortality.[67-69] In a retrospective cohort study, inadequate treatment of major depressive symptoms in patients with recent MI or stroke was associated with higher risk of adverse cardiovascular outcomes.[70,71] In a randomized trial of patients with recent ACS and depression, treatment with escitalopram when compared with matching placebo was associated with significant reduction in major adverse cardiovascular events including MI.[72] Other measures include moderation of alcohol consumption, avoidance of air pollution and marijuana use.[73]

Pharmacological Therapy

Antiplatelet Therapy: Platelet aggregation is an important step in the pathogenesis of MI following plaque rupture and as such antiplatelet therapy is recommended in patients with CCS. Aspirin exerts an antithrombotic effect by irreversibly inhibiting cyclooxygenase-1 and the downstream synthesis of platelet thromboxane A_2. In a meta-analysis of 16 randomized placebo-controlled trials in approximately 17,000 patients with established CAD, treatment with aspirin significantly decreased the rate of major vascular events, particularly MI (4.3% vs 5.3% per year; RR, 0.69; 95% CI, 0.60–0.80) and stroke (2.08% vs 2.54% per year; RR, 0.81; 95% CI, 0.71–0.92), without a significant increase in the risk of hemorrhagic stroke.[74] Daily use of aspirin (75–162 mg/day) for secondary prevention of MI in both men and women with CCS is an AHA/ACC class I recommendation.[11] Low-dose aspirin (75 or 81 mg) is recommended for maintenance therapy in combination with $P2Y_{12}$ inhibitors for patients who undergo percutaneous coronary intervention (PCI).

Clopidogrel, a thienopyridine derivative, inhibits platelet aggregation by irreversible inhibition of the adenosine diphosphate $P2Y_{12}$ receptor and is used in combination with aspirin as part of a strategy of dual antiplatelet therapy (DAPT) following

PCI. The effectiveness of clopidogrel depends on generation of its active metabolite, which is regulated by the enzyme of the cytochrome P450 system, principally *CYP2C19*. Variants of the *CYP2C19* gene that are associated with impaired antiplatelet effects have been identified in up to 30% of patients. Prasugrel and ticagrelor, two other $P2Y_{12}$ inhibitors, have stronger antiplatelet efficacy with reduced inter individual variability, and have been shown to be superior to clopidogrel in randomized trials of patients with ACS. Neither prasugrel nor ticagrelor has been studied in the setting of PCI for CCS. Prasugrel should not be used in patients with prior stroke or transient ischemic attack and is generally avoided in patients aged over 75 years or of low body weight (<60 kg) because of a lack of net clinical benefit.

Few trials have explored the role of extended DAPT (>12 months) in patients with CCS. The Dual Antiplatelet Therapy (DAPT)[75] study randomized 9961 patients who were clinically stable and without bleeding complications 12 months after PCI (38% for stable angina) to an additional 18 months of aspirin plus a thienopyridine (clopidogrel or prasugrel) or aspirin alone. Prolonged DAPT reduced stent thrombosis and MACCE, driven by a reduction in MI related to both stent thrombosis and de novo events in other locations but at the expense of increased bleeding. The Prevention of Cardiovascular Events in Patients with Prior Heart Attack Using

Ticagrelor Compared to Placebo on a Background of Aspirin–Thrombolysis in Myocardial Infarction 54 (PEGASUS-TIMI 54) trial randomized 21,612 post-MI patients (1 to 3 years after MI) to ticagrelor 90 mg twice daily, ticagrelor 60 mg twice daily, or placebo, in addition to aspirin.[76] At a median follow-up of 33 months, for every 10,000 patients treated with ticagrelor 90 mg twice daily, 40 primary endpoints would be prevented at the expense of 41 Thrombolysis in Myocardial Infarction (TIMI) major bleeds; for every 10,000 patients treated with ticagrelor 60 mg twice daily, 42 primary endpoints would be averted at the expense of 31 TIMI major bleeds. In both of these trials, the benefit at reducing ischemic outcomes came at the cost of increased bleeding. Multiple randomized trials and meta-analyses have shown reduced bleeding and no significant increase in ischemic events with short DAPT when compared with extended DAPT.[77] As such, ACC/AHA guidelines recommend a minimal duration of 6 months of DAPT in patients with CCS after PCI with drug-eluting stent (DES) and 1 month of DAPT after PCI with bare metal stent (BMS).[78] In patients at high risk of bleeding, a shorter duration of DAPT (3 months) may be considered.[78] The recommendations for duration of DAPT by ACC/AHA and ESC guidelines are summarized in **Fig. 21–7**. Several randomized trials testing 1 month of DAPT are currently in progress or were recently published. Factors associated with high bleeding risk after PCI are outlined in

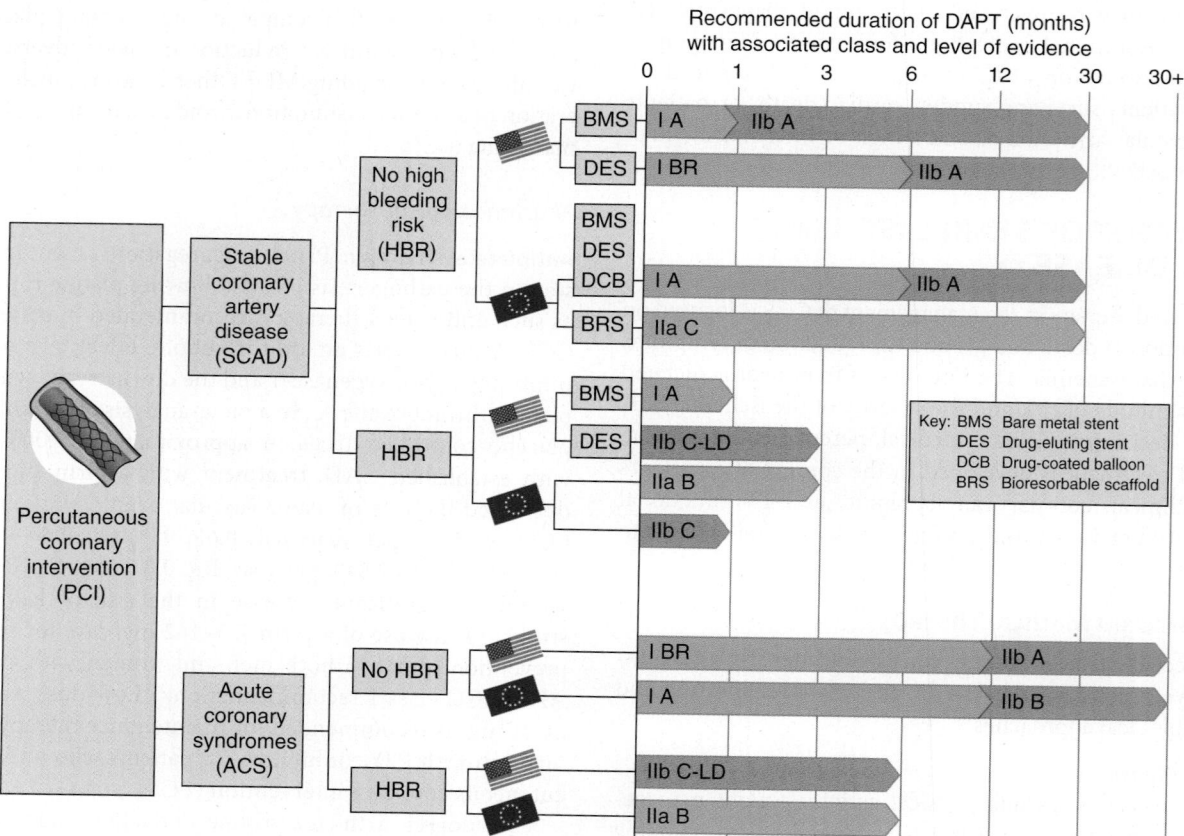

Figure 21–7. Recommendation for duration of DAPT by ACC/AHA and ESC guidelines in patients undergoing PCI. Reproduced with permission from Capodanno D, Alfonso F, Levine GN, et al. ACC/AHA Versus ESC Guidelines on Dual Antiplatelet Therapy: JACC Guideline Comparison. *J Am Coll Cardiol.* 2018 Dec 11;72(23 Pt A):2915-2931.

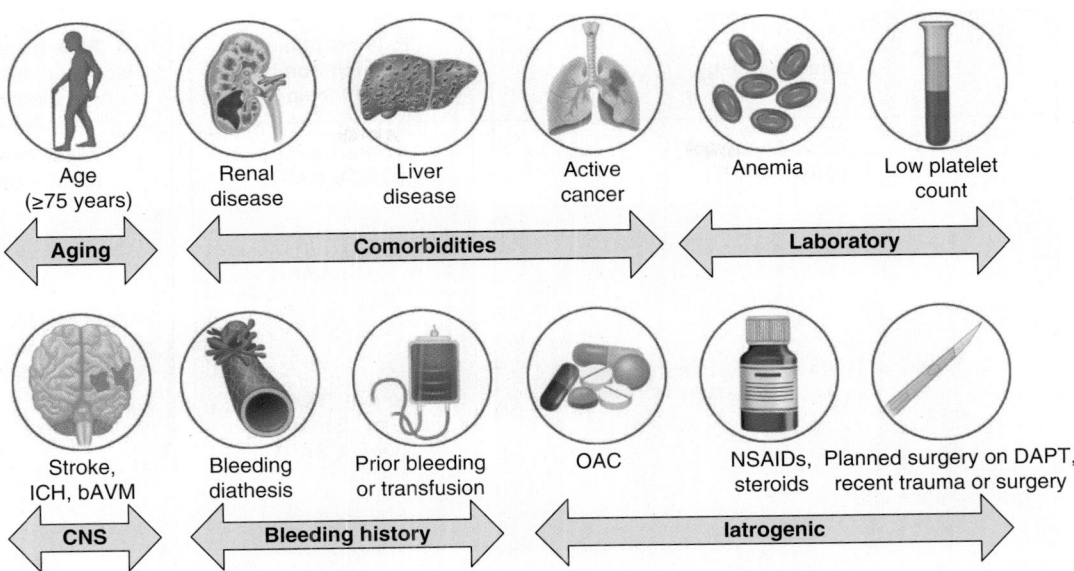

Figure 21–8. Factors associated with an increased bleeding risk after percutaneous coronary intervention. Reproduced with permission from Urban P, Mehran R, Colleran R, et al. Defining High Bleeding Risk in Patients Undergoing Percutaneous Coronary Intervention. *Circulation.* 2019 Jul 16;140(3):240-261.

Fig. 21–8. More recently, monotherapy with a P2Y$_{12}$ inhibitor after a minimum period of DAPT is being tested as an emerging approach to reduce the risk of bleeding after PCI. In the Ticagrelor with Aspirin or Alone in High-Risk Patients after Coronary Intervention (TWILIGHT) trial, 7119 patients were randomized 3 months after PCI (35% for SIHD) to either aspirin or placebo on a background of ticagrelor. Ticagrelor monotherapy reduced bleeding (4.0% vs 7.1%; HR, 0.56; 95% CI, 0.45–0.68; $P < 0.001$) without increase in ischemic endpoints when compared with DAPT with aspirin and ticagrelor.[79] A network meta-analysis of randomized trials confirmed lower bleeding with short DAPT and showed no statistically significant difference between continuing aspirin monotherapy versus P2Y$_{12}$ monotherapy, although the results favored aspirin monotherapy to reduce bleeding and P2Y$_{12}$ monotherapy to reduce stent thrombosis.[77]

Protease-activated receptor (PAR)-1 antagonism with vorapaxar inhibits thrombin-induced platelet aggregation. In the Thrombin Receptor Antagonist in Secondary Prevention of Atherothrombotic Ischemic Events-Thrombolysis in Myocardial Infarction 50 trial (TRA 2°P-TIMI 50),[80] vorapaxar 2.5 mg daily decreased cardiovascular death, MI, stroke, or ischemia requiring revascularization compared to placebo (HR, 0.88; 95% CI, 0.82–0.95; $P = 0.001$) in 26,449 patients with CCS (defined as prior history of MI, ischemic stroke, or peripheral artery disease). However, the risk for moderate or severe bleeding was also increased significantly in the treatment arm (HR, 1.66; 95% CI, 1.43–1.93; $P < 0.001$), and the study was discontinued early for patients with a history of intracranial hemorrhage. For net clinical benefit, there was no difference between groups for the composite endpoint of cardiovascular death, MI, stroke, or moderate/severe bleeding (HR, 0.97; 95% CI, 0.90–1.04; $P = 0.40$). Decisions regarding long-term DAPT with P2Y$_{12}$ inhibitors or use of vorapaxar must be individualized, taking into account ischemic risk versus bleeding hazard.

Anticoagulant Therapy: Anticoagulant therapy inhibits thrombin formation and consequently reduces the risk of arterial thrombosis. In patients with CAD with no compelling indication for oral anticoagulant therapy, low-dose rivaroxaban (a factor Xa inhibitor) has been tested in a number of clinical trials. In the Cardiovascular Outcomes for People Using Anticoagulation Strategies (COMPASS) trial rivaroxaban (2.5 mg twice daily) plus aspirin had better cardiovascular outcomes (reduced the composite of cardiovascular death, stroke, or MI (4.1% vs 5.4%; HR 0.76; 95% CI, 0.66–0.86; $P < 0.001$) but led to more major bleeding events (3.1% vs 1.9%; HR 1.70; 95% CI, 1.40–2.05; $P < 0.001$) when compared with aspirin alone.[81] In a meta-analysis of 5 randomized trials (26,110 patients), low-dose rivaroxaban was associated with reduction in MI (HR 0.85, 95% CI, 0.73–0.99; $P = 0.04$), and stroke (HR 0.59; 95% CI, 0.48–0.73; $P < 0.001$) at the expense of major bleeding (HR 1.64; 95% CI, 1.39–1.94; $P < 0.001$) when compared with control.[82]

In patients post PCI who have a compelling indication for oral anticoagulant therapy (such as atrial fibrillation), triple therapy (aspirin, P2Y$_{12}$, and oral anticoagulant) is associated with significant increase in bleeding. A number of clinical trials (39%–72% SIHD) have tested strategies of dual antithrombotic therapy (Vitamin K antagonist [VKA] or non–vitamin K oral anticoagulant [NOAC] combined with P2Y$_{12}$) when compared with triple therapy.[83] These trials have consistently shown a reduction in bleeding (odds ratio [OR] 0.58; 95% CI, 0.31–1.08 for VKA plus P2Y$_{12}$ inhibitor; OR 0.49; 95% CI, 0.30–0.82 for NOAC plus P2Y$_{12}$ inhibitor) with no increase in ischemic outcomes (OR for MACE 0.96; 95% CI, 0.60–1.46 for VKA plus P2Y$_{12}$ inhibitor; OR 1.02;

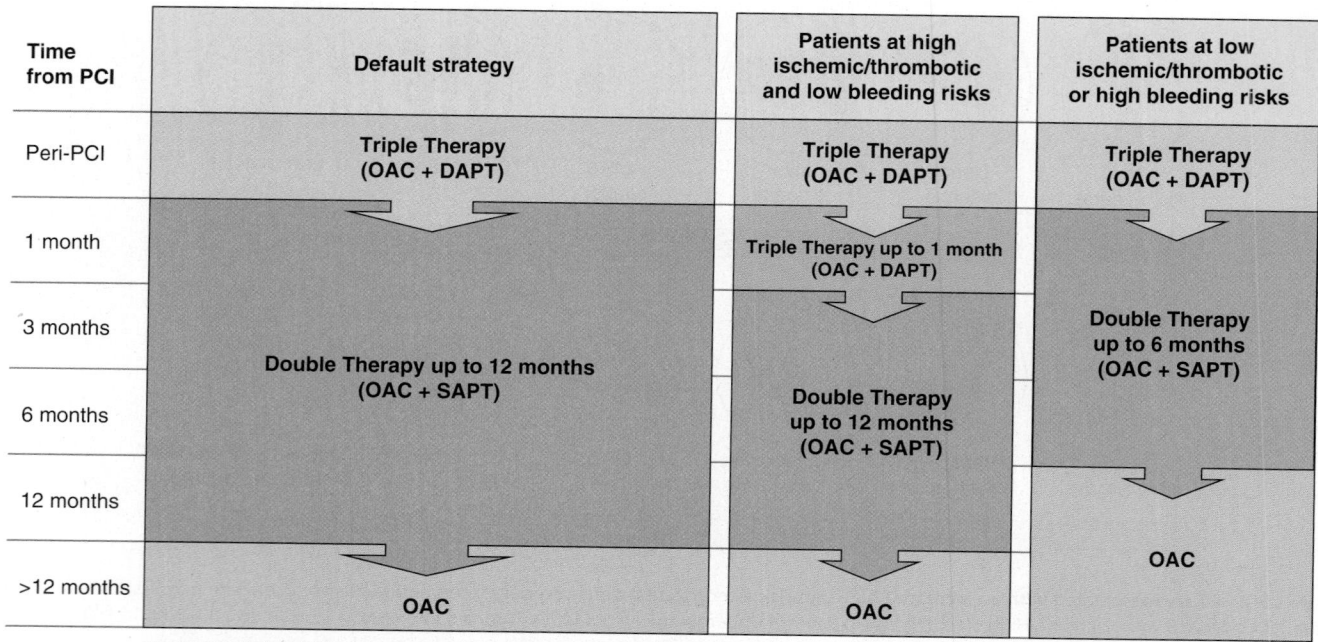

Time from PCI	Default strategy	Patients at high ischemic/thrombotic and low bleeding risks	Patients at low ischemic/thrombotic or high bleeding risks
Peri-PCI	Triple Therapy (OAC + DAPT)	Triple Therapy (OAC + DAPT)	Triple Therapy (OAC + DAPT)
1 month		Triple Therapy up to 1 month (OAC + DAPT)	
3 months	Double Therapy up to 12 months (OAC + SAPT)		Double Therapy up to 6 months (OAC + SAPT)
6 months		Double Therapy up to 12 months (OAC + SAPT)	
12 months			OAC
>12 months	OAC	OAC	

OAC: prefer a NOAC over VKA if no contraindications
SAPT: prefer a $P2Y_{12}$ inhibitor over aspirin
Clopidogrel is the $P2Y_{12}$ inhibitor of choice; ticagrelor may be considered in patients at high ischemic/thrombotic and low bleeding risks; avoid prasugrel
Consider SAPT in addition to OAC after > 12 mo. only in select patients at high ischemic/thrombotic and low bleeding risks

Figure 21–9. Antiplatelet therapy in patients with atrial fibrillation undergoing percutaneous coronary intervention treated with an oral anticoagulant: 2018 North American expert consensus update. Reproduced with permission from Angiolillo DJ, Goodman SG, Bhatt DL, et al. Antithrombotic Therapy in Patients With Atrial Fibrillation Treated With Oral Anticoagulation Undergoing Percutaneous Coronary Intervention: A North American Perspective-2018 Update. *Circulation.* 2018 Jul 31;138(5):527-536.

95% CI, 0.71-1.47, for NOAC plus $P2Y_{12}$ inhibitor) with dual antithrombotic therapy, especially a combination of NOAC with $P2Y_{12}$ (predominantly clopidogrel) when compared with triple therapy.[83] A double-therapy regimen immediately after hospital discharge should be considered for most patients as a default strategy (**Fig. 21–9**). In addition, NOAC should be preferred over a VKA unless contraindicated. Based on the regimen tested in clinical trials, clopidogrel remains the $P2Y_{12}$ inhibitor of choice, but ticagrelor may be considered in selected patients, particularly those at high ischemic/thrombotic and low bleeding risks. In patients with high ischemic/thrombotic and low bleeding risk, it is reasonable to extend low-dose aspirin therapy (ie, triple therapy) up to 1 month after PCI (Fig. 21–9).[84]

Lipid-Lowering Therapy: Serum cholesterol is an important risk factor for CAD. As such, in patients with established CAD, guidelines recommend lipid-lowering therapy irrespective of LDL-C levels. ACC/AHA guidelines recommend high-intensity statin therapy (eg, rosuvastatin 20–40 mg daily or atorvastatin 40–80 mg daily) in patients aged ≤75 years with a history of a prior cardiovascular event and moderate-intensity statin therapy (eg, rosuvastatin 10–20 mg daily or atorvastatin 20–40 mg daily) for patients >75 years of age. The 2019 ESC guidelines recommend lowering LDL-C by at least 50% from the baseline and to <55 mg/dL and a lower target LDL-C of <40 mg/dL for patients who experience a second vascular event within 2 years.[27]

A number of randomized clinical trials have shown the benefit of lipid lowering therapy in primary and secondary prevention of cardiovascular events. These controlled clinical trials have shown that for each 40 mg/dl reduction in LDL-C, there is a 10% reduction in all-cause mortality and 20% reduction in coronary mortality in addition to decreases in nonfatal MI, coronary revascularization, and stroke.[85] LaRosa and colleagues[109] tested the hypothesis that high-dose statin therapy is superior to low-dose statin therapy for the secondary prevention of cardiovascular events in patients with CAD. In the randomized, prospective Treating to New Targets (TNT) trial, 10,001 such patients (enrollment LDL <130 mg/dL) were randomized to receive 80 mg or 10 mg of atorvastatin daily over 6 years. Patients treated with 80 mg of atorvastatin achieved a mean LDL-C level of 77 mg/dL versus 101 mg/dL for those allocated to 10 mg of atorvastatin. High-dose atorvastatin therapy was associated with a 22% relative risk reduction for the combined primary endpoint of death from ischemic heart disease, nonfatal MI, or stroke.[86] While most of these clinical trials are with the use of statin therapy that works by inhibiting cholesterol synthesis in the liver by inhibiting HMG-CoA reductase, ezetimibe that works by inhibiting the absorption of cholesterol by the small intestine has also been shown to improve clinical outcomes. In the Improved Reduction of Outcomes: Vytorin Efficacy International Trial (IMPROVE-IT), simvastatin (40 mg daily) in combination with ezetimibe (10 mg daily), resulted in incremental lowering of LDL-C levels and further reduced cardiovascular outcomes (composite of cardiovascular death, nonfatal MI, unstable angina requiring rehospitalization, coronary revascularization [≥30 days after randomization], or nonfatal stroke) (HR 0.936; 95% CI, 0.89–0.99; $P = 0.016$) when compared with simvastatin alone in patients with recent ACS.[87] More recently, medications that inhibit proprotein convertase subtilisin kexin type 9 (PCSK9), which degrades hepatic LDL receptors and reduces LDL-C by as much as 60%, such as alirocumab and evolocumab, have also shown to improve cardiovascular outcomes. In the FOURIER trial, evolocumab further reduced LDL-C (from a median baseline value of 92 mg/dl to 30 mg/dl) and reduced cardiovascular events (composite of cardiovascular death, MI, stroke, hospitalization for unstable angina, or coronary revascularization) (9.8% vs 11.3%; HR, 0.85; 95% CI, 0.79–0.92; $P < 0.001$) when compared with placebo in 27,564 patients with CCS and LDL-C levels of 70 mg per deciliter or higher who were receiving statin therapy.[88] The 2018 ACC/AHA guidelines on the management of blood cholesterol recommends adding PCSK9 inhibitor in patients at very high-risk of atherosclerotic cardiovascular disease (ASCVD) on clinically judged maximal LDL-C lowering therapy and LDL-C ≥70 mg/dl or non–HDL-C ≥100 mg/dl (class IIa).[89]

β-Adrenergic Receptor Antagonists: β-adrenergic receptor antagonists favorably influence myocardial oxygen supply-demand balance by reducing heart rate, myocardial contractility, systemic arterial pressure, and LV wall stress and can therefore reduce ischemia and angina in the setting of CAD. β-Adrenergic receptor antagonists (when administered orally) are associated with improved short- and long-term survival rates in post-MI patients.[90] However, data to support cardiovascular event reduction in patients with CAD without MI and especially in those with preserved LV systolic function is limited. The REduction of Atherothrombosis for Continued Health (REACH) registry in outpatients with CAD (n = 18,653) and no prior MI showed no difference in the primary outcome (CV death, MI, or stroke) (HR 0.92; 95% CI, 0.79–1.08), higher rate of secondary outcome (primary outcome plus hospitalization) (OR 1.14; 95% CI, 1.03–1.27; $P = 0.01$) and tertiary outcome of hospitalization (OR 1.17; 95% CI, 1.04–1.30; $P = 0.01$) with a β-blocker versus no β-blocker at a median of 3.7 years of follow-up.[91] In the CathPCI registry of 755,215 patients with stable angina (without prior MI, systolic heart failure, or EF <40%) undergoing elective PCI, β-blocker use at discharge was not associated with lower CV events at 3-year follow-up but was associated with a higher rate of the composite of death, MI, stroke, and heart failure (HR_{adj} 1.04; 95% CI, 1.01–1.07; $P = 0.01$) versus the group not discharged on a β-blocker.[92] Other observational studies have shown variable results.[93,94] No adequately powered randomized controlled trial (RCT) has explored the efficacy of β-blockers in this cohort. In general, the efficacy of β-blockers is relatively greater among higher-risk patients, particularly among those with reduced EF, heart failure, or ventricular arrhythmias. In lower-risk patients, however, β-adrenergic receptor antagonists are recommended only for up to 3 years after uncomplicated MI without other relative indications (eg, atrial fibrillation, reduced EF).[11] In patients with CAD and heart failure with reduced ejection fraction (HFrEF), treatment should be restricted to the use of carvedilol, long-acting metoprolol, or bisoprolol, agents shown to reduce adverse outcomes in this population.

In patients with severe angina (ie, CCS class III/IV), full drug efficacy depends largely on dose titration to achieve a heart rate ≤60 bpm at rest or ≤75 bpm with exertion (or ≤75% of the heart rate at which angina occurs). β-Adrenergic receptor antagonists are frequently used in combination with other antianginal medications for maximum benefit and symptom control. Adding a β-adrenergic receptor antagonist to nitrates, for example, appears more effective in controlling anginal symptoms than does monotherapy with either agent alone.[95] Similar observations have been made with combination calcium channel blockers (CCBs); long-acting dihydropyridine derivatives are preferred to avoid excessive bradycardia in this setting.

Calcium Channel Blockers: CCBs decrease vascular smooth muscle cell and cardiac myocyte transmembrane calcium flux. They induce vasodilatation of epicardial coronary arteries to improve CBF and attenuate vasospastic and exertional angina. CCBs also improve angina by lowering systemic vascular resistance and mean arterial blood pressure to decrease LV afterload, thereby decreasing myocardial oxygen demand. The negative inotropic effects of these agents also favorably influence myocardial oxygen supply-demand balance, but may affect cardiac function adversely in patients with significantly impaired LV function. In patients with normal LV systolic function, CCBs may result in increased myocardial contractility as a compensatory response to lowered systemic vascular resistance.

Antianginal efficacy with CCBs is comparable to that obtained with β-adrenergic receptor antagonists.[96] However, the efficacy of CCB monotherapy for reducing MI or cardiac death in patients with CCS has not been demonstrated convincingly. The primary indications for CCB therapy include blood pressure or heart rate control and alleviation of anginal symptoms after optimization with β-adrenergic receptor blockers, nitrate, and angiotensin-converting enzyme (ACE) inhibitor therapy.

Renin-Angiotensin-Aldosterone System Inhibitors: Several randomized controlled trials in support of long-term ACE inhibition for the reduction of cardiovascular death, recurrent MI, and stroke in intermediate- and high-risk patients with CCS have been reported. The Heart Outcomes Prevention Evaluation (HOPE) study tested the efficacy of ramipril (10 mg/day) on cardiovascular outcomes in a large cohort of patients with CAD, stroke, peripheral vascular disease, or diabetes plus at least one other cardiovascular risk factor.[97] Patients with comorbid heart failure were excluded, and participants were not known to a have a decreased LVEF. Compared with placebo, ramipril therapy resulted in a significant reduction in the rate of death from cardiovascular causes, MI, and stroke over 5 years (14.0% vs 17.8%; RR, 0.78; 95% CI, 0.70–0.86). ACE inhibitor therapy also reduced incident diabetes. In the European Trial on Reduction of Cardiac Events With Perindopril in Stable Coronary Artery Disease (EUROPA), a trial that enrolled patients with chronic CAD and relatively lower risk profiles, perindopril therapy was associated with a directionally similar reduction in cardiovascular disease outcomes.[98] The salutary effects of ACE inhibitors were not as firmly established among lower-risk patients enrolled in the Prevention of Events With Angiotensin-Converting Enzyme Inhibitor Therapy (PEACE) trial, especially among patients with normal LV function, optimal lipid profiles, and prior revascularization.[99] In a meta-analysis of 24 randomized trials with 198,275 patient years of follow-up of patients with CAD without heart failure, renin angiotensin system inhibitors reduced cardiovascular events and death only when compared with placebo but not when compared with active controls.[100] ACE inhibitors are a class I recommendation for all CAD patients with LV dysfunction (EF < 0.40), hypertension, diabetes, or CKD and a class IIa recommendation for patients with both CAD and other vascular disease.[11] Angiotensin receptor blockers (ARBs) are an appropriate alternative for patients who cannot tolerate ACE inhibitors. They should not be used in combination with ACE inhibitors.[101] The mineralocorticoid receptor antagonists, spironolactone and eplerenone, have been demonstrated to be beneficial for patients with both advanced (NYHA class III/IV and EF < 0.35) and lesser degrees of HF.[102,103] Initiation of mineralocorticoid receptor antagonists, in addition to the use of β-adrenergic receptor antagonist and ACE inhibitor therapy, is a class I recommendation for treatment of patients after MI with reduced EF (≤0.40) and either symptomatic HF or diabetes.[104]

Organic Nitrates: Organic nitrates (eg, nitroglycerin, isosorbide dinitrate) are nitric oxide donors that activate soluble guanylyl cyclase in vascular smooth muscle cells to increase intracellular cyclic guanosine monophosphate and induce blood vessel relaxation. These medications reduce ischemia by (1) inducing venodilation of capacitance vessels to decrease preload, thus decreasing LV wall stress and myocardial oxygen demand; (2) dilating epicardial coronary arteries to improve CBF; and (3) recruiting coronary collaterals. In patients with CAD, use of nitrates is associated with lower angina frequency and increased time to ischemic ECG findings on treadmill testing.[105] Nitroglycerin also expresses antithrombotic properties, predominantly via attenuation of platelet aggregation. Nitrates do not influence survival or decrease cardiovascular death rates in CAD patients.

Tachyphylaxis to organic nitrate use is common in clinical practice, although the precise mechanisms remain unclear. As such, integrating a nitrate-free interval (8–12 hours) or longer drug holidays has been suggested (ie, intermittent drug cessation for 2- to 3-day periods). Coadministration of nitrates with phosphodiesterase-5 inhibitors (such as sildenafil, tadalafil or vardenafil) greatly increases the risk of potentially life-threatening hypotension because both drugs classes (ie, nitrates and phosphodiesterase-5 inhibitors) increase cyclic guanosine monophosphate bioactivity to potentiate vasodilatation.

Ranolazine: Ranolazine is a selective inhibitor of late sodium influx into myocytes, which in turn leads to decreased myocardial contractility. Early clinical trials established that ranolazine monotherapy is effective in improving exercise tolerance in patients with CAD.[106] In the prospective, randomized, placebo-controlled Combination Assessment of Ranolazine in Stable Angina (CARISA) trial, ranolazine (750–1000 mg twice daily) in combination with standard doses of atenolol, amlodipine, or diltiazem, significantly increased time to onset of angina and exercise performance compared with placebo.[107] Additionally, ranolazine significantly reduced the frequency of angina and nitroglycerin requirements during the 12-week period following randomization. Findings from a meta-analysis of seven randomized controlled trials (including CARISA) comparing ranolazine with placebo or usual care support a benefit with ranolazine on exercise tolerance and angina frequency.[108] Adverse effects include dizziness and constipation; discontinuation rates in large trials have been approximately 1%.[109] Although rare, QT interval prolongation has been seen with ranolazine therapy but not yet linked to clinically important arrhythmias. Drug interactions may be important, however, and the use of ranolazine is not recommended in patients receiving nondihydropyridine CCBs, quinolones, or azole antifungal medications, among others. Ranolazine is best reserved for patients with persistent symptoms despite maximal medical therapy or for patients unable to tolerate other antianginal therapies because of adverse effects.

Vaccination: In patients at high risk of cardiovascular disease, the annual influenza vaccine reduced the risk of major adverse cardiovascular events with greater effect in patients with recent ACS (10.25% vs 23.1%; RR, 0.45 [95% CI, 0.32–0.63]; $P < 0.001$) than patients with stable CAD (6.9% vs 7.4%; RR, 0.94 [95% CI, 0.55–1.61]; $P = 0.81$) ($P_{interaction} = 0.02$) in a meta-analysis of randomized trials of influenza vaccine.[110] It is therefore a class I recommendation by the ACC/AHA guideline committee for annual influenza vaccine for patients with CCS. Meta-analysis of observational studies suggest lower risk of MI in those receiving a pneumococcal vaccine especially in those 65 years or older.[111]

Coronary Artery Revascularization

Intensive lifestyle modification and evidence-based drug therapy remain the cornerstones of treatment for patients with CAD. Patients with refractory symptoms despite optimal medical therapy (OMT) and/or elevated clinical or angiographic risk profiles and suitable coronary anatomy can benefit from revascularization with PCI or coronary artery bypass graft (CABG) surgery. Considerations regarding revascularization in the CAD patient are distinctly different from those in the ACS patient. Indications for coronary artery revascularization in patients with CAD can be considered in terms of those that reduce long-term cardiovascular events including mortality and those that are targeted to symptom relief and improvement

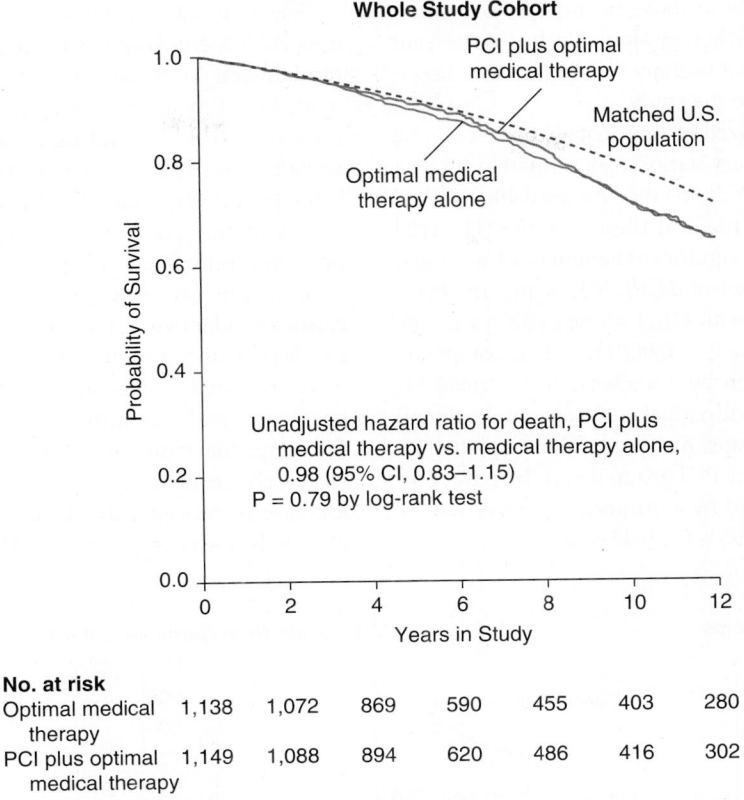

Figure 21–10. Effect of PCI plus OMT versus OMT alone in the long-term follow-up of the COURAGE trial. Reproduced with permission from Sedlis SP, Hartigan PM, Teo KK, et al. Effect of PCI on Long-Term Survival in Patients with Stable Ischemic Heart Disease. *N Engl J Med*. 2015 Nov 12;373(20):1937-1946.

in quality of life. The choice of revascularization strategy (ie, PCI vs CABG) relates to coronary artery anatomy, LV systolic function, systemic factors (eg, diabetes), and patient values and preferences. The benefits of surgical revascularization are generally greater for patients with extensive and complex CAD, as well as when LV systolic dysfunction or diabetes is present. A heart team approach to patient-centered shared decision-making is recommended with left main or multivessel CAD, especially with reduced EF.

Revascularization versus Optimal Medical Therapy

A number of clinical trials have tested a strategy of initial revascularization versus initial medical therapy alone in patients with CCS.

The COURAGE trial enrolled 2287 CAD patients between 1999 and 2004 with symptomatic but stabilized angina (Canadian Cardiovascular System angina class <IV), at least one ≥70% flow obstructing lesion in at least one proximal epicardial coronary artery, and objective evidence of myocardial ischemia.[112] Patients were randomized to receive OMT alone or in combination with PCI (with mainly bare metal stents). There was no significant difference in the primary endpoint of death or MI (19.0% vs 18.5%; HR 1.05; 95% CI, 0.87–1.27; $P = 0.62$), overall survival, survival free of MI, and survival free of ACS at a median follow-up of 4.6 years. However, the OMT plus PCI group was more likely to report freedom from angina and improved quality of life early after randomization but this

was not significantly different between groups 24 months following treatment assignment.[113] Extended survival data on a subgroup of 1211 COURAGE trial patients demonstrated no significant mortality difference between PCI and OMT groups at a mean of 6.2 years (25% vs 24%; HR, 1.03; 95% CI, 0.83–1.21; $P = 0.76$) (**Fig. 21–10**).[114]

The Bypass Angioplasty Revascularization Investigation 2 Diabetes (BARI 2D) trial randomized 2368 type 2 diabetic patients with CAD to receive either prompt revascularization with either PCI or CABG (within 4 weeks) on background of OMT or OMT alone.[115] At 5 years, rates of survival and freedom from major adverse cardiovascular events did not differ between the medical and revascularization arms. Among patients undergoing PCI, 34.7% received a DES, 56.0% received a bare metal stent, and 9.3% did not receive a stent. Patients for whom CABG was the intended method of revascularization (CABG stratum) and who were assigned to revascularization had significantly fewer major cardiovascular events than did patients in the CABG stratum who were assigned to the medical therapy group. Compared with the medical therapy strategy, prompt revascularization at the 3-year follow-up had a lower rate of worsening angina (8% vs 13%; $P < 0.001$), new angina (37% vs 51%; $P = 0.001$), and subsequent coronary revascularizations (18% vs 33%; $P < 0.001$) and a higher rate of angina-free status (66% vs 58%; $P = 0.003$).[116] The difference in freedom from angina was not statistically significant with revascularization after the first year in patients in the PCI stratum but was longer lasting in those in the CABG stratum when compared with medical therapy alone. Forty-two percent of patients assigned to medical therapy crossed over to revascularization over the course of the study.

The FAME 2 trial randomized 888 patients with at least one functionally significant coronary stenosis (as defined by an FFR ≤0.80) to either FFR-guided PCI plus the best available medical therapy or the best available medical therapy alone. The trial was prematurely halted after a significant benefit of FFR-guided PCI on the composite endpoint of death, MI, or urgent revascularization when compared with OMT alone (4.3% vs 12.7%; HR, 0.32; 95% CI, 0.19–0.53; $P < 0.0001$).[117] The composite endpoint reduction was driven by a decrease in the need for urgent revascularization; the individual endpoints of death and MI did not differ between groups. At 5 years follow-up, the primary endpoint was lower in the PCI group driven by reduction in urgent revascularization and by a numerically lower rate of MI (8.1% vs 12.0%; HR, 0.66; 95% CI, 0.43–1.00).[118]

The International Study of Comparative Health Effectiveness With Medical and Invasive Approaches (ISCHEMIA) trial randomized 5179 patients with moderate or severe ischemia to an initial invasive strategy (angiography and revascularization when feasible) and medical therapy or to an initial conservative strategy of medical therapy alone and angiography if medical therapy failed.[119] Most patients underwent blinded CCTA to rule out left main disease or nonobstructive CAD prior to randomization. After a median follow-up of 3.2 years, an initial invasive strategy did not reduce the risk of ischemic cardiovascular events (composite of death from cardiovascular causes, MI, or hospitalization for unstable angina; heart failure; or resuscitated cardiac arrest) or death from any cause when compared with an initial conservative strategy. The curves for the primary outcome and MI crossed at 2 years follow-up with higher event rate with invasive strategy upfront (driven by increase in procedural MI) and lower event rate longer term (driven by lower spontaneous MI) (**Fig. 21–11**). In addition, an

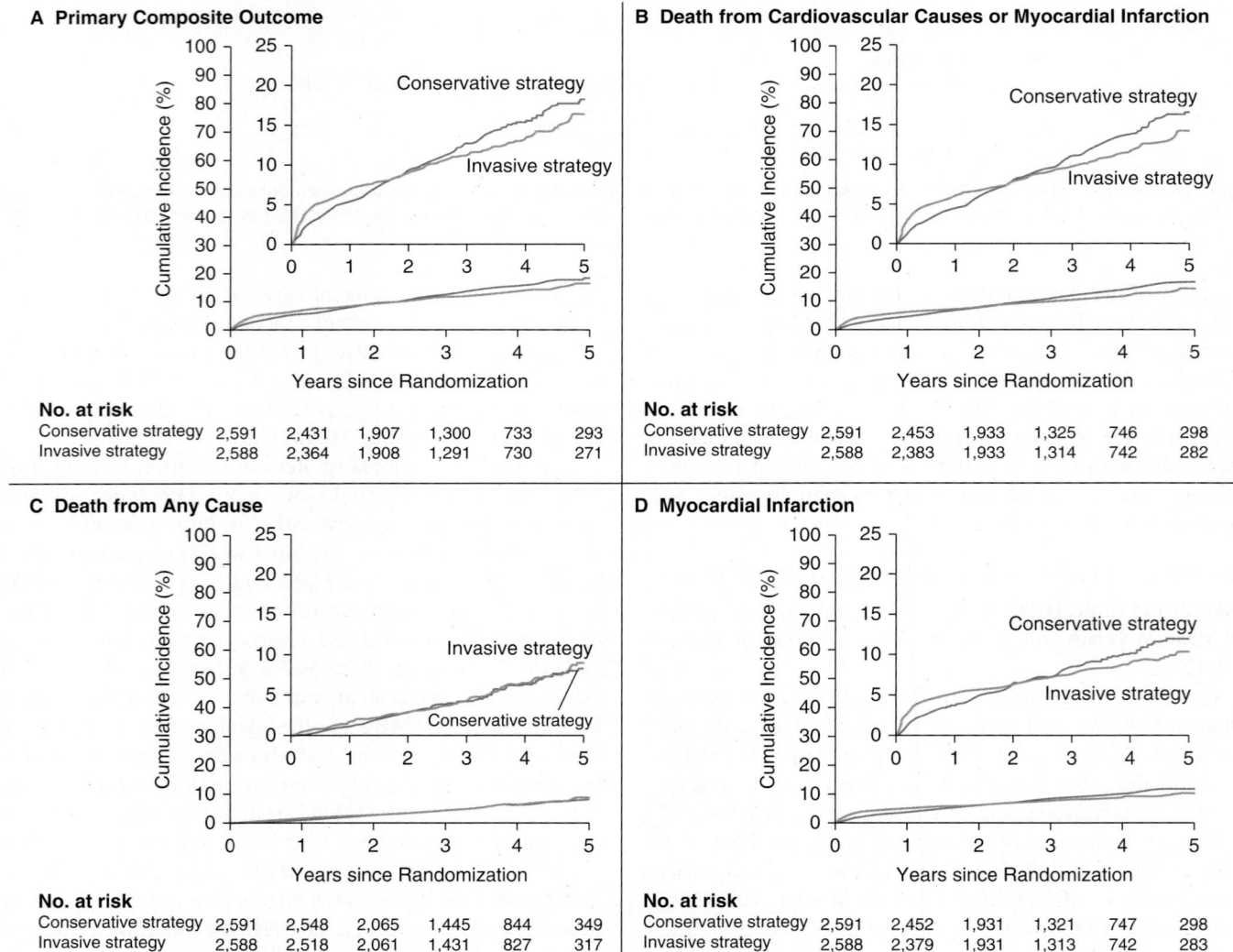

Figure 21–11. Clinical outcomes in the ISCHEMIA trial. (A) Primary composite outcome. **(B)** Death from cardiovascular causes or MI. **(C)** Death from any cause. **(D)** MI. Reproduced with permission from Maron DJ, Hochman JS, Reynolds HR, et al. Initial Invasive or Conservative Strategy for Stable Coronary Disease. *N Engl J Med*. 2020 Apr 9;382(15):1395-1407.

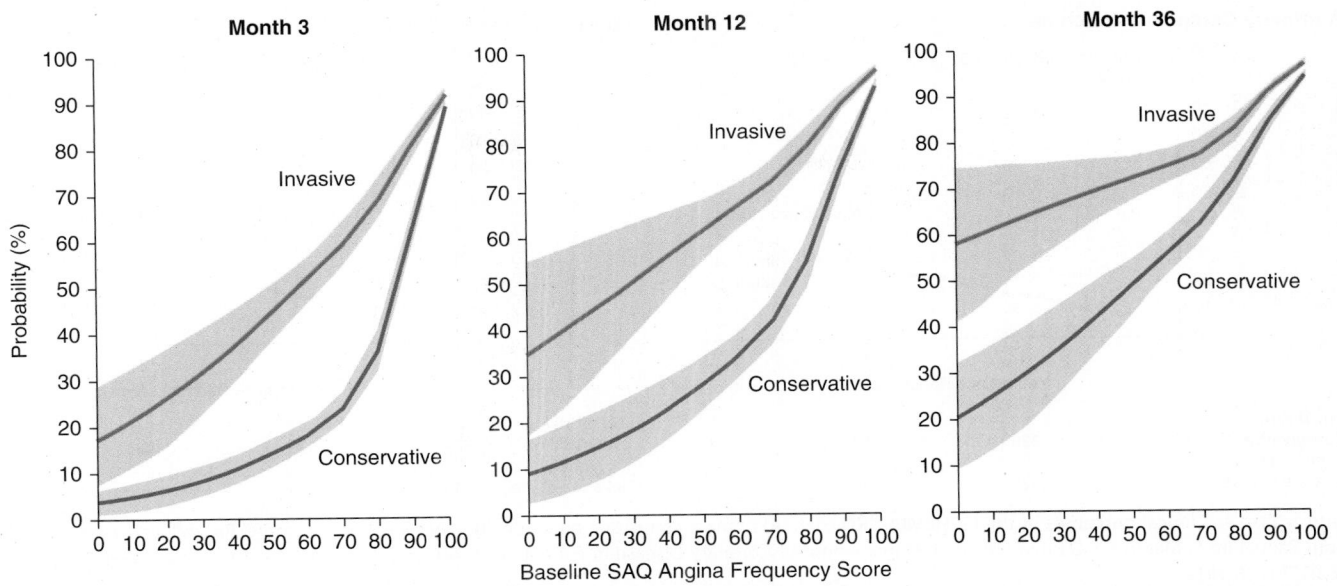

Figure 21–12. Probability of being angina free by treatment as a function of baseline angina frequency score in the ISCHEMIA trial. Reproduced with permission from Spertus JA, Jones PG, Maron DJ, et al. Health-Status Outcomes with Invasive or Conservative Care in Coronary Disease. *N Engl J Med.* 2020 Apr 9;382(15):1408-1419.

initial invasive strategy reduced nonprocedural MI and hospitalization for unstable angina, but increased procedural MI and hospitalization for heart failure. Moreover, patients randomly assigned to the invasive strategy had greater improvement in angina-related health status, which was durable through the length of follow-up than those assigned to the conservative strategy driven largely by differences in the cohort of patients who were symptomatic at baseline (**Fig. 21–12**).[120]

The ISCHEMIA-Chronic Kidney Disease (ISCHEMIA-CKD) trial randomized 777 participants with advanced CKD (eGFR <30 mL/min/1.73 m² or on dialysis) and moderate or severe ischemia to an initial invasive strategy (angiography and revascularization when feasible) and medical therapy or to an initial conservative strategy of medical therapy alone and angiography if medical therapy failed.[121] Over a median follow-up of 2.2 years, an initial invasive strategy did not reduce the risk of the primary endpoint of death or nonfatal MI (36.4% vs 36.7%; HRadj, 1.01; 95% CI, 0.79–1.29; *P* = 0.95) when compared with an initial conservative strategy (**Fig. 21–13**). Moreover, there were no substantial or sustained benefits with regard to angina-related health status with an initially invasive strategy as compared with a conservative strategy in this cohort with 49% of patients without angina at baseline (**Fig. 21–14**).[122]

In a meta-analysis of 14 randomized trials (including the ISCHEMIA trials) with 14,877 patients with CAD followed-up for a median of 4.5 years with 64,678 patient-years of follow-up, routine revascularization was associated with reduced nonprocedural MI, reduced overall MI in the more recent trials, reduced unstable angina, and greater freedom from angina, but at the expense of increased procedural MI with no difference in survival when compared with initial medical therapy alone (**Fig. 21–15**).[123] The trials largely enrolled patients without reduced EF (35% or greater), less angina (Canadian

Cardiovascular System angina class I/II), and without left main disease. Overall, in the routine revascularization group, 71.3% underwent PCI, 16.2% underwent CABG, and 12.5% of patients underwent medical therapy alone. In the initial medical therapy alone group, 31.9% underwent revascularization over the duration of follow-up.[123]

In patients with ischemic cardiomyopathy (EF 35% or less), the Surgical Treatment for Ischemic Heart Failure (STICH) trial randomized 1212 patients to medical therapy alone or medical therapy plus CABG. At a median follow-up of 4.7 years, CABG patients had similar primary outcome (all-cause death) (36% vs 41%; HR, 0.86; 95% CI, 0.72–1.04; *P* = 0.12), numerically lower cardiovascular death (HR 0.81; 95% CI, 0.66–1.00; *P* = 0.05), but significantly lower composite of death or hospitalization for cardiovascular causes (HR 0.74; 95% CI, 0.64–0.85; *P* < 0.001).[124] In the extended follow-up of the trial (median 9.8 years), CABG reduced all-cause death (HR 0.84; 95% CI, 0.73–0.97; *P* = 0.02), cardiovascular death (HR, 0.79; 95% CI, 0.66–0.93; *P* = 0.006), and the composite of death or hospitalization for cardiovascular causes.[125]

PERCUTANEOUS CORONARY INTERVENTION VERSUS CORONARY ARTERY BYPASS GRAFT SURGERY

A number of trials have compared PCI and CABG surgery for patients with multivessel CAD. Evolving technologic advances in stent design, antiplatelet therapies, techniques for chronic total occlusion, and lipid-lowering drugs; improvement in myocardial preservation techniques; and use of arterial conduits at surgery have confounded the application of these older data to contemporary practice.

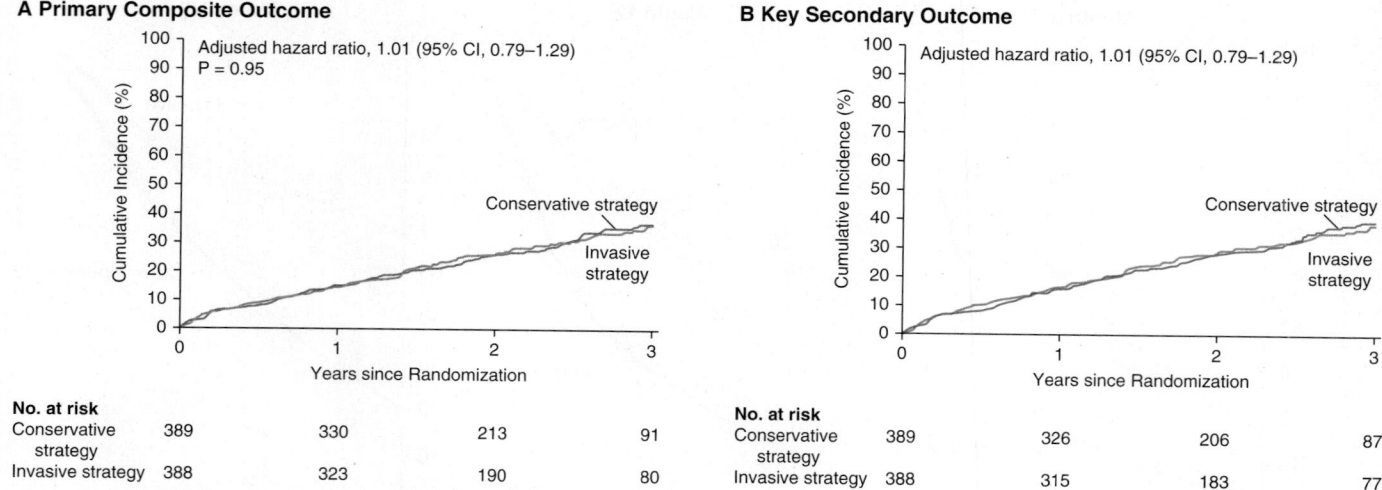

Figure 21–13. Clinical outcomes in the ISCHEMIA-CKD trial. (A) Primary composite outcome. **(B)** Key secondary outcome. Reproduced with permission from Bangalore S, Maron DJ, O'Brien SM, et al. Management of Coronary Disease in Patients with Advanced Kidney Disease. *N Engl J Med.* 2020 Apr 23; 382(17):1608-1618.

In the early 1990s, the Bypass Angioplasty Revascularization Investigation 1 (BARI-1) trial was conducted to test the hypothesis that balloon angioplasty and CABG surgery are equally effective strategies for patients with multivessel CAD and angina.[126] In BARI-1, 1829 multivessel CAD patients were randomly assigned to undergo percutaneous transluminal coronary angioplasty (PTCA) or CABG surgery and were followed for >5 years. No long-term survival advantage was seen for CABG surgery versus PTCA, although a subset of patients with treated diabetes demonstrated improved survival with surgery when the left internal thoracic artery was used for LAD bypass.

The Synergy between PCI with Taxus and Cardiac Surgery (SYNTAX) trial was designed to demonstrate noninferiority between multivessel PCI (with a first-generation paclitaxel-eluting stent) and CABG surgery for patients with multivessel CAD for the primary composite endpoint of death from any cause, stroke, MI, or repeat revascularization during the 12 months following treatment.[127] The results suggested that surgical revascularization resulted in a significantly lower rate of the combined primary endpoint largely driven by the reduced need for revascularization. There was no difference between treatment groups for the combined endpoint of death

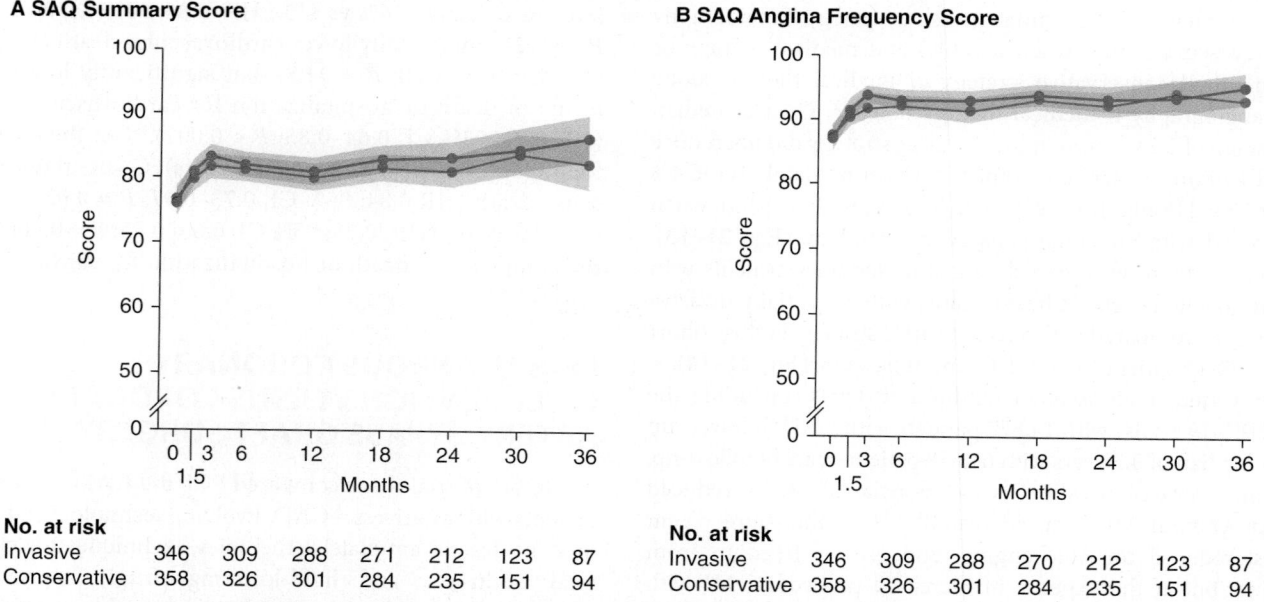

Figure 21–14. Quality of life outcomes in the ISCHEMIA-CKD trial. (A) SAQ summary score. **(B)** SAQ angina frequency score. Reproduced with permission from Spertus JA, Jones PG, Maron DJ, et al. Health Status after Invasive or Conservative Care in Coronary and Advanced Kidney Disease. *N Engl J Med.* 2020 Apr 23;382(17):1619-1628.

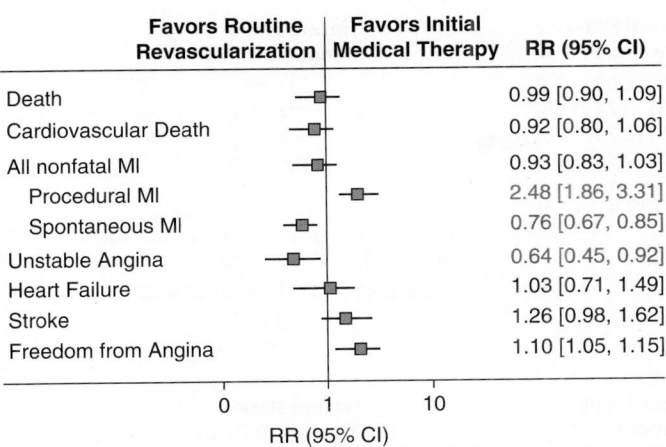

	Favors Routine Revascularization	Favors Initial Medical Therapy	RR (95% CI)
Death			0.99 [0.90, 1.09]
Cardiovascular Death			0.92 [0.80, 1.06]
All nonfatal MI			0.93 [0.83, 1.03]
Procedural MI			2.48 [1.86, 3.31]
Spontaneous MI			0.76 [0.67, 0.85]
Unstable Angina			0.64 [0.45, 0.92]
Heart Failure			1.03 [0.71, 1.49]
Stroke			1.26 [0.98, 1.62]
Freedom from Angina			1.10 [1.05, 1.15]

RR (95% CI)

Figure 21–15. Routine revascularization versus initial medical therapy in SIHD. Meta-analysis of 14 randomized trials. Data from Bangalore S, Maron DJ, Stone GW, et al. Routine Revascularization Versus Initial Medical Therapy for Stable Ischemic Heart Disease: A Systematic Review and Meta-Analysis of Randomized Trials. *Circulation.* 2020 Sep;142(9):841-857.

from any cause, stroke, or MI. Surgery resulted in an increased likelihood of periprocedural stroke. Among the strengths of the SYNTAX trial was the use of a numerical score for the objective evaluation of coronary disease severity and likelihood of revascularization success. The SYNTAX score is generated by summarizing various qualitative plaque features and stenosis locations and serves as an objective measure of coronary disease severity that can be used to stratify anticipated patient outcomes (**Table 21–6**; also see syntaxscore.com).[128] Patients with high (≥33) and intermediate (23–32) SYNTAX scores had lower rates of MACCE with surgery compared with PCI out to

TABLE 21–6. Key Angiographic Characteristics That Influence the SYNTAX Score

Right, left, or codominant coronary circulation
Number of atherosclerotic lesions
Number of artery segments involved per atherosclerotic lesion
Total occlusion:
    Number of segments involved
    Age of total occlusion
    Presence of a blunt stump
    Presence of bridging collateral
    Antegrade vs retrograde filling of the first segment beyond the occlusion
    Side branch involvement
Trifurcation lesion: number of vessel segments diseased
Bifurcation lesion: angulation between the distal main vessel and the side branch <70°
Presence of an aorto-ostial atherosclerotic lesion
Presence of severe vessel tortuosity at lesion site
Atherosclerotic lesion length >20 mm
Presence of heavily calcified plaque
Presence of thrombus
Presence of diffuse or small-vessel disease

Abbreviation: SYNTAX, Synergy between Percutaneous Coronary Intervention with Taxus and Cardiac Surgery.

5 years (high SYNTAX score: 26.8% surgery vs 44.0% PCI; $P < 0.0001$; intermediate SYNTAX score: 25.8% surgery vs 36.0% PCI). Event rates were similar for patients with low (≤22) SYNTAX scores. The trial also established that PCI is noninferior to bypass surgery for treatment of left main CAD (31.0% MACCE rate in the CABG surgery group vs 36.9% in the PCI group; $P = 0.12$).[129] At 10 years follow-up, PCI resulted in similar survival when compared with CABG, with CABG providing a survival benefit in patients with 3-vessel disease but not in patients with left main disease.[130]

Left Main Coronary Artery Disease

Left main CAD is found in approximately 4% of patients undergoing coronary interventions.

The Premier of Randomized Comparison of Bypass Surgery versus Angiogram Trial (PRECOMBAT) randomized 600 patients who had at least a 50% lesion of the left main coronary artery to PCI with DESs versus CABG with a left internal mammary artery graft. The 5-year results showed no significant difference in the primary endpoint of all-cause mortality, MI, stroke, and ischemia-driven target vessel revascularization between PCI and CABG (17.5% vs 14.3%, HR 1.27, 95% CI, 0.84–1.90; $P = 0.26$).[131] Target vessel revascularization was almost double in the PCI group (11.4% vs 5.5%; HR, 2.11; $P = 0.012$). In patients with left main CAD and triple-vessel disease, the results favored bypass surgery. The 10-year follow-up of this trial showed no significant difference between PCI and CABG for MACE and all-cause mortality (14.5% vs 13.8%; HR 1.13; 95% CI, 0.75–1.70).[132]

The NOBLE trial randomized 1201 patients with left main disease to PCI with biomatrix flex stent or to CABG. PCI failed to meet the noninferiority criteria to CABG for the primary endpoint of composite of all-cause mortality, nonprocedural MI, any repeat coronary revascularization, and stroke (28% vs 18%; HR 1·51; 95% CI 1.13–2.00) driven by excess of nonprocedural MI and repeat coronary revascularization with no difference in all-cause death.[133] At 5 years follow-up, PCI was inferior to CABG for the primary endpoint but there was no difference in all-cause mortality between the groups (9% vs 9%; HR 1·08; 95% CI 0.74–1.59; $P = 0.68$).[134]

The Evaluation of XIENCE versus Coronary Artery Bypass Surgery for Effectiveness of Left Main Revascularization (EXCEL) trial randomized 1905 patients with left main disease and SYNTAX score of <32 to PCI with everolimus eluting stent or to CABG. At 3 years, PCI was noninferior to CABG for the primary endpoint of death, MI, or stroke (15.4% vs 14.7%; HR 1.00; 95% CI, 0.79–1.26; $P = 0.98$) with higher event rate with CABG for the secondary endpoint of death, MI, or stroke at 30 days (4.9% vs 7.9%; $P = 0.008$).[135] At 5 years follow-up, PCI was associated with similar rate of primary endpoint, cardiovascular death, and MI, lower rate of cerebrovascular events, but a higher rate of all-cause death and ischemia driven revascularization when compared with CABG.[136]

A meta-analysis of the four trials including a total of 4394 patients with left main disease found similar risk of all-cause death (HR 1.11; 95% CI 0.91–1.35, $P = 0.30$), cardiovascular death, MI, and stroke, but higher rates of

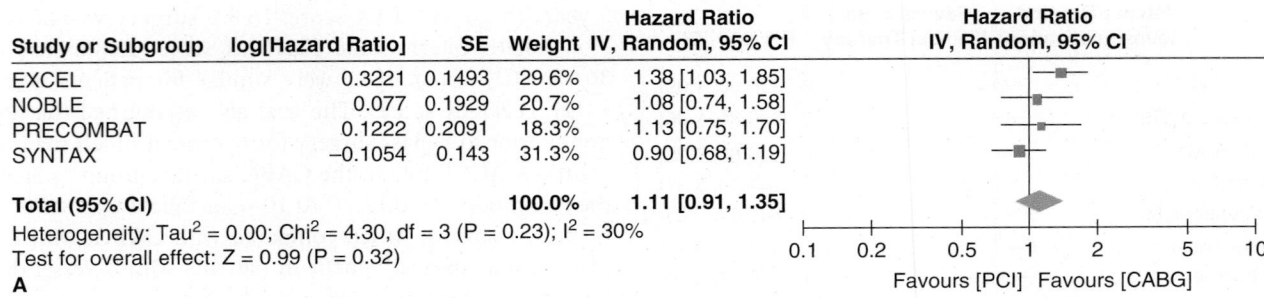

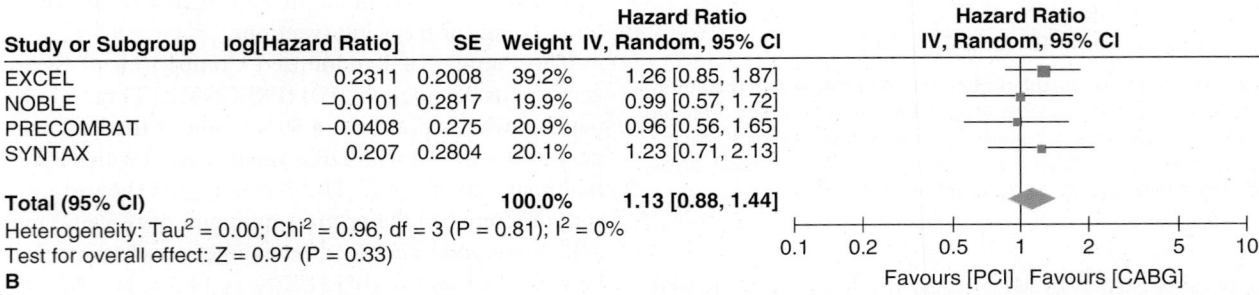

Figure 21–16. Meta-analysis of randomized trial of PCI versus CABG for left main coronary artery disease for the outcome of (A) death and (B) cardiovascular death. Reproduced with permission from Kuno T, Ueyama H, Rao SV, et al. Percutaneous coronary intervention or coronary artery bypass graft surgery for left main coronary artery disease: A meta-analysis of randomized trials. *Am Heart J.* 2020 Sep;227:9-10.

repeat revascularization with PCI when compared to CABG (**Fig. 21–16**). The analysis had 80% power to rule out a 25% or greater reduction in all-cause mortality between the two revascularization strategies.[137]

Diabetes Mellitus

The presence of diabetes at the time of coronary revascularization is one of the strongest predictors of outcome and is a major determinant of the optimal mode of revascularization. The presence of diabetes is a marker of a greater extent of CAD and greater likelihood of important comorbidities such as renal dysfunction, thrombosis, and left ventricular dysfunction. In addition, rates of in-stent restenosis and target vessel revascularization are higher in diabetic patients than they are in non-diabetic patients.

The FREEDOM trial was designed to address the optimal coronary revascularization strategy in 1900 patients with diabetes and multivessel CAD (83% with 3-vessel disease) in the absence of left main disease, prior CABG, prior stenting within 6 months, and current ST-segment elevation MI.[138] In FREEDOM, over a median follow-up of 3.8 years, the primary composite endpoint of death, nonfatal MI, and nonfatal stroke was lower in the CABG group when compared with the first-generation DES group (18.7% vs 26.6%; *P* < 0.005) driven by driven by a decrease in MI (*P* < 0.001), death (*P* = 0.049), but increase in stroke (5.2% vs 2.4%; *P* = 0.03). In the longer-term follow-up of the trial (FREEDOM Follow-on trial), over a median follow-up of 7.5 years, all-cause mortality rate was significantly higher in the PCI-DES group

than in the CABG group (24.3% vs 18.3%; HR 1.36; 95% CI 1.07–1.74; *P* = 0.01).[139] The limitation of the trial is the use of first-generation DES. Data from clinical trials, meta-analysis of clinical trials, and registries consistently show reduction in death and/or MI (driven by decreases in stent thrombosis and restenosis) with newer-generation DES when compared with early generation DES or BMS.[140,141]

In a network meta-analysis of clinical trials, while a mortality benefit of CABG was observed when compared with PCI using first generation DES in patients with diabetes, the mortality gap narrowed to statistical nonsignificance when the comparator was newer generation DES.[142] Similarly, in an analysis of over 16,000 patients with diabetes and multivessel CAD from the New York State registries, PCI with second-generation DES was associated with lower upfront risk of death and stroke when compared with CABG. At long-term follow-up, there was no significant mortality difference between PCI and CABG.[143] Moreover, in a meta-analysis of the only three RCTs of CABG versus PCI using newer-generation DES, major adverse cardiovascular event rate was lower with PCI when compared with CABG at 30 days. Over long-term follow-up (3–5 years) there was no difference in outcomes between the two groups and the diabetes status was not an effect modifier in this analysis (**Fig. 21–17**).[144] The optimal management of patients with diabetes and multivessel disease should be individualized using a heart team to weigh the upfront risk of CABG with potential late benefits, ability to completely revascularize with PCI, ability of patient to be compliant with medication therapies, and most importantly patient preference.[145]

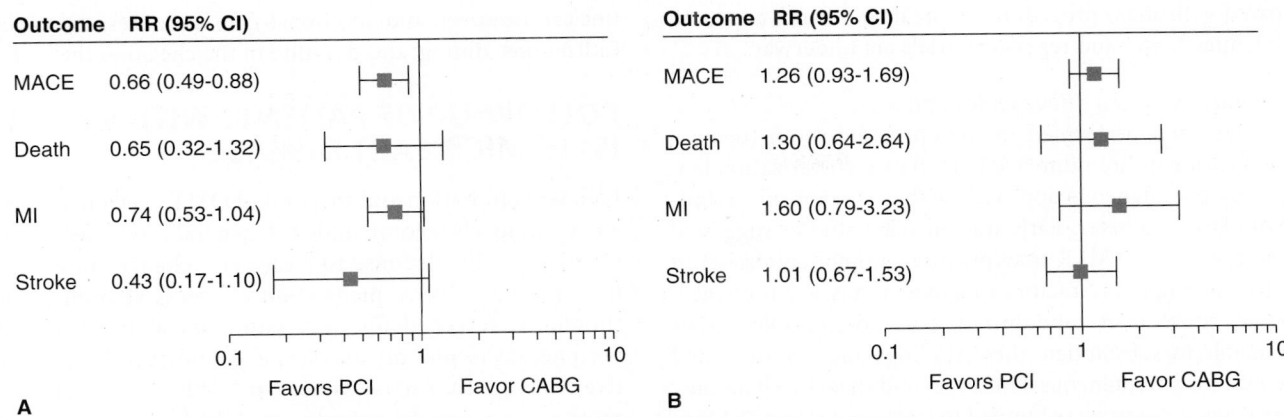

Figure 21–17. Meta-analysis of randomized trials of PCI with second generation DES versus CABG in patients for (A) short-term and (B) long-term outcomes. Diabetes was not an effect modifier in this analysis. Reproduced with permission from Bangalore S, Bhatt DL. Do We Need a Trial of DES Versus CABG Surgery in Diabetic Patients With ACS? *J Am Coll Cardiol.* 2017 Dec 19;70(24):3007-3009.

Left Ventricular Systolic Dysfunction

No randomized trial has compared PCI versus CABG in patients with LV dysfunction. In an analysis of 4616 patients with multivessel disease and severe LV systolic dysfunction (EF ≤35%) who underwent either PCI with everolimus-eluting stent (EES) or CABG from the New York State registries, at a median 2.9 years of follow-up, PCI was associated with similar risk of death (HR, 1.01; 95% CI, 0.81–1.28; $P = 0.91$), a higher risk of MI (HR, 2.16; 95% CI, 1.42–3.28; $P = 0.0003$), a lower risk of stroke (HR, 0.57; 95% CI, 0.33–0.97; $P = 0.04$), and a higher risk of repeat revascularization (HR, 2.54; 95% CI, 1.88–3.44; $P < 0.0001$) when compared with CABG.[146] Randomized trials are awaited.

Less Traditional Therapies in Patients with Refractory Angina

For patients with angina refractory to conventional medical or revascularization therapies, palliative treatment with spinal cord stimulation, enhanced external counterpulsation (EECP), coronary-sinus reducing device, surgical transmyocardial laser revascularization (TMLR), or chelation therapy may be considered.[147]

Spinal Cord Stimulation

The efficacy of spinal cord stimulation depends on the accurate placement of the stimulating electrode in the dorsal epidural space, usually at the C7 to T1 level. Data in favor of spinal cord stimulation as a useful treatment for refractory angina are mainly limited to case series and small clinical trials. The Electrical Stimulation versus Coronary Artery Bypass Surgery in Severe Angina Pectoris (ESBY) study randomized 104 patients with end-stage ischemic heart disease to spinal cord stimulation or CABG surgery.[148] Participants in the ESBY trial were at elevated surgical risk and had preoperative clinical profiles that did not predict a clear prognostic benefit from surgery. Compared with surgery, spinal cord stimulation resulted in lower 6-month mortality with similar improvement in angina

frequency and severity. Subsequent trials have been underpowered or have not shown a compelling benefit with respect to angina, quality-of-life score, or improvement in exercise tolerance with spinal cord stimulation in patients with severe, refractory angina.[149] Nonetheless, spinal cord stimulation appears safe, and speculation remains that this intervention favorably influences sympathetically and parasympathetically mediated neurovascular tone, improves CBF, and exerts anti-ischemic effects in some patients.[150]

Enhanced External Counterpulsation

EECP uses cuff inflation for the application of compressed air-induced pressure to the lower extremities that is synchronized with the cardiac cycle. Specifically, in early diastole, positive pressure is applied sequentially from the lower legs to the lower and upper thighs for the facilitation of increased retrograde aortic blood flow and increased coronary diastolic perfusion pressure. In patients with refractory angina, EECP (~35 hours of treatment time) is associated with a reduction in angina frequency and nitrate use, increased exercise tolerance, and improved quality of life.[151,152] Patients with severely limiting angina and without a smoking history are most likely to benefit.[153] Certain forms of valvular heart disease (eg, aortic regurgitation), recent revascularization, and severe hypertension are contraindications to this form of therapy. Sufficiently powered randomized clinical trials of EECP versus OMT are lacking.

Coronary-Sinus Reducing Device

Coronary-sinus reducing device creates a focal narrowing and increases pressure in the coronary sinus potentially redistributing blood into ischemic myocardium. In the Coronary Sinus Reducer for Treatment of Refractory Angina (COSIRA) trial, implantation of the coronary-sinus reducing device was associated with significant improvement in symptoms and quality of life in 104 patients with refractory angina who were not candidates for revascularization when compared with sham procedure.[154] The device is not approved in the United States and regulatory trials are underway.

Transmyocardial Laser Revascularization

TMLR has been performed in the operating room (using a carbon dioxide or holmium:YAG laser) or catheterization laboratory by percutaneous approach with a specialized (holmium:YAG laser) catheter. Early uncontrolled studies suggested that percutaneous TMLR may provide symptomatic relief in patients with angina refractory to maximal medical therapy.[155] However, subsequent randomized, placebo-controlled trials were unable to substantiate these findings and demonstrated no benefit for percutaneous TMLR beyond that of a sham procedure when patients were blinded to treatment status.[156] Findings from prospective RCTs support surgical TMLR beyond medical therapy alone for symptom relief and decreased hospitalization frequency. Furthermore, in a multicenter randomized trial comparing surgical TMLR with medical therapy in 192 patients with angina refractory to maximal medical therapy, Frazier and colleagues correlated improvements in CCS class from surgical TMLR with a decrease in the number of fixed or reversible perfusion defects evaluated by MPI.[157] These findings have not been widely replicated. The mechanism by which TMLR reduces angina is also not resolved. As a result of discrepancies among reports on efficacy and concern for increased rates of iatrogenic morbidity following surgical or percutaneous TMLR, including ventricular perforation, cardiac tamponade, stroke, and MI, the use of this strategy is infrequent.

Chelation Therapy

Sodium ethylenediamine tetra acetic acid (EDTA) has long been recognized for its capacity to bind di- or trivalent cations, including some implicated in the pathobiology of atherosclerotic CAD, such as calcium (Ca^{2+}). On the heels of promising data from small, uncontrolled trials suggesting a potential benefit with chelation therapy in patients with CAD, the Trial to Assess Chelation Therapy (TACT) was completed and serves as the first sufficiently powered trial studying EDTA therapy in CAD. In this double-blind placebo-controlled 2 × 2 factorial multicenter randomized trial, 1708 patients (>50 years old, >6 weeks post-MI, serum creatinine <2.0 mg/dL) were randomized to receive 40 infusions of 500 mL of chelation solution fortified with B vitamins versus placebo and to an oral vitamin regimen or placebo. A favorable effect on the primary endpoint of total mortality, recurrent MI, stroke, coronary revascularization, or hospitalization for recurrent angina was observed in patients randomized to chelation compared to placebo (HR, 0.82; 95% CI, 0.69–0.99; $P = 0.035$), which did not appear to hinge on randomization to the oral vitamin therapy stratum.[158] The effect of chelation was most pronounced in patients with diabetes or prior anterior MI, setting the framework for the ongoing TACT-2 trial that aims to assess the benefit of combination chelation plus oral vitamin and mineral therapy in diabetic CAD patients specifically. A pathophysiologic mechanism accounting for the benefits of chelation therapy in the original TACT study remains unclear, however, and additional data are necessary to clarify indications, timing, and duration of the chelation therapy.

FOLLOW-UP OF PATIENTS WITH STABLE ISCHEMIC HEART DISEASE

Following initiation and titration of OMT, reevaluation every 4 to 6 months is recommended. A general assessment of functional capacity, response to treatment, changes in quality of life, and any adverse medication effects is advised. Patients should be screened for depression, social isolation, CKD, peripheral vascular disease, sexual dysfunction, and obstructive sleep apnea. An assessment of LVEF and segmental wall motion by echocardiography or MPI is recommended in patients with a change in symptoms or evidence of MI by history or ECG, but not routinely in the absence of these clinical indications. Laboratory assessment of lipids and glucose should be performed in accordance with current guideline recommendations. In the stable patient without weight change or dietary modification, lipids can be assessed every 6 to 12 months.

Guidelines are imprecise regarding the frequency with which routine noninvasive testing should be repeated in patients with SIHD. **Table 21–7** provides the ACC/AHA indications for performing echocardiography, exercise treadmill testing, stress MPI, and coronary angiography in the follow-up setting.

CHEST PAIN WITHOUT SIGNIFICANT EPICARDIAL CORONARY DISEASE

Ischemia and No Obstructive Coronary Artery Disease

INOCA represents patients with chest pain, evidence of ischemia, but no obstructive CAD on coronary angiography. This may reflect microvascular circulatory dysfunction and impaired intramyocardial perfusion. Formerly termed *cardiac syndrome X*, recent investigations have defined more clearly the pathophysiology of microvascular circulatory dysfunction (**Table 21–8**).[159] The original epidemiologic observations that reported a clustering of patient characteristics associated with this clinical phenomenon (eg, female predominance, hypertension, obesity) have been redefined to emphasize the histologic and pathophysiologic processes that increase the probability of disease expression (**Table 21–9**). Abnormal coronary vascular reactivity from impaired endothelial-dependent and -independent signaling likely explains decreased CFR associated with most forms of this condition.[160]

Microvascular ischemia is often difficult to diagnose. Comparison of myocardial blood flow under basal conditions and after intracoronary infusion of adenosine with a Doppler flow wire can be performed once obstructive epicardial CAD has been excluded at angiography.[159] Assessment of CFR or myocardial perfusion reserve using PET or cardiac MRI is the most common and reliable noninvasive method for diagnosing microvascular circulatory dysfunction. Many investigators and clinicians use a cutoff of <3.0 mL/min/g myocardial tissue (quantified at peak hyperemia relative to rest) to diagnose

TABLE 21-7. American College of Cardiology/American Heart Association Recommendations for Work up of Patients With Obstructive Cad Who Present With Stable Chest Pain

COR	LOE	Recommendations
1	A	For patients with obstructive CAD who have stable chest pain despite GDMT and moderate-severe ischemia, ICA is recommended for guiding therapeutic decision-making
1	A	For patients with obstructive CAD who have stable chest pain despite optimal GDMT, those referred for ICA without prior stress testing benefit from FFR or instantaneous wave free ratio
1	B-R	For symptomatic patients with obstructive CAD who have stable chest pain with CCTA-defined ≥50% stenosis in the left main coronary artery, obstructive CAD with FFR with CT ≤0.80, or severe stenosis (≥70%) in all 3 main vessels, ICA is effective for guiding therapeutic decision-making
2a	B-NR	For patients who have stable chest pain with previous coronary revascularization, CCTA is reasonable to evaluate bypass graft or stent patency (for stents ≥3 mm)
1	B-NR	For patients with obstructive CAD who have stable chest pain despite optimal GDMT, stress PET/SPECT MPI, CMR, or echocardiography is recommended for diagnosis of myocardial ischemia, estimating risk of MACE, and guiding therapeutic decision-making
2a	B-R	For patients with obstructive CAD who have stable chest pain despite optimal GDMT, when selected for rest/stress nuclear MPI, PET is reasonable in preference to SPECT, if available, to improve diagnostic accuracy and decrease the rate of nondiagnostic test results
2a	B-NR	For patients with obstructive CAD who have stable chest pain despite GDMT, exercise treadmill testing can be useful to determine if the symptoms are consistent with angina pectoris, assess the severity of symptoms, evaluate functional capacity and select management, including cardiac rehabilitation
2a	B-NR	For patients with obstructive CAD who have stable chest pain symptoms undergoing stress PET MPI or stress CMR, the addition of MBFR is useful to improve diagnosis accuracy and enhance risk stratification

Abbreviations: CAD, coronary artery disease; CCTA, cardiac computed tomographic angiography; CMR, cardiac magnetic resonance imaging; COR, class of recommendation; FFR, fractional flow reserve; GDMT, guideline directed medical therapy; ICA, invasive coronary angiography; LOE, level of evidence; MBFR, myocardial blood flow reserve; MPI, myocardial perfusion imaging; PET, positron emission tomography; SPECT, Single-photon emission computed tomography.
Adapted with permission from Gulati M, Levy PD, Mukherjee D et al. 2021 AHA/ACC/ASE/CHEST/SAEM/SCCT/SCMR guideline for the evaluation and diagnosis of chest pain: a report of the American College of Cardiology/American Heart Association Joint Committee on Clinical Practice Guidelines. *J Am Coll Cardiol*. 78(22):e187-e285.

microvascular circulatory disease provided the patient has cardiac angina and that no epicardial coronary stenosis >50% is present.[161]

Data from the Women's Ischemia Syndrome Evaluation (WISE) study demonstrated a positive association between impaired coronary microvascular reactivity and abnormal functional capacity.[162] In this analysis, 190 women (18% with epicardial coronary luminal stenosis >50%) underwent invasive assessment of coronary flow velocity in response to intracoronary adenosine injection. Women with a decreased coronary

TABLE 21-8. Clinical Causes of Coronary Microvascular Circulatory Disease

Coronary microvascular dysfunction in the absence of obstructive CAD and myocardial diseases	This type represents the functional counterpart of traditional coronary risk factors (smoking, hypertension, hyperlipidemia, and diabetes and insulin-resistant states). It can be identified by noninvasive assessment of coronary flow reserve. This type is at least partly reversible, and coronary flow reserve can also be used as a surrogate end point to assess efficacy of treatments aimed at reducing the burden of risk factors.
Coronary microvascular dysfunction in the presence of myocardial diseases	This type is sustained in most instances by adverse remodeling of intramural coronary arterioles. It can be identified by invasive or noninvasive assessment of coronary flow reserve and may be severe enough to cause myocardial ischemia. It has independent prognostic value. It remains unclear whether medical treatment may reverse some cases. It is found with primary (genetic) cardiomyopathies (eg, dilated and hypertrophic) and secondary cardiomyopathies (eg, hypertensive and valvular).
Coronary microvascular dysfunction in the presence of obstructive CAD	This type may occur in the context of either stable CAD or acute coronary syndromes with or without ST-segment elevation and can be sustained by numerous factors. It is more difficult to identify than the first two types and may be identified through the use of an integrated approach that takes into account the clinical context with the use of a combination of invasive and noninvasive techniques. There is some early evidence that specific interventions might prevent it or limit the resultant ischemia.
Iatrogenic coronary microvascular dysfunction	This type occurs after coronary recanalization and seems to be caused primarily by vasoconstriction or distal embolization. It can be identified with the use of either invasive or noninvasive means on the basis of a reduced coronary flow reserve, which seems to revert spontaneously in the weeks after revascularization. Pharmacologic treatment has been shown to promptly restore coronary flow reserve, and it may also change the clinical outcome. The likelihood of distal embolization can be reduced by the use of appropriate devices during high-risk procedures.

Abbreviation: CAD, coronary artery disease.
Reproduced with permission from Camici PG, Crea F. Coronary microvascular dysfunction. *N Engl J Med*. 2007 Feb 22;356(8):830-840.

TABLE 21–9. Pathogenic Mechanisms of Coronary Microvascular Circulatory Disease

Alterations	Causes
Structural	
Luminal obstruction	Microembolization in acute coronary syndromes or after recanalization
Vascular-wall infiltration	Infiltrative heart disease (eg, Anderson–Fabry cardiomyopathy)
Vascular remodeling	Hypertrophic cardiomyopathy, arterial hypertension
Vascular rarefaction	Aortic stenosis, arterial hypertension
Perivascular fibrosis	Aortic stenosis, arterial hypertension
Functional	
Endothelial dysfunction	Smoking, hyperlipidemia, diabetes
Dysfunction of smooth muscle cell	Hypertrophic cardiomyopathy, arterial hypertension
Autonomic dysfunction	Coronary recanalization
Extravascular	
Extramural compression	Aortic stenosis, hypertrophic cardiomyopathy, arterial hypertension
Reduction in diastolic perfusion time	Aortic stenosis

Reproduced with permission from Camici PG, Crea F. Coronary microvascular dysfunction. *N Engl J Med*. 2007 Feb 22;356(8):830-840.

flow velocity response were significantly more likely to have reduced exercise tolerance compared with women with normal vascular reactivity. Treatment of patients with microvascular disease should focus on pathophysiologic mechanisms that contribute to endothelial dysfunction, with emphasis on smoking cessation, lipid and glycemic management, and blood pressure control. Conventional anti-ischemic therapy may control symptoms in some patients, but overall results are usually mixed.[163] Up to 30% of women diagnosed with microvascular circulatory disease will develop clinically evident CAD within 10 years, and women with this condition experience 5-year cardiovascular disease event rates of approximately 8%.[164] In women with non–flow-limiting epicardial CAD who experience ACS, 30-day mortality of 2% has been reported.[165] As a result of persistent variability in treatment responsiveness to β-adrenergic receptor antagonists, CCBs, ACE inhibitors, and nitrate therapy in this patient population, comprehensive longitudinal studies of novel therapies designed to characterize patient outcome are needed.

Vasospastic Angina

Vasospastic angina should be suspected in younger patients with fewer cardiovascular risk factors who present with chest pain at rest but preserved effort tolerance. Diagnosis is by detecting transient ST-segment changes during an angina attack on ambulatory ECG monitoring. Provocation test with ergonovine or acetylcholine can be done in the cardiac catheterization laboratory to document coronary spasm. CCBs and long-acting nitrates are the treatment of choice.

ACKNOWLEDGMENT

We are thankful to the authors of the previous edition of the chapters on which the current chapter is based:

Bradley A. Maron, Bernard J. Gersh, and Patrick T. O'Gara—The evaluation and management of stable ischemic heart disease.

Michael E. Farkouh, Samin K. Sharma, Matthew I. Tomey, John Puskas, and Valentin Fuster—Coronary artery bypass grafting and percutaneous interventions in stable ischemic heart disease.

SUMMARY

- Myocardial ischemia is mediated by an imbalance between oxygen supply and demand at the cardiomyocyte cellular level.

- Assessment of pretest probability of CAD aids in appropriate risk stratification of patients with suspected CCS. Among the models, the Duke, updated Diamond–Forrester, and CORSCORE risk models were most accurate in predicting CAD.

- The ischemic cascade is based on progressive mismatch between coronary blood flow and myocardial oxygen demand with increasing severity of coronary stenosis with impairment of myocardial perfusion, followed by regional diastolic dysfunction, regional systolic dysfunction, ischemic ECG changes, and finally angina pectoris.

- Since perfusion defects occur earlier than do wall motion abnormalities, tests that rely on detection of perfusion defects (such as SPECT) are more sensitive than are those that detect wall motion abnormalities (such as stress echocardiography), which are more specific for the detection of obstructive CAD.

- Coronary CTA is associated with a reduced incidence of MI driven by an increased incidence of invasive coronary angiography, revascularization, CAD diagnoses, and new prescriptions for aspirin and statins when compared with functional testing.

- Goal-directed medical therapy, the cornerstone of management of chronic CAD, consists of intensive and comprehensive secondary prevention and includes lifestyle and pharmacological approaches.

- Patients with refractory symptoms despite goal-directed medical therapy and/or elevated clinical or angiographic risk profiles and suitable coronary anatomy can benefit from revascularization with PCI or CABG surgery.

- The choice of revascularization strategy (ie, PCI vs CABG) relates to coronary artery anatomy, LV systolic function, systemic factors (eg, diabetes), and patient values and preferences.

REFERENCES

1. Virani SS, Alonso A, Benjamin EJ, et al. Heart disease and stroke statistics-2020 update: a report from the american heart association. *Circulation.* 2020;141:e139-e596.

2. Herberden W. Some account of disorder of the breast. *London: Med Trans R Coll Phys.* 1772;59-67.

3. Campeau L. Letter: grading of angina pectoris. *Circulation.* 1976;54:522-523.

4. Hemingway H, Fitzpatrick NK, Gnani S, et al. Prospective validity of measuring angina severity with Canadian Cardiovascular Society class: the acre study. *Can J Cardiol.* 2004;20:305-309.

5. Rovai D, Neglia D, Lorenzoni V, Caselli C, Knuuti J, Underwood SR, Investigators ES. Limitations of chest pain categorization models to predict coronary artery disease. *Am J Cardiol.* 2015;116:504-507.

6. Saxon JT, Chan PS, Tran AT, et al. Comparison of patient-reported vs physician-estimated angina in patients undergoing elective and urgent percutaneous coronary intervention. *JAMA Netw Open.* 2020;3:e207406.

7. Argulian E, Agarwal V, Bangalore S, et al. Meta-analysis of prognostic implications of dyspnea versus chest pain in patients referred for stress testing. *Am J Cardiol.* 2014;113:559-564.

8. Abidov A, Rozanski A, Hachamovitch R, et al. Prognostic significance of dyspnea in patients referred for cardiac stress testing. *N Engl J Med.* 2005;353:1889-1898.

9. Mackay MH, Ratner PA, Johnson JL, Humphries KH, Buller CE. Gender differences in symptoms of myocardial ischaemia. *Eur Heart J.* 2011;32:3107-3114.

10. Kreatsoulas C, Shannon HS, Giacomini M, Velianou JL, Anand SS. Reconstructing angina: cardiac symptoms are the same in women and men. *JAMA Intern Med.* 2013;173:829-831.

11. Fihn SD, Gardin JM, Abrams J, et al. 2012 ACCF/AHA/ACP/AATS/PCNA/SCAI/STS guideline for the diagnosis and management of patients with stable ischemic heart disease: a report of the American College of Cardiology Foundation/American Heart Association Task Force on practice guidelines, and the American College of Physicians, American Association for Thoracic Surgery, Preventive Cardiovascular Nurses Association, Society for Cardiovascular Angiography and Interventions, and Society of Thoracic Surgeons. *J Am Coll Cardiol.* 2012;60:e44-e164.

12. Cohn PF, Fox KM, Daly C. Silent myocardial ischemia. *Circulation.* 2003;108:1263-1277.

13. Deedwania PC, Carbajal EV. Silent myocardial ischemia. A clinical perspective. *Arch Intern Med.* 1991;151:2373-2382.

14. Zucchelli P, Sturani A, Zuccala A, Santoro A, Degli Esposti E, Chiarini C. Dysfunction of the autonomic nervous system in patients with end-stage renal failure. *Contrib Nephrol.* 1985;45:69-81.

15. Bokhari SRA, Inayat F, Jawa A, et al. Cardiovascular autonomic neuropathy and its association with cardiovascular and all-cause mortality in patients with end-stage renal disease. *Cureus.* 2018;10:e3243.

16. Hage FG, Lusa L, Dondi M, Giubbini R, Iskandrian AE, Investigators ID. Exercise stress tests for detecting myocardial ischemia in asymptomatic patients with diabetes mellitus. *Am J Cardiol.* 2013;112:14-20.

17. Diamond GA, Forrester JS. Analysis of probability as an aid in the clinical diagnosis of coronary-artery disease. *N Engl J Med.* 1979;300:1350-1358.

18. Genders TS, Steyerberg EW, Alkadhi H, et al. A clinical prediction rule for the diagnosis of coronary artery disease: validation, updating, and extension. *Eur Heart J.* 2011;32:1316-1330.

19. Cheng VY, Berman DS, Rozanski A, et al. Performance of the traditional age, sex, and angina typicality-based approach for estimating pretest probability of angiographically significant coronary artery disease in patients undergoing coronary computed tomographic angiography: results from the multinational coronary CT angiography evaluation for clinical outcomes: an international multicenter registry (confirm). *Circulation.* 2011;124:2423-2432, 2421-2428.

20. Shaw LJ, Bairey Merz CN, et al. Insights from the NHLBI-sponsored women's ischemia syndrome evaluation (wise) study: Part i: gender differences in traditional and novel risk factors, symptom evaluation, and gender-optimized diagnostic strategies. *J Am Coll Cardiol.* 2006;47:S4-S20.

21. Fordyce CB, Douglas PS, Roberts RS, et al. Identification of patients with stable chest pain deriving minimal value from noninvasive testing: the promise minimal-risk tool, a secondary analysis of a randomized clinical trial. *JAMA Cardiol.* 2017;2:400-408.

22. Jensen JM, Voss M, Hansen VB, et al. Risk stratification of patients suspected of coronary artery disease: comparison of five different models. *Atherosclerosis.* 2012;220:557-562.

23. Douglas PS, Hoffmann U, Patel MR, et al. Outcomes of anatomical versus functional testing for coronary artery disease. *N Engl J Med.* 2015;372:1291-1300.

24. Investigators S-H, Newby DE, Adamson PD, et al. Coronary CT angiography and 5-year risk of myocardial infarction. *N Engl J Med.* 2018;379:924-933.

25. Foy AJ, Dhruva SS, Peterson B, Mandrola JM, Morgan DJ, Redberg RF. Coronary computed tomography angiography vs functional stress testing for patients with suspected coronary artery disease: a systematic review and meta-analysis. *JAMA Intern Med.* 2017;177:1623-1631.

26. Chest pain of recent onset: assessment and diagnosis (2010 updated 2016) Nice guideline cg95. 2020.

27. Knuuti J, Wijns W, Saraste A, et al. 2019 ESC guidelines for the diagnosis and management of chronic coronary syndromes. *Eur Heart J.* 2020;41:407-477.

28. Greenland P, Bonow RO, Brundage BH, et al. ACCF/AHA 2007 clinical expert consensus document on coronary artery calcium scoring by computed tomography in global cardiovascular risk assessment and in evaluation of patients with chest pain: a report of the American College of Cardiology Foundation clinical expert consensus task force (ACCF/AHA writing committee to update the 2000 expert consensus document on electron beam computed tomography). *Circulation.* 2007;115:402-426.

29. Shaw LJ, Giambrone AE, Blaha MJ, et al. Long-term prognosis after coronary artery calcification testing in asymptomatic patients: a cohort study. *Ann Intern Med.* 2015;163:14-21.

30. Shaw LJ, Raggi P, Berman DS, Callister TQ. Coronary artery calcium as a measure of biologic age. *Atherosclerosis.* 2006;188:112-119.

31. Budoff MJ, Lane KL, Bakhsheshi H, et al. Rates of progression of coronary calcium by electron beam tomography. *Am J Cardiol.* 2000;86:8-11.

32. Ikegami Y, Inoue I, Inoue K, et al. The annual rate of coronary artery calcification with combination therapy with a pcsk9 inhibitor and a statin is lower than that with statin monotherapy. *NPJ Aging Mech Dis.* 2018;4:7.

33. Mittal TK, Pottle A, Nicol E, et al. Prevalence of obstructive coronary artery disease and prognosis in patients with stable symptoms and a zero-coronary calcium score. *Eur Heart J Cardiovasc Imaging.* 2017;18:922-929.

34. Blaha MJ, Cainzos-Achirica M, Greenland P, et al. Role of coronary artery calcium score of zero and other negative risk markers for cardiovascular disease: the multi-ethnic study of atherosclerosis (MESA). *Circulation.* 2016;133:849-858.

35. Mitchell JD, Fergestrom N, Gage BF, et al. Impact of statins on cardiovascular outcomes following coronary artery calcium scoring. *J Am Coll Cardiol.* 2018;72:3233-3242.

36. Uretsky S, Rozanski A, Singh P, et al. The presence, characterization and prognosis of coronary plaques among patients with zero coronary calcium scores. *Int J Cardiovasc Imaging.* 2011;27:805-812.

37. Celeng C, Leiner T, Maurovich-Horvat P, et al. Anatomical and functional computed tomography for diagnosing hemodynamically significant coronary artery disease: a meta-analysis. *JACC Cardiovasc Imaging.* 2019;12:1316-1325.

38. Sandvik L, Erikssen J, Ellestad M, et al. Heart rate increase and maximal heart rate during exercise as predictors of cardiovascular mortality: a 16-year follow-up study of 1960 healthy men. *Coronary Artery Dis.* 1995;6:667-679.

39. Lauer MS, Okin PM, Larson MG, Evans JC, Levy D. Impaired heart rate response to graded exercise. Prognostic implications of chronotropic incompetence in the framingham heart study. *Circulation.* 1996;93:1520-1526.

40. Cole CR, Blackstone EH, Pashkow FJ, Snader CE, Lauer MS. Heart-rate recovery immediately after exercise as a predictor of mortality. *N Engl J Med.* 1999;341:1351-1357.

41. Mark DB, Shaw L, Harrell FE Jr. et al. Prognostic value of a treadmill exercise score in outpatients with suspected coronary artery disease. *N Engl J Med.* 1991;325:849-853.

42. Picano E, Molinaro S, Pasanisi E. The diagnostic accuracy of pharmacological stress echocardiography for the assessment of coronary artery disease: a meta-analysis. *Cardiovasc Ultrasound.* 2008;6:30.

43. Fleischmann KE, Hunink MG, Kuntz KM, Douglas PS. Exercise echocardiography or exercise spect imaging? A meta-analysis of diagnostic test performance. *JAMA.* 1998;280:913-920.

44. Bangalore S, Gopinath D, Yao S-S, Chaudhry FA. Risk stratification using stress echocardiography: incremental prognostic value over historic, clinical, and stress electrocardiographic variables across a wide spectrum of bayesian pretest probabilities for coronary artery disease. *J Am Soc Echocardiogr.* 2007;20:244-252.

45. Bangalore S, Yao SS, Chaudhry FA. Usefulness of stress echocardiography for risk stratification and prognosis of patients with left ventricular hypertrophy. *Am J Cardiol.* 2007;100:536-543.

46. Bangalore S, Yao SS, Puthumana J, Chaudhry FA. Incremental prognostic value of stress echocardiography over clinical and stress electrocardiographic variables in patients with prior myocardial infarction: "Warranty time" of a normal stress echocardiogram. *Echocardiogr-J Cardiovasc Ultrasound Allied Techniq.* 2006;23:455-464.

47. Bangalore S, Yao S-S, Chaudhry FA. Role of right ventricular wall motion abnormalities in risk stratification and prognosis of patients referred for stress echocardiography. *J Am Coll Cardiol.* 2007;50:1981-1989.

48. Bangalore S, Yao S-S, Chaudhry FA. Role of left atrial size in risk stratification and prognosis of patients undergoing stress echocardiography. *J Am Coll Cardiol.* 2007;50:1254-1262.

49. Bangalore S, Yao S-S, Chaudhry FA. Prediction of myocardial infarction versus cardiac death by stress echocardiography. *J Am Soc Echocardiogr.* 2009;22:261-267.

50. Yao S-S, Shah A, Bangalore S, Chaudhry FA. Transient ischemic left ventricular cavity dilation is a significant predictor of severe and extensive coronary artery disease and adverse outcome in patients undergoing stress echocardiography. *J Am Soc Echocardiogr.* 2007;20:352-358.

51. Abidov A, Bax JJ, Hayes SW, et al. Transient ischemic dilation ratio of the left ventricle is a significant predictor of future cardiac events in patients with otherwise normal myocardial perfusion spect. *J Am Coll Cardiol.* 2003;42:1818-1825.

52. Hachamovitch R, Berman DS, Kiat H, et al. Exercise myocardial perfusion spect in patients without known coronary artery disease: Incremental prognostic value and use in risk stratification. *Circulation.* 1996;93:905-914.

53. Abidov A, Bax JJ, Hayes SW, et al. Integration of automatically measured transient ischemic dilation ratio into interpretation of adenosine stress myocardial perfusion spect for detection of severe and extensive cad. *J Nucl Med.* 2004;45:1999-2007.

54. Weiss AT, Berman DS, Lew AS, et al. Transient ischemic dilation of the left ventricle on stress thallium-201 scintigraphy: a marker of severe and extensive coronary artery disease. *J Am Coll Cardiol.* 1987;9:752-759.

55. Bacher-Stier C, Sharir T, Kavanagh PB, et al. Postexercise lung uptake of 99mtc-sestamibi determined by a new automatic technique: validation and application in detection of severe and extensive coronary artery disease and reduced left ventricular function. *J Nucl Med.* 2000;41:1190-1197.

56. Hachamovitch R, Berman DS, Kiat H, Cohen I, Friedman JD, Shaw LJ. Value of stress myocardial perfusion single photon emission computed tomography in patients with normal resting electrocardiograms: an evaluation of incremental prognostic value and cost-effectiveness. *Circulation.* 2002;105:823-829.

57. Hachamovitch R, Berman DS, Kiat H, et al. Incremental prognostic value of adenosine stress myocardial perfusion single-photon emission computed tomography and impact on subsequent management in

patients with or suspected of having myocardial ischemia. *Am J Cardiol.* 1997;80:426-433.

58. Hachamovitch R, Berman DS, Shaw LJ, et al. Incremental prognostic value of myocardial perfusion single photon emission computed tomography for the prediction of cardiac death: differential stratification for risk of cardiac death and myocardial infarction. *Circulation.* 1998;97:535-543.

59. Kang X, Berman DS, Lewin HC, et al. Incremental prognostic value of myocardial perfusion single photon emission computed tomography in patients with diabetes mellitus. *Am Heart J.* 1999;138:1025-1032.

60. Danad I, Raijmakers PG, Driessen RS, et al. Comparison of coronary ct angiography, spect, pet, and hybrid imaging for diagnosis of ischemic heart disease determined by fractional flow reserve. *JAMA Cardiol.* 2017;2:1100-1107.

61. Harnett DT, Hazra S, Maze R, et al. Clinical performance of rb-82 myocardial perfusion pet and tc-99m-based spect in patients with extreme obesity. *J Nuclear Cardiol.* 2019;26:275-283.

62. Nandalur KR, Dwamena BA, Choudhri AF, Nandalur MR, Carlos RC. Diagnostic performance of stress cardiac magnetic resonance imaging in the detection of coronary artery disease: a meta-analysis. *J Am Coll Cardiol.* 2007;50:1343-1353.

63. Gibbons RJ, Abrams J, Chatterjee K, et al. ACC/AHA 2002 guideline update for the management of patients with chronic stable angina–summary article: a report of the American College of Cardiology/American Heart Association Task Force on practice guidelines (committee on the management of patients with chronic stable angina). *J Am Coll Cardiol.* 2003;41:159-168.

64. Patel MR, Peterson ED, Dai D, et al. Low diagnostic yield of elective coronary angiography. *N Engl J Med.* 2010;362:886-895.

65. Anderson L, Oldridge N, Thompson DR, et al. Exercise-based cardiac rehabilitation for coronary heart disease: Cochrane systematic review and meta-analysis. *J Am Coll Cardiol.* 2016;67:1-12.

66. Bangalore S, Fayyad R, Laskey R, DeMicco DA, Messerli FH, Waters DD. Body-weight fluctuations and outcomes in coronary disease. *N Engl J Med.* 2017;376:1332-1340.

67. Hoen PW, Whooley MA, Martens EJ, Na B, van Melle JP, de Jonge P. Differential associations between specific depressive symptoms and cardiovascular prognosis in patients with stable coronary heart disease. *J Am Coll Cardiol.* 2010;56:838-844.

68. van Melle JP, de Jonge P, Spijkerman TA, et al. Prognostic association of depression following myocardial infarction with mortality and cardiovascular events: a meta-analysis. *Psychosom Med.* 2004;66:814-822.

69. Goldstein CM, Gathright EC, Garcia S. Relationship between depression and medication adherence in cardiovascular disease: the perfect challenge for the integrated care team. *Patient Prefer Adherence.* 2017;11:547-559.

70. Bangalore S, Shah R, Gao X, et al. Economic burden associated with inadequate antidepressant medication management among patients with depression and known cardiovascular diseases: insights from a united states-based retrospective claims database analysis. *J Med Econ.* 2020;23:262-270.

71. Bangalore S, Shah R, Pappadopulos E, et al. Cardiovascular hazards of insufficient treatment of depression among patients with known cardiovascular disease: a propensity score adjusted analysis. *Eur Heart J Qual Care Clin Outcomes.* 2018;4:258-266.

72. Kim JM, Stewart R, Lee YS, et al. Effect of escitalopram vs placebo treatment for depression on long-term cardiac outcomes in patients with acute coronary syndrome: a randomized clinical trial. *JAMA.* 2018;320:350-358.

73. DeFilippis EM, Bajaj NS, Singh A, et al. Marijuana use in patients with cardiovascular disease: Jacc review topic of the week. *J Am Coll Cardiol.* 2020;75:320-332.

74. Antithrombotic Trialists C, Baigent C, et al. Aspirin in the primary and secondary prevention of vascular disease: collaborative meta-analysis of individual participant data from randomised trials. *Lancet.* 2009;373:1849-1860.

75. Mauri L, Kereiakes DJ, Yeh RW, et al. Twelve or 30 months of dual antiplatelet therapy after drug-eluting stents. *N Eng J Med.* 2014;371:2155-2166.

76. Bonaca MP, Bhatt DL, Cohen M, et al. Long-term use of ticagrelor in patients with prior myocardial infarction. *N Eng J Med.* 2015;372:1791-1800.

77. Kuno T, Ueyama H, Takagi H, Bangalore S. P2y12 inhibitor monotherapy versus aspirin monotherapy after short-term dual antiplatelet therapy for percutaneous coronary intervention: insights from a network meta-analysis of randomized trials. *Am Heart J.* 2020;227:82-90.

78. Levine GN, Bates ER, Bittl JA, et al. 2016 acc/aha guideline focused update on duration of dual antiplatelet therapy in patients with coronary artery disease: a report of the American College of Cardiology/American Heart Association Task Force on clinical practice guidelines. *J Am Coll Cardiol.* 2016;68:1082-1115.

79. Mehran R, Baber U, Sharma SK, et al. Ticagrelor with or without aspirin in high-risk patients after PCI. *N Eng J Med.* 2019;381:2032-2042.

80. Morrow DA, Braunwald E, Bonaca MP, et al. Vorapaxar in the secondary prevention of atherothrombotic events. *N Eng J Med.* 2012;366:1404-1413.

81. Eikelboom JW, Connolly SJ, Bosch J, et al. Rivaroxaban with or without aspirin in stable cardiovascular disease. *N Eng J Med.* 2017;10.1056/NEJMoa1709118.

82. Khan SU, Khan MZ, Asad ZUA, et al. Efficacy and safety of low dose rivaroxaban in patients with coronary heart disease: a systematic review and meta-analysis. *J Thromb Thrombolysis.* 2020;10.1007/s11239-020-02114-7.

83. Lopes RD, Hong H, Harskamp RE, et al. Safety and efficacy of antithrombotic strategies in patients with atrial fibrillation undergoing percutaneous coronary intervention: a network meta-analysis of randomized controlled trials. *JAMA Cardiol.* 2019;4:747-755.

84. Angiolillo DJ, Goodman SG, Bhatt DL, et al. Antithrombotic therapy in patients with atrial fibrillation treated with oral anticoagulation undergoing percutaneous coronary intervention: a North American perspective-2018 update. *Circulation.* 2018;138:527-536.

85. Cholesterol Treatment Trialists C, Baigent C, Blackwell L, et al. Efficacy and safety of more intensive lowering of ldl cholesterol: a meta-analysis of data from 170,000 participants in 26 randomised trials. *Lancet.* 2010;376:1670-1681.

86. LaRosa JC, Grundy SM, Waters DD, et al. Intensive lipid lowering with atorvastatin in patients with stable coronary disease. *N Eng J Med.* 2005;352:1425-1435.

87. Cannon CP, Blazing MA, Giugliano RP, et al. Ezetimibe added to statin therapy after acute coronary syndromes. *N Eng J Med.* 2015;372:2387-2397.

88. Sabatine MS, Giugliano RP, Keech AC, et al. Evolocumab and clinical outcomes in patients with cardiovascular disease. *N Eng J Med.* 2017;376:1713-1722.

89. Grundy SM, Stone NJ, Bailey AL, et al. 2018 AHA/ACC/AACVPR/AAPA/ABC/ACPM/ADA/AGS/APHA/ASPC/NLA/PCNA guideline on the management of blood cholesterol: a report of the American College of Cardiology/American Heart Association Task Force on clinical practice guidelines. *J Am Coll Cardiol.* 2019;73:e285-e350.

90. Freemantle N, Cleland J, Young P, Mason J, Harrison J. Beta blockade after myocardial infarction: systematic review and meta regression analysis. *BMJ.* 1999;318:1730-1737.

91. Bangalore S, Steg G, Deedwania P, et al. Beta-blocker use and clinical outcomes in stable outpatients with and without coronary artery disease. *JAMA.* 2012;308:1340-1349.

92. Motivala AA, Parikh V, Roe M, Dai D, Abbott JD, Prasad A, Mukherjee D. Predictors, trends, and outcomes (among older patients >/=65 years of age) associated with beta-blocker use in patients with stable angina undergoing elective percutaneous coronary intervention: insights from the NCDR registry. *JACC Cardiovasc Interv.* 2016;9:1639-1648.

93. Zhang H, Yuan X, Zhang H, et al. Efficacy of long-term beta-blocker therapy for secondary prevention of long-term outcomes after coronary artery bypass grafting surgery. *Circulation.* 2015;131:2194-2201.

94. Booij HG, Damman K, Warnica JW, Rouleau JL, van Gilst WH, Westenbrink BD. Beta-blocker therapy is not associated with reductions in angina or cardiovascular events after coronary artery bypass graft surgery: insights from the imagine trial. *Cardiovasc Drugs Ther.* 2015;29:277-285.

95. Waysbort J, Meshulam N, Brunner D. Isosorbide-5-mononitrate and atenolol in the treatment of stable exertional angina. *Cardiology* 1991;79 Suppl 2:19-26.

96. Heidenreich PA, McDonald KM, Hastie T, et al. Meta-analysis of trials comparing beta-blockers, calcium antagonists, and nitrates for stable angina. *JAMA.* 1999;281:1927-1936.

97. Yusuf S, Sleight P, Pogue J, Bosch J, Davies R, Dagenais G. Effects of an angiotensin-converting-enzyme inhibitor, ramipril, on cardiovascular events in high-risk patients. The heart outcomes prevention evaluation study investigators. *N Eng J Med.* 2000;342:145-153.

98. Fox KM, Investigators EUtOrocewPiscAd. Efficacy of perindopril in reduction of cardiovascular events among patients with stable coronary artery disease: randomised, double-blind, placebo-controlled, multicentre trial (the Europa study). *Lancet.* 2003;362:782-788.

99. Braunwald E, Domanski MJ, Fowler SE, et al. Angiotensin-converting-enzyme inhibition in stable coronary artery disease. *N Eng J Med.* 2004;351:2058-2068.

100. Bangalore S, Fakheri R, Wandel S, Toklu B, Wandel J, Messerli FH. Renin angiotensin system inhibitors for patients with stable coronary artery disease without heart failure: systematic review and meta-analysis of randomized trials. *BMJ.* 2017;356:j4.

101. Makani H, Bangalore S, Desouza KA, Shah A, Messerli FH. Efficacy and safety of dual blockade of the renin-angiotensin system: meta-analysis of randomised trials. *BMJ.* 2013;346:f360.

102. Pitt B, Remme W, Zannad F, et al. Eplerenone, a selective aldosterone blocker, in patients with left ventricular dysfunction after myocardial infarction. *N Eng J Med.* 2003;348:1309-1321.

103. Zannad F, McMurray JJ, Krum H, et al. Eplerenone in patients with systolic heart failure and mild symptoms. *N Eng J Med.* 2010;10.1056/NEJMoa1009492.

104. O'Gara PT, Kushner FG, Ascheim DD, et al. 2013 accf/aha guideline for the management of st-elevation myocardial infarction: a report of the American College of Cardiology Foundation/American Heart Association Task Force on practice guidelines. *Circulation.* 2013;127:e362-e425.

105. Wei J, Wu T, Yang Q, Chen M, Ni J, Huang D. Nitrates for stable angina: a systematic review and meta-analysis of randomized clinical trials. *Int J Cardiol.* 2011;146:4-12.

106. Chaitman BR, Skettino SL, Parker JO, et al. Anti-ischemic effects and long-term survival during ranolazine monotherapy in patients with chronic severe angina. *J Am Coll Cardiol.* 2004;43:1375-1382.

107. Chaitman BR, Pepine CJ, Parker JO, et al. Effects of ranolazine with atenolol, amlodipine, or diltiazem on exercise tolerance and angina frequency in patients with severe chronic angina: a randomized controlled trial. *JAMA.* 2004;291:309-316.

108. Banon D, Filion KB, Budlovsky T, Franck C, Eisenberg MJ. The usefulness of ranolazine for the treatment of refractory chronic stable angina pectoris as determined from a systematic review of randomized controlled trials. *Am J Cardiol.* 2014;113:1075-1082.

109. Koren MJ, Crager MR, Sweeney M. Long-term safety of a novel antianginal agent in patients with severe chronic stable angina: the ranolazine open label experience (role). *J Am Coll Cardiol.* 2007;49:1027-1034.

110. Udell JA, Zawi R, Bhatt DL, et al. Association between influenza vaccination and cardiovascular outcomes in high-risk patients: a meta-analysis. *JAMA.* 2013;310:1711-1720.

111. Marra F, Zhang A, Gillman E, Bessai K, Parhar K, Vadlamudi NK. The protective effect of pneumococcal vaccination on cardiovascular disease in adults: a systematic review and meta-analysis. *Int J Infect Dis.* 2020;99:204-213.

112. Boden WE, O'Rourke RA, Teo KK, et al. Optimal medical therapy with or without PCI for stable coronary disease. *N Eng J Med.* 2007;356:1503-1516.

113. Weintraub WS, Spertus JA, Kolm P, et al. Effect of PCI on quality of life in patients with stable coronary disease. *N Eng J Med.* 2008;359:677-687.

114. Sedlis SP, Hartigan PM, Teo KK, et al. Effect of PCI on long-term survival in patients with stable ischemic heart disease. *N Eng J Med.* 2015;373:1937-1946.

115. Frye RL, August P, Brooks MM, et al. A randomized trial of therapies for type 2 diabetes and coronary artery disease. *N Eng J Med.* 2009;360:2503-2515.

116. Dagenais GR, Lu J, Faxon DP, et al. Effects of optimal medical treatment with or without coronary revascularization on angina and subsequent revascularizations in patients with type 2 diabetes mellitus and stable ischemic heart disease. *Circulation.* 2011;123:1492-1500.

117. De Bruyne B, Pijls NH, Kalesan B, et al. Fractional flow reserve-guided PCI versus medical therapy in stable coronary disease. *N Eng J Med.* 2012;367:991-1001.

118. Xaplanteris P, Fournier S, Pijls NHJ, et al. Five-year outcomes with PCI guided by fractional flow reserve. *N Eng J Med.* 2018;379:250-259.

119. Maron DJ, Hochman JS, Reynolds HR, et al. Initial invasive or conservative strategy for stable coronary disease. *N Eng J Med.* 2020;382:1395-1407.

120. Spertus JA, Jones PG, Maron DJ, et al. Health-status outcomes with invasive or conservative care in coronary disease. *N Eng J Med.* 2020;382:1408-1419.

121. Bangalore S, Maron DJ, O'Brien SM, et al. Management of coronary disease in patients with advanced kidney disease. *N Eng J Med.* 2020;382:1608-1618.

122. Spertus JA, Jones PG, Maron DJ, et al. Health status after invasive or conservative care in coronary and advanced kidney disease. *N Eng J Med.* 2020;382:1619-1628.

123. Bangalore S, Maron DJ, Stone GW, Hochman JS. Routine revascularization versus initial medical therapy for stable ischemic heart disease: a systematic review and meta-analysis of randomized trials. *Circulation.* 2020;142:841-857.

124. Velazquez EJ, Lee KL, Deja MA, et al. Coronary-artery bypass surgery in patients with left ventricular dysfunction. *N Eng J Med.* 2011;364:1607-1616.

125. Velazquez EJ, Lee KL, Jones RH, et al. Coronary-artery bypass surgery in patients with ischemic cardiomyopathy. *N Eng J Med.* 2016;374:1511-1520.

126. Comparison of coronary bypass surgery with angioplasty in patients with multivessel disease. The bypass angioplasty revascularization investigation (BARI) investigators. *N Eng J Med.* 1996;335:217-225.

127. Serruys PW, Morice MC, Kappetein AP, et al. Percutaneous coronary intervention versus coronary-artery bypass grafting for severe coronary artery disease. *N Eng J Med.* 2009;360:961-972.

128. Capodanno D, Capranzano P, Di Salvo ME, et al. Usefulness of syntax score to select patients with left main coronary artery disease to be treated with coronary artery bypass graft. *JACC Cardiovasc Interv.* 2009;2:731-738.

129. Mohr FW, Morice MC, Kappetein AP, et al. Coronary artery bypass graft surgery versus percutaneous coronary intervention in patients with three-vessel disease and left main coronary disease: 5-year follow-up of the randomised, clinical syntax trial. *Lancet.* 2013;381:629-638.

130. Thuijs D, Kappetein AP, Serruys PW, et al. Percutaneous coronary intervention versus coronary artery bypass grafting in patients with three-vessel or left main coronary artery disease: 10-year follow-up of the multicentre randomised controlled syntax trial. *Lancet.* 2019;394:1325-1334.

131. Ahn JM, Roh JH, Kim YH, et al. Randomized trial of stents versus bypass surgery for left main coronary artery disease: 5-year outcomes of the precombat study. *J Am Coll Cardiol.* 2015;65:2198-2206.

132. Park DW, Ahn JM, Park H, et al. Ten-year outcomes after drug-eluting stents versus coronary artery bypass grafting for left main coronary disease: extended follow-up of the precombat trial. *Circulation.* 2020;141:1437-1446.

133. Makikallio T, Holm NR, Lindsay M, et al. Percutaneous coronary angioplasty versus coronary artery bypass grafting in treatment of unprotected left main stenosis (noble): a prospective, randomised, open-label, non-inferiority trial. *Lancet.* 2016;388:2743-2752.

134. Holm NR, Makikallio T, Lindsay MM, et al. Percutaneous coronary angioplasty versus coronary artery bypass grafting in the treatment of unprotected left main stenosis: Updated 5-year outcomes from the randomised, non-inferiority noble trial. *Lancet.* 2020;395:191-199.

135. Stone GW, Sabik JF, Serruys PW, et al. Everolimus-eluting stents or bypass surgery for left main coronary artery disease. *N Eng J Med.* 2016;375:2223-2235.

136. Stone GW, Kappetein AP, Sabik JF, et al. Five-year outcomes after PCI or CABG for left main coronary disease. *N Eng J Med.* 2019;381:1820-1830.

137. Kuno T, Ueyama H, Rao SV, et al. Percutaneous coronary intervention or coronary artery bypass graft surgery for left main coronary artery disease: a meta-analysis of randomized trials. *Am Heart J.* 2020;227:9-10.

138. Farkouh ME, Domanski M, Sleeper LA, et al. Strategies for multivessel revascularization in patients with diabetes. *N Eng J Med.* 2012;367:2375-2384.

139. Farkouh ME, Domanski M, Dangas GD, et al. Long-term survival following multivessel revascularization in patients with diabetes: the freedom follow-on study. *J Am Coll Cardiol.* 2019;73:629-638.

140. Kaul U, Bangalore S, Seth A, et al. Paclitaxel-eluting versus everolimus-eluting coronary stents in diabetes. *N Engl J Med.* 2015;373:1709-1719.

141. Bangalore S, Toklu B, Amoroso N, et al. Bare metal stents, durable polymer drug eluting stents, and biodegradable polymer drug eluting stents for coronary artery disease: mixed treatment comparison meta-analysis. *BMJ.* 2013;347:f6625.

142. Bangalore S, Toklu B, Feit F. Outcomes with coronary artery bypass graft surgery versus percutaneous coronary intervention for patients with diabetes mellitus: can newer generation drug-eluting stents bridge the gap? *Circ Cardiovasc Interv.* 2014;7:518-525.

143. Bangalore S, Guo Y, Samadashvili Z, Blecker S, Xu J, Hannan EL. Everolimus eluting stents versus coronary artery bypass graft surgery for patients with diabetes mellitus and multivessel disease. *Circ Cardiovasc Interv.* 2015;8:e002626.

144. Bangalore S, Bhatt DL. Do we need a trial of DES versus CABG surgery in diabetic patients with ACS? *J Am Coll Cardiol.* 2017;70:3007-3009.

145. Bangalore S, Zenati MA. The "fragility" of mortality benefit of coronary artery bypass graft surgery in diabetics. *J Am Coll Cardiol.* 2019;73:639-642.

146. Bangalore S, Guo Y, Samadashvili Z, Blecker S, Hannan EL. Revascularization in patients with multivessel coronary artery disease and severe left ventricular systolic dysfunction: everolimus-eluting stents versus coronary artery bypass graft surgery. *Circulation.* 2016;133:2132-2140.

147. Gibbons RJ, Abrams J, Chatterjee K, et al. ACC/AHA 2002 guideline update for the management of patients with chronic stable angina–summary article: a report of the American College of Cardiology/American Heart Association Task Force on practice guidelines (committee on the management of patients with chronic stable angina). *J Am Coll Cardiol.* 2003;41:159-168.

148. Mannheimer C, Eliasson T, Augustinsson LE, et al. Electrical stimulation versus coronary artery bypass surgery in severe angina pectoris: the ESBY study. *Circulation.* 1998;97:1157-1163.

149. Eldabe S, Thomson S, Duarte R, et al. The effectiveness and cost-effectiveness of spinal cord stimulation for refractory angina (rascal study): a pilot randomized controlled trial. *Neuromodulation.* 2016;19:60-70.

150. Eckert S, Horstkotte D. Management of angina pectoris: the role of spinal cord stimulation. *Am J Cardiovasc Drugs: Drugs Devices Other Intervent.* 2009;9:17-28.

151. Lawson WE, Hui JC, Cohn PF. Long-term prognosis of patients with angina treated with enhanced external counterpulsation: five-year follow-up study. *Clin Cardiol.* 2000;23:254-258.

152. Stys TP, Lawson WE, Hui JC, et al. Effects of enhanced external counterpulsation on stress radionuclide coronary perfusion and exercise capacity in chronic stable angina pectoris. *Am J Cardiol.* 2002;89:822-824.

153. Manchanda A, Soran O. Enhanced external counterpulsation and future directions: step beyond medical management for patients with angina and heart failure. *J Am Coll Cardiol.* 2007;50:1523-1531.

154. Verheye S, Jolicoeur EM, Behan MW, et al. Efficacy of a device to narrow the coronary sinus in refractory angina. *N Eng J Med.* 2015;372:519-527.

155. Mehta S, Johnson RJ, Schofield PF. Staging of colorectal cancer. *Clin Radiol.* 1994;49:515-523.

156. Leon MB, Kornowski R, Downey WE, et al. A blinded, randomized, placebo-controlled trial of percutaneous laser myocardial revascularization to improve angina symptoms in patients with severe coronary disease. *J Am Coll Cardiol.* 2005;46:1812-1819.

157. Frazier OH, March RJ, Horvath KA. Transmyocardial revascularization with a carbon dioxide laser in patients with end-stage coronary artery disease. *N Eng J Med.* 1999;341:1021-1028.

158. Lamas GA, Goertz C, Boineau R, et al. Effect of disodium edta chelation regimen on cardiovascular events in patients with previous myocardial infarction: the tact randomized trial. *JAMA* 2013;309:1241-1250.

159. Camici PG, Crea F. Coronary microvascular dysfunction. *N Eng J Med.* 2007;356:830-840.

160. Lupi A, Buffon A, Finocchiaro ML, Conti E, Maseri A, Crea F. Mechanisms of adenosine-induced epicardial coronary artery dilatation. *Eur Heart J.* 1997;18:614-617.

161. Marinescu MA, Loffler AI, Ouellette M, Smith L, Kramer CM, Bourque JM. Coronary microvascular dysfunction, microvascular angina, and treatment strategies. *JACC Cardiovasc Imaging.* 2015;8:210-220.

162. Handberg E, Johnson BD, Arant CB, et al. Impaired coronary vascular reactivity and functional capacity in women: Results from the NHLBI women's ischemia syndrome evaluation (WISE) study. *J Am Coll Cardiol.* 2006;47:S44-S49.

163. Kaski JC, Rosano GM, Collins P, Nihoyannopoulos P, Maseri A, Poole-Wilson PA. Cardiac syndrome x: clinical characteristics and left ventricular function. Long-term follow-up study. *J Am Coll Cardiol.* 1995;25:807-814.

164. Gulati M, Cooper-DeHoff RM, McClure C, et al. Adverse cardiovascular outcomes in women with nonobstructive coronary artery disease: a report from the women's ischemia syndrome evaluation study and the St James women take heart project. *Arch Intern Med.* 2009;169:843-850.

165. Diver DJ, Bier JD, Ferreira PE, et al. Clinical and arteriographic characterization of patients with unstable angina without critical coronary arterial narrowing (from the timi-iiia trial). *Am J Cardiol.* 1994;74:531-537.

22

Cardiac Rehabilitation
Current Practice and Future Directions

Alan Rozanski, Saman Setareh-Shenas, and Jagat Narula

Cardiac rehabilitation—a multidisciplinary secondary disease prevention program

The five core competencies

Risk factor
management

Aerobic and
resistance
exercises

Patient
education

Psychosocial
interventions

Dietary
counseling

Indications for cardiac rehabilitation

- Following myocardial infarction
- Following CABG or PCI
- Following valve replacement or repair
- Following cardiac transplantation
- Stable angina pectoris
- Peripheral vascular disease
- Heart failure with reduced ejection fraction

Evidence-based medical benefits

Improved clinical outcomes:	Psychosocial benefits:
↓ cardiac death and myocardial infarction	↑ quality of life
↓ all-cause mortality	↓ depressive symptoms
↓ hospitalizations and costs	↓ anxiety symptoms

Current goals and challenges

- Increase referral, enrollment, and adherence
- Increase affordability
- Expand eligibility (eg, older deconditioned adults with evidence of coronary artery disease)
- Develop home-based programs and hybrid programs that provide a combination of center-based and home-based supervision

Chapter 22 Fuster and Hurst's Central Illustration. Cardiac rehabilitation has evolved into a multidimensional secondary prevention program that includes five core competencies and has proven benefits. It usually consists of 36 sessions delivered as 2 to 3 sessions per week over 12 to 18 weeks. Limited insurance coverage currently hinders the use of home-based programs in the United States. Since both center-based and home-based cardiac rehabilitation programs have advantages, hybrid programs may be used in the future. CABG, coronary artery bypass graft; PCI, percutaneous coronary intervention.

CHAPTER SUMMARY

This chapter discusses the indications for referral, evidence-based benefits, utility in specific populations, barriers to participation, and evolving trends in cardiac rehabilitation. Cardiac rehabilitation has evolved into a multidimensional, secondary prevention program that includes five core competencies: exercise training, patient education, dietary counseling, psychosocial interventions, and risk factor modification (see Fuster and Hurst's Central Illustration). Cardiac rehabilitation usually consists of 36 sessions, delivered as 2 to 3 sessions per week over 12 to 18 weeks, and it is indicated for patients following acute myocardial infarction (MI), coronary artery bypass graft surgery, percutaneous coronary intervention (PCI), valvular repair or replacement, and cardiac transplantation, and for patients with chronic angina, peripheral vascular disease, and heart failure. Cardiac rehabilitation is associated with a reduced risk of death, cardiac death, MI, and hospitalization, as well as lower medical costs. In addition, it leads to improved quality of life and reduced depression and anxiety symptoms. Despite these benefits, current referral and enrollment in cardiac rehabilitation is suboptimal. Lower participation is observed among older adults, women, and individuals with less education or fewer socioeconomic resources. Home-based programs, which may reduce costs and increase availability, are currently hindered in the United States due to limited insurance coverage. The future may include the development of hybrid programs that combine center-based and home-based, supervised activities.

Cardiac rehabilitation is a clinically proven, multidisciplinary exercise training and risk factor modification program that enhances survival, reduces the risk of recurrent cardiac events, and improves physical and psychological well-being among patients with cardiovascular disease (CVD). The program is built around the promotion of exercise and associated lifestyle changes, while providing facilitative care for referring physicians' clinical management of cardiac disease and control of CVD risk factors. Despite these broad dimensions, the term *rehabilitation* is still ubiquitously applied to refer to this secondary cardiac prevention program, reflecting its storied and unique origins.

In the early decades of the 20th century, physicians treated myocardial infarction (MI) with as much as 6 to 8 weeks of bedrest due to the concern that early exertion after acute MI could led to recurrent cardiac events or aneurysmal rupture of the left ventricle. Due to this prolonged bedrest, patients became unnecessarily debilitated post-MI, and many never returned to their former employment. In the 1940s, cardiologists began to warn against the dangers of prolonged bedrest post-MI, and by the early 1950s, Levine and Lown called for early "armchair" ambulation, consisting of progressive periods of getting out of bed to sit in a chair within 1 day of acute MI.[1] Data accumulated over the next decade demonstrated that early ambulation was both safe and useful for reducing morbidity following acute MI.

During the 1960s, inpatient cardiac rehabilitation programs became increasingly widespread, but outpatient cardiac rehabilitation programs were still nonexistent. In the late 1960s, Hellerstein described the benefits of exercise training for improving fitness among a small group of patients with known cardiac disease,[2] which was a novel finding at that time. This was then followed by the conduct of small trials that further demonstrated the clinical benefit of initiating exercise training following acute MI. Thereafter, outpatient exercise training programs became commonplace, setting the foundation for cardiac rehabilitation as a new discipline in cardiovascular care.

THE MATURATION OF CARDIAC REHABILITATION

As cardiac rehabilitation emerged, it became organized into two phases, designed to provide a continuity of care for patients following acute MI or myocardial revascularization procedures. Phase 1, the inpatient phase, was provided by a collaborative team of cardiologists, physical and occupational therapists, social workers, and even vocational counselors in some programs. The goal for phase 1 rehabilitation was threefold. First, during hospitalization, patients were instructed on progressive ambulation. Second, there was recognition that patients' hospitalization provided a "teachable moment," induced by patients' feeling of vulnerability after enduring an acute cardiac event or undergoing cardiac surgery. These teachable moments could be used to instruct patients on risk factor modification practices, such as smoking cessation and initiation of a healthier diet. Third, interaction with the phase 1 team created a bridge toward patients' subsequent enrollment in outpatient cardiac

rehabilitation. Formal phase 1 cardiac rehabilitation programs in the United States have now largely devolved due to the current short duration of hospital stays following acute MI and revascularization procedures.

The outpatient portion of cardiac rehabilitation (originally termed *phase 2*) has maintained a relatively routine structure across US medical centers since its initiation: two to three sessions per week of monitored exercise training conducted over 36 sessions. In addition, some cardiac rehabilitation programs offer an optional longer-term (phase 3) exercise maintenance program. These optional programs vary widely in design. They may or may not be medically supervised or conducted within the same facility that houses the phase 2 programs, and they generally do not include electrocardiogram (ECG) monitoring during exercise sessions.

By the 1990s, cardiac rehabilitation programs were commonly addressing all modifiable cardiac risk factors, not just exercise conditioning, leading to the recognition of cardiac rehabilitation as a comprehensive secondary risk factor modification program by the American Heart Association (AHA) in 1994.[3] Subsequent position statements by cardiac societies called for cardiac rehabilitation to address a series of "core competencies" in secondary prevention.[4] These can be grouped into five categories, as shown in **Fig. 22–1**: exercise training, patient education, dietary counseling, psychosocial intervention, and risk factor modification. The bulk of typical cardiac rehabilitation sessions is built around exercise training, which includes supervised aerobic exercise, resistance exercise, and instruction on physical activities and exercise regimens to be conducted at home. Patient education may include personalized instruction to enhance patients' understanding of CVD and the steps that they can take to lead healthier lifestyles. Dietary counseling varies among programs but can include instruction and monitoring of patients' diets; instructions and demonstrations regarding healthy cooking; learning how to read food labels and how to navigate through restaurants, fast food outlets, and supermarkets; and other dietary information. Psychosocial management, which also varies widely among programs, can include screening patients for anxiety and/or depression; instruction regarding stress management; tips on sleep; and instruction on life skills to help address negative

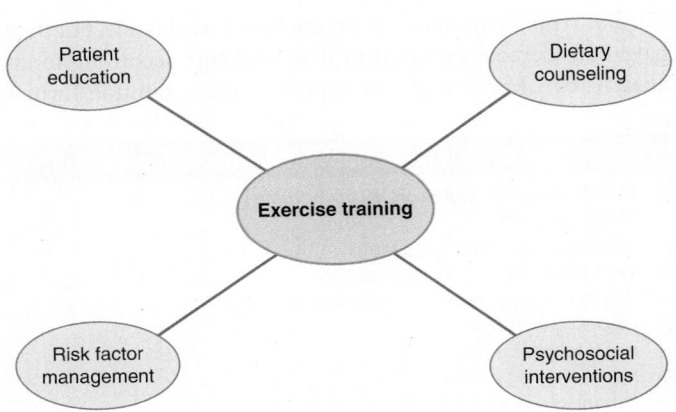

Figure 22–1. The five core components of cardiac rehabilitation.

health behaviors. Some health behaviors and conditions, such as active smoking, poor diet, insomnia, and high levels of stress, may require specialized supervision, necessitating patient referral to stand-alone programs that address each of these issues when necessary. Cardiac rehabilitation staff may help facilitate referring physicians' management of coronary artery disease (CAD) risk factors by encouraging patients' adherence to prescribed medications, amplifying physicians' instructions, or addressing patients' questions regarding their medical management or the results of laboratory and medical testing.

INDICATIONS FOR CARDIAC REHABILITATION

The indications for cardiac rehabilitation cover a wide variety of cardiac conditions and include specified clinical performance and quality measures that were updated by the American College of Cardiology/American Heart Association (ACCAHA) in 2018.[5] As noted in **Table 22–1,** current indications for cardiac rehabilitation include coverage for patients following non-ST elevation acute coronary syndrome, ST-elevation MI, all patients following coronary bypass surgery, as well as patients s/p percutaneous coronary intervention (PCI), valvular repair or replacement, and cardiac transplantation. Cardiac rehabilitation is also available as a treatment modality for patients with chronic angina pectoris or peripheral vascular disease. Finally, heart failure with reduced ejection fraction is a relatively new indication for cardiac rehabilitation in terms of being Medicare-approved (since 2014).

SAFETY OF CARDIAC REHABILITATION

Cardiac rehabilitation is a demonstrably safe program. In 2007, an AHA council reported that supervised exercise within cardiac rehabilitation programs was associated with a very low incidence of adverse clinical events: 1 cardiac arrest per 116,906 patient-hours, 1 MI per 219,970 patient-hours, and 1 fatal event per 752,365 patient-hours.[6] This low rate of events is based on the presumption that patients are first screened for all contraindications for exercise, as listed in **Table 22–2.**

STRUCTURE OF CARDIAC REHABILITATION PROGRAMS

Cardiac rehabilitation programs are found worldwide, but they have considerable variation in their makeup, according to an analysis by Chaves et al.[7] As opposed to the common format

TABLE 22–1. Eligible Indications for Cardiac Rehabilitation

- Non-ST elevation acute coronary syndrome
- ST-elevation MI
- Coronary artery bypass grafting
- Percutaneous coronary intervention
- Valvular surgery (replacement or repair)
- Cardiac transplantation
- Heart-lung transplantation
- Stable angina pectoris
- Peripheral vascular disease
- Heart failure with reduced ejection fraction

TABLE 22–2. Contraindications to Cardiac Rehabilitation

- Inability to exercise due to musculoskeletal conditions
- Inability to comply due to cognitive dysfunction
- Worsening chest pain
- Decompensated heart failure
- Recent stroke or transient ischemic attack
- Atrial arrhythmia with uncontrolled ventricular response
- Complex ventricular arrhythmia
- Severe pulmonary arterial hypertension
- Intracavitary thrombus
- Recent thrombophlebitis
- Pulmonary embolism
- Severe obstructive cardiomyopathy
- Symptomatic or severe aortic stenosis
- Acute infection

of 36 sessions for outpatient cardiac rehabilitation programs in the United States and Canada, the researchers found that the median duration for supervised programs on a worldwide basis was 24 sessions, with 58% of programs offering ≥12 sessions. The median duration of home-based cardiac rehabilitation was only 6 sessions.

Prior to the initiation of rehabilitation, patients may benefit from either a baseline symptom–limited or modified exercise tolerance test, which is best conducted with patients taking their usual medications. Exercise testing, also best conducted with patients taking their usual medications, may be used to identify any inducible symptoms, ischemia, or arrhythmia and to formulate a target training range that is best suited for patients' exercise sessions. When a baseline exercise test is not performed, patients' initial target heart rate may be initiated at approximately 20 beats above the standing heart rate.[8] Ideally, exercise training should seek to achieve a moderate intensity of exercise, equivalent to brisk walking. In practice, initial training heart rates can vary widely according to patients' baseline conditioning, comorbidities, age, motivation, and other factors. Exercise training may often be initiated at low intensity to encourage confidence and an initial sense of success with undertaking physical activity. The establishment of an appropriate intensity of exercise may be greatly aided by having patients evaluate their sense of perceived exertion. The Borg Perceived Exertion Scale has been widely utilized to do this, with patients encouraged to exercise at moderate levels of this exertion scale.

Generally, the staffing of a cardiac rehabilitation program includes a medical director, a nurse to help supervise patient training and medication administration, and other nurses or exercise physiologists to help monitor exercise sessions. A typical cardiac rehabilitation session may involve a period of patient warm-up, monitored and supervised exercise, and cooldown. Educational sessions and other core components of cardiac rehabilitation are integrated into patients' supervision. During the warm-up, patients perform stretching exercises and light calisthenics for 5 to 10 minutes. All exercise sessions are ECG monitored during phase 2 programs; they consist of cross-training on treadmills, stationary bicycles, elliptical machines, and other exercise equipment. Patients are instructed on proper breathing and exercise techniques and monitored for the development of symptoms or abnormal hemodynamic or ECG responses. Upper- and lower-body muscle strengthening (resistance) exercises should be incorporated and applied to patients of all ages, including older ones. Patients should then be monitored for recovery during at least 5 to 10 minutes of cooldown.

CLINICAL BENEFITS OF CARDIAC REHABILITATION

Among its benefits, cardiac rehabilitation can improve physical fitness, decrease the severity of anginal symptoms, reduce the risk for recurrent cardiac events and repeat hospitalizations, lower downstream medical costs, and enhance patients' psychological well-being (**Table 22–3**). The basis for these evidence-based outcomes are multifactorial and synergistic. They include the substantial physiological benefits associated with exercise (see Chapter 12), control of other major CAD risk factors, improved patient adherence to medical regimens, improved medical care fostered by collaboration with patients' primary physicians, and reduction in psychosocial risk factors for disease, including depression.

Among its central benefits, cardiac rehabilitation improves patients' exercise capacity.[9] As patients progress, they may manifest an ability to exercise at higher intensity and/or for longer duration. For patients who are substantially deconditioned, this can translate into significant increase in patients' ability to perform daily activities that previously caused exercise intolerance or dyspnea, as well as an uplifting sensation of increased physical self-efficacy.

The impact of cardiac rehabilitation on clinical outcomes has been extensively studied over recent decades. The conduct of small clinical trials in the 1970s and 1980s led to the first two meta-analyses to assess the efficacy of exercise-based cardiac rehabilitation in the late 1980s.[10–11] These analyses revealed that enrollment in cardiac rehabilitation was associated with a significant reduction in all-cause mortality, and cardiac mortality. Among subsequent studies, a meta-analysis of 34 trials involving randomization of patients to either exercise-based cardiac rehabilitation or usual care found that cardiac rehabilitation was associated with a 26% reduction in all-cause mortality and 36% reduction in cardiac mortality.[12] A division of trials performed before and after 1995 showed similar results. The results of this analysis were paralleled by a systematic review of 47 studies that randomized 10,794 patients to either exercise-based cardiac rehabilitation the usual medical care before 2010.[13] This study also found cardiac rehabilitation to be associated with a lower frequency of both all-cause and cardiac mortality.

More recent meta-analyses provide insights into whether the benefits of cardiac rehabilitation have persisted in our current era of optimized medical therapies. Anderson et al. conducted a meta-analysis of 64 studies that compared cardiac rehabilitation versus usual care.[14] Randomization to cardiac rehabilitation was associated with a 26% reduction in cardiovascular mortality and significant reduction in hospitalizations and medical costs, but no significant reduction in all-cause mortality. In another study, van Halewijn et al. conducted a meta-analysis of 18 trials that randomized patients to cardiac rehabilitation or usual care between 2010 and 2015.[15] Cardiac rehabilitation was associated with a 58% reduction in the risk of cardiovascular mortality, 30% reduction in the risk of MI, and 60% reduction in the risk of cerebrovascular events, but no statistical reduction in all-cause mortality. However, when patients were divided into those who received more versus less intensive management of cardiac risk factors (divided dichotomously into management of more or fewer than six risk factors), there was a significant reduction in all-cause mortality among the patients in whom risk factors were managed more aggressively. A similar pattern was noted in a recent Bayesian network meta-analysis of 134 trials involving 62,322 participants.[16] The analysis compared patients randomized to comprehensive cardiac rehabilitation versus only exercise-based cardiac rehabilitation or usual care. A trial was considered comprehensive if exercise training was combined with other core interventions (ie, education, counseling, risk factor modification, and psychosocial management). Compared to standard care, exercise-only rehabilitation reduced the odds of cardiovascular mortality, MI, and subsequent hospitalization, but not all-cause mortality. By contrast, comprehensive cardiac rehabilitation was associated with a lower odds ratio for all-cause mortality versus usual care, confirming the results of van Halewijn et al.[15]

In conclusion, since its initiation through the current era, cardiac rehabilitation has been consistently associated with a significant reduction in adverse cardiovascular events. It is also associated with a reduction in all-cause mortality when the program is comprehensive in nature. Studies also indicate the presence of a strong dose response relationship between the number of cardiac rehabilitation sessions that patients attend and their subsequent risk for all-cause mortality.[17–20]

TABLE 22–3. Clinical Benefits of Comprehensive Cardiac Rehabilitation

Physical fitness
- Improvement in exercise functional capacity
- Improvement in muscle strength
- Improvement in physical self-efficacy and tolerance for activities of daily living

Reduction in anginal symptoms

Reduction in adverse medical events
- Reduction in all-cause mortality
- Reduction in cardiac mortality
- Reduction in stroke risk
- Reduction in MI
- Reduction in recurrent hospitalizations
- Reduction in downstream medical costs

Improvement in psychological well-being
- Improvement in quality of living
- Reduction in depression and other psychosocial risk factors

INTENSITY OF EXERCISE DURING CARDIAC REHABILITATION

Exercise training is guided by two related tenets. First, low level of maximal aerobic fitness is associated with higher mortality risk.[21-22] Second, improvement in aerobic fitness leads to reduction in mortality risk.[23-24] Importantly, in this regard, patients can manifest substantial variability in their response to exercise training at the levels of intensity commonly prescribed for cardiac rehabilitation, with some patients failing to manifest any significant increase in cardiorespiratory fitness as measured by oxygen consumption (VO_2) max or VO_2 peak.[25-28] This nonresponse is not infrequent. For example, Savage et al. assessed 385 patients who had their VO_2 peak assessed before and after the completion of cardiac rehabilitation.[27] Patients exercised over 36 sessions, with exercise intensity adjusted to maintain the training heart rate within 70% to 85% of the peak heart rate observed on entry treadmill exercise testing, or to a moderate range of self-perceived exertion using the Borg scale. Overall, 21% of patients had no improvement in VO_2 peak following the program. Similarly, De Schutter et al. recently reported that 23% of 1,171 patients had no improvement in maximal oxygen consumption after completing cardiac rehabilitation.[28]

The mortality benefit associated with improvement in aerobic fitness following cardiac rehabilitation has been demonstrated on an objective basis. Martin et al. assessed treadmill exercise performance before and after the completion of cardiac rehabilitation in 5,641 patients.[24] A 13% reduction in mortality risk was noted for each 1–metabolic equivalent of task (MET) increase on repeat treadmill testing. The benefit was more pronounced among patients with low cardiorespiratory fitness at baseline: there was a 30% reduction in mortality for each 1-MET increase. De Schutter et al. noted similar observations among patients divided into high responders, low responders, and nonresponders based on the magnitude of improvement in peak oxygen consumption following cardiac rehabilitation.[28] Compared to the high responders, low responders had a twofold increase in mortality

and nonresponders had a threefold increase in mortality during a mean follow-up of 6.4 years (**Fig. 22–2**).

These observations suggest a need to identify nonresponders, introduce them to exercise training, and attempt to improve their fitness. A study by Ross et al. provides important insights about this.[29] They assessed 121 obese adults who completed exercise sessions 5 times per week over a period of 24 weeks. The patients were randomly split into three groups: (1) a low amount of low-intensity exercise at 50% of VO_2 peak; (2) a high amount of low-intensity exercise at 50% of VO_2 peak; and (3) a high amount of high-intensity exercise at 75% of VO_2 peak. At 24 weeks, nonresponsiveness to exercise (ie, no significant increase in VO_2 peak) was common among the patients exercising at low volume and low intensity, but it was completely eliminated in the group exercising at a high volume and intensity of exercise (**Fig. 22–3**). This study illustrates the important interrelationship between exercise intensity and subsequent nonresponsiveness to exercise training.

This need has led to a growing interest in the potential use of high-intensity interval training (HIIT) for cardiac rehabilitation patients. This training regimen consists of having patients perform repeated bouts of high-intensity exercise, interspersed between periods of lower-intensity exercise or recovery. Studies indicate that HIIT is more effective than moderate-intensity exercise for improving cardiorespiratory fitness[30] and can be conducted safely among patients with CVD.[31] Nevertheless, there is a need for more real-world experience that weighs the benefit versus safety of HIIT among patients with a higher baseline risk (eg, older age, poor cardiorespiratory fitness, or high level of comorbidities).

CARDIAC REHABILITATION FOR HEART FAILURE PATIENTS

Among heart failure patients, cardiac rehabilitation can also enhance health-related quality of life and improve exercise capacity, as recently demonstrated in an individual participant

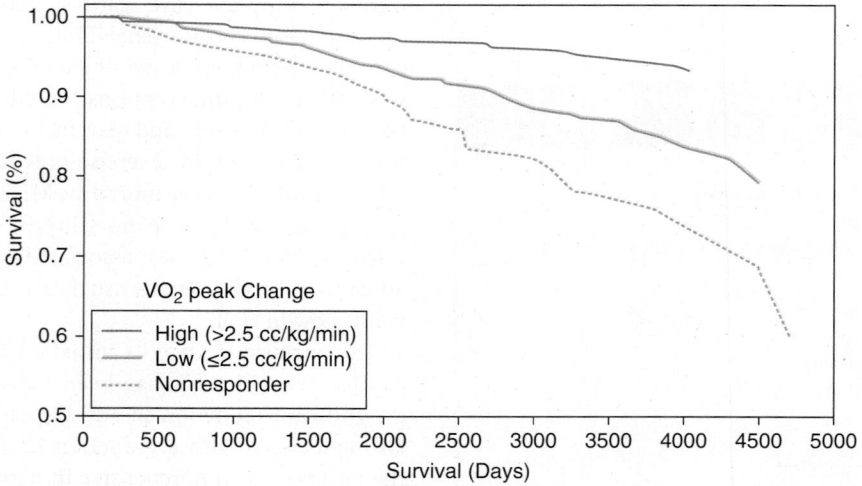

Figure 22–2. Survival curves among 1,171 patients completing a cardiac rehabilitation program. Patients underwent exercise testing before and after completion of the program and were divided into three groups based on their absolute improvement in oxygen consumption (VO_2) peak (none, low, high) on repeat testing, adjusted for predictors of mortality. Those failing to improve oxygen consumption on repeat testing had the lowest survival. Reproduced with permission from De Schutter A, Kachur S, Lavie CJ, et al. Cardiac rehabilitation fitness changes and subsequent survival. *Eur Heart J Qual Care Clin Outcomes.* 2018 Jul 1;4(3):173-179.

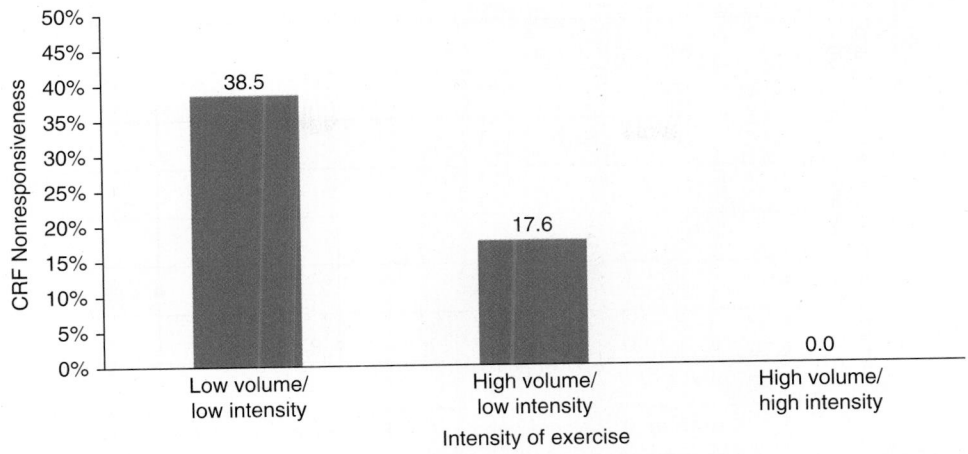

Figure 22–3. **Impact of the intensity and volume of exercise training among 121 obese adults, who were assigned one of three levels of training for 24 weeks.** The vertical axis shows the percentage who failed to improve cardiorespiratory fitness (CRF), as assessed by VO_2 peak on repeat treadmill exercise testing at the end of the exercise trial. CRF nonresponsiveness was common among the subjects exercising at low intensity and volume, but this response was abolished in the group randomized to a high intensity and volume of exercise.

meta-analysis of 13 randomized clinical trials involving heart failure patients.[32] The impact of cardiac rehalitation on hard clinical outcomes was also assessed in a Cochrane meta-analysis of 44 trials (5,783 patients) that randomized heart failure patients to exercise-based cardiac rehabilitation versus a control group.[33] Randomization to cardiac rehabilitation was associated with a subsequent reduction in hospitalizations, especially heart failure–related hospitalizations, but it was not associated with reduction in mortality. Of note, the median follow-up period in the trials constituting this analysis was only 6 months, and the analysis did not consider the patients' degree of improvement in cardiorespiratory fitness during cardiac rehabilitation.

The importance of this latter limitation is illustrated by data from the HF-ACTION (Heat Failure: A Controlled Trail Investigating Outcomes of Exercise Training) trial.[34] In this study, randomization of 2,322 heart failure subjects to either cardiac rehabilitation or usual care yielded no difference in mortality over a median of 30 months. However, there was a low adherence rate to exercise in the training group, resulting in only a 4% improvement in VO_2 peak. In a subsequent analysis of the combined HF-ACTION sample, every 6% increase in VO_2 peak was associated with a 7% decrease in all-cause mortality.[35] Among related studies,[36–37] Bakker et al. found that the combination of low baseline fitness and a lack of improvement in cardiorespiratory fitness was associated with the highest risk of subsequent mortality and/or hospitalization among heart failure patients receiving cardiac rehabilitation[37] (**Fig. 22–4**). The importance of exercise intensity is further supported by a meta-analysis of 74 exercise intervention trials of heart failure patients, which found a proportional relationship between patients' exercise intensity and subsequent improvement in their cardiorespiratory fitness.[38]

Combined, these data suggest a need to focus attention on optimizing improvement in cardiac fitness among heart failure patients. This may be approached by attempting to increase patients' volume of exercise gradually, promoting a combination

of aerobic exercise and resistance training to improve overall fitness, and/or incorporating HIIT in selected patients.

CARDIAC REHABILITATION FOR OLDER ADULTS

Improvements in prevention and therapeutics have led to greater longevity and an increased number of older adults living with CVD. Cardiac rehabilitation may be particularly useful for aiding the medical care of such patients. Aging is associated with an increased frequency of hypertension, insulin resistance, diabetes, visceral obesity, deconditioning, decline in exercise capacity, sarcopenia, and disabilities. These conditions, in combination with the physiological changes associated with primary aging, lead to heightened risk for coronary artery, cerebrovascular, and peripheral vascular disease and heart failure among older adults. Thus, older adults who qualify for cardiac rehabilitation may benefit from its ability to address many of the comorbidities that constitute this accumulated aggregate risk. In addition, older adults tend to have more atypical symptoms, complex medication regimens, and more concerns and questions about their health care, which can be addressed by a supportive cardiac rehabilitation team.

The clinical benefit of cardiac rehabilitation for older adults is supported by large outcomes studies. Hammill et al. evaluated a national sample of 30,161 Medicare beneficiaries with a median age of 74 years who attended one or more cardiac rehabilitation sessions and were followed for 4 years.[19] A strong dose-response relationship was noted between the number of sessions and subsequent mortality (**Fig. 22–5**). In an even larger study, Suaya et al. assessed 601,099 Medicare beneficiaries who were hospitalized for coronary conditions or cardiac revascularization procedures.[20] The patients were then subdivided into those who did and did not participate in subsequent cardiac rehabilitation and propensity matched to compare subgroups with similar clinical profiles. Cumulative mortality was substantially lower among cardiac rehabilitation patients, with

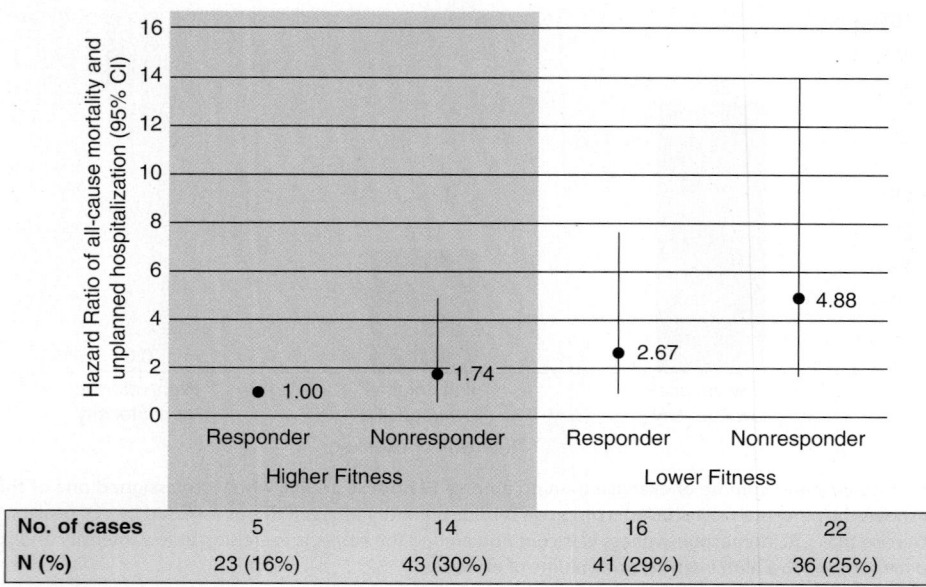

Figure 22–4. **Age, gender, and BMI-adjusted hazard ratios for all-cause mortality and/or unplanned hospitalization among 155 heart failure patients undergoing bicycle exercise before and after completion of a cardiac rehabilitation program.** Patients were assessed for baseline fitness, as well as their improvement in cardiorespiratory fitness (as assessment by improvement of VO$_2$ peak) following the training program. Those patients with both low fitness and a lack of improvement in fitness following cardiac rehabilitation were at highest risk. Reproduced with permission from Bakker EA, Snoek JA, Meindersma EP, et al. Absence of Fitness Improvement Is Associated with Outcomes in Heart Failure Patients. *Med Sci Sports Exerc.* 2018 Feb;50(2):196-203.

those attending more cardiac rehabilitation sessions experiencing lower mortality (**Fig. 22–6**).

CARDIAC REHABILITATION AND PSYCHOLOGICAL WELL-BEING

A variety of psychosocial factors are associated with CVD, including depression, anxiety, pessimism, social isolation and poor social support, lack of life purpose, and certain forms

of chronic stress.[39] Among these, depression is a particularly potent risk factor for CVD and may increase clinical risk even if it is mild.[40] A substantial body of literature links physical inactivity to increased depression risk, and exercise intervention to amelioration of depression.[41] The latter includes randomized control studies that have found exercise intervention to be as effective as antidepressant medication in alleviating depressive symptoms.[42]

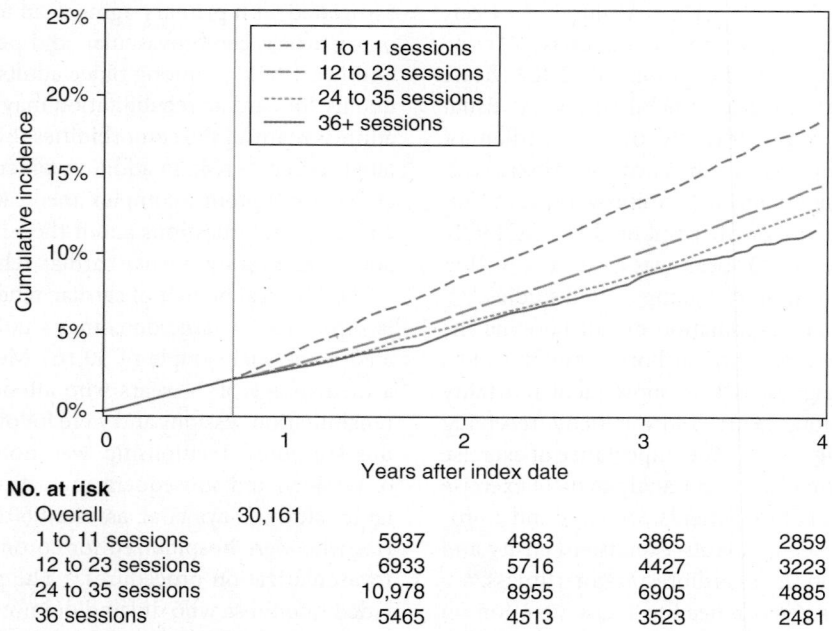

Figure 22–5. **Cumulative incidence of deaths according to the number of sessions attended among 30,161 Medicare beneficiaries participating in cardiac rehabilitation.** A dose-response relationship is present. Reproduced with permission from Hammill BG, Curtis LH, Schulman KA, et al. Relationship between cardiac rehabilitation and long-term risks of death and myocardial infarction among elderly Medicare beneficiaries. *Circulation.* 2010 Jan 5;121(1):63-70.

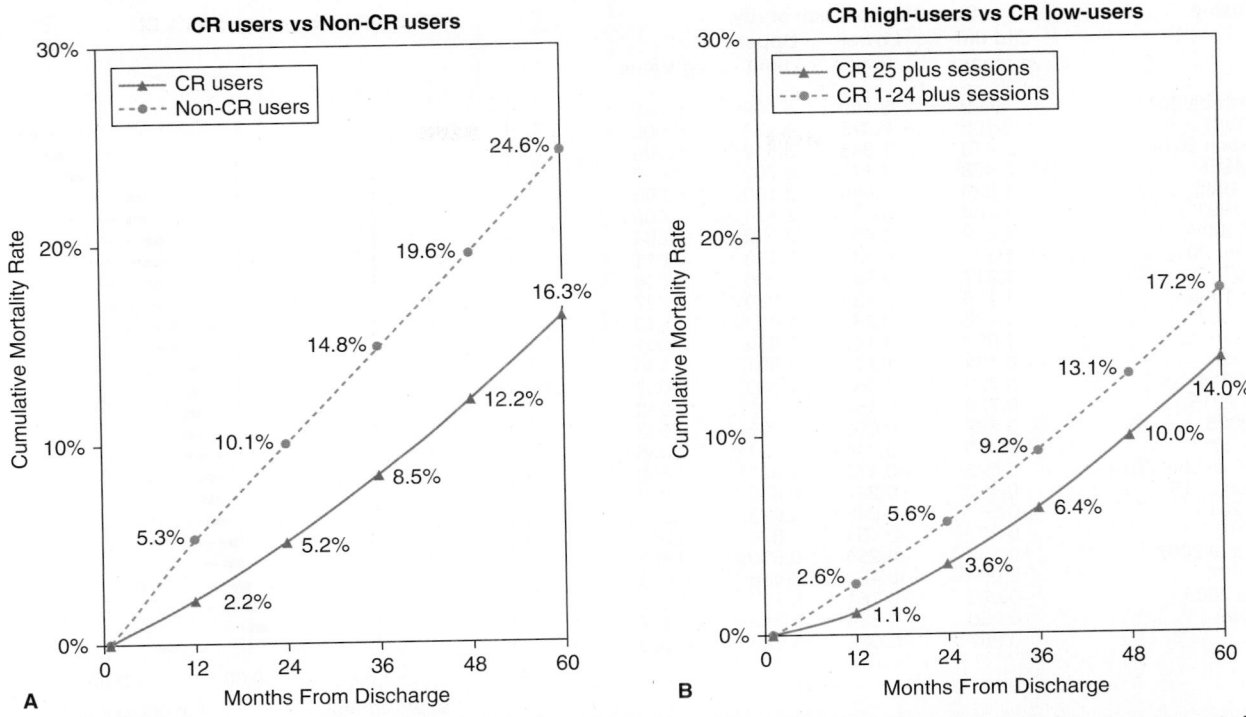

Figure 22-6. (A) Cumulative mortality rates among a propensity matched cohort of eligible older adults following the use or nonuse of cardiac rehabilitation (CR). The mortality rate was higher among nonusers at each time point following discharge from CR. (B) Mortality rate among CR users, divided into those who participated in more or fewer than 25 CR sessions. Reproduced with permission from Suaya JA, Stason WB, Ades PA, et al. Cardiac rehabilitation and survival in older coronary patients. *J Am Coll Cardiol.* 2009 Jun 30;54(1):25-33.

Substantial evidence indicates that exercise training leads to a reduction of depressive symptoms[43-45] and anxiety.[46-47] In a Cochrane meta-analysis of 35 trials involving 1,356 subjects with depressive symptoms who were randomized to exercise versus no treatment or control interventions, exercise training reduced depression to a moderate degree.[43] In another meta-analysis involving 25 exercise trials, randomization of depressed patients to exercise versus a control group reduced depressive symptoms with a large effect (**Fig. 22-7**), including benefits found in 9 trials that studied patients with major depressive disorder.[44] More recently, a similar impact has been noted with resistance training.[45] Exercise training can also reduce depressive symptoms among heart failure patients.[48-49]

A yet insufficiently addressed question is whether there is a dose-response relationship between exercise volume and reduction in depressive symptoms.[50-51] In one study that addressed this issue in quantitative fashion, Milani and Lavie evaluated 522 consecutive patients enrolled in cardiac rehabilitation.[50] VO_2 peak was assessed at baseline and 1 week after completing the program. Reduction in depression was minimal, and subsequent mortality rates were highest among patients with no improvement in fitness, but both parameters decreased substantially among patients with gain in VO_2 peak following the training program (**Fig. 22-8**).

In addition to the potential benefits of exercise training on depressive and anxiety symptoms, cardiac rehabilitation offers the opportunity to apply a wide variety of psychosocial interventions to enhance patient well-being. First, the group nature of cardiac rehabilitation constitutes a useful intervention for promoting social support for patients. This can be augmented by connecting patients to community programs that can further enhance social connectivity. Second, a variety of stress management techniques can also be employed, and preliminary data indicate their effectiveness in improving medical outcomes.[52] Third, epidemiological studies have established that the psychosocial risk factors for CVD exist on a continuum ranging from positive factors that enhance health to negative factors that decrease disease[53] (**Fig. 22-9**). This has led to increasing interest in applying positive psychology techniques for health promotion within medical settings.[54] While the nature of psychological interventions is likely to vary across medical centers, a recent meta-analysis that compared the clinical effectiveness of the five core components of cardiac rehabilitation (shown earlier in Fig. 22-1) found that exercise training and psychosocial interventions were the two most effective interventions for reducing mortality risk.[55]

OVERCOMING BARRIERS TO ENROLLMENT AND PARTICIPATION IN CARDIAC REHABILITATION

Despite its proven benefits, cardiac rehabilitation has been persistently underutilized. For example, an analysis found that only 16.3% of representative Medicare patients and 10.3% of Veterans Administration (VA) patients who were eligible participated in cardiac rehabilitation between 2007 and 2011.[56] Such data have resulted in an increasing demand to improve referral, enrollment, and adherence rates for cardiac rehabilitation. A consensus

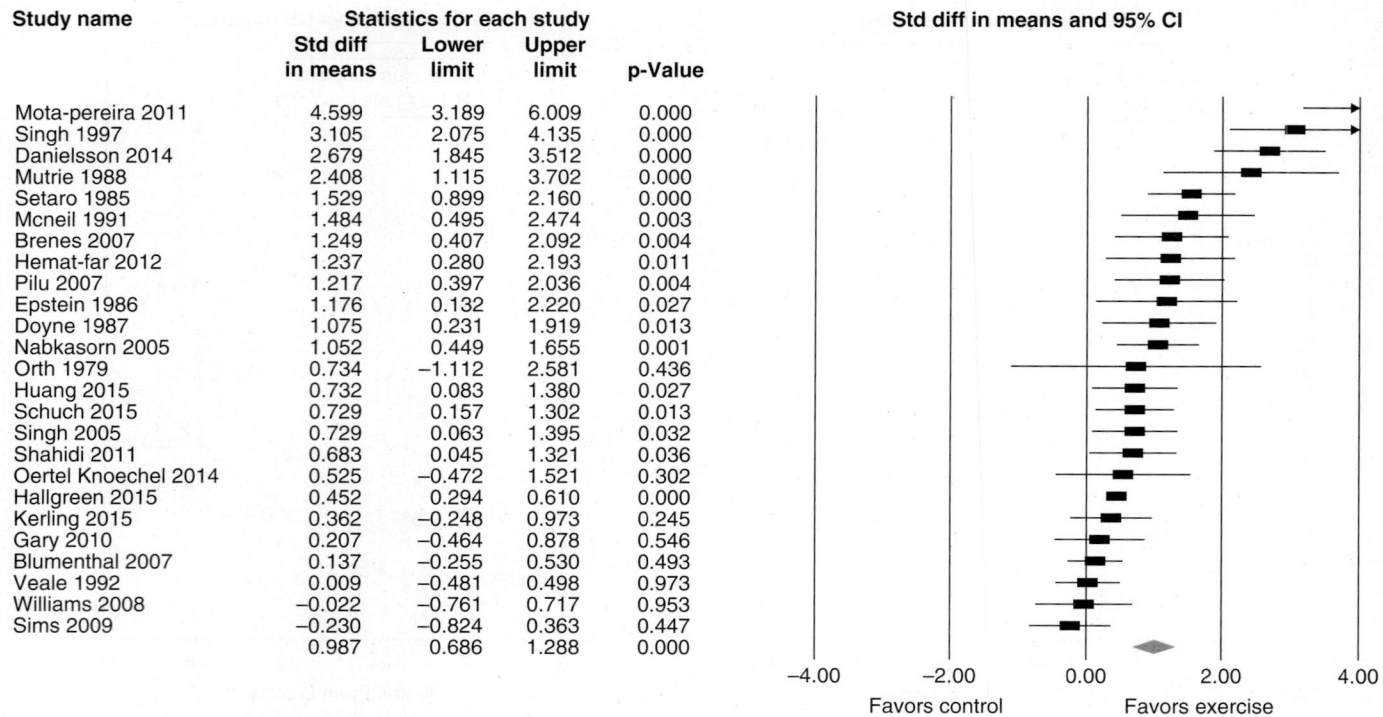

Study name	Statistics for each study				Std diff in means and 95% CI
	Std diff in means	Lower limit	Upper limit	p-Value	
Mota-pereira 2011	4.599	3.189	6.009	0.000	
Singh 1997	3.105	2.075	4.135	0.000	
Danielsson 2014	2.679	1.845	3.512	0.000	
Mutrie 1988	2.408	1.115	3.702	0.000	
Setaro 1985	1.529	0.899	2.160	0.000	
Mcneil 1991	1.484	0.495	2.474	0.003	
Brenes 2007	1.249	0.407	2.092	0.004	
Hemat-far 2012	1.237	0.280	2.193	0.011	
Pilu 2007	1.217	0.397	2.036	0.004	
Epstein 1986	1.176	0.132	2.220	0.027	
Doyne 1987	1.075	0.231	1.919	0.013	
Nabkasorn 2005	1.052	0.449	1.655	0.001	
Orth 1979	0.734	−1.112	2.581	0.436	
Huang 2015	0.732	0.083	1.380	0.027	
Schuch 2015	0.729	0.157	1.302	0.013	
Singh 2005	0.729	0.063	1.395	0.032	
Shahidi 2011	0.683	0.045	1.321	0.036	
Oertel Knoechel 2014	0.525	−0.472	1.521	0.302	
Hallgreen 2015	0.452	0.294	0.610	0.000	
Kerling 2015	0.362	−0.248	0.973	0.245	
Gary 2010	0.207	−0.464	0.878	0.546	
Blumenthal 2007	0.137	−0.255	0.530	0.493	
Veale 1992	0.009	−0.481	0.498	0.973	
Williams 2008	−0.022	−0.761	0.717	0.953	
Sims 2009	−0.230	−0.824	0.363	0.447	
	0.987	0.686	1.288	0.000	

Std diff in means = standardized differences in means, CI = Confidence interval

Figure 22–7. Meta-analysis of 25 trials in which patients were randomized to exercise versus a control group without exercise and assessed for reduction in depression. Shown is the effect size for each study, which cumulatively indicate a substantial reduction in depression with exercise. Reproduced with permission from Schuch FB, Vancampfort D, Richards J, et al. Exercise as a treatment for depression: A meta-analysis adjusting for publication bias. *J Psychiatr Res.* 2016 Jun;77:42-51.

advisory from the AHA has identified a series of patient-oriented, medical, and health-care system–related factors that contribute to the limited referral and enrollment of patients (**Table 22–4**).[57] Lower cardiac rehabilitation participation is observed among older adults, women, and those with lower education, lower socioeconomic status, or lack of adequate medical insurance. Medical factors predicting reduced referral

and enrollment include a high burden of comorbidities and depression. In addition, a variety of health-care system–related factors limit patient referral and enrollment, including lack of programs in certain geographic areas, lack of programs convenient to patients' homes, poor parking, and lack of adequate public transportation. A recent systematic review has observed that these barriers are similar across countries.[58]

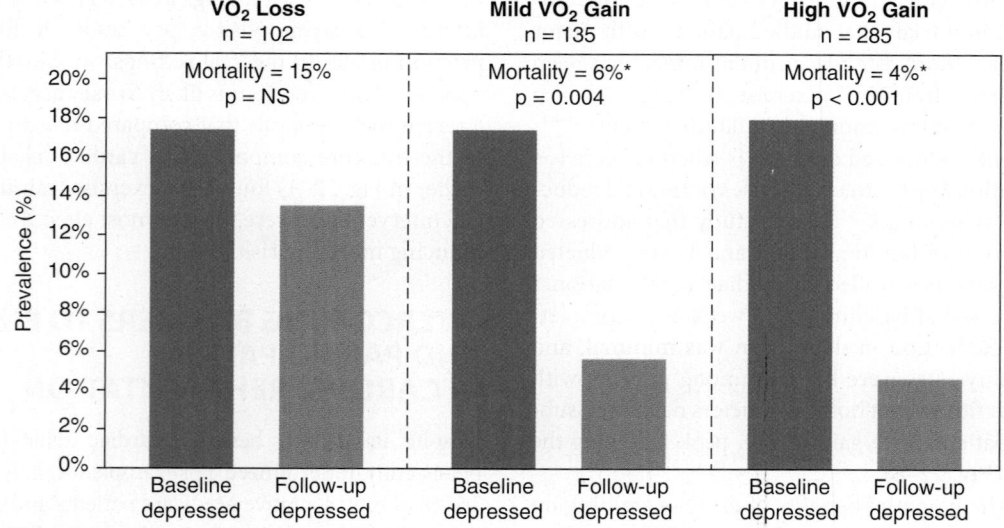

Figure 22–8. Assessment of change in the prevalence of depressive symptoms and subsequent mortality among 522 patients undergoing exercise-based cardiac rehabilitation, divided into three groups based on the change in their VO_2 peak between baseline and repeat testing following completion of the training program. Reproduced with permission from Milani RV, Lavie CJ. Impact of cardiac rehabilitation on depression and its associated mortality. *Am J Med.* 2007 Sep;120(9):799-806.

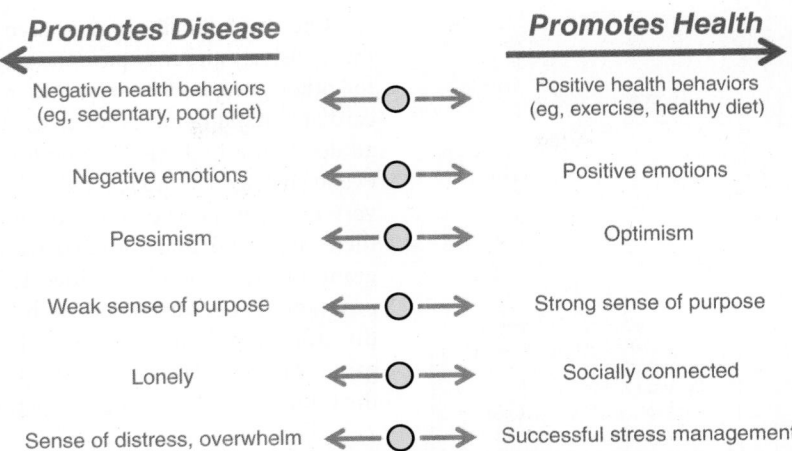

Figure 22–9. Health behaviors and psychosocial factors that can promote CVD exist along a continuum, from positive factors that buffer physiology, enhance well-being, and decrease the likelihood of disease, to negative factors that are pathophysiological, decrease well-being, and promote disease. The cardiac rehabilitation setting provides an opportunity to introduce patients to positive psychological techniques and life skills that can enhance their functioning in each of the domains shown here. Reproduced with permission from Rozanski A. Behavioral cardiology: current advances and future directions. *J Am Coll Cardiol.* 2014 Jul 8;64(1):100-110.

Various recommendations have been made to improve the participation of eligible patients in institutional or center-based cardiac rehabilitation programs. Two of the key ones involve making a patient's referral to cardiac rehabilitation automatic within his or her electronic medical record during hospitalization and designating a liaison to guide his or her enrollment in cardiac rehabilitation prior to hospital discharge.[59] In an analysis of a single center, Grace et al. found that the combination of automatic referral and use of such a liaison was associated with an 85.8% referral rate to cardiac rehabilitation and a 73.5% rate of enrollment, compared to only a 32.2% referral rate and 29.0% of enrollment among patients who received neither step.[60] Other recommendations include making the referral to cardiac rehabilitation a measurable quality-of-care performance outcome, and decreasing or eliminating patient copays for program participation.[59] In support of this finding, Farah et al. observed a dose-response relationship between cost sharing in the form of copays or unmet deductibles and program attendance.[61] Each $10 increase in copays was associated with 1.5 fewer attended sessions.

Alternatively, there has been a growing interest in home-based cardiac rehabilitation. To date, home-based programs are generally not covered by most medical insurance plans in the United States, markedly inhibiting their potential utilization in this country. By contrast, home-based programs are commonly found among various European nations and Australia.[7,59] Home-based programs may vary from unsupervised home exercise to tele-based programs, which attempt to create a form of virtual experience through the direct digital monitoring and supervision of patients.

To date, there are limited and discordant data concerning the effectiveness of home-based cardiac rehabilitation. A Cochrane meta-analysis that evaluated 17 studies in which patients were randomized to either center- or home-based cardiac rehabilitation through 2014[62] found that both programs were comparably effective in reducing CAD risk factors, enhancing health-related quality of life, and reducing subsequent cardiac events. By contrast, a network meta-analysis of 60 randomized trials conducted by Xia et al. found that only center-based, but not home-based cardiac rehabilitation was associated with reduced all-cause mortality and cardiovascular mortality compared to the usual medical care.[63] However, only a small number of these trials involved tele-based programs, which represent a relatively new and particularly innovative way to evaluate and supervise patients in the home setting.

TABLE 22–4. Factors Associated with Limited Referral to and Enrollment of Patients in Cardiac Rehabilitation

Patient-oriented factors
- Female sex
- Older age
- Racial/ethnic minority group
- Limited or lacking health-care insurance
- Low socioeconomic status
- Low educational attainment
- Low health literacy
- Lack of perceived need for cardiac rehabilitation
- Language or cultural barriers
- Lack of understanding of disease and treatment
- Work-related factors (eg, inflexible work hours) or home responsibilities

Limited social support

Medical factors
- Depression
- Musculoskeletal conditions

Health-care system factors
- Limited facilitation of enrollment after referral
- Lack of endorsement by patient's physician
- Lack of programs that serve specific geographic areas
- Inconvenient distance from patient's home
- Poor parking or public transportation access
- Lack of diversity among the cardiac rehabilitation team

Reproduced with permission from Balady GJ, Ades PA, Bittner VA, et al. Referral, enrollment, and delivery of cardiac rehabilitation/secondary prevention programs at clinical centers and beyond: a presidential advisory from the American Heart Association. *Circulation.* 2011 Dec 20;124(25):2951-2960.

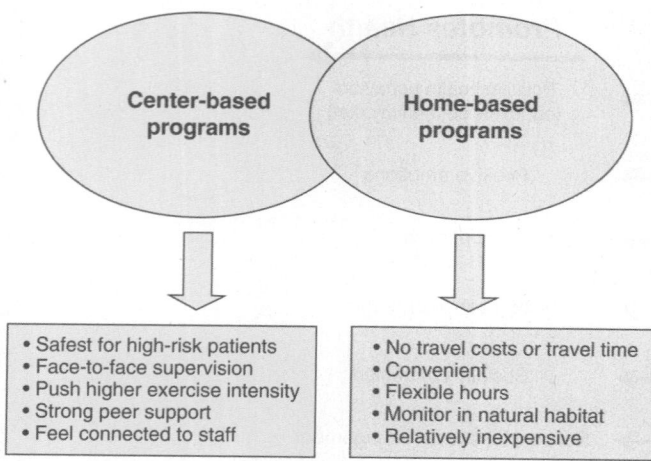

Figure 22–10. Comparison of the advantages of center- versus home-based cardiac rehabilitation. Under a hybrid model, patients could start in a center-based program and then be transitioned to home-based rehabilitation after sufficient exercise instruction and gain in physical self-efficacy.

The future evolution of cardiac rehabilitation is likely to include an increased utility of home-based programs, with recognition that both center- and home-based programs offer advantages and could be combined along a continuum of care (**Fig. 22–10**). Center-based programs offer the greatest degree of safety for the supervision of high-risk patients, such as newly exercising heart failure patients or older deconditioned patients, and the face-to-face supervision provided in this setting may be favored because it initially pushes greater exercise intensity and/or initial introduction to resistance training among untrained subjects. In the recent meta-analysis by Xia et al, none of the stand-alone home-based programs, including the tele-based programs, incorporated strength training with aerobic exercise.[63] Center-based programs also offer patients strong peer support, as well as a strong social connection with the program staff.

However, the potential benefits of home-based programs are considerable, including elimination of travel time and costs, the potential to extend participation into nighttime or weekend hours, and other conveniences. The greater the convenience, the more likely patients are to adhere to an exercise regimen. Home-based training is facilitated by having access to some specialized exercise equipment, such as a treadmill or stationary bicycle, when feasible. Pedometers can be used for tracking overall activity, and heart rate monitors can be employed in order to assess adherence to the prescribed exercise routine. Other monitoring equipment includes bathroom scales, blood pressure monitors, and glucometers.

The 12-week duration of center-based programs is arbitrary; home-based programs could be increased for considerably longer periods of time if prospective studies indicate that this advantage has medical benefits. The lack of face-to-face supervision of patients that is offered by center-based programs could be offset by the advantage of evaluation of patients in their natural habitat using web- and mobile phone–based interactions, text messaging, and application of sensors to provide feedback regarding pertinent health indices such as heart rate and ECG. Finally, home-based programs can be run more inexpensively and may pave the way toward creating programs for other groups of interest that are not currently covered by cardiac rehabilitation guidelines, such as deconditioned older adults with a high-risk profile for CVD but no prior cardiac events. In a hybrid model, higher-risk patients or those who are very deconditioned or unaccustomed to exercise could begin their cardiac rehabilitation participation at a center-based program and then be transitioned to a home-based, supervised program. Thus, further research is indicated to demonstrate the efficacy of home-based and hybrid programs in order to gain critical third-party medical insurance that will help foster the future evolution of these programs.

REFERENCES

1. Levine SA, Lown B. "Armchair" treatment of acute coronary thrombosis. *J Am Med Assoc.* 1952;148:1365-1369.
2. Hellerstein HK. Exercise therapy in coronary disease. *Bull NY Acad Med.* 1968;44:1028-1047.
3. Balady GJ, Fletcher BJ, Froelicher ES, et al. Cardiac rehabilitation programs: a statement for healthcare professionals from the American Heart Association. *Circulation.* 1994;90:1602-1610.
4. Hamm LF, Sanderson BK, Ades PA, et al. Core competencies for cardiac rehabilitation/secondary prevention professionals: 2010 update—position statement of the American Association of Cardiovascular and Pulmonary Rehabilitation. *J Cardiopulm Rehabil Prev.* 2011;31:2-10.
5. Thomas RJ, Balady G, Banka G, et al. 2018 ACC/AHA clinical performance and quality measures for cardiac rehabilitation. *J Am Coll Cardiol.* 2018;71:1814-1833.
6. Thompson P, Franklin BA, Balady GJ, et al. Exercise and acute cardiovascular events: placing the risks in perspective. A scientific statement from the American Heart Association Council on nutrition, physical activity and metabolism and the Council on Clinical Cardiology. *Circulation.* 2007;115:2358-2368.
7. Chaves G, Turk-Adawi K, Supervia M, et al. Cardiac rehabilitation dose around the world: variation and correlates. *Circ Cardiovasc Qual Outcomes.* 2020;13:e005453.
8. Joo KC, Brubaker PH, MacDougall A, et al. Exercise prescription using resting heart rate plus 20 or perceived exertion in cardiac rehabilitation. *J Cardiopulm Rehabil.* 2004;24:178-186.
9. Sandercock G, Hurtado V, Cardoso F. Changes in cardiorespiratory fitness in cardiac rehabilitation patients: a meta-analysis. *Int J Cardiol.* 2013;167:894-902.
10. Oldridge NB, Guyatt GH, Fischer ME, et al. Cardiac rehabilitation after myocardial infarction: combined experience of randomized clinical trials. *JAMA.* 1988;260(7):945-950.
11. O'Connor GT, Buring JE, Yusuf S, et al. An overview of randomized trials of rehabilitation with exercise after myocardial infarction. *Circulation.* 1989;80:234-244.
12. Lawler PR, Filion KB, Eisenberg MJ. Efficacy of exercise-based cardiac rehabilitation post-myocardial infarction: a systematic review and meta-analysis of randomized controlled trials. *Am Heart J.* 2011;162(4):571-584.e2.
13. Heran BS, Chen JM, Ebrahim S, et al. Exercise-based cardiac rehabilitation for coronary heart disease. *Cochrane Database Syst Rev.* 2011;(7):CD001800.
14. Anderson L, Oldridge N, Thompson DR, et al. Exercise-based cardiac rehabilitation for coronary heart disease: Cochrane systematic review and meta-analysis. *J Am Coll Cardiol.* 2016;67:1-12.
15. van Halewijn G, Deckers J, Tay HY, et al. Lessons from contemporary trials of cardiovascular prevention and rehabilitation: a systematic review and meta-analysis. *Int J Cardiol.* 2017;232:294-303.

16. Huang R, Palmer SC, Cao Y, et al. Cardiac rehabilitation programs for chronic heart disease: a Bayesian network meta-analysis. *Can J Cardiol.* 2020;S0828-282X(20)30176-8. Published online ahead of print, February 19, 2020.

17. Kwan G, Balady GJ. Cardiac rehabilitation 2012: advancing the field through emerging science. *Circulation.* 2012;125:e369-e373.

18. Santiago de Araújo Pio C, Marzolini S, Pakosh M, Grace SL. Effect of cardiac rehabilitation dose on mortality and morbidity: a systematic review and meta-regression analysis. *Mayo Clin Proc.* 2017;92:1644-1659.

19. Hammill BG, Curtis LH, Schulman KA, Whellan DJ. Relationship between cardiac rehabilitation and long-term risks of death and myocardial infarction among elderly Medicare beneficiaries. *Circulation.* 2010;121:63-70.

20. Suaya JA, Stason WB, Ades PA, et al. Cardiac rehabilitation and survival in older coronary patients. *J Am Coll Cardiol.* 2009;54:25-33.

21. Kavanagh T, Mertens DJ, Hamm LF, et al. Prediction of long-term prognosis in 12,169 men referred for cardiac rehabilitation. *Circulation.* 2002;106:666-671.

22. Kavanagh T, Mertens DJ, Hamm LF, et al. Peak oxygen intake and cardiac mortality in women referred for cardiac rehabilitation. *J Am Coll Cardiol.* 2003;42:2139-2143.

23. Feuerstadt P, Chai A, Kligfield P. Submaximal effort tolerance as a predictor of all-cause mortality in patients undergoing cardiac rehabilitation. *Clin Cardiol.* 2007;30:234-238.

24. Martin BJ, Arena R, Haykowsky M, et al. Cardiovascular fitness and mortality after contemporary cardiac rehabilitation. *Mayo Clin Proc.* 2013;88:455-463.

25. Bouchard C, Rankinen T. Individual differences in response to regular physical activity. *Med Sci Sports Exerc.* 2001;33(6 Suppl):S446-S453.

26. Sisson SB, Katzmarzyk PT, Earnest CP, et al. Volume of exercise and fitness nonresponse in sedentary, postmenopausal women. *Med Sci Sports Exerc.* 2009;41:539-545.

27. Savage PD, Antkowiak M, Ades PA. Failure to improve cardiopulmonary fitness in cardiac rehabilitation. *J Cardiopulm Rehabil Prev.* 2009;29:284-293.

28. De Schutter A, Kachur S, Lavie CJ, et al. Cardiac rehabilitation fitness changes and subsequent survival. *Eur Heart J Qual Care Clin Outcomes.* 2018;4:173-179.

29. Ross R, de Lannoy L, Stotz PJ. Separate effects of intensity and amount of exercise on interindividual cardiorespiratory fitness response. *Mayo Clin Proc.* 2015;90:1506-1514.

30. Hannan AL, Hing W, Simas V, et al. High-intensity interval training versus moderate-intensity continuous training within cardiac rehabilitation: a systematic review and meta-analysis. *Open Access J Sports Med.* 2018;9:1-17.

31. Wewege MA, Ahn D, Yu J et al. High-intensity interval training for patients with cardiovascular disease—is it safe? A systematic review. *J Am Heart Assoc.* 2018;7:e009305.

32. Taylor RS, Walker S, Smart NA, et al. Impact of exercise rehabilitation on exercise capacity and quality-of-life in heart failure: individual participant meta-analysis. *J Am Coll Cardiol.* 2019;73:1430-1443.

33. Taylor RS, Long L, Mordi IR, et al. Exercise-based rehabilitation for heart failure: Cochrane systematic review, meta-analysis, and trial sequential analysis. *JACC Heart Fail.* 2019;7:691-705.

34. O'Connor CM, Whellan DJ, Lee KL, et al. Efficacy and safety of exercise training in patients with chronic heart failure: HF-ACTION randomized controlled trial. *JAMA.* 2009;301:1439-1450.

35. Swank AM, Horton J, Fleg JL, et al. Modest increase in peak VO$_2$ is related to better clinical outcomes in chronic heart failure patients: results from heart failure and a controlled trial to investigate outcomes of exercise training. *Circ Heart Fail.* 2012;5:579-585.

36. Tabet JY, Meurin P, Beauvais F, et al. Absence of exercise capacity improvement after exercise training program: a strong prognostic factor in patients with chronic heart failure. *Circ Heart Fail.* 2008;1:220-226.

37. Bakker EA, Snoek JA, Meindersma EP, et al. Absence of fitness improvement is associated with outcomes in heart failure patients. *Med Sci Sports Exerc.* 2018;50:196-203.

38. Ismail H, McFarlane JR, Nojoumian AH, et al. Clinical outcomes and cardiovascular responses to different exercise training intensities in patients with heart failure: a systematic review and meta-analysis. *JACC Heart Fail.* 2013; 1:514-522.

39. Rozanski A, Blumenthal JA, Davidson KW, et al. The epidemiology, pathophysiology, and management of psychosocial risk factors in cardiac practice: the emerging field of behavioral cardiology. *J Am Coll Cardiol.* 2005;45:637-651.

40. Bush DE, Ziegelstein RC, Tayback M, et al. Even minimal symptoms of depression increase mortality risk after acute myocardial infarction. *Am J Cardiol.* 2001;88:337-341.

41. Rozanski A. Exercise as medical treatment for depression. *J Am Coll Cardiol.* 2012;60:1064-1066.

42. Blumenthal JA, Sherwood A, Babyak MA, et al. Exercise and pharmacological treatment of depressive symptoms in patients with coronary heart disease: results from the UPBEAT (Understanding the Prognostic Benefits of Exercise and Antidepressant Therapy) study. *J Am Coll Cardiol.* 2012;60:1053-1063.

43. Cooney GM, Dwan K, Greig CA, et al. Exercise for depression. *Cochrane Database Syst Rev.* 2013;(9):CD004366.

44. Schuch FB, Vancampfort D, Richards J, et al. Exercise as a treatment for depression: a meta-analysis adjusting for publication bias. *J Psych Res.* 2016;77:42-51.

45. Gordon BR, McDowell CP, Hallgren M, et al. Association of efficacy of resistance exercise training with depressive symptoms: meta-analysis and meta-regression analysis of randomized clinical trials. *JAMA Psych.* 2018;75:566-576.

46. Herring MP, O'Connor PJ, Dishman RK. The effects of exercise training on anxiety symptoms among patients. A systemic review. *Arch Intern Med.* 2010; 170:321-331.

47. Zheng X, Zheng Y, Ma J, et al. Effect of exercise-based cardiac rehabilitation on anxiety and depression in patients with myocardial infarction: a systematic review and meta-analysis. *Heart Lung.* 2019;48:1-7.

48. Tu RH, Zeng ZY, Zhong GQ, et al. Effects of exercise training on depression in patients with heart failure: a systematic review and meta-analysis of randomized controlled trials. *Eur J Heart Fail.* 2014;16:749-757.

49. Das A, Roy B, Schwarzer et al. Comparison of treatment options for depression in heart failure: a network meta-analysis. *J Psych Res.* 2019;108: 7-23.

50. Milani RV, Lavie CJ. Impact of cardiac rehabilitation on depression and its associated mortality. *Am J Med.* 2007;120:799-806.

51. Smith PJ, Sherwood A, Mabe S, et al. Physical activity and psychosocial function following cardiac rehabilitation: One-year follow-up of the ENHANCED study. *Gen Hosp Psych.* 2017;49:32-36.

52. Blumenthal JA, Sherwood A, Smith PJ, et al. Enhancing cardiac rehabilitation with stress management training: a randomized, clinical efficacy trial. *Circulation.* 2016;133:1341-1350.

53. Rozanski A. Behavioral cardiology: current advances and future directions. *J Am Coll Cardiol.* 2014;64:100-110.

54. Mohammadi N, Aghayousefi A, Nikrhan GR, et al. A randomized trial of optimism training internvention in patients with heart disease. *Gen Hosp Psych.* 2018;51: 46-53.

55. Kabboul NN, Tomlinson G, Francis TA, et al. Comparative effectiveness of the core components of cardiac rehabilitation on mortality and morbidity: a systematic review and network meta-analysis. *J Clin Med.* 2018; 7:514. doi:10.3390/jcm7120514.

56. Beatty AL, Truong M, Schopfer DW, Shen J, Bachman JM, Whooley MA. Geographical variation in cardiac rehabilitation participation in Medicare and Veterans Affairs populations. Opportunity for improvement. *Circulation.* 2018;137:1899-1908.

57. Balady GJ, Ades PH, Bittner VA, et al. Referral, enrollment, and delivery of cardiac rehabilitation/secondary prevention programs at clinical centers and beyond: a presidential advisory from the American Heart Association. *Circulation.* 2011;124:2951-2960.

58. Ruano-Ravina A, Pena-Gil C, Abu-Assi E, et al. Participation and adherence to cardiac rehabilitation programs. A systematic review. *Int J Cardiol.* 2016;223:436-443.

59. Thomas RJ, Beatty AL, Beckie TM, et al. Home-based cardiac rehabilitation: a scientific statement from the American Association of Cardiovascular and Pulmonary Rehabilitation, the American Heart Association, and the American College of Cardiology. *J Am Coll Cardiol.* 2019;74:133-153.

60. Grace SL, Russell KL, Reid RD, et al. Effect of cardiac rehabilitation referral strategies on utilization rates: a prospective, controlled study. *Arch Intern Med.* 2011;171:235-241.

61. Farah M, Abdallah M, Szalai H, et al. Association between patient cost sharing and cardiac rehabilitation adherence. *Mayo Clin Proc.* 2019;94:2390-2398.

62. Buckingham SA, Taylor RS, Jolly K, et al. Home-based versus centre-based cardiac rehabilitation: abridged Cochrane systematic review and meta-analysis. *Open Heart.* 2016;3(2):e000463.

63. Xia TL, Huang FY, Peng Y, et al. Efficacy of different types of exercise-based cardiac rehabilitation on coronary heart disease: a network meta-analysis. *J Gen Intern Med.* 2018;33:2201-2209.

SECTION IV

DISEASES OF THE GREAT VESSELS AND PERIPHERAL VESSELS

Diseases of the Aorta

John A. Elefteriades, Bulat A. Ziganshin, and Jonathan L. Halperin

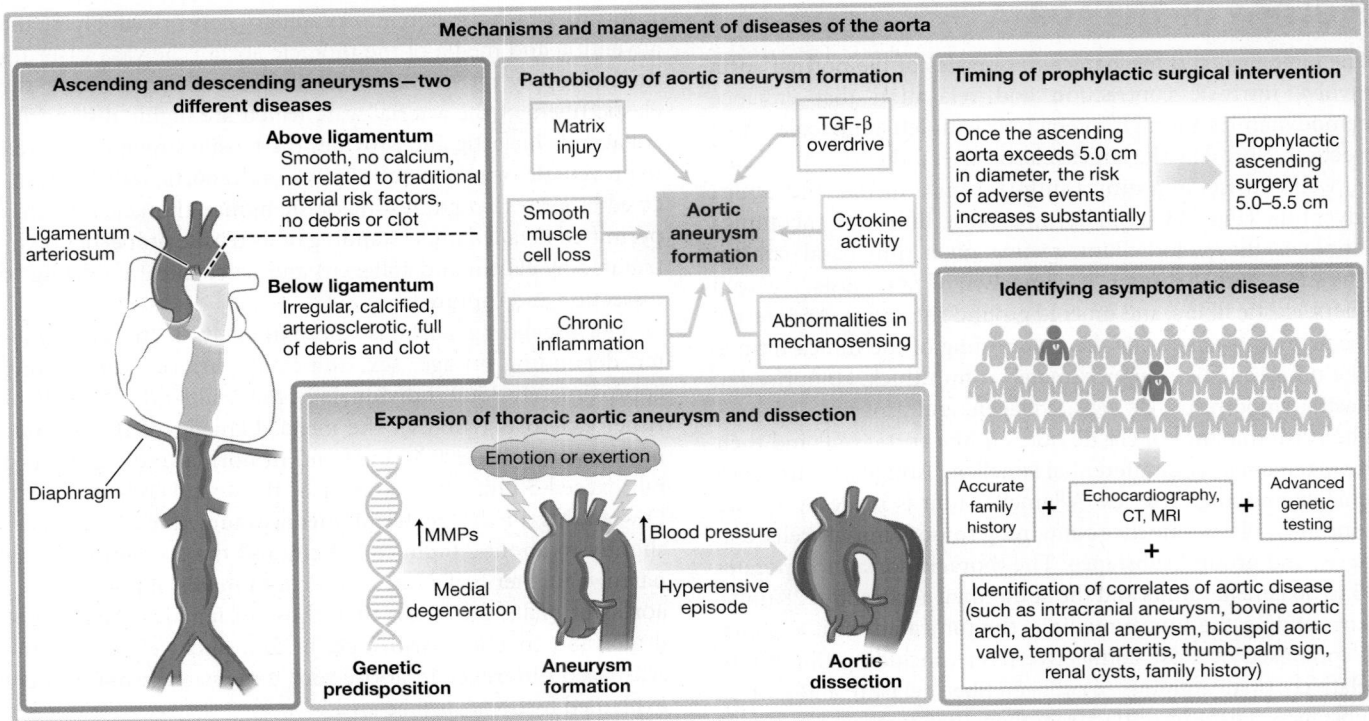

Chapter 23 Fuster and Hurst's Central Illustration. Thoracic aortic aneurysms should be considered as two different diseases, separated by the ligamentum arteriosum. Major mechanisms of aortic aneurysm formation and expansion and progression to aortic dissection are shown. Identification of patients with asymptomatic aortic aneurysm is important to prevent death due to rupture or dissection.

CHAPTER SUMMARY

This chapter discusses the pathophysiology, diagnosis, and management of diseases of the aorta, including both aortic aneurysm and dissection, from the aortic valve to aortic bifurcation. Aneurysmal disease differs between the ascending portion and the descending and thoracoabdominal segments (see Fuster and Hurst's Central Illustration). Genetically mediated degeneration of the aortic wall results in disruption of the normally uniform pattern of regularly spaced aortic lamellae, leading to fluid-filled lacunae and decreased aortic strength. Aneurysmal dilatation ensues. Monitoring by echocardiography, computed tomography (CT), or magnetic resonance imaging (MRI) is recommended. Surgical repair is recommended in patients with symptomatic or rapidly expanding aneurysms or at aortic diameters >5.5 cm. Thresholds for intervention are lower in patients with certain genetic conditions/syndromes. Whole exome sequencing is recommended for affected individuals, and first-order relatives should undergo screening for thoracic aortic aneurysms. Adult male smokers and former smokers should undergo screening for abdominal aortic aneurysm. Aortic dissection occurs catastrophically without premonitory symptoms, often precipitated by conditions that raise blood pressure and hemodynamic stress acting on an enlarged aorta. Urgent surgery is required for ascending (Type A) aortic dissections. Descending (Type B) dissections can usually be managed medically. Endovascular approaches are increasingly employed as alternatives to open surgical repair, but they carry a risk of endoleak, requiring postprocedural imaging surveillance.

BIOLOGY OF THE AORTA

The biological and mechanical properties of the normal aorta involve intrinsic contraction and relaxation that enhance hemodynamics through interaction with left ventricular (LV) ejection. Normally the largest elastic artery, the trilaminar aortic wall consists of a tunica intima, tunica media, and tunica adventitia (**Fig. 23–1**). The innermost lining of the tunica intima is the endothelium, resting on a thin basal lamina. The subendothelial tissue is comprised of fibroblasts, collagen fibers, elastic fibers, and mucoid ground substance. An internal elastic membrane forms the outer lining of the tunica intima. The tunica media is approximately 1 mm thick, comprised of elastin, smooth muscle cells, collagen, and ground substance. The predominance of elastic fibers in the aortic wall and their arrangement as circumferential lamellae distinguish it from the smaller muscular arteries. A lamellar unit is made up of two concentric elastic lamellae containing smooth muscle cells, collagen, and ground substance. The thoracic aorta incorporates 35 to 56 lamellar units and the abdominal aorta about 28 units. Surrounding the tunica media is the tunica adventitia, which is composed of loose connective tissue, including fibroblasts, relatively small amounts of collagen fibers, elastin, and ground substance. The adventitia strengthens the aorta and is essential to aortic surgeons for secure suturing of tissues. Within the tunica adventitia lie the nervi vasorum and vasa vasorum. The arteries arising along the course of the aorta give rise to the vasa

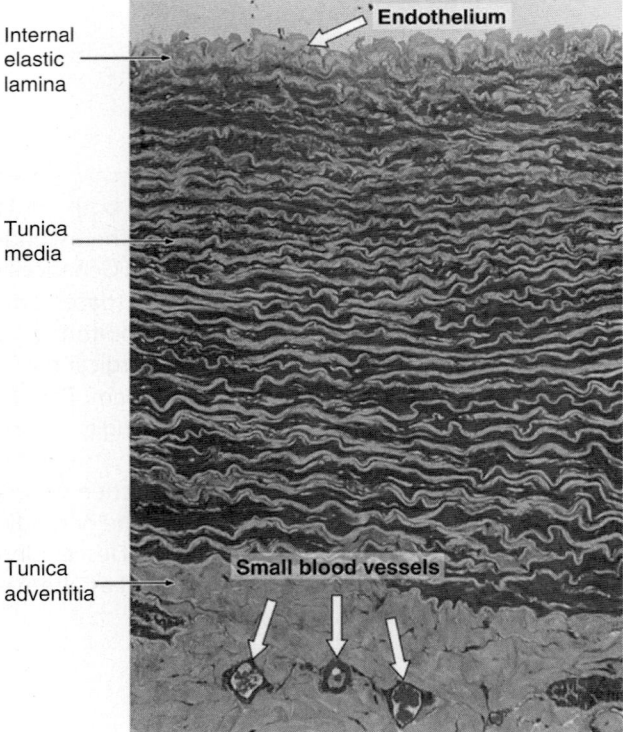

Figure 23–1. Transverse section of the wall of a large elastic artery demonstrating the well-developed tunica media containing elastic lamellae. Pararosaniline–toluidine blue stain; medium magnification. Reproduced with permission from Junqueira LC, Carneiro J. *Basic Histology: Text and Atlas*, 11th ed. New York, NY: McGraw Hill; 2005.

vasorum, which develop into a capillary network supplying the adventitia and media of the thoracic aorta. The vasa vasorum do not supply the media of the abdominal aorta. Unlike the elastic fibers of the arterial wall, which are highly distensible, collagen is inelastic and provides the tensile strength required to prevent deformation and rupture of the aortic wall. Sophisticated bi-axial strength testing of the human thoracic aorta has permitted detailed understanding of its tensile properties (contributed by elastin and collagen) and mechanical modeling of dissection and rupture.[1,2]

The ascending aorta is approximately 3 cm in diameter, depending on age, sex, and body surface area. Among approximately 3500 individuals in the Multi-Ethnic Study of Atherosclerosis (MESA), the mean diameter of the ascending aorta was 3.2 ± 0.4 cm,[3,4] and in normal individuals did not exceed 5 cm. The diameter of the aortic arch is similar. Descending in the posterior mediastinum, the aorta tapers slightly to about 2.0 cm to 2.3 cm and the abdominal aorta narrows further to 1.7 cm to 1.9 cm in its distal portion. The aortas of males are larger than those of females. Aortic root dimension increases with age, height, and weight, but the sex-based difference in aortic root dimension is not entirely explained by body surface area.

Hemodynamic Function of the Aorta

The force of LV ejection creates a pressure wave that traverses the aorta, producing radial expansion and contraction of the wall. Potential energy derived from myocardial contraction and stored in the aortic wall during systole is transformed during diastolic recoil into kinetic energy, which drives blood into the peripheral vessels. The pressure wave is conducted at a velocity of approximately 5 m/s, increasing in amplitude along its course through the aorta. Forward blood flow in the aorta begins when the aortic valve opens, and systolic pressure increases as the pressure wave courses along the length of the aorta. Flow velocity increases rapidly to a peak and then gradually decreases. With aortic valve closure, there is transient backward flow before forward flow resumes during diastole, particularly in the descending thoracic and abdominal aorta, albeit at considerably less than systolic velocity. The incisura in the arterial waveform in the proximal portion of the thoracic aorta gradually disappears and is usually absent in the abdominal aorta.

Changes with Aging and Disease

Each of the four components of the aortic wall—elastic tissue, collagen fibers, smooth muscle cells, and mucoid ground substance—change with age (**Fig. 23–2**). Elastic fibers fragment, collagen content increases at the expense of smooth muscle cells, and glycosaminoglycans accumulate. As a result, the aorta becomes less distensible, reducing its capacity to absorb the forces derived from LV contraction. The increased stiffness of the aortic wall with aging contributes to hypertension.[5] Concurrently, weakening of the aortic wall leads to dilation of the lumen and elongation and uncoiling of the aortic arch, collectively producing ectasia. Accompanying these changes are alterations in aortic wall structure, fragmentation

Labels on Figure 23–1: Internal elastic lamina; Endothelium; Tunica media; Tunica adventitia; Small blood vessels

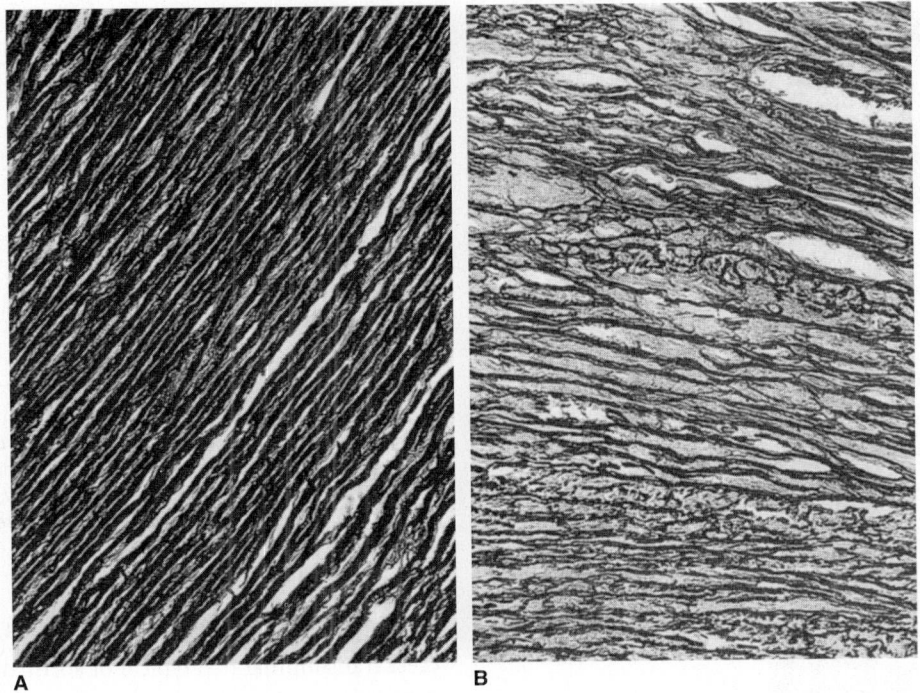

Figure 23-2. Histology of the normal aorta of a child (A) and an elderly adult (B). With aging, elastic fibers fragment, collagen becomes more prominent, smooth muscle cells diminish, and acid mucopolysaccharide ground substance accumulates. Weakening of the aortic wall leads to dilatation of the lumen as well as elongation and uncoiling of the aortic arch. Orcein and van Gieson stain, magnification ×414. Reproduced with permission from Nichols WW, O'Rourke MF, McDonald DA. *McDonald's blood flow in arteries: theoretic, experimental, and clinical principles*, 3rd ed. Philadelphia, PA: Taylor & Francis Group; 1990.

of elastic fibers, loss of smooth muscle cell nuclei (medionecrosis), accumulation of collagenous tissue, and deposition of basophilic ground substance.

When the aorta dilates due to disease of the medial layer, wall stress increases. This is accelerated by hypertension, particularly when pulsatile forces are high. When peripheral vascular resistance is high, the impact of the reflected pressure wave adds to that of antegrade pulsatile flow. The combination of inherited, degenerative, mechanical, and hemodynamic factors adversely affects the medial layer of the aortic wall, leading to dilation and setting the stage for the catastrophes of dissection or rupture.

DEFINITIONS AND CATEGORIES

The aorta can be affected by a variety of pathologic processes leading to *aneurysm*, *dissection*, or *ischemic* syndromes (**Fig. 23-3A**). The term *aneurysm*, derived from the Greek *aneurysma* referring to dilation, is distinguished from *ectasia*, which refers to the modest generalized dilation and elongation of the aorta that occurs with aging. Although the size of the normal aorta varies with gender and body size, most agree that the maximum diameter of the normal thoracic aorta does not exceed 4 cm. For the abdominal aorta, which normally has a smaller diameter than the thoracic segments, aneurysmal dilation refers to diameters exceeding 3 cm or more than 1.5 to 2 times normal.

Aneurysms may be classified according to morphology, location, or etiology. In *true* aneurysms, the wall of the aneurysm is composed of the normal histologic components of the aorta. A *false* aneurysm or *pseudoaneurysm*, on the other hand, represents a contained rupture in which the wall is a fibrous peel around a small perforation, initially controlled by adherence of surrounding tissue and gradually enlarging over time.

A gross morphologic classification distinguishes true aneurysms as *fusiform* (most common) or *saccular*. A fusiform aneurysm is roughly cylindrical and affects the entire circumference of the aorta; a saccular aneurysm is an outpouching of only a portion of the aortic circumference. Frequently, a small neck provides continuity between the aortic lumen and the saccular aneurysm. For aortic aneurysms of specific etiology and diameter, the risk of rupture is generally greater for saccular than for fusiform aneurysms.

Aortic dissection refers to splitting of the medial layer of the aortic wall, permitting longitudinal propagation of blood between the components of aortic wall (**Fig. 23-3B**). Aortic dissection is the most common lethal form of aortic disease. *Atherosclerosis of the aorta* can narrow the ostia of branch vessels or produce mobile atheromatous masses capable of embolism to the brain or other organs and resulting ischemic syndromes.

Several additional types of artic pathology are illustrated in **Fig. 23-4**. *Acute aortic transection*, a consequence of trauma, involves localized disruption of an intrinsically normal aortic wall, which is resistant to propagating dissection. A *ruptured* aortic aneurysm is self-explanatory. *Acute aortic dissection* refers to separation of the layers of the aortic wall. *Intramural hematoma* represents a concentric, circumferentially oriented

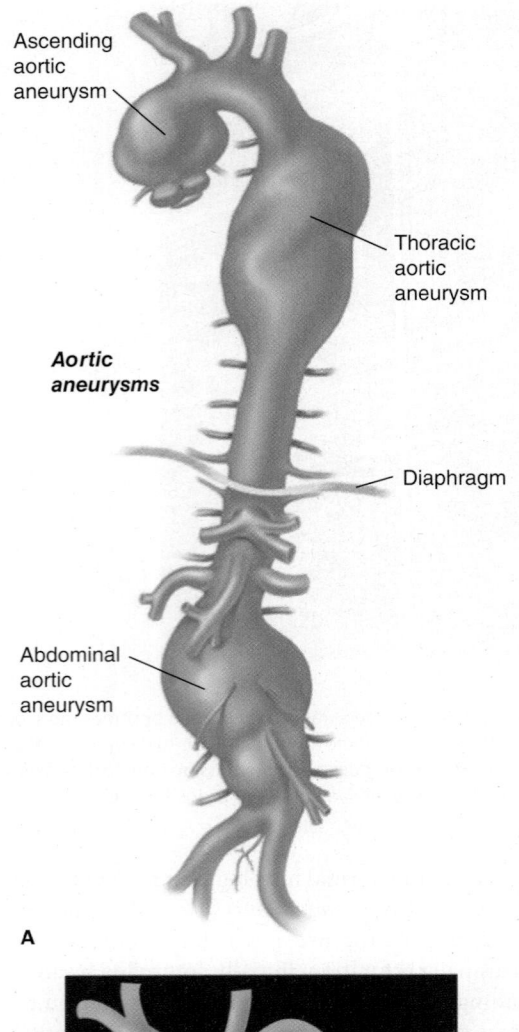

Ascending aortic aneurysm

Thoracic aortic aneurysm

Aortic aneurysms

Diaphragm

Abdominal aortic aneurysm

A

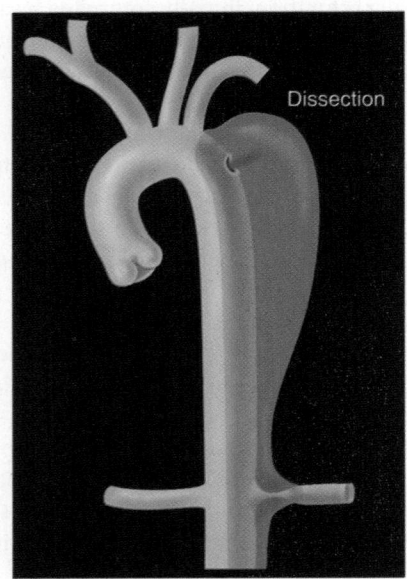

Dissection

B

Figure 23–3. Artist's rendition of aortic aneurysms at various locations (A) and type B aortic dissection (B).

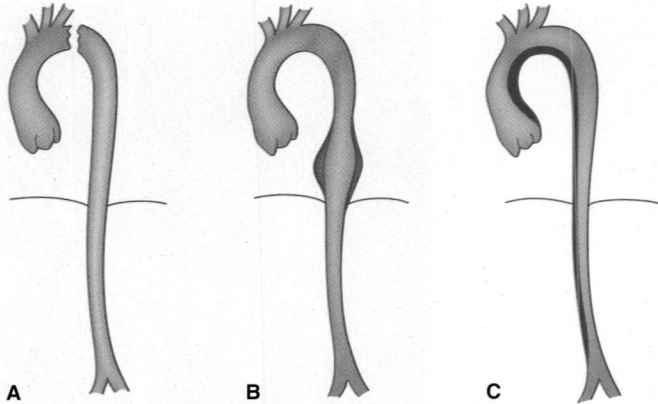

A   B   C

Figure 23–4. Three commonly confused aortic disorders. (A) Acute aortic transection. (B) Degenerative aneurysm of the descending aorta. (C) Type A acute aortic dissection. Reproduced with permissionfrom Elefteriades JA, Geha AS, Cohen LS. *House Officer Guide to ICU Care*. Raven Press; 1994.

collection of thrombi within the aortic wall, without the discrete transluminal flap typical of aortic dissection. *Penetrating aortic ulcer* involves localized perforation of the medial layer of the aortic wall beneath an atherosclerotic plaque.

Aortic aneurysms may also be classified according to the segment involved as thoracic, thoracoabdominal, or abdominal. Aneurysm formation can involve a greater portion of the aorta (**Fig. 23–5**) than obstructive atherosclerotic disease, potentially affecting almost the entire vessel, while atherosclerotic obstruction tends to involve mainly the descending thoracic and abdominal portions of the aorta, when the iliac arteries are often affected as well. Dilation of the aorta may occur as a consequence of atherosclerosis, aging, infection, inflammation, trauma, congenital anomalies, medial degeneration, or combinations of pathologic states. These conditions may cause the aorta to thicken, thin, bulge, tear, rupture, narrow, dissect, or be altered by combinations of these conditions.

With normal aging, degenerative changes occur throughout the aorta, leading to a mild form of *cystic medial necrosis*, in which the normal lamellar structure of the media is disrupted, leaving lakes of amorphous material. Although essentially a normal physiologic process, cystic medial necrosis develops more rapidly in patients with bicuspid aortic valve, during pregnancy, and very markedly in people with Marfan syndrome. Cystic medial necrosis is the most common cause of ascending aortic aneurysms, and although this type of aortic pathology is typical of patients with Marfan syndrome, it may also occur in the absence of other clinical stigmata. The mechanism by which the medial layer of the aorta is subject to this accelerated degeneration is a subject of active molecular genetic investigation. Severe elastic fiber degeneration, necrosis of muscle cells, and cystic spaces filled with mucoid material are most often encountered in the ascending aorta from just above the aortic valve to the brachiocephalic (innominate) artery. Because of accompanying dilation of the aortic root, aortic regurgitation may be a secondary feature, although the valve leaflets themselves are histologically unaffected.

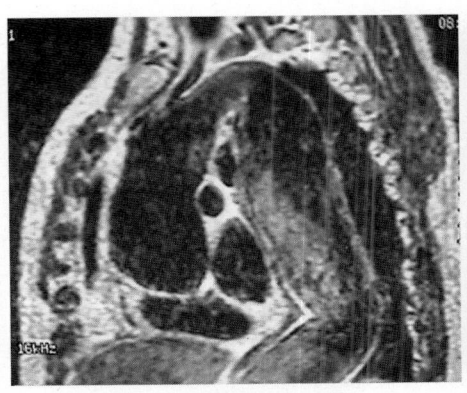 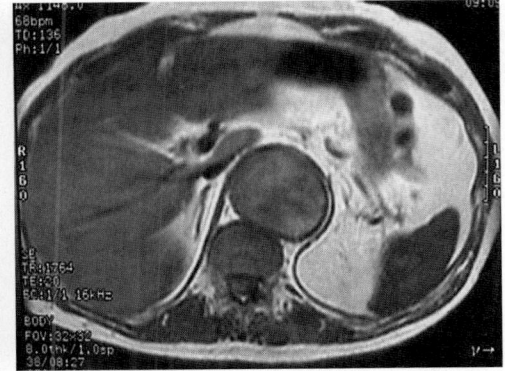

Figure 23–5. **MRI demonstrating aneurysm of the entire aorta viewed in the sagittal thoracic and axial abdominal views.** Reproduced with permission from Elefteriades JA. Thoracic aortic aneurysm: reading the enemy's playbook. *Curr Probl Cardiol.* 2008 May;33(5):203-277.

ETIOLOGY AND PATHOPHYSIOLOGY OF AORTIC ANEURYSMS

Diverse molecular mechanisms contribute to histological disruption of the aortic wall, with disorganization and loss of the lamellar components of the media, and development of fluid-filled cystic spaces within the disrupted lamellar layers.

(**Fig. 23–6**). These mechanisms raise the potential for pharmacologic therapy to prevent aneurysm development.

Up-Regulation of Transforming Growth Factor Beta

Up-regulation of transforming growth factor beta (TGF-β) signaling pathways and interactions with the renin-angiotensin system (RAS) have been implicated in the pathogenesis of

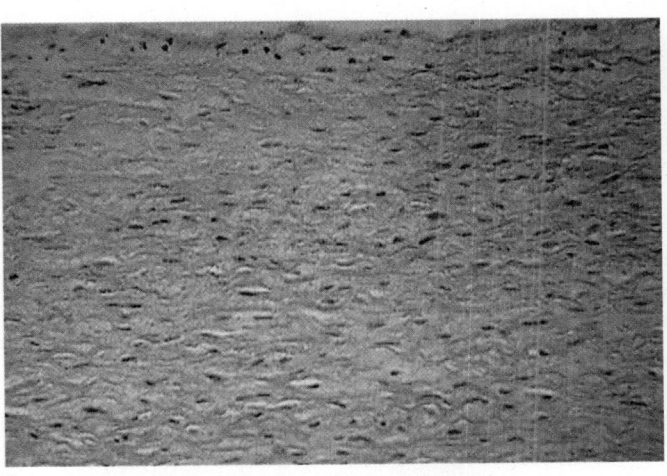 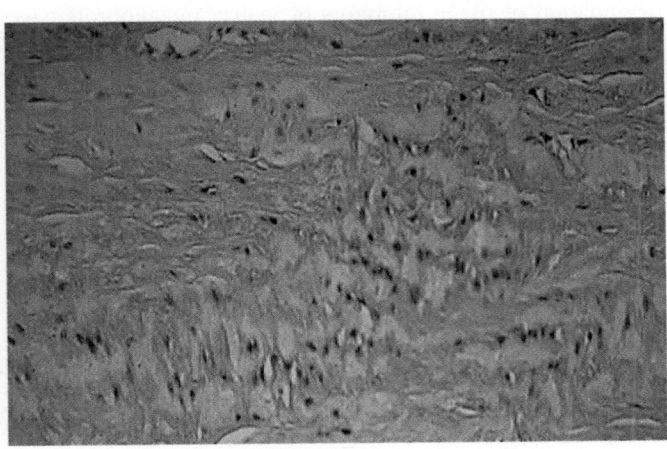

A   B

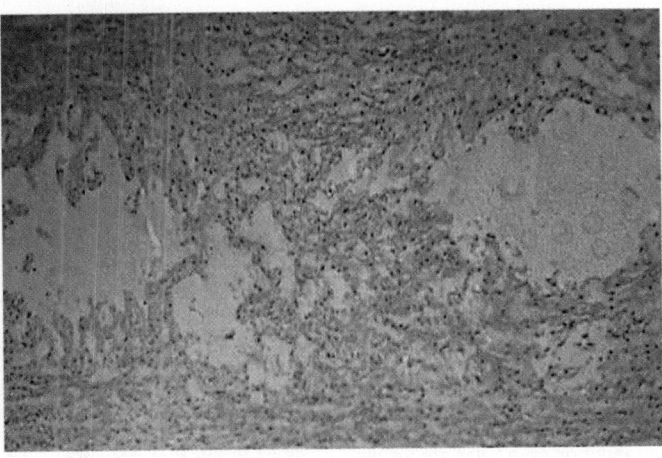

C

Figure 23–6. **Cystic medial necrosis of progressive severity (A to C).** Blood gaining access to one of the cystic spaces through a defect in the intimal layer of the aortic wall can propagate longitudinally along the aorta, initiating dissection.

thoracic aortic aneurysms (TAAs), especially in patients with Marfan syndrome.[6,7] The TGF-β axis regulates several aspects of cell growth, differentiation, and death and plays a pivotal role in extracellular matrix homeostasis. Angiotensin-II receptor blocking drugs inhibit these pathways and may slow the progression of aneurysmal disease. Some aspects of the role of TGF-β in regulation of aortic wall integrity are paradoxical, such as elevation of TGF-β signaling despite loss of function mutations, leaving the true pathologic importance of these pathways incompletely understood.[8]

Abnormalities in Mechanosensing and Transduction

The aortic wall has elaborate inherent mechanisms to respond to ambient blood pressure and remodel in response to mechanical stress.[9,10] Animal and clinical investigations support the view that normal mechanosensory mechanisms that protect the aortic wall from hemodynamic stress become disrupted in certain inherited diseases, representing an important pathway in the pathogenesis and progression of TAAs.

MMP/TIMP Dysregulation

Excess accumulation of matrix metalloproteinases (MMP) and degradation of tissue inhibitors of matrix metalloproteinases (TIMPs) have been implicated in the pathogenesis of TAAs.[11,12] As a result, the aortic wall undergoes net protein degradation, resulting in loss of mechanical integrity (**Fig. 23–7**).

Four main pathophysiologic mechanisms underlying aortic degeneration have been described: proteolysis of the extracellular matrix, inflammation, cytokine activity, and loss of smooth muscle cells (**Fig. 23–8**). After genetic mutations establish the propensity for aneurysm development, lytic MMP enzymes degrade the structural proteins of the aortic wall, leading to aneurysm formation and dissection (**Fig. 23–9**). These enzymes are normally regulated by TIMPs, which antagonize the lytic action of MMPs. An uncertain proportion of patients with aortic aneurysms manifest excessive MMP activity, which

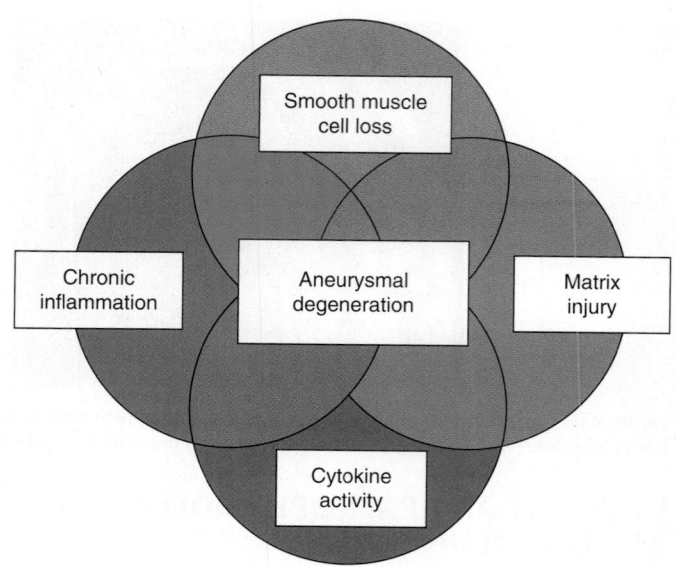

Figure 23–8. Factors involved in the pathogenesis of aortic aneurysms. Reproduced with permission from Elefteriades JA. *Acute aortic disease*. New York, NY: Informa Healthcare; 2007.

can occur in cases of abdominal aortic aneurysms, as well as in cases of ascending aortic aneurysms and aortic dissection. Several dozen specific MMP enzymes and certain TIMPs have been implicated in the pathogenesis of aneurysmal disease.

In addition to proteolysis of the extracellular matrix, the pathogenesis of aortic aneurysms involves inflammation, cytokine activity, and loss of smooth muscle cells. Together, these processes set the stage for aneurysm formation, growth, and rupture. Inflammatory cells participate in the genesis of aneurysms. Smooth muscle cells of the aortic wall normally exhibit reparative properties, and substantial (~75%) reduction

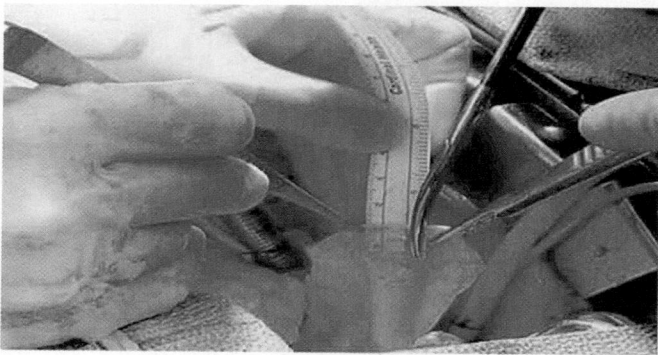

Figure 23–7. The proteins in the wall of this ascending aortic aneurysm were degraded, presumably by MMP–related activity, to the extent that the aortic wall became so thin that the markings on a ruler are visible through the aortic wall.

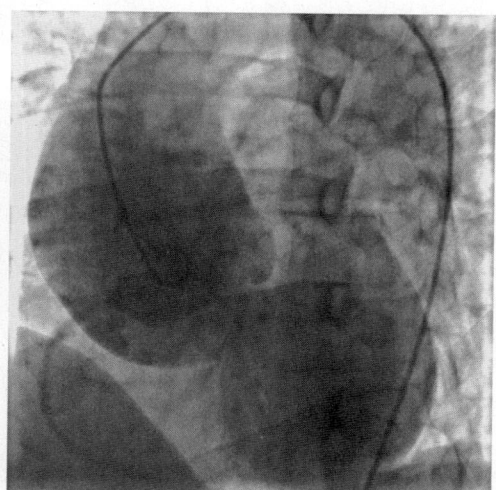

Figure 23–9. Aortogram of a patient with Marfan syndrome. Aortic aneurysms in this disorder are characterized by annuloaortic ectasia involving the sinuses of Valsalva and the ascending aorta produced by degeneration of elastic fibers and the accumulation of mucoid material within the medial layer of the aortic wall, grossly resembling cystic medial necrosis.

in the number of smooth muscle cells in the walls of abdominal aortic aneurysms impairs this function. Aneurysmal smooth muscle cells display a 3-fold increase in apoptosis and impaired growth capacity. Figure 23–8 illustrates the interaction of proteolysis, inflammation, cytokine activation, and deficient smooth muscle cell function in the pathophysiology of aneurysm formation.

Extrinsic Causes of Aortic Aneurysms

Certain extrinsic factors, including the effects of pharmacological agents, have been linked with aortic aneurysm development and dissection. Data from population-based studies and meta-analyses suggest an association between use of fluoroquinolone antibiotics, disclosing a more than double risk of aortic aneurysms and dissection.[13-16]

INHERITED FORMS OF AORTIC ANEURYSMS

TAAs are considered *syndromic* when associated with abnormalities of other organ systems; and *nonsyndromic,* when manifestations are restricted to the aorta. Syndromic cases constitute less than 5% of all patients with thoracic aortic disease, but include Marfan, Loeys-Dietz, Ehlers-Danlos, aneurysm-osteoarthritis, arterial tortuosity, or cutis laxa syndromes, or involve mutations affecting the TGF-β pathway. Approximately 20% of cases of nonsyndromic TAAs are familial; the remainder are sporadic forms.[17-20]

Marfan Syndrome

This inherited disorder, described in 1896, is characterized by dolichostenomelia (long, thin extremities), ligamentous redundancy or laxity, ectopia lentis, ascending aortic dilation, and incompetence of the aortic or mitral valves, or both.[21] According to the Universal Mutation Database,[21] more than 1800 specific mutations in the *FBN1* gene have been identified as potentially causative of Marfan syndrome. Diagnosis is established largely on clinical grounds using the 2010 Revised Ghent criteria summarized in **Table 23–1**.[22] The syndrome is linked to an autosomal dominant anomaly in the genes regulating synthesis of fibrillin type 1 (*FBN1*, chromosome 15), a large glycoprotein that directs and orients elastin in the developing aorta. Marfan syndrome was widely attributed to structural abnormalities and weaknesses of the aortic wall until dysregulation of TGF-β signaling was identified as a correlate.[23,24] TGF-β controls a panoply of cell functions. As fibrillin 1 binds TGF-β in an inactive complex, increased TGF-β signaling develops as a compensatory mechanism and plays a role in the degeneration of elastic fibers, accumulation of mucoid material within the medial layer of the aortic wall and accelerated cystic medial necrosis that characterize this disease.

In patients with the Marfan syndrome, the aortic root tends to enlarge in fusiform fashion in association with aortic valve regurgitation, and about half of patients also have mitral insufficiency (Fig. 23–9). Aneurysms characteristically involve the sinuses of Valsalva and the tubular portion of the ascending aorta, producing annuloaortic ectasia (**Fig. 23–10**). Over time, abnormalities associated with Marfan syndrome typically affect the entire length of the aorta, although dissection most often involves the thoracic portion (especially the ascending aorta).

Ehlers-Danlos Syndrome

Ehlers-Danlos syndrome, first described separately by Edvard Ehlers in Denmark and Henri-Alexandre Danlos in France, is an inherited connective tissue disorder less frequent than Marfan syndrome but also associated with aneurysm formation. While aortic aneurysms and dissections may occur in most types of Ehlers-Danlos syndrome, they are more frequent in the vascular type (Type IV), which results from a mutation of the *COL3A1* gene encoding type III collagen. It is an autosomal dominant disorder with a prevalence of 1 in 10,000 to 25,000 individuals. Sequencing analysis has identified mainly missense mutations in the *COL3A1* gene in 98% of patients diagnosed with Ehlers-Danlos syndrome. Patients with Ehlers-Danlos syndrome present with an initial major medical complication at an average age of 23 years, and the mean age at death is 48 years.[25] Three characteristic clinical features are typical: (1) cutaneous manifestations of thin, translucent skin and easy bruising, (2) visceral manifestations of intestinal or uterine rupture, and (3) arterial aneurysms or dissection.

Loeys-Dietz Syndrome

Loeys-Dietz syndrome is associated with aortic and arterial aneurysms that enlarge rapidly and are prone to rupture. Clinically, it is characterized by hypertelorism (widely spaced eyes), a bifid uvula or cleft palate, arterial tortuosity, and aortic aneurysms, although some patients exhibit features that meet the diagnostic criteria for Marfan syndrome. Loeys-Dietz syndrome is characterized by rapid early onset of TAAs and an early age of death averaging 26 years. Stratification of subtypes is based on delineation of causative genes: Type 1–*TGFBR1*, Type 2–*TGFBR2*, Type 3–*SMAD3*, Type 4–*TGFB2*, Type 5–*TGFB3*, and Type 6–*SMAD2*,[26] with Types 1 and 2 responsible for 75% to 85% of cases. Patients with Loeys-Dietz syndrome and Marfan syndrome have similar degrees of aortic involvement; in both syndromes aortic dilatation affects approximately 80% of patients, and the rate of aortic dissection is similar, as are the age and proportion of patients requiring thoracic aortic surgery.

Aortopathy Associated with Bicuspid Aortic Valve

Patients with congenital bicuspid aortic valve (BAV) have structural abnormalities of the ascending aorta predisposing to aneurysms and dissections. Some have aortic coarctation as well. Aneurysmal enlargement of the aorta in patients with BAV may occur independent of valvular stenosis or regurgitation and is not, therefore, predominantly a consequence of poststenotic dilation, although the aorta expands more rapidly when valvular dysfunction is present. While the embryology has been elucidated in animal models, genetic mutations responsible for human BAV are complex and multifactorial;

TABLE 23–1. Quick Guide to Diagnosis of Marfan Disease

	Cardiovascular	Skeletal System	Ocular System	Pulmonary System	Skin and Integument	Dura	Family History/ Genetics
Major criteria	One required:	Four required:	Ectopia entis	None	None	Dural ectasia	Parent, child, or sibling with Marfan disease
	Dilatation of Asc Ao(+ AI), involving sinuses of Valsalva	Pectus carinatum					FBN1 mutation
		Pectus excavatum (requiring surgery)					
	AAD	Reduced upper-to-lower segment ratio or increased arm span-to-height ratio					
		Positive wrist and thumb signs					
		Elbow extension reduced <170°					
		Pes planus					
		Protrusion acetabulae					
Minor criteria	MVP (± prolapse)	Pectus excavatum (moderate)	Flat corneas	Spontaneous pneumothorax	Striae	None	None
	Dilatation of the main PA (patients younger than 40 y)	Hypermobile joints	Increased axial length of globe	Apical blebs	Recurrent or incisional hernias		
		Crowding of teeth or highly arched palate	Hypoplastic iris or ciliary muscles, causing decreased meiosis				
Involvement (required to say organ system involved)	One major or one minor criterion	Two major or one major and one minor criteria	One major or two minor criteria	One minor criterion	One minor criterion	Major criterion	Major criterion

Diagnosis requires:
• For index case (without documented mutation)
  > Major criteria in two organ systems, plus
  > Involvement of another organ system
• For index case (with documented mutation)
  > Major criterion in one organ system, plus
  > Involvement of another organ system
• For a relative of a known case
  > Major criterion in the family history, plus
  > Major criterion in one organ system, plus
  > Involvement of another organ system
Definitions and reference ranges:
Upper-to-lower segment = Distance from top of head to symphysis pubis/distance symphysis pubis to floor (reference range, 0.89–0.95) arm span-to-height ratio (reference range <1.05).
Wrist sign = Positive if a person's thumb and little finger overlap when gripping own wrist.
Thumb sign = Positive if the entire nail of a person's thumb projects beyond the border of the hand when their fist is closed around the thumb.
Abbreviations: AAD, ascending aortic dissection; AI, aortic insufficiency; Ao, aorta; Asc, ascending; MVP, mitral valve prolapse; PA, pulmonary artery.
Data from Tsipouras P, Silverman DI. The genetic basis of aortic disease. Marfan syndrome and beyond. *Cardiol Clin*. 1999 Nov;17(4):683-696.

abnormalities in the *NOTCH1* gene have been documented in some patients with BAV. The *ROBO4* and *GATA4* genes have also been implicated in BAV with or without evident aortopathy.[27,28] Excess MMP activity has been demonstrated in both valve tissue and aortic wall of patients with BAV. Because bicuspid valves occur in ~2% of the population, the associated aortopathy is responsible for more cases of aortic dissection than Marfan syndrome (which affects 1 in 10,000 people) (**Table 23–2**). It is estimated that bicuspid valves account for more morbidity and mortality than all other congenital cardiac lesions combined. Some authorities believe that every individual with a BAV will eventually develop aortic stenosis, aortic

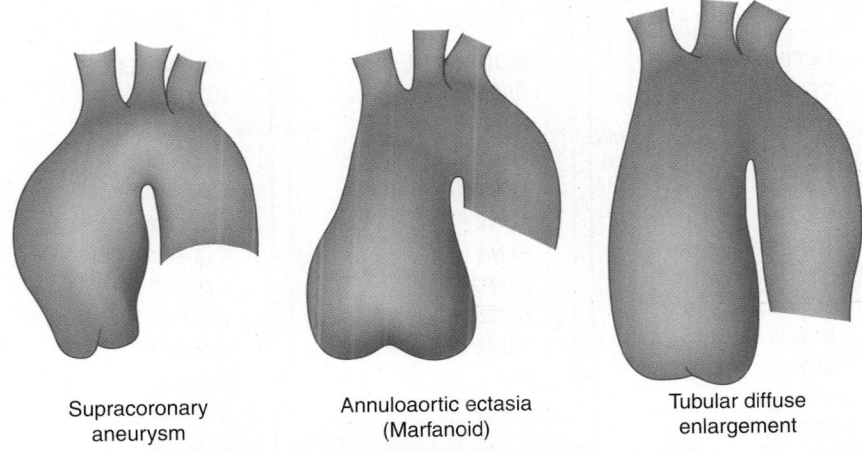

Supracoronary
aneurysm

Annuloaortic ectasia
(Marfanoid)

Tubular diffuse
enlargement

Figure 23–10. Three common patterns of ascending aortic aneurysmal disease: supracoronary, annuloaortic ectasia, and tubular.

insufficiency, aortic aneurysm, or dissection, but this is not a uniform view. Ascending aortic aneurysms in patients with BAV were once considered nearly as dangerous as ascending aortic aneurysms in patients with Marfan syndrome, and elective surgical intervention was offered earlier than in patients without BAVs. Recent consensus statements, however, recommended the same criteria for intervention as for those with trileaflet aortic valves, generally when the diameter of the ascending aorta reaches 5.5 cm.[29,30]

Familial Thoracic Aortic Aneurysms

Many cases of TAAs once classified as atherosclerotic, hypertensive, or idiopathic are now traced to hereditary metabolic abnormalities affecting the aortic wall. There is a family history of aneurysmal disease in 1 of 5 patients with aortic aneurysms. Probands with ascending aortic aneurysms are more likely to have family members with ascending aneurysms, and those with aneurysms involving the descending aorta are more likely to have family members with abdominal aneurysms. Although there are several patterns of inheritance, autosomal dominance with reduced penetrance predominates. Familial TAAs typically follow a more malignant course than sporadic TAAs, presenting at a younger age (mean 58 vs 66 years), and expanding more rapidly (2.1 vs 1.6 mm/year).

TABLE 23–2. Comparison of Epidemiology of Marfan Disease and Bicuspid Aortic Valve with Special Reference to Number of Cases of Aortic Dissection Brought on by Disease[a]

	Incidence	AAD Likelihood (Lifetime) (%)	AAD Caused (as % of Population) (%)
Marfan disease	1/10,000 (0.01%)	40	0.004
Bicuspid aortic valve	2/100 (2%)	5	0.1

Abbreviation: AAD, acute aortic dissection.
[a]Note that bicuspid aortic valve causes 25 times more acute aortic dissections than Marfan disease.

Genetic Testing in Patients with Thoracic Aortic Aneurysms

Approximately 1 in 5 patients with heritable forms of TAAs and dissection can be genetically explained.[31] Multiple genes have been linked with familial or syndromic TAAs and dissection, and the list of new causative genes continues to expand.[32] Functionally, these can be subdivided in to three main groups: (1) genes that encode proteins related to the extracellular matrix (*FBN1, FBN2, COL3A1*, etc.); (2) genes that encode proteins related to the cytoskeleton in smooth muscle cells (*MYH11, ACTA2, MYLK*, etc.); and (3) genes related to the TGF-β signaling pathway (*TGFBR1, TGFBR2, TGFB2*, etc.), among others. Genes associated with TAAs according to the ClinGen framework are classified by level of evidence to support the gene-disease association (**Fig. 23–11**).[31] Most of these mutations predispose to aortic aneurysm formation, but several (eg, *MYLK*) are involved only in aortic dissection or cause dissection at small aortic diameters (*ACTA2*). This near exclusive dissection diathesis poses additional challenges in terms of counseling patients regarding the most appropriate time for preventive surgical intervention, as aneurysm size may not be useful in these subgroups.

Certain genetic mutations influence the natural history of thoracic aneurysmal disease, and in these cases the results of genetic testing may have implications for management. Genetic testing can be accomplished using panels of genes or, increasingly, whole exome sequencing. A potential benefit of routine whole exome sequencing has been reported in patients with TAAs and dissection[33] and genetic testing may lead to detection of asymptomatic aortic disease in family members. Genetic testing is most appropriate in patients with a family history of aortic disease or in those presenting at a relatively young age, although testing should be considered in other patients as well. Exome sequencing establishes the exact DNA sequence of the coding regions of the genome and has advantages over more conventional testing of a panel of genes. It comprehensively and simultaneously evaluates all the genes implicated in aneurysm causation, and by sequencing the entire genome provides

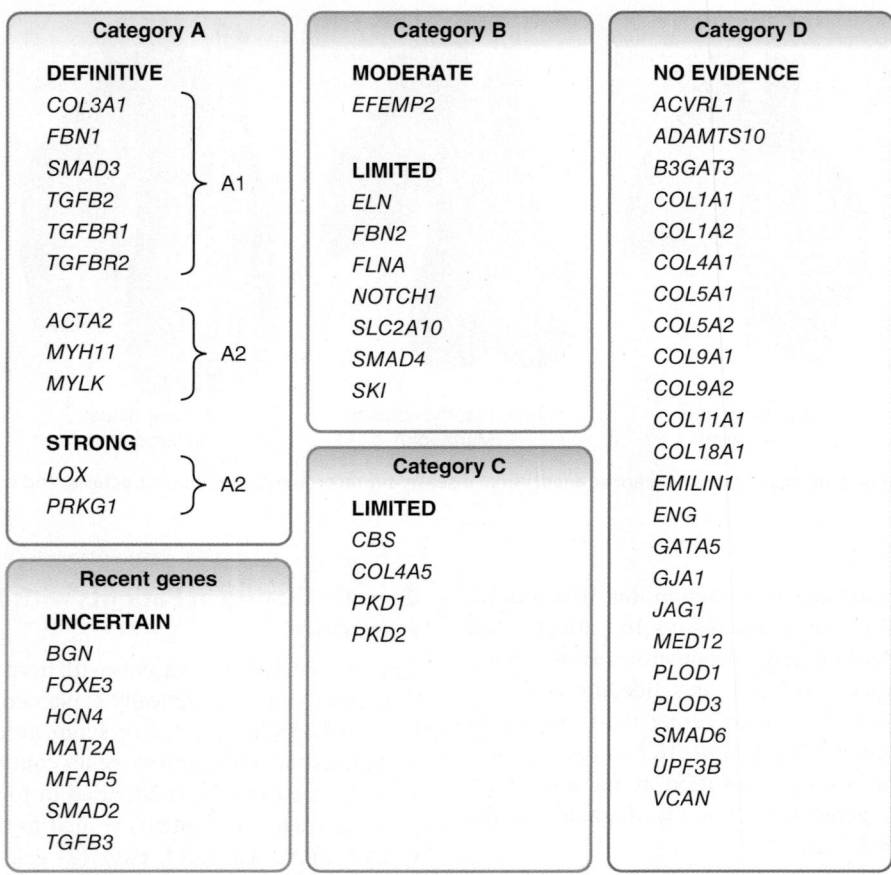

Figure 23–11. Evaluation of the clinical validity of genes for familial thoracic aortic aneurysms and dissections based on the ClinGen framework. Reproduced with permission from Renard M, Francis C, Ghosh R, et al. Clinical Validity of Genes for Heritable Thoracic Aortic Aneurysm and Dissection. *J Am Coll Cardiol.* 2018 Aug 7;72(6):605-615.

an opportunity for subsequent analysis as new causative genes are discovered. Exome sequencing is becoming less expensive and more cost-effective than multiple syndrome- or gene-specific testing in decentralized laboratories and provides data that can be used to search for new disease-associated variants.

Next generation sequencing technologies, including exome sequencing, permits large-scale, in-depth genomic analysis. Thoughtful contextual interpretation of precision genetic testing is necessary when evaluating individual patients. The American College of Medical Genetics and Genomics (ACMG) has established guidelines for reporting sequence variants using a 5-tier standard terminology system—pathogenic, likely pathogenic, uncertain significance, likely benign, and benign variants[34,35]—to clarify the impact of a specific genomic variant for individual patients, but the "variant of uncertain significance" (VUS) category can cause confusion. This category applies to a substantial proportion of results returned from clinical genetic testing. In a study of 102 patients with thoracic aortic disease undergoing exome sequencing, pathogenic or likely pathogenic variants were identified only in 4% of patients, while VUS in genes known to cause thoracic aortic disease were identified in a quarter of all patients.[33] The ACMG recommends that a VUS should not alter the clinical management of a patient. For clinicians, a more practical approach is necessary, based on the frequency of the variant in the general population.

If the variant is common in large population sequencing databases such as the Genome Aggregation Database (gnomAD),[36] it is more likely benign. Some experts recommend a threshold of 1 in 10,000, based on the proportion of the population affected by thoracic aortic diseases. Since thoracic aortic disease is generally dominantly inherited and highly penetrant, a high incidence of a variant in the general population would make the variant more common than the disease. Conversely, rarity suggests that a variant may be pathogenic.

Functional studies of a variant's impact in model organisms can provide strong evidence to reclassify a VUS as pathogenic in the development of aortic disease. Most VUS have not been evaluated in functional studies, which are expensive and time-consuming. Computational prediction of the functional role of genetic variants can be suggestive but generally not confirmatory. In silico predictors account for changes in amino acid composition of the protein coded by a given gene and scale of conservation in phylogeny of the genomic region. Aggregated predictors, such as CADD (Combined Annotation Dependent Depletion) and REVEL (Rare Exome Variant Ensemble), have demonstrated considerable accuracy.[37,38] A combination of multiple predictors classifying a variant as damaging suggests a causative role in the disease process.

In families with multiple affected individuals, segregation analysis of the VUS with the disease phenotype may help determine the role of the variant. If affected individuals do not carry the VUS, it is most likely noncontributory to the patient's condition. However, finding that all or most (depending on penetrance) affected individuals carry the VUS, while unaffected do not, makes a strong case for causal linkage. Since aortic aneurysms typically enlarge over many years, young carriers of a VUS may not have significantly enlarged aortas when first identified yet develop aneurysms over long-term follow-up.

A dictionary of genes and variants causing TAAs will enhance understanding of the natural history for each molecular subtype of aortic disease. Such international collaborations as The Montalcino Aortic Consortium (https://www.montalcinoaorticconsortium.org/) have advanced progress toward that goal. For the clinician, it is important to know the aortic size at which a significant threat of disruption arises, prompting preemptive surgical intervention. Current understanding of the size at which the thoracic aorta should be replaced in the setting of a pathogenic mutation in a specific gene is summarized in **Fig. 23–12.**

Screening for Familial Aortic Aneurysms

Regardless of the genetic findings, family members of patients with thoracic aortic disease (aneurysms or dissections), should be screened radiologically (echocardiogram and/or computed tomography [CT] imaging). If the patient has also been found to harbor a pathogenic genetic variant, then testing family members for that variant is also important to identify asymptomatic individuals at risk of developing aortic aneurysms or dissection. Family members who do not carry the pathogenic variant can forego serial imaging and the emotional burden associated with aneurysm risk. Genetic testing of relatives of patients with VUS can facilitate segregation analysis (see above), to advance knowledge about the behavior of these variants, which is still largely rudimentary.

The multisocietal US Guidelines for the Diagnosis and Management of Patients with Thoracic Aortic Disease[39] recommend aortic imaging for first-degree relatives of patients with TAAs and/or dissection to identify those with asymptomatic disease (Class 1, Level of Evidence B), and for second-degree relatives of patients with thoracic aortic dilatation, aneurysm, or dissection (Class 2, Level of Evidence B). An echocardiogram is usually sufficient, although imaging access is limited to the mid to upper portions of the ascending aorta. Several studies have found that a family history of aortic dissection increases the risk of aortic dissection in a family 3- to 9-fold.[19,40,41] Moreover, dissections tend to cluster in terms of age of onset, with more than 50% of dissection events within a family occurring within ±5 years of that in the index patient.

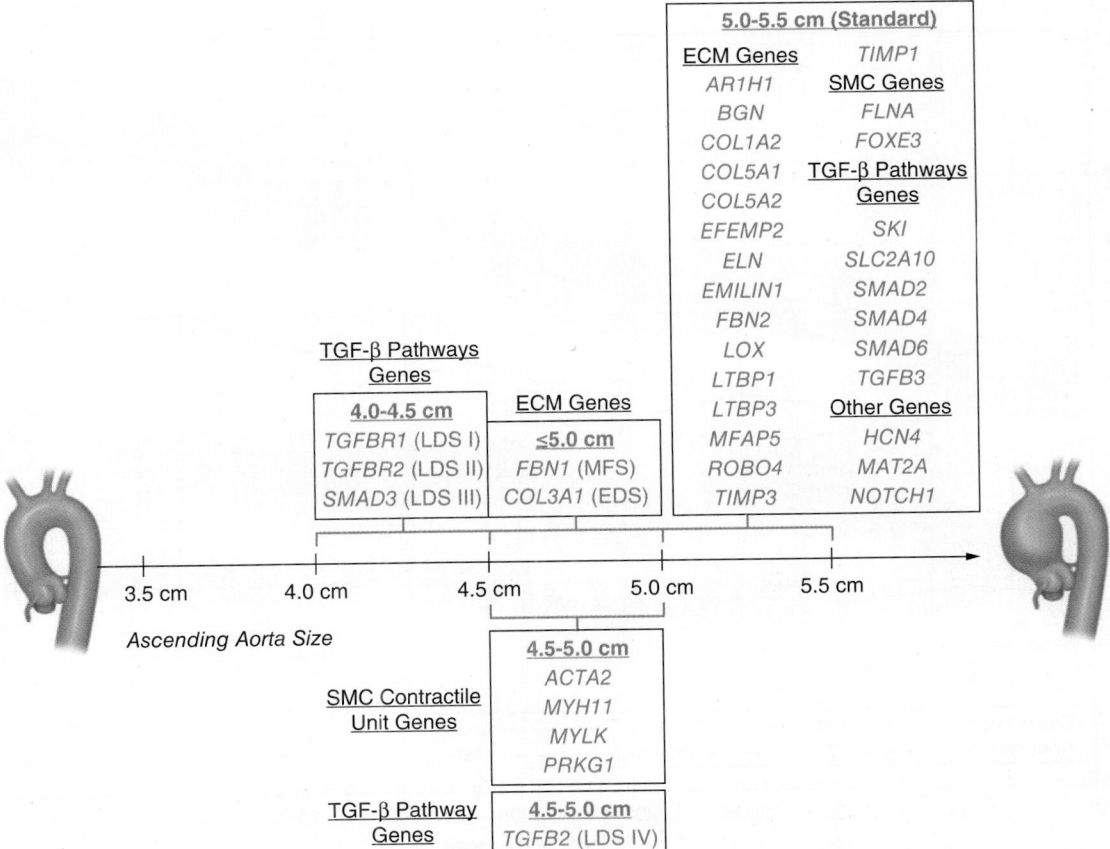

Figure 23–12. Ascending aortic dimensions for prophylactic surgical intervention. ECM, extracellular matrix; SMC, smooth muscle cell; TGF-β, transforming growth factor β. Reproduced with permission from Faggion Vinholo T, Brownstein AJ, Ziganshin BA, et al. Genes Associated with Thoracic Aortic Aneurysm and Dissection: 2019 Update and Clinical Implications. *Aorta (Stamford).* 2019 Jun;7(4):99-107.

Some studies have found intracranial arterial aneurysms in 9% of patients with TAAs (about 9 times the incidence in the general population). Specific reported incidences range from 7% in patients with ascending aortic aneurysms up to 33% in those with descending and thoracoabdominal aneurysms. Conversely, 5% of patients with brain aneurysms patients have been reported to harbor TAAs. Brain imaging for detection of aneurysms may be particularly useful in patients with a family history of stroke or intracranial hemorrhage.

EPIDEMIOLOGY OF AORTIC ANEURYSMAL DISEASE

The epidemiology of aortic aneurysms and the corresponding acute aortic syndromes present challenges because of confusion in terminology, referral bias, unknown incidence of asymptomatic cases, misdiagnosis of aortic rupture or dissection as myocardial infarction (MI), and limitations of administrative databases.[42] The Centers for Disease Control and Prevention (CDC) list aneurysmal disease as the 19th most common cause of death and the 18th most common in those older than 65, contributing to ~10,000 deaths in 2018.[42] Postmortem computerized tomographic studies of victims of out-of-hospital cardiac arrest, in which up to 8% of these deaths were attributable to

type A aortic dissection,[43,44] suggest that in some populations, the mortality resulting from aortic disease may be substantially higher than previously reported.

The incidence of TAAs is approximately 10 per 100,000 population and affects men 2 to 4 times more frequency than females, and the age at diagnosis is a decade higher in women (age 70 to 79). A population-based study from Ontario, Canada, found incidences of TAAs and dissection 7.6 and 4.6 per 100,000 population, respectively,[45] representing an increase over 12 years (**Fig. 23–13**). Similar increasing trends during the last three decades have been reported by analyses of governmental databases in the United States, Scotland, Sweden, the Netherlands, England, and Wales. Clinical data suggest a true increase in incidence rather than more frequent diagnosis due to wider availability of aortic imaging. That a majority of ruptured aneurysms occur in women is notable and unexplained.[46]

Abdominal aortic aneurysms affect approximately 5% of individuals over age 65 years, and the prevalence is considerably higher in men than women. The annual incidence of ruptured abdominal aortic aneurysms is approximately 10 per 100,000 population and is similar in men and women, although the age at diagnosis is a decade higher among women. The rate increases to approximately 50 per 100,000 for men in the seventh decade of life and each year, more than 1 in 1000 men

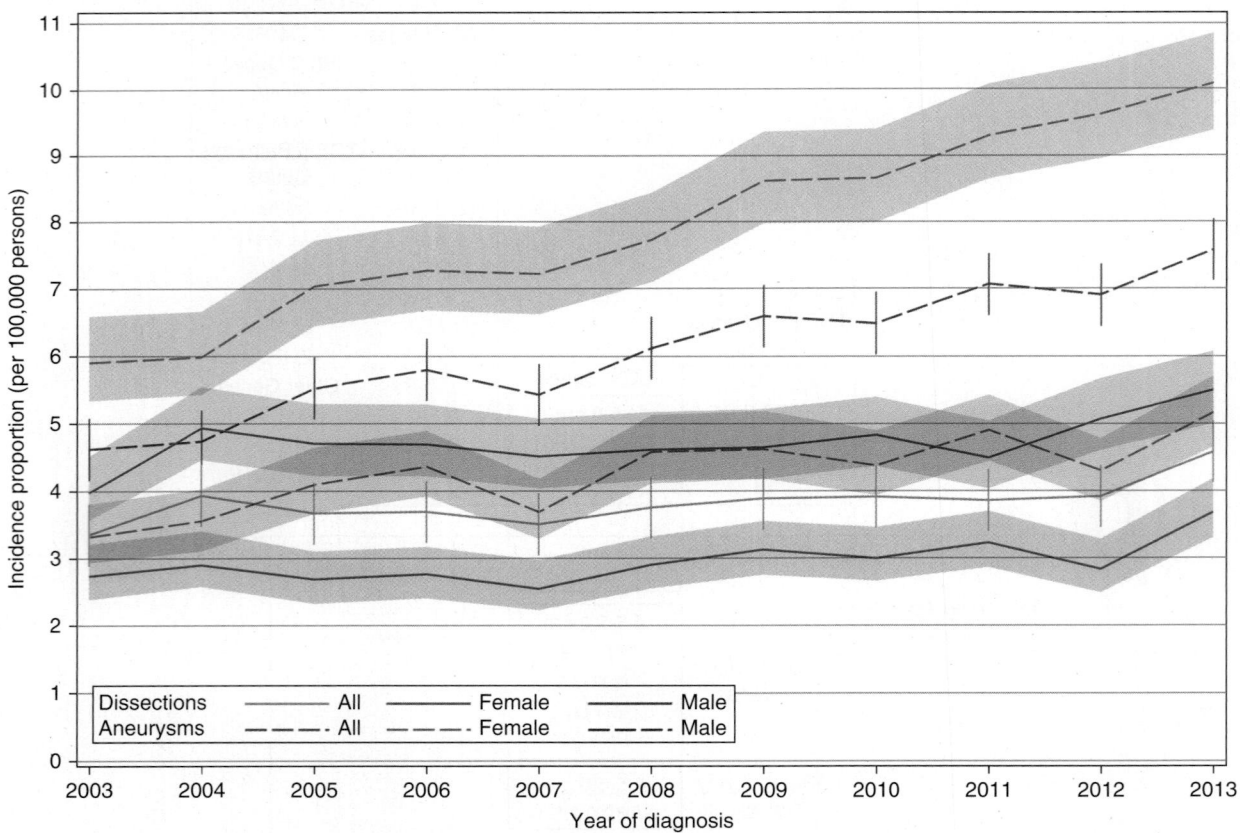

Figure 23–13. **Incidence proportions for thoracic aortic aneurysms and thoracic aortic dissections in Ontario, Canada (2002–2014).** Reproduced with permission from McClure RS, Brogly SB, Lajkosz K, et al. Epidemiology and management of thoracic aortic dissections and thoracic aortic aneurysms in Ontario, Canada: A population-based study. *J Thorac Cardiovasc Surg.* 2018 Jun;155(6):2254-2264.

in the eighth decade experiences rupture of abdominal aortic aneurysms.

CLINICAL CATEGORIES OF AORTIC ANEURYSMS

TAAs may be considered as two distinct diseases, divided at the ligamentum arteriosum (**Fig. 23–14**). Proximal to the ligamentum arteriosum, aneurysms of the ascending aorta and proximal portion of the aortic arch and not strongly associated with arteriosclerotic risk factors, smooth in contour, not calcified, and free of mural thrombus. Distal to the ligamentum arteriosum, aortic aneurysms in the descending and the abdominal aorta have an appearance similar to one another and often develop in patients with risk factors for atherosclerosis (hyperlipidemia, diabetes, hypertension, and smoking); features of

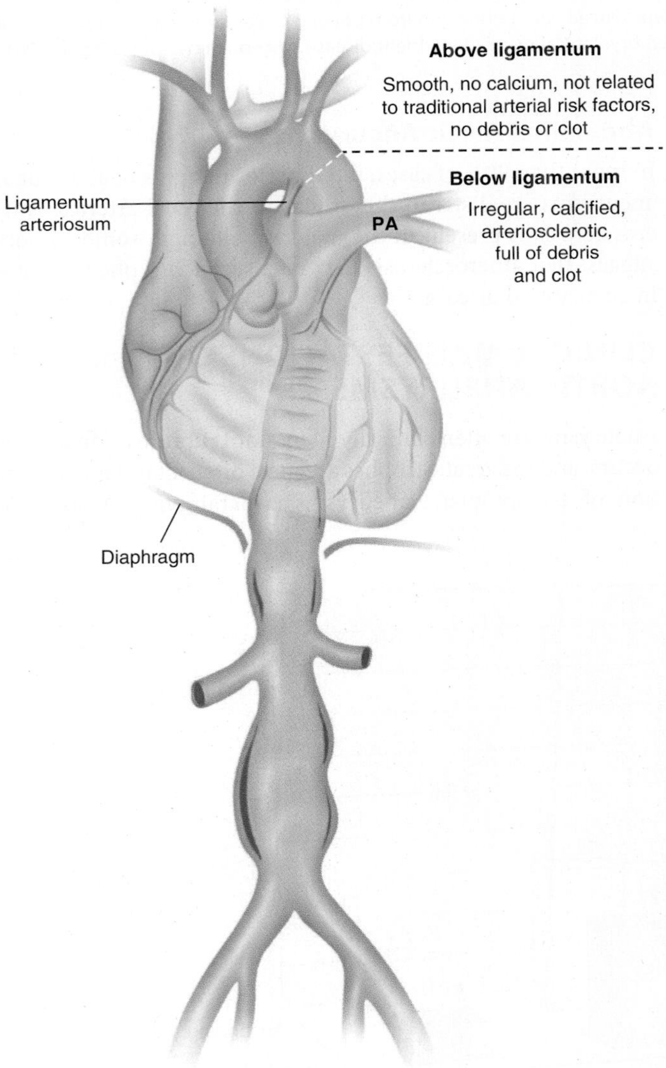

these aneurysms are typical of atherosclerosis, including an irregular contour, calcification, and mural thrombus.

This distinction between the aneurysms in aortic sections parallels differences in their embryological origins. Histological studies have shown that smooth muscle cells in the aortic root derive from the secondary heart field, while the ascending aorta and the aortic arch derive from the neural crest, and the descending aorta arises from the mesoderm (**Fig. 23–15**). This underlies the different pathological characteristics of ascending and descending aortic and abdominal aortic aneurysms. Accordingly, it may be incorrect to think of TAAs as a single entity, and biological differences between aneurysms in these two aortic segments are reflected in the family patterns of disease (**Fig. 23–16**).[47]

Ascending Aortic Aneurysms

Ascending aortic aneurysms occur more frequently in men than in women, are typically fusiform, and often extend into the aortic arch. Consequently, aneurysms of the aortic arch are usually contiguous with aneurysms in the ascending aorta. Ascending aortic aneurysms are categorized according to the pattern of involvement of the aortic root (Fig. 23–10), with direct implications for surgical treatment. In the most common type, *supracoronary aneurysm*, the aortic annulus is normal in diameter, as is the short segment of aorta between the annulus and the coronary ostia. This type of aneurysm is treated by replacement with a tube graft, starting above the coronary arteries and extending cephalad to the end of the aneurysm. The second category, termed *annuloaortic ectasia*, is characterized by enlargement of both the aortic annulus and the proximal portion of the aorta. This type of aneurysm is typical of Marfan syndrome and related disorders characterized by cystic medial necrosis of the aortic wall. Because the annulus and proximal aorta are the most dilated portions, the aneurysmal ascending aorta has a "flask like" shape, requiring replacement of the entire aortic root and valve, usually with a prefabricated composite graft that includes a prosthetic valve and aortic graft in an integrated unit. The third category, the *tubular* type of ascending aortic aneurysm, shares features of the other two configurations. In patients with tubular aortic aneurysms, the annulus and proximal aorta are mildly dilated, and the caliber of the ascending aorta is also uniformly dilated. When surgical repair is necessary, either a supracoronary tube graft or total aortic root replacement may be appropriate based on considerations that include the patient's age. In younger individuals, composite grafting may confer greater protection against late dilation of the proximal portion of the aortic root, while in older patients more limited approaches may be advantageous.

Descending Thoracic Aortic Aneurysms

In contrast to the ascending aorta, the majority of aneurysms of the descending thoracic aorta are atherosclerotic. These are typically fusiform, and often begin distal to the origin of the left subclavian artery and extend to the level of the abdominal aorta. Descending thoracic aneurysms may also develop in patients with aortic coarctation.

Figure 23–14. Aortic aneurysm is really two diseases: Ascending/arch disease differs markedly from descending/abdominal disease. Reproduced with permission from Elefteriades JA, Farkas EA. Thoracic aortic aneurysm clinically pertinent controversies and uncertainties. *J Am Coll Cardiol.* 2010 Mar 2;55(9):841-857.

Labels in figure:
Above ligamentum — Smooth, no calcium, not related to traditional arterial risk factors, no debris or clot
Below ligamentum — Irregular, calcified, arteriosclerotic, full of debris and clot
Ligamentum arteriosum
PA
Diaphragm

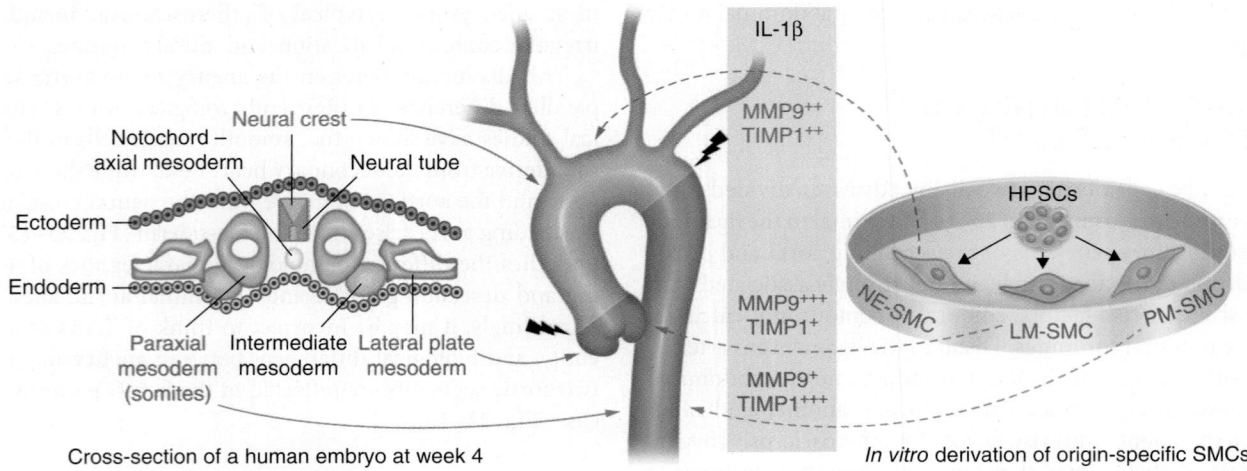

Figure 23–15. The different embryological origins of segments of the thoracic aorta from three distinct cell lineages: the aortic root from the lateral plate, the ascending aorta from the neural crest, and the descending aorta from the mesoderm. These different zones, and their transition points, may contribute to the sites of origin of aortic dissection flaps (jagged bolts). Reproduced with permission from Cheung C, Bernardo AS, Trotter MW, et al. Generation of human vascular smooth muscle subtypes provides insight into embryological origin-dependent disease susceptibility. *Nat Biotechnol.* 2012 Jan 15;30(2):165-173.

Thoracoabdominal Aortic Aneurysms

As the nomenclature indicates, thoracoabdominal aortic aneurysms have features of both thoracic and abdominal aortic aneurysms (**Fig. 23–17**). Although they constitute only approximately 3% of all aortic aneurysms, thoracoabdominal aneurysms are classified separately because of the diffuse and extensive nature of the aortic disease process (usually atherosclerosis) and special considerations for surgical repair, which may entail reimplantation of visceral arteries. Four types of thoracoabdominal aortic aneurysms have been delineated according to the segment and extent of aorta involved (Fig. 23–17).

Abdominal Aortic Aneurysms

In more than 90% of cases, the superior margins of abdominal aneurysms are distal to the origins of the renal arteries. Atherosclerosis is present in the majority, although some authors suggest that atherosclerosis may be a secondary phenomenon in aneurysmal disease.

CLINICAL MANIFESTATIONS OF AORTIC ANEURYSMS

Aneurysms are often clinically silent until rupture or dissection occurs, and these catastrophes are most often fatal. Thus, detection of asymptomatic aneurysms is paramount. A strategic

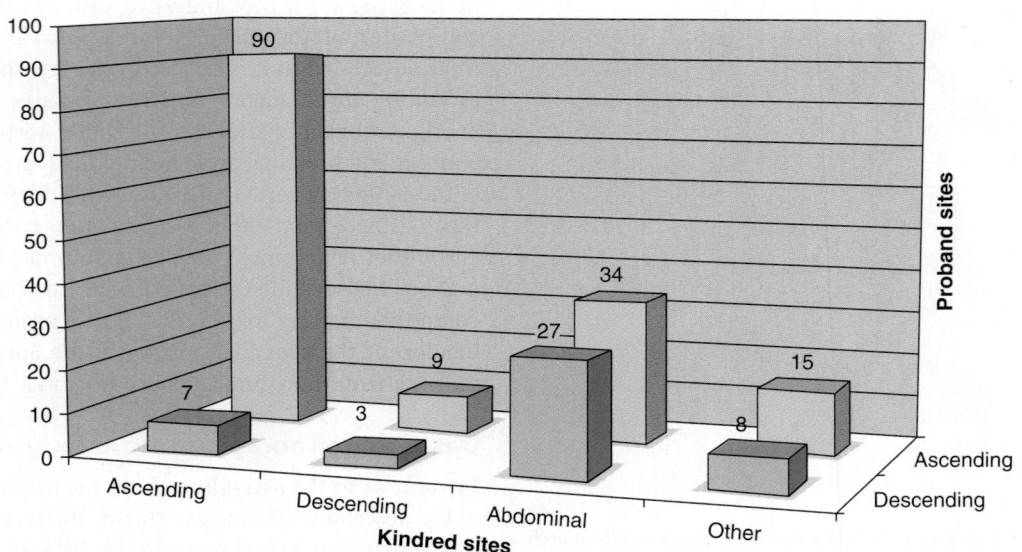

Figure 23–16. Distribution of arterial aneurysm and dissection sites in kindred of familial probands. Note the ascending/ascending and descending/abdominal correlations between probands and kindred. Adapted with permission from Albornoz G, Coady MA, Roberts M, et al. Familial thoracic aortic aneurysms and dissections--incidence, modes of inheritance, and phenotypic patterns. *Ann Thorac Surg.* 2006 Oct;82(4):1400–1405.

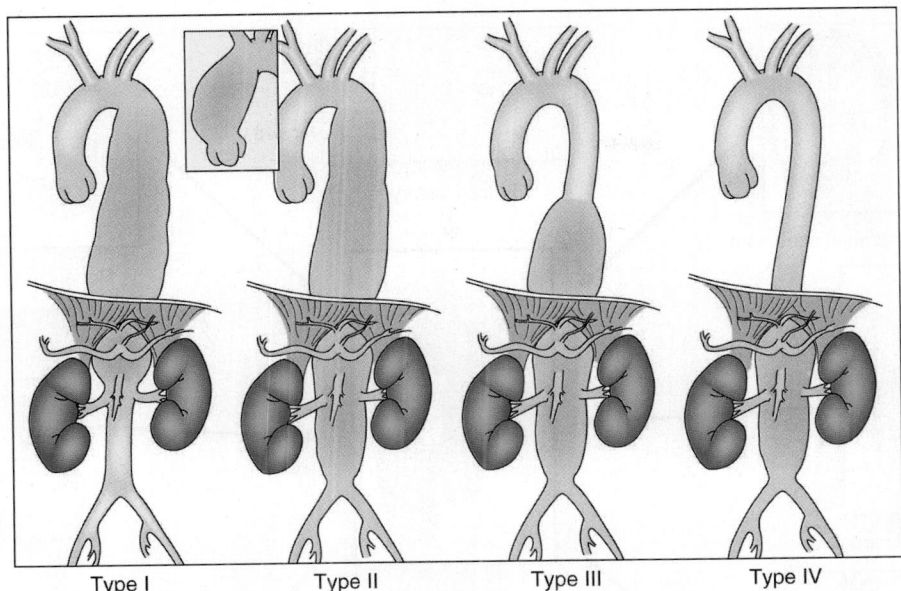

Figure 23–17. Classification of thoracoabdominal aortic aneurysms. Type I aneurysms involve most of the descending aorta from near the origin of the left subclavian artery to the abdominal vessels, but the renal arteries are not involved. **Type II** aneurysms also begin near the origin of the left subclavian artery but extend below the origins of the renal arteries. **Type III** aneurysms arise more distally and involve less of the descending thoracic aorta but often more of the abdominal aorta than types I and II aneurysms. **Type IV** aneurysms arise at the level of the diaphragm and typically extend below the origins of the renal arteries. Reproduced with permission from Crawford ES, Coselli JS. Thoracoabdominal aneurysm surgery. *Semin Thorac Cardiovasc Surg.* 1991 Oct; 3(4):300-322.

approach to detection of a TAA[48] capitalizes on clinical associations with aneurysms in other aortic segments, intracranial aneurysms or aneurysms in other arteries, family history or aneurysmal disease, bovine aortic arch configuration, renal cysts, positive thumb-palm sign, and temporal arteritis (**Fig. 23–18**). Patients with thoracic aneurysms have an approximately 9% likelihood of concurrent intracranial aneurysms (higher for those with descending than ascending aneurysms), probably because of common genetic and pathophysiologic mechanisms. Since the negative prognostic significance of intracranial aneurysms is substantial, and since catheter-based interventions are available to prevent rupture, routine screening for intracranial aneurysms may be warranted in patients with TAAs. Bovine aortic arch and other arch anomalies like direct origin of the left vertebral artery from the aortic arch or aberrant left subclavian artery were previously considered benign variants, but these anomalies occur more frequently in patients with TAAs than in the general population.[49] The association of renal cysts and TAAs may reflect excess matrix metalloproteinase (MMP) activity.[50,51] The significance of family history, the thumb-palm sign, and arteritides are addressed below. The presence of any of these correlates of TAAs may warrant screening by noninvasive imaging.

A minority of patients with thoracic or abdominal aortic aneurysms (5%–10%) experience premonitory symptoms. Aneurysms of any kind can produce pain arising from stretching of the aortic tissue or impingement on adjacent structures. Pain originating in the ascending aorta is usually retrosternal. Pain from the descending aorta is characteristically interscapular. Pain in the lateral or posterior aspects of the chest may occur when an aneurysm compresses surrounding structures

or erodes into adjacent ribs or vertebrae. Pain from the abdominal aorta may occur anywhere in the abdomen, left flank, or lower part of the back. It is often difficult to distinguish from pain of other causes, but patients themselves may distinguish deep visceral pain from superficial or musculoskeletal pain. The interscapular pain of descending aortic enlargement or dissection is less often caused by musculoskeletal disorders.

Rupture of the aorta in any location produces acute symptoms, usually severe pain followed by loss of consciousness or death from internal hemorrhage. Ruptures of abdominal aortic aneurysms usually produce extreme distress similar to that from other intra-abdominal catastrophes. Despite surgical advances, mortality is still the most frequent outcome because abrupt circulatory collapse precludes timely intervention except in unusual circumstances. Patients frequently have severe abdominal or back pain, but the pattern varies considerably. Rupture into the retroperitoneum, peritoneum or pleural cavities leads to tachycardia, hypotension, diaphoresis, pallor, or shock, depending on the extent of rupture and extravasation of blood. On occasion, rupture directly into the duodenum causes aortoduodenal fistula and acute gastrointestinal bleeding. This should be considered when gastrointestinal bleeding is evident along with evidence of aneurysm on physical examination or imaging. Rupture into the inferior vena cava or iliac veins producing arteriovenous fistula is suggested by rapid development of leg swelling or high-output heart failure in a patient with abdominal aortic aneurysm. Rupture of descending or thoracoabdominal aortic aneurysms produces similar physiologic derangements, with pain typically located higher in the trunk, consistent with the anatomical location of the aortic disease.

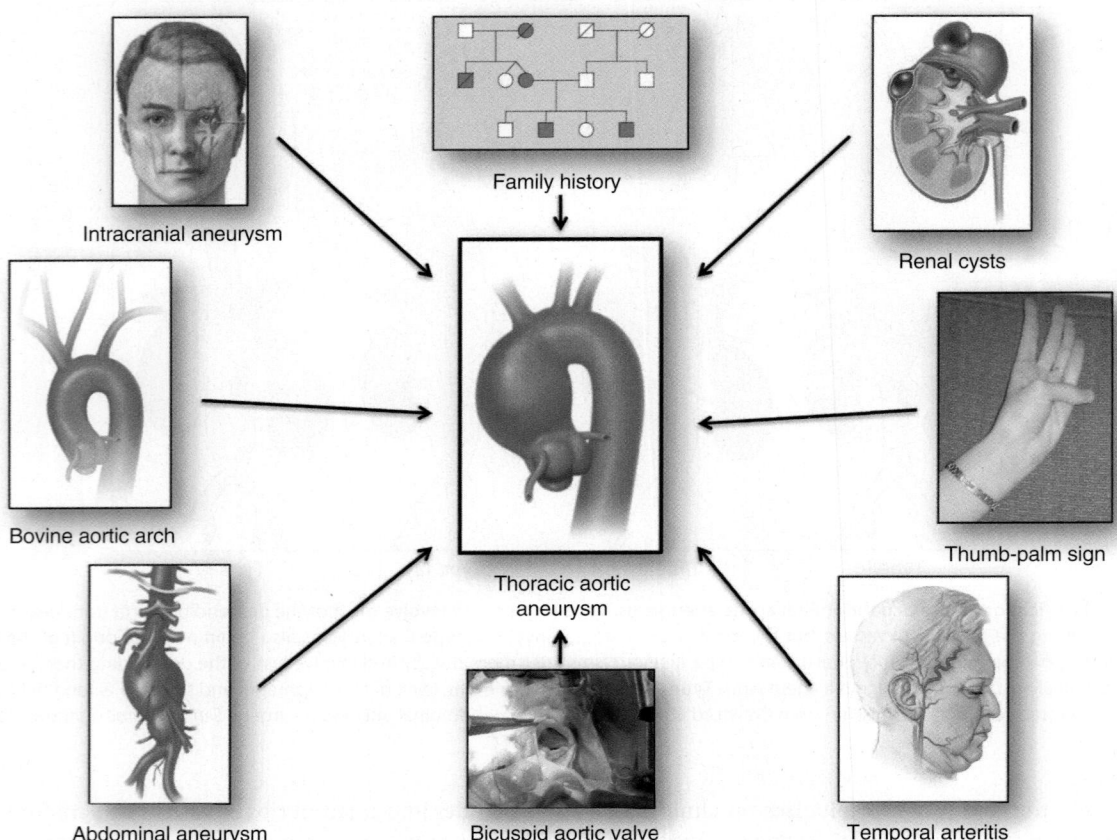

Figure 23–18. Paradigm of "guilt by association" for detection of silent thoracic aortic aneurysm. Reproduced with permission from Elefteriades JA, Sang A, Kuzmik G, et al. Guilt by association: paradigm for detecting a silent killer (thoracic aortic aneurysm). *Open Heart.* 2015 Apr 24;2(1):e000169.

As the aortic root enlarges, diastolic malcoaptation of the aortic valve leaflets causes aortic regurgitation and may lead to heart failure. Aneurysms of the sinuses of Valsalva may rupture into the right ventricular cavity, right atrium, or pulmonary artery, causing heart failure associated with a continuous murmur. Ascending aortic aneurysms can distort or obstruct the trachea, producing respiratory symptoms. Compression of the superior vena cava may produce venous congestion in the head, neck, and upper extremities. Aortic arch aneurysms or descending TAAs may produce hoarseness from distortion of the recurrent laryngeal nerve or dysphagia ("dysphagia lusoria") from impingement on the esophagus. Descending TAAs may cause hemoptysis from erosion into the lung parenchyma or bronchi or hematemesis from esophageal erosion. Because mural thrombosis is common, atherosclerotic aneurysms may be the source of peripheral embolism causing occlusion of distal vessels or clinical features of atheroembolism. Occasionally, patients with abdominal aortic aneurysms become aware of prominent abdominal pulsation. Nausea and vomiting may occur if the aneurysm compresses the duodenum. Compression of the left iliac vein may cause leg swelling, compression of the left ureter may cause hydronephrosis, compression of the testicular veins may cause varicocele, and compression of the bladder may cause urinary frequency or urgency.

Thoracic or abdominal aortic aneurysms are not commonly symptomatic before dissection or rupture and are often found incidentally by imaging performed for other reasons. Chest radiographs may suggest aortic aneurysm, which can be confirmed by CT or magnetic resonance imaging (MRI).

Several clinical conditions should raise suspicion of concurrent TAAs and prompt noninvasive imaging:

- *Intracranial aneurysms,* based upon common genetics and causation.
- *Simple renal cyst,* related to tissue destruction by MMPs.
- *Bovine aortic arch,* as a frequent correlate of ascending TAAs.
- *Positive thumb-palm sign,* as excess bone length and joint laxity are common not only in Marfan syndrome but also in patients with nonsyndromic aortic aneurysmal disease.
- *Abdominal aortic aneurysm,* which often overlap with descending thoracic and thoracoabdominal aortic aneurysms.
- *Bicuspid aortic valve,* as discussed in the text.
- *Temporal aarteritis,* as giant cell arteritis and other arterial inflammatory syndromes may be associated with aneurysms of the aorta and its branch vessels.
- *Family history of aneurysm,* as discussed in the text.

Awareness of these associations among general physicians and cardiovascular specialists may promote detection of asymptomatic cases and reduce the mortality associated with thoracic aortic aneurysmal disease.

SCREENING FOR ABDOMINAL AORTIC ANEURYSMS

The epidemiologic implications of screening for abdominal aortic aneurysms have been extensively studied.[52,53] Screening programs based on abdominal ultrasonography effectively detect aneurysms prior to rupture and reduce the frequency of aneurysm-related deaths. The cost of medical care per single aneurysm-related death prevented is about $10,000. One important benefit of screening is that a single negative ultrasonogram at 65 years of age suffices; patients without aneurysms at this age will not die of aneurysm rupture.[52,53]

Cost-effective screening of the general population is focused on family history of aneurysmal disease, age, male sex, history of cigarette smoking, coronary artery disease, cerebrovascular disease, and hypercholesterolemia as factors linked with incremental risk of aneurysm development. Abdominal aortic aneurysms are 5 times more common in smokers, in whom 89% of all aneurysm ruptures occur.

US Preventive Services Task Force recommendations[53] call for screening by ultrasonography for abdominal aortic aneurysms in men aged 65 to 75 years who have ever smoked. Based on a relatively low yield, the Task Force explicitly recommended against routine screening for abdominal aortic aneurysms in women who have never smoked and have no family history of abdominal aortic aneurysms. Available evidence is insufficient to assess the balance of benefit and harm from screening women aged 65 to 75 years who either have smoked or have a family history of abdominal aortic aneurysms.[53]

EVALUATION OF PATIENTS WITH AORTIC ANEURYSMS

Evaluation of a patient with suspected aneurysmal disease of the aorta requires a multifaceted approach. Aortic aneurysms are usually asymptomatic prior to dissection or rupture, but pain may develop when expansion occurs rapidly, or when the aortic wall becomes inflamed, which is often a harbinger of rupture. Ascending aneurysms may cause anterior chest pain or shortness of breath, while patients with descending TAAs sometimes report interscapular (posterior) thoracic pain. Aneurysmal dilation of the aortic arch and proximal portion of the descending aorta may compress or stretch the recurrent laryngeal branch of the vagus nerve and produce hoarseness. Aneurysms of the abdominal aorta can cause mid-abdominal or low back pain, or radicular symptoms associated with spinal compression or erosion. Other symptoms of aortic aneurysms are described elsewhere in this chapter under Clinical Manifestations of Aortic Aneurysms.

A complete aortic evaluation requires careful recording of the family history with respect to arterial aneurysms, stroke, subarachnoid hemorrhage, or sudden unexpected death in parents, grandparents, siblings, children, and secondary relatives.

Physical Examination: Clinical Signs of Aortic Aneurysms

The ascending aorta, aortic arch, and descending aortas are not palpable except in cases of extreme enlargement or in rare instances when they can be palpated through an attenuated chest wall. The abdominal aorta, in contrast, is easily palpable except in very obese patients. With experience, the diameter of the abdominal aorta can be reliably assessed by palpation. Aortic wall tenderness is generally an ominous finding, portending rupture.

Ascending aortic aneurysms may be associated with the characteristic diastolic blowing murmur of aortic regurgitation, best heard along the right or left sternal border at end-expiration with the patient seated and leaning forward.

Other clues to aneurysmal disease or related syndromes include tall, thin habitus, especially when accompanied by pectus excavatum or carinatum, scoliosis, Marfanoid facies (long, narrow face, with small chin and deep-set eyes), and early-onset myopia. The thumb-palm sign (Fig. 23–18), in which the thumb can cross over and extend beyond the edge of the flat palm, reflects both bone length and joint laxity, common correlates of aortic aneurysmal disease.

Diagnostic Studies

Imaging studies should be employed for evaluation of patients with known or suspected aortic disease to identify aneurysm formation and delineate zones of dissection or rupture. It may be challenging in the emergency department to identify the small proportion of patients with aortic dissection among the larger number presenting with signs and symptoms of chest, abdominal or back pain. The three life-threatening causes of acute chest pain (MI, pulmonary thromboembolism, and aortic dissection) should be front of mind, and the so-called "triple rule-out" CT scan and echocardiographic imaging should be employed judiciously for diagnosis.

On chest roentgenography (CXR), a rounded shadow at the right upper mediastinal border may indicate an ascending aortic aneurysm, but dedicated aortic imaging by ultrasound, CT, or MRI is usually necessary to confirm the diagnosis. The descending aortic stripe is usually clearly apparent on chest x-ray, where adjacent air-filled lung contrasts with the blood density of the aorta to delineate the course and diameter of the descending aorta. Plain chest radiography can be useful in screening for thoracic aortic disease. In the International Registry of Acute Aortic Dissections (IRAD) database,[54] abnormal chest radiography was common in cases of aortic dissection. The general contour of the ascending aorta, the aortic knob, and the stripe of the descending aorta can usually be identified well and evaluated even on a plain chest x-ray.[55]

Transthoracic echocardiography (TTE) is a first-line method for assessment of the ascending aorta, and in thin individuals, the proximal aortic arch can be visualized as well. This method is not suitable, however, for evaluation of the remainder of the thoracic aorta, which requires either CT or MRI. It is usually best to include both the chest and the abdomen in the initial study, as multiple segments of the aorta are often involved in an individual patient. Abdominal ultrasound can accurately assess the abdominal aorta if intestinal gas does not interfere.

Several three-dimensional (3D) imaging modalities applicable to patients with aortic aneurysmal disease include transesophageal echocardiography (TEE), CT, and MRI, each of which offers high sensitivity and specificity. Although CT and MR imaging allow for examination of the structure of the aorta along its entire course, TEE may not fully delineate the aortic arch or abdominal aorta. Conversely, TEE provides detailed information about the ascending and descending portions of the aorta, aortic valve, pericardium and ventricular function. An advantage of TEE is that it can be rapidly performed in the emergency department while the patient receives intensive medical support, but adequate sedation is required to avoid hypertension, which could extend dissection or instigate aortic rupture. The abdominal aorta can be examined by surface ultrasonography, CT, or MRI.

The primary criterion for diagnosis of aortic dissection by CT is demonstration of two contrast-filled lumens separated by an intimal flap. Inaccuracy may result from inadequate contrast opacification, poor visualization of the intimal flap, artifacts extending across the aortic lumen that simulate an intimal flap, misinterpretation of adjacent vessels or a prominent sinus of Valsalva as a flap, atelectasis or pleural thickening, or thrombosis of the false lumen. Modern multidetector-row CT scanners offer rapid image acquisition, electrocardiographic gating, variable section thickness, 3D rendering, diminished helical artifacts, and small contrast requirements. The sensitivity and specificity of CT and MRI imaging for diagnosis of aortic dissection approach 100%. Catheter-based contrast aortography is invasive and does not provide the 3D anatomic information afforded by CT, MR, or TEE imaging. Intravascular ultrasonography using high-frequency transducers, although not widely available, can provide an accurate determination of the location and extent of aortic dissection and assessment of branch vessels and may be a useful adjunct when other imaging studies are not definitive.

Positron emission tomography (PET) has some utility in assessing inflammatory disease of the aorta such as Takayasu's syndrome and other forms of autoimmune or infectious aortitis.[55] Evidence of hypermetabolic activity on a PET scan has also been shown to predict rupture in patients with abdominal and thoracic aortic aneurysms.[57,58]

Assessment of Aortic Dimensions

Management of aortic aneurysms depends to a substantial degree on their size and location, but assessment of diameter using a given modality or with multiple or discrepant modalities can be problematic. Multiple specific sources of error or confusion in aortic measurement are encountered regularly in clinical practice (**Fig. 23–19**).[59]

Resolution of Current Imaging Technologies
Although aortic size is commonly read to the millimeter, available technology does not support that degree of precision; one can have confidence in a measured change of 3 mm or 4 mm after careful review to ascertain that measurements have been obtained at the same anatomical level.

Internal Versus External Diameter of the Aortic Wall
There is no consensus as to whether the thickness of the aortic wall should be included or excluded from measurements of the diameter of the aorta by echocardiography, CT, or MRI, leading to discrepancies of up to several millimeters. Measurements by unenhanced (noncontrast) CT imaging typically involve the external diameter (including the lumen and entire thickness of the aortic wall), whereas measurements based on contrast images are typically limited to the internal luminal diameter. Echocardiography and MRI allow for measurements of the internal or external diameter of the aortic wall.

Limitations of Specific Imaging Modalities
Echocardiography can generate high-quality images of the ascending aorta, but TTE can visualize only the proximal portion of the ascending aorta and sometimes the proximal part of the aortic arch in a patient with suitable anatomy (echo windows) (**Fig. 23–20**). Thus, TTE could fail to identify or lead to inaccurate measurement of aneurysms of the distal portion of the ascending aorta. Even TEE is limited by interposed tracheal air and may fail to visualize a portion of the upper or distal ascending aorta (**Fig. 23–21**).

A CT scan with axial images cannot properly evaluate the proximal portion of the ascending aorta. The aortic valve annulus and coronary artery ostia are usually separated by only one or two centimeters, and it is possible for significant pathology to fall between axial imaging planes. In some cases, it may be difficult to determine the level of a given axial image with respect to the valve plane—a key distinction when measuring the diameter (**Fig. 23–22**). Furthermore, it is naïve to believe that the plane of the aortic valve is confined to the plane of the axial images (perpendicular to the longitudinal axis of the body), since the annulus may normally be skewed. Furthermore, as the ascending aorta elongates, the aortic valve plane becomes more vertically oriented, making assessment of size by axial imaging even more difficult (**Fig. 23–23**). Contemporary CT image reconstructions provide not only axial but also images in the sagittal and coronal planes, but the resolution of nonaxial reconstructions can be insufficient to permit precise assessment of the aortic shape or diameter. Changes in aortic diameter with the cardiac cycle could potentially affect diameter measurements by as much as 17.5%. Electrocardiographically gating CT to synchronize aortic image acquisition with the cardiac cycle mitigates motion artifact and substantially improves diagnostic accuracy (**Fig. 23–24**). The centerline method that utilizes software to automatically set the viewing plane perpendicular to the long axis of the aorta for analysis of CT images enhances precision in assessment of aortic wall morphology and diameter (**Fig. 23–25**). It is important to bear in mind, however, that

Sources of imaging discrepancies

1. Systolic or diastolic measurement?

2. Lumen only or lumen plus aortic wall?

3. Cursor at or just outside aortic wall

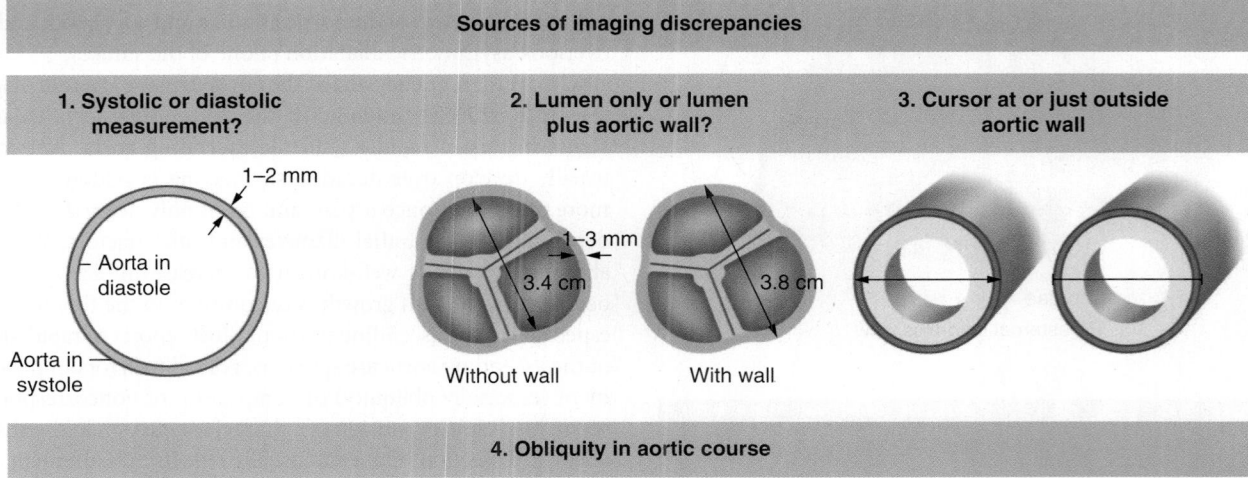

4. Obliquity in aortic course

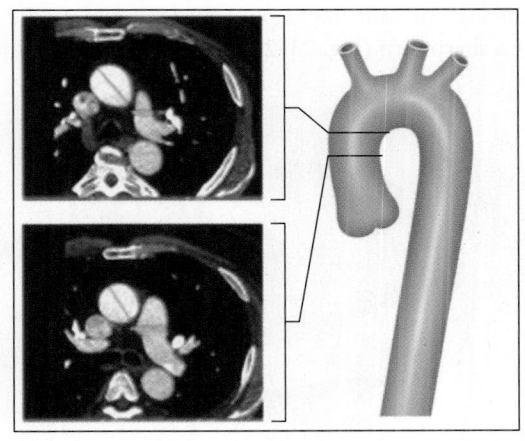

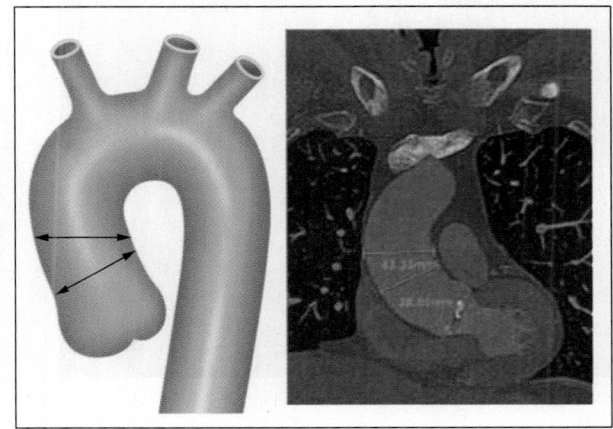

5. Sinus of valsalva: Commissure-to-sinus or sinus to sinus?

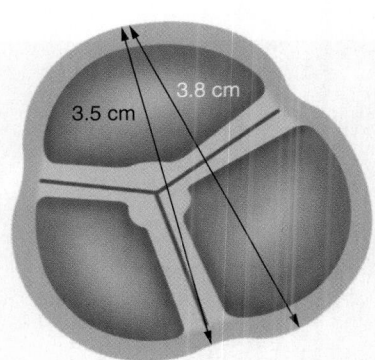

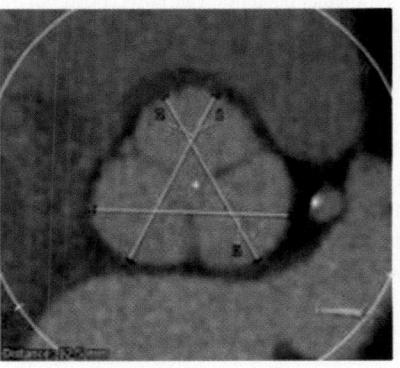

Figure 23–19. Sources of discrepancies in measurement of the ascending thoracic aorta. (1) Systole versus diastole. (2) Wall or no wall. (3) Cursor type and placement. (4) Obliquity at the top of the ascending aorta. (5). Sinus-to-commisure or sinus-to-sinus measurements of the aortic root. Reproduced with permission from Elefteriades JA, Mukherjee SK, Mojibian H. Discrepancies in Measurement of the Thoracic Aorta: JACC Review Topic of the Week. *J Am Coll Cardiol.* 2020 Jul 14;76(2):201-217.

this method may produce smaller diameter measurements than observer-based analysis, and most clinical criteria for selection of patients for aortic surgery have not been based on centerline measurements. Unless criteria for intervention are adjusted to account for this variable, adoption of automated, computerized methods of measurement could potentially lead to underestimation of the risks of dissection and rupture. Evolving micro-CT imaging of the aorta, currently investigational, promises to yield near-histologic clarity regarding the aortic wall (**Fig. 23–26**).[60]

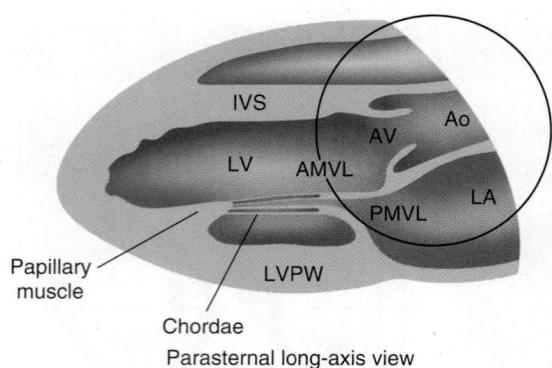

A

Parasternal long-axis view

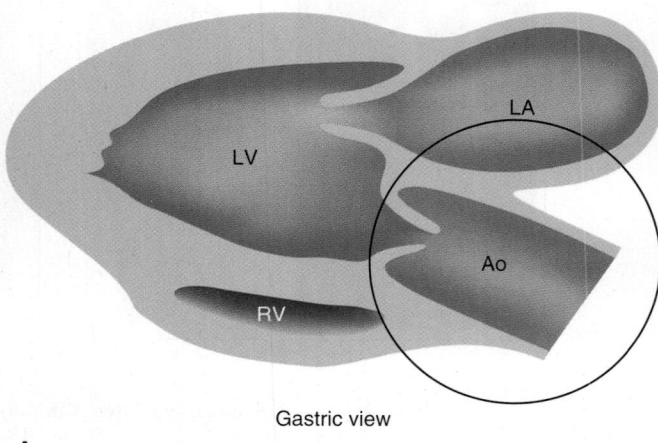

B

Figure 23–20. Limited distance above the aortic valve for which the ascending aorta can be seen on transthoracic echocardiography. **A.** Schematic. **B.** Echocardiographic image. Ao, aorta; AMVL, anterior leaflet of mitral valve; AV, aortic valve; IVS, interventricular septum; LA, left atrium; LV, left ventricle; LVPW, left ventricular posterior wall; PMVL, posterior mitral valve leaflet. Reproduced with permission from Elefteriades JA, Farkas EA. Thoracic aortic aneurysm clinically pertinent controversies and uncertainties. *J Am Coll Cardiol.* 2010 Mar 2;55(9):841-857.

MRI is an inherently multiplane modality that provides axial, sagittal, and coronal images. Depending on resolution, accurate measurements made by this method could overcome some of the limitations of echocardiography and CT imaging arising from imaging windows, planar projection, and vascular calcification.

Geometric Complexity

The human aorta is geometrically complex. The ascending aorta is not vertical, and the aortic arch projects an oblong rather than a circular contour on axial long-axis imaging, making accurate measurements of its diameter technically difficult. The same is true for other curved portions of the aorta, as is often the case where the aorta crosses the diaphragm. When comparing measurements of diameter over time, those obtained from even slightly different longitudinal levels may give a false impression of stability or enlargement. Similarly, at a given cross-sectional level, the aorta may not be circular, and measured girth may vary depending on the geometric diameter selected. Even good

quality transesophageal echocardiography may not accurately assess all diameters of the aortic annulus and aortic root and may overlook asymmetric dilatation of one of the sinuses.

On average, aneurysms of the aorta expand at a rate of about 0.1 cm to 0.2 cm annually,[61-63] the descending aorta enlarging somewhat more rapidly than the ascending aorta. Aneurysms usually develop over decades, so imaging is seldom necessary more often than once a year, and often only every 2 or 3 years, depending on the initial diameter and other factors. While the abdominal aorta is well-known to increase in size quickly on occasion, such rapid growth is uncommon in the thoracic aorta, especially in the ascending portion. Most reports of rapid growth of the ascending aorta are spurious, related to errors in measurement (especially obliquity) or comparison of noncorresponding segments. Rapid expansion of a thoracic aneurysm in the absence of aortic dissection is rare and usually reflects measurement error. One common source of error is oblique measurement of the aorta at the arch or near the diaphragm, where an ectatic aorta may take a sharp turn (**Fig. 23–27**). Current CT and MR technology

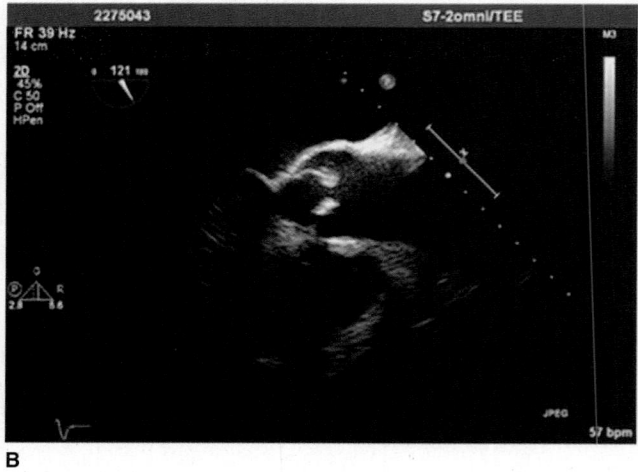

Gastric view

A

B

Figure 23–21. Limited distance above the aortic valve for which the ascending aorta (Ao) can be seen on transesophageal echocardiography; the tracheal air column interferes with visualization of the upper ascending aorta. **A.** Schematic. **B.** Echocardiographic image. LA, left atrium; LV, left ventricle; RV, right ventricle. Reproduced with permission from Elefteriades JA, Farkas EA. Thoracic aortic aneurysm clinically pertinent controversies and uncertainties. *J Am Coll Cardiol.* 2010 Mar 2;55(9):841-857.

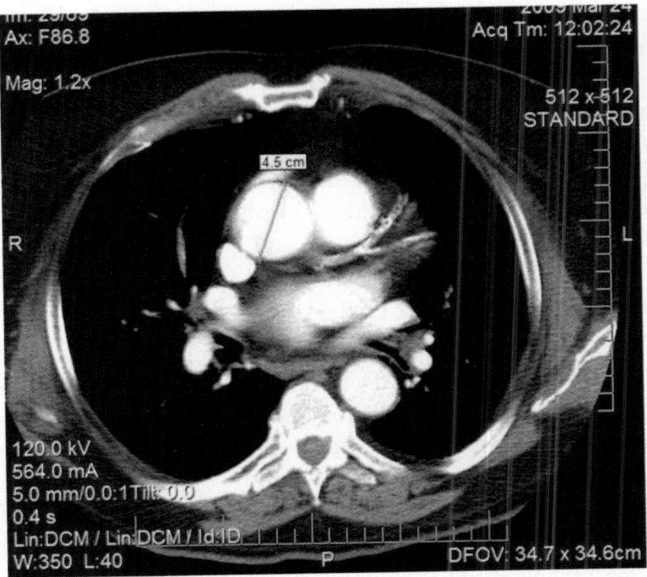

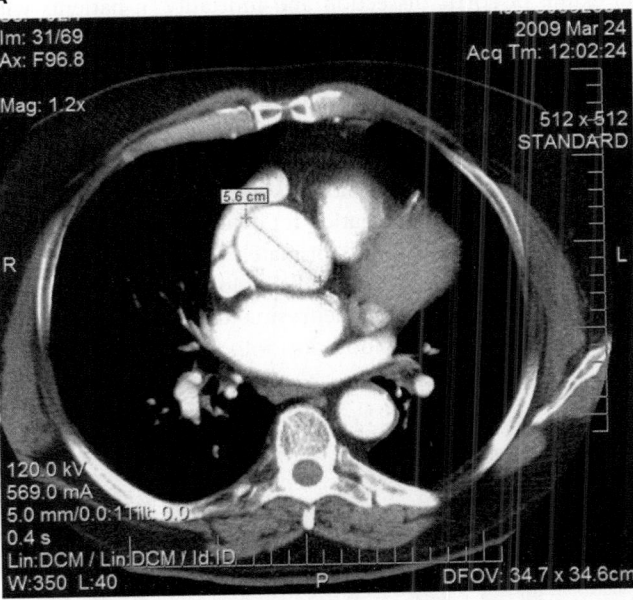

Figure 23–22. Difficulty in determining if a given axial CT image is still in the aorta or passing partially through the aorta and the left ventricular outflow track. This factor can lead to gross misinterpretations of aortic diameter. **A** and **B** differ by only one CT level, yet they yield markedly different diameters. Is the lower frame still in the aorta? Does it represent the dimension of the sinuses, or does it run obliquely through both aorta and left ventricular outflow tract? It can be difficult or impossible to ascertain these answers on a purely axial technique. Reproduced with permission from Elefteriades JA, Farkas EA. Thoracic aortic aneurysm clinically pertinent controversies and uncertainties. *J Am Coll Cardiol.* 2010 Mar 2;55(9):841-857.

can correct for most of these problems in measurement. More important than frequent imaging is to compare the most recent images with the *earliest* image available for a given patient to avoid underestimation of total growth over time.[59]

Studies acquired at narrow intervals of time may fail to identify enlargement. It is therefore imperative to compare measurements over longer intervals to properly appreciate the rate

of change. It is also important to note that size is not the only criterion for intervention; shape, aortic wall integrity, and aortic valve regurgitation, and compromise of the coronary ostia or other branch vessels are additional considerations. Loss of the normal indentation or "waist" of the aorta at the sinotubular junction (so-called "effacement" of the sinuses) is an indication of intrinsic aortic disease that should raise concern about the risk of adverse events (**Fig. 23–28**).

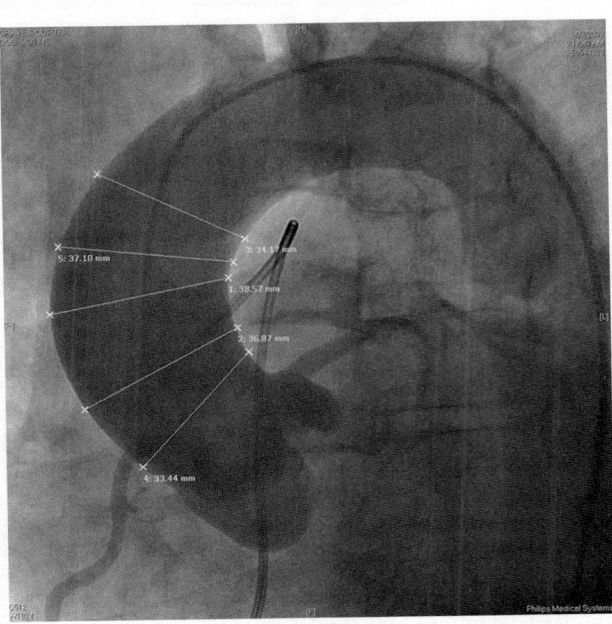

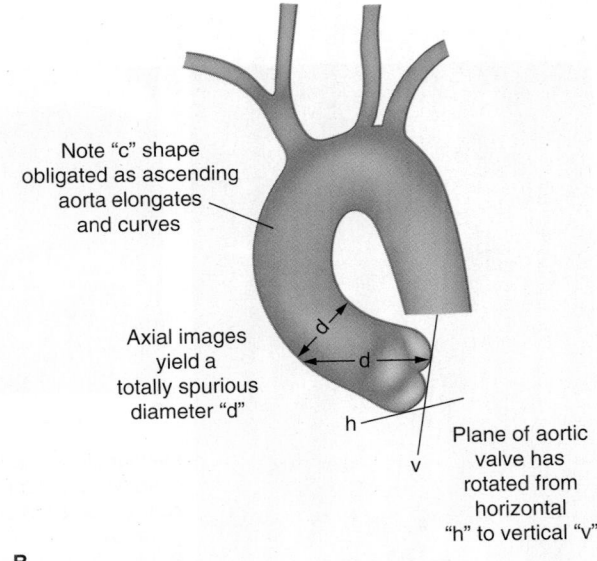

Figure 23–23. Aortogram (A) and schematic (B) showing gross elongation of the ascending aorta, forcing the aorta into a "C" shape and obligating the aortic valve to take a nearly vertical plane of orientation. On an axial computed tomography image, this common anatomy would markedly confound measurement of proximal aortic size. Note the difference between a horizontal diameter (as in an axial image) and a diameter perpendicular to the long axis of the aorta. Reproduced with permission from Elefteriades JA, Farkas EA. Thoracic aortic aneurysm clinically pertinent controversies and uncertainties. *J Am Coll Cardiol.* 2010 Mar 2;55(9):841-857.

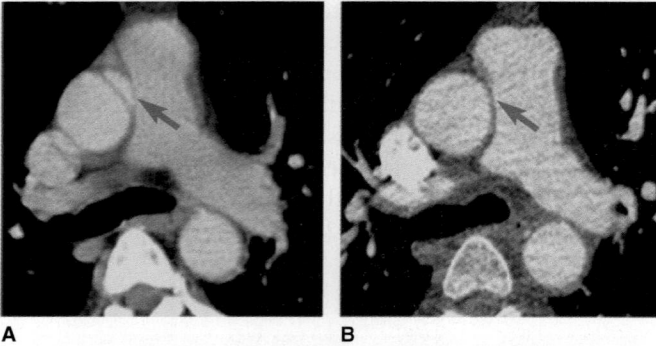

Figure 23–24. Nongated (A) and gated (B) contrast computed tomography angiography demonstrating an imaging artifact suspicious for an intimal flap in a Type A dissection. Reproduced with permission from Chou AS, Ziganshin BA, Elefteraides JA. Computed Tomography Imaging Artifact Simulating Type A Aortic Dissection. *Aorta (Stamford).* 2016 Apr 1;4(2):72-73.

Normalization of Aortic Dimensions for Body Size

Estimating aortic growth rate is not a simple calculation of the difference in aortic size at the same anatomic location between two time-points divided by the time between these points. Sophisticated statistical methods have been developed to accurately assess the rate of aortic growth and minimize sources of statistical error.[61] Furthermore, the rate of expansion of the aorta increases with increasing diameter in all segments.

The z-score can be used to monitor aortic enlargement in growing children. It is calculated by dividing the aortic diameter at specified anatomical levels by body surface area, and employing one of several nomograms to estimate the number of standard deviations of that ratio from the population mean.[64]

The z-score has been used to assess the impact of various treatment regimens (including β-blockers, calcium-channel blockers, angiotensin-inhibitors, and other interventions) over time in children, interpreting a diminishing z-score as evidence of a salutary effect. The validity of this approach has been questioned, however, based on the observation that z-scores decrease normally due to the diminishing leanness associated with maturation.[65]

Biomarkers in Aortic Disease

TAAs are usually silent until lethal complications (dissection or rupture) develop. Detection and monitoring could be enhanced by identification of biomarkers in the blood that correlate with aneurysm development, expansion, and impending disruption[66] (**Table 23–3**). Among those currently employed, D-dimer (a byproduct of fibrin degradation) is usually elevated in cases of acute aortic dissection, with 99% sensitivity. The magnitude of D-dimer elevation correlates with the longitudinal extent of aortic dissection and mortality in patients with aortic dissection. It is nonspecific, however, since elevations also occur in patients with pulmonary embolism, acute coronary syndromes, and other conditions associated with intravascular thrombosis and/or thrombolysis, and because D-dimer rises after the onset of dissection, it is not useful as a predictor.

Several other promising biomarkers, individually or in combination, are under investigation for detection or assessment of aortic aneurysms. MMPs are intimately involved in the pathogenesis of aortic aneurysms and dissection. They may be useful in the early stages of aortic aneurysmal disease, and MMP elevation signals recurrent blood flow into an aneurysm sac after

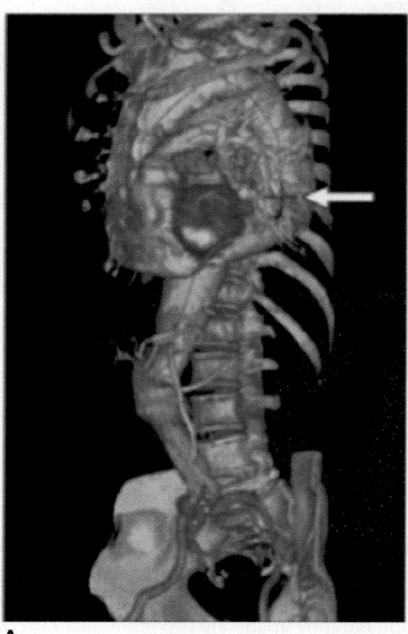

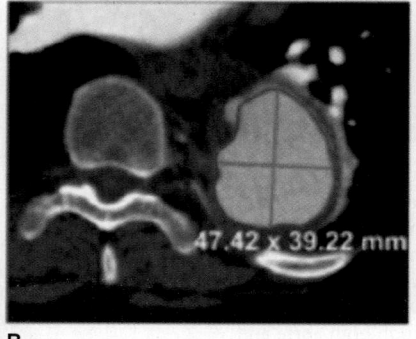

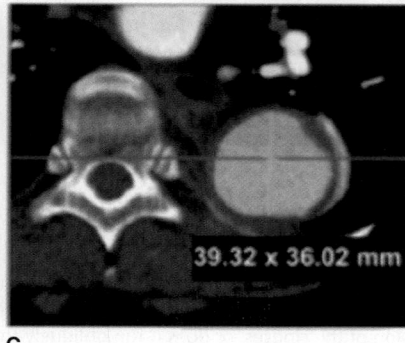

68-year-old woman with thoracoabdominal aortic aneurysm. Comparison of measurements of aortic diameters on axial source image (**B**) and centerline analysis (**C**).
A. Volume-rendered image illustrates pathology and location of performed measurements (*arrow*)
B. Measurement on axial source image results in inaccurate values because image plane is not adjusted perpendicular to course of aorta.
C. Measurement on cross-sectional image plane perpendicular to centerline.

Figure 23–25. Comparison of measurements of aortic diameters on axial source image and centerline analysis. Reproduced with permission from Rengier F, Weber TF, Giesel FL, et al. Centerline analysis of aortic CT angiographic examinations: benefits and limitations. *AJR Am J Roentgenol.* 2009 May;192(5):W255-W263.

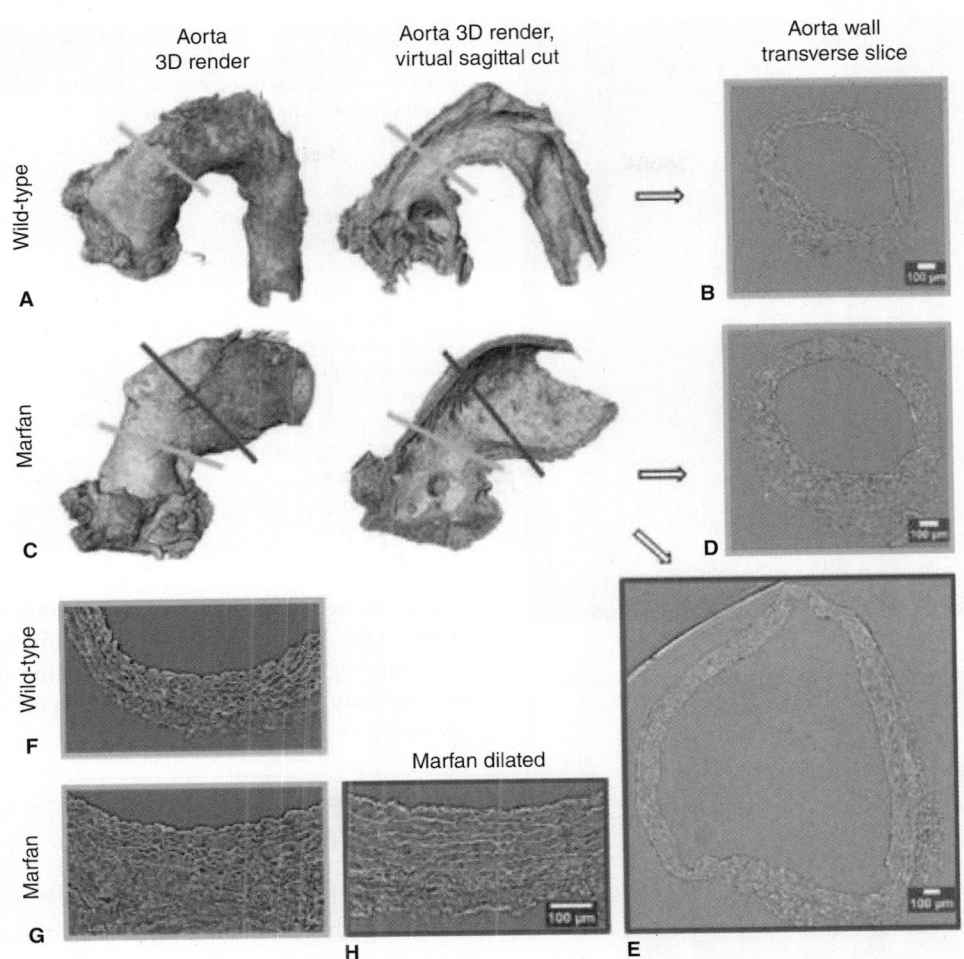

Aorta
3D render

Aorta 3D render,
virtual sagittal cut

Aorta wall
transverse slice

Figure 23–26. Synchrotron-based microCT scan examples of wild type and Marfan syndrome mice aortae. (**A**) Wild-type aorta volumetric rendering. (**B**) Transverse slice of wild-type aorta corresponding to the yellow line in (A). (**C**) Volumetric rendering of a Marfan aorta with a nondilated (yellow line) and a dilated (purple line) zones. (**D**) Transverse slice of the Marfan aorta at the nondilated zone (yellow line in [C]). (**E**) Transverse slice of the Marfan aorta at the dilated zone (purple line in [C]). (**F–H**) Representative transverse sections from microCT scans of 9 month-old wild type and Marfan mice aortae (dilated and nondilated zones). Scale bars in (B, D–E, H), 100 μm. Reproduced with permission from López-Guimet J, Peña-Pérez L, Bradley RS, et al. MicroCT imaging reveals differential 3D micro-scale remodelling of the murine aorta in ageing and Marfan syndrome. *Theranostics*. 2018 Nov 15;8(21):6038-6052.

endovascular repair (endoleak). Inflammation and collagen degradation are involved in the pathogenesis of aortic aneurysms; hence, inflammatory biomarkers and indicators of collagen turnover are under investigation as potential indicators

of aortic diseases. CD4+CD28− T cells and elastin peptide are candidate biomarkers, as is smooth muscle heavy chain myosin. Aneurysm-related RNA may find application for detection and monitoring of aneurysm activity (**Fig. 23–29**). Another

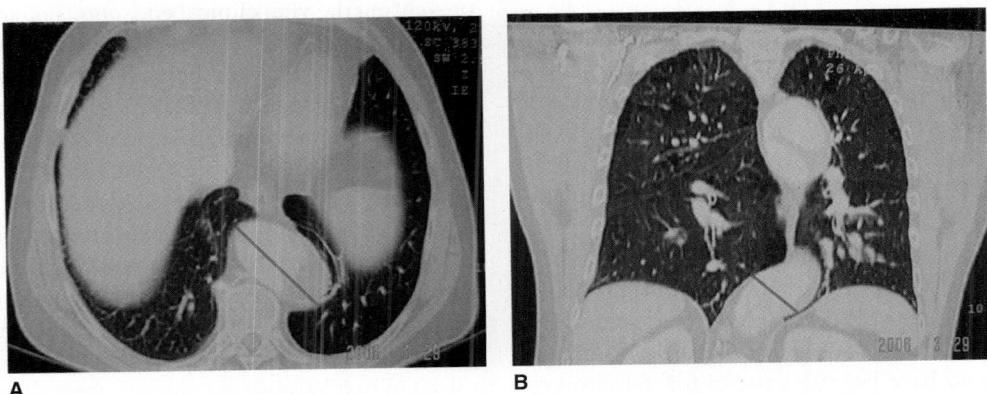

Figure 23–27. Spurious calculation of large aortic dimension (A) caused by measuring an oblique cross section across a tortuous portion of the thoracic aorta (B).

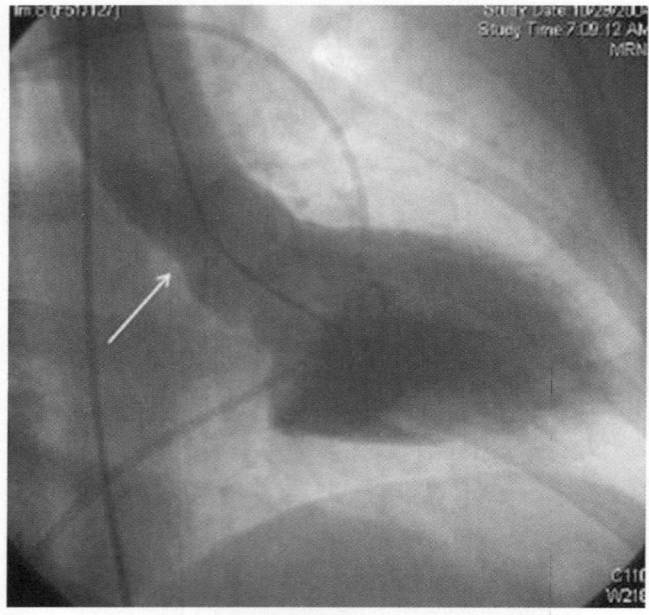

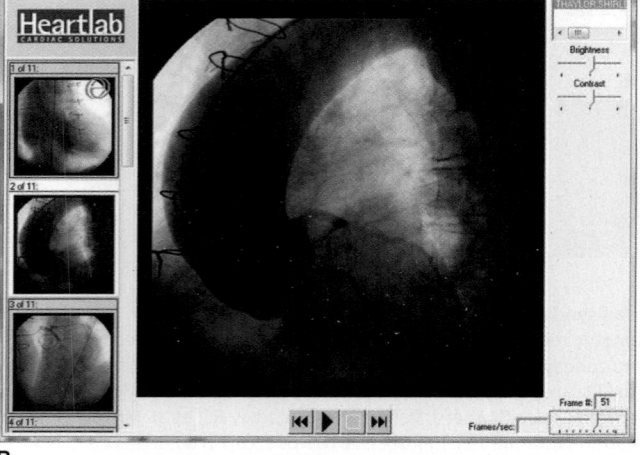

Figure 23–28. Aortograms depicting normal aortic contour with a "waist" (*arrow*) above the coronary arteries (A) and the abnormal aortic contour (with no "waist") of Marfan-like annuloaortic ectasia (B). Reproduced with permission from Elefteriades JA, Farkas EA. Thoracic aortic aneurysm clinically pertinent controversies and uncertainties. *J Am Coll Cardiol.* 2010 Mar 2;55(9):841-857.

potential tool employs advanced glycation end products (AGE) and their soluble receptors (sRAGE), which may be involved in the pathogenesis of TAAs. Low levels of sRAGE and high levels of AGEs seem related to the risk of TAA development and progression.[67] Additional candidates include C-reactive protein, neutrophil/lymphocyte ratio, diamine oxidase (DAO), interleukin 6 (IL-6), tumor necrosis factor alpha (TNF-α), alpha smooth muscle actin (α-SMA), smooth muscle heavy chain (smMHC), and noncoding RNAs (ncRNAs).[68-71] Most of these markers have been found to correlate with aortic dissection after its inception and have been less useful for detection of intact aneurysms or prediction of dissection or rupture. Before or after dissection, molecular genetic evaluation, including

TABLE 23–3. Potential Biomarkers in Aortic Diseases (for Diagnosis and Monitoring)

Indicators of ongoing thrombosis
  D-dimer
  Plasmin
  Fibrinogen
Matrix metalloproteinases
Inflammatory markers
  Cytokines
  CD4+CD28- T-Cells
  C-reactive protein
Markers of collagen turnover
  Elastin peptide
Other
  Endothelin
  Hepatocyte growth factor
  Homocysteine
Genetic markers
  RNA signature

whole exome sequencing has been recommended for patients with TAAs. When a disease-causing mutation or variant of uncertain significance is detected, testing of family members by single-site Sanger sequencing is then focused on the specific variant.

MANAGEMENT OF PATIENTS WITH AORTIC ANEURYSMS

Medical Treatment of Chronic Aneurysms

Patients with aortic aneurysms are commonly treated with β-adrenergic antagonist drugs to decrease systolic arterial wall stress, but the effectiveness of this strategy has been validated in one early long-term study of 70 patients with clinical features of Marfan syndrome. The value of β-adrenergic antagonist drugs in patients with and without Marfan syndrome is controversial.[72-74] Among the concerns, in addition to the potential for side effects, is evidence that β-blockers decrease the elasticity of the aortic wall. The overall effectiveness of β-blockers for TAAs has recently been reviewed.[72-74] As can be seen in **Table 23–4**, the evidence that β-blockers delay aortic dilatation in Marfan patients is quite equivocal and there is, further, simply is no evidence of effectiveness in preventing the vital clinical end-points of aortic dissection or death (Table 23–4).[74]

Angiotensin receptor blocking drugs (ARBs) represent a potential alternative to β-blockers in patients with Marfan syndrome, based on work by Dietz and colleagues, which showed benefit of losartan in a mouse model and in infants with Marfan syndrome. The concept was developed that ARBs (acting on the TGF-β pathway) can attenuate progression of aortic disease in Marfan patients. However, a randomized clinical trial comparing low doses of losartan and atenolol showed no difference in rates of progressive aortic root dilation among children and young adults with Marfan syndrome.[75] The issue remains unresolved in part because of concerns about dose selection.

The antibiotic agent doxycycline, an MMP inhibitor, showed promise in patients with abdominal aortic aneurysms. Other

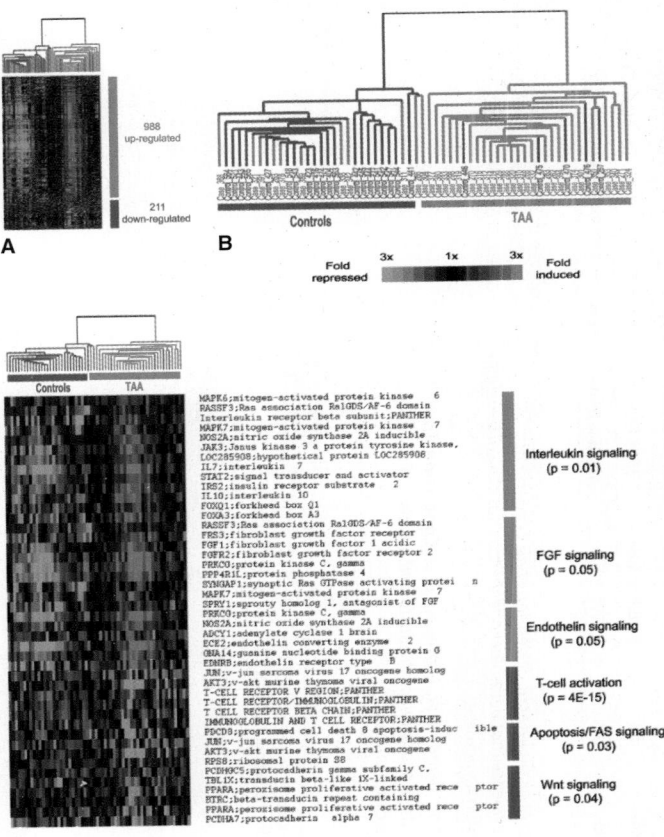

Figure 23–29. The RNA signature test for thoracic aortic aneurysm. In the hierarchical cluster diagram on the left, each *vertical line* represents a patient, and each *horizontal line* represents an RNA. In the grid, the *green* indicates underexpression, and *red* indicates overexpression. Note in the diagram on the left how the overexpression and underexpression cluster, depending on phenotype. In the figure on the right, note that if all the blues were together and all the reds were together, the test would have been 100% accurate. As it turns out, the overall accuracy was more than 82%. Reproduced with permission from Wang Y, Barbacioru CC, Shiffman D, et al. Gene expression signature in peripheral blood detects thoracic aortic aneurysm. *PLoS One.* 2007 Oct 17;2(10):e1050.

drugs that have undergone animal or clinical testing, including cyclooxygenase (COX) 2 inhibitory anti-inflammatory agents, hydroxymethylglutaryl coenzyme A (HMG-CoA) reductase inhibitors (statins), the immunosuppressive agent rapamycin, and the angiotensin receptor inhibitor losartan, have not been associated with consistent clinical benefit. A retrospective study in large numbers of patients with TAAs suggested substantial benefit in meaningful clinical endpoints from statin therapy for TAAs, most pronounced for descending and thoracoabdominal aneurysms.[76]

Observational data from IRAD raise the possibility the β-blockers might be beneficial in some patients with type A aortic dissection and calcium-channel blockers might be useful in those type B aortic dissection, but additional studies are needed to verify these preliminary findings before these agents can be recommended for routine clinical use in these situations.[77,78]

Indications for Surgery

Asymptomatic, Intact Thoracic Aortic Aneurysms

When viewed in terms of cumulative lifetime risk, the natural history of TAAs is characterized by an abrupt increment in the incidence of dissection or rupture at maximum diameter of 6 cm for the ascending aorta; these events tend to occur at a somewhat larger dimension at the level of the descending aorta (**Fig. 23–30**). Yearly risks of rupture, dissection, or death reflect a stepwise increment in risk as the aorta expands, rising most dramatically to 14.1% at a dimension of 6 cm.[61] Based on this observation, patients without overwhelming comorbidities should undergo resection of TAAs before the maximum diameter reaches 5.5 cm to 6.0 cm (**Table 23–5**). Surgical intervention may be considered when the aortic diameter reaches ≥5.0 cm, when aortic expansion occurs at a rate in excess of 0.5 cm annually, or in those with a family history of aortic dissection.[79] For patients with Marfan syndrome or a family history of this disease, a criterion of 5 cm is usually applied because these patients are more prone to rupture or dissection.[61]

It remains controversial whether the anatomical location at which enlargement is greatest (ie, at the level of the sinuses of Valsalva or the tubular portion of the ascending aorta) or body surface area should be considered in determining the threshold for surgical intervention. Analysis of the lifetime risk of experiencing an aortic catastrophe revealed that (for the ascending aorta) 34% of patients will have suffered a rupture or a dissection by the time the size of the aorta reaches 6.0 cm. This size of the ascending aorta represents a "hinge-point" in its behavior (Fig. 23–30). At a diameter of 6 cm, the yearly risk of rupture, dissection, or death in patients with ascending aortic aneurysms is 15% (**Fig. 23–31**). Prophylactic surgical interventions should be carried out prior to the aorta reaching this size, in order to prevent potentially lethal complications.

There are limited data on the aortic diameter at which the risk of dissection is high enough to warrant concomitant aortic resection in patients who already fulfill hemodynamic criteria for aortic valve replacement (AVR) because of severe aortic stenosis or aortic regurgitation. Most authorities suggest that the aorta be resected at 4.5 cm if the surgeon is "already there" for aortic valve replacement.

There has been extensive debate about whether patients with BAVs should undergo surgical intervention for aortic repair at diameters smaller than recommended for patients with tricuspid aortic valves and ascending aortic aneurysms. In general, aortic dissection develops in patients with BAVs at younger ages than in those with tricuspid aortic valve,[80,81] but in some studies the diameters of the aortic root or ascending aorta in patients presenting with acute type A dissection were larger in those with bicuspid than tricuspid valves.[80,81] The latest consensus document suggests that the aorta in BAV not be treated any differently from that in the TAV patient, as there does *not* seem to be increased aortic risk in the BAV setting.[30]

Based on these studies describing the risk of adverse events for patients with TAD, evidence-based intervention criteria have been articulated and included in guidelines for managing patients with thoracic aortic disease.[39,82] For the ascending

TABLE 23-4. Literature on The Effectiveness of β-Blockers in Patients with Marfan Syndrome.

Author name	Year of Publication	Designed to evaluate beta-blocker effect?	β-Blocker Group			Control Group				Study Results	
			Number of patients#	Mean age (years)	Number of clinical end-points*	Number of patients	Mean age (years)	Number of clinical end-points*	Do BBs slow aortic dilatation?	Do BBs prevent clinical end-points?*
Randomized Clinical Trial:											
Shores et al.[147]	1994	Yes	32	15.4	5/32 (15%)	38	14.5	9/38 (24%)	Yes	No (p = 0.399)
Observational Studies:											
Tahernia[349]	1993	Yes	3	10.0 ± 1.0	0/3 (0%)	3	8.3 ± 4.9	0/3 (0%)	Yes	No (p = 1.0)
Roman et al.[350]	1993	No	79	28 ± 15	18/79 (23%)	34	28 ± 15	3/34 (9%)	N/A	No (p = 0.080)
Salim et al.[351]	1994	Yes	100	11.1 ± 3.4	5/100 (5%)	13	10.2 ± 4.6	0/13 (0%)	Yes	No (p = 1.0)
Silverman et al.[352]	1995	No	191	33 ± 14	58/191 (30%)	226	31 ± 17	54/226 (24%)	N/A	No (p = 0.137)
Legget et al.[353]	1996	No	28	21 (median)	9/28 (32%)	55	21 (median)	8/55 (15%)	N/A	No (p = 0.060)
Rossi-Foulkes et al.[354]	1999	Yes	15	11.2 ± 5.3	4/15 (27%)	27	8.0 ± 5.2	0/16 (0%)	Yes	No (p = 0.043)
Tierney et al.[355]	2007	Yes	29	9.2 ± 4.0	1/29 (3%)	34	8.8 ± 4.8	3/34 (9%)	No	No (p = 0.617)
Ladouceur et al.[356]	2007	Yes	77	6.1 ± 3.2	3/77 (4%)	78	7.4 ± 5.2	8/78 (10%)	Yes	No (p = 0.123)
Meta-analyses:											
Gersony et al.[149]	2007	*Includes studies by Tahernia, Roman et al., Shores et al., Salim et al., Silverman et al., Legget et al.* **Conclusions:** *On the basis of this meta-analysis, there is no evidence that beta-blockade therapy has clinical benefit in patients with Marfan's syndrome.*							N/A	No
Gao et al.[150]	2011	*Includes studies by Tahernia, Salim et al., Rossi-Foulkes et al., Tierney et al., Ladouceur et al.* **Conclusion:** *There is evidence that beta-blockade therapy can slow down the rate of dilatation of the aorta and has clinical benefits on children and adolescents with MFS.*							Yes[†]	No

Please note that 4 of the 8 studies involved fewer than 30 patients.
*Clinical end-points included death or related cardiovascular events; N/A, Data not available in study.
†Although the meta-analysis included the Tierney et al. study, the calculations on aortic growth rates did not include their findings.
Reproduced with permission from Ziganshin BA, Mukherjee SK, Elefteriades JA. Atenolol versus Losartan in Marfan's Syndrome. *N Engl J Med.* 2015 Mar 5;372(10):977–978.

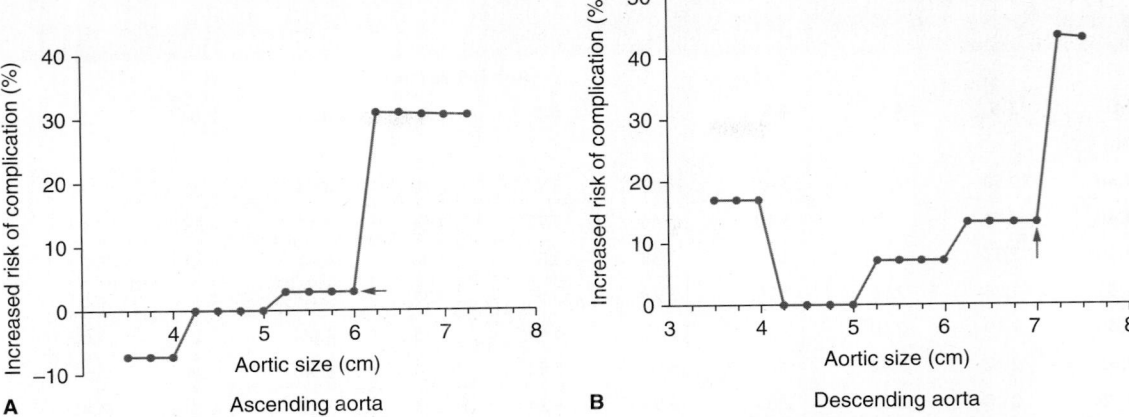

Figure 23–30. Depiction of "hinge points" for lifetime natural history complications at various sizes of the aorta. The *y*-axis lists the probability of complication; *complication* refers to rupture or dissection. The *x*-axis shows aneurysm size. (**A**) The ascending aorta. (**B**) The descending aorta. Reproduced with permission from Coady MA, Rizzo JA, Hammond GL, et al. What is the appropriate size criterion for resection of thoracic aortic aneurysm? *J Thorac Cardiovasc Surg.* 1997 Mar;113(3):476-491.

aorta, prophylactic surgery is recommended when the aorta reaches 5.5 cm, and for the descending aorta at 6.5 cm. When surgery can be delivered at low risk (as at experienced centers), it is appropriate to drop these criteria to 5.0 cm for ascending and 6.0 cm for descending aneurysms. All of these intervention criteria are in the process of being "personalized" based on which specific causative mutation obtains in an individual patient. For patients with Marfan syndrome and other syndromic connective tissue disorders, the recommended criteria are slightly lower than for the general thoracic aortic population—specifically, 5.0 cm and 6.0 cm for ascending and descending, respectively (Table 23–5).

Although the aforementioned intervention criteria are designed for general use, adjustments are necessary for extremes of body size. For example, for a 7-foot-tall athlete, an ascending aorta of 4.4 cm may fall within the range of normal diameters, given the large body and circulatory demand. Conversely, an aorta of the same diameter would represent significant enlargement for a 5-foot-tall woman, placing her at high risk of adverse aortic events. Body size should be included in risk calculations for very large or very small individuals. Tabular guides provide specific risk levels for patients based on body surface area stratified into categories of annual risk, as low (~4%), medium (~8%), or high (~20%), permitting adjustment of recommendations beyond the conventional intervention criteria.

Body surface area has recently been largely replaced by height as the factor against which aortic diameter is normalized.[61] **Table 23–6** presents a nomogram using height alone (rather than body surface area) for aortic prediction. Not only aortic diameter, but also ascending aortic *length* is an important

TABLE 23–5. The Yale Center for Thoracic Aortic Disease Recommended Surgical Intervention Criteria for Thoracic Aortic Aneurysms

1. Rupture
2. Acute aortic dissection
   a. Ascending requires urgent operation
   b. Descending requires a "complication-specific approach"
3. Symptomatic states
   a. Pain consistent with rupture and unexplained by other causes
   b. Compression of adjacent organs, especially the trachea, esophagus, or left main stem bronchus
   c. Significant aortic insufficiency in conjunction with ascending aortic aneurysm
4. Documented enlargement
   a. Growth ≥1 cm/y or substantial growth and aneurysm is rapidly approaching absolute size criteria
5. Absolute size (cm)

	Marfan (cm)	Non-Marfan (cm)
Ascending	5.0	5.5
Descending	6.0	6.5

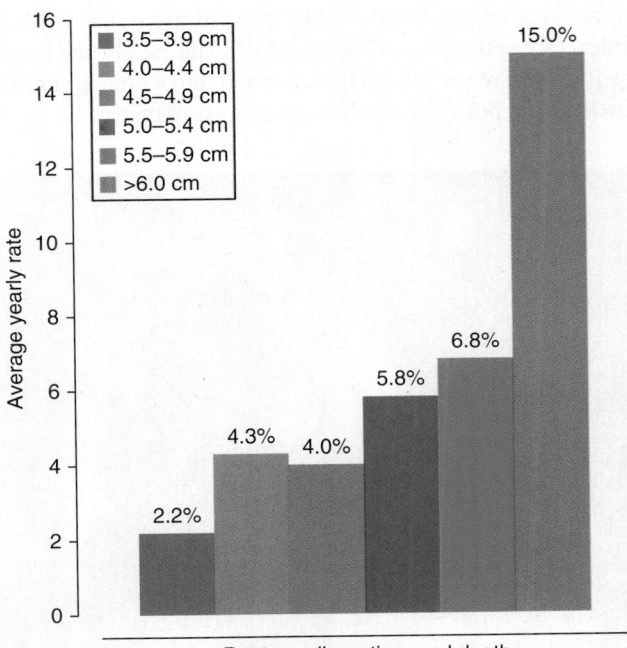

Figure 23–31. Average yearly rates of the composite adverse event endpoint of rupture, dissection, and death related to ascending aortic aneurysm at various aortic sizes. Reproduced with permission from Zafar MA, Li Y, Rizzo JA, et al. Height alone, rather than body surface area, suffices for risk estimation in ascending aortic aneurysm. *J Thorac Cardiovasc Surg.* 2018 May;155(5):1938-1950.

TABLE 23–6. Risk of Complications (Aortic Dissection, Rupture, and Death) in Patients with Ascending aortic Aneurysm as a Function of Aortic Diameter (Horizontal Axis) and Height (Vertical Axis), with the Aortic Height Index Given within the Figure

Height		Aortic Size (cm)									
		3.5	4.0	4.5	5.0	5.5	6.0	6.5	7.0	7.5	8.0
(inches)	(m)										
55	1.40	2.50	2.86	3.21	3.57	3.93	4.29	4.64	5.00	5.36	5.71
57	1.45	2.41	2.76	3.10	3.45	3.79	4.14	4.48	4.83	5.17	5.52
59	1.50	2.33	2.67	3.00	3.33	3.67	4.00	4.33	4.67	5.00	5.33
61	1.55	2.26	2.58	2.90	3.23	3.55	3.87	4.19	4.52	4.84	5.16
63	1.60	2.19	2.50	2.81	3.13	3.44	3.75	4.06	4.38	4.69	5.00
65	1.65	2.12	2.42	2.73	3.03	3.33	3.64	3.94	4.24	4.55	4.85
67	1.70	2.06	2.35	2.65	2.94	3.24	3.53	3.82	4.12	4.41	4.71
69	1.75	2.00	2.29	2.57	2.86	3.14	3.43	3.71	4.00	4.29	4.57
71	1.80	1.94	2.22	2.50	2.78	3.06	3.33	3.61	3.89	4.17	4.44
73	1.85	1.89	2.16	2.43	2.70	2.97	3.24	3.51	3.78	4.05	4.32
75	1.90	1.84	2.11	2.37	2.63	2.89	3.16	3.42	3.68	3.95	4.21
77	1.95	1.79	2.05	2.31	2.56	2.82	3.08	3.33	3.59	3.85	4.10
79	2.00	1.75	2.00	2.25	2.50	2.75	3.00	3.25	3.50	3.75	4.00
81	2.05	1.71	1.95	2.20	2.44	2.68	2.93	3.17	3.41	3.66	3.90

  = low risk (~4% per year)   = moderate risk (~7% per year)   = High risk (~12% per year)   = severe risk (~18% per year)

Light green area indicates low risk, yellow area indicates moderate risk, orange area indicates high risk, and red area indicates severe risk.

Light green indicates low risk; yellow, moderate risk; orange, high risk; red, severe risk.

Reproduced with permission from Zafar MA, Li Y, Rizzo JA, et al. Height alone, rather than body surface area, suffices for risk estimation in ascending aortic aneurysm. *J Thorac Cardiovasc Surg.* 2018 May;155(5):1938-1950.

determinant of malignant aortic events. Ascending aortic length is defined as the distance along a centerline from the aortic annulus to the base of the innominate artery (**Fig. 23–32**). It is anticipated that length will be invoked more commonly in clinical care in the future (**Fig. 23–33**). In fact, height and length together have recently been incorporated into a nomogram that benefits from both those indicators of aortic danger.[83]

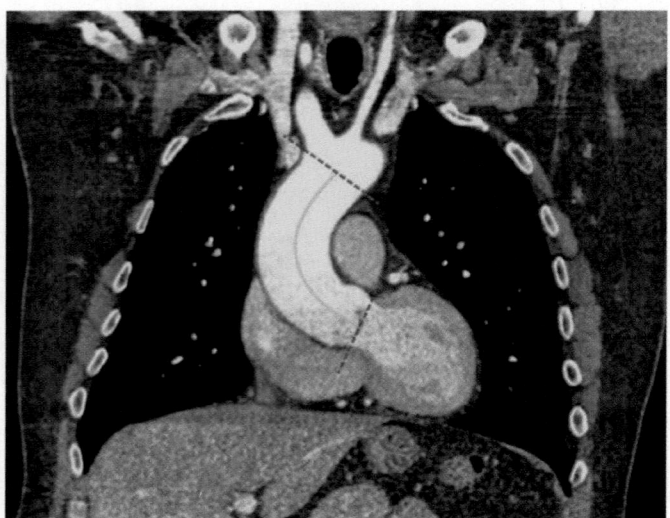

Figure 23–32. Ascending aortic length is measured as distance (*blue*) from the aortic annulus (*red*) to the origin of innominate artery (*red*). Reproduced with permission from Wu J, Zafar MA, Li Y, et al. Ascending Aortic Length and Risk of Aortic Adverse Events: The Neglected Dimension. *J Am Coll Cardiol.* 2019 Oct 15;74(15):1883-1894.

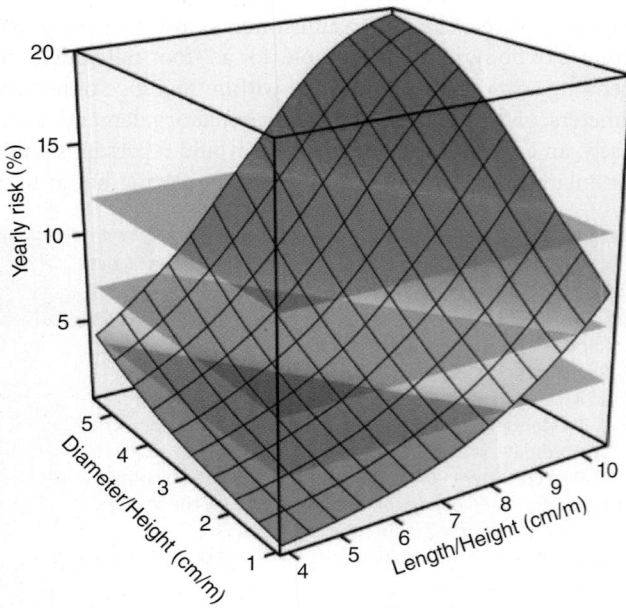

Figure 23–33. Prediction plot as a function of DHI (*x*-axis) and LHI (*y*-axis), with the yearly risk of AAEs presented on the *z*-axis. AAE, aortic adverse events; AHI, aortic height index; DHI, diameter height index; LHI, length height index. Reproduced with permission from Wu J, Zafar MA, Li Y, et al. Ascending Aortic Length and Risk of Aortic Adverse Events: The Neglected Dimension. *J Am Coll Cardiol.* 2019 Oct 15; 74(15):1883-1894.

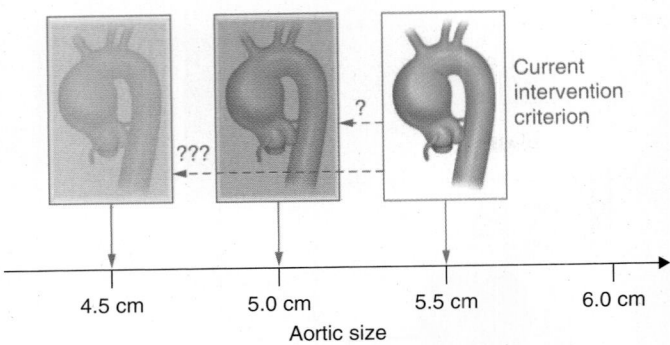

Figure 23–34. **Is it time for a leftward shift in the intervention criteria for ascending aortic aneurysm?** Reproduced with permission from Ziganshin BA, Zafar MA, Elefteriades JA. Descending threshold for ascending aortic aneurysmectomy: Is it time for a "left-shift" in guidelines? *J Thorac Cardiovasc Surg.* 2019 Jan;157(1):37-42.

Morphologic criteria apply only to *asymptomatic* patients. Patients with pain from aneurysms require prompt surgery regardless of diameter or other size criteria. Pain implies impending rupture. Its grave importance must be respected. It may be difficult to determine if pain is aortic or of other origin. Appropriate investigations, supplemented by clinical judgment, can rule out other potential sources (musculoskeletal, costochondritis, esophageal, ischemic, etc). Many patients have died because their pain was underappreciated, dissecting even at criteria below recommended thresholds.

Several evolving factors argue in favor of "shifting left" to a lower size criterion for intervention on the ascending aorta (**Fig. 23–34**).[84] Specifically,

- *Earlier hinge points.* The most recent analyses are showing earlier hinge points in the size at which dissection occurs, more toward the low 5 cm range.[62]
- *Sudden growth at moment of dissection.* It is now recognized that the aorta grows suddenly at the moment of aortic dissection. This has been found courtesy of CT examinations serendipitously performed just before aortic dissection occurs.[85,86] These studies have shown an instantaneous increase in aortic diameter of about 8 mm immediately consequent upon aortic dissection (**Fig. 23–35**).[86] This means that the aorta was considerably smaller when it dissected, meaning that our criteria would need to be moved toward smaller size ranges.[84]
- *Centerline methods yield smaller aortic sizes.* The new computerized algorithms underestimate ascending aortic size compared to the traditional hand measurements on which intervention standards are based.
- *Safety of aortic surgery in the present era.* Aortic surgery has become exceptionally safe, with stroke and deaths rates in the 1% to 2% range, about the same as those for routine coronary artery bypass surgery.
- *Strong impact of a prior family dissection event.* It has been determined that once one dissection has occurred in a family, the risk of dissection in other aneurysm-bearing family members increases by at least 2.7-fold.[40] So, those family members may best be served by very early intervention, as the dissection is "just waiting to happen."
- *Malignant pathologies discovered on genetic analysis.* Genetic analysis often reveals the exact mutation that is causing

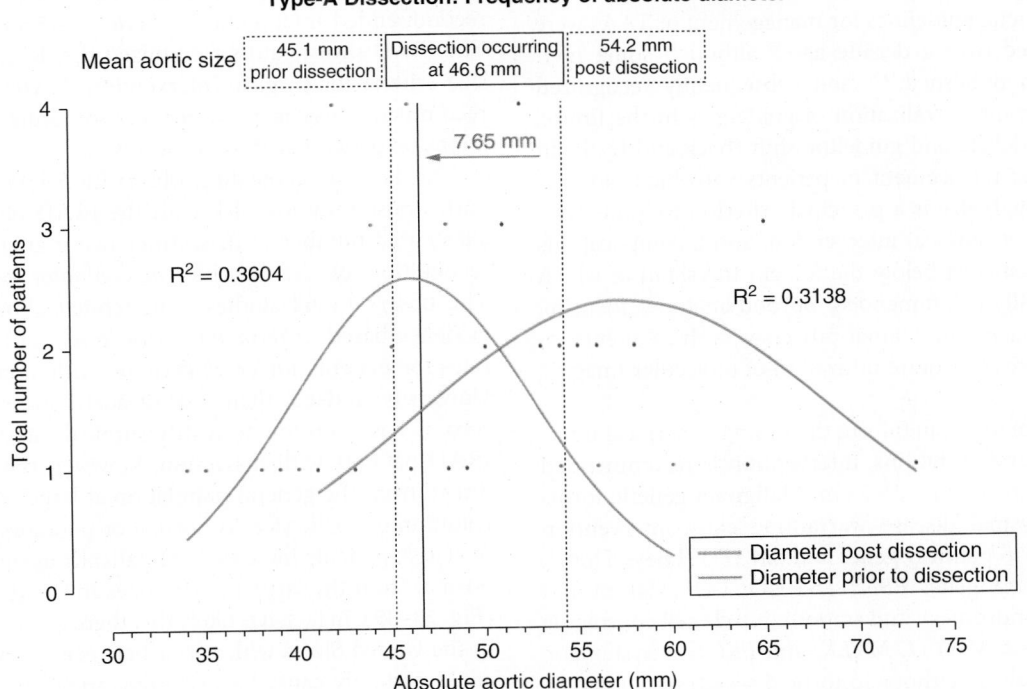

Figure 23–35. **Frequency of aortic sizes before and at the time of aortic dissection.** (Note: In addition to simple arithmetic calculations, regression methods utilizing "aortic dissection" as a variable influencing size mitigated the impact of elapsed time between pre- and post images.) Data from Mansour AM, Peterss S, Zafar MA, et al. Prevention of Aortic Dissection Suggests a Diameter Shift to a Lower Aortic Size Threshold for Intervention. *Cardiology.* 2018;139(3):139-146.

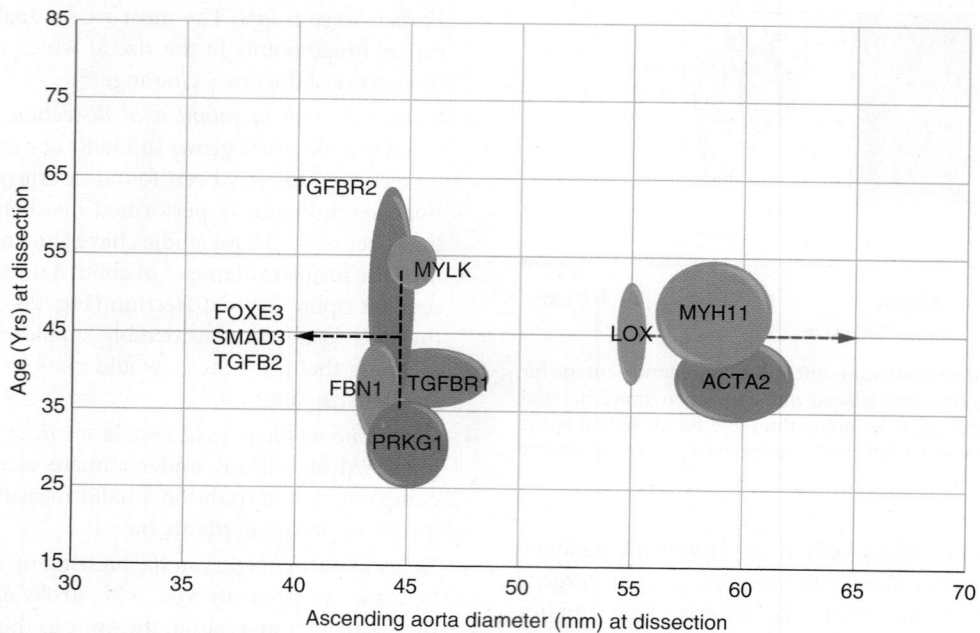

Figure 23–36. Schematic representation of genetic mutations with age and ascending aorta diameter at dissection. The widening of the circles/lines represents SD in terms of age and diameters. Data are obtained from studies included in the systematic review. No numerical data were available for patients affected by aortic dissection regarding the genes *NOTCH1* and *MFAP5*, and patients with *MAT2A* mutation did not experience aortic dissections. Reproduced with permission from Mariscalco G, Debiec R, Elefteriades JA, et al. Systematic Review of Studies That Have Evaluated Screening Tests in Relatives of Patients Affected by Nonsyndromic Thoracic Aortic Disease. *J Am Heart Assoc.* 2018 Aug 7;7(15):e009302.

aortic aneurysms and dissections in a given family. Some of these mutations require early surgery, because genetically mediated aortic dissection may occur with little or no aortic enlargement.

The multisocietal guidelines for management of TAAs were initially published over a decade ago,[39] although some revisions have been published,[29,30] and subsequently recognized factors may warrant liberalization of guidelines in the future. There has been debate and guideline shift (back and forth) in criteria for aortic replacement in patients with bicuspid aortic valves. Although size is a principal criterion to guide timing of prophylactic surgical intervention, aortic complications may occur at diameters below the 5.5 cm threshold at which surgery is generally recommended. Beyond anatomy, focusing on central pathogenic functional processes such as aneurysm disease activity would require utilization of molecular imaging modalities.

Genetic information can inform the timing of surgical intervention. For several mutations, intervention is recommended at aortic diameters less than 5.5 cm. Malignant genetic forms of aortic aneurysmal disease warranting early intervention include the TGF-β pathway genes and *SMAD3* (Loeys-Dietz), extracellular matrix genes *FBN1* and *COL3A1* (Marfan and Ehlers-Danlos syndromes), and smooth muscle cell contractile unit genes *ACTA2*, *MHY11*, *MYLK*, and *PKG1*. A systematic review of nonsyndromic thoracic aortic disease provides additional data on patient age and aortic dimensions at the time of dissection (**Fig. 23–36**).[87]

The "Aortic Size Paradox" in Ascending Aortic Intervention Criteria: Dissections occasionally occur at small aortic sizes, as shown in **Fig. 23–37**. A substantial number of aortic dissections in the IRAD registry occurred at sizes below the currently recommended intervention criterion of 5.5 cm (**Fig. 23–38**). The IRAD investigators recognized the dangers of amending size criteria for surgical intervention downward and did *not* recommend this change for fear of promoting harm from operations on patients with small aortas.

The key to reconciling observational studies that small aortas pose only low risk with the IRAD observation that a substantial number of dissections occur at small sizes lies in recognition of the "at-risk" *denominator* pool of patients. The observational studies (enumerated above in discussing evidence-based criteria for aortic resection) present danger rates for patients *under observation* with small aortas at Yale University; indeed, their risk of aortic events, although not zero, is low—too low to justify surgical intervention. For the IRAD patients with dissection, however, the dissectors were drawn from the general population at large. Whether the distribution of aortic sizes is normal or paranormal, the number of at-risk patients increases dramatically as one moves toward normal from the largest aortic sizes in the distribution curve (**Fig. 23–39**). In fact, it is likely that there are millions of patients in the United States with aortas between 4 cm and 5 cm. One could certainly cause harm by operating on all of them prophylactically. In fact, if one were to divide the numerator of observed dissections in IRAD by a denominator of millions,

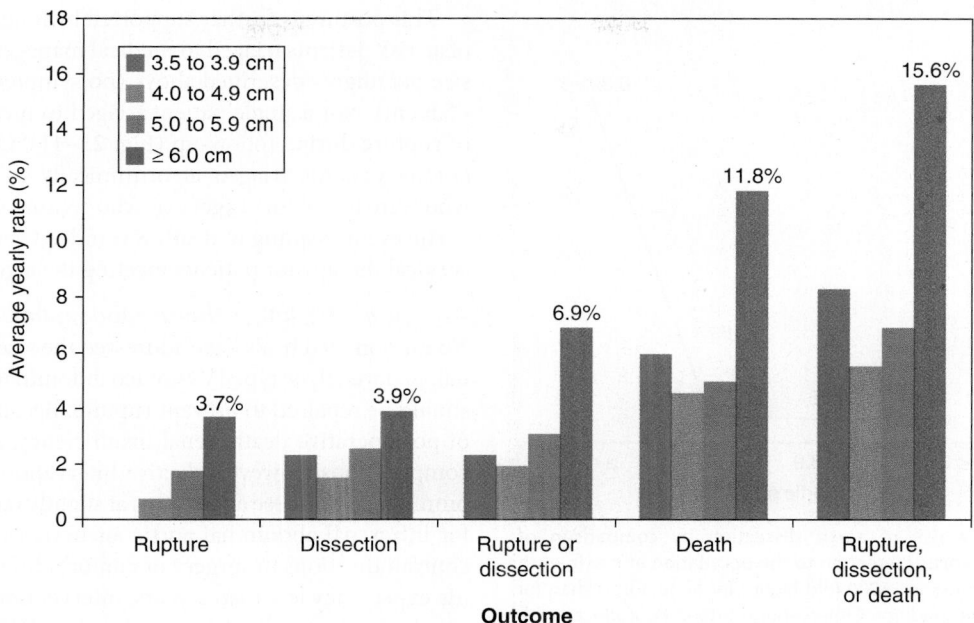

Figure 23–37. Yearly rates of rupture, dissection, or death related to aortic size. Note that the likelihood of rupture, dissection, or death within the coming year also jumps sharply for aneurysms that reach 6 cm or higher. (The rates indicated for "Rupture or Dissection" and for "Rupture, Dissection, or Death" are lower than the sum of the rates in individual categories because patients with multiple complications were counted only once in the combined categories.) These data underlie the conclusion that aneurysms in the ascending aorta need corrective surgery when the artery balloons to 5.5 cm. Reproduced with permission from Alison Kendall.

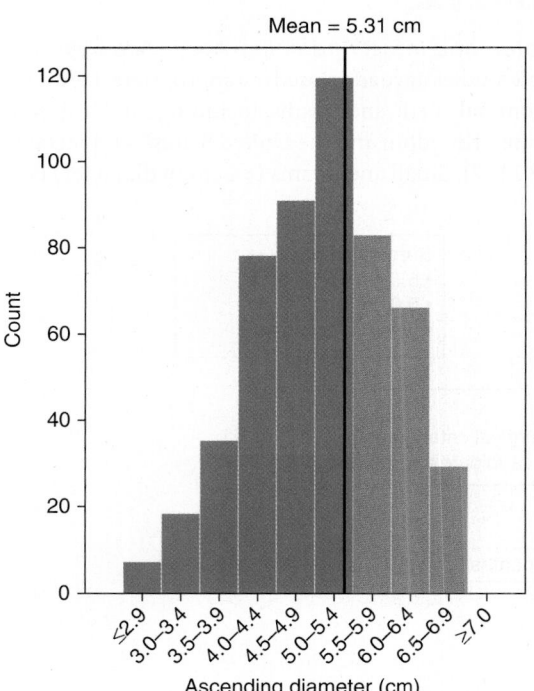

Figure 23–38. Distribution of aortic size at the time of presentation with acute type A aortic dissection (cm). *Orange bars* indicate 50% of patients with diameters smaller than 5.5 cm. Reproduced with permission from Pape LA, Tsai TT, Isselbacher EM, et al. Aortic diameter >or = 5.5 cm is not a good predictor of type A aortic dissection: observations from the International Registry of Acute Aortic Dissection (IRAD). *Circulation.* 2007 Sep 4;116(10): 1120-1127.

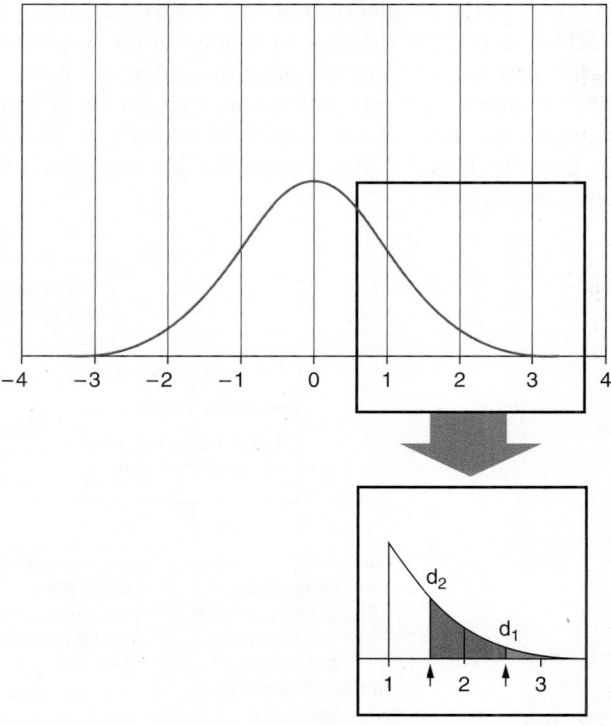

Figure 23–39. Huge general population at risk explains occurrence of some dissections at small sizes. Note how the denominator of individuals increases dramatically. Thus, although dissections do occur at the lower aortic sizes, the likelihood (per population at risk) is very low. Reproduced with permission from Elefteriades JA, Farkas EA. Thoracic aortic aneurysm clinically pertinent controversies and uncertainties. *J Am Coll Cardiol.* 2010 Mar 2;55(9):841-857.

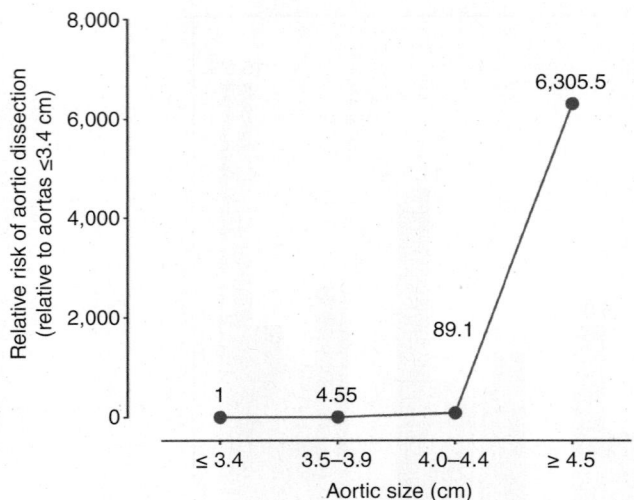

Figure 23–40. Relative risk of aortic dissection by comparison of observed instances of aortic dissection to the population at risk in each size range. The relative risk is >6000-fold higher for large aortas than for small ones. This vindicates traditional intervention criteria. Reproduced with permission from Paruchuri V, Salhab KF, Kuzmik G, et al. Aortic Size Distribution in the General Population: Explaining the Size Paradox in Aortic Dissection. *Cardiology.* 2015;131(4):265-272.

the observed yearly percentage rate of dissection in the small sizes would be very small.

Analysis of the normal distribution of aortic diameters in the MESA[3] and IRAD database in relation to the risk of aortic dissection revealed that although dissection can occur at smaller diameters, patients with aortas ≥4.5 cm are at 6000-fold greater risk of dissection than those with aortas ≤3.4 cm (**Fig. 23–40**).[4] These studies support the current criteria for surgical intervention.

This posture is further supported by longitudinal follow-up of at-risk patients triaged to medical management based on the size paradigms described above (no symptoms and aortic size <5.5 cm). Not a single patient triaged to medical therapy died of rupture during follow-up (**Fig. 23–41**). On the other hand, among patients triaged algorithmically to the surgical arm who were too ill for surgery or who refused surgery, the rate of aortic events leading to death was indeed very high, validating surgical therapy for patients meeting the algorithm criterion.

Asymptomatic, Intact Thoracoabdominal Aortic Aneurysms

No randomized trials have addressed the size at which suprarenal, juxtarenal, or type IV thoracoabdominal aortic aneurysms should be repaired to prevent rupture. Because of the high risk of postoperative death, renal insufficiency, and other surgical complications, however, elective intervention is generally recommended for these aneurysms at slightly larger diameter than for infrarenal abdominal aortic aneurysms. In the absence of contraindications to surgery or comorbidities associated with a life expectancy less than 2 years, intervention is generally indicated in patients with suprarenal or type IV thoracoabdominal aortic aneurysms larger than 5.5 cm to 6.0 cm.

The dimensional criteria for surgical intervention apply only to asymptomatic aneurysms confined to the chest or abdomen. The development of symptoms frequently portends rupture and mandates surgical or endovascular repair. Hence, symptomatic aortic aneurysms at any level should be resected regardless of size.

Asymptomatic, Intact Abdominal Aortic Aneurysms

Multiple studies have addressed the appropriate size for resection of abdominal aortic aneurysms, including randomized trials in the United Kingdom and the United States[88] and meta-analyses (**Table 23–7**). Small aneurysms (<4 cm in diameter) pose a low

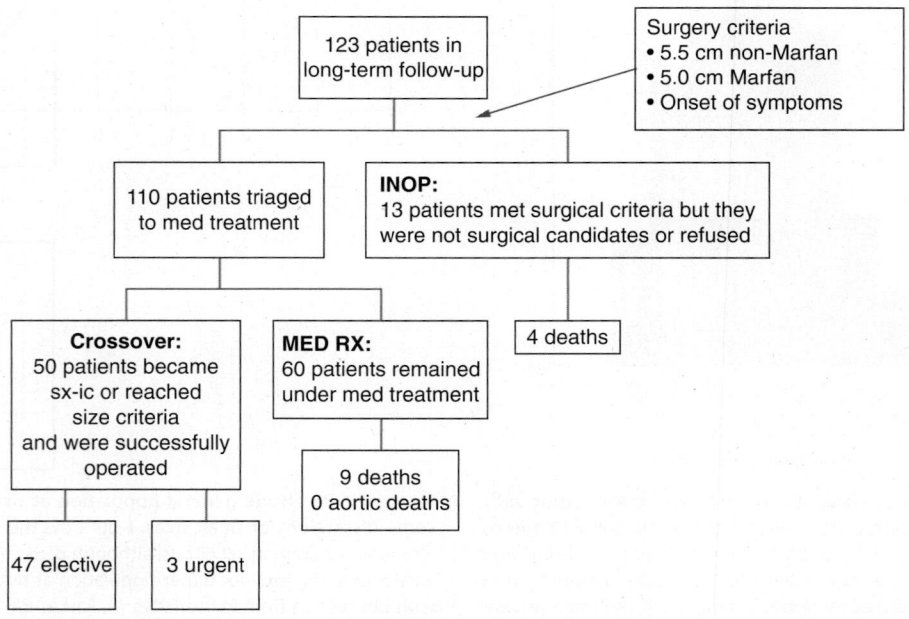

Figure 23–41. Flow diagram of medically treated patients. INOP, inoperable; crossover, crossed-over from medical therapy to surgery; MED RX; medical therapy. Reproduced with permission from Elefteriades JA, Farkas EA. Thoracic aortic aneurysm clinically pertinent controversies and uncertainties. *J Am Coll Cardiol.* 2010 Mar 2;55(9):841-857.

TABLE 23–7. Decision Making for Abdominal Aortic Aneurysms

HSTAT Meta-Analysis of Surgical Intervention Criteria for AAA Leads to the Following Conclusions:		
3.0–3.9 cm AAA	Very low risk of rupture	Yearly ultrasound
4.0–5.4 cm AAA	Yearly rupture rate = 1%	Ultrasound every 6 months
5.5 cm or larger AAA	Substantial rupture risk	Endovascular or open surgery advised

Abbreviations: AAA, abdominal aortic aneurysm; HSTAT, Health Services/Technology Assessment Text.
Data from Elefteriades and Rizzo[91] and Health Services/Technology Assessment Text.[93]

risk of rupture and should be managed with periodic surveillance for enlargement and symptoms. Abdominal aortic aneurysms between 4 cm and 5 cm in diameter are associated with a 1% per year risk of rupture, and decisions regarding surveillance or surgery should be individualized based on age, familial features, and an assessment of surgical risk. Aneurysms 5.5 cm in diameter or larger carry a substantial risk of rupture and should be repaired. As for thoracic aneurysms, the occurrence of symptoms supersedes diameter as a basis for intervention. In general, patients with infrarenal or juxtarenal abdominal aortic aneurysms measuring 4.0 cm to 5.4 cm in diameter should be monitored by ultrasonography or CT scans every 6 months to detect expansion. Repair may be beneficial in selected patients with aneurysms of 5.0 cm to 5.4 cm in diameter at this level. For patients with aneurysms smaller than 4.0 cm in diameter, monitoring by ultrasonography examination yearly is reasonable. Intervention is not recommended for patients with asymptomatic infrarenal or juxtarenal aneurysms smaller than 5.0 cm in diameter in men or 4.5 cm in women. A meta-analysis found that these criteria should be employed as well for *endovascular* treatment of abdominal aortic aneurysms, and that similar size indications for intervention should apply to both endovascular and surgical therapy.[89]

Surgical and Endovascular Therapy of Aortic Aneurysms

The modern era in the treatment of aneurysms and dissections was ushered in by the pioneering innovations of Cooley and DeBakey, which were first reported in 1952.[90] Specific surgical procedures have been developed for resection and graft replacement of aneurysms involving the ascending aorta, transverse (arch), descending thoracic, thoracoabdominal, and abdominal aortic segments. Techniques for elective open surgical treatment of thoracic and abdominal aortic aneurysms that have reached criteria for intervention have been refined over the last 70 years, dating from the efforts of early pioneers including DeBakey, Cooley, Crawford, Cabrol, Dubost, and others. Safe approaches have been standardized for various aneurysmal anatomic patterns,[90] and reliable, durable prosthetic grafts are available in numerous configurations. Dacron grafts do not require long-term anticoagulant therapy. The risks of surgery include bleeding, stroke, paralysis, MI, renal failure, death, and other complications; safety is greatest when surgery is performed electively before aortic rupture or dissection. Due to advances in surgical techniques (specifically myocardial and brain protection), graft materials (impervious), cardiopulmonary bypass, and anesthetic and postoperative care, these operations can be performed electively with outcomes at experienced centers rivaling those of coronary artery bypass and valve replacement surgery.

Aortic Root Aneurysms

The morphology of the aortic root dictates the surgical procedure required for correction of aneurysmal pathology (Fig. 23–10). For supracoronary aneurysms, tube graft replacement is typically used unless stenosis or insufficiency of the aortic valve requires concomitant valve replacement. In patients with annuloaortic ectasia, composite graft replacement of the aortic root and the aortic valve with a prefabricated unit is preferred. When the aortic root is involved in Marfan syndrome or other severe connective tissue disorders, as well as in cases of aortic root aneurysms associated with bicuspid aortic valve, the aortic root is resected, which requires mobilizing, detaching, and re-implanting the coronary artery ostia. The aortic root can be replaced with a valved conduit, which carries either a mechanical or biological valve prefabricated within the graft. In selected cases, valve-sparing procedures can be performed, in which the native valve is implanted within the aortic graft. Yacoub et al.[92] and David et al.[93] have advocated techniques for valve-sparing aortic root replacement. Accumulating data suggest that patient survival and aortic valve function are generally well-maintained following valve-sparing procedures in appropriately selected cases,[94] but caution is warranted because recurrent or progressive aortic insufficiency can occur.[95]

Aortic Arch Aneurysms

When aneurysmal dilatation involves the arch of the aorta beyond the origin of the innominate artery, a more challenging operation is necessary in which the innominate, left carotid, and left subclavian arteries are detached and the aortic arch is resected. The arch structures are then replaced with prefabricated or bespoke neo-aortic arch substitutes. These operations involve interruption of blood supply to the brain, necessitating cerebral protection during attachment of the great vessels to the aortic graft. Carrel patches with a rim of aorta carrying the innominate, left carotid, and left subclavian arteries are commonly used or, alternatively, prefabricated branched grafts are available that permit anastomosis of each great vessel individually. At 18°C, the temperature commonly used, the metabolic rate is below 15% of normal, permitting surgery on the aortic arch. Whole-body cooling slows cerebral metabolism by about 50% for each 6°C drop in temperature, so, at 18°C, the metabolic rate is 12.5% of normal. This allows 45 to 60 minutes to replace the aortic arch with preservation of cognitive function. When longer periods of deep hypothermic circulatory arrest are necessary, or by surgeon preference, direct cerebral perfusion can be provided through cannulae placed individually

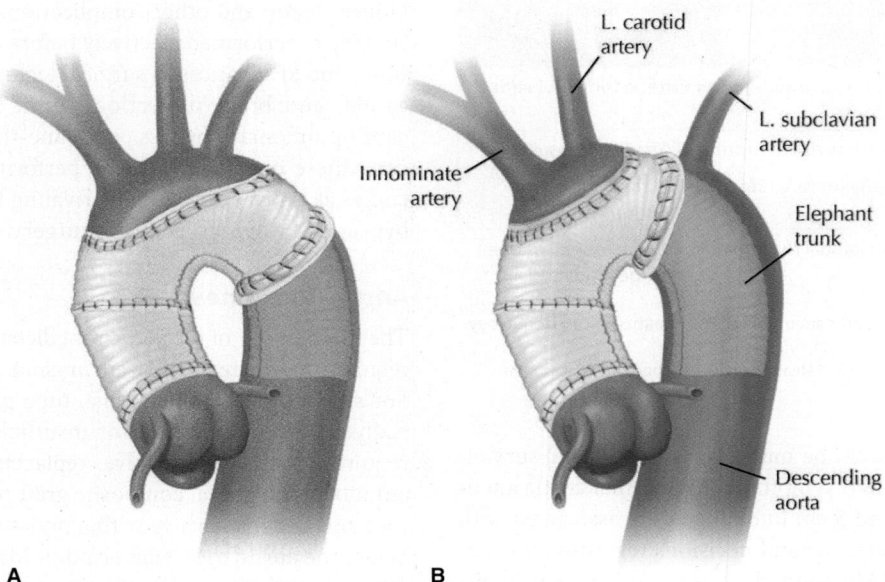

Figure 23–42. **During aortic arch replacement procedures, an "elephant trunk" is placed in the descending aorta to facilitate any future interventions on the descending or thoracoabdominal aorta, should such be necessary.** Reproduced with permission from Ziganshin BA, Rajbanshi BG, Tranquilli M, et al. Straight deep hypothermic circulatory arrest for cerebral protection during aortic arch surgery: Safe and effective. *J Thorac Cardiovasc Surg.* 2014 Sep; 148(3):888-898.

in the great vessels for extraanatomic pump-based antegrade or retrograde cerebral perfusion. An "elephant trunk" placed in the descending aorta facilitates subsequent procedures to address associated disease in the descending or thoracoabdominal aorta (**Fig. 23–42**).

Outcomes of open ascending aortic and aortic arch surgery have also improved over time. Ascending aortic surgery, including aortic root replacement procedures and aortic arch replacements, has become nearly as safe as ordinary cardiac surgical procedures such as coronary artery bypass and aortic valve surgery. Mortality and stroke rates, especially as specialized centers, have fallen into the range of 1% to 2%, respectively (**Table 23–8**). In a retrospective analysis of a large cohort of Medicare beneficiaries, open surgical repair of intact descending TAAs was associated with higher early postoperative mortality but reduced late hazard of death. Despite the late advantage of open repair, net mean survival was superior with endovascular intervention.[96]

Conventional open surgical procedures can lead to dramatically durable long-term results. This is exemplified in the survival of patients after conventional composite graft replacement of the aortic root (**Fig. 23–43**), which is identical to that of an age- and gender-matched population.[97] This demonstrates a simply remarkable beneficial and durable impact on an otherwise lethal disease. This degree of impact on this virulent disease is "almost curative," a statement that can rarely be used in cardiac diseases—almost "like it never happened." Dacron grafts placed by open surgical means last essentially forever.

Infection of surgically placed grafts is rare. When PET-CT imaging is performed (typically for other indications), it is likely that a Dacron graft will appear enhanced. This does not signify infection, but rather reflects a normal inflammatory response to implanted foreign material. Such activity on PET scanning has been described in 92% of uninfected grafts.[98]

Thoracoabdominal Aortic Aneurysms

The key issues in surgery of the thoracoabdominal aorta involve protection of the lower body organs and spinal cord during the period of aortic cross-clamping and attachment of the visceral arteries (superior mesenteric artery, celiac axis, and renal arteries). The arterial supply of the spinal cord is segmental, and viability of spinal cord cells is highly dependent on the artery of Adamkiewicz or arteries arising from the low intercostal or lumbar territory (T8-L2), which are excluded (at least transiently, and at times permanently) during thoracoabdominal aortic surgery. Intraoperative perfusion of the lower body by blood aspirated from the left atrium helps prevent paraplegia, among the most worrisome complications of this procedure. For operations on the descending or thoracoabdominal aorta,

TABLE 23–8. Contemporary Safety of Ascending Aortic, Aortic Root, and Aortic Arch Procedures at Yale University School of Medicine, Reflective of High Safety Levels at Specialized Centers in the Present Era

Location of Surgery	Operative Mortality	Postoperative Stroke
Composite Aortic Root Replacement	1.9%	1.4%
Root Sparing Ascending Aortic Replacement	0%	1.0%
Aortic Arch Replacement with DHCA	1.4%	1.2%

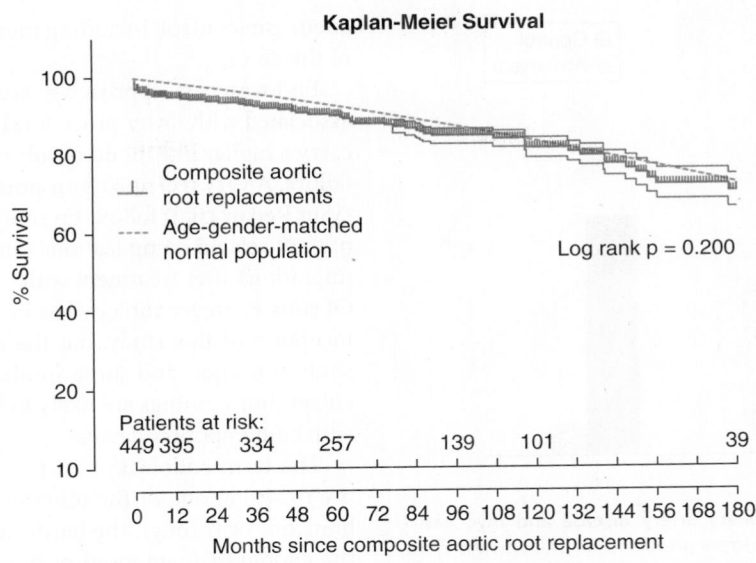

Figure 23–43. Long-term survival after aortic root replacement (biological or mechanical) (blue line) is identical to that of the normal population (red dotted line). Reproduced with permission from Mok SC, Ma WG, Mansour A, et al. Twenty-five year outcomes following composite graft aortic root replacement. *J Card Surg.* 2017 Feb;32(2):99-109.

in which the native aorta may be clamped for considerable periods of time, paraplegia may be permanent and devastating. The incidence of paraplegia varies with aneurysm extent, but in some reports has been as high as 15%.[99,100] Several techniques have been developed to decrease the likelihood of paraplegia, including spinal fluid drainage to decrease the pressure around the spinal cord and encourage collateral blood flow. Intraoperative monitoring of motor evoked potentials (MEPS) helps in detecting spinal cord ischemia in real-time intraoperatively, so that remedial steps can be taken.[101] A novel cooling catheter in an advanced developmental stage (placed by simple lumbar puncture) along the spinal cord can provide topical protective hypothermia to the spinal cord. Other protective techniques include mild systemic hypothermia, aspiration of cerebrospinal fluid to decrease ambient pressure on the spinal cord, and reimplantation of the intercostal arteries.[102]

The technical challenge of attaching the branch vessels of the abdominal aorta has been met by technical advances, most specifically by reimplantation of branch arteries on pedicles of surrounding aorta, often by the inclusion technique (in which the pedicle is not mobilized completely from its bed). Currently, the frequency of mortality or paraplegia with this type of surgery at experienced centers is below 10%, reflecting technical improvements in graft technology, surgical techniques, perfusion, anesthesia, and perioperative care.[103]

Concomitant Coronary Artery Disease

The most important risk factor for cardiac events and death in patients undergoing abdominal aneurysm surgery is coronary artery disease. Because operative mortality is related mainly to myocardial ischemia, it has been suggested that coronary revascularization be performed in selected patients before abdominal aortic aneurysm resection. No well-designed studies are available, however, comparing the

outcome of serial myocardial revascularization and abdominal or TAA repair with aneurysm surgery alone. Even so, an effort should be made to identify preoperatively patients at highest cardiac risk using noninvasive diagnostic methods. Findings of extensive myocardial ischemia may prompt angiography to define the coronary pathoanatomy and LV function. Thereafter, decisions regarding coronary revascularization must be based on symptoms, angiographic findings, and other elements of risk. One anticipates a survival advantage imparted by surgical revascularization in patients with left main coronary artery disease or stenosis greater than 70% involving each of the three major coronary arteries in patients with substantial zones of myocardial ischemia. In those with severe discrete proximal stenosis of a first-order coronary artery and symptomatic or extensive ischemia or reversible LV dysfunction amenable to catheter-based myocardial revascularization, clinical decision making must balance the long-term advantages of drug-eluting intracoronary stents against the need for potent platelet inhibitor therapy that may be difficult to administer in the days before and after aortic aneurysmectomy. Furthermore, in patients soon to undergo aortic reconstructive surgery, coronary balloon angioplasty or bare-metal stenting may be preferred, even though the potential for coronary restenosis may later require a second revascularization procedure after aortic surgery has been completed.

Ascending aortic aneurysms, which are typically nonatherosclerotic, are less often associated with atherosclerotic coronary artery disease than aneurysms located more distally in the aorta. A comparison of patients with ascending aortic aneurysms associated with annuloaortic ectasia or aortic dissection with age- and gender-matched control subjects found less arterial calcification, detected by CT imaging, in those with aneurysms. Patients with ascending aortic aneurysms have lower intimal-medial carotid artery wall thickness (IMT) than control subjects[104] and a low incidence of MI (**Fig. 23–44**).[105]

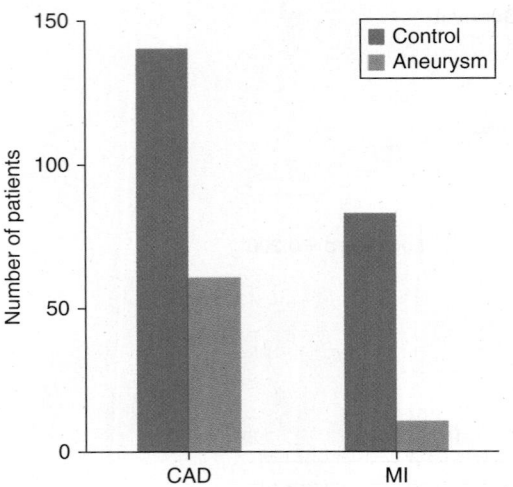

Figure 23–44. Incidence of coronary artery disease and myocardial infarction. There was a significantly lower prevalence of CAD and MIs in the aneurysm group than in the control group. There were 61 patients in the aneurysm group who had CAD (*P* <0.001) versus 140 in the control group. There were 11 patients in the aneurysm group who have had a MI versus 83 in the control group (*P* <0.001). CAD, coronary artery disease; MI, myocardial infarction. Reproduced with permission from Chau K, Elefteriades JA. Ascending thoracic aortic aneurysms protect against myocardial infarctions. *Int J Angiol.* 2014 Sep;23(3):177-182.

Mutations or metabolic pathways such as those involving MMPs or TGF-β that contribute to aortic root or ascending aortic aneurysms might protect against atherosclerosis, MMPs that lead to aortic aneurysm development may have antiatherogenic properties, or the biophysics of atherogenesis could be influenced by changes in pressure or flow dynamics resulting from aneurysmal disease.[106]

Diagnostic cardiac catheterization and angiography are routinely performed as part of the preoperative evaluation of patients undergoing surgical repair of ascending aortic aneurysms to evaluate the morphology of the ascending aorta, function of the aortic valve, and coronary anatomy. Based on the angiographic findings, myocardial revascularization can be readily incorporated into the reparative surgical procedure if warranted. For descending aortic aneurysms, if severe proximal coronary artery disease is found, then options include staged percutaneous or surgical coronary revascularization followed after an interval of several weeks by resection of the aneurysm. Results of such aggressive revascularization via a staged approach were recently reported with favorable outcomes.[107]

Open or Endovascular Correction of Aneurysms

Surgical approaches to management of aortic aneurysms and dissections have traditionally involved large, open procedures. Over the past generation, however, endovascular approaches have rapidly evolved since the first abdominal endovascular graft by Parodi and the first thoracic aortic graft by Dake in 1991 and 1994, respectively. Interventional radiologists, cardiologists, cardiac surgeons, and vascular surgeons have promoted the development of endovascular stents for aneurysm control, including methods to address the branches of the aorta.

Endovascular approaches are less invasive and generally associated with lower procedural risk. On the other hand, they carry a higher likelihood of subsequent reintervention and late failure. A very recent 20-year post-EVAR (Endovascular Aneurysm Repair trial) follow-up study found a staggering 90% rate of graft related complications (endoleak, fracture, thrombosis, migration) after treatment with a first-generation stent graft.[108] Of course, the technology has improved dramatically since the inception of this study, but the duration of follow-up in this study is unique, and some similar, modality related (endovascular) shortcomings are likely to be seen in the long term even with contemporary devices.

The term endoleak itself is a neologism, connoting a failure to seal at one or the other end of the aneurysm or at side branches or through the hardware itself. Also, the sac around the endograft (composed of the wall of the native aorta) can expand over time. The ultimate significance of this persistent or expanding sac is not fully known. Paraplegia can occur during or after endovascular repair of descending and thoracoabdominal aortic aneurysms, although at about less than half the incidence associated with open surgery.[16,109]

A recent large meta-analysis comparing randomized trials open and endovascular treatment of nonruptured abdominal aortic aneurysms found lower 1-month mortality for endovascular therapy but a dramatically sobering higher long-term (8 year) risk of death for the endovascular patients (hazard ratio [HR] 5.12) as well as reintervention (HR 2.13) and aneurysm rupture (odds ratio [OR] 5.08) and death due to rupture (OR 3.57).[110] And, it should be kept in mind that the abdominal aortic aneurysms setting is much more favorable and less complex than other more challenging applications of endovascular therapies, such as the thoracoabdominal or aortic arch settings.

A bottom-line assessment is that endovascular therapy offers lower peri-procedural risks but, accordingly, offers less durability and security in the long term than open therapy.

Furthermore, in certain anatomic and clinical situations, urgent open surgical treatment is preferred. Institutional and personal preferences abound. Even treatment of acute type A dissection by endovascular means is being explored, despite the complexities posed by the adjacent coronary arteries, aortic valve, and great vessels of the aortic arch.[111,112]

AORTIC DISSECTION

Precipitating Factors

MMPs and other pathophysiologic factors leading to degeneration of the aortic wall play an important role in aneurysm formation. Mechanical studies of human aortas in vivo have shown loss of elasticity when expanded to a diameter of 6 cm, beyond which systolic forces cannot be dissipated by further aortic distension and instead accelerate disruption of the integrity of the aortic wall. In addition to diameter, blood pressure plays a major role in determining wall tension. Without aortic enlargement, hypertension alone cannot generate sufficient wall stress to overcome the tensile strength of aortic tissue.

There are case reports of young, ostensibly healthy, athletic men experiencing aortic dissection during isometric weight training or other extreme exertion. All had unknown moderate enlargement of the aorta, and all experienced acute onset of dissection pain during effort. Aortic dissection proved fatal in one-third of these cases. The magnitude of hypertension during weightlifting contributes excess wall stress that exceeds the tolerable aortic load limit, resulting in acute dissection. Nearly three-fourths of patients report either extreme emotion or exertion at the onset of symptomatic dissection, again suggesting a link with hemodynamic forces. Based on these considerations, some authors recommend that individuals embarking on programs involving heavy weightlifting or extreme physical training first undergo echocardiography to exclude ascending aortic aneurysms.

Based on these observations, the following sequence of events is postulated to cause aortic dissection (**Fig. 23–45**):

- *Genetic predisposition* sets the stage for development of aortic aneurysms or dissection;
- *Medial degeneration.* Genetic predisposition results in activation of mechanisms of inflammation, injury to the medial layer of the aorta, loss of smooth muscle cells and histologic damage by cytokines. As a result, the aortic wall is damaged and weakened;
- *Aneurysm formation* results from progressive dilation, increasing mechanical stress on the aortic wall;
- *Hypertensive episode.* At a moment of extreme exertion or emotion, an abrupt rise in blood pressure increases aortic wall stress beyond the tensile strength of aortic tissue;
- *Aortic dissection.* The aorta dissects (and/or ruptures).

These steps hinge on the assumption that dissection originates from an intimal tear, which in turn leads to splitting of the medial layer and creation of the false lumen. However, Humphrey et al.[113] proposed that a pooling of glycosaminoglycans and proteoglycans within the medial layer of the aorta may have a delaminating effect due to localized loss of tensile strength, local stress concentration, and increased swelling pressures—all of which promote dissection.[113,114] Dissection may start with an initial delamination process within the media, which propagates proximally or distally to create an intimal tear. Pooling of glycosaminoglycans and proteoglycans may be related to the dysregulation of TGF-β[114,115] based on the hypothesis that aortic smooth muscle cells increase production of glycosaminoglycans and proteoglycans in response to increased TGF-β activity.[113,114]

Studies of the tensile strength of aortic wall specimens have determined that the aneurysmal wall is susceptible to tearing well below the normal tensile limit of 800 kP (kilo Pascals).[2] The onset of dissection is frequently preceded by physical exertion or emotional stress. Dissection too frequently occurs in young athletes performing weightlifting, an activity associated with abrupt elevation of blood pressure that can exceed 300 mm Hg. Approximately 25% of patients with dissection recall intense exertion, while 40% recall emotional stress at the inception of symptoms.

Many patients with TAAs carry genetic mutations associated with the disease. Through a complex molecular biologic mechanism (as we have seen in this chapter, involving MMP excess, aortic wall smooth muscle cell destruction, disturbances in TGF-β signaling, and other factors), the aortic wall biologically deteriorates (lamellar destruction and lacunar spaces), and the weakening of the aortic wall allows the aorta to dilate substantially. Then, we have found, a specific severe emotion or exertion causes extreme acute hypertension. This hypertensive event exceeds the tensile strength of the aortic wall, and dissection occurs with an intimal tear extending into the media and then propagating longitudinally in a distal direction down the aorta.

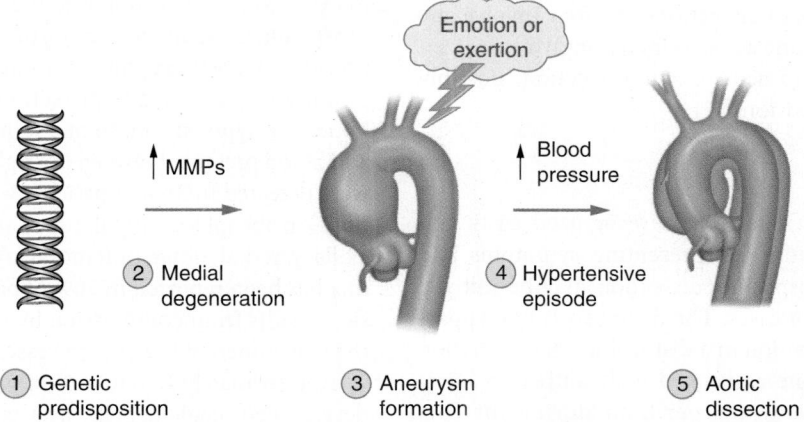

Figure 23–45. Schematic presentation of possible relationships underlying the instigation of an acute aortic dissection at one particular time. Adapted with permission from Hatzaras IS, Bible JE, Koullias GJ, etr al. Role of exertion or emotion as inciting events for acute aortic dissection. *Am J Cardiol.* 2007 Nov 1; 100(9):1470-1472.

Pathophysiology

Clinically, the inciting event responsible for aortic dissection is an intimal tear that permits blood to pass from the true lumen into the middle or outer layer of the aortic media, forming a second or false lumen separated by an intimal flap. In some cases, intramural hematoma precedes perforation of the intima, possibly related to rupture of a vasa vasorum. The dissection may propagate distally (antegrade) or proximally (retrograde) to narrow or occlude the origin of any branch artery arising from the aorta. Antegrade propagation is more common, and the dissection usually has spiral morphology, leaving some aortic branches supplied by the true lumen and others in continuity with the false lumen. Because any branch of the aorta can be affected, dissection can present as disease of any organ system—stroke, paraplegia, abdominal visceral catastrophe, renal failure, or lower limb ischemia. For this reason, aortic dissection has been given the well-earned moniker of "the great masquerader."

The intimal tear originates in the ascending aorta in 65% of cases, transverse arch in 10%, upper descending aorta just beyond the origin of the left subclavian artery in 20%, and more distally in 5% of cases. The false lumen may terminate at any point along the length of the aorta or in the iliac or femoral arteries, and there are sometimes multiple flaps and several sites of reentry. The false lumen can undergo retrograde dissection, thrombotic occlusion, pseudoaneurysm formation, compression, or rupture.

Aortic dissection occurs more often in men than in women, with a 2:1 to 5:1 preponderance, usually in the sixth or seventh decades of life. Systemic hypertension is the major predisposing risk factor. In the IRAD database, 74.4% of 2952 patients with proximal aortic dissections and 80.9% of 1476 with distal dissections had a history of hypertension.[55] Other predisposing conditions include Marfan syndrome, Ehlers-Danlos syndrome, Loeys-Dietz syndrome, BAV, aortic aneurysms, and annuloaortic ectasia associated with cystic medial necrosis. The most common causes of aortic dissection in patients younger than 40 years old are Marfan syndrome and pregnancy. Iatrogenic trauma resulting from intravascular catheterization is the cause in approximately 5% of dissections and may involve any segment of the aorta. Cocaine abuse is increasingly recognized as a factor predisposing to acute aortic dissection, possibly mediated by acute hypertension.[116]

Clinical Presentation

Aortic dissection is often fatal unless recognized early and aggressively treated. Because the presenting symptoms and signs are myriad and nonspecific, dissection may be initially overlooked in up to 40% of cases. The diagnosis is first apparent at postmortem examination in a disturbingly large fraction of cases. The mortality rate associated with untreated aortic dissection approaches 1% to 2% per hour during the first 48 hours, reaching 90% at 3 months; most deaths related to dissection occur within 14 days after onset. Up to 20% of victims die before reaching hospital. With expert care, however, survival rates of more than 70% have been reported for patients reaching the hospital with acute aortic dissection. Most require intensive medical therapy, either as the sole treatment or in conjunction with surgical intervention. Even if the patient survives aortic dissection, expansion of the dissected portion of the aorta (dissecting aortic aneurysm) contributes to mortality beyond the acute phase.

Dissection may occur in the ascending (type A) or descending (type B) segments of the thoracic aorta, defined by the location of the inciting intimal tear. Tears in the ascending aorta generally occur 2 cm to 3 cm above the coronary ostia, and in the descending aorta typically originate 1 cm to 2 cm beyond the origin of the left subclavian artery. The first type produces ascending (type A) dissection and the second descending (type B) dissection, but dissections originating in the ascending aorta commonly extend along the aortic arch to involve the descending and abdominal portions of the aorta as well.

Aortic dissection can cause death in four main ways (Fig. 23–52): (1) hemopericardium with cardiac tamponade caused by retrograde dissection; (2) acute aortic valve insufficiency caused by retrograde dissection; (3) hemothorax caused by rupture of a descending aortic dissection into the pleural space; and (4) tissue ischemia caused by occlusion of a branch artery.

Aortic dissection typically produces sudden intense pain, often described as tearing or shearing in quality. Whereas ascending aortic dissection usually causes anterior, substernal chest pain, dissection of the descending aorta causes posterior, interscapular pain. Pain may migrate inferiorly to the flank or pelvis as the dissection propagates distally. Impending aortic rupture should be considered when pain subsides and later recurs. Painless dissection occurs in as many as 4% to 15% of patients[116] and is commonly detected as an asymptomatic finding on elective CT scans obtained for another purpose. By convention, aortic dissection is considered acute when identified within 2 weeks of onset and chronic when symptoms or other markers of dissection have been present longer.

Most patients with aortic dissection present with hypertension, but 3% to 18% present with shock, sometimes secondary to extension of dissection into the coronary arteries, acute MI, heart failure, acute severe aortic insufficiency, cardiac tamponade, or aortic rupture. Coronary perfusion may be compromised by retrograde dissection, compression by the false lumen, or hypotension. In one series, differential pulse volume and blood pressure between the right and left upper extremities were detected in 38% of patients with ascending aortic dissection. An abrupt loss of pulse may affect the carotid, subclavian, axillary, radial, ulnar, or femoral arteries, and acute limb ischemia has been reported in 20% of patients. Branch vessel occlusion results from compression by the distended false lumen of the true lumen of the branch vessel (**Fig. 23–46**).

Approximately 15% to 20% of patients with aortic dissection develop neurologic deficits, with transient cerebral ischemia or stroke in up to 10% of patients resulting from extension of dissection into the carotid or vertebral arteries. In such cases, brain imaging and neurologic or neurosurgical consultation may be

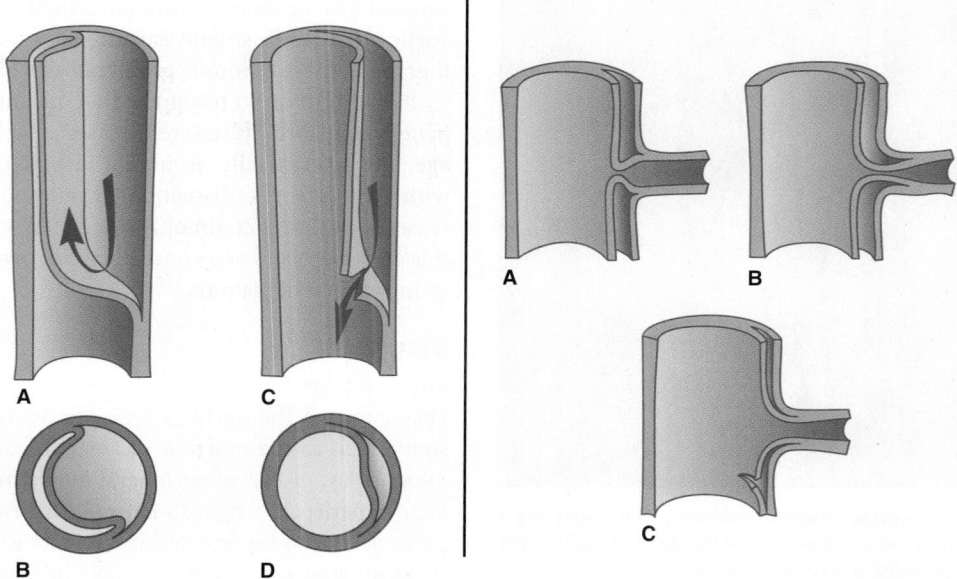

Figure 23–46. Schematic representation of the distended false channel in a case of aortic dissection impinging on the lumen of a branch vessel. Left. Main aortic trunk, with (**A**) and (**B**) before fenestration and (**C**) and (**D**) after fenestration. **Right**. Anatomic events at branch vessel; (**A**) and (**B**) show impingement by a false lumen, and (**C**) shows relief by fenestration. Reproduced with permission from Crawford ES, Coselli JS. Thoracoabdominal aneurysm surgery. *Semin Thorac Cardiovasc Surg*. 1991 Oct;3(4):300-322.

helpful to determine whether cerebral infarction has occurred; surgery is best avoided in such cases for fear of inducing intracerebral bleeding or otherwise extending the zone of infarction. When cerebral infarction is absent or incomplete, urgent operation is generally indicated because repair of the dissection may restore brain perfusion. Similarly, urgent surgical intervention is indicated when interruption of spinal circulation by a dissection of the descending aorta threatens to cause paraplegia.

Studies of the natural history of TAAs using large databases involving thousands of patient-years of observation have established that TAAs are associated with approximately 50% mortality over 5 years, but not all deaths in these cohorts are directly attributable to aneurysms. Aortic rupture is the most common cause of death in patients with aortic dissection. The second most common cause of death in these patients is acute, severe aortic regurgitation, which has been reported in 44% of patients with dissection of the ascending aorta and is poorly tolerated hemodynamically, compared with chronic aortic insufficiency; because sudden volume overload allows no time for LV adaptation, cardiogenic shock typically ensues.

Variants of Aortic Dissection: Intramural Hematoma and Penetrating Aortic Ulcer

Intramural aortic hematoma differs from typical dissection in that there is no flap delineating the true and false lumens, and the hematoma is located circumferentially around the aortic lumen, rather than obliquely (**Fig. 23–47**). Whether the intramural hematoma arises from a small intimal tear that is not radiographically detected or from a rupture of a vasa vasorum within the aortic wall remains controversial. The clinical course is variable: the hematoma may persist, resorb (returning the

aorta to a normal appearance), leave an aneurysm with the possibility of rupture, or later transform into typical dissection.[118]

For intramural hematoma involving the ascending aorta, there is more unanimity favoring immediate surgical intervention, although the Japanese literature challenges the need for routine surgery, even in this anatomic location. Penetrating aortic ulcer (**Fig. 23–48**) involves disruption of the internal elastic lamina and erosion of the medial layer of the aortic wall, resulting in local penetration at the site of an atherosclerotic

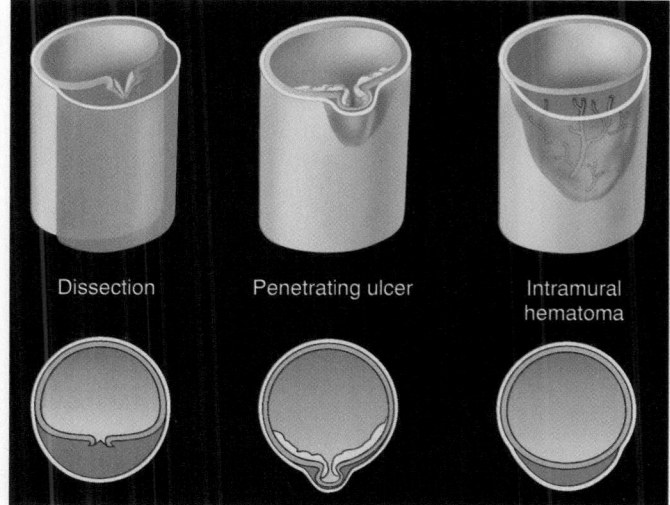

Figure 23–47. Variant forms of aortic dissection. Typical dissection, penetrating aortic ulcer, and intramural hematoma. Reproduce with permission from Elefteriades JA. Thoracic aortic aneurysm: reading the enemy's playbook. *Curr Probl Cardiol*. 2008 May;33(5):203-277.

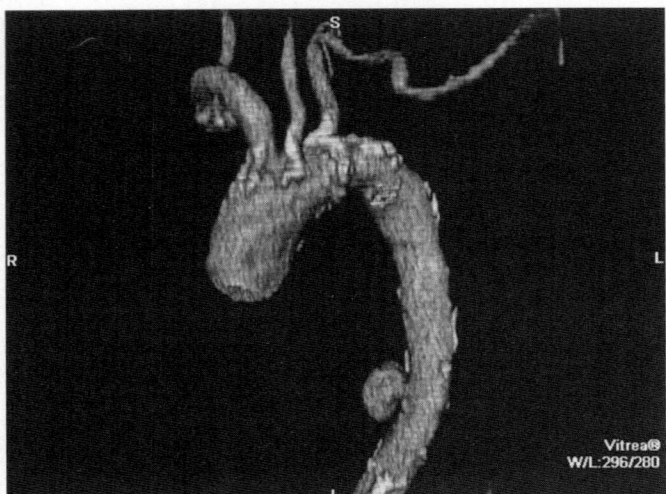

Figure 23–48. MRA with surface-shaded rendering demonstrating a penetrating aortic ulcer in the distal portion of the descending thoracic aorta. Note the severe generalized aortic arteriosclerosis.

plaque. This lesion may mimic or result in aortic dissection, pseudoaneurysm formation, intramural hematoma, or rupture.

Penetrating aortic ulcers usually involve the descending aorta distal to the origin of the left subclavian artery, and for those associated with persistent pain, stent grafting is the treatment of choice. **Figure 23–49** illustrates a dramatic case in which a penetrating ulcer ruptured through the posterior wall of the ascending aorta, mimicking "cryptogenic" pericardial effusion until surgical exploration made the diagnosis clear. Large penetrating ulcers rarely improve, and late surgery is commonly needed. Patients with large, deep penetrating ulcers may benefit from initial surgical management, but whether this applies to intramural hematomas is less clear (**Figure 23–50**).[118] Currently, a conservative, observational approach is often chosen. Endovascular therapy is an alternative to medical or open

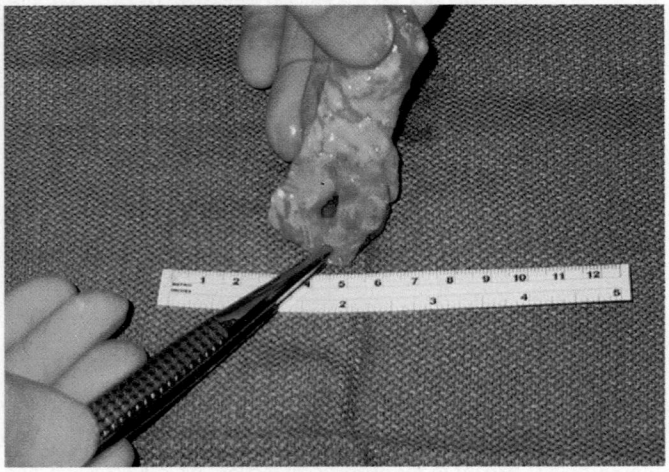

Figure 23–49. Gross specimen of a removed segment of aortic wall harboring a penetrating aortic ulcer. Reproduce with permission from Elefteriades JA. Thoracic aortic aneurysm: reading the enemy's playbook. *Curr Probl Cardiol.* 2008 May;33(5):203-277.

surgical management of intramural hematoma and penetrating aortic ulcer. While still investigational, aggressive endovascular therapy of these lesions is proliferating widely.[119,120]

It is important to recognize that intramural hematoma and penetrating aortic ulcer are diseases associated with advanced age, characteristically occurring in patients older than those with type B aortic dissection. In addition, although branch vessel occlusion is commonly associated with aortic dissection, this does not occur as a consequence of penetrating aortic ulcer or intramural hematoma.[118]

Diagnosis

Physical Signs

Dissection of the aorta is typically associated with physical signs, such as the murmur of aortic regurgitation and decrement, delay, or loss of peripheral pulses in one or more limbs. With experience, a right-to-left radial or right radial-to-femoral pulse delay can be detected in patients with aortic dissection. A substantial difference in blood pressure between the two arms in the appropriate clinical setting should raise suspicion of acute or chronic aortic dissection as well.

Imaging Studies

Several imaging modalities, TTE or TEE, CT, and MRI can be used to identify proximal (type A) thoracic aortic dissection, with accuracies over 95%, but the choice of modality depends on the specific circumstances in a given case. Echocardiography has the advantage of portability to the patient's location in the hospital emergency department, but TEE generally requires patient sedation. CT angiography (CTA) is readily available in many emergency facilities, and contrast-enhanced images are rapidly acquired and processed and extremely informative. MRI is generally less immediately available and requires that the patient be enclosed in the imaging equipment, which can be problematic in hemodynamically unstable situations, making MRI less frequently applied as the initial diagnostic modality for patients with suspected acute aortic dissection.

One technical shortcoming of TTE and TEE, "reverberation artifact,"[121] arises from generation of an artifactual shadow parallel to the aortic wall that can be mistaken for dissection flap (**Fig. 23–51**). The reverberation artifact closely follows the contours of the aortic wall, which is unusual for a dissection flap, and the two can be differentiated by color flow Doppler imaging, since blood flow is not contained by the shadow in the fashion of a true dissection flap.

Differential Diagnosis

Aortic dissection may masquerade as other acute cardiovascular, pulmonary, musculoskeletal, neurologic, or gastrointestinal disorders because it can produce symptoms related to almost any organ (**Fig. 23–52**). Conditions frequently confused with aortic dissection are musculoskeletal chest pain, mediastinal tumors, pericarditis, pleuritis, pneumothorax, pulmonary embolism, cholecystitis, ureteral colic, appendicitis, mesenteric ischemia, pyelonephritis, stroke, transient ischemic attack, and primary limb ischemia. The IRAD database has described the presentation and differential diagnosis of aortic dissection and

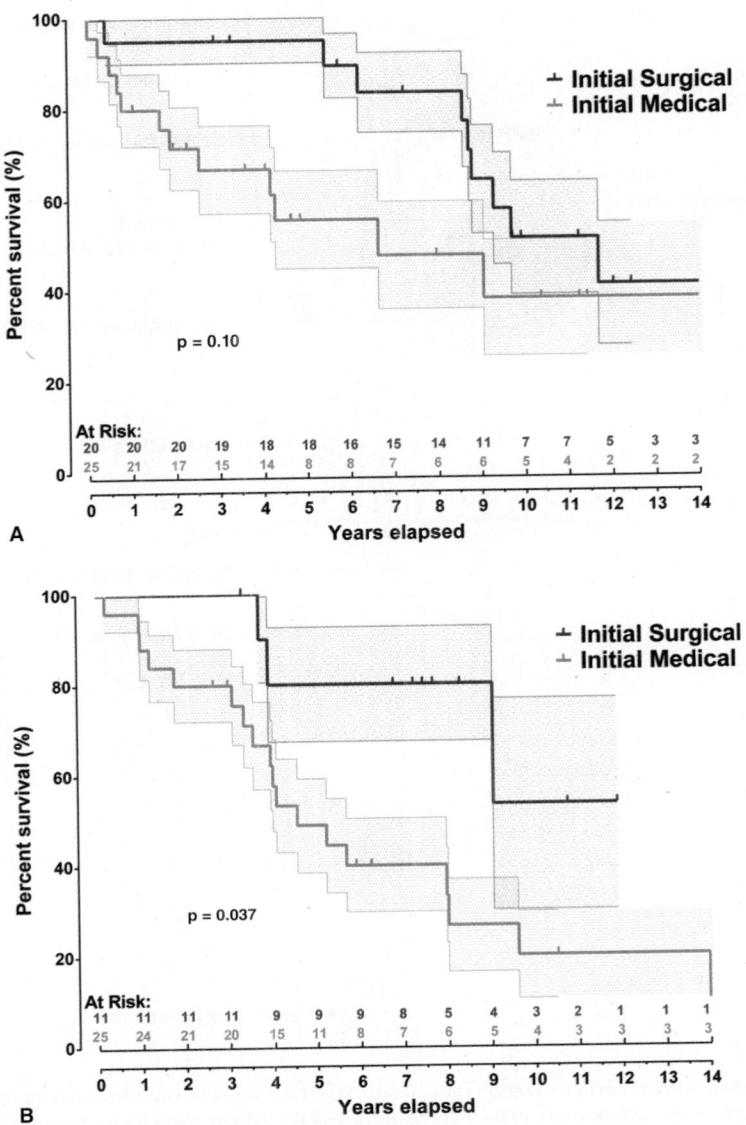

Figure 23–50. (A) Kaplan-Meier survival curve for nonruptured intramural hematoma patients comparing long-term survival between initial surgical and initial medical cohorts. Panel (B) Kaplan-Meier survival curve for patients with nonruptured penetrating ulcers comparing long-term survival between initial surgical and initial medical cohorts. Reproduced with permission from Chou AS, Ziganshin BA, Charilaou P, et al. Long-term behavior of aortic intramural hematomas and penetrating ulcers. *J Thorac Cardiovasc Surg*. 2016 Feb;151(2):361-372.

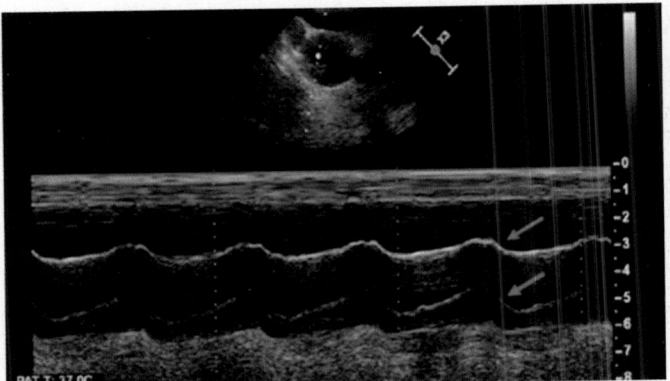

Figure 23–51. **M-mode echocardiography of the aorta in cross section on TEE showing reverberation artifact.** The "dissection flap" (red arrow) shows perfect concordance with the aortic wall (blue arrow), suggesting artifact rather than true dissection.

emphasized its protean potential clinical features.[55,122] The diagnosis is most strongly suggested by migratory chest and back pain of less than 24 hours' duration arising in a patient with a history of hypertension. Aortic dissection should be considered in all patients presenting with chest, back or abdominal pain without another obvious cause, and the aorta should be imaged routinely in such cases. Given the extensive differential diagnosis, prompt diagnosis is essential because without appropriate therapy the clinical course may evolve rapidly to a catastrophic outcome.

256-row multidetector CTA can effectively exclude the major forms of life-threatening thoracic pathology, including acute coronary syndromes, pulmonary thromboembolism, and aortic aneurysm or dissection (including intramural hematoma and penetrating aortic ulcer)—the so-called "triple rule-out" CT scan—but the threshold at which this technology

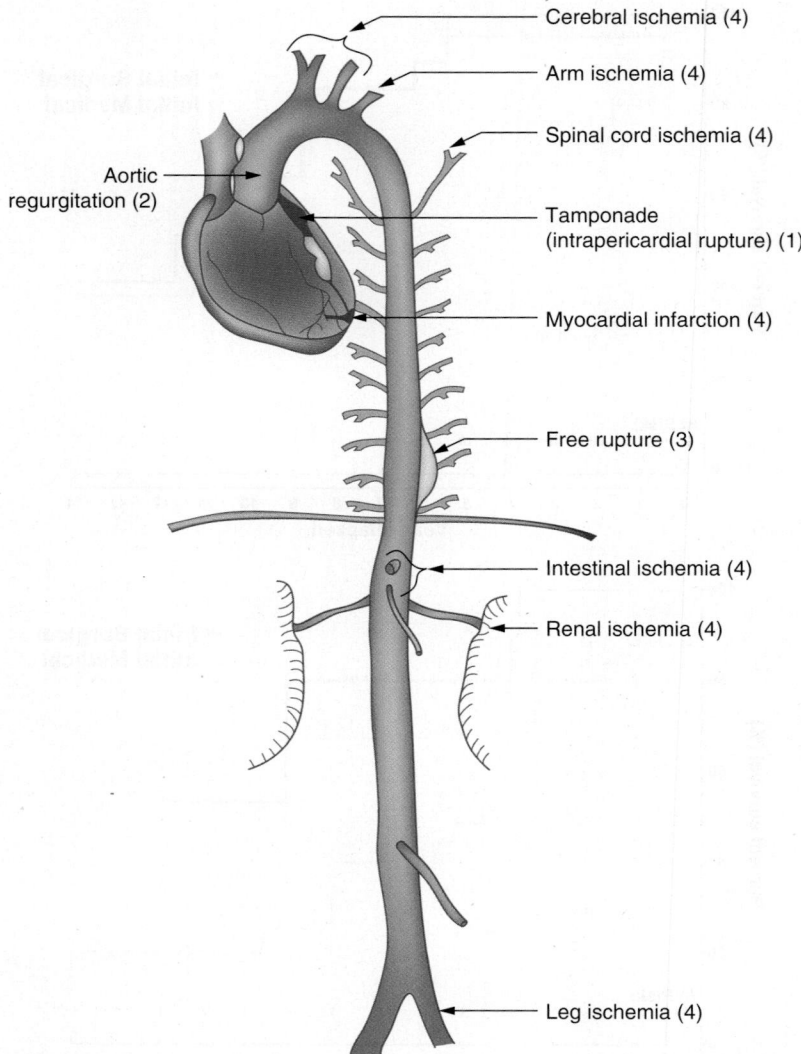

Cerebral ischemia (4)

Arm ischemia (4)

Spinal cord ischemia (4)

Aortic regurgitation (2)

Tamponade (intrapericardial rupture) (1)

Myocardial infarction (4)

Free rupture (3)

Intestinal ischemia (4)

Renal ischemia (4)

Leg ischemia (4)

Figure 23–52. **The mechanisms by which acute aortic dissection cause death. (1) intrapericardial rupture and tamponade, (2) acute aortic insufficiency, (3) free rupture into left pleural space, or (4) occlusion of a branch of the aorta.** Used with permission from Cardiotext Publishing.

can be most cost effectively applied has not been established. The D-dimer assay helps evaluate patients with suspected acute pulmonary embolism, and negative or normal results effectively exclude acute aortic dissection. Thrombosis of the false lumen in cases of aortic dissection typically raises the peripheral blood level of D-dimer levels substantially.[123]

Management of Aortic Dissection

Aortic dissection propagates more vigorously when either blood pressure or the force of cardiac contraction is elevated. Accordingly, control of blood pressure is an important aspect of treatment in patients with acute aortic syndromes, including dissection, rupture, or impending rupture. Intravenous nitroglycerin or sodium nitroprusside are commonly used for this purpose. Lowering blood pressure by administration of vasodilator drugs alone may increase the sheer stress on the aortic wall; however, this can be ameliorated by decreasing the force of cardiac contraction pharmacologically. The objective is to reduce the rate of rise of arterial pressure (dP/dt), reflected in

attenuation of the upslope of the aortic pulse wave, by administering a short-acting β-blocking drug such as esmolol or the β- and α-adrenergic antagonist labetalol by intravenous infusion. When β-blocking drugs are contraindicated, the nondihydropyridine calcium channel blockers diltiazem and verapamil are reasonable alternatives. **Table 23–9** presents specific drug options for the medical management of acute aortic syndrome.

Ascending (Type A) Aortic Dissection

Ascending aortic (type A) dissection requires urgent surgery to avoid death as a consequence of intrapericardial rupture, aortic regurgitation, or MI. Repair involves reapproximation of the aortic wall between layers of Teflon felt. At experienced centers, survival is approximately 85%. Patients with descending aortic (type B) dissections face a better prognosis with initial medical management ("anti-impulse" therapy with β-blockers and vasodilator drugs), withholding surgery unless specific complications develop.[124] Medical management of uncomplicated type B aortic dissections offers long-term survival comparable

TABLE 23–9. Intravenous Agents for Treatment of Ascending Aortic Dissection

Name	Category	Loading dose	Maintenance dose	Adverse effects	Caution
Sodium nitroprusside	Vasodilator	0.3 mcg/kg/min to 3 mcg/kg/min; max. limit for an adult is 10 mcg/kg/min for 10 min	1–3 mcg/kg/min	Nausea, vomiting, agitation, muscle twitching, sweating, cutis anserina and cyanide toxicity, tachycardia	In patients with hepatic or renal dysfunction
Propranalol	β-blocker	1–3 mg (given at 1 mg intervals over 1 min). Can be repeated in not less than every 4 hours	1–3 mg every 4 hours	Hypotension, nausea, dizziness, cold extremities, reversible hair loss, bradycardia	In patients with bradycardia or history of CHF and bronchospasm. Max. initial dose should not exceed 0.15 mg/hr
Esmolol	β-blocker	500 mcg/kg bolus	Continuous 50 mcg/kg/min up to 200 mcg/kg/min	Hypotension, nausea, dizziness, bronchospasm, dyspepsia, constipation, increases digoxin level	In patients with CHF or asthma or on concomitant CCB therapy
Labetolol	α- and β-blocker	20 mg over 2 min, then 40–80 mg every 10–15 min (max. 300)	Continuous IV at 2 mg/min and titrate up to 5–10 mg/min	Vomiting, nausea, scalp tingling, burning in throat, dizziness, heart block, orthostatic hypotension	In patients with lung disease, concomitant CCB therapy
Diltiazem	CCB	0.25 mg/kg IV bolus (up to 25 mg)	5–10 mg/hour by continuous infusion	Heart block, constipation, liver dysfunction	In patients with heart failure, concomitant β-blocker therapy
Enalapril	Vasodilator ACE inhibitor	0.625–1.25 mg bolus	0.625–5 mg every 6 hours	Precipitates fall in BP in high renin states, variable response, renal failure	In patients with high possibility of MI, renal dysfunction
Fenoldopam	Dopamine D1 receptor agonist	0.03–0.1 mcg/kg/min initially	0.1–0.3 mcg/kg/min, max. 1.6 mcg/kg/min	Tachycardia, hypotension, headache, nausea, flushing, hypokalemia, elevation of IOP	In patients with glaucoma
Nicardipine	CCB	5 mg/hour; may increase by 2.5 mg/hour every 5 minutes (for rapid titration) to every 15 minutes (for gradual titration) up to a maximum of 15 mg/hour	For rapidly titrated patients, consider reduction to 3 mg/hour after response is achieved	Flushing, pedal edema, exacerbation of angina pectoris, hypotension, palpitations, tachycardia, headache, dizziness, nausea, vomiting, dyspepsia	In patients with mild to moderate aortic stenosis, severe left ventricular dysfunction (particularly with concomitant β-blockade), hepatic impairment, hypertrophic cardiomyopathy, renal impairment
Clevidipine	CCB	Initial 1–2 mg/hour; dose may be doubled at 90-second intervals toward blood pressure goal. As blood pressure approaches goal, dose may be increased by less than double every 5–10 minutes. For every 1–2 mg/hour increase in dose, an approximate reduction of 2–4 mm Hg in systolic blood pressure may occur	4–6 mg/hour; maximum: 21 mg/hour	Atrial fibrillation, fever, insomnia, nausea, headache, vomiting, postprocedural hemorrhage, acute renal failure, pneumonia, respiratory failure	In patients with heart failure and pheochromocytoma. Avoid abrupt withdrawal of concomitant β-blocker therapy.

Abbreviations: CCB, calcium channel blocker; ACE, angiotensin-converting enzyme; IV, intravenous; BP, blood pressure; IOP, intraocular pressure; CHF, congestive heart failure; MI, myocardial ischemia.
Data from Feldman M, Shah M, Elefteriades JA. Medical management of acute type A aortic dissection. *Ann Thorac Cardiovasc Surg.* 2009 Oct;15(5):286-293.

to that of the general population, whereas patients with an initially complicated course face unfavorable long-term outcomes (**Fig. 23–53**).[124]

After corrective surgery for type A aortic dissection or stabilization on medication therapy for type B dissection, close observation is necessary, with serial aortic imaging during the first month and periodically thereafter. Some patients eventually develop enlargement of the dissected aorta requiring resection, and in these cases, the dimensional criteria for surgical intervention are the same as those used for intact aneurysms.

Descending (Type B) Aortic Dissection
In the 1970s and 1980s, a debate raged regarding the appropriate early management for acute descending aortic dissection

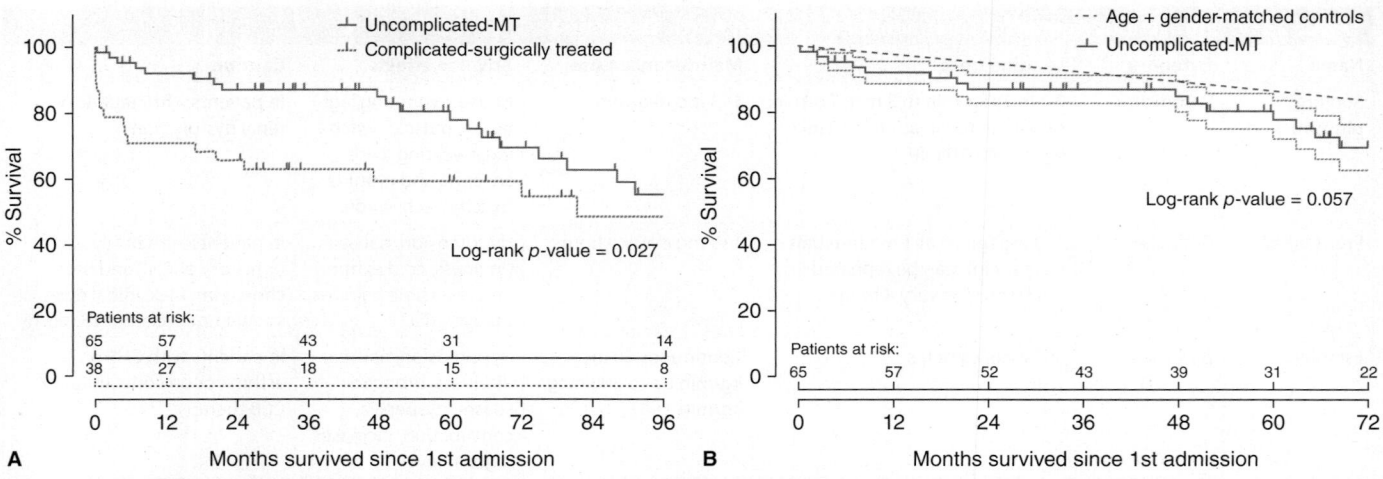

Figure 23–53. **(A)** Kaplan-Meier curves comparing an 8-year follow-up between uncomplicated-medically-treated patients and complicated-surgically treated patients with acute type B aortic dissection (complication-specific approach). **(B)** Kaplan-Meier curves comparing 6-year survival between uncomplicated-medically-treated patients and age + gender-matched control group. Reproduced with permission from Charilaou P, Ziganshin BA, Peterss S, et al. Current Experience With Acute Type B Aortic Dissection: Validity of the Complication-Specific Approach in the Present Era. *Ann Thorac Surg.* 2016 Mar; 101(3):936-943.

(type B). Some surgeons argued for immediate surgery for all patients, others favored nonoperative management because of the very high mortality rate (at or above 50%) associated with early surgery, and others proposed a "complication-specific approach" to type B aortic dissection. Under this last approach, patients presenting with complications underwent surgery, while those without were managed medically. The type of operation was based on the type of complication (**Fig. 23–54**), while medical management for patients without complications was founded upon "anti-impulse therapy," derived from experiments on plastic tubing rather than biological tissue. The experiments demonstrated that decreasing the rate of rise of systolic arterial pressure over time (dP/dT) with various combinations of β-blocker and vasodilator drugs mitigated dissection.

Under the complication-specific paradigm (Fig. 23–54), patients with rupture (usually into the left pleural space) undergo open graft replacement. Patients with organ ischemia undergo fenestration, a relatively noninvasive procedure

usually performed by a retroperitoneal approach, in which the infrarenal abdominal aorta is transected, a communication is created between the true and false lumens, and the aortic wall is reapproximated (**Fig. 23–55**). This simple, relatively safe procedure was reliably effective at restoring organ perfusion above and below the level of fenestration. For impending rupture (manifested by continued pain, radiographic worsening, or, arguably, persistent uncontrolled hypertension), graft replacement is performed.

The complication-specific approach proved effective, overcoming some of the limitation of an all-or-none, surgical non-surgical, strategy, and the majority of patients were treated nonsurgically, with medications alone. Over decades of application in a large number of patients followed long term, the complication-specific approach was associated with favorable early and late outcomes.[124] Most patients were followed expectantly on medical management (**Fig. 23–56**). Many patients initially treated medically ultimately developed substantial aortic dilatation, especially in the proximal portion of the descending aorta just beyond the left subclavian artery. These patients were operated safely, with open descending aortic replacement years after original presentation with acute dissection.[124]

In the modern era, endovascular and stenting techniques have often effectively replaced open surgery for the "complicated" limbs under the complication-specific paradigm (Fig. 23–54). Reasons for this include recognition that rupture can be treated by stent-grafting, development of endovascular methods to achieve fenestration, and application of stent grafting to patients with impending aortic rupture. It has been proposed that even patients with uncomplicated type B aortic dissection should undergo stent grafting, to remodel the dissected aorta and improve long-term outcomes.[125]

Most stent graft devices involve a modular construction consisting of a metallic exoskeleton surrounding an intimal fabric graft to maintain linear stability and prevent kinking. Stent-graft therapy has a valid role in the management of

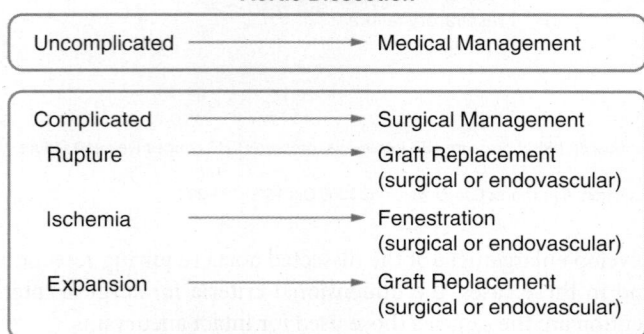

Treatment Strategy for Acute Descending Aortic Dissection

Uncomplicated ⟶ Medical Management

Complicated ⟶ Surgical Management
Rupture ⟶ Graft Replacement (surgical or endovascular)
Ischemia ⟶ Fenestration (surgical or endovascular)
Expansion ⟶ Graft Replacement (surgical or endovascular)

Figure 23–54. The "complication-specific approach" to descending **(type B) aortic dissection.** Reproduced with permission from Elefteriades JA, Lovoulos CJ, Coady MA, et al. Management of descending aortic dissection. *Ann Thorac Surg.* 1999 Jun;67(6):2002-2005.

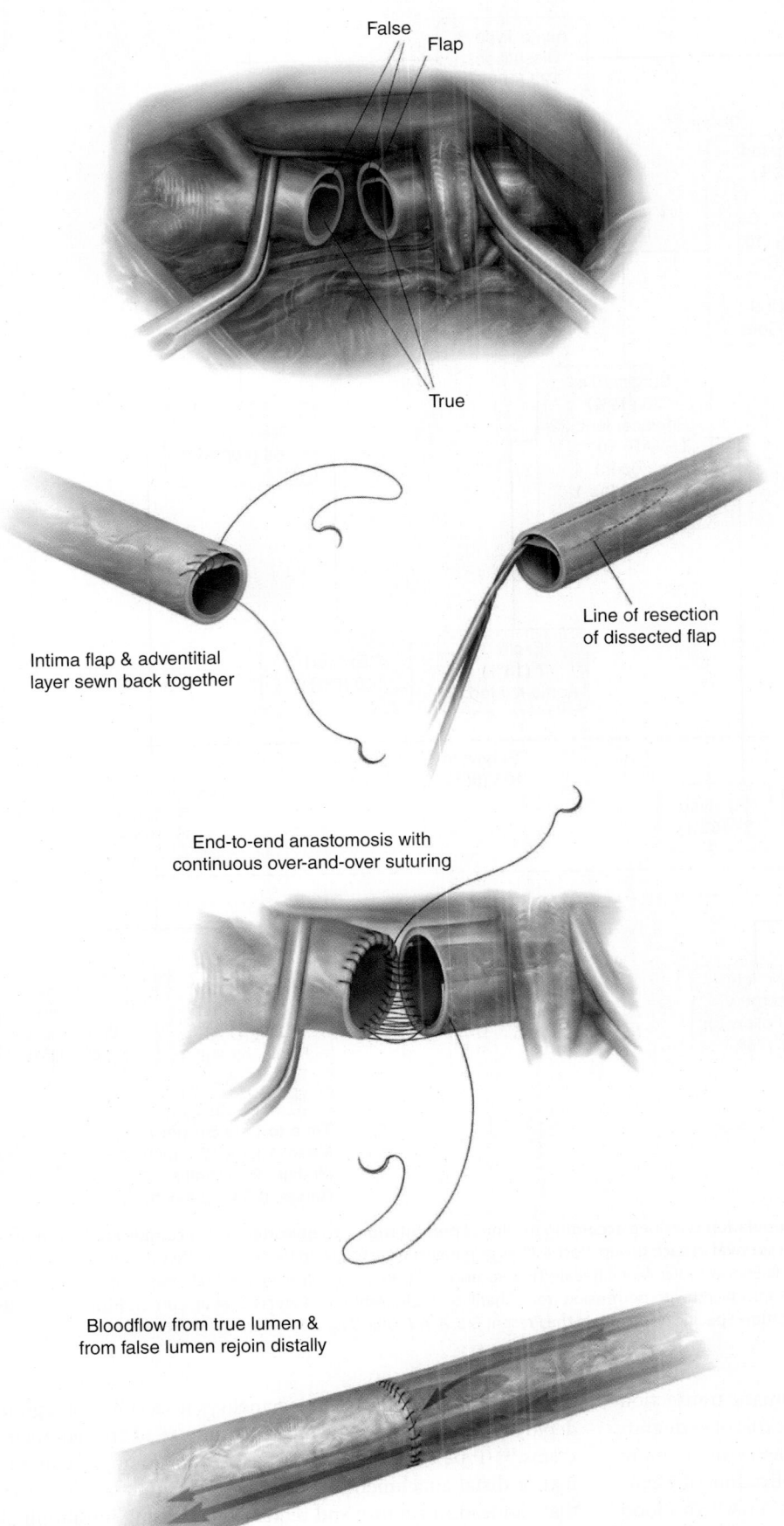

False
Flap

True

Intima flap & adventitial
layer sewn back together

Line of resection
of dissected flap

End-to-end anastomosis with
continuous over-and-over suturing

Bloodflow from true lumen &
from false lumen rejoin distally

Figure 23–55. Fenestration procedure for acute descending (type B) aortic dissection. Reproduced with permission from Elefteriades JA, Escalon JC. Aortic fenestration for dissection. *Oper Tech Thorac Cardiovasc Surg.* 2009 Spring;14(1): 2002-2005.

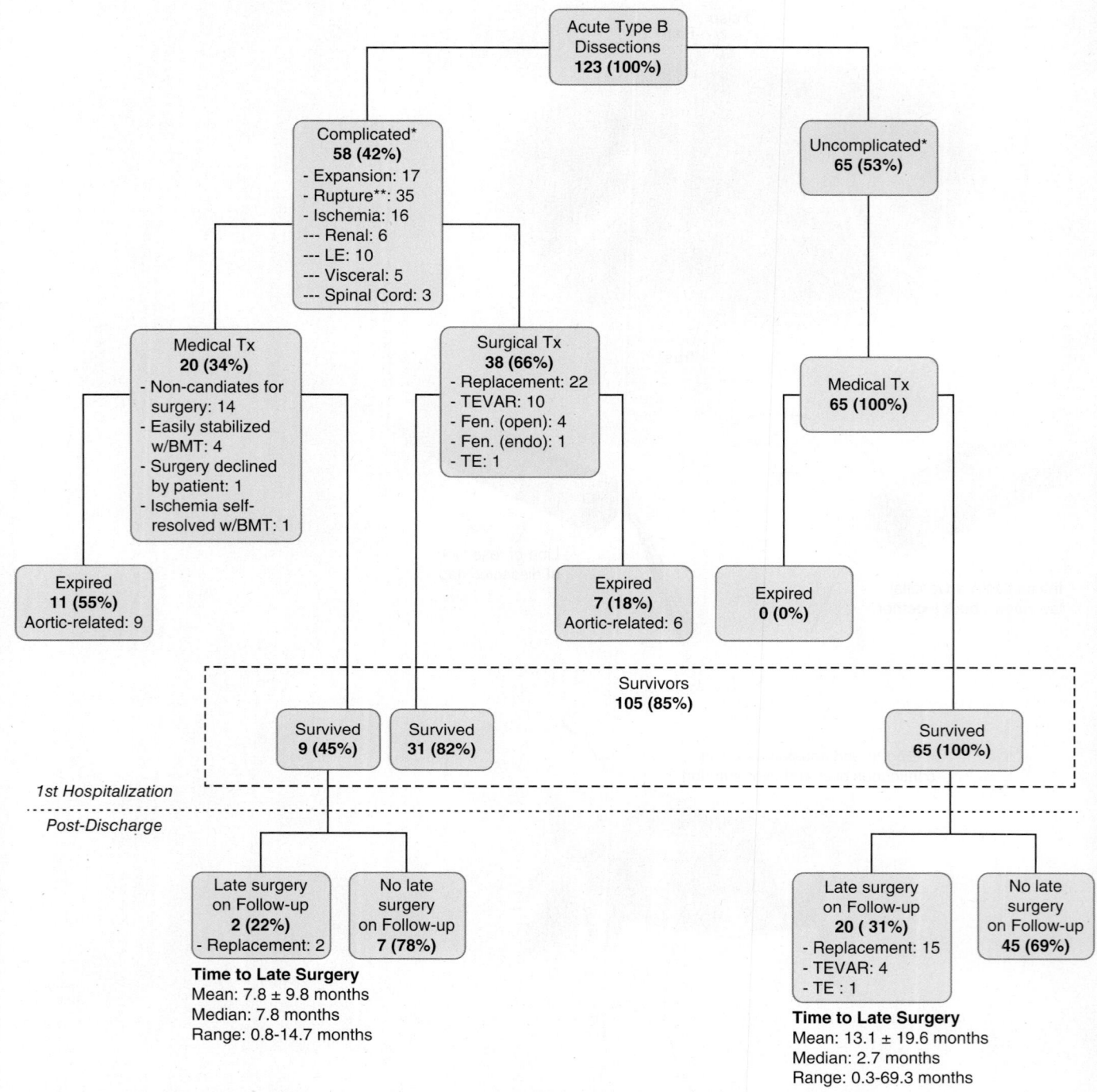

Figure 23–56. **Flow diagram showing the patient population classified according to clinical presentation ("complicated" vs "uncomplicated") and subsequently by treatment received and finally hospital survival in each group.** Postdischarge, patients were followed for need for late surgery. Tx, treatment; Fen, fenestration; LE, lower extremities; TEVAR, Thoracic Endovascular Aortic Repair; TE, thrombo-exclusion; BMT, baseline medical treatment. *At presentation. **Rupture count includes impending ruptures. Reproduced with permission from Charilaou P, Ziganshin BA, Peterss S, et al. Current Experience With Acute Type B Aortic Dissection: Validity of the Complication-Specific Approach in the Present Era. *Ann Thorac Surg.* 2016 Mar;101(3):936-943.

patients with ruptured aortic aneurysms traumatic transection of the aorta, and penetrating aortic ulcers. The role of endograft therapy in typical, fusiform degenerative aneurysms is more controversial. An important limiting complication of stent-graft therapy is the propensity for endoleak, in which blood

flow continues into the excluded aneurysm sac after stent graft deployment. Endoleaks may lead to rupture of treated aneurysms.[126] Type I endoleaks are caused by incompetent proximal or distal attachments, producing high intra-sac pressures that can lead to rupture and require repair using intraluminal extension cuffs or open surgery. Type II endoleaks resulting from retrograde flow from branch vessels (eg, intercostal, lumbar, or inferior mesenteric arteries) occur in as many as 40% of patients after endograft implantation. More than half of these seal spontaneously. Generally, type II endoleaks are followed with surveillance imaging. As long as the aortic sac does not enlarge progressively, usually no treatment is deemed necessary. However, if the aortic sac enlarges, type II endoleaks can usually be corrected by selective arterial embolization. Type III endoleaks are caused by fabric defects, tears, or disruption of modular graft components. These carry the same potential for aneurysm rupture as type I endoleaks and should be promptly repaired. Type IV endoleaks, the least common variety, result from graft porosity and diffuse leakage through interstices and usually develop within 30 days of implantation. Type IV endoleaks do not occur with the device technology that is currently used. Types I and III endoleaks seem the most dangerous and prompt repair is generally recommended.

Other complications of stent-graft repair of abdominal aortic aneurysms include occlusion of the iliac limbs of bifurcation endografts and migration from the proximal attachment as a result of progressive aortic expansion, which can be detected in at least one in five cases. Technical improvements in graft design and deployment techniques are reducing implant complications, but because of the potential for endoleak, graft migration, or graft limb occlusion, periodic follow-up imaging at intervals of 6 to 12 months is recommended after endovascular stent-graft repair.

The effectiveness of endograft therapy in preventing aneurysm growth, rupture, and aneurysm-related mortality compared with open surgical repair remains controversial. Although often ultimately lethal, a TAA is an indolent disease, and even without therapy years may elapse between diagnosis of small- or moderate-size aneurysms and aneurysm-related death. The EUROpean collaborators on Stent-graft Techniques for abdominal aortic Aneurysm Repair (EUROSTAR) survey of endograft repair of abdominal aortic aneurysms exposed cases of late mortality and rupture even after initially successful intervention. Information regarding late outcomes after endograft repair of abdominal aortic aneurysms is more comprehensive than for TAAs, but it appears that the risk of endoleak is ongoing over at least 5 years (**Fig. 23–57**). Endoleak predicted rupture, surgical intervention, or death in 13%, 14%, and 27% of patients, respectively, by 5 years postprocedure in patients originally presenting with large aneurysms. These concerns about long-term effectiveness supported the original view that endograft therapy should be reserved for patients in whom comorbidity precludes direct open surgical repair and emphasize the need for lifelong surveillance. However, more recent data supports an even wider application of endograft therapy, although long-term survival is poor and has not improved much over the years.[127,128] Randomized trials of thoracic endografting versus open surgical repair will be required to provide conclusive evidence regarding the relative merits. Some midterm randomized studies have now come to fruition.

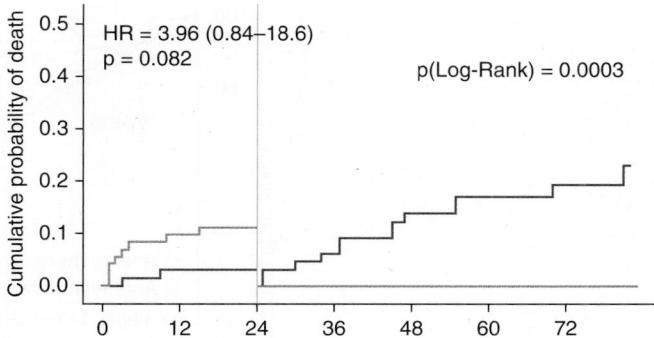

Figure 23–57. Kaplan–Meier estimates of all-cause mortality (death) and Landmark analysis with a breakpoint at 24 months after randomization to the end of the trial are shown for optimal medical treatment (OMT) and OMT + thoracic endovascular aortic repair (TEVAR) groups. Reproduced with permission from Nienaber CA, Kische S, Rousseau H, et al. Endovascular repair of type B aortic dissection: long-term results of the randomized investigation of stent grafts in aortic dissection trial. *Circ Cardiovasc Interv.* 2013 Aug;6(4):407-416.

The Endovascular Aneurysm Repair trials (EVAR-2) compared endovascular aneurysm repair (EVAR) with noninterventional therapy. The key finding (**Fig. 23–58**) was that there was no benefit from stent-grafting of abdominal aortic aneurysms, because the survival curves for all-cause mortality for EVAR and medical therapy were superimposable, as were those for aneurysm-related mortality.

The Dutch Randomized Endovascular Aneurysm Management (DREAM) trial compared EVAR with traditional surgical therapy for abdominal aortic aneurysms. At midterm follow-up (2 years), the survival curves crossed, following which stented patients exhibited poorer survival than surgically treated patients. The early advantage of EVAR reflected the mortality associated with open surgery, but the benefit of EVAR did not prove durable over time.

The Investigation of Stent Grafts in Patients with Type B Aortic Dissection (INSTEAD) trial investigated stent therapy for patients doing well beyond 2 weeks after uncomplicated type B aortic dissection. The hope was that "tacking down" the dissection flap would lead to later benefit. Contrary to expectations, INSTEAD found early mortality and complications subsequent to stent therapy. There was no survival advantage over medical therapy alone. Superiority of routine, early stent grafting was suggested by the results of a landmark analysis of the INSTEAD-XL trial,[125] in which survival beyond 24 months after the stent procedure was demonstrated when early procedure-related complications and deaths were discounted. Limitations of this analysis include the exclusion of earlier events and lack of statistical power for assessment of mortality.[129]

An analysis of data from IRAD also suggested better survival after type B dissection in patients treated by TEVAR (Thoracic Endovascular Aortic Repair), but interpretation is difficult due to potential referral and selection bias.[130,131] Despite lack of convincing evidence, many centers pursue routine stenting of type B aortic dissections, occasionally with more exuberance

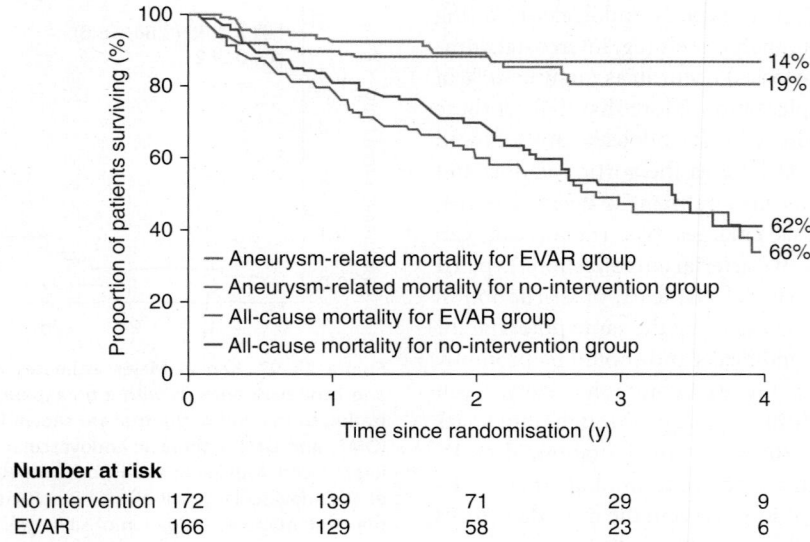

Figure 23–58. Cumulative freedom from aneurysm-related death after endovascular repair of abdominal aortic aneurysm in the EUROSTAR registry. Note low attrition during first 3 years of follow-up followed by rapid attrition in the fourth year. Gp denotes groups defined by increasing initial aneurysm size: Gp A = 4.0 cm to 5.4 cm; Gp B = 5.5 cm to 6.4 cm; Gp C = 6.5 cm or larger. Reproduced with permission from Peppelenbosch N, Buth J, Harris PL. Diameter of abdominal aortic aneurysm and outcome of endovascular aneurysm repair: does size matter? A report from EUROSTAR. *J Vasc Surg.* 2004 Feb;39(2):288-297.

then the available evidence would justify. Carefully planned comparisons between early routine stent therapy and medical management are clearly needed.

More medium-term follow-up is needed to assess the durability of stent therapy. Open surgical repair remains a viable option in terms of both efficacy and durability, and it is essential that the careful consideration be applied in the decision to select between open surgical and less invasive endovascular therapies.

ATHEROSCLEROSIS OF THE AORTA

Pathologic Anatomy

Atherosclerosis of the aorta is common in Western society. The usual risk factors are tobacco smoking, diabetes mellitus, hypertension, hypercholesterolemia, obesity, and a sedentary lifestyle; also, the contribution of elevated levels of plasma homocysteine and C-reactive protein has more recently been suggested.[132] The pathogenesis of atherosclerosis is discussed in Chapter 16.

Atherosclerosis most commonly develops in the infrarenal aorta and may be asymptomatic or produce intermittent claudication, critical limb ischemia, or atheromatous embolism. Typically, atherosclerosis may also involve the aortic arch and the origins of the brachiocephalic, carotid and subclavian vessels, and the descending thoracic aorta. In this era, we usually detect atherosclerosis and calcification on CT scans done for other reasons, or on CT scans done deliberately as screening studies for calcium score. The thoracic aorta is so large that it is distinctly uncommon for calcified atherosclerotic lesions to cause stenosis of the aorta itself. Branch vessels (innominate, left carotid, and left subclavian arteries) are commonly involved and may produce brain or arm symptoms.

Atheromatous Embolism

Embolism of cholesterol-laden atheromatous material and thrombus from the surface of the aorta commonly occurs in patients with severe aortic atherosclerosis. Atheroembolism may be spontaneous, although it more frequently occurs after surgical or arteriographic manipulation, such as catheter-based coronary or peripheral interventions. In a retrospective study of 71 autopsies, the incidence of cholesterol embolism in patients who had undergone arteriography before death was 27% compared with 4.3% in an age- and disease-matched control group that did not undergo angiography.

Whether or not anticoagulant and thrombolytic drugs can exacerbate atheroembolism associated with the "blue-toe syndrome" is controversial.[133] Few cases of this complication were reported in clinical trials of anticoagulation in high-risk patients with atrial fibrillation despite the frequent finding of morphologically complex aortic plaque in this population.

Patients with atheromatous embolism typically have a history of angina pectoris, MI, transient ischemic attack, stroke, intermittent claudication, or peripheral gangrene. Clinical signs and symptoms are variable, depending on the amount, size, and location of origin of the atheromatous material as well as on the tissue affected. Whereas macroembolism may present catastrophically as an acute ischemic limb, patients with microembolism may have milder localized signs or a clinical picture suggesting systemic illness, including fever, weight loss, anorexia, myalgia, headache, nausea, vomiting, or diarrhea. Occasionally, the presentation may suggest vasculitis, infective endocarditis, or malignancy. Cutaneous manifestations are the most frequent findings and include cyanotic toes, gangrenous digits, livedo reticularis, or nodules (**Fig. 23–59**). When atheroembolism affects both lower extremities, the source is generally the aorta, but when only one extremity is involved, it may

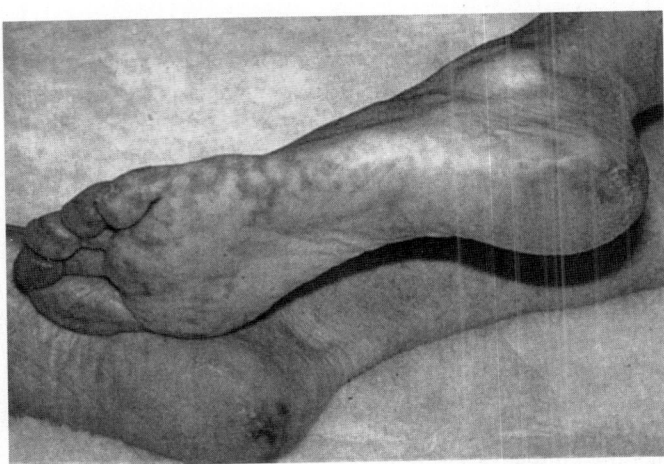

Figure 23–59. Typical appearance of atheromatous embolism involving the feet. The patient has cyanotic toes, livedo reticularis along the lateral portion of the foot, and ischemic lesions on both heels, indicating that the source of embolism is proximal to the aortic bifurcation. Reproduced with permission from Bartholomew JR. *Peripheral Vascular Diseases*, 2nd ed. St. Louis, MO: Mosby; 1996.

be difficult to determine whether the origin is the diseased ipsilateral iliofemoral artery or a more proximal or distal site.

Atheroembolism originating from the suprarenal aorta may involve the kidneys, producing occlusion of multiple small arteries and segmental ischemic atrophy. This small-vessel occlusive disease may cause accelerated hypertension, microscopic hematuria, or renal failure. Pathologically, biconvex cholesterol crystals occlude the interlobular and afferent arterioles (150–200 μm in diameter). A foreign-body reaction leads to small vessel occlusion, reducing glomerular filtration rate, activating the RAS system, and accelerating hypertension. Various patterns of renal insufficiency may develop and progress over weeks or months to irreversible renal failure, requiring dialysis. The differential diagnosis includes renal artery stenosis, renal artery thrombosis, infective endocarditis, vasculitis such as polyarteritis nodosa, and other causes of acute renal failure. No single laboratory test is diagnostic because acceleration of the erythrocyte sedimentation rate, leukocytosis with eosinophilia, and anemia are common in many systemic illnesses. Blood urea nitrogen and creatinine elevations may be early manifestations of renal involvement, and the urine sediment may be abnormal. Elevated serum amylase or hepatic transaminase levels may indicate pancreatic or hepatic involvement, and creatine phosphokinase and aldolase arise from affected muscle. Renal biopsy is rarely required but may reveal pathognomonic needle-shaped cholesterol clefts within small vessels. Atheroembolic renal disease carries a poor prognosis, with a mortality rate of 81% (179 of 221 patients) in one series; the most common causes of death were cardiac, renal, or multiorgan failure.

Atherosclerosis of the Aortic Arch

Atherosclerosis of the thoracic aorta is a strong predictor of initial and recurrent stroke, coronary events, and death. The thickness and morphology (protrusion, ulceration, or mobility) of atheromatous plaque correlate with the prevalence of stroke. Whether this association has a direct atheroembolic mechanism or reflects associated cerebrovascular pathology has not been conclusively determined.

Atheromatous embolism arising from the aortic arch or the carotid and vertebral arteries may cause stroke, transient ischemic attack, amaurosis fugax, blindness, headache, confusion, organic brain syndromes, dizziness, or spinal cord infarction. Retinal artery occlusion may be identified by Hollenhorst plaque visible on ophthalmoscopic examination as yellow, highly refractile atheromatous material at an arteriolar bifurcation.

Treatment

Because treatment of atheroembolism seldom reverses damage, emphasis is on prevention of subsequent ischemic events. When the source of embolism can be confirmed, it is often feasible to isolate or replace a discrete segment of the aorta by surgery, angioplasty and stent, or stent-graft insertion. Treatment should include symptomatic care of affected ischemic tissue and risk factor modification to prevent progression of atheromatous disease and promote plaque stabilization. If embolism affects the lower extremities, this involves local care of ischemic ulcers; when gangrene is present, amputation may be required. The role of sympathectomy is controversial, but this may be helpful when pain is intractable. In cases of renal atheroembolism, dialysis should be performed as necessary and blood pressure controlled pharmacologically.

Optimum antithrombotic therapy (anticoagulants, platelet inhibitors, or a combination of both) for atheromatous embolism has not been defined, but platelet inhibitor drugs generally lessen the risk of cardiovascular ischemic events. Anticoagulation therapy is far from protective, however, with a recurrence rate of cerebral events of 26% in patients with plaques more than 4 mm in thickness despite antiplatelet or warfarin therapy. Case reports of improvement with lipid-lowering therapy are supported by observations in nonrandomized series and evidence in coronary disease that HMG-CoA-reductase inhibitor ("statin") drugs improve plaque stabilization.[134]

The role of surgical therapy for patients with localized atheromata in the aortic arch and cerebral ischemia is controversial because it is seldom possible to determine conclusively whether the cause of symptoms is the aorta or associated cerebrovascular disease.

Aortoiliac Occlusive Disease

Atherosclerotic occlusive disease of the infrarenal aorta and iliac arteries may occur with or without atherosclerosis of the infrainguinal vessels. When isolated, aortoiliac atherosclerosis typically occurs in younger individuals who smoke cigarettes. Almost half the cases are women, many of whom angiographically exhibit the "hypoplastic aortic syndrome," with small-caliber aortic, iliac, and femoropopliteal arteries. The disease in these cases is usually confined to the aortic bifurcation. Disease localized to the distal aorta and common iliac arteries (type I) rarely produces limb-threatening ischemia because of extensive collateral vessels. The classic presentation is Leriche syndrome, a clinical triad of intermittent claudication involving the low back, buttocks, hip, or thigh, which is often mistaken for degenerative joint disease of the low back or hips, impotency (which occurs in 30%–50% of men with aortoiliac occlusive disease), or "global atrophy" of the lower extremities, reflecting the chronicity of low-grade ischemia. The femoral pulses are often weak or absent, but the ankle-brachial index may be normal at rest. A decline in ankle systolic pressure after exercise confirms hemodynamically significant stenosis.

Management

Treatment of patients with occlusive atherosclerosis of the aorta should include measures directed at improving symptoms (eg, claudication or limb ischemia) and thus quality of life, as well as reduction of overall cardiovascular risk. The latter involves the same measures as management of other manifestations of systemic atherosclerosis or peripheral artery disease (see Chapters 16 and 26). Catheter-based interventions to relieve aortic obstruction should be considered in lifestyle interfering claudication or critical limb ischemia.

Patients with aortoiliac occlusive disease should be instructed on a supervised exercise program. The Claudication: Exercise Vs. Endoluminal Revascularization (CLEVER) trial was a randomized prospective trial comparing optimal medical therapy (OMT) alone, supervised exercise plus OMT, and stenting plus OMT. At 6 months and 18 months, those assigned to exercise responded as well as those who received stents.[135] If the patient is not satisfied with the results of an exercise program, revascularization should be performed. In the past, decisions on the type of treatment the patient was offered were based on the location and extent of obstruction as assessed by *The Transatlantic Inter-Societal Consensus (TASC) II* classification. However, the ESC and ACC/AHA guidelines now recommend an endovascular first approach in patients with aortoiliac occlusive disease, independent of the TASC classification.[136] The BRAVISSIMO trial (BelgianeItalian tRial Vascular Iliac StentS In the treatMent of TASC A, B, C, & D iliac lesiOns) reported a 24-month primary patency rate of 87.9% and a technical success of 100% in 325 patients with aorto-iliac lesions.[137] Neither TASC category nor lesion length was predictive of restenosis. At the current time, open surgery is rarely performed for aortoiliac occlusive disease.

ACUTE OBSTRUCTION OF THE TERMINAL AORTA

Etiology

Sudden occlusion of the terminal aorta may result from a large "saddle" embolus, trauma, dissection, or in situ thrombosis superimposed on aneurysmal or atherosclerotic disease. Most emboli large enough to occlude the terminal aorta (saddle embolism) originate in the heart in patients with mitral stenosis, atrial fibrillation, acute anterior MI, infective endocarditis, or paradoxical embolism through a right-to-left intracardiac shunt from a peripheral venous source. When thrombotic occlusion of the aorta develops at a point of atherosclerotic narrowing, collateral perfusion is usually sufficient to prevent acute limb ischemia. Acute aortic occlusion related to thrombosis of abdominal aortic aneurysms is considerably less common than thrombosis of popliteal aneurysms.

Clinical Features

Unlike gradually progressive obstruction, abrupt total or near-total interruption of flow through the terminal aorta or common iliac arteries poses an immediate threat to life and limb. Although the clinical picture varies depending on the collaterals, the full-blown syndrome is characterized by an abrupt onset of pain, typically severe, in the lumbar area, buttocks, perineum, abdomen, and legs. Diffuse cyanosis may be present from the umbilicus to the feet, and the lower limbs may be pale and cold. Numbness, paresthesia, and paralysis dominate the picture. Pulses are absent in the lower limbs and, unless circulation is restored promptly, muscle necrosis may produce myoglobinuria, renal failure, acidosis, hyperkalemia, and death.

Management

In contrast to chronic aortoiliac occlusion, acute aortic occlusion calls for immediate revascularization. The optimum procedure depends on the cause and the strategy for prevention of recurrent embolism. Transfemoral catheter-based embolectomy can extract even large amounts of embolic material from the distal aorta. Even after circulation has been restored, however, mortality is high, related to the underlying disease.

AORTITIS

Inflammation of the aortic wall may occur in noninfectious diseases, such as Takayasu disease, giant cell arteritis, immunoglobulin G (IgG)–related diseases, the spondyloarthropathies, Behçet syndrome, relapsing polychondritis, Cogan syndrome, rheumatoid arthritis, systemic lupus erythematosus, sarcoidosis, idiopathic retroperitoneal fibrosis, as isolated aortitis, drug-induced aortitis, and other disorders.[138] Only the most common of these uncommon entities are discussed in detail. A possible role for infectious agents—including bacteria, viruses, and mycobacterium—in instigating arteritides of various sorts has been postulated.[139]

Takayasu Disease

The prototypical nonspecific aortitis, Takayasu arteritis was named for the Japanese ophthalmologist who first called attention to the funduscopic findings. Because of its predilection for the brachiocephalic vessels, this arteritis has been labeled *pulseless disease* and *aortic arch syndrome*. The classic form occurs with greatest frequency in Asian countries, but patients with a similar nonspecific aortitis are encountered worldwide. The etiology is unknown; no infectious agent has been identified, and identification of endothelial antibodies in 18 of 19 patients with this disease, although nonspecific, supports an autoimmune mechanism. Mutations in *HLA-B* and *IL12B* genes[140,141] suggest that genetic factors predispose to Takayasu disease, and progress in genetics promises to clarify whether Takayasu and other, nonspecific arteritides are the same or different diseases.

Histopathology

Histologic studies of tissue from patients in active stages of the disease disclose a granulomatous arteritis similar to giant cell arteritis and to the aortitis associated with the seronegative spondyloarthropathies and Cogan syndrome. In later stages, medial degeneration, fibrous scarring, intimal proliferation, and thrombosis result in narrowing of the vessel, yet adequate histopathologic criteria for differential diagnosis of noninfectious arteritides, including Takayasu disease and giant cell aortitis are lacking. Aneurysm formation is less common than stenosis, but aneurysm rupture is an important cause of death in patients with Takayasu arteritis. Angiographically, the left subclavian artery is narrowed in approximately 90% of patients. The right subclavian artery, left carotid artery, and brachiocephalic trunk follow closely in frequency of stenosis. Thoracic aortic lesions occur in 66% of patients, the abdominal aorta is involved in 50%, and aortoiliac involvement is seen in approximately 12%. Pulmonary arteritis occurs in about half of patients and may be associated with pulmonary hypertension.

Clinical Features

In 70% to 80% of patients, clinical manifestations of the illness appear during the second or third decade of life, but onset in childhood and in middle life have been reported. Women are affected 8 to 9 times more often than men.[142]

During the early or "prepulseless" phase, symptoms include fever, night sweats, malaise, nausea, vomiting, weight loss, rash, arthralgia, and Raynaud's phenomenon. Splenomegaly may occur, and laboratory findings may include acceleration of the erythrocyte sedimentation rate, elevated levels of C-reactive protein, anemia, and plasma protein abnormalities. A minority of patients, however, may experience none of these signs or symptoms and present with discrepancy of arm blood pressures, absent pulse(s), supraclavicular or cervical bruits, or incidental findings on imaging performed for other reasons.

When arterial obstruction develops, upper-extremity claudication may occur as a consequence of subclavian artery stenosis. Stroke, transient cerebral ischemia, dizziness, or syncope usually indicate stenosis of the brachiocephalic arteries or subclavian steal. The retinopathy that first drew the attention of Takayasu is believed to result from retinal ischemia. Hypertension, observed in more than 50% of the cases, may be severe and occurs due to stenosis of the aorta proximal to the renal arteries or involvement of the renal arteries themselves.

Cardiac manifestations result from severe hypertension, dilatation of the aortic root producing valvular insufficiency, or coronary artery stenosis (**Fig. 23–60**). Angina pectoris, MI, and heart failure have been reported. Clinical pericarditis is infrequent, but healed pericarditis is often encountered at necropsy. Involvement of the visceral arteries may result in splanchnic ischemia, and aortoiliac obstruction may produce lower limb intermittent claudication.

Patients with severe aortitis evident at the time of diagnosis face a 25% to 30% risk of ischemic events or death over the next 5 years. Those without ischemic complications at presentation tend to fare better over 5 to 10 years. Severe hypertension

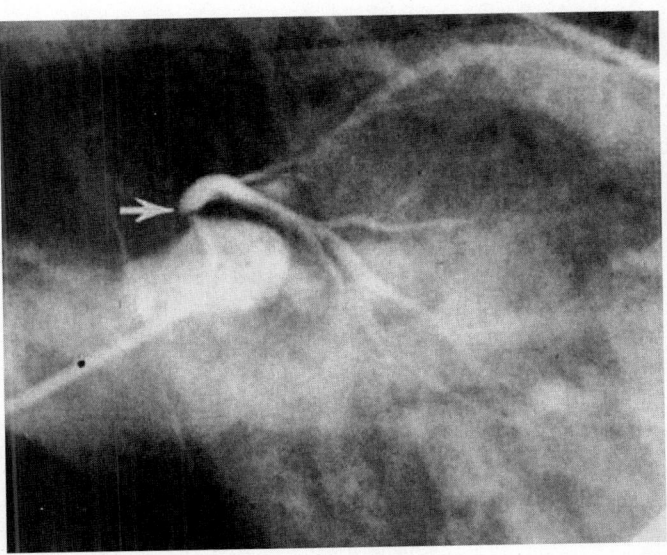

Figure 23–60. Typical angiographic appearance of Takayasu arteritis, showing focal ostial stenosis (*arrow*) of the left main coronary artery. Reproduced with permission from Jolly M, Bartholomew JR, Flamm S, Olin JW. Angina and coronary ostial lesions in a young woman as a presentation of Takayasu's arteritis. *Cardiovasc Surg.* 1999 Jun;7(4):443-446.

and cardiac involvement are associated with a shortened life expectancy.

Diagnosis

The American College of Rheumatology has identified six major criteria for the diagnosis of Takayasu arteritis. Onset of illness by age 40 years avoids overlap with giant cell arteritis. Other criteria include upper-extremity claudication, diminished brachial pulses, greater than 10 mm Hg difference between systolic blood pressure in the arms, subclavian or aortic bruit, and narrowing of the aorta or a major branch. The presence of three of these six criteria carries high diagnostic accuracy.

Arteriography typically shows long areas of smooth narrowing interspersed with areas that appear normal. Aneurysms and occlusions are also common. Duplex ultrasound magnetic resonance angiography (MTA) or CT scans may show wall thickening resulting from inflammation and edema of the media and adventitia. CTA or MRA of the entire aorta and iliac vessels is recommended for all patients with suspected Takayasu disease to define the extent of disease, identify aneurysms, and estimate the activity of disease. A "macaroni sign" on echocardiographic evaluation has recently been described, signifying the thick wall of the vessel with the small, linear residual lumen. PET scanning is showing promise for diagnosis by identifying "hot spots" at sites of active Takayasu lesions.[143]

Management

Corticosteroid therapy appears effective in suppressing inflammation during the active phase, and favorable results have been reported with immunosuppressive and cytotoxic agents. The mainstay of medical treatment continues to be administration of corticosteroids. However, biologic targeted treatments (infliximab, rituximab, tocilizumab) are effective and safe in patients refractory to standard therapy or glucocorticoid-dependent.[144] To date, the only data reported from randomized trials have addressed the use of tocilizumab and abatacept.[145] Operative treatment may be used to relieve symptoms caused by arterial obstruction; percutaneous angioplasty and stenting are associated with mixed results. Restenosis rates are substantial for both surgical and endovascular interventions.[146–148] These procedures are best reserved for patients in whom the acute inflammatory stage of the disease has been controlled.[149,150]

Giant Cell Arteritis

Giant cell arteritis (temporal arteritis, polymyalgia rheumatica) involves extracranial arteries, including the aorta, in 10% to 13% of cases. A peak incidence late in life sets giant cell arteritis apart from other nonspecific arteritides. In recent years, giant cell arteritis is occurring even later in life than in prior decades, although vascular complications generally arise as a consequence of delayed diagnosis and late initiation of treatment.[151] Like Takayasu disease, giant cell arteritis may produce narrowing of the brachiocephalic arteries, aneurysms of the ascending aorta, aortic dissection, and aortic regurgitation. Despite clinical, angiographic, and pathologic similarities to Takayasu arteritis, giant cell arteritis almost always occurs in individuals older than 50 years old. Although the most common presentation involves polymyalgia rheumatica with temporal arteritis, any large artery may be involved.

Treatment of giant cell arteritis usually involves oral prednisone in an initial dose of 40 mg to 60 mg per day. Induction therapy with intravenous steroids has been found beneficial in a randomized trial. During clinical follow-up, CTA, MRA, or [18F]-fludeoxyglucose PET/MRI[152,153] can be of value in monitoring improvement in arterial abnormalities with therapy. In unresponsive cases (<10%) and in those who relapse as the dose is tapered, cytotoxic agents such as cyclosporine, azathioprine, and methotrexate may be helpful. One randomized, double-blind trial found a significant reduction in the rate of relapse and the cumulative mean doses of corticosteroid medication with methotrexate compared with placebo in corticosteroid-treated patients, but another study did not.[154] For patients with symptomatic ascending aortic involvement in giant cell arteritis (pain, inflammation), reports of successful surgical resection have been associated with reduction or withdrawal of corticosteroid treatment. Biological agents are relatively safe and effective corticosteroid-sparing agents for use in treatment of giant call arteritis. Although high-quality data are lacking, tocilizumab is currently considered a standard component of therapy for giant cell arteritis, particularly when relapsing, but the duration of treatment and optimum method for monitoring disease activity remain uncertain.[145,155] Given the limited or in some cases negative data, current clinical practice guidelines do not recommend treatment with azathioprine, mycophenolate mofetil, cyclophosphamide, hydroxychloroquine, dapsone, or cyclosporine.[156]

IgG4-Related Diseases

IgG-related diseases are immune mediated conditions that may involve diverse organ systems.[157] Hallmarks are tumor-like swelling of the involved organs, dense lymphoplasmacytic infiltrate that contains IgG4-positive plasma cells, and storiform fibrosis. Some inflammatory abdominal aortic aneurysms have been linked to IgG4-related sclerosing disease.[158] Serum levels of IgG are usually elevated. A number of conditions are considered part of IgG-related diseases such as autoimmune pancreatitis, sclerosing mesenteritis, Mikulicz's syndrome (salivary and lacrimal glands), Riedel's thyroiditis, eosinophilic angiocentric fibrosis, Küttner's tumor (submandibular glands), inflammatory pseudotumor, mediastinal fibrosis, and hypocomplementemic tubulointerstitial nephritis.[157] The vascular involvement includes IgG4-related retroperitoneal fibrosis, IgG4-related abdominal aortitis, and IgG4-related perianeurysmal fibrosis or inflammatory aortic aneurysms. Clinical manifestations are nonspecific, making presurgical diagnosis difficult. It is now recognized that IgG4-related disease may be the cause of idiopathic retroperitoneal fibrosis (previously called Ormond's disease) in up to two-thirds of cases.[159] Histopathological examination of surgically excised aortic specimens describes IgG4-related disease as among the more common etiologies of aortitis, with a frequency similar to Takayasu's and giant cell arteritis.[160]

Presentations of periaortitis may be nonspecific, leading to a delay in the diagnosis. The most common symptoms are pain in the lower abdomen, flanks, and back. The aorta may be extremely tender to palpation. The thoracic aorta may also be involved leading to aneurysm or dissection. While Takayasu's arteritis and giant cell arteritis affect the primary aortic branches, IgG4-related disease generally spares the branches off the aortic arch.[157]

It is important to diagnose IgG4-related diseases early, as effective therapy is available. Glucocorticoids are first line agents. There are no studies that have evaluated the usual steroid sparing agents (methotrexate, azothioprine). There are no randomized trials using B-cell depletion therapy (targeting a subset of plasma cells that produce the IgG4) with agents such as rituximab but this agent seems to be quite effective in treating some patients with IgG4-related diseases who do not respond to glucocorticoids.[157]

HLA-B27–Associated Spondyloarthropathies

Aortitis is present in a substantial portion of patients with ankylosing spondylitis and Reiter syndrome; more than 90% have the histocompatibility antigen HLA-B27. Aortic involvement is most common in those with spondylitis of long duration, peripheral joint complaints, in addition to spondylitis, and iritis. Inflammation of the aortic root and surrounding tissues, manifest by aortic valve regurgitation or cardiac conduction abnormalities in patients with the HLA-B27 histocompatibility antigen, may also occur without spondyloarthropathies. While the majority of cases occur in the aortic root and ascending aorta, occasionally isolated abdominal aortitis may occur.[161] Histologically, the aortic lesion in this setting resembles the inflammation seen in syphilis, with focal destruction of medial elastic tissue and thickening of the intima and adventitia. Aortic dissection has been reported.

Infectious Aortitis

Primary infection of the aortic wall is a rare cause of aortic aneurysms, which are more often saccular than fusiform. Infectious or "mycotic" aneurysms may arise secondarily from an infection occurring in a preexisting aneurysm of another cause. *Staphylococcus*, *Salmonella*, and *Pseudomonas* species are the most frequent pathogens causing primary aortic infections. Many cases arise as complications of infective endocarditis or arterial catheterization. An intrinsically abnormal aorta, however, may become infected as a consequence of bacteremia. Such infection produces suppurative aortitis, leading to weakness of a portion of the aortic wall. In these cases, aneurysms are typically saccular, yet there is a comparatively high propensity to rupture. Infection of the aorta related to endovascular stents is a new and increasing clinical entity that is difficult to treat.[162]

Syphilitic Aortitis

Treponemal infection produces chronic aortitis in approximately 10% of patients with untreated tertiary syphilis and is the primary cause of death in about the same proportion of cases, but there is evidence of the process at autopsy in about half of patients who have had untreated syphilis for more than 10 years. During the spirochetemic phase of primary syphilis, *Treponema pallidum* organisms lodge in the adventitia of the vasa vasorum and initiate an inflammatory response characterized by perivascular lymphocytic and plasma cell infiltrate. This is followed by obliterative endarteritis, resulting in patchy medial necrosis, elastic fiber fragmentation, weakening of the aortic wall, and aneurysm formation. The intima of the aorta has a characteristic wrinkled appearance, frequently with superimposed atherosclerotic plaques. Because the infection is seeded through the vasa vasorum, the process is most severe in the ascending aorta and the arch, where the density of these vessels is greatest. Luetic aneurysms are typically saccular and involve the ascending aorta whether or not the transverse and descending portions are also affected. Aortic aneurysms resulting from cardiovascular syphilis follow interruption of the elastic fibers as a result of periaortitis and mesoaortitis, which thicken but weaken the aortic wall. Rupture is the major complication, but the enlarging aneurysm may also compress or erode adjacent structures of the mediastinum. Because the inflammatory process tends to interrupt the medial layer by transverse scars, dissection is distinctly uncommon.

Aortic involvement may be asymptomatic or associated with aortic regurgitation, coronary ostial stenosis, or aortic aneurysms. Asymptomatic aortitis may sometimes be identified by linear calcification of the ascending aorta, evident on chest radiographs. Valvular regurgitation, present in 20% to 30% of patients with syphilitic aortitis, is mainly a consequence of aortic root dilatation. Syphilitic coronary ostial stenosis, only a century ago more common than coronary atherosclerosis as a cause of angina pectoris, occurs in 25% to 30% of such patients, most of whom also have aortic regurgitation. MI is rare. The least frequent manifestation of syphilitic aortitis is aneurysm formation, which occurs in 5% to 10% of affected patients. Although the prognosis for patients with uncomplicated syphilitic aortitis is comparable to that of the general population, the outlook is poor when syphilitic aneurysms of the aorta are large enough to produce symptoms. The diagnosis of cardiovascular syphilis may be difficult in patients older than age 50 years, when hypertensive and atherosclerotic disease often coexist.

The frequency of cardiovascular syphilis has fallen dramatically over recent decades as a consequence of early identification and treatment of the disease. However, a recent report indicates that syphilitic ascending aortic aneurysms are still common and must remain in the consciousness of the caring medical and surgical teams.[163]

Adequate antimicrobial therapy of early syphilis is the most important preventive measure, although whether such treatment retards the progression of disease once aortitis has developed has not been clearly established. Without surgical intervention, symptomatic syphilitic aortic aneurysms are associated with a high mortality rate.

Recently, Roberts and colleagues[163] have described the features of syphilitic aortitis at surgery in hopes of permitting intraoperative identification and prompt institution of treatment. The distinguishing features include sparing of the aortic root, involvement of the tubular portion of the ascending aorta, uniform involvement of the surface of the affected aortic portions, and inflammation in all three layers of the aortic wall. The aorta is said to have a "tree bark" appearance characteristic of syphilitic aortitis.

Tuberculous Aortitis

Tuberculous aneurysms usually result from direct extension of infection from hilar lymph nodes and subsequent granulomatous destruction of the medial layer, leading to loss of aortic wall elasticity, although occasional cases of hematogenous spread have been described.[164] The posterior or posterolateral aortic wall is usually the site of saccular aneurysm formation in these cases. Caseating granulomatous lesions affecting the medial layer of the aortic wall characterize the histology. Pseudoaneurysm formation, perforation, or aorto-enteric fistula may result. Infection may occasionally invade the aortic valve ring and adjacent structures, producing a caseating paravalvular abscess. Rupture of tuberculous aortic lesions may occur. It is important to recognize that miliary tuberculous may manifest in a manner similar to Takayasu's arteritis. Therefore, if there is a suspicion of tuberculosis, testing should be performed before starting immunosuppressant medications. Steroids have been used in combination with antituberculosis therapy for inflammatory lesions. Surgery is indicated for aneurysms that expand or remain symptomatic despite drug therapy.[164]

Drug-Induced Aortitis

Several drugs, such as ergot alkaloids, dopaminergic agents, and methysergide, have been observed to cause of acute or chronic aortitis.[165] Aortitis can also develop as a complication of adjuvant/neoadjuvant chemotherapy with human granulocyte-colony stimulating factors (G-CSF) in patients with breast cancer treated with PEGylated filgrastim (incidence 0.3% in one series).[166] The clinical presentation is characterized by fever and chest and/or back pain with high levels of inflammatory markers but no evidence of infection. CTA reveals enhancing wall thickening and periaortic soft tissue infiltration at various levels of the aorta. Rapid improvement followed treatment with prednisolone (0.5 mg/kg/day). Although optimum treatment has not been established, short-term systemic administration of corticosteroid medication and avoidance of G-CSF agents can be effective.

FUTURE PROSPECTS

This is an exciting time in the care of the thoracic aorta. Although clinical trials of ARBs have not revealed the hoped-for medical panacea, other exciting advances are being made.

As the familial nature of aneurysmal diseases becomes familiar to a broader array of physicians, radiologic testing of relatives of affected individuals is likely to become standard practice and reimbursable by insurers. Recognizing an aneurysm in advance of symptoms is the optimal method to enhance survival, and family members represent the most cost-effective candidates for diagnostic testing.

Surgical therapy for the thoracic aorta has become safer and safer, approaching the low mortality rates of conventional cardiac surgical procedures, like coronary artery bypass and valve replacement. This trend is likely to continue, becoming more widespread and proliferating beyond leading large volume centers.

Endovascular devices and technologies are advancing at a rapid rate, providing alternative options, especially for elderly and infirm patients. It is hoped that these endovascular therapies will advance further, perhaps even mimicking the success and durability of open techniques.

The aorta is being understood more and more thoroughly from an engineering standpoint. Engineering calculations are currently on the way toward becoming an integral part of surgical decision-making.[167]

Once a TAA has been identified, we can keep the patient safe by following algorithms based on patient symptoms and aortic size. Perhaps the biggest problem in thoracic aortic disease is the silent nature of TAAs.

Now that whole exome sequencing has become relatively inexpensive, additional genes and variants in known genes are discovered on a regular basis. Genetic screening for family members of patients with aortic aneurysms and dissection are more readily available, and identification of specific genetic mutations permits personalized care at the genetic level. Certain mutations (eg, *ACTA2* and *MYLK*) produce aortic dissection at relatively small aortic diameters. Specific mutations are becoming an integral factor in clinical decision-making. Identification of new pathogenic pathways will open avenues for novel drug development to target deficiencies in the protein structure of the aortic wall.

With the advent and advancement of CRISPR (clustered regularly interspaced short palindromic repeats) techniques, the potential for eventual gene therapy of the genetically susceptible aorta is perhaps the most exciting prospect on the horizon.

More than 100 years ago, Sir William Osler stated: "There is no disease more conducive to clinical humility than aneurysm of the aorta." This is still true today because aneurysms and dissections remain virulent processes that challenge the skill and experience of physicians and surgeons. However, advances in progress at the present time promise to tame this virulent disease.

SUMMARY

Pathogenesis of Aortic Aneurysms

- Aneurysms of the aortic root, ascending aorta, and aortic arch proximal to the ligamentum arteriosum are generally caused by degeneration of the protein structure of the medial layer of the aortic wall, whereas aneurysms of the descending thoracic aorta and abdominal aorta are most often caused by atherosclerosis.

Genetic Causes of Aortic Disease

- Both syndromic and nonsyndromic genetic diseases of the aorta are associated with cystic medial necrosis and may cause aneurysms of other arteries as well.
- Most exhibit autosomal dominant transmission with variable penetrance.

Imaging for Diagnosis and Surveillance of Aortic Aneurysms and Dissection

- Duplex ultrasound is useful for evaluation of aneurysms of the aortic root, ascending aorta and abdominal aorta, but noninvasive evaluation of the uppermost portion of the ascending aorta, aorta arch, and descending thoracic aorta requires contrast-enhanced CTA or MRA.
- Each method is associated with specific advantages and limitations.

Medical Management of Aortic Aneurysmal Disease

- The foundation of medical management of patients with aortic aneurysms is blood pressure reduction, favoring agents that attenuate dynamic circulatory forces (rate of rise in systolic pressure over time).
- Other strategies target pathophysiological factors specific to the various types of aortic diseases (eg, TGF-β, MMPs, atherosclerosis, inflammation, and thrombosis).

Invasive Approaches to Aortic Aneurysms and Dissection

- While open surgical repair of aortic aneurysms or dissections is definitive, endovascular stent-grafting has increased and this trend is likely to continue, although anatomical factors currently limit application to the descending thoracic and abdominal aortic segments.
- Endovascular approaches require postprocedural surveillance at more frequent intervals because of the possibility of endoleaks or incomplete repair, but all patients undergoing aortic interventions require periodic imaging and avoidance or control of hypertension.

ACKNOWLEDGEMENT

The authors would like to acknowledge Jeffrey W. Olin who contributed content to this chapter in the previous edition(s).

REFERENCES

1. Sulejmani F, Pokutta-Paskaleva A, Ziganshin B, et al. Biomechanical properties of the thoracic aorta in Marfan patients. *Ann Cardiothorac Surg.* 2017;6(6):610-624. doi:10.21037/acs.2017.09.12.

2. Martin C, Sun W, Pham T, Elefteriades J. Predictive biomechanical analysis of ascending aortic aneurysm rupture potential. *Acta Biomaterialia.* 2013;9(12):9392-9400. (Research Support, N.I.H., Extramural) (In eng). doi:10.1016/j.actbio.2013.07.044.

3. Turkbey EB, Jain A, Johnson C, et al. Determinants and normal values of ascending aortic diameter by age, gender, and race/ethnicity in the Multi-Ethnic Study of Atherosclerosis (MESA). *JMRI.* 2014;39(2):360-368.doi:10.1002/jmri.24183.

4. Paruchuri V, Salhab KF, Kuzmik G, et al. Aortic size distribution in the general population: explaining the size paradox in aortic dissection. *Cardiology.* 2015;131(4):265-272. doi:10.1159/000381281.

5. AlGhatrif M, Lakatta EG. The conundrum of arterial stiffness, elevated blood pressure, and aging. *Curr Hypertens Rep.* 2015;17(2):12. doi:10.1007/s11906-014-0523-z.

6. van Dorst DCH, de Wagenaar NP, van der Pluijm I, Roos-Hesselink JW, Essers J, Danser AHJ. Transforming growth factor-beta and the renin-angiotensin system in syndromic thoracic aortic aneurysms: implications for treatment. *Cardiovasc Drugs Ther.* 2020. doi:10.1007/s10557-020-07116-4.

7. Andelfinger G, Loeys B, Dietz H. A decade of discovery in the genetic understanding of thoracic aortic disease. *Can J Cardiol.* 2016;32(1):13-25. doi:10.1016/j.cjca.2015.10.017.

8. Mallat Z, Ait-Oufella H, Tedgui A. The pathogenic transforming growth factor-beta overdrive hypothesis in aortic aneurysms and dissections: a mirage? *Circulation Res.* 2017;120(11):1718-1720. doi:10.1161/CIRCRESAHA.116.310371.

9. Humphrey JD, Milewicz DM, Tellides G, Schwartz MA. Cell biology. dysfunctional mechanosensing in aneurysms. *Science.* 2014;344(6183):477-479. doi:10.1126/science.1253026.

10. Humphrey JD, Schwartz MA, Tellides G, Milewicz DM. Role of mechanotransduction in vascular biology: focus on thoracic aortic aneurysms and dissections. *Circulation Res.* 2015;116(8):1448-61. doi:10.1161/CIRCRESAHA.114.304936.

11. Verstraeten A, Luyckx I, Loeys B. Aetiology and management of hereditary aortopathy. *Nature Rev Cardiol.* 2017;14(4):197-208. doi:10.1038/nrcardio.2016.211.

12. Rabkin SW. The role matrix metalloproteinases in the production of aortic aneurysm. *Prog Mol Biol Transl Sci.* 2017;147:239-265. doi:10.1016/bs.pmbts.2017.02.002.

13. Singh S, Nautiyal A. Aortic dissection and aortic aneurysms associated with fluoroquinolones: a systematic review and meta-analysis. *Am J Med.* 2017;130(12):1449-1457.e9. doi:10.1016/j.amjmed.2017.06.029.

14. Lee CC, Lee MG, Hsieh R, et al. Oral fluoroquinolone and the risk of aortic dissection. *J Am Coll Cardiol.* 2018;72(12):1369-1378. doi:10.1016/j.jacc.2018.06.067.

15. Pasternak B, Inghammar M, Svanstrom H. Fluoroquinolone use and risk of aortic aneurysm and dissection: nationwide cohort study. *BMJ.* 2018;360:k678. doi:10.1136/bmj.k678.

16. Hellgren T, Beck AW, Behrendt CA, et al. Thoracic endovascular aortic repair practice in 13 countries: a report from VASCUNET and the International Consortium of Vascular Registries. *Ann Surg.* 2020. doi:10.1097/SLA.0000000000004561.

17. De Backer J, Campens L, De Paepe A. Genes in thoracic aortic aneurysms/dissections—do they matter? *Ann Cardiothorac Surg.* 2013;2(1):73-82. doi:10.3978/j.issn.2225-319X.2012.12.01.

18. Ziganshin BA, Elefteriades JA. Triggers of aortic dissection. In: Stanger OH, Svensson LG, eds. *Surgical management of aortic pathology: current fundamentals for the clinical management of aortic disease.* Springer International Publishing; 2019:191-203.

19. Raunso J, Song RJ, Vasan RS, et al. Familial clustering of aortic size, aneurysms, and dissections in the community. *Circulation.* 2020;142(10):920-928. doi:10.1161/CIRCULATIONAHA.120.045990.

20. Fletcher AJ, Syed MBJ, Aitman TJ, Newby DE, Walker NL. Inherited thoracic aortic disease: new insights and translational targets. *Inherited Thoracic Aortic Dis.* 2020;141(19). doi:10.1161/CIRCULATIONAHA.119.043756.

21. Marfan AB. Un cas de deformation congenitale des quatre membres, plus prononce des extremites, caracterise par r allongement des coeur avec un certain degre d'amincissement. *Bull Mem Soc Med Hop Paris.* 1896;13:220-226.

22. Loeys BL, Dietz HC, Braverman AC, et al. The revised Ghent nosology for the Marfan syndrome. *J Med Genet.* 2010;47(7):476-85. doi:10.1136/jmg.2009.072785.

23. Franken R, Radonic T, den Hartog AW, et al. The revised role of TGF-beta in aortic aneurysms in Marfan syndrome. *Netherlands Heart J.* 2015;23(2):116-121. doi:10.1007/s12471-014-0622-0.

24. Loeys BL. Angiotensin receptor blockers: a panacea for Marfan syndrome and related disorders? *Drug Discovery Today.* 2015;20(2):262-266. doi:10.1016/j.drudis.2014.09.022.

25. Pomianowski P, Elefteriades JA. The genetics and genomics of thoracic aortic disease. *Ann Cardiothorac Surg.* 2013;2(3):271-279. doi:10.3978/j.issn.2225-319X.2013.05.12.

26. Meester JAN, Verstraeten A, Schepers D, Alaerts M, Van Laer L, Loeys BL. Differences in manifestations of Marfan syndrome, Ehlers-Danlos syndrome, and Loeys-Dietz syndrome. *Ann Cardiothorac Surg.* 2017;6(6):582-594. doi:10.21037/acs.2017.11.03.

27. Gould RA, Aziz H, Woods CE, et al. ROBO4 variants predispose individuals to bicuspid aortic valve and thoracic aortic aneurysm. *Nature Genet.* 2019;51(1):42-50. doi:10.1038/s41588-018-0265-y.

28. Yang B, Zhou W, Jiao J, et al. Protein-altering and regulatory genetic variants near GATA4 implicated in bicuspid aortic valve. *Nat Commun.* 2017;8:15481.

29. Hiratzka LF, Creager MA, Isselbacher EM, et al. Surgery for aortic dilatation in patients with bicuspid aortic valves: a statement of clarification from the American College of Cardiology/American Heart Association Task Force on Clinical Practice Guidelines. *J Am Coll Cardiol.* 2016;67(6):724-731. doi:10.1016/j.jacc.2015.11.006.

30. Borger MA, Fedak PWM, Stephens EH, et al. The American Association for Thoracic Surgery consensus guidelines on bicuspid aortic valve-related aortopathy: full online-only version. *J Thoracic Cardiovasc Surg.* 2018;156(2):e41-e74. doi:10.1016/j.jtcvs.2018.02.115.

31. Renard M, Francis C, Ghosh R, et al. Clinical validity of genes for heritable thoracic aortic aneurysm and dissection. *J Am Coll Cardiol.* 2018;72(6):605-615. doi:10.1016/j.jacc.2018.04.089.

32. Faggion Vinholo T, Brownstein AJ, Ziganshin BA, et al. Genes associated with thoracic aortic aneurysm and dissection: 2019 update and clinical implications. *Aorta (Stamford).* 2019;7(4):99-107. doi:10.1055/s-0039-3400233.

33. Ziganshin BA, Bailey AE, Coons C, et al. Routine genetic testing for thoracic aortic aneurysm and dissection in a clinical setting. *Ann Thoracic Surg.* 2015;100(5):1604-1611. doi:10.1016/j.athoracsur.2015.04.106.

34. Richards S, Aziz N, Bale S, et al. Standards and guidelines for the interpretation of sequence variants: a joint consensus recommendation of the American College of Medical Genetics and Genomics and the Association for Molecular Pathology. *Genet Med.* 2015;17(5):405-424. doi:10.1038/gim.2015.30.

35. Nykamp K, Anderson M, Powers M, et al. Sherloc: a comprehensive refinement of the ACMG-AMP variant classification criteria. *Genet Med.* 2017;19(10):1105-1117. doi:10.1038/gim.2017.37.

36. Karczewski KJ, Francioli LC, Tiao G, et al. The mutational constraint spectrum quantified from variation in 141,456 humans. *Nature.* 2020;581(7809):434-443. doi:10.1038/s41586-020-2308-7.

37. Kircher M, Witten DM, Jain P, O'Roak BJ, Cooper GM, Shendure J. A general framework for estimating the relative pathogenicity of human genetic variants. *Nature Genet.* 2014;46(3):310-315. doi:10.1038/ng.2892.

38. Ioannidis NM, Rothstein JH, Pejaver V, et al. REVEL: An ensemble method for predicting the pathogenicity of rare missense variants. *Am J Human Genet.* 2016;99(4):877-885. doi:10.1016/j.ajhg.2016.08.016.

39. Hiratzka LF, Bakris GL, Beckman JA, et al. 2010 ACCF/AHA/AATS/ACR/ASA/SCA/SCAI/SIR/STS/SVM Guidelines for the diagnosis and management of patients with thoracic aortic disease. A Report of the American College of Cardiology Foundation/American Heart Association Task Force on Practice Guidelines, American Association for Thoracic Surgery, American College of Radiology, American Stroke Association, Society of Cardiovascular Anesthesiologists, Society for Cardiovascular Angiography and Interventions, Society of Interventional Radiology, Society of Thoracic Surgeons,and Society for Vascular Medicine. *J Am Coll Cardiol.* 2010;55(14):e27-e129. (Practice Guideline) doi:10.1016/j.jacc.2010.02.015.

40. Ma WG, Chou AS, Mok SCM, et al. Positive family history of aortic dissection dramatically increases dissection risk in family members. *Int J Cardiol.* 2017;240:132-137. doi:10.1016/j.ijcard.2017.04.080.

41. Chen SW, Kuo CF, Huang YT, et al. Association of family history with incidence and outcomes of aortic dissection. *J Am Coll Cardiol.* 2020;76(10):1181-1192. doi:10.1016/j.jacc.2020.07.028.

42. National Center for Injury Prevention and Control. WISQARS leading causes of death reports, 1981–2018. https://webappa.cdc.gov/sasweb/ncipc/leadcause.html

43. Roberts IS, Benamore RE, Benbow EW, et al. Post-mortem imaging as an alternative to autopsy in the diagnosis of adult deaths: a validation study. *Lancet.* 2012;379(9811):136-142. doi:10.1016/S0140-6736(11)61483-9.

44. Moriwaki Y, Tahara Y, Kosuge T, Suzuki N. Etiology of out-of-hospital cardiac arrest diagnosed via detailed examinations including perimortem computed tomography. *J Emergencies Trauma Shock.* 2013;6(2):87-94. doi:10.4103/0974-2700.110752.

45. McClure RS, Brogly SB, Lajkosz K, Payne D, Hall SF, Johnson AP. Epidemiology and management of thoracic aortic dissections and thoracic aortic aneurysms in Ontario, Canada: a population-based study. *J Thorac Cardiovasc Surg.* 2018;155(6):2254-2264.e4. doi:10.1016/j.jtcvs.2017.11.105.

46. Chen JF, Zafar MA, Wu J, et al. Increased virulence of descending thoracic and thoracoabdominal aortic aneurysms in women. *Ann Thorac Surg.* 2020. doi:10.1016/j.athoracsur.2020.08.026.

47. Sherif HM. Heterogeneity in the segmental development of the aortic tree: impact on management of genetically triggered aortic aneurysms. *Aorta (Stamford)* 2014;2(5):186-195. doi:10.12945/j.aorta.2014.14-032.

48. Elefteriades JA, Sang A, Kuzmik G, Hornick M. Guilt by association: paradigm for detecting a silent killer (thoracic aortic aneurysm). *Open Heart.* 2015;2(1):e000169. doi:10.1136/openhrt-2014-000169.

49. Dumfarth J, Chou AS, Ziganshin BA, et al. Atypical aortic arch branching variants: a novel marker for thoracic aortic disease. *J Thorac Cardiovasc Surg.* 2015;149(6):1586-1592. doi:10.1016/j.jtcvs.2015.02.019.

50. Ziganshin BA, Theodoropoulos P, Salloum MN, et al. Simple renal cysts as markers of thoracic aortic disease. *J Am Heart Assoc.* 2016;5(1):e002248. doi:10.1161/JAHA.115.002248.

51. Brownstein AJ, Bin Mahmood SU, Saeyeldin A, et al. Simple renal cysts and bovine aortic arch: markers for aortic disease. *Open Heart* 2019;6(1):e000862. doi:10.1136/openhrt-2018-000862.

52. LeFevre ML, Force USPST. Screening for abdominal aortic aneurysm: U.S. Preventive Services Task Force recommendation statement. *Ann Int Med.* 2014;161(4):281-290. doi:10.7326/M14-1204.

53. U.S. Preventive Services Task Force, Owens DK, Davidson KW, et al. Screening for abdominal aortic aneurysm: US Preventive Services Task Force Recommendation Statement. *JAMA.* 2019;322(22):2211-2218. doi:10.1001/jama.2019.18928.

54. Evangelista A, Isselbacher EM, Bossone E, et al. Insights from the International Registry of Acute Aortic Dissection: a 20-year experience of collaborative clinical research. *Circulation.* 2018;137(17):1846-1860. doi:10.1161/CIRCULATIONAHA.117.031264.

55. Pape LA, Awais M, Woznicki EM, et al. Presentation, diagnosis, and outcomes of acute aortic dissection: 17-year trends from the International Registry of Acute Aortic Dissection. *J Am Coll Cardiol.* 2015;66(4):350-358. doi:10.1016/j.jacc.2015.05.029.

56. Kim J, Song HC. Role of PET/CT in the evaluation of aortic disease. *Chonnam Med J.* 2018;54(3):143-152. doi:10.4068/cmj.2018.54.3.143.

57. Courtois A, Nusgens BV, Hustinx R, et al. 18F-FDG uptake assessed by PET/CT in abdominal aortic aneurysms is associated with cellular and molecular alterations prefacing wall deterioration and rupture. *J Nucl Med.* 2013;54(10):1740-1747. doi:10.2967/jnumed.112.115873.

58. Nchimi A, Couvreur T, Meunier B, Sakalihasan N. Magnetic resonance imaging findings in a positron emission tomography-positive thoracic aortic aneurysm. *Aorta (Stamford).* 2013;1(3):198-201. doi:10.12945/j.aorta.2013.13-022.

59. Elefteriades JA, Mukherjee SK, Mojibian H. Discrepancies in measurement of the thoracic aorta. *J Am Coll Cardiol.* 2020;76(2):212-228. doi:https://doi.org/10.1016/j.jacc.2020.03.084.

60. Lopez-Guimet J, Pena-Perez L, Bradley RS, et al. MicroCT imaging reveals differential 3D micro-scale remodelling of the murine aorta in ageing and Marfan syndrome. *Theranostics.* 2018;8(21):6038-6052. doi:10.7150/thno.26598.

61. Elefteriades JA, Ziganshin BA, Rizzo JA, et al. Indications and imaging for aortic surgery: size and other matters. *J Thorac Cardiovasc Surg.* 2015;149(2 Suppl):S10-S13. doi:10.1016/j.jtcvs.2014.07.066.

62. Zafar MA, Li Y, Rizzo JA, et al. Height alone, rather than body surface area, suffices for risk estimation in ascending aortic aneurysm. *J Thorac Cardiovasc Surg.* 2018;155(5):1938-1950. doi:10.1016/j.jtcvs.2017.10.140.

63. Zafar MA, Chen JF, Wu J, et al. Natural history of descending thoracic and thoracoabdominal aortic aneurysms. *J Thorac Cardiovasc Surg.* 2019;161(2):498-511. doi:10.1016/j.jtcvs.2019.10.125.

64. Curtis AE, Smith TA, Ziganshin BA, Elefteriades JA. The mystery of the z-score. *Aorta (Stamford).* 2016;4(4):124-130. doi:10.12945/j.aorta.2016.16.014.

65. Elkinany S, Weismann CG, Curtis A, et al. Is aortic z-score an appropriate index of beneficial drug effect in clinical trials in aortic aneurysm disease? *Am J Cardiol.* 2021;143:145-153.

66. van Bogerijen GH, Tolenaar JL, Grassi V, et al. Biomarkers in TAA-the Holy Grail. *Prog Cardiovasc Dis.* 2013;56(1):109-15. doi:10.1016/j.pcad.2013.05.004.

67. Prasad K, Sarkar A, Zafar MA, et al. Advanced glycation end products and its soluble receptors in the pathogenesis of thoracic aortic aneurysm. *Aorta (Stamford).* 2016;4(1):1-10. doi:10.12945/j.aorta.2015.15.018.

68. Shalhub S, Dua A, Brooks J. Biomarkers in descending thoracic aortic dissection. *Seminars Vasc Surg.* 2014;27(3-4):196-199. doi:10.1053/j.semvascsurg.2015.01.001.

69. Sbarouni E, Georgiadou P, Analitis A, Voudris V. High neutrophil to lymphocyte ratio in type A acute aortic dissection facilitates diagnosis and predicts worse outcome. *Exp Rev Molecul Diagnost.* 2015;15(7):965-970. doi:10.1586/14737159.2015.1042367.

70. Gu J, Hu J, Qian H, et al. Intestinal barrier dysfunction: a novel therapeutic target for inflammatory response in acute Stanford type A aortic dissection. *J Cardiovasc Pharmacol Therapeut.* 2016;21(1):64-69. doi:10.1177/1074248415581176.

71. Duggirala A, Delogu F, Angelini TG, et al. Non coding RNAs in aortic aneurysmal disease. *Frontiers Genet.* 2015;6:125. doi:10.3389/fgene.2015.00125.

72. Chun AS, Elefteriades JA, Mukherjee SK. Medical treatment for thoracic aortic aneurysm—much more work to be done. *Prog Cardiovasc Dis.* 2013;56(1):103-108. doi:10.1016/j.pcad.2013.05.008.

73. Chun AS, Elefteriades JA, Mukherjee SK. Do beta-blockers really work for prevention of aortic aneurysms?: time for reassessment. *Aorta (Stamford)* 2013;1(1):45-51. doi:10.12945/j.aorta.2013.13.002.

74. Ziganshin BA, Mukherjee SK, Elefteriades JA. Atenolol versus Losartan in Marfan's syndrome. *N Engl J Med.* 2015;372(10):977-978. doi:10.1056/NEJMc1500128#SA1.

75. Lacro RV, Dietz HC, Sleeper LA, et al. Atenolol versus losartan in children and young adults with Marfan's syndrome. *N Engl J Med.* 2014;371(22):2061-2071. doi:10.1056/NEJMoa1404731.

76. Stein LH, Berger J, Tranquilli M, Elefteriades JA. Effect of statin drugs on thoracic aortic aneurysms. *Am J Cardiol.* 2013;112(8):1240-1245. (Comparative Study) doi:10.1016/j.amjcard.2013.05.081.

77. Suzuki T, Isselbacher EM, Nienaber CA, et al. Type-selective benefits of medications in treatment of acute aortic dissection (from the International Registry of Acute Aortic Dissection [IRAD]). *Am J Cardiol.* 2012;109(1):122-127. doi:10.1016/j.amjcard.2011.08.012.

78. Suzuki T, Eagle KA, Bossone E, Ballotta A, Froehlich JB, Isselbacher EM. Medical management in type B aortic dissection. *Ann Cardiothorac Surg.* 2014;3(4):413-417. doi:10.3978/j.issn.2225-319X.2014.07.01.

79. Wojnarski CM, Svensson LG, Roselli EE, et al. Aortic dissection in patients with bicuspid aortic valve-associated aneurysms. *Ann Thorac Surg.* 2015;100(5):1666-1674. DOI:10.1016/j.athoracsur.2015.04.126.

80. Eleid MF, Forde I, Edwards WD, et al. Type A aortic dissection in patients with bicuspid aortic valves: clinical and pathological comparison with tricuspid aortic valves. *Heart.* 2013;99(22):1668-1674. doi:10.1136/heartjnl-2013-304606.

81. Etz CD, von Aspern K, Hoyer A, et al. Acute type A aortic dissection: characteristics and outcomes comparing patients with bicuspid versus tricuspid aortic valve. *Eur J Cardio-Thorac Surg.* 2015;48(1):142-150. doi:10.1093/ejcts/ezu388.

82. Erbel R, Aboyans V, Boileau C, et al. 2014 ESC Guidelines on the diagnosis and treatment of aortic diseases: document covering acute and chronic aortic diseases of the thoracic and abdominal aorta of the adult. The Task Force for the Diagnosis and Treatment of Aortic Diseases of the European Society of Cardiology (ESC). *Eur Heart J.* 2014;35(41):2873-2926. doi:10.1093/eurheartj/ehu281.

83. Wu J, Zafar MA, Li Y, et al. Ascending aortic length and risk of aortic adverse events: the neglected dimension. *J Am Coll Cardiol.* 2019;74(15):1883-1894. doi:10.1016/j.jacc.2019.07.078.

84. Ziganshin BA, Zafar MA, Elefteriades JA. Descending threshold for ascending aortic aneurysmectomy: Is it time for a "left-shift" in guidelines? *J Thoracic Cardiovasc Surg.* 2019;157(1):37-42. doi:10.1016/j.jtcvs.2018.07.114.

85. Rylski B, Branchetti E, Bavaria JE, et al. Modeling of predissection aortic size in acute type A dissection: more than 90% fail to meet the guidelines for elective ascending replacement. *J Thoracic Cardiovasc Surg.* 2014;148(3):944-948.e1. doi:10.1016/j.jtcvs.2014.05.050.

86. Mansour AM, Peterss S, Zafar MA, et al. Prevention of aortic dissection suggests a diameter shift to a lower aortic size threshold for intervention. *Cardiology.* 2018;139(3):139-146. doi:10.1159/000481930.

87. Mariscalco G, Debiec R, Elefteriades JA, Samani NJ, Murphy GJ. Systematic review of studies that have evaluated screening tests in relatives of patients affected by nonsyndromic thoracic aortic disease. *J Am Heart Assoc.* 2018;7(15):e009302. doi:10.1161/JAHA.118.009302.

88. Lederle FA, Wilson SE, Johnson GR, et al. Immediate repair compared with surveillance of small abdominal aortic aneurysms. *N Engl J Med.* 2002;346(19):1437-44. doi:10.1056/NEJMoa012573.

89. Filardo G, Powell JT, Martinez MA, Ballard DJ. Surgery for small asymptomatic abdominal aortic aneurysms. *Cochrane Database Syst Rev.* 2015;2:CD001835. doi:10.1002/14651858.CD001835.pub4.

90. Cooley DA, De Bakey ME. Surgical considerations of intrathoracic aneurysms of the aorta and great vessels. *Ann Surg.* 1952;135(5):660-680.

91. Elefteraides JA, Ziganshin BA. *Practical tips in aortic surgery.* Springer;2021.

92. Yacoub MH, Gehle P, Chandrasekaran V, Birks EJ, Child A, Radley-Smith R. Late results of a valve-preserving operation in patients with aneurysms of the ascending aorta and root. *J Thoracic Cardiovasc Surg.* 1998;115(5):1080-1090. doi:10.1016/S0022-5223(98)70408-8.

93. David TE, Ivanov J, Armstrong S, Feindel CM, Webb GD. Aortic valve-sparing operations in patients with aneurysms of the aortic root or ascending aorta. *Ann Thoracic Surg.* 2002;74(5):S1758-S1761; discussion S1792-S1799.

94. David TE. Aortic valve sparing operations: a review. *Korean J Thoracic Cardiovasc Surg.* 2012;45(4):205-212. doi:10.5090/kjtcs.2012.45.4.205.

95. Kari FA, Doll KN, Hemmer W, et al. Residual and progressive aortic regurgitation after valve-sparing root replacement: a propensity-matched multi-institutional analysis in 764 patients. *Ann Thoracic Surg.* 2016;101(4):1500-1506. doi:10.1016/j.athoracsur.2015.10.002.

96. Chiu P, Goldstone AB, Schaffer JM, et al. Endovascular versus open repair of intact descending thoracic aortic aneurysms. *J Am Coll Cardiol.* 2019;73(6):643-651. doi:10.1016/j.jacc.2018.10.086.

97. Mok SC, Ma WG, Mansour A, et al. Twenty-five year outcomes following composite graft aortic root replacement. *J Cardiac Surg.* 2017;32(2):99-109. doi:10.1111/jocs.12875.

98. Keidar Z, Pirmisashvili N, Leiderman M, Nitecki S, Israel O. 18F-FDG uptake in noninfected prosthetic vascular grafts: incidence, patterns, and changes over time. *J Nucl Med.* 2014;55(3):392-395. doi:10.2967/jnumed.113.128173.

99. Coselli JS, Green SY, Price MD, et al. Spinal cord deficit after 1114 extent II open thoracoabdominal aortic aneurysm repairs. *J Thoracic Cardiovasc Surg.* 2019. doi:10.1016/j.jtcvs.2019.01.120.

100. Coselli JS, LeMaire SA, Preventza O, et al. Outcomes of 3309 thoracoabdominal aortic aneurysm repairs. *J Thoracic Cardiovasc Surg.* 2016;151(5):1323-1337. doi:10.1016/j.jtcvs.2015.12.050.

101. Liu LY, Callahan B, Peterss S, et al. Neuromonitoring using motor and somatosensory evoked potentials in aortic surgery. *J Cardiac Surg.* 2016;31(6):383-389. doi:10.1111/jocs.12739.

102. Ziganshin BA, Elefteriades JA. Surgical management of thoracoabdominal aneurysms. *Heart.* 2014;100(20):1577-1582. doi:10.1136/heartjnl-2013-305131.

103. Coselli JS. Update on repairs of the thoracoabdominal aorta. *Texas Heart Institute J.* 2013;40(5):572-574.

104. Hung A, Zafar M, Mukherjee S, Tranquilli M, Scoutt LM, Elefteriades JA. Carotid intima-media thickness provides evidence that ascending aortic aneurysm protects against systemic atherosclerosis. *Cardiology* 2012;123(2):71-77. doi:10.1159/000341234.

105. Chau K, Elefteriades JA. Ascending thoracic aortic aneurysms protect against myocardial infarctions. *Int J Angiol.* 2014;23(3):177-182. doi:10.1055/s-0034-1382288.

106. Chau KH, Bender JR, Elefteriades JA. Silver lining in the dark cloud of aneurysm disease. *Cardiology* 2014;128(4):327-332. doi:10.1159/000358123.

107. Rajbanshi BG, Charilaou P, Ziganshin BA, Rajakaruna C, Maryann T, Elefteriades JA. Management of coronary artery disease in patients with descending thoracic aortic aneurysms. *J Cardiac Surg.* 2015;30(9):701-706. doi:10.1111/jocs.12596.

108. Vaaramaki S, Salenius J, Pimenoff G, Uurto I, Suominen V. Overall outcome after endovascular aneurysm repair with a first-generation stent graft (Vanguard): a 20-year single-center experience. *J Vasc Surg.* 2020;72(3):896-903. doi:10.1016/j.jvs.2019.11.027.

109. Piazza M, Squizzato F, Milan L, et al. Incidence and predictors of neurological complications following thoracic endovascular aneurysm repair in the global registry for endovascular aortic treatment. *Eur J Vasc Endovasc Surg.* 2019;58(4):512-519. doi:10.1016/j.ejvs.2019.05.011.

110. Antoniou GA, Antoniou SA, Torella F. Editor's choice—endovascular vs. open repair for abdominal aortic aneurysm: systematic review and meta-analysis of updated peri-operative and long term data of randomised controlled trials. *Eur J Vasc Endovasc Surg.* 2020;59(3):385-397. doi:10.1016/j.ejvs.2019.11.030.

111. Roselli EE, Hasan SM, Idrees JJ, et al. Inoperable patients with acute type A dissection: are they candidates for endovascular repair? *Interact Cardiovasc Thoracic Surg.* 2017;25(4):582-588. doi:10.1093/icvts/ivx193.

112. Shah A, Khoynezhad A. Thoracic endovascular repair for acute type A aortic dissection: operative technique. *Ann Cardiothoracic Surg.* 2016;5(4):389-396. doi:10.21037/acs.2016.07.08.

113. Humphrey JD. Possible mechanical roles of glycosaminoglycans in thoracic aortic dissection and associations with dysregulated transforming growth factor-beta. *J Vasc Res.* 2013;50(1):1-10. (Research Support, N.I.H., Extramural Review) doi:10.1159/000342436.

114. Roccabianca S, Ateshian GA, Humphrey JD. Biomechanical roles of medial pooling of glycosaminoglycans in thoracic aortic dissection. *Biomech Model Mechanobiol.* 2014;13(1):13-25. (Research Support, N.I.H., Extramural Research Support, Non-U.S. Gov't). doi: http://dx.doi.org/10.1007/s10237-013-0482-3.

115. Lindsay ME, Dietz HC. Lessons on the pathogenesis of aneurysm from heritable conditions. *Nature.* 2011;473(7347):308-316. doi:10.1038/nature10145.

116. Dean JH, Woznicki EM, O'Gara P, et al. Cocaine-related aortic dissection: lessons from the International Registry of Acute Aortic Dissection. *Am J Med.* 2014;127(9):878-885. doi:10.1016/j.amjmed.2014.05.005.

117. Tolenaar JL, Hutchison SJ, Montgomery D, et al. Painless type B aortic dissection: insights from the International Registry of Acute Aortic Dissection. *Aorta (Stamford).* 2013;1(2):96-101. doi:10.12945/j.aorta.2013.13-014.

118. Chou AS, Ziganshin BA, Charilaou P, Tranquilli M, Rizzo JA, Elefteriades JA. Long-term behavior of aortic intramural hematomas and penetrating ulcers. *J Thoracic Cardiovasc Surg.* 2015;151(2):361-373.e1. doi:10.1016/j.jtcvs.2015.09.012.

119. Rokosh RS, Rockman CB, Patel VI, et al. Thoracic endovascular aortic repair for symptomatic penetrating aortic ulcers and intramural hematomas is associated with poor outcomes. *J Vasc Surg.* 2020. doi:10.1016/j.jvs.2020.11.045.

120. Jiang X, Pan T, Zou L, et al. Outcomes of endovascular stent graft repair for penetrating aortic ulcers with or without intramural hematoma. *J Vasc Surg.* 2020. doi:10.1016/j.jvs.2020.10.022.

121. Upadhyaya K, Ugonabo I, Satam K, Hull SC. Echocardiographic Evaluation of the Thoracic Aorta: Tips and Pitfalls. *Aorta (Stamford).* 2021 Feb;9(1):1-8.

122. Elefteriades JA, Ziganshin BA. Gratitude to the International Registry of Acute Aortic Dissection from the aortic community. *J Am Coll Cardiol.* 2015;66(4):359-362. doi:10.1016/j.jacc.2015.04.073.

123. Gorla R, Erbel R, Kahlert P, et al. Diagnostic role and prognostic implications of D-dimer in different classes of acute aortic syndromes. *Eur Heart J Acute Cardiovasc Care.* 2017 Aug;6(5):379-388.

124. Charilaou P, Ziganshin BA, Peterss S, et al. Current experience with acute type B aortic dissection: validity of the complication-specific approach in the present era. *Ann Thoracic Surg.* 2015;101(6):936-944. doi:10.1016/j.athoracsur.2015.08.074.

125. Nienaber CA, Kische S, Rousseau H, et al. Endovascular repair of type B aortic dissection: long-term results of the randomized investigation of stent grafts in aortic dissection trial. *Circ Cardiovasc Intervent.* 2013;6(4):407-416. doi:10.1161/CIRCINTERVENTIONS.113.000463.

126. Antoniou GA, Georgiadis GS, Antoniou SA, et al. Late rupture of abdominal aortic aneurysm after previous endovascular repair: a systematic review and meta-analysis. *J Endovasc Ther.* 2015;22(5):734-744. doi:10.1177/1526602815601405.

127. Khashram M, Williman JA, Hider PN, Jones GT, Roake JA. Systematic review and meta-analysis of factors influencing survival following abdominal aortic aneurysm repair. *Eur J Vasc Endovascular Surg.* 2016;51(2):203-215. doi:10.1016/j.ejvs.2015.09.007.

128. Bahia SS, Holt PJ, Jackson D, et al. Systematic review and meta-analysis of long-term survival after elective infrarenal abdominal aortic aneurysm repair 1969-2011: 5 year survival remains poor despite advances in medical care and treatment strategies. *Eur J Vasc Endovascular Surg.* 2015;50(3):320-30. doi:10.1016/j.ejvs.2015.05.004.

129. Singh M, Hager E, Avgerinos E, Genovese E, Mapara K, Makaroun M. Choosing the correct treatment for acute aortic type B dissection. *J Cardiovasc Surg.* 2015;56(2):217-229.

130. Goldfinger JZ, Halperin JL, Marin ML, Stewart AS, Eagle KA, Fuster V. Thoracic aortic aneurysm and dissection. *J Am Coll Cardiol.* 2014;64(16):1725-1739. doi:10.1016/j.jacc.2014.08.025.

131. Fattori R, Montgomery D, Lovato L, et al. Survival after endovascular therapy in patients with type B aortic dissection: a report from the International Registry of Acute Aortic Dissection (IRAD). *JACC Cardiovasc Intervent.* 2013;6(8):876-882. doi:10.1016/j.jcin.2013.05.003.

132. McCully KS. Homocysteine and the pathogenesis of atherosclerosis. *Expert Rev Clin Pharmacol.* 2015;8(2):211-219. doi:10.1586/17512433.2015.1010516.

133. Lyaker MR, Tulman DB, Dimitrova GT, Pin RH, Papadimos TJ. Arterial embolism. *Int J Crit Illness Injury Sci.* 2013;3(1):77-87. doi:10.4103/2229-5151.109429.

134. Ueno Y, Yamashiro K, Tanaka Y, et al. Rosuvastatin may stabilize atherosclerotic aortic plaque: transesophageal echocardiographic study in the EPISTEME trial. *Atherosclerosis.* 2015;239(2):476-482. doi:10.1016/j.atherosclerosis.2015.02.021.

135. Murphy TP, Cutlip DE, Regensteiner JG, et al. Supervised exercise, stent revascularization, or medical therapy for claudication due to aortoiliac peripheral artery disease: the CLEVER study. *J Am Coll Cardiol.* 2015;65(10):999-1009. doi:10.1016/j.jacc.2014.12.043.

136. Rooke TW, Hirsch AT, Misra S, et al. Management of patients with peripheral artery disease (compilation of 2005 and 2011 ACCF/AHA Guideline Recommendations): a report of the American College of Cardiology Foundation/American Heart Association Task Force on Practice Guidelines. *J Am Coll Cardiol.* 2013;61(14):1555-1570. doi:10.1016/j.jacc.2013.01.004.

137. de Donato G, Bosiers M, Setacci F, et al. 24-month data from the BRAVISSIMO: a large-scale prospective registry on iliac stenting for TASC A & B and TASC C & D lesions. *Ann Vasc Surg.* 2015;29(4):738-750. doi: 10.1016/j.avsg.2014.12.027.

138. Svensson LG, Arafat A, Roselli EE, et al. Inflammatory disease of the aorta: patterns and classification of giant cell aortitis, Takayasu arteritis, and nonsyndromic aortitis. *J Thoracic Cardiovasc Surg.* 2015;149(2 Suppl):S170-S175. doi:10.1016/j.jtcvs.2014.08.003.

139. van Timmeren MM, Heeringa P, Kallenberg CG. Infectious triggers for vasculitis. *Curr Opinion Rheumatol.* 2014;26(4):416-423. doi:10.1097/BOR.0000000000000068.

140. Terao C. Revisited HLA and non-HLA genetics of Takayasu arteritis–where are we? *J Human Genet.* 2016;61(1):27-32. doi:10.1038/jhg.2015.87.

141. Alibaz-Oner F, Direskeneli H. Update on Takayasu's arteritis. *Presse Medicale.* 2015;44(6 Pt 2):e259-e265. doi:10.1016/j.lpm.2015.01.015.

142. Watanabe Y, Miyata T, Tanemoto K. Current clinical features of new patients with Takayasu arteritis observed from cross-country research in Japan: age and sex specificity. *Circulation* 2015;132(18):1701-1709. doi: 10.1161/CIRCULATIONAHA.114.012547.

143. Angelotti F, Capecchi R, Giorgetti A, et al. 18-FDG PET for large vessel vasculitis diagnosis and follow-up. *Clin Exp Rheumatol.* 2021;39 Suppl 129(2):76-82.

144. Mekinian A, Comarmond C, Resche-Rigon M, et al. Efficacy of biological-targeted treatments in Takayasu arteritis: multicenter, retrospective study of 49 patients. *Circulation.* 2015;132(18):1693-1700. doi:10.1161/CIRCULATIONAHA.114.014321.

145. Hellmich B, Agueda AF, Monti S, Luqmani R. Treatment of giant cell arteritis and Takayasu arteritis-current and future. *Curr Rheumatol Rep.* 2020;22(12):84. doi:10.1007/s11926-020-00964-x.

146. Kim SM, Jung IM, Han A, et al. Surgical treatment of middle aortic syndrome with Takayasu arteritis or midaortic dysplastic syndrome. *Eur J Vasc Endovasc Surg.* 2015;50(2):206-12. doi:10.1016/j.ejvs.2015.04.032.

147. Angle JF, Nida BA, Matsumoto AH. Endovascular treatment of large vessel arteritis. *Tech Vasc Interv Radio.* 2014;17(4):252-257. doi:10.1053/j.tvir.2014.11.006.

148. Labarca C, Makol A, Crowson CS, Kermani TA, Matteson EL, Warrington KJ. Retrospective comparison of open versus endovascular procedures for Takayasu arteritis. *J Rheumatol.* 2016;43(2):427-432. doi:10.3899/jrheum.150447.

149. Agueda AF, Monti S, Luqmani RA, et al. Management of Takayasu arteritis: a systematic literature review informing the 2018 update of the EULAR recommendation for the management of large vessel vasculitis. *RMD Open.* 2019;5(2):e001020. doi:10.1136/rmdopen-2019-001020.

150. Monti S, Agueda AF, Luqmani RA, et al. Systematic literature review informing the 2018 update of the EULAR recommendation for the management of large vessel vasculitis: focus on giant cell arteritis. *RMD Open.* 2019;5(2):e001003. doi:10.1136/rmdopen-2019-001003.

151. Younger DS. Giant cell arteritis. *Neurol Clin.* 2019;37(2):335-344. doi:10.1016/j.ncl.2019.01.008.

152. Einspieler I, Thurmel K, Eiber M. Fully integrated whole-body [18F]-fludeoxyglucose positron emission tomography/magnetic resonance imaging in therapy monitoring of giant cell arteritis. *Eur Heart J.* 2016;37(6):576. doi:10.1093/eurheartj/ehv607.

153. Koster MJ, Matteson EL, Warrington KJ. Large-vessel giant cell arteritis: diagnosis, monitoring and management. *Rheumatology (Oxford).* 2018;57(suppl_2):ii32-ii42. doi:10.1093/rheumatology/kex424.

154. Matteson EL, Buttgereit F, Dejaco C, Dasgupta B. Glucocorticoids for management of polymyalgia rheumatica and giant cell arteritis. *Rheumat Dis Clinics N Am.* 2016;42(1):75-90. doi:10.1016/j.rdc.2015.08.009.

155. Stone JH, Tuckwell K, Dimonaco S, et al. Trial of tocilizumab in giant-cell arteritis. *N Engl J Med.* 2017;377(4):317-328. doi:10.1056/NEJMoa1613849.

156. Mackie SL, Dejaco C, Appenzeller S, et al. British Society for Rheumatology guideline on diagnosis and treatment of giant cell arteritis. *Rheumatology (Oxford).* 2020;59(3):e1-e23. doi:10.1093/rheumatology/kez672.

157. Kamisawa T, Zen Y, Pillai S, Stone JH. IgG4-related disease. *Lancet.* 2015;385(9976):1460-1471. doi:10.1016/S0140-6736(14)60720-0.

158. Oyama-Manabe N, Yabusaki S, Manabe O, Kato F, Kanno-Okada H, Kudo K. IgG4-related cardiovascular disease from the aorta to the coronary arteries: multidetector CT and PET/CT. *Radiographics.* 2018;38(7):1934-1948. doi:10.1148/rg.2018180049.

159. Khosroshahi A, Carruthers MN, Stone JH, et al. Rethinking Ormond's disease: "idiopathic" retroperitoneal fibrosis in the era of IgG4-related disease. *Medicine.* 2013;92(2):82-91. doi:10.1097/MD.0b013e318289610f.

160. Perez-Garcia CN, Olmos C, Vivas D, et al. IgG4-aortitis among thoracic aortic aneurysms. *Heart.* 2019;105(20):1583-1589. doi:10.1136/heartjnl-2018-314499.

161. Grewal GS, Leipsic J, Klinkhoff AV. Abdominal aortitis in HLA-B27+ spondyloarthritis: case report with 5-year follow-up and literature review. *Seminars Arthritis Rheumat.* 2014;44(3):305-308. doi:10.1016/j.semarthrit.2014.05.012.

162. Menna D, Capoccia L, Sirignano P, Esposito A, Rossi M, Speziale F. Infective etiology affects outcomes of late open conversion after failed endovascular aneurysm repair. *J Endovas Ther.* 2015;22(1):110-115. doi:10.1177/1526602814562777.

163. Roberts WC, Barbin CM, Weissenborn MR, Ko JM, Henry AC. Syphilis as a cause of thoracic aortic aneurysm. *Am J Cardiol.* 2015;116(8):1298-1303. doi:10.1016/j.amjcard.2015.07.030.

164. Delaval L, Goulenok T, Achouh P, et al. New insights on tuberculous aortitis. *J Vasc Surg.* 2017;66(1):209-215. doi:10.1016/j.jvs.2016.11.045.

165. Bossone E, Pluchinotta FR, Andreas M, et al. Aortitis. *Vasc Pharmacol.* 2016;80:1-10. doi:10.1016/j.vph.2015.11.084.

166. Lee SY, Kim EK, Kim JY, et al. The incidence and clinical features of PEGylated filgrastim-induced acute aortitis in patients with breast cancer. *Sci Rep.* 2020;10(1):18647. doi:10.1038/s41598-020-75620-6.

167. Gasser TC. Biomechanical rupture risk assessment: a consistent and objective decision-making tool for abdominal aortic aneurysm patients. *Aorta (Stamford).* 2016;4(2):42-60. doi:10.12945/j.aorta.2015.15.030.

168. Chou AS, Ziganshin BA, Elefteriades JA. Computed tomography imaging artifact simulating type A aortic dissection. *Aorta (Stamford).* 2016;4(2):72-73. doi:10.12945/j.aorta.2015.15.021.

169. Ziganshin BA, Rajbanshi BG, Tranquilli M, Fang H, Rizzo JA, Elefteriades JA. Straight deep hypothermic circulatory arrest for cerebral protection during aortic arch surgery: safe and effective. *J Thoracic Cardiovasc Surg.* 2014;148(3):888-898; discussion 898-900. doi:10.1016/j.jtcvs.2014.05.027.

24

Carotid Artery Disease

Christopher J. White

Treatment options for stroke prevention in carotid artery stenosis

Guideline-directed medical therapy

- Lipids at goal (statin therapy)
- Blood pressure control (ACE-Inhibitor)
- Diabetes at goal
- Antiplatelet therapy
- Tobacco cessation
- Exercise program

Benefit in asymptomatic patients

Benefit in symptomatic patients

Revascularization

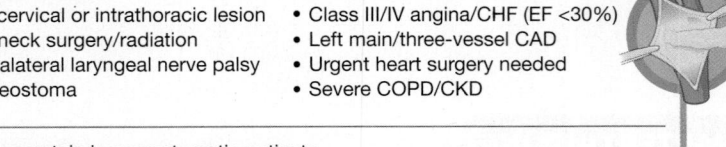

Unfavorable features for stent

Anatomic Criteria
- Type III aortic arch
- Tortuous/Ca^{++} vessel
- Intraluminal thrombus
- Difficult vascular access

Medical Comorbidity
- Age ≥80 years
- Decreased cerebral reserve
- Increased bleeding risk
- Severe CKD

Unfavorable features for surgery

Anatomic Criteria
- High cervical or intrathoracic lesion
- Prior neck surgery/radiation
- Contralateral laryngeal nerve palsy
- Tracheostoma

Medical Comorbidity
- Class III/IV angina/CHF (EF <30%)
- Left main/three-vessel CAD
- Urgent heart surgery needed
- Severe COPD/CKD

Benefit uncertain in asymptomatic patients
(awaiting results from randomized CREST-2 in ≥70% stenosis)

Benefit in symptomatic patients (≥50%–60% stenosis)

Chapter 24 Fuster and Hurst's Central Illustration. Treatment options for stroke prevention in patients with carotid artery stenosis include guideline-directed medical therapy with risk factor modification for both symptomatic and asymptomatic patients. Selected patients with symptomatic carotid artery stenosis benefit from revascularization with either stent or surgery. The benefit of revascularization in addition to guideline-directed medical therapy in asymptomatic patients with carotid artery disease is uncertain and awaits the results of a large international randomized trial (CREST-2). ACE, angiotensin-converting enzyme; Ca^{++}, calcified vessel; CAD, coronary artery disease; CKD, chronic kidney disease; COPD, chronic obstructive pulmonary disease; CREST, Carotid Revascularization Endarterectomy versus Stenting Trial; EF, ejection fraction.

CHAPTER SUMMARY

This chapter discusses the epidemiology, natural history, diagnostic imaging modalities, and treatment options for atherosclerotic carotid artery disease as it relates to acute ischemic stroke. Significant atherosclerotic carotid artery disease (≥50% diameter stenosis) is common in Medicare patients (5%–10%); it is responsible for the vast majority of noncardioembolic acute strokes caused by plaque rupture with atheroembolization. Approximately 90% of the stroke risk is due to modifiable risk factors, such as hypertension, obesity, hyperglycemia, and hyperlipidemia, and 74% can be attributed to behavioral risk factors, such as tobacco smoking, sedentary lifestyle, and unhealthy diet. Doppler ultrasound (DUS) is the preferred noninvasive imaging tool for risk assessment of carotid disease, with cross-sectional multiplanar imaging [either computerized tomographic angiography (CTA) or magnetic resonance angiography (MRA)] reserved for specific cases. The cornerstone of therapy for stroke prevention in patients with carotid artery atherosclerotic disease is risk factor modification and guideline-directed medical therapy (GDMT), with revascularization (stent or surgery) indicated for selected symptomatic patients (see Fuster and Hurst's Central Illustration). Current recommendations regarding revascularization in asymptomatic patients with significant carotid stenosis are uncertain and await the completion of an ongoing international randomized trial (CREST-2).

INTRODUCTION

Epidemiology and Natural History

Atherosclerotic carotid artery disease is responsible for 80% of new noncardioembolic strokes. Cerebrovascular events are most often caused by carotid plaque rupture with atheroembolization, rather than carotid artery occlusion (<20% of ischemic strokes) with thrombosis. Of all strokes, 87% are ischemic, 10% are due to intracranial hemorrhage, and 3% are due to subarachnoid hemorrhage.

Approximately 5% to 10% of patients over age 65 have >50% carotid artery stenosis, with 1% having a stenosis ≥75%. The natural history of patients with carotid artery stenosis is strongly influenced by the presence of focal neurologic symptoms, such as transient ischemic attack (TIA), stroke, and amaurosis fugax. Symptomatic patients have a 5- to 10-fold increased risk of stroke compared to asymptomatic patients, and a TIA is associated with a 20% increased risk of stroke within 90 days.[1] Asymptomatic patients with significant carotid artery stenosis outnumber symptomatic patients by 4:1.

Approximately 90% of stroke risk is due to modifiable factors, such as hypertension, obesity, hyperglycemia, and hyperlipidemia, and 74% can be attributed to behavioral risk factors, such as tobacco smoking, sedentary lifestyle, and unhealthy diet.[1] A small number of all strokes (approximately 12%) are heralded by a TIA, making guideline-directed medical therapy (GDMT) and risk factor modification the keys to stroke prevention in patients with carotid artery disease.

There are no randomized trials to support screening asymptomatic patients (primary prevention) for carotid stenosis to prevent stroke. In 2014, the US Preventive Services Task Force (USPSTF) determined that the potential harms associated with screening for asymptomatic carotid stenosis (leading to unnecessary surgery) far outweighed the potential benefit (stroke prevention). However, there remains debate over *targeted screening* in high-risk groups, such as those with carotid bruits or multiple risk factors for atherosclerosis. Aside from revascularization, the benefit of screening asymptomatic patients without otherwise known atherosclerotic disease is that it can be used to identify candidates for more aggressive secondary strategies to prevent symptomatic cardiovascular disease (CVD).

CAROTID ARTERY IMAGING

Noninvasive Imaging

Doppler Ultrasound

Doppler ultrasound (DUS) of the extracranial carotid arteries to determine lesion severity is safe, cost-effective, accurate, and reproducible by an experienced sonographer (**Fig. 24–1**). Carotid ultrasound can be used to identify the severity of stenosis affecting the carotid artery bifurcation and is the most widely used imaging technique for this purpose. DUS is reported to have a sensitivity of >90% and specificity of >85% for detection of significant (ie, >50%) extracranial stenosis. DUS is the procedure of choice for the initial assessment of patients suspected of carotid artery stenosis.

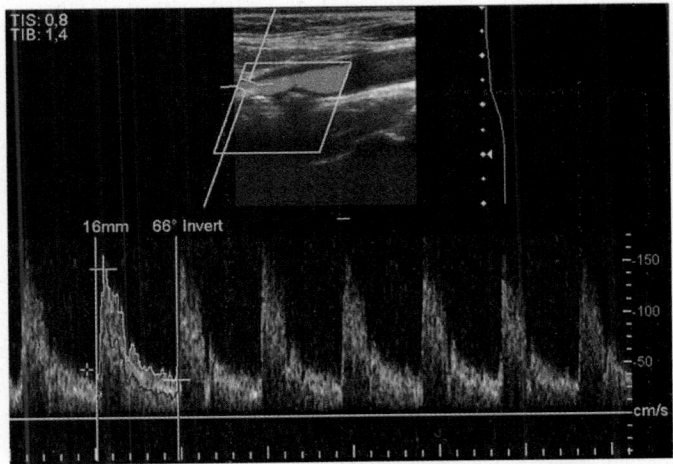

Figure 24–1. Image of a carotid artery DUS.

Ultrasound can also be used to stratify cardiovascular risk. The measurement of carotid plaque burden determined by total plaque area (TPA) has demonstrated significant advantages compared to the traditional measurement of carotid intima-media thickness (IMT) for predicting cardiovascular risk. TPA is as predictive of cardiovascular risk as coronary calcium scores, but it has important advantages over coronary calcium scoring: It is less costly, it does not involve radiation, and plaque burden changes more quickly than IMT or coronary calcium.[2]

The accuracy of carotid DUS is highly dependent on the technician's skill in obtaining images and may be hampered by technical difficulties, such as dense calcification causing acoustic shadowing. DUS may be insensitive when attempting to differentiate high-grade stenosis from complete carotid artery occlusion. In addition, the presence of excessive tortuosity, high bifurcation, or short neck may interfere with obtaining an appropriate ultrasound window.

In patients with prior revascularization, the cost benefits for carotid DUS make it the imaging modality of choice for detection of recurrent carotid stenosis with good sensitivity/specificity, without needing ionizing radiation exposure or radiographic contrast. In subjects with appropriate anatomy without heavy calcification, a nonobstructive (<50%) DUS study will obviate the need for further investigation.

Computerized Tomographic Angiography

Computerized tomographic angiography (CTA) has the ability to examine the carotid artery with serial cross-sectional images that can generate three-dimensional (3D) images of the vessel and intracranial circulation (**Fig. 24–2A**). Compared to conventional angiography, CTA has a 97% concordance for determining lesion severity. The sensitivity and specificity of CTA for carotid stenosis are both >90%. In subjects with a tortuous carotid artery, short neck, or high bifurcation, CTA is the imaging modality of choice.

The disadvantages of CTA include the need for ionizing radiation and the use of intravenous iodinated contrast material. This is of concern in patients at risk for renal insufficiency (ie, patients with diabetes mellitus). CTA imaging should be reserved for patients with indeterminate DUS images.

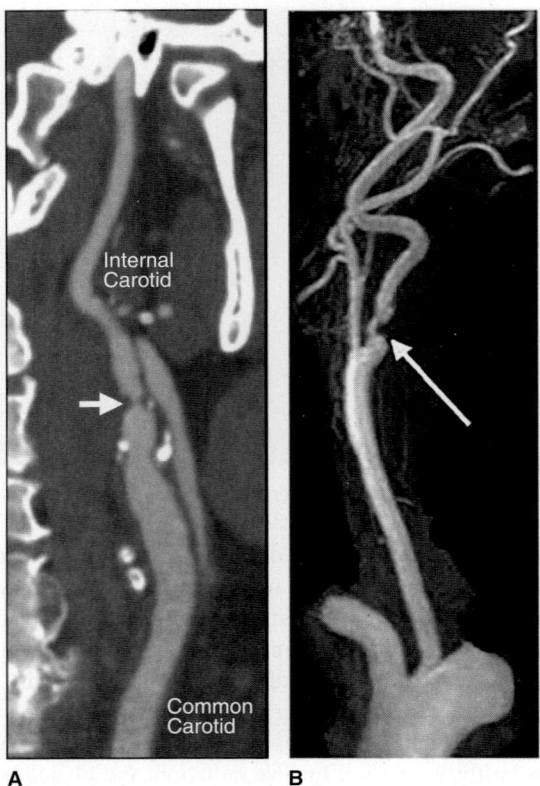

Figure 24–2. (**A**) Carotid artery CTA showing stenosis (arrow). (**B**) Carotid artery MRA showing stenosis (arrow).

Magnetic Resonance Angiography

Another noninvasive cross-sectional imaging alternative that can generate 3D images is magnetic resonance angiography (MRA), which does not require ionizing radiation or iodinated contrast administration and offers high-resolution imaging (**Fig. 24–2B**). MRA has the advantage of providing images of both the cervical and intracranial portions of the carotid artery and its proximal intracranial branches. It may overestimate the degree of stenosis, and as with DUS, there may be errors when attempting to differentiate high-grade stenosis from complete occlusion. Compared to digital subtraction angiography (DSA), discussed later in this chapter, MRA has an accuracy of 95% for determining the severity of a carotid stenosis.

The drawbacks of MRA are imaging time, cost, and the need for gadolinium, which has been associated with nephrogenic systemic fibrosis in patients with renal insufficiency, as a contrast agent. MRA may not be performed in patients with implanted ferromagnetic devices (eg, pacemakers). As MRA imaging improves with larger magnets and improved resolution, this may offer the best opportunity to identify *vulnerable* plaques that would benefit from revascularization. MRA imaging should be reserved for cases with indeterminate DUS images that are not suitable for CTA.

Invasive Imaging

Digital Subtraction Angiography

DSA is an invasive angiographic technique that is considered the gold standard for carotid artery imaging. It provides

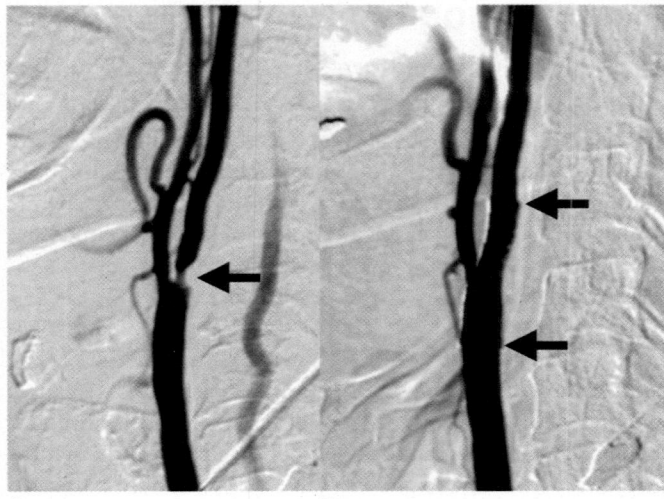

Figure 24–3. Carotid DSA. (**A**) Baseline with internal carotid artery stenois (arrow). (**B**) Postprocedure following CAS placement (arrows).

sensitivity, specificity, and accuracy of 95%, 99%, and 97%, respectively (**Fig. 24–3**). All the revascularization trials in which carotid artery treatment decisions have been tested have used DSA imaging for patient selection.

The major drawback for invasive angiography has been the risk of adverse events associated with the procedure, including access site bleeding, stroke, radiation exposure, and iodinated contrast administration. Operator volume, technical skill, and patient selection are important elements in minimizing the risks for DSA. DSA imaging should not be used to screen patients for carotid artery disease, but it is useful for guiding therapeutic interventions.

THERAPY TO PREVENT STROKE

Guideline-Directed Medical Therapy

GDMT for atherosclerotic carotid artery disease should focus on preventing stroke and stabilizing atherosclerotic lesions in order to prevent plaque rupture and atheroembolization.[3] Hypertension remains the most important and modifiable risk factor for stroke prevention, and treatment of hypertension is among the most effective strategies for preventing both ischemic and hemorrhagic stroke. Blood pressure control is of paramount importance since high blood pressure is a primary risk factor for stroke, as well as atrial fibrillation and myocardial infarction (MI), both of which increase the likelihood of stroke). Angiotensin-converting enzyme inhibitors (ACEIs) and angiotensin receptor blockers (ARBs) seem to be of particular benefit in stroke prevention, particularly for those at higher risk for CVD.

Antiplatelet Therapy

Antiplatelet medications are a critical component of primary stroke prevention. The Antithrombotic Trialists' Collaboration meta-analysis of high-risk patients found that antiplatelet therapy reduced the occurrence of any vascular event by roughly 25%, nonfatal stroke by about 25%, and death due to vascular causes by about 15%. Aspirin was the most widely used drug, with doses of 75 to 150 mg being as beneficial as higher doses. The Women's Health Study found that taking 100 mg of aspirin every other day resulted in a 17% reduction in the risk of stroke over 10 years.

For secondary prevention, aspirin reduces the risk of future strokes by 15% to 25%. High doses of aspirin (160–325 mg daily) provided no more benefit than lower doses, but they were associated with more side effects, including bleeding. Among patients with symptomatic vascular disease, including stroke, the Clopidogrel versus Aspirin in Patients at Risk of Ischemic Events (CAPRIE) trial demonstrated that taking clopidogrel 75 mg daily was associated with an 8.7% relative risk reduction in ischemic stroke, MI, or vascular death, as opposed to taking aspirin 325 mg daily (5.32% vs 5.83% p = 0.043). However, for patients who presented with stroke, the benefit was not significant.

Taking clopidogrel 75 mg daily plus aspirin 75 mg daily was compared to clopidogrel alone in the Management of Atherothrombosis with Clopidogrel in High-risk Patients (MATCH) trial. Among stroke patients, the combination regimen did not improve vascular outcomes but significantly increased the number of major (even life-threatening) bleeding complications.

The Clopidogrel for High Atherothrombotic Risk and Ischemic Stabilization, Management, and Avoidance (CHARISMA) trial included over 4,300 patients with a prior TIA or stroke. It found that aspirin 75–162 mg daily was as effective as aspirin plus clopidogrel in preventing future MI, stroke, or cardiovascular death in patients with multiple risk factors or with clinically evident CVD. This study also found that 81 mg of aspirin is the optimal dose for prevention in terms of safety and efficacy.

The European/Australasian Stroke Prevention in Reversible Ischemia Trial (ESPRIT) compared taking aspirin plus dipyridamole to aspirin alone in patients who had suffered a minor stroke or TIA within 6 months earlier. The primary outcome of vascular death, nonfatal MI, stroke, or major bleeding occurred in 13% of the aspirin/dipyridamole patients and 16% of the aspirin-alone patients (P = NS). The Prevention Regimen for Effectively Avoiding Second Strokes (PRoFESS) study found no difference between clopidogrel and aspirin/dipyridamole in the secondary prevention of stroke.

The American Heart Association (AHA) and American Stroke Association (ASA) guidelines recommend that all patients with carotid atherosclerosis be placed on antiplatelet medications.[3] For stroke prevention, they recommend low-dose aspirin daily, aspirin-dipyridamole in combination, or clopidogrel alone in patients who cannot tolerate aspirin.

Lipid-Lowering Therapy

The efficacy and safety of statins (3-hydroxy-3-methylglutaryl coenzyme A reductase inhibitors) for stroke prevention have been extensively studied. A meta-analysis of 78 lipid-lowering trials involving 266,973 patients reported that statins decreased the risk of total stroke (odds ratio/OR, 0.85; 95% confidence interval/CI, 0.78–0.92), whereas the benefits of other lipid-lowering interventions were not significant, including diet (OR, 0.92; 95% CI, 0.69–1.23); fibrates (OR, 0.98; 95% CI, 0.86–1.12); and other treatments (OR, 0.81; 95% CI, 0.61–1.08). Reduction in the risk of stroke is proportional to the reduction in total and low-density lipoprotein (LDL) cholesterol; each 1% reduction in total cholesterol was associated with a 0.8% reduction in the risk of stroke.

New cholesterol management guidelines recommend that high-intensity statin therapy be initiated or continued as the first-line therapy in patients ≤75 years of age that have clinical atherosclerotic CVD unless contraindicated; and it should be considered in those >75 years of age if the benefits outweigh the risks[4] (**Table 24–1**). The guidelines also recognize the approval by the US Food and Drug Association (FDA) for using statins for stroke prevention in CVD patients and high-risk hypertensive patients.

The Stroke Prevention by Aggressive Reduction in Cholesterol Levels (SPARCL) trial found that high-dose atorvastatin was effective for secondary stroke prevention in patients with an ischemic stroke or TIA. The Justification for the Use of Statins in Prevention: An Intervention Trial Evaluating Rosuvastatin (JUPITER) study showed that rosuvastatin in patients with normal cholesterol levels but elevated levels of c-reactive protein was effective in reducing the rate of stroke. Therefore, statins are an important component of stroke prevention and are indicated for patients with carotid artery disease.

Lifestyle Recommendations

Virtually every multivariable assessment of stroke risk has identified tobacco smoking as a potent risk factor for ischemic

TABLE 24–1. Classification of Statin Drugs Based on Their Efficacy to Reduce LDL[4]

High-Intensity Statin Therapy	Moderate-Intensity Statin Therapy	Low-Intensity Statin Therapy
Lowers cholesterol by ≥50% Atorvastatin 40–80 mg a day Rosuvastatin 20–40 mg a day	Lowers cholesterol by 30%–50% Atorvastatin 10–20 mg a day Rosuvastatin 5–10 mg a day Simvastatin 20–40 mg a day Pravastatin 40–80 mg a day Lovastatin 40 mg a day Fluvastatin XL 80 mg a day Fluvastatin 40 mg twice a day Pitavastatin 2–4 mg a day	Lowers cholesterol by <30% Simvastatin 10 mg a day Pravastatin 10–20 mg a day Lovastatin 20 mg a day Fluvastatin 20–40 mg a day Pitavastatin 1 mg a day

Reproduced with permission from Stone NJ, Robinson JG, Lichtenstein AH, et al: 2013 ACC/AHA guideline on the treatment of blood cholesterol to reduce atherosclerotic cardiovascular risk in adults: a report of the American College of Cardiology/American Heart Association Task Force on Practice Guidelines, *Circulation*. 2014 Jun 24;129(25 Suppl 2):S1-S45.

stroke, associated with an approximate doubling of risk. Dietary recommendations to reduce stroke risk include lower sodium, more fruits and vegetables, lower saturated fat, and the Mediterranean diet with nuts.

A sedentary lifestyle is also associated with an increased risk of stroke. The global vascular risk prediction scale, including the addition of physical activity, waist circumference, and alcohol consumption, showed good prediction of 10-year event rates. Although comparative trials documenting a reduction in risk of a first or recurrent stroke with regular physical activity have not been conducted, the evidence from observational studies is sufficiently strong to make recommendations for routine physical activity to prevent stroke.

Revascularization

Asymptomatic Carotid Stenosis

Carotid Endarterectomy: The purpose of carotid revascularization is to prevent ischemic stroke. There have been three large randomized studies comparing CEA to medical (ie, aspirin) therapy in the treatment of at least moderate (≥50% to 60%) carotid stenosis in asymptomatic patients (ie, without focal neurologic symptoms). All three demonstrated benefits for CEA versus medical therapy (primarily aspirin). Unfortunately, these trials predated the widespread use of modern GDMT and almost certainly underestimated its benefits.

With modern GDMT, the stroke risk for asymptomatic patients with significant carotid artery stenosis is very low (estimated at <1% per year). In a cohort of 3,681 patients with yearly DUS follow-up, 316 (8.6%) asymptomatic patients had carotid artery occlusion that occurred during observation. Of these occlusions, 254 (80%) occurred before the initiation of modern GDMT.[5]

A recent comparative effectiveness study comparing CEA to GDMT in asymptomatic patients was conducted in 5,221 Veteran's Affairs (VA) population.[6] They found that there was a small benefit for CEA over 5 years in reducing stroke and stroke-related death, but when overall mortality was included, there was no benefit for CEA over GDMT. Given the periprocedural risks associated with CEA, the authors suggested that an initial strategy of GDMT was most reasonable in asymptomatic carotid stenosis patients.

To answer the question regarding the safety and efficacy of modern GDMT compared to revascularization for stroke prevention in asymptomatic carotid artery stenosis patients, the second Carotid Revascularization Endarterectomy versus Stenting Trial (CREST) trial is ongoing.[7] CREST-2 is a two-arm randomized controlled trial (RCT) comparing GDMT with CAS versus GDMT alone, and a parallel arm of GDMT with CEA versus GDMT alone (**Fig. 24–4**). CREST-2 medical management goals include systolic blood pressure (SBP) <140 mm Hg (<130 mm Hg for diabetes mellitus patients), LDL <70 mg/dl, hemoglobin A1c <7.0%, smoking cessation, targeted weight management, and more than 30 minutes of moderate exercise three times per week. In funding this trial with parallel, noncomparative revascularization arms, the National Institutes of Health (NIH) has recognized the equipoise of CAS and CEA

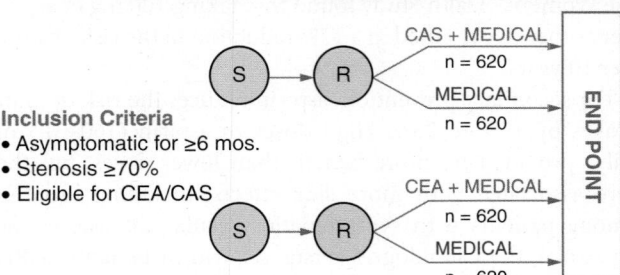

NIH Funded CREST - 2

End point = all 30 day stroke & death plus 4 yr ipsilateral stroke.

Figure 24–4. CREST-2 schematic with parallel arms comparing CAS with GDMT to GDMT alone and CEA with GDMT to GDMT alone. S = screening; R = randomization.

for the safety and efficacy of stroke prevention in asymptomatic carotid stenosis patients.

Current AHA/ASA guidelines state that it is reasonable to consider performing CEA in asymptomatic patients who have >70% stenosis of the internal carotid artery if the risk of perioperative stroke, MI, and death is low (ie, <3%). However, the effectiveness of CEA compared with contemporary GDMT alone is not well established.[3]

Carotid Artery Stenting (CAS): CAS offers a less invasive endovascular approach to revascularize significant carotid artery disease.[8] There are multiple vascular access options for stent delivery, including transfemoral carotid stenting (TFCS), transradial carotid stenting (TRCS), and transcarotid artery revascularization (TCAR). The initial population selected for CAS included patients at increased risk for CEA due to either comorbid conditions or anatomic risk factors (**Table 24–2**). As equipment and operator skill improved, CAS was studied in average surgical risk patients. It is important to remember that patients at higher risk of complications from CEA are not the same patients as those at increased risk of complications for CAS (**Table 24–3**).

The Stenting and Angioplasty with Protection in Patients at High Risk for Endarterectomy (SAPPHIRE) trial is the only randomized trial comparing high-surgical risk (HSR) patients treated with CEA to those treated with CAS. SAPPHIRE

TABLE 24–2. Features Associated with High Risk for CEA

Medical Comorbidity	Anatomic Comorbidity
• Elderly (>75/80 years)	• Surgically inaccessible lesions
• Congestive heart failure (NYHA III/IV)	• At or above second cervical spine (C2)
• Unstable angina (CCS III/IV)	• Below the clavicle
• CAD with ≥2 vessels ≥70% stenosis	• Ipsilateral neck irradiation
• Recent heart attack (≤30 days)	• Spinal immobility of the neck
• Planned open heart surgery (≤30 days)	• Contralateral carotid artery occlusion
• Ejection fraction ≤30%	• Laryngeal nerve palsy
• Severe pulmonary disease (COPD)	• Tracheostoma present
• Severe renal disease	• Prior ipsilateral CEA or neck surgery

Abbreviations: C2, the second cervical spine vertebral body, CEA, carotid endarterectomy, NYHA, New York Heart Association, CCS, Canadian Cardiovascular Society, COPD, chronic obstructive pulmonary disease, CAD, coronary artery disease.

TABLE 24–3. Features That May Increase the Risk of a CAS Procedure

Medical Comorbidity	Anatomic Criteria	Procedural Factor
• Elderly (>75/80 years)	• Aortic arch tortuosity (Type III)	• Inexperienced operator/center
• Symptom status	• Carotid artery tortuosity	• EPD not used
• Bleeding risk/hypercoaguable state	• Heavy calcification	• Lack of femoral access
• Severe aortic stenosis	• Lesion-related thrombus	• Time delay to perform procedure from onset of symptoms
• CKD	• Echolucent plaque	
• Decreased cerebral reserve	• Aortic arch atheroma	

Abbreviations: CKD, chronic kidney disease, EPD, embolic protection device.

enrolled 334 patients with a symptomatic stenosis of ≥50% (~30% were symptomatic) or an asymptomatic stenosis of ≥80% and randomized them to either CEA or CAS. The primary end point of death, stroke, or MI at 30 days, plus ipsilateral stroke or death from neurological causes between day 31 and 1 year, occurred in 12.2% of patients in the CAS group and 20.1% in the CEA group (P = 0.004 for noninferiority). The cumulative incidence of the primary end point at 1 year was 16.8% for CAS, compared with 16.5% for CEA (P = 0.95). In asymptomatic HSR patients, the cumulative incidence of the primary end point at 1 year was lower among those who received a stent (9.9%) than among those who underwent endarterectomy (21.5%, P = 0.02).

The Carotid Revascularization Endarterectomy versus Stenting Trial (CREST) included 1,181 patients with significant asymptomatic carotid artery stenosis who were randomized to CEA or CAS. The primary composite end point (any stroke, MI, or death during the periprocedural period, or ipsilateral stroke thereafter) was 5.4% versus 6.1% (P = 0.95) for CEA and CAS, respectively, at 5 years, and 10.1% versus 9.6% (P = 0.95) for CEA and CAS, respectively, at 10 years (**Fig. 24–5**).

The Asymptomatic Carotid Trial (ACT-1) randomly assigned 1,453 asymptomatic patients with significant carotid stenosis to CAS or CEA in a 3:1 randomization scheme.[9] Like CREST, there was no difference in stroke/death/MI rates between the groups (3.8% for CAS and 3.4% for CEA; P = 0.01 for noninferiority) at 1 year (**Table 24–4**). The cumulative 5-year stroke-free survival was 93.1% for CAS and 94.7% for CEA (P = 0.44).[9]

Current AHA/ASA and specialty guidelines state that prophylactic CAS might be considered in highly selected patients with asymptomatic carotid stenosis (≥60% by DSA, ≥70% by DUS), but its effectiveness compared with medical therapy alone in this situation is not well established (**Table 24–5**).[3,10,11]

Symptomatic Carotid Stenosis

Carotid Endarterectomy: Three large, randomized controlled studies in symptomatic patients with significant carotid artery stenosis have evaluated the benefit of CEA compared to medical therapy (aspirin) in symptomatic patients with moderate to severe carotid artery disease. These three trials were conducted in the 1990s and thus predated the use of modern GDMT. The VA trial screened 5,000 men who presented within 4 months of a minor stroke, TIA, or transient monocular blindness and randomized 189 patients to either CEA with medical therapy or medical therapy alone. The patients had angiographically confirmed carotid stenosis >50% of the time. The trial was ended prematurely when early results from large clinical trials confirmed the significant benefit of CEA. At a mean follow-up of almost 1 year, there was a reduction in ipsilateral stroke or TIA from 19.4% in the medical treatment arm to 7.7% in the CEA arm—an absolute reduction in risk of 11.7%. The benefits of surgery were most profound in patients with stenosis >70% (absolute risk reduction of 17.7%).

The North American Symptomatic Carotid Endarterectomy Trial (NASCET) investigators randomized patients with a TIA or nondisabling stroke within 180 days to CEA with medical therapy (including aspirin) or medical therapy alone. Patients were originally stratified according to the degree of stenosis: <50% (mild), 50% to 69% (moderate), or 70% to 99% (severe).

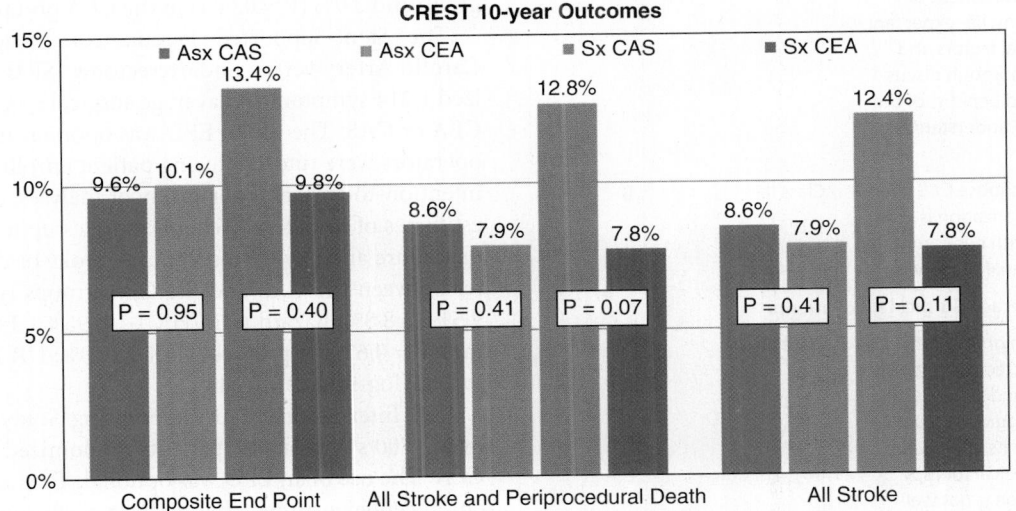

Figure 24–5. The 10-year outcomes of CREST, demonstrating no significant difference between CAS and CEA. Asx, asymptomatic, Sx, symptomatic.

TABLE 24–4. 30-Day Periprocedural Event Rate for Asymptomatic Patients in the ACT-1 Randomized Trial

	CAS N = 1089	CEA N = 364	P- Value
Deaths, strokes, and MI	3.3%	2.6%	0.60
All strokes and deaths	2.9%	1.7%	0.33
Major strokes/deaths	0.6%	0.6%	1.00
Deaths	0.1%	0.3%	0.43
All strokes	2.8%	1.4%	0.23
Major strokes	0.5%	0.3%	1.00
Minor strokes	2.4%	1.1%	0.20
MI	0.5%	0.9%	0.41

Data from Rosenfield K, Matsumura JS, Chaturvedi S, et al: Randomized Trial of Stent versus Surgery for Asymptomatic Carotid Stenosis, *N Engl J Med.* 2016 Mar 17;374(11):1011-1020.

For patients with ≥70% stenosis, CEA demonstrated an absolute risk reduction in the rate of ipsilateral stroke of 17% (26% vs 9%, P < 0.001) at 2 years. CEA lowered the 2-year risk of major or fatal stroke from 13.1% to 2.5%. In patients with 50% to 69% stenosis, the 5-year rate of any ipsilateral stroke was 15.7% for CEA and 22.2% for those treated medically (P = 0.045); to prevent one ipsilateral stroke during the 5-year period, 15 patients would have to be treated with CEA. Among patients undergoing CEA with a 50% to 69% stenosis, the 30-day perioperative stroke or death rate was 6.7%. In patients with <50% stenosis, there was no benefit for stroke prevention with CEA compared to medical therapy alone.

TABLE 24–5. Multidisciplinary Carotid Stent Guidelines: Asymptomatic Lesions

Indication	Recommendation	Level of Evidence
Asymptomatic HSR Patients		
Selection of asymptomatic patients for carotid revascularization should be guided by an assessment of comorbid conditions, life expectancy, and other individual factors and should include a thorough discussion of the risks and benefits of the procedure, with an understanding of patient preferences.	Class I	C
It is reasonable to choose CAS over CEA when revascularization is indicated in patients with neck anatomy unfavorable to arterial surgery.	Class IIa	B
Asymptomatic Average Surgical Risk Patients		
Prophylactic CAS might be considered in highly selected patients with asymptomatic carotid stenosis (minimum 60% by angiography, 70% by validated DUS), but its effectiveness compared with medical therapy alone in this situation is not well established.	Class IIb	B

The European Carotid Surgery Trial (ECST) enrolled 3,024 symptomatic patients with significant carotid stenosis; 60% of the participants were randomized to CEA with medical therapy, and 40% to medical therapy alone that consisted of antihypertensives, antiplatelet agents, and antismoking counseling. The 30-day perioperative risk of major stroke or death with CEA was 7%. While there was an equivocal benefit to surgery for stenosis <70% among patients with a stenosis and ≥70% without near occlusion, the rate of ipsilateral stroke or death at 5 years was 26.7% in the medical therapy group and 11.1% in the CEA group—an absolute reduction of 18.7% (P = 0.0001) favoring CEA. There was no benefit of CEA in patients who had near occlusion (≥99%) of the carotid artery.

A meta-analysis of these three studies found that for carotid stenoses <30% CEA increased the 5-year risk of ipsilateral stroke. CEA provided marginal benefit in patients with 50% to 69% stenosis (absolute risk reduction of 4.6%) and was highly beneficial for patients who had ≥70% stenosis (16% absolute risk reduction, P < 0.001). In patients with near occlusion, defined as a stenosis causing reduced flow to the distal internal carotid artery (ICA) and narrowing of the poststenotic ICA, there was no benefit for CEA. Current AHA/ASA guidelines recommend CEA in symptomatic patients with stenosis of 50% to 99% if the risk of perioperative stroke or death is <6%.

Carotid Artery Stenting (CAS): Four large randomized studies in average surgical risk symptomatic patients have compared CAS to CEA. Three of these trials, conducted in Europe, were compromised by allowing inexperienced CAS operators to participate in the trials and did not require embolic protection devices (EPDs) to be used. The Endarterectomy Versus Angioplasty in Patients with Symptomatic Severe Carotid Stenosis (EVA-3S) trial randomized symptomatic patients with carotid stenosis of ≥60% to either CEA or CAS. All patients had to be suitable candidates for both procedures and had ipsilateral neurological symptoms within 120 days of enrollment. The use of EPD was optional, and many of the CAS operators were tutored while treating patients. The study was terminated early. The 30-day incidence of stroke or death was 9.6% in the CAS group and 3.9% (P = 0.004) in the CEA group.

The Stent-Supported Percutaneous Angioplasty of the Carotid Artery versus Endarterectomy (SPACE) trial randomized 1,214 symptomatic, average surgical risk patients to either CEA or CAS. The use of EPD was optional and inexperienced operators were tutored during patient enrollment. In both the intention-to-treat and per-protocol analyses, the Kaplan-Meier estimates of ipsilateral ischemic strokes up to 2 years after the procedure and any periprocedural stroke or death did not differ between the CAS and the CEA groups (intention to treat 9·5% vs 8·8%; hazard ratio/HR 1·10, 95% CI 0.75 to 1.61; log-rank P = 0.62; per protocol 9·4% vs 7·8%; HR 1·23, 95% CI 0.82 to 1.83; log-rank P = 0.31).

The International Carotid Stenting Study (ICSS) enrolled over 1,700 symptomatic patients randomized to either CAS or CEA. The use of an EPD was optional. To qualify as an experienced center, a surgeon had to have performed 50 CEA procedures, and an interventionalist had to have performed 10 CAS

TABLE 24–6. Multidisciplinary Carotid Stent Guidelines: Symptomatic Lesions

Indication	Recommendation	Level of Evidence
Symptomatic HSR: Among patients with symptomatic severe stenosis (>70%) in whom the stenosis is difficult to access surgically, medical conditions exist that greatly increase the risk for surgery, or when other specific circumstances exist, such as radiation-induced stenosis or restenosis after CEA, CAS may be considered when performed by an experienced operator.	Class IIa	B
It is reasonable to choose CAS over CEA when revascularization is indicated in patients with neck anatomy unfavorable for arterial surgery.	Class IIa	B
Symptomatic Average Surgical Risk		
CAS is indicated as an alternative to CEA for symptomatic patients at average or low risk of complications associated with endovascular intervention when the diameter of the lumen of the internal carotid artery is reduced by more than 70%, as documented by noninvasive imaging, or more than 50%, as documented by catheter angiography, and the anticipated rate of periprocedural stroke or mortality is less than 6%.	Class I	B
CAS is indicated as an alternative to CEA for symptomatic patients at average or low risk of complications associated with endovascular intervention when the diameter of the lumen of the internal carotid artery is reduced by >70% by noninvasive imaging, or >50% by catheter angiography.	Class I	B

procedures. The center was considered to be experienced after randomizing 20 patients if their outcomes were considered acceptable. If the center was less experienced, they were tutored until considered proficient by their proctor. The patients were assigned to CAS or CEA in a 1:1 fashion and followed up for a median of 4.2 years. The number of fatal or disabling strokes and cumulative 5-year risk did not differ significantly between CAS and CEA (6.4% vs 6.5%; HR 1.06, 95% CI 0.72–1.57, P = 0.77). Minor nondisabling strokes occurred at a higher rate in the CAS group. The neurologic functional status (modified Rankin scale scores at 1 year, 5 years, or final follow-up) did not differ for CAS versus CEA.

CREST was the largest randomized trial comparing CAS with EPD to CEA with credentialed operators. There were 1,321 symptomatic average surgical risk patients randomized to either CEA or CAS. The 10-year primary outcome of periprocedural stroke, death, or MI or follow-up ipsilateral stroke was not significantly different between the two groups (13.4% for CAS and 9.8% for CEA, P = 0.40). CAS appeared safer than CEA for patients ≤69 years of age, while CEA yielded better outcomes in those >70 years of age.

CREST differed from the European trials. First, the European trials (EVA-3S, SPACE, and ICSS) allowed inexperienced operators to enroll patients with tutoring. CREST requirements were more stringent, requiring a roll-in period for less experienced operators before they were allowed to participate in the trial. Second, CREST mandated the use of EPD with CAS, whereas the European trials did not.

A recent comparison of post-CREST (2010–2015) symptomatic real-world patients undergoing carotid revascularization found that CEA patients had a higher rate of periprocedural stroke than CAS patients, driven by increased stroke risk in symptomatic CEA patients (8.1% vs 5.6%; OR, 1.47 CI, 1.29–1.68; P < 0.001), but a lower rate of overall inpatient mortality (0.8% vs 1.4%; OR, 0.57, CI, 0.48–0.68; P < 0.001).[12]

Current AHA/ASA and specialty guidelines recommend CAS as an alternative to CEA for symptomatic patients at average or low risk of complications associated with endovascular intervention with significant carotid stenosis if the anticipated rate of 30-day peri-procedural stroke or death is <6% (**Table 24–6**).[3,10,11]

New Developments

Embolic Protection Devices

EPDs were designed to minimize the risk of plaque embolization to the brain during the CAS procedure. There are two classes of EPD in use today, including proximal protection with flow-reversal and distal umbrellalike filters to capture downstream particles (**Fig. 24–6**).

Because of the low incidence of clinical stroke complicating CAS, it has been difficult to demonstrate clinical benefits for any EPD without aggregating data into summary reports.[13] The risk to benefit assessment intuitively favors using a protection device. One has to only retrieve a filter full of debris to realize the empiric benefits relative to the rare complications associated with EPD devices. However, the use of EPDs complicates and prolongs CAS procedures, particularly for inexperienced operators.

There are multiple small (ie, <100 patients) randomized controlled trials comparing EPDs, with divergent results. Because the clinical event rate is so low, these trials rely on surrogate end points, such as the appearance of lesions on diffusion-weighted

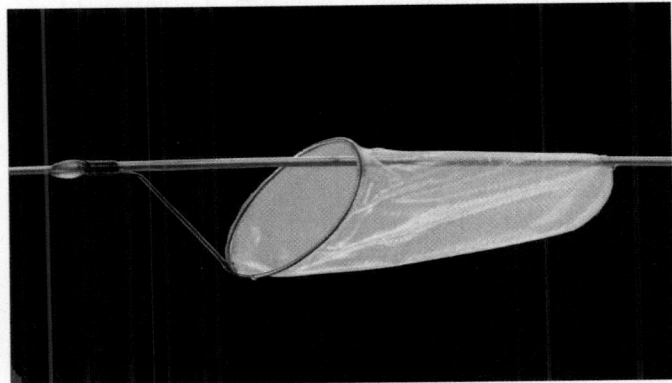

Figure 24–6. EPD; distal filter.

magnetic resonance imaging (DW-MRI) or Doppler transcarotid detection of microembolic signals (MESs). However, these surrogate end points have not been correlated with clinical events, thus leaving us with little evidence to determine the superiority of specific devices.[13,14] A meta-analysis found that proximal occlusion devices were superior to distal filter devices for reducing the surrogate end point of DW-MRI brain lesions after carotid stenting.[15]

These data regarding EPD use and periprocedural stroke prevention are confounded by catheter manipulation of the aortic arch preceding EPD deployment, which can lead to cerebral embolization. Evidence for aortic arch embolization is confirmed by the finding that 15% to 20% of periprocedural strokes involve the contralateral nontarget carotid artery cerebral distribution. At the present time, optimal practice for CAS should include the use of an EPD, one that the operator is most comfortable with using.[13]

Transcarotid Artery Revascularization

TCAR, a specially designed flow-reversal neuroprotection system, was developed as a hybrid technique for carotid stenting to avoid catheter-induced atheroembolization from the aortic arch. TCAR requires a surgical incision to gain access to the common carotid artery (CCA) for the purpose of inserting a catheter system to deliver the carotid stent with carotid artery flow reversal to prevent embolic events. The major advantage of TCAR over TFCS is avoiding catheter manipulation in the aortic arch using direct carotid access with a cerebral embolic protection system employing an extracorporeal arteriovenous shunt from the carotid artery to the femoral vein to reverse carotid flow prior to crossing the carotid stenosis. TCAR mitigates the several anatomic factors that increase embolic risk with TFCS, including those with Type III aortic arches, severe aortic arch calcification or mural thrombus, and ICA features that would preclude distal embolic filter placement.

There are no randomized trials directly comparing TCAR to any other method of carotid revascularization. In 2018, 46% of all CAS procedures were performed with TCAR. A large, retrospective registry (the Vascular Quality Initiative–TCAR Surveillance Project Carotid Artery Stenting Registry) reported outcomes in over 5,000 TCAR patients. TCAR was found to be associated with a significantly lower risk of stroke or death compared with modern transfemoral carotid stenting methods for both in-hospital (1.6% vs 3.1%; RR 0.51, 95%CI 0.37–0.72, P < .001) and 1-year events (5.1% vs 9.6%; HR 0.52, 95%CI 0.41–0.66, P < .001).

Covered Carotid Stents

There is evidence to support postprocedure CAS cerebral embolism due to plaque protrusion through bare metal carotid stent struts. To address this issue, mesh-covered stents have been developed and early clinical trials have demonstrated efficacy in reducing peri-procedural surrogate end points, including a reduction in DW-MRI lesions and Doppler MES. [16-18]

In a two-way comparison of proximal versus distal EPD and covered versus bare metal stents, the combination of proximal protection with a covered stent had the lowest MES count overall.[16] Concerns related to the use of covered versus

bare metal stents include variations in late patency rates with a meta-analysis of covered stents that showed that restenosis rates may vary by specific stent design,[19] and another report raising the concern of increased acute stent thrombosis with covered stents.[20]

CLINICAL DECISION-MAKING

Patient Selection for Revascularization

Symptomatic Carotid Artery Disease

Despite the fact that revascularization with CEA versus medical therapy preceded modern GDMT, the large reduction in events with revascularization is compelling, and it is currently the standard of care and guideline supported. Symptomatic patients have much more to gain than asymptomatic patients regarding stroke prevention with revascularization. The 30-day periprocedural risk of stroke and death should be ≤6% for symptomatic patients. In patients at increased peri-procedural risk for surgery, CAS is generally preferred. For average surgical risk patients, the choice of revascularization methods depends on an informed patient taking into account patient-specific factors (Tables 24–2, 24–3), as well as operator and institutional experience and volume. It is recommended that revascularization be performed within 14 days of the index event.

Asymptomatic Carotid Artery Disease

With the goal of preventing stroke, revascularization should be reserved for patients at the lowest peri-procedural risk of stroke and death and those with the most to gain from the procedure. The 30-day periprocedural risk of stroke and death should be ≤3% for asymptomatic patients. The choice of revascularization methods depends on an informed patient taking into account patient-specific factors (Tables 24–2, 24–3), as well as operator and institutional experience and volume.

The decision to proceed with revascularization to prevent stroke in asymptomatic patients is complex. Current estimates of stroke rates with modern GDMT are ~1% per year. Given a 3% periprocedural complication rate (stroke and death), it takes several years following successful revascularization to realize a net benefit for revascularization. Younger patients have more to gain over their future years than elderly patients. Another factor to consider in making a decision for revascularization is evidence of carotid plaque instability with progression of an asymptomatic stenosis despite GDMT. The decision to proceed with revascularization needs to take into account the patient's wishes once the person has been fully informed about the risks and benefits of the procedure.

There currently is clinical equipoise regarding the management of asymptomatic ≥70% carotid artery stenosis between revascularization (CAS or CEA) and GDMT, which is being tested in the CREST-2 randomized parallel arm trial (Fig. 24–4), and eligible patients should be encouraged to enroll in the trial.

SUMMARY

Atherosclerotic carotid artery disease is common with 5% to 10% of Medicare-eligible patients having a >50% carotid artery stenosis, and 1% having a stenosis ≥75%. Carotid artery disease is responsible for a significant percentage of the 800,000 strokes each year in the United States, and over 130,000 Americans die annually from stroke.[1] Stroke is the fifth-leading cause of mortality in the United States, and 15% to 30% of survivors are permanently disabled.[1]

Symptomatic patients with moderate to severe carotid atherosclerosis are at high risk for stroke that is amenable to treatment with revascularization by either stenting or surgery. The choice of revascularization methods is dependent on the patient's preference, patient and lesion characteristics, and operator skill and institutional experience.

The optimal management to prevent stroke for asymptomatic patients with carotid disease is less clear. The current consensus is that there is equipoise between GDMT alone and revascularization (CEA or CAS) with GDMT. These two strategies are currently being tested in a large multicenter randomized trial called CREST-2. If current patients are not eligible to be enrolled in this trial, then management should be determined by patients' informed preference, patient and lesion characteristics, and operator skill and institutional experience.

REFERENCES

1. Benjamin EJ, Muntner P, Alonso A, et al. Heart disease and stroke statistics—2019 update: a report from the American Heart Association. *Circulation.* 2019;139(10):e56-e528. doi:10.1161/CIR.0000000000000659.

2. Fuster, V. Advantages of measuring carotid plaque burden perspective. Personal communication, 2020.

3. Meschia JF, Bushnell C, Boden-Albala B, et al. Guidelines for the primary prevention of stroke: a statement for healthcare professionals from the American Heart Association/American Stroke Association. *Stroke.* 2014;45(12):3754-3832. doi:10.1161/STR.0000000000000046.

4. Stone NJ, Robinson JG, Lichtenstein AH, et al. 2013 ACC/AHA guideline on the treatment of blood cholesterol to reduce atherosclerotic cardiovascular risk in adults: a report of the American College of Cardiology/American Heart Association Task Force on Practice Guidelines. *Circulation.* 2014;129 (25 Suppl 2):S1-S45. doi:10.1161/01.cir.0000437738.63853.7a.

5. Yang C, Bogiatzi C, Spence JD. Risk of stroke at the time of carotid occlusion. *JAMA Neurol.* 2015;72(11):1261-1267. doi:10.1001/jamaneurol.2015.1843.

6. Keyhani S, Cheng EM, Hoggatt KJ, et al. Comparative effectiveness of carotid endarterectomy vs initial medical therapy in patients with asymptomatic carotid stenosis. *JAMA Neurol.* 2020. doi:10.1001/jamaneurol.2020.1427.

7. Lal BK, Roubin GS, Rosenfield K, et al. Quality assurance for carotid stenting in the CREST-2 registry. *J Am Coll Cardiol.* 2019;74(25):3071-3079. doi:10.1016/j.jacc.2019.10.032.

8. Beckman JA, Ansel GM, Lyden SP, Das TS. Carotid artery stenting in asymptomatic carotid artery stenosis: JACC review topic of the week. *J Am Coll Cardiol.* 2020;75(6):648-656. doi:10.1016/j.jacc.2019.11.054.

9. Rosenfield K, Matsumura JS, Chaturvedi S, et al. Randomized trial of stent versus surgery for asymptomatic carotid stenosis. *N Engl J Med.* 2016;374(11):1011-1020. doi:10.1056/NEJMoa1515706.

10. Furie KL, Kasner SE, Adams RJ, et al. Guidelines for the prevention of stroke in patients with stroke or transient ischemic attack: a guideline for healthcare professionals from the American Heart Association/American Stroke Association. *Stroke.* 2011 2011;42(1):227-276.

11. Brott TG, Halperin JL, Abbara S, et al. ASA/ACCF/AHA/AANN/AANS/ACR/ASNR/CNS/SAIP/SCAI/SIR/SNIS/SVM/SVS guideline on the management of patients with extracranial carotid and vertebral artery disease: executive summary. *Vasc Med.* 2011;16(1):35-77.

12. Cole TS, Mezher AW, Catapano JS, et al. Nationwide trends in carotid endarterectomy and carotid artery stenting in the post-CREST era. *Stroke.* 2020;51(2):579-587. doi:10.1161/STROKEAHA.119.027388.

13. Kobayashi T, Giri J. The role of embolic protection in carotid stenting progress in cardiovascular diseases (PCVD). *Prog Cardiovasc Dis.* 2017;59(6):612-618. doi:10.1016/j.pcad.2017.03.003.

14. Kassavin DS, Clair DG. An update on the role of proximal occlusion devices in carotid artery stenting. *J Vasc Surg.* 2017;65(1):271-275. doi:10.1016/j.jvs.2016.09.048.

15. Stabile E, Sannino A, Schiattarella GG, et al. Cerebral embolic lesions detected with diffusion-weighted magnetic resonance imaging following carotid artery stenting: a meta-analysis of 8 studies comparing filter cerebral protection and proximal balloon occlusion. *JACC Cardiovasc Interv.* 2014;7(10):1177-1183. doi:10.1016/j.jcin.2014.05.019.

16. Montorsi P, Caputi L, Galli S, et al. Carotid wallstent versus roadsaver stent and distal versus proximal protection on cerebral microembolization during carotid artery stenting. *JACC Cardiovasc Interv.* 2020;13(4):403-414. doi:10.1016/j.jcin.2019.09.007.

17. Musialek P, Mazurek A, Trystula M, et al. Novel PARADIGM in carotid revascularisation: prospective evaluation of All-comer peRcutaneous cArotiD revascularisation in symptomatic and Increased-risk asymptomatic carotid artery stenosis using CGuard MicroNet-covered embolic prevention stent system. *EuroIntervention.* 2016;12(5):e658-e670. doi:10.4244/EIJY16M05_02.

18. Gray WA, Levy E, Bacharach JM, et al. Evaluation of a novel mesh-covered stent for treatment of carotid stenosis in patients at high risk for endarterectomy: 1-year results of the SCAFFOLD trial. *Catheter Cardiovasc Interv.* 2020;96(1):121-127. doi:10.1002/ccd.28586.

19. Stabile E, de Donato G, Musialek P, et al. Use of dual-layered stents for carotid artery angioplasty: 1-year results of a patient-based meta-analysis. *JACC Cardiovasc Interv.* 2020;13(14):1709-1715. doi:10.1016/j.jcin.2020.03.048.

20. Abdullayev N, Maus V, Mpotsaris A, et al. Comparative analysis of CGUARD embolic prevention stent with Casper-RX and Wallstent for the treatment of carotid artery stenosis. *J Clin Neurosci.* 2020;75:117-121. doi:10.1016/j.jocn.2020.03.008.

25

Cerebrovascular Disease

Hugo J. Aparicio, Vasileios-Arsenios Lioutas, Thanh N. Nguyen, and Sudha Seshadri

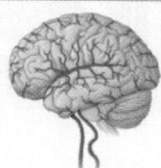

Classification, pathophysiology, and management of cerebrovascular disease

Cerebrovascular diseases: a group of disorders that affect blood vessels supplying the central nervous system

Stroke: sudden signs or symptoms of focal central nervous system dysfunction, with vascular disease as the apparent cause; or symptomatic vascular injury to the brain/retina/spinal cord

Transient ischemic attack (TIA): brief episode (usually <1 hour) of focal brain or retinal dysfunction caused by vascular disease

Subclinical cerebrovascular disease: vascular brain injury observed on neuroimaging, such as covert brain infarction or chronic cerebral small vessel disease, in patients without a clinical history of stroke or TIA

Classification of stroke and TIA

Hemorrhagic stroke

- Intracerebral hemorrhage
- Subarachnoid hemorrhage

Ischemic stroke, by mechanism

- Large artery atherosclerosis
- TIA   Small artery occlusion, "lacunar"
- TIA with brain infarct on MRI/CT
- Cardioembolism
- Other determined source (such as vasculitis, dissection, or venous occlusion)
- Undetermined source or "cryptogenic"
- ESUS

Cardiac sources of embolism

- Left atrial appendage thrombus
- Patent foramen ovale (and paradoxical embolism)
- Atrial or mitral valve prosthesis or vegetation (eg, infective or thrombotic)
- Left atrium
- Atrial fibrillation
- Left ventricle
- Left atrial thrombus
- Cardiomyopathy
- Left ventricular thrombus (after myocardial infarction)

Acute treatment

IV thrombolysis with recombinant tissue-type plasminogen activator (rt-PA or alteplase) or tenecteplase for eligible ischemic stroke patients presenting at the time interval from time last known well before symptom onset:

- Within 4.5 hours
- Between 4.5 and 9 hours, or in eligible patients awakening with stroke, using advanced imaging such as CT perfusion imaging or MRI

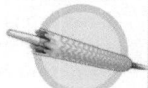

Endovascular mechanical thrombectomy to revascularize a large vessel occlusion in eligible patients presenting within 24 hours from time last known well or with discovery of stroke symptoms upon awakening

Chapter 25 Fuster and Hurst's Central Illustration. The term cerebrovascular disease encompasses ischemic stroke, hemorrhagic stroke, and transient ischemic attack (TIA). Cardioembolism is a common cause of ischemic stroke, accounting for >40% of strokes among persons over age 60 years. Cerebrovascular injury results from embolization from the heart or via a right-to-left shunt or when cardiac dysfunction or arrest result in brain hypoperfusion. Treatments for acute ischemic stroke include intravenous (IV) thrombolysis and endovascular thrombectomy. CT, computed tomography; ESUS, embolic stroke of undetermined source; MRI, magnetic resonance imaging.

CHAPTER SUMMARY

This chapter discusses the classification, pathophysiology, epidemiology, genetics, treatment, and outcomes of stroke and cerebrovascular disease, with an emphasis on cerebrovascular complications of heart disease (see Fuster and Hurst's Central Illustration). Modifiable and nonmodifiable risk factors for stroke overlap with those for ischemic heart disease, including hypertension, diabetes, smoking, age, family history, and certain genetic factors. Heart disease can cause cerebrovascular injury due to embolism of material from the heart, embolism via a right-to-left shunt, and hypoperfusion of the brain resulting from cardiac dysfunction or arrest. The most common etiologies for cardioembolism are atrial fibrillation with thromboembolism from the left atria or left atrial appendage, intracardiac thrombus following anterior myocardial infarction or in the setting of cardiomyopathy, and valvular heart disease causing embolism of thrombotic or infective material. The diagnostic evaluation of cardioembolic stroke includes brain imaging, examination of the blood vessels supplying the brain, electrocardiogram (ECG), and echocardiography (echo). A major focus of acute ischemic stroke management is treatment with intravenous (IV) thrombolysis and the use of endovascular therapy to treat emergent large vessel occlusion stroke. The chapter also discusses secondary stroke prevention using antiplatelet medication and the management of anticoagulation in the setting of intracerebral hemorrhage.

INTRODUCTION

Cerebrovascular diseases are a group of disorders that affect the blood vessels supplying the central nervous system; they include any ischemic or hemorrhagic disease that affects the brain, retina, and spinal cord, caused typically by narrowing, occlusion, or rupture of an artery or arteriole, and less often due to capillary or venous disease. This chapter describes how cerebrovascular and cardiac diseases overlap and interact, with a focus on stroke.

Stroke is a clinical syndrome, recognized as rapidly developing symptoms or signs of focal (at times global) central nervous system dysfunction, lasting more than 24 hours or leading to death, with vascular disease as the apparent cause; stroke may also be defined as a clinically symptomatic, persistent vascular injury to the brain, retina, or spinal cord. This definition traditionally excluded a *transient ischemic attack* (TIA), which is defined as a brief episode (less than 24 hours, but usually less than 1 hour) of focal brain or retinal dysfunction caused by vascular disease. Implicit in this definition was the assumption that the transient and reversible symptoms were due to reversible, rather than permanent, injury to the brain tissue. With the development of sensitive magnetic resonance imaging (MRI) methods, over half of all TIAs were found to be accompanied by evidence of infarction; hence there is now a subset of TIA with evidence of an accompanying brain infarction on imaging that is also considered a stroke. The spectrum of TIA and stroke lie on a continuum, with shared pathophysiological mechanisms and opportunities for secondary stroke prevention. As access to MRI has become more widespread, *subclinical* cerebrovascular disease, including *covert brain infarction* and *chronic cerebral small vessel disease*, are increasingly identified in persons without a stroke or TIA event, and further extend the disease spectrum.[1]

STROKE AND CEREBROVASCULAR DISEASE

Classification of Stroke

Ischemic Stroke

Ischemic stroke is a heterogenous disease. Although the end result is invariably ischemic injury of brain tissue due to thromboembolic vessel obstruction, the source of the thrombus and underlying pathophysiology are diverse. This has important implications for management and secondary prevention. The prototypical stroke subtype classification scheme is the Trial of Org 10 172 in Acute Stroke Treatment (TOAST) classification,[2] which resulted from systematization of prior categorization schemata. TOAST is an intuitive and pragmatic classification that utilizes parenchymal and vascular imaging along with clinical judgment. It reflects real-world assessment of stroke etiology and has face validity. More recent classification schemes such as the Causative Classification System (CCS)[3] and the ASCOD (A: atherosclerosis; S: small-vessel disease; C: cardiac pathology; O: other causes) phenotyping system[4] have introduced more granularity and scoring complexity, but the

underlying principles and categories are the same as those used in the original TOAST classification.

Large Artery Atherosclerosis: These are infarctions due to *hemodynamically significant* (≥50% being necessary but not sufficient) stenosis of a large artery either extracranially (internal carotid or vertebral) or intracranially. The infarctions are in the vascular territory perfused by the affected artery. Coexistent atherosclerosis in other anatomic locations (coronary artery disease, peripheral arterial disease, other cerebral arteries) acts as supportive evidence and conflicting etiologies such as cardioembolism should be excluded.

Small Artery Occlusion (Lacunar Stroke): These are infarcts in the territory of a small penetrating terminal artery (**Fig. 25–1**), often with a unique clinical phenotype of a typical lacunar syndrome (eg, a pure motor hemiparesis, ataxic hemiparesis). Imaging criteria include demonstration of an infarct in the subcortical and brainstem areas supplied by small vessels (basal ganglia, thalamus, internal capsule, corona radiata, pons) and a maximum axial diameter of ≤2 cm in diffusion-weighted brain MRI or ≤1.5 cm in head computed tomography (head CT).[5] Vessel imaging should preclude significant stenosis in the relevant large artery.

Cardioembolism: This category includes infarcts due to established high or low risk cardiac sources. Cardiac sources of embolism include atrial fibrillation, atrial flutter, valvular vegetations, mechanical valves, left ventricular thrombus, intracardiac tumors (eg, atrial myxoma), and depressed ejection fraction (≤35%). Excluding competing etiologies, especially significant luminal stenosis in the vessel supplying the infarcted area is important since the infarcts from both etiologies may be indistinguishable based on clinical presentation or imaging characteristics.

Other Determined Source: These are infarcts due to alternative well-established etiologies. They are less common in the general stroke population but frequent in special subgroups, such as young adults with stroke. This category includes cervical

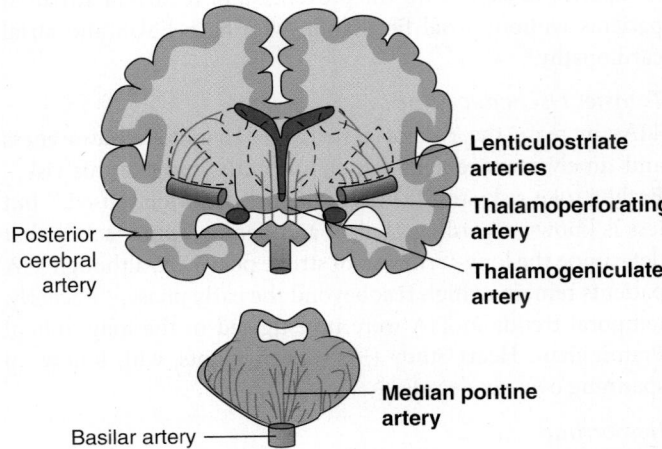

Figure 25–1. Deep penetrating arteries prone to the development of lipohyalinosis and microaneurysms (bold). Occlusion of these arteries causes lacunar infarcts, and rupture of these arteries causes ICH.

artery dissection (carotid or vertebral), other nonatherosclerotic vasculopathies (eg, vasculitis), or prothrombotic states such as cancer-related hypercoagulability and other coagulation disorders.

Undetermined Source: This category includes infarcts whose etiology remains unresolved after completion of the workup. These strokes are also known as cryptogenic. This is a diverse group that includes at least three categories: First, strokes labeled as cryptogenic but not having truly completed a full workup, thus best characterized as "incomplete workup" rather than cryptogenic. Second, patients with more than two coexisting etiologies (eg, a cardioembolic source and ≥50% stenosis in the large artery supplying the infarcted area). In such cases, a clinical judgment call after weighing the totality of clinical and ancillary parameters is necessary. Third, there are strokes that are truly cryptogenic, with no apparent etiology despite a detailed, complete workup.

Embolic Stroke of Undetermined Source: From this latter category, an important subgroup has emerged: embolic stroke of undetermined source (ESUS).[6] ESUS represents a clinical and imaging construct rather than a homogeneous subgroup with distinct underlying pathophysiology. It is mainly defined in negative terms, including the absence of significant large artery atherosclerotic stenosis and cardioembolic source. Imaging characteristics are taken into account to distinguish ESUS from small artery occlusions: ESUS infarcts are by convention cortical and, if subcortical, ≥2 cm in diffusion-weighted brain MRI or ≥1.5 cm in head CT. The true underlying causes are diverse: atrial cardiopathy[7] (which can include atrial fibrosis, dilatation, or impaired contractility) is thought to predispose to cardioembolism, whereas in other patients the culprit is considered to be nonocclusive atherosclerotic disease (atherosclerotic plaque with <50% stenosis). ESUS is a relatively new construct. The definition will likely become more granular and reflective of true underlying pathophysiology as our understanding continues to evolve. For example, the ongoing AtRial Cardiopathy and Antithrombotic Drugs In Prevention After Cryptogenic Stroke (ARCADIA) trial will test if apixaban is superior to aspirin for the prevention of recurrent stroke in patients without atrial fibrillation who have ESUS and atrial cardiopathy.[8]

Transient Ischemic Attack

TIAs increase the risk of a stroke.[9,10] Heightened awareness and timely management can significantly mitigate this risk.[11] Early stroke risk stratification schemes are widely used,[12] but less is known regarding clinical and demographic factors that determine the long-term risk of stroke post-TIA, although TIA patients remain at high risk beyond the early phase.[13] Recently, temporal trends in TIA were investigated in the longitudinal Framingham Heart Study (FHS) participants, with follow-up spanning over six decades.[9]

Hemorrhagic Stroke

Hemorrhagic stroke includes two major subtypes: nontraumatic, spontaneous intracerebral hemorrhage (ICH), and subarachnoid hemorrhage (SAH).

Intracerebral Hemorrhage: ICH is most often a spontaneous event without underlying vascular malformations and this type of event is described as a primary ICH. Anatomical localization of the hemorrhage can help identify the underlying pathophysiology. Hemorrhages in subcortical, deep areas (basal ganglia, thalamus, internal capsule, pons) are typically due to hypertensive microangiopathy of small penetrating arteries (Fig. 25–1). Cortical and juxtacortical hemorrhages, also known as lobar hemorrhages, are more likely to be due to cerebral amyloid angiopathy, although emerging evidence suggests that a considerable proportion might in fact also be due to hypertensive angiopathy.[14] ICH can extend to the ventricular system of the brain (secondary intraventricular hemorrhage) or occur primarily within the ventricles (primary intraventricular hemorrhage).

Subarachnoid Hemorrhage: SAH is a distinct subgroup comprising ~1% of all strokes. The most common etiology is rupture of an intracranial aneurysm. Other, less common etiologies include reversible cerebral vasoconstriction syndrome and underlying cerebral amyloid angiopathy.

Pathophysiology

Ischemic Stroke

Ischemic tissue injury is the end result of deprivation of blood flow for a critical period of time, beyond which irreversible damage occurs. Despite the abrupt symptom onset of stroke, the underlying ischemic process is dynamic and takes place over several hours. Some neurons are irreversibly damaged, comprising the infarct core. Surrounding the core is a zone of oligemia that results in cellular dysfunction and corresponding neurologic deficit, known as the ischemic penumbra. This area is potentially salvageable and is the main target of reperfusion therapies in acute ischemic stroke: a significant anatomical mismatch between the region of the ischemic core and penumbra is a marker of a favorable outcome following restoration of blood flow.[15,16] Without flow restoration, the penumbra ultimately suffers irreversible ischemic damage and the infarct reaches its final size.

Following the occlusion of a vessel and cessation of blood flow, collateral vessels are recruited through various mechanisms: flow diversion in the circle of Willis, leptomeningeal collateral circulation, through pial branches, and via anastomoses between the extracranial and intracranial branches of the carotid artery. Collateral vessels have a crucial role in determining the pathophysiology of an acute ischemic stroke. They influence the size of the initial infarcted core, the rate at which the penumbra progresses to irreversible ischemic injury, and the extent of the final infarct.[17]

Blood flow restoration is the ultimate goal of acute stroke therapies, but this is not always achievable. Augmentation of cerebral perfusion by other means is also important in the acute phase. Given that arterial blood pressure (BP) is the main driver of cerebral perfusion pressure, and it is modifiable, its role in the acute setting is important. Management of elevated BP is temporarily waived, and significantly higher levels are tolerated until neurologic stability is achieved; after which antihypertensive therapy might be gradually introduced,[18] if necessary.

Every infarction is accompanied by a degree of cytotoxic edema. In very large infarcts involving more than two-thirds of the middle cerebral artery territory, this can cause extensive, life-threatening "malignant edema,"[19] which is a leading cause of early death in acute ischemic stroke. The only effective intervention in such cases is decompressive hemicraniectomy.[18]

Intracerebral Hemorrhage

Tissue injury in ICH differs from ischemic stroke, although the clinical presentation is largely indistinguishable and depends on the affected anatomical area. Hematoma formation results in injury primarily due to mechanical disruption; this can be further exacerbated by rapid expansion of the hematoma in the early hours after the bleed occurs. Hematoma evacuation and limitation of hematoma expansion have been treatment targets in clinical trials;[20] although surgical removal of the hematoma has not proven effective, minimally invasive procedures are more promising[21] with several ongoing clinical trials. In addition to primary mechanical injury, ICH is accompanied by formation of perihematomal edema. This is a complex phenomenon occurring in a delayed, subacute fashion over hours to weeks following the primary injury. The process includes inflammation, thrombin-mediated injury, and neurotoxicity, where iron toxicity from heme degradation[22] has a central role. Despite targeted efforts,[23] no effective therapy addressing the secondary injury post-ICH exists.

Subarachnoid Hemorrhage

The pathophysiology of SAH is also complex. Primary injury is induced by a combination of direct effects of the hemorrhage with excitotoxicity, inflammation, and cerebral edema, as well as secondary ischemic injury from vasoconstriction of the microcirculation.[24] Cerebral edema can lead to hydrocephalus, which is a frequent early complication of SAH. Cerebral vasospasm induced by the presence of blood products develops in a delayed fashion, with a peak incidence 5 to 14 days after the event, and leads to delayed cerebral ischemia, further compounding the primary injury. Additionally, SAH, more than any other type of stroke, is likely to induce systemic complications such as hyponatremia due to syndrome of inappropriate antidiuretic hormone (SIADH) or cerebral salt wasting, pulmonary edema, acute respiratory distress syndrome, and systemic inflammatory response.

Epidemiology, Risk Factors, and Brain Health

The Global Burden of Diseases, Injuries, and Risk Factors Study reports that in 2017, there were 11.9 million incident strokes worldwide. Stroke is the second leading cause of mortality, behind ischemic heart disease, with 6.2 million deaths due to stroke annually. Stroke is also the second leading cause of morbidity, leading to loss of an estimated 132 million disability-adjusted life-years. There were 104 million stroke survivors in 2017.[25] Although stroke can occur at any life stage, the risk of stroke increases with age. In older persons, cardioembolic stroke is more frequently the underlying cause because

of the higher prevalence of atrial fibrillation. Among persons over age 60 years, greater than 40% of strokes are secondary to cardioembolism.[26]

Most modifiable and nonmodifiable risk factors for stroke overlap with those for ischemic heart disease. These include hypertension, diabetes mellitus, insulin resistance, obesity, dyslipidemia, chronic kidney disease, physical inactivity, smoking, sleep apnea, substance use disorders, depression, poor diet, air pollution, age, male sex, and familial heritability.[27,28] Hypertension and smoking, in particular, are leading modifiable risk factors for ischemic stroke, ICH, and SAH.[29,30]

Because the modifiable lifestyle and environmental risk factors for ischemic heart disease and stroke overlap, targeting them has drawn emphasis in recent years as a parsimonious route to promote both cardiac and brain health.[31] *Brain health* can be understood as the preserved ability to function adaptively in one's environment, through the contributions of cognition, mood, and physical function. Although the interaction between cerebrovascular disease and neurodegeneration is not well understood, accumulating evidence suggests both stroke and underlying subclinical vascular brain injury contribute to cognitive and functional decline, and to depression.[32,33] The ability to measure the burden of cerebrovascular disease using advanced neuroimaging, including more sensitive MRI measures of occult white matter injury such as diffusion-tensor imaging (DTI) and automated image analytic techniques that measure the number, volume, and locations of ischemic and hemorrhagic brain injury, has improved our understanding of the contribution of vascular disease to cognitive impairment and other perturbations in brain health.[34]

Genetics

Stroke shows strong familial aggregation[35] and moderate heritability of 30% to 40%. Stroke can occur as a result of Mendelian disorders that affect the wall structure of large or small arteries. Some well-known monogenic causes of stroke include autosomal dominant conditions such as cerebral autosomal dominant arteriopathy with subcortical infarcts and leukoencephalopathy (CADASIL; gene: *NOTCH3*) and *COL4A1*-associated small vessel disease; autosomal recessive conditions such as sickle cell disease, cerebral autosomal recessive arteriopathy with subcortical infarcts and leukoencephalopathy (CARASIL; gene: *HTRA1*), hereditary endotheliopathy with retinopathy, nephropathy, and stroke (HERNS; gene: *TREX1*); X-linked conditions such as Fabry's disease (*GLA*); and mitochondrial diseases such as mitochondrial encephalopathy, lactic acidosis, and stroke-like episodes (MELAS). However, to date we have identified the genes explaining only a small proportion of non-Mendelian stroke syndromes. Large genome-wide association studies (GWAS) have identified over 35 loci.[36] Genetic risk factors for stroke may be genetic variants associated with risk factors for stroke (such as hypertension and hyperlipidemia), with subclinical markers of atherosclerosis (such as coronary or carotid atherosclerosis), with genes that determine brain resilience to injury (such as *APOE*), genes that are the target of accepted stroke therapies, or with genes that alter the function

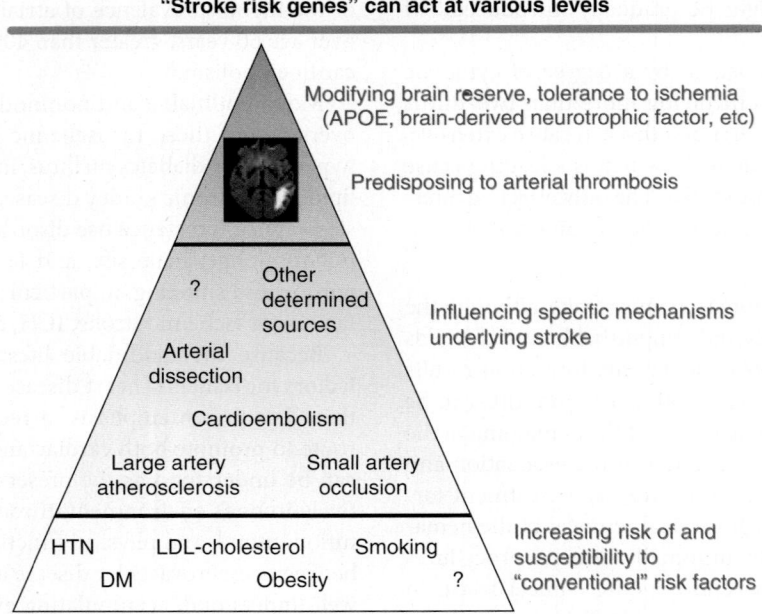

Figure 25-2. Genetic variants and influence on risk of stroke and stroke outcomes. Genes associated with stroke risk can work at various levels, including as genes that determine brain resilience, susceptibility to thrombosis, associated with specific stroke mechanisms or etiologies, or associated with risk and susceptibility to genetic, lifestyle, and environmental risk factors.

of proteins along the coagulation pathway (**Fig. 25–2**). **Figure 25–3** shows the many genes thought to be associated with stroke and the overlap with known stroke risk factors in the MEGA-STROKE consortium. However, genome-wide genetic studies undertaken by these large international consortia have also identified loci whose biological link to known stroke mechanisms is not obvious; these discoveries could potentially lead to novel therapies for stroke, for example genes regulating levels of *HDAC9* that appears to increase the risk of large artery stroke.[37–39] Over 90% of the loci associated with the overall risk of stroke are in nonexonic regions and may have a regulatory function. Most loci underlying the risk of stroke have, as is true for other common, complex genetic disorders, relatively small effects on risk. Some loci appear to be associated with the risk of all types of stroke, whereas most loci are specific altering the risks of large artery stroke, cardioembolic stroke, lacunes, deep or cortical hemorrhages, or the burden of subclinical vascular disease as manifested by white matter hyperintensities.[40–43] Variants in genes associated with the monogenic causes of stroke (such as *NOTCH3* and *COL4A1*) are overrepresented among risk genes for all stroke, albeit the implicated variants appear to result in less extreme biological changes.

To date, the majority of these loci have been identified in persons of European ancestry with only a limited number of studies in Black and Asian groups. Aggregate polygenic risk scores for stroke risk can be used for risk stratification at a population level or enrollment into clinical trials but are not yet sufficiently predictive to be helpful in a clinical setting either for prognostic or differential diagnosis. Recent large collaborative efforts are exploring the genetic determinants underlying stroke recurrence and stroke outcome, integration of multiple

omics to enhance gene discovery, and the conversion of genetic discoveries to novel therapies.[44]

CEREBROVASCULAR COMPLICATIONS OF HEART DISEASE

Direct mechanisms of cerebrovascular injury caused by heart disease include (1) embolism of material originating in the heart or from the venous circulation and associated with a right to left shunt, with occlusion of the extracranial carotid or vertebral arteries, spinal arteries, or intracranial or retinal arteries, and (2) hypoperfusion of the brain resulting from cardiac dysfunction or arrest.

Clinical Presentation

Stroke caused by embolism from the heart typically features sudden, focal neurologic symptoms, with peak deficit at onset. Because embolic occlusion can occur at any of the arteries supplying the cerebrum, cerebellum, retina, or spinal cord, the potential constellation of symptoms (*stroke syndrome*) is varied and can include sudden severe headache or loss of consciousness. **Table 25–1** details the spectrum of neurologic deficits that can occur. Due to acute cortical irritability at the site of the infarction, patients may present with early seizure at the time of stroke or soon after. Focal infarctions can cause symptoms that mimic lacunar syndromes, for example, causing focal motor deficits involving only the face or one limb rather than typical hemiparesis.[45] With very large infarcts (eg, with a malignant middle cerebral artery syndrome), brain edema and swelling can occur over the first 24 to 72 hours. With resulting brainstem compression or herniation, the patient can suffer a

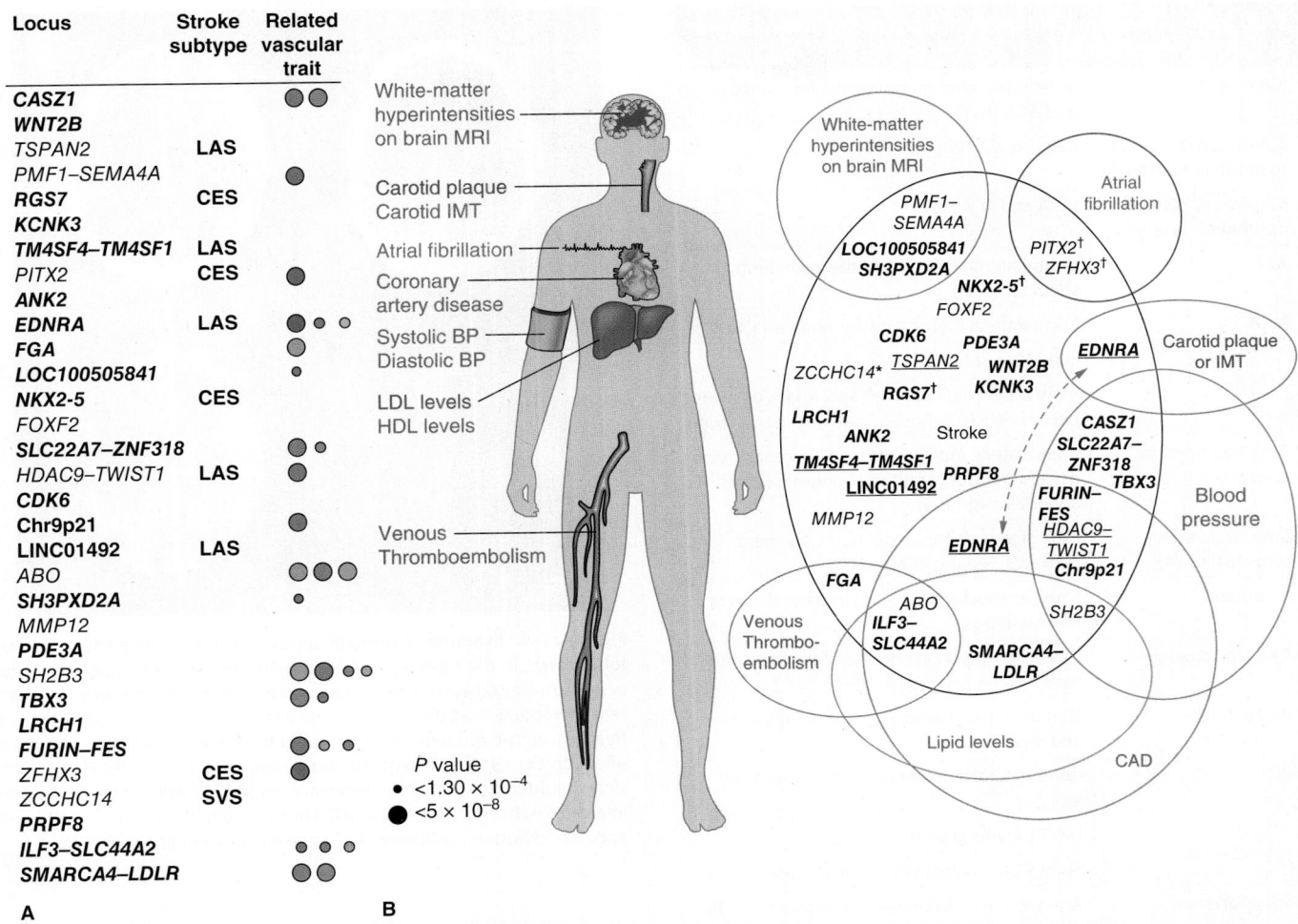

Figure 25–3. **(A)** Association results from the look-ups in published GWAS data for related vascular traits. Symbol sizes reflect *P* values for association with the related trait. **(B)** Venn diagram. Loci reaching genome-wide significance for association with stroke subtypes are marked with a *dagger symbol* (for cardioembolic stroke), *underlined* (for large artery atherosclerotic stroke), or marked with an *asterisk* (for small artery occlusion stroke). Novel loci are in **bold**. *SH3PXD2A, WNT2B, PDE3A,* and *OBFC1* have previously been associated with atrial fibrillation (*SH3PXD2A*), or diastolic (*WNT2B* and *PDE3A*) or systolic (*OBFC1*) BP, but the respective lead single-nucleotide polymorphisms (SNPs) were in low linkage disequilibrium ($r^2 < 0.1$ in the 1000G cosmopolitan panel) with variants associated with stroke in the current GWAS. MRI, magnetic resonance imaging; IMT, intima–media thickness; LDL, low-density lipoprotein; HDL, high-density lipoprotein. The lead variant for *TBX3* is not included in the original datasets for BP traits (systolic and diastolic). Results are based on a perfect proxy SNP (rs35432, $r^2 = 1$ in the European 1000G phase 3 reference). Reproduced with permission from Malik, R, Chauhan, G, Traylor, M, et al. Multiancestry genome-wide association study of 520,000 subjects identifies 32 loci associated with stroke and stroke subtypes. *Nat Genet.* 2018 Apr;50(4):524-537.

deterioration in level of consciousness, weakness of the opposite limbs, pupillary abnormalities, flexor or extensor posturing, and coma.

Key features that distinguish stroke and TIA caused by cardioembolism from other stroke subtypes are highlighted in **Table 25–2.** Clinical findings in patients with brain ischemia due to global hypotension are described in the section "Cardiac Arrest and Brain Hypoperfusion."

Diagnostic Evaluation and Management

In addition to a clinical bedside evaluation, diagnosis requires integration of neuroimaging, vascular examination, and cardiac testing.

Patients with stroke symptoms should undergo urgent *brain imaging*, typically a head CT, to first rule out intracranial

hemorrhage. In patients with no contraindication to contrast material, initial imaging may also include CT angiography (CTA) of the head and neck to evaluate for an abrupt vessel cutoff (or *large vessel occlusion*) that may be treatable with mechanical thrombectomy (see section "Acute Treatment of Stroke"). Cardioembolism is a common cause of large vessel occlusion.[46] In hyperacute stroke, head CT can appear normal, especially with smaller-size infarctions. In the cerebrum, embolic stroke often has the appearance of a distal, cortical, wedge-shaped, or triangular infarction (**Fig. 25–4**); can have a hemorrhagic component; and can involve both superficial and deep structures depending on infarct size. The area of infarction may be large, especially compared to lacunar infarction that is typically <1.5 cm in volume. Multiple or recurrent emboli can infarct multiple neurovascular territories and other organs of the body. MRI is more sensitive for detecting acute cerebral ischemia and

TABLE 25-1. Common Neurologic Signs of Occlusive Disease at Various Arterial Sites

ICA origin	Ipsilateral transient monocular blindness; MCA and ACA signs
ICA siphon (proximal to ophthalmic artery)	Same as ICA origin
ICA siphon (distal to ophthalmic artery)	MCA and ACA signs
ACA	Contralateral weakness of the lower limb and shoulder shrug
MCA	Contralateral motor, sensory, and visual loss
	Left MCA: Aphasia
	Right MCA: Neglect of left space, lack of awareness of deficit (agnosia), apathy, impersistence
Anterior choroidal artery	Contralateral motor, sensory, and visual loss, usually without cognitive changes (such as aphasia or agnosia)
Subclavian artery (proximal to VA)	Lack of arm stamina, cool hand, transient dizziness, veering, diplopia
VA origin	Same as subclavian, but no ipsilateral arm or hand findings
VA intracranially	Lateral medullary syndrome; staggering and veering (cerebellar infarction)
Basilar artery	Bilateral motor weakness; ophthalmoplegia and diplopia
PCA	Contralateral hemianopia and hemisensory loss
	Left PCA: Alexia with agraphia
	Right PCA: Neglect of left visual space
Spinal arteries	Arm weakness, leg weakness, sensory loss, loss of sphincter control, depending on level and extent of infarction

Abbreviations: ACA, anterior cerebral artery; ICA, internal carotid artery; MCA, middle cerebral artery; PCA, posterior cerebral artery; VA, vertebral artery.

can detect hemorrhagic infarction using magnetic resonance (MR) gradient recall echo (GRE) sequences that are sensitive to blood products such as hemosiderin.

A *vascular evaluation* is necessary to rule out large artery disease, such as carotid stenosis, intracranial atherosclerosis,

TABLE 25-2. Clinical and Diagnostic Features That Distinguish Cardioembolic Stroke from Other Stroke Subtypes

Present	Absent
1. Cardiac source for embolic stroke*	1. Stenosis or occlusion of a large artery supplying the vascular territory of the infarction
2. Evidence of systemic embolism	2. Complex aortic atheroma, defined as (1) >4 mm in thickness, (2) ulcerated, or (3) containing a mobile component
3. A clinical syndrome not consistent with small vessel occlusion (*lacunar stroke*)	3. Other evident causes of stroke, which are often less common, such as vasculitis or arterial dissection

*In the context of other features consistent with cardioembolism, the lack of a cardiac source for embolic stroke after a complete initial stroke evaluation designates a patient as having an *embolic stroke of undetermined source*

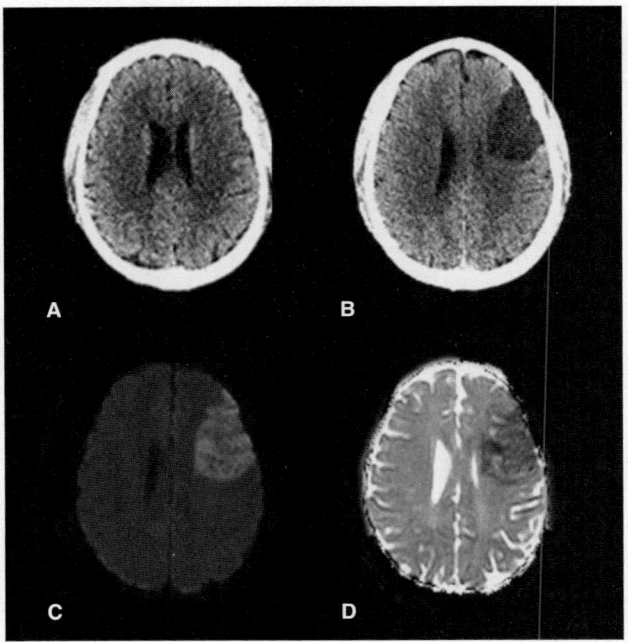

Figure 25-4. Example of embolic-appearing, wedge-shaped left frontal lobe infarct in the territory of the superior division left middle cerebral artery. (A) Day 0 head CT, with very mild loss of gray matter-to-white matter differentiation at the cortex of the left anterior frontal lobe. (B) Day 3 head CT with hypodense area of cerebral infarction and increased mass effect on the left lateral ventricle due to cytotoxic edema. (C) Day 6 diffusion-weighted imaging (DWI) sequence on MRI, showing increased signal in area of ischemic brain tissue. (D) Same Day 6 MRI showing reduction of apparent diffusion coefficient (ADC) signal corresponding with DWI.

or arterial dissection that may be responsible for artery-to-artery embolism or distal hypoperfusion. Vascular evaluation is important in cases where infarction occurs in a single vascular distribution, to determine if there is pathology at a more proximal artery. Imaging modalities such as CTA or MR angiography (MRA), digital subtraction angiography, carotid ultrasound, and transcranial doppler (TCD) are used to evaluate the cervical and intracranial vasculature.

TCD can also be used to monitor for cerebral embolic signals, referred to as HITS (high-intensity transient signals). These transient, short-duration, high-intensity signals are ultrasonic footprints of embolic material moving under the TCD probes (**Fig. 25-5**). TCD with emboli detection studies monitor for HITS in patients with potential cardiac sources, including prosthetic and mechanical heart valves, atrial fibrillation, patent foramen ovale (PFO), left ventricular assist devices, left ventricular thrombi, and in acute myocardial infarction with reduced left ventricular ejection fraction.[47]

Cardiac testing is essential in patients with suspected cardioembolism or embolic stroke of undetermined source. Guidelines for the early management of stroke strongly recommend assessment of cardiac enzymes and electrocardiogram to identify patients with myocardial infarction or sustained atrial fibrillation that may be a source of embolism.[18,48] Inpatient cardiac telemetry and extended (>24-hour) cardiac rhythm monitoring are important for the detection of paroxysmal atrial fibrillation

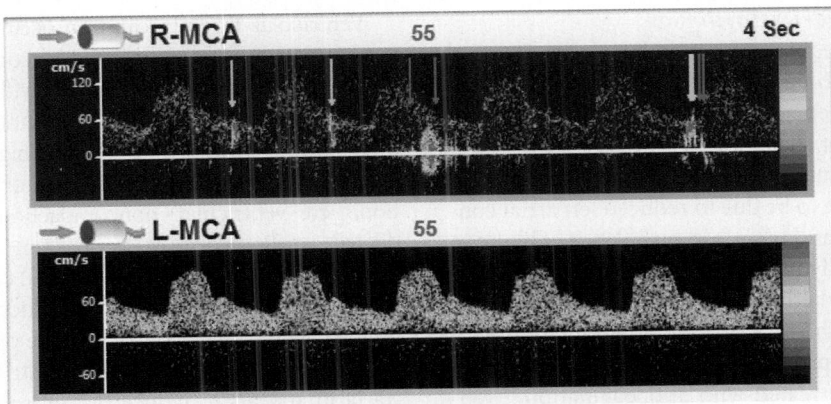

Figure 25–5. Transcranial Doppler recording from the right (R-MCA) and left (L-MCA) middle cerebral arteries. The signals indicated by the yellow arrows in the top panel represent microemboli; blue arrows indicate artifact. Reproduced with permission from Michael Murray, Boston Medical Center and Viken L Babikian, MD, Boston University School of Medicine and the VA Boston Healthcare System.

(PAF). Investigators observed high rates of PAF detection in the 30-Day Cardiac Event Monitor Belt for Recording Atrial Fibrillation After a Cerebral Event (EMBRACE) Trial and the Study of Continuous Cardiac Monitoring to Assess Atrial Fibrillation After Cryptogenic Stroke (CRYSTAL-AF).[49,50] PAF was captured in 16.1% of the EMBRACE group with 30-day monitoring, compared to 3.2% in those who only underwent repeat 24-hour Holter monitoring. In CRYSTAL-AF, up to 30% of patients with an implantable cardiac monitor had PAF detected at 36 months.

In most stroke patients, transthoracic echocardiogram (TTE) is performed to identify high-risk sources of embolism, to assess cardiac function, and to evaluate for structural abnormalities, such as PFO or atrial septal aneurysm. Contrast enhancement can help detect a cardiac mass or thrombus. In younger patients, agitated saline injection is used to screen for intracardiac right-to-left shunt. TTE has limitations, including incomplete visualization of the left ventricle for the presence of a mass or the left atrial appendage for thrombus. Other noninvasive cardiac imaging modalities, such as cardiac CT or MR, may be considered in select patients. Cardiac MR is increasingly used for the diagnosis of left ventricular tumors and certain cardiomyopathies that may be associated with stroke, such as cardiac amyloidosis.[51,52]

Transesophageal echocardiogram (TEE) is a more invasive procedure but has greater sensitivity for abnormalities in the left atrium and appendage, left ventricle, septal regions, and aortic arch. Examples of sources for stroke that would be better detected using TEE include thrombus in the left atrial appendage, atrial septal defects, regional myocardial wall dysfunction, and aortic atherosclerosis.[53] Although TEE appears to increase the diagnostic yield of cardiac lesions in stroke patients,[54] it is debated whether TEE is cost-effective or routinely changes patient management. As with the approach to brain imaging, vascular evaluation, and other cardiac testing, the selection of diagnostics needs to be individualized to each patient, with the foremost goal being to complete the etiologic work up and guide treatment.

Cardioembolism

Table 25–3 summarizes the heart diseases and cardiac structural abnormalities that are associated with increased risk of cardioembolism.

TABLE 25–3. Heart Diseases, Cardiac Structural Abnormalities, and Risk of Cardioembolism

Higher risk etiologies	Potentially higher risk etiologies	Lower or uncertain risk, or rare etiologies
1. Atrial fibrillation and flutter	1. Atrial cardiopathy	1. Lone atrial fibrillation in younger patients
2. Left atrial or ventricular thrombus	2. Sick sinus syndrome	2. Paroxysmal supraventricular tachycardia
3. Recent anterior myocardial infarction (<4 weeks)	3. Systolic heart failure with low ejection fraction (especially <15%)	3. Left ventricular hypokinesis, akinesis, or aneurysm, without thrombus
4. Nonbacterial thrombotic ("marantic") endocarditis	4. Dilated cardiomyopathy	4. Valvular strands
5. Rheumatic valvular disease	5. Papillary fibroelastoma	5. Spontaneous echocardiographic contrast or "smoke" in left atrial cavity
6. Mechanical prosthetic valve	6. Mitral stenosis	6. Bioprosthetic mitral or aortic valve
7. Infective endocarditis	7. High-grade aortic arch atheroma	7. Mitral annular calcification
8. Presence of left ventricular assist device	8. Recent aortic valve replacement or coronary artery bypass graft surgery	8. Mitral valve prolapse
9. Atrial myxoma	9. PFO in selected older stroke patients, with ESUS and lacking vascular risk factors	9. Calcified aortic stenosis
10. Patent foramen ovale (PFO) in selected younger stroke patients (age <60 years, ESUS, lacking vascular risk factors)		10. Low-grade aortic arch atheroma
11. PFO with atrial septal aneurysm		11. Atrial septal aneurysm (no PFO) or defect
		12. PFO in older cryptogenic stroke patients with vascular risk factors

Atrial Fibrillation and Atrial Dysrhythmias

The most common cause of cardioembolic stroke is *atrial fibrillation*. Atrial fibrillation is associated with a nearly 5-fold increased risk of stroke[55] depending on age and major risk factors, such as sex, history of structural heart disease, hypertension, and diabetes.[56] The mechanism of thromboembolism in atrial fibrillation is thought to be due to reduced left atrial contractility, along with stasis and increased turbulence of blood in the left atrial cavity, typically in the left atrial appendage. There is a similar risk of stroke whether atrial fibrillation is sustained or paroxysmal, and as such is treated in either situation with anticoagluation.[57] Only approximately half of eligible patients with atrial fibrillation are treated with anticoagulation,[58] representing a missed opportunity in stroke prevention. Although cases of *secondary paroxysmal atrial fibrillation* triggered by recent cardiovascular surgery or acute illness are not routinely treated with anticoagulation, recent evidence suggests long-term risk of stroke in this population is high.[59,60] The treatment approach for patients with secondary paroxysmal atrial fibrillation warrants further study.

Atrial flutter, which often coexists with atrial fibrillation and likely shares common pathophysiologic mechanisms, is associated with increased risk of stroke and is treated with anticoagulation for stroke prevention.[51,61] *Paroxysmal supraventricular tachycardia* has been associated with a 2-fold increased relative risk of stroke, compared to patients without the condition.[62] The finding of excessive *premature atrial contractions*, perhaps as a precursor to atrial fibrillation, is associated with increased risk of ischemic stroke in observational studies.[63] While patients with symptomatic *sick sinus syndrome* are often treated with insertion of an atrial pacemaker, these patients may undergo routine pacemaker interrogation to evaluate for unrecognized, paroxysmal atrial fibrillation. For further discussion of epidemiology, risk factors, mechanisms, and medical and surgical treatment options for atrial dysrhythmias, please refer to Section 6: Rhythm and Conduction Abnormalities.

Intracavitary Thrombus

Historical case series observed that within 4 weeks of acute myocardial infarction 2.5% of patients suffered a stroke.[64] Patients with large *anterior myocardial infarction* associated with reduced left ventricular ejection fraction and anterior-apical wall-motion abnormalities are at increased risk of developing a mural thrombus. Thrombus forms over areas of ventricular dyskinesis due to stasis of blood as well as endocardial injury with associated inflammation.[65] Stroke is less common among patients with inferior wall myocardial infarction. Thrombus can be visualized with contrast-enhanced echocardiogram. More advanced imaging, such as cardiac MR, is increasingly used to visualize thrombus in cases of cryptogenic stroke.[66] Anticoagulation is typically recommended for 3 to 6 months, although increased risk of stroke may persist after therapy. Rates of stroke after myocardial infarction appear to be decreasing.[67] This may be due to increased use of acute reperfusion therapy, more widespread use of antithrombotic medications, or improved vascular risk factor control after incident cardiovascular disease.

Ventricular thrombi can also occur in patients with chronic ventricular dysfunction caused by coronary disease, hypertension, and *cardiomyopathy*. Patients with *heart failure* have a 2- to 3-fold increased risk of stroke, accounting for approximately 9% of all strokes.[68] Stroke rates may be higher in certain subgroups, including patients with prior stroke or TIA, lower ejection fraction, left ventricular noncompaction, ventricular aneurysm, dilated cardiomyopathy, peripartum cardiomyopathy, Chagas heart disease,[69] and Takotsubo (stress) cardiomyopathy.[70] Multiple trials have investigated the use of anticoagulants versus antiplatelet medications for secondary stroke prevention in patients with reduced ejection fraction and no atrial fibrillation.[68] Although warfarin appears to reduce risk of ischemic stroke, the benefit is offset by an increased risk of major hemorrhage. Secondary analysis of the WARCEF (Warfarin versus Aspirin in Reduced Cardiac Ejection Fraction) trial suggests ejection fraction <15% is associated with higher risk of stroke. Further research is warranted to understand the role of anticoagulation, particularly newer direct oral anticoagulants, to reduce the risk of cardioembolic stroke in heart failure patients with reduced ejection fraction. Left ventricular assist devices used in patients with severe systolic heart failure are associated with a nearly 9% risk of stroke per year;[71] anticoagulation with warfarin with target international normalized ratio (INR) 2.5 to 3.0 is indicated to reduce thromboembolic risk.

Valvular Heart Disease

Rheumatic heart disease is the result of prior streptococcal infection leading to fibrotic changes in the mitral valve, and is the most common cause of mitral stenosis. Up to 2% of patients with rheumatic heart disease suffer a stroke,[72] in large part because the condition is commonly associated with atrial fibrillation. Older age, left atrial enlargement, reduced ejection fraction, and prior embolic events increase risk of stroke and are important factors for considering treatment with an anticoagulant if a stroke patient with rheumatic heart disease is in sinus rhythm.

Atherosclerosis and vascular risk factors contribute to the formation of *mitral annular calcification*, which is a rare cause of stroke.[73] Other valvular diseases, including mitral valve prolapse, mitral regurgitation, and aortic stenosis, are not definitively associated with increased risk of stroke and are generally not treated with antithrombotics, unless coronary artery disease or atrial fibrillation are discovered.

Thrombus can form on *prosthetic valves*, with a higher risk of embolism with placement of a mechanical prosthetic valve, compared to a bioprosthetic valve. The rate of perioperative stroke at 30 days appears to be similar after either surgical or transcatheter aortic valve repair, between 2% and 6%. Covert brain infarcts following these procedures are common.[74] Anticoagulation is recommended for the first 3 months after placement of a bioprosthetic valve, whereas a combination of aspirin and warfarin therapy (target INR 2.5–3.0) is indicated long-term to reduce risk of stroke with mechanical valves.[75] The incidence rate of thromboembolism in patients with mechanical prosthetic valves treated with anticoagulation, compared to no treatment, is reduced from 4 events to 1 event per 100 patient-years.[76] Direct oral anticoagulants are not currently recommended for patients with mechanical valves.[77]

Between 25% and 40% of patients with *infective endocarditis* experience neurologic complications, including ischemic and hemorrhagic stroke, mycotic aneurysm, meningitis, brain abscess, seizures, and spinal cord infection.[78,79] Risk factors for infective endocarditis include intravenous drug use, presence of a bicuspid aortic valve, and recent dental or surgical procedures. Mycotic aneurysms or vascular necrosis of an infected embolus can cause fatal subarachnoid bleeding. Because of the high risk for intracranial hemorrhage in these stroke patients, antithrombotics are typically not recommended. Antibiotics and surgical repair of a severely diseased cardiac valve or abscess are mainstays of treatment; however, surgical valve replacement procedures often require large doses of anticoagulation. Surgery should be delayed at least 4 weeks after a hemorrhagic stroke or major ischemic stroke, although surgical timing in this context has not been well studied and should be individualized with input from multiple specialists.[79]

Nonbacterial thrombotic endocarditis (NBTE), also known as "marantic" endocarditis, is the formation of sterile, fibrous, or fibrinous lesions on heart valves or the endocardium. The vegetations can contain platelet aggregates, are friable, and easily embolised.[80] NBTE occurs in the setting of certain medical conditions that cause changes in the coagulation cascade, such as malignancy or inflammatory disorders. *Libman–Sacks endocarditis* is a subtype of NBTE in patients with systemic lupus erythematosus and antiphospholipid antibody syndrome. Treatment of the underlying condition is essential for management. Anticoagulation is frequently started if stroke has occurred and the patient remains in a hypercoagulable state. The choice of anticoagulant and target INR with warfarin are debated. Recent trials have shown that direct oral anticoagulants (DOACs) are less effective than warfarin for treatment of thrombotic antiphospholipid antibody syndrome.[81]

Mobile, fibrous *valvular strands*, or Lambl's excrescences, are composed of endothelialized connective tissue and are considered a rare source of cardioembolism. There are no guidelines for medical or surgical management of valvular strands associated with cryptogenic stroke.

Cardiac Tumors

The two most common types of cardiac tumors, *atrial myxoma* and *papillary fibroelastomas*, are uncommon sources of cardioembolic stroke. Cardiac myxomas typically form in the left atrium, are friable, and may embolize in 30% of cases.[82] Emboli consist of tumor fragments or secondary thrombi. Antithrombotic medications are not recommended for treatment of myxomas. Papillary fibroelastomas are histologically benign tumors that most commonly affect the valves. Stroke or TIA are the presenting symptom in up to one-third of cases where these tumors were surgically removed.[83] Surgical excision is the standard of care for cardiac tumors that cause cardioembolism.

Paradoxical Embolism

Paradoxical embolism has been strongly implicated as one potential cause of cryptogenic stroke. Although once considered rare, emboli entering the systemic circulation through right-to-left shunting of blood are now often suspected, with shunting identified using agitated saline injection ("bubble study") during TTE, TEE, or transcranial doppler.

Patent Foramen Ovale

By far the most common potential intracardiac shunt is a residual PFO. The high frequency (approximately 25%) of PFOs in the normal adult population has made it difficult to be certain in an individual stroke patient with a PFO whether paradoxical embolism was the cause of the stroke or whether the PFO was merely an incidental finding. Up to 50% of patients with early onset (before age 60 years) cryptogenic stroke have a PFO.[84] A principal mechanism of PFO-associated stroke is migration of a venous thrombus from a leg or pelvic vein through a PFO to the arterial system. PFO associated with an atrial septal aneurysm appears to increase stroke risk.[85]

A detailed history, cardiac and neuroimaging, and assessment for deep venous thrombosis (DVT) are required if there is clinical concern for PFO-associated stroke, such as:

1. Situations that promote thrombosis of the deep veins of the leg or pelvis (eg, sitting for a long duration in one position, such as a transcontinental flight, or recent surgery)

2. Hypercoagulability (eg, the use of oral contraceptives, presence of factor V Leiden mutation, dehydration, and other inherited or acquired thrombophilia)

3. The sudden onset of stroke during Valsalva or other maneuvers that promote right-to-left shunting of blood (eg, sexual intercourse, straining at stool)

4. Pulmonary embolism within a short time before or after the neurologic ischemic event

5. The absence of other putative causes of stroke after thorough evaluation

In addition to assessment with lower extremity doppler imaging to detect DVT, a CT venogram or MR venogram of the pelvic vein should be considered to evaluate for isolated pelvic DVT or iliac vein compression syndrome.[86]

Cases presenting with possible paradoxical embolism may share certain features that increase the likelihood that PFO contributed to the occurrence of a stroke: the Risk of Paradoxical Embolism (RoPE) study performed a patient-level meta-analysis of 12 cryptogenic stroke cohorts. Among 3023 patients with cryptogenic stroke, the prevalence of PFO, and the likelihood that PFO was the cause of the stroke (the PFO-attributable fraction), correlated with the absence of vascular risk factors (ie, hypertension, diabetes, smoking, prior stroke or TIA, older age) and the presence of a cortical (as opposed to subcortical) cryptogenic infarct on imaging suggesting ESUS. Using multivariate modeling, the investigators devised the RoPE score, which estimates the probability that a PFO is either incidental or pathogenic. For each RoPE score stratum, the corresponding PFO prevalence was used to estimate the PFO-attributable fraction: the probability that the index stroke event was related to the PFO. Higher RoPE scores, as found in younger patients who lack vascular risk factors and have a cortical infarct on neuroimaging, suggest pathogenic PFOs, while lower RoPE scores, as found in older patients with vascular risk factors, suggest incidental PFOs. On one hand, in cases where PFO was likely the stroke etiology, the estimated risk of recurrent stroke or TIA was low, 2% over 2 years. On the other hand, cases with low RoPE scores had higher risk of recurrent stroke, up to 20%.

In a subsequent analysis,[87] stroke recurrence was associated with the following three variables only in the high RoPE score group: a history of prior stroke or TIA, a hypermobile interatrial septum (*atrial septal aneurysm*), and a small shunt. The RoPE data did not include shunt size or activity at onset; strokes that develop suddenly during sex, straining at stool, Valsalva maneuvers and sudden exertion are often embolic. The significance of shunt size for stroke risk is currently debated. Large right-to-left shunt was defined in the French PFO-ASA Study as >30 microbubbles observed in the left atrium within 3 cardiac cycles after injection of agitated saline during echocardiogram.[88] Recent positive clinical trials demonstrating the efficacy of endovascular PFO closure were enriched for patients with larger shunt size.[89]

If interdisciplinary clinical assessments and a comprehensive evaluation for stroke etiology determine that the PFO is likely the underlying mechanism, then treatment options include endovascular PFO closure, anticoagulation, or antiplatelet therapy. If there is concomitant hypercoagulability or deep venous thrombosis, anticoagulation is recommended to prevent further ischemic stroke. In younger patients age <60 years with ESUS, PFO closure has shown efficacy in three large randomized trials: CLOSE (Patent Foramen Ovale Closure or Anticoagulants Versus Antiplatelet Therapy to Prevent Stroke Recurrence), REDUCE (Septal Occluder Device for PFO Closure in Stroke Patients), and RESPECT (Randomized Evaluation of Recurrent Stroke Comparing PFO Closure to Established Current Standard of Care Treatment).[90-92] In the CLOSE trial, no strokes occurred among the 238 patients who underwent PFO closure, over a follow-up of 5.3 years, compared to 14 strokes in the arm that received antiplatelet therapy alone (hazard ratio [HR] 0.03; 95% confidence interval [CI], 0–0.26; $P < 0.001$). Subgroup analyses in the RESPECT trial suggested the benefit of PFO closure was greater among patients with atrial septal aneurysm and for those with large shunt size. If there is a contraindication for surgery, anticoagulation remains a treatment option, however their use increases risk for major bleeding events. In shared decision-making with the patient, cumulative exposure to bleeding risk—over potentially decades in younger patients—needs to be considered.

Cardiac Arrest and Brain Hypoperfusion

In the United States, there are more than 325,000 cases of cardiac arrest per year (as of 2017), defined as the cessation of cardiac mechanical activity.[29] After cardiopulmonary resuscitation (CPR), the heart often recovers in individuals whose brain has been irreversibly damaged by ischemic-anoxic damage.[93] The following reviews the pathology, signs, and prognosis of brain dysfunction after periods of circulatory failure.

Different brain regions have selective vulnerability to hypoxic-ischemic damage. Regions that are most remote and at the edges of major vascular supply are more liable to sustain hypoperfusion injury. These zones are referred to as *borderzone* or *watershed* regions. The cerebral cortex and hippocampus are particularly vulnerable to injury.[94] In the cerebral cortex, the border zone regions are between the anterior cerebral artery (ACA) and middle cerebral artery (MCA), and between the MCA and posterior cerebral artery (PCA). The basal ganglia and thalamus are most involved if hypoxia is severe, but some circulation is preserved. Cerebellar neurons, brainstem nuclei, and the spinal cord may also be selectively injured.[95] When cortical damage is severe and protracted, cytotoxic edema causes massive brain swelling, with cessation of blood flow and brain death.

Clinical Findings

Very severe hypoxic-ischemic damage can lead to irreversible coma, and brain death. When initially examined, such patients have no brainstem reflexes and no response to stimuli, except perhaps a decerebration response. These findings do not improve, and respiratory control is absent or lost.

When cerebral cortical damage is very severe, but brainstem reflexes are preserved, there is no meaningful response to the environment. Automatic facial movements such as blinking, tongue protrusion, and yawning usually persist. The eyes may rest slightly up and move from side to side. When this state does not improve, it is referred to as *persistent vegetative state*[93] or *wakefulness without awareness*. Laminar cortical necrosis can cause seizures (multifocal myoclonic twitches or jerks of the facial and limb muscles), which are difficult to control with anticonvulsants.

With severe hypoperfusion ACA-MCA border zone injury, there is weakness of the arms and proximal lower extremities with preservation of face, leg, and foot movement (the "person-in-the-barrel" syndrome). With MCA-PCA ischemia, the symptoms and signs are predominantly visual. Patients describe difficulty seeing and inability to integrate the features of large objects or scenes despite retained capacity to see small objects in some parts of their visual fields. Patients are unable to read. The triad of symptoms including ocular apraxia, simultagnosia, and optic ataxia are the main clinical features of Balint syndrome.[96] Apathy, inertia, and amnesia are also common. Patients cannot make new memories and have patchy, retrograde amnesia for events during and before hospitalization. This Korsakoff-type amnestic syndrome is caused by hippocampal damage and may not be fully reversible. Amnesia may be accompanied by visual abnormalities, apathy, and confusion, or may be isolated.

Treatment and Prognostication

Shortly after resuscitation or arrest, patients with less severe cerebral injuries show some reactivity to the environment. Eye opening and restless limb movements develop. The eyes may fixate on objects. Patients may react to noise or stimuli. Soon patients awaken fully and may begin to speak. Cognitive and behavioral abnormalities may be detected after the patient awakens and over the long term, depending on the degree of injury. These can include deficits in the domains of memory, attention, executive function, and visuospatial perception.

Prognostic signs and variables have been extensively studied.[93,97,98] The initial neurologic findings and their course are helpful in predicting outcome. Patients that are comatose after cardiac arrest have a poor prognosis; however, recovery is difficult to predict due to the advent of therapeutic hypothermia management and intensive care treatment to minimize hypoxic injury and to prevent further complications (ie, by treating fever, maintaining cerebral perfusion with BP support, and identifying and treating seizure). Current American Heart Association (AHA) guidelines for cardiac resuscitation do not recommend examination for prognosis until 72 hours after return to normothermia in patients who undergo targeted temperature management.[99] A multimodal approach to the evaluation is recommended, including clinical exam, neuroimaging (also to rule out other causes of coma), electroencephalogram (EEG), somatosensory evoked potentials, and/or measurement of neuron-specific enolase, a blood biomarker of hypoxic brain injury. Absence of pupillary light reflexes or corneal reflexes on day 3 after cardiac arrest indicate a poor prognosis. The patient's ability to respond to and localize pain may be a sign of good prognosis. Recurrent myoclonus, especially diffuse and sustained (myoclonic status), is another poor prognostic sign. A standardized clinical examination that demonstrates lack of brainstem function, coma, and apnea allows for the determination of brain death.[100]

OTHER CAUSES AND MANIFESTATIONS OF CEREBROVASCULAR DISEASE

Large Artery Atherosclerosis

Extra- and intracranial large artery atherosclerosis are common in patients with coronary artery disease and are among the main causes of stroke.

Figure 25–6 diagrammatically shows the sites of predilection for development of atherosclerosis in the cervicocranial circulation. Note the concentration of these sites at branch points and flow dividers. There are race and sex differences in the distribution of cerebral atherosclerosis.[29] White men more commonly develop lesions of the internal carotid artery (ICA) and vertebral artery (VA) origins. Black individuals and individuals of Asian ancestry have a higher incidence of intracranial occlusive disease and a lower frequency of extracranial disease.[29] Intracranial disease is more prevalent in women and diabetic patients. Interestingly, patients with intracranial occlusive disease do not have a high incidence of coronary or peripheral vascular occlusive disease.

Mechanisms of Ischemia

Ischemia in patients with atherosclerotic occlusive lesions is caused by two different mechanisms: hypoperfusion and embolism. Hypoperfusion develops only when a critical reduction in luminal diameter causes reduced distal perfusion. When flow is reduced slowly, the brain vasculature has a remarkable capacity to develop collateral circulation. Patients with severe ICA-origin occlusive disease can remain asymptomatic despite marked decrease in blood flow. Even when vascular occlusion is abrupt, surprisingly few patients develop persistent brain

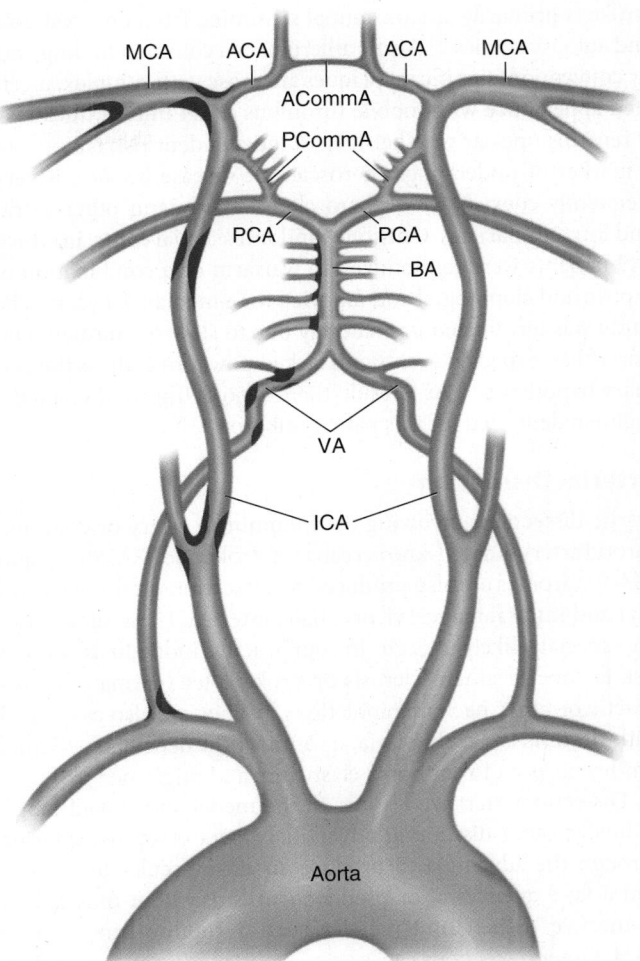

Figure 25–6. Sites of predilection for atherosclerotic narrowing; *darker blue shaded* **areas represent plaques.** ACA, anterior cerebral artery; ACommA, anterior communicating artery; BA, basilar artery; ICA, internal carotid artery; MCA, middle cerebral artery; PCA, posterior cerebral artery; PCommA, posterior communicating artery; VA, vertebral artery.

ischemia. In most patients, within a few days or at most 2 weeks following an arterial occlusion, collateral circulation stabilizes. Intra-arterial embolism from atherosclerotic lesions is probably a much more frequent and important cause of brain infarction than hypoperfusion.

Extracranial Carotid Atherosclerosis

Extracranial carotid atherosclerosis is recognized as a major risk factor for retinal and hemispheric stroke. The risk of stroke increases with higher degree of stenosis and risk of recurrence is high. Plaque characteristics, such as ulceration, presence of soft plaque, or an overlying thrombus, can also be useful in risk stratification. Significant advances in the management of carotid disease have taken place in the last 30 years, including carotid endarterectomy, stenting techniques, and optimization of medical management. The topic is covered in detail in Chapter 24: Carotid Artery Disease.

Aortic Atherosclerosis

The association between aortic arch atherosclerosis and stroke is complex. The evidence linking aortic atherosclerosis and stroke is primarily circumstantial stemming from observational and autopsy studies.[101] Aortic atheroma is a common finding and, by convention, significant plaques are those with complex, ulcerated appearance with mobile thrombus or ≥4 mm in thickness. It remains unclear whether it is an independent risk factor[102] or a marker of underlying atherosclerotic disease because it very frequently coexists with atherosclerotic lesions in other extra- and intracranial sites. Only one randomized trial exists, in which 349 patients were randomized to warfarin or a combination of aspirin and clopidogrel and followed for a median 3.4 years. The study was terminated prematurely due to slow recruitment and lower than expected events and lacked power to address the primary hypothesis.[101] As a result, there is no definitive therapeutic regimen dedicated for this patient subgroup.[103]

Arterial Dissection

Aortic dissections involving the innominate artery or common carotid artery is a well-known cause of stroke and TIA. Stroke and TIA syndromes are also produced by dissections of the extracranial and intracranial cervicocephalic arteries. These dissections are especially likely to occur in young, active individuals without risk factors for atherosclerosis or stroke, after trauma or chiropractic or other neck manipulations.[104] They are also associated with fibromuscular dysplasia, α_1-antitrypsin deficiency, Marfan syndrome, pseudoxanthoma elasticum, and migraine.[105,106]

Dissections start with a tear in the media and spread longitudinally, often disrupting adventitial fibers or even rupturing through the adventitia to produce an extravascular hematoma and a false aneurysm, or pseudoaneurysm, within muscle and connective tissue. Intracranially, such a rupture can produce SAH. Other dissections cause arterial obstruction and secondary thrombosis of the narrowed vascular lumen. Most cerebrovascular dissections occur in the extracranial vessels, particularly the pharyngeal portion of the ICA and the nuchal VA.[105] Extracranial dissections produce sharp pain and throbbing headache; brain and retinal ischemic episodes, which may occur in rapid-fire attacks; and pressure on adjacent structures, especially cranial nerves X through XII, which exit at the skull base. Strokes, usually from embolization of clots, are common but may have a benign course. Intracranial dissections have a poorer prognosis, often with vascular rupture and SAH. The diagnosis is confirmed by digital subtraction angiography, CT, or MRI.

There is debate regarding the appropriate treatment for cervicocephalic arterial dissection. The Cervical Artery Dissection in Stroke Study (CADISS)[107] enrolled 250 participants with cervicocephalic dissection (118 carotid, 132 vertebral), who were randomly assigned to receive antiplatelet or anticoagulants. There was no difference in secondary stroke prevention. It is important to note that the mean time of treatment after symptom onset was 10.8 days (standard deviation 7.0, range 1–31 days) in this study. Published data and expert opinion suggest that most strokes develop within the first 7 days after brain ischemia and the rate of stroke thereafter is low.[108] In addition, strokes are uncommon in patients whose presentation does not include brain ischemia (neck pain, Horner syndrome, compression of nerve roots, or lower cranial nerves). These patients were also included in the trial. In the meta-analysis included in the report, almost all patients were enrolled beyond 5 days after onset. Physicians cannot therefore use the results of this trial to decide on treatment during the acute period after stroke onset. Hence, treatment choice remains highly individualized; both anticoagulant and antithrombotic treatment are considered acceptable. An ongoing randomized clinical trial will assess the noninferiority of aspirin versus vitamin K antagonists, incorporating serum and imaging biomarkers.[109] Follow-up vessel imaging is commonly obtained within 6 to 12 weeks to monitor for recanalization that often occurs spontaneously, while in other patients, only partial or no reconstitution of blood flow is achieved.

Coagulopathies

Hypercoagulability and bleeding caused by decreased coagulability affect most body organs, including the brain and heart. An increased tendency for clotting can be caused by abnormalities of the formed blood elements or serologic factors.[110,111] Increased numbers of red blood cells and platelets and qualitative abnormalities such as sickle cell disease can cause intravascular clotting, especially in the presence of dehydration. Serologic abnormalities may be congenital or acquired. Decreased amounts of natural anticoagulants (antithrombin III, protein C, and protein S), resistance to activated protein C, and prothrombin gene mutations can cause hypercoagulability.[110–112] In many of these patients—those on high-dose estrogen birth control pills, pregnant patients, and patients with cancer—serologic and standard coagulation tests (in vitro) do not clarify the mechanism of the excessive clotting in vivo.

Measurement of various serum antiphospholipid antibodies (APLAs) is usually part of the work-up, including measurement of lupus anticoagulant,[113] anticardiolipin antibodies, and β_2-glycoprotein 1 antibodies. Increased activity of APLAs is found in patients with systemic lupus erythematosus, acquired immunodeficiency syndrome (AIDS), giant cell arteritis, and Sneddon syndrome[114] (livedo reticularis and strokes). When the APLAs are not associated with other conditions and the patient has clinical evidence of excess clotting, the disorder is considered to be primary and is referred to as the *primary APLA syndrome*. Patients with APLAs can have increased incidence of spontaneous abortions, venous occlusive disease of the legs and pulmonary embolism, brain infarcts (often multiple), thrombocytopenia, and false-positive syphilis serologic tests.

Patients with systemic illnesses often have elevated erythrocyte sedimentation rates. Strokes and pulmonary emboli often follow and complicate myocardial infarction. Customarily, such brain infarcts have been attributed to cardiogenic embolism, but some undoubtedly are related to thromboses precipitated by increased levels of acute-phase reactant coagulation proteins. Cancer, especially mucinous adenocarcinoma of the lung, breast, and gastrointestinal tract, has been associated with multiple vascular occlusions, large and tiny brain infarcts, and venous and arterial occlusions.[115]

Subarachnoid Hemorrhage

The most frequent lesions causing SAH are abnormal vessels such as aneurysms and vascular malformations on or near the surface of the brain. An abrupt increase in BP (eg, caused by use of drugs such as cocaine or amphetamines) can sometimes lead to SAH, as can a bleeding diathesis, trauma, and cerebral amyloid angiopathy. SAH describes bleeding directly into the subarachnoid space with rapid dissemination into the cerebrospinal fluid (CSF) pathways.

There may be a past history of a *warning leak or sentinel hemorrhage*, presenting as a sudden-onset headache unusual for the patient that lasts days and prevents normal activities.[24] Aneurysms are usually located at bifurcations of major intracranial arteries. CTA and MRA are useful tests for screening and detecting aneurysms,[116] although the gold standard remains digital subtraction angiography. In patients who present with thunderclap headache yet head CT negative for hemorrhage, lumbar puncture is important in the diagnosis of SAH. The absence of blood in the CSF effectively excludes the diagnosis of SAH if the fluid is examined within 24 hours of the onset of the headache, but bleeds that are very small in volume or older than 72 hours can be missed.

The two most important neurologic complications of aneurysmal SAH are rebleeding and brain ischemia caused by vasoconstriction (vasospasm). Aneurysm rebleeding is highest in the first day (4%) and then is estimated 1% to 2% per day in the first month[23] or cumulatively 20% to 30% in the first month, and then 3% per year.[24] Endovascular coiling or surgical clipping of the aneurysmal sac or obliteration of the aneurysm by endovascular use of balloons or other devices should be attempted before rebleeding occurs.

In patients with SAH secondary to ruptured intracranial aneurysm, two randomized trials demonstrated improved clinical outcome in patients who underwent endovascular coiling of the aneurysm compared with neurosurgical clipping. Decreased death or dependence at 1 year was observed with use of coiling compared with clipping in both trials. National inpatient trends toward increased utilization of endovascular coiling have been observed for unruptured aneurysms compared to clipping since the publication of these two landmark trials, demonstrating lower complication rates and shorter length of stay with coiling.[25]

Cerebral vasospasm of the intracranial arteries is thought to be caused by blood or blood products that bathe the adventitia of arteries. Vasospasm usually has its onset 3 to 5 days after hemorrhage, peaks on days 5 to 9, and usually improves after day 14. It is an angiographic phenomenon, and increases the risk of resultant brain ischemia and infarction, which is a clinical manifestation.[117] The clinical findings in patients with delayed cerebral ischemia due to vasospasm are often those of diffuse brain swelling, such as headache, decreased alertness, and confusion. When vasoconstriction is focal, the clinical findings are those of focal ischemia, such as hemiparesis, aphasia, hemianopia.

Cerebral vasospasm is detected by angiography in 30% to 70% of patients with SAH, depending on the timing of the study. TCD is effective in monitoring for the presence of vasoconstriction.[116] Many treatments have been tried to prevent or treat cerebral vasospasm after SAH. At present, the most common approaches are early securing of the aneurysm, nimodipine (a calcium channel blocker), euvolemic and hypertensive therapy, with intra-arterial rescue in the setting of patients with neurological deficit refractory to medical management. Hypovolemia is common after SAH, as is hyponatremia. Euvolemia does not reverse the vasospasm but helps maintain brain perfusion.

Functional Outcomes after Stroke

Early and aggressive physical, occupational, cognitive, and speech therapies, as indicated, improve function after stroke. Functional outcomes after stroke are usually graded using a modified Rankin scale (mRS) where scores range from 0 (no symptoms) or 1 (minimal symptoms, no disability) to 2 (slight disability but functioning independently), 3 (moderate disability requiring some assistance, but able to walk independently), 4 (needing assistance for ambulation), 5 (bedridden), and 6 (dead).[118]

Vascular Contributions to Cognitive Impairment and Dementia

At the start of the 20th century, most persons with late-onset dementia were thought to have "hardening of the arteries" as the underlying reason. Over time, as the importance of Alzheimer pathology of amyloid plaques and neurofibrillary tangles became clear, the concept of vascular dementia shrank to dementia resulting from multiple infarcts or hemorrhages or very extensive white matter hyperintensities (Binswanger disease).[119] However, as this century began and the continuum of cognitive decline from normal to mild cognitive impairment (clear decline or impairment compared to peers but compensating to function normally) to clinical dementia (also called major neurocognitive disorder) became widely recognized, a broader concept of *vascular cognitive impairment* (VCI) reemerged.[120,121] The term VCI is now used to describe any syndrome of cognitive and behavioral impairment, affecting at least one cognitive domain, and consequent to vascular factors affecting the brain.

The documentation of disease affecting the blood vessels or blood flow to part or all of the brain, and clinical or radiologic evidence of structural damage to the brain due to these vascular factors establishes the structural basis for a diagnosis of VCI; since subclinical vascular brain injury is 5 times more common than clinical strokes, VCI typically shows covert brain infarcts, usually lacunes, white matter hyperintensities, microhemorrhages, enlarged perivascular spaces (around deep arterioles, venules), and cortical microinfarcts.[120] The presence of some degree of vascular copathology becomes extremely common in older persons with neurodegenerative diseases and the frequency with which such vascular injury is detected has increased as our brain MRI methods improve (to include diffusion weighted imaging, diffusion tensor imaging, 7T magnet strengths and measurements of cerebrovascular reactivity, and blood–brain barrier integrity, for example). Hence, the current emphasis is on independently understanding the "vascular contributions to cognitive impairment and dementia (VCID)," which is thought to include an acceleration of neurodegenerative processes such as amyloid and tau accumulation.

The proportion of all persons diagnosed with dementia in whom the etiology is partly or wholly attributable to vascular causes appears to vary by age, ethnicity, geography, and definition used.[122] The clinical profile of VCID can be extremely varied but patients are more often younger, male with a pattern of multifocal deficits, presence of focal neurologic signs (including gait abnormalities), an early and disproportionately greater involvement of psychomotor speed, executive dysfunction when compared to memory loss, and relatively preserved recognition (improved performance when clues are offered) in comparison with spontaneous recall.[123] Depression and emotional lability are also more frequently seen.

The Harmonizing Brain Imaging Methods for Vascular Contributions to Neurodegeneration (HARNESS) group has provided MR protocols and analysis tools (https:// harness-neuroimaging.org/)[124] and the Standards for Reporting Vascular Changes on Neuroimaging (STRIVE) criteria are widely used to define and describe common cerebrovascular pathologies on brain MRI.[125] Similarly, the MarkVCID initiative funded by the National Institute of Neurological Disorders and Stroke (NINDS) currently aims to establish and validate both neuroimaging and serum- or fluid-based biomarkers for VCI (https://markvcid.partners.org/), the DISCOVERY (Determinants of Incident Stroke Cognitive Outcomes and Vascular Effects on RecoverY) study will explore the blood and imaging predictors of VCID after an acute stroke and the INDEED (The Clinical Significance of Incidental White Matter Lesions on MRI Amongst a Diverse Population With Cognitive Complaints) study will explore the cognitive consequences of MRI white matter hyperintensities. Risk factors for VCID are the same as those for clinical stroke.[126] The Hachinski Ischemic Score based on the presence or absence of vascular risk factors and on the clinical course and signs is a quick bedside screening test to consider if vascular brain injury plays an important role in a patient's cognitive decline and dementia. In an abbreviated version, a score of 7 or more out of a possible 12 points is considered diagnostic of VCID, whereas a score less than 4 is thought to exclude VCID. There is strong evidence that lowering BP among persons with hypertension preserves cognition[127] by preventing stroke and perhaps through improved cerebral blood flow, but the optimal level of BP for preserving cognition, may be higher in persons over age 80 compared to younger persons. VCID is managed mainly by control of vascular risk factors to prevent a second stroke. The memory symptoms in this setting may improve with the use of acetylcholinesterase inhibitors used for Alzheimer's disease. Other symptomatic treatments may be required.

ACUTE TREATMENT OF STROKE

Intravenous Thrombolysis

Thrombolytic drugs, especially recombinant tissue-type plasminogen activator (or alteplase) and tenecteplase, have been given intravenously and intra-arterially in patients with acute brain ischemia. In the classic NINDS study in which the arterial lesions were undefined, intravenous therapy with rt-PA given within 90 minutes and 3 hours of ischemia onset, in the aggregate, provided a statistically significant benefit.[128]

The European Cooperative Acute Stroke Study (ECASS) showed extended benefit of intravenous t-PA when given 3 to 4.5 hours after ischemic stroke symptom on set.[129,130] In these studies, up to 6% of patients treated with thrombolytic agents developed intracranial bleeding. Patients with embolic ICA occlusions in the neck and intracranially rarely reperfuse after intravenous thrombolytic therapy, especially if collateral circulation is poor. Brain imaging should precede administration of thrombolytic agents to ensure there is no intracranial hemorrhage or large infarct that would preclude its administration.

Intravenous Thrombolysis in the Extended Time Window

The treatment window for thrombolysis can be extended to 9 hours, or treatment can be considered for patients with unknown time of symptom onset, with the addition of advanced perfusion imaging showing ischemic but not yet infarcted tissue. The EXTEND (Extending the Time for Thrombolysis in Emergency Neurological Deficits) study randomized patients presenting between 4.5 and 9 hours after the onset of stroke, or on awakening with stroke (if within 9 hours from the midpoint of sleep) to IV alteplase versus placebo.[131] The primary outcome of no or minor neurological deficits, defined as a mRS score of 0 or 1 at 90 days, was present in more patients in the alteplase compared to placebo group (35.4% vs 29.5%, absolute risk reduction [ARR] 1.44; 95% CI, 1.0–2.1, $P = 0.04$). The WAKE-UP trial was a European study that randomly assigned patients with unknown time of onset of stroke, with ischemic lesion visible on diffusion-weighted MRI sequences but without corresponding FLAIR (fluid-attenuated inversion recovery) changes (indicating stroke had occurred approximately within 4.5 hours), to receive intravenous alteplase versus placebo.[132] Thrombectomy patients were excluded. Favorable outcome at 90 days was higher in the rt-PA versus placebo group (53.3% vs 41.8%, odds ratio [OR] 1.61; $P = 0.003$). Numerically, more intracranial hemorrhages were seen in the rt-PA versus placebo group for both studies, at 2% to 6%.

Endovascular Therapy of Large Vessel Occlusion Stroke

Early Time Window Trials, 0 to 8 Hours

The recent results of multiple randomized clinical trials across the world demonstrating the benefit of endovascular therapy compared to medical management heralds a new paradigm and standard of care for patients with large vessel occlusion stroke.[133-139] This paradigm is robust not only in highly resourced countries but also in low- and middle-income countries such as Brazil.[140] CT brain, CTA, and occasionally CT perfusion were the imaging modalities used to select patients into these early trials of patients presenting in the early window of stroke symptom onset, generally up to 6 to 8 hours. In these studies, patients received IV alteplase where eligible and stent retrievers were the main devices used for clot retrieval of mechanical thrombectomy (**Fig. 25–7**). A pooled HERMES meta-analysis of five randomized trials (MR CLEAN, ESCAPE, REVASCAT, SWIFT PRIME, EXTEND-IA) including 1287 individual data of patients with occlusion of the proximal anterior artery circulation within 12 hours of symptom onset

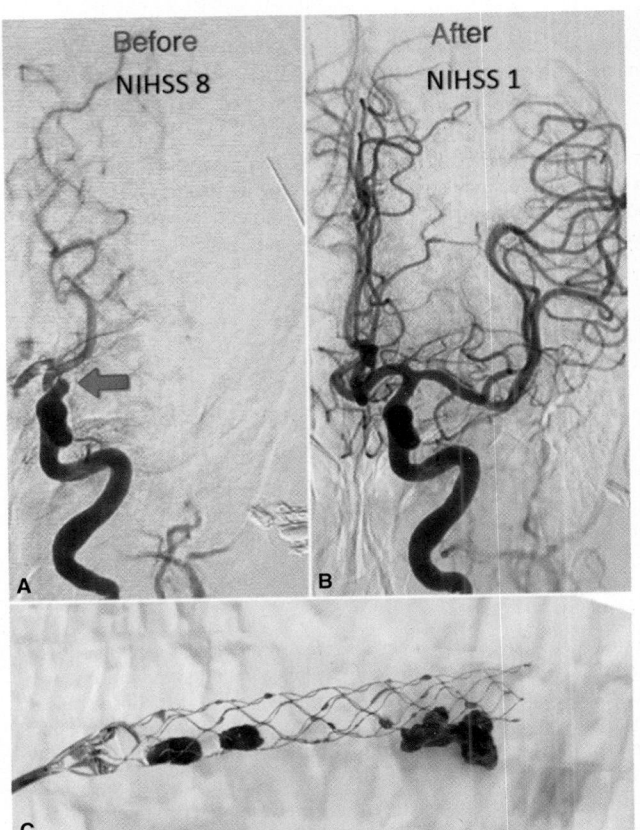

Figure 25–7. Endovascular mechanical thrombectomy for treatment of a large vessel embolic occlusion. (A) Digital subtraction angiography image of an abrupt cut off at the distal intracranial left ICA. **(B)** Reconstitution of flow in the anterior cerebral artery and middle cerebral artery territories subsequent to thrombectomy, with improvement of symptoms to near-resolution. **(C)** Stentriever device with clot/embolus fragments. NIHSS, National Institutes of Health Stroke Scale.

showed endovascular thrombectomy significantly reduced disability at 90 days compared to control (adjusted crude odds ratio [COR] 2.49; 95% CI, 1.76–3.53; $P < 0.0001$), with a number needed to treat to reduce disability by at least one level on mRS of 2.6. Subgroup analysis demonstrated benefit in patients 80 years or older (COR 3.68; 95% CI, 1.95–6.92), patients randomized more than 50 hours after symptom onset, and patients who were not eligible for IV alteplase (COR 2.43, 95% CI, 2.43–4.55).

Postmarketing registries have replicated outcomes of large vessel occlusion therapy clinical trials showing that these results can be reproduced in "real life," as with the NASA[141] and TRACK[142] registries. The notion of "first pass effect," defined as complete recanalization with a single thrombectomy device pass, correlates with good clinical outcome and has gained momentum as a measure upon which devices are benchmarked for success.[143] Compared to conventional guide catheters, balloon guide catheters have been demonstrated to be associated with better reperfusion scores and clinical outcomes, likely due to reduced distal emboli with balloon inflation of the guide catheter in the neck, and interruption of antegrade flow with each retrieval pass.[144,145] With technological advances, large bore aspiration catheters were shown

to have similar results as stent retriever in opening up large vessel occlusion arteries in two randomized trials.[146,147] Rescue intra-arterial thrombolysis[148] and intracranial stenting[149] are alternative techniques in the setting of failed mechanical thrombectomy with better reperfusion scores and similar clinical outcomes.

Late Time Window Thrombectomy, 6 to 24 Hours

Another paradigm shift in stroke care is the definition of a "late window" based on results of the DAWN trial in 2018, and later the DEFUSE-3 trial.[150,151] Patients who present in this delayed or extended window are thought to be slow progressors, with leptomeningeal collaterals that help sustain salvageable brain tissue in the presence of a large vessel occlusion yet small core infarct.[152] These trials studied patients with large vessel anterior circulation occlusion presenting within the late time window, from 6 to up to 24 hours from when they were last known to be normal, and who were selected by clinical imaging mismatch or perfusion imaging mismatch. Both studies showed significant benefit in functional independence at 90 days in favor of endovascular thrombectomy compared to medical management (DAWN: 49% vs 13%, DEFUSE-3: 45% vs 17%, $P < 0.001$); symptomatic ICH risk was similar between the two study groups for both studies, and was up to 7%.

Beyond 24 hours from symptom onset of stroke, two nonrandomized studies showed that clinical benefit could still be achieved if patients were selected based on target mismatch profiles.[153,154] In a propensity score-matched analysis of a Korean single center study, endovascular therapy was associated with better odds of good clinical outcome defined by mRS 0 to 2 (adjusted OR 11.1; 95% CI, 1.9–108.6) or 90-day mRS score shift (COR 5.2; 95% CI, 1.8–15.6).[154]

Table 25–4 summarizes and compares the United States, Canadian, and European guidelines for management of acute ischemic stroke with intravenous thrombolysis and endovascular mechanical thrombectomy. Because of ongoing clinical trials and the evolving data since these guidelines were published in 2018 and 2019, stronger recommendations are likely to be made in future guidelines with regards to alternative thrombolytics (ie, tenecteplase) and treatments in the late window.

Intra-Arterial Thrombolysis

In the current era of mechanical thrombectomy, intra-arterial thrombolysis has transitioned to a secondary rather than primary role for opening proximal large vessel occlusions. As stent-retrievers were the primary devices utilized in the majority of the aforementioned landmark trials, the evidence is weighted in favor of mechanical over chemical means in opening up vessel blockages. Intra-arterial thrombolysis, however, continues to play an important role for rescue therapy in the setting of failed mechanical thrombectomy and with distal occlusions.[148,155] The intra-arterial doses utilized for alteplase usually range from 3 mg to 10 mg. The time window of administration of intra-arterial thrombolytic is typically within 6 hours of last known well. The benefit of intra-arterial thrombolysis beyond this time window is unknown, but may, in part, be supported by the recent studies demonstrating benefit of

TABLE 25–4. Comparison of United States, Canadian, and European Guidelines for Management of Acute Ischemic Stroke

	American Heart Association/American Stroke Association Guidelines (2019)[18]	Canadian Stroke Best Practice Recommendations (2018)[190]	European Stroke Organisation[191] and Karolinska Stroke Update Conference (2019)[48]
Intravenous (IV) thrombolysis with recombinant tissue-type plasminogen activator (rt-PA or alteplase) or tenecteplase to treat eligible adult ischemic stroke patients who present within 3 to 4.5 hours last known well before symptom onset	Yes, although recommendations for treatment in the 3- to 4.5-hour window for (1) severe stroke and (2) history of stroke and diabetes are considered "weak" with only nonrandomized or limited data available. Recommendations for use of tenecteplase were also considered "weak" with only moderate-quality evidence: (1) tenecteplase may be considered as an alternative to alteplase in patients with minor neurological impairment and no major intracranial occlusion and (2) may be considered over alteplase in patients who are eligible to undergo mechanical thrombectomy.	Yes, except use of tenecteplase is not recommended until further evidence from ongoing clinical trials is available.	Yes, except tenecteplase as an alternative to alteplase is not recommended in routine practice.
IV thrombolysis to eligible adult ischemic stroke patients who present within 4.5 to 9 hours from time last known well, or with unknown time from symptom onset, with the use of advanced perfusion imaging or MRI to show ischemic, but not yet infarcted tissue at risk	Yes, based on moderate-quality evidence from a single randomized trial,[133] a "moderate"-strength recommendation is made to treat eligible patients who have unclear time of onset, using MRI to identify ischemic but not yet infarcted tissue. No recommendation is made for the specific 4.5- to 9-hour delayed time window.	Yes, treatment time windows after 4.5 hours with IV alteplase can be considered using MRI selection criteria; consultation with a physician with stroke expertise is recommended. No recommendation is made for the specific 4.5- to 9-hour delayed time window.	Yes, IV alteplase is recommended in eligible patients who present with an unknown time of onset, guided by MRI imaging to show ischemic, but not yet infarcted tissue. For the 4.5- to 9-hour time window a preliminary recommendation was made because peer-reviewed trial results were not yet available[131]: IV alteplase may be considered, guided by MRI or CT perfusion imaging.
Endovascular mechanical thrombectomy to revascularize a large vessel occlusion in patients who present within the early window up to 6 hours from time last known well before symptom onset	Yes, for patients with no preexisting stroke disability and: - small-to-moderate ischemic core on neuroimaging - occlusion of the intracranial internal carotid artery or middle cerebral artery segment 1 - at least moderate-severity stroke symptoms (National Institutes of Health Stroke Scale [NIHSS] >6) - Outside of these indications (eg, large core infarct or occlusion of the middle cerebral artery segment 2 or posterior circulation artery), benefits are uncertain, with a "weak" recommendation to treat carefully selected patients, based on randomized trials and limited data.	Yes, for functionally independent patients with life expectancy >3 months and: - small-to-moderate ischemic core on neuroimaging - proximal intracranial anterior circulation artery occlusion - disabling stroke symptoms Outside of these indications (eg, large core infarct or posterior circulation occlusion), decision to treat should be made by a physician with expertise in stroke, in consultation with the neuro-interventionalist and the patient and/or substitute decision maker.	Yes, for patients with: - small-to-moderate ischemic core on neuroimaging - intracranial anterior circulation artery occlusion - at least moderate-severity (NIHSS >6) stroke symptoms Outside of these indications (eg, large core infarct or patients with disabling stroke and NIHSS <6), treatment is reasonable based on expert opinion. Treatment of posterior circulation occlusion should strongly be considered.
Guided by advanced imaging, patients presenting between 6 and 24 hours may be eligible to undergo endovascular mechanical thrombectomy	Yes, in selected patients that meet eligibility criteria from clinical trials[15,151] that used either: Mismatch between (1) the clinical score (NIHSS) and (2) core infarct volume as assessed by findings on CT perfusion or diffusion weighted MRI or, A combination of (1) perfusion-core mismatch on perfusion CT or MRI and (2) a maximum core infarct volume		

intravenous therapy in patients with favorable imaging mismatch profile.[132]

Reversal of Anticoagulation in Setting of Intracerebral Hemorrhage

Warfarin

Warfarin-associated ICH tends to present with larger baseline hematoma volumes[156] and has higher likelihood of hematoma growth[157] resulting in higher mortality and worse functional outcome.[157,158] It accounts for an increasing proportion of ICH, owing to the addition of new classes of anticoagulants in the last decade and more widespread use.[159] Previous studies in patients with warfarin-associated ICH have clearly shown that reversal of coagulopathy (measured by the INR),[160] is associated with significantly lower rates of hematoma growth.[161] The effect is particularly time-sensitive, vanishing ~5.5 hours from symptom onset. The threshold of achieved INR below which a benefit is apparent was determined at 1.3.[161]

Several studies have demonstrated the superiority of 4-factor prothrombin complex concentrate (PCC) over fresh frozen plasma (FFP). It achieves anticoagulation reversal significantly faster (within 30 minutes to 1 hour) without need for thawing and complications from volume overload.[162,163] PCC is the preferred means for rapid coagulation reversal.

In patients who have been exposed to vitamin K antagonists like warfarin, vitamin K should be given as well, although its effect is biologically apparent 1 to 3 days later; it is not suitable as the sole reversal agent.

Direct Oral Anticoagulants

DOACs, including dabigatran, rivaroxaban, apixaban, and edoxaban, have a superior safety profile compared to warfarin, especially with regards to ICH risk.[164] Their main benefit (no need for routine monitoring) presents a relative drawback in the context of a hemorrhagic complication as there is no widely available laboratory test, analogous to INR, to confirm the presence and intensity of anticoagulant effect and monitor the reversal. New specific antidotes have been developed and clinically tested: for dabigatran, a monoclonal antibody (idarucizumab) achieves rapid removal of dabigatran from the blood, restoration of the clotting mechanism, and satisfactory hemostasis.[165] For the factor Xa inhibitors (rivaroxaban, apixaban, edoxaban) andexanet alfa[166] is recommended; it has been shown to rapidly restore the disrupted coagulation cascade and achieve good or excellent hemostasis in most patients.[167]

Although FDA-approved for clinical use, there are issues with widespread availability and cost, especially for andexanet. In the absence of specific antidotes, use of PCC or FFP is recommended as the only available option, although clinical efficacy in such cases is unproven. If ingestion is very recent, activated charcoal might be used to remove the medication before it is fully absorbed.

Subacute Medical Management of Stroke and Transient Ischemic Attack

Because most patients with ischemic stroke, TIA, and ICH are at increased risk of developing recurrent events, including stroke and myocardial infarction, control of risk factors is very important and should begin in the hospital. Risk factor modification can include treatment plans to address smoking, poor diet, hyperlipidemia, diabetes, and hypertension. BP should not be excessively lowered during the acute ischemic period because this may decrease flow in collateral arteries. Although the benefit of treating severe hypertension (>220/120) in acute stroke is not well established, it is likely reasonable in this scenario to carefully decrease BP by 15% in the first 24 hours.[18] Excessive reduction in BP in the acute period may be detrimental for patients with severe vascular stenosis or occlusion, and for patients with early neurologic worsening. Rehabilitation must also begin early.

ANTITHROMBOTICS FOR SECONDARY STROKE PREVENTION

Antiplatelet Monotherapy

Aspirin

Aspirin monotherapy is the mainstay of short- and long-term secondary stroke prevention, based on landmark trials that showed an unequivocal but modest effect with a relative risk reduction of approximately 15%.[168] Doses ranging from 30 mg to 1300 mg have been used in various trials with favorable clinical effect observed starting at 30 mg without clear increase in benefit with higher doses. Hence, low-dose aspirin is routinely recommended for secondary stroke prevention in clinical practice.[168] There is no benefit of aspirin for primary stroke prevention in patients with vascular disease and its use is not recommended.[169]

Alternative Antiplatelet Classes

Clopidogrel[170] and the combination of aspirin/dipyridamole[171,172] have both been tested against aspirin and against one another[173] with comparable efficacy and safety; all three are considered equally acceptable choices.[104] There is paucity of evidence to address the question whether transitioning to a different antiplatelet class is beneficial in the case of a stroke occurring in patients already on antiplatelet therapy.[104] A recent trial found no significant difference in the efficacy and safety of ticagrelor monotherapy versus aspirin in the early recurrence of stroke in patients with minor stroke or TIA.[174]

Antiplatelet versus Anticoagulation Therapy in Noncardioembolic Stroke and ESUS

Most of the initial secondary prevention studies were all-inclusive, without accounting for stroke subtype. After the superiority of anticoagulation for cardioembolic strokes and carotid endarterectomy for extracranial internal carotid atherosclerotic stenosis were established, subsequent studies were performed on more focused patient populations. A large randomized trial compared aspirin and dose-adjusted warfarin in patients with noncardioembolic stroke[175] and found no significant difference in recurrent stroke or major hemorrhage; hence, empiric anticoagulation is not recommended unless a cardioembolic source is established.

More recently, the clinical and imaging construct of ESUS[6] has attracted considerable attention. It was postulated that a majority of these infarcts are due to occult atrial fibrillation and other cardioembolic sources and anticoagulation was expected to be beneficial. However, two recent randomized controlled trials failed to show superiority of rivaroxaban[176] and dabigatran[177] over aspirin. This failure was attributed to presence of noncardiac embolic sources such as nonstenotic atherosclerotic plaques in a considerable proportion of the patients. Two randomized trials of apixaban versus aspirin in selective populations with ESUS and atrial cardiopathy[7] anticipated to derive benefit from anticoagulation are currently under way.

Dual Antiplatelet Therapy

Large-scale clinical trials using combinations of aspirin and clopidogrel showed a decrease in recurrent ischemic stroke that was offset by increased hemorrhage risk.[178,179] The same approach in a study that focused specifically on patients with recent small vessel (lacunar) stroke yielded similar results.[180] Therefore, long-term dual antiplatelet therapy is not recommended for secondary stroke prevention. However, a consistent observation was that the risk of stroke recurrence is front-loaded with the majority occurring in the first 3 months after the index stroke. This led to recent clinical trials of short-term dual antiplatelet regimens. Two studies using an aspirin–clopidogrel combination[11,181] showed a significant reduction in ischemic stroke recurrence without reciprocal increase in hemorrhage risk; this finding was replicated in a study using a ticagrelor–aspirin combination.[182] Therefore, a short-course regimen of aspirin and clopidogrel or ticagrelor for up to 90 days is an accepted practice in patients with minor ischemic strokes and TIAs categorized as high risk for subsequent stroke.

Cilostazol merits a separate mention: Several studies have examined its efficacy as monotherapy or in combination with aspirin against aspirin monotherapy, with favorable effects in general, especially for the combination treatments.[183] A major caveat is that all the cilostazol clinical trials have been conducted in Asia and their generalizability to non-Asian populations remains to be studied.

Intracranial Large Artery Atherosclerosis

The effectiveness of anticoagulation with dose-adjusted warfarin versus high-dose aspirin was examined in a population of patients with ischemic strokes attributed to significant (>50%) atherosclerotic stenosis of large intracranial arteries.[184] The study was terminated prematurely due to a higher rate of complications in the warfarin group and anticoagulation is not routinely used in these patients. A subsequent study examined the effectiveness of intracranial stenting against best medical management, consisting of a 3-month combination of high-dose aspirin and clopidogrel and high-intensity statin. This study was also terminated prematurely due to a higher complication rate in the stenting group. A 90-day regimen of aspirin and clopidogrel is the treatment of choice for patients with strokes from intracranial atherosclerotic stenosis.

Anticoagulation in Patients with Cardioembolic Risk and Intracerebral Hemorrhage

Initiation or resumption of anticoagulation in patients with ICH is a common conundrum in clinical practice. The most frequent scenario is that of patients with high-risk atrial fibrillation with a CHA_2DS_2-VASc score ≥ 2 who have suffered a recent ICH and the question is safety and timing of anticoagulation. There is very little randomized clinical trial data to guide these decisions. In one recent, open-label trial, 537 patients with occlusive vascular disease and ICH were randomized to resume or withhold antiplatelet therapy.[185] No difference in the rate of recurrent ICH was observed over a median follow-up of 2 years, offering reassurance regarding the use of antiplatelets in this population. However, the issue of therapeutic anticoagulation remains inadequately addressed; all relevant studies are observational and subject to bias and confounding. Several randomized controlled trials are underway: The EdoxabaN foR IntraCranial Hemorrhage Survivors With Atrial Fibrillation (ENRICH-AF-NCT03950076) and Anticoagulation in ICH Survivors for Stroke Prevention and Recovery (ASPIRE-NCT03907046) clinical trials randomize patients with high-risk atrial fibrillation and recent ICH to edoxaban and apixaban versus antiplatelet, respectively. The Avoiding Anticoagulation After IntraCerebral Haemorrhage (A3ICH-NCT03243175) is a three-arm study with similar design with an additional third group of patients randomized to left atrial appendage closure. These trials should be completed between 2022 and 2024.

In this patient population, direct oral anticoagulants are preferred due to their superior safety profile over vitamin K antagonists.[166] Given the central role of hypertension in the pathogenesis of ICH,[186] it is advisable to ensure adequate and sustained control of BP before commencing anticoagulation. MRI markers of ICH risk such as cerebral microbleeds[187] and cortical superficial siderosis[188] are potentially useful in risk stratification. However, their association with recurrent ICH and ischemia in patients with cardioembolic stroke and embolic stroke of undetermined source remains controversial.[187,189] Their interpretation should be individualized and context-specific.

SUMMARY

Cardioembolic stroke etiologies and approach to secondary stroke prevention

- Anticoagulation considered standard of care:
  - Atrial fibrillation or flutter
  - Thrombus in the left atrium, left atrial appendage, or left ventricle
  - Recent anterior myocardial infarction (<4 weeks) with left ventricular thrombus
  - Presence of a left ventricular assist device
  - Mitral stenosis, when associated with rheumatic heart disease and recurrent embolic events, and where paroxysmal atrial fibrillation is suspected
- Anticoagulation + antiplatelet considered standard of care:
  - Mechanical aortic or mitral prosthetic valve

- Anticoagulation may be of value or warrants further study:
  - Systolic heart failure with low ejection fraction (<15%), without visualized thrombus
  - Nonbacterial thrombotic endocarditis, especially with coexistent hypercoagulability
  - Papillary fibroelastoma, if surgical resection is contraindicated
  - Atrial cardiopathy in setting of embolic stroke of undetermined source
- Anticoagulation contraindicated:
  - Infective endocarditis, treated with antibiotics
  - Atrial myxoma, treated with surgical resection
- Antiplatelet considered standard of care:
  - Bioprosthetic aortic or mitral valve
  - Aortic arch atheroma
- Surgical closure of PFO in cryptogenic stroke patients in whom it is determined the PFO has a likely causative role (ie, a combination of early onset stroke age <60 years, embolic appearing stroke on imaging, lack of vascular risk factors)

ACKNOWLEDGMENT

The authors wish to acknowledge Megan C. Leary, Jeffrey S. Veluz, and Louis R. Caplan, the previous edition's authors, for their contributions to this new chapter.

REFERENCES

1. Smith EE, Saposnik G, Biessels GJ, Doubal FN, et al. Prevention of stroke in patients with silent cerebrovascular disease: a scientific statement for healthcare professionals from the American Heart Association/American Stroke Association. *Stroke*. 2017;48:e44-e71.

2. Adams HP, Jr., Bendixen BH, Kappelle LJ, et al. Classification of subtype of acute ischemic stroke. Definitions for use in a multicenter clinical trial. TOAST. Trial of Org 10172 in Acute Stroke Treatment. *Stroke*. 1993;24:35-41.

3. Ay H, Furie KL, Singhal A, Smith WS, Sorensen AG, Koroshetz WJ. An evidence-based causative classification system for acute ischemic stroke. *Ann Neurol*. 2005;58:688-697.

4. Amarenco P, Bogousslavsky J, Caplan LR, Donnan GA, Wolf ME, Hennerici MG. The ASCOD phenotyping of ischemic stroke (Updated ASCO Phenotyping). *Cerebrovasc Dis*. 2013;36:1-5.

5. Wardlaw JM, Smith EE, Biessels GJ, et al. Neuroimaging standards for research into small vessel disease and its contribution to ageing and neurodegeneration. *Lancet Neurol*. 2013;12:822-838.

6. Hart RG, Diener HC, Coutts SB, et al. Embolic strokes of undetermined source: the case for a new clinical construct. *Lancet Neurol*. 2014;13:429-438.

7. Kamel H, Bartz TM, Elkind MSV, et al. Atrial cardiopathy and the risk of ischemic stroke in the CHS (Cardiovascular Health Study). *Stroke*. 2018;49:980-986.

8. Kamel H, Longstreth WT, Jr, Tirschwell DL, et al. The AtRial Cardiopathy and Antithrombotic Drugs In prevention After cryptogenic stroke randomized trial: rationale and methods. *Int J Stroke*. 2019;14:207-214.

9. Lioutas VA, Ivan CS, Himali JJ, et al. Incidence of Transient Ischemic Attack and Association With Long-term Risk of Stroke. *JAMA*. 2021;26; 325:373-381.

10. Kleindorfer D, Panagos P, Pancioli A, et al. Incidence and short-term prognosis of transient ischemic attack in a population-based study. *Stroke*. 2005;36:720-723.

11. Johnston SC, Easton JD, Farrant M, et al. Clopidogrel and aspirin in acute ischemic stroke and high-risk TIA. *N Engl J Med*. 2018;379:215-225.

12. Johnston SC, Rothwell PM, Nguyen-Huynh MN, et al. Validation and refinement of scores to predict very early stroke risk after transient ischaemic attack. *Lancet*. 2007;369:283-292.

13. Amarenco P, Lavallee PC, Monteiro Tavares L, et al. Five-year risk of stroke after TIA or minor ischemic stroke. *N Engl J Med*. 2018;378:2182-2190.

14. Rodrigues MA, Samarasekera N, Lerpiniere C, et al. The Edinburgh CT and genetic diagnostic criteria for lobar intracerebral haemorrhage associated with cerebral amyloid angiopathy: model development and diagnostic test accuracy study. *Lancet Neurol*. 2018;17:232-240.

15. Albers GW, Marks MP, Kemp S, et al. Thrombectomy for stroke at 6 to 16 hours with selection by perfusion imaging. *N Engl J Med*. 2018;378: 708-718.

16. Campbell BCV, Majoie C, Albers GW, et al. Penumbral imaging and functional outcome in patients with anterior circulation ischaemic stroke treated with endovascular thrombectomy versus medical therapy: a meta-analysis of individual patient-level data. *Lancet Neurol*. 2019;18:46-55.

17. Marks MP, Lansberg MG, Mlynash M, et al. Effect of collateral blood flow on patients undergoing endovascular therapy for acute ischemic stroke. *Stroke*. 2014;45:1035-1039.

18. Powers WJ, Rabinstein AA, Ackerson T, et al. Guidelines for the early management of patients with acute ischemic stroke: 2019 update to the 2018 guidelines for the early management of acute ischemic stroke: a guideline for healthcare professionals from the American Heart Association/American Stroke Association. *Stroke*. 2019;50:e344-e418.

19. Huttner HB, Schwab S. Malignant middle cerebral artery infarction: clinical characteristics, treatment strategies, and future perspectives. *Lancet Neurol*. 2009;8:949-958.

20. Hanley DF, Thompson RE, Rosenblum M, et al. Efficacy and safety of minimally invasive surgery with thrombolysis in intracerebral haemorrhage evacuation (MISTIE III): a randomised, controlled, open-label, blinded endpoint phase 3 trial. *Lancet*. 2019;393:1021-1032.

21. Sondag L, Schreuder F, Boogaarts HD, et al. Neurosurgical intervention for supratentorial intracerebral hemorrhage. *Ann Neurol*. 2020;88:239-250.

22. Wagner KR, Sharp FR, Ardizzone TD, Lu A, Clark JF. Heme and iron metabolism: role in cerebral hemorrhage. *J Cereb Blood Flow Metab*. 2003;23:629-652.

23. Selim M, Foster LD, Moy CS, et al. Deferoxamine mesylate in patients with intracerebral haemorrhage (i-DEF): a multicentre, randomised, placebo-controlled, double-blind phase 2 trial. *Lancet Neurol*. 2019;18:428-438.

24. Macdonald RL, Schweizer TA. Spontaneous subarachnoid haemorrhage. *Lancet*. 2017;389:655-666.

25. Krishnamurthi RV, Ikeda T, Feigin VL. Global, regional and country-specific burden of ischaemic stroke, intracerebral haemorrhage and subarachnoid haemorrhage: a systematic analysis of the Global Burden of Disease Study 2017. *Neuroepidemiology*. 2020;54:171-179.

26. Ay H, Arsava Ethem M, Andsberg G, et al. Pathogenic ischemic stroke phenotypes in the NINDS-Stroke Genetics Network. *Stroke*. 2014;45:3589-3596.

27. Seshadri S, Debette S. *Risk factors for cerebrovascular disease and stroke*. Oxford; New York: Oxford University Press; 2016.

28. Sharma P, Meschia JF. *Stroke genetics*. 2nd ed. Cham, Switzerland: Springer; 2017.

29. Virani SS, Alonso A, Aparicio HJ, et al. Heart disease and stroke statistics-2021 update: A report from the American Heart Association. *Circulation*. 2021;23;143:e254-e743.

30. Andreasen Trine H, Bartek J, Andresen M, Springborg Jacob B, Romner B. Modifiable risk factors for aneurysmal subarachnoid hemorrhage. *Stroke*. 2013;44:3607-3612.

31. Gorelick PB, Furie KL, Iadecola C, et al. Defining optimal brain health in adults: a presidential advisory from the American Heart Association/American Stroke Association. *Stroke.* 2017;48:e284-e303.

32. Kuźma E, Lourida I, Moore SF, Levine DA, Ukoumunne OC, Llewellyn DJ. Stroke and dementia risk: a systematic review and meta-analysis. *Alzheimers Dement.* 2018;14(11):1416-1426.

33. Snyder HM, Corriveau RA, Craft S, et al. Vascular contributions to cognitive impairment and dementia including Alzheimer's disease. *Alzheimers Dement.* 2015;11:710-717.

34. Debette S, Schilling S, Duperron M, Larsson SC, Markus HS. Clinical significance of magnetic resonance imaging markers of vascular brain injury: a systematic review and meta-analysis. *JAMA Neurol.* 2018.

35. Seshadri S, Beiser A, Pikula A, et al. Parental occurrence of stroke and risk of stroke in their children: the Framingham study. *Circulation.* 2010;121:1304-1312.

36. Dichgans M, Pulit SL, Rosand J. Stroke genetics: discovery, biology, and clinical applications. *Lancet Neurol.* 2019;18:587-599.

37. Chauhan G, Debette S. Genetic risk factors for ischemic and hemorrhagic stroke. *Curr Cardiol Rep.* 2016;18:124.

38. Malik R, Chauhan G, Traylor M, et al. Multiancestry genome-wide association study of 520,000 subjects identifies 32 loci associated with stroke and stroke subtypes. *Nat Genet.* 2018;50:524-537.

39. Georgakis MK, Malik R, Bjorkbacka H, et al. Circulating monocyte chemoattractant protein-1 and risk of stroke: meta-analysis of population-based studies involving 17 180 individuals. *Circ Res.* 2019;125:773-782.

40. Jian X, Satizabal CL, Smith AV, et al. Exome chip analysis identifies low-frequency and rare variants in MRPL38 for white matter hyperintensities on brain magnetic resonance imaging. *Stroke.* 2018;49:1812-1819.

41. Armstrong NJ, Mather KA, Sargurupremraj M, et al. Common genetic variation indicates separate causes for periventricular and deep white matter hyperintensities. *Stroke.* 2020;51:2111-2121.

42. Falcone GJ, Woo D. Genetics of spontaneous intracerebral hemorrhage. *Stroke.* 2017;48:3420-3424.

43. Bakker MK, van der Spek RAA, van Rheenen W, et al. Genome-wide association study of intracranial aneurysms identifies 17 risk loci and genetic overlap with clinical risk factors. *Nat Genet.* 2020.

44. Woo D, Anderson CD, Maguire J, et al. Top research priorities for stroke genetics. *Lancet Neurol.* 2018;17:663-665.

45. Topcuoglu MA, Rocha EA, Siddiqui AK, et al. Isolated upper limb weakness from ischemic stroke: mechanisms and outcome. *J Stroke Cerebrovasc Dis.* 2018;27:2712-2719.

46. Inoue M, Noda R, Yamaguchi S, et al. Specific factors to predict large-vessel occlusion in acute stroke patients. *J Stroke Cerebrovasc Dis.* 2018;27:886-891.

47. Babikian VL, Wijman CA. Brain embolism monitoring with transcranial Doppler ultrasound. *Curr Treat Opt Cardiovasc Med.* 2003;5:221-232.

48. Ahmed N, Audebert H, Turc G, et al. Consensus statements and recommendations from the ESO-Karolinska Stroke Update Conference, Stockholm 11-13 November 2018. *Eur Stroke J.* 2019;4:307-317.

49. Gladstone DJ, Spring M, Dorian P, et al. Atrial fibrillation in patients with cryptogenic stroke. *N Engl J Med.* 2014;370:2467-2477.

50. Sanna T, Diener H-C, Passman RS, et al. Cryptogenic stroke and underlying atrial fibrillation. *N Engl J Med.* 2014;370:2478-2486.

51. Sacchetti DC, Furie KL, Yaghi S. Cardioembolic stroke: mechanisms and therapeutics. *Seminars Neurol.* 2017;37:326-338.

52. Agha AM, Parwani P, Guha A, et al. Role of cardiovascular imaging for the diagnosis and prognosis of cardiac amyloidosis. *Open Heart.* 2018;5:e000881.

53. Saver JL. Clinical practice. Cryptogenic Stroke. *N Engl J Med.* 2016;374:2065-2074.

54. McGrath ER, Paikin JS, Motlagh B, Salehian O, Kapral MK, O'Donnell MJ. Transesophageal echocardiography in patients with cryptogenic ischemic stroke: a systematic review. *Am Heart J.* 2014;168:706-712.

55. Wolf PA, Abbott RD, Kannel WB. Atrial fibrillation as an independent risk factor for stroke: the Framingham Study. *Stroke.* 1991;22:983-988.

56. Lip GY, Nieuwlaat R, Pisters R, Lane DA, Crijns HJ. Refining clinical risk stratification for predicting stroke and thromboembolism in atrial fibrillation using a novel risk factor-based approach: the euro heart survey on atrial fibrillation. *Chest.* 2010;137:263-272.

57. Link MS, Giugliano RP, Ruff CT, et al. Stroke and mortality risk in patients with various patterns of atrial fibrillation: results from the ENGAGE AF-TIMI 48 trial (Effective Anticoagulation With Factor Xa Next Generation in Atrial Fibrillation-Thrombolysis in Myocardial Infarction 48). *Circ Arrhythm Electrophysiol.* 2017;10.

58. Hsu JC, Maddox TM, Kennedy KF, et al. Oral anticoagulant therapy prescription in patients with atrial fibrillation across the spectrum of stroke risk: insights from the NCDR PINNACLE Registry. Oral anticoagulant therapy in patients with atrial fibrillation. *JAMA Cardiol.* 2016;1:55-62.

59. Benedetto U, Gaudino Mario F, Dimagli A, et al. Postoperative atrial fibrillation and long-term risk of stroke after isolated coronary artery bypass graft surgery. *Circulation.* 2020;142:1320-1329.

60. Walkey AJ, Hammill BG, Curtis LH, Benjamin EJ. Long-term outcomes following development of new-onset atrial fibrillation during sepsis. *Chest.* 2014;146:1187-1195.

61. Vadmann H, Nielsen PB, Hjortshoj SP, Riahi S, Rasmussen LH, Lip GY, Larsen TB. Atrial flutter and thromboembolic risk: a systematic review. *Heart.* 2015;101:1446-1455.

62. Rujirachun P, Wattanachayakul P, Winijkul A, Ungprasert P. Paroxysmal supraventricular tachycardia and risk of ischemic stroke: a systematic review and meta-analysis. *J Arrhythm.* 2019;35:499-505.

63. Binici Z, Intzilakis T, Nielsen OW, Køber L, Sajadieh A. Excessive supraventricular ectopic activity and increased risk of atrial fibrillation and stroke. *Circulation.* 2010;121:1904-1911.

64. Cardiogenic brain embolism. The second report of the Cerebral Embolism Task Force. *Arch Neurol.* 1989;46:727-743.

65. Kernan WN, Ovbiagele B, Black HR, et al. Guidelines for the prevention of stroke in patients with stroke and transient ischemic attack: a guideline for healthcare professionals from the American Heart Association/American Stroke Association. *Stroke.* 2014;45:2160-2236.

66. Takasugi J, Yamagami H, Noguchi T, et al. Detection of left ventricular thrombus by cardiac magnetic resonance in embolic stroke of undetermined source. *Stroke.* 2017;48:2434-2440.

67. Wang Y, Lichtman JH, Dharmarajan K, et al. National trends in stroke after acute myocardial infarction among Medicare patients in the United States: 1999 to 2010. *Am Heart J.* 2015;169:78-85.e4.

68. Kim W, Kim EJ. Heart Failure as a risk factor for stroke. *J Stroke.* 2018;20:33-45.

69. Nunes Maria Carmo P, Beaton A, Acquatella H, et al. Chagas cardiomyopathy: an update of current clinical knowledge and management: a scientific statement from the American Heart Association. *Circulation.* 2018;138:e169-e209.

70. Templin C, Ghadri JR, Diekmann J, et al. Clinical features and outcomes of takotsubo (stress) cardiomyopathy. *N Engl J Med.* 2015;373:929-938.

71. Parikh NS, Cool J, Karas MG, Boehme AK, Kamel H. Stroke risk and mortality in patients with ventricular assist devices. *Stroke.* 2016;47:2702-2706.

72. Zühlke L, Karthikeyan G, Engel ME, et al. Clinical outcomes in 3343 children and adults with rheumatic heart disease from 14 low- and middle-income countries: two-year follow-up of the global rheumatic heart disease registry (the REMEDY study). *Circulation.* 2016;134:1456-1466.

73. Benjamin EJ, Plehn JF, D'Agostino RB, et al. Mitral annular calcification and the risk of stroke in an elderly cohort. *N Engl J Med.* 1992;327:374-379.

74. Davlouros PA, Mplani VC, Koniari I, Tsigkas G, Hahalis G. Transcatheter aortic valve replacement and stroke: a comprehensive review. *J Geriatr Cardiol.* 2018;15:95-104.

75. Nishimura Rick A, Otto Catherine M, Bonow Robert O, et al. 2017 AHA/ACC focused update of the 2014 AHA/ACC guideline for the

management of patients with valvular heart disease: a report of the American College of Cardiology/American Heart Association Task Force on Clinical Practice Guidelines. *Circulation.* 2017;135:e1159-e1195.

76. Cannegieter SC, Rosendaal FR, Briët E. Thromboembolic and bleeding complications in patients with mechanical heart valve prostheses. *Circulation.* 1994;89:635-641.

77. Eikelboom JW, Connolly SJ, Brueckmann M, et al. Dabigatran versus warfarin in patients with mechanical heart valves. *N Engl J Med.* 2013;369:1206-1214.

78. Sotero FD, Rosário M, Fonseca AC, Ferro JM. Neurological complications of infective endocarditis. *Curr Neurol Neurosci Rep.* 2019;19:23.

79. Yanagawa B, Pettersson Gosta B, Habib G, et al. Surgical management of infective endocarditis complicated by embolic stroke. *Circulation.* 2016;134:1280-1292.

80. Asopa S, Patel A, Khan OA, Sharma R, Ohri SK. Non-bacterial thrombotic endocarditis. *Eur J Cardio-Thoracic Surg.* 2007;32:696-701.

81. Pengo V, Denas G, Zoppellaro G, et al. Rivaroxaban vs warfarin in high-risk patients with antiphospholipid syndrome. *Blood.* 2018;132:1365-1371.

82. Wang Z, Chen S, Zhu M, et al. Risk prediction for emboli and recurrence of primary cardiac myxomas after resection. *J Cardiothorac Surg.* 2016;11:22-22.

83. Tamin SS, Maleszewski JJ, Scott CG, et al. Prognostic and bioepidemiologic implications of papillary fibroelastomas. *J Am Coll Cardiol.* 2015;65:2420.

84. Kent DM, Dahabreh IJ, Ruthazer R, et al. Device closure of patent foramen ovale after stroke: pooled analysis of completed randomized trials. *J Am Coll Cardiol.* 2016;67:907-917.

85. Sung YJ, de Las Fuentes L, Winkler TW, et al. A multi-ancestry genome-wide study incorporating gene-smoking interactions identifies multiple new loci for pulse pressure and mean arterial pressure. *Hum Mol Genet.* 2019.

86. Cramer SC, Rordorf G, Maki JH, et al. Increased pelvic vein thrombi in cryptogenic stroke: results of the Paradoxical Emboli from Large Veins in Ischemic Stroke (PELVIS) study. *Stroke.* 2004;35:46-50.

87. Thaler DE, Ruthazer R, Weimar C, et al. Recurrent stroke predictors differ in medically treated patients with pathogenic vs. other PFOs. *Neurology.* 2014;83:221-226.

88. Mas JL, Arquizan C, Lamy C, et al. Recurrent cerebrovascular events associated with patent foramen ovale, atrial septal aneurysm, or both. *N Engl J Med.* 2001;345:1740-1746.

89. Kamel H. Evidence-based management of patent foramen ovale in patients with ischemic stroke. *JAMA Neurol.* 2018;75:147-148.

90. Saver JL, Carroll JD, Thaler DE, et al. Long-term outcomes of patent foramen ovale closure or medical therapy after stroke. *N Engl J Med.* 2017;377:1022-1032.

91. Mas JL, Derumeaux G, Guillon B, et al. Patent foramen ovale closure or anticoagulation vs. antiplatelets after stroke. *N Engl J Med.* 2017;377:1011-1021.

92. Sondergaard L, Kasner SE, Rhodes JF, et al. Patent foramen ovale closure or antiplatelet therapy for cryptogenic stroke. *N Engl J Med.* 2017;377:1033-1042.

93. Caplan LR. Cardiac arrest and other hypoxic ischemic insults. In: LR Caplan, JW Hurst, MI Chimowitz, eds. *Clinical neurocardiology.* New York: Marcel Dekker; 1999:1-34.

94. Cummings JL, Tomiyasu U, Read S, Benson DF. Amnesia with hippocampal lesions after cardiopulmonary arrest. *Neurology.* 1984;34:679-681.

95. Caronna JJ, Finklestein S. Neurological syndromes after cardiac arrest. *Stroke.* 1978;9:517-520.

96. Liu GT, Volpe NJ, Galetta S. Disorders of higher cortical visual function. In: *Liu, Volpe, and Galetta's neuro-ophthalmology: diagnosis and management.* 3rd ed. Edinburgh; New York: Elsevier Inc.; 2019:352-354.

97. Weathered NR. Cardiac and pulmonary disorders and the nervous system. *Continuum (Minneap Minn).* 2020;26:556-576.

98. Cronberg T, Greer DM, Lilja G, Moulaert V, Swindell P, Rossetti AO. Brain injury after cardiac arrest: from prognostication of comatose patients to rehabilitation. *Lancet Neurol.* 2020;19:611-622.

99. Panchal Ashish R, Bartos Jason A, Cabañas José G, et al. Part 3: Adult basic and advanced life support: 2020 American Heart Association Guidelines for Cardiopulmonary Resuscitation and Emergency Cardiovascular Care. *Circulation.* 2020;142:S366-S468.

100. Greer DM, Shemie SD, Lewis A, et al. Determination of brain death/death by neurologic criteria: the world brain death project. *JAMA.* 2020;324:1078-1097.

101. Amarenco P, Davis S, Jones EF, et al. Clopidogrel plus aspirin versus warfarin in patients with stroke and aortic arch plaques. *Stroke.* 2014;45:1248-1257.

102. Ntaios G, Pearce LA, Meseguer E, et al. Aortic arch atherosclerosis in patients with embolic stroke of undetermined source: an exploratory analysis of the NAVIGATE ESUS Trial. *Stroke.* 2019;50:3184-3190.

103. Kernan WN, Ovbiagele B, Black HR, et al. Guidelines for the prevention of stroke in patients with stroke and transient ischemic attack: a guideline for healthcare professionals from the American Heart Association/American Stroke Association. *Stroke.* 2014;45:2160-2236.

104. Biller J, Sacco RL, Albuquerque FC, et al. Cervical arterial dissections and association with cervical manipulative therapy: a statement for healthcare professionals from the American Heart Association/American Stroke Association. *Stroke.* 2014;45:3155-3174.

105. Blum CA, Yaghi S. Cervical artery dissection: a review of the epidemiology, pathophysiology, treatment, and outcome. *Arch Neurosci.* 2015;2.

106. Touze E, Southerland AM, Boulanger M, et al. Fibromuscular dysplasia and its neurologic manifestations: a systematic review. *JAMA Neurol.* 2019;76:217-226.

107. Markus HS, Levi C, King A, Madigan J, Norris J, Cervical Artery Dissection in Stroke Study I. Antiplatelet therapy vs anticoagulation therapy in cervical artery dissection: the cervical artery dissection in stroke study (CADISS) randomized clinical trial final results. *JAMA Neurol.* 2019;76:657-664.

108. Biousse V, D'Anglejan-Chatillon J, Touboul PJ, Amarenco P, Bousser MG. Time course of symptoms in extracranial carotid artery dissections. A series of 80 patients. *Stroke.* 1995;26:235-239.

109. Traenka C, Gensicke H, Schaedelin S, et al. Biomarkers and antithrombotic treatment in cervical artery dissection—Design of the TREAT-CAD randomised trial. *Eur Stroke J.* 2020;5:309-319.

110. de Lau LM, Leebeek FW, de Maat MP, Koudstaal PJ, Dippel DW. Screening for coagulation disorders in patients with ischemic stroke. *Expert Rev Neurother.* 2010;10:1321-1329.

111. Pezzini A, Grassi M, Lodigiani C, et al. Predictors of long-term recurrent vascular events after ischemic stroke at young age: the Italian Project on Stroke in Young Adults. *Circulation.* 2014;129:1668-1676.

112. Soare AM, Popa C. Deficiencies of proteins C, S and antithrombin and factor V Leiden and the risk of ischemic strokes. *J Med Life.* 2010;3:235-238.

113. Levine SR, Welch KM. The spectrum of neurologic disease associated with antiphospholipid antibodies. Lupus anticoagulants and anticardiolipin antibodies. *Arch Neurol.* 1987;44:876-883.

114. Samanta D, Cobb S, Arya K. Sneddon syndrome: a comprehensive overview. *J Stroke Cerebrovasc Dis.* 2019;28:2098-2108.

115. Navi BB, Iadecola C. Ischemic stroke in cancer patients: a review of an underappreciated pathology. *Ann Neurol.* 2018;83:873-883.

116. Connolly ES, Jr., Rabinstein AA, Carhuapoma JR, et al. Guidelines for the management of aneurysmal subarachnoid hemorrhage: a guideline for healthcare professionals from the American Heart Association/American Stroke Association. *Stroke.* 2012;43:1711-1737.

117. Vergouwen MD, Vermeulen M, van Gijn J, et al. Definition of delayed cerebral ischemia after aneurysmal subarachnoid hemorrhage as an outcome event in clinical trials and observational studies: proposal of a multidisciplinary research group. *Stroke.* 2010;41:2391-2395.

118. Saposnik G, Di Legge S, Webster F, Hachinski V. Predictors of major neurologic improvement after thrombolysis in acute stroke. *Neurology.* 2005;65:1169-1174.

119. Roman GC. Senile dementia of the Binswanger type. A vascular form of dementia in the elderly. *JAMA.* 1987;258:1782-1788.

120. Hachinski V, Iadecola C, Petersen RC, et al. National Institute of Neurological Disorders and Stroke-Canadian Stroke Network vascular cognitive impairment harmonization standards. *Stroke.* 2006;37: 2220-2241.

121. Skrobot OA, Black SE, Chen C, et al. Progress toward standardized diagnosis of vascular cognitive impairment: guidelines from the Vascular Impairment of Cognition Classification Consensus Study. *Alzheimers Dement.* 2018;14:280-292.

122. Petrovitch H, White LR, Ross GW, et al. Accuracy of clinical criteria for AD in the Honolulu-Asia Aging Study, a population-based study. *Neurology.* 2001;57:226-234.

123. Lopez OL, Kuller LH, Becker JT, et al. Classification of vascular dementia in the Cardiovascular Health Study Cognition Study. *Neurology.* 2005;64:1539-1547.

124. Smith EE, Biessels GJ, De Guio F, et al. Harmonizing brain magnetic resonance imaging methods for vascular contributions to neurodegeneration. *Alzheimers Dement (Amst).* 2019;11:191-204.

125. Wardlaw JM, Smith EE, Biessels GJ, et al. Neuroimaging standards for research into small vessel disease and its contribution to ageing and neurodegeneration. *Lancet Neurology.* 2013;12:822-838.

126. Pase MP, Satizabal CL, Seshadri S. Role of improved vascular health in the declining incidence of dementia. *Stroke.* 2017;48:2013-2020.

127. Ding J, Davis-Plourde KL, Sedaghat S, et al. Antihypertensive medications and risk for incident dementia and Alzheimer's disease: a meta-analysis of individual participant data from prospective cohort studies. *Lancet Neurol.* 2020;19:61-70.

128. Tissue plasminogen activator for acute ischemic stroke. *N Engl J Med.* 1995;333:1581-1588.

129. Hachinski V, Oveisgharan S, Romney AK, Shankle WR. Optimizing the Hachinski Ischemic Scale. *Arch Neurol.* 2012;69:169-175.

130. Hacke W, Kaste M, Bluhmki E, et al. Thrombolysis with alteplase 3 to 4.5 hours after acute ischemic stroke. *N Engl J Med.* 2008;359:1317-1329.

131. Ma H, Campbell BCV, Parsons MW, et al. Thrombolysis guided by perfusion imaging up to 9 hours after onset of stroke. *N Engl J Med.* 2019;380:1795-1803.

132. Thomalla G, Simonsen CZ, Boutitie F, et al. MRI-guided thrombolysis for stroke with unknown time of onset. *N Engl J Med.* 2018;379:611-622.

133. Berkhemer OA, Fransen PS, Beumer D, et al. A randomized trial of intraarterial treatment for acute ischemic stroke. *N Engl J Med.* 2015;372:11-20.

134. Bracard S, Ducrocq X, Mas JL, et al. Mechanical thrombectomy after intravenous alteplase versus alteplase alone after stroke (THRACE): a randomised controlled trial. *Lancet Neurol.* 2016;15:1138-1147.

135. Campbell BC, Mitchell PJ, Kleinig TJ, et al. Endovascular therapy for ischemic stroke with perfusion-imaging selection. *N Engl J Med.* 2015;372:1009-1018.

136. Eskey CJ, Meyers PM, Nguyen TN, et al. Indications for the performance of intracranial endovascular neurointerventional procedures: a scientific statement from the American Heart Association. *Circulation.* 2018;137:e661-e689.

137. Goyal M, Demchuk AM, Menon BK, et al. Randomized assessment of rapid endovascular treatment of ischemic stroke. *N Engl J Med.* 2015;372:1019-1030.

138. Jovin TG, Chamorro A, Cobo E, et al. Thrombectomy within 8 hours after symptom onset in ischemic stroke. *N Engl J Med.* 2015;372:2296-2306.

139. Saver JL, Goyal M, Bonafe A, et al. Stent-retriever thrombectomy after intravenous t-PA vs. t-PA alone in stroke. *N Engl J Med.* 2015;372:2285-2295.

140. Martins SO, Mont'Alverne F, Rebello LC, et al. Thrombectomy for stroke in the public health care system of Brazil. *N Engl J Med.* 2020;382:2316-2326.

141. Zaidat OO, Castonguay AC, Gupta R, et al. North American solitaire stent retriever acute stroke registry: post-marketing revascularization and clinical outcome results. *J Neurointerv Surg.* 2018;10:i45-i49.

142. Zaidat OO, Castonguay AC, Nogueira RG, et al. TREVO stent-retriever mechanical thrombectomy for acute ischemic stroke secondary to large vessel occlusion registry. *J Neurointerv Surg.* 2018;10:516-524.

143. Zaidat OO, Castonguay AC, Linfante I, et al. First pass effect: a new measure for stroke thrombectomy devices. *Stroke.* 2018;49:660-666.

144. Nguyen TN, Castonguay AC, Nogueira RG, et al. Effect of balloon guide catheter on clinical outcomes and reperfusion in Trevo thrombectomy. *J Neurointerv Surg.* 2019;11:861-865.

145. Nguyen TN, Malisch T, Castonguay AC, et al. Balloon guide catheter improves revascularization and clinical outcomes with the Solitaire device: analysis of the North American Solitaire Acute Stroke Registry. *Stroke.* 2014;45:141-145.

146. Lapergue B, Blanc R, Gory B, et al. Effect of endovascular contact aspiration vs stent retriever on revascularization in patients with acute ischemic stroke and large vessel occlusion: the ASTER randomized clinical trial. *JAMA.* 2017;318:443-452.

147. Turk AS, 3rd, Siddiqui A, Fifi JT, et al. Aspiration thrombectomy versus stent retriever thrombectomy as first-line approach for large vessel occlusion (COMPASS): a multicentre, randomised, open label, blinded outcome, non-inferiority trial. *Lancet.* 2019;393:998-1008.

148. Zaidi SF, Castonguay AC, Jumaa MA, et al. Intraarterial thrombolysis as rescue therapy for large vessel occlusions. *Stroke.* 2019;50:1003-1006.

149. Stracke CP, Fiehler J, Meyer L, et al. Emergency intracranial stenting in acute stroke: predictors for poor outcome and for complications. *J Am Heart Assoc.* 2020;9:e012795.

150. Albers GW, Marks MP, Kemp S, et al. Thrombectomy for stroke at 6 to 16 hours with selection by perfusion imaging. *N Engl J Med.* 2018;378:708-718.

151. Nogueira RG, Jadhav AP, Haussen DC, et al. Thrombectomy 6 to 24 hours after stroke with a mismatch between deficit and infarct. *N Engl J Med.* 2018;378:11-21.

152. Rocha M, Jovin TG. Fast versus slow progressors of infarct growth in large vessel occlusion stroke: clinical and research implications. *Stroke.* 2017;48:2621-2627.

153. Desai SM, Haussen DC, Aghaebrahim A, et al. Thrombectomy 24 hours after stroke: beyond DAWN. *J Neurointerv Surg.* 2018;10:1039-1042.

154. Kim BJ, Menon BK, Kim JY, et al. Endovascular treatment after stroke due to large vessel occlusion for patients presenting very late from time last known well. *JAMA Neurol.* 2020.

155. Castonguay AC, Jumaa MA, Zaidat OO, et al. Insights into intra-arterial thrombolysis in the modern era of mechanical thrombectomy. *Front Neurol.* 2019;10:1195.

156. Flaherty ML, Tao H, Haverbusch M, et al. Warfarin use leads to larger intracerebral hematomas. *Neurology.* 2008;71:1084-1089.

157. Flibotte JJ, Hagan N, O'Donnell J, Greenberg SM, Rosand J. Warfarin, hematoma expansion, and outcome of intracerebral hemorrhage. *Neurology.* 2004;63:1059-1064.

158. Biffi A, Battey TW, Ayres AM, et al. Warfarin-related intraventricular hemorrhage: imaging and outcome. *Neurology.* 2011;77:1840-1846.

159. Liotta EM, Prabhakaran S. Warfarin-associated intracerebral hemorrhage is increasing in prevalence in the United States. *J Stroke Cerebrovasc Dis.* 2013;22:1151-1155.

160. Curtze S, Strbian D, Meretoja A, et al. Higher baseline international normalized ratio value correlates with higher mortality in intracerebral hemorrhage during warfarin use. *Eur J Neurol.* 2014;21:616-622.

161. Kuramatsu JB, Gerner ST, Schellinger PD, et al. Anticoagulant reversal, blood pressure levels, and anticoagulant resumption in patients

with anticoagulation-related intracerebral hemorrhage. *JAMA.* 2015;313:824-836.

162. Goldstein JN, Refaai MA, Milling TJ, Jr, et al. Four-factor prothrombin complex concentrate versus plasma for rapid vitamin K antagonist reversal in patients needing urgent surgical or invasive interventions: a phase 3b, open-label, non-inferiority, randomised trial. *Lancet.* 2015;385:2077-2087.

163. Steiner T, Poli S, Griebe M, et al. Fresh frozen plasma versus prothrombin complex concentrate in patients with intracranial haemorrhage related to vitamin K antagonists (INCH): a randomised trial. *Lancet Neurol.* 2016;15:566-573.

164. Ruff CT, Giugliano RP, Braunwald E, et al. Comparison of the efficacy and safety of new oral anticoagulants with warfarin in patients with atrial fibrillation: a meta-analysis of randomised trials. *Lancet.* 2014;383:955-962.

165. Pollack CV, Jr., Reilly PA, van Ryn J, et al. Idarucizumab for dabigatran reversal—full cohort analysis. *N Engl J Med.* 2017;377:431-441.

166. Siegal DM, Curnutte JT, Connolly SJ, et al. Andexanet Alfa for the reversal of factor Xa inhibitor activity. *N Engl J Med.* 2015;373:2413-2424.

167. Connolly SJ, Crowther M, Eikelboom JW, et al. Full Study report of Andexanet Alfa for bleeding associated with factor Xa inhibitors. *N Engl J Med.* 2019;380:1326-1335.

168. Algra A, van Gijn J. Aspirin at any dose above 30 mg offers only modest protection after cerebral ischaemia. *J Neurol Neurosurg Psychiatry.* 1996;60:197-199.

169. Antithrombotic Trialists C, Baigent C, Blackwell L, et al. Aspirin in the primary and secondary prevention of vascular disease: collaborative meta-analysis of individual participant data from randomised trials. *Lancet.* 2009;373:1849-1860.

170. Committee CS. A randomised, blinded, trial of clopidogrel versus aspirin in patients at risk of ischaemic events (CAPRIE). CAPRIE Steering Committee. *Lancet.* 1996;348:1329-1339.

171. Verro P, Gorelick PB, Nguyen D. Aspirin plus dipyridamole versus aspirin for prevention of vascular events after stroke or TIA: a meta-analysis. *Stroke.* 2008;39:1358-1363.

172. Group ES, Halkes PH, van Gijn J, Kappelle LJ, Koudstaal PJ, Algra A. Aspirin plus dipyridamole versus aspirin alone after cerebral ischaemia of arterial origin (ESPRIT): randomised controlled trial. *Lancet.* 2006;367:1665-1673.

173. Sacco RL, Diener HC, Yusuf S, et al. Aspirin and extended-release dipyridamole versus clopidogrel for recurrent stroke. *N Engl J Med.* 2008;359:1238-1251.

174. Johnston SC, Amarenco P, Albers GW, et al. Ticagrelor versus aspirin in acute stroke or transient ischemic attack. *N Engl J Med.* 2016;375:35-43.

175. Mohr JP, Thompson JL, Lazar RM, et al. A comparison of warfarin and aspirin for the prevention of recurrent ischemic stroke. *N Engl J Med.* 2001;345:1444-1451.

176. Hart RG, Sharma M, Mundl H, et al. Rivaroxaban for stroke prevention after embolic stroke of undetermined source. *N Engl J Med.* 2018;378:2191-2201.

177. Diener HC, Sacco RL, Easton JD, et al. Dabigatran for prevention of stroke after embolic stroke of undetermined source. *N Engl J Med.* 2019;380:1906-1917.

178. Bhatt DL, Fox KA, Hacke W, et al. Clopidogrel and aspirin versus aspirin alone for the prevention of atherothrombotic events. *N Engl J Med.* 2006;354:1706-1717.

179. Diener HC, Bogousslavsky J, Brass LM, et al. Aspirin and clopidogrel compared with clopidogrel alone after recent ischaemic stroke or transient ischaemic attack in high-risk patients (MATCH): randomised, double-blind, placebo-controlled trial. *Lancet.* 2004;364:331-337.

180. Investigators SPS, Benavente OR, Hart RG, et al. Effects of clopidogrel added to aspirin in patients with recent lacunar stroke. *N Engl J Med.* 2012;367:817-825.

181. Wang Y, Wang Y, Zhao X, et al. Clopidogrel with aspirin in acute minor stroke or transient ischemic attack. *N Engl J Med.* 2013;369:11-19.

182. Johnston SC, Amarenco P, Denison H, et al. Ticagrelor and aspirin or aspirin alone in acute ischemic stroke or TIA. *N Engl J Med.* 2020;383:207-217.

183. Kim SM, Jung JM, Kim BJ, Lee JS, Kwon SU. Cilostazol mono and combination treatments in ischemic stroke: an updated systematic review and meta-analysis. *Stroke.* 2019;50:3503-3511.

184. Chimowitz MI, Lynn MJ, Howlett-Smith H, et al. Comparison of warfarin and aspirin for symptomatic intracranial arterial stenosis. *N Engl J Med.* 2005;352:1305-1316.

185. Collaboration R. Effects of antiplatelet therapy after stroke due to intracerebral haemorrhage (RESTART): a randomised, open-label trial. *Lancet.* 2019;393:2613-2623.

186. Lioutas VA, Beiser AS, Aparicio HJ, et al. Assessment of incidence and risk factors of intracerebral hemorrhage among participants in the Framingham Heart Study Between 1948 and 2016. *JAMA Neurol.* 2020.

187. Wilson D, Ambler G, Lee KJ, et al. Cerebral microbleeds and stroke risk after ischaemic stroke or transient ischaemic attack: a pooled analysis of individual patient data from cohort studies. *Lancet Neurol.* 2019;18:653-665.

188. Charidimou A, Linn J, Vernooij MW, et al. Cortical superficial siderosis: detection and clinical significance in cerebral amyloid angiopathy and related conditions. *Brain.* 2015;138:2126-2139.

189. Shoamanesh A, Hart RG, Connolly SJ, et al. Microbleeds and the effect of anticoagulation in patients with embolic stroke of undetermined source: an exploratory analysis of the NAVIGATE ESUS randomized clinical trial. *JAMA Neurol.* 2020.

190. Boulanger JM, Lindsay MP, Gubitz G, et al. Canadian stroke best practice recommendations for acute stroke management: prehospital, emergency department, and acute inpatient stroke care, 6th Edition, Update 2018. *Int J Stroke.* 2018;13:949-984.

191. Turc G, Bhogal P, Fischer U, et al. European Stroke Organisation (ESO) - European Society for Minimally Invasive Neurological Therapy (ESMINT) guidelines on mechanical thrombectomy in acute ischaemic stroke. Endorsed by Stroke Alliance for Europe (SAFE). *Eur Stroke J.* 2019;4:6-12.

Diagnosis and Management of Diseases of the Peripheral Arteries

26

Hillary Johnston-Cox, Daniella Kadian-Dodov, and Jeffrey W. Olin

Diagnosis and management of diseases of the peripheral arteries

Risk factors

• Age
• Diabetes
• Smoking
• Chronic kidney disease

Anatomic hallmark

• Atherosclerotic plaque in arteries of the lower extremities

Clinical manifestations

• Vague symptoms of leg dysfunction
• Claudication: Exertional, reproducible discomfort; resolves with standing in 2–5 mins
• Acute limb ischemia: an abrupt event due to an arterial occlusion, usually resulting from an embolic event or thrombosis of a stent or bypass graft
• Chronic limb-threatening ischemia: rest pain, ischemic ulceration of the lower extremity for >2 weeks or gangrene

Risk of PAD

• Patients with PAD have a markedly increased risk for future MI, stroke, and cardiovascular death.

Clinical assessment

If history and physical exam are suggestive of PAD without evidence of rest pain or history of nonhealing ulcer or gangrene, start with ABI:

$$ABI = \frac{\text{Highest ankle (PT/DP) systolic blood pressure of each leg}}{\text{Highest brachial systolic blood pressure (right or left)}}$$

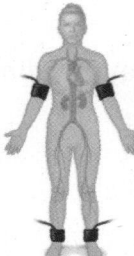

• PAD present if ABI ≤0.90
• Borderline ABI 0.90–0.99
• Normal ABI 1.00–1.40
• ABI >1.4, calcified blood vessels

If symptoms persist despite guideline-directed medical therapy, get a duplex ultrasound, CTA or MRA for anatomical assessment.

If there is evidence of PAD with rest pain and/or nonhealing ulcer, gangrene:

• ABI
• Perfusion assessment: TBI with waveforms, TcPO2, skin perfusion pressure
• Anatomic assessment: Duplex ultrasound, CTA, MRA, or invasive angiography

Guideline-directed medical therapy that decreases the risk of MI, stroke, and cardiovascular death

• Smoking cessation
• Exercise walking program
• Blood pressure control
• High intensity statin
• Antiplatelet and anticoagulant agents

Guideline-directed medical therapy that improves symptoms, quality of life and limb preservation

• Smoking cessation
• Exercise walking program
• Cilostazol
• Focused podiatry care
• Revascularization
• Antiplatelet and anticoagulation agents

Acute limb ischemia management for viable limbs

• Revascularization
• Anticoagulation

Chapter 26 Fuster and Hurst's Central Illustration. Peripheral artery disease (PAD) is defined as any arterial disease (other than aneurysms) from the abdominal aorta to the feet and toes. The clinical manifestations of PAD are determined by the anatomical location and severity of arterial stenosis. The ankle-brachial index (ABI) is key to diagnosis of PAD. Medical management is key for reduction in cardiovascular morbidity and mortality as well as preservation of limb function and survival from amputation. Acute arterial occlusion management for viable limbs should focus on revascularization and anticoagulation. CTA, computed tomographic angiography; MI, myocardial infarction; MRA, magnetic resonance angiography; TBI, toe-brachial index; TcPO2, transcutaneous oxygen pressure measurement.

CHAPTER SUMMARY

This chapter discusses peripheral artery disease (PAD), focusing on risk factors, clinical assessment, classification, and management. The most common cause of PAD is atherosclerotic plaque formation in arteries of the lower extremities. Risk factors for PAD include age, diabetes, smoking, and kidney disease. Patients with PAD have increased risk for future cardiovascular events. Clinical manifestations of patients with PAD depend on location and severity of stenosis. Typical claudication is only present in a minority of patients with PAD; many patients present with vague leg symptoms. Other manifestations of PAD include acute limb ischemia (ALI) and chronic limb-threatening ischemia (CLTI). A systemic and comprehensive approach should be applied to the diagnosis and management of PAD. Diagnostic testing for suspected PAD and CTLI is key to guiding further assessment and revascularization management. The ankle-brachial index (ABI) is key to diagnosis of PAD, with use of exercise to reveal claudication in specific cases. Other testing modalities can be helpful in patients with normal ABIs but high clinical suspicion for PAD. Medical management is key for reduction in cardiovascular morbidity and mortality as well as preservation of limb function and survival from amputation. Acute arterial occlusion management for viable limbs should focus on revascularization and anticoagulation.

INTRODUCTION

Peripheral vascular diseases are a diverse set of processes that can affect the arteries, veins, and lymphatic circulations. This chapter will focus on peripheral artery disease (PAD), which is defined as any arterial disease (other than aneurysms) from the abdominal aorta to the feet and toes. A systemic and comprehensive approach will be applied to the diagnosis and management of PAD. We will focus on the most common cause of PAD: atherosclerosis. Nonatherosclerotic causes of PAD such as vasospastic diseases, inflammatory diseases, and entrapment syndromes are beyond the scope of this chapter.

PERIPHERAL ARTERY DISEASE

The anatomic hallmark of PAD is atherosclerotic plaque formation in arteries of the lower extremities. PAD is the most common cause of lower extremity ischemia in Western societies.[1] The Global Burden of Disease study estimated more than a 30% increase in deaths and disability related to PAD between 2005 and 2015.[2,3] Although many patients are asymptomatic, the most common presentations are complaints of vague symptoms of leg dysfunction, with only 10% to 30% of individuals experiencing classic claudication (leg discomfort brought on by walking and relieved by standing for 2–5 minutes).[4–6] Limb dysfunction significantly impacts the quality of life for those patients who suffer from PAD.[7–10] Progression of leg symptoms to rest pain, ulceration, and gangrene further compounds PAD-associated morbidity and mortality.

Age, smoking, diabetes, and chronic kidney disease (CKD) are the strongest risk factors for PAD. Patients with PAD have a markedly increased risk of future cardiovascular events.[11,12] A low ankle-brachial index (ABI) predicted a 2-fold increased risk in all-cause mortality, cardiovascular death, and major coronary events at all ranges of the Framingham Risk Score.[11,12] Both asymptomatic and symptomatic patients are at elevated risk.[11,12] Those with disease in more than one vascular territory have worse outcomes.[13] In the REACH registry, the prevalence of the combined endpoint of cardiovascular death, myocardial infarction (MI), stroke, or hospitalization was highest in patients with PAD. Several medical therapies have been shown to reduce cardiovascular morbidity and mortality in patients with PAD.[14,15]

Prevalence

PAD affects a large and increasing number of individuals worldwide. The specific numbers for prevalence and incidence vary due to differences in assessment and criteria for diagnosis. PAD affects 8 to 12 million individuals in the United States and more than 200 million individuals worldwide.[16,17] Across Europe and North America, there is an estimated 27 million patients with PAD and approximately 413,000 inpatient admission associated with PAD.[18] The prevalence of PAD in females is at least equivalent to that of males across all age groups and increases in females to a greater extent after the age of 70.[19–21]

In a study of over 3 million participants in the Life Line screening program, the prevalence of PAD was found to be 3.6%.[22] In the Framingham Offspring Study, PAD was defined as an ABI ≤0.9 and the mean age at diagnosis was 58 years old. PAD was found in 1554 males and 1759 females between 1995 and 1998.[23] The prevalence of PAD was 3.9% in males and 3.3% in females, while the prevalence of claudication was only 1.8% in males and 0.8% in females. This discrepancy suggests that only a fraction of the participants with PAD had symptoms that were recognized by their healthcare providers.

The PAD Awareness, Risk, and Treatment: New Resources for Survival (PARTNERS) study studied the prevalence of PAD in 6979 patients aged 70 years or older and those between the age of 50 and 69 years old with diabetes or smoking history.[4] PAD was classified as ABI of 0.9 or less and using this definition, 29% of patients had PAD. Only 13% had PAD only, 16% had PAD and cardiovascular disease (CVD), and 24% had CVD only. Forty-seven percent had neither CVD nor PAD.[4]

The Rotterdam Study evaluated 7000 European participants for PAD; of those older than 55 years, 20% of patients were found to have PAD compared to those over the age of 85 years where 60% were found to have PAD.[24] Only 1.6% of patients with PAD in this study self-reported symptoms or claudication by using the Rose questionnaire, suggestive again that only a small percentage of patients are symptomatic for classic claudication. It is estimated that 10% to 30% of patients have classic claudication, 20% to 40% of patients have atypical leg pain, and approximately 50% of patients are asymptomatic. Additionally, approximately 10% of asymptomatic patients have advanced PAD with significant obstruction to blood flow to the lower extremities.[25]

Natural History and Prognosis

The clinical manifestations of PAD are determined by the anatomical location and severity of arterial stenosis and can range from mild leg discomfort with ambulation (claudication) to limb-threatening acute limb ischemia. Patients with unmanaged risk factors such as smoking or diabetes can have rapid progression of disease. Morbidity and mortality associated with PAD is due to concomitant cerebrovascular or coronary disease. The relative risk of all cause death is 2- to 6-fold higher in patients with PAD compared to the general population.[26–28] The ABI is inversely proportional to mortality so that rates of death increase as the ABI goes down.[29–30] The relative risk for all-cause mortality associated with PAD was 2.36 compared to an ABI <0.4, which was 4.49 in a mortality study of a cohort of PAD patients over a 10-year period.[31] An ABI between 0.91 and 0.99 is not normal, in that it carries increased risk of MI, stroke, and cardiovascular death and an increased risk of future walking impairment.[9,32] An ABI >1.4 (indicative of calcified blood vessels) has also been shown to be associated with an increase in mortality and morbidity.[33,34]

The rate of limb loss and amputation due to progression of disease is low compared to the prevalence of PAD.[35] The need for revascularization due to nonhealing ulcers or rest pain is about 5% per year.[36] Amputation rates have been reported at about 1% per year.[37] In those patients that present with acute limb ischemia, the 30-day amputation rate is 10% to 30%, with a 15% 1-year mortality rate.[38] Those with acute limb ischemia that is present for more than 24 hours tend to do worse with a reported 30-day amputation rate of 25.7%, 1-year amputation rate of 37.1%, and 1-year mortality rate of 34%.[39]

Risk Factors

Multiple risk factors have been identified for PAD[42,43] but the strongest four risk factors are age, current or former smoking, diabetes, and CKD. Hyperlipidemia, hypertension, homocysteinemia, sex, ethnicity, and C-reactive protein are also risk factors but play a lesser role. In 2010, a project looking at the global burden of PAD compiled data investigating the epidemiology of PAD and associated risk factors.[16] The analyses suggest that globally cigarette smoking and diabetes are strong risk factors for PAD. There is also a strong overlap of PAD with other CVD.

Age

The prevalence of PAD progressively increases with age after the age of 40.[23,43–48] Thus, the aging populations of the United States and developed countries are associated with an increased prevalence of PAD. Only about half of older patients are symptomatic from PAD; many have limited mobility due to other comorbidities such as arthritis, cardiac disease, or pulmonary disease.[49]

The United States National Health and Nutrition Examination Survey (NHANES) illustrated the relationship between PAD prevalence and age.[48,50] The prevalence of PAD was reported as 0.9% between the ages of 40 and 49; 2.5% between the ages of 50 and 59; 4.7% between the ages of 60 and 69; 14.5% age 70 and older; and 23.2% for those over 80. Traditional risk factors for patients that are over the age of 80 years old might be absent.[51]

Tobacco

Cigarette smoking significantly correlates with CVD. The diagnosis of PAD is made on average a decade sooner in cigarette smokers compared to nonsmokers.[52] The Erfurt Male Cohort (ERFORT) Study associated smoking with an increased risk of incident claudication.[53] Ongoing cigarette smoking is associated with the largest decline in ABI over time relative to other risk factors.[54]

Smoking appears to be a more significant risk factor for PAD than for CAD.[55–57] In the Edinburgh Artery Study, the adjusted relative risk for PAD in heavy smokers compared with nonsmokers was 2.72, but lower for coronary heart disease at 1.61.[55,57]

There is a significant relationship between cigarette dose and risk for PAD.[4,58,59] The Framingham Heart Study found the risk for developing claudication was directly related to the number of cigarettes smoked; there was a 1.4-fold risk increase for every 10 cigarettes smoked per day.[59] A greater number of pack-years of smoking is associated with worsening disease severity, poorer patency post-revascularization, and an increased risk of amputation and cardiovascular mortality post-revascularization.[52]

Smoking cessation reduces morbidity related to PAD. The risk of progression of PAD is significantly greater in prior smokers compared with never smokers.[58,60,61] The Edinburgh Arterial Study found a decreased risk of claudication for patients who stopped smoking compared with patients who continued to smoke.[25] Smoking cessation is associated with a decreased risk of graft failure following lower extremity bypass surgery.[62] These effects are limited if the patient only reduces cigarette consumption rather than complete cessation.[63]

Diabetes

Patients with diabetes present with more advanced arterial disease at initial diagnosis and have poorer outcomes compared to nondiabetics.[64,65] In the NHANES study, there was an increased risk for PAD in patients with diabetes.[48] In a prospective cohort study with more than 20 years follow-up, there was an increased risk of death for patients with diabetes and PAD, compared to nondiabetic patients with PAD.[66]

Poor glycemic control incrementally increases the risk of atherosclerosis. There is a 26% increase in risk for every 1% increase in HbA1c.[67] In the Framingham Heart Study, diabetes increases the risk for developing symptomatic PAD. There is an increased mortality and amputation rate in patients with diabetes.[68–71] PAD alone conferred a 13.9-fold increased risk of amputation. A combination of PAD and microvascular disease (retinopathy, neuropathy, and nephropathy) was associated with a 22.7-fold increased risk of amputation.[69] Patients with microvascular disease had a 2-fold increased risk of major adverse cardiovascular events. The combination of PAD and microvascular disease conferred a 3.9-fold risk increased risk of major adverse cardiovascular events and was associated with more amputations.

Chronic Kidney Disease

CKD is a coronary disease equivalent. Reduced kidney function has been associated with increased prevalence of PAD and a future risk for developing PAD.[72–74] Patients with low glomerular filtration rate (GFR) and/or albuminuria have a higher prevalence of abnormal ABI (≤0.9, >1.4).[75–80] In patients on dialysis, the prevalence of PAD ranges from 15% to 25%[81–83] and even higher in older dialysis patients.[84] In mild-to-moderate CKD, there is an increased risk of incident PAD; albuminuria is associated with amputation.[85] Patients with end-stage renal disease can develop vascular calcification, which increases the risk of cardiovascular morbidity and mortality.[86,87]

Hypertension

Hypertension is strongly associated with the development of atherosclerosis. The prevalence of hypertension in adults in the United States is 108 million or nearly half of the US adult population.[88] PAD has a strong association comparative to other CVDs with pulse pressure[89] and elevated systolic blood pressure.[90]

In the Rotterdam study, the prevalence of hypertension was 60% in those with an abnormal ABI.[24] In the Framingham study, the risk of developing symptoms of PAD (ie, claudication) was twice that of those without hypertension.[59,91]

Hyperlipidemia

Patients with various lipid and lipoprotein disorders have an increased risk for CVD in addition to adverse long-term cardiovascular outcomes. Patients with PAD are more likely to have elevated levels of cholesterol and/or triglycerides, lipo-protein(a) (Lp[a]), apolipoprotein B, and very low-density lipoprotein when compared to non-PAD patients.[92-94] Levels of "protective" lipoproteins (high-density lipoprotein [HDL]) cholesterol, and apolipoprotein AI and AII levels are lower in PAD patients.[95]

Lp(a) is an independent risk factor for PAD. Lp(a) is genet-ically determined as well as controlled by a single gene locus. In the Québec Cardiovascular Study, there was a doubling of the risk of claudication in men with higher concentrations of plasma Lp(a).[96-98] Patients with early onset PAD have 4-fold higher levels of Lp(a) compared to controls.[99] In the Physicians Health Study, the ratio of total to HDL cholesterol was the best independent predictor of occurrence of PAD.[100]

Homocysteinemia
Homocysteine was one of the early biomarkers studied in the context of atherosclerosis.[101] Elevated homocysteine is associ-ated with early presence of atherosclerosis; elevated levels are present in up to 40% in PAD patients.[102] The effect of homo-cysteine is thought to be mediated through promotion of smooth muscle cell proliferation, increase in inflammation of the arterial wall, and increase in levels of plasminogen activator inhibitor. Nitric oxide release from endothelial cells is altered by homocysteine. An elevated level of homocysteine leads to vessel wall thickening, luminal narrowing, and thrombus formation.

Although a more rapid progression of PAD in patients with elevated homocysteine has been described,[103,104] this finding is not uniform across all studies.[105] However, there has yet to be a study demonstrating that homocysteine-lowering therapy reduces PAD progression or improves outcomes.[106]

CLINICAL ASSESSMENT OF PERIPHERAL ARTERY DISEASE

The clinical manifestations of PAD depend on anatomical locations and severity of arterial stenosis or occlusion; they can range from discomfort in lower extremities when walk-ing (claudication) to limb-threatening ischemia. Claudication can vary from patient to patient.[6,107] Specifics of the symptoms should be elucidated, including onset, character of discomfort, aggravating and alleviating factors, and specific location. The clinical picture can be complicated with the presence of mul-tiple comorbidities and multiple causes of discomfort (such as having vascular claudication and pseudoclaudication due to spinal stenosis) **Table 26-1**.[10,108]

Asymptomatic
The majority of patients with PAD have no lower extremity symptoms[107] and the diagnosis will be missed if ABI testing is restricted to solely individuals with classic claudication. It is a clinical challenge to identify those with PAD without classic claudication.[109] Screening individuals for PAD includes a his-tory of walking impairment, claudication, ischemic rest pain,

TABLE 26-1. Differentiating Vascular Claudication* from Pseudoclaudication**

	Intermittent Claudication	Pseudoclaudication
Character of discomfort	Pain, discomfort, cramping, tightness, tiredness, heaviness	Same, or tingling, weakness, clumsiness
Location of discomfort	Buttock, hip, thigh, calf, arch of the foot or toes	Same
Exercise induced	Yes	Yes or no
Distance to claudication	Same each time	Distance to discom-fort is variable
Occurs with standing	No	Yes
Relief	Stop walking and stand still	Often must lean on something, sit, or change body positions
Time to obtain relief	2–5 minutes	10–20 minutes

*Vascular claudication may be due to arterial disease or venous disease. Venous claudication may occur with a proximal venous obstruction. It is brought on by walking and causes severe pain in thigh as though the thigh muscle is going to continue expanding. Relief is obtained by lying down with leg elevation.
**Pseudoclaudication may be caused by spinal stenosis, nerve root compression, or impingement on the sciatic nerve.

and nonhealing ulcers.[110] Screening for PAD with an ABI is rec-ommended in patients who are 65 years and older, and those who are 50 years and older and have a history of diabetes or tobacco use.[111]

Claudication
Claudication is a discomfort in single or multiple muscle groups in the lower extremities that is brought on by walking and relieved with rest (usually standing) (Table 26-1). The dis-comfort can be described as cramping, pain, heaviness, tired-ness, or weakness. If you ask the patient if they have pain, they often will say no. However if you ask if there is any discomfort, they will then describe exactly what they are feeling.[112] If the workload (and thus oxygen demand) is augmented by increase in pace or walking uphill, the distance or time to symptom onset will decrease. If there is a sudden decrease in the distance or time to onset of symptoms, an embolic or thrombotic event should be considered. Symptoms generally occur one segment distal to the level of occlusion or stenosis. For example, if there is iliac artery obstruction, one may experience buttock, hip, or thigh discomfort; if there is superficial femoral artery obstruc-tion, the symptoms will be in the calf. In patients with multi-level disease, the symptoms often occur distal to the most distal obstruction. Relief with rest should not depend on position; time to relief can vary by patient but should occur within 5 minutes. If specific positions are required for relief, the differ-ential diagnosis should include neurological or musculoskele-tal disorders (Table 26-1). Resting ABI and ABI with exercise will assist in confirmation of diagnosis and establish a baseline walking time to claudication onset.

TABLE 26-2. Acute Limb Ischemia Etiology

Native Arterial Thrombosis	Arterial Thrombosis Following Intervention	Arterial Embolus	Arterial Injury
Atherosclerotic plaque	Vein bypass graft	*Cardiac source:*	*Iatrogenic:* Thromboembolism
Aneurysm thrombosis	Prosthetic bypass graft	Atrial fibrillation Myocardial infarction	Closure devices Device embolization
Arterial dissection	Angioplasty site	Endocarditis,	*Traumatic*
Arterial compression	Stent/stent-graft site	Valvular disease Atrial myxoma	
Popliteal entrapment syndrome		Prosthetic valves	
Thrombophilia		*Arterial source:* Aneurysm	
Low flow state		Atherosclerotic plaque	
		Paradoxical embolus	

Acute Limb Ischemia

Acute limb ischemia (ALI) is an abrupt event due to an arterial occlusion (**Table 26-2**) This usually results from either an embolic event, or thrombosis of a stent or bypass graft. Clinical history should be focused on sudden appearance of a cold, painful toe, or forefoot, especially in the setting of any notable skin changes. Associated symptoms and signs to assess for include the 6Ps: pain, paralysis, paresthesia, pulselessness, pallor, and poikilothermia.[113] Ischemic rest pain should lessen in the dependent position and is usually localized to the foot and toes. Early changes in ALI include loss of light touch sensation, vibratory sensation, and proprioception. Temperature or color change may occur in the lower extremity affected by the acute occlusion.

Chronic Limb-Threatening Ischemia

Chronic limb-threatening ischemia (CLTI), formerly known as critical limb ischemia, is a clinical syndrome in patients with PAD that is characterized by rest pain, ischemic ulceration of the lower extremity for longer than 2 weeks, or gangrene.[114] About 1% to 2% of symptomatic PAD patients manifest CTLI. Many of these patients undergo a surgical or endovascular procedure as well as intensifying their medical therapy to preserve the limb, decrease the cardiovascular event rate and prolong survival. In a systematic review and meta-analysis of 35 studies with a sample size between 109 and 16,440 subjects, the 5-year cumulative incidence of PAD patients with intermittent claudication that progressed to worsening claudication or CLTI has been reported to be as high as 21%.[42] The main limitation of this systematic review is the variability in study cohorts and outcome measures of the included studies, creating significant heterogeneity among the studies.

Patients with CTLI are at risk for limb loss. Amputation rates are as high as 25% and overall survival is poor.[4,115] At the time of initial diagnosis, about 25% of patients with CTLI will suffer a cardiovascular death within 1 year of diagnosis. It has been reported that only 50% of patients with CTLI are alive with intact lower extremities at the end of 1 year.[4] In patients with CTLI and no viable option for revascularization, approximately 40% undergo amputation and 20% die within 6 months.[18] Diabetes and continued smoking lead to worse limb salvage and long-term survival.[116]

Pseudoclaudication

Pseudoclaudication is often due to a neurologic etiology such as spinal stenosis or nerve root compression (Table 26-1). Neurogenic claudication usually presents with an abnormal sensation or sense of touch that is elicited with ambulation that usually requires a specific posture for relief (hips flexed).[117] If ambulation continues, a sense of clumsiness may develop. These symptoms may also develop with prolonged standing (whereas claudication from PAD never occurs with standing).[118]

Venous Claudication

Venous claudication is described as a fullness or tightness, usually in the thighs brought on by walking or running. Rest results in slow relief; elevation of the legs results in alleviation of symptoms more quickly. Iliocaval obstruction is usually present in the setting of venous claudication. On physical exam, there are signs of venous hypertension in the lower abdomen and legs.[119]

Arterial Examination

Blood pressure in each upper extremity should be documented and the higher of the two should be noted for calculation of the ABI. The vascular exam should be performed with the patient supine on the exam table; this should be done after allowing the patient to rest for 15 minutes or warm up if coming in from cold weather. Patients with advanced ischemia who will not tolerate foot elevation can briefly be placed in the supine position to assess abdominal and femoral vessels. The physical examination should include inspection of the skin of the extremities, examination of the abdomen, palpation of all peripheral pulses, auscultation for bruits, and a neurologic examination.

A red or purplish discoloration of the forefoot during dependency (dependent rubor) is frequently seen with severe ischemia. An easy way to determine if there is severe circulatory impairment on physical exam is to elevate the legs (in which case the feet will become quite pale) and then let the legs hang down (in which the feet will become red). This is called pallor on elevation and rubor on dependency. Also at this time, one can determine how long it takes for the veins to fill. The more severe the arterial disease, the longer it takes. While these are useful physical examination findings, they are rarely used since the vascular laboratory is readily available in most clinical settings.

Lower extremity ulcerations have a characteristic appearance based on their origin (**Fig. 26-1, Table 26-3**). Ulcerations

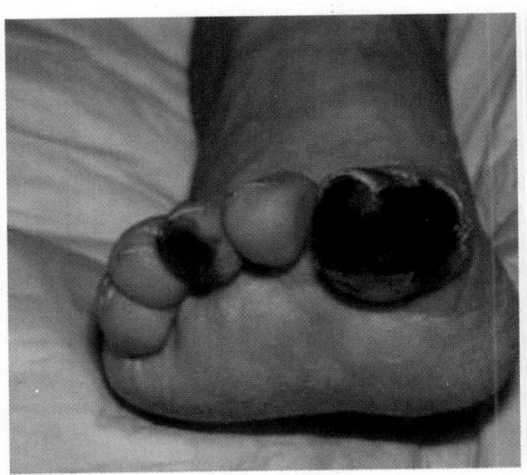
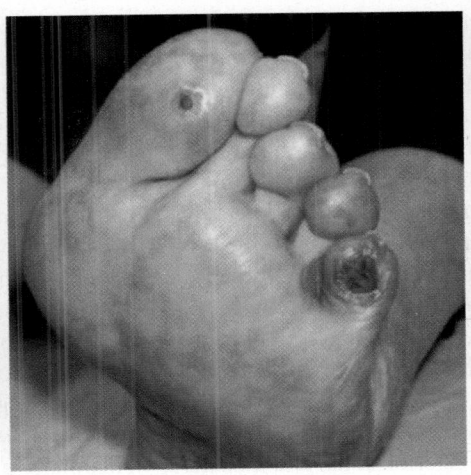
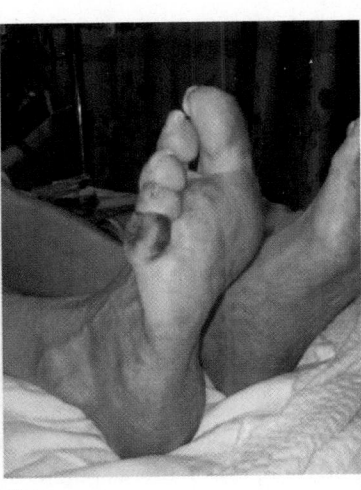

A   B   C

Figure 26–1. (A) Gangrene of the great toe and distal gangrene of the 3rd toe due to thromboembolism from the heart. **(B)** Ischemic ulcers on the great toe and 5th toe. Note the livedo pattern on the plantar surface of the foot suggesting that the etiology is atheromatous embolization. **(C)** Ischemic 5th toe. This patient had CLTI due to severe PAD.

that are caused by ischemia distally or over bony prominence appear dry and punched out and are painful. Typically, there is not significant bleeding.

Patients can also present with gangrene of a digit, forefoot, or hindfoot. Gangrene can either be wet or dry. Dry gangrene has a hard, dry texture and is seen on the distal aspects of toes. There is a clear demarcation between the viable and black

necrotic tissue. Dry gangrene is common in PAD patients. Wet gangrene has a moist appearance, swelling, and blistering.[120] Wet gangrene is associated with infection and is a surgical emergency.

Livedo reticularis is a transient bluish discoloration often described as a lacy pattern in the extremities that varies with extent and intensity. It is most often seen after exposure to cold

TABLE 26–3. Differentiation of Foot Ulcers

Characteristic	Arterial Ulcer	Venous Ulcer	Neuropathic Ulcer
Location	Over body prominences like the malleoli, toe joints, anterior shin, base of the heel, pressure points	Medial and lateral malleolar area *above* a bony prominence; posterior calf; can be large and circumferential	Plantar surface of the foot metatarsal heads, pressure points, heels
Appearance	Irregular margins, the base is dry, appears pale or necrotic **(Figure 1)**	Irregular margins, pink or red base that can be covered with yellow fibrinous tissue; exudate can be present	Punched out ulcer; that may be superficial with a red, deep base. If left untreated, often leads to osteomylytis.
Ulcer within a callus	Rare	No	Ulcer can be underlying a callus
Foot temperature	Warm or cool	Warm	Warm
Pain	Yes	Yes	No
Arterial pulses	Absent	Present	Absent or Present
Sensation	Variable	Present	Absent tactile, pain, temperature, and vibratory sensation
Foot deformities	No	No	Often
Skin changes	Dependent rubor of the leg and foot that becomes pale with elevation of the lower extremities	Erythema, brown-blue Hyperpigmentation that can be diffuse or localized Atrophie blanche (white sclerotic areas) Edema Dry skin Varicose veins Lipodermatosclerosis Bilateral extremities can be involved	Waxy or shiny, Dry skin
Reflexes	Present	Present	Absent

Data from Dormandy JA, Rutherford RB. Management of peripheral arterial disease (PAD). TASC Working Group. TransAtlantic Inter-Society Consensus (TASC). *J Vasc Surg.* 2000 Jan;31(1 Pt 2):S1-S4.

or emotion and dissipates with warming or exercise. It is more common in women, or individuals with fair skin. The pathophysiology is thought to be secondary to spasm of cutaneous arterioles and secondary dilation of capillaries and venules. This leads to slow flow, increased oxygen uptake, and reduced oxygenation of hemoglobin, which leads to the noted color change. Primary livedo often occurs in young, trim healthy woman and is nothing to be concerned about.

Livedo reticularis may be secondary to a host of different diseases and when it takes on the appearance of a patchy, focal, and asymmetric discoloration that is usually fixed in appearance, it is called livedo racemosa. This can be complicated by a local ulceration or infarction.

On exam, the aorta, radial, ulnar, subclavian, carotid, superficial temporal, femoral, popliteal, posterior tibial, and dorsalis pedis arteries should be palpated. We prefer a simple grading system for pulses consisting of normal, reduced, absent. If the pulse feels "full," an underlying aneurysm should be considered. In 12% of young healthy individuals, the dorsalis pedis is absent.[121] In the medical record, it should be noted that the aorta was palpable and of normal size or increased size or the aorta was not able to be palpated (in obese persons). The importance of feeling for the popliteal pulse is 2-fold: (1) it helps to determine the level of obstruction and (2) it allows for the detection of a popliteal artery aneurysm which is quite common in individuals with abdominal aortic aneurysms, with prevalence reported as high as 19%.[122] Unlike abdominal or thoracic aneurysms, popliteal artery aneurysms rarely rupture. However, they may thrombose or embolize, resulting in acute limb ischemia.

Blood pressure should be measured in both arms and should be similar. Pressure variation can be due to respiratory variation, arm positioning, and atrial fibrillation. If there is a significant difference (>20 mm Hg), the blood pressures should be rechecked.[123-125] The femoral, iliac, aortic, carotid, and subclavian arteries should be auscultated. An epigastric bruit that varies with respiration (increases with expiration and decreases with inspiration) is most often due to compression of the celiac artery by the median arcuate ligament.

Vascular Laboratory and Imaging Assessment

Diagnostic Testing

Figs. 26–2A and **26–2B** show an algorithm for diagnostic testing for suspected PAD and diagnostic testing for suspected CLTI. The cornerstone of PAD diagnosis is the ABI, which can be measured using a handheld continuous wave (CW) Doppler and using the higher of the two systolic blood pressures in the dorsalis pedis or posterior tibial artery in each leg divided by the higher of the brachial artery systolic blood pressures. A normal resting ABI generally excludes arterial occlusive disease in most patients; however, PAD may be revealed with exercise testing if the symptoms are suggestive of claudication.[126] A normal ABI ranges from 1.00 to 1.40. An ABI from 0.91 to 0.99 is considered borderline, and values ≤0.90 are considered abnormal with 90% sensitivity and 95% specificity for PAD diagnosis.[127] If the ABI is >1.4, the toe-brachial index (TBI) must be used due to the presence of calcification and

noncompressibility of the arteries, which renders the ABI inaccurate. In this setting, an abnormal TBI is <0.7.[111-117] Patients with diabetes and/or CKD Stage ≥4 are particularly high risk for calcific disease and may have a falsely normal ABI due to the presence of calcification. Thus, TBI should be measured in patients at risk for calcified arteries or those in whom clinical suspicion for more severe PAD exists (eg, patients with a nonhealing wound and a normal ABI).[128] In fact, up to 21% of patients with CLTI undergoing revascularization had a normal ABI in one series.[129] Other testing modalities that may be helpful in these patients include pulse volume recording (PVR) and transcutaneous oximetry.[111,128]

PVR (**Fig. 26–3**) measures the volume displacement of blood flow into the limb. This requires partial inflation of the pneumatic pressure cuff (40–60 mm Hg), which is connected to a pressure transducer. During systole, the pulsatile flow from the arterial system causes distension of the limb being interrogated. This modality provides meaningful information even in the setting of poorly compressible blood vessels.[130] Transcutaneous oxygen pressure measurement ($TCPO_2$) and skin perfusion pressure (SPP) (Fig. 26–2B) measures oxygen tension as compared to capillary perfusion in the skin after cuff deflation, respectively.[131,132] These techniques are not widely available but can be utilized to monitor response post-revascularization.[133] It is also useful in assessment of cutaneous perfusion and likelihood for healing postamputation.[134] Values greater than 40 mm Hg are generally sufficient for healing; values less than 20 mm Hg are not likely to heal.[135] Higher values are required for healing in patients with diabetes. A value less than 20 mm Hg is severely ischemic and will likely require revascularization for adequate wound healing.

Lower extremity arterial exercise testing is performed using a standardized protocol on a treadmill.[136] Protocols may be fixed (2 miles per hour at 10% incline) or graded (increased speed and/or incline at specific intervals, similar to the protocol used in cardiac testing).[137] ABIs are completed pre- and postexercise. During exercise, the systolic blood pressure increases as peripheral vascular resistance decreases, resulting in a larger pressure gradient across the stenosis, a lower ABI, and an abnormal Doppler signal distal to the level of stenosis (Fig. 26–3). Even if resting ABIs are normal at rest, a decrease in ABI following exercise is abnormal and indicates that the patient has PAD. This postexercise pressure decrease peripheral is also a predictor of an increase in mortality.[138-140] Exercise testing provides additional information (overall functional status of the patient) such as distance to onset of symptoms, absolute walking distance, and blood pressure response to exercise. Exercise also allows one to correlate symptoms to hemodynamic testing, which provides evidence of disease.[141] An alternative to treadmill exercise testing is toe tip exercise testing; this is an alternative for patients who are unable to safely walk on a treadmill or where a treadmill is not readily available. Toe tip exercise testing has good correlation with treadmill testing.[126]

When considering revascularization, it is important to identify the level and extent of PAD. Options for diagnostic testing include segmental pressures with the ABI, as well as imaging with duplex ultrasonography, computed tomographic

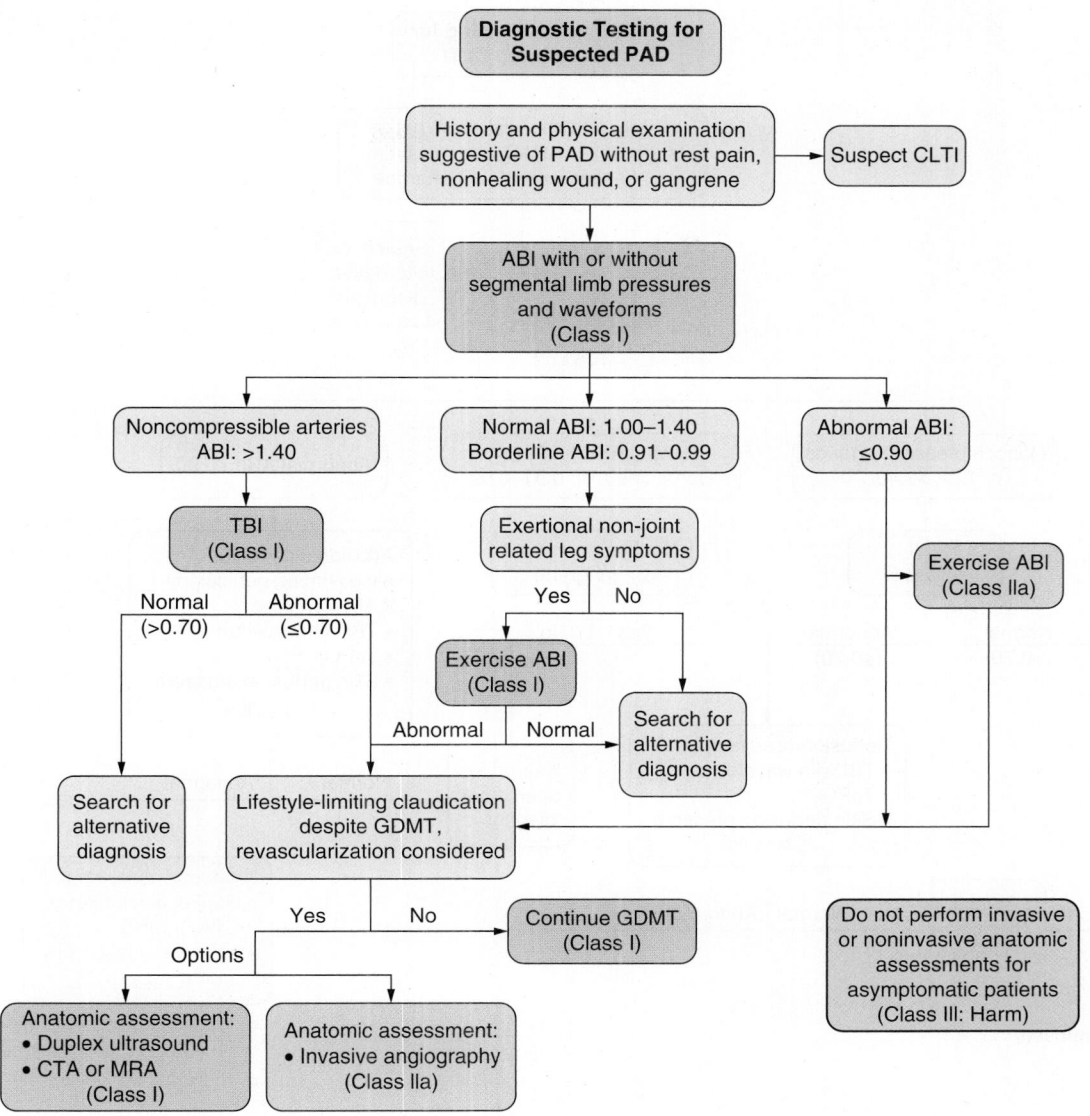

Figure 26–2. (A) Diagnostic testing for suspected PAD. **(B)** Diagnostic testing for suspected CLTI. **A & B,** Reproduced with permission from Gerhard-Herman MD, Gornik HL, Barrett C, et al. 2016 AHA/ACC Guideline on the Management of Patients With Lower Extremity Peripheral Artery Disease: Executive Summary: A Report of the American College of Cardiology/ American Heart Association Task Force on Clinical Practice Guidelines. *J Am Coll Cardiol.* 2017 Mar 21; 69(11):1465-1508.

angiography (CTA), magnetic resonance angiography (MRA), and catheter-based angiography. Although catheter-based angiography is the traditional gold-standard, contemporary management of PAD patients reserves this modality for planned intervention and not diagnostic testing alone. Local expertise will ultimately determine the best approach for imaging approach; however, all modalities have performed with excellent sensitivity and specificity (**Table 26–4**). Segmental pressures are taken with a pneumatic cuff and handheld CW Doppler device at the level of the thigh, calf, and ankle (3-cuff method), which is paired with a continuous wave Doppler interrogation at the femoral artery to assess for inflow disease. Alternatively, segmental pressures may be taken at the high thigh, low thigh, calf, and ankle levels (4-cuff method) to identify the level of disease. The ABI of each leg is obtained, and

then each leg is examined for a pressure drop between levels of ≥20 mm Hg. Segmental pressures are not reliable in patients with noncompressible, seen commonly in patients with diabetes, end-stage kidney disease, or of advanced age.[142-144]

Duplex Ultrasound

Duplex ultrasound allows for assessment of arterial anatomy and hemodynamic effects of stenosis (**Fig. 26–4**). There is no use of contrast or ionizing radiation. Ultrasound is portable and captures images in real time. Body habitus, overlying structures such as bowel gas, and other tissues may interfere with imaging and limit data acquisition. Duplex ultrasound is a useful imaging modality to determine the anatomic location and severity of stenosis in patients with symptomatic PAD in whom revascularization is being considered.[111]

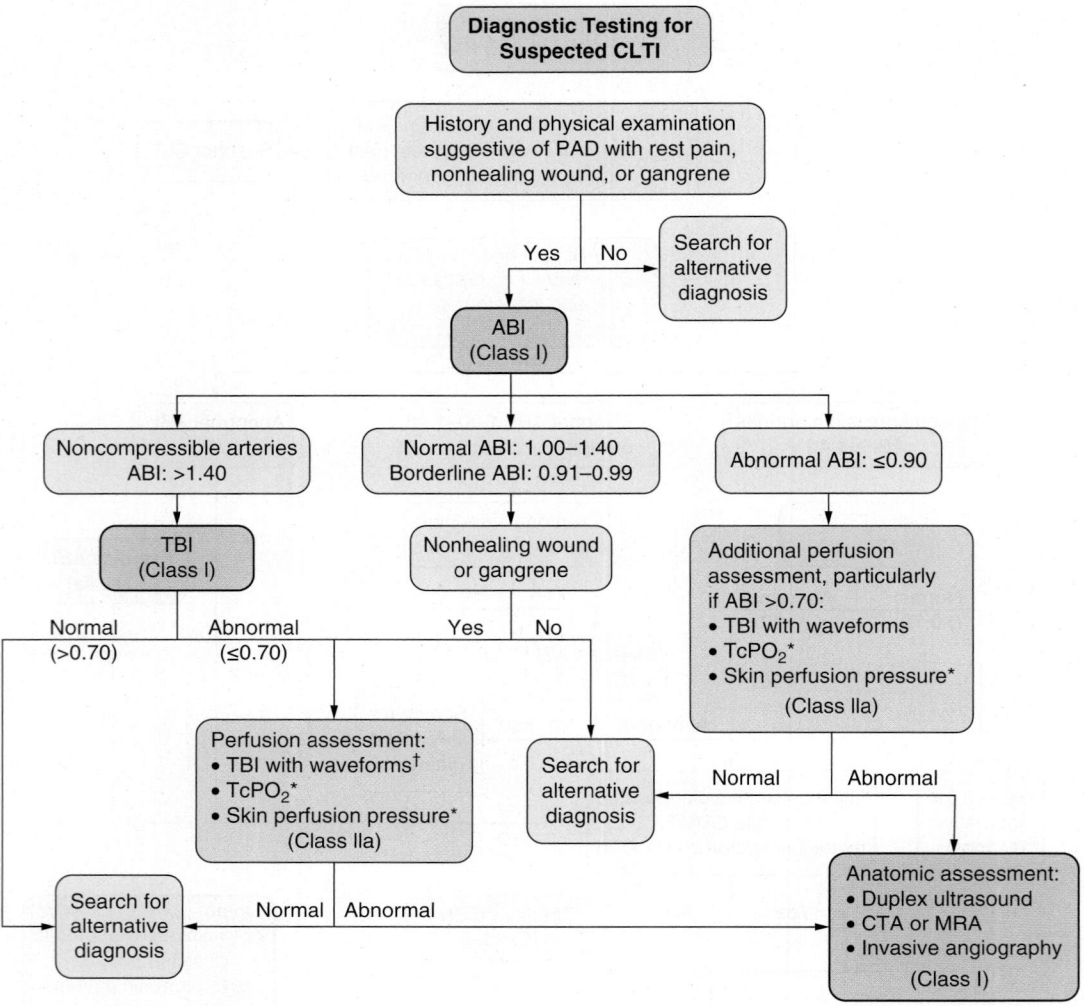

Figure 26–2. (Continued)

Computed Tomography Angiography

CTA provides detailed anatomic information and is noninvasive. Iodinated contrast is required (**Fig. 26–5**). Three-dimensional (3D) reformatting allows for the image to be visualized in multiple planes. The resolution is superior to MRA and this technique is very helpful for determining anatomic assessment and severity of the lesion(s) as well as provide the interventionist information regarding the best access location. Furthermore, the information gained from CTA helps the patient understand the likelihood of technical success of the procedure and information on the durability of the revascularization.[111]

Magnetic Resonance Angiography

MRA provides similar information to a CTA but does not require iodinated contrast but does require gadolinium contrast for optimal images. MRA is another useful imaging modality that provides 3D images and allows for the anatomic location and severity of stenosis in patients with symptomatic PAD in whom revascularization is being considered.[111] For those with a risk for anaphylactoid reaction or contrast nephropathy, it an accurate and safe alternative.[145,146] When gadolinium is in

patients with an eGFR of less than 30, there is an increased risk of gadolinium induced nephrogenic fibrosing dermopathy (or nephrogenic systemic fibrosis).[145,146] Patients with implantable devices will need to be screened for MRI compatibility prior to being put in the magnetic field.

Catheter-Based Angiography

Contrast angiography is the gold standard for evaluation when revascularization is planned.[111] In patients with CTLI or a threatened limb, full anatomic assessment can be done with invasive angiography (**Fig. 26–6**). Most patients with CTLI or lifestyle-limiting claudication have a duplex ultrasound or other imaging modality performed prior to proceeding with invasive angiography because this can provide information key to planning and approach.[111] It is important to assess inflow (aorta and iliac arteries) as well as outflow (common femoral, profunda femoral, superficial femoral, popliteal, tibial-peroneal trunk, anterior tibial, posterior tibial, and peroneal arteries) as well as detailed assessment of the circulation in the foot. While catheter-based angiography can be carried out safely in the large majority of patients, risks of access site injury, contrast

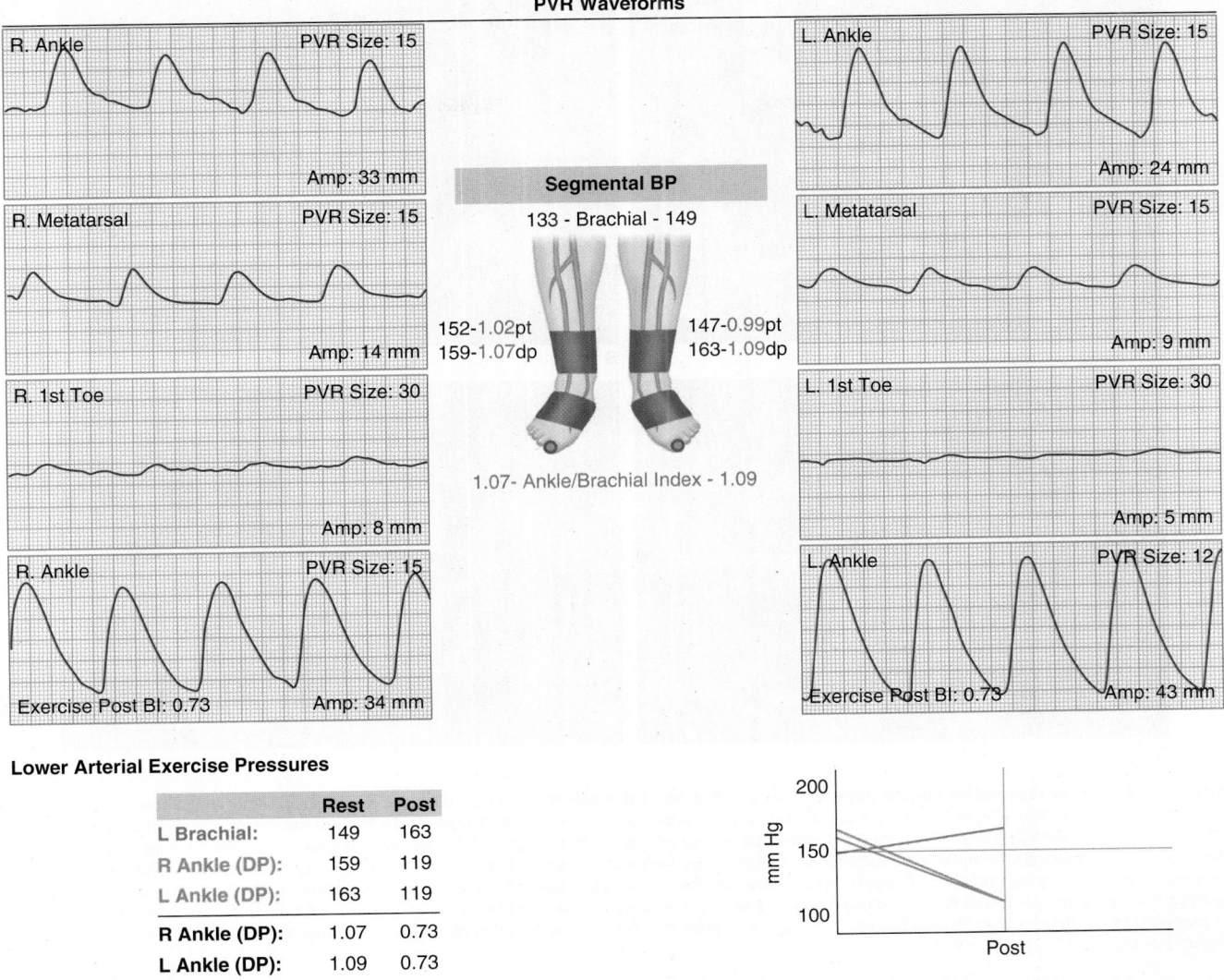

PVR Waveforms

R. Ankle — PVR Size: 15 — Amp: 33 mm

R. Metatarsal — PVR Size: 15 — Amp: 14 mm

R. 1st Toe — PVR Size: 30 — Amp: 8 mm

R. Ankle — PVR Size: 15 — Exercise Post BI: 0.73 — Amp: 34 mm

L. Ankle — PVR Size: 15 — Amp: 24 mm

L. Metatarsal — PVR Size: 15 — Amp: 9 mm

L. 1st Toe — PVR Size: 30 — Amp: 5 mm

L. Ankle — PVR Size: 12 — Exercise Post BI: 0.73 — Amp: 43 mm

Segmental BP
133 - Brachial - 149

152-1.02pt
159-1.07dp

147-0.99pt
163-1.09dp

1.07- Ankle/Brachial Index - 1.09

Lower Arterial Exercise Pressures

	Rest	Post
L Brachial:	149	163
R Ankle (DP):	159	119
L Ankle (DP):	163	119
R Ankle (DP):	1.07	0.73
L Ankle (DP):	1.09	0.73

Figure 26–3. Ankle-brachial index pre- and postexercise testing. Normal resting ankle-brachial index (ABI) and pulse volume waveforms in a 72-year-old male with bilateral calf cramping with exercise. He has a history of CAD, 25-pack year of tobacco use, and diabetes. The ABIs are normal at rest. In the lower panel, note that the arm blood pressure increased while the ankle blood pressures decreased after 3:45 minutes of exercise (2 mph, 12% incline). When the resting ABIs are normal and the ankle pressures and ABIs decrease to a similar degree, one needs to consider aortoiliac disease.

TABLE 26–4. Imaging

	Sensitivity	Specificity	Limitations
Duplex ultrasonography	85%–90%	>95%	Operator dependent Multilevel stenoses Heavily calcified vessels
Magnetic resonance angiography	93%–100%	93%–100%	Renal disease (Gd contrast) In-stent restenosis Critical Limb Ischemia Time
Computed tomography angiography	90%–95%	>90%	Iodinated contrast Ionizing radiation Heavily calcified vessels
Catheter-based angiography		Traditional gold standard	Invasive Iodinated contrast Ionizing radiation May underestimate stenosis (2D)

*Imaging should be performed when considering a revascularization procedure; ie, short-distance claudication or CLTI.
Data from Collins R, Burch J, Cranny G, et al. Duplex ultrasonography, magnetic resonance angiography, and computed tomography angiography for diagnosis and assessment of symptomatic, lower limb peripheral arterial disease: systematic review. *BMJ.* 2007 Jun 16;334(7606):1257 and Pollak AW, Norton PT, Kramer CM. Multimodality imaging of lower extremity peripheral arterial disease: current role and future directions. *Circ Cardiovasc Imaging.* 2012 Nov;5(6):797-807.

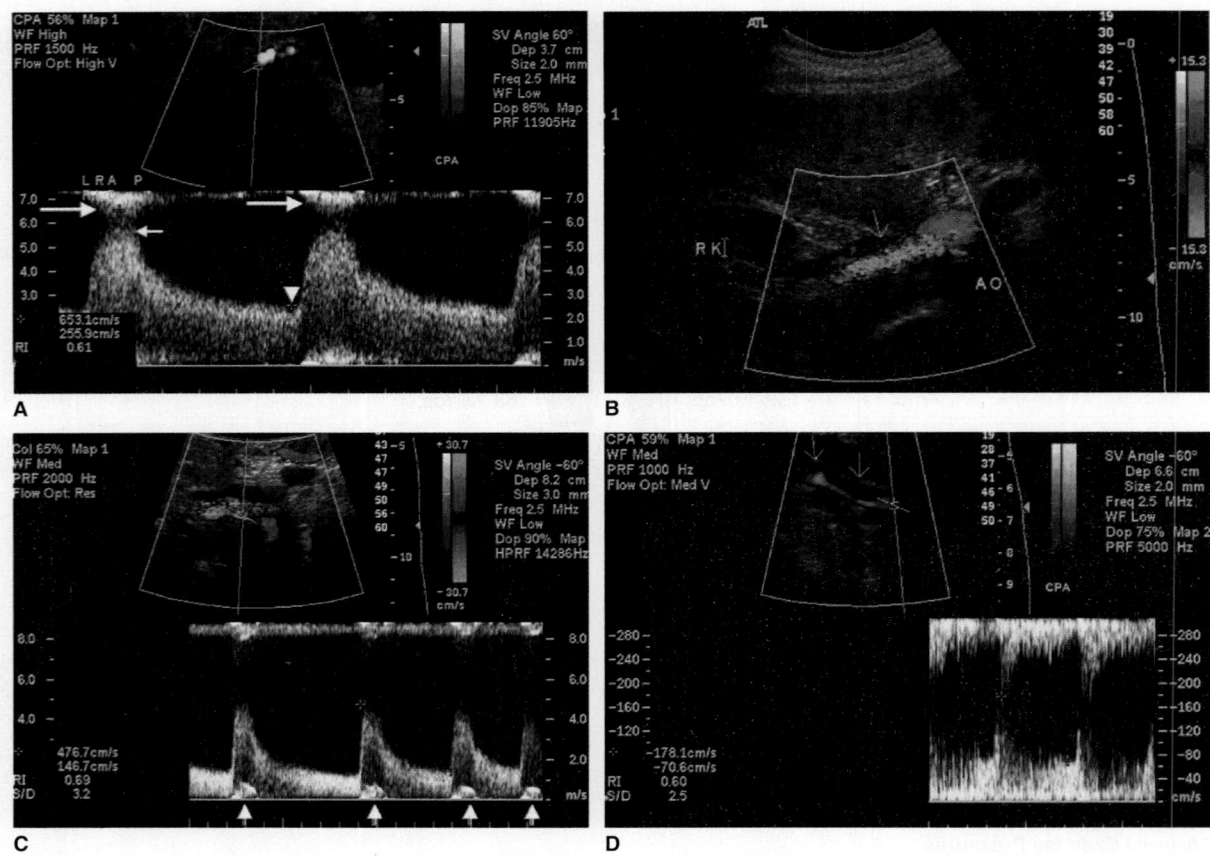

Figure 26–4. Duplex ultrasound findings in patients with severe arterial stenosis. (A) The spectral Doppler waveform appears to "wrap around" to the opposite side of the baseline, an example of aliasing (*large arrows*). Also note that the peak systolic velocity (PSV) is markedly elevated (653 cm/s) (*small arrow*) but this is an underestimation of the true velocity because the Nyquist limit has been exceeded and thus the true velocity cannot be measured. The end diastolic velocity (*arrowhead*) is extremely high at 256 cm/s confirming a severe stenosis. **(B)** The mosaic color pattern is another example of aliasing indicative of high-velocity stenotic color-jets (*arrow*). **(C)** The peak systolic velocity and end diastolic velocity are very high indicative of sever stenosis in this artery. There is also a spectral bruit known as a visual bruit (*arrows*). **(D)** This is an example of turbulent flow as demonstrated by the multiple speeds that the red blood cells are traveling in the spectral waveform. If this is shown in an artery, the ultrasonographer should go back and look more proximally for a high-velocity jet that was missed. Reproduced with permission from Gustavson S, Olin JW. Images in vascular medicine. Clues to severe arterial stenosis by duplex ultrasound. *Vasc Med.* 2003;8(1):59-61.

reactions, contrast nephropathy, and distal embolization can rarely occur.

CLASSIFICATION OF PERIPHERAL ARTERY DISEASE

Classification schemes that are useful for guiding management of acute and chronic lower extremity ischemia are reviewed in this section. There is a wide spectrum of clinical presentations for PAD, ranging from claudication to acute limb ischemia. These classification schemes are distinguished by anatomic and symptom-based criteria.

Anatomic Lesion Classification

Trans-Atlantic Inter-Society Consensus

Trans-Atlantic Inter-Society Consensus (TASC II) classifies arterial lesions as Type A, B, C, or D based on anatomic distribution, number and nature of lesion (stenosis, occlusion), as well as according to the success rates of treatment of the lesion

with endovascular or surgical approach.[18] Short segments are more likely to be successfully treated with an endovascular intervention compared to long segments of occlusion. This classification scheme is limited in focusing on single lesions; most patients with peripheral arterial disease have more than one lesion at more than one level. Scoring systems that take into account multifocal disease have been used in research studies.[95,147] The original TASC I classification scheme included aortoiliac, femoropopliteal, and tibial runoff. TASC II does not include tibial runoff (**Table 26–5**).

Global Limb Anatomic Staging System

Global Limb Anatomic Staging System (GLASS) was proposed in the 2019 global vascular guidelines to help with management in CLTI.[114] This comprehensive classification scheme stratifies anatomic severity and provides a much-needed framework for evidence-based lower extremity revascularization of CLTI. GLASS grades the level of disease at the femoropopliteal and infrapopliteal segments of the anticipated target arterial path

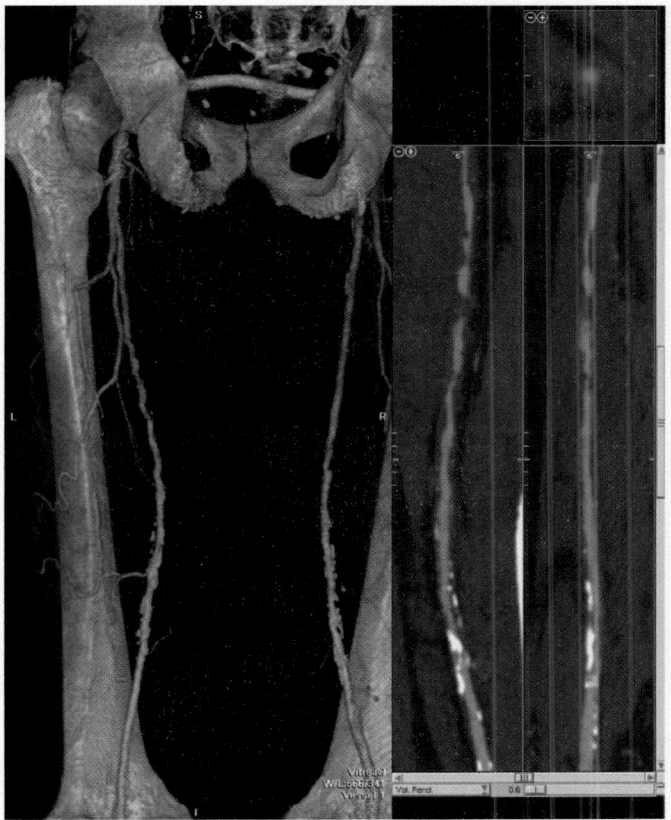

Figure 26–5. CT Angiogram of the femoral arteries. The image on the left is a volume-rendered view that demonstrates severe bilateral atherosclerosis of the superficial femoral arteries. The right-hand images are maximal intensity projections showing three views demonstrating multiple areas of stenosis and occlusion with diffuse atherosclerosis of the right superficial femoral artery. Reproduced with permission from Robert Lookstein, MD.

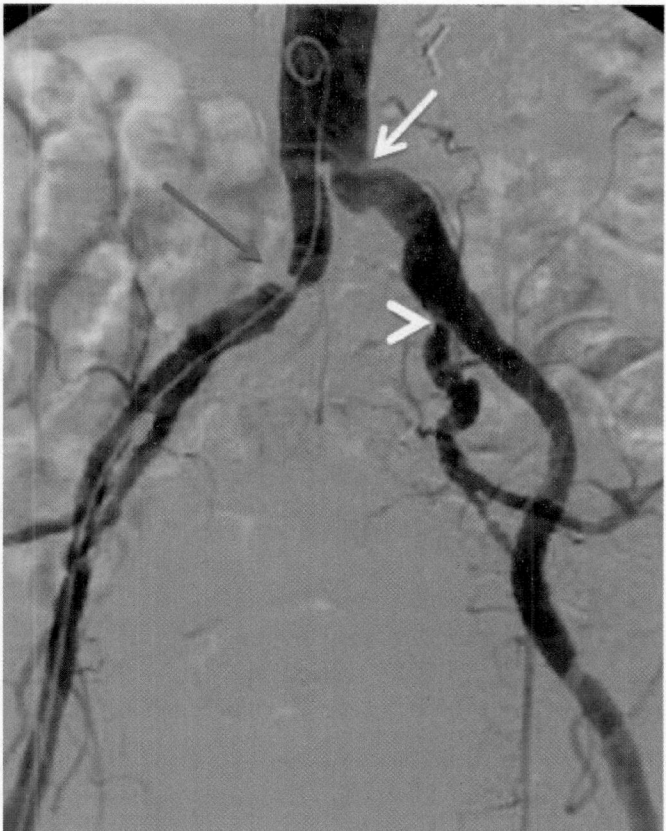

Figure 26–6. Catheter-based angiography of the aortoiliac segments. There is a stenosis at the origin of the left common iliac artery (*white arrow*) and the left internal iliac artery (*white arrowhead*). There is a severe stenosis in the midportion of the right common iliac artery (*blue arrow*).

for revascularization; these grades are combined to provide a level of complexity that is thought to estimate patency of lower extremity interventions in CTLI. The details of this staging system are beyond the scope of this chapter.

Symptom Classification

Chronic extremity ischemia: Rutherford and Fontaine symptom classification systems have been widely used for decades.[148,149]

Rutherford and Fontaine

The Rutherford and Fontaine classifications provide descriptors of various degrees of walking impairment (mild, moderate, and severe claudication) and more severe degrees of limb ischemia (rest pain, ischemic ulcers, and gangrene) (**Table 26–6**).

Wound, Ischemia, Foot Infection

The Society of Vascular Surgery (SVS) Lower Extremity Threatened Limb Classification System, Wound, Ischemia, foot Infection (Wlfl) is an updated system for the classification of threatened limb. It is thought to more accurately reflect the significant clinical considerations that are important for management and amputation risk and allow for analysis of outcomes.[114,150] This classification scheme has been validated in multiple studies and allows one to assess the likelihood of

wound healing and amputation risk for a patient with chronic limb ischemia.[151-155] With this scheme, the patient can be placed into one of four amputation risk categories (very low, low, moderate, and high) that correspond to clinical stage. Wlfl stages at initial presentation correlate with wound healing time and wound healing rate at 1 year.[156-160] This system is also intended to be used for restaging postintervention. Studies have demonstrated wound, ischemia, and infection grades at 1 and 6 months correlated with amputation-free survival as well as staging and restaging identified a cohort high risk for amputation that timely reintervention might be advantageous.[161,162]

ALI can also be classified based on symptoms. The SVS/ISCVS (Rutherford) classification stratifies limb ischemia based on sensorimotor deficits and Doppler findings (Table 26–2).[149,163,164]

TREATMENT OF PERIPHERAL ARTERY DISEASE

It has been shown that patients with PAD are not treated optimally from a medical standpoint when compared to those with coronary artery disease (CAD). **Tables 26–7A** and **26–7B** compare the United States and European guidelines for the management of PAD. In understanding the role of medical management, distinctions must be made between those

TABLE 26–5. TASC Classification

	TASC A	TASC B	TASC C	TASC D
Aortoiliac	Unilateral or bilateral stenoses of CIA Unilateral or bilateral single short (#3 cm) stenosis of EIA	Short (#3 cm) stenosis of infrarenal aorta Unilateral CIA occlusion Single or multiple stenoses totaling 3–10 cm involving the EIA, not extending into the CFA Unilateral EIA occlusion not involving the origins of internal iliac or CFA	Bilateral CIA occlusions Bilateral EIA stenoses 3–10 cm long, not extending into the CFA Unilateral EIA stenosis extending into the CFA Unilateral EIA occlusion that involves the origins of internal iliac and/or CFA Heavily calcified unilateral EIA occlusion with or without involvement of origins of internal iliac and/or CFA	Infrarenal aortoiliac occlusion Diffuse disease involving the aorta and both iliac arteries Diffuse multiple stenoses involving the unilateral CIA, EIA, and CFA Unilateral occlusions of both CIA and EIA Bilateral occlusions of EIA Iliac stenoses in patients with AAA not amenable to endograft placement
Femoral-popliteal	Single stenosis #10 cm in length Single occlusion #5 cm in length	Multiple lesions (stenoses or occlusions), each #5 cm Single stenosis or occlusion #15 cm, not involving the infrageniculate popliteal artery Heavily calcified occlusion #5 cm in length Single popliteal stenosis	Multiple stenoses or occlusions totaling >15 cm, with or without heavy calcification Recurrent stenoses or occlusions after failing treatment	Chronic total occlusions of CFA or SFA (>20 cm, involving the popliteal artery) Chronic total occlusion of popliteal artery and proximal trifurcation vessels
Infrapopliteal	Single focal stenosis, #5 cm in length, in the target tibial artery, with occlusion or stenosis of similar or worse severity in the other tibial arteries	Multiple stenoses, each #5 cm in length, or total length #10 cm, or single occlusion #3 cm in length, in the target tibial artery with occlusion or stenosis of similar or worse severity in the other tibial arteries	Multiple stenoses in the target tibial artery and/or single occlusion with total lesion length >10 cm with occlusion or stenosis of similar or worse severity in the other tibial arteries	Multiple occlusions involving the target tibial artery with total lesion length >10 cm, or dense lesion calcification or nonvisualization of collaterals; the other tibial arteries occluded or with dense calcification

Abbreviations: AAA, abdominal aortic aneurysm; CFA, common femoral artery; CIA, common iliac artery; EIA, external iliac artery; SFA, superficial femoral artery; TASC, Trans-Atlantic Inter-Society Consensus.
Data from TASC Steering Committee, Jaff MR, White CJ, et al. An Update on Methods for Revascularization and Expansion of the TASC Lesion Classification to Include Below-the-Knee Arteries: A Supplement to the Inter-Society Consensus for the Management of Peripheral Arterial Disease (TASC II). *Vasc Med.* 2015 Oct;20(5):465-478.

therapies that improve cardiovascular morbidity and mortality and those that improve limb function and survival from amputation. The PAD prescription as recommended in the guidelines is shown in **Fig. 26–7**.[165]

Claudication and CTLI

Smoking Cessation
Smoking cessation is recommended across multiple guidelines for the management of patients with PAD. Patients should be strongly advised to stop smoking and the healthcare provider should offer methods that may help the patient achieve this goal (referral to a smoking cessation program, pharmacotherapy). At every office visit, the patient should be asked in a nonjudgmental way if they have stopped smoking and reinforce the benefits of smoking cessation. Stress that smoking cessation will not only decrease the risk of MI, stroke, and death but also help prevent the progression of PAD, help to keep a stent or bypass patent, and prevent amputation.[15,166–169]

Exercise Therapy
An exercise regimen is recommended as part of the initial treatment for patients with PAD and claudication based on

TABLE 26–6. Fontaine and Rutherford Stages in Patients with Peripheral Artery Disease

Fontaine		Rutherford		
Stage	Clinical	Grade	Category	Clinical
I	Asymptomatic	0	0	Asymptomatic
IIa	Mild claudication >200 m	I	1	Mild claudication
IIb	Moderate-severe claudication <200 m	I	2 3	Moderate claudication Severe claudication
III	Ischemic rest pain	II	4	Ischemic rest pain
IV	Ulceration or gangrene	III	5	Minor tissue loss
		IV	6	Ulceration or gangrene

TABLE 26–7. Overview of Major Differences

	AHA/ACC	ESC
Focus	In-depth review of single disease location.	Extends to all noncoronary atherosclerotic vascular disease.
Audience	All practitioners.	Predominantly cardiologists and vascular surgeons.
Treatment Approach	Requires evidence for each treatment, specifically for PAD.	Orientated for systemic atherosclerosis generally more than PAD alone.
Selection of Evidence	Inclusive of smaller, well-done nonrandomized studies.	Relegates small studies to level of evidence C.
Medical Management	Clopidogrel = ASA to reduce cardiovascular events.	Clopidogrel > ASA to reduce cardiovascular events.
Management of Symptoms	Recommend cilostazol (class I).	Does not recommend cilostazol.
Revascularization	Emphasis on postprocedure surveillance and wound care.	Greater attention on revascularization strategies and contemporary therapies.

Guidelines for Antiplatelet and Anticoagulation in PAD:

Class	AHA/ACC	ESC
I	Antiplatelet therapy with aspirin alone (range 75–325 mg/day) or clopidogrel alone (75 mg/day) is recommended to reduce MI, stroke, and vascular death in patients with symptomatic PAD.	Long term single antiplatelet therapy is recommended in symptomatic patients. In patients with PADs and AF, oral anticoagulation is recommended when the CHA2DS2-VASc score is ≥2.
IIa	In asymptomatic patients with PAD (ABI ≤ 0.90), antiplatelet therapy is reasonable to reduce the risk of MI, stroke, or vascular death.	Dual antiplatelet therapy with aspirin and clopidogrel for at least 1 month should be considered after infra-inguinal stent implantation.
IIb	In asymptomatic patients with borderline ABI (0.91–0.99), the usefulness of antiplatelet therapy to reduce the risk of MI, stroke, or vascular death is uncertain. Dual antiplatelet therapy (aspirin and clopidogrel) may be reasonable to reduce the risk of limb-related events in patients with symptomatic PAD after lower extremity revascularization.	In patients requiring antiplatelet therapy, clopidogrel may be preferred over aspirin.
	The effectiveness of dual antiplatelet therapy (aspirin and clopidogrel) to reduce the risk of cardiovascular ischemic events in patients with symptomatic PAD is not well established. The overall clinical benefit of vorapaxar adding to existing antiplatelet therapy in patients with symptomatic PAD is uncertain.	
III	Anticoagulation should not be used to reduce the risk of cardiovascular ischemic events in patients with PAD. **NOTE: These guidelines were written before the publication of the COMPASS and VOYAGER Trials (see text) were published. No longer is low-dose rivaroxaban considered harmful in patients with PAD.**	Because of lack of proven benefit, antiplatelet therapy is not routinely indicated in patients with isolated asymptomatic LEAD.

studies that have demonstrated significant improvements in walking parameters. Exercise training is thought to improve claudication through various mechanisms, the contribution of each is not yet clearly established. These mechanisms are as follows: increased calf blood flow; improved endothelial function and subsequent improved vasodilatation; reduced inflammation through reduction in free radicals; improvements in muscle structure, strength, and endurance; vascular angiogenesis; improved mitochondrial function; skeletal muscle metabolism; and reduced red cell aggregation and blood viscosity.[170–177]

The optimal regimen for exercise rehabilitation is still being evaluated;[178,179] recent guidelines provide a guide for implementation of supervised exercise therapy in patients with PAD, including a protocol, outcome measurement, and transition to home based exercise.[180] Ideally, a supervised exercise program should be utilized and continued for a minimum of 12 weeks.[168] In 2017, the Centers for Medicare and Medicaid Services (CMS) established coverage for supervised exercise programs in patients with symptomatic PAD. Those that are post-revascularization with symptoms are also eligible. Those who are still symptomatic after completion of supervised exercise therapy are eligible for an additional 36 sessions.[180]

During these exercise sessions, the intensity of exercise should elicit claudication. Supervised exercise programs follow these parameters with a one-to-one supervision by an exercise physiologist, physical therapist, or a nurse. This individual will monitor claudication threshold and cardiovascular parameters.

Since a supervised exercise program is not available in most centers in the United States, the patient should be counseled on a home exercise program. In our recommended home exercise program, exercise spans for 50 minutes, 3 to 5 times a week (**Fig. 26–8**).[181]

Decrease the Risk of MI, Stroke, and CV Death	Improve Symptoms, Quality of Life, and Prevent Amputation
• Discontinue Tobacco Use	• Discontinue Tobacco Use
• Walking Program	• Walking Program
• Control Blood Pressure to Goal - ACE Inhibitor	• Cilostazol

• High-Dose Statin Therapy	• Good Foot Care
	  - Moisturizing cream, nail care, treat
	    and prevent tinea, orthotics to
	    prevent abnormal pressure points

• Antiplatelet Therapy	• Revascularization

Figure 26–7. PAD prescription. Reproduced with permission from Olin JW, White CJ, Armstrong EJ, et al. Peripheral Artery Disease: Evolving Role of Exercise, Medical Therapy, and Endovascular Options. *J Am Coll Cardiol.* 2016 Mar 22;67(11):1338-1357.

While it is difficult for many patients to adhere to such a program, when they do it properly, it greatly increases maximum walking distance and walking speed and is associated with an improved quality of life. It is important to emphasize that if the patient stops exercising, they often return to their pre-exercise state. Exercise does not increase the collateral circulation as initially thought; it does however increase oxygen utilization in the mitochondria so that the muscle can function on lower levels of oxygen delivery.

Frequency
3–5 days per week

Modality
Treadmill (this program can be adapted for walking outside)

Method
1. Begin at 2 mph and a gradient of 0 (flat)

2. Stop exercise when pain is 3–4 on claudication pain scale*

3. When the pain has ceased, resume exercise at the same intensity

4. Repeat rest/exercise cycles

5. Progress to a higher work load when the patient can walk for 8 min without having to stop for leg symptoms:

   (a) Increase speed by 0.2 mph each time the patient can walk for 8 min

   (b) Once the patient can walk at 3.4 mph, or reaches a speed at which they can no longer keep up, begin increasing the grade by 1–2%

Duration
The total exercise period, including rest periods, should equal 50 min per day

*Claudication pain scale: 1 = no pain; 2 = onset of claudication; 3 = mild pain or discomfort; 4 = moderate pain or discomfort; 5 = severe pain or discomfort. Abbreviations: mph, miles per hour; PAD, peripheral artery disease.

Figure 26–8. Instructions for a home walking program. Reproduced with permission from Weinberg MD, Lau JF, Rosenfield K, et al. Peripheral artery disease. Part 2: medical and endovascular treatment. *Nat Rev Cardiol.* 2011 Jun 14;8(8):429-441.

Exercise rehabilitation reduces symptoms of claudication in patients with PAD.[182,183] In a meta-analysis of nine trials, exercise was shown to improve pain-free walking distance and maximum walking distance; there was no improvement in ABI.[184] Exercise and survival in PAD patients could be associated. A meta-analysis demonstrated a shorter maximum walking distance was associated with an increased 5-year cardiovascular and all-cause mortality.[185-186]

Lipid Lowering

Despite guideline recommendations for patients with PAD, these patients are undertreated when compared to patients with CAD.[187-189] Lipid lowering therapy with at least a moderate intensity statin, irrespective of baseline LDL, is recommended for patients with clinical atherosclerosis.

The effect of lipid lowering therapy on the natural history of PAD has been studied in multiple trials.[190-193] These studies have demonstrated a regression or reduction in progression of femoral atherosclerosis with lipid modifying therapy.[194-198] A meta-analysis from 2007 demonstrated that lipid lowering therapy in patients with PAD reduced progression of disease as visualized on angiography, improved claudication symptoms, as well as improvement in walking times and pain-free distance.[191] In the Heart Protection Study, the use of simvastatin decreased overall mortality by 12% and specifically vascular mortality by 17%.[199]

The effect of proprotein convertase subtilisin/kexin type 9 (PCSK9) inhibition with evolocumab was studied in PAD patients in the FOURIER trial. The primary composite endpoint (cardiovascular death, MI, stroke, hospital admission for stable angina, coronary revascularization) was significantly reduced in patients with PAD compared to those randomized to placebo. The absolute reduction in the primary end point was greater in those with PAD (3.5%) compared to those without PAD (1.6%). This in all likelihood is due to the higher risk of patients with PAD. Evolocumab also reduced the risk of major adverse limb events in all groups.[200]

Antiplatelet/Antithrombotic Therapy

Long-term antithrombotic therapy has been shown to be beneficial in secondary prevention of atherosclerotic CVD. Early randomized trials demonstrated a significant reduction in risk for future adverse cardiovascular events for symptomatic PAD patients with long-term antiplatelet therapy (aspirin, clopidogrel).[111,201,202] The indication for antiplatelet therapy (Clopidogrel or Aspirin) is to reduce the risk for future adverse cardiovascular events (MI, stroke, and cardiovascular death) in patients with symptomatic PAD.[15,40,201] Follow-up studies have demonstrated that aspirin is not as effective in PAD. In the Clopidogrel Versus Aspirin in Patients of Ischemic Events (CAPRIE) trial, clopidogrel (75 mg/day) had a significant advantage over ASA (325 mg/day) with a reduction in risk for combined outcome of ischemic stroke, MI, or vascular death (relative risk reduction 8.7%, $P = 0.043$) in 19,815 patients with a recent stroke, MI, or asymptomatic PAD. In a subgroup analysis, the benefit of clopidogrel over aspirin was predominantly driven by patients with PAD with a 23.8% relative risk reduction.[203]

No benefit over aspirin has been demonstrated in respect to vitamin K antagonists for reducing mortality in PAD patients. In the Warfarin and Antiplatelet Vascular Evaluation (WAVE) trial, the combination of warfarin (INR 2–3) plus antiplatelet therapy was not more effective when compared to solely aspirin in the prevention of cardiovascular morbidity in PAD patients.[204] Recent data suggests a benefit for low-dose factor Xa inhibition in PAD in addition to antiplatelet therapy.[205–207] In the Cardiovascular Outcomes for People Using Anticoagulation Strategies (COMPASS) trial, 27,395 patients were randomized to rivaroxaban 2.5 mg twice a day and ASA 81 mg daily (n = 9152) versus rivaroxaban 5 mg twice daily alone (n = 9117) versus ASA alone (n = 9126). The inclusion criteria were stable atherosclerosis in ≥2 vascular beds or two additional risk factors (current smoking, diabetes, renal insufficiency, heart failure, or nonlacunar ischemic stroke ≥1 month). The primary outcome (MI, stroke, cardiovascular death) occurred in 4.1% of combination therapy as compared to 4.9% in the rivaroxaban alone group and 5.4% in the aspirin alone group ($P < 0.001$). Among 7470 subjects in the COMPASS PAD group, 4129 patients had symptomatic PAD, 1919 had carotid disease, and 1422 had CAD plus and ABI <0.9. In those with PAD, combination therapy reduced composite end point of cardiovascular death, MI, or stroke compared to Aspirin alone, in addition to reduction in major adverse limb events. This was at the expense of a higher incidence of major bleeding with combination and monotherapy with rivaroxaban (**Table 26–8**).[207]

The Vascular Outcomes Study of Aspirin (ASA) Along with Rivaroxaban in Endovascular or Surgical Limb Revascularization for PAD (VOYAGER PAD) trial randomized 6564 PAD patients post-revascularization to rivaroxaban (2.5 mg twice a day) plus ASA 81 mg versus placebo plus ASA.[208] Low-dose rivaroxaban plus ASA reduced the composite endpoint of acute limb ischemia, major amputation, MI, ischemic stroke, or death from a cardiovascular cause (**Fig. 26–9**). It also reduced the incidence of ALI and the need for index-limb revascularization for recurrent limb ischemia. Thrombolysis in myocardial infarction (TIMI) major bleeding in the rivaroxaban arm was 2.7% compared to 1.9% in the placebo group ($P = 0.07$). The incidence of International Society on Thrombosis and Haemostasis (ISTH) major bleeding was 5.94% in the rivaroxaban

TABLE 26–8. Comparison of MACE, MALE, and Major Bleeding in COMPASS*

	Major Adverse Cardiac Events (MACE)	Major Adverse Limb Events (MALE)	Major Bleeding
Rivaroxaban + ASA	5%	1.5%	3.0%
Rivaroxaban	6%	1.9%	3.0%
ASA	7%	2.6%	2.0%

$P = 0.005$ for rivaroxaban plus aspirin vs. aspirin alone; $P = 0.19$ for rivaroxaban alone vs. aspirin alone
$P = 0.01$ for rivaroxaban plus aspirin vs. aspirin alone; $P = 0.07$ for rivaroxaban alone vs. aspirin alone
$P = 0.009$ for rivaroxaban plus aspirin vs. aspirin alone; $P = 0.004$ for rivaroxaban alone vs. aspirin alone

Data from Eikelboom JW, Connolly SJ, Bosch J, et al. Rivaroxaban with or without Aspirin in Stable Cardiovascular Disease. *N Engl J Med.* 2017 Oct 5;377(14):1319-1330 and Anand SS, Bosch J, Eikelboom JW, et al. Rivaroxaban with or without aspirin in patients with stable peripheral or carotid artery disease: an international, randomised, double-blind, placebo-controlled trial. *Lancet.* 2018 Jan 20;391(10117):219-229.

group versus 4.06% in the placebo group, $P = 0.007$). In a pre-specified subgroup analysis, half of the patients received clopidogrel at the time of randomization for up to 6 months. The patients receiving clopidogrel were more likely to undergo endovascular procedures (90.7%) versus surgery (9.3%). There was no additional benefit to adding clopidogrel. There was a small increase in ISTH major bleeding (6.5% in the clopidogrel group) versus 5.4% in those not taking clopidogrel. There was no difference in intracranial bleeds.

The results of the COMPASS trial and Voyager PAD trial are so striking, the paradigm of how PAD patients are treated should be incorporated into the new guidelines.

Vorapaxar is an antagonist of the protease-activated receptor (PAR-1).[209] In the Trial to Assess the Effects of Vorapaxar in Preventing Heart Attack and Stroke in Patients with Atherosclerosis-Thrombolysis in Myocardial Infarction 50 (TRAP®P-TIMI 50) in patients with symptomatic lower extremity PAD, Vorapaxar plus antiplatelet therapy reduced the rate of first acute limb ischemia events, most notable in patients post-revascularization.[210–213] However, the risk of bleeding in this trial was substantial and thus, it will not ever be used widely in patients with PAD.

Antihypertensive Therapy
Hypertension is a risk factor for PAD and atherosclerosis in other locations. Therefore, blood pressure should be well controlled to reduce morbidity from cerebrovascular and CVD.[18] In the Heart Outcomes Prevention Evaluation (HOPE) trial, ramipril significantly reduced the rates of death, MI, and stroke, including patients with asymptomatic and symptomatic PAD.[214] A follow-up study found similar results in patients subdivided by ABI. Event rates were higher in patients with ABI <0.9; this group had absolute benefit that was about twice as large compared to those with an ABI >0.9.[215]

Glycemic Control
It is unknown if intensive glucose control decreases the likelihood of adverse cardiovascular events in patients with diabetes

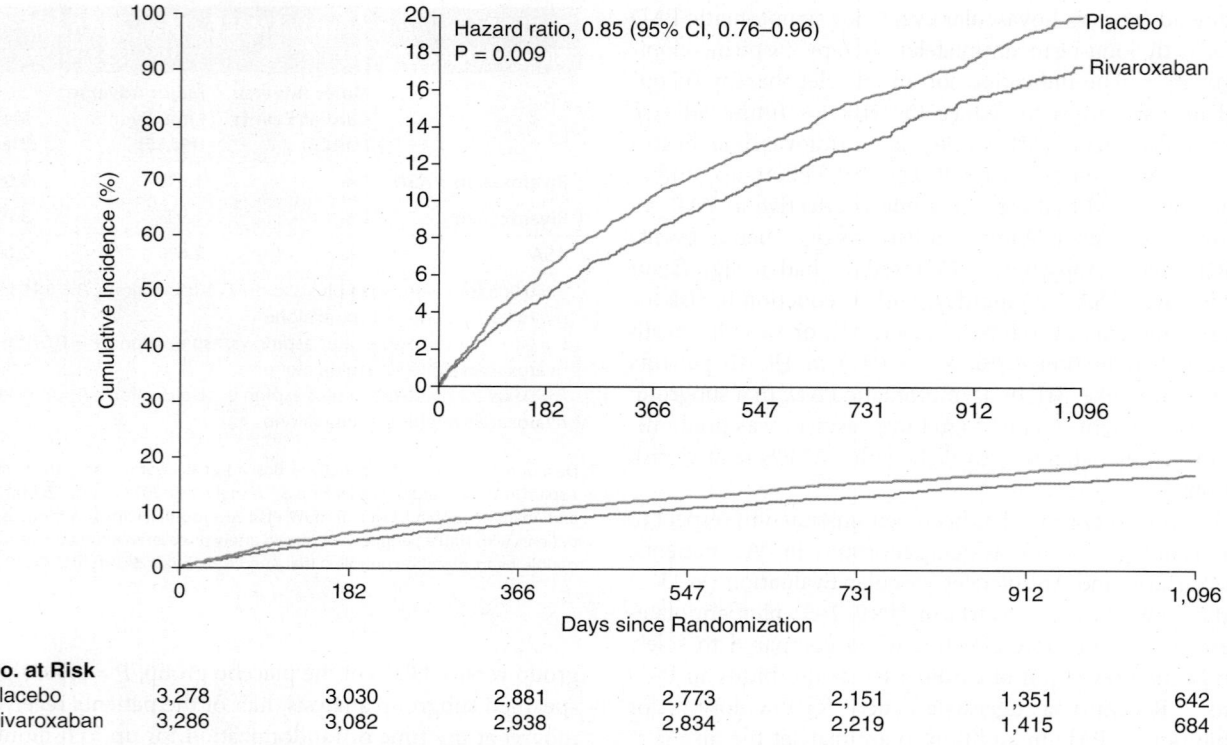

No. at Risk							
Placebo	3,278	3,030	2,881	2,773	2,151	1,351	642
Rivaroxaban	3,286	3,082	2,938	2,834	2,219	1,415	684

Figure 26–9. Kaplan–Meier analysis of the primary composite efficacy outcome. The primary efficacy outcome was a composite of ALI, major amputation for vascular causes, MI, ischemic stroke, or cardiovascular death. The inset shows the same data on an expanded y axis. Reproduced with permission from Bonaca MP, Bauersachs RM, Anand SS, et al. Rivaroxaban in Peripheral Artery Disease after Revascularization. *N Engl J Med.* 2020 May 21;382(21):1994-2004.

and PAD. It is known that treatment of diabetes is effective for reducing microvascular complications.[216] A HbA1c of <7% should be targeted; this may be tailored to specific patient demographics and comorbidities.[217]

Two new classes of agents, the sodium-glucose co-transporter 2 inhibitors (SGLT2-i) and the glucagon-like peptide-1 receptor agonists (GLP1-RA) have demonstrated reductions in cardiovascular events focused predominantly on patients with CVD and diabetes. Both agents were studied in trials that included patients with diabetes and PAD.[218–221] There is specific interest in SGLT2-I in patients with PAD and diabetes mellitus. The CANagliflozin cardiovascular Assessment Study (CANVAS) identified safety concerns for amputations in patients with PAD and prior amputations.[220,222] Another population cohort-based study demonstrated a 2-fold risk of below-the-knee amputation with greatest risk in patients with known diagnosis of PAD.[223–225] This study used medications across the SGLT2-I class. Other studies that used SGLT2-i do not report an increased risk of amputation. The EMPA-REG evaluated the use of empagliflozin; in the PAD subgroup there were significant reductions in cardiovascular and all-cause mortality in addition to major adverse cardiovascular outcomes.[226] There was not a significant difference in amputations across treatment and placebo arms. There was no increased risk in amputation with dapagliflozin versus placebo in the DECLARE-TIMI 58 trial.[227] The black box warning has been subsequently lifted based on newer safety data suggesting lower risk of amputation.

Cilostazol

Among pharmacological therapy options to improve symptoms of PAD (claudication), cilostazol has been demonstrated to be beneficial. Cilostazol is a type III phosphodiesterase inhibitor that suppresses platelet aggregation and is an arterial vasodilator, although the mechanism by which it improves claudication remains unknown.[228] It has been shown to have benefits as early as 4 weeks of therapy but can take up to 4 months to reach full effect. The most effective dose is 100 mg twice a day.[229,230] Several meta-analyses have demonstrated the efficacy of this pharmacologic therapy.[231–234] For example, in a meta-analysis of 2702 patients with moderate-to-severe PAD with claudication who were randomized to Cilostazol or placebo, there was an increase in maximal walking distance and pain-free walking distance in patients in the cilostazol arm.[234] There is a black box warning against the use of cilostazol in patients with heart failure with reduced ejection fraction.

Combination Therapy

Prior studies have compared supervised exercise programs to revascularization in patients with PAD and exercise limiting claudication, with a benefit demonstrated in both interventions. An early study comparing bypass surgery and exercise therapy to each intervention alone showed that combination therapy was superior to individual therapy.[235] The Claudication: Exercise Versus Endoluminal Revascularization (CLEVER) study compared stenting of aortoiliac disease with supervised exercise therapy in a patient population with PAD, symptomatic claudication, and on optimal medical therapy.[236] At 6 months of follow-up, peak walking time on a graded treadmill test was improved in both the exercise and stent groups compared to optimal medical therapy; although the peak walking time was higher in the exercise group compared to the revascularization group. Quality-of-life questionnaires demonstrated improvement in the exercise or stenting groups, relative to optimal medical therapy.[237] This study demonstrated the long-term benefit of both revascularization through stenting and a supervised exercise program in PAD patients with claudication symptoms. Limitations of this study included a very small sample size and difficulties getting patients to agree to randomization; therefore, it took a much longer time to complete the study than planned, and lack of long-term follow-up. The arm of the trial in CLEVER that slotted to look at the combination of exercise and stenting was not completed because of difficulties with enrollment.

A subsequent trial, the Endovascular Revascularization and Supervised Exercise (ERASE) trial, compared combination therapy to supervised exercise therapy alone. At 1-year of follow-up, the combination therapy had a greater improvement in maximum walking distance and reported quality of life scores compared to supervised exercise therapy alone. Although both groups demonstrated improvement in maximum walking distance, pain-free walking distance, and quality of life.[238] This study combination of endovascular revascularization and supervised exercise therapy was the most effective therapy for PAD patients with claudication.

Revascularization Considerations

Guidelines have identified important criteria to be met when considering percutaneous or surgical intervention in patients with claudication.[15,18,40,163,166,167,169,239] The following are criteria to take into consideration when determining the role for an revascularization: (1) claudication is causing significant disability for the patient, in that they cannot perform daily activities of living or other activities that are important to the individual and they feel that it is affecting the quality of their life; (2) exercise therapy and maximum pharmacological therapy provides results that are not satisfactory to the patient; (3) the characteristics of the lesion are amenable to an intervention with a low risk and a high success rate; and (4) the patient will derive a benefit in claudication symptoms (symptoms are not from another etiology, ie, spinal stenosis, osteoarthritis, or shortness of breath limiting exercising capacity).

Options for revascularization depends on the level of obstruction (**Table 26–9**). However, most experts now agree that for claudication, an endovascular first approach should be used. Surgical revascularization should only be used to treat claudication in very unusual circumstances. In general, surgery should be reserved for cases limb salvage where arterial anatomy is not favorable for a percutaneous approach and the surgical risk is acceptable.[18,163,167,169]

Lesions that are unfavorable for percutaneous approach have been identified as the following: long-segment stenosis, multi-focal stenosis, eccentric, calcified stenosis, and long segment occlusions. These characteristics are found in patients

TABLE 26–9. Revascularization Considerations Determined by Anatomy

Level of Disease	Characteristic Symptoms	Treatment
Aortoiliac disease (inflow disease)	Claudication in the thigh, hip, or buttock.	Iliac artery angioplasty and stenting. Rarely is aortoiliac bypass, or aortofemoral bypass, performed since endovascular therapy is so effective.
Femoropopliteal disease, lesions below the inguinal ligament (outflow disease)	Calf claudication	Balloon angioplasty and/or stenting. At times, surgical bypass such as femoral to above-knee or below knee popliteal or tibal bypass. For infrapopliteal disease, angioplasty is generally reserved for patients with chronic limb-threatening ischemia (rest pain and ischemic ulcers).

with severe disease and symptoms. TASC II classifies iliac, femoral, and popliteal lesions as type A, B, C, or D (Table 26–5). Short segments (type A) were more likely to be successfully treated with endovascular intervention when compared to long segment occlusions (type D).[18,167] In addition to the TASC II general guidelines, the location of the lesion, patient comorbidities, patient preference, operator's experience, and long-term success rates all contribute to treatment recommendations.

Endovascular therapy is the preferred therapy for TASC type A and B lesions. Those with Type B lesions who fail endovascular management might also benefit from surgery. Previously, surgery was preferred for patients with TASC type C lesions who are good risk candidates; however, with advances in balloon and stent technology and delivery systems, many physicians will use the endovascular first approach. The choice generally depends on inflow or outflow lesions. Type D lesions are generally treated with surgery; the location of the lesion and the availability of autogenous vein may also influence the choice of intervention. Endovascular interventions, when compared to lower extremity bypass, are associated with fewer periprocedural complications but a higher rate of restenosis; repeat interventions can usually be successful if restenosis occurs.[240] Risk factors for restenosis of the femoropopliteal lesions include diabetes, no stent use, chronic total occlusion, and poor three vessel run-off below the knee.[241] In patient cohorts where percutaneous intervention does not provide adequate revascularization, surgical bypass may be an option for low-risk patients with disabling symptoms and life expectancy that would be long enough to improve quality of life. Patients who derive the most benefit from elective surgical intervention are under the age of 70, nondiabetic, and absence of significant disease distal to the primary lesion.[242]

Open versus Endovascular Therapy in CLTI

The primary goal in patients with CLTI is to preserve limb function and prevent amputation. The optimal treatment strategy, endovascular versus open surgery, depends on anatomic features, comorbidities, patient preference, and operator skill and experience. The NIH-sponsored trial entitled *The Best Endovascular Versus Best Surgical Therapy in Patients With Critical Limb Ischemia (BEST-CLI)* is evaluating open surgery versus endovascular revascularization in CLTI. This trial is still enrolling patients.[243] The Bypass versus Angioplasty in Severe Ischemia of the Leg (BASIL) trial was the only multicenter, randomized controlled trial to compare endovascular-first versus surgery-first revascularization strategy in patients with CTLI.[244] In the follow-up period (1999–2004), there was no significant difference in amputation-free or overall survival between the two groups with an intention to treat analysis. In those that survived greater than 2 years, those who underwent open surgery had an improved overall survival and a trend toward improved amputation free survival. This study found that prosthetic bypass grafts performed worse than angioplasty. Limitations of this study include single intervention endovascular approach (balloon angioplasty), low statistical power, and lack of generalizability of the study patient cohort.[244] There are two trials, BASIL-2 and BASIL-3, that are currently ongoing to address these limitations.[245,246] BASIL-2 is focused on infra-popliteal CLTI and will randomize patients to either vein graft bypass first or best endovascular treatment first.[246] BASIL-3 is focused on femoropopliteal CLTI; patients will be randomized between three groups: balloon angioplasty with or without bare metal stent, drug coated balloon angioplasty with or without bare metal stent, or drug eluting stent.[245] Both studies will follow-up patient cohorts for 24 to 60 months to characterize amputation-free survival, overall-survival, and clinical outcomes, in addition to quality-of-life metrics.

Paclitaxel

The local delivery of paclitaxel in PAD has been shown to improve longevity of interventions through prevention of restenosis. The overall safety of paclitaxel coated balloons and stents underwent review recently. Review of long-term data by the US Food and Drug Administration (FDA) led to the recommendation of health providers discussing the late mortality possibly associated with use of paclitaxel.[247] A meta-analysis of premarket trials demonstrated that mortality at 5 years was significantly increased for patients who underwent therapy with paclitaxel coated devices compared to noncoated devices.[248] This data was consistent with previously published other meta-analyses.[249–251] The mechanism potential increased risk in mortality was unexplainable and dose associated with mortality was also not clear. The interpretation of this data should be done with caution given the limitations of the available data.[248,252] Follow-up studies of high quality and large patient cohorts refuted the increased mortality signal in patients treated with paclitaxel.[253,254] In an analysis of 8367 patients from Vascular Quality Initiative data, the mortality was significantly lower in patients with claudication who were treated with paclitaxel balloon or stent compared to control.[254] For CTLI, the mortality difference was not significant. In a retrospective analysis of 37,914 patients from insurance claims, the use of paclitaxel stents or balloons in patients with CTLI was associated with improved outcomes at 5 years.[253]

ACUTE ARTERIAL OCCLUSION

Presentation

Acute arterial ischemia is a quickly developing or sudden decrease in perfusion to the limb; this presents with new or worsening symptoms and can threaten limb viability.[18] Morbidity, mortality, and limb loss rates are high for acute limb ischemia; a 20-day mortality of 25%.[255,256] Clinical presentation was previously discussed in clinical assessment of PAD. If flow is not restored quickly, limb viability is at risk. Severe ischemia may be present if pallor at rest, profound coolness, tense and/or tender muscles, and loss of sensory and/or motor functions. Acute arterial occlusion can be due to acute thrombosis of a diseased but previously patent atherosclerotic artery, acute thrombosis of a stent or bypass graft, thrombosis of an aneurysm (ie, popliteal), arterial dissection, trauma to the artery, or embolus from a proximal source (Table 26–2).

Native arterial thrombosis is most likely to occur at a site of preexisting atherosclerotic plaque;[257] it can also occur at the site of an aneurysm or sites previously affected by dissection. Recent arterial manipulation can lead to acute occlusion due to mechanical disruption of plaque. Hypercoagulability can lead to thrombosis of stents or vascular grafts, areas of preexisting atherosclerotic plaque, and areas of low flow.[258] Iatrogenic injury due to a complication of a vascular or cardiac procedure can lead to acute arterial occlusion at the arterial access site. Blunt or penetrating trauma can lead to acute lower extremity ischemia either from direct arterial injury or traumatic arterial dissection with thrombosis or thromboembolism. Thrombosis post-endovascular or open procedures can occur due to immediate failure of bypass graft. The majority of arterial emboli are cardiac in origin, with lower extremities more affected than upper extremities.[259] Thromboemboli lodge at an area of narrowing, such as an atherosclerotic plaque or branch point. Bifurcations of the common iliac, common femoral, and popliteal arteries are the most frequent locations.[260] Cardiac sources include atrial thrombus formation due to atrial fibrillation, left ventricular thrombus formation, or septic embolic from infected valves. Arterial-to-arterial embolization of a thrombus or plaque originating from atherosclerotic lesions or aneurysms makes up 20% of peripheral emboli. Paradoxical emboli can cause acute lower extremity ischemia, although they are more often associated with cryptogenic stroke.

Treatment

Immediate management should focus on protecting the limb and restoring blood flow. Heparin should be initiated to prevent further thrombus propagation and for stabilization of embolic sources. Catheter angiography is required to plan repair when there is preexisting occlusive or aneurysmal disease or if the etiology is not clear. All occlusions should be considered for reestablishing flow; urgency should be based on severity of ischemia. If the limb is not viable, amputation should be performed to prevent further complications. For critical ischemia, repair should be done emergently for limb salvage.[261] Thrombolysis of acute thrombus can be effective, although risks of bleeding and stroke should be discussed.[262,263] The period of time that the leg was severely ischemic will determine whether a fasciotomy will be required at the time of revascularization.

SUMMARY

Pathogenesis

- The most common cause of PAD is atherosclerotic plaque formation in arteries of the lower extremities.

Risk Factors

- Age, smoking, diabetes, and CKD are the strongest risk factors for PAD. Those with unmanaged risk factors may have rapid progression of disease.
- Patients with PAD are at a markedly increased risk for future MI, stroke, and cardiovascular death.

Diagnosis

- The clinical manifestations of PAD are determined by the anatomical location as well as severity of arterial stenosis, ranging from leg discomfort with ambulation to CLTI with pain at rest and the presence of ischemic ulcers.
- The cornerstone of diagnosis of PAD is the ABI (normal 1.0–1.4, borderline 0.91–0.99, abnormal ≤0.9)) with the use of TBI to in the presence of noncompressible or calcified blood vessels (ABI >1.4).
- Exercise testing provides additional information about the functional status of patient and allows correlation of symptoms to hemodynamics.
- For interventional planning, a CTA, MRA, or catheter-based angiography are helpful to determine approach.

Treatment/Management

- Claudication and CTLI are managed with risk factor modification.
- Smoking cessation, exercise therapy, high-dose intensity statin, optimal blood pressure control, and antiplatelet therapy decrease the risk of MI, stroke, cardiovascular death, and major adverse limb events.
- Smoking cessation, exercise therapy, cilostazol, podiatry care, and revascularization improve symptoms and quality of life, and prevent limb amputation.
- Acute arterial occlusion management for viable limbs should focus on revascularization and anticoagulation.

ACKNOWLEDGMENT

In the previous edition(s), this chapter was written by Kevin P. Cohoon, Paul W. Wennberg, and Thom W. Rooke, and portions of that chapter have been retained.

REFERENCES

1. Sampson UK, et al. Global and regional burden of death and disability from peripheral artery disease: 21 world regions. 1990 to 2010. *Glob Heart*. 2014;9(1):145-158.e21.

2. Vos T, et al. Prevalence. Global, regional, and national incidence, prevalence, and years lived with disability for 310 diseases and injuries.

1990–2015: a systematic analysis for the Global Burden of Disease Study 2015. *Lancet*. 2016;388(10053):1545-1602.

3. Wang H, et al. Causes of death. Global, regional, and national life expectancy, all-cause mortality, and cause-specific mortality for 249 causes of death. 1980–2015: a systematic analysis for the Global Burden of Disease Study 2015. *Lancet*. 2016;388(10053):1459-1544.

4. Hirsch AT, et al. Peripheral arterial disease detection, awareness, and treatment in primary care. *JAMA*. 2001;286(11):1317-1324.

5. McDermott MM, et al. Leg symptoms in peripheral arterial disease: associated clinical characteristics and functional impairment. *JAMA*. 2001;286(13):1599-1606.

6. McDermott MM, Mehta S, Greenland P. Exertional leg symptoms other than intermittent claudication are common in peripheral arterial disease. *Arch Intern Med*. 1999;159(4):387-392.

7. McDermott. MM. et al. The ankle brachial index is associated with leg function and physical activity: the Walking and Leg Circulation Study. *Ann Intern Med*. 2002. 136(12):873-83.

8. McDermott MM, et al. Functional decline in peripheral arterial disease: associations with the ankle brachial index and leg symptoms. *JAMA*. 2004;292(4):453-461.

9. McDermott MM, et al. Associations of borderline and low normal ankle-brachial index values with functional decline at 5–year follow-up: the WALCS (Walking and Leg Circulation Study). *J Am Coll Cardiol*. 2009;53(12):1056-1062.

10. McDermott MM, et al. Leg symptom categories and rates of mobility decline in peripheral arterial disease. *J Am Geriatr Soc*. 2010;58(7): 1256-1262.

11. Fowkes FGR, et al. Ankle brachial index combined with Framingham Risk Score to predict cardiovascular events and mortality: a meta-analysis. *JAMA*. 2008;300(2):197-208.

12. Criqui MH, Aboyans V. Epidemiology of peripheral artery disease. *Circ Res*. 2015;116(9):1509-1526.

13. Bhatt DL, et al. Comparative determinants of 4–year cardiovascular event rates in stable outpatients at risk of or with atherothrombosis. *JAMA*. 2010;304(12):1350-1357.

14. Bonaca MP, MA Creager. Pharmacological treatment and current management of peripheral artery disease. *Circ Res*. 2015;116(9):1579-1598.

15. Gerhard-Herman MD, et al. 2016 AHA/ACC guideline on the management of patients with lower extremity peripheral artery disease: a report of the American College of Cardiology/American Heart Association Task Force on Clinical Practice Guidelines. *Circulation*. 2017;135(12):e726-e779.

16. Fowkes FG, et al. Comparison of global estimates of prevalence and risk factors for peripheral artery disease in 2000 and 2010: a systematic review and analysis. *Lancet*. 2013;382(9901):1329-1340.

17. Benjamin EJ, et al. Heart Disease and stroke statistics-2017 update: a report from the American Heart Association. *Circulation*. 2017;135(10): e146-e603.

18. Norgren L, et al. inter-society consensus for the management of peripheral arterial disease (TASC II). *J Vasc Surg*. 2007;45 Suppl S:S5-67.

19. Brevetti G, et al. Women and peripheral arterial disease: same disease, different issues. *J Cardiovasc Med (Hagerstown)*. 2008;9(4):382-388.

20. Hirsch AT, et al. A call to action: women and peripheral artery disease: a scientific statement from the American Heart Association. *Circulation*. 2012;125(11):1449-1472.

21. Meadows TA, et al. Ethnic differences in the prevalence and treatment of cardiovascular risk factors in US outpatients with peripheral arterial disease: insights from the reduction of atherothrombosis for continued health (REACH) registry. *Am Heart J*. 2009;158(6):1038-1045.

22. Berger JS, et al. Modifiable risk factor burden and the prevalence of peripheral artery disease in different vascular territories. *J Vasc Surg*. 2013;58(3):673-681.e1.

23. Murabito JM, et al. Prevalence and clinical correlates of peripheral arterial disease in the Framingham Offspring Study. *Am Heart J*. 2002;143(6): 961-965.

24. Meijer WT, et al. Peripheral arterial disease in the elderly: the Rotterdam Study. *Arterioscler Thromb Vasc Biol.* 1998;18(2):185-192.

25. Fowkes FG, et al. Edinburgh Artery Study: prevalence of asymptomatic and symptomatic peripheral arterial disease in the general population. *Int J Epidemiol.* 1991;20(2):384-392.

26. Criqui MH, et al. Mortality over a period of 10 years in patients with peripheral arterial disease. *N Engl J Med.* 1992;326(6):381-386.

27. Hooi JD, et al. Risk factors and cardiovascular diseases associated with asymptomatic peripheral arterial occlusive disease. The Limburg PAOD Study, peripheral arterial occlusive disease. *Scand J Prim Health Care.* 1998;16(3):177-182.

28. Newman AB, Tyrrell KS, Kuller LH. Mortality over four years in SHEP participants with a low ankle-arm index. *J Am Geriatr Soc.* 1997;45(12):1472-1478.

29. Cleven AH, et al. Cardiovascular outcome stratification using the ankle-brachial pressure index. *Eur J Gen Pract.* 2005;11(3–4):107-112.

30. Natsuaki C, et al. Association of borderline ankle-brachial index with mortality and the incidence of peripheral artery disease in diabetic patients. *Atherosclerosis.* 2014;234(2):360-365.

31. McKenna M, Wolfson S, Kuller L. The ratio of ankle and arm arterial pressure as an independent predictor of mortality. *Atherosclerosis.* 1991;87(2–3):119-128.

32. Jones WS, et al. Association of the ankle-brachial index with history of myocardial infarction and stroke. *Am Heart J.* 2014;167(4):499-505.

33. Allison MA, et al. A high ankle-brachial index is associated with increased cardiovascular disease morbidity and lower quality of life. *J Am Coll Cardiol.* 2008;51(13):1292-1298.

34. Wattanakit K, et al. Clinical significance of a high ankle-brachial index: insights from the Atherosclerosis Risk in Communities (ARIC) Study. *Atherosclerosis.* 2007;190(2):459-464.

35. McDaniel MD, JL Cronenwett. Basic data related to the natural history of intermittent claudication. *Ann Vasc Surg.* 1989;3(3):273-277.

36. Garcia LA. Epidemiology and pathophysiology of lower extremity peripheral arterial disease. *J Endovasc Ther.* 2006;13(Suppl 2):II3-II9.

37. Feinglass J, et al. Rates of lower-extremity amputation and arterial reconstruction in the United States. 1979 to 1996. *Am J Public Health.* 1999;89(8):1222-1227.

38. Dormandy J, Heeck L, Vig S. Acute limb ischemia. *Semin Vasc Surg.* 1999;12(2):148-153.

39. Duval S, et al. The impact of prolonged lower limb ischemia on amputation, mortality, and functional status: the FRIENDS registry. *Am Heart J.* 2014;168(4):577-587.

40. Conte MS, Pomposelli FB. Society for Vascular Surgery Practice guidelines for atherosclerotic occlusive disease of the lower extremities management of asymptomatic disease and claudication. Introduction. *J Vasc Surg.* 2015;61(3 Suppl):1S.

41. Go AS, et al. Executive summary: heart disease and stroke statistics—2014 update: a report from the American Heart Association. *Circulation.* 2014;129(3):399-410.

42. Sigvant B, Lundin F, Wahlberg E. The risk of disease progression in peripheral arterial disease is higher than expected: a meta-analysis of mortality and disease progression in peripheral arterial disease. *Eur J Vasc Endovasc Surg.* 2016;51(3):395-403.

43. Criqui MH, et al. The prevalence of peripheral arterial disease in a defined population. *Circulation.* 1985;71(3):510-515.

44. Kroger K, et al. Prevalence of peripheral arterial disease—results of the Heinz Nixdorf recall study. *Eur J Epidemiol.* 2006;21(4):279-285.

45. Ostchega Y, et al. Prevalence of peripheral arterial disease and risk factors in persons aged 60 and older: data from the National Health and Nutrition Examination Survey 1999–2004. *J Am Geriatr Soc.* 2007;55(4):583-589.

46. Pasternak RC, et al. Atherosclerotic Vascular Disease Conference: Writing Group I: epidemiology. *Circulation.* 2004;109(21):2605-2612.

47. Reeder BA, Liu L, Horlick L. Sociodemographic variation in the prevalence of cardiovascular disease. *Can J Cardiol.* 1996;12(3):271-277.

48. Selvin E, Erlinger TP. Prevalence of and risk factors for peripheral arterial disease in the United States: results from the National Health and Nutrition Examination Survey. 1999–2000. *Circulation.* 2004;110(6):738-743.

49. McDermott MM, et al. Sex differences in peripheral arterial disease: leg symptoms and physical functioning. *J Am Geriatr Soc.* 2003;51(2):222-228.

50. Agarwal S. The association of active and passive smoking with peripheral arterial disease: results from NHANES 1999–2004. *Angiology.* 2009;60(3):335-345.

51. Hylton JR, et al. Octogenarians develop infrapopliteal arterial occlusive disease in the absence of traditional risk factors. *Ann Vasc Surg.* 2014;28(7):1712-1718.

52. Powell JT, Greenhalgh RM. Continued smoking and the results of vascular reconstruction. *Br J Surg.* 1994;81(8):1242.

53. Kollerits B, et al. Intermittent claudication in the Erfurt Male Cohort (ERFORT) Study: its determinants and the impact on mortality. A population-based prospective cohort study with 30 years of follow-up. *Atherosclerosis.* 2008;198(1):214-222.

54. Aboyans V, et al. Risk factors for progression of peripheral arterial disease in large and small vessels. *Circulation.* 2006;113(22):2623-2629.

55. Fowkes FG, et al. Smoking, lipids, glucose intolerance, and blood pressure as risk factors for peripheral atherosclerosis compared with ischemic heart disease in the Edinburgh Artery Study. *Am J Epidemiol.* 1992;135(4):331-340.

56. Lu L, Mackay DF, Pell JP. Meta-analysis of the association between cigarette smoking and peripheral arterial disease. *Heart.* 2014;100(5):414-423.

57. Price JF, et al. Relationship between smoking and cardiovascular risk factors in the development of peripheral arterial disease and coronary artery disease: Edinburgh Artery Study. *Eur Heart J.* 1999;20(5):344-353.

58. Conen D, et al. Smoking, smoking cessation, [corrected] and risk for symptomatic peripheral artery disease in women: a cohort study. *Ann Intern Med.* 2011;154(11):719-726.

59. Murabito JM, et al. Intermittent claudication. A risk profile from The Framingham Heart Study. *Circulation.* 1997;96(1):44-49.

60. Fowler B, et al. Prevalence of peripheral arterial disease: persistence of excess risk in former smokers. *Aust N Z J Public Health.* 2002;26(3):219-224.

61. Howard G, et al. Cigarette smoking and progression of atherosclerosis: the Atherosclerosis Risk in Communities (ARIC) Study. *JAMA.* 1998;279(2):119-124.

62. Willigendael EM, et al. Smoking and the patency of lower extremity bypass grafts: a meta-analysis. *J Vasc Surg.* 2005;42(1):67-74.

63. Noike H, et al. Changes in cardio-ankle vascular index in smoking cessation. *J Atheroscler Thromb.* 2010;17(5):517-525.

64. Bundo M, et al. Asymptomatic peripheral arterial disease in type 2 diabetes patients: a 10–year follow-up study of the utility of the ankle brachial index as a prognostic marker of cardiovascular disease. *Ann Vasc Surg.* 2010;24(8):985-993.

65. Jude EB, et al. Peripheral arterial disease in diabetic and nondiabetic patients: a comparison of severity and outcome. *Diabetes Care.* 2001;24(8):1433-1437.

66. Leibson CL, et al. Peripheral arterial disease, diabetes, and mortality. *Diabetes Care.* 2004;27(12):2843-2849.

67. Selvin E, et al. Meta-analysis: glycosylated hemoglobin and cardiovascular disease in diabetes mellitus. *Ann Intern Med.* 2004;141(6):421-431.

68. Beckman JA, Creager MA. Vascular complications of diabetes. *Circ Res.* 2016;118(11):1771-1785.

69. Beckman JA, et al. Microvascular disease, peripheral artery disease, and amputation. *Circulation.* 2019;140(6):449-458.

70. Dosluoglu HH, et al. Insulin use is associated with poor limb salvage and survival in diabetic patients with chronic limb ischemia. *J Vasc Surg.* 2010;51(5):1178-1189; discussion 1188-1189.

71. Melliere D, et al. Influence of diabetes on revascularisation procedures of the aorta and lower limb arteries: early results. *Eur J Vasc Endovasc Surg.* 1999;17(5):438-441.

72. O'Hare AM, et al. High prevalence of peripheral arterial disease in persons with renal insufficiency: results from the National Health and Nutrition Examination Survey 1999–2000. *Circulation.* 2004;109(3):320-323.

73. O'Hare AM, et al. Renal insufficiency and the risk of lower extremity peripheral arterial disease: results from the Heart and Estrogen/Progestin Replacement Study (HERS). *J Am Soc Nephrol.* 2004;15(4):1046-1051.

74. Wattanakit K, et al. Kidney function and risk of peripheral arterial disease: results from the Atherosclerosis Risk in Communities (ARIC) Study. *J Am Soc Nephrol.* 2007;18(2):629-636.

75. Leskinen Y, et al. The prevalence of peripheral arterial disease and medial arterial calcification in patients with chronic renal failure: requirements for diagnostics. *Am J Kidney Dis.* 2002;40(3):472-479.

76. Mostaza JM, et al. Relationship between ankle-brachial index and chronic kidney disease in hypertensive patients with no known cardiovascular disease. *J Am Soc Nephrol.* 2006;17(12 Suppl 3):S201-S205.

77. O'Hare AM, et al. Renal insufficiency and use of revascularization among a national cohort of men with advanced lower extremity peripheral arterial disease. *Clin J Am Soc Nephrol.* 2006;1(2):297-304.

78. Shlipak MG, et al. Cardiovascular disease risk status in elderly persons with renal insufficiency. *Kidney Int.* 2002;62(3):997-1004.

79. Wattanakit K, et al. Albuminuria and peripheral arterial disease: results from the multi-ethnic study of atherosclerosis (MESA). *Atherosclerosis.* 2008;201(1):212-216.

80. Wu CK, et al. Association of low glomerular filtration rate and albuminuria with peripheral arterial disease: the National Health and Nutrition Examination Survey. 1999–2004. *Atherosclerosis.* 2010;209(1):230-234.

81. Cheung AK, et al. Atherosclerotic cardiovascular disease risks in chronic hemodialysis patients. *Kidney Int.* 2000;58(1):353-362.

82. O'Hare AM, et al. Peripheral vascular disease risk factors among patients undergoing hemodialysis. *J Am Soc Nephrol.* 2002;13(2):497-503.

83. Rajagopalan S, et al. Peripheral arterial disease in patients with end-stage renal disease: observations from the Dialysis Outcomes and Practice Patterns Study (DOPPS). *Circulation.* 2006;114(18):1914-1922.

84. Lamping DL, et al. Clinical outcomes, quality of life, and costs in the North Thames Dialysis Study of elderly people on dialysis: a prospective cohort study. *Lancet.* 2000;356(9241):1543-1550.

85. Matsushita K, et al. Measures of chronic kidney disease and risk of incident peripheral artery disease: a collaborative meta-analysis of individual participant data. *Lancet Diabetes Endocrinol.* 2017;5(9):718-728.

86. Jablonski KL, Chonchol M. Vascular calcification in end-stage renal disease. *Hemodial Int.* 2013;17(Suppl 1):S17-S21.

87. Ogawa T, Nitta K. Pathogenesis and management of vascular calcification in patients with end-stage renal disease. *Contrib Nephrol.* 2018;196:71-77.

88. Benjamin EJ, et al. Heart disease and stroke statistics-2019 update: a report from the American Heart Association. *Circulation.* 2019;139(10):e56-e528.

89. Rapsomaniki E, et al. Blood pressure and incidence of twelve cardiovascular diseases: lifetime risks, healthy life-years lost, and age-specific associations in 1.25 million people. *Lancet.* 2014;383(9932):1899-1911.

90. Emdin CA, et al. Usual blood pressure, peripheral arterial disease, and vascular risk: cohort study of 4.2 million adults. *BMJ.* 2015;351:h4865.

91. Kannel WB, McGee DL. Update on some epidemiologic features of intermittent claudication: the Framingham Study. *J Am Geriatr Soc.* 1985;33(1):13-18.

92. Greenhalgh RM, et al. Serum lipids and lipoproteins in peripheral vascular disease. *Lancet.* 1971;2(7731):947-950.

93. Vitale E, et al. Lipoprotein abnormalities in patients with extra-coronary arteriosclerosis. *Atherosclerosis.* 1990;81(2):95-102.

94. Vogelberg KH, et al. Primary hyperlipoproteinemias as risk factors in peripheral artery disease documented by arteriography. *Atherosclerosis.* 1975;22(2):271-285.

95. Bradby GV, Valente AJ, Walton KW. Serum high-density lipoproteins in peripheral vascular disease. *Lancet.* 1978;2(8103):1271-1274.

96. Banerjee AK, et al. A six year prospective study of fibrinogen and other risk factors associated with mortality in stable claudicants. *Thromb Haemost.* 1992;68(3):261-263.

97. Cantin B, et al. Lipoprotein(a) distribution in a French Canadian population and its relation to intermittent claudication (the Quebec Cardiovascular Study). *Am J Cardiol.* 1995;75(17):1224-1228.

98. Lowe GD, et al. Blood viscosity. fibrinogen. and activation of coagulation and leukocytes in peripheral arterial disease and the normal population in the Edinburgh Artery Study. *Circulation.* 1993;87(6):1915-1920.

99. Valentine RJ, et al. Lp(a) lipoprotein is an independent, discriminating risk factor for premature peripheral atherosclerosis among white men. *Arch Intern Med.* 1994;154(7):801-806.

100. Ridker M, Stampfer MJ, Rifai N. Novel risk factors for systemic atherosclerosis: a comparison of C-reactive protein, fibrinogen, homocysteine, lipoprotein(a), and standard cholesterol screening as predictors of peripheral arterial disease. *JAMA.* 2001;285(19):2481-2485.

101. McCully KS. Vascular pathology of homocysteinemia: implications for the pathogenesis of arteriosclerosis. *Am J Pathol.* 1969;56(1):111-128.

102. Asfar S, Safar HA. Homocysteine levels and peripheral arterial occlusive disease: a prospective cohort study and review of the literature. *J Cardiovasc Surg (Torino).* 2007;48(5):601-605.

103. Taylor SM. Current status of heroic limb salvage for critical limb ischemia. *Am Surg.* 2008;74(4):275-284.

104. Valentine RJ, et al. Late outcome of amputees with premature atherosclerosis. *Surgery.* 1996;119(5):487-493.

105. Allison MA, et al. Ethnicity and risk factors for change in the ankle-brachial index: the Multi-Ethnic Study of Atherosclerosis. *J Vasc Surg.* 2009;50(5):1049-1056.

106. Khandanpour N, et al. Peripheral arterial disease and methylenetetrahydrofolate reductase (MTHFR) C677T mutations: a case-control study and meta-analysis. *J Vasc Surg.* 2009;49(3):711-718.

107. McDermott, MM. Lower extremity manifestations of peripheral artery disease: the pathophysiologic and functional implications of leg ischemia. *Circ Res.* 2015;116(9):1540-1550.

108. Collins TC, Petersen NJ, Suarez-Almazor M. Peripheral arterial disease symptom subtype and walking impairment. *Vasc Med.* 2005;10(3):177-183.

109. Lin JS, et al. The ankle-brachial index for peripheral artery disease screening and cardiovascular disease prediction among asymptomatic adults: a systematic evidence review for the US Preventive Services Task Force. *Ann Intern Med.* 2013;159(5):333-341.

110. Rooke TW, et al. 2011 ACCF/AHA focused update of the guideline for the management of patients with peripheral artery disease (updating the 2005 guideline): a report of the American College of Cardiology Foundation/American Heart Association Task Force on Practice Guidelines. *J Am Coll Cardiol.* 2011;58(19):2020-2045.

111. Gerhard-Herman MD, et al. 2016 AHA/ACC guideline on the management of patients with lower extremity peripheral artery disease: executive summary: a report of the American College of Cardiology/American Heart Association Task Force on Clinical Practice Guidelines. *J Am Coll Cardiol.* 2017;69(11):1465-1508.

112. Olson KW, Treat-Jacobson D. Symptoms of peripheral arterial disease: a critical review. *J Vasc Nurs.* 2004;22(3):72-77.

113. Creager MA, Kaufman JA, Conte MS. Clinical practice. Acute limb ischemia. *N Engl J Med.* 2012. 366(23):2198-2206.

114. Conte MS, et al. Global vascular guidelines on the management of chronic limb-threatening ischemia. *Eur J Vasc Endovasc Surg.* 2019; 58(1S):S1-S109.e33.

115. Wolfe JH, Wyatt MG. Critical and subcritical ischaemia. *Eur J Vasc Endovasc Surg.* 1997;13(6):578-582.

116. Ouriel. K. Peripheral arterial disease. *Lancet.* 2001;358(9289):1257-1264.

117. Kavanaugh GJ, et al. "Pseudoclaudication" syndrome produced by compression of the cauda equina. *JAMA.* 1968;206(11):2477-2481.

118. Goodreau JJ, et al. Rational approach to the differentiation of vascular and neurogenic claudication. *Surgery.* 1978;84(6):749-757.

119. Delis KT, Bountouroglou D, Mansfield AO. Venous claudication in iliofemoral thrombosis: long-term effects on venous hemodynamics, clinical status, and quality of life. *Ann Surg.* 2004;239(1):118-126.

120. Toe and foot amputation. In: *Current therapy in vascular surgery.* Stanley, JC Ernst CB, eds. St Louis, MO: Mosby; 1995.

121. Barnhorst DA, Barner HB. Prevalence of congenitally absent pedal pulses. *N Engl J Med.* 1968;278(5):264-265.

122. Tuveson V, Lofdahl HE, Hultgren R. Patients with abdominal aortic aneurysm have a high prevalence of popliteal artery aneurysms. *Vasc Med.* 2016;21(4):369-375.

123. Clark CE, et al. Association of a difference in systolic blood pressure between arms with vascular disease and mortality: a systematic review and meta-analysis. *Lancet.* 2012;379(9819):905-914.

124. Shadman R, et al. Subclavian artery stenosis: prevalence, risk factors, and association with cardiovascular diseases. *J Am Coll Cardiol.* 2004;44(3):618-623.

125. Singh S, et al. Simultaneously measured inter-arm and inter-leg systolic blood pressure differences and cardiovascular risk stratification: a systemic review and meta-analysis. *J Am Soc Hypertens.* 2015;9(8):640-650 e12.

126. McPhail IR, et al. Intermittent claudication: an objective office-based assessment. *J Am Coll Cardiol.* 2001;37(5):1381-1385.

127. Aboyans V, et al. Measurement and interpretation of the ankle-brachial index: a scientific statement from the American Heart Association. *Circulation.* 2012;126(24):2890-2909.

128. Misra S, et al. Perfusion assessment in critical limb ischemia: principles for understanding and the development of evidence and evaluation of devices: a scientific statement from the American Heart Association. *Circulation.* 2019;140(12):e657-e672.

129. Sukul D, et al. Heterogeneity of ankle-brachial indices in patients undergoing revascularization for critical limb ischemia. *JACC Cardiovasc Interv.* 2017;10(22):2307-2316.

130. Halperin JL. Evaluation of patients with peripheral vascular disease. *Thromb Res.* 2002;106(6):V303-V311.

131. Rossi M, Carpi A. Skin microcirculation in peripheral arterial obliterative disease. *Biomed Pharmacother.* 2004;58(8):427-431.

132. Yip WL. Evaluation of the clinimetrics of transcutaneous oxygen measurement and its application in wound care. *Int Wound J.* 2015;12(6):625-629.

133. Ubbink DT, et al. The best TcpO(2) parameters to predict the efficacy of spinal cord stimulation to improve limb salvage in patients with inoperable critical leg ischemia. *Int Angiol.* 2003;22(4):356-363.

134. Chiriano J, et al. Management of lower extremity wounds in patients with peripheral arterial disease: a stratified conservative approach. *Ann Vasc Surg.* 2010;24(8):1110-1116.

135. Arsenault KA, et al. The use of transcutaneous oximetry to predict complications of chronic wound healing: a systematic review and meta-analysis. *Wound Repair Regen.* 2011;19(6):657-663.

136. Labs KH, et al. Reliability of treadmill testing in peripheral arterial disease: a comparison of a constant load with a graded load treadmill protocol. *Vasc Med.* 1999;4(4):239-246.

137. Regensteiner JG, Gardner A, Hiatt WR. Exercise testing and exercise rehabilitation for patients with peripheral arterial disease: status in 1997. *Vasc Med.* 1997;2(2):147-155.

138. Arain FA, et al. Survival in patients with poorly compressible leg arteries. *J Am Coll Cardiol.* 2012;59(4):400-407.

139. Diehm C, et al. Prognostic value of a low post-exercise ankle brachial index as assessed by primary care physicians. *Atherosclerosis.* 2011;214(2):364-372.

140. Feringa HH, et al. The long-term prognostic value of the resting and postexercise ankle-brachial index. *Arch Intern Med.* 2006;166(5):529-535.

141. McDermott MM, et al. Leg symptoms. the ankle-brachial index. and walking ability in patients with peripheral arterial disease. *J Gen Intern Med.* 1999;14(3):173-181.

142. Kroger K, et al. Toe pressure measurements compared to ankle artery pressure measurements. *Angiology.* 2003;54(1):39-44.

143. Wukich DK, et al. Noninvasive arterial testing in patients with diabetes: a guide for foot and ankle surgeons. *Foot Ankle Int.* 2015;36(12):1391-1399.

144. Wang JC, et al. Exertional leg pain in patients with and without peripheral arterial disease. *Circulation.* 2005;112(22):3501-3508.

145. Pollak AW., Norton T, Kramer CM. Multimodality imaging of lower extremity peripheral arterial disease: current role and future directions. *Circ Cardiovasc Imaging.* 2012;5(6):797-807.

146. Sommerville RS, et al. 3-D magnetic resonance angiography versus conventional angiography in peripheral arterial disease: pilot study. *ANZ J Surg.* 2005;75(6):373-377.

147. Morris DR, et al. Assessment and validation of a novel angiographic scoring system for peripheral artery disease. *Br J Surg.* 2017;104(5):544-554.

148. Fontaine R, Kim M, Kieny R. Surgical treatment of peripheral circulation disorders. *Helv Chir Acta.* 1954;21(5–6):499-533.

149. Rutherford RB, et al. Recommended standards for reports dealing with lower extremity ischemia: revised version. *J Vasc Surg.* 1997;26(3):517-538.

150. Zhan LX, et al. The Society for Vascular Surgery lower extremity threatened limb classification system based on Wound, Ischemia, and foot Infection (WIfI) correlates with risk of major amputation and time to wound healing. *J Vasc Surg.* 2015;61(4):939-944.

151. Beropoulis E, et al. Validation of the Wound, Ischemia, foot Infection (WIfI) classification system in nondiabetic patients treated by endovascular means for critical limb ischemia. *J Vasc Surg.* 2016;64(1):95-103.

152. Cull DL, et al. An early validation of the Society for Vascular Surgery lower extremity threatened limb classification system. *J Vasc Surg.* 2014;60(6):1535-1541.

153. Darling JD, et al. Predictive ability of the Society for Vascular Surgery Wound, Ischemia, and foot Infection (WIfI) classification system following infrapopliteal endovascular interventions for critical limb ischemia. *J Vasc Surg.* 2016;64(3):616-622.

154. Mills JL Sr. The application of the Society for Vascular Surgery Wound, Ischemia, and foot Infection (WIfI) classification to stratify amputation risk. *J Vasc Surg.* 2017;65(3):591-593.

155. Mills JL Sr, et al. The Society for Vascular Surgery Lower Extremity Threatened Limb Classification System: risk stratification based on wound, ischemia, and foot infection (WIfI). *J Vasc Surg.* 2014;59(1):220-234.e1-2.

156. Darling JD, et al. Predictive ability of the Society for Vascular Surgery Wound, Ischemia, and foot Infection (WIfI) classification system after first-time lower extremity revascularizations. *J Vasc Surg.* 2017;65(3):695-704.

157. Hicks CW. et al. The Society for Vascular Surgery Wound, Ischemia, and foot Infection (WIfI) classification independently predicts wound healing in diabetic foot ulcers. *J Vasc Surg.* 2018;68(4):1096-1103.

158. Iida O, et al. Three-year outcomes of surgical versus endovascular revascularization for critical limb ischemia: The SPINACH Study (Surgical Reconstruction Versus Peripheral Intervention in Patients With Critical Limb Ischemia). *Circ Cardiovasc Interv.* 2017;10(12).

159. Kobayashi N, et al. Characteristics and clinical outcomes of repeat endovascular therapy after infrapopliteal balloon angioplasty in patients with critical limb ischemia. *Catheter Cardiovasc Interv.* 2018;91(3): 505-514.

160. Okazaki J, et al. Analysis of wound healing time and wound-free period as outcomes after surgical and endovascular revascularization for critical lower limb ischemia. *J Vasc Surg.* 2018;67(3):817-825.

161. Leithead C, et al. Importance of postprocedural Wound, Ischemia, and foot Infection (WIfI) restaging in predicting limb salvage. *J Vasc Surg.* 2018;67(2):498-505.

162. Ramanan B, et al. Determinants of midterm functional outcomes, wound healing, and resources used in a hospital-based limb preservation program. *J Vasc Surg.* 2017;66(6):1765-1774.

163. Hirsch AT, et al. ACC/AHA 2005 Practice Guidelines for the management of patients with peripheral arterial disease (lower extremity. renal.

mesenteric. and abdominal aortic): a collaborative report from the American Association for Vascular Surgery/Society for Vascular Surgery. Society for Cardiovascular Angiography and Interventions. Society for Vascular Medicine and Biology. Society of Interventional Radiology. and the ACC/AHA Task Force on Practice Guidelines (Writing Committee to Develop Guidelines for the Management of Patients With Peripheral Arterial Disease): endorsed by the American Association of Cardiovascular and Pulmonary Rehabilitation; National Heart, Lung, and Blood Institute; Society for Vascular Nursing; TransAtlantic Inter-Society Consensus; and Vascular Disease Foundation. *Circulation.* 2006;113(11):e463-e654.

164. Katzen BT. Clinical diagnosis and prognosis of acute limb ischemia. *Rev Cardiovasc Med.* 2002;3(Suppl 2):S2-S6.

165. Olin JW, et al. Reply: endovascular-first treatment of peripheral arterial disease remains controversial. *J Am Coll Cardiol.* 2016;68(13):1493.

166. Aboyans V, et al. 2017 ESC Guidelines on the Diagnosis and Treatment of Peripheral Arterial Diseases, in collaboration with the European Society for Vascular Surgery (ESVS): document covering atherosclerotic disease of extracranial carotid and vertebral. mesenteric, renal, upper and lower extremity arteries. Endorsed by: the European Stroke Organization (ESO), The Task Force for the Diagnosis and Treatment of Peripheral Arterial Diseases of the European Society of Cardiology (ESC) and of the European Society for Vascular Surgery (ESVS). *Eur Heart J.* 2018;39(9):763-816.

167. European Stroke Organization, et al. ESC guidelines on the diagnosis and treatment of peripheral artery diseases: document covering atherosclerotic disease of extracranial carotid and vertebral, mesenteric, renal, upper and lower extremity arteries: the Task Force on the Diagnosis and Treatment of Peripheral Artery Diseases of the European Society of Cardiology (ESC). *Eur Heart J.* 2011;32(22):2851-2906.

168. Smith SC Jr, et al. AHA/ACCF secondary prevention and risk reduction therapy for patients with coronary and other atherosclerotic vascular disease: 2011 update: a guideline from the American Heart Association and American College of Cardiology Foundation endorsed by the World Heart Federation and the Preventive Cardiovascular Nurses Association. *J Am Coll Cardiol.* 2011;58(23):2432-2446.

169. Rooke TW, et al. ACCG/AHA Task Force. 2011 ACCF/AHA Focused Update of the Guideline for the Management of patients with peripheral artery disease (updating the 2005 guideline): a report of the American College of Cardiology Foundation/American Heart Association Task Force on practice guidelines. *Circulation.* 2011;124(18):2020-2045.

170. Brendle DC, et al. Effects of exercise rehabilitation on endothelial reactivity in older patients with peripheral arterial disease. *Am J Cardiol.* 2001;87(3):324-329.

171. Ernst EE, Matrai A. Intermittent claudication, exercise, and blood rheology. *Circulation.* 1987, 76(5):1110-1114.

172. Gustafsson T, Kraus WE. Exercise-induced angiogenesis-related growth and transcription factors in skeletal muscle, and their modification in muscle pathology. *Front Biosci.* 2001;6:D75-D89.

173. Harwood AE, et al. A review of the potential local mechanisms by which exercise improves functional outcomes in intermittent claudication. *Ann Vasc Surg.* 2016;30:312-320.

174. Hiatt WR, et al. Effect of exercise training on skeletal muscle histology and metabolism in peripheral arterial disease. *J Appl Physiol (1985).* 1996;81(2):780-788.

175. McDermott MM, et al. Physical performance in peripheral arterial disease: a slower rate of decline in patients who walk more. *Ann Intern Med.* 2006;144(1):10-20.

176. Parmenter BJ, Dieberg G, Smart NA. Exercise training for management of peripheral arterial disease: a systematic review and meta-analysis. *Sports Med.* 2015;45(2):231-244.

177. Tisi V, Shearman CP. The evidence for exercise-induced inflammation in intermittent claudication: should we encourage patients to stop walking? *Eur J Vasc Endovasc Surg.* 1998;15(1):7-17.

178. Fakhry F, et al. Supervised walking therapy in patients with intermittent claudication. *J Vasc Surg.* 2012;56(4):1132-1142.

179. Gardner AW, Montgomery S, Parker DE. Optimal exercise program length for patients with claudication. *J Vasc Surg.* 2012;55(5):1346-1354.

180. Treat-Jacobson D. et al. Implementation of supervised exercise therapy for patients with symptomatic peripheral artery disease: a science advisory from the American Heart Association. *Circulation.* 2019;140(13):e700-e710.

181. Weinberg MD, et al. Peripheral artery disease. Part 2: medical and endovascular treatment. *Nat Rev Cardiol.* 2011;8(8):429-441.

182. Vemulapalli S, et al. Supervised vs unsupervised exercise for intermittent claudication: a systematic review and meta-analysis. *Am Heart J.* 2015;169(6):924-937.e3.

183. Watson L, Ellis B, Leng GC. Exercise for intermittent claudication. *Cochrane Database Syst Rev.* 2008;4:CD000990.

184. Lane R, et al. Exercise for intermittent claudication. *Cochrane Database Syst Rev.* 2017;12:CD000990.

185. Garg K, et al. Physical activity during daily life and mortality in patients with peripheral arterial disease. *Circulation.* 2006;114(3):242-248.

186. Morris DR, et al. Association of lower extremity performance with cardiovascular and all-cause mortality in patients with peripheral artery disease: a systematic review and meta-analysis. *J Am Heart Assoc.* 2014;3(4).

187. Pande RL, et al. Secondary prevention and mortality in peripheral artery disease: National Health and Nutrition Examination Study. 1999 to 2004. *Circulation.* 2011;124(1):17-23.

188. Subherwal S, et al. Missed opportunities: despite improvement in use of cardioprotective medications among patients with lower-extremity peripheral artery disease. underuse remains. *Circulation.* 2012;126(11):1345-1354.

189. Skeik N, et al. Lipid-lowering therapies in peripheral artery disease: a review. *Vasc Med.* 2020;1358863X20957091.

190. Aronow WS, et al. Effect of simvastatin versus placebo on treadmill exercise time until the onset of intermittent claudication in older patients with peripheral arterial disease at six months and at one year after treatment. *Am J Cardiol.* 2003;92(6):711-712.

191. Aung P, et al. Lipid-lowering for peripheral arterial disease of the lower limb. *Cochrane Database Syst Rev.* 2007;4:CD000123.

192. Mohler ER 3rd, Hiatt WR, Creager MA. Cholesterol reduction with atorvastatin improves walking distance in patients with peripheral arterial disease. *Circulation.* 2003;108(12):1481-1486.

193. Mondillo S, et al. Effects of simvastatin on walking performance and symptoms of intermittent claudication in hypercholesterolemic patients with peripheral vascular disease. *Am J Med.* 2003;114(5):359-364.

194. Barndt R Jr, et al. Regression and progression of early femoral atherosclerosis in treated hyperlipoproteinemic patients. *Ann Intern Med.* 1977;86(2):139-146.

195. Blankenhorn DH, et al. Effects of colestipol-niacin therapy on human femoral atherosclerosis. *Circulation.* 1991;83(2):438-447.

196. de Groot E, et al. B-mode ultrasound assessment of pravastatin treatment effect on carotid and femoral artery walls and its correlations with coronary arteriographic findings: a report of the Regression Growth Evaluation Statin Study (REGRESS). *J Am Coll Cardiol.* 1998;31(7):1561-1567.

197. Duffield RG, et al. Treatment of hyperlipidaemia retards progression of symptomatic femoral atherosclerosis. A randomised controlled trial. *Lancet.* 1983;2(8351):639-642.

198. Hiatt WR, et al. Effect of niacin ER/lovastatin on claudication symptoms in patients with peripheral artery disease. *Vasc Med.* 2010;15(3):171-179.

199. Collins R, et al. MRC/BHF Heart Protection Study of cholesterol lowering with simvastatin in 20,536 high-risk individuals: a randomised placebo-controlled trial. *Lancet.* 2002;360(9326):7-22.

200. Bonaca MP, et al. Low-density lipoprotein cholesterol lowering with evolocumab and outcomes in patients with peripheral artery disease: insights from the FOURIER trial (Further Cardiovascular Outcomes Research With PCSK9 Inhibition in Subjects With Elevated Risk). *Circulation.* 2018;137(4):338-350.

201. Alonso-Coello, et al. Antithrombotic therapy in peripheral artery disease: Antithrombotic Therapy and Prevention of Thrombosis. 9th ed:

American College of Chest Physicians Evidence-Based Clinical Practice Guidelines. *Chest.* 2012;141(2 Suppl):e669S-e690S.

202. Conte MS, et al. Society for Vascular Surgery practice guidelines for atherosclerotic occlusive disease of the lower extremities: management of asymptomatic disease and claudication. *J Vasc Surg.* 2015;61 (3 Suppl):2S-41S.

203. Gent M, et al. A randomised, blinded, trial of clopidogrel versus aspirin in patients at risk of ischaemic events (CAPRIE). CAPRIE Steering Committee. *Lancet.* 1996;348(9038):1329-1339.

204. Anand S, et al. Oral anticoagulant and antiplatelet therapy and peripheral arterial disease. *N Engl J Med.* 2007;357(3):217-227.

205. Anand SS, et al. Rivaroxaban with or without aspirin in patients with stable peripheral or carotid artery disease: an international, randomised, double-blind, placebo-controlled trial. *Lancet.* 2018;391(10117):219-229.

206. Anand SS, et al. Major adverse limb events and mortality in patients with peripheral artery disease: the COMPASS trial. *J Am Coll Cardiol.* 2018;71(20):2306-2315.

207. Eikelboom JW, et al. Rivaroxaban with or without aspirin in stable cardiovascular disease. *N Engl J Med.* 2017;377(14):1319-1330.

208. Bonaca MP, et al. Rivaroxaban in peripheral artery disease after revascularization. *N Engl J Med.* 2020;382(21):1994-2004.

209. Vorapaxar. *Am J Cardiovasc Drugs.* 2010;10(6):413-418.

210. Bonaca MP, et al. Peripheral revascularization in patients with peripheral artery disease with vorapaxar: insights from the TRA 2 degrees P-TIMI 50 trial. *JACC Cardiovasc Interv.* 2016;9(20):2157-2164.

211. Bonaca MP, et al. Acute limb ischemia and outcomes with vorapaxar in patients with peripheral artery disease: results from the trial to assess the effects of Vorapaxar in preventing heart attack and stroke in patients with atherosclerosis-thrombolysis in myocardial infarction 50 (TRA2 degrees P-TIMI 50). *Circulation.* 2016;133(10):997-1005.

212. Bonaca MP, et al. Vorapaxar in patients with peripheral artery disease: results from TRA2{degrees}P-TIMI 50. *Circulation.* 2013;127(14):1522-1529.e1-e6.

213. Morrow DA, et al. Vorapaxar in the secondary prevention of atherothrombotic events. *N Engl J Med.* 2012;366(15):1404-1413.

214. Heart Outcomes Prevention Evaluation Study, et al. Effects of an angiotensin-converting-enzyme inhibitor, ramipril, on cardiovascular events in high-risk patients. *N Engl J Med.* 2000;342(3):145-153.

215. Ostergren J, et al. Impact of ramipril in patients with evidence of clinical or subclinical peripheral arterial disease. *Eur Heart J.* 2004;25(1):17-24.

216. Group AC, et al. Intensive blood glucose control and vascular outcomes in patients with type 2 diabetes. *N Engl J Med.* 2008;358(24):2560-2572.

217. American Diabetes. A. 2. classification and diagnosis of diabetes. *Diabetes Care.* 2016;39 Suppl 1:S13-S22.

218. Marso SP, et al. Semaglutide and cardiovascular outcomes in patients with type 2 diabetes. *N Engl J Med.* 2016;375(19):1834-1844.

219. Marso SP, et al. Liraglutide and cardiovascular outcomes in type 2 diabetes. *N Engl J Med.* 2016;375(4):311-322.

220. Neal B, Perkovic V, Matthews DR. Canagliflozin and cardiovascular and renal events in type 2 diabetes. *N Engl J Med.* 2017;377(21):2099.

221. Zinman B, et al. Empagliflozin, cardiovascular outcomes, and mortality in type 2 diabetes. *N Engl J Med.* 2015;373(22):2117-2128.

222. Bethel, MA, McMurray JJV. Class effect for sodium glucose-cotransporter-2 inhibitors in cardiovascular outcomes: implications for the cardiovascular disease specialist. *Circulation.* 2018;137(12):1218-1220.

223. Udell JA, et al. Cardiovascular outcomes and risks after initiation of a sodium glucose cotransporter 2 inhibitor: results from the EASEL population-based cohort study (Evidence for Cardiovascular Outcomes With Sodium Glucose Cotransporter 2 Inhibitors in the Real World). *Circulation.* 2018;137(14):1450-1459.

224. Bonaca MP, Beckman JA. Sodium glucose cotransporter 2 inhibitors and amputation risk: Achilles' heel or opportunity for discovery? *Circulation.* 2018;137(14):1460-1462.

225. Udell JA, et al. Fibroblast growth factor-23, cardiovascular prognosis, and benefit of angiotensin-converting enzyme inhibition in stable ischemic heart disease. *J Am Coll Cardiol.* 2014;63(22):2421-2428.

226. Verma S, et al. Cardiovascular outcomes and safety of empagliflozin in patients with type 2 diabetes mellitus and peripheral artery disease: a sub-analysis of EMPA-REG OUTCOME. *Circulation.* 2018;137(4):405-407.

227. Wiviott SD, et al. Dapagliflozin and cardiovascular outcomes in type 2 diabetes. *N Engl J Med.* 2019;380(4):347-357.

228. Reilly MP, Mohler ER 3rd. Cilostazol: treatment of intermittent claudication. *Ann Pharmacother.* 2001;35(1):48-56.

229. Beebe HG, et al. A new pharmacological treatment for intermittent claudication: results of a randomized, multicenter trial. *Arch Intern Med.* 1999;159(17):2041-2050.

230. O'Donnell ME, et al. The vascular and biochemical effects of cilostazol in patients with peripheral arterial disease. *J Vasc Surg.* 2009;49(5):1226-1234.

231. Bedenis R, et al. Cilostazol for intermittent claudication. *Cochrane Database Syst Rev.* 2014;10:CD003748.

232. Pande RL, et al. A pooled analysis of the durability and predictors of treatment response of cilostazol in patients with intermittent claudication. *Vasc Med.* 2010;15(3):181-188.

233. Stevens JW, et al. Systematic review of the efficacy of cilostazol. naftidrofuryl oxalate and pentoxifylline for the treatment of intermittent claudication. *Br J Surg.* 2012;99(12):1630-1638.

234. Thompson D, et al. Meta-analysis of results from eight randomized. placebo-controlled trials on the effect of cilostazol on patients with intermittent claudication. *Am J Cardiol.* 2002;90(12):1314-1319.

235. Lundgren F, et al. Intermittent claudication–surgical reconstruction or physical training? A prospective randomized trial of treatment efficiency. *Ann Surg.* 1989;209(3):346-355.

236. Murphy TP, et al. The Claudication: Exercise Vs. Endoluminal Revascularization (CLEVER) study: rationale and methods. *J Vasc Surg.* 2008;47(6):1356-1363.

237. Murphy TP, et al. Supervised exercise versus primary stenting for claudication resulting from aortoiliac peripheral artery disease: six-month outcomes from the claudication: exercise versus endoluminal revascularization (CLEVER) study. *Circulation.* 2012;125(1):130-139.

238. Fakhry F, et al. Endovascular revascularization and supervised exercise for peripheral artery disease and intermittent claudication: a randomized clinical trial. *JAMA.* 2015;314(18):1936-1944.

239. van Pul KM, et al. Effect of supervised exercise therapy for intermittent claudication in patients with diabetes mellitus. *Ann Vasc Surg.* 2012;26(7):957-963.

240. Tsai TT, et al. The contemporary safety and effectiveness of lower extremity bypass surgery and peripheral endovascular interventions in the treatment of symptomatic peripheral arterial disease. *Circulation.* 2015;132(21):1999-2011.

241. Iida O, et al. Shared and differential factors influencing restenosis following endovascular therapy between TASC (Trans-Atlantic Inter-Society Consensus) II class A to C and D lesions in the femoropopliteal artery. *JACC Cardiovasc Interv.* 2014;7(7):792-798.

242. Zannetti S, L'Italien GJ, Cambria RP. Functional outcome after surgical treatment for intermittent claudication. *J Vasc Surg.* 1996;24(1):65-73.

243. Menard MT, et al. Design and rationale of the best endovascular versus best surgical therapy for patients with critical limb ischemia (BEST-CLI) trial. *J Am Heart Assoc.* 2016;5(7).

244. Bradbury AW, et al. Bypass versus Angioplasty in Severe Ischaemia of the Leg (BASIL) trial: an intention-to-treat analysis of amputation-free and overall survival in patients randomized to a bypass surgery-first or a balloon angioplasty-first revascularization strategy. *J Vasc Surg.* 2010; 51(5 Suppl):5S-17S.

245. Hunt BD, et al. BAlloon versus Stenting in severe Ischaemia of the Leg-3 (BASIL-3): study protocol for a randomised controlled trial. *Trials.* 2017;18(1):224.

246. Popplewell MA, et al. Bypass versus angio plasty in severe ischaemia of the leg-2 (BASIL-2) trial: study protocol for a randomised controlled trial. *Trials.* 2016;17:11.

247. UPDATE: Treatment of peripheral arterial disease with paclitaxel-coated balloons and paclitaxel-eluting stents potentially associated with increased mortality—letter to health care providers. https://www.fda.gov/medical-devices/letters-health-care-providers/ update-treatment-peripheral-arterial-disease-paclitaxel-coated-balloons-and-paclitaxel-eluting. 2019.

248. Correction to: durable clinical effectiveness with paclitaxel-eluting stents in the femoropopliteal artery 5–year results of the Zilver PTX randomized trial. *Circulation.* 2019;139(8):e42.

249. Beckman JA, White CJ. Paclitaxel-coated balloons and eluting stents: is there a mortality risk in patients with peripheral artery disease? *Circulation.* 2019;140(16):1342-1351.

250. Katsanos K, et al. Risk of death following application of paclitaxel-coated balloons and stents in the femoropopliteal artery of the leg: a systematic review and meta-analysis of randomized controlled trials. *J Am Heart Assoc.* 2018;7(24):e011245.

251. Rocha-Singh KJ, et al. Mortality and paclitaxel-coated devices: an individual patient data meta-analysis. *Circulation.* 2020;141(23):1859-1869.

252. Misra S, Dake MD. Paclitaxel-based therapies for patients with peripheral artery disease. *Circulation.* 2019;139(13):1565-1567.

253. Behrendt CA, et al. Editor's choice—long term survival after femoropopliteal artery revascularisation with paclitaxel coated devices: a propensity score matched cohort analysis. *Eur J Vasc Endovasc Surg.* 2020;59(4):587-596.

254. Bertges DJ, et al. Mortality after paclitaxel coated balloon angioplasty and stenting of superficial femoral and popliteal artery in the vascular quality initiative. *Circ Cardiovasc Interv.* 2020;13(2):e008528.

255. Clason AE, et al. Morbidity and mortality in acute lower limb ischaemia: a 5–year review. *Eur J Vasc Surg.* 1989;3(4):339-343.

256. Emmerich J. Current state and perspective on medical treatment of critical leg ischemia: gene and cell therapy. *Int J Low Extrem Wounds.* 2005;4(4):234-241.

257. Callum K, Bradbury A. ABC of arterial and venous disease: acute limb ischaemia. *BMJ.* 2000;320(7237):764-767.

258. Warkentin TE. Ischemic limb gangrene with pulses. *N Engl J Med.* 2015;373(24):2386-2388.

259. Clagett GP, et al. Antithrombotic therapy in peripheral arterial occlusive disease: the Seventh ACCP Conference on Antithrombotic and Thrombolytic Therapy. *Chest.* 2004;126(3 Suppl):609S-626S.

260. Abbott WM, et al. Arterial embolism: a 44 year perspective. *Am J Surg.* 1982;143(4):460-464.

261. Blaisdell FW, Steele M, Allen RE. Management of acute lower extremity arterial ischemia due to embolism and thrombosis. *Surgery.* 1978;84(6):822-834.

262. Giannini D, Balbarini A. Thrombolytic therapy in peripheral arterial disease. *Curr Drug Targets Cardiovasc Haematol Disord.* 2004;4(3):249-258.

263. Ouriel K, Veith FJ, Sasahara AA. A comparison of recombinant urokinase with vascular surgery as initial treatment for acute arterial occlusion of the legs. Thrombolysis or Peripheral Arterial Surgery (TOPAS) Investigators. *N Engl J Med.* 1998;338(16):1105-1111.

Acute Rheumatic Fever

Liesl Zühlke, Jagat Narula, Mark Engel, and Jonathan R. Carapetis

CHAPTER OUTLINE

Cardiac involvement in rheumatic fever

Pericarditis

Pericarditis with small pericardial effusion is equally supportive of diagnosis in primary and recurrent rheumatic fever episodes and best identified by pericardial friction rub.

'Bread-and-butter pericarditis'

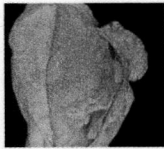

Shaggy fibrinous exudates on the epicardium (left). Fibrin deposits associated with cellular infiltrates containing lymphocytes, histiocytes, plasma cells and occasionally Aschoff cells (right).

Roentgenographic evidence of cardiac enlargement

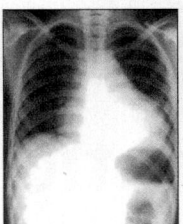

At admission   After improvement

Echocardiographic evidence of pericardial effusion

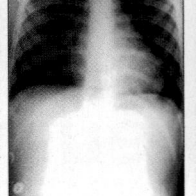

Myocarditis

Rheumatic myocarditis occurs as interstitial carditis and is predominantly represented by areas of fibrinous debris associated with cells of mononuclear and macrophage lineage, and histiocytes.

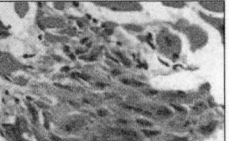
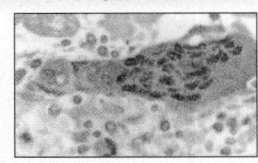

Endomyocardial biopsies: 30-40% of patients have well formed Aschoff Nodules with central ill-defined area of edematous interstitial connective tissue and fibrinoid degeneration (left); multinucleated Aschoff giant cell stained with anti-α1chymotrypsin antibody (right). Interstitial alteration is associated with infiltration of mononuclear cells. Myocytes are not injured.
Thus, left ventricular systolic function remains normal throughout the course of the acute episode.

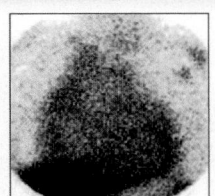
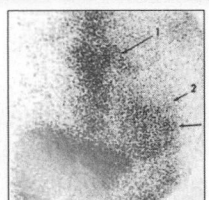

Abnormal antimyosin antibody scans are sometimes seen only with pericardial effusion when the radiolabeled antibody is secreted in exudate, or with gross subendo-cardial stress in volume overload (left). Gallium scans are more frequently abnormal and suggest interstitial inflammation (right).

Endocarditis

Endocarditis or valvulitis constitutes the most important component of rheumatic fever, as it leads to permanent deformity.

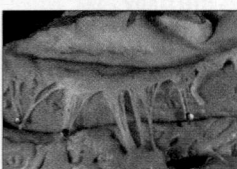
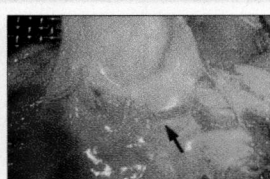

Tiny, wart-like verrucae/vegetations on atrial side of mitral valve (left) and ventricular surface of aortic valve (right); the verrucae are sterile and almost never embolize (unlike bacterial endocarditis).

The thrombotic vegetation has altered collagen and fibrinoid, and is associated with palisading mononuclear cell infiltration and occasionally Aschoff cells at the base of fibrinoid region; the inflammation extends throughout the valve leaflet.

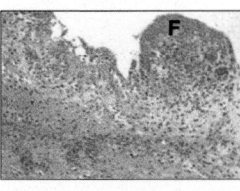

Echo-Doppler: valvular regurgitation of mitral valve (left) and aortic valve (right)

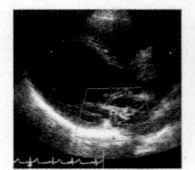
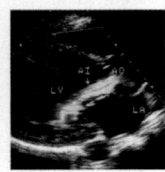

Mitral valve is almost always involved; tricuspid and pulmonary valve involvement is less common and never occurs without left-sided valvular involvement. Nodularity of the mitral valve is seen in a quarter of cases on echocardiographic and magnetic resonance imaging. Although definitively diagnostic in a primary episode, for the diagnosis of recurrence of valvulitis, previous echocardiographic findings are required to document a change in the degree of valvular regurgitation or additional valvular involvement. Valvular regurgitation may resolve or persist and may cicatrize to result in stenosis in the long term.

Chapter 27 Fuster and Hurst's Central Illustration. Cardiac involvement in rheumatic fever involves all three layers—pericarditis, myocarditis, and endocarditis. Reproduced with permission from Narula J, Virmani R, Reddy KS, et al. *Rheumatic Fever*. Washington, DC: American Registry of Pathology. Armed Forces Institute of Pathology; 1999.

CHAPTER SUMMARY

This chapter discusses the pathogenesis, clinical presentation, diagnosis, and management of acute rheumatic fever (ARF) and rheumatic heart disease (RHD). Group A *Streptococcal* disease can infrequently result in ARF when it goes untreated or unrecognized. Postinfective immunologic phenomena may cause multisystem involvement. All three layers of the heart may be affected as fibrinous pericarditis, interstitial myocarditis, and verrucous endocarditis or valvulitis. The endocardial affliction could evolve into severe, even life-threatening heart failure in the acute stages and may progress to permanent heart valve damage. Over 40 million people, largely living in low- and middle-income countries, live with and are affected by this disease. The 2015 revised Jones criteria have helped improve the diagnostic accuracy of ARF in moderate- to high-risk populations, while increased awareness and global advocacy will improve case detection, foster research, and determine the global burden of both ARF and RHD. The pathogenesis of ARF development remains poorly understood, and disease awareness and prevention remain the cornerstones for the eradication of this disease, which primarily afflicts the productive years of life.

INTRODUCTION

Acute rheumatic fever (ARF) is a multisystem autoimmune response to untreated or partially treated group A Streptococcus (GAS) pharyngitis. A single severe episode of ARF or recurrent episodes of ARF can result in permanent heart valve damage known as rheumatic heart disease (RHD). Despite a marked decline in ARF and RHD in high-income regions of the world, ARF and RHD persist as major public health problems in low- and middle-income regions of the world, indicative of inadequate access to health care, poorly functioning health systems, and continued social inequality.

EPIDEMIOLOGY OF ACUTE RHEUMATIC FEVER AND RHEUMATIC HEART DISEASE

The incidence of ARF began to decline in developed countries toward the end of the 19th century, and by the second half of the 20th century, ARF had become rare in most affluent populations. This decline is attributed to more hygienic and less crowded living conditions, better nutrition, improved access to medical care, and, to a lesser extent, the advent of antibiotics in the 1950s. The decline in prevalence of RHD in wealthy countries has followed a similar pattern, albeit with a delay compared to ARF incidence, which is explained by the chronic nature of RHD. However, these diseases continue largely unabated in resource-poor countries and in some populations living in relative poverty in industrialized countries.[1]

It was previously estimated that approximately 470,000 individuals acquire ARF each year, of whom 97% are in developing countries, where the incidence of ARF exceeds 50 per 100,000 children per year.[2] Estimates from the 2015 Global Burden of Disease study put the RHD burden at 33 million prevalent cases, causing 275,000 deaths and more than 9 million disability-adjusted life-years lost each year.[3,4] More recent data from the Institute of Health Metrics and Evaluation website show that this number is increasing with 40 million prevalent cases, despite some declines in mortality (https://vizhub.healthdata.org/gbd-compare/).[5] The major burden of ARF and RHD is in Central Africa, South Asia, and the Pacific region, and the heterogeneity of the disease is clearly depicted in the Years Lived with Disability in **Fig. 27-1** that shows the vast difference between Africa, Americas, Asia, and Europe.

The peak incidence of ARF occurs in those aged 5 to 15 years, with a decline thereafter such that cases are rare in adults aged >35 years.[1] First attacks are rare in the very young; only 5% of first episodes arise in children aged <5 years, and the disease is almost unheard of in those aged <2 years. Recurrent attacks are most frequent in adolescence and young adulthood and are diagnosed infrequently after 45 years of age. By contrast, RHD, which usually represents the accumulated damage from multiple ARF episodes in childhood, is most highly prevalent in the young adult years.[6]

ARF is equally common in males and females, but RHD is more common in females in almost all populations.[6,7] Whether this trend is a result of innate susceptibility, increased exposure to GAS because of greater involvement of women in child rearing, or reduced access to preventive medical care for females is unclear.[1] No association with ethnic origin has been found. There is some evidence that between 3% and 6% of any population is susceptible to ARF.[8]

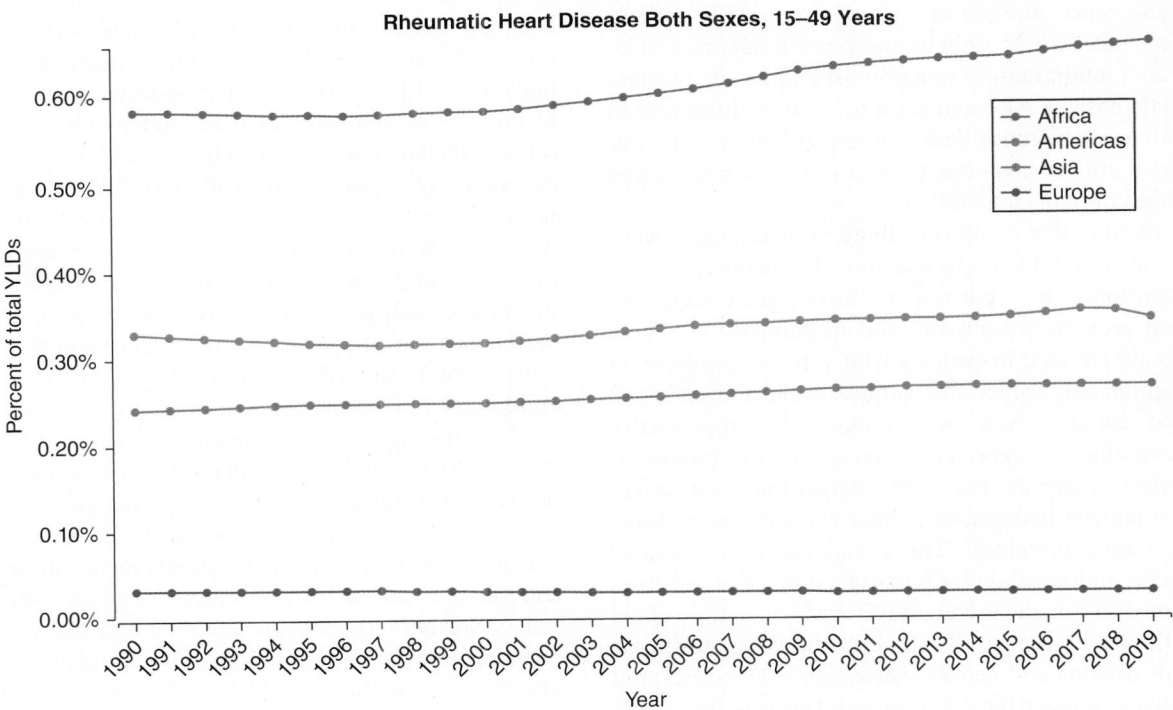

Figure 27–1. Heterogeneity in the global burden of rheumatic heart disease. The graph shows vast differences in Years Lived with Disability between Africa, Americas, Asia, and Europe. Data from The Institute of Health Metrics and Evaluation.

PATHOGENESIS

Epidemiologic and immunologic evidence clearly implicates GAS in the initiation of ARF in a susceptible host.[7,8] Most patients with ARF have elevated titers of plasma antistreptococcal antibodies, such as antideoxyribonuclease B (anti-D-Nase B) and antistreptolysin O (ASO), which are included amongst diagnostic criteria.[9] Outbreaks of ARF usually follow epidemics of GAS pharyngitis. Adequate treatment of GAS pharyngitis reduces the incidence of subsequent ARF, and appropriate antimicrobial prophylaxis prevents recurrences after initial attacks. It has generally been considered that certain strains of GAS are more prone to result in ARF, and this "rheumatogenicity" was thought to be a feature of strains belonging to certain M serotypes. The M protein is encoded by the *emm* gene and is a major virulence factor involved in resisting phagocytosis.[10] To date, in excess of 240 *emm* types have been characterized, of which 175 are considered to be clinically relevant.[11,12] More recent studies, however, suggest that rheumatogenicity may not be serotype specific. The long-held opinion that only streptococcal pharyngitis, and not streptococcal skin infections such as impetigo, may be followed by ARF has also been challenged.[13] Studies in populations where ARF is common find no definite association between GAS sequence type and site of infection or ability to cause disease.[14,15] Thus, the distinction between rheumatogenic and nonrheumatogenic strains, and between those trophic for the skin or throat, is considered by some to become blurred in areas where ARF is common and multiple different GAS strains circulate within small populations.[1]

The streptococcal M protein shares an α-helical coiled structure with cardiomyocyte contractile proteins such as myosin, and since antibodies isolated from ARF patients cross-react both with M protein and heart tissue, molecular mimicry and autoimmunity was proposed to be the primary pathogenetic basis of ARF and carditis.[13] The pathogenesis of RHD continues to be considered an interplay between multiple streptococcal antigens, various cross-reactive antibodies, and multipronged immune targets.[16]

The antibodies that could contribute to rheumatic valvulitis target the *N*-acetyl-β-D-glucosamine–dominant epitope of the GAS carbohydrate,[14] but might also recognize sequences in α-helical proteins (eg, myosin and tropomyosin).[15] These antibodies are elevated in patients with valvular involvement in ARF, significantly reduce after surgical removal of inflamed valves, and correlate with poor prognosis.[17] Cross-reactive M-protein antibodies expected to recognize the intracellular biomarker antigen cardiac myosin target the valve surface endothelial antigen laminin, or similar extracellular or basement membrane proteins.[18] The initial antibody-mediated damage to the endocardium leads to expression of vascular cell adhesion protein 1 on the valvular surface which, in turn, could facilitate the infiltration of T cells into the valve substance, resulting in scarring and neovascularization.[19] The concept of the target that resides on the cell surface and initiates the disease process in response to, or in association with, an intracellular biomarker antigen has also been proposed in the manifestation of ARF Sydenham's chorea, wherein the biomarker antigen in the brain is tubulin and the antigen target on the cell surface leads to calcium/calmodulin-dependent kinase II activation and dopamine release.[17]

Host factors have been considered to be important ever since familial clustering was reported last century. Associations between disease and human leukocyte antigen (HLA) class II alleles have been identified, but the alleles associated with susceptibility or protection differ depending on the population investigated.[20] High concentrations of circulating mannose-binding lectin and polymorphisms of transforming growth factor-β_1 and immunoglobulin genes also are associated with ARF.[21–23] Despite an association having been reported in individual studies, a recent systematic review failed to show a significant overall association between the TNF-α -308G>A (rs1800629) SNP and RF cases.[24] Certain B-cell alloantigens are expressed to a greater level in patients with ARF or RHD than controls, with family members having intermediate expression, suggesting that these antigens are markers of inherited susceptibility. The best characterized is D8/17, which has been associated with ARF and RHD in several populations worldwide.[25] Further investigation is needed before B-cell alloantigen markers can be used to identify individuals with, or at risk for, ARF or RHD, because expression appears to vary in population.[26] There is, currently, no specific investigation that reliably identifies individuals who are at risk of ARF or who will develop chronic rheumatic valvular heart disease.

The histopathologic manifestations of ARF are characterized by connective tissue alterations and are essentially similar in various organs. Collagen is a recognized target for autoantibodies in various autoimmune diseases, and on the basis of histopathologic characteristics, systemic involvement, and complete healing in most tissues, it has been alternatively proposed that collagen could be the primary site for inflammation in ARF.[27] It has been demonstrated that streptococcal M proteins form a complex with human collagen type IV in subendothelial basement membranes and might initiate an autoantibody response to the collagen.[28–30] This appears somewhat similar to pathogenesis of Goodpasture syndrome and Alport syndrome wherein the autoantibodies are directed at the basement membrane collagen type IV. The autoantigen is the mutated collagen IV (COL4 A3/A4/A5/A6) in Alport syndrome and the altered quaternary structure of the NC1 subunits of the α3 and α5 chains of collagen type IV of the lung and kidney in Goodpasture syndrome.[30,31] In ARF, M protein binds to the collagen IV through an octapeptide motif (**Fig. 27–2**); mice immunized with the collagen-binding octapeptide produced anticollagen antibodies[28,29,32] that did not cross-react with inducing M proteins, excluding the likelihood of molecular mimicry. Sera from ARF patients demonstrates collagen antibodies as well as increased titers for M proteins.[33] In Australia's Northern Territory, where rheumatic fever is endemic, prevalence of GAS is low and pharyngeal isolation of group G infections is common, the M-like fibrinogen-binding protein of group G streptococci (FOG) has been shown to interact with the collagen family, similar to M protein.[33,34]

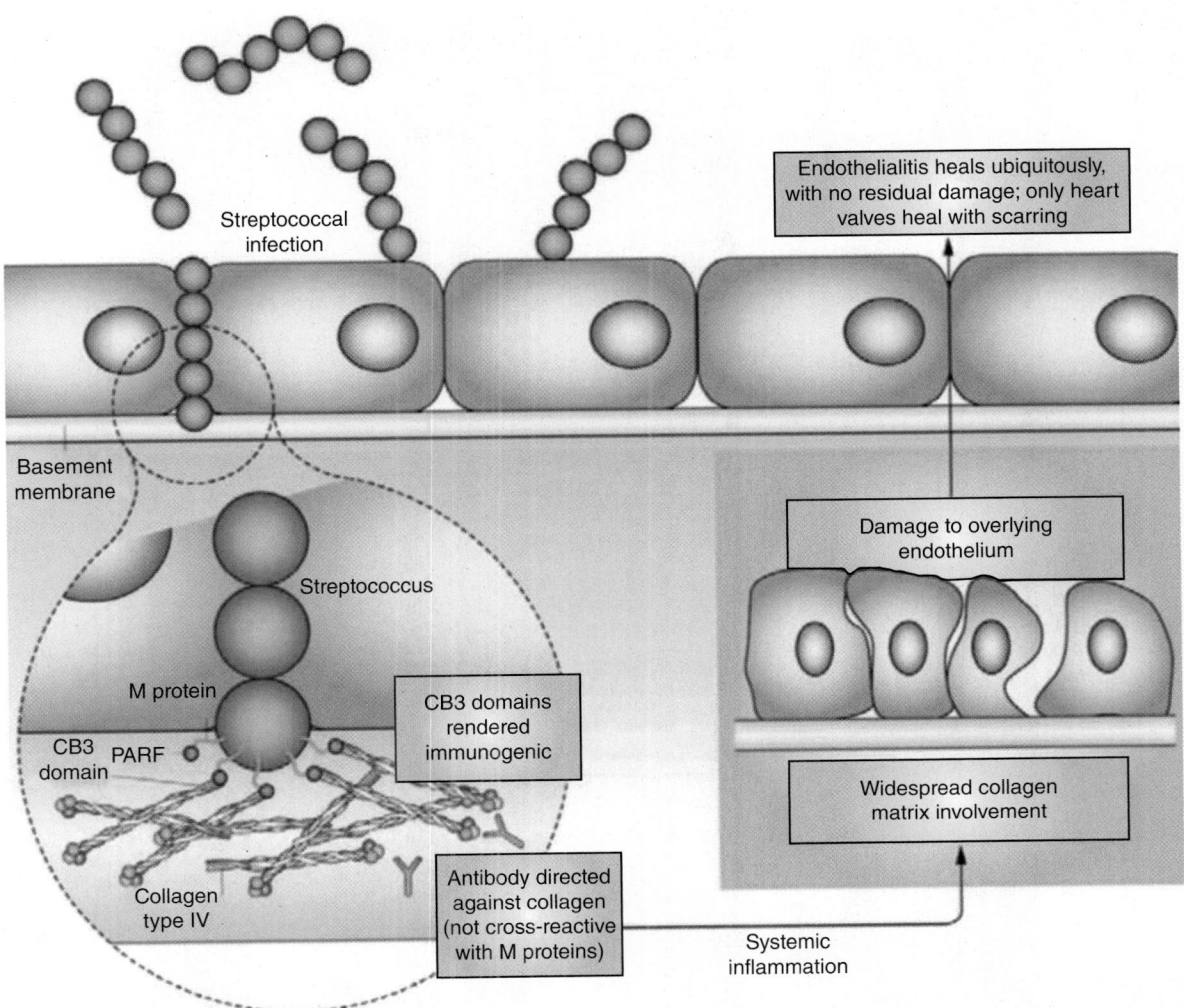

Figure 27–2. **Proposed pathogenesis of rheumatic fever**. Reproduced with permission from Tandon R, Sharma M, Chandrashekhar Y, et al. Revisiting the pathogenesis of rheumatic fever and carditis. *Nat Rev Cardiol*. 2013 Mar;10(3):171-177.

The long-term clinical consequence of ARF is related to permanent cardiac damage. Although rheumatic carditis involves the pericardium, myocardium, and endocardium, fibrinous pericarditis and interstitial myocardial involvement resolve without residual damage, whereas verrucous valvulitis is associated with permanent damage. Notably, the pathologic changes also indicate that, unlike in the more common lymphocytic form of myocarditis, heart muscle cells are spared in rheumatic carditis (**Fig. 27–3**).[27]

Despite the widespread endothelial activation and the diffuse collagen alterations in ARF, the endothelium has an immense capacity to heal, and the subendothelial damage is mostly limited to a shallow depth resulting in healing, but the endothelial cells demonstrate substantial structural and functional variability and may be responsible for the differential response in the valves. Endothelial-cell heterogeneity is best exemplified in the valvular endothelial cells; endothelial cells on the aortic side of the aortic valve have different expression profiles on microarrays from those on the ventricular side.

With valvulitis, neoangiogenesis develops within the substance of the valve tissue, which introduces more vascular endothelium and more collagen inflammation, leading to a vicious cycle of valvular damage, healing, and progressive scarring.[35]

CLINICAL PRESENTATION

The protean manifestations of this condition were well described in the early 20th century with a set of diagnostic criteria proposed by Duckett Jones in 1944[36] and subsequently modified and updated.[37-41] These revisions increased specificity but decreased sensitivity, particularly in endemic populations with potential missed diagnoses and failure to provide secondary prophylaxis to deserving patients.[42] Local guidelines have been adapted to the Jones criteria to reflect the pattern of disease in high-prevalence regions, local evidence, and current best practice, particularly relating to contemporary echocardiographic techniques.[43,44] The Jones criteria recently underwent an extensive revision.[45] This revision has aligned itself

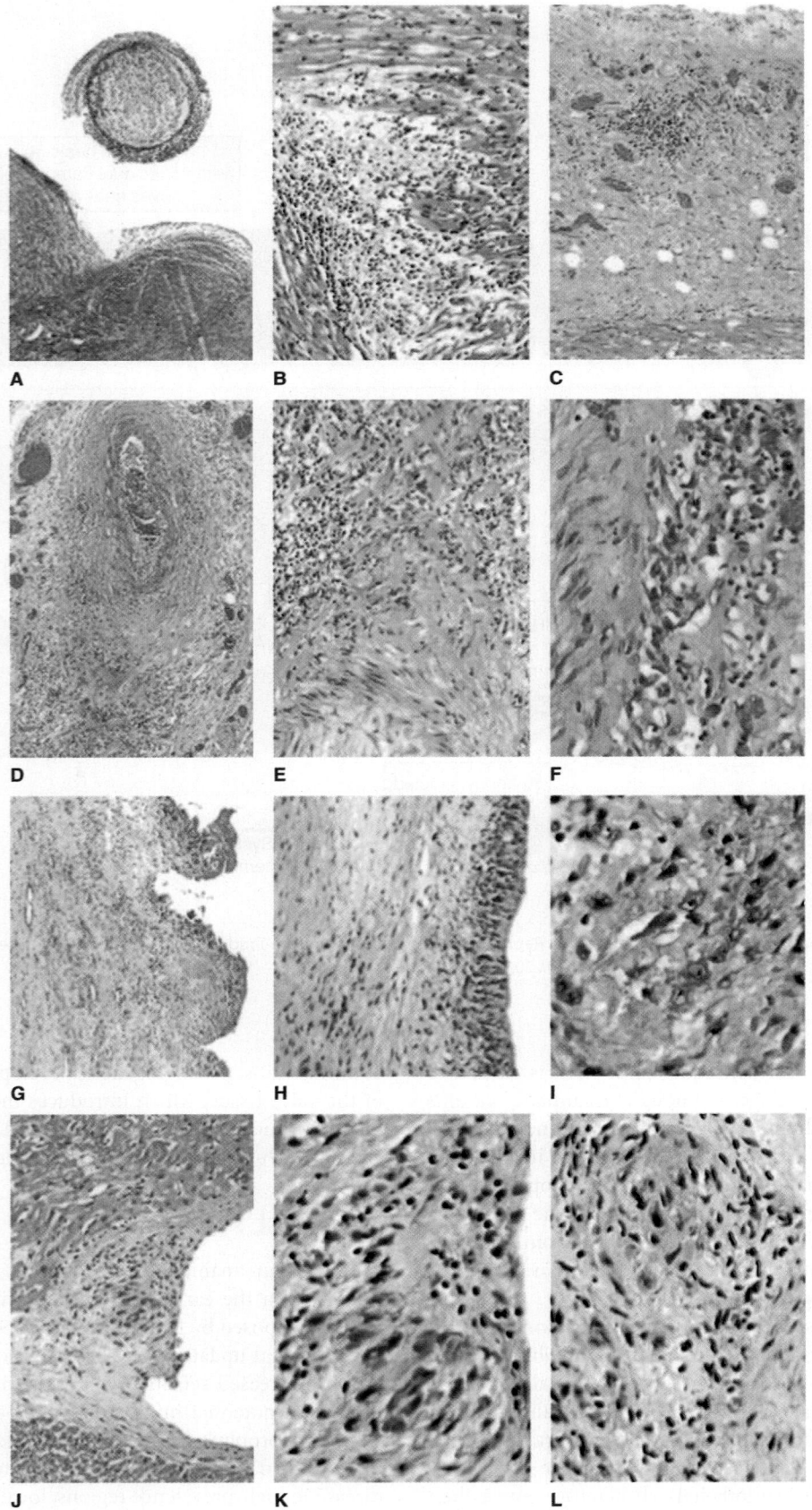

Figure 27–3. Hematoxylin and eosin staining of the heart and vasculature suggests connective tissue involvement in rheumatic fever. Reproduced with permission from Narula J, Virmani R, Reddy KS, et al. *Rheumatic Fever.* Washington, DC: American Registry of Pathology, Armed Forces Institute of Pathology; 1999.

with international guidelines by defining high-risk populations, recognizing the variability in disease burden and presentation, categorizing recommendations according to the favored Classification of Recommendations and Level of Evidence categories, and reflecting the era of Doppler echocardiography[46] (**Table 27–1**). The evolution of the Jones Criteria over the years is summarized in **Figure 27–4**.

The disease usually has an acute febrile onset and presents with variable combinations of major and minor manifestations. The diagnosis of ARF is made when the patient develops two major manifestations, or one major manifestation and at least two minor manifestations; in addition, evidence of preceding infection with GAS must be demonstrated using streptococcal serology. The exceptions are patients who present with chorea or indolent carditis, because these manifestations may only become apparent months after the inciting streptococcal infection so that additional manifestations may not be present and streptococcal serology testing may be normal.[47]

Carditis

Carditis is the single most important component of the disease in determining prognosis. The carditis of ARF occurs in >50% of patients and is almost always characterized by valvulitis of the mitral valve (mitral regurgitation) and, less frequently, the aortic valve (aortic regurgitation).[48–50] Pathologically, ARF produces a pancarditis, with involvement of the pericardium, myocardium, and endocardium. Clinical manifestations may vary widely and range from subclinical to life-threatening heart failure. Pericarditis may manifest with typical pericardial pain and a friction rub. Auscultation may reveal new murmurs or changing murmurs. Stenotic lesions are rare in the early stages of the disease, but a transient apical mid-diastolic murmur (Carey Coombs) may occur in association with the murmur of mitral regurgitation. This murmur occurs in patients with mitral valvulitis due to ARF. It is a short, mid-diastolic rumble best heard at the apex, which disappears as the valvulitis improves. It can be distinguished from the diastolic murmur of mitral stenosis by the absence of an opening snap before the murmur. The murmur is caused by increased blood flow across a thickened mitral valve.[51]

Atrioventricular conduction delay, resulting in a prolonged PR interval, is an important and helpful diagnostic clue. Recent data strongly substantiates the importance of subclinical carditis based on Doppler echocardiography.[50,52–55] Hence, echocardiographic evaluation for all patients with suspicion of ARF is recommended in the 2015 Jones criteria, and both clinical and subclinical carditis fulfil a major criterion, even in the absence of classical auscultatory findings.[45] Subclinical carditis of the mitral or aortic valves requires all four criteria to be met in order to fulfil the major criterion. Additional morphologic features may also be present. The updated Jones criteria also allow for epidemiological assessment of individuals at different risk,[57] longitudinal review of subclinical carditis, and new data regarding progression (worsening) and regression (improving) of subclinical valve lesions are an important advancement to the field.[58]

Arthritis and Arthralgia

The conventional description is of a polyarthritis affecting large joints, with the lower limb joints involved first, and involvement of each joint overlapping giving the impression that the process "flits." The arthritis of ARF responds promptly to anti-inflammatories, and thus, the classical presentation may be uncommon where medication with nonsteroidal anti-inflammatory drugs before the diagnosis is considered or confirmed.

The differential diagnosis of polyarticular arthritis in children and adolescents is wide (**Table 27–2**).[59] Monoarticular arthritis is increasingly recognized to be important in populations where ARF is common. The arthritis of ARF presents

TABLE 27–1. The Revised Jones Critieria[45] for the Diagnosis of Acute Rheumatic Fever		
Primary episode of rheumatic fever	Two major or one major and two minor manifestations **plus** evidence of a preceding group A streptococcal infection[a]	
Recurrent attack of rheumatic fever	Two major or one major and two minor manifestations or three minor **plus** evidence of a preceding group A streptococcal infection[a]	
Risk stratification	**Low-risk population** ARF incidence <2 per 100,000 school-aged children (usually 5–15 years) per year or an all-age prevalence of RHD of ≤1 per 1000 population per year	**Moderate-/high-risk population** Not clearly from a low-risk population depending on their reference population
Major criteria		
Carditis	Clinical and/or subclinical	Clinical and/or subclinical
Arthritis	Polyarthritis only	Monoarthritis or polyarthritis Polyarthralgia
	Chorea	Chorea
	Erythema marginatum	Erythema marginatum
	Subcutaneous nodules	Subcutaneous nodules
Minor criteria		
Arthralgia	Polyarthralgia	Monoarthralgia
Fever	≥38.5°C	≥38°C
ESR	ESR ≥60 mm in the first hour	ESR ≥30 mm/h
	CRP ≥3.0 mg/dL	CRP ≥3.0 mg/dL
	Prolonged PR interval, after accounting for age variability (unless carditis is a major criterion)	Prolonged PR interval, after accounting for age variability (unless carditis is a major criterion)

[a]Supporting evidence of a preceding streptococcal infection within the last 45 days: elevated or rising antistreptolysin-O or other streptococcal antibody, or a positive throat culture, rapid antigen test for group A streptococci, or recent scarlet fever.
Abbreviations: ARF, acute rheumatic fever; CRP, C-reactive protein; ESR, erythrocyte sedimentation rate; RHD, rheumatic heart disease.

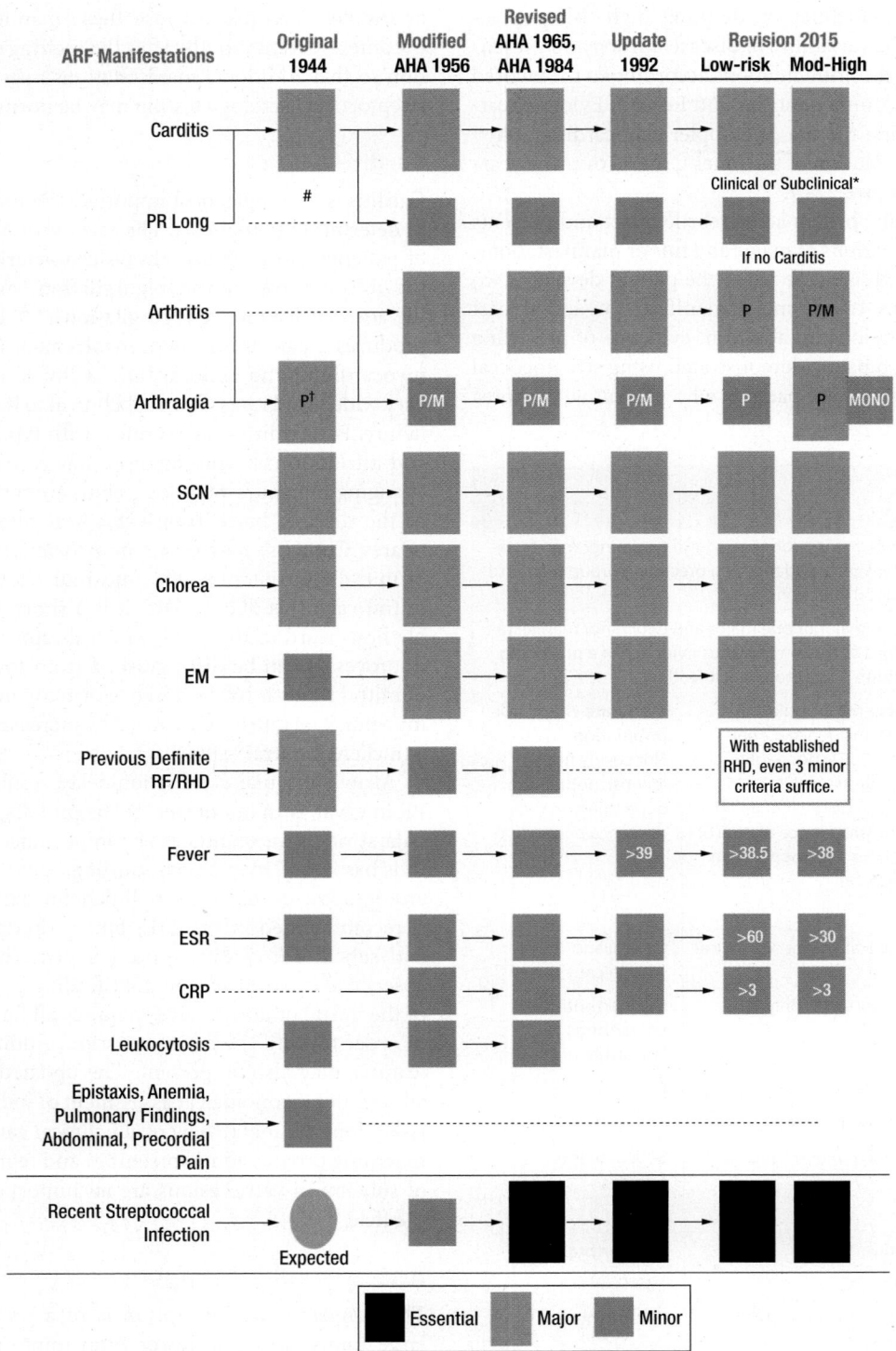

Figure 27–4. Evolution of Jones Criteria. In 1944, T. Duckett Jones first proposed the clinical algorithm for the diagnosis of acute rheumatic fever (ARF). The diagnosis of RF was entertained with 2 major or 1 major + 2 minor manifestations; a combination of multiple minor manifestations was considered suggestive but not diagnostic. Various revisions of the Jones Criteria were made in 1956, 1965, and 1984. The major limitation of the Jones criteria was the diagnosis of recurrence of activity in a patient with established rheumatic heart disease (RHD) because a new carditis needed demonstration of increase/change in pre-existing murmur or definite pericarditis. Therefore, the 1992 update precluded the application of Jones Criteria to recurrences and maintained that it only be employed to define the primary episode of ARF. While it was acceptable for the western countries, it left a big void for the low- and middle-income countries where RHD and ARF recurrences continue to be prevalent, hence local modifications were proposed. The 2015 revision of the Jones Criteria brought it closer to International Guidelines recognizing the high-risk populations and this revision also formally included Doppler echocardiography as a tool to help diagnose cardiac involvement. Low-risk regions included where RF incidence was <2/100K per year in 5-14 year old school going children, or overall RHD prevalence was <1/1K population. AHA, American Heart Association; CRP, C-reactive protein; EM, erythema marginatum; ESR, erythrocyte sedimentation rate; SCN, subcutaneous nodules; P, polyarthritis/arthralgia; †Polyarthralgia or arthritis; M, monoar thritis/arthralgia. Fever in °C, ESR in mm/h, CRP in mg/dL. *Subclinical carditis includes echocardiographic valvulitis; #PR prolongation included in Carditis. Reproduced with permission from Narula J, Virmani R, Reddy KS, et al. *Rheumatic Fever*. Washington, DC: American Registry of Pathology, Armed Forces Institute of Pathology; 1999.

TABLE 27–2. Differential Diagnosis[a] of Carditis and Polyarthritis in Children and Adolescents

Carditis	Polyarthritis
Physiologic mitral regurgitation	Connective tissue and other auto-immune diseases such as juvenile idiopathic arthritis
Mitral valve prolapse	
Myxomatous mitral valve	
Fibroelastoma	Reactive arthropathy
Congenital mitral valve disease	Septic arthritis
Congenital aortic valve disease	Poststreptococcal reactive arthritis
Infective endocarditis	Infective endocarditis
Cardiomyopathy	Lyme disease
Myocarditis, viral or idiopathic	Lymphoma/leukemia
Kawasaki disease	Viral arthropathy
	Sickle cell disease
	Gout and pseudogout
	Henoch-Schönlein purpura

[a]Excludes presentations with chorea.

Data from Gewitz MH, Baltimore RS, Tani LY, et al. Revision of the Jones Criteria for the diagnosis of acute rheumatic fever in the era of Doppler echocardiography: a scientific statement from the American Heart Association. *Circulation*. 2015 May 19; 131(20):1806-1818.

a difficult diagnostic challenge, especially in the patient presenting with an initial monoarthritis.[60] The arthritis of ARF is highly responsive to anti-inflammatory drugs (both aspirin and nonsteroidal anti-inflammatory drugs), and if the patient does not respond within 48 to 72 hours, alternate diagnoses should be considered. Poststreptococcal reactive arthritis is diagnosed in patients who have an arthritis that is not typical of ARF but who recently had streptococcal infection. This condition is said to occur after a shorter latent period than ARF, responds less well to anti-inflammatories, and may be associated with renal manifestations, and evidence of carditis is usually not seen. The distinction between post-streptococcal reactive arthritis and ARF is unclear, and many would recommend that a diagnosis of post-streptococcal reactive arthritis not be made in populations in which ARF is common.[59] Even if the diagnosis is considered, it is appropriate to offer a period of secondary penicillin prophylaxis, as for episodes of ARF in such populations.

Chorea

Sydenham's chorea may be associated with other manifestations of ARF but may also be the sole expression of the disease. It is a neurologic disorder characterized by involuntary, purposeless, rapid, and abrupt movements associated with muscular weakness and emotional lability. Chorea occurs in up to 30% of cases of ARF. The abnormal movements disappear during sleep.

Mild chorea may best be demonstrated by asking the patient to squeeze the examiner's hand. This results in repetitive irregular squeezes labeled as *the milking sign*. Emotional lability manifests in personality changes, with inappropriate behavior, restlessness, and outbursts of anger or crying.[61]

Erythema Marginatum

Erythema marginatum is a nonitchy, evanescent rash that is pink or slightly red and that affects the trunk predominantly. The rash extends centrifugally, and the skin in the center returns toward normal. The rash may be fleeting and disappear within hours. It may be brought out by a warm bath or shower. It is reported to be found in only 4% to 15% of cases and may be difficult to detect in dark-skinned patients.

Subcutaneous Nodules

These nodules generally appear later in the course of the disease after several weeks of illness and are seen most commonly in patients with carditis. They are firm and painless; the overlying skin is not inflamed and may vary in size from a few millimeters to several centimeters. They are most commonly located over bony surfaces or tendons such as elbows, wrists, knees, occiput, and spinous processes of the vertebrae. These occur in less than 10% of cases of ARF.

DIAGNOSIS AND INVESTIGATIONS

There is no definitive laboratory test for ARF, with the diagnosis based on a combination of clinical manifestations and laboratory evidence of previous streptococcal infection. Evidence of preceding streptococcal infection may be demonstrated by a positive throat swab culture or rapid antigen test for group A β-hemolytic streptococci (noting that nucleic acid amplification tests are highly sensitive and specific, whereas older generation antigen detection tests are less reliable), or increased titers of antistreptolysin O or other streptococcal antibodies; given the variability in the elevation of titers following infection, a combination of antibody tests is desirable.[62] The revised Jones critieria[45] present two distinct decision paths depending on the risk category (high and moderate risk vs. low risk) of the population (see Table 27–1 and Fig 27–4). The changes to the major and minor criteria represent a significant attempt at weighing sensitivity versus specificity in its diagnostic acumen in both low- and moderate-/high-risk populations. The three key changes are the risk stratification, adaptation of both major (carditis and arthritis/arthralgia) and minor (arthralgia, fever, and erythrocyte sedimentation rate [ESR] cutoffs) criteria, and the definition of recurrent ARF episodes.

Risk Stratification

Recent data have emphasized the disproportionate burden, pattern, and presentation of ARF and RHD.[63–65] The 2015 iteration of the Jones criteria defines low risk as coming from a population with an ARF incidence of <2 per 100,000 per year for school-aged children or an all-age RHD prevalence of <1 per 1000 population per year, with those not clearly coming from a low-risk population considered to be a moderate-to-high risk with the modified major and minor criteria applying (Class IIa, Level of Evidence C). This has important practical implications for clinicians working in countries with mixed risk populations.[66,67]

Changes in Major and Minor Criteria

Carditis

Subclinical carditis or clinically silent but echocardiographically evident valvulitis has long been recognized as a manifestation of ARF with a weighted pooled prevalence of 16.8%.[68–71] As a result, the comprehensive evaluation of all cases of confirmed and suspected ARF includes echocardiography with Doppler, regardless of the findings on auscultation (Class I, Level of Evidence B).

Arthritis

In moderate-/high-risk populations, monoarthritis in addition to the more classic polyarthritis has been demonstrated to be an important clinical manifestation of ARF.[72,73] Previously reflected in the Australian and New Zealand guidelines,[74,75] the consideration of monoarthritis as part of the ARF spectrum is now included, although limited to moderate- to-high risk populations (Class I, Level of Evidence C). Monoarthralgia is now also included as a minor criterion in moderate-/high-risk populations, although this will only apply when arthritis (monoarthritis/polyarthritis and/or polyarthralgia) has not been used as a major criterion.

Fever and Erythrocyte Sedimentation Rate

Finally, revised cutoffs have been introduced for three of the minor criteria in order to improve sensitivity in the higher risk populations. The cutoff for fever has been lowered to 38.0°C (compared to 38.5°C in low-risk patients), and the ESR has been lowered to >30 mm/h (compared to 60 mm/h in moderate-/high-risk patients).

Definition of Rheumatic Fever Recurrences

Prior to the 2015 iteration, there were no specific diagnostic criteria for ARF recurrences. The new criteria now state that with a reliable past history of ARF or RHD and in the face of documented GAS infection, two major, or one major and two minor, or three minor manifestations may be sufficient for a presumptive diagnosis of an ARF recurrence (Class IIb, Level of Evidence C).

The current guidelines seek to increase sensitivity in populations that have a high incidence of ARF and maintain high specificity in low-risk populations. They rely on considerable diagnostic and echocardiographic acumen complemented by laboratory testing to confirm and monitor disease activity. Table 27–2 presents the differential diagnoses for polyarthritis and carditis in children and adolescents. The Doppler findings in rheumatic valvulitis are presented in **Table 27–3**. Laboratory investigations, other than those to confirm GAS exposure and ESR and C-reactive protein, are otherwise nonspecific. Modest normochromic normocytic anemia of chronic inflammation is frequent.

The electrocardiogram may be unhelpful apart from reflecting sinus tachycardia. Prolongation of the PR interval serves as a useful minor criterion and may be particularly helpful in recurrences where previous electrocardiograms are available.

TREATMENT

Management of the Acute Episode

The aims of treatment of ARF are to suppress the inflammatory response to minimize cardiac damage, to provide symptomatic

TABLE 27–3. Findings on Echocardiogram in Rheumatic Valvulitis

Doppler Findings in Rheumatic Valvulitis of Either the Mitral or the Aortic Valve
(All four Doppler echocardiographic criteria must be met in each category)

Pathologic Mitral Regurgitation	Pathologic Aortic Regurgitation
Seen in two views In at least one view, jet length ≥1 cm Velocity ≥3 m/s for one complete envelope Pansystolic jet in at least one envelope	Seen in two views In at least one view, jet length ≥2 cm Velocity ≥3 m/s in early diastole Pandiastolic jet in at least one envelope

Morphologic Findings on Echocardiogram in Rheumatic Valvulitis Morphological Features of Rheumatic Heart Disease

Acute Mitral Valve Changes	Chronic Mitral Valve Changes (Not Seen in Acute Carditis)	Aortic Valve Changes (Acute or Chronic)
Annular dilatation	Leaflet thickening	Irregular or focal thickening
Chordal elongation	Chordal thickening and fusion	Coaptation defect
Chordal rupture resulting in flail leaflet	Restricted leaflet motion	Restricted leaflet motion
Anterior (or less commonly posterior) leaflet tip prolapse Beading/nodularity of leaflet tips	Calcification	Leaflet prolapse

Adapted with permission from Gewitz MH, Baltimore RS, Tani LY, et al. Revision of the Jones Criteria for the diagnosis of acute rheumatic fever in the era of Doppler echocardiography: a scientific statement from the American Heart Association. *Circulation.* 2015 May 19;131(20):1806-1818.

relief, and to eradicate pharyngeal streptococcal infection.[61] Patients are usually hospitalized, and the long-standing recommendation of bedrest or chair rest is appropriate if heart failure is present. Ambulation is usually started once fever has subsided and joint pain and heart failure are controlled.

Although evidence of active infection is unusual during the acute phase, it is recommended that patients receive a single dose of benzathine penicillin G or a 10-day course of penicillin V (or erythromycin if penicillin allergic) to curtail exposure to streptococcal antigens. After completion of the course, secondary prophylaxis should be commenced. This recommendation is based on observational and longitudinal data.[6]

Anti-inflammatory agents, including salicylates or nonsteroidal anti-inflammatories provide dramatic improvement in symptoms such as arthritis and fever soon after starting treatment. Initial analgesia should be restricted to paracetamol (15 mg/kg 4 hourly) during the diagnostic work-up followed by Naproxen 250 mg to 500 mg (children 10–20mg/kg/d) or ibuprofen 200 mg to 400 mg (5–10mg/kg/d). Doses of aspirin of 80 mg to 100 mg/kg/d in children and 4 g to 8 g/d in adults may be needed initially.[9] The usual dose of prednisone or prednisolone is 1 mg to 2 mg/kg/d. There is no good evidence that steroids are superior to aspirin in terms of altering the natural history of the disease. Some believe that they do result in more rapid resolution of carditis and can be lifesaving, but this is unproven.[59,76]

Sydenham's chorea, the debilitating neurologic condition, remains the most prevalent form of chorea in children. There are many suggested treatments, most without a strong evidence base. Symptomatic management include antipsychotic and anticonvulsant medications, while data on immunomodulatory therapy (steroids, intravenous immunoglobulin [IVIG], and plasma exchange) are limited to individual case reports or series and rare comparison studies. In a meta-analysis, the efficacy of steroid use was supported by a single placebo-controlled study and several case series, while only sparse information was available on other immunomodulatory therapies such as IVIG and plasmapheresis, not including any robust trials.[77]

Patients with severe heart failure require usual antifailure treatment. When carditis complicated by marked valvular regurgitation causes severe hemodynamic compromise, valve surgery is life-saving and should not be delayed by trials of anti-inflammatory medication. Valve repair rather than replacement is the preferred option for RHD surgery, considering the concerns regarding the need for anticoagulation[78] especially in women with reproductive intent.[79,80] However, repair should be performed by a surgeon experienced in rheumatic valvular surgery.[81,82]

PREVENTION

Primary prevention refers to antibiotic treatment of GAS pharyngitis to prevent subsequent attacks of ARF. A single intramuscular injection of 600,000 or 1.2 million units of benzathine penicillin (depending on weight) or 10-day course of penicillin V is advised (**Table 27–4**). Efforts at primary prevention are confounded by the fact that many patients who develop ARF are not aware of preceding sore throat, there are no simple specific clinical signs diagnostic of streptococcal pharyngitis, and throat swabs and cultures are expensive. Even more, robust microdiagnostics are expensive and largely not available in RHD-endemic countries of the world, outside high-incomes countries. In an individual patient, antibiotic treatment for streptococcal sore throat is effective in reducing the occurrence of subsequent attacks of ARF by 70% to 80%.[83] While it is important in populations with a high incidence of ARF to promote presentation to primary health care with sore throat and proper diagnosis and management by the health system,[84] there is no definitive proof that this approach is effective in reducing overall ARF incidence in the population.[85,86]

Secondary prevention, the long-term administration of antibiotics to prevent recurrences, is of proven benefit and is cost-effective.[87] Benzathine penicillin 600,000 or 1.2 million units intramuscularly every 4 weeks is the standard recommendation.[60,88] An injection once every 2 or 3 weeks is more effective but may be more difficult to implement.[87] Oral penicillin V 250 mg orally twice daily is preferred by some practitioners, particularly in very thin patients who are on warfarin anticoagulation after valve replacement surgery, when deep intramuscular injections may be undesirable.[89] However, no studies have compared oral penicillin V with intramuscular benzathine penicillin in the prevention of rheumatic fever.

Prophylaxis is usually advised until age 21 years or for at least 10 years after the last attack of ARF, whichever is longer, with longer durations for individuals who have persistent and significant valvular damage. Duration of secondary prophylaxis should be individualized, taking into account factors

TABLE 27–4. Prevention of Acute Rheumatic Fever

Agent	Dose	Route	Duration
Primary prevention (treatment of group A streptococcal pharyngitis)			
Benzathine penicillin G	≥27 kg: 1.2 million units	Intramuscular (IM) injection	Once
	<27 kg: 600,000 units		
Penicillin V	Children 250 mg × 2–3/d	Oral	10 d
	Adults 500 mg × 2–3/d		
If penicillin allergy, options include narrow-spectrum cephalosporin, clindamycin, azithromycin, and clarithromycin. Consult local guidelines or see American Heart Association guideline.			
Secondary prevention (prevention of recurrent attacks)[a]			
Benzathine penicillin G	≥20 kg: 1.2 million units (<20 kg: 600,000 units) every 4 wk[b]	IM injection	
Penicillin V	250 mg × 2/d	Oral	
Erythromycin	250 mg × 2/d	Oral	

[a]Duration of secondary prophylaxis depends on history of carditis and if valvular involvement persists. In most cases, minimum duration is 10 years since last acute rheumatic fever (ARF) episode or until age 21 years, whichever is longer, with prolongation until age 35 to 40 years in individuals with significant valvular disease.
[b]Although injections every 4 weeks are effective, if good adherence can be assured, benzathine penicillin G may be given more frequently (every 3 or every 2 weeks) if there is a desire to further increase the efficacy in preventing recurrent ARF.
Data from Rutstein DD. Report of the committee on standards and criteria for programs of care of the council of rheumatic fever and congenital heart disease of the American Heart Association: Jones criteria (modified) for guidance in the diagnosis of rheumatic fever. *Circulation.* 1956;13:617-620 and Vijayalakshmi IB, Mithravinda J and Deva AN. The role of echocardiography in diagnosing carditis in the setting of acute rheumatic fever. *Cardiol Young.* 2005;15:583-588.

influencing risk of recurrence. Prophylaxis until age 35 to 40 years, or sometimes for life, is recommended for patients with severe valve disease or after valve replacement surgery.

Vaccines efforts are underway, with a recent Phase I trial of a recombinant 30-valent M protein-based vaccine demonstrating immunogenicity in adults with no laboratory evidence of tissue cross-reactive antibodies.[90] Other vaccines are approaching clinical trials, and there are increasing efforts to coordinate global efforts to accelerate development of these vaccines (see https://savac.ivi.int/). This provides considerable promise for addressing the ARF burden, particularly given the realities of poor availability of penicillin and lack of adherence to prophylaxis.

PROGNOSIS

Cardiac involvement remains the most serious manifestation of ARF with severe life-threatening heart failure in the acute stages due to the acute valvulitis.[91,92] Inadequate coverage with antibiotic prophylaxis to prevent future attacks of ARF puts patients at risk for repeated episodes of ARF, scarring of the heart valves, chronic valvular heart disease, heart failure, and death, usually before middle age. The revised Jones criteria provide an important opportunity to improve the diagnostic accuracy of ARF, in moderate-/high-risk populations. These, together with increased awareness and global advocacy, will improve case detection, foster research, and accurately determine the global burden of ARF and RHD.

SUMMARY

Pathogenesis

- GAS disease can infrequently result in ARF when untreated or unrecognized.
- The pathogenesis of ARF development remains poorly understood.
- Postinfective immunologic phenomenon may cause multisystem involvement. All three layers of the heart may be affected as fibrinous pericarditis, interstitial myocarditis and verrucous endocarditis, or valvulitis.
- The endocardial affliction could evolve into severe heart failure in the acute stages and may progress to permanent heart valve damage.

Epidemiology

- Over 40 million people, largely living in low-and middle-income countries live with and are affected by the disease, in terms of disability-adjusted life-years and years lived with disability.

Diagnosis

- The 2015 revised Jones criteria have helped improve the diagnostic accuracy of ARF, in moderate-/high-risk populations, while increased awareness and global advocacy will improve case detection, foster research, and determine the global burden of ARF and RHD.

Management

- Disease awareness and prevention remain the cornerstones for the eradication of this disease that primarily afflicts the productive years of life.

ACKNOWLEDGMENTS

We would like to acknowledge the contribution and legacy of Professor Bongani M. Mayosi, whose impact on the science and advocacy of ARF/RHD is unparalleled.

REFERENCES

1. Carapetis JR, McDonald M, Wilson NJ. Acute rheumatic fever. *Lancet.* 2005;366:155-168.
2. Carapetis JR, Steer AC, Mulholland EK, Weber M. The global burden of group A streptococcal diseases. *Lancet Infect Dis.* 2005;5:685-694.
3. Global Burden of Disease Study Collaborators. Global, regional, and national incidence, prevalence, and years lived with disability for 301 acute and chronic diseases and injuries in 188 countries, 1990-2013: a systematic analysis for the Global Burden of Disease Study 2013. *Lancet.* 2015;386:743-800.
4. GBD 2013 Mortality and Causes of Death Collaborators. Global, regional, and national age-sex specific all-cause and cause-specific mortality for 240 causes of death, 1990-2013: a systematic analysis for the Global Burden of Disease Study 2013. *Lancet.* 2015;385:117-171.
5. Roth GA, Mensah GA, Johnson CO, et al. Global burden of cardiovascular diseases and risk factors, 1990-2019: update from the GBD 2019 Study. *J Am Coll Cardiol.* 2020;76(25):2982-3021.
6. Lawrence JG, Carapetis JR, Griffiths K, Edwards K, Condon JR. Acute rheumatic fever and rheumatic heart disease: incidence and progression in the Northern Territory of Australia, 1997 to 2010. *Circulation.* 2013;128:492-501.
7. Rothenbuhler M, O'Sullivan CJ, Stortecky S, et al. Active surveillance for rheumatic heart disease in endemic regions: a systematic review and meta-analysis of prevalence among children and adolescents. *Lancet Glob Health.* 2014;2:e717-e726.
8. Carapetis JR, Currie BJ, Mathews JD. Cumulative incidence of rheumatic fever in an endemic region: a guide to the susceptibility of the population? *Epidemiol Infect.* 2000;124:239-244.
9. Anna P, Ralph SN, Vicki Wade, Bart J Currie. The 2020 Australian guideline for prevention, diagnosis and management of acute rheumatic fever and rheumatic heart disease. *Med J Aust.* 2020. 214(5):220-227.
10. Fischetti VA. Streptococcal M protein: molecular design and biological behavior. *Clin Microbiol Rev.* 1989;2(3):285-314.
11. Bessen DE, Smeesters PR, Beall BW. Molecular epidemiology, ecology, and evolution of group A streptococci. *Microbiol Spectr.* 2018;6(5).
12. Dale JB, Smeesters PR, Courtney HS, et al. Structure-based design of broadly protective group a streptococcal M protein-based vaccines. *Vaccine.* 2017;35(1):19-26.
13. Fischetti VA, Vashishta A, Pancholi V. *Rheumatic Fever.* Washington, DC: Armed Forces Institute of Pathology; 1999.
14. Goldstein I, Rebeyrotte P, Parlebas J, Halpern B. Isolation from heart valves of glycopeptides which share immunological properties with *Streptococcus haemolyticus* group A polysaccharides. *Nature.* 1968;219:866-868.
15. Galvin JE, Hemric ME, Ward K, Cunningham MW. Cytotoxic mAb from rheumatic carditis recognizes heart valves and laminin. *J Clin Invest.* 2000;106:217-224.
16. Carapetis JR, Beaton A, Cunningham MW, et al. Acute rheumatic fever and rheumatic heart disease. *Nature Rev Dis Primers.* 2016;2:15084.
17. Ellis NM, Kurahara DK, Vohra H, et al. Priming the immune system for heart disease: a perspective on group A streptococci. *J Infect Dis.* 2010;202:1059-1067.

18. Ellis NM, Li Y, Hildebrand W, Fischetti VA, Cunningham MW. T cell mimicry and epitope specificity of cross-reactive T cell clones from rheumatic heart disease. *J Immunol.* 2005;175:5448-5456.

19. Roberts S, Kosanke S, Terrence Dunn S, Jankelow D, Duran CM, Cunningham MW. Pathogenic mechanisms in rheumatic carditis: focus on valvular endothelium. *J Infect Dis.* 2001;183:507-511.

20. Bessen DE, Carapetis JR, Beall B, et al. Contrasting molecular epidemiology of group A streptococci causing tropical and nontropical infections of the skin and throat. *J Infect Dis.* 2000;182:1109-1116.

21. Berdeli A, Celik HA, Ozyurek R, Aydin HH. Involvement of immunoglobulin FcgammaRIIA and FcgammaRIIIB gene polymorphisms in susceptibility to rheumatic fever. *Clin Biochem.* 2004;37:925-929.

22. Chou HT, Chen CH, Tsai CH, Tsai FJ. Association between transforming growth factor-beta1 gene C-509T and T869C polymorphisms and rheumatic heart disease. *Am Heart J.* 2004;148:181-186.

23. Schafranski MD, Stier A, Nisihara R, Messias-Reason IJ. Significantly increased levels of mannose-binding lectin (MBL) in rheumatic heart disease: a beneficial role for MBL deficiency. *Clin Exp Immunol.* 2004;138:521-525.

24. Muhamed B, Shaboodien G, Engel ME. Genetic variants in rheumatic fever and rheumatic heart disease. *Am J Med Genet C Semin Med Genet.* 2020;184(1):159-177.

25. Khanna AK, Buskirk DR, Williams RC Jr, et al. Presence of a non-HLA B cell antigen in rheumatic fever patients and their families as defined by a monoclonal antibody. *J Clin Invest.* 1989;83:1710-1716.

26. Walker KG, Cooper M, McCabe K, et al. Markers of susceptibility to acute rheumatic fever: the B-cell antigen D8/17 is not robust as a marker in South Africa. *Cardiol Young* 2011;21(3):328-33.

27. Tandon R, Sharma M, Chandrashekhar Y, Kotb M, Yacoub MH, Narula J. Revisiting the pathogenesis of rheumatic fever and carditis. *Nat Rev Cardiol.* 2013;10:171-177.

28. Dinkla K, Nitsche-Schmitz DP, Barroso V, et al. Identification of a streptococcal octapeptide motif involved in acute rheumatic fever. *J Biol Chem.* 2007;282:18686-18693.

29. Dinkla K, Rohde M, Jansen WT, Carapetis JR, Chhatwal GS, Talay SR. *Streptococcus pyogenes* recruits collagen via surface-bound fibronectin: a novel colonization and immune evasion mechanism. *Mol Microbiol.* 2003;47:861-869.

30. Pedchenko V, Bondar O, Fogo AB, et al. Molecular architecture of the Goodpasture autoantigen in anti-GBM nephritis. *N Engl J Med.* 2010;363:343-354.

31. Hudson BG, Tryggvason K, Sundaramoorthy M, Neilson EG. Alport's syndrome, Goodpasture's syndrome, and type IV collagen. *N Engl J Med.* 2003;348:2543-2556.

32. Dinkla K, Talay SR, Morgelin M, et al. Crucial role of the CB3-region of collagen IV in PARF-induced acute rheumatic fever. *PLoS One.* 2009;4:e4666.

33. Vasan RS, Shrivastava S, Vijayakumar M, Narang R, Lister BC, Narula J. Echocardiographic evaluation of patients with acute rheumatic fever and rheumatic carditis. *Circulation.* 1996;94:73-82.

34. Nitsche DP, Johansson HM, Frick IM, Morgelin M. Streptococcal protein FOG, a novel matrix adhesin interacting with collagen I in vivo. *J Biol Chem.* 2006;281:1670-1679.

35. Butcher JT, Simmons CA, Warnock JN. Mechanobiology of the aortic heart valve. *J Heart Valve Dis.* 2008;17:62-73.

36. Jones TD. The diagnosis of rheumatic fever. *J Am Med Assoc.* 1944;126:481-484.

37. Committee of Rheumatic Fever and Bacterial Endocarditis of the American Heart Association. Jones criteria (revised) for guidance in the diagnosis of rheumatic fever. *Circulation.* 1984;69:204A-208A.

38. Guidelines for the diagnosis of rheumatic fever. Jones Criteria, 1992 update. Special Writing Group of the Committee on Rheumatic Fever, Endocarditis, and Kawasaki Disease of the Council on Cardiovascular Disease in the Young of the American Heart Association. *JAMA.* 1992;268:2069-2073.

39. Special Writing Group of the Committee on Rheumatic Fever, Endocarditis, and Kawasaki Disease of the Council on Cardiovascular Disease in the Young of the American Heart Association. Guidelines for the diagnosis of rheumatic fever: Jones Criteria, 1992 update. *JAMA.* 1992;268:2069-2073.

40. Rutstein DD. Report of the committee on standards and criteria for programs of care of the council of rheumatic fever and congenital heart disease of the American Heart Association: Jones criteria (modified) for guidance in the diagnosis of rheumatic fever. *Circulation.* 1956;13:617-620.

41. Stollerman GH, Markowitz M, Taranta A, Wannamaker LW, Whittemore R. Committee report: Jones criteria (revised) for guidance in the diagnosis of rheumatic fever. *Circulation.* 1965;32:664-668.

42. World Health Organization. *Rheumatic Fever and Rheumatic Heart Disease. Report of a WHO Expert Consultation.* Geneva, Switzerland: World Health Organization; 2004.

43. Wilson N. Echocardiography and subclinical carditis: guidelines that increase sensitivity for acute rheumatic fever. *Cardiol Young.* 2008;18:565-568.

44. RHDAustralia (ARF/RHD Writing Group) National Heart Foundation of Australia and the Cardiac Society of Australia and New Zealand. *The Australian Guideline for Prevention, Diagnosis and Management of Acute Rheumatic Fever and Rheumatic Heart Disease.* 2nd ed. Casuarina, Australia: RHDAustralia; 2012.

45. Gewitz MH, Baltimore RS, Tani LY, et al. Revision of the Jones criteria for the diagnosis of acute rheumatic fever in the era of Doppler echocardiography: a scientific statement from the American Heart Association. *Circulation.* 2015;131:1806-1818.

46. Gibbons RJ, Smith S, Antman E. American College of Cardiology/American Heart Association clinical practice guidelines: part I: where do they come from? *Circulation.* 2003;107:2979-2986.

47. Taranta A, Stollerman GH. The relationship of Sydenham's chorea to infection with group A streptococci. *Am J Med.* 1956;20:170-175.

48. Veasy LG, Tani LY, Hill HR. Persistence of acute rheumatic fever in the intermountain area of the United States. *J Pediatr.* 1994;124:9-16.

49. Veasy LG, Wiedmeier SE, Orsmond GS, et al. Resurgence of acute rheumatic fever in the intermountain area of the United States. *N Engl J Med.* 1987;316:421-427.

50. Vijayalakshmi I, Vishnuprabhu RO, Chitra N. The efficacy of echocardiographic criterions for the diagnosis of carditis in acute rheumatic fever. *Cardiol Young.* 2008;18:586-592.

51. Cheng TO. Should the Carey Coombs murmur be called the Richard Caton murmur? *Int J Cardiol.* 2007;120:268.

52. Narula J, Kaplan EL. Echocardiographic diagnosis of rheumatic fever. *Lancet.* 2001;358:2000.

53. Abernethy M, Bass N, Sharpe N, et al. Doppler echocardiography and the early diagnosis of carditis in acute rheumatic fever. *Aust N Z J Med.* 1994;24:530-535.

54. Figueroa FE, Fernandez MS, Valdes P, et al. Prospective comparison of clinical and echocardiographic diagnosis of rheumatic carditis: long term follow up of patients with subclinical disease. *Heart.* 2001;85:407-410.

55. Minich L, Tani LY, Pagotto LT. Doppler echocardiography distinguishes between physiologic and pathologic "silent" mitral regurgitation in patients with rheumatic fever. *Clin Cardiol.* 1997;20:924-926.

56. Beaton A, Carapetis J. The 2015 revision of the Jones Criteria for diagnosis of acute rheumatic fever: implications for practice in low-income and middle-income countries. *Heat Asia.* 2015;7:7-11.

57. Licciardi F, Scaioli G, Mulatero R, et al. Epidemiologic impact of the new guidelines for the diagnosis of acute rheumatic fever. *J Pediatr.* 2018;198:25-28.e1.

58. Guler M, Laloglu F, Ceviz N. Changes in valvular regurgitation in mid-term follow-up of children with first attack acute rheumatic fever: first evaluation after the updated Jones criteria. *Cardiol Young.* 2020;30(3):369-371.

59. Cilliers A, Manyemba J, Adler AJ, Saloojee H. Anti-inflammatory treatment for carditis in acute rheumatic fever. *Cochrane Database Syst Rev.* 2012;6:CD003176.

60. Carapetis J, Brown A, Walsh W, Noonan S. *Australian Guideline for Prevention, Diagnosis and Management of Acute Rheumatic Fever and Rheumatic Heart Disease.* 2nd ed. Casuarina, Australia: RHDAustralia; 2012.

61. Cilliers AM. Rheumatic fever and its management. *Br Med J.* 2006;333: 1153-1156A.

62. Wannamaker LW, Ayoub EM. Antibody titers in acute rheumatic fever. *Circulation.* 1960;21:598-614.

63. Zuhlke L, Engel ME, Karthikeyan G, et al. Characteristics, complications, and gaps in evidence-based interventions in rheumatic heart disease: the Global Rheumatic Heart Disease Registry (the REMEDY study). *Eur Heart J.* 2015;36:1115-1122.

64. Sliwa K, Carrington M, Mayosi BM, Zigiriadis E, Mvungi R, Stewart S. Incidence and characteristics of newly diagnosed rheumatic heart disease in urban African adults: insights from the heart of Soweto study. *Eur Heart J.* 2010;31:719-727.

65. Tibazarwa KB, Volmink JA, Mayosi BM. Incidence of acute rheumatic fever in the world: a systematic review of population-based studies. *Heart.* 2008;94:1534-1540.

66. Engel ME, Haileamlak A, Zühlke L, et al. Prevalence of rheumatic heart disease in 4720 asymptomatic scholars from South Africa and Ethiopia. *Heart.* 2015;101(17):1389-1394.

67. Roberts K, Maguire G, Brown A, et al. Echocardiographic screening for rheumatic heart disease in high and low risk Australian children. *Circulation.* 2014;129:1953-1961.

68. Lanna CC, Tonelli E, Barros MV, Goulart EM, Mota CC. Subclinical rheumatic valvitis: a long-term follow-up. *Cardiol Young.* 2003;13:431-438.

69. Vijayalakshmi IB, Mithravinda J, Deva AN. The role of echocardiography in diagnosing carditis in the setting of acute rheumatic fever. *Cardiol Young.* 2005;15:583-588.

70. Tubridy-Clark M, Carapetis JR. Subclinical carditis in rheumatic fever: a systematic review. *Int J Cardiol.* 2007;119:54-58.

71. Beg A, Sadiq M. Subclinical valvulitis in children with acute rheumatic Fever. *Pediatr Cardiol.* 2008;29:619-623.

72. Harlan GA, Tani LY, Byington CL. Rheumatic fever presenting as monoarticular arthritis. *Pediatr Infect Dis J.* 2006;25:743-746.

73. Mataika R, Carapetis JR, Kado J, Steer AC. Acute rheumatic fever: an important differential diagnosis of septic arthritis. *J Trop Pediatr.* 2008;54:205-207.

74. National Heart Foundation of New Zealand, Cardiac Society of Australia and New Zealand. *Evidence-Based, Best Practice New Zealand Guidelines for Rheumatic Fever 1. Diagnosis, Management and Secondary Prevention.* Auckland, New Zealand: National Heart Foundation of New Zealand; 2006.

75. National Heart Foundation of Australia (RF/RHD Guideline Development Working Group), Cardiac Society of Australia and New Zealand. *Diagnosis and Management of Acute Rheumatic Fever and Rheumatic Heart Disease in Australia: An Evidence-Based Review.* Casuarina, Australia: RHDAustralia; 2006.

76. Cilliers A, Adler AJ, Saloojee H. Anti-inflammatory treatment for carditis in acute rheumatic fever. *Cochrane Database Syst Rev.* 2015;5:CD003176.

77. Dean SL, Singer HS. Treatment of Sydenham's chorea: a review of the current evidence. *Tremor Other Hyperkinet Mov (N Y).* 2017;7:456.

78. Zühlke L, Engel ME, Karthikeyan G, et al. Characteristics, complications, and gaps in evidence-based interventions in rheumatic heart disease: the Global Rheumatic Heart Disease Registry (the REMEDY study). *Eur Heart J.* 2015;36(18):1115-1122a.

79. Chang AY, Nabbaale J, Nalubwama H, et al. Motivations of women in Uganda living with rheumatic heart disease: A mixed methods study of experiences in stigma, childbearing, anticoagulation, and contraception. *PLoS One.* 2018;13(3):e0194030.

80. Chang AY, Nabbaale J, Okello E, et al. Outcomes and care quality metrics for women of reproductive age living with rheumatic heart disease in Uganda. *J Am Heart Assoc.* 2020;9(8):e015562.

81. Essop MR, Peters F. Contemporary issues in rheumatic fever and chronic rheumatic heart disease. *Circulation.* 2014;130:2181-2188.

82. Nishimura RA, Otto CM, Bonow RO, et al. 2014 AHA/ACC Guideline for the management of patients with valvular heart disease: a report of the American College of Cardiology/American Heart Association Task Force on Practice Guidelines. *Circulation.* 2014;130(13):e120.

83. Robertson KA, Volmink JA, Mayosi BM. Antibiotics for the primary prevention of rheumatic fever: a meta-analysis. *BMC Cardiovasc Disord.* 2005;5:11.

84. Karthikeyan G, Mayosi BM. Is primary prevention of rheumatic fever the missing link in the control of rheumatic heart disease in Africa? *Circulation.* 2009;120:709-713.

85. Kerdemelidis M, Lennon DR, Arroll B, Peat B, Jarman J. The primary prevention of rheumatic fever. *J Paediatr Child Health.* 2010;46:534-548.

86. Carapetis J, Steer A. Prevention of rheumatic fever. *Pediatr Infect Dis J.* 2010;29:91-92; author reply 92.

87. Manyemba J, Mayosi BM. Intramuscular penicillin is more effective than oral penicillin in secondary prevention of rheumatic fever—a systematic review. *S Afr Med J.* 2003;93:212-218.

88. WHO Expert Consultation on Rheumatic Fever and Rheumatic Heart Disease. *Rheumatic Fever and Rheumatic Heart Disease: Report of a WHO Expert Consultation, Geneva, 29 October–1 November 2001. WHO Technical Report Series; 923.* Geneva, Switzerland: World Health Organization; 2004.

89. Cilliers A, Manyemba J, Adler AJ, Saloojee H. Anti-inflammatory treatment for carditis in acute rheumatic fever. *Cochrane Database Syst Rev.* 2012;6:CD003176.

90. Pastural E, McNeil SA, MacKinnon-Cameron D, et al. Safety and immunogenicity of a 30-valent M protein-based group a streptococcal vaccine in healthy adult volunteers: A randomized, controlled phase I study. *Vaccine* 2020;38(6):1384-1392.

91. Tani LY, Veasy LG, Minich LL, Shaddy RE. Rheumatic fever in children under 5 years. *Pediatrics.* 2004;114:906.

92. Williams RV, Minich LL, Shaddy RE, Veasy LG, Tani LY. Evidence for lack of myocardial injury in children with acute rheumatic carditis. *Cardiol Young.* 2002;12:519-523.

28

Aortic Stenosis

Marie-Annick Clavel, Marc R. Dweck, Martin Leon, and Philippe Pibarot

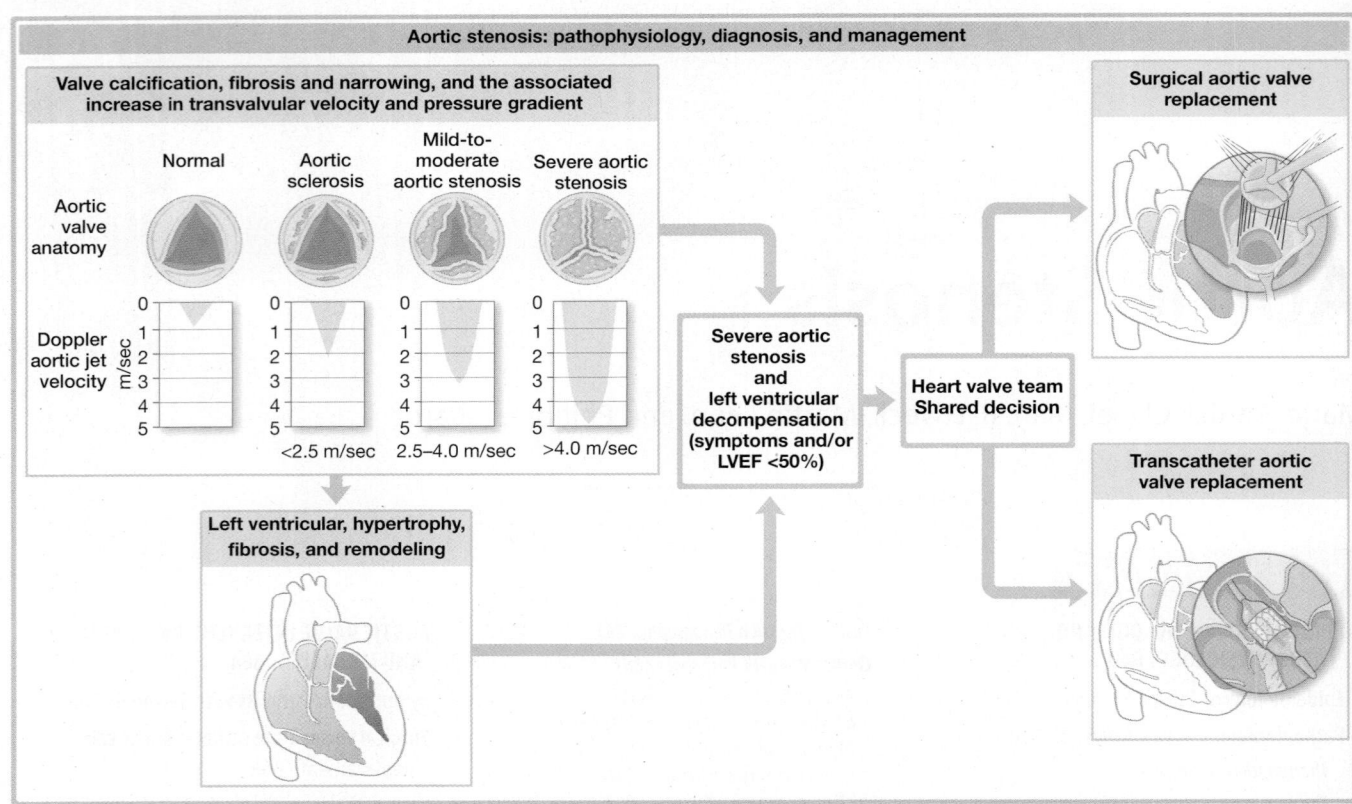

Chapter 28 Fuster and Hurst's Central Illustration. The natural history of aortic stenosis is characterized by a long latent period, during which the stenosis progresses in stages from mild, to moderate, to severe. The patient usually remains asymptomatic in the early stages; however, when cardiac symptoms develop in a patient with severe aortic stenosis, the prognosis in the absence of treatment is extremely poor. The increased afterload imposed by aortic stenosis on the left ventricle triggers a hypertrophic response that restores wall stress and maintains systolic performance for many years, but ultimately this process decompensates and patients transition from hypertrophy to heart failure. Patients with severe aortic stenosis and left ventricular decompensation (symptoms or left ventricular systolic dysfunction) should be considered for aortic valve replacement. Management decisions should involve patients, referring physicians, and a multidisciplinary heart team.

CHAPTER SUMMARY

This chapter discusses the epidemiology, pathophysiology, diagnosis, and management of calcific aortic valve stenosis (AS), a progressive fibro-calcific remodeling of the aortic valve leaflets that eventually impairs leaflet mobility and significantly obstructs blood flow. In high-income countries, AS is the third-most-frequent cardiovascular disease, with a prevalence of up to 5% in those aged >65 years. The first suspicion of AS is often raised by auscultation of a systolic murmur. Confirmation and evaluation of the disease are based on Doppler-echocardiography but may require an additional imaging modality in association with blood biomarkers. In addition to assessing the valve lesion and dysfunction, evaluating the AS-associated damage to the left ventricle and other cardiac chambers is essential to optimize risk stratification and therapeutic decision-making. Routine clinical and Doppler-echocardiography follow-up should be performed every 1–2 years to detect changes in AS severity, left ventricular systolic function, and/or the patient's symptomatic status. No pharmacological approach has yet proven effective to slow the progression of AS. Patients with severe AS and symptoms or left ventricular systolic dysfunction should be considered for aortic valve replacement (see Fuster and Hurst's Central Illustration). The decision to intervene and the choice of surgical versus transcatheter intervention should involve patients, referring physicians, and a multidisciplinary heart team.

Calcific aortic valve disease is a slowly progressive disease that starts with mild fibrosis, calcification and thickening of the valve leaflets without obstruction of blood flow, ie. aortic sclerosis.[1] This disease then evolves over the years to severe calcification with impaired leaflet mobility and significant obstruction to blood flow, ie. aortic stenosis (AS). Doppler-echocardiography is the method of choice for the diagnosis and follow-up of AS and multi-modality imaging provides incremental value for the risk stratification and management of the disease. The natural history of AS is characterized by a long latent period during which, the stenosis progresses in stages from mild, to moderate, to severe, and the patient usually remains asymptomatic in the early stages. However, once cardiac symptoms develop in a patient with severe AS, the prognosis in the absence of treatment is extremely poor with 40% to 50% all-cause mortality at 2 years.[1] There are currently no validated pharmacotherapies that can halt or delay the progression of AS or its resulting adverse effects on cardiac function and patient outcomes. Hence, aortic valve replacement (AVR) currently is the sole effective option for the treatment of severe AS. In the past 15 years, transcatheter AVR (TAVR) has emerged as an alternative to surgical AVR (SAVR) in appropriately selected patients.

EPIDEMIOLOGY, ETIOLOGY, AND PATHOPHYSIOLOGY

Calcific aortic valve disease is, by far, the most prevalent form of AS in high income countries. In low-income countries, AS may also be caused by rheumatic heart disease (**Fig. 28–1**). In this section, we will review the pathophysiology and epidemiology of calcific AS.

Epidemiology of Calcific AS

Calcific AS is the third most common cardiovascular disease and the most common valvular heart disease.[2] Its prevalence

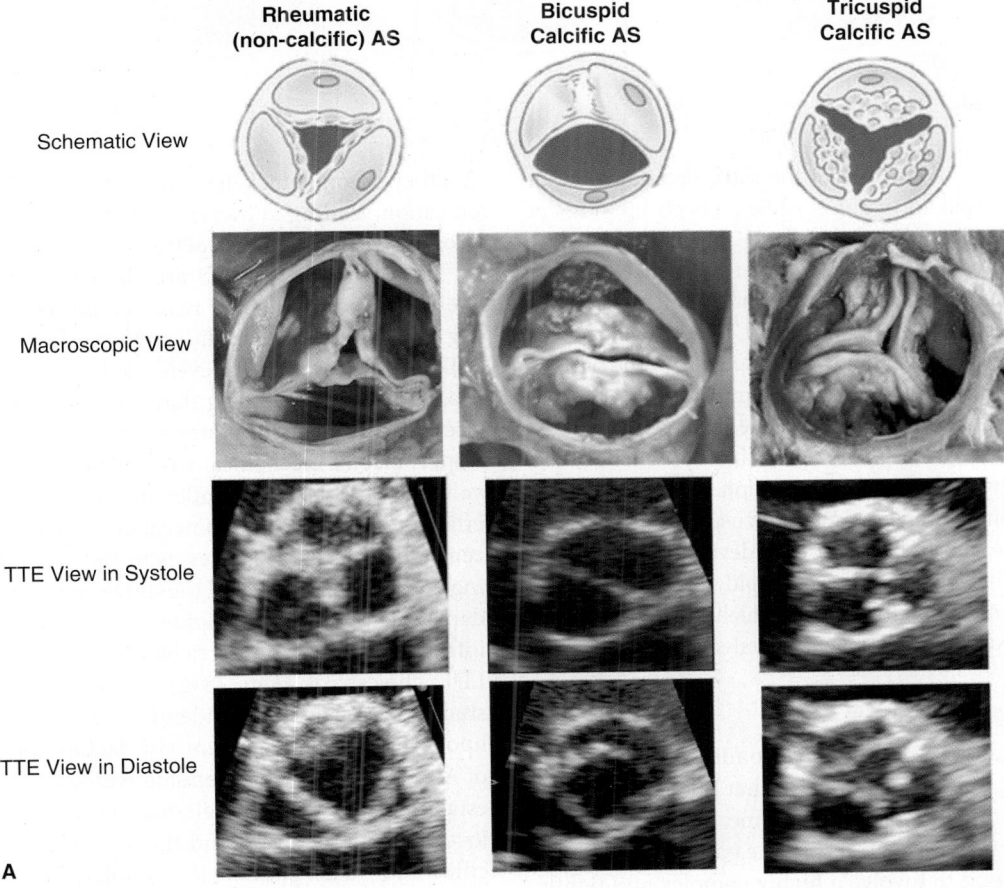

Figure 28–1. Etiologies of Aortic Stenosis. (A) Schematic, macroscopic, and transthoracic echocardiographic views of the 3 main etiologies of AS: rheumatic, non-calcific AS, bicuspid calcific AS, and tricuspid calcific AS. **(B)** Schematic of bicuspid aortic valve phenotypes as seen by transthoracic echocardiogram. The standard imaging technique for BAV diagnosis is transthoracic echocardiogram. The diagnosis is based on parasternal long- and short-axis imaging of the aortic valve. The schematics presented represent the parasternal short-axis echocardiographic view. Bicuspid valves are classified as type 1 (right-left coronary cusp fusion), type 2 (right-noncoronary cusp fusion), and type 3 (left-noncoronary cusp fusion). The figure demonstrates BAV phenotypes. **Top left** shows a type 1 BAV (commissures at 10 and 5 o'clock) with complete raphe, asymmetrical (the nonfused cusp [noncoronary] is smaller than the conjoined anterior cusp). **Top middle** shows a type 2 BAV (commissures at 1 and 7 o'clock) with complete raphe and asymmetrical (the nonfused cusp [left] is larger than the conjoined cusp). **Top right** shows a type 3 BAV (shown with commissures at 2 and 8 o'clock, but could be 1 and 7 o'clock) with complete raphe, asymmetrical (the nonfused cusp [right] is larger than the conjoined one). **Bottom left** shows a symmetrical type 1 BAV with complete raphe. **Bottom middle** shows a symmetrical type 1 BAV without raphe (true BAV). **Bottom right** shows a type 1 BAV with incomplete raphe, partially fused. BAV indicates bicuspid aortic valve; L, left cusp; N, noncoronary cusp; and R, right cusp. Panel B, reproduced with permission from Michelena HI, Prakash SK, Della Corte A, et al. Bicuspid aortic valve: identifying knowledge gaps and rising to the challenge from the International Bicuspid Aortic Valve Consortium (BAVCon). *Circulation*. 2014 Jun 24;129(25):2691-2704.

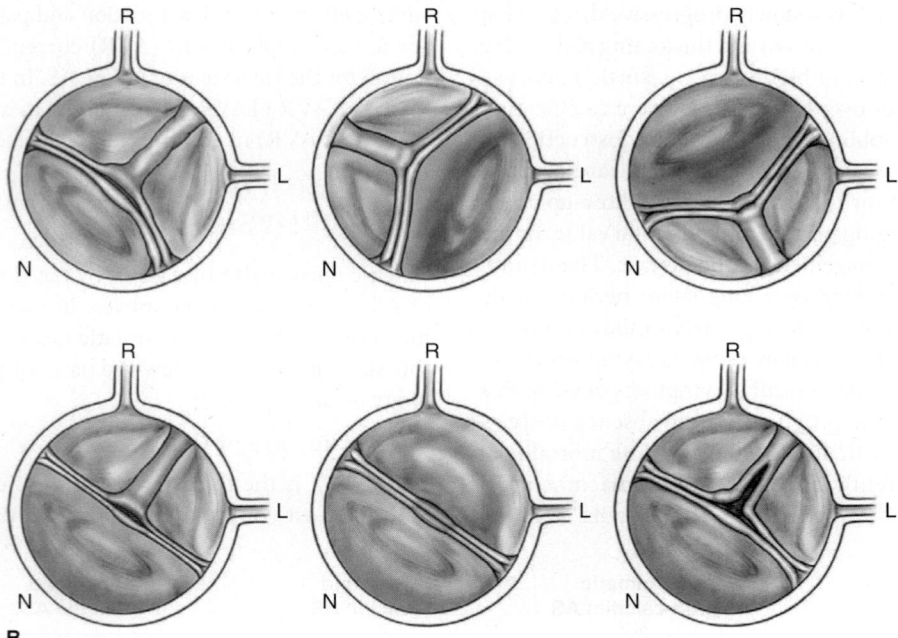

Figure 28–1. (Continued)

increase with age; AS is rare before the sixth decade of life in patients with a tricuspid aortic valve, while it affects up to 5% of the population older than 65 years and 10% in those older than 80 years.[3] Due to aging of the population, the prevalence of severe AS and thus the number of aortic valve interventions, are projected to double by 2050.[4] Without treatment, the estimated 5-year survival with severe symptomatic AS is between 15 % and 50%.[5]

Bicuspid aortic valves are the most common congenital heart defect, with a prevalence of 1%–2% in the general population (Fig. 28–1).[6] There are several phenotypes of bicuspid aortic valves depending on the type of cusp fusion and raphe (Fig. 28–1). During their lifetime, most individuals with bicuspid valves develop aortic valve disease, mostly AS, and they develop stenosis 1 or 2 decades earlier than those with a tricuspid valve. AS is more often diagnosed in men than in women[2], which may be explained by the 3:1 male predominance of bicuspid valve disease.

Pathophysiology of Calcific AS

AS was long considered a degenerative condition, the inevitable result of "wear and tear" in a valve that opens and closes many billions of times in a patient's lifetime. Whilst mechanical stress and injury play a central role, the pathophysiology of AS is now understood to involve a highly complex and tightly regulated series of processes each of which may be amenable to medical intervention (**Fig. 28–2**). Valvular pathology in AS can be divided in to two distinct phases: an early initiation phase and a later propagation phase[7], but it is also important to consider the pathophysiological responses of the myocardium to valve narrowing.

The initiation phase

In healthy individuals, the three aortic valve leaflets are smooth, flexible, and mobile structures less than 1 mm in thickness, in AS, they become thickened, due to progressive fibrosis and calcification, leading to increased stiffness, reduced mobility and progressive valvular obstruction.[7]

The early stages of AS are similar to atherosclerosis and the two conditions share many common risk factors including smoking, age, metabolic syndrome, low-density lipoprotein (LDL) cholesterol, Lp(a) levels and hypertension.[8–10] As in atherosclerosis, the initiating injury is believed to be mechanical stress and subsequent injury to endothelium (Fig. 28–2). The importance of mechanical stress is best illustrated in bicuspid valve disease. The two-leaflet structure of these valves is less efficient in dissipating biomechanical forces to the aorta, concentrating mechanical stresses in the valve thereby accelerating endothelial injury and the development of AS. Endothelial damage allows the same lipids implicated in atherosclerosis to infiltrate the valve: in particular lipoprotein (a) and oxidized LDL cholesterol (Fig. 28–2).[11] Consequently observational studies have consistently identified cholesterol and its related lipoproteins as independent risk factors for the development of AS.[12] Indeed, a strong genome-wide association was recently established between a single nucleotide polymorphism in the locus of lipoprotein (a) and the incidence of aortic valve calcification.[13] The pathological similarities between the early stages of atherosclerosis and AS led to the hypothesis that statins might be beneficial treatment for AS. However statins have failed to halt or slow AS progression in three randomized controlled trials[14–16], leading investigators to re-examine the underlying pathophysiology AS and to the realization that whilst inflammation and lipid deposition may be important in establishing the disease (the initiation phase), the latter stages are instead characterized by an apparently self-perpetuating cycle of calcium formation, fibrosis, and valvular injury (the propagation phase).[7]

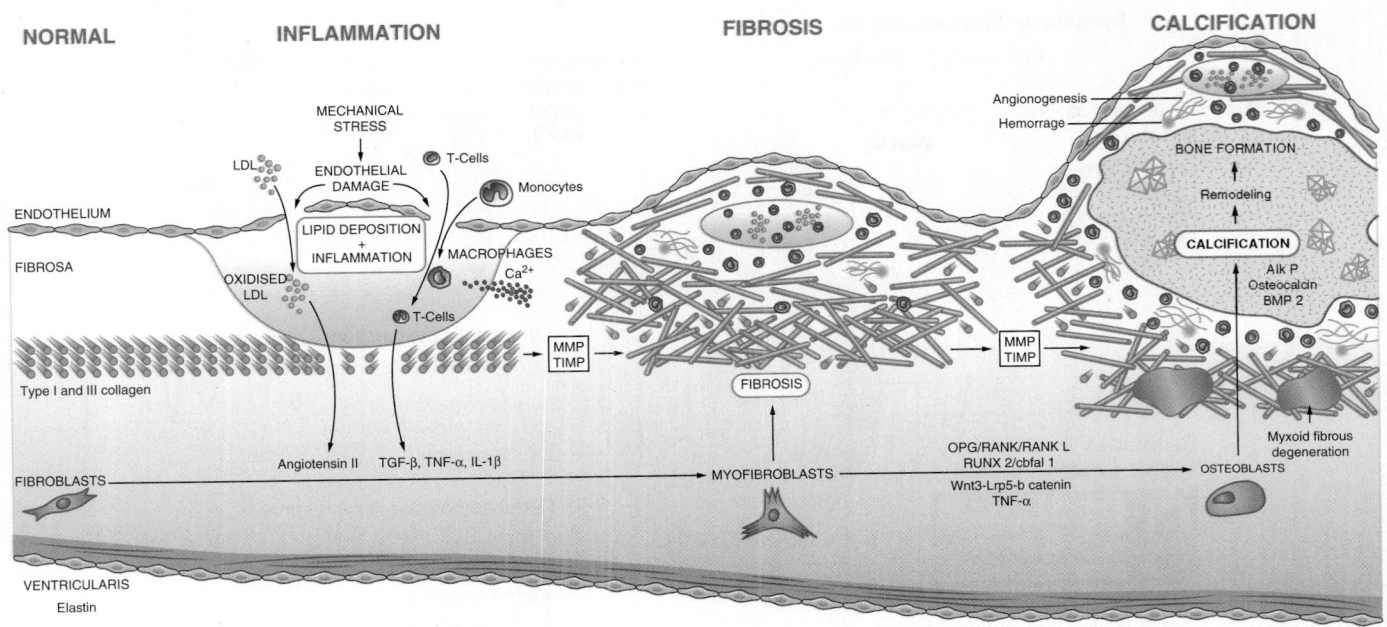

Figure 28–2. Pathological processes occurring within the valve in aortic stenosis. Mechanical stress results in endothelial damage that allows infiltration of lipid and inflammatory cells into the valve. Lipid oxidization further increases inflammatory activity within these lesions and the secretion of proinflammatory and profibrotic cytokines. The latter drives the differentiation of fibroblasts into myofibroblasts that secrete increased collagen under the influence of angiotensin. In combination with the action of matrix metalloproteinases (MMPs) and tissue inhibitors of metalloproteinases (TIMPs), disorganized fibrous tissue accumulates within the valve. This leads to thickening and increased stiffness of the valve and in the latter stages the development of myxoid fibrous degeneration. Microcalcification begins early in the disease, driven by microvesicle secretion by macrophages. However, calcification accelerates in a proportion of patients because of the differentiation of myofibroblasts into osteoblasts. This occurs under the influence of several procalcific pathways, including osteoprotegerin (OPG)/receptor activator of nuclear factor kappa B (RANK)/RANK ligand (RANKL), Runx 2-cbfal 2, Wnt3-Lrp5-b catenin, and tumor necrosis factor (TNF)-α. Osteoblasts subsequently coordinate calcification of the valve as part of a highly regulated process akin to skeletal bone formation, with expression of many of the same mediators, such as osteocalcin, alkaline phosphatase (Alk P), and bone morphogenic protein (BMP)-2. With time, maturation of valvular calcification occurs so that by the end stages of the disease, lamellar bone, microfractures, and hemopoeitic tissue can all be observed within the valve. These pathogenic processes are sustained by angioneogenesis, with new vessels localizing, in particular, to regions of inflammation surrounding calcific deposits. Hemorrhage in relation to these vessels has also been demonstrated in severe disease and may have a role in accelerating disease progression. IL-1β, interleukin-1βbeta; LDL, low-density lipoprotein; TGF, transforming growth factor. Reproduced with permission from Dweck MR, Boon NA, Newby DE. Calcific aortic stenosis: a disease of the valve and the myocardium. *J Am Coll Cardiol.* 2012 Nov 6;60(19):1854-1863.

The propagation phase

Whilst atherosclerotic risk factors predict the incidence of AS, they do not predict disease progression, pointing to different pathological processes governing this stage of the disease and in particular the importance of calcification and fibrosis (Fig. 28-2). Skeletal bone formation is characterized by collagen deposition, that provides a scaffold upon which progressive calcification can develop. Similar structural processes are believed to occur in the aortic valve with fibrosis and calcification progressing in tandem and many of the same cell mediators and proteins implicated (Fig. 28-2).[17,18]

In the majority of patients with AS, calcification is the dominant pathological process in the valve. Valve calcification is coordinated by osteoblast type cells using an array of proteins more commonly associated with skeletal bone formation (Fig. 28-2). A key step in the transition from the initiation phase to the propagation phase is the differentiation of osteoblastic cells within the valve. These appear to play a key role in driving disease progression, helping to establish a vicious cycle, whereby calcium begets more calcium in a positive feedback loop. This cycle may be explained by calcium increasing mechanical stresses within the valve, thereby inducing further leaflet injury and calcification. Regardless of the mechanism, the most consistent predictors of AS progression are baseline assessments of valve calcification.[19,20] Calcium is therefore a key target for future therapeutic intervention, although it is worth noting that there are important sex differences in the balance between pro-fibrotic and pro-calcific processes occurring in the valve with women requiring relatively less calcium to develop severe AS than men.[21,22]

PATHOPHYSIOLOGY AND ITS RELATIONSHIP WITH LV HYPERTROPHY / DYSFUNCTION AND SYMPTOMS

The increased afterload imposed by AS on the left ventricle triggers a hypertrophic response, characterized by increased myocyte size left ventricular wall thickness and mass (**Fig. 28–3**), that restores wall stress and maintains systolic performance for many years if not decades. However, ultimately this process decompensates, and patients transition from hypertrophy to heart failure, driven by two key pathological processes: myocyte cell death and myocardial fibrosis (Fig. 28–3).[23] Myocyte cell death occurs in response to direct mechanical forces,

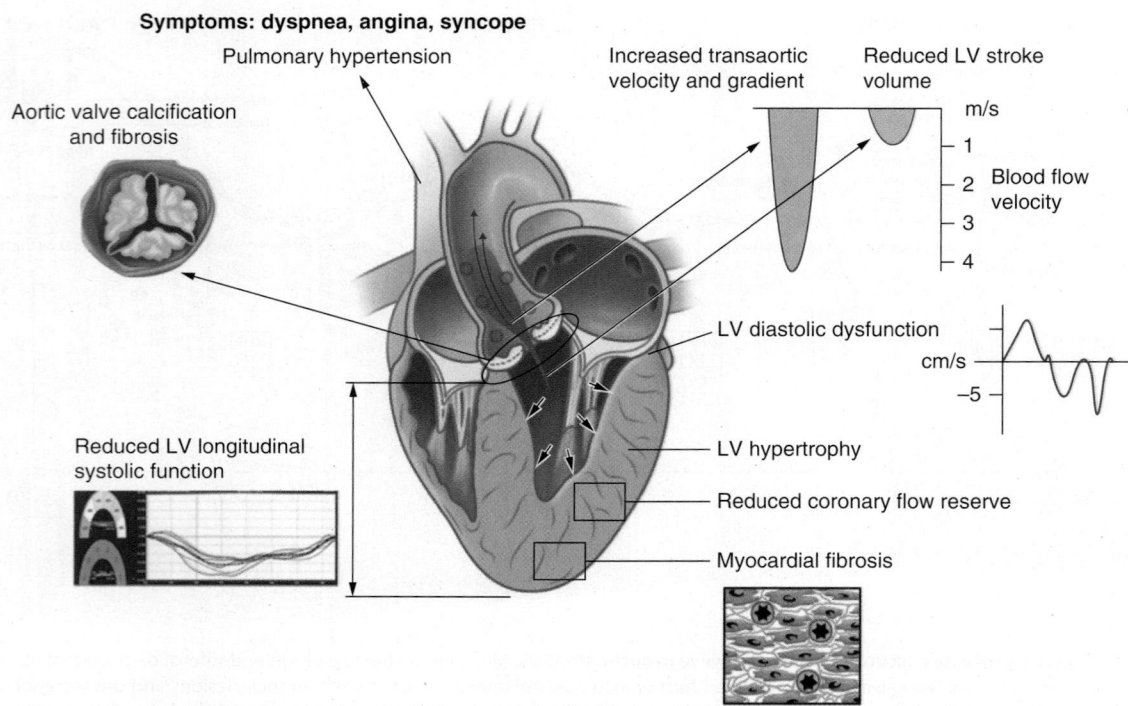

Figure 28–3. Doppler-echocardiographic parameters of AS hemodynamic severity. The narrowing of the aortic valve orifice causes an acceleration of the blood flow velocity with a concomitant decrease in systolic blood pressure between the left ventricular outflow tract (LVOT) and the aorta, and thus an increased transaortic pressure gradient. The increased left ventricular pressure imposed by AS results in left ventricular hypertrophy, reduced coronary flow reserve, myocardial fibrosis, diastolic dysfunction, decreased longitudinal systolic shortening and stroke volume, although the LV ejection fraction remains normal in most patients. Left atrial enlargement is common owing to elevated left ventricular filling pressures, which often lead to secondary pulmonary hypertension and right ventricular dysfunction in the more advanced stages of the disease. LV diastolic dysfunction, reduced coronary flow reserve, and reduced cardiac output may cause symptoms including dyspnea, angina, or syncope.

angiotensin II and myocardial ischemia, the latter reflecting a failure of the myocardial blood supply to increase with the degree of hypertrophy.[24] Consequently, this cell death triggers a healing response and the development of myocardial fibrosis, with similar underlying cellular processes to those regulating fibrosis in the valve leaflets.[23,25]

In AS, myocardial fibrosis exists in two forms: (i) Diffuse interstitial fibrosis, which is distributed evenly across the myocardium and is potentially reversible; and (ii) Replacement fibrosis, which is focal and generally irreversible. Recent imaging studies indicate that diffuse fibrosis begins earlier and replacement fibrosis later in the disease process,[26] although the two are frequently found in association[27]. Together both forms of fibrosis increase myocardial stiffness leading to impaired LV filling and diastolic dysfunction (Fig. 28–3). Moreover, in combination with the reduction in contractile myocytes, myocardial scarring leads to impaired LV systolic function. Hence, myocyte death and fibrosis are the main determinants of LV decompensation in patients with AS and of the occurrence of symptoms, pulmonary hypertension, adverse clinical events, and the need for aortic valve replacement.

The pattern of the LV adaptive response to pressure overload in AS is highly heterogeneous and includes concentric remodeling, concentric hypertrophy and eccentric hypertrophy.[28,29] This pattern is influenced not only by AS severity but also by several other factors including age, sex, genetic factors,

metabolic factors and the coexistence of coronary artery disease or hypertension.

LV Diastolic and Systolic Dysfunction

LV diastolic dysfunction occurs early in the disease course and worsens with progression of stenosis severity and myocardial fibrosis (Fig. 28–3).[30] In the more advanced stages of the disease, increased LV filling pressures (ie, Grade 2 diastolic dysfunction) lead to dyspnea and in some cases pulmonary hypertension.[31] In end-stage disease, LV diastolic dysfunction may occasionally progress to Grade 3, that is, restrictive filling pattern, which is associated with higher risk of treatment futility with SAVR or TAVR.

The LV pressure overload caused by severe AS may lead to an afterload mismatch and thus to a reduction in myocardial contractility and LV ejection fraction (LVEF). This decline in LVEF generally occurs late in the course of the disease and is thus rare in asymptomatic patients with severe AS (~1%).[32] A decrease in LVEF may also be caused by myocardial fibrosis or other concomitant cardiovascular disease, such as coronary artery disease or hypertension, which frequently coexist with AS (Fig. 28–3). Regardless of its cause, reduced LVEF (<50%) is associated with worse outcomes and is a class I indication for AVR in patients with severe AS, regardless of the presence or absence of symptoms.[5,33]

LVEF frequently underestimates the degree of myocardial systolic dysfunction in the presence of LV concentric remodeling/hypertrophy. Hence, a considerable proportion of patients with AS may have subclinical LV systolic dysfunction despite preserved LVEF and absence of symptoms. Several studies have reported that patients with severe AS and an LVEF between 50% and 60% have worse outcomes and may benefit from earlier intervention.[34-36] These findings provide support to consider raising the LVEF threshold proposed in the guidelines to trigger AVR from 50% to 60%. Assessment of LV global longitudinal strain by speckle tracking echocardiography may also help to identify subclinical LV systolic dysfunction and eventually consider earlier AVR in asymptomatic patients with severe AS (Fig. 28–3). LV global longitudinal strain is indeed more sensitive than LVEF in detecting subclinical dysfunction in AS and a cut-point value of <15% has been proposed to identify patients at higher risk for worse outcomes.[37-41] Like LVEF, strain measurement can become impaired due to other pathological co-morbidities most notably coronary artery disease. The LV stroke volume indexed to body surface area is a good marker of the cardiac pump function and the presence of a low flow state (stroke volume index <35 mL/m^2), it is also a powerful predictor of clinical outcomes in patients with AS both prior to and after AVR.[42-44]

Symptoms: Angina, Heart failure, Syncope

Classic symptoms of severe AS include dyspnea and other symptoms of heart failure, angina, and syncope. An important clinical challenge is assessing whether these symptoms are attributable to AS or other co-morbidities. Dyspnea and consequent reduced exercise tolerance are by far, the most frequent symptoms in AS. Angina may also occur due to a mismatch between increased myocardial oxygen demand and reduced oxygen supply. In patients with severe AS, myocardial oxygen demand is increased because of LV pressure overload and hypertrophy and oxygen supply is reduced because of increased LV diastolic pressure, coronary microcirculation dysfunction and reduced coronary blood flow reserve.[45-48] Syncope is the least frequent symptom of AS and generally occurs during exercise because of cerebral hypoperfusion, which could be related to hypotension, arrhythmia and/or imbalance between cardiac output and peripheral resistance.[49,50] In patients with severe AS and an equivocal history or symptoms, exercise testing under careful supervision is recommended to confirm their symptomatic status.[33, 51]

DIAGNOSIS AND RISK STRATIFICATION

Physical Examination

Classic physical findings of AS are a harsh, crescendo-decrescendo systolic murmur, a soft second heart sound, and a delayed carotid upstroke or slow rising pulse (parvus tardus). The auscultation of a murmur at the time of routine physical exam is often the trigger to the first diagnosis of AS by Doppler-echocardiography. Most patients are diagnosed long before the onset of symptoms and are followed prospectively on a regular basis until AVR is indicated.[52] However, a large proportion of the population with AS are never diagnosed and left untreated, while others are identified only late in the course of the disease. The delayed recognition of severe symptomatic AS can result in poor clinical and surgical outcomes, progression to irreversible heart failure, reduced survival, and suboptimal response to AVR.[53,54]

Doppler-Echocardiography

Doppler-echocardiography is the primary modality for the diagnosis and follow-up of AS. In the vast majority of patients, referral to echocardiography is motivated by auscultation of a systolic murmur and/or the development of symptoms including dyspnea, angina, syncope, and dizziness. The visualization of a thickened aortic valve with restricted opening and increased peak aortic velocity/ transvalvular gradient confirms the diagnosis of AS. The purpose of the echocardiographic exam in a patient with a diagnosis of AS is two-fold: (i) grading the stenosis severity; and (ii) staging the extent of cardiac damage related to, or associated with AS.

Grading AS severity

Grading of AS severity (mild, moderate, severe, and very severe) is based on the assessment the anatomic (aortic valve leaflet morphology and mobility) and hemodynamic (peak aortic jet velocity, mean transvalvular gradient, aortic valve area [AVA]) severity of AS (**Table 28–1 and Fig. 28–4**). Severe AS is defined by a peak jet velocity ≥4 m/s, a mean gradient ≥40 mm Hg, and an AVA <1.0 cm^2 or <0.6cm^2/m^2 after indexing to body surface area.[5,55] To avoid underestimation of transvalvular velocity and gradient, and thus AS severity, the continuous-wave Doppler beam must be aligned with the direction of the transvalvular flow.[56] Hence, it is essential to perform multi window imaging including the apical windows but also and importantly the right parasternal window (Fig. 28–4). One limitation of peak aortic velocity and gradients is that they are highly flow-dependent and may thus underestimate AS severity in the presence of low-flow states.

The most widely used "less flow-dependent" measurements include AVA calculated from the continuity equation and the Doppler velocity index (Table 28–1 and Fig. 28–4). These parameters are not strictly flow-independent but they are much less flow dependent than peak jet velocity or mean gradient. However, these parameters, in particular AVA, are more subject to measurement errors. The most important source of error is the measurement of the LV outflow tract area (Fig. 28–4).[57,58] In patients with an ascending aorta diameter <30 mm, it is recommended to calculate the energy loss coefficient and energy loss index to account for the pressure recovery that occurs downstream of the aortic valve (Table 28–1 and **Fig. 28–5**). The consideration of these parameters may reclassify stenosis severity from severe based on AVA to non-severe in a substantial proportion of patient.[59,60]

Up to 40% of patients with severe AS may have discordant echocardiographic assessments of severity, most commonly an AVA <1.0 cm^2, consistent with severe AS and mean gradient <40 mm Hg (or peak jet velocity <4 m/s) consistent with non-severe AS. This subset of patients with "discordant grading" of

TABLE 28–1. Parameters and Criteria for Grading AS Severity

AS Severity Parameter	Imaging Modality	Formula/Method	Concept/Limitations	Mild AS Criteria	Moderate AS Criteria	Severe AS Criteria
Flow-Dependent Parameters			Highly flow dependent			
Peak Aortic Jet Velocity (m/s)	TTE	Direct measure	Velocity increases with AS stenosis severity	2.0–2.9	3.0–3.9	≥4 (≥5.5)*
Mean Transvalvular Gradient (mm Hg)	TTE	$\Delta P = 4 \times V_{AS}^2$	Pressure gradient calculated from velocity using the simplified Bernoulli formula	10–19	20–39	≥40 (≥60)*
Less Flow-Dependent Parameters						
Aortic Valve Area (cm²)	TTE	$AVA = [CSA_{LVOT} \times VTI_{LVOT}]/VTI_{AS}$	Effective AVA calculated by continuity equation/subject to measurement errors	1.51–2.0	1.01–1.50	≤1.0 (≤0.60)*
Aortic Valve Area Index (cm²/m²)	TTE	$AVAi = AVA/BSA$	Accounts for variability in body size by indexing for BSA/may overestimate AS severity in obese people	0.91–1.20	0.59–0.90	≤0.60 ≤0.50†
Doppler Velocity Index (Velocity Ratio)	TTE	$DVI = VTI_{LVOT}/VTI_{AS}$	Simplification of the continuity equation by eliminating $LVOT_{AREA}$ from the continuity equation/may not provide accurate estimation of AS severity in patients with small or large LVOT	≥0.35	0.26–0.35	≤0.25
Energy Loss Coefficient& (cm²)	TTE	$ELC = (AVA \times A_A)/(A_A - AVA)$	Accounts for pressure recovery by correcting the AVA for the size of the aorta/subject to measurement errors	1.51–2.0	1.01–1.50	≤1.0
Energy Loss Index& (cm²/m²)	TTE	$ELI = ELC/BSA$	Indexation of ELC for body size/may overestimate AS severity in obese people	0.91–1.20	0.59–0.90	≤0.60
Flow-Independent Parameters						
Projected aortic valve area at normal flow rate§ (cm²)	DSE	$AVA_{Proj} = AVA_{Rest} + [(AVA_{Peak} - AVA_{Rest})/(Q_{Peak} - Q_{Rest})] \times (250 - Q_{Rest})$	Estimates the AVA at normal flow rate using the AVA/Q linear regression equation/subject to measurement errors. Requires a minimum 15% increase in Q to be calculated	1.51–2.0	1.01–1.50	≤1.0
Aortic Valve calcification (AU)	Non-contrast MSCT	Direct measure	Quantitates valve calcification by counting areas of 4 adjacent pixels with density >130 Hounsfield units/ does not account valvular fibrosis	-		Women¶ ≥1200 Men ≥2000
Aortic Valve calcification density§ (AU)	Non-contrast MSCT	$AVCd = AVC/\text{Aortic annulus area}$	AVC score indexed to the cross-sectional aortic annulus area measured by echocardiography/ does not account valvular fibrosis. Subject to measurement errors			Women ≥300 Men ≥500

*Thresholds for the definition of very severe AS
†Cut-off used in setting of obesity (Body mass index <30 kg/m²).
¶95% specific thresholds are: 1700 AU women and 3400 AU in men and sensitive thresholds are 800 AU in women and 1700 AU in men
§Parameters that are not used in routine practice but that may provide incremental information for therapeutic management in some patients.
&Parameters with limited clinical use.
Abbreviations: A_A, cross-sectional area of the aorta measured 1 cm downstream of the sino-tubular junction; AS, aortic stenosis; AVA, aortic valve area; AVA_{Rest} AVA at rest; AVA_{Peak}, AVA at peak dobutamine stress; AVA_{Proj}, projected AVA at normal flow rate; AVC, aortic valve calcification; AVCd, AVC density; BSA, body surface area; CSA, cross-sectional area; ΔP, mean transaortic pressure gradient; DSE, dobutamine stress echocardiography; DVI, Doppler velocity index; ELC, energy loss coefficient; ELI, energy less index; LV, left ventricle; LVOT, LV outflow tract; MSCT, multi-slice computed tomography; Q, mean transvalvular flow rate (ie, stroke volume divided by LV ejection time); Q_{Rest}, Q at rest; Q_{Peak}, Q at peak dobutamine stress; SV, stroke volume; TTE, transthoracic echocardiography; V_{AS}, peak velocity of the AS jet; VTI_{AS}, velocity-time integral of the AS jet; VTI_{LVOT}, velocity-time integral in the LV outflow tract.

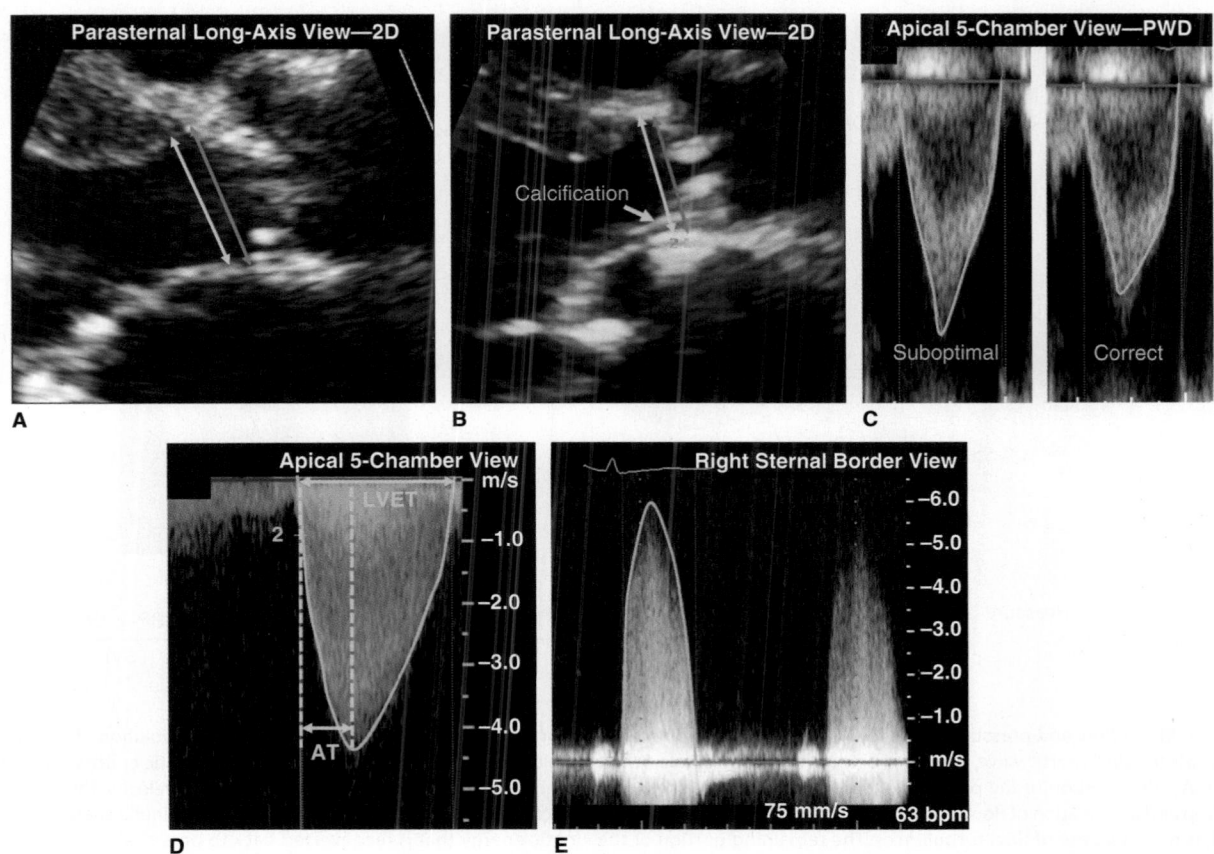

Figure 28–4. Doppler-echocardiographic parameters of AS hemodynamic severity. Aortic valve area (AVA) is calculated using the continuity equation, which is based on the concept of flow conservation: the stroke volume (SV) ejected through the left ventricular outflow tract (LVOT) is equal to SV ejected through the aortic valve orifice:

$$SV = CSA_{LVOT} \times VTI_{LVOT} = AVA \times VTI_{AS}$$

$$AVA = \frac{CSA_{LVOT} \times VTI_{LVOT}}{VTI_{AS}}$$

Where $LVOT_d$ is the diameter of LVOT.

This equation requires the measurement of three echocardiographic parameters: the LVOT velocity time integral (VTI_{LVOT}), the LVOT diameter ($LVOT_d$), and the aortic jet VTI (VTI_{AS}). $LVOT_d$ is a key measure to define AS severity (**Panels A and B**). It should be measured at the aortic annulus level (inner edges of leaflet insertion) from a parasternal long axis view zoomed on the aortic valve during the systolic phase, when the diameter is maximal (**Panel A**) and include LVOT calcification (**Panel B**). VTI_{LVOT} is measured using pulsed-wave Doppler modality from an apical approach, just proximal to the aortic valve, ideally at the same level as the $LVOT_d$ is measured (**Panel C**).

VTI_{AS}, as well as peak jet velocity and mean gradient of the antegrade systolic flow across the narrowed aortic valve are measured using continuous-wave Doppler ultrasound. The maximum velocity is measured at the outer edge of the dark signal, and the outer edge of the spectral Doppler envelope is traced to provide both the velocity-time integral for the continuity equation and mean gradient (using the simplified Bernoulli equation) (**Panel D**).

Velocity or VTI ratio is the ratio V_{Peak} or VTI between LVOT and AV levels. The normal value is 1, while in a severe AS the ratio is <0.25 (or 25%).

$$Velocity\ ratio = \frac{V_{LVOT}}{V_{AS}} \qquad VTI\ ratio = \frac{VTI_{LVOT}}{VTI_{AS}}$$

The analysis of the ejection dynamics transvalvular velocity using CWD may provide additional semi-quantitative parameters to better characterize AS severity. Acceleration time (AT) is the delay between the beginning and the maximal peak of the aortic ejection velocity and ejection time is the overall ejection duration (ET) (**Panel D**). It was demonstrated that an AT >110ms or an AT/ET >0.36 was associated with AS severity and outcomes. However, in low flow patients, these parameters could be increase in non-severe stenosis due to the lack of strength of the flow to open a stenosis that is only moderate.

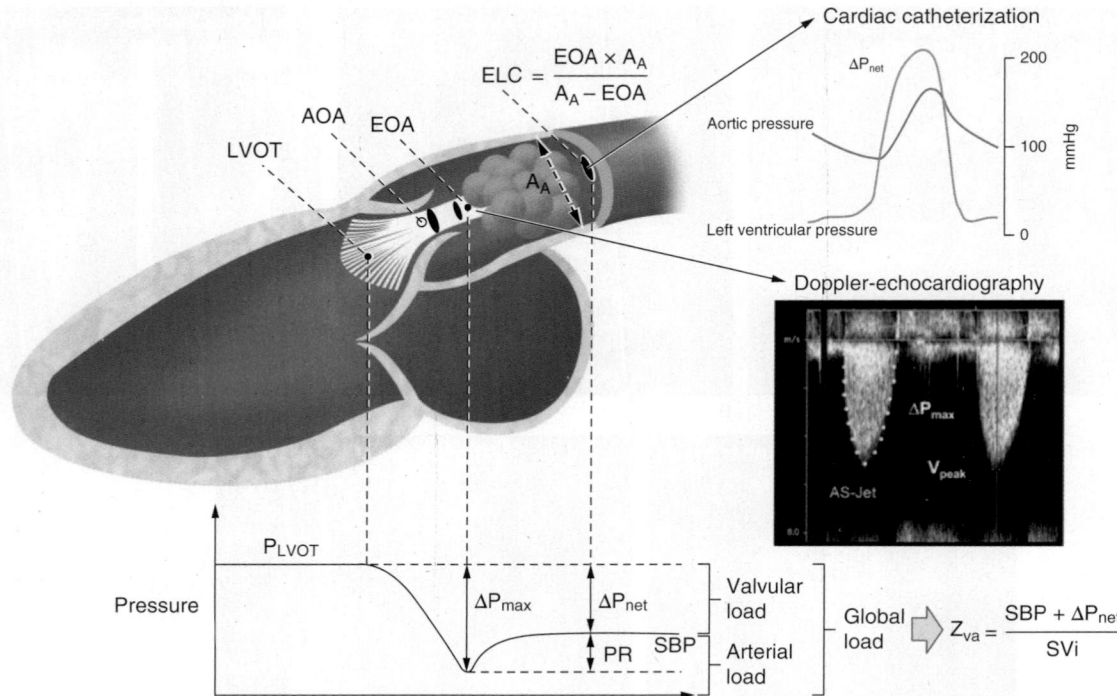

Figure 28–5. Blood flow and pressure across LVOT, aortic valve, and ascending aorta during systole. The figure shows the evolution of blood flow and pressure across the LVOT, aortic valve, and ascending aorta during systole. When the blood flow contracts to pass through a stenotic orifice (ie, the anatomic orifice area [AOA]), a portion of the potential energy of the blood, namely, pressure, is converted into kinetic energy, namely, velocity, thus resulting in a pressure drop and acceleration of flow. Downstream of the vena contracta (ie, the effective orifice area [EOA]), a large part of the kinetic energy is irreversibly dissipated as heat because of flow turbulences. The remaining portion of the kinetic energy that is reconverted back to potential energy is called the "pressure recovery" (PR). The magnitude of the PR is essentially determined by the ratio of the EOA to the size of the aorta. The energy loss coefficient (ELC; see **Table 28–1**) allows to correct the EOA measured by Doppler-echocardiography for the size of the aorta in order to account for PR. The ELC thus provides an estimate the EOA that would be obtained by cardiac catheterization using the Gorlin formula. The global hemodynamic load imposed on the left ventricle results from the summation of the valvular load and the arterial load. This global load can be estimated by calculating the valvulo-arterial impedance. In patients with medium or large size ascending aorta, the impedance can be calculated with the standard Doppler mean gradient in place of the net mean gradient. A_A: cross-sectional area of the aorta at the level of the sino-tubular junction; ELI: energy loss index; ΔP_{max}: maximum transvalvular pressure gradient recorded at the level of vena contracta (ie, mean gradient measured by Doppler); ΔP_{net}: net transvalvular pressure gradient recorded after pressure recovery (i.e., mean gradient measured by catheterization); LVOT: left ventricular outflow tract; P_{LVOT}: pressure in the LVOT; SBP: systolic blood pressure; SVi: stroke volume index; Vpeak: peak aortic jet velocity; Z_{va}: valvulo-arterial impedance. Reproduced with permission from Pibarot P, Dumesnil JG. Improving assessment of aortic stenosis. *J Am Coll Cardiol.* 2012 Jul 17;60(3):169-180.

AS severity" at echocardiography raises challenges from both a diagnostic and therapeutic standpoint and includes 3 categories **(Fig. 28–6)**: (i) "Classical" low-flow, low-gradient with reduced LVEF (<50%) (D2 Stage in American Guidelines); (ii) "Paradoxical" low-flow (stroke volume index <35 ml/m²), low-gradient AS with preserved LVEF (≥50%) (D3 Stage); and (iii) Normal-flow (stroke volume index ≥35 ml/m²), low-gradient AS.[61] Classical low-flow, low-gradient AS corresponds to the heart failure with reduced LVEF (HFrEF) form of AS and is found in about 5% to 10% of the AS population (Fig. 28–6). This entity is more prevalent in men and is very often associated with coronary artery disease.[61] The depressed LVEF may be caused by LV afterload mismatch and/or concomitant intrinsic myocardial disease, the most frequent being an ischemic cardiomyopathy. Paradoxical low-flow, low-gradient corresponds to the heart failure with preserved LVEF (HFpEF) form of AS and is observed in 5% to 15% of AS patients (Fig. 28–6). This entity is more prevalent in women and in elderly people. These patients typically harbor a small LV cavity with pronounced LV concentric remodeling, a restrictive physiology

pattern, and reduced longitudinal systolic function, leading to a decrease in stroke volume despite a preserved LVEF. Other factors may also contribute to the low flow state including significant mitral regurgitation, mitral stenosis, tricuspid regurgitation, and atrial fibrillation. Normal-flow, low-gradient AS is observed in up to 25% of AS patients and is thus the most prevalent type of discordant AS (Fig. 28–6). Although the European guidelines suggest that the stenosis is unlikely to be severe in patients with normal-flow, low gradient AS[5], several studies and one meta-analysis report that approximately 50% of these patients may have a severe stenosis and may thus benefit from intervention.[62,63]

The first step in patients with discordant grading on echocardiography is to rule out measurement errors and consider other parameters of AS severity including the Doppler velocity index (<0.25 being consistent with severe AS) and the ratio of LV outflow acceleration time to LV ejection time (>0.37 consistent with severe) to corroborate AS severity (Table 28–1 and Figs. 28–4 and 28–6).[64] If the discordant grading cannot be reconciled and thus the stenosis severity cannot be confirmed, additional tests such as dobutamine stress echocardiography or aortic valve scoring by CT should be considered.

Dobutamine Stress Echocardiography: In patients with classical low-flow, low-gradient AS, low-dose (up to 20 µg/kg/min) dobutamine stress echocardiography (or dobutamine stress catheterization) may be performed (Fig. 28–6). Various parameters have been proposed to define true severe AS (Table 28–1). A peak stress mean gradient ≥40 mm Hg and/or an AVA ≤1.0 cm² are the main criteria proposed in the guidelines to confirm the presence of severe AS in patients with classical low-flow, low-gradient AS.[55,65] A large proportion of patients, however, have no or limited LV contractile reserve and thus remain in a low flow state with discordant grading during dobutamine stress echocardiography.[66] In these patients, dobutamine stress echocardiography remains inconclusive and other tests such as aortic valve calcium scoring by CT may be used to corroborate AS severity.

Staging cardiac damage
The current decision algorithm for aortic valve replacement presented in the guidelines[5,67] does not take into consideration the cardiac consequences of AS with the exception of reduced LV systolic function, defined as a LVEF <50%. Several recent studies[34,35,68] suggest that the cut-off of LVEF (<50%) proposed in the guidelines to identify LV systolic dysfunction in patients with AS is too low and that this value should be raised to <60% to improve the sensitivity of LVEF to identify LV dysfunction. Furthermore, several other Doppler-echocardiographic parameters may be used, besides LVEF, to assess the extent of cardiac damage related to—or associated with—AS (**Fig. 28–7**). Recently, a novel anatomic and functional staging classification that incorporates several of these parameters measured during routine echocardiographic examinations has been proposed to assess the extent of extra-valvular cardiac damage: Stage 1: LV damage; Stage 2: left atrial or mitral valve damage; Stage 3: pulmonary vasculature or tricuspid valve damage; and Stage 4: right ventricular damage.[69,70] This classification was prospectively validated in both symptomatic and asymptomatic patients with moderate or severe AS.[69–72] Again, consideration should be made as to whether such damage is attributable to AS or other co-morbidities (eg, ischemic heart disease, chronic obstructive pulmonary disease, etc)

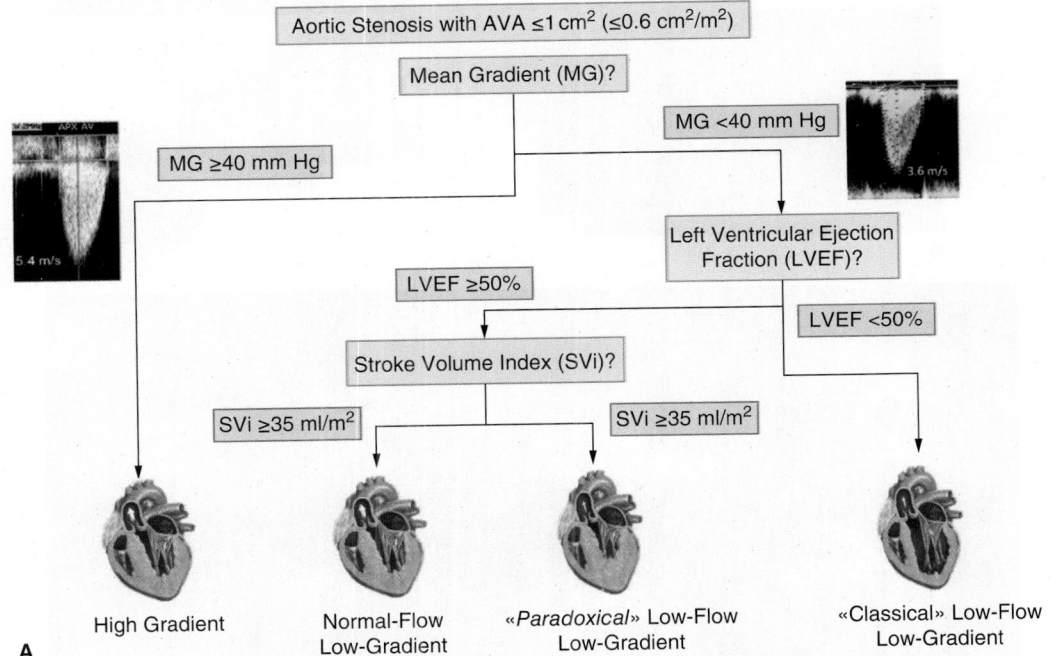

Figure 28–6. **Low-gradient patterns of aortic stenosis. (A)** Classification of the different patterns of low-gradient AS. **(B)** Echocardiographic and computed tomographic images in a patient with classical (low LVEF), low-flow, low-gradient AS. This 78-year-old woman presented with symptomatic aortic stenosis on a known bicuspid aortic valve. At transthoracic echocardiography, LVEF was very low at 20%, with discordant assessments of aortic stenosis severity: peak aortic jet velocity (V_{Peak}) 2.1 m/s, mean gradient 15 mm Hg, and AVA 0.71 cm² (indexed AVA: AVAi at 0.37 cm²/m²). The patient underwent a dobutamine stress echocardiography that demonstrated an increase in LVEF to 30%, and a 32% increase in stroke volume and a slight increase in velocity (2.6m/s) and mean gradient 21 mmHg; AVA did not change significantly and remained severe. Hence, discordance in assessment of AS severity was still present at DSE. Then the patient underwent computed tomography: Aortic valve calcification was scored at 1,033 AU, demonstrating non-severe aortic stenosis (according to the thresholds <1200 AU in women). **(C)** Echocardiographic and computed tomographic images in a patient with paradoxical (preserved LVEF), low-flow, low-gradient AS patient. This 82-year-old man presented with symptomatic aortic stenosis. At transthoracic echocardiography, LVEF was preserved at 60%, with discordant assessments of aortic stenosis severity: peak aortic jet velocity (V_{Peak}) 3.2 m/s, mean gradient (MG) 27 mm Hg, and AVA 0.70 cm² (indexed AVA: AVAi at 0.35 cm²/m²). The patient underwent computed tomography: Aortic valve calcification was scored at 2,837 AU, demonstrating a severe aortic stenosis (according to the thresholds ≥2000 AU in men). **(D)** Echocardiographic and computed tomographic images in a patient with patient with normal-flow, low-gradient AS with preserved LVEF. Aortic valve calcification was scored at 2,314 AU, demonstrating severe aortic stenosis.

AU, arbitrary unit; AVA, aortic valve area; AVC, aortic valve calcification; LVOT, left ventricular outflow tract; LVOTd, LVOT diameter; MG, mean transaortic pressure gradient; SV, stroke volume; V_{Peak}, peak aortic jet velocity; VTI, velocity time integral.

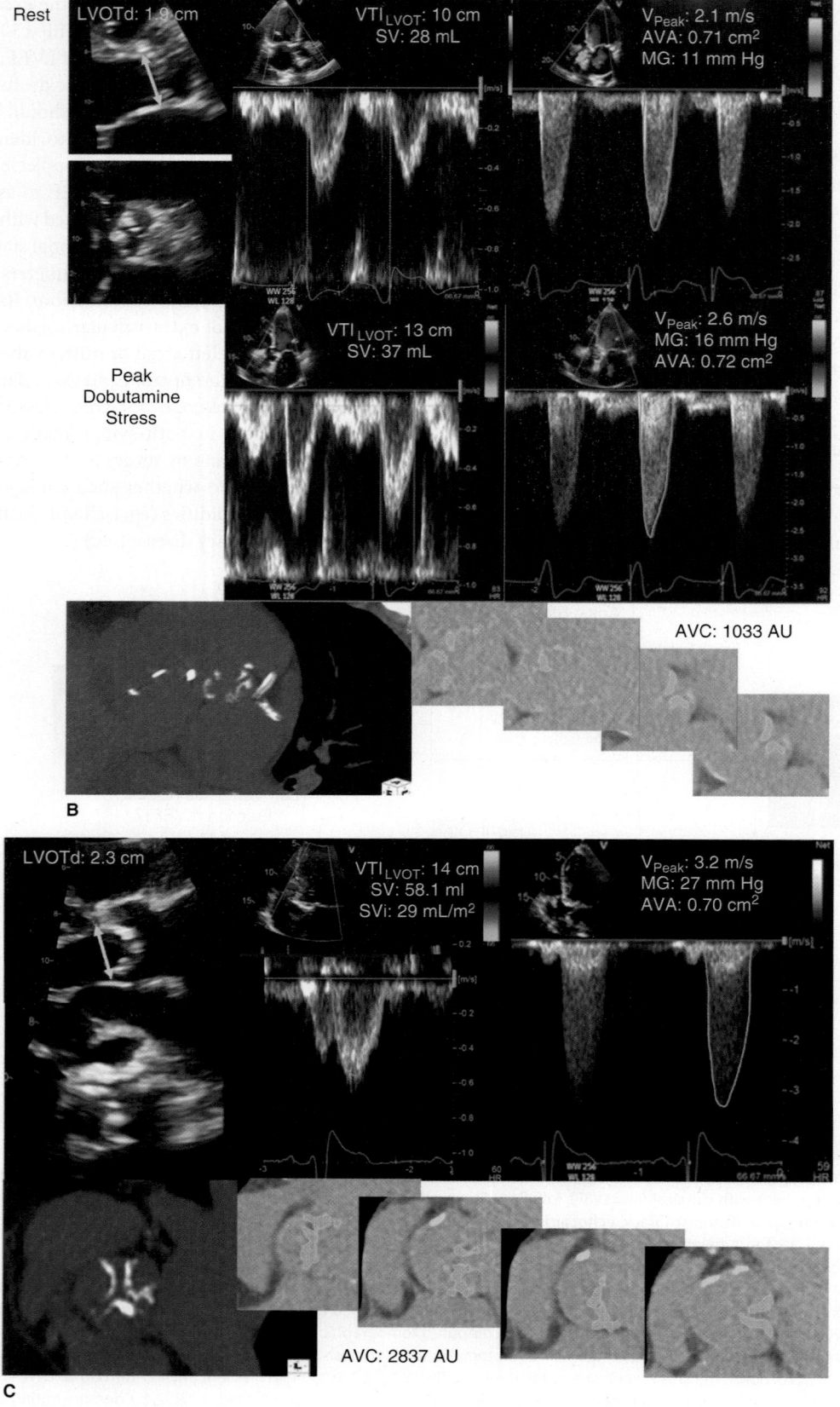

Rest

LVOTd: 1.9 cm

VTI_LVOT: 10 cm
SV: 28 mL

V_Peak: 2.1 m/s
AVA: 0.71 cm²
MG: 11 mm Hg

Peak
Dobutamine
Stress

VTI_LVOT: 13 cm
SV: 37 mL

V_Peak: 2.6 m/s
MG: 16 mm Hg
AVA: 0.72 cm²

AVC: 1033 AU

B

LVOTd: 2.3 cm

VTI_LVOT: 14 cm
SV: 58.1 ml
SVi: 29 mL/m²

V_Peak: 3.2 m/s
MG: 27 mm Hg
AVA: 0.70 cm²

AVC: 2837 AU

C

Figure 28–6. (Continued)

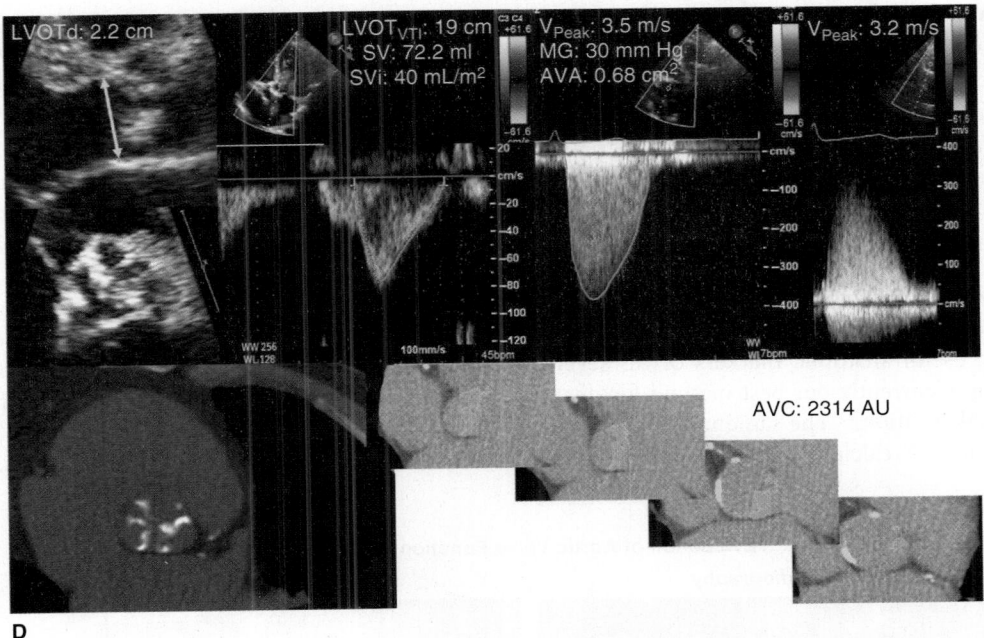

D

Figure 28–6. (Continued)

Multimodality Imaging in AS

Echocardiography remains the cornerstone investigation in patients with AS. However, we increasingly appreciate how other imaging modalities provide complementary information to echocardiography and may be used to aid clinical decision making. Indeed, CT imaging in patients with AS is now widely employed in the clinical arena whilst cardiac magnetic resonance (CMR) and positron emission tomography (PET) techniques

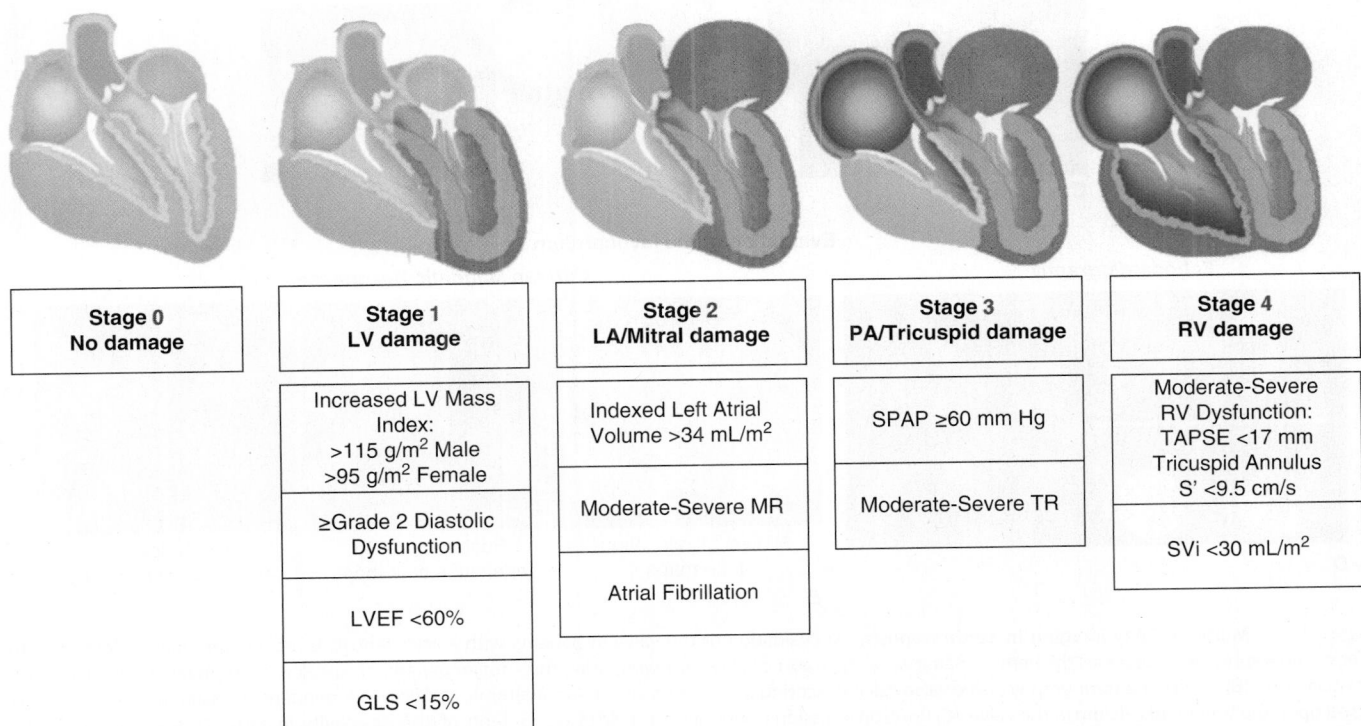

Figure 28–7. Staging of cardiac damage in aortic stenosis. The patient is classified in a given stage if any of the proposed criteria for this stage is met. GLS: global longitudinal strain; LA: left atrial; LV: left ventricular; LVEF: left ventricular ejection fraction; MR: mitral regurgitation; PA: pulmonary arterial; SPAP: systolic pulmonary arterial pressure; RV: right ventricular; SVi: stroke volume index; TAPSE: tricuspid annulus plane systolic excursion; TR: tricuspid regurgitation.

have made important contributions in the research field, aiding our understanding of the pathogenesis of AS (Fig. 28–7).

Computed Tomography

Computed tomography is used in the investigation of patients with AS, both to assess AS severity using CT aortic valve calcium (CT-AVC) scoring and for pre-procedural planning in patients undergoing TAVR.

CT Aortic Valve Calcium Scoring: Given the central role of calcification in AS, assessments of the valve calcium burden provide potentially useful anatomic markers of AS severity. CT calcium scoring is currently our best method for quantifying aortic valve calcification.[73] The same imaging protocols are used for coronary CT calcium scoring (noncontrast CT,

ECG gating in diastole at 60%–80% of the R-R interval, 3mm slice thickness, tube potential of 120–140 kV, and a tube current adjusted according to body size) and are widely available, as well as inexpensive, and are associated with a low radiation burden (1–2 mSv). CT-AVC scans are well tolerated by patients, highly reproducible and demonstrate good agreement with hemodynamic echocardiographic assessments but with the advantage of being independent of flow status and other hemodynamic confounders.

CT-AVC is measured using the modified Agatston method,[74] with the cut off for positive calcium deposit set at ≥130 Hounsfield units (HU).[75] In the axial plane, regions of interest are drawn to include aortic valve calcification, taking care to exclude calcium originating from the aorta, mitral valve, coronary arteries, or the LV outflow tract (**Figs.** 28–6 and **28–8**).

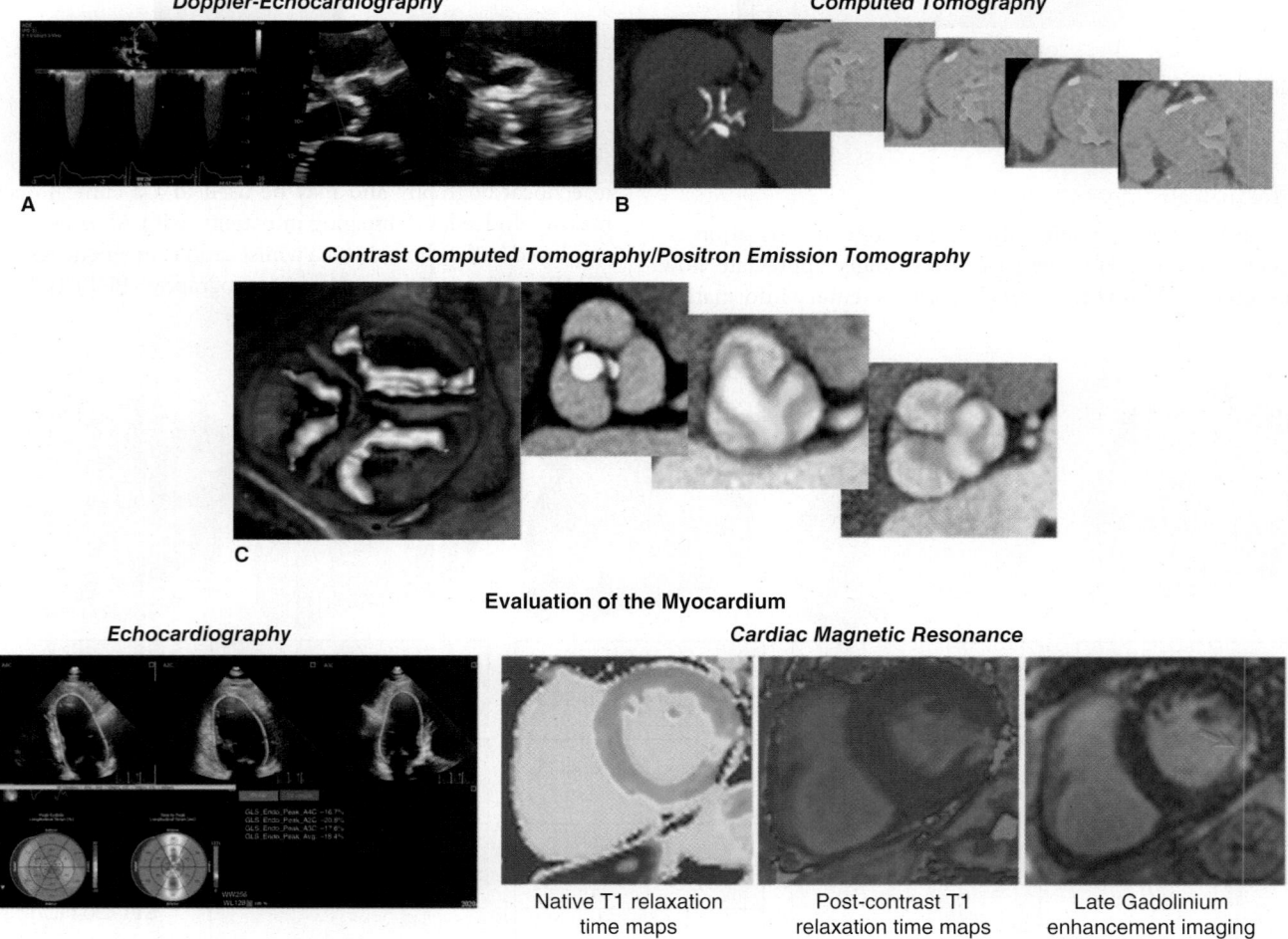

Figure 28–8. Multi-modality imaging in aortic stenosis. (A) Evaluation of the valve in patients with aortic stenosis is most commonly performed with echocardiography, which assesses the hemodynamic severity of aortic valve narrowing using three major parameters (peak velocity, mean gradient and aortic valve area). **(B)** Computed tomography aortic valve calcium scoring provides an alternative anatomic and flow independent assessment of valve severity based upon the burden of calcium in the valve. **(C)** Positron emission tomography provides assessments of disease activity, in particular assessment of valve calcification activity using the tracer 18F-fluoride. **(D)** Echocardiography is commonly used to the functional status of the myocardium in patients with aortic stenosis using ejection fraction, global longitudinal strain and markers of diastolic dysfunction. **(E)** Cardiovascular magnetic resonance provides assessment of replacement myocardial fibrosis using late gadolinium enhancement and interstitial fibrosis with T1 mapping techniques. These fibrosis assessments provide objective markers of left ventricular decompensation.

It is important not to perform quantification after re-orientating the images away from the axial plane, as this can cause large variability in the results.[73]

A key milestone in the development of CT-AVC was the realization that women develop severe stenosis with less aortic valve calcification than men, even after accounting for differences in body size.[21,76,77] Sex-specific CT-AVC thresholds for severe AS are therefore required. Clavel et al. demonstrated that a threshold of 2065 AU in men (sensitivity 86%, specificity 89%) and 1275 in women (sensitivity 89%, specificity 80%) demonstrated the clearest association with hemodynamic assessments in patients with concordant echocardiographic findings (and therefore no controversy as to the true severity of AS).[21,77] These were then validated in a large international, multicenter study of more than 900 patients scanned on a variety of different scanners[78] in whom the optimal severe disease thresholds were very similar to those proposed by Clavel: women 1377 AU; men 2062 AU.

In addition to its diagnostic accuracy, CT-AVC has consistently provided powerful prediction of future disease progression as well as prognostic information, demonstrating a close association with future aortic valve replacement independent of age, sex, and echocardiographic assessments of disease severity—even though the latter, not CT, were used to make such decisions.[77–79] On the basis of these data the most recent European Society of Cardiology Guidelines recommend CT-AVC as an arbitrator of AS severity in low-flow states when echocardiographic assessment are discordant and diagnostic uncertainty persists.[5] With CT-AVC use in clinical practice expanding it is important to note that this approach does not quantify valve fibrosis and can therefore infrequently underestimate AS severity in certain patients such as younger female patients in whom calcium is not the major disease process.[22,80]

Positron Emission Tomography

While CT-ACV assesses the burden of macroscopic calcium that has already developed, 18F-fluoride PET provides an assessment of valve calcification activity. Early studies demonstrated increased valvular 18F-NaF PET activity in patients with AS compared to controls, which increased progressively with disease severity (Fig. 28–8). Importantly, the baseline PET signal also predicted where new macroscopic deposits of calcium on the CT would develop (Fig. 28–8). Indeed a strong correlation was observed between baseline 18F-NaF uptake and the increase in CT-AVC over the next 1 to 2 years, as well as future need for AVR.[81,82] In the research setting, 18F-NaF can provide important insights into the pathophysiology of AS and the triggers to calcification.[83] 18F-NaF PET is also being used as an efficacy endpoint in several randomized clinical trials testing the ability of novel therapies to reduce valve calcification activity (BASIK2 Trial NCT02917525), (SALTIRE 2 trial NCT02132026). Whether 18F-NaF PET might find a clinical role remains to be determined.

Cardiac Magnetic Resonance

Cardiac magnetic resonance (CMR) is an emerging technology that offers excellent spatial resolution, functional assessment, and an unrivaled ability to provide myocardial tissue characterization.

Aortic Valve Function: CMR can provide high resolution images of the aortic valve and can help identify patients with bicuspid valve disease where this is not possible on echocardiography. It can also provide accurate assessments of the aorta and identify aortic dilatation or coarctation associated with aortic valve disease. Planimetry of the AVA is possible on short axis views of the valve,[84] however as with other planimetered anatomic AVA measurements these results should be interpreted in the knowledge that results and severity thresholds differ from effective AVA measurements calculated using the continuity equation. CMR also allows measurement of the velocities through the aortic valve with the advantage that alignment can be optimized and is not limited by the available echocardiographic windows. However, the temporal resolution of CMR is less than echocardiography. Therefore, CMR is unlikely to sample the true peak velocity through the valve, thereby underestimating AS.

LV Mass and Wall Thickening: CMR provides gold-standard assessments of LV volumes, wall thickness and mass, allowing detailed investigation of the LV hypertrophic response and its transition to heart failure. Importantly the degree of hypertrophy is only weakly correlated with the hemodynamic severity of AS[28], with males generally displaying increased LV mass even after correction for body size. Most commonly wall thickening occurs in a concentric pattern but recent studies have shown that asymmetrical patterns also exist in approximately 25% of patients assessed by CMR[28] and that this pattern of remodeling may be associated with adverse outcomes.[85]

Myocardial Fibrosis: Myocardial fibrosis is a key mechanism driving the progression from LV hypertrophy to heart failure in AS. CMR allows noninvasive assessment of fibrosis using two techniques; late gadolinium enhancement (LGE) for replacement fibrosis and T1 mapping for diffuse interstitial fibrosis (Fig. 28–8).[86]

Late Gadolinium Enhancement: Replacement Fibrosis: This technique involves the intravenous administration of gadolinium-based contrast agents (Fig. 28–8), which accumulate in the extracellular space due to delayed wash-out and label regions of replacement fibrosis. Patients with AS demonstrate areas of mid-wall late gadolinium enhancement, which appears as bright white areas in contrast to the surrounding black myocardium.[87,88] This mid-wall LGE has been validated against histological fibrosis assessment[27] and can be clearly differentiated from regions of subendocardial or transmural myocardial infarction. Mid-wall LGE provides an objective marker of LV decompensation in AS, demonstrating a consistent association with an exaggerated hypertrophic response, markers of myocardial injury, impaired systolic and diastolic function, patient exercise capacity and symptoms.[86]

Recent longitudinal studies have investigated the natural history and reversibility of replacement fibrosis. Once developed, mid-wall LGE appears to progress rapidly unless and until aortic valve replacement is performed, which halts further LGE accumulation. However, the replacement fibrosis that develops whilst waiting for surgery is irreversible. This is potentially important because LGE/replacement fibrosis is associated with an adverse long-term prognosis and when advanced, identifies patients that do not gain symptomatic benefit or improved systolic function following surgery.[89,90] Multiple studies have now confirmed the dose dependent increase in mortality and cardiovascular mortality associated with mid-wall LGE in AS.[91-93]

T1 Mapping (Diffuse Fibrosis): The detection of diffuse fibrosis is important because it is widely believed to be reversible[94] and is the precursor to irreversible forms of replacement fibrosis. However, the homogeneous nature of diffuse fibrosis means that it is not well detected by the LGE technique, which relies on regional contrast between areas of scar and normal myocardium. Several myocardial T1 mapping techniques have now been developed to overcome this problem.

Native T1 values (milliseconds) are measured without the use of contrast agents and reflect the combined intracellular and extracellular compartments (Fig. 28-8). Values increase with a greater burden of fibrosis, but also with other factors such as myocardial edema, infiltration as well as myocardial perfusion. Recent studies have demonstrated a correlation between native T1 and both histological fibrosis and the extent of ventricular remodeling.[95-97] A major limitation in native T1 is the variability in measurements made on different scanners. Moreover, even within the same scanner and protocol, substantial overlap exists in T1 values across different severities of AS and with healthy control subjects.[98] Consequently, there are no universal cut-offs for health and disease in AS.[99]

The extracellular volume fraction (ECV%) is calculated using the formula $ECV\% = (\Delta(1/T1_{myo})/\Delta(1/T1_{blood})) \times (1 - hematocrit)$, where $\Delta(1/T1)$ is the difference in myocardial or blood T1 pre- and post contrast.[100] ECV% has been investigated as a method for detecting diffuse myocardial fibrosis in a range of cardiovascular conditions including myocardial infarction, non-ischemic cardiomyopathy and AS.[101,102] As with native T1 and LGE, ECV% values can be influenced by other factors that expand the extracellular space such as myocardial infiltration and edema. However, an important advantage of ECV% is that it corrects for variation in T1 values on different scanners and sequences, making comparison of values acquired at different centers more feasible and potentially allowing for multi-center research.

A number of clinical studies have validated ECV% against histology in AS and have demonstrated the association between ECV% and other markers of LV decompensation (eg, ECG changes of hypertrophy and strain and elevation in biomarkers such as troponin and N-terminal pro-brain natriuretic peptide).[27,103-105] A recent international multicenter study demonstrated the powerful prognostic information it can provide, with ECV% emerging as an independent predictor of all cause and cardiovascular death in patients with AS.[106] However, further prognostic data is required, and we still lack clear ECV% thresholds to guide management decisions.

Cardiac Catheterization

Cardiac catheterization is recommended only when all non-invasive evaluation of AS (ie, CT and echocardiography) are inconclusive. Mean transaortic gradient should be based on simultaneous LV and aortic pressure measurements (Fig. 28-5). AVA should be calculated with the Gorlin formula, using a Fick or thermodilution cardiac output measurement.[55]

In some patients, Doppler-echocardiographic measurement and catheterization measurements of gradients and AVA could differ, as they are not measured at the same level in the aorta (Fig. 28-5). Indeed, Doppler-echocardiography measures the maximum velocity or gradient across the aortic valve at the level of the vena contracta. However, catheterization measurements are generally performed at a few centimeters downstream of the vena contracta, where the blood flow jet re-expands and decelerates whereas blood pressure increases.[59,107] The extent of pressure recovery generally becomes clinically relevant in patients with smaller aortas, ie, with an aorta diameter at the sino-tubular junction ≤30 mm, and especially in those with moderate or moderate-to-severe AS.[59,107,108]

These discrepancies can in large part be reconciled by taking into account the pressure recovery phenomenon by calculating the "energy loss coefficient" (ELC), that adjusts the Doppler AVA for the size of the aorta (Table 28-1 and Fig. 28-5)[59]: The ELC is easily measurable by Doppler-echocardiography and provides an estimate of catheter-derived AVA calculated with the use of the Gorlin formula. Several studies have demonstrated that the energy loss coefficient is superior to the Doppler AVA in predicting the actual energy loss and the occurrence of LV dysfunction and adverse outcomes in patients with AS.[59,60] Not accounting for pressure recovery in patients with small aortas may lead to overestimation of severity by Doppler-echocardiography and unwarranted investigations or interventions.

Blood Biomarkers

Several blood biomarkers of myocardial impairment and heart failure have been applied to the management of patients with AS.

Brain natriuretic peptides

B-type natriuretic peptide (BNP) and its biologically inactive N-terminal-proBNP (NT-proBNP) form are useful predictors of the onset of symptoms and adverse events in patients with severe AS.[109-114] However, elevated plasma of BNP/NT-proBNP is not specific to AS and could be related to several variables including age, female sex, chronic renal disease, and other hemodynamic stimuli.[115] A BNP ratio >1 (or clinical activation of BNP), which is the measured BNP value divided by its expected value according to age and sex[112] was associated with increased long-term mortality, incrementally and independently of classical risk factors.[112] BNP/NT-proBNP are thus useful for identifying left ventricular decompensation in AS in clinical practice.

High sensitivity cardiac troponins

Elevated plasma levels of cardiac troponin have traditionally been used to diagnose myocardial infarction.[116] However, high sensitivity assays now allow detection of cardiac damage in a range of cardiac conditions including AS.[117] Indeed in AS populations, plasma concentrations of high-sensitivity troponin are not associated with markers of coronary artery disease but rather to the degree of LV hypertrophy and the presence of mid-wall fibrosis, provide powerful prediction of AVR or cardiac death.[104] High-sensitivity troponins could thus be an early biomarker of myocardial fibrosis deposition and LV dysfunction, and a potential clinical tool in the management of AS patients.

Other potential biomarkers

Many other blood biomarkers have been proposed to identify early LV dysfunction and outcomes in AS. These include plasma level of soluble interleukin-1 receptor-like-1 which has been associated with symptoms status, AS severity and several parameters of cardiac remodelling.[118] Similarly, growth-differentiation-factor-15 and Galectin-3 showed some prognostic value in patients undergoing TAVR.[119–121] Recent evidence shows an incremental value of increased number of elevated biomarkers beyond classical clinical risk scores alone to predict excess of mortality after AVR.[121]

SEX AND ETHNIC DIFFERENCES IN THE PATHOPHYSIOLOGY AND DIAGNOSIS OF AS

Sex-Related Differences in AS

For years, AS was considered to be the same disease in men and women. However, recent studies have revealed important sex-specific differences related to the pathophysiology, diagnosis, and response to treatment in this condition (**Fig. 28–9**).

Prevalence of AS

Nationwide studies showed a similar proportion of men and women hospitalized for AS with 55% patients hospitalized with AS being men in US[122], while 52% being women in Sweden[123] and 53% in Scotland.[124] Interestingly, 60% of the young patients (≤75 years old) were men as bicuspid aortic valve is more prevalent in men (3:1 men vs women) and more than 50% of the elderly with AS were women.[2] However, given that older women are more frequent that older men, the percentage of men with AS (0.37%) is slightly higher than the percentage of women with AS (0.34%).[2]

Biological sexual differences in pathophysiology

As mentioned, women reach a similar hemodynamic degree of AS severity with a lower amount of aortic valve calcification and consequently, sex-specific thresholds have been proposed to identify severe AS, as well as predicting disease progression, and adverse clinical events.[21,76,77,79] This relatively smaller amount of valve leaflet calcium in women appears to be compensated by fibrosis, which contributes largely to the development of valvular stenosis (Fig. 28–9).[22,80] Thus, sex seems to have an impact on AS pathobiology, but very few studies investigated the sex-specific signaling pathways leading to these observations. Cellular proliferation, apoptosis, migration, ossification, angiogenesis, lipid management, inflammation, and extracellular matrix reorganization were some of the pathways and processes that may be different between women and men.[125–127]

LV remodeling and fibrosis

Several studies have described sex-specific differences in the remodeling response of the left ventricle to AS, with women having more concentric remodeling than men (Fig. 28–9).[128] Moreover, concentric LV hypertrophy in women has been associated with worse outcome (60% increased risk) in women but not in men.[129] Women are also more likely to develop LV restrictive physiology pattern and heart failure in pressure overload cardiomyopathies when compared to men.[130,131] A recent CMR study reported that women have similar replacement myocardial fibrosis (as assessed by late gadolinium enhancement) but higher LV extracellular volume fraction (as assessed by T1 mapping) than men, indicating more pronounced diffuse fibrosis in women independent of the degree of AS severity (Fig. 28–9).[26] Similar results were observed in an analysis of the Multi-Ethnic Study of Atherosclerosis (MESA).[132,133] The major confounder to consider when comparing myocardial fibrosis in men vs. women is coronary disease, as men generally have higher prevalence of coronary artery diseases.[134]

Management and outcomes

Management of AS seems to be different between sexes, with women undergoing fewer diagnostic tests and less likely to be seen by a specialist or proceeding to aortic valve replacement.[135]

After isolated SAVR, women have worse outcomes, with longer post-operative stay, higher 30-day and long-term mortality, higher rates of postoperative stroke and lower LV mass regression than men.[136–139] However, women are often referred to surgery with a worse risk profile as they are older and more hypertensive than men and they are also at higher risk of patient-prosthesis mismatch than men.[140–147] Thus, part of the worsened outcomes after surgical aortic valve replacement in women is probably explained by pre-operative and operative risk factors and delays in their referral for intervention.[148]

Interestingly, it appears women have a better outcome after TAVR than SAVR[149], in any risk strata[150–153], and probably better outcomes than men.[154–156] This may be explained by the smaller aortic annulus in women, which is problematic in SAVR increasing the risk of patient-prosthesis mismatch, but potentially beneficial in TAVR[140,157] reducing the risk of paravalvular leak[158,159] (Fig. 28–9). In addition, the lower burden of valve calcium observed in women would also reduce the risk of paravalvular leak[160,161] and pacemaker implantation post-TAVR.[162] On the other, the smaller femoral artery diameter observed in women makes them more likely to encounter peripheral vascular complications.[135]

Race-Related Differences in AS

There are very few data on ethnic differences associated with AS. Black American population may have a lower prevalence of severe AS compared to Caucasians, even after adjustment for traditional risk factors.[163,164] In addition, Black American population are less likely to be admitted to hospital for AS and are less likely to undergo aortic valve replacement.[165,166] Black American population also have a lower frequency of congenital bicuspid aortic valves, reduced aortic dimensions and less aortic valve calcium determined by pathology.[167] There is increasing evidence in Asian populations, especially notable

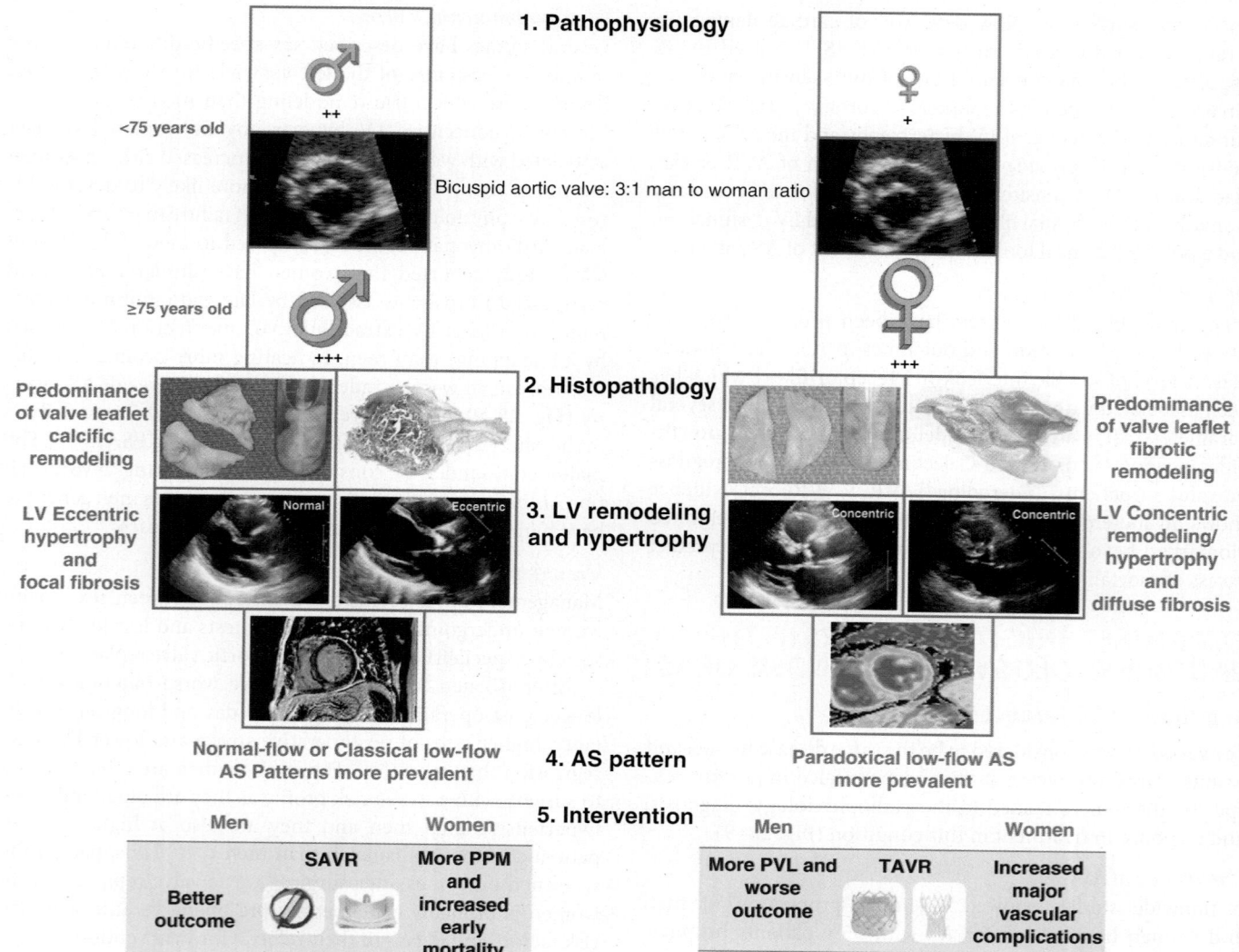

Figure 28–9. Sex-differences in the pathophysiology, presentation and treatment of aortic stenosis. This figure represents five different observation areas between men and women developing AS. **1.** A higher rate of men (younger than 75 years) tends to develop AS when compared to women, linked to bicuspid valve. However, in population over 75 years old the percentage is similar slightly higher in women. **2.** Histological observation of explanted aortic valve specimens and Trichrome Masson staining (calcium and fibrosis/collagen staining) show a more calcific AS (purple) in men and a fibrotic AS (blue) in women, for the same hemodynamic severity. **3.** Left ventricular remodeling to pressure overload in AS is sex-specific. Men have more normal pattern or eccentric hypertrophy, as demonstrated by echocardiographic parasternal long-axis view, and late-gadolinium enhancement measured by cardiac magnetic resonance, is increased demonstrating the presence of focal fibrosis. In women, echocardiographic findings point towards a more concentric remodeling/hypertrophy and diffuse fibrosis deposition is found with T1 mapping by cardiac magnetic resonance. **4.** These left ventricular patterns lead to more classical low-flow AS in men and a higher rate of paradoxical low-flow AS in women when AS does not have normal flow pattern. **5.** Men benefit more from a surgical aortic valve replacement whilst women have better outcomes following a transcatheter aortic valve implantation despite more bleeding than men. Surgical aortic valve replacement leads to more patient-prosthesis mismatch in women while men have higher rates of paravalvular leakage with transcatheter aortic valve replacement.

AS, aortic stenosis; LV, left ventricle; SAVR, surgical aortic valve replacement; TAVR, transcatheter aortic valve replacement; PPM, patient-prosthesis mismatch; PVL, paravalvular leak.

in China, that bicuspid AS is more common and is associated with greater magnitude of valve leaflet calcification.[168,169]

AORTIC VALVE INTERVENTION: TIMING AND MODALITY

Despite major progress in understanding AS pathophysiology, there is still no known beneficial medical treatment. The only meaningful therapy is to replace the aortic valve by surgical or transcatheter approaches (**Fig. 28–10**), resulting in survival improvement, decrease or disappearance of symptoms, improvement in exercise capacity, LV mass regression, and improved LV function, in patients with reduced LV ejection fraction before AVR.

Symptomatic Patients with Severe AS

Survival during the asymptomatic phase of AS is comparable to age-matched populations with a low risk of sudden death

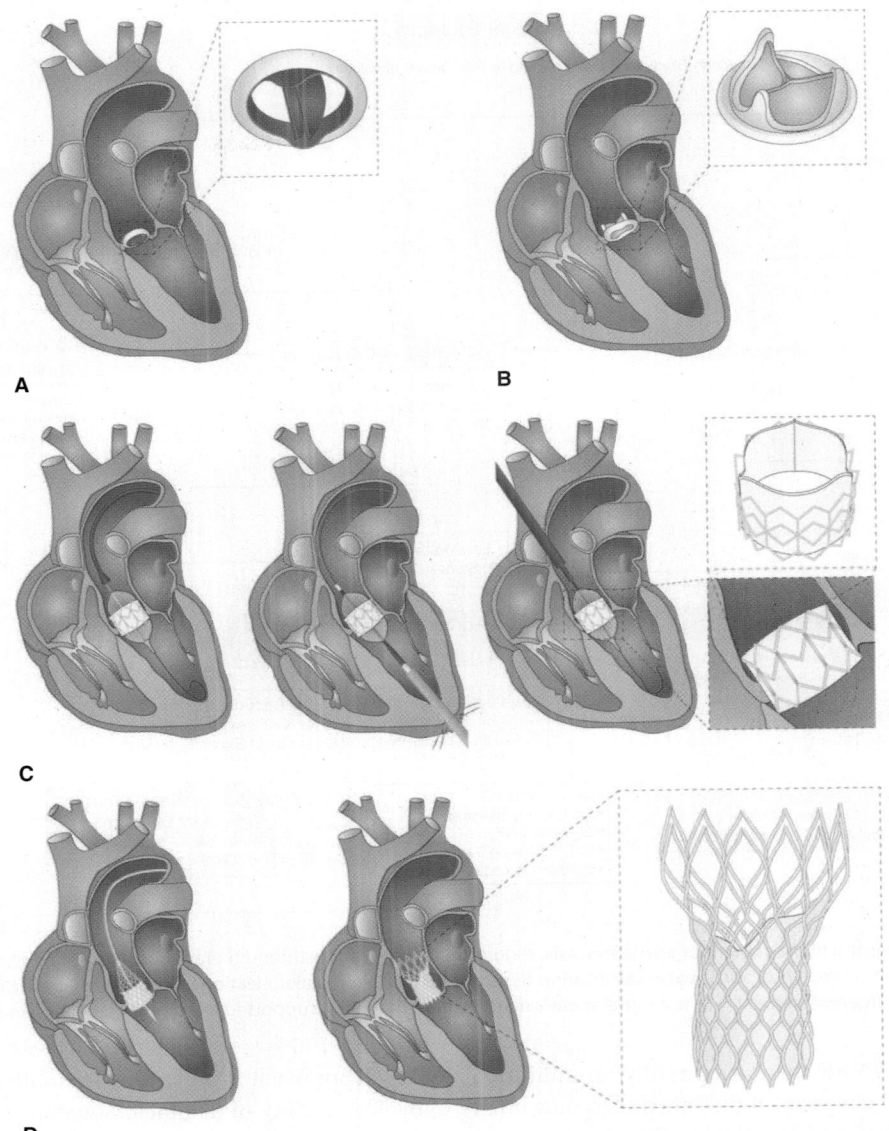

Figure 28–10. Different types of aortic valve replacement. (A) Surgical aortic valve replacement with a bileaflet mechanical valve. (B) Surgical aortic valve replacement with a bioprosthetic valve. (C) Transcatheter aortic valve replacement with a balloon expandable valve via the transfemoral, transapical or transaortic approach. (D) Transcatheter aortic valve replacement with a self-expanding valve via the transfemoral approach. Reproduced with permission from Lindman BR, Clavel MA, Mathieu P, et al. Calcific aortic stenosis. *Nat Rev Dis Primers*. 2016 Mar 3;2:16006.

(<1% per year) when patients are followed prospectively and promptly report symptom onset.[170] However, as symptoms occur, the mortality rate increases rapidly. The occurrence of symptoms has been shown to be correlated with the severity of the stenosis, with 20% to 25% 2-year onset of symptoms in moderate AS patients compared with 50% to 70% in severe AS patients. On the other hand, the symptoms are not specific of AS and, as the AS population ages and comorbidities increase, it often difficult to ascertain that the stenosis is the cause of the symptoms. Nevertheless, symptoms remains a class I indication for aortic valve replacement in patients with severe high gradient AS (American Guidelines Stage D1) **(Fig. 28–11)**[5,55], and intervention should be performed promptly after the onset of symptoms. In severe AS patients without clear symptoms and/or low daily activity, symptoms could be unmasked by exercise stress testing and symptoms occurrence at exercise, a decrease in exercise tolerance, or an exercise fall in blood pressure are triggers for intervention (Class I or IIa).

In symptomatic low-flow, low-gradient AS patients with or without decreased LVEF (American guidelines Stage D2 or D3), intervention is reasonable if the stenosis is confirmed to be severe and the symptoms are related to the stenosis (Class IIa) (Fig. 28–11). In patients with discordant AS, ie, low AVA (<1cm²) and low mean gradient (<40 mm Hg) but normal flow, current guidelines consider AS unlikely to be severe. However, if the severity of AS is confirmed (by CT or echo assessments) and the patient is symptomatic, one should strongly consider intervention. In patients with moderate AS (Stage B), even

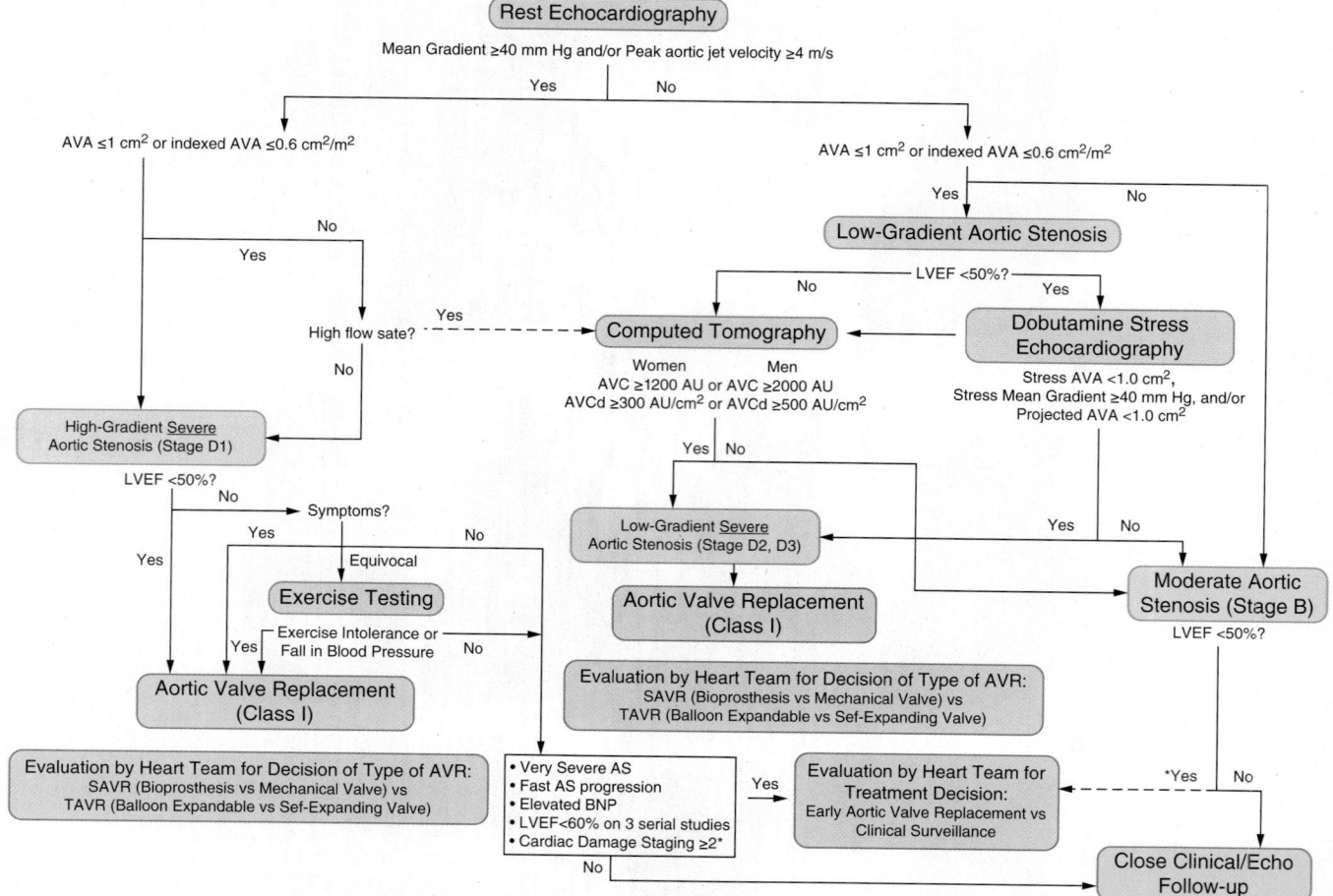

Figure 28–11. Algorithm for the management of aortic stenosis. Algorithm for the diagnostic and therapeutic management of AS. AVA, aortic valve area; AVC, aortic valve calcification score; AVCd, aortic valve calcification density; LVEF, left ventricular ejection fraction; TAVR, transcatheter aortic valve replacement; SAVR, surgical aortic valve replacement. *: denotes therapeutic management that is not supported by current guidelines and requires further validation.

with symptoms or low LVEF, there is currently no indication for aortic valve replacement except if they are undergoing other cardiac surgery (Class IIa[55] or Class I[5]) (Fig. 28–11).

Surgical versus Transcatheter Aortic Valve Replacement

TAVR has transformed the treatment strategy of patients with severe AS. TAVR is now the standard-of-care for patients who are not candidates for surgery or are at high surgical risk and is an alternative to surgery for appropriately selected intermediate and low-risk patients (Fig. 28–10). Indeed, randomized controlled trials and large registries in elderly patients at increased surgical risk show that TAVR is superior to conservative management in extreme-risk patients[171], non inferior or superior to surgery in high-risk patients[150,151,172], non inferior, or superior when performed via transfemoral access to surgery in intermediate-risk patients[152,173–175], and non inferior or superior to surgery in low risk patients.[153,176]

The choice between SAVR and TAVR in a patient with severe AS having an indication for AVR requires evaluation by a Heart Valve Team (**Table 28–2,** Fig. 28–11). The first step is to assess clinical factors, including the surgical risk of the patient. The higher the surgical risk, the more suitable a less-invasive

TAVR approach is preferred. The online calculator developed by The Society of Thoracic Surgeons (STS) is the most used tool to estimate a patient's surgical risk (http://riskcalc.sts.org). High risk is considered when the STS all-cause mortality score within 30 days after surgery is >8%, intermediate risk between 3% and 8%, and low risk <3%. However, risk scores do not take into account other important clinical factors such as frailty, cognitive capabilities, or chest wall deformities which impact surgical outcomes. Thus, a multi disciplinary heart valve team is required to make customized patient-based assessments, considering all co-morbidities. Similarly, the age of the patient deserves special attention, as the shorter recovery time after TAVR is more impactful in elderly patients. Moreover, the knowledge gaps regarding long-term durability (>5 years) of TAVR bioprosthetic valves will be less concerning in elder patients but must be carefully considered in younger (especially <70 years old) patients.

In addition to surgical risk scores and age, specific co-morbidities deserve notable attention, such as significant coronary artery disease (including the need for coronary artery revascularization), mitral valve disease requiring intervention, peripheral arterial disease (especially femoral artery disease that prohibits transfemoral access), significant hepatic disease, and

TABLE 28–2. Conditions to be Considered by the Heart Team for Recommending TAVR Versus SAVR

	Favors TAVR	Favors SAVR
Risk of surgical mortality or morbidity of intermediate or greater risk (eg, STS score ≥3)	Yes	
Advanced age (>75 years), frailty, limited mobility	Yes	
Classical, low-flow, low-gradient AS	Yes	
Advanced cardiac damage staging (≥3)	Yes	
Small annulus requiring a small surgical valve (prosthesis size 21 mm)	Yes	
Longevity unlikely (minimum 2 years required)	Yes	
Mediastinal anatomy unfavorable for surgery (Porcelain aorta, previous thoracotomy, patent grafts, hostile root)	Yes	
Aortic root anatomy unfavorable for TAVR (inadequate or excessive calcification, annulus size out of range, aortic dilation, coronary obstruction risk)		Yes
Advanced atrioventricular block, especially RBBB		Yes
Non-femoral access required		Yes
Congenital bicuspid valve		Yes
Risk of coronary obstruction or coronary access concerns		Yes
Concomitant conditions requiring surgery (eg, multivalve disease, aorta aneurysm, coronary bypass)		Yes
Endocarditis		Yes

Abbreviations: RBBB, right bundle branch block; SAVR, surgical aortic valve replacement; STS, Society of Thoracic Surgeons; TAVR, transcatheter aortic valve replacement.

dementia. Importantly, there are also anatomic factors which may be unfavorable for optimal TAVR, including too small or large aortic annulus size, excessive calcification patterns of the aortic valvar complex (eg, extension of calcium into the LV outflow tract), low coronary arteries at higher risk for coronary obstruction after TAVR (especially with effaced sinuses), and the presence of a bicuspid aortic valve (Table 28–2).[177] In patients with bicuspid aortic valve disease, SAVR remains the gold standard for many patients who are younger, those with significant aortopathy, or with unfavorable anatomy of the aortic annulus or calcified leaflets. Although bicuspid aortic valves were excluded from the randomized controlled trials, several registries have recently challenged a categorical approach to contra-indicating TAVR therapy in carefully selected bicuspid valves. These registries have demonstrated similar clinical outcomes when compared with matched tricuspid valve patients and to bicuspid patients undergoing SAVR.[178–180] Undoubtedly, TAVR for bicuspid aortic valves is more complex with a higher rate of moderate or severe para-valvular regurgitation and aortic root injury due to excessive LV outflow tract calcium, bulky leaflet calcification, or calcified raphes.[181]

When evaluating patients for SAVR or TAVR, one should attempt to avoid futile interventions in patients with irreversible co-morbidities. In this case, irrespective of procedural technical success, patients do not derive sufficient benefit to justify the procedure. A simplified ABCDE mnemonic is helpful to identify patients in whom TAVR may be futile: Advanced dementia, Bedbound or non mobile, Cachexia or severe sarcopenia, Disability for most or all basic activities of daily living, End-stage lung, liver, renal, or malignant disease.[182]

Bioprosthetic versus Mechanical Valves

The choice of valve replacement technology is of utmost importance when SAVR is planned but could also be part of the SAVR versus TAVR discussion (Fig. 28–10). Unfortunately, the ideal replacement aortic valve with excellent hemodynamics, long-term durability, high thrombo-resistance, and reliable implantation does not exist and all available prosthetic valves have inherent limitations.[183] Mechanical valves are nowadays mostly represented by bileaflet valves and have excellent implantability, hemodynamics, and durability. However, they are highly thrombogenic and thus require life-long systemic anticoagulation. Bioprostheses mimic the characteristics of a normal native valve with three leaflets, very good hemodynamics and high thrombo-resistance. However, they are limited by reduced long-term durability. Indeed durability is the Achilles' heel of all bioprosthesis with half of such valves demonstrating evidence of structural valve deterioration within 10 years after implantation.[184] In addition, there are newer bioprosthetic surgical valves with either facilitated implantation methods (so-called "suture-less" valves) or expandable frames, which allow for optimal subsequent implantation of TAVR devices to treat bioprosthetic valve failure.[185–187] The most important factors when considering mechanical versus biological prosthesis will be the patient's age, life expectancy, indication/contraindication for warfarin therapy (especially lifestyle activities), comorbidities, and especially the patient's personal preferences (**Table 28–3**). Finally, the choice of the prosthesis should include the avoidance of prosthesis-patient mismatch (ie, the implantation of a smaller than desirable prosthesis for the cardiac output requirements of the patient), as this condition is not infrequent, especially after SAVR and is associated with worse outcomes.[188,189]

HEART VALVE CLINIC AND HEART VALVE TEAM

The heart valve clinic and the heart team are two distinct entities that may overlap but intervene at different time points along the patient's journey with AS (**Fig. 28–12**).

Follow-Up Before and After Intervention

Patients are generally first diagnosed with AS when cardiac auscultation reveals a systolic murmur or after a Doppler-echocardiogram is requested for another indication. Periodic monitoring with Doppler-echocardiographic examination is recommended for patients with known AS. In patients with AS and normal LV function, the frequency of routine follow-up should be based on the severity of the valve lesion: every 3 to 5 years for mild AS, every 1 to 2 years for moderate AS, and every 6 to 12 months in asymptomatic severe AS patients.[5,55]

TABLE 28-3. Conditions to be Considered by the Heart Team for Selecting a Bioprosthetic Valve versus a Mechanical Valve in Patients Undergoing SAVR

	Favors Mechanical Valve	Favors Bioprosthetic Valve
Desire of the patient	Yes	Yes
Patients at risk of accelerated structural valve deterioration	Yes	
Age <60 years	Yes	
Patients with a reasonable life expectancy for whom future redo valve surgery would be at high risk	Yes	
Patients already on long-term anticoagulation due to the high risk for thromboembolism	Yes	
Good-quality anticoagulation is unlikely		Yes
Patient's life expectancy is lower than the expected durability of the bioprosthesis		Yes
Reoperation for mechanical valve thrombosis despite good long-term anticoagulation		Yes
Low likelihood and/or low operative risk of future redo valve surgery		Yes
Young women contemplating pregnancy		Yes
Age >65 years		Yes

Population-based studies have demonstrated that about two thirds of people with AS are not diagnosed and thus not followed.[53]

In patients with known AS, Doppler-echocardiography should be repeated in addition to routine clinical follow-up to detect: (i) changes in physical examination (systolic murmur or second heart sound or signs of heart failure) because valve obstruction may have progressed since the last evaluation; (ii) the subtle appearance of new symptoms relating to AS, especially if the patient is exposed to increased hemodynamic demands (non cardiac surgery, pregnancy, systemic infection, etc).

The assessment of AS has become more complex and multifaceted (Figs. 28-6, 28-8, and 28-11) necessitating specialized and dedicated heart valve clinics (Fig. 28-12) to coordinate patient follow-up, imaging studies and closer monitoring. The roles of the heart valve clinic before intervention are to: (i) assess and follow the severity of AS and the extent of cardiac damage; (ii) optimize the medical treatment of co-morbidities; (iii) educate the patient and family about early reporting of symptoms; (iv) determine the best timing for intervention and refer the patient for final decisions and choices regarding valve intervention. The heart valve clinic thus should include cardiologists, imaging specialists, geriatricians, and nurses, with expertise and interest in valvular heart disease. After intervention, the roles of the heart valve clinic are to: (i) assess the results of intervention; (ii) educate the patient about anti-thrombotic therapy and endocarditis prophylaxis; (iii) follow the evolution of the structure and function of the prosthesis (Fig. 28-12).

Heart Valve Team and Shared Decision-Making for Intervention

When intervention is necessary, the patient is referred to an expanded version of the heart valve team including heart valve surgeons and structural interventionalists, for the purpose of: (i) confirming the indication for intervention; (ii) selecting the type of intervention (TAVR vs SAVR) and prosthesis (bioprosthetic vs mechanical valve; balloon-expandable vs self-expanding valve) and explaining in detail the risk and benefits of the procedure alternatives; (iii) performing the chosen

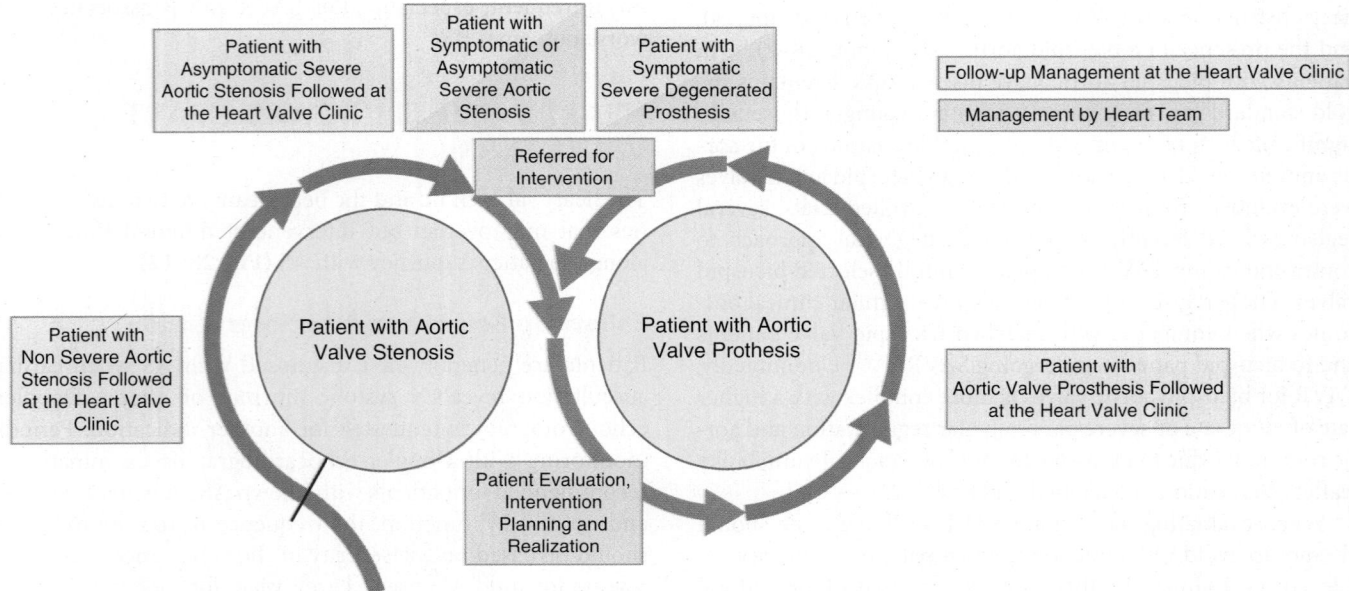

Figure 28-12. **The roles of heart valve clinic and heart valve team.** Role of heart valve clinic and heart team in the patients' pathway.

intervention (Figs. 28–10, 28–11, and 28–12). All individuals attending the heart valve clinic are a part of the enlarged heart valve team which also includes individuals focusing on the procedure itself and post-procedure in-hospital patient care (imaging specialists, anesthesiologists, intensivists, and nurses). In the modern era of complex cardiac disease management, there is a shared decision-making process for all therapy decisions which includes comprehensive discussions with patients and their families to account for lifestyle desires and personal preferences.

Medical Treatment

During the follow-up of patients with native valve AS or aortic prostheses, the heart valve clinic should monitor and adjust medical treatments for the patient. In particular, hypertension often coexists with AS and may contribute to LV afterload excess, low flow state (and thus low gradient AS pattern) symptoms and adverse events.[190] Moreover, high systolic blood pressure may interact with Doppler echocardiographic assessment of AS and has been associated with faster progression of AS.[191-193] In patients with concomitant coronary artery disease, and/or dyslipidemia patients should be treated with statins according to guidelines standards. However, the presence of AS per se is not an indication for lipid lowering therapy. In patients with AS requiring anticoagulation therapy, direct anticoagulant may be preferred to warfarin, as anti-vitamin K drugs may accelerate

the progression of aortic valve calcification and AS hemodynamic severity.[194,195]

FUTURE PERSPECTIVES

Potential Disease Modifying Treatments in Clinical Development

Currently, we lack any medical therapies to effectively prevent or retard disease progression in AS. While valve replacement techniques continue to improve, the development of novel treatments to prevent or slow down AS would be ideal, potentially obviating the need for valve replacement altogether. Achieving this goal will require reappraisal and further investigation of the pathogenesis underlying AS followed by randomized controlled trials to test the efficacy of novel treatment strategies including: (i) Lp(a) lowering therapy with antisense oligonucleotide targeted against apolipoprotein(a); (ii) Inhibition of ectopic valvular calcification using bisphosphonates and denosumab, a monoclonal antibody against RANKL; (iii) Vitamin K supplementation; (iv) Inhibition of valvular fibrosis using Renin Angiotensin Aldosterone System Inhibitors (**Fig. 28–13**).

Physical and Mechanical Interventions for Aortic Valvuloplasty

For patients with symptomatic severe AS who are not suitable candidates for AVR (SAVR or TAVR), mechanical or novel

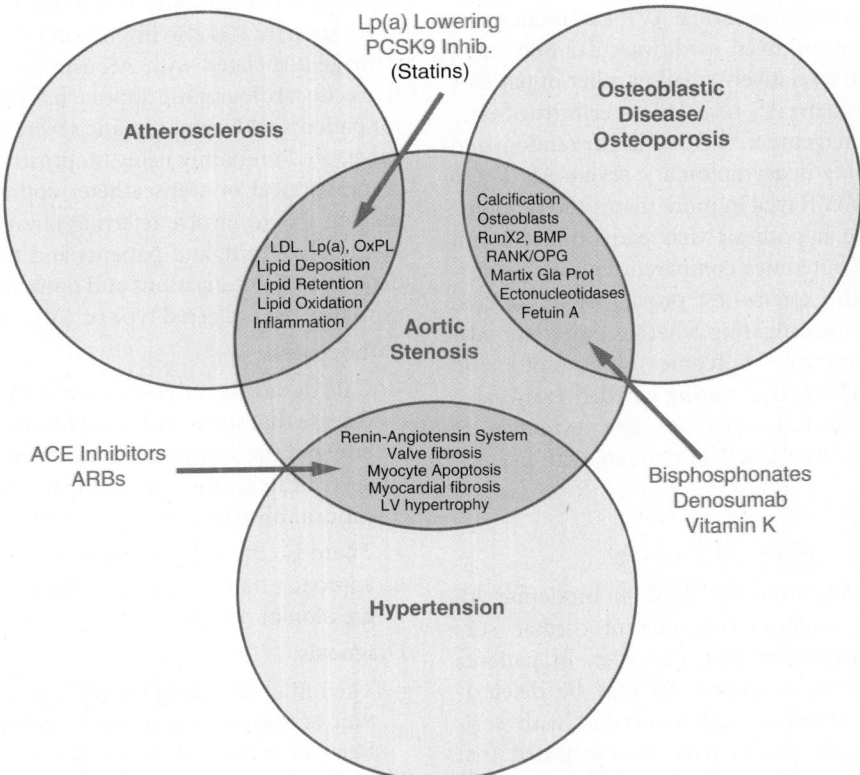

Figure 28–13. Potential pharmacotherapies of aortic stenosis according to pathological mechanism. AS shares several common factors and mechanisms with atherosclerosis, hypertension, and osteoblastic disease/osteoporosis. Hence, potential candidate drugs to slow the progression of AS target these factors/mechanisms. Statins have been tested in several previous randomized trials and failed to slow the progression of AS. ACE, angiotensin conversion enzyme; ARBs, angiotensin 2 receptor blockers; Lp(a), lipoprotein a. Reproduced with permission from Dweck MR, Boon NA, Newby DE. Calcific aortic stenosis: a disease of the valve and the myocardium. *J Am Coll Cardiol.* 2012 Nov 6;60(19):1854-1863.

valvuloplasty devices can improve hemodynamics and quality of life, either as a short-term therapy bridge to AVR, as a palliative therapy, and potentially with longer-term benefits. Balloon aortic valvuloplasty has been used for several decades to reduce the transvalvular pressure gradients in patients with severe AS not eligible for AVR, but most patients (approximately 80%) have clinical and hemodynamic recurrence within 6 months. New techniques of mechanical valvuloplasty are currently being investigated, such as a transfemoral mechanical leaflet scoring device that fractures calcified tissue in multiple locations and improves leaflet mobility to significantly reduce transvalvular gradients.[196] Pulsed cavitational high intensity ultrasound can also be used to soften calcified leaflets to improve valve hemodynamics.[197,198]

Early AVR in Asymptomatic Severe AS

As the risks of SAVR have diminished and the role of transfemoral TAVR without the need for general anesthesia has become established, there is a growing consideration for earlier AS intervention to improve clinical outcomes and prevent irreversible cardiac dysfunction during an asymptomatic waiting phase. Several studies have suggested that earlier AVR is associated with better survival compared to the current standard strategy of active surveillance in patients with asymptomatic severe AS.[199,200] This more aggressive approach may also improve earlier access to definitive AVR in patients with equivocal symptoms. Ultimately, randomized controlled trials will be required to assess whether earlier AVR can reduce cardiac damage and lead to improved cardiovascular outcomes. The RECOVERY trial, in a relatively small number of patients with very severe asymptomatic AS, revealed superiority of early AVR vs. conservative management.[201] Other larger randomized trials are currently ongoing in asymptomatic severe AS. These include: (i) the EARLY TAVR trial in more than 1100 randomized patients testing the hypothesis that early transfemoral TAVR improves clinical outcomes compared with active surveillance in patients with exercise-test proven asymptomatic severe AS; (ii) EASY-AS investigating whether either surgical or transcatheter AVR improves outcomes in asymptomatic severe AS; (iii) the EVOLVED trial testing whether early valve intervention improves clinical outcomes and evidence of replacement fibrosis (LGE) on CMR in patients with asymptomatic severe AS.

AVR for Moderate AS and Heart Failure

There is currently no indication for AVR in moderate AS patients, except if they undergo concomitant cardiac surgery (eg, coronary revascularization). However, in patients with impaired LV function, moderate AS may be deleterious, increasing cardiac afterload and associated with serious adverse events. Recent studies have demonstrated that moderate AS may have a detrimental impact on outcomes, particularly in the presence of reduced LVEF and with clinical evidence of heart failure.[202-204] These findings suggest that although moderate AS may be relatively well tolerated in patients with preserved LV systolic function, it may be poorly

tolerated in patients with depressed systolic function.[61,203,205] The cornerstone of many pharmacological treatments for systolic heart failure is to reduce LV afterload. Unfortunately, in patients with moderate AS, the afterload excess imposed by the AS is fixed and cannot be safely further reduced by pharmacotherapy. The hypothesis that early TAVR may improve outcomes of patients with moderate AS and systolic heart failure is being tested in the TAVR-UNLOAD trial. In this study, patients with systolic heart failure and moderate AS confirmed by rest and/or dobutamine stress echocardiography are randomized to optimized heart failure therapy alone versus optimized heart failure therapy plus TAVR (https://clinicaltrials.gov/ct2/show/NCT02661451).[206]

SUMMARY

Calcific AS is associated with a major healthcare and socioeconomic burden, which is growing sharply due to an aging global population. There is currently no preventive or pharmaco-therapeutic approach that has proven effective to slow or halt the progression of AS. The initial screening for AS is generally based on auscultation of a systolic murmur by primary care physicians and Doppler-echocardiography is the primary modality to diagnose AS severity as well as follow progression over time. Quantitation of aortic valve calcium by non-contrast CT may be useful to confirm stenosis severity in patients with an inconclusive echocardiographic exam, such as the case of patients with low-gradient AS. Besides the grading of AS severity, it is also important to assess the extent of cardiac damage associated with AS using a multi-parameter integrative echocardiographic approach. The only effective treatment for patients with symptomatic severe AS is to replace the aortic valve, predominantly using bioprostheses which are implanted using surgical or transcatheter approaches. Shared decision-making should involve referring physicians, a multi-disciplinary heart valve team, and patients and this process is essential to determine the indications and optimal timing for intervention, as well as the preferred type of AVR (TAVR vs SAVR).

Pathogenesis:

- Calcific aortic valve stenosis (AS) is a slowly progressive disease that starts with mild fibrosis, calcification and thickening of the valve leaflets and then evolves over the years to severe calcification with impaired leaflet mobility and significant obstruction to blood flow.

- There is currently no preventive or pharmaco-therapeutic approach that has proven effective to slow or halt the progression of AS.

Diagnosis:

- The initial screening for AS is generally based on auscultation of a systolic murmur by primary care physicians and Doppler-echocardiography is the primary modality to diagnose AS severity as well as follow progression over time.

- Quantitation of aortic valve calcium by non contrast CT may be useful to confirm stenosis severity in patients with an inconclusive echocardiographic exam, such as the case of patients with low-gradient AS.

- Besides the grading of AS severity, it is also important to assess the extent of cardiac damage associated with AS using a multi parameter integrative echocardiographic approach.

Management

- In patients with known AS, Doppler-echocardiography should be repeated every 1 to 2 years in addition to routine clinical follow-up to detect changes in AS severity, LV systolic function, and/or patient's symptomatic status.
- Patients with severe AS and symptoms or LV systolic dysfunction should be referred for aortic valve replacement.

Treatment:

- The only effective treatment for patients with symptomatic severe AS is to replace the aortic valve, predominantly using bioprostheses which are implanted using surgical or transcatheter approaches.
- Shared decision-making should involve referring physicians, a multi-disciplinary heart valve team, and patients and this process is essential to determine the indications and optimal timing for intervention.

REFERENCES

1. Lindman BR, Clavel MA, Mathieu P, et al. Calcific aortic stenosis. *Nat Rev Dis Primers.* 2016;2:16006.
2. Andell P, Li X, Martinsson A, et al. Epidemiology of valvular heart disease in a Swedish nationwide hospital-based register study. *Heart.* 2017;103(21):1696-1703.
3. Eveborn GW, Schirmer H, Heggelund G, Lunde P, Rasmussen K. The evolving epidemiology of valvular aortic stenosis. The Tromso Study. *Heart.* 2013;99(6):396-400.
4. Osnabrugge RL, Mylotte D, Head SJ, et al. Aortic stenosis in the elderly: disease prevalence and number of candidates for transcatheter aortic valve replacement: a meta-analysis and modeling study. *J Am Coll Cardiol.* 2013;62(11):1002-1012.
5. Vahanian A, Beyersdorf F, Praz F, et al. ESC/EACTS Scientific Document Group. 2021 ESC/EACTS. Guidelines for the management of valvular heart disease. *Eur Heart J.* 2021. Epub ahead of print.
6. Fedak PW, Verma S, David TE, Leask RL, Weisel RD, Butany J. Clinical and pathophysiological implications of a bicuspid aortic valve. *Circulation.* 2002;106(8):900-904.
7. Pawade TA, Newby DE, Dweck MR. Calcification in aortic stenosis: The skeleton key. *J Am Coll Cardiol.* 2015;66(5):561-577.
8. Stewart BF, Siscovick D, Lind BK, et al. Clinical factors associated with calcific aortic valve disease. Cardiovascular Health Study. *J Am Coll Cardiol.* 1997;29(3):630-634.
9. Stritzke J, Linsel-Nitschke P, Markus MR, et al. Association between degenerative aortic valve disease and long-term exposure to cardiovascular risk factors: results of the longitudinal population-based KORA/MONICA survey. *Eur Heart J.* 2009;30(16):2044-2053.
10. Yan AT, Koh M, Chan KK, et al. Association between cardiovascular risk factors and aortic stenosis: The CANHEART aortic stenosis study. *J Am Coll Cardiol.* 2017;69(12):1523-1532.
11. O'Brien KD, Reichenbach DD, Marcovina SM, Kuusisto J, Alpers CE, Otto CM. Apolipoproteins B, (a), and E accumulate in the morphologically early lesion of "degenerative" valvular aortic stenosis. *Arterioscler Thromb Vasc Biol.* 1996;16(4):523-532.
12. Côté C, Pibarot P, Després JP, et al. Association between circulating oxidised low-density lipoprotein and fibrocalcific remodelling of the aortic valve in aortic stenosis. *Heart.* 2008;94(9):1175-1180.
13. Thanassoulis G, Campbell CY, Owens DS, et al. Genetic associations with valvular calcification and aortic stenosis. *N Engl J Med.* 2013;368(6):503-512.
14. Chan KL, Teo K, Dumesnil JG, Ni A, Tam J. Effect of lipid lowering with rosuvastatin on progression of aortic stenosis. Results of the aortic stenosis progression observation: measuring effects of rosuvastatin (ASTRONOMER) trial. *Circulation.* 2010;121(2):306-314.
15. Cowell SJ, Newby DE, Prescott RJ, et al. A randomized trial of intensive lipid-lowering therapy in calcific aortic stenosis. *N Engl J Med.* 2005;352(23):2389-2397.
16. Rossebo AB, Pedersen TR, Boman K, et al. Intensive lipid lowering with simvastatin and ezetimibe in aortic stenosis. *N Engl J Med.* 2008;359(13):1343-1356.
17. Guauque-Olarte S, Messika-Zeitoun D, Droit A, et al. Calcium signalings pathway genes RUNX2 and CACNA1C are associated with calcific aortic valve disease. *Circ Cardiovasc Genet.* 2015;8(6):812-822.
18. Mohler ER, III, Gannon F, Reynolds C, Zimmerman R, Keane MG, Kaplan FS. Bone formation and inflammation in cardiac valves. *Circulation.* 2001;103(11):1522-1528.
19. Rosenhek R, Binder T, Porenta G, et al. Predictors of outcome in severe, asymptomatic aortic stenosis. *N Engl J Med.* 2000;343(9):611-617.
20. Jenkins WS, Vesey AT, Shah AS, et al. Valvular (18)F-fluoride and (18)F-fluorodeoxyglucose uptake predict disease progression and clinical outcome in patients with aortic stenosis. *J Am Coll Cardiol.* 2015;66(10):1200-1201.
21. Clavel MA, Messika-Zeitoun D, Pibarot P, et al. The complex nature of discordant severe calcified aortic valve disease grading: New insights from combined Doppler-echocardiographic and computed tomographic study. *J Am Coll Cardiol.* 2013;62(24):2329-2338.
22. Simard L, Côté N, Dagenais F, et al. Sex-related discordance between aortic valve calcification and hemodynamic severity of aortic stenosis: is valvular fibrosis the explanation? *Circ Res.* 2017;120(4):681-691.
23. Hein S, Arnon E, Kostin S, et al. Progression from compensated hypertrophy to failure in the pressure-overloaded human heart: structural deterioration and compensatory mechanisms. *Circulation.* 2003;107(7):984-991.
24. Galiuto L, Lotrionte M, Crea F, et al. Impaired coronary and myocardial flow in severe aortic stenosis is associated with increased apoptosis: a transthoracic Doppler and myocardial contrast echocardiography study. *Heart.* 2005.
25. Travers JG, Kamal FA, Robbins J, Yutzey KE, Blaxall BC. Cardiac fibrosis: The fibroblast awakens. *Circ Res.* 2016;118(6):1021-1040.
26. Everett RJ, Tastet L, Clavel MA, et al. Progression of hypertrophy and myocardial fibrosis in aortic stenosis: A multicenter cardiac magnetic resonance study. *Circ Cardiovasc Imaging.* 2018;11(6):e007451.
27. Treibel TA, López B, González A, et al. Reappraising myocardial fibrosis in severe aortic stenosis: an invasive and non-invasive study in 133 patients. *Eur Heart J.* 2018;39(8):699-709.
28. Dweck MR, Joshi S, Murigu T, et al. Left ventricular remodeling and hypertrophy in patients with aortic stenosis: insights from cardiovascular magnetic resonance. *J Cardiovasc Magn Reson.* 2012;14:50.
29. Dweck MR, Boon NA, Newby DE. Calcific aortic stenosis: a disease of the valve and the myocardium. *J Am Coll Cardiol.* 2012;60(19):1854-1863.
30. Dahl JS, Christensen NL, Videbaek L, et al. Left ventricular diastolic function is associated with symptom status in severe aortic valve stenosis. *Circ Cardiovasc Imaging.* 2014;7(1):142-148.
31. Zaid RR, Barker CM, Little SH, Nagueh SF. Pre- and post-operative diastolic dysfunction in patients with valvular heart disease: diagnosis and therapeutic implications. *J Am Coll Cardiol.* 2013;62(21):1922-1930.
32. Henkel DM, Malouf JF, Connolly HM, et al. Asymptomatic left ventricular systolic dysfunction in patients with severe aortic stenosis: characteristics and outcomes. *J Am Coll Cardiol.* 2012;60(22):2325-2329.
33. Otto CM, Nishimura RA, Bonow RO, et al. 2020 ACC/AHA Guideline for the Management of Patients With Valvular Heart Disease: A Report

of the American College of Cardiology/American Heart Association Joint Committee on Clinical Practice Guidelines. *J Am Coll Cardiol.* 2021;2;77(4):e25-e197.

34. Capoulade R, Le Ven F, Clavel MA, et al. Echocardiographic predictors of outcomes in adults with aortic stenosis. *Heart.* 2016;102:934-942.

35. Dahl JS, Eleid MF, Michelena HI, et al. Effect of left ventricular ejection fraction on postoperative outcome in patients with severe aortic stenosis undergoing aortic valve replacement. *Circ Cardiovasc Imaging.* 2015;8(4).

36. Ito S, Miranda WR, Nkomo VT, et al. Reduced left ventricular ejection fraction in patients with aortic stenosis. *J Am Coll Cardiol.* 2018;71(12):1313-1321.

37. Herrmann S, Stork S, Niemann M, et al. Low-gradient aortic valve stenosis: Myocardial fibrosis and its influence on function and outcome. *J Am Coll Cardiol.* 2011;58(4):402-412.

38. Vollema EM, Sugimoto T, Shen M, et al. Association of left ventricular global longitudinal strain with asymptomatic severe aortic stenosis natural course and prognostic value. *JAMA Cardiol.* 2018;3(9):839-847.

39. Dahou A, Bartko PE, Capoulade R, et al. Usefulness of global left ventricular longitudinal strain for risk stratification in low ejection fraction, low-gradient aortic stenosis: results from the multicenter True or Pseudo-Severe Aortic Stenosis study. *Circ Cardiovasc Imaging.* 2015;8(3):e002117.

40. Yingchoncharoen T, Gibby C, Rodriguez LL, Grimm RA, Marwick TH. Association of myocardial deformation with outcome in asymptomatic aortic stenosis with normal ejection fraction. *Circ Cardiovasc Imaging.* 2012;5(6):719-725.

41. Magne J, Cosyns B, Popescu BA, et al. Distribution and prognostic significance of left ventricular global longitudinal strain in asymptomatic significant aortic stenosis: an individual participant data meta-analysis. *JACC Cardiovasc Imaging.* 2019;12(1):84-92.

42. Clavel MA, Magne J, Pibarot P. Low-gradient aortic stenosis. *Eur Heart J.* 2016;37(34):2645-2657.

43. Pibarot P. Low flow low gradient aortic stenosis. *JACC Journals.* 2015.

44. Hachicha Z, Dumesnil JG, Bogaty P, Pibarot P. Paradoxical low flow, low gradient severe aortic stenosis despite preserved ejection fraction is associated with higher afterload and reduced survival. *Circulation.* 2007;115(22):2856-2864.

45. Rajappan K, Rimoldi O, Camici PG, Pennell DJ, Sheridan DJ. Factors influencing coronary microcirculatory function in patients with aortic stenosis after aortic valve replacement. *Circulation.* 2002;106(19):II-640.

46. Marcus ML, Doty DB, Hiratzka LF, Wright CB, Eastham CL. Decreased coronary reserve: a mechanism for angina pectoris in patients with aortic stenosis and normal coronary arteries. *N Engl J Med.* 1982;307(22):1362-1366.

47. Gould KL, Carabello BA. Why angina in aortic stenosis with normal coronary arteriograms? *Circulation.* 2003;107(25):3121-3123.

48. Galderisi M, de Simone G, D'Errico A, et al. Independent association of coronary flow reserve with left ventricular relaxation and filling pressure in arterial hypertension. *Am J Hypertens.* 2008;21(9):1040-1046.

49. Carabello BA. Syncope in aortic stenosis: Is it too late to wait? *JACC Cardiovasc Imaging.* 2019;12(2):233-235.

50. Park SJ, Enriquez-Sarano M, Chang SA, et al. Hemodynamic patterns for symptomatic presentations of severe aortic stenosis. *JACC Cardiovasc Imaging.* 2013;6(2):137-146.

51. Das P, Rimington H, Chambers J. Exercise testing to stratify risk in aortic stenosis. *Eur Heart J.* 2005;26(13):1309-1313.

52. Siliste RN, Siliste C. Physical examination in aortic valve disease: do we still need it in the modern era? *e-Journal of Cardiology Practice.* 2020;18(12).

53. d'Arcy JL, Coffey S, Loudon MA, et al. Large-scale community echocardiographic screening reveals a major burden of undiagnosed valvular heart disease in older people: the OxVALVE Population Cohort Study. *Eur Heart J.* 2016;37(47):3515-3522.

54. Gardezi SKM, Myerson SG, Chambers J, et al. Cardiac auscultation poorly predicts the presence of valvular heart disease in asymptomatic primary care patients. *Heart.* 2018;104(22):1832-1835.

55. Nishimura RA, Otto CM, Bonow RO, et al. 2014 AHA/ACC guideline for the management of patients with valvular heart disease: a report of the American College of Cardiology/American Heart Association Task Force on Practice Guidelines. *J Am Coll Cardiol.* 2014;63(22):e57-e185.

56. Thaden JJ, Nkomo VT, Lee KJ, Oh JK. Doppler imaging in aortic stenosis: the importance of the nonapical imaging windows to determine severity in a contemporary cohort. *J Am Soc Echocardiogr.* 2015;28(7):780-785.

57. Delgado V, Clavel MA, Hahn RT, et al. How do we reconcile echocardiography, computed tomography, and hybrid imaging in assessing discordant grading of aortic stenosis severity? *JACC Cardiovasc Imaging.* 2019;12(2):267-282.

58. Hahn RT, Pibarot P. Accurate measurement of left ventricular outflow tract diameter: comment on the updated recommendations for the echocardiographic assessment of aortic valve stenosis. *J Am Soc Echocardiogr.* 2017;30(10):1038-1041.

59. Garcia D, Pibarot P, Dumesnil JG, Sakr F, Durand LG. Assessment of aortic valve stenosis severity: A new index based on the energy loss concept. *Circulation.* 2000;101(7):765-771.

60. Bahlmann E, Gerdts E, Cramariuc D, et al. Prognostic value of energy loss index in asymptomatic aortic stenosis. *Circulation.* 2013;127(10):1149-1156.

61. Clavel MA, Fuchs C, Burwash IG, et al. Predictors of outcomes in low-flow, low-gradient aortic stenosis: results of the multicenter TOPAS Study. *Circulation.* 2008;118(14 Suppl):S234-S242.

62. Dayan V, Vignolo G, Magne J, Clavel MA, Mohty D, Pibarot P. Outcome and impact of aortic valve replacement in patients with preserved LV ejection fraction and low gradient aortic stenosis: a meta-analysis. *J Am Coll Cardiol.* 2015;66(23):2594-2603.

63. Namasivayam M, He W, Churchill TW, et al. Transvalvular flow rate determines prognostic value of aortic valve area in aortic stenosis. *J Am Coll Cardiol.* 2020;75(15):1758-1769.

64. Baumgartner H, Hung J, Bermejo J, et al. Recommendations on the echocardiographic assessment of aortic valve stenosis: a focused update from the European Association of Cardiovascular Imaging and the American Society of Echocardiography. *J Am Soc Echocardiogr.* 2017;30(4):372-392.

65. Vahanian A, Alfieri O, Andreotti F, et al. Guidelines on the management of valvular heart disease (version 2012). *Eur Heart J.* 2012;33(19):2451-2496.

66. Annabi MS, Touboul E, Dahou A, et al. Dobutamine stress echocardiography for management of low-flow, low-gradient aortic stenosis. *J Am Coll Cardiol.* 2018;71(5):475-485.

67. Nishimura RA, Otto CM, Bonow RO, et al. 2017 AHA/ACC focused update of the 2014 AHA/ACC guideline for the management of patients with valvular heart disease: a report of the American College of Cardiology/American Heart Association Task Force on clinical practice guidelines. *J Am Coll Cardiol.* 2017;70(2):252-289.

68. Lancellotti P, Magne J, Dulgheru R, et al. Outcomes of patients with asymptomatic aortic stenosis followed up in heart valve clinics. *JAMA Cardiol.* 2018;3(11):1060-1068.

69. Généreux P, Pibarot P, Redfors B, et al. Staging classification of aortic stenosis based on the extent of cardiac damage. *Eur Heart J.* 2017;38(45):3351-3358.

70. Tastet L, Tribouilloy C, Maréchaux S, et al. Staging cardiac damage in patients with asymptomatic aortic valve stenosis. *J Am Coll Cardiol.* 2019;74(4):550-563.

71. Vollema EM, Amanullah MR, Ng ACT, et al. Staging cardiac damage in patients with symptomatic aortic valve stenosis. *J Am Coll Cardiol.* 2019;74(4):538-549.

72. Fukui M, Gupta A, Abdelkarim I, et al. Association of structural and functional cardiac changes with transcatheter aortic valve replacement outcomes in patients with aortic stnosis. *JAMA Cardiol.* 2019;4(3):215-222.

73. Pawade T, Sheth T, Guzzetti E, Dweck MR, Clavel MA. Why and how to measure aortic valve calcification in patients with aortic stenosis. *JACC Cardiovasc Imaging.* 2019;12(9):1835-1848.

74. Agatston AS, Janowitz WR, Hildner FJ, Zusmer NR, Viamonte M, Detrano R. Quantification of coronary artery calcium using ultrafast computed tomography. *J Am Coll Cardiol.* 1990;15(4):827-832.

75. Agatston AS, Janowitz WR, Hildner FJ, Zusmer NR, Viamonte M, Jr, Detrano R. Quantification of coronary artery calcium using ultrafast computed tomography. *J Am Coll Cardiol.* 1990;15(4):827-832.

76. Aggarwal SR, Clavel MA, Messika-Zeitoun D, et al. Sex differences in aortic valve calcification measured by multidetector computed tomography in aortic stenosis. *Circ Cardiovasc Imaging.* 2013;6(1):40-47.

77. Clavel MA, Pibarot P, Messika-Zeitoun D, et al. Impact of aortic valve calcification, as measured by MDCT, on survival in patients with aortic stenosis: results of an international registry study. *J Am Coll Cardiol.* 2014;64(12):1202-1213.

78. Pawade T, Clavel MA, Tribouilloy C, et al. Computed tomography aortic valve calcium scoring in patients with aortic stenosis. *Circ Cardiovasc Imaging.* 2018;11(3):e007146.

79. Tastet L, Enriquez-Sarano M, Capoulade R, et al. Impact of aortic valve calcification and sex on hemodynamic progression and clinical outcomes in AS. *J Am Coll Cardiol.* 2017;69(16):2096-2098.

80. Voisine M, Hervault M, Shen M, et al. Age, sex, and valve phenotype differences in fibro-calcific remodeling of calcified aortic valve. *J Am Heart Assoc.* 2020:e015610.

81. Dweck MR, Jenkins WS, Vesey AT, et al. 18F-NaF uptake Is a marker of active calcification and disease progression in patients with aortic stenosis. *Circ Cardiovasc Imaging.* 2014;7(2):371-378.

82. Nakamoto Y, Kitagawa T, Sasaki K, et al. Clinical implications of (18) F-sodium fluoride uptake in subclinical aortic valve calcification: Its relation to coronary atherosclerosis and its predictive value. *J Nucl Cardiol.* 2019.

83. Zheng KH, Tsimikas S, Pawade T, et al. Lipoprotein(a) and oxidized phospholipids promote valve calcification in patients with aortic stenosis. *J Am Coll Cardiol.* 2019;73(17):2150-2162.

84. Myerson SG. Heart valve disease: investigation by cardiovascular magnetic resonance. *J Cardiovasc Magn Reson.* 2012;14:7.

85. Kwiecinski J, Chin CWL, Everett RJ, et al. Adverse prognosis associated with asymmetric myocardial thickening in aortic stenosis. *Eur Heart J Cardiovasc Imaging.* 2018;19(3):347-356.

86. Bing R, Cavalcante JL, Everett RJ, Clavel MA, Newby DE, Dweck MR. Imaging and impact of myocardial fibrosis in aortic stenosis. *JACC Cardiovasc Imaging.* 2019;12(2):283-296.

87. Rudolph A, Abdel-Aty H, Bohl S, et al. Noninvasive detection of fibrosis applying contrast-enhanced cardiac magnetic resonance in different forms of left ventricular hypertrophy relation to remodeling. *J Am Coll Cardiol.* 2009;53(3):284-291.

88. Wu E, Judd RM, Vargas JD, Klocke FJ, Bonow RO, Kim RJ. Visualisation of presence, location, and transmural extent of healed Q-wave and non-Q-wave myocardial infarction. *Lancet.* 2001;357(9249):21-28.

89. Weidemann F, Herrmann S, Stork S, et al. Impact of myocardial fibrosis in patients with symptomatic severe aortic stenosis. *Circulation.* 2009;120(7):577-584.

90. Azevedo CF, Nigri M, Higuchi ML, et al. Prognostic significance of myocardial fibrosis quantification by histopathology and magnetic resonance imaging in patients with severe aortic valve disease. *J Am Coll Cardiol.* 2010;56(4):278-287.

91. Dweck MR, Joshi S, Murigu T, et al. Midwall fibrosis is an independent predictor of mortality in patients with aortic stenosis. *J Am Coll Cardiol.* 2011;58(12):1271-1279.

92. Barone-Rochette G, Pierard S, de Meester de Ravenstein C, et al. Prognostic significance of LGE by CMR in aortic stenosis patients undergoing valve replacement. *J Am Coll Cardiol.* 2014;64(2):144-154.

93. Musa TA, Treibel TA, Vassiliou VS, et al. Myocardial scar and mortality in severe aortic stenosis. *Circulation.* 2018;138(18):1935-1947.

94. Krayenbuehl HP, Hess OM, Monrad ES, Schneider J, Mall G, Turina M. Left ventricular myocardial structure in aortic valve disease before, intermediate, and late after aortic valve replacement. *Circulation.* 1989;79(4):744-755.

95. Bull S, White SK, Piechnik SK, et al. Human non-contrast T1 values and correlation with histology in diffuse fibrosis. *Heart.* 2013;99(13):932-937.

96. Lee SP, Lee W, Lee JM, et al. Assessment of diffuse myocardial fibrosis by using MR imaging in asymptomatic patients with aortic stenosis. *Radiology.* 2015;274(2):359-369.

97. Kockova R, Kacer P, Pirk J, et al. Native T1 relaxation time and extracellular volume fraction as accurate markers of diffuse myocardial fibrosis in heart valve disease- comparison with targeted left ventricular myocardial biopsy. *Circ J.* 2016;80(5):1202-1209.

98. Chin CW, Semple S, Malley T, et al. Optimization and comparison of myocardial T1 techniques at 3T in patients with aortic stenosis. *Eur Heart J Cardiovasc Imaging.* 2014;15(5):556-565.

99. Podlesnikar T, Delgado V, Bax JJ. Cardiovascular magnetic resonance imaging to assess myocardial fibrosis in valvular heart disease. *International J Cardiovasc Imaging.* 2018;34(1):97-112.

100. Flett AS, Hayward MP, Ashworth MT, et al. Equilibrium contrast cardiovascular magnetic resonance for the measurement of diffuse myocardial fibrosis: preliminary validation in humans. *Circulation.* 2010;122(2):138-144.

101. Wong TC, Piehler K, Meier CG, et al. Association between extracellular matrix expansion quantified by cardiovascular magnetic resonance and short-term mortality. *Circulation.* 2012;126(10):1206-1216.

102. Ugander M, Oki AJ, Hsu LY, et al. Extracellular volume imaging by magnetic resonance imaging provides insights into overt and sub-clinical myocardial pathology. *Eur Heart J.* 2012;33(10):1268-1278.

103. Shah AS, Chin CW, Vassiliou V, et al. Left ventricular hypertrophy with strain and aortic stenosis. *Circulation.* 2014;130(18):1607-1620.

104. Chin CW, Shah AS, McAllister DA, et al. High-sensitivity troponin I concentrations are a marker of an advanced hypertrophic response and adverse outcomes in patients with aortic stenosis. *Eur Heart J.* 2014;35(34):2312-2321.

105. Chin CW, Everett RJ, Kwiecinski J, et al. Myocardial fibrosis and cardiac decompensation in aortic stenosis. *JACC Cardiovasc Imaging.* 2017;10(11):1320-1333.

106. Everett RJ, Treibel TA, Fukui M, et al. Extracellular myocardial volume in patients with aortic stenosis. *J Am Coll Cardiol.* 2020;75(3):304-316.

107. Garcia D, Dumesnil JG, Durand LG, Kadem L, Pibarot P. Discrepancies between catheter and Doppler estimates of valve effective orifice area can be predicted from the pressure recovery phenomenon: Practical implications with regard to quantification of aortic stenosis severity. *J Am Coll Cardiol.* 2003;41(3):435-442.

108. Gjertsson P, Caidahl K, Svensson G, Wallentin I, Bech-Hanssen O. Important pressure recovery in patients with aortic stenosis and high Doppler gradients. *Am J Cardiol.* 2001;88(2):139-144.

109. Bergler-Klein J, Klaar U, Heger M, et al. Natriuretic peptides predict symptom-free survival and postoperative outcome in severe aortic Stenosis. *Circulation.* 2004;109:2302-2308.

110. Weber M, Hausen M, Arnold R, et al. Prognostic value of N-terminal pro-B-type natriuretic peptide for conservatively and surgically treated patients with aortic valve stenosis. *Heart.* 2006;92(11):1639-1644.

111. Capoulade R, Magne J, Dulgheru R, et al. Prognostic value of plasma B-type natriuretic peptide levels after exercise in patients with severe asymptomatic aortic stenosis. *Heart.* 2014;100(20):1606-1612.

112. Clavel MA, Malouf J, Michelena HI, et al. B-type natriuretic peptide clinical activation in aortic stenosis: Impact on long-term survival. *J Am Coll Cardiol.* 2014;63(19):2016-2025.

113. Henri C, Dulgheru R, Magne J, et al. Impact of serial B-Type natriuretic peptide changes for predicting outcome in asymptomatic patients with aortic stenosis. *Can J Cardiol.* 2016;32(2):183-189.

114. Bergler-Klein J, Mundigler G, Pibarot P, et al. B-type natriuretic peptide in low-flow, low-gradient aortic stenosis: relationship to hemodynamics and clinical outcome. *Circulation.* 2007;115(22):2848-2855.

115. Bergler-Klein J, Gyöngyosi M, Maurer G. The role of biomarkers in valvular heart disease: Focus on natriuretic peptides. *Can J Cardiol.* 2014;30(9):1027-1034.

116. Mahajan VS, Jarolim P. How to interpret elevated cardiac troponin levels. *Circulation.* 2011;124(21):2350-2354.

117. Rosjo H, Andreassen J, Edvardsen T, Omland T. Prognostic usefulness of circulating high-sensitivity troponin T in aortic stenosis and relation to echocardiographic indexes of cardiac function and anatomy. *Am J Cardiol.* 2011;108(1):88-91.

118. Lancellotti P, Dulgheru R, Magne J, et al. Elevated plasma soluble ST2 Is associated with heart failure symptoms and outcome in aortic stenosis. *PLoS One.* 2015;10(9):e0138940.

119. Krau NC, Lunstedt NS, Freitag-Wolf S, et al. Elevated growth differentiation factor 15 levels predict outcome in patients undergoing transcatheter aortic valve implantation. *Eur J Heart Fail.* 2015;17(9):945-955.

120. Baldenhofer G, Zhang K, Spethmann S, et al. Galectin-3 predicts short- and long-term outcome in patients undergoing transcatheter aortic valve implantation (TAVI). *Int J Cardiol.* 2014;177(3):912-917.

121. Lindman BR, Breyley JG, Schilling JD, et al. Prognostic utility of novel biomarkers of cardiovascular stress in patients with aortic stenosis undergoing valve replacement. *Heart.* 2015;101(17):1382-1388.

122. Badheka AO, Singh V, Patel NJ, et al. Trends of hospitalizations in the United States from 2000 to 2012 of patients >60 years with aortic valve disease. *Am J Cardiol.* 2015;116(1):132-141.

123. Martinsson A, Li X, Andersson C, Nilsson J, Smith JG, Sundquist K. Temporal trends in the incidence and prognosis of aortic stenosis: a nationwide study of the Swedish population. *Circulation.* 2015;131(11):988-994.

124. Berry C, Lloyd SM, Wang Y, Macdonald A, Ford I. The changing course of aortic valve disease in Scotland: temporal trends in hospitalizations and mortality and prognostic importance of aortic stenosis. *Eur Heart J.* 2013;34(21):1538-1547.

125. McCoy CM, Nicholas DQ, Masters KS. Sex-related differences in gene expression by porcine aortic valvular interstitial cells. *PLoS One.* 2012;7(7):e39980.

126. Nordstrom P, Glader CA, Dahlen G, et al. Oestrogen receptor alpha gene polymorphism is related to aortic valve sclerosis in postmenopausal women. *J Intern Med.* 2003;254(2):140-146.

127. Parra-Izquierdo I, Castanos-Mollor I, Lopez J, et al. Calcification Induced by Type I Interferon in Human Aortic Valve Interstitial Cells Is Larger in Males and Blunted by a Janus Kinase Inhibitor. *Arterioscler Thromb Vasc Biol.* 2018;38(9):2148-2159.

128. Cramariuc D, Rieck AE, Staal EM, et al. Factors influencing left ventricular structure and stress-corrected systolic function in men and women with asymptomatic aortic valve stenosis (a SEAS Substudy). *Am J Cardiol.* 2008;101(4):510-515.

129. Capoulade R, Clavel MA, Le Ven F, et al. Impact of left ventricular remodelling patterns on outcomes in patients with aortic stenosis. *Eur Heart J Cardiovasc Imaging.* 2017;18(12):1378-1387.

130. Douglas PS, Katz SE, Weinberg EO, Chen MH, Bishop SP, Lorell BH. Hypertrophy remodeling: gender differences in the early response to left ventrcular pressure overload. *J Am Coll Cardiol.* 1998;32(4):1118-1125.

131. Gjesdal O, Bluemke DA, Lima JA. Cardiac remodeling at the population level–risk factors, screening, and outcomes. *Nat Rev Cardiol.* 2011;8(12):673-685.

132. Liu CY, Liu YC, Wu C, et al. Evaluation of age-related interstitial myocardial fibrosis with cardiac magnetic resonance contrast-enhanced T1 mapping: MESA (Multi-Ethnic Study of Atherosclerosis). *J Am Coll Cardiol.* 2013;62(14):1280-1287.

133. Villar AV, Llano M, Cobo M, Expósito V, Merino R, Martín-Durán R, Hurlé MA, Nistal JF. Gender differences of echocardiographic and gene expression patterns in human pressure overload left ventricular hypertrophy. *J Mol Cell Cardiol.* 2009 Apr;46(4):526-35.

134. Treibel TA, Kozor R, Fontana M, et al. Sex dimorphism in the myocardial response to aortic stenosis. *JACC Cardiovasc Imaging.* 2018;11(7):962-973.

135. Chaker Z, Badhwar V, Alqahtani F, et al. Sex differences in the utilization and outcomes of surgical aortic valve replacement for severe aortic stenosis. *J Am Heart Assoc.* 2017;6(9).

136. Vaturi M, Shapira Y, Rotstein M, et al. The effect of aortic valve replacement on left ventricular mass assessed by echocardiography. *Eur J Echocardiography.* 2000;1:116-121.

137. Onorati F, D'Errigo P, Barbanti M, et al. Different impact of sex on baseline characteristics and major periprocedural outcomes of transcatheter and surgical aortic valve interventions: Results of the multicenter Italian OBSERVANT Registry. *J Thorac Cardiovasc Surg.* 2014;147(5):1529-1539.

138. Stamou SC, Robich M, Wolf RE, Lovett A, Normand S-LT, Sellke FW. Effects of gender and ethnicity on outcomes after aortic valve replacement. *J Thorac Cardiovasc Surg.* 2012;144(2):486-492.

139. Brown JM, O'Brien SM, Wu C, Sikora JA, Griffith BP, Gammie JS. Isolated aortic valve replacement in North America comprising 108,687 patients in 10 years: changes in risks, valve types, and outcomes in the Society of Thoracic Surgeons National Database. *J Thorac Cardiovasc Surg.* 2009;137(1):82-90.

140. Popma JJ, Khabbaz K. Prosthesis-patient mismatch after "high-risk" aortic valve replacement. *J Am Coll Cardiol.* 2014;64(13):1335-1338.

141. Urso S, Sadaba R, Vives M, et al. Patient-prosthesis mismatch in elderly patients undergoing aortic valve replacement: impact on quality of life and survival. *J Heart Valve Dis.* 2009;18(3):248-255.

142. Tasca G, Brunelli F, Cirillo M, et al. Impact of the improvement of valve area achieved with aortic valve replacement on the regression of left ventricular hypertrophy in patients with pure aortic stenosis. *Ann Thorac Surg.* 2005;79(4):1291-1296.

143. Fuster RG, Montero Argudo JA, Albarova OG, et al. Patient-prosthesis mismatch in aortic valve replacement: really tolerable? *Eur J Cardiothorac Surg.* 2005;27(3):441-449.

144. Nozohoor S, Nilsson J, Luhrs C, Roijer A, Sjogren J. The influence of patient-prosthesis mismatch on in-hospital complications and early mortality after aortic valve replacement. *J Heart Valve Dis.* 2007;16(5):475-482.

145. Astudillo LM, Santana O, Urbandt PA, et al. Clinical predictors of prosthesis-patient mismatch after aortic valve replacement for aortic stenosis. *Clinics (Sao Paulo).* 2012;67(1):55-60.

146. Hernandez-Vaquero D, Garcia JM, Diaz R, et al. Moderate patient-prosthesis mismatch predicts cardiac events and advanced functional class in young and middle-aged patients undergoing surgery due to severe aortic stenosis. *J Card Surg.* 2014;29(2):127-133.

147. Kandler K, Moller CH, Hassager C, Olsen PS, Lilleor N, Steinbruchel DA. Patient-prosthesis mismatch and reduction in left ventricular mass after aortic valve replacement. *Ann Thorac Surg.* 2013;96(1):66-71.

148. Ter Woorst JF, Hoff AHT, van Straten AHM, Houterman S, Soliman-Hamad MA. Impact of sex on the outcome of isolated aortic valve replacement and the role of different preoperative profiles. *J Cardiothorac Vasc Anesth.* 2019;33(5):1237-1243.

149. Panoulas VF, Francis DP, Ruparelia N, et al. Female-specific survival advantage from transcatheter aortic valve implantation over surgical aortic valve replacement: Meta-analysis of the gender subgroups of randomised controlled trials including 3758 patients. *Int J Cardiol.* 2018;250:66-72.

150. Smith CR, Leon MB, Mack MJ, et al. Transcatheter versus surgical aortic-valve replacement in high-risk patients. *N Engl J Med.* 2011;364(23):2187-2198.

151. Adams DH, Popma JJ, Reardon MJ, et al. Transcatheter aortic-valve replacement with a self-expanding prosthesis. *N Engl J Med.* 2014;370(19):1790-1798.

152. Leon MB, Smith CR, Mack MJ, et al. Transcatheter or surgical aortic-valve replacement in intermediate-risk patients. *N Engl J Med.* 2016;374(17):1609-1620.

153. Mack MJ, Leon MB, Thourani VH, et al. Transcatheter aortic-valve replacement with a balloon-expandable valve in low-risk patients. *N Engl J Med.* 2019;380(18):1695-1705.

154. Stangl V, Baldenhofer G, Laule M, Baumann G, Stangl K. Influence of sex on outcome following transcatheter aortic valve implantation (TAVI): systematic review and meta-analysis. *J Interv Cardiol.* 2014;27(6):531-539.

155. Connolly HM, Oh JK, Orszulak TA, et al. Aortic valve replacement for aortic stenosis with severe left ventricular dysfunction: prognostic indicators. *Circulation.* 1997;95(10):2395-2400.

156. Williams M, Kodali SK, Hahn RT, et al. Sex-related differences in outcomes following transcatheter or surgical aortic valve replacement in patients with severe aortic stenosis: insights from the PARTNER Trial. *J Am Coll Cardiol.* 2014;63(15):1522-1528.

157. Pibarot P, Weissman NJ, Stewart WJ, et al. Incidence and sequelae of prosthesis-patient mismatch in transcatheter versus surgical valve replacement in high-risk patients with severe aortic stenosis—A PARTNER trial cohort A analysis. *J Am Coll Cardio.* 2014;64(13):1323-1334.

158. Abdel-Wahab M, Zahn R, Horack M, et al. Aortic regurgitation after transcatheter aortic valve implantation: incidence and early outcome. Results from the German transcatheter aortic valve interventions registry. *Heart.* 2011;97(11):899-906.

159. Unbehaun A, Pasic M, Dreysse S, et al. Transapical aortic valve implantation: incidence and predictors of paravalvular leakage and transvalvular regurgitation in a series of 358 patients. *J Am Coll Cardiol.* 2012;59(3):211-221.

160. Akodad M, Lattuca B, Agullo A, et al. Prognostic impact of calcium score after transcatheter aortic valve implantation performed with new generation prosthesis. *Am J Cardiol.* 2018;121(10):1225-1230.

161. Ewe SH, Ng AC, Schuijf JD, et al. Location and severity of aortic valve calcium and implications for aortic regurgitation after transcatheter aortic valve implantation. *Am J Cardiol.* 2011;108(10):1470-1477.

162. Fujita B, Kütting M, Seiffert M, et al. Calcium distribution patterns of the aortic valve as a risk factor for the need of permanent pacemaker implantation after transcatheter aortic valve implantation. *Eur Heart J Cardiovasc Imaging.* 2016;17(12):1385-1393.

163. Patel DK, Green KD, Fudim M, Harrell FE, Wang TJ, Robbins MA. Racial differences in the prevalence of severe aortic stenosis. *J Am Heart Assoc.* 2014;3(3):e000879.

164. Beydoun HA, Beydoun MA, Liang H, et al. Sex, race, and socioeconomic disparities in patients with aortic stenosis (from a nationwide inpatient sample). *Am J Cardiol.* 2016;118(6):860-865.

165. Alkhouli M, Holmes DR, Carroll JD, et al. Racial disparities in the utilization and outcomes of TAVR: TVT registry report. 2019;12(10):936-948.

166. Alqahtani F, Aljohani S, Amin AH, et al. Effect of race on the incidence of aortic stenosis and outcomes of aortic valve replacement in the United States. *Mayo Clin Proc.* 2018;93(5):607-617.

167. Chandra S, Lang RM, Nicolarsen J, et al. Bicuspid aortic valve: inter-racial difference in frequency and aortic dimensions. *JACC Cardiovasc Imaging.* 2012;5(10):981-989.

168. Jilaihawi H, Wu Y, Yang Y, et al. Morphological characteristics of severe aortic stenosis in China: imaging corelab observations from the first Chinese transcatheter aortic valve trial. *Catheter Cardiovasc Interv.* 2015;85 (Suppl 1):752-761.

169. Liu F, Yang YN, Xie X, et al. Prevalence of congenital heart disease in Xinjiang multi-ethnic region of China. *PLoS One.* 2015;10(8):e0133961.

170. Pellikka PA, Sarano ME, Nishimura RA, et al. Outcome of 622 adults with asymptomatic, hemodynamically significant aortic stenosis during prolonged follow-up. *Circulation.* 2005;111(24):3290-3295.

171. Leon MB, Smith CR, Mack M, et al. Transcatheter aortic-valve implantation for aortic stenosis in patients who cannot undergo surgery. *N Eng J Med.* 2010;363(17):1597-1607.

172. Mack MJ, Leon MB, Smith CR, et al. 5-year outcomes of transcatheter aortic valve replacement or surgical aortic valve replacement for high surgical risk patients with aortic stenosis (PARTNER 1): a randomised controlled trial. *Lancet.* 2015;385(9986):2477-2484.

173. Thyregod HG, Steinbruchel DA, Ihlemann N, et al. Transcatheter versus surgical aortic valve replacement in patients with severe aortic valve stenosis: one-year results from the all-comers Nordic Aortic Valve Intervention (NOTION) randomized clinical trial. *J Am Coll Cardiol.* 2015;65(20):2184-2194.

174. Thourani VH, Kodali S, Makkar RR, et al. Transcatheter aortic valve replacement versus surgical valve replacement in intermediate-risk patients: a propensity score analysis. *Lancet.* 2016;387(10034):2218-2225.

175. Reardon MJ, Van Mieghem NM, Popma JJ, et al. Surgical or transcatheter aortic-valve replacement in intermediate-risk patients. *N Engl J Med.* 2017;376(14):1321-1331.

176. Popma JJ, Deeb GM, Yakubov SJ, et al. Transcatheter aortic-valve replacement with a self-expanding valve in low-risk patients. *N Engl J Med.* 2019;380(18):1706-1715.

177. Asgar AW, Ouzounian M, Adams C, et al. 2019 Canadian Cardiovascular Society position statement for aortic valve implantation. *Can J Cardiol.* 2019;35(11):1437-1448.

178. Elbadawi A, Saad M, Elgendy IY, et al. Temporal trends and outcomes of transcatheter versus surgical aortic valve replacement for bicuspid aortic valve stenosis. *JACC Cardiovasc Interv.* 2019;12(18):1811-1822.

179. Forrest JK, Kaple RK, Ramlawi B, et al. Transcatheter aortic valve replacement in bicuspid versus tricuspid aortic valves from the STS/ACC TVT registry. *JACC Cardiovasc Interv.* 2020;13(15):1749-1759.

180. Halim SA, Edwards FH, Dai D, et al. Outcomes of transcatheter aortic valve replacement in patients with bicuspid aortic valve disease: A report from the Society of Thoracic Surgeons/American College of Cardiology Transcatheter Valve Therapy Registry. *Circulation.* 2020;141(13):1071-1079.

181. Yoon SH, Kim WK, Dhoble A, et al. Bicuspid aortic valve morphology and outcomes after transcatheter aortic valve replacement. *J Am Coll Cardiol.* 2020;76(9):1018-1030.

182. Lindman BR, Alexander KP, O'Gara PT, Afilalo J. Futility, benefit, and transcatheter aortic valve replacement. *JACC Cardiovasc Interv.* 2014;7(7):707-716.

183. Pibarot P, Dumesnil JG. Prosthetic heart valves: Selection of the optimal prosthesis and long-term management. *Circulation.* 2009;119(7):1034-1048.

184. Salaun E, Mahjoub H, Girerd N, et al. Rate, timing, correlates, and outcomes of hemodynamic valve deterioration after bioprosthetic surgical aortic valve replacement. *Circulation.* 2018;138:971-985.

185. Tasca G, Vismara R, Mangini A, et al. Comparison of the performance of a sutureless bioprosthesis with two pericardial stented valves on small annuli: an in vitro study. *Ann Thorac Surg.* 2017;103(1):139-144.

186. Takagi H, Umemoto T. A meta-analysis of sutureless or rapid-deployment aortic valve replacement. *Thorac Cardiovasc Surg.* 2016;64(5):400-409.

187. Kamperidis V, van Rosendael PJ, de Weger A, et al. Surgical sutureless and transcatheter aortic valves: hemodynamic performance and clinical outcomes in propensity score-matched high-risk populations with severe aortic stenosis. *JACC Cardiovasc Interv.* 2015;8(5):670-677.

188. Pibarot P, Dumesnil JG. Prosthesis-patient mismatch: definition, clinical impact, and prevention. *Heart.* 2006;92(8):1022-1029.

189. Dayan V, Vignolo G, Soca G, Paganini JJ, Brusich D, Pibarot P. Predictors and outcomes of prosthesis patient mismatch after aortic valve replacement. *JACC Cardiovasc Imaging.* 2016;9(8):924-933.

190. Rieck AE, Cramariuc D, Boman K, et al. Hypertension in aortic stenosis: implications for left ventricular structure and cardiovascular events. *Hypertension.* 2012;60(1):90-97.

191. Côté N, Simard L, Zenses AS, et al. Impact of vascular hemodynamics on aortic stenosis evaluation: new insights into the pathophysiology of normal flow-small aortic valve area-low gradient pattern. *J Am Heart Assoc.* 2017;6(7).

192. Kadem L, Dumesnil JG, Rieu R, Durand LG, Garcia D, Pibarot P. Impact of systemic hypertension on the assessment of aortic stenosis. *Heart.* 2005;91(3):354-361.

193. Tastet L, Capoulade R, Clavel MA, et al. Systolic hypertension and progression of aortic valve calcification in patients with aortic stenosis: results from the PROGRESSA study. *Eur Heart J Cardiovasc Imaging.* 2017;18(1):70-78.

194. Rattazzi M, Faggin E, Bertacco E, et al. Warfarin, but not rivaroxaban, promotes the calcification of the aortic valve in ApoE-/- mice. *Cardiovasc Ther.* 2018;36(4):e12438.

195. Tastet L, Pibarot P, Shen M, et al. Oral anticoagulation therapy and progression of calcific aortic valve stenosis. *J Am Coll Cardiol.* 2019;73(14):1869-1871.

196. Jonas M, Rozenman Y, Moshkovitz Y, et al. The Leaflex Catheter System- a viable treatment option alongside valve replacement? Preclinical feasibility of a novel device designed for fracturing aortic valve calcification. *EuroIntervention.* 2014.

197. Villemain O, Robin J, Bel A, et al. Pulsed cavitational ultrasound softening: A new noninvasive therapeutic approach for calcified bioprosthetic valve stenosis. *JACC Basic Transl Sci.* 2017;2(4):372-383.

198. Messas E, Rémond MC, Goudot G, et al. Feasibility and safety of noninvasive ultrasound therapy (NIUT) on porcine aortic valve. *Phys Med Biol.* 2020.

199. Taniguchi T, Morimoto T, Shiomi H, et al. Initial surgical versus conservative strategies in patients with asymptomatic severe aortic stenosis. *J Am Coll Cardiol.* 2015;66(25):2827-2838.

200. Généreux P, Stone GW, O'Gara PT, et al. Natural history, diagnostic approaches, and therapeutic strategies for patients with asymptomatic severe aortic stenosis. *J Am Coll Cardiol.* 2016;67(19):2263-2288.

201. Kang DH, Park SJ, Lee SA, et al. Early surgery or conservative care for asymptomatic aortic stenosis. *N Engl J Med.* 2020;382(2).

202. Strange G, Stewart S, Celermajer D, et al. Poor long-term survival in patients with moderate aortic stenosis. *J Am Coll Cardiol.* 2019;74(15): 1851-1863.

203. Clavel MA, Burwash IG, Mundigler G, et al. Validation of conventional and simplified methods to calculate projected valve area at normal flow rate in patients with low flow, low gradient aortic stenosis: the multicenter TOPAS (True or Pseudo Severe Aortic Stenosis) study. *J Am Soc Echocardiogr.* 2010;23(4):380-386.

204. Samad Z, Vora AN, Dunning A, et al. Aortic valve surgery and survival in patients with moderate or severe aortic stenosis and left ventricular dysfunction. *Eur Heart J.* 2016;37(28):2276-2286.

205. van Gils L, Clavel MA, Vollema EM, et al. Prognostic implications of moderate aortic stenosis in patients with left ventricular systolic dysfunction. *J Am Coll Cardiol.* 2017;69(19):2383-2392.

206. Spitzer E, Van Mieghem NM, Pibarot P, et al. Rationale and design of the Transcatheter Aortic Valve Replacement to UNload the Left ventricle in patients with ADvanced heart failure (TAVR UNLOAD) trial. *Am Heart J.* 2016;182:80-88.

29

Aortic Regurgitation, Mixed Valvular Heart Disease, and Heart Valve Prostheses

Patrizio Lancellotti, Alexandra Chitroceanu, Simona Sperlongano, Raluca Dulgheru, and Adriana Postolache

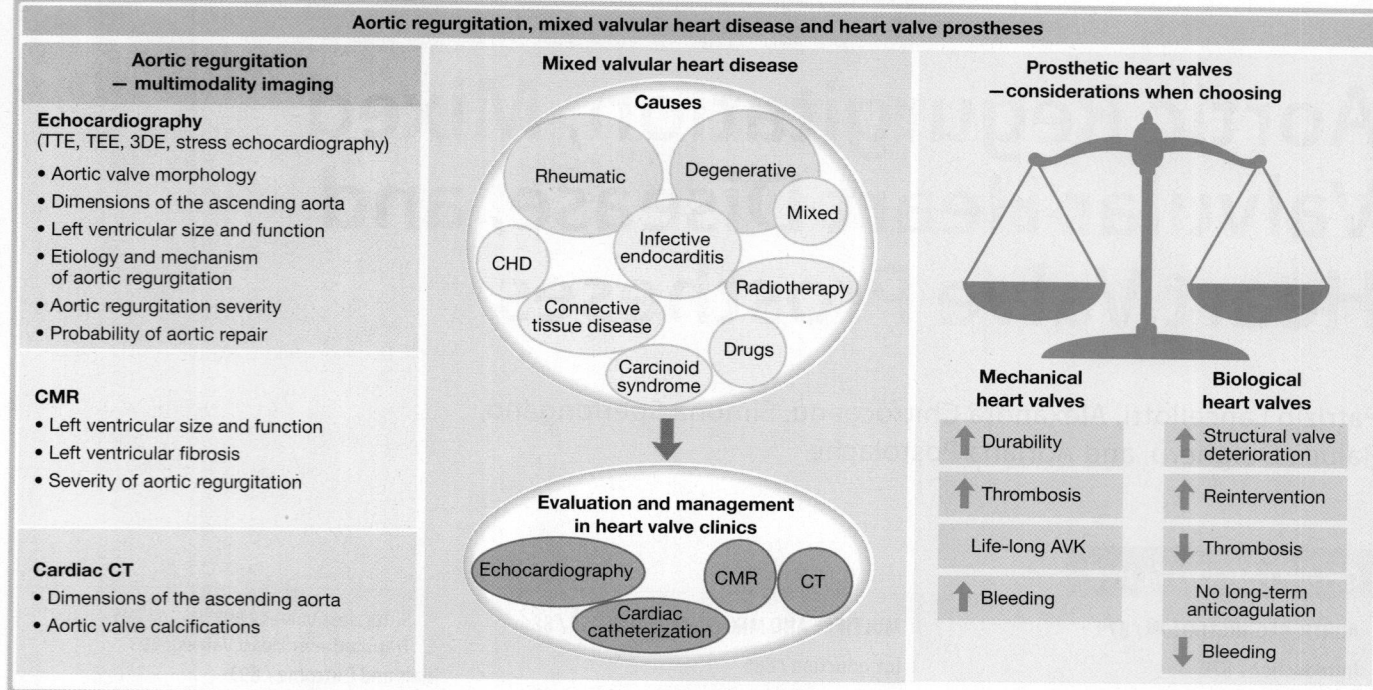

Aortic regurgitation, mixed valvular heart disease and heart valve prostheses

Aortic regurgitation — multimodality imaging

Echocardiography
(TTE, TEE, 3DE, stress echocardiography)
- Aortic valve morphology
- Dimensions of the ascending aorta
- Left ventricular size and function
- Etiology and mechanism of aortic regurgitation
- Aortic regurgitation severity
- Probability of aortic repair

CMR
- Left ventricular size and function
- Left ventricular fibrosis
- Severity of aortic regurgitation

Cardiac CT
- Dimensions of the ascending aorta
- Aortic valve calcifications

Mixed valvular heart disease

Causes
Rheumatic
Degenerative
Mixed
Infective endocarditis
CHD
Radiotherapy
Connective tissue disease
Drugs
Carcinoid syndrome

Evaluation and management in heart valve clinics
Echocardiography
CMR
CT
Cardiac catheterization

Prosthetic heart valves — considerations when choosing

Mechanical heart valves
- ↑ Durability
- ↑ Thrombosis
- Life-long AVK
- ↑ Bleeding

Biological heart valves
- ↑ Structural valve deterioration
- ↑ Reintervention
- ↓ Thrombosis
- No long-term anticoagulation
- ↓ Bleeding

Chapter 29 Fuster and Hurst's Central Illustration. Patients with aortic regurgitation (AR) should be followed up closely and should preferably be evaluated using a multiparametric and multi-imaging approach, with echocardiography being the main imaging modality. The main causes of mixed valvular heart disease worldwide are rheumatic and degenerative valvular disease; other etiologies, such as infective endocarditis or radiotherapy, are less frequent. The evaluation and the management of patients with mixed heart disease is challenging, and these patients should be evaluated in heart valve clinics, where a multimodality investigation can be performed, and which have the required expertise for treating these patients. The choice of implanting a mechanical or a biological prosthetic heart valve is determined mainly by the need for life-long anticoagulation and the higher risk of thrombosis and bleeding with mechanical valves, and the lower durability with a higher risk of valve deterioration and reintervention with biological valves. 3DE, 3-dimensional echocardiography; AVK, antivitamin K antagonists; CHD, congenital heart disease; CMR, cardiac magnetic resonance imaging; CT, computed tomography; LV, left ventricle; TEE, transesophageal echocardiography; TTE, transthoracic echocardiography.

CHAPTER SUMMARY

This chapter discusses three topics in the field of valvular heart disease: aortic regurgitation, mixed valvular heart disease, and prosthetic heart valves. Aortic regurgitation can be caused by a disease of the aortic valve, the ascending aorta, or both. Patients with chronic aortic regurgitation usually develop symptoms in late stages of the disease and should be followed-up closely. Although echocardiography is the main imaging modality for the evaluation of these patients, multimodality imaging should be considered in selected cases (see Fuster and Hurst's Central Illustration). Surgery is recommended in symptomatic patients and in asymptomatic patients with left ventricular dysfunction or marked dilatation. Mixed valvular heart disease is caused mainly by rheumatic and degenerative valvular disease, and has a complex pathophysiological and clinical expression. The evaluation and the management of patients with mixed valvular heart disease are challenging, which is why they should be followed-up in heart valve clinics. Prosthetic heart valve replacement is often the only effective treatment for patients affected by severe valvular heart disease. Mechanical valves require long-term anticoagulation whereas biological valves are associated with a higher risk of structural valve deterioration. Patients with prosthetic heart valves should be followed-up regularly for evaluation of prosthetic function and the occurrence of complications.

AORTIC REGURGITATION

Introduction

Aortic regurgitation (AR) results from inadequate closure of the aortic valve cusps. It may be caused by a disease modifying the aortic valve cusps (primary AR), by distortion or dilation of the aortic root and ascending aorta (secondary AR), or both (mixed AR).[1,2] Severe acute AR leads to acute decompensated heart failure and needs prompt surgical intervention. Severe chronic AR leads to chronic left ventricle (LV) volume and pressure overload, progressive LV dilatation, systolic dysfunction, and if left untreated, to congestive heart failure. Presently, there is no medical treatment to prevent, slow down the progresion of, or cure severe AR. Surgery is the only treatment proven to decrease mortality.

Prevalence

In population-based echocardiographic studies, at least trace AR by color Doppler may exist even in healthy individuals.[3] Depending on the definition used, patient age, and the characterics of the subpopulation examined, the prevalence of AR (whether mild, moderate, or severe) has been estimated between 2% and 30%.[3,4,5]

According to a population-based cohort form the Framingham Heart Study, the prevalence of AR varies with age, gender, and disease severity.[4] AR was unusual before the age of 50 and increased progressively later in life.[4] It was more common in men than women, at least trace AR being reported in 13% of men and 8.5% of women.[4] This could be explained by a higher prevalence of Marfan syndrome and bicuspid aortic valve disease in men.[6] Although the overall prevalence of AR in the Framingham Heart Study was reported to be 4.9%, moderate or severe AR occurred only in 0.5%.[7] The Framingham Heart Study excluded patients with more than mild aortic stenosis (AS) and prosthetic heart valves (PHVs), thus these data do not apply to these groups of patients. Considering that more than 75% of patients with calcific AS have some degree (usually mild) of AR,[8] the prevalence of AR could be higher, but no consistent information is currently available. Moreover, transcatheter aortic valve implantation (TAVI) has emerged as an important treatment for AS. Some degree of paravalvular AR (mild or greater) is common after TAVI, occurring in approximately 20% to 30% of patients and being graded as moderate or severe in approximately 2% to 5%.[1] Assessment of paravalvular AR severity after TAVI currently poses a dilemma for clinicians and requires further investigation to detect the optimal imaging modality for severity grading.

Etiology

Acute AR is mostly caused by infective endocarditis, aortic dissection, or blunt chest trauma.[9] Other causes include iatrogenic complications, such as following percutaneous aortic balloon dilatation or TAVI.[2] *Chronic AR* may result from *primary valvular causes (organic/structural)* from which:

1. *Degenerative tricuspid and bicuspid AR* are the most common causes in Western European countries and in the United States.[10] Some degree of AR (usually mild) coexists with calcific AS in older patients. Although the most frequent complication of congenitally bicuspid aortic valve (BAV) in adults is stenosis, isolated AR due to either incomplete closure of leaflets or valve prolapse, or a combination of AS and AR may also be present;[11]

2. *Infective endocarditis leading to AR,* in which the infection may destroy or perforate a cusp or a vegetation may interfere with the cusp's coaptation, leading to AR;[8]

3. *Rheumatic fever* remains a leading cause of AR in many developing countries;[1]

4. *Trauma, iatrogenic complications* (post–percutaneous balloon aortic valvuloplasty; post-TAVI) or *structural deterioration of a bioprosthetic valve* have become increasingly common causes for AR;

5. Rarely, progressive AR may occur in patients with *myxomatous proliferation of the aortic valve or in association with systemic disease such as systemic lupus erythematosus, rheumatoid arthritis, or ankylosing spondylitis.*[8]

Secondary AR (functional/nonstructural) is due to a marked dilatation of the ascending aorta and is a common cause of isolated AR, found in more than 50% of patients undergoing aortic valve replacement (AVR).[11] Aortic aneurysms with sinotubular junction dilatation may be age-related (degenerative), related to bicuspid aortic valve disease (congenital), due to cystic medial necrosis of the aorta (isolated or associated with syndromes like Marfan syndrome, Loeys–Dietz syndrome, etc.), or may be caused by systemic hypertension, inflammation, or infection.[12]

Pathophysiology

Chronic severe AR leads to chronic LV volume overload because the total stroke volume ejected by the LV (sum of effective stroke volume plus regurgitant volume) is increased.[10] Longstanding LV volume overload leads to eccentric LV hypertrophy and LV enlargement that increases end-diastolic volume (increases preload).[13] Eccentric hypertrophy is necessary to accommodate the rise in wall tension resulting from LV dilation (Laplace's law), with a normal ratio of LV wall thickness to cavity radius in compensated states.[14] The increase in ventricular end-diastolic volume is the major hemodynamic compensatory mechanism to maintain a normal effective stroke volume.[15] In compensated chronic AR, ventricular emptying, end-systolic volume, and LV filling pressure remain normal.[16] However, in accordance with Laplace's law, LV dilation also increases the LV systolic tension required to develop any given level of systolic pressure.[17] Hence, in AR there is an increase in both preload and afterload. During the early phases of chronic AR, the LV ejection fraction (EF) is normal or even increased (due to the increased preload and the Frank–Starling mechanism)[8] but in time these adaptive measures fail. LV emptying deteriorates, end-diastolic volume continues to increase further, and end-systolic wall stress rises.[18] Ultimately, LV end-systolic volume and filling pressure elevate and EF drops.[15] These changes may actually precede the development of clinical symptoms. The increased LV end-systolic volume is an important indicator of progressive myocardial dysfunction.

Patients with severe chronic AR have the largest LV end-diastolic volumes of all types of valvular heart disease (VHD).[8] Total myocardial oxygen requirements are also augmented by LV dilation and hypertrophy.[19] Furthermore, coronary perfusion pressure is reduced in AR as a consequence of lower than normal arterial pressure in diastole. The combination of increased oxygen demand and reduced supply may produce myocardial ischemia, with a reduction of coronary reserve, even in the absence of CAD.[8] In turn, myocardial ischemia may play a role in the deterioration of LV function.[20]

In contrast to the pathophysiological events just described in chronic AR, in acute AR, the compensatory mechanisms cannot develop rapidly enough to avoid hemodynamic deterioration.[8] The same regurgitant volume fills a ventricle of normal size with a limited ability to acutely increase stroke volume, leading to a notable rise in LV end-diastolic pressure and a drop in forward stroke volume.[8] Initially, tachycardia may compensate for the reduced stroke volume, but with little improvement in cardiac output. Usually patients with acute AR present with profound hypotension, cardiogenic shock, and severe dyspnea leading to pulmonary edema.[1]

Phenotypes

A BAV and abnormalities of the aortic root geometry leading to AR are the most common phenotypes of isolated AR requiring AVR.[21] Degenerative trileaflet aortic valve disease is also important, whereas other etiologies are rare.[8] Moreover, since surgical technics may differ, it is important to differentiate between three phenotypes of ascending aortic dilatation leading to AR: aortic root aneurysms (sinuses of Valsalva >45 mm), tubular ascending aorta aneurysms (sinuses of Valsalva <40 mm, but ascending aorta diameter >45 mm), and isolated AR (all diameters <40 mm) (**Fig. 29–1**).[1]

BAV is the most frequent congenital heart disease in humans with a prevalence of 1% to 2%.[22] Some consider BAV as a disease of the entire aortic root because it is frequently associated with aortopathy, resulting in dilation of ascending aorta and/or aortic dissection.[23] The risk of aortic dissection in patients with BAV is 5 to 9 times higher than in the general population, but the absolute risk is still low.[24]

BAV is characterized by fusion of one of the aortic commissures, which results in two functional aortic cusps of different dimensions.[8] The most prevalent BAV subtype is fusion of the right and left coronary cusp (70%–80% of patients), followed by fusion of the noncoronary with the right coronary cusp (20%–30% of cases). Less than 2% of cases are characterized by fusion of the noncoronary with the left coronary cusp.[8] Recently, it has been suggested that the type of BAV dictates the pattern of ascending aorta dilation. The presumed mechanisms are the direction of the systolic transaortic jet and differential parietal pressures on various regions of the ascending aorta.[25] Therefore, BAV type right–left is associated with an eccentric systolic jet that increases parietal pressures on the anterior and right ascending aortic wall and is frequently (87%) associated with dilatation of the aortic sinuses and ascending aorta. In reverse, BAV type noncoronary–left cusp is associated with increased parietal pressures on the right and posterior ascending aortic wall and is rarely associated with aortic dilatation.[21,25]

Abnormalities of the aorta can result in AR even when the leaflets themselves are normal.[8] Annular dilation results in AR because of inadequate coaptation of the stretched cusps.[26] However, mild annular dilation does not necessarily result in AR because an apposition zone is formed between adjacent cusps.[26] A variety of causes may cause annular dilation, including Marfan syndrome, cystic medial necrosis, or chronic hypertension.[12]

Diagnosis
Clinical

History: Acute AR often leads to acute heart failure and shock. Such patients are invariably tachycardic as the heart rate increases to preserve cardiac output. Depending on the etiology of acute AR, signs suggestive of endocarditis or aortic dissection may be present.[27] In contrast, patients with chronic AR typically remain asymptomatic for many years, with symptoms developing in the late stages of the disease, usually after LV dysfunction has occurred.[28] During the initial asymptomatic stage, patients may complain of uncomfortable awareness of a heartbeat and may experience palpitations at minimal exertion.[8]

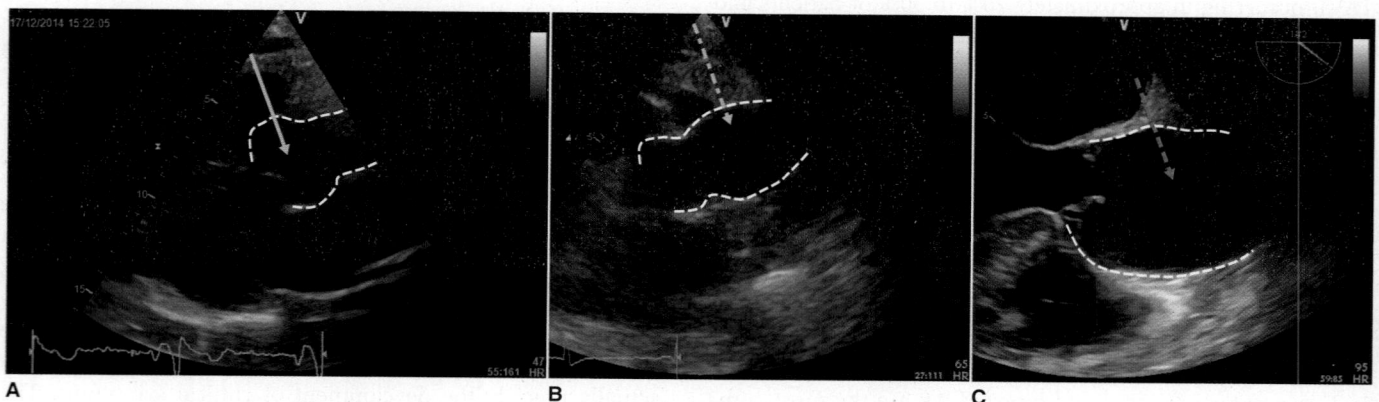

Figure 29–1. Different patterns of ascending aorta dilatation. Root dilatation in (**A**) (*yellow arrow*) with TTE; dilatation of the tubular portion only in (**B**) (TTE) and entire ascending aortic dilatation in (**C**) (TEE).

Shortness of breath is the principal manifestation of diminished cardiac reserve in severe AR, initially occurring during exercise and later also at rest.[15] In some AR patients with concomitant severe AS, exercise-induced angina can be present even in the absence of coronary artery disease. The angina episodes can be prolonged and usually do not respond favorably to sublingual nitroglycerine.[20]

Physical Examination: On physical examination, as soon as AR becomes moderate to severe, systolic blood pressure becomes elevated and diastolic pressure becomes abnormally low. Accordingly, the arterial pulse pressure widens.[8] As heart failure develops, the arterial diastolic pressure may rise through peripheral vasoconstriction.[8]

Numerous signs of AR have been described, despite little evidence, including Hill's sign (greater than normal disparity between upper and lower limb systolic pressure) and Duroziez's sign (systolic murmur heard over the femoral artery).[27] Clinical examination should also be directed toward symptoms and signs associated to conditions predisposing to AR such as Marfan syndrome, endocarditis, and other collagen disorders.[8,20] AR on cardiac auscultation is characterized as a high-pitched, blowing decrescendo diastolic murmur, which may be concomitant with a thrill.[15] However, a diastolic regurgitant murmur is not always audible in patients with mild or moderate AR. Studies have demonstrated that auscultation is highly specific but relatively insensitive for the accurate diagnosis of AR even in the hands of experienced clinicians.[29]

Diagnostic Tests: Multimodality Imaging Diagnosis

Echocardiography: The echo report in a patient with native AR should include information about the morphology of the aortic valve, the etiology (**Fig. 29–2**) plus severity of AR, the mechanism (**Fig. 29–3**) of dysfunction, and the impact on ventricular size and function (**Fig. 29–4**).[12,26] The goal is to determine the optimal timing of surgery.[10] Moreover, the likelihood of valve repair should also be discussed in cases of pure AR.[12]

Transthoracic echocardiography (TTE) and transesophageal echocardiography (TEE) help to evaluate the mechanism and severity of AR, LV size and function, and the diameter of the ascending aorta.[12] Preoperative TEE is also used to define the anatomy of the aortic valve cusps and to assess valve reparability, if valve-sparing surgery is considered.[1] Moreover, three-dimensional (3D) echocardiography may provide better delineation of aortic valve morphology and more precise measurements of ventricular volumes.[30] Loading conditions, technical limitations, and interobserver variability may affect echocardiographic parameters, and thus an integrated approach considering all qualitative, semiquantitative, and quantitative parameters should be used to assess AR severity.[16] Angiography has been used as a comparator to validate echocardiographic criteria for AR severity.[31,32] However, the role of echocardiographic severity criteria in relation to the long-term prognosis of patients with severe, asymptomatic AR was prospectively evaluated only in one study.[33]

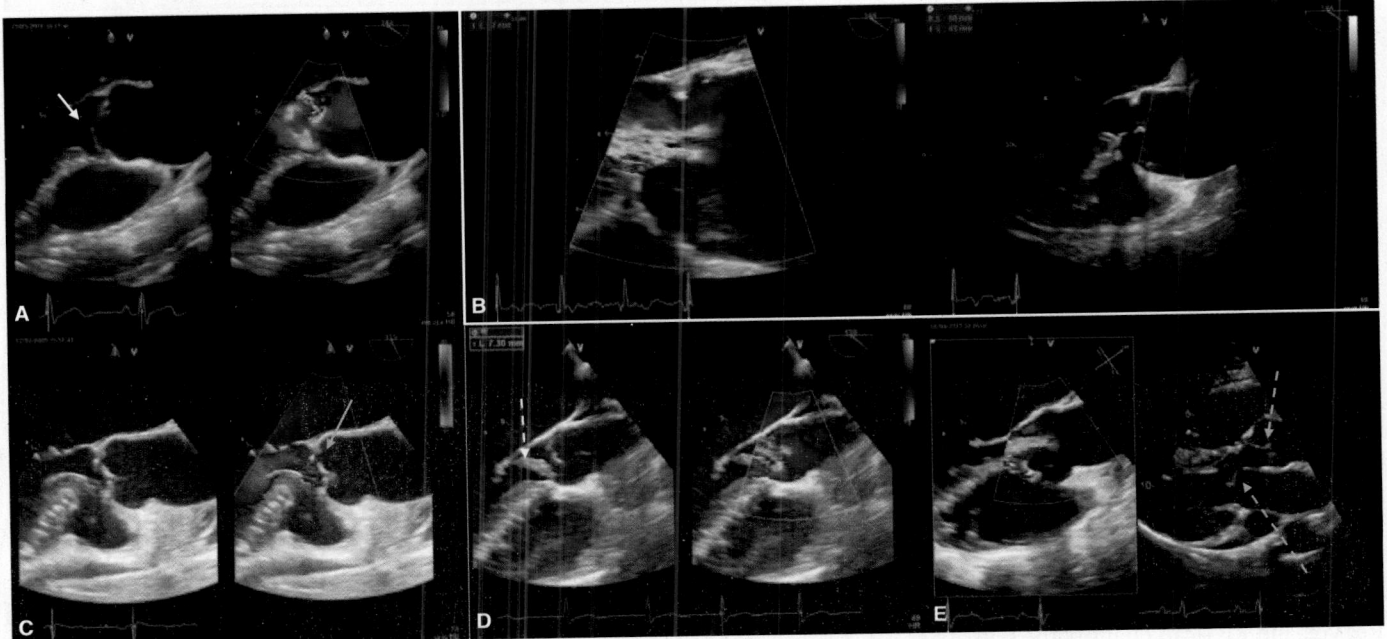

Figure 29–2. TTE and TEE showing different patients with AR of different etiologies. (A) AR due to complete anterior cusp prolapse (*white arrow*) in a patient with bicuspid valve disease; note the eccentric jet oriented away from the prolapsing cusp. **(B)** AR due to enlargement of the ascending aorta and aortic root. **(C)** AR after a car accident with blunt chest trauma related to the perforation of the posterior cusp as seen in TEE (the *yellow arrow* indicates a regurgitant flow through the cusp, which indicates there is a leaflet tear). **(D)** Acute AR due to aortic valve endocarditis; the *dashed white arrow* indicates the presence a voluminous vegetation on the ventricular side of the aortic valve. **(E)** AR in a patient with rheumatic aortic and mitral valve disease; note the doming of the anterior mitral leaflet in diastole indicative of a rheumatic process (*yellow dashed arrow*) and the thickening of the aortic cusps tips (also indicative of a rheumatic process involving the cusps).

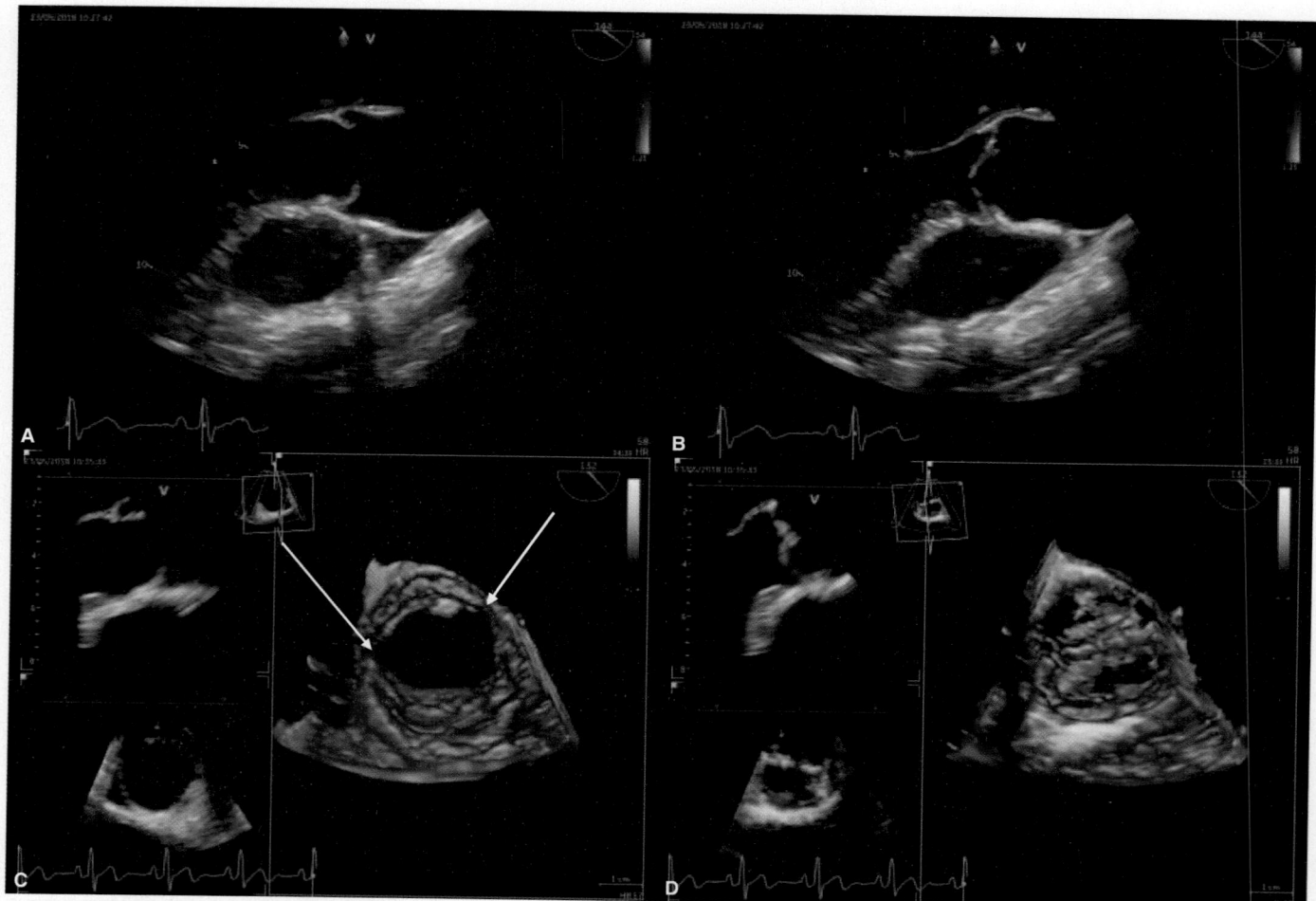

Figure 29–3. **Patient with type 0 BAV and AR due to anterior cusp prolapse as seen with TTE.** Note the doming of the aortic valve in systole with 2D-TEE (**A**), which is suggestive of a BAV. Complete anterior (right) cusp prolapse leading to AR (**B**). Presence of only two commissures (*white arrows*, **C**) with 3D-TEE. Absence of a raphe indicating a type 0 BAV as seen from the unique aortic view of the aortic valve with 3D-TTE (**D**).

Two-dimensional (2D) echocardiography in the parasternal long-axis view is classically used to measure the LV dimensions, LV outflow tract, the aortic annulus, the aortic sinus dimensions, and the maximal diameter of the ascending aorta.[12] In addition, 2D and 3D echocardiography offer information about valve morphology (tricuspid, bicuspid, unicuspid, or quadricuspid valve),[1] cusp pathology (redundancy, mobility, and integrity), and commissure variations (fusion and attachment site).[12]

Assessment of Aortic Regurgitation Severity: There are seven parameters to grade AR severity that can be assessed by TTE.[2] Regurgitant jet width relative to LV outflow tract dimension and vena contracta rely on imaging the regurgitant jet as it crosses the AV and exits into the LV outflow tract. Three others—EROA, RegVol, and RF—can quantify the severity of AR.[16]

- Regurgitant jet width relative to LV outflow tract dimension is measured from parasternal long axis view window but may be inaccurate for eccentric jets.[12]
- Vena contracta (the smallest diameter of regurgitant flow from the aortic valve) may provide an estimate size of the

EROA;[22] it is accurate for simple jets but not clinically validated for multiple jets.[34]

- Regurgitant volume and EROA are obtained using proximal isovolicity flow convergence (PISA) method or pulsed Doppler flow calculations based on comparison of aortic volume at the level of LVOT with mitral or pulmonic stroke volume.[12,34] A regurgitant volume ≥60 mL and EROA ≥0.30 cm² are consistent with severe AR.[10] PISA method has some limitations, including lack of validity for multiple jets, significant interobserver variability, and the measurement feasibility is limited by aortic valve calcification. Importantly, any errors in PISA measurement are squared resulting in large miscalculations.[12,34] Even if pulsed Doppler flow calculations (Doppler quantification from two valves flow) can be used in multiple jets,[16] the approach is time-consuming and is associated with several drawbacks. In general, a regurgitant fraction (regurgitant volume divided by the LVOT stroke volume) >50% indicates severe AR.[16]
- Diastolic flow reversal measured from the pulsed-wave Doppler signal in the proximal descending aorta/abdominal aorta measures whether a flow reversal of blood persists

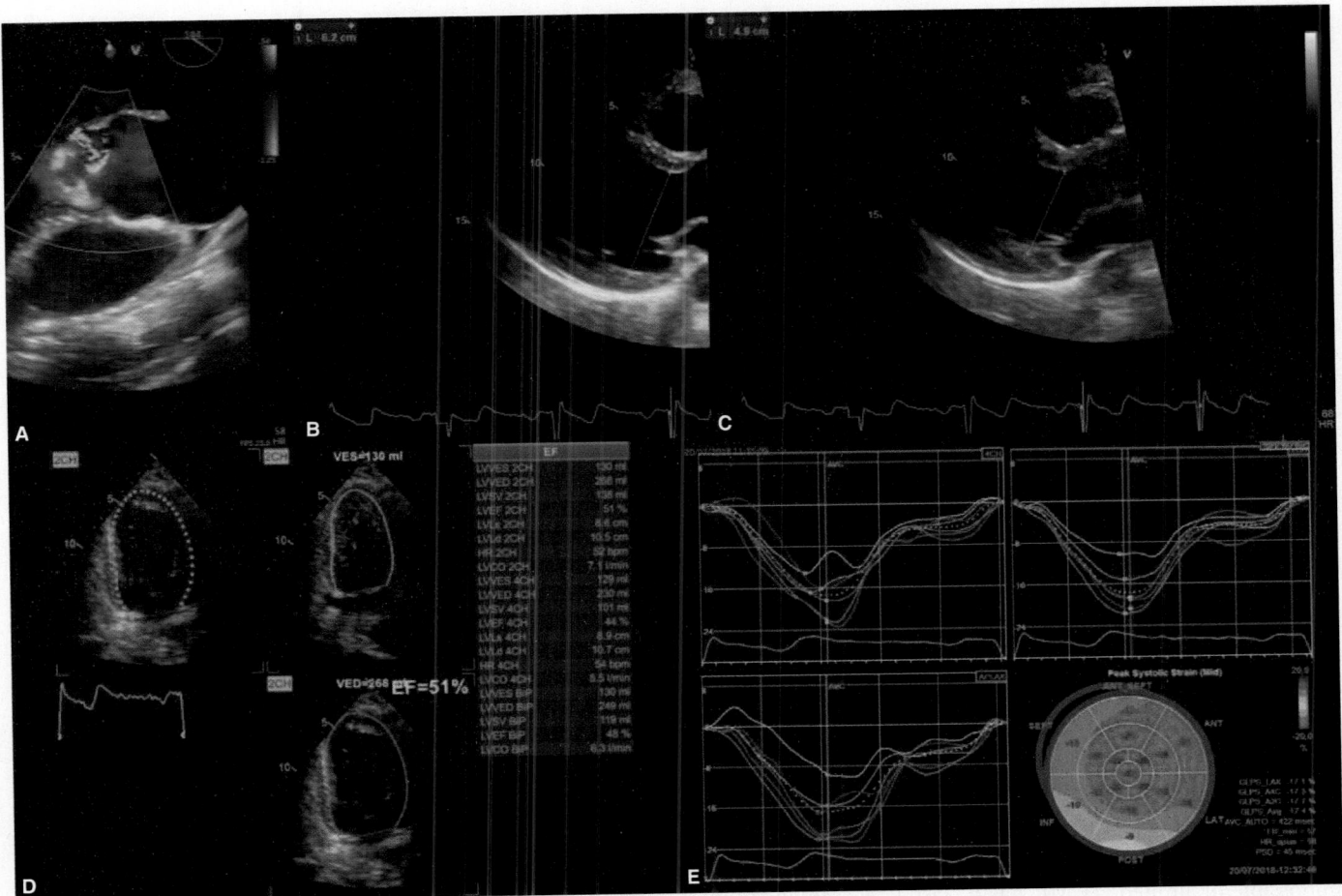

Figure 29–4. **Patient with BAV and a very eccentric jet of AR due to complete prolapse of the right aortic cusp (A).** Note the LV enlargement: end-diastolic diameter measures 62 mm (**B**) and end-systolic diameter measures 49 mm (**C**), while 3D end-diastolic volume is increased at 268 mL (**D**). LVEF is below 50%, measured with 3D-TTE at 48% (**D**). Note also the reduction in GLS = –17.4% (**E**). This patient has a class I indication for aortic valve surgery because LVEF is below 50% and AR is severe.

throughout diastole; a holodiastolic backward flow pattern and a cutoff value of >20 cm/s are indicators of severe AR.[19]

- Pressure half time is a simple, semiquantitative parameter used to assess AR severity.[12] It should be a complementary finding in grading AR severity because it is dependent on LV compliance and arterial pressure.[16] A pressure half-time >500 ms is usually consistent with mild AR, whereas values <200 ms are considered compatible with severe AR.[10] However, pressure half time accuracy depends heavily on the correct alignment of the Doppler beam with the regurgitant jet.

Assessment of Aortic Regurgitation Impact of Ventricular Size and Function: Once severe AR is established, measurements of LV function and dimensions assist in predicting prognosis. Recent studies have suggested that LV end-systolic diameter (LVESD) and volume are strong predictors of adverse clinical outcomes.[35] An LVESD >50 mm is associated with increased risk of developing symptomatic heart failure, whereas a diameter >60 mm or end-diastolic volume greater than 150 mL/m² is associated with a high risk of clinical decompensation.[35] Indexing LV diameters for body surface area (BSA) is recommended

in patients with small body size (BSA <1.68 m²), especially in women, in whom underestimation of chamber enlargement and delayed intervention could contribute to increased mortality.[1] The role of myocardial deformation imaging may be useful in patients with borderline LVEF, where it may help in the decision for surgery.[36] However, no cut-off values are currently validated.

Mechanism of Aortic Regurgitation: Understanding the etiology and mechanisms leading to regurgitation is most accurately discerned using TEE.[15] It is an essential step for proper management, whether aortic valve repair or valve-sparing surgery of the aortic root are considered.[1] Identification of the mechanism follows the same principle as for mitral regurgitation (MR), using Carpentier's classification: normal cusps but insufficient coaptation due to dilatation of the aortic root with central jet (type 1), cusp prolapse with eccentric jet (type 2), or retraction with poor cusp tissue quality and large central or eccentric jet (type 3).[37]

Measurement of the Aortic Root and Ascending Aorta: This is crucial to understand the etiology and mechanism of AR and to determine surgical options. Measurements are performed in the parasternal long axis view, from leading edge to leading edge at four levels: annulus, sinuses of Valsalva, sinotubular junction, and tubular ascending aorta.[1] They should be assessed at end-diastole, except for the annulus that is taken in midsystole.[1] Elective surgical correction of the aorta is recommended when the diameter exceeds 55 mm.[38] However, in some patients, with congenital BAV, aortic root dilatation may be independent of hemodynamics and can progress further even after valve surgery.[15]

Stress Echocardiography: In both the European Society of Cardiology (ESC) and American Heart Association (AHA) recommendations on VHD, the presence of symptoms is a firm indication for aortic valve surgery if AR is severe.[10] Exercise echocardiography is recommended to reveal symptoms in patients with severe AR who report being asymptomatic and in symptomatic patients with nonsevere AR.[39] Because of the small number of patients included in different exercise echocardiographic studies, sometimes with contradictory results, none of the exercise parameters have been included in the ESC/AHA guidelines. They could, together with other tests, like cardiopulmonary exercise testing and B-type natriuretic peptide (BNP), help anticipate surgical timing in patients approaching a surgical indication (LVEF 50%–55%, LVESD approaching 50 mm or 25 mm/m^2) or suggest the need for more frequent follow up in some patients.

Cardiac Magnetic Resonance: Cardiac magnetic resonance imaging (CMR) is an alternative imaging techniques, particularly in rare instances when echocardiography is technically impossible or limited.[15] CMR has a class I recommendation, level of evidence B in AHA/American College of Cardiology (ACC) guidelines on VHD in patients with moderate or severe AR and suboptimal echocardiographic images, in order to assess LV systolic function, systolic and diastolic volumes, and to measure AR severity.[2] An additional indication for CMR is detection of LV myocardial fibrosis.[26] Chronic AR is associated with diffuse reactive fibrosis, which can be detected through T1 mapping.[19] Further studies are still needed to assess the clinical relevance of these findings. Moreover, CMR is the most accurate noninvasive technique for assessing LV volumes and mass. CMR can also measure holodiastolic flow reversal in the descending aorta and can improve discrimination between patients with moderate or severe AR.[40] However, data on prognostic utility is still lacking.

Computed Tomography: Computed tomography (CT) in AR is recommended as an adjunctive examination, when precise measurements of aortic dimensions are needed and there is no (or little) concern for radiation dose.[19] CT is also a method of choice for quantification of leaflet calcification.[19] This is particularly important when contemplating transcatheter aortic valve implantation for inoperable patients with severe AR as the predominant lesion.

Natural History

If left untreated, severe acute AR carries a very high short-term rate of mortality from either the underlying cause (typically infective endocarditis or aortic dissection) or from hemodynamic decompensation of the LV. Moreover, decreased coronary perfusion can cause myocardial ischemia or even sudden death. Prompt surgical intervention is indicated in symptomatic severe acute AR.[8]

Chronic AR usually evolves slowly, with a long-standing asymptomatic period that may last for several years. Patients with mild or moderate AR should be followed clinically and by echocardiography every 12 to 24 months, because the severity of the AR may progress.[8] New-onset dyspnea or angina in these patients may indicate that AR has progressed in severity, highlighting the importance of periodic echocardiographic surveillance.[2]

Chronic severe AR can also remain asymptomatic for a prolonged period until chronic volume overload leads to contractile dysfunction and a decline in the EF.[16] Initially, a compensatory tachycardia may develop to maintain stroke volume. The prognosis for patients with severe AR depends on the presence or absence of symptoms or LV dysfunction.[16] AVR should not be delayed once symptoms or LV dysfunction develop.[10] Echocardiographic measurements of LV dimensions and EF are useful for following progressive LV dysfunction.[1] Moreover, they are the strongest predictors of outcome, highlighting the crucial role of serial echocardiography in asymptomatic patients with chronic severe AR.[35] As LV enlargement often precedes symptoms or a decline in EF, patients with asymptomatic severe AR should be followed at 6 months intervals.[8] A diminished LVEF (below 50%–55%) is associated with reduced prognosis even in asymptomatic patients,[41] particularly since LV dysfunction may become irreversible and may not improve after AVR.[42] However, when LV dysfunction is of short duration (less than 14 months), AVR can lead to full functional recovery.[16] Improvement is less likely after a longer period of LV dysfunction[42] or in the presence of severe LV dilation.[43] It is therefore important to surgically intervene as soon as a drop in EF or LV enlargement occurs. The most commonly used parameters for LV enlargement are echocardiographic end-systolic and end-diastolic diameters.[10]

Among patients with asymptomatic LV dysfunction, more than 25% of them develop symptoms within 1 year.[8] Although symptoms do not necessarily reflect LV function, there is a dramatic change in prognosis harbored by symptom onset in severe AR. Patients with symptomatic severe AR have a mortality rate of 10% to 20% and even moderate AR has been shown to be associated with a 10-year cardiovascular event rate of $34 \pm 6\%$.[33] Congestive heart failure and sudden death may occur in symptomatic patients with previous LV dilation.[8] Without surgical treatment, death usually occurs within 2 years after the development of heart failure and within 4 years after the onset of angina pectoris.[8] Even in the current era, patients with severe AR and New York Heart Association (NYHA) class IV symptoms have a 25% mortality risk at 1 year without surgery.[41]

Management

Medical Therapy

Severely symptomatic patients with acute AR may be stabilized temporarily with intravenous diuretics and vasodilators to control heart failure symptoms, but surgery is indicated urgently.

No specific treatment to prevent disease progression in chronic valvular AR is currently available. Medical therapy can provide symptomatic improvement in early symptoms, such that surgery to be performed in a more controlled setting. Treatment of hypertension is strongly recommended in patients with chronic AR and vasodilators (angiotensin-converting enzyme inhibitors, dihydropyridine calcium channel blockers, hydralazine) are an excellent first choice.[20] However, because of the increased stroke volume, adequate control of blood pressure is difficult to achieve. β-blockers and/or losartan in patients with Marfan syndrome may slow aortic root dilatation and reduce the risk of aortic complications.[1,44] In this regard, they are also commonly used in clinical practice in patients with BAV and aortopathy.[1]

Surgical Management

Severe acute AR is a surgical emergency. Current recommendations for chronic AR management are based on scarce data with no randomized studies to show that surgery is better than conservative therapy in patients with chronic asymptomatic AR.[19] Therefore, guidelines recommendations are based on cut-off values for parameters that indicate poorer outcome in conservatively treated patients.[19,43] A comparison of surgical indications for AVR in chronic AR (ESC/EACTS 2017 vs AHA/ACC 2021) is provided in **Table 29–1**. Although valve replacement is the standard procedure in the majority of patients with AR, ESC/EACTS 2017 guidelines recommend valve repair or

valve sparing surgery in preference to AVR in selected patients (class I, level of evidence C).[1] The indication covers tricuspid or bicuspid valves who have a type I (enlargement of the aortic root with normal cusp motion) or type II (cusp prolapse) mechanism of AR.[1] The recommendation is due to good long-term results obtained in experienced centers, with low rates of valve-related events and good quality of life.[1] However, assessment criteria for the decision between valve replacement and valve repair must still be refined.

Regarding patients with a bicuspid aortic valve and dilatation of the ascending aorta, there are considerable differences between ESC/EACTS and AHA/ACC guidelines (summary provided in **Table 29–2**).[1,45] Recent findings suggest that indexed end-systolic dimension (ESDI) or volume (ESVI) may be more robust indicators for timing of surgical interventions.[33] Patients with ESDI >2.5 cm/m^2 or ESVI >45 mL/m^2 present an increased risk of death and adverse outcomes.[33] However, further data are needed to support these findings.

In summary, the following considerations apply to the selection of patients with chronic severe AR for surgery.[10] Asymptomatic patients with normal and stable LV function do not require prophylactic surgery and should be examined at intervals of 6 months.[8] In asymptomatic patients with LV dilation but no LV dysfunction, the decision should be made based upon several echocardiographic measurements to confirm dilatation, in addition to observations of depressed performance and impaired exercise tolerance.[8] Close follow-up is required to identify the optimal timing for surgery. If evidence is borderline or inconsistent, continued close monitoring is

TABLE 29–1. Indications for Surgery in Chronic Aortic Regurgitation[1,2]

Class of Indication	Level of Evidence	ESC/EACTS 2017	AHA/ACC 2014	Differences between Guidelines
Class I	B	Symptomatic severe AR		None
Class I	B	Asymptomatic chronic severe AR and left ventricular EF (LVEF) ≤50%	Asymptomatic chronic severe AR and left ventricular EF (LVEF) ≤55%	Cut off value for LVEF ≤55% for *AHA/ACC*
Class I	C	Severe AR when undergoing other cardiac surgery (CABG, ascending aorta, other valve)		None
Class IIa	B	Asymptomatic severe AR with normal LVEF (>50%) but with severe LV dilatation	Asymptomatic severe AR with normal LVEF (>55%) but with severe LV dilatation	Definition of LV dysfunction in severe AS: LVEF ≤55% for *AHA/ACC*
Class IIa	C	-	Moderate AR when undergoing other cardiac surgery	Not covered in the ESC/EACTS guidelines
Class IIb	B	-	Asymptomatic severe AR and normal LVEF (≥55%) but with progressive severe LV dilation (LVEDD >65 mm) or progressive LV systolic dysfunction (LVEF 55% to 60% on 3 serial echo examinations) if surgical risk is low	Not covered in the ESC/EACTS guidelines
-	C	Heart Team discussion is recommended in selected patients in whom aortic valve repair may be a feasible alternative to valve replacement.	In patients with BAV and severe AR who meet criteria for AVR, aortic valve repair may be considered in selected patients if the surgery is performed at a Comprehensive Valve Center	AHA/ACC give it a class IIb indication while ESC/EACTS give it a class I

Class I: It is indicated/ recommended; Class IIa: Should be considered; Class IIb: May be considered; Class III: It is contraindicated; Level A: data derived from multiple randomized clinical trials or meta-analyses; Level B: data derived from single randomized clinical trial or large non-radomized studies; Level C: consensus of opinion of experts and/or small studies, retrospective studies, registries.

Abbreviations: ESC/EACTS, European Society of Cardiology/European Association for Cardio-Thoracic Surgery; AHA/ACC, American Heart Association/American College of Cardiology; AR, aortic regurgitation; LVEF, left ventricular ejection fraction; CABG, coronary artery bypass graft; LV, left ventricle; LVEDD, left ventricular end-diastolic volume; LVESV, left ventricular end-systolic volume.

TABLE 29–2. Indication for Surgery in Patients with Bicuspid Aortic Valve and Aortic Root Disease[1,45]

Class of Indication	Level of Evidence	ESC/EACST 2017	AHA/ACC 2016 Consensus on AHA/ACC 2014
Class I	B	No class I indication	Asymptomatic bicuspid aortic valve with dilatation of Valsalva sinuses or the ascending thoracic aortic diameter >55 mm
Class IIa	C (ESC/EACTS) B (AHA/ACC)	Bicuspid aortic valve with an ascending thoracic aortic diameter >50 mm if the patient also has at least one of the followings: -Family history of aortic dissection; -documented increase in the aortic diameter >3 mm/yr (using the same imaging method, at the same level, and with comparative images available); -hypertension; -coarctation of the aorta -severe aortic regurgitation or mitral regurgitation - desire for pregnancy,	In asymptomatic patients with a BAV, a diameter of the aortic sinuses or ascending aorta of 5.0 to 5.5 cm, and an additional risk factor for dissection (eg, family history of aortic dissection, aortic growth rate >0.5 cm per year, aortic coarctation), operative intervention to replace the aortic sinuses and/or the ascending aorta is reasonable if the surgery is performed at a Comprehensive Valve Center
Class IIa	C (ESC/EACTS) B (AHA/ACC)	When surgery is primarily indicated for the aortic valve, replacement of the aortic root or tubular ascending aorta should be considered when >_45 mm, particularly in the presence of a bicuspid valve	

Class I: It is indicated/ recommended; Class IIa: Should be considered; Class IIb: May be considered; Class III: It is contraindicated; Level A: data derived from multiple randomized clinical trials or meta-analyses; Level B: data derived from single randomized clinical trial or large non-randomized studies; Level C: consensus of opinion of experts and/or small studies, retrospective studies, registries.
Abbreviations: AHA/ACC, American Heart Association/ American College of Cardiology; ESC/EACTS, European Society of Cardiology/European Association for Cardio-Thoracic Surgery.

also indicated. If changes are progressive and consistent (at least LVESD >50 mm), AVR is indicated. Symptomatic patients with chronic severe AR should undergo AVR.[10]

MULTIPLE AND MIXED VALVE DISEASE

Introduction

Mixed and multiple valvular disease are highly prevalent forms of VHD, with complex pathophysiological, and clinical expressions related to the different combinations of valvular lesions. Mixed VHD represents the combination of stenotic and regurgitant lesions on the same valve, whereas multiple valvular heart disease (MVD) is the combination of stenotic and regurgitant lesions occurring on ≥2 cardiac valves.[46,47] Despite their prevalence, there are only few data in the literature concerning patients with mixed and multiple valve disease, and as a consequence, no clear recommendations can be made, which makes the management of these patients particularly challenging.

Prevalence

MVD was identified in 20% of patients with native valve disease in the EuroHeart Survey and in over one-third of individuals over 65 years screened by echocardiography in the OxVALVE study.[48,49] Among operated patients with VHD, MVD was present in 15% of cases in the EuroHeart Survey and in 11% of patients from the Society of Thoracic Surgeons (STS) database.[48,50] The most frequent mixed and multiple VHDs are AS plus AR, AS plus MR, and AR plus MR.[46]

There is a growing concern about the presence of MVD in older patients. Twenty percent of TAVR patients have concomitant moderate-to-severe MR, 18% have associated mitral stenosis (MS), and 27% have associated moderate-to-severe

tricuspid regurgitation (TR).[51,52] The presence of moderate-to-severe MR or TR has an important negative clinical impact on the outcome of TAVR patients.[53,54] Moreover, in a recent study, the presence of MS, even if mild, was associated with a 3-fold increased risk of cardiovascular death and disabling stroke in TAVR patients, in particular with rheumatic MS.[52]

Pathogenesis and Particulars of Assessing Mixed and Multiple Valve Disease

Rheumatic and degenerative heart valve diseases are the main causes of MVD, with mitral and aortic valves being involved in most cases. In the EuroHeart Survey, rheumatic heart disease was the etiology of MVD in 51% of cases, followed by degenerative valve disease in 40% of cases.[47] Other, less frequent causes of organic MVD are infective endocarditis, postradiotherapy or drug induced, carcinoid syndrome, congenital heart disease, and connective tissue disorders. Functional and mixed etiologies exist, in particular in older patients (**Table 29–3**).

The most common etiologies of associated AS and AR in industrialized countries are BAV and degenerative VHD, with rheumatic heart disease and infective endocarditis being less frequent. The main causes of mixed mitral valve disease are rheumatic and degenerative.[46,55]

The hemodynamic consequences and the clinical expression of multiple and mixed VHD are dependent on the complex interplay between several factors, including the specific combination of VHD, the severity and timing of onset of each individual lesion, the loading conditions, and the ventricular systolic or diastolic performance.[46,47] In practice, a valvular lesion can be exaggerated or blunted by the presence of another lesion on the same valve or on another valve. For example, the

TABLE 29–3. Etiology of Multivalvular Heart Disease
Rheumatic heart disease
Degenerative
• Prolapse of mitral and tricuspid valves with associated MR and TR
• Degenerative AS + mitral annular calcification with MR or MS
Postradiotherapy on the chest
Drug induced
• Methysergide, ergotamine
• Cabergoline, pergoline
• Fenfluramine, dexfenfluramine, benfluorex
Infective endocarditis
Carcinoid syndrome
• Most commonly on TV and PV, regurgitation > stenosis
• MV and AV involvement rare, in case of intra-cardiac shunts, lung metastasis, or high disease burden with unusually increased levels of serotonin
Congenital
• Schonne syndrome
• Ochronosis
Connective tissue disease
• Marfan Syndrome (associated prolapse, dilatation of the aorta)
• Ehler-Danlos syndrome (prolapse)
Functional
• Functional MR and TR in the context of RV and LV dilatation
• AR caused by aortic dilatation + functional ischemic MR
Mixed
• Degenerative AS + functional MR
• AR caused by infective endocarditis on the AV + ischemic MR

Abbreviations: AR, aortic regurgitation; AS, aortic stenosis; AV, aortic valve; LV, left ventricle; MV, mitral valve; MR, mitral regurgitation; MS, mitral stenosis; PV, pulmonary valve; RV, right ventricle; TR, tricuspid regurgitation; TV, tricuspid valve.

association MR and AR potentiate their effect of volume overload on the LV, whereas MS decreases the volume load posed by the AR on the LV. Also, the severity and clinical effect of one valve lesion can be altered if loading conditions change or the other valve is repaired. More than 50% of functional MR cases are improved after TAVR.

The hemodynamic consequences of multiple and mixed VHDs on blood flow, ventricular size, and function may affect the echocardiographic diagnosis.[47] Low-flow low-gradient stenosis is common in MVD. Severe MR or MS can lead to a decreased flow across the aortic valve and lower gradients, even if EF is preserved (paradoxical low-flow AS, **Fig. 29–5**).

Several methods used for evaluating VHDs have not been validated in multiple or mixed valvular disease. In patients with MS and AR, the continuity equation is not valid for estimating the MVA (the mitral and aortic flows are not equal). Likewise, the pressure half-time method should not be used for estimating mitral valve area in patients with aortic disease or impaired LV diastolic function.

Clinical and Multimodality Assessment

The evaluation of patients with multiple and mixed VHD is challenging, due to the different combinations of valve lesions and their hemodynamic consequences.

The clinical picture depends on the relative severity of each valve lesion. In patients with MVD of similar severity, the proximal (upstream) lesion tends to mask the distal lesion.

For example, in patients with associated mitral and aortic valve disease of similar severity, the manifestation of the mitral valve disease can dominate the presentation, while in patients with associated tricuspid and mitral valve lesions, signs of systemic congestion can dominate the clinical picture. The clinical exam (the intensity and timing of murmurs, changes on pulse pressure, etc.) is also not reliable for estimating the severity of valvular lesions, because of the same reason, one valve masking the other.

Echocardiography is the cornerstone of the diagnosis of multiple and mixed VHD.[46] Similar to single valve disease, it should describe the etiology, the mechanism, and the severity of every valve lesion, assess the hemodynamic consequences of the combined lesion on left and right ventricular size and function, and the pulmonary circulation. The report should also provide information about the suitability for surgical valve repair or transcatheter interventions. However, the echocardiographic examination of patients with mixed and multiple valve disease is more challenging, because of the low-flow conditions frequently encountered and the fact that some parameters which were valid in single valve lesions may not be valid in this subset of patients. An integrative multiparametric approach is recommended and, in general, measurements that are not dependent on loading conditions, such as direct planimetry of a stenotic valve or assessment of the effective regurgitant orifice area or the vena contracta, for a regurgitant valve, are preferred for evaluating the severity of valvular lesions in patients with MVD.

Although there is no data on the potential role of other imaging modalities in patients with mixed and multiple VHD, a multimodality imaging approach can be useful in difficult cases, in particular in low-flow situations.[46]

TEE is useful for evaluating the cause and the mechanism of valvular regurgitation and is the main imaging used for planning and guiding surgical and percutaneous procedures.[56] Three-dimensional echocardiography (on transthoracic or transesophageal images) can be used for measuring the LV outflow area and the MV area and it improves the estimation of LV and RV volumes in comparison with 2D images.[57]

Stress echocardiography should be considered whenever there is a discrepancy between symptoms and the severity of valvular lesions at rest.[1,2,58,59] Exercise echocardiography, preferably using semi supine bicycle exercise, can unmask symptoms in apparently asymptomatic patients and can offer important information for patient management. Earlier intervention might be indicated in patients with an important increase in transvalvular gradients, the absence of LV contractile reserve, or the presence of exercise-induced pulmonary hypertension.[58] Dobutamine stress echocardiography should be considered in low-flow low-gradient AS, for differentiating between pseudo-severe and true severe AS.

CMR imaging should be considered, if available, in patients with inconclusive or discordant echocardiographic evaluation. CMR can assess the severity of valvular regurgitation and is the gold standard for estimating ventricular volumes. In patients with MVD, assessment of regurgitant volume and fraction by calculating ventricular volumes may be misleading (it assumes than only one valve is affected), and alternative methods, such

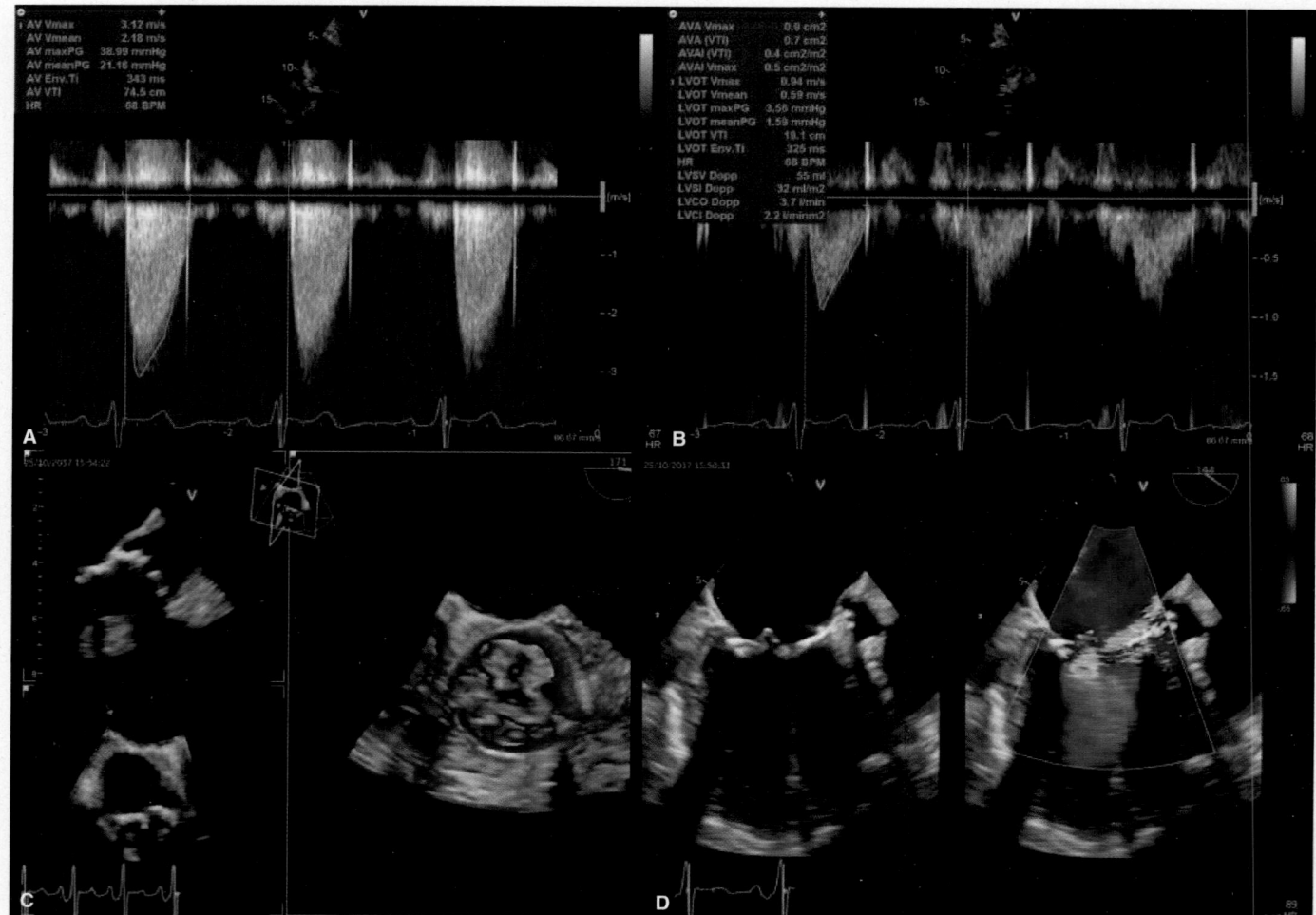

Figure 29–5. Multiple valve disease. Low flow (stroke volume index 32 mL/m²) low gradient (mean pressure gradient across the aortic valve of 21 mm Hg) severe aortic stenosis (aortic valve area by continuity equation of 0.7 cm², aortic valve index area of 0.5 cm²/m²) (**A, B**) in a female patient with severe calcification of a tricuspid aortic valve as seen with 3D-TEE (note the reduced opening of the aortic valve in systole as seen from the aortic root perspective) (**C**). The low flow state is related to the presence of a severe primary mitral regurgitation with ruptured chordae at the level of the P2 scallop (**D**).

as phase-contrast velocity mapping, should be preferred for quantifying valvular regurgitation.[46,60]

Multidetector computed tomography (MDCT) estimation of aortic valve calcium score is useful in patients with paradoxical low-flow AS. High calcium scores (>1200 AU in women and >2000 AU in men) are associated with an increased likelihood of severe AS.[61] Also, MDCT is the preferred imaging for evaluating patients before TAVR.

Cardiac catheterization may be considered in patients with discordant evaluation but has several limitations in patients with MVD. Cardiac output assessment by the thermodilution or the Fick method may be inaccurate in patients with low cardiac output or severe TR. Moreover, the Gorlin formula should not be used in patients with mixed aortic or mixed mitral valve diseases.[46]

Relative Importance of Lesions

Aortic Stenosis and Mitral Regurgitation

The association of AS and MR is the most frequent form of MVD in developed countries, in particular in older patients.

Over 20% of TAVR patients have associated moderate or severe MR and its presence is associated with a significantly increased risk of death.[51,53]

MR in patients with AS can be functional—related to LV and mitral annulus dilatation caused by the afterload mismatch or may be associated with ischemic cardiomyopathy—and organic, mainly degenerative in developed countries, caused by mitral annular calcification or mitral valve prolapse.

Severe AS leads to an increase in MR color Doppler jet and regurgitant volume that overestimate the severity of MR in comparison with the effective regurgitant area. On the other hand, moderate or severe MR can lead to a decrease in stroke volume through the aortic valve and lower gradients, with possible underestimation of AS severity. Dobutamine stress echocardiography is recommended in these patients, but because of MR, the aortic flow might not rise significantly during the Dobutamine infusion for confirming the presence of severe AS. In these patients with low-flow AS and moderate or severe MR, quantification of aortic valve calcium score by MDCT may be more useful for differentiating pseudo-severe from true severe

AS.[46,61] Another consequence of the interaction between the two valvular lesions is that the MR can impede the early detection of LV systolic dysfunction related to the presence of AS if the evaluation is based on LVEF only. Global longitudinal strain (GLS) could prove more useful for estimating the LV systolic function in these patients with apparently preserved LVEF.[62,63]

Aortic Regurgitation and Mitral Stenosis

AR and MS have different, opposing effects on LV loading conditions. In the presence of MS, LV volumes are lower than in isolated AR, the increase in stroke volume typically associated with AR might be blunted and, as a consequence, the clinical signs associated increased pulse pressure might not be observed.[46,47,62] In patients with concomitant, at least moderate AR, the continuity equation and the pressure half-time (PHT) methods are not valid for estimating mitral valve area. Direct planimetry of MV area on 3D transthoracic or transesophageal images should be considered instead.[46]

Aortic Regurgitation and Mitral Regurgitation

MR associated with AR may be primary (rheumatic involvement or prolapse of both valves) or secondary to LV remodeling as a consequence of AR. The association of MR and AR leads to severe volume overload and some pressure overload (related to the presence of AR) of the LV, with important dilation of the LV and progressive contractile dysfunction. This condition is often poorly tolerated and postoperative LV dysfunction is more likely to occur than in isolated MR or AR, which underlines the need for an earlier intervention in these patients.[64] With regard to the echocardiographic examination, the PHT method should be used with caution for estimating the severity of AR in patients with associated MR.

Aortic Stenosis and Mitral Stenosis

The combination of severe AS and MS is rarely seen in developed countries, where the main etiology is degenerative, and is usually poorly tolerated so that patients seek attention earlier and intervention is indicated before both valve lesions become severe.[65] Other less frequent causes are congenital (Shone syndrome), postradiotherapy, or drug induced.

The combination of severe AS and MS leads to an important decrease in cardiac output, with lower transvalvular gradients than expected and possible underestimation of the severity of both valve lesions. The severity of MS can be estimated by measuring the mitral valve area on 3D transthoracic or transesophageal images. Determining the severity of AS is of utmost importance in these patients and all imaging modalities should be used, including aortic valve calcium score on MDCT.[46] Failing to recognize concomitant severe AS and treating only the mitral lesion could have dramatic consequences, because the sudden increase in preload to a small, hypertrophied, and noncompliant LV would result in pulmonary edema.[46,47,62]

Aortic Stenosis and Aortic Regurgitation

Mixed aortic valve disease is characterized by a combination of pressure and volume overload of the LV. Usually, one lesion predominates over the other and symptoms develop early.

Studies have shown that asymptomatic patients with moderate mixed aortic valve disease have a risk of major events similar to patients with isolated severe AS, half of them becoming symptomatic and requiring surgery within 12 months and their outcome without surgery is poor.[66,67]

The transaortic gradients are increased both by the AS and the AR, and the AS leads to an increased pressure of the AR jet. Aortic valve area should be used for evaluating the severity of AS, whereas the effective regurgitant orifice should be used to evaluate the severity of AR, but these parameters do not reflect the overall hemodynamic burden of associated AS and AR. Because the peak aortic jet velocity and mean gradient increase with both AS and AR, these parameters might be useful to assess the overall severity of the mixed aortic valve disease and have been shown to correlate with the outcomes.[66-68] Symptomatic patients with moderate AS plus AR and peak jet velocity ≥4 m/s and mean gradient ≥40 mm Hg should be referred to intervention.[46]

Management

The management of patients with mixed and multiple VHD is challenging. There is little evidence regarding the treatment of these patients and most of the ESC and ACC/AHA recommendations have a level of evidence C (Table 29–4).[1,2,59]

Considering the complexity of this condition, with different combinations of lesions, the many diagnostic pitfalls and the absence of evidence for guiding their management, these patients should be followed-up in heart valve clinics and they should be treated in Heart Valve Centers.[46,69,70] The appropriate timing for follow-up of patients with multiple and mixed VHD is not known. When one lesion is clearly dominant, the follow-up should be made according to the recommendations for that lesion. The association of lesions with similar severity can have more detrimental consequences than the single lesion and patients should be followed-up more closely.[46]

The management of patients with multiple and mixed VHD should be discussed in the heart valve team meeting between cardiologist, imaging specialist, cardiac surgeon, interventional cardiologist, anesthesiologist, and geriatrician. The choice between surgery, transcatheter intervention, and conservative medical treatment should be made on a case-by-case basis. The indications for intervention are based on the presence of symptoms and on the consequences of multiple and mixed VHD on left or right ventricles and the pulmonary circulation.

Surgery is the most recommended treatment for mixed and multiple VHDs by the guidelines but is associated with a higher mortality risk than single valve surgery.[48,50] Whenever possible, repair should be preferred over valvular replacement.[47]

Transcatheter valvular therapies have improved considerably in recent years and represent a less invasive treatment option for selected inoperable or high-risk patients. The dominant lesion is treated first and the severity of the second valvular lesion is reevaluated later. This staged procedure can help to evaluate the need for an intervention on the mitral/tricuspid valve after the treatment of the aortic/left-sided valve lesions. Also, in patients with multiple morbidities, treating only the

TABLE 29–4. Comparison between the ESC/EACTS and the ACC/AHA Recommendations on Multiple Valvular Heart Disease[14-16]

2017 ESC/EACTS Guidelines on VHD	2017 ESC Guidelines on VHD
Aortic stenosis + aortic regurgitation	
In patients with combined stenosis and regurgitation, the indication for interventions should be based on symptoms and objective consequences of the valvular disease. The pressure gradient that reflects the haemodynamic burden of the valve lesion becomes more important than valve area and measures of the regurgitation for the assessment of disease severity.	AVR is recommended in • symptomatic patients with combined AS and AR and a peak transvalvular jet velocity ≥4 m/sec or a mean transvalvular gradient ≥40mmHg • asymptomatic patients with combined AS and AR who have a jet velocity ≥4 m/sec and a LVEF <50%.
Severe aortic stenosis + severe mitral regurgitation	
In patients with severe AS and severe MR and indication for SAVR, concomitant intervention on the mitral valve is, in general non necessary, except in patients with primary MR (flail or prolapse, post-rheumatic changes, signs of infective endocarditis), mitral annulus dilatation or marked abnormalities of LV geometry. Non-severe secondary mitral regurgitation mostly improves after the aortic valve is treated. In patients with severe mitral regurgitation, combined or sequential TAVI and percutaneous mitral edge-to-edge repair can be feasible, but there is not enough experience to make recommendations.	The type of intervention in patients with associated severe AS and severe MR is mainly based on the mechanism of MR, the likelihood of mitral valve repair and the estimated surgical risk of both procedures: • patients with severe AS and severe primary MR are best treated with SAVR and mitral valve surgery (preferably mitral valve repair, if feasible), unless the surgical risk is high or prohibitive, in which case, a staged procedure, with TAVI followed by mitral transcatheter edge-to-edge repair can be effective. • in patients with severe AS and severe primary MR in whom the mitral valve cannot be repaired, the decision between double valve replacement of the aortic and mitral valve vs. SAVR followed by mitral transcatheter edge-to-edge repair should be made by the multidisciplinary team, by taking into consideration the additive risk of a mitral valve replacement. • In patients with severe AS and severe secondary MR, the options are SAVR and mitral valve surgery (in patients at low or intermediate surgical risk and repairable mitral valve) or a staged approach with TAVI followed by mitral transcatheter edge-to-edge repair (in patients at high to prohibitive surgical risk, if symptoms persist after TAVI and if the anatomy is suitable.
Moderate AS + another severe valve disease	
SAVR should be considered in patients with moderate AS undergoing surgery of the ascending aorta or another valve, after Heart Team decision.	In patients with moderate AS who are undergoing cardiac surgery for another indication, concomitant SAVR may be considered.
Severe AR + another valve disease	
If aortic regurgitation requiring surgery is associated with severe mitral regurgitation, both should be addressed during the same operation.	In patients with severe AR who are undergoing cardiac surgery for another indication, concomitant aortic valve surgery is indicated.
Moderate AR + another severe valve disease	
In patients with moderate aortic regurgitation who undergo mitral valve surgery, the decision to treat the aortic valve in more controversial and it should be made by the Heart Team based on the aetiology of AR, other clinical factors, the life expectancy of the patient and the patient's operative risk.	In patients with moderate AR who are undergoing cardiac or aortic surgery for another indication, aortic valve surgery is reasonable.
Mitral stenosis + aortic valve disease	
In patients with severe mitral stenosis combined with severe aortic valve disease, surgery is preferable when it is not contraindicated. The management of patients in whom surgery is contraindicated is difficult and requires a comprehensive and individualized evaluation by the Heart Team. In cases with severe mitral stenosis and moderate aortic valve disease, PMC can be performed to postpone the surgical treatment of both valves.	In patients with MS and AR who have continued severe symptoms not responsive to diuretics, intervention with valve surgery should be pursued. If mitral anatomy is favorable, percutaneous mitral balloon commissurotomy, followed by AVR or SAVR and open mitral commissurotomy should be preferred over double valve replacement.

dominant lesion can be used for symptomatic relief.[71] Some small series have shown good success rates for staged interventional treatment of aortic and mitral valve disease, but data regarding the outcome of staged interventional procedures in MVD are limited.[72]

Two principles guide the management of patients with multiple and mixed VHD: the dominant valve lesion dictates the

management of patients and the association of two moderate lesions can have a similar detrimental effect as a severe lesion, and intervention should be considered earlier if patients are symptomatic or in the presence of ventricular dysfunction/dilation or pulmonary hypertension.[1,2,59]

In patients with MVD, three main clinical scenarios can be encountered in clinical practice:[47]

1. Two or more severe lesions are present. As the likelihood of severe functional intolerance is high if one of the lesions is left untreated, both the European and American guidelines recommend simultaneous surgical correction of both/all severe lesions, if patients are symptomatic or ventricular dysfunction/dilatation are present.[1,2,59] In patients at prohibitive risk for surgery, staged transcatheter interventions may be considered.

2. One severe lesion associated with ≥1 nonsevere lesion(s). The treatment of the most severely diseased valve is recommended by current guidelines, whereas the management of the less-than-severe lesion(s) is less straightforward, but intervention is usually favored.[1,2,59] The surgical risk of a combined valve procedure and the long-term increase in morbidity associated with multiple valve prostheses should be balanced against the risk of eventual reoperation and the prognostic impact of not correcting the less-severe lesion during the initial procedure. In addition, patient's wishes, life expectancy, and comorbidities should be considered, and in elderly patients, incomplete, single valve procedures may be considered for improving quality of life.

3. If ≥2 moderate lesions are present and if the overall hemodynamic burden imposed by these lesions is believed to be the main cause of the symptoms or LV systolic dysfunction, a surgical or transcatheter valve intervention could be considered. In this setting, it is of particular importance to determine the global consequences of the lesions. This includes careful assessment of ventricular volumes and pulmonary pressure, natriuretic peptides measurements, and, in selected cases, the assessment of functional capacity, maximal oxygen consumption, and pulmonary pressure during exercise, although there is only limited literature in the specific setting of multiple valve disease.[46]

In patients with mixed VHD and at least one severe lesion, the management follows the recommendations for the severe lesion. Because patients with moderate mixed VHD seem to have a risk of adverse events similar to patients with isolated single lesion, surgical or transcatheter intervention may be considered.

Areas of Uncertainty

Little evidence exists in the field of multiple and mixed VHD and more studies are needed regarding the use of different imaging modalities for diagnosis, identifying parameters with prognostic importance in patients with associated moderate lesions for guiding intervention or follow-up, and evaluating the outcome of staged interventional therapies.

PROSTHETIC HEART VALVES

Introduction

PHV replacement is often the only effective treatment for patients affected by severe VHD. About 4 million PHV replacements have been performed over the last 50 years, and the total number of replacements is projected to be 850,000 per year by 2050.[73]

Design of Prosthetic Heart Valves

A large number of designs and models of PHVs have been placed on the market over the years, but some were withdrawn or are only rarely implanted nowadays because of a greater risk of complications. PHVs are broadly grouped into two categories: mechanical and biological (**Figs. 29–6 and 29–7**).

Mechanical Heart Valves

There are three types of mechanical heart valves (MHVs): bileaflet, single tilting disc, and caged ball valves (**Fig. 29–6**). Of these, the bileaflet mechanical valves are the most frequently implanted nowadays, followed by low thrombogenicity single tilting disc valves. Although the caged ball valves are practically no longer implanted (because of their high thrombotic risk), due to their long life span they can still be encountered. The bileaflet valve consists of two semilunar discs attached by small hinges to a rigid valve ring. The opening angle of the leaflets relative to the annulus plane ranges from 75° to 90°. When the valve is open, three orifices let the blood pass through: a small, rectangular, central orifice and two larger, semicircular orifices laterally. There is a small amount of normal regurgitation with bileaflet heart valves, designed in part to decrease the risk of thrombosis ("washing jets"), with a small central jet and two lateral converging jets visualized on color-flow Doppler imaging.

Biological Heart Valves

Bioprostheses (tissue valves) can be classified into stented, stentless, sutureless, and transcatheter (**Fig. 29–7**). Based on the origin of the tissue used for making the leaflets, they can be classified into bovine or porcine heterografts (xenografts), homografts (allografts) from human cadaver, and autografts of pericardial or pulmonic valve origine.

Stented Bioprostheses: Stented bioprostheses are the most common biological heart valves (BHVs) implanted. They are composed of fabric-covered polymer or metallic stents with a sewing ring outside and the valve inside.

Porcine stented valves are made of three porcine aortic valve cusps cross-linked with glutaraldehyde and mounted on a fabric-covered metallic or polymer supporting stent. Because there is a muscle bar at the base of the porcine right coronary cusp, making it relatively obstructive, this cusp can be replaced by a single cusp from another pig (eg, Hancock Modified Orifice), or, more frequently, each cusp can be taken from three different pigs to produce a tricomposite valve (eg, Medtronic Mosaic, St. Jude Epic, Carbomedics Synergy).[74]

Stented pericardial bioprostheses have cusps made from pericardium or a sheet of pericardium cut using a template, which is sewn inside and, occasionally, outside of the stent posts (eg, Mitroflow, Trifecta).[74] The pericardium is most commonly bovine, occasionally porcine and, experimentally, from kangaroos.[74] The newer generation bovine pericardial valves (eg, Carpentier-Edwards PERIMOUNT) offer better hemodynamic performance and have a lower rate of structural valve deterioration than earlier-generation porcine bioprostheses.[75] They also seem to have a better hemodynamic performance than the newer generation porcine stented valves.[76]

**Bileaflet Mechanical
Heart Valves**

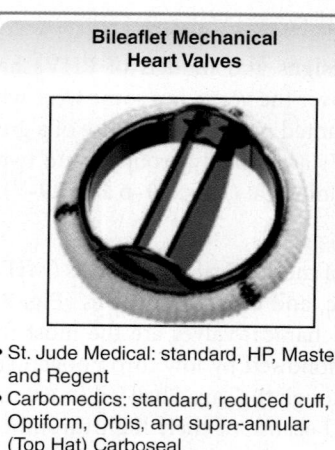

- St. Jude Medical: standard, HP, Masters and Regent
- Carbomedics: standard, reduced cuff, Optiform, Orbis, and supra-annular (Top Hat) Carboseal includes a woven aortic graft
- Edwards Tekna
- Sorin Bicarbon
- Edwards Mira
- ATS
- On-X
- Medtronic Advantage
- Jyros

**Tilting Disc Mechanical
Heart Valves**

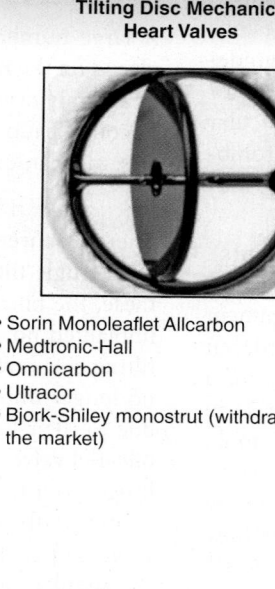

- Sorin Monoleaflet Allcarbon
- Medtronic-Hall
- Omnicarbon
- Ultracor
- Bjork-Shiley monostrut (withdrawn from the market)

**Caged Ball Mechanical
Heart Valves**

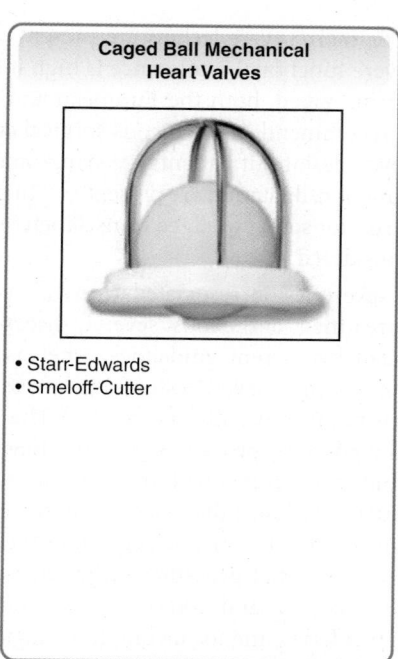

- Starr-Edwards
- Smeloff-Cutter

Figure 29–6. Designs and models of mechanical heart valves. The prostheses represented are the St. Jude Medical bileaflet valve, the Medtronic Hall tilting disc valve, and the Starr–Edwards caged-ball valve. Data from Lancellotti P, Pibarot P, Chambers J, et al. Recommendations for the imaging assessment of prosthetic heart valves: a report from the European Association of Cardiovascular Imaging endorsed by the Chinese Society of Echocardiography, the Inter-American Society of Echocardiography, and the Brazilian Department of Cardiovascular Imaging. *Eur Heart J Cardiovasc Imaging.* 2016 Jun;17(6):589-590. Device images reproduced with permission from Medtronic, Inc., Minneapolis, MN – St. Jude Medical, Inc., Minneapolis, MN – Sorin Group, Inc., Milan, Italy – On-X Life Technologies, Inc., Austin, TX – Edwards Lifesciences, Ltd., Irvine, CA.

Stented Bioprostheses

Stented porcine valves

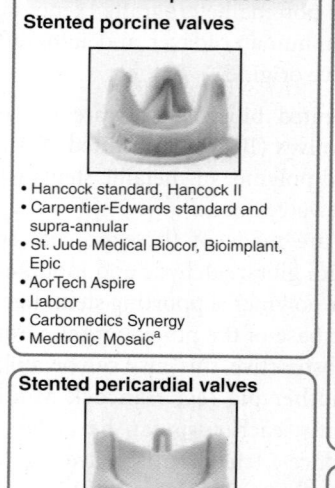

- Hancock standard, Hancock II
- Carpentier-Edwards standard and supra-annular
- St. Jude Medical Biocor, Bioimplant, Epic
- AorTech Aspire
- Labcor
- Carbomedics Synergy
- Medtronic Mosaic[a]

Stented pericardial valves

- Carpentier-Edwards Perimount
- Carpentier Edwards Magna
- Mitroflow Synergy
- St. Jude Biocor pericardia
- St. Jude Trifecta
- Labcor pericardial
- Sorin Pericarbon MORE[a]

Stentless Bioprostheses

Stentless porcine valves

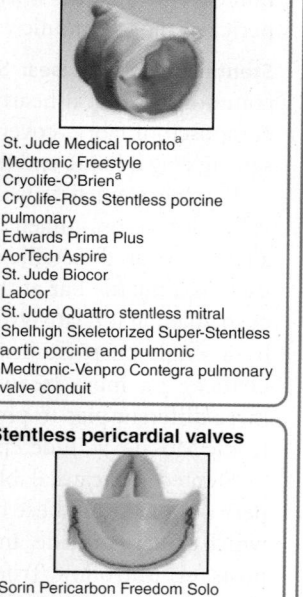

- St. Jude Medical Toronto[a]
- Medtronic Freestyle
- Cryolife-O'Brien[a]
- Cryolife-Ross Stentless porcine pulmonary
- Edwards Prima Plus
- AorTech Aspire
- St. Jude Biocor
- Labcor
- St. Jude Quattro stentless mitral
- Shelhigh Skeletorized Super-Stentless aortic porcine and pulmonic
- Medtronic-Venpro Contegra pulmonary valve conduit

Stentless pericardial valves

- Sorin Pericarbon Freedom Solo
- 3F-SAVR

Sutureless Bioprostheses

- Perceval S (Sorin)
- Edwards Intuity (Edwards Lifesciences)
- 3F Enable (ATS Medical)
- Trilogy (Arbor Surgical Technologies)

Transcatheter Bioprostheses

Balloon-expandable valves

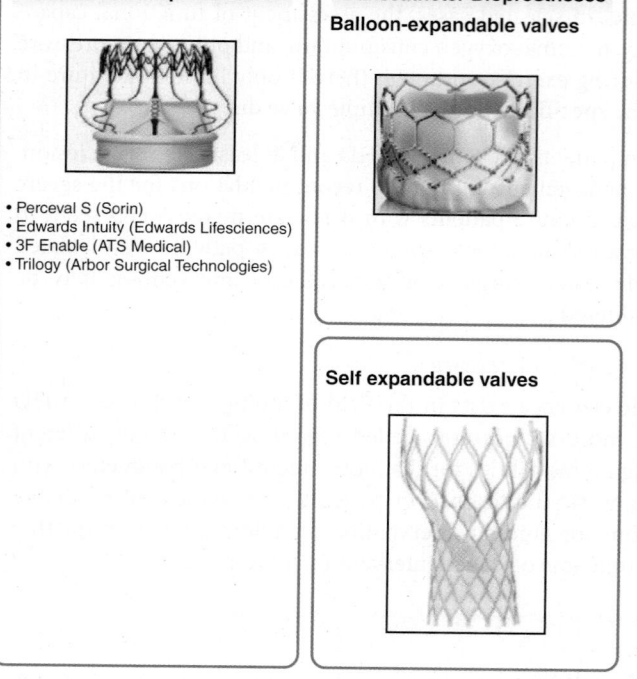

Self expandable valves

Figure 29–7. Designs and models of biological heart valves. The prostheses represented are the Carpentier Edwards standard and the Carpentier Edwards magna ease (stented valves), the Medtronic Freestyle, the Sorin Pericarbon Freedom solo (stentless valves), the Perceval S (sutureless valves), the Sapien 3, and the CoreValve EvolutR (transcatheter valves). [a]Prostheses withdrawn from the market. Data from Lancellotti P, Pibarot P, Chambers J, et al. Recommendations for the imaging assessment of prosthetic heart valves: a report from the European Association of Cardiovascular Imaging endorsed by the Chinese Society of Echocardiography, the Inter-American Society of Echocardiography, and the Brazilian Department of Cardiovascular Imaging. *Eur Heart J Cardiovasc Imaging.* 2016 Jun;17(6):589-590. Device images reproduced with permission from Medtronic, Inc., Minneapolis, MN – St. Jude Medical, Inc., Minneapolis, MN – Sorin Group, Inc., Milan, Italy – On-X Life Technologies, Inc., Austin, TX – Edwards Lifesciences, Ltd., Irvine, CA.

Stentless Bioprostheses: Stentless bioprostheses consist of a preparation of porcine aorta, which can be relatively long (eg, Medtronic Freestyle) or may be made to fit under the coronary arteries (eg, St. Jude Medical Toronto). Some are tricomposite (eg, Cryolife-O'Brien, Biocor) or made from bovine pericardium (eg, Sorin Freedom).[74] They were introduced with the hope of improving the hemodynamic performance and decreasing the risk of complications related to the presence of the stent. The risk of structural vale deterioration of stentless valves is, however, not lower than of the newer generation stented pericardial valves.[77,78] Also, their implantation is more challenging and hence are preferred by only a minority of surgeons. They can be advantageous in patients with small aortic annuli, especially in older patients for whom the risk of structural valve deterioration is lower.[79]

Homografts: Homografts are cryopreserved aortic valves (less often pulmonary valve), harvested from human cadavers within 24 hours of death as blocks of tissue comprising the ascending aorta, aortic valve, a portion of the interventricular septum, and the anterior mitral valve leaflet. They are used especially in cases of aortic valve and root endocarditis, where wide debridement of infection is necessary, allowing the replacement of the aortic root and valve, with the possibility of repairing perforations of the anterior mitral leaflet by using the attached flap of the donor mitral leaflet.[74] Due to their good durability, homographs can also be used as an alternative to MHVs in young patients where anticoagulation can pose a problem.[74] However, more recent trials have shown that long-term durability beyond 10 years of homografts is not superior to that of current generation pericardial valves,[80] the risk of structural valve deterioration being particularly increased in young patients.[81]

Autografts: In the Ross procedure, the patient's own pulmonic valve is harvested as a small tissue block containing the pulmonic valve, annulus, and proximal pulmonary artery, and is inserted in the aortic position with reimplantation of the coronary arteries. An aortic or pulmonic homograft is then implanted in the pulmonary position.[82] It is an infrequently performed surgery, requiring extensive training. Due to the ability of the autograft to increase in size during childhood growth, the Ross procedure is usually preferred in children and young adults with congenital aortic disease. Because the autograft is relatively resistant to infection, it can also constitute an option in cases of aortic valve endocarditis.[74] The use of pericardial autograft valves confectioned in the operating room from the patient's own pericardium has had very limited support but good results in small subsets of patients.[83]

Sutureless Valves: Sutureless valves are biological valves mounted on a stent that expands and attaches to the aortic ring through controlled release under direct vision. Similar to conventional AVR, sutureless AVR requires valve excision and annular decalcification, but avoids the use of permanent sutures. There are three sutureless prostheses on the market: the 3f Enable, the Sorin Perceval S, and the Edwards Intuity. The main advantage of the sutureless valves reside in the reduction of the bypass time, facilitating minimally invasive approaches or concomitant cardiac surgery in high-risk patients.[84] They can also be an alternative to standard surgery in patients with small, calcified aortic root.[84] Current short-term clinical evidence indicates good hemodynamic performance, similar mortality and complication rates as compared to conventional surgical prosthesis,[84] and a lower incidence of paravalvular regurgitation compared to TAVR.[85] However, long-term outcome and durability data are missing.

Transcatheter Heart Valves: Transcatheter heart valves (THVs) are relatively new valves that were first introduced for the treatment of symptomatic patients with severe AS at high risk for surgical aortic valve replacement (SAVR) or considered inoperable for technical reasons.[56] The advances made in recent years in TAVR have led to a significant decrease in complications and have paved the way for the use of this procedure in intermediate- and even low-risk patients with severe AS.

Two main types of THVs are currently available: balloon-expandable and self-expanding valves. Other prostheses are available for TAVR (Lotus valve, Portico, ACURATE Neo, Engager, and JenaValve) but the experience with these valves is more limited.

The third generation of balloon-expandable SAPIEN™ valve (Edwards Lifesciences Corporation, Irvine, California) includes the SAPIEN 3 and the SAPIEN 3 Ultra valves, which are composed of a cobalt-chromium frame cylindrical stent into which three symmetric leaflets made of bovine pericardium are mounted. The sealing skirt is meant to decrease the risk of paravalvular regurgitation, while the short frame height and the open cell geometry of the SAPIEN 3 Ultra valve facilitate coronary access.

The most widely used self-expanding valve is the CoreValve™ (Medtronic, Inc., Minneapolis, Minnesota), which consists of three leaflets of porcine pericardium mounted within an asymmetrical, self-expanding nitinol frame. The frame is anchored within the aortic annulus, but owing to its length also extends superiorly in the supracoronary aorta. The CoreValve™ Evolut™ R can be recaptured and repositioned after deployment and it is the only valve indicated for arterial access diameters down to 5 mm.

Transcatheter replacement for the mitral valve is much less well developed in comparison with the aortic site. Balloon-expandable valves have been implanted through a transapical or transseptal approach in patients with dysfunctional mitral valve bioprosthesis or annuloplasty rings,[86,87] but most of the percutaneous prosthesis designed for the treatment of native MVD (Evoque, Intrepid, Tendyne, Tiara, High Life, Cephea, etc.) are in early clinical trial experiences.

Trials and Outcome

Mortality Rates

Early mortality rates (within 30 days) for surgical valve replacement are similar for mechanical and biological prostheses, in both aortic and mitral position.[88-92] Long-term survival after mitral valve replacement (MVR) and AVR is similar for both older and newer generation biological and mechanical valves,[88-92] but with some studies showing age-dependent differences in long-term mortality rates.[90-94] In a recent, large observational study, long-term mortality was increased in biological versus mechanical PHV in patients with AVR who were <55 years old at the time of surgery, and in patients with MVR who were <70 years old.[95] In a Swedish study on AVR, long-term mortality with a biological prosthesis was significantly increased in patients aged 50 to 59 years, while there was no significant difference in survival between the mechanical and bioprosthetic valve groups in patients aged 60 to 69 years.[93] In contrast, another study on AVR found no significant difference of survival related to the type of prosthesis in patients aged 50 to 69 years.[91]

Valve Durability and Risk of Reoperation

Studies have consistently shown that the risk of structural valve deterioration (SVD) and reoperation is higher in biological versus mechanical valves,[88-95] with failure occurring more commonly and earlier in patients undergoing MVR.[89] The risk of valve failure with consequent reoperation begins to rise 7 years after biological MVR and 10 years after biological AVR, and increases progressively thereafter.[92,95] In a meta-analysis, freedom from SVD post-AVR was 94.0% at 10 years, 81.7% at 15 years, and 52% at 20 years.[96] The risk of structural valve deterioration is higher in younger patients and in certain groups of patients such as those with chronic kidney disease.[90] The mortality associated with reoperation is the main determinant of long-term mortality after BHV replacement.[88] The risk of death related to reoperation for SVD has, however, decreased in recent years, with a 30-day mortality of 7% and 14% after redo-AVR and redo-MVR, respectively.[94] Transcatheter valve-in-valve interventions may offer an alternative to surgical reoperation in case of bioprosthetic valve degeneration, but data on the long-term outcome of this approach is limited.

Thrombotic and Bleeding Complications

Thromboembolism and bleeding are important complications of PHV because the occurrence of stroke or bleeding events is associated with an increased risk of death during follow-up.[90,91]

MHVs are associated with a significantly higher risk of bleeding, related to the use of anticoagulant treatment.[91,93-95] Only one study has shown a similar bleeding risk for biologic and mechanical AVR, but the large number of patients in the BHV group who received anticoagulation for another indication, such as occurrence of atrial fibrillation, could be the reason for the high bleeding risk with BHVs in this trial.[92] With regard to the risk of embolism, several studies have shown a similar risk of embolism and stroke in patients with MHVs and BHVs,[88-90] whereas others have shown an increased incidence of stroke in younger patients with MHVs.[96]

Endocarditis Risk

Prosthetic valve endocarditis (PVE) occurs in 1% to 6% of patients with valve prostheses and is associated with a poor prognosis.[97] Most of the studies have reported similar rates of infective endocarditis in patients with mechanical versus biological valves.[88,89,92] However, some series have suggested a higher incidence of early (<1 year) infection with mechanical

valves than with tissue heterografts[98] and a more recent observational study has suggested higher rates of both early and late infective endocarditis in patients with a bioprosthetic AVR.[99]

Choice of Prosthetic Heart Valve

Whenever there is an indication for valvular intervention and valve repair performed by an experienced surgeon is not an option, the choice of valve intervention (standard or minimally invasive surgery vs. transcatheter intervention) and the choice of prosthesis for valvular replacement (mechanical vs. biological) should be made in the heart valve team meeting. The choice between SAVR and TAVR is discussed in Chapter 28, Aortic Stenosis.

The choice between a mechanical and a biological valve in adults is mainly determined by the risk of anticoagulation-related bleeding and thromboembolism with an MHV versus the risk of SVD and reintervention with a BHV. Both the AHA/ACC guidelines and the ESC guidelines on VHD include recommendations for choice of PHV and both emphasize the importance of a shared decision, which takes into consideration the patient's lifestyle and preferences.[1,59] According to the guidelines, the following factors favor the choice of a MHV: no contraindication to long-term anticoagulation (eg, low risk of bleeding, patient's compliance to treatment); increased risk of accelerated SVD (eg, age <40 years, hyperparathyroidism); presence of an additional indication for anticoagulation (eg, existing mechanical prosthesis in another valve position, high risk of thromboembolism); reasonable patient's life expectancy; and high operative risk in case of redo valve surgery (eg, porcelain aorta, prior radiation therapy).[1,59] On the other hand, the following factors favor the choice of a BHV: contraindication to long-term anticoagulation (eg, high bleeding risk, poor patient's compliance); reoperation for mechanical valve thrombosis despite good long-term anticoagulant control; low operative risk in case of redo valve surgery; young women contemplating pregnancy; and patient's life expectancy lower than the presumed durability of the bioprosthesis.[2,100]

The age cutoffs for choosing a mechanical versus a biological prosthesis are different in the American versus the European guidelines, reflecting contradictory study results. The ACC/AHA guidelines recommend a lower age cutoff (<50 years) compared with the ESC guidelines (<60 years for the aortic position and <65 years for the mitral position) for considering a mechanical rather than a biological valve.[1,2] There has been an increase in the use of biological prosthesis in younger patients,[100] driven by the longer durability of the newer generation bioprostheses and the utilization of transcatheter valve-in-valve procedures for the treatment of degenerated bioprostheses. A shared decision, taking into consideration the factors cited earlier and patient's lifestyle and preferences, is perhaps better than setting arbitrary age limits.

Antithrombotic Therapy for Prosthetic Heart Valves
Mechanical Heart Valves

Vitamin K antagonists (VKAs) are recommended lifelong in patients with MHV in order to prevent valve thrombosis and embolic events, whereas novel oral anticoagulants (NOACs) are contraindicated in patients with MHV.[1,2,101] The initiation of VKAs requires close monitoring of the international normalized ratio (INR). After valve surgery, patients may have a transiently increased sensitivity to warfarin.[102] Measurement of the INR should be performed 2 to 3 times a week as therapy is initiated and at least monthly thereafter, when the target INR is reached. INR monitoring through dedicated anticoagulation clinics results in lower rates of bleeding and thromboembolic complications and improved costs as compared to standard monitoring[103] and should be considered in particular for patients with unstable INR or anticoagulant-related complications.[1] INR self- management with home measurement devices is associated with reduced INR variability and thromboembolic events and can be an option for educated patients.[1,2,104] The target INR is determined by the thrombogenicity of the prosthesis (eg, low for bi-disc and newer generation tilting disc valves, high for Starr–Edwards prosthesis or prosthesis in the mitral position) and patient-related risk factors for thromboembolism (atrial fibrillation, previous thromboembolism, LV dysfunction, or hypercoagulable conditions).[1,2] Both the European and the American guidelines recommend a specific target value for INR, with acceptable values 0.5 units on each side of the target, with the hope of avoiding INR fluctuations and considering extreme values in the target range as valid target INR.[1,2] The target INR for bi-disc and newer generation tilting-disc mechanical prostheses in the aortic position is 2.5 in the absence of risk factors, and 3 in patients with risk factors, whereas the target INR for mechanical valves in the mitral position is 3 in the absence of risk factors.[1,2] In the PRO-ACT study, a lower target INR associated with low-dose aspirin treatment was associated with a significantly lower risk of bleeding, without an increase in thromboembolism, after AVR with the bileaflet On-X mechanical prosthesis.[105] Based on this study, according to the ACC/AHA guidelines, a lower target INR of 1.5 to 2.0 may be reasonable in patients with mechanical On-X AVR and no thromboembolic risk factors after the first 3 months postsurgery.[2]

Aspirin at low-dose (75–100 mg) is recommended along with VKA in all patients with mechanical valves by the ACC/AHA guidelines (class I), whereas the ESC guidelines consider the addition of low-dose aspirin only in the case of concomitant atherosclerotic disease (class IIb) and in patients with thromboembolic events despite an adequate INR (class IIa).[1,2] Because there are no randomized trials with the newer generation, less thrombogenic mechanical prostheses comparing the addition of low-dose aspirin to VKAs in patients without vascular disease or atrial fibrillation, and the studies on atrial fibrillation showing an increased risk of bleeding with the addition of antiplatelet agents to VKAs, perhaps an individualized approach taking into consideration the embolic and hemorrhagic risks of each the patient is more appropriate.[106]

Biological Heart Valves

Several studies have shown an increased risk of ischemic stroke early after bioprosthetic AVR or MVR.[107,108] Anticoagulation early after valve implantation could decrease the embolic

risk until the prosthetic valve is fully endothelized, but at the expense of an increased bleeding risk. While there is general agreement that patients with bioprosthetic mitral valves should be treated with VKAs for at least 3 months, to a target INR of 2.5,[1,2] there is a lack of consensus regrading a clear benefit of anticoagulation over low-dose aspirin early after bioprosthetic AVR.[108-110] Taking into consideration a report from the Danish National Patient Registry that showed an increased risk of cardiovascular death when warfarin was discontinued within 6 months of bioprosthetic AVR, the ACC/AHA guidelines give a class IIa recommendation for the use of VKAs up to 6 months after surgical bioprosthetic AVR in patients at low risk of bleeding.[2] On the other hand, the ESC guidelines favor the use of low-dose aspirin in the first 3 months after biologic AVR.[1]

The recommendations regarding the long-term use of antiplatelet therapy are also different in the European and American Guidelines. According to the ACC/AHA guidelines, low-dose aspirin is reasonable in all patients with a bioprosthetic aortic or mitral valve, whereas the ESC guidelines do not support the use of antiplatelet therapy beyond the first 3 months in patients with surgical bioprostheses who do not have an indication for antiplatelet therapy other than the presence of the bioprosthesis itself.[1,2]

Lifelong oral anticoagulation is recommended for patients with a bioprosthesis and other indications for anticoagulation, such as atrial fibrillation.[1] NOACs can be used after the first 3 months in patients who have atrial fibrillation associated with a bioprosthesis.[101]

Transcatheter Heart Valves

The optimal antithrombotic strategy following TAVR is undetermined. Current guidelines recommend dual antiplatelet therapy (DAPT) with aspirin and clopidogrel for 3 to 6 months, followed by lifelong single antiplatelet treatment (SAPT), while anticoagulant treatment may be considered for the first 3 months post-TAVI in patients at low-bleeding risk.[1,2]

The rationale for prescribing DAPT in TAVR patients has been the prevention of ischemic events, particularly stroke, following the procedure. However, some small randomized studies have suggested the lack of any beneficial effect of DAPT over SAPT for the prevention of cerebrovascular events post-TAVR.[11-113] In the ARTE trial, SAPT (vs DAPT) was associated with a lower risk of major or life-threatening bleeding, without an increased risk of stroke or myocardial infarction at 30 days.[113] More than half of strokes post-TAVR occur in the first 24 hours, caused by embolism related to the procedure itself, and a significant proportion of subacute strokes (>24 hours) are related to atrial arrhythmias.[114] These might be the explanations for the absence of a benefit of DAPT versus SAPT for stroke reduction seen in these small studies. Also, DAPT (vs VKAs) is not effective in preventing valve thrombosis following TAVR, while the bleeding risk of the two treatment options is similar.[115] Large randomized trials comparing SAPT, DAPT, and oral anticoagulant treatment in TAVR patients are ongoing.

For the time being, in the absence of a concurrent indication for anticoagulation, as atrial fibrillation, NOACs should not be used post-TAVR. In the GALILEO trial, rivaroxaban versus antiplatelet treatment post-TVR was associated with an increased risk of death and thromboembolic and bleeding complications.[116]

Follow-Up and Complications

Because there is no ideal PHV, regular lifelong follow-up by a cardiologist is required for evaluating prosthetic function and the occurrence of complications. Both the European and the American guidelines recommend clinical assessment every year or earlier in case symptoms occur.[1,2]

Early postoperative TTE is recommended in all patients to establish the baseline hemodynamic function of the prosthesis, with follow-up imaging at 30 days (ESC), or in between 6 weeks to 3 months after valve implantation (ACC/AHA).[1,2] In the presence of symptoms and signs suggestive of mechanical or biological PHV dysfunction, both guidelines recommend TTE. For MHVs, guidelines do not support regular follow-up imaging for patients who are stable, unless there is another indication for echocardiography. For bioprostheses, the ESC guidelines recommend TTE yearly, while the ACC/AHA guidelines recommend annual TTE only after 10 years from valve implant.[1,2] The ACC/AHA recommendation is based on the observation that bioprosthetic valve failure (BVF) with the newer bioprostheses is rare in the first 10 years. The ESC recommendation is based on the consensus document regarding the standardized definition of SVD and valve failure for surgical and transcatheter bioprosthesis.[117] Because SVD can occur earlier in certain patients, and some complications such as valve thrombosis can occur in the absence of symptoms, routine annual TTE after transcatheter and surgical bioprostheses seems so be a more appropriate follow-up.[106]

The echocardiographic evaluation of PHVs follows the same principles as the evaluation of native valve disease, but the diagnosis and identification of the causes of valvular dysfunction is often more challenging. The parameters that should be evaluated at the echocardiographic follow-up for mitral and aortic prosthesis are synthesized in **Table 29–5**, whereas **Tables 29–6** and **29–7** present the parameters suggesting a dysfunction of mitral and aortic prostheses.

TEE is recommended in all cases of suspected prosthetic dysfunction.[1,2] Three-dimensional echocardiography, in particular on transesophageal images, can improve the evaluation of PHVs through a better visualization of the components of PHVs, offering a more precise localization of thrombus, pannus, vegetations, the regurgitant jets, and the extension of prosthetic valve dehiscence.[74] Stress echocardiography can be useful whenever there is a discordance between patient's symptoms and the hemodynamical evaluation of PHV at rest.[74,39] Cinefluoroscopy (for mechanical valves) and MDCT (for mechanical and biological valves) provide useful additional information in case pannus or thrombus are suspected, and nuclear imaging should be considered when PVE is suspected.[1,74]

Structural Valve Deterioration

SVD represents the dysfunction of the prosthesis caused by changes intrinsic to the valve.[74] The occurrence of SVD is the main limitation of BHVs, being extremely rare in the current

TABLE 29–5. Parameters That Should be Evaluated at the Echocardiographic Follow-Up for Mitral and Aortic Prostheses

Echocardiographic Parameters for Aortic Prostheses	Echocardiographic Parameters for Mitral Prostheses
• Peak velocity • Mean pressure gradient • Velocity time integral (VTI) • Doppler velocity index (DVI) • Effective orifice area (EOA) by the continuity equation • Presence, location, and severity of regurgitation • Evaluation of LV size and function (a hyperdynamic LV is a useful indirect sign of severe aortic regurgitation), LVH, aorta (most likely to continue to dilate if dilated at the time of surgery) • Evaluation of other valves valves: appearance, grade of stenosis, and regurgitation	• Peak velocity • Mean pressure gradient • Velocity time integral (VTI) • Doppler velocity index (DVI) • Effective orifice area (EOA) by the continuity equation • Pressure half time • Presence, location, and severity of regurgitation • Evaluation of LV size and function (a hyperdynamic LV is a useful indirect sign of severe MR), LA size, estimated systolic pulmonary artery pressure (pulmonary hypertension may be a sign of mitral dysfunction) • Evaluation of other valves: appearance, grade of stenosis, and regurgitation.

Abbreviations: LV, left ventricle; LVH, left ventricular hypertrophy; LA, left atrium; MR, mitral regurgitation.
Adapted with permission from Lancellotti P, Pibarot P, Chambers J, et al. Recommendations for the imaging assessment of prosthetic heart valves: a report from the European Association of Cardiovascular Imaging endorsed by the Chinese Society of Echocardiography, the Inter-American Society of Echocardiography, and the Brazilian Department of Cardiovascular Imaging. *Eur Heart J Cardiovasc Imaging.* 2016 Jun;17(6):589-590.

generation MHVs. The risk of SVD is determined by prosthesis related factors—the type of prosthesis and its position, occurring earlier in the mitral than in the aortic position—and patient related factors, with younger age, renal failure, abnormal calcium metabolism, presence of patient–prosthesis mismatch (PPM) being associated with an increased risk of SVD.

In order to better appreciate and compare outcome of bioprosthetic and transcatheter valves between studies, standardized definitions for SVD were provided by the EAPCI (European Association of Percutaneous Cardiovascular Interventions) and VIVID (Valve-in-valve International Data).[117,118] SVD is defined as an acquired, intrinsic, permanent abnormality of the leaflets or supporting structures (calcification, thickening, tear, or flail) leading to degeneration and/or hemodynamic dysfunction, with stenosis or intraprosthetic regurgitation.[117,118] SVD should be differentiated from potentially reversible causes of prosthesis dysfunction (eg, thrombus, endocarditis) and from nonstructural valve dysfunction. Nonstructural valve dysfunction, thrombus and infective endocarditis can subsequently lead to SVD and they can all lead to BVF. **Figure 29–8** represents the relationship between bioprosthetic valve dysfunction and failure.

Echocardiography is the main and first investigation used for the diagnosis of SVD. TTE is especially useful for appreciating the hemodynamic modifications and to a lesser degree the morphologic modifications of the prostheses, which are better appreciated by TEE. TEE, together with CT, can be used for differentiating the causes of prosthetic valve dysfunction in the individual patient.

TABLE 29-6. Echocardiographic Grading of Aortic and Mitral Prosthetic Valve Obstruction

Aortic Prostheses		
Echocardiographic parameters	**Possible obstruction**	**Significant obstruction**
Valve structure and motion	Often abnormal[a]	Abnormal[a]
Vmax	3–3.9 m/s	≥4m/s
MPG	20–34 mm Hg	≥35 mm Hg
ΔMPG (follow-up or during stress echocardiography)	10–19 mm Hg	≥20 mm Hg
EOA	0.8–1.1cm^2	<0.8cm^2
Measured EOA vs. normal reference value	<Reference -1SD	<Reference -2SD
ΔEOA	0.25–0.35 cm^2	>0.35 cm^2
DVI	0.25–0.34	<0.25
Acceleration time	80–100 ms	>100 ms
Acceleration time/LV ejection time ratio	0.32–0.37	>0.37
Transvalvular flow envelope	Triangular to intermediate	Rounded, symmetrical
Mitral Prostheses		
Echocardiographic parameters	**Possible obstruction**	**Significant obstruction**
Valve structure and motion	Often abnormal[a]	Abnormal[a]
Vmax	1.9–2.5 m/s	>2.5 m/s
MPG	6–10 mm Hg	>10 mm Hg
ΔMPG (follow-up)	3–5 mm Hg	>5 mm Hg
ΔMPG (stress echocardiography)	5–12 mm Hg	>12 mm Hg
EOA	1–2 cm^2	<1cm^2
Measured EOA vs. normal reference value	<Reference -1SD	<Reference -2SD
ΔEOA	0.25–0.35 cm^2	>0.35 cm^2
PHT	130–200 ms	>200 ms
DVI	2.2–2.5	>2.5

[a]Abnormal mechanical valves: immobile occluder or with restricted mobility, presence of thrombus/pannus; abnormal biologic valves: leaflet thickening/calcification, presence of thrombus/pannus. Vmax maximum velocity of transvalvular aortic/mitral flow in systole/diastole; MPG mean pressure gradient; ΔMPG is the increase in mean pressure gradient at follow-up (compared to post-operative value) or during stress echocardiography.

Abbreviations: EOA, effective orifice area; ΔEOA, the difference between the reference and the measured EOA; SD, standard deviation; DVI, Doppler velocity index; PHT, pressure half time.

Data from Lancellotti P, Pibarot P, Chambers J, et al. Recommendations for the imaging assessment of prosthetic heart valves: a report from the European Association of Cardiovascular Imaging endorsed by the Chinese Society of Echocardiography, the Inter-American Society of Echocardiography, and the Brazilian Department of Cardiovascular Imaging. Eur Heart J Cardiovasc Imaging. 2016 Jun;17(6):589-590.

The approach to patients with SVD depends on the hemodynamic severity of SVD and patient's symptoms. Patients with evidence of moderate SVD should be followed up more closely, whereas, patients with severe SVD should be evaluated in a similar way as patients with severe native valve stenosis/regurgitation and redo-SAVR or valve-in-valve TAVI should be considered in symptomatic patients.[117,118]

Nonstructural Valve Dysfunction

Nonstructural valve dysfunction represents any abnormality not intrinsic to the valve itself, other than the presence of thrombus or endocarditis, that can lead to stenosis or regurgitation of the prosthesis, or hemolysis.[74] It includes the entrapment of the prosthesis by pannus, tissue, or suture; the presence of paravalvular regurgitation; clinically important intravascular hemolysis; PPM; and AR due to dilatation of the aorta (for stentless prostheses).[74]

Pannus is a nonimmune inflammatory reaction of the organism to the valve prosthesis, with excessive proliferation of fibroelastic tissue and collagen, leading, most often, to obstruction of the prosthesis. Pannus formation starts in the suture/annulus area and has a centripetal extension.

Although it is a rare cause of prosthetic stenosis, pannus formation can have serious consequences, being the second most common cause for MHV reintervention.[119] The incidence of pannus formation causing prosthesis obstruction is similar in BHVs and MHVs, and is higher for the mitral position.[119]

Differentiation of pannus from other causes of prosthetic obstruction, mainly thrombus, remains challenging, but is of paramount importance for patient's treatment. Moreover, pannus and thrombus are often associated, making the task even more difficult. A combination of clinical and imaging parameters can be used for differentiating the two conditions (**Table 29-8**). Pannus develops after the first-year postsurgery, most commonly after 5 years, is associated with a subacute or chronic symptom onset, and, at echocardiography, it presents as a small, dense mass (same echo intensity as the valve housing) firmly fixed to the valve apparatus (valve housing and

TABLE 29–7. Echocardiographic Grading of Aortic and Mitral Prosthetic Valve Regurgitation, According to the EACVI Recommendations for the Evaluation of PHVs

Echocardiographic Parameters	Aortic Prosthesis Regurgitation		
	Mild	Moderate	Severe
Valve structure and motion	Usually normal	Usually abnormal[a]	Usually abnormal[a]
Colour flow AR jet width (for central jets)	Small	Intermediate	Large (>65% of LVOT diameter)
Circumferencial extent of paravalvular regurgitation	<10%	10-29%	≥ 30%
VC width	<3 mm	3-6 mm	>6 mm
EROA	<10 mm²	10-29 mm²	≥ 30 mm²
RVol	<30 mL	30-59 Ml	≥60 Ml
RF	<30 %	30-50%	>50%
Diastolic flow reversal in the descending aorta	Brief, protodiastolic	Intermediate	Holodiastolic, end-diastolic velocity>20 cm/s
PHT	>500 ms	200-500 ms	< 200 ms
CW signal density of the AR jet	Incomplete or faint	Dense	Dense
LV size (for chronic AR, in the absence of other causes).			Dilated LV

Echocardiographic Parameters	Mitral Prosthesis Regurgitation		
	Mild	Moderate	Severe
Valve structure and motion	Usually normal	Usually abnormal[a]	Usually abnormal[a]
Colour flow MR jet	Small	Intermediate	Large central jet or eccentric jet adhering, swirling, and reaching the posterior LA wall
Flow convergence (at Nyquist 50-60cm/s)	No/small	Intermediate	Large (PISA radius ≥9mm at a Nyquist of 40cm/sec)
Circumferential extent of paravalvular regurgitation	<10%	10-29%	≥30%
Mitral inflow	Variable	Variable	Peak E wave >1.9 m/s, MPG >5 mm Hg
VC width	<3 mm	3-5.9 mm	>6 mm
EROA	<20 mm²	20-39 mm²	>40 mm²
RVol	<30 mL	30-59 mL	>60 mL
RF	<30%	30-50%	>50%
Doppler velocity index (VTIPrMV/VTILVOT)	<2.2	2.2-2.5	>2.5
Pulmonary vein flow	Systolic dominance	Systolic blunting	Systolic flow reversal
CW signal of MR jet	Faint, parabolic	Dense, parabolic	Dense, triangular
+LV and LA size, PAP (for chronic prosthetic MR in the absence of another cause)			

Abbreviations: AR aortic regurgitation; LVOT, left ventricular outflow tract; EROA, effective regurgitant orifice area; RVol, regurgitant volume; RF, regurgitant fraction; PHT, pressure half time; LV, left ventricle; MPG, mean pressure gradient; VC, vena contracta; VTI$_{PrMV}$ velocity time integral of the diastolic mitral prosthesis flow; VTILVOT, velocity time integral of the systolic flow of blood at left ventricular outflow tract; LA, left atrium; PAP, pulmonary artery pressure; MR, mitral regurgitation.
Data from Lancellotti P, Pibarot P, Chambers J, et al. Recommendations for the imaging assessment of prosthetic heart valves: a report from the European Association of Cardiovascular Imaging endorsed by the Chinese Society of Echocardiography, the Inter-American Society of Echocardiography, and the Brazilian Department of Cardiovascular Imaging. *Eur Heart J Cardiovasc Imaging*. 2016 Jun;17(6):589-590. [a]Abnormal mechanical valve: immobile occluder, dehiscence or rocking of the prosthesis (paravalvular regurgitation); abnormal biologic valves: cusps thickening/calcification or prolapse, dehiscence or rocking (paravalvular regurgitation).

pivot guards). Fluoroscopy and cardiac CT can be useful for differentiating between the two conditions.[74]

Treatment of patients with severe stenosis due to pannus overgrowth consists in surgical intervention with redo-valve replacement or pannus removal.

Paravalvular Regurgitation or Leak: This occurs external to the prosthetic valve, between the sewing ring and the native valve annulus. Paravalvular regurgitation or leak (PVL) is a common complication of PHVs, occurring in 7% to 17% of mitral and 2% to 10% of aortic prosthesis.[88,120,121] The prevalence of PVL is similar in mechanical and biological valves and, although many patients with TAVR have a small paravalvular regurgitation, the risk of moderate or more regurgitation associated to TAVR has decreased considerably in recent years.

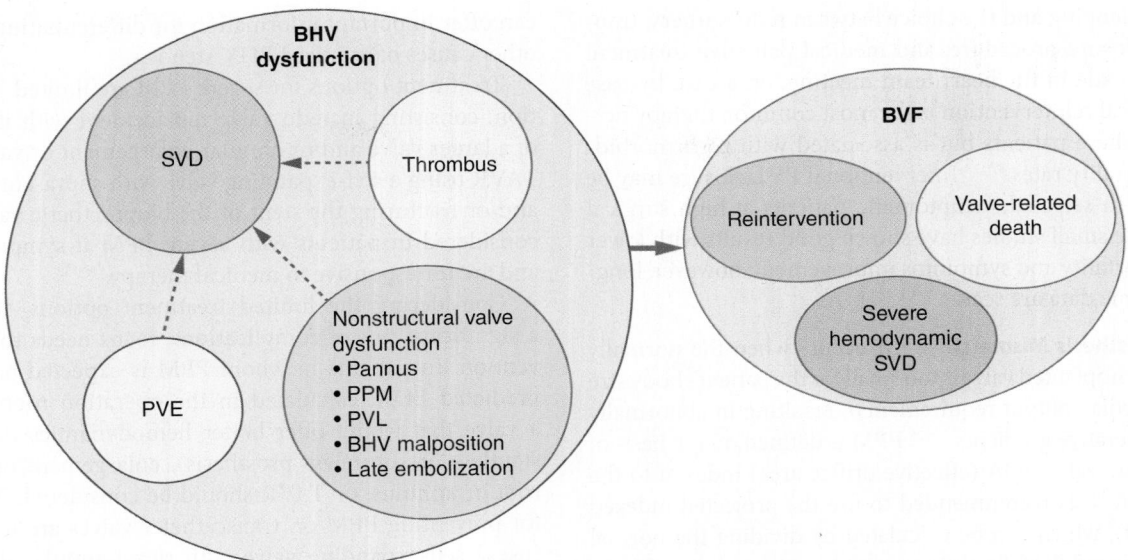

Figure 29–8. Relationship between dysfunction and failure of bioprosthetic heart valves. Bioprosthetic heart valve dysfunction can be caused by SVD, nonstructural valve deterioration, thrombosis, and infection. Thrombus, infection, and nonstructural valve dysfunction can subsequently lead to SVD. Severe BHV dysfunction can lead to BVF. BVF includes patients with severe hemodynamic SVD, patients with reintervention for confirmed BHV dysfunction (redo-surgery, valve-in-valve TAVR, or transcatheter PVL closure) and autopsy findings of BHV dysfunction likely related the cause of death or valve related death (death caused by BHV dysfunction, sudden unexplained death following diagnosis of BHV dysfunction). BHV, bioprosthetic heart valve; BVF, bioprosthetic valve failure; PPM, patient-prosthesis mismatch; PVE, prosthetic valve endocarditis; PVL, paravalvular leak; SVD, structural valve deterioration.

Most PVLs are apparent on the immediate postoperative study being caused by technical problems at the time of surgery (dehiscence or inadequate surgical technique, presence of important calcifications, friable tissue). Late dehiscence is often a consequence of infective endocarditis, and, less commonly, caused to wear- or age-related deterioration of the tissue surrounding the suture line.[74,122]

The diagnosis of PVL is made by echocardiography when the origin of the regurgitant jet is outside the sewing ring. TEE may be needed to appropriately visualize the origin of the jet, especially in the case of mechanical prosthesis and in the mitral position. Nuclear imaging offers important information when infective endocarditis is considered.

The management of patients with PVL depends on the severity of the regurgitant jet and the clinical presentation. Small PVLs, discovered incidentally on the echocardiographic exam, usually do not pose a risk in the absence of infective endocarditis and no treatment is necessary. However, small PVLs can, in some cases, be associated with significant hemolytic anemia and reoperation is recommended in patients who need repeated blood transfusions.[1] Large PVLs lead to volume overload and heart failure. The management of these patients

TABLE 29–8. Differential Diagnosis of Pannus and Thrombus

	Pannus	Thrombus
Chronology	>12 months, commonly >5 years from surgery date	Can occur at any time (if late, associated with pannus)
Relation to anticoagulation (low INR)	Poor relationship	Strong relationship
Location	MV>AV	TV>MV>AV
Morphology	• Small mass • Mostly involve suture lines (ring • Centripetal growth • Confine to the disk plane • Growth beneath the disk	• Larges mass than pannus • Independent motion common • Thin outer ring may be visible • Project into LA for MV position • Mobile elements
Echo density (video intensity ratio)	>0.7 (100% specific)	<0.4
Cardiac CT (attenuation value)	>200 HU	<200 HU
Impact on gradient and valve orifice	AV>MV	MV>AV
Impact on disk motion	Yes/No	Yes

Abbreviations: INR, international normalized ratio; MV, mitral valve; AV, aortic valve; TV, tricuspid valve; LA, left atrium.
Adapted with permission from Lancellotti P, Pibarot P, Chambers J, et al. Recommendations for the imaging assessment of prosthetic heart valves: a report from the European Association of Cardiovascular Imaging endorsed by the Chinese Society of Echocardiography, the Inter-American Society of Echocardiography, and the Brazilian Department of Cardiovascular Imaging. *Eur Heart J Cardiovasc Imaging.* 2016 Jun;17(6):589-590.

can be challenging and the choice between redo-surgery, transcatheter closure procedure, and medical palliative treatment should be made in the heart team meeting, on a case-by-case basis. Surgical reintervention is the most common therapy performed in these patients but is associated with high morbidity and mortality rates.[87,123] Interventional PVL closure may be considered in selected, symptomatic patients at high surgical risk, because small studies have shown good results with lower hospital mortality and symptoms improvement; however, long-term outcome data are scarce.[124,125]

Patient–Prosthesis Mismatch: PPM occurs when the normally functioning implanted valve is too small for the patient's body size (and the cardiac output requirements), resulting in abnormally high postoperative gradients.[74,126] PPM is defined on the basis of the prosthetic valve EOA (effective orifice area) indexed to the patient's BSA. It is recommended to use the projected indexed EOA (EOAi), which can be calculated by dividing the normal reference value of EOA for the implanted model and size of prosthesis by the patient's BSA.[74] Normal reference values of EOA for aortic and mitral mechanical and biological prostheses, and for transcatheter prostheses, can be found in specific papers.[74,127] The projected EOAi is superior to the EOAi calculated based on the continuity equation because it is independent of flow conditions and is not affected by the echocardiographic measurement variability.[74,128,129] PPM is present when EOAi is <0.85 cm^2/m^2 for aortic prostheses and <1.2 cm^2/m^2 for mitral prostheses. PPM is severe if EOAi is <0.65 cm^2/m^2 for aortic prostheses and <0.9 cm^2/m^2 for mitral prosthesis. In obese patients (body mass index ≥30 kg/m^2), the recommended cutoff values for identifying and grading PPM are lower, with EOAi <0.55 cm^2/m^2 and <0.75 cm^2/m^2 being diagnostic for severe PPM in aortic and mitral prostheses, respectively.[74]

PPM is a common complication of PHVs, with a prevalence that ranges in studies from 20% to 70% after SAVR and >50% after MVR.[128–130] The risk of PPM following TAVR is lower than with SAVR, in particular for self-expanding valves with supra-annular design.[130,131] In the STS/ACC TVT registry, 25% of patients had moderate PPM, and 12% had severe PPM following TAVR, whereas the prevalence of severe PPM after SAVR is 2% to 20% in different studies.[128–130]

The risk of PPM following SAVR is higher in small, older women, in bioprostheses, and in the presence of hypertension, diabetes, renal failure, or obesity,[132,133] with some authors suggesting that the increased mortality seen in patients with severe PPM is related to the presence of comorbidities and not to the PPM.[134] Risk factors for severe PPM after TAVR are female sex, young age, non-White/Hispanic race, small prosthesis (diameter <23 mm), and valve-in valve procedures.[131]

The presence of severe PPM is associated with an increased risk of death, worse functional class and exercise capacity, reduced regression of LV hypertrophy, increased risk of heart failure hospitalization, and persistence of pulmonary hypertension.[130,132,135,136] Moreover, PPM can lead to earlier SVD of bioprosthetic valves following SAVR.[137]

The diagnosis of PPM is done by TTE in most cases, but complementary imaging modalities (TEE, CT, fluoroscopy)

can offer important information for differentiating PPM from other causes of acquired PHV stenosis.[74]

Treatment options for severe PPM are limited. Reintervention, consisting in redo valve replacement with implantation of a larger valve and/or annular enlargement or valve-in-valve TAVR using a self-expanding valve with supra-annular design and/or fracturing the stent of the bioprosthetic valve, may be considered in patients with severe PPM if symptoms persist and are unresponsive to medical therapy.[138,139]

Considering the limited treatment options, which carry a significant risk of complications, focus needs to be on prevention. In patients in whom PPM is expected based on the predicted EOAi calculated in the operation room, choosing a valve that would offer better hemodynamics (larger valve, stentless or sutureless prosthesis), enlargement of the aortic root or annulus, or TAVR should be considered. The options for preventing PPM on transcatheter valves are more limited (use of a self-expanding valve with supra-annular design, high implant depth, use of balloon postdilatation) and the benefit of these procedures should be weighed against the risk of complications.[138]

Prosthetic Valve Thrombosis

PHV thrombosis is a feared complication of MHVs, being the main cause of obstruction in MHVs. The annual rate of PHV thrombosis with mechanical valves ranges from 0.1% to 5.7%, with higher rates observed in the early perioperative period, in the mitral and tricuspid positions, with caged ball prosthesis, and in association with subtherapeutic anticoagulation.[140] Although less frequent, thrombosis of BHV is increasingly being recognized (**Fig. 29–9**). In a pathological study from the Mayo Clinic, thrombosis was the cause of BHV dysfunction in 11% of operated patients.[141] Thrombosis is more frequent in mitral than in aortic bioprostheses, in porcine stented valves, and in patients with atrial fibrillation, in particular in the absence of an adequate anticoagulation.[141,142] It is more frequent early after intervention but can occur several years after surgery.[141] TAVR thrombosis is more frequent than thrombosis of surgical bioprosthetic aortic valves and is subclinical in most cases.[143] Subclinical leaflet thrombosis (SLT) is described as a thin layer of thrombus on one or all leaflets, without a significant increase in transvalvular gradients and in the absence of symptoms. The diagnosis of SLT is made on MDCT, with typical appearance of hypo-attenuating defects on the aortic side of the leaflets, also called hypo-attenuating leaflet thickening, which can be associated with a >50% decrease of leaflet motion, or hypo-attenuation affecting motion.[144] In clinical leaflet thrombosis, thrombus leads to an increase in transvalvular gradients, often associated with symptoms of heart failure or systemic embolism. The incidence of clinical valve thrombosis in TAVR is estimated between 0.6% and 2.8%,[145,146] while the incidence of SLT is variable, between 7% and 35%, depending on the frequency of screening.[143,147] Risk factors for the occurrence of thrombosis after TAVR are balloon-expandable valves, in particular for prosthesis of larger size, valve-in-valve-procedures, and absence of anticoagulant treatment.[143,146,147] The presence of thrombus in the sinus of Valsalva can also be detected on

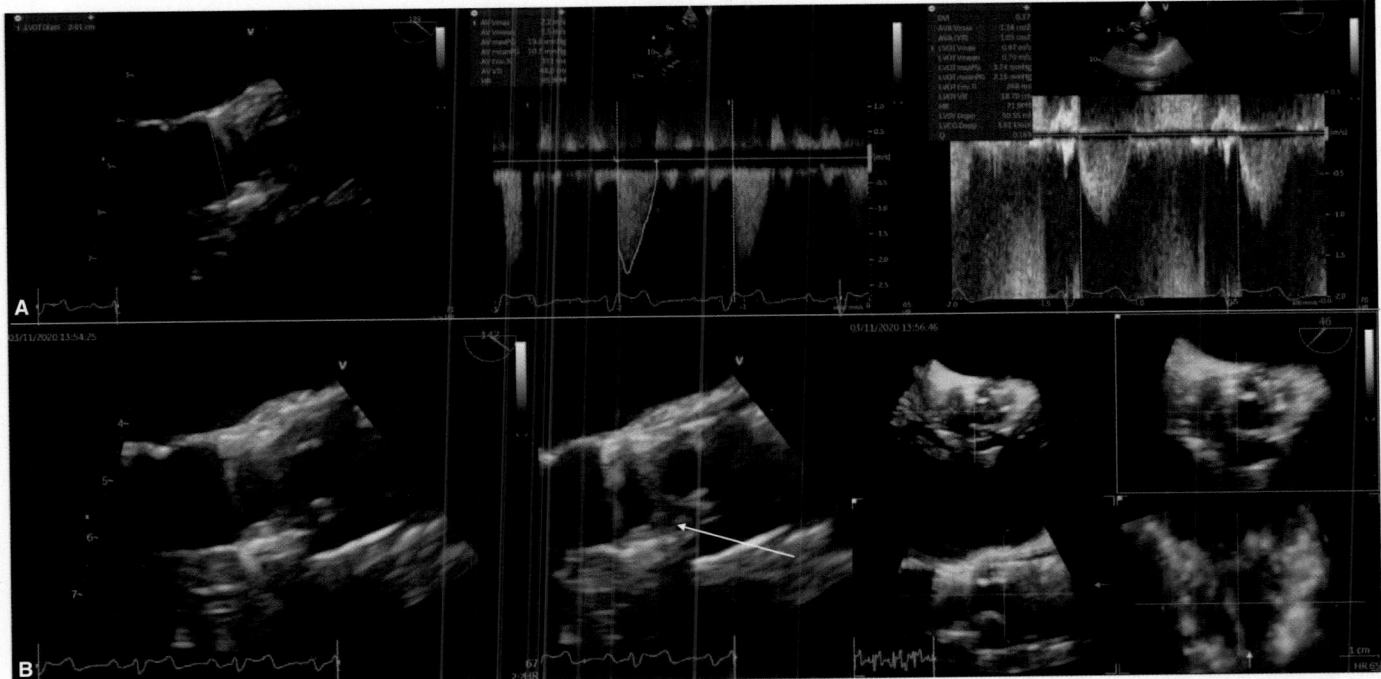

Figure 29–9. Thrombosis of a Perceval valve size S in a patient at 1 month after implantation. Note the slightly elevated transvalvular pressure gradients and reduced aortic valve area by the continuity equation (**A**). The final diagnosis of valve thrombosis is made with TEE showing abnormally thickened aortic valve cusps as well as a hypo echogenic mass (thrombus) on the aortic side of the anterior cusp (*white arrow*). With 3D-TEE, the aortic valve area in systole can be planimetered (**B**, right-hand side).

TABLE 29–9. Comparison between the ESC and the ACC/AHA Recommendations on Prosthetic Heart Valves

ESC Guidelines		ACC/AHA Guidelines	
Choice of prosthesis			
A mechanical prosthesis is recommended according to the desire of the informed patient and if there are no contraindications to long-term anticoagulation.	I	The choice of type of prosthetic heart valve should be a shared decision-making process that accounts for the patient's values and preferences and includes discussion of the indications for and risks of anticoagulant therapy and the potential need for and risk associated with reintervention.	I
A bioprosthesis is recommended according to the desire of the informed patient.	I		
A mechanical prosthesis is recommended in patients at risk of accelerated structural valve deterioration (>40 years, hyperparathyroidism)	I	None	
A mechanical prosthesis should be considered in patients already on anticoagulation because of a mechanical prosthesis in another valve position.	IIa	None	
A mechanical prosthesis should be considered in patients with a reasonable life expectancy (>10 years) for whom future redo valve surgery would be at high risk.	IIa	None	
A bioprosthesis is recommended when good-quality anticoagulation is unlikely (compliance problems, not readily available) or contraindicated because of high bleeding risk (previous major bleed, comorbidities, unwillingness, compliance problems, lifestyle, occupation).	I	A bioprosthesis is recommended in patients of any age for whom anticoagulant therapy is contraindicated, cannot be managed appropriately, or is not desired.	I
A mechanical prosthesis should be considered in patients <60 years of age for prostheses in the aortic position and <65 years of age for prostheses in the mitral position	IIa	An aortic or mitral mechanical prosthesis is reasonable for patients less than 50 years of age who do not have a contraindication to anticoagulation	IIa

(Continued)

TABLE 29–9. Comparison between the ESC and the ACC/AHA Recommendations on Prosthetic Heart Valves (Continued)

ESC Guidelines		ACC/AHA Guidelines	
In patients 60-65 years of age who should receive an aortic prosthesis and those Between 65 and 70 years of age in the case of mitral prosthesis, both valves are acceptable, and the choice requires careful analysis other than the age.		For patients between 50 and 70 years of age, it is reasonable to individualize the choice of either a mechanical or bioprosthetic valve prosthesis on the basis of individual patient factors and preferences, after full discussion of the tradeoffs involved.	IIa
A bioprosthesis should be considered in patients >65 years of age for a prosthesis in the aortic position or >70 years of age in a mitral position or those with a life expectancy lower than the presumed durability of the bioprosthesis.	IIa	A bioprosthesis is reasonable for patients more than 70 years of age.	IIa
A mechanical prosthesis may be considered in patients already on long-term anticoagulation due to the high risk for thromboembolism (atrial fibrillation, previous thromboembolism, hypercoagulable state, severe left ventricle systolic dysfunction).	IIb	None	
A bioprosthesis is recommended for reoperation for mechanical valve thrombosis despite good long-term anticoagulant control.	I	None	
A bioprosthesis should be considered in patients for whom there is a low likelihood and/or a low operative risk of future redo valve surgery.	IIa	None	
A bioprosthesis should be considered in young women contemplating pregnancy.	IIa	None	
None		Replacement of the aortic valve by a pulmonary autograft (the Ross procedure), when performed by an experienced surgeon, may be considered for young patients when VKA anticoagulation is contraindicated or undesirable	IIb
Antithrombotic therapy in patients with mechanical heart valves			
Oral anticoagulation using a VKA is recommended lifelong in all patients with mechanical heart valves.	I	Anticoagulation with a VKA and INR monitoring is recommended in patients with a mechanical prosthetic valve.	I
INR self-management is recommended provided appropriate training and quality control are performed	I	None	
None		Anticoagulation with a VKA to achieve an INR of 2.5 is recommended for patients with a mechanical bileaflet or current-generation single-tilting disc AVR and no risk factors for thromboembolism	I
None		Anticoagulation with a VKA is indicated to achieve an INR of 3.0 in patients with a mechanical AVR and additional risk factors for thromboembolic events (AF, previous thromboembolism, LV dysfunction, or hypercoagulable conditions) or an older-generation mechanical AVR (such as ball-in-cage).	I
None		Anticoagulation with a VKA is indicated to achieve an INR of 3.0 in patients with a mechanical MVR	I
None		A lower target INR of 1.5 to 2.0 may be reasonable in patients with mechanical On-X AVR and no thromboembolic risk factors	IIb
The addition of low-dose aspirin (75–100 mg/day) to VKA should be considered after thromboembolism despite an adequate INR.	IIa	Aspirin 75 mg to 100 mg daily is recommended in addition to anticoagulation with a VKA in patients with a mechanical valve prosthesis	I
The addition of low-dose aspirin (75–100 mg/day) to VKA may be considered in the case of concomitant atherosclerotic disease	IIb		
In patients treated with coronary stent implantation, triple therapy with aspirin (75–100 mg/day), clopidogrel (75 mg/day) and VKA should be considered for 1 month, irrespective of the type of stent used and the clinical presentation (i.e. ACS or stable CAD).	IIa	None	

(Continued)

TABLE 29–9. Comparison between the ESC and the ACC/AHA Recommendations on Prosthetic Heart Valves (Continued)

ESC Guidelines		ACC/AHA Guidelines	
Triple therapy comprising aspirin (75–100 mg/day), clopidogrel (75 mg/day) and VKA for >1 month and up to 6 months should be considered in patients with high ischaemic risk due to ACS or other anatomical/procedural characteristics that outweighs the bleeding risk .	IIa	None	
Dual therapy comprising VKA and clopidogrel (75 mg/day) should be considered as an alternative to 1-month triple antithrombotic therapy in patients in whom the bleeding risk outweighs the ischaemic risk .	IIa	None	
In patients who have undergone PCI, discontinuation of antiplatelet treatment should be considered at 12 months.	IIa	None	
In patients requiring aspirin and/or clopidogrel in addition to VKA, the dose intensity of VKA should be carefully regulated with a target INR in the lower part of the recommended target range and a time in the therapeutic range >65–70%.	IIa		
The use of NOACs is contraindicated.	III	Anticoagulant therapy with oral direct thrombin inhibitors or anti-Xa agents should not be used in patients with mechanical valve prostheses.	III
Antithrombotic treatment in patients with bioprosthetic heart valves			
Oral anticoagulation is recommended lifelong for patients with surgical or transcatheter implanted bioprostheses who have other indications for anticoagulation.	I	None	
Oral anticoagulation using a VKA should be considered for the first 3 months after surgical implantation of a mitral or tricuspid bioprosthesis.	IIa	Anticoagulation with a VKA to achieve an INR of 2.5 is reasonable for at least 3 months and for as long as 6 months after surgical bioprosthetic MVR or AVR in patients at low risk of bleeding	IIa
Oral anticoagulation may be considered for the first 3 months after surgical implantation of an aortic bioprosthesis.	IIb		
Low-dose aspirin (75–100 mg/day) should be considered for the first 3 months after surgical implantation of an aortic bioprosthesis or valve-sparing aortic surgery.	IIa	Aspirin 75 mg to 100 mg per day is reasonable in all patients with a bioprosthetic aortic or mitral valve	IIa
Dual antiplatelet therapy should be considered for the first 3–6 months after TAVI, followed by lifelong single antiplatelet therapy in patients who do not need oral anticoagulation for other reasons.	IIa	Clopidogrel 75 mg daily may be reasonable for the first 6 months after TAVR in addition to life-long aspirin 75 mg to 100 mg daily.	IIb
Single antiplatelet therapy may be considered after TAVI in the case of high bleeding risk.	IIb	None	
None		Anticoagulation with a VKA to achieve an INR of 2.5 may be reasonable for at least 3 months after TAVR in patients at low risk of bleeding	IIb
Management of bioprosthetic valve failure			
Reoperation is recommended in symptomatic patients with a significant increase in transprosthetic gradient (after exclusion of valve thrombosis) or severe regurgitation.	I	Repeat valve replacement is indicated for severe symptomatic prosthetic valve stenosis	I
Reoperation should be considered in asymptomatic patients with significant prosthetic dysfunction if reoperation is at low risk.	IIa	None	
Transcatheter valve-in-valve implantation in the aortic position should be considered by the Heart Team depending on the risk of reoperation and the type and size of prosthesis.	IIa	For severely symptomatic patients with bioprosthetic aortic valve stenosis judged by the heart team to be at high or prohibitive risk of reoperation, and in whom improvement in hemodynamics is anticipated, a transcatheter valve-in-valve procedure is reasonable.	IIa
Management of prosthetic valve regurgitation			
Reoperation is recommended if paravalvular leak is related to endocarditis or causes haemolysis requiring repeated blood transfusions or leading to severe symptoms.	I	Surgery is recommended for operable patients with mechanical heart valves with intractable hemolysis or HF due to severe prosthetic or paraprosthetic regurgitation.	I
None		Surgery is reasonable for asymptomatic patients with severe bioprosthetic regurgitation if operative risk is acceptable	IIa

(Continued)

TABLE 29–9. Comparison between the ESC and the ACC/AHA Recommendations on Prosthetic Heart Valves (Continued)

ESC Guidelines		ACC/AHA Guidelines	
Transcatheter closure may be considered for paravalvular leaks with clinically significant regurgitation in surgical high-risk patients (Heart Team decision).	IIb	Percutaneous repair of paravalvular regurgitation is reasonable in patients with prosthetic heart valves and intractable hemolysis or NYHA class III/IV HF who are at high risk for surgery and have anatomic features suitable for catheter-based therapy when performed in centers with expertise in the procedure	IIa
None		For severely symptomatic patients with bioprosthetic aortic valve regurgitation judged by the heart team to be at high or prohibitive risk for surgical therapy, in whom improvement in hemodynamics is anticipated, a transcatheter valve-in-valve procedure is reasonable	IIa
Management of mechanical prosthesis thrombosis			
None		Urgent evaluation with multimodality imaging is indicated in patients with suspected mechanical prosthetic valve thrombosis to assess valvular function, leaflet motion, and the presence and extent of thrombus .	I
Urgent or emergency valve replacement is recommended for obstructive thrombosis in critically ill patients without serious comorbidity.	I	Urgent initial treatment with either slow-infusion low-dose fibrinolytic therapy or emergency surgery is recommended for patients with a thrombosed leftsided mechanical prosthetic heart valve presenting with symptoms of valve obstruction	I
Surgery should be considered for large (>10 mm) non-obstructive prosthetic thrombus complicated by embolism.	IIa		
Fibrinolysis (using recombinant tissue plasminogen activator 10 mg bolus + 90 mg in 90 min with UFH or streptokinase 1 500 000 U in 60 min without UFH) should be considered when surgery is not available or is very high risk or for thrombosis of right-sided prostheses.	IIa		
Management of bioprosthetic valve thrombosis			
Anticoagulation using a VKA and/or UFH is recommended in bioprosthetic valve thrombosis before considering reintervention.	I	In patients with suspected or confirmed bioprosthetic valve thrombosis who are hemodynamically stable and have no contraindications to anticoagulation, initial treatment with a VKA is reasonable.	IIa

MDCT in TAVR patients and could be associated with systemic embolism.[148]

The presence of PHV thrombosis should be suspected in patients who present with recent onset of heart failure symptoms or an embolic event, independent of the type of PHV.[1,74] The diagnosis should be confirmed by TTE and TEE, with the addition, if necessary, of fluoroscopy (in MHVs) or MDCT (in both MHVs and BHVs).[1,74] Thrombus should be differentiated from other causes of prosthetic valve dysfunction, in particular pannus (**Table 29–8**).

The management of MHV thrombosis is challenging, because both surgery and fibrinolysis are associated with an increased risk of death and complications and there is no randomized trial comparing the two treatment options. The ACC/AHA recommend surgery or slow-infusion low-dose fibrinolysis, as initial approach, depending on individual patient characteristics and the expertise and the capabilities of the institution, with surgery being favored in patients at low surgical risk, in centers with expertise, in severely symptomatic patients (NYHA class IV), in the presence of a large clot burden (>0.8 cm²) or left atrial thrombus, in patients with contraindications to fibrinolysis, and if pannus cannot be ruled

out.[2] The ESC guidelines recommend surgery for obstructive PHV thrombosis in critically ill patients and in patients with large (>10 mm) nonobstructive thrombus complicated by embolism or that persists despite optimal anticoagulation, while standard-dose fibrinolysis can be considered in patients with right-sided valve thrombosis and when surgery poses a high risk or is not available.[1]

With regard to bioprosthetic valves thrombosis, anticoagulant treatment is effective in both clinical and subclinical thrombosis. The ESC guidelines recommend anticoagulant treatment with VKA or intravenous unfractionated heparin in patients with clinical BHV thrombosis.[1] In the absence of a proved impact on outcome of SLT and the increased bleeding risk of the old, often frail TAVR patients, anticoagulant treatment cannot be recommended at this moment. However, closer follow-up is useful in these patients because there is concern of a possible evolution toward an increase in gradients and symptom occurrence in some cases.

Infective Endocarditis

Prosthetic valve endocarditis (PVE) is the most severe form of infective endocarditis, with an in-hospital mortality of 20% to

40%.[149,150] It occurs in 1% to 6% of patients with PHV, having a similar prevalence in mechanical and biological valves. Infective endocarditis after TAVR has a similar incidence as aortic bioprosthetic valve endocarditis and is more common with self-expandable valves and with the use of orotracheal intubation.[151] Early PVE (<1 year) is most commonly a nosocomial infection, with staphylococci, fungi, and Gram-negative bacilli being the primary infectious agents, while late PVE (>1 year) is more often community acquired and is caused by staphylococci, oral streptococci, *Streptococcus bovis*, and enterococci. *Staphylococcus aureus*, coagulase-negative staphylococci, and enterococci are the most common agents of TAVR endocarditis.[152,153]

The diagnosis of PVE remains challenging because the presentation can be atypical and blood cultures and TEE are often negative, rendering the Duke criteria less useful. Other imaging modalities, such as ^{18}F-FDG PET/CT, CT, and CMR can offer valuable information for the detection of cardiac and extracardiac lesions and should be considered whenever there is a suspicion of PVE.[154]

Taking into consideration the severity of the disease, treatment decision should be made by the endocarditis team on a case-by-case basis.[154] Treatment of PVE consists of antibiotic treatment and surgery, which is indicated more often than in native valve endocarditis. The recommended antibiotic treatment is similar to native valve endocarditis, with the exception of *S. aureus* PVE that requires a more prolonged (≥6 weeks) antibiotic regimen (particularly in association with aminoglycosides) and frequent use of rifampin.[1] Surgery is indicated in high-risk patients, *S. aureus*, and fungi infection, PVE complicated by heart failure, severe prosthetic dysfunction, abscess, or persistent fever.[1,2] Noncomplicated late PVE can be managed conservatively, with close follow-up recommended for timely detection of eventual complications.[1]

Future Directions

Important advances have been made in recent years in the field of PHVs, such as the lower thrombogenicity and the longer durability of the newer generation MHVs and, respectively, BHVs, the development of minimally invasive surgery and sutureless valves, and, without a doubt the most important, the development of TAVR, which has revolutionized the treatment of patients with AS. Future large, randomized trials will hopefully bring clarification of some important topics in the field of PHV, such as the optimal antithrombotic strategy after BHV replacement and TAVR, optimal treatment of mechanical PHV thrombosis, the outcome of patients with subclinical leaflet thrombosis, and long-term outcome data for TAVR, sutureless valves, valve-in-valve procedures, or percutaneous PVL closure.

SUMMARY

- PHVs can be classified as mechanical and biological. Transcatheter heart valves are a new type of biological valve that have revolutionized the management of patients with AS.

- The choice between a mechanical and a biological prosthesis is made by taking into consideration the patient preferences and lifestyle and the risk of anticoagulation-related bleeding with a mechanical prosthesis versus the risk of structural valve deterioration and reintervention with a bioprosthesis.

- Anticoagulant treatment with VKAs is recommended lifelong in patients with an MHV. The optimal antithrombotic strategy in patients with biological and transcatheter heart valves is yet to be determined.

- Because there is no ideal PHV, regular follow-up by a cardiologist is recommended in all patients with PHVs.

- The assessment of patients with PHVs is more challenging than the evaluation of native valve disease and a multimodality imaging approach should be used when prosthetic valve dysfunction is suspected.

- **Table 29–9** summarizes the comparison between the ESC and the AHA/ACC guidelines on the management of PHVs.

REFERENCES

1. Baumgartner H, Falk V, Bax JJ, et al. 2017 ESC/EACTS guidelines for the management of valvular heart disease. *Eur Heart J*. 2017;38(36):2739-2786.
2. Otto CM, Nishimura RA, Bonow RO, et al. 2020 ACC/AHA guideline for the management of patients with valvular heart disease: a report of the American College of Cardiology/American Heart Association Joint Committee on Clinical Practice Guidelines. *J Thoracic Cardiovasc Surg*. 2021;143(5).
3. Aronow WS, Ahn C, Kronzon I. Prevalence of echocardiographic findings in 554 men and in 1,243 women aged >60 years in a long-term health care facility. *Am J Cardiol*. 1997;79(3):379-380.
4. Singh JP, Evans JC, Levy D, et al. Prevalence and clinical determinants of mitral, tricuspid, and aortic regurgitation (The Framingham Heart Study). *Am J Cardiol*. 1999;83(6):897-902.
5. Lebowitz NE, Bella JN, Roman MJ, et al. Prevalence and correlates of aortic regurgitation in American Indians: the strong heart study. *J Am Coll Cardiol*. 2000;36(2):461-467.
6. Keane MG, Pyeritz RE. Medical management of Marfan syndrome. *Circulation*. 2008;117:2802-2813.
7. Akinseye OA, Pathak A, Ibebuogu UN. Aortic valve regurgitation: a comprehensive review. *Curr Probl Cardiol*. 2018;43(8):315-334.
8. Libby P, Zipes DP. Aortic valve disease. In: Bonow RO, Mann DL, Tomaselli GF, Bhatt D, eds. *Braunwald's Heart Disease: A Textbook of Cardiovascular Medicine*. 11th ed. Elsevier; 2019.
9. Stout KK, Verrier ED. Acute valvular regurgitation. *Circulation*. 2009;119(25): 3232-3241.
10. Carabello BA. Aortic regurgitation. A lesion with similarities to both aortic stenosis and mitral regurgitation: editorial comment. *Circulation*. 1990;82:1051-1053.
11. Tornos P, Evangelista A, Bonow R. Aortic regurgitation. In: Otto CM, Bonow RO, eds. *Valvular Heart Disease: A Companion to Braunwald's Heart Disease*. Elsevier; 2013.
12. Lancellotti P, Tribouilloy C, Hagendorff A, et al. Recommendations for the echocardiographic assessment of native valvular regurgitation: an executive summary from the European Association of Cardiovascular Imaging. *Eur Heart J Cardiovasc Imaging*. 2013;14(7):611-644.
13. Magid NM, Opio G, Wallerson DC, Young MS, Borer JS. Heart failure due to chronic experimental aortic regurgitation. *Am J Physiol*. 1994;267(2, Pt 2).
14. Kumpuris AG, Quinones MA, Waggoner AD, Kanon DJ, Nelson JG, Miller RR. Importance of preoperative hypertrophy, wall stress and

end-systolic dimension as echocardiographic predictors of normalization of left ventricular dilatation after valve replacement in chronic aortic insufficiency. *Am J Cardiol.* 1982;49(5):1091-1100.

15. Maurer G. Aortic regurgitation. *Heart.* 2006;92:994-1000.

16. Goldbarg SH, Halperin JL. Aortic regurgitation: disease progression and management. *Nature Clin Prac Cardiovasc Med.* 2008;5:269-279.

17. Gaasch WH, Carroll JD, Levine HJ, Criscitiello MG. Chronic aortic regurgitation: prognostic value of left ventricular end-systolic dimension and end-diastolic radius/thickness ratio. *J Am Coll Cardiol.* 1983;1(3):775-782.

18. Wisenbaugh T, Booth D, DeMaria A, Nissen S, Waters J. Relationship of contractile state to ejection performance in patients with chronic aortic valve disease. *Circulation.* 1986;73(1):47-53.

19. Popović ZB, Desai MY, Griffin BP. Decision making with imaging in asymptomatic aortic regurgitation. *JACC: Cardiovascular Imaging.* 2018;11: 1499-1513.

20. O'Gara PT, Loscalzo J. Aortic Regurgitation. In: Jameson JL, Fauci AS, Kasper DL, et al., eds. *Harrison's Principles of Internal Medicine.* 20th ed. McGraw-Hill Medical; 2018.

21. Mărgulescu AD. Assessment of aortic valve disease—a clinician oriented review. *World J Cardiol.* 2017;9(6):481.

22. Siu SC, Silversides CK. Bicuspid aortic valve disease. *J Am Coll Cardiol.* 2010;55:2789-2800.

23. Friedman T, Mani A, Elefteriades JA. Bicuspid aortic valve: clinical approach and scientific review of a common clinical entity. *Expert Rev Cardiovasc Ther.* 2008;6:235–248.

24. Michelena HI, Khanna AD, Mahoney D, et al. Incidence of aortic complications in patients with bicuspid aortic valves. *JAMA.* 2011;306(10): 1104-1112.

25. Mahadevia R, Barker AJ, Schnell S, et al. Bicuspid aortic cusp fusion morphology alters aortic three-dimensional outflow patterns, wall shear stress, and expression of aortopathy. *Circulation.* 2014;129(6):673-682.

26. Otto C. Valvular regurgitation. In: *Textbook of Clinical Echocardiography.* 6th ed. Elsevier; 2018.

27. Babu AN, Kymes SM, Carpenter Fryer SM. Eponyms and the diagnosis of aortic regurgitation: what says the evidence? *Ann Int Med.* 2003;138:736-742.

28. Bonow RO. Chronic mitral regurgitation and aortic regurgitation: have indications for surgery changed? *J Am Coll Cardiol.* 2013;61:693-701.

29. Attenhofer Jost CH, Turina J, Mayer K, et al. Echocardiography in the evaluation of systolic murmurs of unknown cause. *Am J Med.* 2000;108(8):614-620.

30. Lang RM, Badano LP, Tsang W, et al. EAE/ASE recommendations for image acquisition and display using three-dimensional echocardiography. *J Am Soc Echocardiogr.* 2012;25(1):3-46.

31. Borrás X, Carreras F, Augé JM, Pons-Lladó G. Prospective validation of detection and quantitative assessment of chronic aortic regurgitation by a combined echocardiographic and doppler method. *J Am Soc Echocardiogr.* 1988;1(6):422-429.

32. Chen M, Luo H, Miyamoto T, et al. Correlation of echo-Doppler aortic valve regurgitation index with angiographic aortic regurgitation severity. *Am J Cardiol.* 2003;92(5):634-635.

33. Detaint D, Messika-Zeitoun D, Maalouf J, et al. Quantitative echocardiographic determinants of clinical outcome in asymptomatic patients with aortic regurgitation. a prospective study. *JACC Cardiovasc Imaging.* 2008;1(1):1-11.

34. Zoghbi WA, Adams D, Bonow RO, et al. Recommendations for non-invasive evaluation of native valvular regurgitation: a report from the American Society of Echocardiography developed in collaboration with the Society for Cardiovascular Magnetic Resonance. *J Am Soc Echocardiogr.* 2017;30(4):303-371.

35. Siemienczuk D, Greenberg B, Morris C, et al. Chronic aortic insufficiency: factors associated with progression to aortic valve replacement. *Ann Intern Med.* 1989;110(8):587-592.

36. Olsen NT, Sogaard P, Larsson HBW, et al. Speckle-tracking echocardiography for predicting outcome in chronic aortic regurgitation during conservative management and after surgery. *JACC Cardiovasc Imaging.* 2011;4(3):223-230.

37. Le Polain De Waroux JB, Pouleur AC, et al. Functional anatomy of aortic regurgitation: accuracy, prediction of surgical repairability, and outcome implications of transesophageal echocardiography. *Circulation.* 2007;116(11 Suppl. 1).

38. Davies RR, Goldstein LJ, Coady MA, et al. Yearly rupture or dissection rates for thoracic aortic aneurysms: simple prediction based on size. *Ann Thorac Surg.* 2002;73(1):17-28.

39. Lancellotti P, Pellikka PA, Budts W, et al. The clinical use of stress echocardiography in non-ischaemic heart disease: recommendations from the European Association of Cardiovascular Imaging and the American Society of Echocardiography. *J Am Soc Echocardiogr.* 2017;30(2): 101-138.

40. Bolen MA, Popovic ZB, Rajiah P, et al. Cardiac MR assessment of aortic regurgitation: Holodiastolic flow reversal in the descending aorta helps stratify severity. *Radiology.* 2011;260(1):98-104.

41. Dujardin KS, Enriquez-Sarano M, Schaff H V, Bailey KR, Seward JB, Tajik AJ. Mortality and morbidity of aortic regurgitation in clinical practice. A long-term follow-up study. *Circulation.* 1999;99(14):1851-1857.

42. Bonow RO, Picone AL, McIntosh CL, et al. Survival and functional results after valve replacement for aortic regurgitation from 1976 to 1983: impact of preoperative left ventricular function. *Circulation.* 1985;72(6):1244-1256.

43. Bonow RO, Dodd JT, Maron BJ, et al. Long-term serial changes in left ventricular function and reversal of ventricular dilatation after valve replacement for chronic aortic regurgitation. *Circulation.* 1988;78(5 Pt 1): 1108-1120.

44. Forteza A, Evangelista A, Sánchez V, et al. Efficacy of losartan vs. atenolol for the prevention of aortic dilation in Marfan syndrome: a randomized clinical trial. *Eur Heart J.* 2016;37(12):978-985.

45. Hiratzka LF, Creager MA, Isselbacher EM, et al. Surgery for aortic dilatation in patients with bicuspid aortic valves: a statement of clarification from the American College of Cardiology/American Heart Association Task Force on Clinical Practice Guidelines. *J Am Coll Cardiol.* 2016; 67(6):724-731.

46. Unger P, Pibarot P, Tribouilloy C, et al. Multiple and mixed valvular heart diseases. Circulation. *Cardiovasc Imaging.* 2018;11:e007862.

47. Unger P, Clavel MA, Lindman BR, Mathieu P, Pibarot P. Pathophysiology and management of multivalvular disease. *Nature Rev Cardiol.* 2016;13:429-440.

48. Iung B, Baron G, Butchart EG, et al. A prospective survey of patients with valvular heart disease in Europe: the Euro Heart Survey on valvular heart disease. *Eur Heart J.* 2003;24(13):1231-1243.

49. D'Arcy JL, Coffey S, Loudon MA, et al. Large-scale community echocardiographic screening reveals a major burden of undiagnosed valvular heart disease in older people: the OxVALVE Population Cohort Study. *Eur Heart J.* 2016;37(47):3515-3522a.

50. Lee R, Li S, Rankin JS, et al. Fifteen-year outcome trends for valve surgery in North America. *Ann Thorac Surg.* 2011;91(3):677-684.

51. Leon MB, Smith CR, Mack MJ, et al. Transcatheter or surgical aortic-valve replacement in intermediate-risk patients. *N Engl J Med.* 2016; 374(17):1609-1620.

52. Asami M, Windecker S, Praz F, et al. Transcatheter aortic valve replacement in patients with concomitantmitral stenosis. *Eur Heart J.* 2019 May;40(17):1342-1351.

53. Vollenbroich R, Stortecky S, Praz F, et al. The impact of functional vs degenerative mitral regurgitation on clinical outcomes among patients undergoing transcatheter aortic valve implantation. *Am Heart J.* 2017;184:71-80.

54. Lindman BR, Maniar HS, Jaber WA, et al. Effect of tricuspid regurgitation and the right heart on survival after transcatheter aortic valve replacement. *Circ Cardiovasc Interv.* 2015;8(4).

55. Unger P, Rosenhek R, Dedobbeleer C, Berrebi A, Lancellotti P. Management of multiple valve disease. *Heart.* 2011;97:272-277.

56. Zamorano JL, Badano LP, Bruce C, et al. EAE/ASE recommendations for the use of echocardiography in new transcatheter interventions for valvular heart disease. *Eur Heart J.* 2011;32(17):2189-2214.

57. Dorosz JL, Lezotte DC, Weitzenkamp DA, Allen LA, Salcedo EE. Performance of 3-dimensional echocardiography in measuring left ventricular volumes and ejection fraction: a systematic review and meta-analysis. *J Am Coll Cardiol.* 2012;59(20):1799-1808.

58. Lancellotti P, Pellikka PA, Budts W, et al. The clinical use of stress echocardiography in non-ischaemic heart disease: recommendations from the European Association of Cardiovascular Imaging and the American Society of Echocardiography. *Eur Heart J Cardiovasc Imaging.* 2016;17(11):1191-1229.

59. Nishimura RA, Otto CM, Bonow RO, et al. 2017 AHA/ACC Focused Update of the 2014 AHA/ACC guideline for the management of patients with valvular heart disease: a report of the American College of Cardiology/American Heart Association Task Force on Clinical Practice Guidelines. *J Am Coll Cardiol.* 2017;70(2):252-289.

60. Cawley PJ, Maki JH, Otto CM. Cardiovascular magnetic resonance imaging for valvular heart disease. Technique and validation. *Circulation.* 2009;119(3):468-478.

61. Clavel MA, Messika-Zeitoun D, Pibarot P, et al. The complex nature of discordant severe calcified aortic valve disease grading: new insights from combined Doppler echocardiographic and computed tomographic study. *J Am Coll Cardiol.* 2013;62(24):2329-2338.

62. Venneri L, Khattar RS, Senior R. Assessment of complex multi-valve disease and prosthetic valves. *Heart Lung Circ.* 2019;28: 1436-1446.

63. Galli E, Lancellotti P, Sengupta PP, Donal E. LV mechanics in mitral and aortic valve diseases: value of functional assessment beyond ejection fraction. *JACC: Cardiovasc Imaging.* 2014;7:1151-1166.

64. Gentles TL, Finucane AK, Remenyi B, Kerr AR, Wilson NJ. Ventricular function before and after surgery for isolated and combined regurgitation in the young. *Ann Thorac Surg.* 2015;100(4):1383-1389.

65. Unger P, Lancellotti P, de Cannière D. The clinical challenge of concomitant aortic and mitral valve stenosis. *Acta Cardiologica.* 2016;71:3-6.

66. Egbe AC, Poterucha JT, Warnes CA. Mixed aortic valve disease: midterm outcome and predictors of adverse events. *Eur Heart J.* 2016;37(34):2671-2678.

67. Egbe AC, Luis SA, Padang R, Warnes CA. Outcomes in moderate mixed aortic valve disease: Is it time for a paradigm shift? *J Am Coll Cardiol.* 2016;67(20):2321-2329.

68. Zilberszac R, Gabriel H, Schemper M, et al. Outcome of combined stenotic and regurgitant aortic valve disease. *J Am Coll Cardiol.* 2013; 61(14):1489-1495.

69. Lancellotti P, Rosenhek R, Pibarot P, et al. ESC Working Group on Valvular Heart Disease Position Paper-heart valve clinics: organization, structure, and experiences. *Eur Heart J.* 2013;34(21):1597-1606.

70. Chambers JB, Prendergast B, Iung B, et al. Standards defining a "heart valve centre": ESC working group on valvular heart disease and European association for cardiothoracic surgery viewpoint. *Eur Heart J.* 2017;38:2177-2183.

71. Erlebach M, Lange R. Multivalvular disease: percutaneous management in 2019 and beyond. *Intervent Cardiol Rev.* 2019;14:142-146.

72. Kische S, D'Ancona G, Paranskaya L, et al. Staged total percutaneous treatment of aortic valve pathology and mitral regurgitation: institutional experience. *Catheter Cardiovasc Interv.* 2013;82(4).

73. Go AS, Mozaffarian D, Roger VL, et al. Executive summary: heart disease and stroke statistics—2014 update: a report from the American Heart Association. *Circulation.* 2014;29:399-410.

74. Lancellotti P, Pibarot P, Chambers J, et al. Recommendations for the imaging assessment of prosthetic heart valves: a report from the European Association of Cardiovascular Imaging endorsed by the Chinese Society of Echocardiography, the Inter-American Society of Echocardiography, and the Brazilian. *Eur Heart J Cardiovasc Imaging.* 2016;17(6):589-590.

75. Dellgren G, David TE, Raanani E, Armstrong S, Ivanov J, Rakowski H. Late hemodynamic and clinical outcomes of aortic valve replacement with the Carpentier-Edwards perimount pericardial bioprosthesis. *J Thorac Cardiovasc Surg.* 2002;124(1):146-154.

76. Dalmau MJ, González-Santos JM, Blázquez JA, et al. Hemodynamic performance of the Medtronic Mosaic and Perimount Magna aortic bioprostheses: five-year results of a prospectively randomized study. *Eur J Cardio-thoracic Surg.* 2011;39(6):844-852.

77. Kobayashi J. Stentless aortic valve replacement: an update. *Vasc Health Risk Manag.* 2011;7:345-351.

78. Christ T, Claus B, Zielinski C, Falk V, Grubitzsch H. Long-term outcome of the Sorin Freedom SOLO stentless aortic valve. *J Heart Valve Dis.* 2016;25(6):679-684.

79. David TE, Feindel CM, Bos J, Ivanov J, Armstrong S. Aortic valve replacement with Toronto SPV bioprosthesis: optimal patient survival but suboptimal valve durability. *J Thorac Cardiovasc Surg.* 2008;135(1):19-24.

80. Hickey E, Langley SM, Allemby-Smith O, Livesey SA, Monro JL. Subcoronary allograft aortic valve replacement: parametric risk-hazard outcome analysis to a minimum of 20 years. *Ann Thorac Surg.* 2007;84(5):1564-1570.

81. O'Brien MF, Harrocks S, Stafford EG, et al. The homograft aortic valve: a 29-year, 99.3% follow up of 1,022 valve replacements. *J Heart Valve Dis.* 2001;10(3):334-345.

82. Nappi F, Spadaccio C, Chello M, Acar C. The Ross procedure: underuse or under-comprehension? *J Thorac Cardiovasc Surg.* 2015;149:1463-1464.

83. Nunn GR, Bennetts J, Onikul E. Durability of hand-sewn valves in the right ventricular outlet. *J Thorac Cardiovasc Surg.* 2008;136(2):290-297.

84. Phan K, Tsai Y-C, Di Eusanio M, Yan TD. Sutureless aortic valve replacement: a systematic review and meta-analysis. *Hear Lung Circ.* 2015;24:e46.

85. Santarpino G, Vogt F, Pfeiffer S, et al. Sutureless versus transfemoral transcatheter aortic valve implant: a propensity score matching study. *J Heart Valve Dis.* 2017;26(3):255-261.

86. Gaia DF, Palma JH, De Souza JAM, et al. Transapical mitral valve-in-valve implant: an alternative for high risk and multiple reoperative rheumatic patients. *Int J Cardiol.* 2012;154(1):e6.

87. De Weger A, Ewe SH, Delgado V, Bax JJ. First-in-man implantation of a trans-catheter aortic valve in a mitral annuloplasty ring: novel treatment modality for failed mitral valve repair. *Eur J Cardio-thoracic Surg.* 2011;39(6):1054-1056.

88. Hammermeister K, Sethi GK, Henderson WG, Grover FL, Oprian C, Rahimtoola SH. Outcomes 15 years after valve replacement with a mechanical versus a bioprosthetic valve: final report of the Veterans Affairs randomized trial. *J Am Coll Cardiol.* 2000;36(4):1152-1158.

89. Oxenham H, Bloomfield P, Wheatley DJ, et al. Twenty year comparison of a Bjork-Shiley mechanical heart valve with porcine bioprostheses. *Heart.* 2003;89(7):715-721.

90. Peterseim DS, Cen YY, Cheruvu S, et al. Long-term outcome after biologic versus mechanical aortic valve replacement in 841 patients. *J Thorac Cardiovasc Surg.* 1999;117(5):890-897.

91. Chiang YP, Chikwe J, Moskowitz AJ, Itagaki S, Adams DH, Egorova NN. Survival and long-term outcomes following bioprosthetic vs mechanical aortic valve replacement in patients aged 50 to 69 years. *JAMA.* 2014;312(13):1323-1329.

92. Stassano P, Di Tommaso L, Monaco M, et al. Aortic valve replacement. a prospective randomized evaluation of mechanical versus biological valves in patients ages 55 to 70 years. *J Am Coll Cardiol.* 2009;54(20):1862-1868.

93. Glaser N, Jackson V, Holzmann MJ, Franco-Cereceda A, Sartipy U. Aortic valve replacement with mechanical vs. biological prostheses in patients aged 50-69 years. *Eur Heart J.* 2016;37(34):2658-2667.

94. Goldstone AB, Chiu P, Baiocchi M, et al. Mechanical or biologic prostheses for aortic-valve and mitral-valve replacement. *N Engl J Med.* 2017;377(19):1847-1857.

95. Khan SS, Trento A, DeRobertis M, et al. Twenty-year comparison of tissue and mechanical valve replacement. *J Thorac Cardiovasc Surg.* 2001;122(2):257-269.

96. Foroutan F, Guyatt GH, O'Brien K, et al. Prognosis after surgical replacement with a bioprosthetic aortic valve in patients with severe symptomatic aortic stenosis: systematic review of observational studies. *BMJ*. 2016;354.

97. Habib G, Lancellotti P, Antunes MJ, et al. 2015 ESC Guidelines for the management of infective endocarditis: the Task Force for the Management of Infective Endocarditis of the European Society of Cardiology (ESC). Endorsed by: European Association for Cardio-Thoracic Surgery (EACTS), the European Association of Nuclear Medicine (EANM). *Eur Heart J*. 2015;36(44):3075-3128.

98. Mylonakis E, Calderwood SB. Infective endocarditis in adults. *N Engl J Med*. 2001;345(18):1318-1330.

99. Glaser N, Jackson V, Holzmann MJ, Franco-Cereceda A, Sartipy U. Prosthetic valve endocarditis after surgical aortic valve replacement. *Circulation*. 2017;136:329-331.

100. Gammie JS, Sheng S, Griffith BP, et al. Trends in mitral valve surgery in the United States: results from the Society of Thoracic Surgeons Adult Cardiac Database. *Ann Thorac Surg*. 2009;87(5):1431-1439.

101. Steffel J, Verhamme P, Potpara TS, et al. The 2018 European Heart Rhythm Association Practical Guide on the use of non-Vitamin K antagonist oral anticoagulants in patients with atrial fibrillation. *Eur Heart J*. 2018;39(16):1330-1393.

102. Rahman M, BinEsmael TM, Payne N, Butchart EG. Increased sensitivity to warfarin after heart valve replacement. *Ann Pharmacother*. 2006;40(3):397-401.

103. Chiquette E, Amato MG, Bussey HI. Comparison of an anticoagulation clinic with usual medical care: anticoagulation control, patient outcomes, and health care costs. *Arch Intern Med*. 1998;158(15):1641-1647.

104. Heneghan C, Ward A, Perera R. Self-monitoring of oral anticoagulation: systematic review and meta-analysis of individual patient data. *Lancet*. 2012;379(9813):322-334.

105. Puskas J, Gerdisch M, Nichols D, et al. Reduced anticoagulation after mechanical aortic valve replacement: interim results from the Prospective Randomized On-X Valve Anticoagulation Clinical Trial randomized Food and Drug Administration investigational device exemption trial. *J Thorac Cardiovasc Surg*. 2014;147(4).

106. Singh M, Sporn ZA, Schaff H V, Pellikka PA. ACC/AHA versus ESC guidelines on prosthetic heart valve management: JACC Guideline Comparison. *J Am Coll Cardiol*. 2019;73:1707-1718.

107. Heras M, Chesebro JH, Fuster V, et al. High risk of thromboemboli early after bioprosthetic cardiac valve replacement. *J Am Coll Cardiol*. 1995;25(5):1111-1119.

108. Mérie C, Køber L, Skov Olsen P, et al. Association of warfarin therapy duration after bioprosthetic aortic valve replacement with risk of mortality, thromboembolic complications, and bleeding. *JAMA*. 2012;308(20):2118-2125.

109. Brennan JM, Edwards FH, Zhao Y, et al. Early anticoagulation of bioprosthetic aortic valves in older patients: results from the society of thoracic surgeons adult cardiac surgery national database. *J Am Coll Cardiol*. 2012;60(11):971-977.

110. Colli A, Mestres CA, Castella M, Gherli T. Comparing warfarin to aspirin (WoA) after aortic valve replacement with the St. Jude Medical Epic™ heart valve bioprosthesis: results of the WoA epic pilot trial. *J Heart Valve Dis*. 2007;16(6):667-671.

111. Ussia GP, Scarabelli M, Mul M, et al. Dual antiplatelet therapy versus aspirin alone in patients undergoing transcatheter aortic valve implantation. *Am J Cardiol*. 2011;108(12):1772-1776.

112. Stabile E, Pucciarelli A, Cota L, et al. SAT-TAVI (single antiplatelet therapy for TAVI) study: a pilot randomized study comparing double to single antiplatelet therapy for transcatheter aortic valve implantation. *Int J Cardiol*. 2014;174(3):624-627.

113. Rodés-Cabau J, Masson JB, Welsh RC, et al. Aspirin versus aspirin plus clopidogrel as antithrombotic treatment following transcatheter aortic valve replacement with a balloon-expandable valve: the ARTE (Aspirin Versus Aspirin + Clopidogrel Following Transcatheter Aortic Valve Implantation) Randomi. *JACC Cardiovasc Interv*. 2017;10(13):1357-1365.

114. Nombela-Franco L, Webb JG, De Jaegere PP, et al. Timing, predictive factors, and prognostic value of cerebrovascular events in a large cohort of patients undergoing transcatheter aortic valve implantation. *Circulation*. 2012;126(25):3041-3053.

115. Chakravarty T, Søndergaard L, Friedman J, et al. Subclinical leaflet thrombosis in surgical and transcatheter bioprosthetic aortic valves: an observational study. *Lancet*. 2017;389(10087):2383-2392.

116. Dangas GD, Tijssen JGP, Wöhrle J, et al. A controlled trial of rivaroxaban after transcatheter aortic-valve replacement. *N Engl J Med*. 2020;382(2):120-129.

117. Capodanno D, Petronio AS, Prendergast B, et al. Standardized definitions of structural deterioration and valve failure in assessing long-term durability of transcatheter and surgical aortic bioprosthetic valves: a consensus statement from the European Association of Percutaneous Cardiovascular Interven. *Eur J Cardio-thoracic Surg*. 2017;52(3):408-417.

118. Dvir D, Bourguignon T, Otto CM, et al. Standardized definition of structural valve degeneration for surgical and transcatheter bioprosthetic aortic valves. *Circulation*. 2018;137(4):388-399.

119. Rizzoli G, Guglielmi C, Toscano G, et al. Reoperations for acute prosthetic thrombosis and pannus: an assessment of rates, relationship and risk. *Eur J Cardio-thoracic Surg*. 1999;16(1):74-80.

120. Ionescu A, Fraser AG, Butchart EG. Prevalence and clinical significance of incidental paraprosthetic valvar regurgitation: a prospective study using transoesophageal echocardiography. *Heart*. 2003;89(11):1316-1321.

121. Genoni M, Franzen D, Vogt P, et al. Paravalvular leakage after mitral valve replacement: Improved long-term survival with aggressive surgery? *Eur J Cardio-thoracic Surg*. 2000;17(1):14-19.

122. Pallidis LS, Moyssakis IE, Ikonomidis I, Nihoyannopoulos P. Natural history of early aortic paraprosthetic regurgitation: a five-year follow-up. *Am Heart J*. 1999;138(2 I):351-357.

123. Echevarria JR, Bernal JM, Rabasa JM, Morales D, Revilla Y, Revuelta JM. Reoperation for bioprosthetic valve dysfunction a decade of clinical experience. *Eur J Cardio thorac Surg*. 1991;5(10):523-526.

124. Taramasso M, Maisano F, Latib A, et al. Conventional surgery and transcatheter closure via surgical transapical approach for paravalvular leak repair in high-risk patients: results from a single-centre experience. *Eur Heart J Cardiovasc Imaging*. 2014;15(10):1161-1167.

125. Werner N, Zeymer U, Fraiture B, et al. Interventional treatment of paravalvular regurgitation by plug implantation following prosthetic valve replacement: a single-center experience. *Clin Res Cardiol*. 2018;107(12):1160-1169.

126. Pibarot P, Dumesnil JG. Hemodynamic and clinical impact of prosthesis-patient mismatch in the aortic valve position and its prevention. *J Am Coll Cardiol*. 2000;26:1131-1141.

127. Hahn RT, Leipsic J, Douglas PS, et al. Comprehensive echocardiographic assessment of normal transcatheter valve function. *JACC Cardiovasc Imaging*. 2019;12(1):25-34.

128. Pibarot P, Dumesnil JG. Valve prosthesis-patient mismatch, 1978 to 2011: from original concept to compelling evidence. *J Am Coll Cardiol*. 2012;60:1136-1139.

129. Fallon JM, DeSimone JP, Brennan JM, et al. The incidence and consequence of prosthesis-patient mismatch after surgical aortic valve replacement. *Ann Thorac Surg*. 2018;106(1):14-22.

130. Pibarot P, Weissman NJ, Stewart WJ, et al. Incidence and sequelae of prosthesis-patient mismatch in transcatheter versus surgical valve replacement in high-risk patients with severe aortic stenosis: a PARTNER trial cohort-a analysis. *J Am Coll Cardiol*. 2014;64(13):1323-1334.

131. Nombela-Franco L, Ruel M, Radhakrishnan S, et al. Comparison of hemodynamic performance of self-expandable corevalve versus balloon-expandable Edwards SAPIEN aortic valves inserted by catheter for aortic stenosis. *Am J Cardiol*. 2013;111(7):1026-1033.

132. Dayan V, Vignolo G, Soca G, Paganini JJ, Brusich D, Pibarot P. Predictors and outcomes of prosthesis-patient mismatch after aortic valve replacement. *JACC Cardiovasc Imaging.* 2016;9(8):924-933.

133. Hwang H-Y, Sohn S-H, Jang M-J. Impact of prosthesis-patient mismatch on survival after mitral valve replacement: a meta-analysis. *Thorac Cardiovasc Surg.* 2019;67(7):538-545.

134. Dayan V, Soca G, Stanham R, Lorenzo A, Ferreiro A. Is patient-prosthesis mismatch a predictor of survival or a surrogate marker of co-morbidities in cardiac surgery? *Int J Cardiol.* 2015;190:389-392.

135. Bleiziffer S, Eichinger WB, Hettich I, et al. Impact of patient-prosthesis mismatch on exercise capacity in patients after bioprosthetic aortic valve replacement. *Heart.* 2008;94(5):637-641.

136. Tasca G, Brunelli F, Cirillo M, et al. Impact of valve prosthesis-patient mismatch on left ventricular mass regression following aortic valve replacement. *Ann Thorac Surg.* 2005;79(2):505-510.

137. Flameng W, Herregods MC, Vercalsteren M, Herijgers P, Bogaerts K, Meuris B. Prosthesis-patient mismatch predicts structural valve degeneration in bioprosthetic heart valves. *Circulation.* 2010;121(19):2123-2129.

138. Pibarot P, Magne J, Leipsic J, et al. Imaging for predicting and assessing prosthesis-patient mismatch after aortic valve replacement. *JACC: Cardiovasc Imaging.* 2019;12:149-162.

139. Bilkhu R, Jahangiri M, Otto CM. Patient-prosthesis mismatch following aortic valve replacement. *Heart.* 2019;105:S28-33.

140. Lin SS, Tiong IYH, Asher CR, Murphy MT, Thomas JD, Griffin BP. Prediction of thrombus-related mechanical prosthetic valve dysfunction using transesophageal echocardiography. *Am J Cardiol.* 2000;86(10):1097-1101.

141. Egbe AC, Pislaru SV, Pellikka PA, et al. Bioprosthetic valve thrombosis versus structural failure: clinical and echocardiographic predictors. *J Am Coll Cardiol.* 2015;66(21):2285-2294.

142. Brown ML, Park SJ, Sundt TM, Schaff HV. Early thrombosis risk in patients with biologic valves in the aortic position. *J Thorac Cardiovasc Surg.* 2012;144(1):108-111.

143. Hansson NC, Grove EL, Andersen HR, et al. Transcatheter aortic valve thrombosis: incidence, predisposing factors, and clinical implications. *J Am Coll Cardiol.* 2016;68(19):2059-2069.

144. Rosseel L, De Backer O, Søndergaard L. Clinical valve thrombosis and subclinical leaflet thrombosis following transcatheter aortic valve replacement: is there a need for a patient-tailored antithrombotic therapy? *Frontiers Cardiovasc Med.* 2019;6.

145. Latib A, Naganuma T, Abdel-Wahab M, et al. Treatment and clinical outcomes of transcatheter heart valve thrombosis. *Circ Cardiovasc Interv.* 2015;8(4).

146. Jose J, Sulimov DS, El-Mawardy M, et al. Clinical bioprosthetic heart valve thrombosis after transcatheter aortic valve replacement: incidence, characteristics, and treatment outcomes. *JACC Cardiovasc Interv.* 2017;10(7):686-697.

147. Marwan M, Mekkhala N, Göller M, et al. Leaflet thrombosis following transcatheter aortic valve implantation. *J Cardiovasc Comput Tomogr.* 2018;12(1):8-13.

148. Lim SJ, Koo HJ, Jung SC, et al. Sinus of Valsalva thrombosis detected on computed tomography after transcatheter aortic valve replacement. *Korean Circ J.* 2020;50(7):572-582.

149. Habib G, Lancellotti P, Antunes MJ, et al. 2015 ESC guidelines for the management of infective endocarditis: the Task Force for the Management of Infective Endocarditis of the European Society of Cardiology (ESC): Endorsed by: European Association for Cardio-Thoracic Surgery (EACTS), the European. *Russ J Cardiol.* 2016;133(5):65-116.

150. Habib G, Thuny F, Avierinos JF. Prosthetic valve endocarditis: current approach and therapeutic options. *Prog Cardiovasc Dis.* 2008;50(4):274-281.

151. Butt JH, Ihlemann N, De Backer O, et al. Long-term risk of infective endocarditis after transcatheter aortic valve replacement. *J Am Coll Cardiol.* 2019;73(13):1646-1655.

152. Pericas JM, Llopis J, Cervera C, et al. Infective endocarditis in patients with an implanted transcatheter aortic valve: clinical characteristics and outcome of a new entity. *J Infect.* 2015;70(6):565-576.

153. Amat-Santos IJ, Messika-Zeitoun D, Eltchaninoff H, et al. Infective endocarditis after transcatheter aortic valve implantation results from a large multicenter registry. *Circulation.* 2015;131(18):1566-1574.

154. Erba PA, Pizzi MN, Roque A, et al. Multimodality imaging in infective endocarditis: an imaging team within the endocarditis team. *Circulation.* 2019;140:1753-1765.

30

Mitral Regurgitation

Jeroen J. Bax, Nina Ajmone Marsan, Pieter van der Bijl, Hendrik Treede, Michele DeBonis, Bernard Prendergast, Bernard Iung, and Victoria Delgado

CHAPTER OUTLINE

Diagnosis and management of mitral regurgitation

Two major categories

Primary mitral regurgitation
Abnormalities of the valvular apparatus

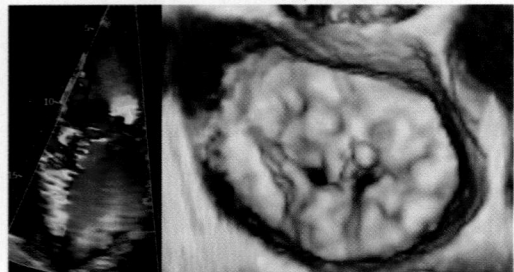

Secondary mitral regurgitation
Left ventricular dysfunction/dilatation, and/or
left atrial enlargement/dysfunction

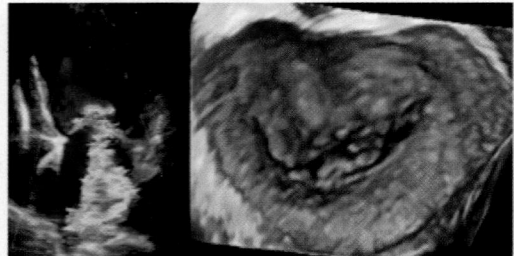

Diagnosis

Routinely performed by 2D or 3D
transthoracic echocardiography

For more precise assessment to
decide therapeutic options
(surgical or transcatheter mitral
valve repair or replacement),
2D and 3D **transesophageal
echocardiography** is mandatory

Detailed anatomical imaging
of the mitral valve (including
assessment of annular
calcification) is now routinely
provided by **cardiac computed
tomography**

Cardiac magnetic resonance
is reserved for selected patient
to precisely quantify severity
of mitral regurgitation

Management

Surgical mitral valve repair/replacement

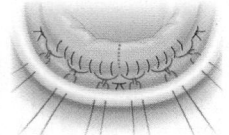

**Transcatheter mitral valve
repair/replacement (e.g. transcatheter
mitral valve repair with MitraClip)**

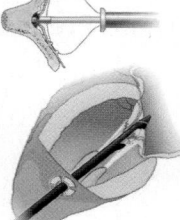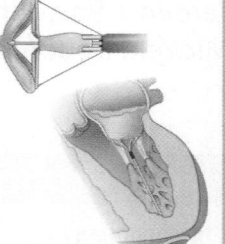

**Guideline-directed medical and device therapies
for heart failure in secondary mitral regurgitation**

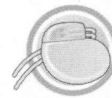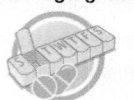

Chapter 30 Fuster and Hurst's Central Illustration. Mitral regurgitation is usually divided into two major categories, based on the underlying etiology. Diagnostic approaches assess the underlying mechanism and the severity of mitral regurgitation. Transcatheter interventions are an emerging alternative for patients with primary mitral regurgitation who are inoperable or at high surgical risk, and those with secondary mitral regurgitation who remain symptomatic despite optimal guideline-directed medical therapy (and cardiac resynchronization therapy when indicated).

CHAPTER SUMMARY

This chapter provides a comprehensive overview of the epidemiology, pathophysiology, diagnosis, and treatment of primary and secondary mitral regurgitation (MR). MR is the most frequent valve disease in the population (estimated prevalence 20%) and, as a disease of the elderly, prevalence will increase steeply over the next few decades. Primary MR results from valvular abnormalities whereas secondary MR is a consequence of left ventricular dysfunction/dilatation or left atrial enlargement/dysfunction (see Fuster and Hurst's Central Illustration). Significant MR is associated with high morbidity/mortality when left untreated, with 5-year survival of 46 ± 3% in secondary MR and 66 ± 3% in primary MR. Still, most MR patients are treated conservatively. MR diagnosis/quantification is performed with two- and three-dimensional transthoracic echocardiography, which provides anatomical and functional information to understand the MR pathophysiology. Cardiac magnetic resonance is ideal for MR quantification. When transcatheter mitral valve repair/replacement is being considered, detailed anatomical imaging of the mitral valve (including annular calcification) can be provided by cardiac computed tomography. Surgical therapies and transcatheter mitral valve repair/replacement are discussed, and a summary of the recommendations from the latest ESC/EACTS and ACC/AHA guidelines for treatment of primary and secondary MR is provided.

INTRODUCTION

Mitral regurgitation (MR) is (together with aortic stenosis) the most frequent heart valve disease in the general population, and particularly is a disease of the elderly. In a nationwide, hospital-based survey in Sweden (including 10,164,211 individuals) performed between 2003 and 2010, the incidence of valvular heart disease was 63.9 per 100,000 person-years, with 24.2% being MR.[1] Importantly, the majority (almost 70%) of heart valve diseases was diagnosed in elderly patients (aged ≥65 years).

More recently, the findings in the OxVALVE Population Cohort Study (OxVALVE-PCS, an ongoing prospective cohort study conducted in Oxfordshire, United Kingdom) were reported.[2] This study is a cross-sectional analysis of a primary care population (n = 2500 patients, aged ≥65 years); the patients were screened for undiagnosed heart valve disease with the use of transthoracic echocardiography (TTE). In 19.8% of the participants, the presence of mild MR was diagnosed, with 2.3% having moderate-to-severe MR. Based on projection of these observations using population data, it is estimated that the prevalence of clinically significant heart valve disease will double before the year 2050, with a major contribution of MR.

It has become clear that MR is associated with significant mortality and morbidity when left untreated. In a nationwide analysis from France, a total of 107,412 patients with MR (68% primary, 32% secondary MR) were admitted to the hospital between 2014 and 2015.[3] Within 1 year, 8% of the patients underwent surgery, whereas 92% were managed conservatively. Readmissions occurred at least once in 63% of patients, and 37% were readmitted two or more times. Moreover, 1-year mortality or heart failure hospitalization was 34%.

Similar findings have been reported in the United States. Dziadzko and colleagues[4] identified 727 patients with isolated, moderate/severe MR in Olmsted County, Minnesota, (between 2000 and 2010); 65% of patients had secondary MR, 32% had primary MR, and 2% had mixed MR. The 5-year survival was 54 ± 2% in all patients, with 46 ± 3% in patients with secondary MR and 66 ± 3% in patients with primary MR. Development of heart failure during the 5-year follow-up occurred in 83 ± 3% of patients with secondary MR, versus 40 ± 3% of patients with primary MR. Importantly, in the time period between 2000 and 2010, mitral valve surgery occurred during patients' lifetime in only 4% of patients with secondary MR, and 37% of patients with primary MR.

This chapter is dedicated to MR. It is important to realize that the mitral valve includes various components (**Table 30–1**). The annulus is a fibrous ring that separates the left atrium (LA) from the left ventricle (LV). The mitral annulus is saddle shaped and changes in shape throughout the cardiac cycle: during systole, the annulus contracts and reduces its surface in order to optimize closure of the leaflets. The valve consists of two leaflets (anterior and posterior), each with three scallops. There are two commissures (anterolateral and posteromedial) where the leaflets insert into the mitral annulus. The chordae tendinae connect the leaflets with the papillary muscles, which insert directly into the LV.

TABLE 30–1. Different Parts of the Mitral Valve

- Mitral annulus
- Two leaflets:
  - anterior leaflet (three scallops: A1 [lateral], A2 [central], A3 [medial])
  - posterior leaflet (three scallops: P1 [lateral] P2 [central], P3 [medial])
- Two commissures: anterolateral and posteromedial
- Chordae tendinae:
  - Primary: attached at the leaflet tips
  - Secondary: attached at the mid part of the leaflets
  - Tertiary: attached at the base of the leaflets
- Two papillary muscles: anterolateral and posteromedial

For the complete evaluation of mitral valve pathology, it is essential to assess the etiology, the mechanism, and the severity of the MR. Patients with MR are usually divided into two major categories, based on the underlying etiology: primary versus secondary MR. Whereas primary MR relates to abnormalities of the valvular apparatus, secondary MR relates to LV dysfunction/dilatation or LA enlargement/dysfunction (ventricular and atrial secondary MR, respectively). In the daily practice, precise distinction between secondary atrial or secondary ventricular MR is often not possible, since LA and LV dilatation/dysfunction often coexist.

The diagnostic assessment of the mechanism and the severity of MR is routinely performed by two-dimensional (2D) TTE, and more recently three-dimensional (3D) TTE, which provides good anatomical and functional information in order to understand the pathophysiology underlying the MR. However, for more precise assessment of the MR to decide therapeutic options (surgical or transcatheter mitral valve repair or replacement), 2D and 3D transesophageal echocardiography (TEE) is mandatory.

While echocardiography is crucial in MR quantification, the advent of transcatheter mitral valve therapies has introduced the need for detailed anatomical imaging of the mitral valve (including assessment of annular calcification), which is now routinely provided by cardiac computed tomography (CT).[5] Cardiac magnetic resonance (CMR) is reserved for selected patients to precisely quantify severity of MR.[6]

In this chapter, the epidemiology and pathophysiology of primary and secondary MR is discussed in depth as well the diagnostic approaches to understand the underlying mechanism and the severity of the MR. Next, the state-of-the-art surgical therapies for both primary and secondary MR are discussed. Thereafter, the many techniques for transcatheter mitral valve repair and replacement are summarized in detail. Finally, the current evidence and recommendations from the latest ESC/EACTS and ACC/AHA guidelines for the treatment of primary and secondary MR are reviewed.

PRIMARY MITRAL REGURGITATION

Epidemiology

Although rheumatic valve disease remains the most common etiology of primary MR globally,[7] degenerative mitral valve disease is the leading cause of primary MR in developed countries.[8] In addition, a number of other etiologies may cause significant primary MR, and a systematic classification of primary MR is

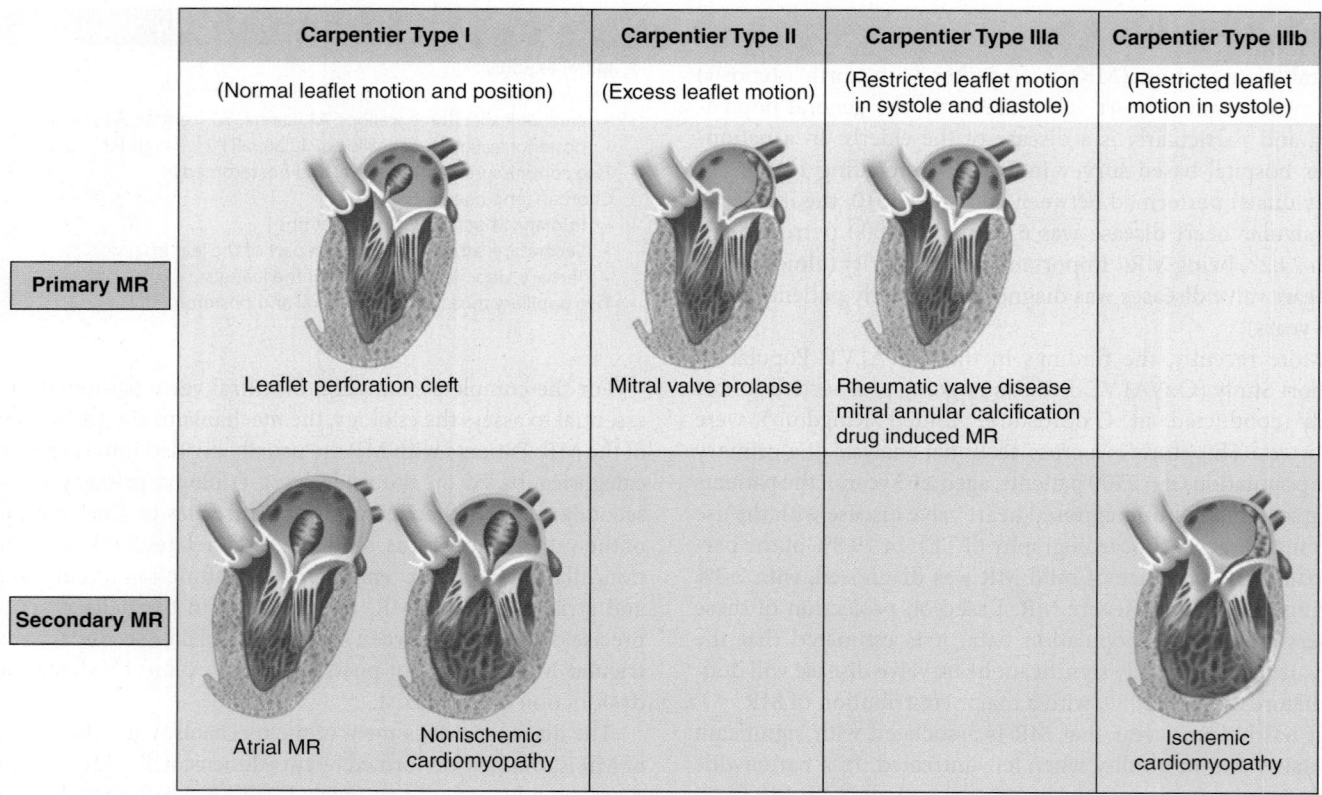

Figure 30–1. Carpentier's classification of primary and secondary MR. Reproduced with permission from El Sabbagh A, Reddy YNV, Nishimura RA. Mitral Valve Regurgitation in the Contemporary Era: Insights Into Diagnosis, Management, and Future Directions. *JACC Cardiovasc Imaging.* 2018 Apr;11(4):628-643.

therefore important not only to identify the underlying mechanism of MR, but also in planning the appropriate management.

Etiology and Lesions: Fibroelastic Deficiency Versus Barlow's Disease

When applying the Carpentier classification for leaflet dysfunction in primary MR (**Fig. 30–1**),[9] leaflet position and motion can be normal (type I), excessive (type II), or restricted in systole and diastole (type IIIa).

Mitral valve leaflet perforation or a cleft are both possible lesions causing type I primary MR, and endocarditis, traumatic injury, or congenital disease (eg, partial atrioventricular septal defect) are the main etiologies (**Fig. 30–2**). Mitral valve prolapse or flail (eversion of the free edge of the leaflet into the left atrium) are the most common lesions underlying Type II primary MR and are caused by degenerative mitral valve disease (Fig. 30–2). Carpentier type II primary MR may also be due to (partial) papillary muscle rupture caused by myocardial infarction or trauma. Finally, the main lesions underlying type IIIa primary MR are leaflet, annulus and subvalvular apparatus thickening, and calcification, mainly caused by rheumatic valve disease (Fig. 30–2), iatrogenic injury (eg, ergotamine or radiation), carcinoid disease, connective tissue diseases (eg, systemic lupus erythematosus), and mucopolysaccharidoses (eg, Hurler syndrome).

Degenerative mitral valve disease is the most common cause of primary MR in developed countries, and is characterized by a spectrum of lesions, varying from simple chordal rupture involving prolapse of an isolated segment (particularly P2) in an otherwise normal valve, to multisegment prolapse involving one or both leaflets in a valve with significant excess tissue and a large annular size (**Fig. 30–3**). It is therefore conventionally further categorized into two main etiologies: fibroelastic deficiency and myxomatous degeneration (**Table 30–2**).[10]

Fibroelastic deficiency occurs most frequently in patients older than 60 years who have a relatively short history of valvular disease. Deficiency of the glycoprotein fibrillin causes loss of structural integrity and rupture of chorda(e), leading to prolapse or flail. Leaflets are usually thin and translucent, although the prolapsing segment often shows myxomatous degeneration with leaflet thickening in case of long-standing regurgitation. The key lesion in fibroelastic deficiency is therefore a chordal rupture with a focal (limited to a single scallop) prolapse/flail, while the segments adjacent to the prolapsing scallop are mostly normal in size, height, and structure. In contrast, patients with myxomatous degeneration are generally younger (<60 years of age) at the time of surgical referral, and often present with long history of follow-up for a murmur. Proteoglycans accumulate in the valve leaflets and subvalvular apparatus, leading to diffuse thickening and redundancy of leaflet tissue and chorda elongation, with multisegment prolapse (and flail). Myxomatous disease is also associated with interscallop separations of the mitral leaflets, varying degrees of annular calcification, fibrosis of the papillary muscles, severe annular

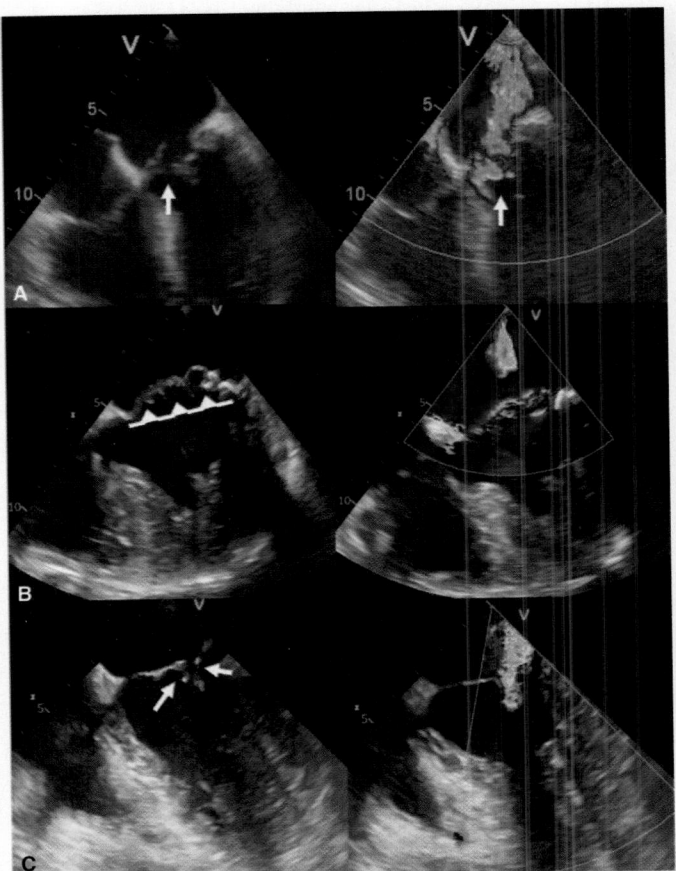

Figure 30–2. Mitral valve lesions causing primary MR. (A) shows the example of a perforation and destruction of the anterior mitral leaflet due to endocarditis (*left, arrow*). The regurgitant jet through the leaflet can be observed on the color Doppler image (*right, arrow*). **(B)** shows an example of a patient with degenerative mitral valve disease with excessive motion of the anterior and posterior mitral valve leaflets that prolapse above the mitral annular plane (*left, dotted line and arrowheads*). On the color Doppler image, the regurgitant jet is central along the line of coaptation. **(C)** shows an example of rheumatic mitral valve disease with thickened leaflets, particularly at the tips (*left, arrows*) with restrictive motion in systole causing mitral valve regurgitation (*right*).

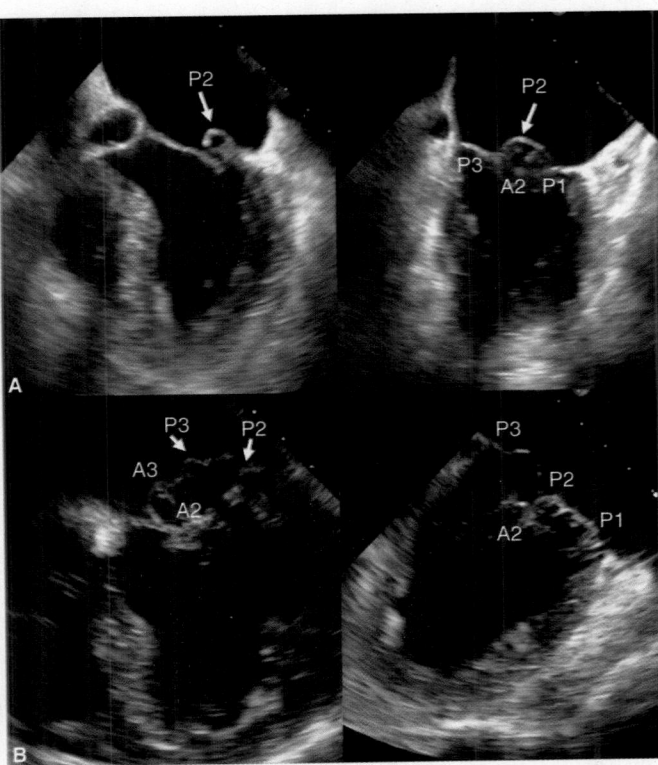

Figure 30–3. Degenerative mitral valve regurgitation. Example of a patient with mitral regurgitation due to prolapse and chorda rupture (flail) of the central scallop of the posterior mitral leaflet (P2, *arrow*). **(A)** on the left shows the TEE mid-esophageal view at 0° where the prolapse of the posterior leaflet can be observed. On the right, the bicommissural view displays the prolapse of the P2 scallop above the plane of the mitral annulus whereas the lateral (P1) and medial (P3) scallops of the posterior mitral leaflet and the central scallop of the anterior mitral leaflet (A2) remain at the annular level. **(B)** shows the example of a patient with Barlow's disease characterized by excessive tissue of the mitral leaflets and prolapse of various scallops. On the left, the TEE mid-esophageal view at 0° shows the prolapse of A3, P3, and P2 while the right panel shows the bicommissural view with the prolapse of all the scallops of the posterior mitral leaflet.

dilatation, and significant mitral annulus abnormalities, such as annular disjunction, decreased anteroposterior contraction, increased intercommissural distance, and attenuation of the saddle shape during systole.[11,12] The term *Barlow's disease* is usually reserved for diffuse myxomatous degeneration of both the anterior and posterior mitral leaflets, while a forme fruste has also been documented, representing the continuum between myxomatous degeneration and fibroelastic deficiency. Numerous disease entities are associated with myxomatous degeneration (eg, Marfan syndrome, Ehlers–Danlos syndrome, osteogenesis imperfecta, pseudoxanthoma elasticum, secundum atrial septal defect, Holt–Oram syndrome, relapsing polychondritis, and genetic hypertrophic cardiomyopathy).

Clinical Presentation

Clinical Symptoms

The typical symptoms of MR are considered dyspnea on exertion, orthopnea, and paroxysmal nocturnal dyspnea. These symptoms may appear abruptly in patients with acute onset of MR, since the LV is suddenly exposed to a large volume overload resulting in high filling pressures and pulmonary congestion. In turn, a more gradual progression to severe MR, such as in patients with myxomatous degeneration, would lead to a chronic compensated phase where the LV develops eccentric hypertrophy and the LA enlarges, ensuring a normal forward stroke volume and LV filling pressures even during exercise. These patients may be referred for cardiological evaluation without any symptoms except for a systolic murmur, and mostly develop dyspnea on exertion only gradually and at a later stage when LV function starts to impair.[13]

Less specific symptoms include palpitations, fatigue, atypical chest pain, or presyncope.[13] Palpitations and thoracic pain are mainly related to development of arrhythmias, such as atrial fibrillation or frequent premature ventricular contractions. In a very small percentage of patients, the first manifestation of mitral valve prolapse may be sudden cardiac death (malignant arrhythmic mitral valve prolapse phenotype).[11,14]

TABLE 30–2. Differences between Fibroelastic Deficiency and Myxomatous Degeneration in Terms of Clinical, Echocardiographic, and Surgical Characteristics

	Fibroelastic Deficiency	Myxomatous Degeneration (Barlow's Disease)
Clinical characteristics		
Age of onset	Older (≥60 years)	Younger (<60 years)
History	No history of murmur	Usually long history of murmur
Duration of the disease	Months (likely <5 years)	Years to decades
Pathology	Connective tissue deficiency	Myxoid infiltration
Auscultation	Holosystolic murmur	Mid-systolic click and late systolic murmur
Echocardiographic characteristics		
Leaflets	No excessive valve tissue Thin leaflets and no billowing in noninvolved segments Single segment involvement	Excessive valve tissue Thickened leaflets Leaflet billowing Multiple segments involvement
Annulus	Normal of moderate dilatation No calcifications	Severe annular dilatation Calcifications could be present
Chordae	Ruptured	Elongated, ruptured
Surgical characteristics		
Annulus	Normal or mildly dilated annulus diameter	Severe annular dilatation; possible calcifications
Leaflets	Thin translucent leaflets without excess tissue Single segment involved, which often shows leaflet thickening No billowing of other segments	Thick leaflets with excess tissue Multiple segments involved, often bi-leaflet Multi-segmental billowing
Chordae	Chordae of the affected segment is mainly ruptured	Chordae elongated or ruptured Chordae thickened and/or calcified
Difficulty to repair	Mostly easy to repair with "respect" techniques (chordal replacement and annuloplasty)	More difficult to repair and with often combined "respect" and "resect" techniques (chordal replacement and annuloplasty + leaflet resection)

On physical examination, the typical murmur is harsh and holosystolic, if the lesion is chordal rupture, and is heard the most at the apex with irradiation to the axilla, with a weak correlation between MR severity and murmur intensity. When MR is severe, the murmur is often accompanied by the third heart sound (S3) produced by the emptying of the large atrial volume against high LV pressure. In patients with Barlow's disease, the murmur is high-pitched and late-systolic, with a mid-to-late systolic click. The click is generated as the elongated chordae are stretched: physical maneuvers that decrease LV volume (and therefore reduce the tension on the mitral valve), such as standing or the Valsalva maneuver, cause the click and the murmur to come earlier in systole and to increase in intensity; maneuvers that increase LV volume, such as squatting or lying down, may cause the opposite effect and make the click and murmur disappear.[13] If pulmonary hypertension has developed, ascites and peripheral edema may also occur.

Laboratory Findings

In patients with primary MR, the electrocardiogram (ECG) and chest x-ray often demonstrate nonspecific abnormalities. The ECG may show evidence of LA enlargement and LV hypertrophy, and T-wave abnormalities in the inferior leads have been associated with malignant arrhythmias in patients with mitral valve prolapse.[15] During palpitations, an ECG should be performed to demonstrate the presence of atrial fibrillation or frequent and complex premature ventricular complexes; the first represents a possible criterium for surgery, and the latter ones have been associated with the malignant arrhythmic phenotype of mitral valve prolapse.

The chest x-ray may show cardiac enlargement and pulmonary congestion in case of decompensated MR. Blood tests are not specific for MR but high brain natriuretic peptide (BNP) levels may help identifying the correct timing for surgery, suggesting high LV filling pressures and indicating increased reliance on preload to maintain an adequate forward cardiac output.[16]

While the aforementioned tests are modestly useful in diagnosing MR, the echocardiogram is the indispensable tool for further diagnostic evaluation.[7,17]

Diagnostic Evaluation

Echocardiography represents the cornerstone in the diagnosis and management of patients with primary MR, but other imaging modalities, such as CMR, may provide important additional information.

Echocardiography

Standard 2D-TTE is the first line diagnostic test in case of suspicion of MR.[17,18] This technique provides crucial information on mitral valve dysfunction and lesions responsible for MR, on the severity of MR, and on the hemodynamic effects of MR on LV remodeling, LA size, pulmonary pressures, and right atrium/ventricle (Table 30–2).

Mitral Valve Dysfunction and Lesion Assessment: Although the majority of mitral valve lesions underlying primary MR can be identified with TTE, TEE can provide more accurate and detailed information of mitral valve abnormalities. Therefore during an initial diagnostic evaluation, TEE is indicated only in patients with inconclusive or technically difficult TTE examinations.[19,20] However, when surgical or transcatheter mitral valve therapy is considered, TEE is routinely performed to evaluate the precise pathophysiology underlying the MR, and to assess the feasibility of the potential treatment (surgery or transcatheter therapy, repair, or replace the mitral valve). Using different 2D views, TTE and TEE can explore all the components of the mitral valve apparatus and describe the type and location of valvular lesions (**Fig. 30–4**).

The typical echocardiographic features of fibroelastic deficiency or Barlow's disease are shown in Fig. 30–3 and described in Table 30–2. An isolated segmental prolapse or flail (most often P2) with chordal rupture and an eccentric regurgitant jet is typical for patients with fibroelastic deficiency with relatively normal appearance of the other valve scallops, with only mild dilatation of the mitral valve annulus. Conversely, echocardiographic findings in patients with Barlow's disease include diffuse redundant leaflet tissue with significant leaflet thickening (>3 mm) and elongated chordae, resulting in multisegmental, often bileaflet prolapse, and multiple regurgitant jets mostly mid-to-late systolic. In addition, significant annular abnormalities are often observed, such as severe annular dilatation (>36 mm), annular calcifications, and mitral annular disjunction, defined as a separation between the LA wall-posterior mitral valve junction and LV attachment (atrial displacement of the mitral valve leaflet hinge point), which leads to annular

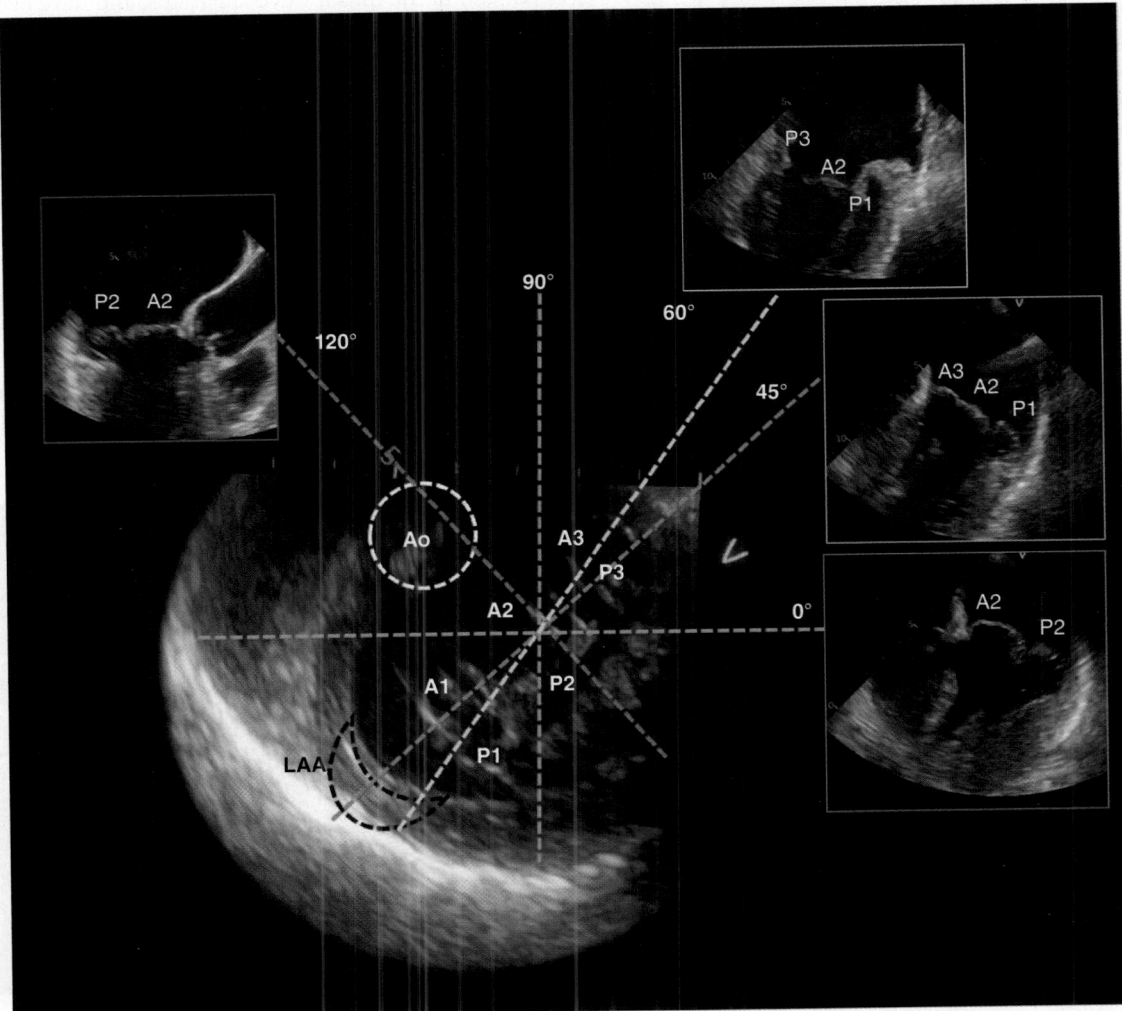

Figure 30–4. Systematic segmental analysis of the mitral valve using TEE for the assessment of the mechanism of MR. From a modified transgastric view of the short-axis of the mitral valve, the landmarks are indicated: the aortic valve (Ao), the left atrial appendage (LAA), and the scallops of the anterior (A1, A2, A3) and posterior (P1, P2, P3) mitral leaflets. The mid-esophageal view at 0° shows the A2 and P2 scallops. By turning the probe to 45°, the P1, A2, and A3 scallops are shown. The 60° view bisects the mitral valve at the level of the commissures and the P1, A2, and P3 scallops can be identified. The 120° view bisects the mitral valve antero-posteriorly and the A2 and P2 scallops can be observed in relation to the aortic valve.

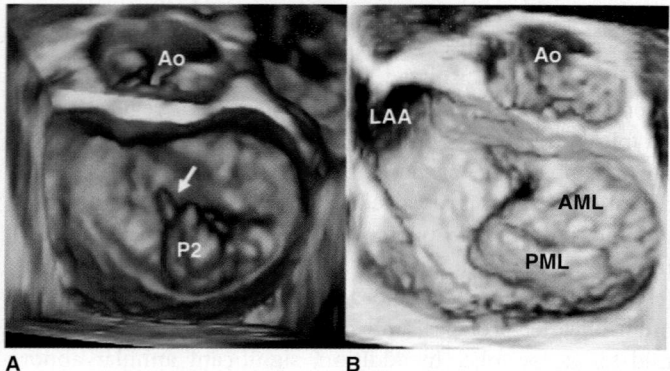

A   **B**

Figure 30–5. 3D-TEE: en face view of the mitral valve. This view resembles the surgical exposure of the mitral valve and permits differentiation between fibroelastic deficiency **(A)** and Barlow's disease **(B)**. **(A)** shows the prolapse of the central scallop of the posterior mitral leaflet (P2) with ruptured chorda (*arrow*). In **(B)**, the prolapse of both the anterior (AML) and posterior (PML) mitral leaflets can be appreciated.

hypermobility with a typical outward movement during systole, and loss of the saddle shape.[11,12]

The introduction of real-time 3D-TTE and particularly 3D-TEE has substantially improved the assessment of mitral valve abnormalities by including both area and depth (volumetric data set) within the imaging plane, and therefore allowing realistic visualization of the mitral valve with any possible orientation (ie, from the LV or the LA point of view) and with minimal probe manipulation.[21] The most commonly used display is the "en face" visualization, also called "the surgical view" **(Fig. 30–5)** since it resembles the intraoperative image of the mitral valve after the surgeon opens the LA. This view allows for a rapid, intuitive but also very complete analysis of mitral valve abnormalities and facilitates the communication between

the echocardiographer and the interventional cardiologist or cardiac surgeon. Complex lesions, such as valvular cleft and commissural involvement, which are often overlooked using 2D echocardiography, can be accurately described with this approach.[21]

Echocardiography is also used to provide quantitative measures of the mitral valve anatomy, such as annular dimensions (anteroposterior diameter, intercommissural diameter, height, etc) or posterior and anterior leaflet lengths and prolapsing height, which may be useful to plan mitral valve procedures.[17,18] However, considering the oval and saddle shape of the mitral valve annulus and the complex geometry of the leaflets and subvalvular apparatus, several limitations and geometric assumptions affect the accuracy of the 2D echocardiographic measures. Commercial software have been recently developed using 3D echocardiographic data sets: mitral annulus and leaflets can be traced to create a 3D model of the mitral valve **(Fig. 30–6)** to provide more accurate (correct 2D alignment) and 3D measures (mitral leaflet surface area, annular perimeter, etc) of the mitral valve apparatus, and have been shown to improve the feasibility of surgical strategies beforehand.[21]

Mitral Regurgitation Severity Assessment: Echocardiography (with color Doppler, pulse- and continuous-wave Doppler) is also the main imaging technique applied to assess the MR severity. Currently, this assessment is recommended using the integration of several quantitative parameters, including measurement of the vena contracta width, regurgitant volume, regurgitant fraction, and effective regurgitant orifice area **(Table 30–3)**.[17,18] This multiparametric approach helps to minimize the effects of technical or measurement errors inherent to each method **(Fig. 30–7)**.

In the case of insufficient or discordant information from TTE and clinical consequences for decision-making, TEE is

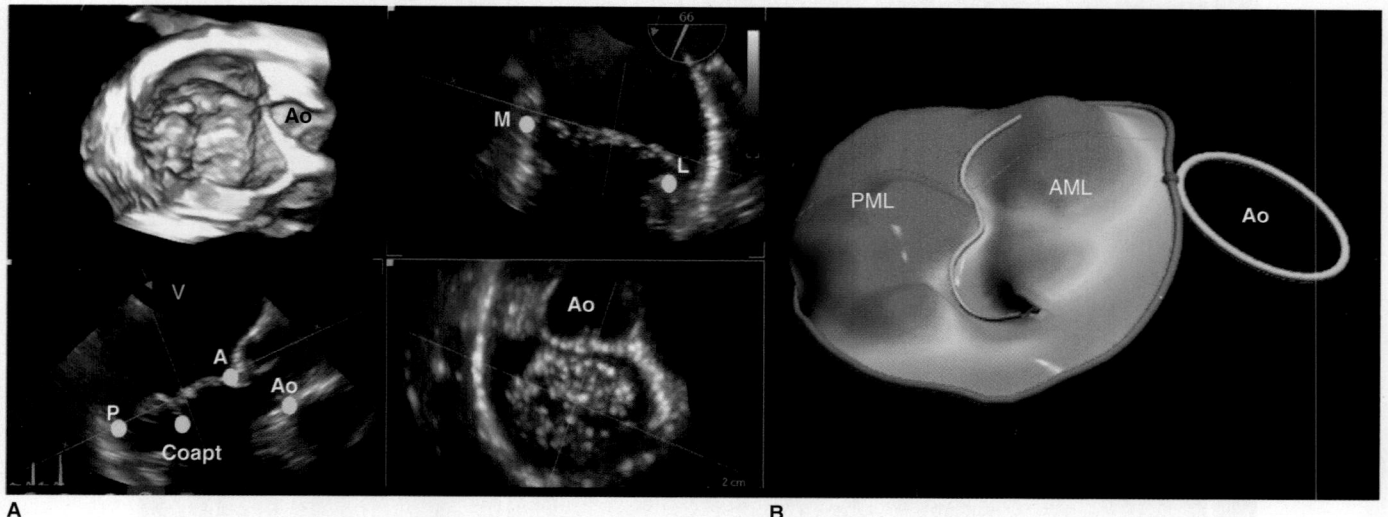

A   **B**

Figure 30–6. Model of the mitral valve from 3D-TEE data sets. On a 3D volume of the mitral valve **(A)**, the multiplanar reformation planes can be aligned and the various anatomical landmarks (anterior [A], posterior [P], medial [M], and lateral [L] points of the mitral annulus, coaptation point [Coapt] and aortic valve [Ao] point) are demarcated; then the software detects automatically the mitral leaflets and creates the model that permits the measurement of the mitral valve annulus, leaflet area and length, prolapse volume, and mitro-aortic angle, among others. The model also displays with elevation colors the segments that are prolapsing above the mitral annulus (in *red*, **B**) facilitating the analysis of the mitral valve.

TABLE 30-3. Echocardiographic Criteria for the Definition of Severe Primary Mitral Regurgitation

	ACC/AHA Guidelines	ESC Guidelines
Qualitative analysis		
Valve morphology	Large mitral valve prolapse Leaflet flail Large coaptation defect Papillary muscle rupture	Large mitral valve prolapse Leaflet flail Large coaptation defect Papillary muscle rupture
Color flow regurgitant jet		Very large central jet or eccentric jet reaching the posterior wall of the LA Large flow convergence zone
CW signal of the regurgitant jet		Dense/Triangular
Semiquantitative analysis		
Regurgitant jet area	Central jet >40% LA or holosystolic eccentric jet	
Vena contracta width	≥0.7 cm	≥0.7 cm (>8 cm for biplane: average between four- and two-chamber apical views)
Mitral valve inflow		Dominant E wave ≥1.5 m/s TVI mitral/TVI aortic >1.4
Pulmonary vein flow		Systolic pulmonary vein flow reversal
Quantitative analysis		
EROA	≥40 mm²	≥40 mm²
Regurgitant volume	≥60 mL/beat	≥60 mL/beat
Regurgitant fraction	≥50%	----
Enlargement of cardiac chambers	LV and LA	LV and LA

Abbreviations: EROA, effective regurgitant orifice area; LA, left atrium; LV, left ventricle; TVI, time-velocity integral

indicated for more accurate assessment of these quantitative parameters, and the introduction of 3D imaging has further improved this evaluation. Several studies[22,23] using 3D echocardiography data sets have proposed quantification of the vena contracta area using orthogonal views optimally aligned to the 3D color mitral regurgitation jets, allowing for a direct planimetry of the regurgitant orifice in the "en face" view (**Fig. 30–8**). This approach showed to be superior to the 2D echocardiographic measures, and is particularly useful in the case of the noncircular regurgitant orifice and multiple regurgitant jets.[22,23]

Hemodynamic Impact of Mitral Regurgitation: TTE also provides important information on the impact of MR on LV size and function, LA size, pulmonary artery pressures, and right ventricular (RV) function, which are crucial for assessing the appropriate timing for surgical/transcatheter intervention. These measures should be performed according to current recommendations for chamber quantification,[24] and when possible using advanced echocardiographic techniques. 3D quantification of LV volumes, and LV ejection fraction (LVEF) has been demonstrated in several cardiac diseases to be superior to 2D biplane Simpson's method and should be considered in centers with the proper expertise.[24] Also, speckle-tracking based measurement of LV global longitudinal strain should be considered, being more sensitive in detecting myocardial dysfunction and less load dependent as compared to standard echocardiographic methods.[19,25] This parameters can be used to improve identification of LV dysfunction before LVEF

becomes impaired and to optimize the timing for mitral valve intervention. Concomitant valvular heart diseases next to primary MR, such as tricuspid regurgitation or aortic stenosis, are also thoroughly assessed with echocardiography at the time of MR analysis. Finally, once an asymptomatic patient has been identified as having severe MR, clinical follow-up and serial echocardiography should be conducted every 6 months to assess the optimal timing for intervention.[19,20]

Exercise Echocardiography
Exercise echocardiography can be performed in patients with moderate-severe primary MR for several purposes. In asymptomatic patients, it might be useful to objectively assess the functional capacity and absence/presence of symptoms during exercise, and therefore help the treating physician in defining the optimal timing for intervention.[19,20] An increase in systolic pulmonary pressure >60 mm Hg during exercise has also been proposed for risk stratification, but this criterium has not been sufficiently well defined to be included in the current recommendations.[19,20] In patients with symptoms but uncertainty about the severity of MR based on the measurements at rest, exercise echocardiography may also be helpful to show a significant worsening of MR during exercise with increasing LV filling pressures, supporting the diagnosis that MR is the cause of patient's symptoms.[19,20]

Cardiac Magnetic Resonance
CMR is considered the gold standard imaging technique for quantification of LV and RV volumes and ejection fractions. It can

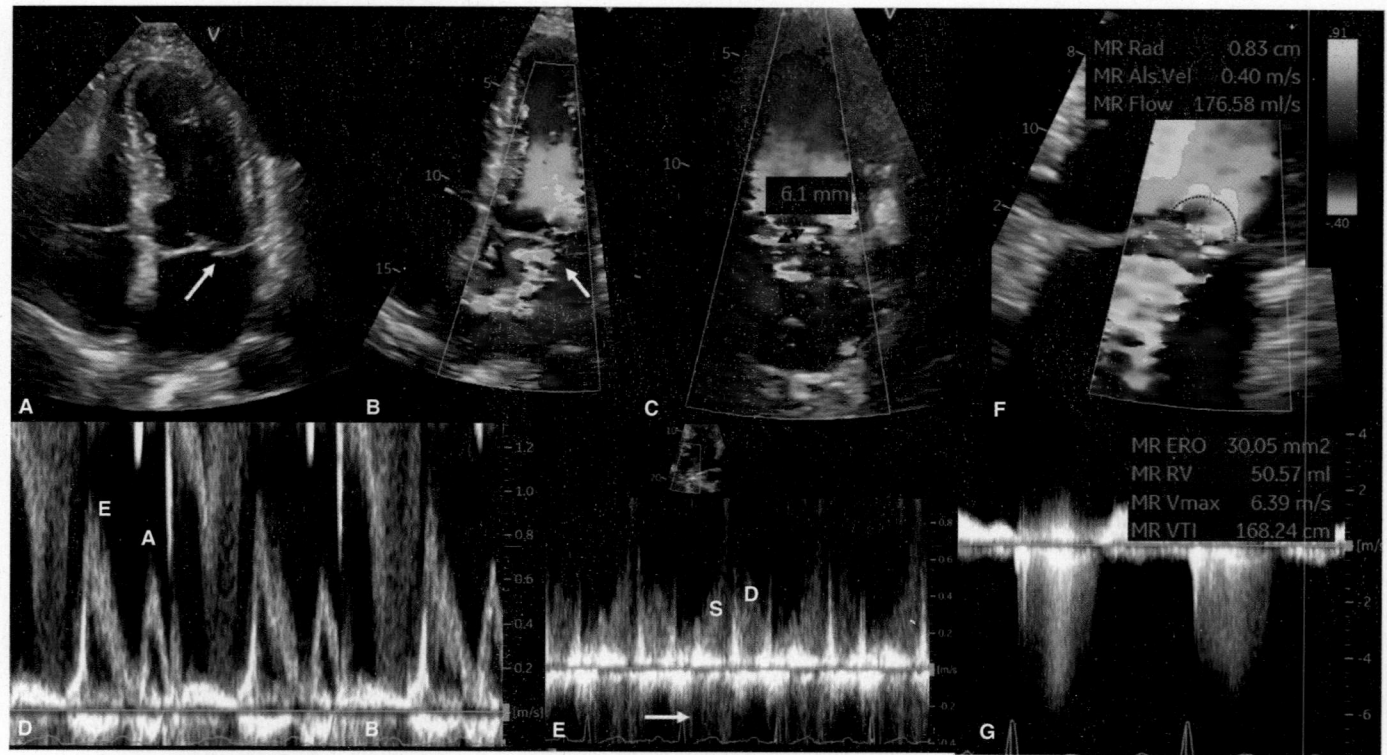

Figure 30–7. **Assessment of MR grade with TTE in a patient with prolapse of the posterior mitral leaflet. (A)** shows the apical four-chamber view where the prolapse of the posterior mitral leaflet can be noted (*arrow*) as well as the dilatation of the left atrium due to volume overload. In **(B)**, the color flow Doppler image shows a regurgitant jet that occupied 50% of the left atrial area. On color Doppler imaging of the apical three-chamber view, the vena contract can be measured (*double arrowhead*, 6.1 mm, **C**). **(D)** displays the pulsed wave Doppler recording of the mitral inflow with a prominent early diastolic peak velocity (E = 1 m/s) while the pulmonary vein flow can be visualized on **(E)** that shows a blunted systolic wave (S) and the mitral regurgitant jet (*arrow*). These qualitative and semiquantative parameters indicate that the MR is moderate. The measurement of the effective regurgitant orifice (ERO) area on a color Doppler zoomed view of the regurgitant jet **(E)** is displayed in **(F)** while the calculation of the regurgitant volume (RV) is presented in **(G)**. Both metrics indicate moderate MR (ERO area 30 mm² and RV 51 mL/beat).

therefore be indicated in patients with primary MR where the image quality of TTE is poor and assessment of the hemodynamic impact of MR on cardiac chambers is crucial.[19,20] Furthermore, CMR can provide accurate quantification of mitral regurgitant fraction using measurements of stroke volume of the RV and LV,[26] and can be useful in assessing MR severity when a discrepancy exists between the clinical assessment and the echocardiography measurements.[19,20] However, outcome data on large numbers of patients have been derived from echocardiography, and it is uncertain whether CMR data can be used interchangeably with echocardiographic data in predicting outcomes.

Finally, CMR has the unique ability of providing myocardial tissue characterization, using T1 mapping to assess LV fibrosis and late gadolinium enhancement to demonstrate areas of LV scar. In patients with primary MR, the detection of focal myocardial fibrosis is of particular interest in patients with mitral valve prolapse and ventricular arrhythmias, since recent studies have suggested the presence of focal fibrosis/scar at the level of the papillary muscles and of the LV inferobasal wall as the structural substrate for the malignant ventricular arrhythmias.[14,15] The fibrosis localization also suggests that excessive mechanical stretch on the mitral valve apparatus due to the prolapsing segment could be the cause of myocardial

fibrosis. In addition, mitral annular disjunction has been also associated with the arrhythmic mitral valve prolapse and can be accurately detected with CMR (**Fig. 30–9**).

Cardiac Catheterization

Noninvasive imaging is adequate for the evaluation of MR severity in most cases. However, in selected cases (ie, with concomitant lung disease), invasive hemodynamic evaluation may be necessary, especially when there is a discrepancy between the symptomatic status and the echocardiographic/CMR measures. Elevated filling pressures support a cardiac cause of dyspnea, while normal LA (or pulmonary artery wedge) pressure and a large transpulmonary gradient suggest pulmonary hypertension secondary to lung disease rather than mitral valve disease.[19,20] Furthermore, when an indication for mitral valve surgery or transcatheter procedure is given, standard screening for significant coronary artery disease is performed by coronary angiography in most patients (cardiac CT angiography can be an alternative).

Prognosis

Primary MR is associated with increased morbidity and mortality. In a large clinical registry, comprising more than 2000 patients with severe primary MR due to flail leaflet, the

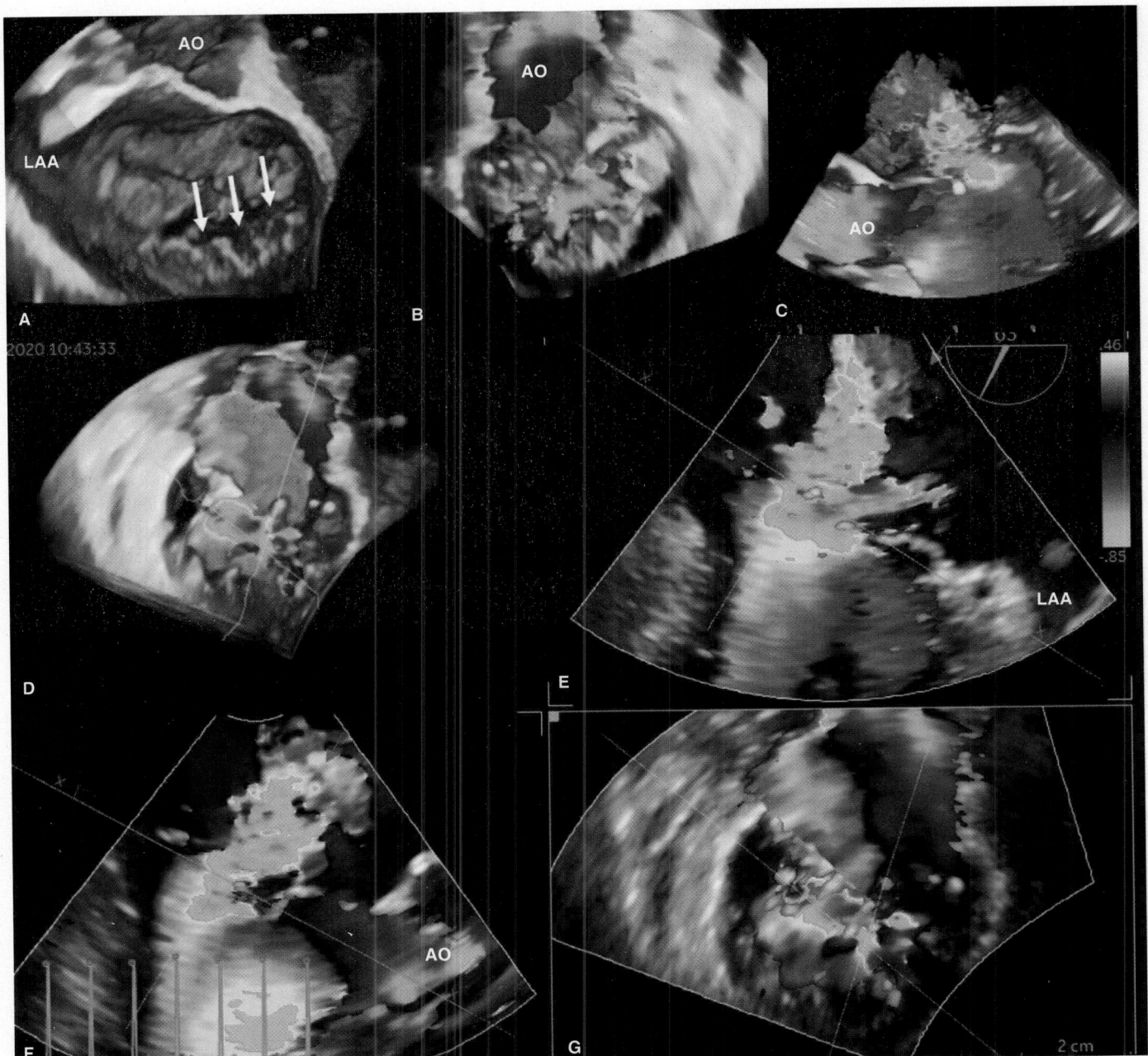

Figure 30–8. 3D-TEE for assessment of primary MR severity. On the en face view of the 3D reconstruction of the mitral valve, a large coaptation defect can be observed due to prolapse of the central and medial scallops of the posterior mitral leaflet (*arrows*, **A**). On color Doppler 3D-TEE, the regurgitant jet along the coaptation line can be visualized (**B**). The plane orthogonal to the line of coaptation permits the 3D reconstruction of the regurgitant jet on color Doppler data (**C**). (**D**) to (**G**) show the assessment of the anatomical regurgitant orifice area from 3D color Doppler data: (**D**) shows the en face view of the mitral valve, (**E**) shows the reconstructed bicommissural plane, while (**F**) shows the orthogonal view. (**G**) is the double oblique plane showing the cross-sectional area of the regurgitant jet, which is severe, along the coaptation line. Ao, aortic valve; LAA, left atrial appendage.

mortality of unoperated patients was 60% after a mean follow-up of 20 years.[27] Also, the incidence of heart failure in the unoperated patients ranged from 30% to 35% after 10 years,[27,28] while a cumulative incidence of 26% new-onset atrial fibrillation has been reported in patients with severe primary MR after 10 years' follow-up.[28] Life-threatening ventricular arrhythmias have also been associated with mitral valve prolapse (malignant arrhythmic phenotype) and mitral annular disjunction

(also without prolapse). The prevalence is estimated at 0.25% to 0.4% per year, and up to 1.8% per year in the presence of a flail leaflet.[11,14]

Various clinical and echocardiographic parameters have demonstrated a significant prognostic value in primary MR. Age was shown to be an independent predictor (hazard ratio [HR], 1.02; 95% confidence interval [CI], 1.01–1.04; $P = 0.005$) of valve surgery in patients with severe primary MR due to

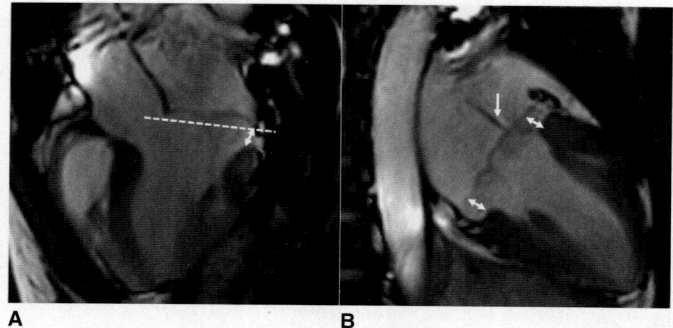

Figure 30–9. Cardiovascular magnetic resonance in primary MR. Example of a patient with moderate MR due to Barlow's disease on echocardiography and symptoms of palpitations. On cardiovascular magnetic resonance, the LV and atrium appear slightly dilated. **(A)** shows the three-chamber view where the prolapse of both mitral leaflets can be visualized. In addition, note the significant separation of the posterior mitral leaflet insertion and the LV myocardium suggesting the presence of mitral annulus disjunction (*double arrowhead*). **(B)** shows the two-chamber views where the prolapse of the mitral valve (*double arrowheads*) and the regurgitant jet (*arrow*) can be visualized.

flail leaflet, possibly due to the decreased ability of the LV to accommodate an increased volume load during senescence.[29] The combined endpoint of heart failure, new-onset atrial fibrillation, an ischemic neurological event, peripheral arterial thromboembolism, and endocarditis was also independently associated (HR, 3.1; 95% CI, 2.0–5.0; P <0.001) with age ≥50 years in patients with mitral valve prolapse.[29] Presence of symptoms, and particularly New York Heart Association (NYHA) functional class, was also associated in patients with severe primary MR with worse outcome, including sudden cardiac death.[30] In contrast, asymptomatic patients with severe primary MR due to mitral valve prolapse showed low all-cause mortality (5.2% after 7 years of follow-up).[29] Atrial fibrillation also showed an independent association with outcome, and sudden cardiac death in primary MR due to flail leaflet (relative risk [RR], 2.40; 95% CI, 0.97–5.95; P = 0.059).[31]

Among the echocardiographic parameters, the severity of MR demonstrated to have significant impact on mortality in mitral valve prolapse patients,[31] being also an independent predictor of valve surgery in asymptomatic individuals (HR, 2.06; 95% CI, 1.11–3.82; P = 0.02).[29] Several studies also showed LV systolic function (and particularly LVEF ≤60% or LV end-systolic diameter ≥40 mm) to be an independent predictor of mortality (RR, 0.94; 95% CI, 0.91–0.97; P = 0.0001) in patients with severe primary MR.[30-32] Finally, the presence of pulmonary hypertension predicted the need for valve surgery in asymptomatic patients with severe primary MR (HR, 1.87; 95% CI, 1.22–2.87; P = 0.003)[29] and an LA diameter ≥40 mm (HR, 2.7; 95% CI, 1.9–3.8; P <0.001) were independently associated with the combined endpoint of heart failure, new-onset atrial fibrillation, ischemic neurological event, peripheral arterial thromboembolism, and endocarditis in patients with flail leaflet.[31]

Accurate characterization and risk stratification of individuals with primary MR, taking into account all the aforementioned

variables, is therefore imperative in clinical decision-making and particularly to timely refer patients for surgical treatment.

Medical Therapy

Drugs with Hemodynamic Effects

Small series have shown short-term benefits of vasodilators in the decrease of regurgitant volume and LV volumes, while long-term results are heterogeneous according to the mechanisms of MR and initial LV remodeling.[33] No medical therapy improves clinical outcome of patients with primary MR. Although MR is associated with adrenergic overstimulation, no consistent hemodynamic benefit of β-blockers has been shown in the absence of LV dysfunction.[34] Therefore, guidelines do not recommend any medical therapy in patients with primary MR, except medications recommended for heart failure with reduced LVEF in patients with LV dysfunction.[19,20]

Infective Endocarditis Prophylaxis

Antibiotic prophylaxis before invasive procedures, in particular dental care, is no longer recommended in patients with native valve disease, but nonspecific hygiene measures are emphasized to prevent bacteremia.[35,36] *Staphylococcus* has become the most frequent responsible microorganism, particularly due to healthcare-related infections. This highlights the need for careful asepsis during all healthcare procedures. Oral *streptococci* still account for 20% to 30% of infective endocarditis cases and oral hygiene remains of importance. Advances in the detection of oral infectious foci and techniques of dental care have changed the management of patients at risk of infective endocarditis.[37] Oral infectious foci should be systematically detected and eradicated before valvular surgery.[38] When anticoagulant therapy is indicated, most dental procedures can and should be performed during oral anticoagulant therapy.[39] After valvular surgery, patients are at high risk of infective endocarditis and require closer dental follow-up and antibiotic prophylaxis before most dental procedures.

Surgical Treatment

Principles of Mitral Valve Repair for Primary Mitral Regurgitation

Mitral valve surgery for primary (degenerative) MR aims for complete elimination of MR and long-term durability of repair/replacement. To reach this goal, a systematic approach to mitral valve repair has to be taken, including thorough evaluation of valve pathology and consideration of various repair techniques. Successful mitral valve repair requires restoration of mitral valve anatomy and function leading to a sufficient area of leaflet coaptation.

After introduction of cardiopulmonary bypass and cardioplegic arrest, the mitral valve is exposed by either opening the left atrium in the Waterston groove or by opening the right atrium and interatrial septum. As a first step, a proper analysis of the mitral valve pathology is performed, using nerve hooks to assess leaflet height in all anterior and posterior segments assessing leaflet prolapse or tethering and leaflet structure. The subvalvular apparatus is examined for ruptured, elongated or fused primary and secondary chords and papillary muscle

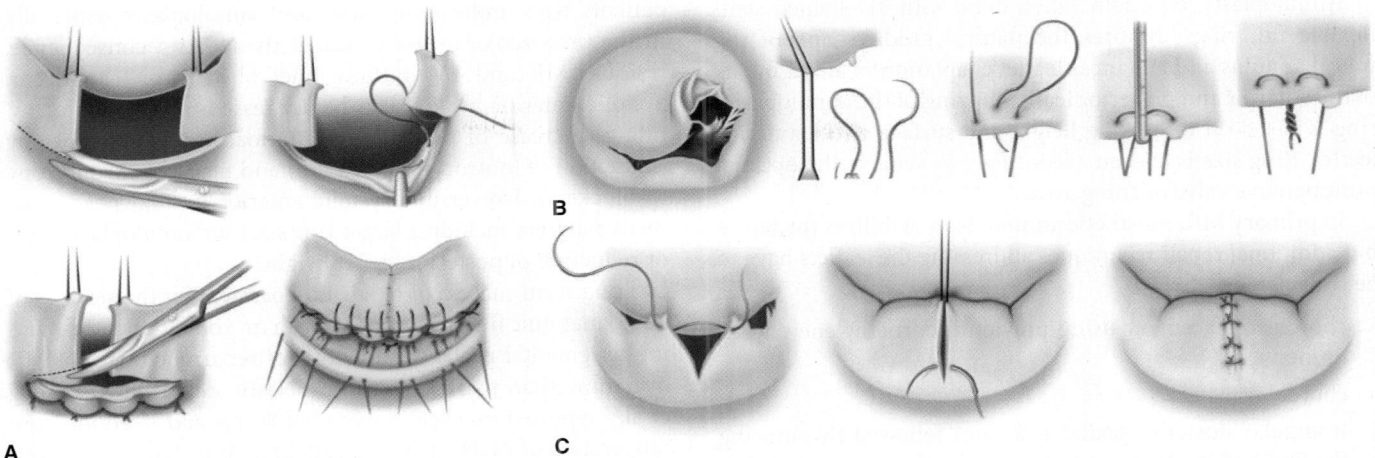

Figure 30–10. Mitral valve repair techniques for primary (degenerative) MR. (A) Quadrangular resection, sliding plasty. **(B)** Chordal replacement. **(C)** Triangular resection.

status and position. Flushing saline into the LV cavity (water test) can help to determine and mark the prolapsing segments. Only after thorough examination of the complete mitral apparatus can a proper repair can be pursued.

Multiple surgical repair techniques have been described over the years and more recently valve sparing techniques are dominating, aiming for the best possible leaflet coaptation height and surface.[40] Carpentier's "French Correction" focused mainly on anatomical restoration of the mitral valve

and included larger quadrangular leaflet resection in prolapsing posterior segments with concomitant sliding plasty techniques (**Fig. 30–10**). Nowadays, leaflet prolapse is more often addressed by chordal replacement only or smaller triangular resection in segments with excessive tissue (Fig. 30–10).

The armentarium of surgical mitral valve repair consists of a variety of techniques. With only very few exceptions, annuloplasty using complete or partial, semi rigid, or flexible prosthetic ring implants, is part of every mitral valve repair (**Fig. 30–11**).

Grade	Pathoanatomic Features	Echocardiography	Operative Findings	Repair Options
1	- Annular dilatation - Isolated posterior leaflet prolapse or single segment flail	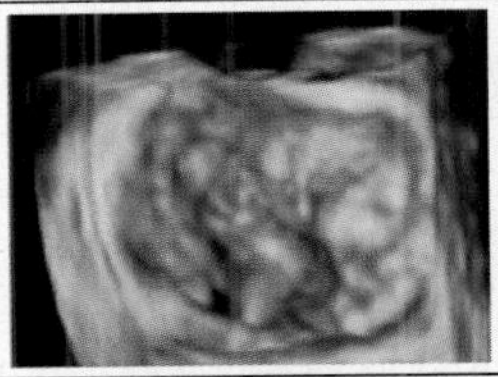	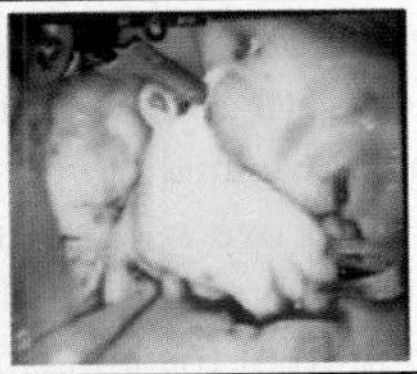	- Focal resection and valvuloplasty with ring annuloplasty - PTFE neochord support - Ring/band annuloplasty
2	- Diffuse myxomatous disease predominantly of posterior leaflet (forme fruste)	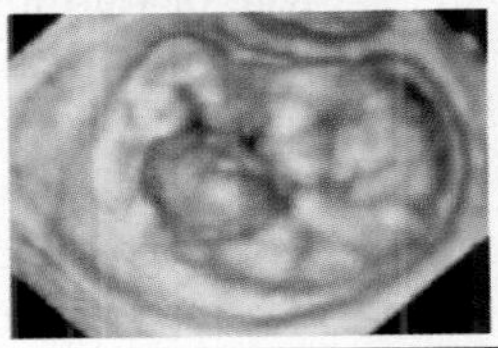	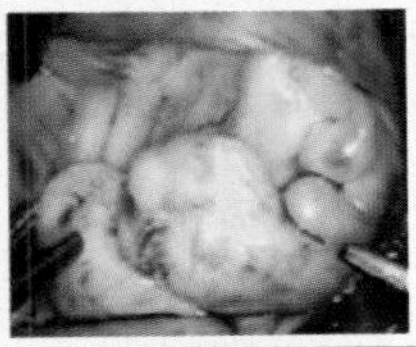	- Partial resection and sliding leaflet valvuloplasty - Multi-segment PTFE neochord support - Ring/band annuloplasty
3	- Diffuse bi-leaflet myxomatous disease (Barlow's) - Anterior leaflet flail - Multi-segment flail - Focal posterior mitral annular calcification	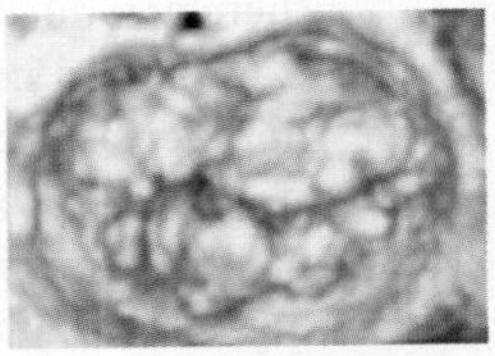	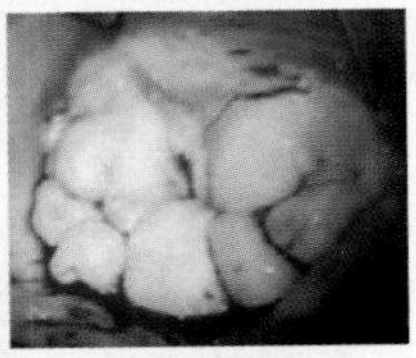	- Partial resection and sliding leaflet valvuloplasty - Multi-segment PTFE neochord support - Secondary chordal transfer - Focal calcium resection - Ring/band annuloplasty
4	- Endocarditis ± leaflet perforation or annular abscess - Rheumatic Type IIIA disease - Secondary Type IIIB disease with severe tethering - Severe mitral annular calcification	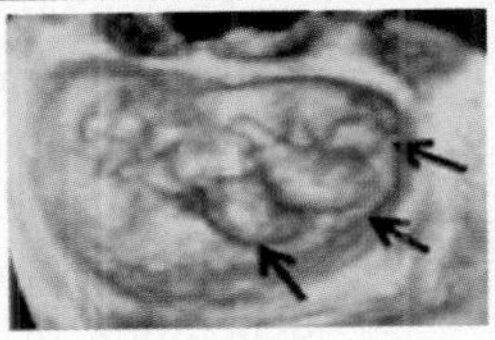	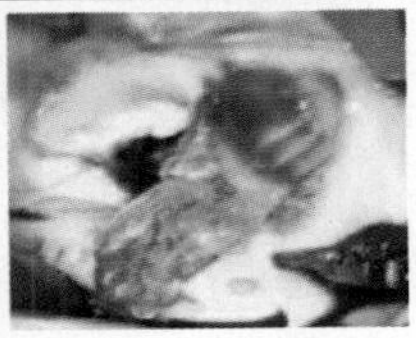	- Reconstruction with patch augmentation - Subvalvular mobilization - Radical annular reconstruction - Ring/band annuloplasty

Figure 30–11. Pathoanatomic findings, echocardiography images, operative findings, and repair options. Reproduced with permission from Alreshidan M, Herron RD, Wei LM, et al. Surgical Techniques for Mitral Valve Repair: A Pathoanatomic Grading System. *Semin Cardiothorac Vasc Anesth.* 2019 Mar;23(1):20-25.

Annuloplasty, especially when done with 3D-shaped semi flexible full rings, restores the natural saddle-shape of the mitral annulus and enhances leaflet coaptation in all segments of the anterior and posterior leaflets. Sizing of the annuloplasty ring is based on measuring height and surface of the anterior leaflet. Ring size is chosen accordingly to achieve the optimal postoperative valve opening area.

In primary MR, prosthetic annuloplasty stabilizes the repair but additional repair techniques addressing the leaflets have to be considered:

- chordal replacement using polytetrafluoroethylene chords or loops
- chordal transfer
- triangular posterior leaflet resection followed by suturing the free leaflet edges
- cleft closure
- commissural prolapse elimination by edge-to-edge sutures
- leaflet augmentation with autologous or bovine pericardial patches
- focal calcium resection
- subvalvular repair techniques

Other valve repair techniques like chordal shortening, papillary muscle shortening, or suture-based annuloplasty have been abandoned due to unsatisfying long-term results. Figure 30–11 provides an overview on pathoanatomic features, echocardiographic presentation, operative findings, and repair options for various degrees of primary mitral valve disease.[41]

After completion of the repair, another saline flush test helps to assess leaflet coaptation and valve competence but can only provide an estimate on the success of the repair.

Final evaluation requires intraoperative TEE and should be assessed before the patient is finally weaned from extracorporeal circulation. TEE is needed to prove successful repair (less than mild MR) and sufficient leaflet coaptation. TEE also helps to rule out systolic anterior motion of the anterior leaflet (**Fig. 30–12**). Systolic anterior motion represents an imbalance between valve area and amount of valve tissue, occurring in patients who underwent undersized annuloplasty, especially in the presence of excessive leaflet tissue. As a consequence, residual MR and LV outflow tract obstruction can occur. Systolic anterior motion can be addressed by increase of LV filling (increase of preload and afterload), negative inotropy (reduction of inotropic medication) and negative chronotropy (β-blockers). Irreversible systolic anterior motion needs corrective surgery including larger ring sizes for annuloplasty and/or reduction of posterior leaflet height.

Long-term success of repair is dependent on the severity of pathoanatomic findings. Patients with myxomatous disease and multisegmental prolapse show higher recurrence rates of MR over time than patients with fibroelastic deficiency. Flameng et al.[42] reported excellent survival of 80.1% and freedom from reoperation of 94.4% at 10 years after repair in 348 patients who underwent mitral valve repair for primary valve incompetence. However, freedom from MR (>2/4) was 98.7% at 1 month, but decreased to 82.2% at 5 years and 64.9% at 10 years, respectively. The linearized recurrence rate of MR (>2/4) was 3.2% per year. Recurrence rate was higher in patients with Barlow's disease (6.0%) and lower in those with fibroelastic deficiency (2.6%) (P = 0.01).[42] Contemporary techniques for mitral valve repair represent an individualized and tailored approach to every single valve. Sophisticated mitral valve repair in the hands of experienced surgeons remains the gold standard treatment for primary MR with excellent short- and long-term results.

Concomitant Tricuspid Valve Repair in Patients with Primary Mitral Regurgitation and Tricuspid Regurgitation

Secondary tricuspid regurgitation is the most common etiology of tricuspid valve disease. It is frequently related to left-sided valve disease causing pulmonary hypertension and RV dilatation and thorough examination is mandatory in patients undergoing mitral valve repair since tricuspid regurgitation does not always regress after correction of mitral valve disease.[43] European Society of Cardiology/European Association for Cardio-Thoracic Surgery (ESC/EACTS) and American College of Cardiology/American Heart Association (ACC/AHA) guidelines recommend mitral valve surgery with concomitant tricuspid valve surgery in patients with tricuspid annulus dilatation and/or at least moderate tricuspid regurgitation.[19,20]

Concomitant tricuspid valve repair can be done on the beating heart in the reperfusion phase of mitral valve surgery thereby reducing cross-clamp time and myocardial damage. In experienced centers, concomitant tricuspid valve repair does not increase surgical risk and can lead to improved functional status and prolonged survival[44] while reoperations for residual or recurrent tricuspid regurgitation are associated with a higher mortality of up to 15%.[45]

The underlying mechanism of secondary tricuspid regurgitation is annular dilatation. The size of the tricuspid annulus seems to be a more reliable indicator of tricuspid valve pathology compared to echocardiographic evaluation of tricuspid regurgitation, since the degree of regurgitation is very much depending on preload and afterload influenced by volume status and right-sided heart function. Correction of tricuspid annular dilatation in addition to mitral valve surgery may

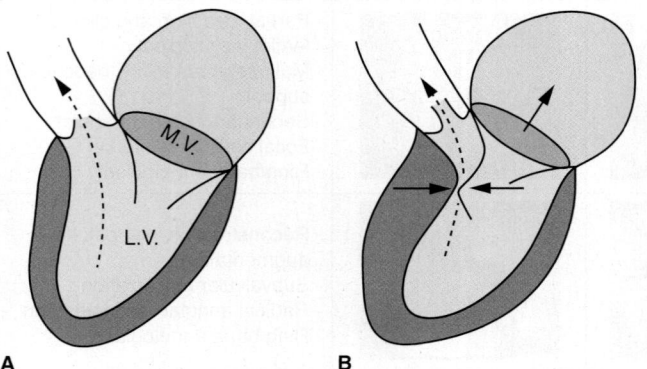

Figure 30–12. Systolic anterior motion of anterior mitral valve leaflet leading to LV outflow tract obstruction.

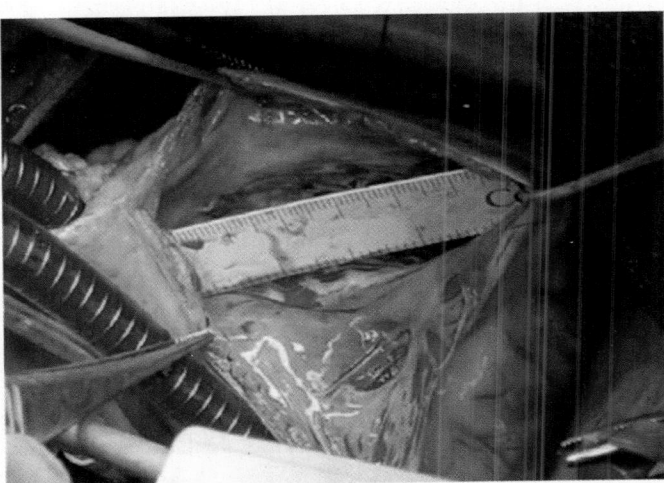

Figure 30–13. Intraoperative measurement of the tricuspid annular diameter from the anteroseptal to the anteroposterior commissure. Reproduced with permission from Dreyfus GD, Corbi PJ, Chan KM, et al. Secondary tricuspid regurgitation or dilatation: which should be the criteria for surgical repair? *Ann Thorac Surg.* 2005 Jan;79(1):127-132.

therefore resolve secondary tricuspid valve pathology. Decision parameters should be an annulus diameter ≥7 cm from the anteroseptal to anteroposterior commissures (**Fig. 30–13**) or 40 mm when measured by echocardiography.[43] Other parameters to be considered are leaflet malcoaptation, presence of atrial fibrillation and pulmonary hypertension, as well as RV dysfunction.

Repair of concomitant secondary tricuspid regurgitation can usually be achieved by prosthetic annuloplasty. The use of open rigid 3D-shaped rings has superior outcome with regards to correction and recurrence of tricuspid regurgitation compared to flexible bands and suture based annuloplasty (DeVega plasty).[46,47] Surgical ring implantation requires special caution to the conducting system to prevent postoperative atrioventricular block. In cases of restricted tricuspid leaflet motion, leaflet augmentation using pericardial patches can help to increase the surface of coaptation. In the presence of cleft related tricuspid regurgitation, suture based cleft closure is recommended.

Concomitant Treatment of Atrial Fibrillation

Atrial fibrillation frequently occurs in patients with primary MR. MR-induced volume overload leads to LA enlargement and, eventually, atrial fibrillation. Although atrial fibrillation is associated with older age and more severe presentation of primary MR, it is independently associated with excess mortality long-term after diagnosis.[48]

Once atrial fibrillation develops, it leads to an increasing degree of atrial fibrosis, which in turn results in an increased substrate for atrial fibrillation.[49] This vicious cycle is likely to lead to continued worsening of the atrial fibrillation burden despite valve surgery and to reduce survival compared to patients free of atrial fibrillation.

In a study among 2425 subjects, Grigioni et al. reported on gradual worsening from sinus rhythm to paroxysmal atrial fibrillation, to persistent atrial fibrillation in patients with primary MR.[50] During follow-up, paroxysmal and persistent atrial fibrillation were associated with excess mortality (10-year survival of patients with sinus rhythm versus paroxysmal and persistent atrial fibrillation was 74 ± 1% vs 59 ± 3% and 46 ± 2%, respectively; *P* <0.0001). This effect persisted 20 years post-diagnosis and was independent from baseline characteristics. Mitral valve surgery led to improved survival in each cardiac rhythm subset, but persistence of excess risk was observed for each type of atrial fibrillation.[50] Notably, only 5.2% of patients with atrial fibrillation underwent concomitant atrial ablation at the time of surgery in this study. The beneficial effect of mitral valve surgery may have therefore been underestimated.

In other studies, concomitant atrial fibrillation ablation has proven to be associated with reduced postoperative mortality and stroke rates in patients undergoing mitral valve surgery.[51,52] The presence of atrial fibrillation in patients with primary MR is currently rated as a class IIa recommendation for mitral valve surgery in both the ESC/EACTS and ACC/AHA guidelines on valvular heart disease.[19,20] In view of the evidence presented by Grigioni at al.,[50] it seems reasonable to recommend concomitant atrial fibrillation ablation in all patients with new-onset atrial fibrillation undergoing mitral valve surgery.

Timing of Mitral Valve Surgery in Primary Mitral Valve Regurgitation

Success and durability of surgical mitral valve repair is dependent on the underlying disease, complexity of repair, and experience of the surgeon. In patients with isolated posterior leaflet prolapse and annular dilatation, repair rates of 100% and perioperative mortality <1% can be achieved in experienced centers.[53,54] In more complex cases like Barlow's disease, early success of repair is even more depending on surgical experience, leading to higher rates of valve replacement in centers with less experience.

When performed in a timely manner, surgical mitral valve repair in severe symptomatic primary MR has proven to ameliorate or prevent heart failure and restore normal life expectancy.[55] However, severe primary MR in asymptomatic patients has long been underestimated and patients were not referred to surgery before symptoms occurred.

Within recent years and in the light of growing evidence,[27] operating on asymptomatic patients with severe MR is now widely accepted, prophylactically avoiding the consequences of chronic MR, such as LV dilatation or functional deterioration, and development of atrial fibrillation and pulmonary hypertension.

The recent ACC/AHA guidelines indicate that surgical mitral valve repair is reasonable in asymptomatic patients with chronic severe primary MR with preserved LV function when the likelihood of a successful and durable repair without residual MR is >95% with an expected mortality rate <1% and when it can be performed at a Primary or Comprehensive Valve Center (class IIa recommendation).[20] Such outcome requirements mandate patient referral to reference centers, which by definition should have a high volume of mitral valve repair patients (≈100 per year) and valid outcome reporting. The unwarranted

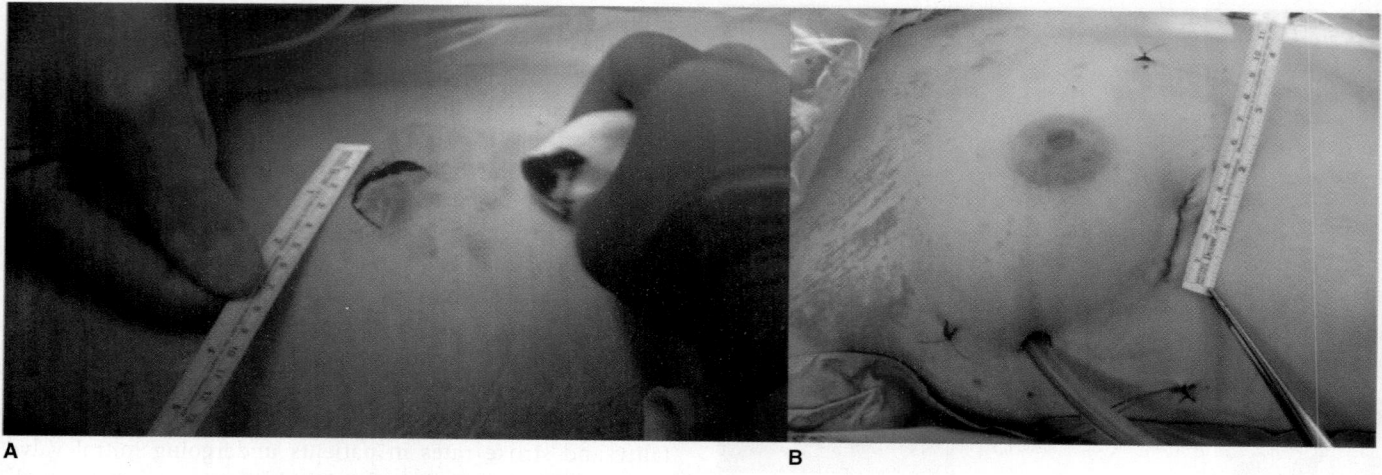

Figure 30–14. Para-areolar (A) and submammary (B) incision for minimally invasive fully endoscopic mitral valve repair.

risk of mitral valve replacement cannot be justified in asymptomatic patients with preserved LV function.

Access for Mitral Valve Repair in Primary Mitral Valve Regurgitation

Median sternotomy is still considered the current standard and remains the most popular approach for mitral valve surgery. It allows central cannulation to establish extracorporeal circulation and cardioplegic arrest and permits direct access in case of complication.

In recent years, video assisted minimally invasive right-sided lateral mini-thoracotomy has become a valid and attractive alternative to median sternotomy. It is performed with or without robotic assistance in rapidly increasing numbers and has the potential to become the new gold standard due to improvements in visualization and instrumentations, allowing for fully endoscopic mitral valve repair using soft-tissue retractors only without any rib-spreading. Cardiopulmonary bypass is accomplished by peripheral cannulation of the femoral artery and vein with retrograde arterial perfusion. This approach is widely preferred by patients due to significantly reduced procedure related pain[56] and optimal cosmetics with periareolar or submammary incisions of less than 5 cm (**Fig. 30–14**).

In addition, the right-sided lateral mini-thoracotomy approach offers excellent visualization of the LA and mitral valve due to a direct line of view if the endoscopic camera is placed through the same intercostal space as the incision. **Figure 30–15** demonstrates the setup of a fully endoscopic mitral valve reconstruction with 3D visualization, femoral cannulation, and periareolar access in the fourth intercostal space. Modern 3D endoscopes allow for uncompromised orientation in the chest cavity offering a high safety profile. Fully endoscopic mitral valve repair is further associated with short intensive care unit and hospital stay, early mobilization, fast recovery, and high patient satisfaction.[56-58] Similar results can be achieved with telemanipulative robotic techniques (da Vinci Surgical System; Intuitive Surgical, Inc.).[59] In experienced centers, minimally invasive fully endoscopic mitral valve repair is

not limited to certain mitral valve pathologies and can even be performed in complex scenarios such as anterior leaflet prolapse or Barlow's disease.

Nevertheless, the most important goal for patients with primary mitral valve disease is to achieve a competent and durable repair of the mitral valve. These goals should be met in all prolapsing valves regardless of the surgical approach and the final cosmetic outcome. Today, minimally invasive fully endoscopic mitral valve repair with or without robotical assistance is restricted to selected, high-volume, specialized centers. It is likely that in the coming years, an increasing number of patients will have access to high-quality minimally invasive mitral valve surgery.

SECONDARY MITRAL REGURGITATION

Epidemiology

Moderate-to-severe MR has a prevalence of 0.46% in the community,[60] 65% of which is secondary.[4] Secondary MR is common in heart failure—a prevalence of 50% has been reported in ischemic cardiomyopathy and 65% in nonischemic cardiomyopathy.[61-63] Mild or moderate secondary MR was present in 49%, and severe secondary MR in 24% of patients in a large cohort of ischemic and nonischemic heart failure.[64]

Etiology and Lesions

The classification of Carpentier characterizing the lesion that causes mitral leaflet malcoaptation and regurgitation is frequently used as a first approach to define the etiology of MR.[9] In secondary MR, the mitral valve leaflets are structurally normal but exhibit restrictive motion during ventricular systole leading to a leaflet coaptation gap (Carpentier IIIb) (**Fig. 30– 16**). This restrictive motion of the leaflets is caused by imbalanced tethering forces exerted by the LV via apical and/or lateral displacement of the papillary muscle(s). The mitral valve coaptation point is displaced away from the mitral annular plane, the third posterior "scallop" (P3) usually being affected most

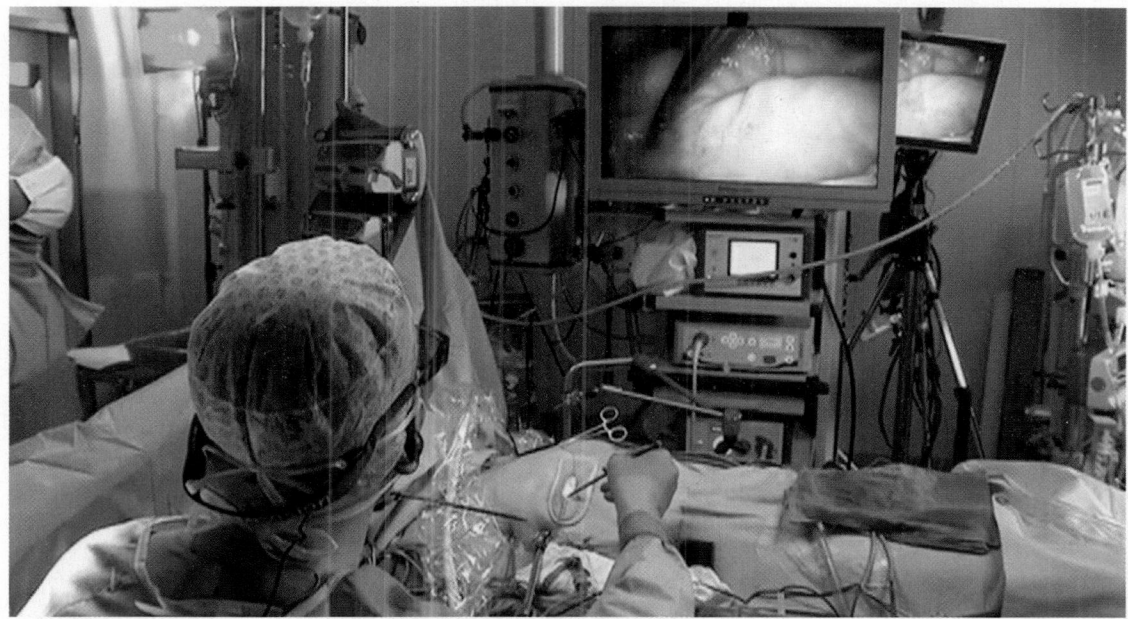

Figure 30–15. Setup of a fully endoscopic mitral valve reconstruction with femoral cannulation and para-areolar access in the fourth intercostal space.

severely.[65] In secondary MR, the movement of the leaflets can also be normal, but the dilatation of the mitral annulus exceeds the area covered by the leaflets, leading to leaflet mal-coaptation (Carpentier I). This mechanism is less frequently observed in isolation than the Carpentier IIIb mechanism. In secondary MR due to a Carpentier I mechanism, mitral annular dilatation may accompany LA enlargement (Fig. 30–16) secondary to increased LV filling pressures or atrial fibrillation. This type of secondary MR, which is caused or worsened by mitral valve annular dilatation secondary to LA enlargement, is termed *atrial functional mitral regurgitation*. The mitral annulus is interrupted posterolaterally with adipose tissue,[66] and it enlarges in a septolateral direction when the LA dilates. A second mechanism of atrial functional MR has also been proposed (ie, atriogenic leaflet tethering) where torque is exerted on the anterior annulus (increased anterior leaflet tethering) and the posterior leaflet is wedged between the LV and the LA.[67,68] Dyssynchrony due to a left bundle branch block can worsen secondary MR by decreasing LV closing forces (dyssynchrony leads to impaired LV contractile function) and increasing LV tethering forces (dyssynchronous contraction, which prevents coordinated closure of the mitral leaflets).[69]

The etiology of secondary MR may be broadly classified as ischemic or nonischemic. In ischemic secondary MR, the mitral valve is most commonly asymmetrically tethered due to displacement of the posteromedial papillary muscle only (**Fig. 30–17**). This papillary muscle is more vulnerable to ischemia and infarction than the anterolateral papillary muscle as a result of its single blood supply from the right coronary artery or a dominant left circumflex coronary artery. Symmetric tethering can also be seen in ischemic secondary MR, when the LV is globally remodeled in the presence of underlying ischemic cardiomyopathy. In nonischemic secondary MR, the valve is typically symmetrically tethered with displacement of both anterolateral and posteromedial papillary muscles secondary to global LV remodeling. Asymmetric tethering can complicate nonischemic secondary MR (eg, with a basal LV aneurysm due to cardiac involvement in sarcoidosis). In a study of moderate and severe secondary MR, mitral annular enlargement in both the intercommissural (3.1 ± 0.1 vs 3.3 ± 0.2 cm; P <0.05) and anteroposterior (2.8 ± 0.2 vs 3.0 ± 0.2 cm; P <0.05) dimensions was found to be less in ischemic secondary MR, compared to nonischemic secondary MR for the same MR grade.[70]

Several experimental and clinical studies have demonstrated that the mitral leaflets are not mere bystanders in secondary MR. Leaflet remodeling is a feature of both ischemic and nonischemic secondary MR.[71,72] Remodeling of the mitral leaflets encompasses increased collagen content, cellularity, glycosaminoglycan deposition, and expansion of the extracellular matrix.[69,71] Leaflet remodeling in secondary MR has been considered as an adaptive response to tethering forces exerted on the valve, and an attempt to increase the coaptation area and reduce the degree of MR.[71] An inadequate remodeling response may lead to worse MR, and the unraveling of the underlying mechanisms in an attempt to therapeutically manipulate the process is a very active area of research.[71,72]

Clinical Presentation

Patients with secondary MR may present with dyspnea on exertion or at rest, palpitations, and symptoms of low cardiac output. Among patients with heart failure, those presenting with severe secondary MR have more severe symptoms (NYHA class III–IV) as compared to patients without MR.[73] On physical examination, a soft holosystolic heart murmur, loudest at the apex, and that radiates to the axilla, can be detected. Bedside maneuvers that increase LV afterload (with the patient lying in the left lateral position and in forced expiration) may

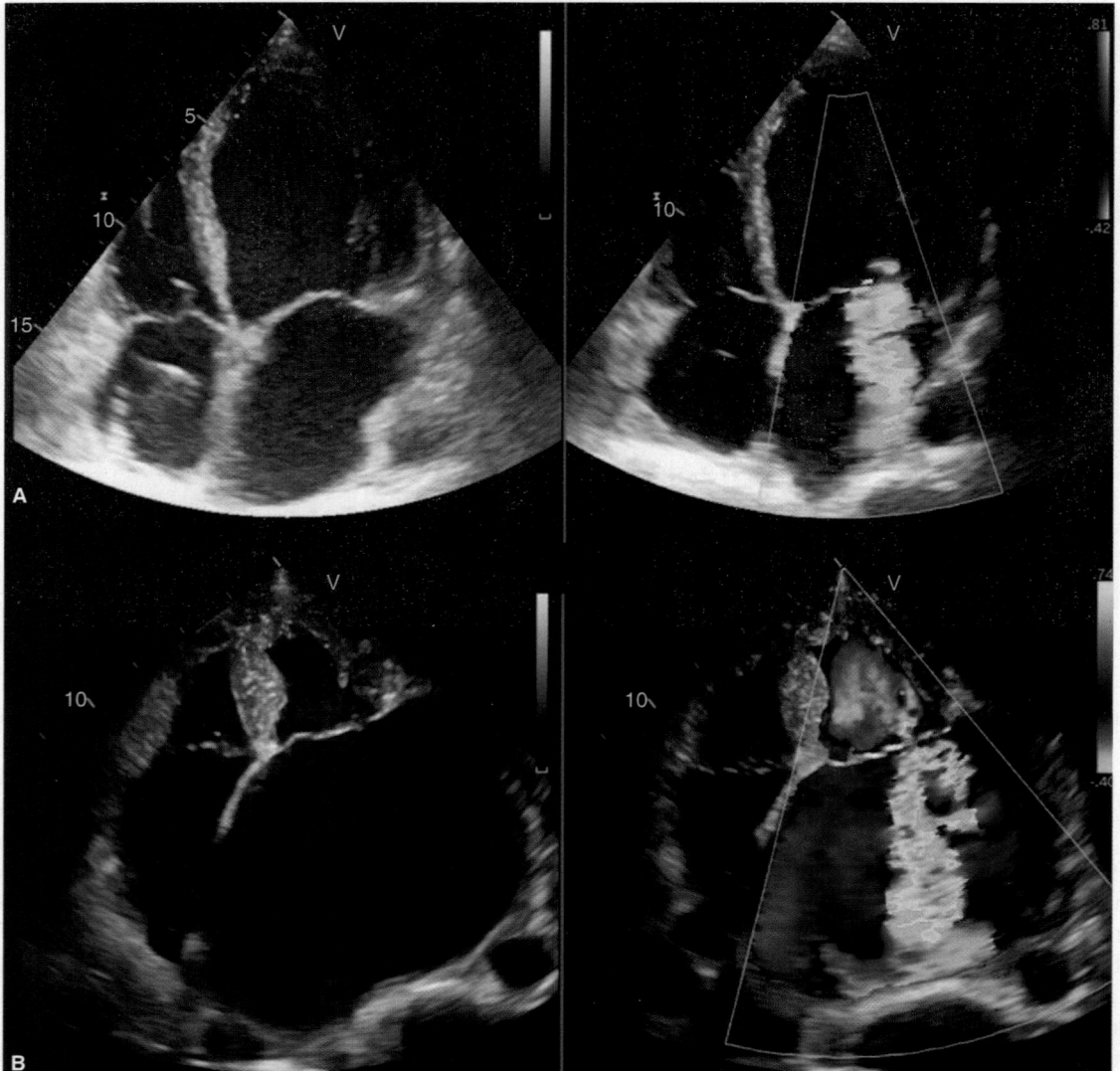

Figure 30–16. Secondary MR. Based on Carpentier's classification two mechanisms of MR can lead to secondary MR. When MR is caused by dilatation of the LV leading to tethering of the mitral leaflets and restrictive motion of the leaflets in systole, the mechanism is known as Carpentier IIIb (**A**). In contrast, when the motion of the leaflets is normal and malcoaption is caused by mitral annulus dilatation due to left atrial dilatation, the mechanism is known as Carpentier I (**B**).

increase its intensity. The pulse may be unremarkable, irregular because of coexistent atrial fibrillation, or rapid because of sympathetic overdrive in the context of heart failure. Systolic blood pressure and pulse pressure may be reduced as a result of reduced forward stroke volume, but this finding is nonspecific and variable. The venous pressure may be elevated. The apex beat is displaced downward and to the left in chronic severe secondary MR as a result of LV dilatation. Severe secondary MR may be accompanied by an S3 produced by rapid emptying of a large LA volume under higher than normal pressure into the LV; in this setting, an S3 may be an indicator of MR severity rather than heart failure severity.

Laboratory Findings

Neurohumoral markers such as N-terminal-pro brain natriuretic peptide (NT-proBNP) are significantly increased in patients with secondary MR as compared to patients with

similar LV systolic function and dimensions but without severe MR.[73,74] Furthermore, elevated levels of NT-proBNP are associated with poor prognosis in patients with even mild secondary MR.[74] However, it has been shown that severe secondary MR is associated with an excess of mortality in patients with intermediate heart failure phenotype (NYHA class II and III heart failure symptoms, moderately reduced LVEF, and within the second quartile of NT-proBNP levels [871–2360 pg/mL]) while in patients with more advanced heart failure, the presence of severe secondary MR did not impact further on survival.[73] These results suggest that current available therapies may be more efficacious in improving survival of patients with severe secondary MR and not very advanced heart failure status.

ECG findings in patients with secondary MR include the presence of Q waves or ST-segment elevation indicating the presence of a LV aneurysm when the underlying cause of heart failure is ischemic. In addition, it is relatively frequent

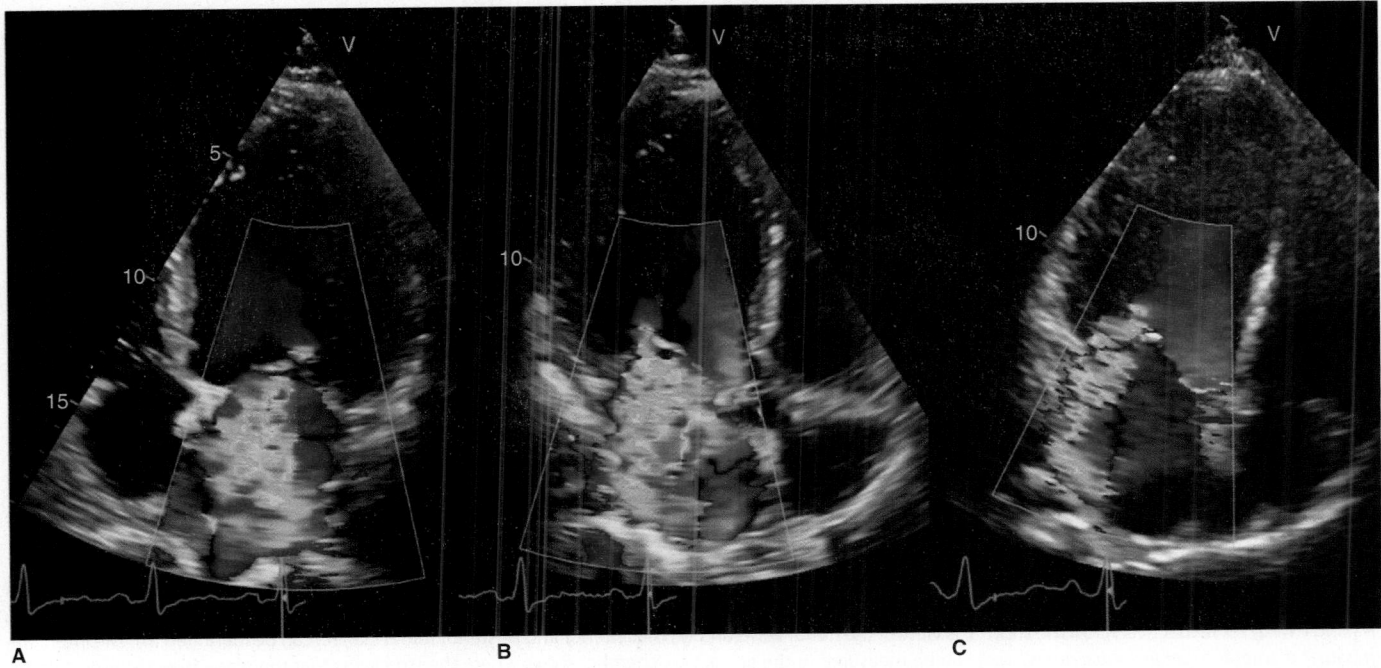

Figure 30–17. **Transthoracic, apical four-chamber view of a central jet of severe secondary MR in a patient with idiopathic dilated cardiomyopathy.** (**A**) The mitral valve is symmetrically tethered due to global LV remodeling. (**B**) Apical three-chamber view of a central, severe secondary MR jet in the same patient as in (**A**). Apical three-chamber view demonstrating a posteriorly directed jet of secondary (ischemic) MR due to asymmetric papillary muscle tethering. (**C**) The posteromedial papillary muscle is displaced by a previous right coronary artery infarction.

to observe conduction abnormalities such as first-degree atrioventricular block and left bundle branch block and atrial fibrillation. On chest radiography, cardiomegaly, prominent pulmonary hila, and Kerley B-lines and pleural effusion can be observed (depending on the hemodynamic and loading conditions of the patient).

Diagnostic Evaluation

Echocardiography
Echocardiography is the imaging technique of first choice to evaluate patients with suspected secondary MR. Echocardiography provides anatomical and functional information that is pivotal for the decision-making. Echocardiographic evaluation of secondary MR comprises the assessment of mitral valve anatomy, considering the size of the mitral annulus, tethering of the mitral leaflets and presence of mitral valve calcifications, as well as the grade of MR using an integrative approach. TTE can provide all this information, although TEE (particularly 3D-TEE) provides particularly better anatomical characterization.

Anatomic Characterization of Secondary Mitral Regurgitation: Secondary MR is characterized by dilatation of the mitral annulus and tethering of the mitral leaflets with restrictive motion in systole. In patients with ischemic heart failure, the tethering is more pronounced at the central and medial scallops of the posterior mitral leaflet while in patients with non-ischemic cardiomyopathy, the tethering is evenly distributed along all the scallops of the anterior and posterior leaflets.[70,75,76] Although not regularly implemented in clinical practice, it has been shown that the measurement of the angles of the mitral

valve leaflets relative to the mitral annulus plane (as a measure of the leaflet tethering) is important to predict the risk of recurrence of MR after surgical mitral valve repair. An angle >25° for the anterior mitral leaflet and >45° for the posterior mitral leaflet have been associated with increased risk of MR recurrence.[77–79] Furthermore, a tenting area (measured as the area enclosed between the mitral leaflets closed and the mitral annulus) >2.5 cm², an interpapillary muscle distance >20 mm, and a distance between the head of the posterior papillary muscle and the mitro-aortic continuity fibrosa >40 mm have been also proposed as markers of severe leaflet tethering and unfavorable characteristics for durable mitral valve repair.

The dimensions of the mitral annulus are important to predict the durability of mitral valve repair. The mitral annulus can be better measured on an apical three-chamber view of the LV where the anteroposterior diameter is shown, and on the apical two-chamber view or bicommissural view where the bicommissural diameter (the largest) can be assessed. However, 3D echocardiography (particularly TEE) allows the construction of a 3D rendering of the mitral annulus providing more accurate measurements of the mitral dimensions (diameters, perimeter, area, and intertrigonal distance) and allowing the visualization of the saddle-shape of the mitral annulus (**Fig. 30–18**). In patients with secondary MR, the saddle-shape of the mitral annulus appears flattened and with restricted dynamism along the cardiac cycle.[80,81]

The presence of severe calcifications on the mitral annulus particularly but also on the leaflets is important to select the most appropriate therapeutic option. Severe calcification of the mitral annulus may challenge surgical mitral valve repair and

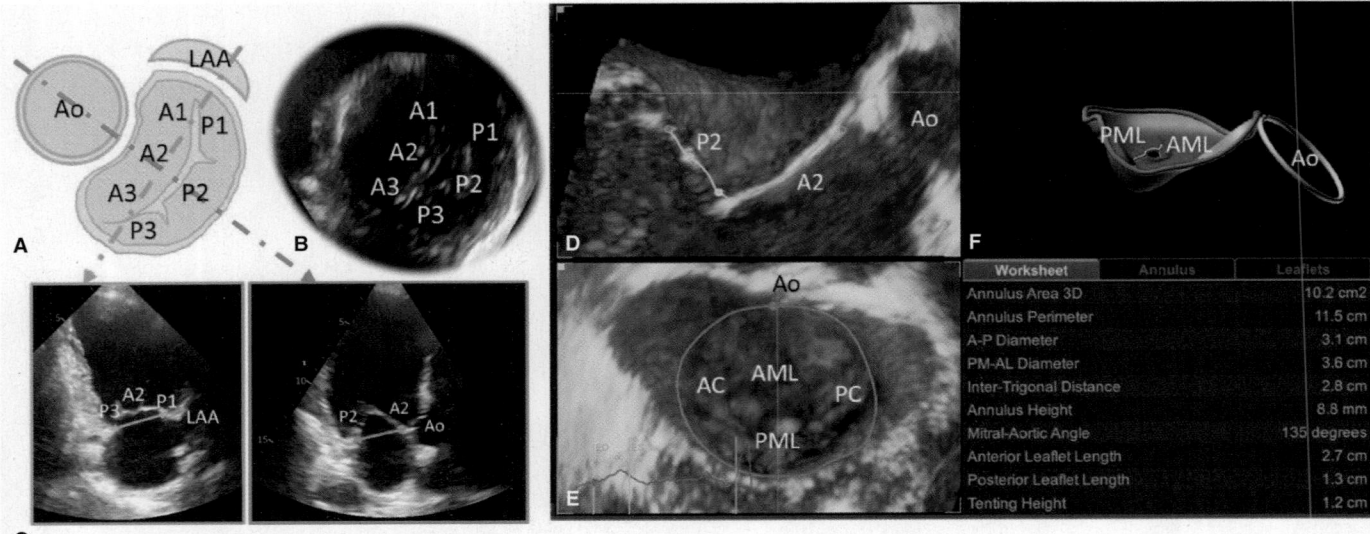

Figure 30–18. Mitral annular dimensions. (A) shows a schematic presentation of the mitral valve in relation to the aortic valve (Ao) and the left atrial appendage (LAA) that are located anterior and anterolateral respectively. The anterior and posterior mitral leaflet can be divided into three scallops (A1, A2, A3 and P1, P2, P3, respectively). On the short-axis view of the mitral valve on TTE, the anterior and posterior mitral leaflets can be identified **(B)**. The intercommissural diameter (*orange double arrowhead*) can be measured in the apical two-chamber views where the structures that the plane bisects (*orange dotted line*) can be observed (from anterolateral to posteromedial commissure: the LAA, and the P1, A2, P3 scallops) **(C, left)**. The anteroposterior diameter (*green double arrowhead*) of the mitral annulus is measured from the apical three-chamber view at the level of the A2-P2 scallops **(C, right)**. **(D)** and **(E)** show the 3D reconstruction of the mitral valve from TEE: the sagittal plane bisecting the mitral valve at the level of the A2-P2 scallops **(D)** and the en face view of the mitral valve with the delineation of the mitral annulus in *red* **(E)**. **(F)** shows the 3D rendering of the mitral valve annulus where its characteristic saddle-shape can be appreciated. The various measurements of the mitral valve annulus and geometry of the mitral valve can be calculated automatically and presented in table.

replacement and is a contraindication for specific transcatheter procedures that target this anatomic structure. In addition, the presence of severe calcifications on the leaflets may challenge transcatheter edge-to-edge repair. These can be visualized with echocardiography but are better defined with CT.

Functional Assessment of Secondary Mitral Regurgitation Grade: Assessment of grade of secondary MR with echocardiography follows the same integrative approach as with primary MR. Qualitative, semiquantitative and quantitative parameters are considered.[18] In severe secondary MR, qualitative parameters

include a large gap of coaptation between the leaflets due to severe tethering or the presence of severely restricted movement of the leaflets, large color flow jet area (>50% of the LA area), large flow convergence area visible throughout the systole, and a holosystolic, dense and triangular shape of the continuous wave spectral Doppler signal **(Fig. 30–19)**.

These parameters are easy to assess but are imprecise, influenced by hemodynamic conditions of the patient and technical aspects and not valid when there are multiple regurgitant jets. Semiquantitative echocardiographic parameters suggesting severe secondary MR include a vena contracta width measured

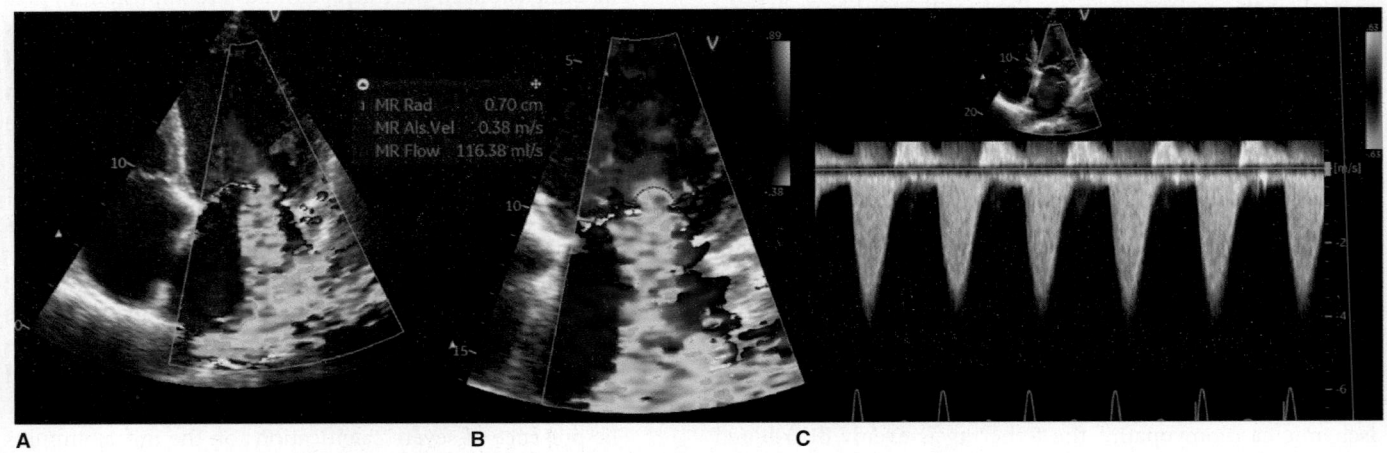

Figure 30–19. Assessment of severity of secondary MR. (A) shows the color Doppler of the mitral regurgitant jet occupying 50% of the left atrium. On a zoomed view of the mitral valve, the color Doppler shows a large flow convergence area (radius 0.7 cm, **B**). On continuous wave Doppler of the regurgitant jet, the spectral signal is dense, **(C)** with a triangular shape. These characteristics indicate severe MR.

on the parasternal long-axis view ≥7 mm, the presence of reversed systolic flow of the pulmonic veins on pulsed wave Doppler, and a prominent early diastolic transmitral wave on pulsed wave Doppler (peak velocity >1.2 m/s). These parameters are rapid to assess but are influenced by image quality, are imprecise when the regurgitant orifice area has a crescentic shape (as often occurs in secondary MR) or eccentric or multiple regurgitant jets, and are influenced by LV relaxation and filling pressures. The use of 3D echocardiography to assess the vena contracta area has provided more accurate grading of secondary MR than 2D echocardiography (**Fig. 30–20**). Current recommendations advocate the use of a quantitative parameter to assess secondary MR grade. An effective regurgitant orifice area ≥0.4 cm², a regurgitant volume ≥60 mL/beat, and regurgitant fraction ≥50% indicate severe secondary MR. The effective regurgitant orifice area and regurgitant volume are calculated with the proximal isovelocity surface area method which assumes a circular regurgitant orifice. Regurgitant fraction is calculated as the difference between the stroke volume

measured at the level of the mitral inflow and the stroke volume through the aortic valve. Mitral and aortic stroke volumes are calculated based on the velocity time integral of the mitral inflow and LV outflow tract respectively obtained with pulsed wave Doppler and calculating the cross-sectional area of the mitral and aortic valve annulus. It is important to note that in secondary MR, an effective regurgitant orifice area ≥0.3 cm² still denotes severe MR, since it is frequent to observe an elliptical or crescent shape of the orifice that cannot be taken into consideration by the proximal isovelocity surface area method. Furthermore, the low flow condition frequently observed in severe heart failure may lead to a regurgitant volume <60 mL/beat. Therefore, a regurgitant volume ≥45 mL/beat can be considered indicative of secondary MR in those situations. Regurgitant fraction takes into account low flow situations. However, the small numbers involved in its calculation lead to larger errors.

Recently, a different framework has been proposed to characterize patients with severe secondary MR, who may benefit from interventions. This framework takes into account the

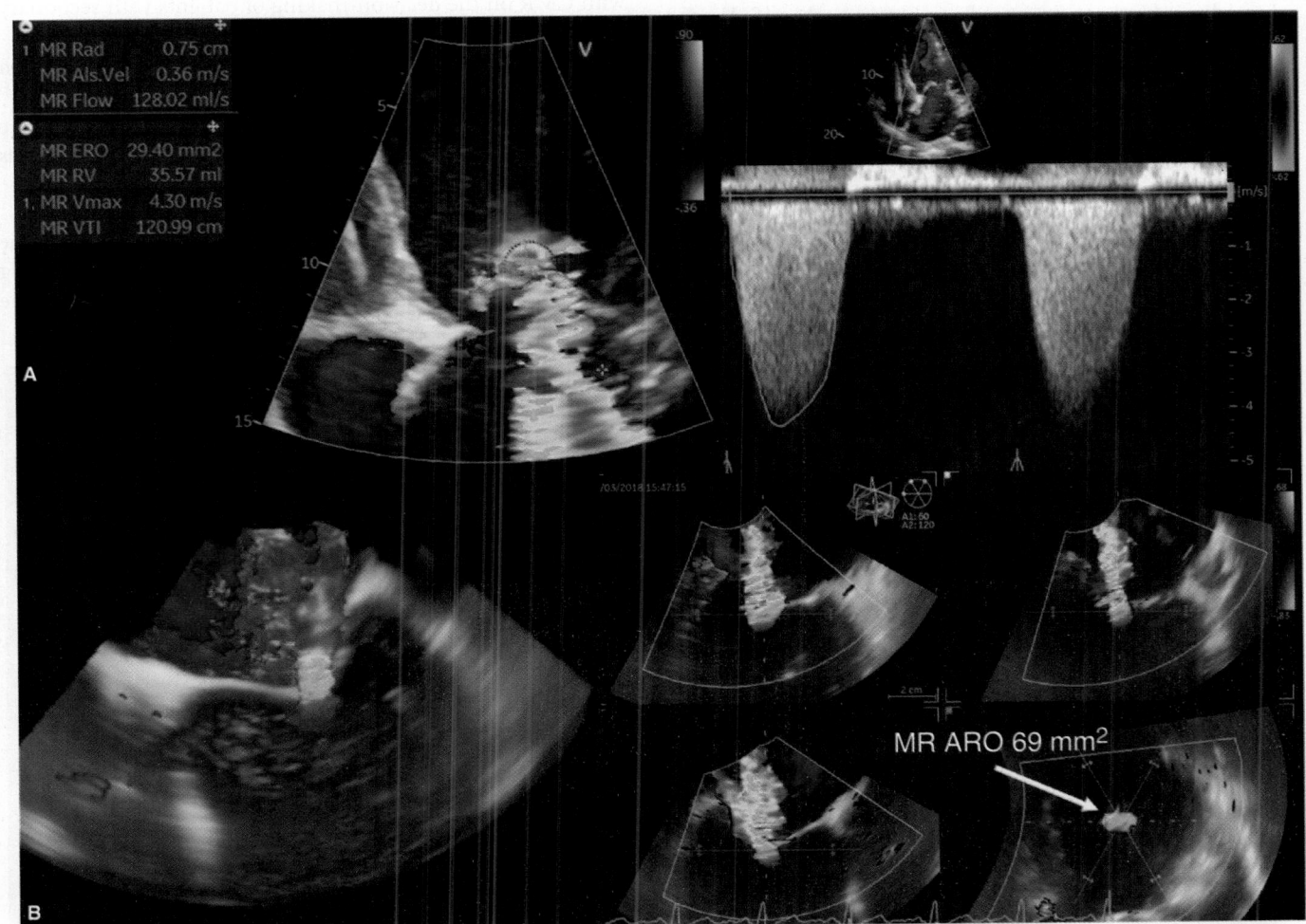

Figure 30–20. Calculation of the effective regurgitant orifice area and regurgitant volume in MR. From 2D color Doppler data (**A**), the effective regurgitant orifice (ERO) area is calculated using the proximal isovelocity surface area method where the radius of the flow convergence zone is measured on a zoomed apical four-chamber view. From the continuous wave Doppler data of the regurgitant jet, the velocity time integral (VTI) and the peak velocity (Vmax) are calculated. Taking into account the aliasing velocity, the ERO area and the regurgitant volume (RV) are calculated. However, on 3D color Doppler TEE data (**B**), the alignment of the multiplanar reformation across the vena contracta demonstrates a noncircular regurgitant orifice area and with planimetry the anatomic regurgitant orifice (ARO) area is larger than on 2D color Doppler data indicating severe MR.

effective regurgitant orifice area and the LV end-diastolic volume and considers disproportionate MR for a given value of LVEF (30%) and regurgitant fraction (50%) when the effective regurgitant orifice area is disproportionally large for the degree of LV dilatation.[82] Those patients may benefit more from mitral valve intervention than patients with smaller effective regurgitant orifice area, for the same extent of LV dilatation.

In addition, assessment of LV dimensions and systolic function as well as assessment of LA volume, estimation of pulmonary pressures, and RV function are important for risk stratification of patients with secondary MR. Echocardiography remains as the mainstay technique to assess these aspects. 3D echocardiography provides more accurate measurements of LV and atrial dimensions and function but it is not frequently used. When the endocardial border cannot be clearly visualized, the use of contrast agents can help to better assess the LV volumes, the wall motion abnormalities and calculation of the LVEF. Recently, the use of LVEF to reflect the LV systolic function of these patients has been questioned. The use of global longitudinal strain, a measure of active deformation of the LV myocardium, has been proposed as a better marker of LV performance in patients with secondary MR. In 75 patients with severe secondary MR, the value of LV global longitudinal strain was significantly reduced compared to patients without MR but similar LV volumes and LVEF (**Fig. 30–21**).[83] In addition, a value of global longitudinal strain <7% has been independently associated with increased all-cause mortality.[84]

Stress Echocardiography

Secondary MR grade depends on the hemodynamic condition of the patient. Patients with symptoms not explained by the severity of MR observed at rest, may have severe MR on exertion. Therefore, exercise echocardiography is a very powerful tool to unmask severe secondary MR. Exercise-induced increase in secondary MR provides additional prognostic information over resting evaluation and identifies patients at higher risk of adverse clinical outcomes (**Fig. 30–22**). For example, an increase in effective regurgitant orifice area ≥13 mm^2 during exercise is associated with increased mortality and heart failure hospitalizations.[85] Exercise echocardiography is preferred over dobutamine stress echocardiography since dobutamine can induce improvement of LV systolic function and closing forces as well as reduced afterload (at low doses) leading to reduction in MR severity (Fig. 30–22).

Cardiac Magnetic Resonance

CMR is the imaging technique of reference to assess chamber dimensions and function. Furthermore, CMR provides information on LV tissue characterization (myocardial scar/fibrosis) by using T1-mapping and late gadolinium contrast-enhanced imaging. However, the impact of LV scar/fibrosis assessment with CMR on the decision-making of patients with secondary MR remains unclear.

Importantly, current guidelines recommend CMR when echocardiography is inconclusive in grading the severity of MR.[86,87] Quantification of the mitral regurgitant volume and fraction are the key parameters to assess the severity of MR. Several methods can be used to quantify the mitral regurgitant volume:[88]

- By calculating the difference between the LV stroke volume measured on cine steady state, free-precession images using planimetry of the LV cavity and the aortic forward volume

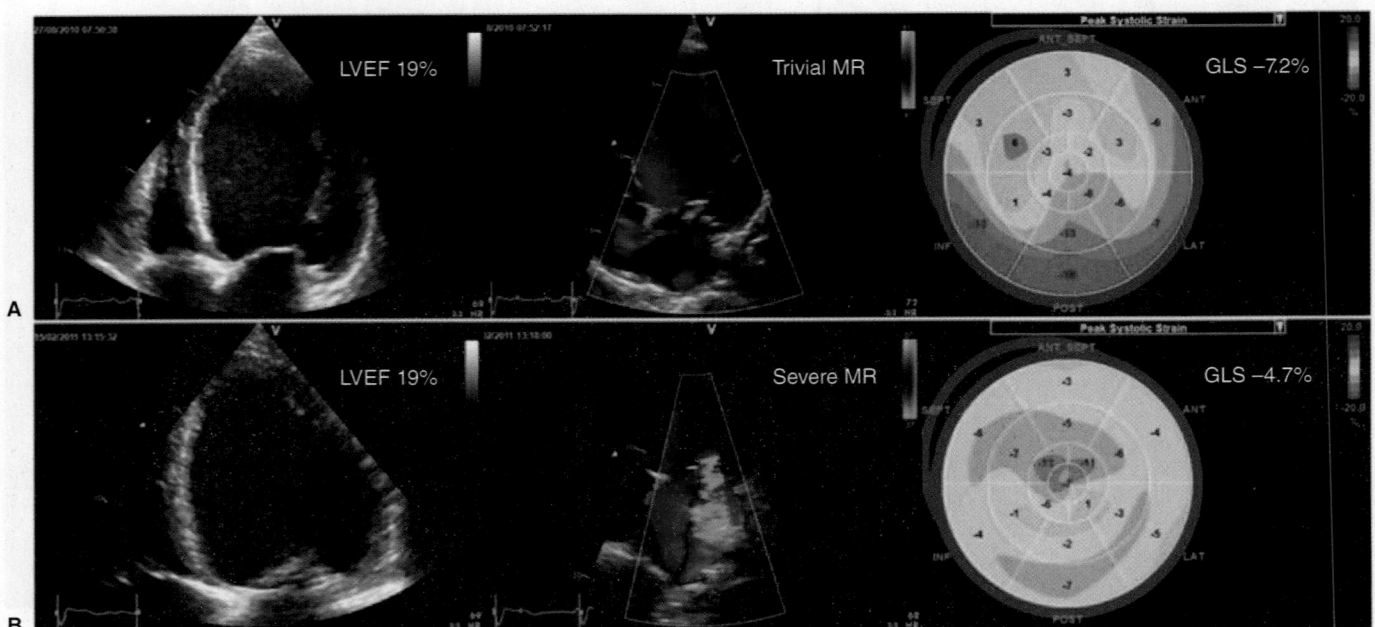

Figure 30–21. Assessment of LV systolic function in severe secondary MR. In (A), the calculated left ventricular ejection fraction (LVEF) of a patient with dilated cardiomyopathy and trivial MR is 19% and the 2D speckle tracking derived global longitudinal strain (GLS) is –7.2%. In (B), a patient with severe MR has the same LVEF, but significantly lower GLS (–4.7%). Reproduced with permission from Kamperidis V, Marsan NA, Delgado V, et al. Left ventricular systolic function assessment in secondary mitral regurgitation: left ventricular ejection fraction vs. speckle tracking global longitudinal strain. *Eur Heart J.* 2016 Mar 7; 37(10):811-816.

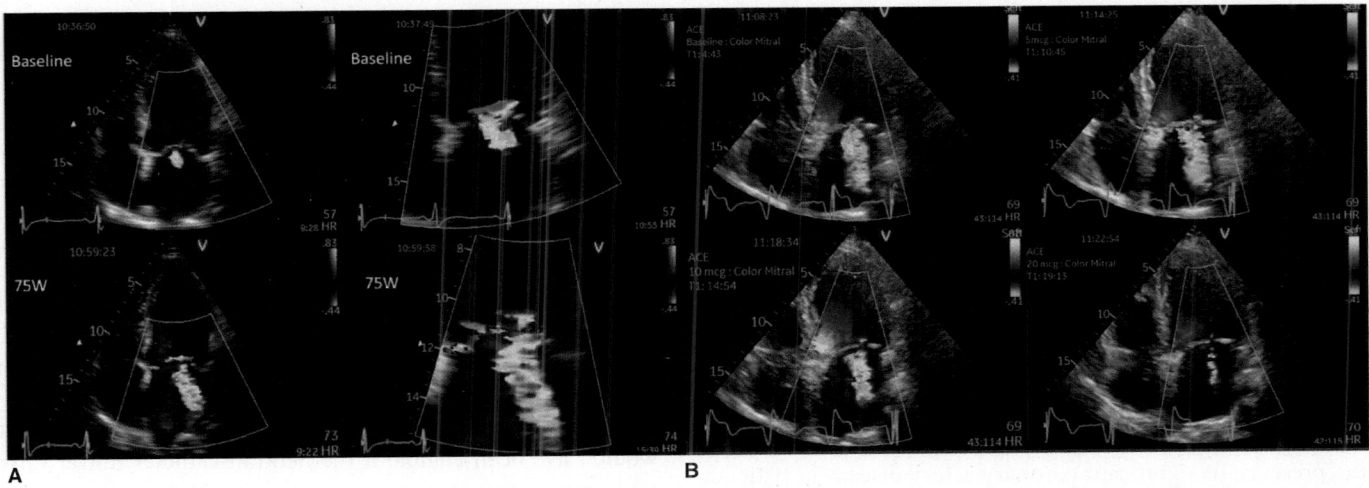

Figure 30–22. Stress echocardiography in secondary MR. Exercise echocardiography can induce an increase in the severity of MR due to an increase in systolic arterial pressure and induction of wall motion abnormalities if a significant coronary artery stenosis exists **(A)**. Note the increase in the regurgitant jet area at 75 watts of exercise load in **(A)**. In contrast, **(B)** shows the dobutamine stress echocardiography of a patient with nonischemic cardiomyopathy and a reduction in MR jet at peak dose (20 mcg/kg/min).

measured on phase-contrast images. This is the most frequently used method and is not affected by the presence of concomitant regurgitant valve lesions.

- By calculating the difference between the LV stroke volume and the RV stroke volume measured using planimetry of the LV and RV cavities on cine steady state, free-precession images. This method cannot be used when concomitant regurgitant valve lesions or significant shunts are present.

- By calculating the difference between the mitral inflow stroke volume and the aortic forward volume measured on phase-contrast images.

- Using 4D flow CMR data with retrospective mitral valve tracking.

In patients with secondary MR where the remodeling and dysfunction of the LV is frequently the underlying pathophysiological mechanism of mitral valve malcoaptation, assessment of extent of myocardial fibrosis/scar has important prognostic implications (**Fig. 30–23**). Cavalcante et al.[89] showed in a cohort of 578 patients with ischemic cardiomyopathy and a mean mitral regurgitant fraction of 18% that patients with significant MR (defined by a regurgitant fraction ≥35%), the presence of a myocardial scar size ≥30% of the LV was associated with a HR of 5.41 for the combined endpoint of all-cause mortality or heart transplantation. However, these results were not corroborated in 441 patients with heart failure (43% with ischemic etiology) where a mitral regurgitant fraction ≥30% was the strongest associate of adverse events and the presence of myocardial scar modulated that association, particularly among patients with moderate burden of myocardial scar.[90]

Dobutamine stress CMR can be used to assess the presence of contractile reserve, a more specific marker of myocardial viability than myocardial scar. However, similarly to dobutamine stress echocardiography, the severity of MR may reduce due to an increase in the leaflet closing forces. The role of this

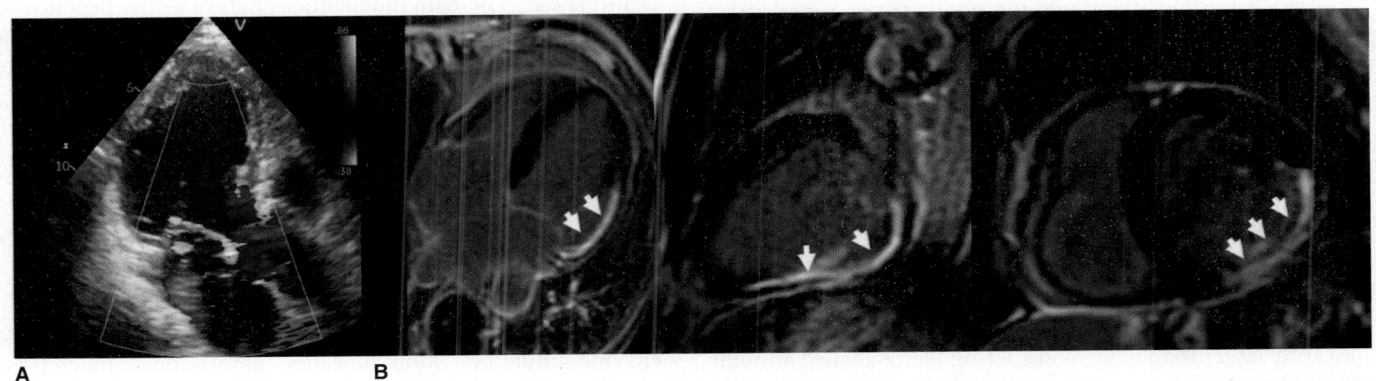

Figure 30–23. Assessment of myocardial scar with late gadolinium contrast-enhanced CMR. Example of a patient with ischemic heart disease and moderate MR due to restriction of the posterior mitral leaflet **(A)**. On late gadolinium contrast-enhanced CMR **(B)**, a large transmural scar can be observed in the basal and mid lateral segments (on the four-chamber view), inferior segments (on the two-chamber view), and the inferoposterior segments at the level of the insertion of the papillary muscles (on the short-axis view).

imaging technique is reserved for patients with ischemic heart failure who may be candidates for revascularization.

Cardiac Catheterization

Assessment of significant coronary artery stenosis as underlying cause of heart failure with secondary MR is frequently performed with invasive coronary angiography. During the same procedure, right heart catheterization can be performed to inform on the severity of secondary MR as well as on the pulmonary pressures and vascular resistances that are critical in selection of patients for heart transplant or LV assist device.

Computed Tomography

In patients with secondary MR, coronary CT angiography can be used instead of invasive coronary angiography to rule out the presence of significant coronary artery disease in patients with low probability of coronary artery disease. In patients with high probability of coronary artery disease and older age, the presence of calcified plaques may challenge the assessment of the severity of the coronary artery lesions and therefore, may need to add a functional imaging test. Currently, the development of transcatheter therapies that can treat MR has increased the demands of CT since it is the imaging technique that provides better anatomical assessment of the mitral valve apparatus. CT is frequently used in direct or indirect transcatheter mitral annuloplasty and in mitral valve replacement.

The key information that needs to be assessed with CT prior to transcatheter mitral annuloplasty (e.g. Cardioband) includes the dimensions of the mitral valve annulus, the location of the coronary sinus and circumflex coronary artery relative to the mitral annulus, and the presence of extensive mitral annular calcifications, particularly at the anterolateral level (P1) where the first three anchors of the Cardioband device are screwed (**Fig. 30–24**). The size of the mitral valve annulus will determine the size of the annuloplasty device. The location of the coronary sinus relative to the mitral annulus is important when considering devices that indirectly cinch the mitral annulus (Carillon Mitral Contour System). In addition, the course of the circumflex coronary artery is important to predict the risk of impingement of this artery by the device (**Fig. 30–25**).

In the selection of patients for transcatheter mitral valve replacement, the dimensions and calcification of the mitral valve annulus should be assessed as well as the LV dimensions and LV outflow tract. The mitral valve annulus has a characteristic saddle shape that may be difficult to conform for a tubular transcatheter expandable valve. Blanke et al.[91] proposed a CT-based simplified annulus description consisting of a D-shaped mitral annulus that is defined as being limited anteriorly by the intertrigonal distance, excluding the aorto-mitral continuity (**Fig. 30–26**). When measuring the mitral valve annulus according to the saddle shape, the area was significantly larger than when considering the D-shaped annulus (13.0 ± 3.0 cm² vs 11.2 ± 2.7 cm²). In addition, the 3D perimeter of the saddle-shaped annulus was significantly larger than the 2D projected perimeter of the D-shaped annulus (136.0 ± 15.5 mm vs 128.2 ± 14.8 mm).

More important is the prediction of LV outflow tract obstruction when considering transcatheter mitral valve replacement; this can be performed by calculating the neo-LV outflow tract area. Blanke et al.[91] noticed that when considering the saddle-shaped mitral valve annulus, the clearance of the LV outflow tract was smaller than when considering the D-shaped annulus. In addition, it is also important to establish how to measure the neo-LV outflow tract. Meduri et al.[92] hypothesized that the current standard CT-assessment performed on end-systolic images might underestimate the neo-LV outflow tract area. Of 33 patients considered for transcatheter mitral valve replacement who were screened for the Intrepid Global Pilot Study and had high risk of transcatheter mitral valve replacement obstruction based on end-systolic measurements,[92] 11 would have been eligible if the neotranscatheter mitral valve replacement area was measured throughout the entire cardiac cycle (multiphase average) or if the neotranscatheter mitral valve replacement area was measured at early systole. Therefore, the potential enrollment would have increased by 33% if multiphase average or early systolic measurements would have been performed. In addition, in nine patients who were considered having high risk of transcatheter mitral valve replacement obstruction based on end-systolic assessment, the Intrepid valve was eventually successfully implanted after the multiphase average measurements showed that the area of the neo-transcatheter mitral valve replacement was acceptable.[92]

Prognosis

The presence of secondary MR is independently associated with all-cause mortality (RR, 1.88; 95% CI, 1.23–2.86; P = 0.003),[62,64,93] and heart failure hospitalization (RR, 3.44; 95% CI, 1.74–6.82; P <0.001).[62,64] This association holds true for both ischemic and nonischemic secondary MR.[63] The severity of secondary MR is correlated with a worse outcome (**Fig. 30–27**),[62,93,94] and secondary MR portends a higher risk at a lower echocardiographic threshold of effective regurgitant orifice area and regurgitant volume than primary MR.[93] In very advanced heart failure (NYHA class IV or LVEF <30%), prognosis is determined primarily by heart failure per se, and the independent contribution of secondary MR diminishes.[73] The true independent nature of the prognostic impact of secondary MR is still debated—most available data are retrospective and multivariable models may fail to adjust for all confounders.

Treatment

Medical Therapy

Patients who have secondary MR and heart failure with reduced LVEF should receive optimal guideline-directed medical therapy and device therapy.[95] Pharmacotherapy (including beta-adrenoreceptor antagonists, angiotensin-converting enzyme inhibitors, loop diuretics, aldosterone antagonists, nitrates, and angiotensin-receptor neprilysin inhibitors) decreases secondary MR in almost 40% of patients with severe secondary MR at baseline.[69,96,97] Lack of improvement or worsening of secondary MR during optimal guideline-directed

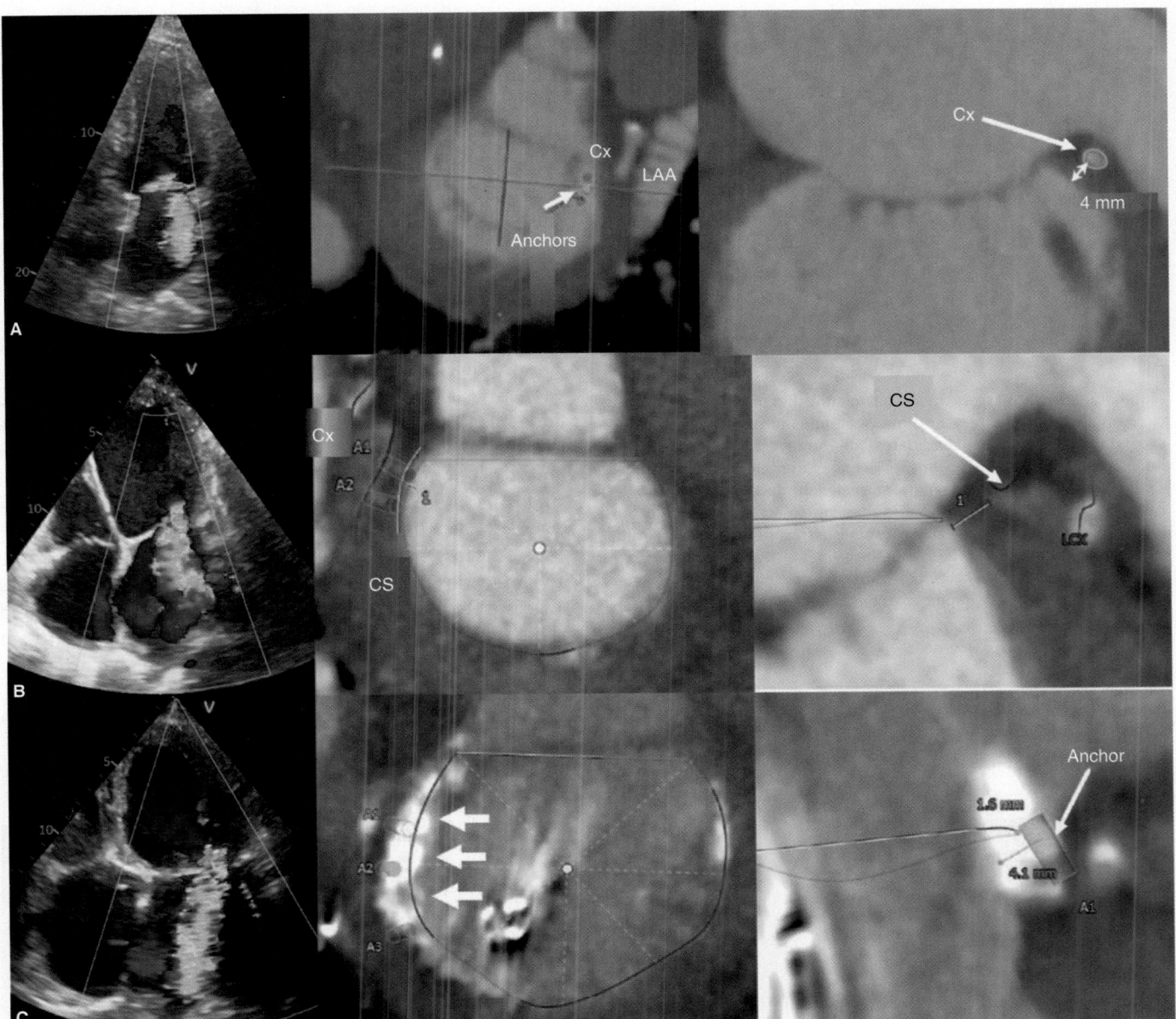

Figure 30–24. CT to assess anatomic suitability for transcatheter direct annuloplasty. The position of the first three anchors is assessed at the level of the P1 scallop of the mitral valve. In **(A)**, an example of a patient with ischemic heart disease and severe secondary MR is shown. On the double oblique transverse view of the mitral annulus, the circumflex coronary artery (Cx) is in close proximity where the first anchor needs to be implanted. On the orthogonal view, the distance between the circumflex coronary artery and the ventricular cavity is only 4 mm, indicating risk of impingement of the coronary artery if the procedure is performed. The spatial relationship of the coronary sinus (CS) with the mitral annulus is shown in **(B)**. Example of a patient with nonischemic cardiomyopathy and severe secondary MR. The distance between the coronary sinus and the mitral annulus is very small, precluding the performance of direct annuloplasty. When the mitral annulus has severe calcification in the area of the P1 scallop, direct annuloplasty is contraindicated **(C)**. Example of a patient with dilated cardiomyopathy and severe MR after failed transcatheter edge-to-edge repair. See the profuse calcification where the anchors should be implanted (*arrows*).

medical therapy, was an independent predictor (odds ratio [OR], 2.5; 95% CI, 1.5–4.3; P <0.05) of a composite endpoint of all-cause mortality, cardiac transplantation, hospitalization for heart failure, or ventricular arrhythmias in a study of patients with secondary MR and heart failure with reduced LVEF.[96] Angiotensin receptor blockers may have beneficial effects on leaflet remodeling in secondary MR, including modulation of cellular proliferation, valvular thickening, and remodeling of the valvular matrix.[68] In the recent Pharmacological Reduction

of Functional Ischemic Mitral Regurgitation trial, use of an angiotensin-receptor neprilysin inhibitor reduced secondary MR to a greater extent than valsartan alone.[97]

The presence of a left bundle branch block was an independent predictor (OR, 3.0; 95% CI, 1.1–8.4; P <0.05) of secondary MR deterioration after pharmacotherapy in a trial comprising 140 patients with LVEF ≤40% at baseline.[96] This underscores the importance of cardiac resynchronization therapy in the presence of underlying electromechanical dyssynchrony.

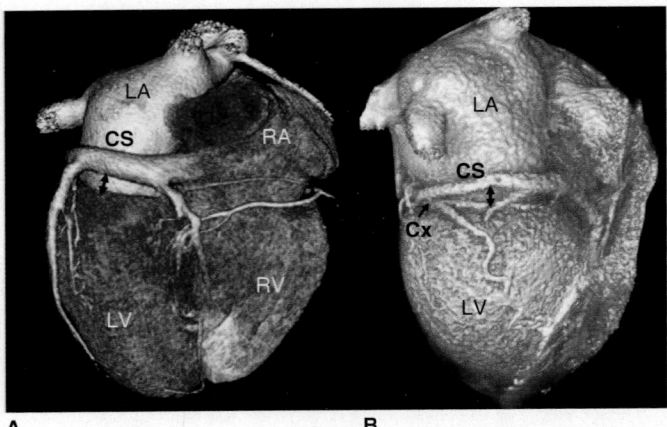

A   **B**

Figure 30-25. CT to assess the spatial relationship of the coronary sinus, circumflex coronary artery, and mitral annulus in patients with severe secondary MR who are candidates for indirect transcatheter annuloplasty. **(A)** shows the 3D volume rendering of the heart with the coronary sinus (CS) coursing above the mitral valve annulus (*double arrowhead*). The caliber of the coronary sinus would be adequate to implant a device for indirect annuloplasty. In **(B)**, the coronary sinus also courses above the mitral valve annulus (*double arrowhead*) but the caliber is smaller compared to **(A)** and in addition, the distal part crosses above the circumflex coronary artery (Cx) increasing the risk of impingement if the procedure is performed.

Device Therapy

Cardiac resynchronization therapy is a well-established therapy for heart failure.[95] The reported effect of cardiac resynchronization therapy on secondary MR is inconsistent, but the preponderance of evidence suggests a reduction of MR grade.[61,86,87] Mechanisms of MR reduction by cardiac resynchronization therapy include an increase in closing forces due to resynchronization and improvement of LV contractility and a decrease in tethering forces.[61] The MR response to cardiac resynchronization therapy is characterized by both a short-term (resynchronization) and long-term (LV reverse remodeling) component.[98] While secondary MR may be subject to dynamic worsening during physical exertion, a study of patients with ischemic and nonischemic cardiomyopathy receiving cardiac resynchronization therapy demonstrated that it maintains its beneficial effect on MR during exercise.[87]

A number of independent predictors of a reduction in MR after cardiac resynchronization therapy have been described: (1) the absence of scar tissue (defined by a wall motion score index ≤2.5) at papillary muscle insertion sites (OR, 2.59; 95% CI, 1.06–6.30; P <0.036); (2) an end-systolic LV dimension index <29 mm/m^2 (OR, 2.53; 95% CI, 1.03–6.20; P <0.042); and (3) an anteroseptal to posterior wall radial strain difference >200 ms (OR, 2.65; 95% CI, 1.11–6.30; P <0.0277).[99] These factors most likely reflect (1) the recruitment of the dynamic closing forces exerted by viable papillary muscles in resynchronization, (2) a limit of LV dilatation beyond which cardiac resynchronization therapy cannot rectify an excessive degree of tethering, and (3) potentially correctable dyssynchrony.[99]

The response of secondary MR to cardiac resynchronization therapy has prognostic significance:[99] moderate-to-severe secondary MR, which does not improve after 6 months of cardiac

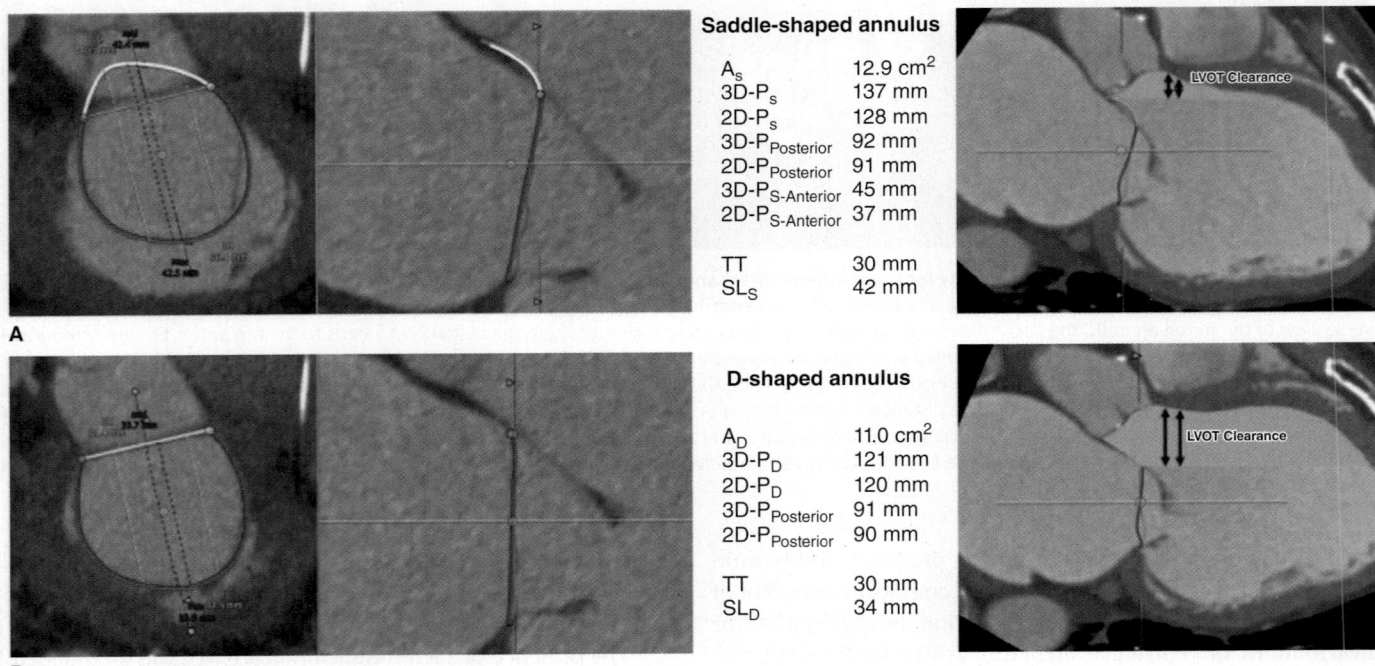

Saddle-shaped annulus

A_S	12.9 cm^2
3D-P_S	137 mm
2D-P_S	128 mm
3D-$P_{Posterior}$	92 mm
2D-$P_{Posterior}$	91 mm
3D-$P_{S-Anterior}$	45 mm
2D-$P_{S-Anterior}$	37 mm
TT	30 mm
SL_S	42 mm

A

D-shaped annulus

A_D	11.0 cm^2
3D-P_D	121 mm
2D-P_D	120 mm
3D-$P_{Posterior}$	91 mm
2D-$P_{Posterior}$	90 mm
TT	30 mm
SL_D	34 mm

B

Figure 30-26. Measurement of the mitral annulus for transcatheter mitral valve implantation. With CT, the mitral valve annulus can be measured considering the saddle shape of the annulus **(A)** or considering the D-shaped annulus **(B)**. When considering the saddle-shaped annulus, the dimensions of the mitral annulus are larger and the clearance of the left ventricular outflow tract (LVOT) is smaller than when considering the D-shaped annulus. Reproduced with permission from Blanke P, Dvir D, Cheung A, et al. A simplified D-shaped model of the mitral annulus to facilitate CT-based sizing before transcatheter mitral valve implantation. *J Cardiovasc Comput Tomogr.* 2014 Nov-Dec;8(6):459-467.

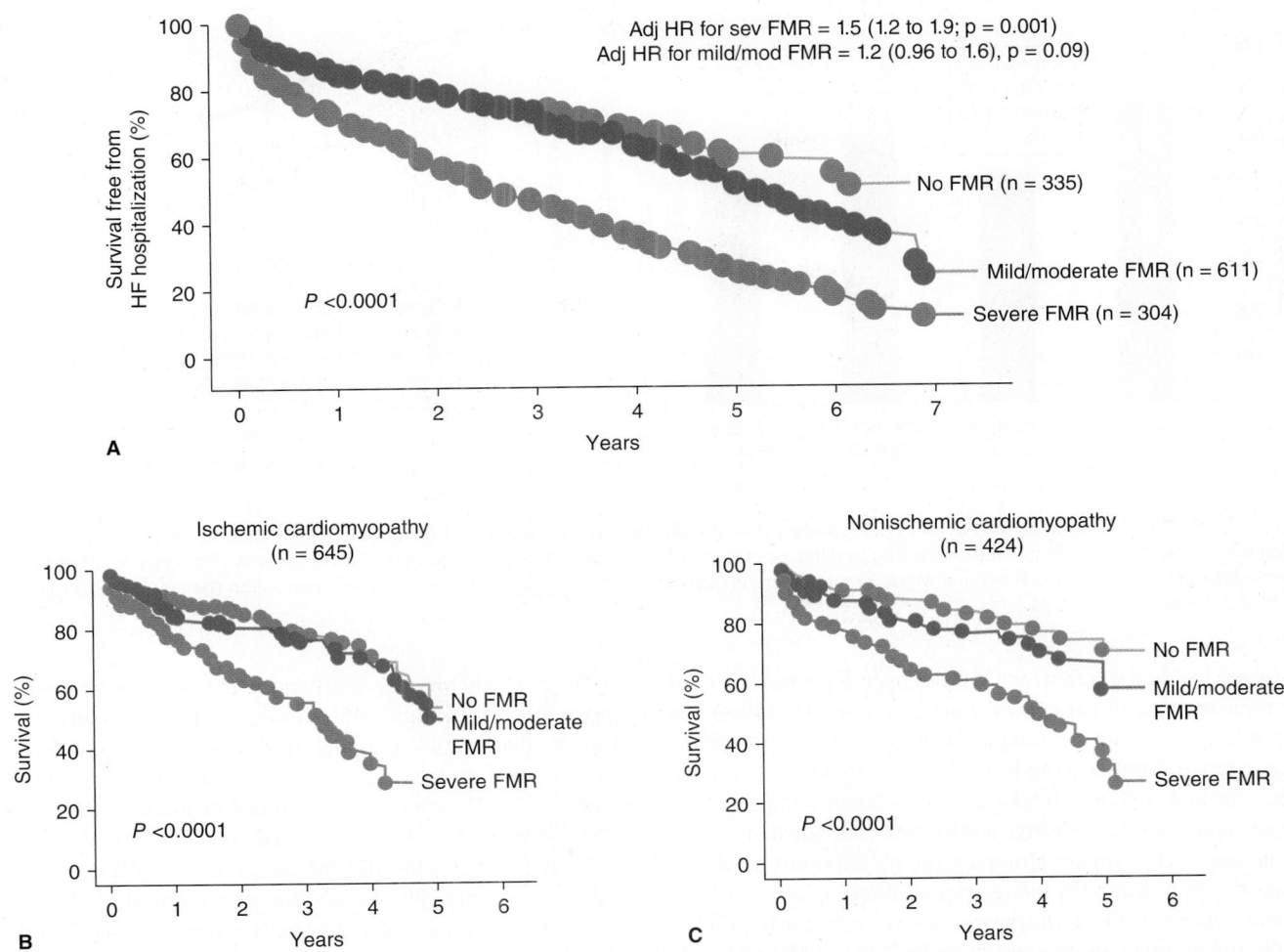

Figure 30–27. Freedom from death or heart failure (HF) hospitalization, according to the degree of secondary (functional) mitral regurgitation (FMR) (A). Freedom from death according to the degree of FMR in ischemic (**B**) and nonischemic (**C**) heart disease. Reproduced with permission from Asgar AW, Mack MJ, Stone GW. Secondary mitral regurgitation in heart failure: pathophysiology, prognosis, and therapeutic considerations. *J Am Coll Cardiol.* 2015 Mar 31; 65(12):1231-1248.

resynchronization therapy, is independently associated with increased all-cause mortality (HR, 1.77; 95% CI, 1.41–2.22; *P* <0.001) (**Fig. 30–28**).[61,86] The treatment of secondary MR, which remains moderate or severe even after cardiac resynchronization therapy, continues to be a clinical challenge. Fifty-one patients who did not respond to cardiac resynchronization therapy and had moderate or severe secondary MR underwent percutaneous edge-to-edge mitral valve repair with the MitraClip device (Abbott Vascular, Santa Clara, CA) in the Percutaneous Mitral Valve Repair in Cardiac Resynchronization Therapy study.[100] Improvement was documented in NYHA class, LV dimensions, and LVEF over the first 12 months postimplant.[100] Even though no control group was included in this analysis, the symptomatic and LV remodeling responses hold promise for structural heart interventional approaches in patients in whom the reduction in secondary MR after cardiac resynchronization therapy is suboptimal. No randomized controlled trial to date, however, has investigated the prevalence, evolution, or impact on mortality of secondary MR before and after cardiac resynchronization therapy.

Surgical Mitral Valve Intervention

Isolated Undersized Annuloplasty: The pathophysiology of secondary MR is complex and its optimal surgical treatment remains the object of ongoing debate. The surgical technique has to be tailored to the stage of the disease. Bolling and Bach[101] introduced the concept of undersized (or restrictive) annuloplasty to treat both ischemic and nonischemic severe secondary MR. After measuring the mitral intertrigonal distance and the surface of the anterior leaflet, an annuloplasty ring at least two sizes smaller than the measured one is chosen and implanted. By significantly reducing the annular dimension, restrictive annuloplasty forces the coaptation of the leaflets and eliminates MR.[101–103] Complete and rigid annuloplasty rings have proved to be more effective than partial and flexible rings[104] and a leaflet coaptation length of at least 8 mm should be obtained at the end of the procedure to ensure a durable repair.[105,106] Restrictive annuloplasty has been used worldwide because of its simplicity and reproducibility and has been associated with a low operative mortality, significant LV reverse remodeling, and clinical improvement in several studies.[103,106,107]

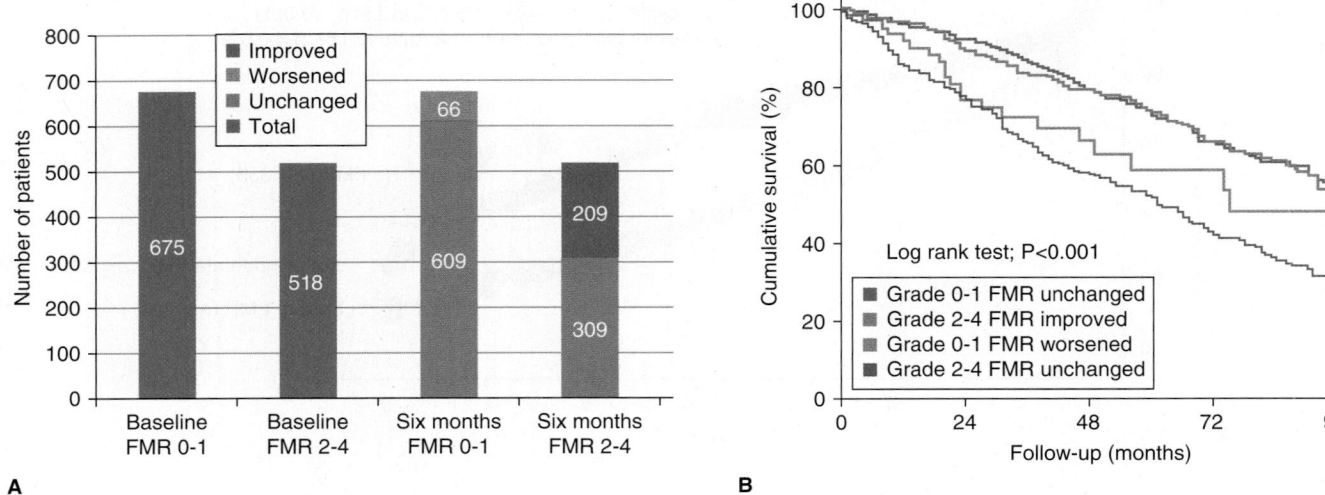

Figure 30–28. Distribution of various degrees of secondary (functional) mitral regurgitation (FMR) at baseline and 6 months after cardiac resynchronization therapy (**A**). Freedom from death, according to different patterns of evolution of FMR (**B**). Reproduced with permission from van der Bijl P, Khidir M, Ajmone Marsan N, et al. Effect of Functional Mitral Regurgitation on Outcome in Patients Receiving Cardiac Resynchronization Therapy for Heart Failure. *Am J Cardiol.* 2019 Jan 1;123(1):75-83.

However, residual or recurrent MR has been reported in a considerable number of patients at short- and midterm follow-up, with a large variability among the centers.[106,108–110] This difference in repair durability can be partly explained by the surgical technique and therefore by the degree of downsizing, the type of ring, and the intraoperative confirmation of adequate coaptation length after repair. However, the most important determinant of the durability of restrictive annuloplasty remains patient selection. Over the years, several echocardiographic predictors of postoperative residual or recurrent MR after isolated undersized annuloplasty have been identified[77–79,111–113] and their presence should be carefully taken into consideration when selecting patients for this procedure (**Table 30–4**). Most

of those predictors are markers of extreme leaflet tethering (posterior leaflet angle >45°, distal anterior leaflet angle >20°) and/or advanced LV remodeling (LV end-diastolic dimension >65 mm, LV end-systolic dimension >100 mL/m², sphericity index >0.7). Whenever one or more of the conditions listed in Table 30–4 are present, isolated restrictive annuloplasty is unlikely to be durable and the recurrence of MR is associated with heart failure episodes and increased mortality.[114]

Therefore, an isolated restrictive annuloplasty is a good solution only in selected patients with a short history of heart failure, small preoperative LV size, significant annular dilatation, and mild-to-moderate degree of leaflet tethering (**Fig. 30–29**), in the absence of predictors of unfavorable outcome. Besides the aforementioned selection criteria, it is important to keep in mind that the occurrence of postoperative reverse LV remodeling remains unpredictable in a significant proportion of patients and that ongoing LV remodeling leads to recurrence of tethering and MR.[106,114] Whenever the clinical and echocardiographic characteristics of the patient are unfavorable for an isolated restrictive annuloplasty, additional valvular/subvalvular techniques or chordal sparing valve replacement should be considered.

Additional Valvular and Subvalvular Mitral Procedures: Patients at high risk of failure of isolated restrictive annuloplasty can be preoperatively identified on the basis of the echocardiographic parameters listed in Table 30–4.[77–79,111–113] In clinical practice, the degree of mitral leaflet tethering as measured by the tenting height (also named coaptation depth), has been commonly used for this purpose. If this parameter exceeds 10 mm, additional procedures at valvular and subvalvular level may be considered to decrease the risk of MR recurrence and favor LV reverse remodeling (**Table 30–5**).

Additional Valvular Procedures: At a valvular level, an additional enlargement of the anterior or posterior leaflet with an

TABLE 30–4. Predictors of MR Recurrence After Mitral Valve Repair Using Restrictive Mitral Annuloplasty, Assessed by TTE[77–79,111–113]
Valvular parameters
MR grade ≥3.5
Central or complex regurgitant jet
Tenting area ≥2.5 cm²
Coaptation depth (= tenting height) ≥10 mm
Posterior leaflet angle ≥45°
Distal anterior leaflet tethering angle ≥20°
Mitral annulus diameter ≥37 mm*
Left ventricular parameters
LV end-diastolic diameter ≥65 mm
LV end-systolic diameter ≥51 mm
LV end-systolic volume ≥145 mL
Presence of a basal aneurysm/dyskinesis
Systolic sphericity index ≥0.7
Myocardial performance index ≥0.9
Wall motion score index ≥1.5
Interpapillary muscle distance >20 mm
Diastolic dysfunction (restrictive filling pattern)

*Assessed by transesophageal echocardiography. LV, left ventricle, MR, mitral regurgitation.

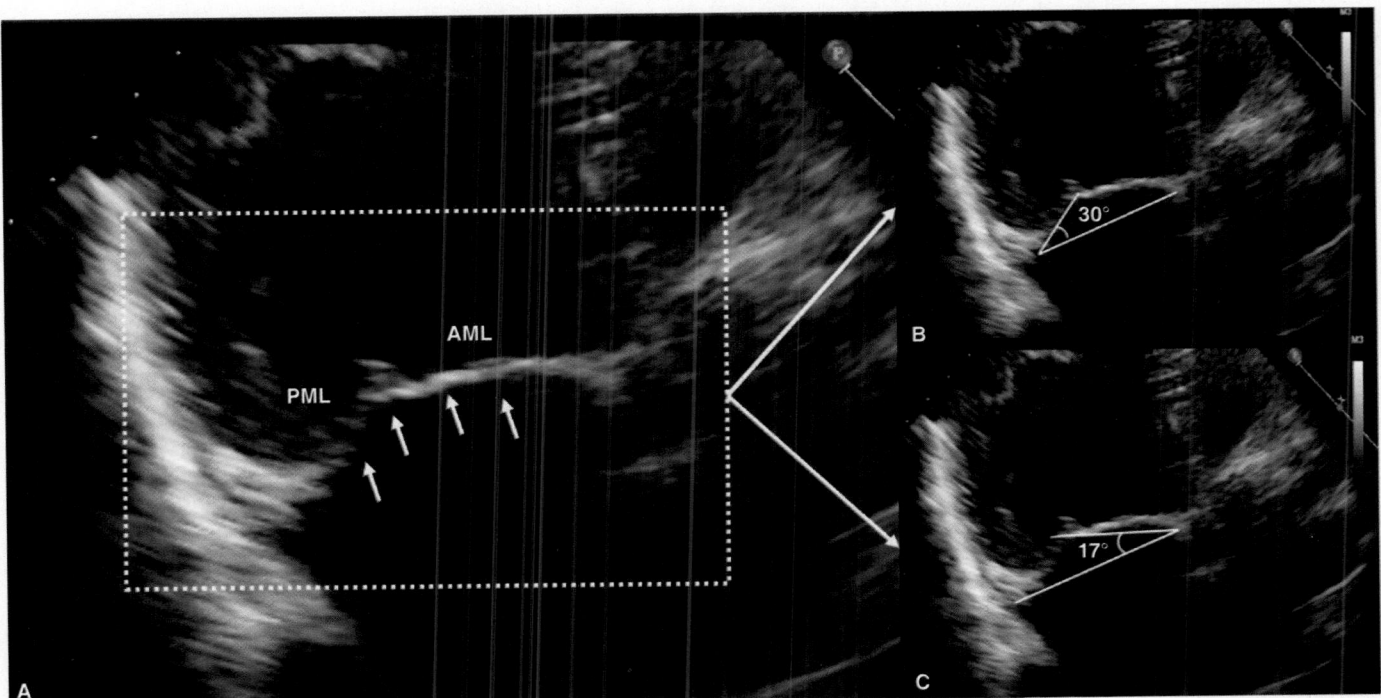

Figure 30–29. Symmetric tethering of both mitral leaflets in a patient with secondary MR. The zoomed view in (**A**) shows the apical four-chamber view of the mitral valve with symmetrical tethering of the anterior (AML) and posterior (PML) mitral leaflets (*arrows*). The measurement of the posterior angle tethering (**B**) and the anterior angle tethering (**C**) indicates that both are below the cut-off values identified as predictors of failure of isolated restrictive annuloplasty.

autologous or bovine pericardial patch or the edge-to-edge procedure can be applied.

Anterior or posterior leaflet augmentation: Augmentation of the anterior leaflet was initially proposed by Kincaid.[115] By augmenting the surface of the anterior leaflet with a pericardial patch, the tension on the chords is relieved and the level of coaptation of the anterior and posterior mitral leaflets falls more posteriorly, toward the direction of the displaced papillary muscles. The increased leaflet area allows the achievement of longer coaptation length in systole, which is important for repair durability. In addition, there is no need of aggressively undersizing the annuloplasty ring, which helps preventing functional mitral stenosis. This technique is simple and reproducible but only early and midterm results in a small number of patients have been reported.

The same principle has been applied to the posterior leaflet that has been expanded with an autologous or bovine

pericardial patch in some series. Tethering has been released and the coaptation significantly improved. Early and midterm encouraging results in limited number of patients are still waiting to be validated in larger studies with longer follow-up.[116]

More recently, a combination of anterior leaflet augmentation and cutting of the secondary chordae, together with ring annuloplasty, has also been reported with good midterm results in patients with secondary (ischemic) MR.[117] Chordal cutting eliminates apical tethering and increases the effective length of the anterior leaflet. In addition, the anatomic expansion of the anterior leaflet surface with a pericardial patch allows the anterior leaflet to freely reach the posterior leaflet. The combination of both repair techniques has a strong rationale and might improve mitral valve competence at long term.

Edge-to-edge procedure: The edge-to-edge technique is another valvular procedure that has been used in combination with ring annuloplasty, mainly in patients with pronounced tethering (tenting height >10 mm). This technique involves suturing the edges of the mitral leaflets together at the site of the main regurgitant jet. In secondary (ischemic) MR due to local remodeling, the regurgitant jet is usually located at the level of the posteromedial commissure. Conversely, in patients with global LV remodeling due to ischemic or nonischemic dilated cardiomyopathy, the MR is located at the level of A2-P2. In the first case, the edge-to-edge suture is performed at the level of the posteromedial commissural area and results in a single orifice mitral valve with a smaller area. In the second case, the edge-to-edge suture is performed at the central portion of the valve, and results in a double orifice mitral valve.

TABLE 30–5. Most Common Valvular and Subvalvular Mitral Procedures That Can Be Added to Restrictive Annuloplasty in Selected Patients

Valvular procedures
Augmentation of the anterior leaflet
Augmentation of the posterior leaflet
Augmentation of both the anterior and posterior leaflets
Edge-to-edge technique
Subvalvular procedures
Cutting of the secondary chordae
Papillary muscle repositioning
Papillary muscle approximation

Outcomes of the edge-to-edge procedure have been disappointing when this technique has been used without concomitant annuloplasty or combined with a flexible band, to prevent further progression of annular dilatation.[118-120] Conversely, when combined with a complete semi-rigid ring annuloplasty, the edge-to-edge procedure has significantly decreased the incidence of recurrent severe MR (grade 3+/4+) both at mid- and long-term follow-up as compared to isolated restrictive annuloplasty.[121,122]

Additional Subvalvular Procedures: Also, at the subvalvular level, several techniques have been proposed in addition to ring annuloplasty in selected patients, including resection of the secondary chordae, papillary muscle repositioning, and papillary muscle approximation. Those subvalvular procedures have been developed as an adjunct to annuloplasty to restore LV geometry, to reduce tethering forces on the mitral valve, to promote LV reverse remodeling, and to improve mitral valve stability after repair. A recent meta-analysis demonstrated that simultaneous subannular techniques are able to increase the durability of restrictive annuloplasty in patients with more pronounced tethering.[123]

Cutting of the secondary chordae: Undersized ring annuloplasty moves the posterior annulus more anterior, thereby worsening tethering of the posterior leaflet. In this situation, the repaired mitral valve remains competent only if the anterior leaflet is mobile enough to cover the entire annular area and coapt with the essentially fixed posterior leaflet.

The mobility of the anterior leaflet depends on the tenting effect caused by the secondary chordae that produces the characteristic seagull sign. If the mobility of the anterior leaflet is significantly restricted, as demonstrated by large distal anterior leaflet angles, residual or recurrent MR is likely to occur after isolated restrictive annuloplasty. Cutting the secondary chordae of the anterior leaflet from both papillary muscles has been proposed and adopted in this subset of patients. Initially, concerns were raised regarding the potential for disruption of the valvular–ventricular continuity and for progressive LV remodeling. However, since this procedure leaves the basal and marginal chordae intact, the continuity between the mitral valve and the LV is preserved and no significant adverse effect on LV function has been demonstrated. Compared to patients undergoing only reduction annuloplasty, patients with concomitant chordal cutting showed significantly lower rate of recurrent MR, improved mitral valve leaflet mobility, and improved NYHA functional class.[124,125]

As aforementioned, this procedure has more recently been proposed in combination with anterior leaflet augmentation with a pericardial patch showing encouraging results.[117]

Papillary muscle repositioning: Papillary muscle repositioning (or relocation) was first reported to alleviate leaflet restriction more than 15 years ago. The original technique consisted of passing a 3.0-prolene suture through the tip of the posterior papillary muscle and then through the mitral annulus immediately posterior to the right fibrous trigone, followed by restrictive annuloplasty. In more recent series, the fixation of both papillary muscles' sutures on the posterior aspect of the annuloplasty ring has been preferred. This approach counteracts subvalvular systolic leaflet tethering and does have the effect of an internal LV restraint. Its combination with ring annuloplasty has been associated with a significantly lower MR recurrence, less leaflet tenting, and improved 1-year outcome compared with annuloplasty alone in patients with tenting height >10 mm.[126]

An original technique of papillary muscle repositioning is the approach named Ring+String, which combines the restrictive annuloplasty (Ring) with the papillary muscle repositioning (String) performed through a horizontal aortotomy. By using this original approach, a pledgeted 3-0 prolene suture is passed through the head of one or both papillary muscles and then exteriorized through the aorto-mitral continuity at the level of the commissure between the noncoronary and left coronary aortic cusps. The suture is tied (guided by TEE) after weaning from cardiopulmonary bypass, until the most physiological shape of the anterior mitral leaflet is achieved. Studies describing the outcomes of this modality of papillary muscle repositioning are limited but report encouraging early and midterm results.[127,128]

Papillary muscle approximation: The aim of papillary muscle approximation is to decrease the anatomical displacement of the papillary muscles and reduce the tethering forces on the mitral leaflets. This subvalvular technique can be applied in different ways depending on the degree of LV remodeling and on the extent of LV scar (if present in patients with ischemic MR).

If the papillary muscles are only partially approximated from the tips to their midparts with pledgeted mattress sutures, a so-called "incomplete papillary muscle approximation" is realized. Less frequently, and usually in presence of a large anterior LV scar, a more aggressive "complete" side-by-side papillary muscle approximation can be performed, through an anterior left ventriculotomy. All patients receive a concomitant ring annuloplasty which does not need to be significantly undersized, thereby decreasing the risk of functional mitral stenosis.[129]

Papillary muscle approximation is usually performed when the tenting height is ≥10 mm and/or when the diastolic interpapillary muscle distance is ≥30 mm.[130]

Several observational studies have described its efficacy.[131-134] Specifically, patients who underwent this combined procedure had significantly decreased mean tenting area and coaptation depth as well as a significantly decreased LV end-systolic and end-diastolic diameter at follow-up, which resulted in a significant decrease of recurrent MR.[131-134] One randomized, controlled trial has demonstrated a lower recurrence of MR ≥grade 3 (27% vs 56%, $P = 0.013$) and superior LV reverse remodeling at 5-year follow-up, as compared to restrictive mitral annuloplasty alone.[135]

Taken together, these results suggest that additional valvular and subvalvular procedures are safe and effective adjunctive procedures to decrease the rate of recurrent MR in selected patients for whom an isolated restrictive annuloplasty is unlikely to be durable. It is nowadays possible to predict the probability of recurrent MR after isolated restrictive annuloplasty by using imaging techniques and focusing on mitral valve configuration and LV size, geometry, and function. When ring annuloplasty provides a suboptimal result, it remains challenging to decide between mitral repair with valvular/subvalvular procedures and mitral valve replacement. Both solutions present advantages and drawbacks and local expertise certainly plays a major role in the final choice.

Mitral Valve Replacement

Besides repair, chordal sparing mitral valve replacement represents another possible surgical option. In older series, mitral replacement for secondary MR, in the presence of significant LV dysfunction, was associated with high hospital mortality, ranging from 10% to 20%. This explains why a low-risk surgical repair, like the undersized annuloplasty, has initially become very popular and successful. In contemporary series however, the adoption of a complete chordal sparing technique has significantly decreased the hospital mortality of mitral valve replacement, which is nowadays around 4% to 5%. Technically a "chordal sparing approach" consists of the implantation of a mitral valve prosthesis with a complete (or almost complete) preservation of the chordae tendineae and their attachment to the leaflets or the annulus. In 1964, Lillehei and colleagues introduced the concept of preserving the attachments between the papillary muscles and the mitral annulus during mitral valve replacement to prevent postoperative LV dysfunction. This concept was initially challenged and largely abandoned until it was noted that mitral valve replacement with preservation of chordae tendineae significantly reduced operative mortality and enhanced late survival in patients with ischemic MR. The main advantage of "chordal sparing" mitral replacement over repair is the avoidance of MR recurrence. Unfortunately, the absence of recurrent MR does not seem to translate into superior LV reverse remodeling or survival as compared to mitral valve repair.[136,137] In a multicenter randomized controlled trial, mitral valve repair using an undersized rigid, complete annuloplasty ring was compared to complete chordal sparing mitral valve replacement.[136,137] The primary endpoint of LV reverse remodeling was similar between the two groups at 1-year and 2-year follow-up. Although the study was not powered to compare mortalities, the incidence was not significantly different at 30 days (1.6% mortality after repair vs 4% after replacement) and at 2 years (19.0% vs 23.2%; $P = 0.39$). Recurrent MR was more frequent in the repair group (59% vs 3.8% at 2 years; $P <0.001$) resulting in a higher rate of cardiovascular re-hospitalization (48.3 vs 32.2 per 100 patient-years; $P = 0.01$). The presence of an infero-basal aneurysm was a predictor of MR recurrence. On the basis of this trial, the 2020 ACC/AHA Guideline for the Management of Patients with Valvular Heart Disease states that it may be reasonable to choose chordal-sparing mitral valve replacement over downsized annuloplasty repair in symptomatic patients with chronic severe ischemic MR (class IIb).[20] However, it is important to emphasize that, in this study, patients referred for mitral valve repair who had no recurrent MR, demonstrated significantly larger reverse LV remodeling 1 year after surgery as compared to those undergoing replacement. This finding supports that an effective and durable repair, in well selected patients, might

be overall more beneficial than replacement. If, according to the preoperative clinical and echocardiographic features, a durable repair is likely to be achieved, this should be pursued. Otherwise a chordal sparing valve replacement should be preferred, since this option is certainly better than a failing repair.

Additional Procedures

Coronary Artery Bypass Grafting: In patients who have severe ischemic MR, coronary arteries suitable for revascularization and evidence of myocardial viability, coronary artery bypass grafting should be combined with mitral valve repair or replacement to address both components of this complex disease.

Tricuspid Valve Repair: In patients with secondary MR, concomitant tricuspid regurgitation of various degrees is often present and usually due to annular dilatation. In presence of significant RV remodeling, leaflet tethering is also contributing to the pathophysiology of tricuspid regurgitation. Observational studies have demonstrated that less than severe tricuspid regurgitation, left untreated at the time of mitral repair for secondary MR, may progress in a significant proportion of patients.[138,139] Factors predisposing to tricuspid regurgitation progression in patients with dilated cardiomyopathy are reduced LVEF, pulmonary hypertension, the high prevalence of RV dysfunction, the need for implantable cardiac defibrillator or cardiac resynchronization therapy, and the possibility of MR recurrence after repair. According to current guidelines, a concomitant tricuspid annuloplasty should be considered at the time of mitral valve surgery, even in the presence of only mild tricuspid regurgitation, if the tricuspid annulus is dilated, or if there is evidence of prior episodes of right-sided heart failure.[19]

Most of the published studies, both randomized controlled trials and observational data, have demonstrated that ring annuloplasty repairs are more durable than suture annuloplasty, particularly in patients with severe tricuspid annular dilatation or pulmonary hypertension.[19] Among the different types of prosthetic rings, the semi rigid or rigid ones should be preferred, since they have been associated with the lowest rate of recurrent tricuspid regurgitation over time.

Left Ventricular Reconstruction: Surgical LV reconstruction is a procedure designed to restore the LV shape and size in patients with large postinfarction areas of akinesia or dyskinesia, associated with wall thinning. The role of concomitant LV reconstruction at the time of restrictive mitral annuloplasty is still controversial and no clear guidelines exist. In clinical practice, surgical LV reconstruction is performed in conjunction with mitral valve repair in selected patients with functional MR, advanced LV remodeling, and large akinetic/dyskinetic areas. Several studies have demonstrated that, under those circumstances, surgical LV reconstruction provides greater reduction of LV end-diastolic and end-systolic volume index as compared to restrictive mitral annuloplasty alone and may improve survival.[140,141]

Kainuma and coworkers[141] compared the efficacy of restrictive mitral annuloplasty alone with restrictive mitral annuloplasty combined with surgical LV reconstruction in patients with MR, secondary to anterior or anteroseptal myocardial infarction and akinesia/dyskinesia ≥35% of the LV circumference. Preoperatively, patients who underwent restrictive mitral annuloplasty plus surgical LV reconstruction had a larger LV end-systolic volume index. After surgery, restrictive mitral annuloplasty plus surgical LV reconstruction reduced LV end-systolic volume index more frequently than restrictive mitral annuloplasty alone (43% vs 22%; P <0.0001), leading to a nearly identical postoperative LV end-systolic volume index (71 ± 17 mL/m^2 vs 78 ± 26 mL/m^2). Interestingly, in patients with preoperative LV end-systolic volume index between 105 and 150 mL/m^2, survival was superior in the restrictive mitral annuloplasty plus surgical LV reconstruction group (73% vs 40%; P = 0.046), accompanied by a greater reduction in plasma BNP.[141] This observation confirms that there may be a specific subgroup of patients who can prognostically benefit from combined restrictive mitral annuloplasty and surgical LV reconstruction. Indeed, in the presence of a severely dilated LV, mitral valve repair alone is associated with a high rate of failure due to severe leaflet tethering and ongoing LV remodeling after surgery. Mitral valve replacement is also unlikely to provide a prognostic benefit considering that severely increased LV end-systolic volume index is the most powerful predictor of survival in patients with impaired LV function.[142] Despite the lack of strong evidence, the data currently available suggest that the combination of surgical LV reconstruction and mitral valve repair may represent a reasonable surgical option in those patients. Further studies are needed to guide patient selection to identify the patients who may benefit most from this combined approach.

Ablation of Atrial Fibrillation: Atrial fibrillation is often observed in patients with secondary MR. It is commonly associated with worsening of symptoms and the underlying LV dysfunction. In patients undergoing mitral valve surgery for secondary MR, a concomitant Cox Maze procedure (with/without LA appendage ligation), may be considered if the likelihood of sinus rhythm restoration is reasonably high. Concomitant atrial fibrillation ablation slightly prolongs the duration of aortic cross-clamp and cardiopulmonary bypass but, if successful, may help counteracting disease progression and improve patients' prognosis. The age of the patient, the duration of atrial fibrillation, the size of the LA, and the severity of LV dysfunction (all predictors of recurrence of atrial fibrillation) should be carefully evaluated during the decision-making process.[143]

Concomitant atrial fibrillation ablation is particularly important in the subset of patients with MR secondary to LA dilatation. In this setting, LVEF is usually normal or only mildly depressed, and LV dilatation less pronounced as compared to MR. Because of the absence of tethering, these patients may be very effectively treated by ring annuloplasty associated with atrial fibrillation ablation. However, evidence is still limited, and more data are needed.

Advanced Heart Failure Therapies

Selecting the patients with secondary MR who will benefit from mitral valve surgery remains challenging and further refinements of imaging tools are needed to better predict the likelihood of reverse LV remodeling and consequently the outcome of the patients. The surgical technique (type of repair or valve replacement) must be tailored to the characteristics of the individual patient. Nevertheless, patients with secondary MR comprise a very heterogeneous group and, in some of them, simply fixing MR would not provide any clinical or prognostic benefit. Indeed, the extent of LV dysfunction, rather than eliminating MR, is the main determinant of their fate. These patients require an intervention addressing the underlying LV dysfunction, and therefore they should be referred to centers with advanced heart failure programs for consideration of implantation of an LV assist device (either as destination therapy or bridge to transplantation) or heart transplantation. Unfortunately, many of these patients will not be eligible for these advanced therapies due to comorbidities and age restrictions. Under those circumstances, adequate support and palliative care should be provided, particularly for patients with severe comorbidities limiting life expectancy to less than 1 year.

TRANSCATHETER TREATMENT OF MITRAL REGURGITATION

Transcatheter interventions are an emerging alternative for patients with primary MR who are inoperable or at high surgical risk, and those with secondary MR who remain symptomatic despite optimal guideline-directed medical therapy (and cardiac resynchronization therapy when indicated). These treatments are rapidly evolving with a number of novel transcatheter techniques whose principles are based on those of surgery, including edge-to-edge leaflet repair, NeoChord placement, direct and indirect annuloplasty, and valve replacement. The complex anatomy and pathophysiology of the mitral valve (and its proximity to the LV outflow tract) provide additional challenges and careful preprocedural imaging assessment is essential.[144,145] The procedures require mastery of multiple transcatheter techniques—many are restricted to a small number of highly specialized centers and are still undergoing assessment within early clinical and preclinical trials.

Techniques and Technologies

Edge-to-Edge Leaflet Repair

Mitral edge-to-edge repair involves grasping and approximating the mitral valve leaflets to create a double orifice, akin to the Alfieri surgical technique (**Fig. 30–30**). The procedure is performed under general anesthesia via transvenous, transseptal approach using TEE guidance. First procedures using the MitraClip device (Abbott, IL, USA) were undertaken in 2003 followed by regulatory approval in Europe and the United States in 2008 and 2013, respectively; this is by far the most widely adopted device, with more than 100,000 procedures performed worldwide. Numerous observational studies have confirmed safety and efficacy,[146-148] clinical improvement (NYHA class, 6-minute walking distance and reverse LV remodeling),[147,149] improved survival,[150,151] and predictors of poor outcome: advanced heart failure (NYHA class IV),

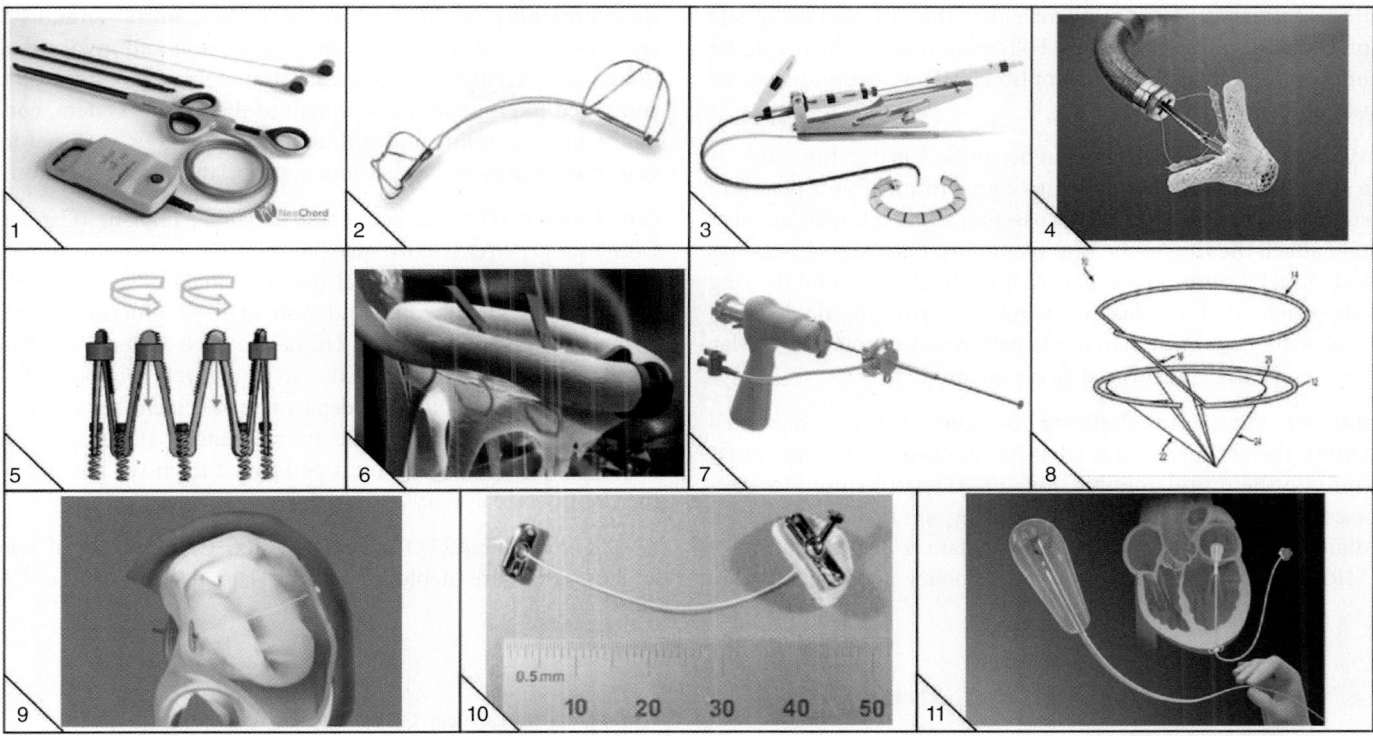

Figure 30–30. Transcatheter mitral valve repair devices: (1) NeoChord DS1000 (NeoChord Inc., St. Louis Park, MN), (2) CARILLON Mitral Contour System (Cardiac Dimensions Inc., Kirkland, WA), (3) Cardioband (Edwards Lifesciences Corp., Irvine, CA), (4) MitraClip (Abbott Vascular, Santa Clara, CA), (5) IRIS (Millipede Inc., Santa Rosa, CA), (6) Amend (ValCare Medical Ltd., Herzlyia Pituach, Israel), (7) TSD-5 (Harpoon Medical, Baltimore, MD), (8) MISTRAL (Mitralix) 9 ARTO (MVRx Inc., Belmont, CA), (10) Trans-Apical Segmented Reduction Annuloplasty (TASRA) (MitraSpan Inc., Belmont, MA), and (11) Mitra-Spacer (Cardiosolutions Inc., West Bridgewater, MA).

severe reduction in LVEF (<30%), extreme NT-proBNP values (>10,000 pg/mL), significant RV dysfunction (tricuspid annular plane systolic excursion <15 mm), severe pulmonary hypertension or tricuspid regurgitation, and the presence of major comorbidities (such as significant renal dysfunction).[146,147,152] As a consequence, international guideline recommendations support the use of MitraClip as a complementary option to medical and surgical treatment of primary and secondary MR.[19,20,153]

Recent results from the global MitraClip EXPAND registry (Contemporary, Prospective Study Evaluating Real-world Experience of Performance and Safety for the Next Generation of MitraClip Devices) enrolling >1000 patients suggest that increasing operator experience and newer MitraClip device iterations may be associated with improved results.[154] Edge-to-edge repair may also be achieved using the PASCAL (Edwards Lifesciences, CA) device consisting of a central spacer that fills the regurgitant orifice area and two paddles and two clasps that allow independent leaflet capture to optimize positioning.[155,156] Further devices adopting similar principles (DRAGONFLY, Hangzhou Valgen Medtech, China) are in the early stages of clinical development.

Artificial NeoChord Placement

Expanded polytetrafluoroethylene (e-PTFE) sutures are routinely used as artificial neochordae to resuspend the prolapsed or flail leaflet margin in conventional surgical mitral valve repair. The NeoChord (NeoChord, Inc., MN) and Harpoon TSD-5 (Edwards Lifesciences, CA) systems allow placement of such sutures as replacement neochordae in the beating heart via transapical access using TEE guidance without need for cardiopulmonary bypass (Fig. 30–30).[157,158] Transfemoral and transseptal delivery systems are under current investigation.

Direct and Indirect Mitral Annuloplasty

Transcatheter annuloplasty techniques differ from surgical annuloplasty in providing both direct and indirect approaches—direct annuloplasty enables closer approximation to the mitral valve whereas indirect annuloplasty is potentially a much simpler procedure (Fig. 30–30).[159-161] Planning for both approaches requires detailed preprocedural multimodality imaging to assess anatomical suitability.[153]

Direct Mitral Annuloplasty Devices:

Cardioband: The Cardioband annuloplasty system (Edwards Lifesciences, CA) consists of a polyester sleeve implant (available in 6 lengths), transseptal steerable sheath, transfemoral delivery system, repositionable and retrievable anchors to fasten the implant to the mitral annulus, and a size adjustment tool.[160] The procedure is performed via transvenous transseptal access under TEE guidance. The first anchor is released close to the anterior commissure and the implant deployed until the radiopaque portion reaches the adjacent marker. The implant catheter is then navigated along the posterior annulus and these actions repeated until reaching the last anchoring site on the posterior commissure. Following final deployment, the implant is tightened to allow optimal MR reduction using the size adjustment tool.

Millipede IRIS: The IRIS (Boston Scientific Corporation, MA) is a semi-rigid complete ring with a zigzag nitinol frame placed in supra-annular position via transseptal approach with anchors that attach the ring to the mitral annulus. Each zigzag peak has individually controlled collars that contract or expand the ring when tightened or released, thereby determining final sizing. Successful first-in-human implantation was announced in May 2017 and early clinical studies are ongoing.[162]

Indirect Mitral Annuloplasty Devices: Devices implanted within the coronary sinus (that lies in close anatomical proximity to the mitral annulus; **Fig. 30–31**) can be used to exert a constraining force, thereby reducing annular septal-lateral diameter with improved leaflet coaptation and reduction of MR. Importantly, the circumflex coronary artery lies within

close proximity of the coronary sinus and mitral annulus[163] and there is a theoretical risk of compression and myocardial infarction. Accurate preprocedural imaging (using cardiac computed tomography) assessment of the venous system, coronary sinus anatomy and mitral annular plane is essential to determine suitability and ensure appropriate patient selection.

Carillon device: The Carillon coronary sinus implant (Cardiac Dimensions, WA) is currently the only CE approved indirect annuloplasty device in clinical use. The main advantage is its simplicity and safety profile, and more than 700 procedures have been performed worldwide.[164] The device is a fixed length nitinol system delivered via the right external jugular vein (Fig. 30–31).[165] Traction is applied following deployment to cinch the posterior periannular tissue and reduce mitral annular dimensions. A selective coronary angiogram is performed to ensure patency of the circumflex coronary artery prior to final device release.

ARTO device: The ARTO system (MVRx, CA) consists of two anchors that are deployed in the lateral wall of the LA

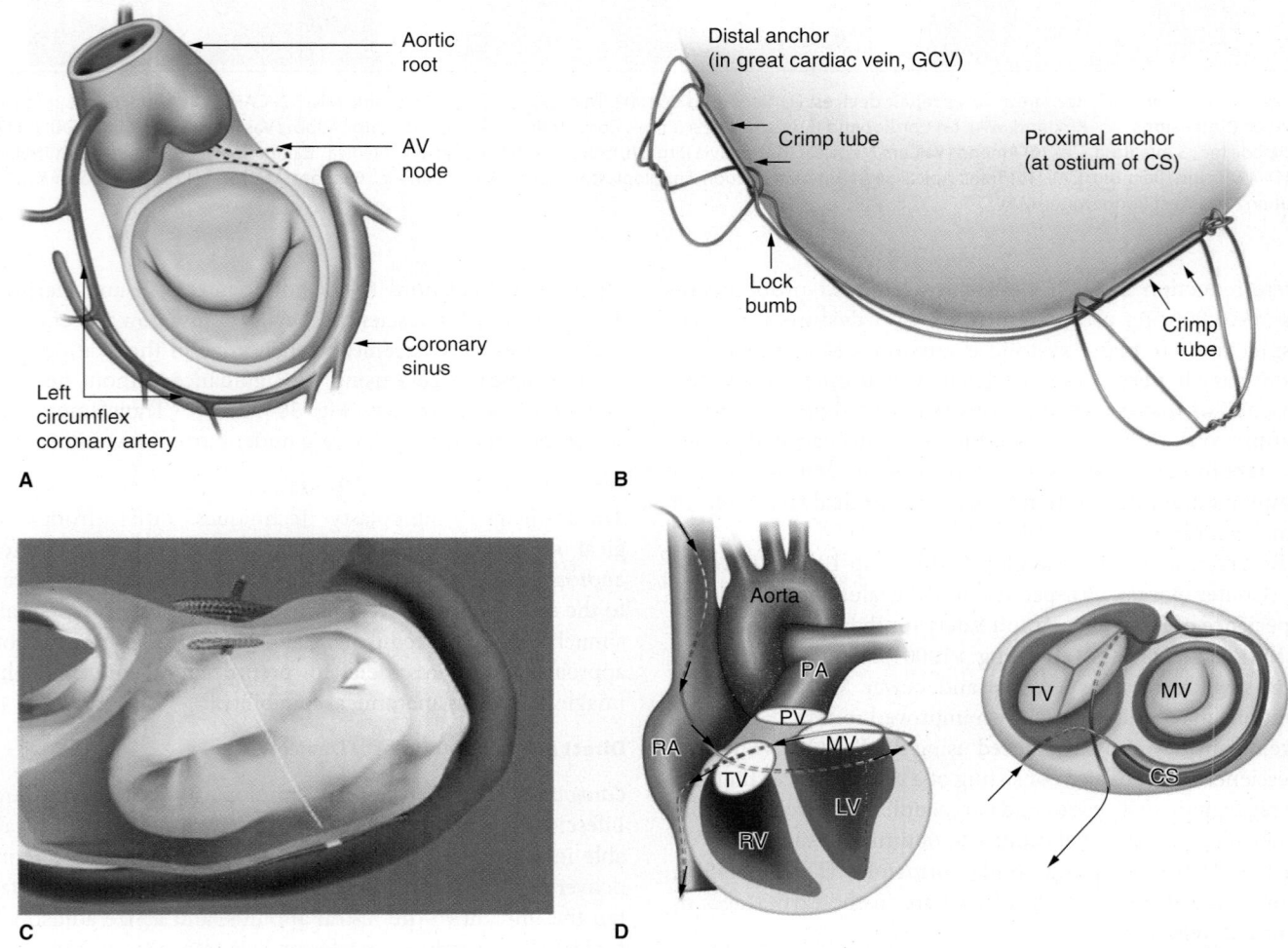

Figure 30–31. Indirect mitral annuloplasty devices. (A) Anatomical relationships (surgeon's view of the mitral valve), demonstrating the close proximity of the mitral annulus, coronary sinus, circumflex artery and conduction system. **(B)** The Carillon coronary sinus implant (Cardiac Dimensions) device. **(C)** Graphical image of the ARTO (MVRx Inc) device following deployment, with two anchors either side of the tether. In this image projection, the T-bar anchor sits inferiorly and the atrial septal anchor (occluder device) sits superiorly. **(D)** Graphical image demonstrating the anatomical course of cerclage annuloplasty to reduce mitral annular dimensions.

(via the coronary sinus) and atrial septum, then connected by a tether traversing the left atrium (Fig. 30–31).[166] Implantation is performed under general anesthesia using TEE guidance. One of two magnetic catheters is positioned in the coronary sinus through right jugular venous access, and the second positioned across the atrial septum via femoral venous access and transseptal puncture. These catheters are then manipulated and linked magnetically in the posterior LA adjacent to the posterior mitral annulus, before connection using a small puncturing wire. Routine catheter exchanges are performed to deliver coronary sinus (T-bar) and atrial septal anchors that are connected by an adjustable suture to reduce the anteroposterior mitral annular diameter until optimal reduction of MR is achieved.

Mitra Loop Cerclage system: This annuloplasty system (Tau-PNU Medical, South Korea) delivered via the left subclavian and right femoral vein is undergoing early clinical assessment and consists of a stainless-steel tension element delivered using a multistep procedure to form a continuous loop from the coronary sinus to a basal septal perforator coronary vein and the RV outflow tract (Fig. 30–31). A coronary sinus tricuspid bridge device (that straddles and protects the septal tricuspid leaflet and coronary conduction system) completes the loop.[167] It is important to note that anatomical variation between individuals may limit the clinical efficacy of indirect annuloplasty—the coronary sinus lies superior to the mitral annulus in a significant number of patients and is often higher posteriorly than anteriorly.[168] Furthermore, the distance between the mitral annulus and coronary sinus is often increased in patients with dilated ventricles and severe MR,[169] potentially explaining the varying clinical efficacy of different devices.

Transcatheter Mitral Valve Replacement

Although transcatheter mitral valve replacement is potentially applicable to a wider of range of pathologies than valve repair, numerous anatomical and engineering challenges have

hampered progress to date, including delivery of often bulky devices, stable positioning, risks of LV outflow tract obstruction and circumflex coronary arterial occlusion, thromboembolic complications (and bleeding related to their prevention), hemodynamic performance, and long-term durability.[170] Current devices are based on nitinol alloy platforms enclosing bovine or porcine leaflets and employ a variety of mechanisms to ensure stable fixation within the mitral annulus (**Fig. 30–32**). Transapical access (requiring general anesthesia) is the norm, although transseptal delivery systems are rapidly emerging. Worldwide experience is currently limited to approximately 500 cases and a number of devices are still undergoing phase I trials. Complications include sepsis, multiorgan failure, device thrombosis, and prolonged recovery from access site complications, reflecting the extensive comorbidity and frailty of currently selected patients.

Intrepid: The Intrepid system (Medtronic, MN) comprises of a self-expanding, nitinol frame, trileaflet bovine pericardial valve, and a transapical hydraulic delivery system for controlled expansion and deployment.[171] The prosthesis has a unique dual structure, consisting of an inner circular stent to house the valve and a conformable outer fixation ring. Fixation and sealing is achieved through a combination of design features: (1) the outer fixation ring is larger in circumference than the native mitral annulus with varying radial stiffness, (2) the atrial portion of the outer ring is flexible (allowing conformation to the native annulus) whereas the stiffer ventricular portion resists compression, producing a final "champagne cork" conformation to resist migration under systolic pressure, and (3) the outer and inner stent frames are covered by a polyester fabric skirt to prevent paraprosthetic leaks and facilitate tissue ingrowth. The prosthesis has minimal subannular protrusion to avoid LV outflow tract obstruction.

Tendyne: The Tendyne system (Abbott Vascular, CA) comprises a transapical, fully repositionable and recapturable

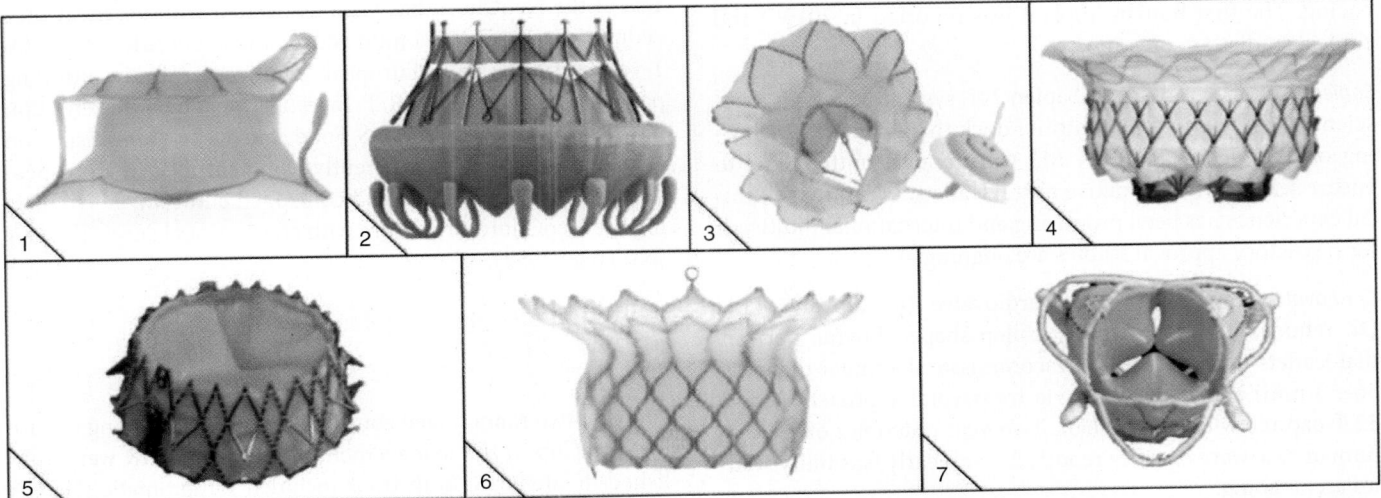

Figure 30–32. Transcatheter mitral valve replacement devices: (1) TIARA (Neovasc Inc., Richmond, BC, Canada), (2) CardiAQ (Edwards Lifesciences Corp., Irvine, CA), (3) Tendyne (Abbott Vascular, Santa Clara, CA), (4) Intrepid (Medtronic Inc., Minneapolis, MN), (5) NaviGate (NaviGate Cardiac Structures Inc., Lake Forest, CA), (6) HighLife (HighLife SAS, Paris, France), and (7) Caisson TMVR (Caisson Interventional LLC, Maple Grove, MN).

trileaflet porcine pericardial valve sewn within two self-expanding nitinol stents, and a LV apical tethering system.[172] The outer stent, available in different sizes, is D-shaped to conform to the native mitral annulus and the inner circular frame is one size, maintaining a large effective orifice area (>3.0 cm²). The apical tethering system is designed to reduce paravalvular regurgitation and assist apical closure. The device received the world's first CE mark for transcatheter mitral valve replacement in 2020 and is currently being investigated in an expanded clinical trial (NCT02321514) recruiting up to 350 subjects at up to 40 centers over 5-year follow-up (projected completion 2024).

TIARA: The TIARA (Neovasc, BC, Canada) is a D-shaped, self-expanding, nitinol frame, trileaflet bovine pericardial valve with a full atrial skirt and three ventricular anchors (one anterior, two posterior) that fix the valve onto the fibrous trigone and posterior annulus.[173] Delivery is via transapical approach and resheathing, repositioning, and retrieval are possible until the final stage of deployment. First-in-human implantation was performed in January 2014[174] and the Early Feasibility Study of the Neovasc Tiara™ Mitral Valve System (TIARA-I) and Tiara™ Transcatheter Mitral Valve Replacement (TIARA-II) trials are ongoing in anticipation of CE mark approval.

Emerging Transseptal Mitral Valve Implantation Devices:

HighLife: The HighLife system (HighLife SAS, France) consists of a nitinol frame, trileaflet, bovine pericardial valve with a preformed annular groove to allow seating within a subannular dock implant.[175] Retrograde advancement of a loop via the aortic valve allows delivery of the subannular implant before insertion of the mitral valve via secondary transseptal access. The subannular implant position and shape of the bioprosthesis ensure stability.

Cephea: The Cephea valve (Abbott Vascular, CA) has a unique design, including a ventricular disc, central leaflet core, and atrial disc allowing transseptal delivery and mitral annular anchoring without using axial compression forces and avoiding the use of subvalvular anchors, pads, tethers, or ventricular pacing. The first human implant was reported in 2019[176] and clinical studies are ongoing.

Sapien M3: The transseptal Sapien M3 system (Edwards Lifesciences, CA) consists of a nitinol dock that facilitates anchoring of the 29 mm SAPIEN M3 valve and a knitted skirt to ensure sealing with the native mitral leaflets. Preliminary clinical experience has been promising and international multicenter regulatory approval studies are ongoing.

Cardiovalve: The low-profile Cardiovalve (Cardiovalve Ltd., Or Yehuda, Israel) has three scallop-shaped bovine pericardial leaflets in three sizes (intracommissural annular diameter 36–53 mm) and is delivered via transseptal approach using a 32-F capsule with a 24-F shaft. Two-year outcomes of the first human case were recently reported[177] and early feasibility studies are ongoing.

AltaValve: The AltaValve (4C Medical Technologies, MN) is a novel supra-annular system consisting of a compliant spherical nitinol frame sized to fit the LA and a 27-mm trileaflet bovine pericardial valve with a fabric skirt at the level of the annular ring to prevent paravalvular regurgitation and enhance tissue growth. First-in-human experience using a transapical approach has recently been reported[178] and a transseptal system is currently in development.

Evidence for Transcatheter Treatment of Primary MR

Edge-to-Edge Repair

The Endovascular Valve Edge-to-Edge Repair Study (EVEREST II) trial randomized 279 patients with severe symptomatic MR to treatment with the MitraClip or conventional surgery in a multicenter, randomized, nonblinded trial. MR was of primary etiology in the majority of patients in both groups (MitraClip 130/178, 73%; surgery 62/80, 78%). At 1-year, conventional surgery was more effective than transcatheter edge-to-edge repair in reducing MR. However, improvements in LV remodeling and clinical outcomes were similar for both approaches, and the percutaneous approach demonstrated a greater level of safety than surgery.[179] At 5 years, freedom from death, surgery, or severe MR (the primary endpoint) was more likely in the surgical group (64.3% vs 44.2%; $P = 0.01$), principally driven by increased rates of severe MR (12.3% vs 1.8%; $P = 0.02$) and the need for redo surgery (27.9% vs 8.9%; $P = 0.003$) in the MitraClip group. This surgery was most likely required (78%) within the first 6 months and rates of surgery and moderate-to-severe MR were comparable thereafter. Five-year mortality rates were equivalent in both groups (20.8% vs 26.8%; $P = 0.4$).[180] Currently, the use of MitraClip in primary MR in the United States has been restricted to patients with favorable anatomy who have prohibitive risk for surgical repair. Recently, additional studies are underway or planned in primary MR patients with lower surgical risk features, including the REPAIR MR study that intends to randomize (1:1) MitraClip versus surgical repair in 500 intermediate risk patients ≥75 years old at 60 centers.

Artificial NeoChord Placement

Use of the NeoChord has been associated with excellent procedural outcomes (97% mild/reduced residual MR, 98% ± 1% 1-year survival) in a European multicenter study enrolling patients with primary MR.[181] Investigational device exemption has been granted by the US Food and Drug Administration (FDA) and subjects are currently being enrolled in a prospective, multicenter, randomized controlled clinical trial comparing the NeoChord procedure with conventional surgical repair (NCT02803957).

Evidence for Transcatheter Treatment of Secondary MR

Edge-to-Edge Repair

The first two randomized controlled trials investigating the use of MitraClip in the management of secondary MR were published in late 2018. Both trials included symptomatic (NYHA II–IV) patients with secondary MR of ischemic and nonischemic etiology, and compared optimal guideline-directed medical therapy alone against optimal guideline-directed medical therapy plus MitraClip. The MITRA-FR (French Multicentre Study of Percutaneous Mitral Valve Repair MitraClip Device in Patients with Severe Secondary Mitral Regurgitation) trial included 304 patients with severe secondary MR (ESC definitions) with a composite primary endpoint of all-cause mortality and hospitalization for heart failure. At 12 months, there was no statistical difference between the MitraClip and control groups (54.6% vs 51.3%; P = NS).[182] In contrast, the US/Canadian COAPT (Cardiovascular Outcomes Assessment of the MitraClip Percutaneous Therapy for Heart Failure Patients with Functional Mitral Regurgitation) study enrolled 614 patients with moderate-severe SMR (AHA definitions) and demonstrated important benefits of MitraClip implantation, with a significant reduction in the primary endpoint of heart failure hospitalization at 24 months (35.8% vs 67.9% per patient year; P <0.001; number needed to treat [NNT] 3.1). The superiority of MitraClip extended to all prespecified secondary endpoints, including all-cause mortality (29.1% vs 46.1%; P <0.001; NNT 5.9) and the composite of death and rehospitalization at 24 months (45.7% vs 67.9%; P <0.001; NNT 4.5).[183] These conflicting results generated considerable discussion attempting to address subtle differences between the studies (**Table 30–6**) and their implementation in clinical practice.[184]

Extended observations from both studies showed no change in the findings of MITRA-FR, with no impact of MitraClip implantation on all-cause mortality or heart failure hospitalization at 24 months follow-up,[185] whilst the benefits of MitraClip implantation in COAPT were even more pronounced at 3-year follow-up (composite endpoint of death and heart failure hospitalization 58.8% vs 88.1%; HR, 0.48 [95% CI, 0.39–0.59];

TABLE 30–6. Key Differences between the COAPT and MITRA-FR Trials

		MITRA-FR	COAPT
	Primary endpoint	All-cause death and hospitalization for CHF at 1 year	All hospitalizations for CHF within 2 years (including recurrent events)
Key exclusion criteria	Heart failure severity	NYHA class <II	NYHA class <II ACC/AHA stage D heart failure
	Left ventricular dimensions	No exclusion criteria	LVESD >70 mm
	Coronary artery disease	CABG or PCI performed within 1 month	Untreated coronary artery disease requiring revascularization
	Right ventricle	No exclusion criteria	Right-sided congestive heart failure with moderate or severe right ventricular dysfunction
	Pulmonary disease	No exclusion criteria	COPD with home oxygen therapy or chronic oral steroid use Estimated or measured PAP >70 mm Hg
Principal baseline characteristics	Number of patients screened	450	1576
	Number of patients enrolled (ITT)	304	614
	Mean age (years)	70 ± 10	72 ± 12
	Mean LVEF (%)	33 ± 7	31 ± 10
	MR severity (EROA, cm²)	0.31 ± 0.10	0.41 ± 0.15
	Mean indexed LVEDV, mL/m²	135 ± 35	101 ± 34
Safety and efficacy endpoints in the intervention arm	Complications* (%)	14.6	8.5
	No implant (%)	9	5
	Implantation of multiple clips (%)	54	62
	Postprocedural MR grade ≤2+ (%)***	92	95
	MR grade ≤2+ at 1 year (%)**	83	95
	Hospitalization for CHF at 1-year (%)	49	38
	30-day mortality (%)	3.3	2.3
	1-year mortality (%)	24	19

*MITRA-FR definition of prespecified serious adverse events: device implant failure, transfusion or vascular complication requiring surgery, ASD, cardiogenic shock, cardiac embolism/stroke, tamponade, urgent cardiac surgery.
**According to ESC/EACTS guidelines[10] in MITRA-FR and AHA/ACC guidelines[11] in COAPT.
Abbreviations: CHF, congestive heart failure; BNP, brain natriuretic peptide; NT-proBNP, N-terminal pro brain natriuretic peptide ACC, American College of Cardiology; AHA, American Heart Association; COPD, chronic obstructive pulmonary disease; PAP, pulmonary artery pressure; ITT, intention to treat; LVEF, left ventricular ejection fraction; EROA, effective regurgitant orifice area; LVESD, left ventricular endsystolic diameter; MR, mitral regurgitation.
Reproduced with permission from Praz F, Grasso C, Taramasso M, et al. Mitral regurgitation in heart failure: time for a rethink. *Eur Heart J.* 2019 Jul 14;40(27):2189-2193.

P <0.001; NNT 3.4 [95% CI, 2.7–4.6]).[186] A proposed patho-physiological model of "proportionate" and "disproportionate" MR[82] based upon the relationship between LV end-diastolic volume and effective regurgitant orifice area, and its disruption in patients with ventricular dyssynchrony or papillary muscle dysfunction, may explain these disparities and awaits prospective validation. Cost-effectiveness analysis of COAPT at 2 years confirmed a higher cost of intervention overall ($73,416 vs $38,345; P <0.001; predominantly related to the price of the MitraClip device) but acceptable economic value based upon current US thresholds (incremental cost-effectiveness ratio $40,361 per life-year gained, $55,600 per quality-adjusted life-year gained).[187] Similarly, use of the PASCAL transcatheter valve repair system in 109 high risk patients (mean STS score 4.7%) with severe MR (33% primary MR, 67% secondary MR) in the Edwards PASCAL Transcatheter Mitral Valve Repair System (CLASP) study resulted in sustained reduction of MR accompanied by high survival and low complication rates, and significant improvements in functional status and quality of life at 1-year follow-up.[188]

These studies confirm the ominous prognosis of secondary MR despite optimal medical therapy, whilst their contrasting outcomes demonstrate varying effects of treatment based on the presenting phenotype. The overarching lesson is that treatment of secondary MR can substantially influence outcomes in carefully selected heart failure patients who remain symptomatic despite optimal guideline-directed medical therapy.

Direct and Indirect Transcatheter Annuloplasty

A single-arm feasibility trial using the Cardioband system in 31 patients with secondary MR demonstrated significant improvement in severity of MR (patients with ≥grade 3 reduced from 77.4% to 13.6%; P <0.001), NYHA class (NYHA III/IV patients reduced from 95.5% to 18.2%; P <0.001) and 6-minute walk test (reduced from 250 ± 107 m to 332 ± 118 m; P <0.001) at 6 months follow up with no periprocedural mortality.[189] The Edwards Cardioband System Pivotal Clinical Trial (ACTIVE) comparing Cardioband plus optimal guideline-directed medical therapy versus guideline-directed medical therapy alone in 375 patients with secondary MR is currently underway.

A randomized sham-controlled study, REDUCE-FMR (Safety and Efficacy of the CARILLON Mitral Contour System® in Reducing Functional Mitral Regurgitation Associated with Heart Failure), investigated the Carillon Mitral Contour system in patients with secondary MR receiving optimal guideline-directed medical therapy.[190] At 12 months, indirect annuloplasty using this system was associated with a significant fall in MR regurgitant volume (the primary endpoint) accompanied by reduction in LV volumes and improvement in paired 6-minute walking distance and NYHA functional class. However, the trial was not powered for clinical endpoints and the reported reduction in MR regurgitant volume (22%) was modest compared to that typically achieved following MitraClip edge-to-edge repair (60%–70%).[191] Indirect annuloplasty devices, including the ARTO and Mitral Loop Cerclage annuloplasty systems, have also demonstrated favorable reduction in regurgitant volume sustained up to 2 years in small clinical studies.[192]

Further high-quality studies will be required to refine selection criteria for the various medical and interventional treatment options in this high-risk group, explore indications for MitraClip beyond the current evidence base, and define the role of hybrid transcatheter procedures (such as edge-to-edge repair plus annuloplasty). The RESHAPE-HF2 (Safety and Effectiveness of the MitraClip System in the Treatment of Clinically Significant Functional Mitral Regurgitation) trial will add to the body of randomized evidence concerning the role of MitraClip implantation in secondary MR whilst the MATTER-HORN (Multicenter, Randomized, Controlled Study to Assess Mitral Valve Reconstruction for Advanced Insufficiency of Functional or Ischemic Origin) study will compare MitraClip with surgery in high-risk patients.

Transcatheter Mitral Valve Replacement

Preliminary experience with transcatheter mitral valve replacement has been predominantly in patients with secondary MR. In a pilot study enrolling 50 high- or extreme-risk patients (84% secondary MR, mean STS score 6.4 ± 5.5%) with severe symptomatic MR, implantation of the Intrepid valve (Medtronic) was successful in 48 (96%) with a 30-day mortality of 14%, only mild or no residual MR at median follow-up of 173 days, and substantial clinical (symptomatic) improvement.[193] The device was previously being compared in a randomized trial with standard mitral valve replacement in high surgical risk patients with moderate-to-severe and severe primary and secondary MR (APOLLO). The original trial design was recently modified and is now focusing on two observational studies: (1) surgically ineligible patients with primary or secondary MR and (2) surgically ineligible patients with symptomatic mitral valve disease due to mitral annular calcification (MAC). Similarly, first reports concerning use of the Tendyne valve in 30 patients (mean STS score 7.3 ± 5.7%, 23 [77%] with severe secondary MR) demonstrated successful device implantation free of cardiovascular mortality, stroke, and device malfunction in 86.6% at 30-day follow-up, with mild (1+) central MR in 1 patient, no residual MR in 26 patients, and substantial symptomatic improvement. One patient died from hospital-acquired pneumonia but there were no other major adverse events.[194] Most recently, the SUMMIT trial was initiated that is a randomized comparison of MitraClip versus Tendyne mitral valve replacement in edge-to-edge eligible patients (both primary and secondary severe MR), with an embedded registry of Tendyne treatment in symptomatic patients with mitral valve disease due to MAC. Careful clinical assessment coupled with detailed pre- and periprocedural multimodality imaging will be essential to the success of these studies and many other transcatheter mitral valve replacement devices that are now undergoing assessment in feasibility or early phase nonrandomized clinical trials.

The Tricuspid Valve

Surgical intervention is the only current guideline-recommended treatment for tricuspid regurgitation, but a relatively low proportion of patients undergo intervention due to the imbalance in inherent risks and uncertain outcomes.[195]

Transcatheter strategies for tricuspid disease remain in their early stages. Anatomical challenges include the large annulus, paucity of valve/annular calcification, adjacency of the right coronary artery, and fragility of the valve tissue. Current approaches under investigation in feasibility and early phase clinical trials include edge-to-edge repair, coaptation enhancement, annuloplasty, heterotopic caval valve implantation and percutaneous tricuspid valve replacement.[195] The supporting data set is substantially smaller than for mitral interventions (which is itself limited), although promising early outcomes have been demonstrated with the MitraClip device.[196,197] Major questions that need to be addressed by future trials include whether earlier intervention for tricuspid regurgitation may be beneficial, and whether combined mitral and tricuspid procedures improve procedural success and clinical outcomes.

Future Perspectives

Transcatheter intervention for mitral valve disease is evolving rapidly with multiple systems under evaluation. The majority of these are based upon well-established surgical techniques (modified to less invasive forms) and it is hoped that they will provide a future alternative for the treatment of patients at high or prohibitive surgical risk. Development of further novel mitral technologies and second- and third-generation devices are anticipated to improve procedural safety and success rates. Such devices will require large-scale clinical validation and Heart Team involvement will be essential to determine patient suitability. Given the complex anatomy and pathophysiology of the mitral valve, Heart Team decision-making will require tailored patient evaluation using novel imaging techniques, including 3D-TEE and CT image fusion (**Fig. 30–33**). Future challenges include the standardized definition of clinical and imaging selection criteria for different devices, and the development of simultaneous and staged approaches using complementary techniques (eg, transcatheter ring followed by valve implant or leaflet clipping). The updated US guidelines

reflect the positive signal from COAPT whilst reaffirming the importance of a multidisciplinary approach, involving imaging cardiologists, heart failure physicians, electrophysiologists, interventional cardiologists, and cardiac surgeons to achieve optimal patient outcomes.[153] A multidisciplinary cooperative approach will ultimately advance the field by generating evidence that can inform guidelines and facilitate adoption of effective and safe technologies.

INTERNATIONAL GUIDELINES FOR THE MANAGEMENT OF MITRAL REGURGITATION

Table 30–7 summarizes the recommendations for surgery in patients with primary MR, as detailed in contemporary international guidelines. The 2020 ACC/AHA guidelines and the 2017 ESC/EACTS guidelines are consistent in the class I recommendation for surgery in symptomatic patients with severe chronic primary MR, with a restriction for severe LV dysfunction in the ESC/EACTS guidelines.[19,20] There is also a consensus for favoring mitral valve repair over prosthetic valve replacement when possible.

The main difference between the ACC/AHA and ESC/EACTS guidelines concerns the indications for surgery in asymptomatic patients with chronic severe primary MR (**Table 30–8**).

In asymptomatic patients, atrial fibrillation or pulmonary hypertension are class IIa recommendations for surgery only in the ESC/EACTS guidelines.[20] More importantly, surgery is considered at an earlier stage in the ACC/AHA guidelines[20] than in the ESC/EACTS guidelines[19] (ie, for LV end-systolic dimension <40 mm in the ACC/AHA guidelines vs 45 mm in the ESC/EACTS guidelines), even when mitral valve replacement is needed. When surgery is at low-risk with a high likelihood of mitral valve repair, there is a class IIa indication for surgery irrespective of LV dimension or LVEF in the ACC/AHA guidelines[20] while the ESC/EACTS guidelines restrict

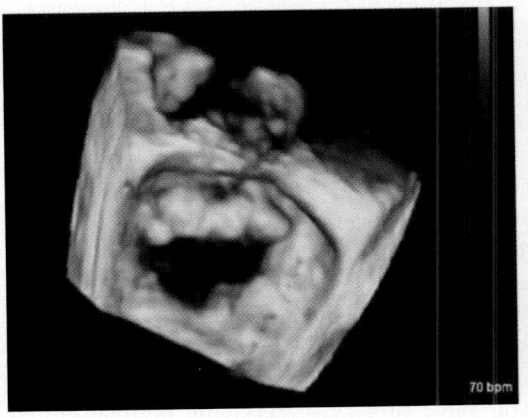
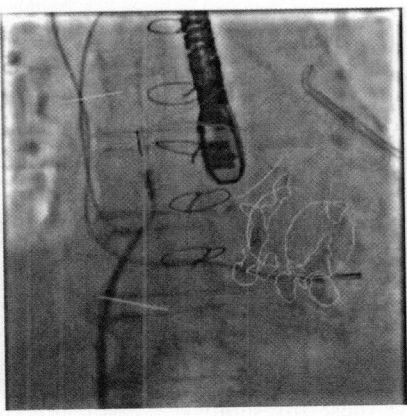
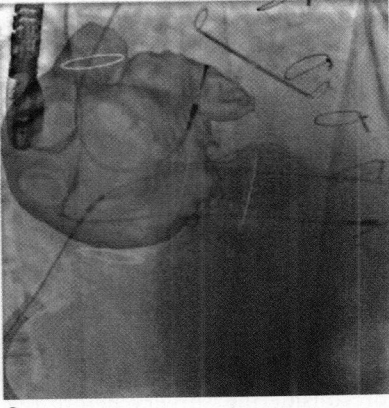

A   **B**   **C**

Figure 30–33. Imaging technique for transcatheter mitral valve repair and replacement techniques. (A) 3D-TEE real-time reconstruction of the mitral valve annulus and leaflets as a preliminary investigation to determine anatomical suitability for transcatheter mitral intervention. **(B)** CT overlay with real-time image fusion to demonstrate the optimal site for transseptal puncture. **(C)** Atrial anatomy and projection of the mitral valve—although this specific example was used for transcatheter mitral valve implantation, it is anticipated that 3D-TEE and CT fusion will be increasingly used for all complex transcatheter mitral interventions in the future.

TABLE 30–7. Recommendations for Isolated Mitral Valve Surgery in Chronic, Severe Primary MR

2020 ACC/AHA Guidelines[3]	2017 ESC/EACTS Guidelines[4]
Surgical technique	
In patients with severe primary MR for whom surgery is indicated, mitral valve repair is recommended in preference to mitral valve replacement when the anatomic cause of MR is degenerative disease, if a successful and durable repair is possible. (1 B-NR)	Mitral valve repair should be the preferred technique when the results are expected to be durable. (IC)
In patients with severe primary MR where leaflet pathology is limited to less than one half the posterior leaflet, MVR should not be performed unless mitral valve repair has been attempted at a Primary or Comprehensive Valve Center and was unsuccessful. (3 B-NR)	
Symptomatic patients	
In symptomatic patients with severe primary MR (Stage D), mitral valve intervention is recommended irrespective of LV systolic function. (1 B-NR)	Surgery is indicated in symptomatic patients with LVEF >30%. (IB)
In symptomatic patients with severe primary MR attributable to rheumatic valve disease, mitral valve repair may be considered at a Comprehensive Valve Center by an experienced team when surgical treatment is indicated, if a durable and successful repair is likely. (2b B-NR)	
Asymptomatic patients	
In asymptomatic patients with severe primary MR and LV systolic dysfunction (LVEF ≤60%, LVESD ≥40 mm) (Stage C2), mitral valve surgery is recommended. (1 B-NR)	Surgery is indicated in asymptomatic patients with LV dysfunction (LVESD ≥45 mm* and/or LVEF ≤60%). (IB)
In asymptomatic patients with severe primary MR and normal LV systolic function (LVEF ≥60% and LVESD ≤40 mm) (Stage C1), mitral valve repair is reasonable when the likelihood of a successful and durable repair without residual MR is >95% with an expected mortality rate of <1%, when it can be performed at a Primary or Comprehensive Valve Center. (2a B-NR) In asymptomatic patients with severe primary MR and normal LV systolic function (LVEF >60% and LVESD <40 mm) (Stage C1) but with a progressive increase in LV size or decrease in EF on ≥3 serial imaging studies, mitral valve surgery may be considered irrespective of the probability of a successful and durable repair. (2b C-LD)	Surgery should be considered in asymptomatic patients with preserved LV function (LVESD <45 mm and LVEF >60%) and AF secondary to MR or pulmonary hypertension (sPAP at rest >50 mmHg**). (IIaB) Surgery should be considered in asymptomatic patients with preserved LVEF (>60%) and LVESD 40-44 mm* when a durable repair is likely, surgical risk is low, the repair is performed in heart valve centres, and at least one of the following findings is present: - flail leaflet or, - presence of significant LA dilatation (volume index ≥60 mL/m² BSA) in sinus rhythm. (IIaC)
Patients with severe LV dysfunction	
	Mitral valve repair should be considered in symptomatic patients with severe LV dysfunction (LVEF <30% and/or LVESD >55 mm) refractory to medical therapy when likelihood of successful repair is high and comorbidity low. (IIaC) MVR may be considered in symptomatic patients with severe LV dysfunction (LVEF <30% and/or LVESD >55 mm) refractory to medical therapy when likelihood of successful repair is low and comorbidity low. (IIbC)

*Cut-offs refer to average-size adults and may require adaptations in patients with unusually small or large stature.
**If an elevated sPAP is the only indication for surgery, the value should be confirmed by invasive measurement.
Abbreviations: AF, atrial fibrillation; BSA, body surface area; LA, left atrium; LVEF, left ventricular ejection fraction; LVESD, left ventricular end-systolic dimension; MR, mitral regurgitation; MVR, mitral valve replacement; sPAP, systolic pulmonary artery pressure.

indications to patients with LV end-systolic dimension ≥40 mm and flail leaflet or LA dilatation.[19] The rationale for surgery in asymptomatic severe primary MR is the prevention of irreversible LV systolic dysfunction after surgery. The sharp increase in the risk of mortality as soon as LVEF is <60% or LV end-systolic dimension is >40 mm may be an incentive for considering surgery before reaching these thresholds.[32] Observational data suggest that early surgery may be associated with better outcome than indications based on symptoms or hemodynamic consequences of MR on the LV.[27,198] Discrepancies between the ACC/AHA and ESC/EACTS guidelines reflect the lack of strong evidence supporting reliable

identification markers of the risk of postoperative irreversible LV dysfunction.[199] Current thresholds of LV dimensions or LVEF have been identified in relatively small observational series and have not been evaluated in randomized controlled trials. Multivariable risk scores seem a promising approach assessing the risk of late mortality in patients with primary MR after mitral valve surgery or receiving optimal guideline-directed medical therapy.[200] Beyond pending concerns regarding the optimal timing of surgery in asymptomatic severe primary MR, prerequisites for early surgery combine low operative risk and high likelihood of durable valve repair. This highlights the need for referring most of these patients

TABLE 30–8. Recommendations for Isolated Mitral Valve Surgery in Chronic, Severe Primary MR. Comparison between ACC/AHA and ESC/EACTS Guidelines

	2020 ACC/AHA guidelines[3]	2017 ESC/EACTS guidelines[4]
Surgical technique		
Mitral valve repair is preferred over valve replacement:		I C
When the results are expected to be durable.		
When the anatomic cause of MR is degenerative disease, if a successful and durable repair is possible.	1 B-NR	
Symptomatic patients		
Symptomatic patients with LVEF >30%.		I B
Symptomatic patients, irrespective of LV function.	1 B-NR	
For rheumatic valve disease when performed at a Comprehensive Valve Center by an experienced team if a durable and successful repair is likely.	2b B-NR	
Asymptomatic patients		
LVESD ≥45 mm and/or LVEF ≤60%.		I B
LVESD ≥40 mm and/or LVEF ≤60%.	1 B-NR	
LVEF >60% and LVESD <45 mm with a high likelihood of a successful and durable repair and new onset of AF or resting pulmonary hypertension (sPAP >50 mm Hg).		IIaB
LVEF >60% and LVESD <40 mm in whom the likelihood of a successful and durable repair without residual MR is >95% with an expected mortality rate <1% when performed at a Primary or Comprehensive Valve Center.	2a B-NR	
LVEF >60% and LVESD 40–44 mm when a durable repair is likely, surgical risk is low, the repair is performed in heart valve centers, and flail leaflet or significant LA dilatation (≥60 mL/m² BSA) in sinus rhythm.		IIaC
LVEF >60% and LVESD <40 mm but with a progressive increase in LV size or decrease in EF on ≥3 serial imaging studies, irrespective of the probability of a successful and durable repair.	2b C-LD	
Symptomatic patients with severe LV dysfunction		
LVEF <30% and/or LVESD >55 mm) refractory to medical therapy when likelihood of successful repair is high and comorbidity low.		IIaB
LVEF <30% and/or LVESD >55 mm) refractory to medical therapy when likelihood of successful repair is low and comorbidity low.		IIbC

Abbreviations: AF, atrial fibrillation; BSA, body surface area; EF, ejection fraction; LV, left ventricle; LVESD, left ventricular end-systolic dimension; MR, mitral regurgitation; sPAP, systolic pulmonary artery pressure.

to specialized centers since operative mortality and the feasibility of valve repair depend on annual case volumes.[201,202] When asymptomatic patients with severe primary MR are not considered for surgery, they should be informed on the need for close clinical and echocardiographic follow-up to avoid progressive deterioration of LV function that may occur without any symptoms.

In patients with LVEF <30%, indications for surgery are more restrictive in the ESC/EACTS guidelines.[19] Patients with severe primary MR and severe LV dysfunction have a worse outcome after surgery than those with moderate LV dysfunction; however, they still derive a clinical benefit as compared with the outcome when treated conservatively (medical therapy), which is particularly poor.[32]

Both ACC/AHA and ESC/EACTS guidelines consider indications of transcatheter edge-to-edge mitral valve repair as an alternative to surgery in patients with primary MR who are contraindicated to or at high risk for surgery, providing anatomical conditions are suitable.

With regards to the adherence to guidelines in current practice, surveys performed in 2007 and 2009 have shown an underuse of mitral valve surgery despite guideline-directed indications for surgery.[203,204] A recent European survey reported a better concordance between class I recommendations and a decision to intervene in patients with severe, symptomatic primary MR who were referred to a hospital.[8] However, the adherence to guidelines was lower for primary MR than for aortic valve disease and almost 30% of patients with a class I indication were denied (or not referred for) surgery. Interventions are even more likely to be underused in the community than in hospitals, as attested in a recent community cohort study showing only 27% rate of intervention in patients with primary MR and a class I indication for surgery.[60] These findings based on patient data are consistent with surveys performed among practitioners, which shows significant gaps between guidelines and the different steps in the management of patients with primary MR.[205,206]

The longstanding debate on the optimal timing of surgery in patients with asymptomatic severe MR should not hide the need for improving guideline implementation so that patients with undisputable indications for intervention are less frequently denied surgery.

REFERENCES

1. Andell P, Li X, Martinsson A, et al. Epidemiology of valvular heart disease in a Swedish nationwide hospital-based register study. *Heart.* 2017;103:1696-1703. doi: 10.1136/heartjnl-2016-310894.

2. d'Arcy JL, Coffey S, Loudon MA, et al. Large-scale community echocardiographic screening reveals a major burden of undiagnosed valvular heart disease in older people: the OxVALVE Population Cohort Study. *Eur Heart J.* 2016;37:3515-3522. doi: 10.1093/eurheartj/ehw229.

3. Messika-Zeitoun D, Candolfi P, Vahanian A, et al. Dismal outcomes and high societal burden of mitral valve regurgitation in France in the recent era: a nationwide perspective. *J Am Heart Assoc.* 2020;9:e016086. doi:10.1161/JAHA.120.016086.

4. Dziadzko V, Dziadzko M, Medina-Inojosa JR, et al. Causes and mechanisms of isolated mitral regurgitation in the community: clinical context and outcome. *Eur Heart J.* 2019;40:2194-2202. doi: 10.1093/eurheartj/ehz314.

5. Weir-McCall JR, Blanke P, Naoum C, Delgado V, Bax JJ, Leipsic J. Mitral valve imaging with CT: relationship with transcatheter mitral valve interventions. *Radiology.* 2018;288:638-655. doi: 10.1148/radiol.2018172758.

6. Fidock B, Archer G, Barker N, et al. Standard and emerging CMR methods for mitral regurgitation quantification. *Int J Cardiol.* 2021;331:316-321. doi: 10.1016/j.ijcard.2021.01.066.

7. Zuhlke L, Engel ME, Karthikeyan G, et al. Characteristics, complications, and gaps in evidence-based interventions in rheumatic heart disease: the Global Rheumatic Heart Disease Registry (the REMEDY study). *Eur Heart J.* 2015;36:1115-1122a. doi: 10.1093/eurheartj/ehu449.

8. Iung B, Delgado V, Rosenhek R, et al. Contemporary presentation and management of valvular heart disease: the EURObservational Research Programme Valvular Heart Disease II Survey. *Circulation.* 2019;140:1156-1169. doi: 10.1161/CIRCULATIONAHA.119.041080.

9. El Sabbagh A, Reddy YNV, Nishimura RA. Mitral valve regurgitation in the contemporary era: insights into diagnosis, management, and future directions. *JACC Cardiovasc Imaging.* 2018;11:628-643. doi: 10.1016/j.jcmg.2018.01.009.

10. Anyanwu AC, Adams DH. Etiologic classification of degenerative mitral valve disease: Barlow's disease and fibroelastic deficiency. *Semin Thorac Cardiovasc Surg.* 2007;19:90-96. doi: 10.1053/j.semtcvs.2007.04.002.

11. Dejgaard LA, Skjolsvik ET, Lie OH, et al. The mitral annulus disjunction arrhythmic syndrome. *J Am Coll Cardiol.* 2018;72:1600-1609. doi: 10.1016/j.jacc.2018.07.070.

12. Antoine C, Mantovani F, Benfari G, et al. Pathophysiology of degenerative mitral regurgitation: new 3-dimensional imaging insights. *Circ Cardiovasc Imaging.* 2018;11:e005971. doi: 10.1161/CIRCIMAGING.116.005971.

13. Adams DH, Rosenhek R, Falk V. Degenerative mitral valve regurgitation: best practice revolution. *Eur Heart J.* 2010;31:1958-1966. doi: 10.1093/eurheartj/ehq222.

14. Basso C, Perazzolo Marra M, Rizzo S, et al. Arrhythmic mitral valve prolapse and sudden cardiac death. *Circulation.* 2015;132:556-566. doi: 10.1161/CIRCULATIONAHA.115.016291.

15. Basso C, Iliceto S, Thiene G, Perazzolo Marra M. Mitral valve prolapse, ventricular arrhythmias, and sudden death. *Circulation.* 2019;140:952-964. doi: 10.1161/CIRCULATIONAHA.118.034075.

16. Pizarro R, Bazzino OO, Oberti PF, et al. Prospective validation of the prognostic usefulness of brain natriuretic peptide in asymptomatic patients with chronic severe mitral regurgitation. *J Am Coll Cardiol.* 2009;54:1099-1106. doi: 10.1016/j.jacc.2009.06.013.

17. Lancellotti P, Tribouilloy C, Hagendorff A, et al. Recommendations for the echocardiographic assessment of native valvular regurgitation: an executive summary from the European Association of Cardiovascular Imaging. *Eur Heart J Cardiovasc Imaging.* 2013;14:611-644. doi: 10.1093/ehjci/jet105.

18. Zoghbi WA, Adams D, Bonow RO, et al. Recommendations for noninvasive evaluation of native valvular regurgitation: a report from the American Society of Echocardiography Developed in Collaboration with the Society for Cardiovascular Magnetic Resonance. *J Am Soc Echocardiogr.* 2017;30:303-371. doi: 10.1016/j.echo.2017.01.007.

19. Baumgartner H, Falk V, Bax JJ, et al. 2017 ESC/EACTS Guidelines for the management of valvular heart disease. *Eur Heart J.* 2017;38:2739-2791. doi: 10.1093/eurheartj/ehx391.

20. Otto CM, Nishimura RA, Bonow RO, et al. 2020 ACC/AHA guideline for the management of patients with valvular heart disease: a report of the American College of Cardiology/American Heart Association Joint Committee on Clinical Practice Guidelines. *Circulation.* 2021;143:e72-e227. doi: 10.1161/CIR.0000000000000923.

21. Lang RM, Badano LP, Tsang W, et al. EAE/ASE recommendations for image acquisition and display using three-dimensional echocardiography. *Eur Heart J Cardiovasc Imaging.* 2012;13:1-46. doi: 10.1093/ehjci/jer316.

22. Thavendiranathan P, Phelan D, Thomas JD, Flamm SD, Marwick TH. Quantitative assessment of mitral regurgitation: validation of new methods. *J Am Coll Cardiol.* 2012;60:1470-1483. doi: 10.1016/j.jacc.2012.05.048.

23. Marsan NA, Westenberg JJ, Ypenburg C, et al. Quantification of functional mitral regurgitation by real-time 3D echocardiography: comparison with 3D velocity-encoded cardiac magnetic resonance. *JACC Cardiovasc Imaging.* 2009;2:1245-1252. doi: 10.1016/j.jcmg.2009.07.006.

24. Lang RM, Badano LP, Mor-Avi V, et al. Recommendations for cardiac chamber quantification by echocardiography in adults: an update from the American Society of Echocardiography and the European Association of Cardiovascular Imaging. *Eur Heart J Cardiovasc Imaging.* 2015;16:233-270. doi: 10.1093/ehjci/jev014.

25. Hiemstra YL, Tomsic A, van Wijngaarden SE, et al. Prognostic value of global longitudinal strain and etiology after surgery for primary mitral regurgitation. *JACC Cardiovasc Imaging.* 2020;13:577-585. doi: 10.1016/j.jcmg.2019.03.024.

26. Myerson SG, d'Arcy J, Christiansen JP, et al. Determination of clinical outcome in mitral regurgitation with cardiovascular magnetic resonance quantification. *Circulation.* 2016;133:2287-2296. doi: 10.1161/CIRCULATIONAHA.115.017888.

27. Suri RM, Vanoverschelde JL, Grigioni F, et al. Association between early surgical intervention vs watchful waiting and outcomes for mitral regurgitation due to flail mitral valve leaflets. *JAMA.* 2013;310:609-616. doi: 10.1001/jama.2013.8643.

28. Ling LH, Enriquez-Sarano M, Seward JB, et al. Early surgery in patients with mitral regurgitation due to flail leaflets: a long-term outcome study. *Circulation.* 1997;96:1819-1825. doi: 10.1161/01.cir.96.6.1819.

29. Kang DH, Kim JH, Rim JH, et al. Comparison of early surgery versus conventional treatment in asymptomatic severe mitral regurgitation. *Circulation.* 2009;119:797-804. doi: 10.1161/CIRCULATIONAHA.108.802314.

30. Grigioni F, Enriquez-Sarano M, Ling LH, et al. Sudden death in mitral regurgitation due to flail leaflet. *J Am Coll Cardiol.* 1999;34:2078-2085. doi: 10.1016/s0735-1097(99)00474-x.

31. Avierinos JF, Gersh BJ, Melton LJ 3rd, et al. Natural history of asymptomatic mitral valve prolapse in the community. *Circulation.* 2002;106:1355-1361. doi: 10.1161/01.cir.0000028933.34260.09.

32. Tribouilloy C, Rusinaru D, Grigioni F, et al. Long-term mortality associated with left ventricular dysfunction in mitral regurgitation due to flail leaflets: a multicenter analysis. *Circ Cardiovasc Imaging.* 2014;7:363-370. doi: 10.1161/CIRCIMAGING.113.001251.

33. Levine HJ, Gaasch WH. Vasoactive drugs in chronic regurgitant lesions of the mitral and aortic valves. *J Am Coll Cardiol.* 1996;28:1083-1091. doi: 10.1016/S0735-1097(96)00288-4.

34. Stewart RA, Raffel OC, Kerr AJ, et al. Pilot study to assess the influence of beta-blockade on mitral regurgitant volume and left ventricular work in degenerative mitral valve disease. *Circulation.* 2008;118:1041-1046. doi: 10.1161/CIRCULATIONAHA.108.770438.

35. Baddour LM, Wilson WR, Bayer AS, et al. Infective endocarditis in adults: diagnosis, antimicrobial therapy, and management of complications: a scientific statement for healthcare professionals from the

American Heart Association. *Circulation.* 2015;132:1435-1486. doi: 10.1161/CIR.0000000000000296.

36. Habib G, Lancellotti P, Antunes MJ, et al. 2015 ESC guidelines for the management of infective endocarditis: the Task Force for the Management of Infective Endocarditis of the European Society of Cardiology (ESC). Endorsed by: European Association for Cardio-Thoracic Surgery (EACTS), the European Association of Nuclear Medicine (EANM). *Eur Heart J.* 2015;36:3075-3128. doi: 10.1093/eurheartj/ehv319.

37. Millot S, Lesclous P, Colombier ML, et al. Position paper for the evaluation and management of oral status in patients with valvular disease: Groupe de Travail Valvulopathies de la Societe Francaise de Cardiologie, Societe Francaise de Chirurgie Orale, Societe Francaise de Parodontologie et d'Implantologie Orale, Societe Francaise d'Endodontie et Societe de Pathologie Infectieuse de Langue Francaise. *Arch Cardiovasc Dis.* 2017;110:482-494. doi: 10.1016/j.acvd.2017.01.012.

38. French Society of Oral Surgery. Management of oral-dental foci of infection. 2012. http://www.societechirorale.com/documents/Recommandations/foyers_infectieux_argument-EN.pdf. Accessed November 20, 2020.

39. French Society of Oral Surgery. Perioperative management of patients treated with antithrombotics in oral surgery. 2015. https://societechirorale.com/documents/Recommandations/recommandations_festion_peri_operatoire_2015_argumentaire-EN.pdf. Accessed November 20, 2020.

40. Perier P, Hohenberger W, Lakew F, Diegeler A. Prolapse of the posterior leaflet: resect or respect. *Ann Cardiothorac Surg.* 2015;4:273-277. doi: 10.3978/j.issn.2225-319X.2014.11.16.

41. Alreshidan M, Herron RD, Wei LM, et al. Surgical techniques for mitral valve repair: a pathoanatomic grading system. *Semin Cardiothorac Vasc Anesth.* 2019;23:20-25. doi: 10.1177/1089253218815465.

42. Flameng W, Meuris B, Herijgers P, Herregods MC. Durability of mitral valve repair in Barlow disease versus fibroelastic deficiency. *J Thorac Cardiovasc Surg.* 2008;135:274-282. doi: 10.1016/j.jtcvs.2007.06.040.

43. Dreyfus GD, Corbi PJ, Chan KM, Bahrami T. Secondary tricuspid regurgitation or dilatation: which should be the criteria for surgical repair? *Ann Thorac Surg.* 2005;79:127-132. doi: 10.1016/j.athoracsur.2004.06.057.

44. Pfannmueller B, Misfeld M, Davierwala P, Weiss S, Borger MA. Concomitant tricuspid valve repair during minimally invasive mitral valve repair. *Thorac Cardiovasc Surg.* 2020;68:486-491. doi: 10.1055/s-0039-1700506.

45. Jeganathan R, Armstrong S, Al-Alao B, David T. The risk and outcomes of reoperative tricuspid valve surgery. *Ann Thorac Surg.* 2013;95:119-124. doi: 10.1016/j.athoracsur.2012.08.058.

46. Adas A, Elnaggar A, Balbaa Y, Elashkar A, Alkady HM. Ring, band or suture in tricuspid annuloplasty for functional tricuspid regurgitation; which is better and more durable? *Heart Surg Forum.* 2019;22:E411-E415. doi: 10.1532/hsf.2517.

47. Navia JL, Nowicki ER, Blackstone EH, et al. Surgical management of secondary tricuspid valve regurgitation: annulus, commissure, or leaflet procedure? *J Thorac Cardiovasc Surg.* 2010;139:1473-1482.e1475. doi: 10.1016/j.jtcvs.2010.02.046.

48. Grigioni F, Avierinos JF, Ling LH, et al. Atrial fibrillation complicating the course of degenerative mitral regurgitation: determinants and long-term outcome. *J Am Coll Cardiol.* 2002;40:84-92. doi: 10.1016/s0735-1097(02)01922-8.

49. Allessie MA. Atrial electrophysiologic remodeling: another vicious circle? *J Cardiovasc Electrophysiol.* 1998;9:1378-1393. doi: 10.1111/j.1540-8167.1998.tb00114.x.

50. Grigioni F, Benfari G, Vanoverschelde JL, et al. Long-term implications of atrial fibrillation in patients with degenerative mitral regurgitation. *J Am Coll Cardiol.* 2019;73:264-274. doi: 10.1016/j.jacc.2018.10.067.

51. Badhwar V, Rankin JS, Ad N, et al. Surgical ablation of atrial fibrillation in the United States: trends and propensity matched outcomes. *Ann Thorac Surg.* 2017;104:493-500. doi: 10.1016/j.athoracsur.2017.05.016.

52. Ad N, Holmes SD, Massimiano PS, Rongione AJ, Fornaresio LM. Long-term outcome following concomitant mitral valve surgery and Cox maze procedure for atrial fibrillation. *J Thorac Cardiovasc Surg.* 2018;155:983-994. doi: 10.1016/j.jtcvs.2017.09.147.

53. Mihaljevic T, Jarrett CM, Gillinov AM, et al. Robotic repair of posterior mitral valve prolapse versus conventional approaches: potential realized. *J Thorac Cardiovasc Surg.* 2011;141:72-80.e71-74. doi: 10.1016/j.jtcvs.2010.09.008.

54. Chikwe J, Toyoda N, Anyanwu AC, et al. Relation of mitral valve surgery volume to repair rate, durability, and survival. *J Am Coll Cardiol.* 2017. doi: 10.1016/j.jacc.2017.02.026.

55. Enriquez-Sarano M, Sundt TM 3rd. Early surgery is recommended for mitral regurgitation. *Circulation.* 2010;121:804-811; discussion 812. doi: 10.1161/CIRCULATIONAHA.109.868083.

56. Casselman FP, Van Slycke S, Dom H, Lambrechts DL, Vermeulen Y, Vanermen H. Endoscopic mitral valve repair: feasible, reproducible, and durable. *J Thorac Cardiovasc Surg.* 2003;125:273-282. doi: 10.1067/mtc.2003.19.

57. Seeburger J, Borger MA, Falk V, et al. Minimal invasive mitral valve repair for mitral regurgitation: results of 1339 consecutive patients. *Eur J Cardiothorac Surg.* 2008;34:760-765. doi: 10.1016/j.ejcts.2008.05.015.

58. Davierwala PM, Seeburger J, Pfannmueller B, et al. Minimally invasive mitral valve surgery: "The Leipzig experience." *Ann Cardiothorac Surg.* 2013;2:744-750. doi: 10.3978/j.issn.2225-319X.2013.10.14.

59. Murphy DA, Moss E, Binongo J, et al. The expanding role of endoscopic robotics in mitral valve surgery: 1,257 consecutive procedures. *Ann Thorac Surg.* 2015;100:1675-1681; discussion 1681-1672. doi: 10.1016/j.athoracsur.2015.05.068.

60. Dziadzko V, Clavel MA, Dziadzko M, et al. Outcome and undertreatment of mitral regurgitation: a community cohort study. *Lancet.* 2018;391:960-969. doi: 10.1016/S0140-6736(18)30473-2.

61. van der Bijl P, Khidir M, Ajmone Marsan N, et al. Effect of functional mitral regurgitation on outcome in patients receiving cardiac resynchronization therapy for heart failure. *Am J Cardiol.* 2019;123:75-83. doi: 10.1016/j.amjcard.2018.09.020.

62. Bursi F, Enriquez-Sarano M, Nkomo VT, et al. Heart failure and death after myocardial infarction in the community: the emerging role of mitral regurgitation. *Circulation.* 2005;111:295-301. doi: 10.1161/01.CIR.0000151097.30779.04.

63. Agricola E, Stella S, Figini F, et al. Non-ischemic dilated cardiopathy: prognostic value of functional mitral regurgitation. *Int J Cardiol.* 2011;146:426-428. doi: 10.1016/j.ijcard.2010.10.096.

64. Rossi A, Dini FL, Faggiano P, et al. Independent prognostic value of functional mitral regurgitation in patients with heart failure. A quantitative analysis of 1256 patients with ischaemic and non-ischaemic dilated cardiomyopathy. *Heart.* 2011;97:1675-1680. doi: 10.1136/hrt.2011.225789.

65. Chan KM, Wage R, Symmonds K, et al. Towards comprehensive assessment of mitral regurgitation using cardiovascular magnetic resonance. *J Cardiovasc Magn Reson.* 2008;10:61. doi: 10.1186/1532-429X-10-61.

66. Muraru D, Guta AC, Ochoa-Jimenez RC, et al. Functional regurgitation of atrioventricular valves and atrial fibrillation: an elusive pathophysiological link deserving further attention. *J Am Soc Echocardiogr.* 2020;33:42-53. doi: 10.1016/j.echo.2019.08.016.

67. Silbiger JJ. Does left atrial enlargement contribute to mitral leaflet tethering in patients with functional mitral regurgitation? Proposed role of atriogenic leaflet tethering. *Echocardiography.* 2014;31:1310-1311. doi: 10.1111/echo.12629.

68. Kagiyama N, Mondillo S, Yoshida K, Mandoli GE, Cameli M. Subtypes of atrial functional mitral regurgitation: imaging insights into their mechanisms and therapeutic implications. *JACC Cardiovasc Imaging.* 2020;13:820-835. doi: 10.1016/j.jcmg.2019.01.040.

69. Packer M, Grayburn PA. Neurohormonal and transcatheter repair strategies for proportionate and disproportionate functional mitral regurgitation in heart failure. *JACC Heart Fail.* 2019;7:518-521. doi: 10.1016/j.jchf.2019.03.016.

70. Kwan J, Shiota T, Agler DA, et al. Geometric differences of the mitral apparatus between ischemic and dilated cardiomyopathy with

significant mitral regurgitation: real-time three-dimensional echocardiography study. *Circulation*. 2003;107:1135-1140. doi: 10.1161/01.cir.0000053558.55471.2d.

71. Debonnaire P, Al Amri I, Leong DP, et al. Leaflet remodelling in functional mitral valve regurgitation: characteristics, determinants, and relation to regurgitation severity. *Eur Heart J Cardiovasc Imaging*. 2015;16:290-299. doi: 10.1093/ehjci/jeu216.

72. Chaput M, Handschumacher MD, Tournoux F, et al. Mitral leaflet adaptation to ventricular remodeling: occurrence and adequacy in patients with functional mitral regurgitation. *Circulation*. 2008;118:845-852. doi: 10.1161/CIRCULATIONAHA.107.749440.

73. Goliasch G, Bartko PE, Pavo N, et al. Refining the prognostic impact of functional mitral regurgitation in chronic heart failure. *Eur Heart J*. 2018;39:39-46. doi: 10.1093/eurheartj/ehx402.

74. Dini FL, Fontanive P, Conti U, Andreini D, Cabani E, De Tommasi SM. Plasma N-terminal protype-B natriuretic peptide levels in risk assessment of patients with mitral regurgitation secondary to ischemic and nonischemic dilated cardiomyopathy. *Am Heart J*. 2008;155:1121-1127. doi: 10.1016/j.ahj.2008.01.003.

75. Delgado V, Tops LF, Schuijf JD, et al. Assessment of mitral valve anatomy and geometry with multislice computed tomography. *JACC Cardiovasc Imaging*. 2009;2:556-565. doi: 10.1016/j.jcmg.2008.12.025.

76. Yu HY, Su MY, Liao TY, Peng HH, Lin FY, Tseng WY. Functional mitral regurgitation in chronic ischemic coronary artery disease: analysis of geometric alterations of mitral apparatus with magnetic resonance imaging. *J Thorac Cardiovasc Surg*. 2004;128:543-551. doi: 10.1016/j.jtcvs.2004.04.015.

77. Ciarka A, Braun J, Delgado V, et al. Predictors of mitral regurgitation recurrence in patients with heart failure undergoing mitral valve annuloplasty. *Am J Cardiol*. 2010;106:395-401. doi: 10.1016/j.amjcard.2010.03.042.

78. Lee AP, Acker M, Kubo SH, et al. Mechanisms of recurrent functional mitral regurgitation after mitral valve repair in nonischemic dilated cardiomyopathy: importance of distal anterior leaflet tethering. *Circulation*. 2009;119:2606-2614. doi: 10.1161/CIRCULATIONAHA.108.796151.

79. Magne J, Pibarot P, Dagenais F, Hachicha Z, Dumesnil JG, Senechal M. Preoperative posterior leaflet angle accurately predicts outcome after restrictive mitral valve annuloplasty for ischemic mitral regurgitation. *Circulation*. 2007;115:782-791. doi: 10.1161/CIRCULATIONAHA.106.649236.

80. van Wijngaarden SE, Kamperidis V, Regeer MV, et al. Three-dimensional assessment of mitral valve annulus dynamics and impact on quantification of mitral regurgitation. *Eur Heart J Cardiovasc Imaging*. 2018;19:176-184. doi: 10.1093/ehjci/jex001.

81. Salgo IS, Gorman JH 3rd, Gorman RC, et al. Effect of annular shape on leaflet curvature in reducing mitral leaflet stress. *Circulation*. 2002;106:711-717. doi: 10.1161/01.cir.0000025426.39426.83.

82. Grayburn PA, Sannino A, Packer M. Proportionate and disproportionate functional mitral regurgitation: a new conceptual framework that reconciles the results of the MITRA-FR and COAPT Trials. *JACC Cardiovasc Imaging*. 2019;12:353-362. doi: 10.1016/j.jcmg.2018.11.006.

83. Kamperidis V, Marsan NA, Delgado V, Bax JJ. Left ventricular systolic function assessment in secondary mitral regurgitation: left ventricular ejection fraction vs. speckle tracking global longitudinal strain. *Eur Heart J*. 2016;37:811-816. doi: 10.1093/eurheartj/ehv680.

84. Namazi F, van der Bijl P, Hirasawa K, et al. Prognostic value of left ventricular global longitudinal strain in patients with secondary mitral regurgitation. *J Am Coll Cardiol*. 2020;75:750-758. doi: 10.1016/j.jacc.2019.12.024.

85. Lancellotti P, Troisfontaines P, Toussaint AC, Pierard LA. Prognostic importance of exercise-induced changes in mitral regurgitation in patients with chronic ischemic left ventricular dysfunction. *Circulation*. 2003;108:1713-1717. doi: 10.1161/01.CIR.0000087599.49332.05.

86. van Bommel RJ, Marsan NA, Delgado V, et al. Cardiac resynchronization therapy as a therapeutic option in patients with moderate-severe functional mitral regurgitation and high operative risk. *Circulation*. 2011;124:912-919. doi: 10.1161/CIRCULATIONAHA.110.009803.

87. Lancellotti P, Melon P, Sakalihasan N, et al. Effect of cardiac resynchronization therapy on functional mitral regurgitation in heart failure. *Am J Cardiol*. 2004;94:1462-1465. doi: 10.1016/j.amjcard.2004.07.154.

88. Garg P, Swift AJ, Zhong L, et al. Assessment of mitral valve regurgitation by cardiovascular magnetic resonance imaging. *Nat Rev Cardiol*. 2020;17:298-312. doi: 10.1038/s41569-019-0305-z.

89. Lopes BBC, Kwon DH, Shah DJ, et al. Importance of myocardial fibrosis in functional mitral regurgitation: from outcomes to decision-making. *JACC Cardiovasc Imaging*. 2021;14:867-878. doi: 10.1016/j.jcmg.2020.10.027.

90. Tayal B, Debs D, Nabi F, et al. Impact of myocardial scar on prognostic implication of secondary mitral regurgitation in heart failure. *JACC Cardiovasc Imaging*. 2021;14:812-822. doi: 10.1016/j.jcmg.2020.11.004.

91. Blanke P, Dvir D, Cheung A, et al. A simplified D-shaped model of the mitral annulus to facilitate CT-based sizing before transcatheter mitral valve implantation. *J Cardiovasc Comput Tomogr*. 2014;8:459-467. doi: 10.1016/j.jcct.2014.09.009.

92. Meduri CU, Reardon MJ, Lim DS, et al. Novel multiphase assessment for predicting left ventricular outflow tract obstruction before transcatheter mitral valve replacement. *JACC Cardiovasc Interv*. 2019;12:2402-2412. doi: 10.1016/j.jcin.2019.06.015.

93. Grigioni F, Enriquez-Sarano M, Zehr KJ, Bailey KR, Tajik AJ. Ischemic mitral regurgitation: long-term outcome and prognostic implications with quantitative Doppler assessment. *Circulation*. 2001;103:1759-1764. doi: 10.1161/01.cir.103.13.1759.

94. Asgar AW, Mack MJ, Stone GW. Secondary mitral regurgitation in heart failure: pathophysiology, prognosis, and therapeutic considerations. *J Am Coll Cardiol*. 2015;65:1231-1248. doi: 10.1016/j.jacc.2015.02.009.

95. Ponikowski P, Voors AA, Anker SD, et al. 2016 ESC guidelines for the diagnosis and treatment of acute and chronic heart failure: The Task Force for the Diagnosis and Treatment of Acute and Chronic Heart Failure of the European Society of Cardiology (ESC) Developed with the special contribution of the Heart Failure Association (HFA) of the ESC. *Eur Heart J*. 2016;37:2129-2200. doi: 10.1093/eurheartj/ehw128.

96. Nasser R, Van Assche L, Vorlat A, et al. Evolution of functional mitral regurgitation and prognosis in medically managed heart failure patients with reduced ejection fraction. *JACC Heart Fail*. 2017;5:652-659. doi: 10.1016/j.jchf.2017.06.015.

97. Kang DH, Park SJ, Shin SH, et al. Angiotensin receptor neprilysin inhibitor for functional mitral regurgitation. *Circulation*. 2019;139:1354-1365. doi: 10.1161/CIRCULATIONAHA.118.037077.

98. Brandt RR, Reiner C, Arnold R, Sperzel J, Pitschner HF, Hamm CW. Contractile response and mitral regurgitation after temporary interruption of long-term cardiac resynchronization therapy. *Eur Heart J*. 2006;27:187-192. doi: 10.1093/eurheartj/ehi558.

99. Onishi T, Onishi T, Marek JJ, et al. Mechanistic features associated with improvement in mitral regurgitation after cardiac resynchronization therapy and their relation to long-term patient outcome. *Circ Heart Fail*. 2013;6:685-693. doi: 10.1161/CIRCHEARTFAILURE.112.000112.

100. Auricchio A, Schillinger W, Meyer S, et al. Correction of mitral regurgitation in nonresponders to cardiac resynchronization therapy by MitraClip improves symptoms and promotes reverse remodeling. *J Am Coll Cardiol*. 2011;58:2183-2189. doi: 10.1016/j.jacc.2011.06.061.

101. Bolling SF, Deeb GM, Brunsting LA, Bach DS. Early outcome of mitral valve reconstruction in patients with end-stage cardiomyopathy. *J Thorac Cardiovasc Surg*. 1995;109:676-682; discussion 682-673. doi: 10.1016/S0022-5223(95)70348-9.

102. Bach DS, Bolling SF. Early improvement in congestive heart failure after correction of secondary mitral regurgitation in end-stage cardiomyopathy. *Am Heart J*. 1995;129:1165-1170. doi: 10.1016/0002-8703(95)90399-2.

103. Bolling SF, Pagani FD, Deeb GM, Bach DS. Intermediate-term outcome of mitral reconstruction in cardiomyopathy. *J Thorac Cardiovasc Surg*. 1998;115:381-386; discussion 387-388. doi: 10.1016/S0022-5223(98)70282-X.

104. Silberman S, Klutstein MW, Sabag T, et al. Repair of ischemic mitral regurgitation: comparison between flexible and rigid annuloplasty

rings. *Ann Thorac Surg.* 2009;87:1721-1726; discussion 1726-1727. doi: 10.1016/j.athoracsur.2009.03.066.

105. Bax JJ, Braun J, Somer ST, et al. Restrictive annuloplasty and coronary revascularization in ischemic mitral regurgitation results in reverse left ventricular remodeling. *Circulation.* 2004;110:II103-II108. doi: 10.1161/01.CIR.0000138196.06772.4e.

106. Braun J, van de Veire NR, Klautz RJ, et al. Restrictive mitral annuloplasty cures ischemic mitral regurgitation and heart failure. *Ann Thorac Surg.* 2008;85:430-436; discussion 436-437. doi: 10.1016/j.athoracsur.2007.08.040.

107. Geidel S, Lass M, Schneider C, et al. Downsizing of the mitral valve and coronary revascularization in severe ischemic mitral regurgitation results in reverse left ventricular and left atrial remodeling. *Eur J Cardiothorac Surg.* 2005;27:1011-1016. doi: 10.1016/j.ejcts.2005.02.025.

108. Gelsomino S, Lorusso R, De Cicco G, et al. Five-year echocardiographic results of combined undersized mitral ring annuloplasty and coronary artery bypass grafting for chronic ischaemic mitral regurgitation. *Eur Heart J.* 2008;29:231-240. doi: 10.1093/eurheartj/ehm468.

109. Crabtree TD, Bailey MS, Moon MR, et al. Recurrent mitral regurgitation and risk factors for early and late mortality after mitral valve repair for functional ischemic mitral regurgitation. *Ann Thorac Surg.* 2008;85: 1537-1542; discussion 1542-1533. doi: 10.1016/j.athoracsur.2008.01.079.

110. Onorati F, Rubino AS, Marturano D, et al. Midterm clinical and echocardiographic results and predictors of mitral regurgitation recurrence following restrictive annuloplasty for ischemic cardiomyopathy. *J Thorac Cardiovasc Surg.* 2009;138:654-662. doi: 10.1016/j.jtcvs.2009.01.020.

111. Hung J, Papakostas L, Tahta SA, et al. Mechanism of recurrent ischemic mitral regurgitation after annuloplasty: continued LV remodeling as a moving target. *Circulation.* 2004;110:II85-II90. doi: 10.1161/01.CIR.0000138192.65015.45.

112. Braun J, Bax JJ, Versteegh MI, et al. Preoperative left ventricular dimensions predict reverse remodeling following restrictive mitral annuloplasty in ischemic mitral regurgitation. *Eur J Cardiothorac Surg.* 2005;27: 847-853. doi: 10.1016/j.ejcts.2004.12.031.

113. Roshanali F, Mandegar MH, Yousefnia MA, Rayatzadeh H, Alaeddini F. A prospective study of predicting factors in ischemic mitral regurgitation recurrence after ring annuloplasty. *Ann Thorac Surg.* 2007;84:745-749. doi: 10.1016/j.athoracsur.2007.04.106.

114. Petrus AHJ, Dekkers OM, Tops LF, Timmer E, Klautz RJM, Braun J. Impact of recurrent mitral regurgitation after mitral valve repair for functional mitral regurgitation: long-term analysis of competing outcomes. *Eur Heart J.* 2019;40:2206-2214. doi: 10.1093/eurheartj/ehz306.

115. Kincaid EH, Riley RD, Hines MH, Hammon JW, Kon ND. Anterior leaflet augmentation for ischemic mitral regurgitation. *Ann Thorac Surg.* 2004;78:564-568; discussion 568. doi: 10.1016/j.athoracsur.2004.02.040.

116. de Varennes B, Chaturvedi R, Sidhu S, et al. Initial results of posterior leaflet extension for severe type IIIb ischemic mitral regurgitation. *Circulation.* 2009;119:2837-2843. doi: 10.1161/CIRCULATIONAHA.108.831412.

117. Calafiore AM, Totaro A, De Amicis V, et al. Surgical mitral plasticity for chronic ischemic mitral regurgitation. *J Card Surg.* 2020;35:772-778. doi: 10.1111/jocs.14487.

118. Umana JP, Salehizadeh B, DeRose JJ Jr., et al. "Bow-tie" mitral valve repair: an adjuvant technique for ischemic mitral regurgitation. *Ann Thorac Surg.* 1998;66:1640-1646. doi: 10.1016/s0003-4975(98)00828-5.

119. Kinnaird TD, Munt BI, Ignaszewski AP, Abel JG, Thompson RC. Edge-to-edge repair for functional mitral regurgitation: an echocardiographic study of the hemodynamic consequences. *J Heart Valve Dis.* 2003;12:280-286.

120. Bhudia SK, McCarthy PM, Smedira NG, Lam BK, Rajeswaran J, Blackstone EH. Edge-to-edge (Alfieri) mitral repair: results in diverse clinical settings. *Ann Thorac Surg.* 2004;77:1598-1606. doi: 10.1016/j.athoracsur.2003.09.090.

121. De Bonis M, Lapenna E, La Canna G, et al. Mitral valve repair for functional mitral regurgitation in end-stage dilated cardiomyopathy: role of the "edge-to-edge" technique. *Circulation.* 2005;112:I402-408. doi: 10.1161/CIRCULATIONAHA.104.525188.

122. De Bonis M, Lapenna E, Barili F, et al. Long-term results of mitral repair in patients with severe left ventricular dysfunction and secondary mitral regurgitation: does the technique matter? *Eur J Cardiothorac Surg.* 2016;50:882-889. doi: 10.1093/ejcts/ezw139.

123. Harmel EK, Reichenspurner H, Girdauskas E. Subannular reconstruction in secondary mitral regurgitation: a meta-analysis. *Heart.* 2018;104:1783-1790. doi: 10.1136/heartjnl-2017-312277.

124. Borger MA, Murphy PM, Alam A, et al. Initial results of the chordal-cutting operation for ischemic mitral regurgitation. *J Thorac Cardiovasc Surg.* 2007;133:1483-1492. doi: 10.1016/j.jtcvs.2007.01.064.

125. Calafiore AM, Refaie R, Iaco AL, et al. Chordal cutting in ischemic mitral regurgitation: a propensity-matched study. *J Thorac Cardiovasc Surg.* 2014;148:41-46. doi: 10.1016/j.jtcvs.2013.07.036.

126. Harmel E, Pausch J, Gross T, et al. Standardized subannular repair improves outcomes in type IIIb functional mitral regurgitation. *Ann Thorac Surg.* 2019;108:1783-1792. doi: 10.1016/j.athoracsur.2019.04.120.

127. Langer F, Kunihara T, Hell K, et al. RING+STRING: successful repair technique for ischemic mitral regurgitation with severe leaflet tethering. *Circulation.* 2009;120:S85-S91. doi: 10.1161/CIRCULATIONAHA.108.840173.

128. Langer F, Schafers HJ. RING plus STRING: papillary muscle repositioning as an adjunctive repair technique for ischemic mitral regurgitation. *J Thorac Cardiovasc Surg.* 2007;133:247-249. doi: 10.1016/j.jtcvs.2006.04.059.

129. Shingu Y, Yamada S, Ooka T, et al. Papillary muscle suspension concomitant with approximation for functional mitral regurgitation. *Circ J.* 2009;73:2061-2067. doi: 10.1253/circj.cj-09-0129.

130. Wakasa S, Shingu Y, Ooka T, Katoh H, Tachibana T, Matsui Y. Surgical strategy for ischemic mitral regurgitation adopting subvalvular and ventricular procedures. *Ann Thorac Cardiovasc Surg.* 2015;21:370-377. doi: 10.5761/atcs.oa.14-00204.

131. Wakasa S, Kubota S, Shingu Y, Ooka T, Tachibana T, Matsui Y. The extent of papillary muscle approximation affects mortality and durability of mitral valve repair for ischemic mitral regurgitation. *J Cardiothorac Surg.* 2014;9:98. doi: 10.1186/1749-8090-9-98.

132. Fattouch K, Lancellotti P, Castrovinci S, et al. Papillary muscle relocation in conjunction with valve annuloplasty improve repair results in severe ischemic mitral regurgitation. *J Thorac Cardiovasc Surg.* 2012;143: 1352-1355. doi: 10.1016/j.jtcvs.2011.09.062.

133. Fattouch K, Castrovinci S, Murana G, et al. Papillary muscle relocation and mitral annuloplasty in ischemic mitral valve regurgitation: midterm results. *J Thorac Cardiovasc Surg.* 2014;148:1947-1950. doi: 10.1016/j.jtcvs.2014.02.047.

134. Roshanali F, Vedadian A, Shoar S, Naderan M, Mandegar MH. Efficacy of papillary muscle approximation in preventing functional mitral regurgitation recurrence in high-risk patients with ischaemic cardiomyopathy and mitral annuloplasty. *Acta Cardiol.* 2013;68:271-278. doi: 10.1080/ac.68.3.2983421.

135. Nappi F, Lusini M, Spadaccio C, et al. Papillary muscle approximation versus restrictive annuloplasty alone for severe ischemic mitral regurgitation. *J Am Coll Cardiol.* 2016;67:2334-2346. doi: 10.1016/j.jacc.2016.03.478.

136. Acker MA, Parides MK, Perrault LP, et al. Mitral-valve repair versus replacement for severe ischemic mitral regurgitation. *N Engl J Med.* 2014;370:23-32. doi: 10.1056/NEJMoa1312808.

137. Goldstein D, Moskowitz AJ, Gelijns AC, et al. Two-year outcomes of surgical treatment of severe ischemic mitral regurgitation. *N Engl J Med.* 2016;374:344-353. doi: 10.1056/NEJMoa1512913.

138. Matsunaga A, Duran CM. Progression of tricuspid regurgitation after repaired functional ischemic mitral regurgitation. *Circulation.* 2005;112:I453-I457. doi: 10.1161/CIRCULATIONAHA.104.524421.

139. De Bonis M, Lapenna E, Pozzoli A, et al. Mitral valve repair without repair of moderate tricuspid regurgitation. *Ann Thorac Surg.* 2015;100: 2206-2212. doi: 10.1016/j.athoracsur.2015.05.108.

140. Shudo Y, Taniguchi K, Takeda K, et al. Restrictive mitral annuloplasty with or without surgical ventricular restoration in ischemic

dilated cardiomyopathy with severe mitral regurgitation. *Circulation.* 2011;124:S107-S114. doi: 10.1161/CIRCULATIONAHA.110.010330.

141. Kainuma S, Taniguchi K, Toda K, et al. Restrictive mitral annuloplasty with or without surgical ventricular reconstruction in ischaemic cardiomyopathy: impacts on neurohormonal activation, reverse left ventricular remodelling and survival. *Eur J Heart Fail.* 2014;16:189-200. doi: 10.1002/ejhf.24.

142. Hamer AW, Takayama M, Abraham KA, et al. End-systolic volume and long-term survival after coronary artery bypass graft surgery in patients with impaired left ventricular function. *Circulation.* 1994;90:2899-2904. doi: 10.1161/01.cir.90.6.2899.

143. Gillinov AM, Sirak J, Blackstone EH, et al. The Cox maze procedure in mitral valve disease: predictors of recurrent atrial fibrillation. *J Thorac Cardiovasc Surg.* 2005;130:1653-1660. doi: 10.1016/j.jtcvs.2005.07.028.

144. Maisano F, Alfieri O, Banai S, et al. The future of transcatheter mitral valve interventions: competitive or complementary role of repair vs. replacement? *Eur Heart J.* 2015;36:1651-1659. doi: 10.1093/eurheartj/ehv123.

145. Regueiro A, Granada JF, Dagenais F, Rodes-Cabau J. Transcatheter mitral valve replacement: insights from early clinical experience and future challenges. *J Am Coll Cardiol.* 2017;69:2175-2192. doi: 10.1016/j.jacc.2017.02.045.

146. Maisano F, Franzen O, Baldus S, et al. Percutaneous mitral valve interventions in the real world: early and 1-year results from the ACCESS-EU, a prospective, multicenter, nonrandomized post-approval study of the MitraClip therapy in Europe. *J Am Coll Cardiol.* 2013;62:1052-1061. doi: 10.1016/j.jacc.2013.02.094.

147. Nickenig G, Estevez-Loureiro R, Franzen O, et al. Percutaneous mitral valve edge-to-edge repair: in-hospital results and 1-year follow-up of 628 patients of the 2011-2012 Pilot European Sentinel Registry. *J Am Coll Cardiol.* 2014;64:875-884. doi: 10.1016/j.jacc.2014.06.1166.

148. Geis NA, Puls M, Lubos E, et al. Safety and efficacy of MitraClip therapy in patients with severely impaired left ventricular ejection fraction: results from the German transcatheter mitral valve interventions (TRAMI) registry. *Eur J Heart Fail.* 2018;20:598-608. doi: 10.1002/ejhf.910.

149. Adamo M, Godino C, Giannini C, et al. Left ventricular reverse remodelling predicts long-term outcomes in patients with functional mitral regurgitation undergoing MitraClip therapy: results from a multicentre registry. *Eur J Heart Fail.* 2019;21:196-204. doi: 10.1002/ejhf.1343.

150. Swaans MJ, Bakker AL, Alipour A, et al. Survival of transcatheter mitral valve repair compared with surgical and conservative treatment in high-surgical-risk patients. *JACC Cardiovasc Interv.* 2014;7:875-881. doi: 10.1016/j.jcin.2014.01.171.

151. Giannini C, Fiorelli F, De Carlo M, et al. Comparison of percutaneous mitral valve repair versus conservative treatment in severe functional mitral regurgitation. *Am J Cardiol.* 2016;117:271-277. doi: 10.1016/j.amjcard.2015.10.044.

152. Kessler M, Seeger J, Muche R, Wohrle J, Rottbauer W, Markovic S. Predictors of rehospitalization after percutaneous edge-to-edge mitral valve repair by MitraClip implantation. *Eur J Heart Fail.* 2019;21:182-192. doi: 10.1002/ejhf.1289.

153. Coats AJS, Anker SD, Baumbach A, et al. The management of secondary mitral regurgitation in patients with heart failure: a joint position statement from the Heart Failure Association (HFA), European Association of Cardiovascular Imaging (EACVI), European Heart Rhythm Association (EHRA), and European Association of Percutaneous Cardiovascular Interventions (EAPCI) of the ESC. *Eur Heart J.* 2021. doi: 10.1093/eurheartj/ehab086.

154. Contemporary outcomes with MitraClip" (NTR/XTR) system in primary mitral regurgitation: results from the global EXPAND study. Presented at ACC.20/WCC. March 28–30, 2020.

155. Praz F, Spargias K, Chrissoheris M, et al. Compassionate use of the PASCAL transcatheter mitral valve repair system for patients with severe mitral regurgitation: a multicentre, prospective, observational, first-in-man study. *Lancet.* 2017;390:773-780. doi: 10.1016/S0140-6736(17)31600-8.

156. Lim DS, Kar S, Spargias K, et al. Transcatheter valve repair for patients with mitral regurgitation: 30-day results of the CLASP study. *JACC Cardiovasc Interv.* 2019;12:1369-1378. doi: 10.1016/j.jcin.2019.04.034.

157. Colli A, Zucchetta F, Torregrossa G, et al. Transapical off-pump mitral valve repair with Neochord Implantation (TOP-MINI): step-by-step guide. *Ann Cardiothorac Surg.* 2015;4:295-297. doi: 10.3978/j.issn.2225-319X.2015.05.01.

158. Gerosa G, D'Onofrio A, Besola L, Colli A. Transoesophageal echo-guided mitral valve repair using the Harpoon system. *Eur J Cardiothorac Surg.* 2018;53:871-873. doi: 10.1093/ejcts/ezx365.

159. Nickenig G, Schueler R, Dager A, et al. Treatment of chronic functional mitral valve regurgitation with a percutaneous annuloplasty system. *J Am Coll Cardiol.* 2016;67:2927-2936. doi: 10.1016/j.jacc.2016.03.591.

160. Maisano F, Taramasso M, Nickenig G, et al. Cardioband, a transcatheter surgical-like direct mitral valve annuloplasty system: early results of the feasibility trial. *Eur Heart J.* 2016;37:817-825. doi: 10.1093/eurheartj/ehv603.

161. Schofer J, Siminiak T, Haude M, et al. Percutaneous mitral annuloplasty for functional mitral regurgitation: results of the CARILLON Mitral Annuloplasty Device European Union Study. *Circulation.* 2009;120:326-333. doi: 10.1161/CIRCULATIONAHA.109.849885.

162. Rogers JH, Boyd WD, Smith TW, Bolling SF. Transcatheter mitral valve direct annuloplasty with the millipede IRIS ring. *Interv Cardiol Clin.* 2019;8:261-267. doi: 10.1016/j.iccl.2019.02.001.

163. Maselli D, Guarracino F, Chiaramonti F, Mangia F, Borelli G, Minzioni G. Percutaneous mitral annuloplasty: an anatomic study of human coronary sinus and its relation with mitral valve annulus and coronary arteries. *Circulation.* 2006;114:377-380. doi: 10.1161/CIRCULATIONAHA.105.609883.

164. Bail DH. Treatment of functional mitral regurgitation by percutaneous annuloplasty using the Carillon Mitral Contour System-Currently available data state. *J Interv Cardiol.* 2017;30:156-162. doi: 10.1111/joic.12370.

165. Maniu CV, Patel JB, Reuter DG, et al. Acute and chronic reduction of functional mitral regurgitation in experimental heart failure by percutaneous mitral annuloplasty. *J Am Coll Cardiol.* 2004;44:1652-1661. doi: 10.1016/j.jacc.2004.03.085.

166. Erglis A, Thomas M, Morice MC, et al. The Arto transcatheter mitral valve repair system. *EuroIntervention.* 2015;11 Suppl W:W47-W48. doi: 10.4244/EIJV11SWA12.

167. Park YH, Chon MK, Lederman RJ, et al. Mitral loop cerclage annuloplasty for secondary mitral regurgitation: first human results. *JACC Cardiovasc Interv.* 2017;10:597-610. doi: 10.1016/j.jcin.2016.12.282.

168. Choure AJ, Garcia MJ, Hesse B, et al. In vivo analysis of the anatomical relationship of coronary sinus to mitral annulus and left circumflex coronary artery using cardiac multidetector computed tomography: implications for percutaneous coronary sinus mitral annuloplasty. *J Am Coll Cardiol.* 2006;48:1938-1945. doi: 10.1016/j.jacc.2006.07.043.

169. Lee MS, Shah AP, Dang N, et al. Coronary sinus is dilated and outwardly displaced in patients with mitral regurgitation: quantitative angiographic analysis. *Catheter Cardiovasc Interv.* 2006;67:490-494. doi: 10.1002/ccd.20616.

170. Goode D, Dhaliwal R, Mohammadi H. Transcatheter mitral valve replacement: state of the art. *Cardiovasc Eng Technol.* 2020;11:229-253. doi: 10.1007/s13239-020-00460-4.

171. Meredith I, Bapat V, Morriss J, McLean M, Prendergast B. Intrepid transcatheter mitral valve replacement system: technical and product description. *EuroIntervention.* 2016;12:Y78-Y80. doi: 10.4244/EIJV12SYA21.

172. Perpetua EM, Reisman M. The Tendyne transcatheter mitral valve implantation system. *EuroIntervention.* 2015;11 Suppl W:W78-W79. doi: 10.4244/EIJV11SWA23.

173. Cheung A, Banai S. Transcatheter mitral valve implantation: Tiara. *EuroIntervention.* 2016;12:Y70-Y72. doi: 10.4244/EIJV12SYA18.

174. Cheung A, Webb J, Verheye S, et al. Short-term results of transapical transcatheter mitral valve implantation for mitral regurgitation. *J Am Coll Cardiol.* 2014;64:1814-1819. doi: 10.1016/j.jacc.2014.06.1208.

175. Lange R, Piazza N. The HighLife transcatheter mitral valve implantation system. *EuroIntervention.* 2015;11 Suppl W:W82-W83. doi: 10.4244/EIJV11SWA25.

176. Modine T, Vahl TP, Khalique OK, et al. First-in-human implant of the cephea transseptal mitral valve replacement system. *Circ Cardiovasc Interv.* 2019;12:e008003. doi: 10.1161/CIRCINTERVENTIONS.119.008003.

177. Maisano F, Benetis R, Rumbinaite E, et al. 2-year follow-up after transseptal transcatheter mitral valve replacement with the cardiovalve. *JACC Cardiovasc Interv.* 2020;13:e163-e164. doi: 10.1016/j.jcin.2020.05.032.

178. Nunes Ferreira-Neto A, Dagenais F, Bernier M, Dumont E, Freitas-Ferraz AB, Rodes-Cabau J. Transcatheter mitral valve replacement with a new supra-annular valve: first-in-human experience with the altavalve system. *JACC Cardiovasc Interv.* 2019;12:208-209. doi: 10.1016/j.jcin.2018.10.056.

179. Feldman T, Foster E, Glower DD, et al. Percutaneous repair or surgery for mitral regurgitation. *N Engl J Med.* 2011;364:1395-1406. doi: 10.1056/NEJMoa1009355.

180. Feldman T, Kar S, Elmariah S, et al. Randomized comparison of percutaneous repair and surgery for mitral regurgitation: 5-year results of EVEREST II. *J Am Coll Cardiol.* 2015;66:2844-2854. doi: 10.1016/j.jacc.2015.10.018.

181. Colli A, Manzan E, Aidietis A, et al. An early European experience with transapical off-pump mitral valve repair with NeoChord implantation. *Eur J Cardiothorac Surg.* 2018;54:460-466. doi: 10.1093/ejcts/ezy064.

182. Obadia JF, Messika-Zeitoun D, Leurent G, et al. Percutaneous repair or medical treatment for secondary mitral regurgitation. *N Engl J Med.* 2018;379:2297-2306. doi: 10.1056/NEJMoa1805374.

183. Stone GW, Lindenfeld J, Abraham WT, et al. Transcatheter mitral-valve repair in patients with heart failure. *N Engl J Med.* 2018;379:2307-2318. doi: 10.1056/NEJMoa1806640.

184. Praz F, Grasso C, Taramasso M, et al. Mitral regurgitation in heart failure: time for a rethink. *Eur Heart J.* 2019;40:2189-2193. doi: 10.1093/eurheartj/ehz222.

185. Iung B, Armoiry X, Vahanian A, et al. Percutaneous repair or medical treatment for secondary mitral regurgitation: outcomes at 2 years. *Eur J Heart Fail.* 2019;21:1619-1627. doi: 10.1002/ejhf.1616.

186. Mack MJ. COAPT: Three-year outcomes from a randomized trial of transcatheter mitral valve leaflet approximation in patients with heart failure and secondary mitral regurgitation. Oral presentation at Transcatheter Cardiovascular Therapeutics (TCT) congress 2019; San Francisco, 2019.

187. Baron SJ, Wang K, Arnold SV, et al. Cost-effectiveness of transcatheter mitral valve repair versus medical therapy in patients with heart failure and secondary mitral regurgitation: results from the COAPT trial. *Circulation.* 2019;140:1881-1891. doi: 10.1161/CIRCULATIONAHA.119.043275.

188. Webb JG, Hensey M, Szerlip M, et al. 1-year outcomes for transcatheter repair in patients with mitral regurgitation from the CLASP study. *JACC Cardiovasc Interv.* 2020;13:2344-2357. doi: 10.1016/j.jcin.2020.06.019.

189. Nickenig G, Hammerstingl C, Schueler R, et al. Transcatheter mitral annuloplasty in chronic functional mitral regurgitation: 6-month results with the cardioband percutaneous mitral repair system. *JACC Cardiovasc Interv.* 2016;9:2039-2047. doi: 10.1016/j.jcin.2016.07.005.

190. Witte KK, Lipiecki J, Siminiak T, et al. The REDUCE FMR trial: a randomized sham-controlled study of percutaneous mitral annuloplasty in functional mitral regurgitation. *JACC Heart Fail.* 2019;7:945-955. doi: 10.1016/j.jchf.2019.06.011.

191. Avenatti E, Mackensen GB, El-Tallawi KC, et al. Diagnostic value of 3-dimensional vena contracta area for the quantification of residual mitral regurgitation after MitraClip procedure. *JACC Cardiovasc Interv.* 2019;12:582-591. doi: 10.1016/j.jcin.2018.12.006.

192. Erglis A, Narbute I, Poupineau M, et al. Treatment of secondary mitral regurgitation in chronic heart failure. *J Am Coll Cardiol.* 2017;70:2834-2835. doi: 10.1016/j.jacc.2017.09.1110.

193. Bapat V, Rajagopal V, Meduri C, et al. Early experience with new transcatheter mitral valve replacement. *J Am Coll Cardiol.* 2018;71:12-21. doi: 10.1016/j.jacc.2017.10.061.

194. Muller DWM, Farivar RS, Jansz P, et al. Transcatheter mitral valve replacement for patients with symptomatic mitral regurgitation: a global feasibility trial. *J Am Coll Cardiol.* 2017;69:381-391. doi: 10.1016/j.jacc.2016.10.068.

195. Rodes-Cabau J, Hahn RT, Latib A, et al. Transcatheter therapies for treating tricuspid regurgitation. *J Am Coll Cardiol.* 2016;67:1829-1845. doi: 10.1016/j.jacc.2016.01.063.

196. Braun D, Rommel KP, Orban M, et al. Acute and short-term results of transcatheter edge-to-edge repair for severe tricuspid regurgitation using the MitraClip XTR system. *JACC Cardiovasc Interv.* 2019;12:604-605. doi: 10.1016/j.jcin.2018.11.028.

197. Nickenig G, Weber M, Lurz P, et al. Transcatheter edge-to-edge repair for reduction of tricuspid regurgitation: 6-month outcomes of the TRILUMINATE single-arm study. *Lancet.* 2019;394:2002-2011. doi: 10.1016/S0140-6736(19)32600-5.

198. Enriquez-Sarano M, Suri RM, Clavel MA, et al. Is there an outcome penalty linked to guideline-based indications for valvular surgery? Early and long-term analysis of patients with organic mitral regurgitation. *J Thorac Cardiovasc Surg.* 2015;150:50-58. doi: 10.1016/j.jtcvs.2015.04.009.

199. Baumgartner H, Iung B, Otto CM. Timing of intervention in asymptomatic patients with valvular heart disease. *Eur Heart J.* 2020;41:4349-4356. doi: 10.1093/eurheartj/ehaa485.

200. Grigioni F, Clavel MA, Vanoverschelde JL, et al. The MIDA Mortality Risk Score: development and external validation of a prognostic model for early and late death in degenerative mitral regurgitation. *Eur Heart J.* 2018;39:1281-1291. doi: 10.1093/eurheartj/ehx465.

201. Chambers JB, Prendergast B, Iung B, et al. Standards defining a "Heart Valve Centre": ESC Working Group on Valvular Heart Disease and European Association for Cardiothoracic Surgery Viewpoint. *Eur Heart J.* 2017;38:2177-2183. doi: 10.1093/eurheartj/ehx370.

202. Nishimura RA, O'Gara PT, Bavaria JE, et al. 2019 AATS/ACC/ASE/SCAI/STS expert consensus systems of care document: a proposal to optimize care for patients with valvular heart disease: a joint report of the American Association for Thoracic Surgery, American College of Cardiology, American Society of Echocardiography, Society for Cardiovascular Angiography and Interventions, and Society of Thoracic Surgeons. *J Am Coll Cardiol.* 2019;73:2609-2635. doi: 10.1016/j.jacc.2018.10.007.

203. Mirabel M, Iung B, Baron G, et al. What are the characteristics of patients with severe, symptomatic, mitral regurgitation who are denied surgery? *Eur Heart J.* 2007;28:1358-1365. doi: 10.1093/eurheartj/ehm001.

204. Bach DS, Awais M, Gurm HS, Kohnstamm S. Failure of guideline adherence for intervention in patients with severe mitral regurgitation. *J Am Coll Cardiol.* 2009;54:860-865. doi: 10.1016/j.jacc.2009.03.079.

205. Wang A, Grayburn P, Foster JA, et al. Practice gaps in the care of mitral valve regurgitation: insights from the American College of Cardiology mitral regurgitation gap analysis and advisory panel. *Am Heart J.* 2016;172:70-79. doi: 10.1016/j.ahj.2015.11.003.

206. Iung B, Delgado V, Lazure P, et al. Educational needs and application of guidelines in the management of patients with mitral regurgitation. A European mixed-methods study. *Eur Heart J.* 2018;39:1295-1303. doi: 10.1093/eurheartj/ehx763.

Acquired Tricuspid Valve Diseases

Luigi P. Badano, Ana Pardo, Denisa Muraru, and Jose Luis Zamorano

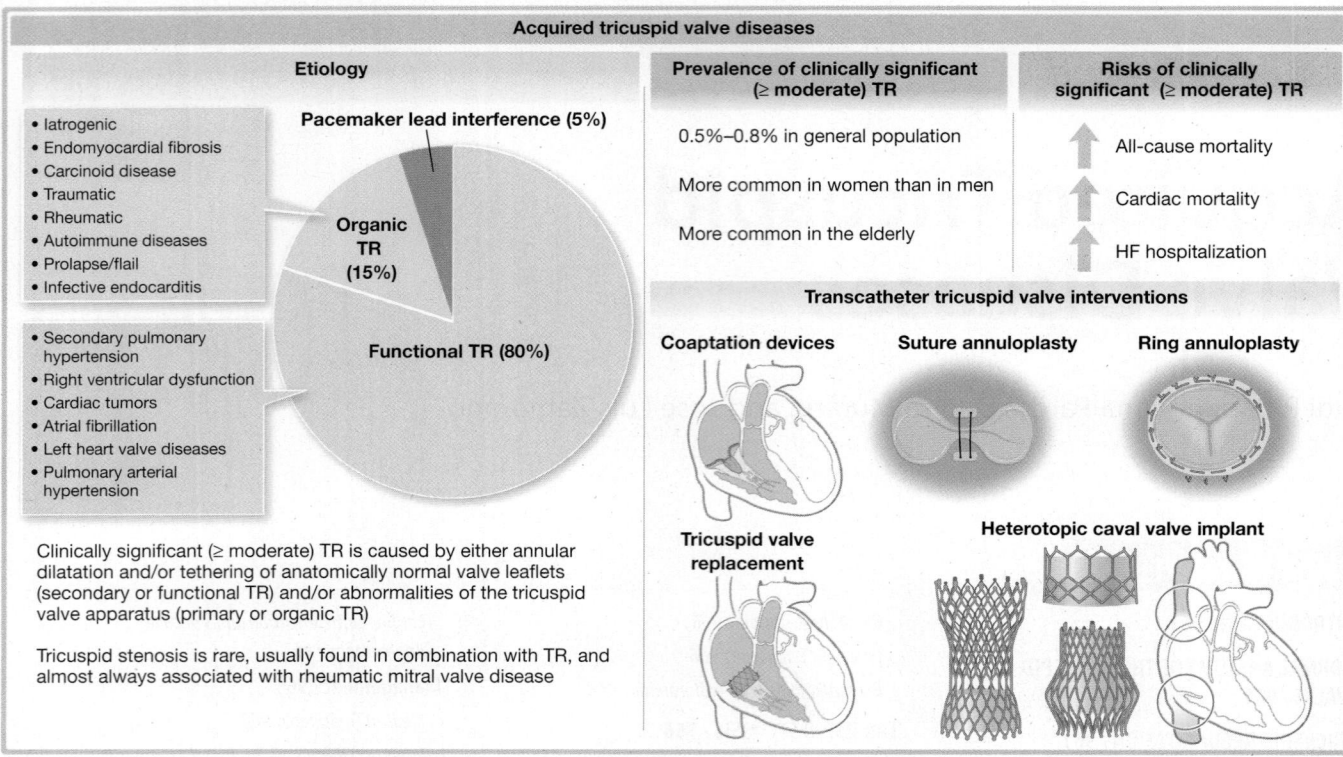

Chapter 31 Fuster and Hurst's Central Illustration. Mild tricuspid regurgitation (TR) in the setting of a structurally normal tricuspid valve apparatus is very common and usually considered a normal variant and benign. Conversely, moderate or severe TR is associated with leaflet abnormalities and/or annular dilation and is an independent predictor of both morbidity and mortality.

CHAPTER SUMMARY

This chapter reviews the prevalence, etiology, clinical presentation, diagnosis, and management of tricuspid regurgitation (TR) and tricuspid stenosis. The tricuspid valve (TV) regulates the blood flow between the right atrium and the right ventricle. During ventricular systole, the TV leaflets coapt to seal the valve orifice, whereas during diastole, they open to allow blood to flow into the right ventricle. Its function as check-valve depends on the integrated and synchronous interplay among the three leaflets, the tricuspid annulus, the subvalvular apparatus, and the surrounding myocardium. The prevalence of clinically significant (ie, moderate or severe) TR in the general population is around 0.5% to 0.8% and the condition is more common in women and in the elderly (see Fuster and Hurst's Central Illustration). Although minimal or trivial TR may be considered a normal variant in structurally normal TVs, moderate and severe TR is associated with increased cardiac and all-cause mortality, independently from pulmonary artery pressure and left and right ventricular function. Moreover, a clear relationship exists between outcome and the severity of TR, making it mandatory to assess TR severity to properly address patients' management. Conversely, tricuspid stenosis is an uncommon valvular abnormality that is usually found in combination with TR and/or other valve lesions.

INTRODUCTION

Tricuspid valve (TV) function depends on the integrated and synchronous interplay among the three leaflets, the tricuspid annulus (TA), the subvalvular apparatus, and the surrounding myocardium. By far, the most frequent acquired TV disease is regurgitation that can be detected in 65% to 85% of the general population.[1] Mild tricuspid regurgitation (TR) in the setting of a structurally normal TV apparatus is usually considered a normal variant and benign. Conversely, moderate or severe TR is associated with leaflet abnormalities and/or annular dilation, it is a pathologic condition, and it has been shown to be an independent predictor of both morbidity and mortality.[2] Approximately 5% to 10% of all acquired TR are organic (or primary) and are caused by abnormalities of one or more components of the tricuspid apparatus (**Table 31–1**). However, the large majority of TR is functional or secondary to conditions that cause right ventricular (RV) and/or right atrial (RA) dilatation/dysfunction, including left-sided heart disease, lung diseases, and chronic atrial fibrillation.

Conversely, stenosis of the TV is a rare condition, usually found in combination with TR, and almost always associated to rheumatic mitral valve disease.

NORMAL ANATOMY OF THE TRICUSPID VALVE

The normal TV area is 7 cm^2 to 9 cm^2; it is the largest of the four cardiac valves. The TV is nearly vertical, oriented at approximately 45° to the sagittal plane, and the most apically located among the cardiac valves. It usually has three leaflets: anterior, septal, and posterior (**Fig. 31–1**). The anterior leaflet is the largest, with a semi-circular shape, whilst the septal one is the

smallest and is inserted ≤10 mm more apically than the mitral valve. The subvalvular apparatus consists of three papillary muscles (anterior, posterior, and septal) and chorda tendineae.[3] However, the anatomy of the valve leaflets, chordae, and papillary muscles is highly variable.[4]

The TA has a saddle shape, with two high points, the antero-septal and postero-lateral, and two lower points, posterior-septal and antero-lateral (**Fig. 31–2**). The high–low distance is approximately 7 mm in healthy subjects, which is considerably less in patients with functional TR.[5] The mediolateral diameter of the TA is normally one-third longer than the anteroposterior one. The TA circumference in healthy subjects is 12 ± 1 cm and its area 11 ± 2 cm^2.[6] The septal part of the TA is considered to be analogous to the intertrigonal portion of the mitral annulus, in that it is relatively spared from annular dilatation.[7]

TRICUSPID REGURGITATION

Several studies have shown that the prevalence of clinically significant (ie, moderate or severe) TR in the general population is approximately 0.5% to 0.8%, and it is more common in women and in the elderly.[1,8] Although minimal or trivial TR may be considered a normal variant in structurally normal TVs and may be detected in 80% to 90% of normal subjects undergoing state-of the-art echocardiography, moderate-to-severe TR is pathological and can be caused by either annular dilatation and/or tethering of anatomically normal valve leaflets (secondary or functional TR) and/or abnormalities of the TV apparatus (primary or organic TR).

The clinical importance of TR and its impact on patients' mortality and morbidity have long been underestimated and has led to undertreatment of patients with severe TR.[9,10]

Prevalence

Using echocardiography, the Framingham Heart study investigators found a prevalence of moderate or severe TR of 0.8%, and an increased prevalence with aging.[1] In 2000, the worldwide population of persons aged >65 years was an estimated 420 million.[11] Between 2000 and 2030, the worldwide population aged >65 years is projected to increase by approximately 550 million to 973 million, and the developing countries' share of the worldwide population aged >65 years is projected to increase from 59% to 71%.[11] Thus, the already notable prevalence of significant TR will most likely dramatically increase in the near future.

Overall, the prevalence of significant TR was 4.3 times greater in women than in men.[1] Recently, in a retrospective, observational study including 16,380 echocardiograms performed at the Mayo Clinic over a 10-year interval, Topilsky et al.[8] found that the prevalence of isolated TR of moderate or greater severity among the inhabitants of the Olmsted County was 0.4%, more commonly in women and elderly persons. Moderate or severe TR accompanied 25% of all left-sided heart valve diseases. The most common etiology of moderate or severe TR in community residents diagnosed by Doppler echocardiography was functional TR secondary to left-sided valvular disease (49.5%), followed by functional TR associated

---

TABLE 31–1. Etiology of Acquired Tricuspid Valve Disease

Structural abnormality of the tricuspid valve apparatus (20% of patients)
- Rheumatic disease (usually with left-sided disease)
- Prolapse, flail
- Infective endocarditis
- Endomyocardial fibrosis
- Carcinoid disease, serotonin active drugs
- Traumatic (blunt chest injury, laceration)
- Iatrogenic
  - Pacemaker/defibrillator lead interference
  - Right ventricular biopsy
  - Drugs (eg, exposure to fenfluramine-phentermine, or methysergide)
  - Radiation therapy of the mediastinum

Functional regurgitation (morphological normal leaflets with annular dilatation) (80% of patients)
- Left heart diseases (left ventricular dysfunction or left heart valve diseases) resulting in pulmonary hypertension
- Primary pulmonary hypertension
- Secondary pulmonary hypertension (eg, chronic lung disease, pulmonary thromboembolism, left-to-right shunt)
- Right ventricular dysfunction from any cause (eg, myocardial diseases, ischemic heart disease, chronic right ventricular pacing)
- Atrial fibrillation
- Cardiac tumors (particularly right atrial myxomas)

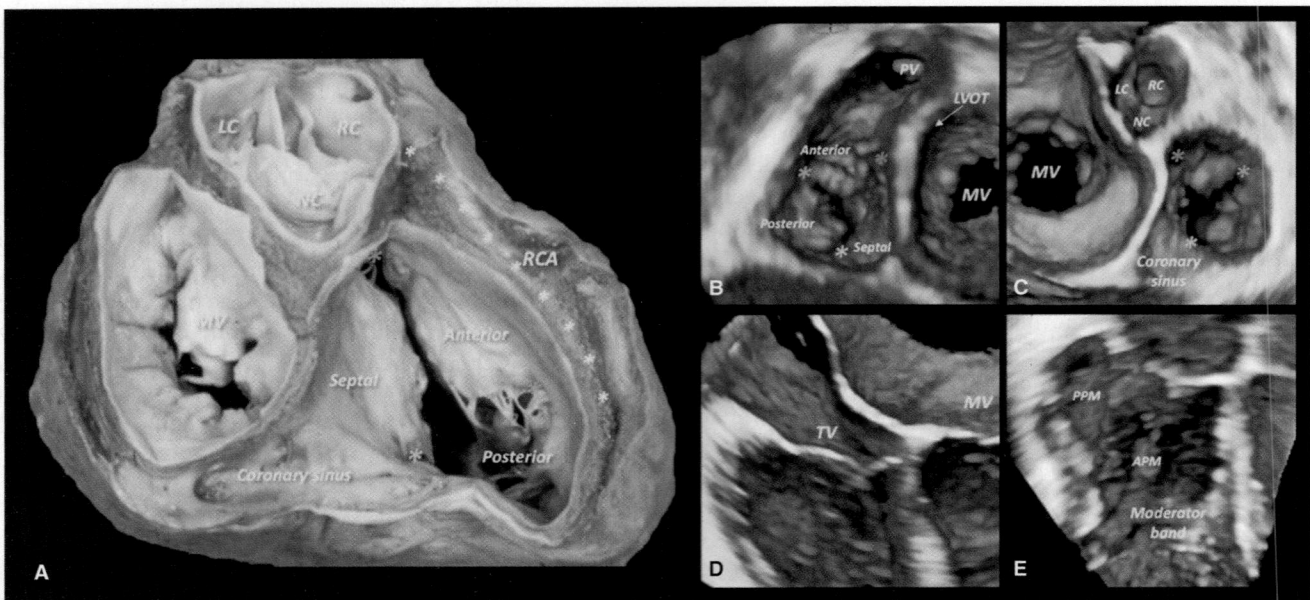

Figure 31–1. The anatomy of the tricuspid valve. (A) Anatomical specimen showing the anterior, septal, and posterior leaflets of the tricuspid valve and their relationships with adjacent anatomical structures: the right coronary artery (RCA, *yellow asterisks*) courses adjacent to the anterior portion of the tricuspid annulus in the right atrioventricular groove; the coronary sinusa; the mitral valve (MV); and the left coronary (LC), right coronary (RC), and noncoronary (NC) aortic cusps. The coronary sinus courtesy of Prof. Cristina Basso, Cardiovascular Pathology, University of Padua, Italy. **(B to E)** 3D echocardiographic views of the tricuspid valve apparatus from the ventricular perspective **(B)**, atrial perspective **(C)**, four-chamber **(D)**, and papillary muscles **(E)**. *Orange asterisk,* anteroseptal commissure; *blue asterisk,* posteroseptal commissure; *green asterisk,* anteroposterior commissure. APM, anterior papillary muscle; LVOT, left ventricular outflow tract; PPM, posterior papillary muscle; PV, pulmonary valve; TV, tricuspid valve. Reproduced with permission from Khalique OK, Cavalcante JL, Shah D, et al. Multimodality Imaging of the Tricuspid Valve and Right Heart Anatomy. *JACC Cardiovasc Imaging.* 2019 Mar;12(3):516-531.

with pulmonary hypertension unrelated to any heart disease (23.0%), functional TR related to left ventricular (LV) dysfunction (12.9%), functional isolated TR (8.1%), organic TR (4.8%), and congenital (1.7%).[8] When the severity of isolated TR was moderate or greater, survival was worse than for matched control subjects with trivial or less TR. Notably, atrial fibrillation is now frequently recognized as an important factor in the etiology of functional TR,[12-16] and its prevalence in the so-called "isolated functional TR" group of the Olmsted County study was 68%.[8]

TR is frequently present in patients with mitral valve disease and more than one-third of patients with mitral stenosis have at least moderate TR.[17] Severe TR has been reported in 23% to 37% of patients after mitral valve replacement for rheumatic valve disease.[18]

The subsequent development of hemodynamically significant TR has been reported in 27% of patients who had only mild TR at the time of left-sided valve surgery.[19] In most cases, TR is diagnosed late after mitral valve replacement.[18,20]

Natural History

Functional TR is an evolving valvulopathy. A recent observational study reported that among 171 patients with heart failure with reduced ejection fraction and nonsevere functional TR at baseline echocardiographic study, 29% experienced progression to at least moderate TR, despite optimal guideline-directed medical therapy, within 3 years after study inclusion.[21] In those patients, progression of functional TR was associated with larger left and right atrial volumes and higher prevalence of atrial fibrillation. Moreover, progression of functional TR was associated with 1.8-fold higher risk of long-term mortality.[21] Prihadi et al.[22] retrospectively analyzed the echocardiography studies of patients with moderate to severe TR and found that

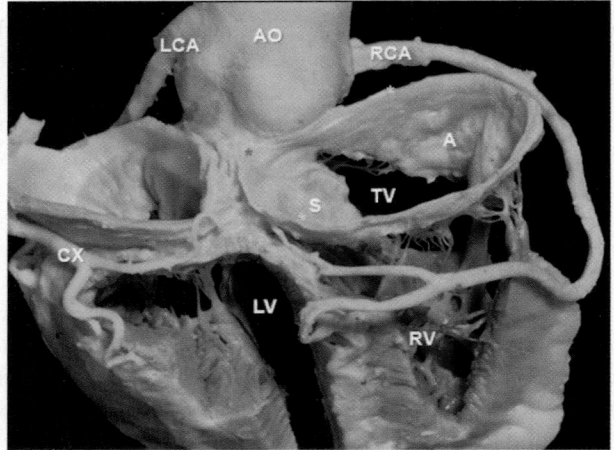

Figure 31–2. Nonplanar geometry of tricuspid annulus. Anatomical specimen showing the complex 3D shape of the tricuspid annulus and its spatial relationships with the surrounding anatomical structures. Abbreviations: A, anterior tricuspid leaflet; Ao, aorta; Cx, circumflex branch of the left coronary artery; LCA, left coronary artery; LV, left ventricle; RCA, right coronary artery; RV, right ventricle; S, septal tricuspid leaflet; TV, tricuspid valve. Reproduced with permission from Dr. Edgardo Bonacina and Dr. Horia Muresian.

older age, presence of either a pace-maker or a defibrillator lead, presence of mild versus no TR at first echocardiography, reduced RV systolic function, larger TA, and any left-sided valvular surgery performed between the first and the index echocardiography were associated with "fast progression" of TR. Moreover, they found that a faster (less than 1.2 years) development of significant TR increased all-cause mortality independent of age, LV ejection fraction, RV systolic pressure, and RV systolic function.[22]

The presence of significant TR has been associated with increased mortality and morbidity,[23-25] and there is a clear relationship between clinical outcomes and the degree of severity of TR[26-29] that may also extend well beyond the conventional definition of severe TR.[30] However, a recent retrospective study of 5886 consecutive patients followed for 10 years found that, although patients with moderate/severe TR without left heart disease had increased risk for heart failure (hazard ratio [HR] = 3.10; 95% CI, 1.41–6.84, P = 0.005) and cardiovascular mortality (HR = 2.75; 95% CI, 1.34–5.63, P = 0.006), after a rigorous propensity matching, there was no significant difference in outcomes between patients with moderate/severe TR and trivial/mild TR.[31] These results are contradictory to most available literature and should be viewed with caution also considering the limitations of the study: retrospective analysis, selection bias of the patients who were followed, and lack of quantitative assessment of TR severity.[9]

The idealized natural clinical and echocardiographic history of patients with functional TR is summarized in **Table 31–2**.[32] Although the proposed staged scheme implies a linear progression of TR, the relationships between morphological and functional alterations of the right heart structures and the severity of TR are quite variable and depend largely on the etiology of functional TR (**Fig. 31–3**).[33] In patients with "*atriogenic*" TR

(ie, patients with atrial fibrillation) there will be little tethering of the leaflets and RV remodeling, whereas the main structural abnormality will be the severe annular dilation mostly related to RA dilation.[25,34] Conversely, in patients with "*ventriculogenic*" TR (ie, patients with pulmonary hypertension) there will be less annular dilation and the main structural abnormalities will be RV dilation and dysfunction, with displacement and reorientation of the papillary muscles, resulting in severe tethering of the TV leaflets. In most of the patients (particularly in the advanced stages of the disease), all the reported morphological and functional abnormalities coexist to varying degrees.[36]

The increase in pulmonary artery pressures and permanent atrial fibrillation have been reported as the most powerful determinants of the progression of the severity of TR.[37,38]

Phenotypes

The etiology of TR is generally divided into primary (or intrinsic) valve disease and secondary (or functional) valve dysfunction (Table 31–1). Primary TR results from structural abnormalities of valve apparatus, may be congenital or acquired, and accounts for only 8% to 10% of all severe TR cases[14,26,39] (**Fig. 31–4**). Secondary or functional TR is usually due to TA dilation that may be primary (atrial fibrillation) or secondary to RV dilation and or dysfunction most frequently caused by pulmonary hypertension that may be either pre- or postcapillary (ie, secondary to diseases affecting the left heart).[40] Although pulmonary artery hypertension from any cause is known to be associated with the occurrence of functional TR, not all patients with pulmonary hypertension develop significant TR. Mutlak et al.[38] assessed the determinants of TR severity in a large cohort (2139 patients) with either mild (<50 mm Hg), moderate (50–70 mm Hg), or severe (>70 mm Hg) elevation of pulmonary artery systolic pressure. In this population, elevated

TABLE 31–2. Clinical and Hemodynamic Stages of Tricuspid Regurgitation

Stage	Definition	Valve Hemodynamics	Hemodynamic Consequences	Clinical Symptoms and Presentation
B	Progressive TR	• Central jet <50% RA • Vena contracta width <0.7 cm • EROA <0.40 cm² • Regurgitant volume <45 mL	• None • None	• None
C	Asymptomatic severe TR	• Central jet ≥50% RA • Vena contracta width ≥0.7 cm • EROA ≥0.40 cm² • Regurgitant volume ≥45 mL • Dense continuous wave signal with triangular shape • Hepatic vein systolic reversal	• Dilated RV and RA • Elevated RA with "c-V" wave	• Elevated venous pressure • No symptoms
D	Symptomatic severe TR	• Central jet ≥50% RA • Vena contracta width ≥0.7 cm • EROA ≥0.40 cm² • Regurgitant volume ≥45 mL • Dense continuous wave signal with triangular shape Hepatic vein systolic reversal	• Dilated RV and RA • Elevated RA with "c-V" wave	• Elevated venous pressure • Dyspnea on exertion, fatigue, ascites, edema

Abbreviations: EROA, effective regurgitant orifice area; RA, right atrium; RV right ventricle; TR tricuspid regurgitation.

Reproduced with permission from Writing Committee Members, Otto CM, Nishimura RA, et al. 2020 ACC/AHA Guideline for the Management of Patients With Valvular Heart Disease: A Report of the American College of Cardiology/American Heart Association Joint Committee on Clinical Practice Guidelines. *J Am Coll Cardiol.* 2021 Feb 2; 77(4):e25-e197.

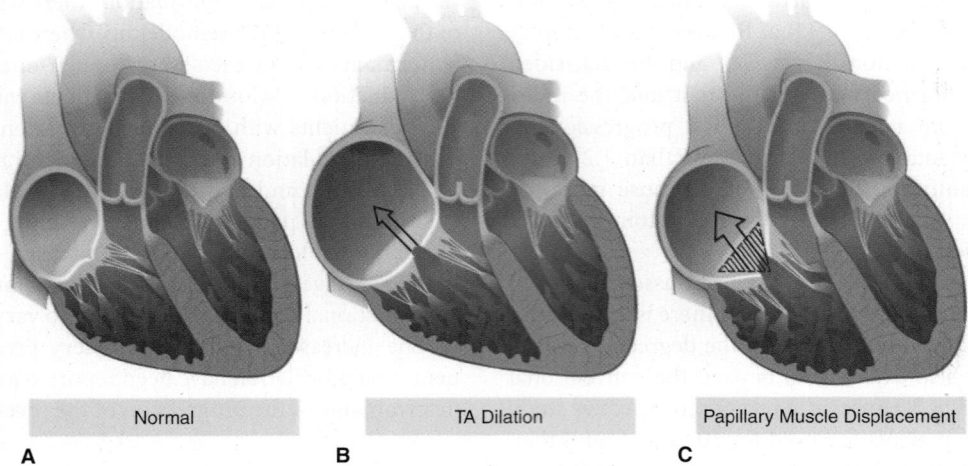

| Normal | TA Dilation | Papillary Muscle Displacement |
| A | B | C |

Figure 31–3. Schematic presentation of the main mechanisms leading to functional tricuspid regurgitation. (A) Normal geometry of the different components of the tricuspid apparatus. **(B)** Tricuspid annulus dilatation, mainly driven by right atrial enlargement with, no or mild right ventricular remodeling (typical pathophysiological model: chronic atrial fibrillation). **(C)** Tricuspid valve leaflet tethering (the *dashed area* shows the tenting area), mainly driven by papillary muscle horizontalization and displacement following right ventricular remodeling (typical pathophysiological model: pulmonary hypertension). During the evolution of the disease, the two mechanisms may coexist at different extent depending on the etiology of functional tricuspid regurgitation.

LA, left atrium; LV, left ventricle; RA, right atrium; RV, right ventricle. Reproduced with permission from Badano LP, Hahn R, Rodríguez-Zanella H, et al. Morphological Assessment of the Tricuspid Apparatus and Grading Regurgitation Severity in Patients With Functional Tricuspid Regurgitation: Thinking Outside the Box. *JACC Cardiovasc Imaging.* 2019 Apr;12(4):652-664.

pulmonary artery systolic pressure was associated with more severe TR (odds ratio 2.26 per 10 mm Hg increase). However, a large number of patients with elevated pulmonary artery systolic pressure showed only mild TR (65.4% of patients with moderate, and 45.6% of patients with severe pulmonary hypertension, respectively). Other factors such as atrial fibrillation, pacemaker leads, and RV remodeling (particularly the increase of the RV transverse mid-diameter) were also significant

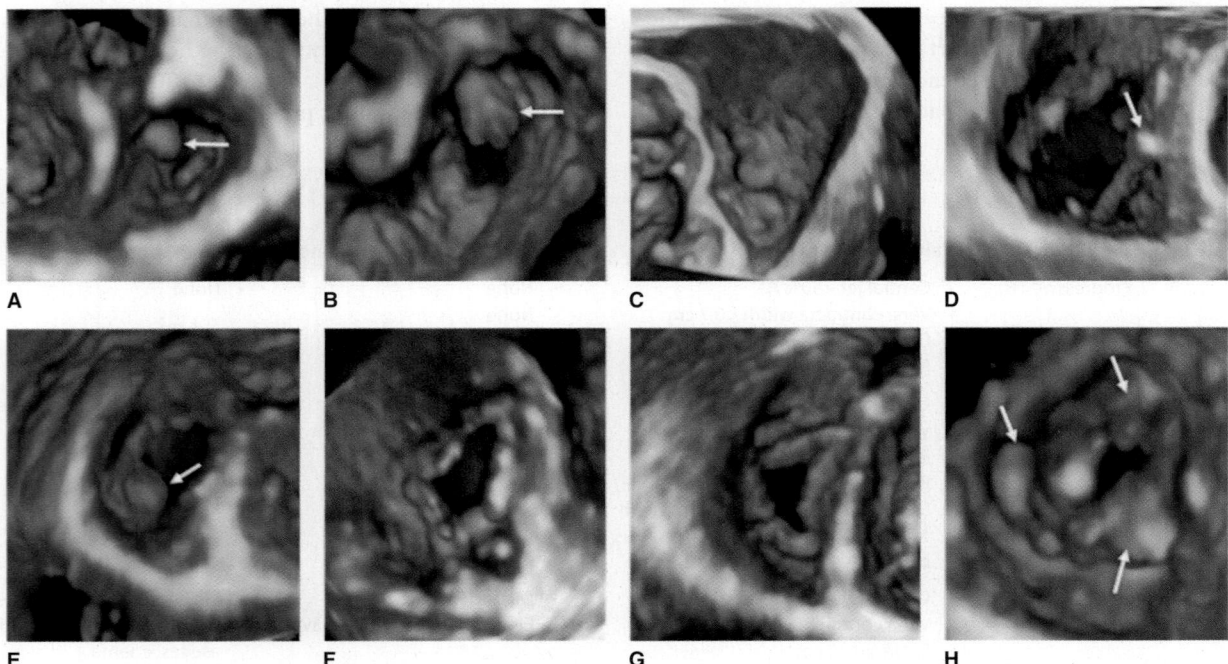

Figure 31–4. Anatomy of acquired tricuspid valve diseases as seen by transthoracic 3D echocardiography. (A) Prolapse of the septal leaflet (*white arrow*) caused by chordal rupture during endomyocardial biopsy in a heart transplant recipient; **(B)** large vegetation and anterior leaflet flail (*white arrow*) due to Staphylococcus infective endocarditis in drug abuser; **(C)** diffuse tricuspid leaflet prolapse with loss of coaptation in Barlow disease; **(D)** pacemaker lead (*white arrow*) impinging upon the septal leaflet and restricting its motion; **(E)** infective endocarditis vegetation on the posterior leaflet; **(F)** tricuspid valve involvement in carcinoid disease, showing the typical "frozen" appearance of leaflets in semi-open position; **(G)** rheumatic tricuspid stenosis with restricted opening due to commissural fusion; **(H)** extensive bioprosthetic valve endocarditis with large vegetations (*white arrows*) and cusp thickening. Reproduced with permission from Muraru D, Hahn RT, Soliman OI, et al. 3-Dimensional Echocardiography in Imaging the Tricuspid Valve. *JACC Cardiovasc Imaging.* 2019 Mar;12(3):500-515.

determinants of the severity of TR. Among them, remodeling of the right heart in response to the increase in pulmonary artery systolic pressure was the most powerful predictor of TR. This data confirms earlier observations that TA dilatation, RV enlargement, or TV tenting, but not pulmonary hypertension itself, are the main determinants of functional TR.[41,42]

Even in the absence of pulmonary hypertension, TA dilatation may cause significant regurgitation.[33,42] In patients with chronic pulmonary thromboembolic hypertension and in patients with mitral stenosis in whom TR resolved after successful pulmonary thromboendoarterectomy or mitral balloon valvuloplasty, there was no change in TA diameter after the resolution of pulmonary hypertension.[43,44] These observations suggest that long-standing TA dilatation could be irreversible and might be the mechanism of late TR encountered in mitral valve disease. Conversely, in patients with short-term TA dilation (such as in patients with persistent atrial fibrillation undergoing successful cardioversion to sinus rhythm) the TA can remodel following the decrease in volume of the RA.[45] Once TR has become significant, progressive RA and/or RV remodeling and dysfunction due to chronic volume overload result in further TA dilation, papillary muscle displacement, and leaflet tethering, which worsen TR and lead to further RA and RV dilatation. Primary acquired TR can result from many different diseases affecting the heart (Table 31–1).

Myxomatous or Degenerative Disease

Myxomatous or degenerative disease of the TV with either a Barlow's or fibroelastic deficiency appearance is rare as isolated TV prolapse, but it can be found in 5% to 52% of patients with TV prolapse.[46] The myxomatous process not only involves the leaflets, but also the chordae, and the annulus. Myxomatous-related TA dilatation contributes not only to the degree of TR, but also to its progressive worsening. The prognosis is related to RV function as well as residual pulmonary hypertension.

Rheumatic Disease

The TV is the third most affected valve by rheumatic disease (after the mitral and the aortic valves). Rheumatic TV disease is characterized by diffuse fibrous thickening of the leaflets and fusion of two or three commissures (Fig. 31–4G). Fibrous leaflet thickening usually occurs in the absence of calcific deposits, and the anteroseptal commissure is the most commonly involved. The rheumatic disease can also involve the chordae, and their fusion and shortening contributes further to restriction of leaflet opening. Rheumatic TV disease may result in both tricuspid stenosis and regurgitation with regurgitation usually predominating.

Infective Endocarditis

Approximately, 90% of TV infective endocarditis is associated with intravenous drug use, and *Staphylococcus aureus* is the predominant causative microorganism (Fig. 31–4A).[47] Other major risk factors are implanted medical devices including valve prostheses (Fig. 31–4H), pacemakers and defibrillators, and vascular access catheters for either dialysis or long-term intravenous treatment. Infective endocarditis can destroy or perforate the TV leaflets and rupture the chordae. Moreover, large vegetations can be associated with relative stenosis, although TR generally predominates. Prognosis depends upon the degree of perivalvular damage, abscess formation, extent of valve destruction, presence of RV failure, emboli, causative organism, removal of a device or a catheter if present, and in the case of drug abusers, changes in behavior.

Cardiac Implantable Electronic Device (CIED)

The incidence of significant TR after CIED implantation varies ranging from 7% to 45%.[48] The large range of the incidence of significant TR after CIED implantation is likely due to the difficulty in identifying the association between the presence of wires/catheters and the resultant TV dysfunction, using conventional two-dimensional (2D) echocardiography. The advent of 3D echocardiography has now allowed the identification of these pathophysiological relationships. Two- and three-dimensional echocardiographic studies, as well as postmortem examinations of hearts with device leads, have shown that CIEDs can interfere with the TV apparatus in various ways: impinging upon a leaflet (Fig. 31–4D), adhering to a leaflet, interfering with the subvalvular apparatus, perforating or lacerating a leaflet, avulsion of a leaflet (which may happen during lead extraction), and transection of papillary muscles or chordae tendineae. Approximately 25% to 29% of patients with permanent pacemakers have TR, roughly double the prevalence in comparison groups.[49] In a population predominantly comprising patients with implantable cardioverter-defibrillators, 38% of patients had a significant increase in severity of TR after CIED implantation, and this was independently associated with increased mortality.

While its clinical importance has gained recognition only recently, it is likely that the prevalence of significant TR after CIEDs implantation will increase in the future due to the progressive aging of the population, and the continued increase in CIED implantation. Patients in whom clinical, hemodynamic, and echocardiographic assessment provides compelling evidence of lead-related severe TR, require corrective intervention in a timely fashion, to avoid the development of severe TA and RV dilation, and severe RV dysfunction.[50] When the latter are present, the lead itself is not the problem any longer, and the condition will no longer be amenable to corrective intervention.

Endomyocardial Biopsy

Another cause of iatrogenic, traumatic TR is represented by repeated endomyocardial biopsies. TR is the most frequent valvular abnormality that occurs after cardiac transplantation.[51] Chordal damage at the time of endomyocardial biopsy leading to TV prolapse is the cause of TR in most of these patients (**Fig. 31–4A**). In 101 patients who underwent orthotopic cardiac transplantation and survived more than 1 year, Nguyen et al.[51] reported that 25% developed severe TR (4% required valve replacement for refractory right-sided heart failure). In their series, there was no case of severe TR in those patients who underwent less than 18 biopsies; conversely, the incidence of severe TR was 60% in those who underwent more than 31 endomyocardial biopsies.

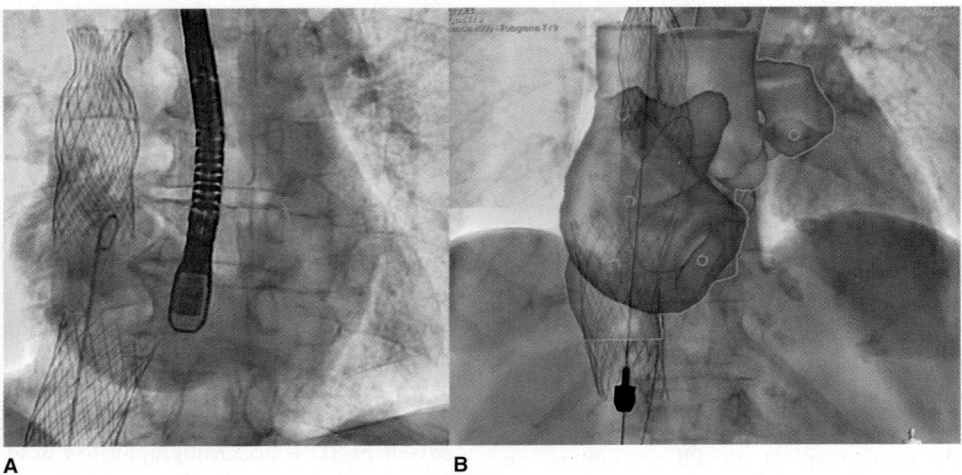

Figure 31–5. Transcatheter implantation of a TricValve in a patient with severe secondary tricuspid regurgitation. (A) The stents are clearly visible in the superior and inferior vena cava. The injection of the contrast media through a pigtail catheter shows no more reflow of blood in the both caval veins. Transesophageal echocardiography is used to monitor the procedure. (B) MSCT-fluoroscopy fusion imaging with surface rendering of anatomical structures in order to facilitate the implantation of the percutaneous bicaval devices.

Blunt Chest Trauma

The incidence of traumatic TV injury has increased because of the increase of traffic accidents, and routine use of airbags as well as technological advances in echocardiography with the introduction of 3D techniques that allow a more accurate assessment of the mechanism of TR.[52] The mechanism of TV injury during blunt chest trauma remains to be clarified. It has been theorized that, during end-diastole, when the RV is particularly sensitive to sagittal shear forces, a severe and sudden anteroposterior compression of the RV from the adjacent sternum can increase the hydrostatic pressure in the RV to a level that causes severe tension on both leaflets and subvalvular structures and can result in a rupture of the TV structures.

The most frequently reported injury is chordal rupture, succeeded by rupture of the anterior papillary muscle, and leaflet tears. After chordal rupture, the valve function is usually relatively preserved, particularly in the anterior leaflet, causing a subacute clinical presentation. The resulting severe TR does not produce symptoms, but the progression is insidious, with right cardiac chambers and the annulus dilating over time.

Conversely, the rupture of a papillary muscle results in severe, immediate TR with an acute presentation characterized by hemodynamic instability and progressive clinical deterioration.

After blunt chest wall trauma, active surveillance, close follow-up, and early surgery in the setting of acute RV failure, can lead to good outcomes.

Carcinoid Syndrome

Carcinoid tumors that produce the carcinoid syndrome can cause thickening, retraction, and hypomobility of the TV leaflets in >50% of cases, with a long latency period. TV leaflets appear short and rigid both at echocardiography and during pathological examination (Fig. 31–4F). The TV can be regurgitant, stenotic, or mixed.[53] Valve damage is related to circulating levels of 5HIAA, which acts on the 5 hydroxytryptamine receptor subtype 5-HT2B, a mediator of mitogenesis and fibroblast proliferation. The presence of high levels of 5HIAA is more likely in patients with hepatic metastases. The TV lesions related to carcinoid are not known to regress, even with control of the disease, but the patient prognosis is still related to the treatment of the underlying disease and timely TV surgery.[54]

Ergot Alkaloids and Fenfluramine

The ergot alkaloid methysergide (used in the past for migraine), diet pills containing fenfluramine, as well as the ergot derived dopamine receptor agonists (cabergoline, utilized to treat pituitary tumors, and pergolide, utilized for Parkinson disease) have been associated with carcinoid-like or 5-HT2B-activated valvular pathology. The effect of these drugs on the TV is related to the dose and the duration of continuous exposure. In patients treated with fenfluramine, the incidence of TV damage is less significant than for left-sided valves.

Other less common causes of primary TR are (1) *radiotherapy*— less common than in the aortic and the mitral valve, and the etiology of TR may be partly functional, related to radiation-induced alterations in RV function, LV systolic or diastolic function, or pulmonary hypertension; (2) *sarcoidosis*—granulomas have been found in the annular region and papillary muscles, as well as on the excised valve; (3) *systemic lupus erythematosus*— valvular pathology includes immune deposition, mononuclear infiltration, fibrous plaque, and calcinosis. Particularly with the IgG antiphospholipid antibody syndrome, thrombi or Libman–Sacks verrucous endocarditis can be found and the bulky thrombi can result in valve stenosis. The fibrotic reaction can result in thickening of both the valve and the chordae causing leaflet fusion and fibrosis with important TR or even tricuspid stenosis.

TRICUSPID STENOSIS

TV involvement in rheumatic disease almost always occurs in conjunction with mitral stenosis, and there are very few case reports of isolated rheumatic tricuspid stenosis in the current literature. The normal TV area is around 4.0 cm² and residual orifice area less than 1.0 cm² is considered severe tricuspid stenosis (Fig. 31–4G).[55]

Clinical Presentation

Many variables may affect the clinical presentation of TV diseases, such as the degree of TR or stenosis, the duration of the disease, the associated underlying etiology, and concomitant cardiac lesions. The symptoms specific to advanced TV disease are related to (1) reduced cardiac output (ie, fatigue, dyspnea, cyanosis), and (2) right atrial hypertension and venous congestion (ie, liver congestion resulting in right upper quadrant discomfort due to stretch of the liver capsule and jaundice, gut congestion with symptoms of dyspepsia and anorexia, and/or fluid retention with leg edema and ascites). However, it should be emphasized that significant TV disease may not be associated with any symptoms until a late stage involving progressive RV dysfunction. Symptoms often direct diagnosis to the underlying etiology (eg, flushing, diarrhea, abdominal pain, and so on, are usually associated with carcinoid heart disease).

Physical findings include both signs related to TV disease and signs secondary to chronic venous congestion (ie, leg edema and ascites). TR results in the jugular venous pulse exhibiting a prominent "C-V" or systolic wave. There is often a parasternal lift due to RV enlargement. The liver is enlarged and often tender, but the pulsatile liver sign of severe TR is a rare finding. Cardiac auscultation can vary according to the etiology of TR. In patients with pulmonary hypertension, the pulmonic component of the S2 becomes accentuated. In these patients, there is a high-pitched holosystolic murmur usually audible in the fourth intercostal space of the left parasternal area. The murmur is accentuated with inspiration (Carvallo sign), leg raise, direct liver compression, and exercise. In patients with no pulmonary hypertension, the pulmonic component of S2 is normal and the murmur is low-pitched and short in duration (early- to midsystole). In patients with RV failure, a S3 and S4 gallop accentuated by inspiration can be detected. In patients with TV prolapse, the murmur is usually mid- or late systolic, and a systolic click may be present. However, it should be emphasized that severe TR may exist without the classic auscultatory findings in the advanced stages of the disease. In those patients, the very large regurgitant orifice makes a single functional chamber of the RV and the RA, and the regurgitant flow becomes laminar. Thus, neither presence nor quantitation of TR can be reliably judged by auscultation only.

Tricuspid stenosis results in characteristic changes in the jugular venous pulse in form of a slow "V" to "Y" descent and prominent "A" waves in patients in sinus rhythm (the A wave is lost in patients with atrial fibrillation). The liver is enlarged with a firm edge, and pulsatile in presystole. Auscultation reveals a low-to-medium-pitched diastolic rumble with inspiratory accentuation, usually localized to the lower sternal border.

Laboratory Tests

Electrocardiogram

There are no specific electrocardiogram findings of TV disease, although some of the following abnormalities may be present: (1) RV hypertrophy and "strain" with right QRS axis, (2) RA enlargement with prominent P waves, (3) incomplete right bundle branch block, and (4) atrial fibrillation.

Chest X-Ray

Chest radiography is usually of limited utility for the diagnosis of TV diseases. However, cardiomegaly associated with prominent right-heart borders can be detected in most patients. Distension of the azygous vain and/or a pleural effusion can be seen in patients with increased RA pressure in whom ascites and diaphragmatic elevation may be present.

Echocardiography

Two-dimensional, and particularly 3D echocardiography,[56] combined with spectral and color-flow Doppler evaluation provides the most accurate diagnostic technique to detect and quantify TV diseases, assess the extent of remodeling of right heart chambers, estimate pulmonary hemodynamics, and identify the etiology of TV diseases.[57] Since the assessment of TR severity is complicated by the peculiar hemodynamics of the right heart and its dependency on respiratory phase and loading conditions,[33] the echocardiographic assessment of TR severity requires a multiparametric approach[57–59] (**Table 31–3**).

Echocardiographic signs of significant tricuspid stenosis are a mean transvalvular gradient higher than 5 mm Hg and/or a TV area derived by the continuity equation smaller than 1.0 cm². Accompanying findings are the presence of extensively thickened leaflets that show limited mobility, retraction, and doming shape during diastole with reduced diastolic opening, and the RA is usually dilated.

Cardiac Magnetic Resonance

In patients with limited acoustic windows, or in patients with a large discrepancy among the echocardiographic parameters, or when the echocardiographic evaluation does not match the clinical presentation, cardiac magnetic resonance (CMR) imaging is indicated. Specific CMR measurements include RV and RA volumes and, combined with phase-contrast-derived pulmonic flow measurements, accurate determinations of the regurgitant volume and fraction.[60] Atrial fibrillation can pose challenges to CMR feasibility and accuracy.

Multidetector Computed Tomography (MDCT)

MDCT is not a routinely used technique for TV assessment due to the significant radiation exposure and the use of iodinated contrast medium. It is usually used when transcatheter procedures are being planned to treat patients with severe TR and there is a need to accurately measure the TV annulus dimensions or to establish anatomical relationships between the TV and adjacent cardiac structures (eg, the right coronary artery). However, MDCT may also be a valuable alternative to CMR in patients with pacemakers, incompatible prosthetic material, and claustrophobia.

Cardiac Catheterization and Selective Angiography

Cardiac catheterization is rarely, if ever, used to diagnose or assess the severity of TV disease. Right heart catheterization is sometimes needed before cardiac surgery to exclude the presence of pulmonary hypertension and selective coronary angiography may be needed to rule out significant coronary artery disease.

TABLE 31-3. Parameters and Relative Threshold Values of Echocardiographic Parameters Used to Assess Tricuspid Regurgitation Severity

| Parameter | TRICUSPID REGURGITATION SEVERITY | | | Limitations |
	Mild	Moderate	Severe	
2D visualization of the leaflets and annulus	Mildly abnormal leaflets (eg, rheumatic disease or mild prolapse) Normal tenting area Normal diastolic annular diameter	Thickened leaflets with or without prolapse Mildly increased tenting area – 0.5–1 cm² Normal or mildly increased diastolic annular diameter	Flail, severely retracted, or papillary muscle rupture Tenting area >1 cm² and large coaptation defect Diastolic annular diameter >40 mm (>21 mm/m²)	Suboptimal acoustic windows Subjectivity Linear metric to estimate a complex 3D structure
2D assessment of chamber and vessel size	RA and RV are usually normal Normal IVC size	RA and RV are usually normal or with mild dilatation IVC 21–25 mm	RA and RV are usually dilated IVC >25 mm	Dilatation is not limited to TR (eg, physiological adaptation, shunts, RV dysfunction, raised PA pressures or concomitant stenosis)
Color Doppler	Small RA penetrance of TR jet Small flow convergence or PISA radius ≤5 mm PISA EROA <20 mm² PISA regurgitant volume <30 mL Jet area <5.0 cm² Jet area: RA area 10–20% Vena Contracta <0.3 cm	Moderate or deep RA penetrance Intermediate size and duration of flow convergence, or PISA radius 6–9 mm PISA EROA 20–39 mm² PISA regurgitant volume 30–44 mL Jet area 6–10 cm² Jet area:RA area 10–33% Vena Contracta 0.3–0.69 cm	Large jet with deep RA penetrance Large flow convergence throughout systole, or PISA radius ≥10 mm PISA EROA ≥40 mm² PISA regurgitant volume ≥45 mL Jet area >10 cm² Jet area:RA area >33% Vena Contracta ≥0.7 cm	Dependent on the momentum and the direction of the jet Multiple jets Non hemispheric shape of PISA (contour flattening) and variable shape of the regurgitant orifice Dependent on the jet momentum, and the direction of the jet (overestimate with central jet or underestimate with eccentric jets) Inaccurate in multiple jets
Pulsed Wave Doppler	Tricuspid E wave <1 m/s or dominant A wave Hepatic vein flow – systolic dominance	Variable tricuspid E wave velocity Hepatic vein flow – systolic blunting	Tricuspid E wave ≥1 m/s Hepatic vein flow – systolic flow reversal	Not reliable in AF or paced rhythms Influenced by concomitant TS Depends on RA compliance
Continuous wave Doppler	Faint / partial contour	Dense/variable contour	Dense, triangular with early peaking	Subjective Direction of jet – may underestimate in eccentric jets Overlap between moderate and severe TR

Abbreviations: AF, atrial fibrillation; EROA, effective regurgitant orifice area; IVC, inferior vena cava; PISA, proximal isovelocity surface area; RA, right atrium; RV, right ventricle; TR, tricuspid regurgitation; TS, tricuspid stenosis.

Data from Zaidi A, et al. Echocardiographic assessment of the tricuspid and pulmonary valves. *Echo Res Pract*. 2021;7(4); Zoghbi WA, et al. Recommendations for noninvasive evaluation of native valvular regurgitation: a report from the American Society of Echocardiography Developed in Collaboration with the Society for Cardiovascular Magnetic Resonance. *J Am Soc Echocardiogr*. 2017;30:303-371; Lancellotti P, et al. European Association of Echocardiography recommendations for the assessment of valvular regurgitation. Part 2: mitral and tricuspid regurgitation (native valve disease). *J Am Soc Echocardiogr*. 2010;11:307-332.

Management

Medical Treatment

The most frequent complaint of patients with severe TR are symptoms related to right-sided heart failure including peripheral edema, ascites, and dyspnea. In addition to low-salt diet and support stockings, diuretics that decrease the volume overload may relieve the venous congestion. However, the use of diuretics should be cautious since they can decrease the RV stroke volume, thus worsening the low-output state and related symptoms such as fatigue and dyspnea. In patients with hepatic congestion that may promote secondary hyperaldosteronism, the addition of aldosterone antagonists may be beneficial.

However, the medical options to manage patients with severe TR are limited and the focus should be the treatment of the underlying conditions that caused secondary TR (ie, restoring sinus rhythm in patients in whom the TR is secondary to TA dilation associated with atrial fibrillation,[61] reducing pulmonary pressure/vascular resistance with specific pulmonary vasomodulators in pulmonary artery hypertension, optimizing the medical treatment of patients with heart failure and reduced LV ejection fraction, etc).

Surgery

Current guidelines (**Table 31-4**)[32,62] recommend surgical TV repair in patients with severe TR when undergoing left-sided valve surgery (Class I recommendations, Level of Evidence: C). Although still debated, TV repair is also recommended at the time of left-sided valve surgery when mild or worse functional TR is associated with TA dilation (at least 40 mm) or right heart failure (Class IIa recommendation, Level of Evidence: B). Adding TV repair, if indicated, during left-sided surgery does not increase operative risk and has been demonstrated to provide reverse remodeling of the RV and improvement of functional status even in the absence of substantial TR when annulus dilatation is present.[63]

TABLE 31-4. Surgical Indication for Tricuspid Valve Repair in Patients with Severe Tricuspid Regurgitation (Stage C or D) According to Current Guidelines

Clinical Condition	ACC/AHA 2021[a]	ESC/EACTS 2017[b]
Primary Tricuspid Regurgitation		
Surgery indicated in patients with severe primary tricuspid regurgitation undergoing left-sided valve surgery	I	I
Surgery is indicated in symptomatic patients with severe isolated primary tricuspid regurgitation without severe right ventricular (RV) dysfunction		I
Surgery should be considered in patients with moderate primary tricuspid regurgitation undergoing left-sided valve surgery	IIb	IIa
Surgery should be considered in asymptomatic or mildly symptomatic patients with severe isolated primary tricuspid regurgitation and progressive RV dilation or deterioration of RV function	IIb	IIa
Secondary Tricuspid Regurgitation		
Tricuspid valve surgery for patients with severe tricuspid regurgitation (TR) undergoing left-sided valve surgery	I	I
Tricuspid valve repair for patients with mild, moderate, or greater functional TR (stage B) at the time of left-sided valve surgery (with either 1. tricuspid annular dilation or 2. prior evidence of right HF)	IIa	IIa
Tricuspid valve surgery for patients with symptoms due to severe primary TR that are unresponsive to medical therapy (stage D)	IIa	
After left-sided valve surgery, surgery for patients with severe TR who are symptomatic or have progressive right ventricular dilatation/dysfunction, in the absence of left-sided valve dysfunction, severe right or left ventricular dysfunction, and severe pulmonary vascular disease	IIb	IIa
In patients with signs and symptoms of right-sided HF and severe isolated secondary TR attributable to annular dilation (in the absence of pulmonary hypertension or left-sided disease) who are poorly responsive to medical therapy (Stage D), isolated tricuspid valve surgery can be beneficial to reduce symptoms and recurrent hospitalizations	IIa	

[a]Data from a Writing Committee M, Otto CM, Nishimura RA, et al. 2020 ACC/AHA guideline for the management of patients with valvular heart disease: a report of the American College of Cardiology/American Heart Association Joint Committee on Clinical Practice Guidelines. *J Am Coll Cardiol.* 2021;77:e25-e197.
[b]Baumgartner H, Falk V, Bax JJ, et al. 2017 ESC/EACTS guidelines for the management of valvular heart diseases. *Eur Heart J.* 2017;38(36):2739-2791.

Reoperation on the TV in cases of persistent or worsening TR after mitral valve surgery carries a high risk, mostly due to delayed surgical presentation in patients with comorbidities and poor clinical status. To improve the prognosis of patients in this challenging scenario, the treatment of severe late TR following left-sided valve surgery should be considered earlier, even in asymptomatic patients, if there are signs of progressive RV dilatation or decline in RV function.

Results from >50,000 patients undergoing TV surgery revealed an overall operative mortality of 9.6%.[64] Since the majority of TR is secondary to left-sided disease, over 80% of TV operations were performed at the time of left-sided surgery. Data concerning isolated TV surgery (either repair or replacement) in the United States were obtained from the National Inpatient Sample.[65] From 2004 to 2013, a total of 5005 isolated TV operations were performed. Operations per year increased from 290 in 2004 to 780 in 2013 and in-hospital mortality was 8.8% and remained stable across the study period. Adjusted in-hospital mortality for TV replacement was significantly higher than TV repair (odds ratio [OR], 1.91; 95% confidence interval [CI], 1.18–3.09; $P < 0.009$). Accordingly, valve repair is generally preferable to valve replacement when sufficient reduction in TR is expected from the repair procedure. Ring annuloplasty, preferably with prosthetic rings, is key to surgery for secondary TR.[66] Valve replacement should be considered when the TV leaflets are significantly tethered and the TA is severely dilated. In the presence of pacemaker leads, the technique used should be adapted to the patient's condition and the surgeon's experience. The lack of pliable leaflet tissue is the main limitation for TV repair. Biological prostheses for valve replacement are usually preferred over mechanical prostheses because of the high risk of thrombosis carried by the latter and the satisfactory long-term durability of the former in the tricuspid position

The optimal timing of surgical intervention during the course of TV disease remains unclear, due to limited availability of natural history data available and the heterogeneous nature of studies.[67] Surgery should be carried out sufficiently early to avoid irreversible RV dysfunction.[62] Use of clinical risk assessment tools can help predict morbidity and mortality for patients, and guide clinical decision-making. Data from the STS Database show several factors which increase the mortality risk of TV surgery: advanced age (>75 years), cardiogenic shock, serum creatinine, urgent or emergent surgical status, and congestive heart failure.[64] Moreover, it has recently been reported that the Model for End-Stage Liver Disease (MELD) score may be useful to stratify the risk of TV surgery since liver and kidney dysfunction accompanies severe TR (stage D), and liver function is not covered in the STS score.

Transcatheter Percutaneous Approach

Due to high surgical mortality for TR, a number of transcatheter devices to reduce TR have recently been developed.[68] There are many challenges associated with transcatheter TR device therapies: (1) large TA diameter (>40 mm) and elliptical TA shape; (2) trabecular structures of the RV; (3) proximity to high-risk cardiac structures (eg, the right coronary artery, coronary sinus, and the conduction system); (4) entry angles across the TA from the SVC to provide coaxial alignment of devices.

In general, there are four categories of new transcatheter tricuspid therapies:

Reduce the Reverse Backflow into Vena Caval System: The rationale for heterotopic transcatheter caval valve implantation in patients with severe TR was to reduce the extent of regurgitant volume and pressure into the vena cava that leads to hepatic, abdominal, and peripheral congestion, to reduce the symptoms of right heart failure. Caval valve implantation has been performed via specifically designed devices such as the self-expandable TricValve®, and the balloon-expandable SAPIEN transcatheter aortic valve, which requires presenting to insure fixation in the IVC. The TricValve® is composed of two biological valve prostheses, both with three cusps of bovine pericardium mounted within a Nitinol scaffold and it can be implanted at the inferior vena cava alone or in combination with a specific valve for superior vena cava implantation (Fig. 31–5). The valves have little radial force and do not require presenting of the vena cava. The main disadvantage of caval valve implantation is that this therapeutic concept does not reduce TR, but only its consequences on the peripheral venous system. No long-term data are available on the safety of both RA ventricularization and the continued RA and RV overload due to persistent severe TR.

Reduce the TA Size: The pathophysiology of functional TR involves progressive TA dilation occurring mainly in the anteroposterior plane, which leads to a lack of leaflet coaptation. Accordingly, transcatheter annular reduction devices are based on a proven surgical background with good long-term outcomes. Moreover, these techniques preserve the anatomy of the TV, allowing future treatment options such as percutaneous edge-to-edge repair or valve replacement, if necessary.

The *Trialign system®* is based on the Kay surgical bicuspidization procedure (conversion of an incompetent TV into a competent bicuspid valve, by plicating the anterior and posterior portion of the TA). Through a transjugular approach, and under fluoroscopy and transoesophageal echocardiography guidance, a set of pledgeted sutures are positioned in proximity of the anteroposterior and posterior commissure at the TA level, and using a connecting suture system, the pledgets are plicated, which reduces the TA circumference. The small footprint of the device, which leaves a significant amount of native anatomy undisturbed for subsequent procedures, is a notable advantage.

TriCinch® is a transcatheter device designed to reduce functional TR by reducing the TA size and restoring leaflet coaptation. A stainless-steel corkscrew is first anchored in the TA next to the anteroposterior commissure. The stent delivery system is locked to the corkscrew via the Dacron band and tension is applied to reduce the septo-lateral diameter and TR severity by pulling the system toward the inferior vena cava. Finally, the stent is deployed in the inferior vena cava to maintain the applied tension.

The *Cardioband®* system (Edwards Lifescience) for the treatment of TR is a percutaneous annuloplasty ring based on the CE-approved Cardioband device for mitral regurgitation

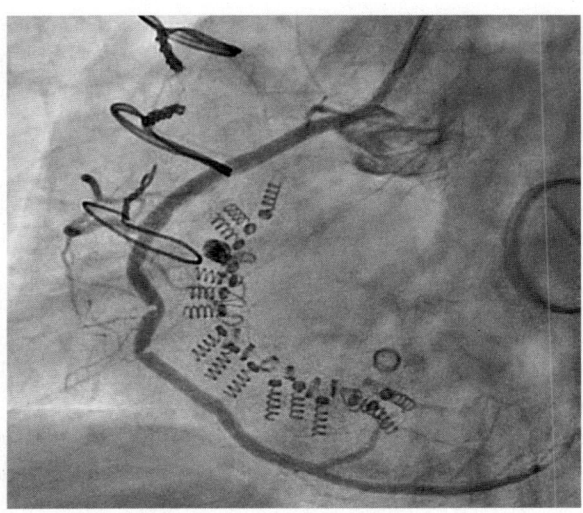

Figure 31–6. Cardioband implantation to perform transcatheter restrictive annuloplasty in a patient with previous mitral valve replacement and severe secondary tricuspid regurgitation. The injection of contrast media in the right coronary artery allows the appreciation of the relationship between tricuspid annulus and the right coronary artery and absence of coronary artery perforation.

(**Fig. 31–6**). The Dacron adjustable band is fixed in a supra-annular position, similar to a surgical annuloplasty ring. The procedure is performed under fluoroscopy and 3D TEE guidance. The Cardioband ring is fastened to the TA via 6-mm-long, stainless steel anchors that are implanted from the anterior to the posterior TA. Once the anchors are fixed, the device is cinched and the TA dimensions are significantly reduced.

Improve TV Leaflet Coaptation and Reduce the Regurgitant Orifice Area: The *FORMA®* device (Edwards Lifescience) is designed to reduce TR by occupying the regurgitant orifice and providing a platform for native leaflet coaptation. It consists of a cylindrical spacer and a rail. The rail tracks the spacer into position and is distally anchored at the RV apex, perpendicular to the TA plane.

MitraClip® (Abbott Vascular) in the tricuspid position mimics the surgical edge-to-edge "clover" technique, which has been validated for the treatment of degenerative and functional mitral regurgitation. However, the edge-to-edge TV repair remains a challenging procedure because of high anatomic variability of the TV, large coaptation gaps between the leaflets that makes grasping more difficult and usually requires multiple clips, and difficulty with echo imaging for guidance. The best results are seen by approximating the anterior and/or posterior leaflet to the septal leaflet, which may also reduce annular dimensions. Clipping the anteroposterior leaflets is generally avoided in functional TR because it may distort the valve and worsen TR. Other edge-to-edge repair devices have recently been developed, including the *PASCAL®* device (Edwards Lifescience).

Tricuspid Valve Replacement: In patients with TR recurrence after prior TV repair (eg, annuloplasty ring failure), or after a degenerated tricuspid bioprosthesis with stenosis or regurgitation, implantation of transcatheter aortic valves or dedicated TVs have been used successfully as an alternative to redo surgery. Importantly, there are anatomic situations not amenable to repair therapies or marked severity of TR (massive or torrential) that can only be effectively treated with complete replacement of the TV. Several transcatheter TV replacement systems are in various stages of development and early clinical trials, including the *EVOQUE*® system (Edwards Lifescience). Challenges confronting these new TV replacement devices include availability of large enough valves to accommodate a dilated TV annulus, imaging limitations with standard echocardiography methods, valve retention and alignment, and requirements for long-term anticoagulation treatment.

There are many ongoing clinical trials designed to test the safety and efficacy of the many devices developed for the percutaneous treatment of TR. The early feasibility study of the Mitralign percutaneous TV annuloplasty system also known as TriAlign" (SCOUT) trial[69] is a prospective, single-arm, multicenter study that enrolled 15 symptomatic patients with moderate or greater functional TR. All patients underwent successful device implantation with no serious complications, but one patient required stent implantation in the right coronary artery. At 30-day follow-up, significant reductions in TA diameter and TR severity were observed, with no differences in estimated systolic pulmonary artery pressure. Reduction of TR severity translated into improvements in NYHA functional class, Minnesota Living with Heart Failure Questionnaire score, and 6-minute walk test.

In the percutaneous treatment of TV regurgitation with the TriCinch System" (PREVENT) trial, 24 patients were treated with the first-generation device. Successful implantation was achieved in 18 patients (75%) with a significant reduction of TR in 94%. Two patients experienced hemopericardium after the procedure and four patients had late detachment of the TA anchor. Follow-up at 6 months showed significantly improved 6-minute walk test and quality of life, with 75% of the patients in NYHA class I or II.

The Cardioband device has been evaluated in the European tricuspid regurgitation repair with Cardioband (TRI-REPAIR) trial and 2-year results have been reported.[70] The Cardioband tricuspid system was safe and in patients with symptomatic and severe functional TR, at 2 years, significant reduction of TR was observed due to a sustained decrease in TA dimensions, and was associated with improvement in heart failure symptoms, quality of life, and exercise capacity.

The first-in-human experience with the FORMA device in 2015 indicated procedural success in 17 (89%) of 19 treated patients. Among 15 successfully implanted patients with at least 24-month follow-up, significant improvements in NYHA functional class (*P* < 0.001), 6-minute walk test (+54 m; *P* = 0.016), and Kansas City Cardiomyopathy Questionnaire score (+16 points; *P* = 0.016) were observed, compared with baseline.[71] Similar results were obtained after 1 year in the US Forma early feasibility study, which enrolled 29 patients. Long-term outcomes at 24 to 36 months of the first-in-human cohort showed significant improvement of functional status and maintained significant reduction of TR.[72]

Extensive operator experiences as well as widespread availability have led to the use of the MitraClip in the tricuspid position in more than 1000 cases of severe TR. In the TriValve registry, which merged data from multiple transcatheter tricuspid repair devices accumulated in 18 international centers, the MitraClip was used in 66% of patients.[73] A multicenter European registry showed reduction of TR by at least one grade in 91% of patients, accompanied by a significant reduction in effective regurgitation orifice area, vena contracta width, and regurgitant volume, as well as an improvement in NYHA class and 6-minute walk test.[74]

A modified version of the MitraClip device and its delivery system to address the specifics of TV anatomy has been tested in the multicenter Evaluation of Treatment With Abbott Transcatheter Clip Repair System in Patients With Moderate or Greater Tricuspid Regurgitation (TRILUMINATE) study.[75] At 1-year follow-up, TR severity was reduced to moderate or less in 71% of patients compared with 8% at baseline (*P* < 0.0001). Patients reported significant functional improvements in NYHA functional class I/II (31%–83%, *P* < 0.0001), 6-minute walk test (272.3 ± 15.6 to 303.2 ± 15.6 meters, *P* = 0.0023), and Kansas City Cardiomyopathy Questionnaire score (improvement of 20 ± 2.61 points, *P* < 0.0001). Significant reverse RV remodeling was also demonstrated. The overall major adverse event rate and all-cause mortality were both 7.1%.

Future Directions

Management of patients with either moderate or severe TR is not supported by evidence-based recommendations (current level of evidence is B or C). Thus, randomized clinical trials comparing medical therapy versus surgery or new transcatheter devices are needed in both symptomatic and asymptomatic patients to provide evidence-based treatment guidance for patients,

Symptomatic patients with severe TR represent a complex and heterogeneous population, in whom the choice of the optimal therapy method and timing of treatment are crucial. Specific treatment strategies adapted to each stage of the disease are needed. Furthermore, both preoperative RV size[76] and function[77] have been associated with postoperative outcomes in severe TR, but threshold values for valve intervention remain to be established. Further research is needed in order to better understand the pathophysiology and underlying mechanisms of TR progression. Finally, there is also a need to develop revised echo criteria for more accurate grading of TR severity that can be validated in clinical trials.[33]

SUMMARY

Epidemiology

- The most frequent acquired tricuspid valve disease is functional (secondary) tricuspid regurgitation.
- The prevalence of significant tricuspid regurgitation is higher in women and increases with age.
- The clinical importance of tricuspid regurgitation and its impact on patients' morbidity and mortality have been underestimated, and this has led to undertreatment of patients with severe tricuspid regurgitation.

Pathogenesis

- In addition to pulmonary artery hypertension, right ventricular cardiomyopathies, heart failure, and left-sided heart valve diseases, atrial fibrillation is a cause of secondary (functional) tricuspid regurgitation.
- Secondary (functional) tricuspid regurgitation is an evolving valvular heart disease. and may progress over decades without symptoms.
- The presence of moderate or severe tricuspid regurgitation is associated with increased morbidity and mortality, and there is a clear relationship between clinical outcomes and the severity of the regurgitation.

Diagnosis

- Significant tricuspid regurgitation may not be associated with any symptoms until a late stage involving progressive right ventricular dysfunction.
- Two- and three-dimensional echocardiography, combined with spectral and color-flow Doppler evaluation, provides the most accurate diagnostic technique to detect and quantify tricuspid valve diseases.

Treatment and Management

- Medical treatment to manage patients with severe, symptomatic tricuspid regurgitation are limited to cautious use of diuretics.
- The focus should be the treatment of the underlying conditions that caused secondary tricuspid regurgitation.
- Surgical treatment of tricuspid regurgitation is recommended either in patients undergoing left-sided valve surgery or in symptomatic patients without severe right ventricular dysfunction.
- Surgical tricuspid valve repair is preferred to valve replacement because of the high risk of prosthesis thrombosis.
- Due to the high surgical mortality for tricuspid regurgitation, a number of transcatheter devices have recently been developed to treat these patients.
- Patients with severe, symptomatic tricuspid regurgitation should be considered for surgical or transcatheter valve repair before the development of severe right ventricular dysfunction, and liver and kidney dysfunction.

REFERENCES

1. Singh JP, Evans JC, Levy D, et al. Prevalence and clinical determinants of mitral, tricuspid, and aortic regurgitation (the Framingham Heart Study). *Am J Cardiol.* 1999;83:897-902.
2. Badano LP, Muraru D, Enriquez-Sarano M. Assessment of functional tricuspid regurgitation. *Eur Heart J.* 2013;34:1875-1885.
3. Huttin O, Voilliot D, Mandry D, Venner C, Juilliere Y, Selton-Suty C. All you need to know about the tricuspid valve: tricuspid valve imaging and tricuspid regurgitation analysis. *Arch Cardiovasc Dis.* 2016;109:67-80.
4. Luxford J, Bassin L, D'Ambra M. Echocardiography of the tricuspid valve: acknowledgements. *Ann Cardiothorac Surg.* 2017;6:223-239.
5. Fukuda S, Saracino G, Matsumura Y, et al. Three-dimensional geometry of the tricuspid annulus in healthy subjects and in patients with functional tricuspid regurgitation: a real-time, 3-dimensional echocardiographic study. *Circulation.* 2006;114:I492-I498.
6. Ton-Nu TT, Levine RA, Handschumacher MD, Dorer DJ, Yosefy C, Fan D, et al. Geometric determinants of functional tricuspid regurgitation: insights from 3-dimensional echocardiography. *Circulation.* 2006;114:143-149.
7. Rogers JH, Bolling SF. The tricuspid valve: current perspective and evolving management of tricuspid regurgitation. *Circulation.* 2009;119:2718-2725.
8. Topilsky Y, Maltais S, Medina Inojosa J, et al. Burden of tricuspid regurgitation in patients diagnosed in the community setting. *JACC Cardiovasc Imaging.* 2019;12:433-442.
9. Hahn RT. Avoiding mistakes of the past with tricuspid regurgitation. *J Am Soc Echocardiogr.* 2019;32:1547-1550.
10. Agarwal S, Tuzcu EM, Rodriguez ER, Tan CD, Rodriguez LL, Kapadia SR. Interventional cardiology perspective of functional tricuspid regurgitation. *Circ Cardiovasc Interv.* 2009;2:565-573.
11. Centers for Disease C, Prevention. Trends in aging–United States and worldwide. *MMWR Morb Mortal Wkly Rep.* 2003;52:101-106.
12. Utsunomiya H, Itabashi Y, Mihara H, et al. Functional tricuspid regurgitation caused by chronic atrial fibrillation: a real-time 3-dimensional transesophageal echocardiography study. *Circ Cardiovasc Imaging.* 2017;10.
13. Muraru D, Guta A-C, Ochoa-Jimenez RC, et al. Functional regurgitation of atrioventricular valves and atrial fibrillation: an elusive pathophysiological link deserving further attention. *J Am Soc Echocardiogr.* 2020;33(1):42-53.
14. Mutlak D, Lessick J, Reisner SA, Aronson D, Dabbah S, Agmon Y. Echocardiography-based spectrum of severe tricuspid regurgitation: the frequency of apparently idiopathic tricuspid regurgitation. *J Am Soc Echocardiogr.* 2007;20:405-408.
15. Najib MQ, Vinales KL, Vittala SS, Challa S, Lee HR, Chaliki HP. Predictors for the development of severe tricuspid regurgitation with anatomically normal valve in patients with atrial fibrillation. *Echocardiography.* 2012;29:140-146.
16. Yamasaki N, Kondo F, Kubo T, et al. Severe tricuspid regurgitation in the aged: atrial remodeling associated with long-standing atrial fibrillation. *J Cardiol.* 2006;48:315-323.
17. Boyaci A, Gokce V, Topaloglu S, Korkmaz S, Goksel S. Outcome of significant functional tricuspid regurgitation late after mitral valve replacement for predominant rheumatic mitral stenosis. *Angiology.* 2007;58:336-342.
18. Izumi C, Iga K, Konishi T. Progression of isolated tricuspid regurgitation late after mitral valve surgery for rheumatic mitral valve disease. *J Heart Valve Dis.* 2002;11:353-356.
19. Dreyfus GD, Corbi PJ, Chan KM, Bahrami T. Secondary tricuspid regurgitation or dilatation: which should be the criteria for surgical repair? *Ann Thorac Surg.* 2005;79:127-132.
20. Matsunaga A, Duran CM. Progression of tricuspid regurgitation after repaired functional ischemic mitral regurgitation. *Circulation.* 2005;112:I453-I457.
21. Spinka G, Bartko PE, Heitzinger G, et al. Natural course of nonsevere secondary tricuspid regurgitation. *J Am Soc Echocardiogr.* 2021;34:13-19.
22. Prihadi EA, van der Bijl P, Gursoy E, et al. Development of significant tricuspid regurgitation over time and prognostic implications: new insights into natural history. *Eur Heart J.* 2018;39:3574-3581.
23. Chorin E, Rozenbaum Z, Topilsky Y, et al. Tricuspid regurgitation and long-term clinical outcomes. *Eur Heart J Cardiovasc Imaging.* 2020;21(2):157-165.
24. Wang N, Fulcher J, Abeysuriya N, et al. Tricuspid regurgitation is associated with increased mortality independent of pulmonary pressures and right heart failure: a systematic review and meta-analysis. *Eur Heart J.* 2019;40:476-484.
25. Benfari G, Antoine C, Miller WL, et al. Excess mortality associated with functional tricuspid regurgitation complicating heart failure with reduced ejection fraction. *Circulation.* 2019;140:196-206.
26. Nath J, Foster E, Heidenreich PA. Impact of tricuspid regurgitation on long-term survival. *J Am Coll Cardiol.* 2004;43:405-409.
27. Bartko PE, Arfsten H, Frey MK, et al. Natural history of functional tricuspid regurgitation: implications of quantitative doppler assessment. *JACC Cardiovasc Imaging.* 2019;12:389-397.

28. Shiran A, Sagie A. Tricuspid regurgitation in mitral valve disease incidence, prognostic implications, mechanism, and management. *J Am Coll Cardiol.* 2009;53:401-408.

29. Muraru D, Previtero M, Ochoa-Jimenez RC, et al. Prognostic validation of partition values for quantitative parameters to grade functional tricuspid regurgitation severity by conventional echocardiography. *Eur Heart J Cardiovasc Imaging.* 2021;22:155-165.

30. Santoro C, Marco Del Castillo A, Gonzalez-Gomez A, et al. Mid-term outcome of severe tricuspid regurgitation: are there any differences according to mechanism and severity? *Eur Heart J Cardiovasc Imaging.* 2019;20:1035-1042.

31. Mutlak D, Khoury E, Lessick J, Kehat I, Agmon Y, Aronson D. Lack of increased cardiovascular risk due to functional tricuspid regurgitation in patients with left-sided heart disease. *J Am Soc Echocardiogr.* 2019;32:1538-1546 e1.

32. Writing Committee M, Otto CM, Nishimura RA, et al. 2020 ACC/AHA guideline for the management of patients with valvular heart disease: a report of the American College of Cardiology/American Heart Association Joint Committee on Clinical Practice Guidelines. *J Am Coll Cardiol.* 2021;77:e25-e197.

33. Badano LP, Hahn R, Rodriguez-Zanella H, Araiza Garaygordobil D, Ochoa-Jimenez RC, Muraru D. Morphological assessment of the tricuspid apparatus and grading regurgitation severity in patients with functional tricuspid regurgitation: thinking outside the box. *JACC Cardiovasc Imaging.* 2019;12:652-664.

34. Guta AC, Badano LP, Tomaselli M, et al. The pathophysiological link between right atrial remodeling and functional tricuspid regurgitation in patients with atrial fibrillation. A three-dimensional echocardiography study. *J Am Soc Echocardiogr.* 2021;34(6):585-594.

35. Muraru D, Addetia K, Guta AC, Ochoa-Jimenez RC, Genovese D, Veronesi F, et al. Right atrial volume is a major determinant of tricuspid annulus area in functional tricuspid regurgitation: a three-dimensional echocardiographic study. *Eur Heart J Cardiovasc Imaging.* 2020;22:660-669.

36. Yucel E, Bertrand PB, Churchill JL, Namasivayam M. The tricuspid valve in review: anatomy, pathophysiology and echocardiographic assessment with focus on functional tricuspid regurgitation. *J Thorac Dis.* 2020;12:2945-2954.

37. Shiran A, Najjar R, Adawi S, Aronson D. Risk factors for progression of functional tricuspid regurgitation. *Am J Cardiol.* 2014;113:995-1000.

38. Mutlak D, Aronson D, Lessick J, Reisner SA, Dabbah S, Agmon Y. Functional tricuspid regurgitation in patients with pulmonary hypetension: is pulmonary artery pressure the only determinant of regurgitation severity? *Chest.* 2009;135:115-121.

39. Ong K, Yu G, Jue J. Prevalence and spectrum of conditions associated with severe tricuspid regurgitation. *Echocardiography.* 2014;31:558-562.

40. Muraru D, Surkova E, Badano LP. Revisit of functional tricuspid regurgitation; current trends in the diagnosis and management. *Korean Circ J.* 2016;46:443-455.

41. Sagie A, Schwammenthal E, Padial LR, et al. Determinants of functional tricuspid regurgitation in incomplete tricuspid valve closure: Doppler color flow study of 109 patients. *J Am Coll Cardiol.* 1994;24:446-453.

42. Porter A, Shapira Y, Wurzel M, Sulkes J, Vaturi M, Adler Y, et al. Tricuspid regurgitation late after mitral valve replacement: clinical and echocardiographic evaluation. *J Heart Valve Dis.* 1999;8:57-62.

43. Song H, Kang DH, Kim JH, et al. Percutaneous mitral valvuloplasty versus surgical treatment in mitral stenosis with severe tricuspid regurgitation. *Circulation.* 2007;116:1246-1250.

44. Sadeghi HM, Kimura BJ, Raisinghani A, et al. Does lowering pulmonary arterial pressure eliminate severe functional tricuspid regurgitation? Insights from pulmonary thromboendarterectomy. *J Am Coll Cardiol.* 2004;44:126-132.

45. Muraru D, Caravita S, Guta AC, Branzi G, Parati G, Badano L. Functional tricuspid regurgitation and atrial fibrillation: which comes first, the chicken or the egg? *CASE (Phila).* 2020;4(5):458-463.

46. Lorinsky MK, Belanger MJ, Shen C, et al. Characteristics and significance of tricuspid valve prolapse in a large multidecade echocardiographic study. *J Am Soc Echocardiogr.* 2021;34:30-37.

47. Hussain ST, Witten J, Shrestha NK, Blackstone EH, Pettersson GB. Tricuspid valve endocarditis. *Ann Cardiothorac Surg.* 2017;6:255-261.

48. Addetia K, Harb SC, Hahn RT, Kapadia S, Lang RM. Cardiac implantable electronic device lead-induced tricuspid regurgitation. *JACC Cardiovascular imaging.* 2019;12:622-636.

49. Al-Bawardy R, Krishnaswamy A, Bhargava M, et al. Tricuspid regurgitation in patients with pacemakers and implantable cardiac defibrillators: a comprehensive review. *Clinical Cardiol.* 2013;36:249-254.

50. Chang JD, Manning WJ, Ebrille E, Zimetbaum PJ. Tricuspid valve dysfunction following pacemaker or cardioverter-defibrillator implantation. *J Am Coll Cardiol.* 2017;69:2331-2341.

51. Nguyen V, Cantarovich M, Cecere R, Giannetti N. Tricuspid regurrgitation after cardiac transplantation: how many biopsies are too many? *J Heart Lung Transplant.* 2005;24:S227-S231.

52. Dounis G, Matsakas E, Poularas J, Papakonstantinou K, Kalogeromitros A, Karabinis A. Traumatic tricuspid insufficiency: a case report with a review of the literature. *Eur J Emerg Med.* 2002;9:258-261.

53. Fox DJ, Khattar RS. Carcinoid heart disease: presentation, diagnosis, and management. *Heart.* 2004;90:1224-1228.

54. Grozinsky-Glasberg S, Grossman AB, Gross DJ. Carcinoid heart disease: from pathophysiology to treatment–"something in the way it moves." *Neuroendocrinology.* 2015;101:263-273.

55. Nishimura RA, Otto CM, Bonow RO, et al. 2014 AHA/ACC guideline for the management of patients with valvular heart disease: a report of the American College of Cardiology/American Heart Association Task Force on Practice Guidelines. *J Am Coll Cardiol.* 2014;63:e57-e185.

56. Muraru D, Hahn RT, Soliman OI, Faletra FF, Basso C, Badano LP. 3-dimensional echocardiography in imaging the tricuspid valve. *JACC Cardiovasc Imaging.* 2019;12:500-515.

57. Zaidi A, Oxborough D, Augustine DX, Bedair R, Harkness A, Rana BS, et al. Echocardiographic assessment of the tricuspid and pulmonary valves. *Echo Res Pract.* 2021;7(4).

58. Zoghbi WA, Adams D, Bonow RO, et al. Recommendations for noninvasive evaluation of native valvular regurgitation: a report from the American Society of Echocardiography Developed in Collaboration with the Society for Cardiovascular Magnetic Resonance. *J Am Soc Echocardiogr.* 2017;30:303-371.

59. Lancellotti P, Moura L, Pierard LA, et al. European Association of Echocardiography recommendations for the assessment of valvular regurgitation. Part 2: mitral and tricuspid regurgitation (native valve disease). *J Am Soc Echocardiogr.* 2010;11:307-332.

60. Khalique OK, Cavalcante JL, Shah D, Guta AC, Zhan Y, Piazza N, et al. Multimodality imaging of the tricuspid valve and right heart anatomy. *JACC Cardiovasc Imaging.* 2019;12:516-531.

61. Muraru D, Caravita S, Guta AC, Mihalcea D, Branzi G, Parati G, et al. Functional tricuspid regurgitation and atrial fibrillation: which comes first, the chicken or the egg? *CASE (Phila).* 2020;4:458-463.

62. Baumgartner H, Falk V, Bax JJ, et al. 2017 ESC/EACTS guidelines for the management of valvular heart diseases. *Eur Heart J.* 2017.

63. Chikwe J, Itagaki S, Anyanwu A, Adams DH. Impact of concomitant tricuspid annuloplasty on tricuspid regurgitation, right ventricular function, and pulmonary artery hypertension after repair of mitral valve prolapse. *J Am Coll Cardiol.* 2015;65:1931-1938.

64. Kilic A, Saha-Chaudhuri P, Rankin JS, Conte JV. Trends and outcomes of tricuspid valve surgery in North America: an analysis of more than 50,000 patients from the Society of Thoracic Surgeons database. *Ann Thorac Surg.* 2013;96:1546-1552; discussion 52.

65. Zack CJ, Fender EA, Chandrashekar P, Reddy YNV, Bennett CE, Stulak JM, et al. National trends and outcomes in isolated tricuspid valve surgery. *J Am Coll Cardiol.* 2017;70:2953-2960.

66. Shinn SH, Schaff HV. Evidence-based surgical management of acquired tricuspid valve disease. *Nat Rev Cardiol.* 2013;10:190-203.

67. Tagliari AP, Perez-Camargo D, Taramasso M. Tricuspid regurgitation: when is it time for surgery? *Expert Rev Cardiovasc Ther.* 2021;19:47-59.

68. Curio J, Demir OM, Pagnesi M, et al. Update on the current landscape of transcatheter options for tricuspid regurgitation treatment. *Interv Cardiol.* 2019;14:54-61.

69. Hahn RT, Meduri CU, Davidson CJ, et al. Early feasibility study of a transcatheter tricuspid valve annuloplasty: SCOUT trial 30-day results. *J Am Coll Cardiol.* 2017;69:1795-1806.

70. Nickenig G, Weber M, Schuler R, et al. Two-year outcomes with the cardioband tricuspid system from the multicentre, prospective TRI-REPAIR study. *Euro Intervention.* 2020.

71. Asmarats L, Perlman G, Praz F, et al. Long-term outcomes of the FORMA transcatheter tricuspid valve repair system for the treatment of severe tricuspid regurgitation: insights from the first-in-human experience. *JACC Cardiovasc Interv.* 2019;12:1438-1447.

72. Perlman GY, Dvir D. Treatment of tricuspid regurgitation with the FORMA repair system. *Front Cardiovasc Med.* 2018;5:140.

73. Taramasso M, Alessandrini H, Latib A, et al. Outcomes after current transcatheter tricuspid valve intervention: mid-term results from the international trivalve registry. *JACC Cardiovasc Interv.* 2019;12:155-165.

74. Nickenig G, Kowalski M, Hausleiter J, et al. Transcatheter treatment of severe tricuspid regurgitation with the edge-to-edge MitraClip technique. *Circulation.* 2017;135:1802-1814.

75. Lurz P, Stephan von Bardeleben R, Weber M, et al. Transcatheter edge-to-edge repair for treatment of tricuspid regurgitation. *J Am Coll Cardiol.* 2021;77:229-239.

76. Perez-Camargo D, Tagliari AP, Taramasso M. Is indexed right ventricular end-diastolic volume a new key for the tricuspid regurgitation puzzle? *Rev Esp Cardiol (Engl Ed).* 2021;74(8):646-647.

77. Bannehr M, Kahn U, Liebchen J, et al. Right ventricular longitudinal strain predicts survival in patients with functional tricuspid regurgitation. *Can J Cardiol.* 2021;37(7):1086-1093.

32

Mitral Stenosis

Vinay K. Bahl and Ravi S. Math

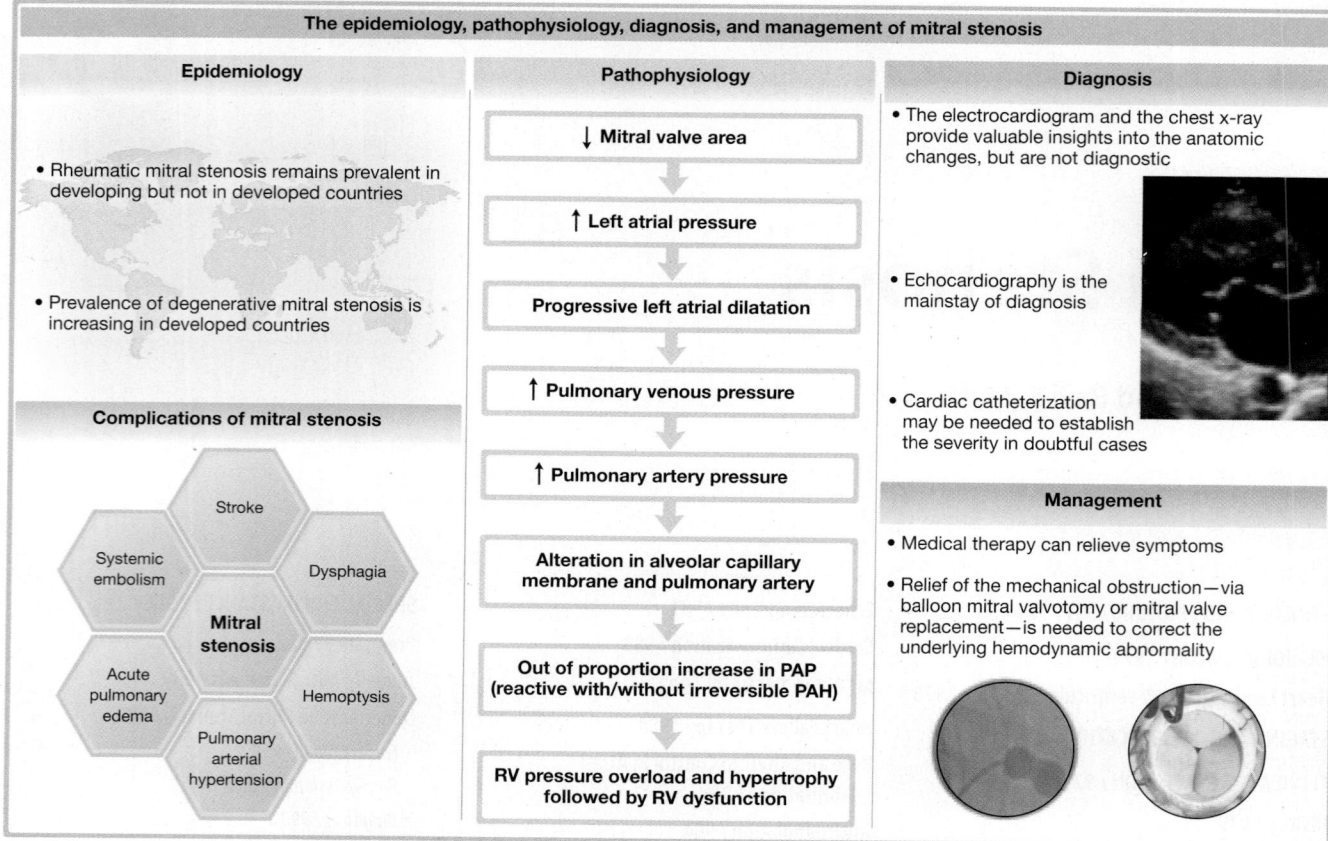

Chapter 32 Fuster and Hurst's Central Illustration. Worldwide, the majority of cases of mitral stenosis are caused by rheumatic heart disease. Echocardiography is the mainstay of diagnosis. It determines the etiology, quantifies the severity of mitral stenosis and its hemodynamic consequences, assesses suitability for balloon mitral valvotomy, and enables serial follow-up. Relief of the mechanical obstruction (by balloon mitral valvotomy or mitral valve replacement) is needed to correct the underlying hemodynamic abnormality. In patients with degenerative mitral stenosis, percutaneous transcatheter mitral replacement is being evaluated. PAH, pulmonary arterial hypertension; PAP, pulmonary artery pressure; RV, right ventricular.

CHAPTER SUMMARY

This chapter discusses the etiology, pathogenesis, clinical presentation, diagnostic modalities, and therapeutic options of mitral stenosis (MS). Rheumatic MS remains prevalent in developing countries whereas prevalence of degenerative MS has increased in developed countries. The hemodynamic hallmark of MS is a persistent diastolic gradient between the left atrium and left ventricle. Exertional dyspnea develops after a long asymptomatic latent period. The course is subsequently complicated by heart failure, atrial fibrillation, thromboembolism, and hemoptysis. Echocardiography is the mainstay of diagnosis, although cardiac catheterization may be needed to establish the severity in doubtful cases. While medical therapy can relieve the symptoms of MS, relief of the mechanical obstruction is needed to correct the underlying hemodynamic abnormality. This is achieved by balloon mitral valvotomy or mitral valve replacement in those with favorable or unfavorable anatomy, respectively. In patients with degenerative MS, newer therapies in the form of percutaneous transcatheter mitral replacement are being evaluated. A concerted global effort to control rheumatic heart disease is needed to reduce the prevalence of rheumatic MS.

ETIOLOGY AND EPIDEMIOLOGY

Worldwide, the majority of cases of mitral stenosis (MS) are caused by rheumatic heart disease (RHD) (**Fig. 32–1**).[1,2] In developed nations, rheumatic fever has become quite rare and so too has MS (0.02% in Sweden).[3] Possible reasons include antibiotic use, improved socioeconomic conditions as well as mutation of the group "A" streptococcus (GAS) to a less rheumatogenic agent. On the other hand, degenerative MS (due to mitral annular calcification) is increasing in developed nations (12.5% in the Euro Heart Survey).[2,4]

RHD remains prevalent in developing countries Using echocardiographic screening, the prevalence of RHD ranged from 20 to 30 per 1000 school children.[5,6] There are an estimated 39 million cases of RHD worldwide,[7] mostly in low- and middle-income countries. Approximately half of the patients with RHD have MS (either isolated or combined with other valve pathologies)[8,9] but only 60% of these patients report a past history of rheumatic fever (RF).[10-12]

Rheumatic MS is a progressive disease with an initial stable course in the early years followed by an accelerated deterioration. The time interval between RF and the clinical appearance of MS varies considerably. In developed countries, the disease has a slow progression with a latency period of 20 to 40 years before symptoms appear.[10-13] Thus, presentation in the West is in the fifth to sixth decades of life.[14] In developing countries, the disease tends to have a more malignant course. Symptoms may appear as early as 20 years of age (juvenile MS), often within 5 years of the initial attack of RF.[15] Usually, the mean age of symptom onset in developing countries is between the third and fourth decades.[16,17] This is likely to be due to recurrent episodes of RF (either clinical or subclinical). Progression from mild to severe disability often takes a decade.[10,12] Once symptoms develop, the prognosis of untreated MS is poor. Among 271 symptomatic patients, the 10-year survival rate of untreated patients in functional class II, III, and IV was 69%, 33%, and 0%, respectively.[13] At 20 years, only half of the

patients in functional class II remained alive while none of the class III patients survived. Overall, the 10-year survival rate was 34% and the 20-year survival rate was only 14%. On the other hand, among asymptomatic or minimally symptomatic patients, the 10-year survival rate is greater than 80%. Echocardiographic studies have demonstrated a progressive reduction in the mitral valve area (MVA) by an average of 0.09 cm^2 per year 18,19 albeit with considerable inter-individual variability (0.0–0.3 cm^2 per year). Some patients showed no change while others had a more rapid decrease (>0.1 cm^2/year) in MVA.[18] Those patients with a larger initial valve area, higher Wilkin's echocardiographic score (>8), higher peak (>10 mm Hg), and mean transmitral gradients had a more progressive course.[19]

The initial attack of RF causes inflammation, thickening, and retraction of the mitral leaflets. This usually causes mild mitral regurgitation (MR), which may disappear as the attack subsides. Why MS develops later is not entirely clear, but at least three factors contribute to the process: gender, the severity of carditis in the first attack, and the number of subsequent attacks. MS is predominantly a disease of women, with a 3:1 female preponderance. The reason for this gender predilection is not clear. It may be due to greater autoimmune susceptibility or due to greater exposure to GAS infection due to closer proximity to children during child rearing. If after the initial attack there is little evidence of valvulopathy and no subsequent attacks occur, the chance of developing severe MS later in life is probably less than 5%.[20] Subsequent attacks can be prevented by faithful adherence to antibiotic prophylaxis. However, what pathologic processes occur between the initial attack of acute rheumatic fever and eventual development of MS (when it does occur) are uncertain. At the time of surgery for MS there are active Aschoff nodules (the pathognomonic lesion of rheumatic fever) in the left atrial appendages (LAAs) of many patients, suggesting that a smoldering rheumatic process persists years after the last acute attack.[21] Alternatively, it may be that after the initial lesion is created by RF, hemodynamic stress on the valve may lead to continued inflammation and scarring. In fact, C-reactive protein is elevated in many MS patients, indicative of ongoing inflammation from either or both processes.[22]

Other rare causes of MS include congenital MS, radiation, infiltrative diseases (eg, mucopolysaccharidosis), multisystemic disorders (eg, systemic lupus erythematosus, rheumatoid arthritis, Fabry's disease, Whipple's disease), drugs (methysergide, pergolide, fenfluramine), and carcinoid heart disease.[17] Sometimes, iatrogenic MS may develop following restrictive surgical mitral valve repair or leaflet-grasping mitraclip implantation.

PATHOPHYSIOLOGY

The main pathology in rheumatic MS is commissural fusion, leaflet thickening, chordal fusion, and shortening leading to a typical "fish-mouth" appearance. Fibrosis may affect leaflets, chordae, as well as papillary muscles. The leaflets and commissures may get calcified. The increased left atrial pressure leads to pathological adaptive modifications in the left atrial wall.

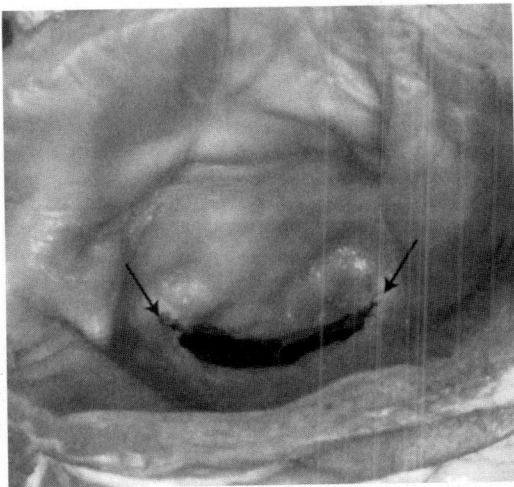

Figure 32–1. The typical "fish mouth" appearance of rheumatic mitral stenosis is shown. Reproduced with permission from Otto CM. *Valvular Heart Disease*. Philadelphia, PA: WB Saunders; 1999.

These include hypertrophy of the atrial muscle fibers and interstitial fibrosis that leads to geometric remodeling and dilatation of the left atria.[23] These, in-turn, lead to development of atrial fibrillation (AF) and thrombus formation in the left atrium (LA) and LAA. Structural changes are also noted in the pulmonary vasculature and lung parenchyma. The small muscular arteries and arterioles show intimal thickening, medial hypertrophy, and muscularization.[24] These changes lead to reactive pulmonary arterial hypertension (PAH).

In normal subjects, the mitral valve area (MVA) is 4 to 6 cm² such that in diastole there is hemodynamically a common chamber of the LA and left ventricle (LV). Thus, as shown in **Fig. 32–2A**, there is an initial small gradient across the mitral valve that rapidly dissipates throughout most of diastole, so that pressures in the LA and LV are equal. However, in MS, as the mitral valve becomes progressively narrowed, a diastolic gradient develops across the valve (**Fig. 32–2B**) so that LA pressure exceeds LV pressure.[25] As MS worsens, the LA pressure becomes progressively higher, in turn creating progressively more pulmonary congestion. The force needed to overcome the increased LA pressure and to drive blood past the stenotic mitral valve is generated by the right ventricle (RV), such that right ventricular pressure (RVSP) and pulmonary pressure (PAP) become elevated. The initial rise in PAP is due to passive retrograde transmission of the elevated left-atrial and pulmonary venous pressures into the pulmonary arterial vasculature. The pulmonary vascular resistance (PVR) is within normal limits (<3 Wood units). The transpulmonary gradient (TPG) and diastolic pulmonary gradient (DFP) are not elevated (<12 and <7 mm Hg, respectively). As MS becomes severe, the PAP pressure rises disproportionate to the increase in LAP and may become extreme. This is termed as reactive PAH, and is due to two mechanisms: (1) pulmonary arteriolar vasoconstriction and (2) morphologic changes in pulmonary vasculature.[26] The PVR, TPG, and DPG are elevated. The exact cause of pulmonary vasoconstriction in MS is unknown. This component of the reactive PAH is almost always reversed by relief of MS[27] and also can be reversed by administration of phosphodiesterase inhibitors such as sildenafil or by nitric oxide inhalation.[28] These data suggest that the nitric oxide pathway is in some way involved in the mechanism of pulmonary vasoconstriction and pulmonary hypertension in MS. The second component (morphologic change) is often described as the "fixed" component and may or may not reverse over years after relief of MS.

The pulmonary hypertension leads to RV pressure overload, RV hypertrophy, and eventually, RV failure. The RV failure in MS is mostly caused by afterload excess rather than contractile dysfunction. As the RV and LV are in series, a reduction in RV output will lead to reduced LV filling (already aggravated by MS) and low cardiac output with a fall in systemic pressure.

PAH creates a "secondary" stenosis at the level of the pulmonary vascular bed that leads to a further decline in cardiac output. This may prevent the development of pulmonary edema at the expense of low cardiac output. However, this is unlikely to be a protective mechanism given the rapidity with which death occurs from congestive heart failure in these patients. The failing RV may lower the PAP leading to an underestimation of the severity of the disease. However, the PVR remains markedly elevated reflecting the true extent of pulmonary vascular disease. Survival of patients with severe PAH (PASP >80 mm Hg) is poor (mean 2.4 years) with half of the patients dying within 1 year of diagnosis.[29]

Heart Failure and Left Ventricular Function

It is generally believed that MS "protects" the LV from damage. That is, unlike other left-sided valve lesions, MS creates no overload on the LV and in fact may decrease preload by impairing LV filling. However, approximately one-third of patients with MS have reduced indices of LV ejection performance.[30,31] Using speckle tracking strain echocardiography, subclinical LV

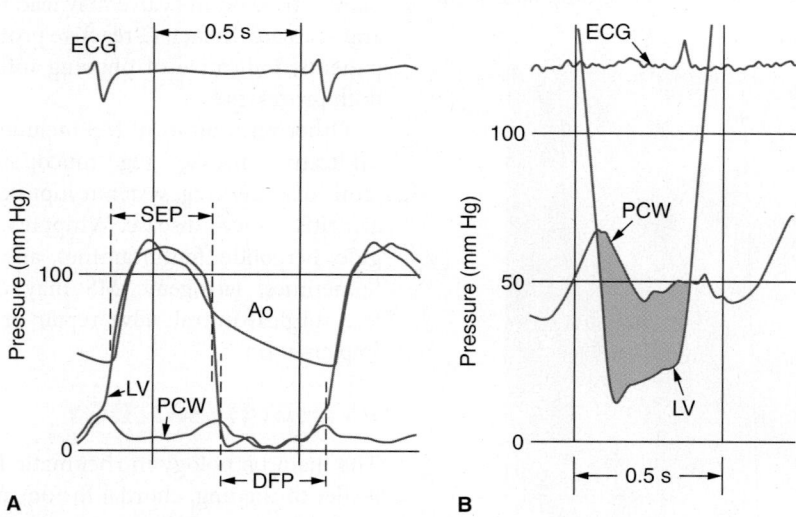

Figure 32–2. **(A)** Normal left ventricle (LV), left atrial, and aortic (Ao) pressure tracings are shown. **(B)** The pressure gradient between pulmonary capillary wedge pressure (PCW) and LV is shown for a patient with mitral stenosis. In this figure, the LV end-diastolic pressure is atypically elevated, consistent with coincident mitral regurgitation. DFP, diastolic filling period; ECG, electrocardiogram; SEP, systolic ejection period. Reproduced with permission from Baim DS, Grossman W. *Grossman's Cardiac Catheterization, Angiography, and Intervention*, 6th ed. Philadelphia, PA: Lippincott Williams & Wilkins; 2000.

TABLE 32-1. Stages and Severity of Mitral Stenosis

Stage	Definition	Valve Anatomy	Valve Hemodynamics	Hemodynamic Consequences	Symptoms
A	At risk of MS	Mild diastolic valve doming	Normal transmitral flow velocity	None	None
B	Progressive MS	1. Rheumatic valve changes with commissural fusion and diastolic doming of the mitral valve leaflets 2. Planimetered MVA >1.5 cm^2	1. Increased transmitral flow velocities 2. MVA >1.5 cm^2 3. Diastolic pressure half-time <150 ms	1. Mild-to-moderate LA enlargement 2. Normal pulmonary pressure at rest	None
C	Asymptomatic severe MS	1. Rheumatic valve changes with commissural fusion and diastolic doming of the mitral valve leaflets 2. Planimetered MVA ≤1.5 cm^2 (MVA ≤1.0 cm^2 with very severe MS)	1. MVA ≤1.5 cm^2 (MVA ≤1.0 cm^2 with very severe MS) 2. Diastolic pressure half-time ≥150 ms (diastolic pressure half-time ≥220 ms with very severe MS)	1. Severe LA enlargement 2. Elevated PASP >30 mm Hg	None
D	Symptomatic severe MS	1. Rheumatic valve changes with commissural fusion and diastolic doming of the mitral valve leaflets 2. Planimetered MVA ≤1.5 cm^2	1. MVA ≤1.5 cm^2 (MVA ≤1.0 cm^2 with very severe MS) 2. Diastolic pressure half-time ≥150 ms (diastolic pressure half-time ≥220 ms with very severe MS)	1. Severe LA enlargement 2. Elevated PASP >30 mm Hg	1. Reduced exercise tolerance 2. Exertional dyspnea

Abbreviations: LA, left atrial; MS, mitral stenosis; MVA, mitral valve area; PASP, pulmonary artery systolic pressure.
Data from Nishimura RA, Otto CM, Bonow RO, et al. 2014 AHA/ACC guideline for the management of patients with valvular heart disease: A report of the American College of Cardiology/American Heart Association Task Force on Practice Guidelines. *J Am Coll Cardiol.* 2014 Jun 10;63(22):2438-2488.

systolic dysfunction was noted in 85% patients despite normal left ventricular ejection fraction (LVEF).[32] A number of factors are responsible for LV dysfunction in MS.[33] First, LV preload is reduced due to reduced LV filling, reduced LV compliance as well as abnormal septal motion from RV pressure overload. Second, myocardial insufficiency from extension of scarring into the subvalvular apparatus or from smoldering rheumatic carditis has been postulated. Third, excessive afterload resulting from increased systemic vascular resistance (arterial vasoconstriction) has been reported. This is further aggravated by reduced LV wall thickness that increases wall stress. Other mechanisms responsible for LV systolic dysfunction include tachycardiomyopathy from an elevated ventricular rate associated with AF and coronary embolism from LA/LAA clot. Acute relief of LV inflow obstruction following balloon mitral valvotomy (BMV) results in rapid correction of LV ejection indices, indicating that loading abnormalities rather than a myocardial factor are the predominant mechanism.[34] However, a minority of patients do not have an improvement in ejection fraction, indicating that intrinsic myocardial dysfunction is also a meaningful contributor.[35]

Diastolic function in MS may also be abnormal. Reverse LV remodeling to smaller than normal LV volumes and regional tethering caused by distortion of the subvalvular apparatus leads to abnormal LV compliance. Like the systolic abnormalities noted earlier, these are also reversed rapidly after balloon valvotomy.[36]

STAGING AND CLASSIFICATION

In 2014, the American College of Cardiology (ACC)/American Heart Association (AHA) guideline committee 37 for the management of valvular heart disease provided a new staging system for rheumatic MS and revised the grading of MS severity (**Table 32-1**). The definition of "severe" MS was revised to the level at which symptoms occurred and when interventional

treatment improved symptoms. Severe MS is now defined as MVA ≤1.5 cm^2, unlike previous guidelines[14] where it was MVA ≤1.0 cm^2 (**Table 32-2**). This may make comparisons with historical cohorts difficult. Further, a large number of patients remain asymptomatic even with MVA of 1.3 to 1.4 cm^2.

CLINICAL PRESENTATION

History

Most patients with mild MS are asymptomatic. Indeed, many women are unaware that they have the disease until the increased cardiac demands of pregnancy cause symptoms to appear. Conditions that increase cardiac output and/or heart

TABLE 32-2. Mitral Stenosis Severity as per ACC/AHA 2006 Guidelines

Mild MS	MVA >1.5 cm^2, Mean gradient <5 mm Hg[a], PASP <30 mm Hg
Moderate MS	MVA 1-1.5 cm^2, Mean gradient 5-10 mm Hg[a], PASP 30-50 mm Hg
Severe MS	MVA <1.0 cm^2, Mean gradient >10 mm Hg[a], PASP >50 mm Hg

[a]Valve gradients are dependent upon transvalvular flow. The gradients suggested in this table assume a normal cardiac output and may not pertain to patients with abnormally high or low transvalvular flows.
Abbreviations: ACC, American College of Cardiology; AHA, American Heart Association; MS, mitral stenosis; MVA, mitral valve area; PASP, pulmonary artery systolic pressure.
Data from American College of Cardiology/American Heart Association Task Force on Practice Guidelines; Society of Cardiovascular Anesthesiologists; Society for Cardiovascular Angiography and Interventions, et al. ACC/AHA 2006 guidelines for the management of patients with valvular heart disease: A report of the American College of Cardiology/American Heart Association Task Force on Practice Guidelines (Writing Committee to Revise the 1998 Guidelines for the Management of Patients With Valvular Heart Disease). Developed in collaboration with the Society of Cardiovascular Anesthesiologists. Endorsed by the Society for Cardiovascular Angiography and Interventions and the Society of Thoracic Surgeons. *Circulation.* 2006 Aug 1;114(5):e84-e231.

rate, such as infection, hyperthyroidism, anemia, or AF, may precipitate symptoms. As MS worsens, symptoms typical of left-sided heart failure occur. Dyspnea on exertion, orthopnea, and paroxysmal nocturnal dyspnea are common. Pulmonary edema may also occur, and if pulmonary hypertension develops, ascites and pedal edema may follow. Fatigue due to low cardiac output and chest pain (angina) from RV hypertrophy with supply-demand mismatch may ensue. The development of pulmonary hypertension may paradoxically reduce dyspnea by creating a proximal obstruction. A symptom seen in MS, but rare in other causes of heart failure, is hemoptysis, usually during activity. As predicted by the Gorlin formula,[38] if exercise causes cardiac output to double, the transmitral gradient will quadruple, causing a sudden increase in LA pressure. This increase is thought to cause rupture of small pulmonary vein anastomoses, leading to frank hemoptysis, to be distinguished from the pink frothy sputum seen in pulmonary edema. Other causes of hemoptysis in MS include pulmonary infarction and chronic bronchitis.[10] In cases where the LA becomes so large that it impinges on the left recurrent laryngeal nerve, hoarseness of voice appears (Ortner syndrome).[39] Not infrequently, an embolic event may be the first symptom of MS. Patients may experience palpitations with episodes of paroxysmal AF.

Physical Examination

Physical examination of the patient with MS may reveal a plethora of signs, many of which are subtle. Therefore, examination should be performed in a quiet, undisturbed setting. In patients with rapid AF, many signs may be inaudible, obscuring the diagnosis. In AF, the pulse is irregularly irregular. The pulse pressure may be reduced, indicating a low stroke volume. The apex beat is usually in its normal position and is tapping in nature. Palpation may reveal a diastolic thrill in the left lateral decubitus position. A left parasternal RV heave and palpable P2 in the second intercostal space may be felt in the presence of pulmonary hypertension. S1 is typically loud because the transmitral gradient holds the valve open throughout diastole and LV systole closes the valve from its fully open (albeit stenotic) position, However, in far advanced disease, the valve may have little motion and S1 becomes soft. S2 may be normal, or its P2 component may be loud, if pulmonary hypertension has developed. S2 is followed by an opening snap (OS), and the S2-OS interval gives a good clue to the severity of the MS. As severity worsens, the LA pressure increases, therefore LA pressure exceeds LV pressure (the force that opens the valve) relatively soon after S2, and the S2-OS interval is short, approximately 80 ms. Conversely, in mild disease, the S2-OS interval is long, approaching 120 ms.[39,40] LV S3 and LV S4 sounds produced by rapid LV filling, are typically absent in MS. However, RV S3 and RV S4 due to RV systolic and diastolic dysfunction may be present. The OS is followed by the typical low-pitched rumbling mid-diastolic murmur of MS. The murmur is heard best at the LV apex using the bell of the stethoscope in the left lateral position with the breath held in expiration. The murmur may be very soft in obese patients, those with emphysema, and those with a low cardiac output and fast ventricular rate.

The duration of the murmur correlates with severity of MS. In mild MS, the murmur is short, while it is heard throughout diastole in severe MS. If the patient is in sinus rhythm, there may be presystolic accentuation of the murmur due to atrial contraction. The OS and diastolic rumble are the hallmarks of MS. In a prospective, blinded study, the diagnostic sensitivity and specificity of clinical examination for MS was 86% and 87%, respectively, whereas the accuracy of assessing moderate or severe MS severity was 92%.[41]

If pulmonary hypertension has ensued, the high-pitched murmur of pulmonary insufficiency (Graham Steell murmur) may be heard in the pulmonic area. However, the concomitant presence of aortic insufficiency is often mistaken for this murmur.[42] In addition, a pansystolic murmur of tricuspid regurgitation (TR) may be heard in the tricuspid area. Both murmurs increase with inspiration. Neck vein distension, ascites, hepatomegaly, and edema all may reflect RV failure.

Complications

AF is the most common complication, developing in approximately 40% of patients.[43] It is initially paroxysmal (often subclinical) and subsequently becomes permanent. Development of AF has a profound effect on the course of MS. The 10-year survival rate of patients with AF is 25% compared to 46% for those who remain in sinus rhythm.[13] AF reduces exercise capacity, precipitates or worsens preexisting symptoms and places the patient at risk of thrombus formation and systemic embolism. The age of the patient and the severity of MS are the most important determinants for development of AF.[43] AF occurs in less than 10% of patients with MS below 30 years of age, but increases to as high as 50% in the sixth and seventh decade. AF is related to LA enlargement, the latter often a result rather than the cause of AF.[43]

Systemic embolism occurs in up to 20%[44–47] of patients, with the majority (60%–75%)[43] occurring to the brain. Eighty percent of patients with thromboembolism and MS are in AF. Increasing age and presence of AF are the main predictors. Previous thromboembolism is positively associated with risk of subsequent embolism. The frequency of recurrence is as high as 15 to 40 events per 100 patient months.[48,49] When embolization occurs in the presence of sinus rhythm (20% cases[44,50]), transient AF and infective endocarditis should be considered.[46] Transient subclinical AF[51] has been shown to be a major predictor for systemic embolic events.

The risk of infective endocarditis in isolated MS is low (2% over 10 years).[47] Other major complications of MS include hemoptysis (sometimes massive), pulmonary embolism, and respiratory infections.[39] In the presurgical era, 62% of the deaths were caused by heart failure, 22% from thromboembolic complications, and 8% from infections.[13] Sudden cardiac death was noted in a significant proportion of cases (14%).[12]

DIAGNOSTIC STUDIES

The electrocardiogram (ECG) and the chest x-ray provide valuable insights into the anatomic changes affecting the various chambers of the heart and the lungs in MS. They are by no means diagnostic.

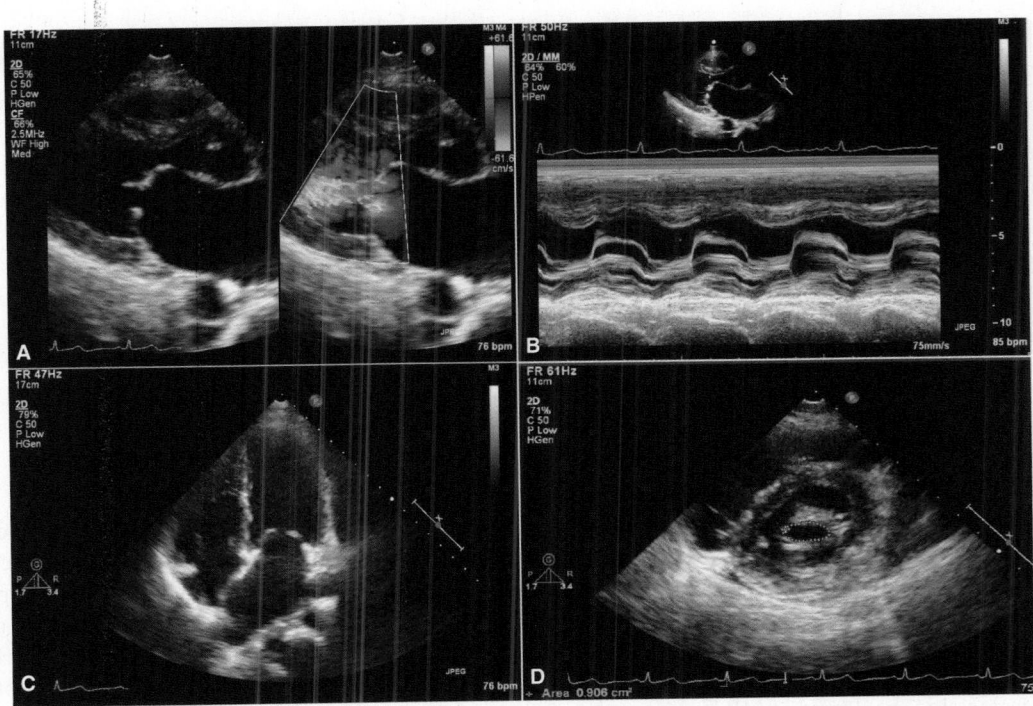

Figure 32–3. **(A)** Transthoracic two-dimensional echocardiogram parasternal long-axis view demonstrating a "hockey-stick" appearance of anterior mitral leaflet. **(B)** M-mode echocardiogram across tips of mitral valve leaflets showing reduced E-F slope and paradoxical anterior motion of posterior leaflet. **(C)** Four-chamber view showing thickening of both leaflets and immobility of posterior mitral leaflet. **(D)** Planimetry of mitral valve in short axis with valve area of 0.9 cm².

Electrocardiogram

Broad and notched P-waves may be present, indicating LA enlargement (P mitrale) in sinus rhythm. Tall "R" waves in the right precordial leads provide a clue to RV hypertrophy. These electrocardiographic findings have high specificity but low sensitivity. AF is often present. In patients with long-standing PAH, right axis deviation and right atrial enlargement may be present.

Chest X-Ray

Before the easy availability of echocardiography, the chest x-ray was often the key diagnostic study. The chest x-ray shows left atrial enlargement, pulmonary arterial hypertension, and varying degrees of pulmonary congestion. Left atrial enlargement causes a retro-cardiac double density (double density sign) along with widening of the subcarinal angle, elevation of left main bronchus and posterior displacement of the esophagus (on lateral view). LAA enlargement leads to straightening of the left heart border or a convexity just below the pulmonary artery segment (third mogul sign).[52]

Echocardiography

The echocardiogram is the diagnostic modality of choice in the evaluation of MS. It establishes the diagnosis, determines the etiology, quantifies the severity of MS and its hemodynamic consequences, detects concomitant valve involvement (including MR), assesses size and function of cardiac chambers, assesses suitability for balloon mitral valvotomy (BMV),

and enables serial follow-up.[53,54] Valve images show restricted opening of mitral leaflets with diastolic doming of the anterior mitral leaflet ("hockey-stick" appearance), immobility of the posterior leaflet, and "fish-mouth" narrowing of the valve orifice (**Fig. 32–3**). Estimation of MVA can be determined by direct planimetry (either two-dimensional [2D] or three-dimensional [3D]), continuity equation, pressure half-time technique (dividing an empirical constant of 220 by the mitral inflow pressure half-time), and the proximal isovelocity surface area (PISA) method. It is important to understand the pitfalls of each of these methods. Often, these measurements are concordant, but sometimes they are not in agreement. In such cases, all measures must be taken into account and clinical judgment is used to decide the severity of MS. The mean transmitral pressure gradient (TMG) across the mitral valve can be determined using the continuous-wave Doppler signal. Although this parameter is affected by flow and heart rate, it correlates well with invasively measured mean TMG.[55] In the presence of AF, an average of 5 beats with least variation should be taken. If tricuspid insufficiency is present, the jet velocity across the tricuspid valve can be used to estimate peak PA pressure. LA dimension and volume also give clues to the impact of the disease on that chamber.

Three-dimensional echocardiography enables accurate en face views of the mitral valve. Planimetry by 3D echocardiography has better reproducibility and intraobserver variability than 2D echocardiography.[56] It has the closest agreement with invasive Gorlin-derived MVA when compared to 2D methods (planimetry, PHT, and PISA).[57] It also provides better

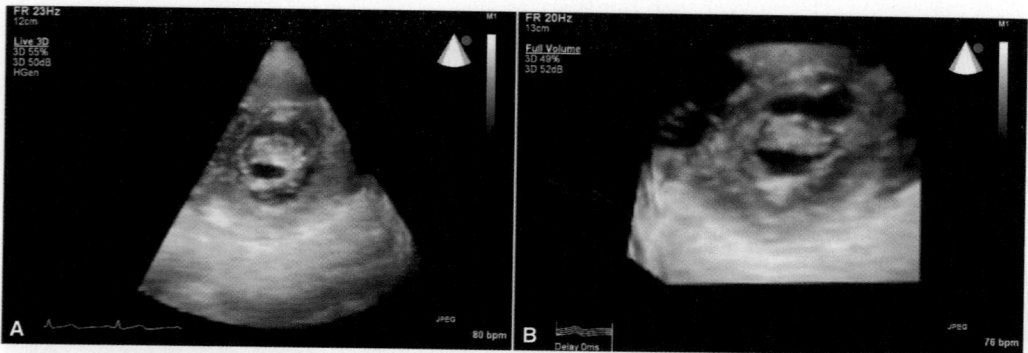

Figure 32–4. (A) Three-dimensional echocardiogram showing typical "fish-mouth" appearance of mitral stenosis. **(B)** Three-dimensional echocardiogram after balloon mitral valvotomy demonstrating a completely split lateral commissure and partially split medial commissure indicative of successful balloon mitral valvotomy.

evaluation of commissural anatomy in patients undergoing BMV[58] (**Fig. 32–4**).

In most patients, transesophageal echocardiography is not routinely necessary because TTE provides the requisite information. TEE is useful when TTE images are suboptimal. TEE is routinely performed prior to BMV to exclude LA/LAA thrombus as well as for reassessing the degree of MR.[37]

Stress echocardiography (by exercise or dobutamine infusion) may be performed if patients are asymptomatic or if symptoms discordant with the severity of MS.[37] Semi-supine echocardiography is preferable to postexercise echocardiography protocols because it allows estimation of hemodynamics throughout the examination.[37] Objective limitation of exercise tolerance accompanied by a rise in MDG greater than 15 mm Hg and an exercise-induced PA systolic pressure (PASP) >60 mm Hg may be an indication for BMV, if valve anatomy is suitable.[59]

Echocardiography plays a pivotal role in selecting patients for BMV, the preferred modality of treatment for MS.[53] Several echocardiographic scores have been developed to select patients best suited for BMV. A combination of variables is used to predict the acute success and complications. The Wilkins' score is the oldest and most commonly used.[60] Valve leaflet thickness, leaflet mobility, valve calcification, and subvalvular apparatus deformity are scored from 0 to 4, with higher values indicating greater morphological abnormality. Valves scored 8 or less generally respond well to BMV (84% good results) whereas those with scores >8 have suboptimal results (58% had suboptimal results). However, this is not a uniform rule, and some patients with higher scores may still achieve a good result with BMV.[61] Other scoring systems using fluoroscopy along with 2D and 3D echocardiographic scores have also been reported.[62,63] A "revised" echocardiographic score[64] was developed to overcome the shortcomings of the Wilkins' score (namely the lack of assessment of commissural pathology). It included four echocardiographic variables: MVA, maximum leaflet displacement, commissural area ratio, and subvalvular involvement. Three groups were identified (low 0–3, intermediate 4–5, and high score 6–11). Suboptimal BMV results were observed in 16.9%, 56.3%, and 73.8%, respectively. It was found to be particularly useful in those with intermediate Wilkins's score of 9 to 11 with net reclassification improvement of 76.8%. However, it must be noted that none of the scores have been proven to be superior to all others.[53] All have limitations in predicting the success (or complications) of BMV and the scoring systems should be considered complementary to one another. Because the mechanism of BMV is splitting of commissures, assessment of commissural calcium is vital. If there is no commissural calcification, there is a >95% chance of a successful BMV procedure with excellent long-term outcome. Thus, in most experienced centers, irrespective of echocardiographic scores, BMV is offered to all patients without commissural calcification. However, bicommissural calcification is an absolute contraindication for BMV.

The presence and severity of concomitant MR is also assessed because BMV may worsen existing MR. Grade 3 to 4 MR is considered an absolute contraindication.[14] More than mild (1+) MR is usually considered a relative contraindication to BMV although BMV may be safely performed in patients with grade 2 MR, if the MR is central. BMV is avoided if the Grade 2 MR is eccentric. If after transthoracic echocardiography, BMV is contemplated, transesophageal echocardiography is usually performed to look for thrombus in the LA and LAA and to reassess the degree of MR. Presence of LA/LAA thrombus has been a contraindication to BMV.[37] If thrombus is detected, warfarin anticoagulation is initiated and the patient is reimaged in 3 months for suitability for BMV.[37] Theoretically, this may entail placing the patient at an increased risk of systemic embolism/hemodynamic decompensation during the 3-month waiting period (as opposed to performing a mitral valve replacement [MVR]/open mitral valvotomy immediately). This needs to be weighed against the potential long-term complications associated with a prosthetic valve. If the thrombus has resolved, BMV may then be performed. On the other hand, persistence of thrombus in the LA/LAA after anticoagulation has traditionally been a contraindication for BMV and such patients are usually offered open mitral valve surgery. Of late, some studies have shown that it is feasible to perform BMV in selected patients with LA/LAA thrombus after 8 to 12 weeks of anticoagulation.[65] The LA/LAA thrombus was classified into five types based on the location (**Table 32–3**). Patients with LA/LAA thrombus type Ia, Ib, and IIa underwent BMV using a

TABLE 32–3. LA/LAA Clot Classification

Type Ia:	LAA clot confined to appendage
Type Ib:	LAA appendage clot protruding into LA cavity
Type IIa:	LA roof clot limited to a plane above the plane of fossa ovalis
Type IIb:	LA roof clot extending below the plane of fossa ovalis
Type III:	Layered clot over the IAS
Type IV:	Mobile clot which is attached to LA free wall or roof or IAS
Type V:	Ball valve thrombus (free floating)

Abbreviations: IAS, interatrial space; LA, left atrium; LAA, left atrial appendage.
Data from Manjunath CN, Srinivasa KH, Ravindranath KS, et al: Balloon mitral valvotomy in patients with mitral stenosis and left atrial thrombus. *Catheter Cardiovasc Interv.* 2009 Oct 1;74(4):653-661.

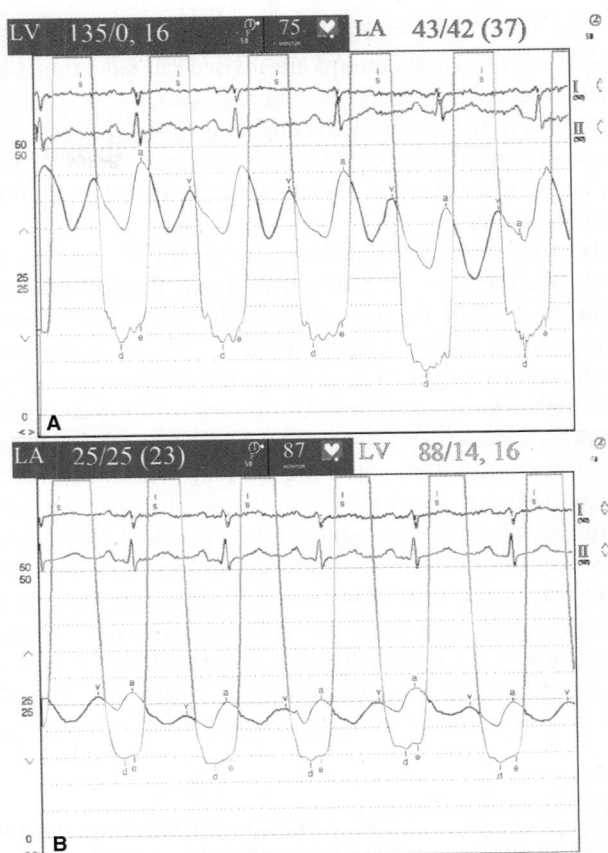

Figure 32–5. (A) Simultaneous left atrial (LA) and left ventricular (LV) pressure tracings in a patient with severe mitral stenosis (mean transmitral gradient 20.4 mm Hg). (B) Simultaneous LA and LV pressure tracings in the same patient after successful balloon mitral valvotomy (mean transmitral gradient reduced to 6.6 mm Hg, reduction in mean LA pressure and V wave height).

modified over the wire technique that virtually excluded the LA from the track of the septal dilator and balloon catheter exchanges.[65] BMV was successfully performed in 98% of cases with only one episode of TIA among 108 patients. However, it is to be noted that BMV was performed by experienced operators (>500 procedures) in this study.

Echocardiography guidance is extremely useful during BMV and for postprocedural assessment. TTE/TEE aids in transseptal puncture. Following each balloon inflation, transmitral gradient, MVA by planimetry, commissural splitting, leaflet mobility; the presence, degree and mechanism of MR, and any complications (pericardial effusion) are assessed. In long-term assessment, echocardiography aids in determining the mechanism of restenosis (commissural vs leaflet stenosis).

Follow-up echocardiography is recommended among asymptomatic individuals at intervals of 3 to 5 years in those with MVA >1.5 cm², every 1 to 2 years with MVA ≤1.5 cm², and yearly in those with MVA <1 cm.[37]

Cardiac Catheterization

In most cases, MS can be completely assessed noninvasively and cardiac catheterization is not required. However, if after echocardiography, the issue of MS severity is still in doubt, the diagnosis may be resolved by cardiac catheterization. This scenario may arise when symptoms are out of proportion to the measured valve area or if the degree of PAH is out of proportion to the transmitral gradient, as measured noninvasively. Invasive hemodynamics are also needed to guide BMV.

The hallmark of MS is a persistent gradient between LV and LA during diastole. In the early phases, there is a prominent "a" wave with increased LA pressure. In long standing cases, the V wave becomes prominent even in the absence of MR due to reduced atrial compliance from fibrosis. Notably, the slope of the Y descent is decreased (unlike in MR) due to obstruction to LV filling. Accurate measurement of the transmitral gradient requires simultaneous LA and LV pressures by means of transseptal puncture (**Figs. 32–5A** and **32–5B**). However, a carefully obtained pulmonary capillary wedge pressure (PCWP, time adjusted) may be substituted for LA pressure in measuring the transvalvular gradient.[66]

Data from invasive hemodynamics are used to calculate the mitral valve area using the Gorlin formula (MVA = CO/*dfp* × *hr*/37.7 $\sqrt{h_2 - h_1}$), where MVA = mitral valve area (cm²), CO = cardiac output (mL/min), *dfp* = diastolic filling period (seconds), *hr* = heart rate, and $h_1 - h_2$ = the mean transmitral gradient.[38]

If resting hemodynamics are unrevealing, dynamic or handgrip exercise may show significant elevation in PCWP and PA pressure, demonstrating the cause of the patient's symptoms (transmitral gradient >15 mm Hg, or a PCWP >25 mm Hg).[37]

A multislice ECG gated computed tomography (CT) scan is useful in detecting calcification, LA/LAA thrombus, and planimetry of the MV. In addition, it provides noninvasive preoperative coronary artery assessment.

MEDICAL THERAPY

MS is a mechanical obstruction. Thus, medical therapy can only ameliorate symptoms. It does not prevent or delay disease progression. Medical therapy aims to relieve heart failure symptoms, reduce thromboembolic events, prevent recurrence of rheumatic fever, and provide infective endocarditis (IE) prophylaxis.

Heart Failure Therapy

Patients with severe symptoms are advised salt reduction, limitation of exercise activity, and diuretic therapy.[39,47] Thiazide and loop diuretics may be used depending on degree of congestion. Potassium sparing diuretic (spironolactone or amiloride) may be added for potassium homeostasis. Overzealous diuresis should be avoided.

Heart rate control improves symptoms in MS patients by prolonging the diastolic filling period and thereby reducing the mean diastolic gradient, PCWP, and mean PAP. Nondihydropyridine calcium channel blockers (CCBs), β-blockers, and digoxin have been used in MS patients with sinus rhythm (with higher heart rates) and AF patients with rapid ventricular rates. Calcium antagonists and β-blockers achieve better heart rate control during exercise but may be associated with reduced exercise capacity. Digoxin is useful in patients with LV and/or RV dysfunction and may be added to β-blockers for added rate control. Ivabradine (a selective sinus node-blocking agent) may have an advantage over β-blockers in patients with sinus rhythm because it has no effect on myocardial contractility. Studies have demonstrated that ivabradine is at least as effective β-blockers in improving exercise tolerance.[67] Anemia, fever, infection, and hyperthyroidism should be corrected.

Rate and Rhythm Control in Atrial Fibrillation

The onset of acute AF with a rapid ventricular response can have markedly severe clinical consequences at times, leading to acute pulmonary edema and shock. In very sick patients, immediate direct current cardioversion is indicated to restore sinus rhythm. If the consequences of rapid AF are less severe, rate control may be accomplished by intravenous administration of a β-blocker such as metoprolol or esmolol, a CCB such as diltiazem, or digoxin. Digoxin gains rate control less rapidly but may be preferable if blood pressure is tenuous. Intravenous amiodarone can be used to control the heart rate in patients where β-blockers or heart-rate–regulating CCBs cannot be used or have not been effective.[37]

In chronic AF, adequate rate control may be achieved with oral β-blockers and CCBs (Class IIa recommendation).[37] Digoxin may be added if optimal heart rate control is not achieved. Heart rate control should be evaluated both at rest and during modest activity. A resting heart rate <80 bpm and an exercise (moderate) heart rate <100 bpm is recommended for symptomatic patients.[68]

Randomized trials of nonvalvular AF have shown that a rhythm control strategy offers no survival advantage over a rate control strategy.[69] However, rheumatic MS patients are younger, with a higher risk of embolism and a structurally abnormal heart. Limited data suggests that rhythm control may be superior to rate control in MS.[70-72] However, as MS severity worsens, sinus rhythm is difficult to achieve and maintain. The decision for cardioversion (electrical or pharmacological) should take into consideration the patient's age, the duration of AF, the hemodynamic response to AF, the LA size, the past history of AF, and the limitation to exercise capacity. A successful BMV enables patients in sinus rhythm to persist in sinus rhythm[73] but it does not promote reversion to sinus rhythm in patients with chronic AF by itself.[74] Studies of successful cardioversion have combined BMV, direct current (DC) cardioversion, and antiarrhythmic therapy.[71] Following successful BMV, patients are loaded with IV amiodarone. Subsequently, they undergo DC cardioversion followed by oral amiodarone therapy for up to 1 year. At 1 year, maintenance of sinus rhythm was achieved in 55% to 96%.[70,71] Those with shorter duration of AF and smaller LA size were more likely to remain in sinus rhythm (LA size <45 mm, duration of AF <1 year).[70] At the time of mitral valve surgery (replacement or repair), the performance of a biatrial maze or pulmonary vein isolation enables more than 60% of patients to remain in sinus rhythm at 1 year.[75] There was, however, a greater need for permanent pacemaker implantation. Catheter-based radiofrequency ablation has been performed in a small number of patients at the time of mitral commissurotomy with limited success.[76] Lastly, AV node ablation with permanent pacemaker implantation may be performed when ventricular rate cannot be controlled by pharmacological methods.[23]

Anticoagulation

The MS patient with AF has a very high risk of stroke (1.5%–4.7% per patient years).[77] The Framingham Heart Study noted that patients with MS and AF have a 17-fold excess risk of stroke as compared to the general population.[76] Although there are no randomized trials, retrospective studies have shown a 4- to 15-fold reduction in incidence of embolic events in MS patients with anticoagulation.[14,48,49] Anticoagulation with vitamin K antagonist (VKA) is recommended for MS patients with AF (paroxysmal, persistent, or permanent), those with a prior embolic event, and those with a left atrial/left atrial appendage thrombus to maintain an international normalized ratio of 2.5 (range 2–3) for an indefinite duration.[37] For patients with an enlarged LA (M-mode diameter >50mm or LA volume >60mL/m^2 or those with spontaneous echo contrast, the ESC guidelines have given a class IIa recommendation (level of evidence C) for anticoagulation (**Table 32–4**), but this has not been adequately studied.[77] Use of aspirin as an alternative is not recommended but low-dose aspirin (81 mg/d) may be added to anticoagulation to further reduce the risk of stroke.[78] Non–vitamin K oral anticoagulants (NOAC) have been approved for prevention of systemic embolism in nonvalvular AF. The pivotal trials of NOACs excluded patients with moderate-to-severe MS and hence these agents remain contraindicated in MS patients with indications for anticoagulation.[77,79] A retrospective analysis of approximately 2000 patients with MS with AF receiving off-label DOACs found reduced rates of thromboembolism and ICH as compared to warfarin.[80]

Infective Endocarditis and Rheumatic Fever Prophylaxis

Among valve lesions, patients with MS are at relatively low risk for developing IE. The ACC/AHA[79] and the ESC[81] guidelines do not recommend preprocedural antibiotic therapy for the prevention of IE in patients with MS unless the patient has had

TABLE 32–4. Comparison of US and European Guidelines for the Management of Mitral Stenosis

	ACC/AHA 2014 Guidelines	Class	ESC 2017 Guidelines	Class
INVESTIGATIONS	TTE is indicated in patients with signs or symptoms of MS to establish the diagnosis, quantify severity, and determine suitability for BMV	I B	No recommendations	
	TEE should be performed before BMV to assess the presence or absence of left atrial thrombus and to further evaluate the severity of MR	I B	No recommendations	
	Exercise testing with Doppler or invasive hemodynamic assessment to evaluate the response of the mean MG and PASP when there is a discrepancy between resting Doppler echocardiographic findings and clinical symptoms or signs	I C	No recommendations	
MEDICAL THERAPY	Anticoagulation (vitamin K antagonist or heparin) is indicated in patients with AF (paroxysmal, persistent, or permanent), a prior embolic event, or left atrial thrombus	I B	Anticoagulation with vitamin K antagonist for new onset, paroxysmal, and persistent AF	I C
			Anticoagulation is recommended if TEE shows dense spontaneous echocardiographic contrast or an enlarged LA (M-mode diameter >50 mm or LA volume >60 mL/m^2)	IIa C
			The use of NOACs is not recommended in patients with AF and moderate to severe MS	III C
	Heart rate control can be beneficial in patients with MS and AF and fast ventricular response	IIa C		
	Heart rate control may be considered for patients with MS in normal sinus rhythm and symptoms associated with exercise	IIb B		
BALLOON MITRAL VALVOTOMY (BMV)	BMV is recommended for symptomatic patients (NYHA II-IV) with severe MS (MVA ≤1.5 cm^2, stage D) and favorable valve morphology in the absence of left atrial thrombus or moderate-to-severe MR	I A	BMV is indicated in symptomatic patients without unfavorable characteristics for BMV	I B
	BMV is reasonable for asymptomatic patients with very severe MS (MVA ≤1.0 cm^2, stage C) and favorable valve morphology	IIa C		
	BMV may be considered for asymptomatic patients with severe MS (MVA ≤1.5 cm^2, stage C) and favorable valve morphology with new onset of AF.	IIb C		
	BMV may be considered for symptomatic patients with MVA >1.5 cm^2 if there is evidence of hemodynamically significant MS based on PAWP >25 mm Hg or mean MVG >15 mm Hg during exercise	IIb C		
	BMV may be considered for severely symptomatic patients (NYHA class III-IV) with severe MS (MVA ≤1.5 cm^2, stage D) who have a suboptimal valve anatomy and who are not candidates for surgery or at high risk for surgery	IIb C	BMV is indicated in any symptomatic patients with a contraindication or a high risk for surgery.	I C
			BMV should be considered as initial treatment in symptomatic patients with suboptimal anatomy but no unfavorable clinical characteristics for BMV	IIa C
			BMV in asymptomatic patients with favorable anatomy and high thromboembolic risk (history of systemic embolism, dense spontaneous contrast in the LA, new-onset, or paroxysmal AF)	IIa C
			BMV in asymptomatic patients with favorable anatomy and high risk of hemodynamic decompensation (PASP >50 mm Hg at rest, need for major noncardiac surgery, desire for pregnancy)	IIa C
			BMV should be considered in pregnant patients with severe symptoms or PASP >50 mm Hg despite medical therapy#	IIa C

(Continued)

TABLE 32–4. Comparison of US and European Guidelines for the Management of Mitral Stenosis (Continued)

	ACC/AHA 2014 Guidelines	Class	ESC 2017 Guidelines	Class
MITRAL VALVE SURGERY	Mitral valve surgery (repair, commissurotomy, or valve replacement) is indicated in severely symptomatic patients (NYHA class III–IV) with severe MS (MVA ≤1.5 cm², stage D) who are not high risk for surgery and who are not candidates for or who have failed previous BMV	I B	Mitral valve surgery is indicated in symptomatic patients who are not suitable for BMV	I C
	Concomitant mitral valve surgery is indicated for patients with Severe MS (MVA ≤ 1.5 cm², stage C or D) undergoing cardiac surgery for other indications	I C		
	Mitral valve surgery is reasonable for severely symptomatic patients (NYHA class III–IV) with severe MS (MVA ≤1.5 cm², stage D), provided there are other operative indications (eg, aortic valve disease, CAD, TR, aortic aneurysm)	IIa C		
	Concomitant mitral valve surgery may be considered for patients with moderate MS (MVA 1.6–2.0 cm²) undergoing cardiac surgery for other indications	IIb C		
	Mitral valve surgery and excision of the left atrial appendage may be considered for patients with severe MS (MVA ≤1.5 cm², stages C and D) who have had recurrent embolic events while receiving adequate anticoagulation	IIb C		

Abbreviations: ACC, American College of Cardiology; AHA, American Heart Association; ESC, European Society of Cardiology; TTE, transthoracic Echocardiography; TEE, transesophageal echocardiography; BMV, Balloon mitral valvotomy; MR, mitral regurgitation; MG, mean gradient; PASP, pulmonary artery systolic pressure; AF, atrial fibrillation; LA, left atrial; MS, mitral stenosis; NYHA, New York Heart Association; MVA, mitral valve area; PAWP, pulmonary artery wedge presssure; CAD, coronary artery disease; TR, tricuspid regurgitation

Data from Nishimura RA, Otto CM, Bonow RO, et al. 2014 AHA/ACC guideline for the management of patients with valvular heart disease: a report of the American College of Cardiology/American Heart Association Task Force on Practice Guidelines. *J Am Coll Cardiol.* 2014;63(22):2438-2488; Baumgartner H, Falk V, Bax J, et al. ESC/EACTS Guidelines for the management of valvular heart disease: the Task Force for the Management of Valvular Heart Disease of the European Society of Cardiology (ESC) and the European Association for Cardio- Thoracic Surgery (EACTS). *Eur Heart J.* 2017;2017:2939-2991; Regitz-Zagrosek V, Roos-Hesselink JW, Bauersachs J, et al. 2018 ESC Guidelines for the management of cardiovascular diseases during pregnancy. *Eur Heart J.* 2018;39:3165-3241.

a previous episode of IE. However, not all international societies are in agreement with this recommendation. The Brazilian,[82] South African,[83] and the Australian guidelines[84] continue to recommend antibiotic prophylaxis for RHD. This is because RHD is still rampant in these areas and has high morbidity and mortality associated with IE. In addition, many of these patients would have poor oral hygiene. Finally, recent studies have raised a concern that IE incidence has increased in countries with reduced IE prophylaxis following the guideline changes.[85,86] As such, individual judgment should be used in advising antibiotic prophylaxis.

Secondary prevention of rheumatic fever (preferably long-acting benzathine penicillin G) should be continued for rheumatic MS. Patients should receive prophylaxis for 10 years after the last episode of acute rheumatic fever or until 40 years of age, whichever is longer.[87] Some high-risk patients may require longer (even lifelong) prophylaxis, depending upon the severity of valvular disease and the potential for exposure to GAS. The risk of recurrence of rheumatic fever declines with increasing age and the number of years from the last attack.

MECHANICAL THERAPY

Three procedures are routinely practiced for the relief of MS: BMV, open commissurotomy (OMV), and MVR. In some areas, closed commissurotomy (CMV) is still practiced quite effectively and does not entail the cost of the catheters and balloons needed for BMV. Because BMV is less morbid and

carries a lower mortality than surgery, the timing for BMV is more liberal than for surgical procedures at both ends of the clinical spectrum. BMV may be applied for mild symptoms caused by severe MS or in late-stage disease in patients at high risk for surgery from various comorbidities. Advanced symptoms worsen prognosis (**Fig. 32–6**), and thus BMV or surgery should be performed before the patients reaches New York Heart Association (NYHA) class III.[88] Additionally, pulmonary hypertension defined as a peak systolic pressure >50 mm Hg at rest also worsens prognosis and increases surgical risk.[89] Thus mechanical relief of obstruction should ideally take place before this degree of severity has developed.

Balloon Mitral Valvotomy

BMV was first performed by Inoue in 1984[90] followed by Lock in 1985.[91] A metanalysis of seven randomized controlled trials comparing BMV with surgical commissurotomy (OMV/CMV) found no difference in immediate results in terms of MVA achieved and postprocedural severe MR as well as restenosis/reintervention at 30 months.[92] Given the greater procedural morbidity of cardiac surgery, BMV is the procedure of choice for relieving MS.[37] Surgery is reserved for patients who are not candidates for BMV.

BMV is recommended for the following groups of patients:[37]

1. Symptomatic patients (class II–IV) with severe MS (MVA ≤1.5 cm²) (class I indication) or asymptomatic patients with very severe MS (MVA ≤1.0 cm²) (class IIa indication) with a

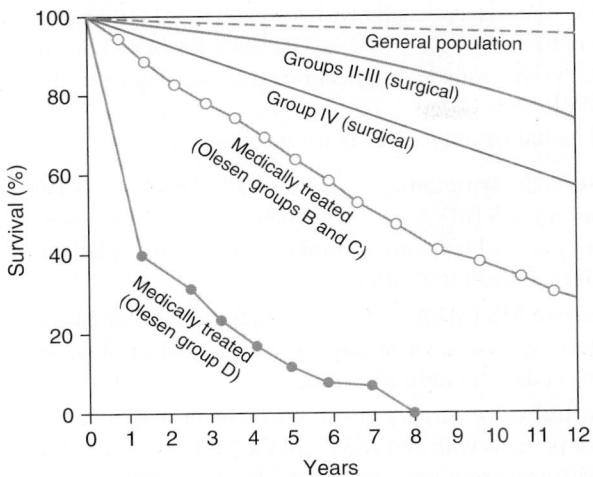

Figure 32–6. Survival according to therapy and symptomatic status for patients with mitral stenosis is shown. New York Heart Association classes II, III, and IV are roughly equivalent to Olesen groups B, C, and D, respectively. Reproduced with permission from Roy SB, Gopinath N. Mitral Stenosis. *Circulation.* 1968 July;38(1 Suppl):68-76.

favorable valve morphology in the absence of LA thrombus and moderate-to-severe MR;

2. Asymptomatic patients with severe MS (MVA ≤1.5 cm²) with new-onset AF and suitable valve anatomy (class IIb indication);

3. Symptomatic patients with MVA >1.5 cm² and hemodynamically significant MS during exercise (mean mitral valve gradient >15, PCWP >25 mm Hg, class IIb indication); and

4. Severely symptomatic patients (NYHA class III–IV) with severe MS (MVA ≤1.5 cm²) with suboptimal valve anatomy and high risk for surgery (class IIb indication).

In addition, BMV may be considered in asymptomatic severe MS (MVA <1.5 cm²) patients if they are at high risk of hemodynamic decompensation (eg, those needing major surgery or desire for pregnancy).[77] Absolute contraindications for the BMV are LA/LAA thrombus, Grade 3 to 4 MR, severe or bicommissural calcification, and absence of commissural fusion.

BMV can be performed using an hourglass-shaped balloon (triple lumen Inoue balloon[90] or double lumen Accura balloon[93]), a single[91] or double peripheral angioplasty balloon,[94] or a reusable valvulotome.[95] Although the three techniques produce a similar outcome,[94,96] the hourglass-shaped balloons are preferred. The steps for BMV are depicted in **Figs. 32–7A, 32–7B, 32–7C, 32–7D.** First, a transseptal puncture is performed (Fig. 32–7A), and the inter-atrial septum is dilated with a dilator (Fig. 32–7B). A balloon is then advanced across the septum, into the LA and across the mitral valve. Stepwise inflation of the balloon (distal, proximal, and then middle portion) causes commissural splitting (Fig. 32–7C, D; Fig. 32–5B), permitting a dramatic increase in leaflet motion and valve area. The procedure has a steep learning curve and hence should be performed

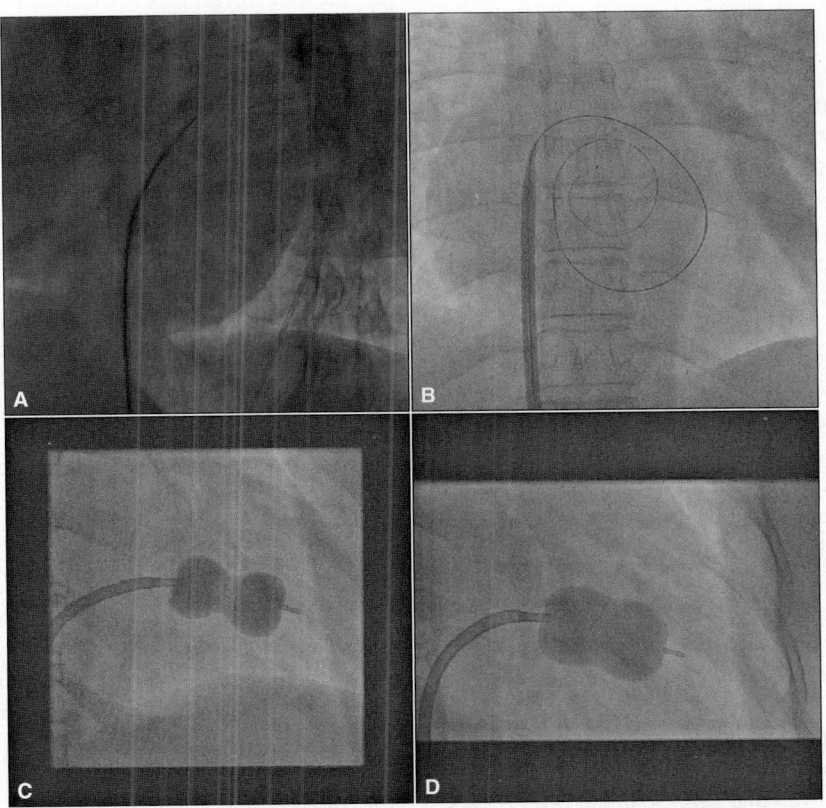

Figure 32–7. The steps for balloon mitral valvotomy are shown. (A) Transeptal puncture. (B) Dilatation of interatrial septum with dilator. (C) Balloon inflation creating a waist at the site of the stenosis. (D) Full balloon inflation with giving of waist.

by experienced, skilled operators. Large cohorts have reported success rates in excess of 90% (95% in experienced centers).[65,97,98] Although successful BMV is usually defined as a postprocedure valve area >1.5 cm^2 (without >grade 2 MR), valve area often exceeds 1.8 cm^2 and is durable for a decade or more. There is an immediate reduction in transmitral gradient, LA mean pressure, and PA pressure. Even patients with systemic or suprasystemic PA pressure have an immediate significant drop in PA pressure after successful BMV.[99] Reduction in PA pressure is associated with improvement in tricuspid regurgitation (TR) in some, but not all, patients. Successful BMV has been shown to reduce systemic embolism,[46] but does not revert AF.[74] Mortality is rare (<1%) in experienced centers. Other complications include severe MR requiring surgery (2%), embolic events (1%), and cardiac perforation (1%).[14,65,97,98]

Following successful BMV, the 10-year survival rate ranges from 87% to 97% with reintervention required in 12% to 16% (redo BMV/surgery).[97,100] At 20 years, the overall survival rate was 75% to 86%, but event rates begin to rise with reintervention rates of 33% to 38%.[101,102] Thus, even at 20 years, about 50% remain free of a repeat procedure.[101,102]

The BMV technique and hardware has remained essentially unchanged over the last three decades, but the indications of BMV have expanded to encompass patients with difficult MV anatomies. In patients, with unfavorable anatomy, previous studies indicated low success rates of 50% to 60%, but with accumulating experience and the use of the stepwise balloon dilatation technique, rates have improved to 75% to 80% even in this high-risk group.[103,104]

Cardiac Surgery

Relief of MS by surgery may be done either by CMV, OMV, or MVR. CMV, via transatrial or transventricular route, is still practiced successfully in many developing countries. The selection criteria of patients for CMV is the same as for BMV (ie, pliable valves). However, the results of BMV are superior to CMV (with larger postprocedural MVA), with lower morbidity. As such, CMV is indicated only if BMV is not available. A study of 3724 consecutive CMV patients (99% in NYHA class III–IV) reported an actuarial survival rate of 89% and 84% at 18 and 24 years, respectively with an in-hospital mortality of 3.8%.[105] Contraindications for CMV are the presence of a LA/LAA thrombus and grade 3 to 4 MR.

OMV is performed under cardiopulmonary bypass. It allows direct visual inspection of the mitral valve, enabling splitting of commissures, splitting of fused chordae tendineae and papillary muscles, and debridement of calcific deposits. LA thrombi may be removed and the LAA amputated to reduce future thromboembolic events. Further, moderate-to-severe TR can be repaired. The results are dependent on the surgical skills. The main advantage of OMV is that it avoids a prosthetic valve. The rates of in-hospital mortality and 10-year survival are 1% to 3% and 80% to 90%, respectively. When extensive calcification and severe subvalvular disease make BMV/OMV unfeasible, MVR is the surgical treatment of choice. Although MVR is a much simpler and more durable operation than

OMV, MVR is associated with lower survival (10-year survival rate of 92%–98% for OMV vs 87%–93% for MVR) due to prosthetic valve-related complications that outweigh the durability of MVR.[106,107]

The indication for MVR are as follows:[37]

1. Severely symptomatic patients (NYHA class III/IV) with severe MS (MVA <1.5 cm^2) who are not high risk for surgery and who are not candidates for, or have failed, previous BMV (class I indication);

2. Severe MS (MVA <1.5 cm^2) undergoing other cardiac surgery (eg, aortic valve surgery, coronary artery bypass grafting) (class IIa indication); and

3. Mitral valve surgery and LAA excision may be considered for patients with severe MS (MVA ≤1.5 cm^2, stages C and D) with recurrent embolic events despite adequate anticoagulation (class IIb indication).

Patients with associated moderate-to-severe TR do better after surgery that includes a tricuspid valve repair as compared to BMV especially in the presence of AF or dilated RV.[108] Given the morbidity and mortality associated with MVR and the potential long-term complications associated with a prosthetic valve (prosthetic valve thrombosis, infective endocarditis, prosthesis mismatch, bleeding complications with anticoagulation), the threshold for MVR is higher than for BMV and is limited to NYHA class III and IV patients. The operative mortality is 3% to 8%, but it may reach as high as 10% to 20% in NYHA class IV patients.[109] Therefore, the patient should not be allowed to reach NYHA class IV during postponement of surgery. Even if the patient does present in NYHA class IV, surgery should not be denied, as the outlook without surgery is very poor. BMV can be an alternative in such cases after careful discussion.[37] The type of valve inserted will depend on the patient's age and the risk of anticoagulation but is often dictated by patient choice. However, if the patient has long-standing AF and must be anticoagulated anyway, a mechanical valve may be preferred. On the other hand, a young patient in sinus rhythm may opt for a bioprosthetic valve to avoid the hazards of anticoagulation, with an understanding of the need for future redo surgery for valve deterioration. If AF is less chronic, a maze procedure may be used at the time of MVR.[110]

SPECIAL CIRCUMSTANCES

Pregnancy

Rheumatic MS primarily affects females of reproductive age. It is thus the most commonly encountered valve lesion during pregnancy especially in developing countries (up to 50% of valve lesions).[111,112] In fact, MS may become manifest for the first time during pregnancy. Pregnancy is associated with an increase in cardiac output (by 70%) and heart rate and reduction in systemic vascular resistance. As predicted by the Gorlin formula, an increase in cardiac output of 1.7-fold would increase the transvalvular gradient by a factor of 2.89. Thus, a small pregravid transmitral gradient of 4 mm Hg might become 11 mm Hg during the second trimester and cause symptoms to appear.

Typically, symptomatic status follows the *rule of one class*. That is, the patient's symptoms will increase by one NYHA class during pregnancy. Thus, the asymptomatic patient may develop class II symptoms, whereas a class II patient may become class III. Cardiac complications of MS in pregnancy include pulmonary edema, AF, cerebrovascular accidents, and death.[113] Most patients worsen during the second trimester. Labor and delivery can also precipitate decompensation. Severity of MS and the NYHA class before pregnancy are the predictors of maternal outcomes. Maternal mortality ranges from 0% to 3% (1% moderate MS, 3% severe MS).[114] In the current era, the rate of heart failure for mild, moderate, and severe MS is 16%, 32%, and 48% respectively.[115] One-third of patients may develop heart failure in the first week after delivery. Effects on the fetus include intrauterine growth retardation, low birth weight, preterm delivery, and fetal loss. Ideally, asymptomatic patients with severe MS (MVA ≤1.5 cm^2) planning for pregnancy with suitable valve should undergo BMV before conception.[77] Loop diuretics can be used safely to control symptoms. But, overaggressive use of diuretics should be avoided because it can lead to placental hypoperfusion. Aldosterone antagonists are contraindicated. Therapy is targeted to reduce heart rate and prolongation of diastolic filling. This includes restriction of physical activity and use of β-blockers (those with selective β-1 activity are preferred). Metoprolol is preferred over atenolol because it has a lower incidence of intrauterine growth retardation.[37,116] Pregnant patients with severe MS (MVA ≤ 1.5 cm^2) who continue to remain symptomatic (NYHA class III–IV) and/or those with systolic pulmonary artery pressure >50 mm Hg despite optimal medical therapy should undergo BMV if the valve is suitable.[116] Technical aspects include use of minimal fluoroscopy with avoidance of right heart study and LV angiogram, utilization of echo guidance, stepwise dilation technique, and use of pelvic and abdominal shield. A combined analysis of 515 patients who underwent BMV during pregnancy found a success rate of 98% (94%–100% in large-volume centers).[117] Maternal mortality was 1%. In the largest of these studies, the average fluoroscopic time was 3.6 ± 3.2 minutes.[118] The radiation to fetus is estimated to be less than 0.2 rad. Long-term follow-up of these children up to 7 years revealed no fetal anomalies.[119] The procedure should be performed by experienced operators. It is best performed after 20 weeks in the second trimester if the patient's symptoms permit, because organogenesis is complete at this stage.[116] However, the procedure is not contraindicated at any time during pregnancy. CMV is indicated if BMV is not available.

For symptomatic patients with valve anatomy unsuitable for BMV, mitral valve surgery is indicated for refractory NYHA class IV heart failure symptoms when the mother's life is threatened. Mitral valve surgery is associated with a significant fetal mortality risk of 20% to 30%.[113,116]

DC cardioversion should be considered for patients with acute AF and hemodynamic decompensation. Amiodarone should be avoided due to risk of IUGR and fetal thyropathy. For patients in chronic AF, digoxin and β-blockers are indicated for rate control. Therapeutic anticoagulation is required for patients in paroxysmal or permanent AF, left atrial thrombosis,

or prior embolism. Options include VKAs, low molecular weight, or unfractionated heparin. The decision regarding the choice of the anticoagulation should be made after a thorough discussion with the patient.[116]

Juvenile Mitral Stenosis

Given the long latent period between RF and symptom onset of MS (two decades), it is extremely rare to encounter symptomatic severe MS in childhood or adolescence in developed countries. In 1963, Sujoy Roy drew attention to the occurrence of symptomatic severe MS of rheumatic etiology among individuals below 20 years of age and coined the term "juvenile mitral stenosis."[15] It has been predominantly reported from developing countries in Southeast Asia, Africa, and the Middle East.[120] It may constitute up to a quarter of cases of all rheumatic MS in developing countries.[15] Studies of juvenile MS have noted a short latent time interval with rapid progression of MS leading to serious disability early in life. The youngest reported patient was a 4-year-old boy who underwent BMV.[121] Unlike the female preponderance in adults, juvenile MS affects both sexes equally or has a slight male preponderance (1.2–1.6:1).[15] Heart failure/pulmonary edema and severe pulmonary hypertension are a frequent finding. AF is uncommon whereas LA thrombi and MV calcification are rare. The MV is often tightly stenosed (<0.5 cm^2) with severe subvalvular disease and thickened leaflets. BMV is the treatment of choice with acute success rates of 94% to 100%,[122,123] which is comparable to adult series. There is an immediate significant drop in the PA pressure after the procedure[122] followed by further substantial regression over long-term follow-up.[124] Event-free survival at intermediate to long-term follow-up ranged from 75% to 79% at 5- to 10-years follow-up. Restenosis rates were 14% to 16%.[122,124] Important procedural aspects include the use of stepwise graded dilatation, the use of a balloon size 2 to 4 mm less than the calculated size, and indexing the MVA to BSA to define procedural success (MVA >1.0 cm^2/m^2 BSA). Long-term continuous penicillin prophylaxis is essential. With improvement in socioeconomic conditions, some studies have shown a reduction in the pathologic severity of juvenile MS.[125]

Degenerative Mitral Stenosis

Degenerative mitral stenosis (DMS) results from chronic noninflammatory degeneration and subsequent calcification of the fibrous mitral annulus.[126] It predominantly affects the elderly. In developed countries, there has been a steady rise in the incidence of DMS due to an aging population and increasing risk factors along with a decline in rheumatic MS.[2]

Epidemiology

The underlying pathological precursor of DMS is mitral annular calcification (MAC).[126-128] MAC is often asymptomatic, but when severe, it may lead to MS. The prevalence of MAC and DMS varies depending on the population characteristics and the imaging modality used. The prevalence of MAC is between 8% and 14%,[129-131] increasing significantly with age (40% in those above 65 years[132]). However, only 6% to 8% of these patients develop significant MS.[133,134] While the exact prevalence of DMS is not known, it comprised 0.22% in an echocardiography database[135] and approximately 10% to 12.5% of all MS cases in the Euro Heart Survey I and II.[2,4] DMS increases with age. Degenerative MS was responsible for ~10%, 30%, and 60% of all MS cases in the age groups 60–70, 70–80, and >80 years of age.[4,127]

Pathophysiology

Calcification predominantly affects the mitral annulus, the posterior annulus being more involved than the anterior annulus.[126,127] Rarely, the entire circumference is involved. This process may extend to the base of leaflets, thereby reducing their mobility and decreasing annular dilatation during diastole. This leads to inflow restriction and MS. Unlike, rheumatic MS, the commissures are not involved. The stenosis is at the annulus and leaflet base. The shape of the MV is tubular in DMS whereas it is funnel shaped in rheumatic MS.

The etiology is not well understood and is multifactorial. It appears to be a combination of atherosclerosis, abnormal calcium and phosphorus metabolism, and increased valve stress.[134] Older age, female sex, chronic kidney disease, diabetes mellitus, hypertension, smoking, dyslipidemia, obesity, metabolic disorders like hurler syndrome, and osteoporosis have been identified as risk factors.

Patients are asymptomatic for a prolonged period and subsequently develop exertional dyspnea, chest pain, and fatigue. Pulmonary hypertension and AF are common. The characteristic mid-diastolic murmur may be difficult to appreciate.

DMS is a slowly progressive disease with a reduction in MVA of 0.05 cm^2 per year[136] and increase in mean MV gradient of 0.8 +/− 2.4 mm Hg per year.[137] Those with diabetes mellitus and milder stenosis have faster progression rates.[137] Patients with DMS have increased cardiovascular morbidity and mortality. The 1- and 3-year survival rates of severe calcific MS (MVA <1.5 cm^2) were 72% and 52%, respectively, which is 2.5 times less than the general population.[136] Inactivity, Charlson Comorbidity Index >5, TMG ≥8 mm Hg, RVSP ≥50 mm Hg, LVEF <50%, and AF are independently associated with all-cause mortality.[136]

Diagnosis

MAC may be visualized on chest x-ray or cinefluoroscopy.[126] Echocardiography is the imaging modality of choice for DMS. It provides anatomic and physiologic data assessment of valve function.[138,139] Calcification is seen as an echodense band-like structure with acoustic shadowing at the junction of AV groove and posterior mitral leaflet. Commissural fusion is not seen. If TTE images are suboptimal, TEE may be helpful. Severity of DMS may be assessed by MVA and TMG. Assessment of MVA in DMS is challenging. The classic echocardiographic techniques used in rheumatic MS have not been validated for DMS. The pressure half-time method tends to overestimate the MVA due to concomitant diastolic dysfunction in elderly patients. Direct planimetry is difficult due to acoustic shadowing and difficulty in identifying the limiting orifice. Three-dimensional (color-coded) planimetry provides en face views and is more reliable.[140] The preferred method for assessment

of MVA in DMS is the continuity equation.[136,138,139,141] The PISA method may be used but is technically challenging and operator dependent. The TMG correlates closely with invasively measured gradient at catheterization. The TMG cutoffs of <5 and >10 mm Hg used to diagnose mild and severe rheumatic MS, respectively, have not been validated for DMS. As in rheumatic MS, an integrated approach is required taking into consideration all echo parameters (including PASP) for assessing DMS severity.

In cases of echocardiography uncertainty, cardiac catheterization with directly measured LA and LV pressures may be required for accurate MVA calculation. Coronary arteries can also be evaluated simultaneously.

Cardiac CT has emerged as an important adjunct to echocardiography in the evaluation of MAC and DMS. It provides quantification and detailed spatial assessment of extent of MAC and DMS. MVA by multislice CT planimetry is compatible with that obtained by cardiac catheterization. It also plays an important role in selection of the type of intervention/surgery for DMS, because it facilitates anatomic reconstruction for assessing the feasibility of transcatheter mitral valve replacement (TMVR).[139] Extension of MAC into extra-annular structures makes surgical debridement risky.

Treatment

The main stay of treatment for DMS is medical management with heart rate control and diuretic therapy.[126,127] Heart rate control may be achieved by β-blockers/CCBs to reduce transmitral gradient. Judicious use of diuretic therapy to optimize volume status is needed to avoid hypotension and electrolyte abnormalities in elderly patients. A retrospective analysis found a possible protective effect of renin-angiotensin system blockers and statins.[142] In those with refractory symptoms, the option of surgical/percutaneous therapy needs to be individualized on an individual basis due to the high morbidity and mortality associated with these invasive procedures. Many patients are debilitated with multiple comorbidities. Traditionally, surgical MVR with or without annular debridement of MAC has been the treatment of choice for low- and intermediate-risk patients with acceptable risk anatomy.[126,127,143] Ultrasonic pulverization for decalcification in MAC has been attempted with limited success. Severe MAC makes surgery challenging even in the most experienced hands. Potentially devastating complications include atrioventricular disruption, LV free wall rupture, paravalvular leak, left circumflex coronary artery injury, heart block, and stroke, all of which increase the surgical mortality. Other surgical options include left-atrial to left-ventricular apical conduit (mitral valve bypass) and intratrial placement of a mitral valve prosthesis. BMV is not indicated in DMS because there is no commissural fusion.

Given the excessive surgical morbidity and mortality in patients with severe MAC, TMVR has been attempted on a compassionate basis (transfemoral or transapical route). Currently, there is no transcatheter device specifically designed for MV. Most of the studies have used balloon-expandable valves designed for the aortic position (most commonly, the SAPIEN family) for TMVR. The procedural success rate is between

62% to 76%.[144,145] Despite the minimally invasive technique, 30-day and 1-year mortality ranges from 25% to 34% and 54% to 63%, respectively.[144,145] Important complications of TMVR include left ventricular outflow tract obstruction (LVOTO), valve embolization, and paravalvular leak. LVOTO was the strongest predictor of 30-day and 1-year mortality in the MAC Global Registry.[145] Preprocedural CT angiography plays an important role in identifying patients at risk for developing LVOTO by measuring the LVOT area before and after "virtual" mitral valve implantation. Strategies to prevent LVOTO include intentional percutaneous laceration of the anterior mitral leaflet (LAMPOON technique), prophylactic alcohol septal ablation, use of self-expanding retrievable aortic valves, and the hybrid surgical approach. The hybrid surgical approach involves transatrial deployment of a transcatheter balloon-expandable SAPIEN valve under direct vision.[146] This overcomes some of the surgical issues and allows resection of the anterior mitral leaflet to reduce the risk of LVOTO. The major drawback remains the need for thoracotomy and cardiopulmonary bypass.

CONCOMITANT VALVE DISEASE

As noted, RF may affect all four heart valves. Perhaps, the most common lesion is mixed MS and MR. The presence of concomitant MR worsens the hemodynamic burden of MS because the regurgitant volume has to pass into the LV with each diastole raising the mean LAP further. The lesions are almost never balanced, with one more prominent than the other. From the standpoint of management, LV remodeling gives the best clue regarding which lesion is dominant and, therefore, which to treat. If the LV is dilated (or if LVS3 is present), MR is the dominant lesion, and strategies for MR therapy are recommended, whereas if the LV volume is normal, MS likely predominates, and the patient should be treated accordingly.

AR is the next most common accompanying lesion with MS. Some degree of AR is seen in 30% to 50% of patients of MS undergoing intervention, but severe AR is found in only 10% of patients. The combination of severe MS and severe AR has the opposite loading effect on the LV.[147] MS reduces cardiac output and LV volume. Thus, clinical clues to AR severity (eg, wide pulse pressure, LV S3, LV dilatation) may be missing in the MS patient, both on clinical and echocardiographic examination.[148] The apical mid-diastolic murmur of MS may be mistaken for an Austin Flint murmur. Further, AR leads to significant shortening of pressure half-time and overestimation of the MVA. Hence, planimetry rather than pressure half-time should be used to assess the MVA. For patients with mild-moderate AR with severe MS, BMV alone is recommended. In patients with severe AR and severe MS, it is preferable to perform BMV first rather than refer the patient for double valve replacement, given the morbidity/mortality associated with the later. If symptomatic improvement occurs, the patient can be followed closely and AVR can be delayed. However, if LV dysfunction (LVEF <50%) or LV dilatation (LV end systolic diameter >50 mm) is present with severe AR, both valves need to be addressed (double valve replacement or AVR with OMV).

Combined mitral and aortic stenosis is quite uncommon and poorly tolerated. The low cardiac output in severe MS leads to a state of low-flow, low-gradient AS potentially leading to underestimation of the severity of AS. Patients with combined AS and MS tend to become symptomatic earlier and the symptoms of MS predominate.[149] From a management point of view, the recognition of severe AS is important before the patient undergoes mitral valvotomy. Sudden relief of MS may place a hemodynamic burden on the unprepared and previously protected LV, leading to heart failure.[150] Thus, it is imperative to accurately assess the aortic valve area either by TTE (continuity equation) or cardiac catheterization. For patients with severe AS and severe MS, both valves need to be addressed (DVR or AVR/OMC or percutaneous interventions). For patients with less than severe AS, BMV alone is sufficient.

Perhaps, the most important concomitant valve lesion is TR. More than one-third of MS patients have at least moderate TR. Although rheumatic deformity of the tricuspid valve does occur, most TR is functional, resulting from RV dilatation secondary to pulmonary hypertension. Regression of PAH following correction of MS often leads to improvement in functional TR. TR fails to improve if there is structural damage of the tricuspid valve and may paradoxically worsen if unattended.[151] The need to address TR surgically as a second operation after successful mitral surgery carries a high operative risk.[152] Thus, at the time of mitral valve surgery, TV annuloplasty is recommended in patients with severe TR as well as for those with mild-moderate TR when the tricuspid annulus is dilated (>40 mm or >21 mm/m² BSA) or there is a prior recent history of right-heart failure.[37] Whether patients with significant functional TR do better with BMV alone or mitral valve surgery with TV annuloplasty has been a matter of debate. While surgery addresses both the valves, BMV does not directly correct TR. Following successful BMV, 50% to 80% of patients with moderate to severe TR show no improvement in TR.[152] On the other hand, MV surgery is associated with increased morbidity and mortality. One retrospective analysis found no difference in survival,[108] but noted lower incidence of heart failure and greater improvement in TR in the surgical group. Multivariate analysis revealed baseline sinus rhythm and TV annuloplasty as independent predictors for improvement in TR. Thus, the surgical option may be preferred in the presence of AF or RV enlargement. Another option would be to closely follow patients for regression of TR after successful BMV and if TR does not improve, TV annuloplasty as a first cardiac surgery should be considered.

SUMMARY

- Rheumatic MS is the most important cause of MS in developing countries while degenerative MS is increasing in developed countries.
- Rheumatic MS has a long asymptomatic latent period followed by an accelerated symptomatic phase. The appearance of symptoms is earlier in developing countries.
- Important complications include heart failure, AF, thromboembolism, hemoptysis, and, at times, sudden death.

- Clinically, the most important diagnostic features are a loud S1, a mididastolic murmur, and an opening snap.
- Echocardiography is the mainstay for diagnosis of MS.
- In those with favorable anatomy, BMV is the treatment modality of choice. MV surgery is recommended for severely symptomatic patients with unfavorable anatomy.
- Patients with degenerative MS are often elderly with multiple comorbidities. Newer therapies in the form of percutaneous transcatheter mitral replacement are being evaluated.

ACKNOWLEDGMENTS

We would like to thank Dr Blasé A. Carabello who contributed to the previous version of this chapter in the 14th edition.

REFERENCES

1. Zühlke L, Engel ME, Karthikeyan G, et al. Characteristics, complications, and gaps in evidence-based interventions in rheumatic heart disease: the Global Rheumatic Heart Disease Registry (the REMEDY study). *Eur Heart J*. 2015;36:1115-1122.
2. Iung B, Delgado V, Rosenhek R, et al. Contemporary presentation and management of valvular heart disease: the EUrobservational research programme valvular heart disease II survey. *Circulation*. 2019;140:1-38.
3. Andell P, Li X, Martinsson A, et al. Epidemiology of valvular heart disease in a Swedish nationwide hospital-based register study. *Heart*. 2017;103:1696-1703.
4. Iung B, Baron G, Butchart EG, et al. A prospective survey of patients with valvular heart disease in Europe: the Euro Heart Survey on valvular heart disease. *Eur Heart J*. 2003;24:1231-1243.
5. Saxena A, Ramakrishnan S, Roy A, et al. Prevalence and outcome of subclinical rheumatic heart disease in India: the RHEUMATIC (Rheumatic Heart Echo Utilisation and Monitoring Actuarial Trends in Indian Children) study. *Heart*. 2011;97:2018-2022.
6. Marijon E, Ou P, Celermajer DS, et al. Prevalence of rheumatic heart disease detected by echocardiographic screening. *N Engl J Med*. 2007;357:470-476.
7. James SL, Abate D, Abate KH, et al. Global, regional, and national incidence, prevalence, and years lived with disability for 354 diseases and injuries for 195 countries and territories, 1990-2017: a systematic analysis for the Global Burden of Disease Study 2017. *Lancet*. 2018;392:1789-1858.
8. Manjunath CN, Srinivas P, Ravindranath KS, Dhanalakshmi C. Incidence and patterns of valvular heart disease in a tertiary care high-volume cardiac center: a single center experience. *Indian Heart J*. 2014;66:320-326.
9. Negi PC, Mahajan K, Rana V, et al. Clinical characteristics, complications, and treatment practices in patients with RHD: 6-year results from HP-RHD registry. *Glob Heart*. 2018;13:267-274.e2.
10. Wood P. An appreciation of mitral stenosis. I. Clinical features. *Br Med J*. 1954;1:1051-1063.
11. Rowe JC, Bland EF, Sprague HB, et al. The course of mitral stenosis without surgery: ten- and twenty-year perspectives. *Ann Intern Med*. 1960;52:741-749.
12. Horstkotte D, Niehues R, Strauer BE. Pathomorphological aspects, aetiology and natural history of acquired mitral valve stenosis. *Eur Heart J*. 1991;12:55-60.
13. OLESEN KH. The natural history of 271 patients with mitral stenosis under medical treatment. *Br Heart J*. 1962;24(3):349-357.
14. Bonow RO, Carabello BA, Chatterjee K, et al. 2008 focused update incorporated into the ACC/AHA 2006 guidelines for the management of patients with valvular heart disease. A report of the American College of Cardiology/American Heart Association Task Force on Practice Guidelines (Writing Committee to. *J Am Coll Cardiol*. 2008;52:e1-e142.
15. Roy S, Bhatia M, Lazaro E, Ramalingaswami V. Juvenile mitral stenosis in India. *Lancet*. 1963;282:1193-1196.
16. Marijon É, Iung B, Mocumbi A O, et al. What are the differences in presentation of candidates for percutaneous mitral commissurotomy across the world and do they influence the results of the procedure? *Arch Cardiovasc Dis*. 2008;101:611-617.
17. Chandrashekhar Y, Westaby S, Narula J. Mitral stenosis. *Lancet*. 2009;374:1271-1283
18. Sagie A, Freitas N, Padial LR, et al. Doppler echocardiographic assessment of long-term progression of mitral stenosis in 103 patients: valve area and right heart disease. *J Am Coll Cardiol*. 1996;28:472-479.
19. Gordon SPF, Douglas PS, Come PC, Manning WJ. Two-dimensional and Doppler echocardiographic determinants of the natural history of mitral valve narrowing in patients with rheumatic mitral stenosis: implications for follow-up. *J Am Coll Cardiol*. 1992;19:968-973.
20. Feinstein AR, Stern EK, Spagnuolo M. The prognosis of acute rheumatic fever. *Am Heart J*. 1964;68:817-834.
21. Bhan A, Das B, Venugopal P, Sampathkumar A, Chopra P. Immunohistochemical characterization of Aschoff nodules and endomyocardial inflammatory infiltrates in resected left atrial appendages. *Indian Heart J*. 1990;42:415-417.
22. Alyan O, Metin F, Kacmaz F, et al. High levels of high sensitivity C-reactive protein predict the progression of chronic rheumatic mitral stenosis. *J Thromb Thrombolysis*. 2009;28:63-69.
23. Iung B, Leenhardt A, Extramiana F. Management of atrial fibrillation in patients with rheumatic mitral stenosis. *Heart*. 2018;104:1062-1068.
24. Tandon HD, Kasturi J. Pulmonary vascular changes associated with isolated MS in India. *Br Heart J*. 1975;37:26-36.
25. Carabello BA, Grossman W. Calculation of stenotic valve orifice area. In: Baim DS, Grossman W, eds. *Grossman's Cardiac Catheterization, Angiography, and Intervention*. 6th ed. Philadelphia, PA: Lippincott Williams & Wilkins; 2000.
26. Ravi S Math. Pulmonary hypertension in mitral stenosis. In. N Parakh, ed. *Mitral Stenosis*. Boca Raton, FL: CRC Press; 2018:319-332
27. Dalen JE, Matloff JM, Evans GL, et al. Early reduction of pulmonary vascular resistance after mitral-valve replacement. *N Engl J Med*. 1967;277:387-394.
28. Mahoney PD, Loh E, Blitz LR, Herrmann HC. Hemodynamic effects of inhaled nitric oxide in women with mitral stenosis and pulmonary hypertension. *Am J Cardiol*. 2001;87:188-192.
29. Ward C, Hancock BW. Extreme pulmonary hypertension caused by mitral valve disease. Natural history and results of surgery. *Br Heart J*. 1975;37:74-78
30. Heller SJ, Carleton RA. Abnormal left ventricular contraction in patients with mitral stenosis. *Circulation*. 1970;42:1099-1110.
31. Gash AK, Carabello BA, Cepin D, Spann JF. Left ventricular ejection performance and systolic muscle function in patients with mitral stenosis. *Circulation*. 1983;67:148-154.
32. Sengupta SP, Amaki M, Bansal M, et al. Effects of percutaneous balloon mitral valvuloplasty on left ventricular deformation in patients with isolated severe mitral stenosis: a speckle-tracking strain echocardiographic study. *J Am Soc Echocardiogr*. 2014;27:639-647.
33. Ravi S Math. Left ventricular dysfunction. In. N Parakh, ed. *Mitral Stenosis*. Boca Raton, FL: CRC Press; 2018:333-344
34. Fawzy ME, Choi WB, Mimish L, et al. Immediate and long-term effect of mitral balloon valvotomy on left ventricular volume and systolic function in severe mitral stenosis. *Am Heart J*. 1996;132:356-360.
35. Lee TM, Su SF, Chen MF et al. Changes of left ventricular function after percutaneous balloon mitral valvuloplasty in mitral stenosis with impaired left ventricular performance. *Int J Cardiol*. 1996;56:211–215.
36. Mayer IV, Fischer A, Jakob M, et al. Reversal of increased diastolic stiffness in mitral stenosis after successful balloon valvuloplasty. *J Heart Valve Dis*. 1999;8:47-56.

37. Nishimura RA, Otto CM, Bonow RO, et al. 2014 AHA/ACC guideline for the management of patients with valvular heart disease: a report of the American College of Cardiology/American Heart Association Task Force on Practice Guidelines. *J Am Coll Cardiol.* 2014;63:2438-2488.

38. Gorlin R, Gorlin SG. Hydraulic formula for calculation of the area of the stenotic mitral valve, other cardiac valves, and central circulatory shunts. I. *Am Heart J.* 1951;41:1-29.

39. Carabello BA. Modern management of mitral stenosis. *Circulation.* 2005;112:432-437.

40. Bayer O, Loogen F, Wolter HH. The mitral opening snap in the quantitative diagnosis of mitral stenosis. *Am Heart J.* 1956;51:234-245.

41. Kawanishi DT, Kotlewski A, McKay CR, et al. The relative value of clinical examination, echo-cardiography with Doppler and cardiac catheterization with angiography in the evaluation of mitral valve disease. In: Bodnar E, ed. *Surgery for Heart Valve Disease.* London: ICR Publishers; 1990:73–78.

42. Runco V, Molnar W, Meckstroth C V, Ryan JM. The Graham Steell murmur versus aortic regurgitation in rheumatic heart disease: results of aortic valvulography. *Am J Med.* 1961;31:71-80.

43. Selzer A, Cohn KE. Natural history of mitral stenosis: a review. *Circulation.* 1972;45:878-890.

44. Coulshed N, Epstein EJ, McKendrick CS, et al. Systemic embolism in mitral valve disease. *Br Heart J.* 1970;32:26-34.

45. Casella L, Abelmann WH, Ellis LB. Patients with mitral stenosis and systemic emboli: Hemodynamic and clinical observations. *Arch Intern Med.* 1964;114:773-781.

46. Chiang CW, Lo SK, Ko YS, et al. Predictors of systemic embolism in patients with mitral stenosis. A prospective study. *Ann Intern Med.* 1998;128:885-889

47. Bruce CJ, Nishimura RA. Newer advances in the diagnosis and treatment of mitral stenosis. *Curr Probl Cardiol.* 1998;23:125-192.

48. Abernathy WS, Willis PW 3rd. Thromboembolic complications of rheumatic heart disease. *Cardiovasc Clin.* 1973;5:131-175.

49. Adams GF, Merrett JD, Hutchinson WM, Pollock AM. Cerebral embolism and mitral stenosis: survival with and without anticoagulants. *J Neurol Neurosurg Psychiatry.* 1974;37:378-383.

50. Manjunath CN, Srinivasa KH, Panneerselvam A, et al. Incidence and predictors of left atrial thrombus in patients with rheumatic mitral stenosis and sinus rhythm: a transesophageal echocardiographic study. *Echocardiography.* 2011;28:457-460.

51. Karthikeyan G, Ananthakrishnan R, Devasenapathy N, et al. Transient, subclinical atrial fibrillation and risk of systemic embolism in patients with rheumatic mitral stenosis in sinus rhythm. *Am J Cardiol.* 2014;11:869-874.

52. Irwin RS, Weg JG. A chest radiograph showing abnormal mediastinal contour. *Chest.* 1996;109:1383-1384.

53. Baumgartner H, Hung J, Bermejo J, et al. Echocardiographic assessment of valve stenosis: EAE/ASE recommendations for clinical practice. *J Am Soc Echocardiogr.* 2009;22:1-23.

54. Wunderlich NC, Beigel R, Siegel RJ. Management of mitral stenosis using 2D and 3D echo-Doppler imaging. *JACC Cardiovasc Imaging.* 2013;6:1191-1205.

55. Nishimura RA, Rihal CS, Tajik AJ, Holmes DR. Accurate measurement of the transmitral gradient in patients with mitral stenosis: a simultaneous catheterization and Doppler echocardiographic study. *J Am Coll Cardiol.* 1994;24:152-158.

56. Dreyfus J, Brochet E, Lepage L, et al. Real-time 3D transoesophageal measurement of the mitral valve area in patients with mitral stenosis. *Eur J Echocardiogr.* 2011;12:750-755.

57. Zamorano J, Cordeiro P, Sugeng L, et al. Real-time three-dimensional echocardiography for rheumatic mitral valve stenosis evaluation: an accurate and novel approach. *J Am Coll Cardiol.* 2004;43:2091–2096.

58. Messika-Zeitoun D, Brochet E, Holmin C, et al. Three-dimensional evaluation of the mitral valve area and commissural opening before and after percutaneous mitral commissurotomy in patients with mitral stenosis. *Eur Heart J.* 2007;28:72-79.

59. Picano E, Pibarot P, Lancellotti P, Monin JL, Bonow RO. The emerging role of exercise testing and stress echocardiography in valvular heart disease. *J Am Coll Cardiol.* 2009;54:2251-2260.

60. Wilkins GT, Weyman AE, Abascal, et al. Percutaneous balloon dilatation of the mitral valve: an analysis of echocardiographic variables related to outcome and the mechanism of dilation. *Br Heart J.* 1998;60:299-308.

61. Palacios IF, Sanchez PL, Harrell LC, et al. Which patients benefit from percutaneous mitral balloon valvuloplasty? Prevalvuloplasty and postvalvuloplasty variables predict long-term outcome. *Circulation.* 2002;105:1465-1472.

62. Iung B, Cormier B, Ducimetiere P, et al. Immediate results of percutaneous mitral commissurotomy. A predictive model on a series of 1514 patients. *Circulation.* 1996;94:2124-2130.

63. Anwar AM, Attia WM, Nosir YF, et al. Validation of a new score for the assessment of mitral stenosis using real-time three-dimensional echocardiography. *J Am Soc Echocardiogr.* 2010;23:13-22.

64. Nunes MCP, Tan TC, Elmariah S, et al. The echo score revisited: impact of incorporating commissural morphology and leaflet displacement to the prediction of outcome for patients undergoing percutaneous mitral valvuloplasty. *Circulation.* 2014;129:886-895.

65. Manjunath CN, Srinivasa KH, Ravindranath KS, et al. Balloon mitral valvotomy in patients with mitral stenosis and left atrial thrombus. *Catheter Cardiovasc Interv.* 2009;74:653-656.

66. Lange RA, Moore DM, Cigarroa RG, et al. Use of pulmonary capillary wedge pressure to assess severity of mitral stenosis: is true left atrial pressure needed in this condition? *J Am Coll Cardiol.* 1989;13:825-831.

67. Parakh N, Chaturvedi V, Kurian S, et al. Effect of ivabradine vs atenolol on heart rate and effort tolerance in patients with mild to moderate mitral stenosis and normal sinus rhythm. *J Card Fail.* 2012;18:282-288.

68. January CT, Wann LS, Alpert JS, et al. 2014 AHA/ACC/HRS guideline for the management of patients with atrial fibrillation: a report of the American College of Cardiology/American Heart Association Task Force on Practice Guidelines and the Heart Rhythm Society. *J Am Coll Cardiol.* 2014;64:e1-e76.

69. Al-Khatib SM, Allen LaPointe NM, Chatterjee R, et al. Rate- and rhythm-control therapies in patients with atrial fibrillation: a systematic review. *Ann Intern Med.* 2014;160:760-773.

70. Hu CL, Jiang H, Tang QZ, et al. Comparison of rate control and rhythm control in patients with atrial fibrillation after percutaneous mitral balloon valvotomy: a randomised controlled study. *Heart.* 2006;92:1096-1101.

71. Vilvanathan VK, Srinivas, Prabhavathi Bhat BC, Nanjappa MC, et al. A randomized placebo-controlled trial with amiodarone for persistent atrial fibrillation in rheumatic mitral stenosis after successful balloon mitral valvuloplasty. *Indian Heart J.* 2016;68:671-677.

72. Vora A, Karnad D, Goyal V, et al. Control of heart rate versus rhythm in rheumatic atrial fibrillation: a randomized study. *J Cardiovasc Pharmacol Ther.* 2004;9:65-73.

73. Eid Fawzy M, Shoukri M, Al Sergani H, et al. Favorable effect of balloon mitral valvuloplasty on the incidence of atrial fibrillation in patients with severe mitral stenosis. *Catheter Cardiovasc Interv.* 2006;68:536-541.

74. Langerveld J, van Hemel NM, Kelder JC, et al. Long-term follow-up of cardiac rhythm after percutaneous mitral balloon valvotomy. Does atrial fibrillation persist? *Europace.* 2003;5:47-53.

75. Gillinov AM, Gelijns AC, Parides MK, et al. Surgical ablation of atrial fibrillation during mitral-valve surgery. *N Engl J Med.* 2015;372:1399-1409.

76. Wolf PA, Dawber TR, Thomas HE Jr, Kannel WB. Epidemiologic assessment of chronic atrial fibrillation and risk of stroke: the Framingham study. *Neurology.* 1978;28:973-977.

77. Baumgartner H, Falk V, Bax J, et al. ESC/EACTS Guidelines for the management of valvular heart disease: the Task Force for the Management of Valvular Heart Disease of the European Society of Cardiology (ESC) and the European Association for Cardio- Thoracic Surgery (EACTS). *Eur Heart J.* 2017;2017:2939-2991.

78. Perez-Gomez F, Alegria E, Berjon J, et al. Comparative effects of antiplatelet, anticoagulant, or combined therapy in patients with valvular and nonvalvular atrial fibrillation: a randomized multicenter study. *J Am Coll Cardiol.* 2004;44:1557-1566.

79. Nishimura RA, Otto CM, Bonow RO, et al. 2017 AHA/ACC focused update of the 2014 AHA/ACC guideline for the management of patients with valvular heart disease: a Report of the American College of Cardiology/ American Heart Association Task Force on Clinical Practice Guidelines. *J Am Coll Cardiol.* 2017;70:252-289.

80. Kim JY, Kim S-H, Myong JP, et al. Outcomes of direct oral anticoagulants in patients with mitral stenosis. *J Am Coll Cardiol.* 2019;73:1123-1131

81. Habib G, Lancellotti P, Antunes MJ, et al. 2015 ESC Guidelines for the management of infective endocarditis: the Task Force for the Management of Infective Endocarditis of the European Society of Cardiology (ESC). Endorsed by: European Association for Cardio-Thoracic Surgery (EACTS), the European Association of Nuclear Medicine (EANM). *Eur Heart J.* 2015;36:3075-3128.

82. Fernandes JR, Grinberg M. Prophylaxis of infective endocarditis: a different Brazilian reality? *Arq Bras Cardiol.* 2013;101:e37-e38.

83. Jankelow D, Cupido BJ, Zühlke LJ, et al. Prevention of infective endocarditis associated with dental interventions. *SA Heart* 2017;14:170-174.

84. RHDAustralia (ARF/RHD writing group). *The 2020 Australian Guideline for Prevention, Diagnosis and Management of Acute Rheumatic Fever and Rheumatic Heart Disease.* 3rd ed. 2020. https://www.rhdaustralia.org.au/arf-rhd-guideline. Accessed August 7, 2020.

85. Cahill TJ, Baddour LM, Habib G, et al. Challenges in infective endocarditis. *J Am Coll Cardiol.* 2017;69:325-344.

86. Dayer MJ, Jones S, Prendergast B, Baddour LM, Lockhart PB, Thornhill MH. Incidence of infective endocarditis in England, 2000-13: a secular trend, interrupted time-series analysis. *Lancet.* 2015;385:1219-1228.

87. Gerber MA, Baltimore RS, Eaton CB, et al. Prevention of rheumatic fever and diagnosis and treatment of acute Streptococcal pharyngitis: a scientific statement from the American Heart Association Rheumatic Fever, Endocarditis, and Kawasaki Disease Committee of the Council on Cardiovascular Disease in the Young, the Interdisciplinary Council on Functional Genomics and Translational Biology, and the Interdisciplinary Council on Quality of Care and Outcomes Research: endorsed by the American Academy of Pediatrics. *Circulation.* 2009;119:1541-1551.

88. Roy SB, Gopinath N. Mitral stenosis. *Circulation.* 1968;38(1s5):V-68.

89. Kim DJ, Lee S, Joo HC, et al. Effect of pulmonary hypertension on clinical outcomes in patients with rheumatic mitral stenosis. *Ann Thorac Surg.* 2020;109:496-503.

90. Inoue K, Owaki T, Nakamura T, et al. Clinical application of transvenous mitral commissurotomy by a new balloon catheter. *J Thorac Cardiovasc Surg.* 1984;87:394-402.

91. Lock JE, Khalilullah M, Shrivastava S, et al. Percutaneous catheter commissurotomy in rheumatic mitral stenosis. *N Engl J Med.* 1985;313:1515-1518.

92. Singh AD, Mian A, Devasenapathy N, et al. Percutaneous mitral commissurotomy versus surgical commissurotomy for rheumatic mitral stenosis: a systematic review and meta-analysis of randomised controlled trials. *Heart.* 2020;106:1094-1101.

93. Manjunath CN, Gerald Dorros, Srinivasa KH, et al. The Indian experience of percutaneous transvenous mitral commissurotomy: comparison of the triple lumen (Inoue) and double lumen (Accura) variable sized single balloon with regard to procedural outcome and cost savings. *J Interv Cardiol.* 1998;11:107-112.

94. Kang DH, Park SW, Song JK, et al. Long-term clinical and echocardiographic outcome of percutaneous mitral valvuloplasty: randomized comparison of Inoue and double-balloon techniques. *J Am Coll Cardiol.* 2000;35:169-175.

95. Cribier A, Eltchaninoff H, Koning R, et al. Percutaneous mechanical mitral commissurotomy with a newly designed metallic valvulotome: immediate results of the initial experience in 153 patients. *Circulation.* 1999;99:793-799.

96. Sharieff S, Aamir K, Sharieff W, et al. Comparison of Inoue balloon, metallic commissurotome and multi-track double-balloon valvuloplasty in the treatment of rheumatic mitral stenosis. *J Invasive Cardiol.* 2008;20:521-525.

97. Ben-Farhat M, Betbout F, Gamra H et al. Predictors of long-term event-free survival and of freedom from restenosis after percutaneous balloon mitral commissurotomy. *Am Heart J.* 2001;142:1072-1079.

98. Chen CR, Cheng TO. Percutaneous balloon mitral valvuloplasty by the Inoue technique: a multicenter study of 4832 patients in China. *Am Heart J.* 1995;129:1197-1203.

99. Bahl VK, Chandra S, Talwar KK, et al. Balloon mitral valvotomy in patients with systemic and suprasystemic pulmonary artery pressures. *Cathet Cardiovasc Diagn.* 1995;36:211-215.

100. Iung B, Garbarz E, Michaud P, et al. Late results of percutaneous mitral commissurotomy in a series of 1024 patients. Analysis of late clinical deterioration: frequency, anatomic findings, and predictive factors. *Circulation* 1999;99:3272-3278.

101. Bouleti C, Iung B, Himbert D, et al. Reinterventions after percutaneous mitral commissurotomy during long-term follow-up, up to 20 years: the role of repeat percutaneous mitral commissurotomy. *Eur Heart J.* 2013;34:1923-1930.

102. Tomai F, Gaspardone A, Versaci F, et al. Twenty year follow-up after successful percutaneous balloon mitral valvuloplasty in a large contemporary series of patients with mitral stenosis. *Int J Cardiol.* 2014;177:881-885.

103. Bouleti C, Iung B, Himbert D, et al. Relationship between valve calcification and long-term results of percutaneous mitral commissurotomy for rheumatic mitral stenosis. *Circ Cardiovasc Interv.* 2014;7:381-389.

104. Desnos C, Iung B, Himbert D, et al. Temporal trends on percutaneous mitral commissurotomy: 30 years of experience. *J Am Hear Assoc.* 2019;8(13):e012031

105. John S, Bashi VV, Jairaj PS et al. Closed mitral valvotomy: early results and longterm follow-up of 3724 consecutive patients. *Circulation* 1983;68:891-896.

106. Cotrufo M, Renzulli A, Vitale N, et al. Long-term follow-up of open commissurotomy versus bileaflet valve replacement for rheumatic mitral stenosis. *Eur J Cardiothorac Surg.* 1997;12:335-340.

107. Kim JB, Kim HJ, Moon DH, et al. Long-term outcomes after surgery for rheumatic mitral valve disease: valve repair versus mechanical valve replacement. *Eur J Cardiothorac Surg.* 2010;37:1039-1046.

108. Song H, Kang DH, Kim JH, et al. Percutaneous mitral valvuloplasty versus surgical treatment in mitral stenosis with severe tricuspid regurgitation. *Circulation.* 2007;116:I246–I250.

109. O'Brien SM, Shahian DM, Filardo G, et al. The Society of Thoracic Surgeons 2008 cardiac surgery risk models. Part 2: isolated valve surgery. *Ann Thorac Surg.* 2009;88:S23.

110. Kim WK, Kim HJ, Kim JB, et al. Concomitant ablation of atrial fibrillation in rheumatic mitral valve surgery. *J Thorac Cardiovasc Surg.* 2019;157:1519-1528.e5.

111. Bhatla N, Lal S, Behera G, et al. Cardiac disease in pregnancy. *Int J Gynaecol Obstet.* 2003;82:153-159.

112. Lumsden R, Barasa F, Park LP, et al. High burden of cardiac disease in pregnancy at a national referral hospital in Western Kenya. *Glob Heart.* 2020;15:10.

113. Elkayam U, Goland S, Pieper PG, Silverside CK. High-risk cardiac disease in pregnancy: part I. *J Am Coll Cardiol.* 2016;68:396-410.

114. Ducas RA, Javier DA, D'Souza R, et al. Pregnancy outcomes in women with significant valve disease: a systematic review and meta-analysis. *Heart.* 2020;106:512-519.

115. van Hagen IM, Thorne SA, Taha N, et al. Pregnancy outcomes in women with rheumatic mitral valve disease: results from the Registry of Pregnancy and Cardiac Disease. *Circulation.* 2018;137:806-816.

116. Regitz-Zagrosek V, Roos-Hesselink JW, Bauersachs J, et al. 2018 ESC Guidelines for the management of cardiovascular diseases during pregnancy. *Eur Heart J.* 2018;39:3165-3241.

117. Hameed AB, Mehra A, Rahimtoola SH. The role of catheter balloon commissurotomy for severe mitral stenosis in pregnancy. *Obstet Gynecol.* 2009;114:1336-1340.

118. Mishra S, Narang R, Sharma M. Percutaneous transseptal mitral commissurotomy in pregnant women with critical mitral stenosis. *Indian Hear J.* 2001;53:192-196.

119. Sivadasanpillai H, Srinivasan A, Sivasubramoniam S. Long-term outcome of patients undergoing balloon mitral valvotomy in pregnancy. *Am J Cardiol.* 2005;95:1504-1506.

120. Bahl VK, Math RS. Juvenile mitral stenosis and Lutembacher's syndrome. *E-J Cardiol Prac.* 2018;16:16.

121. Sarkar A, Patil S, Ahmed I. Balloon mitral valvotomy in youngest documented rheumatic mitral stenosis patient. *Catheter Cardiovasc Interv.* 2015;86:E213-E216.

122. Kothari SS, Ramakrishnan S, Kumar CK, et al. Intermediate-term results of percutaneous transvenous mitral commissurotomy in children less than 12 years of age. *Catheter Cardiovasc Interv.* 2005;64(4):487-490.

123. Joseph PK, Bhat A, Francis B, et al. Percutaneous transvenous mitral commissurotomy using an Inoue balloon in children with rheumatic mitral stenosis. *Int J Cardiol.* 1997;62:19-22.

124. Fawzy ME, Stefadouros MA, Hegazy H, et al. Long term clinical and echocardiographic results of mitral balloon valvotomy in children and adolescents. *Heart.* 2005;91:743-748.

125. Stephen SJ. Changing patterns of mitral stenosis in childhood and pregnancy in Sri Lanka. *J Am Coll Cardiol.* 1992;19:1276-1284.

126. Abramowitz Y, Jilaihawi H, Chakravarty T, Mack MJ, Makkar RR. Mitral annulus calcification. *J Am Coll Cardiol.* 2015;66:1934-1941.

127. Sud K, Agarwal S, Parashar A, et al. Degenerative mitral stenosis: unmet need for percutaneous interventions. *Circulation.* 2016;133:1594-1604.

128. Banovic M, DaCosta M. Degenerative mitral stenosis: from pathophysiology to challenging interventional treatment. *Curr Probl Cardiol.* 2019;44:10-35.

129. Fox CS, Vasan RS, Parise H, et al. Mitral annular calcification predicts cardiovascular morbidity and mortality: the Framingham Heart Study. *Circulation.* 2003;107:1492-1496.

130. Kanjanauthai S, Nasir K, Katz R, et al. Relationships of mitral annular calcification to cardiovascular risk factors: the Multi-Ethnic Study of Atherosclerosis (MESA). *Atherosclerosis.* 2010;213:558-562.

131. Allison MA, Cheung P, Criqui MH, et al. Mitral and aortic annular calcification are highly associated with systemic calcified atherosclerosis. *Circulation.* 2006;113:861-866.

132. Barasch E, Gottdiener JS, Larsen EK, Chaves PH, Newman AB, Manolio TA. Clinical significance of calcification of the fibrous skeleton of the heart and aortosclerosis in community dwelling elderly. The Cardiovascular Health Study (CHS). *Am Heart J.* 2006;151:39-47.

133. Labovitz AJ, Nelson JG, Windhorst DM, et al. Frequency of mitral valve dysfunction from mitral anular calcium as detected by Doppler echocardiography. *Am J Cardiol.* 1985;55:133-137.

134. Aronow WS, Schwartz KS, Koenigsberg M. Correlation of murmurs of mitral stenosis and mitral regurgitation with presence or absence of mitral anular calcium in persons older than 62 years in a long-term health care facility. *Am J Cardiol.* 1987;59:181-182.

135. Ukita Y, Yuda S, Sugio H et al. Prevalence and clinical characteristics of degenerative mitral stenosis. *J Cardiol.* 2016;68:248-252.

136. Kato N, Padang R, Scott CG, et al. The natural history of severe calcific mitral stenosis. *J Am Coll Cardiol.* 2020;75:3048-3057.

137. Tyagi G, Dang P, Pasca I, et al. Progression of degenerative mitral stenosis: insights from a cohort of 254 patients. *J Heart Valve Dis.* 2014;23:707-712.

138. Oktay AA, Gilliland YE, Lavie CJ, et al. Echocardiographic assessment of degenerative mitral stenosis: a diagnostic challenge of an emerging cardiac disease. *Curr Probl Cardiol.* 2017;42:71-100.

139. Eleid MF, Foley TA, Said SM, et al. Severe mitral annular calcification: multimodality imaging for therapeutic strategies and interventions. *JACC Cardiovasc Imaging.* 2016;9:1318-1337.

140. Chu JW, Levine RA, Chua S, et al. Assessing mitral valve area and orifice geometry in calcific mitral stenosis: a new solution by real-time three-dimensional echocardiography. *J Am Soc Echocardiogr.* 2008;21:1006-1009.

141. Sengupta SP, Mohan JC. Calcific mitral stenosis: echoes of aging. *J Am Coll Cardiol.* 2020;75:3058-3060.

142. Pasca I, Dang P, Tyagi G, Pai RG. Survival in patients with degenerative mitral stenosis: results from a large retrospective cohort study. *J Am Soc Echocardiogr.* 2016;29:461-469.

143. Pizano A, Hirji SA, Nguyen TC. Severe mitral annular calcification and mitral valve surgery: an algorithmic approach to management. *Semin Thorac Cardiovasc Surg.* 2020;S1043-0679:30148-30149.

144. Yoon SH, Whisenant BK, Bleiziffer S, et al. Outcomes of transcatheter mitral valve replacement for degenerated bioprostheses, failed annuloplasty rings, and mitral annular calcification. *Eur Heart J.* 2019;40:441-451.

145. Guerrero M, Urena M, Himbert D, et al. 1-year outcomes of transcatheter mitral valve replacement in patients with severe mitral annular calcification. *J Am Coll Cardiol.* 2018;71:1841-1853.

146. Russell HM, Guerrero ME, Salinger MH, et al. Open atrial transcatheter mitral valve replacement in patients with mitral annular calcification. *J Am Coll Cardiol.* 2018;72:1437-1448.

147. Unger P, Rosenhek R, Dedobbeleer C, Berrebi A, Lancellotti P. Management of multiple valve disease. *Heart* 2011;97:272-277.

148. Gash, AK, Carabello BA, Kent RL, et al. Left ventricular performance in patients with coexistent mitral stenosis and aortic insufficiency. *J Am Coll Cardiol.* 1984;3:703-711.

149. Katznelson G, Jreissaty RM, Levinson GE, et al. Combined aortic and mitral stenosis: a clinical and physiological study. *Am J Med.* 1960;29:242-256.

150. Uricchio JF, Likoff W. Effect of mitral commissurotomy on coexisting aortic-valve lesions. *N Engl J Med.* 1957;256:199-204.

151. Porter A, Shapira Y, Wurzel M, et al. Tricuspid regurgitation late after mitral valve replacement: clinical and echocardiographic evaluation. *J Heart Valve Dis.* 1999;8:57-62.

152. Shiran A, Sagie A. Tricuspid regurgitation in mitral valve disease incidence, prognostic implications, mechanism, and management. *J Am Coll Cardiol.* 2009;53:401-408.

33

Infective Endocarditis

Ann F. Bolger

Pathogenesis, epidemiology, diagnosis, and management of infective endocarditis

Pathogenesis

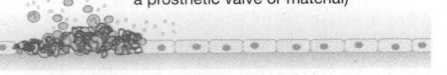

Niche for infection = Cardiac endothelium damaged by hemodynamic or mechanical stress, OR the surface of an implanted cardiac device (including a prosthetic valve or material)

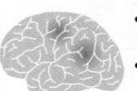

- Transient bacteremia may lead to vegetation, a macroscopic infective mass.
- Vegetations are associated with high-grade bacteremia and damage to the underlying valvular endothelium

  - Embolization of micro or macroscopic pieces of vegetative tissue can result in septic emboli, including to the brain
  - Deposits of immune complexes and complement components may lead to such extravalvular complications as glomerulonephritis

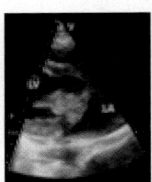

- Common cardiovascular complications include destruction of valvular tissue, heart failure, and conduction disturbances

Diagnosis

- Initial clinical suspicion arises with fever without an alternate etiology, constitutional symptoms (fatigue; anorexia; weight loss; night sweats; or pain in the joints, abdomen or back), and often with identifiable risk factors (eg, intravenous drug use)
- Blood cultures are critical to identifying infection and guiding treatment

  - Evidence of infection on histology and cultures of explanted valve tissue is definitive proof of endocardial infection
  - Usually, evidence is taken from echocardiographic findings of vegetations, perivalvular extension of infection such as abscess, and new valvular regurgitation
  - Echocardiography should be obtained as soon as possible for any patient with suspected infective endocarditis
  - The modified Duke criteria comprise the standard for diagnosis

Epidemiology

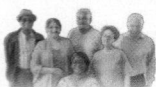

- Incidence is 2 to 10 cases per 100,000 person-years
- 6-month mortality is ~25%
- More than half of all cases in the US and Europe occur in patients aged >60 years

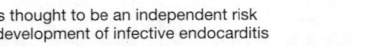

- Among persons who inject drugs, infective endocarditis occurs in 2–5% per year
- HIV infection is thought to be an independent risk factor for the development of infective endocarditis

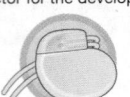

  - Among patients on chronic hemodialysis, incidence is 308 per 100,000 patient-years
  - Cardiovascular implantable electronic devices infection rates range from 0.8% to 5.7%

- Recurrence rates in survivors of infective endocarditis are 2.5–9%
- Heart failure is the most frequent major complication and cause of death

Management

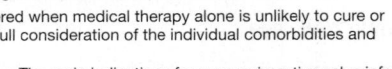

- Rapid use of parenteral antibiotic therapy is critical to limiting valve destruction and risk of emboli
- Neither anticoagulant therapy nor aspirin reduce the risk of embolism in patients and should be used with caution as there is a risk for hemorrhagic conversion of septic emboli
- Surgery should be considered when medical therapy alone is unlikely to cure or control the infection, with full consideration of the individual comorbidities and risk/benefit

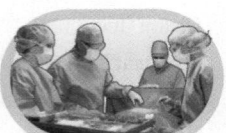

  - The main indications for surgery in native valve infective endocarditis include heart failure, complicated or persistent infections, vegetation size (>1cm), and avoidance or control of embolization
  - The patient is best served by a multispecialty team—including specialists from infectious disease, cardiology, and cardiac surgery—that can determine surgical indication and timing

- Valve repair is preferable to replacement when possible to minimize prosthetic tissue, need for anticoagulation and risk of recurrence

Chapter 33 Fuster and Hurst's Central Illustration. Infection of intracardiac endothelial surfaces results in infective endocarditis, a condition with stubbornly high mortality of ~25% at 6 months. Rapid diagnosis, staging, and careful collaboration between infectious disease, cardiology, and surgical teams to determine the best medical and surgical treatment are important to give the patient their best chance of recovery.

CHAPTER SUMMARY

This chapter discusses the pathogenesis and epidemiology of infective endocarditis (IE), as well as the diagnosis and management of patients with this condition (see Fuster and Hurst's Central Illustration). Cardiac endothelium is normally resistant to infection; endothelial damage, via hemodynamic or mechanical stress, is required for establishment of infection in most cases. The surface of an implanted cardiac device can also be a locus of infection. Bacteria circulating in the bloodstream due to remote infection or transient bacteremia interact with platelets, tissue factors, and endothelium to establish an infective site and form a macroscopic infective mass. Continuous high-grade bacteremia, fragmentation, and direct damage to underlying endocardial tissue and/or valves results. Risk for the development of IE is increased in older adults, persons who inject drugs, individuals with HIV, hemodialysis patients, individuals with cardiovascular implantable electronic devices, and people with prior history of endocarditis. In cases of IE, 6-month mortality is ~25%. Echocardiography should be obtained as soon as possible for any patient with suspected IE. Rapid diagnosis, staging, and careful collaboration between infectious disease, cardiology, and surgical teams to determine the best medical and surgical treatment are important to give the patient their best chance of recovery.

INTRODUCTION

Infection of intracardiac endothelial surfaces results in infective endocarditis (IE), a dreaded disease with many short- and long-term complications and a stubbornly high mortality that approaches 25% at 6 months.[1,2,3] Without treatment, IE is fatal and can wreak havoc with heart valves, chordae, mural surfaces, or deeper myocardium and pericardium. The impact is systemic, with preferential effects on the central nervous system (CNS) and pulmonary systems. Implanted intracardiac devices (ICDs) such as prosthetic valves and rhythm devices amplify vulnerability to infections, which are often complicated and difficult to eradicate. The patient's best chances for recovery result from rapid diagnosis, staging, and careful collaboration between infectious disease, cardiology, and surgical teams to determine the best medical and surgical treatment.[3,4] Prevention of IE in patients at risk hinges on patient education, maintenance of good oral hygiene, and prophylactic antibiotics for a limited spectrum of procedures that may induce bacteremia with organisms known to be associated with endocarditis.

PATHOGENESIS

The natural cardiac endothelium is resistant to infection. In animal models of endocarditis, damage to the endothelium is required to establish infections, despite a large inoculum of bacteria.[5] In most clinical endocarditis involving native tissues, an injury resulting from hemodynamic or mechanical stresses disrupts the endothelium, exposing underlying collagen and other matrix molecules. Fibrin and platelets adhere to these elements, creating a sterile vegetation. Bacteria circulating in the bloodstream due to remote infection or transient bacteremia may then bind to and replicate in this microthrombus, amplifying the extrinsic clotting pathway, monocyte release of cytokines, and local deposition of fibronectin by activated endothelial cells. The result is a macroscopic infective mass that promotes further deposition of platelets and fibrin, resulting in increasing vegetation size and fragility.[6,7] Not all bacteria can establish endovascular infections; organisms commonly associated with endocarditis share an avidity for adherence to valve tissue. Some highly virulent organisms such as *Staphylococcus aureus* may not require underlying trauma to establish infection.

Bacteria may enter the bloodstream from many sources, including skin wounds, indwelling vascular catheters, genitourinary, and gastrointestinal tracts. The periodontal tissues of the mouth are commonly replete with organisms capable of causing endocarditis, and bacteremia often follows mechanical trauma to the oral mucosa from eating, brushing, flossing, or dental procedures.[8]

The infective microorganisms may interact with platelets and become trapped in extracellular neutrophil "traps";[9] some bacteria, including streptococci, generally form sessile, layered communities of cells irreversibly attached to cardiac surfaces that are enclosed in a protective matrix of exopolymeric products called biofilm.[3,10,11] Biofilms are up to 1000-fold more resistant to antibiotic therapy than planktonic cells,

and are particularly associated with endocarditis on prosthetic material, which carry a worse prognosis than native valve infections.

Infection of implanted prosthetic materials is mediated by properties of the device surface.[12] Coagulase-negative staphylococci (CoNS) may adhere directly to plastic polymers on a device. Bacterial adherence may target fibrinogen, fibronectin, and collagen deposited on newly implanted biomaterials.[13] A device surface that has become endothelialized can be infected by bacteria, particularly gram-positive cocci, which can adhere to and be engulfed by endothelial cells.

Infected vegetations are avascular and contain bacteria in great density, often with 10^9 to 10^{10} colony forming units per gram.[14] Neutrophils and host defense molecules have limited penetration into these lesions, allowing them to grow relatively unchecked and resulting in continuous high-grade bacteremia, fragmentation, and direct damage to underlying endocardial tissue and/or valves.

Many cardiac conditions, including congenital heart disease and acquired valvular disease, are associated with an increased risk of endocarditis. High velocity jets may traumatize the endothelium, as occurs in the left ventricular outflow tract in hypertrophic obstructive cardiomyopathy. In other situations, risk is related to turbulent, disorganized flow downstream from an orifice where flow velocities first increase and then decelerate in a lower pressure zone (**Fig. 33–1**). The disorganization of flow that results increases regional platelet and endothelial activation, and the slower eddy zones in proximity to the endothelium, increase the potential for bacterial interaction with the wall.[15]

The most common sites of infection on the atrioventricular valves are therefore on the atrial surface of the valve leaflets or on the mural endocardium in the path of the jet of mitral regurgitation, including on the calcified mitral annulus (**Table 33–1**).[16] For the aortic and pulmonic valves, infections are formed on the ventricular side of the leaflets. The diastolic jet of aortic valve insufficiency may promote an infective nidus on the ventricular surface of the anterior mitral leaflet or the mitral chordae (the kissing lesion). For ventricular septal defects, the edges of the lower pressure right side of the defect or the right heart valves are most likely sites of infection. Regional heterogeneity of flow is a predictor of infection, and valvular insufficiency that fluctuates in extent and turbulence may expand the zones at risk. Examples of this include mitral regurgitation in degenerative disease, where both afterload and ventricular volume status alter the extent and turbulence of mitral regurgitation. Increased afterload related to use of cocaine or methamphetamine may increase the amount or aortic and mitral regurgitation concurrent with an injection-induced bacteremia, for example, just as opioid-induced hypoventilation and pulmonary hypertension may transiently increase the severity of tricuspid regurgitation.[17]

Embolization of micro or macroscopic pieces of vegetative tissue can result in abscesses throughout the body, often in lungs, spleen, and bone; microemboli to the distal arteries of the fingers and toes, or to the palms and soles, can result in dermal microabscesses referred to as Osler and Janeway

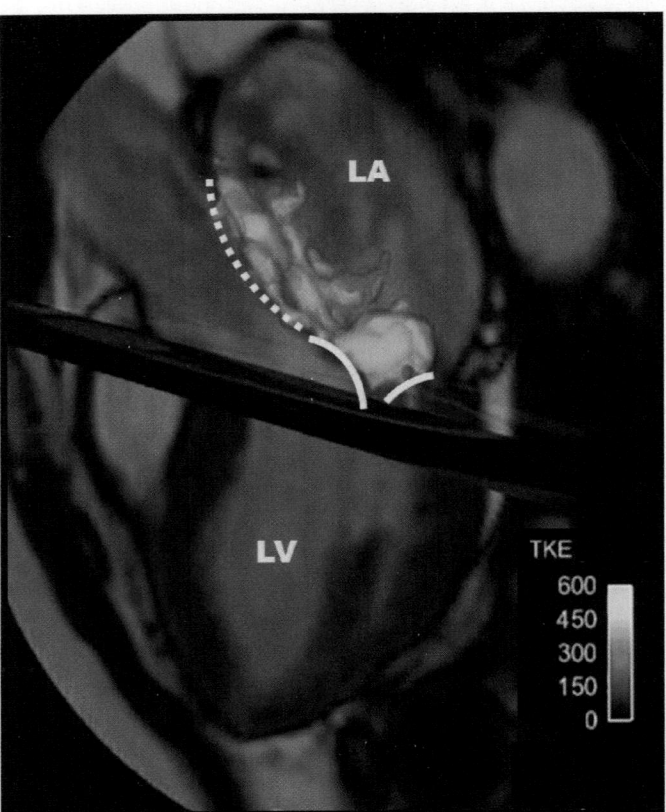

Figure 33–1. Distribution of turbulent flow due to mitral regurgitation. Cardiac MRI demonstration of turbulent kinetic energy (TKE) in the left atrium (LA) due to mitral regurgitation (*orange jet*). The endothelial surfaces exposed to this disorganized flow are the atrial sides of the mitral leaflets (*solid lines*) and the atrial wall washed by the regurgitant jet (*dotted line*). Endocarditis on the mitral valve occurs in these regions due to endothelial and platelet activation and increased time of endothelial exposure to circulating bacteria in the disorganized eddies in the jet's periphery.

lesions, respectively.[18] Emboli to the brain are frequent even in the absence of clinical symptoms.[19]

EPIDEMIOLOGY

The epidemiology of IE has evolved with medical advances and the changing susceptibility of the population. The aging of our population, a success story that introduces the use of many implantable devices, has been shadowed by an increase in the burden of IE in the elderly. Resistance to antimicrobials has created an arms race with infecting organisms, demanding newer agents and reassessment of older ones.

Immunosuppression related to HIV, malignancy, renal disease, and diabetes is also increasingly prevalent and results in infections that are complicated in ways quite different from classic descriptions of IE. In many under-resourced regions rheumatic heart disease (RHD) remains the most common underlying condition in patients with IE.[20] In other regions, IE more commonly complicates degenerative or congenital valve disease or the presence of implanted devices. In all areas, endocarditis without underlying predisposing cardiac conditions can occur.

The incidence of IE has been estimated at 2 to 10 cases per 100,000 person-years.[20-23] The incidence has seen an increase in multiple regions; in the United States, the incidence of IE increased from 11 per 100,000 population to 15 per 100,000 population between 2000 and 2011.[24,25] The prevalence of underlying predisposing cardiac conditions has also varied over time.[26] Infections that develop in the context of recent contact with a healthcare setting with onset of symptoms ≥48 hours after exposure constitute 27% to 38% of IE cases.[2,27]

INFECTIVE ENDOCARDITIS IN SELECTED PATIENT POPULATIONS

Older Adults

Over half of all IE cases in the United States and Europe occur in patients over the age of 60. The median age of IE has trended up in parallel with overall age of the population and decline in rheumatic valvular disease in many regions.[23,28] Older adults have a 5-fold higher risk of IE than the general population.[28,29] Senescent valve changes increase with age, and those findings may interfere with echocardiographic identification of IE. Older adults tend to have smaller and fewer vegetations than younger adults and a higher rate of intracardiac abscess and prosthetic perivalvular complications.[28]

The bacteriology of IE in older adults includes an increase in *Enterococcus faecalis* related to gastrointestinal and genitourinary sources of bacteremia, and staphylococcal species in the setting of implanted cardiac devices.[30] IE mortality is increased in the older adult, particularly with *S. aureus* infection.[31]

Persons Who Inject Drugs

Among persons who inject drugs (PWID), IE occurs in 2% to 5% per year. IE accounts for 5% to 20% of the hospital

TABLE 33–1. Common Sites of Vegetation Attachment				
Aortic Valve	**Mitral Valve**	**Tricuspid Valve**	**Pulmonic Valve**	**VSD with Left-to-Right Shunt**
Ventricular side of AV leaflets	Atrial side of MV leaflets	Atrial side of TV leaflets	Ventricular side of PV leaflets	RV side of VSD rim
Ventricular side of anterior MV leaflet or chordae—seen with aortic valve regurgitation	LA wall (MacCallum patch)	In-dwelling catheter or lead in RA or RV		Ventricular side of TV valve leaflets or chordae

Abbreviations: LA, left atrium; RV, right ventricle; VSD, ventricular septal defect.

admissions and 5% to 10% of overall mortality among PWID.[32] The distinctive feature of IE in PWID is that it frequently involves the right heart, with 60% to 70% of cases involving the tricuspid valve.[3-] Left sided valve infections occur in 20% to 30% cases and a combination of right and left valves in the remainder.

Injecting drugs with contaminants and diluents into vascular or subcutaneous spaces provides entry for bacterial and fungal organisms. Organisms can come from the surface of the skin, the drug itself, injection apparatus, or in diluents including saliva complete with oropharyngeal flora.

The mechanisms underpinning the proclivity of IE in PWID to affect the tricuspid valve have not been clearly established. The most often quoted theory is that substances in the injectate do direct mechanical damage to the valvular endothelium. Absence of tricuspid valve thickening in chronic intravenous heroin users in one study did not support the bombardment mechanism, but chronic valve thickening has been seen in other series.[34,35] Additional underlying mechanisms include drug-induced valvular vasospasm, intimal damage, thrombus formation, and pulmonary hypertension causing right-sided cardiac turbulence. In PWID, increased right-side expression of matrix molecules capable of binding microorganisms and immune dysregulation with or without coexistent HIV infection may also influence the siting of IE infections on the tricuspid valve.[36]

Staphylococcus aureus is the most common etiologic agent of IE in PWID, and gram-negative bacilli (notably *Pseudomonas aeruginosa*) and fungi are also more common.[32] Septic pulmonary emboli often occur in tricuspid infections in PWID. Isolated right heart involvement in PWID partially explains the lower mortality in this population (4%) compared to broader IE cohorts, despite the high frequency of *S. aureus* infection. Uncomplicated right-sided IE may be eligible for short-course parenteral antibiotic therapy (2–4 weeks). Surgery is considered for severe refractory right heart failure caused by tricuspid regurgitation, uncontrolled bacteremia, and persistent tricuspid vegetations >20 mm with recurrent septic pulmonary emboli or left-sided valve involvement. Critical to the success of medical or surgical treatment of IE is a focus on modifying addiction and drug use behaviors. Opioid substitution therapy is associated with a 50% reduction in addiction relapse. This should be addressed in concert with addiction specialists beginning during hospitalization and then carefully addressed in discharge planning and follow-up.

HIV Infection and the Immunocompromised Host

It has been suggested that HIV infection is an independent risk factor for the development of IE.[37] In situations where HIV infection and intravenous drug use coexist, the risk and incidence of IE are similar in PWID with or without HIV.[38] HIV patients with low CD4 counts (<200 cells/mL) tend to have an increased risk of IE, as well as a higher associated mortality.[39]

The characteristics of IE in patients with AIDS and other non–HIV-infected immunocompromised hosts reflect their greater vulnerability to unusual opportunistic organisms.

Atypical IE organisms in HIV positive patients have included *Bartonella* species as well as *Salmonella* and *Listeria*. In HIV and other immunocompromised patients, gram-negative bacteremia or fungemia create the risk for developing IE with those organisms.

Hemodialysis Patients

More than 500,000 patients in the United States receive chronic hemodialysis (HD). Patients on chronic HD are at significant risk for IE, with an incidence of 308 per 100,000 patient-years.[40] Vascular access via central venous catheters, arteriovenous (AV) grafts, or AV fistulae are potential portals of entry for staphylococcal species or other organisms. Primary AV fistulae and indwelling central venous catheters have the lowest and highest rates of infection, respectively.[41] Removal of infected catheters or grafts is necessary for successful IE treatment in most circumstances.

HD patients experience one episode of bacteremia per 100 patient-care months. Few other medical conditions are associated with such high rates of bacteremia. IE occurs in approximately 2% to 6% of patients receiving HD and causes nearly 10% of deaths (second only to ischemic heart disease) in this patient population.[42] Overall mortality due to IE is 22% in-hospital and 51% at 1 year.[41]

Dystrophic calcification of the mitral and aortic valves is very common in patients with chronic renal disease and is often accompanied by flow abnormalities that are audible as murmurs and which increase the valves' risk of infection. Detecting vegetations on a calcified valve with echocardiography is difficult, and transesophageal imaging is often required. The index of suspicion for IE must remain high.

Cardiac Device–Related Infective Endocarditis

The use of cardiovascular implantable electronic devices (CIEDs) is expanding, and CIED infection rates range from 0.8% to 5.7%.[43,44] IE related to CIED is most frequently a right-sided infection, primarily involving the intracardiac portion of leads along their route through the right atrium and tricuspid valve.

The clearest risk factor for CIED infection is recent implantation or manipulation of the device or generator. Approximately three-quarters of infections occur within the first year and result from pocket site contamination at the time of device placement.[45] Devices that have been in place for longer periods of time are less vulnerable to secondary infection from bacteremia arising from a distant focus. Bacteremic seeding primarily involves the intracardiac lead and is due to staphylococcal species in more than 70% of cases.[46]

Early-onset CIED infections (within 3 to 6 months of CIED implantation or generator change) comprise approximately one-third of cases and generally present with marked systemic symptoms and associated generator pocket infection.[47,48] Two-thirds of infections are late-onset (more than 6 months after CIED manipulation). The average time from procedure to symptom onset is 25 months. CIED-IE may involve the lead, a valve (right or left), or present as an occult bacteremia of unclear source.[49] IE may occur in patients with a CIED in the absence of device infection.

The clinical presentation of CIED infection mimics right-sided IE. Acute infections may present with sepsis and shock. More often, the presentation is subacute and may be atypical, with prominent respiratory or rheumatologic symptoms. The modified Duke criteria do not perform as well in diagnosis of CIED-IE as in other endocarditis types.

Manifestations of CIED-IE include fever in 84% to 100% of patients and pulmonary infections or embolism in 20% to 45%. Tricuspid regurgitation develops in about 25% of patients, and metastatic seeding of mitral or aortic valve, bone, joints, liver, and spleen can occur.

Suspicion of intracardiac device infections requires prompt imaging. Valvular vegetation, generally of the tricuspid valve, will be detected on up to 50% of patients with CIED-IE with the use of transthoracic echocardiography (TTE), transesophageal echocardiography (TEE), or intraoperative echocardiography.[47]

In noninfected patients, thrombotic tissue in the form of fibrin strands and organized clots are commonly found attached to intracardiac leads, and clinical pulmonary embolization is rare.[50] Differentiation of these sterile findings from infected vegetation is often not possible and relies on the clinical setting. A goal of echocardiography in this situation is to visualize all components of the device and leads throughout their entire course including into the coronary sinus and vena cava. TTE is often able to provide good views of the tricuspid valve and right atrium, while TEE provides better views of left heart and vascular structures.

Management of CIED-IE requires prolonged treatment with parenteral antibiotics. Complete device removal, including leads and generator, is the standard of care.[51] When valvular IE occurs in a patient with an implanted device in place, there is a high likelihood of concomitant device infection even when no lead vegetation is visualized. This usually necessitates extraction of the full device.[12]

Lead extraction is a complex procedure due to endothelialization and the presence of attached vegetation or thrombus. Pulmonary embolism of vegetative debris is frequent during lead extraction.[52] Mobile vegetations on transvenous leads are common but thankfully rarely associated with acute major adverse outcomes when the vegetation size is less than 2 cm.[53] With vegetations that are larger than 2.5 cm, open extraction should be considered.[51] Decisions regarding optimal timing and site of subsequent device reimplantation are complex and individualized. At the time of CIED placement or replacement, prophylaxis with an antistaphylococcal agent should be administered. Antimicrobial prophylaxis for the prevention of CIED infections is not recommended for dental or other invasive procedures not directly related to device manipulation.[12]

Patients with Prior Infective Endocarditis

A patient with a prior history of endocarditis remains at high risk of another episode of IE. Recurrence rates in survivors of IE range from 2.5% to 9%. The drivers of their initial risk may still be present (congenital or acquired valve disease) and

valvular dysfunction may have worsened due to the prior infection. Ongoing use of injectable illicit drugs is a powerful driver of recurrent IE episodes in PWID. Despite successful treatment of IE, patients also remain at risk for late complications, including heart failure, ischemic and hemorrhagic stroke, myocardial infarction, and sudden death.[53]

MICROBIOLOGY

Microorganisms have variable intrinsic competence for establishing endocardial infection. The likely microbiology of a given infection varies with the route of acquisition, site of infection, and presence of prosthetic materials. Three species account for most cases of IE. *Staphylococcus aureus* is the predominant organism in the United States and developed countries and particularly in healthcare-associated infections. Historically, streptococcal species were the most common group of pathogens causing IE overall, and they remain common causative agents of community acquired IE.[22,27,54] Among PWID, *S. aureus* is the cause of right-sided IE in up to 70%, with streptococci, enterococci, fungi, and gram-negative bacilli as less-common causes.

Data from the International Collaboration on Endocarditis-Prospective Cohort Study representing 2781 adults from 25 countries identified the proportion of infective agents in IE (**Table 33–2**).[2] This series is based on patients referred from tertiary care centers and may not reflect the spectrum of infections found in other settings.

In the international ICE cohort, among infections of known source, 71% were community acquired rather than healthcare associated. Among those with healthcare-associated IE, staphylococcal infections were responsible for almost 70%.[2]

TABLE 33–2. Spectrum of Infectious Agents in Infective Endocarditis (IE)

Organism	Percent of IE Cases
Staphylococcus aureus	31
Viridans group streptococci	17
Enterococci	11
Coagulase-negative staphylococci	11
Streptococcus gallolyticus	6
Other *streptococci* (including nutritionally variant *streptococci*)	6
Non-HACEK gram-negative bacteria	2
Fungi/yeast	2
HACEK	2
Culture-negative endocarditis	10
Polymicrobial	1
Other	4

HACEK includes fastidious gram-negative bacilli: *Haemophilus aphrophilus* (subsequently called *Aggregatibacter aphrophilus* and *Aggregatibacter paraphrophilus*); *Actinobacillus actinomycetemcomitans* (subsequently called *Aggregatibacter actinomycetemcomitans*); *Cardiobacterium hominis*; *Eikenella corrodens*; and *Kingella kingae*.[2]

Native Valve Infective Endocarditis

Streptococci

The viridans group streptococci are normal flora of the oropharynx and are a frequent cause of community acquired NVE in adults.[3,55] Among the viridans group, *Streptococcus sanguinis*, *Streptococcus gallolyticus* (formerly *bovis*), *Streptococcus mutans*, and *Streptococcus mitior* are often associated with IE.

Endocarditis due to *S. gallolyticus* should prompt consideration of gastrointestinal sources of bacteremia, as gastrointestinal (GI) malignancy, polyps, and inflammatory disease have been associated with up to 60% of cases.[56]

The nutritionally variant streptococci *Abiotrophia* and *Granulicatella* species require specialized techniques for growth and diminished susceptibility to penicillins and cephalosporins often requiring addition of aminoglycosins.[27,57]

The enterococcal species (previously known as Group D streptococci) are part of the normal GI and genitourinary (GU) flora and bacteremia with these organisms may follow GU and GI instrumentation. Given its frequent association with prosthetic materials and indwelling catheters, it is a frequent cause of healthcare-associated IE. High-level antibiotic resistance is increasingly common among hospital-acquired enterococcal infections. *Enterococcus faecalis* is more common and more virulent in native valve IE than *E. faecium*.

Group A *Streptococcus* rarely causes IE. *Streptococcus pneumoniae* IE is an acute, fulminant illness with severe valve damage and high mortality.[18] *Streptococcus pyogenes* is not associated with IE in adults.

Group B streptococci such as *Streptococcus agalactiae* are infrequent causes of IE and are most frequently seen in the setting of obstetric complications, diabetes, carcinoma, liver failure, alcoholism, and injection of illicit drugs.[58]

Staphylococci

Worldwide, the most common etiologic agent in acute IE is *Staphylococcus*, and 80% to 90% is due to *S. aureus*, which possesses virulence factors that allow it to adhere to endothelial and prosthetic surfaces and evade host defenses.[2] Nosocomial *S. aureus* infections are prevalent in patients receiving both inpatient and outpatient medical therapy. The risk that *S. aureus* bacteremia is associated with IE is increased among patients with hemodialysis, diabetes, HIV infection, or recent surgery.[32,42] Community-acquired infections appear to be an independent risk factor for the development of IE and metastatic disease.[59]

CoNS species are present on normal skin and, in contrast to *S. aureus*, do not often infect undamaged endothelium. *Staphylococcus epidermidis* is an important infective agent on prosthetic or damaged valves and intracardiac devices, with rates of heart failure and death equivalent to *S. aureus* infections on native valves. It can cause recalcitrant infections on implanted devices.[60] Of the other CoNS occasionally detected in IE, community-acquired *Staphylococcus lugdunensis* has been associated with an increasingly common and virulent form of IE.[61]

Gram-Negative Bacilli

A small proportion of IE cases are caused by gram-negative bacilli. The HACEK group comprises *Haemophilus* species, *Actinobacillus*, *Cardiobacterium hominis*, *Eikenella corrodens*, and *Kingella* species. These fastidious gram-negative rods are residents of the oropharynx and may take 3 to 4 weeks to grow in culture, although modern BACTEC methods have accelerated this to 5 to 7 days. Immunocompromised patients, patients with advanced liver disease or with illicit injection drug use, and prosthetic heart valve recipients are at particular risk. *Haemophilus parainfluenzae*, *Haemophilus aphrophilus*, and *Haemophilus paraphrophilus* are the most common IE agents from this group, and are known to form large, friable vegetations that tend to embolize. *Salmonella* infections of atherosclerotic plaque and *Pseudomonas aeruginosa* endocarditis in PWID are other rare infections.

Q fever, due to the rickettsial organism *Coxiella burnetii*, is seen in areas with cattle, sheep, and goat farming and is associated with IE in those areas.[62] IE due to *Bartonella* species have been recognized in homeless men and HIV-infected patients. Serologic and polymerase chain reaction (PCR) are among special approaches to the diagnosis.[63] Brucellosis is often due to consumption of unpasteurized dairy products or handling livestock. In Spain, brucella has been estimated to cause 4% of cases of IE. Surgery is usually required for cure.[64]

Fungi

Fungal endocarditis, most often with *Candida* and *Aspergillus* species, (52% and 24%, respectively) generally affects the immunocompromised host or patients with indwelling devices.[65-67] Bulky fungal vegetations are prone to embolization and even local obstruction of valves. While *Candida* can be identified on blood culture, cultures in *Aspergillus* infections are rarely positive. The mortality is extremely high and usually requires a combined medical/surgical strategy, including replacement of an infected prosthetic valve and chronic suppressive therapy.[68]

Culture-Negative Infective Endocarditis

The definition of blood culture-negative IE is an endocarditis illness with no known etiology 7 days following inoculation and subculturing of three independent blood samples in a standard blood culture system.[69] A long list of noninfectious causes of vegetations and inflammation must also be considered. Failed detection of IE may be the result of inadequate culture technique, highly fastidious organisms or a nonbacterial pathogen, or acquisition of blood cultures after antimicrobial therapy is given. Despite all efforts, cultures remain negative in 2% to 7% of patients with IE.[70]

Coxiella burnetii and *Bartonella* spp. are common agents of culture-negative endocarditis.[71] *Tropheryma whipplei* may be a more important cause of culture-negative IE than previously recognized, and *Cutibacterium* (formerly *Propionibacterium*) *acnes* is a rare cause of IE with time to positivity of valve cultures of 3 to 28 days (median 5.5 days). Careful questioning regarding possible exposure to fastidious organisms is important in assessment (**Table 33–3**).[69]

Serology and PCR on blood or explanted valve tissue may identify fastidious pathogens. *Coxiella burnetii*, *Bartonella* spp., *Legionella* spp., and *Brucella* spp. are best identified by serology.[72] PCR has identified streptococci, enterococci,

TABLE 33–3. Historical Details Useful in Suspected Culture-Negative Infective Endocarditis

Exposure	Organism
Farm animals	*Brucella* spp *Coxiella* *Tropheryma whipplei*
Body louse	*Bartonella quintana*
Cats	*Bartonella henselae*
Unpasteurized milk or cheese	*Brucella* spp *Coxiella*
Incompletely cooked meat	*Brucella* spp
Immunosuppression/HIV	Fungi *Coxiella*
Alcoholism	*Bartonella quintana*
Soil	*Tropheryma whipplei*
Abattoirs	*Coxiella*
Travel to endemic areas	*B. quintana*—North Africa *Brucella* spp—Middle East, other
Recent or prolonged antibiotic use	

staphylococci, *Bartonella* spp., and *T. whipplei* as culprit organisms.[73,74] Positron emission tomography (PET) has been used to identify infected cardiac devices, periprosthetic valve abscesses, mycotic aneurysms, and heart valve infections and may contribute to diagnosis of fastidious organisms, such as *T. whipplei* and *C. burnetii*.[75]

Prosthetic Valve Endocarditis

Infection of an implanted valve occurs in up to 6% of patients at 5 years. The microbiology of prosthetic infections relates strongly to the time since surgery. The immediate postoperative period (within 2 months) reflects nosocomial exposures with a preponderance of *S. aureus* and CoNS. Over the remaining months of the first postoperative year, a combined spectrum of nosocomial and community-acquired organisms is seen. After the first year, for patients who do not inject illicit drugs, infecting organisms are resemble native valve infections, including sporadic cases of fungi and the less common bacteria. The microbiology of endocarditis affecting percutaneously inserted aortic valve prostheses is generally similar to surgically implanted valves, although enterococcal infections are more frequent after transcatheter aortic valve replacement.[76]

APPROACH TO THE PATIENT WITH SUSPECTED INFECTIVE ENDOCARDITIS

Initial clinical suspicion of IE arises in a patient with fever without obvious etiology, other worrisome symptoms, and often with identifiable risk factors. Given the seriousness of the illness, a high index of suspicion and rapid assessment is important.

Clinical Clues

IE may present with a spectrum of symptoms and findings. A careful history targeting a patient's predisposing factors that make IE more likely and/or more dangerous should be quickly obtained. Congenital heart disease or acquired valvular disease, presence of an intracardiac device or in-dwelling central venous catheter, intravenous drug use, or a prior history of IE are all important. More uncommon details of exposure are relevant to unusual and often culture negative IE infections. With respect to symptoms, the IE patient may report fever (present in up to 90% of IE patients), fatigue, anorexia, weight loss, night sweats, or pain in the joints, abdomen, or back.[21] A fulminant illness with high fever and sepsis is often associated with *S. aureus* infection, for example, while streptococcal infections may be more indolent. On examination, the presence of fever, a new heart murmur indicative of valvular insufficiency (noted in approximately 85% of patients), signs of heart failure, and peripheral vascular phenomena all support the suspicion of IE. Physical examination findings of mucosal or conjunctival petechiae, splinter hemorrhages of the nail beds, palpable purpuric skin rashes, Janeway lesions (small, flat, irregular erythematous spots on the palms and soles, most often seen with acute infections), Osler nodes (tender, erythematous nodules occurring in the pad portion of the fingers), and Roth spots (cytoid bodies and associated hemorrhage caused by microinfarction of retinal vessels) should be sought. Routine laboratory results may include nonspecific elevations of erythrocyte sedimentation rate and/or elevated C-reactive protein, normocytic/normochromic anemia, positive rheumatoid factor, and false-positive serologic tests for syphilis. Urinalysis may reveal hematuria, proteinuria, and/or pyuria; red cell casts are consistent with glomerulonephritis. Imaging may detect findings consistent with splenomegaly, pulmonary emboli (with right-sided IE), or mycotic brain aneurysms with intracranial hemorrhage.

To solidify suspicion based on history and findings into an actionable diagnosis of IE, efforts must shift to demonstration of persistent bacteremia and evidence of endocardial infection.

Persistent Bacteremia

Blood cultures are critical to identifying the infection and guiding treatment. Patients with IE typically have continuous bacteremia regardless of whether fever is present at the time of blood sampling, and at least three sets of blood cultures should be obtained from separate venipuncture sites prior to initiation of antibiotic therapy. The volume of blood for each blood culture set in adults is 20 mL (10 mL into each bottle). The diagnostic yield of more than three sets of blood cultures is minimal in the absence of recent antimicrobial therapy.

Most clinically significant bacteremias are evident in cultures within 48 hours. For fastidious pathogens such as the HACEK group, blood cultures often turn positive after five days of incubation, and still others may take even longer or never grow in routine culture at all. One explanation for culture-negative IE is antecedent antibiotic use. For the most commonly encountered bacterial pathogens (staphylococci, streptococci, enterococci), the first two sets of blood cultures will be positive in the vast majority of cases.

Evidence of Endocardial Infection

Evidence of infection on histology and cultures of explanted valve tissue is definitive proof of endocardial infection. Most of the time, evidence is taken from echocardiographic findings of vegetations, perivalvular extension of infection such as abscess, and new valvular regurgitation.

Modified Duke Criteria

The modified Duke criteria comprise the standard for diagnosis and clinical research and have been validated across many different patient groups.[77,78] Application of these criteria in clinical practice captures the vast majority of cases of IE. These criteria evolved from earlier diagnostic schema, including the von Reyn criteria and the initial Duke criteria, to include echocardiographic data and improve performance particularly in cases due to S. aureus bacteremia and culture-negative IE.[79]

The modified Duke criteria (**Tables 33–4** and **33–5**) outline a strategy that combines major and minor criteria to classify cases as "Definite" or "Possible" IE.[77]

According to these criteria, a diagnosis of *definite IE* is established by evidence of two major criteria, one major plus three minor criteria, or five minor criteria. *Possible IE* patients with one major criterion plus one minor criterion or three minor criteria should be treated for IE until the diagnosis is excluded by other means. Cases without sufficient evidence by these criteria can be rejected as endocarditis.

ECHOCARDIOGRAPHY IN INFECTIVE ENDOCARDITIS

Echocardiography findings are core in the use of the modified Duke criteria.[77,80] Echocardiography should be obtained as soon as possible for any patient with suspected endocarditis. Evidence of vegetation, abscess, prosthetic valve dehiscence, or new valvular regurgitation are major diagnostic criteria for detection of definite or possible IE, and detection of high-risk features suggesting need for early surgery can expedite urgent management decisions. Expeditious imaging of the patient with possible IE is endorsed by the European Society of Cardiology (ESC) and the American College of Cardiology/American Heart Association (ACC/AHA) guidelines.[3,4,81] The specific choice, sequence and repetition among echocardiographic modality is influenced by factors of the individual case including patient characteristics such as acuity and risk for complicated infections (**Tables 33–6** and **33–7**).

The echo findings of valvular or perivalvular findings consistent with infection are not qualified according to study quality, and using echocardiography effectively within this construct requires a careful imaging plan and high standards for image quality. Low-quality images cannot be relied upon to rule out signs of endocardial infection, and if neither TTE nor TEE can provide clear views of all valves from multiple windows, other imaging modalities can be brought to bear.

Echocardiographic Signs of Endocarditis

A valvular vegetation is defined as a discrete mass of echogenic material adherent to a leaflet surface and distinct in character

TABLE 33–4. Definition of Terms Used in the Proposed Modified Duke Criteria for the Diagnosis of Infective Endocarditis

Major criteria

Blood culture positive for IE

Typical microorganisms consistent with IE from two separate blood cultures:

Viridans streptococci, *Streptococcus bovis,* HACEK group, *Staphylococcus aureus*; or

Community-acquired enterococci in the absence of a primary focus; or

Microorganisms consistent with IE from persistently positive blood cultures, defined as follows:

At least two positive cultures of blood samples drawn more than 12 h apart; or

All of three or a majority of greater than four separate cultures of blood (with first and last sample drawn at least 1 h apart)

Single positive blood culture for *Coxiella brunetti* or anti–phase 1 IgG antibody titer greater than 1:800

Evidence of endocardial involvement

Echocardiogram positive for IE (TEE recommended in patients with prosthetic valves, rated at least "possible IE" by clinical criteria, or complicated IE [paravalvular abscess]; TTE as first test in other patients), defined as follows:

Oscillating intracardiac mass on valve or supporting structures, in the path of regurgitant jets, or on implanted material in the absence of an alternative anatomic explanation; or

Abscess; or

New partial dehiscence of prosthetic valve

New valvular regurgitation (worsening or changing of pre-existing murmur not sufficient)

Minor criteria

Predisposition, predisposing heart condition, or injection drug use

Fever, temperature >100.4°F (38°C)

Vascular phenomena, major arterial emboli, septic pulmonary infarcts, mycotic aneurysm, intracranial hemorrhage, conjunctival hemorrhages, and Janeway lesions

Immunologic phenomena; glomerulonephritis, Osler nodes, Roth spots, and rheumatoid factor

Microbiologic evidence: positive blood culture but does not meet a major criterion,[a] or serologic evidence of active infection with organism consistent with IE

Echocardiographic minor criteria eliminated

Abbreviations: HACEK, *Haemophilus* species, *Actinobacillus*, *Cardiobacterium hominis, Eikenella corrodens,* and *Kingella* species; IE, infective endocarditis; Ig, immunoglobulin; TEE, transesophageal echocardiography; TTE, transthoracic echocardiography.

[a]Excludes single positive cultures for coagulase-negative staphylococci and organisms that do not cause endocarditis.

Reproduced with permission from Li JS, Sexton DJ, Mick N, et al. Proposed modifications to the Duke criteria for the diagnosis of infective endocarditis. *Clin Infect Dis.* 2000 Apr;30(4):633-638.

from the remainder of the leaflet.[82] An irregular mass with independent oscillating motion is consistent with vegetation, particularly at sites known to be commonly affected by infection (**Table 33–8**).

In a patient with blood cultures positive for a likely organism, and with a clinical presentation consistent with IE, a mass must be assumed to be infected unless and until more information, including higher resolution echocardiography, can be obtained. Review of prior echocardiographic images can

TABLE 33–5. Definition of Infective Endocarditis According to the Proposed Modified Duke Criteria

Definite infective endocarditis
Pathologic criteria
(1) Microorganisms demonstrated by culture or histologic examination of a vegetation, a vegetation that has embolized, or an intracardiac abscess specimen; or
(2) Pathologic lesions, vegetation, or intracardiac abscess confirmed by histologic examination showing active endocarditis

Clinical criteria
(1) Two major criteria; or
(2) One major criterion and three minor criteria; or
(3) Five minor criteria

Possible infective endocarditis
(1) One major criterion and One minor criterion; or
(2) Three minor criteria

Rejected
(1) Firm alternate diagnosis explaining evidence of infective endocarditis; or
(2) Resolution of infective endocarditis syndrome with antibiotic therapy for less than 4 days; or
(3) No pathologic evidence of infective endocarditis at surgery or autopsy, with antibiotic therapy for less than 4 days; or
(4) Does not meet criteria for possible infective endocarditis, as noted above

Reproduced with permission from Li JS, Sexton DJ, Mick N, et al. Proposed modifications to the Duke criteria for the diagnosis of infective endocarditis. *Clin Infect Dis.* 2000 Apr;30(4):633-638.

TABLE 33–6. Indications for Transthoracic Echocardiography in Endocarditis

Class I
1. Transthoracic echocardiography to detect valvular vegetations with or without positive blood cultures is recommended for the diagnosis of infective endocarditis. *(Level of Evidence: B)*
2. Transthoracic echocardiography is recommended to characterize the hemodynamic severity of valvular lesions in known infective endocarditis. *(Level of Evidence: B)*
3. Transthoracic echocardiography is recommended for assessment of complications of infective endocarditis (eg, abscesses, perforations, and shunts). *(Level of Evidence: B)*
4. Transthoracic echocardiography is recommended for reassessment of high-risk patients (eg, those with a virulent organism, clinical deterioration, persistent or recurrent fever, new murmur, or persistent bacteremia). *(Level of Evidence: C)*

Class IIa
Transthoracic echocardiography is reasonable to diagnose infective endocarditis of a prosthetic valve in the presence of persistent fever without bacteremia or a new murmur. *(Level of Evidence: C)*

Class IIb
Transthoracic echocardiography may be considered for the re-evaluation of prosthetic valve endocarditis during antibiotic therapy in the absence of clinical deterioration. *(Level of Evidence: C)*

Class III
Transthoracic echocardiography is not indicated to re-evaluate uncomplicated (including no regurgitation on baseline echocardiogram) native valve endocarditis during antibiotic treatment in the absence of clinical deterioration, new physical findings, or persistent fever. *(Level of Evidence: C)*

Data from Baddour LM, Wilson WR, Bayer AS, et al. Infective endocarditis in adults: diagnosis, antimicrobial therapy, and management of complications: a scientific statement for healthcare professionals from the American Heart Association. *Circulation.* 2015 Oct 13;132(15):1435-1486.

TABLE 33–7. Indications for Transesophageal Echocardiography in Endocarditis

Class I
1. Transesophageal echocardiography is recommended to assess the severity of valvular lesions in symptomatic patients with infective endocarditis, if transthoracic echocardiography is nondiagnostic. *(Level of Evidence: C)*
2. Transesophageal echocardiography is recommended to diagnose infective endocarditis in patients with valvular heart disease and positive blood cultures, if transthoracic echocardiography is nondiagnostic. *(Level of Evidence: C)*
3. Transesophageal echocardiography is recommended to diagnose complications of infective endocarditis with potential impact on prognosis and management (eg, abscesses, perforation, and shunts). *(Level of Evidence: C)*
4. Transesophageal echocardiography is recommended as first-line diagnostic study to diagnose prosthetic valve endocarditis and assess for complications. *(Level of Evidence: C)*
5. Transesophageal echocardiography is recommended for preoperative evaluation in patients with known infective endocarditis, unless the need for surgery is evident on transthoracic imaging and unless preoperative imaging will delay surgery in urgent cases. *(Level of Evidence: C)*
6. Intraoperative transesophageal echocardiography is recommended for patients undergoing valve surgery for infective endocarditis. *(Level of Evidence: C)*

Class IIa
Transesophageal echocardiography is reasonable to diagnose possible infective endocarditis in patients with persistent staphylococcal bacteremia without a known source. *(Level of Evidence: C)*

Class IIb
Transesophageal echocardiography might be considered to detect infective endocarditis in patients with nosocomial staphylococcal bacteremia. *(Level of Evidence: C)*

Data from Baddour LM, Wilson WR, Bayer AS, et al. Infective endocarditis in adults: diagnosis, antimicrobial therapy, and management of complications: a scientific statement for healthcare professionals from the American Heart Association. *Circulation.* 2015 Oct 13;132(15):1435-1486.

be invaluable in determining the acuity of concerning echo findings.

There is a long list of other etiologies of masses associated with the endocardium, including Lambl's excrescences, redundant or ruptured mitral chordae, a billowing section of a dystrophic mitral valve, and mitral annular calcification. A chronic healed vegetation from a prior episode of IE may appear bright and sessile without the dynamic motion of an acute vegetation, but differentiation is difficult. Comparison with prior images is helpful.

Vegetation is more likely when a mass is located at a likely site for vegetation and has tissue quality similar to myocardium. Fine oscillation of the mass can often be demonstrated clearly with use of high temporal resolution and slow play-back on review. Tethered excursion that does not mirror the motion of the subtending valve is another clue.[83] Masses with bright reflection similar to calcium, attachment at atypical sites, or with a fine strand-like structure are less likely to be vegetation.

Other echocardiographic features of infection are important indicators of high risk. Periannular extension of infection in the form of abscess, fistula, aneurysm, or prosthetic valve dehiscence is evidence of severe infection. Valvular destruction

TABLE 33–8. Typical Echocardiographic Findings in Infective Endocarditis

Finding	Description
Vegetation	Irregularly shaped, discrete echogenic mass.
	Adherent to, yet distinct from, endocardial surface.
	High-frequency oscillation of the mass with motion that is independent of that of normal cardiac structures is a supportive, but not mandatory, finding.
Abscess	Thickened area or mass within the myocardium or annular region.
	Appearance is nonhomogeneous, often with both echogenic and echolucent areas in the lesion.
	Evidence of flow (by Doppler interrogation) within the area is strongly supportive, but not mandatory.
Aneurysm	Echolucent space that is contiguous with the cavity of origin and that is completely bounded by a thin layer of tissue extending from the cavity of origin.
Fistula	Connection between two distinct cardiac blood spaces through a nonanatomic channel.
Leaflet perforation	Defect in the body of a cardiac valve leaflet with evidence of blood flow through the defect.
Prosthetic valvular dehiscence	Rocking motion of a prosthetic valve with excursion of more than 15 degrees in any single plane.

Data from Sachdev M, Peterson GE, Jollis JG. Imaging techniques for diagnosis of infective endocarditis. *Cardiol Clin.* 2003 May;21(2):185-195.

with leaflet perforation or flail is usually associated with significant valvular incompetence and often heart failure, requiring careful quantification of regurgitant volumes and ventricular function.

Prognostic Features

High-risk features on echo relate to vegetation characteristics, extension of the infection into perivalvular regions, and the presence of significant valvular dysfunction or heart failure. Vegetation size (generally measured as its longest dimension in any echo view) correlates with embolization and risk for other IE complications. A vegetation length of more than 15 mm was associated with complications in 100% of patients, versus 50% for lengths of 6 mm.[83] Length more than 10 mm increased the incidence of emboli from 19% to 47% in another series.[84] Surgery during the initial IE hospitalization should be considered for native valve aortic or mitral vegetations >10 mm with low operative risk or for very large vegetations >30 mm.[4] An increase in vegetation size despite appropriate medical therapy is evidence of a complicated course associated with need for surgery.[85]

Perivalvular extension of infection is most commonly evidenced by the presence of abscess. Imaging early in the course of an infection may miss an incipient abscess, which can appear as nonspecific thickening of the periannular tissues. As an abscess organizes and expands, it may create local effects such as interruption of the conduction system in the septum with progressive block of atrioventricular conduction. The growing abscess may eventually break through and connect with a great vessel or cardiac chamber, creating a fistula.

Perivalvular involvement is a dominant feature in prosthetic valve infections, and abscess can lead to dehiscence of the valve. In one series of 26 cases of prosthetic valve endocarditis, 54% had valve dehiscence at surgery.[87]

Symptomatic heart failure or echocardiographic signs of poor hemodynamic tolerance associated with left-sided severe regurgitation, valvular obstruction, or fistula formation are additional indicators for surgery.

Echocardiographic Approaches to Infective Endocarditis

All echocardiographic modalities can be limited by issues of resolution and interference. TTE uses lower ultrasound frequencies compared to TEE, which accounts for its poorer resolution for very small structures such as minimal vegetations. TTE is also subject to interference from lung and chest wall structures, as well as artifactual interference from implanted devices. TEE can similarly be hampered by nonsonolucent structures in its imaging path. The initial echo modality and subsequent imaging choices are determined by individual case details (**Fig. 33–2**).

Transthoracic

TTE is generally the most rapidly available and most common initial cardiac ultrasound test. The sensitivity of TTE for detection of vegetations on a native valve is 50% to 90%, with 95% specificity (**Fig. 33–3**).[88] On a prosthetic valve, the sensitivity of TTE for vegetation is 50%. TTE is even less sensitive for detection of abscess, approximately 30% to 50% in native and as low as 15% to 35% with prosthetic valves.[89]

In a patient with a low pretest likelihood of IE, a negative TTE may suffice. In a series of low-risk patients with moderate- or better-quality studies, TTE had a negative predictive value of 97% when the studies confirmed normal anatomy without valvular stenosis or sclerosis, less than mild valvular regurgitation, no significant pericardial effusion, no catheter or pacemaker leads, and no evidence of vegetation.[90] A positive TTE may also be sufficient for diagnosis and early management. For example, in a patient with mitral valve endocarditis caused by a penicillin-sensitive viridans streptococcal species and no predictors of a complications, antibiotic therapy could be initiated with careful follow-up and complementary imaging as clinically indicated if a high-quality TTE demonstrated an isolated posterior leaflet vegetation of less than 1 cm in length with mild mitral regurgitation but no suggestion of other valvular abnormality.

One-fifth of patients have technically inadequate TTE images for proper resolution of valvular and endocardial structures which should prompt TEE assessment if the patient is at increased risk for complications. Even in those cases, TTE may assist in early risk assessment by determining valvular competence, ventricular size and function, and pulmonary pressures. TTE also creates a baseline to which sequential imaging studies can be compared to assess response to treatment.

Point of care ultrasound (POCUS) is increasingly available and commonly used in emergency rooms and in hospital, often by nonechocardiography staff. POCUS is not equivalent to TTE. Detection of vegetation falls outside the nonexpert

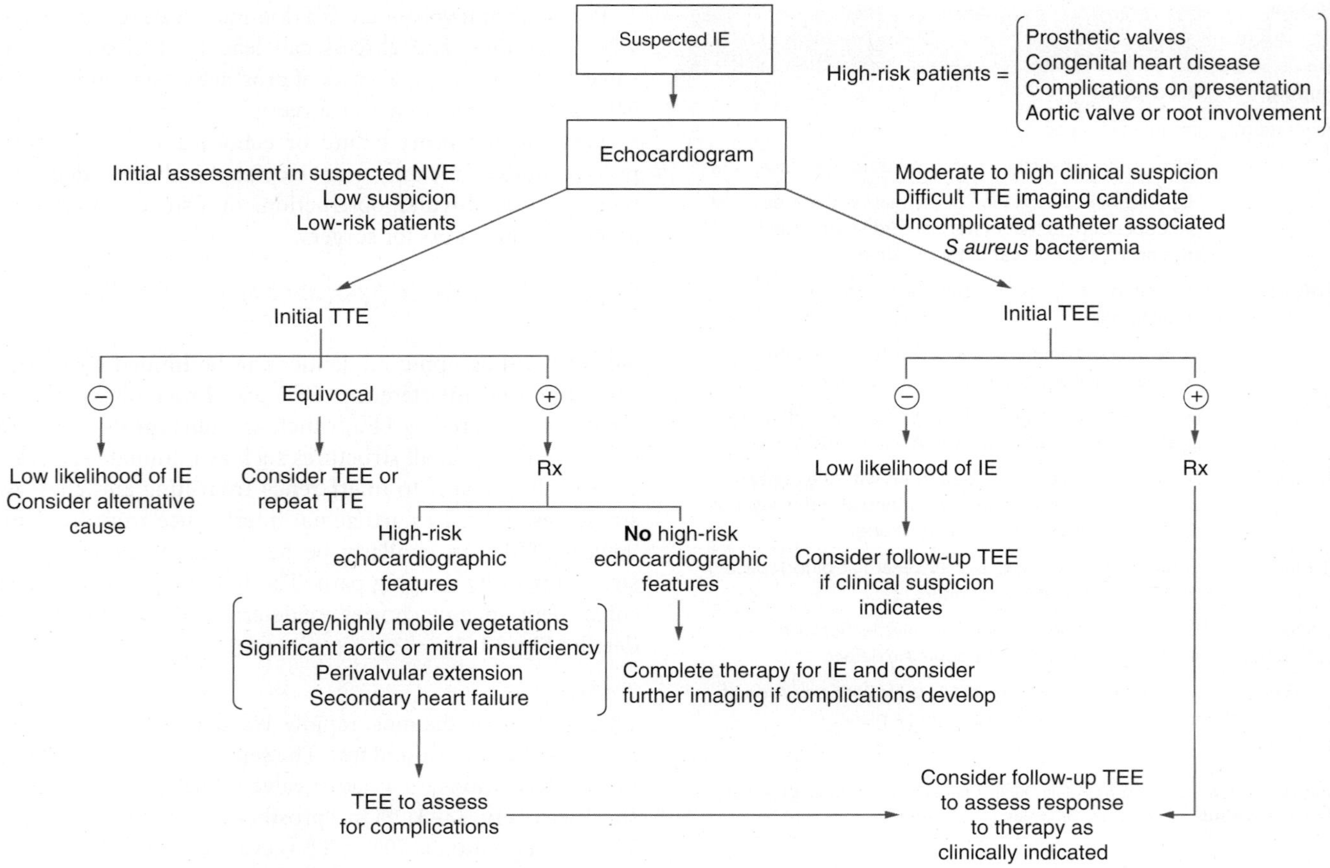

```
                                    ┌──────────────┐
                                    │ Suspected IE │                    ┌ Prosthetic valves
                                    └──────────────┘     High-risk      │ Congenital heart disease
                                           │             patients =     │ Complications on presentation
                                           ▼                            └ Aortic valve or root involvement
                                    ┌──────────────┐
                                    │Echocardiogram│
                                    └──────────────┘
    Initial assessment in suspected NVE                      Moderate to high clinical suspicion
              Low suspicion                                  Difficult TTE imaging candidate
             Low-risk patients                               Uncomplicated catheter associated
                                                                    S aureus bacteremia

                    Initial TTE                                        Initial TEE

        ⊖          Equivocal          ⊕                     ⊖                            ⊕
        │              │              │                     │                            │
        ▼              ▼              ▼                     ▼                            ▼
  Low likelihood   Consider TEE      Rx              Low likelihood of IE               Rx
     of IE         or repeat TTE
    Consider                    High-risk      No high-risk       Consider follow-up TEE
   alternative                echocardiographic echocardiographic   if clinical suspicion
     cause                       features         features               indicates

                         ┌ Large/highly mobile vegetations ┐        │
                         │ Significant aortic or mitral     │        ▼
                         │      insufficiency               │  Complete therapy for IE and consider
                         │ Perivalvular extension           │  further imaging if complications develop
                         └ Secondary heart failure          ┘

                                      │                                    Consider follow-up TEE
                                      ▼                                     to assess response
                              TEE to assess ──────────────────────────────→  to therapy as
                             for complications ←───────────────────────────  clinically indicated
```

Figure 33–2. Use of echocardiography in diagnosis and management of infective endocarditis (IE). NVE, native valve endocarditis; TEE, transesophageal echocardiography; TTE, transthoracic echocardiography. Reproduced with permission from Bayer AS, Bolger AF, Taubert KA, et al. Diagnosis and management of infective endocarditis and its complications. *Circulation*. 1998 Dec 22-29;98(25):2936-2948.

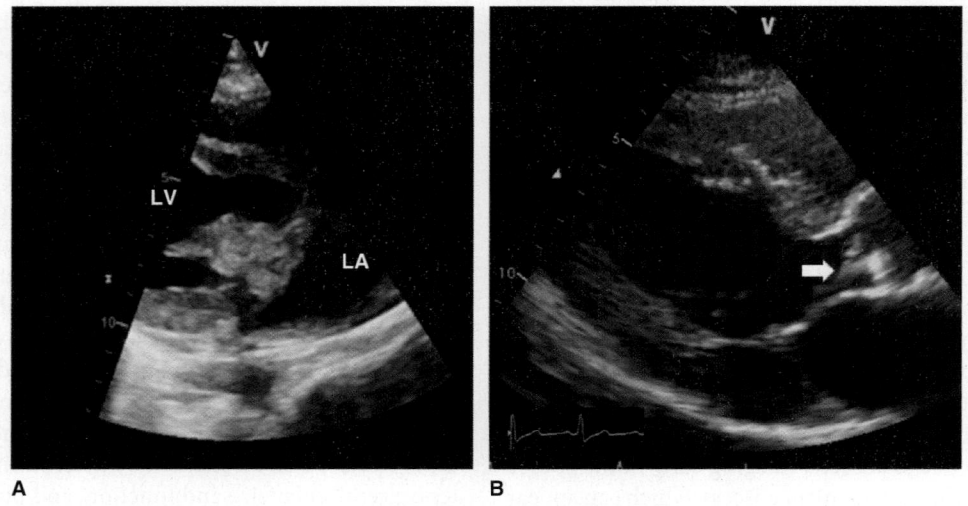

A   B

Figure 33–3. Transthoracic echocardiography (TTE) images of *Staphylococcus aureus* IE. (A) Large, complex vegetation attached to the left atrial (LA) surface of the anterior mitral valve leaflet and causing obstruction of flow through the mitral valve into the left ventricle (LV). Image quality is excellent and TTE can provide full hemodynamic assessment of the vegetation's impact. Vegetation size and organism indicates a high risk of IE complications, and subsequent TEE should be performed to further assess for perivalvular extension of infection. **(B)** In a different patient, a pendant vegetation (*white arrow*) that was highly mobile and associated with mild aortic valve regurgitation is attached to the ventricular side of the thickened aortic valve. Image quality is marginal, and while these TTE results fulfill the diagnostic criteria for echocardiographic evidence of endocardial infection, TEE should be performed as soon as possible to assess for high-risk features that would impact therapy, including perivalvular abscess.

examination of a patient suspected of IE, because complete visualization of valves from multiple views with the best possible quality images is required. A negative examination is not reassuring that the patient does not have IE, and great care should be taken to avoid communication to other providers that "the echo is negative" in a patient who has undergone POCUS but not a complete echocardiogram. Similarly, a large vegetation detected with POCUS may guide early strategies, but additional views of all valves and functional assessment of valvular competence and ventricular function are critical to early risk stratification. Miscommunication about POCUS findings is common, and rapid initial echocardiographic assessment of the patient suspected of IE with full TTE remains critical.

Transesophageal

TEE is indicated as the initial echo study when TTE will be inadequate for detection of diagnostic findings or in the presence of high-risk features such as prosthetic valves, poor quality prior TTE, complex congenital heart disease, new heart block, or thoracic trauma. The procedural risks of TEE are very low. A different form of risk in a TEE-first strategy in some settings are delays in time to first echo investigation. This can result from time required to mobilize staff and resources, to the patient not being nil by mouth, to time required to obtain informed consent from patients or their responsible family member. In addition, TEE provides less thorough investigation of associated hemodynamically important findings. A thorough TTE should be performed close to the time of the TEE in order to address those gaps, and also to establish a baseline set of transthoracic images to which subsequent TTE studies may be compared.

The sensitivity of TEE for vegetation is 96% for native valves and 92% for prosthetic valves with a specificity of 90% in both settings. For detection of abscess, the sensitivity and specificity of TEE have been reported at 87% and 90%.[86] Other intracardiac complications including valve perforation, aneurysm, kissing lesion (the ventricular surface infection of the anterior mitral valve leaflet that occurs in the path of a jet of aortic regurgitation), and mural vegetation are all more reliably detected with TEE than TTE.[84,87,91] Differentiation of vegetation from flail leaflet is also improved.

Several scenarios present difficulties for TEE. An early abscess may appear as nonspecific perivalvular thickening without a central lucent area (**Fig. 33–4**). Repeat echo after 3 to 5 days may demonstrate the evolution of the abscess. An abscess involving the posterior mitral annulus in the setting of mitral annular calcification may be obscured by the bright reflections from the annulus. Another problematic site is the anterior aspect of the sewing ring of an aortic valve prosthesis, which may be shielded from a TEE perspective by the interference from the prosthesis. In that situation, a transthoracic view of the region may be able to visualize the abscess since the interference then projects away from the chest wall. A single negative TEE cannot rule out IE in a high-risk patient with ongoing suspicion of IE and repeat imaging in 4 to 5 days may be indicated.[92]

For both TEE and TTE, detection of vegetation in a patient who has had episodes of embolization can be difficult if most of the infected mass has recently broken off. This often leaves an irregular attachment point with thickening and sometimes fine fibrillar structures that can be seen with the use of high frame rates. Since vegetations are dynamic structures that shed and reform, unlucky timing of an echo may result in uncertainty regarding the presence

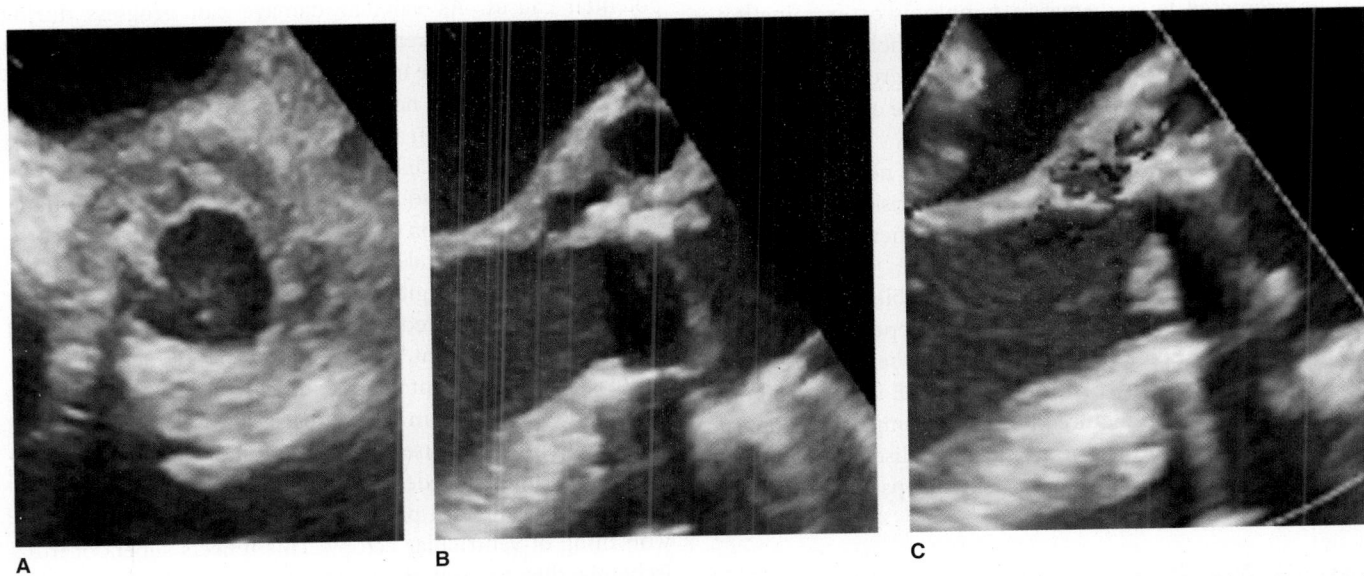

A **B** **C**

Figure 33–4. Transesophageal echocardiography (TEE) images of perivalvular abscess. (A) Inhomogeneous thickening surrounds the sewing ring of a prosthetic aortic valve, seen in the short axis view. This "moth eaten" appearance is consistent with abscess, despite the absence of clear cavities. **(B)** In a different patient, a perivalvular abscess posterior to the aortic valve prosthesis is seen, with clear cavitation (*white arrow*). The anterior aspect of the sewing ring is not seen well in this view due to interference from prosthetic shadowing. **(C)** Flow from the cavity into the LV outflow tract (LVOT) is consistent with transition of abscess to perivalvular fistula.

of a valvular infection. Subsequent re-imaging may demonstrate partial recurrence of the amorphous mass.

Three-dimensional (3D) echo images constructed from TEE data may improve the characterization of an abscess and its relationship to fistulae, aneurysms, and prosthetic valve dehiscence. However, the 3D images have significantly lower spatial and temporal resolution.[93]

Intraoperative TEE performed at the time of surgery is an important reassessment of the extent of endocarditis damage to valves that may have progressed during the preoperative treatment phase. It is not uncommon for perivalvular fistulae or abscesses to have progressed in the interim, or for other valves to have become involved. Following completion of the procedure, intraoperative TEE can assess surgical results.[94]

TEE in *Staphylococcus aureus* Bacteremia: *Staphylococcus aureus* can affect normal valves with few physical stigmata. *Staphylococcus aureus* bacteremia (SAB) of uncertain source is a common problem that raises appropriate concerns regarding possible IE. SAB is of great concern in high-risk cardiac conditions such as prosthetic heart material, congenital heart disease, cardiac transplantation, history of endocarditis, or presence of a cardiac device.[95] TEE is appropriate for SAB; in patients without those high-risk conditions, TEE is also reasonable if SAB is prolonged more than >72 hours.[96] In patients with an intermediate pretest likelihood of IE, an initial TEE is cost-effective in guiding the duration of therapy in patients with SAB and intravascular catheters, intracardiac electronic devices, or prosthetic valves.[2,97]

Repeat Studies

Repeat echocardiography can be useful in further assessing unresolved suspicions for IE and clarifying the evolution of findings such as valvular incompetence, abscess, and vegetation dimensions after an interval of 3 to 7 days.[4,81] A repeat echo can be prompted by a change in symptoms or examination, including a new or changing murmur, embolism, persistent fever, signs of heart failure, or new or progressive atrioventricular heart block. A follow-up echo in the absence of such changes is of limited use.[98]

A repeat TEE 4 to 5 days after an initial negative study is appropriate for ongoing suspicion in a high-risk situation such as community-acquired bacteremia in a patient with a prosthetic valve.[92]

At the end of treatment, a TTE will establish a new baseline for the patient for future follow-up. Repeat TEE maybe the modality of choice in circumstances where the relevant findings are best seen by that mode, but TTE images of those finding should also be acquired for future comparison. Repeat TEE has been used to determine safety of discontinuation of treatment in special circumstances, such as partial outpatient treatment of endocarditis.[99]

OTHER IMAGING

Several imaging methods are highly useful in the diagnosis and care of endocarditis patients. In patients with ongoing suspicion of IE after inconclusive echocardiography, 18-FDG PET/computed tomography (CT) may indicate an infection of cardiac or vascular tissues.[100] Suspected perivalvular extension of infection can be further assessed with electrographically gated CT that may identify abscesses and other sequelae.[101] The systemic consequences of IE are important to detect, and cerebral imaging with CT or magnetic resonance imaging (MRI) is obtained in many IE patients to assess for evidence of brain embolization and formation of mycotic aneurysms (**Fig. 33–5**).[102]

COMPLICATIONS

Complications of IE occur in up to 57% of cases.[103] They can generally be related to destruction of or interference with intracardiac structures (eg, leaflet destruction or valvular obstruction), local extension of infection (eg, valve ring abscess, fistulae, conduction block), embolization (eg, stroke, septic pulmonary emboli), disseminated infection/sepsis (eg, osteomyelitis), and immune complex disease (eg, glomerulonephritis).

Cardiac Complications

Cardiac complications are the most common complications in IE; they occur in up to half of patients. These include destruction of cardiac and great vessel tissues, and heart failure.

Heart Failure

Heart failure is the most frequent major complication and cause of death due to IE. Due to its high mortality, it is the most common motivator for cardiac surgery during treatment of IE. Heart failure in IE is most often due to destruction of the aortic or mitral valves with subsequent new or progressive insufficiency. Rupture of infected mitral chordae, valve obstruction caused by bulky vegetations, development of intracardiac shunts, or prosthetic valve dehiscence are other potential causes. As valvular damage can progress during apparently successful treatment, monitoring for incipient signs of heart failure (change in heart murmurs, pulmonary congestion, volume overload, new arrhythmia, hypotension) needs to be thoughtfully done on a very frequent basis. IE with *S. aureus* infection increases the likelihood of heart failure.

Heart failure can also reflect myocardial ischemia or infarction due to embolization of vegetation fragments into the coronary ostia or more distal arteries.

Acute aortic regurgitation (AR) underlies 29% of heart failure episodes followed by mitral valve (20%) and tricuspid valve (8%) involvement.[104] In acute severe AR, sudden delivery of a large regurgitant volume into an unprepared LV results in a marked increase in left ventricle diastolic and left atrial pressures, and a decrease in stroke volume. Patients may present with pulmonary edema and progress to shock. A highly concerning event in a patient with AR in IE is the onset or worsening of ventricular ectopy. This reflects subendocardial ischemia due to wall stress and impaired coronary perfusion; sustained ventricular tachycardia causes abrupt further increase in LVEDP and ischemia, often resulting in recalcitrant arrhythmias. Patients should be maintained on telemetry during their acute phase, and orders written to notify the care team

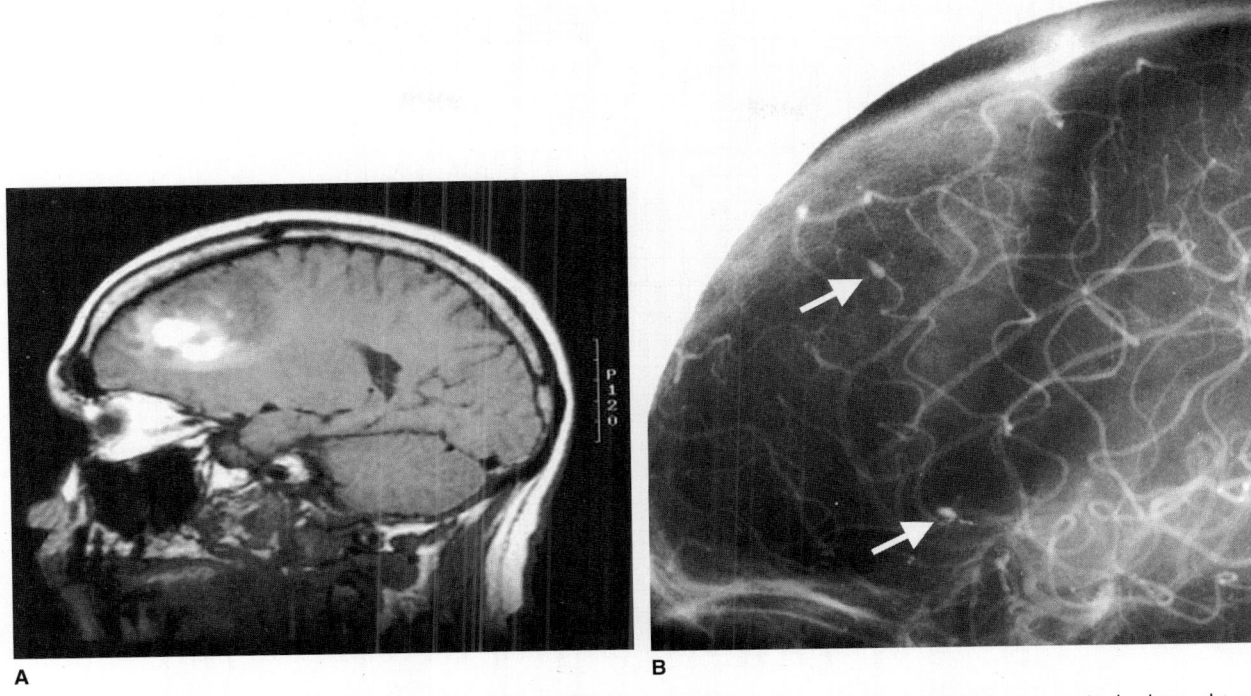

Figure 33–5. Neurological consequences of IE. (A) Large right frontal hemorrhage in a patient with *Staphylococcus aureus* mitral valve endocarditis. **(B)** Mycotic aneurysms (*arrows*) along the course of the branches of the middle cerebral artery. Reproduced with permission from Mauri L, de Lemos JA, O'Gara PT. Infective endocarditis. *Curr Probl Cardiol.* 2001 Sep;26(9):562-610.

if ventricular ectopy appears or increases. The physical examination of acute severe AR is not dramatic. The pulse pressure is not widened, the first heart sound is soft, and the diastolic murmur is of relatively short duration. Inappropriate bradycardia may arise due to extension of infection into the conduction system and subsequent AV block. The longer diastolic filling time, and lower heart rate can combine to prompt more ventricular ischemia and further depression of the cardiac output. Any of these worrisome changes should prompt emergent surgery. Patients with acute severe mitral regurgitation (MR) may present with pulmonary edema, low cardiac output, and/or rapid atrial fibrillation. Surgery should be pursued promptly, but medical treatment may offer some temporary margin of safety in contrast to acute AR. Acute tricuspid regurgitation may cause right heart failure, which generally improves with medical management. Less severe valvular dysfunction may be associated with heart failure if preexisting cardiac disease is present.

Perivalvular Extension of Infection

Extension of infection beyond the valve annulus (PVEI) into the surrounding structures is a marker of complicated infection with a high risk of needing early surgery. Such infections are rarely cured with medical therapy alone. In native valve infections, PVEI develops in 30% to 40%, and most commonly affects the aortic valve.[105] In prosthetic heart valves where infections begin in the annular sewing ring, 50% of IE cases involve PVEI. Persistent fever and bacteremia despite antibiotic therapy, heart failure, or new conduction block raise suspicion

of PVEI. New AV block in the setting of aortic valve IE has a high positive predictive value for the presence of perivalvular abscess (**Fig. 33–6**). PVEI includes abscess formation, fistula, or aneurysm. The resolution of TTE is inadequate to assess regions at risk for PVEI, and TEE should be performed as soon as possible. In one study, the sensitivity, specificity, and positive and negative predictive values of TEE for perivalvular abscess were 87%, 95%, 91%, and 92%, respectively.[105] The presence of perivalvular abscess has been associated with significantly increased rates of embolization and death.[106] Surgery in this situation aims for complete eradication of the infection, often requiring extensive debridement and reconstruction of tissues around a new prosthetic valve.

Embolism

Embolization of infected vegetative matter is extremely common in IE and may occur before or during treatment. Emboli with clinical sequelae have been documented in up to 44% of IE patients.[84,107,108]

Any systemic or pulmonary arterial vessel is vulnerable to occlusion with infected emboli.[3] Signs of arterial occlusion to brain and spinal cord, retina, extremities, heart, lungs, spleen and kidneys, and myocardium may all be clues to IE. Brain and spleen are most common in left-sided IE, and pulmonary arteries in right-sided IE. Neurological complications are subsequently discussed.

Splenic abscess does not always present with significant abdominal pain or splenomegaly; persistent fever and/or

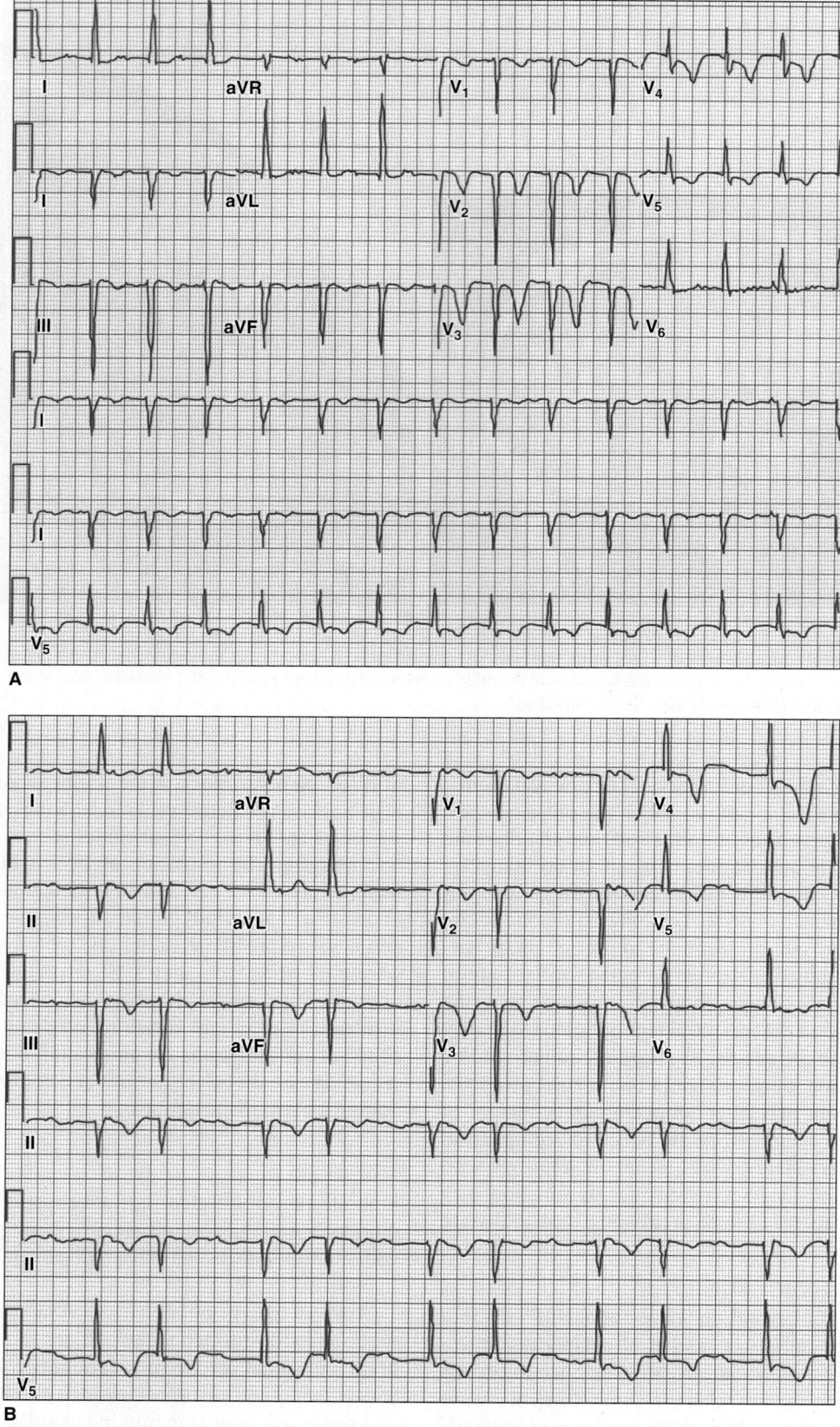

Figure 33–6. Complications of the conduction system. Serial electrocardiograms of a patient with methicillin-resistant Staphylococcus aureus (MRSA) aortic valve endocarditis complicated by root abscess and ventricular septal rupture. Note progressive degrees of high-grade atrioventricular (AV) block. **(A)** First-degree AV block. **(B)** Second-degree AV block. **(C)** Complete heart block.

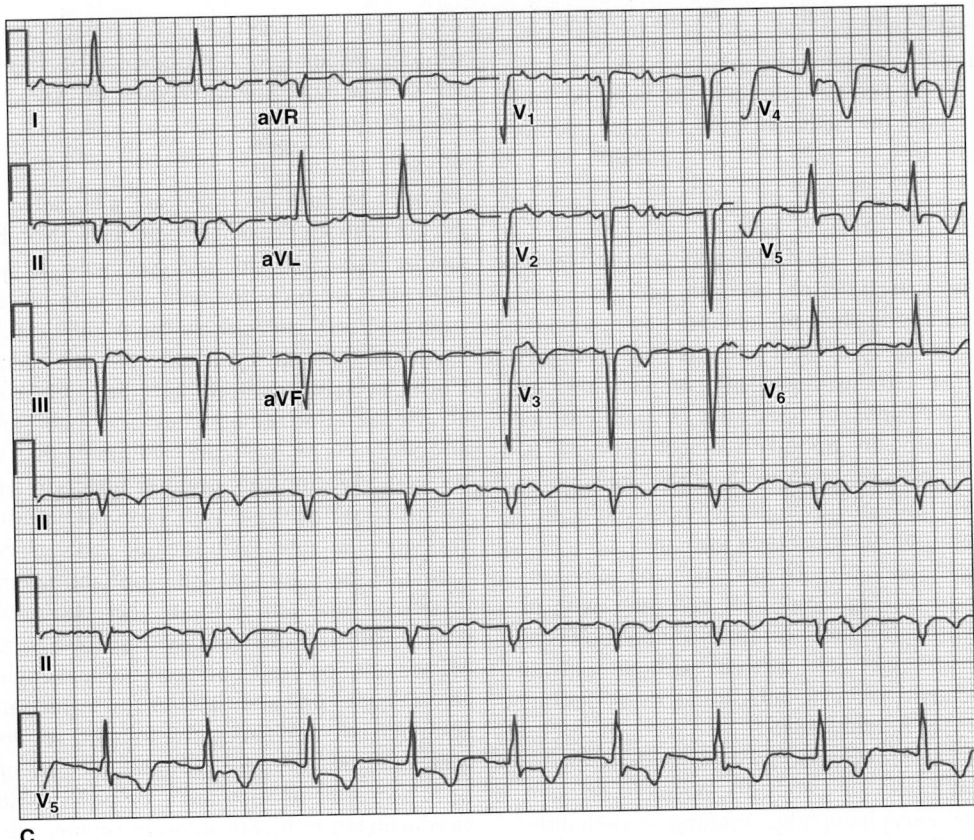

Figure 33–6. (Continued)

recurrent bacteremia during or after completion of antimicrobial therapy may be clues to its presence. Splenic abscess has a high mortality, and frequently requires splenectomy for cure. Other metastatic sites of infection include the spine and paraspinous spaces. Cutaneous findings including Janeway and Osler lesions are evidence of embolization of vegetative material to the far periphery.[18]

Embolization risk appears to decrease rapidly with initiation of appropriate antibiotic therapy, and serious events are rare after 2 weeks.[107,109,110] Embolic stroke fell from 4.8 to 1.7 events per 1000 patient-days between the first and second week of therapy in a study from the ICE group.[110] This time course emphasizes the importance of expeditious surgery when the goal Is to minimize emboli in high-risk situations.

The risk of embolization is usually gauged according to vegetation size, response to treatment, and microbiology. Vegetations larger than 10 mm with marked mobility are associated with more embolic episodes. Supporting this is the finding that patients whose vegetations were only seen on TEE but not on TTE had lower risk of embolization.[111] Vegetations on the anterior mitral leaflet are associated with more emboli than other sites; the proposed mechanism has been the mechanical effects of the leaflet's flinging motion due to abrupt leaflet excursion in early diastole.[55] Of causative organisms, fungi, *S. aureus,* and *S. gallolyticus* have been Identified as risk factors for emboli.[112] Other atypical organisms can also cause bulky vegetations prone to embolization. Increasing or unchanged vegetation size on TEE during appropriate antimicrobial therapy has been associated with higher embolic rates.[113]

Antiphospholipid antibodies have been associated with risk of embolization (62% vs 23%).[114] Possible mechanisms include thrombin generation and defective fibrinolysis.

Renal Dysfunction

Acute renal failure occurs in up to one-third of IE patients. Potential causes include septic embolization with renal infarction or abscess, glomerulonephritis due to immune complex deposition, and drug-induced interstitial nephritis. Toxicity from aminoglycosides and other agents may also damage renal function, as well as low cardiac output and systemic congestion. The impact of all of these is worse in the setting of preexisting renal disease. A series of 62 IE patients detected renal infarction in 31%, acute glomerulonephritis in 26%, acute interstitial nephritis in 10%, and renal cortical necrosis in 10%.[115]

Musculoskeletal Complications

Vertebral osteomyelitis, particularly common in *S. aureus* IE, results in back pain that should prompt imaging. Septic arthritis due to IE is generally polyarticular and often involves sacroiliac, pubic, or manubriosternal joints. An aspirate from septic joint may be a clue to the diagnosis of IE and its causative organism.

Pulmonary Complications

Right-sided endocarditis is frequently associated with septic pulmonary emboli. These can have direct hemodynamic consequences, and may result in pneumonia, lung abscess, pleural effusion, or pneumothorax.

Neurologic Complications

Cerebrovascular complications in IE may be clinically evident (with focal neurological deficit, headache, confusion, or seizures), or may be silent in their presentation. Symptomatic complications occur in up to 35% of patients.[108,116–118] Eighty percent of IE patients demonstrate silent complications on imaging.[19,102,108,119] Microbleeds (round T2* hypointensities with a diameter ≤10 mm) are frequently detected with MRI in patients with IE. These do not correlate with parenchymal hemorrhage or postoperative neurological complications; surgery should not be postponed due to their presence.[119]

Cerebral imaging is mandatory for any suspicion of neurological complication of IE (**Fig. 33–7**). CT scanning, with or without contrast agent, is the most common initial modality, while the higher sensitivity of MRI, with or without contrast gadolinium enhancement, more detailed analysis of lesions and higher sensitivity for microbleeds.

The spectrum of cerebrovascular complications is broad. Embolic stroke, brain abscess or cerebritis, purulent or aseptic meningitis, acute encephalopathy, meningoencephalitis, cerebral hemorrhage (due to stroke or a ruptured mycotic aneurysm), and seizures (secondary to abscess or embolic infarction) may all occur with IE and may portend a poor prognosis.[120] In one series of patients with stroke due to IE, the 1-year mortality rate was 50%.[121] These complications may be the presenting symptom in some patients with IE and should prompt evaluation. An unexplained fever accompanying a stroke in a patient with valvular disease can be an important clue pointing to IE.

Mycotic Aneurysms

Mycotic aneurysms (MA) are a dreaded complication that occurs in about 1 to 5 of IE patients with emboli.[3,122] MA, which can be solitary or multiple, can evolve anywhere in the circulation but are most frequent in the intracranial arteries (66% in one series), particularly the middle cerebral artery and its branches, followed by arteries of the viscera or extremities.[123] Coronary MA have been described.[124] MA are general located at arterial bifurcations, sites at which flow disorganization and eddy currents occur.[3,123] Emboli that become lodged in the vasa-vasorum can establish infection with weakening and distortion of the vessel wall. Features pointing to an infectious etiology of an aneurysm include saccular, eccentric, or multilobulated shape surrounded by inflammatory mass, intramural or perivascular air, or fluid. These features are well demonstrated with CT angiography (Fig. 33–5).[125] Angiography with MR can also be used, and conventional angiography is reasonable if high clinical suspicion for intracranial mycotic aneurysm persists despite negative imaging results. Imaging for MA is generally reserved for symptomatic patients.

MA may be asymptomatic or present with a small sentinel bleed with headache. Spontaneous rupture with intracranial hemorrhage and dense deficits may occur during or after treatment; progressive MA enlargement on therapy may portent this event.

Mortality among IE patients with intracranial MAs is 60% overall, and 80% if rupture occurs. Spontaneous resolution of MA with antibiotic therapy can occur.[126]

MEDICAL TREATMENT

Antimicrobial Therapy

Rapid institution of appropriate parenteral antibiotic therapy is critical to limiting valve destruction and risk of emboli due to IE. After presumptive diagnosis or determination of a high level of suspicion for IE but before culture results are available, empiric therapy is generally begun as soon as possible once at least two (and preferably three) sets of blood cultures have been obtained from separate venipunctures and ideally spaced over 30 to 60 minutes. In a patient with low suspicion of IE and without high-risk features, antibiotic initiation may await culture results with careful monitoring and a plan to initiate treatment if circumstances change. Blood cultures will be positive in more than 90% of IE patients. The choice of an initial empiric regimen depends on the likely bacteriology and resistance patterns. Risk of *S. aureus* IE is increased with a history of chronic hospitalization, in-dwelling central venous catheters or prosthetic devices, surgical wounds, and intravenous drug use. In general, empiric therapy should cover staphylococci (both methicillin susceptible and resistant), streptococci, and enterococci. Vancomycin plus ceftriaxone is an appropriate choice for initial therapy in most patients but should be guided by institutional patterns of infection.

```
┌──────────────────────────────────────────┐
│ Suspected neurological complication in     │
│ an IE patient being considered for surgery │
└──────────────────────────────────────────┘
                    │
                    ▼
┌──────────────────────────────────────────┐
│        Cerebral imaging: CT or MRI          │
└──────────────────────────────────────────┘
                    │
                    ▼
┌──────────────────────────────────────────┐
│        Intracranial hemorrhage              │
│ (not including asymptomatic microbleeds)    │
│        Stroke with severe deficit           │
│                Coma                         │
└──────────────────────────────────────────┘
         │                          │
         ▼                          ▼
┌──────────────────┐      ┌──────────────────┐
│  Delay surgery    │      │  Consider surgery │
│ Continue treatment│      │                   │
│  and monitoring   │      │                   │
└──────────────────┘      └──────────────────┘
```

Figure 33–7. Impact of neurological complications on patient candidacy for surgery. CT, computed tomography; MR, magnetic resonance. Data from Habib G, Lancellotti P, Antunes MJ, et al. 2015 ESC Guidelines for the management of infective endocarditis: The Task Force for the Management of Infective Endocarditis of the European Society of Cardiology (ESC). Endorsed by: European Association for Cardio-Thoracic Surgery (EACTS), the European Association of Nuclear Medicine (EANM). *Eur Heart J.* 2015 Nov 21;36(44):3075-3128.

Detailed antibiotic therapy recommendations are maintained by several professional organizations including the AHA and the ESC. These are subject to update and revision based on evolving antibiotic effectiveness and organism resistance data. There are several key overarching discriminators that defining the appropriate regimen for the individual patient's circumstances and that will assist in accessing the relevant published guidelines. The causative organism and its sensitivity are the most important details driving antibiotic selection. Regimens for streptococcal species, staphylococcal species, enterococci, HACEK organisms, and culture-negative infections are available. Those regimens will be further parsed by resistance to penicillins or methicillin (streptococcal spp. and staphylococcal spp., respectively) or to vancomycin (for enterococci). A second critical component is the presence or absence of prosthetic materials, which may influence choice of therapy as well as its duration. Third, availability and safety of different strategies for inpatient or outpatient infusion or even conversion to oral antibiotics is considered. The need for postoperative continuation of antibiotics or chronic suppressive therapy is another consideration in patients who require surgery.

Organism-specific treatment regimens are outlined in consensus guidelines (**Tables 33–9** through **33–15**).[3,4,127] Current online versions of regimens should always be reviewed

TABLE 33–9. Therapy of Native Valve Endocarditis Caused by Highly Penicillin-Susceptible Viridans Group *Streptococci* and *Streptococcus gallolyticus* (Formerly Known as *Streptococcus bovis*)

Regimen	Dosage[a] and Route	Duration (wk)	Comments
Aqueous crystalline penicillin G sodium	12–18 million U per 24 h IV either continuously or in 4–6 equally divided doses	4	Preferred in most patients >65 y of age or patients with impairment of 8th cranial nerve function or renal function
			Ampicillin 2 g IV every 4 h is an alternative if penicillin not available
or			
Ceftriaxone sodium	2 g per 24 h IV/IM in 1 dose	4	
	Pediatric dose[b]: penicillin 200,000 U/kg per 24 h IV in 4–6 equally divided doses or ceftriaxone 100 mg per 24 h IV/IM in 1 dose		
Aqueous crystalline penicillin G sodium	12–18 million U per 24 h IV either continuously or in 6 equally divided doses	2	Two-week regimen not intended for patients with known cardiac or extracardiac abscess or for those with creatinine clearance of <20 mL/min, impaired 8th cranial nerve function, or *Abiotrophia*, *Granulicatella*, or *Gemella* spp. infection. Gentamicin dosage should be adjusted to achieve peak serum concentration of 3–4 µg/mL and trough serum concentration of <1 µg/mL when 3 divided doses are used; nomogram used for single-daily dosing.
or			
Ceftriaxone sodium	2 g per 24 h IV/IM in 1 dose	2	
plus			
Gentamicin sulfate[c]	3 mg/kg per 24 h IV/IM in 1 dose	2	
	Pediatric dose: penicillin 200,000 U/kg per 24 h IV in 4–6 equally divided doses or ceftriaxone 100 mg/kg per 24 h IV/IM in 1 dose; gentamicin 3 mg/kg per 24 h IV/IM in 1 dose or 3 equally divided doses[d]		
Vancomycin hydrochloride[e]	30 mg/kg per 24 h IV in 2 equally divided doses not to exceed 2 g per 24 h unless concentrations in serum are inappropriately low	2	Vancomycin therapy recommended only for patients unable to tolerate penicillin or ceftriaxone; vancomycin dosage should be adjusted to a trough concentration range of 10–15 µg/mL
	Pediatric dose: 40 mg/kg per 24 h IV in 2–3 equally divided doses		

Minimum inhibitory concentration ≤0.12 µg/mL.
Abbreviations: IM, intramuscular; IV, intravenous.
[a]Dosages recommended are for patients with normal renal function.
[b]Pediatric dose should not exceed that of a normal adult.
[c]Other potentially nephrotoxic drugs (eg, nonsteroidal anti-inflammatory drugs) should be used with caution in patients receiving gentamicin therapy.
[d]Data for once-daily dosing of aminoglycosides for children exist, but no data for treatment of infective endocarditis exist.
[e]Vancomycin dosages should be infused during course of at least 1 hour to reduce risk of histamine-release "red man" syndrome.
Reproduced with permission from Baddour LM, Wilson WR, Bayer AS, et al. Infective endocarditis in adults: diagnosis, antimicrobial therapy, and management of complications: a scientific statement for healthcare professionals from the American Heart Association. *Circulation*. 2015 Oct 13;132(15):1435-1486.

TABLE 33–10. Therapy of Native Valve Endocarditis Caused by Strains of Viridans Group Streptococci and *Streptococcus gallolyticus* (*bovis*) Relatively Resistant to Penicillin

Regimen	Dosage[a] and Route	Duration (wk)	Comments
Aqueous crystalline penicillin G sodium	24 million U per 24 h IV either continuously or in 4–6 equally divided doses	4	Patients with endocarditis caused by penicillin-resistant (MIC > 0.5 µg/mL) strains should be treated with regimen recommended for enterococcal endocarditis
or			
Ceftriaxone sodium	2 g per 24 h IV/IM in 1 dose	4	If isolate is susceptible to ceftriaxone
plus			
Gentamicin sulfate	3 mg/kg per 24 h IV/IM in 1 dose	2	
	Pediatric dose[b]: penicillin 200,000–300,000 U per 24 h IV in 4–6 equally divided doses or ceftriaxone 100 mg/kg per 24 h IV/IM divided every 12 h; gentamicin 3 mg/kg per 24 h IV/IM in 1 dose or 3 equally divided doses		
Vancomycin hydrochloride[c]	30 mg/kg per 24 h IV in 2 equally divided doses not to exceed 2 g per 24 h, unless serum concentration are inappropriately low	4	Vancomycin therapy is recommended only for patients unable to tolerate penicillin or ceftriaxone therapy
	Pediatric dose: 40 mg/kg per 24 h in 2 or 3 equally divided doses		

MIC > 0.12 µg/mL to ≤0.5 µg/mL.
Abbreviations: IM, intramuscular; IV, intravenous; MIC, minimum inhibitory concentration.
[a]Dosages recommended are for patients with normal renal function.
[b]Pediatric dose should not exceed that of a normal adult.
Reproduced with permission from Baddour LM, Wilson WR, Bayer AS, et al. Infective endocarditis in adults: diagnosis, antimicrobial therapy, and management of complications: a scientific statement for healthcare professionals from the American Heart Association. *Circulation*. 2015 Oct 13;132(15):1435-1486.

because updated versions may be available. Treatment tables are dense and should be considered carefully. Multiple provisos to the recommendations are included in the tables and footnotes. Given the rising rate of antimicrobial resistance among causative organisms, guidance from infectious disease specialists is invaluable in informing the dose, duration, and method of delivery of antimicrobial therapy during and after hospitalization.

All patients should have surveillance blood cultures obtained 2 to 3 days after the initiation of antibiotic therapy to ensure efficacy. Serum antibiotic levels should be monitored where appropriate and renal, hepatic, and auditory function assayed when indicated.

Most regimens require 4 to 6 weeks of treatment to eradicate infections, since they exist in sequestered areas that impede host defenses. Drugs with bactericidal activity are most effective, and more rapid bactericidal effect can often be gained by synergistic combinations of antimicrobial agents. Two-week IE treatment may sometimes be appropriate with uncomplicated native valve endocarditis caused by highly penicillin-susceptible viridans group streptococci and *S. gallolyticus*. Long-term venous access via peripherally inserted catheters is necessary for intravenous infusion of medications. Patients should remain in an inpatient setting during the initial phase of treatment when complications are most likely to occur. Selected patients can be considered for outpatient parenteral antibiotic therapy.

A strategy for shortened duration of parenteral therapy in favor of treatment completion with oral agents in selected stable patients with left-sided native valve endocarditis was examined in the Partial Oral Treatment of Endocarditis (POET)

trial. Patients who completed at least 10 days of intravenous therapy were randomly assigned to normal intravenous treatment or to oral treatment with a two-drug antibiotic regimen for an equivalent total duration. Infecting organisms included streptococci (54%), *E. faecalis* (25%), methicillin-susceptible *S. aureus* (23%), or CoNS (13%).[128] In comparison to conventional intravenous therapy, the partial oral regimen was noninferior with respect to treatment completion and outcomes including all-cause mortality, unplanned cardiac surgery, embolic events, or relapse of bacteremia at 6 months. At 3.5-year follow-up, no indication of worse outcomes was detected.[99] The generalizability of these findings has not been substantiated to date, and such regimens have not been incorporated in the treatment guidelines.

Antiplatelet and Antithrombotic Therapy

Despite the role of thrombogenesis in establishing endocardial infection and formation of vegetations, neither anticoagulant therapy nor aspirin reduce the risk of embolism in patients with IE.[129,130] IE patients are at high risk for bleeding complications, including intracerebral hemorrhage, and as such, anticoagulants and antiplatelet agents should not be given. Warfarin therapy should be discontinued at initial presentation because of the risk of hemorrhagic stroke and the potential need for invasive procedures or early surgery. Unfractionated intravenous heparin may be considered for cautious substitution if the need for continuous anticoagulation (for mechanical mitral valve or mitral stenosis patients who are in atrial fibrillation, for example) is deemed to be sufficiently high relative to the risk of hemorrhage. The acute phase of IE is the period of highest

TABLE 33–11. Therapy for Endocarditis Caused by *Enterococcus*

Regimen	Dosage[a] and Route	Duration (wk)	Comments
Therapy for native valve or prosthetic valve enterococcal endocarditis caused by strains susceptible to penicillin and gentamicin and in patients who can tolerate β-lactam therapy			
Ampicillin sodium	2 g every 4 h IV in 6 equally divided doses	4–6	Native valve: 4-wk therapy recommended for patients with symptoms of illness ≤3 mo; 6-wk therapy recommended for patients with symptoms >3 mo
Or			
Aqueous crystalline penicillin G sodium	18–30 million U per 24 h IV either continuously or in 6 equally divided doses	4–6	Prosthetic valve or other prosthetic cardiac material: minimum of 6-wk therapy recommended
Plus			
Gentamicin sulfate[b]	3 mg/kg per 24 h IV/IM in 3 equally divided doses	4–6	
	Pediatric dose[c]: ampicillin 200–300 mg/kg per 24 h IV in 4–6 equally divided doses up to 12 g daily or penicillin 200,000–300,000 U/kg per 24 h IV in 4–6 equally divided doses; gentamicin 3–6 mg/kg per 24 h IV/IM in 3 equally divided doses		
Or			
Ampicillin	2 g IV every 4 h		
Plus			
Ceftriaxone			Recommended for patients with creatinine clearance <50 mL/min before or after gentamicin therapy
	2 g IV every 12 h		
Therapy for endocarditis involving a native or prosthetic valve or other prosthetic material resulting from *Enterococcus* species caused by a strain susceptible to penicillin and resistant to aminoglycosides or streptomycin-susceptible gentamicin-resistant in patient able to tolerate β-lactams			
Ampicillin	2 g IV every 4 h	6	
Plus			
Ceftriaxone	2 g IV every 12 h	6	
For streptomycin-susceptible, gentamicin-resistant patients			
Ampicillin sodium	2 g IV every 4 h	4-6	
Or			
Aqueous penicillin G	18-30 million U per 24 h IV either continuously or in 6 divided doses		
Plus			
Streptomycin sulfate	15 mg/kg per 24 h IV or two doses IM		
Vancomycin-containing regimens for vancomycin- and aminoglycoside-susceptible penicillin-resistant *Enterococcus* species for native or prosthetic valve IE in patients unable to tolerate β-lactams			
Vancomycin	30 mg/kg per 24 h IV in 2 equally divided doses	6	
Plus			
Gentamicin	3 mg/kg per 24 h IV or IM in 3 doses	6	
Penicillin resistance; intrinsic or β-lactamase producer			
Vancomycin plus aminoglycoside	30 mg/kg per 24 h IV in 2 equally divided doses		
Therapy for endocarditis involving a native or prosthetic valve or other prosthetic material resulting from *Enterococcus* species caused by strains resistant to penicillin, aminoglycosides, and vancomycin			
Linezolid	600 mg IV or orally every 12h	>6	
Or			
Daptomycin	10–12 mg/kg per dose	>6	

Abbreviations: IE, infective endocarditis; IM, intramuscular; IV, intravenous.
[a]Dosages recommended are for patients with normal renal function.
[b]Dosage of gentamicin should be adjusted to achieve peak serum concentration of 3 to 4 µg/mL and a trough concentration of less than 1 µg/mL. Patients with a creatinine clearance of <50 mL/min should be treated in consultation with an infectious diseases specialist.
[c]Pediatric dose should not exceed that of a normal adult.
Reproduced with permission from Baddour LM, Wilson WR, Bayer AS, et al. Infective endocarditis in adults: diagnosis, antimicrobial therapy, and management of complications: a scientific statement for healthcare professionals from the American Heart Association. *Circulation*. 2015 Oct 13;132(15):1435-1486.

TABLE 33-12. Therapy for Endocarditis Caused by Staphylococci in the Absence of Prosthetic Materials

Regimen	Dosage[a] and Route	Duration (wk)	Comments
Oxacillin-susceptible strains: Nafcillin or oxacillin[b]	12 g per 24 h IV in 4–6 equally divided doses	6	For complicated right-sided IE and for left-sided IE; for uncomplicated right-sided IE, 2 wk
For penicillin-allergic (nonanaphylactoid type) patients:			Consider skin testing for oxacillin-susceptible staphylococci and questionable history of immediate-type hypersensitivity to penicillin
Cefazolin	6 g per 24 h IV in 3 equally divided doses	6	Cephalosporins should be avoided in patients with anaphylactoid-type hypersensitivity to β-lactams; vancomycin should be used in these cases
Oxacillin-resistant strains: Vancomycin	30 mg/kg per 24 h IV in 2 equally divided doses	6	Adjust vancomycin dosage to achieve trough concentration of 10–20 µg/mL
	Pediatric dose: 40 mg/kg per 24 h IV in 2 or 3 equally divided doses up to 2 g/day		
Daptomycin	≥8 mg/kg dose		

Abbreviations: IE, infective endocarditis; IV, intravenous.
[a]Dosages recommended are for patients with normal renal function.
[b]Pediatric dose should not exceed that of a normal adult.
Reproduced with permission from Baddour LM, Wilson WR, Bayer AS, et al. Infective endocarditis in adults: diagnosis, antimicrobial therapy, and management of complications: a scientific statement for healthcare professionals from the American Heart Association. *Circulation*. 2015 Oct 13;132(15):1435-1486.

TABLE 33-13. Therapy for Prosthetic Valve Endocarditis Caused by Staphylococci

Regimen	Dosage[a] and Route	Duration (wk)	Comments
Oxacillin-susceptible strains			
Nafcillin or oxacillin	12 g per 24 h IV in 6 equally divided doses	At least 6	Penicillin G 24 million U per 24 h IV in 4–6 equally divided doses may be used in place of nafcillin or oxacillin if strain is penicillin susceptible (minimum inhibitory concentration ≤0.1 µg/mL) and does not produce β-lactamase; vancomycin should be used in patients with immediate-type hypersensitivity reactions to β-lactam antibiotics; cefazolin may be substituted for nafcillin or oxacillin in patients with non–immediate-type hypersensitivity reactions to penicillins
plus			
Rifampin	900 mg per 24 h IV/PO in 3 equally divided doses	At least 6	
plus			
Gentamicin[b]	3 mg/kg per 24 h IV/IM in 2 or 3 equally divided doses	2	
	Pediatric dose[c]: nafcillin or oxacillin 200 mg/kg per h IV in 4–6 equally divided doses; +/– rifampin 20 mg/kg per 24 h IV/PO in 3 equally divided doses if prosthetic material present; gentamicin 3 mg/kg per 24 h IV/IM in 3 equally divided doses		
Oxacillin-resistant strains			
Vancomycin	30 mg/kg per 24 h in 2 equally divided doses	At least 6	Adjust vancomycin to achieve 1-h serum concentration of 30-45 µg/mL and trough concentration of 10–15 µg/mL
	Pediatric dose: vancomycin 40 mg/kg per 24 h IV in 2 or 3 equally divided doses; +/– rifampin 20 mg/kg per 24 h IV/PO in 3 equally divided doses if prosthetic material present (up to adult dose); gentamicin 3 mg/kg per 24 h IV or IM in 3 equally divided doses		

Abbreviations: IM, intramuscular; IV, intravenous; PO, by mouth.
[a]Dosages recommended are for patients with normal renal function.
[b]Gentamicin should be administered in close proximity to vancomycin, nafcillin, or oxacillin dosing.
[c]Pediatric dose should not exceed that of a normal adult.
Reproduced with permission from Baddour LM, Wilson WR, Bayer AS, et al. Infective endocarditis in adults: diagnosis, antimicrobial therapy, and management of complications: a scientific statement for healthcare professionals from the American Heart Association. *Circulation*. 2015 Oct 13;132(15):1435-1486.

TABLE 33–14. Therapy for Both Native and Prosthetic Valve Endocarditis Caused by HACEK[a] Microorganisms

Regimen	Dosage and Route	Duration (wk)	Comments
Ceftriaxone sodium	2 g per 24 h IV/IM in 1 dose[b]	4	Cefotaxime or another third- or fourth-generation cephalosporin may be substituted
or			
Ampicillin-sodium	2 g IV every 4 h	4	
or			
Ciprofloxacin[c,d]	1000 mg per 24 h PO or 800 mg per 24 h IV in 2 equally divided doses	4	Fluoroquinolone therapy recommended only for patients unable to tolerate cephalosporin and ampicillin therapy; levofloxacin or moxifloxacin may be substituted; fluoroquinolones generally not recommended for patients <18 y old. Prosthetic valve: patients with endocarditis involving prosthetic cardiac valve or other prosthetic cardiac material should be treated for 6 wk
	Pediatric dose[e]: Ceftriaxone 100 mg/kg per 24 h IV/IM every 12 h; or ampicillin-sulbactam 200–300 mg/kg per 24 h IV divided into 4 or 6 equally divided doses		

Abbreviations: IM, intramuscular; IV, intravenous; PO, by mouth.
[a]*Haemophilus parainfluenzae, Haemophilus aphrophilus, Actinobacillus actinomycetemcomitans, Cardiobacterium hominis, Eikenella corrodens,* and *Kingella kingae.*
[b]Patients should be informed that intramuscular injection of ceftriaxone is painful.
[c]Dosage recommended for patients with normal renal function.
[e]Pediatric dose should not exceed that of a normal adult.
Modified with permission from Baddour LM, Wilson WR, Bayer AS, et al. Infective endocarditis in adults: diagnosis, antimicrobial therapy, and management of complications: a scientific statement for healthcare professionals from the American Heart Association. *Circulation.* 2015;132(15):1435-1486.

hemorrhagic risk, so delaying anticoagulation for this earliest period, if possible, may improve safety. Low-molecular-weight heparins should be avoided.[131] If neurologic symptoms develop, anticoagulant therapy should be stopped immediately pending CNS imaging. In the event of a CNS bleed, a rupture of a mycotic aneurysm should be suspected, and neurosurgical and interventional neuroradiologic consultation sought urgently.

SURGERY

In contemporary studies of predominantly left-sided IE, surgery is performed in nearly 50%.[132] Early surgery in IE has been broadly defined as surgery performed before completion of a full course of antibiotics; in many cases, early surgery is performed within days of a diagnosis or recognition of a severe complication.[133] Surgery should be considered when medical therapy alone is unlikely to cure or control the infection, with full consideration of the individual comorbidities and risk/benefit. The online Society of Thoracic Surgeons' (STS) Risk Calculator (https://riskcalc.sts.org) includes a variable for treated or active IE and is useful in calculating operative risk. Nearly 1 in 4 patients with a surgical indication for IE will not undergo surgery due to their level of operative risk.[132]

The main indications for surgery in native valve IE include heart failure, complicated or persistent infections, and avoidance or control of embolization (**Tables 33–16** and **33–17**). The decision to intervene surgically must be made in the absence of data from large randomized trials. Studies based on propensity scoring and/or subset analysis of patients with high-risk features suggest that surgery is associated with reduced mortality in IE patients with HF, intracardiac abscess or fistula, native valve *S. aureus* IE, or systemic embolization.[3,134–136] The patient is best served by a multispecialty team that can determine surgical indication and timing. Team members should include specialists from infectious disease, cardiology, and cardiac surgery.

Heart failure is the indication for surgery in 65% to 75% of patients. The mortality of medical therapy alone is greater than 75%, compared to less than 25% with surgery.[137] A prospective multicenter study of more than 4000 IE patients demonstrated that both in-hospital and 1-year mortality were significantly reduced in patients undergoing surgery.[134] It is important to move quickly to surgery once signs or symptoms of heart failure appear, or symptoms out of proportion to preexisting ventricular dysfunction are noted.

Perivalvular extension of infection is rarely curable with medical therapy, particularly in the setting of prosthetic valves. Complex repair procedures are generally required. Similarly, difficult-to-treat pathogens including fungi and multidrug-resistant organisms such as vancomycin-resistant *Enterococcus* often require surgery for cure. Persistent bacteremia or fever lasting >7 days after initiation of appropriate antibiotic therapy, if other causes of fever have been excluded, is another indication for surgery.

Large vegetations (>10 mm) are less firmly assigned as a stand-alone indication for surgery. Large vegetations are associated with higher rates of embolization; other risk factors for embolization include vegetation mobility, location on the anterior mitral leaflet, prior embolization, and infection with *S. aureus, S. gallolyticus,* or fungus. A large observational study suggested that higher mortality was observed in patients with large vegetations managed medically (hazard ratio [HR] 1.86; 95% confidence interval [CI] 1.48–2.34) but not in those managed surgically (HR 1.01; 95% CI 0.69–1.49) compared with patients with smaller vegetations.[138]

In contrast to left-sided infections, right-sided IE rarely requires surgery for heart failure because severe tricuspid valve

TABLE 33–15. Therapy for Culture-Negative Endocarditis Including *Bartonella* Endocarditis

Regimen	Dosage[a] and Route	Duration (wk)	Comments
Native valve			
Ampicillin-sulbactam	12 g per 24 h IV in 4 equally divided doses	4–6	Patients with culture-negative endocarditis should be treated with consultation with an infectious diseases specialist
plus			
Gentamicin sulfate[b]	3 mg/kg per 24 h IV/IM in 2 equally divided doses	4–6	
Vancomycin[c]	30 mg/kg per 24 h IV in 2 equally divided doses	4–6	Vancomycin recommended only for patients unable to tolerate penicillins
plus			
Gentamicin sulfate	3 mg/kg per 24 h IV/IM in 3 equally divided doses	4–6	
plus			
Ciprofloxacin	1000 mg per 24 h PO or 800 mg per 24 h IV in 2 equally divided doses	4–6	
	Pediatric dose[d]: ampicillin-sulbactam 200–300 mg/kg per 24 h IV in 4–6 equally divided doses; gentamicin 3 mg/kg per 24 h IV/IM in 3 equally divided doses; vancomycin 60 mg/kg per 24 h in 2 or 3 equally divided doses; ciprofloxacin 20–30 mg/kg per 24 h IV/PO in 2 equally divided doses		
Prosthetic valve (early: ≤1y)			
Vancomycin	30 mg/kg per 24 h IV in 2 equally divided doses	6	
plus			
Gentamicin sulfate	3 mg/kg per 24 h IV/IM in 3 equally divided doses	2	
plus			
Cefepime	6 g per 24 h IV in 3 equally divided doses	6	
plus			
Rifampin	900 mg per 24 h PO/IV in 3 equally divided doses	6	
	Pediatric dose: vancomycin 60 mg/kg per 24 h IV in 2 or 3 equally divided doses; gentamicin 3 mg/kg per 24 h IV/IM in 3 equally divided doses; cefepime 150 mg/kg per 24 h IV in 3 equally divided doses; rifampin 20 mg/kg per 24 h PO/IV in 3 equally divided doses		
Prosthetic valve (late: >1 y)		6	Same regimens as listed above for native valve endocarditis
Suspected Bartonella, culture negative			
Ceftriaxone sodium	2 g per 24 h IV/IM in 1 dose	6	Patients with *Bartonella* endocarditis should be treated in consultation with an infectious diseases specialist
plus			
Gentamicin sulfate	3 mg/kg per 24 h IV/IM in 3 equally divided doses	2	
with/without			
Doxycycline	200 mg/kg per 24 h IV/PO in 2 equally divided doses		
Documented *Bartonella* culture positive			
Doxycycline	200 mg per 24 h IV or PO in 2 equally divided doses	6	If gentamicin cannot be given, then replace with rifampin 600 mg per 24 h PO/IV in 2 equally divided doses
plus			
Gentamicin sulfate	3 mg/kg per 24 h IV/IM in 3 equally divided doses	2	
	Pediatric dose: ceftriaxone 100 mg/kg per 24 h IV/IM every 12 h; gentamicin 3 mg/kg per 24 h IV/IM in 3 equally divided doses; doxycycline 2–4 mg/kg per 24 h IV/PO in 2 equally divided doses; rifampin 20 mg/kg per 24 h PO/IV in 2 equally divided doses		

Abbreviations: IM, intramuscular; IV, intravenous; PO, by mouth.
[a]Dosages recommended are for patients with normal renal function.
Reproduced with permission from Baddour LM, Wilson WR, Bayer AS, et al. Infective endocarditis in adults: diagnosis, antimicrobial therapy, and management of complications: a scientific statement for healthcare professionals from the American Heart Association. *Circulation.* 2015 Oct 13;132(15):1435-1486.

TABLE 33-16. Indications for Surgery for Native Valve Endocarditis

Class I

1. Early surgery (during initial hospitalization and before completion of a full course of antibiotics) is indicated in patients with IE who present with valve dysfunction resulting in symptoms of heart failure. CLASS I
2. Early surgery should be considered particularly in patients with IE caused by fungal or highly resistant organisms (eg, vancomycin-resistant *Enterococcus*, multidrug-resistant gram-negative bacilli). CLASS I
3. Early surgery is indicated in patients with IE complicated by heart block, annular or cardiac or aortic abscess, or destructive penetrating lesions. CLASS I
4. Early surgery is indicated for evidence of persistent infection (manifested by persistent bacteremia or fever lasting >5–7 days and provided that other sites of infection and fever have been excluded) after the start of appropriate antibiotics. CLASS I

Class II

5. Early surgery is reasonable in patients who present with recurrent emboli and persistent or enlarging vegetations despite appropriate antibiotic therapy. CLASS IIa
6. Early surgery is reasonable in patients with severe valve regurgitation and mobile vegetations >10 mm. CLASS IIa
7. Early surgery may be considered in patients with mobile vegetations >10 mm, particularly when involving the anterior leaflet of the mitral valve and associated with other relative indications for surgery. CLASS IIb

Valve Surgery in Patients with Right-Sided IE

1. Surgical intervention is reasonable for patients with certain complications (eg, heart failure, recurrent emboli, resistant organisms). CLASS IIa
2. Valve repair rather than replacement should be performed when feasible. CLASS I
3. If valve replacement is performed, then an individualized choice of prosthesis by the surgeon is reasonable. CLASS IIa
4. It is reasonable to avoid surgery when possible in patients who are IV drug users. CLASS IIa

Valve Surgery in Patients with Prior Emboli/Hemorrhage/Stroke

1. Valve surgery may be considered in IE patients with stroke or subclinical cerebral emboli and residual vegetation without delay if intracranial hemorrhage has been excluded by imaging studies and neurologic damage is not severe. CLASS IIb
2. In patients with major ischemic stroke or intracranial hemorrhage, it is reasonable to delay valve surgery for at least 4 weeks. CLASS IIa

Abbreviations: IE, infective endocarditis; IV, intravenous.
Data from Baddour LM, Wilson WR, Bayer AS, et al. Infective endocarditis in adults: diagnosis, antimicrobial therapy, and management of complications: a scientific statement for healthcare professionals from the American Heart Association. *Circulation*. 2015 Oct 13;132(15):1435-1486.

regurgitation is better tolerated than severe left-sided regurgitation. Very large vegetations (≥20 mm), recurrent septic pulmonary emboli, presence of a difficult-to-treat organism, and persistent bacteremia may prompt surgery in right-sided IE.

In most cases of complicated IE, there is no advantage to delaying intervention in the setting of surgical indications.[3] Among patients with cerebral emboli, surgery does not need to be delayed for silent microembolism, transient ischemic attack, cerebral abscess, or ischemic stroke with no hemorrhagic conversion and without severe neurological impairment

or decreased level of consciousness. A 4-week delay is indicated for major ischemic stroke or intracerebral hemorrhage.[139] ESC guidelines provide recommendations for management of neurologic complications and the timing of surgery (**Table 33–18**).[4]

Valve repair is preferable to replacement when possible to minimize prosthetic tissue, need for anticoagulation, and risk of recurrent IE.[53] Postoperatively, antimicrobial therapy should be continued for at least 2 weeks. The "first day" of postoperative antibiotic therapy should be considered to be the first day of negative blood cultures or the day of surgery itself (whichever is later).[3,4]

TABLE 33-17. Indications for Surgery for Prosthetic Valve Endocarditis

Class I

1. Early surgery is indicated in patients with symptoms or signs of heart failure resulting from valve dehiscence, intracardiac fistula, or severe prosthetic valve dysfunction. CLASS I
2. Early surgery should be done in patients who have persistent bacteremia despite appropriate antibiotic therapy for 5 to 7 days in whom other sites of infection have been excluded. CLASS I
3. Early surgery is indicated when IE is complicated by heart block, annular or aortic abscess, or destructive, penetrating lesions. CLASS I
4. Early surgery is indicated in patients with PVE caused by fungi or highly resistant organisms. CLASS I

Class II

5. Early surgery is reasonable for patients with PVE who have recurrent emboli despite appropriate antibiotic therapy. CLASS IIa
6. Early surgery is reasonable for patients with relapsing PVE IE. CLASS IIa
7. Early surgery may be considered in patients with mobile vegetations >10 mm. CLASS IIb.

Abbreviation: IE, infective endocarditis; PVE, prosthetic valve endocarditis.
Data from Baddour LM, Wilson WR, Bayer AS, et al. Infective endocarditis in adults: diagnosis, antimicrobial therapy, and management of complications: a scientific statement for healthcare professionals from the American Heart Association. *Circulation*. 2015 Oct 13;132(15):1435-1486.

TABLE 33-18. Management of Neurologic Complications of Infective Endocarditis

1. After a silent cerebral embolism or transient ischemic attack, surgery is recommended without delay if an indication still remains. CLASS I
2. Neurosurgery or endovascular therapy is indicated for very large, enlarging, or ruptured intracranial aneurysms. CLASS I
3. After a stroke, surgery is indicated for heart failure, uncontrolled infection, abscess, or persistent high embolic risk and should not be delayed. Surgery should be considered as long as coma is absent and cerebral hemorrhage has been excluded by cranial CT or MRI. CLASS IIa
4. Intracranial aneurysm should be looked for in patients with IE and neurologic symptoms—CT or MRI angiography should be considered for diagnosis. If noninvasive techniques are negative and the suspicion of intracranial aneurysm remains, conventional angiography should be considered. CLASS IIa
5. After intracranial hemorrhage, surgery must be postponed for at least 1 month. CLASS IIa

Abbreviations: CT, computed tomography; IE, infective endocarditis; MRI, magnetic resonance imaging.
Data from Habib,G, Lancellotti P, Antunes MJ, et al. 2015 ESC guidelines for the management of infective endocarditis. *Eur Heart J*. 2015 Nov 21;36(44):3075-3128.

In contrast to native valve infections, prosthetic valve infections occur at the interface between the sewing ring and surrounding tissues, resulting in a high likelihood of perivalvular extension of infection and resistance to cure with medical therapy alone. Indications for surgery in patients with prosthetic valve endocarditis (PVE) are similar to those for patients with native valve IE. Heart failure, difficult-to-treat microorganism, perivalvular extension, or prosthetic valve dehiscence are indications for early surgery. Early surgery may also be considered for patients with PVE due to *S. aureus* in the absence of perivalvular extension or heart failure. These infections are rarely eradicated with antibiotics alone, and retrospective analysis suggests that combined medical and surgical therapy is more effective than medical therapy alone.[140] In patients with uncomplicated PVE due to less virulent organisms, antibiotic therapy alone is often successful. Such infections generally occur more than 12 months after prosthesis implantation.

Complex reconstruction of the aortic or mitral valve apparatus and the supporting structures may be required during surgery for PVE. Operative mortality rates for such procedures range from 10% to 30%. After surgery, the rate of recurrent PVE is 6% to 15%; repeat surgery is required for recurrent PVE or for dysfunction of the newly implanted prosthesis in 18% to 26%.[141] Relapse of PVE after appropriate antibiotic therapy should lead to a careful search for perivalvular extension or for metastatic foci of infection.

FOLLOW-UP

During therapy, the patient should be monitored closely for complications, especially during the first week. Repeat blood cultures on antibiotics should be obtained to ensure clearance of bacteremia. Fever persisting beyond 1 week of appropriate therapy should raise the suspicion for complications including perivalvular extension of infection, peripheral abscess, or antibiotic-resistant organism. Patients should be maintained on telemetry while in hospital; the need for surveillance electrocardiograms (ECGs) during outpatient therapy is dictated by the location of the infection and the predicted likelihood of conduction disturbances. Patients should be monitored for antimicrobial toxicity, particularly with aminoglycoside use.

At the completion of therapy, the intravenous catheter used for antibiotic administration should be removed promptly. TTE should be performed to establish a new "post-IE baseline" that defines valvular and ventricular function as well as anatomic distortions remaining after infection. Vegetations often remain visible after resolution of infection. Follow-up monitoring is indicated with a frequency based on the severity of valvular regurgitation, following standard recommendations for chronic valve regurgitation. Posttreatment baseline white cell count, erythrocyte sedimentation rate, and C-reactive protein should also be obtained.

After resolution of IE, patients remain at high risk for recurrent IE. The patient and providers must maintain a high index of suspicion for possible re-infection. Routine surveillance blood cultures are not indicated in the absence of clinical symptoms of infection. Patient education is critical in this effort

and should be reinforced at every encounter. Modification of controllable exposures should be stressed, including maintenance of good oral hygiene and dental care, and abstinence from injection in PWID with support from addiction treatment programs. All patients with prior IE should be carefully reminded about possible symptoms and signs of IE for which to notify care providers before any exposure to antibiotics. In addition, signs or symptoms of worsening valve disease should be explained. Patients with prior IE are considered candidates for antibiotic prophylaxis for IE prevention during relevant procedures as outlined in professional guidelines.[142]

OUTCOME

The in-hospital mortality rate of IE is 18% to 23% and the 6-month mortality rate is 22% to 27%.[1,23,31,143,144] Given the spectrum of patients, organisms, and complications, as well as the individualized need for early surgery, the variability of IE outcomes is not surprising.

Many characteristics of IE patients and disease features have been correlated with increased risk of mortality. Among infecting organisms, *S. aureus* infection has a higher risk than streptococcal infections,[23,143] as does evidence of uncontrolled infection such as persistent bacteremia or positive valve culture.[144,145] Direct complications of infection such as larger vegetation size,[112] heart failure,[1,144] embolization,[143] and perivalvular abscess[144,146] increase mortality. Patient factors such as diabetes mellitus,[143] low serum albumin,[31] and abnormal mental status[23] also contribute to poor outcomes. Poor surgical candidacy portends poor outcome.[23,147] Three risk factors (heart failure, periannular complications, and *S. aureus* infection) during the first 72 hours of hospitalization were predictive of in-hospital mortality or the need for urgent surgery in one study of IE patients. The presence of all three risk factors predicted 100% risk of adverse outcome.[148] Longer term outcomes in IE survivors were assessed in a population-based study in Taiwan. Higher rates of ischemic stroke, hemorrhagic stroke, myocardial infarction, readmission for heart failure, and sudden and all-cause death were noted in IE survivors compared to matched controls without IE.[53]

ANTIBIOTIC PROPHYLAXIS FOR THE PREVENTION OF INFECTIVE ENDOCARDITIS

Endocarditis can affect normal hearts as well as those with preexisting congenital or acquired disease. Bacteremias with organisms known to cause endocarditis are extremely common, occurring with daily activities of life such as chewing, tooth brushing and flossing. Prophylactic use of antimicrobials to avoid episodes of IE resulting from every predictable bacteremia with common culprit organisms is therefore impossible. It has never been proven that antibiotic prophylaxis is effective at preventing IE, as no individual episode can be linked to a single bacteremic episode against the backdrop of thousands of such episodes. While IE is a potentially mortal infection in anyone, the incidence of the worst IE outcomes is higher in

TABLE 33–19. Cardiac Conditions Associated with the Highest Risk of Adverse Outcome from Infective Endocarditis for Which Antibiotic Prophylaxis Is Recommended

A. Prosthetic cardiac valve
B. Previous IE
C. Specific patients with CHD (except for the conditions listed below, antibiotic prophylaxis is no longer recommended for any other form of CHD):
  1. Unrepaired cyanotic CHD, including palliative shunts and conduits
  2. Completely repaired congenital heart defect with prosthetic material or device, whether placed by surgery or catheter intervention, during the first 6 months after the procedure (prophylaxis is recommended because endothelialization of prosthetic material occurs within 6 months after the procedure)
  3. Repaired CHD with residual defects at the site of or adjacent to the site of a prosthetic patch or prosthetic device (which inhibit endothelialization)
D. Cardiac transplant recipients who develop cardiac valvulopathy

Abbreviations: CHD, congenital heart disease; IE, infective endocarditis.
Data from Baddour LM, Wilson WR, Bayer AS, et al. Infective endocarditis in adults: diagnosis, antimicrobial therapy, and management of complications: a scientific statement for healthcare professionals from the American Heart Association. *Circulation*. 2015 Oct 13;132(15):1435-1486.

TABLE 33–20. Procedures for Which Antibiotic Prophylaxis Is Recommended for High-Risk Patients

A. Dental: All dental procedures that involve manipulation of gingival tissue or the periapical region of teeth or perforation of the oral mucosa. The following procedures and events do not need antibiotic prophylaxis: routine anesthetic injections through noninfected tissue, taking dental radiographs, placement of removable prosthodontic or orthodontic appliances, adjustment of orthodontic appliances, placement of orthodontic brackets, shedding of deciduous teeth, and bleeding from trauma to the lips or oral mucosa.
B. Respiratory tract: Invasive procedures of the respiratory tract that involve incision or biopsy of the respiratory mucosa, such as tonsillectomy or adenoidectomy. Routine prophylaxis for bronchoscopy is not recommended unless the procedure involves incision of the respiratory tract mucosa.
C. Infected skin or musculoskeletal: Surgical procedures that involve infected skin, skin structure, or musculoskeletal tissue.

Data from Baddour LM, Wilson WR, Bayer AS, et al. Infective endocarditis in adults: diagnosis, antimicrobial therapy, and management of complications: a scientific statement for healthcare professionals from the American Heart Association. *Circulation*. 2015 Oct 13;132(15):1435-1486.

patients with certain preexisting cardiac conditions, potentially altering the risk/benefit for the small proportion of the population with those disorders.

Assuming any benefit from prophylaxis would require that it has been proven effective. A meta-analysis of 36 studies of the impact of antibiotic prophylaxis on risk for IE concluded that the evidence base for use of antibiotic prophylaxis is limited and heterogeneous, and the methodological quality of many studies is poor.[149] It has been estimated that, even if antimicrobial prophylaxis were 100% effective, less than 10% of all cases of endocarditis could be prevented by use of antimicrobial therapy prior to procedures.[150] Most cases of IE do not occur after a procedure; 5% or less of IE cases are preceded by a dental procedure.[151,152]

The 2007 AHA guidelines on prevention of endocarditis, in light of the paucity of evidence of effectiveness, suggested restricting the use of prophylaxis to the patient groups with the highest rick of poor outcomes. The cardiac conditions associated with the highest risk of adverse outcomes from IE for which antibiotic prophylaxis is recommended are listed in **Table 33–19**.[3,142] The specific procedures for which antibiotic prophylaxis is recommended are listed in **Table 33–20**.

TABLE 33–21. Prophylactic Regimens for a Dental Procedure

Situation	Agent	Regimen: Single Dose 30–60 min Before Procedure	
		Adults	**Children**
Oral	Amoxicillin	2 g	50 mg/kg
Unable to take oral medication	Ampicillin *or*	2 g IM or IV	50 mg/kg IM or IV
	Cefazolin or Ceftriaxone	1 g IM or IV	50 mg/kg IM or IV
Allergic to penicillins or ampicillin–oral	Cephalexin[a,b] *or*	2 g	50 mg/kg
	Clindamycin	600 mg	20 mg/kg
	Or		
	Azithromycin *or*	500 mg	15 mg/kg
	Clarithromycin		
Allergic to penicillins or ampicillin and unable to take oral medication	Cefazolin or Ceftriaxone[b] *or*	1 g IM or IV	50 mg/kg IM or IV
	Clindamycin	600 mg IM or IV	20 mg/kg IM or IV

Abbreviations: IM, intramuscular; IV, intravenous.
[a]Or other first- or second-generation cephalosporin in equivalent adult or pediatric dosage.
[b]Cephalosporins should not be used in an individual with a history of anaphylaxis, angioedema, or urticaria with penicillins or ampicillin.
Data from Baddour LM, Wilson WR, Bayer AS, et al. Infective endocarditis in adults: diagnosis, antimicrobial therapy, and management of complications: a scientific statement for healthcare professionals from the American Heart Association. *Circulation*. 2015 Oct 13;132(15):1435-1486.

TABLE 33–22. Comparison of the US, European, and Canadian Guidelines

	Diagnosis and Management	Antibiotic Regimens	Surgical Indications	Antibiotic Prophylaxis for Prevention of IE
American				
AHA	2015 Baddour LM, et al. Infective endocarditis in adults: diagnosis, antimicrobial therapy, and management of complications.[3]	2015 Baddour LM, et al. Infective endocarditis in adults: diagnosis, antimicrobial therapy, and management of complications.[3]	2015 Baddour LM, et al. Infective endocarditis in adults: diagnosis, antimicrobial therapy, and management of complications.[3]	2007 Wilson W, et al. Prevention of infective endocarditis.[142]
ACC/AHA	2014 Nishimura RA, et al. 2014 AHA/ACC guideline for the management of patients with valvular heart disease.[158]		2014 Nishimura RA, et al. 2014 AHA/ACC guideline for the management of patients with valvular heart disease.[158] 2017 Nishimura RA, et al. 2017 AHA/ACC focused update of the 2014 AHA/ACC Guideline for the Management of Patients with Valvular Heart Disease.[81]	2014 Nishimura RA, et al. 2014 AHA/ACC guideline for the management of patients with valvular heart disease.[158] 2017 Nishimura RA, et al. 2017 AHA/ACC focused update of the 2014 AHA/ACC Guideline for the Management of Patients with Valvular Heart Disease.[81]
AATS	2016 The American Association for Thoracic Surgery consensus guidelines: surgical treatment of infective endocarditis.[159]		2016 The American Association for Thoracic Surgery consensus guidelines: surgical treatment of infective endocarditis.[159]	
Canadian				
CPS				2010, 2018 Canadian Paediatric Society (CPS): practice point on prevention of infective endocarditis—Updated guidelines.[160]
European				
ESC	2015 Habib G, Lancellotti P, Antunes MJ, et al. 2015 ESC Guidelines for the management of infective endocarditis.[4]	2015 Habib G, Lancellotti P, Antunes MJ, et al. 2015 ESC Guidelines for the management of infective endocarditis.[4]	2015 Habib G, Lancellotti P, Antunes MJ, et al. 2015 ESC Guidelines for the management of infective endocarditis.[4]	2015 Habib G, Lancellotti P, Antunes MJ, et al. 2015 ESC Guidelines for the management of infective endocarditis.[4]
British				
NICE				2008 Prophylaxis against infective endocarditis. National Institute for Health and Care Excellence (UK) 2015: Modified recommendations against any Prophylaxis to "not routinely."[161]
BSAC	2012 Gould FK, Denning DW, Elliott TSJ, et al. Guidelines for the diagnosis and antibiotic treatment of endocarditis in adults.[127]	2012 Gould FK, Denning DW, Elliott TSJ, et al. Guidelines for the diagnosis and antibiotic treatment of endocarditis in adults.[127]		

Many international guidelines address different aspects of IE treatment and prevention. The Guidelines are highly concordant in specific recommendations but vary in their focus and emphasis. The NICE guidelines differ from other societies' prevention guidelines in not recommending routine antibiotic prophylaxis for any procedure or with any preexisting cardiac condition.

Abbreviations: AHA, American Heart Association; ACC, American College of Cardiology; AATS, American Association for Thoracic Surgery; CPS, Canadian Paediatric Society; NICE, National Institute for Health and Care Excellence; BSAC, British Society for Antimicrobial Chemotherapy.[3,4,81,127,142,158–161]

The shift from providing antibiotic prophylaxis to patients at high risk for the lifetime acquisition of IE to patients at highest risk for the development of an adverse outcome from IE was controversial. An excellent summary of the data informing this ongoing debate is presented by Sexton and Chu.[153] The decision to proceed with use of prophylaxis outside of guideline recommendations remains with the individual provider and patient.

Concerns have been raised by observational studies that suggest that increases in IE incidence have followed on the heels of more restricted use of IE prophylaxis.[153–156] Studies of IE incidence in different regions and patient groups have shown that, while the incidence of IE continues an upward trend that began years before changes in prophylaxis strategy, much of this may be due to the increasing proportion of infections due to staphylococcal species. The aging of the population and the prevalence of ICDs and other healthcare-associated risks likely underpin this trend in IE.[155]

High-risk patient groups are listed in Table 14–19.[142] Notable exclusions include patients with coronary artery bypass grafting, percutaneous coronary intervention (with or without a stent), or implanted pacemaker or ICD. An important area of ongoing discussion is the exclusion of patients with bicuspid aortic valve and mitral valve prolapse from the group of patients at highest risk of IE complications. In one study, patients with those two conditions had similar rates of intracardiac complications as the high-risk patients in the study.[157] While methodologic challenges with this and other studies have been pointed out, it highlights the difficulty categorizing patients in the highest risk category.

Recommended antibiotic regimens for prophylaxis are listed in **Table 33–21**.

Prophylactic antibiotics for IE prevention should be administered in a single dose 30 to 60 minutes prior to the procedure. Intravenous vancomycin, when used for prophylaxis, should be administered 120 minutes prior to the procedure. The preferred regimen is oral amoxicillin 2 grams; alternative regimens and regimens for children are also provided in Table 33–21. If patients are receiving antibiotics for other indications at the time that dental or invasive procedures are undertaken, an alternate antibiotic of a different class is often chosen. If the dosage is inadvertently not administered before the procedure, it may be given up to 2 hours after the procedure.

There is general agreement between recommendations presented in the AHA Statement on Prevention of Infective Endocarditis, the 2015 ESC guidelines for the management of infective endocarditis, and the 2017 AHA/ACC focused update of the 2014 valvular heart disease guidelines.[4,81] The guidelines issued in 2008 by the National Institute for Health and Care Excellence (NICE) in the United Kingdom differed from other organizations in that they did not recommend antibiotic prophylaxis for patients despite any preexisting cardiac condition. Those guidelines were subsequently updated in 2015 to suggest that prophylaxis should not be used "routinely."[127]

International guidelines regarding treatment, surgery, and prophylaxis issues in IE are listed in **Table 33–22**.[3,4,81,127,142,158–161]

SUMMARY

PATHOGENESIS

- Endothelial injury exposing underlying collagen and matrix molecules

  Direct mechanical injury: Intracardiac leads

  Turbulent flow and high velocity jets due to congenital or acquired valve disease

  Fibrin and platelet adherence create a sterile vegetation

- Infective organisms circulating in bacteremia bind to the sterile vegetation via extracellular neutrophil "traps" or biofilm, creating an infective vegetation

- The vegetation is a macroscopic infective mass that promotes further deposition of platelets and fibrin, resulting in increasing vegetation size and fragility.

- Vegetation impact

  Continuous bacteremia and potential for sepsis and immune complex disease.

  Local destruction of valvular or perivalvular tissues

  Embolization of micro or macroscopic pieces of vegetative tissue to systemic and/or pulmonary circulations

  Disseminated infection

  Visceral and vascular infarction or infection

MEDICAL TREATMENT
Antimicrobial Therapy

- Blood culture results are critical to diagnosis and treatment planning.

  At least two (and preferably three) sets of blood cultures should be obtained from separate venipunctures and ideally spaced over 30 to 60 minutes

- Empiric therapy can be initiated after blood cultures obtained.

- The initial empiric regimen depends on likely bacteriology and resistance patterns empiric therapy should cover staphylococci (both methicillin susceptible and resistant), streptococci, and enterococci.

  Vancomycin and ceftriaxone is an appropriate choice for initial therapy in most patients but should be guided by institutional patterns of infection.

- Detailed and current antibiotic therapy recommendations are maintained in guidelines from the AHA and ESC, among others.

  Discriminators that define the appropriate regimen for the individual patient include:

  Infecting organism and sensitivity

  Streptococcal spp.: Sensitive or relatively resistant to penicillin

  Staphylococcal spp.: Sensitive or resistant to methicillin

  Enterococcal spp.: Sensitive or resistant to vancomycin

  Native versus prosthetic valve IE

  Availability and safety of options for outpatient completion of antibiotic infusions

- Surveillance blood cultures should be obtained 2 to 3 days after antibiotic initiation
- Antibiotic levels and renal, hepatic, and auditory function should be assessed during treatment as indicated.
- Most regimens require 4 to 6 weeks of treatment to eradicate infection
- Two-week IE treatment may sometimes be appropriate with uncomplicated native valve IE caused by highly penicillin-susceptible viridans group streptococci and Str*eptococcus gallolyticus*
- Drugs with bactericidal activity or synergistic combinations of antimicrobial agents are most effective

Antiplatelet and Antithrombin Therapy

- Neither anticoagulant therapy nor aspirin reduce the risk of embolism in patients with IE
- IE patients are at high risk for bleeding complications, particularly in the acute phase
- Warfarin therapy should be discontinued at initial presentation due to the risk of hemorrhagic stroke and the potential need for invasive procedures or early surgery
- Unfractionated intravenous heparin may be considered for cautious substitution when risk of cessation of anticoagulation are high (eg, mechanical mitral valve or mitral stenosis patients in atrial fibrillation). Low-molecular-weight heparins should be avoided.
- If neurologic symptoms develop, anticoagulant therapy should be stopped immediately, and urgent CNS imaging obtained. Neurosurgical and interventional neuroradiologic consultation if rupture of a mycotic aneurysm is suspected

SURGERY

- Early surgery in IE, performed before completion of a full course of antibiotics, is performed in nearly 50% of left-sided IE
- Indications for surgery in IE

    Heart failure—indication in up to 75% of surgeries

    Perivalvular extension of infection

    Difficult-to-treat pathogens, including fungi and vancomycin-resistant Enterococcus

    Persistent bacteremia or fever lasting >7 days after initiation of appropriate antibiotic therapy

    Avoidance or control of embolization—usually in combination with another factor favoring surgery, including eventual need for surgery to address valve destruction

    Large vegetations (>10 mm)

    Marked mobility

    Location on the anterior mitral leaflet

    Prior embolization

    Infection with Staphylococcus aureus, Streptococcus gallotly*ticus*, or fungus

- Surgical timing

    Cerebral emboli

Without severe neurological impairment or decreased level of consciousness, do not delay surgery:

    Silent microembolism

    Transient ischemic attack

    Cerebral abscess

    Ischemic stroke with no hemorrhagic conversion

Delay surgery for ≥4 weeks

    Major ischemic stroke

    Intracerebral hemorrhage

- Antibiotic timing

Continue antimicrobial therapy ≥2 weeks post operatively for native valve infection

    The "first day" of postoperative antibiotic therapy should be considered the first day of negative blood cultures or the day of surgery itself (whichever is later)

Continue antimicrobial therapy up to 6 weeks post operatively for prosthetic valve infections

    Recurrent prosthetic valve IE occurs in 6% to 15%

- A multispecialty team including specialists from infectious disease, cardiology, and cardiac surgery should determine surgical indication, timing, and approach

ACKNOWLEDGMENT

The author would like to thank Dr. Joseph S. Alpert and Dr. Stephen A. Klotz, who contributed to the previous version of this chapter in the 14th edition.

REFERENCES

1. Hasbun R, Vikram HR, Barakat LA, Buenconsejo J, Quagliarello VJ. Complicated left-sided native valve endocarditis in adults: risk classification for mortality. *JAMA.* 2003;289(15):1933-1940.
2. Murdoch DR, Corey GR, Hoen B, et al. Clinical presentation, etiology, and outcome of infective endocarditis in the 21st century: the International Collaboration on Endocarditis-Prospective Cohort Study. *Arch Intern Med.* 2009;169:463.
3. Baddour LM, Wilson WR, Bayer AS, et al. Infective endocarditis in adults: diagnosis, antimicrobial therapy, and management of complications: a scientific statement for healthcare professionals from the American Heart Association [published correction appears in *Circulation.* 2015;132(17):e215] [published correction appears in *Circulation.* 2016;134(8):e113] [published correction appears in *Circulation.* 2018;138(5): e78-e79]. *Circulation.* 2015;132(15):1435-1486.
4. Habib G, Lancellotti P, Antunes MJ, et al. 2015 ESC Guidelines for the management of infective endocarditis: the Task Force for the Management of Infective Endocarditis of the European Society of Cardiology (ESC). Endorsed by: European Association for Cardio-Thoracic Surgery (EACTS), the European Association of Nuclear Medicine (EANM). *Eur Heart J.* 2015;36(44):3075-3128.
5. Garrison PK, Freedman LR. Experimental endocarditis I. Staphylococcal endocarditis in rabbits resulting from placement of a polyethylene catheter in the right side of the heart. *Yale J Biol Med.* 1970;42:394.
6. Durack DT, Beeson PB. Experimental bacterial endocarditis. I. Colonization of a sterile vegetation. *Br J Exp Pathol.* 1972;53:44.
7. Chambers HF, Bayer AS. Native-valve infective endocarditis. *N Engl J Med.* 2020;383:567-576.
8. Lockhart PB, Brennan MT, Sasser HC, Fox PC, Paster BJ, Bahrani-Mougeot FK. Bacteremia associated with toothbrushing and dental extraction. *Circulation.* 2008;117:3118-3125.

9. Jung CJ, Yeh CY, Hsu RB, Lee CM, Shun CT, Chia JS. Endocarditis pathogen promotes vegetation formation by inducing intravascular neutrophil traps through activated platelets. *Circulation.* 2015;131:571-581.

10. Sousa C, et al. Infective endocarditis in intravenous drug abusers: an update. *Eur J Clin Microbiol Infect Dis.* 2012;31:2905-2910.

11. Jung CJ, Yeh CY, Shun CT, et al. Platelets enhance biofilm formation and resistance of endocarditis-inducing streptococci on the injured heart valve. *J Infect Dis.* 2012;205:1066.

12. Baddour LM, et al. Update on cardiovascular implantable electronic device infections and their management: a scientific statement from the American Heart Association. *Circulation.* 2010;121:458-477.

13. Francois P, Vaudaux P, Lew PD. Role of plasma and extracellular matrix proteins in the pathophysiology of foreign body infections. *Ann Vasc Surg.* 1998;12:34-40.

14. Werdan K, Dietz S, Löffler B, et al. Mechanisms of infective endocarditis: pathogen-host interaction and risk states. *Nat Rev Cardiol.* 2014;11:35.

15. Rodbard S. Blood velocity and endocarditis. *Circulation* 1963;27:18-28.

16. Pressman GS, Rodriguez-Ziccardi M, Gartman CH, et al. mitral annular calcification as a possible nidus for endocarditis: a descriptive series with bacteriological differences noted. *J Am Soc Echocardiogr.* 2017;30:572.

17. Jain V, Yang M-H, Kovacicova-Lezcano G, et al. Infective endocarditis in an urban medical center: association of individual drugs with valvular involvement. *J Infect.* 2008;57(2):132-138.

18. Alpert JS, Krous HF, Dalen JE, O'Rourke RA, Bloor CM. Pathogenesis of Osler's nodes. *Ann Intern Med.* 1976;85:471-473.

19. Cooper HA, Thompson EC, Laureno R, et al. Subclinical brain embolization in left-sided infective endocarditis: results from the evaluation by MRI of the brains of patients with left-sided intracardiac solid masses (EMBOLISM) pilot study. *Circulation.* 2009;120(7):585-591.

20. Bin Abdulhak AA, Baddour LM, Erwin PJ, et al. Global and regional burden of infective endocarditis, 1990-2010: a systematic review of the literature. *Glob Heart.* 2014;9:131-143.

21. Cahill TJ, Prendergast BD. Infective endocarditis. *Lancet.* 2016;387:882-893.

22. Tleyjeh IM, Abdel-Latif A, Rahbi H, et al. A systematic review of population-based studies of infective endocarditis. *Chest.* 2007;132(3):1025-1035.

23. Hill EE, Herijgers P, Claus P, Vanderschueren S, Herregods MC, Peetermans WE. Infective endocarditis: changing epidemiology and predictors of 6-month mortality: a prospective cohort study. *Eur Heart J.* 2007;28(2):196-203.

24. Pant S, Patel NJ, Deshmukh A, et al. Trends in infective endocarditis incidence, microbiology, and valve replacement in the United States from 2000 to 2011. *J Am Coll Cardiol.* 2015;65(19):2070-2076.

25. Toyoda N, Chikwe J, Itagaki S, Gelijns AC, Adams DH, Egorova NN. Trends in Infective Endocarditis in California and New York State, 1998-2013. *JAMA.* 2017;317(16):1652-1660.

26. Ambrosioni J, Hernandez-Meneses M, Téllez A, et al. The changing epidemiology of infective endocarditis in the twenty-first century. *Curr Infect Dis Rep.* 2017;19(5):21.

27. Selton-Suty C, Célard M, LeMoing V, et al. Preeminence of Staphylococcus aureus in infective endocarditis: a 1-year population-based survey. *Clin Infect Dis.* 2012;54(9):1230-1239.

28. Durante-Mangoni E, Bradley S, Selton-Suty C, et al. Current features of infective endocarditis in elderly patients: results of the International Collaboration on Endocarditis Prospective Cohort Study. *Arch Intern Med.* 2008;168:2095.

29. Ursi MP, Durante Mangoni E, Rajani R, Hancock J, Chambers JB, Prendergast B. Infective endocarditis in the elderly: diagnostic and treatment options. *Drugs Aging.* 2019;36(2):115-124.

30. Fernandez-Guerrero ML, Herrero L, Bellver M, et al. Nosocomial enterococcal endocarditis: a serious hazard for hospitalized patients with enterococcal bacteraemia. *J Intern Med.* 2002;252:510-515.

31. Wallace SM, Walton BI, Kharbanda RK, Hardy R, Wilson AP, Swanton RH. Mortality from infective endocarditis: clinical predictors of outcome. *Heart.* 2002;88(1):53-60.

32. Miro JM, del Rio A, Mestres CA. Infective endocarditis in intravenous drug abusers and HIV-1 infected patients. *Infect Dis Clin North Am.* 2002;16:273-295, vii-viii.

33. Chahoud J, Sharif Yakan A, Saad H, Kanj SS. Right-sided infective endocarditis and pulmonary infiltrates: an update. *Cardiol Rev.* 2016;24(5):230-237.

34. Pons-Lladó G, Carreras F, Borrás X, et al. Findings on Doppler echocardiography in asymptomatic intravenous heroin users. *Am J Cardiol.* 1992;69(3):238-241.

35. Sande MA, Lee BL, Mills J, et al. Endocarditis in intravenous drug users. In: Kaye D, ed, *Infective Endocarditis.* New York City: Raven Press; 1992:345.

36. Frontera JA, Gradon JD. Right-side endocarditis in injection drug users: review of proposed mechanisms of pathogenesis. *Clin Infect Dis.* 2000;30(2):374-379.

37. Nahass RG, Weinstein MP, Bartels J, Gocke DJ. Infective endocarditis in intravenous drug users: a comparison of human immunodeficiency virus type 1-negative and -positive patients. *J Infect Dis.* 1990;162(4):967-970.

38. Gebo KA, Burkey MD, Lucas GM, Moore RD, Wilson LE. Incidence of, risk factors for, clinical presentation, and 1-year outcomes of infective endocarditis in an urban HIV cohort. *J Acquir Immune Defic Syndr.* 2006;43(4):426-432.

39. Cecchi E, Imazio M, Tidu M, et al. Infective endocarditis in drug addicts: role of HIV infection and the diagnostic accuracy of Duke criteria. *J Cardiovasc Med (Hagerstown).* 2007;8(3):169-175.

40. Nucifora G, Badano LP, Viale P, et al. Infective endocarditis in chronic haemodialysis patients: an increasing clinical challenge. *Eur Heart J.* 2007;28(19):2307-2312.

41. Chaudry MS, Carlson N, Gislason GH, et al. Risk of infective endocarditis in patients with end stage renal disease. *Clin J Am Soc Nephrol.* 2017;12(11):1814-1822.

42. Sexton DJ. Vascular access infections in patients undergoing dialysis with special emphasis on the role and treatment of Staphylococcus aureus. *Infect Dis Clin North Am.* 2001;15:731-742, vii.

43. Dai M, Cai C, Vaibhav V, et al. Trends of cardiovascular implantable electronic device infection in 3 decades: a population-based study. *JACC Clin Electrophysiol.* 2019;5(9):1071-1080.

44. Greenspon AJ, Patel JD, Lau E, et al. 16-year trends in the infection burden for pacemakers and implantable cardioverter-defibrillators in the United States 1993 to 2008. *J Am Coll Cardiol.* 2011;58(10):1001-1006.

45. Sandoe JA, Barlow G, Chambers JB, et al. Guidelines for the diagnosis, prevention and management of implantable cardiac electronic device infection. Report of a joint Working Party project on behalf of the British Society for Antimicrobial Chemotherapy (BSAC, host anization), British Heart Rhythm Society (BHRS), British Cardiovascular Society (BCS), British Heart Valve Society (BHVS) and British Society for Echocardiography (BSE). *J Antimicrob Chemother.* 2015;70(2):325-359.

46. Chambers ST. Diagnosis and management of staphylococcal infections of pacemakers and cardiac defibrillators. *Intern Med J.* 2005;35(suppl 2):S63-S71.

47. Duval X, Selton-Suty C, Alla F, et al. Endocarditis in patients with a permanent pacemaker: a 1-year epidemiological survey on infective endocarditis due to valvular and/or pacemaker infection. *Clin Infect Dis.* 2004;39(1):68-74.

48. Tarakji KG, Chan EJ, Cantillon DJ, et al. Cardiac implantable electronic device infections: presentation, management, and patient outcomes. *Heart Rhythm.* 2010;7(8):1043-1047.

49. Huang XM, Fu HX, Zhong L, et al. Outcomes of transvenous lead extraction for cardiovascular implantable electronic device infections in patients with prosthetic heart valves. *Circ Arrhythm Electrophysiol.* 2016;9(9):e004188.

50. Noheria A, Ponamgi SP, Desimone CV, et al. Pulmonary embolism in patients with transvenous cardiac implantable electronic device leads. *Europace.* 2016;18:246-252.

51. Kusumoto FM, Schoenfeld MH, Wilkoff BL, et al. 2017 HRS expert consensus statement on cardiovascular implantable electronic device lead management and extraction. *Heart Rhythm.* 2017;14(12):e503-e551.

52. Ho G, Bhatia P, Mehta I, et al. Prevalence and short-term clinical outcome of mobile thrombi detected on transvenous leads in patients undergoing lead extraction. *JACC Clin Electrophysiol.* 2019;5(6):657-664.

53. Shih CJ, Chu H, Chao PW, et al. Long-term clinical outcome of major adverse cardiac events in survivors of infective endocarditis: a nationwide population-based study. *Circulation.* 2014;130(19):1684-1691.

54. Correa de Sa DD, Tleyjeh IM, Anavekar NS, et al. Epidemiological trends of infective endocarditis: a population-based study in Olmsted County, Minnesota. *Mayo Clin Proc.* 2010;85:422.

55. Bayer AS, Bolger AF, Taubert KA, et al. Diagnosis and management of infective endocarditis and its complications. *Circulation.* 1998;98(25):2936-2948.

56. Klein RS, Recco RA, Catalano MT, et al. Association of Streptococcus bovis with carcinoma of the colon. *N Engl J Med.* 1977;297:800.

57. Téllez A, Ambrosioni J, Llopis J, et al. Epidemiology, clinical features, and outcome of infective endocarditis due to Abiotrophia species and Granulicatella species: report of 76 cases, 2000-2015. *Clin Infect Dis.* 2018;66:104.

58. Sambola A, Miro JM, Tornos MP, et al. Streptococcus agalactiae infective endocarditis: analysis of 30 cases and review of the literature, 1962-1998. *Clin Infect Dis.* 2002;34:1576-1584.

59. Lesens O, Hansmann Y, Storck D, et al. Risk factors for metastatic infection in patients with Staphylococcus aureus bacteremia with and without endocarditis. *Eur J Intern Med.* 2003;14:227-231.

60. Chu VH, Cabell CH, Abrutyn E, et al. Native valve endocarditis due to coagulase-negative staphylococci: report of 99 episodes from the International Collaboration on Endocarditis Merged Database. *Clin Infect Dis.* 2004;39:1527-1530.

61. Anguera I, Del Rio A, Miro JM, et al. Staphylococcus lugdunensis infective endocarditis: description of 10 cases and analysis of native valve, prosthetic valve, and pacemaker lead endocarditis clinical profiles. *Heart* 2005;91:e10.

62. Peter O, Flepp M, Bestetti G, et al. Q fever endocarditis: diagnostic approaches and monitoring of therapeutic effects. *Clin Investig.* 1992;70:932-937.

63. Maguina C, Gotuzzo E. Bartonellosis. New and old. *Infect Dis Clin North Am.* 2000;14:1-22, vii.

64. Solera J. Treatment of human brucellosis. *J Med Liban.* 2000;48:255-263.

65. Ellis ME, Al-Abdely H, Sandridge A, et al. Fungal endocarditis: evidence in the world literature, 1965-1995. *Clin Infect Dis.* 2001;32:50.

66. Rivoisy C, Vena A, Schaeffer L, et al. Prosthetic valve candida spp. endocarditis: new insights into long-term prognosis-the ESCAPE study. *Clin Infect Dis.* 2018;66:825.

67. Meshaal MS, Labib D, Said K, et al. Aspergillus endocarditis: diagnostic criteria and predictors of outcome, a retrospective cohort study. *PLoS One.* 2018;13:e0201459.

68. El-Hamamsy I, Dürrleman N, Stevens LM, et al. Aspergillus endocarditis after cardiac surgery. *Ann Thorac Surg.* 2005;80:359.

69. Raoult D, Sexton DJ. Culture-negative endocarditis: epidemiology, microbiology, and diagnosis. *UpToDate.* 2019. https://uptodate.com. Accessed on October 1, 2020.

70. Lamas CC, Fournier PE, Zappa M, et al. Diagnosis of blood culture-negative endocarditis and clinical comparison between blood culture-negative and blood culture-positive cases. *Infection.* 2016;44:459.

71. Erbay AR, Erbay A, Canga A, et al. Risk factors for in-hospital mortality in infective endocarditis: five years' experience at a tertiary care hospital in Turkey. *J Heart Valve Dis.* 2010;19:216.

72. Raoult D, Casalta JP, Richet H, et al. Contribution of systematic serological testing in diagnosis of infective endocarditis. *J Clin Microbiol.* 2005;43:5238.

73. Rampini SK, Bloemberg GV, Keller PM, et al. Broad-range 16S rRNA gene polymerase chain reaction for diagnosis of culture-negative bacterial infections. *Clin Infect Dis.* 2011;53:1245.

74. Fournier PE, Gouriet F, Casalta JP, et al. Blood culture-negative endocarditis: Improving the diagnostic yield using new diagnostic tools. *Medicine (Baltimore).* 2017;96:e8392.

75. Thuny F, Gaubert JY, Jacquier A, et al. Imaging investigations in infective endocarditis: current approach and perspectives. *Arch Cardiovasc Dis.* 2013;106:52.

76. Karchmer AW, Chu VH. Prosthetic valve endocarditis: epidemiology, clinical manifestations, and diagnosis. *UpToDate.* 2020. https://uptodate.com. Accessed on October 1, 2020.

77. Li JS, Sexton DJ, Mick N, et al. Proposed modifications to the Duke criteria for the diagnosis of infective endocarditis. *Clin Infect Dis.* 2000;30:633-638.

78. Cecchi E, Parrini I, Chinaglia A, et al. New diagnostic criteria for infective endocarditis. A study of sensitivity and specificity. *Eur Heart J.* 1997;18:1149-1156.

79. von Reyn CF, Levy BS, Arbeit RD, et al. Infective endocarditis: an analysis based on strict case definitions. *Ann Intern Med.* 1981;94:504-518.098.

80. Durack DT, Lukes AS, Bright DK. New criteria for diagnosis of infective endocarditis: utilization of specific echocardiographic findings. Duke Endocarditis Service. *Am J Med.* 1994;96:200-209.

81. Nishimura RA, Otto CM, Bonow RO, et al. 2017 AHA/ACC focused update of the 2014 AHA/ACC guideline for the management of patients with valvular heart disease: a report of the American College of Cardiology/American Heart Association Task Force on Clinical Practice Guidelines. *J Am Coll Cardiol.* 2017;70(2):252-289.

82. Sachdev M, Peterson GE, Jollis JG. Imaging techniques for diagnosis of infective endocarditis. *Cardiol Clin.* 2003;21(2):185-195.

83. Sampedro MF, Patel R. Infections associated with long-term prosthetic devices. *Infect Dis Clin North Am.* 2007;21:785.

84. De Castro S, Magni G, Beni S, et al. Role of transthoracic and transesophageal echocardiography in predicting embolic events in patients with active infective endocarditis involving native cardiac valves. *Am J Cardiol.* 1997;80(8):1030-1034.

85. Rohmann S, Erbel R, Darius H, et al. Prediction of rapid versus prolonged healing of infective endocarditis by monitoring vegetation size. *J Am Soc Echocardiogr.* 1991;4:465-474.

86. Leung DY, Cranney GB, Hopkins AP, Walsh WF. Role of transoesophageal echocardiography in the diagnosis and management of aortic root abscess. *Br Heart J.* 1994;72:175.

87. Anguera I, Miro JM, Cabell CH, et al. Clinical characteristics and outcome of aortic endocarditis with periannular abscess in the International Collaboration on Endocarditis Merged Database. *Am J Cardiol.* 2005;96:976.

88. Bai AD, Steinberg M, Showler A, et al. Diagnostic accuracy of transthoracic echocardiography for infective endocarditis findings using transesophageal echocardiography as the reference standard: a meta-analysis. *J Am Soc Echocardiogr.* 2017;30(7):639-646.e8.

89. Daniel WG, Mugge A, Grote J, et al. Comparison of transthoracic and transesophageal echocardiography for detection of abnormalities of prosthetic and bioprosthetic valves in the mitral and aortic positions. *Am J Cardiol.* 1993;71:210-215.

90. Sivak JA, Vora AN, Navar AM, et al. An approach to improve the negative predictive value and clinical utility of transthoracic echocardiography in suspected native valve infective endocarditis. *J Am Soc Echocardiogr.* 2016;29:315.

91. Habib G, Erba PA, Iung B, et al. Clinical presentation, aetiology and outcome of infective endocarditis. Results of the ESC-EORP EURO-ENDO (European infective endocarditis) registry: a prospective cohort study. *Eur Heart J.* 2019;40:3222.

92. Ryan EW, Bolger AF. Transesophageal echocardiography (TEE) in the evaluation of infective endocarditis. *Cardiol Clin.* 2000;18:773-787.

93. Anwar AM, Nosir YF, Alasnag M, Chamsi-Pasha H. Real time three-dimensional transesophageal echocardiography: a novel approach for the assessment of prosthetic heart valves. *Echocardiography.* 2014;31:188.

94. Eltzschig HK, Rosenberger P, Löffler M, Fox JA, Aranki SF, Shernan SK. Impact of intraoperative transesophageal echocardiography on surgical decisions in 12,566 patients undergoing cardiac surgery. *Ann Thorac Surg.* 2008;85(3):845-852.

95. Showler A, et al. Use of transthoracic echocardiography in the management of low-risk staphylococcus aureus bacteremia: results from a retrospective multicenter cohort study. *JACC Cardiovasc Imaging.* 2015;8(8):924.

96. Palraj BR, et al. Predicting risk of endocarditis using a clinical tool (predict): scoring system to guide use of echocardiography in the management of Staphylococcus aureus bacteremia. *Clin Infect Dis.* 2015;61(1):18.

97. Rosen AB, Fowler VG Jr, Corey GR, Downs SM, Biddle AK, Li J, Jollis JG. Cost-effectiveness of transesophageal echocardiography to determine the duration of therapy for intravascular catheter-associated Staphylococcus aureus bacteremia. *Ann Intern Med.* 1999;130(10):810-820.

98. Vieira ML, Grinberg M, Pomerantzeff PM, et al. Repeated echocardiographic examinations of patients with suspected infective endocarditis. *Heart.* 2004;90:1020-1024.

99. Bundgaard H, Ihlemann N, Gill SU, et al. Long-term outcomes of partial oral treatment of endocarditis. *N Engl J Med.* 2019;380(14):1373-1374.

100. de Camargo RA, Sommer Bitencourt M, Meneghetti JC, et al. The role of 18F-fluorodeoxyglucose positron emission tomography/computed tomography in the diagnosis of left-sided endocarditis: native vs prosthetic valves endocarditis. *Clin Infect Dis.* 2020;70(4):583-594.

101. Feuchtner GM, Stolzmann P, Dichtl W, et al. Multislice computed tomography in infective endocarditis: comparison with transesophageal echocardiography and intraoperative findings. *J Am Coll Cardiol.* 2009;53(5):436-444.

102. Duval X, Iung B, Klein I, et al. Effect of early cerebral magnetic resonance imaging on clinical decisions in infective endocarditis. A prospective study. *Ann Intern Med.* 2010;152:497-504.

103. Mansur AJ, Grinberg M, da Luz PL, Bellotti G. The complications of infective endocarditis. A reappraisal in the 1980s. *Arch Intern Med.* 1992;152(12):2428-2432.

104. Mills J, Utley J, Abbott J. Heart failure in infective endocarditis: predisposing factors, course, and treatment. *Chest.* 1974;66:151-157.

105. Omari B, Shapiro S, Ginzton L, et al. Predictive risk factors for periannular extension of native valve endocarditis. Clinical and echocardiographic analyses. *Chest.* 1989;96(6):1273-1279.

106. Daniel WG, Mügge A, Martin RP, et al. Improvement in the diagnosis of abscesses associated with endocarditis by transesophageal echocardiography. *N Engl J Med.* 1991;324(12):795-800.

107. Steckelberg JM, Murphy JG, Ballard D, et al. Emboli in infective endocarditis: the prognostic value of echocardiography. *Ann Intern Med.* 1991;114(8):635-640.

108. Snygg-Martin U, Gustafsson L, Rosengren L, et al. Cerebrovascular complications in patients with left-sided infective endocarditis are common: a prospective study using magnetic resonance imaging and neurochemical brain damage markers. *Clin Infect Dis.* 2008;47(1):23-30.

109. Fabri J Jr, Issa VS, Pomerantzeff PM, Grinberg M, Barretto AC, Mansur AJ. Time-related distribution, risk factors and prognostic influence of embolism in patients with left-sided infective endocarditis. *Int J Cardiol.* 2006;110(3):334-339.

110. Dickerman SA, Abrutyn E, Barsic B, et al. The relationship between the initiation of antimicrobial therapy and the incidence of stroke in infective endocarditis: an analysis from the ICE Prospective Cohort Study (ICE-PCS). *Am Heart J.* 2007;154(6):1086-1094.

111. Fowler VG Jr, Sanders LL, Kong LK, et al. Infective endocarditis due to Staphylococcus aureus: 59 prospectively identified cases with follow-up. *Clin Infect Dis.* 1999;28(1):106-114.

112. Thuny F, Di Salvo G, Belliard O, et al. Risk of embolism and death in infective endocarditis: prognostic value of echocardiography: a prospective multicenter study [published correction appears in *Circulation.* 2005;112(9):e125. Disalvo, Giovanni [corrected to Di Salvo, Giovanni]; Calabro, Raffaello [corrected to Calabró, Raffaele]. *Circulation.* 2005;112(1):69-75.

113. Rohmann S, Erbel R, Darius H, Makowski T, Meyer J. Effect of antibiotic treatment on vegetation size and complication rate in infective endocarditis. *Clin Cardiol.* 1997;20(2):132-140.

114. Kupferwasser LI, Hafner G, Mohr-Kahaly S, Erbel R, Meyer J, Darius H. The presence of infection-related antiphospholipid antibodies in infective endocarditis determines a major risk factor for embolic events. *J Am Coll Cardiol.* 1999;33(5):1365-1371.

115. Majumdar A, Chowdhary S, Ferreira MA, et al. Renal pathological findings in infective endocarditis. *Nephrol Dial Transplant.* 2000;15:1782-1787.

116. Habib G, Hoen B, Tornos P, et al. Guidelines on the prevention, diagnosis, and treatment of infective endocarditis (new version 2009): the Task Force on the Prevention, Diagnosis, and Treatment of Infective Endocarditis of the European Society of Cardiology (ESC). *Eur Heart J.* 2009;30(19):2369-2413.

117. García-Cabrera E, Fernández-Hidalgo N, Almirante B, et al. Neurological complications of infective endocarditis: risk factors, outcome, and impact of cardiac surgery: a multicenter observational study. *Circulation.* 2013;127(23):2272-2284.

118. Ruttmann E, Willeit J, Ulmer H, et al. Neurological outcome of septic cardioembolic stroke after infective endocarditis. *Stroke.* 2006;37(8):2094-2099.

119. Klein I, Iung B, Labreuche J, et al. Cerebral microbleeds are frequent in infective endocarditis: a case-control study. *Stroke.* 2009;40(11):3461-3465.

120. Spelman D. Complications and outcome of infective endocarditis. *UpToDate.* 2020. https://uptodate.com. Accessed on October 1, 2020.

121. Anderson DJ, Goldstein LB, Wilkinson WE, et al. Stroke location, characterization, severity, and outcome in mitral vs aortic valve endocarditis. *Neurology.* 2003;61(10):1341-1346.

122. Monteleone PP, Shrestha NK, Jacob J, et al. Clinical utility of cerebral angiography in the preoperative assessment of endocarditis. *Vasc Med.* 2014;19(6):500-506.

123. González I, Sarriá C, López J, et al. Symptomatic peripheral mycotic aneurysms due to infective endocarditis: a contemporary profile. *Medicine (Baltimore).* 2014;93(1):42-52.

124. Negishi K, Ono Y, Kurosawa K, et al. Infective endocarditis complicated by mycotic aneurysm of a coronary artery with a perforated mitral valvular aneurysm. *J Am Soc Echocardiogr.* 2009;22(5):542.e1-542.e5424.

125. Lee WK, Mossop PJ, Little AF, et al. Infected (mycotic) aneurysms: spectrum of imaging appearances and management. *Radiographics.* 2008;28(7):1853-1868.

126. Wu FZ, Lai PH. Evolution and regression of intracranial infectious aneurysm diagnosed by brain computed tomographic angiography. *Arch Neurol.* 2010;67(9):1147.

127. Gould FK, Denning DW, Elliott TSJ, et al. Guidelines for the diagnosis and antibiotic treatment of endocarditis in adults: a report of the Working Party of the British Society for Antimicrobial Chemotherapy. *J Antimicrob Chemother.* 2012;67:269–289.

128. Iversen K, Ihlemann N, Gill SU, et al. Partial oral versus intravenous antibiotic treatment of endocarditis. *N Engl J Med.* 2019;380(5):415-424.

129. Chan KL, Dumesnil JG, Cujec B, et al. A randomized trial of aspirin on the risk of embolic events in patients with infective endocarditis. *J Am Coll Cardiol.* 2003;42(5):775-780.

130. Anavekar NS, Tleyjeh IM, Anavekar NS, et al. Impact of prior antiplatelet therapy on risk of embolism in infective endocarditis [published correction appears in *Clin Infect Dis.* 2007;44(10):1398]. *Clin Infect Dis.* 2007;44(9):1180-1186.

131. Ortel TL and Gaasch WH. Antithrombotic therapy in patients with infective endocarditis. *UpToDate*. 2019. https://uptodate.com. Accessed on October 1, 2020.

132. Chu VH, Park LP, Athan E, et al. Association between surgical indications, operative risk, and clinical outcome in infective endocarditis: a prospective study from the International Collaboration on Endocarditis. *Circulation*. 2015;131(2):131-140.

133. Park LP, Chu VH, Peterson G, et al. Validated Risk Score for Predicting 6-Month Mortality in Infective Endocarditis. *J Am Heart Assoc*. 2016;5(4):e003016.

134. Kiefer T, Park L, Tribouilloy C, et al. Association between valvular surgery and mortality among patients with infective endocarditis complicated by heart failure. *JAMA*. 2011;306(20):2239-2247.

135. Bannay A, Hoen B, Duval X, et al. The impact of valve surgery on short- and long-term mortality in left-sided infective endocarditis: do differences in methodological approaches explain previous conflicting results? *Eur Heart J*. 2011;32(16):2003-2015.

136. Lalani T, Cabell CH, Benjamin DK, et al. Analysis of the impact of early surgery on in-hospital mortality of native valve endocarditis: use of propensity score and instrumental variable methods to adjust for treatment-selection bias. *Circulation*. 2010;121(8):1005-1013.

137. Blaustein AS, Lee JR. Indications for and timing of surgical intervention in infective endocarditis. *Cardiol Clin*. 1996;14(3):393-404.

138. Fosbøl EL, Park LP, Chu VH, et al. The association between vegetation size and surgical treatment on 6-month mortality in left-sided infective endocarditis. *Eur Heart J*. 2019;40(27):2243-2251.

139. Yanagawa B, Pettersson GB, Habib G, et al. Surgical management of infective endocarditis complicated by embolic stroke: practical recommendations for clinicians. *Circulation*. 2016;134:1280.

140. Sohail MR, Martin KR, Wilson WR, et al. Medical versus surgical management of Staphylococcus aureus prosthetic valve endocarditis. *Am J Med*. 2006;119:147-154.

141. Pansini S, di Summa M, Patane F, Forsennati PG, Serra M, Del Ponte S. Risk of recurrence after reoperation for prosthetic valve endocarditis. *J Heart Valve Dis*. 1997;6(1):84-87.

142. Wilson W, Taubert KA, Gewitz M, et al. Prevention of infective endocarditis: guidelines from the American Heart Association: a guideline from the American Heart Association Rheumatic Fever, Endocarditis, and Kawasaki Disease Committee, Council on Cardiovascular Disease in the Young, and the Council on Clinical Cardiology, Council on Cardiovascular Surgery and Anesthesia, and the Quality of Care and Outcomes Research Interdisciplinary Working Group [published correction appears in *Circulation*. 2007;116(15):e376-e377]. *Circulation*. 2007;116(15):1736-1754.

143. Chu VH, Cabell CH, Benjamin DK Jr, et al. Early predictors of in-hospital death in infective endocarditis. *Circulation*. 2004;109(14): 1745-1749.

144. Wang A, Athan E, Pappas PA, et al. Contemporary clinical profile and outcome of prosthetic valve endocarditis. *JAMA*. 2007;297(12): 1354-1361.

145. García-Granja PE, López J, Vilacosta I, et al. Impact of valve culture in the prognosis of active left-sided infective endocarditis. *Clin Infect Dis*. 2019;68(6):1017-1023.

146. Cosmi JE, Tunick PA, Kronzon I. Mortality in patients with paravalvular abscess diagnosed by transesophageal echocardiography. *J Am Soc Echocardiogr*. 2004;17(7):766-768.

147. Lauridsen TK, Park L, Tong SY, et al. Echocardiographic findings predict in-hospital and 1-year mortality in left-sided native valve Staphylococcus aureus endocarditis: analysis from the International Collaboration on Endocarditis-Prospective Echo Cohort Study. *Circ Cardiovasc Imaging*. 2015;8(7):e003397.

148. López J, Fernández-Hidalgo N, Revilla A, et al. Internal and external validation of a model to predict adverse outcomes in patients with left-sided infective endocarditis. *Heart*. 2011;97(14):1138-1142.

149. Cahill TJ, Harrison JL, Jewell P, et al. Antibiotic prophylaxis for infective endocarditis: a systematic review and meta-analysis. *Heart*. 2017;103(12): 937-944.

150. van der Meer JT, Thompson J, Valkenburg HA, Michel MF. Epidemiology of bacterial endocarditis in The Netherlands. II. Antecedent procedures and use of prophylaxis. *Arch Intern Med*. 1992;152(9):1869-1873.

151. Duval X, Leport C. Prophylaxis of infective endocarditis: current tendencies, continuing controversies. *Lancet Infect Dis*. 2008;8(4):225-232.

152. Tubiana S, Blotière PO, Hoen B, et al. Dental procedures, antibiotic prophylaxis, and endocarditis among people with prosthetic heart valves: nationwide population-based cohort and a case crossover study. *BMJ*. 2017;358:j3776.

153. Sexton DJ, Chu VH. Antimicrobial prophylaxis for the prevention of bacterial endocarditis. *UpToDate*. 2020. https://uptodate.com. Accessed on October 1, 2020.

154. Warnes CA, Williams RG, Bashore TM, et al. ACC/AHA 2008 guidelines for the management of adults with congenital heart disease: a report of the American College of Cardiology/American Heart Association Task Force on Practice Guidelines (writing committee to develop guidelines on the management of adults with congenital heart disease). *Circulation*. 2008;118(23):e714-e833.

155. Dayer MJ, Jones S, Prendergast B, Baddour LM, Lockhart PB, Thornhill MH. Incidence of infective endocarditis in England, 2000-13: a secular trend, interrupted time-series analysis. *Lancet*. 2015;385(9974):1219-1228.

156. Thornhill MH, Gibson TB, Cutler E, et al. Antibiotic prophylaxis and incidence of endocarditis before and after the 2007 AHA recommendations. *J Am Coll Cardiol*. 2018;72(20):2443-2454.

157. Zegri-Reiriz I, de Alarcón A, Muñoz P, et al. Infective endocarditis in patients with bicuspid aortic valve or mitral valve prolapse. *J Am Coll Cardiol*. 2018;71(24):2731-2740.

158. Nishimura RA, Otto CM, Bonow RO, et al. 2014 AHA/ACC guideline for the management of patients with valvular heart disease: a report of the American College of Cardiology/American Heart Association Task Force on Practice Guidelines [published correction appears in *J Thorac Cardiovasc Surg*. 2014;64(16):1763. Dosage error in article text]. *J Thorac Cardiovasc Surg*. 2014;148(1):e1-e132.

159. AATS Surgical Treatment of Infective Endocarditis Consensus Guidelines Writing Committee Chairs, Pettersson GB, Coselli JS, et al. 2016 The American Association for Thoracic Surgery (AATS) consensus guidelines: Surgical treatment of infective endocarditis: Executive summary. *J Thorac Cardiovasc Surg*. 2017;153(6):1241-1258.e29.

160. Canadian Paediatric Society (CPS): Practice point on prevention of infective endocarditis—updated guidelines (2010, reaffirmed 2018).

161. Prophylaxis against infective endocarditis: antimicrobial prophylaxis against infective endocarditis in adults and children undergoing interventional procedures. London: National Institute for Health and Care Excellence (UK); July 2016.

SECTION VI

RHYTHM AND CONDUCTION ABNORMALITIES

Electrophysiologic Anatomy, Mechanisms of Arrhythmias and Conduction Disturbances, and Genetics

34

Peng-Sheng Chen, Siew Yen Ho, Silvia G. Priori, and Charles Antzelevitch

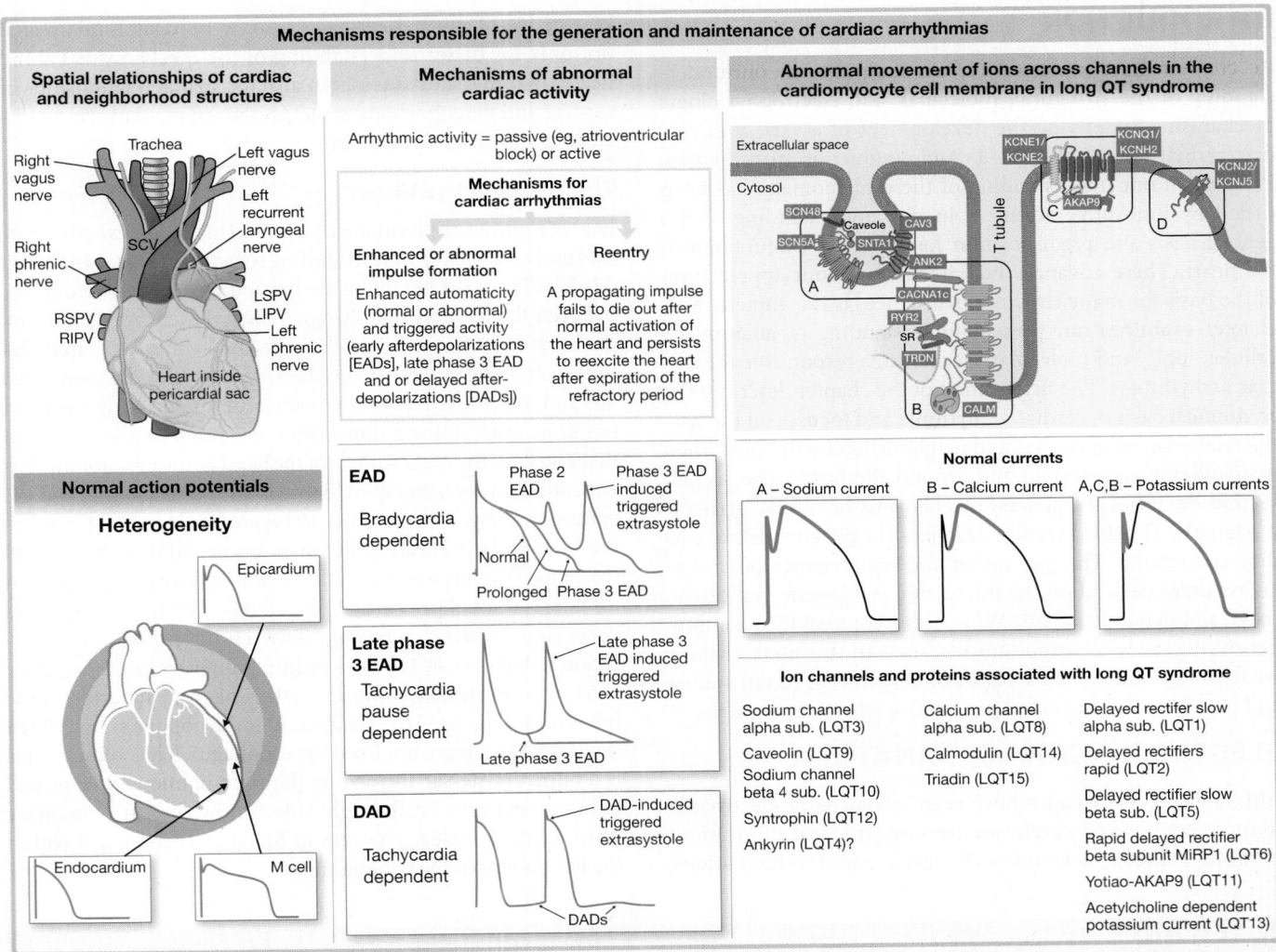

Chapter 34 Fuster and Hurst's Central Illustration. The heart is structurally and electrophysiologically heterogeneous. The heart rate and ion channel functions are controlled by the two arms of the autonomic nervous system. Genetic abnormalities further complicate the ion channel responses to autonomic stimulation while the disease processes lead to structural, electrophysiological, and neural remodeling. The interactions among these factors underlie the mechanisms of cardiac arrhythmogenesis and conduction disturbances. DAD, delayed afterdepolarization; EAD, early afterdepolarization; LIPV, left inferior pulmonary vein; LQT, long QT syndrome genetic variant; LSPV, left superior pulmonary vein; RIPV, right inferior pulmonary vein; RSPV, right superior pulmonary vein; SCV, superior caval vein.

CHAPTER SUMMARY

This chapter examines our present understanding of anatomical, cellular, ionic, and molecular mechanisms responsible for cardiac arrhythmias (see Fuster and Hurst's Central Illustration). The anatomical basis of cardiac arrhythmia is first discussed, with focus on the spatial relationships of cardiac and neighborhood structures when maneuvering catheters in and around the heart. The generation and maintenance of cardiac arrhythmias and conduction disturbances depend on the interactions of various genetic, molecular, fixed, and dynamic factors. Recent years have witnessed important advances in our understanding of the structural, molecular, and electrophysiologic mechanisms, fueled by innovative research into the genetic basis and predisposition for electrical dysfunction of the heart. These advances notwithstanding, our appreciation of the basis for many rhythm disturbances is still incomplete. While it is not possible to comprehensively review all important literature in this book chapter, we tried to examine new insights obtained from recent studies and put them into historical perspective whenever possible.

INTRODUCTION

Recent years have witnessed important advances in our understanding of the structural, molecular, and electrophysiologic mechanisms underlying the development of a variety of cardiac arrhythmias (**Table 34–1**) and conduction disturbances. Progress in our understanding of these phenomena has been fueled by innovative advances in our understanding of the genetic basis and predisposition for electrical dysfunction of the heart. These advances notwithstanding, our appreciation of the basis for many rhythm disturbances is incomplete. This chapter examines our present understanding of anatomical, cellular, ionic, and molecular mechanisms responsible for cardiac arrhythmias. The first section of the chapter describes the anatomical basis of cardiac arrhythmia and focuses on the spatial relationships of cardiac and neighborhood structures when maneuvering catheters in and around the heart. The second section describes the general mechanisms of cardiac arrhythmogenesis. The third section describes the genetic basis of cardiac arrhythmia. The generation and maintenance of cardiac arrhythmias depend on the interactions of genetic, molecular, fixed, and dynamic factors. While it is not possible to comprehensively review all important literature in this book chapter, we tried to examine new insights obtained from recent studies and put them into historical perspective whenever possible.

ELECTROPHYSIOLOGIC ANATOMY

Although recent decades have seen advances in electroanatomic mapping and cardiovascular imaging and innovations in both catheter ablation and device-based interventions, knowledge of normal cardiac anatomy remains fundamental not only for better understanding of the mechanisms behind heart rhythm disturbances, but also for spatial relationships of cardiac and neighborhood structures when maneuvering catheters in and around the heart.

The Heart in the Chest

For the clinician, the heart must be viewed in the context of its location and relationship to surrounding structures (**Figs. 34–1A** and **34–1B**). The heart lies in the mediastinum of the thoracic cavity, between the left and right lungs. When viewed from the front, the heart has a trapezoidal silhouette. Two-thirds of its bulk lies to the left of the midline of the chest, with its apex directed to the left and inferiorly. The fibrous pericardium enclosing the heart has as its inner lining a thin membrane, the serous pericardium that also lines the outer surface of the heart as the epicardium. The pericardial cavity is the space between the parietal lining and the epicardium (Fig. 34–1A). These layers are continuous at two cuffs, one around the aorta and pulmonary trunk and the other around the veins. Two recesses within the pericardial cavity are important for interventional pericardial procedures. The first is the transverse sinus, which is a passage between the superior and posterior reflections of the pericardium, anterior to the superior vena cava, posterior to the arterial trunk, and superior to the left atrium (Fig. 34–1B). The second is the oblique sinus, which separates the left atrium from the esophagus. The oblique sinus is a blind cul-de-sac formed by the right pulmonary veins and inferior vena cava on the right side and by the left pulmonary veins on the left side. The vein of Marshall is contained within the left margin of the oblique sinus.

TABLE 34–1.   Characteristics and Presumed Mechanisms of Cardiac Arrhythmia

Tachycardia	Mechanism	Origin	AV or VA Conduction
Sinus tachycardia	Automatic (normal)	Sinus node	1:1
Sinus node reentry	Reentry	Sinus node and right atrium	1:1 or variable
Atrial fibrillation	Reentry, automatic, triggered activity	Atria, thoracic veins, pulmonary veins, SVC, vein of Marshall	Variable
Atrial flutter	Reentry	RA, LA (infrequent)	Variable
Atrial tachycardia	Reentry, automatic, triggered activity	Atria	1:1, 2:1, or variable
AV nodal reentry tachycardia	Reentry	AV junction	1:1 or variable
AV reentry (WPW or concealed accessory AV connection)	Reentry	Circuit includes accessory AV connection, atria, AV node, His-Purkinje system, ventricles	1:1
Accelerated AV junctional tachycardia	Automatic	AV junction (AV node and His bundle)	1:1 or variable
Accelerated idioventricular rhythm	Abnormal automaticity	Purkinje fibers	Variable, 1:1, or AV dissociation
Ventricular tachycardia	Reentry, automatic, triggered	Ventricles	AV dissociation, variable
Bundle branch reentrant tachycardia	Reentry	Bundle branches and ventricular septum	AV dissociation, variable, or 1:1
RVOT	Automatic, triggered activity	RVOT	AV dissociation, variable, or 1:1
TdP tachycardia	Reentry, triggered activity	Ventricles	AV dissociation
Bidirectional tachycardia	Triggered activity	Purkinje cells	AV dissociation

Abbreviations: AV, atrioventricular; LA, left atrium; RA, right atrium; RVOT, right ventricular outflow tract; SVC, superior vena cava; TdP, torsades de pointes; VA, ventriculoatrial; WPW, Wolff-Parkinson-White.

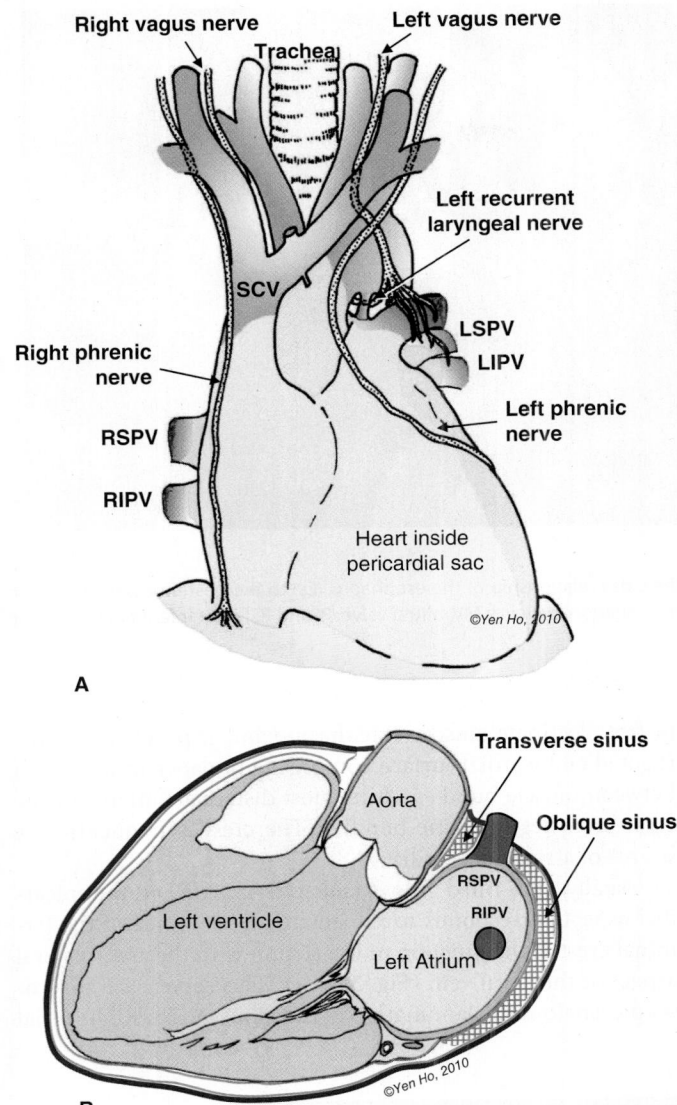

Figure 34–1. Diagrams showing the arrangement of the pericardium. (**A**) The right phrenic nerve runs on the surface of the fibrous pericardium in relation to the lateral aspect of the superior caval vein (SCV) and the orifices of the right superior and inferior pulmonary veins (RS and RIPV) while the left phrenic nerves courses in the area over the LV. (**B**) The locations of the transverse and oblique pericardial sinuses. LI and LSPV, left inferior and superior pulmonary veins.

On the frontal silhouette, the left atrium is barely seen; only its appendage curling round the edge of the pulmonary trunk is visible. The left atrium is the most posterior cardiac chamber (closest to the spine), and the esophagus descends behind it (**Figs. 34–2A** and **34–2B**). Understanding this spatial relationship is crucial to reduce the risk of the postprocedural complication of atrioesophageal fistula.

In the context of pulmonary vein isolation, it is important to note that the right phrenic nerve descends along the anterolateral aspect of the superior caval vein to pass in front of the hilum of the right lung and then along the fibrous pericardium lateral to the right atrium to reach the diaphragm (Fig. 34–1A). Its course in front of the hilum can be as little as 1 mm or 2 mm

from the right upper pulmonary vein, although it is frequently 0.5 cm to 1 cm or more distant.

The left phrenic nerve descends on the left side close to the aortic arch and onto the pericardium over the left atrial appendage and the left ventricle (LV). It takes one of three courses over the LV, passing over the anterior surface, leftward over the obtuse margin, or more posteriorly over the left atrial appendage and the basal lateral wall. Most commonly, the course of the left phrenic nerve is close to the lateral branches of the great cardiac vein and, thus, can be stimulated during left ventricular pacing for cardiac resynchronization therapy (Fig. 34–1A).[1]

Relationships of Cardiac Chambers

Noninvasive imaging can exquisitely demonstrate the three-dimensional spatial relationships between right heart chambers and left heart chambers, the locations and orientations of the valves, the planes of the cardiac septum, and much more than an endocast can. Nevertheless, an endocast still has its use in unraveling the intricate relationships of left and right heart chambers to each other and to the great arteries (**Fig. 34–3**). Briefly, the plane of the right atrioventricular junction is oriented nearly vertically, hence the right atrium is posterior and to the right of the right ventricle (RV). The plane of the pulmonary valve is nearly horizontal and located well cephalad, making the pulmonary valve the most superiorly situated of the cardiac valves. Thus, the RV sweeps from posterior to anterior and passes cephalad such that its outflow tract lies superior to that of the LV. From the left lateral perspective, the inflow tract of the LV can be seen projecting anteriorly and leftward with its apex directed inferiorly. Its outflow tract then passes cephalad and rightward underneath the right ventricular outflow tract (Fig. 34–3). The plane of the aortic valve is inferior and at an angle to that of the pulmonary valve. Understanding the central location of the aortic root and this "crossover" relationship between right and left ventricular outflow tracts is fundamental to spatial relationships between cardiac chambers.

The Atria

The relationship between the right and left atria is highlighted in Fig. 34–3. When viewed from the frontal plane, the right atrium is rightward and anterior, whereas the left atrium is leftward and posterior. Consequently, the atrial septum runs obliquely from the front extending rightward and posteriorly. The posterior part of the left atrium receives the pulmonary veins. The orifices of the left pulmonary veins are more superiorly located than those of the right pulmonary veins. Coursing close to the lateral and posterior mitral annulus is the coronary sinus/great cardiac vein. The oblique vein of Marshall enters the coronary sinus; it passes from superiorly to inferiorly, between the left atrial appendage and the left superior pulmonary vein (Fig. 34–3). The mitral valve orifice and left atrial appendage are the anterior structures of the left atrium (Fig. 34–3).

The Right Atrium

From the epicardial aspect, the right atrium is dominated by its large, triangular-shaped appendage, which extends anteriorly

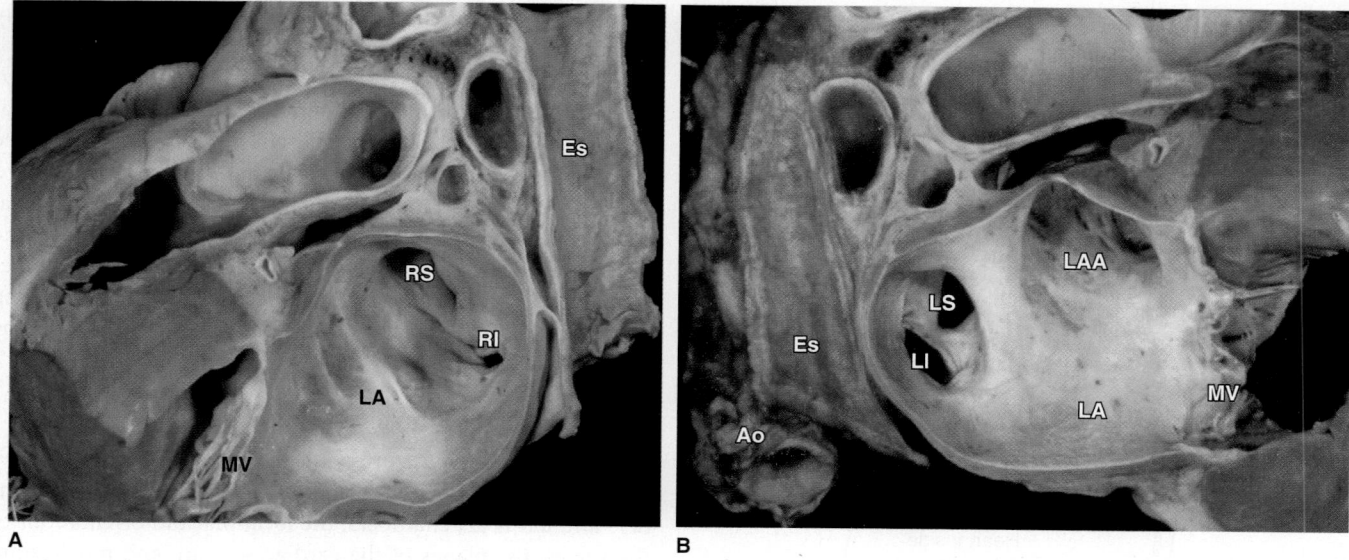

Figure 34–2. **(A)** and **(B)** are two halves of the same heart specimen showing the close relationship of the esophagus (Es) to the posterior wall of the left atrium (LA). Ao, aorta; LAA, left atrial appendage; LI and LS, left inferior and superior pulmonary veins; MV, mitral valve; RI and RS, right inferior and superior pulmonary veins.

and laterally (**Fig. 34–4A**). Endocardially, a muscular ridge termed the terminal crest (*crista terminalis*) demarcates the border between the appendage and the smooth-walled posterior part of the atrium that receives the caval veins. The crest arises medially from the septal aspect, curves around the anterior quadrant of the entrance of the superior caval vein, and then descends along the postero-lateral wall of the atrium toward the entrance of the inferior caval vein (**Fig. 34–4B**). Along the way, it gives off an array of pectinate muscles terminating at the smooth-walled vestibule leading to the tricuspid

orifice. Pectinate muscles line the appendage producing a corrugated endocardial surface comprising of paper-thin walls in between muscle bundles. At its most distal part inferiorly, the crest branches into fine bundles. The crest is frequently the source of atrial tachycardia.

Usually, a fat-filled groove (*sulcus terminalis*) on the epicardial aspect corresponds to the anterolateral course of the terminal crest at the junction of the atrium with the anterolateral aspect of the caval vein (Fig. 34–4A). This serves as a macroscopic anatomical landmark for the sinus node. Right atrial

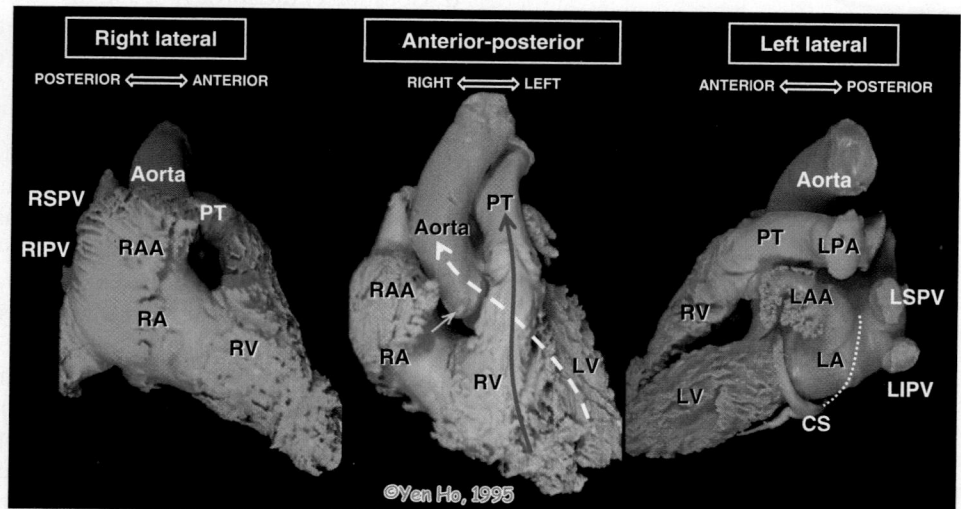

Figure 34–3. A cast of the inner surfaces of a human heart specimen displays the relationship between left (*red*) and right (*blue*) heart chambers viewed from three perspectives. The left ventricular outflow tract (*white arrow with dashed line*) passes rightward and postero-inferior to that of the right ventricular outflow tract (*blue arrow*). Note the imprints of the semilunar valves in the middle panel show the aortic and pulmonary valves are at different levels and angles to one another. The *yellow arrow* indicates the origin of the right coronary artery. The *dotted line* represents the course of the vein/ligament of Marshall. CS, coronary sinus; LPA, left pulmonary artery; PT, pulmonary trunk; RA, right atrium; RAA, right atrial appendage; RV, right ventricle. Other abbreviations as in Figs. 34-1 and 34-2.

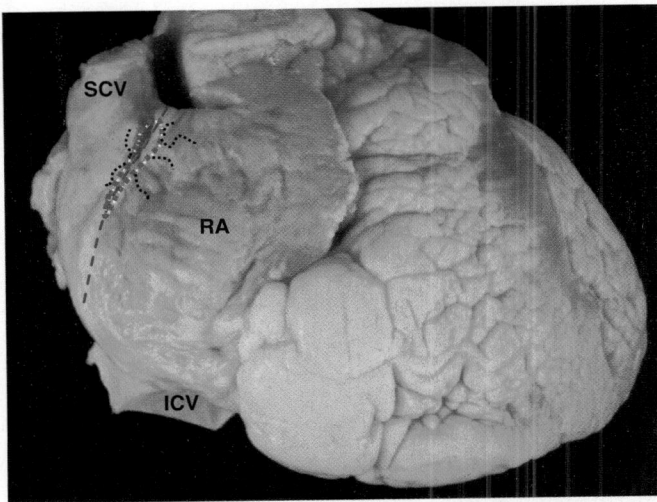

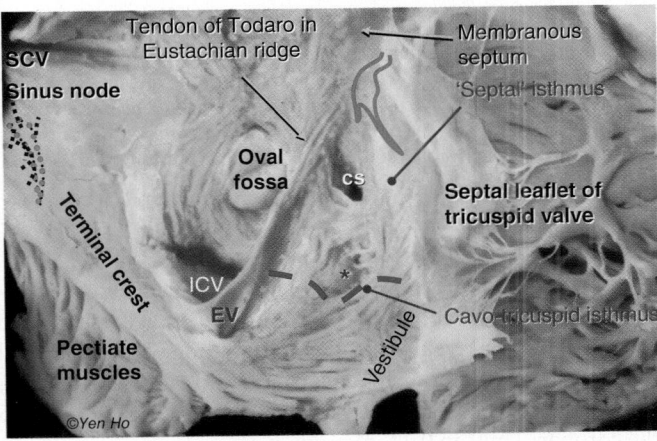

Figure 34–4. (A) Right lateral view showing the epicardial surface of the right atrium dominated by its triangular-shaped atrial appendage. The groove of the terminal crest (*blue broken line*) is filled with epicardial fat. The shape outlined by red dots represents the sinus node with prongs of nodal tissue (*black dotted lines*). (B) The septal aspect of the right atrium and RV viewed from similar perspective as (A) prepared to show the arrangement of the atrial musculature, the borders of the triangle of Koch, and the location of the membranous septum adjacent to the atrioventricular node that continues into the atrioventricular conduction bundle (*irregular red line*). Note the right inferior extension of the atrioventricular node runs toward the hinge line of the tricuspid valve and its relationship to the septal isthmus for slow pathway ablation. The inferior cavo-tricuspid isthmus (*blue broken line*) may traverse through a pouch (*asterisk*) in some patients. ICV, inferior caval vein. Other abbreviations as in Figs. 34-1 and 34-2.

musculature often extends a short distance into the superior vena cava and can be another source of focal atrial arrhythmias.

The Eustachian valve guarding the entrance of the inferior caval vein is variably developed between individuals. In most hearts, it appears as a triangular flap of fibrous tissue. In some cases, the Eustachian valve is particularly large and muscular and can pose an obstacle to passage of catheters from the inferior caval vein to the inferior part of the right atrium where lies the cavotricuspid isthmus. Sometimes, the valve is perforated or net-like and is often described as a Chiari network.

The free border of the Eustachian valve continues as the fibrous tendon of Todaro that passes within the musculature of the Eustachian ridge (also known as sinus septum) as one of the borders of the triangle of Koch, which is the location of the atrioventricular node (Fig. 34–4B). The other borders of the triangle of Koch include the septal leaflet of the tricuspid valve anteriorly and the coronary sinus ostium inferiorly. The tendon of Todaro inserts into the central fibrous body at the apex of the triangle of Koch (see section The Cardiac Conduction System). The region between the coronary sinus ostium and tricuspid valve, also known as the paraseptal isthmus, is the area often targeted for ablation of the slow pathway in atrioventricular nodal reentrant tachycardia. Inferior extensions of the atrioventricular node have been observed in this area (Fig. 34–4B). The so-called *fast pathway*, which usually forms the retrograde limb in patients with slow-fast atrioventricular nodal tachycardia (eg, typical atrioventricular nodal reentrant tachycardia), corresponds to the area of musculature immediately posterior and adjacent to the apex of the triangle of Koch.

The coronary sinus is a structure of critical importance in cardiac electrophysiology, particularly relevant in cardiac mapping, catheter ablation, and placement of leads for cardiac resynchronization. A small crescentic flap, the besian valve, often partially guards the orifice of the coronary sinus. Frequently, the thebesian valve is fenestrated. A complete or imperforate thebesian valve is rare but can be a cause of inability to cannulate the coronary sinus.

The anteroinferior wall between the inferior caval vein and the tricuspid valve (Fig. 34–4B) is the cavotricuspid isthmus containing the terminal ramifications of the terminal crest. This area has a critical role in atrial flutter as it is a site of functional block, which is necessary to facilitate reentry in cavotricuspid-dependent flutter. During catheter ablation of typical flutter, electrophysiologists tend to target the central aspect of the isthmus. However, this part of the isthmus wall bears a pouch like (subeustachian sinus of Keith) in some patients, making it difficult to achieve transmurality. A slightly more lateral isthmus line is longer and may pass through pectinate muscles whereas the septal or medial isthmus is closer to the inferior parts of the atrioventricular node and the right coronary artery.

The Atrial Septum

During transseptal catheterization, the left atrium is accessed from the right atrium. Transseptal catheterization requires an appreciation of the extent of the true atrial septum. Importantly, transseptal maneuvers across the so-called *anterior septum* will lead to inadvertently puncturing the aortic root (**Figs. 34–5A** and **34–5B**). Although inspection of the septum from the right atrium suggests an extensive septal area, the true septum separating the right and left atrial cavities is much smaller. This is due to an infolding of the atrial wall in the septal plane between the caval vein openings and the orifices of the right pulmonary veins forming a muscular rim around the thin valve of the oval fossa.[2] Enclosed within this fold is epicardial fat. The left aspect of the atrial septum lacks the crater-like feature of the right side. The true septum that can be safely crossed

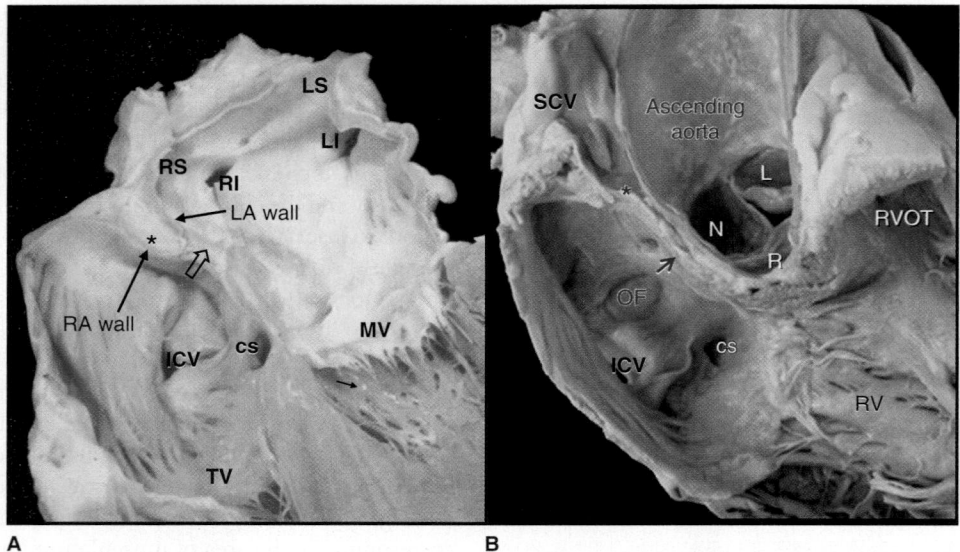

Figure 34–5. (**A**) Longitudinal section through the atrial and ventricular chambers showing the atrial septum in profile. The floor of the oval fossa (*open arrow*) is surrounded by a muscular rim that is an infolding of the atrial wall enclosing epicardial fat (*asterisk*). Note the proximity of the orifices of the right pulmonary veins to the plane of the atrial septum. (**B**) This normal heart viewed from the anterior perspective has been prepared with window dissections to show the aortic root, right atrium, and ventricle. The noncoronary aortic sinus bulges toward the anterior wall of the right atrium (*blue arrow*). The transverse pericardial sinus (*asterisk*) lies between them. L, N, R, left, non-, right coronary aortic sinus respectively; RVOT, right ventricular outflow tract; OF, oval fossa; TV, tricuspid valve. Other abbreviations as in Figs. 34-1 and 34-2.

is limited to the fossa ovalis and its immediate muscular rim as seen on the right atrial aspect (Fig. 34–5A). Most hearts have a well-defined muscular rim on the right atrial aspect, allowing the operator to "feel" and observe (in the left anterior oblique view) the "jump" from firm muscular rim to tenting of the fossa ovalis as the transseptal access sheath is withdrawn from the superior caval vein to the right atrium.

In approximately 20% to 25% of normal hearts, the fossa is patent, even though on the left atrial side, the valve is large enough to overlap the rim. This is because the adhesion of the valve to the rim is incomplete, leaving a gap usually in the anterosuperior margin corresponding to a C-shaped mark in the left atrial side just behind the anterior atrial wall. The gap in adhesion allows a catheter in the right atrium to slip between the rim and the valve into the left atrial chamber. In so doing, if the crevice is narrow, the tip of the catheter will be directed antero-cephalad toward a region of the left atrial wall that is particularly thin. This increases the risk of perforating the heart wall and entering into the pericardial sinus and the aortic root.

The Left Atrium

The atrial appendage is a narrow crenelated blind ending tube with a variety of forms. In fibrillating atria, thrombi may form in the appendage as a result of low flow and stasis. The lumen of the appendage is lined by a network of muscular ridges and intervening membranes that form its wall. Its tip can be directed anteriorly overlying the pulmonary trunk, superiorly behind the arterial pedicle, or posteriorly. When its tip is directed anteriorly, the body of the appendage usually also overlies the main stem of the left coronary artery. As previously

described, the remnant of the vein of Marshall runs on the lateral epicardial aspect of the neck of the appendage, anterior to the left pulmonary veins, which is an infolding of the atrial wall described as the lateral ridge or Coumadin ridge (Fig. 34–3). The vein persists as the left superior caval vein draining into the coronary sinus in 0.3% of individuals. In the majority, however, it is a ligament with patency up to approximately 0.5 cm to 3 cm from the coronary sinus. Its wall has multiple muscle bundles connecting it with the walls of the left atrium, left pulmonary veins, and the coronary sinus. Moreover, it is richly supplied with sympathetic and parasympathetic nerve fibers and ganglion cells.

The venous component of the left atrium receives the pulmonary veins posteriorly. The orifices of the right pulmonary veins are directly adjacent to the plane of the atrial septum (Fig. 34–5A). The musculature of the atrial wall extends into the veins to varying lengths, with the longest sleeves along the upper or superior veins. Close to the venous orifices, the sleeves are thicker and surround the epicardial aspect of the vein. The veins often have electrical continuity with bridging muscle fibers between the superior and inferior veins, which are present in approximately half of left vein pairs and one-third of right vein pairs. The distal margins of the sleeves, however, are usually thinner and irregular as the musculature fades out. The composition of the muscle sleeves is complex with abrupt changes in myoarchitecture resulting in chaotic conduction. Diverse cell types including Cajal cells, P cells, transitional cells, and Purkinje cells have been reported in the sleeves suggesting their role as potential triggers for atrial fibrillation (AF). These sources of ectopic activity are targeted during pulmonary vein isolation procedures for the treatment of drug-refractory AF.

The anterior vestibular component leads to the mitral valve. There are no surface anatomic landmarks that separate the venous left atrium from the vestibule. The region between the left inferior pulmonary vein and the mitral valve annulus is the mitral isthmus and is frequently a zone of slow conduction that favors the development of atypical left atrial flutter, particularly in patients with prior left atrial ablation. The mitral isthmus is occasionally targeted in substrate ablation during ablation procedures in patients with advanced AF. The tissue of the mitral isthmus can be very thick and may require access via the coronary sinus to achieve complete transmural ablation.

The Atrioventricular Junctions

In the normal heart, the epicardial tissues of the atrioventricular grooves and the fibrous tissues of the hinge lines of the tricuspid and mitral leaflets provide electrical separation of the atrial and ventricular tissue. The only site of muscular continuity is via the specialized myocardium of the atrioventricular conduction system. However, anomalous muscular atrioventricular connections at the atrioventricular junctions (accessory pathways or bypass tracts) can lead to atrioventricular reentry and preexcitation, including Wolff-Parkinson-White syndrome. Description of the location of accessory pathways in the literature and clinical arena has been complicated by the use of heterogeneous terminology. This terminology has been particularly complicated by the interchangeable use of the terms *anterior* and *superior* and the terms *posterior* and *inferior*. Anatomically, the term *superior* is more accurate and is preferred to *anterior*, whereas *inferior* is more accurate and preferred to *posterior* (**Figs. 34–6A** and **34–6B**).

The true septal component is limited to the area of the central fibrous body and immediate musculature. The so-called *anterior septum* is contiguous with part of the supraventricular crest of the RV, whereas the *posterior septum* is formed by the muscular floor of the coronary sinus overlying the diverging posterior walls of the ventricular mass and the vestibule of the right atrium overlapping tissues of the atrioventricular groove that overlie the ventricular septum. Anatomically, the atrioventricular junction can be described as comprising extensive right and left parietal junctions that meet with a small true-septal component (Figs. 34–6A and 34–6B). The right parietal junction is relatively circular and occupies a near vertical plane in the heart marked by the course of the right coronary artery in the atrioventricular groove. The superior and most medial part of the junction abuts directly on the membranous septum.

The left parietal junction surrounds the orifice of the mitral valve, and part of it is the area of fibrous continuity between the mitral and aortic valves (Figs. 34–6A and 34–6B). On the left side, because of the nature of the aorto-mitral continuity, accessory atrioventricular connections are mainly limited to the hinge line of the posterior leaflet of the mitral valve. This portion of the mitral hinge line runs from posterosuperior to posterior and inferior when the heart is viewed in left anterior oblique projection (Figs. 34–6A and 34–6B). The inferior area harbors the coronary sinus and its tributary, the great cardiac vein. The inferior paraseptal region, the so-called *posterior*

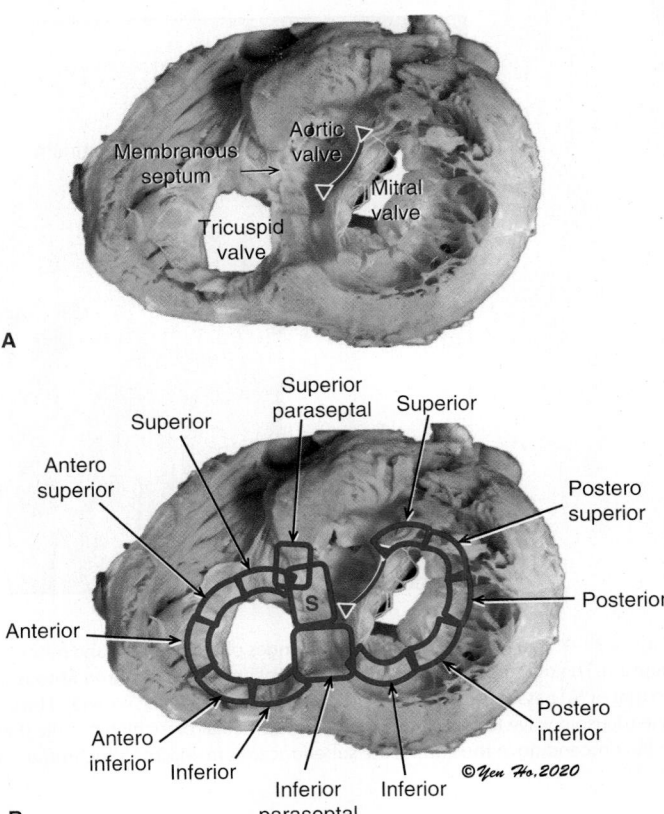

Figure 34–6. The base of the heart displaying the ventricles viewed from the cardiac apex in approximately LAO perspective. (**A**) There is continuity of fibrous tissue (*blue line*) between the hinge line of the anterior leaflet of the mitral valve and the aortic valve with fibrous trigones at each end (*triangles*). (**B**) The *blue outlines* mark the various segments of the right and left atrioventricular junctions with attitudinally appropriate terminology. Note the septal component (S) is a relatively small segment.

septum, is the inferior pyramidal space that contains epicardial fibrofatty tissues together with the artery supplying the atrioventricular node.[5] Maintaining a more ventricular position when ablating septal pathways is important to avoid injury to the compact atrioventricular node and subsequent complete heart block. Because the tricuspid valve hinge line is more caudal than the mitral valve (Fig. 34–5A), there is a tiny portion of the right atrium that shares a common wall with the LV—the atrioventricular portion of the membranous septum (**Figs. 34–7A** and **34–7B**). The atrioventricular membranous septum is immediately adjacent to the apex of Koch's triangle, which is formed by the central fibrous body (Fig. 34–4B). More extensive than the atrioventricular membranous septum is the so-called *atrioventricular muscular septum*, which is formed by the right atrial wall in part overlying the left side of the ventricular septum in the medial portion of the atrioventricular junction, and sandwiched in between is epicardial fat of the pyramidal space inferiorly and the central fibrous body with atrioventricular node lying superiorly (Figs. 34–7A and 34–7B). Appreciation of this atrioventricular septum is important because a catheter at this location may record a large ventricular signal from the basal LV, leading the electrophysiologist to think the

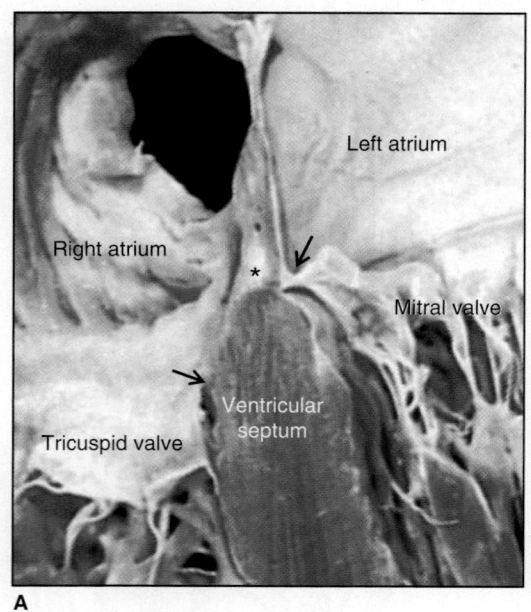
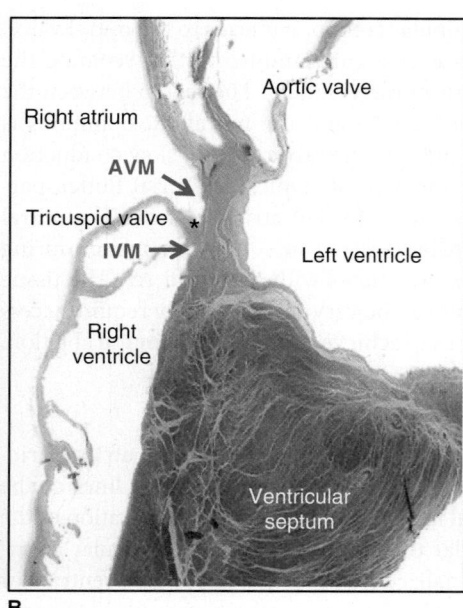

Figure 34–7. **(A)** The offset between the hinges of the tricuspid and mitral valves (*arrows*) results in a sandwich arrangement of the muscular atrioventricular septum. The right atrial wall overlies a plane of epicardial fatty and fibrous tissues (*asterisk*). **(B)** This histological section from a heart cut in a plane cephalad to that of (A) passes through the membranous septum which is divided into an atrioventricular (AVM) and an interventricular portion (IVM) by the insertion of the tricuspid valve (*asterisk*). Note the atrioventricular branching bundle (BB) on the left side of the crest of the muscular septum and the left bundle branch (LBB) descending in the immediate subendocardium. Masson's trichrome stains myocardium red and fibrous tissue green.

catheter is more ventricular with little risk of heart block during attempted ablation of a septal accessory pathway. In fact, a catheter on the atrioventricular septum is on the atrial side of the junction, with significant risk of iatrogenic heart block.

The Ventricles

Viewing the heart from the front, the RV overlaps much of the LV, allowing only a small portion that forms the left margin and cardiac apex to be visible. When viewed from the side, the RV is more-or-less triangular. The tricuspid and pulmonary valves separated by muscle of the supraventricular crest gives a wider angle between inflow and outflow tracts than in the LV. The LV, being more conical in shape, has an inflow tract that makes a sharp angle with the outflow that is sandwiched between the ventricular septum and the anterior leaflet of the mitral valve. The curvature of the ventricular septum places the right ventricular outflow tract anteriorly and cephalad to that of the LV.

The Right Ventricle

Being the most anteriorly situated cardiac chamber (Fig. 34–3), the RV is located immediately behind the sternum. This is an important relationship to bear in mind when performing pericardiocentesis. Using an anterior approach, if the needle continues through and past the pericardial space, the needle will encounter the right ventricular free wall, thus creating potential for right ventricular puncture or laceration. The leaflets of the tricuspid valve guarding the inlet to the RV can be distinguished as septal, anterosuperior, and inferior (mural). The septal leaflet, with its cords inserting directly to the ventricular septum, is characteristic of the tricuspid valve. The medial

papillary muscle, a small out-budding from the septum, supports the commissure between the septal and anterosuperior leaflets (**Figs. 34–8A** and **34–B**). A larger papillary muscle, the anterior papillary muscle, supports the extensive anterosuperior leaflet and its junction with the inferior leaflet. The inferior leaflet and its junction with the anterosuperior and inferior leaflets are usually supported by a group of small papillary muscles, the inferior papillary muscles.

The apical portion is characterized by coarse crisscrossing muscular trabeculations and a distinctive muscle bundle, the moderator band, that bridges the ventricular cavity between the body of the septomarginal trabeculation and the parietal wall (Fig. 34–8A). The anterior papillary muscle arises from the moderator band close to the parietal wall. Within its musculature runs a major subbranch from the right bundle branch. The septomarginal trabeculation itself is a y-shaped muscular band that is adherent to the septal surface. In between its limbs lies the infolding of the heart wall forming the ventricular roof, an area also known as the supraventricular crest. This crest separates the two right heart valves and is an integral part of the outlet, continuous with the freestanding subpulmonary muscular infundibulum, which is a tube-like structure supporting the pulmonary valve (Fig. 34–8B). Owing to the semilunar attachments of the leaflets crossing the border between the infundibulum and the arterial wall, infundibular muscle is enclosed in the nadirs of the pulmonary sinuses. The right ventricular outflow tract is a frequent origin of adenosine-sensitive triggered ventricular extrasystoles and ventricular tachycardia (VT) in patients without structural heart disease. Most outflow tract VTs arise in the perivalvular tissue. Although electrophysiologists

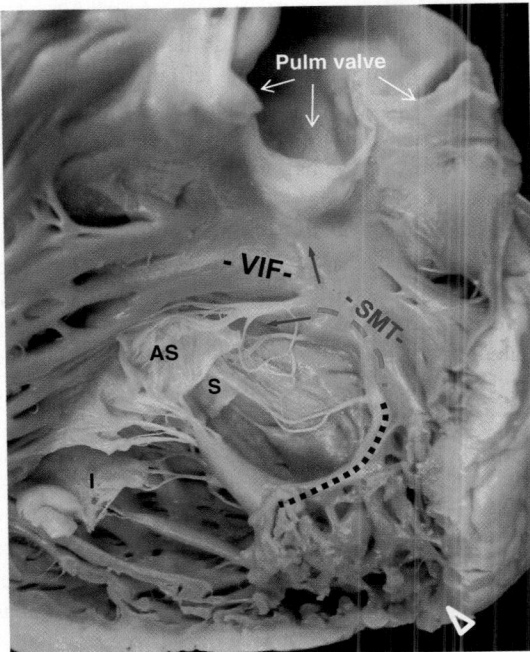

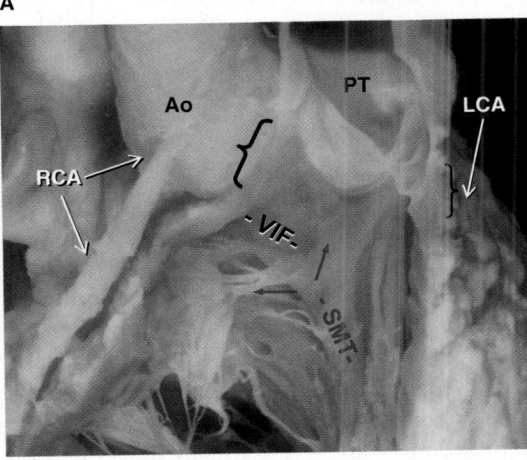

Figure 34–8. (A) Right ventricle opened along the inflow and outflow tracts shows its normal thin wall, especially at the apex (*open triangle*). The pulmonary and tricuspid valves are separated by the muscle of the supraventricular crest comprising of the ventriculo-infindibuar fold (VIF) and the arms (*blue arrows*) of the septomarginal trabeculation (SMT). The right bundle branch (*red broken line*) emerges from the septum to travel apically on the SMT and sends a branch along the moderator band (*dotted line*) to the parietal wall of the ventricle. **(B)** This dissection cutting through the VIF shows it is not septal. It contributes to the muscular infundibulum (brace) that accounts for the higher level of the pulmonary valve relative to the aortic valve. Note the relationship of the coronary arteries (LCA, RCA) to the outflow tract. AS, S, I, antero-superior, septal and inferior leaflets of the tricuspid valve respectively; Ao, aorta; PT, pulmonary trunk.

frequently refer to septal and free wall portions of the right ventricular outflow tract, it should be noted that the infundibulum does not have a true septal component (Fig. 34–8B) because the pulmonary valve is located more cephalad than the aortic valve. Thus, the aortic root lies immediately posterior and to the right of the "septal" right ventricular outflow tract

(Fig. 34–3). Two of the pulmonary sinuses are adjacent to the right and left coronary sinuses of the aortic valve, although the planes of the aortic and pulmonary valves are at an angle to one another. Consequently, the main coronary arteries can also be at risk when ablating in the so-called septal part of the right ventricular outflow tracts (see Fig. 34–8B).

The Left Ventricle

Guarding the entrance to the LV, the mitral valve hinge line has limited attachment to the ventricular septum. The larger portion of its hinge line is to the parietal atrioventricular junction, whereas a third is the span of fibrous continuity with the aortic valve (Figs. 34–6A and 34–6B). The aortomitral continuity very rarely contains muscle but has been reported as another site from which triggered idiopathic ventricular arrhythmias can originate. At the septal end of valvar fibrous continuity is the right fibrous trigone, and at the parietal end is the left fibrous trigone. The right trigone in continuity with the membranous septum forms the central fibrous body (**Fig. 34–9A**). The two leaflets of the mitral valve are disproportionate in size. The *anterior* leaflet in continuity with the aortic valve is deep, whereas the *posterior* (or mural) leaflet is shallow. The mitral leaflets are attached via tendinous cords exclusively to two groups of papillary muscles: anterolateral and posteromedial papillary muscles. The papillary muscles can also be sources for ventricular arrhythmias that are often difficult to ablate given their location and motion within the left ventricular cavity as well as their thickness.

The normal LV has a thicker wall than the RV but at its apex the thickness of the wall tapers to 1 mm to 2 mm (Fig. 34–9A). The apical third of the ventricle is characterized by trabeculations that are finer than those found in the RV. Occasionally, fine fibrous, muscular, or fibromuscular strands, or so-called *false tendons*, extend between the septum and the papillary muscles or the parietal wall. About 30% have been found to carry the distal ramifications of the left bundle branch or Purkinje fibers and have been implicated in idiopathic left VT.

The left ventricular outlet is bordered by the muscular ventricular septum anterosuperiorly and the anterior leaflet of the mitral valve posteroinferiorly (**Fig. 35-9B**). The common atrioventricular conduction bundle emerges from the central fibrous body to pass between the membranous septum and the crest of the muscular ventricular septum (**Fig. 35-9A**). The landmark for the site of the atrioventricular conduction bundle is the fibrous body that adjoins the crescentic hinge lines of the right and noncoronary leaflets of the aortic valve. From here, the left bundle branch descends in the subendocardium and usually branches into three main fascicles that interconnect and further divide into finer and finer branches as the Purkinje network (see section The Cardiac Conduction System).

In the outlet, the nadirs of two sinuses of the aortic valve have ventricular muscle, these being the right sinus and the medial half of the left coronary aortic sinuses. These sinuses are nearest to the pulmonary valve. The third sinus, the noncoronary sinus, does not contain muscle because it is an integral part of the fibrous continuity with the mitral leaflet.

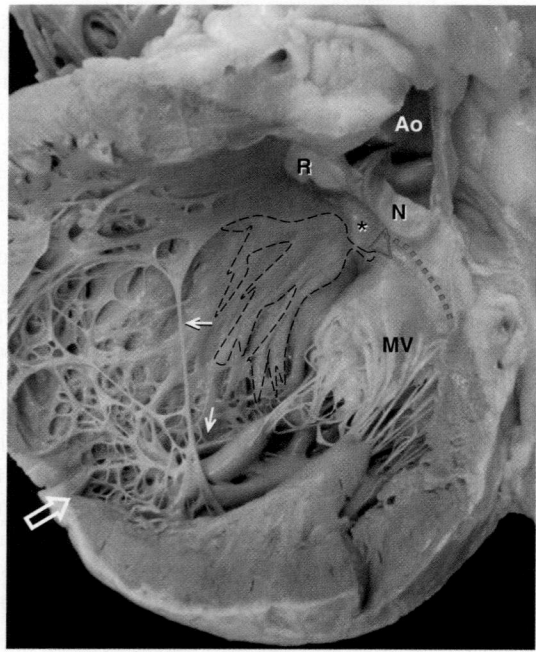

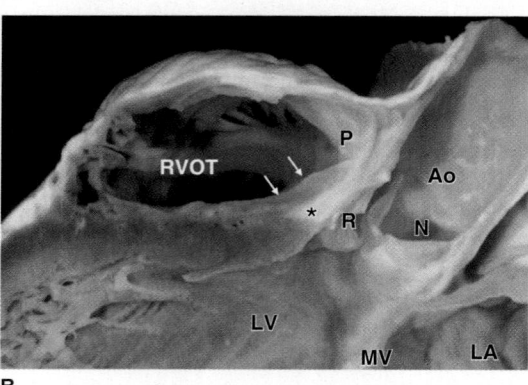

Figure 34–9. (**A**) The LV opened from apex through to the aortic valve. The right (R) and noncoronary (N) leaflets are closely related to the membranous septum (*asterisk*), the right fibrous trigone (*triangle*), and the atrioventricular conduction bundle giving origin to the left bundle branch (*black broken lines*). *Red dotted line* marks the fibrous continuity between aortic and mitral valves. Strands of false tendons (*white arrows*) cross the cavity. Note the thick ventricular wall tapers to become extremely thin at the apex. (**B**) This longitudinal cut through the LV shows the relationship between the pulmonary valve (P) and the aortic valve. The so-called septal component (*arrows*) of the right ventricular outflow tract (RVOT) overlaps the left and right (R) coronary aortic sinuses through epicardial fat (*asterisk*). The noncoronary aortic sinus is anterior to the atrial walls. Abbreviations as in Figs. 34–1 and 34–2.

Thus, ventricular arrhythmias emanating from the aortic sinuses are limited to the right and left coronary sinuses. Owing to the spatial relationship of the subpulmonary infundibulum with the left ventricular outlet (**Fig. 34–9B**), the foci may be ablated from within the part of the right ventricular outlet that overlies the adjacent aortic sinuses. Since the main coronary arteries usually arise from the arterial part of the sinuses, they are not in the immediate field, and thus ablations can be performed

relatively safely without significant risk of injury to the coronaries. The noncoronary aortic sinus, being immediately adjacent to the paraseptal region of the left and right atriums and close to the superior atrioventricular junction, may be used to map and ablate focal atrial tachycardias that have earliest activation in the vicinity of the His bundle area—so-called "parahisian" atrial tachycardias (Fig. 34–5B, Fig. 34–9B).

In the last decade or so, the left ventricular summit has come into prominence owing to it being the site to target for ablation of a proportion of ventricular arrhythmias. This is the most superior part of the LV viewed from the epicardial aspect demarcated anteriorly by the left anterior descending coronary artery and posteriorly by the circumflex artery where it enters the atrioventricular groove. Passing through this area is the anterior interventricular vein as it turns laterally and posteriorly to become the great cardiac vein. The apical portion of the summit toward the coronary arterial bifurcation is usually covered with abundant epicardial fat limiting access for direct contact. Septal and diagonal branches of the arteries and veins in this area may be utilized for access. On the endocardial aspect, the summit corresponds to the region between the left aortic coronary sinus to the septal-anterior wall of the ventricular outlet.

The Coronary Veins

The venous return from the myocardium is channeled either via small the besian veins that open directly into the cardiac chambers or, more significantly, is collected by the greater coronary venous system, which drains 85% of the venous flow. The main coronary veins in the greater system are the great, middle, and small cardiac veins. The great cardiac vein is a continuation of the anterior interventricular vein that ascends parallel to the anterior descending coronary artery. It turns into the left atrioventricular groove to continue into the coronary sinus. The middle cardiac vein runs alongside the posterior descending coronary artery and usually drains into the coronary sinus. The small cardiac vein receives tributaries from the right atrium and the inferior wall of the RV before coursing in the right atrioventricular groove to open to the right margin of the coronary sinus orifice or into the middle cardiac vein. Several other veins from the anterior surface of the RV drain directly into the right atrium. The coronary veins may be surrounded by a cuff of myocardium that gives the potential for accessory atrioventricular connection as the vein passes through the atrioventricular groove.

The coronary sinus is a critical structure in electrophysiology. It is a tubular structure with an ostium diameter of between 5 mm and 15 mm. Its transition to the great cardiac vein is marked by the valve of Vieussens and the entrance of the vein/ligament of Marshall. The latter is an embryonic remnant of the left superior vena cava. Even when a lumen is present, the vein of Marshall rarely exceeds 3 cm in length before tapering to a blind end. If adequately wide, this channel may be used for ablating the left atrial wall, including the use of alcohol instillation. The valve of Vieussens found in 80% to 90% of hearts, is flimsy but can provide some resistance to potential catheter placement. Once past Vieussens valve, a sharp bend in the great cardiac vein can cause further obstruction in 20% of patients. There is a muscular sleeve around the proximal portion of the coronary sinus. Bundles from the sleeve often extend into the left atrial wall, the vein of Marshall, and may also cover the walls of adjacent coronary arteries.

As the great cardiac vein begins its course in the atrioventricular groove, it passes underneath the left atrial appendage. Further along, it collects tributaries draining the LV, including the lateral (obtuse marginal) veins and inferior veins, which are important targets for left ventricular pacing in cardiac resynchronization therapy (**Figs. 34–10A** to **34–10C**). The distribution, courses, and calibers of the left ventricular veins vary from individual to individual. When using these veins for pacing lead implants, it is worth noting that the left phrenic nerve running in the pericardium may pass across or very close to the lateral or posterolateral veins. Thus, pacing from these veins can cause phrenic capture and diaphragmatic stimulation. The left ventricular veins may be accessed for ablating VT from a

source close to the epicardium. When deploying catheters or wires in superficial veins, it is important to note that venous walls are thin and "unprotected" by muscle on the epicardial side.

The orifice of the middle cardiac vein usually opens just within the coronary sinus orifice. Occasionally it opens directly into the right atrium. At the cardiac crux the middle cardiac vein passes immediately superficial to the right coronary artery. It is a useful portal for ablating epicardial inferior paraseptal ("posteroseptal") accessory atrioventricular pathways located in the inferior pyramidal space. Ablations at this site can cause injury to the right coronary artery or posterior descending artery, given its close proximity (Figs. 34–10A to 34–10C). Rarely, the entrance of the middle vein is dilated (or aneurysmal) and surrounded by a cuff of muscle, giving the potential for accessory atrioventricular connections. Tributaries from the middle cardiac vein with a lateral course can also be used to access the lateral wall for lead placement in biventricular pacing.

The Cardiac Conduction System

The cardiac conduction system is composed of specialized myocytes that are histologically different from ordinary working myocytes. The cardiac conduction system comprises of the sinus node that generates the cardiac impulse that is received by the atrioventricular node and transmitted along the atrioventricular conduction system to be distributed by the Purkinje fiber network to the ordinary myocardium.

Although much has been written about *specialized internodal tracts* (anterior, middle, and posterior) connecting the sinus node to the atrioventricular node, their existence in the form as originally defined by early anatomists has never been demonstrated. Instead, the arrangement of muscle bundles such as the terminal crest, the rim of the oval fossa, Bachmann's bundle, have the architecture to facilitate transmission within and between the atria. Bachmann's bundle is a prominent interatrial muscle bridge that extends across the roof of the atria anterosuperior to the fossa ovalis (**Fig. 34–11A**). Conduction over Bachmann's bundle leads to early endocardial activation in the anterior left atrium in order to help facilitate interatrial synchrony. Some interatrial muscle bundles, however, may be relevant in rhythm disorders. Multiple smaller interatrial bridges are frequently present, giving the potential for macroreentry. Some connect the muscular sleeves of the right pulmonary veins to the right atrium, and the superior caval vein to the left atrium (**Fig. 34–11B**).

The Sinus Node

The sinus node is tadpole-like in shape, with a mean length of 13.5 mm in the adult heart.[3] The "head" of the sinus node is located close to the epicardium of the terminal crest at the anterolateral aspect of the junction between the right atrium and superior caval vein (Fig. 34–4A). The "tail" of the node lies deeper, toward the endocardium of the terminal crest. The sinus node can extend down more than 50% of the length of the crest toward the inferior caval vein. The node is richly supplied with nerves from both the sympathetic chains and the vagus

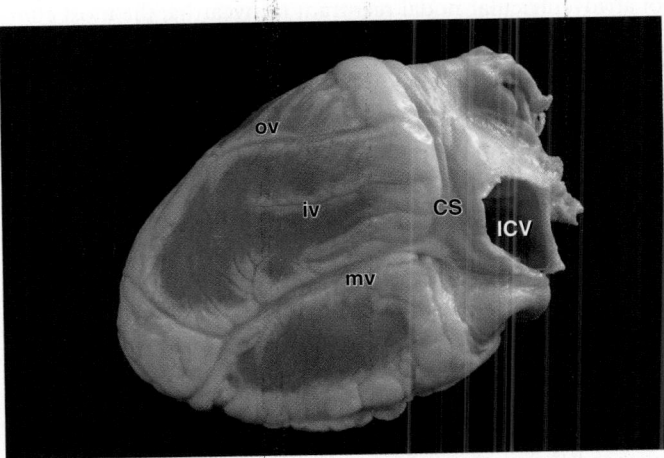

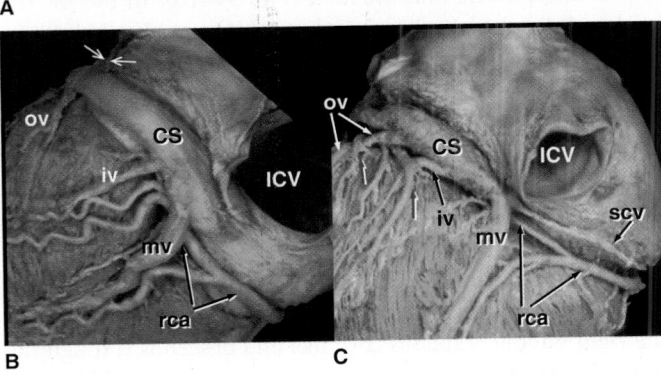

Figure 34–10. Diaphragmatic aspects of a sample of hearts to show some of the variations in distribution of left ventricular veins. (A) The epicardial surface shows the thin translucent walls of the coronary sinus (CS) and veins. (B) and (C) are prepared by removing epicardial tissues and fatty tissues in the atrioventricular groove to show the differing shapes of the CS and angle of origins and courses of the left ventricular inferior (IV) and oblique veins (OV). Veins are typically superficial to arteries but the heart in (C) shows branches (*blue arrows*) of the circumflex artery passing over the OV and IV. *Double arrows* in (B) mark insertion of ligament of Marshall. ICV, inferior caval vein; MV, middle cardiac vein, RCA, right coronary artery; SCV, small cardiac vein.

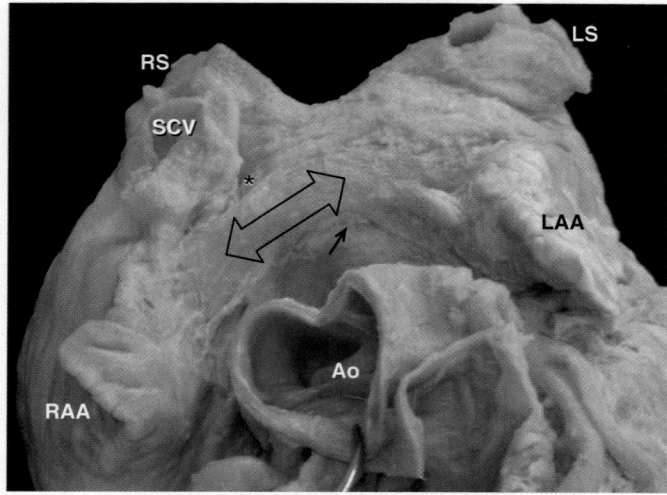

A

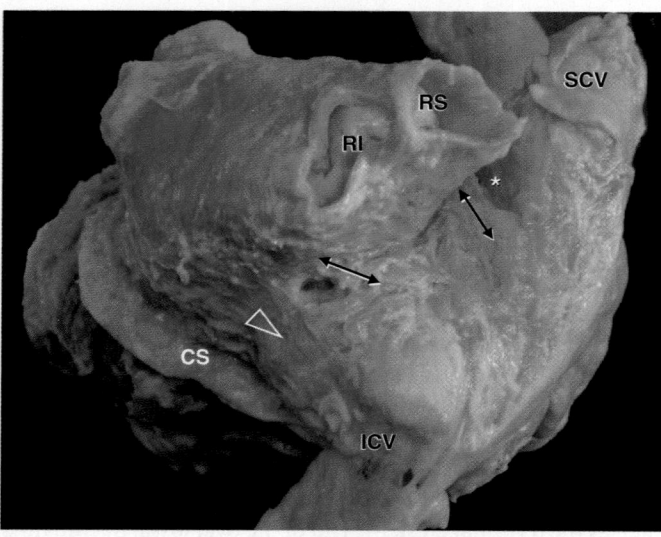

B

Figure 34–11. (**A**) Anterior perspective of the atria after removal of epicardial tissues. The aorta (Ao) is pulled forward to display a particularly thin area (*small arrow*) in the left atrial wall. Bachmann's bundle (*open double arrows*) crosses the interatrial groove (*asterisk*). (**B**) Tilted view of the posterior aspect showing muscle bridges (double-headed arrows) crossing the interatrial groove (*asterisk*) superiorly and inferiorly. This heart is unusual in having a broad band (*triangle*) connecting the inferior wall of the left atrium to the right atrium close to the orifice of the inferior caval vein (ICV). Abbreviations as in Figs. 34-1 and 34-2.

nerve. Nodal tissues are accompanied by the nodal artery, which arises from the right coronary artery in 65% of individuals. The tissue surrounding the sinus node is dominated by calcium channel activation (as opposed to Na^+), and therefore, sinus node exit conduction is slow and decremental, similar to the atrioventricular node. The borders of the node are irregular with frequent interdigitations between nodal and ordinary atrial myocytes, facilitating communication between the node and right atrial wall.

The Atrioventricular Conduction System
In the normal heart (without accessory pathway connections), the atrioventricular conduction system provides the only pathway of muscular continuity between atrial and ventricular myocardium. There is an interface of transitional cells between ordinary atrial myocardium and the histologically specialized cells that make up the atrioventricular node. The compact atrioventricular node is located near the apex of the triangle of Koch (see Fig. 34–4B). In the adult, the compact atrioventricular node is approximately 5 mm long and wide. The atrioventricular nodal artery mostly arises from the dominant coronary artery. Inferior extensions from the compact node pass to the right and left sides of the artery.[5] The right extension courses adjacent to the septal leaflet hinge line, whereas the left extension projects toward the mitral vestibule. The distance of the right inferior extension to the endocardial surface is approximately 1 mm to 5 mm. With reference to the triangle of Koch, the compact node (Fig. 34–4B) is near the apex, but the right inferior extensions reach to the midlevel of the triangle and may even extend to the vicinity of the coronary sinus in hearts with small nodal triangles. This area is the location at which catheter ablation targets the slow pathway in patients with evidence of dual atrioventricular nodal physiology and evidence of atrioventricular nodal reentrant tachycardia, the most common form of supraventricular tachycardia.

The Atrioventricular Conduction Bundles
Superiorly, at the apex of the triangle of Koch, the penetrating bundle of His passes through the central fibrous body coursing anterocephalad. This short bundle of specialized myocardium is a direct extension of the compact atrioventricular node, enabling atrial activity to be conveyed to the ventricles.[4] From the fibrous body, a thin sheath of fibrous tissue continues to surround the atrioventricular conduction bundle, its bundle branches and their continuations and ramifications into the Purkinje system until their terminations into ordinary ventricular myocardium. The atrioventricular bundle leaves the fibrous body to be directly related to the membranous septum and the aortic outflow tract (Fig. 34–4B). In the LV, the landmark for the membranous septum is immediately inferior to the fibrous area between the right and noncoronary aortic sinuses (Fig. 34–9A). The bundle is sandwiched between the membranous septum and the crest of the muscular ventricular septum. Although the bundle commonly passes to the left side of the septal crest, there are variations relevant to His bundle pacing.[3] After a short distance, the bundle bifurcates into the left and right bundle branches. The left bundle branch fans out into interconnecting fascicles as it descends in the subendocardium of the septal surface of the LV (Fig. 34–9A). By contrast, the right bundle branch is cord like and descends through the musculature of the ventricular septum to reach the RV where it emerges in the subendocardium at the base of the medial papillary muscle to run in the septomarginal trabeculation (Fig. 34–8A). Along its descent, it divides into further branches, one of which crosses to the parietal wall within the moderator band. Toward the apical portion of the heart, both the left and right bundle branches continue into finer and finer branches, eventually ramifying into a network of the Purkinje fibers, running in the subendocardium and through the thickness of the ventricular walls and septum to contact working myocardium.

Fat Pads and Innervation

The heart is heavily influenced by autonomic innervation. Moreover, cardiac innervation includes both extrinsic innervation as well as influence from the intrinsic cardiac nervous system. The intrinsic cardiac nervous system is largely an atrial network of neural ganglia. The vagal inputs to the heart arise from various nuclei in the medulla. Sympathetic inputs come from the paravertebral, superior cervical, middle cervical, cervicothoracic (stellate), and thoracic ganglia. The stellate ganglion is the primary source of cardiac sympathetic innervation. If targeting it for neuromodulation, it is worth bearing in mind its proximity to structures such as the brachial plexus, spinal nerve roots, prevertebral portion of the vertebral artery, subclavian artery, and cervical pleura.

Generally speaking, the innervation of the atria is predominantly parasympathetic, while the innervation of the ventricles is predominantly sympathetic. The extrinsic cardiac nerves course through the hilum at the base of the heart and branch into different autonomic ganglia. These ganglionated plexuses contain neuronal inputs from the atrial myocardium and the extrinsic cholinergic and adrenergic neurons. Between 6 and 10 collections of ganglia or ganglionated plexuses have been described in the human heart. Approximately half of the plexuses are located on the atria and the other half on the ventricles. Occasional ganglia are located in other atrial and ventricular regions of the epicardium. The ganglionated plexuses are generally associated with islands of adipose tissue referred to as fat pads that serve as visual landmarks to cardiac surgeons (**Figs. 35-12A and 35-12B**). The atrial fat pads are located in the interatrial groove, at the cavoatrial junctions, and on the left atrial wall in the vicinity of the venoatrial junctions. The ligament of Marshall is densely innervated with both parasympathetic and sympathetic inputs. During catheter ablation of AF, ablation of ganglionated plexi in the ligament of Marshal often results in vagal events during radiofrequency application.

The posterior and posterolateral surfaces of the left atrium and areas adjacent to the sinus and atrioventricular nodes have the largest populations of ganglia. The ganglia within each plexus are interconnected by thin nerves, whereas ganglia of adjacent plexuses are also interconnected, forming the meshwork of the epicardiac neural plexus. Further nerves penetrate into the myocardium to become thinner and thinner and devoid of ganglia. Autonomic influences from cardiac ganglia are known to exert important roles in both atrial and ventricular arrhythmogensis.

Conclusion

Whereas the structure of the human heart has not changed, understanding of its anatomy has evolved over time as electrophysiologic diagnostic and therapeutic strategies have evolved, each calling for a revisit of cardiac anatomy. In recent decades, the development of electrophysiologic mapping and catheter ablation techniques has outpaced the work of cardiac anatomists in many ways. Nevertheless, better understanding of detailed anatomy is relevant to clinical electrophysiologists, not only to improve outcomes and therapeutic efficacy and avoid or minimize complications during interventional procedures, but also to provide the anatomic background for different substrate and mechanisms behind many heart rhythm disorders.

MECHANISMS OF ARRHYTHMIAS AND CONDUCTION DISTURBANCES

Cardiac activation and repolarization are controlled by movement of ions across channels in the cell membrane of cardiomyocytes, which in turn are strongly influenced by the activity of the autonomic nervous system. Abnormal activity of these ionic movements is important in cardiac arrhythmogenesis. Arrhythmic activity can be categorized as passive (eg, atrioventricular [AV] block) or active. The mechanisms responsible for

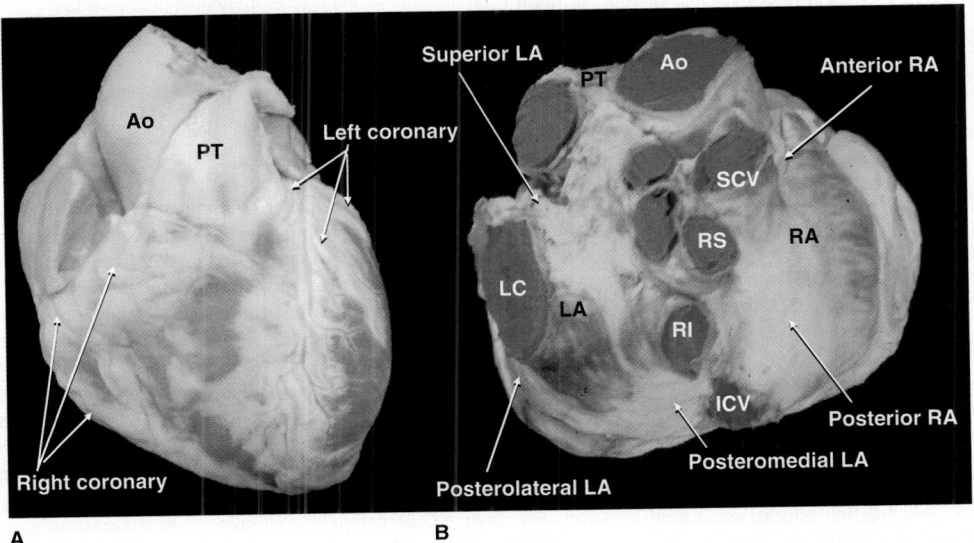

Figure 34–12. (A) Anterior view showing fat pads relating to coronary arteries. (B) Right posterior view of atrial fat pads and relationship to pulmonary veins and insertions of superior (SCV) and inferior (ICV) caval veins. Ao, aorta; LA, left atrium; RA, right atrium; PT, pulmonary trunk; LC, RI, and RS, left common, right inferior, and right superior pulmonary veins respectively.

active cardiac arrhythmias are generally divided into two major categories: (1) enhanced or abnormal impulse formation, and (2) reentry (**Fig. 34–13**). Reentry occurs when a propagating impulse fails to die out after normal activation of the heart and persists to reexcite the heart after expiration of the refractory period. Evidence implicating reentry as a mechanism of cardiac arrhythmias stems back to the turn of the last century. Multichannel mapping studies subsequently documented that reentrant wavefronts may underlie the mechanisms of atrial and ventricular tachyarrhythmias. *Phase 2 reentry, spiral waves of excitation, mother rotors, and fibrillatory conduction* are interesting concepts advanced to explain the development cardiac

fibrillation.[5] Mechanisms responsible for abnormal impulse formation include enhanced automaticity and triggered activity. Automaticity can be further subdivided into normal and abnormal. Triggered activity consists of: (1) early afterdepolarizations (EADs), (2) *late phase 3 EAD*, and (3) delayed afterdepolarizations (DADs). We will briefly discuss each of these factors below.

Abnormal Impulse Formation

Normal Automaticity

Automaticity is the property of cardiac cells to generate spontaneous action potentials. Spontaneous activity is the result of

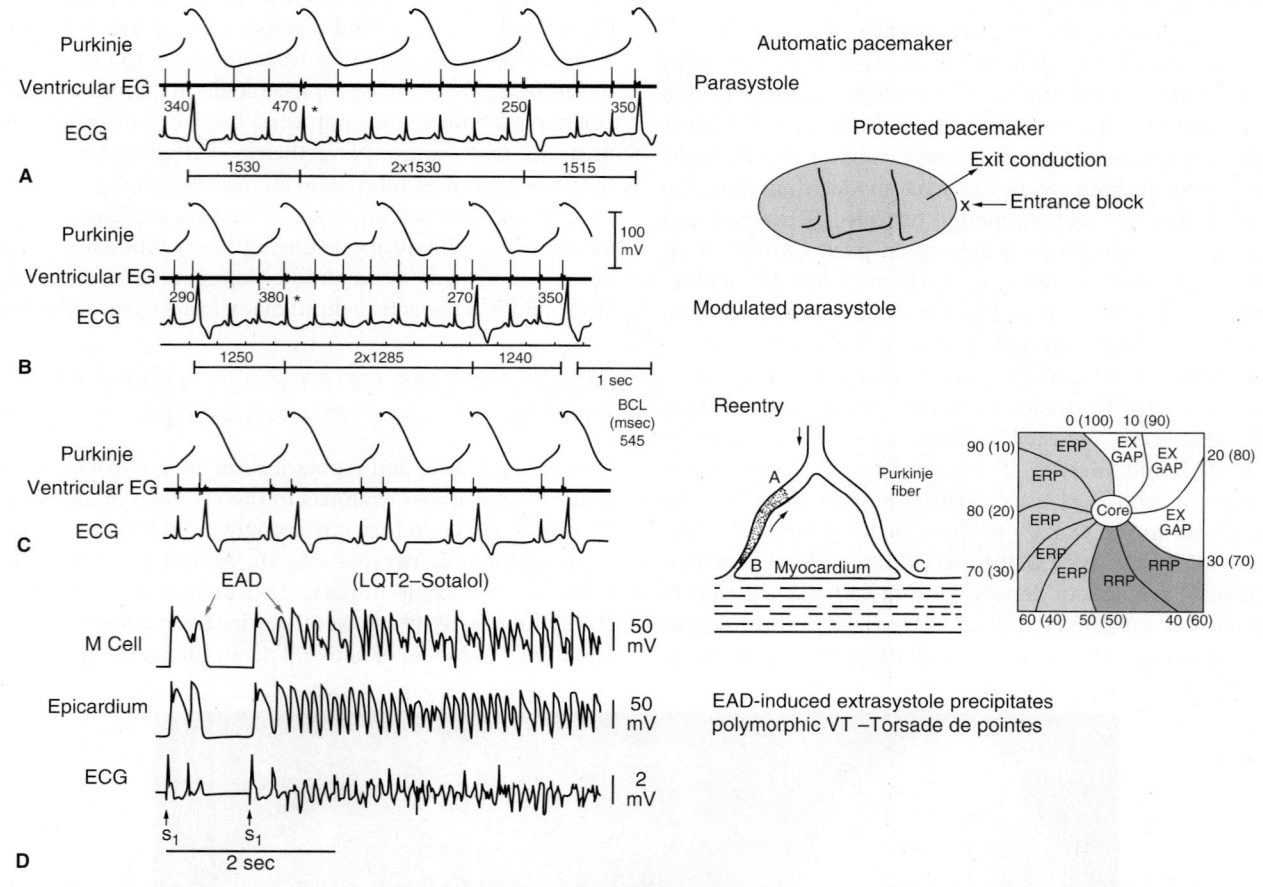

Figure 34–13. Examples of the main classes of active cardiac arrhythmias. (**A**) Automaticity. Shown is an example of an automatic pacemaker firing independently of ventricular activity. This classical parasystolic behavior is characterized by variable coupling intervals of the ectopic extrasystoles and inter ectopic intervals that are multiples of the pacemaker cycle length (1530 ms). Complete entrance block into the pacemaker focus is seen but unencumbered exit conduction out of the protected focus. (**B**) The pacemaker activity in the protected focus is electrotonically modulated by ventricular activity in this example. This modulated parasystolic activity is characterized by variable couple intervals at some rates (panel B) and fixed coupling intervals at select rates (panel C) due to the incomplete entrance block. (**C**) Reentry. Reentrant activity is characterized by fixed coupling intervals of the premature extrasystoles to the beat of sinus origin. Such activity can be due to modulated parasystole, to circus movement reentry with or without an anatomical obstacle, reflection or phase 2 reentry. The first schematic to the right illustrates reentry around an anatomical obstacle, in the Purkinje fiber-muscle junction. The one on the far right shows reentry around a functional obstacle. The number in the latter schematic represents the times (ms) of activation, while the number in the parenthesis is the times (ms) of recovery. Reentry may be associated with an excitable gap (EX GAP), a relative refractory period (RRP), and an effective refractory period (ERP). (**D**) Triggered activity. Shown is an example of sotalol-mediated early afterdepolarization (EAD)–induced triggered extrasystole giving rise to a polymorphic VT characteristic of TdP. In this experimental model of LQT2 (coronary-perfused wedge), the EAD generally arises from the M cell layer in the deep subendocardium of the ventricular wall. A-C, Reproduced with permission from Antzelevitch C, Bernstein MJ, Feldman HN, et al: Parasystole, reentry, and tachycardia: a canine preparation of cardiac arrhythmias occurring across inexcitable segments of tissue, *Circulation.* 1983 Nov;68(5):1101-1115. **D**, Reproduced with permission from Shimizu W, Antzelevitch C. Differential effects of beta-adrenergic agonists and antagonists in LQT1, LQT2 and LQT3 models of the long QT syndrome, *J Am Coll Cardiol.* 2000 Mar 1;35(3):7787-7786. **Square box far right side**, Reproduced with permission from Bonometti C, Hwang C, Hough D, et al: Interaction between strong electrical stimulation and reentrant wavefronts in canine ventricular fibrillation, *Circ Res.* 1995 Aug;77(2):407-716.

diastolic depolarization caused by a net inward current during phase 4 of the action potential, which progressively brings the membrane potential to threshold. The sinoatrial (SA) node normally displays the highest intrinsic rate. All other pacemakers are referred to as subsidiary or latent pacemakers because they take over the function of initiating excitation of the heart only when the SA node is unable to generate impulses or when these impulses fail to propagate. There is a hierarchy of intrinsic rates of subsidiary pacemakers that have normal automaticity: atrial pacemakers have faster intrinsic rates than AV junctional pacemakers, and AV junctional pacemakers have faster rates than ventricular pacemakers.

Wit and Cranefield[6] defined automatic activity as activity that arose in the absence of an external cause (ie, activity that did not have to be triggered by a stimulated action potential). The prototypical example of automaticity is the spontaneous beating of the SA node. On the other hand, triggered activity was the activity in which nondriven action potentials were initiated by one or more driven action potentials. The authors used the term "triggered" to explain the mechanisms by which quiescent fibers remained quiescent until driven at fast rate. However, more recent studies have shown that automaticity and triggered activity may share a common mechanism (ie, activation of the sodium–calcium exchange current [I_{NCX}]).

The Voltage Clock and Automaticity: Lakatta, Maltsev, and their collaborators used the terms *membrane clocks* and *calcium (Ca) clocks* to describe the mechanisms of SA node automaticity. These two clocks were mutually entrained to form a robust, stable, coupled-clock system that drives normal cardiac pacemaker cell automaticity. The membrane clock is formed by voltage-sensitive membrane currents, such as the hyperpolarization-activated pacemaker current (I_f). This current is also referred to as a "funny" current because, unlike the majority of voltage-sensitive currents, it is activated by hyperpolarization (from –40/–50 mV to –100/–110 mV) rather than depolarization. At the end of the action potential, the I_f is activated and is responsible for early diastolic depolarization that gradually depolarizes the sarcolemmal membrane. The I_f is a mixed sodium–potassium (Na–K) inward current modulated by the autonomic nervous system through cAMP. Sympathetic stimulation (isoproterenol) increases the I_f while parasympathetic stimulation (acetylcholine) reduces I_f. These findings suggest that I_f is responsible for heart rate control by the autonomic nervous system. The depolarization activates L-type Ca current ($I_{Ca,L}$) which provides Ca to activate the type 2 (cardiac) ryanodine receptor (RyR2). The activation of RyR2 initiates sarcoplasmic reticulum Ca release (Ca induced Ca release), leading to contraction of the heart, a process known as EC coupling. The intracellular Ca (Ca$_i$) is then pumped back into sarcoplasmic reticulum by the sarcoplasmic reticulum Ca-ATPase (SERCA2a), which completes this Ca cycle. Because of the discovery of I_f in cardiac pacemaking, the I_f current inhibitor ivabradine has been developed as a heart rate reducing agent.[7]

In addition to I_f, multiple time- and voltage-dependent ionic currents have been identified in cardiac pacemaker cells, which contribute to diastolic depolarization. These currents include (but are not limited to) I_{Ca-L}, T-type Ca current (I_{Ca-T}) and various types of delayed rectifier potassium currents. Many of these membrane currents are known to respond to β-adrenergic stimulation. All these membrane ionic currents contribute to the regulation of SA node automaticity by changing the membrane potential. In addition to the contribution of voltage-gated ionic currents, the small conductance Ca-activated K (SK) current also plays an important role in modulating automaticity both in the SA node and in the AV node.[8] The SK current could be a novel target for modulating the heart rate.

The Calcium Clock and Automaticity: The I_f is not the only depolarizing current active in late phase 3 or phase 4 of the action potential. Another important ionic current that can depolarize the cell is the I_{NCX}.[9] In its forward mode, the I_{NCX} exchanges 3 extracellular Na$^+$ with one intracellular Ca^{2+}, resulting in a net intracellular charge gain. This electrogenic current is active during late phase 3 and phase 4 because the Ca$_i$ decline outlasts the SA node action potential duration (APD). Multiple studies showed that I_{NCX} may participate in normal pacemaker activity. The sequence of events includes spontaneous rhythmic sarcoplasmic reticulum Ca release, Ca$_i$ elevation, the activation of I_{NCX}, and membrane depolarization. This process is highly regulated by the cAMP and the autonomic nervous system. Sympathetic stimulation accelerates heart rate by phosphorylation of proteins that regulate Ca$_i$ balance and spontaneous sarcoplasmic reticulum Ca cycling. These proteins include phospholamban (PLB, a sarcoplasmic reticulum membrane protein regulator of SERCA2a), L-type Ca channels, and RyR2. Phosphorylation of these proteins controls the phase and size of subsarcolemmal sarcoplasmic reticulum Ca releases. The resultant I_{NCX} is crucial for both basal and reserve cardiac pacemaker function. Spontaneous diastolic Ca^{2+} release and I_{NCX} activation also underlie the mechanisms of DADs and triggered activity,[10] the automaticity and triggered activity are in fact due to the same mechanism. The difference is that the nonpacemaking cells such as ventricular myocytes or Purkinje cells have a highly negative diastolic membrane potential that usually prevents DADs from reaching the threshold to cause triggered activity. On the other hand, the SA node had a less negative diastolic potential to begin with. It also develops spontaneous early diastolic depolarization due to the membrane clock. When DADs occur during late diastole, they reliably trigger a propagated depolarization. Nevertheless, DADs (without propagation) are occasionally observed in the canine SA node under the right experimental conditions.

Many studies on automaticity were performed in isolated SA node cells. However, the SA node is a complex structure and that many factors interact with each other to ensure the initiation of the heart beats. Activation maps in intact canine RA have shown that the SA node impulse origin is multicentric and sympathetic stimulation predictably results in a cranial (superior) shift of the pacemaking site in humans and dogs. Based on evidence from isolated SA node myocytes, late diastolic Ca$_i$ elevation prior to the membrane action potential upstroke is a key signature of pacemaking by the Ca clock. Simultaneous mapping of membrane potential and

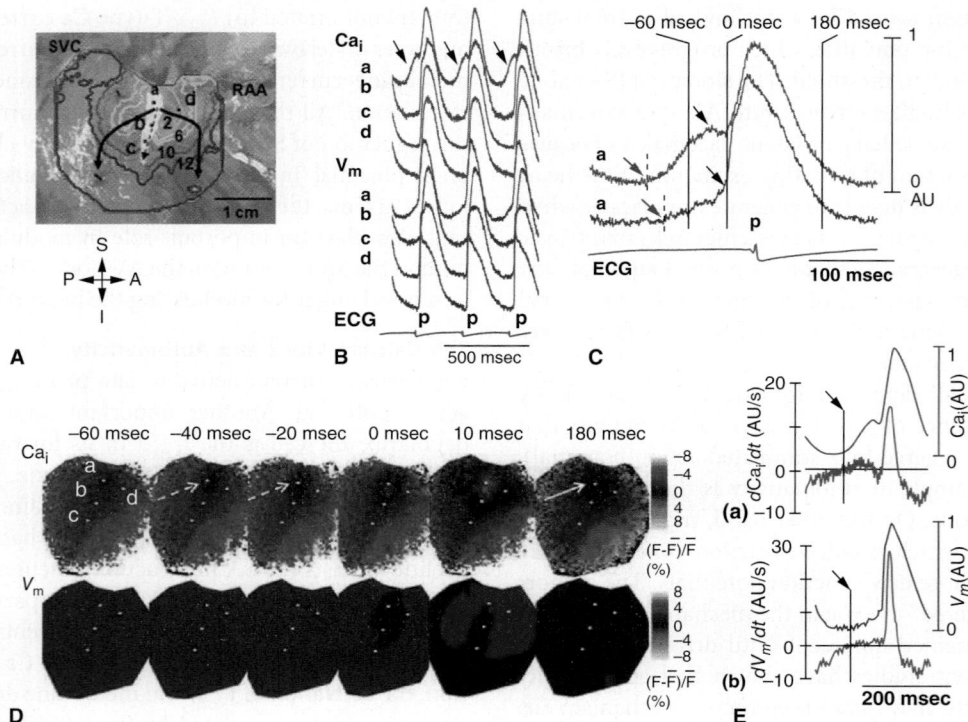

Figure 34–14. Activation pattern of sinoatrial (SA) node and surrounding RA during isoproterenol infusion of 0.3 μmol/L. This study was done in an isolated Langendorff-perfused RA preparation. (**A**) Isochronal map of V_m. The number on each isochronal line indicates time (ms). *White shaded area* is the SA node identified by the presence of spontaneous phase 4 depolarization. (**B**) The V_m (*blue*) and Ca_i (*red*) recordings from the superior (a), middle (b), inferior (c) SA node, and RA (d) presented in (**A**). (**C**) Magnified view of Ca_i and V_m tracings of superior SA node. Note the robust late diastolic Ca elevation before phase 0 of action potential (0 ms), which in turn was much earlier than onset of p wave on ECG. (**D**) The V_m and Ca_i ratio maps at times from –60 ms before to 180 ms after phase 0 AP of C. The late diastolic Ca^{2+} elevation (*broken arrows* in frame –40 and –20 ms) was followed by the Ca_i sinkhole during early diastole (*solid arrow* in frame 180 ms). (**E**) (a) Ca_i and dCa_i/dt. (b) V_m and dV_m/dt. The onset of late diastolic Ca^{2+} elevation and diastolic depolarization were (*arrows*) identified by the time when dCa_i/dt and dV_m/dt, respectively, crossed the baseline. Reproduced with permission from Joung B, Tang L, Maruyama M, et al: Intracellular calcium dynamics and acceleration of sinus rhythm by beta-adrenergic stimulation, *Circulation.* 2009 Feb 17;119(6):788-796.

Ca_i transient in Langendorff-perfused canine RA preparation showed changes consistent with Ca clock mechanism of impulse generation (**Figs. 34–14A** to **34–14E**). In that study, sympathetic stimulation (isoproterenol) induced spontaneous sarcoplasmic reticulum Ca release during phase 4 depolarization of intact canine SA node. The spontaneous Ca release then induces upward (cranial) shift of the leading pacemaker site and heart rate acceleration. Studies performed in human electrophysiological laboratories have confirmed the presence of multiple early sites in the right atrium during sinus rhythm, consistent with multicentric origin of SA nodal rhythm. In contrast, unresponsiveness of superior SA node to sympathetic stimulation is a characteristic finding in patients with AF and symptomatic bradycardia (**Figs. 34–15A** to **34–15C**).

Subsidiary Pacemakers: In addition to SA node, AV nodes and the Purkinje system are also capable of generating automatic activity. The contribution of I_f and I_K differs in SA node/AV nodes and Purkinje fiber because of the different potential ranges of these two pacemaker types (ie, –70 to –35 mV and –90 to –65 mV, respectively). The contribution of other voltage-dependent currents can also differ among the different cardiac cell types. Similar to the SA node, the Ca clock also contributes significantly to the automaticity of the AV node.

Cells in the SA node possess the fastest intrinsic rates. Thus, the SA node is the primary pacemaker in the normal heart. When impulse generation or conduction within or out of the SA node is impaired, latent or subsidiary pacemakers within the atria or ventricle are capable of taking control of pacing the heart. The intrinsically slower rates of these latent pacemakers result in bradycardia. Subsidiary atrial pacemakers with more negative diastolic potentials (–75 to –70 mV) than SA nodal cells are located at the junction of the inferior right atrium and the inferior vena cava, near or on the Eustachian ridge. Other atrial pacemakers have been identified in the crista terminalis, the orifice of the coronary sinus and in the atrial muscle that extends into the tricuspid and mitral valves. The cardiac muscle sleeves that extend into the cardiac veins (venae cavae and pulmonary veins) can also have the property of normal automaticity. Latent pacemaking cells in the AV junction are responsible for AV junctional rhythms. Both atrial and AV junctional subsidiary pacemakers are under autonomic control, with the sympathetic system increasing and parasympathetic system slowing the pacing rate.

The slowest subsidiary pacemakers are found in the His-Purkinje system in the ventricles of the heart.[11] In the His-Purkinje system, parasympathetic effects are less apparent than those of the sympathetic system. Although acetylcholine

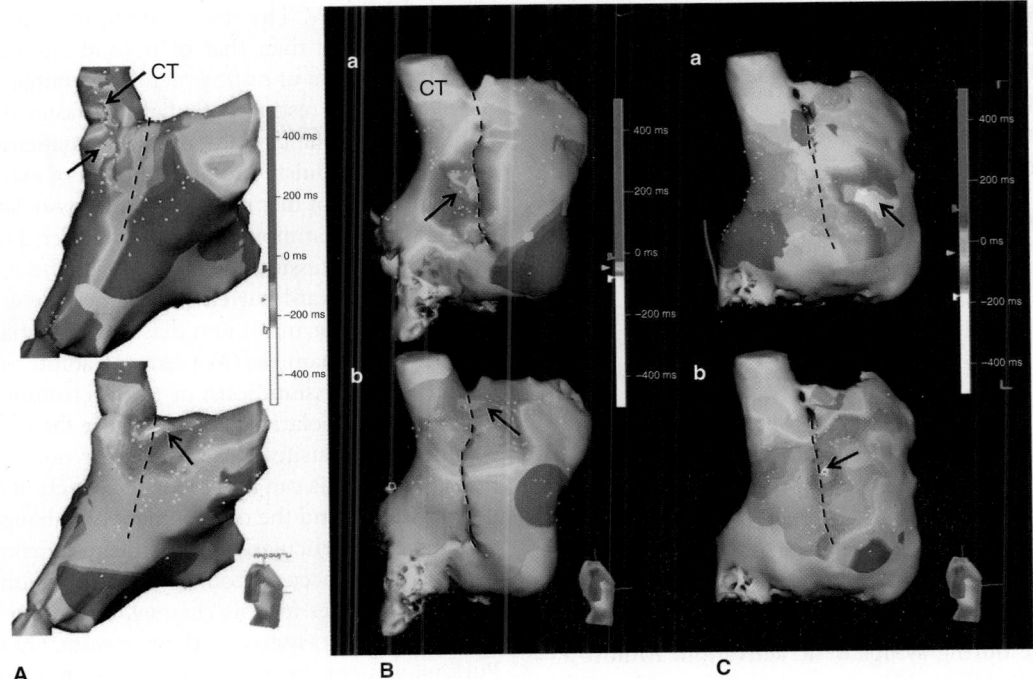

Figure 34–15. Effects of isoproterenol infusion on early activation site (EAS) in humans. (**A**) is from a patient without SA nodal diseases. The most cranial EAS at baseline (a) was in the superior vena cava (*arrows*). The EAS during isoproterenol infusion (b) was at the superior one-third of crista terminalis, consistently with cranial shift of pacemaking site. (**B**) Cranial shift of the EAS in a patient with AF but no symptomatic bradycardia. The EAS at baseline (a) and during isoproterenol infusion (b) were at the mid and superior part of crista terminalis, respectively. (**C**) Impaired cranial shift of the EAS in a patient with AF and symptomatic bradycardia. The EAS at baseline (a) was ectopic (at the right atrial free wall). The EAS during isoproterenol infusion (b) was located at the mid one-third of crista terminalis. The superior SA node in this patient was inactive with or without isoproterenol. The *dashed line* in each panel marks the crista terminalis.

produces little in the way of a direct effect, it can significantly reduce Purkinje automaticity by means of the inhibition of the sympathetic influence, a phenomenon termed *accentuated antagonism*. Simultaneous recording of cardiac sympathetic and parasympathetic activity in ambulatory dogs confirmed that sympathetic activation followed by vagal activation may be associated with profound bradycardia. Accentuated antagonism is also important in abnormal automaticity in the His-Purkinje system. Adenosine has no effects on His-Purkinje system activation rate at baseline, but reduces its activation rate during isoproterenol infusion. These findings suggest that adenosine's effects on the human His-Purkinje system are primarily antiadrenergic and are thus consistent with the concept of accentuated antagonism. These effects of adenosine may serve as a counter-regulatory metabolic response that improves the oxygen supply-demand ratio perturbed by enhanced sympathetic tone. Some catecholamine-mediated ventricular arrhythmias that occur during ischemia or enhanced adrenergic stress may be due to an imbalance in this negative feedback system.

Biological Pacemakers: Biological pacemakers, generated by somatic gene transfer, cell fusion, or cell transplantation, provide an alternative to electronic devices.[12] *The gene-based approach* uses gene therapy methods to suppress or activate ionic current, such as inward rectifier potassium current (I_{K1}) to enhance automaticity of ventricular myocytes. It is also possible to insert hyperpolarization-activated cyclic nucleotide-gated

(HCN) channels into cells using viral gene transfer, cell fusion, or stem cell technologies. Successful HCN expression in the myocytes leads to the activation of I_f, enabling nonpacemaking cells to generate automaticity. The *cell-based approaches* alter the gene expression during embryonic stem cell development to upregulate pacemaker gene program, and enhance automaticity.[13] *Hybrid gene-cell approaches* is the delivery of cells carrying pacemaker genes into the heart to generate biological pacemaker activity. *The somatic reprogramming approaches,* which involve transfer of genes encoding transcription factors to transform working myocardium into a surrogate sinoatrial node, are furthest along in the translational pipeline. In spite of these developments, the biological pacemakers are unlikely to compete with the electronic pacemakers in reliability, longevity, and programmability in the near future. More work is clearly needed before the biological pacemakers are clinically useful.

Automaticity as a Mechanism of Cardiac Arrhythmias
Abnormal automaticity includes both reduced automaticity, which causes bradycardia, and increased automaticity, which causes tachycardia. Arrhythmias caused by abnormal automaticity can result from diverse mechanisms (see Table 34–1). Alterations in sinus rate can be accompanied by shifts of the origin of the dominant pacemaker within the sinus node or to subsidiary pacemaker sites elsewhere in the atria. Impulse conduction out of the SA mode can be impaired or blocked as

a result of disease or increased vagal activity leading to development of bradycardia. AV junctional rhythms occur when AV junctional pacemakers located either in the AV node or in the His bundle accelerate to exceed the rate of SA node, or when the SA nodal activation rate was too slow to suppress the AV junctional pacemaker.

Hereditary Bradycardia: Bradycardia can occur in structurally normal hearts due to genetic mutations that result in abnormalities of either membrane clock or Ca clock mechanism of automaticity. One example is the mutation of subtype 4 of HCN channel (HCN4), which is part of the channels that carry I_f. Mutations of the HCN4 cause changes of the HCN4 channel expression and kinetics,[14] leading to familial bradycardia. However, the bradycardia caused by HCN4 mutations may be entirely asymptomatic. While HCN4 mutations cause baseline bradycardia, the heart rate responses to exercise may be either suboptimal with a maximum rate of 100 bpm or entirely normal with maximum rates of >150 bpm. The presence of normal heart rate response in patients with HCN4 mutation can be explained by the intact Ca clock, which can accelerate the sinus rate during sympathetic activation. Almost all of the ion channels affected by the various types of long QT syndrome (LQTS) gene mutations are also expressed in the human sinoatrial node. It is therefore not surprising that sinus bradycardia has been reported in relation to a large number of LQTS mutations, especially in patients with LQT3.[15] In addition to abnormal membrane ion currents, diseases associated with abnormal calcium handling may also be associated with sinus bradycardia. For example, catecholaminergic polymorphic ventricular tachycardia (CPVT) due to ryanodine receptor type 2 (RyR2) mutation is commonly associated with sinus bradycardia.

Secondary SA Node Dysfunction: Common diseases, such as heart failure and AF, may be associated with significant SA node dysfunction. Malfunction of membrane voltage clocks and Ca clocks might be both present in these common diseases. Zicha et al. reported that downregulation of HCN4 expression contributes to heart failure–induced sinus node dysfunction and upregulation of atrial HCN4 may help to promote atrial arrhythmia formation. Heart failure is also known to be associated with significant abnormalities of Ca_i regulation.[16] It is likely that abnormalities of both membrane voltage clock and Ca clock are responsible for the SA node dysfunction in heart failure. Similarly, AF is also associated with malfunction of both membrane and Ca clocks. The SA node malfunction is reversible after successful radiofrequency catheter ablation of AF, supporting the notion that AF is the cause of the sinus node dysfunction rather than the other way around.

Enhanced Automaticity: Atrial and ventricular myocardial cells do not display spontaneous diastolic depolarization or automaticity under normal conditions, but can develop these characteristics when depolarized, resulting in the development of repetitive impulse initiation, a phenomenon termed *depolarization-induced automaticity*. The membrane potential at which abnormal automaticity develops ranges between

–70 and –30 mV. The rate of abnormal automaticity is substantially higher than that of normal automaticity and is a sensitive function of resting membrane potential (ie, the more depolarized the resting potential, the faster the rate). Similar to normal automaticity, abnormal automaticity is enhanced by β-adrenergic agonists and by reduction of external potassium. Depolarization of membrane potential associated with disease states is most commonly a result of either: (1) an increase in extracellular potassium, which reduces the reversal potential for I_{K1}, the outward current that largely determines the resting membrane or maximum diastolic potential; (2) a reduced number of I_{K1} channels; (3) a reduced ability of the I_{K1} channel to conduct potassium ions; or (4) electrotonic influence of a neighboring depolarized zone. Because the conductance of I_{K1} channels is a sensitive to extracellular potassium concentration, hypokalemia can lead to major reduction in I_{K1}, leading to depolarization and the development of enhanced or abnormal automaticity, particularly in Purkinje pacemakers. A reduction in I_{K1} can also occur secondary to a mutation in *KCNJ2*, the gene that encodes for this channel, leading to increased automaticity and extrasystolic activity presumably arising from the Purkinje system. Interestingly, because β-adrenergic stimulation is effective in augmenting I_{K1}, sympathetic stimulation can produce a paradoxical slowing of automaticity and ectopy in this setting.

Autonomic Mechanisms SA Nodal Tachycardia and Atrial Tachycardia: Normal or subsidiary pacemaker activity can also be enhanced, leading to sinus tachycardia or a shift to ectopic sites within the atria, giving rise to atrial tachycardia. One cause can be abnormal autonomic nerve activity, including sympathetic activation and parasympathetic withdrawal. Direct recording from the stellate ganglion and vagal nerves show that stellate ganglion nerve activity (SGNA) and vagal nerve activity (VNA) are both important in controlling sinus rate and in triggering atrial tachycardia in ambulatory dogs. **Figures 34–16A** and **34–16B** show an example of heart rate acceleration induced by SGNA. The SGNA consists of two types of activity. The vast majority of activity was in the form of low amplitude burst discharge activity (LABDA). A second form of activity is the high amplitude spike discharge activity (HASDA), which occurs less than 10 times daily in normal dogs and the incidence may more than double in dogs with heart failure or myocardial infarction. Vagal nerve activation, on the other hand, induces sinus bradycardia. **Figure 34–17** shows an example of bradycardia associated with increased vagal nerve activity. The same figure shows that simultaneous sympathovagal discharges are common triggers of atrial tachyarrhythmia. It is difficult to directly record vagal nerve activity in humans. However, it is possible to record skin sympathetic nerve activity (SKNA) using standard electrocardiogram (ECG) patch electrodes.[17,18] Consistent with the results of the canine studies, the SKNA recordings showed active SKNA prior to the onset of human atrial tachycardia episodes[19] (**Figs. 34–18A** and **34–18B**). In addition, there is SKNA discharges immediately prior to termination of the atrial tachycardia in that same patient. These findings indicate that sympathetic nerve activities are important both in the initiation

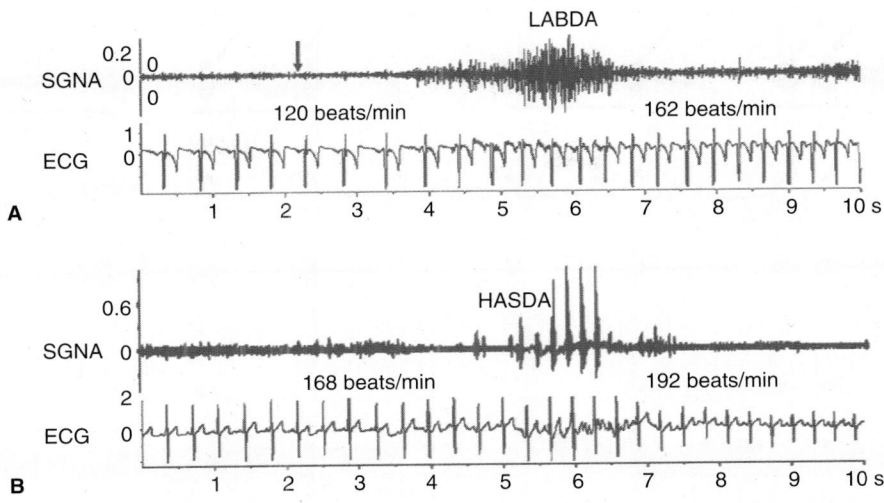

Figure 38-16. Sympathetic control of heart rate. Stellate ganglion nerve activity (SGNA) was recorded simultaneously with electrocardiogram (ECG) in a normal ambulatory dog with an implanted radiotransmitter. (**A**) shows low amplitude burst discharge activity (LABDA), which induced heart rate acceleration. (**B**) shows high amplitude spike discharge activity (HASDA) that occurred during LABDA. HASDA further accelerated the heart rate. The unit for SGNA and ECG is mV. bpm. Reproduced with permission from Zhou S, Jung BC, Tan AY, et al: Spontaneous stellate ganglion nerve activity and ventricular arrhythmia in a canine model of sudden death, *Heart Rhythm.* 2008 Jan;5(1):131-139.

and termination of atrial tachycardia in canine models and in humans.

Overdrive Suppression of Automaticity: The automaticity of all pacemakers within the heart is inhibited when they are overdrive paced. This inhibition is called *overdrive suppression*. Under normal condition, all subsidiary pacemakers are overdrive-suppressed by SA nodal activity. The mechanisms of overdrive suppression are thought to be related to pacing-induced intracellular accumulation of Ca and Na. The Na accumulation leads to enhanced activity of the sodium pump (sodium–potassium adenosine triphosphatase [Na+–K+ ATPase]), which generates a hyperpolarizing electrogenic current that opposes phase 4 depolarization. The faster the overdrive rate or the longer the duration of overdrive, the greater the enhancement of sodium pump activity, so that the period of quiescence after cessation of overdrive is directly related to the rate and duration of overdrive.

Parasystole and Modulated Parasystole
Latent pacemakers throughout the heart are generally reset by the propagating wavefront initiated by the dominant pacemaker and are therefore unable to activate the heart. An exception to

this rule occurs when the pacemaking tissue is protected from the impulse of sinus origin. A region of entrance block arises when cells exhibiting automaticity are surrounded by ischemic, infarcted, or otherwise compromised cardiac tissues that prevent the propagating wave from invading the focus, but which permit the spontaneous beat generated within the automatic focus to exit and activate the rest of the myocardium. A pacemaker region exhibiting entrance block and exit conduction defines a parasystolic focus. The ectopic activity generated by a parasystolic focus is characterized by premature ventricular complexes with variable coupling intervals, fusion beats, and interectopic intervals that are multiples of a common denominator.

Afterdepolarization and Triggered Activity
Oscillatory depolarizations that attend or follow the cardiac action potential and depend on preceding transmembrane activity for their manifestation are referred to as *afterdepolarizations*. Two subclasses are traditionally recognized: (1) early and (2) delayed. EADs interrupt or retard repolarization during phase 2 and/or phase 3 of the cardiac action potential, whereas DADs occur after full repolarization. When EAD or

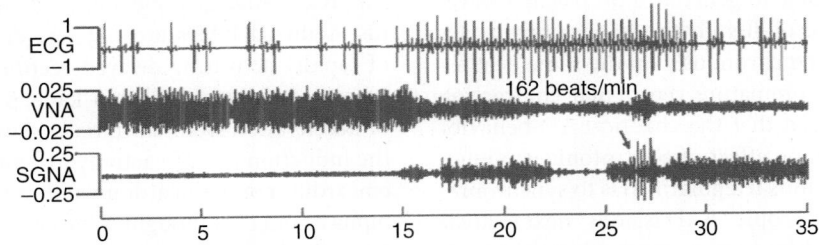

Figure 38-17. Vagal control of heart rate. This figure was obtained from a normal ambulatory dog with implanted transmitter. Vagal nerve activity (VNA) is associated with slow heart rate response (left part of the figure) while sympathovagal coactivation was associated with atrial tachycardia, followed by irregular heartbeats and sinus bradycardia toward the end of the tracing. *Arrows* point to an episode of HASDA amid continuous LABDA. Reproduced with permission from Ogawa M, Zhou S, Tan AY, et al: Left stellate ganglion and vagal nerve activity and cardiac arrhythmias in ambulatory dogs with pacing-induced congestive heart failure, *J Am Coll Cardiol.* 2007 Jul 24;50(4):335-343.

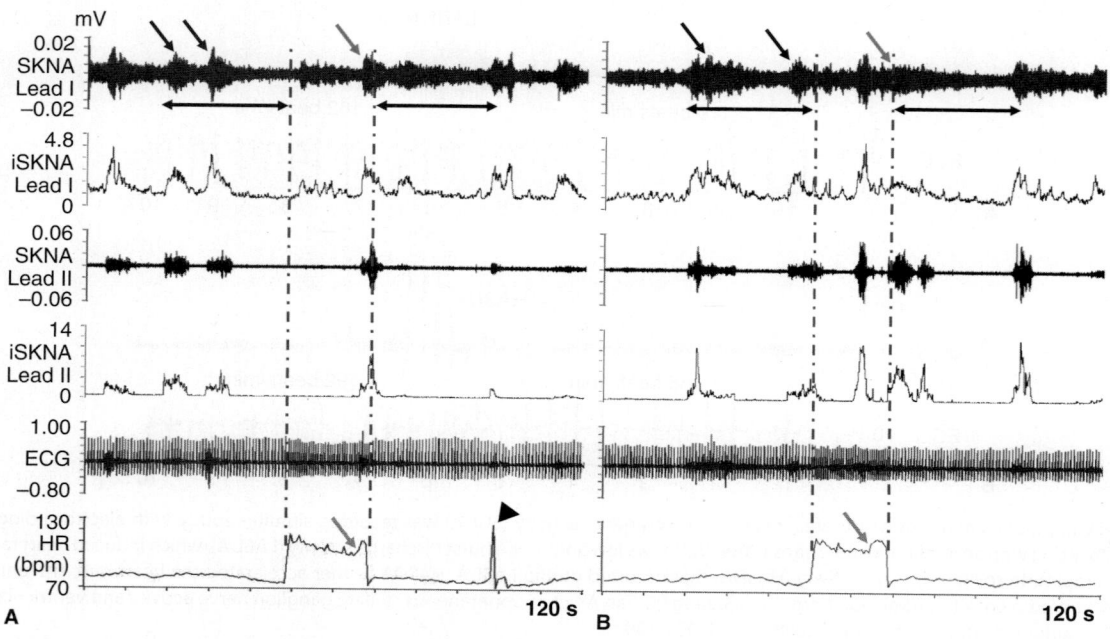

Figure 38-18. Skin sympathetic nerve activity (SKNA) characteristics before onset and after termination of atrial tachycardia. Signals were bandpass filtered from 500 Hz to 1000 Hz to reveal SKNA and from 0.5 Hz to 150 Hz to reveal ECG. Integrated SKNA (iSKNA) was obtained by integrating the voltage of digitized data over 100 ms windows. **(A)** Multiple episodes of SKNA bursts (*black arrows*) were present within 30 s (*double-headed arrows*) prior to atrial tachycardia onset. Heart rate acceleration (*green arrows*) associated with SKNA burst (*blue arrows*) was observed prior to atrial tachycardia termination (*red dotted line*). This phenomenon was present in all 32 atrial tachycardia termination episodes analyzed for this patient. SKNA continues to be elevated during the 30 s after termination. SKNA was also increased during premature atrial contraction (*arrowhead*). **(B)** Similar findings in a separate atrial tachycardia episode, consistent with **(A)**. Reproduced with permission from Uradu A, Wan J, Doytchinova et al: Skin sympathetic nerve activity precedes the onset and termination of paroxysmal atrial tachycardia and fibrillation, *Heart Rhythm.* 2017 Jul;14(7):964-971.

DAD amplitude suffices to bring the membrane to its threshold potential, a spontaneous action potential referred to as a triggered response is the result. These triggered events can be responsible for extrasystoles and tachyarrhythmias that develop under conditions predisposing to the development of afterdepolarizations.

Early Afterdepolarizations and Triggered Activity: EADs generally occurs when the APD is prolonged. They are observed in isolated cardiac tissues exposed to injury, altered electrolytes, hypoxia, acidosis, catecholamines, and pharmacologic agents, including antiarrhythmic drugs. Congenital LQTS, ventricular hypertrophy, and heart failure also predispose to the development of EADs. However, because of source–sink mismatch in well-coupled cardiac tissues, it is unlikely that the EAD of a single cardiomyocyte will be able to generate a propagated wavefront. Rather, a critical mass of literally thousands of myocytes needs to develop an EAD synchronously on the same beat for an overt EAD to trigger a premature ventricular contraction (PVC). Weiss et al. proposed that the chaotic EAD behavior combined with the smoothing effect of electrotonic gap junction coupling normally permits irregular EADs to synchronize regionally, producing macroscopic "EAD islands" next to areas without EADs. This synchronization mechanism produces shifting focal activations, mixed with reentry, which arise suddenly from normal or bradycardic heart rates and produce characteristic features of polymorphic and torsades de pointes (TdP) VT.

EAD characteristics vary as a function of animal species, tissue, or cell type, and the method by which the EAD is elicited. Although specific mechanisms of EAD induction can differ, a critical prolongation of repolarization accompanies most, but not all, EADs. Drugs that block potassium currents may reduce repolarization reserve, and predispose the cells to EADs. **Figures 34–19A** to **34–19C** illustrate the two types of EAD generally encountered in Purkinje fibers. Oscillatory events appearing at potentials positive to –30 mV, are generally referred to as phase 2 EADs. Those occurring at more negative potentials are termed phase 3 EADs. Phase 2 and phase 3 EADs sometimes appear in the same preparation.

EAD-induced triggered activity is sensitive to stimulation rate. Antiarrhythmic drugs with class III action generally induce EAD activity at slow stimulation rates and totally suppress EADs at rapid rates. In contrast, β-adrenergic agonist–induced EADs are fast rate-dependent. In the presence of rapidly activating delayed rectifier current (rapid outward potassium current [I_{Kr}]) blockade, β-adrenergic agonists, and/or acceleration from an initially slow rate transiently facilitate the induction of EAD activity in ventricular M cells, but not in epicardium or endocardium and rarely in Purkinje fibers. This biphasic effect is thought to be caused by an initial priming of I_{NCX}, which provides an electrogenic inward current that facilitates EAD development and prolongs APD. This early phase is followed by recruitment of slowly activating delayed rectifier current (slow outward potassium current [I_{Ks}]), which abbreviates APD and suppresses EAD activity.

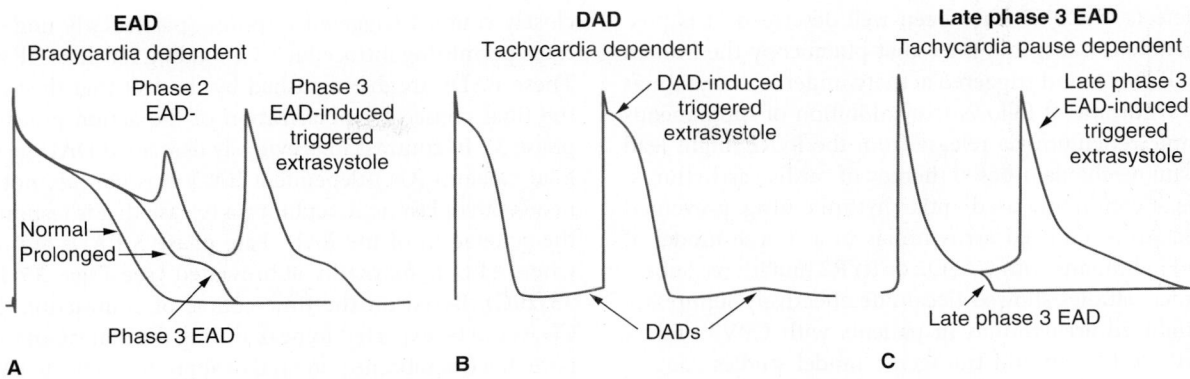

Figure 38-19. Examples of EAD, DAD, and late phase 3 EAD.

Cellular Origin of Early Afterdepolarizations: EADs develop more in midmyocardial M cells and Purkinje fibers than in epicardial or endocardial cells when exposed to APD-prolonging agents. This is in part due to the presence of a weaker I_{Ks} and the apamin-sensitive small conductance calcium activated potassium (I_{KAS}) in M cells. Because I_{KAS} current is low, the M cell myocytes are not able to shorten the APD in conditions associated with increased Ca_i. The reduced I_{KAS} current can therefore contribute to the development of EADs in the M cells. Chromanol 293B, which blocks both the I_{Ks} and the I_{KAS}, permits the induction of EADs in canine epicardial and endocardial tissues in response to I_{Kr} blockers such as E-4031 or sotalol. The predisposition of cardiac cells to the development of EADs depends principally on the reduced availability of I_{Kr}, I_{Ks}, and I_{KAS} as occurs in many forms of cardiomyopathy and heart failure. Under these conditions, EADs can appear in any part of the ventricular myocardium.

Ionic Mechanisms Responsible for the EAD: An EAD occurs when the balance of current active during phase 2 or 3 of the action potential shifts in the inward direction. If the change in current-voltage relation results in a region of net inward current during the plateau range of membrane potentials, it leads to a depolarization or EAD. Most pharmacological interventions or pathophysiological conditions associated with EADs can be categorized as acting predominantly through one of four different mechanisms: (1) a reduction of repolarizing potassium currents (I_{Kr}, class IA and III antiarrhythmic agents; I_{Ks}, chromanol 293B or I_{K1}); (2) an increase in the availability of calcium current (Bay K 8644, catecholamines); (3) an increase in the I_{NCX} caused by augmentation of Ca_i activity or upregulation of the I_{NCX}; and (4) an increase in late Na current (I_{NaL}) (aconitine, anthoplexurin-A, and ATX-II). Combinations of these interventions (ie, calcium loading and I_{Kr} reduction) or pathophysiological states can act synergistically to facilitate the development of EADs.

A sustained component of sodium channel current (I_{Na}) active during the action potential plateau, originating from channels that fail to inactivate and a nonequilibrium component arising from channels recovering from inactivation during phases 2 and 3, has been shown to contribute prominently the APD and induction of EADs. Reactivation of $I_{Ca,L}$ may contribute to the development of EADs when there was persistent late I_{Na} and reduced repolarization reserve. Calcium-calmodulin kinase II (CaMKII) has been linked to the development of EAD in mouse models of cardiac hypertrophy. Ranolazine, which suppresses late I_{Na}, is a promising antiarrhythmic agent.[20,21]

Delayed Afterdepolarization-Induced Triggered Activity: DADs occur because of spontaneous sarcoplasmic reticulum Ca release, which activates the I_{NCX} and result in oscillations of transmembrane potentials that occur after full repolarization of the action potential. When there is spontaneous sarcoplasmic reticulum Ca release, it activates the I_{NCX} and depolarizes the cell membrane. DADs may reach the threshold and give rise to spontaneous action potentials generally referred to as triggered activity. However, whether or not spontaneous sarcoplasmic reticulum Ca releases can cause a DAD depends in part on the cell type. Maruyama et al. used the term "diastolic Ca_i-voltage coupling gain" to describe membrane potential (V_m) responses to elevated Ca_i during diastole. This concept is based on the finding that the same magnitude of sarcoplasmic reticulum Ca release may induce DADs in the Purkinje fibers but not in the epicardial cells. The reduced I_{K1} in the Purkinje cells was thought to underlie the higher diastolic Ca_i-voltage coupling gain than other myocardial cells. As discussed, recent studies suggest that rhythmic spontaneous sarcoplasmic reticulum Ca release (Ca clock) is also a mechanism of SA nodal automaticity. Therefore, while spontaneous sarcoplasmic reticulum Ca release is an arrhythmogenic mechanism, it also contributes significantly to the normal automaticity.

Role of Delayed Afterdepolarization-Induced Triggered Activity in the Development of Cardiac Arrhythmias: An excellent example of DAD-induced arrhythmia is CPVT, which may be caused by mutation of the type 2 ryanodine receptor (RyR2), calsequestrin (CSQ2), *CALM1*, and *CALM2*. The fundamental mechanism of these arrhythmias is the "leaky" ryanodine receptor, which is aggravated during catecholamine stimulation to induce DADs. A typical clinical phenotype of CPVT is bidirectional VT, which is also seen in digitalis toxicity and long QT type 7 (KCNJ2 mutation). Alternans of Ca_i may play a role in the development of bidirectional VT. Because the genetic defects of CPVT have been well described, it is possible to generate transgenic mice that phenocopy the human genotype. If DADs and triggered activity underlie arrhythmias in CPVT syndrome, it follows that inhibition of spontaneous sarcoplasmic reticulum Ca release from the RyR2 might lead to successful mechanism-based therapy of cardiac arrhythmia. Flecainide, a commonly used antiarrhythmic drug, prevented adrenergic stress–induced arrhythmias in a mouse model of CPVT and in humans with CASQ2 or RYR2 mutations. Subsequent clinical studies showed flecainide effectively suppresses exercise-induced arrhythmias in patients with CPVT. Taken together, these human and transgenic model studies suggest that spontaneous sarcoplasmic reticulum Ca release, DAD and triggered arrhythmias underlie the mechanisms of CPVT. However, in order for DAD to induce triggered activity, there is a need for Na channel activation. Therefore, the effects of flecainide in suppressing CPVT could also be explained by its action on Na channels.[22] Other studies indicate that the epicardial origin of these ectopic beats increases transmural dispersion of repolarization, thus providing the substrate for the development of reentrant tachyarrhythmias, which underlie rapid polymorphic VT/ventricular fibrillation (VF). In addition to CPVT, DADs may also contribute significantly to arrhythmogenesis in common arrhythmias, such as premature ventricular contractions from the peri-infarct zone in rabbit hearts with subacute myocardial infarction. Heart failure is associated with structural and electrophysiological remodeling, leading to tissue heterogeneity that enhances arrhythmogenesis and the propensity of sudden cardiac death (SCD). The mechanisms of arrhythmogenesis in heart failure may be attributed to the upregulation of I_{NCX} activity, abnormal Ca_i handling, and non-reentrant ventricular arrhythmias due to triggered activity. DADs occur in heart failure due to sarcoplasmic reticulum Ca overload and spontaneous sarcoplasmic reticulum Ca release that activates electrogenic I_{NCX} during phase 4 of the action potential. Because DADs are often induced by rapid activation and Ca_i accumulation, the best time to observe DADs is at the cessation of rapid pacing or tachycardia such as immediately after ventricular defibrillation. **Figures 34–20A** to **34–20F** show an example of spontaneous VF in a Langendorff-perfused failing heart. Figure 34–20A shows a baseline recording. The arrow in Fig. 34–20C shows spontaneous Ca_i elevation, associated with a DAD on the epicardium.

Late Phase 3 Early Afterdepolarizations and Their Role in the Initiation of Cardiac Fibrillation: Figures 34–20C and 34–20D show Vm and Cai at termination and at the onset of spontaneous VF, respectively. Note the presence of short APD in the immediate postshock period (Fig. 34–20C) and that the first ectopic beat that initiated VF occurred from late phase 3 of the preceding action potential (Fig. 34–20D). The mechanism of VF is best explained by the late phase 3 EAD and triggered activity. This arrhythmogenic mechanism combines properties of both EAD and DAD, but has its own unique character (Fig. 34–19C). Late phase 3 EAD-induced triggered extrasystoles occur because abbreviated repolarization permits *normal sarcoplasmic reticulum Ca release* to induce an EAD-mediated

closely coupled triggered response, particularly under conditions permitting intracellular Ca loading (such as AF and VF). These EADs are distinguished by the fact that they interrupt the final phase of repolarization of the action potential (late phase 3). In contrast to previously described DAD or intracellular calcium (Ca_i)-dependent EAD, it is *normal,* not spontaneous sarcoplasmic reticulum Ca release that is responsible for the generation of the EAD. Late phase 3 EADs are observed when APD is markedly abbreviated (see **Figs. 35-19C** and **35-20C**). Based on the time-course of contraction, levels of Ca_i would be expected to peak during the plateau of the action potential (membrane potential of approximately –5 mV) under control conditions but during the late phase of repolarization (membrane potential of approximately –70 mV) when there is an abbreviated APD. As a consequence, the two principal Ca-mediated currents—I_{NCX} and calcium-activated chloride conductance ($I_{Cl(Ca)}$)—would be expected to be weakly inward or even outward ($I_{Cl(Ca)}$) when APD is normal (control), but strongly inward when APD is very short (such as during acetylcholine infusion). Thus, abbreviation of the atrial APD allows for a much stronger recruitment of both I_{NCX} and $I_{Cl(Ca)}$ in the generation of late phase 3 EADs. In the isolated canine atria, late phase 3 EAD-induced extrasystoles have been shown to initiate AF, immediately following the termination of the arrhythmia. The same mechanisms may play an important role in the development of triggered activity within the pulmonary veins, where the APD is short even at baseline. In addition to the atrial arrhythmias, late phase 3 EAD may also be responsible for the development of recurrent VF in failing hearts. As shown in Figs. 34–20A to 34–20F, Langendorff-perfused failing hearts develop acute and transient APD shortening immediately after successful defibrillation. Because of Ca_i accumulation during fibrillation, a combination of short APD and large Ca_i allows late phase 3 EAD to occur. Subsequent studies showed that I_{KAS} is upregulated during heart failure and may play an important role in modulating cardiac memory.[23] VF results in the Ca_i elevation, which activates I_{KAS} and shortens the postshock APD. A combination of high Ca_i and short APD results in spontaneous VF as shown in Figs. 34–20A to 34–20F. Apamin, a specific blocker of I_{KAS}, prevents the spontaneous recurrences of VF. Therefore, in addition to recurrent atrial arrhythmias, late phase 3 EADs may also be the mechanism responsible for ventricular arrhythmias associated with heart failure.

Reentrant Arrhythmias

Reentry is a fundamentally different mechanism of arrhythmogenesis than automaticity or triggered activity. Circus movement reentry occurs when an activation wavefront propagates around an anatomical or functional core, and reexcites the site of origin. In this type of reentry, all cells recover from excitation and are ready to be excited again when the next wavefront arrives. In comparison, reflection and phase 2 reentry occur when there are large differences of recovery from one site to another. The site with delayed recovery serves as a virtual electrode that excites its already recovered neighbor, resulting in

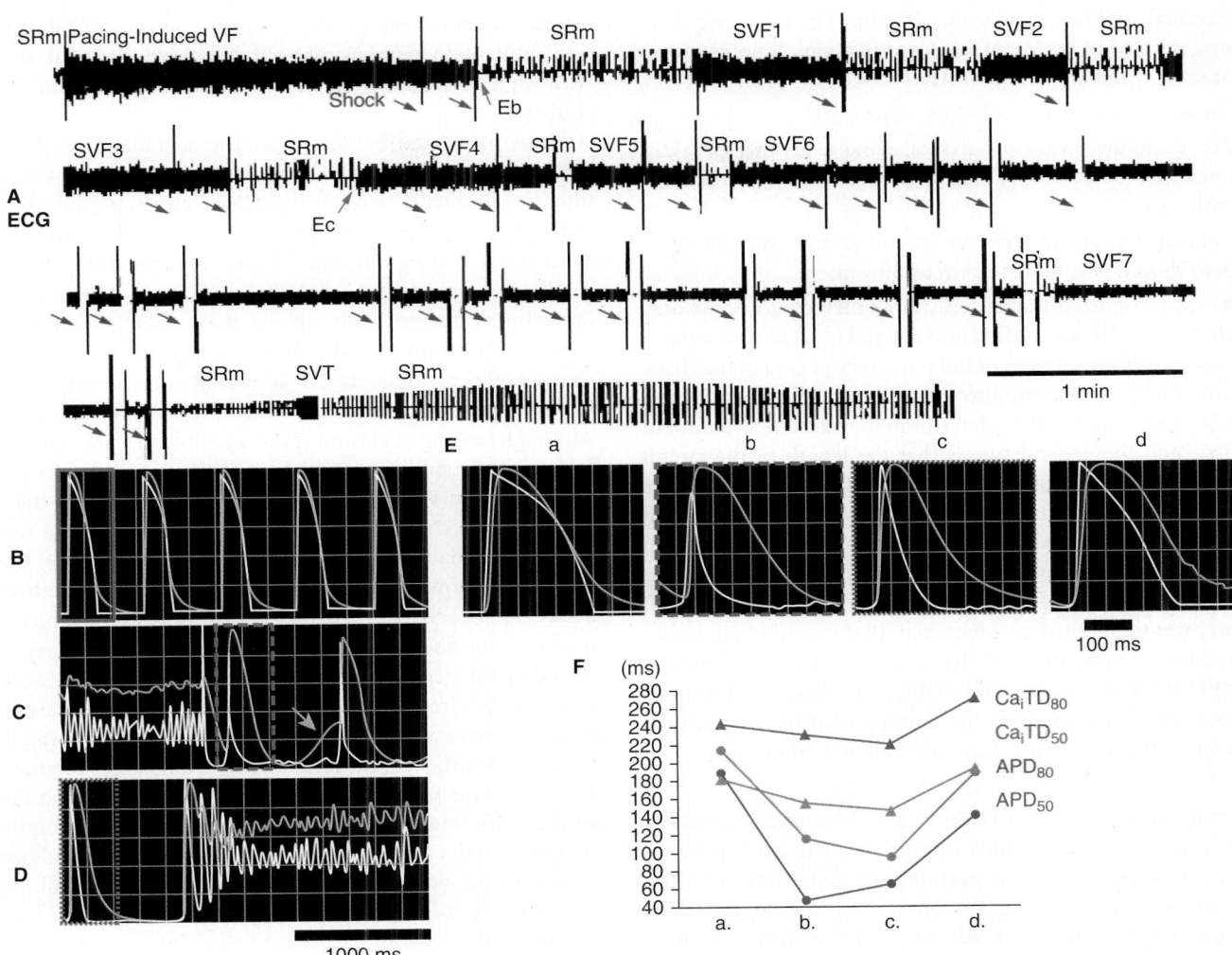

Figure 34–20. Ventricular fibrillation (VF) storm in a failing heart. A total of seven episodes of spontaneous VF occurred within 20 minutes after initial successful defibrillation. (**A**) Continuous recording of pseudo-ECG. (**B**) Baseline membrane potential (Vm, *white line*) and intracellular calcium (Ca$_i$, *yellow line*) recordings. (**C**) and (**D**) Vm and Ca$_i$ at termination and at onset of spontaneous VF, respectively. Note presence of spontaneous Ca$_i$ elevation with DAD (*arrow*) and short action potential duration (APD) in the immediate postshock period (**C**) and that the first ectopic beat that initiated VF occurred from late phase 3 of the preceding action potential (**D**). Tracings in red boxes in (**B–D**) are also shown in (**E**), which highlights the Vm and Ca$_i$ changes at different time points during the study. There was transient shortening of APD and, to a lesser extent, Ca$_i$ transient duration after defibrillation. (**F**) Measurements of APD and Ca$_i$ transient duration, showing the transient nature of these changes. Time points (b) and (c) are marked as Eb and Ec, respectively, in (**A**). Time points (a) and (d) are from baseline and 31 minutes after the last episode of spontaneous VF, respectively. Time point (d) is outside of the range and is not part of the figure. SRm, sinus rhythm. Reproduced with permission from Ogawa M, Morita N, Tang L: Mechanisms of recurrent ventricular fibrillation in a rabbit model of pacing-induced heart failure, *Heart Rhythm.* 2009 Jun;6(6):784-792.

reentry. A circus movement is not observed. In addition, reentry can also be classified as anatomical and functional, although there is a gray zone in which both functional and anatomical factors are important in determining the characteristics of reentrant excitation.

Circus Movement Reentry Around an Anatomical Obstacle

The ring model is the prototypical example of reentry around an anatomical obstacle. It first emerged as a concept at the beginning of the 20th century, when Mayer reported the results of experiments involving the subumbrella tissue of a jellyfish (*Sychomedusa cassiopeia*). The muscular disk did not contract until ring-like cuts were made and pressure and a stimulus applied. This caused the disc to "spring into rapid rhythmical

pulsation so regular and sustained as to recall the movement of clockwork."[24] His experiments proved valuable in identifying two fundamental conditions necessary for the initiation and maintenance of circus movement excitation: (1) unidirectional block—the impulse initiating the circulating wave must travel in one direction only; and (2) for the circus movement to continue, the circuit must be long enough to allow each site in the circuit to recover before the return of the circulating wave. GR Mines[25] was the first to develop the concept of circus movement reentry as a mechanism responsible for cardiac arrhythmias. The clinical importance of reentry was reinforced with the discovery by Kent of an accessory pathway connecting the atrium and ventricle of a human heart, and that successful surgical ablation of the accessory pathway results in the cure of the paroxysmal supraventricular tachycardia. The following three criteria developed by Mines for identification of circus movement reentry remains in use today:

1. An area of unidirectional block must exist.
2. The excitatory wave progresses along a distinct pathway, returning to its point of origin and then following the same path again.
3. Interruption of the reentrant circuit at any point along its path should terminate the circus movement.

It was recognized that successful reentry could occur only when the impulse was sufficiently delayed in an alternate pathway to allow for expiration of the refractory period in the tissue proximal to the site of unidirectional block. Both conduction velocity and refractoriness determine the success or failure of reentry, and the general rule is that the length of the circuit (pathlength) must exceed or equal that of the wavelength, the wavelength being defined as the product of the conduction velocity and the refractory period or that part of the pathlength occupied by the impulse and refractory to reexcitation. The theoretical minimum path length required for development of reentry was therefore dependent on both the conduction velocity and the refractory period. Reduction of conduction velocity or APD can both significantly reduce the theoretical limit of the pathlength required for the development of reentry, thus facilitating the development of reentrant arrhythmias.

Circus Movement Reentry Without an Anatomical Obstacle

That reentry could be initiated without the involvement of anatomic obstacles and that "natural rings are not essential for the maintenance of circus contractions"[26] was first suggested by Garrey in 1914. Years later, Allessie and coworkers provided direct evidence in support of this hypothesis in experiments in which they induced a tachycardia in isolated preparations of rabbit left atria by applying properly timed premature extrastimuli. Using multiple intracellular electrodes, they showed that although the basic beats elicited by stimuli applied near the center of the tissue spread normally throughout the preparation, premature impulses propagate only in the direction of shorter refractory periods. An arc of block thus develops around which the impulse is able to circulate and reexcite its site of origin. Recordings near the center of the circus movement showed only subthreshold responses. The authors proposed the term *leading circle* to explain their observation. They argued that the functionally refractory region that develops at the vortex of the circulating wavefront prevents the centripetal waves from short-circuiting the circus movement and thus serves to maintain the reentry. The authors also proposed that the refractory core was maintained by centripetal wavelets that collide with each other. Because the head of the circulating wavefront usually travels on relatively refractory tissue, a fully excitable gap of tissue may not be present; unlike other forms of reentry, the leading circle model may not be readily influenced by extraneous impulses initiated in areas outside the reentrant circuit and thus may not be easily entrained. Although leading circle reentry for a while was widely accepted as a mechanism of functional reentry, there is significant conceptual limitation

to this model of reentry. For example, the centripetal wavelet was difficult to demonstrate either by experimental studies with high resolution mapping or with computer simulation studies.[27]

First introduced by Wiener and Rosenblueth in 1946, the concept of spiral waves (rotors) has attracted a great deal of interest. Originally used to describe reentry around an anatomic obstacle, the term *spiral wave reentry* was later adopted to describe circulating waves in the absence of an anatomic obstacle. Because spiral waves of excitation is a well-described phenomenon in many excitable media, the application of the spiral waves of excitation to cardiac tissues was met with great enthusiasm. Spiral wave theory has advanced our understanding of the mechanisms responsible for the functional form of reentry. Although leading circle and spiral wave reentry are considered by some to be similar, a number of distinctions have been suggested. The curvature of the spiral wave is the key to the formation of the core. The curvature of the wave forms a region of high impedance mismatch (source-sink mismatch), where the current provided by the reentering wavefront (source) is insufficient to charge the capacity and thus excite larger volume of tissue ahead (sink). The ability of impulse propagation to succeed depends critically on the ability of source current generated by already activated cells to excite the cells ahead that have not been activated as yet, generally referred to as the sink. When the source current generated by a few cells is required to activate a large number of cells in the sink, the dilution of the current may lead to conduction failure or block. A prominent curvature of the spiral wave is generally encountered following a wave break, where the wavefront meets the wavetail and a large curvature (and short action potential) is present. Due to a very small source in part related to a short action potential (wavefront and wavetail meets), the broken end of the wave moves most slowly. **Figures 34–21A** to **34–21C** show the formation of the spiral wave by wave front interaction with the refractory tail of a previous activation. This three-dimensional (3D) computer simulation study reproduced the wavebreak observed in the optical mapping studies of VF in swine ventricle. The wavebreak occurs when the wavefront encounters refractory tail of a previous activation, inducing two spiral waves (Fig. 34–21A). A 3D view of the scroll wave is shown in Fig. 34–21B. Figure 34–21C is a blow up of the wavebreak. Note that the newly formed wavebreak has a very high curvature. As curvature decreases along the more distal parts of the spiral, propagation speed increases. The high curvature prevents the wave from propagating in the direction of wavebreak. The wavefront (*red*) then circles around the wavebreak site to form circus movement. In three dimensions, there are two new scroll waves formed by these interactions.[28]

The term *spiral wave* is usually used to describe reentrant activity in two dimensions. The center of the spiral wave is called the *core* and the distribution of the core in three dimensions is referred to as the *filament*. The 3D form of the spiral wave forms a scroll wave (**Fig. 34–21B**). In its simplest form, the scroll wave has a straight filament spanning the ventricular wall (ie, from epicardium to endocardium). Theoretical studies have described three major scroll wave configurations with

Wavebreak, phase singularity, rotors, vortex and scroll waves

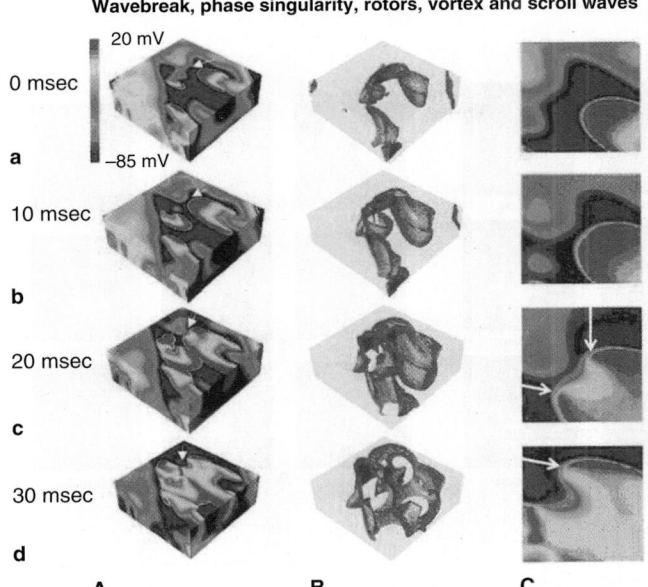

Figure 34–21. 3D simulation of wavebreak by a wave front running into the trailing edge of refractoriness. **(A)** Surface activation patterns (*red* = wave front, *green* = wave back) at the times indicated. The *white arrows* indicate the region where this mechanism of wave break occurs. **(B)** Corresponding scroll wave fronts in the tissue (*red* = rising membrane voltage). **(C)** Blowup of the region of wave break on the upper surface (near the *white arrows* in [A]). Residual refractoriness (*green*) was left over by a previous wave front, and when the next wave (*red*) encountered this refractory region, wave break occurred, generating two new scroll waves. *White arrows* point to the new wave breaks. At that site, the curvature of the wave is high and the source-sink ration is low, preventing the wave front from propagating. The wavefront (*red*) then circles around the wavebreak and forms circus movement. Reproduced with permission from Lee MH, Qu Z, Fishbein GA, et al: Patterns of wave break during ventricular fibrillation in isolated swine right ventricle, *Am J Physiol Heart Circ Physiol*. 2001 Jul;281(1):H253-H265.

curved filaments (L-, U-, and O-shaped), although numerous variations of these 3D filaments in space and time are assumed to exist during cardiac arrhythmias.

Spiral wave activity has been used to explain the electrocardiographic patterns observed during monomorphic and polymorphic cardiac arrhythmias as well as during fibrillation. Monomorphic VT results when the spiral wave is anchored and not able to drift within the ventricular myocardium. In contrast, a meandering or drifting spiral wave causes polymorphic VT- and VF-like activity. VF seems to be the most complex representation of rotating spiral waves in the heart. VF is often preceded by VT. One of the theories suggests that VF develops when a single spiral wave responsible for VT breaks up, leading to the development of multiple spirals that are continuously extinguished and recreated.

Stability of Circus Movement Reentry

The stability of reentry is critical to the understanding of the electrocardiographic manifestations of arrhythmias. If only a single stable reentrant wavefront is present, the ECG is likely to show consistent beat-to-beat QRS morphology (such as during monomorphic VT) or a consistent beat-to-beat P-wave morphology (such as during cavotricuspid isthmus dependent atrial flutter). On the other hand, if the reentrant circuit either

meanders or breaks down into multiple reentrant circuits, then the electrocardiographic manifestation becomes polymorphic or fibrillatory.

Size of the Anatomical Obstacle: While circus movement reentry can be conveniently classified as anatomical and functional, there is a gray zone in which the features of these two mechanisms are both present. Ikeda et al. performed a study in isolated superfused canine atria.[29] The authors punched holes with 2-mm to 10-mm diameters in the center of the tissue. **Figures 34–22A** to **34–22C** show the effects of a central hole (anatomical obstacle) on reentrant wavefronts (spiral waves). In the absence of a lesion (Fig. 34–22A), the induced single (functional) reentrant wave front, in the form of a spiral wave, meandered irregularly from one site to another before terminating at the tissue border. Holes with 2-mm to 4-mm diameters (Fig. 34–22B) had no effect on meandering. However, when the hole diameters were increased to 6 mm to 10 mm (Fig. 34–22C), the tip of the spiral wave attached to the holes, and reentry became stationary. This model shows that a critically sized anatomic obstacle converts a nonstationary meandering reentrant wave front to a stationary one. This electrical activation changed from irregular "fibrillation-like" activity into regular monomorphic activity. However, there was not an abrupt transition from functional reentry to anatomical reentry. Rather, with a small anatomical obstacle, the reentrant wavefront exhibits the characteristics of both functional and anatomical reentry. Many previous studies showed that the functional reentrant wavefronts tend to have a very short life span and is frequently unstable in whole hearts. For example, electrically induced reentry in the ventricles usually has a life span averaging a few seconds in the whole heart. Under normal conditions, it is unlikely for the initial reentrant wavefronts to persist and continue to serve as the source of rapid excitation to induce sustained ventricular arrhythmia. To induce sustained arrhythmia in the whole heart, these initial spiral waves will need to breakdown and induce multiple spiral waves to induce VF or to anchor to a large anatomical barrier to induce VT.

Figure-Eight Reentry: Figure-eight reentry was first described by El-Sherif and coworkers in the surviving epicardial layer overlying infarction produced by occlusion of the left anterior descending artery in canine hearts in the late 1980s.[30] The same patterns of activation can also be induced by creating artificial anatomical obstacles in the ventricles, or during functional reentry induced by a single premature ventricular stimulation. In the figure-eight model, the reentrant beat produces a wavefront that circulates in both directions around a long line of conduction block (**Fig. 34–23**) rejoining on the distal side of the block. The wavefront then breaks through the arc of block to reexcite the tissue proximal to the block. The reentrant activation continues as two circulating wavefronts that travel in clockwise and counterclockwise directions around the two arcs in a pretzel-like configuration. The diameter of the reentrant circuit in the ventricle can be as small as a few millimeters or as large as a several centimeters. When the line of block is short and functional, the reentrant circuits are unstable and the

Anatomical obstacles

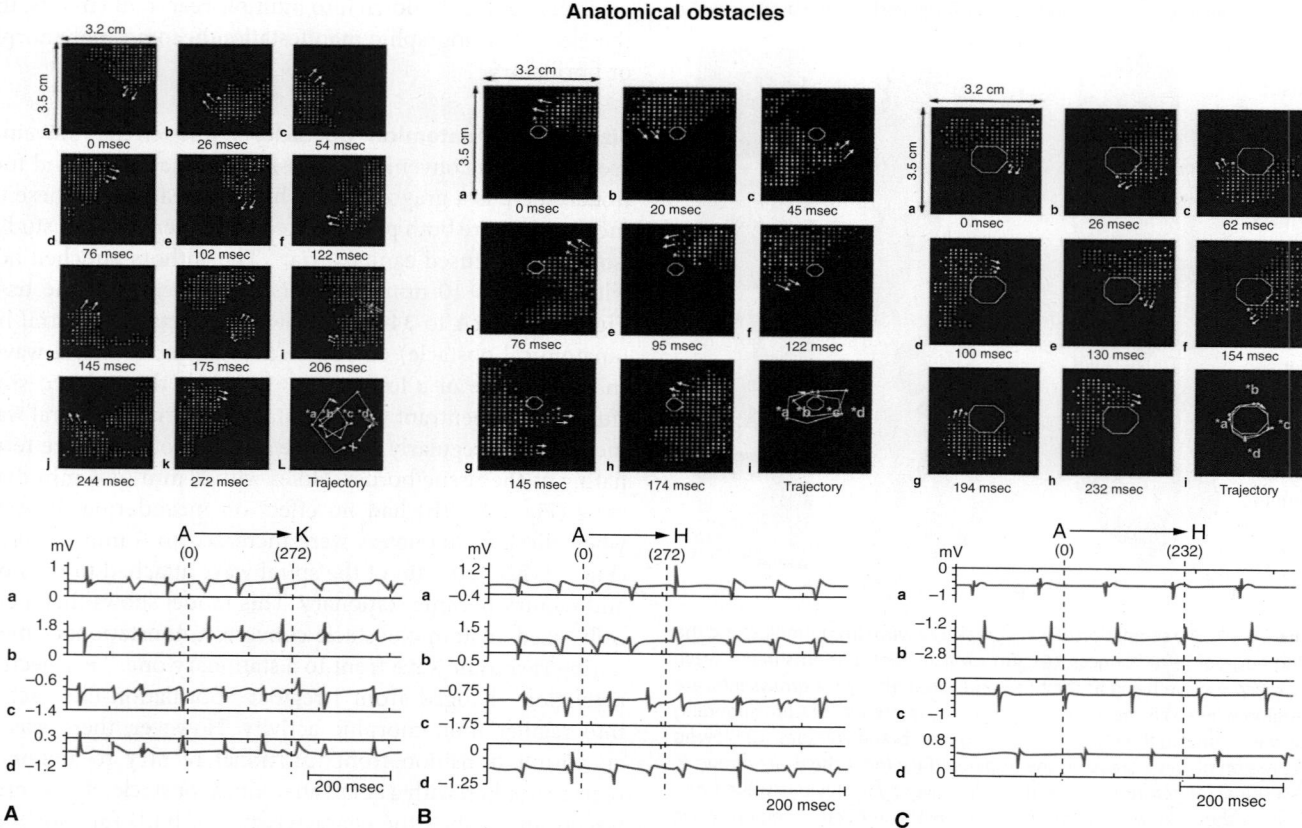

Figure 34–22. Functional and anatomical reentry in isolated superfused canine right atrium. Reentry was induced by electrical stimulation. The *red dots* represent activation wavefront. The color then changed every 10 ms from *yellow* to *green* to *light blue* and *purple* before becoming *black* (background color). **(A)** shows reentry without a functional obstacle. The reentrant wavefronts (*spiral waves*) meandered in the preparation. Bipolar electrogram showed irregular activations. **(B)** shows reentry after a 4-mm-diameter hole was created in the middle of the preparation (*white circle*). There is less meandering, and the activation cycle length was irregular but slower. **(C)** shows the effects of a 10-mm-central hole on reentrant wavefront. The reentry is no longer meandering, and the bipolar electrogram showed regular activations consistent with sustained monomorphic tachycardia. Reproduced with permission from Ikeda T, Yashima M, Uchida T, et al. Attachment of meandering reentrant wave fronts to anatomic obstacles in the atrium. Role of the obstacle size. *Circ Res.* 1997 Nov;81(5):753-764.

figure-eight pattern may soon terminate. However, more sustained figure-eight reentry can be induced when large anatomical obstacles are present in the preparation.

Critical Mass: A second factor that determines the stability of circus movement reentry is the tissue size. As first documented by Garrey, a critical mass is present for VF to sustain. If the tissue mass reduces to below that critical mass, VF invariably terminates. Kim et al. induced VF in isolated and perfused swine right ventricular free wall.[31] The tissue mass was then progressively reduced by sequential cutting. The critical mass to sustain VF in this preparation was around 20 grams. As tissue mass was decreased, the number of wave fronts decreased, the life span of reentrant wave fronts increased, and the cycle length, the diastolic interval, and the duration of action potential lengthened. When the mass is small enough, the remaining wavefront might anchor to the papillary muscle and convert VF into VT. **Figures 34–24A** to **34–24C** show typical examples of activation patterns after progressive tissue mass reduction. In addition, the APD progressively lengthened and the average activation rate progressively reduced with the tissue size reduction. There was a parallel decrease in the dynamical complexity of VF as measured by Kolmogorov entropy and Poincaré

plots. A period of quasiperiodicity became more evident before the conversion from VF (chaos) to a more regular arrhythmia (periodicity). Therefore, reducing tissue size is antifibrillatory. It causes a decrease in the number of wave fronts in VF by tissue mass reduction causes a transition from chaotic to periodic dynamics via the quasiperiodic route. This observation might explain the ameliorative effects of the Maze procedure in the setting of an AF.[32]

Action Potential Duration Restitution and Effective Refractory Period: A third important factor in determining the stability of circus movement reentry is the APD restitution properties of the cardiac tissue. The APD restitution describes the relationship between APD and the preceding diastolic interval (DI). The slope of APD restitution in theory determines the stability of cardiac activation. When the slope is less than 1.0, repeated pacing of the system will induce APD alternans and dynamic instability, leading to fibrillation. On the other hand, flattening the restitution might be an antifibrillatory strategy. **Figures 34–25A** to **34–25F** illustrate this concept with the help of computer simulation and a rabbit heart experiment. A shows APD shortening and APD alternans as pacing cycle length decreases. Figure 34–25B shows two different APD restitution curves;

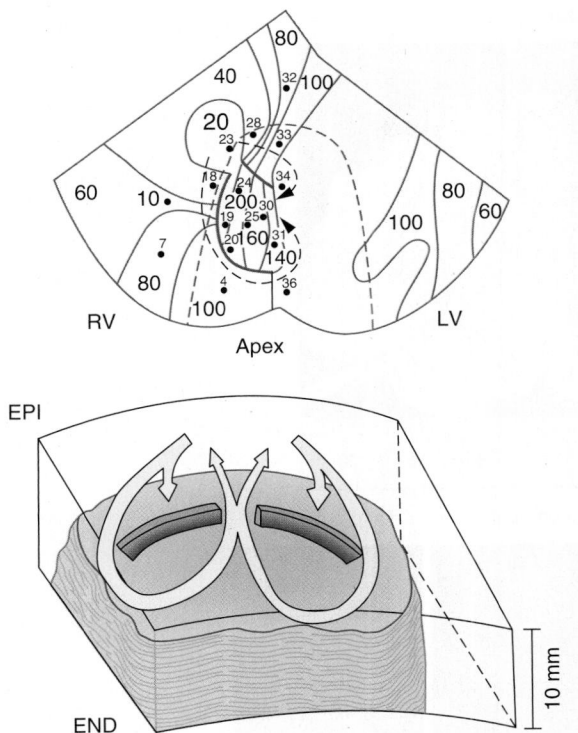

Figure 34–23. Figure-of-eight model of reentry. Isochronal activation map during monomorphic reentrant VT occurring in the surviving epicardial layer overlying an infarction. Recordings were obtained from the epicardial surface of a canine heart 4 days after ligation of the left anterior descending coronary artery. Activation isochrones are drawn at 20 ms intervals. The reentrant circuit has a characteristic figure-of-eight activation pattern. Two circulating wavefronts advance in clockwise and counterclockwise directions, respectively, around two zones (*arcs*) of conduction block (*heavy solid lines*). The epicardial surface is depicted as if the ventricles were unfolded following a cut from the crux to the apex. A 3D diagrammatic illustration of the ventricular activation pattern during the reentrant tachycardia is shown in the lower panel. END, endocardium; EPI, epicardium; LV, left ventricle; RV, right ventricle. Reproduced with permission from El-Sherif N. Reentry revisited. *Pacing Clin Electrophysiol.* 1988 Sep;11(9):1358-1368.

one with slope >1 (*solid line*) or one <1 (*dashed line*, obtained with 50% block of the calcium current). Figures 34–25C and 34–25D are results of computer simulation studies while Figs. 34–25E and 34–25F are actual experimental data from a Langendorff perfused rabbit heart. Flattening of the restitution curves in both simulation studies and in rabbit hearts resulted in the conversion of VF to VT.

In normal hearts, the atrial effective refractory period (ERP) approximates action potential duration at 70% repolarization in atria and at 90% repolarization in the ventricle (APD70-90). Abbreviation of ERP is associated with increased susceptibility for development of reentry. In experimental models of AF, without cardiovascular disease, abbreviation of atrial ERP, secondary to pharmacological interventions or sustained rapid atrial activation, is associated with a significant increase in AF vulnerability. In structurally remodeled atria or following exposure to sodium channel blockers, ERP can outlast APD70-90 secondary to reduced excitability leading to development of post-repolarization refractoriness. Prolongation of ERP, whether by prolongation of APD or development of post

repolarization refractoriness can terminate and/or prevent the development of reentry and is an effective treatment for paroxysmal AF.

In addition to APD restitution, the conduction velocity (CV) restitution is also an important factor that determines the stability of the reentrant wavefronts. **Figures 34–26A** to **34–26C** show that at baseline, the activation rate was fast, and the dominant frequency of VF was around 16 Hz. D600 (Ca channel blocker) flattened the APD restitution curve and converted baseline fast (Type I) VF to VT. Further increasing the D600 concentration to 2.5 mg/L or 5.0 mg/L converted VT to slow (Type II) VF with an average dominant frequency around 11 Hz. Because high concentrations of D600 block Na channels as well as Ca channels, the authors hypothesized that reduced excitability might underlie Type II VF, which was not driven by steep APD restitution, but was due to broad CV restitution. Whereas steep APD restitution drives wave instability by making the *waveback* sensitive to small changes in diastolic interval, CV can drive wave instability by making the *wavefront* sensitive to small changes in diastolic interval, especially if structural and electrophysiological heterogeneities are present.

Calcium Dynamics: Electrical activation and calcium dynamics are closely coupled. However, the coupling between the two can be variable, which results in additional complex dynamics that affect the APD restitution and the stability of the reentrant wavefronts. Positive Ca_i –V coupling refers to the mode in which a larger Ca_i transient produces a longer APD. This occurs when the large Ca_i transient enhances net inward current during the action potential plateau by potentiating inward I_{NCX} to a greater extent than it reduces the $I_{Ca,L}$ (by facilitating Ca-induced inactivation). On the other hand, negative Ca–V coupling refers to the mode in which a larger Ca_i transient causes a shorter APD. While increased $I_{Ca,L}$ can increase the Ca_i and prolong the APD through I_{NCX} activation, the increased $I_{Ca,L}$ can also activate the calcium-sensitive potassium currents such as I_{KS} and I_{KAS} to shorten the APD.[33] When the balance between the two favors the APD shortening, then larger Ca_i transient is coupled to shorter APD and vice versa (negative coupling). Apamin, a specific I_{KAS} blocker, can prevent negative coupling in rabbit ventricles.[34] In addition to complex coupling, the cardiac Ca handling has its own dynamics. It is possible to have a large discrepancy between the Ca_i transient duration and the APD in pathological conditions. The dynamic Vm–Ca_i coupling underlies the development of repolarization instability and increases the probability of ventricular arrhythmias.[35] Dynamic coupling could also affect the stability of the spiral waves and contribute to the degeneration of VT into VF.

Reflection

One noncircus movement reentry mechanism is reflected reentry (or reflection). The concept of reflection was first suggested by studies of the propagation characteristics of slow action potential responses in K+-depolarized Purkinje fibers. In strands of Purkinje fiber, Wit and coworkers demonstrated a phenomenon similar to that observed by Schmitt and Erlanger in which slow anterograde conduction of the impulse was

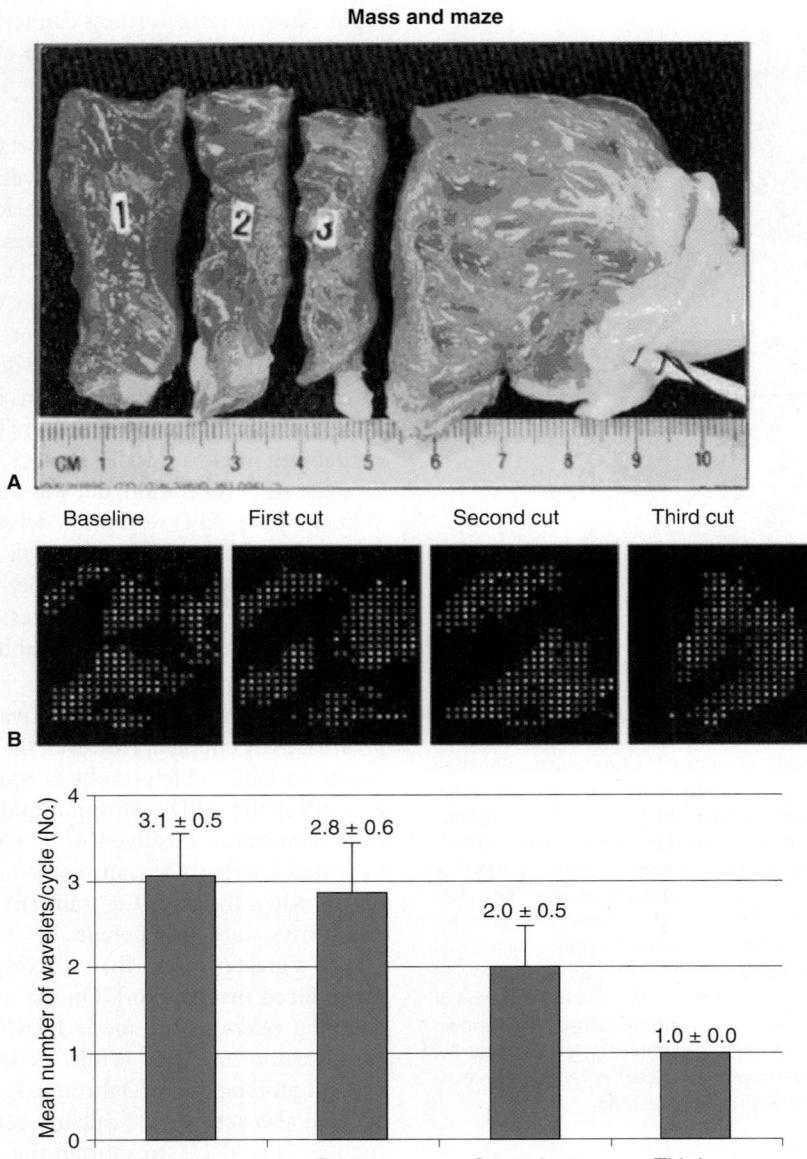

Figure 34–24. Effects of tissue mass reduction on reentrant wavefronts in VF. (**A**) shows an isolated perfused swine RV preparation. (**B**) shows the patterns of activation in the RV at baseline and after first, second and third cuts. (**C**) shows the average number of wavefronts after each cut in six different preparations. After third cut, a single reentrant wavefront (*spiral wave*) is present. Reproduced with permission from Kim YH, Garfinkel A, Ikeda T, et al: Spatiotemporal complexity of ventricular fibrillation revealed by tissue mass reduction in isolated swine right ventricle. Further evidence for the quasiperiodic route to chaos hypothesis *J Clin Invest.* 1997 Nov 15;100(10):2486-2500.

at times followed by a retrograde wavefront that produced a "return extrasystole." They proposed that the nonstimulated impulse was caused by circuitous reentry at the level of the syncytial interconnections, made possible by longitudinal dissociation of the bundle, as the most likely explanation for the phenomenon but also suggested the possibility of reflection. Direct evidence in support of reflection as a mechanism of arrhythmogenesis was provided by Antzelevitch and coworkers in the early 1980s. A number of models of reflection have been developed. The first of these involves use of *ion-free* isotonic sucrose solution to create a narrow (1.5–2 mm) central inexcitable zone (gap) in unbranched Purkinje fibers mounted in a three-chamber tissue bath (**Figs. 34–27A** to **34–27C**). In the sucrose-gap model, stimulation of the proximal (P) segment

elicits an action potential that propagates to the proximal border of the sucrose gap. Active propagation across the sucrose gap is not possible because of the ion-depleted extracellular milieu, but local circuit current continues to flow through the intercellular low resistance pathways (an Ag/AgCl extracellular shunt pathway is provided). This local circuit or electrotonic current, very much reduced on emerging from the gap, gradually discharges the capacity of the distal (D) tissue thus giving rise to a depolarization that manifests as either a subthreshold response (last distal response) or a foot-potential that brings the distal excitable tissue to its threshold potential (**Fig. 34–28**). Active impulse propagation stops and then resumes after a delay that can be as long as several hundred milliseconds. When anterograde (P to D) transmission time is sufficiently

APD restitution

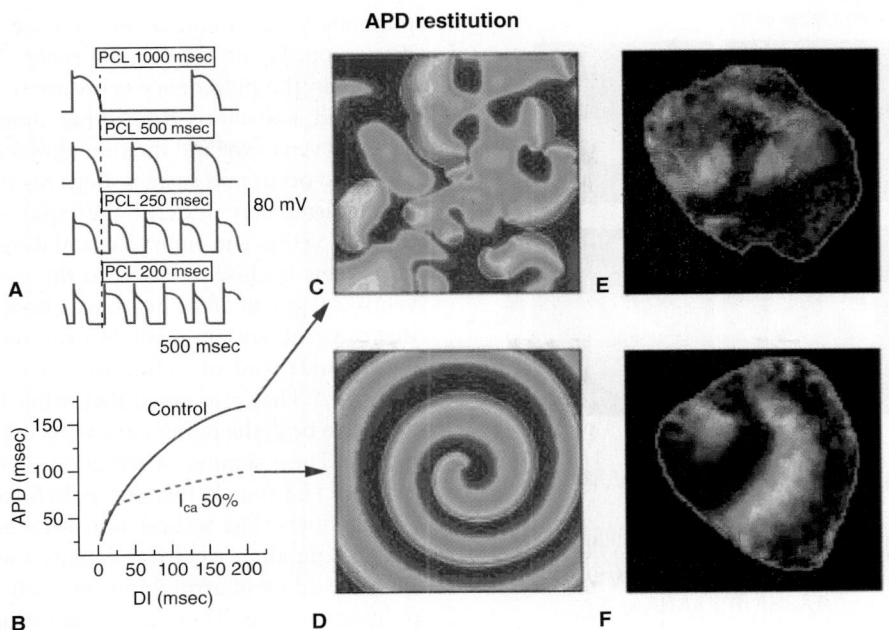

Figure 34–25. Action potential duration (APD) restitution and stability of reentrant activity. (**A**) APD shortening and APD alternans as pacing cycle length (PCL) decreases (computer simulation). Diastolic interval (DI) is measured from the end of the preceding action potential to the onset of phase zero of the present action potential. As shown in these examples, the shorter the preceding DI, the shorter the APD. (**B**) APD restitution curves with slope >1 (solid line) or <1 (*dashed line*, obtained with 50% block of the calcium current). (**C**) and (**D**) Spiral wave behavior several seconds after initiating a spiral wave in homogeneous 2D tissue. All cells are identical, with either a steep (**C**) or shallow (**D**) APD restitution slope. (**E**) and (**F**) Optically measured surface voltage maps in an intact Langendorff rabbit heart before (**E**) and after (**F**) partially blocking the L-type calcium current with D600 (0.5 mg/mL) to flatten the APD restitution slope to >1. In (**E**), multiple wavefronts move in a complex VF pattern. In (**F**), VF has converted to VT, manifested as a stable double armed rotor. Reproduced with permission from Weiss JN, Qu Z, Chen PS, Lin SF, Karagueuzian HS, Hayashi H, Garfinkel A, Karma A. The dynamics of cardiac fibrillation, *Circulation.* 2005 Aug 23;112(8):1232-1240.

delayed to permit recovery of refractoriness at the proximal end, electrotonic transmission of the impulse in the retrograde direction is able to reexcite the proximal tissue, thus generating a closely coupled reflected reentry. Reflection therefore results from the to-and-fro electrotonically mediated transmission of the impulse across the same inexcitable segment; neither longitudinal dissociation nor circus movement need be invoked to explain the phenomenon.

A second model of reflection involved the creation of an inexcitable zone permitting delayed conduction by superfusion of a central segment of a Purkinje bundle with a solution designed to mimic the extracellular milieu at a site of ischemia. The gap was shown to be largely comprised of an inexcitable cable across which conduction of impulses was electrotonically mediated.

Phase 2 Reentry
Another reentrant mechanism that does not depend on circus movement and can appear to be of focal origin is Phase 2 reentry. Phase 2 reentry occurs when the dome of the action potential, most commonly epicardial, propagates from sites at which it is maintained to sites at which it is abolished, causing local reexcitation of the epicardium and the generation of a closely coupled extrasystole. Accentuated spatial dispersion of repolarization is needed for phase 2 reentry to occur.

Spatial Dispersion of Repolarization
Studies conducted over the last three decades have established that ventricular myocardium is not homogeneous but is comprised of at least three electrophysiologically and functionally

distinct cell types: epicardial, M, and endocardial cells. These three principal ventricular myocardial cell types differ with respect to phase 1 and phase 3 repolarization characteristics (**Fig. 34–29**). Ventricular epicardial and M, but not endocardial, cells generally display a prominent phase 1, because of a large 4-aminopyridine (4-AP) sensitive transient outward current (I_{to}), giving the action potential a spike and dome or notched configuration. These regional differences in I_{to} have now been directly demonstrated in ventricular myocytes from a wide variety of species including canine, guinea pig, swine, rabbit, and humans. Differences in the magnitude of the action potential notch and corresponding differences in I_{to} have also been described between right and left ventricular epicardium. Similar interventricular differences in I_{to} have also been described for canine ventricular M cells. This distinction is thought to form the basis for why Brugada syndrome (BrS), a channelopathy-mediated form of sudden death, is a right ventricular disease.

Recent optical mapping studies using normal and failing human ventricles confirmed the presence of M cell islands in the midmyocardial layer. These M cell islands are characterized by long APDs. A large APD gradient is present between the APD within the island and the surrounding myocardium. Apamin, a specific I_{KAS} blocker, prolonged APDs in the surrounding myocardium to a greater extent than within the M cell island.[36] These findings suggest a highly heterogeneous transmural distribution of the I_{KAS}. The I_{KAS} deficiency may contribute to the long APD of the M cells.

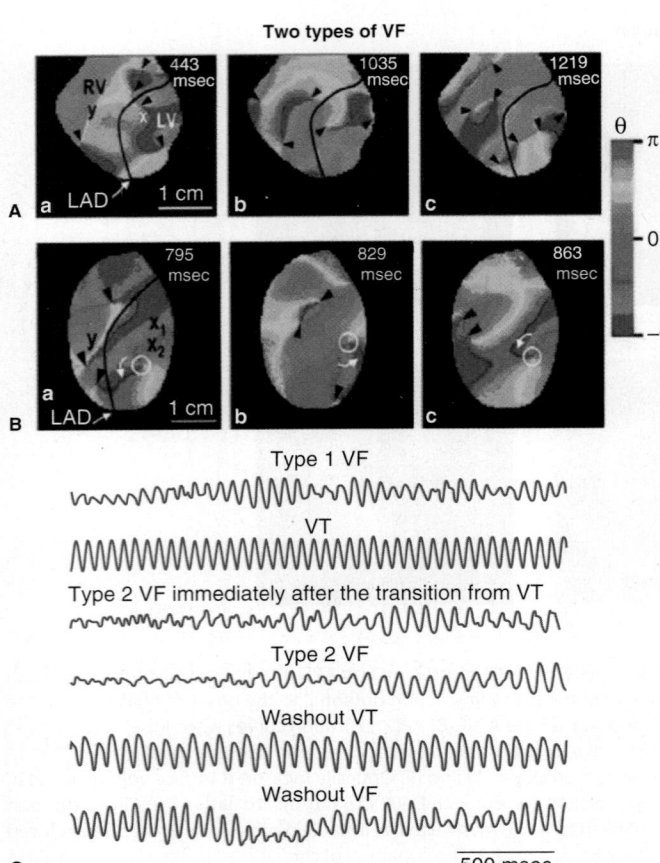

Two types of VF

Type 1 VF

VT

Type 2 VF immediately after the transition from VT

Type 2 VF

Washout VT

Washout VF

500 msec

Figure 34–26. Two types of VF. (**A**) shows phase maps of type 1 VF, which is characterized by a steep APD restitution but narrow conduction velocity (CV) restitution curve. (**B**) shows type 2 VF, with a single meandering mother rotor (*white circle*) which meandering on the epicardium. This type of VF is characterized by flat APD restitution (which prevents spiral breakup) and broad CV restitution (which facilitates wavebreak). (**C**) shows the electrograms corresponding to types 1 and 2 VF. Note that there is a period of monomorphic VT between types 1 and 2 VF. Reproduced with permission from Wu TJ, Lin SF, Weiss JN, et al: Two types of ventricular fibrillation in isolated rabbit hearts: Importance of excitability and action potential duration restitution, *Circulation*. 2002 Oct 1;106(14):1859-1866.

Between the surface epicardial and endocardial layers are transitional and M cells. M cells are distinguished by the ability of their action potential to prolong disproportionately relative to the action potential of other ventricular myocardial cells in response to a slowing of rate and/or in response to APD-prolonging agents. In the dog, the ionic basis for these features of the M cell include the presence of a smaller I_{Ks}, a larger late I_{Na}, and a larger I_{NCX}. In the canine heart, the I_{Kr} and I_{K1} currents are similar in the three transmural cell types. Transmural and apical-basal differences in the density of I_{Kr} channels have been described in the ferret heart. Amplification of transmural heterogeneities normally present in the early and late phases of the action potential can lead to the development of a variety of genetic arrhythmias.

Thoracic Veins as an Arrhythmogenic Structure

Because of the discovery that pulmonary veins are important sources of AF, the arrhythmogenic mechanisms of the pulmonary veins and other thoracic veins deserve separate discussion. While the original report showed that rapid activations in the pulmonary veins are responsible for triggering AF, rapid activations from other thoracic veins, such as the superior vena cava and the vein of Marshall, are also important for AF to occur and sustain. Both reentrant and non-reentrant mechanisms may underlie the rapid activations within these thoracic veins. The embryological development of the pulmonary veins is closely related to the development of the sinus venosus segment of the heart, which are known to be structures that can generate automaticity. Brunton and Fayer first demonstrated independent pulmonary vein contractions in rabbits and cats.[37] They also noted that, while both atria subsequently ceased to beat, the pulmonary veins in both lungs continued to pulsate. These seminal observations have two important implications: The first is that the pulmonary vein has contractile muscle fibers. The second is that the pulmonary vein is capable of generating electrical activity independent of the atria. Multiple different arrhythmogenic cell types are present in the pulmonary veins. These cell types include Purkinje-like cells,[38] interstitial Cajal-like cells, and Melanocyte-like cells. All these cells are potentially electrically active and can contribute to the generation of either automaticity or triggered activity.

Cheung demonstrated that ouabain infusion or norepinephrine infusion could trigger the onset of repetitive rapid responses from the distal pulmonary vein.[39] Several types of electrical activity within the pulmonary veins, including silent electrical activity, fast response action potentials driven by electrical stimulation, and spontaneous fast or slow response action potentials with or without early afterdepolarizations can be observed in the cells from the pulmonary veins. The incidence of action potentials with an EAD and of spontaneous tachycardias is much greater in dogs subjected to chronic rapid pacing than in normal dogs. Because of the short APD, the pulmonary veins are also prone to the development of late phase 3 EADs and triggered arrhythmias. In addition to increased propensity for automaticity and triggered activity, the complex myocardial fiber orientation in the pulmonary veins and at the pulmonary vein–left atrial junction can cause conduction blocks and facilitate reentrant excitations in that region. In addition, increased fibrosis at the pulmonary vein–left atrial junction in heart failure may play an important role in determining the characteristics of the reentrant wavefronts, and thereby perpetuate AF.

Remodeling and the Mechanisms of Cardiac Arrhythmia

While genetic arrhythmias often occur in structurally normal hearts, most of the common cardiac arrhythmias (such as AF, VF, and SCD) occur primarily in diseased hearts. Therefore, cardiac remodeling associated with heart diseases plays an important role in cardiac arrhythmogenesis. Remodeling in diseased hearts includes structural remodeling, electrophysiological remodeling, and neural remodeling. Neural remodeling may include both reduced innervation (denervation) and increased innervation through cardiac nerve sprouting.

Reflection (reflected reentry)

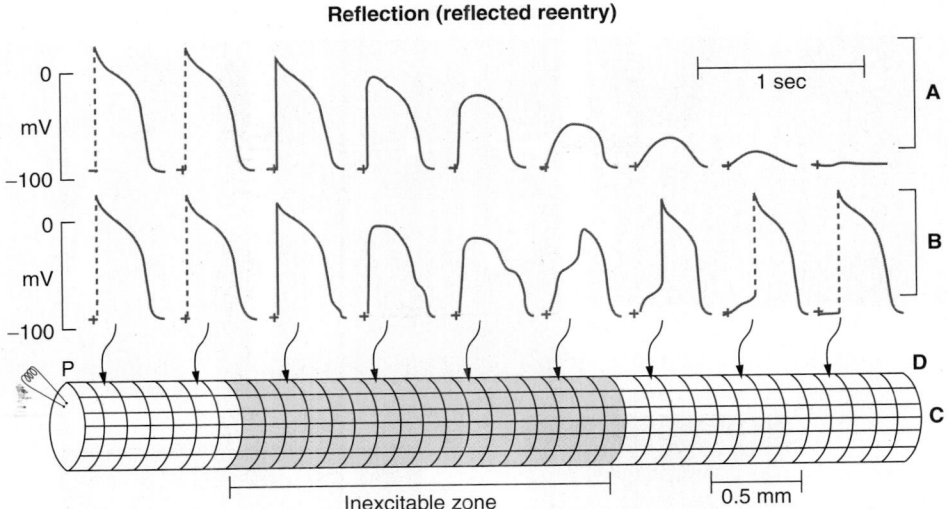

Figure 34–27. Conduction block (**A**) and discontinuous conduction (**B**) in a Purkinje strand with a central inexcitable zone (**C**). The schematic illustration is based on transmembrane recordings obtained from canine Purkinje fiber-sucrose gap preparations. An action potential elicited by stimulation of the proximal (P) side of the preparation conducts normally up to the border of the inexcitable zone. Active propagation of the impulse stops at this point, but local circuit current generated by the proximal segment continues to flow through the preparation encountering a cumulative resistance (successive gap junctions). Transmembrane recordings from the first few inexcitable cells show a response not very different from the action potentials recorded in the neighboring excitable cells, in spite of the fact that no ions may be moving across the membrane of these cells. The responses recorded in the inexcitable region are the electrotonic images of activity generated in the proximal excitable segment. The resistive-capacitive properties of the tissue lead to an exponential decline in the amplitude of the transmembrane potential recorded along the length of the inexcitable segment and to a slowing of the rate of change of voltage as a function of time. If, as in (**B**), the electrotonic current is sufficient to bring the distal excitable tissue to its threshold potential, an action potential is generated after a step delay imposed by the slow discharge of the capacity of the distal (**D**) membrane by the electrotonic current (foot-potential). Active conduction of the impulse therefore stops at the proximal border of the inexcitable zone and resumes at the distal border after a step delay that can range from a few to tens or hundreds of milliseconds. Modified wiith permission from Antzelevitch C, Rosen MR, Janse MJ, et al: Electrotonus and reflection. Cardiac electrophysiology: A textbook. Mount Kisco, NY: Futura Publishing Company, Inc; 1990.

Myocardial Remodeling

A common structural remodeling in diseased hearts is increased fibrosis, which occurs in both ischemic and nonischemic cardiomyopathy. Histological studies of human hearts have shown a strong association between myocardial scars and VT. Computerized mapping studies of human hearts with dilated cardiomyopathy showed that reentrant wavefronts and

transmural scroll waves were present during VF. Although the coronary arteries are open, these diseased hearts have increased fibrosis, and that these fibrotic tissues provide a site for conduction block, leading to the continuous generation of reentry. **Figures 34–30A** to **34–30E** show an example of increased fibrosis in a human heart with nonischemic dilated cardiomyopathy. The patient underwent cardiac transplantation, and the heart was Langendorff perfused and mapped. Trichrome staining showed significantly increased fibrosis, which was a consistent finding in all hearts at two different levels of sections.

Reflection (reflected reentry)

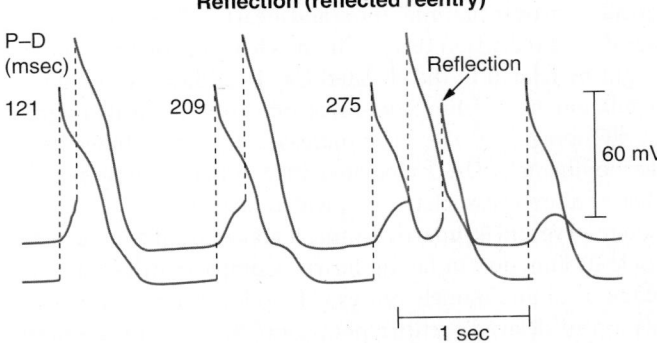

Figure 34–28. Delayed transmission and reflection across an inexcitable gap created by superfusion of the central segment of a Purkinje fiber with an *ion-free* isotonic sucrose solution. The two traces were recorded from proximal (P) and distal (D) active segments. P–D conduction time (indicated in the upper portion of the figure, in ms) increased progressively with a 4:3 Wenckebach periodicity. The third stimulated proximal response was followed by a reflection. Reproduced wtih permission from Antzelevitch C: Clinical application of new concepts of parasystole, reflection, and tachycardia, *Cardiol Clin.* 1983 Feb;1(1):39-50.

Heterogeneity

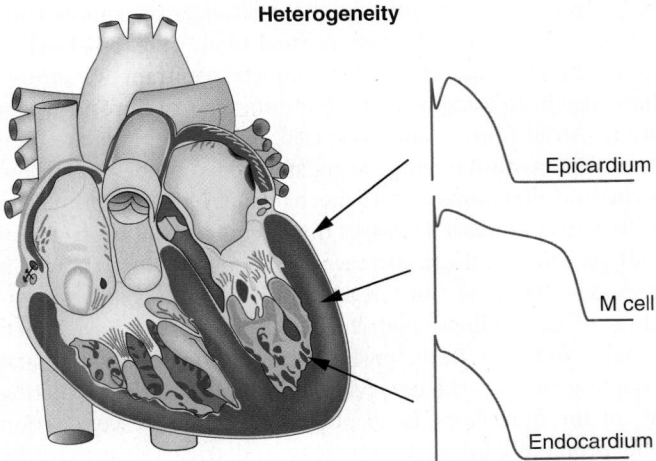

Figure 34–29. Action potential characteristics recorded from epicardial, M, and endocardial regions of the canine LV.

Reentry and fibrosis

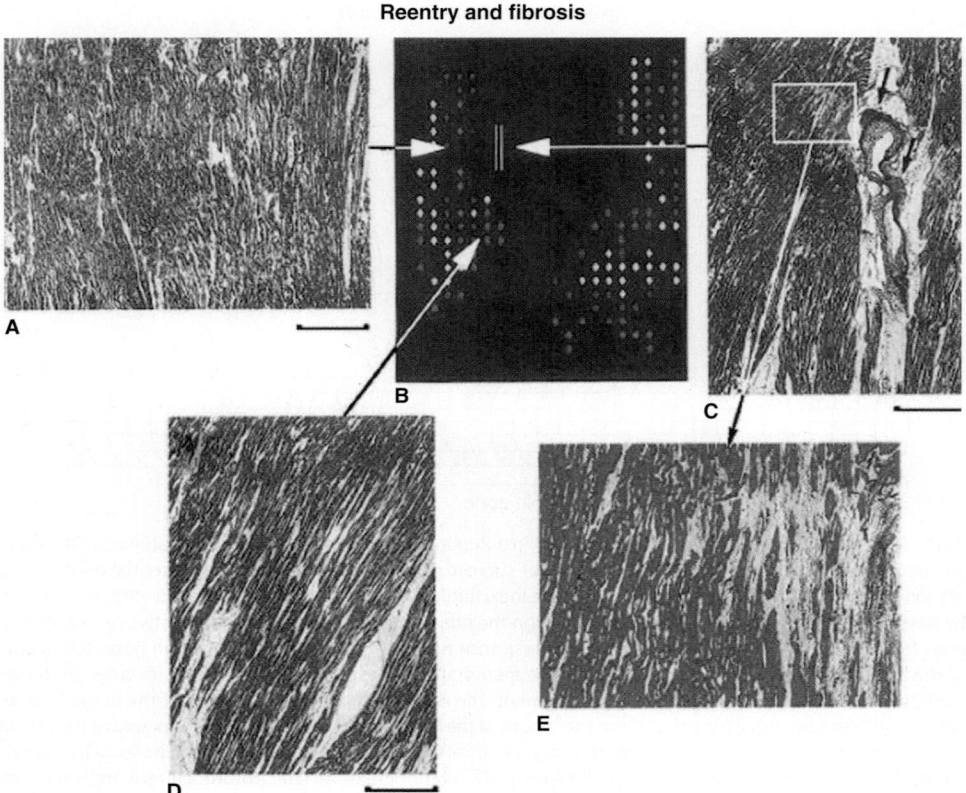

Figure 34–30. Fibrosis and conduction block in human hearts. (**A**), (**C**), (**D**), and (**E**) show sections of the left ventricular myocardium parallel to the epicardium in heart no. 1. With trichrome stain, small veins with perivascular fibrosis (*blue areas*) were clearly seen in (**C**) (*arrows*). The magnified view (**E**) also showed interstitial and replacement fibrosis. The areas of fibrosis in (**C**) and (**E**) corresponded to the line of conduction block in (**B**), which showed computerized mapping of wavefronts in VF. The *red color* is the wavefront. The color then changed every 10 ms to *orange, yellow, green, blue, purple* and then *black* (background). It shows propagation block (*double white line* segments) and wavefront circling around the lower end of the block in a counterclockwise direction. The wavefront then continues to form a complete circus movement around the site of block (not shown). However, in the areas without conduction block, histological examination showed either normal tissue (**A**) or mild fibrosis (**D**). Calibration line segments are 1 mm long. Reproduced with permission from Wu TJ, Ong JJ, Hwang C, et al: Characteristics of wave fronts during ventricular fibrillation in human hearts with dilated cardiomyopathy: role of increased fibrosis in the generation of reentry, *J Am Coll Cardiol*. 1998 Jul;32(1):187-196.

However, these fibrotic tissues were distributed unevenly. As shown in this figure, significant interstitial, replacement, and perivascular fibrosis are presents in Figs. 34–30C and 34–30E. These fibrotic tissues corresponded to the area of conduction block shown (Fig. 34–30B). In comparison, areas without conduction block showed either normal tissue (Fig. 34–30A) or mild fibrosis (Fig. 34–30D). Complete reentrant wavefronts have also been documented around the sites of fibrosis in that study. Atrial fibrosis and increased atrial fibroblasts are seen in patients with AF,[40] suggesting an association between these structural alterations and AF mechanisms. One possible reason is that atrial fibrosis decreases the safety factor of propagation and promotes anisotropic reentry, similar to that shown in Figs. 34–30A to 34–30E. In addition to synthesis and remodeling of extracellular matrix (ECM), fibroblasts have much broader functions in the myocardium. Through the functional coupling between the myocytes and fibroblasts, the oscillating V_m of the fibroblasts could potentially modulate conduction and promote cardiac automaticity and triggered activity by raising the diastolic V_m toward depolarization.

In addition to structural remodeling, electrophysiological remodeling is also important in the development of cardiac arrhythmia. As previously described in this chapter, reduction of I_{K1} significantly increases the incidence of DADs. Both chronic myocardial infarction and heart failure can result in significant reduction of I_{K1}. The mechanisms of I_{K1} reduction might be related to the elevated Ca_i. In addition to I_{K1} downregulation, heart failure and myocardial infarction also significantly upregulates I_{NCX}. The increased I_{NCX} contributes to the developments of DAD-mediated arrhythmias in these settings. Heart failure is associated I_{NaL}, which helps reduce repolarization reserve and is proarrhythmic. It may also contribute to diastolic dysfunction in failing hearts. Complete atrioventricular block in canine models causes QT prolongation by downregulation of delayed rectifier potassium currents. Ionic current remodeling help reduce repolarization reserve and promote arrhythmias in diseased conditions. However, recent findings indicate that heart failure, myocardial infarction, complete AV block, and hypokalemia can upregulate the I_{KAS}, which serve as a countermeasure to preserve the repolarization reserve. Blocking I_{KAS} with apamin can further reduce repolarization reserve, leading to EADs and ventricular arrhythmias.[41]

In summary, myocardial remodeling in diseased states includes both structural and electrophysiological remodeling.

These changes significantly increase the propensity of arrhythmia through both reentrant and non-reentrant mechanisms.

Neural Remodeling and Cardiac Nerve Sprouting

Static myocardial remodeling by itself does not provide a trigger for arrhythmia to occur. Additional remodeling of the autonomic nervous system in diseased states might also be important in triggering cardiac arrhythmia. In the central nervous system, nerve sprouting is an important mechanism of seizure disorder. Vracko et al. first demonstrated an increased number and complexity of cardiac nerve fibers in human myocardial scars and in animal models, suggesting that myocardial ischemia and infarction can also induce nerve sprouting.[42] Compatible with this hypothesis, necrotic injury to the rat myocardium results in denervation followed by proliferative regeneration of both Schwann cells and nerve axons. Cao et al. performed immunocytochemical studies of the native hearts of the transplant recipients. In some patients, there was strong evidence of cardiac nerve sprouting and neural regenerative activity.[43] Abundant nerve twigs are also present in tissues resected from the origin of VT **(Fig. 34–31)**. There was a correlation between nerve density and a clinical history of ventricular arrhythmia. Subsequent studies in dogs confirmed that increased cardiac nerve sprouting and sympathetic hyperinnervation may be responsible for the initiation of VT, VF, and SCD. In addition to histological evidence, I-123-metaiodobenzylguanidine scanning showed that myocardial infarction can lead to both denervation and reinnervation of the heart. A potential benefit of cardiac reinnervation is improved hemodynamic performance, as has been demonstrated in recipients of cardiac transplantation. These data suggest that nerve sprouting and sympathetic hyperinnervation occur after myocardial infarction and cardiac transplantation, which may contribute to the increased hemodynamic performance of the surviving myocardium. Excessive and heterogeneous nerve sprouting, however, may result in abnormal patterns of myocardial innervation, leading to cardiac arrhythmia and SCD.

The mechanisms of nerve sprouting after myocardial infarction are not completely understood. However, it is known that multiple neurotrophic factors are overexpressed after myocardial infarction. Among them, nerve growth factor (NGF) promotes the survival and differentiation of sympathetic nerves and maintains the catecholamine phenotype, as well as participates in axonal collateral sprouting after injury. An increase in the number and size of neurons in the sympathetic ganglia, as well as a marked elevation of catecholamine level in the heart, were demonstrated in transgenic mice that overexpressed NGF. Enlarged ganglion cells have also been observed in the stellate ganglia after myocardial infarction.[44] NGF is increased in both the myocardium and the left stellate ganglion after myocardial infarction. These findings suggest that retrograde axonal transport from the myocardium to the left stellate ganglion might be responsible for the increased growth associated protein 43 (GAP43) and nerve sprouting within the left stellate ganglion. **Figure 34–32** illustrates the involvement of the stellate ganglia in cardiac nerve sprouting after acute myocardial infarction. The figure shows that nerve sprouting is a process that involves not only the site of infarction but also the entire heart. Therefore, a small-to-medium sized myocardial infarction in the left anterior descending artery distribution can cause nerve sprouting in the atria and increase atrial vulnerability to arrhythmia. Remodeling of nerve structures, such as the stellate ganglia, are associated with increased sympathetic nerve activities for at least 2 months after myocardial infarction. The increased cardiac sympathetic outflow might contribute to the cardiac arrhythmia and sudden death after myocardial infarction.

Sympathetic Nerve Activity and Ventricular Arrhythmia

Myocardial infarction and heart failure both increase sympathetic nerve activity. Using neuECG recordings,[17] it is possible to simultaneously record the skin sympathetic nerve activity

Cardiac nerve sprouting

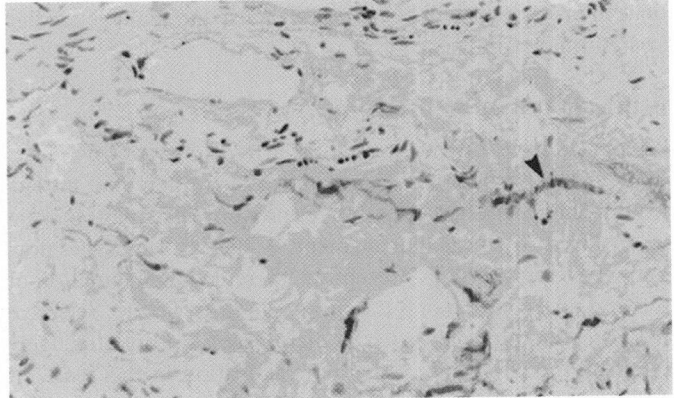

Figure 34–31. S100 positive nerve fibers in VT origin of patients with coronary artery disease who underwent surgical ablation of VT. The S100 protein staining in the heart identifies Schwann cells. There are abundant positive stains located in perivascular area and areas with fibrosis. Reproduced with permission from Cao JM, Fishbein MC, Han JB, et al: Relationship between regional cardiac hyperinnervation and ventricular arrhythmia, *Circulation.* 2000;Apr 25;101(16):1960-1969.

Mechanisms of nerve sprouting

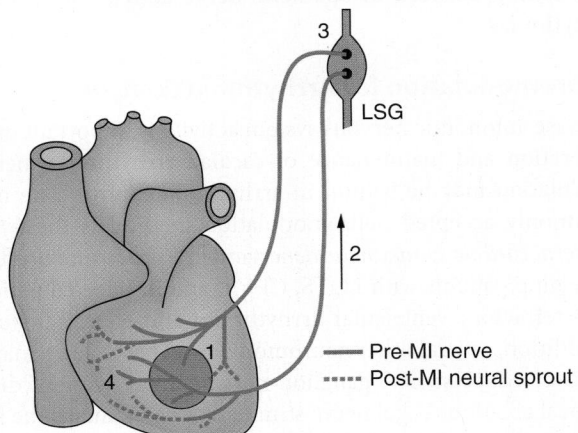

Figure 34–32. Cardiac nerve sprouting after myocardial infarction. Myocardial injury results in the overexpression of multiple neurotrophic factors, including (but not limited to) NGF. After binding with the high affinity NGF receptor (Trk A) on the axons, the NGF is transported to the stellate ganglia via axonal retrograde transport system. NGF then triggers cardiac nerve sprouting and sympathetic hyperinnervation that occur not only in the infarcted region but also throughout the heart.

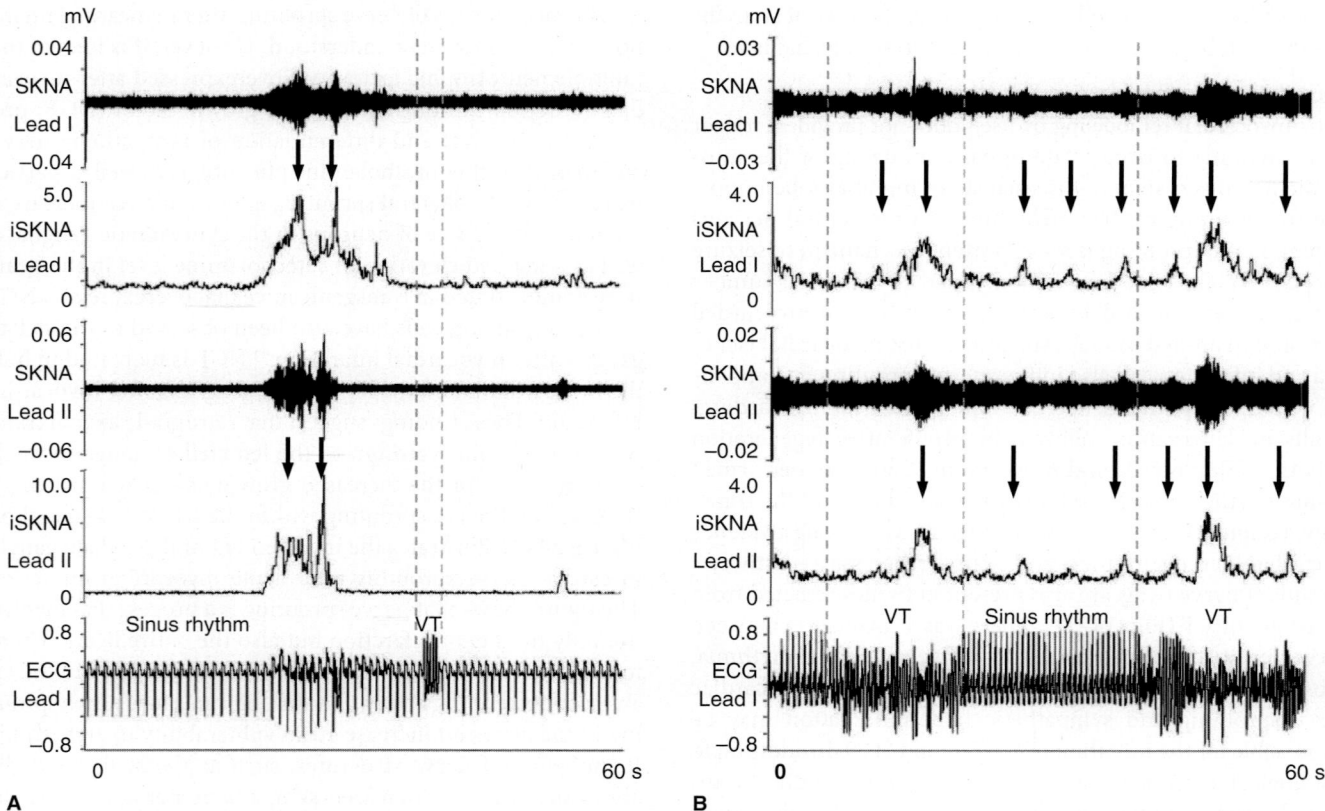

Figure 34–33. Relationship between SKNA and VT. (**A**) Actual recording of the SKNA in Lead I and ECG in the patient with single VT episode. The onsets of VT are indicated by *red dotted lines* and the terminations of VT by *blue dotted lines*. The baseline heart rhythm of this patient was atrial fibrillation. SKNA discharges (*downward arrows*) were observed before VT onset. (**B**) Actual recording in the patient with early recurrence of VT episodes. Multiple SKNA bursts occurred during sinus rhythm between VT episodes and also during VT. SKNA, skin sympathetic nerve activity; Iskna, integrated SKNA; VT, ventricular tachycardia; ECG, electrocardiogram; HR, heart rate. Reproduced with permission from Kusayama T, Wan J, Doytchinova A, et al: Skin sympathetic nerve activity and the temporal clustering of cardiac arrhythmias, *JCI Insight.* 2019 Feb 21;4(4):e125853.

(SKNA) and ECG in patients with recurrent VT and VF. There is an association between SKNA bursts and VT and VF (**Figs. 34–33A** and **34–33B**).[45] Similarly SKNA bursts are also associated with AF clusters. These findings further support the relationship between sympathetic nerve activity and cardiac arrhythmias.

Neuromodulation for Arrhythmia Control

Because autonomic nervous system activity is important in the generation and maintenance of cardiac arrhythmias, neuromodulation may be helpful in arrhythmia control. The most commonly accepted neuromodulation method is the *left or bilateral cardiac sympathetic denervation*, a procedure useful in managing patients with LQTS, CPVT, and in selected patients with refractory ventricular arrhythmias and electrical storm. In addition, several other neuromodulation procedures may be used to reduce stellate ganglion nerve activity without direct surgical ablation. Vagal nerve stimulation can damage the stellate ganglion, reduces stellate ganglion nerve activity, and controls the ventricular rate during AF.[46] Ganglionated plexi and ligament of Marshall ablation have similar effects on the stellate ganglion.[47] These data suggest that stellate ganglion damage may underlie the beneficial effects of ganglionated plexi ablation in controlling AF. Bilateral *renal denervation* causes

significant central and peripheral sympathetic nerve remodeling and reduced stellate ganglion nerve activity in ambulatory dogs.[48] Among patients with paroxysmal AF and hypertension, renal denervation added to catheter ablation, compared with catheter ablation alone, significantly increased the likelihood of freedom from AF at 12 months.[49] It is likely that neuromodulation procedures will be increasingly used to manage cardiac arrhythmias in the near future.

β-Blockers and Arrhythmia Control

β-blockers have long been used for arrhythmia control. However, there is growing appreciation of the differential antiarrhythmic effects between selective and nonselective β-blockers in cardiac arrhythmia management. While cardiac tissues normally have primarily β-1 receptors, there is downregulation of β-1 and upregulation of β-2 receptors in heart failure. Selective β-1 receptors blockers (such as metoprolol) do not effectively block all the effects of sympathetic activation in the heart. In addition to cardiac actions, sympathetic stimulation also has significant extracardiac effects. Skeletal muscle, the largest muscle mass in the body, has abundant β-2 receptors. Selective activation of β-2 receptors in the skeletal muscle induces hypokalemia, increases QT interval and dispersion of repolarization in the ventricular myocardium. Because hypokalemia inhibits the Na-K pump, even moderate hypokalemia can play a critical role in EAD-mediated cardiac arrhythmias.[50] Therefore, a second major antiarrhythmic action of β-2 blockade is to prevent systemic hypokalemia during sympathetic stimulation. Consistent with the theoretical importance of β-2 blockade in arrhythmia control, a recent randomized clinical trial[51] found that patients with electrical storm (recurrent VT/VF) treated with propranolol had much better outcomes than patients treated with metoprolol. Note that neuromodulation methods which reduce sympathetic outflow also reduce the activation of both β-1 and β-2 receptors in the heart to achieve its antiarrhythmic effects.

Summary

In summary, the mechanism of cardiac arrhythmia includes automaticity, triggered activity, and reentry. Myocardial infarction, heart failure, and cardiac hypertrophy are associated with significant structural, electrophysiological, and neural remodeling. Disease-induced cardiac remodeling may facilitate the development of both reentrant and non-reentrant arrhythmias. Understanding these arrhythmogenic mechanisms is important to providing mechanism-based therapy for cardiac arrhythmia.

GENETIC, IONIC, AND CELLULAR MECHANISMS UNDERLYING THE J-WAVE SYNDROMES

Introduction

The J-wave syndromes, consisting of the Brugada (BrS) and Early Repolarization Syndromes (ERS), have intrigued the cardiology community since the initial presentation of BrS as a clinical entity in 1992.[52] The clinical impact of ERS was not fully realized until 2008, when publication of the now classical studies of Haïssaguerre and coworkers,[53] Nam and coworkers,[54] and Rosso et al.[55] appeared. The genetic basis for BrS and ERS has progressed, but the Mendelian nature of their inheritance has been questioned by recent studies. The cellular mechanisms underlying the J-wave syndromes have also been a matter of debate.

The appearance of prominent J waves in the ECG was first reported in clinical cases of hypothermia and hypercalcemia. Accentuation of the J wave has been associated with life-threatening ventricular arrhythmias.[56] Under these circumstances, the accentuated J wave typically may be so broad as to appear as an ST-segment elevation, as in cases of BrS. The normal J wave in humans often appears as a J point elevation, with part of the J wave buried inside the QRS. An early repolarization (ER) pattern in the ECG, characterized by a distinct J wave, J point elevation, a notch or slur of the terminal part of the QRS with and without an ST-segment elevation has traditionally been viewed as benign. In 2000, Gussak and Antzelevitch[57] challenged this view on the basis of experimental data showing that this ECG manifestation predisposes to the development of polymorphic VT/VF in coronary-perfused wedge preparations. This hypothesis was validated 8 years later by Haïssaguerre et al.,[53] Nam et al.,[54] and Rosso et al.[55] These formative

studies coupled with many additional case control and population-based studies have provided clinical evidence for an increased risk for development of life-threatening arrhythmic events and SCD among patients presenting with an ER pattern, particularly in inferior and infero-lateral leads. This field has been marred by inconsistent reporting of data due to lack of agreement regarding terminology relative to ER. An expert consensus statement published by MacFarlane and coworkers provided recommendations of measurement and reporting of ER and J waves. The task force recommended that peak of an end QRS notch and/or the onset of an end QRS slur be designated as J_p and that J_p should exceed 0.1 mV in ≥2 contiguous inferior and/or lateral leads of a standard 12-lead ECG for early repolarization to be present.[58] It was further recommended that the start of the end QRS notch or J wave be designated as J_o and the termination as J_t.

Both BrS and ERS have been associated with vulnerability to development of polymorphic VT and VF leading to SCD in young adults and occasionally to sudden infant death syndrome (SIDS).[56] The region generally most affected in ERS is the inferior LV and in BrS it is the anterior right ventricular outflow tract. BrS is characterized by accentuated J waves, appearing as a coved-type ST-segment elevation in the right precordial leads, V1-V3, whereas ERS is characterized by J waves, J_o elevation, notch or slur of the terminal part of the QRS, and ST-segment or J_t elevation in the lateral (type I), infero-lateral (type II) or in infero-lateral + anterior or right ventricular leads (type III).[59] ER pattern (ERP) is often encountered in healthy individuals, particularly in young, Black individuals and athletes. ERP is also observed in acquired conditions, including hypothermia and ischemia. When associated with VT/VF, ERP is referred to as early repolarization syndrome (ERS).

Prevalence of the J-wave syndromes varies widely based on geographic location. The prevalence of type 1 BrS ECG is higher in Asian countries, such as Japan (0.15%–0.27%), the Philippines (0.18%), and among Japanese Americans in North America (0.15%) than in Western countries, including Europe (0%–0.017%) or North America (0.005%–0.1%). The prevalence of an ERP in the inferior and/or lateral leads with a J_o elevation of ≥0.1 mV ranges between 1% and 24% and for J_o of ≥0.2 mV, it ranges between 0.6% and 6.4%. An ERP is significantly more common in Blacks than in Caucasians. Early repolarization appears to be more common in Aboriginal Australians than in Caucasian Australians.[60]

Similarities and Differences Between BRS and ERS

ERS and BrS share several phenotypic features, suggesting similar pathophysiology (**Table 34-2**).[56,61] Males predominate in both syndromes: in BrS, presenting in males in 71% to 80% among Caucasians and in 94% to 96% among Japanese. BrS and ERS patients may be totally asymptomatic until presenting with sudden cardiac arrest. In both syndromes, the highest incidence of VF or SCD occurs in the third decade of life, thought to be tied to testosterone levels in males. In both syndromes, the appearance of accentuated J waves and ST-segment elevation is generally associated with bradycardia or pauses,

TABLE 34-2. Similarities and Differences Between Brugada Syndrome (BrS) and Early Repolarization Syndrome (ERS) and Possible Underlying Mechanisms

	BrS	ERS	Possible Mechanism(s)
Similarities between BrS and ERS			
Male predominance	Yes (>75%)	Yes (>80%)	Testosterone modulation of ion currents underlying the epicardial AP notch
Average age of first event	30–50	30–50	
Associated with mutations or rare variants in *SCN5A*	Yes	Yes	Loss of function in inward currents (I_{Na})
Relatively short QT intervals in subjects with Ca channel mutations	Yes	Yes	Loss of function of I_{Ca}
Dynamicity of ECG	High	High	Autonomic modulation of ion channel currents underlying early phases of the epicardial AP
VF often occurs during sleep or at a low level of physical activity	Yes	Yes	Higher level of vagal tone and higher levels of I_{to} at the slower heart rates
VT/VF trigger	Short-coupled PVC	Short-coupled PVC	Phase 2 reentry
Ameliorative response to quinidine and bepridil	Yes	Yes	Inhibition of I_{to} and possible vagolytic effect
Ameliorative response to Isoproterenol denopamine and milrinone	Yes	Yes	Increased I_{Ca} and faster heart rate
Ameliorative response to cilostazol	Yes	Yes	Increased I_{Ca}, reduced I_{to}, and faster heart rate
Ameliorative response to pacing	Yes	Yes	Reduced availability of I_{to} due to slow recovery from inactivation
Vagally mediated accentuation of ECG pattern	Yes	Yes	Direct effect to inhibit I_{Ca} and indirect effect to increase I_{to} (due to slowing of heart rate)
Effect of sodium channel blockers on unipolar epicardial electrogram	Augmented J waves	Augmented J wave	Outward shift of balance of current in the early phases of the epicardial action potential
Fever	Augmented J waves	Augmented J waves (rare)	Accelerated inactivation of I_{Na} and accelerated recovery of I_{to} from inactivation
Hypothermia	Augmented J waves mimicking BrS	Augmented J waves	Slowed activation of I_{Ca}, leaving I_{to} unopposed. Increased phase 2 reentry, but reduced pVT due to prolongation of APD[246]
Differences between BrS and ERS			
Region most involved	RVOT	Inferior LV wall	Higher levels of I_{to} and/or differences in conduction
Leads affected	V1-V3	II, II aVF V4, V5, V6; I, aVL Both: infero-lateral	
Regional difference in prevalence			Europe: BrS = ERS Asia: BrS > ERS
Incidence of late potential in SAECG	Higher	Lower	
Inducibility of VF during an EPS	Higher	Lower	
Prevalence of atrial fibrillation	Higher	Lower	
Effect of sodium channel blockers on the surface ECG	Increased J wave manifestation	Reduced J wave Manifestation	Reduction of J wave in the setting of ER is thought to be due largely to prolongation of QRS. Accentuation of repolarization defects predominates in BrS, whereas accentuation of depolarization defects predominates in ERS

Abbreviations: AP, action potential; PVC, premature ventricular contraction, RVOT, right ventricular outflow tract.

Adapted with permission from Antzelevitch C, Yan GX, Ackerman MJ, et al: J-Wave syndromes expert consensus conference report: Emerging concepts and gaps in knowledge. *Heart Rhythm.* 2016 Oct;13(10):e295-e324.

explaining why VF in both syndromes often occurs during sleep or at a low level of physical activity.[62] The QT interval is relatively short in patients with ERS and BrS who carry mutations in calcium channel genes.[63]

BrS and ERS also show similar responses to pharmacological therapy. In both syndromes, electrical storms and associated J-wave manifestations can be suppressed using β-adrenergic agonists. Chronic oral pharmacological therapy using quinidine, cilostazol, denopamine, and bepridil is reported to suppress the development of VT/VF in both syndromes secondary to inhibition of I_{to}, augmentation of I_{Ca}, I_{Na}, or both (see [64] for references).

Differences between the two syndromes include: (1) the region of the heart most affected (RVOT vs. inferior LV); (2) greater incidence of late potentials in signal-averaged ECGs in BrS (60%) versus ERS; (3) greater inducibility of VF during electrophysiological study in BrS than in ERS; (4) greater elevation of J_O, J_P, or J_t (ST-segment elevation) in response to sodium channel blockers in BrS versus ERS; and (5) higher prevalence of AF in BrS versus ERS. Some early studies suggested different pathophysiological bases for ERS and BrS because sodium channel blockers were shown to unmask or accentuate J-wave manifestation in BrS, but to reduce J-wave amplitude in ERS. Nakagawa et al. recently reported that J waves recorded using unipolar LV epicardial leads introduced into the left lateral coronary vein in ERS patients are indeed augmented, even though J waves recorded in the lateral precordial leads are diminished. The latter were diminished due widening of the QRS leading to engulfment of the surface J wave. Also in support of the thesis that these ECG patterns and syndromes are closely related are reports of cases in which ERS transitions into ERS plus BrS.[65]

J waves have been reported to be accentuated or induced by both hypothermia and fever. However, the development of arrhythmias in ERS is much more sensitive to hypothermia and arrhythmogenesis in BrS appears to be promoted exclusively by fever. Hypothermia is reported to increase the risk of VF in ERS and fever is well recognized as a major risk factor in BrS. Wu and coworkers recently reported cases of COVID-19 patients in which fever unmasked the Brugada phenotype.[66] It is noteworthy that hypothermia can actually diminish the manifestation of a BrS ECG when a prominent J wave or ST-segment elevation is already present.

An ER pattern is associated with an increased risk for VF in patients with acute myocardial infarction and hypothermia. A concomitant ER pattern in the infero-lateral leads has also been reported to be associated with an increased risk of arrhythmic events in patients with BrS. Kawata et al. reported that the prevalence of ER in infero-lateral leads was high (63%) in BrS patients with documented VF.[67]

Genetics

Candidate gene, Next Generation, whole genome and exome sequencing, as well as genome wide association studies (GWAS) have associated variants in 23 different genes in the case of BrS and 10 different genes in the case of ERS (**Table 34–3**) (see 68 for references). To date more than 300 BrS-related variants in *SCN5A* have been described. The available evidence suggests that the presence of a prominent I_{to} determines whether loss of function mutations resulting in a reduction in I_{Na} will manifest as BrS/ERS as opposed to conduction disease.[69-72] Variants in *CACNA1C* ($Ca_v1.2$), *CACNB2b* (Cavβ2b), and *CACNA2D1* (Cavα2δ) have been reported in up to 13% of probands. Variants in glycerol-3-phophate dehydrogenase 1-like enzyme gene (*GPD1L*), *SCN1B* (β1-subunit of Na channel), *KCNE3* (MiRP2), *SCN3B* (β3-subunit of Na channel), *KCNJ8* (Kir 6.1), *KCND3* (Kv4.3), *RANGRF* (MOG1), *SLMAP*, *ABCC9* (SUR2A), (Navβ2), *PKP2* (Plakophillin-2), *FGF12* (FHAF1), *HEY2*, *SEMA3A* (Semaphorin), and *KCNAB2* (Kvβ2) are relatively rare. An association of BrS with *SCN10A*, a neuronal sodium channel, has been reported. A wide range of yields were reported by the two studies that examined the prevalence of pathogenic *SCN10A* mutations and rare variants (5% vs 16.7%). Like Hu et al.,[73] Monasky and coworkers recently reported that the yield of SCN10A variants associated with BrA is second to that of SCN5A and that BrS ECG pattern, family history of sudden death, and arrhythmic substrate are not significantly different between probands harboring SCN10A or SCN5A variants.[74] Abnormal myocardial expression of the synapse-associated protein 97 (SAP97) has recently been associated with arrhythmogenic risk in patients with BrS.[75] SAP97 is a *DLG1*-encoded scaffolding protein that plays a critical role in functional expression of several cardiac ion channels. Alterations in the functional expression of SAP97 can modify the ionic currents underlying the cardiac action potential and consequently confer susceptibility for cardiac arrhythmogenesis as well as schizophrenia.[76] Shimizu et al. recently reported association of mutations in TMEM168 encoding the transmembrane protein 168 with familial cases of BrS.[77]

Variants in *KCNH2*, *KCNE5*, and *SEMA3A*, although not causative, have been identified as capable of modulating the substrate for the development of BrS (see 68 for references). Loss-of-function mutations in *HCN4* causing a reduction in pacemaker current, I_f, can unmask BrS by reducing heart rate.

Mutations in the aforementioned genes lead to loss of function in sodium (I_{Na}) and calcium (I_{Ca}) channel currents, as well as to a gain of function in transient outward potassium current (I_{to}), delayed rectifier potassium channel current (I_{Kr}), or ATP-sensitive potassium current (I_{K-ATP}).[78]

An ER pattern in the ECG is also known to be familial (see 68 for references). Consistent with the findings that I_{K-ATP} activation can generate an ER pattern in canine ventricular wedge preparations, variants in genes responsible for the pore forming and ATP-sensing subunits of the I_{K-ATP} channel, *KCNJ8* and *ABCC9*, have been reported in patients with ERS. Loss of function variations in the α-1, β-2, and α2δ subunits of the cardiac L-type calcium channel (*CACNA1C*, *CACNB2*, and *CACNA2D1*) and the α-1 subunit of Nav1.5 and Nav1.8 (*SCN5A* and *SCN10A*) have been reported in BRS patients. In 2018, Cheng et al.[79] reported a novel mutation, K801T, in *hERG* in a Chinese family with ERS. The authors showed that the K801T variant leads to a significant increase in hERG current (I_{Kr}), a significant negative shift in the voltage dependence of activation, faster rate of activation and deactivation, and a positive shift in the voltage dependence of inactivation, suggesting that

TABLE 34–3. Gene Defects Associated with the Early Repolarization Syndrome (ERS) and Brugada Syndrome (BrS)

	Genetic Defects Associated with ERS		
	Locus	**Gene/Protein**	**Ion Channel**
ERS1	12p11.23	*KCNJ8*, Kir6.1	$\uparrow I_{K\text{-}ATP}$
ERS2	12p13.3	*CACNA1C*, Ca$_v$1.2	$\downarrow I_{Ca}$
ERS3	10p12.33	*CACNB2b*, Ca$_v$β2b	$\downarrow I_{Ca}$
ERS4	7q21.11	*CACNA2D1*, Ca$_v$a2d1	$\downarrow I_{Ca}$
ERS5	12p12.1	*ABCC9*, SUR2A	$\uparrow I_{K\text{-}ATP}$
ERS6	3p21	*SCN5A*, Na$_v$1.5	$\downarrow I_{Na}$
ERS7	3p22.2	*SCN10A*, Na$_v$1.8	$\downarrow I_{Na}$
ERS8	7q35	*KCNH2*, hERG	$\uparrow I_{Kr}$
ERS9	19q13.1	*SCN1Bβ*, Na$_v$β1	$\uparrow I_{to}$
ERS10	1p13.2	*KCND3*, K$_v$4.3	$\uparrow I_{to}$
	Locus	**Gene/Protein**	**Ion Channel**
BrS1	3p21	*SCN5A*, Na$_v$1.5	$\downarrow I_{Na}$
BrS2	3p24	*GPD1L*	$\downarrow I_{Na}$
BrS3	12p13.3	*CACNA1C*, Ca$_v$1.2	$\downarrow I_{Ca}$
BrS4	10p12.33	*CACNB2b*, Ca$_v$β2b	$\downarrow I_{Ca}$
BrS5	19q13.1	*SCN1B*, Na$_v$β1	$\downarrow I_{Na}$
BrS6	11q13-14	*KCNE3*, MiRP2	$\uparrow I_{to}$
BrS7	11q23.3	*SCN3B*, Na$_v$β3	$\downarrow I_{Na}$
BrS8	12p11.23	*KCNJ8*, Kir6.1	$\uparrow I_{K\text{-}ATP}$
BrS9	7q21.11	*CACNA2D1*, Ca$_v$a2d1	$\downarrow I_{Ca}$
BrS10	1p13.2	*KCND3*, K$_v$4.3	$\uparrow I_{to}$
BrS11	17p13.1	*RANGRF*, MOG1	$\downarrow I_{Na}$
BrS12	3p21.2-p14.3	*SLMAP*	$\downarrow I_{Na}$
BrS13	12p12.1	*ABCC9*, SUR2A	$\uparrow I_{K\text{-}ATP}$
BrS14	11q23	*SCN2B*, Na$_v$β2	$\downarrow I_{Na}$
BrS15	12p11	*PKP2*, Plakophillin-2	$\downarrow I_{Na}$
BrS16	3q28	*FGF12*, FHAF1	$\downarrow I_{Na}$
BrS17	3p22.2	*SCN10A*, Na$_v$1.8	$\downarrow I_{Na}$
BrS18	6q	*HEY2 (transcriptional factor)*	$\uparrow I_{Na}$
BrS19	1p36.3	*KCNAB2*, Kvβ2	$\uparrow I_{to}$
BrS20	7q31.1	*TMEM168*, trans-membrane protein 168 *168168.*	$\downarrow I_{Na}$
BrS21	3q29	*SLG1/SAP97*	$\uparrow I_{to}$
BrS22	17q12	*TCAP*- Z-disk cytoskeletal protein	$\downarrow I_{Na}$
BrS23	1p13.3	*GSTM3*–Glutathione S-transferase transferase	$\downarrow I_{Na}$

Listed in chronological order of their discovery. Adapted with permission from Antzelevitch C, Yan GX, Ackerman MJ, et al: J-Wave syndromes expert consensus conference report: Emerging concepts and gaps in knowledge. *Heart Rhythm.* 2016 Oct;13(10):e295-e324.

the gain-of-function mutation of hERG channel was responsible for the ERS phenotype. The hERG channel blockers, including quinidine, disopyramide, sotalol, and flecainide, were effective in inhibiting the K801T-*hERG* channel current. Also in 2018, Yao et al.[80] reported two mutations (S248R and R250T) in *SCN1Bβ* associated with ERS. The *SCN1Bβ* variant produced a gain of function in I$_{to}$, similar to the *SCN1Bβ* variants previously associated with BrS, which also produced a loss

of function I$_{Na.}$ In 2019, Takayama et al. identified another ERS susceptibility gene. The authors found a novel heterozygous mutation in *KCND3* associated with ERS as a result of a gain of function in I$_{to}$.[81]

It is fundamentally important to recognize that very few variants in the genes associated with BrS and ERS have been evaluated using functional expression studies or other modalities to ascertain causality and to establish pathogenicity. Very few variants have been studied in genetically engineered animal models, native cardiac cells or in induced pluripotent stem cell-derived cardiac myocytes isolated from ERS and BrS patients. In silico tools developed to predict the functional consequences of mutations are helpful, but have not been rigorously tested. The lack of functional validation remains a severe limitation of genetic test interpretation. Recent technological advances have resulted in expansion of disease specific-panels, which have challenged our understanding of the extent of background genetic variation within cardiac channelopathy-susceptibility genes. These issues suggest that the results of the genetic test should be treated as probabilistic, rather than binary or deterministic. Additional evidence can be obtained from cosegregation, studies, in silico prediction tools, and variant frequency in cases and control databases. Despite these aids, a large number of variants remain in "genetic purgatory." Kapplinger et al. recently reported the synergistic use of up to seven in silico tools to help promote or demote a variant's pathogenic status and alter its relegation to genetic purgatory.[82]

Le Scouarnec and coworkers calculated the burden of rare coding variations in arrhythmia-susceptibility genes among 167 BrS index patients and compared this with 167 individuals aged over 65 years old with no history of cardiac arrhythmia.[83] The authors concluded that, except for *SCN5A*, rare coding variations in all previously reported BrS-susceptibility genes do not contribute significantly to the occurrence of BrS in a population with European ancestry, emphasizing that caution should be taken when interpreting genetic variations in these other genes because rare coding variants are observed to a similar extent in both cases and controls.[83]

Hosseini et al. subsequently published a full reappraisal of reported genes for BrS.[84] The authors evaluated the clinical validity of genes tested by diagnostic and academic laboratories for BrS using an evidence-based semi-quantitative scoring system of genetic and experimental evidence for gene-disease associations. The reappraisal of reported BrS-susceptibility genes whether by application of these ClinGen evidence-based gene curation frameworks[84] or by means of testing for the increased burden of rare genetic variants in BrS patients compared to controls,[83] supported only the involvement of rare variations in *SCN5A*, found in ~20% of probands.

As a consequence, the sole gene thus far unequivocally implicated in BrS is *SCN5A*. Moreover, the often-sporadic presentation of the disorder and the low disease penetrance in families with rare variants in *SCN5A*, as well as the observation of phenotype-positive genotype-negative individuals in such families, suggests that BrS may be a disease with complex genetics and that inheritance is likely not Mendelian. These data suggest that in individual cases, BrS and the susceptibility to SCD may not be due to a single mutation, but rather to inheritance of multiple BrS-susceptibility variants (oligogenic). The multifactorial nature of the genetics, may be further confounded by the fact that expressivity of the syndrome may be multifactorial in that the phenotype is importantly modulated by hormonal (testosterone, thyroxine) and other environmental factors.

Cellular Mechanisms Underlying BRS and ERS

The J-wave syndromes are so named because they involve accentuation of the electrocardiographic J wave.[70] The J wave is believed to be inscribed as a consequence of transmural differences in the manifestation of the action potential notch between epicardium and endocardium secondary to heterogeneous transmural distribution of I_{to}. The transmural gradient and associated J wave is much greater in the RV versus LV, particularly in the region of the RVOT, because of the more prominent I_{to}-mediated AP notch in right ventricular epicardium. This distinction is the basis for why BrS is a right ventricular disease. An end of QRS notch, resembling a J wave, has been proposed to be caused by intramural conduction delays. The distinction can be made on the basis of the response to heart rate, with the latter showing accentuation at faster rates.[85-87]

The J wave is thus a reflection of early repolarization of the epicardial action potential in both RVs and LVs. It can manifest as a J point elevation (Fig 34–34A), a distinct J wave (Fig. 34–34B), a slurring of the terminal portion of the QRS (Fig. 34–34C), a distinct J wave with an ST-segment elevation (Fig. 34–34D), or as a gigantic J wave appearing as an ST-segment elevation (due to the influence of the I_{to} agonist NS5806; Fig. 34–34E). It is under these last set of conditions that we see the development of phase 2 reentry and polymorphic VT (Fig. 34–34F).

The cellular mechanisms underlying the J-wave syndromes have long been a matter of debate.[88,89] Two principle hypotheses have been advanced in the case of BrS: (1) the *repolarization hypothesis* maintains that an outward shift in the balance of currents in the right ventricular epicardium leads to repolarization abnormalities, resulting in the development of phase 2 reentry, which generates closely-coupled premature beats capable of precipitating VT/VF (**Figs. 34–35A to 34–35F**); (2) the *depolarization hypothesis* maintains that delayed conduction in the RVOT plays a primary role in the development of the electrocardiographic and arrhythmic manifestations of the syndrome and that the J wave or ST-segment elevation is due to a difference in activation time of RVOT versus the remainder of RV. Contributing to the outward shift in the balance of current responsible for the J wave is the presence of small-conductance calcium (Ca^{2+})-activated potassium (SK) channel current (I_{SK}) in ventricular myocardium. Landaw et al.[90] recently suggested that colocalization of SK channels with L-type Ca^{2+} channels may preferentially sense Ca^{2+} in the subsarcolemmal or junctional space resulting in a "spiky" I_{SK}, which can functionally play a role similar to that of I_{to} in promoting J-wave syndrome and ventricular arrhythmias.

In support of the repolarization hypothesis is the observation that in patients with BrS acceleration of heart rate leads to a reduction of the ST-segment elevation, which is due to reduced availability of I_{to} and smaller RV epicardial AP notches at the faster rate. In contrast, in the depolarization hypothesis, acceleration of rate is expected to have the opposite effect (ie, exacerbation of the ST-segment elevation at fast rates) since acceleration is usually associated with slowing of conduction.[88,91]

Also in support of the repolarization hypothesis is the report of Zhang et al. who used noninvasive ECG imaging

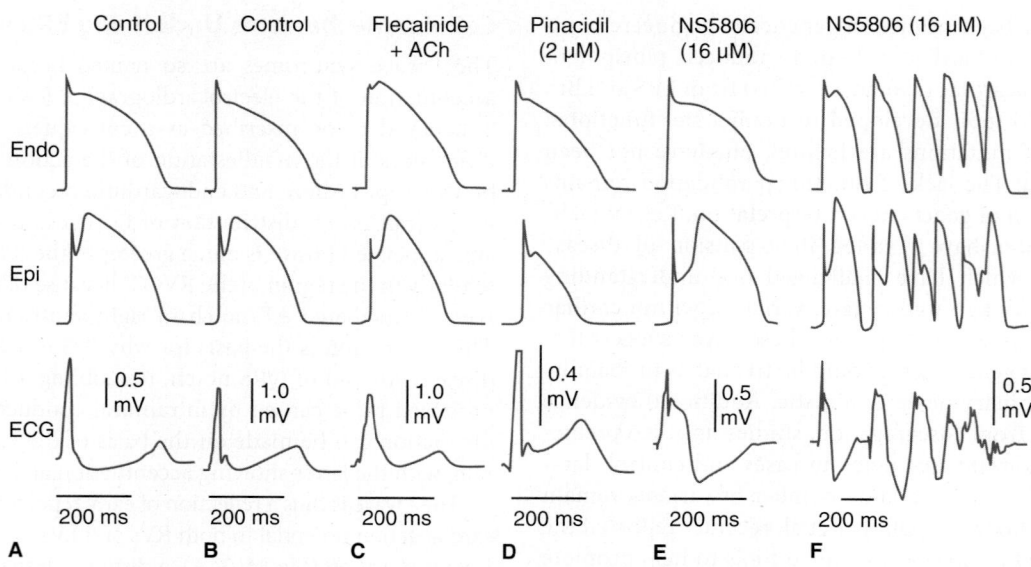

Figure 34–34. Electrocardiographic manifestations of early repolarization recapitulated in coronary perfused canine ventricular wedge preparations. Each panel shows action potential recordings from epicardium (Epi) and endocardium (Endo) and a transmural ECG. J waves are a reflection of early repolarization of ventricular epicardium and can manifest as **(A)** a J point elevation, **(B)** a distinct J wave, **(C)** a slurring of the terminal part of the QRS recorded following exposure to flecainide + acetylcholine, **(D)** a distinct J wave with an ST segment recorded following exposure to pinacidil, and **(E)** a gigantic J wave appearing as an ST-segment elevation recorded following exposure to the Ito agonist NS5806. It is under these conditions that we observe the development of polymorphic VT **(F)**.

techniques (ECGI) to study 25 BrS and 6 right bundle branch block (RBBB) patients.[92] The authors concluded that both slow, discontinuous conduction and steep dispersion of repolarization are present in the RVOT of BrS patients. Unlike BrS, RBBB showed delayed activation in the entire RV (not just in the RVOT as in BrS patients), without ST-segment elevation, fractionation, or repolarization abnormalities shown on the electrograms. Increasing the heart rate in 6 of the BrS patients led to augmented fractionation of the electrograms *but* to a reduction of the ST-segment elevation in the right precordial ECG leads, indicating that the conduction impairment was not the principal cause of the BrS ECG phenotype.

In 2011, Nademanee et al.[93] reported a seminal study showing that radiofrequency (RF) ablation of epicardial sites displaying fractionated bipolar electrograms (EGs) and late potentials (LP) in the RVOT of patients with BrS suppresses the electrocardiographic and arrhythmic manifestations of BrS. These authors hypothesized that LP and fractionated electrogram activity are due to conduction delays within the RVOT.[93] Similar results and conclusions were reported by Sacher and coworkers and Brugada et al.[94,95] Szél and coworkers[71] provided a direct test of this hypothesis and showed, using experimental models of BrS, that the electrophysiologic and arrhythmic manifestations are due to repolarization defects rather than depolarization or conduction defects.

Figures 34–36A and **34–36B** show the similarity between the low voltage fractionated electrical bipolar electrogram activity recorded by Nademanee and coworkers from the RVOT epicardium of patients with BrS with low voltage fractionated electrical activity recorded by Szel et al. from RV epicardium of a coronary-perfused wedge model of BrS. The study by Szel

et al. clearly showed that such fractionated electrical activity in these cases is not due to conduction delay within the RV but rather to temporal heterogeneities in the appearance of the epicardial action potential dome giving rise to undulations in the bipolar electrogram appearing as fractionated epicardial electrical activity.[71]

In some regions of the wedge model of BrS, Szel et al. recorded late potentials very similar to those recorded by Nademanee et al. in the RVOT of patients with BrS (**Figs. 34–37A** and **34–37B**). Here again, the late potentials were not due to delayed conduction but rather to concealed phase 2 reentry.

It remained to be explained why ablation of regions of the RVOT exhibiting fractionated electrogram activity and late potentials is effective in suppressing the ECG and arrhythmic manifestations of BrS. Patocskai et al.[96] demonstrated that ablation was effective because it eliminated the cells in the surface of the RVOT responsible for the repolarization defects giving rise to a BrS phenotype (**Fig. 34–38**).

Recent studies have endeavored to create whole-heart models of BrS and used these to provide a further test of the repolarization versus depolarization hypotheses (**Figs. 34–39A** to **34–39D**).[97] Adult canine hearts were perfused in Langendorff mode after removal of the atria. The hearts, allowed to beat spontaneously or paced from the septum, were immersed in a volume-conducting chamber with preset electrodes to record a 12-lead ECG as well as vector cardiogram (VCG). Epi unipolar EGs were recorded from the RVOT, RV inferior wall, LV antero-basal region, and LV apex. Transmembrane APs were recorded from the RVOT using floating glass microelectrodes. The I_{to} agonist NS5806 (5–10 μM, NS), ajmaline (10 μM), or hypothermia (30–32°C) were used to elicit J waves.

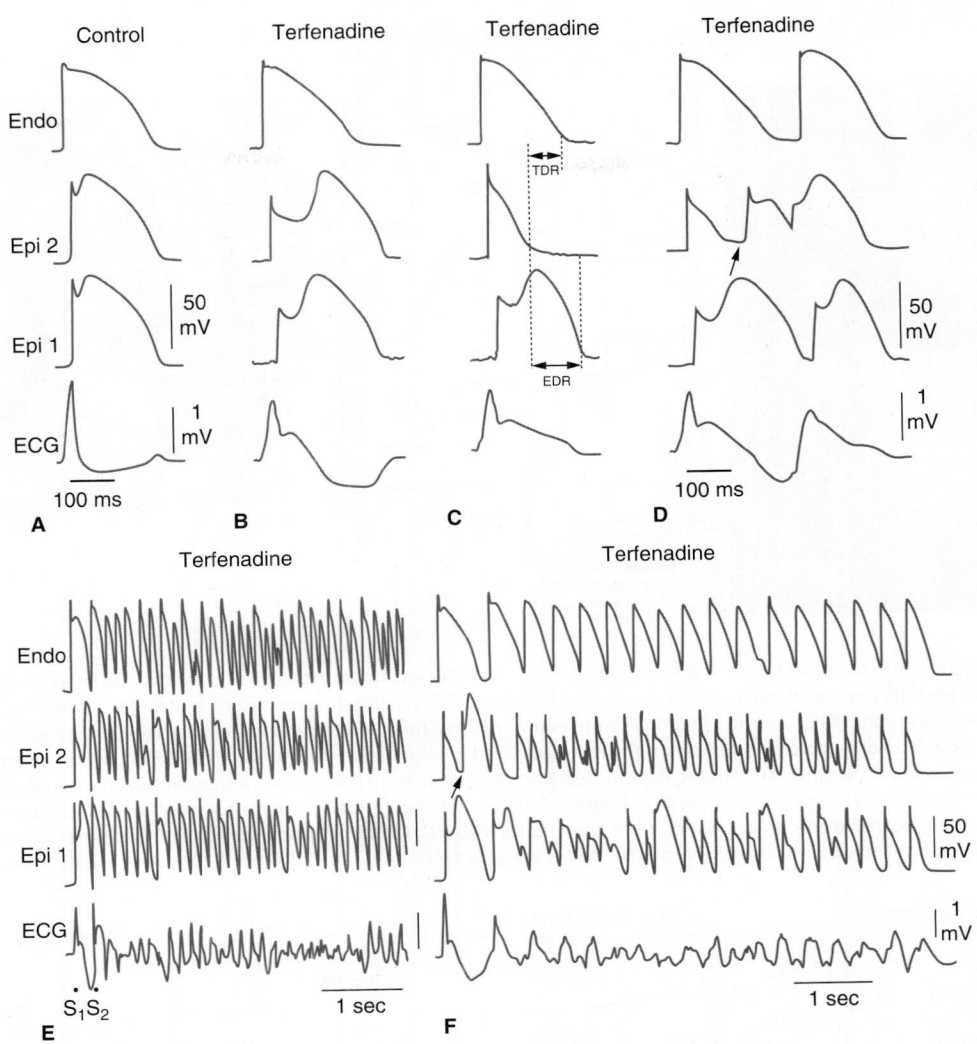

Figure 34–35. Cellular basis for electrocardiographic and arrhythmic manifestation of BrS. Each panel shows transmembrane APs from one endocardial (*top*) and two epicardial sites together with a transmural ECG recorded from a canine coronary-perfused right ventricular wedge preparation. **(A)** Control (Basic cycle length [BCL] 400 ms). **(B)** Combined sodium and calcium channel block with terfenadine (5 μM) accentuates the epicardial AP notch creating a transmural voltage gradient that manifests as an ST-segment elevation or exaggerated J wave in the ECG. **(C)** Continued exposure to terfenadine results in all-or-none repolarization at the end of phase 1 at some epicardial sites but not others, creating a local epicardial dispersion of repolarization (EDR) as well as a transmural dispersion of repolarization (TDR). **(D)** Phase 2 reentry occurs when the epicardial AP dome propagates from a site where it is maintained to regions where it has been lost giving rise to a closely coupled extrasystole. **(E)** Extra-stimulus (S1–S2 = 250 ms) applied to epicardium triggers a polymorphic VT. **(F)** Phase 2 reentrant extrasystole triggers a brief episode of polymorphic VT. Reproduced with permission from Fish JM, Antzelevitch C. Role of sodium and calcium channel block in unmasking the Brugada syndrome. *Heart Rhythm.* 2004 Jul;1(2):210-217.

The I_{to} agonist and sodium channel blocker served to mimic the genetic defects associated with BrS. In the example illustrated in Figs. 34–39A to 34–39D, NS increased the Epi AP notch in the RVOT (compare Figs. 34–39A to 34–39B) leading to a prominent J wave in V1. Activation of the RVOT (Vmin; circled) of the EGs clearly did not contribute to inscription of the J wave. Figure 34–39C, recorded 4 minutes later, shows loss of the AP dome at one site but not the other and the development of a closely-coupled extrasystole arising from the RVOT, consistent with a phase 2 reentry mechanism, which, 1 minute later, precipitated VT/VF (Fig. 34–39D).

In similar studies, inhibition of I_{to} with 4-AP (0.5–1 mM) or acacetin (5 μM) was found to greatly reduce or eliminate the J wave and to prevent arrhythmogenesis. Moreover, activation

delay in the RVOT (relative to RV inferior wall) induced by ajmaline and/or hypothermia did *not* contribute to inscription of the J wave.

These findings provide compelling evidence against the depolarization hypothesis showing that the electrocardiographic and arrhythmic manifestations of BrS can be due exclusively to dispersion of repolarization and refractoriness secondary to accentuated *repolarization* during the early phases of the RV epicardial action potential. These data notwithstanding, it stands to reason that the repolarization and depolarization hypotheses are not necessarily mutually exclusive and may indeed be synergistic.

In an attempt to create an in vivo model of BrS, Park et al. genetically engineered Yucatan minipigs to heterozygously

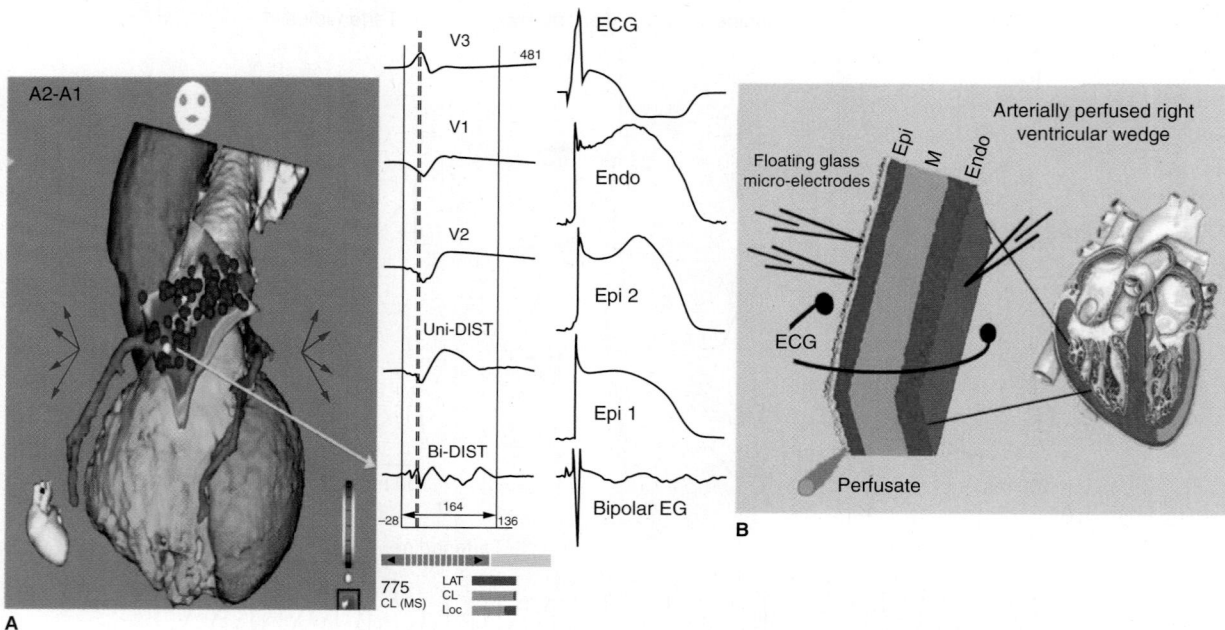

Figure 34–36. Heterogeneities in the appearance of the epicardial action potential second upstroke gives rise to fractionated epicardial EG activity in the setting of BrS. **(A)** Shown are right precordial lead recordings, unipolar and bipolar EGs recorded form the right ventricular outflow tract of a BrS patient (from Nademanee et al.[81] with permission). **(B)** ECG, action potentials from endocardium (Endo) and two epicardial (Epi) sites, and a bipolar epicardial EG (Bipolar EG) all simultaneously recorded from a coronary-perfused right ventricular wedge preparation treated with NS5806 (5 μM) and verapamil (2 μM) to induce the Brugada phenotype. Basic cycle length = 1000 ms. **A,** Reproduced with permission from Nademanee K, Veerakul G, Chandanamattha P, et al: Prevention of ventricular fibrillation episodes in Brugada syndrome by catheter ablation over the anterior right ventricular outflow tract epicardium, *Circulation*. 2011 Mar 29;123(12):1270-1279. **B,** Reproduced with permission from Szél T, Antzelevitch C. Abnormal repolarization as the basis for late potentials and fractionated electrograms recorded from epicardium in experimental models of Brugada syndrome, *J Am Coll Cardiol*. 2014 May 20;63(19):2037-2045.

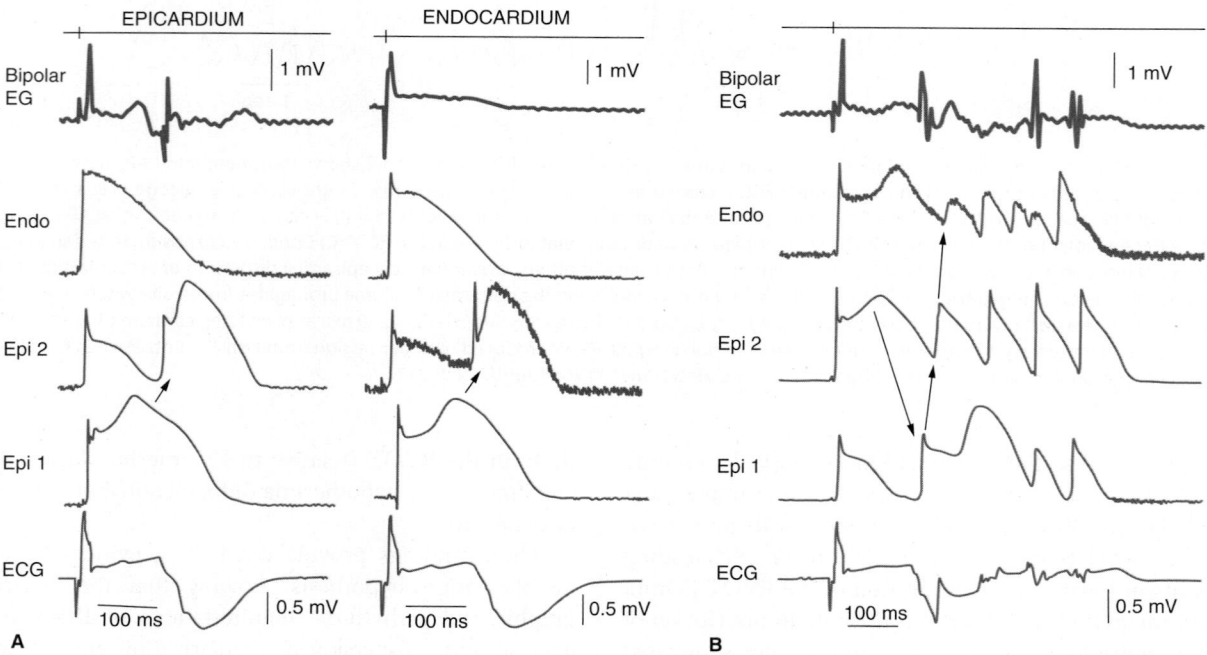

Figure 34–37. **(A)** Concealed phase 2 reentry gives rise to late potentials and fractionated bipolar electrogram (Bipolar EG) activity recorded from epicardium but not endocardium (Endo) in an experimental model of BrS. Each panel shows (from top to bottom) a bipolar epicardial (Epi) EG, action potentials recorded from Endo and two Epi sites and an ECG all simultaneously recorded from a coronary-perfused right ventricular (RV) wedge preparation exposed to NS5806 (5 μM) and verapamil (2 μM) to induce the Brugada phenotype. Heterogeneous loss of the dome at epicardium caused local reexcitation via a concealed phase 2 reentry mechanism, leading to the development of late potentials and fractionated bipolar epicardial EGs. Basic cycle length = 1000 ms. **(B)** Phase 2 Reentry-induced ventricular fibrillation. All traces were simultaneously recorded from a coronary-perfused RV wedge preparation exposed to NS5806 (5 μM) and verapamil (2 μM). The phase 2 reentrant beat produced a closely coupled extrasystole that precipitated an episode of polymorphic tachycardia. Reproduced with permission from Szél T, Antzelevitch C. Abnormal repolarization as the basis for late potentials and fractionated electrograms recorded from epicardium in experimental models of Brugada syndrome, *J Am Coll Cardiol*. 2014 May 20;63(19):2037-2045.

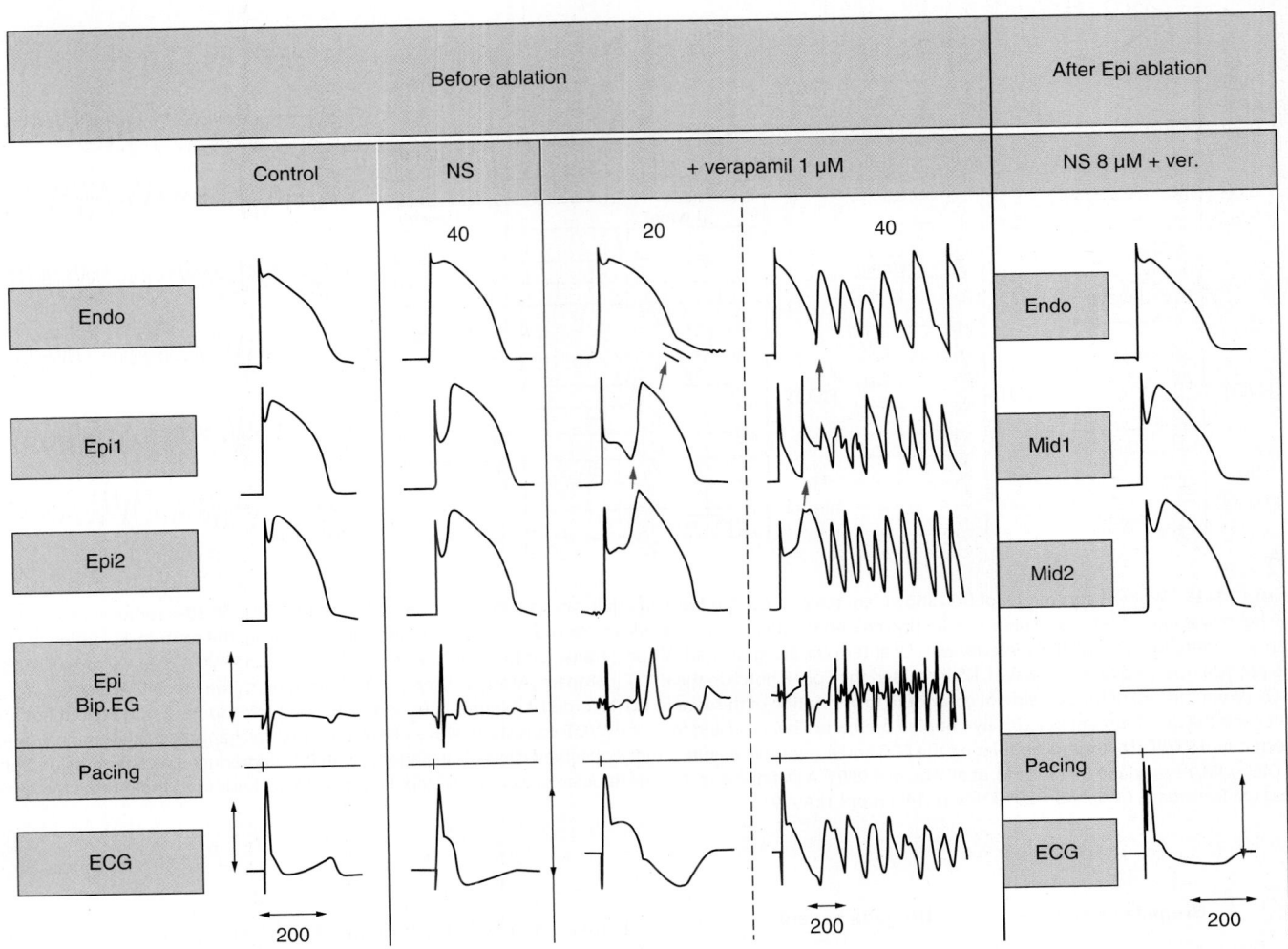

Figure 34–38. Radiofrequency ablation of epicardium (Epi) suppresses the electrocardiographic and arrhythmic manifestations of BrS in coronary-perfused canine RV wedge model generated using a combination of the I_{to} blocker NS806 (8 μM) and the calcium channel blocker verapamil (1 μM). Column 1: Control. 2: Recorded 40 min after the addition of NS5806; 3–4: Recorded 20 and 40 min after the addition of verapamil. The addition of NS5806 and verapamil to the coronary perfusate induced pronounced J waves, phase 2 reentry, and polymorphic VT. Bipolar electrogram recorded from RV epicardium shows late potentials and fractionated electrogram activity. 5: Recorded following 45 reintroduction of provocative agents following ablation of RV epicardium. AP recordings were obtained from midmyocardial (Mid) and subepicardial layers due to inactivation of the epicardium. Ablation of the outermost layer of the RV epicardium totally suppressed all ECG and arrhythmic manifestations of BrS. Calibrations of Bipolar EG and ECG at 1 and 2 mV, respectively. Modified with permission from Patocskai B, Yoon N, Antzelevitch C. Mechanisms Underlying Epicardial Radiofrequency Ablation to Suppress Arrhythmogenesis in Experimental Models of Brugada Syndrome, *JACC Clin Electrophysiol.* 2017 Apr;3(4):353-363.

express a nonsense mutation in *SCN5A* (E558X) originally identified in a child with BrS.[69] Atrial myocytes isolated from the SCN5A[E558X/+] pigs showed a loss of function of I_{Na}. Consistent with the loss of function of sodium channel activity, the minipigs displayed conduction abnormalities consisting of prolongation of the P wave, QRS complex, and PR interval. A BrS phenotype was never observed, not even after the administration of flecainide. These observations are expected owing to the lack of I_{to} in the pig, which is a prerequisite for the development of the repolarization abnormalities associated with BrS. These observations provide additional strong evidence for the repolarization hypothesis and against the depolarization hypothesis.

These experiments also provide the first test in a large mammal of the hypothesis that a slowly conducting embryonic phenotype is maintained in the adult RVOT and is unmasked when cardiac sodium channel function is reduced.[98] The hypothesis is not supported since conduction in the RVOT of the SCN5A[E558X/+] pigs was no different from conduction in the rest of RV. Both were equally depressed by the loss of function of sodium channel activity.[69]

Further evidence in support of the repolarization hypothesis derives from the observation that monophasic action potentials recorded from the epicardial and endocardial surfaces of the RVOT of a patient with BrS are nearly identical to transmembrane action potentials recorded from the epicardial and endocardial surfaces of the wedge model of BrS.[99,100] In both cases, the action potential displays a prominent accentuation of the notch in epicardium, but not endocardium without any major transmural conduction delays (**Figs. 34–40A** and **34–40B**). It is noteworthy that these electrophysiologic distinctions were not observed in an isolated heart explanted from a BrS patient after

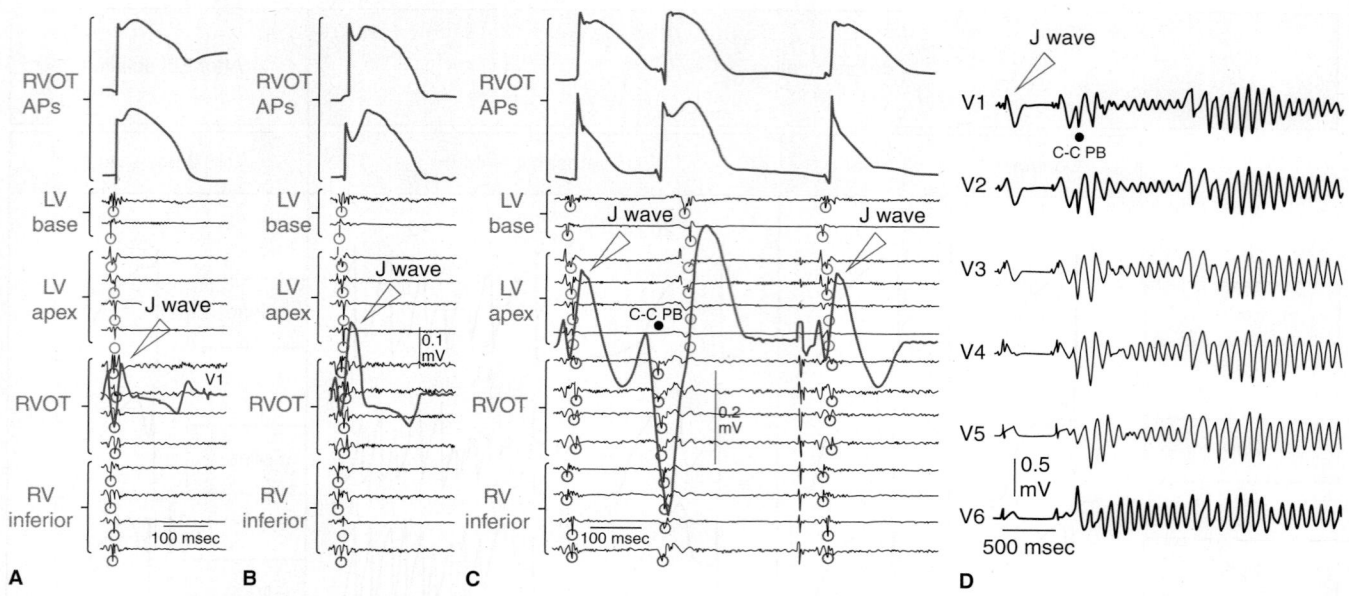

Figure 34–39. Whole-heart model of BrS. Shown are traces recorded from an adult canine heart perfused in Langendorff mode after removal of the atria. The heart was immersed in a volume-conducting chamber with preset electrodes to record a 12-lead ECG and was paced from the septum. Epi unipolar EGs were recorded from the RVOT, RV inferior wall, LV antero-basal region, and LV apex. Transmembrane APs were recorded from the RVOT. The I_{to} agonist NS5806 (7.5 μM, NS) was used to elicit J waves. NS increased the Epi AP notch in the RVOT [compare **(A)** and **(B)**] leading to a prominent J wave in V1. Activation of the RVOT (Vmin; circled) of the EGs did not contribute to inscription of the J wave. **(C)** Recorded 4 minutes later, shows loss of the AP dome at one site but not the other and the development of a closely-coupled premature beats arising from the RVOT, consistent with a phase 2 reentry mechanism which, 1 minute later, precipitated VT/VF **(D)**, thus recapitulating the ECG and arrhythmic manifestations observed clinically in patients with BrS. Reproduced with permission from Di Diego JM, Argenziano M, Tabler M, et al. Abstract 9991: A Definitive Test of the Repolarization versus Depolarization Hypothesis in a Whole-heart Model of Brugada Syndrome, *Circulation.* 2019 Nov 19;140(Suppl 1):A9991.

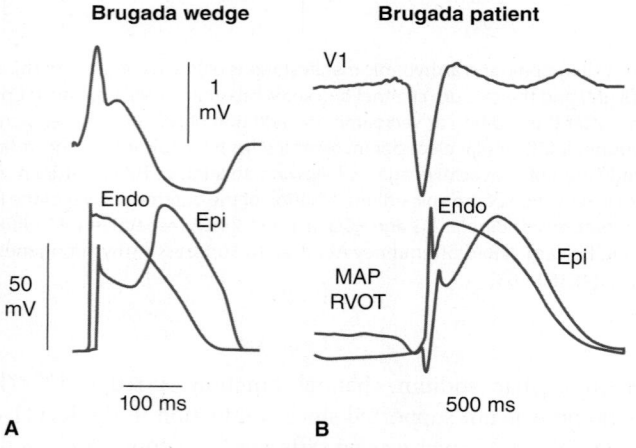

Figure 34–40. Comparison of transmembrane and monophasic action potentials and ECGs recorded from a wedge model of BrS and a patient diagnosed with BrS. **(A)** shows a pseudo-ECG and transmembrane action potentials recorded from the epicardium and endocardium of a right ventricular wedge preparation in which the Brugada phenotype was elicited using 5 uM terfenadine to block I_{Na} and I_{Ca}, thus mimicking the genetic variants associated with BrS. **(B)** shows lead V1 and monophasic action potentials recorded from epicardium and endocardium of the RVOT of a patient with BrS. Note that the apparent notch in the endocardial MAP is an "intrinsic potential" and not a true notch. **A**, Adapted with permission from Fish JM, Antzelevitch C. Role of sodium and calcium channel block in unmasking the Brugada syndrome, Heart Rhythm. 2004 Jul;1(2):210-217. **B**, Reproduced with permission from Antzelevitch C, Brugada P, Brugada J, et al: Brugada syndrome: a decade of progress. *Circ Res.* 2002 Dec 13;91(12):1114-1148.

transplantation of a new heart. The epicardium of this heart was very depressed, perhaps as a result of the 129 shocks delivered by the implantable cardioverter defibrillator (ICD) in an attempt to control the multiple electrical storms.[101]

Zhang et al. recently reported the results of noninvasive ECG imaging (ECGI) of 25 BrS and 6 right bundle branch block (RBBB) patients.[92] The authors concluded that both slow discontinuous conduction and steep dispersion of repolarization are present in the right ventricular outflow tract of patients with BrS. ECGI was able to differentiate between BrS and right bundle-branch block. Unlike BrS, RBBB showed delayed activation in the entire RV, without ST-segment elevation, fractionation, or repolarization abnormalities on the electrograms. The response to an increase in rate was studied in 6 BrS patients. The increase in heart rate increased fractionation of the electrogram *but reduced* ST-segment elevation, indicating that the conduction impairment was not the principal cause of the BrS ECG.

The strong similarity between BrS and ERS with respect to clinical manifestations and response to treatment lend further support for the repolarization hypothesis. Using an experimental model of ERS, Koncz et al.[102] provided evidence in support of the hypothesis that, similar to the mechanism operative in BrS, an accentuation of transmural gradients in the LV wall is responsible for the repolarization abnormalities underlying ERS, giving rise to J point elevation, distinct J waves, or slurring of the terminal part of the QRS. The repolarization defect was shown to be accentuated by cholinergic agonists and reduced by quinidine, isoproterenol, cilostazol, and milrinone, accounting for the ability of these agents to reverse the repolarization abnormalities responsible in patients with ERS.[102-104] Greater intrinsic levels of I_{to} in the inferior LV were shown to underlie the greater vulnerability of the inferior LV wall to VT/VF.[102] Using ECGI, Rudy and coworkers provided additional evidence in support of the repolarization abnormalities by identifying abnormally short activation-recovery intervals (ARI) in the inferior and lateral regions of LV and a marked dispersion of repolarization.[105] Recent ECGI mapping studies performed in an ERS patient during VF demonstrated VF rotors anchored in the inferior-lateral left ventricular wall.[106]

Conduction delays are known to give rise to notching of the QRS complex. When it occurs on the rising phase of the R wave, it can be demonstrated to be due to a conduction defect within the ventricular myocardium. When the notching occurs at the terminal portion of the QRS, thus masquerading as a J wave, it may be due either to a conduction or repolarization defects.[107] The response to prematurity or to an increase in rate can differentiate between the two.[70] Delayed conduction with very rare exceptions becomes more exaggerated at faster rates or during premature beats thus leading to an accentuation of the QRS notch, whereas repolarization defects are usually moderated resulting in a diminution of the J wave at faster rates. Although typical J waves are usually accentuated with bradycardia or long pauses, the opposite has also been described.[108,109] J waves are often seen in young males with no apparent structural heart diseases, whereas intra-ventricular conduction delay is often observed in older individuals or in cases of postmyocardial infarction or cardiomyopathy.[107,108] The prognostic value of a fragmented QRS has been demonstrated in BrS, although fragmentation of the QRS is not associated with increased risk in the absence of cardiac disease.[110]

The mechanism underlying ERS has been shown to be very similar to that of BrS, and also to be amenable to suppression with radiofrequency ablation. Using a canine ventricular wedge model of ERS, Koncz et al.[102] provided evidence in support of the hypothesis that in ERS, as in the BrS, accentuation of transmural gradients in the LV wall is responsible for the repolarization abnormalities underlying the ECG phenotype. Additional evidence for repolarization abnormalities in ERS patients was provided by Rudy and colleagues who used noninvasive ECGI techniques to demonstrate short activation-recovery intervals and marked dispersion of repolarization in the inferior and lateral regions of the LV in ERS patients.[105]

Because the mechanisms underlying BrS and ERS are closely related, it is not surprising that the response to pharmacologic agents is similar. Quinidine, Phosphodiesterase III inhibitors (cilostazol and milrinone), and isoproterenol all suppress arrhythmogenesis associated with both ERS and BrS. Quinidine by virtue of its ability to inhibit I_{to} was recommended as therapy for BrS over two decades ago (see 68 and 65 for references). Agents that augment the L-type calcium channel current, such as β-adrenergic agents like isoproterenol or orciprenaline, are useful as well. Increasing I_{Ca} is believed to prevent the arrhythmogenesis associated with J-wave syndrome by opposing the relative augmented repolarization forces and thus restoring

the epicardial AP dome in both BrS and ERS. Isoproterenol, sometimes in combination with quinidine, has been used to successfully control VF storms and normalizing ST elevation. Isoproterenol has been shown to be effective in quieting electrical storms developing in patients with both BrS and ERS. All of these agents have been shown to correct the repolarization defects responsible for development of phase 2 reentry and VT/VF in experimental models of BrS and ERS.[102]

Cilostazol, a phosphodiesterase (PDE) III inhibitor, normalizes the ST segment by augmenting I_{Ca} as well as by reducing I_{to} secondary to an increase in cAMP and heart rate. Of note, failure of cilostazol in the treatment of BrS has been described in a single case report.

Milrinone, another PDE III inhibitor, was recently identified as a more potent alternative to cilostazol in suppressing ST-segment elevation and arrhythmogenesis in an experimental model of BrS, although there are no clinical data available as yet. *Wenxin Keli,* a traditional Chinese medicine, has also been shown to inhibit I_{to} and to suppress arrhythmogenesis in experimental models of BrS when combined with low concentrations of quinidine (5 μM) (see 64 for references). Agents that augment peak and late I_{Na}, including *bepridil* and *dimethyl lithospermate B* (dmLSB), are suggested to be of value in BrS. Bepridil has been reported to suppress VT/VF in several studies of patients with BrS. The drug's actions are thought to be mediated by: (1) inhibition of I_{to}; (2) augmentation of I_{Na} via upregulation of the sodium channels; and (3) prolongation of QT interval at slow rates, thus increasing the QT/RR slope. Dimethyl lithospermate B, an extract of Danshen, a traditional Chinese herbal remedy, slows inactivation of I_{Na}, thus increasing I_{Na} during the early phases of the AP, thereby reducing the AP notch and restoring the epicardial AP dome and, in the process, suppressing arrhythmogenesis in experimental models of BrS. Finally, *acacetin,* a natural flavone, has recently been shown to inhibit I_{to} in human atrial myocytes in a frequency-dependent manner.[111] The drug produces inhibition of I_{to} in ventricular myocardium and has recently been shown to produce an ameliorative effect in experimental models of BrS and ERS.[112]

GENETICS OF CHANNELOPATHIES AND CLINICAL IMPLICATIONS

Introduction

Genetic mutations that destabilize the cardiac electrical substrate, predispose to malignant arrhythmias, and sudden death are a group of diseases defined as cardiac channelopathies or *inherited arrhythmogenic diseases* (IADs). IADs typically manifest with peculiar electrocardiographic manifestation in structurally intact hearts.[113]

Some of these conditions (eg, LQTS, CPVT) have been clinically described as typical Mendelian traits before the identification of their causative genes. They are generally well-characterized conditions and molecular analysis is able to identify the culprit mutations in the majority of cases. Other forms of IAD (BrS, short QT syndrome [SQTS]) have more heterogeneous presentation with some cases showing clear

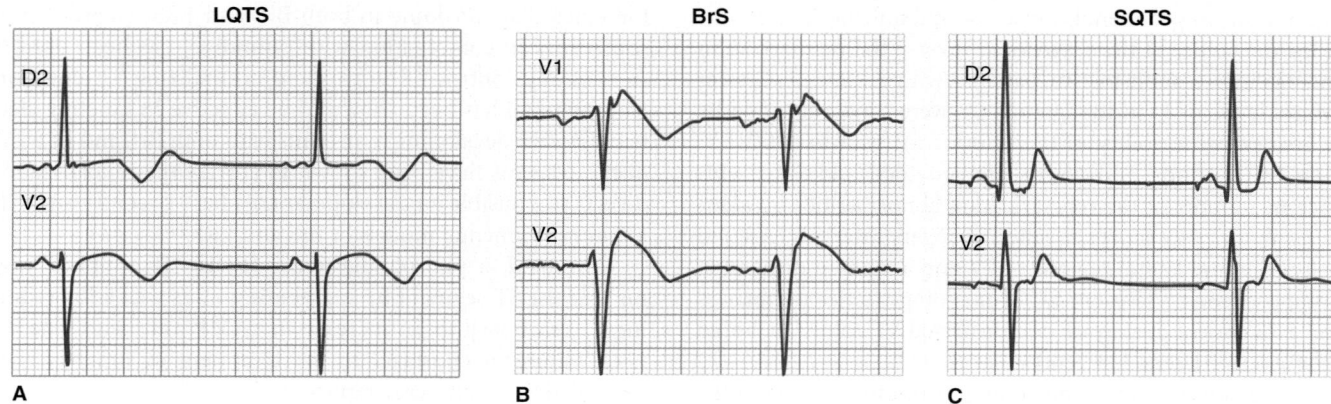

Figure 34–41. Electrocardiographic abnormalities in inherited arrhythmias. LQTS **(A)**: the ECG shows and example of QT prolongation and diphasic T wave in a LQT2 (KCNH2 gene) patient. BrS **(B)** example of type 1 ECG pattern in V1 and V2 leads, which are the ECG leads that usually manifest the ST elevation (<2.0 mm) followed by negative T wave that allows to diagnose the disease this pattern may be present in second, third, and fourth intercostal space. SQTS **(C)**: lead D2 and V2 of a SQTS patient.

familial distribution but also a significant percentage of sporadic cases, suggesting complex and possibly multifactorial pathogenesis (eg, oligogenic inheritance). In this chapter, we will review the clinical and genetic features of the most relevant cardiac channelopathies.

Long QT Syndrome

Definition

LQTS (or Romano–Ward syndrome) is a repolarization disorder. It usually presents with autosomal dominant inheritance of typical ECG phenotypes characterized by prolonged QT and morphologic abnormalities of the T wave (**Figs. 34–41A** to **34–41C**). It predisposes to recurrent syncopal spells and sudden death due to ventricular arrhythmias. The estimated prevalence of LQTS is 1:2000.[114]

Rare LQTS variants have been also described which manifest with the common feature of QT prolongation and arrhythmic risk but also include extracardiac abnormalities: Jervell and Lange-Nielsen syndrome (sensorineural deafness, autosomal recessive inheritance); and Timothy syndrome (syndactyly, autism spectrum disorders, congenital cardiac defects, metabolic abnormalities, with sporadic presentation or parental mosaicism). Another repolarization disorder, namely the Andersen–Tawil syndrome (ATS) is characterized by facial dysmorphisms, periodic paralysis, and ECG abnormalities in the context of normal QT interval.

Genetic Basis and Pathophysiology

The common consequence of LQTS gene mutations is the disruption of one or more ionic currents that contribute to the cardiac action potential. It is interesting to note that similar electrophysiological abnormalities in specific ionic currents may result from mutations of different genes (Table 34–2). Thus, the genetic heterogeneity of LQTS can be reconciled in a reduced spectrum of physiological functions controlled by the dysfunctional gene products.

It is also relevant to note that three genetic variants (LQT1, LQT2, LQT3, see Table 34–4) are largely more prevalent and that the interpretation of the genetic testing is far more easy for these well-known variants than for all the "minor" LQTS

genetic forms.[115] This is a clinically important concept since the "minor" LQTS genes (Table 34–2) have been reported in the literature with few evidences of pathogenicity: few cases, no or questionable co segregation, and unclear in vitro findings. As a consequence, true causative role of these genes has been recently questioned.[116]

Another important concept is that the probability of finding a pathogenic genetic mutation when testing a LQTS case is proportional to the accuracy of the clinical diagnosis and the yield of testing drops dramatically from ≈65% of genetic substrates identified in clinically overt forms to a meager ≈14% of conclusive genetic analysis among patients with borderline QT prolongation.[117]

However, given that knowing the specific genetic mutation is relevant to LQTS clinical management,[118] genetic testing has a key role and it is important to outline the electrophysiological mechanisms of the disease on the basis of the specific ionic current affected (**Fig. 34–42, Table 34–4**).

Potassium Currents and LQTS: There are four cardiac potassium currents that can cause LQTS: the slow (I_{Ks}) and rapid (I_{Kr}) components of the delayed rectifier, and the acetylcholine-dependent potassium current (I_{KAch}).[119] Another current, I_{K1}, is associated with the repolarization disorder, ATS.[120] This was initially considered a genetic variant of long QT syndrome, but now is considered as a channellopathy with unique characteristics.[120]

KCNQ1 is the gene encoding the channel that conducts the I_{Ks} current (slow component of the delayed rectifier current). It represents the most common variant of LQTS (LQT1) that accounts for 40% to 50% of patients.[121] I_{Ks} is active during terminal plateau and early phase 3 of the action potential and LQTS mutations reduce the activity of this current (loss of function). It is a catecholamine-sensitive current and therefore its role in the control of repolarization becomes more evident during adrenergic stimulation. This explains why LQT1 hearts are unable to properly shorten the action potential duration/QT interval during increased sympathetic tone (I_{Ks} cannot be properly activated), and why most of the arrhythmic events in patients occur during exercise or acute emotional stress.

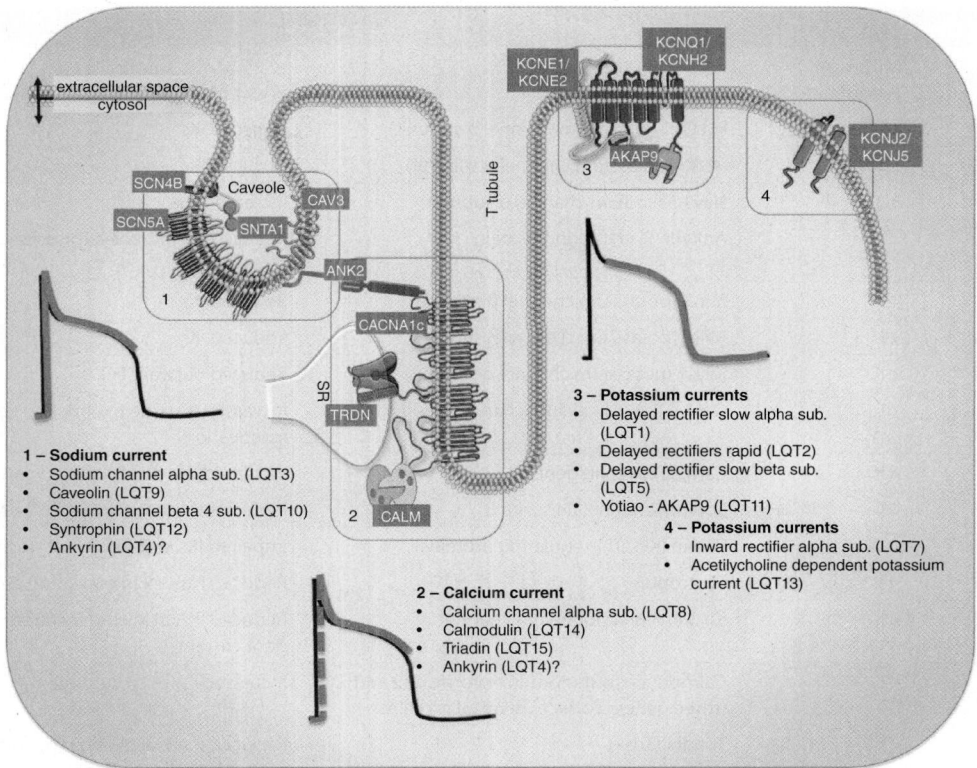

Figure 34–42. Cartoon showing the LQTS genes and proteins grouped by function. Four major groups can be identified. Genes that alter the cardiac sodium current (group 1), genes affecting cardiac calcium channel and intracellular calcium handling (group 2), genes controlling the early repolarization (group 3) including phase 2–3 of the cardiac action potential, and genes that affect mainly the resting membrane potential (group 4). The action potential phases involved for each functional group are highlighted with a *red line* on the action potential. *Dotted line* indicates the fact that I_{Ca} is partially active, during phase 0.

The second most common variant of LQTS, LQT2 is due to loss of function mutations in the *KCNH2* gene. *KCNH2* encodes for the α subunit (pore-forming protein) of the I_{Kr} (the rapid component of the delayed rectifier) channel, which participates in the control of cardiac repolarization during phase 3. Adrenergic activation plays an arrhythmogenic role also for LQT2 patients who are at particularly high risk during acute emotional stresses.

Overall, LQT1 (50%–60%) and LQT2 (30%–35%) represent the majority of LQTS patients with identified mutations.

I_{Ks} and I_{Kr} currents can be affected in two other LQTS variants: *KCNE1-LQT5* (which coassembles with *KCNQ1*) and *KCNE2-LQT6* (which is thought to coassemble mainly with *KCNH2*, but also with other potassium channels) are beta-subunits of I_{Ks} and I_{Kr}. Initial reports have linked these two genes to overt LQTS. However, recent data,[122] that confirm previous observations,[118] show that *KCNE1*-dependent LQTS has a very low penetrance (only 20% with prolonged QT interval) and it causes a mild form of LQTS with a rate of definitive arrhythmic episodes of 16.9% of cases.[122]

In a similar fashion, a meta-analysis of published *KCNE2* mutations[123] shows that the high allelic frequencies of LQT6 mutations (ExAC database) and the absence of documentation of Mendelian inheritance shed doubts on the causal link between *KCNE2* and LQTS. Instead, *KCNE2* variants may confer susceptibility to drug-induced QT prolongation.

Both *KCNQ1* and *KCNE1* mutations, when present in "double dose" (homozygosity) and inherited as recessive traits

cause the Jervell and Lange-Nielsen syndrome. Interestingly, *KCNE1*-related Jervell and Lange-Nielsen syndrome is also associated with mild clinical presentation.[122]

In rare cases, I_{Ks} current can be reduced by mutations in the *AKAP9* gene (Yotiao–LQT11) that binds in the carboxyl-terminal region of *KCNQ1* protein to transduce the adrenergic signal to the channel. Only a small number of mutations in few families with unclear cosegregation have been described and therefore, the causative role of this gene LQTS remains unclear.

The *KCNJ2* gene encoding for the cardiac inward rectifier I_{K1} current (*Kir2.1*) causes the LQT7 variant, also known as ATS.[124] LQT7 is a rare variant (estimated population prevalence < 1:10,000) that includes variable extracardiac manifestations (periodic paralysis and dysmorphic features). I_{K1} participates in the control of the late repolarization phase and resting membrane potential. Although the inward rectifier current is involved in the regulation of action potential duration,[125,126] when mutated it induces a typical ECG abnormality with prominent U waves that are distinct from the T wave. Furthermore, the QTc is not prolonged in all patients,[120] which questions its classification among LQTS variants. Nonetheless, ATS is a very severe arrhythmogenic condition with a 5-year cumulative probability of life-threatening arrhythmic events of 7.9%, which is similar to that observed among LQT2 and LQT3 patients.[127]

Sodium Current and LQTS: *Gain-of-function SCN5A mutations cause LQT3*, the third most frequent LQTS variant.

TABLE 34–4. LQTS Genes

Variant	Gene	Mutation Frequency (%)	Protein	Effect of Mutations
LQT1/JLN1*	KCNQ1	45–55	KvLQT1 (potassium channel α subunit)	Reduced IKs
LQT2	KCNH2	30–45	HERG (potassium channel α subunit)	Reduced IKr
LQT3	SCN5A	8-15	Nav1.5 (sodium channel α subunit)	Increased INa
LQT4	ANK2	<1	Ankyrin B, anchoring protein	Reduced membrane expression of Na$^+$ and Ca^{2+} channels
LQT5/JLN2*	KCNE1	<1	MinK (potassium channel β subunit)	Reduced IKs
LQT6	KCNE2	<1	MiRP (potassium channel β subunit)	Reduced IKr
LQT7 (ATS)	KCNJ2	<1	Kir2.1 (potassium channel α subunit)	Reduced outward IK1
LQT8 (TS)	CACNA1c	<1	Cav1.2 (L-type calcium channel α subunit)	Increased ICα due to impaired voltage-dependent inactivation
LQT9	CAV3	<1	Cardiac caveolin gene	Increased INa due to altered gating kinetic
LQT10	SCN4B	<1	Sodium channel β4 subunit	Reduced subunit expression causing increased INa
LQT11	AKAP9	<1	Yotiao (KvLQT1 regulating proteins)	Impaired IKs activation by catecholamines
LQT12	SNTA1	<1	Syntrophin	Reduced NaV1.5 nitrosylation an increased current
LQT13	KCNJ5	<1	Kir 3.4/GIRK4 potassium channel	Reduced IKAch inward rectified acetilycholine dependent current
LQT14	CALM	<1	Calmodulin mutations in isoforms 1, 2 and 3 (three genes produce identical proteins)	Increased Calcium current
LQT15	TRDN	<1	Triadin (Trisk)	Reduced ICa inactivation (hypothesized but not experimentally verified)

Abbreviations: ATS, Andersen–Tawil syndrome; JLN, Jervell and Lange-Nielsen syndrome; TS, Timothy syndrome.
*Heterozygous mutations cause LQT1, homozygous mutations cause JLN.

Interestingly, loss of function mutations in *SCN5A*, cause the BrS phenotype.

LQT3 mutations associated with LQTS impair the inactivation of the I_{Na} current leading to an increase in the late component of I_{Na} resulting in prolongation of the plateau of the action potential. It is important to keep in mind that some *SCN5A* mutations with complex biophysical consequences can generate the so-called "overlap syndromes." In these cases, it is possible to observe, within the same family, subjects with QT interval prolongation and others with ST elevation suggesting BrS.

With due caveats regarding the uncertainties of the pathogenic role of the mutations that have been identified, a gain of function of I_{Na} is also present in LQT9 associated in mutations in the Caveolin 3 gene (*CAV3*), LQT10 associated with mutations in the beta four subunit of the sodium channel (*SCN4B*), and LQT12 associated with mutations in syntrophin (*SNTA1*). Overall mutations in these latter variants are rare (<5%) and it is currently unclear if the associated outcome is similar to that of LQT3.

L-Type Calcium Current and LQTS: The initial mutations of the gene encoding for the cardiac calcium channel (*CACNA1c*) were identified in patients with Timothy syndrome (TS), a complex, extremely severe, and rare disease, including QT prolongation, syndactyly, congenital heart defects, cardiac hypertrophy, atrioventricular block, paroxysms of hypoglycemia, autism-spectrum of disorders, reduced immune response, and developmental delay.[128]

CACNA1C encodes the alpha subunit of the CaV1.2 calcium channel that conducts the I_{Ca} current, the main component of the plateau of the cardiac action potential. Experimental studies have demonstrated that *CACNA1c* mutations cause a gain-of-function type of defect with loss of voltage-dependent inactivation of the channel leading to increase of I_{Ca}.[128]

While the experimental findings have described how CaV1.2 mutations prolong action potential duration and QT interval, the role of these in the pathogenesis of the extracardiac phenotypes of TS remains less clear. The remarkable clinical variability of the extracardiac manifestations probably reflects the complexity of splicing, regulation, and distribution of tissue expression of *CACNA1c*.

More recently, the number of *CACNA1c* mutations associated with typical TS but also with isolated nonsyndromic QT prolongation has progressively grown. Interestingly, all *CACNA1c* mutations that cause QT prolongation are predominantly located in the intracellular portion of the protein. In other cases, "mild"[129] or nontypical [130] extracardiac manifestations may occur suggesting that calcium channel mutations can create a continuum of clinical manifestations between TS and nonsyndromic QT prolongation. Thus, the identification of a *CACNA1c* mutation in a patient with QT prolongation requires careful investigations to exclude the possibility of a subclinical manifestation of the other phenotypes.

Infrequent LQTS Variants: *CALM1, 2, 3* (LQT14), and *TRDN* (LQT15) (Table 34–4) have been linked with rare and severe LQTS. The Calmodulin protein is encoded by three identical genes (*CALM1*, *CALM2*, and *CALM3*). Available data show that the clinical presentation is similar among the affected individuals, including a markedly prolonged QTc, T-wave alternans, 2:1 functional atrioventricular block, and high incidence of malignant arrhythmias.[131] Of note, *CALM1* and *CALM3* mutations have also been associated with CPVT.[131,132]

The triadin gene (*TRDN*) can cause a rare arrhythmogenic syndrome that presents with QT prolongation in approximately half of the patients and with adrenergic-dependent arrhythmias.[133] Other features are mild skeletal myopathy and T-wave inversions. Ninety-five percent of the 21 cases recently reported[133] had cardiac arrest or syncope at an average age of 3 years. Whether or not this can be considered an LQTS variant is a matter of discussion.

Diagnosis and Risk Stratification

The diagnosis of LQTS is based on the evaluation of QT interval on resting ECG. Current guidelines[134] indicate that LQTS can be diagnosed under the following conditions: (1) either QTc ≥480 ms at rest on 12-lead ECGs or LQTS risk score >3; (2) confirmed pathogenic LQTS mutation, irrespective of the QT duration; and (3) a QTc ≥460 ms in repeated 12-lead ECGs in patients with unexplained syncope in the absence of secondary causes for QT prolongation. Subjects without family members with prolonged QTc who have a borderline QTc (440 ms to 479 ms) do not meet the diagnostic criteria.[134] Exercise stress test and Holter monitoring are helpful to support the diagnosis in borderline cases with the assessment of QTc at different heart rates to quantify QT adaptation to RR interval.

Triggers and Risk Factors for Arrhythmias in LQTS

Syncope and sudden death in LQTS are due to the onset of rapid polymorphic VT defined as torsade de pointes (TdP) that may degenerate into VF. In LQTS, cardiac arrhythmias are often precipitated by physical or emotional stress (predominantly in LQT1 and LQT2), although in 10% to 15% of patients, cardiac events occur at rest (predominantly LQT3).

Accurate assessment of QTc is an independent predictor. When QTc is consistently ≥500 ms, there is a 5-fold increased risk of events with a rate of 4% to 5% per year.[118] Other risk factors are the presence of a LQT2 or LQT3 genotype (approximately 1.8-fold increase), female sex (approximately 2-fold increased risk), the postpartum period, the occurrence of a first cardiac event in early childhood, and the presence of a pore region mutation of *KCNH2* (LQT2).

By combining QT duration and genotype, it is possible to further improve risk stratification in LQTS. Indeed, the 5-year life-threatening events in LQTS can be defined with high granularity using only these two variables (**Fig. 34–43**), which substantially improves the clinical management.[127] Electrophysiologic study with programmed electrical stimulation is not recommended for risk stratification in LQTS.[135]

Therapy

Lifestyle and cautionary behavior are absolutely important for a correct approach to LQTS: avoidance of QT prolonging drugs, correction of any electrolyte disturbance (especially reduced potassium levels), and the avoidance of gene-specific triggers (swimming in LQT1 and loud noises in LQT2) have a class I indication. In parallel, β-blockers are recommended (class I) in all patients with a clinical diagnosis of LQTS[134] and in those with QTc above 470 ms with history of syncope.[135] The use of β-blockers should also be considered (class IIa) in carriers of LQTS mutations with normal QT interval[134,135] (**Table 34–5**).

Among β-blockers, nadolol at a dose of 1 mg/kg/day has demonstrated its superiority in the prevention of arrhythmic events with a hazard ratio of 0.38 (95% confidence interval [CI], 0.15–0.93)[127] and should be considered the β-blocker of choice in this disease.

The use of ICDs, always in conjunction with β-blockers, is indicated in all patients surviving cardiac arrest (secondary prevention) and those who experience recurrence of syncope despite β-blockade (class IIa); in these subjects, left cardiac sympathetic denervation should be also considered (class IIa).[135] Finally ICD can be considered for primary prevention of cardiac arrest in high-risk genotypes (class IIb, Table 34–4).[134]

Gene-specific therapy in LQT3 with mexiletine was proposed several years ago due to its favorable effect of QTc shortening in a few patients and an experimental model. More recently, mexiletine has been definitively shown to shorten QTc by approximately 60 ms in LQT3 patients and to reduce the annual rate of cardiac events from 10.3% to 0.7%[137] (**Figs. 34–44A** and **34–44B**). Based on this evidence, mexiletine should be given in all LQT3 patients. Preliminary observations also suggest that mexiletine could be beneficial by shortening QTc by ≥40 ms in approximately 60% of LQT2 patients.[137]

Catecholaminergic Polymorphic Ventricular Tachycardia

Definition

In 1978, CPVT was described by Philippe Coumel as an inherited disorder characterized by a structurally normal heart, an unremarkable resting ECG, a typical and reproducible pattern of bidirectional adrenergic-dependent VT, and a high incidence of sudden death and arrhythmic syncope (**Fig. 34–45**).

Genetic Basis and Pathophysiology

Genetic Variants Associated with Typical CPVT: In 2001, we discovered that mutations in the gene encoding for the cardiac ryanodine receptor (*RyR2*) cause the autosomal dominant form of CPVT (CPVT1).[138] RyR2 is a tetrameric Ca^{2+} release channel spanning the membrane of the junctional sarcoplasmic reticulum (jSR) where it releases calcium from the jSR to the cytoplasm where it is required for initiating cardiac contraction.

RyR2 is the most important causative gene in CPVT and pathogenic mutations in the *RyR2* gene are present in 50% to 60% of CPVT patients.

Shortly after our discovery of the role of *RyR2* in dominant CPVT, Lahat et al. discovered that mutations in the cardiac calsequestrin 2 gene (*CASQ2*) cause the autosomal recessive form of CPVT (CPVT2).[139] Calsequestrin is a calcium-buffering protein located in the jSR where it controls the SR Ca^{2+} concentration and modulates the opening probability of *RyR2*. Two other proteins, triadin and junctin, interact with *CASQ2* and

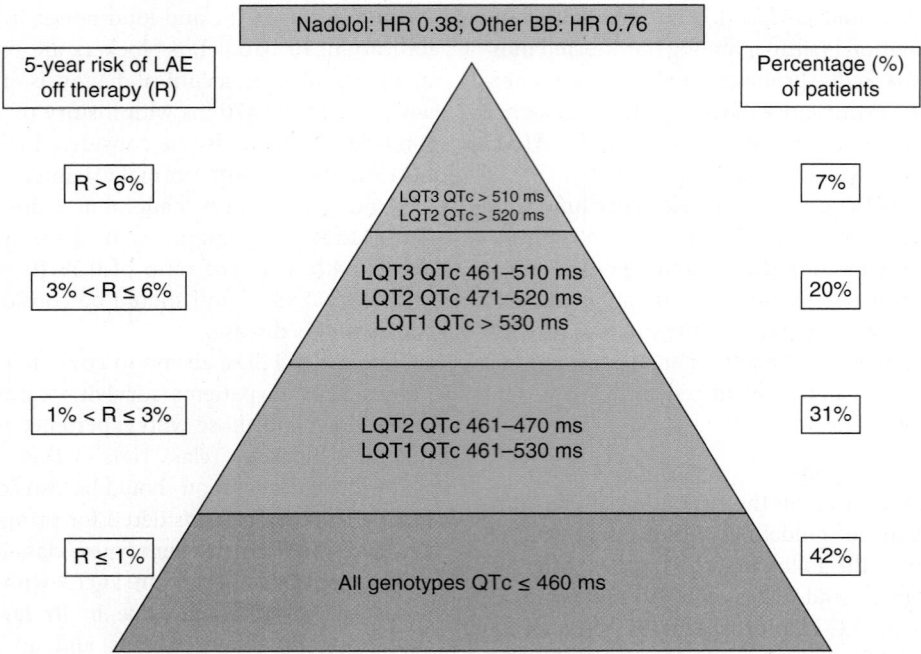

Figure 34–43. Risk stratification in LQTS. Visualization of 5-year risk of LAEs by genotype and QTc interval before therapy. The column to the left indicates the cutoff of the 5-year risk of LAEs that corresponds to each color-coded group of patients characterized by QTc duration and genotype (from *green* [lower risk] to *red* [higher risk]). The column to the right indicates the percentage of patients in each color-coded category present in the cohort. The bar on the top shows the hazard ratio (HR) of patients treated with nadolol (HR: 0.38) and other BBs (selective BBs and propranolol; HR: 0.76) and can be used to estimate the residual risk for each group of patients when treated with BBs. Modified with permission from Mazzanti A, Maragna R, Vacanti G, et al: Interplay Between Genetic Substrate, QTc Duration, and Arrhythmia Risk in Patients With Long QT Syndrome, *J Am Coll Cardiol.* 2018 Apr 17;71(15):1663-1671.

concur to form the *RyR2* macromolecular complex (Fig. 34–38).

Experimental evidence obtained in cellular models and transgenic mice demonstrates that in the presence of gain of function mutations in *RyR2* that facilitate the opening of *RyR2* in response to catecholamines and in the presence of loss of function mutations in *RyR2* that disrupt the stabilizing effect on the closed state of *RyR2*, the heart becomes prone to release calcium in the cytosol during diastole. As a consequence, DADs develops leading to triggered ventricular arrhythmias that may degenerate into VF.[140]

Atypical CPVT Variants: Other genes have been linked with adrenergically induced polymorphic of bidirectional VTs including: (1) two of the three genes that encode calmodulin (*CALM1, CALM3*), (2) the genes that encode Triadin (*TRDN*), (3) the gene that encodes Ankiryn B (*ANK2*), and (4) the *KCNJ2* gene that encodes the channel for the inward rectifier current.

CALM1 and *CALM3* mutations are associated with adrenergic-dependent arrhythmias and sudden death. These mutations reduce the calcium binding affinity of calmodulin [141] and lower the threshold for the SR calcium release. As outlined earlier in this chapter, other studies have associated *CALM1, CALM2,* or *CALM3* mutations with LQTS.[142] Experimental studies have suggested that the functional/cellular effects of *CALM1* mutations associated with CPVT and LQTS are not substantially different.[141,143] Therefore, it is possible that overlap CPVT-LQTS phenotypes are generated in the presence of *CALM* mutations, irrespectively from the gene isoform (the produced protein is identical).

Recessive (homozygous) *TRDN* mutations were found in families with cases of syncope and sudden death during exercise but without evidence of inducible typical bidirectional VT.[144,145] Cardiac triadin, also known as Trisk32, has a single transmembrane segment spanning the SR membrane (Fig. 34–45) where it participates in the formation of SR calcium releasing macromolecular complex. *TRDN* knock out results in reduced SR Ca²⁺ release, impaired I_{Ca} inactivation, and intracellular Ca²⁺ overload. As mentioned, a mild QT prolongation has been observed in *TRDN* mutation carriers.[133]

Ankyrins are adapter proteins with key modulatory and targeting roles in membrane protein targeting, including the cardiac sodium channel and the sodium-calcium exchanger (NCX). Ankyrin-B mutation are associated with "mixed" phenotypes including mild QT prolongation, sinus node dysfunction, and adrenergic arrhythmias resembling CPVT.[146]

Finally, *KCNJ2*, the gene of ATS, causes repolarization abnormalities (U waves) and bidirectional VTs similar to those of CPVT. Since U waves can also be present in CPVT, the differential diagnosis between CPVT and ATS can be difficult in the absence of genetic testing.

Clinical Presentation in CPVT

CPVT patients have unremarkable resting ECGs with the exception of sinus bradycardia and prominent U waves reported in some cases. A distinctive pattern of arrhythmias is observed during exercise or acute emotion: an alternating 180-degree QRS axis on a beat-to-beat basis, the so-called *bidirectional ventricular tachycardia* (Fig. 34–45). In the typical CPVT, this pattern is reproduced upon repeated exercise stress

TABLE 34–5. Recommendations for LQTS

Recommendations – Diagnosis	Class
LQTS is diagnosed with either – QTc ≥480 ms in repeated 12-lead EKG or – LQTS risk score >3	I
LQTS is diagnosed in the presence of a confirmed pathogenic LQTS mutation, irrespective of the QT duration.	I
EKG diagnosis of LQTS should be considered in the presence of a QTc ≥460 ms in repeated 12-lead EKG in patients with an unexplained syncopal episode in the absence of secondary causes for QT prolongation.	IIa
Recommendations – Management	
The following lifestyle changes are recommended in all patients with a diagnosis of LQTS: (a) Avoidance of QT-prolonging drugs (b) Correction of electrolyte abnormalities (hypokalemia, hypomagnesaemia, hypocalcemia) that may occur during diarrhea, vomiting or metabolic conditions. (c) Avoidance of genotype-specific triggers for arrhythmias (strenuous swimming, especially in LQTS1, and exposure to loud noises in LQTS2 patients).	I
Beta-blockers are recommended in patients with a clinical diagnosis of LQTS – QTc >470 ms	I
ICD implantation with the use of beta-blockers is recommended in LQTS patients with previous cardiac arrest	I
Beta-blockers should be considered in carriers of a causative LQTS mutation and normal QT interval.	IIa
In patients with suspected long QT syndrome, ambulatory electrocardiographic monitoring, recording the EKG lying and immediately on standing, and/or exercise treadmill testing can be useful for establishing a diagnosis and monitoring the response to therapy	IIa
ICD implantation in addition to beta-blockers should be considered in LQTS patients who experienced syncope and/or VT while receiving an adequate dose of beta-blockers.	IIa
Left cardiac sympathetic denervation should be considered in patients with symptomatic LQTS when **(a)** Beta-blockers are either not effective, not tolerated or contraindicated; **(b)** ICD therapy is contraindicated or refused; **(c)** Patients on beta-blockers with an ICD experience multiple shocks.	IIa
Sodium channel blockers (mexiletine, flecainide or ranolazine) may be considered as add-on therapy to shorten the QT interval in LQTS3 patients with a QTc >500 ms.	IIb
*In asymptomatic patients with long QT syndrome and a resting QTc greater than 500 ms while receiving a beta-blocker, intensification of therapy with medications (guided by consideration of the particular long QT syndrome type), left cardiac sympathetic denervation or an ICD may be considered	IIb
Implant of an ICD may be considered in addition to beta-blocker therapy in asymptomatic carriers of a pathogenic mutation in KCNH2 or SCN5A when QTc is >500 ms.	IIb
*Invasive EPS with PVS is not recommended for SCD risk stratification.	III
*In patients with long QT syndrome, QT-prolonging medications are potentially harmful	III

*recommendation present in AHA/ACC[123] guidelines only.

Data from Priori SG, Blomström-Lundqvist C, Mazzanti A, et al: 2015 ESC Guidelines for the management of patients with ventricular arrhythmias and the prevention of sudden cardiac death: The Task Force for the Management of Patients with Ventricular Arrhythmias and the Prevention of Sudden Cardiac Death of the European Society of Cardiology (ESC). Endorsed by: Association for European Paediatric and Congenital Cardiology (AEPC). Eur Heart J. 2015 Nov 1;36(41):2793-2867 and Al-Khatib SM, Stevenson WG, Ackerman MJ, et al: 2017 AHA/ACC/HRS Guideline for Management of Patients With Ventricular Arrhythmias and the Prevention of Sudden Cardiac Death: A Report of the American College of Cardiology/American Heart Association Task Force on Clinical Practice Guidelines and the Heart Rhythm Society. J Am Coll Cardiol. 2018 Oct 2;72(14):e91-e220.

test with a threshold for the onset of arrhythmias that, in the absence of therapy, is reproducible for the individual patient. Supraventricular arrhythmias (supraventricular tachycardia and AF) are also observed.[147,148]

The mean age of onset of symptoms in CPVT patients is 12 years of age. Syncope, triggered by exercise or acute emotion, is the typical manifestation. Sudden death can be the first manifestation of the disease.[147] Available data show that 75% to 80% of patients experience at least one life-threatening event before the age of 40 years if left without therapy.[147,149] The presence of a normal resting ECG is often the cause of a dangerous delay in the diagnosis of CPVT,[147,150] and may expose patients to unnecessary risk of life-threatening events. The exercise stress test is the most important diagnostic tool to identify CPVT in subjects with normal ECG and history of syncope, presyncope, or dizziness triggered by exercise or acute emotions. Programmed electrical stimulation is not recommended for risk stratification in CPVT.

Therapy

CPVT management include as class I indications for all patients the use of β-blockers and lifestyle modifications (avoidance of competitive sports, strenuous exercise, and stressful environments).[134] Nonspecific β-blockers (nadolol and propranolol) are preferable over selective compounds.[151] Given to its favorable pharmacodynamics with stable plasma levels and long half-life, nadolol (1.5–3 mg/kg/day) is the drug of choice; the dose should be always individualized to demonstrate the absence of repetitive arrhythmias during exercise stress testing. β-blockers are also indicated for genetically positive, phenotype negative subjects (class IIa).[134] Despite optimal use of β-blockers, there is a 25% to 35% risk of recurrent cardiac events.[147,150]

In these subjects, the addition of flecainide has proven effective.[152] This drug should be considered in patients with recurrence of syncope and/or repetitive ventricular during exercise stress test in the presence of optimized (maximally tolerated dose) β-blockers (class IIa). The average dose is 100 mg to

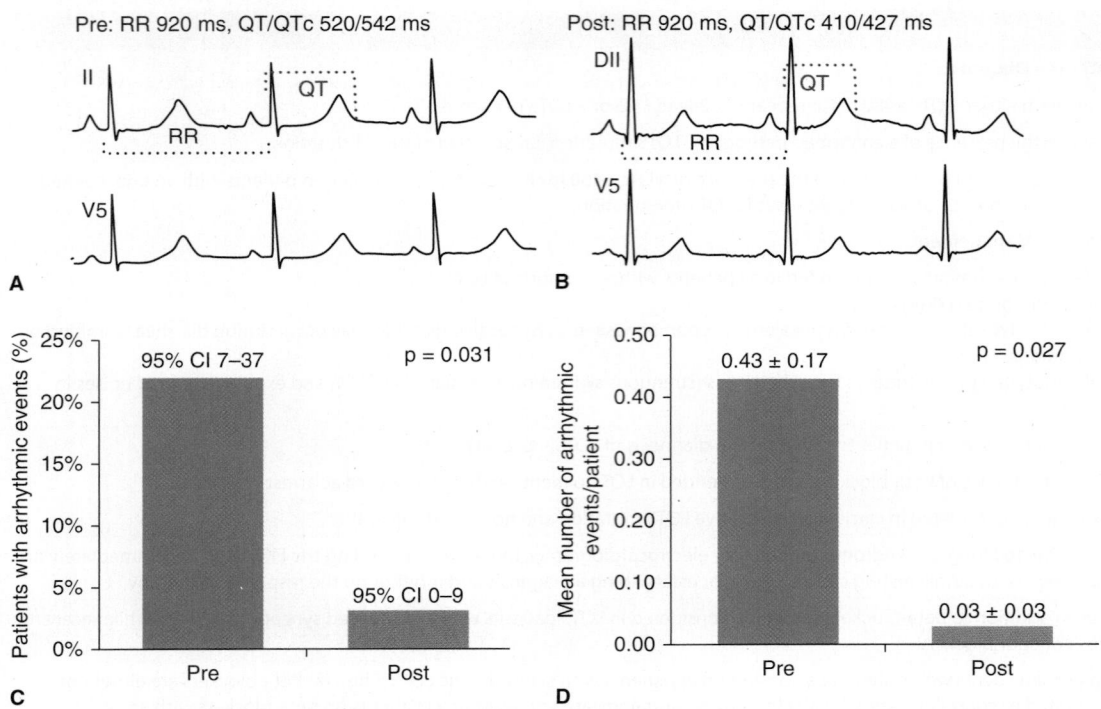

Figure 34–44. Therapeutic effect of mexiletine in LQT3. **(A)** Example of QTc normalization in LQT3 patients after mexiletine treatment. **(B)** Arrhythmic burden in LQT3 patients treated with mexiletine during matched periods of a median of 35 months. **(C)** The percentage of patients with arrhythmic events declined from 22% (95% CI, 7–37) to 3% (95% CI, 0–9; $p = 0.031$). **(D)** The mean number of arrhythmic events per patient decreased from 0.43 ± 0.17 to 0.03 ± 0.03 ($p = 0.027$). Reproduced with permission from Mazzanti A, Maragna R, Faragli A, et al: Gene-Specific Therapy With Mexiletine Reduces Arrhythmic Events in Patients With Long QT Syndrome Type 3, *J Am Coll Cardiol.* 2016 Mar 8;67(9):1053-1058.

200 mg per day. Flecainide may also be considered as monotherapy in the few patients who are intolerant to β-blockers, but its efficacy is less defined.

Current guidelines recommend the use of ICD, in addition to β-blockers with or without flecainide, in patients with a diagnosis of CPVT who experience cardiac arrest, recurrent syncope, or polymorphic/bidirectional VT despite optimized β-blockers therapy (class I). However, it is important to mention here that the usefulness of ICD in CPVT can be reduced limited by high rate of complications, including inappropriate shocks, and does not appear to significantly improve survival.[153,154] Therefore, the optimization of medical therapy remains the most important goal for CPVT management.

Left cardiac sympathetic denervation (LCSD) has been proposed for CVPT patients; however, since arrhythmic recurrences after LCSD are reported,[150,155] LCSD should be considered as a means to lower arrhythmic burden in high-risk patients with optimized therapy but not as a replacement of drug therapy or ICD (despite its limitations).

Brugada Syndrome

Definition

BrS is characterized by a peculiar pattern of ST-segment elevation in leads V_1 to V_2 (Figs. 34–41A to 34–41C) and incomplete or complete RBBB in the absence of signs of acute myocardial ischemia. Syncope and sudden death are the typical symptoms.

Genetic Basis and Pathophysiology

BrS has a complex genetic background. Several decades after the identification of the first mutations in the *SCN5A* gene

(BrS1 variant), still no more than 30% of patients are eventually genotyped event after extensive screening of the known genes (**Table 34–6**). Besides *SCN5A*, which accounts for approximately 20% of cases, the remaining BrS genes explain only a minority. Furthermore, a systematic analysis of the reported mutations has shown that with the exception of *SCN5A*, little evidence exists to definitely[148] associate the other putative BrS genes with the disease.[156] This concern about the true pathogenic role of several genes attributed to the disease in the published literature raises concerns on how which genes should be screened in clinical practice.

This observation together with the high percentage of nonfamilial cases and highly incomplete penetrance has led to hypothesize that BrS may also be an oligogenic trait. This hypothesis has found initial confirmation in studies that have identified a set of genetic polymorphisms (common genetic variants in the population) significantly associated with presence on the ECG of the typical Brugada pattern.[157]

Sodium Current and Brugada Syndrome: I_{Na} is conducted by the Nav1.5 channel that is encoded by the *SCN5A* gene: loss of function mutations in this gene is considered to have a causative role in the manifestation of BrS. Loss of I_{Na} also results in negative bathmotropic and dromotropic effects that contribute to the high prevalence of atrioventricular and intraventricular conduction defects in BrS.[158]

Several other putative BrS genes may alter I_{Na} (*GPD1-L, SCN1B, SCN3B, SLMAP, TRPM4, SCN2B, RANGRF, TCAP,* and *GSTM3*) (Table 34–6); however, as previously described, their causative role in BrS has been questioned.

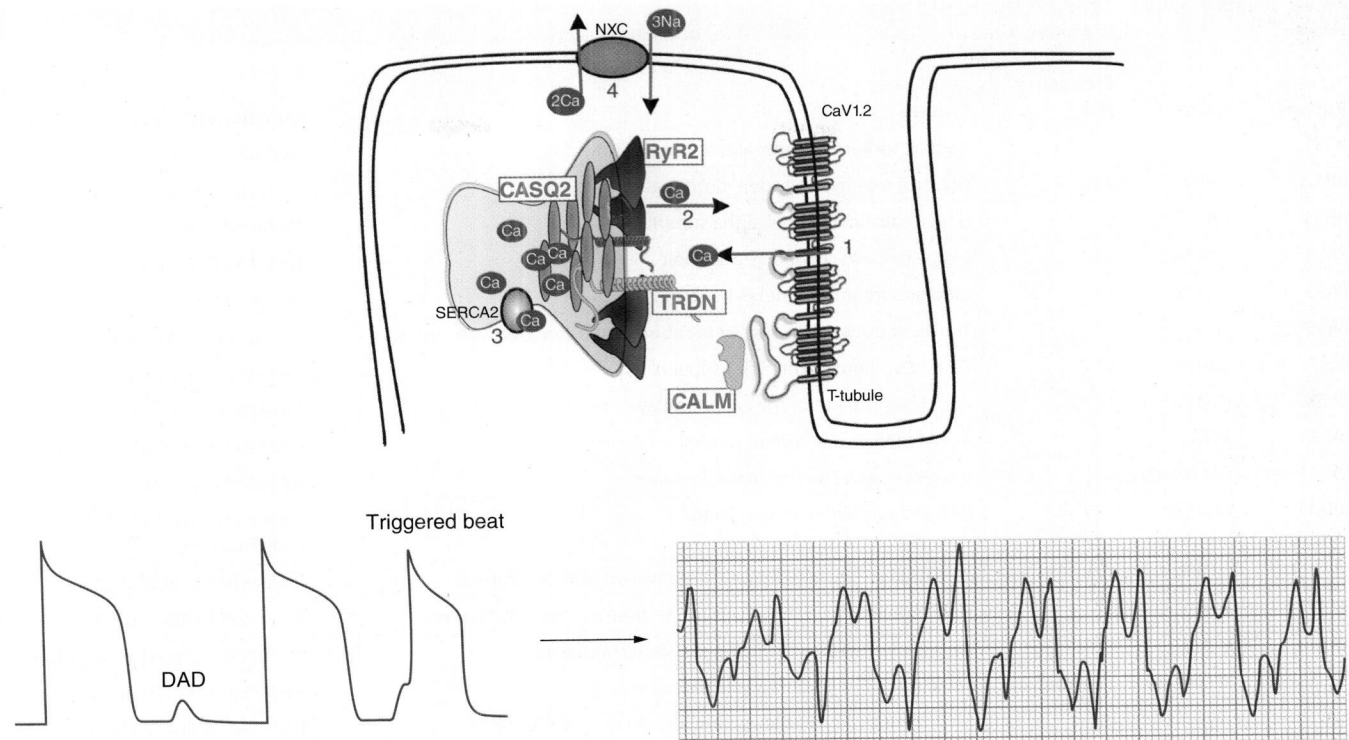

Figure 34–45. Pathophysiology and arrhythmias in CPVT. The normal process of calcium-induced calcium release (CICR) includes three steps (*blue numbers 1 to 3*): (1) the calcium entering the cell through the voltage-dependent L-type channels triggers further calcium release from the sarcoplasmic reticulum (3) through the ryanodine receptors. After contraction the calcium reuptake from the cytosol to the SR is an active process controlled by the Calcium ATPase pump (SERCA). In the presence of CPVT mutations, the ryanodine receptor releases an excessive amount of calcium and it is "leaky" during the electrical diastole. This leads to cytosolic calcium overload that is removed from the cells by an abnormal hyperactivation of the sodium-calcium exchanger (NCX) that extrudes calcium (4). However, NCX generates a net inward current because it transports three sodium ions (three positive charges) for one calcium ion (two positive charges). This current is called *transient inward* current and is visible as a depolarizing "hump," (DAD) on the action potential. When large enough, DADs may trigger extrasystolic action potential(s) that generate the typical bidirectional VT (lower-right ECG).

More recently, using genome-wide copy number variation analysis, a 5.5 Kb deletion in the *GSTM3* gene deletion that reduces I_{Na} has been found in 23% of *SCN5A* negative probands (vs 1% of controls). This promising finding awaits confirmation but it can potentially represent a significant cause of the BrS phenotype.[159]

Calcium and Potassium Channels in Brugada Syndrome: Loss of function cardiac calcium channel mutations have been reported in a few BrS patients and three genes have been involved: *CACNA1c, CACNB2,* and *CACNA2D1.* They all encode for subunits that cooperate to form the multimeric structure of the channel. *CACNA1C* and *CACNB2* constitute the α and β subunits, *CACNA2D1* produces a preprotein that is cleaved into multiple chains that comprise the α-2 and delta subunits. A common feature of BrS associated with calcium channel mutations may be the presence of a short QT interval.

I_{to} can also be involved in the pathogenesis of BrS. I_{to} is the current controlling the phase 1 of the cardiac action potential (initial fast repolarization). Mutations have been found in BrS patients that directly or indirectly affect I_{to} are: *KCNE3, KCND3, KCNE5. KCNE3, KCNE5,* and *KCND3.* In general, the effect of mutations in these gene is to increase I_{to}, which shortens the action potential and increases transmural dispersion of

repolarization. Gain of function mutations in the ATP-dependent potassium channel, in the cardiac delayed rectifier channel, and in the pacemaker channel have been reported (Table 34–6), but their pathogenetic role has been questioned.

Brugada Syndrome ECG and Arrhythmias: Mechanistic Insights: Two hypotheses have been proposed to explain the presence of ST-segment elevation and polymorphic VT in BrS: repolarization and depolarization.[160]

Repolarization Hypothesis: According to this hypothesis, either the reduction of the depolarizing currents I_{Na}, and I_{Ca}, or the increase of the repolarizing current I_{to} lead to loss of the action potential dome thus causing a shortening of the action potential duration in the epicardium of the RVOT, where I_{to} is more expressed. This process generates a transmural repolarization gradient/dispersion that causes ST-segment elevation and arrhythmias through the so-called phase 2 re entry.

Depolarization Hypothesis: According to this hypothesis, the ST-segment elevation in the right precordial leads of the ECG is attributable to slowing of conduction and delayed activation in the RVOT thus promoting the development of reentrant arrhythmias.

Surface mapping studies[161] provided evidence in support of both hypotheses. Indeed, ST elevation, delayed and

TABLE 34–6. Brugada Syndrome Genes

Variant	Gene	Mutation Frequency (%)	Protein	Functional Defect
BRS1	SCN5A	20	Cardiac sodium channel alpha subunit (Nav1.5)	Reduced Na+ current
BRS2	GPD1-L	<1	Glycerol-6-phosphate-dehydrogenase	Reduced Na+ current
BRS3	CACNA1c	5	L-type calcium channel alpha subunit (Cav1.2)	Reduced Ca2+ current
RRS4	CACNB2	<1	L-type calcium channel β-2 subunit	Reduced Ca2+ current
BRS5	SCN1B	<1	Cardiac sodium channel β-1 subunit	Reduced Na+ current
BRS6	KCNE3	<1	Transient outward current beta subunit- transient outward current	Increased K+ Ito current
BrS7	SCN3B	<1	Cardiac sodium channel β-3 subunit	Reduced Na+ current
BRS8	KCNH2	<1	Rapid component of the cardiac delayed rectifier current	Increased K+ IKr current
BRS9	KCNJ8	<1	Acetylcholine-dependent potassium current	Increased IK ATP-sensitive current
BRS10	CACNA2D1	<1	L-type calcium channel delta-2 subunit	Reduced Ca2+ current
BRS11	RANGRF	<1	RAN protein GTP releasing factor	Unknown (possible effect on sodium current)
BRS12	KCNE5	<1	Potassium channel β-5 subunit – transient outward current	Increased K+ Ito current
BRS13	KCND3	<1	SHAL potassium channel isoform 3 – transient outward current	Increased K+ Ito current
BRS14	HCN4	<1	Hyperpolarization activated potassium channel (If)	No functional studies available.
BRS15	SLMAP	<1	Sarcolemmal membrane associated protein	Reduced Na+ current
BRS16	TRPM4	<1	Calcium activated cationic channel subfamily M isoform 4	Reduced sodium current*
BRS17	SCN2B	<1	Cardiac sodium channel β-2 subunit	Reduced Na+ current
BRS18	SCN10A	<1	Voltage gated sodium channel alpha subunit 10	Reduced NaV1.8 current
BRS19	MOG1	<1	Guanine nucleotide release factor, control of NaV1.5 trafficking	Reduced Na+ current
BRS21	ABCC9	<1	SUR2A (sulfonylurea receptor subunit 2 A)	Increased outward current
BRS22	TCAP	<1	Z-disk protein that maintains cytoskeletal integrity	Reduced Na+ current
BRS23	GSTM3	?*	Glutathione S-transferase (anti oxidant enzyme). A 5.5 Kb deletion found in all subjects	Reduced Na+ current

*23% of SCN5A patients reported in a single study; the results await for confirmation.

fractionated EGs (depolarization abnormality), and repolarization gradients (dispersion of repolarization) have been simultaneously detected. Thus, the RVOT of BrS patients is prone to arrhythmias due to transmural dispersion of repolarization or due to epicardial reentry favored by localized slow conduction. These data provide a robust rationale for the use of ablation in the treatment of the disease.

Diagnosis

BrS is diagnosed in the presence of a "type 1 ECG," consisting of a coved J point elevation ≥2 mm with descending ST segment and negative T wave in the right precordial leads V1 and V2 (**Fig. 34–46**). On the basis of electro-anatomical studies[162] the current guidelines[163] suggest recording right precordial leads (V1 and V2) also in the third and second intercostal spaces to improve the diagnostic sensitivity.

If patients present with an ST-segment elevation in V1-V3 that is not coved but rather it has a saddle-back morphology (Fig. 34–46), the term "type 2 ECG" is used when the elevation exceeds 2 mm and the term "type 3 ECG" is used when the saddle back elevation is less than 2 mm.

In the presence of type 2 and type 3 patterns, it is indicated to perform a provocative test with the intravenous administration

of sodium channel blockers (flecainide 2 mg/kg or ajmaline 1 mg/kg) with the objective of investigating whether a type 1 ECG can be pharmacologically induced.

Determining whether patients have a spontaneous or an induced type 1 pattern has important prognostic implications because patients with spontaneous type 1 are at higher risk of developing VT/VF.

For these reasons, the use of 12-lead Holter monitoring has a relevant diagnostic and prognostic role because, given the intermittent presence of the type 1 ECG pattern, a single 12-lead recording may miss the diagnosis, thus underestimating the risk of life-threatening arrhythmias.

Natural History and Cardiac Events

BrS manifests with syncope and cardiac arrest occurring at rest or during sleep. Specific triggers for events are fever, abundant meals leading to distension of the stomach, excessive alcohol consumption, and several drugs (www.brugadadrugs.org). Avoiding such conditions is recommended as class I by clinical practice guidelines (**Table 34–7**). The first arrhythmic manifestation of the disease typically occurs in the third or fourth decade of life. However, the occurrence of arrhythmic events in the pediatric BrS population is emerging as a previously

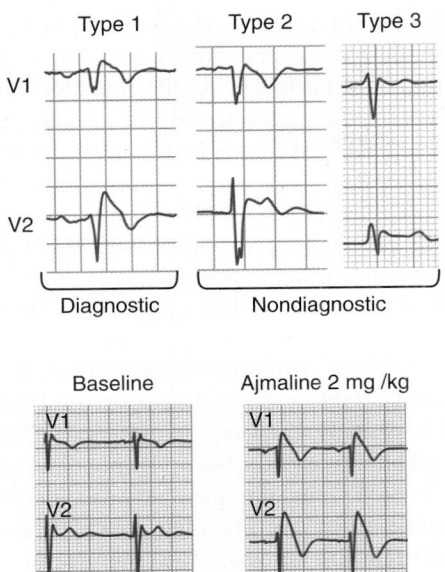

Figure 34–46. ECG patterns in BrS. Ajmaline test in BrS. The possible ECG presentation is shown in the upper panels depicting the type 1 (diagnostic) and the "possible" BrS ECGs defined as type 2 (≥2.0 mm ST elevation) or type 3 (<2.0 ST elevation). The lower panels show a type 3 ECG converted into a type 1 during IV injection of ajmaline.

unrecognized clinical problem.[164] In a recent survey of the Italian database TRIAD, among 129 children, 2.4% had life-threatening arrhythmic events and 8.6% syncope.[165] These data support the view that ECG should be performed in children of parents with BrS.

Risk Stratification

The recommendations for risk stratification as management of BrS are summarized in **Table 34–7**. ICD is the only proven effective treatment to reduce mortality in BrS. ICD is clearly indicated in cardiac arrest survivors (class I)[134] who have a 4% to 5% year risk of recurrence, the highest among the BrS patient population.[166] In this group of patients, the use of the subcutaneous ICD (S-ICD) avoiding lead-related complications (malfunction and infections) may be preferred. On the opposite end of the spectrum of severity of the disease, asymptomatic patients with drug-induced type 1 ECG only have a very low rate of events, 0.2% to 0.4% year.[166,167] In these patients, monitoring the ECG with annual 12-lead holter recording seems to be a reasonable approach to identify the appearance of a spontaneous type 1 pattern that would require the adoption of a more structured risk stratification protocol.[135] Agreement also exists to support ICD use in patients with history of syncope and a spontaneous type 1 ECG with an AHA/ACC class I and ESC class IIa indication.[134,135] These patients have approximately 1.5% to 2.0% yearly risk of arrhythmic events.[166,168,169]

The patients with a spontaneous type 1 pattern without history of syncope (approximately 40% of the cases), represent the most difficult scenario. Their risk of life-threatening events is approximately 0.8% to 1.0% per year.[166] The inducibility of arrhythmias (VT/VF) at programmed electrical stimulation (PES) has been proposed as a marker of increased risk, but

TABLE 34–7. Recommendations for Brugada Syndrome

Recommendations – diagnosis	Class
Brugada syndrome is diagnosed in patients with ST-segment elevation with type 1 morphology ≥2 mm in one or more leads among the right precordial leads V1 and/or V2 positioned in the second, third, or fourth intercostal space, occurring either spontaneously or after provocative drug test with intravenous administration of sodium channel blockers (such as ajmaline, flecainide, procainamide, or pilsicainide	I
Recommendations – Management	
The following lifestyle changes are recommended in all patients with a diagnosis of Brugada syndrome: (a) Avoidance of drugs that may induce ST-segment elevation in right precordial leads (http://www.brugadadrugs.org) (b) Avoidance of excessive alcohol intake and large meals (c) Prompt treatment of any fever with antipyretic drugs.	I
ICD implantation is recommended in patients with a diagnosis of Brugada syndrome who (a) Are survivors of an aborted cardiac arrest and/or (b) Have documented spontaneous sustained VT.	I
*In patients with Brugada syndrome experiencing recurrent ICD shocks for polymorphic VT, intensification of therapy with quinidine or catheter ablation is recommended	
*In asymptomatic patients with only inducible type 1 Brugada electrocardiographic pattern, observation without therapy is recommended.	I
*Quinidine should be considered in patients who qualify for an ICD but present a contraindication or refuse it and in patients who require treatment for supraventricular arrhythmias.	IIa – I **
ICD implantation should be considered in patients with a spontaneous diagnostic type 1 EKG pattern and history of syncope.	IIa
*In patients with suspected Brugada syndrome in the absence of a spontaneous type 1 Brugada electrocardiographic pattern, a pharmacological challenge using a sodium channel blocker can be useful for diagnosis	
Quinidine or isoproterenol should be considered in patients with Brugada syndrome to treat electrical storms	IIa
ICD implantation may be considered in patients with a diagnosis of Brugada syndrome who develop VF during PVS with two or three extrastimuli at two sites.	IIb
Catheter ablation may be considered in patients with a history of electrical storms or repeated appropriate ICD shocks.	IIb
*In patients with asymptomatic Brugada syndrome and a spontaneous type 1 Brugada electrocardiographic pattern, an electrophysiological study with programmed ventricular stimulation using single and double extrastimuli may be considered for further risk stratification	IIb

*recommendation present in AHA/ACC[139] guidelines only; **class IIa ESC guidelines, class I AHA/ACC guidelines that also add catheter ablation as alternative to quinidine.

Data from Priori SG, Blomström-Lundqvist C, Mazzanti A, et al: 2015 ESC Guidelines for the management of patients with ventricular arrhythmias and the prevention of sudden cardiac death: The Task Force for the Management of Patients with Ventricular Arrhythmias and the Prevention of Sudden Cardiac Death of the European Society of Cardiology (ESC). Endorsed by: Association for European Paediatric and Congenital Cardiology (AEPC). *Eur Heart J.* 2015 Nov 1;36(41):2793-2867 and Al-Khatib SM, Stevenson WG, Ackerman MJ, et al: 2017 AHA/ACC/HRS Guideline for Management of Patients With Ventricular Arrhythmias and the Prevention of Sudden Cardiac Death: A Report of the American College of Cardiology/American Heart Association Task Force on Clinical Practice Guidelines and the Heart Rhythm Society. *J Am Coll Cardiol.* 2018 Oct 2;72(14):e91-e220.

conflicting results have been published. The limitation of PES relies on the fact that while a positive test is associated with approximately 3-fold higher risk, a negative PES does not exclude a risk due to the unsatisfactory negative predictive value (30%–40% of events occur in PES negative patients).[170] Thus, ICD implant strategy based on results of PES has limitations and PES results have to be used with caution. Among other proposed risk markers, the analysis of QRS fragmentation is a promising approach.[171,172]

Therapy

Drug therapy of BrS is based on the use of quinidine, a class IA antiarrhythmic drug that in small studies showed to be able to prevent arrhythmia inducibility during PES,[173] to reduce burden of events in symptomatic patients[173] and recurrence of arrhythmic events.[168,174] In order to gather more insights on this promising role of quinidine, two clinical trials were designed (clinicaltrials.org ID: NCT00927732 and NCT00927732) but unfortunately both were early-terminated due to an insufficient number of cardiac events. Currently, quinidine has received a class I indication for the treatment of patients with ICD and recurrent shocks and for patients with spontaneous type 1 ECG and symptomatic VA who either are not candidates for or decline an ICD.[135] Quinidine is also indicated for the treatment of electrical storm (class IIa) or in patients with contraindications for ICD (class IIa).[134] The prophylactic use of quinidine in patients with drug-induced type 1 ECG, is a reasonable approach but it is not yet recommended by clinical practice guidelines.

A most promising therapeutic approach in BrS is catheter ablation of the arrhythmogenic substrate that may encompass PVC, endocardial, and epicardial ablation. Epicardial ablation is currently at the core of investigation by several groups. The approach was originally proposed by Nademanee.[175] Low voltage, fragmented electrical activity was identified in the right ventricular outflow tract patients. Ablation of these areas prevented induction of VT/VF with PES and was associated with the loss of the type 1 ECG pattern during provocation with ajmaline or flecainide. According to AHA/ACC guidelines, ablation has the same recommendation (class I) as quinidine for the treatment of patients with recurrent ICD shocks and for patients with spontaneous type 1 ECG and symptomatic arrhythmias who either are not candidates for or decline an ICD.[134] It is currently unknown whether ablation can effectively reduce the future risk of events in asymptomatic patients.

Short QT Syndrome

Definition

SQTS is a rare disorder causing arrhythmias and sudden death in the setting of a short QT interval and structurally normal heart (Figs. 34–41A to 34–41C). Although the disease has been defined as clinical entity for several decades, there is still limited experience (approximately 250 cases described worldwide) and risk stratification schemes are lacking.

Genetic Basis and Pathophysiology

The prevalence of SQTS in the population is undefined but it is likely to be <1:10 000. To date, eight genes have been identified (*CACNA1C*, *CACNA2D1*, *CACNB2*, *KCNH2*, *KCNJ2*, *KCNQ1*, *SCN5A*, and *SLC4A*). Genetic screening of all eight genes leads to identification of likely pathogenic mutations in approximately 20% of the clinically affected and screened individuals. *KCNH2*-related SQTS seems to be the most frequent genetic form of the disease.[176]

A short QT interval (QTc <340 ms) may also be found in patients with BrS and specifically in carriers of pathogenic or likely pathogenic mutations in the genes encoding subunits of the L-Type cardiac calcium channels, *CACNA1C* and *CACNB2*.

The shortening of ventricular repolarization, the hallmark of SQTS, translates into a short refractory period that has been recognized in patients[177] and reproduced in a *KCNH2*-N588K transgenic rabbit model.[176] In silico 3D modeling and in vitro expression of SQTS, mutants have revealed increased tissue temporal vulnerability for initiating reentry[178] and reduced minimal substrate size necessary to sustain reentry. This may explain both the high susceptibility to ventricular arrhythmias and AF observed in several SQTS patients.

Clinical Presentation and Management

SQTS can be diagnosed in the presence of QTc <340 ms (class I)[134] and can also be considered (class IIa) in the presence of a QTc ≤360 ms and one or more of the following: (1) confirmed pathogenic mutation, (2) family history of SQTS, (3) family history of sudden death at age <40 years, and (4) survival from a VT/VF episode in the absence of heart disease.[134]

The measurement of QT interval for SQTS diagnosis can be complicated by the lack or markedly reduced QT adaptation to heart rate (ie, a flat QT/RR relationship). Therefore, Bazett correction may lead to bias with a tendency for overdiagnosis during bradycardia and underdiagnosis when the QT is measured during tachycardia. It has been suggested that QT interval measurements should be made at heart rates between 55 bpm and 65 bpm.[179] Tall and peaked T waves (hyperkalemic-like pattern) or asymmetrical T waves with a normal ascending phase and a rapid descending limb are commonly observed in patients with SQTS.

The average cardiac event rate in SQTS is approximately 1% per year,[177] but cardiac arrests and SCD events seem to peak in the first 1 to 2 years of life and subsequently after 25 years of age. AF occurs in more than half of SQTS cases.[180]

Unfortunately, no correlation has been found between the QT duration and the risk of events and programmed electrical stimulation has no prognostic value since the majority of patients are inducible. Therefore, risk stratification is difficult in asymptomatic patients.

Treatment options for SQTS include the use of ICD and quinidine. ICD is indicated (class I) for all subjects with an established diagnosis and documented cardiac arrest or sustained ventricular arrhythmias.[134,135] Currently, there is no indication for the use of ICD in asymptomatic patients.

Quinidine should be considered for patients with recurrent sustained arrhythmias (class IIa)[135] and can be considered (class IIb) for subjects with contraindications of technical limitations to ICD use (eg, young children).

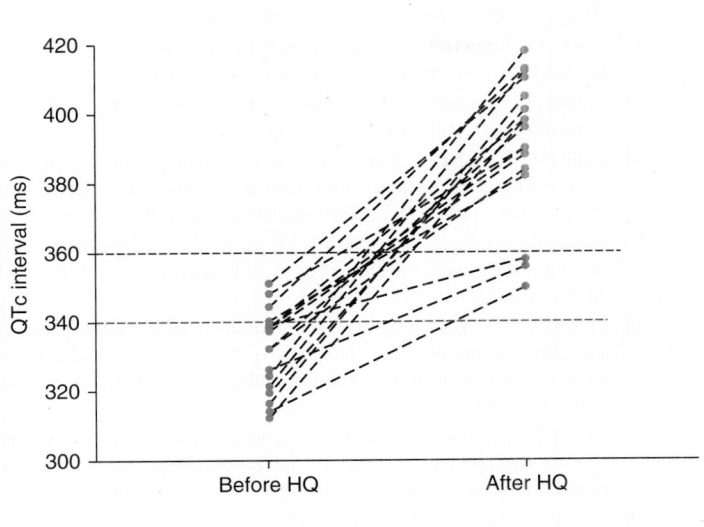

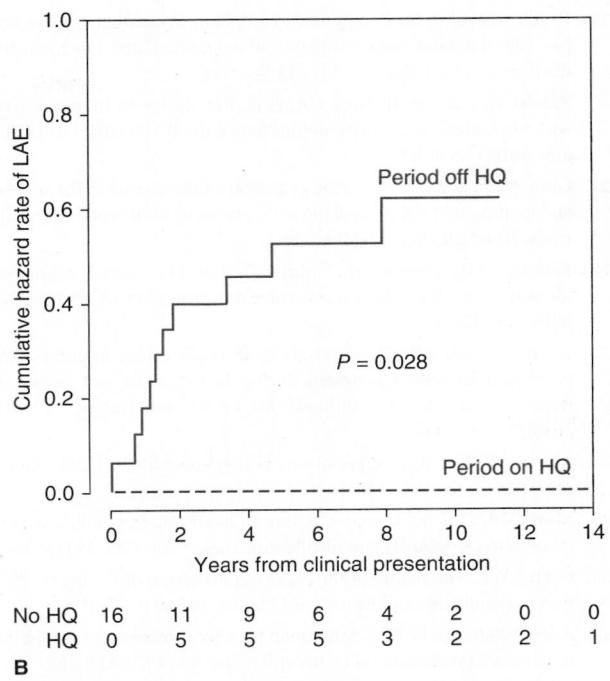

No HQ	16	11	9	6	4	2	0	0
HQ	0	5	5	5	3	2	2	1

A   **B**

Figure 34–47. Effect of quinidine in SQTS. **(A)** After starting hydroquinidine (HQ), the number of patients with QTc <340 ms, *orange dotted line*) dropped from 76% to 0%, and 82% of the patients normalized their QTc values (*orange dots*). *Blue dots* represent QTc values before HQ; *gray dots* represent QTc interval values that persisted below 360 ms during HQ therapy. The *purple dotted line* represents the threshold of "normal" QTc (ie, >360 ms). **(B)** Risk of LAE in SQTS with a previous cardiac arrest (Kaplan-Meier analysis). All patients at the beginning of observation were included in the nontreatment group (*continuous blue line*), and the assignment to the treatment group (*orange dashed line*) was updated at the time of HQ initiation. Overall, in the group of symptomatic SQTS patients, the annual rate of LAE dropped from 12% while off HQ (10 LAE over 82 person-years) to 0% while on HQ. Reproduced with permission from Mazzanti A, Maragna R, Vacanti G, et al: Hydroquinidine Prevents Life-Threatening Arrhythmic Events in Patients With Short QT Syndrome, *J Am Coll Cardiol.* 2017 Dec 19;70(24):3010-3015.

We have recently[181] demonstrated for the first time the efficacy of quinidine: the occurrence of arrhythmic events (documented VA, cardiac arrest or appropriate ICD shocks) during 6 years of follow-up was significantly reduced from 0.73 ± 0.3 events per patient to 0 (*P* = 0.026) (**Fig. 34–47A** and **34–47B**). Furthermore, the annual rate of LAE in the 16 patients with a previous cardiac arrest dropped from 12% before to 0% on hydroquinidine therapy (*P* = 0.028). Based on these results, it appears reasonable to consider the use of quinidine for primary prevention in patients with SQTS.

REFERENCES

1. Ho SY, Ernst S. *Anatomy for Electrophysiologists: A Practical Handbook.* Cardiotext Publishing; 2012.

2. Ho SY, Cabrera JA, Sanchez-Quintana D. Left atrial anatomy revisited. *Circ Arrhythm Electrophysiol.* 2012;5:220-228.

3. Ho SY, Sanchez-Quintana D. Anatomy and pathology of the sinus node. *J Interv Card Electrophysiol.* 2016;46:3-8.

4. Nagarajan VD, Ho SY, Ernst S. Anatomical considerations for His bundle pacing. *Circ Arrhythm Electrophysiol.* 2019;12:e006897.

5. Calkins H, Hindricks G, Cappato R, et al. 2017 HRS/EHRA/ECAS/APHRS/SOLAECE expert consensus statement on catheter and surgical ablation of atrial fibrillation. *Heart Rhythm.* 2017;14:e275-e444.

6. Wit AL, Cranefield PF. Triggered and automatic activity in the canine coronary sinus. *Circ Res.* 1977;41:434-445.

7. DiFrancesco D. A brief history of pacemaking. *Front Physiol.* 2019;10:1599.

8. Torrente AG, Zhang R, Wang H, et al. Contribution of small conductance K+ channels to sinoatrial node pacemaker activity: insights from atrial-specific Na+/Ca2+ exchange knockout mice. *J Physiology.* 2017;595:3847-3865.

9. Kohajda Z, Loewe A, Toth N, Varro A, Nagy N. The cardiac pacemaker story-fundamental role of the Na(+)/Ca(2+) exchanger in spontaneous automaticity. *Front Pharmacol.* 2020;11:516.

10. Boyden PA, Smith GL. Ca(2+) leak-What is it? Why should we care? Can it be managed? *Heart Rhythm.* 2018;15:607-614.

11. Boyden PA, Dun W, Robinson RB. Cardiac Purkinje fibers and arrhythmias; The GK Moe Award Lecture 2015. *Heart Rhythm.* 2016;13:1172-1181.

12. Cingolani E, Goldhaber JI, Marban E. Next-generation pacemakers: from small devices to biological pacemakers. *Nat Rev Cardiol.* 2018;15:139-150.

13. Ionta V, Liang W, Kim EH, et al. SHOX2 overexpression favors differentiation of embryonic stem cells into cardiac pacemaker cells, improving biological pacing ability. *Stem Cell Reports.* 2015;4:129-142.

14. Verkerk AO, Wilders R. Pacemaker activity of the human sinoatrial node: an update on the effects of mutations in HCN4 on the hyperpolarization-activated current. *Int J Mol Sci.* 2015;16:3071-3094.

15. Wilders R, Verkerk AO. Long QT syndrome and sinus bradycardia–a mini review. *Front Cardiovasc Med.* 2018;5:106.

16. Bers DM, Chen-Izu Y. Sodium and calcium regulation in cardiac myocytes: from molecules to heart failure and arrhythmia. *J Physiol.* 2015;593:1327-1329.

17. Kusayama T, Wong J, Liu X, et al. Simultaneous noninvasive recording of electrocardiogram and skin sympathetic nerve activity (neuECG). *Nat Protoc.* 2020;15:1853-1877.

18. Doytchinova A, Hassel JL, Yuan Y, et al. Simultaneous noninvasive recording of skin sympathetic nerve activity and electrocardiogram. *Heart Rhythm.* 2017;14:25-33.

19. Uradu A, Wan J, Doytchinova A, et al. Skin Sympathetic nerve activity precedes the onset and termination of paroxysmal atrial tachycardia and fibrillation. *Heart Rhythm.* 2017;14:964-971.

20. Zareba W, Daubert JP, Beck CA, et al. Ranolazine in high-risk patients with implanted cardioverter-defibrillators: the RAID trial. *J Am Coll Cardiol.* 2018;72:636-645.

21. Gong M, Zhang Z, Fragakis N, et al. Role of ranolazine in the prevention and treatment of atrial fibrillation: a meta-analysis of randomized clinical trials. *Heart Rhythm.* 2017;14:3-11.

22. Bannister ML, Thomas NL, Sikkel MB, et al. The mechanism of flecainide action in CPVT does not involve a direct effect on RyR2. *Circ Res.* 2015;116:1324-1335.

23. Chan YH, Tsai WC, Ko JS, et al. Small-conductance calcium-activated potassium current is activated during hypokalemia and masks short-term cardiac memory induced by ventricular pacing. *Circulation.* 2015;132:1377-1386.

24. Mayer AG. Rhythmical pulsations is scyphomedusae. *Publication 47 of the Carnegie Institute.* 1906:1-62.

25. Mines GR. On circulating excitation in heart muscles and their possible relation to tachycardia and fibrillation. *Trans R Soc Can.* 1914;4:43-53.

26. Garrey WE. The nature of fibrillatory contruction of the heart - its relation to tissue mass and form. *Am J Physiol.* 1914;33:397-414.

27. Allessie MA, Bonke FIM, Schopman JG. Circus movement in rabbit atrial muscle as a mechanism of tachycardia. *Circ Res.* 1973;33:54-62.

28. Wiener N, Rosenblueth A. The mathematical formulation of the problem of conduction of impulses in a network of connected excitable elements, specifically in cardiac muscle. *Arch Inst Cardiol Mex.* 1946;16:205-265.

29. Ikeda T, Yashima M, Uchida T, et al. Attachment of meandering reentrant wave fronts to anatomic obstacles in the atrium. Role of the obstacle size. *Circ Res.* 1997;81:753-764.

30. El-Sherif N, Smith RA, Evans K. Canine ventricular arrhythmias in the late myocardial infarction period. Epicardial mapping of reentrant circuits. *Circ Res.* 1981;49:255-265.

31. Kim YH, Xie F, Yashima M, et al. Role of papillary muscle in the generation and maintenance of reentry during ventricular tachycardia and fibrillation in isolated swine right ventricle. *Circulation.* 1999;100:1450-1459.

32. Ruaengsri C, Schill MR, Khiabani AJ, Schuessler RB, Melby SJ, Damiano RJ, Jr. The Cox-maze IV procedure in its second decade: still the gold standard? *Eur J Cardiothorac Surg.* 2018;53:i19-i25.

33. Kennedy M, Bers DM, Chiamvimonvat N, Sato D. Dynamical effects of calcium-sensitive potassium currents on voltage and calcium alternans. *J Physiol.* 2017;595:2285-2297.

34. Chen M, Yin D, Guo S, et al. Sex-specific activation of SK current by isoproterenol facilitates action potential triangulation and arrhythmogenesis in rabbit ventricles. *J Physiol.* 2018;596:4299-4322.

35. Nemec J, Kim JJ, Salama G. The link between abnormal calcium handling and electrical instability in acquired long QT syndrome – Does calcium precipitate arrhythmic storms? *Prog Biophys Mol Biol.* 2016;120:210-221.

36. Yu CC, Corr C, Shen C, et al. Small conductance calcium-activated potassium current is important in transmural repolarization of failing human ventricles. *Circ Arrhythm Electrophysiol.* 2015;8:667-676.

37. T. L. Brunton and J. Fayer. Note on independent pulsation of the pulmonary veins and vena cava. *Proc Roy Soc Lond.* 1876;25:174-176.

38. Kugler S, Nagy N, Racz G, Tokes AM, Dorogi B, Nemeskeri A. Presence of cardiomyocytes exhibiting Purkinje-type morphology and prominent connexin45 immunoreactivity in the myocardial sleeves of cardiac veins. *Heart Rhythm.* 2018;15:258-264.

39. Cheung DW. Electrical activity of the pulmonary vein and its interaction with the right atrium in the guinea-pig. *J phys.* 1981;314:445-456.

40. Krul SP, Berger WR, Smit NW, et al. Atrial fibrosis and conduction slowing in the left atrial appendage of patients undergoing thoracoscopic surgical pulmonary vein isolation for atrial fibrillation. *Circ Arrhythm Electrophysiol.* 2015;8:288-295.

41. Chang PC, Chen PS. SK channels and ventricular arrhythmias in heart failure. *Trends Cardiovasc Med.* 2015;25:508-514.

42. Vracko R, Thorning D and Frederickson RG. Fate of nerve fibers in necrotic, healing, and healed rat myocardium. *Lab Invest.* 1990;63:490-501.

43. Vracko R, Thorning D and Frederickson RG. Nerve fibers in human myocardial scars. *Hum Pathol.* 1991;22:138-146.

44. Ajijola OA, Yagishita D, Reddy NK, et al. Remodeling of stellate ganglion neurons after spatially targeted myocardial infarction: neuropeptide and morphologic changes. *Heart Rhythm.* 2015;12:1027-1035.

45. Kusayama T, Wan J, Doytchinova A, et al. Skin sympathetic nerve activity and the temporal clustering of cardiac arrhythmias. *JCI Insight.* 2019;4:e125853.

46. Chinda K, Tsai WC, Chan YH, et al. Intermittent left cervical vagal nerve stimulation damages the stellate ganglia and reduces ventricular rate during sustained atrial fibrillation in ambulatory dogs. *Heart Rhythm.* 2016;13:771-780.

47. Zhao Y, Jiang Z, Tsai WC, et al. Ganglionated plexi and ligament of Marshall ablation reduces atrial vulnerability and causes stellate ganglion remodeling in ambulatory dogs. *Heart Rhythm.* 2016;13:2083-2090.

48. Tsai W-C, Chan YH, Chinda K, et al. Effects of renal sympathetic denervation on the stellate ganglion and the brain stem in dogs. *Heart Rhythm.* 2017;14:255-262.

49. Steinberg JS, Shabanov V, Ponomarev D, et al. Effect of renal denervation and catheter ablation vs catheter ablation alone on atrial fibrillation recurrence among patients with paroxysmal atrial fibrillation and hypertension: the ERADICATE-AF randomized clinical trial. *JAMA.* 2020;323:248-255.

50. Pezhouman A, Singh N, Song Z, et al. Molecular basis of hypokalemia-induced ventricular fibrillation. *Circulation.* 2015;132:1528-1537.

51. Chatzidou S, Kontogiannis C, Tsilimigras DI, et al. Propranolol versus metoprolol for treatment of electrical storm in patients with implantable cardioverter-defibrillator. *J Am Coll Cardiol.* 2018;71:1897-1906.

52. Brugada P, Brugada J. Right bundle branch block, persistent ST segment elevation and sudden cardiac death: a distinct clinical and electrocardiographic syndrome: a multicenter report. *J Am Coll Cardiol.* 1992;20:1391-1396.

53. Haissaguerre M, Derval N, Sacher F, et al. Sudden cardiac arrest associated with early repolarization. *N Engl J Med.* 2008;358:2016-2023.

54. Nam GB, Kim YH, Antzelevitch C. Augmentation of J waves and electrical storms in patients with early repolarization. *N Engl J Med.* 2008;358:2078-2079.

55. Rosso R, Kogan E, Belhassen B, et al. J-point elevation in survivors of primary ventricular fibrillation and matched control subjects: incidence and clinical significance. *J Am Coll Cardiol.* 2008;52:1231-1238.

56. Antzelevitch C, Yan GX, Ackerman MJ, et al. J-Wave syndromes expert consensus conference report: emerging concepts and gaps in knowledge. *Heart Rhythm.* 2016.

57. Gussak I, Antzelevitch C. Early repolarization syndrome: clinical characterstics and possible cellular and ionic mechanisms. *J Electrocardiol.* 2000;33:299-309.

58. Macfarlane P, Antzelevitch C, Haissaguerre M, et al. Consensus paper – early repolarization pattern. *J Am Coll Cardiol.* 2015;66:470-477.

59. Antzelevitch C, Yan GX. J wave syndromes. *Heart Rhythm.* 2010;7:549-558.

60. Brosnan MJ, Kumar S, LaGerche A, et al. Early repolarization patterns associated with increased arrhythmic risk are common in young non-Caucasian Australian males and not influenced by athletic status. *Heart Rhythm.* 2015;12:1576-1583.

61. Priori SG, Napolitano C. J-wave syndromes: electrocardiographic and clinical aspects. *Card Electrophysiol Clin.* 2018;10:355-369.

62. Nademanee K. Sudden unexplained death syndrome in southeast Asia. *Am J Cardiol.* 1997;79(6A):10-11.

63. Antzelevitch C, Pollevick GD, Cordeiro JM, et al. Loss-of-function mutations in the cardiac calcium channel underlie a new clinical entity

characterized by ST-segment elevation, short QT intervals, and sudden cardiac death. *Circulation.* 2007;115:442-449.

64. Argenziano M, Antzelevitch C. Recent advances in the treatment of Brugada syndrome. *Expert Rev Cardiovasc Ther.* 2018;16:387-404.

65. Nakagawa K, Nagase S, Morita H, Ito H. Left ventricular epicardial electrogram recordings in idiopathic ventricular fibrillation with inferior and lateral early repolarization. *Heart Rhythm.* 2014;11:314-317.

66. Wu CI, Postema PG, Arbelo E, et al. SARS-CoV-2, COVID-19, and inherited arrhythmia syndromes. *Heart Rhythm.* 2020;17(9):1456-1462.

67. Kawata H, Morita H, Yamada Y, et al. Prognostic significance of early repolarization in inferolateral leads in Brugada patients with documented ventricular fibrillation: a novel risk factor for Brugada syndrome with ventricular fibrillation. *Heart Rhythm.* 2013;10:1161-1168.

68. Di Diego JM, Antzelevitch C. J wave syndromes as a cause of malignant cardiac arrhythmias. *Pacing Clin Electrophysiol.* 2018:684-699.

69. Park DS, Cerrone M, Morley G, et al. Genetically engineered SCN5A mutant pig hearts exhibit conduction defects and arrhythmias. *J Clin Invest.* 2015;125:403-412.

70. Antzelevitch C, Yan GX. J-wave syndromes: Brugada and early repolarization syndromes. *Heart Rhythm.* 2015;12:1852-1866.

71. Szel T, Antzelevitch C. Abnormal repolarization as the basis for late potentials and fractionated electrograms recorded from epicardium in experimental models of brugada syndrome. *J Am Coll Cardiol.* 2014;63:2037-2045.

72. Patocskai B, Szel T, Yoon N, Antzelevitch C. Cellular mechanisms underlying the fractionated and late potentials on epicardial electrograms and the ameliorative effect of epicardial radiofrequency ablation in an experimental model of Brugada syndrome. *Heart Rhythm.* 2014;11(5S):S464.

73. Hu D, Barajas-Martinez H, Pfeiffer R, et al. Mutations in *SCN10A* are responsible for a large fraction of cases of Brugada syndrome. *J Am Coll Cardiol.* 2014;64:66-79.

74. Monasky MM, Micaglio E, Vicedomini G, et al. Comparable clinical characteristics in Brugada syndrome patients harboring SCN5A or novel SCN10A variants. *Europace: Eur Pacing Arrhythmias Cardiac Electrophysiol.* 2019;21:1550-1558.

75. Musa H, Marcou CA, Herron TJ, et al. Abnormal myocardial expression of SAP97 is associated with arrhythmogenic risk. *Am J Physiol Heart Circulat Physiol.* 2020;318:H1357-H1370.

76. Uezato A, Yamamoto N, Jitoku D, et al. Genetic and molecular risk factors within the newly identified primate-specific exon of the SAP97/DLG1 gene in the 3q29 schizophrenia-associated locus. *Am J Med Genet B Neuropsychiatr Genet.* 2017;174:798-807.

77. Shimizu A, Zankov DP, Sato A, et al. Identification of transmembrane protein 168 mutation in familial Brugada syndrome. *FASEB J.* 2020;34:6399-6417.

78. Behr ER, Savio-Galimberti E, Barc J, et al. Role of common and rare variants in SCN10A: results from the Brugada syndrome QRS locus gene discovery collaborative study. *Cardiovasc Res.* 2015.

79. Cheng YJ, Yao H, Ji CC, et al. A heterozygous missense hERG mutation associated with early repolarization syndrome. *Cell Physiol Biochem.* 2018;51:1301-1312.

80. Yao H, Fan J, Cheng YJ, et al. SCN1Bβ mutations that affect their association with Kv4.3 underlie early repolarization syndrome. *J Cell Mol Med.* 2018;22:5639-5647.

81. Takayama K, Ohno S, Ding WG, et al. A de novo gain-of-function KCND3 mutation in early repolarization syndrome. *Heart Rhythm.* 2019;16:1698-1706.

82. Kapplinger JD, Giudicessi JR, Ye D, et al. Enhanced classification of Brugada syndrome-associated and long-QT syndrome-associated genetic variants in the SCN5A-encoded Nav1.5 cardiac sodium channel. *Circ Cardiovasc Genet.* 2015;8:582-595.

83. Le Scouarnec S, Karakachoff M, Gourraud JB, et al. Testing the burden of rare variation in arrhythmia-susceptibility genes provides new insights into molecular diagnosis for Brugada syndrome. *Human Molecul Genet.* 2015;24(10):2757-2763.

84. Hosseini SM, Kim R, Udupa S, et al. Reappraisal of reported genes for sudden arrhythmic death: an evidence-based evaluation of gene validity for Brugada syndrome. *Circulation.* 2018. 138(12):1195-1205.

85. Antzelevitch C, Patocskai B. Brugada syndrome: clinical, genetic, molecular, cellular, and ionic aspects. *Curr Probl Cardiol.* 2016;41:7-57.

86. Macfarlane PW, Antzelevitch C, Haissaguerre M, et al. The early repolarization pattern: a consensus paper. *J Am Coll Cardiol.* 2015;66:470-477.

87. Huikuri HV, Juhani Junttila M. Clinical aspects of inherited J-wave syndromes. *Trends Cardiovasc Med.* 2015;25:24-30.

88. Wilde AA, Postema PG, Di Diego JM, et al. The pathophysiological mechanism underlying Brugada syndrome: depolarization versus repolarization. *J Mol Cell Cardiol.* 2010;49:543-553.

89. Morita H, Zipes DP, Wu J. Brugada syndrome: insights of ST elevation, arrhythmogenicity, and risk stratification from experimental observations. *Heart Rhythm.* 2009;6:S34-S43.

90. Landaw J, Zhang Z, Song Z, et al. Small-conductance Ca(2+)-activated K(+) channels promote J-wave syndrome and phase-2 reentry. *Heart Rhythm.* 2020;17(9):1582-1590.

91. Antzelevitch C, Gan-Xin Y. J wave syndrome: Brugada and early repolarization syndromes. *Heart Rhythm.* 2015;12:1852-1866.

92. Zhang J, Sacher F, Hoffmayer K, et al. Cardiac electrophysiological substrate underlying the ECG phenotype and electrogram abnormalities in Brugada syndrome patients. *Circulation.* 2015;131:1950-1959.

93. Nademanee K, Veerakul G, Chandanamattha P, et al. Prevention of ventricular fibrillation episodes in Brugada syndrome by catheter ablation over the anterior right ventricular outflow tract epicardium. *Circulation.* 2011;123:1270-1279.

94. Sacher F, Derval N, Horlitz M, Haissaguerre M. J wave elevation to monitor quinidine efficacy in early repolarization syndrome. *J Electrocardiol.* 2014;47:223-225.

95. Brugada J, Pappone C, Berruezo A, et al. Brugada syndrome phenotype elimination by epicardial substrate ablation. *Circ Arrhythm Electrophysiol.* 2015;8(6):1373-1381.

96. Patocskai B, Yoon N, Antzelevitch C. Mechanisms underlying epicardial radiofrequency ablation to suppress arrhythmogenesis in experimental models of Brugada syndrome. *JACC: Clin Electrophysiol.* 2017;3:353.

97. Di Diego JM, Argenziano M, Chen K, Tabler M, Antzelevitch C. In a whole-heart model of the Brugada syndrome, delayed conduction in the RVOT "does not" contribute to inscription of the electrocardiographic J wave / ST segment elevation. *Heart Rhythm.* 2018;15:S242.

98. Boukens BJ, Sylva M, de Gier-de VC, et al. Reduced sodium channel function unmasks residual embryonic slow conduction in the adult right ventricular outflow tract. *Circ Res.* 2013;113:137-141.

99. Antzelevitch C, Brugada P, Brugada J, et al. Brugada syndrome: a decade of progress. *Circ Res.* 2002;91:1114-1119.

100. Kurita T, Shimizu W, Inagaki M, et al. The electrophysiologic mechanism of ST-segment elevation in Brugada syndrome. *J Am Coll Cardiol.* 2002;40:330-334.

101. Coronel R, Casini S, Koopmann TT, et al. Right ventricular fibrosis and conduction delay in a patient with clinical signs of Brugada syndrome: a combined electrophysiological, genetic, histopathologic, and computational study. *Circulation.* 2005;112:2769-2777.

102. Koncz I, Gurabi Z, Patocskai B, et al. Mechanisms underlying the development of the electrocardiographic and arrhythmic manifestations of early repolarization syndrome. *J Mol Cell Cardiol.* 2014;68C:20-28.

103. Gurabi Z, Koncz I, Patocskai B, Nesterenko VV, Antzelevitch C. Cellular mechanism underlying hypothermia-induced ventricular tachycardia/ventricular fibrillation in the setting of early repolarization and the protective effect of quinidine, cilostazol, and milrinone. *Circ Arrhythm Electrophysiol.* 2014;7:134-142.

104. Patocskai B, Barajas-Martinez H, Hu D, Gurabi Z, Koncz I, Antzelevitch C. Cellular and ionic mechanisms underlying the effects of cilostazol, milrinone, and isoproterenol to suppress arrhythmogenesis in an experimental model of early repolarization syndrome. *Heart Rhythm.* 2016;13:1326-1334.

105. Ghosh S, Cooper DH, Vijayakumar R, et al. Early repolarization associated with sudden death: insights from noninvasive electrocardiographic imaging. *Heart Rhythm.* 2010;7:534-537.

106. Mahida S, Derval N, Sacher F, et al. History and clinical significance of early repolarization syndrome. *Heart Rhythm.* 2015;12:242-249.

107. Huikuri HV. Separation of benign from malignant J waves. *Heart Rhythm.* 2015;12:384-385.

108. Aizawa Y, Sato M, Kitazawa H, et al. Tachycardia-dependent augmentation of "notched J waves" in a general patient population without ventricular fibrillation or cardiac arrest: not a repolarization but a depolarization abnormality? *Heart Rhythm.* 2015;12:376-383.

109. Badri M, Patel A, Yan G. Cellular and ionic basis of J-wave syndromes. *Trends Cardiovasc Med.* 2015;25:12-21.

110. Terho HK, Tikkanen JT, Junttila JM, et al. Prevalence and prognostic significance of fragmented QRS complex in middle-aged subjects with and without clinical or electrocardiographic evidence of cardiac disease. *Am J Cardiol.* 2014;114:141-147.

111. Li GR, Wang HB, Qin GW, et al. Acacetin, a natural flavone, selectively inhibits human atrial repolarization potassium currents and prevents atrial fibrillation in dogs. *Circulation.* 2008;117:2449-2457.

112. Di Diego JM, Argenziano M, Tabler M, et al. A definitive test of the repolarization versus depolarization hypothesis in a whole-heart model of Brugada syndrome. *Circulation.* 2019;Abstract.

113. Priori SG, Remme CA. Inherited conditions of arrhythmia: translating disease mechanisms to patient management. *Cardiovasc Res.* 2020;116:1539-1541.

114. Schwartz PJ, Stramba-Badiale M, Crotti L, et al. Prevalence of the congenital long-QT syndrome. *Circulation.* 2009;120:1761-1767.

115. Napolitano C, Novelli V, Francis MD, Priori SG. Genetic modulators of the phenotype in the long QT syndrome: state of the art and clinical impact. *Curr Opin Genet Dev.* 2015;33:17-24.

116. Adler A, Novelli V, Amin AS, et al. An international, multicentered, evidence-based reappraisal of genes reported to cause congenital long QT syndrome. *Circulation.* 2020;141:418-428.

117. Bai R, Napolitano C, Bloise R, Monteforte N, Priori SG. Yield of genetic screening in inherited cardiac channelopathies: how to prioritize access to genetic testing. *Circ Arrhythm Electrophysiol.* 2009;2:6-15.

118. Priori SG, Schwartz PJ, Napolitano C, et al. Risk stratification in the long-QT syndrome. *New Engl J Med.* 2003;348:1866-1874.

119. Yang Y, Yang Y, Liang B, et al. Identification of a Kir3.4 mutation in congenital long QT syndrome. *Am J Hum Genet.* 2010;86:872-880.

120. Mazzanti A, Guz D, Trancuccio A, et al. Natural history and risk stratification in Andersen-Tawil syndrome type 1. *J Am Coll Cardiol.* 2020;75:1772-1784.

121. Napolitano C, Priori SG, Schwartz PJ, et al. Genetic testing in the long QT syndrome: development and validation of an efficient approach to genotyping in clinical practice. *JAMA.* 2005;294:2975-2980.

122. Roberts JD, Asaki SY, Mazzanti A, et al. An international multicenter evaluation of type 5 long QT syndrome: a low penetrant primary arrhythmic condition. *Circulation.* 2020;141:429-439.

123. Roberts JD, Krahn AD, Ackerman MJ, et al. Loss-of-function KCNE2 variants: true monogenic culprits of long-QT syndrome or proarrhythmic variants requiring secondary provocation? *Circ Arrhythm Electrophysiol.* 2017;10.

124. Tristani-Firouzi M, Etheridge SP. Kir 2.1 channelopathies: the Andersen-Tawil syndrome. *Pflugers Arch.* 2010;460:289-294.

125. Klein MG, Shou M, Stohlman J, et al. Role of suppression of the inward rectifier current in terminal action potential repolarization in the failing heart. *Heart Rhythm.* 2017;14:1217-1223.

126. Hibino H, Inanobe A, Furutani K, Murakami S, Findlay I, Kurachi Y. Inwardly rectifying potassium channels: their structure, function, and physiological roles. *Physiol Rev.* 2010;90:291-366.

127. Mazzanti A, Maragna R, Vacanti G, et al. Interplay between genetic substrate, QTc duration, and arrhythmia risk in patients with long QT syndrome. *J Am Coll Cardiol.* 2018;71:1663-1671.

128. Splawski I, Timothy KW, Sharpe LM, et al. Ca(V)1.2 calcium channel dysfunction causes a multisystem disorder including arrhythmia and autism. *Cell.* 2004;119:19-31.

129. Boczek NJ, Ye D, Jin F, et al. Identification and functional characterization of a novel CACNA1C-mediated cardiac disorder characterized by prolonged QT intervals with hypertrophic cardiomyopathy, congenital heart defects, and sudden cardiac death. *Circ Arrhythm Electrophysiol.* 2015;8:1122-1132.

130. Gillis J, Burashnikov E, Antzelevitch C, et al. Long QT, syndactyly, joint contractures, stroke and novel CACNA1C mutation: expanding the spectrum of Timothy syndrome. *Am J Med Genet A.* 2012;158A:182-187.

131. Crotti L, Johnson CN, Graf E, et al. Calmodulin mutations associated with recurrent cardiac arrest in infants. *Circulation.* 2013;127:1009-1017.

132. Gomez-Hurtado N, Boczek NJ, Kryshtal DO, et al. Novel CPVT-associated calmodulin mutation in CALM3 (CALM3-A103V) activates arrhythmogenic Ca waves and sparks. *Circ Arrhythm Electrophysiol.* 2016;9.

133. Clemens DJ, Tester DJ, Giudicessi JR, et al. International Triadin Knockout Syndrome Registry. *Circ Genom Precis Med.* 2019;12:e002419.

134. Priori SG, Blomstrom-Lundqvist C, Mazzanti A, et al. 2015 ESC Guidelines for the management of patients with ventricular arrhythmias and the prevention of sudden cardiac death: the Task Force for the Management of Patients with Ventricular Arrhythmias and the Prevention of Sudden Cardiac Death of the European Society of Cardiology (ESC). Endorsed by: Association for European Paediatric and Congenital Cardiology (AEPC). *Eur Heart J.* 2015;36:2793-867.

135. Al-Khatib SM, Stevenson WG, Ackerman MJ, et al. 2017 AHA/ACC/HRS guideline for management of patients with ventricular arrhythmias and the prevention of sudden cardiac death: a report of the American College of Cardiology/American Heart Association Task Force on Clinical Practice Guidelines and the Heart Rhythm Society. *J Am Coll Cardiol.* 2018;72:e91-e220.

136. Priori SG, Napolitano C, Schwartz PJ, et al. Association of long QT syndrome loci and cardiac events among patients treated with beta-blockers. *JAMA.* 2004;292:1341-1344.

137. Mazzanti A, Maragna R, Faragli A, et al. Gene-specific therapy with mexiletine reduces arrhythmic events in patients with long QT syndrome Type 3. *J Am Coll Cardiol.* 2016;67:1053-1058.

138. Priori SG, Napolitano C, Tiso N, et al. Mutations in the cardiac ryanodine receptor gene (hRyR2) underlie catecholaminergic polymorphic ventricular tachycardia. *Circulation.* 2001;103:196-200.

139. Lahat H, Pras E, Olender T, et al. A missense mutation in a highly conserved region of CASQ2 is associated with autosomal recessive catecholamine-induced polymorphic ventricular tachycardia in Bedouin families from Israel. *Am J Human Genet.* 2001;69:1378-1384.

140. Priori SG, Chen SR. Inherited dysfunction of sarcoplasmic reticulum Ca2+ handling and arrhythmogenesis. *Circ Res.* 2011;108:871-883.

141. Sondergaard MT, Tian X, Liu Y, et al. Arrhythmogenic calmodulin mutations affect the activation and termination of cardiac ryanodine receptor-mediated Ca2+ release. *J Biol Chem.* 2015;290:26151-26162.

142. Limpitikul WB, Dick IE, Joshi-Mukherjee R, et al. Calmodulin mutations associated with long QT syndrome prevent inactivation of cardiac L-type Ca(2+) currents and promote proarrhythmic behavior in ventricular myocytes. *J Mol Cell Cardiol.* 2014;74:115-124.

143. Vassilakopoulou V, Calver BL, Thanassoulas A, et al. Distinctive malfunctions of calmodulin mutations associated with heart RyR2-mediated arrhythmic disease. *Biochim Biophys Acta.* 2015;1850:2168-21676.

144. Roux-Buisson N, Cacheux M, Fourest-Lieuvin A, et al. Absence of triadin, a protein of the calcium release complex, is responsible for cardiac arrhythmia with sudden death in human. *Human Molecul Genet.* 2012;21:2759-2767.

145. Rooryck C, Kyndt F, Bozon D, et al. New family with catecholaminergic polymorphic ventricular tachycardia linked to the triadin gene. *J Cardiovasc Electrophysiol.* 2015;26:1146-1150.

146. Koenig SN, Mohler PJ. The evolving role of ankyrin-B in cardiovascular disease. *Heart Rhythm*. 2017;14:1884-1889.

147. Priori SG, Napolitano C, Memmi M, et al. Clinical and molecular characterization of patients with catecholaminergic polymorphic ventricular tachycardia. *Circulation*. 2002;106:69-74.

148. van der Werf C, Nederend I, Hofman N, et al. Familial evaluation in catecholaminergic polymorphic ventricular tachycardia: disease penetrance and expression in cardiac ryanodine receptor mutation-carrying relatives. *Circ Arrhythm Electrophysiol*. 2012;5:748-756.

149. Hayashi M, Denjoy I, Extramiana F, et al. Incidence and risk factors of arrhythmic events in catecholaminergic polymorphic ventricular tachycardia. *Circulation*. 2009;119:2426-2434.

150. Roston TM, Vinocur JM, Maginot KR, et al. Catecholaminergic polymorphic ventricular tachycardia in children: analysis of therapeutic strategies and outcomes from an international multicenter registry. *Circ Arrhythm Electrophysiol*. 2015;8:633-642.

151. Leren IS, Saberniak J, Majid E, Haland TF, Edvardsen T, Haugaa KH. Nadolol decreases the incidence and severity of ventricular arrhythmias during exercise stress testing compared with beta-selective beta-blockers in patients with catecholaminergic polymorphic ventricular tachycardia. *Heart Rhythm*. 2015;15:S1547-S5271.

152. Kannankeril PJ, Moore JP, Cerrone M, et al. Efficacy of flecainide in the treatment of catecholaminergic polymorphic ventricular tachycardia: a randomized clinical trial. *JAMA Cardiol*. 2017;2:759-766.

153. Roston TM, Jones K, Hawkins NM, et al. Implantable cardioverter-defibrillator use in catecholaminergic polymorphic ventricular tachycardia: a systematic review. *Heart Rhythm*. 2018;15:1791-1799.

154. van der Werf C, Lieve KV, Bos JM, et al. Implantable cardioverter-defibrillators in previously undiagnosed patients with catecholaminergic polymorphic ventricular tachycardia resuscitated from sudden cardiac arrest. *Eur Heart J*. 2019;40:2953-2961.

155. De Ferrari GM, Dusi V, Spazzolini C, et al. Clinical management of catecholaminergic polymorphic ventricular tachycardia: the role of left cardiac sympathetic denervation. *Circulation*. 2015;131:2185-2193.

156. Hosseini SM, Kim R, Udupa S, et al. Reappraisal of reported genes for sudden arrhythmic death: evidence-based evaluation of gene validity for Brugada syndrome. *Circulation*. 2018;138:1195-1205.

157. Bezzina CR, Barc J, Mizusawa Y, et al. Common variants at SCN5A-SCN10A and HEY2 are associated with Brugada syndrome, a rare disease with high risk of sudden cardiac death. *Nature Genet*. 2013;45:1044-1049.

158. Probst V, Allouis M, Sacher F, et al. Progressive cardiac conduction defect is the prevailing phenotype in carriers of a Brugada syndrome SCN5A mutation. *J Cardiovasc Electrophysiol*. 2006;17:270-275.

159. Juang JJ, Binda A, Lee SJ, et al. GSTM3 variant is a novel genetic modifier in Brugada syndrome, a disease with risk of sudden cardiac death. *EBioMedicine*. 2020;57:102843.

160. Wilde AA, Postema PG, Di Diego JM, et al. The pathophysiological mechanism underlying Brugada syndrome: depolarization versus repolarization. *J Mol Cell Cardiol*. 2010;49:543-553.

161. Zhang J, Sacher F, Hoffmayer K, et al. Cardiac electrophysiologic substrate underlying the ECG phenotype and electrogram abnormalities in Brugada syndrome patients. *Circulation*. 2015;131:1950–1959.

162. Veltmann C, Papavassiliu T, Konrad T, et al. Insights into the location of type I ECG in patients with Brugada syndrome: correlation of ECG and cardiovascular magnetic resonance imaging. *Heart Rhythm*. 2012;9:414-421.

163. Priori SG, Wilde AA, Horie M, et al. HRS/EHRA/APHRS expert consensus statement on the diagnosis and management of patients with inherited primary arrhythmia syndromes: document endorsed by HRS, EHRA, and APHRS in May 2013 and by ACCF, AHA, PACES, and AEPC in June 2013. *Heart Rhythm*. 2013;10:1932-1963.

164. Michowitz Y, Milman A, Andorin A, et al. Characterization and management of arrhythmic events in young patients with Brugada syndrome. *J Am Coll Cardiol*. 2019;73:1756-1765.

165. Mazzanti A, Ovics P, Shauer A, et al. Unexpected risk profile of a large pediatric population with Brugada syndrome. *J Am Coll Cardiol*. 2019;73:1868-1869.

166. Adler A, Rosso R, Chorin E, Havakuk O, Antzelevitch C, Viskin S. Risk stratification in Brugada syndrome: clinical characteristics, electrocardiographic parameters, and auxiliary testing. *Heart Rhythm*. 2016;13:299-310.

167. Rattanawong P, Kewcharoen J, Kanitsoraphan C, et al. The utility of drug challenge testing in Brugada syndrome: a systematic review and meta-analysis. *J Cardiovasc Electrophysiol*. 2020;31(9):2474-2483.

168. Hernandez-Ojeda J, Arbelo E, Jorda P, et al. The role of clinical assessment and electrophysiology study in Brugada syndrome patients with syncope. *Am Heart J*. 2020;220:213-223.

169. Priori SG, Gasparini M, Napolitano C, et al. Risk stratification in Brugada syndrome: results of the PRELUDE (PRogrammed ELectrical stimUlation preDictive valuE) registry. *J Am Coll Cardiol*. 2012;59:37-45.

170. Sroubek J, Probst V, Mazzanti A, et al. Programmed ventricular stimulation for risk stratification in the Brugada syndrome: a pooled analysis. *Circulation*. 2015;132:A10920.

171. Rattanawong P, Riangwiwat T, Prasitlumkum N, et al. Baseline fragmented QRS increases the risk of major arrhythmic events in Brugada syndrome: systematic review and meta-analysis. *Ann Noninvasive Electrocardiol*. 2018;23:e12507.

172. Morita H, Zipes DP, Fukushima-Kusano K, et al. Repolarization heterogeneity in the right ventricular outflow tract: correlation with ventricular arrhythmias in Brugada patients and in an in vitro canine Brugada model. *Heart Rhythm*. 2008;5:725-733.

173. Belhassen B, Rahkovich M, Michowitz Y, Glick A, Viskin S. Management of Brugada Syndrome: thirty-three-year experience using electrophysiologically guided therapy with class 1A antiarrhythmic drugs. *Circ Arrhythm Electrophysiol*. 2015;8:1393-1402.

174. Anguera I, Garcia-Alberola A, Dallaglio P, et al. Shock reduction with long-term quinidine in patients with Brugada syndrome and malignant ventricular arrhythmia episodes. *J Am Coll Cardiol*. 2016;67:1653-1654.

175. Nademanee K, Veerakul G, Chandanamattha P, et al. Prevention of ventricular fibrillation episodes in Brugada syndrome by catheter ablation over the anterior right ventricular outflow tract epicardium. *Circulation*. 2011;123:1270-1279.

176. Campuzano O, Sarquella-Brugada G, Cesar S, Arbelo E, Brugada J, Brugada R. Recent advances in short QT syndrome. *Front Cardiovasc Med*. 2018;5:149.

177. Mazzanti A, Kanthan A, Monteforte N, et al. Novel insight into the natural history of short QT syndrome. *J Am Coll Cardiol*. 2014;63:1300-1308.

178. Deo M, Ruan Y, Pandit SV, et al. KCNJ2 mutation in short QT syndrome 3 results in atrial fibrillation and ventricular proarrhythmia. *Proc Natl Acad Sci U S A*. 2013;110:4291-4296.

179. Mazzanti A, Underwood K, Nevelev D, Kofman S, Priori SG. The new kids on the block of arrhythmogenic disorders: short QT syndrome and early repolarization. *J Cardiovasc Electrophysiol*. 2017;28:1226-1236.

180. Gollob MH, Redpath CJ, Roberts JD. The short QT syndrome: proposed diagnostic criteria. *J Am Coll Cardiol*. 2011;57:802-812.

181. Mazzanti A, Maragna R, Vacanti G, et al. Hydroquinidine prevents life-threatening arrhythmic events in patients with short QT syndrome. *J Am Coll Cardiol*. 2017;70:3010-3015.

182. Antzelevitch C, Bernstein MJ, Feldman HN, Moe GK. Parasystole, reentry, and tachycardia: a canine preparation of cardiac arrhythmias occurring across inexcitable segments of tissue. *Circulation*. 1983;68:1101-1115.

183. Shimizu W, Antzelevitch C. Differential effects of beta-adrenergic agonists and antagonists in LQT1, LQT2 and LQT3 models of the long QT syndrome. *J Am Coll Cardiol*. 2000;35:778-786.

184. Shimizu W, Antzelevitch C. Sodium channel block with mexiletine is effective in reducing dispersion of repolarization and preventing torsade des pointes in LQT2 and LQT3 models of the long-QT syndrome. *Circulation*. 1997;96:2038-2047.

185. Bonometti C, Hwang C, Hough D, et al. Interaction between strong electrical stimulation and reentrant wavefronts in canine ventricular fibrillation. *Circ Res.* 1995;77:407-416.

186. Joung B, Tang L, Maruyama M, et al. Intracellular calcium dynamics and acceleration of sinus rhythm by beta-adrenergic stimulation. *Circulation.* 2009;119:788-796.

187. Zhou S, Jung BC, Tan AY, et al. Spontaneous stellate ganglion nerve activity and ventricular arrhythmia in a canine model of sudden death. *Heart Rhythm.* 2008;5:131-139.

188. Ogawa M, Zhou S, Tan AY, et al. Left stellate ganglion and vagal nerve activity and cardiac arrhythmias in ambulatory dogs with pacing-induced congestive heart failure. *J Am Coll Cardiol.* 2007;50:335-343.

189. Ogawa M, Morita N, Tang L, et al. Mechanisms of recurrent ventricular fibrillation in a rabbit model of pacing-induced heart failure. *Heart Rhythm.* 2009;6:784-792.

190. Lee MH, Qu Z, Fishbein GA, et al. Patterns of wave break during ventricular fibrillation in isolated swine right ventricle. *Am J Physiol Heart Circ Physiol.* 2001;281:H253-H265.

191. El-Sherif N. Reentry revisited. *Pacing and Cardiac Electrophysiology.* 1988;11:1358-1368.

192. Kim YH, Garfinkel A, Ikeda T, et al. Spatiotemporal complexity of ventricular fibrillation revealed by tissue mass reduction in isolated swine right ventricle. Further evidence for the quasiperiodic route to chaos hypothesis. *J Clin Invest.* 1997;100:2486-2500.

193. Weiss JN, Qu Z, Chen PS, et al. The dynamics of cardiac fibrillation. *Circulation.* 2005;112:1232-1240.

194. Wu TJ, Lin SF, Weiss JN, Ting CT, Chen PS. Two types of ventricular fibrillation in isolated rabbit hearts: importance of excitability and action potential duration restitution. *Circulation.* 2002;106:1859-1866.

195. Antzelevitch C, Rosen MR, Janse MJ, Wit AL. Electrotonus and reflection. In: *Cardiac Electrophysiology: A Textbook.* Mount Kisco, NY: Futura Publishing Company, Inc.; 1990:491-516.

196. Antzelevitch C. Clinical applications of new concepts of parasystole, reflection, and tachycardia. *Cardiol Clin.* 1983;1:39-50.

197. Wu TJ, Ong JJ, Hwang C, et al. Characteristics of wave fronts during ventricular fibrillation in human hearts with dilated cardiomyopathy: role of increased fibrosis in the generation of reentry. *J Am Coll Cardiol.* 1998;32:187-196.

198. Cao JM, Fishbein MC, Han JB, et al. Relationship between regional cardiac hyperinnervation and ventricular arrhythmia. *Circulation.* 2000;101:1960-1969.

199. Antzelevitch C, Yan GX. Ionic and cellular basis for arrhythmogenesis. In: GX Yan, PR Kowey, eds. *Management of Cardiac Arrhythmias.* 2nd. ed. New York, NY: Springer; 2011:41-64.

200. Fish JM, Antzelevitch C. Role of sodium and calcium channel block in unmasking the Brugada syndrome. *Heart Rhythm.* 2004;1:210-217.

Supraventricular Tachycardia: Atrial Tachycardia, Atrioventricular Nodal Reentry, and Wolff-Parkinson-White Syndrome

David Spragg and Hugh Calkins

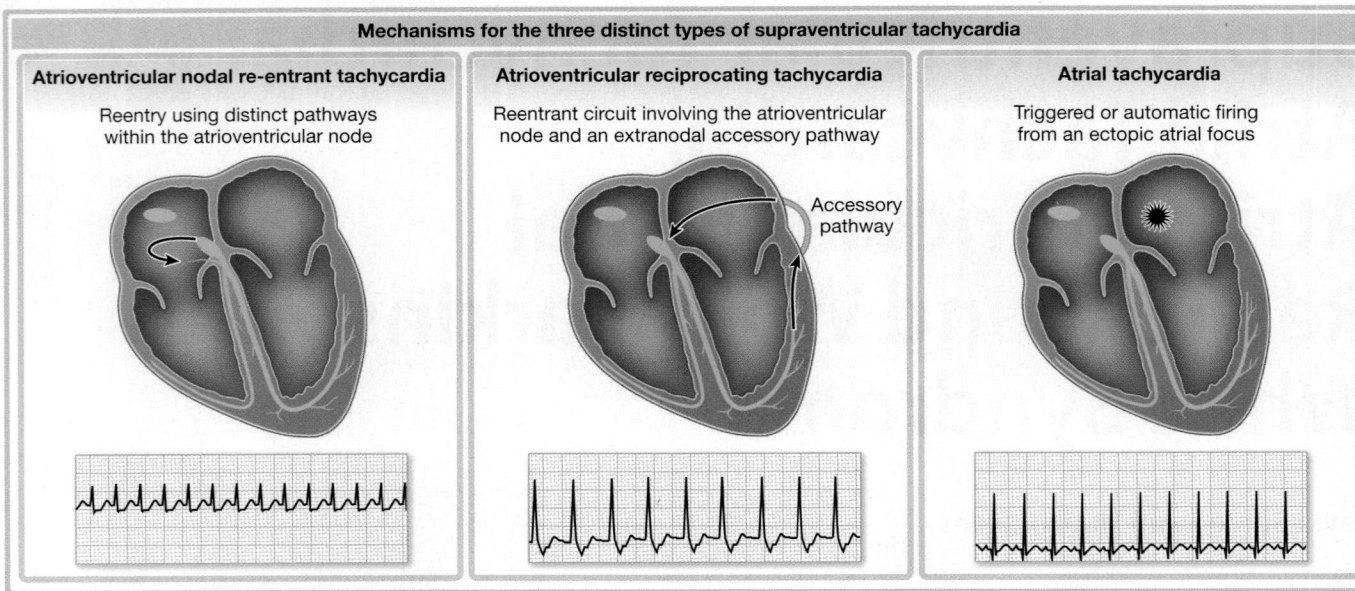

Chapter 35 Fuster and Hurst's Central Illustration. Shown are the three mechanisms for supraventricular tachycardias, including that for atrioventricular reentrant tachycardia (AVNRT), atrioventricular reciprocating tachycardia (AVRT), and atrial tachycardia (AT). AVNRT is due to reentry using distinct pathways within the atrioventricular node. Antegrade ventricular activation and retrograde atrial activation occur nearly simultaneously in typical AVNRT, such that P waves are often fused with the QRS complex on surface ECG (and may be indistinguishable). AVRT is due to a reentrant circuit involving the atrioventricular node and an extranodal accessory pathway. Antegrade ventricular and retrograde atrial activation happen in series, allowing for discernment of the P wave shortly after ventricular activation on surface ECG. AT is due to triggered or automatic firing from an ectopic atrial focus. AT is typically a "long RP" tachycardia, with atrial activation occurring well after the preceding QRS complex. Examples of typical ECG findings for AVNRT, AVRT, and AT are provided.

CHAPTER SUMMARY

This chapter discusses the mechanisms and treatment of supraventricular tachycardia (SVT), a term that encompasses three distinct arrhythmias: atrioventricular nodal reentrant tachycardia (AVNRT), atrioventricular reciprocating tachycardia (AVRT), and atrial tachycardia (AT). These arrhythmias, while not life threatening, can cause significant symptoms in afflicted patients including palpitations, dizziness, and syncope. AVNRT accounts for roughly two-thirds and AVRT for nearly one-third of SVT cases. AVNRT and AVRT are reentrant rhythms, while AT can be due to triggering or automaticity (see Fuster and Hurst's Central Illustration). The reentrant circuit for AVNRT includes pathways with distinct electrophysiological properties within the atrioventricular node, while the circuit for AVRT includes the atrioventricular node and an extranodal accessory pathway. Frequently, SVTs can be terminated acutely with vagal maneuvers. Long-term management options include chronic suppression with antiarrhythmic medications or definitive therapy with catheter ablation.

INTRODUCTION

Supraventricular tachycardias (SVTs) include all tachyarrhythmias that either originate from supraventricular tissue or that incorporate supraventricular tissue in a reentrant circuit. The ventricular rate may be the same or less than the atrial rate, depending on atrioventricular (AV) nodal conduction. The term *paroxysmal supraventricular tachycardia* (PSVT) refers to a clinical syndrome characterized by a rapid, regular tachycardia with an abrupt onset and termination. Approximately two-thirds of cases of PSVT result from AV nodal reentrant tachycardia (AVNRT). Orthodromic AV reentrant tachycardia (AVRT), which involves an accessory pathway (AP), is the second most common cause of PSVT, accounting for approximately one-third of cases. The term *Wolff-Parkinson-White* (WPW) *syndrome* designates a condition comprising both preexcitation and tachyarrhythmias. Atrial tachycardias, which arise exclusively from atrial tissue, account for approximately 5% of all cases of PSVT.[1] The purpose of this chapter is to review the mechanism, clinical features, and approach to diagnosis and treatment of patients with AVNRT and AP-mediated tachycardias (including WPW syndrome). Particular attention is focused on reviewing management guidelines developed by the American Heart Association (AHA), American College of Cardiology (ACC), European Society of Cardiology (ESC), and Heart Rhythm Society (HRS; formerly known as the North American Society of Pacing and Electrophysiology).[1,2] We will also provide a brief overview of atrial tachycardia.

ATRIOVENTRICULAR NODAL REENTRANT TACHYCARDIA

AVNRT is an important arrhythmia for several reasons. First, AVNRT is extremely common. The incidence of SVT is approximately 35 cases per 100,000 person-years, and the prevalence is 2.25 per 1000; AVNRT accounts for roughly two-thirds of these cases.[3] Although AVNRT can occur at any age, it is extremely uncommon before 5 years of age. The usual age of onset is beyond the fourth decade of life and is later than the usual age of onset of AP-mediated tachycardias. Women are affected twice as often as men. A second reason for the importance of AVNRT is the fact that it can result in significant debility and decreased quality of life.

Pathophysiologic Basis of Atrioventricular Nodal Reentrant Tachycardia

Anatomic Considerations of the Atrioventricular Node

The AV node is located subendocardially, anterior to the nodal artery and between the coronary sinus (CS) and medial tricuspid valve leaflet. It comprises three different components: the transitional cell zone, the compact node, and the penetrating bundle of His (**Figs. 35–1A and 35–1B**). The *compact* AV node

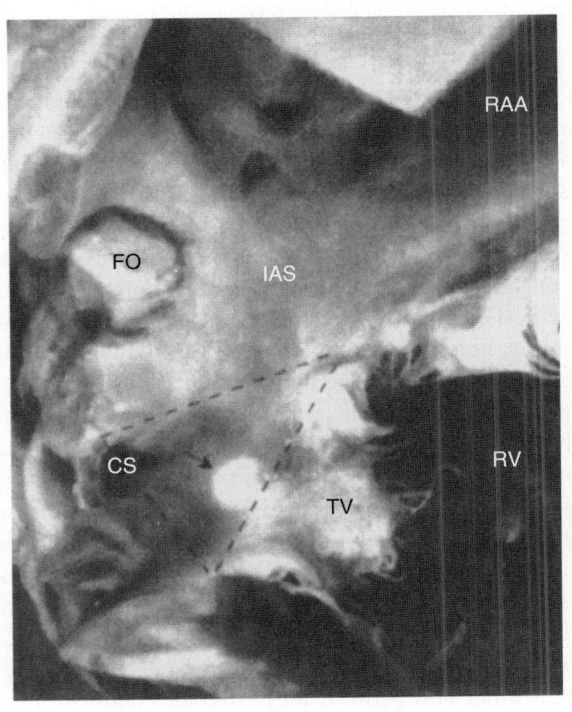

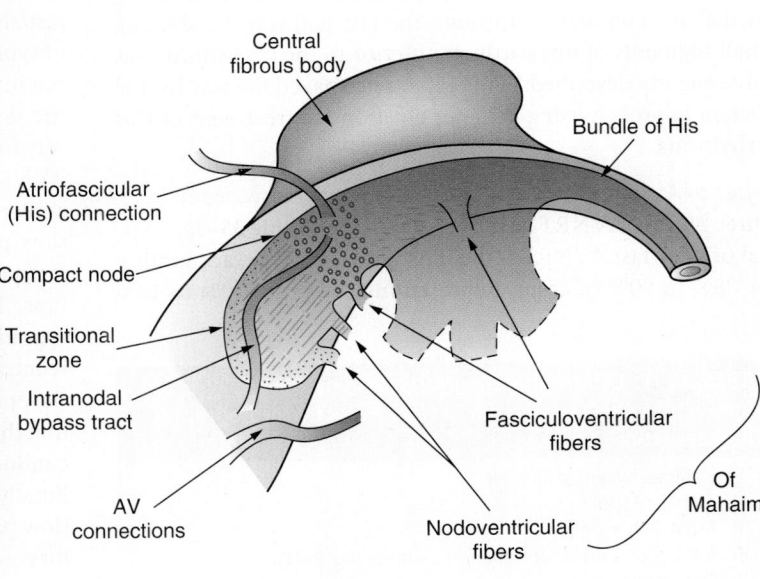

A   **B**

Figure 35–1. Structure of the atrioventricular (AV) node. **(A)** Heart specimen from patient with atrioventricular nodal reentrant tachycardia (AVNRT). The Koch triangle is formed by tendon of Todaro, coronary sinus (CS), ostium, and septal attachment of tricuspid valve (TV). *Arrow* represents site of successful ablation. **(B)** Schematic drawing depicting the three zones of the AV node and various types of perinodal and atrioventricular bypass tracts. FO, fossa ovalis; IAS, interatrial septum; RAA, right atrial appendage; RV, right ventricle. **(A)** Reproduced with permission from Olgin JE, Ursell P, Kao AK, et al. Pathological findings ollowing slow pathway ablation for AV nodal reentrant tachycardia. *J Cardiovasc Electrophysiol.* 1996 Jul;7(7):625-631; **(B)** Reproduced with permission from Singer I. *Interventional Electrophysiology*, 2nd ed. New York, NY: Lippincott Williams & Wilkins; 2001.

refers to the most easily histologically distinguishable tissue located at the apex of the triangle of Koch (TOK). A zone of transitional cells is interposed between the compact node and the atrial myocardium. Transitional cells enter the TOK to join the compact node superiorly, inferiorly, posteriorly, and from the left. At its distal extent, the AV node is distinguished from the penetrating bundle, not so much by cellular characteristics as by the presence of a fibrous collar surrounding the specialized cells. Systematic anatomic investigation of the AV node in patients with AVNRT is lacking. No obvious histologic abnormalities have been identified among patients with AVNRT versus patients without AVNRT. Several recent autopsy studies have reported that the sites of successful slow pathway ablation were clearly away from the histologic compact AV node, approximately 1 cm or 2 cm inferior and posterior to it.

Concept of Dual Pathways

The concept of dual AV nodal physiology was introduced in the 1950s in an effort to explain AVNRT. It was proposed that dual AV node physiology results from functional dissociation within the compact node into fast and slow pathways, with the fast pathway characterized by rapid conduction velocity and relatively prolonged refractoriness, and the slow pathway characterized by slower conduction velocity and more rapid repolarization. AVNRT was postulated to result from reentry within the AV node involving these two pathways. Subsequently, several investigators developed a catheter-based ablative technique that used direct current shocks or radiofrequency (RF) energy to target the fast AV pathway and permanently eliminate AVNRT. Despite the excellent results of this procedure, it was complicated by a small, but definite, risk of AV block. A technique to interrupt slow pathway conduction without affecting normal AV conduction through the fast pathway, by ablating small segments of myocardium anterior to the CS ostium, was subsequently described.[4] This experience paved the way for the current approach using catheter ablation for treatment of this arrhythmia.

Types of Atrioventricular Nodal Reentrant Tachycardia

Three types of AVNRT have been described (**Table 35–1**).[5] Typical or slow/fast AVNRT is the most prevalent type, accounting for 85% to 90% of cases. Representing the other 10% to 15%

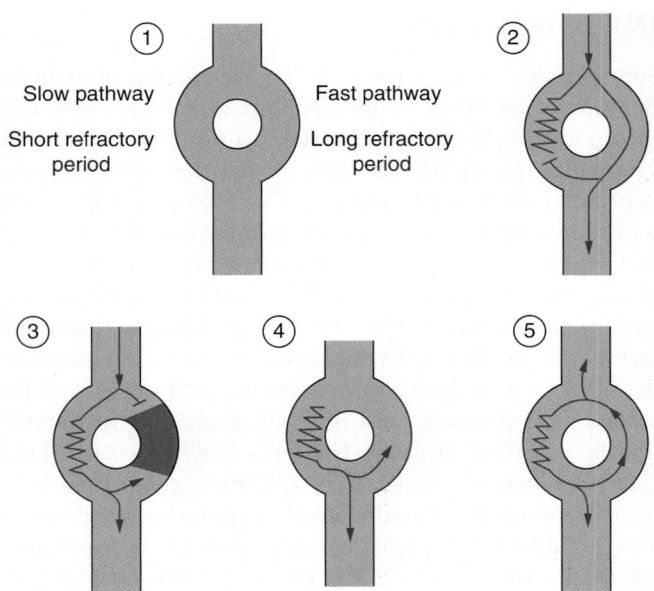

Figure 35–2. Schematic drawing showing dual atrioventricular (AV) nodal conduction. **1.** The two AV nodal pathways, one with fast conduction and a relatively long refractory period and a second with slower conduction and shorter refractory period. **2.** During sinus rhythm, impulses are conducted over both pathways but reach the bundle of His through the fast pathway. **3.** A premature atrial impulse finds the fast pathway still refractory and is conducted over the slow pathway. **4, 5.** If the fast pathway has enough time to recover excitability, the impulse may reenter the fast pathway retrogradely and establish reentry. Modified with permission from Podrid PJ, Kowey PR. *Cardiac Arrhythmia: Mechanisms, Diagnosis and Management*, 2nd ed. New York, NY: Lippincott Williams & Wilkins; 2001.

of cases, atypical AVNRT can be further differentiated into fast/slow and slow/slow (or intermediate) AVNRT. Induction of typical and atypical AVNRT in the same patient is possible, but unusual. The typical or slow/fast AVNRT is thought to use the slow pathway for antegrade conduction and the fast pathway for retrograde conduction (**Fig. 35–2**). Initiation of typical AVNRT may occur when an atrial premature complex blocks antegrade in the fast pathway but conducts (slowly) along the slow pathway; antegrade conduction is slow enough that the fast pathway has enough time to recover from its refractoriness. This allows the impulse to activate the fast pathway retrogradely and return to the atrium, giving rise to an AV nodal reentrant echo beat. The impulse then travels down along the slow pathway again, giving rise to AVNRT. It has been proposed that the fast/slow AVNRT uses the fast pathway for anterograde conduction and the slow pathway for retrograde conduction. Finally, slow/slow AVNRT requires presence of two or more slow pathways with different conduction properties and refractory periods; one slow pathway is used for antegrade conduction and the other slow pathway for retrograde conduction.

Diagnosis

Clinical Features

Patients with AVNRT typically present with the clinical syndrome of paroxysmal SVT. Episodes may last from seconds to several hours. Patients often learn to use certain maneuvers

---

TABLE 35–1. Differential Diagnosis for Types of Supraventricular Tachycardia Based on Electrocardiographic Characteristics

I. Long-RP tachycardia: RP ≥ PR
   i. Atypical AVNRT
   ii. Atrial tachycardia
   iii. AVRT with a slowly conducting pathway (eg, PJRT)
   iv. Sinus node reentry
   v. Sinus tachycardia
II. Short-RP tachycardia RP < PR
   i. Typical AVNRT
   ii. AV reentry

Abbreviations: AV, atrioventricular; AVRT, atrioventricular reciprocating tachycardia; AVNRT, atrioventricular nodal reentrant tachycardia; PJRT, permanent junctional reciprocating tachycardia.

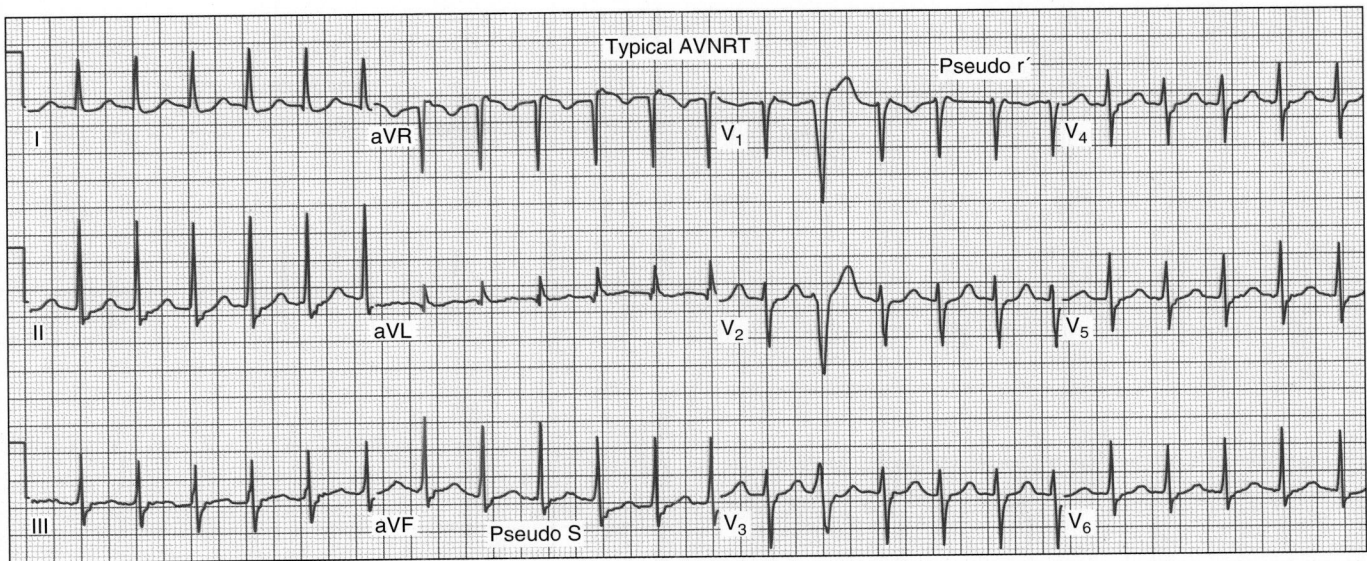

Figure 35–3. Twelve-lead electrocardiogram of a patient with typical atrioventricular nodal reentrant tachycardia (AVNRT). Note the pseudo r′ and pseudo S waves, which are very typical of this arrhythmia.

such as carotid sinus massage or the Valsalva maneuver to terminate the arrhythmia, but many patients require pharmacologic treatment to achieve this. There is no significant association of AVNRT with other types of structural heart disease. The physical examination is usually remarkable only for a rapid, regular heart rate. At times, because of the simultaneous contraction of atria and ventricles, cannon A-waves can be seen. Clinical variables that are predictive of AVNRT rather than AVRT as the cause of paroxysmal SVT include older age at onset of symptoms (>30 years), the presence of palpitations in the neck during tachycardia, and female gender.

Electrocardiographic Characteristics

AVNRT is characterized by a tachycardia with a narrow QRS complex with sudden onset and termination generally at regular rates between 120 bpm and 200 bpm. Uncommonly, the rate can be as low as 110 bpm; occasionally, especially in children, it may exceed 200 bpm. The rate of tachycardia may vary from episode to episode. In typical or slow/fast AVNRT, anterograde AV node conduction usually exceeds 200 ms. Because the retrograde conduction is through the fast pathway, the ventriculoatrial (VA) interval is short, resulting in superimposition of the P wave onto the QRS complex on the surface electrocardiogram (ECG). Usually, the P wave is obscured by the QRS or may be seen slightly before or after the QRS complex. The presence of a pseudo r′ wave in lead V_1 or pseudo S wave in leads II, III, and aVF suggests typical AVNRT (**Fig. 35–3**). Because of fast retrograde conduction, the RP interval is shorter than the PR interval.

In atypical fast/slow or slow/slow AVNRT, the atrial to His bundle (AH) interval is relatively short and the His bundle to atrial (HA) interval long. The P wave on surface ECG hence can be well delineated and is inverted in II, III, and aVF. The RP interval is equal to or longer than the PR interval (**Fig. 35–4**). This is one of the causes of *long R–P tachycardia* (see Table 35–1).

Functional bundle branch block (BBB) may develop during an episode of AVNRT, producing a wide QRS tachycardia. However, functional BBB should not affect the rate of tachycardia. Less commonly, dual pathways can be manifest on the ECG during sinus rhythm by sudden prolongation of the PR interval, PR alternans, and two QRS complexes in response to a single P wave (**Fig. 35–5**).

Other ECG changes may be seen during or after the termination of AVNRT. Significant ST-segment depressions can be observed during tachycardia in nearly 25% to 50% of patients with AVNRT, and this is not predictive of ischemia.

Newly acquired T-wave inversions after termination of AVNRT, commonly in anterior or inferior leads, can be seen in nearly 40% of patients. They may be seen immediately after termination of tachycardia or may develop within 6 hours, and they can persist for a variable duration. This occurrence is also not related to rate or duration of tachycardia. This is also not the result of coronary artery disease, but is caused by repolarization abnormalities, probably because of ionic current alterations resulting from the rapid rate.

A beat-to-beat oscillation in the QRS amplitude (ie, QRS alternans) can be observed, although uncommonly, during episodes of AVNRT. Studies have reported that QRS alternans is observed more frequently in association with AP-mediated tachycardias than during AVNRT.

Electrophysiologic Testing

Dual AV nodal physiology can be demonstrated by two pacing techniques. Atrial pacing with introduction of premature atrial contractions (PACs) with increasing prematurity shows a gradual and progressive conduction delay in the AH interval. At a critical atrial coupling interval, a 10-ms decrement in the A_1A_2 results in a marked (>50-ms) prolongation of the A_2H_2 interval, suggesting antegrade block in the fast pathway, but preserved and unmasked antegrade conduction in the slow pathway (with an attendant "jump" in AH interval). It is a well-accepted

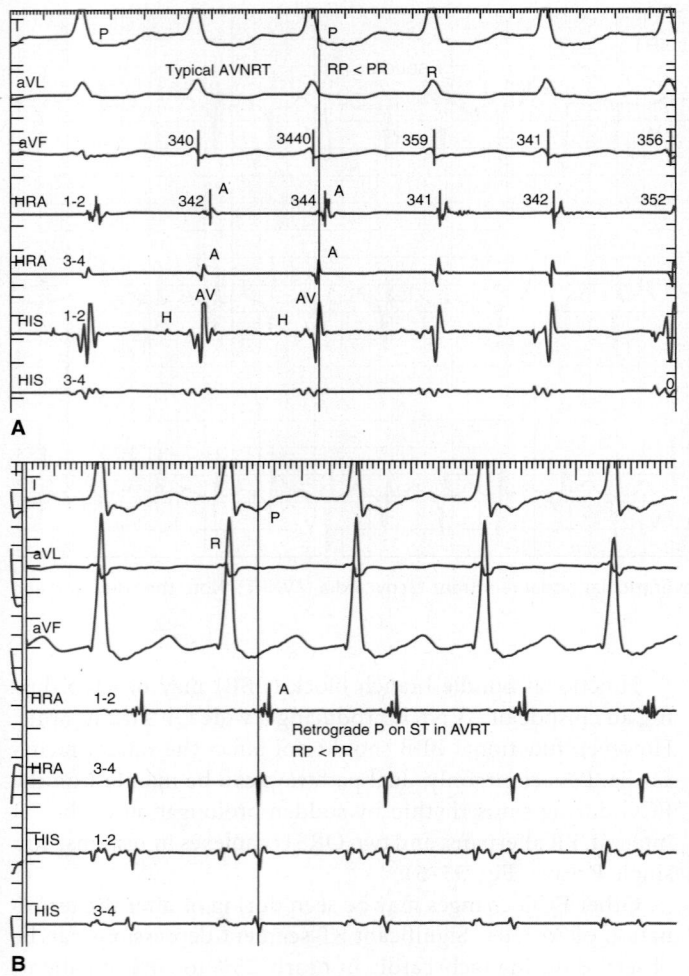

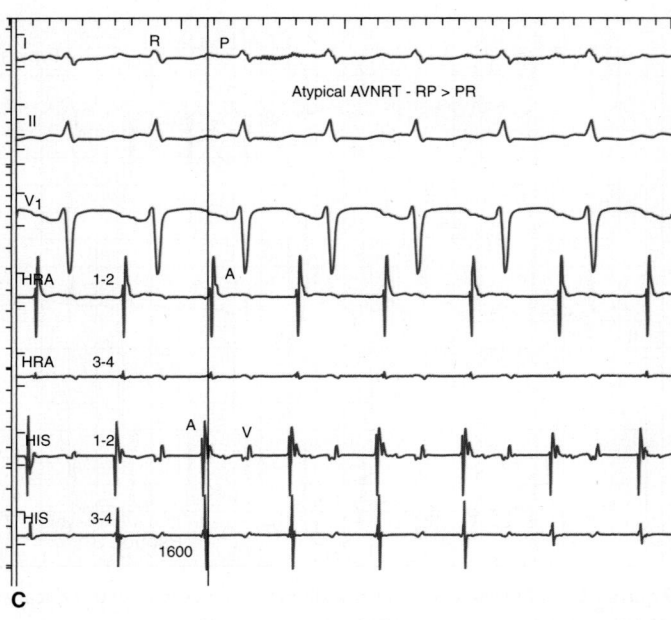

Figure 35–4. Surface electrocardiogram and intracardiac electrograms shown simultaneously in three different paroxysmal supraventricular tachycardias. The vertical line in each of the panels shows the onset of atrial depolarization to indicate the timing of the P wave relative to the QRS. (**A**) Typical atrioventricular nodal reentrant tachycardia (AVNRT). (**B**) Atrioventricular reciprocating tachycardia (AVRT) involving an accessory pathway. (**C**) Atypical AVNRT. *R* and *P* denote the corresponding waves on the surface ECG. A, atrial; HRA, high right atrium; V, ventricular deflection.

convention that a 50-ms or greater increase in the AH interval in response to a 10-ms shortening of the A_1A_2 is considered evidence of dual AV node physiology. A plot of the A_1A_2 versus the A_2H_2 or the A_2H_2 versus the H_1H_2 shows a discontinuous curve (**Fig. 35–6**). The fast pathway has a shorter conduction time and longer refractory period, and the slow pathway has a longer conduction time and shorter refractory period. The abrupt increase in AV nodal conduction time is caused by block in the conduction of fast pathway with a selective conduction over the slow pathway (**Fig. 35–7**). Some patients with AVNRT may not have discontinuous refractory period curves, and some

patients without AVNRT exhibit discontinuous refractory period curves. It has been estimated that *dual AV node physiology* is present in approximately 10% of the general population. Such existence in the latter patients is a benign finding. Multiple AV nodal pathways can be demonstrated in occasional patients. More than one pathway may be involved in clinical tachycardia. The development of a PR interval that is greater than the atrial pacing cycle length during stable 1:1 AV conduction is a quite specific sign of slow AV nodal conduction.

Whereas typical AVNRT is usually not inducible with ventricular pacing, this is the rule with atypical AVNRT. Lack of reproducible arrhythmia induction is most often caused by a block in retrograde fast pathway. Other causes include slow-pathway block and an inability to achieve a critical delay in the AH interval.

During typical AVNRT, the atrial and ventricular activation is nearly simultaneous, resulting in short HA intervals. An HA interval below 70 ms is virtually diagnostic of AVNRT (see Fig. 35–7). Differentiation of AVNRT, particularly of the atypical type, from other forms of SVT can be challenging, requiring the use of several maneuvers during the electrophysiologic study (EPS).

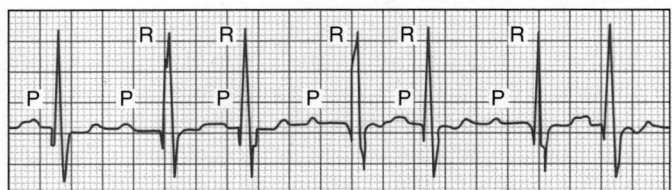

Figure 35–5. Rhythm strip of a patient during sinus rhythm. Note the sudden alternation of the PR interval from beat to beat. PR alternans is a manifestation of dual atrioventricular node physiology.

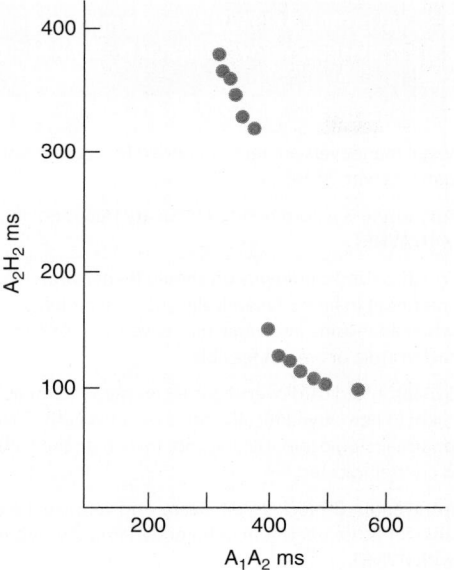

Figure 35-6. Atrioventricular (AV) nodal function curve in a patient with dual AV nodal physiology. As the coupling interval of A_1A_2 is progressively decreased, there is a progressive prolongation of A_2H_2 intervals. At a coupling interval of around 360 ms, there is a large jump in the A_2H_2 interval. This is caused by the fast pathway effectively reaching refractoriness at 360 ms and conduction proceeding over the slow pathway, which has a shorter refractory period but slower conduction. Modified with permission from Josephson M. *Clinical Cardiac Electrophysiology: Technique and Interpretation*, 3rd ed. New York, NY: Lippincott Williams & Wilkins; 2002.

Management

Because AVNRT is generally a benign arrhythmia that does not influence survival, the main reason for treating it is to alleviate symptoms. The threshold for initiation of therapy varies based on patient preference and on the frequency and duration of the episodes of tachycardia as well as the associated symptoms. The threshold for treatment also reflects whether the patient is a competitive athlete, a woman considering pregnancy, or someone participating in high-risk activities such as scuba diving. The ACC/AHA/HRS and the ESC have recently published updated guidelines on the management of supraventricular arrhythmias. The recommendations made by these task forces are reviewed at the end of this section.[1,2]

Acute Management

The dependence of AVNRT on AV nodal conduction has important therapeutic implications. Because of the known influence of autonomic tone on AV nodal conduction, maneuvers that increase vagal tone, such as the Valsalva and Mueller maneuvers, gagging, carotid sinus massage, and occasionally exposing the face to ice water, can be used to terminate the tachycardia. The effect of vagal maneuvers is most pronounced on the slow pathway. Hence, in the slow/fast form of AVNRT, the tachycardia typically terminates in the anterograde direction; in the fast/slow type of AVNRT, the block is in the retrograde limb of the tachycardia circuit.

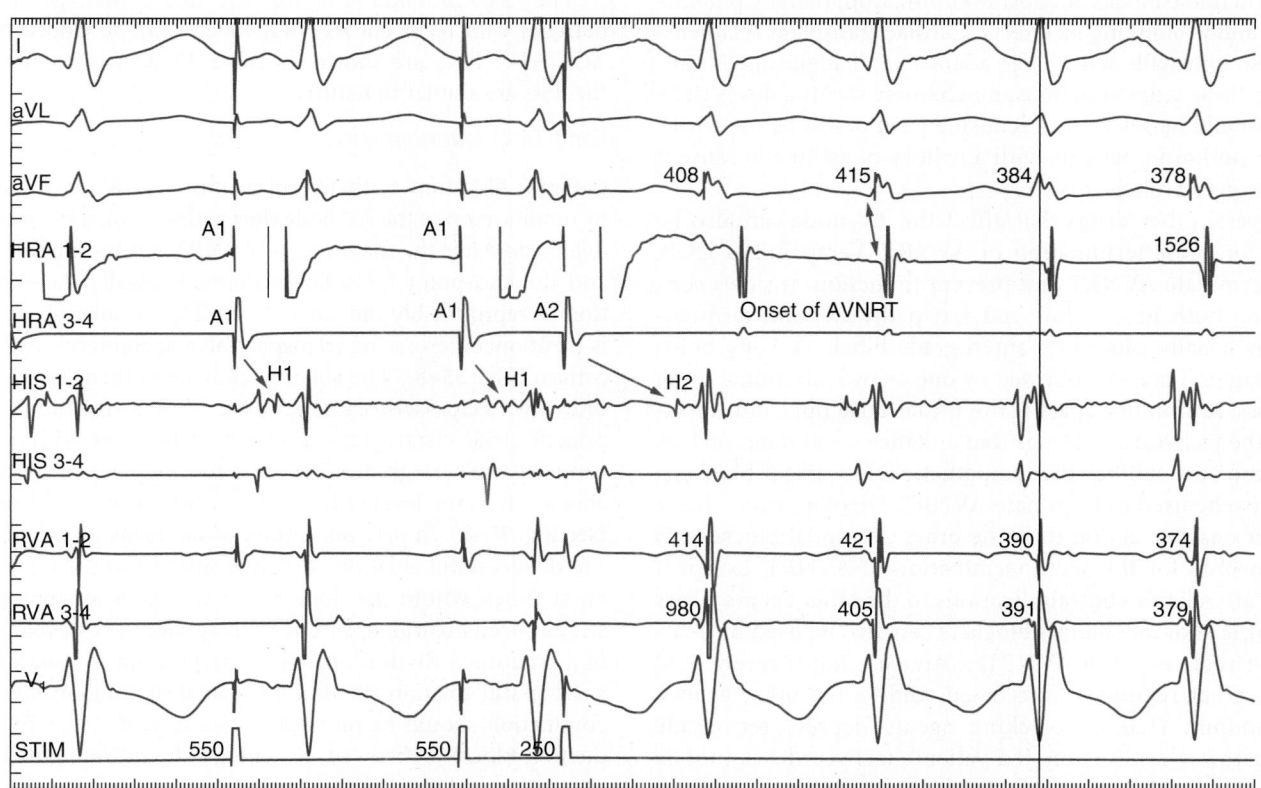

Figure 35-7. Electrophysiologic demonstration of dual atrioventricular nodal physiology and initiation of atrioventricular nodal reentrant tachycardia (AVNRT). At an A_1A_2 coupling interval of 350 ms, there is a jump in the A_2H_2 interval (*arrows*). This is followed by initiation of tachycardia. Note the very short VA conduction time. A, atrial; HRA, high right atrium; RVA, right ventricular apex.

Adenosine, a purinergic blocking agent that causes acute and transient AV nodal blockade, is the drug of choice for acute termination of AVNRT. Adenosine is nearly 100% effective in terminating AVNRT. It has a rapid onset of action (seconds) and a short half-life (<10 seconds); moreover, it does not impair contractility. When used for termination of a narrow-complex tachycardia, an initial dose of 6 mg may be followed by 12 mg if the first dose is ineffective. Because of its short duration of action, it is essential that adenosine be administered as a rapid bolus. This is best achieved by having a syringe with adenosine and a 5-mL flush attached to the patient using a stopcock. In this fashion, the dose of adenosine can be followed immediately by a saline flush to ensure rapid delivery of the drug. Minor side effects, including transient dyspnea or chest pain, are common with adenosine. Sinus arrest or bradycardia may occur but resolve quickly if appropriate upward dosing is used. Adenosine shortens the atrial refractory period, and atrial ectopy may induce atrial fibrillation. This may be dangerous if the patient has an AP capable of rapid antegrade conduction. Because adenosine is cleared so rapidly, reinitiation of tachycardia after initial termination may occur. Either repeat administration of the same dose of adenosine or substitution of a calcium channel blocker (CCB) will often be effective. Adenosine mediates its effects via a specific cell-surface receptor, the A_1 receptor. Theophylline and other methylxanthines block the A_1 receptor. Caffeine levels achieved after beverage ingestion may be overcome by increased doses of adenosine to treat patients with PSVT. Dipyridamole blocks adenosine elimination, thereby potentiating and prolonging its effects. Cardiac transplant recipients are also unusually sensitive to adenosine. If adenosine is chosen in these latter situations, much lower starting doses (ie, 1 mg) should be selected. Adenosine should also be used with great caution in patients with a history of asthma because it may trigger bronchospasm.

Several other drugs that affect the AV node can also be used for acute termination of AVNRT. Verapamil, a CCB, can terminate AVNRT and prevent induction. It slows conduction both in the slow and fast pathways, and termination is usually caused by anterograde block. A 5-mg bolus of verapamil may be followed by one or two additional 5-mg boluses 10 minutes apart if the initial dose does not terminate the tachycardia. Drugs that enhance vagal tone, such as digoxin, or that block the sympathetic effect, like β-blockers, can also be used to terminate AVNRT. Digoxin, which has a slower onset of action than the other AV nodal blockers, is not favored for the acute termination of AVNRT, except if there are relative contraindications to the other agents. Class Ia and Ic sodium channel blockers can also be used in treating an acute event of AVNRT, a strategy that is rarely used when other regimens have failed. Unlike the other agents, the sodium channel blocking agents depress retrograde fast-pathway conduction. If a patient's tachycardia cannot be terminated with intravenous drugs, direct-current shock cardioversion can always be used. Energies in the range of 10 J to 50 J are usually adequate.

TABLE 35–2. AHA/ACC/HRS 2015 Recommendations for the Acute Treatment of Atrioventricular Nodal Reentrant Tachycardia[1]

Class	
I	Vagal maneuvers are recommended for acute treatment in patients with AVNRT.
I	Adenosine is recommended for acute treatment in patients with AVNRT.
I	Synchronized cardioversion should be performed for acute treatment in hemodynamically unstable patients with AVNRT when adenosine and vagal maneuvers do not terminate the tachycardia or are not feasible.
I	Synchronized cardioversion is recommended for acute treatment in hemodynamically stable patients with AVNRT when pharmacologic therapy does not terminate the tachycardia or is contraindicated.
IIa	Intravenous β-blockers, diltiazem, and verapamil are reasonable for acute treatment in hemodynamically stable patients with AVNRT.
IIb	Oral β-blockers, diltiazem, or verapamil may be reasonable for acute treatment in hemodynamically stable patients with AVNRT.
IIb	Intravenous amiodarone may be considered for acute treatment in hemodynamically stable patients with AVNRT when other therapies are ineffective or contraindicated.

Abbreviation: AVNRT, atrioventricular nodal reentrant tachycardia.

The recommendations for the acute management of patients with recurrent AVNRT, which were developed by the ACC/AHA/HRS, are shown in **Table 35–2**.[1] Guidelines from the ESC are similar in nature.[2]

Long-Term Management

Catheter Ablation: Catheter ablation of AVNRT is performed by modification of the AV node slow pathway using the *posterior approach*. After the diagnosis of AVNRT has been established and the end point for ablation defined (ideally the elimination of reproducibly inducible AVNRT), the ablation catheter is positioned across the tricuspid valve at the level of the CS ostium (**Fig. 35–8**). The ablation catheter is then slowly withdrawn with clockwise catheter torque until a small multicomponent atrial electrogram is observed together with a large ventricular electrogram.[5] The most common site of successful ablation is at the level of the superior aspect of the CS ostium (see Fig. 35–8). In patients with unusual forms of AVNRT, the site of successful ablation is slightly inferior to the CS ostium or, at times, within the floor of the CS. After an appropriate site has been identified, RF energy is applied. The development of a junctional rhythm during RF application is a marker for a successful ablation site. If a junctional rhythm develops, VA conduction should be monitored carefully; if VA or AV conduction block is observed, RF energy should immediately be discontinued. Some centers, including ours, use an even more conservative strategy for RF energy delivery in an effort to further reduce the risk of AV block.[6]

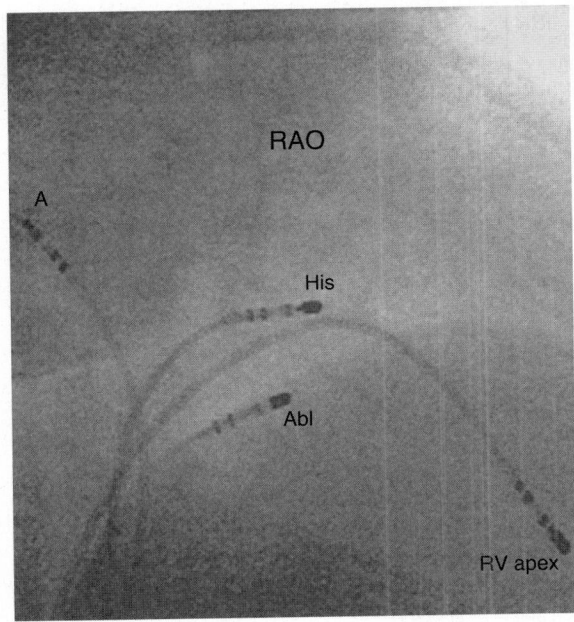

A

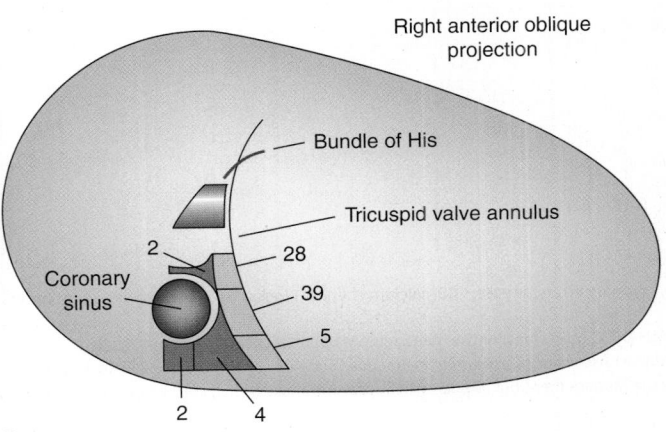

Right anterior oblique
projection

Bundle of His

Tricuspid valve annulus

Coronary
sinus

2   28
39
5
2   4

B

Figure 35–8. Site of slow-pathway ablation for atrioventricular nodal reentrant tachycardia. (**A**) Accessory pathway and left lateral fluoroscopic images showing the alignment of the catheters during slow-pathway ablation. Note that the site of the slow pathway is a considerable distance from the site of the His bundle or compact atrioventricular node. (**B**) Schematic showing the orientation of heart during corresponding fluoroscopic projection. The numbers represent the sites of successful slow-pathway ablation in corresponding patients. A, atrial catheter; Abl, ablation catheter; RAO, right anterior oblique; RV, right ventricle. (**A**) Modified with permission from Meininger GR, Calkins H. One method to reduce heart block risk during catheter ablation of atrioventricular nodal reentrant tachycardia. *J Cardiovasc Electrophysiol.* 2004 Jun;15(6):727-728.

Successful ablation of AVNRT with the posterior approach is usually characterized by an increase in the AV block cycle length and in the AV nodal effective refractory period; a normal PR interval on ECG and lack of inducibility of AVNRT, both at baseline and during isoproterenol infusion, are also seen. Retrograde conduction is generally not affected. The presence of more than one AV nodal echo beat or a PR prolongation that exceeds the paced atrial cycle length during stable

1:1 AV conduction suggests that the AVNRT is likely to recur and will require further RF applications.

Calkins and colleagues[7] reported the largest multicenter experience with the posterior approach. In this trial of more than 1000 patients with AV tachycardias, 373 patients had AVNRT. The overall success rate of ablation was 97%. AV block was the most common complication, occurring in 0.5% to 1% of patients. The incidence of recurrence after successful ablation was approximately 3%. Because of the higher efficacy and lower incidence of AV block and arrhythmia recurrence, and the greater likelihood of maintaining a normal PR interval during sinus rhythm, the posterior approach is now considered the preferred approach to ablation of AVNRT.[6]

Cryoablation has become available as an alternative energy source for creation of myocardial lesions that can be used for treatment of AVNRT.[8] The main advantage of cryoenergy as compared with RF energy is that the risk of heart block appears to be lower.[9-12] This potential, but unproven, benefit must be balanced against longer procedure times and lower acute and long-term efficacy. Because of the implications of heart block in children, cryoablation is used by an increasing number of pediatric electrophysiologists.[10] In contrast, RF energy has remained the dominant ablation energy source for treatment of AVNRT in adults.

Medical Therapy: Most pharmacologic agents that depress AV nodal conduction may be demonstrated to reduce the frequency of recurrences of AVNRT. These pharmacologic agents include β-blockers, CCBs, class Ia antiarrhythmic agents such as procainamide and disopyramide, class Ic antiarrhythmic agents such as flecainide and propafenone, and class III antiarrhythmic agents such as sotalol and amiodarone. The best studied among these have been the class Ic antiarrhythmic agents. Although the 1c antiarrhythmic agents are effective for treatment of AVNRT, they are used rarely because of the curative nature of catheter ablation.

Management Strategy

Patients with AVNRT typically present with the clinical syndrome of PSVT. The diagnosis of PSVT can be made with a high degree of certainty based on the clinical history alone, even if the tachycardia has never been documented by an ECG. Physicians may try to document the tachycardia with an ECG using either a 30-day event monitor or by instructing the patient to go to an emergency department or physician's office if another episode of tachycardia occurs. Because AVNRT is not a life-threatening arrhythmia, the primary indication for its treatment relates to its impact on the patient's quality of life. Patients who develop a highly symptomatic episode of PSVT, particularly if it requires an emergency room visit for termination, may elect to initiate therapy after a single episode. By contrast, a patient who presents with minimally symptomatic episodes of PSVT that terminate spontaneously or with a Valsalva maneuver may elect to be followed clinically without specific therapy.

After it has been decided to initiate treatment for AVNRT, the question arises of whether to initiate pharmacologic therapy

TABLE 35–3. Recommendations for Long-Term Management of Patients with Recurrent Atrioventricular Nodal Reentrant Tachycardia

Clinical Presentation	Recommendation	Classification	Level of Evidence
Poorly tolerated AVNRT with hemodynamic intolerance	Catheter ablation	I	B
	Verapamil, diltiazem, β-blockers	IIa	C
	Sotalol, amiodarone	IIa	C
	Flecainide, propafenone	IIa	C
Recurrent symptomatic AVNRT	Catheter ablation	I	B
	Verapamil	I	B
	Diltiazem, β-blockers	I	C
	Digoxin	IIb	C
	Verapamil, diltiazem, digoxin	III	C
Recurrent AVNRT unresponsive to β-blockade or CCB and patients not desiring RF ablation	Flecainide, propafenone, sotalol	IIa	B
	Amiodarone	IIb	C
AVNRT with infrequent or a single episode in patients desiring complete control of arrhythmia	Catheter ablation	I	B
Documented PSVT with only dual AV-nodal pathways or single echo beats demonstrated during EPS and no identified cause of arrhythmia	Verapamil, diltiazem, β-blockers	I	C
	Flecainide, propafenone	I	C
	Catheter ablation	I	B
Infrequent, well-tolerated AVNRT	No therapy	I	C
	Vagal maneuvers	I	B
	Pill in the pocket	I	B
	Verapamil, diltiazem, β-blockers	I	B
	Catheter ablation	I	B

Abbreviations: AV, atrioventricular; AVNRT, atrioventricular nodal reentrant tachycardia; CAD, coronary artery disease; CCB, calcium channel blocker; EPS, electrophysiology study; RF, radiofrequency; LV, left ventricle; PSVT, paroxysmal supraventricular tachycardia.
Adapted with permission from Blomström-Lundqvist C, Scheinman MM, Aliot EM, et al: ACC/AHA/ESC guidelines for the management of patients with supraventricular arrhythmias—executive summary: a report of the American College of Cardiology/American Heart Association Task Force on Practice Guidelines and the European Society of Cardiology Committee for Practice Guidelines (Writing Committee to Develop Guidelines for the Management of Patients With Supraventricular Arrhythmias). *Circulation*. 2003 Oct 14;108(15):1871-1890.

or to use catheter ablation (**Table 35–3**). Because of its greater than 95% efficacy and low incidence of complications, catheter ablation is now considered first-line therapy. The ACC/AHA/HRS and ESC SVT Guidelines include catheter ablation of AVNRT using the posterior approach as a class I indication for catheter ablation.[1,2] It is therefore reasonable to discuss catheter ablation with all patients suspected of having AVNRT. Depending on the frequency and severity of tachycardia episodes as well as the patient's lifestyle and preferences, an individual may elect to be followed clinically without specific therapy, to begin a trial of pharmacologic therapy with a β-blocker or CCB, or to undergo EPS and catheter ablation.

The recommendations for the long-term management of patients with recurrent AVNRT, which were developed by the ACC/AHA/HRS, are shown in **Table 35–4**.[1] Catheter ablation is considered class I therapy for treatment of patients with symptomatic AVNRT. The indications for pharmacologic management are also provided.

ATRIOVENTRICULAR REENTRANT TACHYCARDIA AND WOLFF-PARKINSON-WHITE SYNDROME

APs are important because they provide a substrate for antidromic and orthodromic AV reciprocating tachycardia, are associated with sudden cardiac death, and may be detected in asymptomatic patients on a routine screening ECG. The sections that follow cover the pathophysiology, diagnosis, and management of this fascinating clinical entity.

Pathophysiology

APs are anomalous, typically extranodal connections that connect the atrium and ventricle along the AV groove. Accessory bypass tracts, which conduct antegrade from the atrium to the ventricle and, therefore, are detectable on an ECG, are reportedly present in 0.15% to 0.25% of the general population. A higher

TABLE 35-4. AHA/ACC/HRS 2015 Recommendations for Ongoing Management of Atrioventricular Nodal Reentrant Tachycardia[1]

Class	
I	Oral verapamil or diltiazem is recommended for ongoing management in patients with AVNRT who are not candidates for, or prefer not to undergo, catheter ablation.
I	Catheter ablation of the slow pathway is recommended in patients with AVNRT.
I	Oral β-blockers are recommended for ongoing management of AVNRT patients who are not candidates for, or prefer not to undergo, catheter ablation.
IIa	Flecainide or propafenone is reasonable for ongoing management in patients without structural heart disease or ischemic heart disease who have AVNRT and are not candidates for, or prefer not to undergo, catheter ablation and in whom β-blockers, diltiazem, and verapamil are ineffective or contraindicated.
IIa	Clinical follow-up without pharmacologic therapy or ablation is reasonable for ongoing management of minimally symptomatic patients with AVNRT.
IIb	Oral sotolol or dofetiline may be reasonable for ongoing management in patients with AVNRT who are not candidates for, or prefer not to undergo, catheter ablation.
IIb	Oral digoxin or amiodarone may be reasonable for ongoing treatment of AVNRT in patients who are not candidates for, or prefer not to undergo, catheter ablation.
IIb	Self-administered ("pill-in-the-pocket") acute doses of oral β-blockers, diltiazem, or verapamil may be reasonable for ongoing management in patients with infrequent, well-tolerated episodes of AVNRT.

Abbreviations: ACC, American College of Cardiology; AHA, American Heart Association; AVNRT, atrioventricular nodal reentrant tachycardia; HRS, Heart Rhythm Society.

prevalence of 0.55% has been reported in first-degree relatives of patients with WPW syndrome.

Classification

APs can be classified based on their site of origin and insertion, location along the mitral or tricuspid annulus, type of conduction, and properties of conduction (decremental or nondecremental). APs usually exhibit rapid, nondecremental conduction, similar to that which is present in normal His-Purkinje tissue or atrial and ventricular myocardium. Approximately 8% of APs display decremental antegrade or retrograde conduction. Whereas APs that are capable only of retrograde conduction are referred to as *concealed*, those capable of antegrade conduction are referred to as *manifest*, demonstrating preexcitation on a standard ECG (**Fig. 35–9**). Concealed APs account for approximately 15% of all APs. APs capable of antegrade conduction usually also can conduct retrogradely. Antegrade-only APs are particularly uncommon. When present, they are usually right sided and frequently demonstrate

δ+ Manifest   Concealed

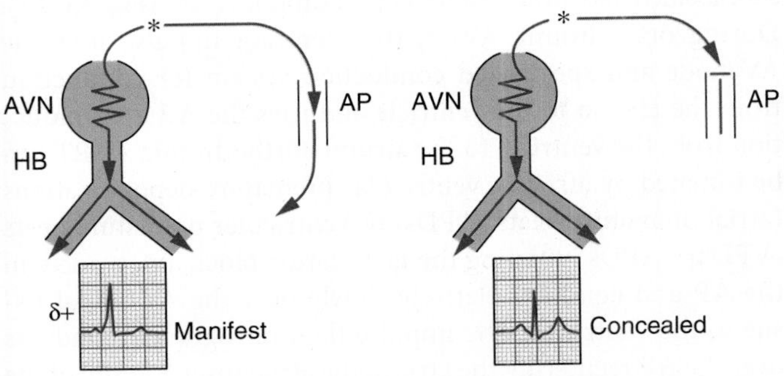

Figure 35–9. Atrioventricular conduction patterns and QRS morphologies during sinus rhythm for manifest and concealed accessory pathways (APs). AVN, atrioventricular node; HB, His bundle. Modified with permission from Cain ME, Luke RA, Lindsay BD. Diagnosis and localization of accessory pathway. *Pacing Clin Electrophysiol*. 1992 May;15(5):801-824.

decremental conduction between the atrium and the distal right bundle of the His-Purkinje system. Some patients exhibit retrograde-only conducting pathways that exhibit decremental conduction and sensitivity to nodal agents including CCBs and adenosine. These pathways are typically located in the posterosptal region and mediate a long-RP form of AVRT (sometimes referred to by the misnomer "permanent junctional reciprocating tachycardia [PJRT]"). Patients with Ebstein anomaly who also have WPW syndrome frequently have more than one AP.

Variant APs include those that connect the atrium to the distal or compact AV node (James fibers), the atrium to the His bundle (the Brechenmacher fiber), and the AV node or His bundle to the distal Purkinje fibers or ventricular myocardium (the Mahaim fibers) (see Fig. 35–1B).

Concept of Preexcitation

The hallmark of antegrade AP conduction during sinus rhythm is depolarization of all or part of the ventricles earlier than expected if conduction had occurred only over the normal AV conduction system, resulting in ventricular preexcitation (**Fig. 35–10**).

The degree of shortening of the PR interval and the extent of ventricular preexcitation depends on several factors, including location of the AP, the relationship between antegrade conduction times and refractory periods of the AV bypass tract, and the normal AV conduction system. A bypass tract that crosses the AV groove in the left lateral region may also result in inapparent preexcitation and minimal PR interval shortening during sinus rhythm because of greater interatrial distance for impulse propagation from the sinus node to this site of atrial input into the AP. Conversely, an AP on the right side is more likely to demonstrate marked preexcitation. Preexcitation may be less apparent during sinus tachycardia, when sympathetic tone is high and vagal tone low, resulting in relatively faster AV node

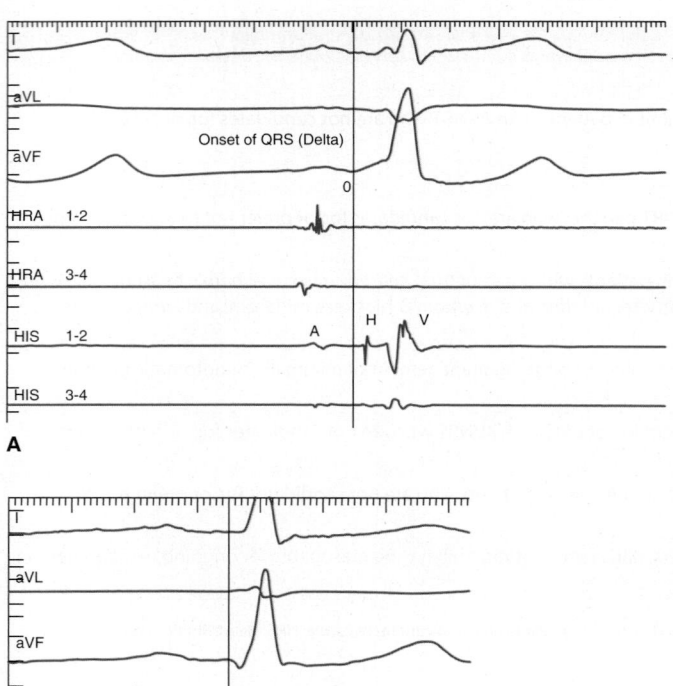

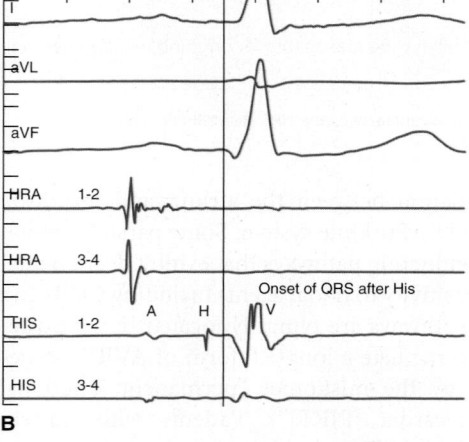

Figure 35–10. Electrophysiologic confirmation of preexcitation. **(A)** Pre-excited QRS complex in Wolff-Parkinson-White syndrome. Onset of QRS or delta wave is clearly before the His electrogram before ablation. **(B)** Loss of preexcitation and shift of onset of QRS after His deflection postablation. A, atrial electrogram; H, His electrogram; HRA, high right atrium; HIS, His bundle electrogram; V, ventricular electrogram.

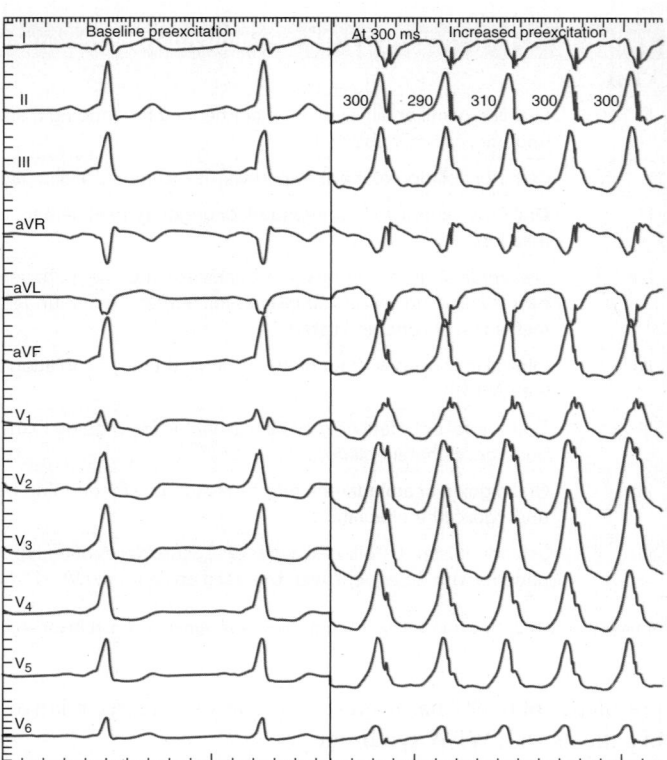

Figure 35–11. Increase in degree of preexcitation with atrial pacing. Left panel shows 12-lead electrocardiogram during sinus rhythm. Note the obvious increase in preexcitation in the right panel with atrial pacing at a cycle length of 300 ms (200 bpm). Increase in atrial input causes decremental conduction in the atrioventricular node, resulting in increased conduction over the accessory pathway.

conduction time. On the other extreme, during conditions of slowed conduction through the AV node by intrinsic nodal factors, withdrawal of sympathetic tone, or increased vagal tone, the amount of preexcitation apparent on the 12-lead ECG is maximized because of relatively greater contribution through the AP. Rapid intravenous administration of adenosine causing blocking or slowing of AV node conduction and exposing the anterograde AP conduction has been used as a diagnostic maneuver. The degree of preexcitation can also be enhanced with atrial pacing directly over the AP, eliminating the intra-atrial conduction delay from the sinus node to the atrial insertion site of AP (**Fig. 35–11**).

Intermittent preexcitation is characterized by abrupt loss of delta wave, normalization of the QRS duration, and an increase in the PR interval during a continuous ECG recording, often despite only minor variations in resting sinus rhythm heart rate. This should be distinguished from day-to-day variability in preexcitation or inapparent preexcitation caused by factors described above. The presence of intermittent preexcitation

has been considered to suggest that the refractory period in the AP is long, making them very unlikely to mediate a rapid, pre-excited ventricular response during atrial fibrillation.

Tachycardias Associated with Accessory Pathways

Tachycardias associated with APs can be subdivided into those in which the AP is necessary for initiation and maintenance of tachycardia and those in which the AP acts as a bystander.

AVRT is a macro-reentrant tachycardia involving the atrium, the AP, the AV node, and the ventricle. AVRT is further subclassified into orthodromic and antidromic AVRT (**Fig. 35–12**). During orthodromic AVRT, the reentrant impulse uses the AV node and specialized conduction system for conduction from the atrium to the ventricle and uses the AP for conduction from the ventricle to the atrium. Orthodromic AVRT can be initiated by atrial or ventricular premature depolarizations (atrial premature beats [APDs] or ventricular premature beats [VPDs]). APDs initiating the tachycardia block antegradely in the AP and conduct relatively slowly over the AV nodal tissue to the ventricles. The impulse then retrogradely conducts over the AP reentering the atria at the atrial insertion site of the pathway, thus completing the reentrant loop (**Fig. 35–13**). A VPD, conversely, blocks in the His-Purkinje system and retrogradely reaches the atria through retrogradely conducting AP. The impulse then antegradely conducts through the AV nodal

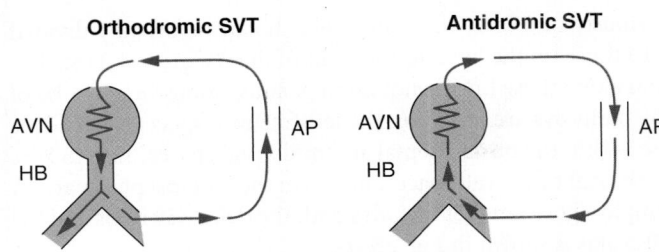

Figure 35–12. Schematic representation of the patterns of conduction through an accessory pathway (AP) and the normal conduction system during orthodromic atrioventricular reentrant tachycardia (AVRT) and antidromic AVRT. AVN, atrioventricular node; HB, His bundle; SVT, supraventricular tachycardia. Modified with permission from Cain ME, Luke RA, Lindsay BD. Diagnosis and localization of accessory pathway. *Pacing Clin Electrophysiol.* 1992 May;15(5):801-824.

tissue, completing the circuit. The QRS complex during orthodromic AVRT hence is not preexcited.

During antidromic AVRT, however, the reentrant impulse travels in the reverse direction, with conduction from the atrium to the ventricle occurring via the AP. Antidromic AV reciprocating tachycardia is rare, occurring in only 5% to 10% of patients with WPW syndrome. APDs that occur at a coupling interval that is longer than the refractory period of the AP and shorter than the AV nodal refractory period can initiate the antidromic AVRT; the converse is true with a VPD. Susceptibility of antidromic AVRT appears to depend on the existence of adequate separation between the AP and the AV nodal tissue. Hence, most of the antidromic AVRTs seem to occur only with left-sided bypass tracts.

Other forms of SVTs, including atrial tachycardia, junctional tachycardia, AVNRT, and even ventricular tachycardia, may occur in patients with bypass tracts. Dual AV nodal physiology has been noted in nearly 12% of patients with WPW syndrome. Coexisting ventricular tachycardia is less likely because patients with WPW syndrome tend to present at a younger age and have less structural heart disease.

Atrial fibrillation is a less common than other types of SVTs, but potentially more serious, arrhythmia in patients with the WPW syndrome. If an AP has a short antegrade refractory period, atrial fibrillation may result in a rapid ventricular response with subsequent degeneration to ventricular fibrillation.[13-15] The risk of sudden death has been shown to be higher if the shortest R-R interval is less than 250 ms during spontaneous or induced atrial fibrillation.[13] It has been estimated that one-third of patients with WPW syndrome also have atrial fibrillation. APs appear to play a pathophysiologic role in the development of atrial fibrillation in these patients, because most are young and do not have structural heart disease. Furthermore, surgical or catheter ablation of APs usually results in elimination of atrial fibrillation as well.

Diagnosis

Clinical Features

Preexcitation occurs in the general population at a frequency of around 1.5 per 1000. Of these, 50% to 60% of patients become symptomatic. Approximately one-third of all patients with PSVT are diagnosed as having an AP-mediated tachycardia. Patients with AP-mediated tachycardias most commonly present with the syndrome of PSVT. Population-based studies have

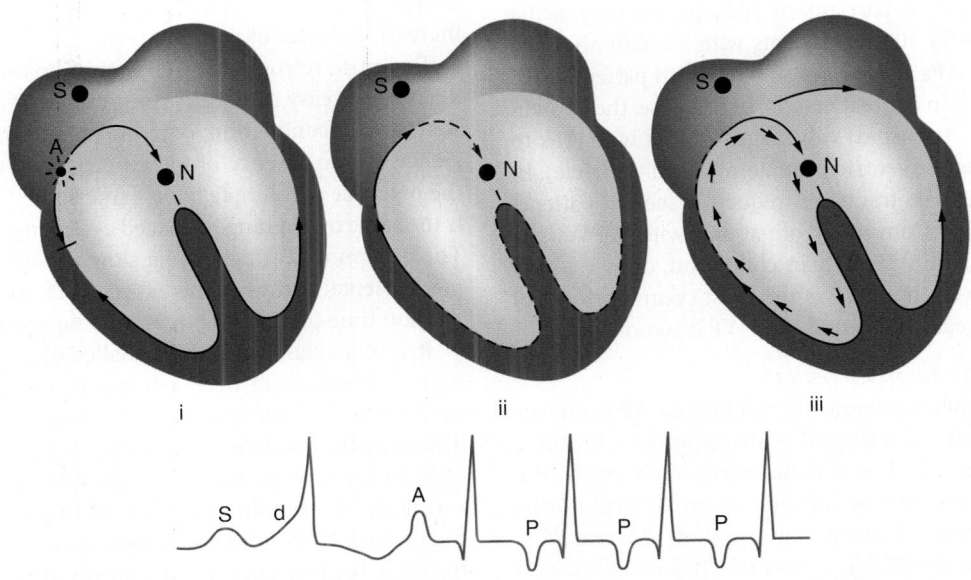

Figure 35–13. Schematic of initiation of orthodromic atrioventricular (AV) reentrant tachycardia (AVRT). A diagrammatic electrocardiograph recording shows the first P wave of sinus node (S) origin yielding a preexcited QRS complex with a delta wave (d) and short PR interval (I). An ectopic atrial impulse (A) blocks antegradely in the bypass tract, but still conducts over the AV node (N) and His-Purkinje system to the ventricles. This causes the second QRS complex to appear nonpreexcited (ii). The premature impulse continues to conduct retrogradely over the bypass tract because the latter had time to recover excitability while the impulse was conducting over the node (iii). The retrogradely conducted impulse has activated the atria from the bypass tracts' atrial insertion point and generated the first retrograde P wave (P) of AVRT. Reentrance of impulse through the node then occurs, causing AVRT to perpetuate. Modified with permission from Chung EK. Wolff-Parkinson-White syndrome: current views. *Am J Med.* 1977 Feb;62(2):252-266.

demonstrated a bimodal distribution of symptoms for patients with preexcitation, with a peak in early childhood followed by a second peak in young adulthood. Nearly 25% of patients will become asymptomatic over time. More than half the patients with an episode will experience a recurrence.

Symptoms range from palpitations to syncope. As in AVNRT, episodes of tachycardia may be associated with dyspnea, chest pain, decreased exercise tolerance, anxiety, dizziness, or syncope. Although syncope is often considered a bad prognostic sign, the evidence is not clear. Physical examination demonstrates a fast, regular pulse with a constant-intensity first heart sound. The jugular venous pressure waveform is usually constant, but it can sometimes be elevated. The incidence of sudden cardiac death in patients with WPW syndrome has been estimated to range from 0.15% to 0.39%.[13–15] It is distinctly unusual for cardiac arrest to be the first symptomatic manifestation of WPW syndrome. A recent report by Bunch et al. compared the outcomes of 872 WPW patients who underwent ablation, 1461 WPW patients who did not have ablation, and 11,175 control patients.[16] Among all WPW patients, the mortality and incidence of sudden death was no different than in the control population. However, the risk of atrial fibrillation was greater in WPW patients. It is also notable that patients with WPW who underwent ablation had a lower mortality than those who did not. Surprisingly, however, there was no difference in the incidence of sudden death in these two groups. Given the high prevalence of atrial fibrillation among patients with WPW syndrome and the concern for sudden cardiac death resulting from rapid preexcited atrial fibrillation, the low annual incidence of sudden death among patients with WPW syndrome is reassuring.

Patients with functioning AV bypass tracts may have certain congenital abnormalities, particularly Ebstein anomaly of the tricuspid valve. Nearly 10% of patients with Ebstein anomaly have preexcitation. APs also commonly occur in patients with corrected transposition of great vessels. In this case, the Ebstein anomaly of the left (tricuspid) valve is associated with APs to the functioning systemic ventricle (anatomic right ventricle). In addition, multiple bypass tracts are frequently seen in patients with Ebstein anomaly. Conversely, of patients with WPW syndrome presenting with SVT early in childhood, only 5% have Ebstein anomaly, even though it is the most common form of congenital heart disease associated with WPW syndrome.

Electrocardiographic Characteristics

The ECG hallmark of an antegradely conducting AP is unusually short PR interval and a slurred upstroke to the QRS complex (frequently described as a delta wave). Conversely, the presence of retrograde conduction only in an AP will not be apparent on a surface ECG during sinus rhythm. Whereas ECG during orthodromic AVRT has a normal QRS complex with retrogradely conducting P wave after the completion of the QRS complex in the ST segment or early in the T wave (see Fig. 35–4), the QRS during antidromic AVRT is fully preexcited.

Numerous algorithms have been described to localize the site of the AP using the axis of the delta wave and QRS morphology. The location of the AP along the AV ring is classified

variously into 5 or 10 regions, which can be broadly divided into those on the left and the right of the AV groove. Distribution along these lines is not homogenous. Some 46% to 60% of the pathways are found on the left free wall space. Nearly 25% are within the posteroseptal and midseptal spaces, 15% to 20% in the right free wall space, and 2% in the anteroseptal space. A simple algorithm that includes both the delta wave axis and the QRS axis is shown in **Fig. 35–14**.

ST-segment depression may also occur during orthodromic AVRT. It may occur even in young individuals, who are unlikely to have coronary artery disease. The location of the ST-segment depression may vary with the location of the AP. ST-segment depression in V_3 to V_6 is almost invariably seen with a left lateral pathway; a negative T wave in the inferior leads is associated with a posteroseptal or posterior pathway; and a negative or notched T wave in V_2 or V_3 with a positive retrograde P wave in at least two inferior leads suggests an anteroseptal pathway. However, ST-segment depression occurring during orthodromic AVRT episodes in older patients or associated with symptoms of ischemia mandate the consideration of coexisting coronary artery disease.

Electrophysiologic Testing

EPS in patients with AVRT is done to not only confirm the presence of an AP and differentiate this condition from other forms of SVT, but also to find the pathway participating in the tachycardia and aid in ablative therapy.

By definition, if an AP is present and conducting antegradely, some part of the ventricle begins activation earlier than expected, so that the HV interval is shorter than normal at rest (see Fig. 35–10). Because the QRS complex is a fusion complex of conduction down both the AV node and the AP, slowing of conduction down the normal pathway results in an increasing degree of preexcitation.

Eccentric retrograde atrial activation with ventricular pacing makes it easy to identify the presence of an AP (**Fig. 35–15**). Retrograde conduction over most APs is nondecremental. Hence, in the absence of intraventricular conduction delay or the presence of multiple bypass tracts, the VA conduction time is the same over a range of paced cycle lengths (see Fig. 35–15). The exception to this are the slowly conducting decremental posteroseptal pathways mediating PJRT, in which the VA conduction time increases with increasing ventricular pacing rate.

It is important and often challenging to differentiate retrograde conduction over a septal pathway from conduction over the normal AV system. One maneuver that can make this differentiation is *differential pacing* (ie, pacing both from the right ventricular apex and the right ventricular base) and measuring the VA conduction time. Retrograde conduction over the normal AV conduction system is fastest when pacing from the apex because conduction can occur rapidly over the His-Purkinje system. VA intervals are longer when the pacing site is moved from the apex to the base. The converse is true in the presence of an AP, with VA intervals shortest when pacing from the base, closer to the site of pathway insertion, than from the apex. The technique of *para-Hisian pacing* is useful in determining whether a septal AP is present. In the *absence*

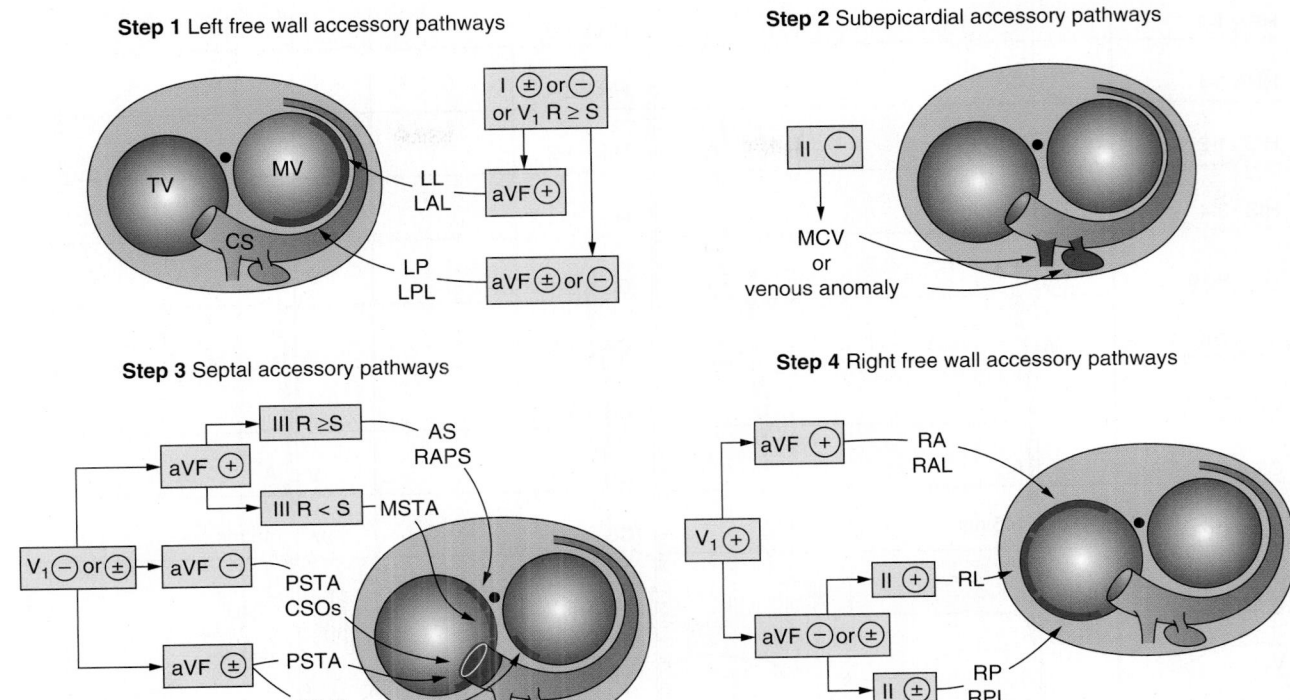

Figure 35–14. Localization of accessory pathways in patients with Wolff-Parkinson-White syndrome. The line drawings illustrate the anatomic relationships between the tricuspid valve (TV), mitral valve (MV), coronary sinus (CS), atrioventricular conducting system, and accessory pathways. For each accessory pathway location indicated, the combination of QRS vectors most likely to result are shown based on upright (+) or inverted (–) QRS waveforms. These vectorial guidelines are generally useful, but not necessarily precise because activation patterns from specific sites may vary in individual patients. AS, anteroseptal; CSOs, coronary sinus ostium; LAL, left anterolateral; LL, left lateral; LP, left posterior; LPL, left posterolateral; MCV, middle cardiac vein (coronary vein); MSTA, midseptal tricuspid annulus; PSMA, posteroseptal mitral annulus; PSTA, posteroseptal tricuspid annulus; RA, right anterior; RAL, right anterolateral; RAPS, right anterior paraseptal; RL, right lateral; RP, right posterior; RPL, right posterolateral. Adapted with permission from Arruda MS, McClelland JH, Wang X, et al: Development and validation of an ECG algorithm for identifying accessory pathway ablation site in Wolff-Parkinson-White syndrome. *J Cardiovasc Electrophysiol.* 1998 Jan;9(1):2-12.

of an AP, high-output pacing at the His region will result in His capture and prompt retrograde activation of the atrium via the AV node. Reduction in pacing amplitude will lead to loss of His capture (but continued ventricular capture). Retrograde activation of the atrium will prolong significantly, as the paced impulse must propagate to the distal right bundle, and then retrogradely over the His-Purkinje system to the AV node and atrium. In the *presence* of a septal AP, both high- and lower-output pacing are immediately conducted retrogradely to the atrium via the AP; no prolongation in stimulation to retrograde atrial activation is seen with decremental pacing output.

Development of BBB aberration during tachycardia can be useful in determining both presence of, and participation of, an AP in tachycardia (**Fig. 35–16**). An increase in tachycardia cycle length caused by an increase in VA conduction time with functional BBB is consistent with the presence of an AP ipsilateral to the BBB.

Management

Catheter Ablation of Accessory Pathways

Catheter ablation of APs is performed in conjunction with a diagnostic EPS. After the AP has been localized to a region of the heart, precise mapping and ablation are performed using a steerable ablation catheter. No prospective, randomized clinical trials have evaluated the safety and efficacy of catheter ablation of APs. However, the results of catheter ablation of APs have been reported in a large number of other trials.[7,10,11,17–23] The largest prospective, multicenter clinical trial to evaluate the safety and efficacy of RF ablation was reported by Calkins and colleagues.[7] This study involved analysis of 1050 patients, of whom 500 had APs. Overall success of catheter ablation in curing APs was 93%. The success rate for catheter ablation of left free wall APs was slightly higher than for catheter ablation of right-sided APs (95% vs 90%, *P* = 0.03). After an initially successful procedure, recurrence of AP conduction was found in approximately 5% of patients. The recurrence-free interval postablation was also best with left-sided pathways (**Fig. 35–17**). APs that recur can usually be successfully ablated again. Complications associated with catheter ablation of APs may result from obtaining vascular access (hematomas, deep venous thrombosis, perforation of the aorta, arteriovenous fistula, and pneumothorax), catheter manipulation (valvular damage, microemboli, perforation of the CS or myocardial wall, and coronary dissection or thrombosis), or delivery of RF energy (AV block, myocardial perforation, coronary artery spasm or occlusion, transient ischemic attacks, or cerebrovascular accidents).

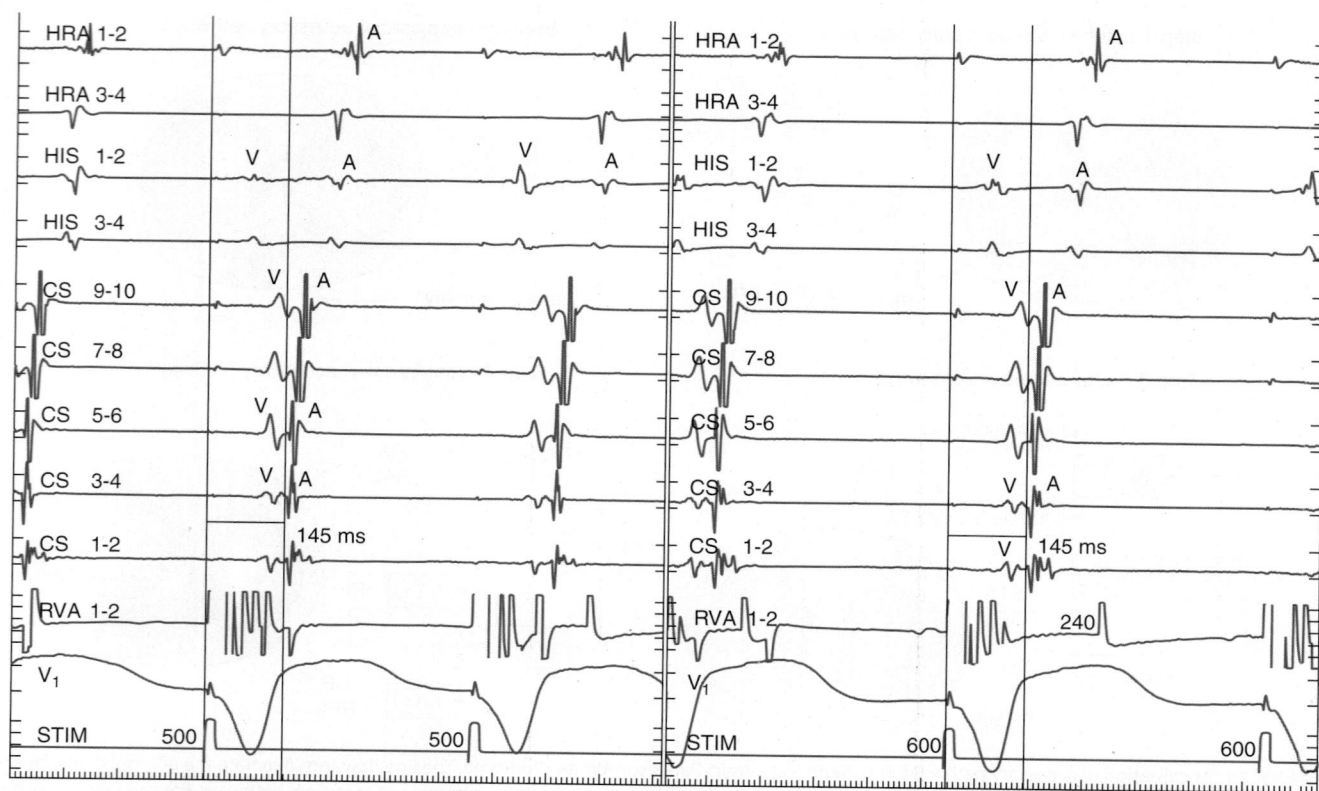

Figure 35-15. Nondecremental retrograde conduction in the accessory pathway. Note the eccentric activation of the atrium with pacing from the ventricle, with earliest atrial depolarization at the distal coronary sinus (CS) lead (CS 1-2). The left panel shows right ventricular pacing at a 120 bpm (cycle length, 500 ms), and the right panel shows the same at 100 bpm (cycle length, 600 ms). Note that the ventriculoatrial (VA) conduction time shown between the vertical lines remains the same with varying pacing rates. 1-2, distal electrodes; 3-4, proximal electrodes in each catheter; A, atrial electrogram; CS 9-20, the most proximal electrode in the CS catheter; HIS, His bundle electrogram; HRA, high right atrium; RVA, right ventricular apex; V, ventricular electrogram.

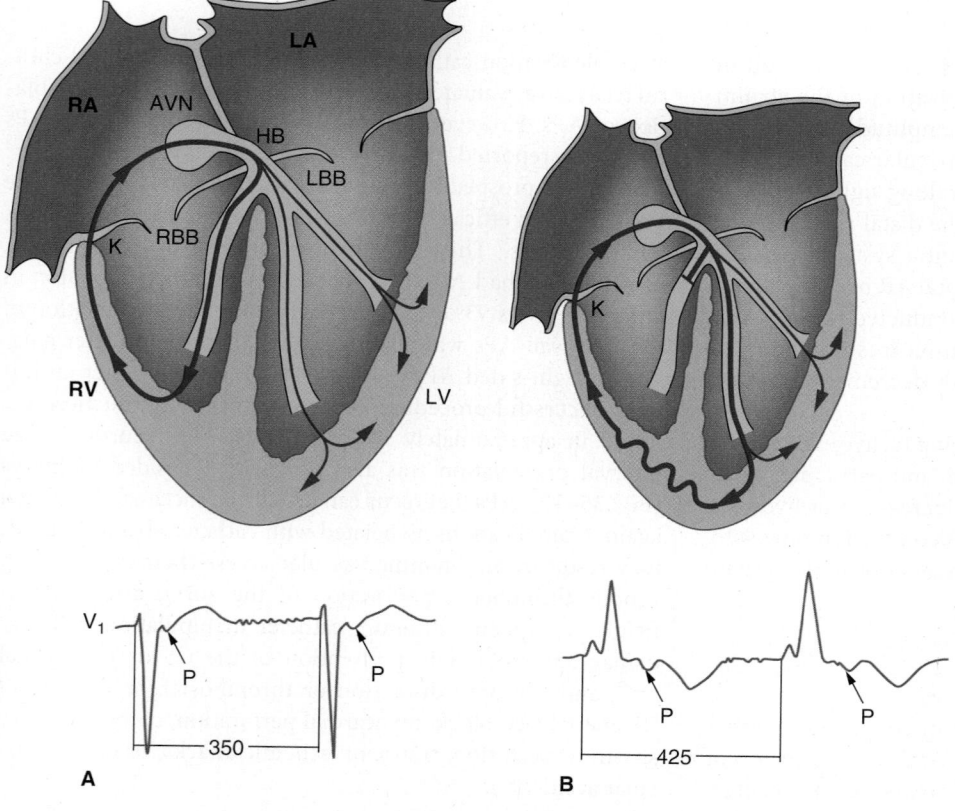

Figure 35-16. Effect of bundle-branch block (BBB) on atrioventricular reentrant tachycardia (AVRT). **(A)** AVRT involving a right-sided accessory pathway. Schematic at the bottom shows the electrocardiographic appearance of the tachycardia at a cycle length of 350 ms. **(B)** Appearance of BBB on the same side leads to increase in the cycle length of the tachycardia to 425 ms. See text for discussion. AVN, atrioventricular node; HB, His bundle; LA, left atrium; LBB, left bundle branch; LV, left ventricle; RA, right atrium; RBB, right bundle branch; RV, right ventricle. Modified with permission from Josephson M. *Clinical Cardiac Electrophysiology: Technique and Interpretation*, 3rd ed. New York, NY: Lippincott Williams & Wilkins; 2002.

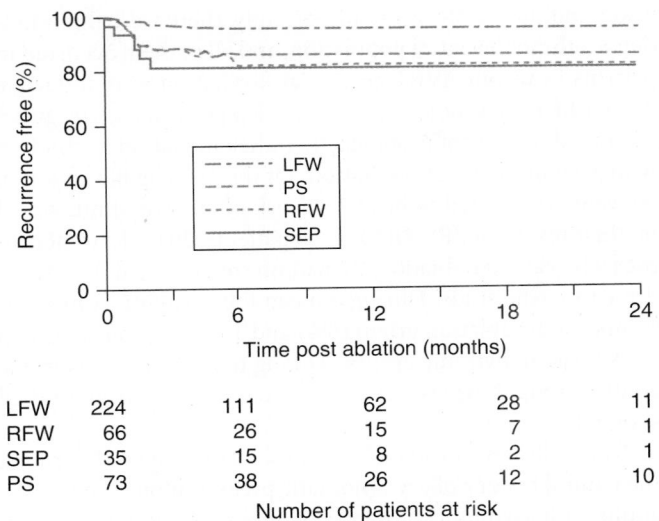

LFW	224	111	62	28	11
RFW	66	26	15	7	1
SEP	35	15	8	2	1
PS	73	38	26	12	10

Number of patients at risk

Figure 35–17. Kaplan–Meier curve showing freedom from arrhythmia recurrence among patients who underwent successful ablation of an accessory pathway subclassified by its location. This analysis was confined to patients in whom successful ablation was achieved with the investigational ablation system. LFW, left free wall; PS, posteroseptal; RFW, right free wall; SEP, septal. Reproduced with permission from Calkins H, Yong P, Miller JM, et al. Catheter ablation of accessory pathways, atrioventricular nodal reentrant tachycardia, and the atrioventricular junction: final results of a prospective, multicenter clinical trial. The Atakr Multicenter Investigators Group. *Circulation.* 1999 Jan 19;99(2):262-270.

Calkins and coworkers[7] reported the incidence of major complications in their trial to be 3% and of minor complications around 8%. The procedure-related mortality associated with catheter ablation of APs has ranged from 0% to 0.2%. The two most common types of major complications reported during catheter ablation of APs are inadvertent complete AV block and cardiac tamponade. The incidence of inadvertent complete AV block ranges from 0.17% to 1.0%. Most instances of

complete AV block occur in the setting of the ablation of septal and posteroseptal APs. The frequency of cardiac tamponade as a result of the ablation of APs varies between 0.13% and 1.1%.

In the last few years, cryoablation has become available as an alternative energy source for creation of myocardial lesions, which can be used for catheter ablation of APs. The main advantage of cryoenergy compared with RF energy is that the risk of heart block appears to be lower.[18] This potential benefit must be balanced against longer procedure times and lower acute and long-term efficacy.[18] Because of the lower acute and long-term success rates of catheter ablation of APs using cryoenergy, this energy source is generally used only for ablation of APs located in the anteroseptal and para-Hisian locations.

Medical Therapy

Antiarrhythmic drugs represent one therapeutic option for management of patients with AP-mediated arrhythmias (see **Table 35–5**). Antiarrhythmic drugs that primarily modify conduction through the AV node include verapamil, β-blockers, and adenosine. In contrast, the antiarrhythmic drugs, which primarily modify conduction across the AP, consist of class I drugs such as procainamide, propafenone, and flecainide as well as class III antiarrhythmic drugs such as sotalol and amiodarone. The approach to acute termination of these arrhythmias generally differs from that used for long-term suppression and prevention of further episodes of SVT. In general, the approach used does not vary based on the specific tachycardia mechanism, which generally is unknown when the patient first presents to an emergency department. Pharmacologic agents are in general more effective in terminating an acute episode of tachycardia than in preventing future recurrences. Verapamil or diltiazem should not be administered intravenously to patients with atrial fibrillation and preexcitation because they may accelerate conduction through the AP and precipitate a cardiac arrest.

Class	
TABLE 35–5. AHA/ACC/HRS 2015 Recommendations for Acute Management of Patients with Accessory Pathway-Mediated Arrhythmias[1]	
Class	
I	Vagal maneuvers are recommended for acute treatment in patients with orthodromic AVRT.
I	Adenosine is beneficial for acute treatment in patients with orthodromic AVRT.
I	Synchronized cardioversion should be performed for acute treatment in hemodynamically unstable patients with AVRT if vagal maneuvers or adenosine are ineffective or not feasible.
I	Synchronized cardioversion is recommended for acute treatment in hemodynamically stable patients with AVRT when pharmacologic therapy is ineffective or contraindicated.
I	Synchronized cardioversion should be performed for acute treatment in hemodynamically unstable patients with preexcited AF.
I	Ibutlide or intravenous procainamide is beneficial for acute treatment in patients with preexcited AF who are hemodynamically stable.
IIb	Intravenous diltiazem, verapamil, or β-blockers can be effective for acute treatment in patients with orthodromic AVRT who do not have preexcitation on their resting ECG during sinus rhythm.
IIb	Intravenous β-blockers, diltiazem, or verapamil might be considered for acute treatment in patients with orthodromic AVRT who have preexcitation on their resting ECG and have not responded to other therapies.
III	Intravenous digoxin, intravenous amiodarone, intravenous or oral β-blockers, and verapamil are potentially harmful for acute treatment in patients with pre-excited AF.

Abbreviations: ACC, American College of Cardiology; AF, atrial fibrillation; AHA, American Heart Association; AVRT, atrioventricular reentrant tachycardia; ECG, electrocardiogram; HRS, Heart Rhythm Society.

There have been no controlled trials of drug prophylaxis involving patients with AV reentry. However, a number of small, nonrandomized trials have been performed that have demonstrated reasonable effectiveness of propafenone, flecainide, and amiodarone.

Management Considerations

Management of Asymptomatic Preexcitation

Most patients with asymptomatic preexcitation have a good prognosis. Because of the small, but real, risks associated with invasive procedures, EPS is not mandated for risk stratification or ablative therapy. The ACC/AHA/HRS Guidelines for Management of Patients with Supraventricular Arrhythmias and the 2019 ESC Guidelines for the Management of Patients with Supraventricular Tachycardia both give electrophysiologic testing and catheter ablation when indicated a IIa classification for treatment of patients with asymptomatic preexcitation.[1] A IIa designation means that it is reasonable to offer EPS with or without ablation in selected patients after a thorough discussion of the risks and benefits of the procedure. Similar recommendations have been made in the PACES/HRS Expert Consensus Statement on the Management of Asymptomatic Young Patients with a WPW ECG Pattern.[16]

Several noninvasive and invasive tests have been proposed as useful in stratifying patients for the risk of sudden death.[1,18] The detection of intermittent preexcitation—which is characterized by an abrupt loss of the delta wave, normalization of the QRS complex, and an increase in the PR interval during a continuous ECG recording—is evidence that an AP has a relatively long refractory period and is unlikely to precipitate ventricular fibrillation. The loss of preexcitation after administration of antiarrhythmic drugs such as procainamide or ajmaline has also been used to indicate a low-risk subgroup. These noninvasive tests are generally considered inferior to EPS in the assessment of risk of sudden cardiac death. In the ESC Guidelines, for instance, noninvasive testing to assess AP conduction properties was given a IIb indication. Because of the relatively limited information provided by noninvasive studies, they play little role in patient management at present.

When screening studies are performed in patients with asymptomatic preexcitation, approximately 20% of those who are asymptomatic will demonstrate a rapid ventricular rate during atrial fibrillation induced at EPS. Studies have identified markers that identify patients at increased risk. These include (1) a short preexcited R-R interval below 250 ms during spontaneous or induced atrial fibrillation, (2) a history of symptomatic tachycardia, (3) multiple APs, and (4) Ebstein anomaly.[1,19,20] A short preexcited R-R interval during atrial fibrillation above 250 ms has been reported to have a negative predictive value greater than 95%.

More recent evidence makes a stronger case for the use of EPS in risk stratifying all asymptomatic patients with preexcitation.[25] Pappone and coworkers[25] studied 212 consecutive asymptomatic WPW patients after a baseline EPS over 5 years. After a mean follow-up of 37.7 months, 33 patients became symptomatic. Of these, 29 had inducible SVT on EPS, and only 4 were not inducible. More importantly, there were three sudden deaths in the entire population, and all of them occurred in patients in whom AVRT and atrial fibrillation were inducible during EPS. In a more recent study, Pappone and colleagues[26] examined the role of prophylactic catheter ablation in children with asymptomatic preexcitation. Of the 165 eligible children, 60 were determined to be at high risk of an arrhythmia based on their results of EPS. Of these 60 patients, 20 underwent prophylactic catheter ablation, 27 had no treatment, and 13 withdrew from the study. During a mean follow-up of 34 months, 1 child in the ablation group (5%) and 12 in the control group (44%) had arrhythmic events. Among these 12 patients in the control group, 2 experienced ventricular fibrillation, and 1 died suddenly.

Santinelli and coworkers[27,28] published two papers describing the natural history of asymptomatic preexcitation. Among 293 adults with asymptomatic preexcitation followed for a median of 67 months, 31 patients (10.6%) developed a first arrhythmic event. Among these patients, the event was classified as potentially life threatening in 17 patients. One of these patients experienced a cardiac arrest. Multivariate analysis identified inducibility and an anterograde AP effective refractory period shorter than 250 ms as predictive of potentially life-threatening arrhythmias.[26] And among 184 children with asymptomatic preexcitation followed for a median of 57 months, 51 patients (28%) developed a first arrhythmic event. Among these patients, the event was classified as potentially life threatening in 19 patients. Three of these patients experienced a cardiac arrest. Multivariate analysis identified an anterograde effective refractory period shorter than 240 ms and the presence of multiple APs as predictive of potentially life-threatening arrhythmias.[27,28] Pappone et al. went on to publish an outcome registry involving 2169 WPW patients followed for 8 years[29]; among this group, 1001 (550 asymptomatic) did not undergo ablation and 1168 (206 asymptomatic) did have ablation. VF occurred during follow-up in 1.5% of patients who did not have catheter ablation. In contrast, no patients with WPW who underwent ablation experienced VF during follow-up. Based on the results of these studies, as well as the well-established safety and efficacy of catheter ablation of APs, an increasing proportion of electrophysiologists, particularly pediatric electrophysiologists, now advocate screening EPS and prophylactic catheter ablation when a high-risk AP is uncovered. EPS and ablation of an AP if appropriate is a class IIa recommendation in both the ACC/AHA/HRS and the ESC Guidelines. The European Guidelines go even further, giving EPS and AP ablation (if appropriate) in asymptomatic patients with high-risk occupations or hobbies a class I recommendation.[2] The recommendations made for management of asymptomatic preexcitation in the AHA/ACC/HRS 2015 and the ESC 2019 SVT Guidelines are summarized in **Table 35–6.**

Management of Symptomatic Wolff-Parkinson-White Syndrome

The ACC/AHA/HRS Guidelines for Management of Patients with SVT states that catheter ablation is considered first-line therapy (class I) and the treatment of choice for patients with

TABLE 35–6. AHA/ACC/HRS 2015 and ESC 2019 Recommendations for Management of Patients with Asymptomatic Manifest Accessory Pathways[1]

Class	
I	In asymptomatic patients with preexcitation, the findings of abrupt loss of conduction over a manifest pathway during exercise in sinus rhythm or intermittent loss of preexcitation during electrocardiogram or ambulatory monitoring are useful to identify patients at low risk of rapid conduction over the pathway.
I	Performance of an EPS, with the use of isoprenaline, is recommended to risk stratify individuals with asymptomatic pre-excitation who have high-risk occupations/hobbies, and those who participate in competitive athletics.*
IIa	An electrophysiology study is reasonable in asymptomatic patients with preexcitation to risk stratify for arrhythmic events.
IIa	Catheter ablation of the accessory pathway is reasonable in asymptomatic patients with preexcitation if an electrophysiology study identifies a high risk of arrhythmic events including rapidly conducting preexcited atrial fibrillation.
IIa	Catheter ablation of the accessory pathway is reasonable in asymptomatic patients if the presence of preexcitation precludes specific employment (such as pilots).
IIa	Observation, without further evaluation or treatment, is reasonable in asymptomatic patients with preexcitation.

Abbreviations: ACC, American College of Cardiology; AHA, American Heart Association; HRS, Heart Rhythm Society; ESC, European Society of Cardiology. *ESC 2019 guideline

WPW syndrome (ie, patients with manifest preexcitation along with symptoms).[1,21,22] It is curative in more than 95% of patients and has a low complication rate. It also obviates the unwanted side effects of antiarrhythmic agents. Catheter ablation is also considered first-line therapy (class I) for patients with PSVT involving a concealed AP. However, because concealed APs are not associated with an increased risk of sudden cardiac death in these patients, catheter ablation can be presented as one of a number of potential therapeutic approaches, including pharmacologic therapy and clinical follow-up alone (see discussion of management of AVNRT). When pharmacologic therapy is selected for patients with concealed APs, it is reasonable to consider a trial of β-blocker therapy, CCB therapy, or a class Ic antiarrhythmic agent. It is important to note that β-blockers and CCBs generally are not recommended for the management of patients who have evidence of preexcitation.

The recommendations for the acute and long-term management of patients with AP-mediated arrhythmias developed by the ACC/AHA/HRS are shown in **Tables** 36–5 and **36–7**.[1] Catheter ablation is considered class I therapy for treatment of patients with WPW syndrome and for those with AVRT in the absence of preexcitation.

ATRIAL TACHYCARDIA

Atrial tachycardia is an arrhythmia that arises from the left or right atrium or the musculature of the great cardiac veins.[1] There are many types of atrial tachycardias. Some are paroxysmal while others are continuous. The mechanisms of atrial tachycardias vary widely and include enhanced automaticity, triggered activity, and reentry. Although atrial fibrillation and atrial flutter can be considered under the broad umbrella of atrial tachycardias, in our opinion it is best to consider atrial flutter and atrial fibrillation as distinct arrhythmias, in part because of the marked increase in stroke risk that accompanies atrial fibrillation and atrial flutter.

TABLE 35–7. AHA/ACC/HRS 2015 Recommendations for Management of Patients with Symptomatic Manifest or Concealed Accessory Pathways[1]

Class	
I	Catheter ablation of the accessory pathway is recommended in patients with AVRT and/or preexcited AF
I	Oral β-blockers, diltiazem, and verapamil are indicated for ongoing management of AVRT in patients without preexcitation on their resting ECG.
IIa	Oral flecainide or propafenone is reasonable for ongoing management in patients without structural heart disease or ischemic heart disease who have AVRT and/or preexcited AF and are not candidates for, or prefer not to undergo, catheter ablation.
IIb	Oral dofetilide or sotolol may be reasonable for ongoing management in patients with AVRT and/or preexcited AF who are not candidates for, or prefer not to undergo, catheter ablation.
IIb	Oral amiodarone may be considered for ongoing management in patients with AVRT and/or preexcited AF who are not candidates for, or prefer not to undergo, catheter ablation and in whom β-blockers, diltiazem, flecainide, propafenone, and verapamil are ineffective or contraindicated.
IIb	Oral β-blockers, diltiazem, or verapamil may be reasonable for ongoing management of orthodromic AVRT in patients with pre excitation on their resting ECG who are not candidates for, or prefer not to undergo, catheter ablation.
IIb	Oral digoxin may be reasonable for ongoing management of orthodromic AVRT in patients without preexcitation on their resting ECG, who are not candidates for, or prefer not to undergo, catheter ablation.
III	Oral digoxin is potentially harmful for ongoing management in patients with AVRT or AF and preexcitation on their resting ECG.

Abbreviations: ACC, American College of Cardiology; AF, atrial fibrillation; AHA, American Heart Association; AVRT, atrioventricular reentrant tachycardia; ECG, electrocardiogram; HRS, Heart Rhythm Society.

Atrial tachycardias are generally benign arrhythmias where the main indication for treatment is symptom relief. One important exception is incessant atrial tachycardia with a rapid rate. It is well established that incessant atrial tachycardias that result in a persistently rapid ventricular response can lead to a rate related cardiomyopathy. It is important to recognize that this potentially serious condition is reversible once the atrial tachycardia is eliminated with an associated return of the ventricular rate to normal.

There are many approaches to treatment of atrial tachycardia. Pharmacologic therapy with β-blockers or CCBs is effective in a proportion of patients. If these first-line medications fail, membrane active antiarrhythmic medications such as flecainide, propafenone, sotolol, or rarely amiodarone can be considered. Catheter ablation is an important treatment strategy that is appropriate to use as first-line therapy based on patient's values and preferences. With the use of three-dimensional computerized mapping systems, the cure rate associated with ablation of atrial tachycardia exceeds 90%. One important exception to this rule is multifocal atrial tachycardia, which is far more difficult to approach with ablation because of its multifocal origin.

SUMMARY

- SVT encompasses three distinct arrhythmias: AVNRT; AVRT; and AT.
- AVNRT accounts for roughly two-thirds of SVT cases. AVRT accounts for nearly one-third of cases.
- Both AVNRT and AVRT are due to reentry. AVNRT arises from a reentrant circuit using distinct pathways within the AV node, while AVRT arises from a reentrant circuit using the AV node and an accessory pathway.
- Acute management of SVT can include vagal maneuvers, therapy with β-blockers or calcium channel blockers, or catheter ablation.
- Chronic management of SVTs can be achieved by catheter ablation in most patients, or by suppressive medical therapy in patients for whom procedures are not desirable.

REFERENCES

1. Page RL, Joglar JA, Caldwell MA, et al. 2015 ACC/AHA/HRS Guideline for the Management of Adult Patients with Supraventricular Tachycardia: a report of the American College of Cardiology/American Heart Association Task Force on Clinical Practice Guidelines and the Heart Rhythm Society. *J Am Coll Cardiol.* 2016 Apr 5;67(13):e27-e115. doi: 10.1016/j.jacc.2015.08.856. Epub 2015 Sep 24.
2. 2019 ESC Guidelines for the Management of Patients with Supraventricular Tachycardia. *Eur Heart J.* 2019;41:655-720.
3. Orejarena LA, Vidaillet H Jr, DeStefano F, et al. Paroxysmal supraventricular tachycardia in the general population. *J Am Coll Cardiol.* 1998;31:150-157.
4. Jackman WM, Beckman KJ, McClelland JH, et al. Treatment of supraventricular tachycardia due to atrioventricular nodal reentry by radiofrequency catheter ablation of slow-pathway conduction. *N Engl J Med.* 1992;327:313-318.
5. Katritsis DG, Josephson ME. Classification of electrophysiological types of atrioventricular nodal re-entrant tachycardia: A reappraisal. *Europace.* 2013;15(9):1231-1240. Epub 2013 Apr 23.
6. Haissaguerre M, Gaita F, Fischer B, et al. Elimination of atrioventricular nodal reentrant tachycardia using discrete slow potentials to guide application of radiofrequency energy. *Circulation.* 1992;85:2162-2175.
7. Calkins H, Yong P, Miller JM, et al. Catheter ablation of accessory pathways, atrioventricular nodal reentrant tachycardia, and the atrioventricular junction: final results of a prospective, multicenter clinical trial. The Atakr Multicenter Investigators Group. *Circulation.* 1999;99:262-270.
8. Sandilands A, Boreham P, Pitts-Crick J, et al. Impact of cryoablation catheter size on success rates in the treatment of atrioventricular nodal re-entry tachycardia in 160 patients with long-term follow-up. *Europace.* 2008;10(6):683-686.
9. Opel A, Murray S, Kamath N, et al. Cryoablation versus radiofrequency ablation for treatment of atrioventricular nodal reentrant tachycardia: Cryoablation with 6-mm-tip catheters is still less effective than radiofrequency ablation. *Heart Rhythm.* 2010;7(3):340-343.
10. Pieragnoli P, Paoletti Perini A, Checchi L, et al. Cryoablation of typical AVNRT: younger age and administration of bonus ablation favor long-term success. *Heart Rhythm.* 2015;12(10):2125-2131.
11. Rodriguez-Entem FJ, Expósito V, Gonzalez-Enriquez S, Olalla-Antolin JJ. Cryoablation versus radiofrequency ablation for the treatment of atrioventricular nodal reentrant tachycardia: Results of a prospective randomized study. *J Interv Card Electrophysiol.* 2013;36(1):41-45.
12. de Sisti A, Tonet J. Cryoablation of atrioventricular nodal reentrant tachycardia: a clinical review. *Pacing Clin Electrophysiol.* 2012;35(2):233-240. Epub 2011 Oct 20.
13. Klein GJ, Bashore TM, Sellers TD, et al. Ventricular fibrillation in the Wolff-Parkinson-White syndrome. *N Engl J Med.* 1979;301:1080-1085.
14. Timmermans C, Smeets JL, Rodriguez LM, et al. Aborted sudden death in the Wolff-Parkinson-White syndrome. *Am J Cardiol.* 1995;76:492-494.
15. Pappone C, Santinelli V, Rosanio S, et al. Usefulness of invasive electrophysiologic testing to stratify the risk of arrhythmic events in asymptomatic patients with Wolff-Parkinson-White pattern: results from a large prospective long-term follow-up study. *J Am Coll Cardiol.* 2003;41(2):239-244.
16. Bunch TJ, May HT, Bair TL, et al. Long-term natural history of adult Wolff-Parkinson-White syndrome patients treated with and without catheter ablation. *Circ Arrhythm Electrophysiol.* 2015;8(6):1465-1471. Epub 2015 Oct 19.
17. Sacher F, Wright M, Tedrow UB, et al. Wolff-Parkinson-White ablation after a prior failure: a 7-year multicentre experience. *Europace.* 2010;12(6):835-841.
18. Bar-Cohen Y, Cecchin F, Alexander ME, Berul CI, Triedman JK, Walsh EP. Cryoablation for accessory pathways located near normal conduction tissues or within the coronary venous system in children and young adults. *Heart Rhythm.* 2006;3(3):253-258.
19. Cohen MI, Triedman JK, Cannon BC, et al. PACES/HRS expert consensus statement on the management of the asymptomatic young patient with a Wolff-Parkinson-White (WPW, ventricular preexcitation) electrocardiographic pattern: developed in partnership between the Pediatric and Congenital Electrophysiology Society (PACES) and the Heart Rhythm Society (HRS). Endorsed by the governing bodies of PACES, HRS, the American College of Cardiology Foundation (ACCF), the American Heart Association (AHA), the American Academy of Pediatrics (AAP), and the Canadian Heart Rhythm Society (CHRS). *Heart Rhythm.* 2012;9(6):1006-1024.
20. Lesh MD, Van Hare GF, Schamp DJ, et al. Curative percutaneous catheter ablation using radiofrequency energy for accessory pathways in all locations: results in 100 consecutive patients. *J Am Coll Cardiol.* 1992 May;19(6):1303-1309.
21. Jackman WM, Wang X, Friday KJ, et al. Catheter ablation of accessory atrioventricular pathways (Wolff-Parkinson-White syndrome) by radiofrequency current. *N Engl J Med.* 1991;324:1605-1611.

22. Calkins H, Langberg J, Sousa J, et al. Radiofrequency catheter ablation of accessory atrioventricular connections in 250 patients: abbreviated therapeutic approach to Wolff-Parkinson-White syndrome. *Circulation.* 1992;85:1337-1346.

23. Drago F, DeSantis A, Grutter G, Silverti MS. Transvenous cryothermal catheter ablation of re-entry circuit located near the atrioventricular junction in pediatric patients. *J Am Coll Cardiol.* 2005;45:1096-1103.

24. Fitzsimmons PJ, McWhirter PD, Peterson DW, et al. The natural history of Wolff-Parkinson-White syndrome in 228 military aviators: a long-term follow-up of 22 years. *Am Heart J.* 2001;142(3):530-536.

25. Pappone C, Santinelli V, Rosanio S. Usefulness of invasive electrophysiology testing to stratify the risk of arrhythmic events in asymptomatic patients with Wolff-Parkinson-White pattern: results from a large prospective long-term follow-up study. *J Am Coll Cardiol.* 2003;41:239-244.

26. Pappone C, Manguso F, Santinelli R, et al. Radiofrequency ablation in children with asymptomatic Wolff-Parkinson-White syndrome. *N Engl J Med.* 2004;351:1197-1205.

27. Santinelli V, Radinovic A, Manguso F, et al. Asymptomatic ventricular pre-excitation: a long-term prospective follow-up study of 293 adult patients. *Circ Arrhythm Electrophysiol.* 2009;2(2):102-107.

28. Santinelli V, Radinovic A, Manguso F, et al. The natural history of asymptomatic ventricular pre-excitation: a long-term prospective follow-up study of 184 asymptomatic children. *J Am Coll Cardiol.* 2009;53(3):275-280.

29. Pappone C, Vicedomini G, Manguso F, et al. Wolff-Parkinson-White syndrome in the era of catheter ablation: insights from a registry study of 2169 patients. *Circulation.* 2014;130(10):811-819. Epub 2014 Jul 22.

36

Atrial Fibrillation and Atrial Flutter

Anne B. Curtis, Tina Baykaner, and Sanjiv M. Narayan

CHAPTER OUTLINE

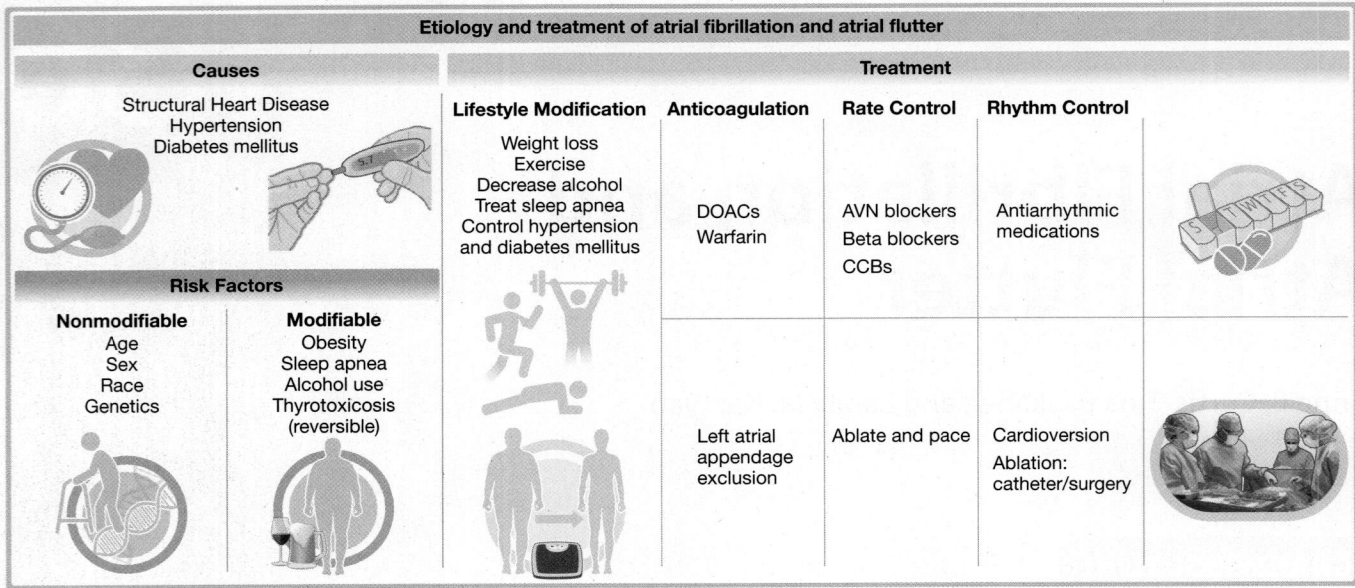

Etiology and treatment of atrial fibrillation and atrial flutter

Causes

Structural Heart Disease
Hypertension
Diabetes mellitus

Risk Factors

Nonmodifiable	Modifiable
Age	Obesity
Sex	Sleep apnea
Race	Alcohol use
Genetics	Thyrotoxicosis (reversible)

Treatment

Lifestyle Modification	Anticoagulation	Rate Control	Rhythm Control
Weight loss Exercise Decrease alcohol Treat sleep apnea Control hypertension and diabetes mellitus	DOACs Warfarin	AVN blockers Beta blockers CCBs	Antiarrhythmic medications
	Left atrial appendage exclusion	Ablate and pace	Cardioversion Ablation: catheter/surgery

Chapter 36 Fuster and Hurst's Central Illustration. Atrial fibrillation has multiple potential causes, including structural heart disease and conditions such as hypertension; nonmodifiable risk factors such as age, sex, and genetics; and modifiable factors such as obesity and sleep apnea. The three pillars of treatment of atrial fibrillation include anticoagulation in patients at risk for thromboembolism; rate control, mainly with beta blockers and CCBs; and rhythm control with antiarrhythmic drugs or catheter ablation. Lifestyle modification may help in preventing recurrences of atrial fibrillation. Atrial flutter has many of the same risk factors as atrial fibrillation. It is treated in a similar fashion, although catheter ablation is often used as a first line therapy for typical atrial flutter. AVN, atrioventricular node; CCBs, calcium channel blockers; DOACs, direct oral anticoagulants.

CHAPTER SUMMARY

This chapter discusses the epidemiology, pathophysiology, and classification of atrial fibrillation (AF) and atrial flutter, as well as the clinical presentation, evaluation, and management of patients with these arrhythmias (see Fuster and Hurst's Central Illustration). Patients may have a range of presentations from asymptomatic, with the arrhythmia detected only by electrocardiography or other monitoring, to highly symptomatic. Management approaches should be individualized to patient symptoms and comorbidities. Management of AF may require cardioversion acutely for symptomatic patients, followed by strategies to prevent recurrent AF and minimize sequelae such as stroke. An important consideration in the management of AF is lifestyle modification, because conditions such as sleep apnea, obesity, excessive alcohol intake, and lack of exercise may contribute to the development or maintenance of AF. Long-term management includes anticoagulation for the prevention of thromboembolism in patients deemed to be high risk. The other pillars of management of AF are rate control and rhythm control. Emerging data support early rhythm control by antiarrhythmic drugs or catheter ablation, especially in certain subpopulations such as those with concurrent heart failure. The management of atrial flutter is analogous in most respects to that of AF, although typical atrial flutter is curative in most cases with catheter ablation.

INTRODUCTION

Atrial fibrillation (AF) is the most common sustained arrhythmia in the world, affecting at least 33 million individuals.[1] This is likely an underestimate because it is expected to double over the next 40 years in parallel with the aging of the population and an increasing worldwide prevalence of the contributory comorbidities of obesity and the metabolic syndrome.[2] While the impact of AF was historically underestimated, AF is now clearly linked with heart failure (HF),[3] stroke, potentially dementia, mortality, and loss of productive life Patients treated with catheter ablation for AF have long-term rates of death, stroke, and dementia similar to patients without AF, is now clearly linked with heart failure (HF),[3] stroke, and potentially dementia. Patients treated with catheter ablation for AF have long-term rates of death, stroke, and dementia similar to patients without AF, mortality, and loss of productive life. Aside from its human costs, the economic cost of AF is vast. Annually, 454,000 patients with a primary diagnosis of AF are hospitalized in the United States at a cost of $6 to $26 billion in 2011.

The foundations of AF management are the robust identification of reversible etiologies, such as thyrotoxicosis; the institution of lifestyle choices, such as controlling obesity, hypertension, and limiting alcohol ingestion; and the timely initiation of therapy to reduce the risk for stroke, to control heart rate, or to restore sinus rhythm.[4]

The field of AF is moving rapidly in multiple directions. Because the noninvasive electrocardiogram (ECG) is central to detection, AF is a prototypical disease for which wearable monitors coupled to a digital health infrastructure could change the paradigm for disease diagnosis and tracking before and during therapy. The epidemiology of AF has been directly linked with global demographic trends in aging and obesity, and lifestyle modifications have been shown to attenuate both the pathophysiology and clinical presentation of AF. New options for stroke prevention have been developed that include novel anticoagulants and devices to exclude the left atrial appendage (LAA) for nonpharmacological stroke prevention in certain populations. A plethora of recent studies have advanced our understanding of AF mechanisms using omics and biochemical studies at the cellular level, gene and pharmacological therapy at the whole heart level, and bioengineering innovations that span biological scales from the cell to the patient. These findings have enabled new approaches to ablation, surgical therapy, and prevention of AF-related stroke.

This chapter provides a broad overview of the clinical presentation, pathophysiology, and management of AF. The goal is to emphasize established strategies while outlining promising future areas of clinical relevance.

EPIDEMIOLOGY

The overall prevalence of AF in United States is 1% to 2%[1] and growing. About one-third of patients with AF are asymptomatic (termed "silent AF"). The worldwide burden of AF is rising rapidly[1] for many reasons (**Fig. 36–1**).[2] First, AF is increasingly detected due to growing awareness and the broader application of portable event monitors, smartphones, and wearables. Second, AF burden is growing due to shifts in global demographics and increases in the prevalence of risk factors.

Nonmodifiable risk factors for AF include age, sex, genetics, and racial differences. Advancing age is the predominant independent risk factor for AF. Beyond the age of 80 years, the prevalence of AF reaches 10% to 17%, contributing to the epidemic of AF as the population ages. Individuals with European ancestry have a higher prevalence and incidence of AF than those with Asian and African ancestry, for which genetic bases has been uncovered. The lifetime risk of developing AF is estimated to reach about 1 in 3 in White Americans and 1 in 5 for Black Americans.

Modifiable risk factors for AF identified from the Framingham Heart Study include hypertension, congestive HF,

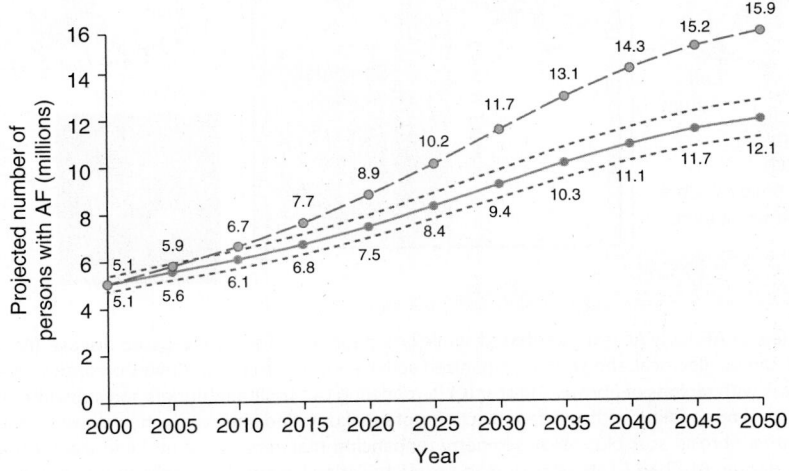

Figure 36–1. Current and projected prevalence of AF in the United States. Projected number of persons with AF in the United States between 2000 and 2050, assuming no further increase in age-adjusted AF incidence (*solid curve*); and assuming a continued increase in incidence rate as was evident from 1980 to 2000 (*dotted curve*), projecting 15.9 million persons with AF by 2050. Other parts of the world show similar projected increases in AF prevalence over the next several decades. Reproduced with permission from Miyasaka Y, Barnes ME, Gersh BJ, et al. Secular trends in incidence of atrial fibrillation in Olmsted County, Minnesota, 1980 to 2000, and implications on the projections for future prevalence. *Circulation.* 2006 Jul 11;114(2):119-125.

coronary artery disease, valvular heart disease, and diabetes mellitus. Several additional risk factors are now recognized, including left ventricular (LV) hypertrophy, excessive alcohol use,[5] and obesity. Obstructive sleep apnea is highly prevalent in the AF population and appears to lead to an increased risk of developing AF. While physical inactivity and poor cardiorespiratory fitness contribute to the growing burden of AF, there is an increasingly recognized converse association between high-intensity endurance training and increased AF risk (**Table 36–1**).

PATHOPHYSIOLOGY

AF has a complex pathophysiology that spans abnormalities at the heart, organ system, cellular, and molecular levels. AF is initiated by triggers and then sustained by distinct mechanisms for days, weeks, or longer. The best understood triggers are rapidly firing ectopic foci or rapid tachycardias near the pulmonary veins (PV), although others exist. Sustaining mechanisms or "substrates" are less well defined, but broadly reflect altered atrial electrophysiology (electrical remodeling) and architecture (structural remodeling). Substrates and triggers are likely interrelated and can be influenced in some patients by the neuroendocrine and other organ systems. These dynamic alterations

TABLE 36–1. Modifiable Risk Factors in Atrial Fibrillation

Physical Activity	Moderate exercise decreases incidence of AF; endurance exercise may increase incidence
Obesity	Sustained weight loss reduces AF burden; fluctuations in weight increase AF burden; bariatric surgery decreases incidence of AF
Obstructive sleep apnea	Continuous positive airway pressure treatment lowers risk of progression to more permanent AF
Hypertension	Poorly controlled hypertension increases risk of AF
Diabetes	Treatment with metformin lowers incidence of AF
Alcohol	Reduction in alcohol intake lowers risk of recurrence of AF and lowers AF burden
Smoking	Smoking increases risk of AF, but no specific study has demonstrated that smoking cessation directly decreases AF

Abbreviation: AF, atrial fibrillation.

result from AF but also facilitate it, a vicious circle often termed "AF begets AF." As the clinical picture of AF progresses from paroxysmal to persistent AF, underlying mechanisms often progress from a trigger-driven to a substrate-maintained disease (**Fig. 36–2**). Mechanisms for AF likely vary among patients to explain their diverse clinical presentations.

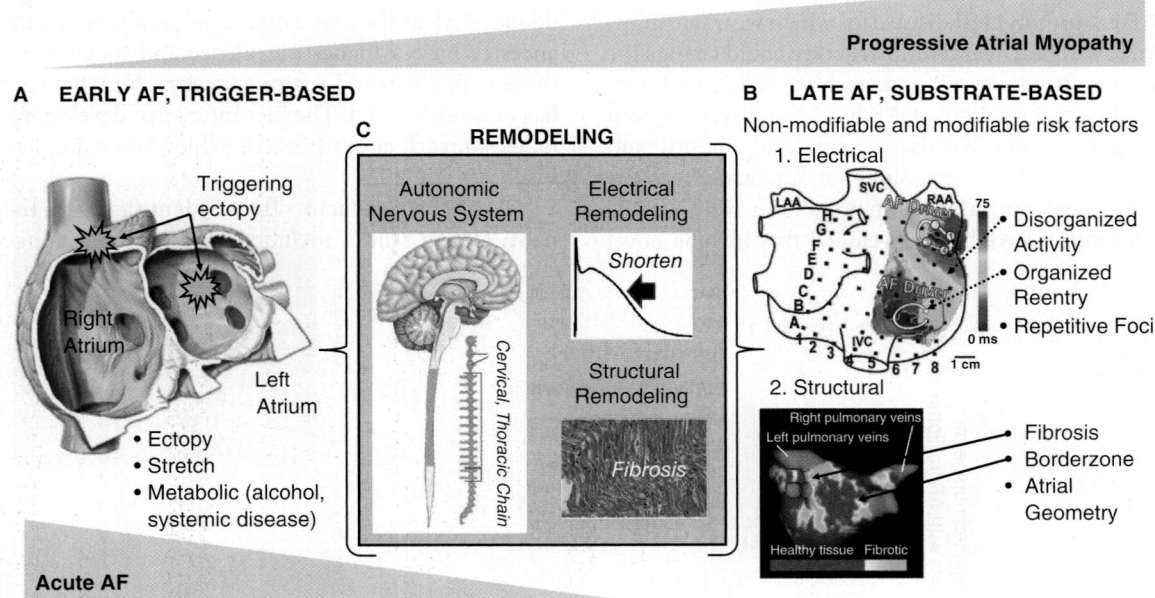

Figure 36–2. Mechanistic overview of AF. Early AF is trigger-based, while late stage AF is a substrate-based disease. **(A)** Triggers lie near pulmonary veins, but also elsewhere. **(B)** Substrates can be electrical, shown as disorganized activity and/or organized drivers on optical dye fluorescence imaging of human AF. Substrates can also be structural, with regions of fibrosis and scar **(C)** Remodeling can facilitate triggers and substrate, and spans the autonomic nervous system (promoting triggers), electrical remodeling with shortened action potential duration and conduction slowing (enhancing maintenance of reentry), and structural remodeling with atrial fibrosis, scar plus atrial geometry (enhancing maintenance of multiple electrical mechanisms for AF).[18,19] Panel B1 reproduced with permission from Hansen BJ, Zhao J, Li N, et al. Human Atrial Fibrillation Drivers Resolved With Integrated Functional and Structural Imaging to Benefit Clinical Mapping. *JACC Clin Electrophysiol.* 2018 Dec;4(12):1501-1515. Panel B2 (Electrical) reproduced with permission from Hansen BJ, Zhao J, Li N, et al. Human Atrial Fibrillation Drivers Resolved With Integrated Functional and Structural Imaging to Benefit Clinical Mapping. *JACC Clin Electrophysiol.* 2018 Dec;4(12):1501-1515; (Structural) Reproduced with permission from Siebermair J, Kholmovski EG, Marrouche N. Assessment of Left Atrial Fibrosis by Late Gadolinium Enhancement Magnetic Resonance Imaging: Methodology and Clinical Implications. *JACC Clin Electrophysiol.* 2017 Aug;3(8):791-802.

Systemic Diseases and AF Mechanisms

AF can occur across a wide range of ages in healthy individuals without comorbidities. More commonly, however, AF coexists with comorbidities such as diabetes, hypertension, and HF. Nontraditional risk factors for AF are increasingly recognized such as sleep apnea and obesity. It is not yet defined how AF mechanistically differs between these clinical scenarios.

AF may be secondary to reversible causes, and it may resolve when the inciting cause resolves. Hyperthyroidism confers an AF incidence of >16%, which resolves when patients become euthyroid. Supraventricular tachycardia such as Wolff-Parkinson-White syndrome (with pre-excitation on the ECG) or atrioventricular (AV) nodal reentrant tachycardia can trigger AF, and AF may not recur if the precipitating tachycardias are eliminated. AF may also follow inflammatory conditions such as viral illnesses, likely due to myopericarditis.[6] The impact of coronavirus infection on AF is uncertain.[7] Postoperative AF is another inflammatory condition that resolves in two-thirds of patients. In this case, there is debate about the extent to which such patients experience adverse events on long-term follow-up. Accepted therapies for AF such as PV isolation are ineffective for postoperative AF,[8] supporting a distinct mechanistic phenotype.

Finally, AF may be aggravated by systemic conditions, treatment of which unfortunately may not eliminate AF. Treatment of sleep apnea by positive airway pressure devices, reduction in obesity by weight loss, and reduction of alcohol consumption[5] may attenuate yet not fully eliminate AF. AF associated with sinus node dysfunction, valvular disease, HF, or congenital heart disease also may not fully resolve when these conditions are treated.

AF and Atrial Myopathy

Patients with nonreversible causes of AF, both paroxysmal and persistent, show electrical, structural, and contractile abnormalities of the atrium that support the concept of "atrial myopathy" or "atrial failure."[9]

Triggers

AF is typically initiated when single or salvoes of ectopic beats interact with baseline rhythm to produce disordered AF. Haïssaguerre et al. reported that ectopic impulses near the PV ostia may trigger paroxysmal AF[10] (Fig. 36–2). Pathological studies show that myocardial sleeves in the PVs have electrophysiological, anatomic, and geometric nonuniformities that may predispose to focal or reentrant activity. Other sites of triggered activity include the superior vena cava, the ligament of Marshall, and the LAA, although these are less clearly linked to AF initiation. It is unclear what factors activate triggers for AF, but they likely relate in different patients to comorbidities such as atrial stretch, HF, and autonomic imbalance.

Autonomic Nervous System

The electrophysiology of the heart is influenced by its rich autonomic nervous system, with efferent nerves and atrial mixed ganglionated plexi (GP) supplied by the parasympathetic nervous system (the vagus nerve) and the cervical sympathetic chain (**Figs. 36–2** and **36–3**). Some patients give a clear history of AF initiation at times of sympathetic dominance such as stress, or vagal dominance such as swallowing. At the whole heart and cellular levels, autonomic modulation has been shown to produce early or late after-depolarizations that create trigger beats for AF. In animal models of AF, autonomic stimulation can trigger and sustain AF. However, ablation of GP

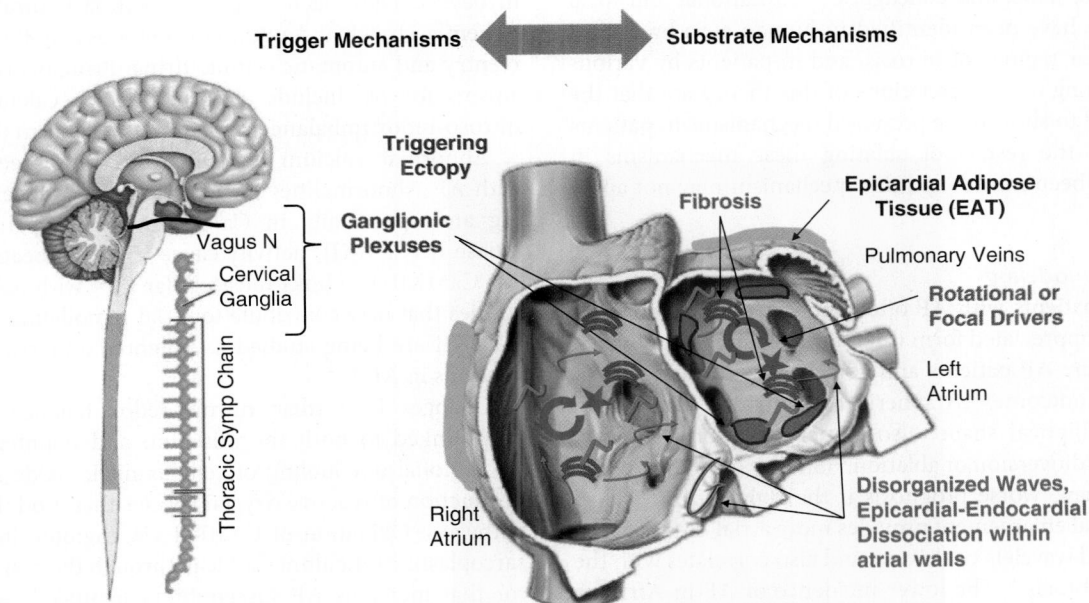

Figure 36–3. Mechanisms of human AF at the whole-heart level. Trigger mechanisms include rapid ectopic foci that may reflect autonomic innervation, stretch, and metabolic factors. Substrate mechanisms include electrical elements (focal and rotational drivers, disorganized waves), anatomical elements such as fibrosis and scar, metabolic components including altered nitroso-redox balance related to epicardial adipose tissue (EAT), and neuroendocrine components.

regions has had mixed success in eliminating AF.[11] Emerging strategies are to ablate the renal autonomic ganglionic plexuses,[12] or to apply low-level vagal nerve stimulation to modulate rather than denervate the heart. Stimulus strengths lower than those required to slow the sinus node applied to the tragus of the ear have recently been shown to modestly reduce AF burden in patients with paroxysmal AF.[13]

Substrates for Maintaining AF

Disorganized wavelets in AF self-terminate, such as by colliding with anatomic boundaries, and they must be replenished for AF to sustain. Distinct mechanistic schools of thought have been proposed as to how waves are replenished and sustain AF (Figs. 36–2 and 36–3).

In the first theory, disordered wavelets self-replenish. This concept was developed in computer modeling studies by Gordon Moe then supported by mapping of induced AF in canine atria by Allessie et al. Replenishment can occur by collision of unstable reentrant waves or foci. This mechanism has been supported by intraoperative mapping in patients with permanent AF undergoing cardiac surgery. Wavelets may replenish in many ways, facilitated by structural obstacles such as dissociation between the endocardial and epicardial surfaces of the atrial wall. This theory does not require "special regions" of the atria, and it implies that extensive ablation is required to treat AF. It is not clear from this theory how limited ablation of the pulmonary vein regions can be effective in many patients.[14,15]

The second theory proposes that localized "special regions" in AF in the form of drivers activate too rapidly for surrounding tissue to keep up and thus cause AF. The concept of small rapidly rotating circuits in the heart was pioneered by Krinsky and Winfree then shown in optical mapping of a sheep heart by Davidenko, Jalife, and colleagues.[16,17] Rotational and focal drivers of AF have been identified in human atria by optical mapping[18] near regions of fibrosis, and in patients by various clinical mapping tools. Limitations of this theory are that the tools required to show these proposed mechanisms in patients are complex, the results of ablating these mechanisms in patients have been mixed, and this mechanism may not apply to all patients.[19]

Structural Remodeling

The atria of patients with AF often show structural remodeling. The best appreciated form is left atrial enlargement, which is seen in many AF patients and correlates with disease progression and outcome.[11] A spherical left atrium, rather than the normal elliptical shape, also confers risk for AF recurrence after cardioversion or ablation.[20] Studies have shown that AF patients have worse prognosis if the right atrium is also enlarged. Atrial enlargement provides more atrial tissue to harbor disordered wavelets or drivers, and also correlates with the presence of fibrosis.[21] The lower incidence of AF in Africans and Asians compared to Caucasians may be attributable to a smaller size and altered geometry of the left atrium.

There is increasing interest in the link between AF and atrial fibrosis. Fibrosis was initially considered a bystander of aging, but there is autopsy evidence that fibrosis co-migrates with AF rather than age per se.[21] Atrial fibrosis causes heterogeneous electrical repolarization and conduction, and in optical mapping studies of human AF may facilitate multiple wavelet reentry or anchor driver regions.[22] There is active investigation into the optimal approaches to identify atrial fibrosis in vivo. Promising techniques include increased signal intensity on gadolinium-enhanced magnetic resonance imaging (MRI),[23] or low amplitude electrical signals at invasive electrophysiology study.

Periatrial Epicardial Adipose Tissue

The mechanisms that explain the association between obesity and AF are unclear. Pericardial fat comprises *paracardial adipose tissue* that lies outside visceral pericardium, and *epicardial adipose tissue* (EAT; Fig. 36–3) that lies between the visceral pericardium and epicardium. EAT may contribute to the pathophysiology of AF through secreted adipokines, inflammatory cytokines, and reactive oxygen species leading to fibrotic remodeling.[24] In the Framingham Heart cohort of 3217 participants, pericardial fat volume quantified by computed tomography (CT) associated independently with AF. EAT volume is associated with the incidence of persistent AF, with recurrent AF after cardioversion, and potentially with recurrent AF after ablation.[24] It is unclear if EAT relates to dietary fat intake or if EAT is a therapeutic target.

AF Mechanisms at the Cellular and Molecular Level

Electrical remodeling in AF patients takes the form of shortened atrial refractory periods from downregulation of Ca^{2+} currents, shortened repolarization and hyperpolarization of atrial cells from increased outward K^+ currents,[25] and conduction slowing from altered expression and localization of connexins between myocytes. These factors interact with structural remodeling, ischemia, stretch and autonomic nervous activity, and promote reentry and automatic ectopic firing. Principal cellular mechanisms for AF include abnormalities in calcium signaling, nitroso-redox imbalance, and atrial metabolism (**Fig. 36–4**).

Abnormal calcium signaling has long been associated with AF. Abnormalities in subcellular Ca^{2+}-dependent signaling and specifically in Ca^{2+}/calmodulin-dependent protein kinase II (CaMKII) activity cause triggered beats that initiate AF. CaMKII also links intracellular Ca^{2+} with reactive oxygen species that may contribute to atrial remodeling. Inhibitors of CaMKII are being studied as potential antiarrhythmic interventions in AF.[26]

Changes in cardiac nitroso-redox balance are increasingly linked to both the initiation and maintenance of AF, via regional uncoupling of cellular nitric oxide synthase and production of reactive oxygen species that modulate signaling pathways. Oxidation of CaMKII via angiotensin-II increases sarcoplasmic reticulum Ca^{2+} leak through the ryanodine receptor that increases AF susceptibility in mice.[27] Atrial-specific upregulation of small noncoding RNAs may disrupt neuronal nitric oxide signaling, shorten refractoriness, and predispose to AF.[28] Again, these pathways are being investigated as novel therapeutic targets.

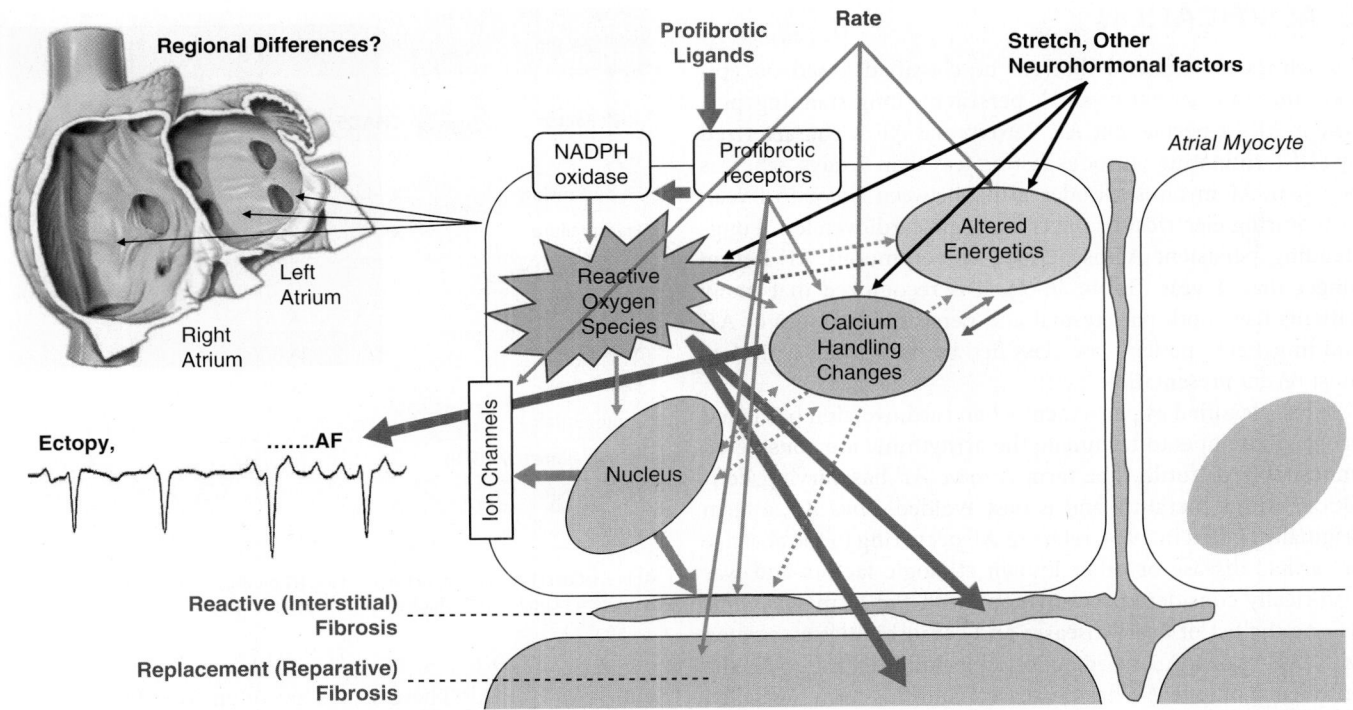

Figure 36–4. Cellular and molecular mechanisms for human AF. Inputs of profibrotic ligands, increased rate, stretch, and other neurohumoral factors engage with several potential mechanisms for AF, each of which vary regionally. Profibrotic ligands of angiotensin II, transforming growth factor 1b (TGF1b), and others drive cytosolic and nuclear mechanisms promoting reactive (interstitial) and replacement (reparative) fibrosis. Reactive oxygen species (ROS) are important contributors. Fibrosis can slow conduction velocity, contribute to wave fractionation and promote AF. Increased activation rate leads to electrical remodeling via altered ion channel function, altered intracellular calcium handling, and altered energetics. These factors cause the formation of early and late afterdepolarizations that can cause AF triggers, and also promote AF maintaining mechanisms. Genetic factors contribute to each mechanism via mutations with large effect sizes and multiple variants with smaller effect sizes.

Abnormal atrial metabolism is a novel mechanistic avenue in AF. Aerobic metabolism in the heart is essential to prevent acidosis and pump fatigue, and each sinus rhythm beat expends 2% of myocardial ATP stores.[29] Accordingly, rapid atrial and ventricular rates in AF introduce considerable metabolic challenges. Clinically, diabetes mellitus, obesity, HF, and thyroid abnormalities comigrate with AF and have been shown to affect atrial metabolism. Such metabolic abnormalities may drive abnormalities in calcium homeostasis, abnormal nitroso-redox state, and electrical and structural remodeling.[29]

AF Mechanisms at the Genetic Level

The heritability of AF, which indicates the proportion of phenotypic variability in AF that is explainable by genetic factors, is estimated to be as high as 62%.[30] In families with an inherited tendency to AF, so-called *familial AF*, individuals have a 40% risk of developing AF.[30] The lower incidence of AF in Africans and Asians versus Caucasians may also be attributable to specific single nucleotide polymorphisms such as one identified on chromosome 10.[31]

The mechanisms for this heritability in AF likely fall into three categories. Rare coding variations with a large effect size occur in families with AF. These include germline mutations that can be passed on to offspring and somatic mutations such as in the connexin gene *GJA5*, which impairs cell-to-cell connectivity and conduction and may facilitate reentrant AF. However, most mutations have a less clear functional role. While monogenic or polygenic variants that confer a large AF risk may be discovered in the future, they would be expected to be family-specific and not broadly generalizable.

Common variations identified by genome-wide association studies (GWAS) confer a smaller additive risk. The first reported example in AF was a region at the 4q25 locus, upstream of the transcription factor gene *PITX2c*. This region regulates chirality in the heart and other organs, although its precise contribution to AF is unclear. Many GWAS-identified variants in AF have been reported, with over 100 susceptibility signals in a recent biobank-based GWAS study in more than 1 million individuals.[32] Linking them to clinical AF phenotypes is an ongoing challenge. While specific variants may correlate with racial predispositions to AF, genetic susceptibility signals for AF appear to correlate poorly with response to therapy.[33]

Other ongoing lines of investigation are focusing on undiscovered genetic mechanisms for AF such as inherited or acquired epigenetic modifications, somatic variations and mosaicisms, rare variants with strong effects, or large or small copy number variants.

CLASSIFICATION

Guidelines recommend that AF be classified based on episode duration as paroxysmal, persistent, long-standing persistent AF, or permanent AF. Paroxysmal AF is characterized by self-terminating episodes lasting less than 7 days, whereas persistent AF involves episodes lasting between 7 days to 1 year, or requiring electrical or pharmacologic cardioversion. Long-standing persistent AF is defined as continuous AF lasting longer than 1 year (**Table 36-2**). It is recognized that many patients have both paroxysmal and persistent episodes of AF, and in general, patients are classified by their more typical or most recent presentation.[34]

AF is classified as permanent when cardioversion has failed or when attempts to terminate the arrhythmia are considered undesirable or futile. The term *chronic AF* has varying definitions in the literature and is best avoided. *Lone AF*, a term originally coined in 1954, refers to AF occurring in the absence of cardiac disease or other known etiologic factors and was historically considered synonymous with the term *idiopathic AF*. As the list of heart diseases and comorbidities associated with AF expands, and diagnostic techniques improve, the prevalence of lone AF has decreased, and this term has fallen out of favor. *Subclinical AF* can be defined as atrial high-rate episodes (AHRE, defined as atrial tachyarrhythmia episodes with rate >190 bpm) of >6 minutes and <24 hours with a lack of correlated symptoms in patients with implantable cardiac devices.[35] This group may have a lower rate of clinical events than patients with traditionally established clinical AF. In ASSERT (Asymptomatic Atrial Fibrillation and Stroke Evaluation in Pacemaker Patients and the AF Reduction Atrial Pacing Trial), patients with subclinical AF had a rate of thromboembolic events similar to individuals without subclinical AF, while patients with AF of ≥24 hours duration had a rate similar to those with clinical AF.[35]

Classification of AF based on 7-day and 1-year time points has been criticized as having limited utility in disease management and little pathophysiologic basis. Clinical risk scores are often used to classify AF patients based on risk for thromboembolic stroke, such as the CHA_2DS_2-VASc score, or risk for bleeding, the more common being ATRIA, $HEMORR_2HAGES$,

TABLE 36-3. Risk Factor Scoring Systems for Stroke in Patients with AF

Risk Factor	$CHADS_2$	CHA_2DS_2-VASc	ABC	ATRIA
Age	X	X	X	X
Hypertension	X	X		X
Heart failure	X	X		X
Diabetes mellitus	X	X		X
Prior stroke/TIA	X	X	X	
Vascular disease		X		
Female sex		X		X
Proteinuria				X
Renal failure (by eGFR)				X
NT-proBNP			X	
cTn-hs			X	

Abbreviations: TIA, transient ischemic attack; NT-proBNP, N terminal pro b-type natriuretic peptide; cTn-hs, high sensitivity cardiac troponin

and HAS-BLED.[36] These scores are often used to guide therapy, such as prescribing oral anticoagulant therapy for patients with CHA_2DS_2-VASc ≥2, or assigning elevated bleeding risk in patients with HAS-BLED ≥2. However, these risks typically compete in the same patient, since each is associated with similar comorbidities. The CHA_2DS_2-VASc score for thromboembolic risk assigns points (in parentheses) for *Cardiac* failure (1), *Hypertension* (1), *Age* ≥75 years (2), *Diabetes* mellitus (1), prior *Stroke* or thromboembolic event (2), *Vascular* disease including coronary arterial disease (1), *Age* ≥65 years (1), and female *Sex* category (1). A score ≥ 2, recently modified to be a score of ≥3 in women, is a typical indication for systemic oral anticoagulation. The ATRIA (AnTicoagulation and Risk factors In AF) score for bleeding assigns points for anemia (3), age ≥75 years (2), severe renal disease (3), prior bleeding (1), and Hypertension (1). A score <4 indicates a low risk for bleeding (**Table 36-3**). The $HEMORR_2HAGES$ score for bleeding risk comprises *Hepatic* or renal disease (1), *Ethanol* abuse (1), *Malignancy* (1), *Older* age (1), *Reduced* platelet count or function (1), *Rebleeding* (2), *Hypertension* (1), *Anemia* (1), *Genetic* factors (1), *Excessive* fall risk (1), and *Stroke* (1). A score of 0 to 1 is low risk, 2 to 3 is intermediate risk, and ≥4 indicates high risk. The HAS-BLED score for bleeding assigns points for *Hypertension* (1), *Abnormal* renal/liver function (1–2), *Stroke* (1), *Bleeding* history or predisposition (1), *Labile* international normalized ratio (1), *Elderly* ≥65 years (1), and *Drugs*/alcohol (1–2). A score ≥2 indicates a higher risk for bleeding (**Table 36-4**).

Several other classification schemes have been proposed, including those based on EHRA (European Heart Rhythm Association) symptom scores or CCS-SAF (Canadian Cardiovascular Society Severity in Atrial Fibrillation) symptom scores. In a recent randomized trial, a simple index of AF episode duration <24 hours identified patients with better outcomes from catheter ablation than those with episodes ≥24 hours.[37]

TABLE 36-2. Classification of Atrial Fibrillation

Classification	Definition
Paroxysmal AF	Self-terminating AF episodes <7 days
Persistent AF	AF episodes lasting 1 week to 1 year, or requiring cardioversion
Longstanding persistent AF	Continuous AF >1year
Permanent AF	AF when attempts to restore sinus rhythm have been abandoned or are futile
Subclinical AF	AHRE >6min <24hrs on CIED without correlated symptoms[31]

Abbreviations: AHRE, Atrial high-rate episodes; ^CIED, Cardiac implantable electronic device.

TABLE 36–4. Calculation of Bleeding Risk Estimation Scores

ATRIA		HAS-BLED		HEMORR₂HAGES	
Anaemia[1]	3	Hypertension[4]	1	Hepatic[10] or renal disease[2]	1 1
Severe renal disease[2]	3	Abnormal renal[5] or liver function[6]	1 1	Ethanol abuse	1
Age ≥75 yrs	2	Stroke	1	Malignancy	1
Any prior hemorrhage	1	Bleeding	1	Older age (>75 yrs)	1
Hypertension[3]	1	Labile INR[8]	1	Reduced platelet number or function[11]	1
		Elderly (>65 yrs)	1	Rebleeding[12]	2
		Drugs[9] or alcohol	1 1	Hypertension[4]	1
				Anaemia[13]	1
				Genetic factors[18]	1
				Excessive fall risk[19]	1
				Stroke	1

Table superscripts:
[1]Defined as hemoglobin <13 g/dl in men and <12 g/dl in women. [2]Defined as estimated glomerular filtration rate <30 ml/min or dialysis-dependent. [3]Defined as diagnosed hypertension. [4]Defined as systolic blood pressure >160 mmHg. [5]Defined as the presence of chronic dialysis or renal transplantation or serum creatinine ≥200 mmol/L. [6]Defined as chronic hepatic disease (eg cirrhosis) or biochemical evidence of significant hepatic derangement (eg bilirubin 2 × upper limit of normal, in association with aspartate aminotransferase/alanine aminotransferase/alkaline phosphatase >3 × upper limit normal, etc). [8]Refers to unstable/high INRs or poor time in therapeutic range (eg <60%). [9]Refers to concomitant use of drugs, such as antiplatelet agents, nonsteroidal anti-inflammatory drugs, or alcohol abuse etc. [10]Defined as cirrhosis, two-fold or greater elevation of AST or APT, or albumin <3.6 g/dl. [11]Platelets <75,000, use of antiplatelet therapy (eg, daily aspirin) or NSAID therapy; or blood dyscrasia. [12]Prior hospitalization for bleeding. [13]Defined as most recent hematocrit <30 or hemoglobin <10 g/dl. [14]CYP2C9*2 and/or CYP2C9*3. [15]Alzheimer's dementia, Parkinson disease, schizophrenia, or any condition predisposing to repeated falls.

Imaging-based classifications using MRI in another randomized trial showed that patients with more regions of abnormal delayed gadolinium uptake in the atria have lower success after AF ablation.[23]

CLINICAL PRESENTATION AND EVALUATION

Symptoms

Patients with AF may or may not present with symptoms.[34, 35] Typical symptoms include palpitations, rapid heartbeats, shortness of breath, dyspnea on exertion, exercise intolerance, fatigue, dizziness, and chest pain. New onset AF with a rapid ventricular response will often cause a patient to seek urgent medical attention. However, other patients may be unaware of changes in rhythm and may not seek medical attention for weeks or months until complications such as HF (from tachycardia-induced cardiomyopathy) occur. In other patients, the first indication that a patient has AF may be presentation with a stroke or transient ischemic attack.

AF may be the primary problem that brings a patient to medical attention. It also may be a complicating factor of other conditions, such as HF or acute coronary syndromes. Some patients are truly asymptomatic, particularly the elderly, some patients with AF episodes after catheter ablation, and if ventricular response is well controlled. A moderate ventricular rate may reflect intrinsic disease in the AV conduction system or concurrent use of β-blockers or calcium channel blockers for reasons such as hypertension that then moderate the ventricular response. Some patients may deny symptoms, or ascribe symptoms such as exercise intolerance to aging, only to realize a much better sense of well-being if sinus rhythm can be restored. This observation is supported by several studies showing that quality of life is adversely affected by AF.

Hemodynamic consequences of AF due to rapid heart rates, loss of atrial contraction, irregularity of the rhythm, bradycardia upon conversion to sinus rhythm from AF, or long pauses while in AF may all contribute to symptoms.

Clinical Evaluation

Clinical evaluation starts with a comprehensive history and physical examination. Aside from presenting symptoms, any history of cardiovascular disease should be elicited. Hypertension, diabetes, obesity, and sleep apnea are all associated with AF. Heavy alcohol intake may promote AF. A history of thyroid disease is relevant, as hyperthyroidism may cause AF. Any past history of cerebrovascular disease is also important, due to the propensity for AF to be associated with stroke or transient ischemic attacks.

On physical examination, attention should be paid to the irregularity of the pulse or heart sounds, to determine whether the patient is currently in AF. Auscultation of the heart is performed to detect evidence of valvular heart disease that may lead to AF. Mitral stenosis and regurgitation are the conditions most likely to be associated with AF, as both may eventually result in marked enlargement of the left atrium. Mitral stenosis may be associated with a malar flush. Due to the loss of atrial contraction in AF, an S4 will not be present. Evidence of fluid overload such as rales and peripheral edema may be present if the patient is in HF.

Patients should have basic laboratory tests such as a blood count, serum electrolytes, and assessment of renal, hepatic, and thyroid function. A chest x-ray may be indicated if the patient has pulmonary disease or signs of HF. If the latter is present, then measurement of B-type natriuretic peptide is indicated as well. An echocardiogram is performed to assess the patient for valvular heart disease, LV hypertrophy and ejection fraction, cardiomyopathy, and left atrial size. A high left atrial "sphericity index," which can be determined by transthoracic echocardiography, is associated with recurrence of AF after cardioversion or ablation.[16,40]

Assessment of a patient for ischemic heart disease should not be pursued solely because the patient has been diagnosed with AF, but only if it is suspected from other aspects of the history, physical examination, ECG, or echocardiogram. An exercise treadmill test may be reasonable if a patient, especially middle-aged or older, is being considered for therapy with Class Ic antiarrhythmic drugs (flecainide, propafenone) that are contraindicated in, or ablation or surgical therapies that may be influenced by, the presence of ischemic heart disease.

Other imaging studies such as cardiac MRI are not routinely indicated in the evaluation of a patient with AF. However, there is interest in the finding that greater abnormalities in delayed gadolinium enhancement on MRI, which may indicate atrial scar, can identify patients at higher risk of recurrence after AF ablation.[19] Left atrial 4D flow cardiac MRI has been used to demonstrate reduced left atrial blood flow velocities in patients with AF that may be predictive of the risk of stroke.[41]

Electrocardiography and Rhythm Monitoring

Every patient suspected of having AF should have an ECG (**Fig. 36–5**). The ECG may confirm the diagnosis of AF, and it may also provide evidence of structural heart disease such as left atrial enlargement or prior myocardial infarction. Because AF is often paroxysmal at initial presentation and an ECG only gives a 10-second snapshot of rhythm, longer monitoring is often necessary for further evaluation. The decision as to the type of monitor to use depends on the frequency of a patient's symptoms, the typical duration of symptoms when they occur, whether they are symptomatic or not, and whether the goal is diagnosis or monitoring for recurrence of AF after procedures such as catheter ablation. Options for monitoring are summarized in **Table 36–5**.

An ambulatory Holter monitor is usually worn for 24 to 48 hours and captures all rhythm data for that period of time. It requires the use of electrodes attached to the patient's skin that are connected to a portable device that records the ECG rhythm continuously. The data are analyzed after the Holter is removed and thus monitoring is not real time. If a patient has frequent

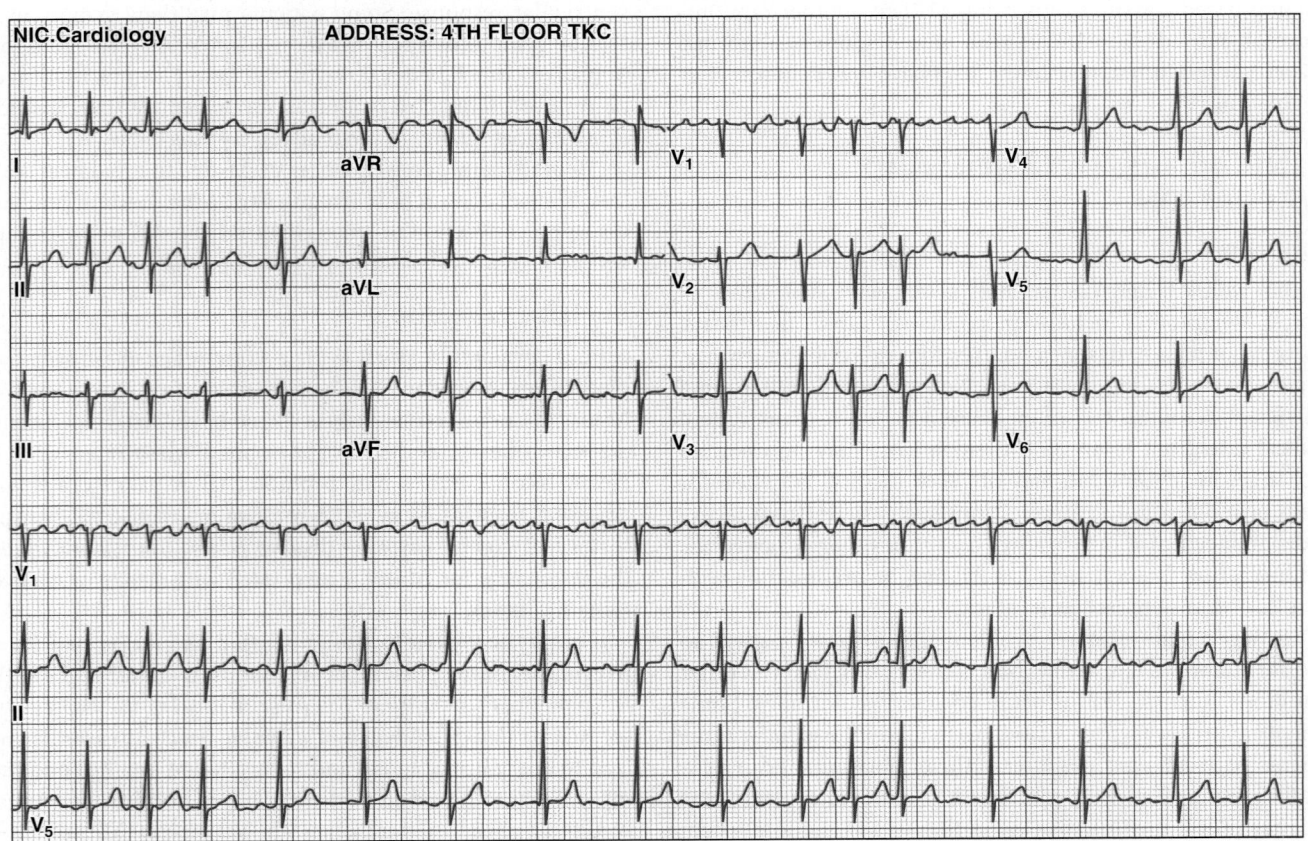

Figure 36–5. Twelve-lead ECG of atrial fibrillation. Note the rapid, irregular, low-amplitude fibrillatory waves with varying morphology and an irregularly irregular ventricular response.

TABLE 36–5. Rhythm Diagnosis and Monitoring Options for Atrial Fibrillation

Type	Description	Advantages	Disadvantages
ECG	12-leads; 10 second duration	Immediate diagnosis of rhythm; provides evidence of other structural heart disease	Not useful alone for detecting paroxysmal AF or for assessing AF burden
Holter monitor	External monitor with electrodes worn for 24 hours	Confirms diagnosis when AF is frequent; correlates symptoms with rhythm; provides heart rate range and mean heart rate for assessing rate control	Unlikely to provide diagnosis for patients with infrequent symptoms
Event monitor	External monitor with electrodes worn up to 30 days	Continuous loop recording of rhythm; stores events when activated by patient or automatically as programmed	No real-time assessment; more cumbersome for patient to use over duration of recording
Mobile cardiac outpatient telemetry	External monitor with electrodes; rhythm transmitted via receiver to monitoring station	Continuous monitoring of heart rhythm with constant oversight to detect and act on abnormalities in real time	More expensive; not practical for monitoring over periods longer than 30 days
ECG Patch	~5 x 14 cm patch attached by adhesive to infraclavicular area for 14 days	ECG electrodes are imbedded in patch; relatively unobtrusive for continuous monitoring	No real time analysis; uncomfortable for some; patch is mailed back for subsequent interpretation
Photoplethysmography	In many wearables such as fitness trackers; detects rate and regularity of rhythm	May alert a patient to an irregular or fast rhythm that could represent a new diagnosis or recurrence of AF	No ECG; AF needs to be confirmed independently by other monitoring technologies
Portable ECG electrodes/app; KardiaMobile	Lightweight, handheld device with electrodes to record rhythm on app	Easy for patient to use; unobtrusive; no electrodes attached to patient	Only records rhythm when patient opens app and applies fingers to electrodes
Smart Watch	Records single-lead ECG by holding finger on crown of watch	Watch is always on patient and ready to use; irregular rhythm alert can prompt patient to record ECG	Only records rhythm when patient opens app and applies fingers to electrodes
Insertable loop recorder	Device implanted via a small incision in prepectoral area	Provides continuous monitoring of rhythm for up to 3 years, including AF burden; download events during clinic visits or remotely	Requires minimally invasive procedure; Lacks immediate feedback; slight risk of infection
Pacemakers, ICDs	Continuous monitoring of rhythm including elevated atrial rates	Easy for specialist to follow rhythm and results of interventions such as ablation without additional monitoring device	Only applicable to patients who already have implanted devices; Lacks immediate feedback.

Abbreviations: AF, atrial fibrillation; ECG, electrocardiogram; ICDs, implantable cardioverter defibrillators

episodes of AF, a Holter may be sufficient for diagnosis. If a patient is in persistent AF, a Holter will provide information on the minimum, maximum, and mean ventricular rates. This information is most useful for assessing the adequacy of rate control, maximum heart rates during daily exertion, and minimum rates and pauses during the night, at the time of highest vagal tone. However, for patients with infrequent symptoms, a Holter is often not the best monitoring technology to use. While one can use Holters for up to 72 hours, the incremental benefit beyond 24 hours is low.

If monitoring for longer periods is needed, there are ambulatory monitors, also known as event recorders or external loop recorders, that are set up similarly to a Holter monitor but can be used for 14 to 30 days. They perform continuous loop recording of cardiac rhythm and will save a 1- to 3-lead rhythm strip encompassing the time before and after patient activation for symptoms, or whenever predetermined parameters are exceeded (tachycardia or bradycardia). When detecting AF in patients who have had a cryptogenic stroke or transient ischemic attack, the yield of AF lasting longer than 30 seconds with a 24-hour Holter monitor was 2.2%, increasing to 11.6% with 2 weeks of recording, and 14.8% with 4 weeks

of monitoring.[42] Other devices monitor the patient actively throughout the recording period and use a portable receiver to transmit rhythm data to a remote receiving center, an approach called mobile cardiac outpatient telemetry. A newer technology uses a patch applied to the infraclavicular area. Separate electrodes are not necessary, nor is there a separate recording device that must be worn by the patient, making this approach more convenient and unobtrusive for the patient. The patch is removed after 14 days and returned for analysis. While real-time monitoring is not possible with this system, it can provide information on AF burden (amount of time in AF divided by the total monitoring time period). Any of these types of monitors are useful for capturing short episodes of arrhythmias, as no action by the patient is necessary at the time they occur. Patients are asked to keep track of symptoms while wearing these monitors to correlate them with the cardiac rhythm at the time of analysis.

Newer wearable technologies have begun to revolutionize the way we diagnose and monitor AF.[43,44] One approach to record the heart rhythm directly uses a small, lightweight set of two electrodes that allow recording of a lead I rhythm strip when the patient places their fingers on each electrode. The device stores the ECG via an app on the patient's smart phone and can provide an instant analysis of "normal," "possible AF," or "indeterminate" based on an algorithm. The rhythm tracing can be uploaded to the cloud and then accessed for review by the physician. There is now a version of this device that uses a third electrode and records all six limb leads. While this technology is very easy for a patient to use, it is only useful for assessing the rhythm at the time of a patient's symptoms, because it only captures 30 seconds of the cardiac rhythm for any one recording. Also, any symptoms need to last long enough to allow a patient to open the app, take out the device and apply the fingers to it, and then wait 30 seconds. More transient symptoms require more constant monitoring to capture them.

Other smartphone-based solutions use an app to analyze the pulsatile signal acquired by illuminating the fingertip using a smart phone light-emitting diode and imaging-reflected light with a camera (photoplethysmography) to detect pulsatile fluctuations and AF in real time.[43,45] A meta-analysis of smart phone photoplethysmography apps for detecting AF found a positive predictive value ranging from 19.3% to 37.5%, and a negative predictive value of 99.8% to 99.9%.[41] Another wearable technology uses a smart watch to analyze the regularity of the heart rhythm and provide an alert if irregularity is detected. The Apple Watch Study enrolled 419,297 participants with no history of AF and found that 2161 (0.52%) received a notification of an irregular pulse. Patients were advised to wear a patch monitor to confirm the diagnosis. Of the 450 participants who did so, AF was confirmed in 34%.[46] Other reasons for irregularity can be frequent ectopic atrial or ventricular beats or even artifact, and paroxysmal AF, being transient by definition, may be absent in any subsequent 2-week period, which collectively may explain why confirmation of arrhythmia was fairly low. In contrast, the MAFA II Study (Mobile Health Technology for Improved Screening, Patient Involvement and Optimizing Integrated Care in Atrial Fibrillation) confirmed AF by subsequent ECG monitoring in 87% of patients who had received a notification of "possible AF" by photoplethysmography.[47] The

patients who received an irregular rhythm notification constituted 0.23% of the 187,912 patients screened. The latest generation smart watch not only detects irregularity of rhythm, but it can also record a 1-lead rhythm strip simply by placing one's fingers on the crown and the side of the watch. The rhythm is shown on the watch face with a preliminary interpretation for the patient.

The use of wearable technologies is accelerating rapidly.[43] Areas of active investigation include identification of the optimal population to monitor, the high false positive rate in unselected populations that leads to further testing that may concern a patient unnecessarily, and what to do with results if AF is, indeed, detected. Currently, no study has shown that diagnosis of AF at an early, asymptomatic stage and initiation of treatment such as anticoagulation in high risk patients can effectively prevent future strokes.

For longer-term monitoring over more than 1 year, insertable loop recorders are very useful (**Fig. 36–6A**). These small devices are implanted under the skin in the left infraclavicular or parasternal areas (**Fig. 36–6B**) to record and store tachy- and brady-arrhythmias according to programmable parameters, and to record when a patient presses an activation button such as at the time of symptoms. These devices are used in some patients after catheter ablation to detect recurrences, especially in the course of a clinical trial where outcomes such as recurrences of asymptomatic AF or AF burden would otherwise be difficult to determine. Another use for insertable loop recorders is after cryptogenic stroke. When patients appear to have had an embolic stroke, but they are in sinus rhythm upon presentation, the possibility arises that the patient has had episodes of AF that have not previously been diagnosed. The use of insertable loop recorders has been shown to have a diagnostic yield within six months for AF lasting >30 seconds of 8.9% compared to conventional monitoring at 1.4% (hazard ratio [HR] 6.4; 95% confidence interval [CI], 1.9–21.7; $P < 0.001$).[48]

The yield of different monitoring strategies must be considered when selecting a device to evaluate a specific patient

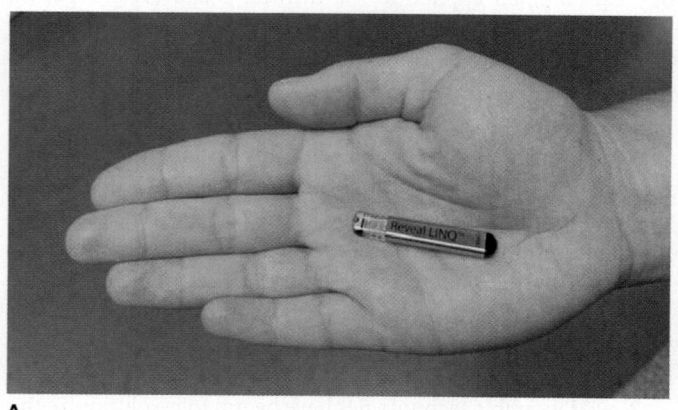

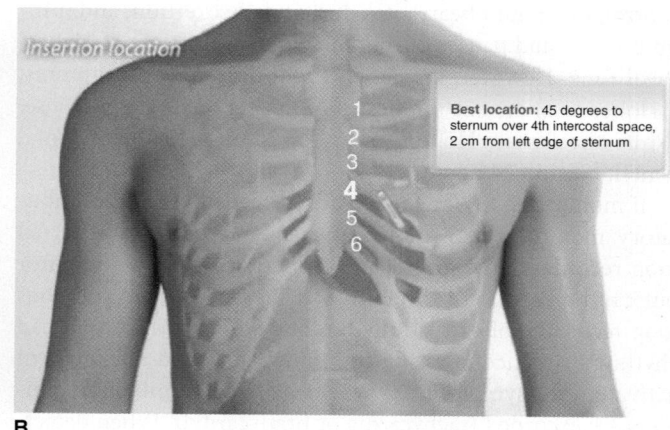

A   **B**

Figure 36–6. (A) Insertable loop recorders are small devices that are implanted under the skin in the prepectoral area. They provide continuous monitoring of cardiac rhythm for up to 3 years. Events are saved either by patient activation during symptoms, or automatically based on programmed parameters. **(B) Optimal location of an insertable loop recorder.** Best location is 45 degrees to sternum over the fourth intercostal space, 2 cm from the left edge of the sternum. Reproduced with permission from AliveCor, Inc.

for AF. A recent study involved implantation of insertable loop recorders in 590 patients with risk factors for stroke but no history of AF. The patients were followed for at least 3 years for AF lasting at least 6 minutes. Random sampling was applied to the complete data set to determine the expected yield for AF from different durations of monitoring. The sensitivity of a 10-second single ECG was 1.5%; it was 8.3% for twice daily 30-second ECGs over 14 days, and 11%, 13%, 15%, 21%, and 34% for a single 24-hour, 48-hour, 72-hour, 7-day, or 30-day continuous monitor. AF detection improved if the same monitoring duration was spread out over a longer period of time compared with a single time period (that is, 3–24 hour Holter monitors at different times rather than one 72-hour monitor).[49]

Any patient with an implanted pacemaker or cardioverter defibrillator effectively has built-in monitoring for AF, as tachyarrhythmias are routinely recorded by these devices.[43] As long as an atrial lead is in place, tachyarrhythmias can be determined to be supraventricular in origin by an atrial rate that is substantially higher than the ventricular rate. Without an atrial lead, rapid, irregular ventricular rhythms may be presumed to represent AF, but with a lesser degree of certainty. One can also determine total AF burden. Many studies of antiarrhythmic drugs and other therapeutic approaches have used patients with these implantable cardiac electrical devices because no separate technology or device is needed in order to collect information on the cardiac rhythm.

Complications

Stroke

Ischemic strokes constitute 85% of all strokes with an identifiable cause. AF substantially increases the risk for ischemic stroke, representing approximately 36% of all strokes in individuals aged 80 to 89 years. Stroke may actually be the first manifestation of previously undiagnosed AF. In cryptogenic strokes (ie, with no cause elucidated on extensive poststroke diagnostic testing), prolonged rhythm monitoring can reveal previously unknown AF in 30% of patients.[48] Individuals with AF are not all at equal risk for stroke, and several predisposing clinical factors may identify those patients at higher risk (subsequently discussed).

Ischemic strokes related to AF usually result from embolism of a thrombus from the left atrium to a large cerebral artery, and therefore they tend to be larger and more frequently fatal or associated with greater disability than strokes from other causes.[50] Most thrombi associated with AF leading to cardioembolic stroke are presumed to arise within the LAA. Flow velocity within the LAA is reduced during AF because of the loss of organized mechanical contraction. Compared with transthoracic echocardiography (TTE), transesophageal echocardiography (TEE) is more sensitive and specific for assessing LAA thrombi and is the most commonly used test to evaluate for their presence. Magnetic resonance angiography (MRA) and contrast CT are emerging imaging modalities to assess for LAA thrombi, and may have comparable sensitivity and specificity to TEE.

Several mechanisms contribute to enhanced thrombogenicity in AF. During AF, hypoxia, stretch, inflammation, and oxidative stress are likely to promote increased endothelial dysfunction and apoptotic cell death, leading to the externalization of normally internalized procoagulant aminophospholipids on the cell membrane. Nitric oxide production in the left atrial endocardium is reduced in experimental AF, with increased levels of the prothrombotic protein plasminogen activator inhibitor 1 (PAI-1), Von Willebrand Factor (vWF), soluble thrombomodulin (sTM), and fibrinogen.[51]

Patients undergoing radiofrequency ablation for AF treatment have an additional increase in platelet- and leukocyte-derived procoagulant microparticles, which is also assumed to be the case for cryoenergy ablative sources. It is therefore important to continue uninterrupted anticoagulation during and after such procedures. A decrease in several apoptotic markers months after the restoration of sinus rhythm has been observed, suggesting that the extent of apoptosis is reversible and that robust rhythm control could potentially normalize thromboembolic risk.[52]

Peripheral Thromboembolism

Patients with AF also have an increased risk of thromboembolic events in the aorta and the renal, mesenteric, pelvic, and extremity arteries, compared with the population not carrying a diagnosis of AF, although at a lower incidence than for stroke. One possible explanation for this observation is that many cerebral arteries are functional end arteries, whereas other arterial systems are protected by collateral circulation and occlusion may not lead to clinical manifestations. Despite their lower overall prevalence, the majority of patients with acute peripheral thromboembolic events may have AF. This includes 60% to 95% of patients undergoing surgical therapy for acute limb ischemia, 31% of patients with splenic arterial emboli, 55% with acute renal ischemia, and 47% with acute mesenteric ischemia. Extracerebral AF-related thromboembolic events are associated with serious clinical consequences, including a high mortality rate.[53]

Dementia

Although the pathophysiology of dementia has several unknowns, there is increasing evidence from registries and databases that AF is an independent risk factor for cognitive dysfunction and dementia compared to similar individuals without AF.[54] The increased rate of dementia in patients with AF is seen across strata of CHA_2DS_2-VASc scores and may be independent of the presence of prior clinical stroke or transient ischemic attack.[55] Some observational studies show that patients with AF who received oral anticoagulant therapy had a lower prevalence of dementia than those who did not, supporting the presence of multi-infarct (vascular) dementia at least in some cases. This is the basis for an ongoing randomized trial using oral anticoagulants to reduce incident dementia in patients with AF.[56] Overall, AF appears to be associated with a general increase in risk for dementia, including nonvascular phenotypes. The impact of rhythm control is uncertain. In large registry studies, patients who received catheter ablation for AF had a lower rate of dementia than those who did not.[57] Whether this reflects selection bias or a real benefit of rhythm

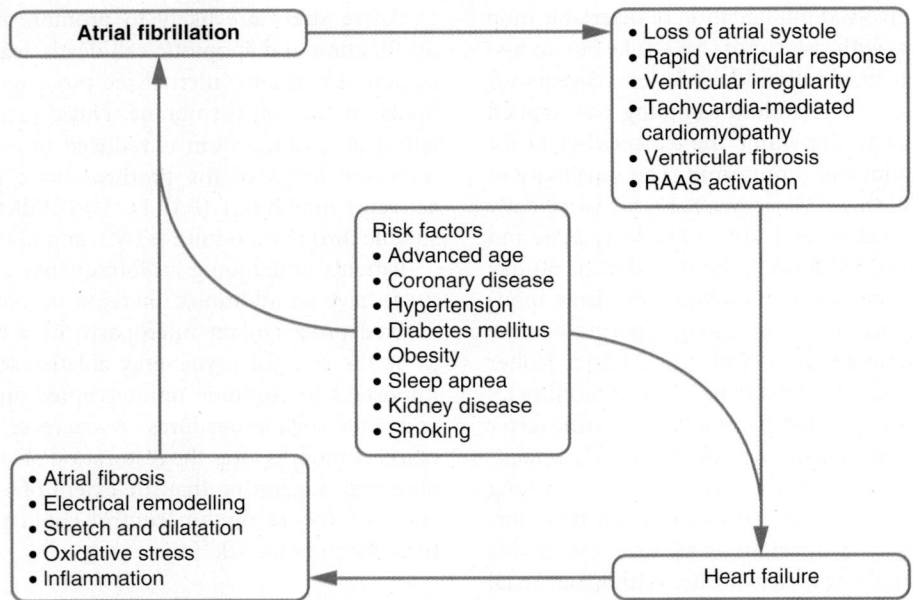

Figure 36–7. Pathophysiological interactions between AF and HF. AF and HF can perpetuate each other through shared risk factors, hemodynamic changes, and structural changes. AF, atrial fibrillation; HF, heart failure; RAAS, renin–angiotensin–aldosterone system.[58] Reproduced with permission from Ling LH, Kistler PM, Kalman JM, et al. Comorbidity of atrial fibrillation and heart failure. *Nat Rev Cardiol.* 2016 Mar;13(3):131-147.

control on the pathophysiology of dementia remains to be determined.

Adverse Hemodynamic Effects

Adverse hemodynamic effects of AF include loss of atrial contraction, loss of AV synchrony, and rapid and irregular ventricular rhythm. All of these effects impair diastolic filling. Atrial systole normally increases ventricular end-diastolic volume by up to 25%, with a corresponding increase in end-diastolic pressure and stroke volume through the Frank–Starling mechanism. The loss of mechanical AV synchrony may have a dramatic impact on ventricular filling and cardiac output when there is reduced ventricular compliance, as is the case with diastolic dysfunction, restrictive cardiomyopathy, mitral stenosis, constrictive pericarditis, or right ventricular failure. In all these conditions, patients typically experience marked hemodynamic deterioration when in AF. In addition to the loss of atrial systole, rapid ventricular rates also result in limited diastolic ventricular filling. The irregular ventricular contraction has adverse hemodynamic effects that are independent of the ventricular rate at the same heart rate, further contributing to reduced stroke volume.[58]

Heart Failure

AF and HF coexist in up to 30% of patients, and the combination may result in particularly poor clinical outcomes. In patients with existing HF, the development of AF doubles mortality, and in patients with existing AF, the development of HF triples mortality.[58]

In occasional patients, the first clinical manifestation of AF may be HF secondary to tachycardia. The clinical syndrome of *tachycardia-mediated cardiomyopathy* generally occurs in patients who have minimal other symptoms from AF and who present with shortness of breath and overt signs of HF. Patients typically have high ventricular rates (usually >120 bpm) for prolonged periods often of months to years, which leads to deterioration of LV function. In the absence of other concurrent causes of cardiomyopathy, LV dysfunction is reversible with improved rate control or rhythm control within weeks to months.[58]

Although epidemiological data suggest that AF and HF tend to coexist, insights into causal relationships between these two conditions are lacking (**Fig. 36-7**).[58]

MANAGEMENT

The management of AF should assess the multiple potential comorbidities of AF and their sequelae, which should ideally involve a multidisciplinary team approach (**Fig. 36–8**).

Acute Management

When a patient presents with AF, hemodynamic status and the severity of symptoms dictate how urgently one must slow the heart rate or restore sinus rhythm. Hypotension, markedly elevated heart rates, severe chest pain, shortness of breath, decompensated HF, or evidence of ischemia are all observations that may prompt consideration of urgent cardioversion (**Fig. 36–9**). AF in association with Wolff-Parkinson-White syndrome may be associated with particularly rapid heart rates with wide, preexcited QRS complexes on the ECG that may degenerate to ventricular fibrillation, and urgent cardioversion should be considered (**Fig. 36–10**).

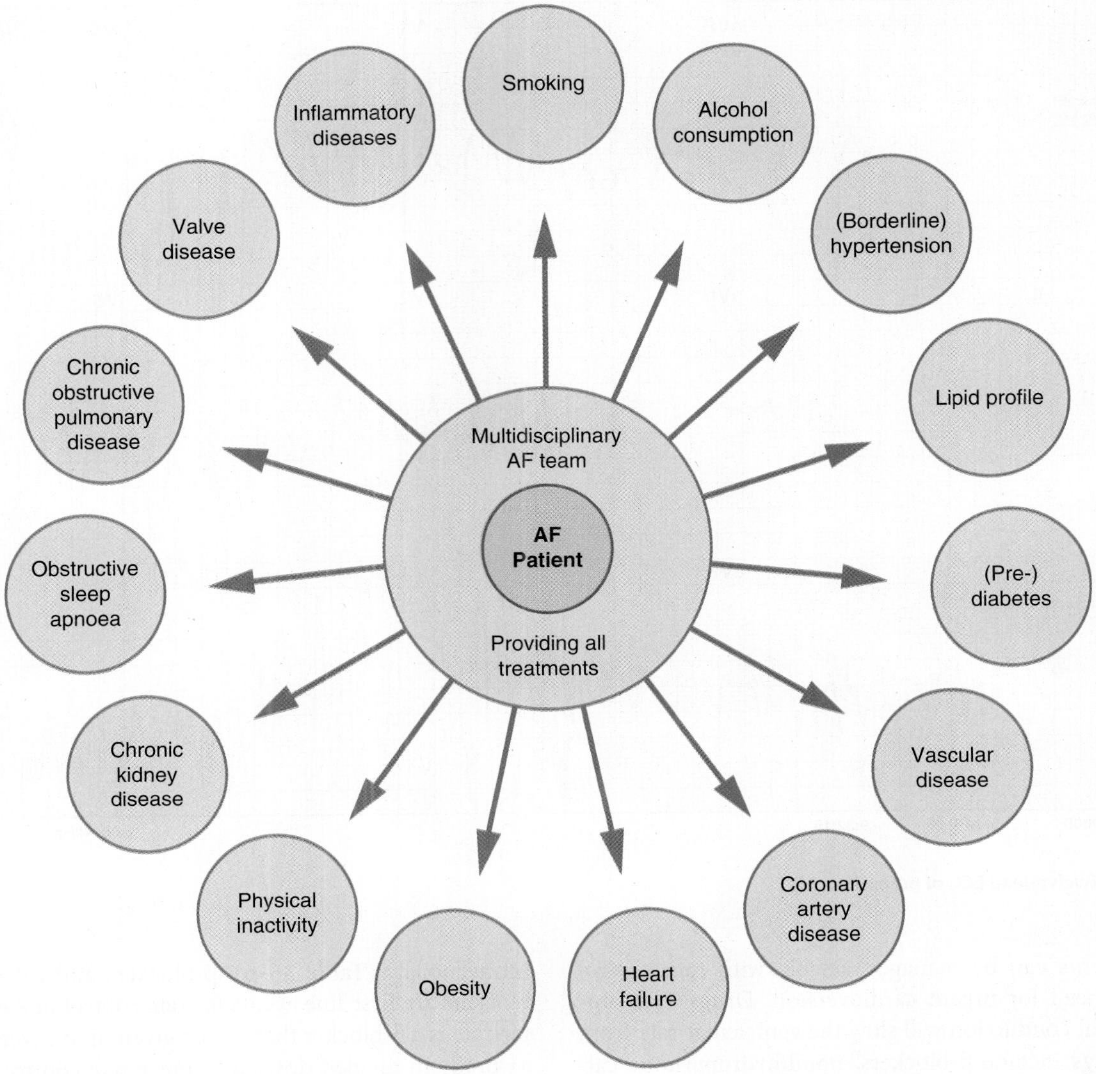

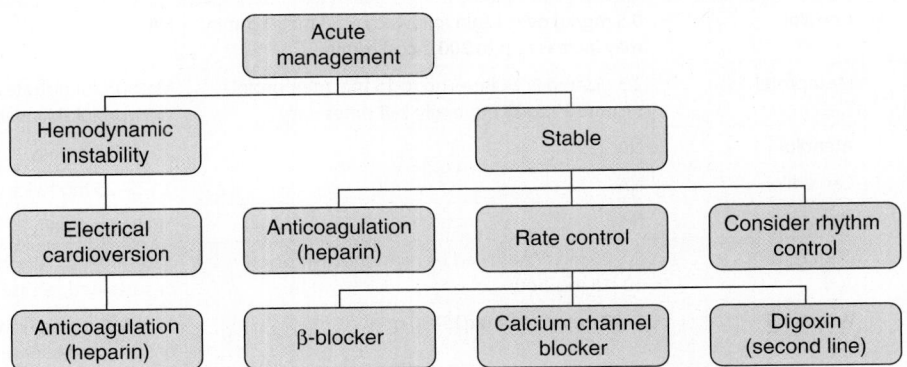

Figure 36–8. Risk factors and underlying comorbidities to be addressed in chronic comprehensive management of AF. Reproduced with permission from Brandes A, Smit MD, Nguyen BO, et al. Risk Factor Management in Atrial Fibrillation. *Arrhythm Electrophysiol Rev.* 2018 Jun;7(2):118-127.

Figure 36–9. Acute management of AF. Initial assessment should focus on the hemodynamice stability of the patient and associated conditions. If a patient presents with AF with a rapid ventricular response and exhibits findings such as severe hypotension, ischemia, or decompensated HF, urgent electrical cardioversion may be necessary. The patient should be adequately sedated first if at all possible. Anticoagulation with heparin should be started as well. For patients who are more stable, anticoagulation can be initiated at the same time as drugs to slow the ventricular rate. β-blockers and nondihyropyridine calcium channel blockers are first line agents for this indication, with digoxin used only if rate control is still not adequate.

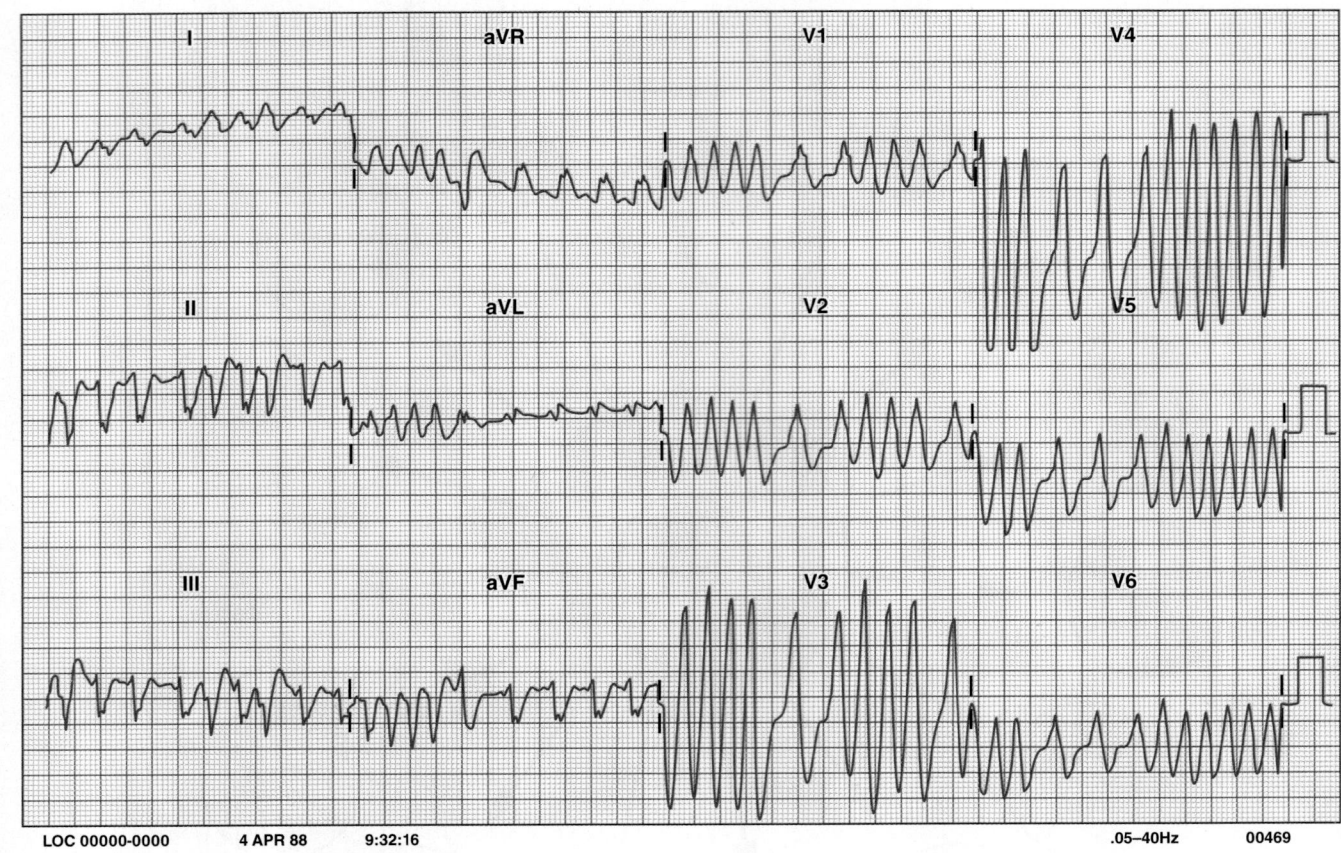

Figure 36–10. Twelve-lead ECG of preexcited AF.

Most patients can be managed acutely with rate control without the need for urgent cardioversion. Drugs that suppress AV nodal conduction will slow the ventricular rate from AF. Such drugs include β-blockers, nondihydropyridine calcium channel blockers, and digoxin, all of which can be given intravenously (**Table 36–6**). β-blockers and calcium channel blockers are first-line agents for rate control in AF. Metoprolol tartrate is a β-blocker that can be given in intravenous boluses, or orally in divided doses to achieve rate control. It is best to avoid metoprolol succinate in the acute setting, as the onset

TABLE 36–6. Pharmacologic Rate Control in Atrial Fibrillation

Drug Category	Drug	Acute Rate Control	Chronic Rate Control
β-Blockers	Esmolol	0.5 mg/kg over 1 min followed by 50 mcg/kg/min; may increase up to 200 mcg/kg/min	NA
	Metoprolol	2.5–5.0 mg IV boluses up to 15 mg; metoprolol tartrate 12.5–25 mg orally 2–4 times daily	Metoprolol tartrate 25–100 mg twice daily; metoprolol succinate 25–200 mg daily
	Atenolol	NA	25–100 mg daily
	Carvedilol	NA	3.125–25 mg twice daily
	Nadolol	NA	10–240 mg daily
Calcium Channel Blockers	Diltiazem	20–25 mg IV followed by continuous infusion 10–15 mg/hour	120–480 mg daily in divided doses, or sustained release daily
	Verapamil	5–10 mg IV; repeat q15–30 min	120–360 mg daily in divided doses, or sustained release daily
Cardiac Glycoside	Digoxin	0.125–0.25 mg IV; repeat q6h up to 1.0 mg	0.125 mg daily*
Multichannel Antiarrhythmic Drug	Amiodarone	150–300 mg IV; 1 mg/min for 6 h, then 0.5 mg/min	100–200 mg daily

Abbreviations: IV, intravenous; NA, not applicable.
*Dose adjustment necessary for abnormal renal function.

of action is too slow. Patients who are treated with metoprolol tartrate in the inpatient setting can be converted to metoprolol succinate for long-term use. Esmolol is a short acting intravenous β-blocker administered as a bolus followed by an infusion that can be increased sequentially to 200 mcg/kg/min if rate control is not achieved by lower doses. Diltiazem is administered as an initial bolus intravenously followed by a constant infusion. Verapamil is another calcium channel blocker that is effective in slowing AV nodal conduction. It is administered in divided doses every 15 to 30 minutes, provided that blood pressure remains stable. Digoxin is used infrequently in contemporary practice, but it may be added to either calcium channel blockers or β-blockers for better rate control, especially in patients with HF with reduced ejection fraction, acknowledging that its onset of action is slower in the acute setting. When used, it is typically administered in divided doses every 6 hours to a total dose of 1.0 mg to 1.5 mg. While intravenous amiodarone can help to slow the heart rate, it is not a first-line drug for this purpose. In addition, it could lead to chemical cardioversion to sinus rhythm and risk for a thromboembolic event if a patient is not adequately anticoagulated prior to its use.

Cardioversion

Electrical Cardioversion

If there are urgent reasons to restore sinus rhythm, one should proceed with cardioversion regardless of the anticoagulation status of the patient. Anticoagulation should be started as soon as possible and continued for at least 4 weeks after cardioversion. If cardioversion is less urgent, it is important to consider whether anticoagulation is necessary in order to avoid a thromboembolic event at the time of or after cardioversion. Key factors to consider are the duration of AF and the CHA_2DS_2-VASc score of the patient. For AF or atrial flutter of more than 48 hours duration or in patients with a CHA_2DS_2-VASc score of ≥ 2 in men and ≥ 3 in women, transesophageal echocardiography is usually performed to exclude the presence of thrombus in the left atrium if a patient is not already on chronic oral anticoagulation. In the latter case, patients should be started on heparin or a direct oral anticoagulant as soon as possible before cardioversion. If thrombus is found, cardioversion should be postponed and the patient treated for at least 3 weeks with oral anticoagulation before performing cardioversion preceded by repeat imaging to assess resolution of thrombus. If no atrial thrombus is detected, then cardioversion may proceed immediately.

Electrical cardioversion is performed using adhesive gel electrodes placed anteriorly over the sternum and posteriorly to the left of the spine. If cardioversion is not successful, other electrode positions such as to the right or lateral to the sternum can be tried. Shocks must be synchronized to the R wave, so it is important to ensure that adequate sensing of the R wave is present before proceeding. Adequate sedation of the patient is necessary before proceeding with cardioversion. Biphasic shocks are used routinely, usually starting around 200 joules. If the initial shock is unsuccessful, shock energy may be increased sequentially to the maximum output of the

defibrillator, 360 joules. A recent study that compared using 360 joule shocks up to three times if necessary compared to lower dose, escalating shocks of 125–150–200 joules showed that the high energy shocks more often restored sinus rhythm (88% vs. 66%, $P < 0.001$).[59] If sinus rhythm is still not restored after several shocks, one can apply direct pressure to the anterior electrode (or both electrodes in the anterior-lateral configuration) to lower impedance. Another option is to administer ibutilide intravenously, because this drug has been shown to facilitate cardioversion when shocks alone are unsuccessful. In patients considered at high risk for recurrent AF, particularly those with persistent AF, it may be prudent to consider loading the patient with an antiarrhythmic drug prior to cardioversion, in an attempt to prevent early recurrence of AF.

After cardioversion, all patients should be treated with anticoagulation for a minimum of 4 weeks. Decisions about long-term treatment with anticoagulation should be based on the thromboembolic risk profile of the patient (CHA_2DS_2-VASc score) and the bleeding risk profile (HAS-BLED score and others)[60] (Tables 36–3 and 36–4). If warfarin is used in a patient who is going to undergo elective cardioversion, the patient needs to have a therapeutic INR (international normalized ratio) of at least 2.0 for at least 3 consecutive weeks prior to performing cardioversion, and at least 4 weeks after cardioversion. The need to continue anticoagulation after cardioversion for at least this amount of time reflects the fact that atrial hypocontractility may occur from a combination of the duration of time in AF, the presence of atrial substrates including fibrosis, and the acute effects of cardioversion ("stunning"). Normal atrial function may take up to a month to recover after cardioversion, and thromboembolic events have been reported if anticoagulation is discontinued early within this period.

It was previously thought that patients with AF of less than 48 hours' duration may be cardioverted without the need for anticoagulation before or after cardioversion. There are actually limited data to support that approach, and recent studies show that this approach should be modified at least in patients with comorbidities. In the Finnish Cardioversion Study (FinCV), embolic complications were analyzed after 5116 cardioversions in 2481 patients with AF lasting <48 hours. Patients had neither had oral anticoagulation prior to cardioversion nor periprocedural heparin therapy. There were 38 (0.7%) definite thromboembolic events (31 strokes) within 30 days (median 2 days, mean 4.6 days) after cardioversion, and four patients suffered transient ischemic attacks. Age, female sex, HF, and diabetes were the independent predictors of definite embolic events, with the highest risk of thromboembolism (9.8%) in patients with HF and diabetes. Patients with no HF and age <60 years had the lowest risk of thromboembolism (0.2%). A subsequent analysis from the same study showed that cardioversion more than 12 hours since the onset of symptoms was associated with a higher risk of thromboembolism than when cardioversion was performed in less than 12 hours (1.1% vs 0.3%).[61]

Pharmacologic Cardioversion

Cardioversion can also be accomplished with antiarrhythmic drugs. The thromboembolic risk is similar whether a patient is cardioverted electrically or chemically. Thus, one should not start any antiarrhythmic drug, including amiodarone, in a patient with persistent AF unless one has considered the need for anticoagulation and initiated it as indicated for at least 3 weeks before starting the antiarrhythmic drug; or until confirming the absence of thrombus with transesophageal echocardiogram. Pharmacologic cardioversion is much more likely to be successful if AF has been present for a short duration of time, with AF duration <1 week more likely to terminate.

A recent meta-analysis of randomized controlled trials of pharmacologic cardioversion of AF of less than 48 hours duration found that ranolazine plus intravenous amiodarone, vernakalant, flecainide, oral or intravenous amiodarone, ibutilide, and propafenone were significantly more likely than placebo to lead to cardioversion to sinus rhythm. While the overall quality of the studies was low, the authors were able to conclude that vernakalant and flecainide appeared to be relatively more efficacious, and propafenone and intravenous amiodarone were somewhat less so, in converting recent onset AF to sinus rhythm.[62]

Ibutilide is a class III antiarrhythmic drug that is effective for acute cardioversion of AF. It is given as a 1-mg intravenous bolus followed by a second 1 mg intravenously within 10 to 30 minutes if the first dose is ineffective. This is an attractive option if a patient cannot undergo electrical cardioversion immediately because of, for example, recent ingestion of food. As ibutilide can prolong the QT interval and lead to torsades de pointes, ECG monitoring of the patient for at least four hours after administration is necessary. It is also prudent to check potassium and magnesium levels and correct any deficiencies before proceeding.

Intravenous amiodarone is most useful for cardioversion in patients in the postoperative setting or when conditions such as HF are present and restoration of sinus rhythm is desired. Because it is often prudent to continue an antiarrhythmic drug to prevent further recurrences of AF in these settings, the ability to switch the patient from intravenous to oral amiodarone is helpful. Typical dosing would be an intravenous bolus of 150 mg followed by infusion of 1 mg/min for 6 hours and 0.5 mg/min for 18 hours. The drug can also be given orally from the start if rapid cardioversion is not essential. In that case, loading doses of 600 mg to 800 mg daily in divided doses are given for approximately 10 days, followed by a maintenance dose of 200 mg daily.

Flecainide or propafenone, both of which are class Ic antiarrhythmic drugs, are useful for rapid cardioversion of AF in the outpatient setting. The term "pill-in-the-pocket" has been used to indicate that patients may use the drug on their own to terminate occasional episodes of AF without the need to seek medical attention. Typical doses would be 300 mg of flecainide or 600 mg of propafenone as a single oral dose. In addition, the drugs should usually be administered concomitantly with an AV nodal blocker such as metoprolol in order to avoid the possibility of an actual acceleration of the ventricular rate if atrial activity becomes organized and slows down enough to allow 1:1 AV conduction at rapid rates. For select patients, having the first administration in a monitored setting may be prudent, as

sinus arrest might occur in some patients at the time of conversion to sinus rhythm. It should be noted that these drugs are only used in patients without structural heart disease, because adverse outcomes have been observed in patients with previous myocardial infarction or HF.

Ranolazine is a drug that was developed as an antianginal agent. However, because of its inhibitory effects on the late and fast sodium currents, it has also been investigated as an antiarrhythmic drug. Ranolazine reduces the incidence of AF after cardiac surgery and in acute coronary syndromes. It has been investigated for the conversion of recent onset of AF in combination with intravenous amiodarone. The combination of the two drugs is more effective than amiodarone alone in converting AF to sinus rhythm, and the time to conversion is also shorter.[63]

Vernakalant is a multichannel blocker that has been studied as an intravenous formulation for the conversion of recent onset AF. A recent systematic review and meta-analysis found that vernakalant was superior to placebo and comparable in efficacy to amiodarone or ibutilide, with no significant difference in adverse events between drug groups.[64] Vernakalant is still not available in the United States, at least in part because of previous safety concerns regarding cases of bradycardia and hypotension upon conversion of AF to sinus rhythm.

Lifestyle Modification

Given the known association of AF with various risk factors such as obesity and sleep apnea, studies have examined whether risk factor modification could reduce the burden of AF[61] (**Fig. 36–11**). The link between risk factors and AF is not linear, and U-shaped and J-shaped curves can be seen. Endurance exercise such as running marathons can increase the incidence of AF as much as 5-fold, possibly due to mechanisms such as left atrial enlargement, fibrosis, inflammation, hemodynamic stress, and increased vagal tone.[62] On the other hand, moderate exercise decreases the incidence of AF compared to a sedentary lifestyle. In the CARDIO-FIT Study (Impact of CARDIOrespiratory FITness on Arrhythmic Recurrence in Obese Individuals with Atrial Fibrillation), obese individuals with a body mass index ≥27 kg/m² participated in a tailored exercise program. AF burden and symptom severity decreased significantly in those with a cardiorespiratory fitness gain ≥2 METS compared to <2 METs, and arrhythmia-free survival with or without rhythm control strategies was also greatest in those who gained the most in fitness ($P < 0.001$)[63] (Table 36–1).

The LEGACY Study (Long-Term Effect of Goal-Directed Weight Management in an Atrial Fibrillation Cohort: A Long-Term Follow-Up Study) and ARREST-AF (Aggressive Risk Factor Reduction Study for Atrial Fibrillation and Implications for the Outcome of Ablation) both showed that exercise and weight loss could reduce AF burden.[68] LEGACY showed that patients who had weight loss ≥10% had better arrhythmia-free survival compared to patients who lost lesser amounts of weight. Importantly, weight fluctuation >5% partially offset the benefit of weight loss.[68] ARREST-AF examined the effects of risk factor modification on recurrence of AF after ablation. Patients who underwent risk factor modification had better

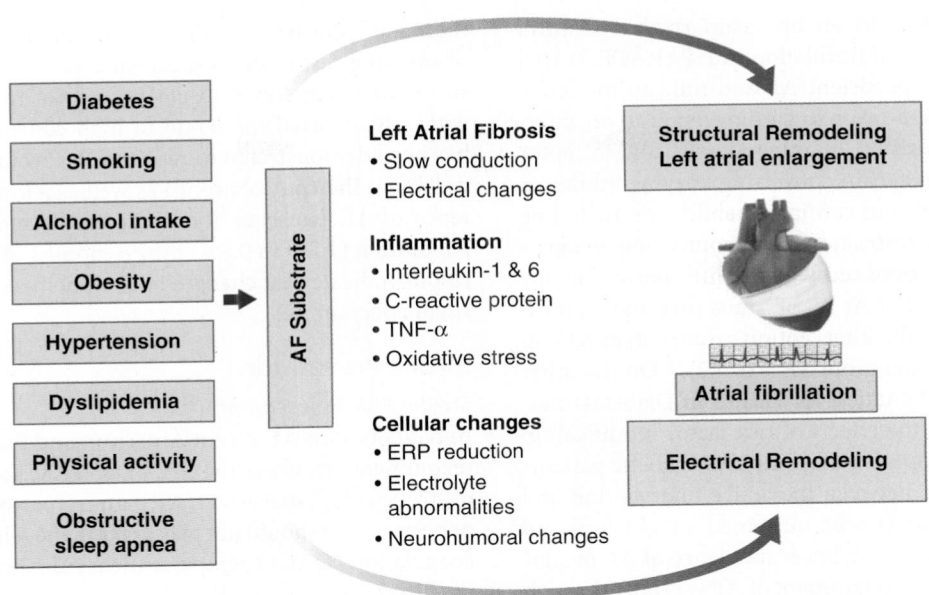

Figure 36–11. **Difference possible mechanisms through which modifiable risk factors may contribute to AF.** Reproduced with permission from Shamloo AS, Dagres N, Arya A, et al. Atrial fibrillation: A review of modifiable risk factors and preventive strategies. *Rom J Intern Med.* 2019 Jun 1;57(2):99-109.

drug-free arrhythmia survival after ablation (*P* < 0.001) as well as a decrease in AF frequency, duration, symptoms, and symptom severity. In addition to exercise and weight loss, risk factor modification in this study included control of hypertension, glucose intolerance/diabetes, hyperlipidemia, sleep apnea, smoking, and alcohol use (**Fig. 36–12**).

The beneficial effects of broad risk factor modification in AF patients have been confirmed in other studies.[69] The Routine

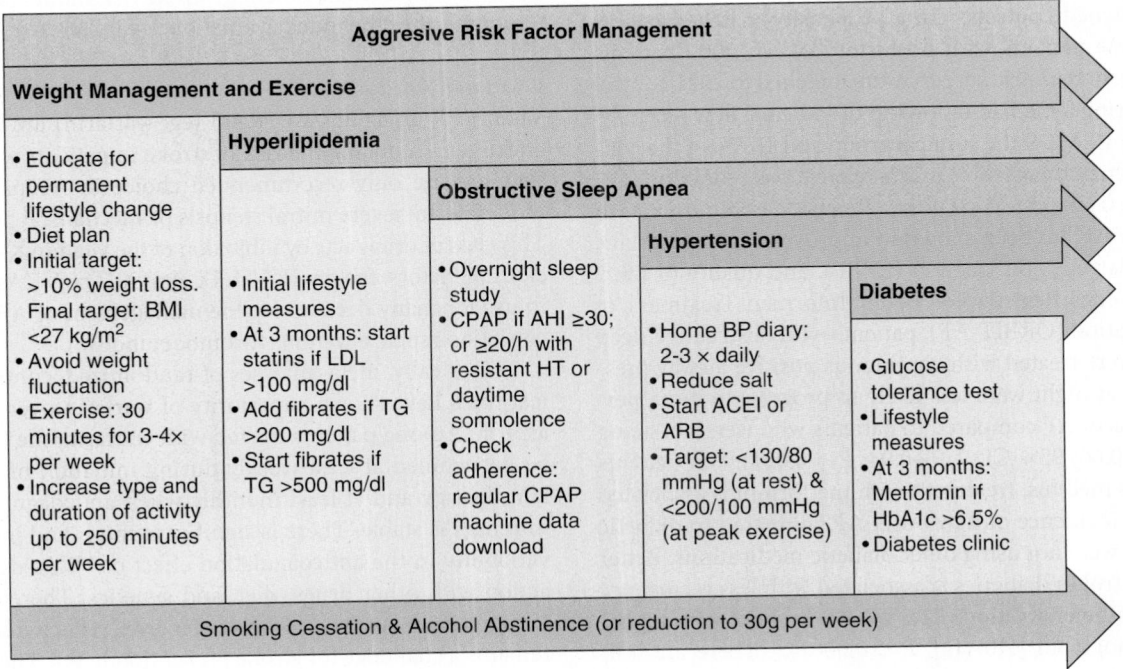

Figure 36–12. **Components of risk factor management from the ARREST-AF and LEGACY studies.** Note that the threshold or target for the various risk factors was specific to these studies in the absence of dedicated clinical trial evidence or guideline recommendations. ACEI indicates angiotensin-converting enzyme inhibitor; AHI, apnea-hypopnea index; ARB, angiotensin II receptor blocker; BMI, body mass index; BP, blood pressure; CPAP, continuous positive airway pressure; HbA1c, hemoglobin A1c; HT, hypertension; LDL, low-density lipoprotein; and TG, triglycerides. Reproduced with permission from Lau DH, Schotten U, Mahajan R, et al. Novel mechanisms in the pathogenesis of atrial fibrillation: practical applications. *Eur Heart J.* 2016 May 21;37(20):1573-1581.

vs. Aggressive risk factor driven upstream rhythm Control for prevention of Early atrial fibrillation in HF (RACE 3) trial took patients with early persistent AF and mild to moderate HF and randomized them prior to cardioversion to an intervention group that consisted of mineralocorticoid receptor antagonists, statins, angiotensin converting enzyme inhibitors and/or receptor blockers, and cardiac rehabilitation including physical activity, dietary restrictions, and counselling versus a usual care group. Both groups received rhythm control therapy and standard therapy for HF. At 1 year, sinus rhythm was present in 75% of patients in the intervention group versus 63% of patients in the conventional group ($P = 0.042$).[69] On the other hand, the Look AHEAD (Action for Health in Diabetes) randomized trial examined the effects of risk factor modification on the subsequent development of AF in 5067 diabetic patients and found no difference between the active intervention and the control groups. Patients who sustained weight loss and exercise at 1 year did not have a lower incidence of AF in subsequent years. However, ascertainment of AF was only through ECGs at study visits and hospital discharge summaries, and it is unclear whether patients maintained adherence to strict risk factor modification over the prolonged follow-up (mean 9 years).[70] Nonadherence to risk factor protocols and/or suboptimal ascertainment of AF could explain the apparent failure of this strategy to influence AF.

In addition to comprehensive risk factor modification, other studies have addressed individual risk factors and the impact of modification/control on AF. Patients who underwent bariatric surgery for morbid obesity were found to have a 29% lower incidence of AF (0.8% vs 2.9%, $P = 0.0001$) in follow-up compared to matched controls.[71] In a propensity-matched cohort study in obese patients with no history of AF, 2000 patients who underwent bariatric surgery were matched to 2021 control subjects. During a median follow-up of 19 years, new onset AF developed in 12.4% of the surgical group and 16.8% of the control group, which represented a 29% relative risk reduction (HR 0.71; 95% CI, 0.60–0.83; $P < 0.001$).[68] Regular aerobic exercise in patients with AF has been shown to improve exercise capacity, left ventricular ejection fraction (LVEF), and quality of life.[73] In the Outcomes Registry for Better Informed Treatment of Atrial Fibrillation (ORBIT-AF), patients with obstructive sleep apnea who were treated with continuous positive airway pressure (CPAP) at night were less likely to progress to more permanent forms of AF compared to patients who were not being treated (HR 0.66; 95% CI, 0.46–0.94; $P = 0.021$).[74] In patients with diabetes mellitus, treatment with metformin is associated with a lower incidence of new onset AF compared to diabetic patients who were not using other diabetic medications. Better glycemic control in diabetics is associated with less recurrence of AF after catheter ablation (32% vs 69% in those with higher glycated hemoglobin [HbA1c], $P < 0.0001$).[71] There are limited studies that have targeted blood pressure control alone in the prevention of recurrences of AF. In the Substrate Modification with Aggressive Blood Pressure Control (SMAC AF) study, tight blood pressure control in patients with hypertension and AF did not improve outcomes after catheter ablation.[76] While cessation of smoking is important for cardiovascular health,

there have not been studies specifically addressing the effect of smoking cessation on recurrence of AF. On the other hand, substantial reductions in alcohol intake in patients with AF with self-reported moderate to high consumption of alcohol has been demonstrated to result in less recurrence of AF (53% vs 73% in the control group) as well as a longer time to recurrence of AF. However, there was only a modest reduction in AF burden (1.2% vs 0.5%) over 6 months of follow-up.[5] These results indicate that changes in alcohol intake may have only a small effect on AF.

Stroke Prevention

Stroke Risk Assessment

In patients with AF, recent American and European guidelines recommend the use of the CHA_2DS_2-VASc score for assessment of stroke risk (Table 36–3). AF pattern (paroxysmal, persistent, or permanent) should not play a role in the selection of oral anticoagulation (OAC) therapy. Anticoagulation with warfarin or the direct non–vitamin K oral anticoagulants (DOACs) reduces the risk for stroke with a net clinical benefit against the potential for serious bleeding for patients with CHA_2DS_2-VASc score of ≥ 2 in men and ≥ 3 in women. For patients with a CHA_2DS_2-VASc score of 1 in men and 2 in women, prescribing an oral anticoagulant to reduce thromboembolic stroke risk may be considered. Stroke risk reassessment at periodic intervals is recommended to identify patients no longer at low risk of stroke for initiation of OAC, along with repeated assessment of bleeding risk scores to address potentially modifiable bleeding risk factors. In patients with AF initially at low risk of stroke, the first reassessment of stroke risk should be made 4 to 6 months after the index evaluation[73] (**Fig. 36–13**).

Vitamin K Antagonists

Vitamin K antagonists (VKAs) (eg, warfarin) are remarkably effective in reducing the risk of stroke in patients with AF, and they are the only recommended choice in AF patients with moderate-to-severe mitral stenosis or mechanical heart valves. This class of drugs acts by inhibition of the vitamin K–dependent clotting factors: factors II, VII, IX, and X. The VKAs have been in use for many decades for the management of AF and other conditions such as venous thromboembolism.

Historically, meta-analyses of randomized, controlled clinical trials have shown superiority of warfarin over placebo or aspirin. Among patients treated with warfarin, the INR should be determined at least weekly during initiation of anticoagulant therapy and at least monthly when anticoagulation (INR in range) is stable. There is significant inter- and intra-patient variability in the anticoagulation effect of VKAs due to interaction with other drugs, diet, and genetics. Therefore, maintaining an adequate anticoagulation level, reflected by the INR, remains a challenge for stroke prevention in AF. The therapeutic range is 2.0 to 3.0 for most patients with AF, while 2.5 to 3.5 is the target in patients with specific types and locations of mechanical valves. Time in therapeutic INR range (2.0–3.0 for AF) of >65% to 70% is recommended, which can be improved by education and counselling. The SAMe-TT2R2 (sex, age, medical history, treatment, tobacco, race) score was developed

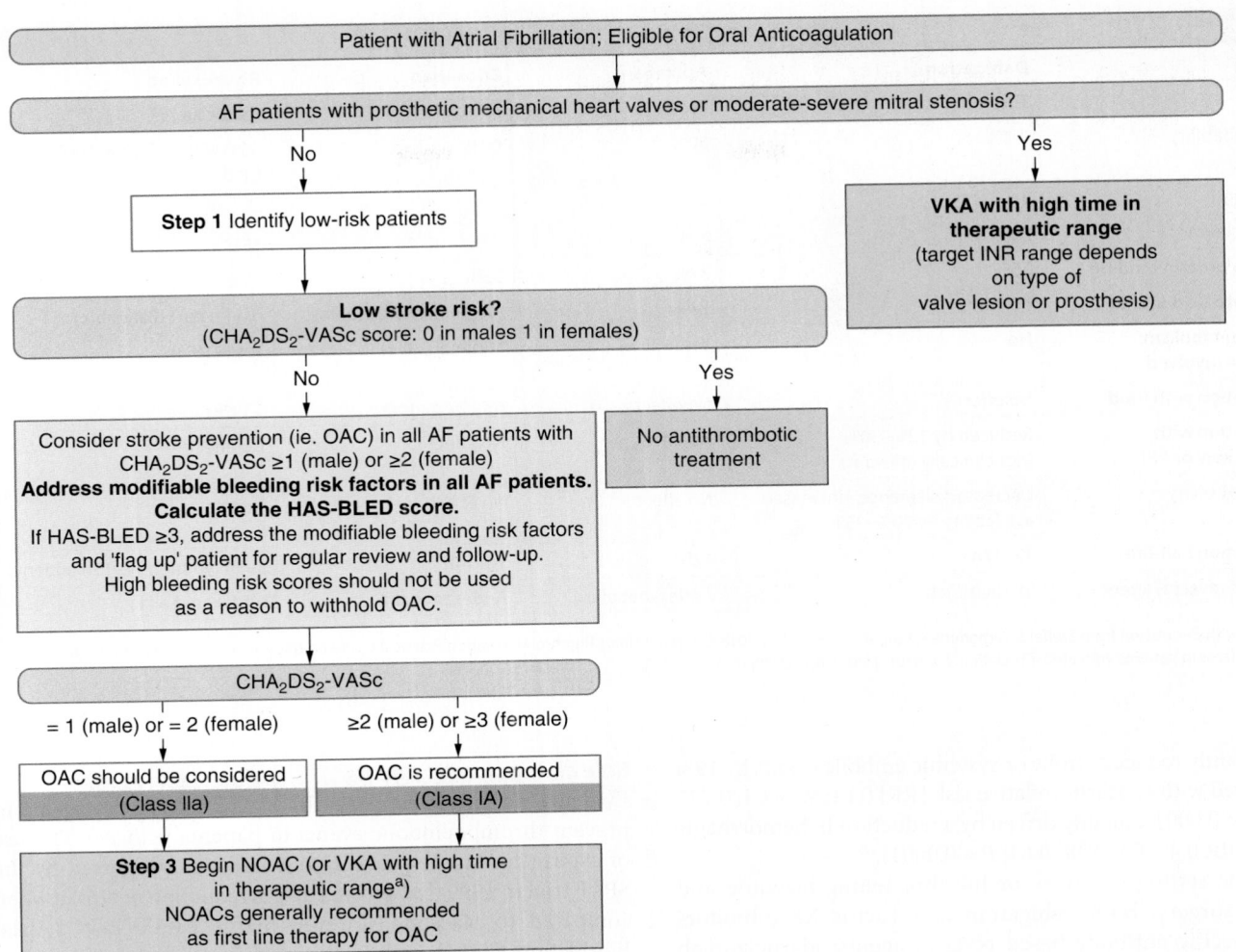

Figure 36–13. Decision pathway for anticoagulation use in patients with AF. Key: AF, atrial fibrillation; CHA2DS2-VASc, Congestive heart failure, Hypertension, Age >_75 years, Diabetes mellitus, Stroke, Vascular disease, Age 65–74 years, Sex category (female); HAS-BLED, Hypertension, Abnormal renal/liver function, Stroke, Bleeding history or predisposition, Labile INR, Elderly (>65 years), Drugs/alcohol concomitantly; INR, international normalized ratio; NOAC, non–vitamin K antagonist oral anticoagulant; OAC, oral anticoagulant; SAMe-TT2R2, Sex (female), Age (<60 years), Medical history, Treatment (interacting drug(s)), Tobacco use, Race (non-Caucasian) (score); TTR, time in therapeutic range; VKA, vitamin K antagonist. If a VKA is being considered, calculate SAMe-TT2R2 score: if score 0–2, may consider VKA treatment (eg, warfarin) or NOAC; if score >2, should arrange regular review/frequent INR checks/counselling for VKA users to help good anticoagulation control, or reconsider the use of NOAC instead; TTR ideally >70%. Reproduced with permission from Hindricks G, Potpara T, Dagres N, et al. 2020 ESC Guidelines for the diagnosis and management of atrial fibrillation developed in collaboration with the European Association for Cardio-Thoracic Surgery (EACTS): The Task Force for the diagnosis and management of atrial fibrillation of the European Society of Cardiology (ESC) Developed with the special contribution of the European Heart Rhythm Association (EHRA) of the ESC. *Eur Heart J.* 2021 Feb 1;42(5):373-498.

to determine the likelihood of whether a patient would achieve a good TTR. A score of >2 is indicative of patients who are less likely to maintain a good TTR and who might require additional measures such as more frequent INR checks, counseling, or transitioning to a DOAC.[77]

Direct Oral Anticoagulants

DOACs (dabigatran, rivaroxaban, apixaban, and edoxaban) are recommended over warfarin for stroke prevention in patients with AF, except for those with moderate-to-severe mitral stenosis or a mechanical heart valve.[60] DOACs act by direct inhibition of thrombin (dabigatran) or activated Factor X (rivaroxaban, apixaban and edoxaban). They offer similar efficacy and safety and increased convenience compared with the VKAs.

Unlike VKAs, DOACs do not require routine INR monitoring and have favorable pharmacological properties in that they act rapidly and have stable and predictable dose-related anticoagulant effects with less clinically relevant drug–drug interactions. All the DOACs have a moderate half-life (8–15 hours) necessitating drug adherence and persistence (**Table 36–7**). Renal function and hepatic function should be evaluated before initiation of a DOAC and should be reevaluated at least annually.

Individual phase III trials comparing DOACs to warfarin for stroke prevention in patients with nonvalvular AF demonstrated that they are at least as efficacious and safe as warfarin. A meta-analysis of these four pivotal trials (42,411 participants on DOACs and 29,272 on warfarin) found that DOACs

TABLE 36–7. Absorption and Metabolism of Direct Oral Anticoagulants

	Dabigatran	**Apixaban**	**Edoxaban**	**Rivaroxaban**
Target	Thrombin	Factor Xa	Factor Xa	Factor Xa
Bioavailability	3–7%	50%	62%	66% without, 80%–100% with food
Prodrug	+	–	–	–
Renal clearance	80%	27%	50%	35%
Plasma protein binding	35%	87%	55%	95%
Ability to be dialyzed	50–60%	14%	n/a (in part dialysable)	n/a (in part dialysable)
Liver metabolism: CYP3A4 involved	No	Yes (~25%)	Minimal (<4%)	Yes (~18%)
Absorption with food	No effect	No effect	6%–22% more	>39% more
Absorption with H$_2$-Blockers or PPI	Reduced by 12%–30% (not clinically relevant)	No effect	No effect	No effect
Asian ethnicity	Decreased clearance / increased availability by 20%–25%	No effect	No effect	No effect
Elimination half-life	12–17h	12h	10–14h	5–9h (young), 11–13h (elderly)
Specific reversal agent	Idarucizimab	Andexanet alfa	Andexanet alfa	Andexanet alfa

Modified with permission from Steffel J, Verhamme P, Potpara TS, et al. The 2018 European Heart Rhythm Association Practical Guide on the use of non-vitamin K antagonist oral anticoagulants in patients with atrial fibrillation. *Eur Heart J.* 2018 Apr 21;39(16):1330-1393.

significantly reduced stroke or systemic embolic events by 19% compared with warfarin (relative risk [RR] 0.81; 95% CI, 0.73–0.91; $P < 0.0001$), mainly driven by a reduction in hemorrhagic stroke (RR 0.49; CI, 0.38–0.64; $P < 0.0001$).[60]

In the setting of severe or life-threatening bleeding and urgent surgery, both dabigatran and Factor Xa inhibitors have specific antibody-based reversal agents: idarucizumab and andexanet alfa, respectively. However, their use could be associated with increased thromboembolic events. If these specific reversal agents are not available, the use of prothrombin complex concentrate (PCC) can be considered as an alternative treatment for reversing the anticoagulant effect of Factor Xa inhibitors, although specific evidence is limited [77] (**Table 36–8**).

Absolute contraindications to OAC include active serious bleeding, recurrent bleeding events without a reversible etiology, severe thrombocytopenia (ie, platelets <50 k/µL), severe anemia under investigation, or a recent high-risk bleeding event such as intracranial hemorrhage. In chronic conditions prohibiting OAC use, nondrug options may be considered.

Role of Antiplatelet Agents

Evidence no longer supports the use of antiplatelet agents to prevent thromboembolic events in patients with AF. The use of aspirin for stroke prevention in AF was supported by the SPAF trial in 1999 that showed a 22% reduction of stroke when compared to placebo. However, in the ACTIVE-W (Atrial Fibrillation Clopidogrel Trial with Irbesartan for Prevention of Vascular Events) trial, dual antiplatelet therapy with aspirin and clopidogrel was less effective than warfarin for prevention of stroke, systemic embolism, myocardial infarction, and vascular death. In the AVERROES [Apixaban Versus Acetylsalicylic Acid (ASA) to Prevent Stroke in Atrial Fibrillation Patients Who Have Failed or Are Unsuitable for Vitamin K Antagonist Treatment] trial, apixaban significantly reduced stroke risk compared to aspirin with no significant difference in major bleeding.

Stroke Prevention in Patients With Renal Dysfunction

For patients with moderate-to-severe chronic kidney disease (CKD), the dosage of DOACs should be adjusted (**Table 36–9**).

TABLE 36–8. Specific Reversal Agents for DOACs

Reversal agent	Description	Landmark Study	Main Results	Cost	Shelf Life
Idarucizumab	Monoclonal antibody that binds dabigatran, resulting in a rapid reversal of its anticoagulant effect	REVERSE-AD	Idarucizumab stopped bleeding in a median time of 2.5 h and hemostasis was achieved in median time 1.6 h in 93.4% of patients.	US $3,483	36 months
Andexanet alfa	Catalytically inactive recombinant modified human factor Xa protein that binds to factor Xa inhibitors	ANNEXA-4	Anti-factor Xa activity was reduced by 92% in patients on rivaroxaban or apixaban. Effective hemostasis at 12 h was achieved in 82% of patients.	US $58,000	12 months

TABLE 36–9. Dose Selection Criteria for Direct Oral Anticoagulants

	Dabigatran	Apixaban	Edoxaban	Rivaroxaban
Standard dose	150 mg bid	5 mg bid	60 mg daily	20 mg daily
Reduced dose	75 mg bid	2.5 mg bid	30 mg daily	15 mg daily
Dose reduction criteria	Any of the following: -Creatinine clearance (CrCl) 15–30 mL/min -Concomitant use of p-glycoprotein inhibitors dronedarone or ketoconazole	At least 2 of the following: -Age ≥80 years -Weight ≤60 kg -Creatinine ≥1.5 mg/dL	CrCl: 15–50 mL/min	CrCl: 15–49 mL/min

For patients with end-stage CKD (creatinine clearance [CrCl] <15 mL/min) or who are on dialysis, it might be reasonable to prescribe warfarin (INR 2.0–3.0) or apixaban for oral anticoagulation as its major elimination is through hepatic metabolism. In a retrospective analysis, apixaban was associated with superior safety and comparable effectiveness for stroke prevention as warfarin, in patients with AF on dialysis.[78]

Interruptions in Anticoagulation and Bridging Therapy
Bridging therapy with unfractionated heparin or low-molecular-weight heparin is recommended for patients with AF and a mechanical heart valve undergoing procedures that require interruption of warfarin. For patients with AF without mechanical heart valves who require interruption of warfarin for procedures, decisions about bridging therapy should balance the risks of stroke and bleeding. Absence of bridging was found to be noninferior to bridging with low-molecular-weight heparin for prevention of arterial thromboembolism and was found to decrease the risk of bleeding. Bridging anticoagulation may be appropriate only in warfarin-treated patients with a very high thromboembolic risk.[79]

Anticoagulation for Cardioversion and Catheter Ablation
For patients with AF or atrial flutter undergoing cardioversion or ablation, anticoagulation with warfarin (INR 2.0–3.0) or a DOAC is recommended for at least 3 weeks before and at least 4 weeks after cardioversion. Details on antithrombotic strategies for patients undergoing cardioversion are provided in the section on acute management.

In patients undergoing catheter ablation as part of a rhythm control strategy, therapeutic OAC with a VKA or DOAC is recommended for ≥3 weeks preprocedure. The ablation procedure is commonly performed on uninterrupted OAC, an approach that has been demonstrated to result in fewer adverse events compared to an interrupted strategy.[11] Randomized studies have shown fewer complications in patients undergoing ablation procedures with an uninterrupted DOAC strategy compared to uninterrupted warfarin.[80] Preprocedure TEE may be used for patients not on adequate OAC and/or for higher-risk patients. OAC should be continued after ablation for ≥2 months. As with cardioversion, the decision to continue long-term OAC postablation should be based on stroke risk factors, rather than the apparent maintenance (or not) of sinus rhythm. At 1 year after ablation, European guidelines suggest that it is reasonable to discuss discontinuation of OAC if there is no recurrence of AF.[77]

Antithrombotic Therapy in AF Patients With Acute or Chronic Coronary Syndromes
Patients with AF undergoing coronary stenting should be managed with a brief initial period of triple therapy (OAC plus aspirin plus clopidogrel), following which the patient should be treated with dual therapy (OAC plus a single antiplatelet agent, preferably clopidogrel) for the first 12 months after percutaneous coronary intervention (PCI) for acute coronary syndrome (ACS), or 6 months after PCI in patients with chronic coronary syndromes (CCS). In patients with coronary artery disease without recurrent medically managed ACS, PCI, or coronary artery bypass surgery in the past ≥1 year, patients can be managed with OAC alone, without aspirin or clopidogrel (Fig. 36–14).[77]

Left Atrial Appendage Occlusion Devices
The LAA is the most common source of thrombi in patients with AF who have suffered a stroke. As an alternative to pharmacologic therapy, a percutaneous device to occlude the LAA may be considered for stroke prevention in patients with AF if they have contraindications for long-term anticoagulant treatment. In addition to stroke prevention, there are early data that epicardial LAA occlusion with the LARIAT device may decrease arrhythmia burden and have a significant impact on systemic homeostasis, including blood pressure and fluid and electrolyte balance.[81] The results of the Percutaneous alternative to the Maze procedure for the treatment of persistent or long-standing persistent AF (aMAZE) trial, a randomized trial evaluating elimination of persistent or long-standing persistent AF with or without the addition of a LARIAT device to AF ablation procedures in 600 patients, are pending.[82]

Percutaneous LAA occlusion with the WATCHMAN™ device has been compared with warfarin in patients with AF (in the absence of moderate to severe mitral stenosis or a mechanical heart valve) at increased risk of stroke in two randomized clinical trials: the PROTECT AF (WATCHMAN™ Left Atrial Appendage System for Embolic Protection in Patients With Atrial Fibrillation) and the PREVAIL (Evaluation of the WATCHMAN™ LAA Closure Device in Patients With Atrial Fibrillation Versus Long Term Warfarin Therapy) trials. A meta-analysis combining data from these trials and their registries demonstrated that patients receiving the device had significantly fewer hemorrhagic strokes than did those receiving warfarin, but there was an increase

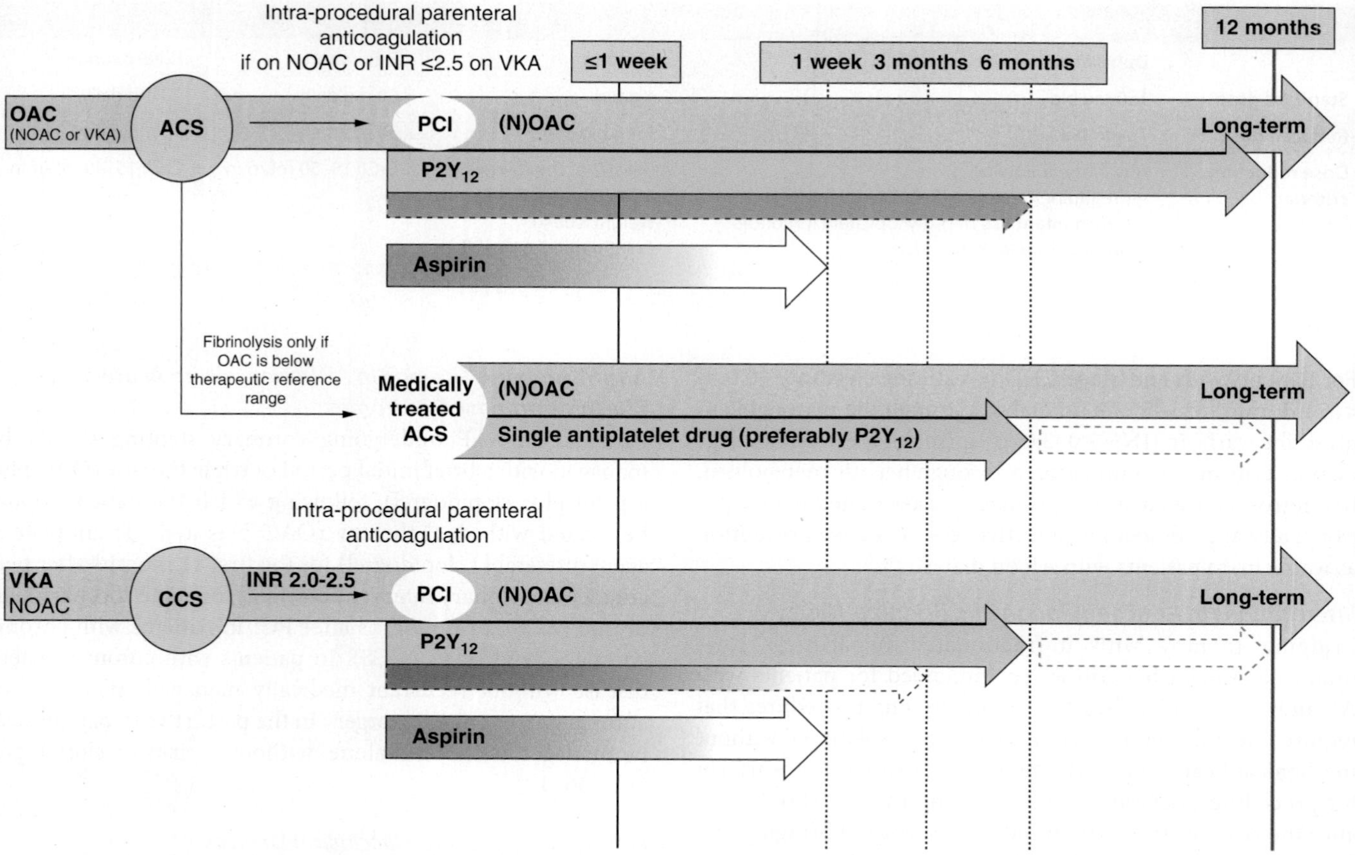

Intra-procedural parenteral anticoagulation if on NOAC or INR ≤2.5 on VKA

≤1 week

1 week　3 months　6 months

12 months

OAC (NOAC or VKA)

ACS

PCI

(N)OAC

Long-term

P2Y₁₂

Aspirin

Fibrinolysis only if OAC is below therapeutic reference range

Medically treated ACS

(N)OAC

Long-term

Single antiplatelet drug (preferably P2Y₁₂)

Intra-procedural parenteral anticoagulation

VKA NOAC

CCS

INR 2.0-2.5

PCI

(N)OAC

Long-term

P2Y₁₂

Aspirin

Figure 36–14. Postprocedural Management of Patients with AF and ACS/PCI. (*Full-outlined arrows* represent a default strategy; *graded/dashed arrows* show treatment modifications depending on individual patient's ischemic and bleeding risks). ACS, acute coronary syndromes; ASA, acetylsalicylic acid; CAD, coronary artery disease; CCS, chronic coronary syndromes; CKD, chronic kidney disease; DAPT, dual antithrombotic therapy; eGFR, estimated glomerular filtration rate; ICH, intracranial hemorrhage; INR, international normalized ratio; LMWH, low-molecular-weight heparin; MI, myocardial infarction; NOAC, non–vitamin K antagonist oral anticoagulant; OAC, oral anticoagulant; PCI, percutaneous coronary intervention; PPI, proton-pump inhibitor; VKA, vitamin K antagonist. Reproduced with permission from Hindricks G, Potpara T, Dagres N, et al. 2020 ESC Guidelines for the diagnosis and management of atrial fibrillation developed in collaboration with the European Association for Cardio-Thoracic Surgery (EACTS): The Task Force for the diagnosis and management of atrial fibrillation of the European Society of Cardiology (ESC) Developed with the special contribution of the European Heart Rhythm Association (EHRA) of the ESC. *Eur Heart J.* 2021 Feb 1;42(5):373-498.

in ischemic strokes in the device group.[83] Other epicardial and endovascular LAA occlusion devices are currently under investigation (**Fig. 36–15**).

Periprocedural antithrombotic and anticoagulation management after LAA occlusion has been poorly defined and is based on historical studies (**Table 36–10**). For patients who do not tolerate any antiplatelet therapy, either an epicardial catheter approach (eg, Lariat system) or surgical thoracoscopic clipping of the LAA may be an option. Surgical exclusion of the LAA may also be considered for stroke prevention in patients with AF undergoing cardiac surgery for other reasons.

Pharmacologic Management for Rate and Rhythm Control

Aside from a decision about anticoagulation, it is important to determine whether a rate control approach or a rhythm control

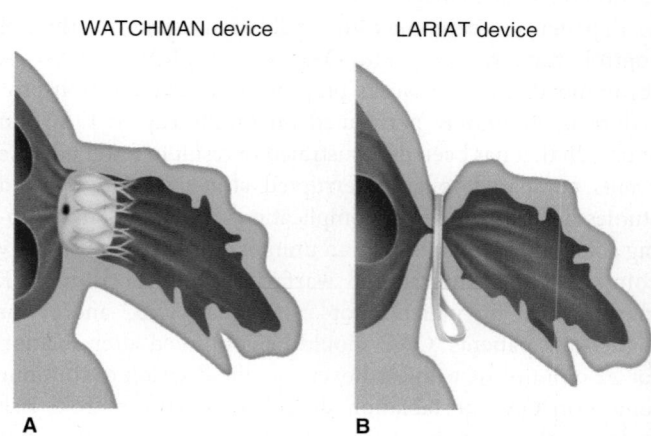

WATCHMAN device

LARIAT device

A

B

Figure 36–15. Examples of percutaneous left atrial appendage closure devices with schematics of left atrial appendage placement for the (**A**) endocardial WATCHMAN device and (**B**) the epicardial LARIAT device.

TABLE 36–10. Left Atrial Appendage Occlusion Devices

Device/patient	Aspirin	OAC	Clopidogrel
Watchman/low bleeding risk	75–325 mg/day indefinitely	Start warfarin after procedure (target INR 2–3) until 45 days or continue until adequate LAA sealing* is confirmed by TEE. NOAC is a possible alternative.	Start 75 mg/day when OAC is stopped, continue for 6 months after the procedure.
Watchman/high bleeding risk	75–325 mg/day indefinitely	None	75 mg/day for 1–6 months while ensuring adequate LAA sealing*
Amplatzer Amulet Occluder	75–325 mg/day indefinitely	None	75 mg/day for 1–6 months while ensuring adequate LAA sealing*

Abbreviations: LAA, left atrial appendage; OAC, oral anticoagulation.

*less than 5-mm leak.

Reproduced with permission from Hindricks G, Potpara T, Dagres N, et al. 2020 ESC Guidelines for the diagnosis and management of atrial fibrillation developed in collaboration with the European Association for Cardio-Thoracic Surgery (EACTS): The Task Force for the diagnosis and management of atrial fibrillation of the European Society of Cardiology (ESC) Developed with the special contribution of the European Heart Rhythm Association (EHRA) of the ESC. *Eur Heart J.* 2021 Feb 1;42(5):373-498.

approach is best for the patient (**Fig. 36–16**). This question has been the subject of multiple studies with conflicting results that may reflect the types of patients studied, the interventions used to achieve rhythm control and the outcomes assessed.[4,84] In general, the decision should be based on the type and frequency of AF episodes, the symptoms the patient has, and any comorbidities. A patient with occasional, self-limited episodes of AF may need no treatment unless anticoagulation is indicated because of an elevated risk of stroke. For infrequent episodes, the pill-in-the-pocket approach is worth considering.

If a patient is asymptomatic from AF, whether it is paroxysmal or persistent, again no specific treatment may be indicated beyond anticoagulation if indicated. Lack of symptoms may be more likely in patients with some degree of AV conduction

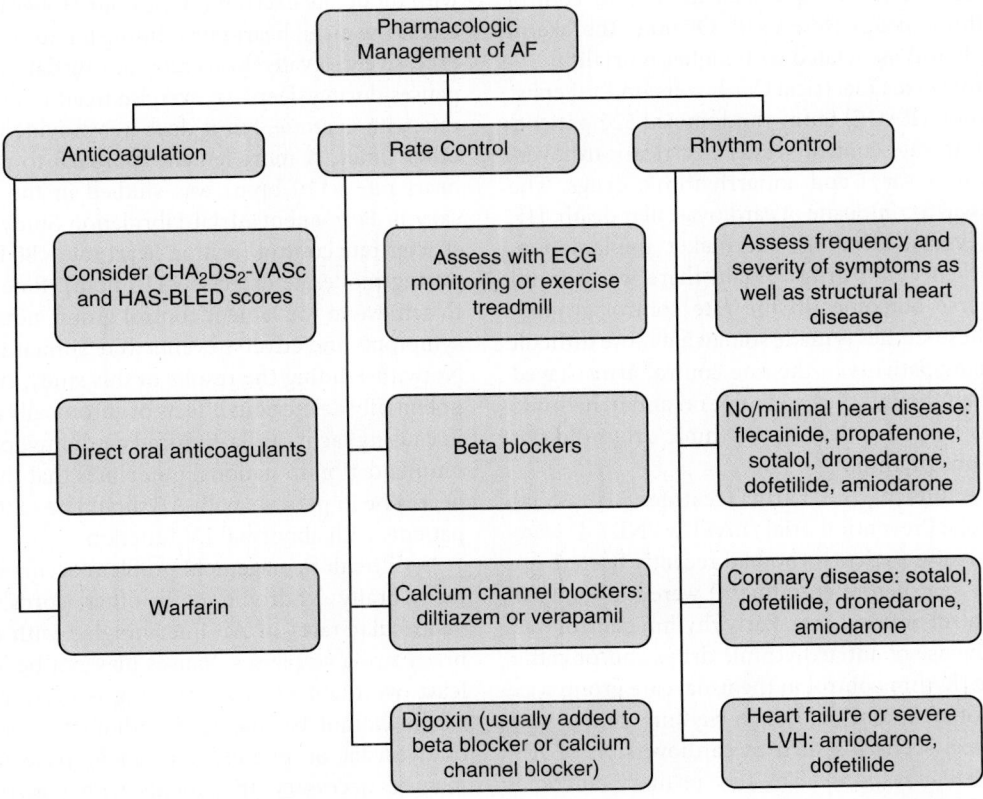

Figure 36–16. Pharmacologic management of AF. The three pillars of management of AF are anticoagulation, rate control, and rhythm control. The decision on anticoagulation is based on the CHA$_2$DS$_2$-VASc and HAS-BLED scores. Direct oral anticoagulants are preferred over warfarin except in specific situations, such as the presence of a mechanical heart valve. Rate control is best accomplished with β-blockers or calcium channel blockers, with digoxin added in selected cases when rate control is not adequate. Rate control should be assessed with 24-hour ambulatory monitoring, and in some cases, exercise treadmill testing. The choice of an antiarrhythmic drug is based on the presence or absence of underlying heart disease. Flecainide and propafenone may only be used in patients without structural heart disease. Amiodarone is a second-line agent in patients with no or minimal heart disease, whereas it is a first-line agent in patients with HF and severe LV hypertrophy.

disease resulting in moderate heart rates when the patient is in AF. This is most likely to be true in an elderly population. True lack of symptoms is not always straightforward to determine. In patients with nonspecific symptoms that may be related to persistent AF, performing cardioversion to assess the patient's physical well-being in a "trial of sinus rhythm" may reveal marked improvement and support a rhythm control strategy in that individual.

For symptomatic patients, pharmacologic rate and/or rhythm control is usually attempted before considering more invasive means of management. The Atrial Fibrillation Follow-up Investigation of Rhythm Management (AFFIRM) study examined outcomes with rate versus rhythm control in patients with AF and found that there was no difference in survival with either approach, although there was a trend toward lower mortality in the rate control group (HR 0.87, $P = 0.08$).[84] An "on treatment" analysis from that trial found that patients who maintained sinus rhythm had improved survival compared to patients in AF. On the other hand, the use of antiarrhythmic drugs was not associated with improved survival, suggesting that the beneficial effects of antiarrhythmic drugs in maintaining sinus rhythm were offset by adverse effects from the drugs.[85] These findings suggested that maintenance of sinus rhythm would be better for patients if safer antiarrhythmic drugs could be developed, or an alternative approach to rhythm control besides antiarrhythmic drugs were used. Of note, the use of digoxin in this study was associated with higher mortality.

The Rate Control versus Electrical Cardioversion for Persistent Atrial Fibrillation (RACE) Study randomized 522 patients with persistent AF to rate control versus electrical cardioversion (repeated as necessary) and antiarrhythmic drugs. The primary endpoint was a composite of cardiovascular death, HF, thromboembolic events, bleeding, pacemaker implantation, and severe adverse effects of drugs. Again there was a trend toward fewer adverse outcomes in the rate control group.[86] Interpretation of these studies is made somewhat more difficult by the fact that many patients in the rate control arms stayed in sinus rhythm even though they were not on antiarrhythmic drugs, and patients treated with antiarrhythmic drugs did not always maintain sinus rhythm.

Recently, the results of the Early Treatment of Atrial Fibrillation for Stroke Prevention Trial (EAST-AFNET 4) were published.[4] In this study, patients who had recently been diagnosed with AF (≤1 year before enrollment) were randomized to early rhythm control or usual care. Early rhythm control was accomplished by the use of antiarrhythmic drugs and/or catheter ablation, while rhythm control in the usual care group was limited to control of symptoms, although rhythm control was permitted for clinical scenarios such as cardioversion of AF with a rapid ventricular response. The first primary outcome was a composite of death from cardiovascular causes, stroke, or hospitalization with worsening HF or acute coronary syndrome. Of the 2789 patients randomized (median time since diagnosis of 36 days), the first primary outcome occurred in 249 patients assigned to early rhythm control (3.9 per 100 person-years) and in 316 patients in the usual care group (5.0 per 100 person-years) (HR 0.79; 95% CI, 0.66–0.94; $P = 0.005$). The improvement in outcomes demonstrated in this trial may indicate that early and more aggressive rhythm control in patients with recently diagnosed AF is warranted, which would represent a shift from a more symptom-oriented approach.

Rate Control

Rate control is a reasonable first approach to the long-term management of AF, especially in older patients who tend to be less symptomatic. β-blockers are usually the first choice for heart rate control, but the nondihydropyridine calcium channel blockers diltiazem or verapamil are also useful. Calcium channel blockers should not be used in patients with decompensated HF. Digoxin is not used as a first line agent for rate control in AF. It can help to lower resting heart rate, but it is less effective during exertion, making it less useful in young, active patients. However, digoxin can be used as an adjunct to obtain better rate control if a β-blocker or calcium channel blocker alone is insufficient, especially in patients with HF. While there have been conflicting data on the effect of digoxin on mortality, it can be used safely in lower doses with monitoring of renal function. Oral amiodarone can help to control the ventricular rate in AF, but it should rarely be used for this indication alone (Table 36–6).

Acceptable heart rate control in AF is usually considered to be a resting heart rate of 60 to 80 bpm and a rate of 90 to 115 bpm with moderate exertion. A 24-hour Holter monitor is useful to assess the mean heart rate (aiming for around 80 bpm), without excessively elevated heart rates during daily activities or marked pauses during sleep. An exercise treadmill test can assess heart rate with exercise, but it does not provide information during other times. A more lenient approach to rate control (resting heart rate <110 bpm) was studied in the Rate Control Efficacy in Permanent Atrial Fibrillation Study (RACE II) against stricter rate control (resting heart rate <80 bpm and heart rate during moderate exercise <110 bpm). Rate control was easier to achieve in the lenient control group, not surprisingly, while symptoms and adverse events were similar in the two groups.[87] Notwithstanding the results of this study, consideration of the potentially deleterious effects of chronically elevated heart rates in causing tachycardia-induced cardiomyopathy led to the recommendation in national guidelines that the target for resting heart rate in patients with AF should be <80 bpm, especially in patients with abnormal LV function.

A difficult management problem occurs when patients have tachy-brady syndrome, or in other words, episodes of rapid ventricular rates in AF intermingled with episodes of severe bradycardia or pauses. Pauses may not be identified unless at least overnight ECG monitoring is performed. When tachycardia cannot be managed without the risk of symptomatic bradycardia or pauses, permanent pacemaker implantation may be necessary. In patients with paroxysmal AF, a dual-chamber pacemaker can provide heart rate support, continuous monitoring of AF to provide information on AF burden, and mode switching to transition from dual-chamber pacing to ventricular-only pacing when AF occurs. If pauses are infrequent, an attractive option may be a leadless pacemaker to provide heart rate support when needed. Any pacing option is more often considered in elderly patients, especially those

TABLE 36–11. Antiarrhythmic Drugs for Atrial Fibrillation

Drug	Vaughn-Williams Class	Dosing
Flecainide	Ic	50–150 mg twice daily
Propafenone	Ic	150–300 mg 3x daily; sustained release 225–425 mg twice daily
Sotalol	III	80–160 mg twice daily
Dronedarone	Multichannel blocker	400 mg twice daily
Dofetilide	III	125–500 mcg twice daily
Amiodarone	Multichannel blocker	600–800 mg daily in divided doses to 10 g, then 200 mg daily

Class Ic drugs are sodium channel blockers; Class III drugs are potassium channel blockers; amiodarone and dronedarone have effects on multiple channels, including β-blocking effects, calcium channel blocking effects, and Class I and III effects.

with comorbidities, as a simpler approach than ablation. For patients who are good candidates for catheter ablation of AF, this potentially curative approach should be considered before moving on to permanent pacing.

Rhythm Control

While medications to control heart rate may be sufficient in some patients, others will benefit from antiarrhythmic drugs to control AF and maintain sinus rhythm. Most are used in conjunction with rate control agents. Antiarrhythmic drugs exert their effects by acting on cardiac ion channels to alter their excitability, refractoriness, conduction, or automaticity (**Table 36–11**).

Class Ic Antiarrhythmic Drugs: Flecainide and propafenone are class Ic antiarrhythmic drugs, which indicates that they are potent sodium channel blockers. They have few extracardiac side effects, which make them attractive for initial therapy in many patients. Because they do not block potassium channels, they are not associated with QT prolongation and torsades de pointes. On the other hand, they can prolong the PR and QRS intervals on the ECG. For very infrequent episodes of AF, flecainide or propafenone can be used just when AF occurs, as described under pharmacologic cardioversion. Either drug can lead to termination of AF in under 2 hours in most patients. The potent conduction-slowing properties of these drugs can lead to relatively slow atrial rates in atrial flutter, which can promote 1:1 A:V conduction if they are not used with an AV nodal blocker. Flecainide is administered twice daily. Propafenone has an immediate release formulation that is given three times daily, and a sustained release preparation that is dosed twice daily. Use of either of these drugs in patients with structural heart disease, in particular coronary artery disease and HF, has led to adverse outcomes, and so these drugs are contraindicated in such patients.

Sotalol: Sotalol is a class III antiarrhythmic drug with β-blocking properties in addition to its class III effect of potassium channel blockade. It is a reasonable choice for antiarrhythmic drug therapy in most patients with AF, except for those with advanced HF. It is eliminated by the kidneys, so dose

adjustment is necessary in patients with abnormal renal function. As a potassium channel blocker, sotalol may cause QT prolongation and torsades de pointes. It is prudent to be sure that serum potassium and magnesium levels are normal before starting the drug. The drug can be started as an outpatient, if the patient is in sinus rhythm and has minimal or no heart disease and a normal QTc. An ECG should be obtained at steady state (after approximately five doses) before titrating the dose upward. Some physicians hospitalize all patients for initiation of sotalol for continuous ECG monitoring. The target dose in patients with normal renal function is 120 mg twice daily. Sotalol is ineffective for chemical conversion of AF.

Dronedarone: Dronedarone was one of the more recent antiarrhythmic drugs to become available. It has some similarities to amiodarone with respect to its multichannel blocking action. It does not contain iodine, as amiodarone does, and so it does not cause thyroid abnormalities. Initially, there was a great deal of enthusiasm with this drug, particularly as one study showed that cardiovascular outcomes were improved with dronedarone, suggesting favorable actions separate from a pure antiarrhythmic drug effect. However, a subsequent study that randomized patients in permanent AF (and thus any effects could not be due to antiarrhythmic actions) to dronedarone or placebo found that patients on the active drug had worse outcomes. There were higher event rates for both co-primary outcomes (stroke, myocardial infarction, systemic embolism or death from cardiovascular causes, and the second co-primary outcome of hospitalization for a cardiovascular cause or death) in patients on active drug. The drug is therefore contraindicated in persistent or permanent AF. Patients should be monitored periodically to be sure that their arrhythmia burden has not increased from paroxysmal to persistent or permanent AF. If so, the drug must be discontinued. Dronedarone is also contraindicated in patients with recently decompensated HF. The fact that dronedarone is no more effective than other antiarrhythmic drugs and that it cannot be used in certain patient populations has led to less use than in the past. More recently, dronedarone was studied in combination with ranolazine, both in reduced doses (ranolazine 750 mg twice daily with dronedarone at 150 mg or 225 mg twice daily) for reduction in AF burden in patients with implanted pacemakers. Either set of doses significantly reduced AF burden and was well tolerated.

Dofetilide: Dofetilide is a class III antiarrhythmic drug that is effective for maintenance of sinus rhythm, and it can also be effective for pharmacologic cardioversion of AF in a small percentage of patients in whom dofetilide is initiated while in persistent AF. It can be used safely in patients including those with structural heart disease such as HF. In fact, only dofetilide and amiodarone have been shown to be safe in patients with advanced structural heart disease, as cardiovascular outcomes are not worsened when these drugs are used. The requirement that dofetilide only be initiated during a 3-day inpatient hospitalization stems from the initial clinical studies with the drug, as dose adjustment is necessary if QT prolongation is observed on ECGs obtained after each dose. Dose adjustment is also necessary for patients with renal insufficiency. The mandate for inpatient initiation has undoubtedly led to less use of the drug than might otherwise be the case, as it has reasonably good efficacy. One situation in which dofetilide has been used more often is in the postablation setting, particularly in patients undergoing catheter ablation for persistent AF, as the patient may already be in an inpatient setting. It can be used to suppress recurrences of AF or convert AF postablation.

Amiodarone: Possibly the most used drug for AF is amiodarone, despite the fact that it is not approved in the United States for that indication. Amiodarone has effects attributed to all four classes of antiarrhythmic drugs, which makes it quite unique compared to the others (aside from dronedarone). In addition to its antiarrhythmic effects, it can slow the ventricular response to AF. While that is useful as an adjunct to AV nodal blockers, it would be unusual to use amiodarone solely for heart rate control. Amiodarone is safe to use in patients with advanced structural heart disease. It has an intravenous formulation, so it is easy to start in patients in the postoperative setting, for example, or any situation in which rhythm control is desired and the patient cannot take drugs orally. Patients given amiodarone for AF require higher doses in the initial weeks of administration because of the pharmacologic properties of the drug, and steady state is not reached for several weeks after initiation. Amiodarone has multiple potential side effects, some of which can be quite serious, such as pulmonary and hepatic toxicity. The drug is also associated with thyroid abnormalities (hyper- and hypothyroidism), neurologic effects, corneal deposits, skin photosensitivity, and others. With proper monitoring, most patients can take the drug safely at least over the first few years. Changes in patients' conditions or the development of side effects lead to discontinuation in many patients over the long term.

While amiodarone is more effective than any of the other antiarrhythmic drugs, the number and seriousness of the potential side effects indicate that the drug should not be used as a first line agent except in specific circumstances, such as advanced age of the patient or serious structural heart disease. Other situations in which amiodarone can be considered is when it is intended for short-term use only, but there is a strong need or desire to get the patient back to sinus rhythm. Examples include the postoperative setting, an admission for rapid AF during which rate control and restoration of sinus rhythm quickly is desired, or there are other potentially reversible conditions promoting AF and use of the drug is only intended until the underlying condition is brought under control. Amiodarone can convert AF to sinus rhythm, as can dofetilide, flecainide, and propafenone.

The choice of an antiarrhythmic drug for AF depends on the presence and severity of underlying structural heart disease (**Fig. 36–16**). Most of the available drugs have comparable efficacy, while amiodarone has superior efficacy, as mentioned. For patients without structural heart disease, initial therapy for rhythm control can include flecainide, propafenone, sotalol, or dronedarone. Dofetilide can be used as well, but the

inconvenience of inpatient initiation means that it is not often selected first. At least one of these drugs is often tried before recommending catheter ablation to a patient as an option to cure the arrhythmia. For mild-moderate heart disease, flecainide and propafenone are not used, which leaves sotalol, dronedarone, or dofetilide as initial agents. For more advanced heart disease, dofetilide or amiodarone are options. For patients with substantial LV hypertrophy, amiodarone would usually be the initial choice for antiarrhythmic therapy. The ease of initiation of amiodarone (oral administration as an outpatient rather than a 72-hour hospital stay) makes it a more attractive option in most cases.

Catheter Ablation and Other Nonpharmacologic Strategies

Nonpharmacological therapies for AF aim to modify etiological mechanisms; clinical approaches apply focused destruction of atrial tissue by catheter ablation or surgery (**Fig. 36–17**). Experimental strategies include functional modification of structural or electrical substrates by pacing, stem cell, or gene therapy.

Identifying Candidate Populations for Nonpharmacologic Therapy of AF

There is currently no approach to accurately identify a priori which AF patients will or will not respond to ablation or surgery. Notably, the clinical labels of paroxysmal or nonparoxysmal AF, and CHA_2DS_2-VASc, APPLE, and HATCH scores predict ablation success with only ~60% to 70% accuracy. Extensive atrial scarring by MRI[19] may portend failure of ablation, based on structural remodeling that is not targeted by empirical ablation or surgical lesions. Such patients may be triaged for more extensive therapy.

The rationale for AF ablation in patient groups underrepresented in randomized trials is based on observational series. Such groups include individuals older than 75 years, who derived less benefit from ablation in the CABANA trial,[88] competitive athletes, individuals with hypertrophic cardiomyopathy, and others. Clinical judgment should be used in each case to weigh the potential benefits and risks.

Catheter Ablation

Catheter ablation for AF is based on pulmonary vein isolation (PVI) as a cornerstone.[11] PVI historically evolved to eliminate PV triggers, but it could also eliminate other mechanisms at these sites, including fibrotic regions, drivers, or ganglionic plexi (see Fig. 36–3). Depending on specific features of the patient undergoing ablation, other lesion sets are often added to improve success rates. Patients with paroxysmal AF typically undergo PVI alone, which eliminates AF in 60% to 70% of patients at 12 to 18 months and relieves symptoms.[89] Patients with persistent or long-standing persistent AF have a lower success rate from PVI alone of 40% to 60% at 12 to 18 months,[90] and additional lesion sets are sometimes added in an attempt to improve success rates. However, consensus guidelines recommend PVI alone as the initial approach to

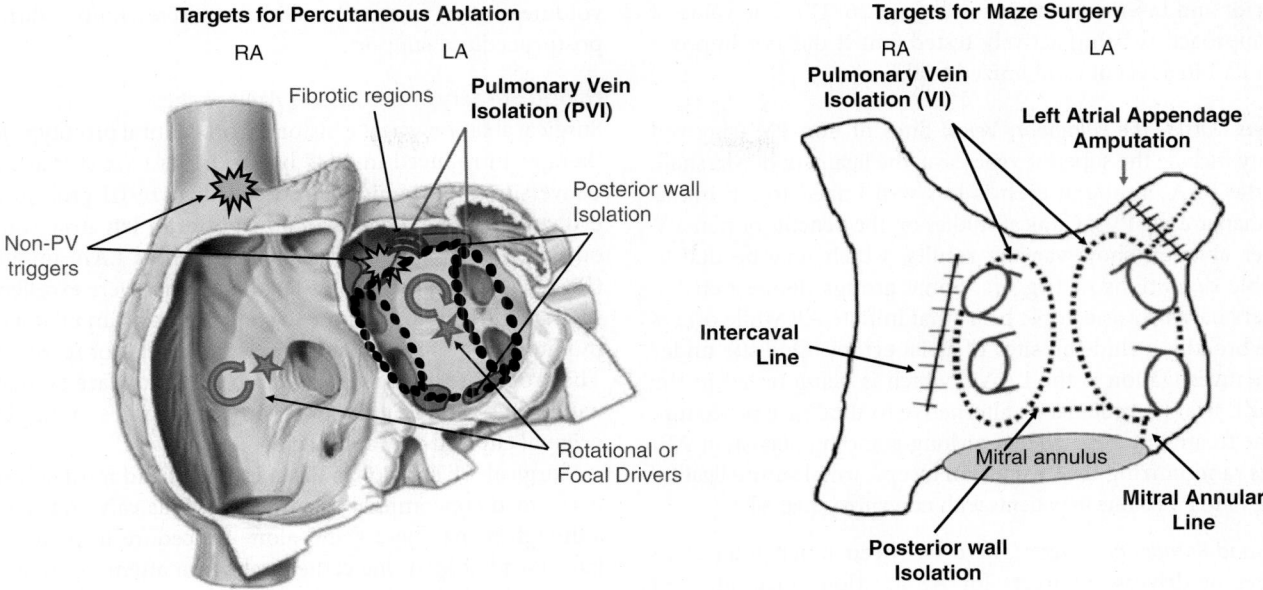

Figure 36–17. Nonpharmacological therapy for AF by percutaneous ablation or surgical maze. Consensus elements of each procedure are shown in *bold black font*, and proposed strategies are in *gray*. LA, left atrium; RA, right atrium.

ablation of persistent AF. Compared to antiarrhythmic drugs, ablation has been shown to reduce the burden (extent) of AF[90] and improve quality of life.[88] In patients with concomitant HF, ablation improved survival compared to pharmacological therapy in the Catheter Ablation versus Standard Conventional Therapy in Patients with Left Ventricular Dysfunction and Atrial Fibrillation (CASTLE-AF)[91] trial and subpopulations of the Catheter Ablation vs. Antiarrhythmic Drug Therapy for Atrial Fibrillation (CABANA) trial.[88] At the current time, AF ablation has not been shown to prolong survival in broader populations of AF patients.[88] Whether AF ablation can eliminate the need for long-term anticoagulation or reduce the risk for dementia is under investigation.[92]

Pulmonary Vein Isolation: As shown in Fig. 36–17, two right and two left pulmonary veins typically drain into the left atrium, although variations exist. PVI aims to electrically isolate the PVs from the left atrium using lesions to block electrical connection. PVI is typically percutaneous, with catheters passed via the femoral veins to the right atrium, then to the left atrium via trans-septal puncture. There are several technical approaches. Contemporary PVI includes ablation of a wide cuff of PV antral tissue that is more effective than ablating near the ostia, and PVs can be isolated individually or in pairs. Several tools exist for PVI, including catheters with tips that emit radiofrequency energy to heat or cryo-energy to freeze local tissue in a point-by-point fashion, causing necrosis at these sites. Spheroidal balloons that fit the PV antrum can rapidly isolate each PV in turn by delivering cryo-(freezing), radiofrequency, or laser[2] energy. Each strategy produces comparable results.[89]

AF may recur postablation and is associated with PV reconnection, especially in patients with paroxysmal AF.[93] Several strategies can increase the durability of PVI (ie, prevent PV reconnection), including ensuring sufficient contact between the catheter and the atrium or by using respiratory ventilator settings to reduce thoracic movement and improve catheter stability. Success rates are also enhanced by pacing maneuvers to confirm entrance and exit block from the PVs or by the use of pharmacological maneuvers.

Ablation Targets Outside the Pulmonary Vein Antra: Several efforts are underway to identify additional ablation targets for patients who do not respond to PVI alone, which includes patients in whom AF recurs even with intact PVI.[93] Several techniques have been proposed, although none have yet been shown to improve upon PVI alone in multicenter randomized trials.[90]

Empirical Lines and Complex Fractionated Atrial Electrograms: The STAR AF II (Substrate and Trigger Ablation for Reduction of Atrial Fibrillation) trial randomized 589 patients with nonparoxysmal AF and found no reduction and a trend for lower success in groups receiving either linear ablation or ablation of complex fractionated electrograms in addition to PVI compared to PVI alone.[94] Success rates ranged from 50% to 60% when considering patients on or off antiarrhythmic drugs, but they dropped to 38% to 50% when considering success as the elimination of AF without the use of antiarrhythmic drugs. This result has been supported by multiple randomized trials.[90,95]

Isolation of the Posterior Left Atrial Wall: The posterior wall is a component of the Cox Maze surgical procedure, and its possible mechanistic role is supported by its embryological origin from the sinus venosus similar to the PVs.[96] Posterior wall isolation can be achieved by encircling all four PVs in a box, or connecting the isolated PVs by horizontal linear lesions at the superior and inferior posterior wall (Fig. 36–17). The value of this approach is being actively tested, but it did not improve upon PVI in a recent randomized trial.[97]

Triggers Outside the Pulmonary Veins: Sites of non-PV triggered activity include the superior vena cava, the ligament of Marshall, and the LAA, although each is less well linked to AF initiation than are the PVs. Clinical studies on the benefits of non-PV trigger ablation show varying results, which may be due to variable definitions of triggers. Some groups define non-PV triggers narrowly as ectopic beats that initiate AF, while others more broadly include all sites of atrial ectopy. One site under active investigation is the LAA,[98] which is being tested in the aMAZE trial (Percutaneous alternative to the Maze procedure for the treatment of persistent or long-standing persistent AF) that is randomizing LAA exclusion by epicardial suture ligation plus PVI to PVI alone in patients with nonparoxysmal AF.[82]

Focal and Rotational Drivers: There has been much interest in sources or drivers as targets for AF ablation. Such sites are seen by optical mapping of human AF with high concordance with clinical mapping.[99] A multitude of clinical systems are now available, most of which reveal two to five AF drivers per patient of which two-thirds lie in the left atrium, near and remote from PVs, and one-third in the right atrium. Ablation outcomes are mixed, with results that are promising overall but disappointing in some reports.[15,100] As with all other AF ablation approaches, randomized trials have yet to demonstrate benefit over PVI alone. A possible cause of divergent results for driver ablation is a lack of standardization between mapping methods, advances to eliminate subjectivity in reading AF maps, identification of which patients may benefit, and some standardization of ablation lesion sets.

Scar and Low Voltage Regions: Fibrotic and scar border zone sites may contribute to wavefront disorganization and also anchor driving regions. Proposed ablation strategies have been to homogenize sites to reduce nonuniformity, and to connect fibrotic sites to nonconducting boundaries. Data from early small series are promising,[101] and they are currently being tested widely in the ongoing Delayed-Enhancement MRI Determinant of Successful Radiofrequency Catheter Ablation of Atrial Fibrillation (DECAAF-2) trial of PVI with or without ablation of fibrotic atrium defined by delayed enhanced MRI.[23]

Complications of Percutaneous Ablation: Recent analyses of US Medicare databases show overall complication rates of 2% to 5% from percutaneous AF ablation, comprising pericardial effusion and cardiac tamponade (~1%), coronary artery occlusion and stenosis, stroke and TIA (~0.3%), silent microemboli that may explain asymptomatic silent emboli on brain scanning, atrial-esophageal fistula that is often fatal (0.1%), PV stenosis, gastric hypomotility, phrenic nerve palsy, stiff left atrial syndrome, radiation injury, and death. Mortality from AF ablation is uncommon, with a rate of <0.5%[102] that is inversely related to operator volume. These observations emphasize that AF ablation, as with all procedures, should be performed by experienced operators and teams at high volume centers who can provide intensive preprocedural and postprocedural support.

Hybrid Surgery and Catheter Approaches

Surgical ablation was the historical procedural prototype for AF therapy, introduced in 1987 by Dr. James Cox at Washington University in St. Louis. The so-called Maze-III procedure has evolved to isolate the PVs and the posterior left atrial wall with other left and right atrial lesions as well as LAA amputation (Fig. 36–17). Reported long-term outcomes were excellent, but they are difficult to compare to contemporary ambulatory ECG monitoring strategies that increase sensitivity for recurrent AF. The procedure has been adapted to the Cox-Maze IV that uses handheld radiofrequency or cryothermy clamps to simplify the original cut-and-sew approach.

Surgical AF ablation is FDA-approved and most commonly performed concomitant to surgery such as valve replacement, although it may be a stand-alone procedure in patients who have failed at least one catheter ablation attempt.[11] In a recent multicenter study of 260 patients with persistent or long-standing persistent AF undergoing mitral valve surgery, patients were randomized to surgical ablation or no ablation.[103] Patients in the ablation group were further randomized to PVI or a biatrial maze, and all had LAA closure. Patients in the ablation group were more likely than those in the control group to be free of AF at 12 months (63.2% vs 29.4%; $P < 0.001$), with no significant difference between those who underwent PVI or a biatrial maze (61.0% and 66.0%, respectively; $P = 0.60$). One-year mortality was 6.8% in the ablation group and 8.7% in the control group ($P = 0.55$). Implantation of a permanent pacemaker implantation was more common in the ablation than the nonablation limb (21.5 vs 8.1 per 100 patient-years; $P = 0.01$).

Ongoing studies are combining AF surgery with percutaneous ablation to improve the results of either alone. This hybrid approach provides the ability to touch up incomplete lines and add lesion sets that may be difficult to deliver by either approach alone. This so-called convergent or hybrid surgery is increasingly performed, but again success is variable, ranging from 40%[104] to 80%. Future advances in surgical therapy for AF will likely include continued improvements in thoracoscopy tools and autonomic modulation by epicardial ganglion plexus ablation.

Catheter Ablation of the Atrioventricular Node With Pacemaker/Cardiac Resynchronization Therapy

AV node ablation is designed to eliminate rapid ventricular rates from AF, using permanent ventricular pacing for heart rate support. This approach may be appropriate for patients with tachycardia-induced cardiomyopathy, when AF ablation has failed, and if pharmacological rate control is difficult to achieve. AV node ablation can improve symptoms, quality of life, healthcare utilization, and mortality. Limitations are that AV node ablation does not eliminate AF with its indications for anticoagulation, patients do not regain the atrial kick, may thus remain symptomatic, and are rendered pacemaker dependent. In patients with a reduced LVEF, cardiac resynchronization therapy rather than right ventricular pacing is indicated.

In a small randomized study of patients with AF and HF with reduced ejection fraction, AV node ablation with cardiac resynchronization therapy was still inferior to PVI in improving symptoms of HF and LVEF.

Pacemaker Therapies/Programming

Two pacing strategies have been proposed to reduce AF burden. The first, in patients with dual-chamber pacemakers, is to reduce the burden of right ventricular pacing using programming such as managed ventricular pacing, which decreases the percentage of ventricular pacing by promoting atrial pacing alone and only pacing the ventricle when AV conduction fails. The second strategy uses atrial antitachycardia pacing during periods of atrial ectopy. In a recent meta-analysis of randomized trials, a low versus a high burden of right ventricular pacing (<10% vs >10%) was associated with a nonsignificant reduction in AF progression (HR 0.80; 95% CI 0.57–1.13; $P = 0.21$). While atrial pacing reduced the burden of atrial ectopy, it did not decrease AF burden or the number of AF episodes, and did not alter AF progression.[105] These data show that pacemaker strategies appear safe, but may not significantly reduce AF in patients with existing indications for dual-chamber pacing.

Specific Scenarios

Postoperative AF

AF is well recognized as a complication after cardiothoracic surgery, occurring in approximately one-third of patients. Mechanisms are incompletely defined but may include ischemia, inflammation, and sympathetic activation.[106] Postoperative AF is associated with an increased risk of mortality, stroke, and other complications, and it prolongs hospitalization. β-blockers are recommended as first-line treatment for AF that occurs after cardiothoracic surgery, with nondihydropyridine calcium channel blockers an alternative if β-blockers are ineffective. Both amiodarone and sotalol have been studied and found to be effective in reducing the incidence of postoperative AF, provided that they are started before surgery.[107] However, these drugs are not commonly used in clinical practice for this purpose. Statins, with atorvastatin being the most often studied, have been shown to reduce the incidence of postoperative AF when they are started preoperatively.[108] While most patients who undergo coronary artery bypass surgery should already be on statin drugs, these drugs have proven to be effective in patients undergoing valve and ascending aortic surgery. Anticoagulation and antiarrhythmic drugs should be used as in nonpostoperative patients with AF, although the risk of bleeding in the postoperative setting should be factored into treatment decisions.

In a study of patients undergoing cardiac surgery, AF developed in 33% of patients who had no history of the arrhythmia preoperatively.[109] Of these patients, 523 underwent randomization to a rate or a rhythm control strategy. Amiodarone was used for rhythm control. There were no differences in length of hospitalization, death rate, or serious adverse event rates in the two arms of the trial. At 60 days, 93.8% of the patients in the rate control group and 97.9% of those in the rhythm control group had a stable rhythm with no AF for the previous 30 days

($P = 0.02$), and 84.2% and 86.9%, respectively, had been free of AF from discharge to 60 days ($P = 0.41$).[109] The results of this study indicate that AF after cardiac surgery is likely to be short-lived, and antiarrhythmic drug therapy, if used, may not be necessary long term.

Not only does postoperative AF increase morbidity short term in patients after cardiac surgery, but it is also associated with an increased risk of stroke and mortality long term. In a meta-analysis of 35 studies including 2.5 million patients, postoperative AF was associated with a HR of 1.37 (95% CI, 1.07–1.77) for long-term stroke and 1.37 (95% CI, 1.27–1.49) for long-term mortality.[110] In addition, postoperative AF is an independent predictor of the late development of AF, with a 4- to 5-fold increased risk. Using propensity score matching in a retrospective analysis of a large hospital system database, postoperative AF after coronary artery bypass surgery was found to be associated with a higher incidence of total AF (18.9% vs 2.9%; $P < 0.001$) and long-term AF recurrence (10.2% vs 1.6%; $P < 0.001$) compared to patients without postoperative AF.[111] In a large, observational cohort study of 7145 patients after isolated coronary artery bypass surgery, patients who developed postoperative AF (33% of patients undergoing surgery; no history of preoperative AF) were compared to patients who did not developed AF after surgery and to matched controls. During a median follow-up of 9.8 years, patients with postoperative AF had a 3-fold higher incidence of AF compared with matched controls. Postoperative AF was also associated with a significantly higher risk of ischemic stroke, HF, and mortality in follow-up, although the association with mortality appears to be explained partly by comorbidities.[112] Thus, postoperative AF should not be viewed as a benign problem, even if it usually does not persist in the immediate postoperative period. These patients are at higher risk of future AF and complications and should be monitored carefully.

The incidence of AF after noncardiac surgery is lower than after cardiac surgery; it occurs in 10% to 20% of noncardiac thoracic operations.[106] The risk is approximately 3% in unselected patients undergoing noncardiothoracic surgery, with the majority of patients having a preoperative history of AF.[113] Mortality is higher and hospital length of stay longer in patients who develop AF after noncardiac surgery. Of interest, postoperative AF appears to be more strongly associated with a long-term risk of stroke in patients undergoing noncardiac surgery (HR 2.00; 95% CI, 1.70–2.35) than cardiac surgery (HR 1.20; 95% CI, 1.07–1.34).[110]

AF and Heart Failure

AF and HF often coexist. In the Framingham Heart Study, among patients with new onset AF, 37% had HF, and among patients with new onset HF, 57% had AF.[114] Prevalent AF was more strongly associated with HF with a preserved ejection fraction (HR 2.34; 95% CI, 1.48–3.70) compared to HF with a reduced ejection fraction (HR 1.32; 95% CI, 0.83–2.10). HF may cause AF via inflammation leading to fibrosis, neurohormonal changes, elevated filling pressures, and changes in cardiac ion channels leading to calcium overload and action potential prolongation.[115] AF can cause HF because of elevated ventricular rates (tachycardia-mediated cardiomyopathy). It is well recognized that ventricular function may recover if heart rate is controlled, whether by rate control medications, ablation of the AV junction with permanent pacing, or curative ablation of AF. In addition to the effects of rate itself, the irregularity of the rate in AF is detrimental to ventricular function. Loss of atrial systole contributes to HF as well.

AF in patients with HF is associated with a worse prognosis; attempts to improve outcomes in patients with these conditions have involved both rate and rhythm control strategies. In the Atrial Fibrillation and Congestive Heart Failure (AF-CHF) trial, a rhythm control strategy, primarily with amiodarone, did not reduce the rate of death from cardiovascular causes compared to a rate control strategy with AV nodal blockers or ablation of the AV junction with permanent pacing.[112] Studies of catheter ablation of AF have shown more promising results. In the CASTLE-AF trial, patients who failed antiarrhythmic drug therapy, had unacceptable side effects, or were unwilling to take antiarrhythmic drugs were randomized to catheter ablation of AF or medical rate or rhythm control. The primary endpoint, all-cause mortality or hospitalization for HF, was lower in the ablation arm compared to the medical therapy arm (28.5% vs 44.6%; HR 0.62; 95% CI, 0.43–0.87; $P = 0.007$).[91] In the CABANA trial, patients with AF, 57.1% of whom had persistent AF, were randomized to catheter ablation or standard therapy with rate and/or rhythm control drugs. The primary endpoint was a composite of death, disabling stroke, serious bleeding, or cardiac arrest. There was no significant difference in the primary endpoint between the two strategies, although there was a trend in favor of ablation among patients with HF.[88]

Association of AF With Other Supraventricular Tachycardias
Patients with Wolff-Parkinson-White syndrome who develop AV reentrant supraventricular tachycardia (SVT) using the accessory pathway may experience transition of the rhythm to AF at a fast rate. If the accessory pathway is capable of rapid conduction, AF may degenerate to ventricular fibrillation and cause sudden death. If a patient is hemodynamically unstable, electrical cardioversion is indicated. In stable patients, intravenous procainamide or ibutilide may be used to restore sinus rhythm or slow the ventricular response. β-blockers and calcium channel blockers are contraindicated in this setting, because they may cause hypotension and yet have no impact on slowing antegrade conduction over the accessory pathway. Digoxin is also contraindicated in this setting, because it might suppress conduction over the AV node, effectively accelerating conduction over the accessory pathway and leading to faster ventricular rates. If a patient has AF associated with Wolff-Parkinson-White syndrome, definitive treatment by ablation of the accessory pathway is the best course of action.

AF may occasionally be found in conjunction with other supraventricular tachycardias. In one series from a high volume ablation center, AV nodal reentrant tachycardia was found in 4.3% of patients referred for ablation of AF. Patients with AV nodal reentrant tachycardia and AF were younger than patients with AF alone (36.8±13.8 vs. 48.2±11.7 years; P <0.01). Thirteen patients underwent slow pathway modification alone, and 12 remained free of AF long-term without the need for PVI. In addition to AV nodal reentrant tachycardia and SVT associated with Wolff-Parkinson-White syndrome, other tachycardias such as atrial tachycardia may rarely be found in patients with AF who have never previously undergone ablation, although the most common correlation remains atrial flutter.

ATRIAL FLUTTER

Pathophysiology
Atrial flutter is a form of atrial tachycardia characterized by rapid stable reentry circuits. It is less common than AF. Atrial flutter, like AF, may be triggered by inflammation, postoperatively, by conditions such as acute HF exacerbation, or metabolic derangements such as acute alcohol exposure or thyrotoxicosis. It is a macro-reentrant circuit that requires an area of slow conduction and a region of functional conduction block for initiation and propagation.

The ECG appearance in atrial flutter reflects circuit location and electrical propagation to the remainder of the atrium (**Fig. 36-18**). *Typical* atrial flutter is defined by *counterclockwise* reentry around the tricuspid valve annulus in the right atrium, or a *clockwise* circuit in *reverse typical* atrial flutter (**Fig. 36-19**). The negative sawtooth pattern in ECG leads II, III, and aVF represents activation superiorly up the interatrial septum, followed by inferiorly directed activation down the right atrial free wall anterior to the crista terminalis, and then across the tricuspid annulus. In reverse typical flutter, this circuit occurs in a clockwise direction. Lead V1 is perpendicular to this frontal plane and so does not show a sawtooth pattern, but instead discrete upright P waves. This morphology may confuse the diagnosis when only a limited number of ECG leads are used, such as on telemetry. Atypical atrial flutter reflects circuits in other right or left atrial regions (**Fig. 36-20**). Left atrial circuits result in electrical activation from the left to the right atrium with positive flutter waves in ECG lead V1.

Strong clues to the location of atypical flutter circuits can be gleaned from a history of right atriotomy for cardiopulmonary bypass, incision lines for surgical correction of congenital heart disease or heart transplant, or prior ablation lines for AF. Right atrial circuits[117] may lie around the superior vena cava and superior right atrium (upper loop reentry), or around the inferior vena cava and right atrium (lower loop reentry). However, atypical right atrial flutter is most often due to prior incisions rather than upper or lower loop reentry. Common left atrial circuits lie near gaps in AF ablation lines, reentry around the mitral isthmus or around the pulmonary veins, or around large areas of scar. Multiple atrial flutter circuits, in which one circuit simultaneously "entrains" the other(s), may occur in patients with prior atrial procedures. Importantly, typical atrial flutter circuits are still common in patients with prior left and right atrial instrumentation, including correction of congenital defects.

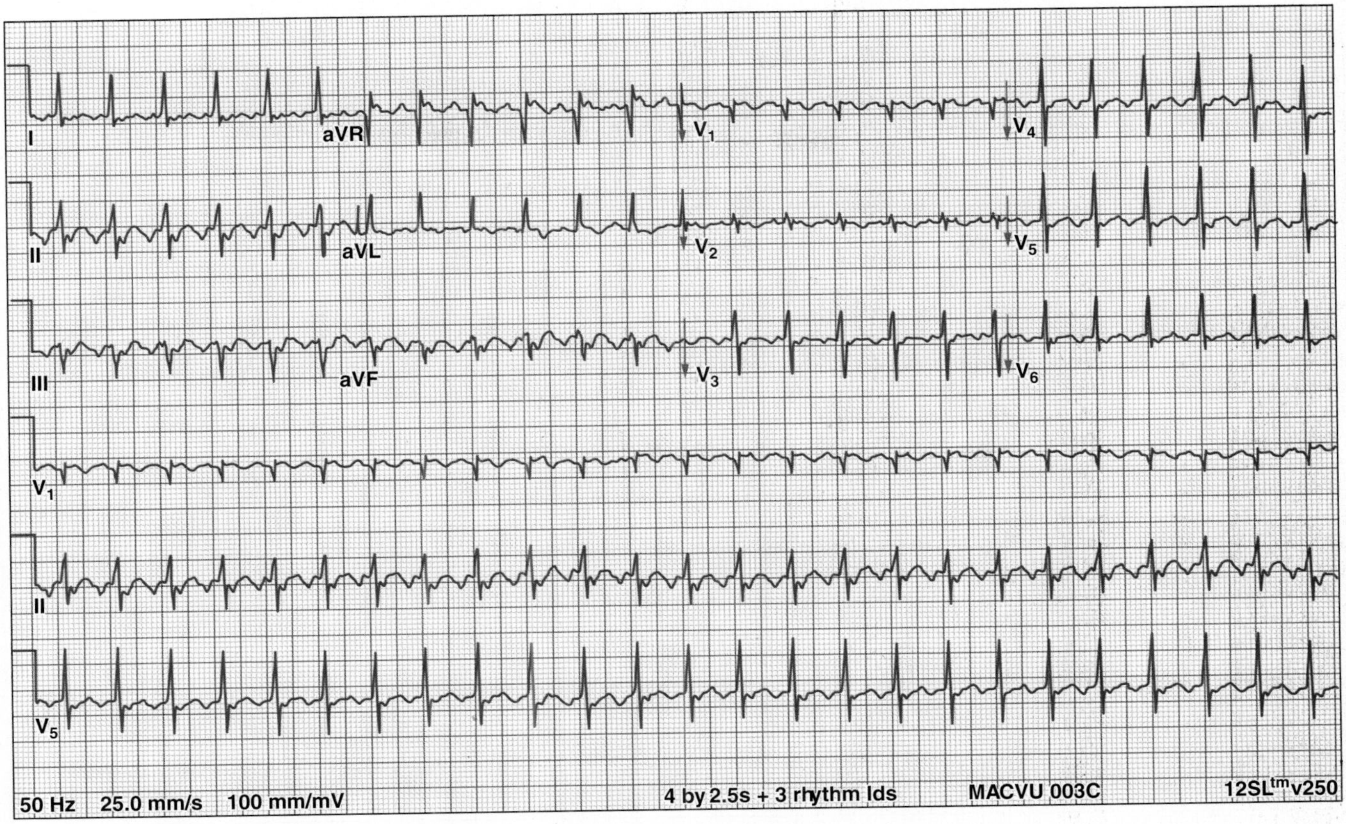

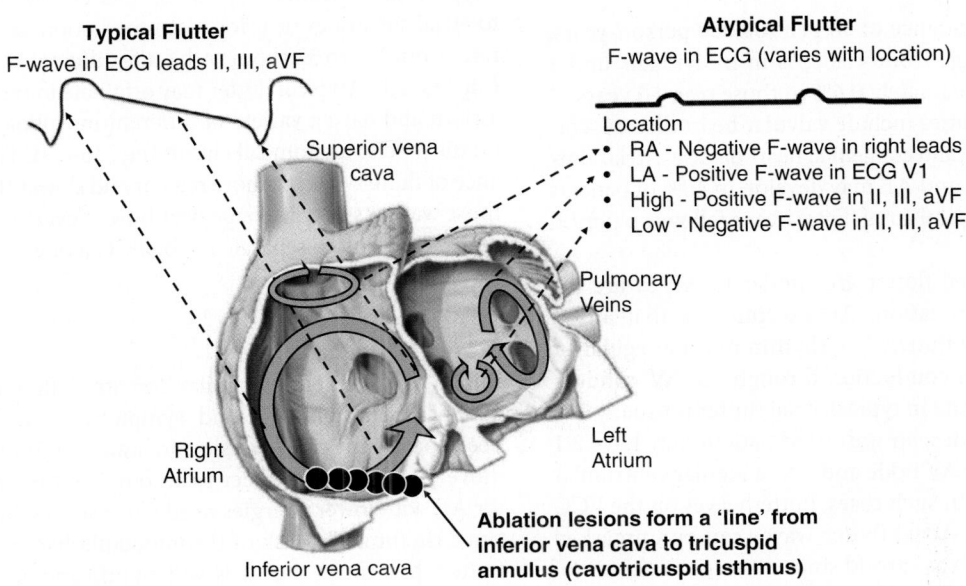

Figure 36–18. Twelve-lead ECG of typical atrial flutter. Note the negative flutter waves in leads II, III, and aVF and the upright flutter waves in lead V1. This is characteristic of counterclockwise, isthmus-dependent atrial flutter. This example shows a 2:1 atrioventricular block pattern, which is quite common.

Typical Flutter
F-wave in ECG leads II, III, aVF

Atypical Flutter
F-wave in ECG (varies with location)

Location
- RA - Negative F-wave in right leads
- LA - Positive F-wave in ECG V1
- High - Positive F-wave in II, III, aVF
- Low - Negative F-wave in II, III, aVF

Superior vena cava

Pulmonary Veins

Right Atrium

Left Atrium

Ablation lesions form a 'line' from inferior vena cava to tricuspid annulus (cavotricuspid isthmus)

Inferior vena cava

Figure 36–19. Mechanisms and ablation approach for atrial flutter. Typical atrial flutter shows counterclockwise reentry (reverse typical flutter shows clockwise reentry) on the atrial border of the tricuspid annulus. The ECG appearance in leads II, III, and aVF is stereotypical and generated as shown. Atypical flutter has several variants, which may arise from surgical incisions, gaps in prior ablation lines, or other atrial substrates. Its ECG appearances depend on its location and the extent of substrates, but left atrial circuits typically produce positive F-waves in lead V1, right atrial circuits may produce negative F-waves in right-facing ECG leads, and superiorly and inferiorly located circuits may produce positive and negative F-waves, respectively, in ECG leads II, III, and aVF. Ablation aims to bisect the circuit by connecting nonconducting boundaries. Cavotricuspid isthmus ablation for typical atrial flutter is shown.

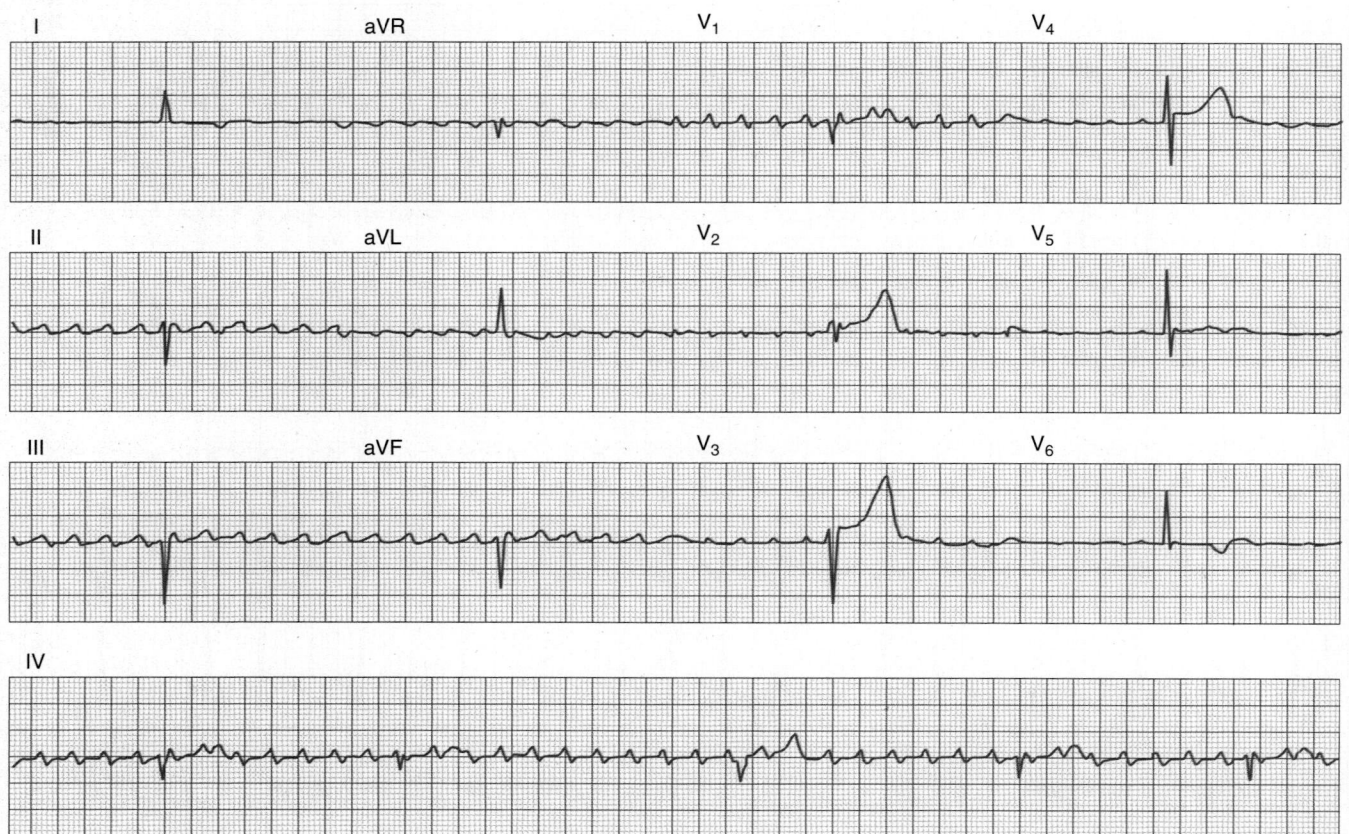

Figure 36–20. Twelve-lead ECG of a left atrial flutter that did not involve the usual cavotricuspid isthmus. Note the upright flutter waves in leads II, III, and aVF and the upright flutter waves in lead V1.

Clinical Presentation

Atrial flutter has an incidence of 88 per 100,000 person-years, which increases with age from <0.005% in individuals under 50 years of age to approximately 0.6% in those over 80 years.[118] Predisposing comorbidities include valvular heart disease, coronary artery disease, HF, and congenital heart disease. Atrial flutter comigrates with AF, and AF may develop in 40% of patients with newly diagnosed typical atrial flutter over a follow-up period of 3 years.[119]

Symptoms from atrial flutter are similar to AF, as are the signs on physical examination. An exception is that an S4 may be present in atrial flutter. The rhythm may be regular or irregular, depending on conduction through the AV conduction system. The atrial rate in typical atrial flutter is usually 250 to 300 bpm. At these rates, an untreated patient may have 2:1 conduction through the AV node and thus a regular ventricular rate of 125 to 150 bpm. In such cases, flutter waves on the ECG may be difficult to see. Atrial flutter waves can be unmasked by vagal maneuvers such as carotid sinus massage or the use of adenosine to block the AV node transiently (**Fig. 36–21**).

The key to the diagnosis of atrial flutter is the ECG. The ECG in typical or type 1 atrial flutter (also known as counterclockwise flutter), in which there is a large single reentry circuit in the right atrium, produces a classical negative sawtooth pattern in ECG leads II, III, and aVF (Fig. 36–18). The reverse circuit, clockwise atrial flutter, has positive flutter waves in the inferior leads.

Atypical atrial flutter reflects circuits elsewhere, often related to atrial substrates or prior instrumentation, at a wide range of rates from 180 to 320 bpm with quite different ECG flutter waves (Fig. 36–20). Atypical flutter may originate in the left or the right atrium and have a variety of different morphologies depending on the precise anatomical circuit (Fig. 36–19). The ECG appearance of flutter waves is more regular and slower than AF, because those wavelets vary in shape over time. Nevertheless, some cases may be difficult to separate by the ECG alone.

Management

Acute Management

Initial management is similar for atrial flutter and AF. The patient's hemodynamic and symptomatic status dictate the need for urgent cardioversion to sinus rhythm. Electrical cardioversion is usually easier to accomplish for atrial flutter than for AF, with lower energies needed for successful conversion to sinus rhythm. The risk of thromboembolism is lower in atrial flutter than in AF, but it is still significant, and patients with atrial flutter often have AF at other times. Therefore, patients should be treated with anticoagulation and evaluated with TEE prior to cardioversion in the same way one would approach a patient with AF. Ibutilide can be used for chemical conversion of atrial flutter and, in fact, the success rate for ibutilide converting AF or atrial flutter to sinus rhythm is highest with new-onset atrial flutter. Flecainide, dofetilide, and propafenone

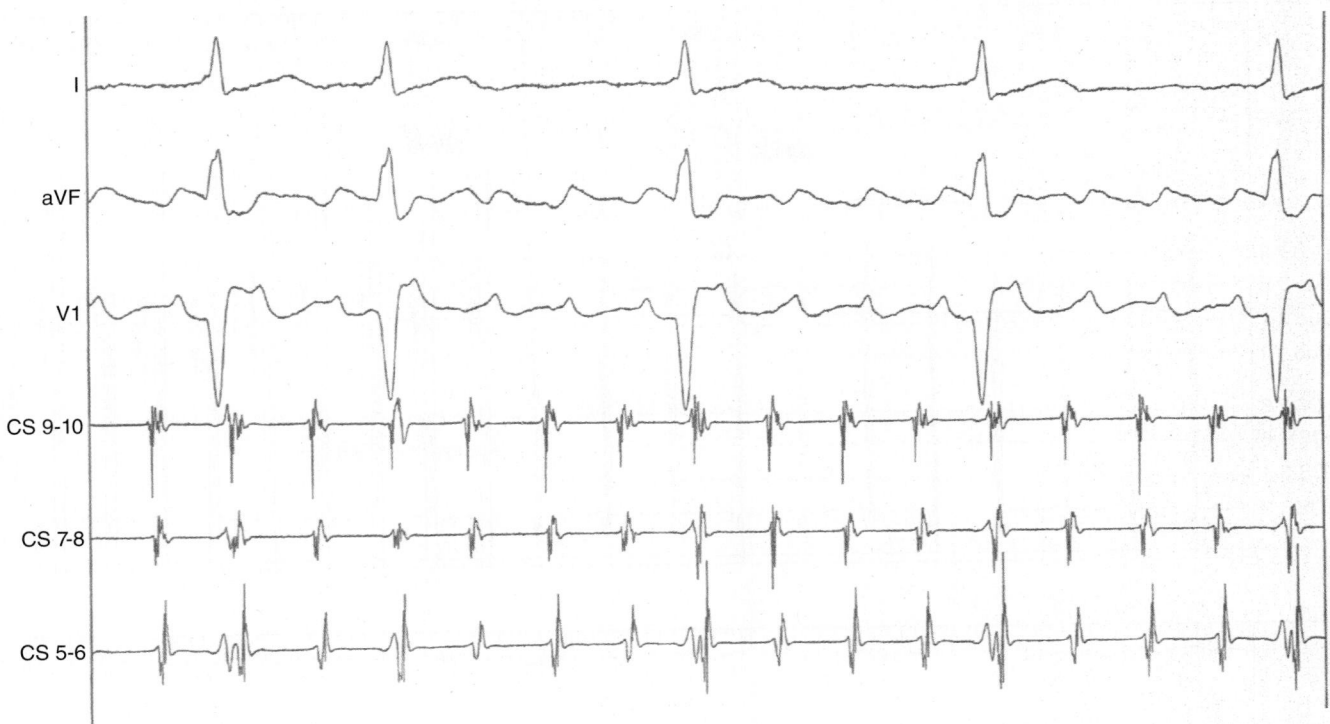

Figure 36–21. Unmasking of flutter waves after administration of adenosine 6 mg intravenously. Top three tracings are ECG leads I, aVF, and V1. Atrial flutter changes from 2:1 conduction to 4:1, at which point the flutter waves are easier to see. Bottom three tracings are intracardiac recordings from paired electrodes on a coronary sinus (CS) catheter, with CS 9-10 being the most proximal pair and CS 7-8 and 5-6 progressively closer to the tip of the catheter and therefore recording from a more distal position in the coronary sinus. These intracardiac electrograms show regular atrial flutter waves.

can also be used for pharmacologic cardioversion of atrial flutter, although their onset of action is slower than ibutilide.

Because atrial flutter is a macro-reentrant circuit, an option for termination that is not possible with AF is rapid atrial pacing. Short bursts of atrial pacing at a rate faster than the flutter rate may abruptly terminate the rhythm to sinus (**Fig. 36–22**). This approach is most often used in patients with cardiac implantable electrical devices such as pacemakers or implantable cardioverter defibrillators, as long as the patient has an atrial lead. If so, rapid atrial pacing through the programmer may terminate the arrhythmia. This technique can also be used in patients who are in the postoperative period after cardiac surgery, if temporary pacing wires are in place.

If cardioversion or pace termination is not needed immediately, rate slowing with AV nodal blockers should be initiated. The same options of β-blockers, calcium channel blockers, and digoxin are used as in AF. Amiodarone can be used acutely for rate control as well.[120] A distinct difference in atrial flutter is that rate control may often be *more* difficult than in AF. The reason for this observation is that the fixed atrial rate in flutter will require sufficient AV nodal blockade to drop a 2:1 ventricular response to 3:1 or 4:1. Anything less than that will allow the faster ventricular response to continue. In contrast, AF has more rapid atrial rates and more concealed conduction to the AV node, rendering moderation of the ventricular rate easier to achieve.

Chronic Management

For chronic management, the need for anticoagulation should be determined. The CHA$_2$DS$_2$-VASc score is used for

decision-making, as in AF. Lone atrial flutter appears to have a lower risk of stroke than AF, but thromboembolic events may still occur, necessitating attention to anticoagulation.[121]

The choice of rate or rhythm control is analogous to that in AF, with the major difference that ablation is more often considered a first line therapy for atrial flutter.[120] Reasons for this include the relatively high success rate of ablation, particularly for typical atrial flutter, as well as the common difficulty of achieving good rate control. If ablation is not feasible or successful, then a rhythm control strategy may be pursued, with the same options for antiarrhythmic drugs as in AF. One key point to remember concerns the use of flecainide or propafenone in atrial flutter. As both have a potent effect in slowing conduction in the atrium, the result could be an atrial flutter circuit that slows down from a typical rate near 300 bpm to somewhere closer to 200 to 250 bpm. At 300 bpm, conduction through the AV conduction system is typically 2:1, resulting in a ventricular rate of 150 bpm. If the atrial rate slows down, conduction may become 1:1, resulting in a *faster* ventricular rate. This problem may be avoided by insuring that any patient on these drugs is also prescribed an AV nodal blocker.

Catheter Ablation

Catheter ablation for typical atrial flutter is often highly successful, with a 90% or greater success rate on long-term follow-up, a relatively straightforward procedural approach, and a <1% complication rate. Ablation is designed to bisect the stable electrical circuit at its shortest point. For typical flutter, ablation targets the cavotricuspid isthmus by drawing a series of

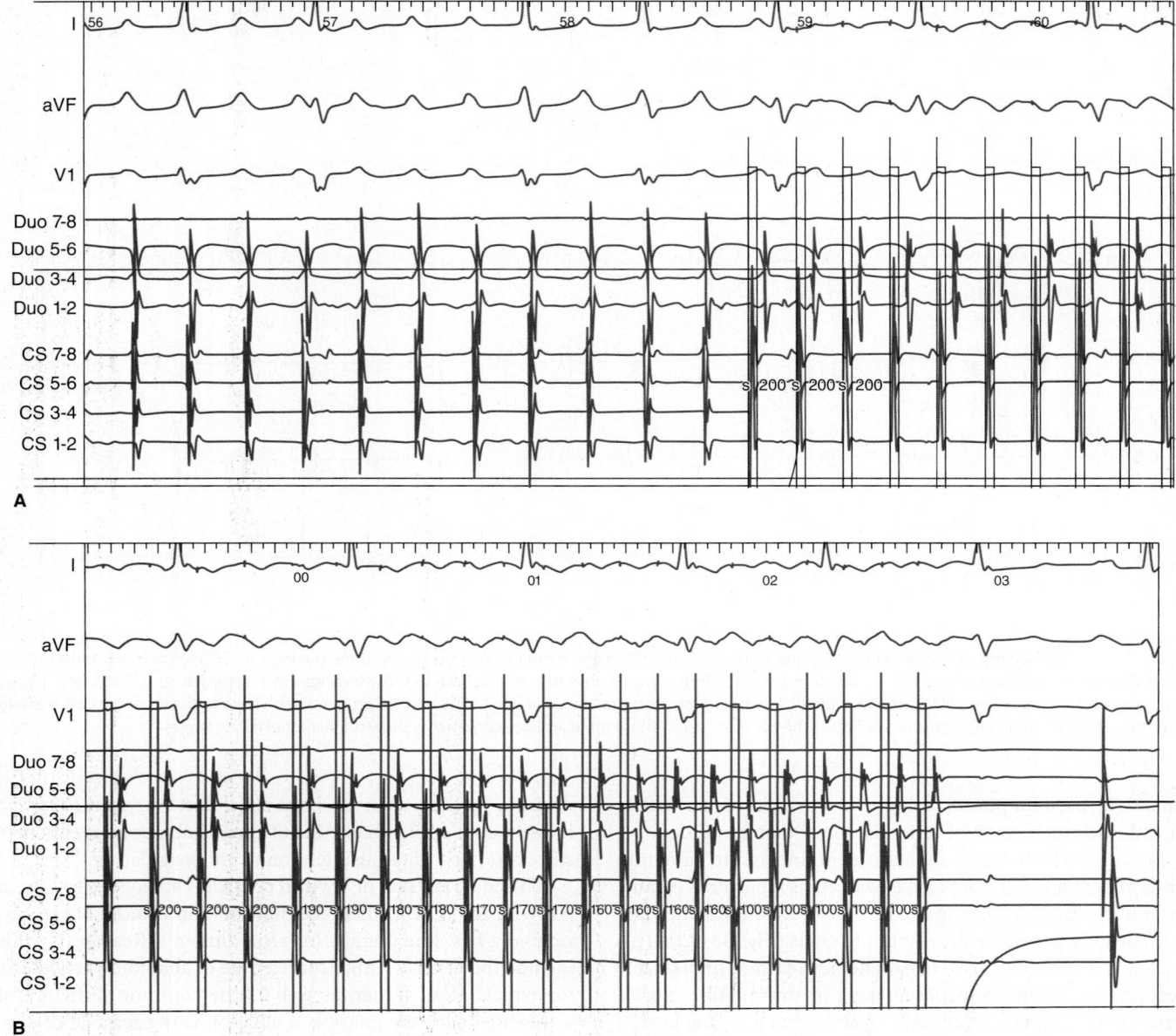

Figure 36–22. **(A) Pace termination of clockwise atrial flutter.** Top three leads are ECG leads I, aVF, and V1. Bottom tracings are from a coronary sinus catheter (CS) and a mapping catheter (Duo), which show the flutter waves. On the right, pacing is initiated at a slightly faster rate than the flutter rate. **(B) Pacing is abruptly terminated and sinus rhythm** is restored on the right side of the recording.

nonconducting lesions (a "line") from the tricuspid annulus anteriorly to the inferior vena cava posteriorly (Fig. 36–19).[11]

Catheter ablation for patients with atypical atrial flutter has mixed success. Some variants, such as upper and lower loop right atrial flutters, also have success rates >90%. Other types are more challenging, such as left atrial flutters in patients with prior surgical incisions. The most challenging are atypical left (or right) atrial flutters in the milieu of prior AF ablation, which may be multiple and coexisting, for which the success rate at 1 year is ~70%.[11]

It is important to recognize that atrial flutter and AF comigrate. New onset or first detection of AF has been reported in 25% to 80% of patients after successful elimination of atrial

flutter by ablation. New documentation of AF is particularly likely to occur in patients with *a priori* risk factors for AF, such as those with higher CHA_2DS_2-VASc scores. Indeed, AF ablation by PVI concomitant with typical atrial flutter ablation has been shown to reduce the incidence of new onset AF compared to atrial flutter ablation alone. In patients who present with both AF and atrial flutter, ablation can thus target both atrial flutter and AF via PVI. However, empirical PVI is not standard of care in patients who present with atrial flutter alone, because it would introduce additional procedural risks to patients who may never develop AF or in whom AF may be relatively asymptomatic and who would therefore not necessarily proceed to AF ablation in the future.

PRACTICE GUIDELINES

Guidelines for the management of AF and atrial flutter are constantly evolving. Key areas of alignment and differences among the American College of Cardiology/American Heart Association/Heart Rhythm Society, European Heart Rhythm Association, and Canadian Cardiovascular Society guidelines are shown in **Table 36–12**.[60, 122-124] Many of the salient areas that have been updated include the definition of nonvalvular AF, stroke risk stratification algorithms, recommendations for prevention of thromboembolism, antithrombotic regimens in the setting of AF and coronary artery disease/procedures, anticoagulation for cardioversion, and periprocedural anticoagulation. There are minor differences in the recommendations for rate and rhythm control. Treatment of atrial flutter is generally handled the same as for AF.

TABLE 36–12. Comparison of US, European, and Canadian Guidelines for the Management of Atrial Fibrillation

	AHA/ACC/HRS[60,122]	European Society of Cardiology[73]	Canadian Cardiovascular Society[123,124]
Classification	Paroxysmal, persistent (>7 days), longstanding persistent (>1 year), permanent	First diagnosed, paroxysmal, persistent (>7 days), longstanding persistent (>1 year), permanent; clinical AF: symptomatic or asymptomatic documented by ECG, ambulatory monitor, or wearable; subclinical: asymptomatic, detected by implantable device such as pacemaker	Newly detected/diagnosed, paroxysmal, persistent (>7 days), longstanding persistent (>1 year), permanent
Symptom score	No recommendation	Modified EHRA Score, grades 1 (asymptomatic) to 4 (disabling symptoms)	CCS-SAF Score, grades 0 (asymptomatic) to 4 (severe effect on QOL)
Definition of nonvalvular AF for use of DOACs	Absence of moderate-to-severe MS or mechanical heart valve	Absence of moderate-to-severe MS or mechanical heart valve	Absence of rheumatic MS (any severity), moderate to severe MS, or mechanical heart valve
Stroke risk stratification algorithm	CHA$_2$DS$_2$-VASc	Modified CHA$_2$DS$_2$-VASc (female sex not counted in the absence of other risk factors)	CCS (CHADS-65): no points for vascular disease or female sex; one point for ≥65 years; no additional point ≥75 years
Stroke risk score: 0 (or 1 in women) 1 (or 2 in women) ≥2 ≥3	Antithrombotic recommendations and class: None (IIa) OAC, ASA, none (IIb) Men: OAC (I) Women: OAC (I)	Antithrombotic recommendations and class: None (III) OAC (IIa) OAC for men (I) OAC for men and women (I)	Antithrombotic recommendations and class: None (conditional) OAC (strong) OAC (strong)
Role of ASA in stroke prevention	CHA$_2$DS$_2$-VASc = 1	None	CCS = 0 and coronary or vascular disease
OAC recommendation	DOAC preferred (Class I)	DOAC preferred (Class I)	DOAC preferred (strong)
Antithrombotic regimens for CAD, ACS, and PCI (DOAC lifelong in all after 1 year)	OAC (VKA, low-dose rivaroxaban, dabigatran) +clopidogrel post PCI (IIa); if ASA added, stop at 4-6 weeks (IIb)	DOAC+clopidogrel+ASA for 1 week (I) (1 month if high risk of stent thrombosis (IIa)); DOAC+clopidogrel for 1 year	DOAC and clopidogrel for 1 year for PCI; add ASA for 6 months if ACS; OAC+clopidogrel for ACS without PCI
Cardioversion for AF or atrial flutter <48 hours	CHA$_2$DS$_2$-VASc=0 (men) or 1 (women): OAC not needed post cardioversion ((IIb)	No specific recommendation	CHADS$_2$<2 (or <12 hours and no recent stroke or TIA: no OAC needed (weak)
Periprocedural anticoagulation	Interruption of OAC not needed for procedures with low risk of bleeding (eg, CIEDs); bridging therapy for patients with mechanical heart valves	Interruption of OAC not needed for procedures with low risk of bleeding (eg, CIEDs); bridging therapy for patients with mechanical heart valves	Interruption of OAC not needed for procedures with low risk of bleeding (eg, CIEDs); no bridging for patients on VKA unless mechanical heart valve or high risk of bleeding (CHADS$_2$≥4); no bridging needed for patients on DOACs if interruption of therapy necessary
Prevention of thromboembolism in atrial flutter	Use same risk profile as for AF	Use same risk profile as for AF	Use same risk profile as for AF
Target heart rate for rate control	<80 bpm (IIa) <110 bpm (IIb)	<110 bpm (IIa)	<100 bpm (strong)
Medications for rate control	β-blocker or CCB; digoxin second line	β-blocker, CCB, or digoxin	β-blocker or CCB; β-blocker first in MI or LV dysfunction; digoxin second line

(Continued)

TABLE 36–12. Comparison of US, European, and Canadian Guidelines for the Management of Atrial Fibrillation (Continued)

	AHA/ACC/HRS[60,122]	European Society of Cardiology[73]	Canadian Cardiovascular Society[123,124]
Antiarrhythmic drugs			
Normal heart	All (amiodarone second line)	All except amiodarone and dofetilide	All except dofetilide (amiodarone second line)
CAD	All except IC (flecainide, propafenone)	All except IC and dofetilide	Sotalol, dronedarone, amiodarone
LVH	Dronedarone, amiodarone	Dronedarone, sotalol, amiodarone	All except dofetilide
Valvular	Not specified	Dronedarone, sotalol, amiodarone	Not specified
Heart failure	Dofetilide, amiodarone	Amiodarone	Amiodarone; sotalol or dronedarone if EF>35%
Catheter ablation when antiarrhythmic drug(s) failed for			
Paroxysmal AF	Class I	Class I	Strong
Persistent AF	Class IIa	Class I	After 2 AAD failures
Long-standing persistent AF	Class IIb	Class IIb	After 3 AAD failures
Catheter ablation prior to trying antiarrhythmic drug			
Paroxysmal AF	Class IIa	Class IIa	Selected patients
Persistent AF	Class IIa	Class IIa	Not recommended
Long-standing persistent AF	Class IIb	Class IIb	Not recommended
Ablation during cardiac surgery	Class IIa	To improve symptoms (IIa) Asymptomatic (IIb)	Conditional when symptomatic benefit is expected
Stand-alone surgical AF ablation	Class IIb	Failed catheter ablation (IIa)	Failed catheter ablation
Surgical left atrial appendage excision	Class IIb during cardiac surgery	"Should be considered" during cardiac surgery	Class IIb during cardiac surgery
Left atrial appendage occlusion	Increased risk of stroke and contraindications to long-term anticoagulation (IIb)	High risk patients in systematic protocols when OAC contraindicated	Increased risk of stroke and contraindications to long-term anticoagulation (IIb)

Abbreviations: AAD, antiarrhythmic drug; ACC, American College of Cardiology; ACS, acute coronary syndrome; AF, atrial fibrillation; AHA, American Heart Association; ASA, aspirin; CAD, coronary artery disease; CCB, calcium channel blocker; CCS, Canadian Cardiovascular Society; CCS-SAF, Canadian Cardiovascular Society-Severity of Atrial Fibrillation; CIED, cardiac implantable electrical device; CHADS-65, congestive heart failure, hypertension, age ≥65 years, diabetes, history of stroke or transient ischemic attack; CHA_2DS_2-VASc, congestive heart failure, hypertension, age≥75 years, diabetes, history of stroke or transient ischemic attack, vascular disease, age 65–74 years, female sex; DOAC, direct oral anticoagulant; EHRA, European Heart Rhythm Association; EF, ejection fraction; LV, left ventricular; LVH, left ventricular hypertrophy; MI, myocardial infarction; MS, mitral stenosis; OAC, oral anticoagulant (DOAC or vitamin K antagonist); PCI, percutaneous coronary intervention; QOL, quality of life; TIA, transient ischemic attack; VKA, vitamin K antagonist.

SUMMARY

Epidemiology

- The prevalence of AF is 1% to 2%, with a lifetime risk of developing AF of 1 in 3 in White individuals and 1 in 5 for Black individuals.

- Advancing age is the most prominent risk factor associated with AF; other important risk factors include male sex, diabetes mellitus, HF, coronary artery disease, valvular heart disease, alcohol and tobacco consumption, obesity, and sleep apnea.

Pathophysiology

- AF is initiated by triggers. Over time, an atrial myopathy may develop that enables AF to sustain, once initiated, by the electrical substrates of reentry and focal activity, modulated by the autonomic nervous system and structural substrates such as atrial myocardial scar.

- The electrical substrate for AF is mediated by cellular electrical remodeling, with abnormalities in calcium signaling, nitroso-redox pathways, and metabolism that shorten repolarization.

- The structural substrate for AF is mediated by altered connexin biology and fibrosis, which impair cell-to-cell electrical propagation and slow conduction.

- Genetic mechanisms explain the heritability of AF via a complex network of genes with small effect sizes and rare coding variants with large effect sizes.

Classification

- AF may occur acutely (first occurrence) in the setting of conditions such as metabolic derangements, hyperthyroidism, or surgery; it is often reversible in such settings.

- AF is commonly classified as paroxysmal, persistent, long-standing persistent, and permanent.

- Silent AF denotes AF in the absence of any symptoms or prior diagnosis, often presenting as a complication related to AF.

- Subclinical AF refers to atrial high rate episodes >6 minutes with a lack of correlated symptoms in patients with cardiac implantable electronic devices such as pacemakers and no prior AF diagnosis.

Clinical Presentation

- Typical symptoms include palpitations, rapid heart rates, shortness of breath, dyspnea on exertion, fatigue, exercise intolerance, dizziness, and chest discomfort.
- AF is asymptomatic in about one-third of patients, especially in the elderly and after catheter ablation.
- Stroke may be the first manifestation of AF, even if the arrhythmia is not present on admission.

Initial Evaluation

- A history of valvular heart disease, thyroid disease, hypertension, diabetes, obesity, stroke, obstructive sleep apnea, and alcohol intake should be elicited.
- On physical examination, irregularity of the pulse or heart sounds, murmurs indicative of valvular heart disease, evidence of HF, and signs of hyperthyroidism such as exophthalmos and unexplained sinus tachycardia should be assessed.
- Basic laboratory tests such as complete blood count, serum electrolytes, and assessment of renal, hepatic, and thyroid function should be obtained as well as B-type natriuretic peptide if HF is suspected.
- A chest x-ray may be indicated in some patients.
- An echocardiogram should be obtained to assess ventricular function, left atrial size, and left ventricular hypertrophy, as well as the presence of valvular heart disease or cardiomyopathy.
- Other imaging studies such as cardiac magnetic resonance are not routinely indicated but may be helpful in selected patients.

Electrocardiographic Diagnosis and Monitoring of Atrial Fibrillation

- An ECG should be obtained in all patients; it may confirm the diagnosis of AF and also provide evidence of other structural heart disease.
- The longer the duration of monitoring, the greater the likelihood of detecting AF.
- A 24- to 48-hour ambulatory ECG monitor is useful for assessment of the adequacy of rate control in AF; it can also correlate symptoms with arrhythmia if symptoms are frequent.
- Event monitors worn for 14 to 30 days are a good option for noninvasive monitoring if symptoms are infrequent or for detecting asymptomatic episodes, but rare episodes of AF may be missed.
- Insertable loop recorders are implanted devices that can monitor rhythm for up to 3 years. They are useful for patients with infrequent symptoms, and they are also used in patients who have had thromboembolic strokes for detection of occult AF.
- Wearable technologies range from wrist bands and watches that can alert the patient to a fast or irregular rhythm and prompt further testing, to recording of electrocardiographic rhythm strips using a portable set of electrodes and/or a smart watch.

Complications

- Stroke, peripheral thromboembolism, dementia, tachycardia-mediated cardiomyopathy, and other adverse hemodynamic effects constitute the main complications associated with AF.
- Ischemic stroke related to AF is thought to be cardioembolic in origin, arising in the LAA due to stasis of blood flow and increased thrombogenicity in the setting of AF.
- Increased risk of dementia secondary to AF is independent from a history of prior stroke or anticoagulation use.

Acute Management

- The hemodynamic status of the patient (eg, hypotension, decompensated HF, ischemia) should dictate the urgency of restoring sinus rhythm.
- Rate control may be required to improve hemodynamics and/or symptoms. β-blockers and nondihydropyridine calcium channel blockers are preferred as first-line drugs.
- Transesophageal echocardiography should be performed before electrical or chemical cardioversion in most patients with AF unless the patient has been effectively anticoagulated for a minimum of three weeks prior to presentation.
- Ibutilide, flecainide, propafenone, and amiodarone may be effective for chemical cardioversion.
- Flecainide and propafenone can be used in a "pill-in-the-pocket" approach to cardioversion in patients with AF and no structural heart disease.

Lifestyle Modification

- Lifestyle choices may have a U-shaped or J-shaped relationship to AF. Compared to a sedentary lifestyle, moderate exercise decreases the incidence of AF while extreme exercise can increase the incidence of AF.
- Weight loss decreases the recurrence of AF, while obesity or fluctuations in weight can increase the rate of recurrence.
- Bariatric surgery in severe obesity may prevent the development of AF as well as decrease recurrences of AF.
- Treatment of obstructive sleep apnea and reduction of heavy alcohol use may reduce the frequency of AF recurrences.

Stroke Prevention

- The CHA_2DS_2-VASc score is used to assess stroke risk and guide anticoagulation management.
- Oral anticoagulation is recommended for patients with CHA_2DS_2-VASc scores of ≥ 2 in men and ≥ 3 in women and may be considered for patients with a CHA_2DS_2-VASc score of 1 in men and 2 in women.
- Direct oral anticoagulants are recommended over warfarin, except for patients with moderate-to-severe mitral stenosis or mechanical heart valves.
- Evidence does not support the use of aspirin as monotherapy for the prevention of thromboembolic events in patients with AF with any CHA_2DS_2-VASc score.
- Patients undergoing coronary stenting should have a brief initial period of triple therapy (aspirin plus another

antiplatelet drug plus an oral anticoagulant), following by dual therapy (oral anticoagulant plus preferably clopidogrel) for the first 12 months after percutaneous coronary intervention (PCI) for acute coronary syndrome, or 6 months after PCI otherwise.

- LAA occlusion may be considered in patients at increased risk of stroke who have contraindications for oral anticoagulation.

Rate and Rhythm Control

- Decisions as to a rate or rhythm control strategy for an individual patient should take into consideration the patient's symptoms or lack thereof, the type and frequency of AF episodes, and comorbidities such as HF.
- Recent evidence suggests that early rhythm control (maintaining sinus rhythm) can prevent downstream cardiovascular hospitalizations and mortality.
- Control of the ventricular rate during AF using rate control drugs should be instituted whether or not antiarrhythmic drugs will be prescribed as well.
- Adequate rate control is considered to be a mean ventricular rate of approximately 80 bpm over 24 hours without excessively elevated heart rates during exercise or marked pauses during sleep.
- The choice of antiarrhythmic drug should be based on the presence and type of underlying structural heart disease.
- Flecainide and propafenone are good choices for rhythm control in patients without structural heart disease.
- Dronedarone and sotalol can be used in patients with mild-moderate heart disease as well as in patients without structural heart disease; dronedarone is contraindicated in patients with persistent AF.
- Dofetilide and amiodarone are the two antiarrhythmic drugs that have been demonstrated to be safe to use in patients with HF.

Catheter Ablation and Other Nonpharmacologic Approaches

- PVI is the mainstay of ablation therapy; it involves electrically isolating the common trigger regions near the pulmonary veins from the rest of the left atrium.
- Additional sites are often ablated in patients in whom PVI is insufficient, including nonpulmonary vein trigger sites or sites of localized drivers, autonomic innervation, or scar.
- Ablation may be performed endocardially, surgically by an epicardial approach, or using a combined (hybrid) approach.

Atrial Flutter

- Atrial flutter is a macro-reentrant electrical circuit in the atria that requires an area of slow conduction and a region of functional conduction block for initiation and propagation.
- Typical atrial flutter is defined by counterclockwise reentry in the right atrium parallel to the tricuspid annulus.

- Atypical flutter may be found in the left or the right atrium and may be related to incisions or scars from previous procedures such as surgery or catheter ablation.
- Symptoms, clinical evaluation and initial management are similar for AF and atrial flutter.
- Rate control may be more difficult in atrial flutter than AF because of the fixed, macro-reentrant atrial circuit with less concealed conduction in the AV node.
- The choice of antiarrhythmic drugs, if pharmacologic management is chosen, is similar to AF.
- Catheter ablation is often a first-line strategy in typical atrial flutter because the procedure is usually relatively straightforward with a high success rate and low complication rate.

REFERENCES

1. Chugh SS, Havmoeller R, Narayanan K, et al. Worldwide epidemiology of atrial fibrillation: a Global Burden of Disease 2010 Study. *Circulation.* 2014;129:837-847.
2. Miyasaka Y, Barnes ME, Gersh BJ, et al. Secular trends in incidence of atrial fibrillation in Olmsted County, Minnesota, 1980 to 2000, and implications on the projections for future prevalence. *Circulation.* 2006;114:119-125.
3. Packer M, Lam CSP, Lund LH, Redfield MM. Interdependence of atrial fibrillation and heart failure with a preserved ejection fraction reflects a common underlying atrial and ventricular myopathy. *Circulation.* 2020;141:4-6.
4. Kirchhof P, John CA, Goette A, et al. E-AT. Early rhythm-control therapy in patients with atrial fibrillation. *New Engl J Med.* 2020;383:1305-1316.
5. Voskoboinik A, Kalman JM, De Silva A, et al. Alcohol abstinence in drinkers with atrial fibrillation. *N Engl J Med.* 2020;382:20-28.
6. Packer M. Characterization, pathogenesis, and clinical implications of inflammation-related atrial myopathy as an important cause of atrial fibrillation. *J Am Heart Assoc.* 2020;9:e015343.
7. Kochi AN, Tagliari AP, Forleo GB, Fassini GM, Tondo C. Cardiac and arrhythmic complications in Covid-19 patients. *J Cardiovasc Electrophysiol.* 2020;31:1003-1008.
8. Kiaii B, Fox S, Chase L, et al. Postoperative atrial fibrillation is not pulmonary vein dependent: results from a randomized trial. *Heart Rhythm* 2015;12:699-705.
9. Bisbal F, Baranchuk A, Braunwald E, Bayes de Luna A, Bayes-Genis A. Atrial failure as a clinical entity: JACC Review Topic of the Week. *J Am Coll Cardiol.* 2020;75:222-232.
10. Haissaguerre M, Jais P, Shah DC, et al. Spontaneous initiation of atrial fibrillation by ectopic beats originating in the pulmonary veins. *N Eng J Med.* 1998;339:659-666.
11. Calkins H, Hindricks G, Cappato R, et al. 2017 HRS/EHRA/ECAS/APHRS/SOLAECE expert consensus statement on catheter and surgical ablation of atrial fibrillation. *Europace.* 2018;20:e1-e160.
12. Steinberg JS, Shabanov V, Ponomarev D, et al. Effect of renal denervation and catheter ablation vs catheter ablation alone on atrial fibrillation recurrence among patients with paroxysmal atrial fibrillation and hypertension: the ERADICATE-AF randomized clinical trial. *JAMA.* 2020;323:248-255.
13. Stavrakis S, Stoner JA, Humphrey MB, et al. TREAT AF (Transcutaneous Electrical Vagus Nerve Stimulation to Suppress Atrial Fibrillation): a randomized clinical trial. *JACC Clin Electrophysiol.* 2020;6:282-291.
14. Moe GK and Abildskov JA. Atrial fibrillation as a self-sustaining arrhythmia independent of focal discharge. *Am Heart J.* 1959;58:59-70.

15. Allessie MA, de Groot NM, Houben RP, Schotten U, Boersma E, Smeets JL, Crijns HJ. Electropathological substrate of long-standing persistent atrial fibrillation in patients with structural heart disease: longitudinal dissociation. *Circ Arrhythm Electrophysiol.* 2010;3:606-615.

16. Krinsky, V. Spread of excitation in an inhomogeneous medium (state similar to cardiac fibrillation. *Biophysics.* 1966;11:676-683.

17. Davidenko, JM, Pertsov AV, Salomonsz R, Baxter W, Jalife J. Stationary and drifting spiral waves of excitation in isolated cardiac muscle. *Nature.* 1992;355(6358): 349-351.

18. Hansen BJ, Zhao J, Csepe TA, et al. Atrial fibrillation driven by micro-anatomic intramural re-entry revealed by simultaneous sub-epicardial and sub-endocardial optical mapping in explanted human hearts. *Eur Heart J.* 2015;36:2390-2401.

19. Baykaner T, Rogers AJ, Meckler GL, et al. Clinical implications of ablation of drivers for atrial fibrillation: a systematic review and meta-analysis. *Circ Arrhythm Electrophysiol.* 2018;11:e006119.

20. Bisbal F, Alarcon F, Ferrero-de-Loma-Osorio A, et al. Left atrial geometry and outcome of atrial fibrillation ablation: results from the multicentre LAGO-AF study. *Eur Heart J Cardiovasc Imaging.* 2018;19:1002-1009.

21. Platonov PG, Mitrofanova LB, Orshanskaya V, Ho SY. Structural abnormalities in atrial walls are associated with presence and persistency of atrial fibrillation but not with age. *J Am Coll Cardiol.* 2011;58: 2225-2232.

22. Fedorov VV, Hansen BJ. A secret marriage between fibrosis and atrial fibrillation drivers. *JACC Clin Electrophysiol.* 2018;4:30-32.

23. Marrouche NF, Wilber D, Hindricks G, et al. Association of atrial tissue fibrosis identified by delayed enhancement MRI and atrial fibrillation catheter ablation: the DECAAF study. *JAMA.* 2014;311:498-506.

24. Hatem SN, Redheuil A, Gandjbakhch E. Cardiac adipose tissue and atrial fibrillation: the perils of adiposity. *Cardiovasc Res.* 2016;109:502-509.

25. Heijman J, Voigt N, Nattel S, Dobrev D. Cellular and molecular electrophysiology of atrial fibrillation initiation, maintenance, and progression. *Circ Res.* 2014;114:1483-1499.

26. Mesubi OO, Anderson ME. Atrial remodelling in atrial fibrillation: CaMKII as a nodal proarrhythmic signal. *Cardiovasc Res.* 2016;109:542-557.

27. Purohit A, Rokita AG, Guan X, et al. Oxidized Ca(2+)/calmodulin-dependent protein kinase II triggers atrial fibrillation. *Circulation.* 2013; 128:1748-1757.

28. Reilly SN, Liu X, Carnicer R, et al. Up-regulation of miR-31 in human atrial fibrillation begets the arrhythmia by depleting dystrophin and neuronal nitric oxide synthase. *Sci Transl Med.* 2016;8:340ra74.

29. Opacic D, van Bragt KA, Nasrallah HM, Schotten U, Verheule S. Atrial metabolism and tissue perfusion as determinants of electrical and structural remodelling in atrial fibrillation. *Cardiovasc Res.* 2016;109:527-541.

30. Tucker NR, Clauss S, Ellinor PT. Common variation in atrial fibrillation: navigating the path from genetic association to mechanism. *Cardiovasc Res.* 2016;109:493-501.

31. Roberts JD, Hu D, Heckbert SR, et al. Genetic investigation into the differential risk of atrial fibrillation among black and white individuals. *JAMA Cardiol.* 2016;1:442-450.

32. Nielsen JB, Thorolfsdottir RB, Fritsche LG, et al. Biobank-driven genomic discovery yields new insight into atrial fibrillation biology. *Nat Genet.* 2018;50:1234-1239.

33. Shoemaker MB, Husser D, Roselli C, et al. Genetic susceptibility for atrial fibrillation in patients undergoing atrial fibrillation ablation. *Circ Arrhythm Electrophysiol.* 2020;13:e007676.

34. ACC/AHA/HRS. 2014 AHA/ACC/HRS guideline for the management of patients with atrial fibrillation: a Report of the American College of Cardiology/American Heart Association Task Force on Practice Guidelines and the Heart Rhythm Society. *J Am Coll Cardiol.* 2014;64:e1-76.

35. Gorenek BC, Bax J, Boriani G, et al. Device-detected subclinical atrial tachyarrhythmias: definition, implications and management-an European Heart Rhythm Association (EHRA) consensus document, endorsed by Heart Rhythm Society (HRS), Asia Pacific Heart Rhythm Society (APHRS) and Sociedad Latinoamericana de Estimulacion Cardiaca y Electrofisiologia (SOLEACE). *Europace.* 2017;19:1556-1578.

36. Yao X, Gersh BJ, Sangaralingham LR, et al. Comparison of the CHA2DS2-VASc, CHADS2, HAS-BLED, ORBIT, and ATRIA risk scores in predicting non-vitamin k antagonist oral anticoagulants-associated bleeding in patients with atrial fibrillation. *Am J Cardiol.* 2017;120:1549-1556.

37. Andrade JG, Deyell MW, Verma A, et al. Association of atrial fibrillation episode duration with arrhythmia recurrence following ablation: a secondary analysis of a randomized clinical trial. *JAMA Netw Open.* 2020;3:e208748.

38. Dilaveris PE, Kennedy HL. Silent atrial fibrillation: epidemiology, diagnosis, and clinical impact. *Clin Cardiol.* 2017;40:413-418.

39. Boriani G, Laroche C, Diemberger I, et al. Asymptomatic atrial fibrillation: clinical correlates, management, and outcomes in the EORP-AF Pilot General Registry. *Am J Med.* 2015;128:509-518 e2.

40. Osmanagic A, Moller S, Osmanagic A, Sheta HM, Vinther KH, Egstrup K. Left atrial sphericity index predicts early recurrence of atrial fibrillation after direct-current cardioversion: an echocardiographic study. *Clin Cardiol.* 2016;39:406-412.

41. Lee DC, Markl M, Ng J, Carr M, Benefield B, Carr JC, Goldberger JJ. Three-dimensional left atrial blood flow characteristics in patients with atrial fibrillation assessed by 4D flow CMR. *Eur Heart J Cardiovasc Imaging.* 2016;17:1259-1268.

42. Gladstone DJ, Spring M, Dorian P, et al. Atrial fibrillation in patients with cryptogenic stroke. *N Engl J Med.* 2014;370:2467-2477.

43. Krittanawong C, Rogers AJ, Johnson KW, et al. Integration of novel monitoring devices with machine learning technology for scalable cardiovascular management. *Nat Rev Cardiol.* 2021;18:75-91.

44. Sana F, Isselbacher EM, Singh JP, Heist EK, Pathik B, Armoundas AA. Wearable devices for ambulatory cardiac monitoring: JACC State-of-the-Art Review. *J Am Coll Cardiol.* 2020;75:1582-1592.

45. O'Sullivan JW, Grigg S, Crawford W, et al. Accuracy of smartphone camera applications for detecting atrial fibrillation: a systematic review and meta-analysis. *JAMA Netw Open.* 2020;3:e202064.

46. Perez MV, Mahaffey KW, Hedlin H, et al. Large-scale assessment of a smartwatch to identify atrial fibrillation. *N Engl J Med.* 2019;381:1909-1917.

47. Guo Y, Wang H, Zhang H, et al. Mobile photoplethysmographic technology to detect atrial fibrillation. *J Am Coll Cardiol.* 2019;74:2365-2375.

48. Sanna T, Diener HC, Passman RS, et al. Cryptogenic stroke and underlying atrial fibrillation. *N Engl J Med.* 2014;370:2478-2486.

49. Diederichsen SZ, Haugan KJ, Kronborg C, et al. Comprehensive evaluation of rhythm monitoring strategies in screening for atrial fibrillation: insights from patients at risk monitored long term with an implantable loop recorder. *Circulation.* 2020;141:1510-1522.

50. Freedman B, Potpara TS, Lip GY. Stroke prevention in atrial fibrillation. *Lancet.* 2016;388:806-817.

51. Khan AA, Lip GYH. The prothrombotic state in atrial fibrillation: pathophysiological and management implications. *Cardiovasc Res.* 2019;115: 31-45.

52. Rewiuk K, Grodzicki T. Osteoprotegerin and TRAIL in acute onset of atrial fibrillation. *Biomed Res Int.* 2015;2015:259843.

53. Wasilewska M, Gosk-Bierska I. Thromboembolism associated with atrial fibrillation as a cause of limb and organ ischemia. *Adv Clin Exp Med.* 2013;22:865-873.

54. Kim D, Yang PS, Yu HT, et al. Risk of dementia in stroke-free patients diagnosed with atrial fibrillation: data from a population-based cohort. *Eur Heart J.* 2019;40:2313-2323.

55. Chen LY, Norby FL, Gottesman RF, et al. Association of atrial fibrillation with cognitive decline and dementia over 20 years: the ARIC-NCS (Atherosclerosis Risk in Communities Neurocognitive Study). *J Am Heart Assoc.* 2018;7.

56. Bunch TJ, Jacobs V, May H, et al. Rationale and design of the impact of anticoagulation therapy on the Cognitive Decline and Dementia in Patients with Nonvalvular Atrial Fibrillation (CAF) Trial: a Vanguard study. *Clin Cardiol*. 2019;42:506-512.

57. Bunch TJ, Crandall BG, Weiss JP, et al. Patients treated with catheter ablation for atrial fibrillation have long-term rates of death, stroke, and dementia similar to patients without atrial fibrillation. *J Cardiovasc Electrophysiol*. 2011;22:839-845.

58. Ling LH, Kistler PM, Kalman JM, Schilling RJ, Hunter RJ. Comorbidity of atrial fibrillation and heart failure. *Nat Rev Cardiol*. 2016;13:131-147.

59. Schmidt AS, Lauridsen KG, Torp P, Bach LF, Rickers H, Lofgren B. Maximum-fixed energy shocks for cardioverting atrial fibrillation. *Eur Heart J*. 2020;41:626-631.

60. January CT, Wann LS, Calkins H, et al. 2019 AHA/ACC/HRS focused update of the 2014 AHA/ACC/HRS guideline for the management of patients with atrial fibrillation: a report of the American College of Cardiology/American Heart Association Task Force on Clinical Practice Guidelines and the Heart Rhythm Society. *J Am Coll Cardiol*. 2019;74:104-132.

61. Nuotio I, Hartikainen JE, Gronberg T, Biancari F, Airaksinen KE. Time to cardioversion for acute atrial fibrillation and thromboembolic complications. *JAMA*. 2014;312:647-649.

62. deSouza IS, Tadrous M, Sexton T, Benabbas R, Carmelli G, Sinert R. Pharmacologic cardioversion of recent-onset atrial fibrillation: a systematic review and network meta-analysis. *Europace*. 2020;22:854-869.

63. Gong M, Zhang Z, Fragakis N, et al. Role of ranolazine in the prevention and treatment of atrial fibrillation: a meta-analysis of randomized clinical trials. *Heart Rhythm*. 2017;14:3-11.

64. McIntyre WF, Healey JS, Bhatnagar AK, et al. Vernakalant for cardioversion of recent-onset atrial fibrillation: a systematic review and meta-analysis. *Europace*. 2019;21:1159-1166.

65. Chung MK, Refaat M, Shen WK, et al. Atrial fibrillation: JACC council perspectives. *J Am Coll Cardiol*. 2020;75:1689-1713.

66. Flannery MD, Kalman JM, Sanders P, La Gerche A. State of the art review: atrial fibrillation in athletes. *Heart Lung Circ*. 2017;26:983-989.

67. Pathak RK, Elliott A, Middeldorp ME, et al. Impact of CARDIOrespiratory FITness on Arrhythmia Recurrence in Obese Individuals With Atrial Fibrillation: the CARDIO-FIT study. *J Am Coll Cardiol*. 2015;66:985-96.

68. Pathak RK, Middeldorp ME, Meredith M, et al. Long-term effect of goal-directed weight management in an atrial fibrillation cohort: a long-term follow-up study (LEGACY). *J Am Coll Cardiol*. 2015;65:2159-2169.

69. Brandes A, Smit MD, Nguyen BO, Rienstra M, Van Gelder IC. Risk factor management in atrial fibrillation. *Arrhythm Electrophysiol Rev*. 2018;7:118-127.

70. Alonso A, Bahnson JL, Gaussoin SA, et al. Effect of an intensive lifestyle intervention on atrial fibrillation risk in individuals with type 2 diabetes: the Look AHEAD randomized trial. *Am Heart J*. 2015;170:770-777 e5.

71. Lynch KT, Mehaffey JH, Hawkins RB, Hassinger TE, Hallowell PT, Kirby JL. Bariatric surgery reduces incidence of atrial fibrillation: a propensity score-matched analysis. *Surg Obes Relat Dis*. 2019;15:279-285.

72. Jamaly S, Carlsson L, Peltonen M, Jacobson P, Sjostrom L, Karason K. Bariatric surgery and the risk of new-onset atrial fibrillation in Swedish obese subjects. *J Am Coll Cardiol*. 2016;68:2497-2504.

73. Kato M, Kubo A, Nihei F, Ogano M, Takagi H. Effects of exercise training on exercise capacity, cardiac function, BMI, and quality of life in patients with atrial fibrillation: a meta-analysis of randomized-controlled trials. *Int J Rehabil Res*. 2017;40:193-201.

74. Holmqvist F, Kim S, Steinberg BA, et al. Heart rate is associated with progression of atrial fibrillation, independent of rhythm. *Heart*. 2015;101:894-9.

75. Donnellan E, Aagaard P, Kanj M, et al. Association between pre-ablation glycemic control and outcomes among patients with diabetes undergoing atrial fibrillation ablation. *JACC Clin Electrophysiol*. 2019;5:897-903.

76. Parkash R, Wells GA, Sapp JL, et al. Effect of aggressive blood pressure control on the recurrence of atrial fibrillation after catheter ablation: a randomized, open-label clinical trial (SMAC-AF [Substrate Modification With Aggressive Blood Pressure Control]). *Circulation*. 2017;135:1788-1798.

77. Hindricks G, Potpara T, Dagres N, et al. 2020 ESC Guidelines for the diagnosis and management of atrial fibrillation developed in collaboration with the European Association of Cardio-Thoracic Surgery (EACTS). *Eur Heart J*. 2021;42(5):373-498.

78. Siontis KC, Zhang X, Eckard A, et al. Outcomes associated with apixaban use in patients with end-stage kidney disease and atrial fibrillation in the United States. *Circulation*. 2018;138:1519-1529.

79. Douketis JD, Spyropoulos AC, Kaatz S, et al. Perioperative bridging anticoagulation in patients with atrial fibrillation. *N Eng J Med*. 2015;373:823-833.

80. Calkins H, Willems S, Gerstenfeld EP, et al. Uninterrupted dabigatran versus warfarin for ablation in atrial fibrillation. *N Eng J Med*. 2017;376:1627-1636.

81. Turagam MK, Vuddanda V, Verberkmoes N, et al. Epicardial left atrial appendage exclusion reduces blood pressure in patients with atrial fibrillation and hypertension. *J Am Coll Cardiol*. 2018;72:1346-1353.

82. Sharples L, Everett C, Singh J, et al. Amaze: a double-blind, multicentre randomised controlled trial to investigate the clinical effectiveness and cost-effectiveness of adding an ablation device-based maze procedure as an adjunct to routine cardiac surgery for patients with pre-existing atrial fibrillation. *Health Technol Assess*. 2018;22:1-132.

83. Kheiri B, Kumar K, Simpson TF, et al. Meta-analysis of left atrial appendage closure versus anticoagulation in patients with atrial fibrillation. *Am J Cardiol*. 2020;132:181-182.

84. Wyse DG, Waldo AL, DiMarco JP, et al. A comparison of rate control and rhythm control in patients with atrial fibrillation. *N Engl J Med*. 2002;347:1825-1833.

85. Corley SD, Epstein AE, DiMarco JP, et al. Relationships between sinus rhythm, treatment, and survival in the Atrial Fibrillation Follow-Up Investigation of Rhythm Management (AFFIRM) Study. *Circulation*. 2004;109:1509-1513.

86. Van Gelder IC, Hagens VE, Bosker HA, et al. A comparison of rate control and rhythm control in patients with recurrent persistent atrial fibrillation. *N Engl J Med*. 2002;347:1834-1840.

87. Van Gelder IC, Groenveld HF, Crijns HJ, et al. Lenient versus strict rate control in patients with atrial fibrillation. *N Engl J Med*. 2010;362:1363-1373.

88. Packer DL, Mark DB, Robb RA, et al. Effect of catheter ablation vs antiarrhythmic drug therapy on mortality, stroke, bleeding, and cardiac arrest among patients with atrial fibrillation: the CABANA randomized clinical trial. *JAMA*. 2019;321:1261-1274.

89. Kuck KH, Brugada J, Furnkranz A, et al. Cryoballoon or radiofrequency ablation for paroxysmal atrial fibrillation. *N Eng J Med*. 2016;74:2235-2245.

90. Clarnette JA, Brooks AG, Mahajan R, et al. Outcomes of persistent and long-standing persistent atrial fibrillation ablation: a systematic review and meta-analysis. *Europace*. 2018;20:f366-f376.

91. Marrouche NF, Brachmann J, Andresen D, et al. Catheter ablation for atrial fibrillation with heart failure. *N Engl J Med*. 2018;378:417-427.

92. Bunch TJ, Bair TL, Crandall BG, et al. Stroke and dementia risk in patients with and without atrial fibrillation and carotid arterial disease. *Heart Rhythm*. 2020;17:20-26.

93. Nery PB, Belliveau D, Nair GM, et al. Relationship between pulmonary vein reconnection and atrial fibrillation recurrence: a systematic review and meta-analysis. *JACC Clin Electrophysiol*. 2016;2:474-483.

94. Verma A, Jiang CY, Betts TR, et al. Approaches to catheter ablation for persistent atrial fibrillation. *N Eng J Med*. 2015;372:1812-1822.

95. Fink T, Schluter M, Heeger CH, et al. Stand-alone pulmonary vein isolation versus pulmonary vein isolation with additional substrate modification as index ablation procedures in patients with persistent and long-standing persistent atrial fibrillation: the randomized

Alster-Lost-AF trial (Ablation at St. Georg Hospital for Long-Standing Persistent Atrial Fibrillation). *Circ Arrhythm Electrophysiol.* 2017;10.

96. Elbatran AI, Anderson RH, Mori S, Saba MM. The rationale for isolation of the left atrial pulmonary venous component to control atrial fibrillation: a review article. *Heart Rhythm* 2019;16:1392-1398.

97. Lee JM, Shim J, Park J, et al. The electrical isolation of the left atrial posterior wall in catheter ablation of persistent atrial fibrillation. *JACC Clin Electrophysiol.* 2019;5:1253-1261.

98. Di Biase L, Burkhardt JD, Mohanty P, et al. Left atrial appendage isolation in patients with longstanding persistent AF undergoing catheter ablation: BELIEF trial. *J Am Coll Cardiol.* 2016;68:1929-1940.

99. Hansen BJ, Zhao J, Li N, et al. Human atrial fibrillation drivers resolved with integrated functional and structural imaging to benefit clinical mapping. *JACC Clin Electrophysiol.* 2018;4:1501-1515.

100. Ramirez FD, Birnie DH, Nair GM, et al. Efficacy and safety of driver-guided catheter ablation for atrial fibrillation: a systematic review and meta-analysis. *J Cardiovasc Electrophysiol.* 2017;28:1371-1378.

101. Kottkamp H, Schreiber D, Moser F, Rieger A. Therapeutic approaches to atrial fibrillation ablation targeting atrial fibrosis. *JACC: Clinical Electrophysiol.* 2017;3:643–653.

102. Cheng EP, Liu CF, Yeo I, et al. Risk of mortality following catheter ablation of atrial fibrillation. *J Am Coll Cardiol.* 2019;74:2254-2264.

103. Gillinov AM, Gelijns AC, Parides MK, et al. Surgical ablation of atrial fibrillation during mitral-valve surgery. *N Eng J Med.* 2015;372:1399-1409.

104. Maclean E, Yap J, Saberwal B, et al. The convergent procedure versus catheter ablation alone in longstanding persistent atrial fibrillation: a single centre, propensity-matched cohort study. *Int J Cardiol.* 2020;303:49-53.

105. Munawar DA, Mahajan R, Agbaedeng TA, et al. Implication of ventricular pacing burden and atrial pacing therapies on the progression of atrial fibrillation: a systematic review and meta-analysis of randomized controlled trials. *Heart Rhythm* 2019;16:1204-1214.

106. Dobrev D, Aguilar M, Heijman J, Guichard JB, Nattel S. Postoperative atrial fibrillation: mechanisms, manifestations and management. *Nat Rev Cardiol.* 2019;16:417-436.

107. Yadava M, Hughey AB, Crawford TC. Postoperative atrial fibrillation: incidence, mechanisms, and clinical correlates. *Heart Fail Clin.* 2016;12:299-308.

108. Yuan X, Du J, Liu Q, Zhang L. Defining the role of perioperative statin treatment in patients after cardiac surgery: a meta-analysis and systematic review of 20 randomized controlled trials. *Int J Cardiol.* 2017;228:958-966.

109. Gillinov AM, Bagiella E, Moskowitz AJ, et al. Rate control versus rhythm control for atrial fibrillation after cardiac surgery. *N Engl J Med.* 2016;374:1911-1921.

110. Lin MH, Kamel H, Singer DE, Wu YL, Lee M, Ovbiagele B. Perioperative/postoperative atrial fibrillation and risk of subsequent stroke and/or mortality. *Stroke.* 2019;50:1364-1371.

111. Lee SH, Kang DR, Uhm JS, et al. New-onset atrial fibrillation predicts long-term newly developed atrial fibrillation after coronary artery bypass graft. *Am Heart J.* 2014;167:593-600.e1.

112. Thoren E, Wernroth ML, Christersson C, Grinnemo KH, Jideus L, Stahle E. Compared with matched controls, patients with postoperative atrial fibrillation (POAF) have increased long-term AF after CABG, and POAF is further associated with increased ischemic stroke, heart failure and mortality even after adjustment for AF. *Clin Res Cardiol.* 2020;109:1232-1242.

113. Bhave PD, Goldman LE, Vittinghoff E, Maselli J, Auerbach A. Incidence, predictors, and outcomes associated with postoperative atrial fibrillation after major noncardiac surgery. *Am Heart J.* 2012;164:918-924.

114. Santhanakrishnan R, Wang N, Larson MG, et al. Atrial fibrillation begets heart failure and vice versa: temporal associations and differences in preserved versus reduced ejection fraction. *Circulation.* 2016;133:484-492.

115. Sugumar H, Nanayakkara S, Prabhu S, et al. Pathophysiology of atrial fibrillation and heart failure: dangerous interactions. *Cardiol Clin.* 2019;37:131-138.

116. Roy D, Talajic M, Nattel S, et al. Rhythm control versus rate control for atrial fibrillation and heart failure. *N Engl J Med.* 2008;358:2667-2677.

117. Bun SS, Latcu DG, Marchlinski F, Saoudi N. Atrial flutter: more than just one of a kind. *Eur Heart J.* 2015;36:2356-2363.

118. Manolis AS. Contemporary diagnosis and management of atrial flutter: a continuum of atrial fibrillation and vice versa? *Cardiol Rev.* 2017;25:289-297.

119. Gula LJ, Redfearn DP, Jenkyn KB, et al. Elevated incidence of atrial fibrillation and stroke in patients with atrial flutter-a population-based study. *Can J Cardiol.* 2018;34:774-783.

120. Page RL, Joglar JA, Caldwell MA, et al. 2015 ACC/AHA/HRS guideline for the management of adult patients with supraventricular tachycardia: a report of the American College of Cardiology/American Heart Association Task Force on Clinical Practice Guidelines and the Heart Rhythm Society. *J Am Coll Cardiol.* 2016;67:e27-e115.

121. Vadmann H, Nielsen PB, Hjortshoj SP, et al. Atrial flutter and thromboembolic risk: a systematic review. *Heart.* 2015;101:1446-1455.

122. January CT, Wann LS, Alpert JS, et al. 2014 AHA/ACC/HRS guideline for the management of patients with atrial fibrillation: a report of the American College of Cardiology/American Heart Association Task Force on Practice Guidelines and the Heart Rhythm Society. *J Am Coll Cardiol.* 2014;64:e1-76.

123. Macle L, Cairns J, Leblanc K, et al. 2016 focused update of the Canadian Cardiovascular Society Guidelines for the Management of Atrial Fibrillation. *Can J Cardiol.* 2016;32:1170-1185.

124. Andrade JG, Verma A, Mitchell LB, et al. 2018 Focused Update of the Canadian Cardiovascular Society Guidelines for the Management of Atrial Fibrillation. *Can J Cardiol.* 2018;34:1371-1392.

Ventricular Arrhythmias and Sudden Cardiac Death

37

Justin Hayase, Kalyanam Shivkumar, and Jason S. Bradfield

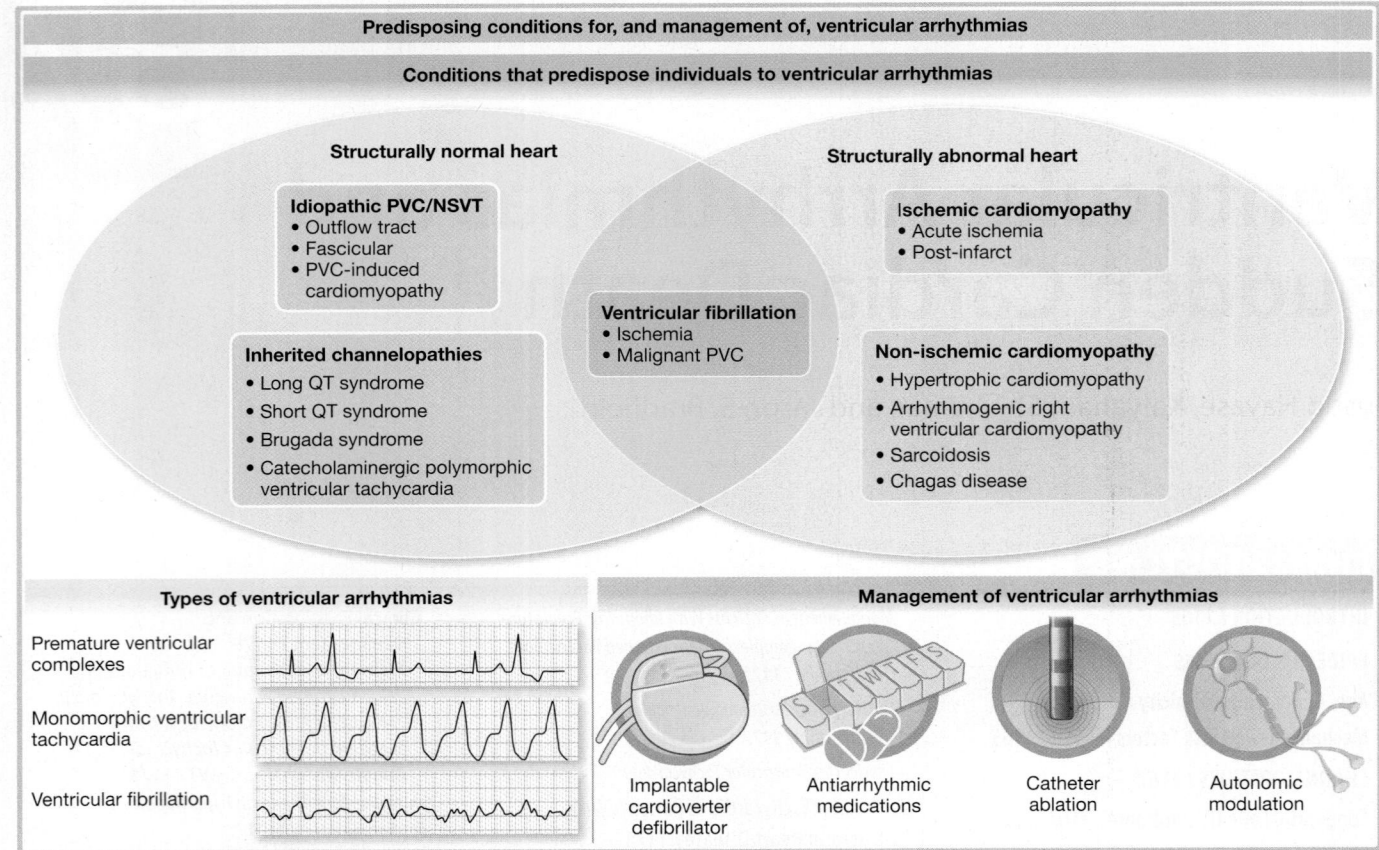

Chapter 37 Fuster and Hurst's Central Illustration. Major risk factors for developing ventricular arrhythmias include cardiac structural abnormalities and coronary artery disease. A number of inherited channelopathies can also predispose to these arrhythmias and should be considered in the context of a structurally normal heart. Management may involve multiple types of therapy. NSVT, non-sustained ventricular tachycardia; PVC, premature ventricular complex.

CHAPTER SUMMARY

This chapter discusses the epidemiology and pathophysiology of sudden cardiac death (SCD), which is most often caused by ventricular arrhythmias, and addresses some of the key considerations for the evaluation and treatment of ventricular arrhythmias. Major risk factors for developing these arrhythmias include cardiac structural abnormalities and coronary artery disease (CAD) (see Fuster and Hurst's Central Illustration). Moreover, a number of inherited channelopathies can predispose to these arrhythmias and should be considered in the context of a structurally normal heart. Ventricular arrhythmias can range from idiopathic premature ventricular complexes, to monomorphic ventricular tachycardia (VT), to ventricular fibrillation (VF). Management of ventricular arrhythmias requires a comprehensive approach that may involve multiple therapies, including an implantable cardioverter defibrillator (ICD), antiarrhythmic medications, catheter ablation, and/or autonomic modulation. The decision-making process for management depends highly upon the presence of underlying structural abnormalities.

INTRODUCTION

Sudden cardiac death (SCD) is defined as an unexpected death resulting from a cardiac cause within a short time period after the onset of symptoms. It is most often caused by a sustained ventricular tachyarrhythmia (ventricular tachycardia [VT] and ventricular fibrillation [VF]). Although many cardiovascular disorders increase the risk of SCD, the presence of preexisting overt cardiovascular disease is not necessary, and SCD may be the first manifestation of otherwise phenotypically silent cardiac disease.

Ventricular arrhythmias commonly occur in clinical practice and range from benign asymptomatic premature ventricular complexes (PVCs) to sustained VT or VF resulting in SCD. The presence of structural heart disease plays a major role in risk stratification; however, it is important to recognize that potentially lethal arrhythmias can occur in structurally normal-appearing hearts. Management depends on the associated symptoms, underlying pathologic substrate, hemodynamic consequences, and associated long-term prognosis. Given the complexity of these arrhythmias, initial management, risk stratification, and treatment of ventricular arrhythmias pose a significant challenge to clinicians.

This chapter provides an overview of the epidemiology, mechanisms, clinical presentation, natural history, diagnosis, and therapeutic options for ventricular arrhythmias encountered in clinical practice.

EPIDEMIOLOGY

Roughly half of all deaths due to cardiovascular disease are estimated to be due to SCD. Because 80% of sudden deaths occur in the home environment and up to 40% are unwitnessed, the cardiac rhythm that precipitated onset of symptoms are frequently unknown. Therefore, precise measurement of SCD rates and understanding of associated mechanisms is difficult. Estimates for SCD range between 180,000 and over 450,000 deaths yearly in the United States. Global estimates for the incidence of SCD range widely from 15 to 150 per 100,000 for adults age ≥18 years old, depending on the region.[1] In autopsy-based studies, a cardiac etiology of sudden death has been reported in 60% to 70% of sudden death victims. More recent data from the United States, Europe, and Asia have demonstrated an incidence of approximately 40 to 100 SCDs per 100,000 persons,[1] with significant geographical variation. While arrhythmic related cause of death continues to comprise the majority of causes of sudden death, there can be discrepancy between emergency medical services reported cause of death and the etiology revealed by comprehensive autopsy, which may be determined to be due to neurologic, toxicologic, or gastrointestinal in nature.[2] This further complicates epidemiological data regarding SCD mechanisms and outcomes.

Age, Gender, and Ethnicity

The incidence of SCD increases with age, coinciding with the rising prevalence of ischemic heart disease with advancing age

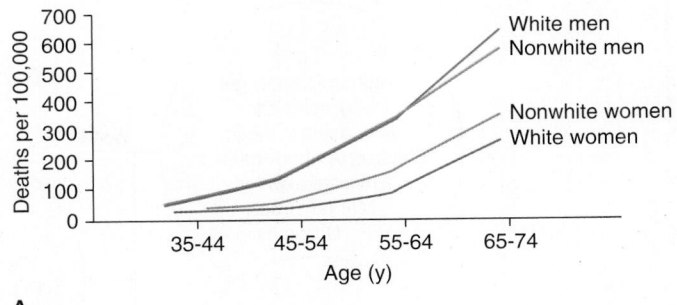

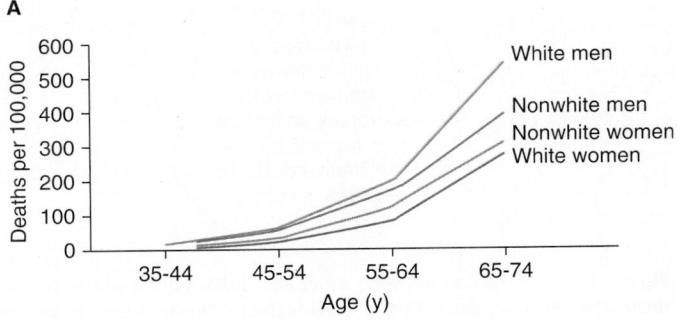

Figure 37–1. Plots of mortality (deaths per 100,000 persons) for ischemic heart disease occurring **(A)** out of hospital or in an emergency department (an estimate for sudden cardiac death rate) and **(B)** occurring in the hospital, by age, sex, and race in 40 states during 1985. From the National Center for Health Statistics. Reproduced with permission from the National Center for Health Statistics.

(**Fig. 37–1**). Among sudden natural deaths, the proportion with cardiac causes also increases with age. Age-adjusted SCD rates are significantly higher in men than in women. As is the case with coronary artery disease (CAD), however, this gender disparity decreases with advancing age, with a male:female ratio for SCD incidence of 7:1 in 45- to 64-year-olds, but only 2:1 in 65- to 74-year-olds. Women are more likely than men (64% vs 50%) to suffer SCD without prior evidence of CHD. With regards to ethnicity, numerous studies have demonstrated high incidence of SCD and poorer outcomes in Black Americans compared to White Americans.[2-4]

Mechanisms and Risk Factors for SCD

The majority of patients who have experienced SCD have cardiac structural abnormalities. In the adult population, these consist predominantly of CHD, cardiomyopathies, valvular heart disease, and abnormalities of the conduction system. These structural changes provide the substrate for ventricular tachyarrhythmias, the cause of SCD in most cases. It is important to recognize the role of triggering factors such as ischemia, hemodynamic changes, fluctuations in the autonomic nervous system, electrolyte abnormalities, and proarrhythmic effects of drugs in the initiation of ventricular arrhythmias resulting in SCD (**Fig. 37–2**).

As the majority of patients who experience SCD do not have cardiac rhythm monitoring at the time of their event, it is frequently difficult to determine the cardiac rhythm that initiated SCD. Ventricular fibrillation is the first recorded rhythm by first

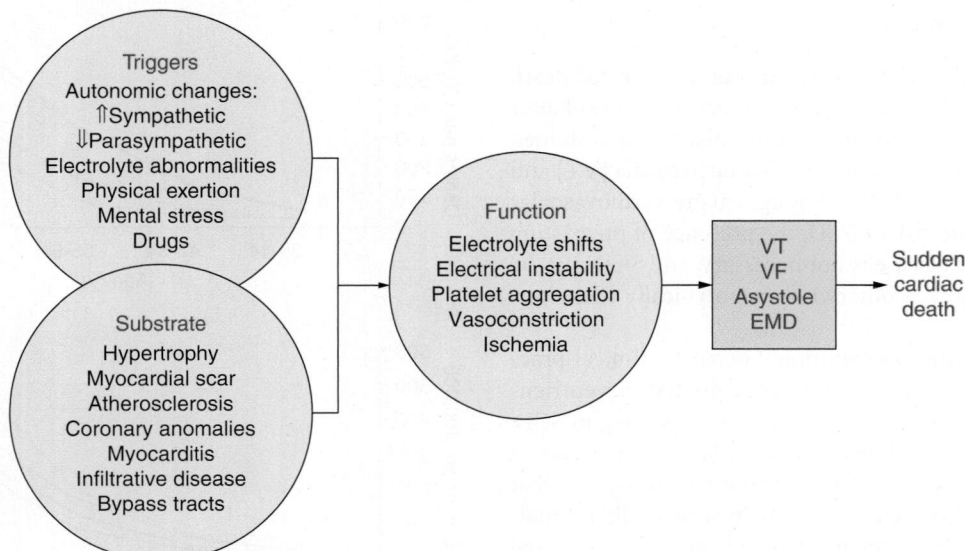

Figure 37–2. Interaction between structural cardiac abnormalities, functional changes, and triggering factors in the pathophysiology of sudden cardiac death. The role of triggering factors, such as changes in autonomic tone or reflexes, is increasingly being recognized. EMD, electromechanical dissociation; VF, ventricular fibrillation; VT, ventricular tachycardia.

responders in the majority of patients who have cardiac arrest. Sustained monomorphic VT is only rarely (< 2%) documented as the initial rhythm, but it is unknown how often it precedes and precipitates VF. In a series of 157 ambulatory patients who were wearing an electrocardiogram (ECG) monitor at the time of their cardiac arrest, primary VF was documented in 8%, VT degenerating into VF in 63%, and torsades de pointes (TdP) in 13%; however, it should be noted that selection bias may influence these numbers in comparison to the general population. Electromechanical dissociation and asystole are found in approximately 30% of patients experiencing cardiac arrest, and this finding is usually related to the time interval from collapse to first monitoring of the rhythm, suggesting that it is often a later manifestation of cardiac arrest. In patients who have died suddenly while wearing an ambulatory ECG monitor, bradyarrhythmias as the initial rhythm were documented infrequently, and ventricular tachyarrhythmias were most often the mode of

cardiac arrest, even in patients with preexisting atrioventricular (AV) or intraventricular conduction defects.[5]

Traditional risk factors for CAD also increase the risk of SCD among men and women. Higher prevalence of hypertension, hyperlipidemia, diabetes mellitus, smoking, and obesity all correlate with increasing incidence of SCD. CAD is thought to be the underlying structural abnormality in roughly 70% to 80% of SCD cases (**Fig. 37–3**).

Acute myocardial ischemia leads to intracellular and extracellular acidosis and loss of myocellular membrane integrity with efflux of potassium and influx of calcium. These biochemical abnormalities have electrophysiological consequences, including decreases in the amplitude and upstroke velocity of the cardiac action potential, inhomogeneous depolarization of the resting membrane potential, and shortening of action potential duration.[6] Fast sodium and slow calcium channels in partially depolarized fibers may remain inactive, thereby

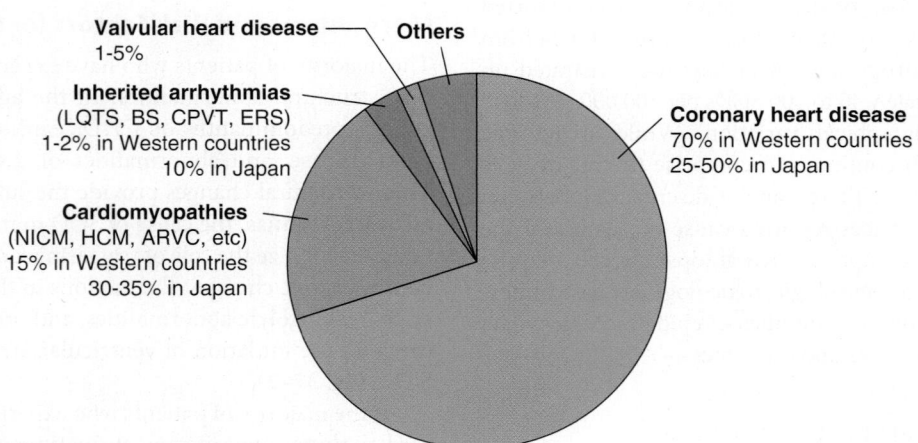

Figure 37–3. Causes of sudden cardiac death. Reproduced with permission from Wong CX, Brown A, Lau DH, et al. Epidemiology of Sudden Cardiac Death: Global and Regional Perspectives. *Heart Lung Circ.* 2019 Jan;28(1):6-14.

prolonging refractoriness even after completion of repolarization. This may further contribute to electrical heterogeneities within and around the ischemic zone, causing conduction delays and unidirectional block, which promote reentrant arrhythmias. In the late phases after MI, when the infarction is healed, macroreentry is the principal mechanism of ventricular arrhythmias. Critical areas of the reentrant circuit are formed by surviving myocardial cells in the epicardial and endocardial border zone of a healed infarction, as well as surviving intramural fibers within the infarct zone.

Although it is an imperfect marker of SCD risk, left ventricular (LV) dysfunction has been identified as the strongest independent predictor of SCD. The assessment of left ventricular ejection fraction (LVEF) has become the major criterion in patient selection for implantation of a primary prevention implantable cardioverter defibrillator (ICD) in those with structural heart disease.[7] This will be discussed in further detail later in the chapter. It is important to note that while low LVEF identifies patients at elevated risk of SCD, this patient group comprises only a small fraction of the total disease burden of SCD (**Fig. 37–4**). Much work has been done with regard to additional risk stratification tools to identify elevated SCD risk such as heart rate variability, baroreceptor sensitivity, signal averaged ECG, or microvolt T wave alternans; however, these have not proved effective in broad application.

CHANNELOPATHIES

Congenital Long QT Syndrome

Congenital long QT syndrome (LQTS) is a heterogeneous channelopathy with associated increased risk of arrhythmic SCD. As the name implies, the hallmark of LQTS is a prolonged QT interval on ECG once alternative etiologies for prolonged QT are excluded. The long QT interval reflects abnormal prolongation of repolarization caused predominantly by defects in outward currents (potassium) or impaired inactivation of inward currents (sodium). Prolonged repolarization enhances the propensity to develop early after-depolarizations, leading to triggered activity that is the initiating mechanism for TdP. Irregular rhythms with "long-short" R-R intervals are frequent triggers of TdP.

There are currently 17 genes that have been identified as causative for the condition, with the number of identified genes continually increasing.[8] The first 3 genes involving *KCNQ1*, *KCNH2*, and *SCN5A*, initially reported in 1995, comprise over 92% of patients with genetically confirmed LQT1, LQT2, and LQT3.[9] Certain triggers for arrhythmias tend to correlate with specific LQTS genotypes. Physical or emotional stress typically initiates events in LQT1, and auditory stimulation tends to trigger events in LQT2. In LQT3, events most often occur during rest or sleep. The risk of overall cardiac events is significantly higher in patients with LQT1 or LQT2, but the percentage of lethal cardiac events is significantly higher in patients with LQT3. Risk of SCD correlates positively with the QT interval. A corrected QT interval (QTc) greater than 500 ms portends higher risk and even higher risk at over 600 ms. Specific genotype variants such as the autosomal recessive Jervell and Lange–Nielsen syndrome, which is associated with deafness, also portends higher risk. Other factors such as gender, age of first arrhythmia event, and continued events in spite of medical therapy also inform as to a patient's risk.

The mainstay of treatment for LQTS, aside from avoidance of QT prolonging agents and arrhythmic triggers, is β-blocker therapy, based on observational data. Left cardiac sympathetic

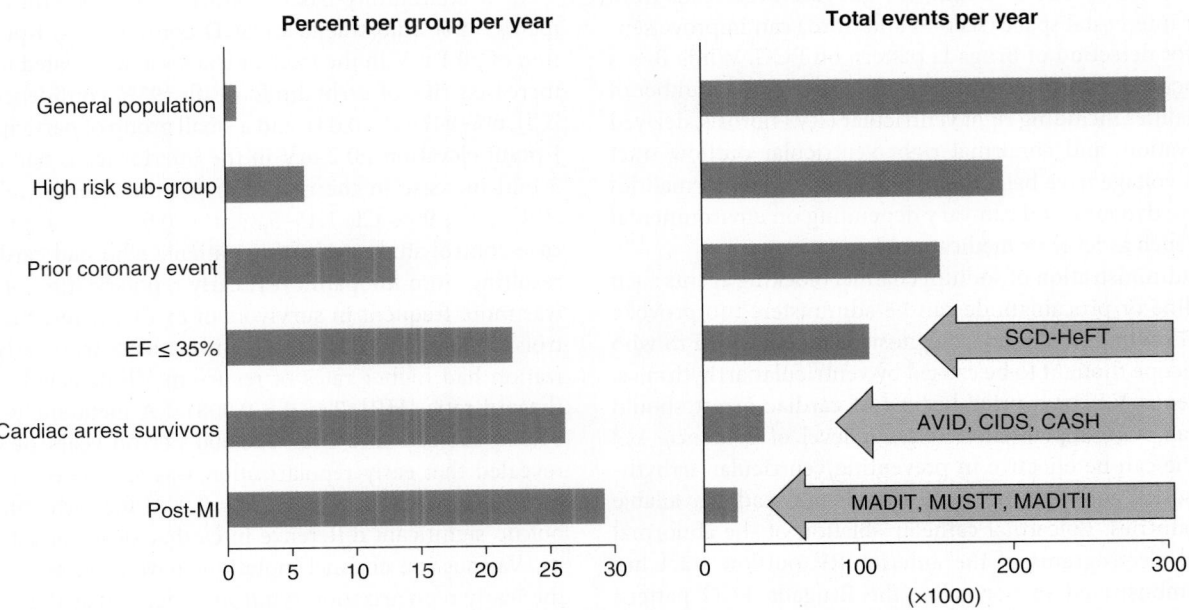

Figure 37–4. Incidence of SCD within different risk groups. While risk is highest in certain identified patients such as survivors of cardiac arrest or patients with low EF, these at-risk groups comprise only a small fraction of the total events/year of SCD. Modified with permission from Myerburg RJ, Interian A Jr, Mitrani RM, et al. Frequency of sudden cardiac death and profiles of risk. *Am J Cardiol.* 1997 Sep 11;80(5B):10F-19F.

denervation (LCSD) can be considered for patients who continue to have events in spite of medical therapy. In LQTS patients who have survived SCD, an ICD is recommended (Class I), and in patients who continue to experience events while on medical therapy, an ICD can be considered (class IIa).[9]

Short QT Syndrome

Short QT syndrome (SQTS) is a rare channelopathy with known association with atrial and ventricular fibrillation, typically identified by QTc less than 330 ms. Several genes have been implicated in SQTS with *KCNH2, KCNQ1,* and *KCNJ2* gain of function mutations (loss of function mutations in these genes have been associated with LQTS). Mutations in the *CACNA1C* and *CACNB2* genes, which encode the alpha- and beta-subunits of the L-type cardiac calcium channels have also been described.[10] An ICD is recommended for patients with SQTS who have survived SCD.[9]

Brugada Syndrome

Brugada syndrome (BrS) is an autosomal dominant inherited channelopathy with original descriptions in 1992 of patients with aborted SCD with right bundle branch block (RBBB) and ST-segment elevations in leads V1 to V3.[11] Loss of function mutation in the gene *SCN5A* is the most common genetic abnormality, although other genes explain the majority of BrS. The type 1 ECG pattern which is characterized by coved ST-segment elevation ≥2 mm (0.2 mV) followed by a negative T-wave in >1 lead from V1 to V3 is the only diagnostic ECG finding for BrS. Type 2, which has ≥2 mm J-point elevation, ≥1 mm ST-segment elevation, and a saddleback appearance, and type 3, which has either a saddleback or coved appearance with an ST-segment elevation of <1 mm, are suggestive but not diagnostic of BrS. The recording of right precordial leads from a higher intercostal space (second and third) can improve sensitivity for detection of Brugada pattern on ECG. While BrS is not associated with structural heart disease per se, a number of abnormalities including right ventricular (RV) fibrosis, delayed RV activation, and abnormal right ventricular outflow tract (RVOT) voltage have been described. The ECG abnormalities in BrS are dynamic and can vary depending on environmental factors (such as fever or medications).

The administration of sodium channel blocking agents such as ajmaline or procainamide can be administered to provoke the ECG findings and aid in diagnosis. Patients with BrS who have syncope thought to be caused by ventricular arrhythmias, spontaneous VT, or a prior history of cardiac arrest should receive an ICD implantation (class I, level of evidence A).[9] Quinidine can be effective in preventing ventricular arrhythmia episodes, although the medication is not readily available in all countries. Epicardial catheter ablation of the abnormal electrical electrograms of the anterior RV outflow tract has been demonstrated to normalize the Brugada ECG pattern and potentially reduce risk of arrhythmic events. Endocardial ablation has also been performed, although with more limited efficacy possibly due to the presence of epicardial substrate.[12]

However, large clinical trial data supporting catheter ablation for BrS are lacking.

Catecholaminergic Polymorphic Ventricular Tachycardia

Catecholaminergic polymorphic ventricular tachycardia (CPVT) is a rare idiopathic ventricular arrhythmia characterized by polymorphic or bidirectional VT triggered by increased adrenergic tone. The more common autosomal dominant form of CPVT is characterized by a mutation in the ryanodine receptor (*RyR2*) gene. The less common autosomal recessive form is caused by a mutation in the calsequestrin (*CASQ2*) gene. Patients with CPVT have normal resting ECG with no structural abnormalities, and exercise testing can commonly elicit the arrhythmia. Drug challenge with epinephrine or isoproterenol can be useful in patients unable to exercise. β-blockers are the mainstay therapy for CPVT, with flecainide as a second-line agent.[9] If patients remain refractory to medical management, LCSD can also be an effective treatment option. ICD implantation is only recommended for patients who experience cardiac arrest, recurrent syncope, or polymorphic/bidirectional VT in spite of β-blockers and/or LCSD. ICD shocks can result in increased sympathetic tone and lead to worsening arrhythmias.[9]

Early Repolarization Syndrome

Early repolarization is characterized by elevation of the QRS complex-ST segment (J-point) above the baseline or slurring of the terminal part of the QRS complex into the ST segment. Early repolarization can be present in up to 19% of the population. Although early repolarization has been historically considered a benign ECG finding, data have suggested that it may be associated with an increased risk of SCD.

In a community-based cohort of 10,864 Finnish participants, after adjustment for SCD confounders, J-point elevation of ≥0.1 mV in the inferior leads was associated with a 43% increased risk of arrhythmic death (95% confidence interval [CI], 6%–94%; $P = 0.03$), and a small group of participants with J-point elevation ≥0.2 mV in the inferior leads had an almost 3-fold increase in the risk of arrhythmic death (relative risk [RR], 2.92; 95% CI, 1.45–5.89; $P = 0.01$).[13] In a retrospective case-control study evaluating patients who had cardiac arrest resulting from idiopathic VF, early repolarization of ≥0.1 mV was more frequent in survivors of cardiac arrest than in controls (31% vs 5%; $P < 0.001$), and patients with early repolarization had higher rates of recurrent VF detected with ICDs (hazard ratio [HR], 2.1; $P = 0.008$).[14] A meta-analysis of over 31,000 subjects and over 726,000 person-years of follow-up revealed that early repolarization was associated with an RR of 1.70 (95% CI, 1.19–2.42; $P = 0.003$) for arrhythmic death, but no significant difference in cardiac death or total mortality. Various ion channel mutations have been associated with the "early repolarization syndrome" defined as the presence of early repolarization ECG pattern and idiopathic VF.

In patients with early repolarization but no ventricular arrhythmias, no specific treatment is recommended, because the ECG finding is highly prevalent and benign in the vast majority of cases.[7] Secondary prevention of SCD in patients with early repolarization and VF/cardiac arrest is managed the same way as in patients without early repolarization. Further study of the interplay between early repolarization and SCD is needed.

THERAPIES TO REDUCE SCD

The primary aim in patients who have presented with sustained VT is to reduce recurrence of VT and prevent SCD. LV function is a well-established independent risk factor for SCD in patients with ventricular arrhythmias. In a subanalysis of the Candesartan in Heart Failure Assessment of Reduction in Mortality and Morbidity (CHARM) study, evaluation of the impact of LVEF quartiles on long-term survival revealed a 39% increase in the HR for mortality for every 10% reduction in LVEF.[15]

Patients who present with sustained VT and a structural heart disease should be considered for an ICD (**Table 37–1**). Patients with a history of cardiac arrest have clear benefit from ICD implantation across many trials, as shown in a meta-analysis of secondary prevention ICD versus antiarrhythmic drug trials. In this meta-analysis ICD therapy was associated with a 50% reduction in arrhythmic death (25% all-cause mortality decrease). Before implantation of an ICD, it is important that VT is clinically well controlled to minimize the risk of multiple shocks from the ICD. Reversible causes of VT should be corrected.

In patients with preserved LV function, the data for implantation of an ICD is less robust. A meta-analysis of the secondary-prevention ICD trials revealed that the patients who benefited from ICD therapy over amiodarone therapy had an EF <35%. Amiodarone was equivalent to ICD in patients with EF >35%. However, most patients with sustained VT, not likely to be idiopathic in origin, should receive an ICD. In some patients with preserved LV function, antiarrhythmic therapy or catheter ablation alone can be considered. Long-term amiodarone toxicity (eg, pulmonary, hepatic, thyroid, neurological, and skin) and the high rate of drug cessation as a result of intolerance remain practical limitations for chronic amiodarone therapy.

Once an ICD is implanted, numerous studies have demonstrated the efficacy of antiarrhythmic agents in reducing ICD shocks. In a randomized study of patients with ICDs implanted for inducible or spontaneously occurring VT or VF, 412 patients were randomized to β-adrenergic blockers alone (n = 140), sotalol alone (n = 134), or amiodarone plus β-blocker (n = 140). After a mean follow-up of 359 days, ICD shocks occurred in 38.5% of patients assigned to the β-blocker group, 24.3% of patients in the sotalol group, and 10.3% of patients in the amiodarone plus β-blocker group. Amiodarone plus β-blocker resulted in significantly fewer shocks compared with β-blocker alone (P = 0.006).[16] The decision for empiric therapy with antiarrhythmic agents at the time of ICD implantation depends on numerous clinical factors, including recent VT burden and likelihood or recurrence. The current consensus is

that β-adrenergic blocking agent should be administered in all patients unless contraindicated.

When antiarrhythmic agents are initiated in patients with an ICD, care must be taken in programming the device because antiarrhythmic medications can have varying effects on defibrillation thresholds and may slow the rate of the VT below a programmed detection zone. Further, both appropriate and inappropriate shocks can be detrimental[17-19] and associated with increased mortality. ICD programming with longer VT detection times and more ATP therapies can help minimize shocks for nonsustained episodes of VT or inappropriate shocks from supraventricular arrhythmias.

VENTRICULAR ARRHYTHMIAS

Ventricular Tachyarrhythmias in the Setting of a Structurally Normal Heart

Premature Ventricular Complexes/Nonsustained Ventricular Tachycardia in the Absence of Organic Heart Disease
PVCs and nonsustained ventricular tachycardia (NSVT) are commonly seen in clinical practice in patients with structurally normal hearts. NSVT is defined as ventricular tachycardia lasting for at least 3 consecutive beats but less than 30 seconds (**Table 37–2**). The significance of PVCs/NSVT depends on the frequency, the presence and severity of structural heart disease, and the presence of associated symptoms.

PVCs occur frequently in the general population. In patients without structural heart disease, PVCs are not associated with any excess risk of sudden death. Kennedy and coworkers studied 73 patients with frequent ventricular ectopy and no structural heart disease on a 24-hour ambulatory (Holter) monitor.[20] Patients were followed for an average of 6.5 years with no excess in mortality. These findings were reaffirmed in a meta-analysis. PVCs that occur in patients with a structurally normal heart may not warrant therapy, unless significant symptoms are present or there is concern for PVC-induced cardiomyopathy. NSVT is also very common, occurring in up to 6% of patients in Holter studies.

The RVOT is the most common site of origin of idiopathic PVCs/NSVT. PVCs/NSVT originating from this region are characterized on the 12-lead ECG by a left bundle branch block (LBBB) pattern in V1 and tall, monophasic R waves in the inferior leads. Although most outflow tract PVCs/NSVT originate from the RVOT, in at least 25% of cases the site of origin is reported to be from other sites (coronary cusps, mitral annulus, LV summit, papillary muscles, moderator band, or within or adjacent to the epicardial coronary venous structures) based on mapping studies (**Fig. 37–5**). For most patients with structurally normal hearts who have idiopathic outflow tract PVCs/NSVT, the prognosis is good. This group of patients may manifest with frequent single PVCs, bigeminy, trigeminy, NSVT, or as repetitive salvos of nonsustained monomorphic VT.

Premature Ventricular Complexes as a Cause of Cardiomyopathy
Clinical evidence of an association between frequent PVCs and a dilated cardiomyopathy has been demonstrated. A higher

TABLE 37–1. Implantable Cardioverter-Defibrillator Indications

Class I Indications

1. ICD therapy is recommended for secondary prevention of SCD in patients who are survivors of cardiac arrest due to VF or hemodynamically unstable sustained VT not due to reversible causes, if meaningful survival greater than 1 year is expected. *(Level of Evidence: A)*
2. ICD therapy is indicated in patients with structural heart disease and spontaneous sustained VT whether hemodynamically stable or unstable. *(Level of Evidence: B)*
3. ICD therapy is indicated in patients with syncope of undetermined origin with clinically relevant, hemodynamically significant sustained VT or VF induced at electrophysiologic study. *(Level of Evidence: B)*
4. ICD therapy is recommended in patients with LVEF <35% due to prior myocardial infarction who are at least 40 days post–myocardial infarction and at least 90 days post-revascularization and are in NYHA functional class II or III. *(Level of Evidence: A)*
5. ICD therapy is recommended in patients with nonischemic dilated cardiomyopathy who have an LVEF ≤35% and who are in NYHA functional class II or III. *(Level of Evidence: A)*
6. ICD therapy is indicated in patients with LV dysfunction due to prior myocardial infarction who are at least 40 days post–myocardial infarction and 90 days post-revascularization, have an LVEF <30%, and are in NYHA functional class I. *(Level of Evidence: A)*
7. ICD therapy is indicated in patients with nonsustained VT due to prior myocardial infarction, LVEF <40% and inducible VF or sustained VT at electrophysiologic study. *(Level of Evidence: B)*
8. ICD implantation is recommended for the prevention of SCD in patients with arrhythmogenic right ventricular dysplasia/cardiomyopathy who have one or more risk factors for SCD. *(Level of Evidence: B)*
9. ICD implantation is recommended to reduce SCD in patients with long QT syndrome who are experiencing syncope and/or VT while receiving β-blockers. *(Level of Evidence: B)*
10. ICD implantation is recommended for patients with catecholaminergic polymorphic VT who have syncope and/or documented sustained VT while receiving β-blockers. *(Level of Evidence: B)*
11. ICD implantation is recommended for patients with spontaneous type 1 Brugada pattern who have had sustained VA or syncope due to presumed VA. *(Level of Evidence: B)*

Class IIa Indications

1. ICD implantation is reasonable for patents with unexplained syncope, significant LV dysfunction, and nonischemic dilated cardiomyopathy. *(Level of Evidence: C)*
2. Implantation of an ICD is reasonable in patients with sustained VT and normal or near-normal ventricular function, *(Level of Evidence: C)*
3. ICD implantation is reasonable in non-hospitalized patients with NYHA class IV symptoms who are candidates for cardiac transplantation or an LVAD, if meaningful survival greater than 1 year is expected. *(Level of Evidence: B)*
4. ICD implantation is reasonable in patients with nonischemic cardiomyopathy due to Lamin A/C mutation who have 2 or more risk factors (NSVT, LVEF <45%, nonmissense mutation, and male sex). *(Level of Evidence: B)*
5. ICD implantation is reasonable for patients with hypertrophic cardiomyopathy who have one or more major risk factors for SCD. *(Level of Evidence: B)*
6. ICD implantation is reasonable for the prevention of SCD in patients with arrhythmogenic right ventricular dysplasia/cardiomyopathy and syncope. *(Level of Evidence: B)*
7. ICD implantation is reasonable for patients with cardiac sarcoidosis, giant-cell myocarditis, or Chagas disease. *(Level of Evidence: C)*

Class IIb Indications

1. ICD therapy may be considered in patients with nonischemic heart disease who have an LVEF of <35% and who are in NYHA functional class I. *(Level of Evidence: C)*
2. ICD therapy may be considered for patients with long QT syndrome and risk factors for SCD. *(Level of Evidence: B)*
3. ICD therapy may be considered in patients with syncope and advanced structural heart disease in whom thorough invasive and noninvasive investigations have failed to define a cause. *(Level of Evidence: C)*
4. ICD therapy may be considered in patients with a familial cardiomyopathy associated with sudden death. *(Level of Evidence: C)*
5. ICD therapy may be considered in patients with LV noncompaction. *(Level of Evidence: C)*

Class III Indications

1. ICD therapy is not indicated for patients who do not have a reasonable expectation of survival with an acceptable functional status for at least 1 year, even if they meet ICD implantation criteria specified in the classes I, IIa, and IIb recommendations above. *(Level of Evidence: C)*
2. ICD therapy is not indicated for patients with incessant VT or VF until sufficient control of the VA is achieved to prevent repeated ICD shocks. *(Level of Evidence: C)*
3. ICD therapy is not indicated in patients with significant psychiatric illnesses that may be aggravated by device implantation or that may preclude systematic follow-up. *(Level of Evidence: C)*
4. ICD therapy is not indicated for NYHA class IV patients with drug-refractory congestive heart failure who are not candidates for cardiac transplantation or implantation of a CRT device that incorporates both pacing and defibrillation capabilities. *(Level of Evidence: C)*
5. ICD therapy is not indicated for syncope of undetermined cause in a patient without inducible ventricular tachyarrhythmias and without structural heart disease. *(Level of Evidence: C)*

Abbreviations: CRT, cardiac resynchronization therapy; ICD, implantable cardioverter-defibrillator; LV, left ventricular; LVEF, left ventricular ejection fraction; NYHA, New York Heart Association; SCD, sudden cardiac death; VF, ventricular fibrillation; VT, ventricular tachycardia.
Data from Epstein AE, DiMarco JP, Ellenbogen KA, et al. ACC/AHA/HRS 2008 guidelines for device-based therapy of cardiac rhythm abnormalities: a report of the American College of Cardiology/ American Heart Association Task Force on Practice Guidelines (writing committee to revise the ACC/AHA/NASPE 2002 guideline update for implantation of cardiac pacemakers and antiarrhythmia devices) developed in collaboration with the American Association for Thoracic Surgery and Society of Thoracic Surgeons. J Am Coll Cardiol. 2008 May 27;51(21):e1-e62 and Al-Khatib SM, Stevenson WG, Ackerman MJ, et al. 2017 AHA/ACC/HRS guideline for management of patients with ventricular arrhythmias and the prevention of sudden cardiac death: executive summary: a report of the American College of Cardiology/ American Heart Association Task Force on Clinical Practice Guidelines and the Heart Rhythm Society. J Am Coll Cardiol. 2018 Oct 2;72(14):1677-1749.

TABLE 37-2. Ventricular Tachycardia Definitions

Sustained VT: Duration of VT is >30 seconds or <30 seconds associated with hemodynamic collapse.

Nonsustained VT: Duration ≥3 beats and <30 seconds, not associated with hemodynamic collapse.

VT Storm: More than three separate episodes of VT in 24 hours requiring intervention to terminate.

Monomorphic VT: All beats have same QRS morphology (some variation may be seen at initiation).

Polymorphic VT: Continuously changing morphology of the VT is seen from beat to beat.

Pleomorphic VT: More than one distinct morphology during the same episode of VT.

burden of PVCs over a 24-hour period is associated with higher risk, but development of cardiomyopathy associated with a burden as low as 10% has been described.

In a study by Niwano and associates,[21] 239 patients with frequent PVCs and no evidence of primary cardiomyopathy by echocardiography and cardiac magnetic resonance imaging (MRI) were followed for >4 years. Forty-six patients had highly frequent PVCs (>20,000/24 h), 105 patients had moderately frequent PVCs (5000–20,000/24 h), and 88 patients had less frequent PVCs (1000–5000/24 h). A significant negative correlation was observed between PVC frequency and LVEF at 4 years and 5.6 years.

Several studies have further demonstrated that elimination of PVCs among patients with depressed LV function may improve EF. In a series of 60 consecutive patients with frequent PVCs (>10 PVCs/h), reduced LV function (mean LVEF 34% ± 13%) was present in 22 patients (37%). Patients with depressed LV function had more frequent PVCs than patients with normal LV function (37% ± 13% vs. 11% ± 10% of all QRS complexes, respectively; $P = 0.0001$). Radiofrequency catheter ablation was successful in eliminating PVCs in 48 (80%) of 60 patients. Among the 22 patients with abnormal LV function, LV function assessed 6 months after the procedure returned to normal in 18 (82%) of 22 patients (LVEF of 34% ± 10% to LVEF of 59% ± 7%; $P < 0.0001$). Among patients with LV dysfunction

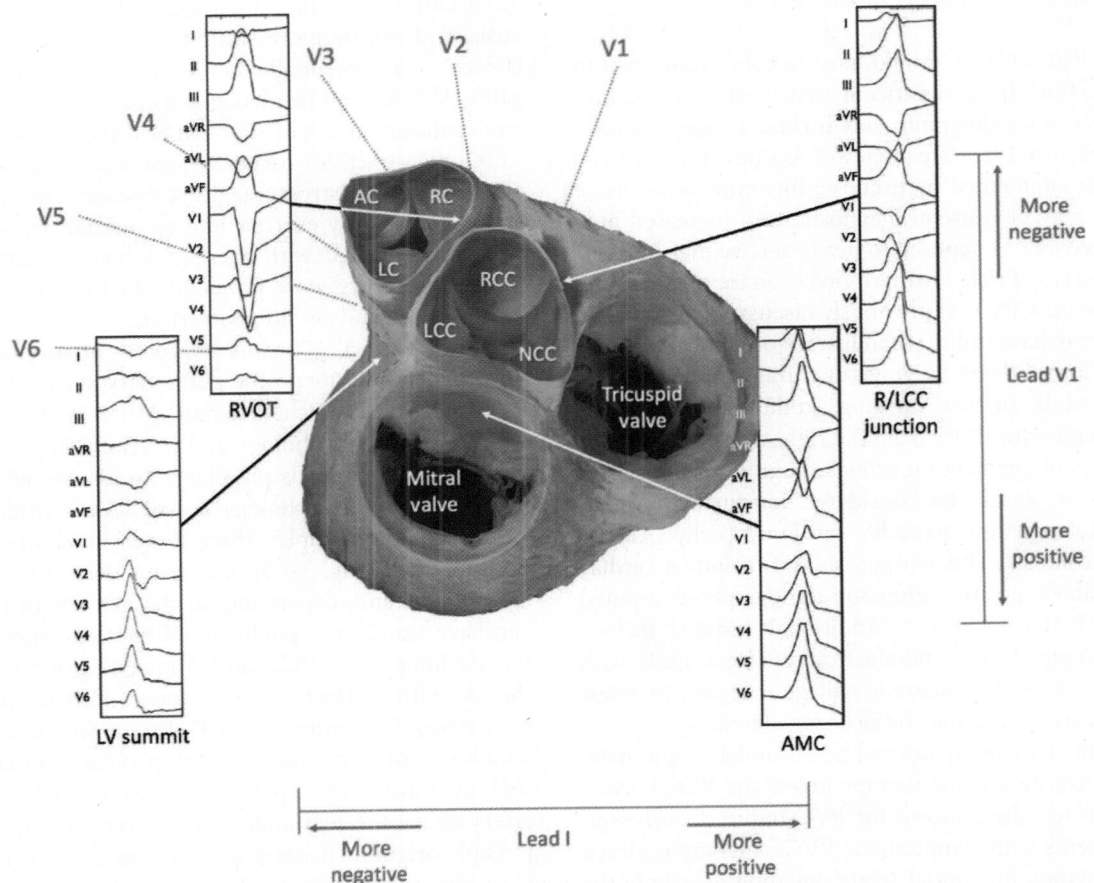

Figure 37-5. Idiopathic PVCs of variable origin. Top left: RVOT origin PVC with LBBB morphology, inferior axis, and "late" transition (R > S after V3) in precordial leads. Top right: A right coronary cusp/left coronary cusp (RCC/LCC) junction origin PVC with LBBB morphology with "W"-shaped V1, inferior axis, and earlier precordial transition then the RVOT PVC. Bottom right: Aorto-mitral continuity (AMC) origin PVC with an RBBB morphology pattern, inferior axis, and "qR" V1 morphology. Bottom left: An LV summit origin PVC with an RBBB morphology, inferior axis. *White arrows* indicate the anatomic location of these PVCs in an anatomic specimen from a superior view with the atria removed. Outflow-origin ventricular tachycardia/PVCs can originate below the pulmonary or aortic valve, or they can also arise from strands of myocardium above the valve. *Blue triangle* demonstrates area of LV summit between the left anterior descending and circumflex coronary arteries. AV, aortic valve; MA, mitral annulus; PV, pulmonic valve; TA, tricuspid valve. Illustration courtesy UCLA Cardiac Arrhythmia Center, Wallace A. McAlpine MD collection.

at baseline who were not successfully ablated, the LV function further declined (LVEF of 34% ± 10% to LVEF of 25% ± 7%; $P = 0.06$).

In summary, current studies regarding the role of PVCs in the development of a CM demonstrate the following: (1) LV dysfunction can occur when PVCs are present for a prolonged period of time; (2) LV dysfunction occurs among patients with a high frequency of PVCs; and (3) among patients with a PVC-induced cardiomyopathy, LVEF improves in the majority of patients when the PVCs can be eliminated with radiofrequency catheter ablation.

A number of electrocardiographic and other factors have been associated with increased risk of PVC-induced cardiomyopathy, but further assessment is ongoing. A higher burden, LV dyssynchrony,[22] retrograde ventriculoatrial (VA) conduction, PVC QRS duration, site of origin,[23,24] interpolation, male gender, PVCs throughout the day,[24,25] epicardial origin,[26] coupling interval dispersion,[27,28] and post-extrasystolic potentiation[29] have been described as potential contributing factors.

Management of Patients With Idiopathic Premature Ventricular Complexes/Nonsustained Ventricular Tachycardia

Patients with PVCs/NSVT should have an echocardiogram to assess LV function. If no significant structural abnormalities are noted on echocardiography, no further imaging studies are typically required. The frequency of "outflow tract" PVCs/NSVT is often augmented by exercise; therefore, an exercise treadmill test may be a useful diagnostic test. Increased burden during recovery as opposed to peak exercise may be associated with increased risk. Furthermore, exercise stress testing can help assess for CPVT, as previously discussed. In addition, cardiac MRI may have utility when history or clinical findings raise concern for subtle underlying structural pathology.

However, while further imaging studies are often not required, patients with PVCs from the right ventricle, with RV dysfunction or enlargement on echocardiogram or multiform RV-origin PVCs, should be considered for further evaluation to exclude arrhythmogenic RV cardiomyopathy (ARVC) or cardiac sarcoidosis. This workup should include a cardiac MRI and possibly a positron emission tomography-computed tomography (PET-CT) scan.[30] Additional testing, including a signal-averaged ECG and electrophysiologic study with three-dimensional electroanatomic voltage mapping to assess for early endocardial scar, may be also considered.

Patients with structurally normal hearts and asymptomatic PVCs do not require specific therapy unless the PVC burden is high enough to raise concern for PVC-induced cardiomyopathy. In patients with symptomatic PVCs, therapy is aimed at alleviating symptoms. Initial treatment should include the avoidance of potential exogenous stimulants (such as caffeine, excess alcohol, recreational drugs) or a trial of β-adrenergic blocking or calcium channel-blocking agents. However, the success rate for medical therapy is low (<50%) in this population.

Radiofrequency catheter ablation can be a curative treatment option for patients with symptomatic PVCs/NSVT when

there is a predominant PVC/NSVT morphology, the PVCs are causing symptoms or possible risk of cardiomyopathy, and drug therapy has proven ineffective, is not tolerated, or is not preferred (ACC/AHA/HRS guidelines)[7] (**Fig. 37–6**). Catheter ablation is more effective at decreasing PVC burden than antiarrhythmic medication, and the success rate is consistently over 75% in studies on ablation of PVCs of various locations of origin.

Outflow Tract Sustained Ventricular Tachycardia

Clinically, the percentage of patients presenting with idiopathic VT as compared to VT in the setting of structural heart disease will depend largely on the type of center evaluating the patient. Idiopathic VT likely represents the majority of VT cases in community hospitals and many tertiary care centers. In more specialized referral centers, structural heart disease–related VT may be more common.

The two main clinical entities of idiopathic VT include "outflow tract" VT and "idiopathic LV" VT (also known as fascicular VT or verapamil-sensitive VT). The differentiation of these VTs from VTs associated with structural heart disease is important because they are associated with an excellent prognosis, and can be more easily treated with catheter ablation. However, the potentially subtle differences between an idiopathic VT that can be managed conservatively and a VT with more substantial risk of SCD can be difficult to decipher.

"Outflow tract" VT occurs frequently in young to middle-aged patients without structural heart disease. This arrhythmia is often provoked by exercise and emotional stress. Recurrence may be associated with exercise, stress, or caffeine, and in women, it occurs more frequently during premenstrual, perimenopausal, and gestational periods.

"Outflow tract" VT most commonly arises from the RVOT immediately inferior to the pulmonary valve. Outflow origin PVCs and VT have a characteristic pattern on the 12-lead ECG, with an LBBB morphology and inferior axis.[31,32] This general description often leads physicians to assume all arrhythmias with this ECG morphology are of RVOT origin. However, because of the complex three-dimensional structure of the outflow tracts (Fig. 37–5), numerous sites of potential origin are possible and, depending on the exit site of the PVC/VT, can have similar morphologies. Numerous other sites can be foci for idiopathic PVCs and VT including, but not limited to, the LV outflow tract (LVOT), aortic sinus of Valsalva/coronary cusps, LV summit (Fig. 37–5), mitral annulus, tricuspid annulus, coronary venous system, papillary muscles, moderator band, cardiac crux, para-Hisian region, and the pulmonary artery above the pulmonic valve. Given the multiple sites of possible origin, it is important to have a consistent approach to localizing and mapping these arrhythmias when ablation is considered, and to utilize available published criteria to help differentiate likely sites of origin.

The proposed cellular mechanism of this tachycardia is cyclic adenosine monophosphate–mediated (cAMP) triggered activity from delayed afterdepolarizations. This mechanism is supported by the sensitivity of the arrhythmia to adenosine infusion, which often terminates the arrhythmia. This is

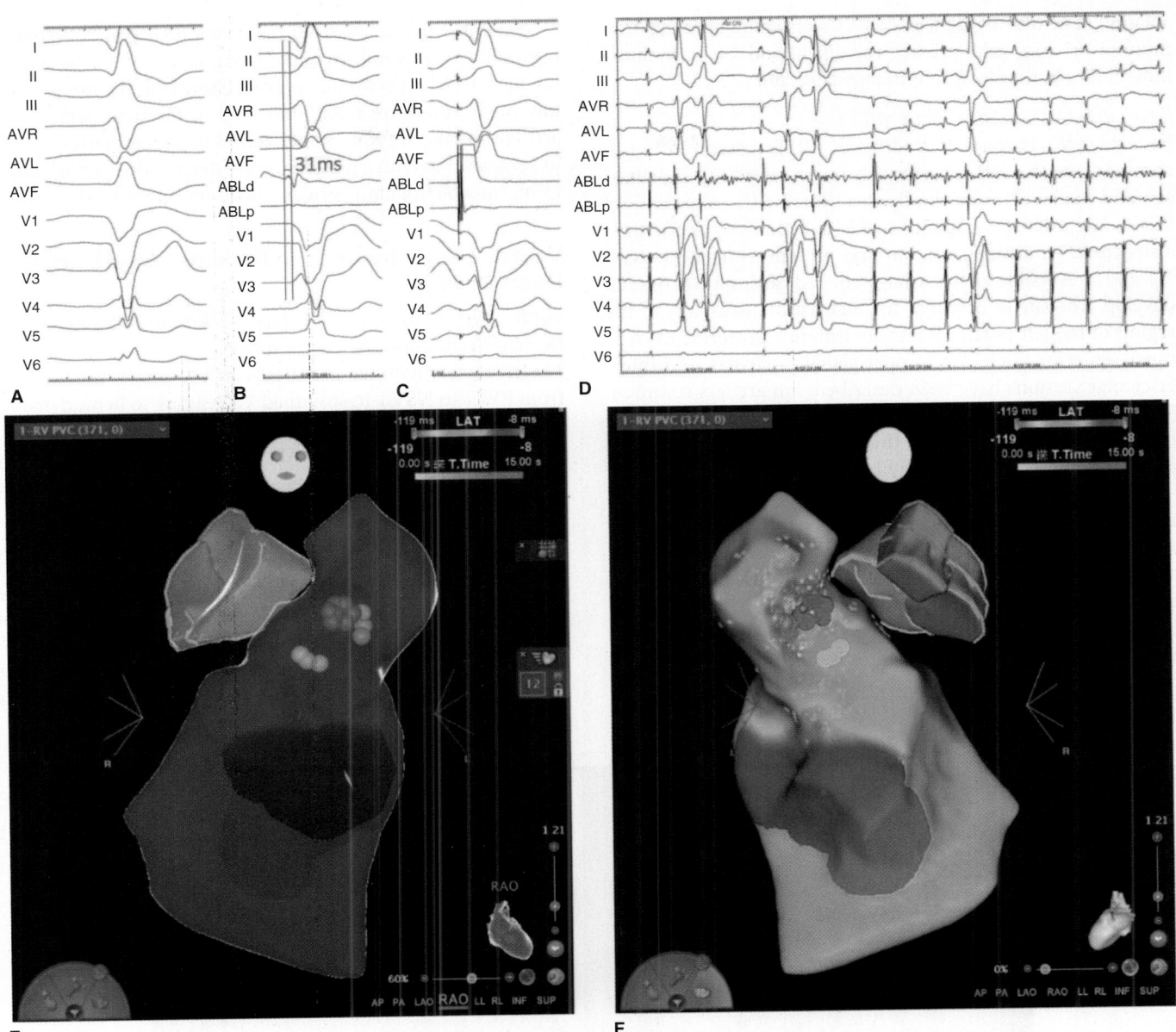

Figure 37–6. A 35-year-old male patient with PVC-mediated cardiomyopathy referred for catheter ablation. **(A)** Twelve-lead ECG of clinical PVC demonstrating LBBB morphology, V4 to V5 transition, inferior axis suggesting RVOT origin. **(B)** An ablation catheter placed in the posterior RVOT recorded an electrogram 31 ms preceding the surface QRS of the clinical PVC. **(C)** Pacing from this site demonstrates a surface 12-lead ECG morphology that matches the clinical PVC. **(D)** Ablation at this location eliminated the PVC after an initial increase in activity. Electroanatomic map (Carto, Biosense Webster, Irvine, CA) of the outflow tracts in right anterior oblique view **(E)** and left posterior oblique view **(F)** demonstrating ablation lesions as *red dots*, site of excellent pace map as *blue dot*. His bundle electrogram recordings at sites of *yellow dots*. The patient's ejection fraction recovered following successful PVC ablation.

consistent with the finding that myocardial cells from RVOT, LVOT, LV epicardium, and aortic sinus of Valsalva share a common embryologic origin in the neural crest.

As with idiopathic PVCs/NSVT, idiopathic VT is associated with an excellent prognosis. Therefore, treatment is again aimed at the alleviation of symptoms. It remains important to consider the diagnosis of ARVC, myocarditis and sarcoidosis in the workup of patients presenting with VT from the RVOT.

β-Adrenergic receptor blockers and calcium channel antagonists are usually the first choice for the treatment of symptomatic VT, but their efficacy in preventing arrhythmia recurrence

is modest. In general, β-blockers and calcium channel blockers are effective in approximately 25% to 50% of patients. Class I or III antiarrhythmic medications can also be considered, but the potential side effects and risk of proarrhythmia is increased with the use of these medications compared to β-blockers and calcium channel blockers.

Radiofrequency catheter ablation of idiopathic VT is an excellent option. Originally described in the 1980s,[33] this technique has continued to evolve, with success rates ranging from 75% to 100%; the major limitation of ablation is the potential lack of PVC activity or inducibility at the time of attempted ablation. The diurnal pattern of PVCs on ambulatory rhythm monitoring can help predict the likelihood of arrhythmia inducibility in the electrophysiology laboratory.

Fascicuclar Ventricular Tachycardia

Fascicular VT is characterized by an RBBB pattern and most commonly with a left superior axis on a 12-lead ECG. Belhassen and Laniado[34] were the first to describe the sensitivity of this tachycardia to verapamil in 1981. Patients typically have a structurally normal heart, but may present with an incessant VT and a reversible tachycardia-mediated cardiomyopathy can develop. The site of origin of the tachycardia is usually in the region of the left posterior fascicle (inferior posterior LV septum). Anterior fascicular,[35] upper septal fascicular, and interfascicular versions have been described, but are less common. The ability to induce fascicular VT using programmed stimulation and the ability to entrain this tachycardia support reentry as the mechanism for this arrhythmia.

The clinical features of this VT include (1) a structurally normal heart; (2) VT with a relatively narrow QRS (<140 ms), an RBBB pattern in V1, and superior axis; (3) sensitivity to verapamil; and (4) induction with atrial pacing. The arrhythmia usually presents in patients between 15 and 40 years of age. False tendons in the left ventricle are found in a most patients with fascicular VT, but their anatomic and functional significance is unknown.

Patients with fascicular VT have a good prognosis, responding well to verapamil for acute termination of VT as well as for long-term arrhythmia control. Class I or III antiarrhythmic medications are rarely indicated in the treatment of this arrhythmia and are usually ineffective. In patients unresponsive to verapamil or with a preference not to take medications longterm, catheter ablation is an excellent option for treatment.[7]

Ventricular Tachycardia in Patients With Structural Heart Disease

Ventricular Tachycardia in Patients With Coronary Artery Disease/Ischemic Cardiomyopathy

Ventricular arrhythmias in patients with coronary disease range from PVCs to NSVT to sustained VT leading to hemodynamic compromise and SCD. The understanding of the pathophysiology of VT in patients with CAD has been greatly enhanced by animal studies, electrophysiologic studies in humans, and the results from multicenter randomized trials.

Pathophysiology: The anatomic substrate from which ischemic VT originates usually involves a healed scar after an acute myocardial infarction (MI) **(Fig. 37–7)**. The interplay of healthy, damaged (border zone), and scarred (fibrotic) myocardium serves as a setting for slowed conduction and reentry. Evolution of the electrophysiologic substrate occurs over weeks

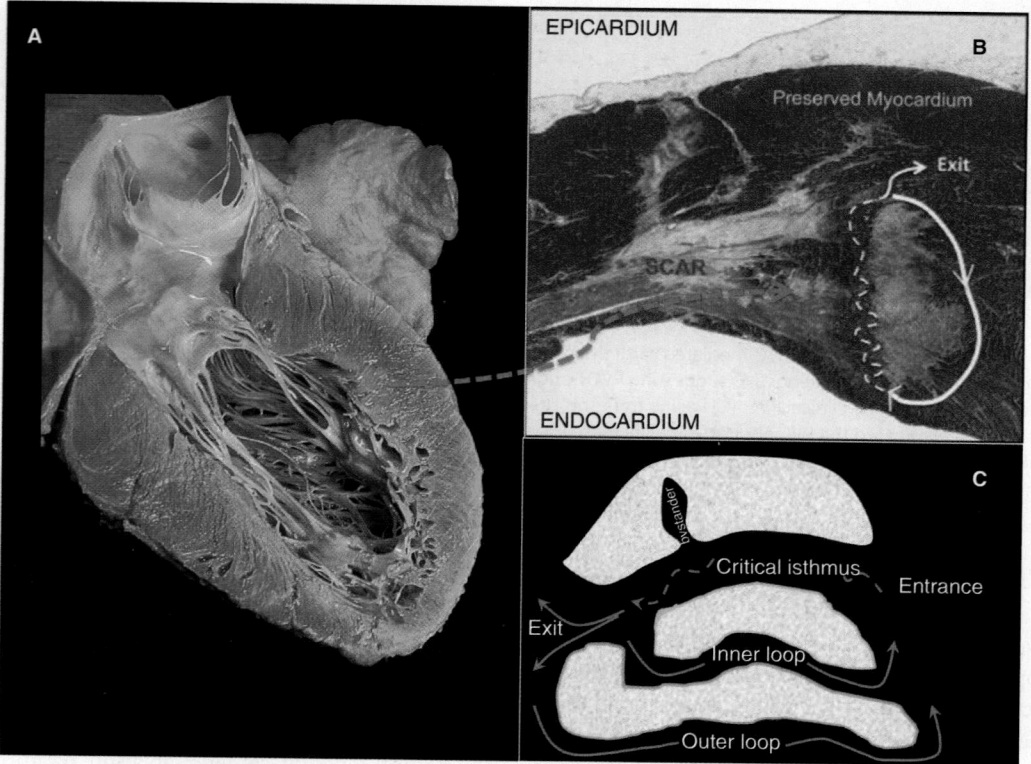

Figure 37–7. Schematic of reentry in patients with myocardial scar tissue/fibrosis. Regions of scar/fibrosis allow for conduction slowing and the potential for a reentrant circuit to form. **(A)** The gross pathologic specimen. **(B)** A representative histologic section shows scar tissue stained *blue*. The *white arrow* represents the potential reentrant circuit and the *dashed white lines* the region of slow conduction within the scar. **(C)** A schematic similar to that proposed by Stevenson et al.[81] of a potential ventricular tachycardia circuit including both critical (isthmus) and noncritical (inner loop, outer loop, bystander) locations. Illustration courtesy UCLA Cardiac Arrhythmia Center, Wallace A. McAlpine MD collection.

to months after an MI and then remains indefinitely. The tissue may continue to be modified by subsequent ischemic insults as well as late ventricular remodeling and worsening pump function. These changes may lead to neurohormonal activation, sympathetic hyperinnervation, and progressive LV dilatation with regional and global elevations in wall tension, all of which may contribute to the proarrhythmic potential.

Patients with VT have a high risk of recurrence even when heart failure and coronary ischemia are controlled. Early data demonstrated that the risk of VT is highest during the first year after an MI (3%–5%), but VT may occur many years later. The mortality benefit of ICDs has been demonstrated over decades, suggesting ongoing risk of ventricular arrhythmias over time, remote from the initial MI event.

Mechanism: The acute and chronic phases of ischemia have distinct mechanisms for ventricular arrhythmias. In acute ischemia, depolarization in the resting membrane potential of myocardial cells occurs. Multiple factors including increase in extracellular potassium, tissue hypoxia, acidosis, and increased catecholamines exert complex derangements on the cardiac action potential. As previously discussed, the inhomogeneity of these effects can establish the substrate whereby wavebreak and functional block can promote reentrant arrhythmia mechanisms. Non-reentrant mechanisms are also supported via either triggered activity or enhanced automaticity, particularly within Purkinje fiber tissue, which can also provoke sustained arrhythmias.

After the acute infarct and healing begins to occur, the formation of scar serves as the basis for a different arrhythmia mechanism in the chronic phase. Multiple findings support reentry as the mechanism of NSVT and sustained VT in most patients with previous MI. Ischemic VT can be initiated, terminated, and reset with programmed electrical stimulation in the electrophysiology laboratory. The reentry circuit most frequently exists within the border zone of the scar with areas of slow conduction or unidirectional block serving as the basis for initiation and perpetuation of monomorphic VT. Importantly, reentrant scars are often three-dimensional and critical regions can exist deep within the infarcted or fibrotic regions. The presence of an infarct does not, however, preclude the possibility of a concomitant focal VT, with recent estimates that focal arrhythmias account for between 9% and 39% of VTs in patients with structural heart disease.

Clinical Presentation and Management: Symptoms associated with ischemic VT are variable. The main determinants of hemodynamic tolerance are the rate of the VT and the degree of LV dysfunction; however, a number of patient factors also predict whether or not hemodynamic collapse will occur during VT. Interestingly, the hemodynamic stability of sustained VT is not necessarily prognostic of risk of death. In the Antiarrhythmics Versus Implantable Defibrillators (AVID) registry, patients with hemodynamically tolerated VT at presentation had similar mortality to patients with syncopal/unstable VT.

A 12-lead ECG should be obtained whenever possible to help localize the origin of the VT (**Fig. 37–8**). Algorithms have

been described to localize the origin and help differentiate endocardial and epicardial sites of origin[36–38]; however, there are limitations to such algorithms, especially in the presence of antiarrhythmic medications or when the VT is sufficiently fast, resulting in fusion of T waves with the initial component of the QRS complex.

Premature Ventricular Complexes after Myocardial Infarction: The relationship between PVCs after MI and SCD has been studied extensively, and patients with larger MIs and lower LVEFs are at the greatest risk of sudden death. Early data from trials of the thrombolytic therapy era have also shown an association between PVCs and sudden death. These observations reflect the contribution of infarct size and, by association, EF to the prognosis of patients who have experienced an MI. However, these studies predate many current advances in management of acute MI such as primary percutaneous coronary intervention, and therefore need to be understood in this context.

While the association between PVCs after MI and adverse events has been established, there is no clear benefit to routinely treating PVCs with antiarrhythmics in this setting. The association of PVCs with SCD previously led to the routine use of intravenous lidocaine in patients following MIs. Subsequent randomized controlled studies demonstrated poorer survival when PVCs were treated with Class Ic antiarrhythmic agents.[39] Based on these findings, the routine prophylactic use of antiarrhythmic agents for patients after an MI is not recommended. The treatment of PVCs and NSVT with antiarrhythmics is also not recommended unless they are associated with hemodynamic compromise or refractory symptoms, or there is evidence of PVC-induced cardiomyopathy. In patients with frequent ventricular ectopy, electrolyte and acid-base imbalance should be corrected. If frequent and persistent ventricular ectopy results in hemodynamic instability (which is rare), a β-adrenergic blocking agent or amiodarone are the preferred pharmacologic interventions in this setting.

The use of amiodarone in patients during and after an acute MI is controversial. Amiodarone has unique pharmacologic properties beyond its effects on the cardiac sodium and potassium channels. It is also a β-adrenergic receptor blocker and a calcium channel blocker and has anti-ischemic effects. The European Myocardial Infarction Amiodarone Trial (EMIAT) was a study that randomized 1486 patients with an EF of <40% and prior MI to amiodarone or placebo. No difference in total mortality was observed after a mean follow-up of 21 months.[40] A meta-analysis of 13 trials of amiodarone after MI or in congestive heart failure reported a reduction in mortality and arrhythmic death in patients treated with amiodarone. Based on the available information, the prophylactic use of amiodarone in patients after an MI is not recommended for primary prevention. However, the use of amiodarone for the treatment of hemodynamically significant ventricular arrhythmias or other arrhythmias, such as atrial fibrillation, in the postinfarct setting appears to be safe.

In patients with chronic ischemic cardiomyopathy (ICM) or nonischemic cardiomyopathy (NICM), there may be benefit to treatment of PVCs in certain clinical circumstances. Patients

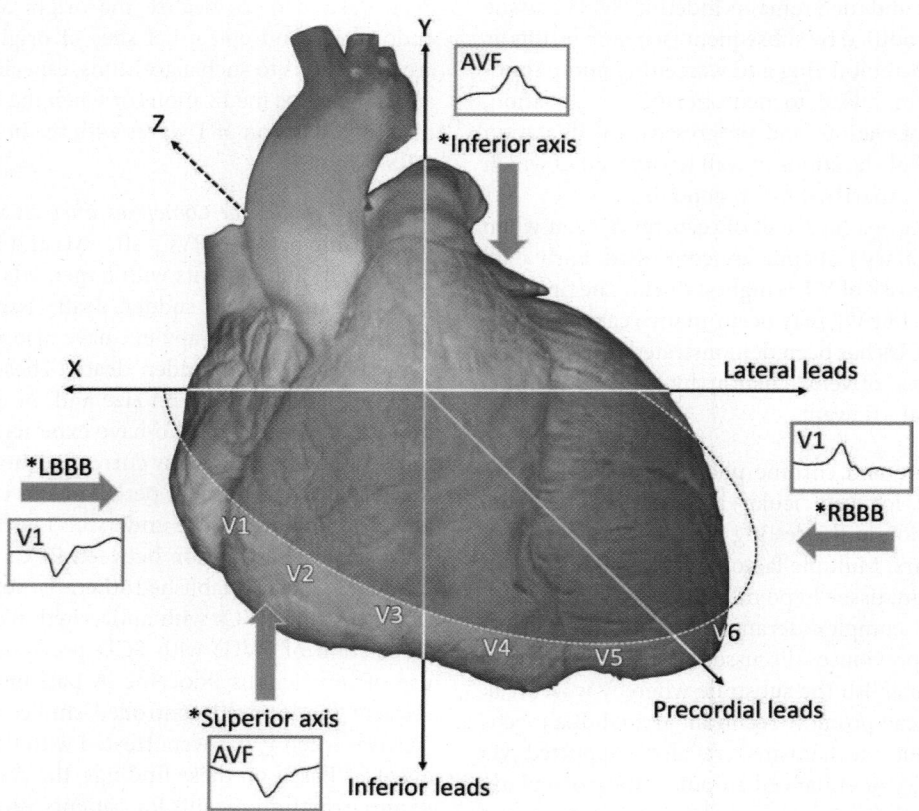

Figure 37–8. Using the 12-lead ECG for localization of ventricular arrhythmias. The X and Y (coronal) plane can be determined by the bundle branch block pattern as well as the limb lead axis. An RBBB morphology (dominant R waves in V1) suggests left ventricle exit. A LBBB pattern suggests right ventricle or interventricular septum exit. A superior axis indicates inferior wall exit and an inferior axis indicates a superior exit. The Z (axial) plane is localized by the predominant forces as well as the transition pattern within the precordial leads (predominantly positive forces indicate basal and negative forces indicate apical exit). Illustration courtesy UCLA Cardiac Arrhythmia Center, Wallace A. McAlpine MD collection.

with previous MI and presumed ICM may have appreciable EF improvement to the point of no longer requiring primary prevention ICD implantation if a high burden of PVCs can be successfully reduced. Further evidence suggests that in cardiac resynchronization therapy (CRT) nonresponders, decreasing a high burden of PVCs may allow for improved percentage of biventricular pacing and potentially improve response to CRT.

Nonsustained Ventricular Tachycardia: The evaluation and management of patients with ischemic heart disease and asymptomatic NSVT begins with the evaluation of the patient's LVEF. Patients with preserved LV function are generally at low risk and often require no further treatment other than β-blockers as part of optimal medical management. Patients with low EF are at risk of SCD. The importance of treating these patients with goal-directed medical therapy including angiotensin-converting enzyme inhibitor (ACEI), aspirin, and a β-adrenergic receptor blocker cannot be overemphasized.

Previously programmed electrical stimulation at electrophysiologic study has been advocated for risk stratification. However, this technique has demonstrated limited utility except in specific circumstances. Spontaneous NSVT and/or inducible VT does not differentiate patients who would benefit

from a primary prevention ICD in this setting. An analysis of the Multicenter Unsustained Tachycardia Trial (MUSTT) registry data demonstrated that patients with a moderately reduced ejection fraction of ≤40% with nonsustained VT and inducible VT or VF during electrophysiologic study had mortality benefit with ICD implantation.[41] Current guidelines provide a class I indication for ICD implantation for this specific patient population.[7]

In patients who already have an ICD and are known to have frequent NSVT, changes in ICD programming should be considered to minimize the risk of inappropriate shocks for arrhythmias that are likely to self-terminate. The detection time should be increased in the VT zones to decrease the likelihood of ICD shocks for NSVT, and anti-tachycardia pacing (ATP) should be utilized as a painless means of terminating ventricular arrhythmias whenever possible. Device programming targeted to minimize the number of ICD shocks have been demonstrated to improve quality of life without increasing risk of SCD in the MADIT-RIT and Pain-FREE Rx II trials.[42,43]

Accelerated Idioventricular Rhythm: Accelerated idioventricular rhythm (AIVR) is typically an automatic rhythm originating in the ventricle with rates between 40 and 120 bpm. It is often seen gradually accelerating beyond the sinus rate, resulting in isorhythmic atrioventricular dissociation. Fusion beats may be seen at the onset and termination of the arrhythmia. AIVR may be associated with ICM, acute coronary syndromes, rheumatic heart disease, dilated cardiomyopathy, and acute myocarditis. Furthermore, AIVR has been described in patients with no apparent heart disease. In the setting of acute coronary syndromes, AIVR is considered to be a nonspecific marker for successful reperfusion after thrombolytic therapy. The incidence of AIVR is not affected by the location of MI or the infarct size. The presence of AIVR after an MI is not associated with an increase in mortality.

The mechanism of AIVR is thought to be increased automaticity in a region of the ventricle; however, in some instances, such as in myocardial ischemia and digitalis toxicity, the mechanism may be caused by triggered activity. AIVR is a benign rhythm; no specific treatment is necessary. In the acute setting, when loss of atrioventricular synchrony results in hemodynamic compromise, atrial overdrive pacing or atropine may reestablish atrioventricular synchrony when the two rhythms are competing. However, one must consider that in the setting of patients with cardiomyopathy already on antiarrhythmic medications, reentry VT can be confused with an automatic rhythm.

Sustained Ventricular Tachycardia: Patients who present in clinically stable VT may be treated with antiarrhythmic drugs, ATP when available, or synchronized direct current (DC) cardioversion. Patients in VT with hemodynamic compromise, congestive heart failure, chest pain, or ischemia should be treated promptly with synchronized DC cardioversion. When antiarrhythmic drug therapy is required for acute termination of VT, amiodarone has historically been the treatment of choice. The efficacy of amiodarone was felt superior to lidocaine or procainamide in this setting based on early data. However, more recent randomized data suggest superiority of procainamide over amiodarone acutely, so procainamide has received a higher level of recommendation for use in recent guidelines.[7] Lidocaine may be considered temporarily when recurrent hemodynamically significant ventricular arrhythmias occur in the setting of acute MI, or in combination with amiodarone.

All patients with VT should be treated with a β-blocker unless prohibited by hypotension, bradycardia, or other clinical factors (ie, reactive airway disease, vasospastic coronary disease). Reversible factors contributing to VT, such as congestive heart failure exacerbation, acute ischemia, or electrolyte abnormalities, should be diagnosed rapidly and treated. However, while concerning in the setting of polymorphic VT, ischemia is rarely a cause of monomorphic VT. Monomorphic VT in the setting of structural heart disease suggests underlying myocardial fibrosis/scar.

In the setting of VT storm (VT requiring more than 3 ICD therapies in a 24-hour period) that cannot be controlled by antiarrhythmics, consideration should be given to intubation and sedation and possibly neuraxial modulation to decrease the sympathetic surge that may be contributing to the electrical

TABLE 37–3. Management of VT/VF Storm

Intensive care unit/coronary care unit admission
ICD reprogramming to maximize use of ATP and minimize shocks
Correct ischemia and electrolyte imbalance
Consider potential for drug proarrhythmia
β-blockade
Antiarrhythmic drugs (amiodarone, lidocaine, procainamide)
Sedation, intubation
Hemodynamic support (intra-aortic balloon pump, Impella)
Catheter ablation (when feasible)
Neuraxial modulation (thoracic epidural anesthesia, cardiac sympathetic denervation)

storm (see **Table 37–3**). In patients who have refractory VT despite aggressive treatment, patients may be treated successfully with an emergent or elective radiofrequency catheter ablation procedure (Table 37–3). If this intervention fails, mechanical ventricular assist devices and/or cardiac transplantation may be treatment options in specialized centers.

As previously discussed, ICD implantation is integral to reduce risk of SCD in selected patients with structural heart disease and those with history of ventricular arrhythmias. Patients with ICM and recurrent VT refractory to medications may be successfully treated with radiofrequency catheter ablation techniques.[7,44–49] When performed in experienced centers, the 1-year freedom from VT is approximately 70% in retrospective studies. Ablation has demonstrated benefit in the setting of electrical storm (VT requiring more than three ICD therapies in a 24-hour period). Additionally, studies have shown that ablation decreases the risk of future ICD therapies and is superior to escalation in antiarrhythmic therapy, particularly in patients already taking amiodarone.[50]

Ventricular Tachycardia in Patients With Nonischemic Cardiomyopathy

NICM includes a heterogeneous group of conditions resulting in LV and/or RV dysfunction. Causes of NICM include idiopathic, valvular heart disease, chronic ethanol/drug abuse, viral infections, Chagas disease, and cardiac sarcoidosis, among others. Sudden death in dilated cardiomyopathy is usually caused by VT/VF and may account for up to 30% of deaths in this population, although bradyarrhythmias must also be a cause.

Pathophysiology: The pathogenesis of ventricular arrhythmias in NICM is not well understood and may reflect a variety of mechanisms. In a study of the autopsy findings in 152 patients with NICM, subendocardial scarring was present in 33% of patients. Histologic sectioning revealed multiple patchy areas of fibrosis in 57% of patients. These patchy areas of fibrosis, intermingled with viable myocardium, may serve as the substrate for reentry and associated VT, and were predominantly found in the LV basal lateral wall and anteroseptum. These patterns do not follow any coronary distribution, unlike fibrotic scars in ICM. Subsequent studies have reinforced the predominance of basal lateral and septal scars in NICM, and demonstrated frequent involvement of the mid-myocardium and epicardium.[51]

Clinical Presentation and Management:

Premature Ventricular Contractions and Nonsustained Ventricular Tachycardia In Nonischemic Cardiomyopathy: The association between PVCs and NSVT in NICM and SCD is unclear. NSVT is common in patients with NICM and is seen on 24-hour ambulatory and telemetry monitoring in 50% to 60% of these patients. The prevalence of NSVT increases with worsening heart failure symptoms. In patients with class I to II congestive heart failure, the prevalence of NSVT is 15% to 20%; and in patients with class IV heart failure, the prevalence is 50% to 70%.[52,53] Based on available studies, the clinical significance of asymptomatic NSVT in patients with NICM remains uncertain.

Sustained Ventricular Tachycardia: Patients with NICM should be treated with optimal medical therapy for LV dysfunction.

If sustained VT or cardiac arrest occurs, the data for benefit from secondary prevention ICDs is clear from analysis of trials such as AVID,[54] CIDS,[55] and CASH.[56] Radiofrequency catheter ablation in patients with drug-refractory VT may offer an additional treatment option for patients with NICM suffering from recurrent VT and/or frequent ICD therapies.[7] As a result of the frequent epicardial substrates, a combined endocardial-epicardial approach is often required in NICM patients and is safe in experienced centers. In patients with prior cardiac surgery, pericardial adhesions can limit percutaneous access, so a hybrid surgical approach via either subxiphoid window or anterolateral thoracotomy can be performed with similar outcomes to percutaneous procedures[57] (**Fig. 37–9**).

Bundle Branch Reentry VT: Bundle branch reentry (BBR) VT is a reentrant ventricular arrhythmia utilizing the conduction

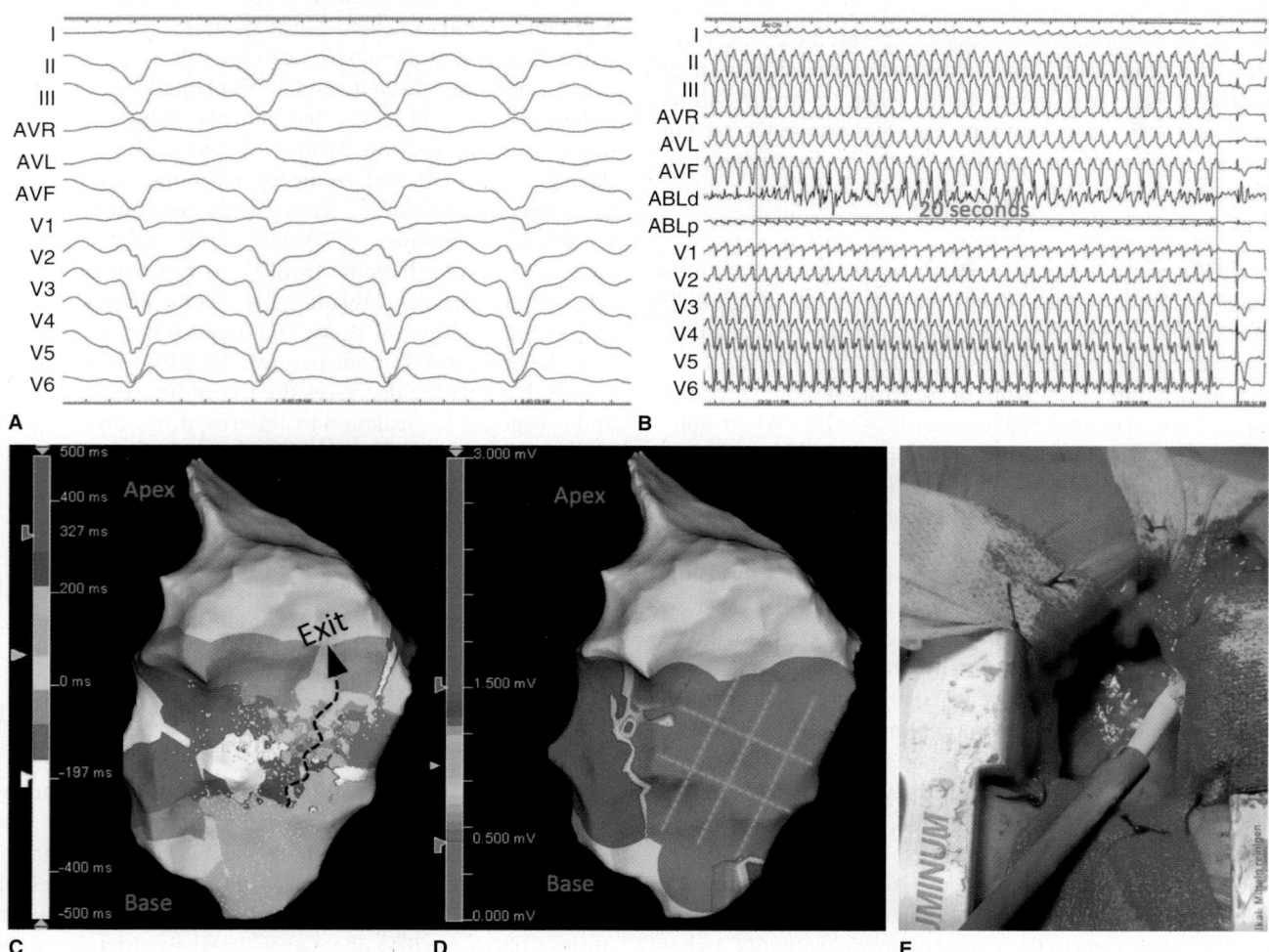

Figure 37–9. A 71-year-old male with history of prior coronary artery bypass surgery suffering repeated ICD shocks in spite of high dose amiodarone was referred for catheter ablation. Epicardial access was obtained via anterolateral thoracotomy by the cardiac surgical team. **(A)** Twelve-lead ECG of monomorphic, slow VT at a rate of 115 bpm with right bundle branch morphology, superior axis, V2 transition. QS pattern in inferior leads with prolonged pseudodelta interval in the precordial leads suggests epicardial exit site at the apical inferior LV. **(B)** Radiofrequency ablation at the apical inferior epicardial surface resulted in termination of VT after 20 seconds. **(C)** Epicardial isochronal late activation map (Ensite, Abbott, Minneapolis, MN) during sinus rhythm from a caudal view demonstrating area of isochronal crowding in the inferolateral epicardium. Likely VT isthmus site indicated with *black hatched arrow* through a region of slow conduction. **(D)** Postablation voltage map demonstrating homogenization of substrate in the inferolateral epicardium. *Blue hatched lines* indicate cryoablation lesions. **(E)** Photograph of anterolateral thoracotomy during cryoablation on the exposed epicardial surface (CryoIce Probe, Atricure, West Chester, OH). Radiofrequency ablation is challenging in the region exposed to free air due to impedance limitations.

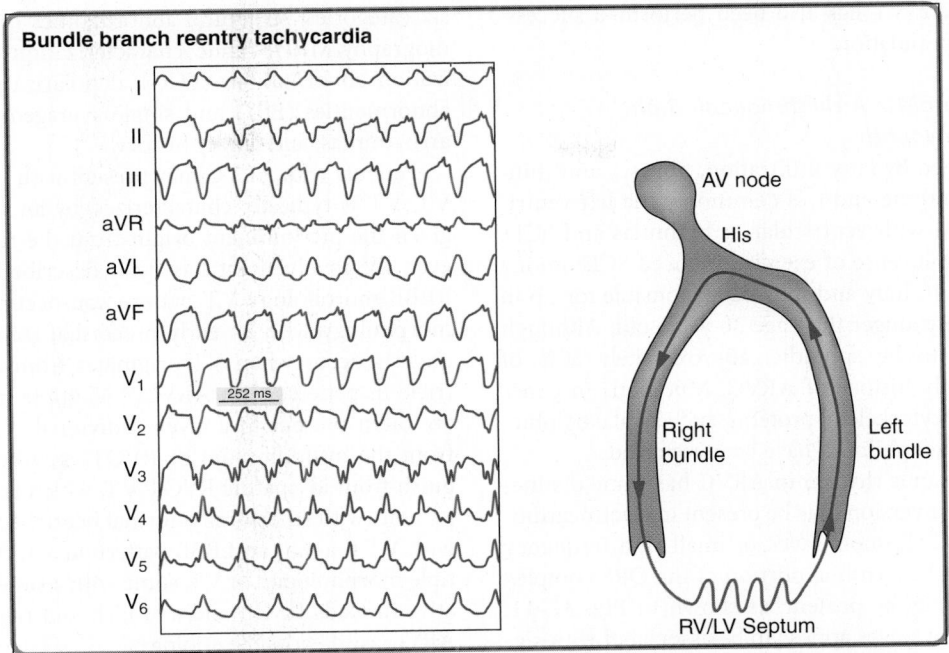

Figure 37–10. Representative 12-lead ECG and schematic of BBR VT. In typical BBR VT, the morphology is LBBB as the conduction blocks in the left bundle antegrade and is able to conduct antegrade down the right bundle and retrograde back up the left bundle to form the circuit. An RBBB version has been described, but is less common. LV, left ventricular; RV, right ventricular.

system, most commonly with antegrade conduction over the right bundle fibers and retrograde conduction over the left bundle. The 12-lead ECG during VT typically has an LBBB configuration in lead V1 (**Fig. 37–10**). Rarely, if anterograde conduction is over the left bundle branch, then RBBB QRS morphology will be seen in V1. The clinical recognition of BBR VT is essential because this arrhythmia can easily be cured by ablation.[58] The rate of BBR VT is usually rapid and may be associated with syncope. The sinus rhythm 12-lead ECG usually demonstrates an intraventricular conduction delay or an LBBB. The treatment of choice for this arrhythmia is radiofrequency ablation of the right bundle branch. Antiarrhythmic drugs for BBR are associated with a high recurrence rate. Patients with BBR with an EF <35% should receive an ICD even after successful ablation of the right bundle because they remain at risk for other lethal ventricular arrhythmias. The role of an ICD in patients with an EF >35%, who have had a successful ablation for BBR, is less clear.

Ventricular Arrhythmias in Hypertrophic Cardiomyopathy

Hypertrophic cardiomyopathy (HCM) is the most common genetic cardiomyopathy and is associated with ventricular hypertrophy with or without outflow tract obstruction, atrial and ventricular arrhythmias, myocardial ischemia, stroke, heart failure, and SCD. HCM is discussed in detail in Chapter 42. SCD is relatively uncommon in patients with HCM, although HCM is the cause of SCD in approximately 10% of cases,[59,60] and is among the most common causes of SCD among young athletes.

Based on observational studies of patients with HCM, six clinical risk factors have been found to be associated with an increased risk of SCD: (1) a history of sudden cardiac arrest or spontaneous sustained VT, (2) unexplained syncope, (3) NSVT, (4) abnormal blood pressure response to exercise, (5) family history of SCD, and (6) extreme LV hypertrophy (septal thickness >3.0 cm).[7,61] Antiarrhythmic agents do not appear to provide protection against sudden death, and the only clinically proven primary and secondary treatment option against sudden death is an ICD.

In a large international registry of ICDs implanted in 506 patients with HCM at risk for SCD, appropriate ICD shocks were observed at a rate of 5.5% per year. In the secondary prevention cohort, appropriate ICD shocks occurred at a rate of 11% per year, and in the primary prevention cohort, it was 4% per year. An interesting observation in this study was that in the primary prevention group, the event rate was the same in the subset of patients with one, two, or three risk factors of SCD. Overall, 25% of patients experienced an appropriate ICD shock for ventricular arrhythmias after a follow-up of 5 years.

For primary prevention, the decision to implant an ICD is individualized with the recognition that complications from inappropriate shocks caused by atrial arrhythmias and lead fractures may occur in up to 23% of patients, and that given the young age of the population, many lead revisions may be required over time. The ACC/AHA/HRS guidelines recommend implantation of an ICD in patients with HCM with a prior history of cardiac arrest, sustained VT (class I), or one or more major risk factors for SCD[7] (see Table 37–1). An additional risk stratification tool is scar quantification with delayed-enhancement cardiac MRI. Patients with larger areas of delayed enhancement on cardiac MRI have a higher incidence of ventricular arrhythmias. Catheter ablation for the treatment of recurrent VT has also been performed successfully in this patient population.

Ventricular Tachycardia in Arrhythmogenic Right Ventricular Cardiomyopathy

ARVC is characterized by fatty infiltration, fibrosis, and thinning of the right ventricle and less commonly the left ventricle, and is associated with ventricular arrhythmias and SCD. It is the most common cause of exercise-induced SCD among young male athletes in Italy and may be responsible for up to 20% of SCD in men younger than age 30 years old. Although most cases appear to be sporadic, approximately 30% of patients have a family history of ARVC. Mutations in genes encoding for several cytoskeletal proteins, such as plakoglobin, desmoplakin, and plakophilin-2, have been reported.

The ECG during sinus rhythm in ARVC has some distinctive features. T-wave inversion may be present in electrocardiographic leads V1 to V3. Epsilon waves, or small high-frequency deflections found in the terminal portion of the QRS complex in leads V1 to V3, may be present, as shown in **Fig. 37–11**. When present, epsilon waves appear to be associated with significant conduction delays and scarring and may correlate with electrical activation of the subtricuspid region.[62]

The diagnosis of ARVC can be difficult. In 1994, a task force proposed several criteria for the diagnosis of ARVC, which were updated in 2015.[63] Several major and minor diagnostic criteria are described, and the presence of two major, or one major and two minor, criteria are needed to make a definite diagnosis of ARVC. Major and minor criteria fall into one of six categories: structural abnormalities on imaging (echocardiography/MRI), tissue characterization on biopsy, repolarization abnormalities (ECG), depolarization and conduction abnormalities (ECG and single averaged ECG), documented arrhythmias, and family history.

Patients with ARVC may present with stable monomorphic VT. VT is typically characterized by an LBBB pattern in V1 given the predominant origin from the right ventricle. However, LV involvement has been described, in which case an RBBB morphology VT pattern can occur. Notably, an RBBB morphology with an early precordial transition can also frequently occur when VT originates from a dilated right ventricle in patients with ARVC.[64] Multiple morphologies of VT are often present in a given individual. VT, which originates from the infundibulum or RVOT, may be difficult to distinguish from idiopathic RVOT VT, which is a benign disease in patients with structurally normal hearts. Among these patients with VT that has an LBBB pattern in V1, the presence of multiple morphologies of VT, some with a superior QRS axis (negative in leads II, III, and aVF), should raise the suspicion for ARVC as the possible etiology.

Treatment of ventricular arrhythmias arising from ARVC is aimed at preventing SCD and palliation of the clinical burden of VT. β-blockers are generally recommended in treatment of patients with ARVC, in addition to goal-directed medical therapy for cardiomyopathy.[65] However, registry data suggested that β-adrenergic blocking agents do not have a protective effect on recurrent VT and ICD shocks. Patients on amiodarone had a significantly lower risk of clinically relevant ventricular

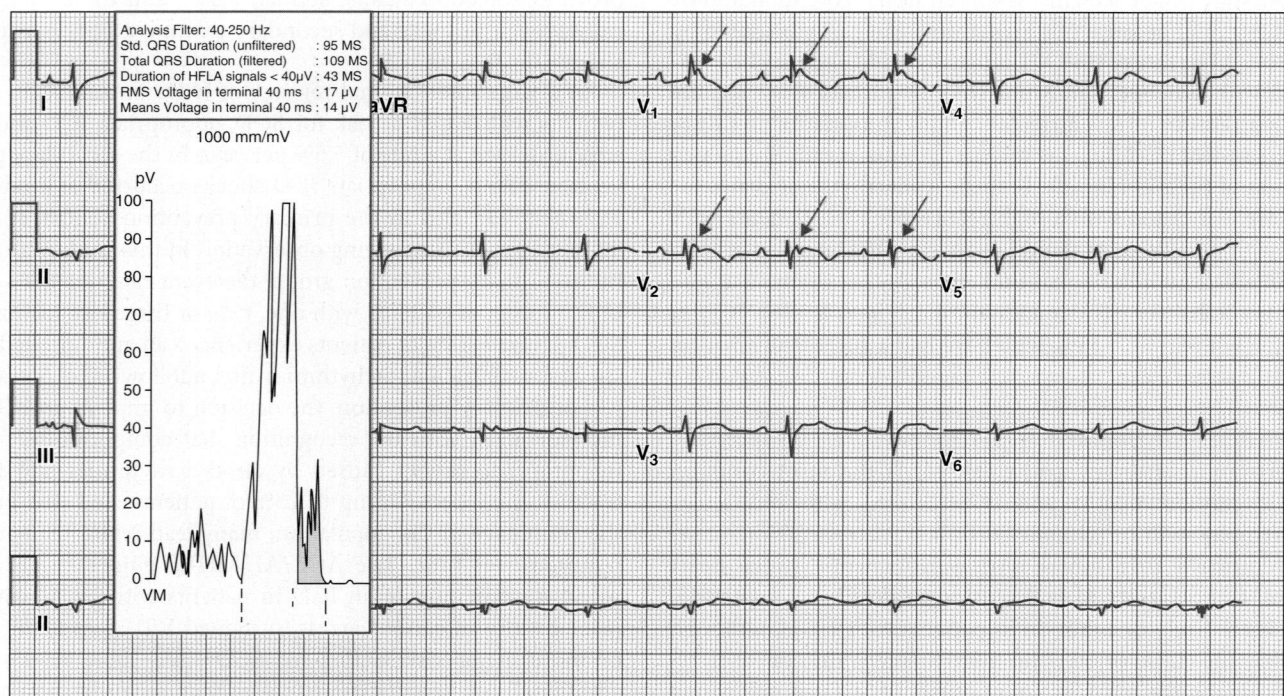

Figure 37–11. Epsilon waves (*arrows*) in a patient with ARVC. Epsilon waves meet a major criterion for the diagnosis of ARVC. Inset shows results from a signal-averaged electrocardiogram (SAECG) demonstrating a duration of the terminal <40 μV, which was >38 ms and the root-mean square (RMS) voltage of the terminal 40 ms ≤20 μV. SAECG provides a minor criterion for ARVC.

arrhythmias (HR = 0.25; 95% CI, 0.07–0.95; $P = 0.041$), which was superior to sotalol or β-blockers alone; however, the use of amiodarone must be weighed against the increased risk for adverse effects.

Patients who have had sustained VT or a history of cardiac arrest from VF should receive an ICD. Recurrent VT, not responsive to antiarrhythmic medications, can be treated with ablation.[65] Mapping guided by classic entrainment techniques can often be utilized as most patients with ARVC have preserved LVEF and, therefore, are more likely to have hemodynamically tolerated VT. If not, a substrate-based approach can be utilized. Although ablation of one clinical VT may be successful, an ICD is often implanted, as multiple VT morphologies typically occur with progression of disease. Evidence demonstrates that the arrhythmogenic substrate for reentry is more often accessible from the RV epicardium, because VT mapping studies demonstrate that many patients have VT mapped in the epicardium that is associated with normal adjacent endocardial voltages. Epicardial radiofrequency ablation at these sites can successfully eliminate and prevent long-term VT recurrence when endocardial ablation is unsuccessful.

Ventricular Tachycardia in Cardiac Sarcoidosis

Sarcoidosis is a granulomatous disease involving multiple organ systems. The incidence of cardiac symptoms in patients with sarcoidosis is relatively low; however, 20% to 30% of patients with sarcoidosis are found to have evidence of cardiac involvement.[66,67] Myocardial involvement may be diffuse, but is frequently focal or patchy with a propensity for the basal free wall and the basal septum. The most common cardiac arrhythmias associated with cardiac sarcoidosis are VT and heart block (LBBB, RBBB, hemi-blocks, and complete heart block). VT can be of LV or RV origin. The mechanism of VT is reentry within areas of patchy fibrosis, scarring, and granulomatous involvement of the myocardium. Diagnosis of cardiac sarcoidosis often relies on 18-FDG (fluoro-2-deoxyglucose) PET/CT scans and cardiac MRI because tissue diagnosis is most often not available. However, recent data suggest that occult inflammation is often present in patients referred for VT ablation with NICM, and therefore clinicians must differentiate patients with true cardiac sarcoidosis from those with an alternative etiology for their NICM.

Because of the increased risk of sudden death from VT/VF in patients with sarcoidosis, the ACC/AHA/HRS guidelines give primary prevention with an ICD in patients with sarcoidosis a class IIa recommendation.[7] In addition to an ICD, patients with sustained VT may be treated initially with a β-adrenergic blocking agent with the potential addition of amiodarone or sotalol as needed.

Catheter ablation of VT is a reasonable option for those patients with VT recurrence refractory to antiarrhythmic medications. Because of the frequent RV involvement and associated RV-origin VTs, one must always consider the potential crossover of electrophysiologic properties for VT resulting from sarcoidosis and that resulting from ARVC. The success rate of VT ablation in sarcoidosis, however, may be mitigated by multiple morphologies and active inflammation and associated substrate progression occurring during active disease. Therefore, if evidence of active inflammation is present by PET scan, initial anti-inflammatory medical therapy in addition to antiarrhythmics should be considered. Acute success rates for ablation in this setting in one study were 78%; however, freedom from VT at 1 year was lower, at 37%. Because of the complexity of the arrhythmia substrate in sarcoidosis, a combined endocardial-epicardial approach may be needed and even when acutely successful, residual VTs may be present and require continued antiarrhythmic therapy. Importantly, the relative contribution of myocardial fibrosis in conjunction with active inflammation in cardiac sarcoidosis is incompletely understood and remains the subject of ongoing clinical research.

Ventricular Tachycardia in Chagas Disease

Chagas disease is the major cause of cardiomyopathy and VT in Central and South America, and has a rising incidence in the United States as a result of immigration patterns. The protozoan *Trypanosoma cruzi* is transmitted to humans via triatome insect vectors. The etiology of chronic Chagas cardiomyopathy and associated VT is likely a combined effect of direct-parasitism, autoimmune reaction, inflammatory effects, microvascular destruction, and autonomic dysregulation. Recurrent monomorphic VT is common in chronic Chagas cardiomyopathy. Most VTs can be induced with programmed stimulation and entrained during VT favoring reentry as the predominant mechanism.

Histologic examination of patients with Chagas disease reveals focal and diffuse fibrosis of the myocardium, predominantly in the subepicardium and interspersed with surviving myocardial fibers. Regional wall-motion abnormalities are present often in the inferolateral wall of the left ventricle. Apical septal and apical inferior aneurysms also frequently occur. Sudden death is the most common cause of death in Chagas disease, accounting for 55% to 65% of deaths. A systematic review demonstrated that EF, heart failure class, and NSVT predicted risk of cardiac events.

Chagas patients with sustained VT have a high mortality, and patients with Chagas disease and depressed EF or previous sustained VT benefit from ICD insertion. Cardiac MRI may have predictive value with regards to VT risk in this population; patients with two or more regions of transmural delayed enhancement are at increased risk of clinical VT. The ACC/AHA/HRS guidelines provide a class IIa recommendation for ICD implantation for primary prevention of sudden death in patients with Chagas disease.[68]

Amiodarone has modest benefit (62% suppression of VT at 1 year) in this patient population. Radiofrequency catheter ablation may be considered for the treatment of recurrent VT. This often requires epicardial mapping and ablation because Chagas patients often have more epicardial substrate than endocardial.[69]

Ventricular Fibrillation and Polymorphic Ventricular Tachycardia

Ventricular fibrillation (VF) is characterized by rapid, chaotic, and asynchronous contraction of the left ventricle. The surface electrogram of VF reveals a rapid, irregular, dysmorphic pattern with no clearly defined QRS complex. VF is associated with rapid hemodynamic collapse and is the most common arrhythmia resulting in out-of-hospital cardiac arrest. Furthermore, patients who suffer a cardiac arrest have significant risk of subsequent arrest.

Polymorphic VT, unlike VF, has clearly defined QRS complexes, but they are constantly changing with no clear pattern. TdP is polymorphic VT, often self-terminating, in the setting of a prolonged QT interval. It is characterized by a rapid polymorphic VT that constantly changes (cycle length, axis, and morphology), in a pattern that appears to twist around a central axis.

Mechanism

The exact mechanism underlying VF continues to be enigmatic. Experimental studies suggest functional reentry plays a role in VF and an excitable gap has been demonstrated. In mathematical models, these functional reentry wavelets have the appearance of nonstationary rotating spiral waves. The ever-changing pathways of these wavelets through the complex three-dimensional geometry of the ventricle accounts for the chaotic appearance of this rhythm on a rhythm strip or 12-lead ECG.

CAD and resultant MI is the most common etiology of VF, polymorphic VT, and cardiac arrest, as previously discussed. Other causes of VF/polymorphic VT include dilated cardiomyopathies, HCM, myocarditis, valvular heart disease, congenital heart disease,[70,71] proarrhythmia from drugs, acid-base and electrolyte abnormalities, inherited arrhythmia syndromes, and atrial fibrillation in a patient with Wolff-Parkinson-White syndrome with an anterograde rapidly conducting bypass tract.

Identification of the etiology of VF/polymorphic VT is essential in the risk stratification and prevention of further episodes. For example, revascularization of patients with myocardial ischemia caused by coronary disease, ablation of a bypass tract in a patient with VF as a result of Wolff-Parkinson-White syndrome, or elimination of proarrhythmic drugs decreases the risk of future VF episodes. However, even patients thought to have a reversible cause of cardiac arrest may continue to be at risk for further episodes of VF/polymorphic VT.

Clinical Characteristics and Management

In the early stages of cardiac arrest, VF is the most common arrhythmia encountered. Patients with VF require immediate defibrillation. Early defibrillation is essential, as with every minute of delay in defibrillation for VF, the chance of survival decreases by 7% to 10%. Determinants of successful defibrillation include time to defibrillation, energy delivered, defibrillation waveform, transthoracic impedance, shock electrode placement, surface area of the shock electrodes, and the patient's metabolic status (acid-base and electrolytes). Biphasic waveforms appear to have an advantage over monophasic waveforms in that less energy is required for defibrillation. In the setting of VF, a nonsynchronized shock should be delivered.

The management of patients presenting with a resuscitated VF arrest is aimed at determining its cause and treating potential recurrence. As most cardiac arrests occur in patients with CAD, all patients should have serial cardiac enzymes monitored and be evaluated for the presence of epicardial coronary disease (usually via coronary angiography).[72,73] However, recent data suggest that a strategy of delayed coronary angiography, after neurologic recovery, is noninferior to an immediate coronary assessment in patients who suffer VF arrest who don't have ST-segment elevation present.[74] Aside from evaluation for ischemia, an echocardiogram should be performed to assess LV function. In patients with structurally normal–appearing hearts without evidence of ischemia or MI, other etiologies of VF should be considered, including coronary artery spasm, Wolff-Parkinson-White syndrome, proarrhythmia from medications, LQTS, BrS, SQTS, and CPVT.

When VF occurs during an acute MI, it usually occurs within the first 4 hours following onset of coronary occlusion. It is important to emphasize that all patients with an acute MI should undergo revascularization (if appropriate) and be treated with aspirin, a P2Y12 receptor antagonist, a β-adrenergic receptor blocker, and a statin. An angiotensin-converting enzyme (ACE) inhibitor and mineralocorticoid receptor antagonist should be added in the presence of LV dysfunction.

Identification and treatment of reversible causes of VF, such as removal of proarrhythmic medications and correcting electrolyte abnormalities, should be performed without delay. Patients with LQTS should be treated with a β-adrenergic receptor blocker as a long-term treatment to decrease the risk of TdP; however, for acute therapy for incessant torsades, isoproterenol infusion, or temporary pacing should be considered to increase the heart rate and shorten the QT interval.

When the patient's evaluation is complete and all reversible causes or contributions to VF are corrected, most patients presenting with VF arrest should undergo implantation of an ICD. ICD implantation has become the mainstay of therapy for cardiac arrest survivors. Recent early data suggest the potential benefit of left and bilateral[75-78] cardiac sympathetic denervation as an additional treatment modality, both for recurrent VF/polymorphic VT in channelopathies as well as for monomorphic VT in the setting of structural heart disease. In select cases, focal triggers of VF can be mapped and ablated (**Fig. 37–12**). These PVCs tend to originate in the border zones between scars and normal myocardium.

Malignant Premature Ventricular Complexes: Rarely, "idiopathic" PVCs thought to be benign, with no known underlying pathological substrate, can have a more malignant clinical course. "Short-coupled" PVCs inducing polymorphic VT have been demonstrated, in patients with structural/electrical heart disease and those without. Patients developing recurrent syncope or seizures with frequent PVCs on ambulatory monitoring warrant closer evaluation. This should include longer-term monitoring and a careful evaluation to rule out inherited arrhythmia syndromes and subtle structural heart abnormalities. When a monomorphic PVC is the trigger for VT or VF, catheter ablation is an excellent treatment option (Table 37–3). However, recurrent VF after apparently successful ablation has been observed, and ICD therapy is warranted in the majority of these patients.

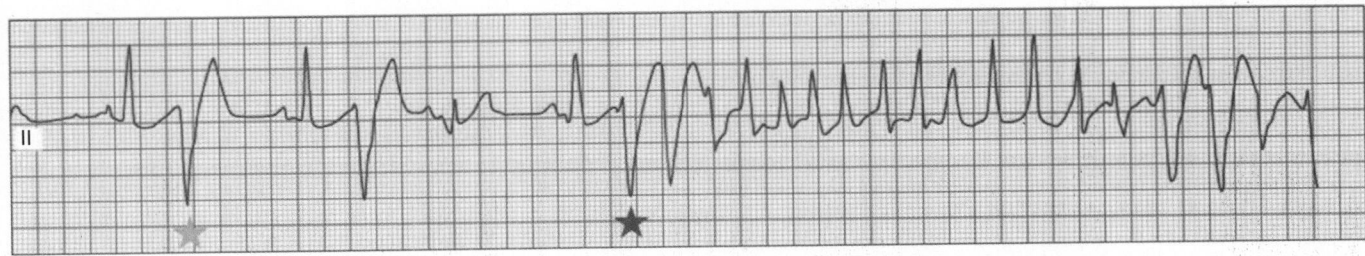

A

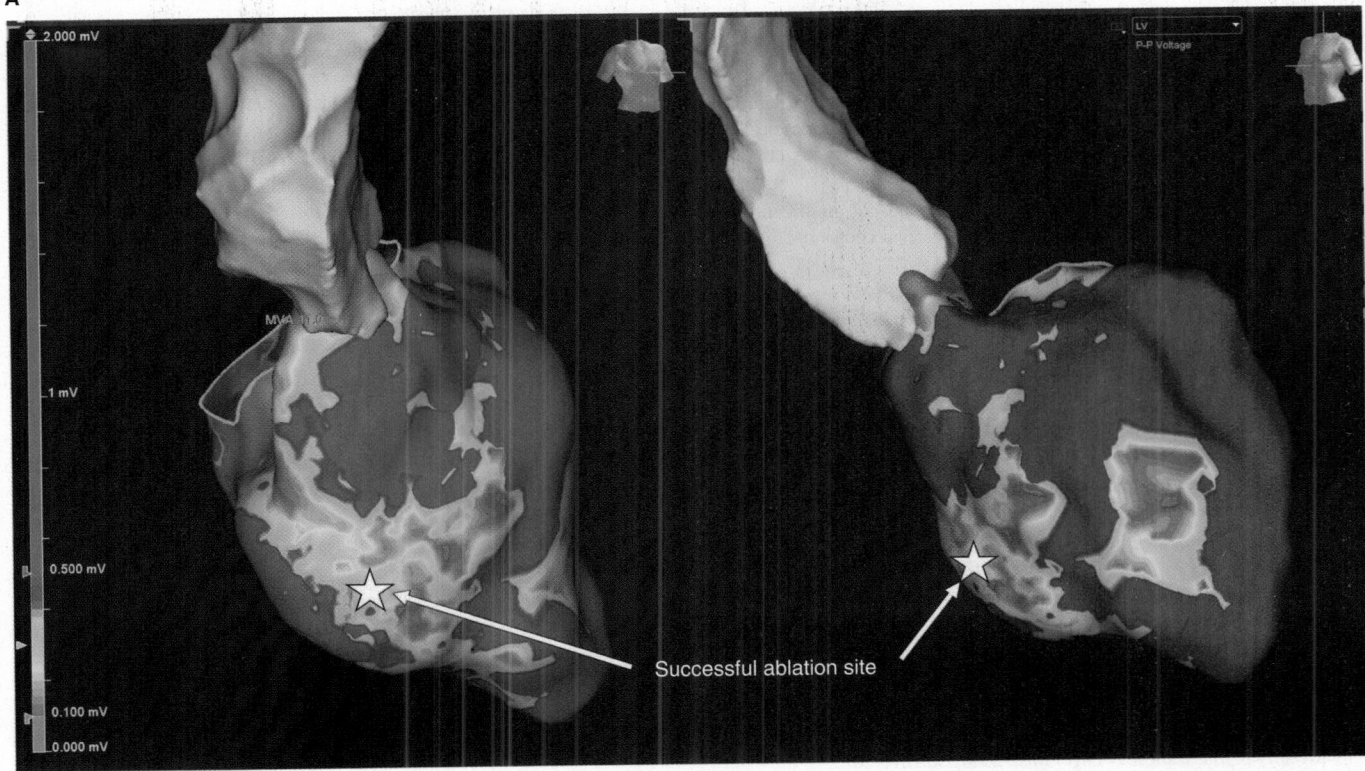

B

Figure 37–12. **(A)** Rhythm strip of recurrent PVC that repeatedly triggered VF. (*Orange star* = PVC, and *blue star* = PVC-initiated VF.) **(B)** Three-dimensional anatomic map (Ensite, Abbott, Minneapolis, MN) of the site of origin of the PVC within the scar "border zone." *Purple* represents normal tissue, *other colors* indicate abnormal tissue. Left anterior oblique view on the left, right anterior oblique view on the right.

SUMMARY

- SCD is unexpected death resulting from a cardiac cause most often due to ventricular tachyarrhythmia (VT or VF).
- SCD may be the first manifestation of otherwise phenotypically silent cardiac disease.
- Ventricular arrhythmias occur commonly and range from benign asymptomatic PVCs to sustained VT or VF resulting in SCD.
- Structural heart disease is the most important factor in risk stratification for ventricular arrhythmias; however, potentially lethal arrhythmias can occur in structurally normal–appearing hearts, particularly with underlying congenital conditions such as cardiac ion channelopathies.
- Idiopathic PVCs or VT in the absence of structural abnormalities is associated with excellent prognosis, but catheter ablation can be an effective treatment option in select patients.

- Ventricular arrhythmia management is multifaceted and depends on the associated symptoms, underlying pathologic substrate, hemodynamic consequences, and associated long-term prognosis.

ACKNOWLEDGMENTS

We would like to thank Dr. Jonathan Waks and Dr. Mark Josephson, who contributed to the previous version of the Sudden Cardiac Death chapter in the 14th edition. We would also like dedicate this chapter to Dr. Josephson, for his monumental contributions to the field of cardiac electrophysiology.

REFERENCES

1. Wong CX, Brown A, Lau DH, et al. Epidemiology of sudden cardiac death: global and regional perspectives. *Heart Lung Circ.* 2019;28:6-14.
2. Tseng ZH, Olgin JE, Vittinghoff E, et al. Prospective countywide surveillance and autopsy characterization of sudden cardiac death: POST SCD Study. *Circulation.* 2018;137:2689-2700.

3. Zheng ZJ, Croft JB, Giles WH, Mensah GA. Sudden cardiac death in the United States, 1989 to 1998. *Circulation*. 2001;104:2158-2163.

4. Becker LB, Han BH, Meyer PM, et al. Racial differences in the incidence of cardiac arrest and subsequent survival. The CPR Chicago Project. *N Engl J Med*. 1993;329:600-606.

5. Bayes de Luna A, Coumel P, Leclercq JF. Ambulatory sudden cardiac death: mechanisms of production of fatal arrhythmia on the basis of data from 157 cases. *Am Heart J*. 1989;117:151-159.

6. Janse MJ, Wit AL. Electrophysiological mechanisms of ventricular arrhythmias resulting from myocardial ischemia and infarction. *Physiol Rev*. 1989;69:1049-1169.

7. Al-Khatib SM, Stevenson WG, Ackerman MJ, et al. 2017 AHA/ACC/HRS guideline for management of patients with ventricular arrhythmias and the prevention of sudden cardiac death: executive summary: a report of the American College of Cardiology/American Heart Association Task Force on Clinical Practice Guidelines and the Heart Rhythm Society. *J Am Coll Cardiol*. 2017.

8. Adler A, Novelli V, Amin AS, et al. An international, multicentered, evidence-based reappraisal of genes reported to cause congenital long QT syndrome. *Circulation*. 2020;141:418-428.

9. Priori SG, Wilde AA, Horie M, et al. HRS/EHRA/APHRS expert consensus statement on the diagnosis and management of patients with inherited primary arrhythmia syndromes: document endorsed by HRS, EHRA, and APHRS in May 2013 and by ACCF, AHA, PACES, and AEPC in June 2013. *Heart Rhythm* 2013;10:1932-1963.

10. Bjerregaard P. Diagnosis and management of short QT syndrome. *Heart Rhythm*. 2018;15:1261-1267.

11. Brugada P, Brugada J. Right bundle branch block, persistent ST segment elevation and sudden cardiac death: a distinct clinical and electrocardiographic syndrome. A multicenter report. *J Am Coll Cardiol*. 1992;20:1391-1396.

12. Talib AK, Takagi M, Shimane A, et al. Efficacy of endocardial ablation of drug-resistant ventricular fibrillation in Brugada syndrome: long-term outcome. *Circ Arrhythm Electrophysiol*. 2018;11:e005631.

13. Tikkanen JT, Anttonen O, Junttila MJ, et al. Long-term outcome associated with early repolarization on electrocardiography. *N Engl J Med*. 2009;361:2529-2537.

14. Haissaguerre M, Derval N, Sacher F, et al. Sudden cardiac arrest associated with early repolarization. *N Engl J Med*. 2008;358:2016-2023.

15. Solomon SD, Anavekar N, Skali H, et al. Influence of ejection fraction on cardiovascular outcomes in a broad spectrum of heart failure patients. *Circulation*. 2005;112:3738-3744.

16. Connolly SJ, Dorian P, Roberts RS, et al. Comparison of beta-blockers, amiodarone plus beta-blockers, or sotalol for prevention of shocks from implantable cardioverter defibrillators: the OPTIC Study: a randomized trial. *JAMA*. 2006;295:165-171.

17. Sweeney MO, Sherfesee L, DeGroot PJ, Wathen MS, Wilkoff BL. Differences in effects of electrical therapy type for ventricular arrhythmias on mortality in implantable cardioverter-defibrillator patients. *Heart Rhythm*. 2010;7:353-360.

18. Poole JE, Johnson GW, Hellkamp AS, et al. Prognostic importance of defibrillator shocks in patients with heart failure. *N Engl J Med*. 2008;359:1009-1017.

19. Sears SF, Rosman L, Sasaki S, et al. Defibrillator shocks and their effect on objective and subjective patient outcomes: Results of the PainFree SST clinical trial. *Heart Rhythm*. 2018;15:734-740.

20. Kennedy HL, Whitlock JA, Sprague MK, Kennedy LJ, Buckingham TA, Goldberg RJ. Long-term follow-up of asymptomatic healthy subjects with frequent and complex ventricular ectopy. *N Engl J Med*. 1985;312:193-197.

21. Niwano S, Wakisaka Y, Niwano H, et al. Prognostic significance of frequent premature ventricular contractions originating from the ventricular outflow tract in patients with normal left ventricular function. *Heart*. 2009;95:1230-1237.

22. Walters TE, Rahmutula D, Szilagyi J, et al. Left ventricular dyssynchrony predicts the cardiomyopathy associated with premature ventricular contractions. *J Am Coll Cardiol*. 2018;72:2870-2882.

23. Del Carpio Munoz F, Syed FF, Noheria A, et al. Characteristics of premature ventricular complexes as correlates of reduced left ventricular systolic function: study of the burden, duration, coupling interval, morphology and site of origin of PVCs. *J Cardiovasc Electrophysiol*. 2011;22:791-798.

24. Voskoboinik A, Hadjis A, Alhede C, et al. Predictors of adverse outcome in patients with frequent premature ventricular complexes: the ABC-VT risk score. *Heart Rhythm*. 2020.

25. Hasdemir C, Ulucan C, Yavuzgil O, et al. Tachycardia-induced cardiomyopathy in patients with idiopathic ventricular arrhythmias: the incidence, clinical and electrophysiologic characteristics, and the predictors. *J Cardiovasc Electrophysiol*. 2011;22:663-668.

26. Sadron Blaye-Felice M, Hamon D, Sacher F, et al. Premature ventricular contraction-induced cardiomyopathy: related clinical and electrophysiologic parameters. *Heart Rhythm*. 2016;13:103-110.

27. Kawamura M, Badhwar N, Vedantham V, et al. Coupling interval dispersion and body mass index are independent predictors of idiopathic premature ventricular complex-induced cardiomyopathy. *J Cardiovasc Electrophysiol*. 2014;25:756-762.

28. Hamon D, Rajendran PS, Chui RW, et al. Premature ventricular contraction coupling interval variability destabilizes cardiac neuronal and electrophysiological control: insights from simultaneous cardioneural mapping. *Circ Arrhythm Electrophysiol*. 2017;10.

29. Kowlgi GN, Ramirez RJ, Kaszala K, et al. Post-extrasystolic potentiation as a predictor of premature ventricular contraction-cardiomyopathy in an animal model. *Europace*. 2020.

30. Lakkireddy D, Turagam MK, Yarlagadda B, et al. Myocarditis causing premature ventricular contractions: insights from the MAVERIC Registry. *Circ Arrhythm Electrophysiol*. 2019;12:e007520.

31. Van Herendael H, Garcia F, Lin D, et al. Idiopathic right ventricular arrhythmias not arising from the outflow tract: prevalence, electrocardiographic characteristics, and outcome of catheter ablation. *Heart Rhythm*. 2011;8:511-518.

32. Enriquez A, Baranchuk A, Briceno D, Saenz L, Garcia F. How to use the 12-lead ECG to predict the site of origin of idiopathic ventricular arrhythmias. *Heart Rhythm*. 2019;16:1538-1544.

33. Davis MJ, Murdock C. Radiofrequency catheter ablation of refractory ventricular tachycardia. *Pacing Clin Electrophysiol*. 1988;11:725-729.

34. Belhassen B, Rotmensch HH, Laniado S. Response of recurrent sustained ventricular tachycardia to verapamil. *Br Heart J*. 1981;46:679-682.

35. Nogami A, Naito S, Tada H, et al. Verapamil-sensitive left anterior fascicular ventricular tachycardia: results of radiofrequency ablation in six patients. *J Cardiovasc Electrophysiol*. 1998;9:1269-1278.

36. Josephson ME, Callans DJ. Using the twelve-lead electrocardiogram to localize the site of origin of ventricular tachycardia. *Heart Rhythm*. 2005;2:443-446.

37. Berruezo A, Mont L, Nava S, Chueca E, Bartholomay E, Brugada J. Electrocardiographic recognition of the epicardial origin of ventricular tachycardias. *Circulation*. 2004;109:1842-1847.

38. Bazan V, Bala R, Garcia FC, et al. Twelve-lead ECG features to identify ventricular tachycardia arising from the epicardial right ventricle. *Heart Rhythm*. 2006;3:1132-1139.

39. Echt DS, Liebson PR, Mitchell LB, et al. Mortality and morbidity in patients receiving encainide, flecainide, or placebo. The Cardiac Arrhythmia Suppression Trial. *N Engl J Med*. 1991;324:781-788.

40. Julian DG, Camm AJ, Frangin G, et al. Randomised trial of effect of amiodarone on mortality in patients with left-ventricular dysfunction after recent myocardial infarction: EMIAT. European Myocardial Infarct Amiodarone Trial Investigators. *Lancet*. 1997;349:667-674.

41. Buxton AE, Lee KL, DiCarlo L, et al. Nonsustained ventricular tachycardia in coronary artery disease: relation to inducible sustained ventricular tachycardia. MUSTT Investigators. *Ann Intern Med.* 1996;125:35-39.

42. Moss AJ, Schuger C, Beck CA, et al. Reduction in inappropriate therapy and mortality through ICD programming. *N Engl J Med.* 2012;367:2275-2283.

43. Wathen MS, DeGroot PJ, Sweeney MO, et al. Prospective randomized multicenter trial of empirical antitachycardia pacing versus shocks for spontaneous rapid ventricular tachycardia in patients with implantable cardioverter-defibrillators: Pacing Fast Ventricular Tachycardia Reduces Shock Therapies (PainFREE Rx II) trial results. *Circulation.* 2004;110:2591-2596.

44. Marchlinski FE, Callans DJ, Gottlieb CD, Zado E. Linear ablation lesions for control of unmappable ventricular tachycardia in patients with ischemic and nonischemic cardiomyopathy. *Circulation.* 2000;101:1288-1296.

45. Soejima K, Suzuki M, Maisel WH, et al. Catheter ablation in patients with multiple and unstable ventricular tachycardias after myocardial infarction: short ablation lines guided by reentry circuit isthmuses and sinus rhythm mapping. *Circulation.* 2001;104:664-669.

46. Stevenson WG, Wilber DJ, Natale A, et al. Irrigated radiofrequency catheter ablation guided by electroanatomic mapping for recurrent ventricular tachycardia after myocardial infarction: the multicenter thermocool ventricular tachycardia ablation trial. *Circulation.* 2008;118:2773-2782.

47. Di Biase L, Santangeli P, Burkhardt DJ, et al. Endo-epicardial homogenization of the scar versus limited substrate ablation for the treatment of electrical storms in patients with ischemic cardiomyopathy. *J Am Coll Cardiol.* 2012;60:132-141.

48. Calkins H, Epstein A, Packer D, et al. Catheter ablation of ventricular tachycardia in patients with structural heart disease using cooled radiofrequency energy: results of a prospective multicenter study. Cooled RF Multi Center Investigators Group. *J Am Coll Cardiol.* 2000;35:1905-1914.

49. Kuck KH, Schaumann A, Eckardt L, et al. Catheter ablation of stable ventricular tachycardia before defibrillator implantation in patients with coronary heart disease (VTACH): a multicentre randomised controlled trial. *Lancet.* 2010;375:31-40.

50. Sapp JL, Wells GA, Parkash R, et al. Ventricular tachycardia ablation versus escalation of antiarrhythmic drugs. *N Engl J Med.* 2016;375:111-121.

51. Zeppenfeld K. Ventricular tachycardia ablation in nonischemic cardiomyopathy. *JACC Clin Electrophysiol.* 2018;4:1123-1140.

52. Stevenson LW, Fowler MB, Schroeder JS, Stevenson WG, Dracup KA, Fond V. Poor survival of patients with idiopathic cardiomyopathy considered too well for transplantation. *Am J Med.* 1987;83:871-876.

53. Kjekshus J. Arrhythmias and mortality in congestive heart failure. *Am J Cardiol.* 1990;65:42I-48I.

54. A comparison of antiarrhythmic-drug therapy with implantable defibrillators in patients resuscitated from near-fatal ventricular arrhythmias. The Antiarrhythmics versus Implantable Defibrillators (AVID) Investigators. *N Engl J Med.* 1997;337:1576-1583.

55. Connolly SJ, Gent M, Roberts RS, et al. Canadian implantable defibrillator study (CIDS) : a randomized trial of the implantable cardioverter defibrillator against amiodarone. *Circulation.* 2000;101:1297-1302.

56. Kuck KH, Cappato R, Siebels J, Ruppel R. Randomized comparison of antiarrhythmic drug therapy with implantable defibrillators in patients resuscitated from cardiac arrest: the Cardiac Arrest Study Hamburg (CASH). *Circulation.* 2000;102:748-754.

57. Li A, Hayase J, Do D, et al. Hybrid surgical versus percutaneous access epicardial ventricular tachycardia ablation. *Heart Rhythm.* 2017.

58. Chien WW, Scheinman MM, Cohen TJ, Lesh MD. Importance of recording the right bundle branch deflection in the diagnosis of His-Purkinje reentrant tachycardia. *Pacing Clin Electrophysiol.* 1992;15:1015-1024.

59. Ullal AJ, Abdelfattah RS, Ashley EA, Froelicher VF. Hypertrophic cardiomyopathy as a cause of sudden cardiac death in the young: a meta-analysis. *Am J Med.* 2016;129:486-496 e2.

60. Corrado D, Basso C, Thiene G. Sudden cardiac death in young people with apparently normal heart. *Cardiovasc Res.* 2001;50:399-408.

61. Maron BJ, Maron MS. Contemporary strategies for risk stratification and prevention of sudden death with the implantable defibrillator in hypertrophic cardiomyopathy. *Heart Rhythm.* 2016;13:1155-1165.

62. Tanawuttiwat T, Te Riele AS, Philips B, et al. Electroanatomic correlates of depolarization abnormalities in arrhythmogenic right ventricular dysplasia/cardiomyopathy. *J Cardiovasc Electrophysiol.* 2016;27:443-452.

63. Corrado D, Wichter T, Link MS, et al. Treatment of arrhythmogenic right ventricular cardiomyopathy/dysplasia: an International Task Force consensus statement. *Circulation.* 2015;132:441-453.

64. Marchlinski DF, Tschabrunn CM, Zado Pac ES, Santangeli P, Marchlinski FE. Right bundle branch block ventricular tachycardia in arrhythmogenic right ventricular cardiomyopathy more commonly originates from the right ventricle: Criteria for identifying chamber of origin. *Heart Rhythm.* 2020.

65. Towbin JA, McKenna WJ, Abrams DJ, et al. 2019 HRS expert consensus statement on evaluation, risk stratification, and management of arrhythmogenic cardiomyopathy. *Heart Rhythm.* 2019;16:e301-e372.

66. Birnie DH, Sauer WH, Bogun F, et al. HRS expert consensus statement on the diagnosis and management of arrhythmias associated with cardiac sarcoidosis. *Heart Rhythm.* 2014;11:1305-1323.

67. Lynch JP, 3rd, Hwang J, Bradfield J, Fishbein M, Shivkumar K, Tung R. Cardiac involvement in sarcoidosis: evolving concepts in diagnosis and treatment. *Semin Respir Crit Care Med.* 2014;35:372-390.

68. Epstein AE, DiMarco JP, Ellenbogen KA, et al. ACC/AHA/HRS 2008 guidelines for device-based therapy of cardiac rhythm abnormalities: a report of the American College of Cardiology/American Heart Association Task Force on Practice Guidelines (writing committee to revise the ACC/AHA/NASPE 2002 guideline update for implantation of cardiac pacemakers and antiarrhythmia devices) developed in collaboration with the American Association for Thoracic Surgery and Society of Thoracic Surgeons. *J Am Coll Cardiol.* 2008;51:e1-e62.

69. Henz BD, do Nascimento TA, Dietrich Cde O, et al. Simultaneous epicardial and endocardial substrate mapping and radiofrequency catheter ablation as first-line treatment for ventricular tachycardia and frequent ICD shocks in chronic chagasic cardiomyopathy. *J Interv Card Electrophysiol.* 2009;26:195-205.

70. Downar E, Harris L, Kimber S, et al. Ventricular tachycardia after surgical repair of tetralogy of Fallot: results of intraoperative mapping studies. *J Am Coll Cardiol.* 1992;20:648-655.

71. Stout KK, Daniels CJ, Aboulhosn JA, et al. 2018 AHA/ACC guideline for the management of adults with congenital heart disease: a report of the American College of Cardiology/American Heart Association Task Force on Clinical Practice Guidelines. *J Am Coll Cardiol.* 2019;73:e81-e192.

72. Nolan JP, Neumar RW, Adrie C, et al. Post-cardiac arrest syndrome: epidemiology, pathophysiology, treatment, and prognostication. A scientific statement from the International Liaison Committee on Resuscitation; the American Heart Association Emergency Cardiovascular Care Committee; the Council on Cardiovascular Surgery and Anesthesia; the Council on Cardiopulmonary, Perioperative, and Critical Care; the Council on Clinical Cardiology; the Council on Stroke. *Resuscitation.* 2008;79:350-379.

73. Field JM, Hazinski MF, Sayre MR, et al. Part 1: executive summary: 2010 American Heart Association Guidelines for Cardiopulmonary Resuscitation and Emergency Cardiovascular Care. *Circulation.* 2010;122:S640-S656.

74. Lemkes JS, Janssens GN, van der Hoeven NW, et al. Coronary angiography after cardiac arrest without ST-segment elevation. *N Engl J Med.* 2019;380:1397-1407.

75. Ajijola OA, Lellouche N, Bourke T, et al. Bilateral cardiac sympathetic denervation for the management of electrical storm. *J Am Coll Cardiol.* 2012;59:91-92.

76. Vaseghi M, Gima J, Kanaan C, et al. Cardiac sympathetic denervation in patients with refractory ventricular arrhythmias or electrical storm: Intermediate and long-term follow-up. *Heart Rhythm.* 2014;11:360-366.

77. Vaseghi M, Barwad P, Malavassi Corrales FJ, et al. Cardiac sympathetic denervation for refractory ventricular arrhythmias. *J Am Coll Cardiol.* 2017;69:3070-3080.

78. Bourke T, Vaseghi M, Michowitz Y, et al. Neuraxial modulation for refractory ventricular arrhythmias: value of thoracic epidural anesthesia and surgical left cardiac sympathetic denervation. *Circulation.* 2010;121:2255-2262.

79. Gillum RF. Sudden coronary death in the United States: 1980-1985. *Circulation.* 1989;79:756-765.

80. Myerburg RJ, Interian A, Jr., Mitrani RM, Kessler KM, Castellanos A. Frequency of sudden cardiac death and profiles of risk. *Am J Cardiol.* 1997;80:10F-19F.

81. Stevenson WG, Friedman PL, Sager PT, et al. Exploring postinfarction reentrant ventricular tachycardia with entrainment mapping. *J Am Coll Cardiol.* 1997;29:1180-1189.

Conduction System Disturbances and Bradyarrhythmias

38

Pugazhendhi Vijayaraman, Jeffrey Arkles, Jayanthi N. Koneru, and David J. Callans

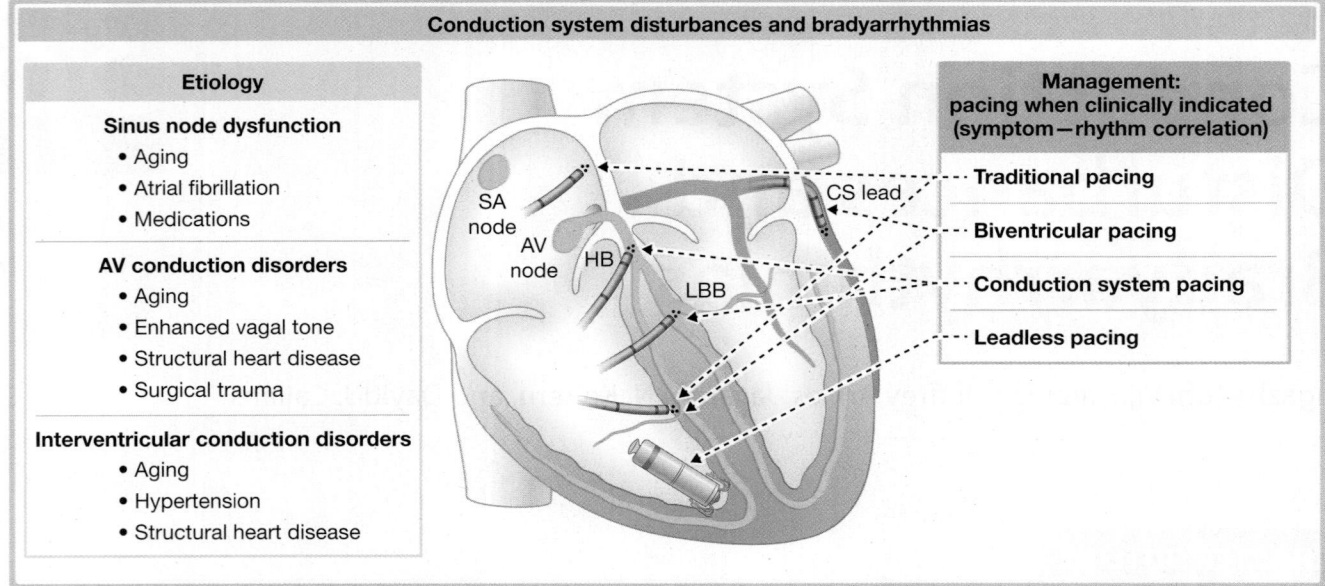

Chapter 38 Fuster and Hurst's Central Illustration. Conduction system dysfunction can occur at any level of the electrical system, sinus node, AV conduction axis (AV node/HB), and intraventricular conduction (right and left bundle branches), with variable clinical effects. Treatment primarily involves pacemaker implantation when appropriate. AV, atrioventricular; CS, coronary sinus; HB, His bundle; LBB, left bundle branch; SA, sinoatrial.

CHAPTER SUMMARY

This chapter examines the pathophysiology of various clinical forms of conduction system disturbances and sinus node dysfunction (SND) (see Fuster and Hurst's Central Illustration). The conduction system serves as the "translator" between the autonomic nervous system's various demands for heart rate and coordinates electrical activation to provide efficient excitation–contraction coupling. Dysfunction can occur at any level of the electrical system, sinus node, atrioventricular (AV) conduction axis (AV node/His bundle), and intraventricular conduction (right and left bundle branches), with variable clinical effects. Many disease processes affect the electrical system, but the most prominent are aging and concomitant structural heart disease. Genetic disorders, although rare, are important to discover because they may be syndromic and can affect other family members. AV block caused by surgical trauma, particularly during transcatheter aortic valve procedures, is increasing in incidence and often requires complex decision making. Treatment primarily involves pacemaker implantation when appropriate, and the indications for pacing are reviewed. Novel technologies, including leadless pacing, conduction system pacing, and the promise of biological pacing, are also discussed.

SINUS NODE DYSFUNCTION

The sinus node serves as the dominant pacemaker of the heart. Its role is to provide adequate rates at rest as well as increased rate during periods of exercise or other metabolic stressors (chronotropic competence). The function of the sinus node is modulated by unique anatomic features, rich autonomic nervous system innervation, and distinctive aspects of its cellular electrophysiology. Failure of the sinus node may be due to abnormalities in impulse formation or conduction block, as will be discussed in this chapter. Incident sinus node dysfunction (SND) occurs in approximately 0.8 per 1000 person-years and is highly age-related, representing an indication for more than 50% of pacemakers implanted in the United States. SND and atrial fibrillation (AF) commonly coexist ("tachy-brady syndrome"), with a lifetime incidence of AF in patients with SND as high as 50%.

Anatomy and Physiology

There are several unique anatomic features of the sinus node that relate to its function. The sinus node is a "tadpole-shaped" structure, 8 mm to 22 mm in length, located subepicardially within the sulcus terminalis (**Fig. 38–1**).[1] It receives blood from the sinus node artery, which arises from the right (60%) or left circumflex (40%) coronary artery. It is relatively electrically insulated anatomically (fibrosis, fat, blood vessels) and functionally (limited connexins), linked by a finite number of sinoatrial conduction pathways to surrounding atrial myocytes.[2] This isolation is thought to be important, to protect hyperpolarization of the sinus node cells by the larger atrial mass (with more negative resting potential), allowing the smaller "source" to activate the larger "sink."[2,3] The location of impulse generation is in the superior portion of the sinus node during faster rates and more inferior during slower rates.[3] A related concept is the presence of more widely distributed pacemaker regions within the atria, with the same hierarchy of rates based on superior versus inferior location. These sites range from the sulcus terminalis to the area bordering the Eustachian ridge, as well as involving left atrial and venous sites. These observations lead to the concept that multiple layers of protection and redundancy are protective to the essential function of continuous and uninterrupted function of the sinus node.[4]

The cellular electrophysiology of the sinus node has several unique features: (1) resting membrane potential –50 to –60 mV (less negative than surrounding atrial cells); (2) absence of fast inward sodium current (action potential phase 0 is mediated by slow inward calcium current [I_{CaL}]); (3) absence of inward rectifier potassium current (I_{k1}); and most importantly (4) phase 4 automaticity, which is the direct cause of its prominence in determining rate. The differences in central (location of primary pacemaker cells) and peripheral sinus nodal and surrounding atrial cellular electrophysiology are shown in **Fig. 38–2**. Current thinking about the mechanism of phase 4 depolarization supports the interaction of two forces, including the membrane "clock" and the calcium "clock."[3,5] Phase 4 depolarization is initiated by the membrane clock, which represents the balance between the decay of outward potassium repolarizing currents (I_k) and the activation of depolarizing currents, particularly the "funny" current I_f primarily carried by Na+. I_k was named the funny current because it is activated by hyperpolarization, whereas most voltage-gated currents are activated by depolarization. The membrane clock depolarizes the membrane to a level where the Ca^{2+} inward current results in phase 0 of the action potential. The sarcolemmal calcium clock can also initiate phase 4 depolarization in the sinus node due to spontaneous, rhythmic release of Ca^{2+} from the sarcoplasmic reticulum (SR) via the ryanodine type 2 receptor (RYR2). Elevation in intracellular calcium concentration activates the electrogenic sodium-calcium exchange current (I_{NCX}), which transfers one calcium ion outward for three sodium ions inward. This net increase in positive charge results in membrane depolarization.

The relative contribution of the membrane clock and the calcium clock to phase 4 depolarization continues to be debated. It is clear from the effects of drugs (eg, ivabradine, which blocks I_f) or specific genetic alterations that affect one system or the other that both systems may mediate the pacemaker role of the sinus node. Perhaps this is another expression of the biological necessity of redundancy. Automaticity in subsidiary pacemakers (atrial and nodal tissue) is thought to arise from similar electrophysiologic mechanisms, but at a slower rate, so they are naturally entrained by the sinus node. Interestingly, in the setting of clinically important SND, subsidiary pacemakers also fail. This is thought to be due to a more diffuse loss of electrically active myocytes, involving not only the sinus node but also the surrounding atrial tissue.

The sinus node region is richly innervated with postganglionic adrenergic and cholinergic nerves. Neural and hormonal factors influence the sinus rate based on several mechanisms. Parasympathetic tone reduces heart rate, caused by G-protein activation of I_{KACh} (acetylcholine-activated inward rectifying current). This results in membrane hyperpolarization, lengthening the time required to depolarize to threshold, thus slowing the heart rate. Sympathetic tone and the accompanying systemic catecholamine release leads to increase in heart rate by at least three mechanisms: (1) cAMP (cyclic adenosine 3′,5′-monophosphate) medicated increase in calcium current (I_{Ca}), (2) increase in I_f, and (3) superior shift of the site of impulse formation in the sinus node (which may allow different and more favorable exit pathways to the atrium).

Pathophysiology

Theoretically, SND could be caused by either failure of impulse generation or sinoatrial exit block. Despite electrocardiographic patterns that may suggest the latter mechanism, in most cases it is difficult to decipher which mechanism predominates. It is certainly easy to understand how many of the pathological conditions subsequently discussed would affect sinus node automaticity and the transmission of the pacemaker current to the perinodal atrium. As aforementioned, these same conditions can affect the atrium more diffusely, leading to dysfunction of subsidiary pacemakers.

Traditionally, causes of SND have been categorized as *intrinsic*: processes that directly alter the anatomy or physiology of the

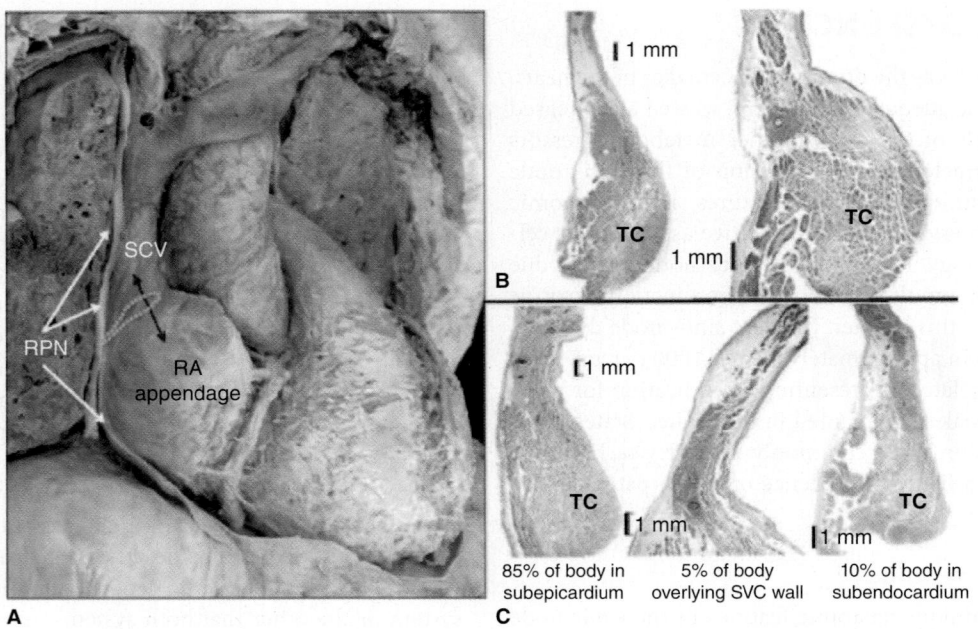

Figure 38–1. **(A)** Anterior view of a pathologic specimen demonstrating the subepicardial location of the sinus node (outlined in *green dots*) near the intersection of the right atrial appendage, right atrium, and superior vena cava. The *double-headed arrow* marks the sectioning plane for the histologic sections **(B)** and **(C).** RPN and white arrows: right phrenic nerve; SVC: superior vena cava **(B)** The histological sections demonstrate the fibrous matrix of the sinus node, stained in *green* (Masson's trichrome stain) and its relationship to the crista terminalis; **(C)** shows nodal relationships to the epicardial and endocardial surfaces. Reproduced with permission from Ho SY, Sánchez-Quintana D. Anatomy and pathology of the sinus node, *J Interv Card Electrophysiol.* 2016 Jun;46(1):3-8.

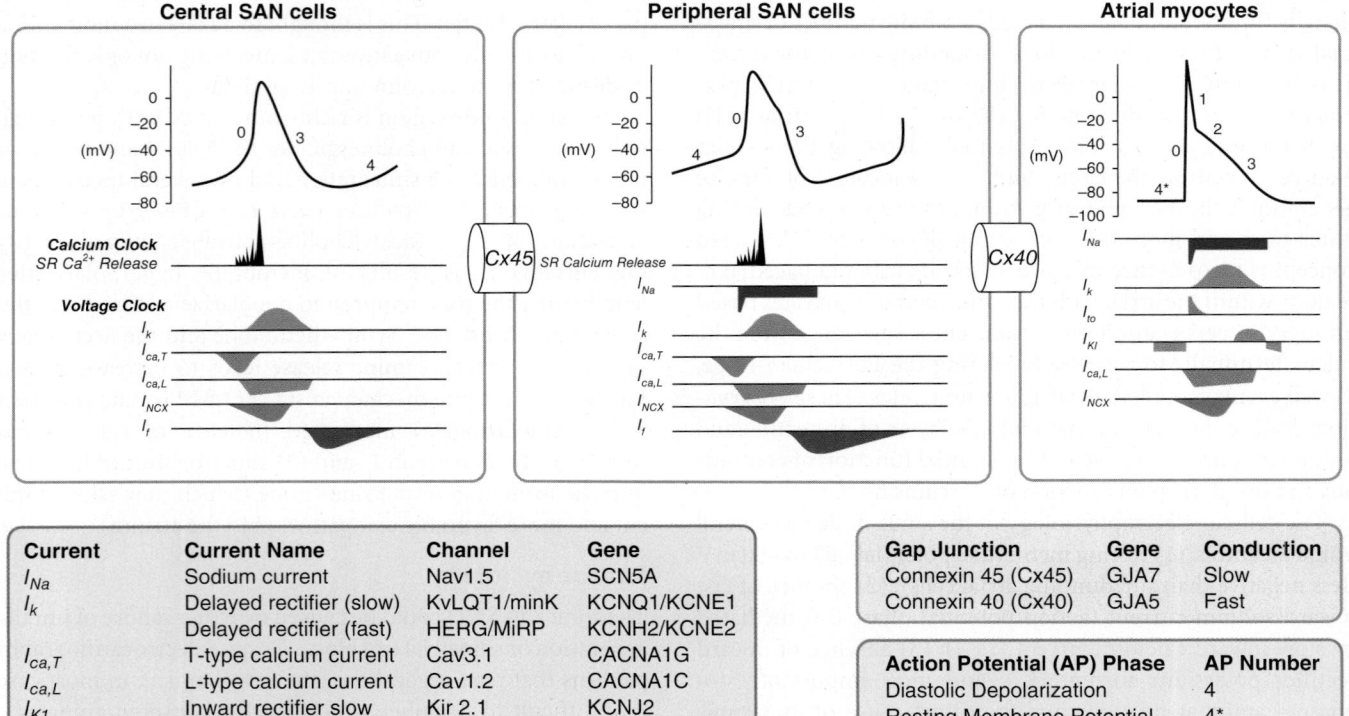

Current	Current Name	Channel	Gene
I_{Na}	Sodium current	Nav1.5	SCN5A
I_k	Delayed rectifier (slow)	KvLQT1/minK	KCNQ1/KCNE1
	Delayed rectifier (fast)	HERG/MiRP	KCNH2/KCNE2
$I_{ca,T}$	T-type calcium current	Cav3.1	CACNA1G
$I_{ca,L}$	L-type calcium current	Cav1.2	CACNA1C
I_{K1}	Inward rectifier slow	Kir 2.1	KCNJ2
I_f	Funny current	HCN4	HCN4
$I_{NCX\,(Iti)}$	Na+-Ca2+ exchanger	NCX1	SLC8A1
I_{to}	Transient outward	Kv4.2/Kv4.3	KCND2/KCND3

Gap Junction	Gene	Conduction
Connexin 45 (Cx45)	GJA7	Slow
Connexin 40 (Cx40)	GJA5	Fast

Action Potential (AP) Phase	AP Number
Diastolic Depolarization	4
Resting Membrane Potential	4*
Depolarization	0
Fast Repolarization	1
Plateau	2
Terminal Repolarization	3

Figure 38–2. Electrophysiological heterogeneity of the SAN. The central SAN, the site of dominant pacemaking, is electronically insulated from the hyperpolarizing atrial myocardium through the differential expression of connexins and ion channels. Peripheral SAN cells are electrophysiologically intermediate between central cells and atrial cardiomyocytes. SR, sarcoplasmic reticulum. Reproduced with permission from Park DS, Fishman GI. The cardiac conduction system, *Circulation* 2011 Mar 1;123(8):904-915.

TABLE 38-1. Causes of Sinus Node Dysfunction

Intrinsic
Idiopathic degenerative disorder
Atrial arrhythmias
Ischemic heart disease
Heart failure
Trauma (surgical)
    repair of congenital lesions
    heart transplantation (atrial–atrial anastomosis)
    AF catheter ablation (disruption of arterial supply)
Genetic
    SCN5A
    HCN4
    GJA5
    RYR2 and *CASQ2*
    ANKB
Neuromuscular disorders
Infiltrative cardiomyopathy
    amyloidosis
    sarcoidosis
Hypertensive heart disease
Inflammation
    collagen vascular disease
    rheumatic heart disease
    pericarditis
Infectious
    Lyme disease
    viral myocarditis
Athletic training
Extrinsic
Autonomic effects
Medications
    antiarrhythmic agents
    ivabradine
    antihypertensive agents (clonidine)
    antipsychotic drugs (lithium, phenothiazines, amitriptyline)
Obstructive sleep apnea
Hypoxia
Hyperkalemia
Hypothermia
Cushing reflex (intracranial hypertension)

sinus node, or *extrinsic*: conditions that affect SN function in the absence of structural abnormalities (**Table 38–1**). In many patients, SND is multifactorial (eg, aging plus the negative effects of cardiovascular medications).

Intrinsic Sinus Node Dysfunction

Idiopathic Degenerative Disorder

SND is strongly age-related, and even normal aging is accompanied by progressive loss in peak heart rate, which has important consequences for exercise performance. The major cause of both normal and pathologic reduction in sinus node function with aging is idiopathic degenerative disorder, representing a loss of electrically functioning myocytes with progressive fibrosis (structural remodeling).[1] Electrical remodeling may contribute as well, with decreased expression of connexin-45 (which connects the primary pacemaker complexes to the peripheral sinus node cells) as well as ion channel remodeling causing decreased function of the membrane and calcium clocks. When SND occurs in younger patients in the absence

of anatomic causes, idiopathic degenerative disorder is often a default diagnosis; in some patients, genetic causes are operative (see Genetic Abnormalities), whether recognized or not.

Atrial Arrhythmias

The pathophysiology of SND and atrial arrhythmias are intricately linked on multiple mechanistic levels. Chronic overdrive suppression of the sinus node by atrial tachyarrhythmias causes electrical remodeling, including downregulation of I_f and malfunction of the calcium clock, caused by downregulation of ryanodine receptors and decreased sarcoplasmic reticular calcium release. These changes are probably reversible as sinus node function improves in many patients following successful ablation for AF and atrial flutter. Similar mechanisms and recovery are observed in animal models of pacing-induced SND. Alternatively, significant structural abnormalities within the sinus node are observed in patients with SND and AF, with progressive cell loss and degeneration. Furthermore, unselected patients with SND without AF were demonstrated to have an atrial myopathy characterized by left atrial enlargement, abnormal and fragmented atrial electrograms, and diffuse right atrial voltage abnormalities.

Ischemic Heart Disease

Coronary heart disease is common in patients with SND. Although partially explained by the common demographic, it is thought that chronic ischemia, presumably through direct effects on sinus node blood supply, may be responsible for one-third of SND. SND is seen in 15% to 20% of patients with acute myocardial infarction (MI), typically inferior and posterior infarction, again implicating direct effects on sinus node blood supply. Other mechanisms such as increased vagal tone secondary to the Bezold–Jarisch reflex also contribute to SND in acute infarction, but these effects are usually transient.

Heart Failure

SND occurs in some patients with clinical heart failure (HF), which is almost certainly multifactorial given known changes in neurohormonal activation, and the negative chronotropic medications used as treatment. Prolongation of the intrinsic sinus cycle length, increase in sinoatrial conduction time and sinus node recovery time, as well as an inferior shift of sinus node pacemaker activity have been observed clinically and in various animal models. In addition, indirect evidence of structural remodeling has been observed, suggested by diffuse atrial myopathy in the region of the sinus node.

Surgical Trauma

SND is common in patients with congenital heart disease, mostly associated with corrective surgery, such as Mustard, Senning, Glenn, and Fontan procedures, due to direct trauma or interruption of sinus node blood supply and/or innervation. Heart transplantation, particularly with an atrial-atrial anastomosis is also a cause of SND, presumably due to direct sinus node trauma. Acute or subacute SND has been observed in catheter ablation of inappropriate sinus tachycardia, isolation of the superior vena cava (adjuvant ablation for AF), and anterior mitral isthmus linear ablation for atypical flutter (due to effects on sinus node arterial supply).[6]

Genetic Abnormalities

Although genetic causes of SND are recognized only rarely, they are worthy of consideration for three reasons. First, characterization of genetic causes of SND has greatly informed our understanding of normal sinus node physiology. Second, these are often heritable and cascade screening is important. Third, some genetic causes of SND are not isolated to effects on the sinus node but have important cardiac or extracardiac manifestations. *SCN5A*, which codes for the alpha subunit of the cardiac sodium channel, has been implicated in SND even though central nodal cells do not express sodium current (I_{Na}). Peripheral sinus nodal cells do express I_{Na}, which appears to counterbalance hyperpolarizing effects of repolarizing currents in the surrounding atrial myocytes. In the absence of peripheral cell I_{Na}, pacemaker activity is slowed, and sinoatrial conduction is threatened. Importantly, in addition to SND, mutations in *SCN5A* are also implicated in progressive conduction system disease, Brugada syndrome, and long QT syndrome type 3. I_f is generated by the hyperpolarization-activated cyclic nucleotide-gated channel (HCN). Mutations in *HCN4* cause reduction in pacemaker current and resultant SND. Other recognized genetic causes of SND include mutations of the *GJA5* gene (which encodes for connexin 40), *RYR2* and *CASQ2* (ryanodine and calsequestrin, involved in sarcoplasmic reticular calcium handling; also implicated in catecholaminergic polymorphic ventricular tachycardia [VT]), and *ANK2* (ankyrin, which links membrane proteins to the cytoskeleton). There is also an important association between SND and muscular dystrophy. Mutations in the *EMD* gene can cause SND as well as Emery–Dreifuss muscular dystrophy when concurrent *LMNA* mutation (also an important cause of cardiomyopathy) is present.

Extrinsic Sinus Node Dysfunction

The most important extrinsic causes of SND are autonomic influences (excessive vagal tone) and medications (**Table 38–2**). Virtually all membrane active antiarrhythmic drugs (except quinidine and dofetilide) and well as cardiac glycosides, beta adrenergic antagonists, and calcium channel blockers effect sinus node function directly or indirectly by influence on the autonomic nervous system.

Electrocardiographic Manifestations

Sinus Bradycardia

Sinus bradycardia is broadly defined as a heart rate less than 60 bpm. Mean heart rate is variable throughout the day and with sympathetic stimulation and it also varies by age and gender. Therefore, a clinical context is important when diagnosing sinus bradycardia. Sinus bradycardia of less than 40 bpm is more specific for significant SND.

Sinus Pause or Sinus Arrest

Sinus pause or arrest is the failure of the sinus node to discharge and subsequent lack of atrial depolarization (**Fig. 38–3**). This is evident by periods of atrial asystole with or without escape beats from other pacemakers. It is distinct from sinoatrial block, which is characterized by absent P waves in multiple of prior P-P cycle lengths. Sinus pauses can be seen in normal hearts related to autonomic influences and are frequently seen in trained athletes.[7]

Sinoatrial Exit Block

Sinoatrial (SA) exit block is failure of electrical conduction of the SA node (SAN) discharge to the atria (**Fig. 38–4**). Although it is difficult to distinguish sinus pause (failure of impulse

TABLE 38–2. Recommendations and Choice of Pacing for Permanent Pacing in Sinus Node Dysfunction

COR	LOE	RECOMMENDATIONS
I	C-LD	1. In patients with symptoms that are directly attributable to SND, permanent pacing is indicated to increase heart rate and improve symptoms.
I	C-EO	2. In patients who develop symptomatic sinus bradycardia as a consequence of guideline-directed management and therapy for which there is no alternative treatment and continued treatment is clinically necessary, permanent pacing is recommended to increase heart rate and improve symptoms.
IIa	C-EO	3. For patients with tachy-brady syndrome and symptoms attributable to bradycardia, permanent pacing is reasonable to increase heart rate and reduce symptoms attributable to hypoperfusion.
IIa	C-EO	4. In patients with symptomatic chronotropic incompetence, permanent pacing with rate-responsive programming is reasonable to increase exertional heart rates and improve symptoms.
IIb	C-LD	5. In patients with symptoms that are likely attributable to SND, a trial of oral theophylline may be considered to increase heart rate, improve symptoms, and help determine the potential effects of permanent pacing.
Choice of Pacing		
I	B-R	1. In symptomatic patients with SND, atrial-based pacing is recommended over single-chamber ventricular pacing.
I	B-R	2. In symptomatic patients with SND and intact atrioventricular conduction without evidence of conduction abnormalities, dual-chamber or single-chamber atrial pacing is recommended.
IIa	B-R	3. In symptomatic patients with SND who have dual-chamber pacemakers and intact atrioventricular conduction, it is reasonable to program the dual-chamber pacemaker to minimize ventricular pacing.
IIa	C-EO	4. In symptomatic patients with SND in which frequent ventricular pacing is not expected or the patient has significant comorbidities that are otherwise likely to determine the survival and clinical outcomes, single-chamber ventricular pacing is reasonable

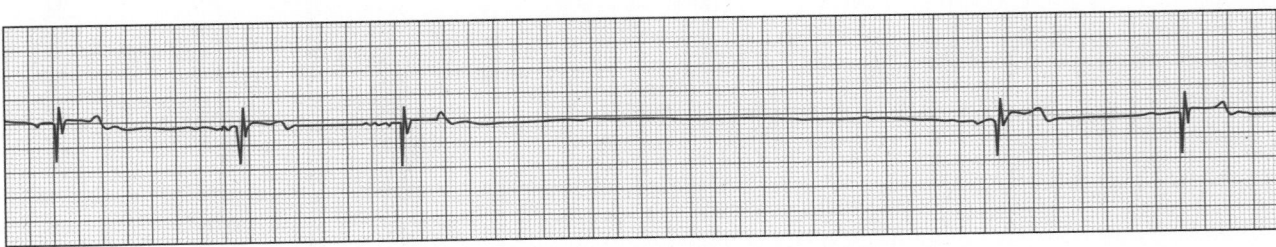

Figure 38–3. Telemetry recording demonstrating sinus bradycardia followed by a 4.5-second sinus pause.

generation) from SA exit block (failure of the impulse to propagate from the sinus node to the atrium), the traditional electrocardiographic manifestation of the latter is a pause interval of twice the sinus cycle length. First-degree SA exit block reflects delay from the SAN to the atria and cannot be detected on a surface electrocardiogram (ECG). Second-degree type I is seen with a Wenckebach type pattern of prolonging P-P intervals, absent P wave followed by a shorter P-P interval. Second-degree type II is unpredictable with little variability in P-P intervals. Third degree is complete absence of P waves for long periods.

Tachy-Brady Syndrome

As mentioned, there is a complex interaction between atrial tachyarrhythmias and SND. Atrial arrhythmias predispose to sinus bradycardia and after the termination of an atrial arrhythmia, a pause in sinus rhythm may occur (**Fig. 38–5**). These pauses can result in significant symptoms including syncope or presyncope due to the sudden change in heart rate.

Chronotropic Incompetence

An inability to appropriately augment heart rate with physical activity defines chronotropic incompetence. Generally, a cutoff of 70% to 85% of the age-predicted maximal heart rate

(APMHR) while at peak exercise is used, although other definitions have been proposed.

Atrial Standstill

Atrial standstill is a rare finding where there are no discernible P waves or evidence of atrial electrical activation (including retrograde conduction). This may be due to extensive fibrosis of the atrium sometimes seen with amyloidosis.

Clinical Presentation

SND affects patients of all ages but generally occurs in patients over 50 and is often benign associated with only mild symptoms. SND leading to syncope is highly concerning because falls and trauma that are associated with syncope are morbid especially in the elderly population that is most affected by SND.

Symptoms can be divided into those related to sudden bradycardia and those related to chronic sinus bradycardia and chronotropic incompetence. Acute bradycardia can manifest as syncope or presyncope with symptoms such as "dizzy spells" or lightheadedness. Patients with sinus bradycardia and chronotropic incompetence often present with vague complaints of exercise intolerance and fatigue. Palpitations related to atrial

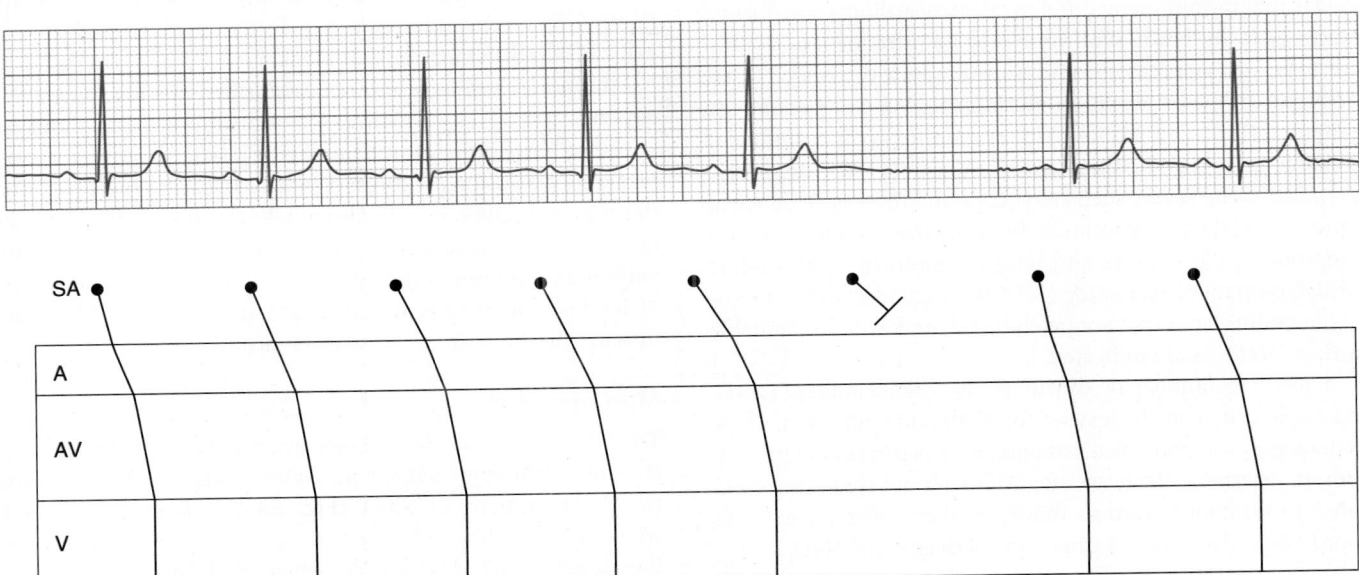

Figure 38–4. Telemetry recording demonstrating transient sinoatrial exit block. The ladder diagram illustrates block between the site of impulse generation in the sinus node and the surrounding atrium, causing a pause of twice the interval between preceding and following P waves. A, atrium; AV, atrioventricular conduction system; S, sinus node; V, ventricle.

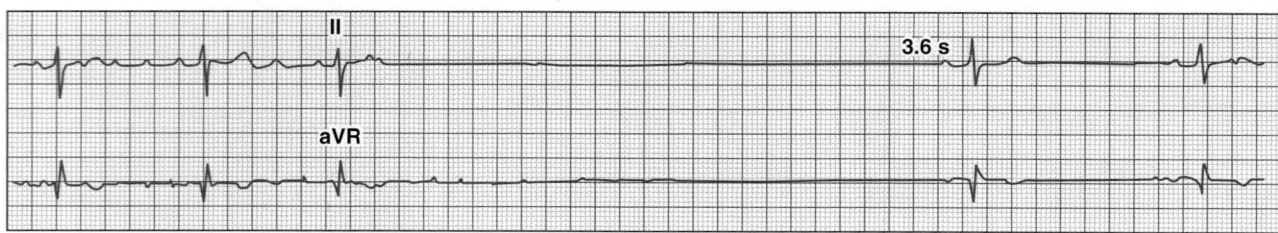

Figure 38–5. Tachy-brady syndrome. Telemetry recordings showing AF that terminates spontaneously. Sinus bradycardia returns following a 3.6-second pause.

arrhythmias are common as well given the overlap of SND and atrial arrhythmias.

Sinus bradycardia, pauses, and atrioventricular (AV) block are associated with vasovagal or neurocardiogenic syncope. Often, these episodes are preceded by a prodrome or noxious stimulation and have rapid resolution. Another form of autonomically mediated SND is carotid sinus hypersensitivity where autonomic influences can depress SAN and AV node (AVN) function. History taking is important for evaluating these forms of SND.

Diagnostic Evaluation

A diagnostic flow diagram is proposed in the ACC/AHA 2018 guidelines (**Fig. 38–6**).[8] Symptoms of SND are frequently non-specific and correlation with heart rhythm is critical. Physical examination, including carotid sinus massage and sitting and standing vital signs, is useful to assess for autonomic dysfunction. If there is suspicion for obstructive sleep apnea, testing for this is reasonable because some studies have shown improvement in SND with treatment.

Electrocardiography

Electrocardiographic recordings are the primary tool used to assess for SND. There is a multitude of monitors available and more technologies rapidly emerging. As aforementioned, SND is manifest in many different electrocardiographic forms. Pauses or tachy-brady syndrome may be infrequent and difficult to record whereas chronic sinus bradycardia is well characterized with short duration monitoring. When assessing for symptomatic SND, a 24-hour Holter monitor is often sufficient to characterize chronic sinus bradycardia and assess for pauses. If symptoms are severe such as syncope and there is evidence of significant SND, a diagnosis can be easily made. In many cases, symptoms are less severe and longer monitoring with mobile cardiac outpatient telemetry (MCOT), extended event monitors including ones that are patch based, and even implantable cardiac monitors are indicated.

A growing number of consumer devices including "Kardia and Apple Watch" are being used for rhythm identification. These technologies use photoplethysmography, electrocardiography, or both, to determine the heart rate. Although not rigorously compared to traditional cardiac monitors, these offer an exciting, affordable, and accessible technology for diagnosing SND.

Exercise Testing

Exercise testing can be performed through several protocols. The most common is exercise treadmill testing using the Bruce

or modified Bruce protocols where a patient walks on a treadmill at specific speeds and graded elevations. Exercise testing is a useful tool with significant utility in predicting cardiovascular outcomes. For assessing SND it is typically used to assess chronotropic incompetence. As mentioned, most testing uses percentage cutoffs based on the APMHR. The ability to quantitatively determine patient effort and ability to exercise is useful in evaluating heart rate response and can increase the specificity of the treadmill findings. Those patients who provide maximal effort without appropriate increase in heart rate or who have significant fluctuations in heart rate may benefit from implantation of a permanent pacemaker.

Electrophysiology Study

Despite a rich history of invasive electrophysiology studies (EPS) for the diagnosis of SND, its utility for the evaluation of SAN remains limited due to questionable prognostic value. As such, recent guidelines recommended against EPS as a primary tool for the assessment of SND.[8] However, evaluation of the sinus node during EPS that is indicated for other reasons such as assessing atrioventricular block or syncope can be performed and may add diagnostic information. The properties of the sinus node including sinus node recovery time can be determined by overdrive atrial pacing, and measuring the longest resultant pause in excess of the sinus cycle. Sinoatrial conduction time measurement can quantify the physiology that is exhibited in the sinoatrial exit block.

Autonomic testing is another established method to identify patients with SND. It involves the infusion of medications to affect the autonomic stimulation of the heart. Atropine and isoproterenol infusions will result in a tachycardic response, but this may be blunted in patients with SND. Autonomic blockade or a simultaneous infusion of vagolytic (ie, atropine) and sympatholytic (propranolol) medications allows for the assessment of intrinsic heart rate, which is also reduced in SND. These invasive methods are rarely used clinically.

Management

The 2018 American Heart Association (AHA)/American College of Cardiology (ACC) guidelines suggest an algorithm for the treatment of SND (**Fig. 38–7**).[8] Reversible causes when present should be treated (see Table 38–1, extrinsic). Frequently, SND is worsened when medications exacerbate preexisting intrinsic SAN pathology. β-blockers and nondihydropyridine calcium channel blockers are commonly prescribed medications for the treatment of AF and can often

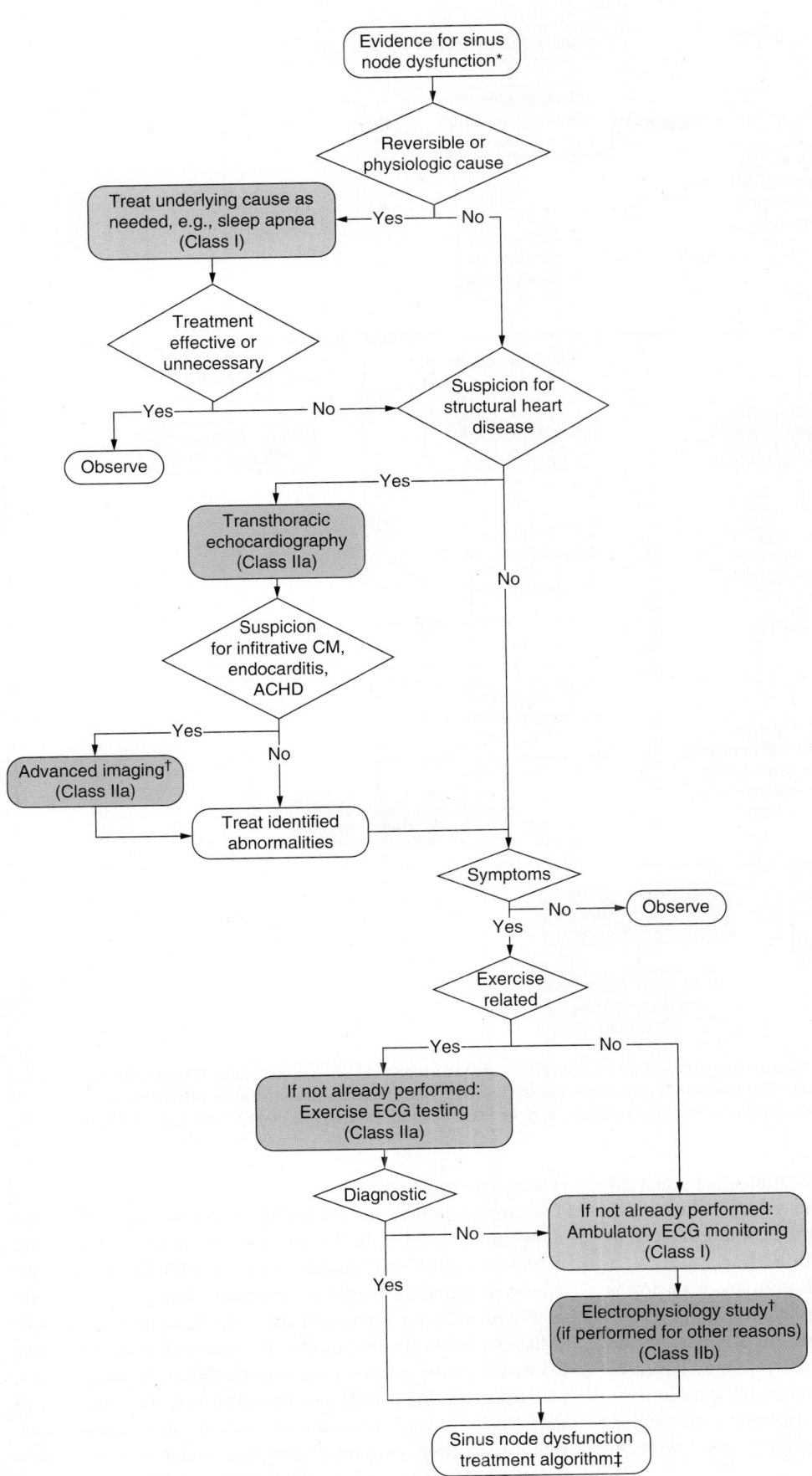

Figure 38–6. A flowchart for evaluation of SND. Reproduced with permission from Kusumoto FM, Schoenfeld MH, Barrett C, et al: 2018 ACC/AHA/HRS Guideline on the Evaluation and Management of Patients With Bradycardia and Cardiac Conduction Delay: Executive Summary: A Report of the American College of Cardiology/ American Heart Association Task Force on Clinical Practice Guidelines, and the Heart Rhythm Society, *Circulation* 2019 Aug 20; 140(8):e333-e381.

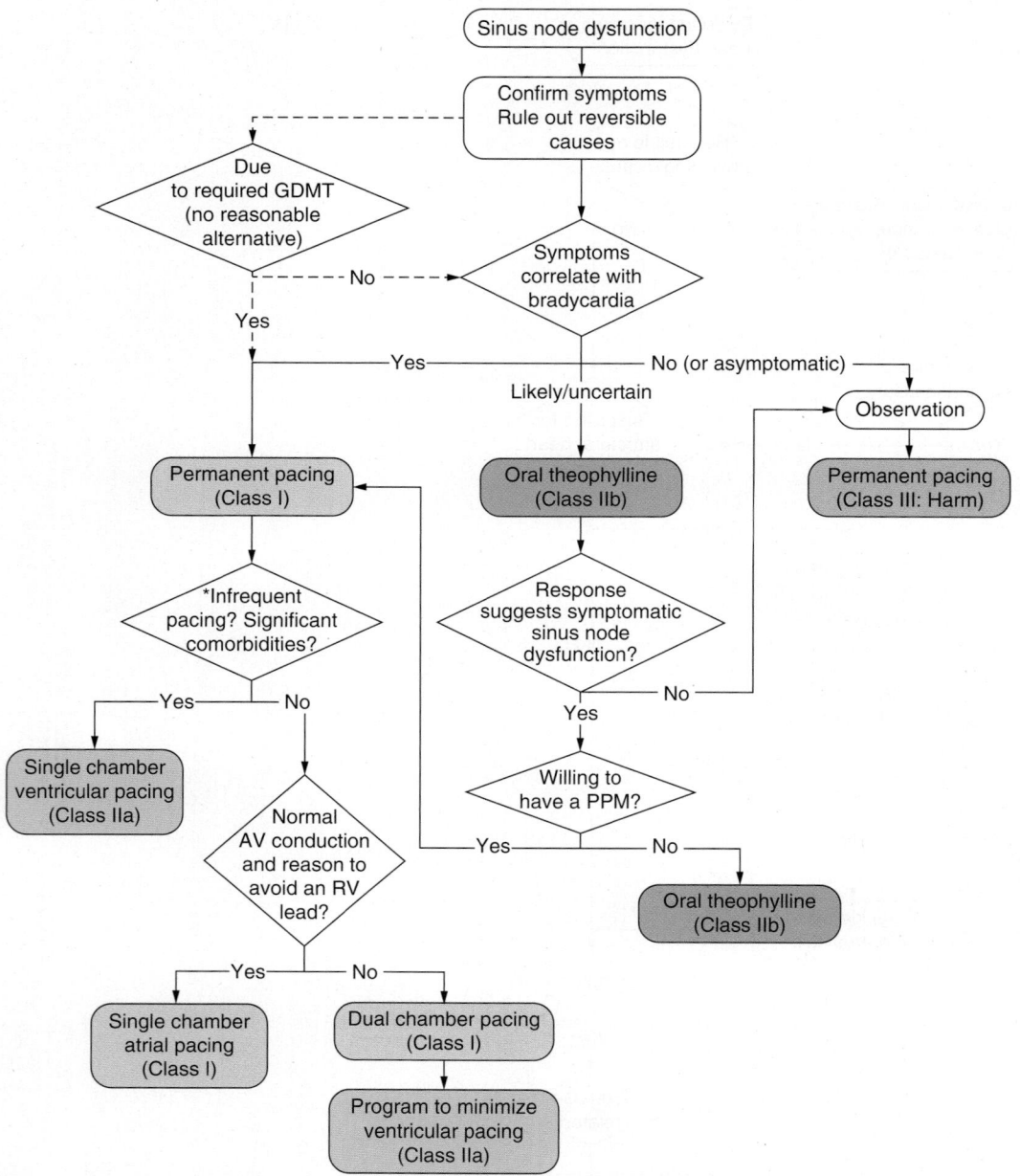

Figure 38–7. A flowchart for treatment of SND. Reproduced with permission from Kusumoto FM, Schoenfeld MH, Barrett C, et al: 2018 ACC/AHA/HRS Guideline on the Evaluation and Management of Patients With Bradycardia and Cardiac Conduction Delay: Executive Summary: A Report of the American College of Cardiology/American Heart Association Task Force on Clinical Practice Guidelines, and the Heart Rhythm Society, *Circulation* 2019 Aug 20;140(8):e333-e381.

exacerbate underlying SND. Other medications that affect the sinus node should also be considered and reduced when possible. Treatment of sleep apnea and endocrine conditions such as hypothyroidism can improve SAN function.

After reversible causes are excluded, permanent pacing is indicated when symptoms are clearly related to SND. When symptoms are uncertain, further observation or a trial of oral theophylline is reasonable to better assess symptoms. The 2018 guidelines removed indications for minimally symptomatic SND based on heart rate <40 bpm. Instead, there is an emphasis in the guidelines in avoiding pacing for patients with no attributable symptoms.

Pacing Therapy

The current indications for pacing in the setting of SND are shown in Table 38–2. In this and subsequent tables, the format used for the AHA/ACC guidelines is used, with class I to III indications denoting the degree of agreement for a given procedure or treatment that is useful and effective.[8] In asymptomatic individuals with sinus bradycardia or sinus pauses that are secondary to physiologically elevated parasympathetic tone, or sleep-related, permanent pacing should not be performed. In patients with sleep-related sinus bradycardia or transient sinus pauses occurring during sleep, permanent pacing should not be performed unless other indications for pacing are present (class III: Harm).

SND is the most common indication for permanent pacemaker implantation in North America, accounting for more than 42% to 60% of new pacemaker implants. The optimal pacemaker choice is influenced by several factors. At the time of diagnosis of SND, 17% of patients have been reported to have AV conduction abnormalities in the form of a PR interval >240 ms, bundle branch block (BBB), HV interval prolongation, AV Wenckebach rates <120 bpm, and second- or third-degree AV block. The annual incidence of change in pacing mode from AAIR to DDDR in the Danish Multicentre Randomized Trial on Single Lead Atrial versus Dual Chamber Pacing in Sick Sinus Syndrome (DANPACE) trial was observed to be 4.5% during long-term follow-up.[9] Generally, if the patient has persistent AF, a rate-responsive single-chamber ventricular pacemaker (VVIR) is recommended. In all other situations, a rate-responsive dual-chamber pacemaker (DDDR) is used, whereas a single-chamber atrial pacemaker (AAIR) can be implanted if no evidence of AV conduction disease is present.

Many nonprospective, nonrandomized studies have suggested significant survival benefits with atrial-based pacing compared with ventricular demand pacing (VVI mode) in patients with SND. This led to randomized, large-scale prospective trials as well as a meta-analysis of randomized pacing modes where atrial-based pacing was associated with a significant reduction in AF of approximately 20% (95% confidence interval [CI], 0.77–0.89; $P = 0.00003$) and a borderline significant reduction in the risk of stroke of 19% (95% CI, 0.67–0.99; $P = 0.035$). The use of atrial-based pacing did not, however, reduce mortality or the incidence of congestive HF.[10]

It is now well accepted that long-term right ventricular (RV) pacing causes a deterioration of left ventricular (LV) function through complex effects on regional ventricular wall strain and loading conditions. This deterioration is thought to result from intraventricular dyssynchrony between different regions of the left ventricle induced by RV apical pacing. Sweeney and coworkers demonstrated, by careful review of data from the Mode Selection Trial (MOST), that an increase in the frequency of ventricular pacing in patients with sick sinus syndrome who had a narrow native QRS complex was associated with an increased incidence of AF and congestive HF.[11] These observations were confirmed by Wilkoff and colleagues in the Dual Chamber and VVI Implantable Defibrillator (DAVID) study, in which backup ventricular pacing and dual-chamber pacing were prospectively compared in patients with dual-chamber defibrillators.[12] The primary end point was a composite of congestive HF, hospitalization, and death, which was increased by a factor of 1.6 in patients with an increased frequency of ventricular pacing. Thus, RV pacing is a double-edged sword, conferring atrioventricular synchrony but at the same time possibly negating its benefit by inducing ventricular dysfunction. It is recommended that patients with SND have the pacemaker programmed to either AAIR or DDDR with an algorithm that minimizes unnecessary ventricular pacing or utilizes ventricular conduction system pacing (see section Management of AV Block and Interventricular Conduction Disease).

ATRIOVENTRICULAR CONDUCTION ABNORMALITIES

The atrioventricular conduction system, comprised of the AV node and His bundle, provide the only route of electrical continuity between the atrium and the ventricle. The normal slow conduction within the AV node is essential for the coordination of atrial filling and ventricular systole. In addition, the decremental conduction properties of the AV node provide a natural defense against rapid ventricular rates during atrial flutter and fibrillation. Traditionally, AV conduction, when abnormal, is classified into three categories, namely, first, second, and third degrees corresponding to: (1) prolonged AV conduction, (2) intermittent AV conduction, and (3) no AV conduction, respectively. Conduction block within the AV system can be benign or malignant and is characterized by the site at which the block occurs.

Anatomy and Physiology

The compact AV node measures 5 mm in length and width and 0.8 mm in thickness. It is an atrial structure, located subendocardially at the apex of the triangle of Koch. The AV node and perinodal area are comprised of three regions (atrionodal, nodal, and nodal-His), denoting the transitions between cellular anatomy and electrophysiology between these regions. The His bundle connects to the distal portion of the AV node complex to penetrate the central fibrous body; it courses for 1 cm to 2 cm and divides to become the left and right bundle branches (**Figs. 38–8 and 38–9**).[5,13] Of great significance for His bundle pacing (HBP), the His bundle contains "committed fibers" destined to become the right and left bundle (see section Anatomy and Physiology of the His-Purkinje System).[14,15]

Blood supply to the AVN and His bundle is from the AV nodal artery (arising from the right coronary artery in 90%); the His bundle is also supplied by the first septal branch of the left anterior descending artery. The conduction system axis is richly innervated by sympathetic and parasympathetic nerves. AV nodal conduction is dramatically affected by autonomic tone, in terms of conduction velocity, safety factor for conduction, and the rate of phase 4 automaticity. Conduction velocity and escape rate of the His bundle are less affected by innervation.

Within the nodal region, action potentials are similar to those of the central sinus node: (1) phase 4 automaticity has a similar mechanism (with a slower rate), (2) sodium channel density is low, and (3) the action potential upstroke is primarily due to Ca^{2+} current. AV nodal cells are poorly coupled due to relatively sparse gap junctions with low conductance (primarily connexin 45) and conduction through the AV node is slow (0.03 m/sec). Conduction is much more rapid in the His bundle (2.3 m/sec, faster than ventricular myocardium) due to a high density of high capacitance gap junctions (connexins 43 and 40) and sodium-dependent action potentials.

Pathophysiology of AV Block

As aforementioned, the autonomic nervous system has a profound effect on AV nodal conduction. Slowed conduction or

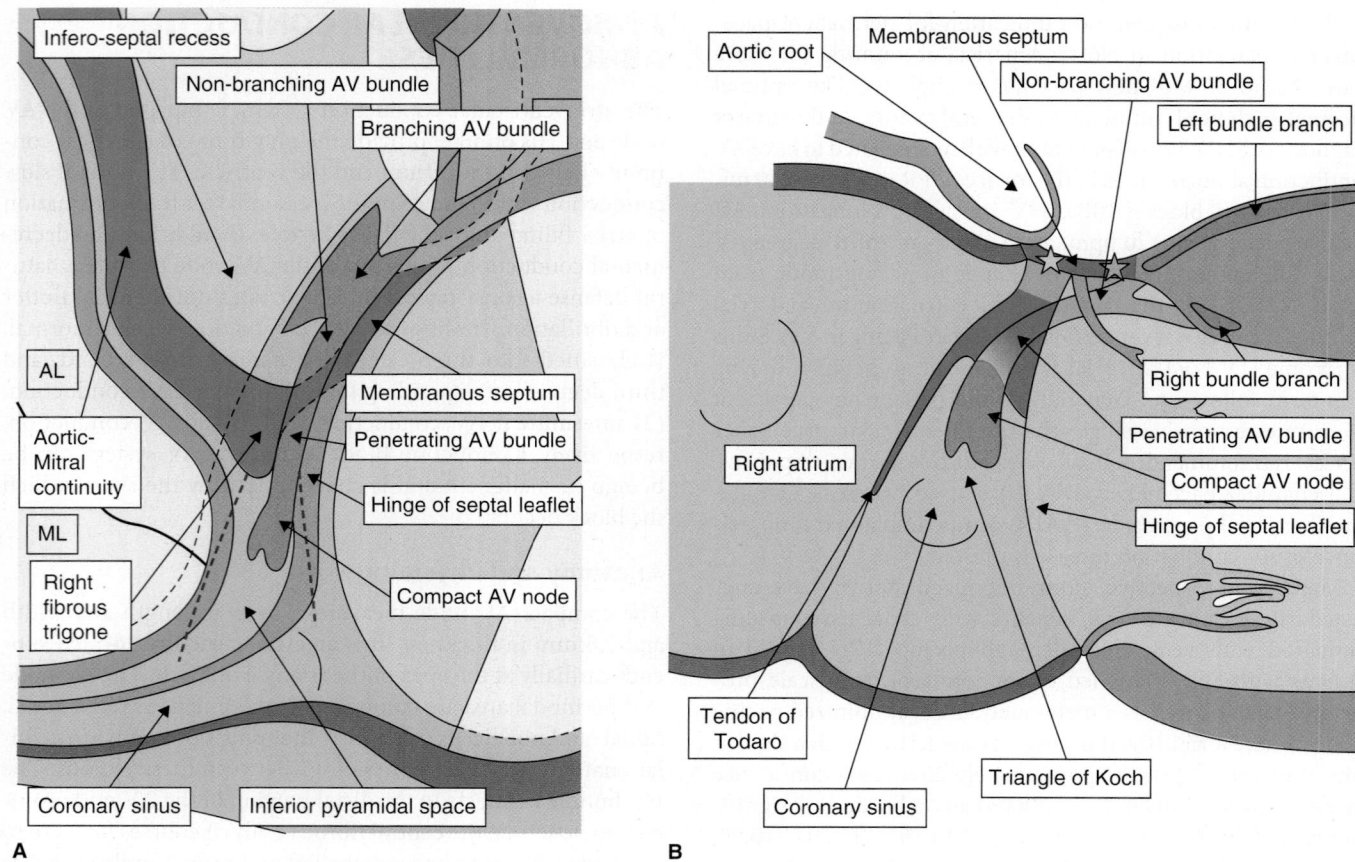

Figure 38–8. The normal atrioventricular conduction axis in humans. Schematic drawings representing the arrangement of the AV conduction axis in the inferior pyramidal space and the inferoseptal recess of the left ventricle **(A)** and at the level of the Koch triangle **(B)**. Note the inferoseptal recess located between the leaflets of the mitral valve and the muscular interventricular septum. The AV conduction axis is made up of the compact node, the penetrating AV bundle, the nonbranching AV bundle, the branching AV bundle, and the right and left bundle branches. Note that when viewed from the right atrial cavity, the triangle of Koch **(B)** overlies the inferior pyramidal space and is delimited by the hinge line of the septal tricuspid leaflet, the tendon of Todaro, and the mouth of the coronary sinus forming its base. The fibrous membranous septum forms the apex of the triangle. The hinge of the septal leaflet of the tricuspid valve provides the dividing line between the AV (*yellow star*) and interventricular (*pink star*) components of membranous septum **(B)**. *Red dashed lines* indicate the anatomical limits of the inferior pyramidal space. *Black dashed lines* indicate structures that are out of the schematic plane (ie, inferior to the right AV groove). AL, aortic leaflet; ML, mural leaflet.

Reproduced with permission from Cabrera JÁ, Anderson RH, Macías Y, et al: Variable Arrangement of the Atrioventricular Conduction Axis Within the Triangle of Koch: Implications for Permanent His Bundle Pacing, *JACC Clin Electrophysiol* 2020 Apr;6(4):362-377.

block at the level of the AV node is common and physiologic under conditions of heightened vagal tone, such as sleep, sleep apnea episodes, nausea, in highly trained athletes, and during acute inferior MI. Inherited and acquired causes of AV block are next discussed (**Table 38–3**).

Inherited Causes of AV Block

Progressive Cardiac Conduction Disease

Progressive cardiac conduction disease (PCCD), originally described as Lev and Lenégre disease, has many causes, some heritable and some related to aging and/or associated with progressive structural heart disease. Disease can occur at any level of the conduction system (sinus node exit block, AV block, BBB). Lev originally described fibrosis within the proximal His bundle, and Lenégre more distal conduction system disease. Although most cases of PCCD are related to aging, heritable forms are important to recognize because many have syndromic

manifestations. Loss of function mutations in *SCN5A* causes most inherited forms of PCCD, which may be isolated or combined with manifestations of Brugada syndrome or long QT type 3. The *TRPM4* gene mediates a Ca^{2+}-activated nonelective cationic current (I_{NSCca}) involved in cardiac conduction, phase 4 depolarization, and action-potential repolarization. Mutations in *TRPM4* cause isolated PCCD. The *KCNJ2* gene encodes a critical component of I_{k1} and mutations are associated with PCCD and long QT7 (Anderson–Tawil syndrome). Mutations in the *PRKAG2* gene are implicated in patients with Wolff-Parkinson-White syndrome and PCCD. Lamin A and C encode for nuclear envelope proteins; mutations can cause PCCD as well as progressive LV dysfunction with prominent atrial and ventricular arrhythmias; Lamin A/C abnormalities are also associated with muscular dystrophy. Although unusual, patients with long QT syndrome with marked QT prolongation can have functional block between the conduction system and ventricular

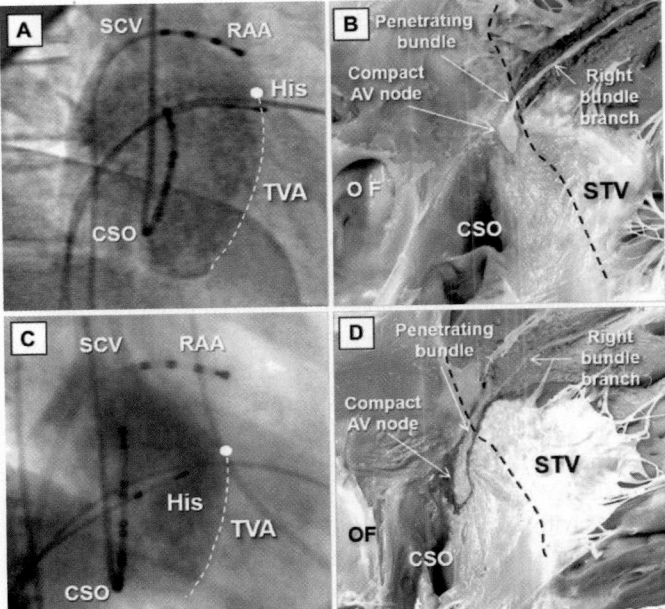

Figure 38–9. His bundle and the landmarks of the triangle of Koch (**A, C**) Right atrial angiography in right anterior oblique projection displays the tricuspid valvar annulus (TVA) and the relation between the site of recording of the largest His bundle potential (His) and the landmarks of the triangle of Koch. In (**A**), the His bundle was recorded superiorly at the vertex of the triangle, whereas (**C**) shows the arrangement with an inferior location of the recording. (**B, D**) The images show gross dissections of the human AV conduction axis relative to the triangle of Koch, revealing the variable position of the atrioventricular node and the penetrating bundle relative to the tendon of Todaro and the hinge line of the septal leaflet of the tricuspid valve (STV), which is represented by the *dashed black line*. (**B**) In the heart shown, there is a superior location of the conduction axis, with a shorter length of the penetrating bundle. (**D**) The heart shown illustrates an inferior location within the triangle of Koch, accompanied by a longer length of the penetrating bundle. The more inferior location of the penetrating bundle was linked to a greater distance from the endocardium and from the hinge line of the tricuspid valve to the bundle itself, and this may be a partial explanation why many His bundle pacing operators find that the superior location is associated with easier selective pacing. CSO, coronary sinus orifice; OF, oval fossa; RAA, right atrial appendage; SCV, superior caval vein. Reproduced with permission from Cabrera JÁ, Anderson RH, Macías Y, et al: Variable Arrangement of the Atrioventricular Conduction Axis Within the Triangle of Koch: Implications for Permanent His Bundle Pacing, *JACC Clin Electrophysiol* 2020 Apr;6(4):362-377.

myocardium caused by prolonged refractoriness, leading to 2:1 AV block.

Congenital Complete AV Block

Isolated congenital complete heart block is thought to result from failure of development at the level of the AV node. The incidence is estimated between 1 in 15,000 and 1 in 22,000 live births. Its pathophysiology is often linked with neonatal lupus (in the setting of overt or subclinical autoimmune disease in the mother) with damage of the AV node by maternal autoantibodies to intracellular ribonucleoproteins Ro and La. Typically, this condition is associated with a stable, narrow complex escape rhythm which augments with exercise and, thus, may be asymptomatic.[16] Congenital complete heart block is associated with complex congenital heart disease, particularly in lesions involving formation and orientation of the AV rings.

Acquired AV Block

Degenerative Diseases

As aforementioned, fibrotic replacement of electrically active conduction system tissue can be caused by specific gene mutations but is more often caused by aging and may be accelerated by various forms of structural heart disease (annular calcification, hypertension, atherosclerosis affecting blood supply to the conduction system). PCCD is the cause of approximately 50% of clinically significant AV block in adults.

Acute Myocardial Infarction

The incidence of high-grade heart block during acute MI has decreased with improvements in acute care of patients with this condition; however, the incidence is still 2.2% in patients with acute ST elevation MI. High-grade block can occur in either inferior or anterior infarction. In the setting of inferior MI, the level of block is usually at the level of the AV node and the escape rate is narrow and 40 bpm to 60 bpm. Heart block in acute inferior MI may be secondary to vagotonia and may resolve within several days. However, when heart block develops later in the course, it is more likely to be permanent and caused by ischemia (hypoperfusion of the AV nodal artery). In the setting of anterior MI, the level of block is subnodal and the escape pacemaker rhythm is wide, slower, and less reliable. High-grade AV block complicating acute MI is associated with poor prognosis, because it is associated with larger infarct size.

Infiltrative Cardiomyopathies

Infiltrative cardiomyopathies (sarcoidosis, amyloidosis, hemochromatosis) may be associated with AV block, which may represent the presenting manifestation. Cardiac sarcoidosis, in particular, occurs in approximately 25% of patients with systemic sarcoidosis and can cause AV block or BBB; importantly, cardiac sarcoidosis can also cause malignant ventricular arrhythmias and progressive LV dysfunction. AV block may be reversible with immunosuppressive agents in early stages of the condition.

Infectious Diseases

A variety of infectious diseases can affect AV conduction. Infectious endocarditis of the aortic valve with perivalvular abscess can cause varying degrees of conduction abnormalities including complete heart block or BBB. Lyme disease can involve the heart in 1% to 2% of cases. Importantly, intranodal block caused by Lyme carditis is typically transient and recovers over 1 to 6 weeks with appropriate antibiotic treatment.

Surgical Trauma

Complete heart block occurs as a complication of cardiac surgery in 15% of patients, particularly during valve replacement procedures; although recovery is seen over 6 months in 12% of patients.[17] Of recent concern is the incidence of heart block following transcatheter aortic valve replacement (TAVR), which is estimated to be as high as 17% and may occur suddenly following hospital discharge. The incidence of heart block varies greatly between different valves but is higher in self-expanding than balloon-expandable models; however, the incidence of heart block during implantation of the mechanically

TABLE 38–3. Causes of Atrioventricular Block

Enhanced vagal tone
Inherited causes
Progressive cardiac conduction disorder
   SCN5A
   TRPM4
   KCNJ2
   PRKAG2
   neuromuscular disorders (eg, lamin A/C)
   long QT syndrome with functional block
Congenital complete heart block
   autoimmune mediated
   associated with complex congenital heart disease
Acquired causes
Progressive cardiac conduction disorder
   idiopathic, age related
   associated with structural heart disease (eg, aortic valve calcification)
Acute myocardial infarction
Infiltrative cardiomyopathies
   sarcoidosis
   amyloid
   hemochromatosis
Infectious diseases
   endocarditis
   Lyme carditis
   Chagas disease
   myocarditis
Surgical trauma
   cardiac surgery, especially valve replacement
   transcatheter aortic valve replacement (TAVR)
   catheter ablation
Drugs
   beta adrenergic antagonists
   calcium channel blockers,
   digitalis
   class I and III antiarrhythmic agents
Collagen vascular disease
Miscellaneous
   hyperkalemia
   hypermagnesemia
   hyperthyroidism
Paroxysmal atrioventricular block
   vagally mediated
   intrinsic
   idiopathic

expandable Lotus valve was 34.2% in the REPRISE III trial.[18] Prediction models for the development of heart block after TAVR implicate male sex, previous conduction system abnormalities (1° AV block, right BBB [RBBB]), intraprocedural AV block, preoperative bradycardia or permanent AF, advanced age, and postoperative left BBB [LBBB]. Heart block is also a recognized complication of catheter ablation procedures, including those for supraventricular tachycardia involving the midseptal space and VT involving the septum.

Drugs

Many cardiovascular medications (beta adrenergic antagonists, calcium channel blockers, digitalis, class I and III antiarrhythmic agents) affect AV nodal conduction either by direct effects or indirectly through their effects on the autonomic nervous system. Class I and III antiarrhythmic agents can affect His

bundle conduction and cause heart block, although this is unusual in patients without preexisting conduction system abnormalities. Other medications that can also affect AV conduction include clonidine, lithium, and donepezil.

Electrocardiographic Manifestations

First-Degree Atrioventricular Block

Prolongation of the PR interval >200 ms constitutes first-degree AV block (**Fig. 38–10**), although technically speaking, represents delay rather than block. It is most commonly caused by conduction delay within the AV node and occasionally caused by intra-atrial, intra-Hisian, or *balanced* infra-Hisian conduction delay. If the QRS duration is normal, the site of conduction delay is almost always within the AV node. If first-degree AV block occurs in the presence of BBB, the conduction delay can be in the AV node (60% of cases), His-Purkinje system, or both. Patients with first-degree AV block have an excellent prognosis even when associated with chronic bifascicular block, because the rate of progression to third-degree AV block is low, warranting no specific therapy. A prolonged PR interval can be detrimental to cardiac hemodynamics, particularly in patients with HF because it may result in elevated LV end-diastolic pressure, diastolic mitral regurgitation, and reduced LV systolic function. This seems especially the case in patients with heart disease, as it is associated with an increased risk for AF, advanced AV heart block, HF, and death.[19]

Second-Degree Atrioventricular Block

Second-degree AV block is characterized by intermittent failure of conduction from the atria to the ventricles. If the AV block occurs with the atrial rate in the physiologic range, it is considered a pathological arrhythmia. AV block in the setting of atrial tachyarrhythmias could be a normal response. Based on the electrocardiographic patterns, second-degree AV block is classified into Mobitz types I and II.

Mobitz Type I: Second-degree AV block of the Wenckebach type (Mobitz type I) is characterized by the following features: (1) progressive prolongation of the PR interval before a nonconducted P wave, (2) PR interval prolongation at progressively decreasing increments, (3) progressive shortening of R-R intervals, (4) pause encompassing the blocked P wave shorter than the sum of two P-P cycles, and (5) the last conducted PR interval before the blocked P wave longer than the next conducted PR interval (**Fig. 38–11**). All features are not necessary to qualify the rhythm as Mobitz type I because variations do occur frequently. The PR might not sequentially lengthen in all cases of Mobitz type I block, but the conducted PR interval after a dropped beat is always the shortest: *This is the sine qua non of Mobitz I AV block.*

Mobitz Type II: Mobitz type II second-degree AV block is characterized by (1) constant P-P intervals and R-R intervals, (2) constant PR intervals before a nonconducted P wave, and (3) pause encompassing the nonconducted P wave equal to two P-P cycles. Type II AV block usually occurs in the presence of BBB and is almost always caused by a block in the intra and/or

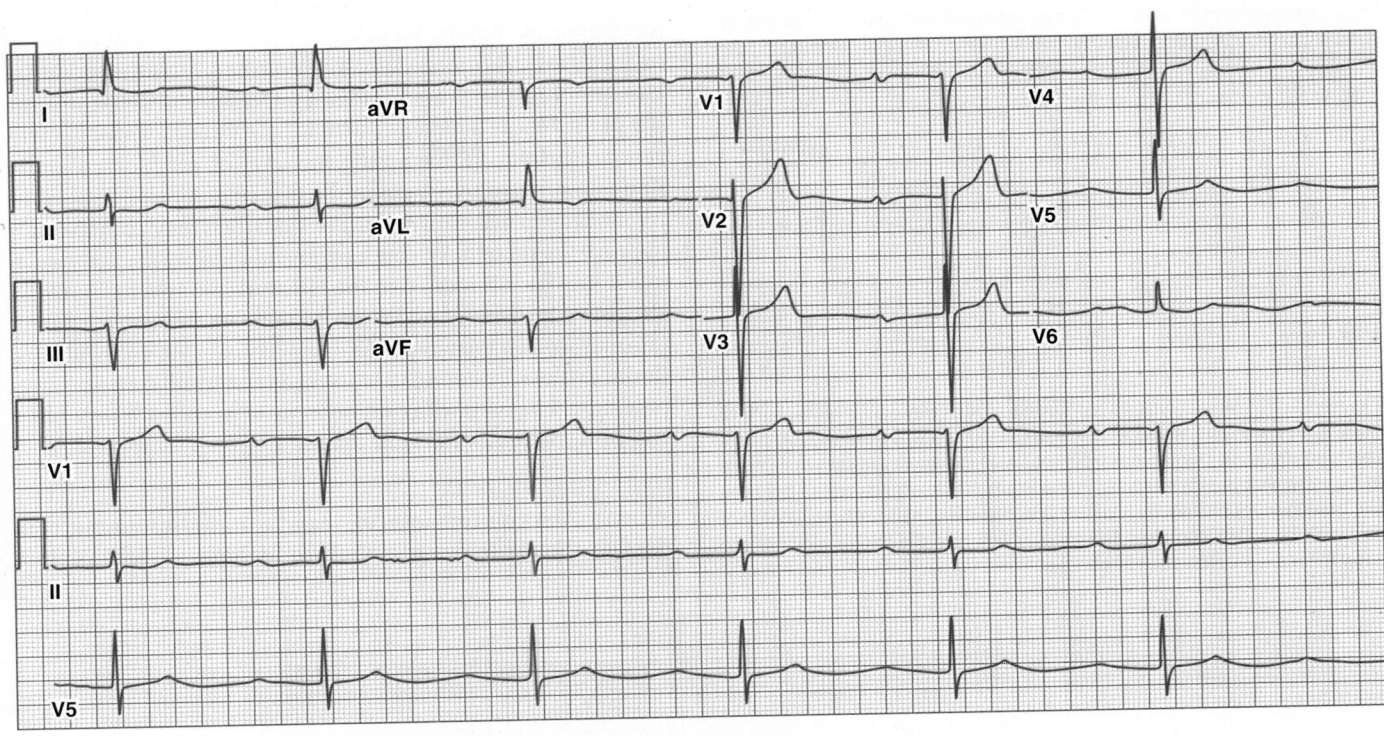

Figure 38–10. First degree AV block. Surface ECG shows a prolonged PR interval (520 ms).

infra-Hisian-Purkinje system (**Fig. 38–12**). Type II AV block rarely occurs in patients with normal QRS duration. When Mobitz type II block occurs in the setting of a normal QRS duration, the site of block is most likely to be intra-Hisian. Mobitz Type II AV block frequently progresses to complete AV block and may result in recurrent syncope, warranting permanent pacing upon diagnosis.

2:1 AV Block: In this form of second-degree AV block, every other P wave is not conducted, making it difficult to diagnose

the level of AV block (**Figs. 38–13A** and **38–13B**). 2:1 AV block pattern with normal QRS duration and a normal conducted PR interval (<160 ms) suggests intra-Hisian block and 2:1 block with a prolonged PR interval generally suggests block in the AV node. 2:1 AV block pattern in the presence of widened QRS duration favors block below the AV node, but is not diagnostic (Fig. 38–13B). A prolonged electrocardiographic recording may sometimes reveal a transition to varying degrees of AV block (3:2 or 4:3), with type I or type II features that aid in

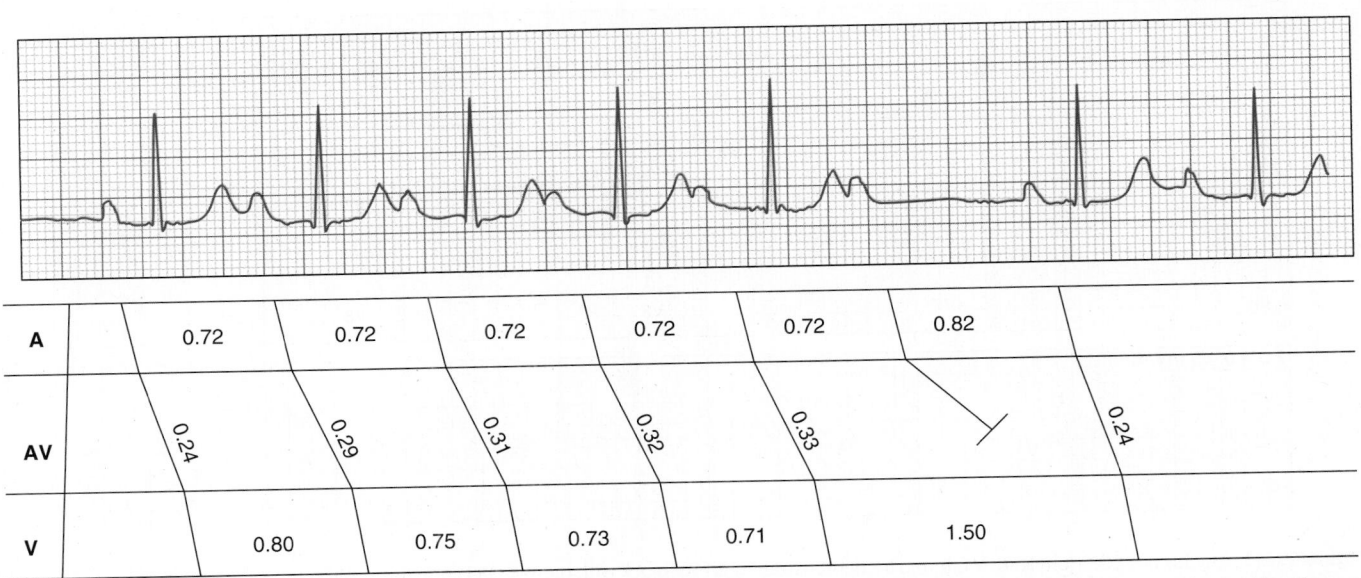

A	0.72	0.72	0.72	0.72	0.72	0.82		0.24
AV	0.24	0.29	0.31	0.32	0.33			
V		0.80	0.75	0.73	0.71	1.50		

Figure 38–11. Mobitz I second-degree AV block. A 6:5 AV Wenkebach periodicity is shown. Note that the PR interval progressively lengthens with a decreasing increment. This results in a shortening of the intervals between successive QRS complexes. The last conducted PR interval before the block is longer (0.33 seconds) than the PR interval after the block (0.24 seconds).

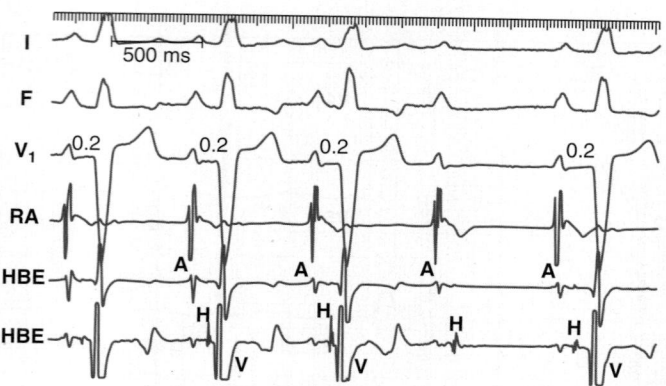

Figure 38–12. Mobitz type II second-degree atrioventricular block. Surface ECG, leads I, aVF, and V1, and intracardiac electrograms from the RA, proximal, and distal His bundle electrogram (HBE) catheters are shown. Surface ECGs show that the PR intervals are constant at 0.2 seconds with a left bundle branch block morphology of the QRS complex; the fourth P wave is not followed by a QRS complex. The HBEs reveal that the site of block of the fourth P wave is below the His bundle.

the diagnosis. Rarely, Wenckebach periodicity may be noted in the His-Purkinje system. Intracardiac recordings with a His-bundle catheter are sometimes necessary to determine the site of the block. In patients with a 2:1 AV block, vagal maneuvers are helpful in diagnosing the level of AV block. Carotid sinus stimulation may worsen the degree of block if it is in the AV node, whereas slowing of the sinus rate may paradoxically improve the ratio of AV conduction and increase the ventricular rate if the block is located in the His-Purkinje system. Similarly, atropine improves AV nodal conduction, but the increased sinus rate may worsen the ratio of AV conduction in patients with His-Purkinje block, resulting in worsened bradycardia. Hence, atropine should be used with caution in patients with a 2:1 AV block and BBB where His-Purkinje disease is strongly suspected.

High-Grade AV Block

When two or more consecutive atrial impulses do not conduct to the ventricle, it is defined as high-grade AV block

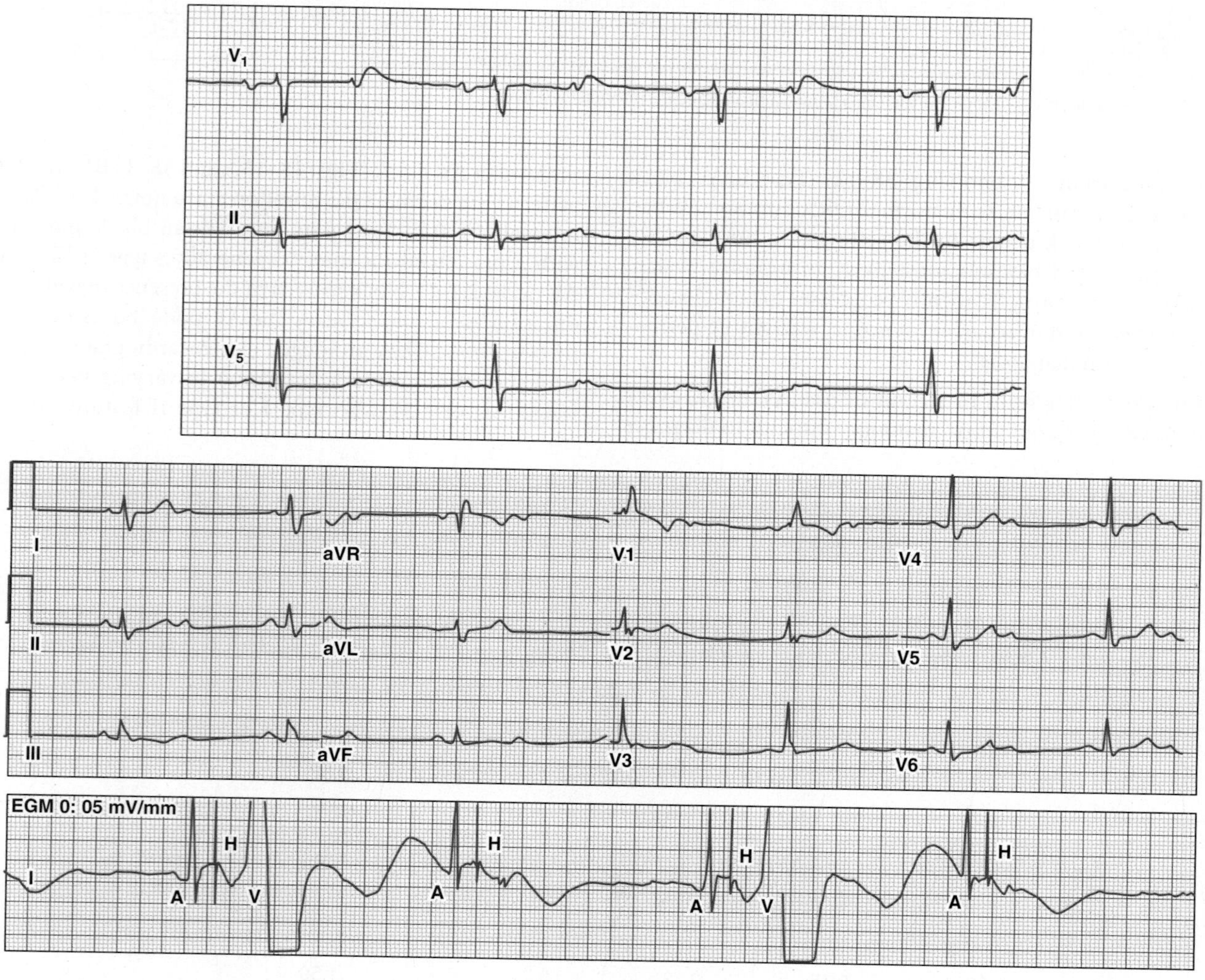

Figure 38–13. (A) Surface ECG from leads V1, II, and V5 demonstrating 2:1 AV block with narrow QRS complexes. Although a definite diagnosis of type I or type II AV block cannot be made, longer rhythm strip recordings might reveal Wenckebach periodicity. Vagal maneuvers or exercise might assist further in the final diagnosis. **(B)** Twelve-lead surface ECG shows 2:1 AV block in the presence of normal PR interval and RBBB. His bundle electrogram in the lower panel demonstrates that the level of block is below the His bundle. A, atrial; H, His; V, ventricle.

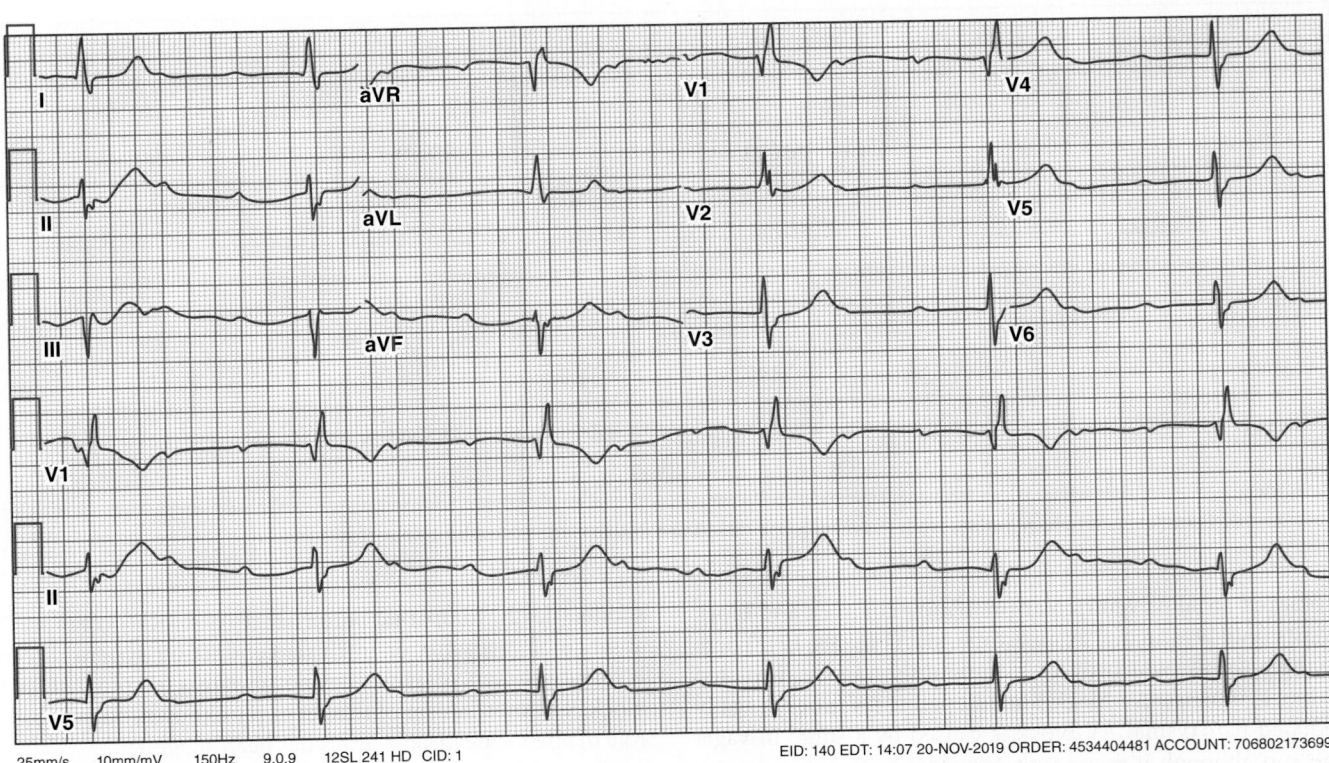

25mm/s   10mm/mV   150Hz   9.0.9   12SL 241 HD   CID: 1   EID: 140 EDT: 14:07 20-NOV-2019 ORDER: 4534404481 ACCOUNT: 706802173699

Figure 38–14. Sinus tachycardia with 3:1 AV conduction, RBBB, and left anterior fascicular block. The third P wave is "buried" within the QRS complex. Note that the AV interval on the conducted beat is constant, although long (540 ms).

(**Fig. 38–14**) and may be associated with a junctional or ventricular escape rhythm. Unless a clearly defined reversible etiology is identified, permanent pacing is indicated.

Third-Degree AV Block

Complete or third-degree AV block is characterized by complete and absolute failure of conduction from the atria to the ventricle. This results in complete dissociation of P waves and QRS complexes. Complete AV block may occur as a result of block in the AV node or at the His-Purkinje level. In patients with block at the AV node level, the escape rhythm is usually junctional, with a narrow QRS complex (unless associated with preexisting bundle branch block), (**Fig. 38–15**). In complete heart block resulting from His-Purkinje disease, the escape rhythm is ventricular in origin, with a wide QRS interval and a ventricular escape rhythm at 20 bpm to 40 bpm (**Fig. 38–16**).

Atrioventricular Dissociation

This phenomenon is characterized by atrial and ventricular activity independent of each other. AV dissociation may be secondary to AV block (complete heart block) or physiologic refractoriness. AV dissociation can occur when the sinus rate is slower than the secondary junctional or ventricular pacemaker as in patients with sinus bradycardia. In contrast, AV dissociation can also occur in the presence of normal sinus rhythm and accelerated junctional (junctional tachycardia) or VT rhythm with retrograde conduction block. In patients with complete heart block, the atrial rate is faster than the ventricular rate, whereas in AV dissociation, the ventricular rate is faster than

the atrial rate. Although AV dissociation is present in complete heart block, it is not synonymous. AV dissociation is usually a manifestation of another rhythm abnormality, such as complete heart block, sinus bradycardia, or VT.

In isorhythmic AV dissociation, the atria and ventricles are depolarized by separate and independent foci that have similar rates. There is no block in either AV or VA direction—the P wave can conduct to the QRS and the ventricular impulse can reach the atria, given time. Thus, the 4 types of AV dissociation can be due to (1) AV block, (2) VA block (as occurs in VT or V pacing), (3) isorhythmic AV dissociation where there is no AV or VA block, and (4) the slowing of the primary rhythm and emergence of subsidiary pacemaker rhythm.

Bifascicular/Trifascicular Block

Traditionally, there has been an assumption that the left bundle has two fascicles. Many investigators subsequently have presented evidence of various degrees to suggest that there are more than two divisions and therefore the terms fascicular and/or divisional block has been preferred over the term hemiblock. However, trifascicular LBBB should not be confused with so-called *trifascicular AV block*. The latter term evolved when there was a combination of two fascicles showing conduction delay and/or block and additional PR interval prolongation.

Paroxysmal AV Block

Paroxysmal AV block describes the sudden development of transient complete heart block, followed by resumption of normal AV conduction. AV block is usually initiated by a conducted

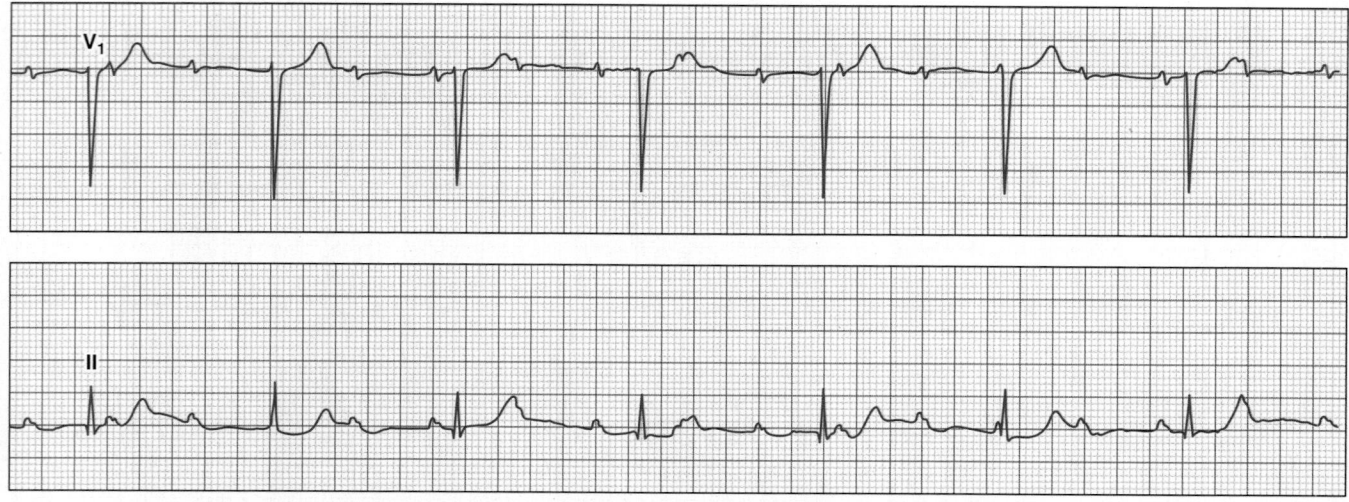

Figure 38–15. Complete heart block. Surface leads show complete heart block with a narrow complex escape rhythm.

or blocked atrial or ventricular premature complex and block persists until terminated by an escape beat (**Fig. 38–17**). There are three forms, which differ in prognosis: vagally mediated AV block, intrinsic AV block, and idiopathic AV block. Vagally mediated paroxysmal AV block is caused by a surge in vagal tone and although it may result in syncope, its course is typically benign. Intrinsic paroxysmal AV block is sudden heart block following premature beats or an abrupt decrease in heart rate, which persists unless it is interrupted by an escape beat. This mechanism is thought secondary to phase 4 depolarization and subsequent inexcitability due to decrease in the transmembrane potential below which there is capacity to conduct. This physiology is found in diseased His-Purkinje system tissue and can be malicious, resulting in recurrent syncope or

sudden death. Idiopathic paroxysmal AV block occurs in the absence of vagotonia or intrinsic conduction system disease. It may cause syncope but does not progress to complete heart block. The mechanism of this form is unknown, but a possible role of adenosine plasma levels has been suggested.

Diagnostic Evaluation

The prognosis and treatment of AV block depend on its association with symptoms and the level of block. Routine 12-lead surface ECGs adequately establish the diagnosis of varying degrees of AV block in many patients. Analyzing the PR interval, QRS duration, Wenckebach phenomenon, and ventricular rates on the surface ECG provides important clues to the level of AV block. In certain situations, such as 2:1 AV block,

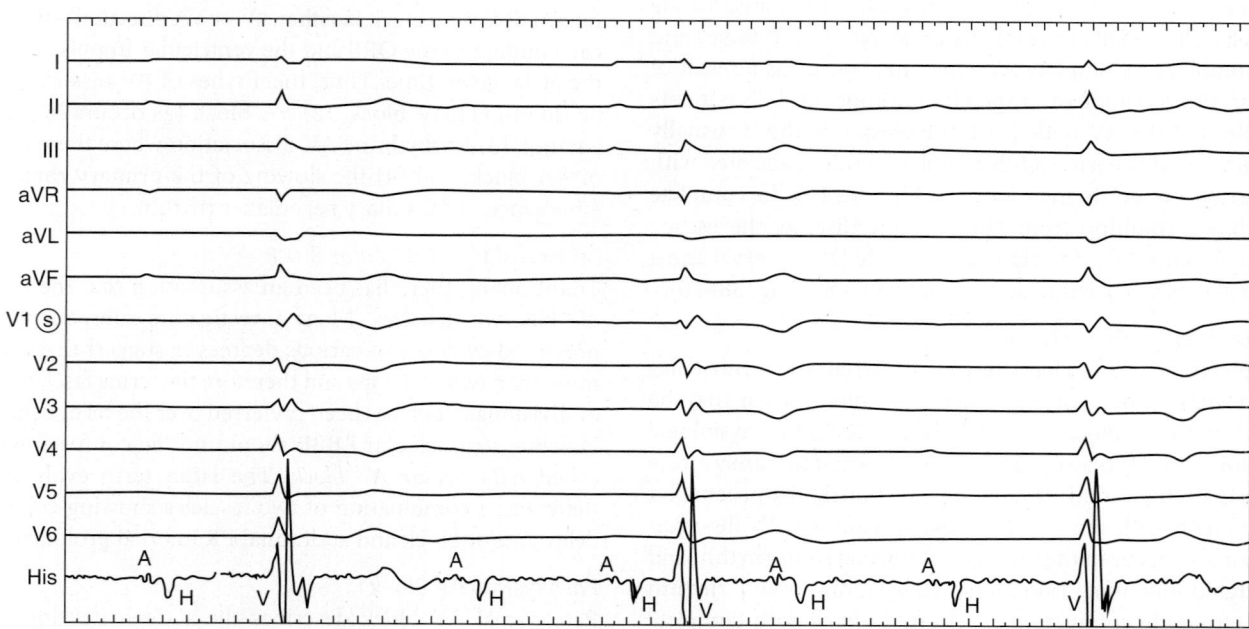

Figure 38–16. Complete heart block. Surface leads show complete heart block with an RBB morphology escape rhythm. Simultaneous His bundle electrogram demonstrates block below the level of the His. A, atrial; H, His; V, ventricle. (Recorded at 100 ms/cm).

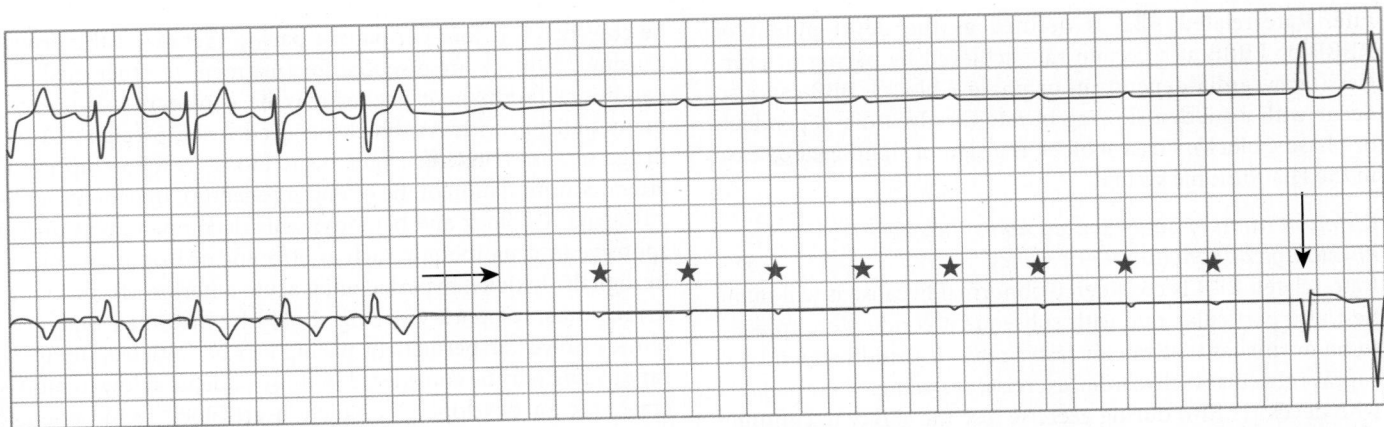

Figure 38–17. Paroxysmal AV block. Telemetry strip demonstrating paroxysmal AV block. There is a brief sinus pause (*horizontal black arrow*) followed by multiple, nonconducted P waves (*red stars*) with associated sinus acceleration, reflecting an intrinsic failure of AV nodal conduction. The nearly 7-second pause is eventually interrupted by a junctional escape complex (*vertical black arrow*).

additional maneuvers may be necessary to establish the level of block. Response to carotid sinus massage, atropine, and exercise is often very helpful. In patients with paroxysmal symptoms of near syncope or syncope and no significant conduction abnormalities on the surface ECG, prolonged electrocardiographic monitoring with 24- to 48-hour Holter recordings or 30-day event monitors may be helpful. Newer event monitors with automatic detection algorithms and remote capabilities have increased the yield of these monitors. An implantable loop recorder may be necessary to establish the diagnosis, particularly in patients with infrequent symptoms. Electrophysiology study is indicated in patients with syncope or near syncope in whom high-grade AV block is suspected as the cause. Importantly, in patients with structural heart disease, in addition to AV conduction disease, VT can also be a major etiology for syncope, and electrophysiology study can be useful in establishing the diagnosis.

INTRAVENTRICULAR CONDUCTION DISEASE

The role of the distal His-Purkinje network is to provide rapid (within 80–100 ms) and coordinated activation of the ventricular endocardium. Intraventricular conduction disturbances slow this conduction, either at the level of the bundle branches or ventricular myocardium. Abnormalities can be functional/transient or fixed.

Anatomy and Physiology of the His-Purkinje System

The right bundle (RB) is a cord-like direct continuation of the His bundle and progresses subendocardially down the right side of the intraventricular septum to the moderator band before subdividing into a rich network of Purkinje fibers. The left bundle (LB) leaves the distal His bundle as a fan-like structure and proceeds under the septal endocardium to divide into separate divisions: the left anterior fascicle (LAF), left posterior fascicle (LPF) and the left septal fascicle (in 65% of hearts). The LAF and LPF continue to their respective papillary muscles and afterward ramify to form the Purkinje network. The bundle branches are isolated from the underlying ventricular

myocardium allowing activation of the apex of the ventricles first. The His-Purkinje system is designed for rapid conduction, with sodium-dependent action potentials and abundant, high capacitance gap junctions allowing for each Purkinje fiber to conduct to thousands of ventricular myocytes.[5] Blood supply to the His bundle and the proximal LB are from the septal branches of the anterior and posterior descending coronary arteries. The RB and the LAF are supplied by the septal branches of the LAD and the LPF is usually supplied by the conus branch of the RCA. This is clinically important in that right bundle branch (RBB) or LAF block can occur with LAD occlusion, but LBBB requires occlusion of both the RCA and the LAD.

Pathophysiology of the His-Purkinje System

The electrocardiographic patterns associated with bundle branch and fascicular block may be caused by fixed conduction block in these structures (or within the His bundle, as already discussed) or delay. In any case, the physiology is the same and BBB (or the underlying causes associated with it) results in an increase in all-cause mortality. LBBB causes significant ventricular dyssynchrony and, like RV pacing, is a potential independent cause of LV dysfunction and HF. LBBB can be caused by lesions within the His bundle, the proximal left bundle branch (LBB) or more peripherally. This distinction is important for HBP but is poorly made using traditional electrocardiography.[20]

Etiologies of BBB include factors that are important in AV block, such as PCCD, hypertension, MI, chronic ischemic heart disease, valvular heart disease, or other cardiomyopathies. Given their subendocardial location, they are also susceptible to mechanical stress and trauma. Nonspecific intraventricular conduction disturbances are related to dysfunction of the distal Purkinje network or ventricular myocardium; they typically occur in the setting of significant myocardial hypertrophy or in various cardiomyopathies.

Electrocardiographic Manifestations of Interventricular Conduction Disease

RBBB or LBBB on the baseline ECG with sinus rhythm signifies His-Purkinje system delay or block at the recorded heart rate. Rate-related BBB is defined as the development of RBBB or LBBB at a certain rate achieved by pacing or exercise (tachycardia-dependent, or phase 3 block). BBB can also occur with a sudden slowing in rate (bradycardia-dependent, or phase 4 block). Phase 4 block is a sign of significant disease in the His-Purkinje system.

Differentiation of Rate-Related Aberrancy Versus Physiological/Functional Aberrancy

Rate-related BBB is considered abnormal because it will manifest at a particular rate with subsequent conduction unlikely to be normal at that rate or faster rates. It could happen with supraventricular tachycardia, exercise, or pacing. Some patients who develop LBBB during exercise lose the ability to continue the exercise at the same intensity and may even have chest pain. With physiologic or functional BBB, in contrast, the BB or fascicle can conduct normally in time at the same or faster rate at which it conducts aberrantly.

The Site of Block in Bundle Branch Block

The exact site of block in patients with pathologic BBB is not consistently known, but certain seminal observations have been made. El-Sherif and colleagues[14] in an experimental model and Narula[21] in humans showed that a lesion in the His bundle produced classic changes of a BBB downstream. These investigators explained these finding on the basis of longitudinal dissociation in the His bundle. In essence, certain fibers within the His bundle are committed to become the bundle branches. Pacing proximal to the lesion produced an aberrant QRS morphology and axis exactly as the baseline sinus rhythm, whereas pacing a few millimeters distally completely normalized the QRS. The current accepted explanation for these findings is more likely to involve anisotropic conduction providing sufficient delay to produce a BBB because the HPS impulse feed distal to the lesion may be delayed sufficiently and can be overcome by pacing distally.

Differentiating LBBB from Nonspecific Interventricular Conduction Delay

One of the criteria used to interpret LBBB versus nonspecific interventricular conduction delay (IVCD) is based on the absence of a Q wave in lead I, AVL, and V6. Anatomic studies have indicated that the septal division of the LBB can frequently be a separate and the largest division. Incomplete LBBB, which essentially means a loss of Q wave in lead I with minimal QRS widening may simply be a pure form of septal divisional block. Many patients with nonspecific IVCD of the LBB type have long HV intervals, suggesting HPS disease.

MANAGEMENT OF ATRIOVENTRICULAR BLOCK AND INTRAVENTRICULAR CONDUCTION DISORDERS

Although there is no specific pharmacologic therapy for chronic AV block or intraventricular block, identifying transient or reversible causes is the first step in management. Withdrawal of any offending drugs, correction of any electrolyte abnormalities, or treatment of any infectious processes should

be considered before permanent pacing therapy. If the drugs causing AV block are essential for treatment of other medical conditions, permanent pacing may be considered. However, many patients with AV block believed to be precipitated by drugs may develop recurrent heart block in follow-up even after discontinuation of the offending agent(s). In patients with advanced AV block and hemodynamic decompensation unresponsive to drug therapy such as atropine or isoproterenol, as in digitalis toxicity, hyperkalemia, acute anterior MI, or Lyme myocarditis, temporary pacing should be instituted until AV block resolves or permanent pacing can be initiated. Temporary pacing may be considered in those patients at low to moderate risk for developing complete heart block or in patients with complete heart block and hemodynamically stable escape rhythms. Transcutaneous pacing for prolonged periods, however, is uncomfortable and transvenous pacing should be performed in patients with need for continuous active pacing.

Pacing Therapy in Atrioventricular Block

Permanent pacemaker implantation is indicated in most patients with advanced heart block associated with symptoms. Permanent pacemakers are also indicated in asymptomatic patients with complete heart block and infra-Hisian second-degree AV block because permanent pacing has clearly been shown to decrease mortality in patients with advanced heart block and syncope. The indications for pacing in adults with acquired heart block are described in **Table 38–4**.[8]

Most patients with complete AV block require dual-chamber pacemakers to maintain AV synchrony and prevent the development of pacemaker syndrome. In patients with associated SND, DDDR is the preferred mode of choice (**Figs. 38–18 and 38–19**). In patients with normal sinus node function and AV block, VDD pacing using a single lead with a series of electrodes for atrial sensing and ventricular pacing and sensing is an ideal mode of pacing, because it provides AV synchrony and rate responsiveness and is superior to single-chamber VVI pacing. In patients with chronic AF and bradycardia, VVIR is adequate. Prospective, randomized, large-scale trials showed that dual-chamber pacing provided little benefit over ventricular pacing for the prevention of death while the incidence of pacemaker syndrome was as high as 26% in patients with ventricular pacing, necessitating crossover to dual-chamber pacing.

Right Ventricular Pacing-Induced Cardiomyopathy

The adverse effects of RVA pacing are well substantiated, and while the majority of patients who receive pacemakers for standard bradycardia indications do not experience HF, about 12% to 22% of patients with significant RV pacing develop pacing-induced cardiomyopathy.[22,23] Growing recognition of the long-term adverse effects of RVA pacing has stimulated interest in strategies to promote physiologic pacing and to minimize or eliminate the deleterious effects. There is no consensus, however, regarding the optimal ventricular pacing sites and approach in patients undergoing permanent pacemaker implantation for AV block in whom ventricular pacing cannot be avoided. Alternative RV pacing sites (ie, non-RVA), including the RV septum, RV outflow tract (RVOT), and dual-site

TABLE 38–4. Recommendations and Choice of Pacing for Permanent Pacing in Acquired Atrioventricular Block

COR	LOE	RECOMMENDATIONS
I	B-NR	1. In patients with acquired second-degree Mobitz type II atrioventricular block, high-grade atrioventricular block, or third-degree atrioventricular block not attributable to reversible or physiologic causes, permanent pacing is recommended regardless of symptoms.
I	B-NR	2. In patients with neuromuscular diseases associated with conduction disorders, including muscular dystrophy (such as myotonic dystrophy type 1) or Kearns-Sayre syndrome, who have evidence of second-degree atrioventricular block, third-degree atrioventricular block, or an HV interval of 70 ms or greater, regardless of symptoms, permanent pacing, with additional defibrillator capability if needed and meaningful survival of greater than 1 year is expected, is recommended.
I	C-LD	3. In patients with permanent atrial fibrillation (AF) and symptomatic bradycardia, permanent pacing is recommended.
I	C-LD	4. In patients who develop symptomatic atrioventricular block as a consequence of guideline-directed management and therapy for which there is no alternative treatment and continued treatment is clinically necessary, permanent pacing is recommended to increase heart rate and improve symptoms.
IIa	B-NR	5. In patients with an infiltrative cardiomyopathy, such as cardiac sarcoidosis or amyloidosis, and second-degree Mobitz type II atrioventricular block, high-grade atrioventricular block, or third-degree atrioventricular block, permanent pacing, with additional defibrillator capability if needed and meaningful survival of greater than 1 year is expected, is reasonable.
IIa	B-NR	6. In patients with Lamin A/C gene mutations, including limb-girdle and Emery-Dreifuss muscular dystrophies, with a PR interval greater than 240 ms and LBBB, permanent pacing, with additional defibrillator capability if needed and meaningful survival of greater than 1 year is expected, is reasonable.
IIa	C-LD	7. In patients with marked first-degree or second-degree Mobitz type I (Wenckebach) atrioventricular block with symptoms that are clearly attributable to the atrioventricular block, permanent pacing is reasonable.
IIb	C-LD	8. In patients with neuromuscular diseases, such as myotonic dystrophy type 1, with a PR interval greater than 240 ms, a QRS duration greater than 120 ms, or fascicular block, permanent pacing, with additional defibrillator capability if needed and meaningful survival of greater than 1 year is expected, may be considered.
Choice of Pacing		
I	A	1. In patients with SND and atrioventricular block who require permanent pacing, dual-chamber pacing is recommended over single-chamber ventricular pacing.
I	A	2. In select patients with atrioventricular block who require permanent pacing in whom frequent ventricular pacing is not expected, or who have significant comorbidities that are likely to determine clinical outcomes and that may limit the benefit of dual-chamber pacing, single-chamber ventricular pacing is effective.
I	B-R	3. For patients in sinus rhythm with a single-chamber ventricular pacemaker who develop pacemaker syndrome, revising to a dual-chamber pacemaker is recommended.
IIa	B-R	4. In patients with atrioventricular block who have an indication for permanent pacing with LVEF between 36% and 50% and are expected to require ventricular pacing more than 40% of the time, it is reasonable to choose pacing methods that maintain physiologic ventricular activation (eg, cardiac resynchronization therapy [CRT] or His bundle pacing) over right ventricular pacing.
IIa	B-R	5. In patients with atrioventricular block who have an indication for permanent pacing with LVEF between 36% and 50% and are expected to require ventricular pacing less than 40% of the time, it is reasonable to choose right ventricular pacing over pacing methods that maintain physiologic ventricular activation (eg, CRT or His bundle pacing).
IIb	B-R	6. In patients with atrioventricular block at the level of the atrioventricular node who have an indication for permanent pacing, His bundle pacing may be considered to maintain physiologic ventricular activation.
III: Harm	C-LD	7. In patients with permanent or persistent AF in whom a rhythm control strategy is not planned, implantation of an atrial lead should not be performed.

right ventricle have been investigated, but the benefits of alternative-site pacing remain unresolved. Conduction system pacing is increasingly being used in this application (see section His-Purkinje Conduction System Pacing).

In a study of 101 patients with RV pacing-induced cardiomyopathy, cardiac resynchronization therapy with biventricular (BiV) pacing in 29 patients resulted in significant echocardiographic and clinical improvement.[22] In another study of 69 patients with pacing-induced cardiomyopathy who received cardiac resynchronization therapy (CRT), 59 (85.5%) responded with an absolute improvement of ≥5% in the left ventricular ejection fraction (LVEF), a mean change in LVEF from 29.3% to 45.3%, or an absolute increase in LVEF of 16%.[24]

Recently, HB has also been shown to improve LV function and clinical outcomes in RV pacing-induced cardiomyopathy. In a multicenter observational study, HBP was associated with improvement in QRS duration and LVEF in a group of 60 patients with pacing-induced cardiomyopathy.[25]

Bundle Branch Block

Conduction disturbances that occur at various levels of the branches of the His-Purkinje system are described as BBB or IVCDs. In patients with isolated chronic RBBB or LBBB, the progression to advanced AV block is rare. Patients with bifascicular block (RBBB and left anterior or posterior fascicular block) or LBBB and left axis deviation have a 6% annual

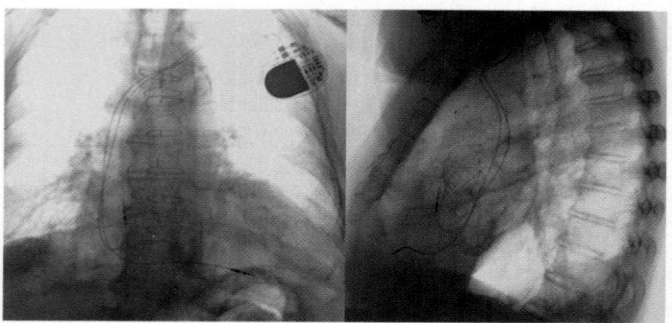

Figure 38–18. Posteroanterior and lateral chest radiographs of RA and RV pacing leads in a patient with a dual-chamber pacemaker.

incidence of progression to complete heart block. Alternating BBB, even in asymptomatic patients, is a sign of advanced conduction disturbance in the His-Purkinje system and is considered a class I indication for permanent pacing. In patients with BBB, His-bundle recordings can occasionally be helpful in identifying patients at high risk for progression to high-grade AV block. The incidental findings of markedly prolonged HV interval (>100 ms) or atrial-pacing–induced infra-Hisian block that is not physiologic during an electrophysiology study are considered to indicate high risk for progression to advanced AV block, and prophylactic permanent pacing is recommended (**Table 38–5**). Intraventricular conduction disturbances are

usually associated with significant structural heart disease, especially dilated (ischemic or idiopathic) cardiomyopathies, and are a marker of poor prognosis both in terms of advanced HF and increased mortality in these patients. LBBB in patients with cardiomyopathy is associated with significant ventricular dyssynchrony, worsening HF, and increased mortality. BiV pacing in these patients have been shown to improve HF and decrease mortality. In a subgroup of patients with nonischemic cardiomyopathy, BiV pacing can normalize LV function (hyper-responders) raising the possibility of LBBB-induced cardiomyopathy. Evidence also suggests that BBB is often due to disease in the proximal His bundle and may be amenable to correction by permanent HBP.[20,26]

Current guideline-based indications for permanent pacing in patients following cardiac surgery and in adults with congenital heart disease are described in **Tables 38–6** and **38–7**. In patients undergoing transcatheter aortic valve replacement, there is a high incidence of AV block depending on preexisting RBBB, type of valve used, and relationship of the valve to the membranous septum. In patients who have new atrioventricular block after transcatheter aortic valve replacement associated with symptoms or hemodynamic instability that does not resolve, permanent pacing is recommended before discharge. In patients who develop new LBBB, careful monitoring for AV block is recommended while permanent pacing may be considered in select patients.

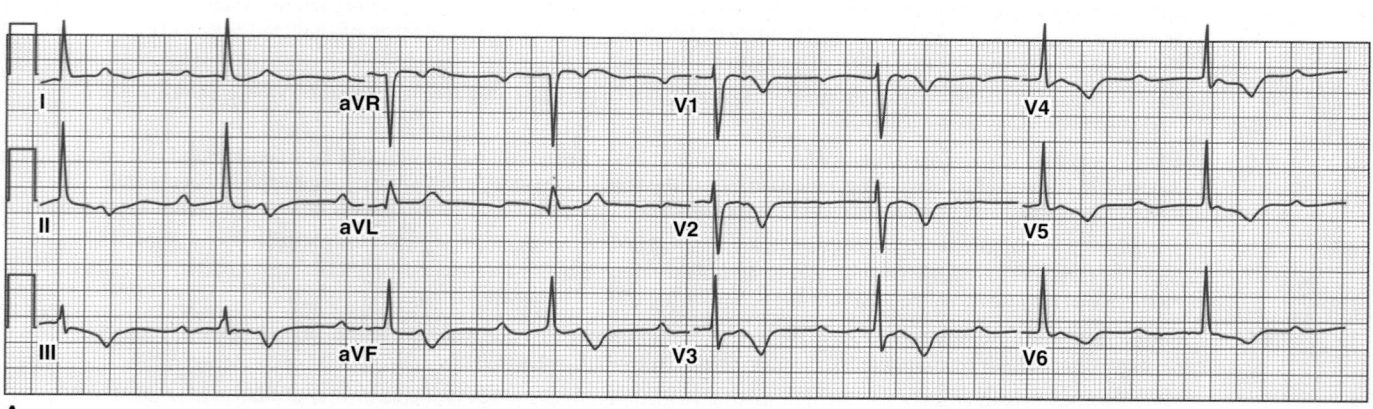

A

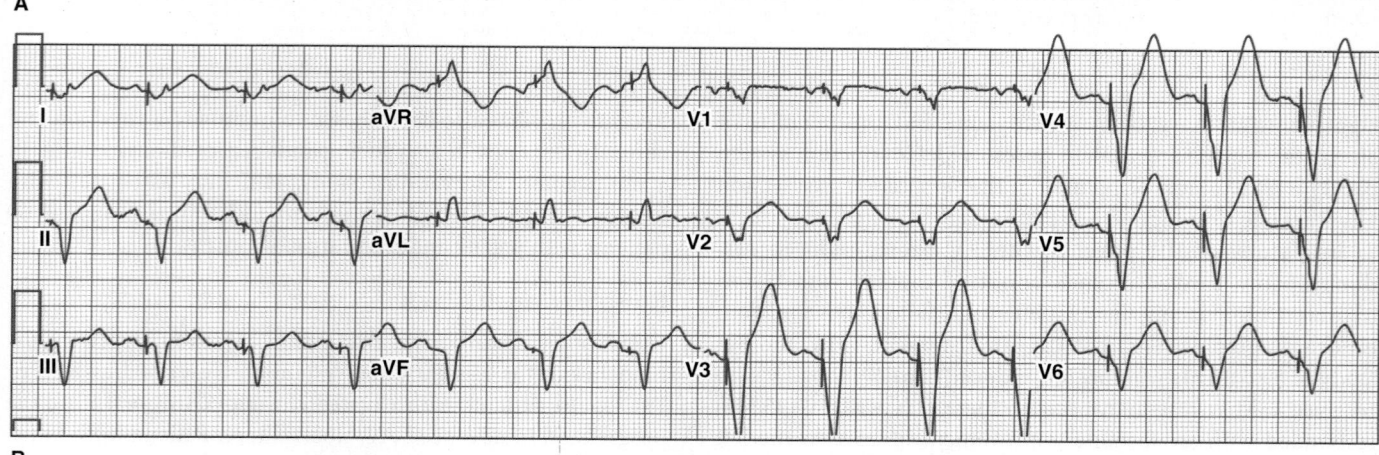

B

Figure 38–19. ECGs of a patient with complete AV nodal block at baseline (**A**) and following RV pacing (**B**) are shown.

TABLE 38–5. Recommendations for Pacing in Bundle Branch Block and 1:1 Atrioventricular Conduction

COR	LOE	RECOMMENDATIONS
I	C-LD	1. In patients with syncope and bundle branch block who are found to have an HV interval 70 ms or greater or evidence of infranodal block at EPS, permanent pacing is recommended.
I	C-LD	2. In patients with alternating bundle branch block, permanent pacing is recommended.
IIa	C-LD	3. In patients with Kearns–Sayre syndrome and conduction disorders, permanent pacing is reasonable, with additional defibrillator capability if appropriate and meaningful survival of greater than 1 year is expected.
IIb	C-LD	4. In patients with Anderson–Fabry disease and QRS prolongation greater than 110 ms, permanent pacing, with additional defibrillator capability if needed and meaningful survival of greater than 1 year is expected, may be considered.
IIb	C-LD	5. In patients with heart failure, a mildly to moderately reduced LVEF (36%–50%), and LBBB (QRS ‡150 ms), CRT therapy may be considered.
III: Harm	B-NR	6. In asymptomatic patients with isolated conduction disease and 1:1 atrioventricular conduction, permanent pacing is not indicated (in the absence of other indications for pacing).

Leadless Pacing

Integrated pulse generator and sensing/pacing systems that are fully self-contained (and are therefore "leadless") are commercially available. These devices overcome some of the limitations of the conventional transvenous lead-based systems, including the early risk of acute complications such as pneumothorax, upper extremity thrombosis, or frozen shoulder, as well as mitigating longer-term risks such as lead-associated infection, fracture, or need for extraction. Indeed, some have argued that the lead is the "Achilles' heel" of a pacing system. Two fully integrated pulse generator and sensing/pacing systems have now been studied in human trials: the Nanostim leadless cardiac pacemaker (LCP, St. Jude Medical) and the Micra transcatheter pacing system (TCP, Medtronic) (**Figs. 38–20** and **38–21**). Both devices rely on a catheter-based deployment tool and are delivered to the RV. The LCP utilizes an active helix fixation mechanism whereas the TCP employs self-expanding nitinol tines delivered into the RV apical septum. Both devices are tethered to the delivery catheter and "tug-tested" before final release.

The LEADLESS II study was a prospective, nonrandomized, multicenter analysis of 526 patients receiving LCP with a primary outcome of efficacy and safety.[27] Pacemaker implant success was achieved in 95.8% of patients, with an average procedural time of 28.6±17.8 minutes and an average hospital stay of 1.1±1.7 days. The primary efficacy end point of an acceptable pacing threshold (≤2.0 V at 0.4 ms) and an acceptable sensing amplitude (R wave ≥5.0 mV, or a value equal to or greater than the value at implantation) through 6 months was achieved in 270 of 300 patients (90%). Efficacy failure resulted predominantly from inadequately sensed R waves. The primary safety end point of freedom from device-related serious adverse events through 6 months was observed in 6.7% over a 6-month period, and included device dislodgement (1.7%), cardiac perforation (1.3%), and vascular complications (1.3%).

The Micra TCP trial was a prospective, nonrandomized study of 725 patients whose primary indication for enrollment was persistent or permanent atrial tachyarrhythmia (64%), SND (17.5%), and AV block (14.8%).[28] Implant success was achieved in 99.2% and freedom from major complication was 96% at 6 months. Cardiac perforation or effusion (1.6%) and vascular access complication (0.7%) were the most common complications. No radiographic device dislodgements were noted, but three patients required system revision as a result of elevated pacing threshold, symptoms of pacemaker syndrome, or intermittent loss of capture. In a 12-month follow-up study of Micra Post Approval Registry involving 1817 patients, implant success was 99.1% with a major complication rate of 2.7% (66% less than the IDE study).[29]

TABLE 38–6. Recommendations for Pacing after Cardiac Surgery or Valve Replacement

COR	LOE	RECOMMENDATIONS
I	B-NR	1. In patients who have new postoperative SND or atrioventricular block associated with persistent symptoms or hemodynamic instability that does not resolve after coronary artery bypass surgery, aortic valve replacement, mitral valve repair/replacement, or tricuspid valve repair/replacement permanent pacing is recommended before discharge.
IIb	C-EO	2. In patients undergoing coronary artery bypass, aortic, mitral, or tricuspid valve surgery who will likely require future CRT or ventricular pacing, intraoperative placement of a permanent epicardial left ventricular lead may be considered.
I	B-NR	3. In patients who have new atrioventricular block after transcatheter aortic valve replacement associated with symptoms or hemodynamic instability that does not resolve, permanent pacing is recommended before discharge.
IIa	B-NR	4. In patients with new persistent bundle branch block after transcatheter aortic valve replacement, careful surveillance for bradycardia is reasonable.
IIb	B-NR	5. In patients with new persistent LBBB after transcatheter aortic valve replacement, implantation of a permanent pacemaker may be considered.

TABLE 38–7. Recommendations for Pacing in Adults with Congenital Heart Disease

COR	LOE	RECOMMENDATIONS
I	B-NR	1. In adults with adult congenital heart disease (ACHD) and symptomatic SND or chronotropic incompetence, atrial based permanent pacing is recommended.
I	B-NR	2. In adults with ACHD and symptomatic bradycardia related to atrioventricular block, permanent pacing is recommended.
I	B-NR	3. In adults with congenital complete atrioventricular block with any symptomatic bradycardia, a wide QRS escape rhythm, mean daytime heart rate below 50 bpm, complex ventricular ectopy, or ventricular dysfunction, permanent pacing is recommended.
I	B-NR	4. In adults with ACHD and postoperative second-degree Mobitz type II atrioventricular block, high-grade atrioventricular block, or third-degree atrioventricular block that is not expected to resolve, permanent pacing is recommended.
IIa	B-NR	5. In asymptomatic adults with congenital complete atrioventricular block, permanent pacing is reasonable.
IIa	B-NR	6. In adults with repaired ACHD who require permanent pacing for bradycardic indications, a bradycardia device with atrial anti-tachycardia pacing capabilities is reasonable.
IIa	C-EO	7. In adults with ACHD with preexisting sinus node and/or atrioventricular conduction disease who are undergoing cardiac surgery, intraoperative placement of epicardial permanent pacing leads is reasonable.
IIb	B-NR	8. In adults with ACHD and pacemakers, atrial-based permanent pacing for the prevention of atrial arrhythmias may be considered.
III: Harm	B-NR	9. In selected adults with ACHD and venous to systemic intracardiac shunts, placement of endocardial pacing leads is potentially harmful.

With relatively short implant times, low rate of dislodgement, and projected longevity lasting 10 to 14 years, there is growing enthusiasm and increased adoption of fully self-contained cardiac implantable electronic devices (CIEDs) for pacing. Although they do not expand the indication for pacing, they may be associated with fewer adverse events, particularly those resulting from late infection or extraction, as compared with conventional transvenous systems. The Micra Atrial Tracking Using A Ventricular Accelerometer (MARVEL) study was a prospective, nonrandomized, multicenter clinical feasibility study designed to characterize the closed-loop performance of an AV synchronous algorithm downloaded into previously implanted Micra devices.[30] The MARVEL study demonstrated the feasibility of tracking atrial contractions and providing AV synchrony in 87% of subjects at rest using a mechanical accelerometer-based sensor in the Micra ventricular pacemaker during a 30-minute test period. This feature allows VDD mode pacing and maintains AV synchrony in patients with AV block and sinus rhythm. The MARVEL2 study enrolled 75 patients; in the 40 patients with sinus rhythm and AV block, the mean percentage of AV synchrony increased from 26.8% (median: 26.9%) during VVI pacing to 89.2% (median: 94.3%) during VDD pacing.[31] With ongoing research and innovation it is likely that dual-chamber leadless pacemakers capable of pacing and sensing in both chambers will become a reality in the near future.

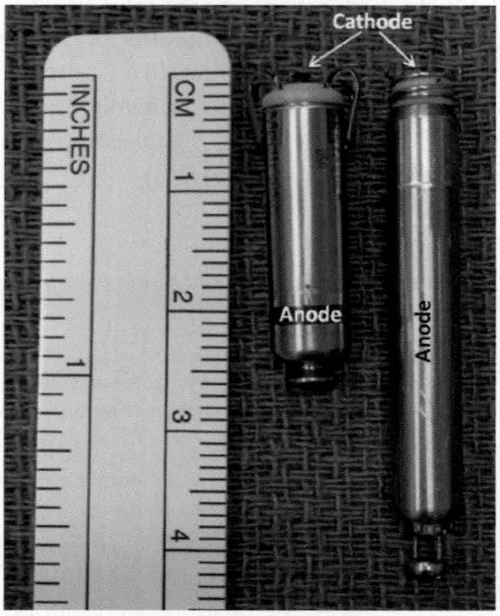

Biventricular Pacing

The role of BiV pacing in patients with AV block and a normal LVEF or only modest depression of LV function remains unsettled. During RV pacing, the LV contraction pattern is dyssynchronous resulting in disproportionate workload of the LV lateral wall. In BiV pacing, a LV pacing lead is placed in the branches of the coronary sinus (preferably in a lateral vein) in addition to the RV lead (**Figs. 38–22** and **38–23**). By simultaneous or sequential stimulation of the LV and RV, ventricular dyssynchrony can be prevented. In a study of 177 patients with bradycardia and a normal EF in whom a BiV pacemaker had been successfully implanted, patients randomized to undergo RV pacing had a lower mean LVEF (54.8 ± 9.1% vs 62.2 ± 7.0%; $P < .001$) and a larger LV end-systolic volume (35.7 ± 16.3 mL vs. 27.6 ± 10.4 mL; $P < 0.001$) than patients in the BiV pacing group at 12 months.[32] In the RV apical pacing group, LVEF further decreased from the first to the second year, but it remained unchanged in the BiV pacing group, leading to a significant difference of 9.9 percentage points between groups at 2-year follow-up ($P < 0.001$).[33] The Biventricular versus RV

Figure 38–20. Leadless pacemakers: the St. Jude Nanostim (right) and the Medtronic Micra (center, next to ruler). Reproduced with permission from Miller MA, Neuzil P, Dukkipati SR, et al: Leadless cardiac pacemakers: back to the future, *J Am Coll Cardiol.* 2015 Sep 8;66(10):1179-1189.

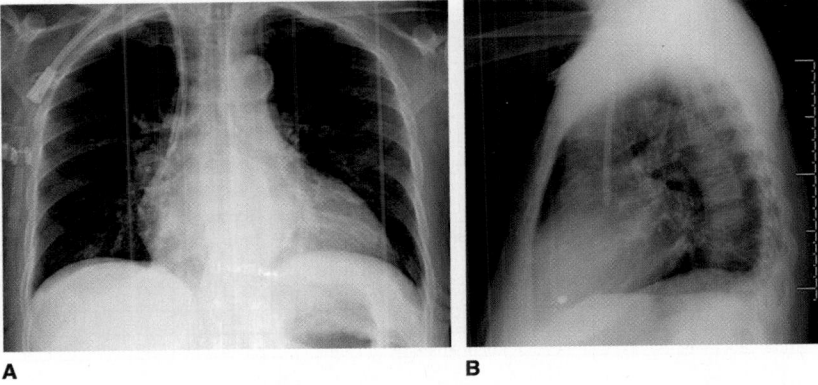

Figure 38–21. **(A)** Posteroanterior and **(B)** lateral chest films of patient with leadless cardiac pacemaker.

Pacing in Heart Failure Patients with Atrioventricular Block (BLOCK HF) study was a prospective trial that randomized 691 patients with mild to moderate HF (NYHA Class I, II, or III), LV dysfunction (LVEF ≤0.50), and AV block to RV pacing versus BiV pacing with an average follow-up of 37 months.[34] The primary outcome was the time to death from any cause, an urgent care visit for HF that required intravenous therapy, or a 15% or more increase in the LV end-systolic volume index. The primary outcome occurred in 190 of 342 patients (55.6%) in the RV-pacing group, as compared with 160 of 349 (45.8%) in the BiV-pacing group. Patients randomly assigned to BiV pacing had a significantly lower incidence of the primary outcome over time than did those assigned to RV pacing (hazard ratio [HR], 0.74; 95% credible interval, 0.60–0.90). An important limitation to this trial was the inclusion of patients with LVEF ≤35%, and an indication for an ICD comprising 30% of the study population. Differences in the primary outcome between the two pacemaker subgroups with LVEF ≥35% were driven predominantly by an increase in LV end-systolic volume index. A secondary outcome of HF hospitalizations was higher in the conventional pacemaker group when compared with that in the BiV pacing group. The Biventricular Pacing for Atrioventricular Block to Prevent Cardiac Desynchronization (BioPace) trial randomized 1810 patients with AV block (mean age 73.5 years) to either RV pacing (n = 908) or BiV pacing (n = 902). After a mean follow-up of 5.6 years, the groups had a similar rate of the composite endpoint that included time-to-death or first hospitalization due to HF, with a nonsignificant trend in favor of BiV (HR 0.87; P = 0.08) [Blanc JJ: European Society of Cardiology Congress, 2014]. This trend persisted, without reaching statistical significance, when patients were stratified according to their LVEF. For patients with an LVEF of 50% or less, the HR was 0.92 (P = 0.47) and for patients with an LVEF of more than 50% it was 0.88 (P = 0.21). It is important to note that 14.8% of patients in the BiV group failed initial implant. Current AHA/ACC/HRS guidelines recommend physiologic pacing in the form of BiV pacing or HBP as class IIa indication for pacing in patients with AV block and LVEF of 35% to 50% (Table 38–4).

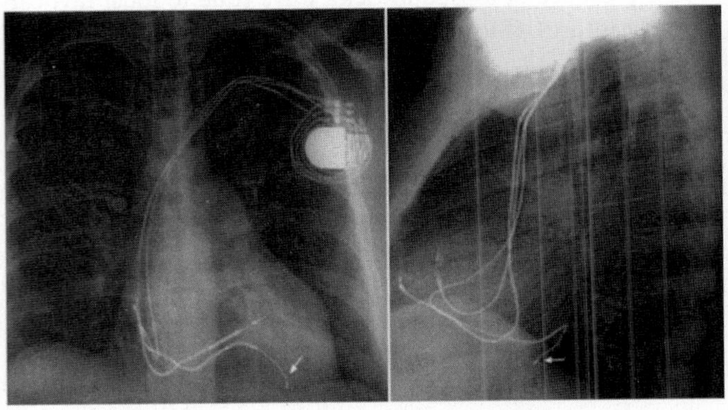

His-Purkinje Conduction System Pacing

An ideal physiologic approach to ventricular stimulation should engage the His-Purkinje conduction system. By preserving normal electrical activation of the ventricles, His-Purkinje conduction system pacing prevents ventricular dyssynchrony and its long-term consequences. While the concept of pacing the main body of the bundle of His is not new, directly pacing the His bundle with a permanent pacemaker was initially described in 2000.[35] Leads and delivery systems specific for HBP have enabled increasing adoption of HBP into clinical practice. Since then, several studies have demonstrated the feasibility and safety of permanent HBP. Recent studies have also demonstrated the feasibility of pacing the LBB region, intraseptally via the RV.[36–38]

The His bundle is a cylindrical fascicle extending inferiorly and leftward from the AV node. The bundle of His and has two segments: the penetrating portion and the branching portion. The penetrating His bundle is about 5 mm to 10 mm in length overlying the atrial portion of the membranous septum while the branching portion extends for about 5 mm to 10 mm from the point where the posterior fibers of the LBB arise to the point where the LBB completely branches out and the RBB begins. The proximal LBB fans out beneath the LV subendocardium to form a wider target for pacing as compared to the

Figure 38–22. **(A)** Posteroanterior and **(B)** lateral chest films of patient with biventricular pacemaker. The LV lead in the coronary sinus branch is shown.

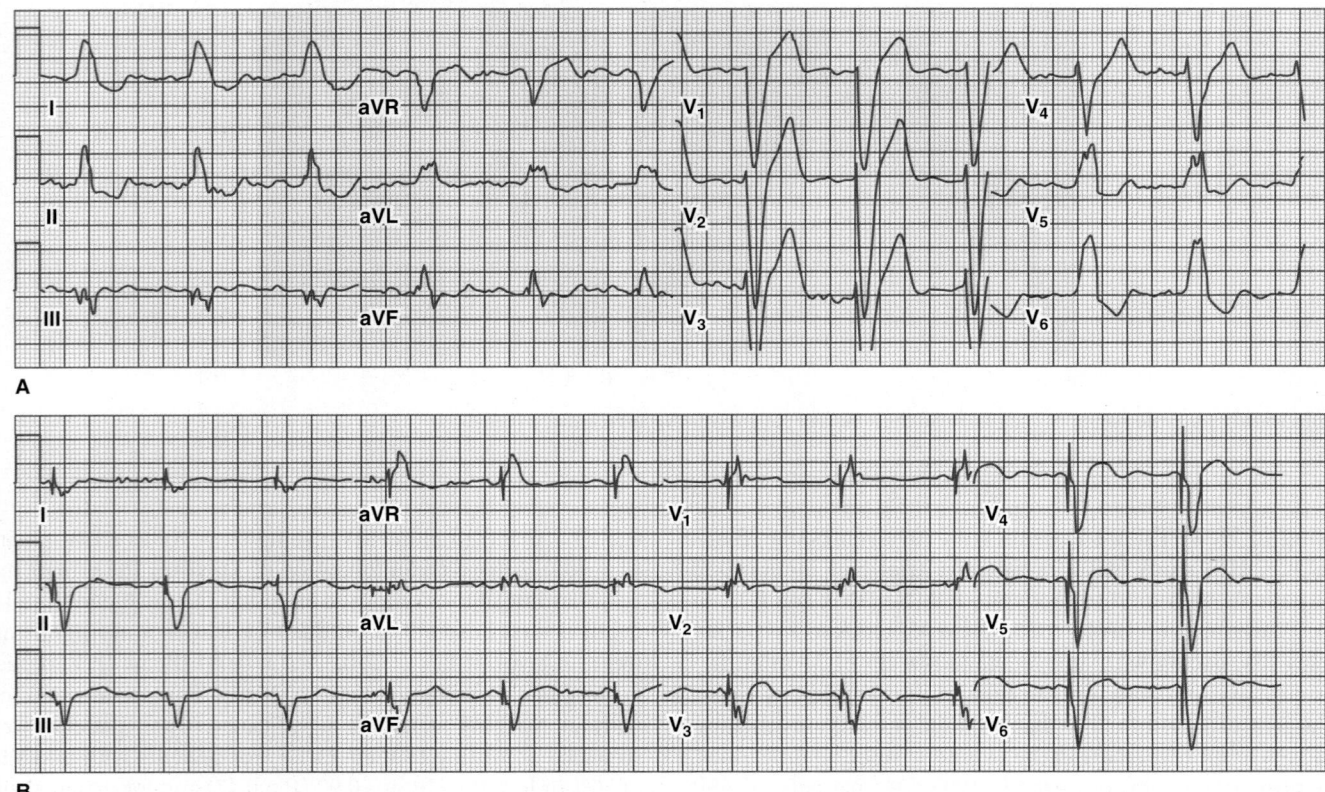

Figure 38–23. ECGs of a patient with LBBB (**A**) at baseline and following BiV pacing (**B**) are shown.

narrow His bundle. It divides into anterior and posterior fascicles each heading toward the corresponding papillary muscle head. The left posterior fascicle is composed of multiple bands of fibers as compared to thin tendon-like anterior fascicle. Subsequently, the fascicles give rise to Purkinje fibers that arborize into the ventricular myocardium.

Definitions and Criteria of His Bundle Pacing

A multicenter HBP collaborative working group proposed a refined set of criteria to define HBP in patients with normal His-Purkinje conduction and in those with His-Purkinje conduction disease (HPCD) (**Table 38–8**).[39] The authors broadly defined two forms of His bundle capture: Selective capture in which the His bundle is the only tissue captured by the pacing stimulus and nonselective capture in which there is fusion of the His bundle and adjacent RV tissue.

Selective His Bundle Pacing (S-HBP): During S-HBP, ventricular activation occurs directly and completely over the HPS and is accompanied by the following criteria:

1. The pacing stimulus to QRS (S-QRS) onset interval is equal to the native His-QRS onset interval (H-QRS). However, in patients with HPCD, the S-QRS interval can be shorter than the H-QRS intervals as in patients with BBB or HV block due to capture of latent fascicular tissue. (**Figs. 38–24** and **38–25**).

2. The local ventricular electrogram on the pacing lead will be discrete from the pacing artifact.

3. The paced QRS morphology is the same as the native QRS morphology. In patients with HPCD, paced QRS duration may be narrower than the native QRS with BBB or an escape rhythm.

4. Usually a single capture threshold (His capture) is observed; particularly at typical outputs. However, in patients with HPCD, two distinct His capture thresholds, with and without correction of underlying BBB, may be seen.

Nonselective His Bundle Pacing (NS-HBP): During NS-HBP, in addition to direct His bundle capture, there is capture of adjacent RV septal myocardium.

1. S-QRS interval is usually equal to zero, as there is no isoelectric interval between the pacing stimulus and QRS due to the presence of a pseudo-delta wave (due to local myocardial capture). (**Fig. 38–26**)

2. The local ventricular electrogram is directly captured by the pacing stimulus and is not seen as a late discrete component.

3. The paced QRS duration will usually be longer than the native QRS duration by the H-QRS interval and the overall electrical axis of the paced QRS will be concordant with the electrical axis of the intrinsic QRS. In patients with HPCD, the paced QRS duration may be narrower than the native QRS due to correction of underlying BBB.

4. There will usually be two distinct capture thresholds: RV capture and His capture. The His capture threshold may be lower or higher than the RV capture threshold. The output difference between the two thresholds (RV and His) is usually small

TABLE 38–8. Criteria for His Bundle Pacing

| Baseline | Normal QRS | His-Purkinje Conduction Disease | |
		With correction	Without correction
Selective HBP	• S-QRS = H-QRS with isoelectric interval • Discrete local ventricular electrogram in HBP lead with S-V=H-V • Paced QRS = native QRS • Single capture threshold (His bundle)	• S-QRS ≤ H-QRS with isoelectric interval • Discrete local ventricular electrogram in HBP lead • Paced QRS < native QRS • 2 distinct capture thresholds (HBP with BBB correction, HBP without BBB correction)	• S-QRS ≤ or > H-QRS with isoelectric interval • Discrete local ventricular electrogram in HBP lead • Paced QRS = native QRS • Single capture threshold (HBP with BBB)
Nonselective HBP	• S-QRS < H-QRS (S-QRS usually 0, S-QRS$_{end}$ = H-QRS$_{end}$) with or without isoelectric interval (Pseudodelta wave +/−) • Direct capture of local ventricular electrogram in HBP lead by stimulus artifact (local myocardial capture) • Paced QRS > native QRS with normalization of precordial and limb lead axes with respect to rapid dV/dt components of the QRS • 2 distinct capture thresholds (His bundle capture, RV capture)	• S-QRS < H-QRS (S-QRS usually 0, S-QRS$_{end}$ < H-QRS$_{end}$) with or without isoelectric interval (Pseudodelta wave +/−) • Direct capture of local ventricular electrogram in HBP lead by stimulus artifact • Paced QRS ≤ native QRS • 3 distinct capture thresholds possible (HBP with BBB correction, HBP without BBB correction, RV capture)	• S-QRS < H-QRS (S-QRS usually 0) with or without isoelectric interval (Pseudodelta wave +/−) • Direct capture of local ventricular electrogram in HBP lead by stimulus artifact • Paced QRS > native QRS • 2 distinct capture thresholds (HBP with BBB, RV capture)

Abbreviations: BBB, bundle branch block; dV/dt, rate oc change in voltage; H-V, His-ventricular; H-QRS, His-QRS; RV, right ventricle; S-QRS, stimulus-QRS; S-V, stimulus-ventricular.
Data from Vijayaraman P, Dandamudi G, Zanon F, et al. Permanent his bundle pacing (HBP): recommendations from International HBP Collaborative Group for Standardization of Definitions, Implant Measurements and Follow-up. *Heart Rhythm* 2018;15:460-468.

and the final programmed output including the safety margin would result in nonselective His capture. In patients with HPCD, three distinct capture thresholds may be observed in varying combination (RV capture, His capture with correction of BBB, His capture without correction of BBB).

The technical feasibility and safety outcomes of HBP have been demonstrated in several clinical studies [**Table 38–9**].[40-47] Preliminary data suggest that permanent HBP is associated with an improvement in exercise capacity, myocardial perfusion,

ventricular synchrony, and LVEF compared to RV pacing.[23] In observational, case-control studies, HBP was associated with significant reduction in the combined endpoint of death, HF hospitalization, or upgrade to BiV pacing when compared to RV pacing.[23,48] Overall success rates with dedicated implant tools range from 80% to 95%. The average pacing threshold for His bundle capture is above 1 V and may lead to premature battery depletion. In a long-term study of HBP, generator changes were required in 9% of patients at 5 years, while lead related

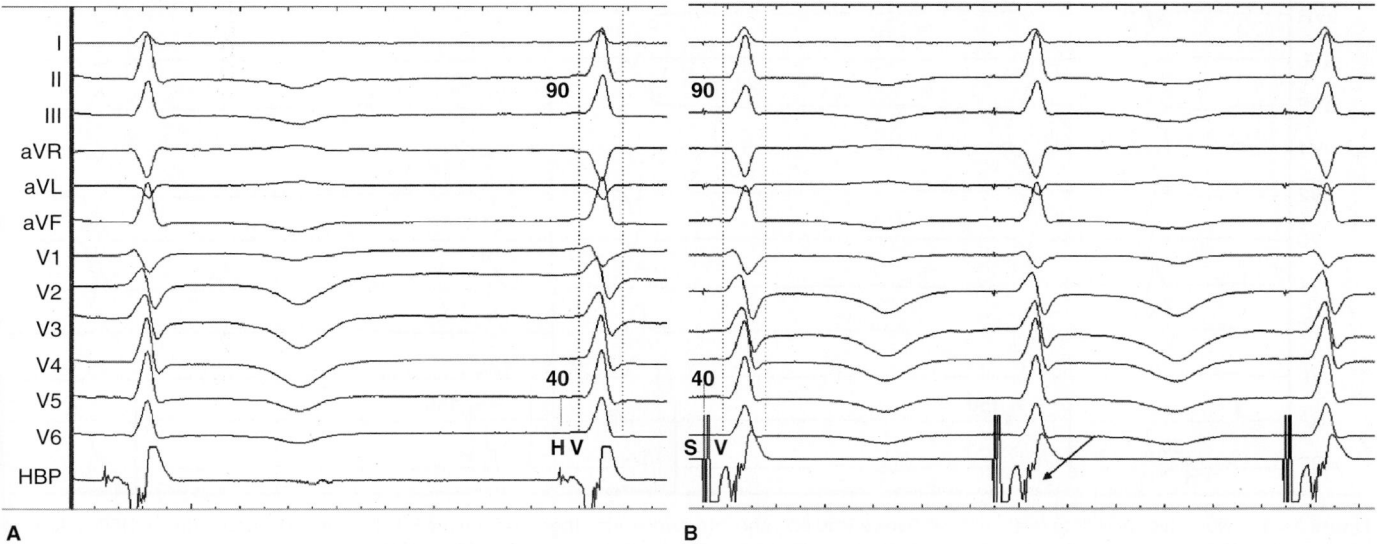

Figure 38–24. Selective His bundle pacing: twelve-lead ECG and intracardiac electrograms from the HBP lead at baseline and during HBP are shown at a sweep speed of 100 mm/s. His-QRS and the stimulus-QRS intervals are identical at 40 ms. The QRS morphology during HBP is same as baseline. The local ventricular electrogram (*arrow*) is discrete from the pacing stimulus suggesting absent local ventricular capture. Reproduced with permission from Vijayaraman P, Dandamudi G, Zanon F, et al: Permanent His bundle pacing: Recommendations from a Multicenter His Bundle Pacing Collaborative Working Group for standardization of definitions, implant measurements, and follow-up, *Heart Rhythm* 2018 Mar;15(3):460-468.

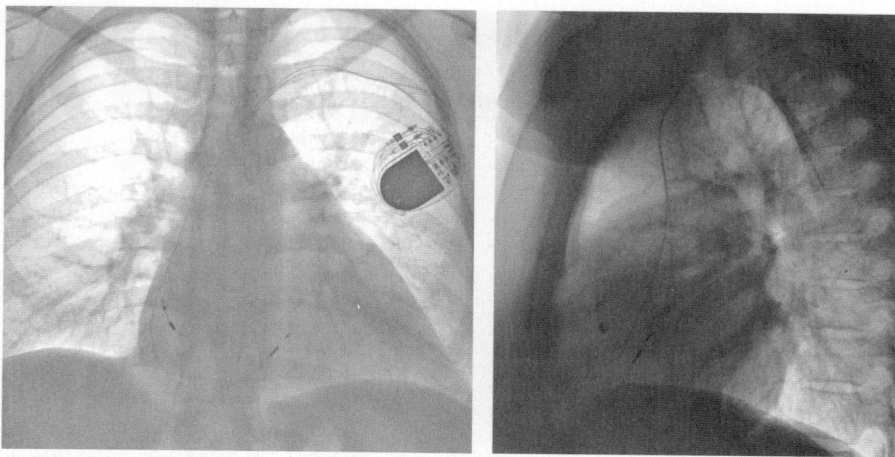

Figure 38–25. **(A)** Posteroanterior and **(B)** lateral chest films of patient with HBP lead.

complications such as significant increase in threshold requiring lead revisions were observed in 6.7% of patients.[22] While HBP is successful in both AV nodal and infranodal AV block, concerns regarding progression of conduction disease remain. Additionally, undersensing of ventricular signals and atrial oversensing can occasionally be problematic.

Left Bundle Branch Pacing

Huang and coworkers first demonstrated the direct capture of the LBB by placing the lead deep inside the septum beyond the

site of block in a patient with LBBB resulting in synchronized ventricular activation.[37] Since then, left bundle branch pacing (LBBP) has emerged as an alternate modality to deliver physiological pacing because it overcomes many of the limitations of the HBP. Several studies have demonstrated the feasibility of LBBP in patients with SND, AV block, and those with indications for cardiac resynchronization therapy (**Table 38–10**).[37,49–59] LBBP is defined as the direct capture of the LBB or one of its fascicles along with the LV septal myocardium at low output (<1 V at 0.5 ms pulse width). Commonly, the 4.1F diameter

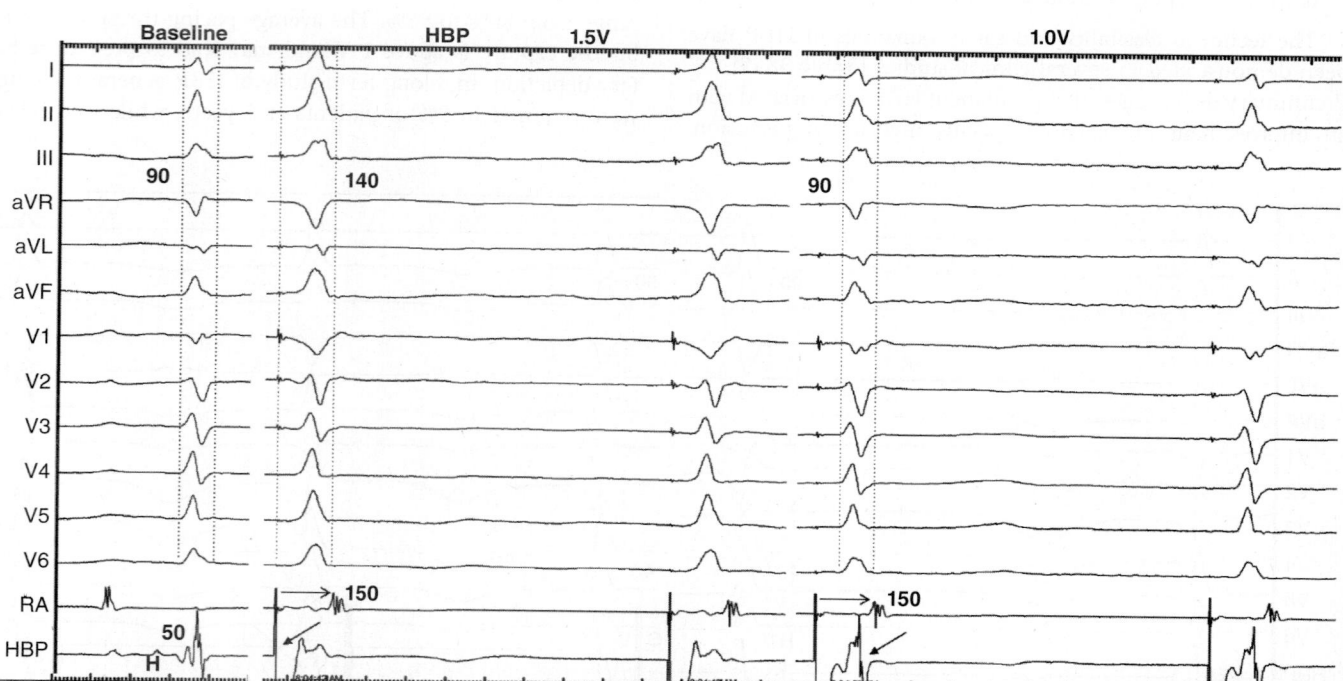

Figure 38–26. Nonselective HBP to selective HBP: Twelve-lead ECG and intracardiac electrograms from the HBP lead at baseline and during HBP at decreasing output are shown at a sweep speed of 100 mm/s. During HBP at 1.5 V, the paced QRS duration is 140 ms due to fusion between conduction via the His-Purkinje system and ventricular capture. There is no isoelectric interval between the stimulus and QRS onset (S-QRS = 0). There is no discrete local ventricular electrogram noted following the pacing artifact (*arrow*) in the HBP lead. As the pacing output is decreased to 1 V, there is selective His bundle capture and loss of ventricular capture (see the discrete local ventricular electrogram in the HBP lead–*arrow*) resulting in QRS morphology identical to baseline QRS (90 ms). Reproduced with permission from Vijayaraman P, Dandamudi G, Zanon F, et al: Permanent His bundle pacing: Recommendations from a Multicenter His Bundle Pacing Collaborative Working Group for standardization of definitions, implant measurements, and follow-up, *Heart Rhythm* 2018 Mar;15(3):460-468.

TABLE 38–9. Permanent His Bundle Pacing for Bradycardia

Author	Design	Follow-up (Months)	Number	Indication	Success (%)	Important Characteristics	Outcomes
Deshmukh et al. 2000 (35)	Observational	36	18	AV node ablation	66%	Chronic AF, LVEF <40%, QRS duration <120 ms	Improvement in LV dimensions, NYHA class, and LVEF
Deshmukh et al. 2004 (63)	Observational	42	54	AV node ablation	72%	Chronic AF, LVEF <40%, QRS duration <120 ms	Improved LVEF, NYHA class, peak VO2
Occhetta et al. 2006 (64)	Randomized, 6-months, crossover RVP vs HBP	12	18	AV node ablation	94%	Chronic AF, QRS <120 ms	Improvement in NYHA FC, 6MWT, QOL and hemodynamics
Huang et al. 2017 (38)	Observational	20	52	AV node ablation	81%	Chronic AF, CHF	Improvement in LV dimensions, NYHA class and LVEF
Vijayaraman et al. 2017 (41)	Observational	19	42	AV node ablation	95%	Paroxysmal or persistent AF, CHF	Improvement in NYHA class, LVEF
Barba-Pichardo et al. (65)	Prospective	>3	91	AV Nodal–65 Infra-nodal–26	68% 57%	182 patients with AV block mapped with EP catheter	5% lead failure
Kronborg et al. 2014 (66)	Randomized crossover HBP vs RVSP	24	38	AV nodal block	84%	AV block, baseline narrow QRS, LVEF >40%	Improvement in LVEF, no significant improvement in FC, 6MWT, QOL
Pastore et al. 2015 (67)	Retrospective	12	148	AV nodal 100 Infra-nodal 48		High grade AVB, Paroxysmal AF	HBP associated with lower risk of AF progression compared with RV pacing
Vijayaraman et al. 2015 (15)	Observational	19	100	AV nodal–46 Infra-nodal–54	93% 76%	High-grade AV block, no back-up RV pacing	High success in infranodal block. Lead failure 5%
Abdelrahman et al. 2018 (48)	Case control	24	332	SSS–118 AVB–214	91.6%	Clinical outcomes compared to RVP	Relative risk reduction of 29% in combined endpoint of death, HFH or upgrade to BiVP (P = 0.02)
Vijayaraman et al. 2018 (68)	Case control	60	94	SSS 41% AVB 59%	80%	Clinical outcomes compared to RVP	Significant reduction in death or HFH in patients with >40% ventricular pacing (P = 0.02)
Zanon et al. 2018 (42)	Meta-analysis	16.9	1438	AVB 62%	84.8%	Included patients with standard leads and dedicated HBP systems	In patients with reported LVEF, 5.9% improvement in EF was noted in follow-up
Keene et al. 2019 (44)	Multicenter, observational	7	571	SSS, AVB, and CRT indications	81%		Threshold increase in 7.5% of implants. Learning curve plateaued after 40 cases.
Zanon et al. 2019 (43)	Multicenter, observational	36	844	AVB 41% AF 40%	Only successful patients	Long-term outcomes	Freedom from lead related complications 91.6%
Wang et al. 2019 (47)	Retrospective, case control	30	86	AVN ablation in cardiomyopathy	95%	Clinical outcomes	Reduction in inappropriate ICD therapy, improvement in NYHA class, LVEF and dimensions
Vijayaraman et al. 2020 (46)	Multicenter, prospective	12	69	AVB 45%	88%	Imaging correlation of lead location and type of HBP	Freedom from lead complications 93%. Atrial location in 22%. Ventricular location in 78%
Vijayaraman et al. 2020 (45)	Multicenter, retrospective	12	65	AVB, post TAVR 100%	HBP 63% LBBP 93%	Feasibility of HBP and LBBP in patients with AV block, post-TAVR	HBP was more successful in patients with Sapien valves than Corevalve.

Abbreviations: AF, atrial fibrillation; AVB, AV block; AV node, atrioventricular; CHF, congestive heart failure; HBP, His bundle pacing; LBBP, left bundle branch pacing; LVEF, left ventricle ejection fraction; NYHA, New York Heart Association; QOL, quality of life; RVSP, right ventricle septal pacing; SSS, sick sinus syndrome; TAVR, transcatheter aortic valve replacement; 6MWT, 6 minute walk test.

Modified with permission from Vijayaraman P, Chung MK, Dandamudi G, et al: His Bundle Pacing, *J Am Coll Cardiol.* 2018 Aug 21;72(8):927-947.

TABLE 38–10. Permanent Left Bundle Branch Pacing for Bradycardia Indications

	Study	Number of patients[n]	Implant success [%]	Paced QRS [ms]	Threshold V@0.5ms	R wave [mV]	Lead revision	Objectives
Bradycardia								
1	Vijayaraman et al. 2019 (36)	100	93%	136±17	0.6 ± 0.4	10 ± 6 mV	3% (3)	Prospective study in patients requiring pacing for bradycardia or heart failure indications
2	Li et al. 2019 (49)	87	80.5%	113.2 ± 9.9	0.76±0.22	11.99±5.36	0	Prospective study in patients requiring pacing for bradycardia indications
4	Hou et al. 2019 [51]	56	NR	117.8 ± 11.0	0.5±0.1	17±6.7	0	Prospective study assessing LV synchrony in HBP vs. LBBP vs. RVP
5	Li et al. 2019 [50]	33	90.9%	112.8 ± 10.9	0.76±0.26	14.4	3.03 (1)	Prospective study of LBBP in AV block
6	Zhang et al. 2019 [52]	23	95%	112.6 ± 12.14	0.68 ± 0.2	9.28 ± 5.00	0	Prospective comparative study of LBBP over RVP in 44 consecutive patients
7	Hasumi et al. 2019 [53]	21	81%	116 ± 8.3	0.7 ±0.07	9.1 ± 1.4	0	Retrospective study assessed the feasibility of LBBP in failed HBP for AV block
8	Chen et al. 2019 [54]	20	NR	111.8 ± 10.7	0.73 ± 0.2	NR	0	Prospective study to compare the feasibility and ECG patterns during LBBP vs. RVP
9	Jastrzebski et al. 2020 [55]	143	NR	111.9 ± 15.1	0.6 ± 0.3	9.0 ± 5.1	NR	Prospective study to analyze the programmed deep septal stimulation in regard to diagnosis of LBB capture
10	Su et al. 2020 [56]	115	NR	111.4 ± 10.3	0.6 ± 0.2	11.3 ± 5.4	0	Retrospective study to assess LB current of injury in LBBP
11	Cai et al. 2020 (57)	40	90%	101 ± 8.7	0.49±0.22	11.7 ± 5.3	0	Prospective study to assess the cardiac synchrony in SSS patients undergoing LBBP vs. RVP
12	Wang et al. 2020 [58]	66	94%	121.4 ± 9.8	0.94±0.21	12.1 ± 3.6	4.5% (3)	Prospective randomized study to compare the depolarization and repolarization measures between LBBP vs. RVP
13	Vijayaraman et al. 2020 [45]	28	93%	125 ±15	0.64 ± 0.3	14 ± 8	0	Retrospective study to assess the feasibility of HPCSP pacing after TAVR (LBBP and HBP)
14	Ponnsuamy SS et al. 2020 [60]	99	94%	110.8 ±12.4	0.59± 0.22	14.1± 7.1	0	Prospective study to assess the efficacy and midterm outcomes of LBBP in Indian population

Abbreviations: AF, atrial fibrillation; AV, atrioventricular; AVJ, atrioventricular junction; BBB, bundle branch block; BiV, biventricular; CRT, cardiac resynchronization therapy; ECG, electrocardiogram; HBP, His bundle pacing; HF, heart failure; HPCSP, His-Purkinje conduction system pacing; ICD, implantable cardioverter-defibrillator; LB, left bundle; LBB, left bundle branch; LBBP, left bundle branch pacing; LV, left ventricular; LVEF, left ventricular ejection fraction; NICM, nonischemic cardiomyopathy; RVP, right ventricular pacing; SSS, sick sinus syndrome; TAVR, transcatheter aortic valve replacement.

Reproduced with permission with Ponnusamy SS, Arora V, Namboodiri N, et al: Left bundle branch pacing: A comprehensive review, *J Cardiovasc Electrophysiol*. 2020 Sep; 31(9):2462-2473.

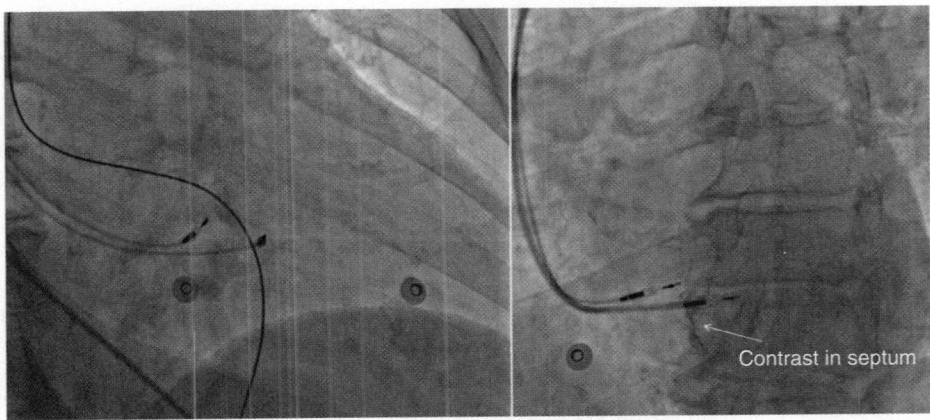

Figure 38–27. Fluoroscopic localization for left bundle branch area pacing (LBBAP): HBP and LBBAP lead locations in right anterior oblique (RAO) and left anterior oblique (LAO) 30° fluoroscopic views are shown. A thin layer of contrast is seen layering the RV septal wall in the LAO projection demonstrating the lead depth in the septum. Reproduced with permission from Vijayaraman P, Subzposh FA, Naperkowski A, et al: Prospective evaluation of feasibility and electrophysiologic and echocardiographic characteristics of left bundle branch area pacing, *Heart Rhythm.* 2019 Dec;16(12):1774-1782.

3830 SelectSecure™ pacing lead (Medtronic Inc, Minneapolis, MN) is positioned deep inside the interventricular septum 1 cm to 1.5 cm below the His bundle at the LV subendocardium adjacent to the LBB or its branches (**Figs. 38–27** and **38–28**). In addition to demonstrating a paced QRS of RBB conduction delay pattern, at least one of the following criteria should be demonstrable to confirm direct capture of the LB or its branches[36,60]:

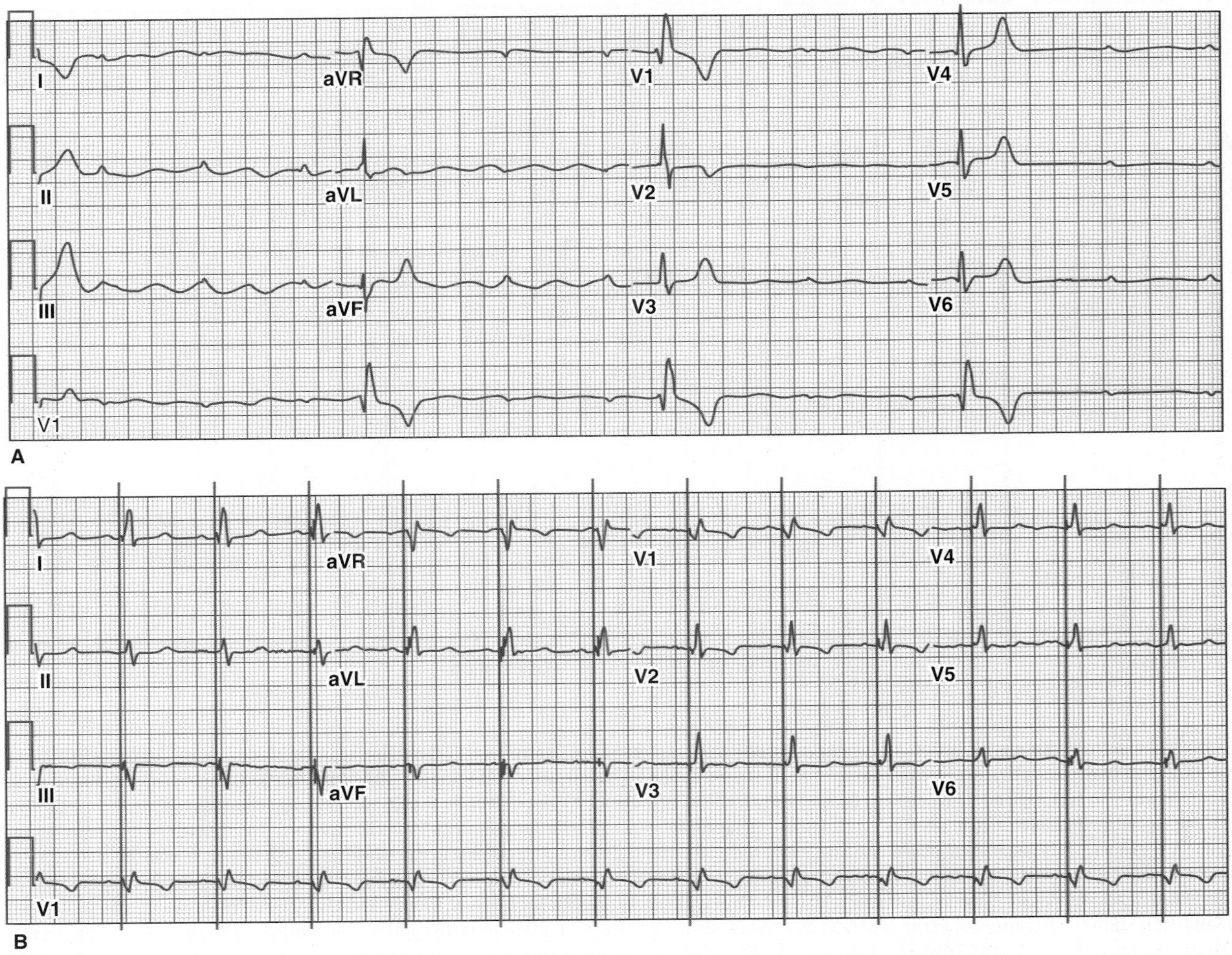

A

B

Figure 38–28. ECGs of a patient with complete heart block and RBBB escape rhythm (**A**) and during LBB pacing (**B**) are shown.

1. Demonstration of LBB potential with LB-V interval of 20 ms to 35 ms. If an LBBB is present, meeting this criterion first requires the placement of a temporary HBP lead with LBBB correction in order to identify the LBB potential.

2. Demonstration of transition in QRS morphology from non-selective to selective LB capture or nonselective to LV septal capture during threshold testing with decrementing output (**Fig. 38–29**).

3. Peak LV activation time as measured in lead $V_{5,6}$ <80 ms.

4. Programmed stimulation to demonstrate differences in refractory period of LB and septal myocardium.

During LBBP, capture thresholds are consistently <1 V and result in an RBBB morphology pattern with rapid LV activation. Sensing R wave amplitudes are similar to those observed with RV pacing. In patients with infranodal AV block and LBBB, the pacing site is consistently beyond the site of block allaying concerns for progression of conduction disease. Studies have shown preservation of ventricular synchrony and/or improvement of dyssynchrony in patients with LBBB. During medium-term follow-up, capture thresholds are stable with

infrequent lead-related complications. Potential concerns for migration of the lead into the LV cavity and unknown risks of lead extraction in the long-term remain. There are no major randomized controlled clinical trials other than prospective and retrospective observational or case-control studies demonstrating the efficacy and safety of His-Purkinje conduction system pacing.

Biological Pacemakers

Several approaches have been studied in animal models to develop biological pacemakers.[61] These include (1) stem cell-based approach, (2) cell and gene therapy-based approach (hybrid), (3) functional reengineering using gene therapy overexpressing single or combination of ion channels, and (4) somatic reprogramming using gene therapy.

Embryonic stem cells or induced pluripotent cells capable of differentiating into spontaneously beating pacemaker cells have been studied. Stem cells "loaded" with ion channel genes, have also been used; human mesenchymal stem cells have been loaded with the HCN family of genes responsible for generating I_f. Overexpressing a dominant negative mutant

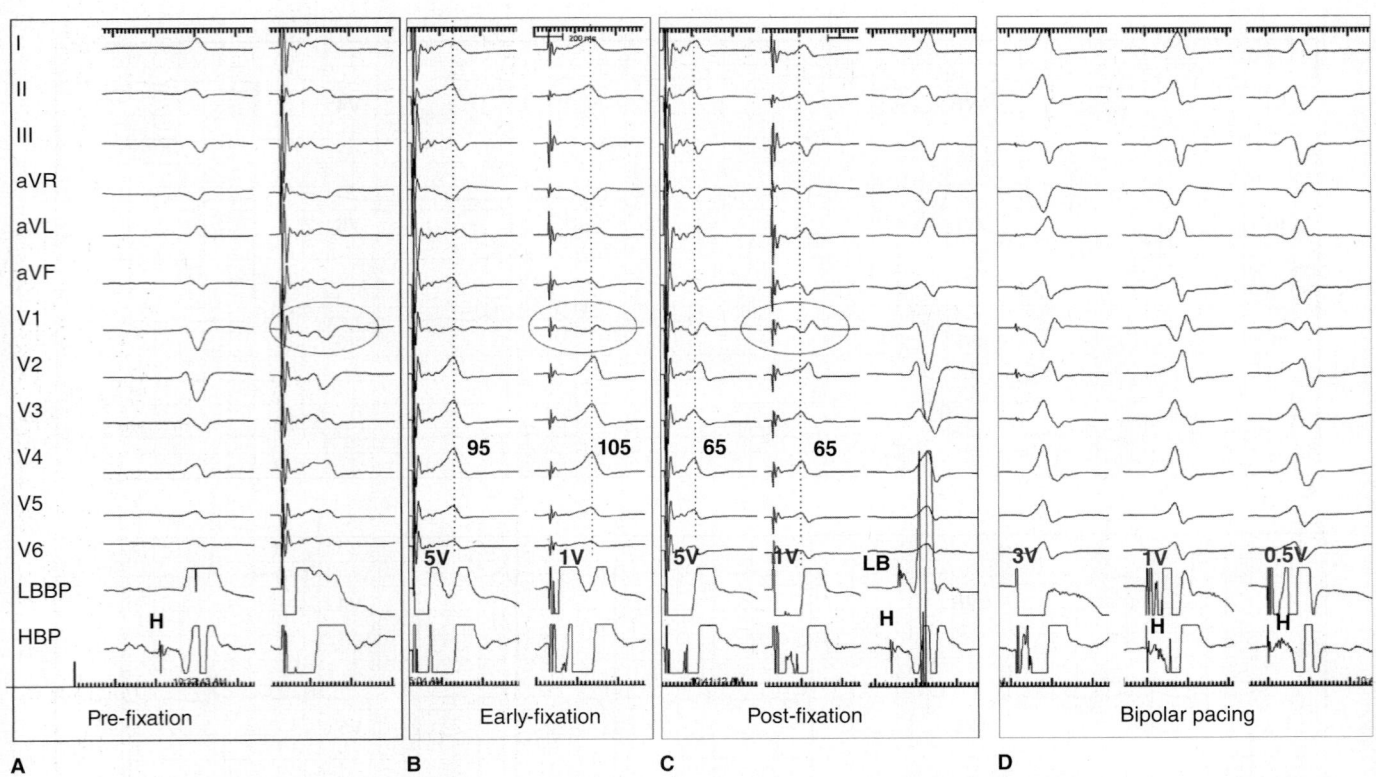

Figure 38–29. Electrocardiographic observations during LBBAP lead implantation: Twelve-lead ECG and intracardiac electrograms from the HBP and LBBAP lead are shown at sweep speed of 100 mm/s during various stages of LBBAP lead fixation. (A) Prior to LBBAP lead fixation, pacing from the lead at demonstrates a QS pattern in surface lead V1 (*circle*). (B) During early fixation as the lead is driven deeper, the QS morphology changes to Qr pattern (*circle*) during unipolar pacing. Note the difference in peak left ventricular activation time (pLVAT) during pacing at 5 V and 1 V (95 and 105 ms). (C) At final fixation, unipolar pacing at 5 V and 1 V results in identical pLVAT of 65 ms. Note the LBB potential with injury current in the LBBAP lead. (D) During bipolar pacing at 3 V there is anodal (RV septal) capture and at 1 V there is nonselective LBBAP. Note the subtle changes in QRS morphology in leads V1 and V2 and the intracardiac electrograms in LBBAP lead. Pacing at 0.5 V demonstrates selective LBBAP with a short isoelectric interval. More importantly note the presence of retrograde His (H) potentials (short stimulus-His interval) in the HBP lead during LBBAP at 1 V and 0.5 V confirming LBB capture. Reproduced with permission from Vijayaraman P, Subzposh FA, Naperkowski A, et al: Prospective evaluation of feasibility and electrophysiologic and echocardiographic characteristics of left bundle branch area pacing, *Heart Rhythm*. 2019 Dec;16(12):1774-1782.

(Kir2.1AAA) of the inward rectifier current (I_{k1}) converted a normally-quiescent myocyte into one capable of generating spontaneous action potentials and biological pacemaker activity in vivo. Somatic programming appears promising wherein sinus node tissue is recreated from ordinary cardiac myocytes. The *TBX18* gene (involved in the development of embryonic sinoatrial node) injected into a rodent model of heart block was able to generate biological pacemaker activity from the injected site by reprogramming normal working myocytes into pacemaker cells.[62] In pigs with complete AV nodal block (AV node ablation), adenoviral vectors expressing *TBX18* were injected into the His region. Biological pacing initiated by this approach was shown to result in superior chronotropic support, lower pacemaker utilization, and improved ejection fraction. By this approach, pacemaker-induced cardiomyopathy could also be reversed. Transfer of genes encoding transcription factors to change working myocardium into a surrogate sinoatrial node may also become a reality. This approach may be of value in children with congenital heart block and patients with recurrent device infections. Biological pacemakers may expand the therapeutic armamentarium for conduction system disorders. While these approaches are promising, they are very early in their development and require further study.

SUMMARY

Sinus Node Dysfunction (SND)

Pathogenesis

- Multifactorial: multiple intrinsic and extrinsic causes.
- Age-related fibrosis and ion channel remodeling as common causes.
- Structural heart disease, particularly ischemic heart disease and infiltrative cardiomyopathies.
- Monogenetic and polygenetic associations involving genes mediating sodium (*HCN4*, *SCN5A*) and calcium (*RYR2*, *CASQ2*) handling.

Clinical Presentation

- Most patients are asymptomatic or mildly symptomatic at diagnosis.
- In general, SND is relatively benign causing mild symptoms such as fatigue and exercise intolerance.
- Symptoms related to sudden changes in heart rate due to sinus pauses or arrest can be more severe and result in syncope or presyncope.
- There is significant overlap of atrial arrhythmias such as AF and SND. Often, there are symptoms related to these concomitant arrhythmias.

Evaluation

- Symptomatic correlation to SND is key to treatment.
- The main tool to evaluate SND is electrocardiographic monitoring.
- Wearable cardiac monitors are a useful tool in quantifying SND and correlating with symptoms.

- Longer duration monitors or implantable cardiac monitors are frequently needed to make a diagnosis.
- Exercise testing is a useful tool for assessing chronotropic incompetence.
- Electrophysiologic study has limited utility and is not used as a primary method to evaluate SND.

Treatment

- Reversible causes such as obstructive sleep apnea, hypothyroidism, and negative chronotropic medications should be identified and treated.
- Pacemaker therapy is the main treatment for symptomatic SND.
- In most cases, atrial pacing with a single-chamber atrial or dual-chamber pacemaker is preferable.
- In some cases where only intermittent pacing is required, a single-chamber ventricular pacemaker is reasonable.
- Pacemaker therapy for asymptomatic SND is contraindicated.

Atrioventricular Block

Pathogenesis

- Age-related fibrosis is the most common cause; inherited causes can present earlier in life and may have syndromic manifestations.
- Coronary heart disease, infiltrative cardiomyopathy (especially sarcoidosis), infectious processes.
- Surgical trauma, particularly during valvular surgery including transcatheter procedures.
- Benign forms of AV block can be caused by high levels of vagal tone.

Clinical Presentation

- Symptoms with AV block are variable, ranging from asymptomatic to abrupt syncope.
- The symptoms and prognosis related to AV block depend on the degree of block (ie, first degree, second degree, third degree) and the anatomic site of block (AV node, subnodal).
- In patients with high grade AV block, symptoms may depend on the rate of the escape rhythm, which varies with the site of block.
- Paroxysmal AV block is potentially dangerous and often difficult to diagnose.

Evaluation

- Most abnormalities in AV conduction can be diagnosed using ECG.
- The level of block (particularly in 2:1 AV block) can be deduced using changes with autonomic tone or electrocardiographic characteristics.
- Wearable cardiac monitors are a useful tool in detecting transient AV block and establishing symptom/rhythm correlation.
- Longer duration monitors or implantable cardiac monitors are sometimes necessary when symptoms are rare.
- Electrophysiologic studies may be useful, particularly for evaluation of patients with syncope.

Management of AV Block and Interventricular Conduction Disease

- There is no chronic medical therapy to improve AV conduction; withdrawal of medications that contribute to AV block may be helpful.
- Pacemaker therapy is indicated in most patients with advanced AV block and associated symptoms.
- Traditional RV pacing for AV block can cause progressive pacing-related cardiomyopathy in 11% to 22% of patients.
- Physiologic pacing (His bundle pacing, left bundle pacing) prevents RV pacing cardiomyopathy.
- Cardiomyopathy related to RV pacing and LBBB typically responds to BiV pacing, HBP, or LB pacing
- Leadless pacing allows ventricular pacing without the complications associated with pacing leads (lead dysfunction, systemic infection, need for extraction).
- Biological pacing using gene therapy techniques have demonstrated promise in animal models.

ACKNOWLEDGMENT

The authors would like to acknowledge Dr. Robert Schaller for his careful and thorough review, which greatly improved this chapter.

REFERENCES

1. Ho SY, Sanchez-Quintana D. Anatomy and pathology of the sinus node. *J Interv Card Electrophysiol.* 2016;46:3-8.
2. Fedorov VV, Glukhov AV, Chang R. Conduction barriers and pathways of the sinoatrial pacemaker complex: their role in normal rhythm and atrial arrhythmias. *Am J Physiol Heart Circ Physiol.* 2012;302:H1773-H1783.
3. Murphy C, Lazzara R. Current concepts of anatomy and electrophysiology of the sinus node. *J Interv Card Electrophysiol.* 2016;46:9-18.
4. Li N, Hansen BJ, Csepe TA, et al. Redundant and diverse intranodal pacemakers and conduction pathways protect the human sinoatrial node from failure. *Sci Transl Med.* 2017;9.
5. Dobrzynski H, Anderson RH, Atkinson A, et al. Structure, function and clinical relevance of the cardiac conduction system, including the atrioventricular ring and outflow tract tissues. *Pharmacol Ther.* 2013;139:260-288.
6. Barra S, Gopalan D, Baran J, Fynn S, Heck P, Agarwal S. Acute and subacute sinus node dysfunction following pulmonary vein isolation: a case series. *Eur Heart J Case Rep.* 2018;2:ytx020.
7. Boyett MR, Wang Y, Nakao S, et al. Point: exercise training-induced bradycardia is caused by changes in intrinsic sinus node function. *J Appl Physiol (1985).* 2017;123:684-685.
8. Kusumoto FM, Schoenfeld MH, Barrett C, et al. 2018 ACC/AHA/HRS Guideline on the Evaluation and Management of Patients with Bradycardia and Cardiac Conduction Delay: Executive Summary: a report of the American College of Cardiology/American Heart Association Task Force on Clinical Practice Guidelines, and the Heart Rhythm Society. *Circulation* 2019;140:e333-e381.
9. Brandt NH, Kirkfeldt RE, Nielsen JC, et al. Single lead atrial vs. dual chamber pacing in sick sinus syndrome: extended register-based follow-up in the DANPACE trial. *Europace* 2017;19:1981-1987.
10. Healey JS, Toff WD, Lamas GA, et al. Cardiovascular outcomes with atrial-based pacing compared with ventricular pacing: meta-analysis of randomized trials, using individual patient data. *Circulation* 2006;114:11-17.
11. Sweeney MO, Hellkamp AS, Ellenbogen KA, et al. Adverse effect of ventricular pacing on heart failure and atrial fibrillation among patients with normal baseline QRS duration in a clinical trial of pacemaker therapy for sinus node dysfunction. *Circulation* 2003;107:2932-2937.
12. Wilkoff BL, Cook JR, Epstein AE, et al. Dual-chamber pacing or ventricular backup pacing in patients with an implantable defibrillator: the Dual Chamber and VVI Implantable Defibrillator (DAVID) trial. *JAMA* 2002;288:3115-3123.
13. Kawashima T, Sasaki H. Gross anatomy of the human cardiac conduction system with comparative morphological and developmental implications for human application. *Ann Anat.* 2011;193:1-12.
14. El-Sherif N, Amay YLF, Schonfield C, et al. Normalization of bundle branch block patterns by distal His bundle pacing. Clinical and experimental evidence of longitudinal dissociation in the pathologic his bundle. *Circulation* 1978;57:473-483.
15. Vijayaraman P, Naperkowski A, Ellenbogen KA, Dandamudi G. Electrophysiologic insights into site of atrioventricular block: lessons from permanent His bundle pacing. *JACC Clin Electrophysiol.* 2015;1:571-581.
16. de Caluwe E, van de Bruaene A, Willems R, et al. long-term follow-up of children with heart block born from mothers with systemic lupus erythematosus: a retrospective study from the Database Pediatric and Congenital Heart Disease in University Hospitals Leuven. *Pacing Clin Electrophysiol.* 2016;39:935-943.
17. Kiehl EL, Makki T, Matar RM, et al. Incidence and predictors of late atrioventricular conduction recovery among patients requiring permanent pacemaker for complete heart block after cardiac surgery. *Heart Rhythm* 2017;14:1786-1792.
18. Feldman TE, Reardon MJ, Rajagopal V, et al. Effect of mechanically expanded vs self-expanding transcatheter aortic valve replacement on mortality and major adverse clinical events in high-risk patients with aortic stenosis: the REPRISE III randomized clinical trial. *JAMA* 2018;319:27-37.
19. Salden F, Kutyifa V, Stockburger M, Prinzen FW, Vernooy K. Atrioventricular dromotropathy: evidence for a distinctive entity in heart failure with prolonged PR interval? *Europace* 2018;20:1067-1077.
20. Upadhyay GA, Cherian T, Shatz DY, et al. Intracardiac delineation of septal conduction in left bundle-branch block patterns. *Circulation* 2019;139:1876-1888.
21. Narula OS. Longitudinal dissociation in the His bundle. Bundle branch block due to asynchronous conduction within the His bundle in man. *Circulation* 1977;56:996-1006.
22. Kiehl EL, Makki T, Kumar R, et al. Incidence and predictors of right ventricular pacing-induced cardiomyopathy in patients with complete atrioventricular block and preserved left ventricular systolic function. *Heart Rhythm* 2016;13:2272-2278.
23. Vijayaraman P, Naperkowski A, Subzposh FA, et al. Permanent His-bundle pacing: long-term lead performance and clinical outcomes. *Heart Rhythm* 2018;15:696-702.
24. Khurshid S, Obeng-Gyimah E, Supple GE, et al. Reversal of pacing-induced cardiomyopathy following cardiac resynchronization therapy. *JACC Clin Electrophysiol.* 2018;4:168-177.
25. Vijayaraman P, Herweg B, Dandamudi G, et al. Outcomes of His-bundle pacing upgrade after long-term right ventricular pacing and/or pacing-induced cardiomyopathy: insights into disease progression. *Heart Rhythm* 2019;16:1554-1561.
26. Lustgarten DL, Crespo EM, Arkhipova-Jenkins I, et al. His-bundle pacing versus biventricular pacing in cardiac resynchronization therapy patients: a crossover design comparison. *Heart Rhythm* 2015;12:1548-1557.
27. Reddy VY, Exner DV, Cantillon DJ, et al. Percutaneous implantation of an entirely intracardiac leadless pacemaker. *N Engl J Med.* 2015;373:1125-1135.
28. Reynolds D, Duray GZ, Omar R, et al. A leadless intracardiac transcatheter pacing system. *N Engl J Med.* 2016;374:533-541.
29. El-Chami MF, Al-Samadi F, Clementy N, et al. Updated performance of the Micra transcatheter pacemaker in the real-world setting: a comparison to the investigational study and a transvenous historical control. *Heart Rhythm* 2018;15:1800-1807.

30. Chinitz L, Ritter P, Khelae SK, et al. Accelerometer-based atrioventricular synchronous pacing with a ventricular leadless pacemaker: results from the Micra atrioventricular feasibility studies. *Heart Rhythm* 2018;15:1363-1371.

31. Steinwender C, Khelae SK, Garweg C, et al. Atrioventricular synchronous pacing using a leadless ventricular pacemaker: results from the MARVEL 2 Study. *JACC Clin Electrophysiol.* 2020;6:94-106.

32. Yu CM, Chan JY, Zhang Q, et al. Biventricular pacing in patients with bradycardia and normal ejection fraction. *N Engl J Med.* 2009;361:2123-2134.

33. Chan JY, Fang F, Zhang Q, et al. Biventricular pacing is superior to right ventricular pacing in bradycardia patients with preserved systolic function: 2-year results of the PACE trial. *Eur Heart J.* 2011;32:2533-2540.

34. Curtis AB, Worley SJ, Adamson PB, et al. Biventricular pacing for atrioventricular block and systolic dysfunction. *N Engl J Med.* 2013;368: 1585-1593.

35. Deshmukh P, Casavant DA, Romanyshyn M, Anderson K. Permanent, direct His-bundle pacing: a novel approach to cardiac pacing in patients with normal His-Purkinje activation. *Circulation* 2000;101:869-877.

36. Vijayaraman P, Subzposh FA, Naperkowski A, et al. Prospective evaluation of feasibility and electrophysiologic and echocardiographic characteristics of left bundle branch area pacing. *Heart Rhythm* 2019;16:1774-1782.

37. Huang W, Su L, Wu S, et al. A novel pacing strategy with low and stable output: pacing the left bundle branch immediately beyond the conduction block. *Can J Cardiol.* 2017;33:1736 e1-e3.

38. Huang W, Chen X, Su L, Wu S, Xia X, Vijayaraman P. A beginner's guide to permanent left bundle branch pacing. *Heart Rhythm* 2019;16:1791-1796.

39. Vijayaraman P, Dandamudi G, Zanon F, et al. Permanent His bundle pacing: recommendations from a Multicenter His Bundle Pacing Collaborative Working Group for standardization of definitions, implant measurements, and follow-up. *Heart Rhythm* 2018;15:460-468.

40. Huang W, Su L, Wu S, et al. Benefits of permanent his bundle pacing combined with atrioventricular node ablation in atrial fibrillation patients with heart failure with both preserved and reduced left ventricular ejection fraction. *J Am Heart Assoc.* 2017;6.

41. Vijayaraman P, Subzposh FA, Naperkowski A. Atrioventricular node ablation and His bundle pacing. *Europace* 2017;19:iv10-iv6.

42. Zanon F, Ellenbogen KA, Dandamudi G, et al. Permanent His-bundle pacing: a systematic literature review and meta-analysis. *Europace* 2018;20: 1819-1826.

43. Zanon F, Abdelrahman M, Marcantoni L, et al. Long term performance and safety of His bundle pacing: a multicenter experience. *J Cardiovasc Electrophysiol.* 2019;30:1594-1601.

44. Keene D, Arnold AD, Jastrzebski M, et al. His bundle pacing, learning curve, procedure characteristics, safety, and feasibility: insights from a large international observational study. *J Cardiovasc Electrophysiol.* 2019;30:1984-1993.

45. Vijayaraman P, Cano O, Koruth JS, et al. His-Purkinje conduction system pacing following transcatheter aortic valve replacement: feasibility and safety. *JACC Clin Electrophysiol.* 2020;6:649-657.

46. Vijayaraman P, Dandamudi G, Subzposh FA, et al. Imaging-based localization of his bundle pacing electrodes: results from the prospective IMAGE HBP Study. *JACC Clin Electrophysiol.* 2021;7(1):73-84.

47. Wang S, Wu S, Xu L, et al. Feasibility and efficacy of his bundle pacing or left bundle pacing combined with atrioventricular node ablation in patients with persistent atrial fibrillation and implantable cardioverter-defibrillator therapy. *J Am Heart Assoc.* 2019;8:e014253.

48. Abdelrahman M, Subzposh FA, Beer D, et al. clinical outcomes of his bundle pacing compared to right ventricular pacing. *J Am Coll Cardiol.* 2018;71:2319-2330.

49. Li X, Li H, Ma W, et al. Permanent left bundle branch area pacing for atrioventricular block: feasibility, safety, and acute effect. *Heart Rhythm* 2019;16:1766-1773.

50. Li Y, Chen K, Dai Y, et al. Left bundle branch pacing for symptomatic bradycardia: implant success rate, safety, and pacing characteristics. *Heart Rhythm* 2019;16:1758-1765.

51. Hou X, Qian Z, Wang Y, et al. Feasibility and cardiac synchrony of permanent left bundle branch pacing through the interventricular septum. *Europace* 2019;21:1694-1702.

52. Zhang J, Wang Z, Cheng L, et al. Immediate clinical outcomes of left bundle branch area pacing vs conventional right ventricular pacing. *Clin Cardiol.* 2019;42:768-773.

53. Hasumi E, Fujiu K, Nakanishi K, Komuro I. Impacts of left bundle/peri-left bundle pacing on left ventricular contraction. *Circ J.* 2019;83:1965-1967.

54. Chen K, Li Y, Dai Y, et al. Comparison of electrocardiogram characteristics and pacing parameters between left bundle branch pacing and right ventricular pacing in patients receiving pacemaker therapy. *Europace* 2019;21:673-680.

55. Jastrzebski M, Moskal P, Bednarek A, et al. Programmed deep septal stimulation: a novel maneuver for the diagnosis of left bundle branch capture during permanent pacing. *J Cardiovasc Electrophysiol.* 2020;31:485-493.

56. Su L, Xu T, Cai M, et al. Electrophysiological characteristics and clinical values of left bundle branch current of injury in left bundle branch pacing. *J Cardiovasc Electrophysiol.* 2020;31:834-842.

57. Cai B, Huang X, Li L, et al. Evaluation of cardiac synchrony in left bundle branch pacing: Insights from echocardiographic research. *J Cardiovasc Electrophysiol.* 2020;31:560-569.

58. Wang J, Liang Y, Wang W, et al. Left bundle branch area pacing is superior to right ventricular septum pacing concerning depolarization-repolarization reserve. *J Cardiovasc Electrophysiol.* 2020;31:313-322.

59. Ponnusamy SS, Muthu G, Kumar M, Bopanna D, Anand V, Kumar S. Mid-term feasibility, safety and outcomes of left bundle branch pacing-single center experience. *J Interv Card Electrophysiol.* 2021;60(2):337-346.

60. Ponnusamy SS, Arora V, Namboodiri N, Kumar V, Kapoor A, Vijayaraman P. Left bundle branch pacing: a comprehensive review. *J Cardiovasc Electrophysiol.* 2020;31(9):2462-2473.

61. Cingolani E, Goldhaber JI, Marban E. Next-generation pacemakers: from small devices to biological pacemakers. *Nat Rev Cardiol.* 2018;15:139-150.

62. Dawkins JF, Hu YF, Valle J, et al. Antegrade conduction rescues right ventricular pacing-induced cardiomyopathy in complete heart block. *J Am Coll Cardiol.* 2019;73:1673-1687.

63. Deshmukh P, Romanyshyn M: Direct His-Bundle pacing: present and future. *PACE* 2004;27:862-887.

64. Occhetta E, Bortnik M, Magnani A, et al. Prevention of ventricular desynchronization by permanent para-Hisian pacing after atrioventricular node ablation in chronic atrial fibrillation: A crossover, blinded, randomized study versus apical right ventricular pacing. J Am Coll Cardiol. 2006;47:1938-1945.

65. Barba-Pichardo R, Morina-Vaquez P, Fernandez-Gomez JM, Venegas-Gamero J, Herrera-Carranza M: Permanent His-bundle pacing: seeking physiological ventricular pacing. *Europace* 2010;12:527-533.

66. Kronberg MB, Mortensen PT, Poulsen SH, et al. His or para-His pacing preserves left ventricular function in AV block: a double-blind, randomized, crossover study. *Europace* 2014 ;16:1033-1039.

67. Pastore G, Aggio S, Baracca E, at al. Hisian area and right ventricular apical pacing differently affect left atrial function: an intra-patient evaluation. *Europace* 2014;16:1033-1039.

68. Vijayaraman P, Chung M, Dandamudi G, et al. His bundle pacing. *J Am Coll Cardiol.* 2018;72:927-947.

39

Diagnosis and Management of Syncope

Zachary D. Goldberger, Mohammed Ruzieh, and Blair P. Grubb

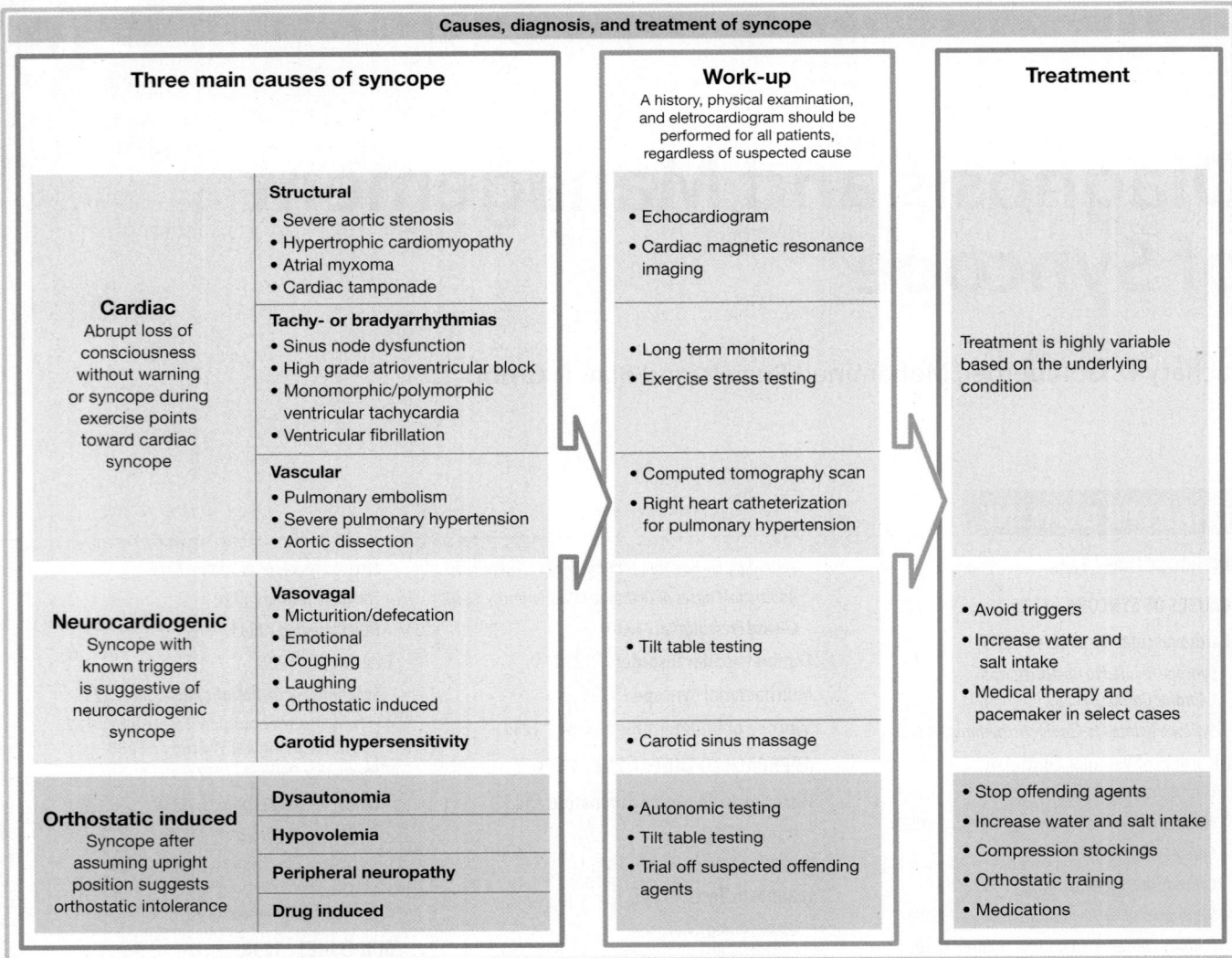

Causes, diagnosis, and treatment of syncope

Three main causes of syncope

Work-up
A history, physical examination, and eletrocardiogram should be performed for all patients, regardless of suspected cause

Treatment

Cardiac
Abrupt loss of consciousness without warning or syncope during exercise points toward cardiac syncope

Structural
- Severe aortic stenosis
- Hypertrophic cardiomyopathy
- Atrial myxoma
- Cardiac tamponade

Tachy- or bradyarrhythmias
- Sinus node dysfunction
- High grade atrioventricular block
- Monomorphic/polymorphic ventricular tachycardia
- Ventricular fibrillation

Vascular
- Pulmonary embolism
- Severe pulmonary hypertension
- Aortic dissection

- Echocardiogram
- Cardiac magnetic resonance imaging

- Long term monitoring
- Exercise stress testing

- Computed tomography scan
- Right heart catheterization for pulmonary hypertension

Treatment is highly variable based on the underlying condition

Neurocardiogenic
Syncope with known triggers is suggestive of neurocardiogenic syncope

Vasovagal
- Micturition/defecation
- Emotional
- Coughing
- Laughing
- Orthostatic induced

Carotid hypersensitivity

- Tilt table testing

- Carotid sinus massage

- Avoid triggers
- Increase water and salt intake
- Medical therapy and pacemaker in select cases

Orthostatic induced
Syncope after assuming upright position suggests orthostatic intolerance

Dysautonomia

Hypovolemia

Peripheral neuropathy

Drug induced

- Autonomic testing
- Tilt table testing
- Trial off suspected offending agents

- Stop offending agents
- Increase water and salt intake
- Compression stockings
- Orthostatic training
- Medications

Chapter 39 Fuster and Hurst's Central Illustration. Cardiac syncope tends to increase the risk of sudden cardiac death if left untreated, whereas neurocardiogenic and orthostatic causes usually follow a more benign course. Regardless of the cause, syncope may impair quality of life and confer serious physical injury if not properly treated. Treatment will vary based on the underlying etiology.

CHAPTER SUMMARY

This chapter summarizes the pathophysiology, etiology, diagnosis, and management of syncope (see Fuster and Hurst's Central illustration). Syncope is a common symptom, characterized by an abrupt, transient, and complete loss of consciousness, followed by spontaneous recovery. The incidence of syncope increases with age, with a lifetime prevalence of 40% and a recurrence rate of 14%. Given the myriad causes and protean manifestations of syncope, the diagnosis is often elusive, and the treatment will vary based on the underlying etiology. There are three main causes of syncope: cardiac (primarily due to arrhythmia or structural heart disease), neurocardiogenic (vasovagal syncope and carotid hypersensitivity), and orthostatic hypotension (dysautonomia, hypovolemia, and medication-induced). Cardiac syncope generally increases the risk of sudden cardiac death if left untreated, whereas neurocardiogenic and orthostatic causes usually follow a more benign course. Syncope, regardless of the cause, may impair quality of life and confer serious physical injury if not properly treated.

INTRODUCTION

Syncope is characterized by an abrupt, transient, and complete loss of consciousness. The presumed mechanism is cerebral hypoperfusion, which leads to the inability to maintain postural tone. Recovery after a syncopal episode is spontaneous.

Syncope can occur suddenly, without warning, or may be preceded by a prodrome of presyncope, including lightheadedness, dizziness but not true vertigo, nausea, a feeling of warmth, diaphoresis, and blurred or tunnel vision. Self-limited episodes of presyncope can occur in the absence of loss of consciousness. Syncope can significantly impact quality of life for patients and their families, particularly when it occurs abruptly without warning, is recurrent, or when it is likely to occur in relation to certain activities. In such cases, patients may need to adjust their lifestyle or even change occupation.

The prevalence of syncope in the general population, as reflected in the Framingham Study, was estimated at 3.0% in men and 3.5% in women over a 26-year follow-up.[1] In general, the incidence of syncope increases with age, with a lifetime prevalence of 40%, with a recurrence rate of 14%. Syncope accounts for 1% to 3% of emergency department visits and 6% of hospital admissions.[2] As a result, management of syncope is associated with significant resource use and expense—indeed, the annual cost of syncope hospitalizations is approximately $1.7 billion, with up to $26,000 per hospitalization.[3]

CAUSES OF SYNCOPE

The causes of syncope can be broadly classified into *cardiovascular disorders, disorders of vascular tone or blood volume,* and *cerebrovascular disorders.* The relative incidence of these categories varies with the clinical site from which the patients are selected; in hospitalized patients, syncope is most often a result of a cardiovascular disorder, whereas in the emergency room, other causes of syncope predominate.[4] In many cases, the cause of syncope may be multifactorial. Furthermore, in up to 50% of cases, the cause of syncope remains elusive even after an extensive, and often expensive evaluation.

Recent studies document the widely divergent risks of death that are associated with an episode of syncope, ranging from those that are benign to cardiac arrhythmias that are potentially lethal.[2] Data from the Framingham Heart Study suggests that the risk of all-cause mortality is increased by approximately 31% among all patients with syncope, but doubled with cardiac syncope.[2] Other studies find that syncope caused by cardiovascular disorders is associated with the highest risk for death, approaching 50% over 5 years and 30% in the first year after diagnosis.[4,5] The mortality is lower among patients with syncope from other causes (30% over 5 years and <10% in the first year), but still substantial. Syncope that is not associated with cardiac disease and is of undetermined cause is usually associated with the lowest mortality (6%–10% over 3 years and 24% over 5 years).[6]

For prognostic and therapeutic reasons, it is important to distinguish syncope from other causes of transient loss of consciousness, including seizures, psychogenic seizures, hypoglycemia, pharmacologic agents, and trauma. In some cases, this may prove difficult because reduced cerebral blood flow associated with syncope can cause tonic-clonic movements similar to those that occur with certain seizures. In one study, syncope had been misdiagnosed as seizures in 38% of patients who continued to have episodes despite adequate anticonvulsant therapy.[7] It is also important to differentiate between syncope and cardiac arrest. In the latter, there is loss of consciousness without spontaneous recovery.

Cardiovascular Disorders

Cardiac syncope can occur from either severe obstruction of cardiac output or disturbances of cardiac rhythm. Obstructive lesions and arrhythmias frequently coexist; indeed, one abnormality may accentuate the effects of the other. **Table 39–1** lists the cardiovascular disorders that may be associated with syncope.

Syncope Related to Obstruction of Cardiac Output

Obstruction to cardiac output in the left or right side of the heart may cause syncope. The relationship of syncope to exertion may provide clues to the etiology. Loss of consciousness during or immediately after exertion can occur with any of the cardiac causes of syncope, but is particularly common and may be the presenting symptom in patients with certain obstructive lesions, including aortic stenosis and hypertrophic cardiomyopathy. Studies suggest that in such patients, failure of cardiac output to increase adequately during exercise together with a reflex decrease in peripheral vascular resistance may play a role.[8,9] Nonexertional syncope related to acute decreases in preload or afterload, or to inotropic stimulation, may also occur in either aortic stenosis or hypertrophic cardiomyopathy (see Chapters 28 and 42). Transient arrhythmias can also induce syncope in patients with obstructive lesions. Syncope is an ominous sign in patients with hypertrophic cardiomyopathy, portending a significant risk for sudden cardiac death.[10] Syncope in patients with aortic stenosis suggests that the obstruction is severe and is associated with poor prognosis.

Malfunction of a left-sided prosthetic heart valve can produce transient and profound obstruction to blood flow resulting

TABLE 39–1. Cardiac Disorders Associated with Syncope

Obstructive
  Aortic stenosis
  Hypertrophic cardiomyopathy
  Mitral stenosis
  Prosthetic mitral or aortic valve malfunction
  Atrial myxoma
  Pulmonary embolism
  Pulmonary hypertension
  Unrepaired Tetralogy of Fallot
  Cardiac tamponade
Arrhythmic
  Sinus node dysfunction
  Atrioventricular block
  Supraventricular tachyarrhythmias
  Ventricular tachycardia
  Pacemaker disorders

in syncope. Mitral stenosis can produce cardiac syncope, but usually does so only when tachycardia or other arrhythmias occur (see Chapter 32). A left atrial myxoma may cause syncope by obstructing left ventricular (LV) filling. In some cases, the obstruction of LV inflow is posturally induced.

Obstruction in the pulmonary vasculature as a result of pulmonary artery hypertension, pulmonary stenosis, pulmonary embolism, or malfunction of a right-sided prosthetic valve can cause syncope. Pulmonary embolism as a cause of syncope should be suspected in paraplegic patients and in those who have been at prolonged bedrest.[11] In tetralogy of Fallot, because the right ventricular (RV) outflow obstruction is often fixed, the magnitude of flow through the right-to-left shunt increases when systemic resistance falls during exertion. This shunting can result in marked arterial hypoxemia, which may precipitate syncope. Cardiac tamponade, which affects both the right and the left sides of the heart, rarely causes syncope. The likelihood of syncope is increased by concomitant arrhythmias.

Syncope Related to Cardiac Arrhythmia

Arrhythmias are a common cause of syncope and must be considered in any patient, particularly when cardiac disease is present. Either extreme of ventricular rate (bradycardia or tachycardia) can depress cardiac output to the point of critical hypotension with cerebral hypoperfusion and syncope. The arrhythmias that produce syncope most often are due to sinus node dysfunction (bradycardia, exit block, or pauses), high-grade atrioventricular (AV) block, and ventricular tachycardia. Although arrhythmias are usually secondary to disorders such as ischemic heart disease, cardiomyopathy, valvular heart disease, or primary conduction system disease, they can, on occasion, occur in the absence of apparent heart disease.

Primary degenerative disease of the sinus node and the specialized conduction tissue is the most common cause of sinus node dysfunction (*sick sinus syndrome;* see Chapter 38). The sick sinus syndrome may be manifested by persistent or episodic sinus bradycardia or sinoatrial exit block, often with impaired subsidiary pacemakers. The presence of alternating sinus bradycardia or sinoatrial block with atrial tachyarrhythmias is referred to as the *bradycardia-tachycardia syndrome.* Syncope often occurs with asystole or bradycardia at the termination of tachycardia because of overdrive suppression of the sinoatrial and junctional pacemakers.[12] AV and intraventricular conduction defects are more prevalent in the sick sinus syndrome and, along with ventricular tachyarrhythmias, may be responsible for syncope in these patients.[13]

High-grade AV block may be a result of disease of either the AV node or the His-Purkinje system. Conduction block in the AV node is usually associated with a junctional pacemaker, a normal QRS complex, and a heart rate that can sustain blood pressure adequate to maintain consciousness, whereas AV block as a result of His-Purkinje system disease is usually associated with a wide-complex idioventricular escape rhythm that may be too slow to maintain adequate blood pressure. Bifascicular block in the presence of a prolonged PR interval suggests that His-Purkinje system disease is present and is associated with a substantial risk of developing high-grade AV block and

syncope. Progression to high-grade AV block in patients with bifascicular block and a normal PR interval is less common. Alternating bundle branch block (BBB) patterns (ie, right and left BBB [RBBB/LBBB]), or alternating left hemiblock patterns with an RBBB is termed trifascicular block, and should signal a cause of syncope.

Sinus bradycardia, AV block, or cardiac asystole may be mediated by reflex vagal mechanisms and have been observed in a variety of disease states or during diagnostic procedures.[14] For example, transient sinus bradycardia or AV block also can occur in apparently healthy young individuals, and may be due to mitral valve prolapse.[15]

Supraventricular tachyarrhythmias rarely cause syncope unless they occur in the presence of other abnormalities that decrease cerebral perfusion (decreased cardiac output because of structural heart disease, a neurocardiogenic reaction, disorders of vascular control, or reduced blood volume). Indeed, even in young patients, palpitations followed by syncope should raise the suspicion for ventricular, not supraventricular, tachyarrhythmias. As is the case for other causes of syncope, a neurocardiogenic reaction may be precipitated by the hemodynamic effects of arrhythmias. In such cases, syncope may be related to vasomotor factors and not be solely a result of heart rate.[12] Syncope can occur in patients with Wolff-Parkinson-White (WPW) syndrome who experience atrial fibrillation (AF) and a very rapid ventricular rate as a consequence of rapid anterograde conduction of AF across an accessory atrioventricular connection.

Ventricular tachycardia is the most common arrhythmic cause of syncope and often occurs in the setting of structural heart disease (especially coronary artery disease or prior revascularization). In the United States, ventricular tachycardia is usually associated with previous myocardial infarction (MI) and depressed left ventricular ejection fraction (LVEF), but it can also occur in nonischemic cardiomyopathy.

Ventricular tachycardia may also cause syncope in patients with normal LV function (ie, hypertrophic cardiomyopathy, long QT syndrome, short QT syndrome, Brugada syndrome, outflow tract ventricular tachycardia, arrhythmogenic right ventricular cardiomyopathy [ARVC], and idiopathic LV tachycardia).[16,17] Syncope is considered to be an ominous sign, portending a high risk for sudden cardiac arrest in patients with long QT syndrome, Brugada syndrome, and ARVC.

Torsades de pointes (TdP) ventricular tachycardia can cause syncope in patients with either congenital or acquired long QT syndrome (see Chapter 34). A normal QT interval does not preclude the diagnosis of long QT syndrome, because prolongation of repolarization can be intermittent. In some heritable forms of the syndrome, QT prolongation and ventricular tachycardia can be triggered by exercise or a startle response.[18] Although a number of drugs can prolong ventricular repolarization, the most frequent causes of acquired long QT syndrome are antiarrhythmic drugs (Vaughan Williams Class Ia and III) and electrolyte disorders (hypokalemia and hypomagnesemia). High grade or complete AV block can also lead to TdP (so-called brady-induced TdP). A pause preceding the onset of tachycardia is common, because the early afterdepolarizations thought to be responsible for TdP in some long QT syndrome patients are bradycardia dependent.

A variety of other drugs may produce or aggravate arrhythmias, resulting in syncope or presyncope. Type Ic antiarrhythmic drugs (eg, flecainide, propafenone) may cause ventricular arrhythmias in patients with structural heart disease, particularly known coronary artery disease with prior MI and low LVEF. β-adrenoceptor antagonists, calcium-channel blockers, digoxin, sotalol, and amiodarone are some of the agents that most commonly cause significant sinus bradycardia or AV block. Theophylline and β agonists, used for therapy of chronic obstructive pulmonary disease, may precipitate ventricular or supraventricular arrhythmias. Therapy with diuretics can cause hypokalemia and hypomagnesemia. Both caffeine and alcohol may precipitate either atrial or ventricular tachyarrhythmias.

In the patient who has an artificial ventricular pacemaker, near-syncope or syncope may be secondary to pacemaker malfunction or to the pacemaker syndrome. Dual-chamber pacemakers can produce pacemaker-mediated tachycardias when there is retrograde conduction of the ventricular impulse to the atria. Improvements in technology have reduced the incidence of this complication.

Disorders of Vascular Control or Blood Volume

Disorders of vascular control or blood volume that can cause syncope include reflex syncope (numerous etiologies) and a number of causes for orthostatic intolerance (**Table 39–2**).[19] Under normal circumstances, systemic blood pressure is regulated by a complex process that includes the musculature, the venous valves, the autonomic nervous system, and the renin-aldosterone-angiotensin system. Knowledge of these processes is a prerequisite to understanding the disorders of vascular control or blood volume that can cause syncope.

Maintenance of Postural Blood Pressure

A principal stress imposed while standing is produced by gravity displacing venous blood downward to a level below the heart. Although the renin-aldosterone-angiotensin system regulates long-term blood pressure responses to upright posture, the autonomic nervous system provides the majority of the short- and medium-term responses to postural change.[20]

In the normal supine individual, approximately one-quarter of the blood volume is in the thorax. On standing, there is a gravity-mediated displacement of between 300 and 800 mL of blood to both the dependent extremities and the inferior mesenteric area.[21] Approximately 50% of this displacement occurs within the first few seconds of standing, resulting in a drop in venous return to the heart and a mean fall in stroke volume of approximately 40%.[21] In the normal subject, accommodation to this change in posture occurs in less than 1 minute.

Immediately on standing, muscle contractions in the legs, abdomen, and arms, in concert with the venous valvular system, support blood pressure by facilitating venous return.[21] However, this alone is insufficient to maintain venous return and systemic blood pressure. The reduction in venous return with upright posture is followed by a slow progressive fall in arterial pressure and cardiac filling that produces less stretch

TABLE 39–2. Disorders of Vascular Control and Blood Volume

Reflex syncope
  Neurocardiogenic (vasovagal)
  Situational
  Carotid sinus hypersensitivity
Orthostatic intolerance
  Autonomic nervous system disorders
    Primary autonomic failure
      Pure autonomic failure
      Multiple system atrophy
      Postural orthostatic tachycardia syndrome
        Peripheral or partial dysautonomic
        Hyperadrenergic
        Autoimmune
      Acute autonomic failure
    Secondary autonomic failure
      Amyloidosis
      Diabetes
      Sarcoidosis
      Renal failure
      Cancer
      Nerve growth factor deficiency
      β-Hydroxylase deficiency
    Pharmacologic agents
    Certain heavy metals
      Mercury
      Lead
      Arsenic
      Iron
  Intravascular volume depletion
    Anemia
    Blood loss
    Dehydration
    Diuretics
  Venous pooling/vasodilation
    Prolonged bed rest
    Prolonged weightlessness
    Pregnancy
    Hypermobility
    Venous varicosities
    Pharmacologic agents
    Hyperbradykininism
    Mastocytosis
    Carcinoid syndrome

and reduces the discharge rate of aortic arch and carotid sinus baroreceptors. Fibers from these mechanoreceptors travel with unmyelinated vagal fibers from the atria and the ventricles to the nucleus tractus solitarii and other areas of the medulla that modulate vascular tone. In the resting supine position, impulses from these fibers increase efferent parasympathetic activity and have an inhibitory effect on efferent sympathetic activity to the heart. After standing, the drop in arterial pressure receptor firing in the carotid sinuses decreases efferent vagal activity and increases efferent sympathetic activity, producing a reflex increase in heart rate and peripheral vasoconstriction. As a result, assumption of upright posture results in a 10 to 15 bpm increase in heart rate, minimal change in systolic blood pressure, and an approximately 10 mm Hg increase in diastolic blood pressure.[22]

Any inability of this complex process to respond adequately or in a coordinated manner may result in varying degrees of postural hypotension and ultimately loss of consciousness. Failure of one component may be compensated for by increased action of another component. For example, a failure of the peripheral vasculature to constrict during upright posture may be compensated for by increased heart rate and myocardial contractility sufficient to maintain blood pressure. Nonetheless, compensatory mechanisms may not be sufficient, or may not be sustainable over long periods of time. Furthermore, compensatory mechanisms, if not modulated, may result in orthostatic hypertension and inappropriate sinus tachycardia.

Reflex Syncope

In each of the causes of reflex syncope, there is a sudden failure of the autonomic nervous system to maintain sufficient vascular tone during periods of gravitational stress resulting in hypotension (and sometimes bradycardia). The two types most commonly encountered are neurocardiogenic (vasodepressor or vasovagal) syncope and the carotid sinus syndrome.[23] The other forms of reflex syncope are frequently grouped together under the term *situational* because they occur in association with specific activities or conditions (such as micturition, defecation, swallowing, coughing, postprandial). It is important to realize that the reflexes responsible for neurocardiogenic syncope are normal; healthy individuals will experience neurocardiogenic syncope in the setting of a stimulus that is sufficiently strong and prolonged. However, some individuals develop neurocardiogenic syncope frequently and with relatively little provocation, suggesting that disorders of autonomic control exist.

Neurocardiogenic syncope can be quite diverse in presentation and tends to occur more often in young people.[24] The episodes often include three stages: a prodrome (nausea, sweating, lightheadedness, or visual alterations), abrupt loss of consciousness, and rapid recovery without a postictal state, although fatigue may be present after the episode. However, close to one-third of patients (often elderly) experience little if any prodrome and report a sudden loss of consciousness (drop attack).

The etiology of neurocardiogenic syncope is poorly understood. It can be provoked by prolonged standing, warm environments, emotional distress, and pain, although episodes can also occur without an identifiable trigger.[24] Many episodes of neurocardiogenic syncope are provoked by prolonged orthostatic stress. Gravity-mediated displacement of blood and venous pooling in dependent areas decreases venous return to the heart, resulting in a reflex-mediated increase in myocardial contractility that activates ventricular mechanoreceptors that would normally fire only during stretch.[25] This sudden increase in neural traffic to the medulla appears to mimic the conditions seen in hypertension, resulting in a "paradoxic" decrease in sympathetic activity that results in hypotension (vasodepressor response), and in some cases, an increase in vagal efferent activity that results in bradycardia (cardioinhibition). Other nonorthostatic stimuli (such as fear, fright, or epileptic discharges) can provoke virtually identical responses, suggesting that these patients may have an inherent predisposition to these events.[24]

During head upright tilt-table testing, individuals susceptible to neurocardiogenic syncope demonstrate a precipitous fall in blood pressure that is frequently (but not always) followed by a fall in heart rate (on occasion to the point of asystole).[26]

Carotid Sinus Hypersensitivity

Syncope caused by carotid sinus hypersensitivity is most common in men ≥50 years old and is precipitated by pressure on the carotid sinus baroreceptors, typically in the setting of shaving, a tight collar, or turning the head to one side. Activation of carotid sinus baroreceptors gives rise to impulses to the medulla oblongata that, in turn, activate efferent sympathetic nerve fibers to the heart and blood vessels, cardiac vagal efferent nerve fibers, or both. In patients with carotid sinus hypersensitivity, these responses may cause sinus arrest or AV block (a cardioinhibitory response), vasodilatation (a vasodepressor response), or both (a mixed response). The underlying mechanisms responsible for the syndrome are not clear, and validated diagnostic criteria do not exist.[27]

Some investigators have noted that the hemodynamic responses observed in neurocardiogenic syncope and carotid sinus hypersensitivity are similar, suggesting that the two syndromes may represent different aspects of the same condition.[28] Others have proposed that each of the reflex syncopes may occur in predisposed individuals when rapid activation of neuroreceptors from multiple sites (esophagus, bladder, rectum, or cough) activates a similar response.[29] Recent observations concerning defecation syncope support this.[26] What seems to distinguish the reflex syncopes from the other autonomic syndromes is that between episodes of syncope, these patients rarely complain of symptoms referable to the autonomic nervous system. Consequently, in the reflex syncopes, the autonomic nervous system functions normally, despite being at times "hypersensitive," in contrast to other conditions wherein the autonomic system appears to "fail," operating at a level sufficient for the body's needs, and thereby resulting in persistent levels of orthostatic intolerance.[26]

Syndromes of Orthostatic Intolerance

Orthostatic hypotension may occur as a result of hypovolemia or disturbances in vascular control (see Table 39-2). The latter may occur because of agents that affect the vasculature directly or to primary or secondary abnormalities of autonomic control. During the last two decades, several autonomic disorders have been identified that can impact vascular control and cause syncope. The schema presented here corresponds with that developed by the American Autonomic Society and the Heart Rhythm Society and attempts to present these disorders in a clinically useful framework.[19,30] Primary autonomic disorders that affect vascular control are often idiopathic, occur in the absence of other disease states that affect the autonomic nervous system, and may follow either an acute or chronic course. In contrast, the secondary forms occur in conjunction with another illness (such as amyloidosis or diabetes), in the setting of a known biochemical or structural alteration, or following exposure to various drugs or toxins (heavy metals, alcohol, or some chemotherapeutic agents) (**Tables** 39-2 and **39-3**).

TABLE 39–3. Pharmacologic Agents That May Cause or Worsen Orthostatic Intolerance

Angiotensin-converting enzyme inhibitors
α-Receptor blockers
Calcium channel blockers
β-Blockers
Phenothiazines
Tricyclic antidepressants
Bromocriptine
Opiates
Diuretics
Hydralazine
Ganglionic-blocking agents
Nitrates
Sildenafil citrate
Monoamine oxidase inhibitors
Chemotherapeutic agents
    Vincristine
    Vinblastine

Primary Causes of Autonomic Failure

Pure Autonomic Failure: Bradbury and Eggleston first reported an autonomic failure syndrome in 1925, coining the term *idiopathic orthostatic hypotension* to describe the disorder.[31] In the interim, it has become apparent that this term insufficiently describes the diffuse state of autonomic failure present in these patients, as evidence by impaired bladder, bowel, thermoregulatory, motor, and sexual function (all in the absence of somatic nerve involvement). Currently, the condition is referred to as *pure autonomic failure* (PAF).[32] Onset of symptoms in PAF is usually between ages 50 and 75 years, and affects twice as many men as women. PAF is manifested by orthostatic hypotension, syncope, and near syncope, neurocardiogenic bladder, constipation, heat intolerance, inability to sweat, and erectile dysfunction. Typically, the onset of symptoms is gradual and insidious, often with sensations of positional weakness, lightheadedness, and dizziness. Male patients often report that the earliest signs of PAF were erectile dysfunction and diminished libido; women often report that their earliest symptoms were urinary retention and incontinence. Although not the initial symptom, syncope may be the event that prompts the patient to seek medical attention. Whereas PAF may result in severe functional impairment, it infrequently leads to death.

Multiple System Atrophy: Multiple system atrophy (MSA) is a more severe form of autonomic failure, first reported by Shy and Drager in 1960.[33] In contrast to PAF, these patients display not only significant orthostatic hypotension, but also urinary and rectal incontinence, anhidrosis, iris atrophy, external ocular palsy, erectile dysfunction, rigidity, and tremor. As with PAF, the condition is twice as common in men as women, and usually starts in the fifth and sixth decades of life.[34] Although MSA may initially be indistinguishable from PAF, patients with MSA eventually experience somatic nervous system involvement.

MSA is subclassified into three groups according to the somatic system involvement.[35] Group I patients exhibit a muscle tremor similar to that seen in Parkinson disease (also referred to by some as suffering from striatonigral degeneration).[36] As opposed to patients with true Parkinson disease, MSA patients display more rigidity than tremor and the rigidity usually lacks the "lead pipe" or "cogwheel" character observed in Parkinson disease. Patients with the parkinsonism form of MSA often show a loss of facial expression as well as limb akinesia.

Group II (olivopontocerebellar degenerative atrophy) patients demonstrate pronounced cerebellar and/or pyramidal signs and symptoms. These patients display both gait disturbance and a truncal ataxia severe enough to prevent standing without assistance. They may have a mild intention tremor and severe slurring of speech with impaired diction. Group III (mixed) patients display features of both the parkinsonian and cerebellar groups.

The frequency of MSA may be underappreciated, as an autopsy study found that between 7% and 22% of patients thought to have Parkinson disease during life had neuropathologic changes consistent with the disorder. MSA is relentlessly progressive, with the vast majority of patients dying within 5 to 8 years after onset of the illness (although occasional patients have been reported to have lived up to 20 years).[35] Aspiration, apnea, and respiratory failure are the most frequent terminal events.

Postural Tachycardia Syndrome: Postural (orthostatic) tachycardia syndrome (POTS) is a somewhat less severe autonomic insufficiency in which heart rate increases excessively in response to upright posture.[37] POTS is a syndrome characterized by symptoms (often palpitations, near-syncope, weakness, fatigue) when moving from the supine to standing position, with concomitant increase in heart rate >30 bpm, and the absence of orthostatic hypotension (<20 mm Hg drop in systolic blood pressure).[19] There are two primary forms of the disorder. The more common type is referred to as the peripheral (or partial) dysautonomic form. These individuals appear to suffer from an inability to increase adequately peripheral vascular resistance in the face of continuing orthostatic stress. This leads to a greater than normal amount of blood pooling in the dependent areas of the body (including the mesenteric vasculature), which is then compensated for by an excessive increase in both heart rate and myocardial contractibility.

Patients with dysautonomic POTS experience constant tachycardia (up to 160 bpm) while standing, and often complain of palpitations, exercise intolerance, fatigue, lightheadedness, cognitive impairment, visual disturbances, dizziness, near-syncope, and syncope. Patients may complain of heat intolerance and that they constantly feel cold. Heart rate increases greater than 30 bpm or to a rate greater than 120 bpm, usually with minimal drop in blood pressure during the first 10 minutes of upright tilt.[37] Approximately 10% of dysautonomic POTS patients progress to PAF. Dysautonomic POTS often occurs following a viral infection, surgery, or trauma. Multiple studies suggest a link between POTS and the joint hypermobility syndrome.[38]

A second primary form of POTS is referred to as the *hyperadrenergic*, *β-hypersensitivity*, or *central* form. This form is thought to be associated with a failure of normal feedback mechanisms above the level of the baroreflex. Whereas the initial heart rate response to postural changes is adequate, the brain appears to be unable to discontinue the response, allowing heart rate to continue to rise. These patients may also be noted to have significant orthostatic *hypertension*. Although supine serum catecholamine levels are normal, upright levels are often quite elevated (over 600 mg/dL) and these patients often display an excessive response to an infusion of isoproterenol (greater than 30 bpm increase in response to 1 µg/min).

In contrast to patients with the peripheral dysautonomic form, patients with hyperadrenergic POTS complain more often of tremor, hyperhidrosis, diarrhea, panic attacks, and severe migraines headaches. Recent studies in a family with several affected members identified genes that appear to be responsible for hyperadrenergic POTS.[39] A defect was found in the genetic code for a protein that functions to recycle norepinephrine in the intra-synaptic cleft, allowing for excessively high serum levels of norepinephrine. Additional studies suggest that there may be several different genetic forms of the disorder. Most recently, a growing body of evidence suggests that POTS could be an autoimmune disorder, with a high proportion of POTS patients having adrenergic and/or muscarinic antibodies that affect heart rate, blood pressure, or both.[40,41]

Acute Autonomic Failure: Although less common than the other autonomic disorders, acute autonomic failure is dramatic in presentation.[42] The onset is surprisingly rapid and is characterized by severe widespread failure of both parasympathetic and sympathetic components of the autonomic nervous system, while the somatic system is unaffected. Patients may have profound orthostatic hypotension, and syncope may manifest simply by attempting to sit up in bed. Many suffer from complete anhidrosis and disturbances in bowel and bladder function that result in abdominal pain, cramping, bloating, nausea, and vomiting. Cardiac denervation is common, resulting in a fixed heart rate of 45 to 50 bpm and chronotropic incompetence. Most of these patients have high circulating levels of antibodies to adrenergic receptors within the ganglia of the autonomic nervous system, supporting the idea that the disorder is autoimmune in nature.[40]

Secondary Causes of Autonomic Dysfunction

A wide variety of conditions may cause orthostatic hypotension by disturbing normal autonomic function (see Table 39–2).[19,30] Almost any systemic illness that affects multiple organ systems (such as diabetes mellitus, amyloidosis, sarcoidosis, renal failure, and certain cancers) may disrupt autonomic function sufficiently so as to result in orthostatic hypotension and syncope. A subgroup of patients with autonomic failure syndrome (especially diabetic patients) have a combination of supine hypertension and orthostatic hypertension, thought to be caused by a failure to properly vasoconstrict when upright or properly vasodilate when supine. It is not uncommon for these patients to exhibit a fall in systolic blood pressure up to 100 mm Hg upon standing. In some hypertensive patients, a rapid fall in blood pressure may exceed the brain's autoregulatory ability to maintain perfusion, causing syncope even though the systemic blood pressure may at the time be in a

relatively normal range. Some investigators suggest that there may be an association between Alzheimer's disease and orthostatic hypotension as a consequence of effects on autonomic control.[43] Isolated enzyme abnormalities may also cause orthostatic hypotension, examples of which are nerve growth factor deficiency and β-hydroxylase deficiency.[44] In addition, certain pharmacologic agents may either produce or contribute to orthostatic hypotension by interfering with autonomic control (see Table 39–3).

Additional Causes of Orthostatic Intolerance

Intravascular volume depletion, venous pooling, certain pharmacologic agents, and a number of endogenous vasodilators may cause orthostatic hypotension and syncope. Anemia, acute blood loss, and dehydration may cause intravascular volume depletion. Venous pooling is more common in older individuals who have incompetent venous valves in the lower extremities. Individuals subjected to prolonged periods of bedrest or weightlessness often experience orthostatic hypotension. In addition to those pharmacologic agents that interfere with autonomic vascular control, a number of pharmacologic agents can cause orthostatic hypotension by reducing intravascular volume or causing vasodilatation. Certain endogenous vasodilators may cause syncope when they are present in high concentrations.

Clinical Presentation

The principal feature shared by the syndromes of orthostatic intolerance is a disturbance in cardiovascular regulation sufficient enough to result in orthostatic hypotension. Symptoms, the response to tilt testing (see section Diagnostic Tests), and associated comorbidities may assist in differentiating among the autonomic nervous system disorders. Symptoms are related to both the rate and magnitude of change in blood pressure. However, it may be difficult to fully distinguish between these disorders because there is a considerable degree of overlap between them and because our understanding of mechanisms remains incomplete.

In addition, these disorders should be distinguished from neurocardiogenic syncope. Patients with neurocardiogenic syncope tend to experience an abrupt fall in blood pressure that is commonly associated with definitive prodrome. In dysautonomic syncope, the drop in blood pressure tends to be slow and may not be perceived, resulting in a "drop attack" with little or no warning, particularly in older patients.[44] Those who experience a prodrome report feeling lightheaded, dizzy, and blurred or tunnel vision. In contrast to reflex syncope, dysautonomic syncope is seldom associated with either bradycardia or diaphoresis.[35] Patients with the dysautonomic forms of syncope find that symptoms are more common in the morning after waking from sleep and are made worse by situations that enhance peripheral venous pooling (extreme heat, fatigue, dehydration, and alcohol). Patients suffering from PAF and MSA may display severe chronotropic incompetence with a relatively fixed heart rate (usually around 50 to 70 bpm).[45]

Cerebrovascular Disorders

A number of cerebrovascular disorders can cause syncope. Syncope can occur in patients with extensive occlusive disease of the origins of the brachiocephalic vessels, such as pulseless disease (eg, aortic arch syndrome and Takayasu arteritis).[46] With lesser degrees of cerebral occlusive disease, as with atherosclerotic narrowing, transient lowering of arterial pressure such as that immediately following assumption of the upright posture may be followed by vague symptoms suggesting impaired cerebral blood flow. In patients with cerebrovascular occlusive disease, a transient decrease in cardiac output and arterial pressure may provoke syncope at levels of arterial pressure that would otherwise be tolerated (see section Multifactorial Syncope).

Impairment in, or loss of, consciousness in relation to changing positions of the head, particularly hyperextension and lateral rotation, has been attributed to mechanical narrowing of the vertebral arteries by skeletal deformities of the cervical spine. Such symptoms have been observed in patients with Klippel–Feil deformity, cervical spondylosis, and severe cervical osteoarthritis. Altered consciousness is often preceded by vestibular symptoms. However, when vertigo is a predominant symptom, the syndrome of benign postural vertigo must be considered.

Syncope in the *subclavian steal syndrome* is caused by major occlusive disease of the subclavian artery proximal to the origin of the vertebral artery. During upper extremity exercise, blood flow is shunted retrograde, by the circle of Willis, to the distal subclavian artery. The consequent decrease in cerebral circulation induces cerebral ischemia.[46] This syndrome is suggested by the findings of diminished brachial arterial pressure on the affected side, a bruit that is maximal over the supraclavicular area adjacent to the origin of the vertebral artery, and the induction of symptoms by exercise of the involved extremity.

Although focal neurologic symptoms and signs are the usual neurologic manifestations of cerebral emboli, transient loss of consciousness can be a primary presenting symptom. Syncopal episodes are more likely to occur when atherosclerotic occlusive disease involves the vertebrobasilar system, with compromised perfusion to the medullary arousal center. In vertebrobasilar vascular insufficiency, syncope or presyncope is nearly always preceded by symptoms of vertigo, diplopia, dysarthria, and ataxia. The episodes are generally attributed to micro emboli arising from an atherosclerotic plaque, although vasospasm or postural hypotension may contribute.

Multifactorial Syncope

The cause of syncope is often multifactorial. Patients with structural heart disease or cerebrovascular disease may be predisposed to lose consciousness when blood pressure is compromised because of other causes, such as orthostatic hypotension, a neurocardiogenic reaction, cerebrovascular disease, or an arrhythmia. In addition, patients may have more than one abnormality that alone can cause syncope. In these patients, the history may provide clues that enable the clinician to identify the cause of a particular event.

Syncope of Undetermined Cause

Unfortunately, despite careful diagnostic evaluation, the cause of syncope often remains elusive in as many as 50% of patients.

Furthermore, it is important to note that an abnormality discovered on testing may not be responsible for syncope. Unexplained syncope has a broad spectrum of etiologies. The varying mortality among patients with syncope of undetermined cause likely reflects the varying incidence of undetected cardiac syncope. A certain number of these patients may have experienced syncope from multiple causes.[47]

APPROACH TO THE PATIENT

The diagnosis of syncope can be challenging, in part because the cause, like the event, may be only transiently apparent. In addition, it is often difficult to discern between syncope or another causes for transient loss of consciousness.[48] Once syncope is suspected, risk stratification is paramount. This is particularly important because many of the life-threatening causes for syncope can be treated effectively to prolong and improve the quality of life. However, exclusion of a life-threatening cause is not the only goal. The efficacy of therapy depends to a great extent on an accurate diagnosis. Furthermore, a decision should be made to whether admit the patient to the hospital or evaluate in the outpatient settings. Admission to the hospital to expedite evaluation and treatment is appropriate if the cause of syncope is suspected to be due to serious condition such as arrhythmias, or obstructive cardiac disorders (see Table 39-1), if the syncope resulted in major trauma, or if there is persistent vital signs abnormality such as persistent hypotension despite appropriate treatment.[48,49] In the Syncope Evaluation in the Emergency Department Study (SEEDS), a syncope unit in the emergency room reduced hospital admission and total length of hospital stay without affecting recurrent syncope or mortality.[50] On the other hand, patients who have a normal heart and for whom the history strongly suggests vasovagal or situational syncope may be treated in the outpatient setting if the episodes are neither frequent nor severe.

History and Physical Examination

The history and physical examination remain of paramount importance in evaluating a patient with syncope, and may alone diagnose the etiology or reveal an alternative cause for loss of consciousness.[48,49]

History
The history should include questions about when and in what settings the event occurred. Medications should be carefully reviewed—including supplements, diet pills, and illicit drugs. Symptoms, the patient's posture, and activities preceding the event may provide clues to the cause. Elderly patients who experience lightheadedness or syncope immediately after assuming upright posture may have orthostatic hypotension. Bradycardia, caused by sinus node dysfunction or AV block, should be suspected in the elderly who experience abrupt loss of consciousness without warning. Syncope during exercise may be due to AV block, but should also raise concern for ventricular arrhythmias, especially in the setting of type 1 long QT syndrome, hypertrophic obstructive cardiomyopathy, or possibly catecholaminergic polymorphic ventricular tachycardia

(more common in children). Arrhythmic events are often (but not always) preceded by palpitations.

Exertional syncope may be seen in the context of obstructive lesions due to aortic stenosis (which may also engender potentially lethal arrhythmias). Of importance, neurocardiogenic syncope rarely occurs postexertion, or when the patient is supine, and arrhythmic etiologies should be suspected. Subclavian steal syndrome should be considered when syncope is provoked by upper extremity exercises.

Neurocardiogenic syncope should be suspected in young patients without apparent structural heart disease who lose consciousness after a particular trigger (ie, standing for a prolonged period or after venipuncture). Syncope while shaving or after turning one's head to the side suggests that carotid sinus hypersensitivity may be the cause.

Typically, neurocardiogenic syncope is associated with spontaneous recovery of consciousness within seconds when the patient becomes supine. One of the most valuable historical clues in trying to discern between a cardiac or neurocardiogenic cause for syncope is what the symptoms were after the event. Patients often experience prolonged fatigue, confusion, or disorientation after an episode of neurocardiogenic syncope.[51]

Whenever possible, the history should include observations of the patient during an episode. Video recordings of the patient made by bystanders using smartphone technology during an event can be particularly useful. Tonic-clonic movements may accompany loss of postural tone if cerebral anoxia is prolonged. Although trauma can occur with syncope, tongue biting and incontinence are more commonly associated with seizures.[51] The time course of the event may suggest an etiology of syncope. Most episodes of syncope are brief, seconds to minutes, although episodes in patients with dysautonomias may be more prolonged.

Patients should be asked whether a family history exists for cardiovascular disease, neurologic disorders, and early sudden death. Questions centering upon family members who had unexplained car accidents, died due to drowning, or even sudden infant death syndrome may provide valuable insight. Furthermore, it is difficult, but important to have a family member clarify if a relative's death was truly due to a "heart attack," given cardiac arrest is often is distinct from succumbing to an acute coronary syndrome. Secondary causes of orthostatic intolerance and autonomic failure should be sought (see Table 39-2).

The Evaluation of Guidelines in Syncope Study 2 (EGSYS) trial[52] derived a risk model that employed historical elements as a means of determining a cardiac cause of syncope in the emergency department setting. A score >3 identified cardiac syncope with a sensitivity of 95% and specificity of 61% (see **Table 39-4**).

Physical Examination

The physical examination should include evaluation of orthostatic blood pressure and heart rate measurements. Specifically, taken in the supine, sitting, and upright positions, and again in the upright position 3 to 5 minutes after standing to determine if abnormal changes in orthostatic control are present.

TABLE 39-4. Risk Score to Determine a Cardiac Cause of Syncope

Variable	P Value	OR (95% CI)	Score
Palpitations preceding syncope	<0.001	64.8 (8.94–69.8)	4
Heart disease or abnormal ECG, or both	<0.001	11.8 (7.7–42.3)	3
Syncope during effort	<0.001	17.0 (4.1–72.2)	3
Syncope while supine	0.007	7.6 (1.7–33.0)	2
Precipitating or predisposing factors, or both	0.01	0.3 (0.1–0.8)	−1
Autonomic prodromes	0.02	0.4 (0.2–0.9)	−1

Abbreviation: CI, confidence interval; ECG, electrocardiogram; OR, odds ratio

Blood pressure should be determined with the arm extended horizontally so as to diminish the hydrostatic effect that occurs when the arm is in a dependent position. Traditionally, orthostatic hypotension is defined as a fall in systolic blood pressure of at least 20 mm Hg or at least a 10 mm Hg fall in diastolic blood pressure during the first 2 minutes of standing. However, in some patients, a less dramatic fall in blood pressure may be associated with symptoms.[26]

Cardiac auscultation, especially when combined with appropriate physical maneuvers, may reveal evidence for structural heart disease. When the cause of syncope is unknown, an attempt to reproduce the event may assist in determining the cause. A Valsalva maneuver may reproduce cough syncope; hyperventilation for 2 to 3 minutes may reproduce episodes that are related to anxiety. Although carotid sinus massage may induce significant bradycardia in susceptible individuals, it is not recommended in elderly patients, and/or for those who may have carotid atherosclerotic disease, because the procedure may cause plaque to embolize. The absence of a carotid bruit does not exclude the presence of an atheroma that could be dislodged during carotid sinus massage. In a patient with syncope, a pause of longer than 3 seconds during carotid sinus massage suggests that carotid sinus hypersensitivity may be the cause.[53]

Diagnostic Tests

The history and physical examination guide the choice of diagnostic tests.

Blood Testing

Blood tests may sometimes be helpful in the initial evaluation of a syncopal patient. A complete blood count can evaluate for anemia, or suggest occult infection or systemic disease. Serum electrolytes, including potassium and magnesium, may suggest a metabolic abnormality, or increase the risk of arrhythmia (ie, hypo/hyperkalemia). More advanced testing could include supine and upright serum catecholamine levels when hyperadrenergic postural orthostatic tachycardia is suspected; drug levels can be measured when the patient's medication or an illicit drug has the potential to precipitate an arrhythmia (ie, digoxin, tricyclic antidepressants), although an electrocardiogram (ECG) is usually the first signal of drug toxicity. The role of troponin and brain natriuretic peptide is not well established for patients with syncope and is unlikely to affect decision-making.[54]

Electrocardiogram and Electrocardiographic Monitoring

Because of their transient nature, arrhythmic causes of syncope may be very difficult to diagnose. **Figure 39–1** lists the various diagnostic tests used for the evaluation of arrhythmic syncope. Although it is unlikely alone to provide a diagnosis, almost all patients should undergo a 12-lead surface ECG because it may identify abnormalities that can predispose to syncope. Specifically, Q waves suggestive of prior infarction; ventricular preexcitation (WPW syndrome); AV or BBB (especially alternating), or bifascicular block; short or long QT interval; RBBB with right precordial ST-segment elevation (Brugada syndrome); epsilon waves and/or right precordial T-wave inversion suggestive of ARVC; voltage and/or ST-T wave abnormalities

criteria suggestive of hypertrophic cardiomyopathy; or fragmented QRS complexes suggestive of scar. Certain patterns of early repolarization have also been implicated in sudden death (although most often a benign variant). Macrovolt/microvolt T-wave alternans and QT dispersion are two examples of many other signals that may suggest the substrate for an arrhythmia, which are harder to detect without computerized software. The signal-averaged ECG, which was developed to detect late potentials following MI, is rarely used for that purpose in light of the several clinical trials that demonstrated that LVEF ≤35% and the presence of heart failure predict benefit from an implantable cardioverter-defibrillator (ICD).

Since many arrhythmias are intermittent, continuous ECG monitoring (Holter monitor) is a widely used screening test for suspected arrhythmic syncope, but it has a low yield in unselected patients. One 24-hour monitoring period may not be sufficient for detecting transient rhythm disturbances. However, the diagnostic yield increases only slightly with more

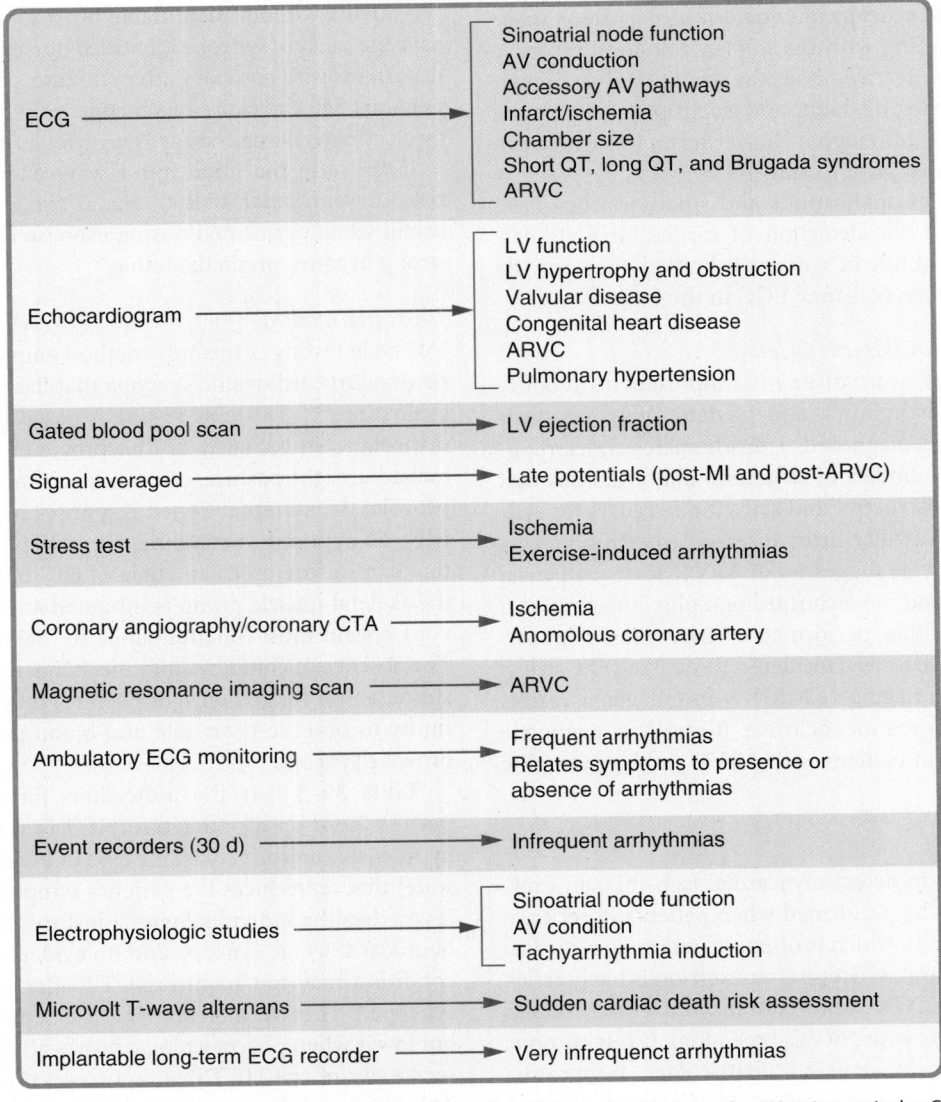

Figure 39–1. Diagnostic tests for arrhythmic syncope. ARVC, arrhythmogenic right ventricular cardiomyopathy; AV, atrioventricular; CT, computed tomography; CTA, computed tomography angiography; ECG, electrocardiogram; LV, left ventricular; MI, myocardial infarction.

prolonged monitoring. When a Holter monitor does not document an arrhythmia, a patient-activated ECG device (event recorder) may prove efficacious, particularly if the episodes are infrequent (days to weeks).[55] In patients without ICDs, event recorders should not be used when significant arrhythmias are thought to be the likely cause of symptoms. In those situations, mobile cardiac outpatient telemetry monitoring may be appropriate, given patient- or auto-triggering of a significant arrhythmia will be remotely transmitted to technicians who will see the arrhythmia in real time. It should be remembered that any device is most useful with symptom-correlation; indeed, the absence of an arrhythmia associated with a syncopal event may be as "diagnostic" as identifying one.

Patients in whom syncope is very infrequent (weeks to months between episodes) may benefit from an implantable loop recorder (ILR), which is a small device inserted subcutaneously in the chest near the sternum that can store up to 45 minutes of retrospective electrocardiographic data, and can record automatically or be activated by the patient. Implantable loop recorders provide diagnostic information in up to two-thirds of patients with syncope of undetermined cause. A diagnostic strategy beginning with the implantable loop recorder may be more cost-effective than the traditional approach (external event recorder, tilt-table, and electrophysiologic testing) in some patients (although a shorter term, less expensive monitor may be needed prior to an ILR).[56]

Lately, smartphones applications and smart watches have gained popularity for the detection of cardiac arrhythmias. Although their current role in syncope is limited, they provide hope for a cost-effective, real-time ECG in the future.[57]

Evaluation for Structural Heart Disease
Testing for structural heart disease is important to identify patients at risk for arrhythmia and to determine prognosis when an arrhythmia is diagnosed. Transthoracic echocardiography can identify a number of structural abnormalities that are associated with obstructive and arrhythmic causes for syncope such as severe valvular heart disease, hypertrophic cardiomyopathy, and may be suggestive of ARVC. Rarely, an atrial myxoma can be found on echocardiographic imaging. An echocardiogram should be performed whenever the diagnosis of structural heart disease is considered to be likely.[58] Cardiac magnetic resonance imaging (CMRI) is useful when results from echocardiogram are inconclusive. It also has diagnostic and prognostic value in patients with ARVC and hypertrophic cardiomyopathy.[16,59]

Cardiac Stress Testing
In addition to its use to detect myocardial ischemia, an exercise stress test should be performed when patients experience syncope during exertion, which is often secondary to a cardiac cause. On the other hand, syncope after exertion is likely reflex mediated.[60] Exercise ECG treadmill test may unveil ventricular arrhythmias in patients with ARVC, type I long QT syndrome, catecholaminergic polymorphic ventricular tachycardia (CPVT), or hypertrophic cardiomyopathy. Cases of exercise-induced high-grade AV block have also been reported.[61] In

addition, exercise can be used to assess hemodynamic response with exertion in patients with aortic stenosis and hypertrophic cardiomyopathy.

Electrophysiological Study
When noninvasive testing does not diagnose arrhythmic causes, an electrophysiologic study may be useful in high-risk patients (those with structural heart disease, suspicious arrhythmia by ECG monitoring, or recurrent syncope) to assess sinus and AV node function and susceptibility to supraventricular and ventricular tachyarrhythmias (see Chapters 35 and 37). The yield of electrophysiologic testing in patients with an otherwise normal evaluation for syncope is approximately 3%.[56] Furthermore, the sensitivity of electrophysiologic testing for bradyarrhythmias is low.[62] However, electrophysiologic testing can be useful in stratifying risk among symptomatic patients with BBB and in those with bifascicular block.[63] Patients who receive a permanent pacemaker on the basis of electrophysiologic testing also have a favorable prognosis, with a low rate of symptom recurrence.[63]

Patients without identifiable heart disease are less likely to have the cause of syncope identified by electrophysiologic study. In patients with coronary artery disease, particularly those with previous MI, the cause of syncope most commonly identified by electrophysiologic study is ventricular tachycardia.[62]

The use of the microvolt T-wave alternans test to stratify risk for ventricular arrhythmias is evolving. The test is most useful when performed during exercise and appears to have a strong negative predictive value.[64]

Tilt-Table Testing
Tilt-table testing is the only method employed for the diagnosis of neurocardiogenic syncope that has undergone extensive evaluation.[48,49] Tilt-table testing is based on the principle that orthostatic stress, such as that provided by a period of prolonged upright posture, can produce venous pooling and thus provoke the aforementioned responses in susceptible individuals. As opposed to standing, the patient is placed on a table that can incline up to an angle of 60° to 70°. In this position, the skeletal muscle pump is inhibited and the autonomic nervous system must function alone to maintain blood pressure. The absence of compensatory mechanisms in the presence of a stimulus (prolonged upright posture) may provide the opportunity to observe heart rate and blood pressure patterns that provoke syncope.

Table 39–5 lists the indications for tilt-table testing. A positive head up tilt-table test (HUTT) is one that provokes a hypotensive episode (or in the case of POTS, a tachycardic episode) that reproduces the patient's symptoms.[48] A young, otherwise healthy individual with a history that strongly suggests neurocardiogenic syncope and no evidence of life-threatening condition may not require HUTT after an initial episode of syncope.[49] The specificity of HUTT is reported to be near 90%, but lower when pharmacologic provocation is employed.[65] The sensitivity of the HUTT is reported to be between 20% and 74%, the variability a result of differences in study populations, protocols, and the absence of a true "gold standard" to which

TABLE 39–5. Head-Up Tilt-Table Testing

Indications for head-up tilt-table testing

1. Unexplained recurrent syncope or single syncopal episode associated with injury (or significant risk of injury) in absence of organic heart disease.
2. Unexplained recurrent syncopal episodes or a single syncopal episode associated with injury (or significant risk of injury) in setting of organic heart disease after exclusion of potential cardiac cause of syncope.
3. After identification of a cause of recurrent syncope in situations in which determination of an increased predisposition to neurocardiogenic syncope could alter treatment.

Conditions in which tilt-table testing may be useful

1. Differentiating convulsive syncope from epilepsy.
2. Evaluation of recurrent near syncope or dizziness.
3. Evaluation of syncope in autonomic failure syndromes.
4. Exercise- or postexercise-induced syncope in absence of organic heart disease in whom exercise stress testing cannot reproduce an episode.
5. Evaluation of recurrent unexplained falls.
6. Educating patients about syncope/presyncope symptoms, and teaching counterpressure maneuvers.

the results of the test can be compared.[66,67] The reproducibility of the test (in a time frame ranging from several hours to weeks) is 80% to 90% for an initially positive response, but less for an initially negative response (ranging from 30% to 90%).

It is important to remember that the type of autonomic stress provided by tilt-table testing is different from that which the patient encounters clinically. The International Study of Syncope of Unknown Etiology (ISSUE) compared heart rates during syncopal episodes induced during tilt-table testing with those that occurred spontaneously (as documented by an implantable loop recorder) and showed that spontaneous events were more likely to be associated with significant bradycardia.[68]

Abnormal tilt-table responses can be classified into five groups.[66] The first is referred to as a *classic neurocardiogenic response*, which is characterized by an abrupt drop in blood pressure. When accompanied by a significant drop in heart rate, this is referred to as a *vasovagal response*; in the absence of a decrease in heart rate, a *vasodepressor response*. A second pattern, referred to as a *dysautonomic* (or *delayed orthostatic*), is characterized by a gradual progressive fall in blood pressure with relatively little change in heart rate. This pattern is often noted in the autonomic failure syndromes. The third pattern, termed a *postural tachycardic response*, is associated with a >30 bpm increase in heart rate (or a heart rate of >120 bpm) during the first 10 minutes of the baseline tilt. The fourth pattern is called *cerebral syncope*. These patients experience syncope in the absence of systematic hypotension concomitant with intense cerebral vasoconstriction (as determined by transcranial Doppler), as well as cerebral hypoxia (as determined by electroencephalogram). The fifth response pattern is *psychogenic*. These patients are noted to experience loss of consciousness in the absence of systemic hypotension or any observable change in electroencephalogram or transcranial Doppler recording.[69] These patients are often found to suffer

from psychiatric disorders that range from conversion reactions to severe depression. Patients suffering from conversion reactions are not consciously aware of these events.[70] Many patients with psychogenic syncope are young women who have been victims of sexual abuse.

Other Imaging

Due to its low yield in providing diagnostic information that would alter management, brain imaging using computed tomography (CT) or magnetic resonance imaging (MRI) is not routinely recommend in the absence of head trauma, focal neurological deficits, parkinsonism, or cognitive impairment. Similarly, carotid ultrasound has low yield in patients with syncope.[49,71] Pulmonary embolism (PE) is not a common cause of syncope, and thus screening for PE is not warranted in all patients,[72,73] but may be considered in those with other symptoms or signs of PE who are at high risk for it such as active malignancy, recent immobilization, or hypercoagulable state.

Treatment

Treatment of syncope depends to a great extent on the cause. However, regardless of the etiology, patients should be counseled to minimize exposure to factors that have or are likely to provoke a syncopal episode. This is particularly important for individuals with neurocardiogenic syncope in whom prolonged standing or specific environmental factors have played a role in initiating syncope. Patients should be counseled to avoid situations in which they or others could be injured where they lose consciousness, particularly when syncope occurs frequently, abruptly, and without warning.

A patient who has lost consciousness should be placed in a position that maximizes cerebral blood flow, offers protection from trauma, and secures the airway. Whenever possible, the patient should be placed supine with the head turned to the side to prevent aspiration and the tongue from blocking the airway. Assessment of the pulse and direct cardiac auscultation may assist in determining if the episode is associated with a bradyarrhythmia or tachyarrhythmia. Clothing that fits tightly around the neck or waist should be loosened.

Syndromes of Orthostatic Intolerance

Therapies for the syndromes of orthostatic intolerance target the various components of the complex mechanisms responsible for control of systemic blood pressure including blood volume, the skeletal muscle pump, heart rate, and central and peripheral components of the autonomic nervous system. **Table 39–6** lists therapies and the syndromes for which they are used.

Nonpharmacological Treatment: Moderate aerobic and isometric exercises are of paramount importance because these therapies enhance skeletal muscle pump function and thereby venous return to the heart. Patients with orthostatic hypotension should be instructed to move their legs prior to rising in order to facilitate venous return and to rise slowly and systematically (supine to seated, seated to standing) from the bed or a chair. Whenever possible, medications that aggravate the problem (eg, vasodilators, diuretics) should be discontinued.

TABLE 39–6. Orthostatic Intolerance Syndrome Therapies

Treatment	Application	Form Effective In				Problems
		NCS	PD	HA	OH	
Reconditioning	Aerobic exercise 20 min 3 times/wk	X	X	X	X	If done too vigorously may worsen symptoms
Physical maneuvers (tilt training, etc)	30 min 3 times/d	X				Noncompliance is common
Sleeping with head tilted upright	During sleep	X		X	X	
Hydration	2 L PO/d	X	X		X	Edema
Salt	2–4 g/d	X	X		X	Edema
Fludrocortisone	0.1–0.2 mg PO qd	X	X		X	Hypokalemia, hypomagnesemia, edema
Metoprolol	25–100 mg bid	X				Fatigue
Labetalol	100–200 mg PO bid			X		Fatigue
Midodrine	5–10 mg PO tid	X	X		X	Nausea, scalp itching, supine hypertension
Methylphenidate	5–10 mg PO tid	X	X	X		Anorexia, insomnia, dependency
Bupropion	150–300 mg XL/qd		X	X	X	Tremor, agitation, insomnia
Clonidine	0.1–0.3 mg PO bid			X		Dry mouth, blurred vision
	0.1–0.3 mg patch qwk					
Pyridostigmine	30–60 mg PO/d		X		X	Nausea, diarrhea
SSRI-escitalopram	10 mg PO/d	X	X		X	Tremor, agitation, sexual problems
Erythropoietin	10,000–20,000 µg SC qwk	X	X		X	Pain at injection site, expensive
Octreotide	50–200 µg SC tid		X	X	X	Nausea, diarrhea, gallstone
Permanent pacing Ivabradine	5–7.5 mg PO bid	X	X		X	Nausea, flashing lights
Droxidopa	100–600 mg PO tid	X				Nausea, supine hypertension

Abbreviations: BID, twice daily; HA, hyperadrenergic postural orthostatic tachycardia syndrome; NCS, neurocardiogenic syncope; OH, orthostatic hypotension; PD, partial dysautonomia; PO, orally; qd, once daily; qwk, every week; SC, subcutaneously; SSRI, selective serotonin reuptake inhibitor; tid, three times per day; XL, extended release.

A variety of physical maneuvers have been employed to treat the syndromes of orthostatic intolerance. Tilt training has been advocated; for neurocardiogenic syncope, however, long-term compliance is often poor.[74] Isometric counter maneuvers, such as tensing of the arm and leg muscle, can sometimes prevent neurocardiogenic syncope if used at the first onset of symptoms.[75] Sleeping with the head of the bed elevated 15 cm above the feet is reported to be useful in neurocardiogenic syncope and the autonomic failure syndromes. Elastic support stockings can be helpful in some patients; to be truly effective, however, they must be waist high and provide a minimum of 30 mm Hg of ankle counterpressure. In some patients, salt and water loading increase intravascular volume and are effective in controlling syncope.[76]

Pharmacological Therapy: Stopping or reducing vasoactive agents can reduce syncope specially in older patients and should be attempted whenever possible.[77] Nonetheless, many patients require pharmacologic therapy. β-adrenoceptor antagonists were one of the first agents used to prevent neurocardiogenic syncope. The postulated mechanism is from the negative inotropic effect of these drugs reducing the degree of cardiac mechanoreceptor activation provoked by a sudden drop in venous return. However, randomized trials of β-blockers have yielded mixed results. In the Prevention of Syncope Trial (POST), metoprolol was ineffective in patients who were younger than 42 years of age, but decreased the incidence of syncope in patients who were older than 42 years of age, raising the possibility that there may be important age-related differences in response to pharmacotherapy.

The mineralocorticoid fludrocortisone, in addition to promoting sodium and fluid retention, appears to enhance peripheral α-receptor sensitivity (promoting vasoconstriction). In patients with vasovagal syncope, fludrocortisone can be helpful specially when a dose of 0.2 mg/day is achieved, and patients are volume replete.[78]

Several vasoconstrictive agents have been employed as treatments. The first of these were ephedra alkaloids such as dexedrine and methylphenidate, both of which are α-receptor stimulants.[79] Midodrine, another α-agonist, has been approved by the US Food and Drug Administration for the treatment of symptomatic orthostatic hypotension and was shown to be effective in preventing neurocardiogenic syncope.[80] Bupropion is a norepinephrine and dopamine reuptake inhibitor that has been useful in certain patients. It tends to have fewer sexual side effects, but may aggravate hypertension. Other vasoconstrictive substances, such as theophylline, ephedrine, and yohimbine, also are reported to be effective; however, tolerance of these agents is often poor.

The α_2-receptor agonist clonidine causes a paradoxic increase in blood pressure in patients with autonomic failure and a high degree of postganglionic sympathetic impairment. These individuals appear to have reduced peripheral sympathetic stimulation, but increased density of postjunctional α_2 receptors throughout the vasculature. Whereas clonidine causes a reduction in central sympathetic output with subsequent blood pressure reduction in normal subjects, in patients with autonomic failure, the vasoconstrictive effects of the drug seem to predominate.[44] Clonidine may be most useful in patients with both hyper- and hypotensive episodes.

Recent investigations suggest that the acetylcholinesterase inhibitor pyridostigmine may be an effective agent for both orthostatic hypotension and postural tachycardia syndrome.[81] Randomized, double-blind, placebo-controlled trials show that the agent is safe and effective and seems to be able to prevent falls in blood pressure without exacerbating supine hypertension.[82]

Evidence that serotonin plays a vital role in regulation of heart rate and blood pressure and the postulated role of serotonin in neurocardiogenic syncope has led to the investigation of selective serotonin reuptake inhibitors as a treatment for the disorder. Several open-label studies and one double-blind, randomized, placebo-controlled trial have demonstrated that the serotonin reuptake inhibitors prevent recurrent neurocardiogenic syncope.

It has been observed that many patients suffering from the autonomic failure syndromes have some degree of anemia. In 1993, Hoeldtke and Streeten published a landmark study demonstrating that erythropoietin given by subcutaneous injection would not only raise red cell counts, but would also prevent orthostatic hypotension. Other studies have confirmed these findings, demonstrating that erythropoietin is an effective treatment for orthostatic hypotension. Erythropoietin has vasoconstrictive effects (related to its effects on peripheral metric oxide) that are independent of its effect on red cell production.

Octreotide, a synthetic somatostatin analogue, causes splanchnic mesenteric vasoconstriction, thus enhancing venous return to the heart.[83] Ivabradine, a selective sinus node slowing agent, can reduce heart rate without affecting blood pressure. It is an approved medication to lower the heart rate in patients with heart failure, and has been employed for inappropriate sinus tachycardia. However, studies have reported that ivabradine may be useful in the management of both POTS and neurocardiogenic syncope, especially when β-adrenoceptor antagonists are ineffective or not tolerated.[84–86] Droxidopa is a synthetic amino acid precursor that acts as a prodrug to the neurotransmitter norepinephrine, resulting in peripheral vasoconstriction.[87] It has been approved in the United States for the treatment of neurogenic orthostatic hypotension. In patients with low circulating levels of adenosine, theophylline may be effective.[88] Recently, sibutramine, a norepinephrine transport inhibitor, was effective in treating a small group of patients who failed other therapies.[89] Biofeedback therapy also has been useful in preventing neurocardiogenic syncope provoked by a variety of psychogenic stimuli.[24]

Pacemaker Therapy

Despite several trials evaluating its efficacy, the role of permanent cardiac pacing for neurocardiogenic syncope remains somewhat controversial. Initial randomized trials reported that pacing was effective in preventing syncope.[90–92] However, because all patients who received a pacemaker were paced and patients in the control group did not receive a pacemaker, there were concerns that the observed benefit could be a result of placebo effect. In two ensuing studies, pacemakers were implanted in all patients who were then randomized to having the pacemaker programmed to an "on" or "off" mode. The Vasovagal Pacemaker Study II (VPS 2) reported no significant reduction in the time to a first recurrence of syncope during dual-chamber pacing over 6 months of follow-up.[93] The Vasovagal Syncope and Pacing Trial (SYNPACE) also reported that there was no significant difference between the "on" and "off" groups.[94] However, they did observe that the subgroup of patients who had demonstrated asystole during tilt-table testing had a significant increase in time to first syncope recurrence compared to those with bradycardia alone (91 vs 11 days). The ISSUE II trial reported that permanent pacing in patients with periods of asystole had a significant reduction in the frequency of syncope.[95] This observation leads to the ISSUE III trial, in which implantable loop recorders were used to identify asystole during the patient's syncopal events. Each patient with documented asystole then received a dual-chamber pacemaker, with half of them being randomly assigned to the pacemaker being "on" and half being "off."[96] After 1 year, the patients were crossed over (the ones who had pacing "off" were converted to "on" and vice versa). They reported a 57% relative risk reduction of syncope for pacemaker "on" patients at 2 years, with 25% of "on" versus 57% of "off" patients having had syncope recurrence. In many patients, however, a fall in blood pressure precedes the decline in heart rate; therefore, the increase in heart rate will not prevent the loss of postural tone. Newer systems using continuous RV impedance measurements have been developed that can provide an indirect measurement of blood pressure by the pacemaker. Preliminary observational studies have suggested that this technology may be superior to standard pacing methods in patients suffering from vasovagal syncope, particularly if they demonstrate cardioinhibitory response on tilt table test.[97] These findings were recently supported by the double blinded, controlled SPAIN study which demonstrated significant benefit with dual-chamber closed-loop stimulation pacing compared to sham pacing in patients with cardioinhibitory vasovagal syncope.[98] Patients with the cardioinhibitory or mixed forms of carotid sinus hypersensitivity may also benefit from permanent pacing.[99] In SAFE PACE, permanent pacing reduced falls, recurrent syncope, and injuries in elderly patients with frequent nonaccidental falls and cardioinhibitory carotid sinus hypersensitivity.[100]

For patients who suffer from syncope with little or no prodrome, in whom other forms of therapy have failed, permanent pacing can potentially reduce the frequency of syncope or prolong the time from onset of symptoms to loss of consciousness. This may allow the patient sufficient time to take evasive action (ie, lie down) and prevent injury if not loss of consciousness.

In contrast to reflex syncope, the autonomic failure syndromes can be associated with symptoms in addition to hypotension, some of which are easier to control than others. In addition, some of the autonomic disorders are chronic and progressive necessitating treatment alterations to meet the patient's changing needs. The patient with a severe form of autonomic neuropathy may encounter a wide range of both personal and social difficulties that may include psychosocial problems that necessitate a multidisciplinary approach, including social work, psychological therapy, and physical therapy.

Cerebrovascular Disorders

The treatment of recurrent syncope in cerebrovascular disease is predicated on an accurate diagnosis. In this regard, it is essential to segregate the potential contribution of cardiac and vascular factors and their interplay. Anticoagulants and/or platelet antiaggregant agents are recommended for the prevention of embolic disease from the heart or central vessels. Endarterectomy or percutaneous dilatation should be considered in carotid arterial occlusive disease.

Cardiovascular Disorders

Obstructive heart disease: Open cardiac surgery or minimally invasive interventions are often the treatment of choice for patients with syncope caused by obstructive heart disease. Patients with hypertrophic cardiomyopathy and syncope may respond well to pharmacologic therapy, but certain patients may respond to AV sequential pacing. However, in patients with severe obstruction and persistent symptoms, septal myectomy or alcohol septal ablation should be considered. High-risk patients with hypertrophic cardiomyopathy benefit from placement of an ICD.[101] Among all patients with obstructive heart disease and recurrent syncope, the diagnosis of fixed pulmonary hypertension is most difficult to treat because effective therapeutic options are limited (see Chapter 57).

Arrhythmic Syncope: Detailed discussions of therapy for cardiac arrhythmias are presented in Chapters 34 to 38 of this book. General principles of arrhythmia management as they apply to patients with syncope are summarized here. Treatment of arrhythmic syncope requires accurate definition of the arrhythmia associated with syncope or presyncope.

The bradycardic rhythm disturbances responsible for syncope, primarily AV and sinoatrial pauses or exit block, usually require the implantation of a permanent pacemaker. However, patients who are receiving drugs that cause or contribute to the bradyarrhythmia may benefit from withdrawal or substitution of the offending agent.[102] Patients with bradycardia-tachycardia syndrome usually require pacemaker therapy, because the antiarrhythmic agents required for control of the tachycardia often further suppress sinoatrial function; at times, catheter ablation is performed in concert with pacemaker implantation. A select group of patients with symptomatic sick sinus syndrome may benefit from oral theophylline.[103]

Implicit in the approach to the tachycardias causing syncope is the accurate diagnosis of a specific tachycardia. The definition of the tachycardia and the response to antiarrhythmic therapy are often achieved best in the electrophysiologic laboratory. Patients with syncope caused by supraventricular tachycardia associated with an atrioventricular accessory pathway are most often treated with catheter ablation. Catheter ablation is also a successful mode of therapy in patients with AV nodal reentry supraventricular tachycardia, atrial flutter, and some atrial tachycardias (see Chapter 35) (although supraventricular tachycardia rarely causes syncope).

ICDs are the first-line therapy for ventricular tachycardia in the setting of structural heart disease. It is important to recognize that some patients may continue to experience presyncope or even syncope if cerebral hypoperfusion occurs before the ICD terminates the arrhythmia. Some patients may require additional antiarrhythmic drugs to reduce the frequency of shocks from the ICD. Ventricular tachycardia ablation may be palliative for ventricular tachycardia, which requires frequent ICD shocks. Catheter ablation also may be effective for outflow tract tachycardias, bundle branch reentrant tachycardia, fascicular tachycardias, and LV tachycardia.

In patients with polymorphic ventricular tachycardia in the setting of a long QT interval (TdP), the potential offending drug(s) (usually an antiarrhythmic drug) should be stopped. Acute therapy includes intravenous magnesium and measures to increase the heart rate and shorten electrical diastole (ie, cardiac pacing). Long-term therapy for congenital long QT syndrome may include β-blockers, permanent pacing, an implantable defibrillator, and lifestyle changes.

Pacemaker-induced hypotension and syncope are rectified by changing from RV pacing to AV sequential pacing (if possible) when hypotension is a result of loss of atrial transport or neurocardiogenic response is responsible for symptoms. Pacemaker-mediated tachycardia can usually be corrected by reprogramming the pacemaker. Pacemaker malfunction or myopotential inhibition requires a change in programming or replacing the defective system component.

Syncope of Unknown Cause

Treatment of syncope can be particularly challenging when the cause is unknown. Often, treatment must be targeted to the most likely cause and to prolong life. This is particularly true for patients in whom an arrhythmia is the likely (but undocumented) cause of syncope. Certain patients who are at high risk for sudden cardiac arrest may benefit from an ICD even when it is not clear that a ventricular arrhythmia caused syncope. Patients with certain cardiac conduction abnormalities may benefit from a permanent pacemaker.

GUIDELINES

The European Society of Cardiology (ESC) released its first set on guidelines the diagnosis and management of syncope in 2001,[104] which was followed by three additional iterations, the most recent update in 2018.[48,105,106] The American College of Cardiology (ACC), in association with the American Heart Association (AHA) and Heart Rhythm Society (HRS), issued its first set of syncope guidelines in 2017.[49] These guidelines from the ESC and the ACC/AHA/HRS have important similarities in recommendations, largely centered upon cardiac syncope, reflex-mediated syncope, and orthostatic (neurogenic hypotension). There are also notable differences, which are due to several factors—specifically, differences in the writing group selection and composition, differences in defining classes of recommendations, interpretation of evidence cited, and socioeconomic and cultural differences in clinical practice between North America and Europe.[107] These guidelines are valuable documents that serve to inform the multidisciplinary management of syncope, and are not meant to supplant clinical judgment.

SUMMARY

Syncope, transient loss of consciousness and postural tone as a result of decreased cerebral blood flow with spontaneous recovery, is common and can occur as a result of a number of underlying mechanisms and disorders, some of which may be normal or benign and do not require therapy (a single episode of neurocardiogenic syncope), and others that are life-threatening and require intervention (eg, ventricular arrhythmias, aortic stenosis). Identifying the cause for syncope is important for establishing a prognosis and to guide therapy. In addition, syncope must be distinguished from other causes of loss of consciousness (eg, seizures, trauma, metabolic abnormalities, certain drugs). Syncope can be classified as cardiac, noncardiac, unknown origin, or multifactorial. The history, physical examination, and certain tests can be used to identify the likely cause and guide therapy in many cases. Yet in many cases, the cause may remain obscure, more than one explanation may exist, or syncope may have occurred as a result of more than one process. In these cases, clinical judgment and assessment of the risks and benefits of therapies are required for effective management.

ACKNOWLEDGMENTS

The authors are indebted to Dr. Mark D. Carlson, who contributed to a previous version of this chapter in the 13th edition.

REFERENCES

1. Savage DD, Corwin L, McGee DL, Kannel WB, Wolf PA. Epidemiologic features of isolated syncope: the Framingham Study. *Stroke.* 1985;16(4):626-629.

2. Soteriades ES, Evans JC, Larson MG, et al. Incidence and prognosis of syncope. *N Eng J Med.* 2002;347(12):878-885.

3. Sandhu RK, Tran DT, Sheldon RS, Kaul P. A population-based cohort study evaluating outcomes and costs for syncope presentations to the emergency department. *JACC Clin Electrophysiol.* 2018;4(2):265-273.

4. Kapoor WN, Karpf M, Wieand S, Peterson JR, Levey GS. A prospective evaluation and follow-up of patients with syncope. *N Eng J Med.* 1983;309(4):197-204.

5. Kofflard MJM, Ten Cate FJ, van der Lee C, van Domburg RT. Hypertrophic cardiomyopathy in a large community-based population: clinical outcome and identification of risk factors for sudden cardiac death and clinical deterioration. *J Am Coll Cardiol.* 2003;41(6):987-993.

6. Olshansky B. Syncope: overview and approach to management. In: Grubb BP, Olshansky B, eds. *Syncope: Mechanisms and Management.* Armonk, NY: Futura; 1998:15-71.

7. Zaidi A, Clough P, Cooper P, Scheepers B, Fitzpatrick AP. Misdiagnosis of epilepsy: many seizure-like attacks have a cardiovascular cause. *J Am Coll Cardiol.* 2000;36(1):181-184.

8. Frenneaux MP, Counihan PJ, Caforio AL, Chikamori T, McKenna WJ. Abnormal blood pressure response during exercise in hypertrophic cardiomyopathy. *Circulation.* 1990;82(6):1995-2002.

9. Grech ED, Ramsdale DR. Exertional syncope in aortic stenosis: evidence to support inappropriate left ventricular baroreceptor response. *Am Heart J.* 1991;121(2, Part 1):603-606.

10. O'Mahony C, Elliott P, McKenna W. Sudden cardiac death in hypertrophic cardiomyopathy. *Circulation: Arrhyth Electrophysiol.* 2013;6(2):443-451.

11. Prandoni P, Lensing AW, Prins MH, et al. Prevalence of pulmonary embolism among patients hospitalized for syncope. *N Eng J Med.* 2016;375(16):1524-1531.

12. Chen PS, Chen LS, Fishbein MC, Lin SF, Nattel S. Role of the autonomic nervous system in atrial fibrillation: pathophysiology and therapy. *Circulation Res.* 2014;114(9):1500-1515.

13. Brignole M, Menozzi C, Moya A, et al. Mechanism of syncope in patients with bundle branch block and negative electrophysiological test. *Circulation.* 2001;104(17):2045-2050.

14. Frink RJ, Merrick B, Lowe HM. Mechanism of the bradycardia during coronary angiography. *Am J Cardiol.* 1975;35(1):17-22.

15. Miller MA, Dukkipati SR, Turagam M, Liao SL, Adams DH, Reddy VY. Arrhythmic mitral valve prolapse. *Review Topic of the Week.* 2018; 72(23 Part A):2904-2914.

16. Corrado D, Link MS, Calkins H. Arrhythmogenic right ventricular cardiomyopathy. *N Eng J Med.* 2017;376(1):61-72.

17. Brugada J, Campuzano O, Arbelo E, Sarquella-Brugada G, Brugada R. Present status of Brugada syndrome. *J Am Coll Cardiol.* 2018;72(9): 1046-1059.

18. Goldenberg I, Moss AJ. Long QT syndrome. *J Am Coll Cardiol.* 2008; 51(24):2291-2300.

19. Sheldon RS, Grubb BP 2nd, Olshansky B, et al. 2015 heart rhythm society expert consensus statement on the diagnosis and treatment of postural tachycardia syndrome, inappropriate sinus tachycardia, and vasovagal syncope. *Heart Rhythm.* 2015;12(6):e41-e63.

20. Lombard J, Cowley A. Neural control of the blood vessels. In: Robertson D, Biaggioni I, Low P, Paton J, eds. *A Primer on the Autonomic Nervous System, 3rd ed.* San Diego: Elsevier Academic Press; 2012:187-191.

21. Streeten D. Physiology of the microcirculation. In: Streeten D, ed. *Orthostatic Disorders of the Circulation.* New York: Plenum; 1987:1-12.

22. Wieling W, van Lieshout JJ. Maintenance of postural normotension in humans. In: Low P, Benarroch E, eds. *Clinical Autonomic Disorders, 3rd ed.* Philadelphia: Lippincott-Williams & Wilkins; 2008:57-67.

23. Grubb BP. Clinical practice. Neurocardiogenic syncope. *N Eng J Med.* 2005;352(10):1004-1010.

24. Grubb BP. Neurocardiogenic syncope. In: Grubb BP, Olshanski B, eds. *Syncope: Mechanisms and Management.* Malden, MA: Blackwell-Futura; 2005:47-71.

25. Kosinski D, Grubb BP, Temesy-Armos P. Pathophysiological aspects of neurocardiogenic syncope: current concepts and new perspectives. *PACE* 1995;18(4 Pt 1):716-724.

26. Grubb BP. Neurocardiogenic syncope and related disorders of orthostatic intolerance. *Circulation.* 2005;111(22):2997-3006.

27. O'Mahony D. Pathophysiology of carotid sinus hypersensitivity in elderly patients. *Lancet (London, England).* 1995;346(8980):950-952.

28. Sutton R, Petersen MEV. The clinical spectrum of neurocardiogenic syncope. *J Cardiovas Electrophysiol.* 1995;6(7):569-576.

29. Morillo CA, Ellenbogen A, Pava LF. Pathophysiologic basic for vasodepressor syncope. In: Klein G, ed. *Syncope: Cardiology Clinics of North America.* Philadelphia: Saunders; 1997:233-250.

30. Consensus statement on the definition of orthostatic hypotension, pure autonomic failure, and multiple system atrophy. The Consensus Committee of the American Autonomic Society and the American Academy of Neurology. *Neurology.* 1996;46(5):1470.

31. Bradbury S, Eggleston C. Postural hypotension: a report of three cases. *Am Heart J.* 1925;1:73-86.

32. Freeman R. Pure autonomic failure. In: Robertson D, Biaggiona I, eds. *Disorders of the Autonomic Nervous System.* Luxembourg: Harwood Academic; 1995:83-106.

33. Shy GM, Drager GA. A Neurological syndrome associated with orthostatic hypotension: a clinical-pathologic study. *AMA Arch Neurol.* 1960;2(5):511-527.

34. Low PA, Banister R. Multiple system atrophy and pure autonomic failure. In: Low P, ed. *Clinical Autonomic Disorders, 2nd ed.* Philadelphia: Lippincott-Raven; 1997:555-575.

35. Bannister R, Iodice V, Vichayanrat E, Mathias C. Clinical features and evaluation of the primary chromic autonomic failure syndromes. In: Mathias C, Bannister R, eds. *Autonomic Failure: A Textbook of Clinical Disorders of the Autonomic Nervous System, 5th ed.* Oxford, UK: Oxford University Press; 2013:485-497.

36. Fearnley JM, Lees AJ. Striatonigral degeneration. A clinicopathological study. *Brain* 1990;113 (Pt 6):1823-1842.

37. Grubb BP. Postural tachycardia syndrome. *Circulation.* 2008;117(21): 2814-2817.

38. Roma M, Marden CL, De Wandele I, Francomano CA, Rowe PC. Postural tachycardia syndrome and other forms of orthostatic intolerance in Ehlers-Danlos syndrome. *Autonomic Neurosci: Basic Clin.* 2018;215:89-96.

39. Shannon JR, Flattem NL, Jordan J, et al. Orthostatic intolerance and tachycardia associated with norepinephrine-transporter deficiency. *N Eng J Med.* 2000;342(8):541-549.

40. Ruzieh M, Batizy L, Dasa O, Oostra C, Grubb B. The role of autoantibodies in the syndromes of orthostatic intolerance: a systematic review. *Scandinavian Cardiovasc J.* 2017;51(5):243-247.

41. Gunning WT, 3rd, Kvale H, Kramer PM, Karabin BL, Grubb BP. Postural orthostatic tachycardia syndrome is associated with elevated G-protein coupled receptor autoantibodies. *J Am Heart Assoc.* 2019;8(18):e013602.

42. Grubb BP, Kosinski DJ. Acute pandysautonomic syncope. *Eur J Cardiac Pacing Electrophysiol.* 1997;7:10–14.

43. Freidenberg DL, Shaffer LE, Macalester S, Fannin EA. Orthostatic hypotension in patients with dementia: clinical features and response to treatment. *Cognitive Behavior neurol.* 2013;26(3):105-120.

44. Grubb BP, Kanjwal Y, Karabin B, Imran N. Orthostatic hypotension and autonomic failure: a concise guide to diagnosis and management. *Clinical Med Cardiol.* 2008;2:279-291.

45. Coon EA, Singer W, Low PA. Pure autonomic failure. *Mayo Clinic Proc.* 2019;94(10):2087-2098.

46. Bousser MG, Dubois B, Castaigne P. Transient loss of consciousness in ischaemic cerebral events. A study of 557 ischaemic strokes and transient ischaemic attacks (author's trans.). *Annales de medecine interne.* 1981;132(5):300-305.

47. Krahn AD, Klein GJ, Fitzpatrick A, et al. Predicting the outcome of patients with unexplained syncope undergoing prolonged monitoring. *PACE.* 2002;25(1):37-41.

48. Brignole M, Moya A, de Lange FJ, et al. 2018 ESC Guidelines for the diagnosis and management of syncope. *Eur Heart J.* 2018;39(21):1883-1948.

49. Shen W-K, Sheldon RS, Benditt DG, et al. 2017 ACC/AHA/HRS guideline for the evaluation and management of patients with syncope: a report of the American College of Cardiology/American Heart Association Task Force on Clinical Practice Guidelines and the Heart Rhythm Society. *Circulation.* 2017;136(5):e60-e122.

50. Shen WK, Decker WW, Smars PA, et al. Syncope Evaluation in the Emergency Department Study (SEEDS): a multidisciplinary approach to syncope management. *Circulation.* 2004;110(24):3636-3645.

51. Sheldon R, Rose S, Ritchie D, et al. Historical criteria that distinguish syncope from seizures. *J Am Coll Cardiol.* 2002;40(1):142-148.

52. Del Rosso A, Ungar A, Maggi R, et al. Clinical predictors of cardiac syncope at initial evaluation in patients referred urgently to a general hospital: the EGSYS score. *Heart (British Cardiac Society).* 2008;94(12):1620-1626.

53. Puggioni E, Guiducci V, Brignole M, et al. Results and complications of the carotid sinus massage performed according to the "method of symptoms". *Am J Cardiol.* 2002;89(5):599-601.

54. Thiruganasambandamoorthy V, Ramaekers R, Rahman MO, et al. Prognostic value of cardiac biomarkers in the risk stratification of syncope: a systematic review. *Intern Emerg Med.* 2015;10(8):1003-1014.

55. Locati ET, Moya A, Oliveira M, et al. External prolonged electrocardiogram monitoring in unexplained syncope and palpitations: results of the SYNARR-Flash study. *Europace* 2016;18(8):1265-1272.

56. Krahn AD, Klein GJ, Yee R, Hoch JS, Skanes AC. Cost implications of testing strategy in patients with syncope: randomized assessment of syncope trial. *J Am Coll Cardiol.* 2003;42(3):495-501.

57. Perez MV, Mahaffey KW, Hedlin H, et al. Large-scale assessment of a smartwatch to identify atrial fibrillation. *N Eng J Med.* 2019;381(20):1909-1917.

58. Sarasin FP, Junod AF, Carballo D, Slama S, Unger PF, Louis-Simonet M. Role of echocardiography in the evaluation of syncope: a prospective study. *Heart (British Cardiac Society).* 2002;88(4):363-367.

59. Ramchand J, Fava AM, Chetrit M, Desai MY. Advanced imaging for risk stratification of sudden death in hypertrophic cardiomyopathy. *Heart (British Cardiac Society).* 2020;106(11):793-801.

60. Colivicchi F, Ammirati F, Biffi A, Verdile L, Pelliccia A, Santini M. Exercise-related syncope in young competitive athletes without evidence of structural heart disease. Clinical presentation and long-term outcome. *Eur Heart J.* 2002;23(14):1125-1130.

61. Wissocq L, Ennezat PV, Mouquet F. Exercise-induced high-degree atrioventricular block. *Arch Cardiovasc Dis.* 2009;102(10):733-735.

62. Brembilla-Perrot B, Suty-Selton C, Beurrier D, et al. Differences in mechanisms and outcomes of syncope in patients with coronary disease or idiopathic left ventricular dysfunction as assessed by electrophysiologic testing. *J Am Coll Cardiol.* 2004;44(3):594-601.

63. Kalscheur MM, Donateo P, Wenzke KE, et al. Long-term outcome of patients with bifascicular block and unexplained syncope following cardiac pacing. *PACE.* 2016;39(10):1126-1131.

64. Verrier RL, Klingenheben T, Malik M, et al. Microvolt T-wave alternans physiological basis, methods of measurement, and clinical utility–consensus guideline by International Society for Holter and Noninvasive Electrocardiology. *J Am Coll Cardiol.* 2011;58(13):1309-1324.

65. Parry SW, Gray JC, Newton JL, Reeve P, O'Shea D, Kenny RA. 'Front-loaded' head-up tilt table testing: validation of a rapid first line nitrate-provoked tilt protocol for the diagnosis of vasovagal syncope. *Age Ageing.* 2008;37(4):411-415.

66. Grubb BP, Kosinski D. Tilt table testing: concepts and limitations. *PACE.* 1997;20(3 Pt 2):781-787.

67. Benditt DG, Ferguson DW, Grubb BP, et al. Tilt table testing for assessing syncope. American College of Cardiology. *J Am Coll Cardiol.* 1996;28(1):263-275.

68. Krahn AD, Klein GJ, Yee R, Skanes AC. Randomized assessment of syncope trial: conventional diagnostic testing versus a prolonged monitoring strategy. *Circulation.* 2001;104(1):46-51.

69. Tannemaat MR, van Niekerk J, Reijntjes RH, Thijs RD, Sutton R, van Dijk JG. The semiology of tilt-induced psychogenic pseudosyncope. *Neurology.* 2013;81(8):752-758.

70. Kouakam C, Lacroix D, Klug D, Baux P, Marquié C, Kacet S. Prevalence and prognostic significance of psychiatric disorders in patients evaluated for recurrent unexplained syncope. *Am J Cardiol.* 2002;89(5):530-535.

71. Pournazari P, Oqab Z, Sheldon R. Diagnostic value of neurological studies in diagnosing syncope: a systematic review. *Can J Cardiol.* 2017;33(12): 1604-1610.

72. Costantino G, Ruwald MH, Quinn J, et al. Prevalence of pulmonary embolism in patients with syncope. *JAMA Intern Med.* 2018;178(3):356-362.

73. Badertscher P, du Fay de Lavallaz J, Hammerer-Lercher A, et al. Prevalence of pulmonary embolism in patients with syncope. *J Am Coll Cardiol.* 2019;74(6):744-754.

74. Zeng H, Ge K, Zhang W, Wang G, Guo L. The effect of orthostatic training in the prevention of vasovagal syncope and its influencing factors. *Int Heart J.* 2008;49(6):707-712.

75. Krediet CT, van Dijk N, Linzer M, van Lieshout JJ, Wieling W. Management of vasovagal syncope: controlling or aborting faints by leg crossing and muscle tensing. *Circulation.* 2002;106(13):1684-1689.

76. El-Sayed H, Hainsworth R. Salt supplement increases plasma volume and orthostatic tolerance in patients with unexplained syncope. *Heart (British Cardiac Society).* 1996;75(2):134-140.

77. Solari D, Tesi F, Unterhuber M, et al. Stop vasodepressor drugs in reflex syncope: a randomised controlled trial. *Heart (British Cardiac Society).* 2017;103(6):449-455.

78. Sheldon R, Raj SR, Rose MS, et al. Fludrocortisone for the prevention of vasovagal syncope: a randomized, placebo-controlled trial. *J Am Coll Cardiol.* 2016;68(1):1-9.

79. Grubb BP, Kosinski D, Mouhaffel A, Pothoulakis A. The use of methylphenidate in the treatment of refractory neurocardiogenic syncope. *PACE.* 1996;19(5):836-840.

80. Izcovich A, González Malla C, Manzotti M, Catalano HN, Guyatt G. Midodrine for orthostatic hypotension and recurrent reflex syncope: a systematic review. *Neurology.* 2014;83(13):1170-1177.

81. Singer W, Opfer-Gehrking TL, McPhee BR, Hilz MJ, Bharucha AE, Low PA. Acetylcholinesterase inhibition: a novel approach in the treatment of neurogenic orthostatic hypotension. *J Neurol Neurosurg Psychiat.* 2003;74(9):1294-1298.

82. Raj SR, Black BK, Biaggioni I, Harris PA, Robertson D. Acetylcholinesterase inhibition improves tachycardia in postural tachycardia syndrome. *Circulation.* 2005;111(21):2734-2740.

83. Kanjwal K, Saeed B, Karabin B, Kanjwal Y, Grubb BP. Use of octreotide in the treatment of refractory orthostatic intolerance. *Am J Therapeut.* 2012;19(1):7-10.

84. Sutton R, Salukhe TV, Franzen-McManus AC, Collins A, Lim PB, Francis DP. Ivabradine in treatment of sinus tachycardia mediated vasovagal syncope. *Europace.* 2014;16(2):284-288.

85. McDonald C, Frith J, Newton JL. Single centre experience of ivabradine in postural orthostatic tachycardia syndrome. *Europace.* 2011;13(3):427-430.

86. Ruzieh M, Sirianni N, Ammari Z, et al. Ivabradine in the treatment of postural tachycardia syndrome (POTS), a single center experience. *PACE.* 2017;40(11):1242-1245.

87. Kaufmann H, Freeman R, Biaggioni I, et al. Droxidopa for neurogenic orthostatic hypotension: a randomized, placebo-controlled, phase 3 trial. *Neurology.* 2014;83(4):328-335.

88. Brignole M, Solari D, Iori M, Bottoni N, Guieu R, Deharo JC. Efficacy of theophylline in patients affected by low adenosine syncope. *Heart Rhythm.* 2016;13(5):1151-1154.

89. Sheldon RS, Ritchie D, McRae M, Raj S. Norepinephrine transport inhibition for treatment of vasovagal syncope. *J Cardiovasc Electrophysiol.* 2013;24(7):799-803.

90. Connolly SJ, Sheldon R, Roberts RS, Gent M. The North American Vasovagal Pacemaker Study (VPS). A randomized trial of permanent cardiac pacing for the prevention of vasovagal syncope. *J Am Coll Cardiol.* 1999;33(1):16-20.

91. Sutton R, Brignole M, Menozzi C, et al. Dual-chamber pacing in the treatment of neurally mediated tilt-positive cardioinhibitory syncope: pacemaker versus no therapy: a multicenter randomized study. The Vasovagal Syncope International Study (VASIS) Investigators. *Circulation.* 2000;102(3):294-299.

92. Ammirati F, Colivicchi F, Santini M. Permanent Cardiac pacing versus medical treatment for the prevention of recurrent vasovagal syncope. *Circulation.* 2001;104(1):52-57.

93. Connolly SJ, Sheldon R, Thorpe KE, et al. Pacemaker therapy for prevention of syncope in patients with recurrent severe vasovagal syncope: Second Vasovagal Pacemaker Study (VPS II): a randomized trial. *JAMA.* 2003;289(17):2224-2229.

94. Raviele A, Giada F, Menozzi C, et al. A randomized, double-blind, placebo-controlled study of permanent cardiac pacing for the treatment of recurrent tilt-induced vasovagal syncope. The vasovagal syncope and pacing trial (SYNPACE). *Eur Heart J.* 2004;25(19):1741-1748.

95. Brignole M, Sutton R, Menozzi C, et al. Early application of an implantable loop recorder allows effective specific therapy in patients with recurrent suspected neurally mediated syncope. *Eur Heart J.* 2006;27(9):1085-1092.

96. Brignole M, Menozzi C, Moya A, et al. Pacemaker therapy in patients with neurally mediated syncope and documented asystole. *Circulation.* 2012;125(21):2566-2571.

97. Ruzieh M, Ghahramani M, Nudy M, et al. The benefit of closed loop stimulation in patients with cardioinhibitory vasovagal syncope confirmed by head-up tilt table testing: a systematic review and meta-analysis. *J Intervention Cardiac Electrophysiol.* 2019;55(1):105-113.

98. Baron-Esquivias G, Morillo CA, Moya-Mitjans A, et al. Dual-chamber pacing with closed loop stimulation in recurrent reflex vasovagal syncope: the SPAIN study. *J Am Coll Cardiol.* 2017;70(14):1720-1728.

99. Brignole M, Menozzi C. The natural history of carotid sinus syncope and the effect of cardiac pacing. *Europace.* 2011;13(4):462-464.

100. Kenny RA, Richardson DA, Steen N, Bexton RS, Shaw FE, Bond J. Carotid sinus syndrome: a modifiable risk factor for nonaccidental falls in older adults (SAFE PACE). *J Am Coll Cardiol.* 2001;38(5):1491-1496.

101. Maron BJ, Shen WK, Link MS, et al. Efficacy of implantable cardioverter-defibrillators for the prevention of sudden death in patients with hypertrophic cardiomyopathy. *N Eng J Med.* 2000;342(6):365-373.

102. Kusumoto FM, Schoenfeld MH, Barrett C, et al. 2018 ACC/AHA/HRS guideline on the evaluation and management of patients with bradycardia and cardiac conduction delay: a report of the American College of Cardiology/American Heart Association Task Force on Clinical Practice Guidelines and the Heart Rhythm Society. *Circulation.* 2019;140(8): e382-e482.

103. Alboni P, Menozzi C, Brignole M, et al. Effects of permanent pacemaker and oral theophylline in sick sinus syndrome the THEOPACE study: a randomized controlled trial. *Circulation.* 1997;96(1):260-266.

104. Brignole M, Alboni P, Benditt D, et al. Guidelines on management (diagnosis and treatment) of syncope. *Eur Heart J.* 2001;22(15):1256-1306.

105. Brignole M, Alboni P, Benditt DG, et al. Guidelines on management (diagnosis and treatment) of syncope-update 2004. Executive summary. *Eur Heart J.* 2004;25(22):2054-2072.

106. Moya A, Sutton R, Ammirati F, et al. Guidelines for the diagnosis and management of syncope (version 2009). *Eur Heart J.* 2009;30(21):2631-2671.

107. Goldberger ZD, Petek BJ, Brignole M, et al. ACC/AHA/HRS versus ESC guidelines for the diagnosis and management of syncope: JACC guideline comparison. *J Am Coll Cardiol.* 2019;74(19):2410-2423.

SECTION VII

HEART FAILURE

40

Classification of Cardiomyopathies

Eloisa Arbustini, Barry J. Maron, Navneet Narula, and Jagat Narula

Cardiomyopathies: more than half a century of history towards a universal classification				
The roots	The evolution: from phenotype-based to phenotype-cause integration			The future
History	**2006, AHA**	**2008, ESC**	**2013, WHF-endorsed MOGE(S)**	**Towards a universal classification**
1956, Blankenhorn & Gall: myocardiosis and myocarditis **1957,** Brigden & Cantab: cardiomyopathy—noncoronary heart muscle disease **1972,** Goodwin and Oakley: hypertrophic, congestive, obliterative **1980,** WHO added specific heart muscle diseases **1996,** WHO/ISFC: addition of ARVC	Genetically driven, subgrouped as: • Genetic • Mixed • Acquired Channelopathies: included LVNC: included	Phenotypically-driven subgroups, subdivided as familial/genetic and nonfamilial/nongenetic Channelopathies: excluded LVNC: not specified	The genotype-to-phenotype attributes; combines ACC/AHA and ESC principles: (M) morphofunctional characteristics (O) organ involvement (G) genetic/familial with inheritance pattern vs nongenetic/nonfamilial (E) etiology (S) functional status	Any further evolution will have to include both phenotype and cause and be applicable to all forms of cardiomyopathy. At present, MOGE(S) is the closest to a universal classification, and define wherein the affected myocardium is the cause of the observed phenotype.

Chapter 40 Fuster and Hurst's Central Illustration. The evolving classification of cardiomyopathies. ACC, American College of Cardiology; AHA, American Heart Association; ARVC, arrhythmogenic right ventricular cardiomyopathy; ESC, European Society of Cardiology; ISFC, International Society and Federation of Cardiology; LVNC, left ventricular noncompaction; WHF, World Heart Federation; WHO, World Health Organization.

CHAPTER SUMMARY

This chapter reviews the evolving classification of cardiomyopathies over the last 65 years, which were first defined in 1957 as noncoronary cardiomyopathies or isolated noncoronary myocardial diseases (see Fuster and Hurst's Central Illustration). In 2013, the World Heart Federation (WHF) endorsed a systematic classification referred to as MOGE(S), which combined two complementary concepts from the previous American Heart Association (AHA) and European Society of Cardiology (ESC) recommendations. The system of classification describes morphofunctional presentation (M), organ involvement (O), genetic basis (G), precise description of (genetic or acquired) etiology (E) and functional New York Heart Association (NYHA) class and American College of Cardiology (ACC)–AHA status (S). In the 2019 classification of cardiomyopathies in children, the AHA incorporated the elements of MOGE(S) in a hierarchy system based on the structural and functional phenotype with genetic and nongenetic causes as subcategories. Going forward, each new formula for reporting the classification will have to realize the need for short and rapid communication tools that can be universally adopted, but we must also recognize that the acceptance of every new proposal by the clinical community takes time. Any commitment of the clinical community has to go beyond the phenotype and include the cause as mandatory information, so that all cardiologists share a common diagnostic language.

As any classification is necessarily incomplete and acts as a bridge between complete ignorance and total understanding in any biological system, ... further modification and changes are likely to occur.

— *John Goodwin, London, 1982*

INTRODUCTION

Clinical taxonomy aids understanding and facilitates appropriate categorization of diseases through the use of logical groups and hierarchies on the basis of predefined criteria that are useful for the diagnosis and management of human ailments. Disease classifications result in standardization of disease nomenclature. In the premolecular era, this process was driven by clinical phenotypes (eg, heart failure, cardiomyopathies, and arrhythmias) and pathology (eg, cancer). For etiologically heterogeneous diseases such as cardiomyopathies, the principles of classification have been historically based on morphofunctional characteristics shared by phenotypically similar disorders. Traditionally, the cardiomyopathies have been considered *idiopathic* diseases. In the last two decades, clinical and molecular genetics and advanced imaging have contributed to elucidate the etiology of cardiomyopathies, to the point that the term *idiopathic* is gradually becoming obsolete. Most cardiomyopathies have a genetic basis, and for many of those that are not heritable, the mechanisms are now known.

CLASSIFICATION OF CARDIOMYOPATHIES: A HISTORICAL PERSPECTIVE

Heart muscle disorders are relatively young diseases. In a famous editorial published in *Heart* in 1982, John F. Goodwin reviewed the 30-year history of cardiomyopathies,[1] starting from the early 1950s, when Brigden published the St. Cyres lecture on "Uncommon Myocardial Diseases: The Non-coronary Cardiomyopathies."[2] The evolution from description to definition and clustering of similar cardiomyopathies led to the first classification of cardiomyopathies in 1972, when Goodwin and Oakley defined cardiomyopathies as the heart muscle diseases of unknown cause and described them as congestive (or dilated) (DCM), hypertrophic (HCM), and restrictive (or obliterative) (RCM) cardiomyopathy types.[3] In 1980, the World Health Organization (WHO) adopted the classification of cardiomyopathies as "heart muscle diseases of unknown cause" (**Fig. 40–1**) to distinguish cardiomyopathy from cardiac dysfunction as a result of known cardiovascular entities such as hypertension, ischemic heart disease, or valvular disease.[4] In 1995, the WHO/International Society and Federation of Cardiology (ISFC) Task Force on the Definition and Classification of the Cardiomyopathies expanded the classification to include all diseases affecting heart muscle and to take into consideration etiology as well as the dominant pathophysiology.[5] The WHO/ISFC task force added two more classes: arrhythmogenic

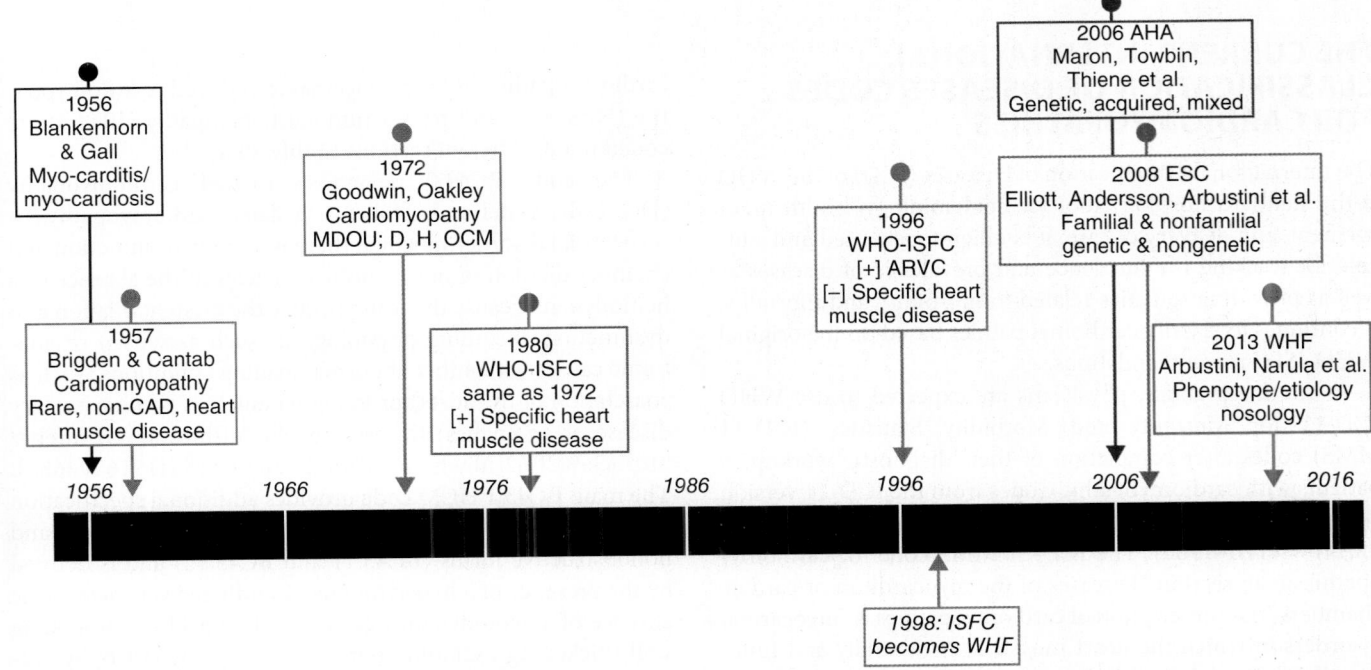

Figure 40–1. Classification of cardiomyopathies: A historical perspective. Cardiomyopathies were described only about 60 years ago. Their classifications have gone through many contentious iterations. The classification has traditionally been provided by the World Health Organization (WHO) and International Society and Federation of Cardiology (ISFC; which latter evolved into the World Heart Federation [WHF]) in 1998, the American Heart Association (AHA) in 2006, the European Society of Cardiology (ESC) in 2008, and the comprehensive phenotype-to-genotype classification of the WHF in 2013. ARVC, arrhythmogenic right ventricular cardiomyopathy; CAD, coronary artery disease; D, H, OCM, dilated, hypertrophic, other cardiomyopathy; MDOU, muscle diseases of unknown causes.

cardiomyopathy (ACM; ie, arrhythmogenic right ventricular cardiomyopathy [ARVC]) and unclassified cardiomyopathy.[5] In 1998, the ISFC evolved as the World Heart Federation (WHF) and, until recently, did not indulge in developing scientific statements for both diagnosis and management of cardiomyopathies. The morphofunctional phenotype has continued to be the unique basis for classification of cardiomyopathy.

During this period, a substantial increase in the knowledge of the genetic etiology of cardiomyopathy led the American Heart Association (AHA) to propose revisions to the classification of cardiomyopathy. In a valiant departure from the original definition, Maron et al.[6] classified cardiomyopathy on the genetic basis. The European Society of Cardiology (ESC)[7] retained the description in original morphofunctional categories, but added subclassification into familial and nonfamilial forms. Both AHA and ESC classifications excluded specific heart muscle diseases from consideration as cardiomyopathic disorders. In 2013, the WHF endorsed a novel classification of cardiomyopathies.[8,9] This update combined the best of both the AHA and ESC classifications. The proposed nomenclature, MOGE(S) (which stands for morphofunctional phenotype, organ involvement, genetic inheritance, underlying etiology, and functional status), is descriptive, flexibly modifiable, and expandable (see section, The World Heart Federation [2013] Classification). The recently released scientific statement of the AHA on the classification and diagnosis of cardiomyopathy in children used a classification system based on a hierarchy incorporating the required elements of the MOGE(S) classification.[9]

THE CURRENT INTERNATIONAL CLASSIFICATION OF DISEASES CODES FOR CARDIOMYOPATHIES

The International Classification of Diseases (ICD) of the WHO is the standard nosology tool for epidemiology, health management, and delivery of care. It is ubiquitously used and suitable for tracking the incidence and prevalence of diseases as well as providing statistics related to morbidity and mortality. It continues to classify cardiomyopathies based on the original WHO-ISFC recommendations.

In routine practice, physicians are expected to use WHO ICD-11 for Mortality and Morbidity Statistics (ICD-11 MMS) codes after completion of their diagnostic workup in patients with cardiomyopathy. Codes from the ICD-11 version September 2020 are available at the ICD website (https://icd.who.int/browse11/l-m/en). The ICD-11 MMS code for cardiomyopathies is in section "Diseases of the myocardium or cardiac chambers." The description of cardiomyopathies is "myocardial disorders in which the heart muscle is structurally and functionally abnormal, in the absence of coronary artery disease, hypertension, valvular disease and congenital heart disease sufficient to cause the observed myocardial abnormality." The cardiomyopathy code is BC43; inflammatory cardiomyopathy (BC42) and myocarditis (BC42) are excluded while ischemic

TABLE 40–1. ICD-11 for Mortality and Morbidity Statistics (Version: September 2020)

DISEASES OF THE MYOCARDIUM OR CARDIAC CHAMBERS

BC40 ACQUIRED ATRIAL ABNORMALITY
BC41 ACQUIRED VENTRICULAR ABNORMALITY
BC42 MYOCARDITIS
BC43 CARDIOMYOPATHY
  BC43.0 DILATED CARDIOMYOPATHY
    BC43.00 FAMILIAL–GENETIC DILATED
    BC43.01 NONFAMILIAL DILATED CARDIOMYOPATHY
    BC43.0Z DILATED CARDIOMYOPATHY, UNSPECIFIED
  BC43.1 HYPERTROPHIC CARDIOMYOPATHY
    BC43.10 FAMILIAL–GENETIC HYPERTROPHIC CARDIOMYOPATHY
    BC43.11 NON-OBSTRUCTIVE HYPERTROPHIC CARDIOMYOPATHY
    KB60.1 S. INFANT OF A DIABETIC MOTHER, TYPE 1 OR 2, NONGESTATIONAL, INSULIN DEPENDENT
    BC43.1Y OTHER SPECIFIED HYPERTROPHIC CARDIOMYOPATHY
    BC43.1Z HYPERTROPHIC CARDIOMYOPATHY, UNSPECIFIED
  BC43.2 RESTRICTIVE CARDIOMYOPATHY
    BC43.20 NON FAMILIAL RESTRICTIVE
    BC43.2Y OTHER SPECIFIED RESTRICTIVE CARDIOMYOPATHY
    BC43.2Z RESTRICTIVE CARDIOMYOPATHY, UNSPECIFIED
  BC43.3 ENDOCARDIAL FIBROELASTOSIS
  BC43.4 CARDIOMYOPATHY DUE TO DRUGS OR OTHER EXTERNAL AGENTS
  BC43.5 STRESS-INDUCED CARDIOMYOPATHY
  BC43.6 ARRHYTHMOGENIC VENTRICULAR CARDIOMYOPATHY
  BC43.7 DIABETIC CARDIOMYOPATHY
BC44 NONCOMPACTION CARDIOMYOPATHY
BC45 CARDIOMEGALY
BC46 INTRACARDIAC THROMBOSIS
BC4Y OTHER SPECIFIED DISEASES OF THE MYOCARDIUM OR CARDIAC CHAMBERS
BC4Z DISEASES OF THE MYOCARDIUM OR CARDIAC CHAMBERS, UNSPECIFIED

Data from World Health Organization, ICD-11 for Mortality and Morbidity Statistics.

cardiomyopathy (BA51), pacemaker-induced cardiomyopathy (NE82.03), and peripartum cardiomyopathy (JB44.3) are coded under different sections (**Table 40-1**).

The code BC43.0 recognizes dilated cardiomyopathy (DCM) that is defined as follows: "Dilated cardiomyopathy is a myocardial disorder in which there is systolic dysfunction and chamber dilation of one or both ventricles in the absence of a hemodynamic cause that can produce the existent dilation and dysfunction, including physiological (such as sepsis) or anatomic causes with either abnormal loading conditions (such as coarctation of the aorta) or ischemia (such as coronary artery disease or anomalies) (https://icd.who.int/browse11/l-m/en#/http%3a%2f%2fid.who.int%2ficd%2fentity%2f1916294688). The main BC43.1 HCM code provides additional specification codes for familial-genetic HCM (BC43-10), obstructive and nonobstructive forms (BC43.11 and BC43.12) and is defined by the presence of a hypertrophied, nondilated ventricle in the absence of a hemodynamic cause that is capable of producing wall thickening excluding both physiologic hypertrophy secondary to physical activity, and pathologic hypertrophy due to systemic hypertension, aortic valvular stenosis, and coarctation. The BC43.2 code is for restrictive cardiomyopathy that is defined as the presence of impaired ventricular function related to reduced rate and/or extent of relaxation and/or compliance in the absence of another predominant phenotype of dilated or HCM. Although the BC43.20 describes nonfamilial restrictive cardiomyopathy, no specific codes are available for the familial forms. The ICD-11BC43.6 recognizes *arrhythmogenic ventricular cardiomyopathy* as a cardiomyopathy characterized by myocardial cell loss with partial or total replacement of right ventricular muscle by adipose and fibrous tissue, beginning subepicardially to becoming transmural over time, sparing the papillary muscles and trabeculae, and often associated with aneurysms particularly of the right ventricular outflow tract. The description includes the classical form mainly affecting the right ventricle, as well as the biventricular and predominantly left ventricular forms, that are included in the main descriptor BC43.6. The code ICD11-BC46.5 describes *stress-induced or Takotsubo cardiomyopathy*, a disease of the myocardium characterized by episodes of acute onset, reversible left ventricular apical wall motion abnormalities mimicking acute myocardial infarction, but with nonspecific electrocardiographic ST elevation and T wave changes, and minimal myocardial enzyme release, in the absence of coronary stenosis. The endocardial fibroelastosis ICD11-BC43.3 specifies "the formation of a marked fibro-elastic thickening of the subendocardium in one or both ventricles." It is described as "a disorder of fetuses and infants, secondary causes include congenital left-sided obstructive cardiac lesions, metabolic disorders, autoimmune disease (anti-Ro/ anti-La antibodies), and transplacental viral infection such as mumps."

An unexpected independent descriptor is ICD11-BC44, that is excluded from the main ICD-11BC43 for cardiomyopathies but addresses *noncompaction cardiomyopathy* defined as "a morphologic abnormality of the myocardium predominantly affecting the apex of the ventricle characterized by hypertrabeculation and deep inter-trabecular recesses, usually accompanied by an abnormally thin subepicardial layer of compacted myocardium, that is generally but not always associated with ventricular dysfunction. Noncompaction cardiomyopathy typically manifests in the left ventricle; the right ventricle is less commonly affected. It can occur as an isolated finding (LVNC) or in the context of a cardiomyopathy (dilated, hypertrophic, etc.). It has been described in association with complex congenital heart disease, coronary artery anomalies, and as an isolated finding, with and without musculoskeletal and other system abnormalities." Given the still-missing univocal definition of LVNC (left ventricular noncompaction) (at present, it only describes a morphological trait of the trabecular myocardium), the use of this code is unlikely to contribute to the epidemiology of LVNC (see Chapter 45, LVNC).

Other codes cover all unaccounted cardiomyopathies. Overall, the statistics based on ICD codes are unlikely to be useful for any practical purposes (https://www.who.int/classifications/en/).

Heart failure, that commonly manifests in cardiomyopathies, is coded as a distinct entity (ICD-11 BD10 for congestive heart failure) and further BD11, BD12, BD13, and BD14 for left ventricular failure, high output syndromes, right ventricular failure, and biventricular failure, respectively. For epidemiology purposes it could be useful to integrate the cardiomyopathy code with a specification of the type of heart failure: heart failure with reduced ejection fraction (HFrEF) and heart failure with preserved ejection fraction (HFpEF).[10]

The WHO works to keep the classification system aligned with current scientific knowledge and it is compatible with contemporary information systems. The future WHO-ICD system for cardiomyopathies should probably be expanded to provide a realistic and clinically useful epidemiologic tool for cardiomyopathies.

THE AMERICAN HEART ASSOCIATION (2006) CLASSIFICATION

The Basis

The diverse cardiomyopathy classifications presented through the years have been designed either for clinicians or biomedical scientists, and have been based on etiology, anatomy, physiology, primary treatment, method of diagnosis (including histopathology), and patient symptoms. The AHA classification[6] was developed in response to the following drawbacks of the traditional WHO-ISFC classification:

1. *The traditional WHO-ISFC classification admixes morphologic with functional traits.* The AHA authors pointed out that the clinical classification HCM-DCM-RCM was fraught with major limitations. The classification combines anatomic and functional traits, wherein the same disease could legitimately cross over to two or even three of the phenotypes. In HCM, the key descriptor is morphologic (ie, thickened left ventricular [LV] walls are present, and diastolic dysfunction is common). Similarly, in DCM, the key descriptor is morphologic (ie, LV dilation). However, systolic dysfunction is an obligatory part of the definition of the disease and functionally more relevant than simple ventricular dilatation. The myocardial dysfunction is so relevant that a recent ESC-endorsed consensus document has introduced the variant "hypokinetic non-dilated cardiomyopathy."[11] On the other hand, the key property in RCM is mechanical (ie, diastolic dysfunction, generally with preserved systolic function). However, the disease has a precise morphologic phenotype characterized by dilated atria in the absence of LV hypertrophy or dilatation. Although in ARVC, the original key descriptor was primarily right-sided morphologic involvement with a prominent arrhythmogenic profile, biventricular and predominantly left-sided variants are increasingly recognized. LV involvement complicates the clinical diagnosis, and it may be challenging to distinguish between ARVC with LV involvement from DCM with right ventricular involvement. To solve the increasing risk of misdiagnosis resulting from the 2010 Task Force (TF2010) criteria, an International Expert Report was released with the major aims of critically revising the clinical performance and highlighting the potential limitations of TF2010 criteria; proposing possible solutions for their better clinical use; identifying potential areas of improvement, with particular

reference to the diagnosis of left-sided phenotypes and identification of early disease in the pediatric population. The International Expert Report maintained the original designation of ARVC because the novel document is a critical appraisal of the 2010 International Task Force (ITF) criteria that were specifically designed to diagnose the "classic" ARVC phenotype. The current classification of ARVC includes the following clinical variants: (1) the classic ARVC phenotype (ie, the originally reported and most common disease variant, characterized by isolated right ventricular [RV] involvement); (2) the "biventricular disease variants" (ie, "balanced," "dominant-right," or "dominant-left" characterized by the parallel, predominant RV, and predominant LV involvement, respectively); and (3) the LV phenotype characterized by isolated LV involvement (ie, without clinically demonstrable RV involvement).[12]

2. *The overlapping phenotypes render traditional classification difficult.* The HCM-DCM-RCM classification also failed to consider the heterogeneous clinical expression and natural history of the diseases. For example, storage cardiomyopathies are characterized by substantial LV hypertrophy with increased wall thickness. These conditions are also frequently associated with restriction to diastolic filling, whereas purely restrictive forms of cardiomyopathy (without LV hypertrophy) are exceedingly rare. Investigation into the genetic basis of HCM and other cardiomyopathies has led to the identification of individuals who do not develop LV hypertrophy. Dilated forms of cardiomyopathy show a considerably increased cardiac mass with myocyte enlargement indicative of cardiac hypertrophy, although absolute LV wall thicknesses might remain normal. The end-stage phase of HCM could demonstrate hypertrophic, dilated, and restrictive components. Furthermore, some patients may evolve from one category to another as a consequence of remodeling during their natural clinical course. For example, HCM, cardiac amyloidosis, and other HCM phenocopies may progress from a nondilated (often hyperdynamic) state with ventricular stiffness to a dilated form with systolic dysfunction and heart failure. Finally, because quantitative assessments of ventricular size represent a continuum and patients can vary widely in the degree of chamber enlargement (and dimensional cutoff values are arbitrary), it can be difficult to discriminate dilated from nondilated hypokinetic forms of cardiomyopathy.

3. *Etiologically/genetically diverse cardiomyopathies present with similar phenotypes.* Etiologic classification of cardiomyopathies also appears problematic, given that diseases with the same (or similar) phenotypes can harbor different etiology and, vice versa, similar causes (eg, defects in same genes) may be associated with different phenotypes (eg, defects of *TNNT2* may cause HCM, DCM, and RCM). For example, DCM may have genetic, infectious, autoimmune, and toxic causes (and in some cases still be designated as *idiopathic just because of an "undetected" cause*); all may lead to the final common pathway of ventricular dilatation with systolic dysfunction.

The Definition

A heterogeneous group of diseases of the myocardium associated with mechanical and/or electrical dysfunction, which usually exhibit inappropriate ventricular hypertrophy or dilatation, and are due to a variety of etiologies that frequently are genetic. Cardiomyopathies are either confined to the heart or are part of generalized systemic disorders, often leading to cardiovascular death or progressive heart failure-related disability.[6]

Within this broad definition, cardiomyopathies are usually associated with failure of myocardial performance, which may be mechanical (eg, diastolic or systolic dysfunction) or a primary electrical dysfunction that increases susceptibility to life-threatening arrhythmias. The ion channelopathies (long and short QT syndromes, Brugada syndrome, and catecholaminergic polymorphic ventricular tachycardia, among others) are primary electrical diseases without gross or histopathologic abnormalities. The basic pathologic abnormality in these diseases is not identifiable by either conventional noninvasive imaging or myocardial biopsy during life, even by electron microscopy, or autopsy examination. This is because there are no known specific pathology markers pertinent to the defects of different disease-genes. The ion channelopathies are included in the AHA classification of cardiomyopathies based on the assertion that ion channel mutations are responsible for altering biophysical properties and protein structure of the cardiomyocyte, thereby creating structurally abnormal ion channel interfaces and architecture with electrical dysfunction and risk of primary life-threatening ventricular tachyarrhythmias.

The Classification

Cardiomyopathies were divided into two major groups based on predominant organ involvement. The *primary* cardiomyopathies were those solely or predominantly confined to heart muscle (**Fig. 40–2A**).[6] The categorization into genetic, acquired, and mixed varieties represented the novelty of the AHA classification. The *secondary* cardiomyopathies showed pathologic myocardial involvement as part of systemic (multiorgan) disorders. In prior classifications, the primary cardiomyopathies represented idiopathic processes while the systemic diseases associated with secondary forms of cardiomyopathies were previously referred to as *specific cardiomyopathies*[4] or *specific heart muscle diseases*.[5] Such vague nomenclature was abandoned in the AHA classification.

The Major Attributes of the AHA Classification

The AHA classification introduced the concept of classification of primary cardiomyopathy based on *genetic* origin. A large body of evidence had become available in 2006 that supported the genetic basis of cardiomyopathies, and the writing group asserted that it was time that cardiomyopathies be appropriately classified on the basis of their cause (ie, genetic, acquired, or mixed). The genotype hierarchically preceded the phenotype description and underlined substantial evolution of knowledge of the genetic etiology of cardiomyopathies. The AHA classification was a welcome change, even though it has

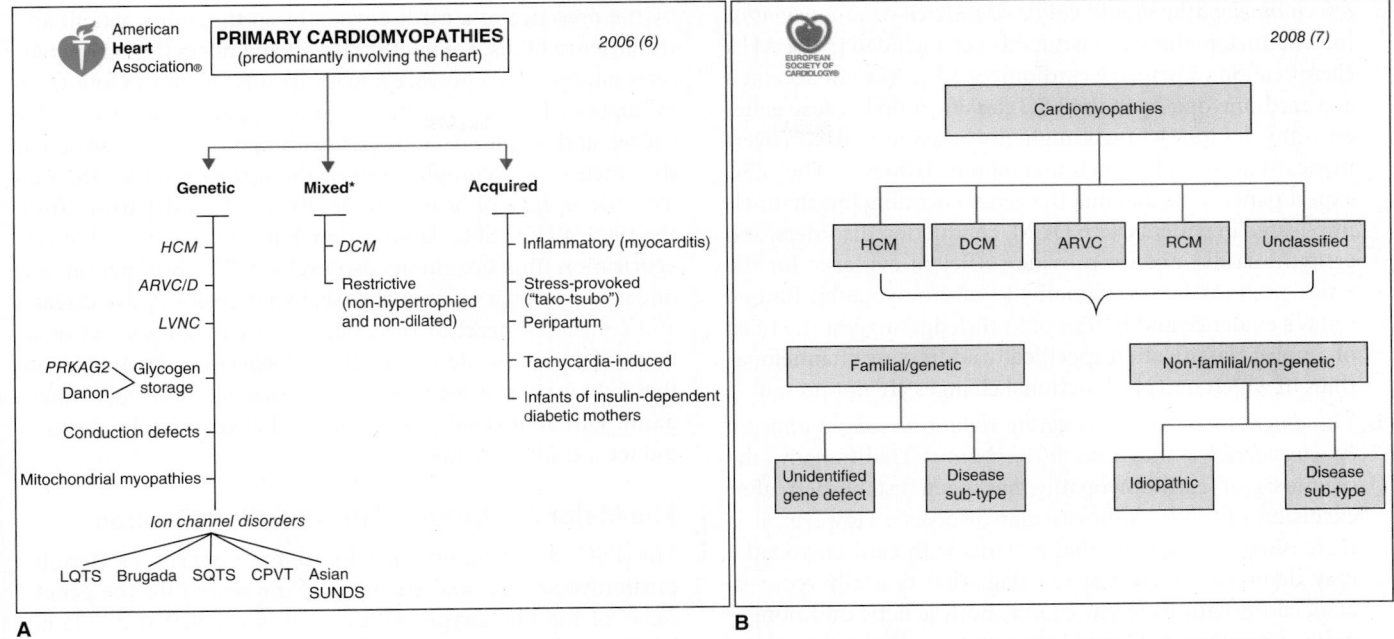

Figure 40-2. Graphical presentation of the AHA classification (2006). Primary cardiomyopathies in which the clinically relevant disease processes solely or predominantly involve the myocardium. The conditions have been segregated according to their genetic or nongenetic etiologies. *Predominantly nongenetic; familial disease with a genetic origin has been reported in a minority of cases. **Graphical presentation of the European Society of Cardiology classification (2008).** ARVC/D, arrhythmogenic right ventricular cardiomyopathy/dysplasia; CPVT, catecholaminergicpolymorphic ventricular tachycardia; DCM, Dilated cardiomyopathy; HCM, hypertrophic cardiomyopathy; LQTS, long QT syndrome; LVNC, left ventricularnoncompaction; RCM, restrictive cardiomyopathy; SQTS, short QT syndrome; SUNDS, sudden unexpected nocturnal death syndrome. (**A**, Reproduced with permission from Maron BJ, Towbin JA, Thiene G, et al. Contemporary definitions and classification of the cardiomyopathies: an American Heart Association Scientific Statement from the Council on Clinical Cardiology, Heart Failure and Transplantation Committee; Quality of Care and Outcomes Research and Functional Genomics and Translational Biology Interdisciplinary Working Groups; and Council on Epidemiology and Prevention. *Circulation.* 2006 Apr 11;113(14):1807-1816. **B**, Reproduced with permission from Elliott P, Andersson B, Arbustini E, et al. Classification of the cardiomyopathies: a position statement from the European Society Of Cardiology Working Group on Myocardial and Pericardial Diseases. *Eur Heart J.* 2008 Jan;29(2):270-276).

been somewhat difficult to translate the classification recommendation into clinical reality.

THE EUROPEAN SOCIETY OF CARDIOLOGY (2008) CLASSIFICATION

The Basis

The 2008 position paper of the ESC proposed the classification of cardiomyopathies that aimed at providing an algorithm for daily clinical practice.[7] The following were key tenets of the proposal, specifically in response to the original WHO-ISFC classification and 2006 AHA classification:

1. *Phenotypic characterization should precede genetic characterization.* Although the ESC endorsed the necessity for identifying the causative genetic defect, as proposed by the AHA, the ESC scheme retained the morphofunctional phenotype as the basis of the classification and management of cardiomyopathy. Cardiomyopathy was grouped into morphofunctional phenotypes including DCM, HCM, RCM, ACM, and unclassified varieties. Each of these types was further divided into familial (genetic) and nonfamilial (nongenetic) forms. The insistence on the morphofunctional classification was based on the fact that the pathway from diagnosis

to treatment in clinical practice rarely begins with the identification of the causative genetic mutation; instead, patients present with symptoms, clinical signs, or abnormal screening test results. Even if the genetic defect is identified in probands, offspring or siblings, the clinical diagnosis relies on the presence of a morphofunctional phenotype.

2. *The broad classification between primary and secondary cardiomyopathy should not be necessary.* The original WHO-ISFC classification system had distinctly defined the cardiomyopathies as primary myocardial disorders (when the cause of the myocardial involvement was unknown) and secondary or specific-heart muscle diseases (when the etiology was known). However, in the AHA classification, the term *primary cardiomyopathy* was applied when the heart was the sole (or predominantly) involved organ, and the term *secondary cardiomyopathy* described heart muscle disease as an integral part of a systemic disorder.[6] It was further contended that the application of the terms *primary* and *secondary cardiomyopathy* per AHA recommendation would be difficult when primary cardiomyopathy was associated with major extracardiac manifestations, or secondary cardiomyopathy predominantly (or exclusively) involved the heart. Therefore, ESC panelists abandoned the distinction between primary and secondary cardiomyopathies.

3. *Ion channelopathy should not be considered cardiomyopathy.* Ion channelopathies, a genetic subtype included in the AHA classification of primary cardiomyopathy, was not accepted as a cardiomyopathy in the ESC classification because genes encoding for ion channels might not be associated with overt myocardial morphofunctional abnormalities.[13] The ESC expert panel contested that the genes encoding ion channels implicated in patients with DCM, conduction disorders, and arrhythmia did not yet provide sufficient evidence for the redesignation of channelopathy as cardiomyopathy. Rather, today's evidence and bodies of knowledge suggest the need of a novel classification specifically addressing channelopathies in which morphofunctional changes are not present.

4. *The diagnosis of cardiomyopathy should be sought and not be considered a diagnosis of exclusion.* Traditionally, the diagnosis of cardiomyopathy has been established after exclusion of other cardiovascular disorders. However, it is increasingly recognized that patients with cardiomyopathy may demonstrate clinical red flags that typically recur in association with different causes, both genetic and nongenetic. Therefore, ESC panelists recommended a diagnostic workup toward a positive, logical deep phenotyping searching for disease-specific markers and differentiating clinical traits and outcome on the basis of the cause rather than on the exclusion of common causes of heart failure or LV hypertrophy. The aim has been to promote a greater appreciation of the broad spectrum of diseases that can result in cardiomyopathy and to abandon the differentiation between cardiomyopathies and specific heart muscle diseases (noncoronary, valvular, hypertensive, or congenital).

The Definition

The 2008 ESC classification defined cardiomyopathy as a myocardial disorder in which the heart muscle is structurally and functionally abnormal, which, in the absence of coronary artery, hypertensive, valvular, and congenital disease, is sufficient to cause the observed myocardial abnormality.

The Classification

In the 2008 ESC classification, cardiomyopathies are grouped into specific morphologic and functional phenotypes; each phenotype is then subclassified into familial and nonfamilial forms (**Fig. 40–2B**).[7] In this context, familial refers to the occurrence in more than one family member of either the same disorder or a phenotype that is (or could be) caused by the same genetic mutation and not a result of acquired cardiac or systemic diseases in which the clinical phenotype is influenced by a genetic polymorphism. Most familial cardiomyopathies are monogenic disorders wherein the gene defect is sufficient by itself to cause the observed phenotype. A monogenic cardiomyopathy can appear as sporadic when the causative mutation is de novo (ie, has occurred in an individual for the first time within the family). In this classification system, patients with identified de novo mutations are assigned to the familial category because their disorder can be subsequently transmitted to their offspring. Nonfamilial cardiomyopathies are clinically defined

by the presence of a cardiomyopathy in the index patient and the absence of disease in other family members (based on pedigree analysis and clinical evaluation) at baseline and follow-up evaluation. They are subdivided into idiopathic (no identifiable cause) and acquired cardiomyopathies in which ventricular dysfunction is a complication of the disorder rather than an intrinsic feature of heart muscle disease. In a departure from the 1995 WHO-ISFC classification, but similar to the AHA categorization, this taxonomy also excludes LV dysfunction secondary to coronary artery disease, hypertension, valve disease, and congenital heart disease, because the diagnosis and treatment of these disorders generally involve clinical management that may vary in some ways from management of cardiomyopathy. Different familial and nonfamilial genetic diseases may induce a similar phenotype.

The Major Attributes of the ESC Classification

The ESC classification introduced the concept of "familial cardiomyopathies" and encouraged the search for the genetic cause of the phenotype. Although it is implicit that a familial disease has a genetic origin, the definition of familial cardiomyopathy was directed at motivating physicians to elicit a detailed family history and execute thorough phenotyping assessment of probands and relatives to establish the diagnosis within the clinical encounter, independent of genetic testing that might not be universally available. In clinical practice, cardiologists still use the morphofunctional classification of cardiomyopathies (HCM, RCM, DCM, ARVC, and unclassified varieties) followed by further characterization into genetic or nongenetic subtypes. The subsequent documents of the ESC Working Group reinforced the recommendations for screening of relatives as the most powerful clinical tool for the recognition of familial cardiomyopathies[14] and clinical monitoring of families in a phenotype-driven mindset to formulate a pretest hypothesis of specific gene defects.[15]

THE WORLD HEART FEDERATION (2013) CLASSIFICATION

The Basis

The classifications by the AHA and ESC have advanced the field substantially. The writing group of the AHA classification promulgated the importance of the genetic basis of cardiomyopathy. The ESC writing group recognized the importance of the heritability of the cardiomyopathies and retained the practicality of their taxonomy for routine clinical use. The WHF-endorsed classification represents a stepwise union of the two characteristics of phenotype and genotype into a cogent classification system.[8,9] The WHF writing group integrates the deep clinical phenotyping and the identification of genetic defects to provide comprehensive information about the precise diagnosis (phenotype and genotype) in cardiomyopathies. A substantially large number of disease genes have been either confirmed or suspected as candidate genes; genetic heterogeneity has been established, and the wider use of next-generation sequencing is continuously increasing our understanding of the manifestations of the disease. The WHF classification adds value to both preceding classifications and is based on the following principles:

1. *Most cardiomyopathies are familial diseases.* The epidemiology of cardiomyopathies is derived from clinical family studies performed in the pregenetic era. In this context, the traditionally accepted prevalence of cardiomyopathy based on the diagnosis of overt phenotypes may be a gross underestimation of the actual prevalence of cardiomyopathies. Familial cardiomyopathies are predominantly inherited as autosomal dominant traits and, less frequently, as autosomal recessive, X-linked recessive or dominant, and matrilineal disorders. Familial cardiomyopathy is diagnosed when two or more family members are affected. The age dependence of the phenotype may require long-term follow-up for a comprehensive evaluation of the family. The diagnosis of familial cardiomyopathy is easily established in families where more members are contemporaneously affected. However, the diagnostic assumption of nonfamilial cardiomyopathy should rely either on the evidence of a nongenetic cause or should remain labeled as unknown wherein systematic screening is limited by family size, adoption, or deceased relatives. After comprehensive assessment of pedigree, cascade family screening is undertaken to allow for identification of all affected family members, including healthy carriers of genetic variants causally linked to the disease.

2. *Familial cardiomyopathies have a genetic origin and display clinical and genetic heterogeneity.* The list of candidate genes as the cause of cardiomyopathies is still progressing. Such genes are identified through linkage analyses, genome-wide association studies, and whole exome sequencing. With more than 100 genes identified, the list still remains incomplete, but the most common genes associated with the different types of cardiomyopathies are well known, and genetic testing is translated into clinical reality.

Although all cardiomyopathies are broadly classified as five major morphofunctional phenotypes, a careful clinical evaluation demonstrates high phenotypic variability.[9] Various cardiomyopathy subsets show variations in gender predisposition, age of onset, rate of progression, complications, and risk of developing end-stage heart failure or life-threatening ventricular arrhythmias. For example, DCM patients with *LMNA* mutations may develop life-threatening ventricular arrhythmias[16] even in the presence of only mild LV enlargement and dysfunction,[11] whereas those with dystrophin mutations may carry only low arrhythmogenic risk even with extreme LV dilatation or dysfunction.[17] Similarly, there are HCM patients with severe LV hypertrophy (>30 mm) but low arrhythmogenic risk and those with mild or moderate hypertrophy but high arrhythmogenic risk. In addition, gene-specific traits and diagnostic markers (red flags) may be reproducibly associated with subgroups of cardiomyopathy patients; such red flags include atrioventricular block (AVB), preexcitation syndrome (eg, Wolff-Parkinson-White [WPW] pattern or syndrome), repolarization abnormalities, or attenuated QRS voltage.[9] Furthermore, noninvasive imaging may reveal variable severity, distribution, and extent of myocardial hypertrophy, valve pathology, LV noncompaction, varying extents of ventricular dilatation and dysfunction, and variations in extent and distribution of myocardial fibrosis, or fatty infiltration within the myocardium. An integrated multidisciplinary workup including ascertainment of inheritance pattern, determination of major clinical phenotype (eg, DCM or HCM), identification of cardiac markers (eg, AVB, short PR interval, or WPW), characterization of extracardiac organ involvement (eg, ocular, muscle, skeletal, or neurologic traits), or measurement of biomarkers (eg, increased serum creatinine phosphokinase or lactic acidemia as markers of associated myopathy) provides a preliminary filter for selecting genes for testing. For instance, cardiolaminopathies are associated with AVB in up to 80% of cases[18]; dystrophinopathies are inherited in male patients in the absence of male-to-male transmission of the disease and are associated with increased serum creatinine phosphokinase (80%)[17]; and myocardial storage diseases typically demonstrate concentric LV hypertrophy with short PR interval and/or WPW pattern or syndrome. The presence of clinical red flags in probands and/or relatives guides genetic testing and provides for a sustainable strategy for clinical translation.[19] After the conclusion of the clinical workup, genetic testing is offered to patients and families.

The genetic heterogeneity (more genes, similar phenotype) complicates the overall diagnostic workup of familial cardiomyopathies: several genes influencing the same or different pathway(s) may be associated with similar clinical manifestations, and identical gene mutations may result in altogether different phenotypes. For instance, the sarcomeric gene defects may be associated with HCM and DCM; desmosome gene defects, which are typically associated with the classical ARVC, may cause DCM; genes encoding intermediate filaments such as nuclear lamins may also be associated with ARVC; and nonsarcomeric genes are also known to be associated with HCM. An increasing number of cardiomyopathies are recognized to be associated with complex genetics. Studies interrogating panels of genes in single patients have demonstrated a higher-than-expected rate of patients who are carriers of more than one mutation in the same or in different genes, which might imply that the incomplete genetic penetrance or variable expressivity of gene mutations represents incomplete genotyping or that the presumptive disease-causing role has erroneously been assigned to a wrong gene and mutation. Although in vitro functional studies can contribute to elucidating the role of protein mutations in a given cardiomyopathy, the detection of mutations will continue to be faster than developing animal models or performing in vitro studies for confirmation of their functional roles. An approach to genetic testing could be clinically guided or broader based (eg, large panels of disease-associated/candidate genes). It is becoming evident that interpreting the results, rather than performing the tests, is the greater challenge in the modern era of next-generation sequencing.[20-23]

3. *The knowledge of genetic background would allow an improved management strategy.* The major clinical decisions (eg, implantable cardioverter-defibrillator implantation) are still based on mechanical (eg, LV ejection fraction in DCM) or morphologic (eg, maximal LV wall thickness in HCM) characteristics, regardless of the intrinsic disease risk related to the underlying genotype.[24,25] However, such risk stratification based on anatomic and/or mechanical features has limitations. For example, patients with laminopathies may not always demonstrate substantial LV dysfunction and dilatation when their arrhythmogenic risk first manifests,[26] and those with dystrophinopathies may be significantly less susceptible to the risk of malignant arrhythmias even when the left ventricle is dramatically enlarged and dysfunctional.[17] Similarly, patients with troponinopathies may not manifest severe LV wall thickness, but may display a high arrhythmogenic potential.[27]

4. *Ever-increasing knowledge of genetic background may result in random nomenclature.* Based on the underlying gene mutations,[8] numerous new terms (eg, desmosomalopathies, cytoskeletalopathies, sarcomyopathies, channelopathies, cardiodystrophinopathies, cardiolaminopathies, zaspopathies, myotilinopathies, dystrophinopathies, αB-crystallinopathies, desminopathies, or caveolinopathies) are being proposed. These are likely to cloud the description of cardiomyopathy, and it has become important that a uniform nomenclature be developed.

5. *The taxonomy should be a flexible, user-friendly system that can be used at the bedside.* As was the case for the universal TNM staging for malignant tumors, an improved taxonomy for classification of cardiomyopathy should be comprehensive and user-friendly, allowing for easier communication among physicians and facilitating the development of multicenter/multinational registries to promote research in diagnosis and management of cardiomyopathies. Various investigators suggested additional integrations, and modifications have been proposed for AVRC,[28] endomyocardial fibrosis,[29,30] and HCM.[31]

The applicability and prognostic relevance of the MOGE(S) classification was investigated in 213 consecutive patients with DCM who underwent a complete diagnostic work-up, including genetic evaluation and endomyocardial biopsy.[32] Organ involvement was demonstrated in 35 (16%) patients and genetic or familial DCM in 70 (33%) patients. At least one cause was found in 155 (73%) patients, of whom 48 (23%) had more than one possible cause. After a median follow-up of 47 months, organ involvement and higher New York Heart Association (NYHA) functional class were associated with adverse outcome. Worse outcome was observed when genetic or familial DCM was accompanied by additional environmental etiologic factors (significant viral load, immune-mediated factors, rhythm disturbances, or toxic triggers) (*P* = 0.03). A higher presence of MOGE(S) attributes (≥2 vs ≤1 attributes) showed an adverse outcome (*P* = 0.007). The authors concluded that the MOGE(S) classification in DCM is applicable, and each attribute or the gene-environment interaction is associated with outcome.[32]

The clinical applicability of MOGE(S) nomenclature was tested in 181 HCM patients with HCM.[31] Gene testing was performed in 125 subjects with HCM phenotype. A significant percentage (24.3%) of the participants was at NYHA class III/IV, while all participants underwent the routine clinical evaluation for HCM patients and were under the guideline-based medical treatment. Study participants were divided into two MOGE(S) categories: $M_H O_H G_{AD} E_{G-}$ were gene-negative HCM patients (*n* = 67) and $M_H O_H G_{AD} E_{G+}$ were gene-positive (*n* = 57). Gene-positive patients were younger at the baseline evaluation and more likely to be female and have a family history of HCM or sudden cardiac death, as well as ventricular tachycardia. There were no significant differences in other clinical or imaging characteristics between the two groups. The authors suggested that the MOGE(S) classification should include information regarding the presence or absence of obstruction and the location of hypertrophy, given the role of these data on the clinical course of the disease. It was proposed that HCM could be further categorized as nonobstructive HCM ([obs-neg] HCM) and obstructive HCM ([obs] HCM), or (obs-NA) HCM when this information is not yet available.[31] An updated review on HCM acknowledges that the MOGE(S) approach enables a standardized classification of cardiomyopathies, including HCM.[33] MOGE(S) was applied to a large series of patients diagnosed with Anderson Fabry disease to provide details on the organ involvement in carriers of different mutations of the GLA gene.[34] Westphal et al.[35] critically revised the MOGE(S) criteria and suggested that in the case of myocarditis, it would be useful to differentiate between MCrEF (myocarditis with reduced LVEF), MCmrEF (myocarditis with mid-range LVEF), and MCpEF (myocarditis with preserved LVEF). This differentiation could have clinical implications for use of neurohumoral antagonists as well as for the indication for EMB.[35]

The Definition

The cardiomyopathies in the WHF classification are described as disorders characterized by morphologically and functionally abnormal myocardium in the absence of any other disease that is sufficient, by itself, to cause the observed phenotype.[8] In this classification, although the conventional phenotypic subtype of the cardiomyopathy continues to provide the basis for the classification, an etiology-based assessment dictates the diagnostic workup and, when possible, treatment decisions in probands and relatives, as well as the follow-up plan. Once the genetic cause of the cardiomyopathy has been established, the cascade family screening can help identify healthy mutation carriers who may eventually develop the phenotype over the ensuing years.[13] Avoidance of competitive sport activity and tailored monitoring with early medical treatment may favorably influence the natural history of the disease and the development of the manifest phenotype, as well as the risk of life-threatening arrhythmias. Identification of genetic diseases may also help subjects and alert physicians to refrain from the use of injurious agents. For instance, agents triggering malignant hyperthermia (succinylcholine) or volatile anesthetics (halothane and isoflurane) are to be avoided in emerinopathies and laminopathies causing muscular dystrophy.[36] Statins should be administered with caution in patients with genetic cardiomyopathies with possible involvement of the skeletal muscle, even when markers of myopathy are negative.[37] Patients with disorders of the respiratory chain may need surgeries in the long term, but anesthetics may interfere with metabolism and may trigger unexpected complications.[38] Patients with mitochondrial cardiomyopathy and epilepsy should not receive valproate because it could cause pseudoatrophy of the brain.[39] Common indications for heart transplantation in patients with end-stage cardiomyopathy should take into account the specific diagnosis; conditions such as Danon disease or other comorbidities, such as mental retardation, are a matter of debate regarding indication for heart transplantation.[40] Finally, genotype-based diagnoses can be pooled in large international databases for future clinical trials and validation of novel management strategies.

The Classification

The most effective nosology system should encompass clinical presentation, organ involvement, genetic inheritance, and precise etiologic information. This could be optionally supplemented by the functional class/stage/status and should use universally adopted terms. The WHF's MOGE(S) classification system is the first attempt to integrate morphofunctional phenotype-based description, information on the involvement of extracardiac organs/tissues, clinical genetics in familial diseases (pattern of inheritance), and molecular genetics (disease gene and mutation). MOGE(S) can also describe "sporadic" nongenetic cardiomyopathies and specify their etiology if known. In the case of phenotypically sporadic cardiomyopathies, a genetic origin of the disease (in case of de novo mutation or still unknown disease genes) cannot be excluded unless a nongenetic cause is proven and clinical family screening has ruled out a familial disease. When not certain, each cardiomyopathy should be considered as a potentially genetic disease, allowing families to receive the same screening options offered to families with known familial cardiomyopathy.

MOGE(S) classification is inspired by the TNM (tumor, nodes, metastases) staging system; it is a descriptive nosology algorithm that includes five essential descriptors of cardiomyopathies (**Fig. 40–3**), both inherited and noninherited.[8] These five attributes are morphofunctional phenotype (M), organ involvement (O), genetic or familial inheritance pattern (G), etiologic (E) description of genetic defect or nongenetic cause, and functional status (S), using the American College of Cardiology (ACC)/AHA stage (stage A–D) and NYHA (class I–IV). The "S" notation becomes especially useful when

SUBSCRIPT NOTATION	M MORPHO-FUNCTIONAL PHENOTYPE	O ORGAN/SYSTEM INVOLVEMENT	G GENETIC INHERITANCE PATTERN		E ETIOLOGY	S STAGE
	D Dilated	H Heart *LV=left ventricle* *RV=right ventricle* *RLV=biventricular*	N Family history negative	G Genetic cause	ACC-AHA stage represented as letter A, B, C, D
	H Hypertrophic		U Family history unknown	OC Obligate carrier	
	R Restrictive		AD Autosomal dominant	ONC Obligate noncarrier	
	R EMF Endomyocardial fibrosis *LV=left ventricle* *RV=right ventricle* *RLV=biventricular*	M Muscle (skeletal)	AR Autosomal recessive	DN *De novo*	NA not applicable
		N Nervous	XLD X-linked dominant	Neg Genetic test negative for the known familial mutation	NU not used
		C Cutaneous	XLR X-linked recessive	N Genetic defect not identified	
		E Eye, ocular	XL X-linked	O No genetic test, any reason*	
		A Auditory	M Matrilineal	G-A-TTR Genetic amyloidosis	*followed by*
	A ARVC *M=major* *m=minor* *c=category* *LV= left ventricle* *RV=right ventricle* *RLV=biventricular*	K Kidney	O Family history not investigated*	G-HFE Hemochromatosis	NYHA class represented as Roman numeral I, II, III, IV
		G Gastrointestinal	Undet Inheritance still undetermined	*Nongenetic etiologies:*	
		Li Liver	S Phenotypically sporadic (apparent or real)	M Myocarditis	
		Lu Lung		V Viral infection (add the virus identified in affected heart)	
	NC LVNC	S Skeletal		AI Autoimmune/immune-mediate; suspected (AI-S), proven (AI-P)	
	E Early, with type in parentheses	O Absence of organ/system involvement,* e.g. in family members who are healthy mutation carriers; the mutation is specified in E and inheritance in G		A Amyloidosis (add type: A-K, A-L, A-SAA)	
	NS Nonspecific phenotype			I Infectious, nonviral (add the infectious agent)	
	NA Information non available			T Toxicity (add cause/drug)	
	O Unaffected*			Eo Hypereosinophilic heart disease	
				O Other	

Figure 40–3. MOGE(S): classification of cardiomyopathies. It is a descriptive nosology algorithm that includes five descriptors of cardiomyopathies, both inherited and noninherited. The five attributes of MOGE(S) are morphofunctional phenotype (M), organ involvement (O), genetic or familial inheritance pattern (G), etiologic (E) description of genetic defect or nongenetic cause, and the functional status (S) using the American College of Cardiology (ACC)/American Heart Association (AHA) stage (stage A–D) and New York Heart Association (NYHA) class (class I–IV). ARVC, arrhythmogenic right ventricular cardiomyopathy; LVNC, left ventricular noncompaction. Reproduced with permission from Arbustini E, Narula N, Tavazzi L, et al. The MOGE(S) classification of cardiomyopathy for clinicians. *J Am Coll Cardiol.* 2014 Jul 22;64(3):304-301.

mutation carriers are healthy (phenotypically unaffected) or if they demonstrate preclinical imaging-verified early abnormalities suggestive of the cardiomyopathy.[9] The cardiac phenotype description precedes genetic information. The approach to the evaluation of cardiomyopathies should involve a comprehensive family history and identification of other accompanying disease characteristics (red flags) that may predict candidate gene involvement. Even if genetic information is not available, consideration of heritability allows conceptualizing of the disease as a familial process.

Morphofunctional Phenotype, or M

The morphofunctional presentation is described as a subscript to the notation M; for example, M_D (DCM), M_H (HCM), M_A (ACM), M_R (RCM), and M_{NC} (LV noncompaction). ACM is categorized in three major subtypes: classical right ventricular ACM (ARVC or RV-ACM), biventricular ACM (BV-ACM), and predominantly left ventricular ACM (LV-ACM). This terminology will be revised considering the recent expert document that reintroduces the term ARVC but classifies the disease as classical right ventricular, biventricular, and predominantly left ventricular.[12] Unlike previous classifications, the mixed or

overlapping phenotypes can be easily presented, such as HCM that evolves into dilated congestive phenotype (M_{H+D}) or HCM presenting with predominant restrictive pattern (M_{H+R}). Other combinations are possible, such as M_{D+NC}, M_{A+NC}, M_{H+NC}, and M_{H+R+D}. The M notation can add key clinical red flags such as short PR interval ($\downarrow$PR), WPW pattern or syndrome, and AVB (displayed as $M_{H[\downarrow PR]}$, $M_{H[WPW]}$, and $M_{D[AVB]}$, respectively), or nonspecific or noncoded traits (such as hypertrabeculation when criteria for LV noncompaction are not fulfilled, or any other trait specifically associated with the disease) can be added (**Fig. 40–4**). Most importantly, M allows the description of *early* phenotypes (M_E) or variants (mildly dilated cardiomyopathy, [M_{MD}]), such as when the diagnostic criteria for the suspected clinical phenotype (such as DCM or HCM) are not fulfilled and imaging data indicate an increased LV diameter and a borderline LV function ($M_{E[D]}$) or possible LV hypertrophy ($M_{E[H]}$).[11] Clinically healthy mutation carriers are described as $M_{0[H]}$ or $M_{0[D]}$ (0 is for zero). When the information about the cardiac phenotype is not available, such as with deceased relatives, the description is M_{NA}. Overall, the M notation is flexible and suitable for any clinical combination of disease phenotypes and clinical traits.

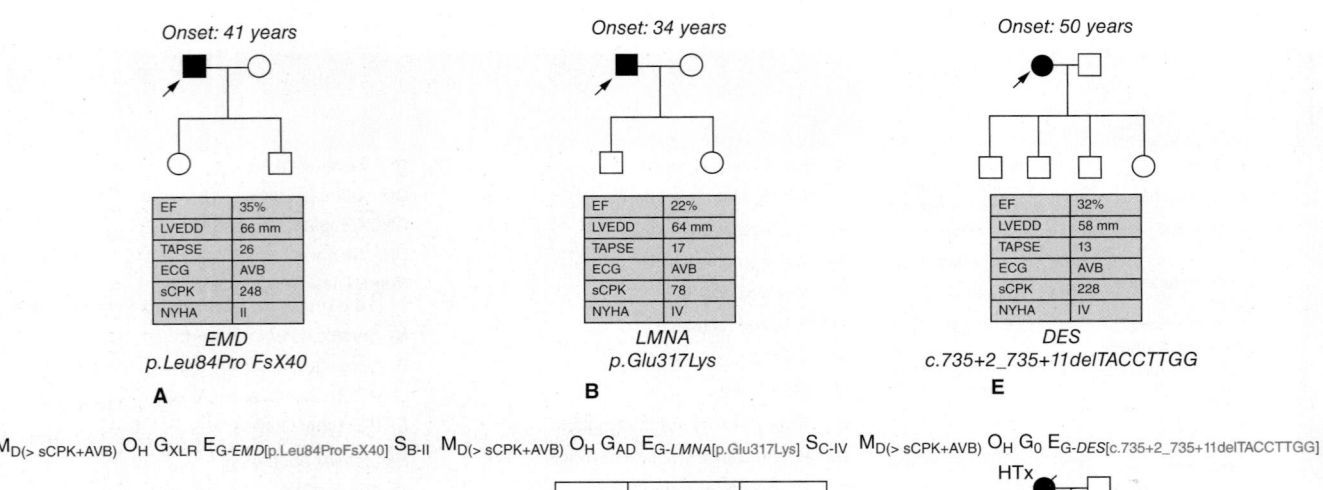

Figure 40–4. Morphologic descriptor and genotypic interaction. Three pedigrees with probands (*arrows*) demonstrating similar dilated cardiomyopathy (DCM) phenotypes (A–D) in the first two and restrictive cardiomyopathy (RCM; E–F) in the third patient. The identification of the causative genes and mutations underscores the importance of the genetic diagnosis on the management of the three families. The identification of a mutation in the *Emerin* (*EMD*) gene provides information about the genetic status of the offspring. The son of the proband is obligate negative because a male cannot transmit an X-linked defect to his son. However, the daughters of affected males in X-linked diseases are obligate carriers of the paternal mutations. The identification of a mutation in the lamin AC (*LMNA*) gene (*middle panel*) or desmin (*DES*) gene (*right panel*) provides evidence that offspring can inherit the mutation with 50% probability for each pregnancy. All patients had advanced atrioventricular block and increases in serum creatinine phosphokinase (sCPK) levels. Pedigree symbols are as follows: *circles* represent females, *squares* represent males, *diagonal lines* represent deceased, and *solid-filled symbols* denote the presence of the phenotype. ECG, electrocardiogram; EF, ejection fraction; HF, heart failure; HTx, heart transplantation; LVEDD, left ventricular end diastolic diameter; NYHA, New York Heart Association; PM, pace-maker; SD, sudden death; TAPSE, tricuspid annular plane systolic excursion.

Organ Involvement, or O

The notation O describes organ involvement in the subscript. The comprehensive presentation of the involved organs helps identify syndromes. The cardiomyopathy, that is cardiac involvement, is represented as O_H. The involvement of other organs is added on the cardiac involvement, such as skeletal muscle involvement in dystrophin defect (O_{H+M}); involvement of kidney, gastrointestinal system, skin/cutaneous, and eye in classical Anderson-Fabry disease ($O_{H+K+G+C+E}$) and, less commonly, in Fabry patients carriers of late-onset cardiac variants (**Fig. 40–5**); or involvement of auditory system, nervous system, liver, lungs, and mental retardation in mitochondrial DNA–related diseases (O_{H+A}, O_{H+N}, O_{H+L}, O_{H+Lu}, and O_{H+MR}, respectively). The involvement of uncommon organs can be adopted on the basis of anatomic terms in the Systematized Nomenclature of Medicine topography (eg, thyroid [O_{H+T}] and adrenal glands [O_{H+AD}]). Healthy mutation carriers are described as (O_0) because the heart is still clinically unaffected (M_0). "O" is similarly represented in nongenetic disorders (eg, the liver involvement and hypereosinophilia [$O_{H+L+\uparrow Eo}$] in endomyocardial fibrosis).

Genetic Inheritance, or G

The notation G describes the genetic or familial inheritance as clinically identified from the family screening, with inheritance including autosomal dominant (G_{AD}), autosomal recessive (G_{AR}), X-linked (G_{XL}), X-linked recessive (G_{XLR}) or dominant (G_{XLD}), and matrilineal (G_M). A solitary involvement is described as sporadic (G_S) cardiomyopathy after the family screening and review of medical records of deceased relatives of the proband. The patient with unknown (G_U) or negative (G_N) family history should also be described.

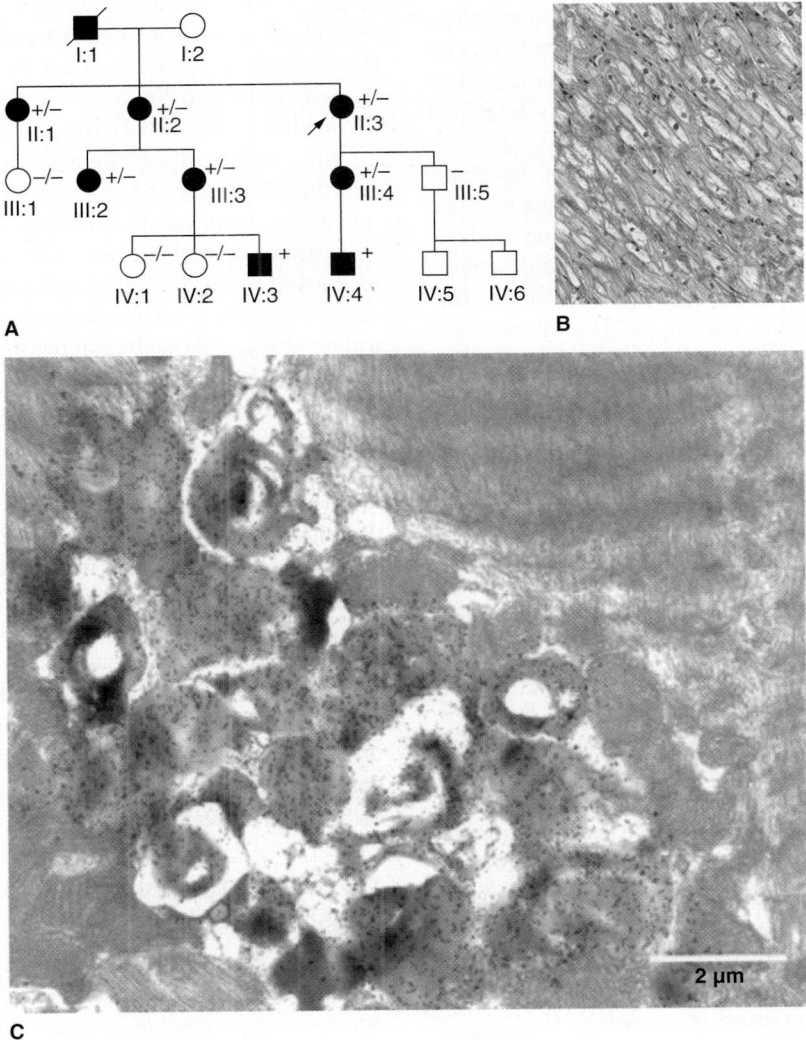

Figure 40–5. X-linked Anderson-Fabry disease (AFD). The pedigree (A) shows a typical family with Anderson-Fabry disease caused by the cardiac variant p.(Asn215Ser) in *a-galactosidase gene.* In the bottom half of the figure, the pathologic features of AFD in endomyocardial biopsy are shown. **B. The hematoxylin and eosin stain shows a large number of vacuolated myocytes (glycosphingolipids are extracted in formalin-fixed, paraffin-embedded tissues). C. Immuno-electron microscopy view shows typical lamellar and dense osmiophilic bodies specifically immuno-labeled by anti-GB3 antibodies.** Pedigree symbols are as follows: *circles* represent females, *squares* represent males, *diagonal lines* represent deceased, and *solid-filled symbols* denote the presence of the phenotype.

Underlying Etiology, or E

The notation E is represented in two steps. The first step is presented as a coupled subscript for the genetic (E_G), or nongenetic nature (E_{NG}) of the disease. For the genetic background (E_G), if the genetic defect is identified and characterized, then the second step provides complete information on the gene mutation, such as in the case of HCM ($E_{G-MYH7[p.Arg403Glu]}$), familial amyloidosis ($E_{G-ATTR[p.Val122Ile]}$), or hemochromatosis ($E_{G-HFE[p.Cys282Tyr\ Homozygous]}$). When the mutation is identified or when more than one mutation/genetic variant is identified, it is described by the standard colors used for characterizing pathologic mutations in human mutations databases. The color code describes possible and probable pathologic mutations in red; genetic variants of unknown significance in yellow; and single-nucleotide polymorphisms with possible functional significance in green. If the genetic characterization is not available, but the clinical and genetic family screening provides the necessary information, the (E_G) notation is to be specified as obligate carrier (E_{G-OC}), obligate noncarrier (E_{G-ONC}), or the sporadic/de novo occurrence of mutation (E_{G-DN}). These are important notations because they complement the data on inheritance in the G descriptor. A genetic test negative for the known family mutation is described as (E_{G-NEG}); a negative genetic test is described as (E_{G-N}). When the genetic test could not be done for any reason, the descriptor is (E_{G-0}). Reporting on healthy family members who test negative for the *culprit* mutation(s) is essential for segregation study in the family. When all members of a single family are described, the MOGE(S) nomenclature system highlights mutations that do not fully segregate with the phenotype. The international nomenclature of genetic variants provides the principles for their description (https://varnomen.hgvs.org/). The in silico evaluation supports the interpretation of the significance of each variant (e.g. http://genetics.bwh.harvard.edu/pph2/, http://provean.jcvi.org/index.php/, https://evs.gs.washington.edu/EVS/, https://www.internationalgenome.org/, http://www.umd.be/HSF/). The family studies provide the segregation data, and the pathologic or in vitro studies may contribute to document the abnormal expression of the mutated protein.

Similar to the genetic diseases (E_G), the cause of the underlying disease in the nongenetic cardiomyopathies (E_{NG}) is specified in two steps, with the first notation being a couplet. The first notation (E_{NG}) is coupled as predominantly toxic/degenerative, inflammatory, infiltrative, or hypersensitivity disease or others, as presented in Fig. 40-3. The second step should detail the exact cause if known. Some specific examples include a viral myocarditis caused by the Coxsackie B3 virus, human cytomegalovirus, or the Epstein–Barr virus using the taxonomy system as coded by the International Committee on Taxonomy of Viruses (https://talk.ictvonline.org/) may be presented as $E_{NG-M[HCMV]}$, $E_{NG-M[CB3]}$, or $E_{NG-M[EBV]}$, respectively. Inflammatory myocarditis suggestive of sarcoidosis ($E_{NG-M[Sarcoid]}$) or giant cell myocarditis ($E_{NG-M[Giant\ cell]}$) can be specifically addressed. Other examples of nongenetic inflammatory variety include autoimmune etiology ($E_{NG-AI[TYPE]}$), hypersensitivity ($E_{NG-Hs[TYPE]}$), or eosinophilic disease as from a parasitic process ($E_{NG-Eo[Type\ of\ Parasitic\ Disease]}$). Eosinophilic Loeffler endomyocarditis

may be described, according to the cause, as either being idiopathic or part of a myeloproliferative disorder associated with the somatic chromosomal rearrangement of the *PDGFRα* or *PDGFRβ* genes that generate a fusion gene encoding constitutively active PDGFR tyrosine kinases. Nonheritable amyloidosis with kappa ($E_{NG-A[K]}$), lambda ($E_{NG-A[L]}$), or serum amyloid A protein ($E_{NG-A[SAA]}$) characterization can be easily presented and distinguished from the genetic varieties ($E_{G-A[TTR]}$). Similarly, the toxic cardiomyopathies, such as pheochromocytoma-related ($E_{NG-T[Pheo]}$) or drug-induced ($E_{NG-T[Chloroquine]}$) cardiomyopathy, are classifiable; when the former is in the context of a syndrome (eg, von Hippel-Lindau, multiple endocrine neoplasia type 2A/2B, or neurofibromatosis type 1), the name of the syndrome could be added ($E_{NG-T[Pheo-VHL]}$).

Functional Status, or S

The notation S describes the heart failure ACC/AHA stage A to D and NYHA functional class I to IV, combined such as S_{A-I} or S_{C-III}.[41] Although there has been some resistance to the universal application of ACC/AHA and NYHA staging, we believe that this allows the most practical solution to the description of early cardiomyopathies and mutation-carrying healthy family members. The ACC/AHA guidelines include patients with a family history of cardiomyopathy in stage A heart failure, and there has never been a way to include them in a cardiomyopathy classification. Although criteria for early diagnosis of cardiomyopathy are not systematically documented, the increasing family screening and monitoring have revealed that cardiomyopathies such as laminopathies reveal a long preclinical or subclinical incubation before the onset of manifest clinical disease.

The MOGE(S) nosology combines morphofunctional trait and organ (system) involvement with familial inheritance pattern, while characterizing heritable and nonheritable mechanisms of disease. ACC/AHA staging with NYHA class description offers special value for the inclusion of genetically mutated but yet unaffected individuals in the classification. Just as was the case for the universal TNM staging for malignant tumors, it is expected that this description will be improved, revised, modified, and made more comprehensive and user-friendly in years to come. It will allow for a better understanding of the disease process and easier communication among providers and help develop multicenter and multinational registries to promote research in diagnosis and management of cardiomyopathies.

The Major Attributes of the WHF-Endorsed Classification

MOGE(S) is an example of a coding system that has a sound basis and retains the phenotypic classification of cardiomyopathies (as in the ESC classification) but also incorporates the innovative soul of the AHA classification. Furthermore, because of its flexibility, MOGE(S) can be conveniently modified, adapted, and implemented.

The MOGE(S) system of classification of cardiomyopathies not only allows the possibility of retaining a phenotype-based description, but also allows inclusion of information about extracardiac organ involvement, the heritability of the disease, and data on both genetic and nongenetic contributors. Addition of information pertaining to functional status and disease state also allows description of mutation carriers who are clinically healthy or show subclinical or early disease. One of the main barriers encountered today in drawing reliable epidemiologic and clinical information from large, international databases lies in the difference in adopted definitions of the same object in various settings.[42] Descriptive definitions such as MOGE(S) might help to overcome such obstacles. If universally adopted, the cardiology community would have enough data to group cardiomyopathies based on their causes to herald an open era for the development of disease-specific drugs and clinical trials.

THE AHA CLASSIFICATION AND DIAGNOSIS OF CARDIOMYOPATHY IN CHILDREN

The need for an appropriate nomenclature for cardiomyopathies is particularly felt for the pediatric age.[43] The AHA scientific statement "Cardiomyopathy in Children: Classification and Diagnosis"[44] was recently released and addressed two issues: (1) the most current understanding of the causes of cardiomyopathy in children and (2) the optimal approaches to the diagnosis of cardiomyopathy in children. Although cardiomyopathies are rare in children, once diagnosed, they carry a substantial risk of morbidity and mortality and are the primary indication for heart transplantation, particularly among children >1 year of age. "Children are not small adults" and cardiomyopathy classifications in children, although adopting the same diagnostic descriptors that are used for adult cardiomyopathies, should consider specific requirements such as very rare, often malignant, extreme etiology heterogeneity, more common in syndromes, highly demanding diagnostic work-up, and timely and precise diagnoses for appropriate treatments, especially for metabolic diseases.

The proposed classification of the cardiomyopathies is hierarchical, based on the structural and functional phenotype with genetic and nongenetic causes as subcategories. The consensus of the authors is to use a system incorporating the required elements of MOGE(S) that is a hierarchy system based on the structural and functional phenotype with genetic and nongenetic causes as subcategories. In this novel classification, the main structural and functional phenotypes correspond to the dilated, hypertrophic, and restrictive cardiomyopathies. A new entry in the DCM group is the "cardiomyopathy associated with pulmonary conditions" acknowledging that the RV dysfunction most commonly occurs from factors causing pulmonary hypertension (PH). The writing group links the novel causal classification of PH with the RV hypertrophy or dilation secondary to non–group 2 PH.[45] Again, "secondary forms" of HCM, both syndromic and nonsyndromic, predominate with respect to sarcomeric ones. Among the RCM, amyloidosis is included, which is

unlikely to occur in children. However, children with heritable autoinflammatory diseases may develop systemic AA amyloidosis at a young/young-adult age, which is more typically localized at renal than at cardiac level.[46] As for LVNC, the writing group acknowledges that controversy remains as to whether the finding of trabeculations in the LV fulfilling imaging criteria for LVNC is cardiomyopathy (disease) or simply a morphological trait; in fact, LVNC in children has been described in association with complex congenital heart disease and coronary artery anomalies and as an isolated finding in the heart, with and without musculoskeletal and other system abnormalities. Finally, it is considered prudent to include both ARVC and "Cardiomyopathy Caused by Channelopathies" in a subgroup of arrhythmia substrate–associated cardiomyopathies.

CLASSIFICATION IN THE ERA OF PRECISION AND PERSONALIZED MEDICINE

This is the time of the precision medicine. Tonight, I'm launching a new Precision Medicine Initiative to bring us closer to curing diseases like cancer and diabetes—and to give all of us access to the personalized information we need to keep ourselves and our families healthier. —President Barack Obama, addressing the United States on January 20, 2015, in a State of the Union Address.

Although the major emphasis was placed on cancer and diabetes[47] in the 2015 State of the Union Presidential Address, the concept of *precision* applied to the entire field of medicine. We are in progressive transition from pathology-based descriptive medicine to specific etiology–driven medicine. *Precision medicine* and *personalized medicine* are often used interchangeably, but they represent two sides of the same coin wherein the precision is directed at the specific diagnosis and the personalized management is directed at an individually tailored approach.[48] Precision cardiology aims at detecting the primary causes of heart diseases and developing targeted, personalized therapies.[49,50] The impact of such an approach is expected to be almost immediate for the diseases caused by a unique factor, noxa, or genetic defect. Cardiomyopathies are paradigmatic examples of feasible and sustainable precision diagnostic workup. Their genetic origin and convenient genetic testing offer an ideal platform for providing patients and families with clinical and etiologic diagnosis. In most cardiomyopathy families, the most common autosomal dominant transmission lends itself to a precise diagnosis and plays a major role in family health for preimplantation, prenatal, preclinical, and presymptomatic assessment. Personalized medical therapy guided by pharmacogenetics and inducible pluripotent stem cells are also becoming an emerging application for the clinical practice.[51] Precision data would remain underused if they are not incorporated in classifications and coding systems that can make meaningful contributions in etiology-based epidemiology of diseases.

REFERENCES

1. Goodwin JF. The frontiers of cardiomyopathy. *Br Heart J.* 1982;48:1-18.

2. Brigden W. Uncommon myocardial diseases: the non-coronary cardiomyopathies. *Lancet.* 1957;273:1179-1184, 1243-1249.

3. Goodwin JF, Oakley CM. The cardiomyopathies. *Br Heart J.* 1972;34:54-5552.

4. Brandenbourg RO, Chazov E, Cherian G, et al. Report of the WHO/ISFC task force on the definition and classification of cardiomyopathies. *Br Heart J.* 1980;44:672-673.

5. Richardson P, McKenna W, Bristow M, et al. Report of the 1995 World Health Organization/International Society and Federation of Cardiology Task Force on the Definition and Classification of Cardiomyopathies. *Circulation.* 1996;93:841-842.

6. Maron BJ, Towbin JA, Thiene G, et al. American Heart Association; Council on Clinical Cardiology, Heart Failure and Transplantation Committee; Quality of Care and Outcomes Research and Functional Genomics and Translational Biology Interdisciplinary Working Groups; Council on Epidemiology and Prevention. Contemporary definitions and classification of the cardiomyopathies: an American Heart Association Scientific Statement from the Council on Clinical Cardiology, Heart Failure and Transplantation Committee; Quality of Care and Outcomes Research and Functional Genomics and Translational Biology Interdisciplinary Working Groups; and Council on Epidemiology and Prevention. *Circulation.* 2006;113:1807-1816.

7. Elliott P, Andersson B, Arbustini E, et al. Classification of the cardiomyopathies: a position statement from the European Society of Cardiology Working Group on Myocardial and Pericardial Diseases. *Eur Heart J.* 2008;29:270-276.

8. Arbustini E, Narula N, Dec WG, et al. The MOGE(S) Classification for a phenotype–genotype nomenclature of cardiomyopathy. Endorsed by the World Heart Federation. *J Am Coll Cardiol.* 2013;62:2046-2072.

9. Arbustini E, Narula N, Tavazzi L, et al. The MOGE(S) classification of cardiomyopathy for clinicians. *J Am Coll Cardiol.* 2014;64:304-318.

10. Seferović PM, Polovina M, Bauersachs J, et al. Heart failure in cardiomyopathies: a position paper from the Heart Failure Association of the European Society of Cardiology. *Eur J Heart Fail.* 2019;21(5):553-576.

11. Pinto YM, Elliott PM, Arbustini E et al. Proposal for a revised definition of dilated cardiomyopathy, hypokinetic non-dilated cardiomyopathy, and its implications for clinical practice: a position statement of the ESC working group on myocardial and pericardial diseases. *Eur Heart J.* 2016;37(23):1850-1858.

12. Corrado D, van Tintelen PJ, McKenna WJ et al. Arrhythmogenic right ventricular cardiomyopathy: evaluation of the current diagnostic criteria and differential diagnosis. *Eur Heart J.* 2020;41(14):1414-1429.

13. Adler E, Fuster V. SCN5A: a mechanistic link between inherited cardiomyopathies and a predisposition to arrhythmias? *JAMA.* 2005;293:491-493.

14. Charron P, Arad M, Arbustini E, et al. Genetic counselling and testing in cardiomyopathies: a position statement of the European Society of Cardiology Working Group on Myocardial and Pericardial Diseases. *Eur Heart J.* 2010;31:2715-2726.

15. Rapezzi C, Arbustini E, Caforio AL, et al. Diagnostic work-up in cardiomyopathies: bridging the gap between clinical phenotypes and final diagnosis. A position statement from the ESC Working Group on Myocardial and Pericardial Diseases. *Eur Heart J.* 2013;34:1448-1458.

16. Pasotti M, Klersy C, Pilotto A et al. Long-term outcome and risk stratification in dilated cardiolaminopathies. *J Am Coll Cardiol.* 2008;52(15):1250-1260.

17. Diegoli M, Grasso M, Favalli V et al. Diagnostic work-up and risk stratification in X-linked dilated cardiomyopathies caused by dystrophin defects. *J Am Coll Cardiol.* 2011;58(9):925-934.

18. Captur G, Arbustini E, Bonne G et al. Lamin and the heart. *Heart.* 2018;104(6):468-479.

19. Favalli V, Serio A, Grasso M, Arbustini E. Genetic causes of dilated cardiomyopathy. *Heart.* 2016;102(24):2004-2014.

20. Bennett JS, Bernhardt M, McBride KL et al. Reclassification of variants of uncertain significance in children with inherited arrhythmia syndromes is predicted by clinical factors. *Pediatr Cardiol.* 2019;40(8):1679-1687.

21. El Mecky J, Johansson L, Plantinga M, et al. Reinterpretation, reclassification, and its downstream effects: challenges for clinical laboratory geneticists. *BMC Med Genomics.* 2019;12(1):170.

22. Costa S, Medeiros-Domingo A, Gasperetti A et al. Impact of genetic variant reassessment on the diagnosis of arrhythmogenic right ventricular cardiomyopathy based on the 2010 Task Force criteria. *Circ Genom Precis Med.* 2020. doi: 10.1161/CIRCGEN.120.003047.

23. Tsai GJ, Rañola JMO, Smith C et al. Outcomes of 92 patient-driven family studies for reclassification of variants of uncertain significance. *Genet Med.* 2019;21(6):1435-1442.

24. Arbustini E, Disertori M, Narula J. Primary prevention of sudden arrhythmic death in dilated cardiomyopathy: Current guidelines and risk stratification. *JACC Heart Fail.* 2017;5(1):39-43.

25. Disertori M, Masè M, Rigoni M et al. Implantable cardioverter-defibrillator in dilated cardiomyopathy after the DANISH-trial lesson. A poly-parametric risk evaluation is needed to improve the selection of patients. *Front Physiol.* 2017;8:873.

26. van Rijsingen IA, Arbustini E, Elliott PM, et al. Risk factors for malignant ventricular arrhythmias in lamin A/C mutation carriers a European cohort study. *J Am Coll Cardiol.* 2012;59:493-500.

27. Mogensen J, Hey T, Lambrecht S. A systematic review of phenotypic features associated with cardiac troponin I mutations in hereditary cardiomyopathies. *Can J Cardiol.* 2015;31(11):1377-1385.

28. Arbustini E, Narula N, Dec GW, et al. MOGE(S) nosology in low-to-middle-income countries. *Nat Rev Cardiol.* 2014;11:307.

29. Arbustini E, Narula N, Dec GW, et al. The MOGE(S) classification for a phenotype-genotype nomenclature of cardiomyopathy: more questions than answers? *J Am Coll Cardiol.* 2014;63:2584-2586.

30. Mayosi BM. Cardiomyopathies: MOGE(S): a standardized classification of cardiomyopathies? *Nat Rev Cardiol.* 2014;11(3):134-135.

31. Agarwal A, Yousefzai R, Jan MF, et al. Clinical application of WHF-MOGE(S) classification for hypertrophic cardiomyopathy. *Glob Heart.* 2015;10:209-219.

32. Hazebroek MR, Moors S, Dennert R et al. Prognostic relevance of gene-environment interactions in patients with dilated cardiomyopathy: applying the MOGE(S) classification. *J Am Coll Cardiol.* 2015;66(12):1313-1323.

33. Makavos G, 9Aairis C, Tselegkidi M et al. Hypertrophic cardiomyopathy: an updated review on diagnosis, prognosis, and treatment. *Heart Fail Rev.* 2019;24(4):439-459.

34. Favalli V, Disabella E, Molinaro M et al. Genetic screening of Anderson-Fabry disease in probands referred from multispecialty clinics. *J Am Coll Cardiol.* 2016;68(10):1037-1050.

35. Westphal JG, Rigopoulos AG, Bakogiannis C et al. The MOGE(S) classification for cardiomyopathies: current status and future outlook. *Heart Fail Rev.* 2017;22(6):743-752.

36. Bonne G, Leturcq F, Ben Yaou R. Emery Dreifuss muscle dystrophy. In: Pagon RA, Bird TD, Dolan CR, Stephens K, Adam MP, eds. *Gene Reviews [Internet].* Updated January 17, 2013. Seattle, WA: University of Washington Seattle; 2013.

37. Piccolo G, Azan G, Tonin P, et al. Dilated cardiomyopathy requiring cardiac transplantation as initial manifestation of Xp21 Becker type muscular dystrophy. *Neuromuscul Disord.* 1994;4:143-146.

38. Niezgoda J, Morgan PG. Anesthetic considerations in patients with mitochondrial defects. *Paediatr Anaesth.* 2013;23:785-793.

39. Galimberti CA, Diegoli M, Sartori I, et al. Brain pseudoatrophy and mental regression on valproate and a mitochondrial DNA mutation. *Neurology.* 2006;67:1715-1717.

40. Van Der Starre P, Deuse T, Pritts C, Brun C, Vogel H, Oyer P. Late profound muscle weakness following heart transplantation due to Danon disease. *Muscle Nerve.* 2013;47:135-137.

41. Yancy CW, Jessup M, Bozkurt B, et al. 2013 ACCF/AHA Guideline for the Management of Heart Failure: a report of the American College of Cardiology Foundation/American Heart Association Task Force on Practice Guidelines. *J Am Coll Cardiol.* 2013;62:e-147-239.

42. Califf RM. The new era of clinical research: using data for multiple purposes. *Am Heart J.* 2014;168(2):133-134.

43. Lipshultz SE, Law YM, Asante-Korang A et al. Cardiomyopathy in children: classification and diagnosis: a scientific statement from the American Heart Association. *Circulation.* 2019;140(1):e9-e68.

44. Konta L, Franklin RC, Kaski JP. Nomenclature and systems of classification for cardiomyopathy in children. *Cardiol Young.* 2015;25 (Suppl 2): 31-42.

45. Simonneau G, Montani D, Celermajer DS et al. Haemodynamic definitions and updated clinical classification of pulmonary hypertension. *Eur Respir J.* 2019;53(1):1801913.

46. Ter Haar NM, Jeyaratnam J, Lachmann HJ et al. The phenotype and genotype of mevalonate kinase deficiency: a series of 114 cases from the Eurofever registry. *Arthritis Rheumatol.* 2016;68(11):2795-2805.

47. Fox JL. Obama catapults patient-empowered precision medicine. *Nat Biotechnol.* 2015;33:325.

48. Collins FS, Varmus H. A new initiative on precision medicine. *N Engl J Med.* 2015;372:793-795.

49. Blaus A, Madabushi R, Pacanowski M, et al. Personalized cardiovascular medicine today: a Food and Drug Administration/Center for Drug Evaluation and Research Perspective. *Circulation.* 2015;132:1425-1432.

50. Kirchhof P, Sipido KR, Cowie MR, et al. The continuum of personalized cardiovascular medicine: a position paper of the European Society of Cardiology. *Eur Heart J.* 2014;35:3250-3257.

51. Panguluri SK, Sneed KB, Pathak Y, Zhou S. Editorial: current topics in pharmacogenomics. *Recent Pat Biotechnol.* 2014;8(2):109.

41

Dilated Cardiomyopathy

Eloisa Arbustini, Alessandro Di Toro, Lorenzo Giuliani, Mario Urtis, G. William Dec, and Jagat Narula

Dilated cardiomyopathy: a wide spectrum of heart muscle disease phenotypes

Inherited DCM (up to 50%)

Modes of inheritance:

- Autosomal dominant (majority)
- Autosomal recessive
- X-linked recessive, including DCM in neuromuscular diseases
- X-linked dominant (rare)
- Matrilineal, syndromic in most cases; end phenotype of symmetrical non-obstructive hypertrophic cardiomyopathy

Disease genes encoding proteins of:

- Sarcomere
- Nuclear envelope
- Z-disc
- Sarcolemma Golgi
- Sarcoplasmic reticulum
- Mitochondria,
- Both mt-DNA and nuclear genes

Nondilated hypokinetic cardiomyopathy in familial DCM:

Diagnostic criteria: Major (M) (N=2) and minor (m) (N=6).

Diagnostic levels:
- Definite diagnosis: when the DCM criteria are met
- Probable HNDC: when one M criterion is associated with at least one m criterion
- Possible HNDC: either two M criteria; or one M criterion plus being the carrier of the causative mutation; or one M criterion in the absence of M criteria and genetic data

Autoimmune/immune-mediated DCM

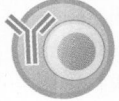

Antibody- and T-cell-mediated

Cardiomyopathy: not a diagnostic criterion of autoimmune diseases

Nonetheless, the heart is commonly involved in:
- Systemic autoimmune diseases, possible organ-dominant phenotypes
- Organ-specific autoimmune diseases

Cardiomyopathy can complicate treatments for autoimmune diseases (e.g., chloroquine)

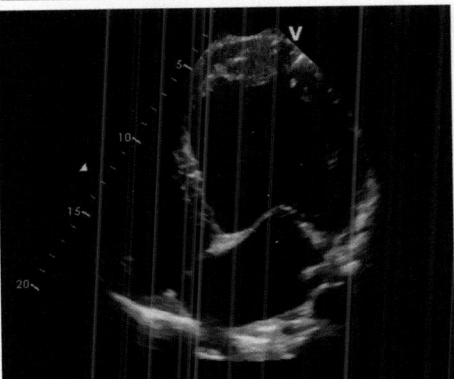

Peripartum DCM

Multifactorial pathogenic hypothesis

Rare life-threatening cardiomyopathy of unknown cause that occurs in the peripartum period in previously healthy women:
- The diagnosis is confined to a narrow period
- Requires echocardiographic evidence of LV systolic dysfunction
- Potentially reversible

Can unmask pre-existing genetic DCM

Inflammatory DCM

Usually following infectious myocarditis

Multifactorial pathogenesis

Chronic myocardial inflammation and fibrosis associated with persistent LV dysfunction and ventricular remodeling

Diagnosis requires the presence of myocardial inflammation

The viral cause has to be demonstrated

To be distinguished from auto-inflammatory genetic diseases

Alcoholic cardiomyopathy

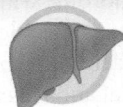

Chronic, heavy alcohol consumption is associated with DCM

Ethanol induces toxic effects that weaken the heart muscle

Cirrhotic cardiomyopathy

Chronic cardiac dysfunction with impaired contractile responsiveness to stress and/or altered diastolic relaxation with electrophysiological abnormalities

Cardiotoxicity

Endogenous and exogenous
In patients with previously healthy cardiovascular system
In patients with pre-existing cardiovascular diseases

Spectrum of toxic myocardial and vascular effects:
- DCM, myocarditis, arrhythmias,
- Accelerated vascular disease, thrombotic complications

Cardio-oncotoxicity — past definition:
- Type 1 nonreversible injury e.g., anthracycline; type 2 reversible, e.g., trastuzumab
- Caused by different classes of drugs: e.g., anti-Her2; fluoropyrimidines; tyrosine kinase inhibitors; proteasome inhibitors. Immunotherapies: immune checkpoint inhibitors and chimeric antigen receptor t-cell therapy

Chapter 41 Fuster and Hurst's Central Illustration. The term dilated cardiomyopathy (DCM) covers a wide spectrum of heart muscle disease phenotypes characterized by dilatation and systolic impairment of the left or both ventricles unexplained by abnormal loading conditions or coronary artery disease sufficient to induce the observed phenotype. The causes of DCM are heterogeneous. LV, left ventricular.

CHAPTER SUMMARY

This chapter summarizes the pathogenesis, diagnosis, and management of dilated cardiomyopathy (DCM). The term DCM covers a wide spectrum of heart muscle disease phenotypes characterized by dilatation and systolic impairment of the left or both ventricles unexplained by abnormal loading conditions (such as hypertensive, diabetic, valvular, or congenital heart disease) or coronary artery disease sufficient to induce the observed phenotype (see Fuster and Hurst's Central Illustration). The causes of DCM are heterogeneous; genetic in up to 50% (familial DCM), autoimmune/immune-mediated and inflammatory (usually postmyocarditic), and, less commonly, cardiotoxicity (anticancer drugs, alcohol abuse, and cirrhosis). DCM is diagnosed by clinical presentation and morphofunctional echocardiographic and magnetic resonance imaging. Tissue diagnosis is needed for inflammatory cardiomyopathies. The genetic diagnosis is based on testing of genes coding for proteins of the sarcomere, nuclear lamina, intermediate filaments, sarcolemma, sarcoplasmic reticulum and Golgi, desmosomes, and mitochondria. Familial DCM is considered when two or more family members are affected, and diagnosed by family history, clinical screening of relatives, and cascade genetic testing. Early diagnosis in relatives can be framed in the context of nondilated hypokinetic cardiomyopathy based upon the recommended major or minor criteria.

DILATED CARDIOMYOPATHY: DEFINITION

In 2006, the American Heart Association (AHA) defined dilated forms of cardiomyopathy as "characterized by ventricular chamber enlargement and systolic dysfunction with normal left ventricular (LV) wall thickness."[1] In 2008, the European Society of Cardiology (ESC) defined dilated cardiomyopathy (DCM) as a chronic heart muscle disease characterized by "the presence of dilatation and systolic impairment of the left or both ventricles unexplained by abnormal loading conditions or coronary artery disease sufficient to cause the observed myocardial dilation and dysfunction."[2] In 2016, a position statement of the ESC working group on myocardial and pericardial diseases proposed the definition of hypokinetic nondilated cardiomyopathy (HNDC), and its implications for clinical practice to bridge the gap between recent understanding of the disease spectrum and its clinical presentation in relatives.[3] The last universal definition and classification of heart failure (HF) distinguished HF from cardiomyopathy: "HF is a clinical syndrome with different etiologies and pathophysiology rather than a specific disease." 'Cardiomyopathy' is a term, itself with widely differing definitions, that describes features of structural and functional heart muscle dysfunction."[4]

In this chapter, DCM is intended as a disease of heart muscle defined by structural (dilation) and functional (systolic dysfunction) descriptors. DCM is proven to be familial with identifiable genetic defects in more than 50% of cases.[5] Acquired disorders manifesting with the DCM phenotype, or DCM phenocopies (defined as environmentally induced phenotypes mimicking one usually produced by a specific genotype) are sporadic and are categorized as nongenetic DCM. This distinction is essential to separate heritable nonreversible DCM from acquired, nongenetic, and potentially reversible phenotypes arising from protean causes. The therapeutic options for acquired DCM often differ from those for familial DCM (FDCM).

In its descriptive definition, overt DCM represents the *end phenotype* of heart muscle damage induced by heterogeneous causes whose pathogenic mechanisms are increasingly being identified by the implementation of molecular and genetic assays for patients and families, high-resolution and functional imaging, and novel biomarkers. In end-stage, most DCMs look phenotypically alike (**Fig. 41–1**). *Intermediate phenotypes* are manifest by borderline, persistent LV dilation and/or dysfunction and may present with arrhythmias and/or conduction disease, now recognized as "early DCM" or HNDC.[3] In genotyped families, the *preclinical phase* of the disease can be diagnosed in phenotypically healthy, but genetically affected, relatives of probands with DCM. Overall, DCM can be grouped mechanistically as genetic and nongenetic.

THE BURDEN OF DILATED CARDIOMYOPATHY

Current estimates of incidence are not derived from population-based studies but rather from heterogeneous cohorts (surveys on a voluntary basis, cross-sectional surveys, or statistics from hospitalized patients and necropsy data)[6] collected far before the publication of the last guidelines for DCM (**Table 41–1**). Generally accepted estimates are 6.0 per 100,000 person-years and prevalence is 36.5 per 100,000 person-years (about 1:2500).[7] These epidemiology data are based on clinical diagnoses and have been obtained in the pregenetic era. New estimates are expected,[8] based on data obtained with early diagnoses, systematic family screening and monitoring, genetic testing, and advanced diagnostics for nongenetic DCM.[9-17] As the long-term follow-up of FDCM increases, the overall prevalence of the disease is anticipated to increase.

When DCM is defined by etiology, the prevalence data of each specific subgroup is far less common, placing most DCM subtypes in the context of rare diseases (<1:2000). Therefore, the burden of DCM in general, and of FDCM in particular, is a dynamic issue that should be regarded as evolving and deserving further efforts to generate precise etiology-based epidemiology of DCM.

CLINICAL PRESENTATION AND DIAGNOSTIC WORK-UP IN INDEX PATIENTS

DCM typically manifests with systolic HF. The spectrum of symptoms is wide and nonspecific; it includes fatigue, breathlessness, palpitations, and signs of congestion/fluid retention in the presence of structural cardiac abnormalities corresponding to the diagnostic definition.[2,18] The key diagnostic tool is the *two-dimensional transthoracic echocardiography* (2D-TTE) that demonstrates LV systolic dysfunction (LVSD; impaired LV ejection fraction [LVEF]) and dilatation (as defined by Z-score >2 standard deviations for LV end-diastolic volumes or diameters, according to nomograms corrected for body surface area, height, and age), normal LV wall thickness, possible LV diastolic dysfunction, and elevation in LV filling pressure. 2D-TTE may also show LV dyssynchrony, right ventricular (RV) dysfunction, atrial dilation, functional mitral and tricuspid regurgitation, and secondary pulmonary hypertension.

New technologies such as three-dimensional (3D) *transthororacic echocardiography* (3D-TTE), *tissue Doppler imaging* (TDI), and *speckle-tracking echocardiography* (STE) add value for LV volume and EF quantification (3D-TEE), cardiac mechanics, and segmental and global LV function (TDI and STE).[19] Three-dimensional echocardiography may add information on valvular anatomy and remodeling, particularly in patients with limited views on 2D echocardiography.[20] The major advantages of 3D echocardiography include the independence from geometric assumption, semiautomatic delineation of the endocardium border, and the absence of errors deriving from "foreshortening" of the LV apex. Regional wall motion can be assessed by calculating the volume change of each segment in the cardiac cycle.[19] New fully automated, fast 3D-TTE software can simultaneously assess left atrial (LA) volumes and LAEF, LV volumes, LV mass, and LVEF.[21] The TDI index of systolic longitudinal function (peak systolic myocardial velocity S'), is a marker of impaired subendocardial fiber contraction and correlates with myocardial fibrosis.[22] STE discriminates

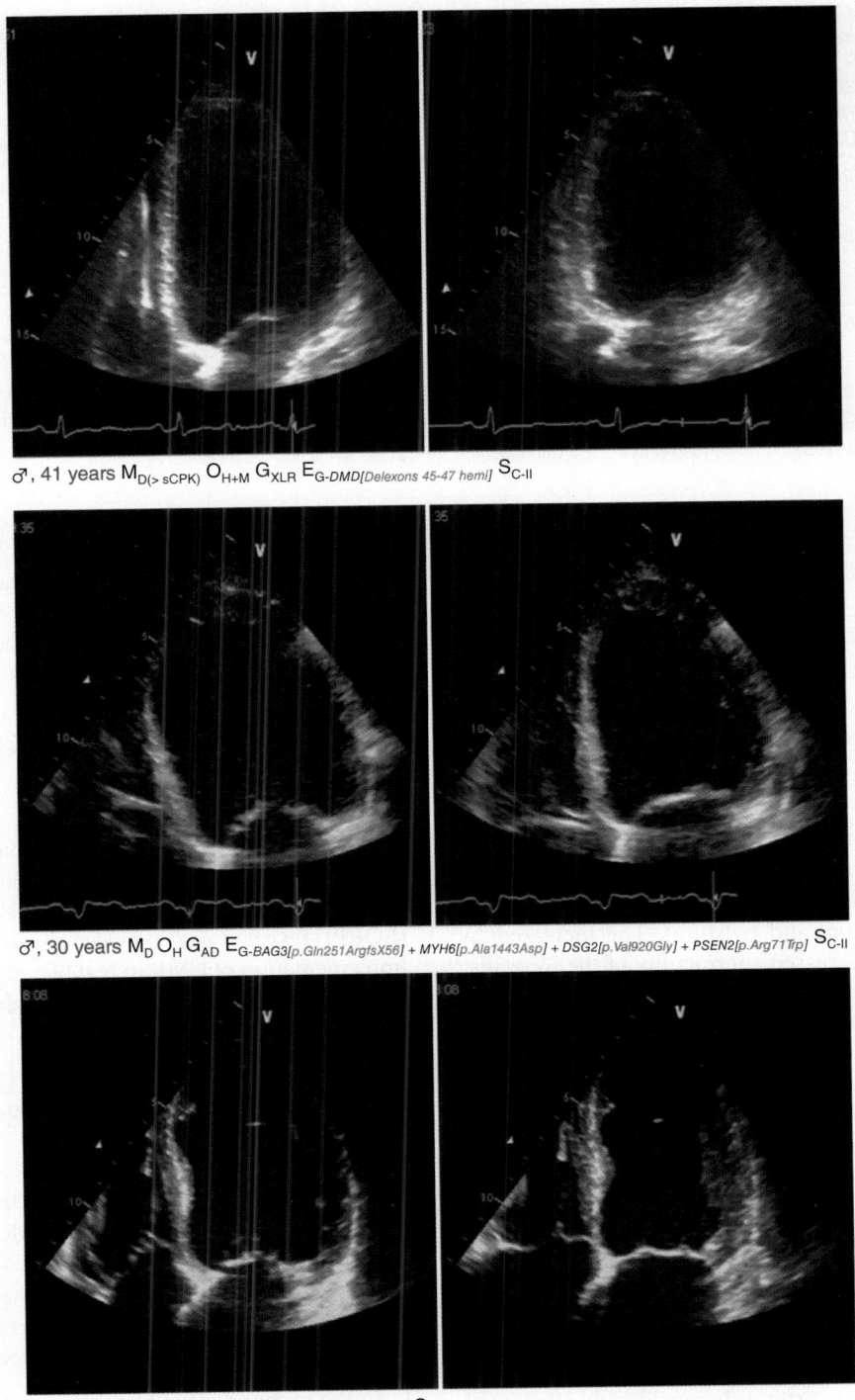

♂, 41 years $M_{D(> sCPK)}$ O_{H+M} G_{XLR} $E_{G-DMD[Delexons\ 45-47\ hemi]}$ S_{C-II}

♂, 30 years M_D O_H G_{AD} $E_{G-BAG3[p.Gln251ArgfsX56]\ +\ MYH6[p.Ala1443Asp]\ +\ DSG2[p.Val920Gly]\ +\ PSEN2[p.Arg71Trp]}$ S_{C-II}

♂, 60 years $M_{D(AVB)}$ O_H G_{AD} $E_{G-LMNA[p.Arg72Cys]}$ S_{C-II}

Figure 41–1. Phenotypically similar DCM caused by defects in different genes: precise description by MOGE(S) nosology system. The figure shows three different examples of DCM; although the clinical diagnosis is the same, the diseases are different. In the MOGE(S) notation,[38] **M** describes the morphofunctional phenotype (HCM, DCM, RCM, ARVC) as defined in current guidelines,[1] eventually adding key markers such as atrioventricular block; **O** describes the organs affected in the given patient (eg, Heart, Skeletal muscle, Auditory, ocular systems); **G** defines whether a cardiomyopathy is genetic or not and includes information on the pattern of inheritance (autosomal dominant, autosomal recessive, X-linked, matrilineal); **E** is the precision diagnostic descriptor and specifies the cause and, in case of genetic diseases, the disease gene(s) and the mutation(s); and **S** includes New York Heart Association functional class and American Heart Association stage.

TABLE 41–1. Epidemiology of Idiopathic Dilated Cardiomyopathy (IDCM)

COUNTRY/YEAR OF PUBLICATION	YRS OBSERVATION/ DATA COLLECTION	STUDY	TYPE OF THE STUDY	INCIDENCE PER 100,000 PERSONS-YEAR	PREVALENCE PER 100,000 PERSONS	AUTHOR
Sweden (Malmo study) (1978)	1970–1977	Retrospective	Clinical, and Autopsy	3 (7,5 when including autopsy data)	NA	Torp A. *Postgrad Med J.* 1978; 54:435–439
Western Denmark (1984)	1980–1981	Retrospective	Clinical, and Autopsy	5,4 (+2 when including autopsy data	NA	Bagger et al. *Br Heart J.* 1984;52:327–331
USA (1986)	1970–1982	Death certificate*	Administrative data	NA	27 (Black men) 11 (White men)	Gillum RF. *Am Heart J.* 1986;111: 752–755
England (1985)	1983–1984	Questionnaire-based	Clinical	NA	8317 (point prevalence)	Williams DG, Olsen EG. *Br Heart J.* 1985;54:153–155
New Zealand (1987)	1974–1983	Prospective	Clinical	2°	NA	Ikram et al. *Br Heart J.* 1987;57:521–527.
USA-Olmstead County study (1989)	1975–1984	Prospective	Clinical, and Autopsy	6	36,5	Codd et al. *Circulation.* 1989;80:564–572
Italy (Trieste) (1997)	1987–1989	Prospective	Clinical, and Autopsy	6,95	NA	Rakar et al. *Eur Heart J.* 1997;18:117 –123.
Japan, nation-wide	2002	Survey	-	NA	17	Miura et al. *Heart.* 2002; 87:126–130.

*Low rate of autopsy and referrals. °Clinically driven study. National Center for Health Statistics.

Data from Pasqualucci D, Iacovoni A, Palmieri V, et al. Epidemiology of cardiomyopathies: essential context knowledge for a tailored clinical work-up. *Eur J Prev Cardiol.* 2020 Nov 7:zwaa035.

between active and passive movements of myocardial segments and separates assessment of distinct components of myocardial deformation (longitudinal and circumferential shortening, radial thickening, rotation, and twisting). The increased LV mass and volume and decreased contractility of the LV walls[23] impair longitudinal, radial, and circumferential strain.[24] *Contrast echocardiography* eventually enhances endocardial border definition, increases accuracy to 2D and 3D volume assessment, and highlights trabecular anatomy; it is not needed in routine evaluations, but may help in cases of suboptimal image quality.[21,25] The detection of "early phenotypes" can be supported by myocardial deformation imaging techniques[26] and myocardial tagging by cardiac magnetic resonance (CMR).[3,27,28]

Coronary angiography is routinely used to exclude coronary atherosclerosis.[1,2,18] Coronary computed tomography (CT) angiography may be considered as an alternative anatomic assessment for the evaluation of obstructive coronary artery disease. The presence of flow-limiting luminal stenosis in one or more epicardial coronary arteries is considered sufficient to assign the cause of DCM to coronary artery disease. However, coronary and/or systemic atherosclerosis and DCM can exist concurrently and be demonstrated in genetic DCM.[29] Individualized decision-making and testing are often necessary to clarify the extent of the contribution made by coronary artery disease in the pathogenesis of DCM. Functional testing, as with myocardial perfusion imaging, may determine the presence and/or extent of ischemia and may be useful in this regard.[30]

CMR is now part of the routine evaluation, both helping to confirm the diagnosis and adding information on the type and extent of myocardial fibrosis.[31–33] CMR may further assess the LV trabecular anatomy with high precision (see Chapter 45). However, a recent report from the ESC cardiomyopathy registry (part of the EURObservational Research Programme [EORP]) revealed a gap between current guidelines and clinical implementation of CMR in real life; in fact, less than one-third of patients enrolled in the registry underwent CMR.[34]

DIAGNOSIS OF FAMILIAL DILATED CARDIOMYOPATHY: THE ROLE OF FAMILY SCREENING

In more than 50% of cases of DCM, the disease is familial, as proven by clinical family screening demonstrating that more than one member is either affected or shows traits that predict the development of the disease.[3,35] The diagnosis of FDCM is formulated when at least two members of the same family are affected. The clinical work-up is a three-step investigation:

1. In the proband, deep phenotyping should include a general medical evaluation of anthropometric features and noncardiovascular traits in syndromic DCM[36] including, in particular, the neuro-musculo-skeletal system because many neuromuscular diseases demonstrate heart involvement.[37] A general phenotype examination can add information about clinical traits potentially associated with the DCM and provides robust clinical data for geno-phenotype correlations and segregation studies in families.

2. The next step in family screening is genetic counseling with pedigree construction and information provided to patients about why family studies are necessary when a genetic

disease is suspected. The collection of the clinical history of relatives and tracing of clinical reports of deceased relatives are uniquely useful for the correct interpretation of fatal events in families.[35,36]

3. The third step is family screening, which is independent of genetic testing. Clinical family screening is based on physical examination, electrocardiography (ECG), TTE, and biochemical testing followed by regular monitoring of relatives. Once completed, information gleaned from the clinical family screening may modify the original pedigree. Determination of the mode of inheritance of the DCM results from the integration of pedigree and family data and is essential for guiding and interpreting data generated by genetic testing.[38,39] Numerous complex and systemic syndromes with clinical manifestations affecting different organs (kidney, brain, gastrointestinal, ocular, auditory, skin) also demonstrate cardiac involvement, and family segregation studies can benefit from clinical observations in relatives. A typical example is MELAS, a mitochondrial disease that, almost invariably, involves the heart with an early hypertrophic symmetrical nonobstructive phenotype that over time evolves toward a dilated phenotype no longer distinguishable from a DCM. The search for the causes stems from deep phenotyping, which is a major contributor to the segregation study.[37]

Data achieved in family screening studies of consecutive patients demonstrate that relatives of patients with DCM can:

- Be affected, and therefore presenting the criteria for diagnosis, but be asymptomatic and unaware of their disease
- Manifest early, persistent (confirmed on more than one clinical occasion) signs of LV remodeling and/or borderline dysfunction[3]
- Demonstrate ECG abnormalities such as conduction disease, short PR interval/Wolff-Parkinson-White pattern, prolonged QT interval, T-wave abnormalities, early repolarization, or abnormally high or low voltages of the QRS[3,36]
- Show abnormal biochemical markers such as increased serum creatinine phosphokinase or lactic acid[37]
- Exhibit extracardiac traits that may also occur in probands, such as hearing loss, diabetes mellitus, cutaneous lesions, skeletal abnormalities, abnormal faces, or ocular defects[36]

Family screening may, by itself, offer added value for family health.[3,5,36,38] Monitoring of family members helps generate reliable data on the natural history of the disease (**Fig. 41–2**). In fact, DCM is often characterized by subtle onset and slow progression; it shows a typical age-dependency of the phenotype. Overall, clinical family screening is integral and indispensable for the diagnosis of FDCM.

GENETIC DILATED CARDIOMYOPATHY

Inheritance and Phenotype Variability

The increasing identification of genetic defects segregating with the phenotype in families confirms the genetic origin of the majority of FDCMs[35] (**Table 41–2**). Mendelian laws and rules of matrilinear inheritance govern the transmission of cardiomyopathies. Most FDCMs are autosomal dominant diseases; a minority shows autosomal recessive, X-linked recessive, and matrilineal inheritance. X-linked dominant forms are exceptional.[38] In autosomal dominant FDCM, each patient has a 50% probability of transmitting the mutation to offspring; in autosomal recessive FDCM, each parent is a healthy carrier of the mutation: the risk of transmission of the mutated allele from both parents is 25%. In X-linked recessive FDCM, the risk is 50% when the carrier is the mother; when the proband is the father, all daughters are obligate carriers, whereas all sons are noncarriers. In families with matrilineal cardiomyopathies, females transmit the mutation to both male and female offspring; accordingly, both genders can be affected. Vice versa, male carriers do not transmit the mutation. Mitochondrial DNA-related cardiomyopathies can demonstrate both dilated and hypertrophic phenotypes, with the latter frequently evolving through dilation and systolic dysfunction, mimicking typical DCM in later stages.[39]

Clinical traits, both cardiac and extracardiac, may help formulate pretest hypotheses.[36] ECG or imaging markers, skeletal muscle disease, auditory defects, ocular abnormalities, gastrointestinal disturbances, renal disease, cutaneous lesions, cognitive impairment, and cryptogenic stroke can be associated with DCM caused by different disease genes. Cardiomyopathies caused by mutations in mitochondrial DNA genes are commonly observed in the clinical context of syndromes with involvement of skeletal muscle (myopathies), brain (cryptogenic stroke), ear (sensorineural hearing loss), and kidney (renal failure); in mitochondrial diseases, diabetes is common and should be considered a phenotypic trait contributing to the characterization of the phenotype in the family[35-37] (**Table 41–3**).

Genetic Heterogeneity

The heterogeneity can be grouped in genetic heterogeneity (mutations in different genes cause similar phenotypes) and allelic diversity (different mutations in the same genes cause similar or different phenotypes). Genetic DCM is the paradigmatic example of how "similar phenotypes" may be caused by "different genes and mutations." More than 100 genes are now included in the list of disease and candidate genes (see Table 41–2). Attempts to group disease genes according to the pathways or structures in which their products are involved may outline macrogroups of disease genes:[40-46]

- Sarcomere genes (*TTN, MYH7, MYBPC3, TNNT2, TNNI3, MYL2, MYL3*) in 25% to 30% of DCM patients.[40] Although truncation predicting mutations in *TTN* have been reported in 25% of DCM patients,[41] confirmatory data are necessary, because 1 in 500 individuals carried truncation-predicting variants in the control series.[42]
- Nuclear envelop genes (*LMNA, EMD, SYNE1, TMPO*) in about 7% to 10% of cases, with *LMNA* mutations accounting for the majority of DCM in this subgroup.[43-45]

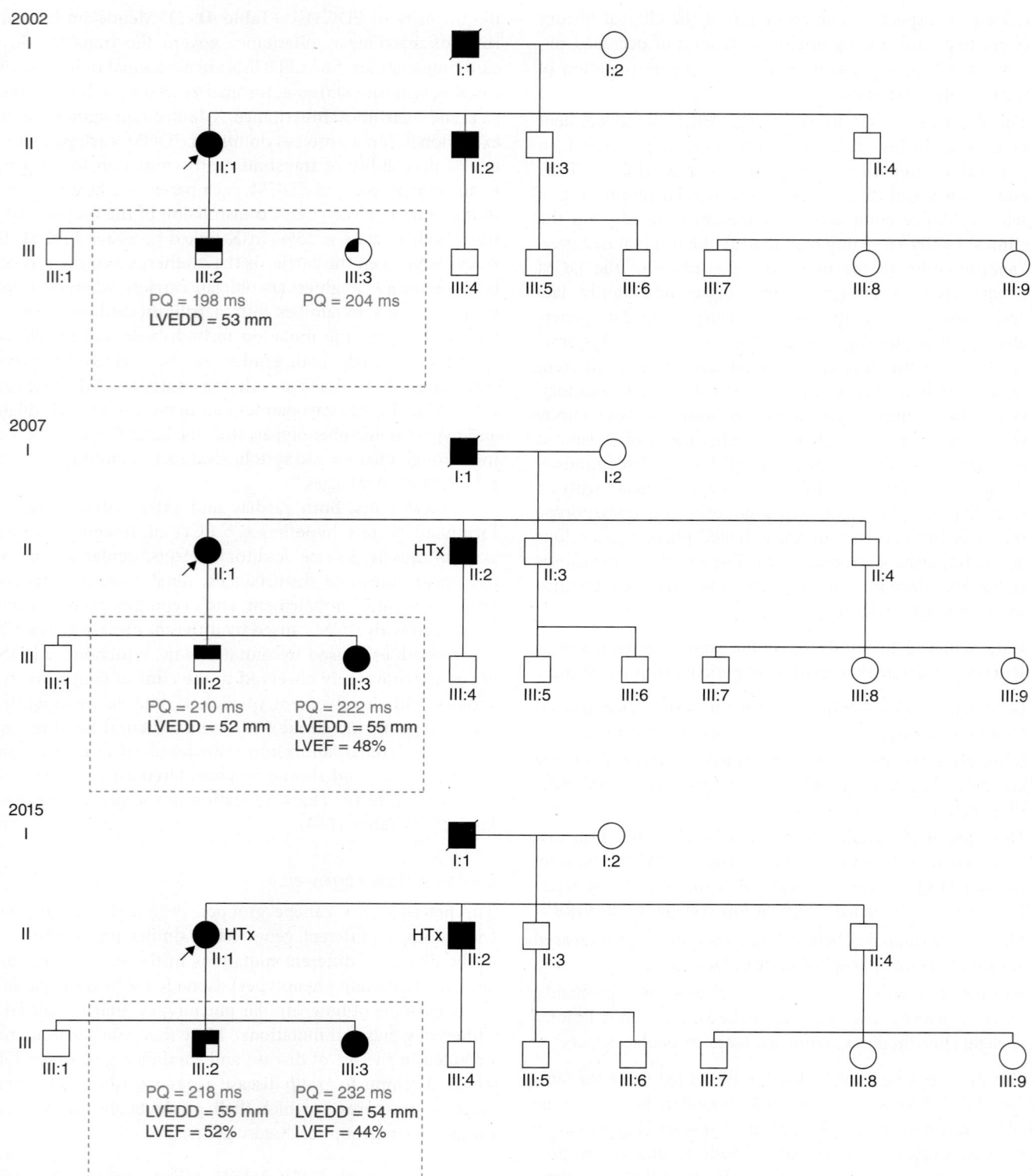

Figure 41–2. DCM. The figure shows the pedigree of a family in which the proband (II:1; *arrow*) was diagnosed with DCM and conduction disease after the younger brother (II:2). Both siblings underwent pacemaker (PM) implantation. The father died of DCM that manifested 9 years after PM implantation; he died at the age of 61 years from congestive heart failure. Clinical family screening included mother (I:2), who was hypertensive and diabetic, and the two siblings (II:3 and II:4) of the proband who showed normal LV function and dimensions and normal PQ interval. The three children of the proband were screened; one (III:1) showed normal electrocardiographic (ECG) and echocardiographic features; one demonstrated borderline PQ interval and slightly increased LV end-diastolic diameter (LVEDD) (III:2), and one showed atrioventricular block (AVB; III:3). Both were asymptomatic. The son of II:2 showed normal ECG and echocardiographic features. The five nephews (III:5, III:6, III:7, III:8, and III:9) of the proband showed normal ECG and echocardiographic features. *LMNA* genetic testing identified the *LMNA* p.(Arg89Leu) mutation in II:1. Cascade genetic screening in the family identified the same mutation in her brother (II:2) and in two of her offspring (III:2 and III:3). II:3, II:4, III:1, III:4 tested negative. During the course of 13 years, the daughter of the proband developed DCM, and the mutated son developed AVB, mild LV dilation, and borderline LV dysfunction. LVEF, LV ejection fraction.

TABLE 41–2. All Genes Reported, at Least Once, as Associated with DCM

Nuclear genes	MIM* Gene	Protein	H: HCM R: RCM A: ARVC NC: LVNC°	Phenotypes/diseases/traits allelic at the same locus	Inheritance
ABCC9	601439	ATP-Binding Cassette, Subfamily C, Member 9, sulfanylurea receptor 2		Cantu syndrome; hypertrichosis: familial atrial fibrillation	AD
ACTC1	102540	Cardiac actin alpha	H / R /NC	Nemaline myopathy	AD
ACTN2	102573	Alpha-actinin 2	H / NC	Distal myopathy 6	AD
ALMS1	606844	ALMS 1		Alstrom syndrome (70%: DCM)	AR
ANO5	608662	Anoctamin 5		Limb girdle muscular dystrophy, gnathodiaphyseal dysplasia, Miyoshi muscular dystrophy 3; dysphagia	AR
ANKRD1	609599	Ankyrin repeat domain-containing protein 1	H		AD
BAG3	603883	BCL2-associated athanogene	H	BAG3-related myofibrillar myopathy, CRYAB-related myofibrillar myopathy, fatal infantile hypertrophy,	AD
CALR3*	611414	Calreticulin 3	H		AD
CAV3	601253	Caveolin3	H	sCPK elevated; long QT syndrome-9; muscular dystrophy, limb-girdle; myopathy, distal, tateyama type; rippling muscle disease.	AD
CHKB	612395	Choline kinase, beta		Muscular dystrophy, congenital, megaconial type	AR
CHRM2	118493	Cholinergic receptor, muscarinic 2		Anti-CHRM2 autoantibodies; atrial and ventricular arrhythmias	AD
CRYAB	123590	Alpha B crystallin	H / R	Posterior polar cataract	AD
CSRP3	600824	Cysteine- and glycine-rich protein 3	H		AD
CTF1	600435	Cardiotrophin 1			AD
CTNNA3	607667	Alpha3-catenin	A		AD
DAG1	128639	Dystrophin-associated Glycoprotein 1		Muscular dystrophy-dystroglycanopathy	AR
DES	125660	Desmin	H / R / A	Des-related myofibrillar myopathy, neurogenic scapuloperoneal syndrome, Kaeser type; AVB, sCPK	AD
DMD	300377	Dystrophin		Duchenne muscle dystrophy, Becker muscle dystrophy; >sCPK/myopathy	XLR
DMPK	605377	Dystrophia myotonica protein kinase gene		(Dystrophia myotonica type 1) or Steinert's disease; AVB	AD
DOLK	610746	Dolichol kinase		Congenital disorder of glycosylation, type Im; Myopathy, possible ichthyosiform dermatitis	AR
DSC2	125645	Desmocollin 2	A	With and without mild palmoplantar keratoderma and woolly hair	AD
DSG2	125671	Desmoglein 2	A		AD
DSP	125647	Desmoplakin	A	Lethal acantholytic epidermolysis bullosa, Keratosis palmoplantaris striata II, Skin fragility-woolly hair syndrome	AD
DTNA	601239	Dystrobrevin, alpha	NC	With or without congenital heart defects	AD
EMD	300384	Emerin		EDMD1, X-linked; AVB, Myopathy, sCPK	XLR
EYA4	603550	Eyes absent 4		Deafness, autosomal dominant	AD
FHL1	300163	Four-and –a-half LIM domains 1	H	EMDM6, X-linked, myopathy, reducing body, childhood-onset and severe early-onset, myopathy with postural muscle atrophy, scapuloperoneal myopathy, XLD	XLR, XLD
FHL2	602633	Four and a half limb domains 2			AD
FKTN	607440	Fukutin		Muscular dystrophy-dystroglycanopathy (with brain and eye anomalies), typeA,4; (without mental retardation), type B, 4; (limb-girdle), type C,4	AR

(Continued)

TABLE 41–2. All Genes Reported, at Least Once, as Associated with DCM (Continued)

Nuclear genes	MIM* Gene	Protein	H: HCM R: RCM A: ARVC NC: LVNC°	Phenotypes/diseases/traits allelic at the same locus	Inheritance
FHOD3	609691	FH1/FH2 domain-containing protein 2			AD
FOXD4	611080	Forkhead box D4-like 3		DCM with obsessive-compulsive disorder, and suicidality	AD
GATA4	600576	GATA-binding protein 4		Congenital heart disease	AD
GATA5	611496	GATA-binding protein 5			AD
GATA6	601656	GATA-binding protein 6		Congenital heart disease	AD, AR
GATAD1	614518	GATA zinc finger domain containing protein 1			AR
HRC	142705	Histidine-rich calcium binding protein		Arrhythmogenic DCM	AD
ILK	602366	Integrin-linked kinase			AD
JUP (DP3)	173325	Plakoglobin, Desmoplakin III	A	Naxos traits	AD, AR
LMNA	150330	Lamin AC	A/NC	DCM with conduction disease plus 11 additional phenotypes; AVB; possible sCPK elevation	AD
LAMA2	156225	Laminin alpha, 2		Congenital merosin-deficient muscular dystrophy type 1A	AR
LAMA4	600133	Laminin alpha, 4			AD
LDB3	605906	LIM domain-binding 3	H/NC	ZASP-related myofibrillar myopathy; LVNC, possible > sCPK; Hypertrabeculation;	AD
LIMS1	607908	LIM and Senescent cell antigen like domains 1			AD
LIMS2	602567	LIM and Senescent cell antigen like domains 2			AD
MIB1	608677	Midbomb, homolog of drosophila	NC	LVNC	AD
MURC	602633	Muscle-related coiled-coil protein, Z-line protein			AD
MYBPC3	600958	Myosin-binding protein C	H / NC		AD
MYH6	160710	Alpha-myosin heavy chain 6	H	Atrial septal defect, Sick sinus syndrome	AD
MYH7	160760	Beta-myosin heavy chain 7	H / R / NC	Laing distal myopathy; myosin storage myopathy; scapuloperoneal syndrome, myopathic type; possible sCPK	AD
MYH7B	609928	Myosin Heavy Chain 7B	H / NC	Congenital myopathy?	AD, AR
MYL2	160781	Myosin Light Chain 2	H		AD
MYL3	160790	Myosin Light Chain 3	H / R		AD, AR
MYOZ1	605603	Myozenin 1	H		AD
MYOZ2	605602	Myozenin 2	H		AD
MYPN	608517	Myopalladin	H / R		AD
NEBL	605491	Nebulette			AD
NEXN	613121	Nexilin	H		AD
NKX2-5	600584	NK2 homeobox 5; cardiac specific homeobox 1		Possible conduction system disease; congenital heart diseases; hypothyroidism; congenital nongoitrous	AD
OBSCN	608616	Obscurin	NC		AD, AR
PDLIM3	605889	PDZ and LIM domain protein 3			AD
PLN	172405	Phospholamban	A		AR
PLEKHM2	609613	Pleckstrin homology domain containing protein, family M, member	NC		AR

(Continued)

TABLE 41-2. All Genes Reported, at Least Once, as Associated with DCM (Continued)

Nuclear genes	MIM* Gene	Protein	H: HCM R: RCM A: ARVC NC: LVNC°	Phenotypes/diseases/traits allelic at the same locus	Inheritance
PKP2	602861	Plakophilin 2	A		AD
PRDM16	605557	PR domain containing 16	NC	LVNC	AD
PSEN1	104311	Presenilin 1		Familial acne inversa, 3; Alzheimer D., 3; Frontotemporal dementia; Pick D	AD
PSEN2	600759	Presenilin 2		Alzheimer disease, type 4	AD
RBM20	613171	RNA-binding motif protein 20			AD
RYR2	180902	Ryanodine receptor 2	A/NC	Ventricular tachycardia, catecholaminergic polymorphic, 1	AD
SCN5A	600163	Sodium channel, voltage gated, type V, alpha subunit		LQT3, Brugada1, atrial fibrillation, Sick sinus syndrome, familial VF,	AD
SDHA	600857	Succinate dehydrogenase subunit A		Leigh syndrome, MT respiratory chain complex II deficiency, Paragangliomas, 5.	AD, AR
SGCA	600119	α-sarcoglycan		Limb-girdle muscular dystrophy, 2D	AR
SGCD	601411	Delta-sarcoglycan		Limb-girdle muscular dystrophy	AD
SYNE1	608441	Nesprin 1, synaptic nuclear envelop protein 1		EMD4, AD; spinocerebellar ataxia, autosomal recessive	AD, AR
SYNE2	608442	Nasprin 2, synaptic nuclear envelope protein 2		EMD5, AD	AD
TBX5	601620	T-Box 5		Holt-Oram syndrome; CHD	AD
TBX20	606061	T-Box 20		Atrial septal defect; CHD	AD
TCAP	604488	Titin-cap; telethonin	H	Muscular dystrophy, limb-girdle, type 2G; sCPK	AD
TCF21	603306	Transcription factor 21, epicardin		Hearing loss	AD
TGFB3	190230	Transforming growth factor b 3	A	Rienhoff syndrome	AD
TMEM43	612048	Transmembrane protein 43	A	Emery-Dreifuss muscular dystrophy, AD	AD
TMPO	188380	Thymopoietin			AD
TNNC1	191040	Cardiac troponin C	H/R		AD
TNNI3	191044	Cardiac troponin I3	H/R/NC		AD
TNNI3K	613932	TNNI3-interacting kinase	R		AD
TNNT2	191045	Cardiac troponin T2	H/R/ NC		AD
TPM1	191010	Tropomyosin 1	H/R/NC	Limb-girdle muscular dystrophy, early-onset myopathy with fatal CMP, proximal myopathy with early respiratory muscle involvement, tardive tibial muscular dystrophy	AD
TTN	188840	Titin	H / A°		AD
VCL	193065	Vinculin	H		AD
AGK	610345	Acylglycerol kinase	H / NC	Cataract, myopathy, Senger syndrome	AR
ANT1 (PEOA2)	103220	Adenin nucleotide translocator 1	H	Mitochondrial DNA depletion syndrome 12 (cardiomyopathic type), AD-PEO with multiple mtDNA deletions	AD, AR
COX10	602125	Cytochrome C oxidase assembly Protein, 10	H	Leigh syndrome due to mitochondrial COX4 deficiency	AR
COX15	603646	Cytochrome C oxidase assembly protein, 15		Cardio-encephalo-myopathy, fatal infantile, due to COX deficiency 2	AR
DNAJC19	608977	DNAJ/HSP40 homolog, subfamily C, member 19	H	3-methylglutaconic aciduria type V	AR
FXN	606829	Frataxin	NC	Friedreich ataxia, Friedreich ataxia with retained reflexes	AR
G4.5	300394	Tafazzin	H	Barth syndrome	XLR

(Continued)

TABLE 41–2. All Genes Reported, at Least Once, as Associated with DCM (Continued)

Nuclear genes	MIM* Gene	Protein	H: HCM R: RCM A: ARVC NC: LVNC°	Phenotypes/diseases/traits allelic at the same locus	Inheritance
NDUFB11	300403	Nadh dehydrogenase 1b, subcomplex 11		Linear skin defects with multiple congenital anomalies	XLR
NDUFS2	602985	NAD-ubiquinone oxidoreductase Fe-S protein 2	H	Encephalopathy, Mt complex I deficiency	AR
NDUFV2	600532	NAD-ubiquinone oxidoreductase flavoprotein 2	H	Hypotonia, encephalopathy, Mt complex I deficiency	AR
POLG (PEOA1)	174763	DNA polymerase γ	H	Alpers-type syndrome, MNGIE-type, AD-PEO and AR-PEO, SANDO syndrome, SCAE	AD, AR
SCO2	604272	Homolog of S cervisiae, 2	H	Fatal infantile cardioencephalomyopathy, due to COX1 deficiency	AR
SDHA	600857	Succinate dehydrogenase complex subunit A	H	Leigh syndrome, mitochondrial respiratory chain complex II deficiency, paragangliomas	AR
TMEM70	612418	Mitochondrial complex V (ATP synthase) deficiency, nuclear type 2		Neonatal mitochondrial encephalocardiomyopathy with ATP synthase deficiency	AR
PTPN11	176876	Protein tyrosin phosphatase, non-receptor type 11	H	Noonan syndrome type 1; LEOPARD type 1	AD
KRAS	190070	V-KI-RAS2 Kirsten rat sarcoma viral oncogene homolog	H	Noonan syndrome type 3; cardio-facio-cutaneous syndrome 2	AD
RAF1	164760	V-RAF-1 Murine leukemia viral oncogene homolog 1	H	Noonan syndrome 5, LEOPARD syndrome 2	AD
NRAS	164790	Neuroblastoma RAS viral oncogene homolog	H	Noonan syndrome 6	AD
RIT1	609591	Ric-like protein without CAAL Motif 1	H	Noonan syndrome 8	AD

Note: Some of these genes are confirmed and replicated in several series. Others have been reported in either small series of single families. The central column shows other cardiomyopathy phenotypes that have been reported as associated with mutations in the same genes.
°In this table, NC or LVNC define the trabecular morphology of the left ventricle (see Chapter 45).
AD, autosomal dominant; AR autosomal recessive; XLR, X-Linked recessive; XLD, X-Linked dominant; sCPK, serum creatin-phosphokinase;

TABLE 41–3. Clinical and Instrumental Markers to be Annotated and Potentially Useful for Formulating Pretest Clinical Hypothesis of Specific Genetic DCMs or Syndromes

	Proband	Feature/marker/trait	Gene/s	Inheritance
ECG	M or F	AVB	LMNA	AD
	M		EMD	XLR
	M or F		DES (Usually RCM)	AD, AR
	M or F	Short PR with or without WPW	MtDNA	Matrilineal
	M or F	Low QRS voltage	PLN*	AR
	M or F	High QRS voltage	Sarcomere genes	AD
	M or F	Increase or decrease QT interval	Ion channel genes	AD
	M	Atrial standstill/giant atria	EMD	XLR
	M or F		NPPA	AR
	M or F	Atrial Standstill	GJA5	AD
	M or F	SSS1/atrial disease with/without DCM	SCN5A	AR
	M or F	SSS2	HCN4	AD
	M	Posterolateral Q waves	DMD	XLR

(Continued)

TABLE 41–3. Clinical and Instrumental Markers to be Annotated and Potentially Useful for Formulating Pretest Clinical Hypothesis of Specific Genetic DCMs or Syndromes (Continued)

	Proband	Feature/marker/trait	Gene/s	Inheritance
TTE and CMR	M	Left ventricular non-compaction Left ventricular hypertrabeculation (nonspecific marker)	G4.5	XLR
	M or F		LDB3	AD
	M or F		MIB1	AD
	M or F		DTNA	AD
	M or F		MtDNA (Multiple variants)	Matrilineal
	M or F		PRDM16	AD
	M or F		ACTN2	AD
	M or F		TNNT2, MYH7, MYBPC3, ACTC1, TPM1, DES	AD
Biochemistry/ Biomarkers	M	>sCPK°	DMD	XLR
	M or F		LMNA	AD, AR
	M or F		FKTN	AR
	M or F		LDB3	AD
	M; M or F		DAG-related genes	AD, AR, XLR
	M		EMD	XLR
	M or F		BAG3	AD
	F	>sCPK	Healthy carriers of DMD defects	XLR
	M	>sCPK°	Muscle dystrophies/myopathies	XLR
	M	>Lactacidemia	Mitochondrial diseases	AD, AR, Matrilineal
	M	Hypocholesterolemia	G4.5	XLR
	M	Methylglutaconic aciduria/organic acuduria	G4.5	XLR
	M or F		DNAJC19	AR
	M	Leukocytopenia	G4.5	XLR
	M or F	Hypomagnesemia	MtDNA	Matrlineal
	M or F	Myoglobinuria	MtDNA	Matrlineal
Extracardiac traits (major, recurrent)	M or F	Neurosensorial hearing loss	MtDNA	Matrlineal
	M or F		Nuclear genes coding Mt proteins	AD, AR
	M or F		Epicardin	AD
	M or F		EYA4	AD
	M or F	Cryptogenic stroke	MtDNA	Matrlineal
	M or F	Fahr's syndrome	MtDNA	Matrlineal
	M or F	Palpebral ptosis	POLG1 and other nuclear genes coding mitochondrial proteins	AD
	M or F		ANT1	AD
	M or F		MtDNA genes	Matrilineal
	M; M or F	Myopathy/dystrophy°	Multiple genes	AD, AR, XLR
	M or F	Cataract	CRYAB	AD
	M or F		AGK	AR
	M or F	Palpebral ptosis	POLG	AD
	M or F	Diabetes^	MtDNA	Matrlineal
	M or F	Renal failure	ALMS1	AR
	M or F	Fingers' anormalities	TBX5	AD

(Continued)

TABLE 41–3. Clinical and Instrumental Markers to be Annotated and Potentially Useful for Formulating Pretest Clinical Hypothesis of Specific Genetic DCMs or Syndromes (Continued)

	Proband	Feature/marker/trait	Gene/s	Inheritance
	M or F	Brachydactyly, mild hand; severe foot involvement	LMNA	AD
	M or F	Learning disability[§]	MtDNA	Matrilineal
	M		LAMP2	XLR
	M or F	Ataxia with & without retained reflexes	FXN	AR
	M or F	Woolly hair and keratoderma	DSP	AR
	M or F	Woolly hair, keratoderma, and tooth agenesis	DSP	AD
	M or F	Cutaneous collagenoma of the occipital scalp	LMNA	AD
	M or F	Hypergonadothropic Hypogonadism (Malouf S.)	LMNA	AD
	M or F	Valproate-induced brain pseudoatrophy	MTATP8	Matrilineal
	F	Corpus callosum agenesis	NDUFB11	XLD
	M or F	Ataxia, 3-methylglutaconic aciduria	DNAJC19	AR
	M or F	Lipodystrophy	LMNA	AD
	M or F	Progeria, and other premature aging syndromes	LMNA	AD
	M or F	Tautness of the skin, restrictive dermopathy	LMNA	AR
	M or F	Hypoplastic mandible with severe dental anomalies	LMNA	AR
	M or F	Hypertrichosis, long, curly eyelashes	ABCC9	AD
EMB	M or F	Histiocytoid cardiomyopathy	MTCYB	Matrilineal
	F		NDUFB11	XLD
	M or F		AARS2	AR
	M or F	Loss of endothelial cell loss**	LAMA4	AD
	M or F	Loss/irregular expression of nuclear Lamin A/C,	LMNA	AD
	M	Loss of expression of dystrophin, sarcolemma	DMD	XLR
	M	Loss of expression of Emerin, nuclear membrane	EMD	XLR
	M or F	Severely reduced activity of complex II	SDHA	AR
	M or F	Decreased desmosomes, intercalate disc "paleness"**	DSG2	AD
	M or F	Desmin positive granulophilamentous material°°	DES	AD, AR
	M	Loss of expression of LAMP2	LAMP2	XL
	M or F	Mitochondrial proliferation and abnormalities	MtDNA genes	Matrilineal
	M		G4.5	XLR
	M or F		Nuclear "mitochondrial" genes	AR, AD
	M or F	Myocyte iron storage	FXTN	AR
	M or F	Sarcoplasmic accumulation of electron-dense granulofilamentous material	BAG3	AD

Up to 15% DCM and ARVC in Netherlands
°The list includes several genes known to cause muscle dystrophies/myopathies.
^Common in families with mitochondrial DNA–related cardiomyopathies.
§More common in patients with HCM. EMB: Endomyocardial biopsy.
**To be confirmed. Never observed to date in DCM phenotypes. DAG, Dystrophin associated glycoproteins. (OMIM and PubMed, last accessed October 28, 2015).

- Z-disc genes (*ACTN2, ANKRD1, BAG3, CRYAB, CSRP3, FHL2, LDB3, MYPN, MURC, NEXN, PGM1, VCL, FLNC*), all together accounting for less than 10% of DCM.[46,47]

- Genes coding intermediate filaments connecting sarcolemma with sarcomeres (*DES*) in about 1% of cases.[48]

- Mitochondrial genes, both nuclear (eg, *G4.5, CTF1, SDHA, DNAJC19*) and mitochondrial DNA genes, in less than 5% of cases.[39]

- Sarcolemma genes, including *DMD* defects in 6% to 7% of DCM in consecutive male series and dystrophin-associated glycoprotein complex (ie, *SGCA, SGCB, SGCD*) in less than 1% of DCM cases.[49-51]

- Ion channels (*SCN5A*)[52,53] or genes such as *ABCC9* or *CHRM2*, in less than 1% of cases.[54]

- Genes whose products are active in Golgi apparatus machinery (eg, *FKTN*) or in the intracellular calcium handling (*RBM20*)[37] or sarcoplasmic reticulum (*PLN*) in less than 1% of cases.[55] The prevalence of *PLN*-related DCM varies in different geographic areas. Founder mutations, such as *PLN* R14del, in the Netherlands account for more than 10% of all DCM among the Dutch population.[56]

Mechanisms of Myocardial Damage

The mechanisms through which mutations in different genes cause functional and structural myocyte damage ending in a similar phenotype depend on the gene and the role of its product(s) in the myocyte, type of mutation and its effects on the protein expression, epistasis (the action of one gene upon another), and epigenetic factors.[53] Mechanisms such as haploinsufficiency (a single functional copy of a gene is insufficient to maintain normal function) have been demonstrated in dilated cardiolaminopathies and dilated cardiodystrophinopathies.[57-59] Two genes (*LMNA* and *DMD*) typically cause DCM, with or without arrhythmias, but do not cause hypertrophic cardiomyopathy (HCM). However, most DCM genes also cause other types of cardiomyopathy (HCM, restrictive cardiomyopathy [RCM], and arrhythmogenic RV cardiomyopathy [ARVC]). The paradigmatic example is DCM caused by mutations in sarcomeric genes such as *MYH7* (**Fig. 41–3**); the understanding of the mechanisms that cause either HCM or DCM in carriers of *MYH7* mutations is still far from being elucidated. It has been proposed that mutant myosins with enhanced contractility lead to HCM, whereas those displaying decreased contractility lead to DCM. Gain or loss of function could be the primary consequence of a specific mutation.[60]

Genetic Testing

Genetic testing is now routinely performed using massive parallel sequencing of multigene panels (next-generation sequencing [NGS]) for both nuclear genes[5] and mitochondrial DNA.[61] The time needed for testing is short, and the costs are lower than with Sanger-based technologies. The mismatch between fast rate of detection and the time needed for developing functional studies that assess the effects of mutations explains the multiple pipelines generated in the last decade to contribute to the interpretation of novel genetic variants including those with uncertain significance.

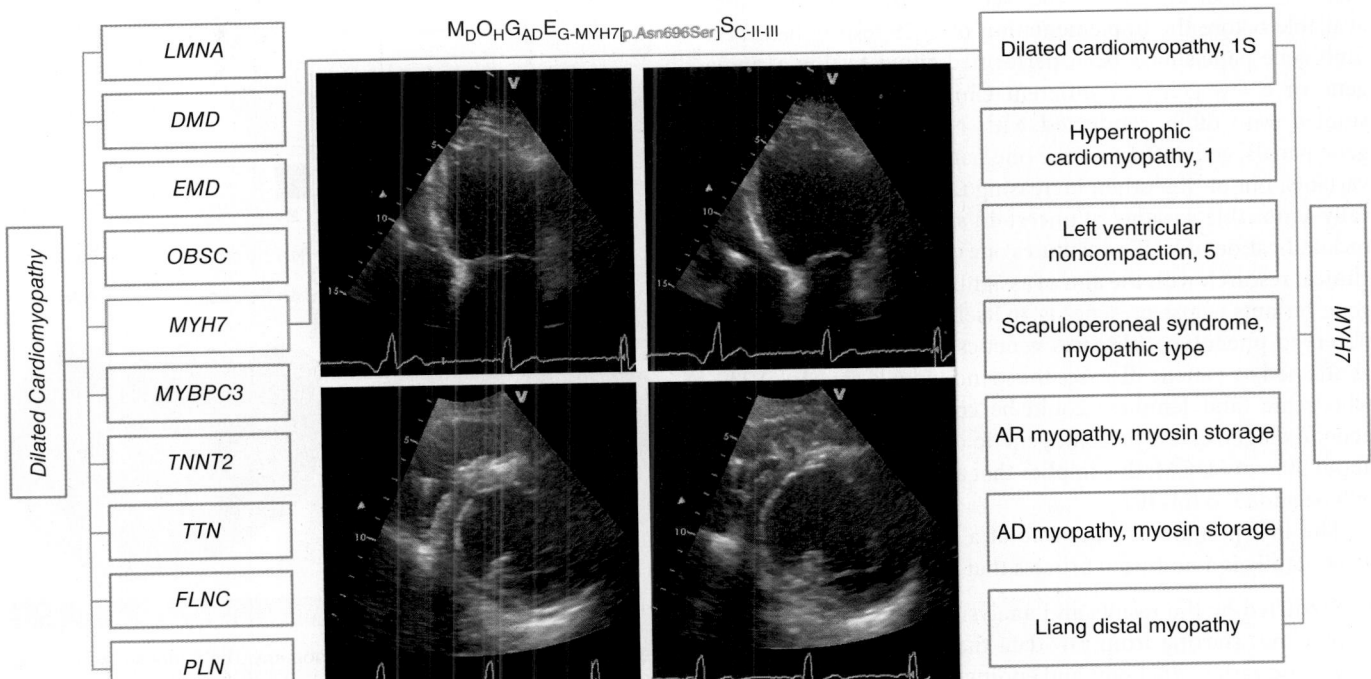

Figure 41–3. The 2D-TTE shows the dilated phenotype in the carrier of a pathogenic variant in *MYH7* gene. This variant has been reported as associated with HCM. Nonetheless, although there is discrepancy between the observed and expected phenotype, the p.(Asn696Ser) variant is likely the disease-causing mutation. The figure shows the list of clinically heterogeneous phenotypes associated with *MYH7* mutations, which also include DCM (MIM # 613426).

For several disease genes, a proven cause-and-effect relationship between gene mutations and disease is now robust enough to assign a diagnostic role to genetic testing; the causal link of the mutation with the disease is still provisional for several other candidate genes, especially those reported in one or a few families and still unconfirmed in larger series. Interpretation of genetic testing is the challenge of the next decade, considering that when multiple genes are tested and the gene panels include giant genes such as *titin* (*TTN*) or large and complex genes such as *Duchenne muscle dystrophy* (*DMD*) and *obscurin*, the probability of finding more than one mutation per individual increases.[5] Further developments are needed to generate efficient tools for exploring the functional effects and pathologic role of mutations, especially when considering that most heritable DCMs are Mendelian diseases transmitted through an autosomal dominant mode, a rule that does not change even in families in which more than one mutation is identified. This implies that one major (or leading) mutation or two mutations inherited from the same affected parent plays a causative role, with other variants potentially acting as phenotype modifiers. Misinterpretation of the role of the mutation in the pathogenesis of the DCM may have severe implications for the patient and family, especially when procreative plans include prenatal diagnosis.

The proportion of DCM causally linked with known genes can be posted as definite (ie, *LMNA*, *DYS*, and sarcomere genes) or considered provisional, especially among genes that have been reported in unique families/cases (see Table 41–2). Ethnic variations and founder mutations may explain different prevalence of mutations in disease genes; for example, *PLN* p.(Arg14Del) is rare in the general population but causes more than 10% of all FDCMs in the Netherlands.[56,62] Most studies available before the implementation of NGS testing based on multigene panels have been performed either testing a single gene or a few genes in different clinical series. Subsequent studies were often conducted with NGS analysis of multigene panels, generating, on the one hand, a greater number of variants, but on the other, increasing the number of nonclinically actionable variants of uncertain significance (VUS). The reclassification of VUS constitutes one of the main objectives of clinical research with the aim of assigning a causal role to those gene variants whose presence is, in itself, sufficient to cause the observed phenotype (diseases genetics) and to avoid labeling as affected by genetic diseases those individuals carrying VUS, whose life (and families) could be conditioned by a wrong genetic diagnosis. At present, genetic defects are identified in about 50% of FDCM; this implies that additional disease genes will be added to this list.

The interpretation of the role of a putative mutation in a given family is a multistep process that is:

1. Predicted by the results and analysis of NGS tests through pipelines starting from raw data that include thousands of genetic variants/patients and ending with one or a few probable or possible disease mutation(s).

2. Based on consolidated evidence of pathogenicity for known mutations: automated collection of information on mutations that have been previously reported and proven as pathogenic requires disease specific expertise and regular monitoring of disease databases. Identification of a mutation, while integral to the assignment of pathogenicity, cannot by itself, at least in some instances, be sufficient to establish pathogenesis. For example, although truncation-predicting mutations are likely to be pathologic, a few of them occur in nonaffected control population and should be considered either nonpathologic or variants of uncertain significance.

3. Confirmed by in vivo or in vitro functional and pathologic studies (**Fig. 41–4**): either endomyocardial biopsy with immunohistochemical study of the protein coded by the mutated gene or in vitro studies on fibroblasts or induced pluripotent stem cell–derived myocytes obtained from circulating cells or fibroblasts from patients who carry the putative mutation.

4. Integrated into a clinical context, based on segregation studies in families (**Fig. 41–5**): mutated family members are affected and nonmutated members are not affected. Healthy mutation carriers are usually younger than affected mutated family members.

The overall evidence gained by the combination of the above criteria should establish whether a mutation is pathologic and, therefore, should be posted as a disease-causing mutation. The American College of Medical Genetics and Genomics (ACMG) guidelines substituted the term *mutation and polymorphism* with the term *variant* and assigned a precise interpretation of each genetic variant on the basis of combined

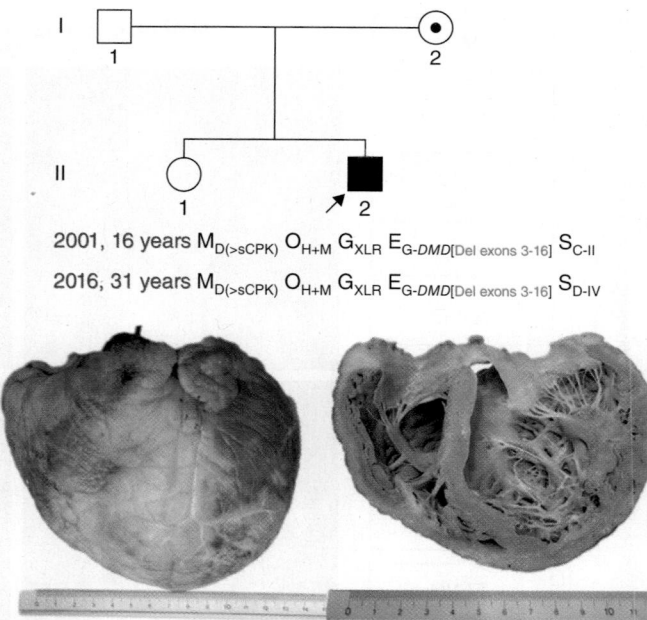

2001, 16 years $M_{D(>sCPK)}$ O_{H+M} G_{XLR} $E_{G\text{-}DMD[Del\ exons\ 3\text{-}16]}$ $S_{C\text{-}II}$

2016, 31 years $M_{D(>sCPK)}$ O_{H+M} G_{XLR} $E_{G\text{-}DMD[Del\ exons\ 3\text{-}16]}$ $S_{D\text{-}IV}$

Figure 41–4. Dilated cardiodystrophinopathy. The figure shows the pedigree and the macroscopic view of a heart with DCM from a young male patient who developed DCM at the age of 16 years; the disease showed slow progression to end-stage heart failure, and the patient underwent heart transplantation 15 years later. The dystrophin defect is not associated with severe muscle dystrophy.

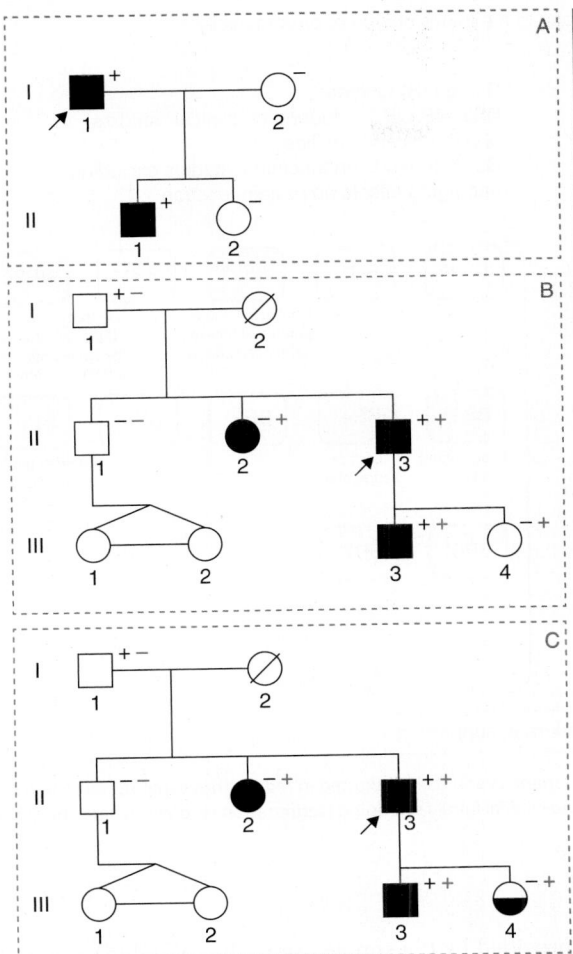

A: The early nucleus of the family in which the p.(Asp117Asn) in *LDB3* (+) gene was identified in the two affected family members.

B: The expansion of family screening, both clinical and genetic, shows that the unaffected father (I:1) of the proband (II:3) carries the same genetic variant and the affected sister (II:2) does not. The affected sister showed signs of LVH in her ECG, mild LV thickening (12 mm), mild LV dilation (LVEDD = 55 mm), and borderline LV dysfunction (LVEF = 49%). Testing of further genes demonstrated the presence of the p.(Arg502Gln) in *MYH7* (+) in the proband (II:3), in his affected son (III:3) and unaffected daughter (III:4), as well as in the affected sister (II:2), but not in the father (I:1). This mutation better segregates with the phenotype in the family. The mother of the proband (I:2) died at the age of 37 years for breast cancer diagnosed during her 3rd pregnancy: she was the obligate carrier of the *MYH7* mutation.

C: 6 years later, the young healthy carrier (III:4) of the p.(Arg502Gln) demonstrated mild HCM (max LV thickness = 13 mm) with normal LV function and borderline LV diameter (LVEDD = 53 mm), further supporting the role of the *MYH7* mutation.

Figure 41-5. Segregation study in families. The figure shows the pedigree of a family in which the first genetic testing in the proband identified a genetic variant in the *LDB3* gene originally considered as the potential cause of the disease (**A**). Clinical and genetic family screening demonstrated that the variant did not segregate with the phenotype (**A** and **B**). Further genetic testing in the proband identified a second mutation in the *MYBPC3* gene (**B** and **C**). Long-term follow-up of the family supported the segregation of this latter mutation in the family (**C**). ECG, electrocardiogram; HCM, hypertrophic cardiomyopathy; LV, left ventricular; LVEDD, left ventricular end-diastolic diameter; LVEF, left ventricular ejection fraction; LVH, left ventricular hypertrophy.

criteria supporting pathogenicity (n = 16) or benignity (n = 12).[63] The ACMG criteria are based on clinical genetics, phenotype information, genetic epidemiology/population data, computational/predictive data, characteristics of the gene, and mutation (**Fig. 41-6**). The strength of each contributor to the interpretation of pathogenicity is classified as very strong, strong, moderate, or supporting. On stringent and rigorous basis, many genetic variants previously interpreted as disease-causing are now being reinterpreted to either confirm or exclude a causative role in DCM.[64]

Grouping Genetic Dilated Cardiomyopathy by Disease Gene

Although to date more than 100 disease and candidate genes have been associated with DCM, only a few of them have been confirmed and replicated in more clinical series and families. In a large sequenced DCM cohort, robust disease association was observed with 12 genes (*TTN, DSP, MYH7, LMNA, BAG3, TNNT2, TNNC1, PLN, ACTC1, NEXN, TPM1,* and *VCL*), highlighting their importance in DCM and translating into

high interpretability in diagnostic testing. The other less common disease genes probably need to be reevaluated in ongoing curation efforts to determine their validity as Mendelian DCM genes.[65]

Clinical markers typically recurring in DCM caused by mutations in these genes are now consolidated contributors in the pretest clinical orientation about the possible disease gene to be tested in the probands.[36] Phenotype-oriented single-gene testing is now superseded by multigene panels' NGS analysis methods; pretest clinical predictors weigh little on the genes to be analyzed. Therefore, today, recurrent phenotypic traits in DCM associated with defects of the different disease genes can emerge more after the test than in the pretest phase. Nevertheless, the goal of phenotypically characterizing DCMs associated with defects in different genes in an ever more specific way remains a cornerstone of the research aims.[66]

The following examples represent ongoing clinical efforts to improve the clinical phenotypic characterization of DCMs associated with defects in different genes. They have been selected based on different criteria: cardiolaminopathies because of

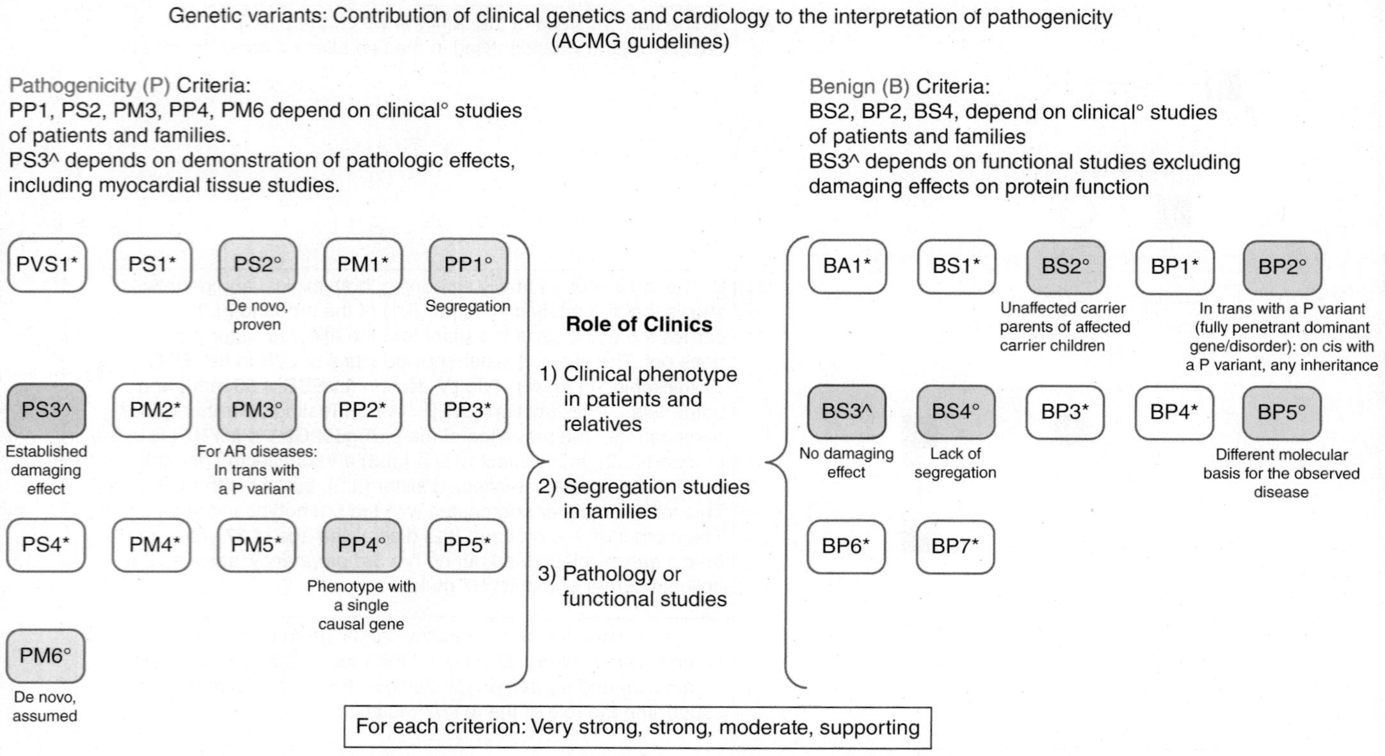

Genetic variants: Contribution of clinical genetics and cardiology to the interpretation of pathogenicity
(ACMG guidelines)

Pathogenicity (P) Criteria:
PP1, PS2, PM3, PP4, PM6 depend on clinical° studies
of patients and families.
PS3^ depends on demonstration of pathologic effects,
including myocardial tissue studies.

Benign (B) Criteria:
BS2, BP2, BS4, depend on clinical° studies
of patients and families
BS3^ depends on functional studies excluding
damaging effects on protein function

Figure 41–6. The figure summarizes the ACMG criteria for interpretation of genetic variants. Variants highlighted in *red* are those that depend on the clinical contribution that cardiologists should provide with deep phenotyping of probands and clinical family screening (segregation studies); in *blue*, the criteria that can demonstrate (or exclude) the functional effects of the mutation.

their high arrhythmogenic risk (they represent the first genetic DCM formally recognized based on the disease gene and types of mutations in guidelines for primary prevention of sudden death with implantable cardioverter-defibrillator [ICD] implantation); cardioemerinopathies because, although very rare, their phenotype may look similar to cardiolaminopathies (DCM with conduction disease and myopathy) but with different pattern of inheritance (X-linked recessive vs autosomal dominant); cardiodystrophinopathies because they may represent the major or unique phenotype in male patients with DCM and are associated with increased serum creatine phosphokinase in >80% of cases; cardiozaspopathies because of the frequent association with prominent trabecular anatomy of the LV; cardiomyosinopathies because defects of the structural and regulatory myosin complex of the sarcomere may cause typical HCM, but also DCM and HCM-DCM (ie, a phenotype that in the end-stage phases is similar to DCM but frequently maintains ECG features suggestive of LV hypertrophy); dilated cardioMITOmyopathies because of their high malignancy and the syndromic context in which the cardiomyopathy is observed; cardiotitinopathies because of their high prevalence in DCM series; and phospholambanopathies because of the high arrhythmogenic risk and peculiar ECG markers.

LAMIN AC (LMNA) DCM

This subgroup of DCM can be described as dilated cardiolaminopathies, or DCM-LMNA; an individual description can

be provided by the simple use of the MOGE(S) system (morphofunctional phenotype, organ involvement, genetic inheritance pattern, etiologic annotation including genetic defect or underlying disease/substrate, and functional status of the disease) (see Chapter 40). DCM-LMNA is phenotypically characterized by the association of the DCM with conduction system disease, which occurs in up to 80% of patients with cardiolaminopathies.[67] In the last 15 years, the association between *LMNA* gene mutations and DCM with conduction system disease has been replicated and confirmed.[68–70] Dilated cardiolaminopathies constitute 6% to 7% of all DCMs in consecutive series.[46] The development of conduction system disease usually precedes the appearance of the DCM;[8,17] the natural history is characterized by a long asymptomatic phase in which regular monitoring demonstrates a progressive prolongation of the PR interval and slowly progressive LV dilation and/or dysfunction. Cardiolaminopathies display high arrhythmogenic potential for both atrial and ventricular arrhythmias. The high risk of life-threatening ventricular arrhythmias is one of the characteristics of cardiolaminopathies, and such arrhythmias may manifest even in mildly dilated and dysfunctioning hearts.[69–71] ESC guidelines on the primary prevention of sudden cardiac death (SCD) recommend ICD implantation in patients with DCM and a confirmed disease-causing *LMNA* mutation and clinical risk factors (class IIa, level of evidence B)[72] such as nonsustained ventricular tachycardia during ambulatory ECG monitoring, LVEF <45% on initial evaluation, male gender, and nonmissense mutations (insertion, deletion, truncation, or mutations affecting splicing). These factors correspond to those previously identified in a large European cohort of patients with dilated cardiolaminopathy.[70]

The biology of lamin A/C heart disease (genetics, structure, and function of lamins), clinical presentation (diagnostic markers, ECG and imaging features), and aspects of screening and management, including current uncertainties, are major matters of current investigation.[73] *LMNA* mutations located upstream versus downstream of the NLS seem to have a more adverse cardiac phenotype, and some missense mutations can be as harmful as nonmissense ones.[74] In a recent meta-analysis aimed at determining predictors of sustained ventricular arrhythmias in patients with DCM, the presence of mutations in the *LMNA* gene (along with mutations in PLN and FLNC) was one of the contributors to arrhythmogenic risk stratification.[75]

Emerin (EMD) DCM

Dilated cardioemerinopathies, or DCM-EMD, constitute a small subgroup of DCM but also provide a paradigmatic example of rare DCM that may phenotypically mimic cardiolaminopathies.[38,43] They are, in fact, typically associated with conduction disease; different from cardiolaminopathies, they are inherited as X-linked recessive diseases and invariably associated with muscle dystrophy. This latter feature is also possible in DCM-LMNA, but less common. Emerin is a ubiquitous protein, a major component of the nuclear envelope, and a member of the nuclear lamina-associated protein family.[76]

Defects in the *EMD* gene cause X-linked recessive Emery–Dreifuss muscular dystrophy. Cardiac involvement is common and manifests with palpitations, presyncope and syncope, poor exercise tolerance, and HF. The clinical management includes treatments for cardiac arrhythmias, atrioventricular conduction disorders, and congestive HF, including antiarrhythmic drugs, cardiac pacemaker, ICD, and heart transplantation for end-stage HF.[43,77] Conduction disease is, therefore, the marker of the disease in patients with X-linked inheritance and DCM; the immediate clinical differential diagnosis with autosomal dominant laminopathies is the inheritance pattern.

X-Linked Dilated Cardiodystrophinopathies

Dilated cardiodystrophinopathies, or DCM-DYS, typically manifest in male patients. Mild cardiac involvement may manifest in females: about 8% of female carriers present with late-onset DCM, though it may vary from 0% to 16.7%, depending on whether the carrier is classified as affected by DMD or BMD. More commonly, female carriers demonstrate variable, asymptomatic, cyclic increase of the sCPK levels.[78] Most patients carry large *DMD* gene rearrangements, both in-frame and out-of-frame deletions (>80%);[49,50] in a minority of cases, mutations are either nonsense or missense or splice. Mutations are associated with loss of protein expression at the level of the cardiomyocyte sarcolemma.[50] *DMD* gene (MIM#300377) mutations cause the following three phenotypes: Duchenne muscular dystrophy (MIM#310200), Becker muscular dystrophy (MIM#300376), and X-linked DCM (MIM#302045). Most

data on cardio-phenotypes have been generated in series of patients with Duchenne muscular dystrophy and Becker muscular dystrophy; single case reports and a few series explored patients presenting with DCM phenotype at onset.[49,50] Milasin et al.[79] first described a family with X-linked DCM associated with a splice donor site mutation in the *DMD* gene. Antidystrophin immunostain showed reduced, but normally distributed, protein in the skeletal muscle and no detectable protein in the myocardium, suggesting that selective heart involvement in DCM-DMD is related to the absence in the heart of a compensatory expression of dystrophin from alternative promoters.[79] This case generated a cardio-specific interest; further reports of single cases demonstrated that mutations in the *DMD* gene may exclusively or predominantly affect the heart, with normal or early involved skeletal muscle.[80,81] The precise diagnosis can be missed and eventually determined after a heart transplant, when muscle dystrophy may manifest and be attributed to statin treatments.[82]

Although rare, these previous studies facilitated the feasibility of heart transplantation in either patient with X-linked DCM or Becker muscular dystrophy with DCM as a major and initial presentation of dystrophinopathy (see Fig. 41–4). The diagnosis of X-linked DCM-DYS is feasible by endomyocardial biopsy, which demonstrates loss of protein expression; genetic testing confirms the diagnosis.[49,50] X-linked DCM-DYS carries a low arrhythmogenic risk even when patients show severely dilated and dysfunctioning hearts, requiring ICD for primary prevention of SCD according to current guidelines. No ICD shock was observed during a median follow-up of 14 months (interquartile range, 5–25 months) in 34 patients with DCM caused by defects of dystrophin.[50] DCM-DMD may show LV noncompaction (LVNC), which occurs in up to 30% of cases and is now proposed as a prognostic marker.[83,84] The recent introduction of ventricular assist device implantation in children affected by DMD opens novel avenues for treatment of the most severe forms of DCM-DMD.[85,86]

Overall, HF, rather than arrhythmia burden, is the strongest cardiac predictor of mortality. Sudden arrhythmic death is rare, even in patients with previously diagnosed arrhythmias.[87] Despite this, recommendations for ICD placement in patients with cardio-dystrophinopathies have been extrapolated from adult HF recommendations based on decreased LVEF <35%.[88] The actual arrhythmogenic risk in these patients and its impact on decisions such as placing an ICD should be reexamined in light of the low arrhythmic risk evident in these cardiomyopathies to date.

Filamin A (FLNA) DCM

Filamin A (FLNA), B (FLNB), and C (FLNC) are structural crosslinkers of actin rods at the sarcomeric Z-disc of both cardiac and skeletal muscle.[47] Whereas FLNA and FLNB are ubiquitously expressed, FLNC is predominantly enriched in cardiac and skeletal muscle.[89] *FLNC* gene (MIM * 102565) maps at 17q31.2 and encodes the sarcomeric protein filamin C. *FLNC* mutations typically cause myofibrillar myopathy 3 (MIM #609524) and distal myopathy 4 (MIM #614065). In the last 5 years, numerous mutations in the *FLNC* gene have been found in both phenotypically different (HCM, RCM, DCM, and ARVC) and overlapping dilated and left-dominant arrhythmogenic cardiomyopathies. Truncation-predicting mutations—stop, frameshift, splice site, and large rearrangements, in particular—are associated with the overlapping phenotypes such as dilated and left-dominant arrhythmogenic cardiomyopathy complicated by frequent and life-threatening arrhythmias and premature sudden death,[90] cardiac-restricted arrhythmogenic DCM phenotype,[91] and ARVC.[92] The prominent interstitial fibrosis commonly observed in these hearts could explain the high arrhythmogenic risk. The phenotype does not manifest in childhood; clinical signs and symptoms appear in young-adult adult age. Experts suggest that implantation of a cardiac defibrillator should be considered in patients harboring truncating mutations in *FLNC*. Family screening is mandatory, to prevent the risk of missing asymptomatic carriers. The ECG may show inferolateral negative T waves. Echocardiography demonstrates mild-to-moderate LVSD, and regional dyskinesia.[90]

Dilated Sarcomeric Cardiomyopathies

Recent studies have focused on the question of why mutations in the *MYH7* gene that typically cause HCM may also be associated with the development of DCM[60] rather than the most common HCM. In murine models investigating the S532P and F764L mutations in the *MYH7* gene and associated with the DCM phenotype, the molecular mechanism leading to DCM may be the depressing molecular function in cardiac myosin, which may initiate heart remodeling and pathologic dilation. Accordingly, mutations that lead to DCM are likely be those that are associated with loss of function; those that are associated with gain of function may be associated with HCM.[60,93] The reconstitution of the entire contractile system (actin and myosin[94] and tropomyosin 1, troponin C, troponin I, and troponin T[95,96]) seems to be necessary to fully understand the effects of *MYH7* mutations in HCM and DCM.[97] Alternative explanations include the possibility of compound mutations in mitochondrial DNA genes and in the *MYH7* gene; patients who carry the sole *MYH7* mutation demonstrate HCM, whereas those carrying both *MYH7* and mitochondrial DNA mutations develop hypertrophic DCM with an end phenotype resembling DCM.[98] Yet another explanation is the presence of more than one mutation in the same patient; depending on the mutation, the DCM phenotype should be explained by a complex genetic make-up when more than one mutation is present and contributing to the final phenotype.[38] Overall, the role of *MYH7* in DCM remains a matter of research and deserves specific investigation for any novel mutation identified in patients with DCM.

Dilated CardioMITOchondrial Diseases

In this subgroup of patients, the DCM is usually observed in the context of multiorgan syndromes with a particular risk of complications such as cryptogenic strokes and intolerance to several drugs.[38,39,61] Mitochondrial cardiomyopathies can be caused by mutations both in mitochondrial DNA genes (maternal inheritance, no male passes down the disease to children) and in

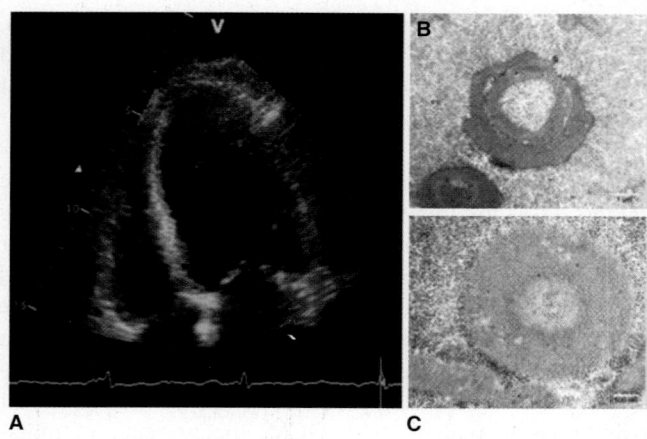

Figure 41–7. Mitochondrial cardiomyopathy. This figure shows the echocardiographic view (**A**) of the dilated cardiomyopathy (DCM) in a 53-year-old woman affected by mitochondrial myopathy, encephalopathy, lactic acidosis, and stroke (MELAS) syndrome. Her endomyocardial biopsy (**B** and **C**) showed typically abnormal mitochondria. The DCM phenotype was associated with hearing loss and mild myopathy.

nuclear genes (Mendelian inheritance) coding mitochondrial proteins. They are characterized by either hypertrophic phenotype evolving through dilated and dysfunctioning hearts or DCM (**Fig. 41–7**). The clinical manifestations associated with mutations in mitochondrial DNA genes depend on the grade of heteroplasmy in affected organs. They are commonly observed in families in which mutation carriers also express noncardiac traits such as hearing loss, palpebral ptosis, myopathy, renal failure, cryptogenic stroke, diabetes, optic neuritis, and/or retinitis pigmentosa. Sequencing of mitochondrial DNA, either by Sanger-based techniques or NGS tools, identifies the causative mutation. Nuclear "mitochondrial" cardiomyopathies are inherited according to Mendelian rules: they can be autosomal dominant or recessive.[37] Typical cardiac phenotypes are primarily DCM, such as in the autosomal recessive DCM caused by *ANT1* mutations[99] or in autosomal dominant DCM and progressive external ophthalmoplegia caused by *POLG1* mutations.[100]

Titin (TTN) DCM

The titin (*TTN*) gene encodes the largest human protein and the third most abundant striated muscle protein. Of the different titin isoforms, the N2B and N2BA isoforms are predominantly expressed at the cardiac level; the cardiac isoform Novex-3 titin (5600 amino acids) is less represented in cardiac tissue than full-length titin.[101] Truncation-predicting mutations have been identified in 25% of FDCMs and in 18% of sporadic DCMs.[41] The penetrance of *TTN* truncating mutations was more than 95% for patients who were older than 40 years of age. Clinical manifestations, morbidity, and mortality were similar to those observed in DCM patients who were noncarriers of *TTN* mutations. DCM was not accompanied by conduction system defects or skeletal muscle disease.[41] A further study in women with peripartum cardiomyopathy (PPCM) showed a distribution of truncating variants remarkably similar to that found in patients with DCM.[102] Missense variants have been further investigated in DCM distinguishing "bioinformatically severe" *TTN* versus nonsevere variants; carriers of "severe *TTN* variants" showed a clinical course similar to that of noncarriers.[103] *TTN* mutations have been involved in HCM (MIM#613765); muscular dystrophy of the Limb-Girdle, type 2J (MIM#608807); autosomal recessive early-onset myopathy with fatal cardiomyopathy (MIM#611705); tardive tibial muscular dystrophy (MIM#600334); and proximal myopathy, with early respiratory muscle involvement (MIM#603689).[42,104] Because 1 in 500 individuals in the general population carries a truncation variant in the *TTN* A-band, the interpretation of such mutations in DCM should be cautious.[42] The definition of the precise role of *TTN* in DCM may contribute to implement research exploring antisense-mediated exon skipping as a therapeutic strategy.[105] Genetics may also contribute to arrhythmogenic risk stratification. In a recent study including 537 individuals (61% men; 317 probands) with baseline LVSD, TTNtv were associated with frequent arrhythmia, but malignant ventricular arrhythmias were observed only in patients with severe LVSD. Male sex and LVSD were independent predictors of outcomes. Mutation location did not impact clinical phenotype or outcomes.[106] Other studies exploring the natural history TTNtv showed a relatively mild disease course with significant excess mortality in elderly patients.[107]

Phopsholamban (PLN) DCM

Dilated phopsholambanopathies are a distinct group of DCM caused by mutations in the phospholamban (*PLN*) gene that encodes a protein expressed in the sarcoplasmic reticulum membrane. Phospholamban inhibits cardiac muscle sarcoplasmic reticulum Ca^{2+}-ATPase (SERCA2a) in the unphosphorylated state. Mutations in *PLN* impair sarcoplasmic reticulum calcium homeostasis and cause DCM.[56,108] Less commonly, mutations in *PLN* cause HCM. p.(Arg14del) is the most frequently identified mutation in Dutch cardiomyopathy patients (10%–15%), both DCM and arrhythmogenic phenotypes.[56] Patients with p.(Arg14del) diagnosed with DCM demonstrate high arrhythmogenic risk and SCD as first disease presentation.[62] A common ECG pattern in *PLN* mutation carriers is a low-voltage QRS complex and inverted T waves in leads V_4 to V_6.[109] In non-Dutch patients, *PLN* mutations are less common but equally malignant.[110,111] Therefore, although rare, *PLN* mutations can be clinically suspected in patients with DCM, high arrhythmogenic risk, and low voltage on ECG.

Desmoplakin Cardiomyopathy

Desmoplakin *(DSP)* defects cause both ARVC and DCM. Arrhythmogenic LV cardiomyopathy (ALVC) and arrhythmogenic DCM are poorly defined and potentially difficult to distinguish. *DSP* defects cause more regionality in LV impairment. The most defining characteristic is a subepicardial ring-like scar pattern in DSP/FLNC, which should be considered in future diagnostic criteria for ALVC.[112] The arrhythmogenic potential seems to be strongly associated with defects in *DSP*, irrespective of their phenotype, either ALVC or arrhythmogenic DCM. In 107 patient carriers of *DSP* defects, LVEF <55% was strongly associated with severe ventricular arrhythmias

(P <0.001, sensitivity 85%, specificity 53%). *DSP* cardiomyopathy is emerging as a distinct form of arrhythmogenic cardiomyopathy characterized by episodic myocardial injury, LV fibrosis that precedes systolic dysfunction, and a high incidence of ventricular arrhythmias.[113]

LDB3 and DCM

This small subgroup of DCM is caused by mutations in the *LDB3* gene that codes the Z-disc Cypher-ZASP protein. *LDB3* mutations were originally reported in adult-onset, isolated, dilated LVNC[114] (OMIM*605906.0007) (see Chapter 45). Therefore, LVNC and LV hypertrabeculation are the clinical markers that characterize DCM hearts of patients who are carriers of mutations in *LDB3*.[115,116] Mutations in the *LDB3* gene seem to also be associated with HCM and myofibrillar myopathy type 4.[117] The more common "variant" in this gene is p.(D117N) has been recently reported to represent a polymorphism in a Bedouin population in which it occurs in 5.2% of nonaffected individuals.[118] The possibility exists that mutations in *LDB3* may influence trabecular anatomy, leading to either prominent trabeculation or LVNC, which, by itself, only describes an anatomic feature and not necessarily a functional phenotype. Although available data are not sufficient to post *LDB3* as a disease gene specifically associated with both DCM and LVNC, this latter marker should be a matter of further investigation in *LDB3* hearts to definitely assess its role in the trabecular anatomy of DCM hearts.

Future Developments in Genetic Dilated Cardiomyopathy

As the number of patients and families diagnosed with DCM caused by different disease genes increases, the possibility of generating large groups of patients with shared genotypes and phenotypes will provide data for both novel and precise genetic epidemiology and for large disease-specific databases. Ideally, precisely diagnosed genetic DCM should be grouped per disease genes and mutations causing similar effects. Genetic epidemiology will help highlight proportions of different genetic DCM, guiding the assignment of clinical priorities and engaging all stakeholders in research and development programs for disease-specific treatments aimed at managing the basic genetic defects and not just the phenotype.

NONGENETIC DILATED CARDIOMYOPATHY

Nongenetic DCM includes etiologically heterogeneous diseases whose onset and progression may largely differ from those of genetic DCM. Theoretically, DCM phenotypes associated with acquired diseases/conditions and/or toxic exposures are potentially reversible with recognition, control, and/or removal of the offending cause. The major subgroups of acquired DCM include the following:

- Autoimmune/immune-mediated DCM may manifest in patients with systemic autoimmune disease such as systemic sclerosis, systemic lupus erythematosus, rheumatoid arthritis, Sjögren syndrome, and polymyositis/dermatomyositis (see Chapter 76). The Churg–Strauss syndrome (historically included in this group of diseases) has been renamed as eosinophilic granulomatosis with polyangiitis and is reviewed in the chapter on myocarditis (see Chapter 46).

- Toxic DCM, both exogenous and endogenous, with the former being mostly caused by drug toxicity leading to structural and persistent myocardial damage and dysfunction and the latter being represented by the presence of noxae that affect the heart. The proof of causality is essential to label the disease as toxic DCM.

- Inflammatory cardiomyopathies that are clinically defined by the presence of diagnostic criteria of DCM and pathologic evidence of myocardial inflammation (see Chapter 46). Despite guidelines and recent consensus documents define the disease criteria, the diagnosis of inflammatory cardiomyopathy is rarely released in clinical reports because it requires endomyocardial biopsy and often overlaps with the diagnosis of myocarditis. This ends up making inflammatory cardiomyopathy an imprecise clinical entity, whose translational clinical benefits or specific treatments are not universally shared, and remain limited to a few highly specialized centers that include EMB in the routine diagnostic path of DCM.[119] On the one hand, it is understandable that consensus documents suggest sending patients to referral centers, on the other hand, relatively simple pathological diagnoses such as those concerning tissue inflammation should be feasible in all pathology centers. Thus, the question remains of what the future perspectives of these diagnoses will be, if more solid evidence of their clinical benefits will no longer emerge.

- PPCM that manifests during the last month of pregnancy or in the 5 months postpartum (see also Chapters 51 and 78). PPCM must be distinguished from genetic DCM whose clinical onset has been triggered by pregnancy.

The current nosology of these entities to nongenetic DCM is subject to future modifications; in fact, new genetic diseases are being described in the setting of autoinflammatory Mendelian disorders and in PPCM. Rare "autoinflammatory diseases" are now recognized as genetic diseases. Accordingly, the collection of family data and genetic counseling should be incorporated in the clinical work-up of all patients with DCM to generate precise data for future research and progression of knowledge to better characterize the mechanism(s) underlying this particular DCM.

AUTOIMMUNE/IMMUNE-MEDIATED DILATED CARDIOMYOPATHY

Introduction

The clinical manifestations of cardiovascular involvement in autoimmune/immune-mediated diseases (AID) are heterogeneous and include cardiomyopathies, "myocardial damage," either showing chronic low-grade inflammation and fibrosis or isolated fibrosis, ischemic heart disease when epicardial or intramural coronary arteries are involved, valve disease with possible dysfunction, conduction defects, arrhythmias, pericarditis, and pulmonary hypertension (see Chapter 76). Myocardial involvement can occur in both T-cell-mediated AID (eg, rheumatoid arthritis [RA], type 1 diabetes mellitus, multiple sclerosis [MS], celiac disease) and antibody-mediated AID (typically systemic lupus erythematosus [SLE]), either systemic, typically RA, SLE, Sjogren's syndrome, scleroderma, or organ-specific (eg, MS, Hashimoto tyroiditis, Graves disease, inflammatory bowel disease, type 1 diabetes mellitus, myasthenia gravis). Although cardiac involvement is common, no diagnostic nosology of autoimmune diseases includes cardiac manifestations among the diagnostic criteria.

Cardiac involvement can either follow a proven diagnosis of autoimmune diseases or be the first manifestation in undiagnosed patients. In this latter case, the diagnostic work-up should go beyond the cardiology evaluation and involve the multidisciplinary collaboration with immunologists, rheumatologists, and other specialists in case of organ-specific AID in order to investigate the entire spectrum of traits potentially associated with each of the suspected diseases: ocular (ie, uveitis), cutaneous (ie, both diffuse cutaneous and limited cutaneous systemic sclerosis), respiratory (ie, pulmonary hypertension and fibrosis), thyroid (common in many autoimmune diseases), renal (either renal failure or acute crises in certain diseases), gastrointestinal (ie, esophagus in systemic sclerosis), and nervous and musculoskeletal systems. Routine cardiologic evaluation includes history and physical examination, ECG, and TTE; myocardial and disease-specific biomarkers, autoimmunity panel, and further imaging investigations are planned according to the diagnostic hypotheses and individual needs.

Familial clustering may manifest with the presence of the same or different autoimmune diseases in more than one family member (**Fig. 41–8**). The emerging autoinflammatory genetic diseases constitute a novel clinical need for differential diagnoses; accordingly, collection of family data may be clinically and scientifically useful for sporadic diseases.

Autoimmune diseases that commonly involve the heart with DCM-like phenotype/HF are systemic sclerosis, RA, SLE, polymyositis/dermatomyositis, and Sjögren syndrome, as well as overlapping syndromes (**Table 41–4**). Iatrogenic "cardiomyopathy" can result from common medications used for AID; the cardiac phenotypes are restrictive/dilated in case of hydroxychloroquine toxicity[120] and dilated in case of tumor necrosis factor (TNF)-α inhibitors (eg, etanercept, infliximab, adalimumab; see also section Cardiovascular Oncotoxicity). Iatrogenic cardiomyopathy has to be distinguished from the intrinsic risk of HF directly related to the different autoimmune diseases because it can reverse with the withdrawal of the cardiotoxic drug.

Systemic Sclerosis (Scleroderma)

Introduction

Systemic sclerosis (SS) is a clinically heterogeneous disorder of the connective tissue characterized by fibrosis of the skin and internal organs, vascular abnormalities, and presence of autoantibodies against various cellular antigens[121] including

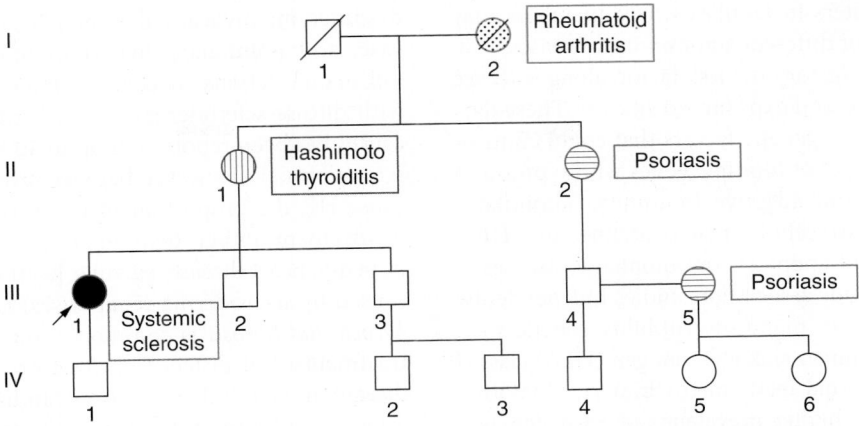

Figure 41–8. Familial clustering of autoimmune diseases. The figure shows the pedigree of a female patient (*arrow*) diagnosed with systemic sclerosis 5 years before developing mild DCM. In her family, different autoimmune diseases occurred in multiple members.

antimitochondrial antibodies (AMAs) whose detection in consecutive non-SS DCM is only 1.1%, of patients, in particular those who suffer from respiratory failure.[122] Main clinical traits include Raynaud phenomenon (98%), sclerodactyly (92%), clinically visible mat-like telangiectasias (78%), skin

TABLE 41–4. The Spectrum of Cardiac Phenotypes in Autoimmune Diseases	
Disease	**Heart involvement may include:**
Systemic sclerosis (SSc)	HF/DCM, MVR, CD, pericarditis
Rheumatoid arthritis (RA)	HF/DCM, MVR, CD, pericarditis
Systemic erythematous lupus	Accelerated atherosclerosis, DCM/myocardial fibrosis/HF
Rhupus: overlapping features of both SLE and RA	HF and pericarditis
Mixed connective tissue disease (MCTD)	Pericarditis, MVR, CD, accelerated atherosclerosis
Undifferentiated connective tissue disease (UCTD)	"Cardiomyopathy"
Sjögren's syndrome	Accelerated atherosclerosis
Vasculites	
• Polyarteritis nodosa (PAN)	Hypertension
• Granulomatosis with polyangiitis (GPA) (Wegener's)	Uncommon
• Microscopic polyangiitis (MPA)	Uncommon
Other autoimmune diseases	
Behçet's syndrome	Pericarditis, endocarditis, intracardiac thrombosis, MI, endomyocardial fibrosis
Dermatomyositis (DM) and polymyositis (PM)	Subclinical cardiac involvement; CAD
Adult Still's disease (AOSD)	Rare myocarditis
Fibromyalgia*	Heart rate variability

Note: Pericarditis, myocarditis, cardiomyopathy (DCM)/heart failure (HF), conduction disease (CD), accelerated atherosclerosis, mitral valve regurgitation (MVR)/prolapse (MVP), intracavitary thrombosis, endomyocardial fibrosis, arrhythmias, and modifications in heart rate variability (HRV). The most common autoimmune diseases are in **bold**.
*Pregabalin-related risk for edema or congestive heart failure.

involvement above the fingers (58%), lung fibrosis (35%), pulmonary hypertension (15%), and gastrointestinal tract involvement. In limited cutaneous scleroderma, fibrosis mainly affects the face, arms, and hands; patients may demonstrate Raynaud phenomenon years before the skin manifestation and may develop pulmonary hypertension (see Chapter 76).[123] In diffuse cutaneous scleroderma, fibrosis involves large cutaneous areas and internal organs, including the heart whose involvement accounts for a significant proportion of systemic sclerosis (SSc)-associated mortality.[124] When the risk of incidental HF is comparatively evaluated in clinical series of patients with autoimmune/inflammatory diseases, SS and SLE are associated with the highest risks of HF, followed by RA.[125] Cardiologists contribute to the clinical work-up, differential diagnosis, characterization of cardiac involvement, treatment of the heterogeneous clinical phenotypes, risk stratification, and decision-making in emergencies (eg, cardiac tamponade) or in chronic management of the disease. In the last decade, better awareness of the disease and early diagnoses have contributed to improve care[121] even though optimal screening for early diagnosis and treatment guidelines are lacking, in particular for very early and early diagnosis of SSc.

Epidemiology

Currently available data indicate a prevalence of SS ranging from 50 to 300 cases per 1 million persons and an incidence ranging from 2.3 to 22.8 cases per 1 million persons per year.[126] This wide range of prevalence variability reflects the diagnostic complexity of multifactorial syndromes with overlapping traits and manifestations and the different diagnostic criteria currently used to establish a precise diagnosis.[127] Classification and diagnostic criteria are a matter of continuous revision by scientific societies and experts.[123,128] Overlap syndromes, as well as silent, asymptomatic, early phases of the disease, impact the prevalence data. The female-to-male ratio ranges from 3:1 to 14:1; susceptibility to scleroderma demonstrates ethnic variations.[129]

Causes and Major Pathology Features

SS is a sporadic multifactorial disease in the majority of cases. Environmental factors and occupational risk factors have been reported in patients with scleroderma-like phenotypes.[121,130]

Less commonly, SS clusters in families where members may show either the same[131] or different autoimmune diseases.[132] In addition, positive family history is a risk factor, along with age (45–64 years), female sex, and exposure to silica.[132] These data suggest the contribution of genetic factors that could contribute with a small dose effect of multiple genes whose products are involved in innate and adaptive immunity, autoinflammation, cell signaling, extracellular matrix architecture, DNA or RNA degradation, and apoptosis or autophagy diseases.[133] Replication of genome-wide association studies independently confirmed the candidacy of many susceptibility genetic variants, including selected human leukocyte antigen (HLA) class II molecules.[134] The maternal-fetal microchimeric hypothesis may help explain the higher prevalence of SS in females. According to this hypothesis, fetal and maternal lymphocytes can cross the placenta during pregnancy and trigger a graft-versus-host-like microreaction that may culminate in scleroderma.[135] This hypothesis is further supported by the presence of allogeneic cells in peripheral blood and in skin biopsy samples obtained from patients with scleroderma,[136] and by the short interval between pregnancy and onset of the disease, in particular in the first year after delivery.[137]

Interstitial fibrosis is the main pathologic feature observed in hearts affected by scleroderma (**Fig. 41–9**). Early features are microvascular damage and mononuclear cell infiltrates. In later stages, the main pathology features are dense fibrosis of the dermis, loss of interstitial cells and vasculature, and tissue atrophy. **Table 41–5** summarizes pathologic tissue and cellular changes as well as the expression of possible markers in affected tissue and autoantibodies.

Cardiac Involvement

The heterogeneous clinical manifestations include HF, myocarditis, pericarditis, and pericardial effusion; conduction disturbances; LV systolic and diastolic dysfunction; valve

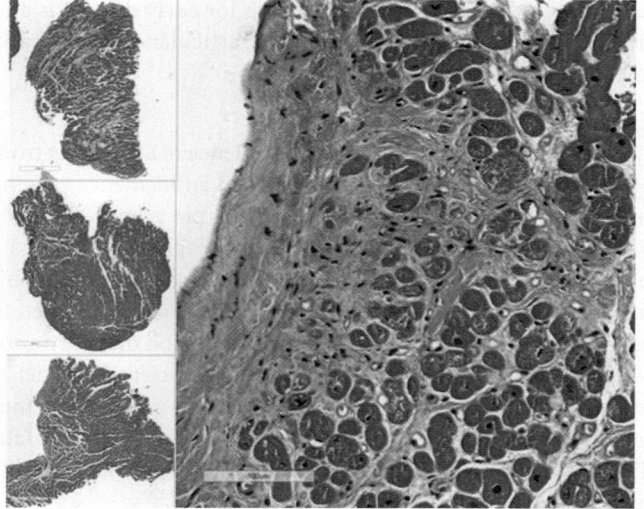

Figure 41–9. Endomyocardial biopsy in systemic sclerosis. The figure shows the endomyocardial biopsy of a 59-year-old woman diagnosed with DCM and systemic sclerosis in the same clinical occasion. The endomyocardial biopsy shows interstitial fibrosis and sparse inflammatory cells in the context of the fibrosis. There is no evidence of vasculitis or active myocarditis.

dysfunction; myocardial ischemia and coronary artery disease; and pulmonary hypertension.[138] Cardiac involvement (all manifestations) occurs in about 15% to 30% of patients with diffuse scleroderma.[139] A *dilated cardiac phenotype* (any cause) has been reported in up to 40% of patients with diffuse scleroderma.[140] However, because several potential causes may cause HF, the proportion of HF attributable to heart muscle involvement rather than to an alternative mechanism (eg, ischemic heart disease, valvular heart disease, or hypertension caused by scleroderma renal crises) is difficult to establish.[141] *Myocardial fibrosis* is common[142] and is a potential target for treatments;[143] it differs from that observed in ischemic heart disease; in fact, it does not occur in tributary areas of affected arteries, and hemosiderin deposits that are typically seen in postischemic myocardium are characteristically absent. *Low-grade inflammation* can involve either small vessels or the myocardial interstitium. In patients with newly developed cardiac manifestations, myocardial inflammation can occur, but with very low inflammatory burden. *The involvement of cardiac vessels* (capillaries, arteriolar and epicardial coronary arteries) can now be well assessed using CMR imaging and coronary angiotomography.[144] *Pericardial involvement* includes fibrinous or fibrous pericardial thickening, and focal adhesions and effusion are common; these abnormalities are often clinically silent and benign (see Chapter 76). In the majority of cases, small pericardial effusions do not cause clinical symptoms or impact prognosis.[145] Hemodynamically significant pericardial effusions can be associated with HF; a small amount of rapidly accumulating pericardial fluid in the rigid, fibrosclerotic pericardium may occasionally cause tamponade.[145] The pericardial fluid is generally noninflammatory and does not contain autoantibodies, immune complexes, or evidence of complement depletion. Histologically, the pericardium shows fibrous thickening and nonspecific inflammation. Valve disease and pulmonary artery hypertension can be part of the complex cardiac involvement in scleroderma.[138,141]

Impact of Precision Diagnosis

The increasing availability of disease- and organ-specific treatments targeting unique biologic networks and signaling pathways[123] makes a precise diagnosis imperative: DCM-like end-phenotypes may benefit from common treatments for HF. Biologic therapies can target molecules involved in the mechanisms of the immune system, such as cytokines (TNF-α, interleukin [IL]-6), immune cells (B cells), or costimulation molecules (cytotoxic T-lymphocyte–associated antigen 4 [CTLA4]), and are currently used in several autoimmune diseases. These drugs provide an alternative to the existing treatment methods of disease-modifying antirheumatic drugs and other immunosuppressive medications.[146] Therefore, confounding scleroderma DCM with genetic DCM or other DCM phenotypes prevents or limits the identification of disease-specific causes and limits potentially beneficial treatments.

Rheumatoid Arthritis

In patients diagnosed with RA, DCM accounts for about 20% of mortality.[147] Compared to the general population, patients

TABLE 41–5. Scleroderma: A Summary of Myocardial and Cellular Changes, Expression of Possible Markers in Affected Tissue and Autoantibodies

PHASE	Vascular changes: small arteriolar vessels	Fibrosis: derma and interstitial spaces	Cells showing abnormalities	Immuno-histochemistry	Autoantibodies against:
Early phase	• Loss of continuity of the endothelial layer with gaps between endothelial cells, cytoplasmic vacuolization of endothelial cells • Replication of basement lamina • Perivascular mononuclear infiltrates with rare lymphocytes • Hyperplastic small vessel disease	• Early fibrosis of the lower dermis and upper subcutaneous layer in parallel with progressive loss of small vessels • Different collagen types, proteoglycans, and elastic fibers including fibrillins	• ET cells • Pericytes • SMC • Fibroblasts	• Overexpression TGF-β • PDGF, which is linked to wound healing and fibrosis • Endothelin-1	• Topoisomerase I (Scl-70) • Centromere-associated proteins • Nucleolar antigens • Cell-surface antigens
Late phase	• Rarefaction of capillaries • Paucity of small blood vessels	Dense fibrosis with prevalence of type I collagen	Cell density decrease		

with RA still demonstrate higher mortality. In autopsy series, heart involvement was present in up to 60% of patients with RA.[147] As with other autoimmune diseases, RA hearts may show a variety of cardiovascular manifestations: DCM; pericarditis in up to 50% of cases (but hemodynamically significant pericardial effusions is uncommon, 0.5% of patients); pericardial calcifications;[148] nodular thickening and calcifications of cardiac valves;[149] and coronary atherosclerosis.[147]

Dilated Cardiomyopathy and Heart Failure
Congestive HF is a major cause of morbidity and mortality in RA patients.[150] The risk of HF remains high after adjustment for underlying coronary artery disease; in long-term follow-up studies, the burden of HF was significantly higher in RA patients than in a control population. Markers such as rheumatoid factor positivity and erythrocyte sedimentation rate, clinical traits such as extra-articular involvement, and treatments such as steroids are associated with risk of congestive HF after adjusting for coronary artery disease and risk factors, suggesting that RA is an independent risk factor for HF.[150] Diastolic dysfunction adds to systolic dysfunction in RA hearts.[151] The modification of cardiac mass in RA hearts is debated, with TTE supporting this hypothesis versus CMR studies that did not confirm an increase in cardiac mass, but rather showed lower LV volumes compared with age-matched controls.[152] The cause of diastolic dysfunction may be ascribed to the effects of inflammatory cytokines such as TNF-α, IL-1, and IL-6, all of which mediate inflammation and fibrosis; cytokine profiles seem to distinguish patients with moderate-to-severe diastolic dysfunction from those with normal heart function;[153] higher myocardial levels of citrullinated proteins compared with controls may partly account for myocardial involvement in RA.[154]

Iatrogenic Myocardial Damage Caused by Rheumatoid Arthritis Treatment
Disease-modifying drugs used to treat RA (and other connective tissue diseases) may lead to iatrogenic myocardial damage. Toxicity may result from long-term use of TNF inhibitors (TNF-I) and antimalarial agents such as hydroxychloroquine.[120,155,156]

Hydroxychloroquine toxicity manifests with either hypertrophic-restrictive cardiomyopathy or DCM and is diagnosed with endomyocardial biopsy demonstrating myelin figures and curvilinear bodies (**Fig. 41–10**) (see Chapters 44 and 76). Scintigraphy 99mTc-99mTc-DPD (3,3-diphosphono-1,2-propanodicarboxylic acid) may show myocardial uptake.[157] The role of TNF-I in causing HF is debated and can differ with different treatments (eg, abatacept, compared to etanercept, is prescribed to patients with a worse cardiovascular profile but does not seem to increase the risk of developing HF).[158]

In the most recent guidelines for treatment of RA, the Voting Panel of the American College of Rheumatology reported that recommendations are conditional because the evidence is of very low quality and noted that "there are no reports of exacerbation of HF using non-TNF biologics; the US Food and Drug Administration (FDA) warns against using TNF-I in this population-based on worsening of congestive HF with TNF-I in the Adverse Event Reporting System database. TNF-I should only be used if there are no other reasonable options, and then, perhaps, only in compensated HF"[159] (see Chapter 76).

Reactive Amyloidosis in Rheumatoid Arthritis
Reactive amyloid A deposition occurs in RA as a result of long-term, uncontrolled inflammation. The rate of pathologic detection is 21% to 30% of patients with RA, with cardiac involvement in 28%.[160] Cardiac amyloidosis causes a restrictive phenotype with myocardial wall thickening and biventricular enlargement and atrial dilation. The diagnosis is suspected by imaging and by demonstration of the involvement of other organs (renal or gastrointestinal tract, heart, spleen, liver, adrenal glands, and, less frequently, lungs, pancreas, thyroid, aorta, muscle, synovial membranes, lymph nodes, peripheral nerves, bones, and skin). The incidence of amyloidosis is likely related to the severity and duration of inflammation.

Accelerated Atherosclerosis in Rheumatoid Arthritis
Vascular heart disease may contribute to HF. Accelerated atherosclerosis is a major cause of morbidity and mortality in RA. A meta-analysis in 41,490 patients with RA from 14 studies showed a 48% increased risk of cardiovascular events

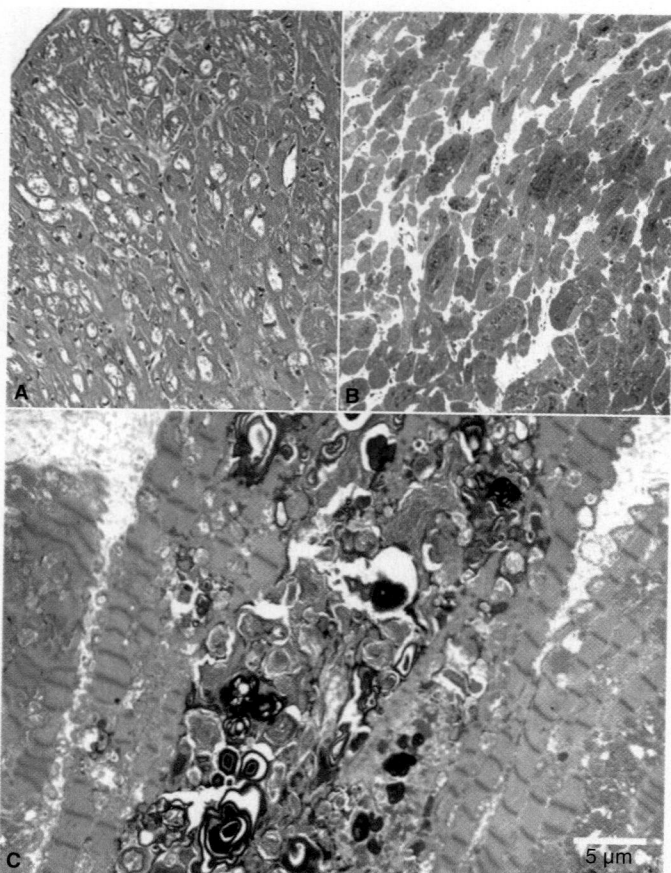

Figure 41–10. Chloroquine cardiotoxicity. The figure shows the endomyo-cardial biopsy of a female patient diagnosed with systemic sclerosis who developed hydroxychloroquine-related cardiotoxicity. (**A**) The hematoxylin and eosin stain of the endomyocardial biopsy with optically empty myo-cytes. (**B**) The toluidine blue semi-thin section shows the intramyocyte accumulation of sphingolipid bodies. (**C**) The electron micrograph shows the typical lamellar and curvilinear bodies that characterize iatrogenic intracellular accumulation of osmiophilic material. The pathologic differen-tial diagnosis in undiagnosed patients includes Anderson–Fabry disease, in which the osmiophilic bodies show a typical lamellar pattern and specifi-cally immune react with anti-GB3 antibodies.

compared with the general population.[161] Both classic risk fac-tors (diabetes, dyslipidemia, obesity, hypertension, and smok-ing) and disease-related factors, such as RA disease duration, RA positivity, and disease activity, contribute to increasing the risk of cardiovascular diseases.[161] Paradoxically, decreased lipid levels may precede the diagnosis of RA,[162] but evolve during and after treatments, when cholesterol increases in particular in treated and responder patients.[163] TNF-I increases total cho-lesterol and high-density lipoprotein levels without an equiva-lent effect on low-density lipoprotein levels;[164] statins may be required in treated patients with high low-density lipoprotein levels,[165] and discontinuation of statins in RA can increase the risk of myocardial infarction.[166]

Rheumatoid Arthritis Heart Can Display a Pancardiac Involvement

Cardiac involvement in RA can clinically manifest with car-diomyopathy, pericarditis, and valve disease, and can further be complicated by the development of reactive amyloidosis. Iatrogenic myocardial damage is proven for hydroxyl-chloroquine, but not confirmed for biologic drugs such as TNF-I, in par-ticular regarding the development of HF. Several disease-specific risk factors and effects of medications must be added to tradi-tional risk factors in the pathogenesis of accelerated coronary atherosclerosis. Cardiovascular risk seems to decrease when combined methotrexate and TNF-I achieve good control of the disease.[167]

Systemic Lupus Erythematosus

Dilated Cardiomyopathy in Systemic Lupus Erythematosus
SLE is a multiorgan autoimmune disease demonstrating higher prevalence in Black than in White individuals, and typically affects women of childbearing age.[168,169] The clinical course is characterized by cyclic evolution, with periods of quiescence alternating with periods of disease activity. The heart is com-monly involved: DCM is one of the most serious forms of organ involvement in SLE,[168,169] and LVSD is associated with poor outcomes. Nonetheless, in 2019, the consensus group of experts on SLE (the Systemic Lupus International Collaborat-ing Clinics) revised the prior American College of Rheumatol-ogy criteria[170] for SLE and established the diagnostic criteria (**Table 41–6**). Similar to prior criteria, myocardial involvement is not included in diagnostic criteria; pericarditis is listed in the context of serositis and occurs in 10% to 30% of patients.[168] Although myocardial involvement does not provide a diagnos-tic contribution, it is common in early and late phases of the disease; diastolic dysfunction is detected in 45% of patients without evidence of cardiac disease;[171] it also accounts for the majority of deaths.[172,173]

Epidemiology
Most SLE manifests between the ages of 16 and 50 years; esti-mated incidence rates in North America, South America, and Europe range from 1 to 23 per 100,000 per year.[173,174] Pediatric-onset SLE represents 10% to 20% of all SLE cases and is asso-ciated with greater disease severity than adult-onset SLE; the majority of pediatric-onset SLE patients will have developed irreversible disease manifestations within 5 to 10 years of dis-ease onset, most commonly involving the musculoskeletal, ocular, renal, and neuropsychiatric systems.[174]

Pathogenesis
The current pathogenic hypothesis integrates the effects of both environmental factors and genetic predisposition; risk factors are both SLE-specific and traditional. Women are more com-monly affected; the role of estrogens (17β-estradiol) and related receptors has been investigated. Estrogens are involved in the regulation of cellular subsets of the immune system through estrogen receptor-dependent and -independent mechanisms; estrogen receptors regulate innate immune cells and signaling pathways,[175] including all subsets of T cells and related cytok-ines,[176] and B cells, influencing B-cell differentiation, activity, function, and survival.[177]

Epigenetic factors (eg, hypomethylation of CpG sites within genes involved in different pathways) seem to be associated

TABLE 41–6. Clinical and Immunologic Criteria Used in the SLICC Classification Criteria

ENTRY CRITERION

Antinuclear antibodies (ANA) at a titer of ≥80 on Hep-2 cells or an equivalent positive test (ever)

If absent, do not classify as SLE

If present, apply additive criteria

ADDITIVE CRITERIA

Do not count a criterion if there is a more likely explanation than SLE.

Occurrence of a criterion on at least one occasion is sufficient.

SLE classification requires at least one clinical criterion and ≥ 10 points.

Criteria need not occur simultaneously.

Within each domain, only the highest weighted criterion is counted toward the total score

TOTAL SCORE

Classify as SLE with a score of 10 or more if entry criterion fulfilled.

CLINICAL DOMAINS, CRITERIA AND (WEIGHT)

CONSTITUTIONAL
Fever (2)

HEMATOLOGIC
Leukopenia (3)
Thrombocytopenia (4)
Autoimmune hemolysis (4)

NEUROPSICHYATRIC
Delirium (2)
Psychosis (3)
Seizure (3)

MUCOCUTANEOUS
Nonscarring alopecia (2)
Oral ulcers (2)
Subacute cutaneous OR discoid lupus (4)
Acute cutaneous lupus (6)

SEROSAL (CARDIOLOGY PERTINENCE)
Pleural or pericardial effusion (5)
Acute pericarditis (6)

MUSCULOSKELETAL
Joint involvement (6)

RENAL
Proteinuria >0.5g/24h (4)
Renal biopsy Class II or V lupus nephritis (8)
Renal biopsy Class III or IV lupus nephritis (10)

IMMUNOLOGY DOMAINS, CRITERIA AND (WEIGHT)

ANTIPHOSPHOLIPID ANTIBODIES
OR
Anti-cardiolipin antibodies (2) OR
Anti-b2GP1 antibodies (2)
Lupus anticoagulant (2)

COMPLEMENT PROTEINS
Low C3 or Low C4 (3)
Low C3 and Low C4 (4)

SLE-SPECIFIC ANTIBODIES
Anti-dsDNA antibody (6)
OR
Anti-Smith antibody (6)

Note: Only pericardial involvement is included in the diagnostic criteria but with high weight (either 5 or 6). Therefore, patients with entry ANA criterion, acute pericarditis, fever, and any other criterion theoretically fulfill diagnostic criteria for SLE.

with increased production of autoantibodies (anti-dsDNA, anti-SSA, anti-Sm, and anti-RNP antibodies)[178] and also influence endothelial-inflammatory cell interactions and inflammatory responses. Among susceptibility alleles identified with genome-wide association studies, *NCF2*, encoding a core component of the multiprotein NADPH oxidase, confers susceptibility to SLE in individuals of European ancestry;[179] *HLA-DRB1*15-DQB1*06* haplotype has recently been proposed as the greatest risk factor for the development of disease in certain ethnic groups. In a recent meta-analysis, the *HLA-G* 14-base pair insertion/deletion polymorphism was associated with susceptibility to a subgroup of autoimmune diseases such as SLE, but not RA.[180] Additional genes/loci have been assigned to SLE: *PTPN22, FCGR2A, FCGR2B, CTLA4, TEX1,* and *DNAS1* are all included in the Mendelian Inheritance in Man (MIM) catalog as associated with increased susceptibility to SLE. However, at present, there is no evidence supporting a Mendelian inheritance of SLE, which thus remains a potential multifactorial autoimmune disorder.

Myocardial Involvement

Heart and vessels are commonly involved in SLE. The major pathology features include HF, accelerated atherosclerosis, myocardial fibrosis.

DCM/HF is common in patients with SLE; although the causes can be related to either systemic (cytokine burden) or local inflammation.[181] The contribution of accelerated atherosclerosis is not easy to dissect from local damage potentially induced by chronic inflammation. However, SLE patients with cardiomyopathy have a prognosis similar to those with idiopathic DCM.

Accelerated atherosclerosis[182] is not explained by traditional risk factors but likely promoted by systemic inflammation.[183] Traditional risk factors (eg, diabetes, hypertension, hyperlipidemia) are common in young SLE patients, often as a side effect of immunosuppressant therapy.[184] SLE-related risk factors include the presence of autoantibodies, such as antiphospholipid antibodies, anticardiolipin antibodies, and lupus anticoagulant,[184] which are produced in 30% to 40% of SLE patients. These antibodies do not fully explain the increased thrombotic risk in SLE; in fact, published data show that only 10% of "positive" patients experience a thrombotic event, and 40% of SLE thrombosis cases are in patients without such antibodies.[185] Treatment-related risk includes the effects of both corticosteroids and immunosuppressant drugs. Risk stratification and modification for cardiovascular events should, therefore, be tailored on individual risk profiles, based on modifiable risk factors and SLE-specific risk factors. Atherosclerosis is associated with increased risk of cardiac, cerebral, or peripheral arterial ischemic events and mortality; in a systematic review and meta-analysis including 17,187 patients from 32 studies, the incidence of cardiovascular events was almost 25%, and 4.5% of the patients had an acute myocardial infarction.[184] Although early subclinical atherosclerosis can manifest as intima-media thickening of carotid arteries, recent studies demonstrated that atherosclerotic plaque lesions can be found frequently in the absence of intima-media thickening in both SLE and

SS patients; sonography of carotid and femoral arteries may identify additional atherosclerotic lesions and detect patients at high risk for cardiovascular events.[186] Coronary contrast enhancement by CMR may detect subclinical disease in the coronary vessel wall, thus providing a novel direct marker of vessel wall disease.[187] Considering that traditional Framingham cardiovascular risk factors do not fully explain the excess of the risk of coronary artery disease in SLE,[182] it is likely that inflammatory and autoimmune mechanisms interact with genetic, environmental, and treatment-related factors.

Myocardial fibrosis represents a significant independent predictor of adverse cardiac outcomes in both ischemic and non-ischemic cardiomyopathies.[188] Recent CMR studies confirmed that mid-wall myocardial fibrosis is frequent in SLE and is associated with age, but not with disease duration or severity; in addition, late gadolinium enhancement comprising >15% of LV mass may be associated with diastolic dysfunction and impaired exercise capacity.[189] The European League Against Rheumatism recommends baseline cardiovascular evaluation and regular, a yearly cardiovascular follow-up to assess common risk factors, vascular events (cerebral/cardiovascular), physical activity, oral contraceptives, hormonal therapies, and family history of cardiovascular disease; to perform blood tests, including blood cholesterol and glucose; and to measure blood pressure and body mass index (and/or waist circumference).[190]

PERIPARTUM CARDIOMYOPATHY

Definition

In the workshop held by the National Heart, Lung, and Blood Institute and the Office of Rare Diseases (2000), PPCM was defined as a "rare life-threatening cardiomyopathy of unknown cause that occurs in the peripartum period in previously healthy women: diagnosis is confined to a narrow period and requires echocardiographic evidence of LV systolic dysfunction."[191] According to the ESC, PPCM is defined as "idiopathic cardiomyopathy presenting with HF secondary to LV systolic dysfunction towards the end of pregnancy or in the months following delivery, where no other cause of HF is found. It is a diagnosis of exclusion"[192] (see also Chapter 51). The LV may not be dilated, but the EF is nearly always reduced below 45%.[192] Both definitions share the following concepts: (1) idiopathic condition (no detectable cause of HF); (2) temporal appearance (the last month of pregnancy or during the first 5 months postpartum according to the National Heart, Lung, and Blood Institute and the Office of Rare Diseases and toward the end of pregnancy or in the months following delivery according to ESC); (3) the absence of preexisting known heart disease; and (4) the presence of LV dysfunction. Therefore, the precise clinical diagnosis of PPCM should be based on these criteria. A further condition that could confirm the diagnosis is the regression of PPCM within 12 months after delivery.[192]

Incidence

PPCM is estimated to occur in 0.1% of all pregnancies. The prevalence of PPCM ranges between 1:4000 and 1:1000 live births in the Western world.[193,194] Approximately 75% of cases are diagnosed within the first month after delivery, and 45% occur in the first week. Regional variation is wide: 1 case per 20,000 live births in Japan; 1 case per 1000 live births in South Africa; 1 case per 40,322 in China; and 1 case per 300 live births in Haiti.[194] A high prevalence in Nigeria is likely caused by the tradition of ingesting kunun kanwa (dried lake salt) while lying on heated mud beds twice a day for 40 days postpartum to stimulate breast milk production. This variable prevalence suggests that regional and cultural factors influence the risk of PPCM.

Risk Factors

Risk factors for PPCM include age (>30 years), multiparity, African race, obesity, substance use, preeclampsia, and chronic hypertension.[195,196] It is unclear whether race is an independent risk factor or whether the increased risk of PPCM results from the interaction of race with hypertension. Factors such as poor nutrition and lack of prenatal care are included in the list of risk factors but are unconfirmed. Climate may also contribute: PPCM seems to be more common in tropical regions with increased heat and humidity.

Etiologic Hypotheses

Etiologic hypotheses include familial/genetic predisposition, maladaptive response to hemodynamic stresses of pregnancy, viral myocarditis, stress-activated cytokines, malnutrition and selenium deficiency, fetal micro-chimerism, prolactin, and prolonged tocolysis[197] (**Fig. 41–11**).

Genetic Hypothesis

In a recent study including 172 women (one-third of African descent) with PPCM versus 332 patients with DCM, sequencing of 43 DCM genes identified 26 heterozygous truncating variants in 8 genes (17 mutations were identified in the *TTN* gene). The prevalence of truncation-predicting variants in PPCM (15%) was similar to that in DCM (17%) and significantly higher than in the reference population (4.7%); 65% of the truncating variants were in the *TTN* gene.[198] This study may have relevant implications for both PPCM and genetic DCM; in fact, *TTN* mutations have been reported in 25% of FDCM and in 18% of nonfamilial, sporadic DCM.[41] The persistence of the DCM phenotype in one-fifth of patients suggests the pathogenic role of the *TTN* mutation and implies that one-fifth of cases of PPCM are actually genetic DCM unmasked by pregnancy.[41] Conversely, if the phenotype regresses after pregnancy among women with mutated PPCM, the role of *TTN* variants could be questioned not only in PPCM but also in DCM associated with the same variants. At present, it appears prudent then to consider a genetic predisposition to PPCM rather than a genetic cause.

Abnormal Hemodynamic Response

During pregnancy, in particular in the last trimester, blood volume and cardiac output increase while afterload decreases because of relaxation of vascular smooth muscle cells; LV mass and arterial compliance also increase, whereas total vascular resistance decreases.[199] The consequent functional and transient LV "hypertrophy" aims at meeting fetal and maternal

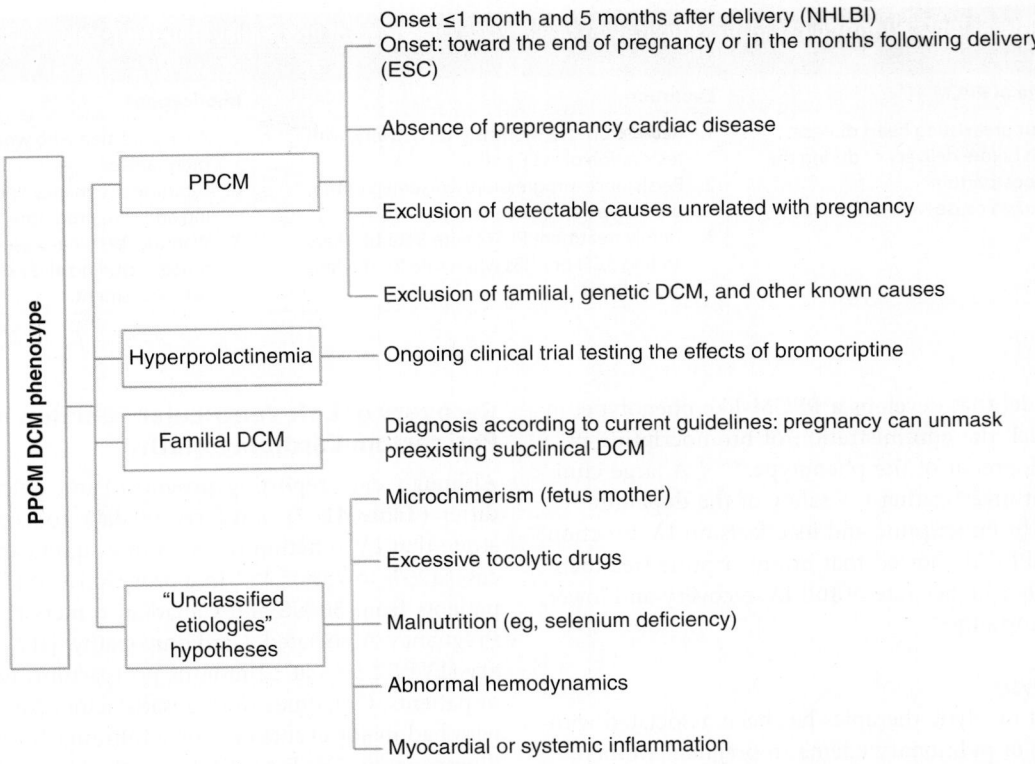

Figure 41–11. Pathogenesis of PPCM. The figure summarizes key diagnostic criteria and pathogenetic hypothesis in PPCM. DCM, dilated cardiomyopathy; ESC, European Society of Cardiology; NHLBI, National Heart, Lung, and Blood Institute.

demands. In normal pregnancies, this transient LV functional and structural remodeling regresses shortly after birth.[199] Although PPCM might, in part, be a result of an exaggerated decrease in LV function when these hemodynamic changes of pregnancy occur, this hypothesis is unlikely to explain, by itself, PPCM.

Viral Myocarditis and Systemic Inflammation

Previous studies proposed viral myocarditis as the main mechanism for PPCM. This hypothesis remains unconfirmed. Clinical outcomes do not seem to differ in women with and without clinically diagnosed myocarditis. Increased levels of plasma inflammatory, apoptosis mediators, and cytokines measured in women with PPCM do not correlate with LV function or outcomes. LVEF at the time of initial diagnosis remains the strongest predictor of outcome.[200]

Malnutrition and Selenium Deficiency

Deficiencies in selenium and other nutrients have also been advocated as causes of PPCM.[201] Selenium deficiency (serum selenium concentration <70 μg/L) is a well-known cause of DCM and of increased susceptibility to viral infections, hypertension, and hypocalcemia.[202] Selenium deficiency is a risk factor for PPCM in Kano, Nigeria, and seems to be related to rural residency.[202]

Fetal Microchimerism

During pregnancy, the trafficking of circulating cells generates bidirectional microchimerism (ie, fetus to mother and vice versa). Cell trafficking from fetus to the mother starts very early; the numbers of fetal cells increase in the maternal circulation in pregnancies affected by preeclampsia and before the onset of preeclampsia symptoms.[203] Adult women may bear chimeric blood cells from multiple sources.[204] For instance, microchimerism is one of the factors advocated in the pathogenesis of autoimmune diseases, which are more common in females than in males. The small shared epitopic-mimetic compound QKRAA has been proposed as a contributor to the pathogenesis of RA by acting as a ligand that activates proarthritogenic signal transduction events.[205] Women who lack RA susceptibility HLA alleles encoding the small QKRAA epitope can acquire RA susceptibility alleles from microchimerism, thus increasing their risk of RA.[206]

Prolactin

Prolactin is one of the key candidates in the pathophysiology of PPCM. Increased levels of prolactin in pregnancy are associated with increased blood volume and levels of circulating erythropoietin and hematocrit and decreased blood pressure, angiotensin responsiveness, and levels of water, sodium, and potassium. In the last trimester of pregnancy, oxidative stress is enhanced; under defective antioxidative mechanisms, prolactin is increasingly cleaved into a 16-kDa fragment (16-kDa prolactin). This fragment may induce microvascular damage, leading to cardiac injury and dysfunction. The dopamine D_2 receptor agonist bromocriptine inhibits prolactin release and may represent a therapeutic option. This hypothesis was tested

TABLE 41–7. Criteria for Diagnosing PPCM and Implication of a Precise Diagnosis of Pregnancy-Related Transient DCM versus Persistent DCM

Diagnostic Criteria of PPCM	Evolution	Implications
1. Women without preexisting heart disease 2. Onset: 1 month before delivery or during the first 5 months postpartum 3. Exclusion of known causes and of familial, genetic DCM 4. LV dysfunction	1. Regression ≤12 months after delivery, with restoration of LVEF ≥50% 2. Persistence, progression/worsening of the phenotype after pregnancy 3. Timely treatment PPCM with Beta-blockers adding ACEI or ARBs when safe for the fetus (guidelines)	1. Advise women who would have new pregnancies 2. Establish pregnancy-specific monitoring and care programs 3. Warning: better assessed risk of recurrence, including all available tools for risk assessment.

in a murine model that develops a PPCM-like phenotype; in this mouse model, the administration of bromocriptine prevented the development of the phenotype.[207,208] A large clinical trial aimed at investigating the safety of the dopamine D_2 receptor agonist bromocriptine and its effects on LV function in women with PPCM showed that bromocriptine treatment is associated with a higher rate of full LV-recovery and lower morbidity and mortality.[209]

Prolonged Tocolysis

Prolonged use of tocolytic therapies has been associated with the development of pulmonary edema in pregnant women;[210] based on this observation, chronic use of β-sympathomimetic medications was linked with PPCM. Prolonged tocolysis refers to the use of β-sympathomimetic drugs for more than 4 weeks. Although these agents are used for the management of various other conditions, the association between tocolytic therapies and HF appears to be unique to pregnancy.

Diagnostic Work-Up and Management

Echocardiography is the first-line imaging test.[211] Ideally, baseline data should be available and demonstrate normal baseline LV size and function. Such baseline data, however, are rarely available because echocardiography is not indicated routinely in pregnancy and the later development of PPCM is unpredictable. However, early diagnosis is possible, and when treated in the early phases, LV SD may normalize in a high percentage of cases.[192] The increasing awareness of PPCM is contributing to earlier diagnosis and better management and outcomes. A major limitation is the absence of baseline echocardiographic evaluation in women who develop PPCM. However, the combined treatment with β-blockers plus angiotensin-converting enzyme (ACE) inhibitors or angiotensin receptor blockers (ARBs) is now recommended (class I) by the AHA and ESC Guidelines[18,212] for treatment of HF with reduced LVEF after delivery. ACE inhibitors and ARBs are highly teratogenic and should be avoided during pregnancy.[213] After delivery, PPCM should be treated in accordance with the current ESC guidelines for HF. During pregnancy, treatment options include hydralazine, long-acting nitrates, and $β_1$-selective β-blockers; diuretics (furosemide and hydrochlorothiazide) should be used sparingly because they can cause decreased placental blood flow[192] (see Chapters 51 and 78).

Recovery of Left Ventricular Function in Peripartum Cardiomyopathy

Although data reporting prognosis and outcome in PPCM differ (**Table 41–7**), most recent data concordantly demonstrate that LV function recovers in a significant percentage of cases (23% to 78%).[214-216] In a prospective study including 100 patients from 30 US and Canadian centers (Investigations of Pregnancy-Associated Cardiomyopathy [IPAC]), full recovery (LVEF ≥50% at 12 months postpartum) occurred in 72% of patients. Outcomes were unsatisfactory for 13% of women, who had major events or evolved through severe chronic cardiomyopathy (LVEF <35%) during the 1-year observation time after delivery. Women of African heritage had more frequent hypertension (preeclampsia, gestational, and chronic) and a later PPCM diagnosis.[217] The most impressive data are from the German PPCM registry, with improvement in 85% of patients; the highest percentage of recovery (96%) was observed in patients treated with bromocriptine, β-blockers, and ACE inhibitors/ARBs, albeit full recovery with an EF >55% was present in only 47% of patients.[218] Event-free survival was significantly worse for women with a baseline LVEF <30% compared with those with LVEF >30% (1-year event-free survival rate, 82% vs 99%; P <0.004) (**Fig. 41–12**).[218] Results recorded in the IPAC registry in women who did not receive bromocriptine were comparable with those reported by German investigators in PPCM patients who received bromocriptine in addition to standard evidence-based treatment.[218]

ALCOHOLIC HEART DISEASE

Introduction

Light-to-moderate alcohol intake is beneficial for cardiovascular health,[219] whereas habitual heavy alcohol consumption is associated with increased risk of LV dilatation and dysfunction (alcoholic cardiomyopathy [A-CMP]),[220] arrhythmias,[220,221] systemic hypertension,[222] ischemic heart disease,[223] stroke,[224] and skeletal muscle abnormalities.[225] Heavy alcohol consumption corresponds to daily ingestion of at least three standard-size drinks or alcohol consumption over 80 g; light-to-moderate alcohol intake corresponds to less than three standard-sized drinks or <80 g/d. Because standard-sized portions of wine, liquor, or beer contain approximately the same amount of alcohol, the daily amount of ethanol is usually measured per number of standard drinks.[220,221]

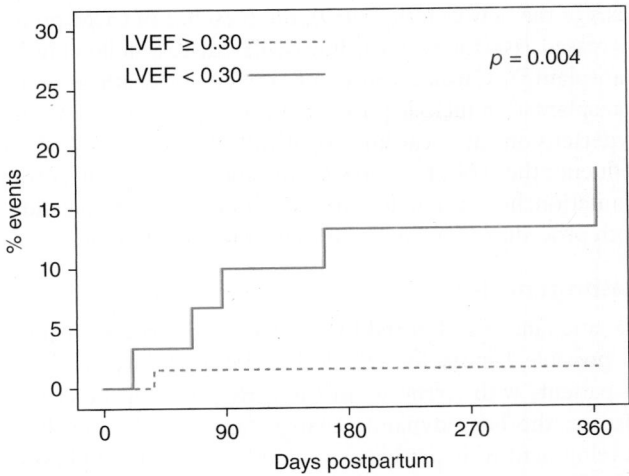

Figure 41–12. Severe impaired LV function influences prognosis in PPCM. Event-free survival is significantly worse in women with PPCM with a baseline LVEF <30% compared with those with an LVEF >30%. Reproduced with permission from McNamara DM, Elkayam U, Alharethi R, et al. Clinical outcomes for peripartum cardiomyopathy in North America: results of the Investigations of Pregnancy Associated Cardiomyopathy (IPAC) study. *J Am Coll Cardiol.* 2015 Aug 25;66(8):905-914.

Alcoholic Cardiomyopathy

A-CMP clinically manifests with DCM phenotype; it is considered a specific disease by both the ESC and AHA.[1,2] In the ESC consensus document on the classification of cardiomyopathies, A-CMP is included among the acquired forms of DCM.[2] Thiamine deficiency (beriberi) is no longer confused with A-CMP; the former fully responds to thiamine administration, whereas the latter does not.[220]

Among alcoholics, the prevalence of DCM is higher in women than in men. An excessive ethanol intake is reported in 3% to 40% of patients with DCM.[226] The three criteria for diagnosing A-CMP include DCM phenotype, absence of other known and detectable causes of DCM, and a long history of heavy alcohol intake. The toxic effect is expected for daily alcohol consumption over 80 g (three or more standard-sized drinks per day) lasting 5 years or more before the onset or diagnosis.[226,227] The symptoms correspond to those of DCM, with patients presenting with HF as a result of reduced cardiac output and atrial and/or ventricular arrhythmias. The LV function ameliorates with either abstinence or reduction of the daily intake of alcohol.[220,226,227] There are no specific guidelines for the treatment of A-CMP; current management should include complete alcohol abstinence and therapies recommended to treat HF as a result of other causes (see Chapter 49).

Mechanisms

The toxic damage of ethanol is attributed to a nonoxidative metabolic pathway for alcohol-related to fatty acid metabolism in the heart, skeletal muscle, pancreas, and brain.[220] Factors that have been involved in the pathogenic mechanisms of A-CMP include apoptosis, abnormal excitation–contraction coupling, functional and structural mitochondrial damage, loss of contractile filaments, deregulation of protein synthesis, ATPase, L-type calcium channels, and activation of the renin-angiotensin and sympathetic nervous systems.[220,221] None of these factors and mechanisms has been confirmed, and they may all contribute. However, alcohol-induced mitochondria toxicity ends in mitochondrial dysfunction, loss of mitochondrial membrane potential, and increase in mitochondrial oxidative stress, eventually culminating in cell death.[221,228] Nonselective mitochondrial damage could link oxidative stress, apoptosis, and mitochondrial loss, and explain the multiorgan damage in those with alcohol use disorders.[228] Recent experimental studies showed that chronic plus binge ethanol feeding in mice causes alcohol-induced cardiomyopathies characterized by increased myocardial oxidative/nitrative stress, impaired mitochondrial function and biogenesis, and enhanced cardiac steatosis.[229]

Genetic predisposition could play a role in the pathogenesis, with a predominant burden of 9.9% TTNtv in patients with alcoholic cardiomyopathy. According to these data, 1 of 10 patients with A-CMP could carry a TTNtv, evidence supporting the indication to genetic testing in these patients. However, the presence of TTNtvs does not seem to predict phenotype, outcome, or functional recovery.[230]

Prognosis

Current knowledge regarding A-CMP is mostly based on historical studies; data on prognosis using contemporary HF pharmacologic agents are not available. Alcohol withdrawal is associated with A-CMP regression in 40% to 50% of cases, but not in all of them, suggesting that factors other than alcohol abuse may contribute to the natural history of the disease.[220] A-CMP seems to have a better prognosis than idiopathic DCM; during a median follow-up of 59 months (interquartile range, 25–107 months), 94 consecutive patients with A-CMP demonstrated higher transplantation-free survival than 188 patients with nonalcoholic DCM. During follow-up, 63% of patients reported remaining abstinent, 32% continued alcohol consumption but had reduced intake to <80 g/d, and only 5% were persistent or heavy alcohol drinkers (>80 g/d). Atrial fibrillation, QRS width >120 ms, and the absence of β-blocker therapy identify patients with a poor outcome. A-CMP patients who reduced their alcohol intake to moderate levels exhibited similar survival ($P = 0.22$) and cardiac function recovery ($P = 0.8$) as abstainers.[221]

CIRRHOTIC CARDIOMYOPATHY

Definition and Impact of Diagnosis

Patients with cirrhosis frequently demonstrate hyperdynamic circulation and increased cardiac output, decreased systemic vascular resistance, and increased compliance of the arterial vessels. This combination of hemodynamic conditions corresponds to latent left HF where any stressor may clinically unmask the LV dysfunction.[231,232] According to the 2005 World Congress of Gastroenterology, cirrhotic cardiomyopathy (CCM) is defined by "chronic cardiac dysfunction in patients with cirrhosis characterized by impaired contractile responsiveness to stress and/or altered diastolic relaxation with electrophysiological abnormalities in the absence of other known cardiac disease."[232] The impaired diastolic relaxation is more common in early phases, whereas systolic dysfunction and LV dilation are manifest in advanced phases; electrophysiologic abnormalities include prolongation of QT interval in more than 50% of cases, electromechanical dyssynchrony, and chronotropic and/or inotropic incompetence[231,233] (Table 41–8). The 2005 criteria have been recently redefined including contemporary cardiovascular imaging parameters with aim of improving clinical outcomes, particularly surrounding liver transplantation.[234] In fact, cardiac evaluation is increasingly relevant for patients who are candidates for liver transplantation and/or transjugular intrahepatic portosystemic shunt (TIPS) implantation. TIPS decompression of the portal hypertension increases the preload to the heart, pulmonary artery pressure, and systemic vascular resistances, thus lowering afterload. Recent data show that TIPS placement successfully resolves not only hepatic encephalopathy but also refractory right HF in most patients.[235] In the complex pathophysiology of cirrhosis-related cardiac and hemodynamic changes, diastolic dysfunction seems to predict death after TIPS implantation.[236]

In addition, pretransplant diastolic dysfunction predisposes patients with hepatic cirrhosis to posttransplant adverse cardiac events.[237] Of 107 patients who received liver transplantation, 24% developed HF in association with diastolic dysfunction prior to liver transplantation, and diastolic dysfunction was a predictor of a poor prognosis.[238] Even when diagnosed on the basis of the new criteria (2019), the presence of CCM predicts increased risk for new cardiovascular disease following liver transplant.[238] Cardiac causes of immediate death after liver transplantation include postreperfusion syndrome, pulmonary hypertension, and cardiomyopathy.[240] Therefore, CCM may influence the evolution of post-TIPS and orthotopic liver transplantation; however, it does not constitute a contraindication to both procedures, in particular to liver transplantation.[241]

Pathogenesis

Hepatic failure and portal hypertension have been considered as possible factors for the development of cardiac changes in patients with cirrhosis. In the early phase of the cirrhotic disease, the hemodynamic changes are compensated by the development of hyperdynamic circulation. In later phases, as splanchnic arterial vasodilation progresses, effective arterial blood volume declines, and there is subsequent activation of the renin-angiotensin-aldosterone system and development of LV dilation and dysfunction. Factors involved in the development of cardiac impairment include inflammation mediated by intestinal bacterial translocation,[242] cytokines that can influence both LV remodeling and function, and the negative inotropic effects of nitric oxide, carbon monoxide, and endogenous cannabinoids.[243] The accumulation of toxic chemicals such as bile acids seems to adversely affect the myocardial function; the major mechanisms of bile acid cytotoxicity are oxidative stress and mitochondrial impairment whose effects could be mitigated by the administration of taurine.[244]

TABLE 41–8. Summary of Morphofunctional Imaging-Based, Electrophysiologic, Electromechanical, and Biochemical Criteria for Cirrhotic Cardiomyopathy

Systolic Dysfunction		Diastolic Dysfunction		Other Criteria	
2005	2019	2005	2019	2005	2019
Any of the following: -Rest LVEF <55% -Systolic dysfunction unmasked during pharmacological or physiological stress (eg, failure of LVEF to increase on stress testing by >5%)	Any of the following: -LVEF ≤50% -Absolute° global longitudinal strain (GLS) <18	Any of the following: -E/A ratio <1.0 (corrected by age) -Prolonged deceleration time (>200 ms) -Prolonged isovolumetric relaxation time (>80 ms)	Advanced diastolic dysfunction: -E/e' ratio ≥15* - LA volume index >34 mL/m² -Septal e' velocity <7 cm/second -TR velocity > 2.8 m/second (In the absence of primary pulmonary hypertension or portopulmonary hypertension)	-Tricuspid valve regurgitation -LA dilation -Increased cardiac mass -Electrophysiological abnormalities - QT interval prolongation - Abnormal chronotropic response -Electromechanical criteria -Ventricular dyssynchrony -Increased natriuretic peptides -Increased hs-TnT -Soluble urokinase-type plasminogen activator receptor (suPAR) -High-sensitive C-reactive protein MR myocardial stress testing	-Chamber enlargement -Abnormal chronotropic or inotropic response -Electrocardiographic changes -Electromechanical uncoupling -Myocardial mass change -Serum biomarkers -CMRI (Myocardial extracellular volume as a surrogate for myocardial fibrosis can be assessed using this modality)

*Only medial annulus velocity is recommended. After applying the modified criteria, filling pressure is first assessed, then diastolic function is graded based on E/A ratio.
°according to criteria established by the American Society of Echocardiography (ASE) and the European Association of Cardiovascular Imaging (EACVI) guidelines.
First Established by World Congress of Gastroenterology Criteria (2005) and Later Refined in Criteria Proposed by the Cirrhotic Cardiomyopathy Consortium (2019).

Diagnosis and Imaging

Cardiac evaluation of patients with cirrhosis requires special attention to clinically latent signs of HF, because it may influence candidacy for TIPS or liver transplantation. The presence of diastolic dysfunction should be recognized before liver transplant because it may be associated with intraoperative complications and may complicate the early postoperative course.[245] Latent cardiac dysfunction, defined by abnormal stroke volume response to unclamping of the portal vein, is common in liver transplant recipients.[246] Preoperative low systemic vascular resistance and LA dilation are independent predictors of inadequate responses.[246] All cardiac imaging modalities contributing to better characterize diastolic dysfunction should be integrated to provide the best assessment of diastolic dysfunction; echocardiography with TDI is the most common method to detect and monitor diastolic dysfunction. A few studies have applied CMR and contrast-enhanced CMR as well as cardiac CT with coronary artery calcification scoring. More studies are needed to establish the clinical contribution of both CMR and CT in patients with CCM.[247] Tests with either physiologically or pharmacologically induced circulatory stress are useful to assess systolic dysfunction; echocardiography with TDI is the most common method to detect diastolic dysfunction (E/A and E/E′ ratio). Strain techniques can offer incremental information. The impaired cardiac pharmacologic response to stress can be additionally investigated with magnetic resonance myocardial stress testing; deformation parameters may be more sensitive in identifying abnormalities in inotropic response to stress than are conventional methods.[248] CCM is, therefore, assuming an increasing relevance considering the negative impact that an unrecognized CCM may have during and after liver transplantation. An early diagnosis of CCM with pretransplant treatment of HF may prevent an acute onset or worsening of cardiac failure after liver transplantation.[249] Pretransplant treatment of HF may improve quality of life before transplantation and reduce perioperative complications after liver transplantation.

TRANSIENT AND REVERSIBLE DILATED CARDIOMYOPATHY

Different types of DCM that have been variably included in past classifications of cardiomyopathies are potentially reversible. In future nosologies of cardiomyopathies, these entities should probably be separated from cardiomyopathies and be part of a disease-specific classification. Apart from PPCM, A-CMP, and CCM, other DCMs that potentially reverse when the cause is controlled and treated are tachycardia-induced cardiomyopathies, premature ventricular contraction (PVC)–induced cardiomyopathy, Takotsubo cardiomyopathy, metabolic cardiomyopathies (both endocrine and nutritional), cardiomyopathies complicating end-stage chronic diseases such as renal failure (uremic cardiomyopathy revised in Chapter 75), and inflammatory and infectious cardiomyopathy. The existence of an independent "obesity cardiomyopathy" characterized by systolic dysfunction fulfilling criterion for the diagnosis of DCM is debated; recent studies highlight the role of obesity as an independent risk factor for the development of HF, but obesity-related HF is thought to be multifactorial.[250]

Arrhythmia-Induced Cardiomyopathy

Tachycardia-induced cardiomyopathy is caused by persistent tachycardia that induces increased ventricular filling pressures, severe biventricular systolic dysfunction, reduced cardiac output, and increased systemic vascular resistance. Arrhythmias include atrial fibrillation, atrial flutter, atrial tachycardia, reentrant supraventricular tachycardia, accessory pathway tachycardia, frequent ectopic beats, and ventricular tachycardia; sustained rates above 115 or 120 bpm may be an important prognostic factor.[251] Sinus tachycardia has also been reported as a cause of cardiomyopathy.[252,253] The diagnosis is based on the absence of other causes of nonischemic cardiomyopathy (eg, hypertension, alcohol or drug use, stress) and on the absence of LV hypertrophy and relatively normal LV diameter (LV end-diastolic dimension <5.5 cm). The recovery of LV function after control of tachycardia (by rate control, cardioversion, or radiofrequency ablation) within 1 to 6 months confirms the diagnosis.[254–256]

Premature Ventricular Contraction–Induced Cardiomyopathy

PVC-induced cardiomyopathy is characterized by LV dilation and/or dysfunction, diastolic dysfunction, and reduced ventricular strain by speckle tracking imaging.[257,258] A dose-response relation has been demonstrated in serial evaluations of LV function among 239 consecutive patients with frequent PVCs and no obvious cardiac disease; >20,000 PVCs per 24 hours were associated with subclinical deterioration in LVEF, whereas >10,000 PVCs per 24 hours showed LV dilation without a change in LVEF.[259] An increasing PVC burden was associated with adverse outcomes in 1139 healthy participants of the Cardiovascular Health Study (≥65 years) with an initial normal LVEF and no history of congestive HF who underwent 24-hour Holter monitoring. Over a median follow-up of >13 years, a PVC burden in the upper quartile was associated with a 3-fold greater odds of a decrease in LVEF, a 48% increased risk of incident congestive HF, and a 31% increased risk of death, compared with the lower quartile.[260] PVC-induced cardiomyopathy appears reversible, with a reduction in ectopy burden. Rapid normalization of LV parameters follows successful radiofrequency ablation of the PVC focus.[261-262] After successful ablation, the rates of improvement in LVEF have varied between 47.1% and 100%.[261,262] Randomized trials are ongoing, aimed at assessing whether therapy for frequent PVCs in patients with idiopathic LV dysfunction modifies clinical outcomes. The Early Elimination of Premature Ventricular Contractions in Heart Failure study (ClinicalTrials.gov identifier: NCT01757067) is testing the effects of ablation versus medical therapy; the Reversal of Cardiomyopathy by Suppression of Frequent Premature Ventricular Complexes study (NCT01566344) is testing conventional HF therapy and PVC suppression therapy (ablation or amiodarone if unsuccessful ablation) versus HF therapy alone. In children, the proportion of PVC-induced cardiomyopathy seems higher than previously expected especially because ectopy tends to persist throughout follow-up. The possibility of radiofrequency ablation of the ectopic ventricular focus could be considered in children who manifest LV ventricular dilation or dysfunction.[263] The pathophysiology of PVC-induced cardiomyopathy remains unknown, and the optimal management of these patients is not yet established.

The Left Apical Ballooning Syndrome

The left apical ballooning syndrome, or Takotsubo cardiomyopathy, is a transient hypocontractility of the mid and apical segments of the LV associated with hyperkinesis of the basal walls. This mismatched contractility causes a balloon-like appearance of the distal ventricular walls in systole. The phenomenon may mimic acute coronary syndrome in the absence of coronary artery disease or spasm (see Chapter 20).[264] The transient dysfunction is most prevalent in older women exposed to emotional or physical stressors. The disease can manifest with atypical phenotypes such as reversed and RV Takotsubo and global hypokinesis.[265,266] Biomarkers include increased levels of circulating catecholamines, especially epinephrine. Takotsubo cardiomyopathy may not follow obvious physical or emotional stress; in addition, it may carry significant early and late serious complication risks. It can occur concomitantly in the presence of subcritical coronary artery disease; patients often demonstrate cardiovascular risk factors and associated comorbidities.[266] Primary Takotsubo cardiomyopathy is frequently related to emotional stress, is largely reversible, and carries a benign prognosis; in contrast, secondary forms are associated with acute potentially severe conditions and may result in a higher event rate.[267] Although included in the cardiomyopathy classification, they do not share the chronic morphologic LV abnormalities and remodeling that characterize DCM.

Metabolic Cardiomyopathies

Metabolic cardiomyopathies are secondary to effects of primary noncardiac defects of energy production leading to impaired cardiac function. They may be caused by several different endocrine diseases and nutritional deprivations. Endocrine cardiomyopathies include growth hormone (GH) excess and GH deficiency and thyroid hypo- and hyperfunction.[268-272]

Excess or Deficiency in Growth Hormone and/or Insulin-Like Growth Factor 1

Excess or deficiency in GH and/or insulin-like growth factor-1 (IGF-1) is deleterious for the cardiovascular system. Acromegaly is an endocrine disease with specific somatic changes caused by an excess of GH; in the majority of cases, the cause is a pituitary tumor producing GH. Chronic GH and IGF-1 excess cause cardiomyopathy that is characterized by early concentric cardiac hypertrophy associated with diastolic dysfunction and by later evolution to systolic dysfunction.[268,273]

The control of GH/IGF-1 excess is accompanied by a decrease in cardiac mass and improvement of cardiac function.[269] In

patients with hypopituitarism, either childhood-onset or adulthood onset, GH deficiency is characterized by a decrease of cardiac mass and impairment of systolic function; other effects include increased cardiovascular risk with changes in body composition, unfavorable lipid profile, insulin resistance, endothelial dysfunction, and atherosclerosis.[269,274]

In patients with GH deficiency, the administration of recombinant GH is followed by an increase in cardiac mass, improvement in cardiac performance, and improvement of the cardiovascular risk factor profile.[269,270] In 51 patients (29 females), 45.9 ± 11.3 years (mean ± standard deviation), median follow-up 36.2 months, the long-term administration of GH-R of GH deficiency (GHD) positively affected interventricular septum diameter and LV posterior wall end diastole. In a subgroup of patients with severe GHD, LV mass index increased concomitantly to the decline in N-terminal-pro B-type natriuretic peptide (NT-proBNP) and this was positively correlated to the final IGF-1 concentration.[275] Therefore, in acromegaly and GH deficiency, the control of GH/IGF-1 secretion reverses cardiomyopathy and risk factors and restores normal life expectancy.[270]

Thyroid Cardiomyopathy

Thyroid dysfunction may be associated with either high cardiac output cardiomyopathy in hyperthyroidism or low cardiac output cardiomyopathy in hypothyroidism.[276] Thyroid hormone effects are exerted on β-adrenergic receptors, contractile apparatus, ion-ATPase pump, and the sarcoplasmic reticulum.[271] Clinically, thyroid function is usually investigated in patients that manifest high-output HF. Hyperthyroidism is characterized by resting tachycardia and increased blood volume, stroke volume, myocardial contractility, and EF. High-output HF may be a result of a tachycardia-mediated cardiomyopathy mechanism. In hypothyroidism, thyroid hormone deficiency is associated with bradycardia, decreased myocardial contractility and relaxation, and prolonged systolic and early diastolic times. Cardiac preload is decreased as a result of impaired diastolic function, cardiac afterload is increased, and chronotropic and inotropic functions are reduced. Subclinical hypothyroidism is associated with increased risk of cardiovascular, events, but not of total mortality.[272] Medical or surgical treatment of either hyper- or hypothyroidism restores cardiac function.[272] Accordingly, thyroid cardiomyopathy is potentially reversible. Recurrent pericarditis and pericardial effusion are well-known complications of hypothyroidism (see Chapter 54); less commonly, pericarditis is observed in thyrotoxic crisis in Graves disease.[277]

Two medical emergencies, thyroid storm and myxedema coma, are unrelated to thyroid cardiomyopathy and may involve cardiologists for the diagnosis and management. *Thyroid storm* presenting with palpitation, atrial arrhythmias, and hypertension is managed according to a multidisciplinary approach aimed at lowering thyroid hormone synthesis and secretion, reducing circulating thyroid hormones and controlling the peripheral effects of the storm up to the resolution of systemic manifestations. In patients presenting with thyroid storm-induced shock the use of β-blockers could exacerbate their condition; the most effective management seems to be therapeutic plasma exchange in order to decrease thyroid hormone levels. Furthermore, the use of extracorporeal membrane oxygenation and Impella is advised to reduce pressure on the heart and ensure the patient's organs are well oxygenated and perfused while the LV function recovers.[278] *Myxedema coma*—incidence of approximately 0.22 per million per year in the Western world—is a rare fatal condition resulting from long-standing hypothyroidism with loss of the adaptive mechanism to maintain homeostasis.[279] It is characterized by somnolence, lethargy, hypotension, and hypothermia. It is precipitated by triggers such as cold exposure, infection, drugs, trauma, stroke, HF, and gastrointestinal bleeding, and is more common in old women presenting with altered consciousness and history of hypothyroidism, neck surgery, or radioactive iodine treatment (www.thyroidmanager.org). Patients should receive thyroid hormone therapy when myxedema coma is highly suspected. To prevent adrenal crises, administration of hydrocortisone is recommended before thyroid hormone therapy, especially in patients with hypotension. Hydrocortisone can be stopped or weaned down based on cortisol when blood levels are back, and hypotension resolves, eventually followed by the administration of IV Levothyroxine. Serial TSH, FT4, and FT3 are needed for dose adjustment.[280] The mortality rate is variable with some reports as high as 60% and others as low as 20% to 25% in the presence of advanced intensive support care.[281]

Uremic Cardiomyopathy

Despite advances in dialysis treatment and in the improved management of hypertension, hypervolemia, anemia, and chronic kidney disease–mineral and bone disorder (CKD-MBD), patients with CKD continue to have abnormal myocardial remodeling, which results in the persistently high rates of cardiovascular events and mortality.[282]

Uremic cardiomyopathy was originally defined by severe uremia accompanied by cardiomegaly, systolic dysfunction, and pericarditis.[283] Uremic cardiomyopathy is a common complication in chronic renal diseases and is considered a risk factor for morbidity and death among patients with CKD or end-stage renal disease.[284] Along with coronary artery disease, LV hypertrophy and congestive HF account for approximately 50% of deaths in patients with CKD. Nontraditional risk factors (eg, uremic toxins, renin-angiotensin-aldosterone system activation, sympathetic nervous system activation, anemia, calcium phosphate imbalance, inflammation) are involved in the pathogenesis of cardiac disease in CKD.[285,286] Two novel factors—the FGF23, and its cofactor, αKlotho—have been identified and investigated in the last few decades in CKD-MBD. Klotho is a beta-glucuronidase that hydrolyzes extracellular sugar residues on the transient receptor potential ion channel TRPV5, entrapping the channel in the plasma membrane.[287] Klotho is encoded by *KL* gene (MIM*604824 – Chr. 13q13.1); homozygous mutations cause the AR Hyperphosphatemic Familial Tumoral Calcinosis type 3 and other pending associations are under investigation. The fibroblast growth factor FGF23 is encoded by the *FGF23* gene (MIM*605380 – Chr.12p13-32); heterozygous mutations cause the autosomal

dominant hypophosphatemic rickets, while homozygous mutations cause tumoral calcinosis, familial hyperphosphatemic tumoral calcinosis type 2. Whereas FGF23 seems to be deleterious to the myocardium, the αKlotho—obligatory cofactor for FGF23 action as the primary phosphaturic hormone in phosphorus homeostasis—is protective. Therefore, FGF23 and αKlotho seem to have independent and antagonistic effects on the myocardium.[288] The triad of hyperphosphatemia, αKlotho deficiency, and elevated FGF23 levels is central in the pathophysiology of uremic cardiomyopathy. Both FGF23 and Klotho, are probably involved in the earliest biochemical abnormality of CKD-MBD syndrome and therefore of the development and progression of cardiovascular complications of uremia, including not only uremic cardiomyopathy but also cardiac hypertrophy, and atherosclerotic and arteriosclerotic vascular lesions.[289] More translational studies are needed to fully unravel the role of these two factors in uremic cardiomyopathy and to implement specific diagnostic paths and target treatments such as small molecules and antibodies.[290]

The "Kidney Disease: Improving Global Outcomes" report emphasized the need for unraveling the origin and mechanism of cardiac dysfunction and diagnosing asymptomatic LV dysfunction in patients with CKD.[291] Recently, texture analysis (TA) of T_1 images and vertical run-length nonuniformity (VRLN) provided better parameters for assessing myocardial fibrosis than T_1 times—increased in dialysis patients indicating fibrosis in uremic cardiomyopathy.[292] Compared with conventional hemodialysis (3 days per week), frequent hemodialysis (nocturnal home hemodialysis, short daily hemodialysis, and peritoneal dialysis) optimizes the ultrafiltration rate with minimal reductions in intravascular volume and cooling the dialysate; this reduces dialysis-induced myocardial stunning and intradialysis hypotension. Kidney transplantation may improve or reverse uremic cardiomyopathy and confers a significant survival advantage over hemodialysis.[293,294] The clinical benefit is extended also to the atrial uremic cardiomyopathy.[295] Early diagnosis of uremic cardiomyopathy and resolution of uremic toxemia contribute to risk stratification and decisions about the proper type of dialysis therapy.[296]

CARDIOVASCULAR ONCOTOXICITY

Introduction

Cardiovascular toxicity during and after chemotherapy and radiotherapy for cancer has been and remains a potential limitation to leveraging the full benefits of most advanced treatments of malignancies in childhood and adulthood.[297] Progression in cancer treatments has significantly increased the number of long-term survivors but has also increased the possibility of toxicity manifesting to the cardiovascular system over time.[298,299] Cardiovascular toxicity includes a range of complications, including involvement of the myocardium (eg, DCM, myocarditis), pericardium (eg, pericarditis, pericardial effusion), and vascular system (eg, coronary atherosclerosis, peripheral arterial disease, acute aortic syndromes, coagulopathy, hypertension, and hypotension)[300,301] (**Table 41–9**).

TABLE 41–9. Examples of Patients Diagnosed with Genetically Proven DCM Who Developed Cancer (Ca) before or after the Diagnosis of Cardiomyopathy

Sex	DCM Age	Cancer Age	MOGE(S) Baseline	MOGE(S) last	Event /Years
M	53	71	$M_{D(AVB)}$ O_H G_{AD} $E_{G\text{-}LMNA[p.\,Glu317Lys]}$ $S_{C\text{-}II}$	$M_{D(AVB)}$ O_H G_{AD} $E_{G\text{-}LMNA[p.\,Glu317Lys]\,+\,Lung\,Cancer\,+\,RX\,therapy}$ $S_{C\text{-}IV}$	Death HF 76
F	40	51	$M_{D(AVB)}$ O_H G_{AD} $E_{G\text{-}DMPK[E2,500\text{-}1000\,CTG]}$ $S_{C\text{-}II}$	$M_{D(AVB)}$ O_H G_{AD} $E_{G\text{-}DMPK[E2,500\text{-}1000\,CTG]\,+\,T\,Doxo\,in\,Breast\,Ca}$ $S_{C\text{-}IIb}$	Alive 56
M	50	55	$M_{D(E)}$ O_H G_{AD} $E_{G\text{-}MYBPC3[p.Q969X]}$ $S_{B\text{-}I}$	$M_{D(E)}$ O_H G_{AD} $E_{G\text{-}MYBPC3[p.Q969X]\,+\,T\,Doxo\,in\,Colon\,Ca}$ $S_{C\text{-}IV}$	Death HF 58
F	66	49	$M_{D(AVB)}$ O_H G_{AD} $E_{G\text{-}LMNA[p.\,Arg335Gln]}$ $S_{C\text{-}IIb}$	$M_{D(AVB)}$ O_H G_{AD} $E_{G\text{-}LMNA[p.\,Arg335Gln]\,+\,T\,Doxo\,in\,Breast\,Ca}$ $S_{C\text{-}III}$	Alive 69
F	61	55	$M_{D(AVB)(>sCPK)}$ O_{H+M} G_{AD} $E_{G\text{-}LMNA[p.\,Lys171Lys]}$ $S_{C\text{-}II}$	$M_{D(AVB)(>sCPK)}$ O_{H+M} G_{AD} $E_{G\text{-}LMNA[p.\,Lys171Lys]\,+\,T\,Doxo\,in\,Breast\,Ca}$ $S_{C\text{-}IV}$	Death HF 67

The genotypes and phenotypes are coded according to the WHF 2013 MOGE(S) classification (see Chapter 40).

Although these possible complications are known, the individual risk of occurrence remains largely unpredictable. Whereas greater risk would be expected in older patients and those with a preponderance of traditional risk factors, clinical evidence across a range of ages indicates that underlying risk does not necessarily correlate with expression of the phenotype. Pretreatment risk stratification requires meticulous consideration to prevent or limit the effects of potentially harmful treatments in patients at high risk while not excluding patients from receiving effective treatments.[302] New cardiovascular imaging tools (ie, strain imaging) and biomarkers (eg, troponin, BNP) are now contributing to early detection, better risk stratification, and monitoring of the cardiovascular toxic effects of chemotherapy.[303,304] None of these markers has been specifically generated for detection or monitoring of cardiovascular toxicity per se; rather, their use represents the extension of standards in cardiovascular diagnosis generally to chemotherapy-induced cardiovascular abnormalities specifically.

The new immunotherapies that harness the native immune system to effectively treat advanced malignancies, also induce immune-related adverse events also affecting the cardiovascular system with a significant risk of morbidity and mortality.[305]

The relevance of oncocardiotoxicity and DCM is related to the paradigmatic and well-known anthracycline-induced DCM, and to the possibility that patients with genetic DCM may develop cancer and therefore require chemotherapy. A detailed discussion of cardiovascular toxicity induced by chemotherapy is provided in Chapter 74.

Myocardial Toxicity

Patients who develop cancer may have either healthy cardiovascular systems or preexisting cardiovascular conditions, including DCM (see Table 41–9). The former is obviously the most common, favorable, and expected condition. The latter requires the involvement of cardiologists, multidisciplinary evaluation, and specific monitoring.[212,299,301,306–308] Heart muscle toxicity is generally characterized by *nonreversible injury* (type 1) as a result of the presence of structural damage (prototyped by the anthracycline or high-dose cyclophosphamide DCM in acute and chronic forms) and *potentially reversible* (on cessation of therapy) dysfunction (type 2) in the absence of structural abnormalities, as with targeted therapies (ie, trastuzumab, sunitinib, lapatinib).[212,307,309–312] In patients first treated with drugs causing type 1 injury and then with drugs causing type 2 injury, the damage may be cumulative. Myocardial toxicity occurs with many agents used in the treatment of cancer; examples are summarized in **Table 41–10**.

Systolic Dysfunction

The substantial difference between the diagnostic criteria in toxic myocardial dysfunction related to cancer therapy (American College of Cardiology Foundation/AHA 5.4.3) versus nontoxic dysfunction (eg, inherited DCM) is the dynamic concept of the diagnosis. The cardio-oncotoxicity is a double-step diagnosis that implies normal baseline cardiovascular function and evidence of the decline of function during or after treatment. Therefore, the definition of cancer therapy–related cardiac dysfunction (CTRCD) or chemotherapy-related cardiac dysfunction (CRCD) seems to better describe both type 1 and type 2 myocardial damage. Anthracyclines (see Table 41–10) are the best-known drugs increasing the risk of CTRCD caused by type 1 injury; the incidence rate is as high as 2.1% in randomized controlled trials and 26% in observational studies.[297] Targeted drugs such as trastuzumab, a monoclonal antibody targeting the human epidermal growth factor receptor-2 in the breast or gastroesophageal malignancies, are associated with CTRCD caused by type 2 injury with a 3-year cumulative incidence of 6.6% when trastuzumab is used with anthracyclines and 5.1% when used without anthracyclines. Higher risk in mid- and long-term follow-up is reported with trastuzumab after anthracycline treatment.[297,299,300] The possibility of CTRCD occurring in FDCM may confound the interpretation of the cause of the myocardial disease (**Fig. 41–13**).

Anti-HER2 Therapy: In 2002, the Review and Evaluation Committee of Trastuzumab-Associated Cardiomyopathy supervising trastuzumab trials defined CRCD as follows: "(1) characterized by a decrease in cardiac LVEF, either global or more severe in the septum; (2) symptoms of HF; (3) associated signs of HF, including but not limited to S3 gallop, tachycardia, or both; and (4) decline in LVEF of at least 5% to less than 55% with accompanying signs or symptoms of HF, or a decline in LVEF of at least 10% to below 55% without accompanying signs or symptoms. The presence of any one of the four criteria is sufficient to confirm a diagnosis of CRCD."[313] From 2002 to the present, these criteria have been repeatedly discussed and applied in clinical trials, but their systematic application is still debated and guidelines for their application are still lacking.[297] Patients treated with trastuzumab should undergo regular echocardiographic monitoring (every 3 months during treatment)[314] (https://www.accessdata.fda.gov/drugsatfda_docs/label/2017/103792s5337lbl.pdf).

TABLE 41–10. Summary Table Showing Major Cardiovascular Toxicity Effects and Phenotypes in Cancer Patients Treated with Different Chemotherapeutic Agents

CLASS	DRUGS AND DOSE DEPENDANT (DD°) EFFECTS	MYO-PERI-ENDO-CARDIAL					RHYTHM AND CONDUCTION EFFECTS AND EVENTS						VASCULAR TOXICITY					
		CARDIOVASCULAR TOXICITY (RANGE %)	LV DYSFUNCTION-DCM	(ENDO)MYOCARDIAL FIBROSIS	MYOCARDITIS	PERICARDITIS/PERICARDIAL EFFUSION	ARRHYTHMIAS	CONDUCTION DEFECTS (NONOTHERWISE DESCRIBED)	QT INTERVAL PROLONGATION	BRADYCARDIA AND AV BLOCK	SUDDEN DEATH/CARDIAC ARREST	VENTRICULAR TACHYCARDIA/FIBRILLATION	VASOSPASM/ARTERIAL CONSTRICTION	ACUTE CORONARY SYNDROMES	ARTERIAL THROMBOSIS	VENOUS THROMBOEMBOLISM	AORTIC DISSECTION	BLOOD PRESSURE
Antracycline	Doxorubicyne°	3–48	•		•	•	•	•	•	•		•						
	Idarubicin, Idarubicin	5–18	•					•										
	Epirubucin	<1–3	•				•	•		•					•			↑
	Mitoxantrone*	<1–30	•				•	•		•								
Alkylating agents	Cyclophosh-amide°	7–28	•			•	•					•						
	Ifosfamide°	17	•				•					•		•				↑or↓
	Busulfan			•			•											
	Mitomycin°	10							•									↑or↓
Antimetabolites	Clofarabine	27	•			•			•									↓
	5-Fluorouracil	1–78					•		•	•			•	•				
	Capecitabine	2–9					•		•	•			•	•	•			
	Cytarabine					•								•				
Mab-tyrosine kinase I	Bevacizumab	4–35	•						•					•	•	•	•	↑↑
	Trastuzumab	2–28	•												•			↑or↓
	Pertuzumab	3–7	•															
	Alemtuzumab						•											↑or↓
	Rituximab^						•											↓
Small molecule tyrosine Kinase I	Dasatinib	2–4	•				•		•			•						↑
	Imatinib mesylate	0.5–2	•										•					↑
	Lapatinib	1.5–16	•				•		•									↑
	Sunitinib°	2.7–11	•				•		•				•	•	•	•	•	↓
	Sorafenib	4–28													•		•	↑
	Pazopanib	7–13												•	•			↑
Proteasome I	Bortezomib	2–5	•				•			•								
	Carfilzomib		•															
AMTA	Paclitaxel	<1–31					•							•				
	Docetaxel	<2–8	•											•				
AAG	Lenalidomide	3–75														•		
	Thalidomide	1–58					•			•						•		
PA	Cisplatin	8.5					•			•	•		•			•	•	↑or↓

(Continued)

TABLE 41–10. Summary Table Showing Major Cardiovascular Toxicity Effects and Phenotypes in Cancer Patients Treated with Different Chemotherapeutic Agents (Continued)

CLASS	DRUGS AND DOSE DEPENDANT (DD°) EFFECTS	MYO-PERI-ENDO-CARDIAL					RHYTHM AND CONDUCTION EFFECTS AND EVENTS						VASCULAR TOXICITY					
		CARDIOVASCULAR TOXICITY (RANGE %)	LV DYSFUNCTION-DCM	(ENDO)MYOCARDIAL FIBROSIS	MYOCARDITIS	PERICARDITIS/PERICARDIAL EFFUSION	ARRHYTHMIAS	CONDUCTION DEFECTS (NONOTHERWISE DESCRIBED)	QT INTERVAL PROLONGATION	BRADYCARDIA AND AV BLOCK	SUDDEN DEATH/CARDIAC ARREST	VENTRICULAR TACHYCARDIA/ FIBRILLATION	VASOSPASM/ARTERIAL CONSTRICTION	ACUTE CORONARY SYNDROMES	ARTERIAL THROMBOSIS	VENOUS THROMBOEMBOLISM	AORTIC DISSECTION	BLOOD PRESSURE
AMTA	Vincristine	25					•							•				↑or↓
Miscellaneous	Interferon-alpha2b	25	•							•	•			•				↓
	Aflibercept	1–7												•	•			↓
	Pentostatin	3–10			•									•	•			
	All Trans retinoic acid	6				•			•									↓
	Arsenic Trioxide	26–93							•									

Note: The prevalence ranges include data from both isolated and combined protocols.
*Mitoxantrone being an antracycline derivative, with immunosuppression effects, used in the past for multiple sclerosis is reported as potentially associated with the risk of acute leukemia.
^angioedema, rare. Abbreviations: PA, platinum agents; AMTA, antimicro-tubule agents; AAG, anti-angio-genesis.

Other HER2 inhibitors (eg, lapatinib) seem to show a more favorable cardiac risk profile compared with trastuzumab.

Fluoropyrimidines: These drugs, such as fluorouracil (FU) and the related prodrug capecitabine, are largely used in solid tumors; their use can be complicated by LVSD and, rarely, by myocarditis.[315]

The Class of Tyrosine Kinase Inhibitors (TKIs): TKIs targeting estimated glomerular filtration rate (EGFR), or vascular endothelial growth factor (VEGF) or ABL, may exert a nondose-dependent cardiotoxicity at any time during treatment, from a few days to months. The risk of cardiotoxicity seems to be higher (up to 10%) using TKIs with anti-VEGF activity, such as sunitinib and sorafenib.[316] The EGFR-directed TKI Osimertinib, used for treatment of the non–small-cell lung cancer, may cause cardiotoxicity in up to 5% of patients early during treatment.[317] Patients to be treated with TKIs should undergo baseline LVEF assessment and regular clinical monitoring.[318] Global longitudinal strain (GLS) and biomarkers may contribute to better monitoring.[316]

Proteasome Inhibitors (PIs): PIs such as carfilzomib and bortezomib, largely used for treating multiple myeloma, may cause cardiotoxicity via unfolded protein effects, with oxidative stress and myocyte death.[319] The cardiac damage seems to be more common and irreversible with Carfilzomib than with Bortezomib[320] (7% vs 2%–5%, respectively), with a dose-dependent

effect,[321] requiring a very close monitoring, especially in those patients previously treated with anthracyclines, doxorubicin, and chest radiation.[322]

The Class of BRAF- and MEK-Inhibitors: These inhibitors are often used in combination to treat metastatic BRAF+ melanoma and may cause myocardial damage and dysfunction in up to 10% of patients. When used in monotherapy, LV dysfunction is less common;[323] the treatment should be discontinued when LVEF declines significantly, especially in the early phase of treatment.[324]

Immune Checkpoint Inhibitors (ICIs): ICIs block negative regulators of the T-cell immune response and are used in breast, renal, and lung cancer. The cardiotoxicity may manifest with "arrhythmogenic" myocarditis or noninflammatory myocardial damage.[325] GLS seems to decrease in myocarditis regardless of the decline of EF.[326] The Cardio-Oncology Study Group of the Heart Failure Association and the Cardio-Oncology Council of the ESC[327] recommends baseline echocardiogram, and biomarker dosage (cardiac troponin, and BNP[proBNP]) before treatment initiation, and monitoring in particular for high-risk patients, to be performed before the administration of each subsequent dose.

Chimeric Antigen Receptor T-Cell (CAR-T) Therapy: This is especially used for treating refractory hematological malignancies. It improves survival, but exerts cardiotoxic effects by cytokine

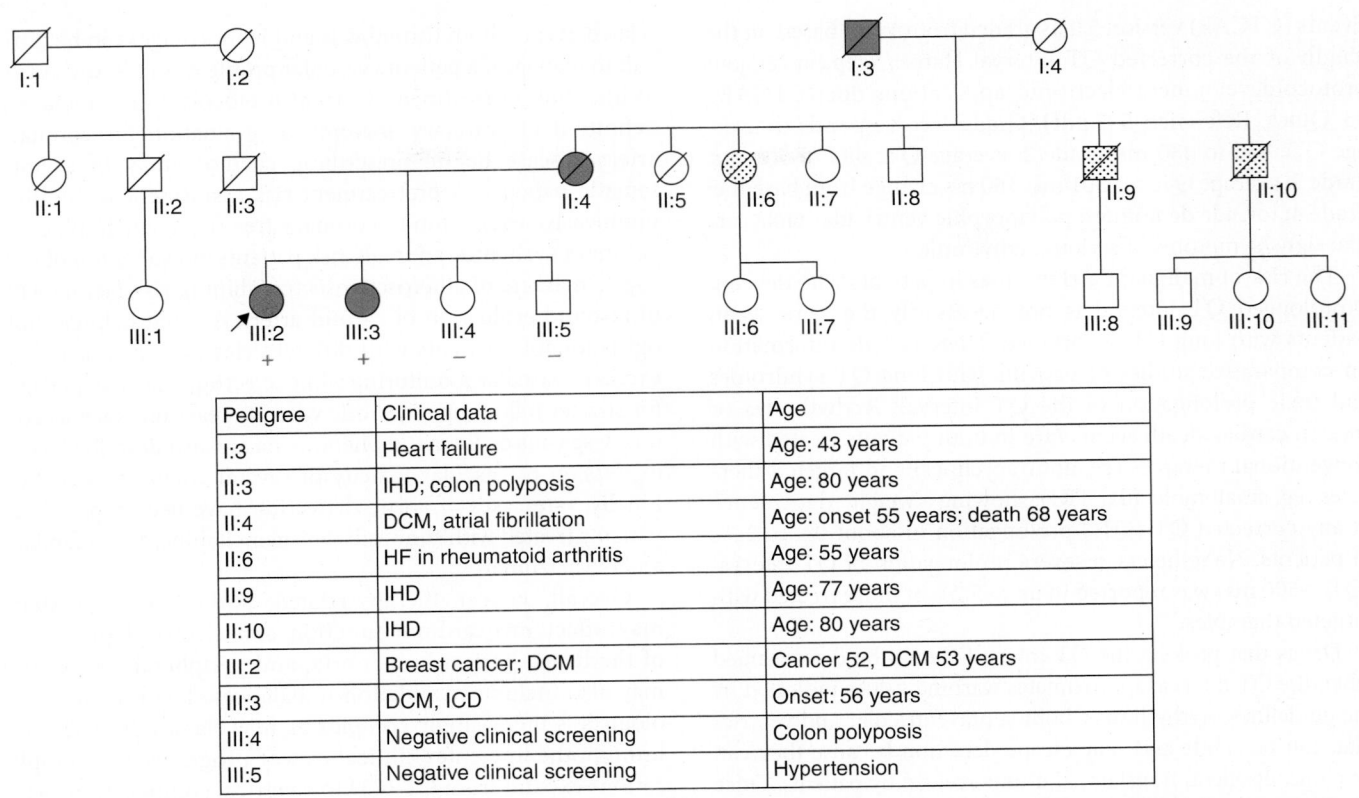

Pedigree	Clinical data	Age
I:3	Heart failure	Age: 43 years
II:3	IHD; colon polyposis	Age: 80 years
II:4	DCM, atrial fibrillation	Age: onset 55 years; death 68 years
II:6	HF in rheumatoid arthritis	Age: 55 years
II:9	IHD	Age: 77 years
II:10	IHD	Age: 80 years
III:2	Breast cancer; DCM	Cancer 52, DCM 53 years
III:3	DCM, ICD	Onset: 56 years
III:4	Negative clinical screening	Colon polyposis
III:5	Negative clinical screening	Hypertension

Figure 41–13. Cancer therapy–related cardiac dysfunction (CTRCD). The figure shows the pedigree of a family in which the proband (III:2) developed breast cancer that was treated with a trastuzumab-based protocol, and 1 year later, she developed DCM. One sister (III:3) is affected by DCM, whereas another sister (III:4) and the brother (III:5) are not affected. Genetic testing demonstrated the presence (+) in both sisters with DCM of the variant p.(Arg634Trp) in the *RBM20* gene; this variant was absent (−) in both nonaffected siblings (III:4 and III:5). The mother (II:4) was affected by DCM, whereas the father died of ischemic heart disease (IHD); none of them could be tested. In the same position of *RBM20*, p.(Arg634Gln) has been described in two families as a disease-causing mutation (Brauch et al. *J Am Coll Cardiol.* 229;54:930–941; Li et al. *Clin Transl Sci.* 2010;3:90–97). The p.(Arg634Trp) identified in the two sisters III:2 and III:3 is pathogenic according to ACMG criteria (PM1, PM2, PM5, PP3, PP5_Strong). The family demonstrates that in patients with cancer and familial DCM, the interpretation of the causative role of CTRCD should be done cautiously. HF, heart failure; ICD, implantable cardioverter-defibrillator.

release syndrome (CRS).[328] In 145 patients treated with CAR-T therapy, the Kaplan-Meier estimates for MACE and CRS at 30 days were 17% and 53%, respectively; survival at 1 year was 71%. MACE included cardiovascular death, symptomatic HF, acute coronary syndrome, ischemic stroke, and de novo cardiac arrhythmia.[329] Cardiac complications include myocarditis, HF, cardiogenic shock, and myocardial injury resulting in troponin elevation, abnormalities in myocardial strain, and asymptomatic drop in LVEF.[330] Patients should receive regular monitoring, both echocardiography and biomarkers because major adverse events seem to be preceded by the manifestations of the CRS. As far as the use of CAR-T therapy expands to include a larger spectrum of malignancies, careful patient selection, pretreatment cardiac evaluation, and cardiovascular risk stratification should be considered within the CAR-T treatment protocol.[331]

Myocarditis

Myocarditis is a rare complication described in patients treated for cancer (ie, cyclophosphamide and hemorrhagic myocarditis). It may present as fulminant myocarditis.[332,333] In a systematic review that included 73 studies, myocarditis (45%) was reported to be the most common manifestation of cardiotoxicity

in patients treated with ICIs.[334] These drugs upregulate T-cell activity triggering an immune response against cancer cells but may also induce autoimmune reactions with high fatality rate. Myocarditis also complicates CAR-T therapies and bispecific T-cell engagers.[335] Overall, ICI-associated myocarditis is the most recognized and potentially fatal cardiotoxicity, with mortality approaching 50%.[305] Compared with previous pharmacovigilance studies the observed absolute risk is higher (eg, 1.8% peri-/myocarditis 1-year risk).[336,337]

Pericardial Involvement

Pericardial effusion and pericarditis (excluding carcinomatous pericarditis) may occur commonly in patients treated with different classes of chemotherapeutic drugs. They may be reliable markers of cardiotoxicity, especially when it can be demonstrated that the pericardial abnormality was not present prior to the administration of chemotherapy (see Chapters 54 and 74).

Rhythm Disturbances

Variations of cardiac rhythm and ECG intervals are common in patients treated with anticancer drugs. Prolongation of the QT interval is a consequence of many classes of anticancer drugs[301] and, according to Common Terminology Criteria for Adverse

Events (CTCAE) version 5.0, is graded from 1 to 4 based on the length of the corrected QT interval (https://ctep.cancer.gov/protocoldevelopment/electronic_applications/docs/CTCAE_v5_Quick_Reference_5x7.pdf). Grade 1 corresponds to average QTc 450 to 480 ms; grade 2: average QTc 481 to 500 ms; grade 3: average QTc >= 501 ms; >60 ms change from baseline; grade 4: torsade de pointes; polymorphic ventricular tachycardia; signs/symptoms of serious arrhythmia.

The risk of malignant arrhythmias in patients who develop a prolonged QT interval is not necessarily the same as in patients with long QT syndromes. There is little information on comparative studies of patients with long QT syndromes and toxic prolongation of the QT interval. Arrhythmias or sudden cardiac death seems rare in both patients treated with conventional therapies (eg, anthracyclines) and targeted therapies (eg, small molecular TKI), showing a weighted incidence of any corrected QT (QTc) prolongation in about 0% to 22% of patients. Nonetheless, a severe prolongation of QT interval (QTc >500 ms) was reported in up to 5.2% of those treated with targeted therapies.[338]

Drugs that prolong the QT interval should be discontinued when the QT interval approximates warning values indicated by the guidelines. Arrhythmias, both supraventricular and ventricular, can be subtle and may escape detection because they can be clinically silent, transient, and unperceived by patients. Once life-threatening arrhythmias are demonstrated in patients treated for cancer, exclusion of noncardiotoxic causes is essential to prevent an incorrect assignment of the event to the chemotherapeutics, to decide about premature termination of chemotherapy, and to appropriately manage the arrhythmias.[338,339]

Arterial Blood Pressure

Chemotherapeutics may either increase or decrease blood pressure (see Table 41–9). Hypertension is common in adult patients; it should be either excluded or recognized with certainty before assigning the hypertensive complication to chemotherapy.[340] The CTCAE version 5.0 grading of hypertension includes four grades (http://evs.nci.nih.gov/ftp1/CTCAE/CTCAE_4.03_2010-06-14_QuickReference_5x7.pdf); grade 1, or prehypertension (systolic blood pressure of 120–139 mm Hg or diastolic blood pressure of 80–90 mm Hg), is very common in the general adult population (see Chapters 5 and 74). In nonhypertensive patients, chemotherapy-induced endothelial dysfunction is associated with loss of vasorelaxant effects and suppression of anti-inflammatory and vascular repair functions. These effects may initiate and further maintain the development of hypertension, thrombosis, and atherogenesis. Hypertension is the most common cardiovascular complication associated with VEGF inhibitors.[341] Effective antihypertensive treatment is mandatory before starting chemotherapy. In addition, drugs such as ACE inhibitors may exert nonspecific protection to cardiotoxicity (see Chapter 74).[298,301,304]

Vascular Toxicity

Atherosclerosis-related events such as ischemic heart disease (both acute and chronic) and coagulation imbalances and related events (both thrombosis and hemorrhage) can be difficult to manage if a patient's vascular profile was unknown prior to initiation of treatment. Current protocols do not include a definition of coronary anatomy or evaluation for coronary artery disease before prescribing chemotherapy in asymptomatic patients. A pretreatment risk assessment with either noninvasive evaluation of coronary tree (eg, angiographic CT coronary evaluation) in high-risk patients or evaluation of surrogate markers of atherosclerosis (combining risk factors with ultrasound evaluation of carotid arteries) could help cardiologists identify patients with different classes of risk, avoiding excess of vascular monitoring while selecting high-risk patients for stricter follow-up. Dynamic vascular reactions such as coronary spasms or Raynaud phenomena are also described as an expression of vascular toxicity of several chemotherapeutics. Finally, rare cases of aortic dissection have been reported in patients treated with sunitinib,[342,343] gemcitabine,[344] sorafenib,[345] and bevacizumab.[346]

Overall, cancer therapy-related cardiovascular toxicity may affect myocardium function and electrical properties of the heart, pericardium, aorta, and peripheral vessels and may also include coagulation imbalances. The role of cardiologists is increasingly complex as new classes of drugs and immunotherapy enter clinical cancer programs and complications expand from CTRCD to electrical complications with variable risk of life-threatening arrhythmias and myocarditis. Cardio-oncology units should regularly operate in all cancer centers and units. (The list of drugs and current protocols is available and regularly updated at http://www.cancer.gov/about-cancer/treatment/drugs/.)

PROGNOSIS IN DILATED CARDIOMYOPATHY

The prognosis of DCM has been largely investigated in nongenotyped series of nonischemic DCM index patients. Prognostic stratification largely coincides with that of systolic HF (see Chapter 48). Currently available data are based on the phenotype and do not systematically include the etiology. Exceptions include small series of genetic DCMs, potentially reversible DCM, PPCM, and DCM in autoimmune diseases.

Over the last three decades, the prognosis of DCM has progressively and significantly improved in the overall population of DCM patients.[347,348] The optimized use of ACE inhibitors, ARBs, β-blockers, antialdosterone therapy, and resynchronization therapy[18,212] has substantially modified the natural history of DCM (see Chapter 48). The annual incidence of major cardiac events (death and cardiac transplantation) declined, and transplant-free survival improved. HF-related deaths have decreased by 40% in the last 20 years.[349] Reasons for better survival and low event rate include early diagnosis, earlier medical treatment, resynchronization therapy, and primary prevention of sudden death with ICD implantation[350,251] (see Chapters 37 and 48). Patients enrolled in the last decade have a shorter history of HF, are less symptomatic for HF, and have fewer previous hospital admissions for HF and less severe heart disease; this modification can partly be attributed to the beneficial impact of systematic familial screening.[350] The enrollment in clinical series of family members (identified as affected in family screening studies) added a proportion of patients who were diagnosed in the early phases of the disease. In a single-center series, the incidence of major events declined to <2 per 100 patients per year, with an 87% survival free from heart transplantation at 8 years in the last decade.[350] Earlier diagnoses imply earlier medical treatments, which are consequent further contributors to improved clinical outcomes.

The pharmacologic and device-based treatments modifying LV remodeling contribute to the improvement of LVEF. Key drugs such as ACE inhibitors and β-blockers[18,30,212] and the use of aldosterone antagonists, improving LV remodeling and systolic function, positively impact prognosis;[352–354] up to 50% of patients receiving cardiac resynchronization therapy demonstrate significant reverse remodeling during the course of 24 months in nonischemic DCM with more evident benefits when follow-up is longer and patients demonstrate mild HF.[355] In patients in New York Heart Association (NYHA) class I/II, cardiac resynchronization therapy decreased all-cause mortality, reduced HF hospitalizations, and improved LVEF.[356]

Early reverse remodeling, achieved with both medical and device-based therapy, positively influences decisions on primary prevention, preventing unnecessary ICD implantation in patients with idiopathic DCM presenting with SCD in Heart Failure Trial criteria.[357] In 131 patients diagnosed with DCM, LV reverse remodeling was independently predicted by hypertension, no family history of DCM, symptom duration <90 days, LVEF <35%, and QRS duration <116 ms.[358] Reverse remodeling influences mitral valve dysfunction, a further relevant negative prognostic contributor.[359] MitraClip can improve symptoms and promote reverse remodeling in nonresponders to cardiac resynchronization therapy.[360] The proportion of super-responders to cardiac resynchronization therapy in the DCM series is difficult to establish; however, the predictors of responsiveness to cardiac resynchronization therapy can be usefully applied to DCM, especially because they include the lack of prior myocardial infarction.[361]

Overall, current prognostic markers and optimized medical and interventional treatments provide evidence that the natural history of DCM substantially improved in the last few decades and can be further ameliorated. The arrhythmogenic risk stratification deserves further research. Even super-responders to cardiac resynchronization therapy remain at risk for ventricular arrhythmias.[362] To this regard, fibrosis is a potential predictor. The association of myocardial fibrosis with mortality and SCD in patients with DCM is known.[363,364] In patients with nonischemic cardiomyopathy, only those with ventricular midwall fibrosis detected by CMR benefited from cardiac resynchronization therapy-defibrillator when compared to cardiac resynchronization therapy-pacing.[365] However, beyond fibrosis, prognostic predictors such as low LVEF have limited sensibility and specificity. Selecting patients according to the current guidelines shows that most DCM patients do not actually benefit from ICD, while suffering collateral effects. In addition, it is now evident that also patients exhibiting mildly depressed LVEF can be at risk of sudden death. In the complex substrates underlying SCD, multiple risk

factors can probably contribute to predict the risk.[71] Genetics can significantly contribute to stratify arrhythmogenic risk, as demonstrated in *LMNA* mutation carriers[69,70] and by the first introduction of genetics in the 2015 ESC guidelines for the management of patients with ventricular arrhythmias and prevention of SCD.[366] Overall, we expect that in time the increased proportion of genotyped patients with DCM will generate data useful for progressing from the phenotype-based prognostic stratification to cause-specific risk stratification, either genetic or nongenetic.

MILDLY DILATED CARDIOMYOPATHY AND HYPOKINETIC NONDILATED CARDIOMYOPATHY

Historical Notes and Concept Evolution

In 1985, Karen et al. first described five patients who underwent cardiac transplantation for NYHA class IV HF with only mildly dilated ventricles (MDCM) but other features typical of congestive cardiomyopathy. The authors concluded that end-stage congestive cardiomyopathy may occur without significant ventricular dilatation and that their clinical, hemodynamic, and pathologic findings are virtually identical to those of patients with typical DCM.[367] In 20 patients with 40 months of follow-up, Lida et al. observed that (1) some patients with MDCM have neither definite histories nor symptoms suggesting HF; (2) the hemodynamic conditions of patients with MDCM do not always deteriorate, but rather stabilize, and even improve during follow-up periods; (3) several types of arrhythmias can be observed, even in standard resting ECGs; and (4) patients with MDCM may die suddenly.[368] In a follow-up study including 12 nontransplant patients, Keren et al. observed variable but negative prognosis after prospective diagnosis of MDCM, with poor survival in patients with persistence of the original diagnostic features during follow-up. Thus, heart transplantation was suggested to be strongly considered in MDCM if signs of severe cardiac dysfunction persisted despite therapy.[369] The MDCM attracted the clinical observation and in 1993, 45 patients with MDCM were compared with 99 patients with typical DCM to address the issues of variability and prognostic role of LV dimensions in DCM. The authors concluded that minimal or mild ventricular dilatation is not uncommon in DCM and that it identifies a heterogeneous group of patients—some who are in the early stages of disease and others with severe pump dysfunction and persistently small hearts. Ventricular dilation was not an independent predictor of prognosis.[370] In 2002, Kitaoka et al. described 21 patients with MDCM and impaired hemodynamics at diagnosis: LV end-diastolic pressure, mean pulmonary artery pressure, and LA dimension at the time of follow-up were significant predictors of poor outcome, suggesting that these patients should be followed carefully even if the LV dilatation is mild.[371]

After first description of MDCM, mild ventricular dilation has often been the subject of research both in terms of the stand-alone entity and extent of negative remodeling in DCM with potential susceptibility to recovery in patients treated with optimal medical treatment. The three decades of research addressing clinical and genetic screening of families have intro-duced not only the culture of clinical genetics in familial DCM, but also the evidence that the early stages of DCM (eg, the mutated children of affected parents) can be associated with early clinical markers. This evidence has led to the clinical need to assign a nosology to the preclinical and early forms of DCM, often observed in young descendants of probands with overt DCM. The 2016 ESC position paper stemmed from the need of addressing the "diagnostic criteria" of HNDC with the aim of assigning a nosology to the early phases of genetic DCM, when diagnostic criteria of DCM are still not fulfilled, to provide both monitoring and early therapeutic interventions.[3]

Epidemiology of HNDC and Significance

The source of epidemiological estimates of HNDC needs pre-cise definition: are patients diagnosed with HNDC relatives of the proband: son or younger siblings identified with family screening? Or are they index patients who meet the diagnostic criteria of HNDC, irrespective of the family history? Or, are they patients who meet the historical criteria of MDCM, with severe LV dysfunction and only mild LV dilation? Without a precise framing of the data source, the concept of hypokinetic nondilated cardiomyopathy versus MDCM risks being con-fusing. Data coming from family screening show that HNDC identifies early stages of disease in genetically predisposed individuals. Given that most FDCMs are autosomal dominant diseases, the future epidemiology of HNDC is expected to reflect prevalence higher than the historical 1:2500 prevalence of DCM (see Table 41–1). Vice versa, data obtained from con-secutive DCM patients with severe LV dysfunction but mildly dilated LVs meet the original description of MDCM.[367] There-fore, the distinction between HNDC and MDCP is essential for the future nosology framework and epidemiology, as well as for early therapeutic decisions, either presymptomatic or preclinical, that can impact the future development of clinical research. The recent universal definition of HF acknowledges the "heart failure with mid-range ejection fraction" (HFmrEF, 40% to <50%), a functional descriptor that could be useful for classify the HF observed in HNDC.[4]

Etiology

At present, the causes are to be referred to the same known causes of DCM.[3] Transient, potentially reversible mild LV dys-function could also recognize exposure to cardiotoxic agents or transient myocardial involvement in flu epidemics, or endo-crine dysfunction that can recover with treatments, prolonged endurance exercise, or tachyarrhythmia, and many other trig-gers whose control is associated with reversal of myocardial dysfunction. Therefore, any diagnosis of HNDC should be supported by serial controls confirming the persistence of the observed instrumental abnormalities.

Diagnostic Criteria

The HNDC position statement distinguishes the diagnostic criteria in probands and relatives. In relatives, diagnostic crite-ria are grouped into major (n = 2) and minor (n = 6). The three

diagnostic levels are *definite diagnosis* when the DCM criteria are met; *probable* HNDC when one major criterion is associ-ated with at least one minor criterion; *possible* HNDC in the presence of either two minor criteria; or one minor criterion plus being the carrier of the causative mutation identified in the proband; or one major criterion in the absence of minor criteria and no genetic data in the family (**Fig. 41–14**).[3]

Clinical Context

The clinical context of HNDC is familial DCM. Systematic clinical screening of families leads to the early identification of the disease when criteria for a conclusive diagnosis of DCM are not yet present. The first screening of the family provides baseline data, which must be considered the starting point for regular monitoring. However, a family member with HNDC in the context of a familial DCM is a patient with the same rights for cardiology care as patients with DCM. Therefore, diagnostic investigations (imaging), biomarkers (eg, natriuretic peptides or troponin levels), arrhythmogenic risk stratification (therefore instrumental investigations such as 24-hour ECG), can be pre-scribed and considered, on a case by case basis, establishing a personalized scheduling plan. A different clinical context with similar possible mild LV dysfunction and minimal or absent LV dilation is that of "arrhythmogenic DCM." For patients with her-itable DCM, mildly impaired or moderate LV dysfunction and ventricular arrhythmias exceeding the extent of underlying mor-phological abnormalities, the possible overlap with left dominant arrhythmogenic cardiomyopathy (LDAC) may be nosologically confounding. In fact, the so-called "arrhythmogenic DCM" may look alike LDAC but genetic causes differ, being *LMNA*, *SCN5A*, *FLNC*, *TTN*, and *RBM20*, rather than desmosomal genes, the genes more commonly associated with arrhythmogenic DCM.[372]

HNDC: Better Prognosis

It seems obvious that the first cases described as MDCM have to be included in the classic DCM, although an important mes-sage remains regarding the prognostic role of LV dilation in DCM. The evolving concept is gathered from the new defini-tion of HNDC that shifts the diagnostic question from patients with DCM to their relatives and early diagnosis and the open question of whether HNDC requires a distinct subnosology in the domain of DCM in order to generate data that could clarify, especially in genetic forms, the natural history of the different genetic DCMs. Use of the terms *MDCM* versus *HNDC* could in the future be confusing or indicating the simple more friendly use of the term *MDCM*. A recent study including 236 patients with MDCM defined these patients as diagnosed in an earlier stage and presenting an apparent better evolution. However, some MDCMs evolved into DCM despite optimal medical therapy, whereas persistent MDCMs with nonsustained ven-tricular arrhythmias and restrictive filling patterns were char-acterized by a very poor outcome.[373]

What's Next?

The next step addresses the clinical significance and the pre-dictive values of mild LV dysfunction with mild or absent

HYPOKINETIC NONDILATED CARDIOMYOPATHY

DIAGNOSIS IN PROBANDS

- **LEFT VENTRICULAR**

  OR

- **BIVENTRICULAR GLOBAL SYSTOLIC DYSFUNCTION* (DEFINED AS LVEF <45%), NOT EXPLAINED BY ABNORMAL LOADING CONDITIONS OR CAD;**

- **NO DILATION^**

*Strictly decreased LVEF is mandatory in index patient with HNDC since no combination with dilatation is mandatory for the diagnosis.
Systolic dysfunction = abnormal LV ejection fraction, measured using any modality and shown either by two independent imaging modalities or on two distinct occasions by the same technique, preferably echocardiography or CMR.
^ LV dilation = LV end-diastolic (ED) volumes or diameters >2SD from normal according to normograms (Z scores >2 standard deviations) corrected by BSA and age, or BSA and gender.

DIAGNOSIS IN RELATIVES

DEFINITE DISEASE: MEETS CRITERIA FOR DCM OR HNDC
PROBABLE DISEASE
ONE MAJOR CRITERION PLUS AT LEAST ONE MINOR CRITERION
OR ONE MAJOR CRITERION PLUS CARRYING THE CAUSATIVE MUTATION IDENTIFIED IN THE PROBAND
POSSIBLE DISEASE (IN FAMILIAL DISEASE)
-TWO MINOR CRITERIA OR ONE MINOR CRITERION PLUS CARRYING THE CAUSATIVE MUTATION IDENTIFIED IN THE PROBAND
-ONE MAJOR CRITERION BUT WITHOUT ANY MINOR CRITERION AND WITHOUT GENETIC DATA WITH IN THE FAMILY

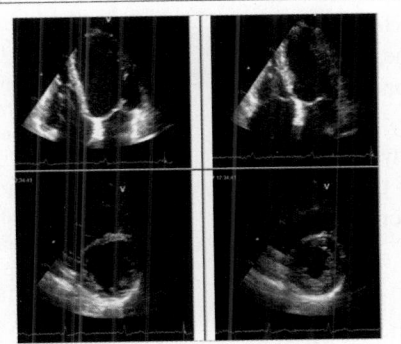

MAJOR CRITERIA

1. Unexplained decrease of LVEF ≤50% but >45%

2. Unexplained LVEF dilatation (diameter or volume) according to nomograms (*LVED diameter/volume >2SD + 5% since this more specific echocardiographic criterion was used in studies that demonstrated the predictive impact of isolated dilatation in relatives*)[a]

MINOR CRITERIA

1. Complete LBBB, or AV block (PR >200 ms or higher degree AV block)

2. Unexplained ventricular arrhythmia (>100 ventricular premature beats per hour in 24 h or nonsustained ventricular tachycardia, ≥3 beats at a rate of ≥120 beats per minute).

3. Segmental wall motion abnormalities in the left ventricle in the absence of intraventricular conduction defect

4. Late enhancement (LGE) of nonischemic origin on cardiac magnetic resonance imaging.

5. Evidence of nonischemic myocardial abnormalities (inflammation, necrosis and/or fibrosis) on EMB.

6. Presence of serum organ-specific and disease-specific AHA by one or more autoantibody tests.

Figure 41–14. Diagnostic criteria of HNDC according to the position statement of the ESC on myocardial and pericardial diseases.[3] The 2D-TTE panels show an example of mildly dilated cardiomyopathy with LVEF 48% and LV end-diastolic diameter = 52 mm.

LV dilation, its role in the DCM progression and prognosis. It will be necessary to distinguish within the clinical series also of genetically characterized DCM, the probands from the younger relatives, starting to separate the early or intermediate phenotypes from the clinically overt disease fulfilling the diagnostic criteria of DCM. Often, to increase the sample size of these series, probands with overt disease and relatives with the earlier disease are included, preventing the real predictive role of early disease markers from being highlighted.

The open questions remain numerous. Can prevention of LV remodeling slow the progression of genetically determined CMPs? In the absence of disease-specific drugs, can ACE inhibitors or ARBs or aldosterone antagonists be considered even before (or in combination with) β-blockers as useful for preventing the progression of LV dysfunction or control LV remodeling? The available studies describe the benefits of optimized therapy in DCM, but do not distinguish between specific effects of drugs on remodeling assessed independently of dysfunction and vice versa.

treatments that influence the phenotype independent of the underlying mechanism. However, knowledge gleaned with novel DNA sequencing technologies, biomarkers, and advanced imaging is demonstrating that different causes of DCM call for different diagnostic and treatment strategies. The majority of DCMs have heterogeneous genetic origins, with more than 100 disease genes discovered to date. Other diseases with end-DCM phenotype are phenocopies of genetic DCM; each subtype is opening novel avenues of disease-specific research and paving the way for novel, targeted treatments. Typical examples are uremic cardiomyopathy and CCM. DCM secondary to metabolic diseases or other potentially treatable causes, such as persistent tachycardia, may reverse with the control or treatment of the primary cause. It is time to separate DCM by cause, generating novel nosology and descriptors useful to improve disease-specific and individually tailored monitoring and treatments. Confounding different etiologies in the broad group of phenotypes is an obstacle to the development and delivery of personalized treatment. Cardiomyopathies in general and DCM in particular can generate precise disease models exportable to other cardiovascular diseases.

CONCLUSION

The current descriptive diagnosis of DCM is based on a common end-phenotype that is functionally characterized by systolic dysfunction and LV remodeling with either mild or severe LV dilation. During the course of the last five decades, several different disorders of myriad origins and causes have been categorized as DCM simply based on shared phenotype. This "nosology strategy" was mainly based on the paucity of information about specific causes and pathophysiologic mechanisms of the different types of diseases that could culminate in a DCM phenotype and on the available, overlapping guideline-based

SUMMARY

Definition

- DCM is characterized by dilatation and systolic impairment of the left or both ventricles unexplained by abnormal loading conditions or coronary artery disease sufficient to cause the observed phenotype.

Etiopathogenesis

- Genetic/familial (up to 50%) (FDCM).

- Autoimmune/immune mediated.

- Inflammatory.

- Onco-cardiotoxic, and other cardiotoxic exogenous and endogenous agents.
- Peripartum cardiomyopathy.
- Alcoholic and cirrhotic cardiomyopathy.

Genetics

- Genetically heterogeneous disease.
- Inheritance: autosomal dominant in most cases.
- Disease genes and defects reported to date are associated with DCM code for proteins of the sarcomere, nuclear lamina, intermediate filaments, sarcolemmal membrane, sarcoplasmic and Golgi reticulum, desmosomes, mitochondria.
- Family screening, both clinical and genetic, is a major contributor to the diagnosis of FDCM; early diagnosis in relatives can be framed in the context of the HNDC based upon the combination of major or minor criteria of the ESC.

Diagnosis

- The diagnosis is based upon clinical data and morpho-functional imaging (2D-TTE, with CMR informing about fibrosis). Tissue diagnosis (endomyocardial biopsy) is needed for inflammatory cardiomyopathies; it may confirm the loss of protein expression in genetic DCM such as those associated with *DMD* or *LMNA* gene defects.

Prognosis

- The prognosis of DCM significantly improved in the last few decades with the optimization of medication and devices.
- Early diagnoses and treatments aimed at reverse remodeling of the LV dilation partly explain a better prognosis.
- Fibrosis impacts both arrhythmogenic risk and progression of LV dysfunction, while the impact of different genetic defects is, with a few well-known arrhythmogenic genes now opening the way for future gene-based risk stratification.

Medical and Device Treatment

- Medical and device treatments are as per HF and arrhythmia guidelines, irrespective of the cause and with little decisions taken on the basis of the different cause.
- Immunosuppression can ameliorate DCM in patients with autoimmune/immune-mediated DCM.
- Removal or discontinuation of the acquired toxic agents/cause/triggers or the treatment of the underlying systemic causes may significantly improve acquired DCM.

Surgical Management

- Mitral valve repair for severe functional mitral valve regurgitation is a possible option in selected patients unsuitable for transplantation.
- Heart transplantation is the only cure for end-stage DCM, genetic in particular.
- Liver transplantation can contribute to the improvement of CCM.

REFERENCES

1. Maron BJ, Towbin JA, Thiene G, et al. Contemporary definitions and classification of the cardiomyopathies: an American Heart Association Scientific Statement from the Council on Clinical Cardiology, Heart Failure and Transplantation Committee; Quality of Care and Outcomes Research and Functional Genomics and Translational Biology Interdisciplinary Working Groups; and Council on Epidemiology and Prevention. American Heart Association; Council on Clinical Cardiology, Heart Failure and Transplantation Committee; Quality of Care and Outcomes Research and Functional Genomics and Translational Biology Interdisciplinary Working Groups; Council on Epidemiology and Prevention. *Circulation.* 2006;113:1807-1816.
2. Elliott P, Andersson B, Arbustini E, et al. Classification of the cardiomyopathies: a position statement from the European Society of Cardiology Working Group on Myocardial and Pericardial Diseases. *Eur Heart J.* 2008;29:270-276.
3. Pinto YM, Elliott PM, Arbustini E, et al. Proposal for a revised definition of dilated cardiomyopathy, hypokinetic non-dilated cardiomyopathy, and its implications for clinical practice: a position statement of the ESC working group on myocardial and pericardial diseases. *Eur Heart J.* 2016;37(23):1850-1858.
4. Bozkurt B, Coats A, Tsutsui H. Universal Definition and Classification of Heart Failure. *J Card Fail.* 2021:S1071-9164(21)00050-6.
5. Haas J, Frese KS, Peil B, et al. Atlas of the clinical genetics of human dilated cardiomyopathy. *Eur Heart J.* 2015;36:1123-1135a.
6. Pasqualucci D, Iacovoni A, Palmieri V, et al. Epidemiology of cardiomyopathies: essential context knowledge for a tailored clinical work-up. *Eur J Prev Cardiol.* 2020 Nov 7:zwaa035.
7. Codd MB, Sugrue DD, Gersh BJ, et al. Epidemiology of idiopathic dilated and hypertrophic cardiomyopathy. A population-based study in Olmsted County, Minnesota, 1975-1984. *Circulation.* 1989;80:564-572.
8. Morales A, Hershberger RE. Genetic evaluation of dilated cardiomyopathy. *Curr Cardiol Rep.* 2013;15:375.
9. Baig MK, Goldman JH, Caforio AL, et al. Familial dilated cardiomyopathy: cardiac abnormalities are common in asymptomatic relatives and may represent early disease. *J Am Coll Cardiol.* 1998;31:195-201.
10. Gruenig E, Tasman JA, Kuecherer H, et al. Frequency and phenotypes of familial dilated cardiomyopathy. *J Am Coll Cardiol.* 1998;31:186-194.
11. Gavazzi A, Repetto A, Scelsi L, et al. Evidence-based diagnosis of familial non-X-linked dilated cardiomyopathy. Prevalence, inheritance and characteristics. *Eur Heart J.* 2001;22:73-81.
12. Crispell KA, Hanson EL, Coates K, et al. Periodic rescreening is indicated for family members at risk of developing familial dilated cardiomyopathy. *J Am Coll Cardiol.* 2002;39:1503-1507.
13. Michels VV, Olson TM, Miller FA, et al. Frequency of development of idiopathic dilated cardiomyopathy among relatives of patients with idiopathic dilated cardiomyopathy. *Am J Cardiol.* 2003;91:1389-1392.
14. Repetto A, Serio A, Pasotti M, et al. Rescreening of "healthy" relatives of patients with dilated cardiomyopathy identifies subgroups at risk of developing the disease. *Eur Heart J Suppl.* 2004;6:F54-F60.
15. Mahon NG, Murphy RT, MacRae CA, et al. Echocardiographic evaluation in asymptomatic relatives of patients with dilated cardiomyopathy reveals preclinical disease. *Ann Intern Med.* 2005;143:108-115.
16. Caforio ALP, Mahon NG, Baig MK, et al. Prospective familial assessment in dilated cardiomyopathy: cardiac autoantibodies predict disease development in asymptomatic relatives. *Circulation.* 2007;115:76-83.
17. Brodt C, Siegfried JD, Hofmeyer M, et al. Temporal relationship of conduction system disease and ventricular dysfunction in LMNA cardiomyopathy. *J Card Fail.* 2013;19:233-239.
18. McDonagh TA, Metra M, Adamo M et al. 2021 ESC Guidelines for the diagnosis and treatment of acute and chronic heart failure. Eur Heart J. 2021 Sep 21;42(36):3599-3726. Erratum in: *Eur Heart J.* 2021 Oct 14;.

19. Lang RM, Badano LP, Mor-Avi V, et al. Recommendation for cardiac chamber quantification by echocardiograph in adults: an update from American Society of Echocardiography and the European Association of Cardiovascular Imaging. *J Am Soc Echocardiogr.* 2015;28:1-39.

20. Tsuburaya RS, Uchizumi H, Ueda M, et al. Utility of real-time three-dimensional echocardiography for Duchenne muscular dystrophy with echocardiographic limitations. *Neuromuscul Disord.* 2014;24:402-408.

21. Levy F, Iacuzio L, Schouver ED et al. Performance of a new fully automated transthoracic three-dimensional echocardiographic software for quantification of left cardiac chamber size and function: comparison with 3 Tesla cardiac magnetic resonance. *J Clin Ultrasound.* 2019;47(9):546-554.

22. Shan K, Bick RJ, Poindexter BJ, et al. Relation of tissue Doppler derived myocardial velocities to myocardial structure and beta-adrenergic receptor density in humans. *J Am Coll Cardiol.* 2011;36:891-896.

23. Takamura T, Dohi K, Onishi K, et al. Left ventricular contraction-relaxation coupling in normal, hypertrophic and failing myocardium quantified by speckle-tracking global strain and strain rate imaging. *J Am Soc Echocardiogr.* 2010;23:747-754.

24. Meluzin J, Spinarova L, Hude P, et al. Left ventricular mechanics in idiopathic dilated cardiomyopathy: systolic-diastolic coupling and torsion. *J Am Soc Echocardiogr.* 2009;22:486-493.

25. Jenkins C, Moir S, Chan J, et al. Left ventricular volume measurement with echocardiography: a comparison of left ventricular opacification, three-dimensional echocardiography, or both with magnetic resonance imaging. *Eur Heart J.* 2009;30:98-106.

26. Mada RO, Lysyansky P, Daraban AM, et al. How to define end-diastole and end-systole? Impact of timing on strain measurements. *JACC Cardiovasc Imaging.* 2015;8:148-157.

27. Moody WE, Taylor RJ, Edwards NC, et al. Comparison of magnetic resonance feature tracking for systolic and diastolic strain and strain rate calculation with spatial modulation of magnetization imaging analysis. *J Magn Reson Imaging.* 2015;41:1000-1012.

28. Jan MF, Tajik AJ. Modern imaging techniques in cardiomyopathies. *Circ Res.* 2017;121:874-891.

29. Repetto A, Dal Bello B, Pasotti M, et al. Coronary atherosclerosis in end-stage idiopathic dilated cardiomyopathy: an innocent bystander? *Eur Heart J.* 2005;26:1519-1527.

30. Seferović PM, Polovina M, Bauersachs J, et al. Heart failure in cardiomyopathies: a position paper from the Heart Failure Association of the European Society of Cardiology. *Eur J Heart Fail.* 2019;21(5):553-576.

31. Barison A, Grigoratos C, Todiere G, Aquaro GD. Myocardial interstitial remodelling in non-ischaemic dilated cardiomyopathy: insights from cardiovascular magnetic resonance. *Heart Fail Rev.* 2015;20:731-749.

32. Kallianos K, Moraes GL, Ordovas KG. Prognostic role of MR imaging in non-ischemic myocardial disease. *Magn Reson Imaging Clin N Am.* 2015;23:89-94.

33. Madanieh R, Mathew S, Shah P, et al. Cardiac magnetic resonance imaging might complement two-dimensional echocardiography in the detection of a reversible nonischemic cardiomyopathy. *Clin Med Insights Case Rep.* 2015;8:109-114.

34. Mizia-Stec K, Charron P, Gimeno Blanes JR, et al. Current use of cardiac magnetic resonance in tertiary referral centres for the diagnosis of cardiomyopathy: the ESC EORP Cardiomyopathy/Myocarditis Registry. *Eur Heart J Cardiovasc Imaging.* 2021:jeaa329.

35. Charron P, Arad M, Arbustini E, et al. Genetic counselling and testing in cardiomyopathies: a position statement of the European Society of Cardiology Working Group on Myocardial and Pericardial Diseases. *Eur Heart J.* 2010;31:2715-2726.

36. Rapezzi C, Arbustini E, Caforio ALP, et al. Diagnostic work-up in cardiomyopathies: bridging the gap between clinical phenotypes and final diagnosis. A position statement from the ESC Working Group on Myocardial and Pericardial Diseases. *Eur Heart J.* 2013;34:1448-1458.

37. Arbustini E, Di Toro A, Giuliani L, et al. Cardiac Phenotypes in Hereditary Muscle Disorders: JACC State-of-the-Art Review. *J Am Coll Cardiol.* 2018;72(20):2485-2506.

38. Arbustini E, Narula N, Dec GW, et al. The MOGE(S) classification for a phenotype-genotype nomenclature of cardiomyopathy: endorsed by the World Heart Federation. *J Am Coll Cardiol.* 2014;64:304-318.

39. Brunel-Guitton C, Levtova A, Sasarman F. Mitochondrial diseases and cardiomyopathies. *Can J Cardiol.* 2015;31:1360-1376.

40. Hershberger RE, Givertz MM, Ho CY, et al. Genetic evaluation of cardiomyopathy: a clinical practice resource of the American College of Medical Genetics and Genomics (ACMG). *Genet Med.* 2018;20(9):899-909.

41. Herman DS, Lam L, Taylor MR, et al. Truncations of titin causing dilated cardiomyopathy. *N Engl J Med.* 2012;366:619-628.

42. Akinrinade O, Koskenvuo JW, Alastalo TP. Prevalence of titin truncating variants in general population. *PLoS One.* 2015;10:e0145284.

43. Finsterer J, Stöllberger C, Sehnal E, Rehder H, Laccone F. Dilated, arrhythmogenic cardiomyopathy in Emery-Dreifuss muscular dystrophy due to the emerin splice-site mutation c.449 + 1G>A. *Cardiology.* 2015;130:48-51.

44. Zhou C, Li C, Zhou B, Sun H, et al. Novel nesprin-1 mutations associated with dilated cardiomyopathy cause nuclear envelope disruption and defects in myogenesis. *Hum Mol Genet.* 2017;26(12):2258-2276.

45. Taylor MR, Slavov D, Gajewski A, et al. Familial Cardiomyopathy Registry Research Group. Thymopoietin (lamina-associated polypeptide 2) gene mutation associated with dilated cardiomyopathy. *Hum Mutat.* 2005;26:566-574.

46. Jordan E, Hershberger RE. Considering complexity in the genetic evaluation of dilated cardiomyopathy. *Heart.* 2021;107(2):106-112.

47. Verdonschot JAJ, Vanhoutte EK, Claes GRF, et al. A mutation update for the FLNC gene in myopathies and cardiomyopathies. *Hum Mutat.* 2020;41(6):1091-1111.

48. Brodehl A, Dieding M, Biere N, et al. Functional characterization of the novel DES mutation p.L136P associated with dilated cardiomyopathy reveals a dominant filament assembly defect. *J Mol Cell Cardiol.* 2015;91:207-214.

49. Arbustini E, Diegoli M, Morbini P, et al. Prevalence and characteristics of dystrophin defects in adult male patients with dilated cardiomyopathy. *J Am Coll Cardiol.* 2000;35:1760-1768.

50. Diegoli M, Grasso M, Favalli V, et al. Diagnostic work-up and risk stratification in X-linked dilated cardiomyopathies caused by dystrophin defects. *J Am Coll Cardiol.* 2011;58:925-934.

51. Guimarães-Costa R, Fernández-Eulate G, Wahbi K, et al. Clinical correlations and long-term follow-up in 100 patients with sarcoglycanopathies. *Eur J Neurol.* 2021;28(2):660-669.

52. Sasaki T, Ikeda K, Nakajima T, et al. Multiple arrhythmic and cardiomyopathic phenotypes associated with an SCN5A A735E mutation. *J Electrocardiol.* 2021;65:122-127.

53. Peters S, Johnson R, Birch S, et al. Familial dilated cardiomyopathy. *Heart Lung Circ.* 2020;29(4):566-574.

54. Bienengraeber M, Olson TM, Selivanov VA, et al. ABCC9 mutations identified in human dilated cardiomyopathy disrupt catalytic KATP channel gating. *Nat Genet.* 2004;36:382-387.

55. Arimura T, Hayashi YK, Murakami T, et al. Mutational analysis of fukutin gene in dilated cardiomyopathy and hypertrophic cardiomyopathy. *Circ J.* 2009;73:158-161.

56. Taha K, Te Rijdt WP, Verstraelen TE, et al. Early mechanical alterations in phospholamban mutation carriers: identifying subclinical disease before onset of symptoms. *JACC Cardiovasc Imaging.* 2020:S1936-878X(20)30918-9.

57. Wolf CM, Wang L, Alcalai R, et al. Lamin A/C haploinsufficiency causes dilated cardiomyopathy and apoptosis-triggered cardiac conduction system disease. *J Mol Cell Cardiol.* 2008;44:293-303.

58. Narula N, Favalli V, Tarantino P, et al. Quantitative expression of the mutated lamin A/C gene in patients with cardiolaminopathy. *J Am Coll Cardiol.* 2012;60:1916-1920.

59. Wahbi K. Cardiac involvement in dystrophinopathies. *Arch Pediatr.* 2015;22:12S37-12S41.

60. Moore JR, Leinwand L, Warshaw DM. Understanding cardiomyopathy phenotypes based on the functional impact of mutations in the myosin motor. *Circ Res.* 2012;111:375-385.

61. Zaragoza MV, Fass J, Diegoli M, et al. Mitochondrial DNA variant discovery and evaluation in human cardiomyopathies through next-generation sequencing. *PLoS One.* 2010;5:e12295.

62. van der Zwaag PA, van Rijsingen IA, de Ruiter R, et al. Recurrent and founder mutations in the Netherlands-Phospholamban p.Arg14del mutation causes arrhythmogenic cardiomyopathy. *Neth Heart J.* 2013;21(6):286-293.

63. Richards S, Aziz N, Bale S, et al. Standards and guidelines for the interpretation of sequence variants: a joint consensus recommendation of the American College of Medical Genetics and Genomics and the Association for Molecular Pathology. *Genet Med.* 2015;17(5):405-424.

64. Richmond CM, James PA, Pantaleo SJ, et al. Clinical and laboratory reporting impact of ACMG-AMP and modified ClinGen variant classification frameworks in MYH7-related cardiomyopathy. *Genet Med.* 2021.

65. Mazzarotto F, Tayal U, Buchan RJ, et al. Reevaluating the genetic contribution of monogenic dilated cardiomyopathy. *Circulation.* 2020;141(5):387-398.

66. Di Toro A, Giuliani L, Favalli V, et al. Genetics and clinics: current applications, limitations, and future developments. *Eur Heart J Suppl.* 2019;21(Suppl B):B7-B14.

67. Fatkin D, MacRae C, Sasaki T, et al. Missense mutations in the rod domain of the lamin A/C gene as causes of dilated cardiomyopathy and conduction system disease. *N Engl J Med.* 1999;341:1715-1724.

68. Arbustini E, Pilotto A, Repetto A, et al. Autosomal dominant dilated cardiomyopathy with atrioventricular block: a lamin A/C defect-related disease. *J Am Coll Cardiol.* 2002;39:981-990.

69. Pasotti M, Klersy C, Pilotto A, et al. Long-term outcome and risk stratification in dilated cardiolaminopathies. *J Am Coll Cardiol.* 2008;52:1250-1260.

70. van Rijsingen IAW, Arbustini E, Elliott PM, et al. Risk factors for malignant ventricular arrhythmias in lamin A/C mutation carriers a European cohort study. *J Am Coll Cardiol.* 2012;59:493-500.

71. Disertori M, Quintarelli S, Mazzola S, Favalli V, Narula N, Arbustini E. The need to modify patient selection to improve the benefits of implantable cardioverter-defibrillator for primary prevention of sudden death in non-ischaemic dilated cardiomyopathy. *Europace.* 2013;15:1693-1701.

72. Priori SG, Blomström-Lundqvist C, Mazzanti A, et al. 2015 ESC Guidelines for the management of patients with ventricular arrhythmias and the prevention of sudden cardiac death: The Task Force for the Management of Patients with Ventricular Arrhythmias and the Prevention of Sudden Cardiac Death of the European Society of Cardiology (ESC) Endorsed by: Association for European Paediatric and Congenital Cardiology (AEPC). *Eur Heart J.* 2015;36(41):2793-2867.

73. Captur G, Arbustini E, Bonne G, et al. Lamin and the heart. *Heart.* 2018;104(6):468-479.

74. Captur G, Arbustini E, Syrris P, et al. Lamin mutation location predicts cardiac phenotype severity: combined analysis of the published literature. *Open Heart.* 2018;5(2):e000915.

75. Sammani A, Kayvanpour E, Bosman LP, et al. Predicting sustained ventricular arrhythmias in dilated cardiomyopathy: a meta-analysis and systematic review. *ESC Heart Fail.* 2020;7(4):1430-1441.

76. Muchir A, Worman HJ. Emery-Dreifuss muscular dystrophy: focal point nuclear envelope. *Curr Opin Neurol.* 2019;32(5):728-734.

77. Bonne G, Leturcq F, Ben Yaou R. Emery-Dreifuss muscular dystrophy. 2004 Sept 29 [updated 2015 Nov 25]. In: Pagon RA, Adam MP, Ardinger HH, et al., eds. GeneReviews® [Internet]. Seattle, WA: University of Washington, Seattle; 1993-2016.

78. Lim KRQ, Sheri N, Nguyen Q, Yokota T. Cardiac involvement in dystrophin-deficient females: current understanding and implications for the treatment of dystrophinopathies. *Genes (Basel).* 2020;11(7):765.

79. Milasin J, Muntoni F, Severini GM, et al. A point mutation in the 5' splice site of the dystrophin gene first intron responsible for X-linked dilated cardiomyopathy. *Hum Mol Genet.* 1996;5:73-79.

80. Kimura S, Ikezawa M, Ozasa S, et al. Novel mutation in splicing donor of dystrophin gene first exon in a patient with dilated cardiomyopathy but no clinical signs of skeletal myopathy. *J Child Neurol.* 2007;22:901-906.

81. Franz WM, Cremer M, Herrmann R, et al. X-linked dilated cardiomyopathy. Novel mutation of the dystrophin gene. *Ann N Y Acad Sci.* 1995;752:470-491.

82. Piccolo G, Azan G, Tonin P, et al. Dilated cardiomyopathy requiring cardiac transplantation as initial manifestation of Xp21 Becker type muscular dystrophy. *Neuromuscul Disord.* 1994;4:143-146.

83. Statile CJ, Taylor MD, Mazur W, et al. Left ventricular noncompaction in Duchenne muscular dystrophy. *J Cardiovasc Magn Reson.* 2013;15:67.

84. Kimura K, Takenaka K, Ebihara A, et al. Prognostic impact of left ventricular noncompaction in patients with Duchenne/Becker muscular dystrophy: prospective multicenter cohort study. *Int J Cardiol.* 2013;168: 1900-1904.

85. Iodice F, Testa G, Averardi M, et al. Implantation of a left ventricular assist device as a destination therapy in Duchenne muscular dystrophy patients with end stage cardiac failure: management and lessons learned. *Neuromuscul Disord.* 2015;25:19-23.

86. Ryan TD, Jefferies JL, Sawnani H, et al. Implantation of the HeartMate II and HeartWare left ventricular assist devices in patients with Duchenne muscular dystrophy: lessons learned from the first applications. *ASAIO J.* 2014;60:246-248.

87. Rajdev A, Groh WJ. Arrhythmias in the muscular dystrophies. *Card Electrophysiol Clin.* 2015;7(2):303-308.

88. Bennett J, Kertesz NJ. Management of rhythm disorders in Duchenne muscular dystrophy: is sudden death a cardiac or pulmonary problem? *Pediatr Pulmonol.* 2021;56(4):760-765.

89. Mao Z, Nakamura F. Structure and function of Filamin C in the muscle Z-disc. *Int J Mol Sci.* 2020;21(8):2696.

90. Ortiz-Genga MF, Cuenca S, Dal Ferro M, et al. Truncating FLNC mutations are associated with high-risk dilated and arrhythmogenic cardiomyopathies. *J Am Coll Cardiol.* 2016;68(22):2440-2451.

91. Begay RL, Graw SL, Sinagra G, et al. Filamin C truncation mutations are associated with arrhythmogenic dilated cardiomyopathy and changes in the cell-cell adhesion structures. *JACC Clin Electrophysiol.* 2018;4(4):504-514.

92. Hall CL, Akhtar MM, Sabater-Molina M, et al. Filamin C variants are associated with a distinctive clinical and immunohistochemical arrhythmogenic cardiomyopathy phenotype. *Int J Cardiol.* 2020;307:101-108.

93. Al-Numair NS, Lopes L, Syrris P, et al. The structural effects of mutations can aid in differential phenotype prediction of beta-myosin heavy chain (Myosin-7) missense variants. *Bioinformatics.* 2016;32(19):2947-2955.

94. Aksel T, Choe Yu E, Sutton S, Ruppel KM, Spudich JA. Ensemble force changes that result from human cardiac myosin mutations and a small-molecule effector. *Cell Rep.* 2015;11:910-920.

95. Gupte TM, Haque F, Gangadharan B, et al. Mechanistic heterogeneity in contractile properties of α-tropomyosin (TPM1) mutants associated with inherited cardiomyopathies. *J Biol Chem.* 2015;290:7003-7015.

96. Sommese RF, Nag S, Sutton S, et al. Effects of troponin T cardiomyopathy mutations on the calcium sensitivity of the regulated thin filament and the actomyosin cross-bridge kinetics of human beta-cardiac myosin. *PLoS One.* 2013;8:e83403.

97. Spudich JA, Aksel T, Bartholomew SR, et al. Effects of hypertrophic and dilated cardiomyopathy mutations on power output by human β-cardiac myosin. *J Exp Biol.* 2016;219:161-167.

98. Arbustini E, Fasani R, Morbini P, et al. Coexistence of mitochondrial DNA and beta myosin heavy chain mutations in hypertrophic cardiomyopathy with late congestive heart failure. *Heart.* 1998;80:548-558.

99. McManus MJ, Picard M, Chen HW, et al. Mitochondrial DNA variation dictates expressivity and progression of nuclear DNA mutations causing cardiomyopathy. *Cell Metab.* 2019;29(1):78-90.e5.

100. Verhoeven WM, Egger JI, Kremer BP, de Pont BJ, Marcelis CL. Recurrent major depression, ataxia, and cardiomyopathy: association with a novel POLG mutation? *Neuropsychiatr Dis Treat.* 2011;7:293-296.

101. Ware JS, Cook SA. Role of titin in cardiomyopathy: from DNA variants to patient stratification. *Nat Rev Cardiol*. 2018;15(4):241-252.

102. Ware JS, Li J, Mazaika E, et al. IMAC-2 and IPAC Investigators. Shared genetic predisposition in peripartum and dilated cardiomyopathies. *N Engl J Med*. 2016;374:233-241.

103. Begay RL, Graw S, Sinagra G, et al. Familial cardiomyopathy registry. Role of titin missense variants in dilated cardiomyopathy. *J Am Heart Assoc*. 2015;4:e002645.

104. Savarese M, Sarparanta J, Vihola A, Udd B, Hackman P. Increasing role of titin mutations in neuromuscular disorders. *J Neuromuscul Dis*. 2016;3(3):293-308.

105. Gramlich M, Pane LS, Zhou Q, et al. Antisense-mediated exon skipping: a therapeutic strategy for titin-based dilated cardiomyopathy. *EMBO Mol Med*. 2015;7:562-576.

106. Akhtar MM, Lorenzini M, Cicerchia M, et al. Clinical phenotypes and prognosis of dilated cardiomyopathy caused by truncating variants in the TTN gene. *Circ Heart Fail*. 2020;13(10):e006832.

107. Jansen M, Baas AF, van Spaendonck-Zwarts KY, Ummels AS, et al. Mortality risk associated with truncating founder mutations in titin. *Circ Genom Precis Med*. 2019;12(5):e002436.

108. Young HS, Ceholski DK, Trieber CA. Deception in simplicity: hereditary phospholamban mutations in dilated cardiomyopathy. *Biochem Cell Biol*. 2015;93:1-7.

109. Corrado D, Wichter T, Link MS, et al. Treatment of arrhythmogenic right ventricular cardiomyopathy/dysplasia: an international task force consensus statement. *Circulation*. 2015;132:441–453.

110. Sanoudou D, Kolokathis F, Arvanitis D, et al. Genetic modifiers to the PLN L39X mutation in a patient with DCM and sustained ventricular tachycardia? *Glob Cardiol Sci Pract*. 2015;2015:29.

111. Liu GS, Morales A, Vafiadaki E, et al. A novel human R25C-phospholamban mutation is associated with super-inhibition of calcium cycling and ventricular arrhythmia. *Cardiovasc Res*. 2015;107:164-174.

112. Augusto JB, Eiros R, Nakou E, et al. Dilated cardiomyopathy and arrhythmogenic left ventricular cardiomyopathy: a comprehensive genotype-imaging phenotype study. *Eur Heart J Cardiovasc Imaging*. 2020;21(3):326-336.

113. Smith ED, Lakdawala NK, Papoutsidakis N, et al. Desmoplakin cardiomyopathy, a fibrotic and inflammatory form of cardiomyopathy distinct from typical dilated or arrhythmogenic right ventricular cardiomyopathy. *Circulation*. 2020;141(23):1872-1884.

114. Vatta M, Mohapatra B, Jimenez S, et al. Mutations in Cypher/ZASP in patients with dilated cardiomyopathy and left ventricular non-compaction. *J Am Coll Cardiol*. 2003;42:2014-2027.

115. Lin X, Ruiz J, Bajraktari I, et al. Z-disc-associated, alternatively spliced, PDZ motif-containing protein (ZASP) mutations in the actin-binding domain cause disruption of skeletal muscle actin filaments in myofibrillar myopathy. *J Biol Chem*. 2014;289(19):13615-13626.

116. Stöllberger C, Finsterer J. Understanding left ventricular hypertrabeculation/noncompaction: pathomorphologic findings and prognostic impact of neuromuscular comorbidities. *Expert Rev Cardiovasc Ther*. 2019;17(2):95-109.

117. Cassandrini D, Merlini L, Pilla F, et al. Protein aggregates and autophagy involvement in a family with a mutation in Z-band alternatively spliced PDZ-motif protein. *Neuromuscul Disord*. 2021;31(1):44-51.

118. Levitas A, Konstantino Y, Muhammad E, et al. D117N in Cypher/ZASP may not be a causative mutation for dilated cardiomyopathy and ventricular arrhythmias. *Eur J Hum Genet*. 2016;24(5):666-671.

119. Bozkurt B, Colvin M, Cook J, et al. Current diagnostic and treatment strategies for specific dilated cardiomyopathies: a scientific statement from the American Heart Association. *Circulation*. 2016;134(23):e579-e646.

120. Tönnesmann E, Kandolf R, Lewalter T. Chloroquine cardiomyopathy: a review of the literature. *Immunopharmacol Immunotoxicol*. 2013;35: 434-442.

121. Denton CP, Khanna D. Systemic sclerosis. *Lancet*. 2017;390(10103): 1685-1699.

122. Yokokawa T, Yoshihisa A, Misaka T, et al. Anti-mitochondrial antibodies in patients with dilated cardiomyopathy. *Intern Med*. 2021;60(2):201-208.

123. Smith V, Scirè CA, Talarico R, et al. Systemic sclerosis: state of the art on clinical practice guidelines. *RMD Open*. 2018;4(Suppl 1):e000782.

124. Bruni C, Ross L. Cardiac involvement in systemic sclerosis: Getting to the heart of the matter. *Best Pract Res Clin Rheumatol*. 2021:101668.

125. Prasada S, Rivera A, Nishtala A, et al. Differential associations of chronic inflammatory diseases with incident heart failure. *JACC Heart Fail*. 2020;8(6):489-498.

126. Calderon LM, Pope JE. Scleroderma epidemiology update. *Curr Opin Rheumatol*. 2021;33(2):122-127.

127. Chatzis L, Vlachoyiannopoulos PG, Tzioufas AG, Goules AV. New frontiers in precision medicine for Sjogren's syndrome. *Expert Rev Clin Immunol*. 2021;17(2):127-141.

128. van den Hoogen F, Khanna D, Fransen J, et al. 2013 classification criteria for systemic sclerosis: an American College of Rheumatology/European League Against Rheumatism Collaborative Initiative. *Ann Rheum Dis*. 2013;72:1747-1755.

129. Moore DF, Steen VD. Racial disparities in systemic sclerosis. *Rheum Dis Clin North Am*. 2020;46(4):705-712.

130. Ouchene L, Muntyanu A, Lavoué J, et al. Toward understanding of environmental risk factors in systemic sclerosis. *J Cutan Med Surg*. 2020.

131. Kurteva EK, Boyadzhieva VV, Stoilov NR. Systemic sclerosis in mother and daughter with susceptible HLA haplotype and anti-topoisomerase I autoantibodies. *Rheumatol Int*. 2020;40(6):1001-1009.

132. Abbot S, Bossingham D, Proudman S, et al. Risk factors for the development of systemic sclerosis: a systematic review of the literature. *Rheumatol Adv Pract*. 2018;2(2):rky041.

133. Orvain C, Assassi S, Avouac J, Allanore Y. Systemic sclerosis pathogenesis: contribution of recent advances in genetics. *Curr Opin Rheumatol*. 2020;32(6):505-514.

134. Chairta P, Nicolaou P, Christodoulou K. Genomic and genetic studies of systemic sclerosis: a systematic review. *Hum Immunol*. 2017;78(2): 153-165.

135. Di Cristofaro J, Karlmark KR, Kanaan SB, et al. Soluble HLA-G expression inversely correlates with fetal microchimerism levels in peripheral blood from women with scleroderma. *Front Immunol*. 2018;14;9:1685.

136. Artlett CM, Smith JB, Jimenez SA. Identification of fetal DNA and cells in skin lesions from women with systemic sclerosis. *N Engl J Med*. 1998;338:1186-1191.

137. Marder W, Somers EC. Is pregnancy a risk factor for rheumatic autoimmune diseases? *Curr Opin Rheumatol*. 2014;26:321-328.

138. Hung G, Mercurio V, Hsu S, et al. Progress in understanding, diagnosing, and managing cardiac complications of systemic sclerosis. *Curr Rheumatol Rep*. 2019;21(12):68.

139. Mohameden M, Vashisht P, Sharman T. Scleroderma and primary myocardial disease. 2020. In: StatPearls [Internet]. Treasure Island (FL): StatPearls Publishing; 2021.

140. Fernandez-Codina A, Simein-Aznar CP, Pinal-Fernandez I, et al. Cardiac involvement in systemic sclerosis: differences between clinical subsets and influence on survival. *Rheumatol Int*. 2015 October 25. doi: 10.1007/ s00296-015-3382-2.

141. Asano Y, Sato S. Vasculopathy in scleroderma. *Semin Immunopathol*. 2015;37:489-500.

142. Sandmeier B, Jäger VK, Nagy G, et al. Autopsy versus clinical findings in patients with systemic sclerosis in a case series from patients of the EUSTAR database. *Clin Exp Rheumatol*. 2015;33:S75-S79.

143. Ishizaki Y, Ooka S, Doi S, et al. Treatment of myocardial fibrosis in systemic sclerosis with tocilizumab. *Rheumatology (Oxford)*. 2020:keaa865.

144. Rodríguez-Reyna TS, Morelos-Guzman M, Hernández-Reyes P, et al. Assessment of myocardial fibrosis and microvascular damage in systemic sclerosis by magnetic resonance imaging and coronary angiotomography. *Rheumatology*. 2015;54:647-654.

145. Fernández Morales A, Iniesta N, Fernández-Codina A, et al. Cardiac tamponade and severe pericardial effusion in systemic sclerosis: report of nine patients and review of the literature. *Int J Rheum Dis.* 2017;20(10):1582-1592.

146. Ciechomska M, Skalska U. Targeting interferons as a strategy for systemic sclerosis treatment. *Immunol Lett.* 2018;195:45-54.

147. Koivuniemi R, Paimela L, Suomalainen R, et al. Cardiovascular diseases in patients with rheumatoid arthritis. *Scand J Rheumatol.* 2013;42:131-135.

148. Corrao S, Messina S, Pistone G, et al. Heart involvement in rheumatoid arthritis: systematic review and meta-analysis. *Int J Cardiol.* 2013;167:2031-2038.

149. Yiu KH, Wang S, Mok MY, et al. Relationship between cardiac valvular and arterial calcification in patients with rheumatoid arthritis and systemic lupus erythematosus. *J Rheumatol.* 2011;38:621-627.

150. Khalid Y, Dasu N, Shah A, et al. Incidence of congestive heart failure in rheumatoid arthritis: a review of literature and meta-regression analysis. *ESC Heart Fail.* 2020;7(6):3745-3753.

151. Mokotedi L, Gunter S, Robinson C, et al. Early wave reflection and pulse wave velocity are associated with diastolic dysfunction in rheumatoid arthritis. *J Cardiovasc Transl Res.* 2019;12(6):580-590.

152. Mavrogeni SI, Markousis-Mavrogenis G, Kolovou GD. Cardiac disease in rheumatoid arthritis—can cardiovascular magnetic resonance imaging depict the Janus duality? *J Rheumatol.* 2018;45(8):1073-1074.

153. Davis J, Knutson K, Strausbauch M, et al. Signature of aberrant immune responsiveness identifies myocardial dysfunction in rheumatoid arthritis. *Arthritis Rheum.* 2011;63:1497-1506.

154. Geraldino-Pardilla L, Russo C, Sokolove J, et al. Association of anti-citrullinated protein or peptide antibodies with left ventricular structure and function in rheumatoid arthritis. *Rheumatology (Oxford).* 2017;56(4): 534-540.

155. Joyce E, Fabre A, Mahon N. Hydroxychloroquine cardiotoxicity presenting as a rapidly evolving biventricular cardiomyopathy. *Eur Heart J Acute Cardiovasc Care.* 2013;2:77.

156. Nadeem U, Raafey M, Kim G, et al. Chloroquine- and hydroxychloroquine-induced cardiomyopathy: a case report and brief literature review. *Am J Clin Pathol.* 2020;14:aqaa253.

157. Wakfie-Corieh CG, Ramos López N, Saiz-Pardo Sanz M, et al. Not all heart uptakes on 99mTc-DPD scintigraphy are amyloidosis: chloroquine-induced cardiomyopathy. *Clin Nucl Med.* 2021;46(4):e188-e189.

158. Generali E, Carrara G, Kallikourdis M, et al. Risk of hospitalization for heart failure in rheumatoid arthritis patients treated with etanercept and abatacept. *Rheumatol Int.* 2019;39(2):239-243.

159. Singh JA, Saag KG, Bridges SL Jr, et al. 2015 American College of Rheumatology guideline for the treatment of rheumatoid arthritis. *Arthritis Rheumatol.* 2016;68:1-26.

160. Okuda Y, Yamada T, Ueda M, Ando Y. First nationwide survey of 199 patients with amyloid A amyloidosis in Japan. *Intern Med.* 2018;57(23): 3351-3355.

161. Løgstrup BB, Ellingsen T, Pedersen AB, et al. Cardiovascular risk and mortality in rheumatoid arthritis compared with diabetes mellitus and the general population. *Rheumatology (Oxford).* 2021;60(3):1400-1409.

162. Halacoglu J, Shea LA. Cardiovascular risk assessment and therapeutic implications in rheumatoid arthritis. *J Cardiovasc Transl Res.* 2020;13(5):878-890.

163. Guevara M, Ng B. Positive effect of hydroxychloroquine on lipid profiles of patients with rheumatoid arthritis: a Veterans Affair cohort. *Eur J Rheumatol.* 2020;8(2):62-66.

164. van Sijl AM, Peters MJ, Knol DL, et al. The effect of TNF-α blocking therapy on lipid levels in rheumatoid arthritis: a meta-analysis. *Semin Arthritis Rheum.* 2011;41:393-400.

165. Svensson AL, Christensen R, Persson F et al. Multifactorial intervention to prevent cardiovascular disease in patients with early rheumatoid arthritis: protocol for a multicentre randomised controlled trial. *BMJ Open.* 2016;6(4):e009134.

166. De Vera MA, Choi H, Abrahamowicz M, et al. Statin discontinuation and risk of acute myocardial infarction in patients with rheumatoid arthritis: a population-based cohort study. *Ann Rheum Dis.* 2011;70:1020-1024.

167. Weinblatt ME, Kremer J, Cush J, et al. Tocilizumab as monotherapy or in combination with nonbiologic disease-modifying antirheumatic drugs: twenty-four-week results of an open-label, clinical practice study. *Arthritis Care Res.* 2013;65:362-371.

168. Miner JJ, Kim AH. Cardiac manifestations of systemic lupus erythematosus. *Rheum Dis Clin North Am.* 2014;40(1):51-60.

169. Pearce FA, Rutter M, Sandhu R, et al. BSR guideline on the management of adults with systemic lupus erythematosus (SLE) 2018: baseline multicentre audit in the UK. *Rheumatology (Oxford).* 2021;60(3):1480-1490.

170. Aringer M, Costenbader K, Daikh D, et al. 2019 European League Against Rheumatism/American College of Rheumatology classification criteria for systemic lupus erythematosus. *Ann Rheum Dis.* 2019;78(9):1151-1159.

171. Gusetu G, Pop D, Pamfil C, et al. Subclinical myocardial impairment in SLE: insights from novel ultrasound techniques and clinical determinants. *Med Ultrason.* 2016;18:47-56.

172. Yurkovich M, Vostretsova K, Chen W, Aviña-Zubieta JA. Overall and cause-specific mortality in patients with systemic lupus erythematosus: a meta-analysis of observational studies. *Arthritis Care Res (Hoboken).* 2014;66:608-616.

173. Izmirly PM, Parton H, Wang L, et al. Prevalence of systemic lupus erythematosus in the United States: estimates from a meta-analysis of the Centers for Disease Control and Prevention National Lupus Registries. *Arthritis Rheumatol.* 2021;73(6):991-996.

174. Charras A, Smith E, Hedrich CM. Systemic lupus erythematosus in children and young people. *Curr Rheumatol Rep.* 2021;23(3):20.

175. Kovats S. Estrogen receptors regulate innate immune cells and signaling pathways. *Cell Immunol.* 2015;294:63-69.

176. Priyanka HP, Krishnan HC, Singh RV, Hima L, Thyagarajan S. Estrogen modulates in vitro T cell responses in a concentration- and receptor-dependent manner: effects on intracellular molecular targets and antioxidant enzymes. *Mol Immunol.* 2013;56:328-239.

177. Hill L, Jeganathan V, Chinnasamy P, Grimaldi C, Diamond B. Differential roles of estrogen receptors α and β in control of B-cell maturation and selection. *Mol Med.* 2011;17:211-220.

178. Chung SA, Nititham J, Elboudwarej E, et al. Genome-wide assessment of differential DNA methylation associated with autoantibody production in systemic lupus erythematosus. *PLoS One.* 2015;10:e0129813.

179. Alarcón-Riquelme ME, Ziegler JT, Molineros J, Howard TD, et al. Genome-wide association study in an Amerindian ancestry population reveals novel systemic lupus erythematosus risk loci and the role of European admixture. *Arthritis Rheumatol.* 2016;68(4):932-943.

180. Lee YH, Bae SC. Association between a functional HLA-G 14-bp insertion/deletion polymorphism and susceptibility to autoimmune diseases: a meta-analysis. *Cell Mol Biol.* 2015;61:24-30.

181. Durrance RJ, Movahedian M, Haile W, et al. Systemic lupus erythematosus presenting as myopericarditis with acute heart failure: a case report and literature review. *Case Rep Rheumatol.* 2019;2019:6173276.

182. Appleton BD, Major AS. The latest in systemic lupus erythematosus-accelerated atherosclerosis: related mechanisms inform assessment and therapy. *Curr Opin Rheumatol.* 2021;33(2):211-218.

183. Awan Z, Genest J. Inflammation modulation and cardiovascular disease prevention. *Eur J Prev Cardiol.* 2015;22:719-733.

184. Ballocca F, D'ascenzo F, Moretti C, et al. Predictors of cardiovascular events in patients with systemic lupus erythematosus (SLE): a systematic review and meta-analysis. *Eur J Prev Cardiol.* 2015;22:1435-1441.

185. Ward NKZ, Linares-Koloffon C, Posligua A, et al. Cardiac manifestations of systemic lupus erythematous: an overview of the incidence, risk factors, diagnostic criteria, pathophysiology and treatment options. *Cardiol Rev.* 2020 Sep 4. doi: 10.1097/CRD.0000000000000358

186. Frerix M, Stegbauer J, Kreuter A, Weiner SM. Atherosclerotic plaques occur in absence of intima-media thickening in both systemic sclerosis

and systemic lupus erythematosus: a duplex sonography study of carotid and femoral arteries and follow-up for cardiovascular events. *Arthritis Res Ther.* 2014;16:R54.

187. Varma N, Hinojar R, D'Cruz D, et al. Coronary vessel wall contrast enhancement imaging as a potential direct marker of coronary involvement: integration of findings from CAD and SLE patients. *JACC Cardiovasc Imaging.* 2014;7:762-770.

188. Jain D, Halushka MK. Cardiac pathology of systemic lupus erythematosus. *J Clin Pathol.* 2009;62:584-592.

189. Seneviratne MG, Grieve SM, Figtree GA, et al. Prevalence, distribution and clinical correlates of myocardial fibrosis in systemic lupus erythematosus: a cardiac magnetic resonance study. *Lupus.* 2016;25(6): 573-581.

190. Aringer M, Brinks R, Dörner T, et al. European League Against Rheumatism (EULAR)/American College of Rheumatology (ACR) SLE classification criteria item performance. *Ann Rheum Dis.* 2021 Feb 10. doi: 10.1136/annrheumdis-2020-219373

191. Sliwa K, Petrie MC, Hilfiker-Kleiner D, et al. Long-term prognosis, subsequent pregnancy, contraception and overall management of peripartum cardiomyopathy: practical guidance paper from the Heart Failure Association of the European Society of Cardiology Study Group on Peripartum Cardiomyopathy. *Eur J Heart Fail.* 2018;20(6):951-962.

192. Bauersachs J, König T, van der Meer P, et al. Pathophysiology, diagnosis and management of peripartum cardiomyopathy: a position statement from the Heart Failure Association of the European Society of Cardiology Study Group on peripartum cardiomyopathy. *Eur J Heart Fail.* 2019;21(7):827-843.

193. Kolte D, Khera S, Aronow WS, et al. Temporal trends in incidence and outcomes of peripartum cardiomyopathy in the United States: a nationwide population-based study. *J Am Heart Assoc.* 2014;3:e001056.

194. Davis MB, Arany Z, McNamara DM et al. Peripartum Cardiomyopathy: JACC State-of-the-Art Review. *J Am Coll Cardiol.* 2020;75(2): 207-221.

195. Grixti S, Magri CJ, Xuereb R, Fava S. Peripartum cardiomyopathy. *Br J Hosp Med (Lond).* 2015;76:95-100.

196. Hameed AB, Lawton ES, McCain CL, et al. Pregnancy-related cardiovascular deaths in California: beyond peripartum cardiomyopathy. *Am J Obstet Gynecol.* 2015;213:379.e1-e10.

197. Jha N, Jha AK. Peripartum cardiomyopathy. *Heart Fail Rev.* 2021;26(4): 781-797.

198. van Spaendonck-Zwarts KY, Posafalvi A, van den Berg MP, et al. Titin gene mutations are common in families with both peripartum cardiomyopathy and dilated cardiomyopathy. *Eur Heart J.* 2014;35:2165-2173.

199. Melchiorre K, Sharma R, Thilaganathan B. Cardiac structure and function in normal pregnancy. *Curr Opin Obstet Gynecol.* 2012;24:413-421.

200. Gad MM, Elgendy IY, Mahmoud AN, et al. Disparities in cardiovascular disease outcomes among pregnant and post-partum women. *J Am Heart Assoc.* 2021;5;10(1):e017832.

201. Karaye KM, Sa'idu H, Balarabe SA, et al. Selenium supplementation in patients with peripartum cardiomyopathy: a proof-of-concept trial. *BMC Cardiovasc Disord.* 2020;20(1):457.

202. Karaye KM, Yahaya IA, Lindmark K, Henein MY. Serum selenium and ceruloplasmin in Nigerians with peripartum cardiomyopathy. *Int J Mol Sci.* 2015;16:7644-7654.

203. Choolani M, Mahyuddin AP, Hahn S. The promise of fetal cells in maternal blood. *Best Pract Res Clin Obstet Gynaecol.* 2012;26:655-667.

204. Nelson JL. The otherness of self: microchimerism in health and disease. *Trends Immunol.* 2012;33:421-427.

205. Rak JM, Maestroni L, Balandraud N, et al. Transfer of the shared epitope through microchimerism in women with rheumatoid arthritis. *Arthritis Rheum.* 2009;60:73-80.

206. Fu J, Ling S, Liu Y, et al. A small shared epitope-mimetic compound potently accelerates osteoclast-mediated bone damage in autoimmune arthritis. *J Immunol.* 2013;191:2096-2103.

207. Hilfiker-Kleiner D, Kaminski K, Podewski E, et al. A cathepsin D-cleaved 16 kDa form of prolactin mediates postpartum cardiomyopathy. *Cell.* 2007;128:589-600.

208. Ricke-Hoch M, Bultmann I, Stapel B, et al. Opposing roles of Akt and STAT3 in the protection of the maternal heart from peripartum stress. *Cardiovasc Res.* 2014;101:587-596.

209. Hilfiker-Kleiner D, Haghikia A, Berliner D, et al. Bromocriptine for the treatment of peripartum cardiomyopathy: a multicentre randomized study. *Eur Heart J.* 2017;38(35):2671-2679.

210. Lampert MB, Hibbard J, Weinert L, et al. Peripartum heart failure associated with prolonged tocolytic therapy. *Am J Obstet Gynecol.* 1993;168: 493-495.

211. Regitz-Zagrosek V, Roos-Hesselink JW, Bauersachs J, et al. 2018 ESC guidelines for the management of cardiovascular diseases during pregnancy: the task force for the management of cardiovascular diseases during pregnancy of the European Society of Cardiology (ESC). *Eur Heart J.* 2018:3165-3241.

212. Yancy CW, Jessup M, Bozkurt B, et al. 2017 ACC/AHA/HFSA Focused Update of the 2013 ACCF/AHA guideline for the management of heart failure: a report of the American College of Cardiology/American Heart Association Task Force on Clinical Practice Guidelines and the Heart Failure Society of America. *J Card Fail.* 2017;23(8):628-651.

213. Polifka JE. Is there an embryopathy associated with first-trimester exposure to angiotensin-converting enzyme inhibitors and angiotensin receptor antagonists? A critical review of the evidence. *Birth Defects Res A Clin Mol Teratol.* 2012;94:576-598.

214. Blauwet LA, Cooper LT. Diagnosis and management of peripartum cardiomyopathy. *Heart.* 2011;97(23):1970-1981.

215. Goland S, Modi K, Hatamizadeh P, Elkayam U. Differences in clinical profile of African-American women with peripartum cardiomyopathy in the United States. *J Card Fail.* 2013;19:214-218.

216. Blauwet LA, Libhaber E, Forster O, et al. Predictors of outcome in 176 South African patients with peripartum cardiomyopathy. *Heart.* 2013;99:308-313.

217. McNamara DM, Elkayam U, Alharethi R, et al. Clinical outcomes for peripartum cardiomyopathy in North America: results of the Investigations of Pregnancy Associated Cardiomyopathy (IPAC) study. *J Am Coll Cardiol.* 2015;66:905-914.

218. Haghikia A, Podewski E, Libhaber E, et al. Phenotyping and outcome on contemporary management in a German cohort of patients with peripartum cardiomyopathy. *Basic Res Cardiol.* 2013;108:366.

219. Fagrell B, De Faire U, Bondy S, et al. The effects of light to moderate drinking on cardiovascular diseases. *J Intern Med.* 1999;246:331-340.

220. Klatsky AL. Alcohol and cardiovascular diseases: where do we stand today? *J Intern Med.* 2015;278:238-250.

221. Guzzo-Merello G, Segovia J, Dominguez F, et al. Natural history and prognostic factors in alcoholic cardiomyopathy. *JACC Heart Fail.* 2015;3(1):78-86.

222. Marchi KC, Muniz JJ, Tirapelli CR. Hypertension and chronic ethanol consumption: what do we know after a century of study? *World J Cardiol.* 2014;6:283-294.

223. Roerecke M, Rehm J. Alcohol consumption, drinking patterns, and ischemic heart disease: a narrative review of meta-analyses and a systematic review and meta-analysis of the impact of heavy drinking occasions on risk for moderate drinkers. *BMC Med.* 2014;12:182.

224. Jimenez M, Chiuve SE, Glynn RJ, et al. Alcohol consumption and risk of stroke in women. *Stroke.* 2012;43:939-945.

225. Urbano-Marquez A, Estrich R, Navarro-Lopez F, Grau JM, Rubin E. Effects of alcohol on cardiac and skeletal muscle. *N Engl J Med.* 1989;320: 409-415.

226. Gavazzi A, De Maria R, Parolini M, Porcu M. Alcohol abuse and dilated cardiomyopathy in men. *Am J Cardiol.* 2000;85:1114-1118.

227. Fauchier L, Babuty D, Poret P, et al. Comparison of long-term outcome of alcoholic and idiopathic dilated cardiomyopathy. *Eur Heart J.* 2000;21:306-314.

228. Varga ZV, Ferdinandy P, Liaudet L, Pacher P. Drug-induced mitochondrial dysfunction and cardiotoxicity. *Am J Physiol Heart Circ Physiol.* 2015;309:H1453-H1467.

229. Mátyás C, Varga ZV, Mukhopadhyay P, et al. Chronic plus binge ethanol feeding induces myocardial oxidative stress, mitochondrial and cardiovascular dysfunction and steatosis. *Am J Physiol Heart Circ Physiol.* 2016;310(11):H1658-H1670.

230. Ware JS, Amor-Salamanca A, Tayal U, et al. Genetic etiology for alcohol-induced cardiac toxicity. *J Am Coll Cardiol.* 2018;71(20):2293-2302.

231. Milić S, Lulić D, Štimac D, Ružić A, Zaputović L. Cardiac manifestations in alcoholic liver disease. *Postgrad Med J.* 2016;92(1086):235-239.

232. Ruiz-del-Árbol L, Serradilla R. Cirrhotic cardiomyopathy. *World J Gastroenterol.* 2015;21:11502-11521.

233. Ruíz-del-Árbol L, Achécar L, Serradilla R, et al. Diastolic dysfunction is a predictor of poor outcomes in patients with cirrhosis, portal hypertension, and a normal creatinine. *Hepatology.* 2013;58:1732-1741.

234. Izzy M, VanWagner LB, Lin G, et al. Cirrhotic cardiomyopathy consortium. redefining cirrhotic cardiomyopathy for the modern era. *Hepatology.* 2020;71(1):334-345.

235. Sarwar A, Esparaz AM, Chakrala N, et al. Efficacy of TIPS reduction for refractory hepatic encephalopathy, right heart failure, and liver dysfunction. *AJR Am J Roentgenol.* 2021:1-6.

236. Cazzaniga M, Salerno F, Pagnozzi G, et al. Diastolic dysfunction is associated with poor survival in cirrhotic patients with transjugular intrahepatic portosystemic shunt. *Gut.* 2007;56:869-875.

237. Carvalheiro F, Rodrigues C, Adrego T, et al. Diastolic dysfunction in liver cirrhosis: prognostic predictor in liver transplantation? *Transplant Proc.* 2016;48:128-131.

238. Dowsley TF, Bayne DB, Langnas AN, et al. Diastolic dysfunction in patients with end-stage liver disease is associated with development of heart failure early after liver transplantation. *Transplantation.* 2012;94:646-651.

239. Izzy M, Soldatova A, Sun X, et al. Cirrhotic cardiomyopathy predicts post-transplant cardiovascular disease: revelations of the new diagnostic criteria. *Liver Transpl.* 2021;27(6):876-886.

240. Fouad TR, Abdel-Razek WM, Burak KW, Bain VG, Lee SS. Prediction of cardiac complications after liver transplantation. *Transplantation.* 2009;87:763-770.

241. EASL Clinical Practice Guidelines: liver transplantation. *J Hepatol.* 2016;64:433-485.

242. Karagiannakis DS, Vlachogiannakos J, Anastasiadis G, Vafiadis-Zouboulis I, Ladas SD. Frequency and severity of cirrhotic cardiomyopathy and its possible relationship with bacterial endotoxemia. *Dig Dis Sci.* 2013;58:3029-3036.

243. Baldassarre M, Giannone FA, Napoli L. The endocannabinoid system in advanced liver cirrhosis: pathophysiological implication and future perspectives. *Liver Int.* 2013;33:1298-1308.

244. Mousavi K, Niknahad H, Ghalamfarsa A, et al. Taurine mitigates cirrhosis-associated heart injury through mitochondrial-dependent and antioxidative mechanisms. *Clin Exp Hepatol.* 2020;6(3):207-219.

245. Gassanov N, Caglayan E, Semmo N, Massenkeil G, Er F. Cirrhotic cardiomyopathy: a cardiologist's perspective. *World J Gastroenterol.* 2014;20:15492-15498.

246. Escobar B, Taurá P, Martínez-Palli G, et al. Stroke volume response to liver graft reperfusion stress in cirrhotic patients. *World J Surg.* 2014;38:927-935.

247. Wiese S, Hove JD, Møller S. Cardiac imaging in patients with chronic liver disease. *Clin Physiol Funct Imaging.* 2017;37(4):347-356.

248. Sampaio F, Lamata P, Bettencourt N, et al. Assessment of cardiovascular physiology using dobutamine stress cardiovascular magnetic resonance reveals impaired contractile reserve in patients with cirrhotic cardiomyopathy. *J Cardiovasc Magn Reson.* 2015;17:61.

249. Zardi EM, Zardi DM, Chin D, Sonnino C, Dobrina A, Abbate A. Cirrhotic cardiomyopathy in the pre- and post-liver transplantation phase. *J Cardiol.* 2016;67:125-130.

250. Khan MF, Movahed MR. Obesity cardiomyopathy and systolic function: obesity is not independently associated with dilated cardiomyopathy. *Heart Fail Rev.* 2013;18:207-217.

251. Huizar JF, Ellenbogen KA, Tan AY, Kaszala K. Arrhythmia-induced cardiomyopathy: JACC State-of-the-Art Review. *J Am Coll Cardiol.* 2019;73(18):2328-2344.

252. Kavanaugh M, McDivitt J, Philip A, et al. Cardiomyopathy induced by sinus tachycardia in combat wounded: a case study. *Mil Med.* 2014;179:e1062-e1064.

253. Mueller KAL, Heinzmann D, Klingel K et al. Histopathological and immunological characteristics of tachycardia-induced cardiomyopathy. *J Am Coll Cardiol.* 2017;69(17):2160-2172.

254. Gupta S, Figueredo VM. Tachycardia mediated cardiomyopathy: pathophysiology, mechanisms, clinical features and management. *Int J Cardiol.* 2014;172:40-46.

255. Ellis ER, Josephson ME. What about tachycardia-induced cardiomyopathy? *Arrhythm Electrophysiol Rev.* 2013;2:82-90.

256. Hékimian G, Paulo N, Waintraub X, et al. Arrhythmia-induced cardiomyopathy: a potentially reversible cause of refractory cardiogenic shock requiring venoarterial extracorporeal membrane oxygenation. *Heart Rhythm.* 2021:S1547-5271(21)00206-X.

257. Hasdemir C, Kartal Y, Sımsek E, Yavuzgıl O, Aydın M, Can LH. Time course of recovery of left ventricular systolic dysfunction in patients with premature ventricular contraction-induced cardiomyopathy. *Pacing Clin Electrophysiol.* 2013;36:612-617.

258. Panizo JG, Barra S, Mellor G, et al. Premature ventricular complex-induced cardiomyopathy. *Arrhythm Electrophysiol Rev.* 2018;7(2):128-134.

259. Niwano S, Wakisaka Y, Niwano H, et al. Prognostic significance of frequent premature ventricular contractions originating from the ventricular outflow tract in patients with normal left ventricular function. *Heart.* 2009;95:1230-1237.

260. Dukes JW, Dewland TA, Vittinghoff E, et al. Ventricular ectopy as a predictor of heart failure and death. *J Am Coll Cardiol.* 2015;66:101-109.

261. Zhong L, Lee YH, Huang XM, et al. Relative efficacy of catheter ablation vs antiarrhythmic drugs in treating premature ventricular contractions: a single-center retrospective study. *Heart Rhythm.* 2014;11:187-193.

262. Yokokawa M, Good E, Crawford T, et al. Recovery from left ventricular dysfunction after ablation of frequent premature ventricular complexes. *Heart Rhythm.* 2013;10:172-175.

263. Spector ZZ, Seslar SP. Premature ventricular contraction-induced cardiomyopathy in children. *Cardiol Young.* 2015;17:1-7.

264. Ahmad SA, Brito D, Khalid N, Ibrahim MA. Takotsubo cardiomyopathy. 2021. In: StatPearls [Internet]. Treasure Island (FL): StatPearls Publishing; 2021.

265. Sharkey SW, Maron BJ. Epidemiology and clinical profile of Takotsubo cardiomyopathy. *Circ J.* 2014;78:2119-2128.

266. Pelliccia F, Parodi G, Greco C, et al. Comorbidities frequency in Takotsubo syndrome: an international collaborative systematic review including 1109 patients. *Am J Med.* 2015;128:654.e11-e19.

267. Desai SK, Shinbane J, Das JR, Mirocha J, Dohad S. Takotsubo cardiomyopathy: clinical characteristics and outcomes. *Rev Cardiovasc Med.* 2015;16:244-252.

268. Mosca S, Paolillo S, Colao A, et al. Cardiovascular involvement in patients affected by acromegaly: an appraisal. *Int J Cardiol.* 2013;167:1712-1718.

269. Lombardi G, Di Somma C, Grasso LF, Savanelli MC, Colao A, Pivonello R. The cardiovascular system in growth hormone excess and growth hormone deficiency. *J Endocrinol Invest.* 2012;35:1021-1029.

270. McCabe J, Ayuk J, Sherlock M. Treatment factors that influence mortality in acromegaly. *Neuroendocrinology.* 2016;103:66-74.

271. Vargas-Uricoechea H, Sierra-Torres CH. Thyroid hormones and the heart. *Horm Mol Biol Clin Investig.* 2014;18:15-26.

272. Seol MD, Lee YS, Kim DK, et al. Dilated cardiomyopathy secondary to hypothyroidism: case report with a review of literatures. *J Cardiovasc Ultrasound.* 2014;22:32-35.

273. Goldberg MD, Vadera N, Yandrapalli S, Frishman WH. Acromegalic cardiomyopathy: an overview of risk factors, clinical manifestations, and therapeutic options. *Cardiol Rev.* 2018;26(6):307-311.

274. Chanson P. The heart in growth hormone (GH) deficiency and the cardiovascular effects of GH. *Ann Endocrinol (Paris).* 2020: S0003-4266(20)30040-8.

275. Ziagaki A, Blaschke D, Haverkamp W, Plöckinger U. Long-term growth hormone (GH) replacement of adult GH deficiency (GHD) benefits the heart. *Eur J Endocrinol.* 2019;181(1):79-91.

276. Khan R, Sikanderkhel S, Gui J, et al. Thyroid and cardiovascular disease: a focused review on the impact of hyperthyroidism in heart failure. *Cardiol Res.* 2020;11(2):68-75.

277. Inami T, Seino Y, Goda H, et al. Acute pericarditis: unique comorbidity of thyrotoxic crisis with Graves' disease. *Int J Cardiol.* 2014;171:e129-e130.

278. Modarresi M, Amro A, Amro M, et al. Management of cardiogenic shock due to thyrotoxicosis: a systematic literature review. *Curr Cardiol Rev.* 2020;16(4):326-332.

279. Kwaku MP, Burman KD. Myxedema coma. *J Intensive Care Med.* 2007;22(4): 224-231.

280. Jonklaas J, Bianco AC, Bauer AJ, et al. Guidelines for the treatment of hypothyroidism: prepared by the American thyroid association task force on thyroid hormone replacement. *Thyroid.* 2014;24(12):1670-751.

281. Elshimy G, Correa R. Myxedema. 2020. In: StatPearls [Internet]. Treasure Island (FL): StatPearls Publishing; 2021.

282. de Albuquerque Suassuna PG, Sanders-Pinheiro H, de Paula RB. Uremic cardiomyopathy: a new piece in the chronic kidney disease-mineral and bone disorder puzzle. *Front Med (Lausanne).* 2018;5:206.

283. Nik-Akhtar B, Khonsari H, Hesabi A, Khakpour M. Uremic cardiomyopathy in hemodialysis patients. *Angiology.* 1978;29(10):758-763.

284. Alhaj E, Alhaj N, Rahman I, Niazi TO, Berkowitz R, Klapholz M. Uremic cardiomyopathy: an underdiagnosed disease. *Congest Heart Fail.* 2013;19:E40-E45.

285. Chinnappa S, Hothi SS, Tan LB. Is uremic cardiomyopathy a direct consequence of chronic kidney disease? *Expert Rev Cardiovasc Ther.* 2014;12: 127-130.

286. Gansevoort RT, Correa-Rotter R, Hemmelgarn BR, et al. Chronic kidney disease and cardiovascular risk: epidemiology, mechanisms, and prevention. *Lancet.* 2013;382:339-352.

287. Kawarazaki W, Fujita T. Kidney and epigenetic mechanisms of salt-sensitive hypertension. *Nat Rev Nephrol.* 2021.

288. Grabner A, Faul C. The role of fibroblast growth factor 23 and Klotho in uremic cardiomyopathy. *Curr Opin Nephrol Hypertens.* 2016;25(4):314-324.

289. Memmos E, Papagianni A. New insights into the role of FGF-23 and klotho in cardiovascular disease in chronic kidney disease patients. *Curr Vasc Pharmacol.* 2021;19(1):55-62.

290. Law JP, Price AM, Pickup L, et al. Clinical potential of targeting fibroblast growth factor-23 and αklotho in the treatment of uremic cardiomyopathy. *J Am Heart Assoc.* 2020;9(7):e016041.

291. Herzog CA, Asinger RW, Berger AK, et al. Cardiovascular disease in chronic kidney disease. A clinical update from Kidney Disease: Improving Global Outcomes (KDIGO). *Kidney Int.* 2011;80:572-586.

292. Zhou H, An DA, Ni Z, et al. Texture analysis of native T1 images as a novel method for noninvasive assessment of uremic cardiomyopathy. *J Magn Reson Imaging.* 2021;51(4):290-300.

293. Zolty R, Hynes PJ, Vittorio TJ. Severe left ventricular systolic dysfunction may reverse with renal transplantation: uremic cardiomyopathy and cardiorenal syndrome. *Am J Transplant.* 2008;8:2219-2224.

294. Hayer MK, Radhakrishnan A, Price AM, et al. Early effects of kidney transplantation on the heart—A cardiac magnetic resonance multiparametric study. *Int J Cardiol.* 2019;293:272-277.

295. Zapolski T, Furmaga J, Wysokiński AP, et al. The atrial uremic cardiomyopathy regression in patients after kidney transplantation—the prospective echocardiographic study. *BMC Nephrol.* 2019;20(1):152.

296. Hassanin N, Alkemary A. Early detection of subclinical uremic cardiomyopathy using two-dimensional speckle tracking echocardiography. *Echocardiography.* 2016;33(4):527-536.

297. Abdel-Qadir H, Amir E, Thavendiranathan P. Prevention, detection, and management of chemotherapy-related cardiac dysfunction. *Can J Cardiol.* 2016;32(7):891-899.

298. Jaworski C, Mariani JA, Wheeler G, Kaye DM. Cardiac complications of thoracic irradiation. *J Am Coll Cardiol.* 2013;61:2319-2328.

299. Truong J, Yan AT, Cramarossa G, Chan KK. Chemotherapy-induced cardiotoxicity: detection, prevention, and management. *Can J Cardiol.* 2014;30:869-878.

300. Bhave M, Akhter N, Rosen ST. Cardiovascular toxicity of biologic agents for cancer therapy. *Oncology (Williston Park).* 2014;28:482-490.

301. Tamargo J, Caballero R, Delpon E. Cancer chemotherapy and cardiac arrhythmias: a review. *Drug Saf.* 2015;38:129-152.

302. Lenihan DJ, Oliva S, Chow EJ, Cardinale D. Cardiac toxicity in cancer survivors. *Cancer.* 2013;119:2131-2142.

303. Davis M, Witteles RM. Cardiac testing to manage cardiovascular risk in cancer patients. *Semin Oncol.* 2013;40:147-155.

304. Singh D, Thakur A, Tang WH. Utilizing cardiac biomarkers to detect and prevent chemotherapy-induced cardiomyopathy. *Curr Heart Fail Rep.* 2015;12:255-262.

305. Stein-Merlob AF, Rothberg MV, Ribas A, Yang EH. Cardiotoxicities of novel cancer immunotherapies. *Heart.* 2021 Mar 15. doi: 10.1136/heartjnl-2020-318083.

306. J.L. Zamorano, P. Lancellotti, D. Rodriguez, et al. 2016 ESC position paper on cancer treatments and cardiovascular toxicity developed under the auspices of the ESC Committee for practice guidelines the task force for cancer treatments and cardiovascular toxicity of the European Society of Cardiology (ESC). *Eur Heart J.* 2016;2768-2801.

307. Poulin F, Thavendiranathan P. Cardiotoxicity due to chemotherapy: role of cardiac imaging. *Curr Cardiol Rep.* 2015;17:564.

308. Curigliano G, Cardinale D, Suter T, et al. Cardiovascular toxicity induced by chemotherapy, targeted agents and radiotherapy: ESMO Clinical Practice Guidelines. *Ann Oncol.* 2012;23(Suppl 7):vii155-66.

309. Salvatorelli E, Menna P, Cantalupo E, et al. The concomitant management of cancer therapy and cardiac therapy. *Biochim Biophys Acta.* 2015;1848:2727-2737.

310. Vejpongsa P, Yeh ET. Prevention of anthracycline-induced cardiotoxicity: challenges and opportunities. *J Am Coll Cardiol.* 2014;64:938-945.

311. Sandoo A, Kitas GD, Carmichael AR. Breast cancer therapy and cardiovascular risk: focus on trastuzumab. *Vasc Health Risk Manag.* 2015;11: 223-228.

312. Lancellotti P, Anker SD, Donal E, et al. EACVI/HFA Cardiac Oncology Toxicity Registry in breast cancer patients: rationale, study design, and methodology (EACVI/HFA COT Registry)-EURObservational Research Program of the European Society of Cardiology. *Eur Heart J Cardiovasc Imaging.* 2015;16:466-470.

313. Seidman A, Hudis C, Pierri MK, et al. Cardiac dysfunction in the trastuzumab clinical trials experience. *J Clin Oncol.* 2002;20:1215-1221.

314. Curigliano G, Lenihan D, Fradley M, et al. Management of cardiac disease in cancer patients throughout oncological treatment: ESMO consensus recommendations. *Ann Oncol.* 2020;31(2):171-190.

315. Sara JD, Kaur J, Khodadadi R, Rehman M, et al. 5-fluorouracil and cardiotoxicity: a review. *Ther Adv Med Oncol.* 2018;10:1758835918780140.

316. Nhola LF, Abdelmoneim SS, Villarraga HR, et al. Echocardiographic assessment for the detection of cardiotoxicity due to vascular endothelial growth factor inhibitor therapy in metastatic renal cell and colorectal cancers. *J Am Soc Echocardiogr.* 2019;32:267-276.

317. Anand K, Ensor J, Trachtenberg B, et al: Osimertinib-induced cardiotoxicity. *JACC CardioOncol.* 2019;1:172-178.

318. Skubitz KM. Cardiotoxicity monitoring in patients treated with tyrosine kinase inhibitors. *Oncologist.* 2019;24:e600-e602.

319. Cole DC, Frishman WH. Cardiovascular complications of proteasome inhibitors used in multiple myeloma. *Cardiol Rev.* 2018;26: 122-129.

320. Chang HM, Moudgil R, Scarabelli T, et al. Cardiovascular complications of cancer therapy. *J Am Coll Cardiol.* 2017;70:2536-2551.

321. Waxman AJ, Clasen S, Hwang WT, et al. Carfilzomib-associated cardiovascular adverse events: A systematic review and meta-analysis. *JAMA Oncol.* 2018;4:e174519.

322. Wu P, Oren O, Gertz MA, Yang EH. Proteasome inhibitor-related cardiotoxicity: mechanisms, diagnosis, and management. *Curr Oncol Rep.* 2020;22(7):66.

323. Mincu RI, Mahabadi AA, Michel L, et al. Cardiovascular adverse events associated with BRAF and MEK inhibitors: a systematic review and meta-analysis. *JAMA Netw Open.* 2019;2(8):e198890.

324. Rassaf T, Totzeck M, Backs J, et al: Onco-cardiology: consensus paper of the German Cardiac Society, the German Society for Pediatric Cardiology and Congenital Heart Defects and the German Society for Hematology and Medical Oncology. *Clin Res Cardiol.* 2020;109:1197-1222.

325. Hu JR, Florido R, Lipson EJ, et al. Cardiovascular toxicities associated with immune checkpoint inhibitors. *Cardiovasc Res.* 2019;115:854-868.

326. Awadalla M, Mahmood SS, Groarke JD, et al. Global longitudinal strain and cardiac events in patients with immune checkpoint inhibitor-related myocarditis. *J Am Coll Cardiol.* 2020;75:467-478.

327. Pudil R, Mueller C, Čelutkienė J, et al. Role of serum biomarkers in cancer patients receiving cardiotoxic cancer therapies: a position statement from the Cardio-Oncology Study Group of the Heart Failure Association and the Cardio-Oncology Council of the European Society of Cardiology. *Eur J Heart Fail.* 2020;22:1966-1983.

328. Alvi RM, Frigault MJ, Fradley MG, et al. Cardiovascular events among adults treated with chimeric antigen receptor T-cells (CAR-T). *J Am Coll Cardiol.* 2019;74:3099-3108.

329. Lefebvre B, Kang Y, Smith AM, et al. Cardiovascular effects of CAR T cell therapy. *JACC CardioOncol.* 2020;2:193-203.

330. Catino AB. Cytokines are at the heart of it. *JACC CardioOncol.* 2020;2(2): 204-206,

331. Ganatra S, Carver JR, Hayek SS, et al. Chimeric antigen receptor T-Cell therapy for cancer and heart: JACC Council Perspectives. *J Am Coll Cardiol.* 2019;74(25):3153-3163.

332. Dhesi S, Chu MP, Blevins G, et al. Cyclophosphamide-induced cardiomyopathy: a case report, review, and recommendations for management. *J Invest Med High Impact Case Rep.* 2013;1:2324709613480346.

333. Katayama M, Imai Y, Hashimoto H, et al. Fulminant fatal cardiotoxicity following cyclophosphamide therapy. *J Cardiol.* 2009;54:330-334.

334. Mir H, Alhussein M, Alrashidi S. Cardiac complications associated with checkpoint inhibition: a systematic review of the literature in an important emerging area. *Can J Cardiol.* 2018;34(8):1059-1068.

335. Stein-Merlob AF, Rothberg MV, Holman P, Yang EH. Immunotherapy-associated cardiotoxicity of immune checkpoint inhibitors and chimeric antigen receptor T cell therapy: diagnostic and management challenges and strategies. *Curr Cardiol Rep.* 2021;23(3):11.

336. D'Souza M, Nielsen D, Svane IM. The risk of cardiac events in patients receiving immune checkpoint inhibitors: a nationwide Danish study. *Eur Heart J.* 2020:ehaa884.

337. Ganatra S, Neilan TG. Immune checkpoint inhibitor-associated myocarditis. *Oncologist.* 2018;23(8):879-886.

338. Porta-Sánchez A, Gilbert C, Spears D, et al. Incidence, diagnosis, and management of QT prolongation induced by cancer therapies: a systematic review. *J Am Heart Assoc.* 2017;6(12):e007724.

339. Alomar M, Fradley MG. Electrophysiology translational considerations in cardio-oncology: QT and beyond. *J Cardiovasc Transl Res.* 2020;13:390-401.

340. Pande A, Lombardo J, Spangenthal E, Javle M. Hypertension secondary to anti-angiogenic therapy: experience with bevacizumab. *Anticancer Res.* 2007;27:3465-3470.

341. Cameron AC, Touyz RM, Lang NN. Vascular complications of cancer chemotherapy. *Can J Cardiol.* 2016;32(7):852-862.

342. Formiga MN, Fanelli MF. Aortic dissection during antiangiogenic therapy with sunitinib. A case report. *Sao Paulo Med J.* 2015;133:275-277.

343. Edeline J, Laguerre B, Rolland Y, Patard JJ. Aortic dissection in a patient treated by sunitinib for metastatic renal cell carcinoma. *Ann Oncol.* 2010;21:186-187.

344. Madden GW, Ishaq MK, Gupta R. Acute aortic dissection in a patient receiving gemcitabine and cisplatin. *Am J Ther.* 2014;21:e21-e25.

345. Serrano C, Suárez C, Andreu J, Carles J. Acute aortic dissection during sorafenib-containing therapy. *Ann Oncol.* 2010;21:181-182.

346. Aragon-Ching JB, Ning YM, Dahut WL. Acute aortic dissection in a hypertensive patient with prostate cancer undergoing chemotherapy containing bevacizumab. *Acta Oncol.* 2008;47:1600-1601.

347. Moretti M, Merlo M, Barbati G, et al. Prognostic impact of familial screening in dilated cardiomyopathy. *Eur J Heart Fail.* 2010;12:922-927.

348. Castelli G, Fornaro A, Ciaccheri M, et al. Improving survival rates of patients with idiopathic dilated cardiomyopathy in Tuscany over 3 decades: impact of evidence-based management. *Circ Heart Fail.* 2013;6: 913-921.

349. Laribi S, Aouba A, Nikolaou M, et al. Trends in death attributed to heart failure over the past two decades in Europe. *Eur J Heart Fail.* 2012;14: 234-239.

350. Merlo M, Pivetta A, Pinamonti B, et al. Long-term prognostic impact of therapeutic strategies in patients with idiopathic dilated cardiomyopathy: changing mortality over the last 30 years. *Eur J Heart Fail.* 2014;16:317-324.

351. Palmiero G, Florio MT, Rubino M, et al. Cardiac resynchronization therapy in patients with heart failure: what is new? *Heart Fail Clin.* 2021;17(2): 289-301.

352. Matsumura Y, Hoshikawa-Nagai E, Kubo T, et al. Left ventricular reverse remodeling in long-term (> 12 years) survivors with idiopathic dilated cardiomyopathy. *Am J Cardiol.* 2013;111:106-110.

353. Ikeda Y, Inomata T, Iida Y, et al. Time course of left ventricular reverse remodeling in response to pharmacotherapy: clinical implication for heart failure prognosis in patients with idiopathic dilated cardiomyopathy. *Heart Vessels.* 2016;31(4):545-554.

354. Gulati A, Ismail TF, Jabbour A, et al. The prevalence and prognostic significance of right ventricular systolic dysfunction in nonischemic dilated cardiomyopathy. *Circulation.* 2013;128:1623-1633.

355. Goldenberg I, Kutyifa V, Klein HU, et al. Survival with cardiac-resynchronization therapy in mild heart failure. *N Engl J Med.* 2014;370:1694-1701.

356. Adabag S, Roukoz H, Anand IS, Moss AJ. Cardiac resynchronization therapy in patients with minimal heart failure: a systematic review and meta-analysis. *J Am Coll Cardiol.* 2011;58:935-941.

357. Zecchin M, Merlo M, Pivetta A, et al. How can optimization of medical treatment avoid unnecessary implantable cardioverter-defibrillator implantations in patients with idiopathic dilated cardiomyopathy presenting with "SCD-HeFT criteria"? *Am J Cardiol.* 2012;109:729-735.

358. Kimura Y, Okumura T, Morimoto R. A clinical score for predicting left ventricular reverse remodelling in patients with dilated cardiomyopathy. *ESC Heart Fail.* 2021;8(2):1359-1368.

359. Stolfo D, Merlo M, Pinamonti B, et al. Early improvement of functional mitral regurgitation in patients with idiopathic dilated cardiomyopathy. *Am J Cardiol.* 2015;115:1137-1143.

360. Kamperidis V, van Wijngaarden SE, van Rosendael PJ, et al. Mitral valve repair for secondary mitral regurgitation in non-ischaemic dilated cardiomyopathy is associated with left ventricular reverse remodelling and increase of forward flow. *Eur Heart J Cardiovasc Imaging.* 2018;19(2):208-215.

361. Hsu JC, Solomon SD, Bourgoun M, et al; MADIT-CRT Executive Committee. Predictors of super-response to cardiac resynchronization therapy and associated improvement in clinical outcome: the MADIT-CRT (Multicenter Automatic Defibrillator Implantation Trial with Cardiac Resynchronization Therapy) study. *J Am Coll Cardiol.* 2012;59:2366-2373.

362. Yuyun MF, Erqou SA, Peralta AO, et al. Risk of ventricular arrhythmia in cardiac resynchronization therapy responders and super-responders: a systematic review and meta-analysis. *Europace*. 2021:euaa414.

363. Gulati A, Jabbour A, Ismail TF, et al. Association of fibrosis with mortality and sudden cardiac death in patients with nonischemic dilated cardiomyopathy. *JAMA*. 2013;309:896-908.

364. Mandawat A, Chattranukulchai P, Mandawat A, at al. Progression of myocardial fibrosis in nonischemic DCM and association with mortality and heart failure outcomes. *JACC Cardiovasc Imaging*. 2021: S1936-878X(20)31005-6.

365. Leyva F, Zegard A, Acquaye E, at al. Outcomes of cardiac resynchronization therapy with or without defibrillation in patients with nonischemic cardiomyopathy. *J Am Coll Cardiol*. 2017;70(10):1216-1227.

366. Priori SG, Blomström-Lundqvist C, Mazzanti A, et al. 2015 ESC Guidelines for the management of patients with ventricular arrhythmias and the prevention of sudden cardiac death: The Task Force for the Management of Patients with Ventricular Arrhythmias and the Prevention of Sudden Cardiac Death of the European Society of Cardiology (ESC). Endorsed by: Association for European Paediatric and Congenital Cardiology (AEPC). *Eur Heart J*. 2015;36(41):2793-2867.

367. Keren A, Billingham ME, Weintraub D, et al. Mildly dilated congestive cardiomyopathy. *Circulation*. 1985;72(2):302-309.

368. Iida K, Sugishita Y, Yukisada K, Ito I. Clinical characteristics of cardiomyopathy with mild dilatation. *J Cardiol*. 1990;20(2):301-310.

369. Keren A, Gottlieb S, Tzivoni D, et al. Mildly dilated congestive cardiomyopathy. Use of prospective diagnostic criteria and description of the clinical course without heart transplantation. *Circulation*. 1990;81(2):506-517.

370. Gavazzi A, De Maria R, Renosto G, et al. The spectrum of left ventricular size in dilated cardiomyopathy: clinical correlates and prognostic implications. SPIC (Italian Multicenter Cardiomyopathy Study) Group. *Am Heart J*. 1993;125(2 Pt 1):410-422.

371. Kitaoka H, Matsumura Y, Yamasaki N, et al. Long-term prognosis of patients with mildly dilated cardiomyopathy. *Circ J*. 2002;66(6):557-560.

372. Zegkos T, Panagiotidis T, Parcharidou D, Efthimiadis G. Emerging concepts in arrhythmogenic dilated cardiomyopathy. *Heart Fail Rev*. 2020;26(5):1219-1229.

373. Gigli M, Stolfo D, Merlo M, et al. Insights into mildly dilated cardiomyopathy: temporal evolution and long-term prognosis. *Eur J Heart Fail*. 2017;19(4):531-539.

42

Hypertrophic Cardiomyopathy

Massimiliano Lorenzini and Perry M. Elliott

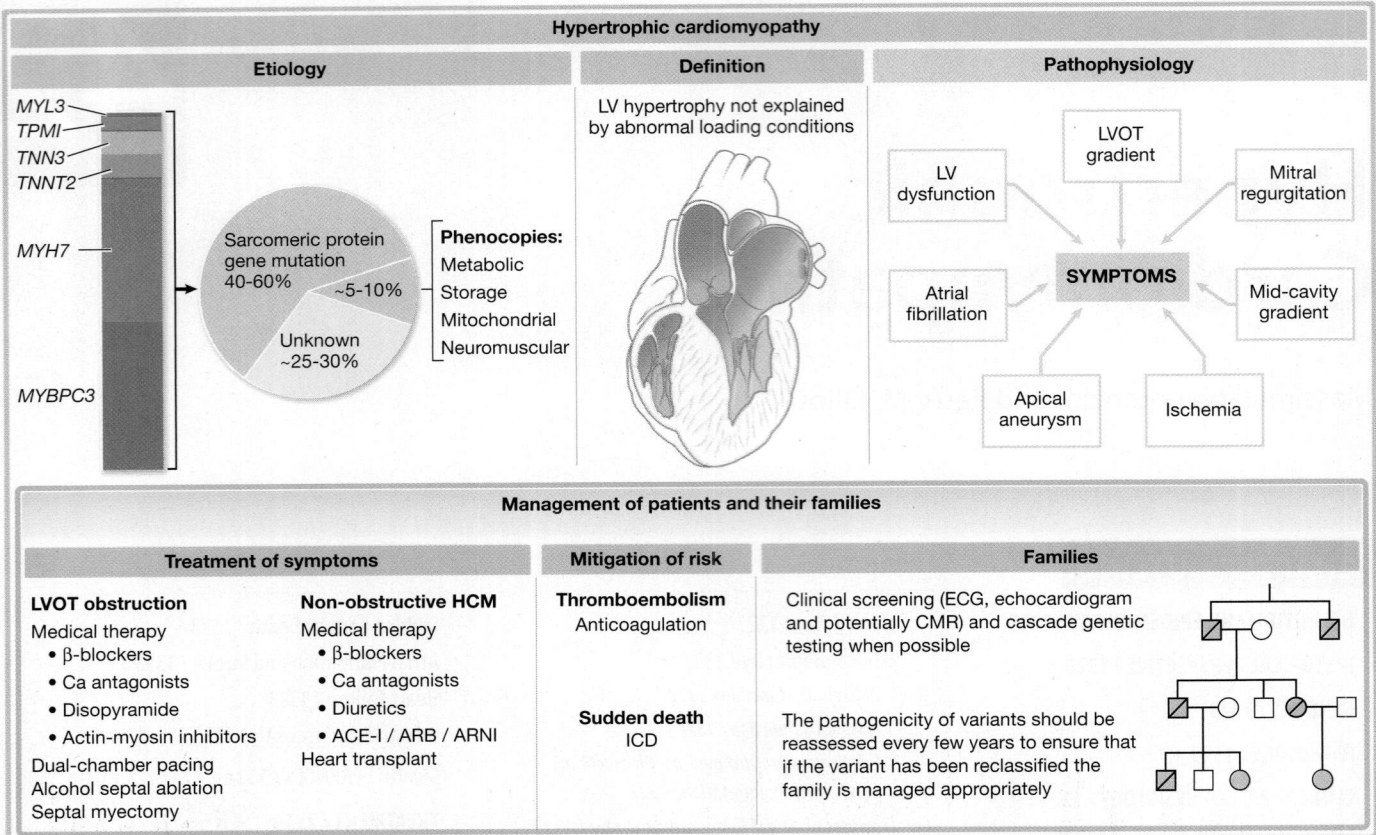

Chapter 42 Fuster and Hurst's Central Illustration. Hypertrophic cardiomyopathy (HCM) is a common inherited condition. The pathophysiology of HCM is complex and consists of multiple interrelated abnormalities. Management involves treatment of symptoms, mitigation of risk, and screening of families with cascade genetic testing when possible. ACE-I, angiotensin-converting enzyme inhibitor; ARB, angiotensin-receptor blocker; ARNI, angiotensin receptor–neprilysin inhibitor; ICD, implantable cardioverter defibrillator; LV, left ventricular; LVOT, left ventricular outflow tract.

CHAPTER SUMMARY

This chapter discusses the epidemiology, pathophysiology, diagnosis, and management of hypertrophic cardiomyopathy (HCM), a common inherited condition. In ~50% of cases, HCM is due to a pathogenic variant in a sarcomere protein gene (see Fuster and Hurst's Central Illustration) and is inherited as an autosomal dominant trait with incomplete penetrance. Phenocopies should be actively ruled out during diagnostic work-up. The pathophysiology is complex and consists of multiple interrelated factors, including myocardial ischemia, diastolic (and rarely systolic) dysfunction, left ventricular outflow tract (and/or midcavity) obstruction (LVOTO), mitral regurgitation, and atrial fibrillation. Symptoms related to LVOTO are managed medically in the first instance but may require invasive treatment with surgical septal myectomy or alcohol septal ablation. Heart failure is an important cause of death and is treated according to the current standard recommendations. Atrial fibrillation carries a high thromboembolic risk and mandates anticoagulation. Defibrillators are the only effective protection from sudden death in high-risk patients.

DEFINITION AND EPIDEMIOLOGY

Hypertrophic cardiomyopathy (HCM) is defined as left ventricular (LV) hypertrophy in the absence of abnormal loading conditions, such as severe hypertension or valve disease, sufficient to cause the observed phenotype.[1,2] Echocardiographic studies in healthy young adults suggest a prevalence of around 1:500, with no significant differences across ethnicities or geographical location. Extrapolation based on the autosomal genetic basis of disease has led to speculation that this may be an underestimate.[3] Conversely, studies based on electronic health records indicate that the clinically evident prevalence may be closer to 1:2500.[4] Large cohorts have a male predominance of 60% to 65%. Ventricular hypertrophy most frequently develops during periods of rapid somatic growth, but can appear de novo at any time from infancy to old age.[5,6]

The term *hypertrophic cardiomyopathy* does not indicate a single condition, but rather describes a phenotype that is shared by a range of disorders that can be grouped into familial/genetic and nonfamilial/nongenetic subtypes.[7,8] In 50% to 60% of adolescents and adults, HCM is inherited as an autosomal dominant trait caused by mutations in cardiac sarcomere protein genes. Overall, 5% to 10% of HCM cases are caused by phenocopies (disorders with the same phenotype but different etiology) that include metabolic or storage disorders (eg, Anderson–Fabry, glycogen storage diseases), mitochondrial disorders, cardiac amyloidosis, neuromuscular disorders, chromosome abnormalities, and genetic syndromes such as cardio-facial-cutaneous syndromes, RASopathies, and LEOPARD syndrome.[9] The prevalence of individual phenocopies varies with age,[10,11] and many have a very different natural history from sarcomeric HCM and a correct diagnosis is of paramount importance for patient management, risk stratification, and in some cases (eg, cardiac amyloidosis and Anderson–Fabry disease) to initiate specific treatment.[12] The remaining 25% to 30% of HCM cases, that are not due to a sarcomeric pathogenic variant or phenocopies, remain unexplained (**Fig. 42–1**).

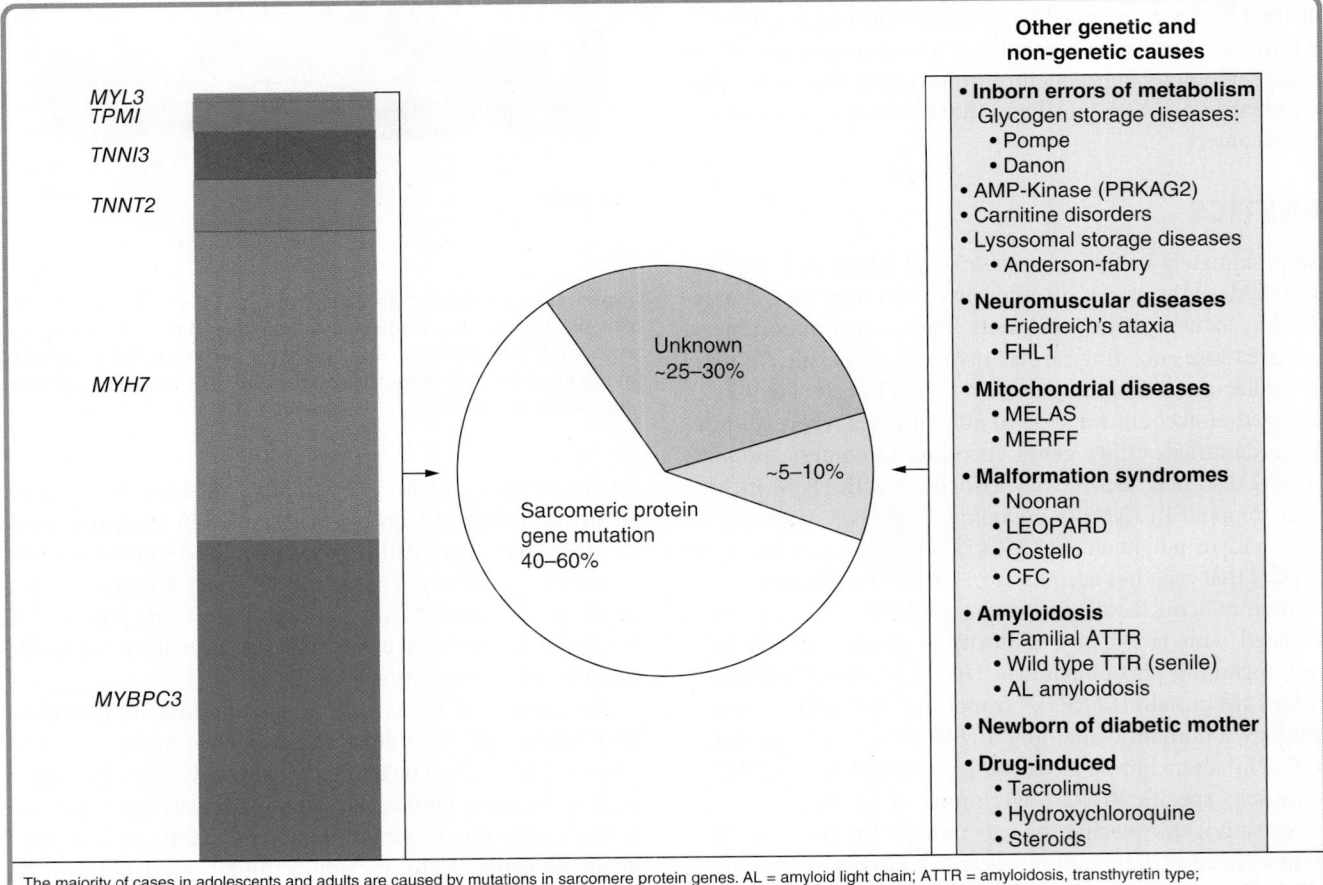

The majority of cases in adolescents and adults are caused by mutations in sarcomere protein genes. AL = amyloid light chain; ATTR = amyloidosis, transthyretin type; CFC = cardiofaciocutaneous; FHL-1 = Four and a half LIM domains protein I; LEOPARD = lentigines, ECG abnormalities, ocular hypertelorism, pulmonary stenosis, abnormal genitalia, Retardation of growth, and sensorineural deafness; MELAS = mitochondrial encephalomyopathy, lactic acidosis, and stroke-like episodes; MERFF = myoclonic epilepsy with ragged red fibres; MYL3 = myosin light chain 3; MYBPC3 = myosin-binding protein C, cardiac-type; MYH7 = myosin, heavy chain 7; TNNI3 = troponin I, cardiac; TNNT2 = troponin T, cardiac, TTR, transthyretin.

Figure 42–1. Causes of hypertrophic cardiomyopathy. Adapted with permission from Authors/Task Force, Elliott PM, Anastasakis A, et al. 2014 ESC Guidelines on diagnosis and management of hypertrophic cardiomyopathy: The Task Force for the Diagnosis and Management of Hypertrophic Cardiomyopathy of the European Society of Cardiology (ESC). *Eur Heart J.* 2014 Oct 14;35(39):2733-2779.

HISTORICAL PERSPECTIVE

Patients with unexplained ventricular hypertrophy have been described for more than 100 years, but it was not until the publication of Sir Russell Brock's paper "Functional Obstruction of the Left Ventricle" in 1957 and Donald Teare's description of asymmetrical myocardial hypertrophy in 1958 that HCM was established as a distinct disease.[13] From the 1960s onward, diagnostic criteria for the disease evolved with the prevailing technologies used to interrogate the heart. An initial focus on clinical signs and symptoms and cardiac catheterization meant that dynamic LV outflow tract obstruction (LVOTO) was central to the diagnosis of the disease. In the 1970s, the asymmetrical distribution of hypertrophy was emphasized by the use of M-mode echocardiography, but with the advent of two-dimensional echocardiographic imaging and cardiac magnetic resonance imaging (CMR), the complex spectrum of ventricular involvement is now better appreciated.

Early clinical reports suggested that HCM is inherited in 30% to 50% of patients. This was confirmed in prospective clinical genetic studies using two-dimensional echocardiography that suggested 50% to 60% of cases are inherited as an autosomal dominant trait. In 1989, the first genetic mutation for HCM was mapped to chromosome 14q and then to the β-myosin heavy chain protein, a major component of the cardiac sarcomere. Subsequently, hundreds of mutations have been identified, mostly involving the myofilaments of the cardiac sarcomere.

GENETICS

In approximately half of adolescents and adults with the disease, HCM is inherited as an autosomal dominant trait, characterized by locus and allelic diversity. The most common causal genes are those encoding cardiac myosin heavy chain (*MYH7*) and cardiac myosin binding protein C (*MYBPC3*) (**Fig. 42–2**), that together account for 75% to 80% of cases where a mutation is identified. Other genes encoding sarcomeric proteins that have also been definitively associated with HCM include cardiac troponin T (*TNNT2*), troponin I (*TNNI3*), α- tropomyosin (*TPM1*), myosin light chains (*MYL2, MYL3*), and cardiac actin (*ACTC1*) that together account for 15% to 20% of cases.[14]

Other noncontractile sarcomere proteins have also been associated with HCM in a minority of cases (<1% for each gene), including phospholamban (*PLN*), filamin C (*FLNC*),[15] cardiac LIM protein (*CSRP3*),[16] troponin C (*TNNC1*),[17] formin homology 2 domain containing 3 (*FHOD3*),[18] alpha actinin 2 (*ACTN2*),[19] alpha kinase 3 (*ALPK3*),[20] junctophilin 2 (*JPH2*),[21] and muscle- specific RING-finger protein 1 (*TRIM63*).[22]

Two pathogenic mechanisms are thought to account for disease associated with mutations in cardiac sarcomere proteins.[23] Pathogenic missense nucleotide variants (a nucleotide change that results in an amino acid being substituted by another amino acid in the protein) predominantly lead to a *dominant negative effect* ("poison peptide" mechanism) in which the mutated protein is not destroyed, but rather integrates into the sarcomere, leading to the disease phenotype; this is thought to

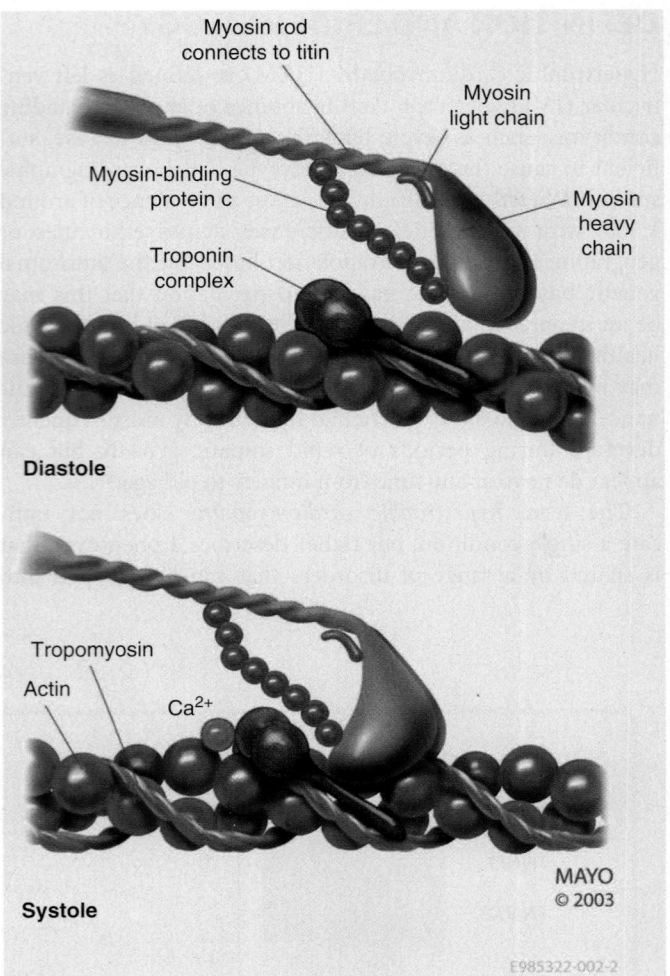

Figure 42–2. Schematic diagram of the sarcomere. In the majority of patients, hypertrophic cardiomyopathy is caused by mutations in genes encoding the thick and thin filaments of the sarcomere. The two most commonly involved are β-myosin heavy chain (*MYH7*) and cardiac myosin binding protein C (*MYBPC3*).

be characteristic of *MYH7* variants.[24] Alternatively, nonsense single nucleotide variants or small frameshift insertion-deletions can introduce a premature stop codon and cause *haploinsufficiency* as a result of nonsense mRNA-mediated decay or proteolysis of a truncated (just partially translated) protein.[24] This mechanism is believed to be typical of the majority of *MYBPC3* disease-causing mutations.[25]

Penetrance of HCM due to sarcomere gene mutations is incomplete, age dependent, and greater in males.[6] The condition is characterized by marked phenotypic heterogeneity even within the same family, that remains largely unexplained but is most likely due to a combination of genetic, epigenetic, and acquired factors.[26] This variability initially hindered clear genotype-phenotype correlations, but contemporary cohort studies have shown that compared to those with negative genetic testing, patients with HCM due to a sarcomere gene mutation are younger, more frequently have a family history, have more pronounced LV hypertrophy, and overall have a worse prognosis.[27,28] Among those with sarcomere gene mutations, patients with

MYH7 mutations probably have a worse outcome, particularly a greater incidence of advanced heart failure compared to patients with *MYBPC3* variants.[27,29]

A small subset of patients (<5% of those with sarcomere gene mutations[30]), have a complex genotype and carry multiple sarcomere gene mutations in the same or different genes. These patients have an adverse prognosis due to both advanced heart failure and ventricular arrhythmias.[26,31,32]

PATHOLOGY

Gross examination of the heart demonstrates asymmetric septal hypertrophy with a small LV cavity (**Fig. 42–3**).[33–35] The mural endocardium may be thickened by fibrous tissue, and if LVOTO is present, there is often a plaque located on septal endocardium where the mitral valve has repeatedly made contact. The mitral valve itself may be abnormal, with elongation of the mitral chordae and anterior displacement of hypertrophied papillary muscles. Abnormal attachments of the mitral valve chordae into the septum, insertion of the papillary muscle head directly onto the mitral leaflets, and myocardial clefts are also common.[36,37] The left (and sometimes the right) atrium is usually dilated in advanced disease as a result of increased filling pressures secondary to LVOTO, mitral regurgitation, and

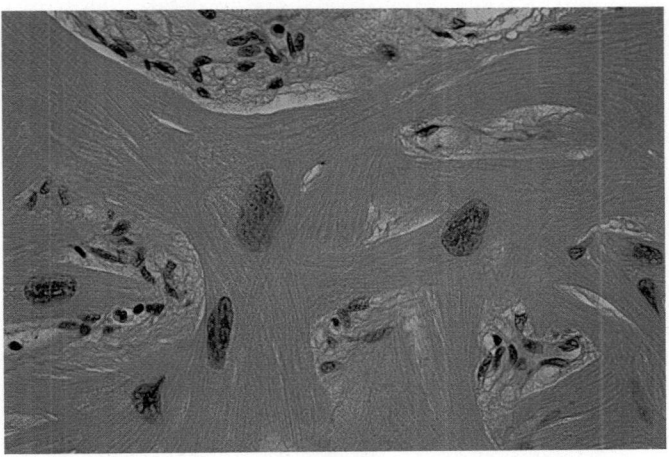

Figure 42–4. Microscopic section of the myocardium from a patient with hypertrophic cardiomyopathy showing myocyte disarray.

diastolic dysfunction. Although the epicardial coronary arteries are usually normal, they can follow an intramural course and be compressed during ventricular systole.[38]

The classical histopathologic appearance of HCM consists of cardiomyocyte hypertrophy and disarray, interstitial and replacement fibrosis, and dysplastic arterioles (**Fig. 42–4**).[38,39] Phenocopies have specific histopathology findings according to etiology, including infiltration and vacuolization.

CLINICAL PATHOPHYSIOLOGY

The pathophysiology of HCM is complex and consists of multiple interrelated abnormalities, including diastolic dysfunction, LVOTO, and mitral regurgitation.

Left Ventricular Dysfunction

Diastolic dysfunction arises from multiple factors that affect both ventricular relaxation and chamber stiffness (**Fig. 42–5**).[40–43] Impairment of ventricular relaxation can result from nonuniformity of ventricular contraction and relaxation, delayed myosin-actin inactivation caused by abnormal intracellular calcium reuptake,[41–43] and disruption of myosin interacting heads motif.[44] Myocardial ischemia caused by supply-demand mismatch may also contribute.[45–48] Patients with HCM have increased oxygen demand as a result of ventricular hypertrophy and abnormal loading conditions, and also have compromised coronary blood flow to the LV myocardium because of abnormally small and partially obliterated intramural coronary arteries.[45,46,49–51] With exercise, diastolic function is further compromised by a decrease in the diastolic filling period and prolongation of the time to peak filling, which increase pulmonary venous pressure and cause dyspnea.[43]

A minority of patients (3%–8%) develop severe LV systolic dysfunction.[30,52–54] In this *burnt-out* phase of the condition (also sometimes called end-stage) the LV cavity enlarges, the LV walls thin, the LVOT gradient (if previously present) disappears, and extensive fibrosis develops.[55,56] This progression is associated with an adverse prognosis, due to both advanced

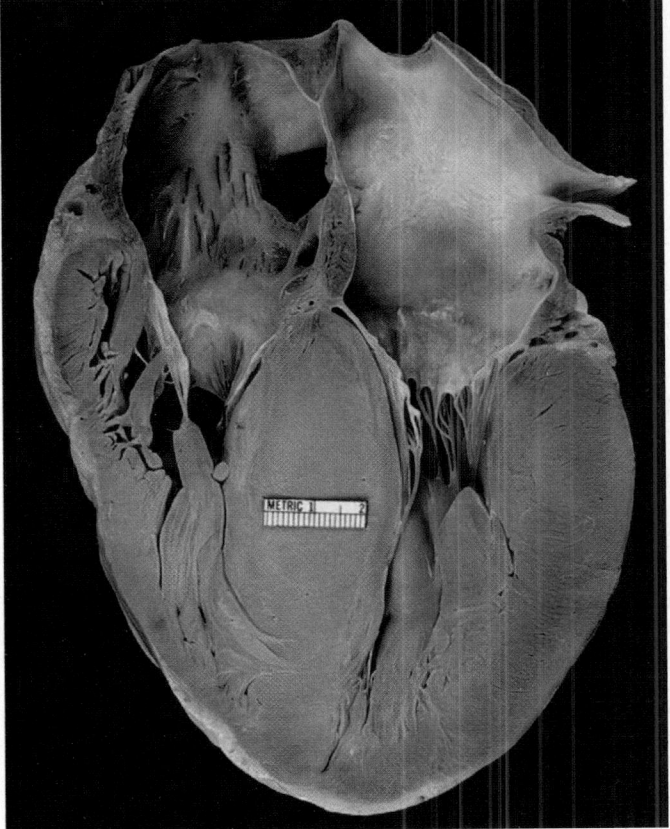

Figure 42–3. Pathologic specimen of a patient who died suddenly with hypertrophic cardiomyopathy. There is severe ventricular hypertrophy and a small left ventricular cavity. The left atrium is enlarged. Reproduced with permission from Dr. WD Edwards. Mayo Clinic, Rochester, MN.

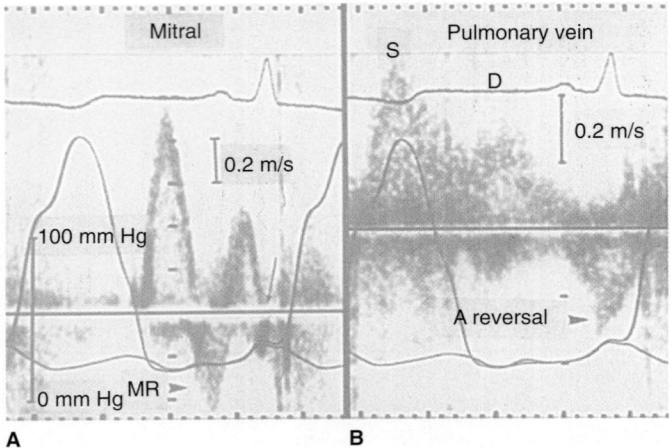

Figure 42–5. Evidence of severe diastolic dysfunction in a patient with hypertrophic cardiomyopathy. The left ventricular and left atrial pressures are shown in both the left and right panels. The mean left atrial pressure is severely elevated to 30 mm Hg. **(A)** The mitral flow velocity curve is shown, demonstrating a high E:A ratio and a short deceleration time. Diastolic mitral regurgitation (MR) is present. There is abrupt cessation of the "a" duration (*arrow*). **(B)** The pulmonary vein velocity curve is shown, with a high velocity at atrial reversal of long duration. The systolic forward flow (S) and diastolic forward flow (D) are shown.

heart failure and an increased risk of sudden cardiac death (SCD).[30,54] LV systolic dysfunction is also a potential red flag for HCM phenocopies.[12]

Another subgroup of patients (~5%) have marked *restrictive pathophysiology*, with diastolic dysfunction dominating the clinical picture, and leading to progressive biatrial enlargement, atrial fibrillation (AF), progressive heart failure, and pulmonary hypertension.[57]

During exercise, approximately 25% of HCM patients have an abnormal blood pressure response defined by either a failure to increase >20 mm Hg or indeed a drop in systolic blood pressure.[58] This was initially proposed as a negative prognostic marker, particularly for SCD,[58] but was subsequently not confirmed in larger cohort and meta-analysis.[59] The pathophysiological mechanism is complex and involves inappropriate systemic vasodilatation during exercise and a reduced cardiac output reserve caused by small LV stroke volume.[60]

Left Ventricular Outflow Tract Obstruction and Mitral Regurgitation

Dynamic LVOTO is present in one-third of patients at rest and a further one-third during exercise or with physical maneuvers that reduce ventricular volume or increase contractility.[61] It is due to systolic anterior movement (SAM) of the mitral valve leaflets that brings them into contact with the interventricular septum. Along with hypertrophy of the septum, a number of other anatomical factors predispose to SAM and LVOTO in HCM, including elongation of the mitral valve leaflets,[62] anterior and apical papillary muscle displacement,[63] and fibrotic, retracted secondary chordae.[64] Historically, the mechanism of obstruction was thought to be the narrowing of the LV outflow tract (LVOT) caused by systolic contraction of the hypertrophied basal septum with the resultant suction force (Venturi effect) pulling the mitral valve leaflets anteriorly.[61] The modern concept is that SAM is initiated by the drag force of flow against the abnormally positioned and elongated mitral valve leaflets in late diastole and early systole, that pushes the leaflets into the LVOT.[65,66] Following initial septal contact, the leaflet is pushed further onto the septum by the pressure difference between the LV cavity and LVOT.[67] LVOTO typically varies with loading conditions and LV contractility, increasing with a reduced preload (Valsalva maneuver, dehydration, postprandial splanchnic hyperemia), a reduced afterload (vasodilators), or increased contractility (positive inotropes) (**Figs. 42–6**, **42–7**, and **42–8**).[61]

Mitral regurgitation is common in patients with LVOTO and contributes to dyspnea. It is generally caused by the distortion of the mitral valve apparatus during SAM, with a jet directed posteriorly and laterally (see Fig. 42–6), predominantly during mid to late systole, and tends to be proportional to the severity of LVOTO.[68] Changes in ventricular load and contractility that

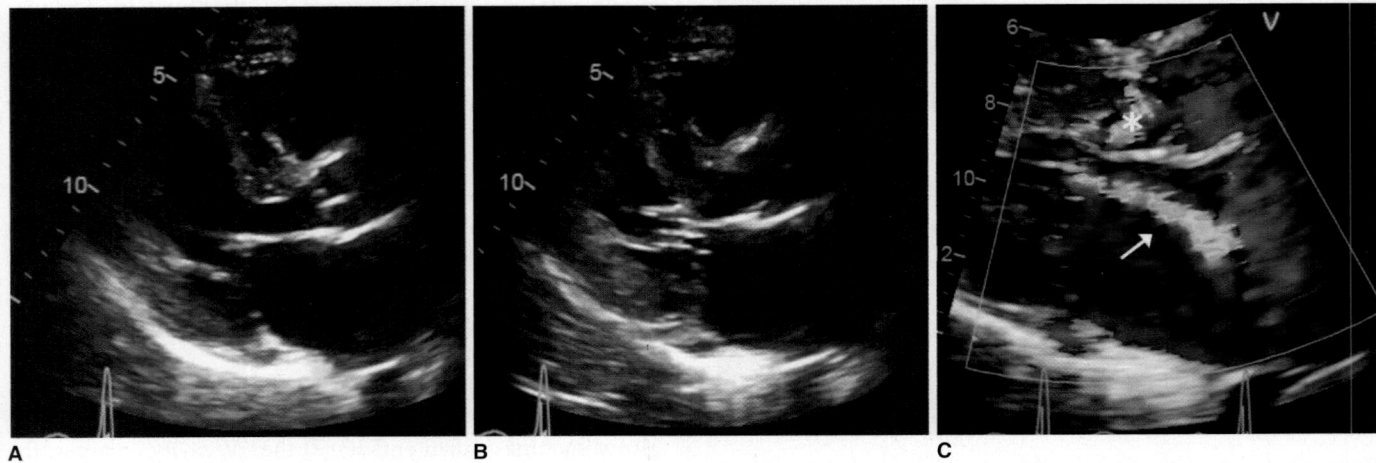

Figure 42–6. Parasternal long axis images from a transthoracic echocardiogram showing asymmetric left ventricular hypertrophy in diastole (**A**), complete systolic anterior movement of the mitral valve (the anterior mitral valve leaflet comes into contact with the septum in systole, (**B**), and color Doppler (**C**) showing accelerated flow in the left ventricular outflow tract (*asterisk*) and mitral regurgitation (*arrow*).

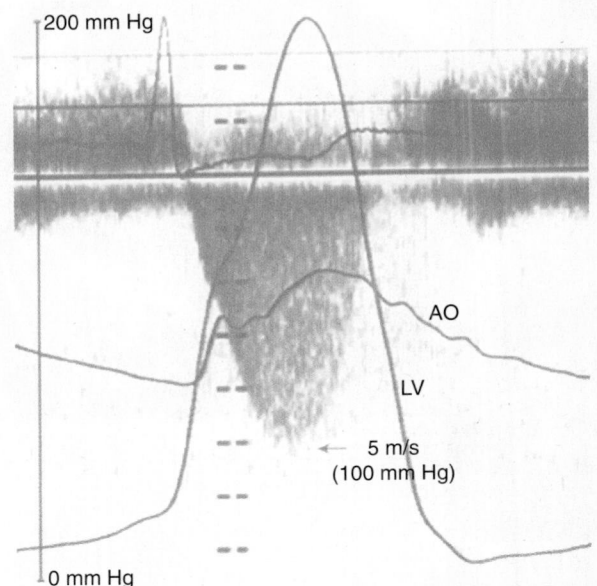

Figure 42–7. Simultaneous Doppler echocardiogram and cardiac catheterization demonstrating the presence of severe left ventricular outflow tract obstruction. The gradient between the left ventricle (LV) and aorta (Ao) at catheterization is 100 mm Hg. A continuous wave Doppler across the left ventricular outflow tract reveals a peak velocity of 5 m/s, which is consistent with a calculated left ventricular outflow tract gradient of 100 mm Hg.

affect the severity of LVOTO will similarly affect the degree of mitral regurgitation. It is important to identify patients in whom mitral regurgitation is not purely SAM-related, who have additional intrinsic mitral valve disease (eg, leaflet prolapse or flail, annular or leaflet calcification), because this will influence subsequent treatment decisions.[1]

Midcavity Obstruction and Apical Aneurysm

In approximately 10% of patients with HCM a midcavity pressure gradient is present.[69] This can coexist with LVOTO and is due to the hypertrophied septum coming in contact with the hypercontractile lateral wall, often with an interposed hypertrophied papillary muscle. Around one-third of patients with midcavity obstruction also have an LV apical aneurysm[69] in the form of a discrete, dyskinetic or akinetic, thin-walled segment of the most distal portion of the LV (**Fig. 42–9**). They are not exclusively associated with midcavity obstruction and can also be found in cases of HCM with an apical distribution of hypertrophy with an overall prevalence around 5% of all HCM cases.[70] They are thought to be the result of regional myocardial scarring due to the increased wall stress secondary to the high intracavity systolic pressure that causes ischemia. Apical aneurysms have been associated with a higher incidence of monomorphic ventricular tachycardia and thromboembolism.[70]

CLINICAL PRESENTATION

Most patients with HCM are asymptomatic and are diagnosed incidentally, following an abnormal electrocardiogram (ECG), detection of a heart murmur, or screening echocardiogram. When symptoms are present, they often vary from day to day and may be exacerbated during hot humid weather, presumably as a result of fluid loss and vasodilation that cause decreases in both preload and afterload. Similarly, symptoms may be more prominent after eating a large meal or drinking alcohol.

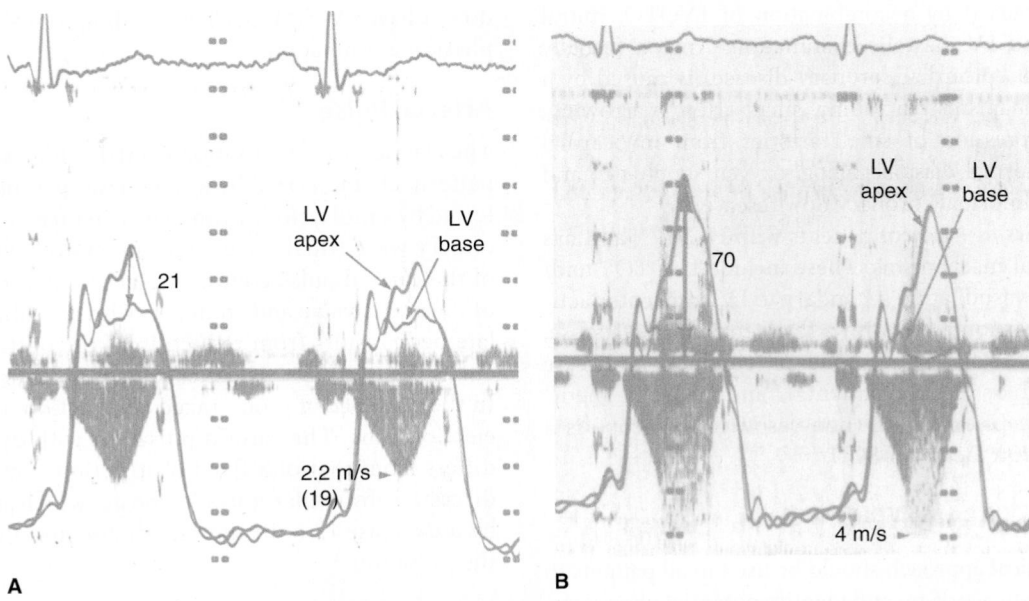

A   **B**

Figure 42–8. The dynamic nature of the left ventricular (LV) outflow tract obstruction is shown by simultaneous Doppler echocardiography and cardiac catheterization. The cardiac catheterization is performed with a pressure measurement of the LV apex and LV base. The gradient occurs during systole between the LV apex and LV base. The continuous wave Doppler velocities through the LV outflow tract are shown. The calculated gradient from the Doppler echocardiogram is shown in parentheses. (**A**) The gradient in the baseline state is 21 mm Hg as assessed by both cardiac catheterization and Doppler echocardiography. (**B**) During inhalation of amyl nitrite, the gradient increases to 70 mm Hg.

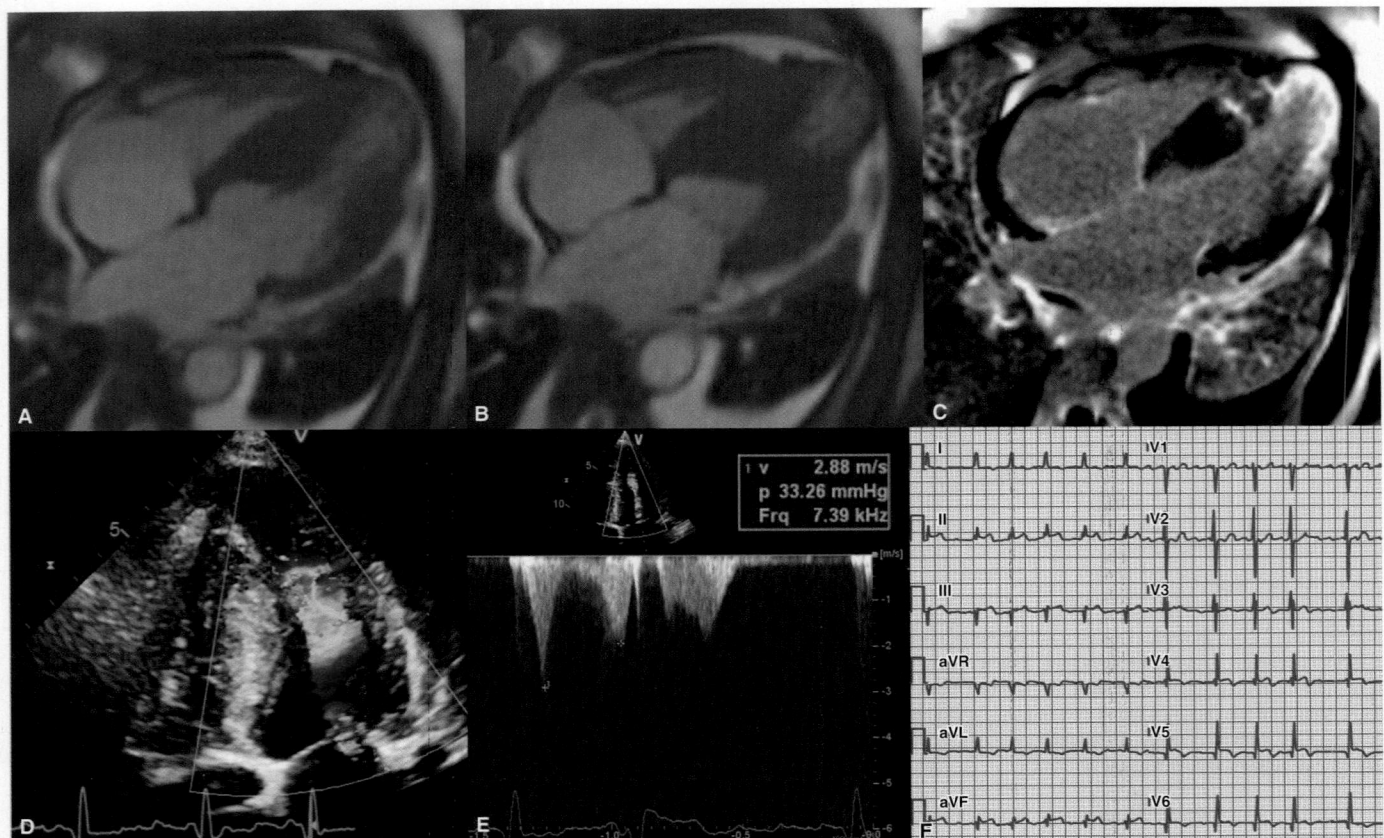

Figure 42–9. Midcavity gradient and apical aneurysm in a patient with hypertrophic cardiomyopathy. The thinned apex is well visualized on the cardiac magnetic resonance cine sequences as a thin-walled dyskinetic segment (**A**, diastole; **B**, systole) with transmural scar on late enhancement sequences (**C**, scar visible in *white*). The echocardiogram demonstrates a midcavity gradient on color Doppler (**D**), and on continuous Doppler, the gradient has a typical forked morphology (**E**) that is due to the flow being interrupted in mid systole when the midventricular cavity is obliterated and is clearly distinct from the classic outflow tract gradient. The ECG shows ST elevation in V4-V6 and the inferior leads that should raise the suspicion of apical aneurysm (**F**).

Dyspnea is caused by a combination of LVOTO, mitral regurgitation, and LV diastolic dysfunction. Angina (usually in the absence of epicardial coronary disease) is caused by a number of mechanisms, including small-artery narrowing, intramural compression of small arteries from myocardial hypertrophy, abnormal diastolic filling, oxygen supply-demand mismatch, and abnormal coronary flow reserve.[49–51]

Syncope occurs in ~15% of patients with HCM[71,72] and has multiple potential mechanisms. These include LVOTO[73] and/ or inappropriate vasodilation secondary to LV baroceptor activation during exertion,[58] AF with a fast ventricular response, ventricular tachycardia, sinus node or conduction disease (in middle aged or elderly patients), and neurally mediated (vasovagal). Unexplained (non-vasovagal) syncope is a well-established risk factor for SCD.[71,72,74–76]

PHYSICAL EXAMINATION

A systematic clinical approach should be used in all patients to guide the diagnostic work-up and identify potential phenocopies.[1,12] **Table 42–1** lists some of the most important diagnostic clues or "red flags."

The classical physical findings of HCM are present in patients who have an LV outflow tract gradient. Patients who do not have LVOTO may have findings of LV hypertrophy on physical examination.

Arterial Pulse

The classic carotid pulsation is brisk with a spike-and-dome pattern, characterized by a rapid rise (percussion wave) followed by a midsystolic drop that is, in turn, followed by a secondary wave (tidal wave). The midsystolic fall in amplitude of the carotid pulse contour is caused by premature closure of the aortic valve and coincides with mitral valve SAM. The late peak results from reduction of the outflow tract gradient as the mitral valve leaflet returns to its original position. In the presence of pronounced obstruction, there is a longer ejection time. The carotid pulsation with dynamic LVOTO differs from that of a fixed obstruction such as valvular or discrete subvalvular aortic stenosis, which is characterized by a decrease in both the rate of rise and the amplitude of the pulsation.

Jugular Venous Pulse

Jugular venous pressure is normal in most patients, but the *a* wave can be prominent, indicating a decrease in ventricular compliance caused by right ventricular (RV) hypertrophy,

TABLE 42–1. Summary of the Main Clinical Features That Can Help Identify Specific Causes of Hypertrophic Cardiomyopathy

Cardiomyopathy	Inheritance	Age at Presentation	Extracardiac Manifestations	ECG	Laboratory Testing	Echocardiogram	CMR
Sarcomeric HCM	AD	Any (most frequent adolescent/young adult)	No	Giant negative T-wave inversion in the precordial and/or inferolateral leads suggests involvement of the LV apex	For general assessment: hemoglobin, renal function; NT-brain natriuretic peptide		Midwall LGE LGE at the insertion zones of the RV in the septum Mildly increased native T1
AFD	X-linked	Childhood for classic disease. In the cardiac forms: >30 years (male), >40 years (female)	Acroparesthesias, hypohidrosis, sensorineural deafness, angiokeratomata, cataracts, lymphedema, others	Short PR AV block LVH	Proteinuria ± impaired GFR Low values or undetectable plasma and leukocyte α-galactosidase A present in male patients Raised plasma lyso-GB3	Increased AV valve thickness RV hypertrophy Concentric LVH Papillary muscle enlargement	Posterolateral LGE Reduced native T1
Cardiac amyloidosis	AD if inherited TTR Sporadic if wild type or AL form	>60 years for wild type TTR, male predominance	Bilateral carpal tunnel syndrome, spinal stenosis, biceps tendon rupture (TTR), peripheral sensory neuropathy	AV block Low QRS voltages (50% of AL and 20% of TTR)	Proteinuria ± impaired GFR Serum immunoglobulin free light chain assay, serum and urine electrophoresis if AL amyloidosis is suspected Disproportionately raised NT-brain natriuretic peptide Raised Troponin	Increased interatrial septum thickness Increased AV valve thickness RV hypertrophy Pericardial effusion Concentric LVH Global hypokinesia Apical sparing (strain imaging)	Widespread subendocardial LGE Abnormal gadolinium kinetics Significantly increased native T1 and extracellular volume
Glycogen storage disease (GSD)	AR	Neonates/infants	Muscle weakness, neurologic involvement	Short PR Pre-excitation Extreme LVH (voltage)	Abnormal liver tests Raised creatine phosphokinase	Extreme concentric LVH	No established markers
Danon (GSD IIB)	X-linked	Neonates/infants	Mental retardation, deafness, muscle weakness	Short PR Pre-excitation AV block Extreme LVH (voltage)	Abnormal liver tests Raised creatine phosphokinase	Extreme concentric LVH Global hypokinesia	No established markers
PRKAG2	AD	Adolescent/young adult		Short PR Pre-excitation AV block	Raised creatine phosphokinase	Concentric LVH Global hypokinesia	No established markers
RASopathies	AD	Infants	Mental retardation, dysmorphic features, lentigines, café-au-lait spots, woolly hair	North-West QRS axis deviation		RV hypertrophy Congenital heart disease (eg, pulmonary stenosis) RV outflow tract obstruction	No established markers
Mitochondrial cardiomyopathy	Matrilinear (mitochondrial DNA) AD/AR/X-linked (nuclear DNA)	Neonates/infants	Wide range (eg, deafness, encephalopathy, diabetes, muscle weakness)	Short PR AV block	Impaired GFR and proteinuria Abnormal liver tests Raised creatine phosphokinase Elevated lactate	Global hypokinesia	No established markers
Desminopathies	AD or AR	Young adult (wide range)	Muscle weakness	AV block			No established markers

Abbreviations: AD, autosomal dominant; AFD, Anderson-Fabry disease; AL, amyloid light-chain; AR, autosomal recessive; AV, atrioventricular; CMR, cardiac magnetic resonance; ECG, electrocardiogram; GFR, glomerular filtration rate; HCM, hypertrophic cardiomyopathy; LGE, late gadolinium enhancement; LV, left ventricle; LVH, left ventricular hypertrophy; NT, N-terminal; RV, right ventricle; TTR, transthyretin.

Data from Rapezzi C, Arbustini E, Caforio AL, et al: Diagnostic work-up in cardiomyopathies: bridging the gap between clinical phenotypes and final diagnosis. A position statement from the ESC Working Group on Myocardial and Pericardial Diseases. *Eur Heart J.* 2013 May;34(19):1448-1458.

pulmonary hypertension from left-sided diastolic pressure elevation, or RV outflow obstruction.

Apical Impulse

The apical impulse is almost always abnormal in patients with HCM. Typically, it is a sustained systolic thrust that continues throughout most of systole and can be bifid as a result of a forceful atrial systole. There may be a triple impulse, with a third component occurring near the end of systole if LVOTO is present. A systolic thrill may be palpable at the apex from severe mitral regurgitation or at the lower left sternal border from LVOTO.

Cardiac Auscultation

Auscultation usually reveals a normal or loud first heart sound. The second heart sound is usually split physiologically, although some patients have a paradoxical split as a result of either a concomitant left bundle branch block or severe LVOTO. A fourth heart sound is usually present, especially if there is severe hypertrophy. In young patients, an early diastolic filling sound is frequently heard, indicating rapid early filling. In the presence of severe mitral regurgitation, the excess flow across the mitral valve may result in a diastolic flow rumble.

The classic murmur from LVOTO is a crescendo-decrescendo murmur located primarily at the left sternal border. The murmur usually ends before the second heart sound. The murmur can radiate to the base of the heart as well as to the apex, but in contrast to valvular aortic stenosis, there is seldom radiation to the carotid arteries. Mitral regurgitation may be a separate murmur audible at the apex and is more holosystolic in nature. The presence of an aortic diastolic decrescendo murmur should suggest another disease, such as aortic valve disease or a discrete subvalvular stenosis.

Dynamic auscultation should be performed to differentiate the murmur of HCM from that of valvular aortic stenosis and mitral regurgitation. Maneuvers that decrease preload (Valsalva) or decrease afterload (stand from squat) will increase the dynamic gradient and increase the intensity of the murmur. Simple exercise, such as walking or climbing stairs, can also be used to provoke the murmur.

DIAGNOSTIC TESTING

Electrocardiography

The ECG is abnormal in the majority (~95%) of patients with HCM,[77,78] with a variable combination of repolarization abnormalities (eg, ST-segment depression and/or T-wave inversion) in 75% of patients, LV hypertrophy in ~50%, and abnormal Q waves that simulate a previous myocardial infarction (pseudo-necrosis) can be found in ~30% of cases (**Fig. 42–10**).[78] In most cases, Q waves are generated by the altered balance of depolarization vectors between the hypertrophied septum and infero-lateral wall, and less frequently they reflect areas of replacement scar.[79]

The ECG can also provide clues to the specific morphology and distribution of hypertrophy, with distinctive deep

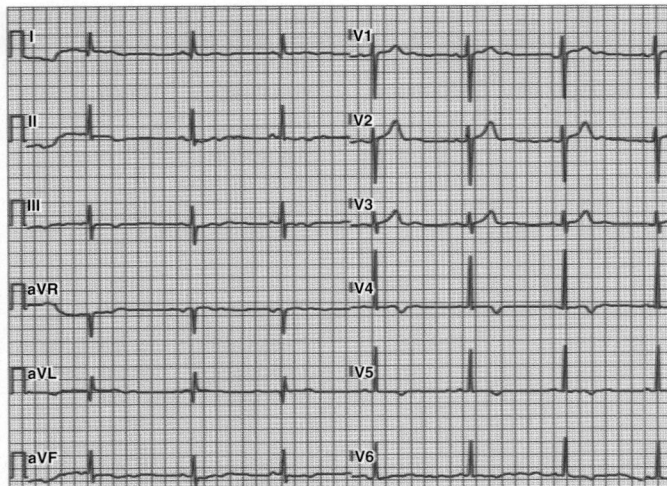

Figure 42–10. Twelve-lead electrocardiogram from a patient with hypertrophic cardiomyopathy showing possible left ventricular hypertrophy, anterior and inferior negative T waves, and lateral pathological Q waves.

symmetric T-wave inversion in V4-V6, the lateral and inferior leads in patients with predominantly apical LV hypertrophy (**Fig. 42–11**). When preceded by ST-segment elevation, this pattern of T-wave inversion suggests an apical aneurysm (see Fig. 42–9F). Additional ECG abnormalities such as preexcitation and atrioventricular (AV) block are potential "red flags" for HCM phenocopies,[12] as summarized in Table 42–1.

The ECG has an important role in the screening of sarcomere mutation carriers and relatives. ECG abnormalities in mutation carriers are a strong risk factor for subsequently developing HCM; however, these abnormalities can precede the development of overt HCM by a number of years (up to 13 in one series).[6,80] It should be noted that a normal ECG does not exclude a diagnosis of HCM with 25% to 50% of carriers found to have a normal ECG at the time they fulfilled diagnostic criteria on cardiac imaging.[6,80]

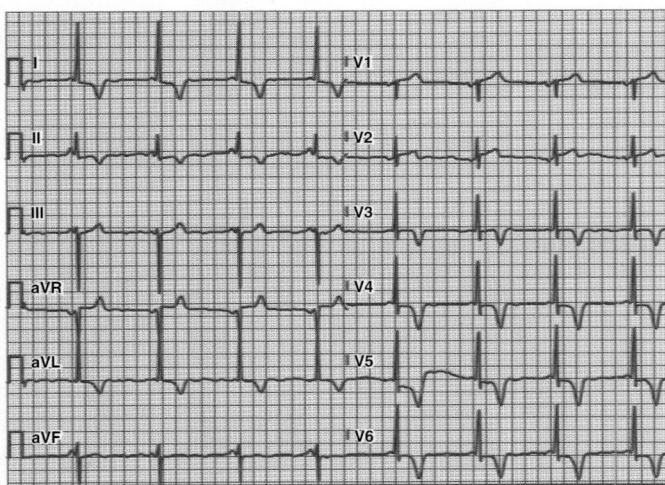

Figure 42–11. Twelve-lead electrocardiogram from a patient with the apical variant of hypertrophic cardiomyopathy showing left ventricular hypertrophy and deep symmetric negative T waves in the antero-lateral leads.

Most patients are in normal sinus rhythm at the time of diagnosis, but AF is common with a prevalence of ~20%.[81-83] Nonsustained ventricular tachycardia is recorded on ambulatory ECG monitoring in ~20% of patients,[84,85] and is associated with an increased risk of SCD in young patients.[85]

Chest X-Ray

The chest x-ray usually shows mild-to-moderate enlargement of the cardiac silhouette. The LV contour is rounded, consistent with LV hypertrophy. There is usually enlargement of the left atrium, and the right-sided chambers are generally normal.

Echocardiography

Echocardiography plays a central role in the diagnosis and management of HCM by providing essential data for risk stratification and the pathophysiology of symptoms, and in guiding septal reduction therapies and pacemaker programing.

Increased LV wall thickness measured by any imaging technique and unexplained by loading conditions is the basis for the diagnosis of HCM. In adults, a wall thickness ≥15 mm at end-diastole in one or more myocardial segments, and in children a wall thickness more than two standard deviations greater than the predicted mean (Z-score >2) are sufficient for a diagnosis.[1,2] In first-degree relatives of patients with unequivocal disease or sarcomere protein mutation carriers, the diagnosis is based on the presence of otherwise unexplained LV hypertrophy ≥13 mm.[1,2] LV hypertrophy most commonly involves the basal septum and anterior wall but can involve any segment, and occasionally has a noncontiguous distribution.[86] Echocardiographic studies should therefore systematically examine all ventricular segments from base to apex. Wall thickness measurements from the short-axis images are considered more accurate, but RV structures (eg, moderator band or *crista supraventricularis*) should not be included.[87] When image quality is poor, intravenous contrast agents can help to visualize the endocardium (this can be particularly useful if the hypertrophy mainly involves the lateral wall or apex).[1,2]

LV wall thickness on echocardiography should be correlated with the ECG findings. For instance, relatively small QRS voltages in the presence of significantly increased wall thickness, should raise suspicion of an infiltrative disorder[12] (**Fig. 42–12**). The opposite can occur in glycogen storage disease (eg, Pompe disease) where ECG voltages are dramatically increased, sometimes in association with ventricular preexcitation.[12]

Diastolic Dysfunction

Diastolic function is assessed through an integrated assessment of left atrial size, transmitral flow pattern, tissue Doppler imaging, pulmonary vein flows, and estimated pulmonary artery systolic pressure.[1,87] However, the correlation between Doppler estimated and invasively measured LV filling pressures is modest.[88]

Systolic Dysfunction

LV ejection fraction is normal or supranormal in the vast majority of HCM cases, although indexed stroke volume is often reduced due to the small cavity size.[87] Longitudinal function measured by tissue Doppler imaging or longitudinal strain is reduced[87] and is an early marker of phenotypic expression that can precede overt LV hypertrophy.[89-91] The progression to a *burn-out* phase that occurs in a minority of HCM patients is defined as LV ejection fraction ≤50%.

Left Ventricular Outflow Tract Obstruction and Mitral Regurgitation

Echocardiography is the primary tool for defining the presence and severity of LVOTO.[1,2,87] It is also essential for ruling out other causes of LVOTO such as a subaortic membrane,[1,2,87,92] and to identify mitral valve structural abnormalities.

Dynamic LVOTO is characterized by a high-velocity, "dagger-shaped" signal on continuous wave Doppler (see Fig. 42–8).[87] Conventionally, LVOTO is defined as an instantaneous peak Doppler LV outflow tract pressure gradient ≥30 mm Hg at rest or during physiologic provocation such as Valsalva maneuver, standing, or exercise. A gradient ≥50 mm Hg is usually considered to be the threshold at which LVOTO becomes hemodynamically significant.[1,87] Latent LVOTO (ie, present only during physiologic provocation) is present in approximately one-third of patients. In patients with outflow tract gradients <50 mm Hg, provocation with the Valsalva maneuver (including on standing if no gradient is provoked at the lateral decubitus or sitting position) is recommended as part of the routine echocardiographic examination. In symptomatic patients with an LVOT gradient <50 mm Hg, exercise stress echocardiography should be considered.[1,2]

The presence of a midcavity obstruction can also be visualized by color flow Doppler (see Fig. 42–9). However, midcavity gradients are underestimated by continuous wave Doppler due to midsystolic flow interruption in the obliterated LV cavity.[93]

Doppler color flow imaging is also used to determine the presence and severity of mitral regurgitation.[87] When mitral regurgitation is secondary to distortion of the mitral valve apparatus by SAM, it occurs mainly during mid-to-late systole with a regurgitant jet directed laterally and posteriorly. In the presence of a holosystolic regurgitation with a central or anterior jet, a primary abnormality of the mitral valve apparatus should be suspected.[1,87] When measuring the LVOT gradient by continuous wave Doppler, care should be taken to ensure it is not contaminated by the jet of mitral regurgitation that would lead to an overestimation of the gradient (**Fig. 42–13**).[87]

Transesophageal Echocardiography

In most patients, transthoracic echocardiography alone is sufficient to obtain the required anatomic and hemodynamic information, but transesophageal echocardiography may be useful in patients in whom discrete subvalvular stenosis or a primary mitral valve abnormality is suspected.[1,2,87] It is also mandatory for the peri- and intraoperative monitoring of septal myectomy to confirm of the mechanism of LVOTO, guide the surgical strategy, and detect postsurgical complications such as ventricular septal defects and residual LVOTO.[1,2,87]

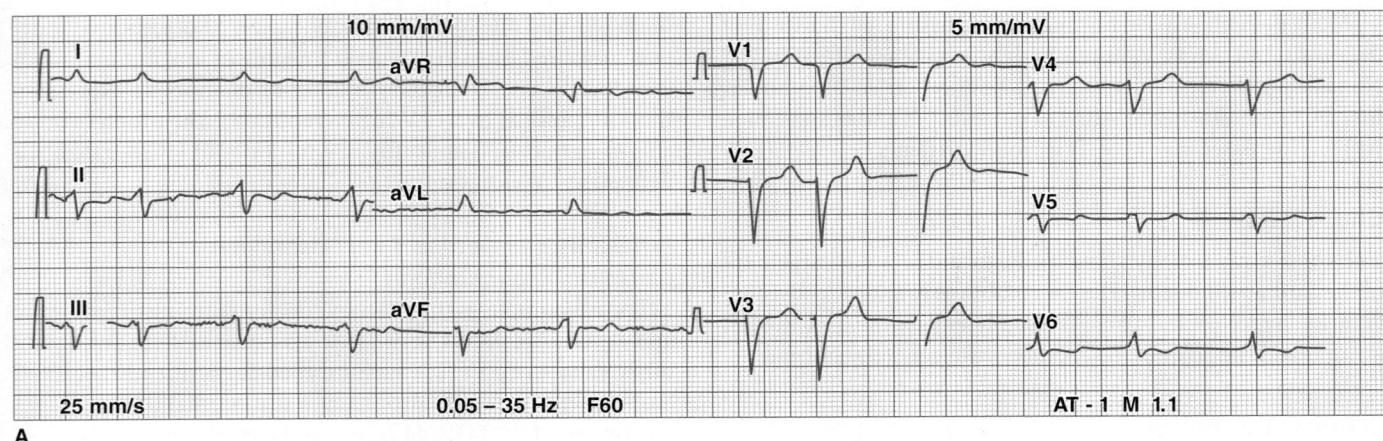

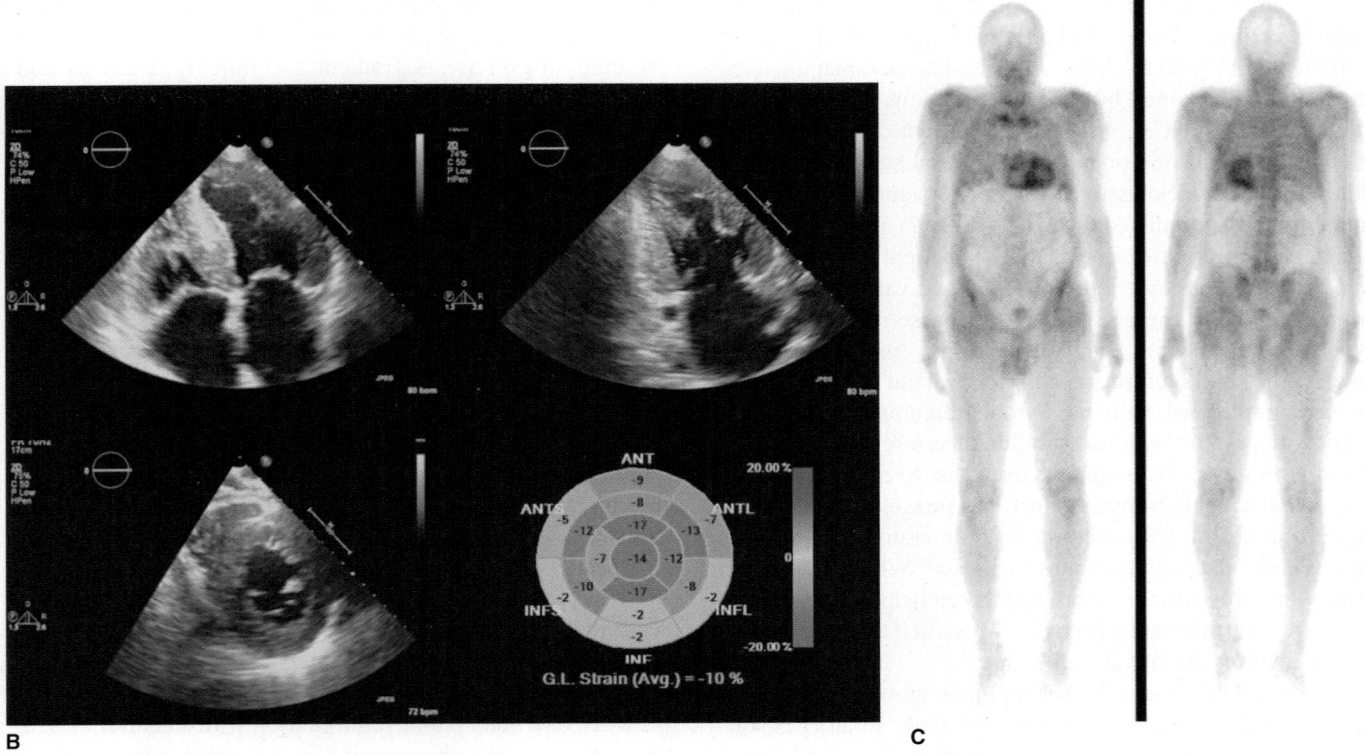

Figure 42–12. Cardiac investigations from a patient with wild-type transthyretin cardiac amyloidosis. **(A)** Twelve-lead electrocardiogram shows low voltage and pseudo-infarct pattern, consistent with infiltrative disease as responsible for the increased left ventricular wall thickness. **(B)** Two-dimensional echocardiogram shows concentric hypertrophy; in the bull's eye plot (*lower-right image*), note the relative apical sparing for the markedly diminished global longitudinal strain. **(C)** Technetium-99m-3,3-diphosphono-1,2-propanodicarboxylic acid (99mTc-DPD) scan showing strong myocardial uptake.

Cardiac Magnetic Resonance Imaging

CMR imaging provides high-resolution images of the myocardium that allow an accurate assessment of the site and degree of LV hypertrophy (**Fig. 42–14**).[87] This is particularly useful in patients with suboptimal echocardiographic images and/or equivocal hypertrophy, especially when it involves the LV apex or basal antero-lateral wall that are not well visualized on echo (**Fig. 42–15**).[86]

Compared to echocardiography, CMR also yields a more precise measurement of the LV ejection fraction and can easily

demonstrate LV apical aneurysms (as well as the thrombus they potentially contain), that can be challenging to visualize on echo.[87]

CMR also provides tissue characterization. In HCM, the most commonly used method for this purpose is late gadolinium enhancement (LGE) that represents areas of replacement fibrosis. LGE is common, but not a constant finding in HCM, being present in 50% to 60% of patients.[94] The pattern of LGE in HCM is variable, but almost always has a nonischemic distribution, most often involving the hypertrophied segments

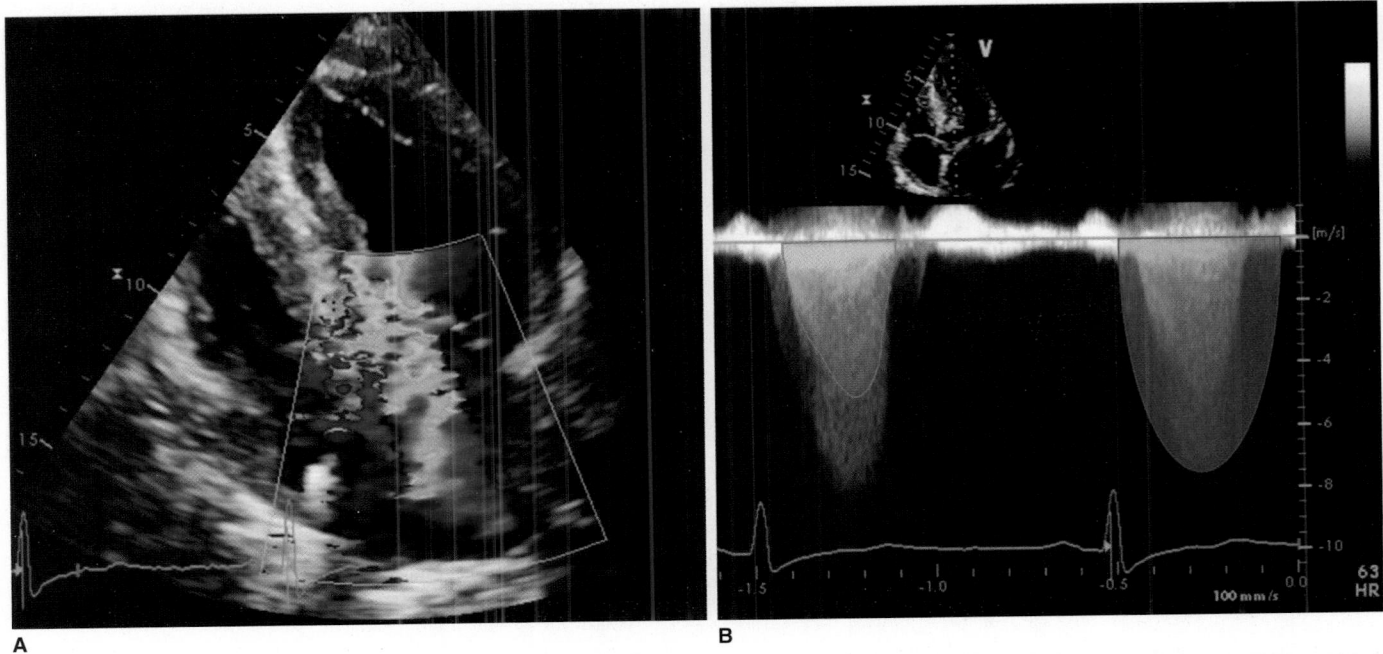

A   **B**

Figure 42–13. Mitral regurgitation and left ventricular outflow tract obstruction in a patient with hypertrophic cardiomyopathy. **(A)** Color Doppler shows accelerated flow in the left ventricular outflow tract and a jet of mitral regurgitation in the left atrium. **(B)** Continuous wave Doppler shows two distinct envelopes, the first is dagger-shaped and late peaking (outflow tract gradient, highlighted in *red*) and the second has a higher maximum velocity and a holosystolic duration (mitral regurgitation, highlighted in *blue*).

and RV insertion points. The presence of LGE is associated with a worse prognosis, specifically a higher risk of progression to a *burn-out* phase[30] and all-cause mortality.[95] Critically however, whether the extent of LGE is independently associated with SCD events remains controversial, and this is at least partially due to the lack of standardization of LGE quantification methods.[96,97]

More recently, the development of T1 mapping has provided a further useful tissue characterization tool. Compared to healthy subjects, native T1 values (and estimated extracellular volume) are mildly increased as a result of interstitial fibrosis.

This finding is not specific, but T1 mapping can be useful in raising the suspicion of specific phenocopies, namely cardiac amyloidosis (where values are markedly increased) and Anderson–Fabry disease (where myocardial T1 is lower than normal) (see Table 42–1).[98]

Perfusion sequences demonstrate defects in most HCM patients both at rest and following adenosine stress despite the absence of epicardial coronary artery disease; these perfusion defects are not necessarily limited to hypertrophied segments. Quantitative perfusion mapping has recently shown that in a subgroup of HCM patients, myocardial blood flow

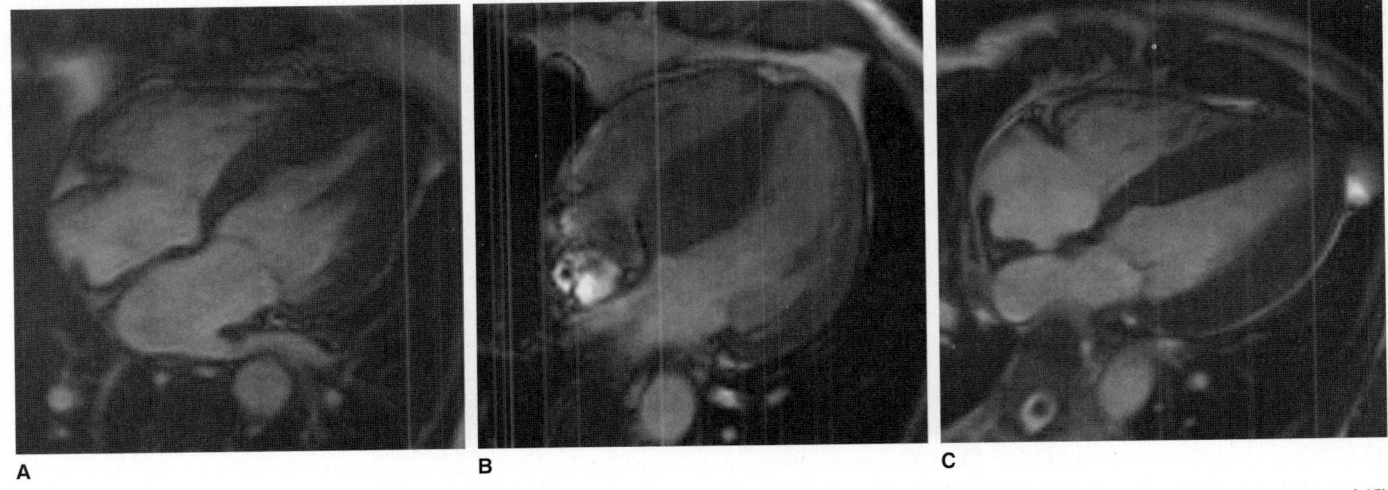

A   **B**   **C**

Figure 42–14. Different distributions of hypertrophy in hypertrophic cardiomyopathy on cardiac magnetic resonance: **(A)** apical, **(B)** asymmetric, and **(C)** concentric.

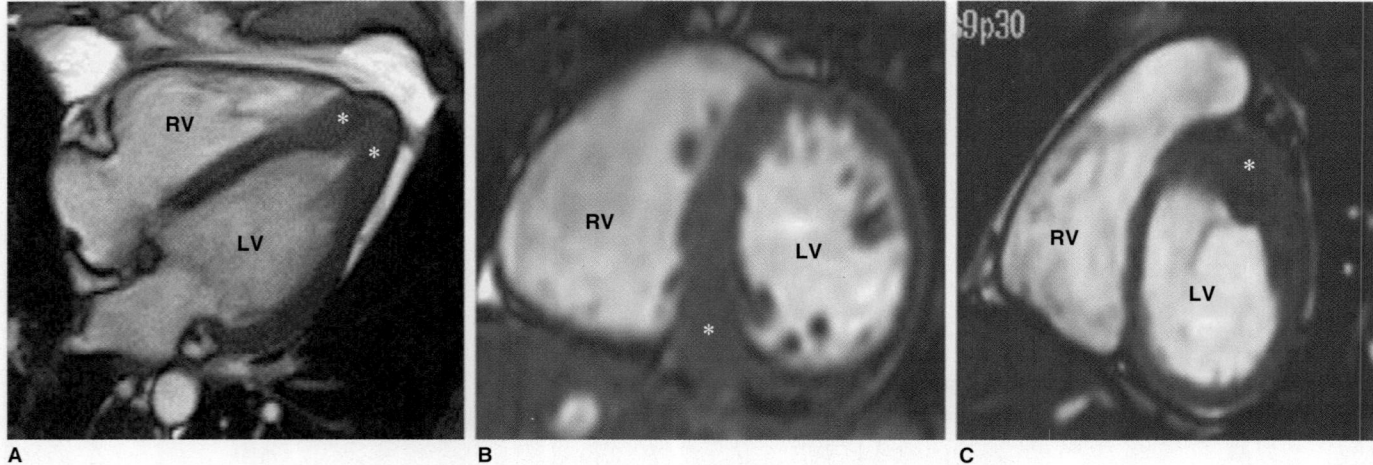

Figure 42–15. In specific segments of the left ventricle, hypertrophy can be very challenging to visualize on echocardiogram but is well appreciated on cardiac magnetic resonance imaging (*asterisk*). These segments include the apex (**A**), the posterior septum where it transitions into the inferior wall (**B**), and the basal anterior wall (**C**). LV, left ventricle; RV, right ventricle. Reproduced with permission from Maron MS, Maron BJ, Harrigan C, Bet al: Hypertrophic cardiomyopathy phenotype revisited after 50 years with cardiovascular magnetic resonance. *J Am Coll Cardiol*. 2009 Jul 14;54(3):220-228.

actually decreases following adenosine (rather than increase as expected).[51]

CMR plays an increasingly important role in screening sarcomere protein mutation carriers, mainly due to the higher sensitivity than echocardiography in detecting mild hypertrophy.[6] It can also demonstrate a number of structural anomalies in mutation carriers, including crypts, anterior mitral valve leaflet elongation, abnormal trabeculae,[99] and increased extracellular volume,[100] although the clinical significance of these findings in predicting subsequent development of HCM has yet to be established.

Finally, CMR images also provide important anatomical detail in patients being considered for invasive septal reduction therapy, by accurately showing the distribution and extent of hypertrophy (particularly in the basal septum), mitral valve leaflet length, and anatomy of the subvalvular apparatus.[87]

Nuclear Imaging

Similar to stress CMR, single-photon emission computed tomography (CT) myocardial perfusion imaging frequently shows reversible and fixed defects in HCM in the absence of epicardial coronary artery disease.[87] Positron emission tomography allows quantification of myocardial blood flow, which typically shows a blunted response to vasodilators.[87]

Scintigraphy with bone-seeking tracers (technetium[99m]-3,3-diphosphono-1,2-propanodicarboxylic acid [DPD] in Europe, and technetium[99m]-pyrophosphate [PYP] in the United States) has emerged as the key noninvasive test for the diagnosis of transthyretin cardiac amyloidosis,[101] a frequent HCM phenocopy in elderly patients (see Fig. 42–12C).

Cardiac Catheterization

Cardiac catheterization to assess LV function and dynamic LVOTO is rarely required in HCM.[1] LVOTO can be assessed by placing an end-hole catheter at the LV apex and pulling it back to the base of the heart and then into the aorta. However,

because the small LV cavity can cause catheter "entrapment" resulting in a falsely increased LV systolic pressure, the gradient is ideally assessed by a simultaneous LV inflow and LV outflow (or aortic) pressure,[40] but this requires a trans-septal approach.

When there is little resting obstruction, provocation using the Valsalva maneuver or infusion of isoproterenol can be performed in the catheterization laboratory. The Brockenbrough phenomenon—the hallmark of latent obstruction—refers to the phenomenon that occurs after a premature contraction, when the increase in the contractility of the ventricle results in a marked increase in the degree of dynamic obstruction (**Fig. 42–16**). This is seen as an increase in the outflow gradient and a decrease in the aortic pulse pressure after the pause. This is in contrast to a fixed obstruction in which the increase in stroke volume leads to an increase in outflow tract gradient, but also an increase in aortic pulse pressure.

Left ventriculography usually reveals a small LV cavity size with hypertrophied papillary muscles further impinging into the cavity. Hyperdynamic radial systolic function causes complete obliteration of the mid and apical cavity in systole (**Fig. 42–17**). In the apical variant of HCM, there is obliteration of the apex by the hypertrophied muscle, causing a "spade-like" configuration. With midventricular obstruction, an apical akinetic or dyskinetic pouch (aneurysm) may be visible.

Coronary angiography should be carried out to exclude coexistent coronary disease in patients with severe exertional angina or sustained ventricular tachycardia, and in cardiac arrest survivors.[1] Myocardial bridging is frequent (prevalence 15%–40%), particularly in younger patients with severe hypertrophy; however, the impact of bridging on outcomes remains unclear.[38,102-104]

Endomyocardial biopsy is only recommended when the noninvasive work-up suggests inflammatory, infiltrative, or metabolic disease that cannot be confirmed by other means (eg, biopsy of another tissue/organ).[1]

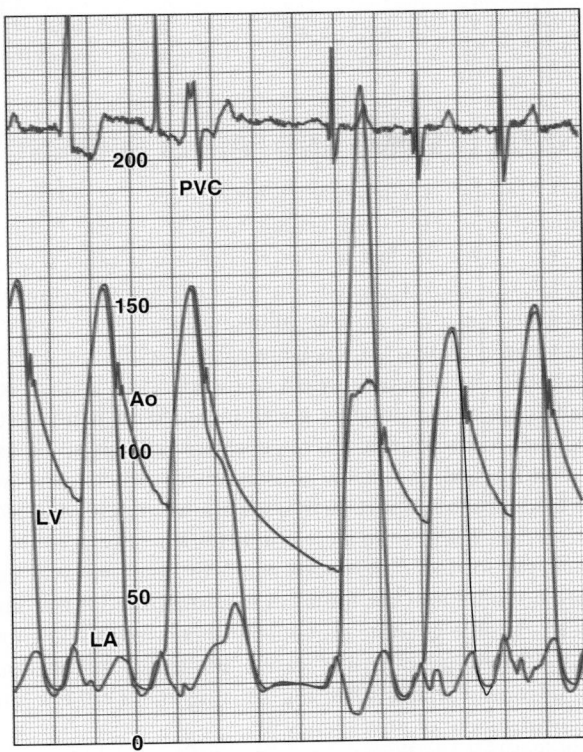

Figure 42–16. Cardiac catheterization from a patient with no resting left ventricular outflow tract obstruction. However, after a premature ventricular contraction (PVC), the left ventricular outflow tract gradient is close to 100 mm Hg. The pulse pressure of the ascending aorta (Ao) is decreased on the beat following the premature ventricular contraction. This phenomenon is termed the Brockenbrough phenomenon. LA, left atrium; LV, left ventricle.

Cardiac Computed Tomography

Coronary artery CT angiogram should be considered in patients with exertional chest pain, based on their atherosclerotic risk profile.[1] Cardiac CT can also be used to evaluate ventricular size, wall thickness and function in patients with poor echocardiographic windows and contraindications or intolerance to CMR.[1]

Stress Testing

Exercise stress testing is of limited value for the diagnosis of epicardial coronary disease in patients with HCM, but is helpful in assessing prognosis and the pathophysiology of symptoms.[105,106] Cardiopulmonary exercise testing provides an objective measurement of exercise tolerance, and parameters such as ventilatory efficiency, anaerobic threshold, and peak oxygen consumption are predictors of death from heart failure.[107]

Laboratory Testing

General laboratory tests are useful in the assessment of comorbidities that can have an impact on symptoms and/or prognosis (eg, renal disease), and in detecting phenocopies (see Table 42–1). N-terminal pro–B-type natriuretic peptide (NT-proBNP) is a strong predictor of all-cause mortality,

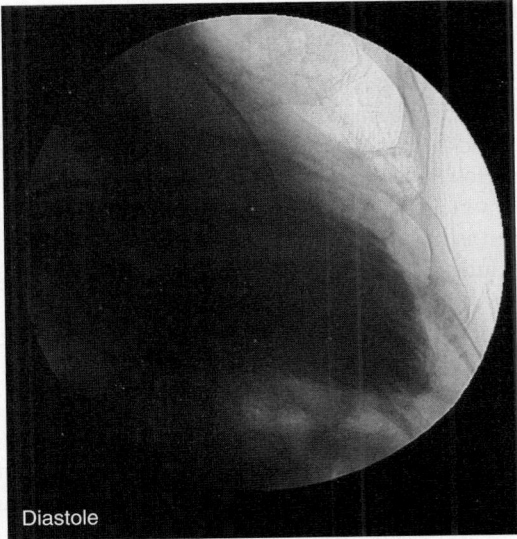

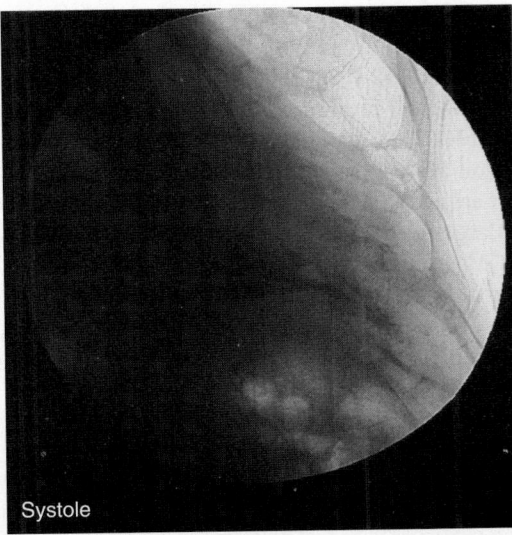

Figure 42–17. Left ventriculography from a patient with hypertrophic cardiomyopathy. There is near-complete systolic obliteration of the left ventricular cavity.

heart failure death, and cardiac transplantation.[108] Measurement of plasma and leukocyte α-galactosidase A is used to screen for Anderson–Fabry disease in male patients. In cases where primary (AL) amyloidosis is suspected, serum and urine immunofixation and serum-free light-chains should be measured.[12] In patients with an HCM phenotype, a raised creatine kinase can be associated with mitochondrial diseases, glycogenosis (Pompe disease or *PRKAG2*-related), Danon disease, and muscular dystrophy (*FHL1*-related).[12]

DIFFERENTIAL DIAGNOSIS

The list of differential diagnoses for LV hypertrophy is considerable and a number of HCM phenocopies including infiltrative, metabolic, and neuromuscular diseases should be considered (Table 42–1).

Hypertensive Heart Disease

The most common differential diagnosis is hypertensive heart disease. Morphology and distribution of hypertrophy are not helpful, but the degree of hypertrophy may be, with maximal LV wall thickness rarely reaching 15 mm in hypertensive heart disease. However, the differential can be very challenging in Black hypertensive patients, in whom a wall thickness of 15 to 20 mm is not uncommon.[109] Other potentially helpful features include dilation of the LV cavity and/or ascending aorta, both suggesting hypertensive heart disease rather than HCM. Importantly, the presence of LVOTO is not helpful because it is found in both.[110]

Athlete's Heart

Differently from HCM, the LV hypertrophy that develops as a physiological adaptation to training is eccentric, being associated with LV cavity dilation.[111] The hypertrophic response is greater in males, reaching 15 mm in White and 16 mm in Black male athletes,[112] while wall thickness never reaches these values in female athletes.

The standard 12-lead ECG is generally very useful with some pathological findings strongly suggesting a diagnosis of HCM (**Table 42–2**).[113] The presence of LVOTO or diastolic dysfunction are also suggestive of HCM because they are not found in athletes.[111] On the other hand, the presence of left atrial enlargement is not helpful because it can be found in both HCM and athletic adaptation (to a degree). CMR can be a useful tool, clearly documenting ventricular cavity size, degree and distribution of hypertrophy, and importantly, the presence of late enhancement that is not present in athletic adaptation.[111]

TABLE 42–2. ECG Abnormalities That Suggest a Diagnosis of HCM in Athletes

ECG Finding	Definition
T-wave inversion	≥1 mm in depth in two or more contiguous leads; excludes leads aVR, III, and V1 Exceptions: - Black athletes with J-point elevation and convex ST segment elevation followed by TWI in V2–V4 - athletes <age 16 with TWI in V1-V3 - biphasic T waves in only V3
ST-segment depression	≥0.5 mm in depth in two or more contiguous leads
Pathologic Q waves	Q/R ratio ≥0.25 or ≥40 ms in duration in two or more leads (excluding III and aVR)
Complete left bundle branch block	QRS ≥120 ms, predominantly negative QRS complex in lead V1 (QS or rS), and upright notched or slurred R wave in leads I and V6
Profound nonspecific intraventricular conduction delay	Any QRS duration ≥140 ms

Abbreviations: TWI, T-wave inversion. Data from Sharma S, Drezner JA, Baggish A, et al: International recommendations for electrocardiographic interpretation in athletes. *Eur Heart J.* 2018 Apr 21;39(16):1466-1480.

Finally, detraining is a potentially helpful tool, HCM being the likely diagnosis in absence of hypertrophy regression.[114,115]

GENETIC TESTING AND FAMILY SCREENING

Genetic testing is currently recommended for all patients diagnosed with HCM, to enable cascade genetic testing of relatives.[1,2] Over the last few years, massive parallel sequencing platforms have replaced conventional Sanger sequencing in diagnostic genetic testing, allowing for a larger panel of genes to be evaluated.[14] Increasing panel size has not however substantially increased the yield of testing.[116] In fact, a recent reevaluation of the putative genes included in panels established that most nonsarcomere genes are unlikely to be associated with HCM.[117] The few nonsarcomere protein genes with good evidence to support their association with HCM (*CSRP3, FHL1, PLN, TNNC1, FLNC,* and *FHOD3*) only account for a small proportion (0.25%–2% each) of "gene-elusive" cases (where no mutations are found in the established 8 sarcomere genes).[117] Whole genome sequencing increases the diagnostic yield (~10% of "gene-elusive" cases), but this is mainly due to deep intronic variants affecting splicing in *MYBPC3* rather than involvement of novel genes.[118]

All probands undergoing genetic testing should be offered genetic counseling.[1,2,119] This includes the construction of a family pedigree, which can be valuable in assessing patterns of inheritance and detecting etiologic clues.[12] When a pathogenic variant is identified in the proband, first-degree relatives may be screened using targeted DNA analysis for the same mutation (predictive testing) along with clinical screening with ECG, echocardiogram, and potentially CMR. Relatives who carry a pathogenic variant but have no overt cardiomyopathy should be kept under regular follow-up, while those who do not carry the pathogenic variant can be discharged because their risk of developing HCM is considered similar to that of the general population.[1,2,119] When no pathogenic variants are identified, family screening will need to be performed using clinical assessment alone.[1,2] Importantly, the pathogenicity of variants should be reassessed every few years to ensure that if the variant has been reclassified (upgraded or downgraded) the family is managed appropriately.[2] Economic modeling studies have suggested that genetic screening strategies are more cost-effective than clinical screening alone.[120]

Current European guidelines recommend clinical screening from the age of 10 to 12 years (in absence of a malignant family history or concerning symptoms),[1] but based on growing evidence of preadolescent penetrance of HCM,[5] the more recent American Heart Association/American College of Cardiology (AHA/ACC) guidelines now recommend screening from childhood.[2] The frequency of follow-up screening visits that is currently recommended by guidelines for both mutation carriers and families with unavailable or negative genetic testing is based solely on age (every 1–3 years in children, adolescents, and teens; every 2–5 years in adults),[1,2] but recent data suggest that follow-up of mutation carriers should be tailored to sex and genotype rather than age.[6] Individuals with an abnormal ECG but no overt hypertrophy should be followed up closely, every 6 to 12 months.[1]

NATURAL HISTORY

The natural history of individual patients with HCM is highly variable. The early literature described a poor prognosis (all-cause mortality ~5% per year) with a high incidence of SCD, but this was influenced by significant referral bias since these small cohorts consisted mainly of younger, severely affected patients who had been referred because they were judged to be at high risk or had severe symptoms requiring specialized care.[121] Contemporary studies report a much lower mortality due to advances in management (particularly implantable cardioverter defibrillators [ICDs], and the wider use of septal myectomy and anticoagulation), and as a result of the inclusion of patients with milder disease.[122,123]

Despite the improved outcome however, an excess mortality in HCM compared to the general population persists, particularly in young patients and women[84] and there are clearly patient subgroups that remain at high risk.[124]

Sudden Cardiac Death

SCD can be the first manifestation of HCM (incidence 0.5%–0.8% per year)[74,125] and is most frequent in young adults.[84] SCD in HCM is most commonly due to ventricular fibrillation and the underlying pathophysiologic mechanisms include myocyte disarray, hypertrophy, and fibrosis that promote reentry arrhythmias, abnormal calcium dynamics causing delayed afterdepolarizations, and increased calcium sensitivity leading to increased dispersion of repolarization.[126] Other arrhythmias that have been reported in association with SCD in HCM include asystole, rapid supraventricular arrhythmias, pulseless electrical activity, and AV block.[126]

Atrial Fibrillation and Stroke

The overall prevalence of paroxysmal and permanent AF in HCM is ~20%,[81-83] with an annual incidence around 3%.[82] The main predictor of AF is left atrial size, but it is also associated with age, female sex, and New York Heart Association (NYHA) functional class.[127] The loss of atrial systole as a consequence of AF is often poorly tolerated, with a reduction in exercise tolerance[83] and increased mortality.[83,127]

Systemic embolism in HCM is usually caused by AF[82] and has a cumulative incidence of ~6% at 10 years.[128] Other predictors of thromboembolism include age, prior thromboembolism, NYHA class, left atrial size, and maximal LV wall thickness. The CHA_2DS_2-VASc score (congestive heart failure, hypertension, age ≥ 75 years, diabetes mellitus, prior stroke or thromboembolism, vascular disease, age 65–74 years, female sex) has a low predictive value in HCM [128] and should not be used to estimate thromboembolic risk.[1,2]

Heart Failure

Patients with *burnt-out* HCM can remain stable for a number of years on optimal medical treatment, but have a poor prognosis, due to both advanced heart failure and an increased risk of SCD, particularly with an LV ejection fraction <35% (**Fig. 42–18**).[30,54] Even though the factors responsible for systolic heart failure have yet to be clarified, the risk appears to be higher in those with a family history of *burn-out* progression,[54] and in those with HCM due to sarcomere gene mutations, particularly thin filament genes (*TNNI3, TNNT2, TPM1,* and *ACTC1*).[30] An association with septal reduction therapies (surgical myectomy and alcohol septal ablation) has also been recently observed, although it remains unclear whether this is a causal relationship or part of the natural history of disease.[30]

Pulmonary hypertension is relatively common in HCM, with a prevalence of 35% to 40% on echocardiography, but is infrequently severe.[129] Increased pulmonary pressures are associated with age and female sex, and pulmonary hypertension has been proposed as an independent prognostic marker in patients with a nonobstructive pathophysiology and those with LVOTO who do not undergo septal reduction treatment.[129]

Infective Endocarditis

National registry data suggests that HCM confers an increased risk of infective endocarditis compared to the general population with a cumulative 10-year risk of 0.5%.[130] Multicenter studies

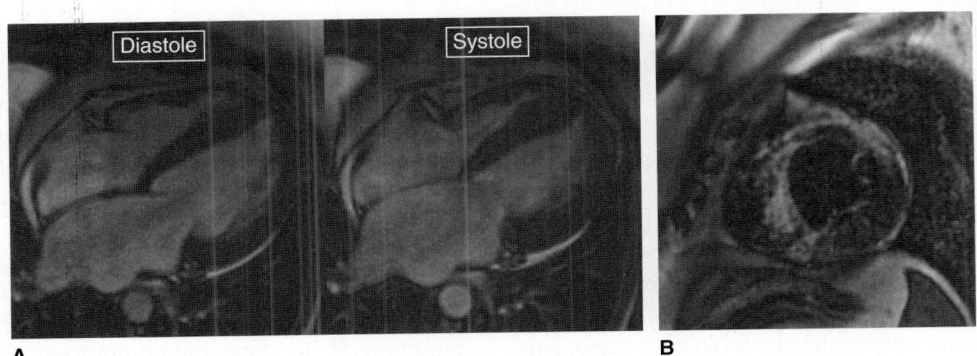

Figure 42–18. Burn-out hypertrophic cardiomyopathy in a patient with a *TNNT2* mutation. **(A)** Four-chamber cine sequence on cardiac magnetic resonance showing a nondilated left ventricle with concentric hypertrophy and severe systolic dysfunction. **(B)** Short axis black-blood late gadolinium enhancement sequence showing very extensive fibrosis (visible in *white*) that has almost entirely replaced the septal myocardium.

suggest the risk is limited to patients with LVOT obstruction, with an incidence of 3.8% person-years in this group.[131] However, the rate of aortic and mitral valve involvement appears to be similar.[132] Current guidelines recommend good routine oral hygiene, but not routine antibiotic prophylaxis for procedures with a risk of bacteremia.[133]

SEX DIFFERENCES

A male predominance around 60% is a constant finding in large HCM cohorts[27,84,122,123,134–136] with a clear sex differences in clinical profile at presentation, females being older more symptomatic, and with a greater degree of LVOT obstruction.[84,134–136] Worse all-cause mortality has been reported in women[84,135,136] and this is probably related to a higher heart failure and stroke-related mortality.[84,134] These differences in baseline profile and outcome have yet to be explained. Some degree of survival bias is possible, with males being affected at a younger age[6] and possibly more severely. In murine models, HCM phenotype (LV hypertrophy, function and fibrosis) appears to be the result of a complex interaction between sex, sex hormones, genotype (specific sarcomeric mutation, but also other genes such as androgen receptors), and hypertrophic stimuli.[137–143] Finally, nonbiological factors may also contribute to the observed sex differences, since women have been shown to have a reduced awareness of cardiovascular risk,[144] a longer delay in seeking medical attention in acute coronary syndromes,[145,146] and less access to screening programs.[147,148]

TREATMENT

Left Ventricular Outflow Tract Obstruction

Medical Therapy

Patients with LVOTO should maintain good hydration at all times, avoid excessive alcohol consumption, and maintain a healthy weight. Arterial and venous vasodilators (including dihydropyridine calcium channel blockers) should be avoided because they worsen the LVOT gradient.[1,2] AF is often poorly tolerated and a rhythm control strategy is generally preferred with amiodarone and ablation procedures used to maintain sinus rhythm as long as possible. Overall, AF catheter ablation has a low complication rate, but is less effective in patients with HCM. It does, however, still have a role, particularly in patients with smaller atria and paroxysmal AF.[149] Rate control can be achieved with β-blockers or nondihydropyridine calcium channel antagonists; digoxin should be avoided in patients with LVOT obstruction due to the positive inotropic effect.[1,2]

Medical therapy is the first-line therapy for the relief of symptoms in patients with obstructive HCM and by consensus β-adrenergic blocking agents are generally the first choice.[1,2,150] The dosage should be titrated to symptom relief or to obtain a resting heart rate <60 bpm.

Nondihydropyridine calcium channel blockers (verapamil and diltiazem) are also of value in the treatment of LVOTO,[41] particularly if β-blockers are contraindicated or ineffective.[1,2] By preventing calcium influx, they not only decrease inotropy and chronotropy, but also improve diastolic relaxation.[41,151] Verapamil has been shown to decrease LVOT gradient,[152] improve exercise capacity,[153] and may improve angina to a greater degree than β-blockers. Verapamil is used most frequently due to the minimal effect on afterload, and the dose should be titrated up to 480 mg/day to obtain a resting heart rate <60 bpm.

A small subset of patients can deteriorate hemodynamically with verapamil, presumably because of a lowering of afterload.[154] This deterioration occurs particularly in the presence of severe outflow tract gradients (≥100 mm Hg), high diastolic filling pressures, and elevated pulmonary artery systolic pressures.

In patients with LVOTO who remain symptomatic despite treatment with β-blockers and/or calcium channel blockers, disopyramide can be used to improve symptoms.[1,2,155] Despite being an antiarrhythmic drug, in this context it is used for its negative inotropic effect. Concomitant β-blockade (or verapamil) is important to prevent rapid AV node conduction, particularly during exercise or with coexistent AF.[1,2,155] The dose of disopyramide required to produce symptomatic benefit is between 300 and 600 mg/day. The corrected QT interval should be monitored at the initiation of disopyramide and dose reduced if it exceeds 480 ms.[1] Contraindications to its use include glaucoma, prostatic hypertrophy, and concomitant use of other QT-prolonging drugs.[1] Anticholinergic adverse effects can limit its usefulness in older patients.

Mavacamten is a cardiac myosin ATPase inhibitor that was specifically developed to target the pathophysiology of HCM by reducing actin–myosin cross-bridge formation, thereby reducing contractility and improving myocardial energetics.[156] In the recently published EXPLORER-HCM trial, it reduced the LVOT gradient and improve exercise capacity when compared to placebo (on top of β-blockers or calcium channel blockers) in patients with HCM and symptomatic LVOTO;[157] 27% of patients on mavacamten had a LVOT gradient reduction to <30 mm Hg and improved to NYHA class I. The drug was well tolerated and has a good safety profile, only a small subset of patients developed transient LV systolic dysfunction that resolved after suspending the drug. A small CMR substudy suggests that mavacamten may also lead to positive myocardial remodeling, with reduction in myocardial mass, LV wall thickness, and left atrial volume.[158]

Septal Reduction Therapy

Patients with a significant LVOTO gradient and severe symptoms despite optimal medical therapy should be considered for invasive treatment.[1,2] The AHA/ACC guidelines also allow consideration of patients with milder symptoms (**Table 42–3**). Invasive options include septal myectomy, alcohol septal ablation, and dual-chamber pacing.

When performed in experienced surgical centers, surgical septal myectomy remains the reference standard therapy for patients with obstruction and severe drug-refractory symptoms.[1,2] To date, no randomized controlled trial has investigated the effect on outcome, but observational data suggest that myectomy may improve survival of patients with LVOTO.[159]

TABLE 42–3. Comparison of Guideline Recommendations for Septal Reduction Therapies in HCM

ESC 2014 Guidelines[1]	AHA/ACC 2020 Guidelines[2]
SRT carried out in experienced centres is recommended to improve symptoms in patients with a resting or provoked LVOT peak gradient ≥50 mm Hg and severe symptoms (NYHA functional class III/IV), despite maximum tolerated medical therapy.	SRT performed at experienced centres is recommended to relieve LVOT obstruction in patients with a resting or provoked LVOT peak gradient ≥50 mm Hg who remain severely symptomatic (NYHA functional class III/IV or exertional syncope/pre-syncope), despite optimal medical therapy.
SRT should be considered in experienced centres in patients with recurrent exertional syncope and a resting or provoked LVOT peak gradient ≥50 mm Hg, despite optimal medical therapy.	Surgical myectomy performed at experienced centres may be reasonable in patients with a resting or provoked LVOT peak gradient ≥50 mm Hg and moderate symptoms (NYHA class II) in the presence of additional clinical factors, including: - Severe and progressive pulmonary hypertension thought to be attributable to LVOT obstruction or associated MR. - Left atrial enlargement with ≥1 episodes of symptomatic AF. - Poor functional capacity attributable to LVOT obstruction as documented on treadmill exercise testing. - Children and young adults with very high resting LVOT gradients (>100 mm Hg).

Abbreviations: HCM, hypertrophic cardiomyopathy; ESC, European Society of Cardiology; AHA/ACC, American Heart Association/American College of Cardiology; SRT, septal reduction therapies; LVOT, left ventricular outflow tract; NYHA, New York Heart Association; MR, mitral regurgitation; AF, atrial fibrillation.

A careful preoperative work-up is paramount and includes transthoracic and transesophageal echocardiography, CMR, and coronary artery imaging. Intraoperative transesophageal echocardiography is essential in achieving an optimal outcome.[87]

Septal myectomy is performed via a transaortic incision and involves resection of a small amount of muscle from the proximal to midseptal region (Morrow procedure). This enlarges the LV outflow tract and significantly decreases or totally abolishes LVOT gradient in 90% of patients.[64,160] Concomitant SAM-related mitral regurgitation usually improves following myectomy (**Fig. 42–19**).[68] Additional mitral valve surgery may be necessary in patients who undergo traditional septal myectomy,[68,160] but it has been recently suggested that resection of thickened secondary mitral valve chordae at the time of myectomy can improve results, particularly in patients with mild hypertrophy.[64] Additionally, anomalous papillary muscles can be resected or repositioned[161] and mitral valvuloplasty or plication can be carried out.[162,163] Mitral valve replacement should be reserved for cases where severe, nonrepairable mitral valve disease is present;[1,2] observational data suggest a worse outcome following mitral valve replacement in HCM compared to myectomy with or without mitral valve repair.[160]

For cases with a significant midcavity obstruction, a midventricular myectomy via a transapical approach has been proposed[164] but the technique is confined to few centers.

In experienced, large-volume centers, the operative mortality for septal myectomy is <1%,[165] but outcomes are not as good in lower volume centers[166] and the risk is higher in elderly patients who require additional procedures, such as aortic valve replacement, mitral valve repair, or coronary artery bypass grafting. The most common surgical complication is AV block requiring permanent pacemaker insertion, the risk being particularly high in patients with a preexisting right bundle branch block,[167] while ventricular septal defect, stroke, and aortic regurgitation are now uncommon in experienced centers.[168]

Alcohol septal ablation (ASA) is a procedure in which alcohol is injected in the septal perforator arteries in order to cause necrosis and scarring of the proximal interventricular septum.[169] The subsequent wall thinning and remodeling of the basal septum leads to widening of the LVOT and reduction of the gradient over 3 to 6 months (**Figs. 42–20** and **42–21**).[170] Prior to the injection of alcohol, contrast is injected in the septal branch to visualize on transthoracic echo the area of myocardium perfused by the selected septal branch.[171] If the basal septum target region is not highlighted by the contrast, a different septal branch is chosen or the procedure aborted. The volume of alcohol injected corresponds with the degree of LVOT gradient reduction and with the most common complication, AV block requiring a permanent pacemaker; a volume of 1.5 to 2.5 mL has been suggested as optimal.[172] The risk of complete AV block is particularly high in patients with a preexisting left bundle branch block.[173] Other procedural complications include ventricular arrhythmias, coronary dissection, extensive infarction from alcohol leakage, ventricular septal defect, and myocardial perforation.[174] Periprocedural mortality is ~1%.[172,175] Historically, the main concern following ASA is the long-term repercussions of a iatrogenic infarction, particularly with regards to ventricular arrhythmias. Large series have now provided reassuring medium-term data[172,175]; however, considering the young age of many HCM patients, follow-up in these studies was relatively brief (3–6 years).[176]

The choice of invasive septal reduction treatment should be discussed by a multidisciplinary team and individualized on the basis of clinical profile, and thorough anatomical evaluation of the septum and mitral valve apparatus.[1,2] No clinical trials have compared myectomy and ASA to date, but observational data provide some useful points to assist decision making. While mortality for the two procedures is similar,[175] recovery following a percutaneous procedure is faster than following a sternotomy. On the other hand, myectomy is probably more effective in relieving symptoms, the likelihood of reintervention after ASA being 5 times higher.[175] The likelihood of requiring a permanent pacemaker is higher following ASA than myectomy (~10% vs ~5%).[175] Finally, it is also worth noting the worse outcome of myectomy following a previous ASA.[177]

Dual-Chamber Pacing

Dual-chamber pacing can decrease the LVOT gradient. The underlying mechanism is not completely understood, but the following have been proposed: reduction of LV hypercontractility, delayed septal activation and thickening, reduction of mitral valve SAM (possibly by early anterior papillary muscle

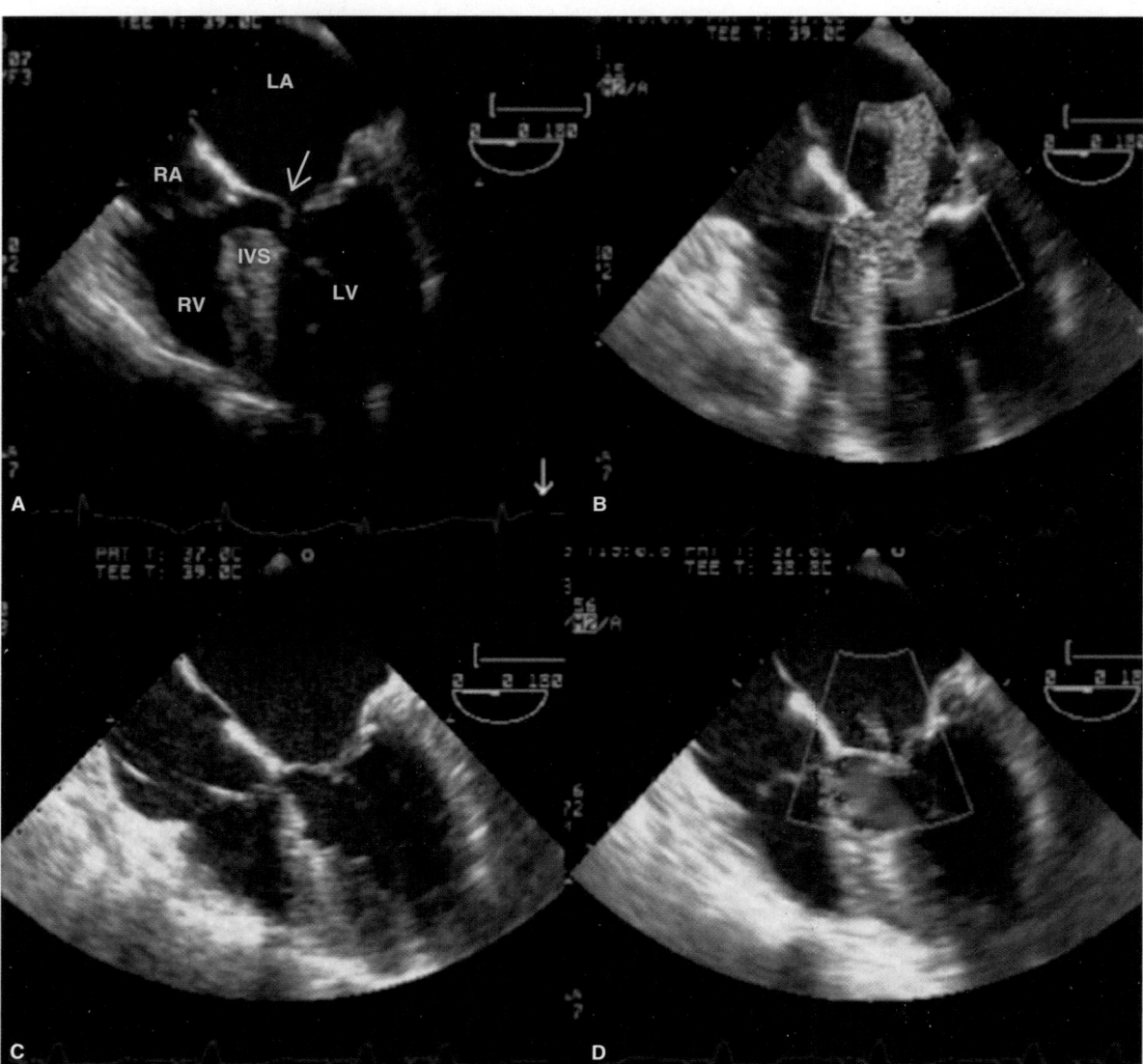

Figure 42–19. Septal myectomy intraoperative monitoring with transesophageal echocardiography. Preoperatively mitral valve systolic anterior movement (SAM) is visible (**A**, *arrow*) with flow acceleration in the left ventricular (LV) outflow tract and SAM-related mitral regurgitation (**B**). Postoperatively, mitral valve SAM is no longer present (**C**) and no flow acceleration is visible in the LV outflow tract with trivial residual mitral regurgitation (**D**). IVS, interventricular septum; LA, left atrium; RA, right atrium; RV, right ventricle. Reproduced with permission from Cardim N, Galderisi M, Edvardsen T, et al: Role of multimodality cardiac imaging in the management of patients with hypertrophic cardiomyopathy: an expert consensus of the European Association of Cardiovascular Imaging Endorsed by the Saudi Heart Association. *Eur Heart J Cardiovasc Imaging.* 2015 Mar;16(3):280.

activation), and chronic LV reverse remodeling.[178] Pacing also allows uptitration or combination treatment with β-blockers and calcium channel blockers.

To date, three small randomized cross-over studies have compared DDD to back-up atrial pacing (AAI mode) and have shown an improvement in LVOT gradient, but no clear effect on exercise capacity or quality of life.[179-181] It is worth noting that these studies showed a significant placebo effect associated with device implantation.[178]

There are some important technical considerations when considering pacing to treat LVOTO symptoms in HCM. First, to obtain a reduction in LVOT gradient, the ventricular lead needs to be placed at the RV apex,[182] however this can be challenging due to hypertrophied RV trabeculae. In addition to

pacing the ventricle, the hemodynamic contribution of atrial systole should be maintained by sensing or pacing the atrium if needed and there is an optimal AV delay for maximizing hemodynamic performance (**Fig. 42–22**).[183] If the paced AV interval is too short, atrial systole may coincide with the mitral valve closure (truncated A wave on pulsed mitral valve Doppler), leading to increased left atrial pressure, reduced preload, and worse exercise tolerance. On the other hand, an overly long AV delay can result in incomplete RV capture with suboptimal gradient reduction.[178]

Pacing may also be considered in selected patients who are in sinus rhythm, have drug-refractory LVOTO symptoms and are not good candidates for surgery or ASA, or have a high risk of developing advanced AV block with either procedure.[1]

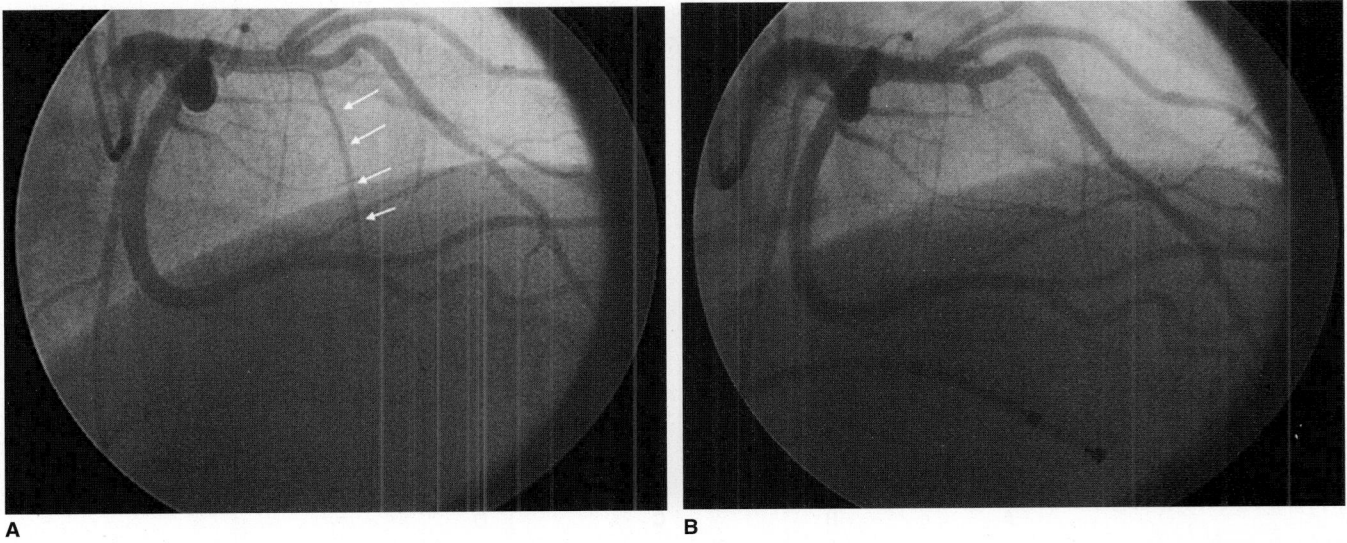

Figure 42–20. Coronary angiogram of a patient undergoing septal ablation. A large first septal perforator artery is shown by the *white arrows* in (**A**). In (**B**), following the septal ablation, there has been complete cessation of flow in the first septal perforator artery.

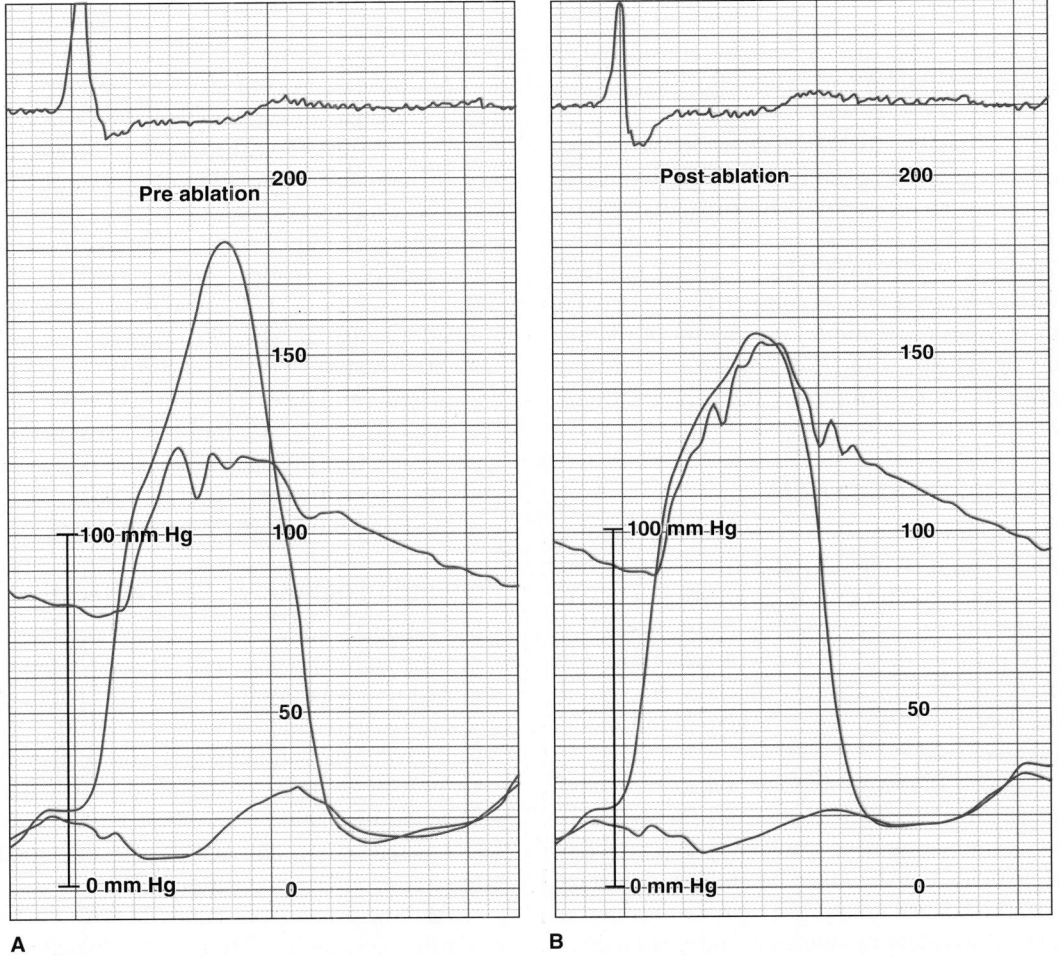

Figure 42–21. (**A**) Cardiac catheterization before ablation, demonstrating left ventricular outflow tract obstruction of 60 mm Hg. (**B**) Following the septal ablation, there has been complete obliteration of the gradient across the left ventricular outflow tract.

HOCM pacing study

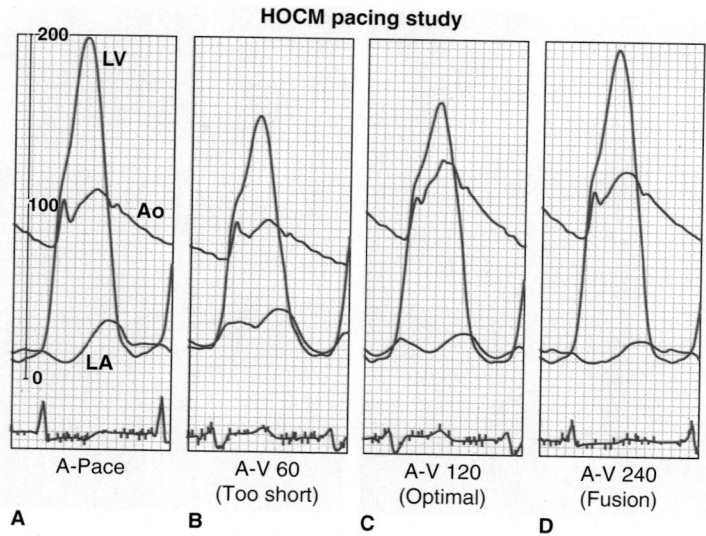

Figure 42–22. Cardiac catheterization study during atrioventricular sequential pacing in a patient with hypertrophic obstructive cardiomyopathy, demonstrating the effect of the differing atrioventricular (AV) intervals. The left ventricular (LV) pressure, aortic (Ao) pressure, and left atrial (LA) pressures are shown. **(A)** In the baseline state (A pace), the patient is undergoing atrial pacing with native antegrade atrioventricular conduction. There is a left ventricular outflow tract obstruction of 100 mm Hg. **(B)** The patient is undergoing atrioventricular pacing with an atrioventricular interval of 60 ms. This interval is too short because atrial contraction is now occurring on top of a closed mitral valve, causing an elevation of LA pressure. Although the gradient is decreased, there is also a decrease in Ao pressure caused by the decreased preload in the left ventricle. **(C)** This is the optimal AV interval of 120 ms. The gradient has been decreased to 35 mm Hg. **(D)** The AV delay is 240 ms. There is fusion between the antegrade conduction and the paced QRS complex with incomplete preexcitation. The gradient across the left ventricular outflow tract is 60 mm Hg.

A dual-chamber transvenous device can be considered in patients with an ICD indication and drug-refractory LVOTO symptoms.[1,2]

Ongoing trials of pacing for LVOTO in HCM include the TRICHAMPION study, a randomized, single-blind trial that will compare the effect of DDD biventricular pacing to placebo (AAI mode) on exercise capacity and quality of life (ClinicalTrials.gov: NCT01614717). Finally, a randomized double-blind cross-over trial is comparing the effect of DDD pacing to placebo (AAI mode) on quality of life and exercise capacity in patients with HCM and a midcavity gradient with drug-refractory symptoms (ClinicalTrials.gov: NCT03450252).

Treatment of Nonobstructive HCM

β-Blockers and calcium channel blockers can be used to improve diastolic filling in symptomatic patients with a normal LV ejection fraction and no resting or provoked LVOTO. Diuretics can be used to reduce elevated filling pressures.[1,2] In patients with chest pain but no LVOTO or epicardial coronary disease, β-blockers or calcium channel blockers are recommended because they improve diastolic function and reduce myocardial oxygen demand.[1,2]

Perhexiline has been shown to improve diastolic function and exercise capacity in a randomized controlled trial;[184] however, clinical use is limited by drug availability and concerns regarding hepatotoxicity. On the other hand, both trimetazidine[185] and ranolazine[186] failed to improve exercise tolerance in nonobstructive HCM in recent randomized controlled trials.

For patients with systolic impairment, the general guidelines for chronic heart failure apply, and treatment is based on diuretics, β-blockers, and renin-angiotensin-aldosterone system inhibitors.[1,2] No data on use of sacubitril/valsartan in HCM are currently available. To date, no dedicated trials have investigated the role of cardiac resynchronization therapy in *burn-out* HCM and the available observation data is conflicting, suggesting a possible symptomatic benefit in some patients,[187] but no evidence of a prognostic benefit.[188] Cardiac transplantation should be considered in patients with refractory, severe symptoms despite conventional treatment; posttransplantation survival is similar or better compared to other conditions (75% at 5 years; 60% at 10 years).[189] Patients with HCM are traditionally not considered candidates for ventricular assist devices due to the small LV cavity size and restrictive pathophysiology, but data suggest that this may be a viable option in selected HCM patients, a recent series reporting ventricular assist device use in almost one-third of HCM patients listed for transplant.[54]

Prevention of Sudden Cardiac Death

Observational studies have suggested amiodarone can suppress nonsustained ventricular tachycardia,[190,191] but there are no randomized trial data to support the use of antiarrhythmic agents to improve survival in patients with HCM. An ICD is the only reliable treatment option for protecting patients from SCD.[192]

A previous episode of sustained ventricular tachycardia or ventricular fibrillation is a well-established marker of high risk for recurrent events and SCD,[193] and these patients should be offered a secondary prevention ICD.[1,2]

Regarding primary prevention of SCD, the European Society of Cardiology (ESC) and AHA/ACC guidelines have a different approach to exercise, the European recommendations being more restrictive (**Table 42–4**).[1,2,194]

TABLE 42–4. Comparison of Guideline Recommendations for Exercise in HCM

ESC 2014 Guidelines [1]	AHA/ACC 2020 Guidelines [2]
Advise against participation in competitive sport and avoid intense physical activity, especially if risk factors for SCD or LVOT obstruction are present.	Participation in high-intensity recreational activities or moderate- to high- intensity competitive sports may be considered after a comprehensive evaluation and shared discussion, repeated annually with an expert provider.
Recreational exercise permitted following expert assessment.[194]	Mild to moderate recreational exercise is beneficial, in line with the recommendations for the general population.

Abbreviations: HCM, hypertrophic cardiomyopathy; ESC, European Society of Cardiology; AHA/ACC, American Heart Association/American College of Cardiology; SCD, sudden cardiac death; LVOT, left ventricular outflow tract.

TABLE 42–5. Comparison of Guideline Recommendations for Primary Prevention ICD Implantation in HCM Patients Aged >16

ESC 2014 Guidelines [1]	AHA/ACC 2020 Guidelines [2]
5-year risk of SCD calculated based on variables listed in Table 42–6 and ICD recommendations based on estimated risk: • ≥6% - ICD should be considered • 4%-6% - ICD can be considered • <4% - ICD generally not recommended	ICD should be considered with one or more of the following: • Family history of SCD • LV wall thickness ≥28-30 mm • Unexplained syncope • Apical aneurysm • EF ≤50% ICD can be considered in the presence of: • Nonsustained VT • Extensive LGE on CMR ICD not recommended if none of the above are present

Abbreviations: ICD, implantable cardioverter defibrillator; HCM, hypertrophic cardiomyopathy; ESC, European Society of Cardiology; AHA/ACC, American Heart Association/American College of Cardiology; SCD, sudden cardiac death; LV, left ventricle; LA, left atrium; LVOT, left ventricular outflow tract; EF, ejection fraction; VT, ventricular tachycardia, LGE, late gadolinium enhancement; CMR, cardiac magnetic resonance.

The two guidelines have a different approach to risk stratification (**Table 42–5**) but are based on similar risk factors. Well-established risk factors for SCD include a family history of SCD in a first degree relative,[72,74] severity of LV hypertrophy,[72,74,85,195,196] unexplained syncope,[71,72,74,76] LVOT gradient,[74,197] and nonsustained ventricular tachycardia (particularly in young patients).[72,74,85] LV systolic dysfunction (EF ≤50%) has also been recognized more recently as an independent major risk factor for SCD.[30,54] Single-center data support the role of LV apical aneurysm in SCD risk stratification,[70] and extensive LGE on CMR has also been proposed as a risk modifier.[120]

The ESC recommendations are based on the estimated 5-year risk of SCD (Table 42–5; online calculator available at https://www.doc2do.com/hcm/webHCM.html);[74] **Table 42–6** summarizes the predictors used in the calculator and their definitions. The risk calculator should not be used in HCM phenocopies (infiltrative/storage diseases or syndromes), or patients aged <16, and does not account for the effect of septal reduction therapies (surgical myectomy or alcohol ablation) and should be used cautiously in such patients. Two separate risk prediction models for pediatric HCM patients have been published very recently.[198,199]

The AHA/ACC recommendations, on the other hand, are based on the presence of one or more risk factors (Table 42–5), but also acknowledge that the 5-year risk calculator can be considered in decision-making discussions.[2]

Most importantly, regardless of the approach to decision-making, the recommendation for an ICD should always be individualized and not based solely on the estimated risk of SCD, but also consider age, general health, socioeconomic

TABLE 42–6. Variables Included in the ESC HCM Sudden Death Risk Calculator

Predictor Variable	Definition	Coding
Age	Age at evaluation.	Continuous, years
Family history of SCD	History of sudden cardiac death in ≥1 first degree relatives aged <40 or SCD in a first degree relative with confirmed HCM at any age (post- or ante-mortem diagnosis).	Binary (yes = 1/no = 0)
Maximal wall thickness	The greatest LV wall thickness measured in parasternal short-axis plane using echocardiography at time of evaluation.	Continuous, mm
Left atrial diameter	Antero-posterior left atrial diameter measured in the parasternal long axis view using echocardiography at time of evaluation.	Continuous, mm
Maximal LVOT gradient	The maximum LVOT gradient determined at rest and with Valsalva provocation (irrespective of concurrent medical treatment) using continuous wave Doppler from the apical three- and five-chamber views.	Continuous, mm Hg
Nonsustained VT	≥3 consecutive ventricular beats at a rate of ≥120 bpm and <30 s in duration on Holter monitoring (minimum duration 24 hours) at or prior to evaluation.	Binary (yes = 1/no = 0)
Unexplained syncope	History of unexplained syncope at or prior to evaluation.	Binary (yes = 1/no = 0)

Abbreviations: ESC, European Society of Cardiology; HCM, hypertrophic cardiomyopathy; LV, left ventricle; LVOT, left ventricular outflow tract; SCD, sudden cardiac death; VT, ventricular tachycardia. Reproduced with permission from O'Mahony C, Jichi F, Pavlou M, et al: A novel clinical risk prediction model for sudden cardiac death in hypertrophic cardiomyopathy (HCM risk-SCD). *Eur Heart J.* 2014 Aug 7;35(30):2010-2020.

factors, and the psychological impact of the device.[1] The negative repercussions of an ICD should also be considered, including the lifetime burden of inappropriate shocks (~5% per year) and device-related complications that are a consequence of the young age and frequent incident AF in patients with HCM.[200]

Stroke Prevention

Guidelines recommend lifelong anticoagulation for patients with paroxysmal or permanent AF and HCM (in absence of a contraindication);[1,2] however, no randomized controlled trials have investigated the role of anticoagulation or antiarrhythmic drugs to reduce thromboembolic risk in HCM. These recommendations are based on observational data that suggest a protective effect of vitamin K antagonists;[82,128] direct oral anticoagulants appear to be at least as effective and potentially safer that vitamin K antagonists in observational studies.[201]

Disease-Modifying Drugs and Novel Treatments

The growing number of preclinical carriers identified through genetic testing and family screening has led to increased interest in the development of new therapeutics that can inhibit or attenuate the development of the HCM phenotype.[202] Diltiazem has shown promising results in preventing ventricular remodeling in sarcomere mutation carriers.[203] The VANISH trial is currently investigating the role of Valsartan on disease progression in sarcomere protein mutation carriers and patients with mild HCM (ClinicalTrials.gov: NCT01912534).

The potential effect of losartan and spironolactone on positive remodeling in HCM has been investigated in randomized controlled trials, but no evidence of a beneficial effect on fibrosis, LV hypertrophy, or exercise capacity was found for either.[204,205]

As well as good results in obstructive HCM, mavacamten has also shown promising results in nonobstructive HCM, reducing NT-proBNP and troponin levels in a phase II trial,[206] but larger studies with clinical endpoints are needed to establish the potential clinical utility.

Pregnancy

All HCM patients who wish to become pregnant should receive prenatal counseling about the risk of transmission of disease to their offspring (autosomal dominant inheritance) and the risks associated with pregnancy.[1,2] Pregnancy is generally not contraindicated in patients with HCM and is usually well tolerated, with the exception of severe LV systolic dysfunction or severe symptomatic LVOTO that are associated with high morbidity and mortality.[1] Echocardiography is recommended each trimester or in the presence of new symptoms. Patients with LV dysfunction, severe LVOTO, or arrhythmias despite medical treatment should be followed up monthly or bimonthly by a specialized team.[1]

Patients on treatment with β-blockers should continue them throughout the pregnancy, monitoring fetal growth.[1,2] β-blockers are also indicated in the presence of new symptoms related to LVOTO. Calcium channel blockers and disopyramide can be used when benefits are judged to outweigh potential risks.[1] Low-dose diuretics may be required if pulmonary congestion occurs. Epidural and spinal anesthesia should be used cautiously given the risks of vasodilation and hypotension in the presence of significant LVOTO, but are not contraindicated.[1,2] Cesarean section should be considered in cases of severe LVOTO, preterm labor in patients receiving oral anticoagulant drugs, and with severe heart failure symptoms.[1]

SUMMARY

- HCM is a common inherited condition.
- Phenocopies should be actively sought during diagnostic work-up because they generally have a different management and treatment.
- ~50% of cases HCM are due to a pathogenic variant in a sarcomere protein gene (*MYBPC3, MYH7, TNNI3, TNNT2, TPM1, MYL2, MYL3,* and *ACTC1*) that is inherited as an autosomal dominant trait with incomplete penetrance.
- The pathophysiology is complex and consists of multiple interrelated abnormalities, including diastolic (and rarely systolic) dysfunction, LVOT (and/or midcavity) obstruction, and mitral regurgitation.
- Genetic testing and screening are central to management of families.
- ESC and AHA/ACC guidelines have a different approach to sudden death risk stratification and ICD recommendations.
- Symptoms related to LVOTO are managed medically in the first instance but may require invasive treatment with surgical septal myectomy or alcohol septal ablation.
- AF mandates anticoagulation and is often poorly tolerated, requiring aggressive rhythm-control.
- Heart failure is an important cause of mortality and is treated according to the current standard recommendations.

ACKNOWLEDGMENTS

We thank Dr. Steve R. Ommen, Dr. Rick A. Nishimura, Dr. A. Jamil Tajik, and Dr Luis R. Lopes who contributed to the previous versions of this chapter.

REFERENCES

1. Elliott PM, Anastasakis A, Borger MA, et al. 2014 ESC Guidelines on diagnosis and management of hypertrophic cardiomyopathy. *Eur Heart J.* 2014;35(39):2733-2779. doi:10.1093/eurheartj/ehu284
2. Ommen SR, Mital S, Burke MA, et al. 2020 AHA/ACC guideline for the diagnosis and treatment of patients with hypertrophic cardiomyopathy. *J Am Coll Cardiol.* 2020;76(25):e159-e240. doi:10.1016/j.jacc.2020.08.045
3. Semsarian C, Ingles J, Maron MS, Maron BJ. New perspectives on the prevalence of hypertrophic cardiomyopathy. *J Am Coll Cardiol.* 2015;65(12):1249-1254. doi:10.1016/j.jacc.2015.01.019
4. Pujades-Rodriguez M, Guttmann OP, Gonzalez-Izquierdo A, et al. Identifying unmet clinical need in hypertrophic cardiomyopathy using national electronic health records. *PLoS One.* 2018;13(1):e0191214. doi:10.1371/journal.pone.0191214
5. Norrish G, Jager J, Field E, et al. Yield of clinical screening for hypertrophic cardiomyopathy in child first-degree relatives. *Circulation.* 2019;140(3):184-192. doi:10.1161/CIRCULATIONAHA.118.038846

6. Lorenzini M, Norrish G, Field E, et al. Penetrance of hypertrophic cardiomyopathy in sarcomere protein mutation carriers. *J Am Coll Cardiol.* 2020;76(5):550-559. doi:10.1016/j.jacc.2020.06.011

7. Elliott P, Andersson B, Arbustini E, et al. Classification of the cardiomyopathies: a position statement from the European Society of Cardiology working group on myocardial and pericardial diseases. *Eur Heart J.* 2007;29(2):270-276. doi:10.1093/eurheartj/ehm342

8. Elliott PM, Anastasakis A, Borger MA, et al. web addenda ESC 2014 HCM guidelines. *Eur Heart J.* 2014;35(39):2733-2779. doi:10.1093/eurheartj/ehu284a

9. Elliott P, Charron P, Blanes JRG, et al. European cardiomyopathy pilot registry: EURObservational research programme of the European Society of Cardiology. *Eur Heart J.* 2016;37(2):164-173. doi:10.1093/eurheartj/ehv497

10. Norrish G, Field E, Mcleod K, et al. Clinical presentation and survival of childhood hypertrophic cardiomyopathy: a retrospective study in United Kingdom. *Eur Heart J.* 2019;40(12):986-993. doi:10.1093/eurheartj/ehy798

11. Rosmini S, Biagini E, O'Mahony C, et al. Relationship between aetiology and left ventricular systolic dysfunction in hypertrophic cardiomyopathy. *Heart.* 2017;103(4):300-306. doi:10.1136/heartjnl-2016-310138

12. Rapezzi C, Arbustini E, Caforio ALP, et al. Diagnostic work-up in cardiomyopathies: bridging the gap between clinical phenotypes and final diagnosis. A position statement from the ESC Working Group on Myocardial and Pericardial Diseases. *Eur Heart J.* 2013;34(19):1448-1458. doi:10.1093/eurheartj/ehs397

13. Coats CJ, Hollman A. Hypertrophic cardiomyopathy: lessons from history. *Heart.* 2007;94(10):1258-1263. doi:10.1136/hrt.2008.153452

14. Mazzarotto F, Olivotto I, Boschi B, et al. Contemporary insights into the genetics of hypertrophic cardiomyopathy: toward a new era in clinical testing? *J Am Heart Assoc.* 2020;9(8):e015473. doi:10.1161/JAHA.119.015473

15. Valdés-Mas R, Gutiérrez-Fernández A, Gómez J, et al. Mutations in filamin C cause a new form of familial hypertrophic cardiomyopathy. *Nat Commun.* 2014;5:5326. doi:10.1038/ncomms6326

16. Geier C, Perrot A, Ozcelik C, et al. Mutations in the human muscle LIM protein gene in families with hypertrophic cardiomyopathy. *Circulation.* 2003;107(10):1390-1395. doi:10.1161/01.cir.0000056522.82563.5f

17. Hoffmann B, Schmidt-Traub H, Perrot A, Osterziel KJ, Gessner R. First mutation in cardiac troponin C, L29Q, in a patient with hypertrophic cardiomyopathy. *Hum Mutat.* 2001;17(6):524. doi:10.1002/humu.1143

18. Ochoa JP, Sabater-Molina M, García-Pinilla JM, et al. Formin homology 2 domain containing 3 (FHOD3) is a genetic basis for hypertrophic cardiomyopathy. *J Am Coll Cardiol.* 2018;72(20):2457-2467. doi:10.1016/j.jacc.2018.10.001

19. Chiu C, Bagnall RD, Ingles J, et al. Mutations in alpha-actinin-2 cause hypertrophic cardiomyopathy: a genome-wide analysis. *J Am Coll Cardiol.* 2010;55(11):1127-1135. doi:10.1016/j.jacc.2009.11.016

20. Almomani R, Verhagen JMA, Herkert JC, et al. Biallelic truncating mutations in ALPK3 cause severe pediatric cardiomyopathy. *J Am Coll Cardiol.* 2016;67(5):515-525. doi:10.1016/j.jacc.2015.10.093

21. Landstrom AP, Weisleder N, Batalden KB, et al. Mutations in JPH2-encoded junctophilin-2 associated with hypertrophic cardiomyopathy in humans. *J Mol Cell Cardiol.* 2007;42(6):1026-1035. doi:10.1016/j.yjmcc.2007.04.006

22. Salazar-Mendiguchía J, Ochoa JP, Palomino-Doza J, et al. Mutations in TRIM63 cause an autosomal-recessive form of hypertrophic cardiomyopathy. *Heart.* 2020;106(17):1342-1348. doi:10.1136/heartjnl-2020-316913

23. Lopes LR, Elliott PM. A straightforward guide to the sarcomeric basis of cardiomyopathies. *Heart.* 2014;100(24):1916-1923. doi:10.1136/heartjnl-2014-305645

24. Seidman JG, Seidman C. The genetic basis for cardiomyopathy: from mutation identification to mechanistic paradigms. *Cell.* 2001;104(4):557-567. doi:10.1016/s0092-8674(01)00242-2

25. Marston S, Copeland O, Jacques A, et al. Evidence from human myectomy samples that MYBPC3 mutations cause hypertrophic cardiomyopathy through haploinsufficiency. *Circ Res.* 2009;105(3):219-222. doi:10.1161/CIRCRESAHA.109.202440

26. Ho CY, Charron P, Richard P, Girolami F, Van Spaendonck-Zwarts KY, Pinto Y. Genetic advances in sarcomeric cardiomyopathies: state of the art. *Cardiovasc Res.* 2015;105(4):397-408. doi:10.1093/cvr/cvv025

27. Ho CY, Day SM, Ashley EA, et al. Genotype and lifetime burden of disease in hypertrophic cardiomyopathy. *Circulation.* 2018;138(14):1387-1398. doi:10.1161/CIRCULATIONAHA.117.033200

28. van Velzen HG, Vriesendorp PA, Oldenburg RA, et al. Value of genetic testing for the prediction of long-term outcome in patients with hypertrophic cardiomyopathy. *Am J Cardiol.* 2016;118(6):881-887. doi:10.1016/j.amjcard.2016.06.038

29. Sedaghat-Hamedani F, Kayvanpour E, Tugrul OF, et al. Clinical outcomes associated with sarcomere mutations in hypertrophic cardiomyopathy: a meta-analysis on 7675 individuals. *Clin Res Cardiol.* 2018;107(1):30-41. doi:10.1007/s00392-017-1155-5

30. Marstrand P, Han L, Day SM, et al. Hypertrophic cardiomyopathy with left ventricular systolic dysfunction: insights from the SHaRe registry. *Circulation.* 2020;141(17):1371-1383. doi:10.1161/CIRCULATIONAHA.119.044366

31. Girolami F, Ho CY, Semsarian C, et al. Clinical features and outcome of hypertrophic cardiomyopathy associated with triple sarcomere protein gene mutations. *J Am Coll Cardiol.* 2010;55(14):1444-1453. doi:10.1016/j.jacc.2009.11.062

32. Ingles J, Doolan A, Chiu C, Seidman J, Seidman C, Semsarian C. Compound and double mutations in patients with hypertrophic cardiomyopathy: implications for genetic testing and counselling. *J Med Genet.* 2005;42(10):e59. doi:10.1136/jmg.2005.033886

33. Davies MJ, Pomerance A, Teare RD. Pathological features of hypertrophic obstructive cardiomyopathy. *J Clin Pathol.* 1974;27(7):529-535. doi:10.1136/jcp.27.7.529

34. Olsen EGJ. The pathology of cardiomyopathies. A critical analysis. *Am Heart J.* 1979;98(3):385-392. doi:10.1016/0002-8703(79)90052-8

35. Davies MJ, McKenna WJ. Hypertrophic cardiomyopathy—pathology and pathogenesis. *Histopathology.* 1995;26(6):493-500. doi:10.1111/j.1365-2559.1995.tb00267.x

36. Klues HG, Proschan MA, Dollar AL, Spirito P, Roberts WC, Maron BJ. Echocardiographic assessment of mitral valve size in obstructive hypertrophic cardiomyopathy. Anatomic validation from mitral valve specimen. *Circulation.* 1993;88(2):548-555. doi:10.1161/01.cir.88.2.548

37. Klues HG, Roberts WC, Maron BJ. Anomalous insertion of papillary muscle directly into anterior mitral leaflet in hypertrophic cardiomyopathy. Significance in producing left ventricular outflow obstruction. *Circulation.* 1991;84(3):1188-1197. doi:10.1161/01.cir.84.3.1188

38. Tavora F, Cresswell N, Li L, Ripple M, Fowler D, Burke A. Morphologic features of exertional versus nonexertional sudden death in patients with hypertrophic cardiomyopathy. *Am J Cardiol.* 2010;105(4):532-537. doi:10.1016/j.amjcard.2009.10.022

39. Varnava AM, Elliott PM, Baboonian C, Davison F, Davies MJ, McKenna WJ. Hypertrophic cardiomyopathy: histopathological features of sudden death in cardiac troponin T disease. *Circulation.* 2001;104(12):1380-1384. doi:10.1161/hc3701.095952

40. Wigle ED, Rakowski H, Kimball BP, Williams WG. Hypertrophic cardiomyopathy. Clinical spectrum and treatment. *Circulation.* 1995;92(7):1680-1692. doi:10.1161/01.cir.92.7.1680

41. Bonow RO, Dilsizian V, Rosing DR, Maron BJ, Bacharach SL, Green MV. Verapamil-induced improvement in left ventricular diastolic filling and increased exercise tolerance in patients with hypertrophic cardiomyopathy: short- and long-term effects. *Circulation.* 1985;72(4):853-864. doi:10.1161/01.cir.72.4.853

42. Bonow RO, Vitale DF, Maron BJ, Bacharach SL, Frederick TM, Green MV. Regional left ventricular asynchrony and impaired global left ventricular filling in hypertrophic cardiomyopathy: effect of verapamil. *J Am Coll Cardiol.* 1987;9(5):1108-1116. doi:10.1016/s0735-1097(87)80315-7

43. Nihoyannopoulos P, Karatasakis G, Frenneaux M, McKenna WJ, Oakley CM. Diastolic function in hypertrophic cardiomyopathy: relation to exercise capacity. *J Am Coll Cardiol.* 1992;19(3):536-540. doi:10.1016/S0735-1097(10)80268-2

44. Yotti R, Seidman CE, Seidman JG. Advances in the genetic basis and pathogenesis of sarcomere cardiomyopathies. *Annu Rev Genomics Hum Genet.* 2019;20(1):129-153. doi:10.1146/annurev-genom-083118-015306

45. Cannon RO, Rosing DR, Maron BJ, et al. Myocardial ischemia in patients with hypertrophic cardiomyopathy: contribution of inadequate vasodilator reserve and elevated left ventricular filling pressures. *Circulation.* 1985;71(2):234-243. doi:10.1161/01.cir.71.2.234

46. Cannon RO, Schenke WH, Maron BJ, et al. Differences in coronary flow and myocardial metabolism at rest and during pacing between patients with obstructive and patients with nonobstructive hypertrophic cardiomyopathy. *J Am Coll Cardiol.* 1987;10(1):53-62. doi:10.1016/s0735-1097(87)80159-6

47. Maron MS, Olivotto I, Maron BJ, et al. The case for myocardial ischemia in hypertrophic cardiomyopathy. *J Am Coll Cardiol.* 2009;54(9):866-875. doi:10.1016/j.jacc.2009.04.072

48. Olivotto I, Girolami F, Sciagrà R, et al. Microvascular function is selectively impaired in patients with hypertrophic cardiomyopathy and sarcomere myofilament gene mutations. *J Am Coll Cardiol.* 2011;58(8):839-848. doi:10.1016/j.jacc.2011.05.018

49. Maron BJ, Wolfson JK, Epstein SE, Roberts WC. Intramural ("small vessel") coronary artery disease in hypertrophic cardiomyopathy. *J Am Coll Cardiol.* 1986;8(3):545-557. doi:10.1016/s0735-1097(86)80181-4

50. Tanaka M, Fujiwara H, Onodera T, et al. Quantitative analysis of narrowings of intramyocardial small arteries in normal hearts, hypertensive hearts, and hearts with hypertrophic cardiomyopathy. *Circulation.* 1987;75(6):1130-1139. doi:10.1161/01.cir.75.6.1130

51. Camaioni C, Knott KD, Augusto JB, et al. Inline perfusion mapping provides insights into the disease mechanism in hypertrophic cardiomyopathy. *Heart.* 2020;106(11):824-829. doi:10.1136/heartjnl-2019-315848

52. Harris KM, Spirito P, Maron MS, et al. Prevalence, clinical profile, and significance of left ventricular remodeling in the end-stage phase of hypertrophic cardiomyopathy. *Circulation.* 2006;114(3):216-225. doi:10.1161/CIRCULATIONAHA.105.583500

53. Thaman R, Gimeno JR, Murphy RT, et al. Prevalence and clinical significance of systolic impairment in hypertrophic cardiomyopathy. *Heart.* 2005;91(7):920-925. doi:10.1136/hrt.2003.031161

54. Rowin EJ, Maron BJ, Carrick RT, et al. Outcomes in patients with hypertrophic cardiomyopathy and left ventricular systolic dysfunction. *J Am Coll Cardiol.* 2020;75(24):3033-3043. doi:10.1016/j.jacc.2020.04.045

55. Galati G, Leone O, Pasquale F, et al. Histological and histometric characterization of myocardial fibrosis in end-stage hypertrophic cardiomyopathy. *Circ Hear Fail.* 2016;9(9):e003090. doi:10.1161/CIRCHEARTFAILURE.116.003090

56. Olivotto I, Cecchi F, Poggesi C, Yacoub MH. Patterns of disease progression in hypertrophic cardiomyopathy: an individualized approach to clinical staging. *Circ Heart Fail.* 2012;5(4):535-546. doi:10.1161/CIRCHEARTFAILURE.112.967026

57. Maron MS, Rowin EJ, Olivotto I, et al. Contemporary natural history and management of nonobstructive hypertrophic cardiomyopathy. *J Am Coll Cardiol.* 2016;67(12):1399-1409. doi:10.1016/j.jacc.2016.01.023

58. Sadoul N, Prasad K, Elliott PM, Bannerjee S, Frenneaux MP, McKenna WJ. Prospective prognostic assessment of blood pressure response during exercise in patients with hypertrophic cardiomyopathy. *Circulation.* 1997;96(9):2987-2991. doi:10.1161/01.cir.96.9.2987

59. Liu Q, Li D, Berger AE, Johns RA, Gao L. Survival and prognostic factors in hypertrophic cardiomyopathy: a meta-analysis. *Sci Rep.* 2017;7(1):11957. doi:10.1038/s41598-017-12289-4

60. Critoph CH, Patel V, Mist B, Elliott PM. Cardiac output response and peripheral oxygen extraction during exercise among symptomatic hypertrophic cardiomyopathy patients with and without left ventricular

outflow tract obstruction. *Heart.* 2014;100(8):639-646. doi:10.1136/heartjnl-2013-304914

61. Maron BJ, Maron MS, Wigle ED, Braunwald E. The 50-year history, controversy, and clinical implications of left ventricular outflow tract obstruction in hypertrophic cardiomyopathy: from idiopathic hypertrophic subaortic stenosis to hypertrophic cardiomyopathy. *J Am Coll Cardiol.* 2009;54(3):191-200. doi:10.1016/j.jacc.2008.11.069

62. Maron MS, Olivotto I, Harrigan C, et al. Mitral valve abnormalities identified by cardiovascular magnetic resonance represent a primary phenotypic expression of hypertrophic cardiomyopathy. *Circulation.* 2011;124(1):40-47. doi:10.1161/CIRCULATIONAHA.110.985812

63. Levine RA, Vlahakes GJ, Lefebvre X, et al. Papillary muscle displacement causes systolic anterior motion of the mitral valve. Experimental validation and insights into the mechanism of subaortic obstruction. *Circulation.* 1995;91(4):1189-1195. doi:10.1161/01.cir.91.4.1189

64. Ferrazzi P, Spirito P, Iacovoni A, et al. Transaortic chordal cutting: mitral valve repair for obstructive hypertrophic cardiomyopathy with mild septal hypertrophy. *J Am Coll Cardiol.* 2015;66(15):1687-1696. doi:10.1016/j.jacc.2015.07.069

65. Sherrid MV, Gunsburg DZ, Moldenhauer S, Pearle G. Systolic anterior motion begins at low left ventricular outflow tract velocity in obstructive hypertrophic cardiomyopathy. *J Am Coll Cardiol.* 2000;36(4):1344-1354. doi:10.1016/s0735-1097(00)00830-5

66. Ro R, Halpern D, Sahn DJ, et al. Vector flow mapping in obstructive hypertrophic cardiomyopathy to assess the relationship of early systolic left ventricular flow and the mitral valve. *J Am Coll Cardiol.* 2014;64(19):1984-1995. doi:10.1016/j.jacc.2014.04.090

67. Sherrid MV, Chu CK, Delia E, Mograder A, Dwyer EM. An echocardiographic study of the fluid mechanics of obstruction in hypertrophic cardiomyopathy. *J Am Coll Cardiol.* 1993;22(3):816-825. doi:10.1016/0735-1097(93)90196-8

68. Yu EHC, Omran AS, Wigle ED, Williams WG, Siu SC, Rakowski H. Mitral regurgitation in hypertrophic obstructive cardiomyopathy: relationship to obstruction and relief with myectomy. *J Am Coll Cardiol.* 2000;36(7):2219-2225. doi:10.1016/s0735-1097(00)01019-6

69. Minami Y, Kajimoto K, Terajima Y, et al. Clinical implications of midventricular obstruction in patients with hypertrophic cardiomyopathy. *J Am Coll Cardiol.* 2011;57(23):2346-2355. doi:10.1016/j.jacc.2011.02.033

70. Rowin EJ, Maron BJ, Haas TS, et al. Hypertrophic cardiomyopathy with left ventricular apical aneurysm: implications for risk stratification and management. *J Am Coll Cardiol.* 2017;69(7):761-773. doi:10.1016/j.jacc.2016.11.063

71. Spirito P, Autore C, Rapezzi C, et al. Syncope and risk of sudden death in hypertrophic cardiomyopathy. *Circulation.* 2009;119(13):1703-1710. doi:10.1161/CIRCULATIONAHA.108.798314

72. Elliott PM, Gimeno JR, Tomé MT, et al. Left ventricular outflow tract obstruction and sudden death risk in patients with hypertrophic cardiomyopathy. *Eur Heart J.* 2006;27(16):1933-1941. doi:10.1093/eurheartj/ehl041

73. McCully RB, Nishimura RA, Tajik AJ, Schaff HV, Danielson GK. Extent of clinical improvement after surgical treatment of hypertrophic obstructive cardiomyopathy. *Circulation.* 1996;94(3):467-471. doi:10.1161/01.cir.94.3.467

74. O'Mahony C, Jichi F, Pavlou M, et al. A novel clinical risk prediction model for sudden cardiac death in hypertrophic cardiomyopathy (HCM Risk-SCD). *Eur Heart J.* 2014;35(30):2010-2020. doi:10.1093/eurheartj/eht439

75. Efthimiadis GK, Parcharidou DG, Giannakoulas G, et al. Left ventricular outflow tract obstruction as a risk factor for sudden cardiac death in hypertrophic cardiomyopathy. *Am J Cardiol.* 2009;104(5):695-699. doi:10.1016/j.amjcard.2009.04.039

76. Kofflard MJM, Ten Cate FJ, van der Lee C, van Domburg RT. Hypertrophic cardiomyopathy in a large community-based population: clinical outcome and identification of risk factors for sudden cardiac death

and clinical deterioration. *J Am Coll Cardiol.* 2003;41(6):987-993. doi:10.1016/s0735-1097(02)03004-8

77. McLeod CJ, Ackerman MJ, Nishimura RA, Tajik AJ, Gersh BJ, Ommen SR. Outcome of patients with hypertrophic cardiomyopathy and a normal electrocardiogram. *J Am Coll Cardiol.* 2009;54(3):229-233. doi:10.1016/j.jacc.2009.02.071

78. Biagini E, Pazzi C, Olivotto I, et al. Usefulness of electrocardiographic patterns at presentation to predict long-term risk of cardiac death in patients with hypertrophic cardiomyopathy. *Am J Cardiol.* 2016;118(3):432-439. doi:10.1016/j.amjcard.2016.05.023

79. Dumont CA, Monserrat L, Soler R, et al. Interpretation of electrocardiographic abnormalities in hypertrophic cardiomyopathy with cardiac magnetic resonance. *Eur Heart J.* 2006;27(14):1725-1731. doi:10.1093/eurheartj/ehl101

80. Maurizi N, Michels M, Rowin EJ, et al. Clinical course and significance of hypertrophic cardiomyopathy without left ventricular hypertrophy. *Circulation.* 2019;139(6):830-833. doi:10.1161/CIRCULATIONAHA.118.037264

81. Rowin EJ, Hausvater A, Link MS, et al. Clinical profile and consequences of atrial fibrillation in hypertrophic cardiomyopathy. *Circulation.* 2017;136(25):2420-2436. doi:10.1161/CIRCULATIONAHA.117.029267

82. Guttmann OP, Rahman MS, O'Mahony C, Anastasakis A, Elliott PM. Atrial fibrillation and thromboembolism in patients with hypertrophic cardiomyopathy: systematic review. *Heart.* 2014;100(6):465-472. doi:10.1136/heartjnl-2013-304276

83. Siontis KC, Geske JB, Ong K, Nishimura RA, Ommen SR, Gersh BJ. Atrial fibrillation in hypertrophic cardiomyopathy: prevalence, clinical correlations, and mortality in a large high-risk population. *J Am Heart Assoc.* 2014;3(3):e001002. doi:10.1161/JAHA.114.001002

84. Lorenzini M, Anastasiou Z, O'Mahony C, et al. Mortality among referral patients with hypertrophic cardiomyopathy vs the general European population. *JAMA Cardiol.* 2020;5(1):73. doi:10.1001/jamacardio.2019.4534

85. Monserrat L, Elliott PM, Gimeno JR, Sharma S, Penas-Lado M, McKenna WJ. Non-sustained ventricular tachycardia in hypertrophic cardiomyopathy: an independent marker of sudden death risk in young patients. *J Am Coll Cardiol.* 2003;42(5):873-879.

86. Maron MS, Maron BJ, Harrigan C, et al. Hypertrophic cardiomyopathy phenotype revisited after 50 years with cardiovascular magnetic resonance. *J Am Coll Cardiol.* 2009;54(3):220-228. doi:10.1016/j.jacc.2009.05.006

87. Cardim N, Galderisi M, Edvardsen T, et al. Role of multimodality cardiac imaging in the management of patients with hypertrophic cardiomyopathy: an expert consensus of the European Association of Cardiovascular Imaging Endorsed by the Saudi Heart Association. *Eur Heart J Cardiovasc Imaging.* 2015;16(3):280. doi:10.1093/ehjci/jeu291

88. Geske JB, Sorajja P, Nishimura RA, Ommen SR. Evaluation of left ventricular filling pressures by Doppler echocardiography in patients with hypertrophic cardiomyopathy: correlation with direct left atrial pressure measurement at cardiac catheterization. *Circulation.* 2007;116(23):2702-2708. doi:10.1161/CIRCULATIONAHA.107.698985

89. Ho CY, Sweitzer NK, McDonough B, et al. Assessment of diastolic function with Doppler tissue imaging to predict genotype in preclinical hypertrophic cardiomyopathy. *Circulation.* 2002;105(25):2992-2997. doi:10.1161/01.cir.0000019070.70491.6d

90. Nagueh SF, Bachinski LL, Meyer D, et al. Tissue Doppler imaging consistently detects myocardial abnormalities in patients with hypertrophic cardiomyopathy and provides a novel means for an early diagnosis before and independently of hypertrophy. *Circulation.* 2001;104(2):128-130. doi:10.1161/01.cir.104.2.128

91. Yiu KH, Atsma DE, Delgado V, et al. Myocardial structural alteration and systolic dysfunction in preclinical hypertrophic cardiomyopathy mutation carriers. *PLoS One.* 2012;7(5):e36115. doi:10.1371/journal.pone.0036115

92. Bruce CJ, Nishimura RA, Tajik AJ, Schaff HV, Danielson GK. Fixed left ventricular outflow tract obstruction in presumed hypertrophic obstructive cardiomyopathy: implications for therapy. *Ann Thorac Surg.* 1999;68(1):100-104. doi:10.1016/s0003-4975(99)00447-6

93. Malcolmson JW, Hamshere SM, Joshi A, et al. Doppler echocardiography underestimates the prevalence and magnitude of mid-cavity obstruction in patients with symptomatic hypertrophic cardiomyopathy. *Catheter Cardiovasc Interv.* 2018;91(4):783-789. doi:10.1002/ccd.27143

94. Neubauer S, Kolm P, Ho CY, et al. Distinct subgroups in hypertrophic cardiomyopathy in the NHLBI HCM registry. *J Am Coll Cardiol.* 2019;74(19):2333-2345. doi:10.1016/j.jacc.2019.08.1057

95. Briasoulis A, Mallikethi-Reddy S, Palla M, Alesh I, Afonso L. Myocardial fibrosis on cardiac magnetic resonance and cardiac outcomes in hypertrophic cardiomyopathy: a meta-analysis. *Heart.* 2015;101(17):1406-1411. doi:10.1136/heartjnl-2015-307682

96. Maron MS. Clinical utility of cardiovascular magnetic resonance in hypertrophic cardiomyopathy. *J Cardiovasc Magn Reson.* 2012;14(1):13. doi:10.1186/1532-429X-14-13

97. Chan RH, Maron BJ, Olivotto I, et al. Prognostic value of quantitative contrast-enhanced cardiovascular magnetic resonance for the evaluation of sudden death risk in patients with hypertrophic cardiomyopathy. *Circulation.* 2014;130(6):484-495. doi:10.1161/CIRCULATIONAHA.113.007094

98. Radenkovic D, Weingärtner S, Ricketts L, Moon JC, Captur G. T1 mapping in cardiac MRI. *Heart Fail Rev.* 2017;22(4):415-430. doi:10.1007/s10741-017-9627-2

99. Captur G, Lopes LR, Mohun TJ, et al. Prediction of sarcomere mutations in subclinical hypertrophic cardiomyopathy. *Circ Cardiovasc Imaging.* 2014;7(6):863-871. doi:10.1161/CIRCIMAGING.114.002411

100. Ho CY, Abbasi SA, Neilan TG, et al. T1 measurements identify extracellular volume expansion in hypertrophic cardiomyopathy sarcomere mutation carriers with and without left ventricular hypertrophy. *Circ Cardiovasc Imaging.* 2013;6(3):415-422. doi:10.1161/CIRCIMAGING.112.000333

101. Gillmore JD, Maurer MS, Falk RH, et al. Nonbiopsy diagnosis of cardiac transthyretin amyloidosis. *Circulation.* 2016;133(24):2404-2412. doi:10.1161/CIRCULATIONAHA.116.021612

102. Sorajja P, Ommen SR, Nishimura RA, Gersh BJ, Tajik AJ, Holmes DR. Myocardial bridging in adult patients with hypertrophic cardiomyopathy. *J Am Coll Cardiol.* 2003;42(5):889-894. doi:10.1016/s0735-1097(03)00854-4

103. Mohiddin SA, Begley D, Shih J, Fananapazir L. Myocardial bridging does not predict sudden death in children with hypertrophic cardiomyopathy but is associated with more severe cardiac disease. *J Am Coll Cardiol.* 2000;36(7):2270-2278. doi:10.1016/s0735-1097(00)00987-6

104. Yetman AT, McCrindle BW, MacDonald C, Freedom RM, Gow R. Myocardial bridging in children with hypertrophic cardiomyopathy–a risk factor for sudden death. *N Engl J Med.* 1998;339(17):1201-1209. doi:10.1056/NEJM199810223391704

105. Frenneaux MP, Porter A, Caforio ALP, Odawara H, Counihan PJ, McKenna WJ. Determinants of exercise capacity in hypertrophic cardiomyopathy. *J Am Coll Cardiol.* 1989;13(7):1521-1526. doi:10.1016/0735-1097(89)90342-2

106. Gimeno JR, Tomé-Esteban M, Lofiego C, et al. Exercise-induced ventricular arrhythmias and risk of sudden cardiac death in patients with hypertrophic cardiomyopathy. *Eur Heart J.* 2009;30(21):2599-2605. doi:10.1093/eurheartj/ehp327

107. Coats CJ, Rantell K, Bartnik A, et al. Cardiopulmonary exercise testing and prognosis in hypertrophic cardiomyopathy. *Circ Hear Fail.* 2015;8(6):1022-1031. doi:10.1161/CIRCHEARTFAILURE.114.002248

108. Coats CJ, Gallagher MJ, Foley M, et al. Relation between serum N-terminal pro-brain natriuretic peptide and prognosis in patients with hypertrophic cardiomyopathy. *Eur Heart J.* 2013;34(32):2529-2537. doi:10.1093/eurheartj/eht070

109. Peterson GE, de Backer T, Contreras G, et al. Relationship of left ventricular hypertrophy and diastolic function with cardiovascular and renal outcomes in African Americans with hypertensive chronic

kidney disease. *Hypertension.* 2013;62(3):518-525. doi:10.1161/HYPERTENSIONAHA.111.00904

110. Zywica K, Jenni R, Pellikka PA, Faeh-Gunz A, Seifert B, Attenhofer Jost CH. Dynamic left ventricular outflow tract obstruction evoked by exercise echocardiography: prevalence and predictive factors in a prospective study. *Eur J Echocardiogr.* 2008;9(5):665-671. doi:10.1093/ejechocard/jen070

111. Pelliccia A, Caselli S, Sharma S, et al. European Association of Preventive Cardiology (EAPC) and European Association of Cardiovascular Imaging (EACVI) joint position statement: recommendations for the indication and interpretation of cardiovascular imaging in the evaluation of the athlete's heart. *Eur Heart J.* 2018;39(21):1949-1969. doi:10.1093/eurheartj/ehx532

112. Basavarajaiah S, Boraita A, Whyte G, et al. Ethnic differences in left ventricular remodeling in highly-trained athletes. *J Am Coll Cardiol.* 2008;51(23):2256-2262. doi:10.1016/j.jacc.2007.12.061

113. Sharma S, Drezner JA, Baggish A, et al. International recommendations for electrocardiographic interpretation in athletes. *Eur Heart J.* 2018;39(16):1466-1480. doi:10.1093/eurheartj/ehw631

114. Pelliccia A, Maron BJ, De Luca R, Di Paolo FM, Spataro A, Culasso F. Remodeling of left ventricular hypertrophy in elite athletes after long-term deconditioning. *Circulation.* 2002;105(8):944-949. doi:10.1161/hc0802.104534

115. Weiner RB, Wang F, Berkstresser B, et al. Regression of "gray zone" exercise-induced concentric left ventricular hypertrophy during prescribed detraining. *J Am Coll Cardiol.* 2012;59(22):1992-1994. doi:10.1016/j.jacc.2012.01.057

116. Alfares AA, Kelly MA, McDermott G, et al. Results of clinical genetic testing of 2,912 probands with hypertrophic cardiomyopathy: expanded panels offer limited additional sensitivity. *Genet Med.* 2015;17(11):880-888. doi:10.1038/gim.2014.205

117. Walsh R, Buchan R, Wilk A, et al. Defining the genetic architecture of hypertrophic cardiomyopathy: Re-evaluating the role of non-sarcomeric genes. *Eur Heart J.* 2017;38(46):3461-3468. doi:10.1093/eurheartj/ehw603

118. Bagnall RD, Ingles J, Dinger ME, et al. Whole genome sequencing improves outcomes of genetic testing in patients with hypertrophic cardiomyopathy. *J Am Coll Cardiol.* 2018;72(4):419-429. doi:10.1016/j.jacc.2018.04.078

119. Charron P, Arad M, Arbustini E, et al. Genetic counselling and testing in cardiomyopathies: a position statement of the European Society of Cardiology Working Group on Myocardial and Pericardial Diseases. *Eur Heart J.* 2010;31(22):2715-2728. doi:10.1093/eurheartj/ehq271

120. Wordsworth S, Leal J, Blair E, et al. DNA testing for hypertrophic cardiomyopathy: a cost-effectiveness model. *Eur Heart J.* 2010;31(8):926-935. doi:10.1093/eurheartj/ehq067

121. Elliott PM, Gimeno JR, Thaman R, et al. Historical trends in reported survival rates in patients with hypertrophic cardiomyopathy. *Heart.* 2006;92(6):785-791. doi:10.1136/hrt.2005.068577

122. Maron BJ, Rowin EJ, Casey SA, et al. Hypertrophic cardiomyopathy in children, adolescents, and young adults associated with low cardiovascular mortality with contemporary management strategies. *Circulation.* 2016;133(1):62-73. doi:10.1161/CIRCULATIONAHA.115.017633

123. Maron BJ, Rowin EJ, Casey SA, et al. Hypertrophic cardiomyopathy in adulthood associated with low cardiovascular mortality with contemporary management strategies. *J Am Coll Cardiol.* 2015;65(18):1915-1928. doi:10.1016/j.jacc.2015.02.061

124. Marian AJ, Braunwald E. Hypertrophic cardiomyopathy: genetics, pathogenesis, clinical manifestations, diagnosis, and therapy. *Circ Res.* 2017;121(7):749-770. doi:10.1161/CIRCRESAHA.117.311059

125. O'Mahony C, Jichi F, Ommen SR, et al. International external validation study of the 2014 European Society of Cardiology guidelines on sudden cardiac death prevention in hypertrophic cardiomyopathy (EVIDENCE-HCM). *Circulation.* 2018;137(10):1015-1023. doi:10.1161/CIRCULATIONAHA.117.030437

126. O'Mahony C, Elliott PM. Prevention of sudden cardiac death in hypertrophic cardiomyopathy. *Heart.* 2014;100(3):254-260. doi:10.1136/heartjnl-2012-301996

127. Guttmann OP, Pavlou M, O'Mahony C, et al. Predictors of atrial fibrillation in hypertrophic cardiomyopathy. *Heart.* 2017;103(9):672-678. doi:10.1136/heartjnl-2016-309672

128. Guttmann OP, Pavlou M, O'Mahony C, et al. Prediction of thromboembolic risk in patients with hypertrophic cardiomyopathy (HCM Risk-CVA). *Eur J Heart Fail.* 2015;17(8):837-845. doi:10.1002/ejhf.316

129. Ong KC, Geske JB, Hebl VB, et al. Pulmonary hypertension is associated with worse survival in hypertrophic cardiomyopathy. *Eur Heart J Cardiovasc Imaging.* 2016;17(6):604-610. doi:10.1093/ehjci/jew024

130. Østergaard L, Valeur N, Wang A, et al. Incidence of infective endocarditis in patients considered at moderate risk. *Eur Heart J.* 2019;40(17):1355-1361. doi:10.1093/eurheartj/ehy629

131. Spirito P, Rapezzi C, Bellone P, et al. Infective endocarditis in hypertrophic cardiomyopathy: prevalence, incidence, and indications for antibiotic prophylaxis. *Circulation.* 1999;99(16):2132-2137. doi:10.1161/01.cir.99.16.2132

132. Sims JR, Anavekar NS, Bhatia S, et al. Clinical, radiographic, and microbiologic features of infective endocarditis in patients with hypertrophic cardiomyopathy. *Am J Cardiol.* 2018;121(4):480-484. doi:10.1016/j.amjcard.2017.11.010

133. Habib G, Lancellotti P, Antunes MJ, et al. 2015 ESC Guidelines for the management of infective endocarditis: the Task Force for the Management of Infective Endocarditis of the European Society of Cardiology (ESC). Endorsed by: European Association for Cardio-Thoracic Surgery (EACTS), the European Association of Nuclear Medicine (EANM). *Eur Heart J.* 2015;36(44):3075-3128. doi:10.1093/eurheartj/ehv319

134. Olivotto I, Maron MS, Adabag AS, et al. Gender-related differences in the clinical presentation and outcome of hypertrophic cardiomyopathy. *J Am Coll Cardiol.* 2005;46(3):480-487. doi:10.1016/j.jacc.2005.04.043

135. Geske JB, Ong KC, Siontis KC, et al. Women with hypertrophic cardiomyopathy have worse survival. *Eur Heart J.* 2017;38:3434-3440. doi:10.1093/eurheartj/ehx527

136. Wang Y, Wang J, Zou Y, et al. Female sex is associated with worse prognosis in patients with hypertrophic cardiomyopathy in China. *PLoS One.* 2014;9(7):e102969. doi:10.1371/journal.pone.0102969

137. Maass AH, Ikeda K, Oberdorf-Maass S, Maier SKG, Leinwand LA. Hypertrophy, fibrosis, and sudden cardiac death in response to pathological stimuli in mice with mutations in cardiac troponin T. *Circulation.* 2004;110(15):2102-2109. doi:10.1161/01.CIR.0000144460.84795.E3

138. Geisterfer-Lowrance AA, Christe M, Conner DA, et al. A mouse model of familial hypertrophic cardiomyopathy. *Science* 1996; 272(5262):731-734.

139. Olsson MC, Palmer BM, Leinwand LA, Moore RL. Gender and aging in a transgenic mouse model of hypertrophic cardiomyopathy. *Am J Physiol Heart Circ Physiol.* 2001;280(3):H1136-44.

140. Xin H-B, Senbonmatsu T, Cheng D-S, et al. Oestrogen protects FKBP12.6 null mice from cardiac hypertrophy. *Nature.* 2002;416(6878):334-338. doi:10.1038/416334a

141. Lind JM, Chiu C, Ingles J, et al. Sex hormone receptor gene variation associated with phenotype in male hypertrophic cardiomyopathy patients. *J Mol Cell Cardiol.* 2008;45(2):217-222. doi:10.1016/j.yjmcc.2008.05.016

142. Najafi A, Schlossarek S, van Deel ED, et al. Sexual dimorphic response to exercise in hypertrophic cardiomyopathy-associated MYBPC3-targeted knock-in mice. *Pflugers Arch Eur J Physiol.* 2015;467(6):1303-1317. doi:10.1007/s00424-014-1570-7

143. McKee LAK, Chen H, Regan JA, et al. Sexually dimorphic myofilament function and cardiac troponin i phosphospecies distribution in hypertrophic cardiomyopathy mice. *Arch Biochem Biophys.* 2013;535(1):39-48. doi:10.1016/j.abb.2012.12.023

144. Mosca L, Ferris A, Fabunmi R, Robertson RM, American Heart Association. Tracking women's awareness of heart disease: an American Heart Association national study. *Circulation.* 2004;109(5):573-579. doi:10.1161/01.CIR.0000115222.69428.C9

145. Kaul P, Armstrong PW, Sookram S, Leung BK, Brass N, Welsh RC. Temporal trends in patient and treatment delay among men and women presenting with ST-elevation myocardial infarction. *Am Heart J*. 2011; 161(1):91-97. doi:10.1016/j.ahj.2010.09.016

146. Diercks DB, Owen KP, Kontos MC, et al. Gender differences in time to presentation for myocardial infarction before and after a national women's cardiovascular awareness campaign: a temporal analysis from the Can Rapid Risk Stratification of Unstable Angina Patients Suppress ADverse Outcomes wi. *Am Heart J*. 2010;160(1):80-87.e3. doi:10.1016/j.ahj.2010.04.017

147. Corrado D, Basso C, Schiavon M, Thiene G. Screening for hypertrophic cardiomyopathy in young athletes. *N Engl J Med*. 1998;339(6):364-369. doi:10.1056/NEJM199808063390602

148. Hada Y, Sakamoto T, Amano K, et al. Prevalence of hypertrophic cardiomyopathy in a population of adult Japanese workers as detected by echocardiographic screening. *Am J Cardiol*. 1987;59(1):183-184. doi:10.1016/S0002-9149(87)80107-8

149. Providencia R, Elliott P, Patel K, et al. Catheter ablation for atrial fibrillation in hypertrophic cardiomyopathy: a systematic review and meta-analysis. *Heart*. 2016;102(19):1533-1543. doi:10.1136/heartjnl-2016-309406

150. Nistri S, Olivotto I, Maron MS, et al. β Blockers for prevention of exercise-induced left ventricular outflow tract obstruction in patients with hypertrophic cardiomyopathy. *Am J Cardiol*. 2012;110(5):715-719. doi:10.1016/j.amjcard.2012.04.051

151. Bonow RO, Frederick TM, Bacharach SL, et al. Atrial systole and left ventricular filling in hypertrophic cardiomyopathy: effect of verapamil. *Am J Cardiol*. 1983;51(8):1386-1391. doi:10.1016/0002-9149(83)90317-x

152. Rosing DR, Kent KM, Borer JS, Seides SF, Maron BJ, Epstein SE. Verapamil therapy: a new approach to the pharmacologic treatment of hypertrophic cardiomyopathy. I. Hemodynamic effects. *Circulation*. 1979;60(6):1201-1207. doi:10.1161/01.cir.60.6.1201

153. Rosing DR, Kent KM, Maron BJ, Epstein SE. Verapamil therapy: a new approach to the pharmacologic treatment of hypertrophic cardiomyopathy. II. Effects on exercise capacity and symptomatic status. *Circulation*. 1979;60(6):1208-1213. doi:10.1161/01.cir.60.6.1208

154. Epstein SE, Rosing DR. Verapamil: its potential for causing serious complications in patients with hypertrophic cardiomyopathy. *Circulation*. 1981;64(3):437-441. doi:10.1161/01.cir.64.3.437

155. Sherrid MV, Barac I, McKenna WJ, et al. Multicenter study of the efficacy and safety of disopyramide in obstructive hypertrophic cardiomyopathy. *J Am Coll Cardiol*. 2005;45(8):1251-1258. doi:10.1016/j.jacc.2005.01.012

156. Anderson RL, Trivedi D V., Sarkar SS, et al. Deciphering the super relaxed state of human β-cardiac myosin and the mode of action of mavacamten from myosin molecules to muscle fibers. *Proc Natl Acad Sci U S A*. 2018;115(35):E8143-E8152. doi:10.1073/pnas.1809540115

157. Olivotto I, Oreziak A, Barriales-Villa R, et al. Mavacamten for treatment of symptomatic obstructive hypertrophic cardiomyopathy (EXPLORER-HCM): a randomised, double-blind, placebo-controlled, phase 3 trial. *Lancet*. 2020;396(10253):759-769. doi:10.1016/S0140-6736(20)31792-X

158. Saberi S, Cardim N, Yamani MH, et al. Mavacamten favorably impacts cardiac structure in obstructive hypertrophic cardiomyopathy: EXPLORER-HCM CMR substudy analysis. *Circulation*. November 2020: doi:10.1161/CIRCULATIONAHA.120.052359

159. Ommen SR, Maron BJ, Olivotto I, et al. Long-term effects of surgical septal myectomy on survival in patients with obstructive hypertrophic cardiomyopathy. *J Am Coll Cardiol*. 2005;46(3):470-476. doi:10.1016/j.jacc.2005.02.090

160. Collis R, Watkinson O, O'Mahony C, et al. Long-term outcomes for different surgical strategies to treat left ventricular outflow tract obstruction in hypertrophic cardiomyopathy. *Eur J Heart Fail*. 2018;20(2):398-405. doi:10.1002/ejhf.1038

161. Lentz Carvalho J, Schaff HV, Morris CS, et al. Anomalous papillary muscles-Implications in the surgical treatment of hypertrophic obstructive cardiomyopathy. *J Thorac Cardiovasc Surg*. April 2020. doi:10.1016/j.jtcvs.2020.04.007

162. Kofflard MJ, van Herwerden LA, Waldstein DJ, et al. Initial results of combined anterior mitral leaflet extension and myectomy in patients with obstructive hypertrophic cardiomyopathy. *J Am Coll Cardiol*. 1996;28(1):197-202. doi:10.1016/0735-1097(96)00103-9

163. McIntosh CL, Maron BJ, Cannon RO, Klues HG. Initial results of combined anterior mitral leaflet plication and ventricular septal myotomy-myectomy for relief of left ventricular outflow tract obstruction in patients with hypertrophic cardiomyopathy. *Circulation*. 1992;86(5 Suppl):II60-II67.

164. Sun D, Schaff HV, Nishimura RA, Geske JB, Dearani JA, Ommen SR. Transapical septal myectomy for hypertrophic cardiomyopathy with mid-ventricular obstruction. *Ann Thorac Surg*. August 2020. doi:10.1016/j.athoracsur.2020.05.182

165. Ball W, Ivanov J, Rakowski H, et al. Long-term survival in patients with resting obstructive hypertrophic cardiomyopathy comparison of conservative versus invasive treatment. *J Am Coll Cardiol*. 2011;58(22):2313-2321. doi:10.1016/j.jacc.2011.08.040

166. Kim LK, Swaminathan RV, Looser P, et al. Hospital volume outcomes after septal myectomy and alcohol septal ablation for treatment of obstructive hypertrophic cardiomyopathy: US Nationwide Inpatient Database, 2003-2011. *JAMA Cardiol*. 2016;1(3):324-332. doi:10.1001/jamacardio.2016.0252

167. Cui H, Schaff HV, Nishimura RA, et al. Conduction abnormalities and long-term mortality following septal myectomy in patients with obstructive hypertrophic cardiomyopathy. *J Am Coll Cardiol*. 2019;74(5):645-655. doi:10.1016/j.jacc.2019.05.053

168. Collis RA, Rahman MS, Watkinson O, Guttmann OP, O'Mahony C, Elliott PM. Outcomes following the surgical management of left ventricular outflow tract obstruction; a systematic review and meta-analysis. *Int J Cardiol*. 2018;265:62-70. doi:10.1016/j.ijcard.2018.01.130

169. Knight C, Kurbaan AS, Seggewiss H, et al. Nonsurgical septal reduction for hypertrophic obstructive cardiomyopathy: outcome in the first series of patients. *Circulation*. 1997;95(8):2075-2081. doi:10.1161/01.cir.95.8.2075

170. van Dockum WG, Beek AM, ten Cate FJ, et al. Early onset and progression of left ventricular remodeling after alcohol septal ablation in hypertrophic obstructive cardiomyopathy. *Circulation*. 2005;111(19):2503-2508. doi:10.1161/01.CIR.0000165084.28065.01

171. Faber L, Seggewiss H, Gleichmann U. Percutaneous transluminal septal myocardial ablation in hypertrophic obstructive cardiomyopathy: results with respect to intraprocedural myocardial contrast echocardiography. *Circulation*. 1998;98(22):2415-2421. doi:10.1161/01.cir.98.22.2415

172. Veselka J, Jensen MK, Liebregts M, et al. Long-term clinical outcome after alcohol septal ablation for obstructive hypertrophic cardiomyopathy: results from the Euro-ASA registry. *Eur Heart J*. 2016;37(19):1517-1523. doi:10.1093/eurheartj/ehv693

173. Qin JX, Shiota T, Lever HM, et al. Conduction system abnormalities in patients with obstructive hypertrophic cardiomyopathy following septal reduction interventions. *Am J Cardiol*. 2004;93(2):171-175. doi:10.1016/j.amjcard.2003.09.034

174. Cooper RM, Stables RH. Non-surgical septal reduction therapy in hypertrophic cardiomyopathy. *Heart*. 2018;104(1):73-83. doi:10.1136/heartjnl-2016-309952

175. Liebregts M, Vriesendorp PA, Mahmoodi BK, Schinkel AFL, Michels M, ten Berg JMJM. A systematic review and meta-analysis of long-term outcomes after septal reduction therapy in patients with hypertrophic cardiomyopathy. *JACC Hear Fail*. 2015;3(11):896-905. doi:10.1016/j.jchf.2015.06.011

176. Sorajja P. Alcohol septal ablation for obstructive hypertrophic cardiomyopathy: a word of balance. *J Am Coll Cardiol*. 2017;70(4):489-494. doi:10.1016/j.jacc.2017.06.011

177. Quintana E, Sabate-Rotes A, Maleszewski JJ, et al. Septal myectomy after failed alcohol ablation: Does previous percutaneous intervention compromise outcomes of myectomy? *J Thorac Cardiovasc Surg*. 2015;150(1):159-167.e1. doi:10.1016/j.jtcvs.2015.03.044

178. Daubert C, Gadler F, Mabo P, Linde C. Pacing for hypertrophic obstructive cardiomyopathy: an update and future directions. *Europace.* 2018;20(6):908-920. doi:10.1093/europace/eux131

179. Nishimura RA, Trusty JM, Hayes DL, et al. Dual-chamber pacing for hypertrophic cardiomyopathy: a randomized, double-blind, crossover trial. *J Am Coll Cardiol.* 1996;29(2):435-441. doi:10.1016/s0735-1097(96)00473-1

180. Kappenberger L, Linde C, Daubert C, et al. Pacing in hypertrophic obstructive cardiomyopathy. A randomized crossover study. PIC Study Group. *Eur Heart J.* 1997;18(8):1249-1256. doi:10.1093/oxfordjournals.eurheartj.a015435

181. Maron BJ, Nishimura RA, McKenna WJ, Rakowski H, Josephson ME, Kieval RS. Assessment of permanent dual-chamber pacing as a treatment for drug-refractory symptomatic patients with obstructive hypertrophic cardiomyopathy. A randomized, double-blind, crossover study (M-PATHY). *Circulation.* 1999;99(22):2927-2933. doi:10.1161/01.cir.99.22.2927

182. Gadler F, Linde C, Juhlin-Dannfeldt A, Ribeiro A, Rydén L. Influence of right ventricular pacing site on left ventricular outflow tract obstruction in patients with hypertrophic obstructive cardiomyopathy. *J Am Coll Cardiol.* 1996;27(5):1219-1224. doi:10.1016/0735-1097(95)00573-0

183. Nishimura RA, Hayes DL, Ilstrup DM, Holmes DR, Tajik AJ. Effect of dual-chamber pacing on systolic and diastolic function in patients with hypertrophic cardiomyopathy. Acute Doppler echocardiographic and catheterization hemodynamic study. *J Am Coll Cardiol.* 1996;27(2):421-430. doi:10.1016/0735-1097(95)00445-9

184. Abozguia K, Elliott P, McKenna W, et al. Metabolic modulator perhexiline corrects energy deficiency and improves exercise capacity in symptomatic hypertrophic cardiomyopathy. *Circulation.* 2010;122(16):1562-1569. doi:10.1161/CIRCULATIONAHA.109.934059

185. Coats CJ, Pavlou M, Watkinson OT, et al. Effect of trimetazidine dihydrochloride therapy on exercise capacity in patients with nonobstructive hypertrophic cardiomyopathy. *JAMA Cardiol.* 2019;4(3):2-7. doi:10.1001/jamacardio.2018.4847

186. Olivotto I, Camici PG, Merlini PA, et al. Efficacy of ranolazine in patients with symptomatic hypertrophic cardiomyopathy: The RESTYLE-HCM randomized, double-blind, placebo-controlled study. *Circ Heart Fail.* 2018;11(1):e004124. doi:10.1161/CIRCHEARTFAILURE.117.004124

187. Rogers DPS, Marazia S, Chow AW, et al. Effect of biventricular pacing on symptoms and cardiac remodelling in patients with end-stage hypertrophic cardiomyopathy. *Eur J Heart Fail.* 2008;10(5):507-513. doi:10.1016/j.ejheart.2008.03.006

188. Cappelli F, Morini S, Pieragnoli P, et al. Cardiac resynchronization therapy for end-stage hypertrophic cardiomyopathy: the need for disease-specific criteria. *J Am Coll Cardiol.* 2018;71(4):464-466. doi:10.1016/j.jacc.2017.11.040

189. Maron MS, Kalsmith BM, Udelson JE, Li W, DeNofrio D. Survival after cardiac transplantation in patients with hypertrophic cardiomyopathy. *Circ Heart Fail.* 2010;3(5):574-579. doi:10.1161/CIRCHEARTFAILURE.109.922872

190. McKenna WJ, Oakley CM, Krikler DM, Goodwin JF. Improved survival with amiodarone in patients with hypertrophic cardiomyopathy and ventricular tachycardia. *Br Heart J.* 1985;53(4):412-416. doi:10.1136/hrt.53.4.412

191. Cecchi F, Olivotto I, Montereggi A, Squillatini G, Dolara A, Maron BJ. Prognostic value of non-sustained ventricular tachycardia and the potential role of amiodarone treatment in hypertrophic cardiomyopathy: assessment in an unselected non-referral based patient population. *Heart.* 1998;79(4):331-336. doi:10.1136/hrt.79.4.331

192. Maron BJ, Shen W-K, Link MS, et al. Efficacy of implantable cardioverter-defibrillators for the prevention of sudden death in patients with hypertrophic cardiomyopathy. *N Engl J Med.* 2000;342(6):365-373.

193. Elliott PM, Sharma S, Varnava A, Poloniecki J, Rowland E, McKenna WJ. Survival after cardiac arrest or sustained ventricular tachycardia in patients with hypertrophic cardiomyopathy. *J Am Coll Cardiol.* 1999;33(6):1596-1601. doi:10.1016/s0735-1097(99)00056-x

194. Pelliccia A, Sharma S, Gati S, et al. 2020 ESC Guidelines on sports cardiology and exercise in patients with cardiovascular disease. *Eur Heart J.* August 2020:1-80. doi:10.1093/eurheartj/ehaa605

195. Spirito P, Bellone P, Harris KM, Bernabo P, Bruzzi P, Maron BJ. Magnitude of left ventricular hypertrophy and risk of sudden death in hypertrophic cardiomyopathy. *N Engl J Med.* 2000;342(24):1778-1785. doi:10.1056/NEJM200006153422403

196. Elliott PM, Gimeno Blanes JR, Mahon NG, Poloniecki JD, McKenna WJ. Relation between severity of left-ventricular hypertrophy and prognosis in patients with hypertrophic cardiomyopathy. *Lancet.* 2001;357(9254):420-424. doi:10.1016/S0140-6736(00)04005-8

197. Maron MS, Olivotto I, Betocchi S, et al. Effect of left ventricular outflow tract obstruction on clinical outcome in hypertrophic cardiomyopathy. *N Engl J Med.* 2003;348(4):295-303. doi:10.1056/NEJMoa021332

198. Norrish G, Ding T, Field E, et al. Development of a novel risk prediction model for sudden cardiac death in childhood hypertrophic cardiomyopathy (HCM Risk-Kids). *JAMA Cardiol.* 2019;4(9):918-927. doi:10.1001/jamacardio.2019.2861

199. Miron A, Lafreniere-Roula M, Steve Fan C-P, et al. A validated model for sudden cardiac death risk prediction in pediatric hypertrophic cardiomyopathy. *Circulation.* 2020;142(3):217-229. doi:10.1161/CIRCULATIONAHA.120.047235

200. O'Mahony C, Lambiase PD, Quarta G, et al. The long-term survival and the risks and benefits of implantable cardioverter defibrillators in patients with hypertrophic cardiomyopathy. *Heart.* 2012;98(2):116-125. doi:10.1136/hrt.2010.217182

201. Lozier MR, Sanchez AM, Lee JJ, Donath EM, Font VE, Escolar E. Thromboembolic outcomes of different anticoagulation strategies for patients with atrial fibrillation in the setting of hypertrophic cardiomyopathy: a systematic review. *J Atr Fibrillat.* 2019;12(4):2207. doi:10.4022/jafib.2207

202. Van Der Velden J, Ho CY, Tardiff JC, Olivotto I, Knollmann BC, Carrier L. Research priorities in sarcomeric cardiomyopathies. *Cardiovasc Res.* 2015;105(4):449-456. doi:10.1093/cvr/cvv019

203. Ho CY, Lakdawala NK, Cirino AL, et al. Diltiazem treatment for preclinical hypertrophic cardiomyopathy sarcomere mutation carriers: a pilot randomized trial to modify disease expression. *JACC Heart Fail.* 2015;3(2):180-188. doi:10.1016/j.jchf.2014.08.003

204. Axelsson A, Iversen K, Vejlstrup N, et al. Efficacy and safety of the angiotensin II receptor blocker losartan for hypertrophic cardiomyopathy: the INHERIT randomised, double-blind, placebo-controlled trial. *Lancet Diabetes Endocrinol.* 2015;3(2):123-131. doi:10.1016/S2213-8587(14)70241-4

205. Maron MS, Chan RH, Kapur NK, et al. Effect of spironolactone on myocardial fibrosis and other clinical variables in patients with hypertrophic cardiomyopathy. *Am J Med.* 2018;131(7):837-841. doi:10.1016/j.amjmed.2018.02.025

206. Ho CY, Mealiffe ME, Bach RG, et al. Evaluation of Mavacamten in symptomatic patients with nonobstructive hypertrophic cardiomyopathy. *J Am Coll Cardiol.* 2020;75(21):2649-2660. doi:10.1016/j.jacc.2020.03.064

Cardiac Amyloidosis

Morie A. Gertz, Jagat Narula, Edgar Argulian, and Sumeet S. Mitter

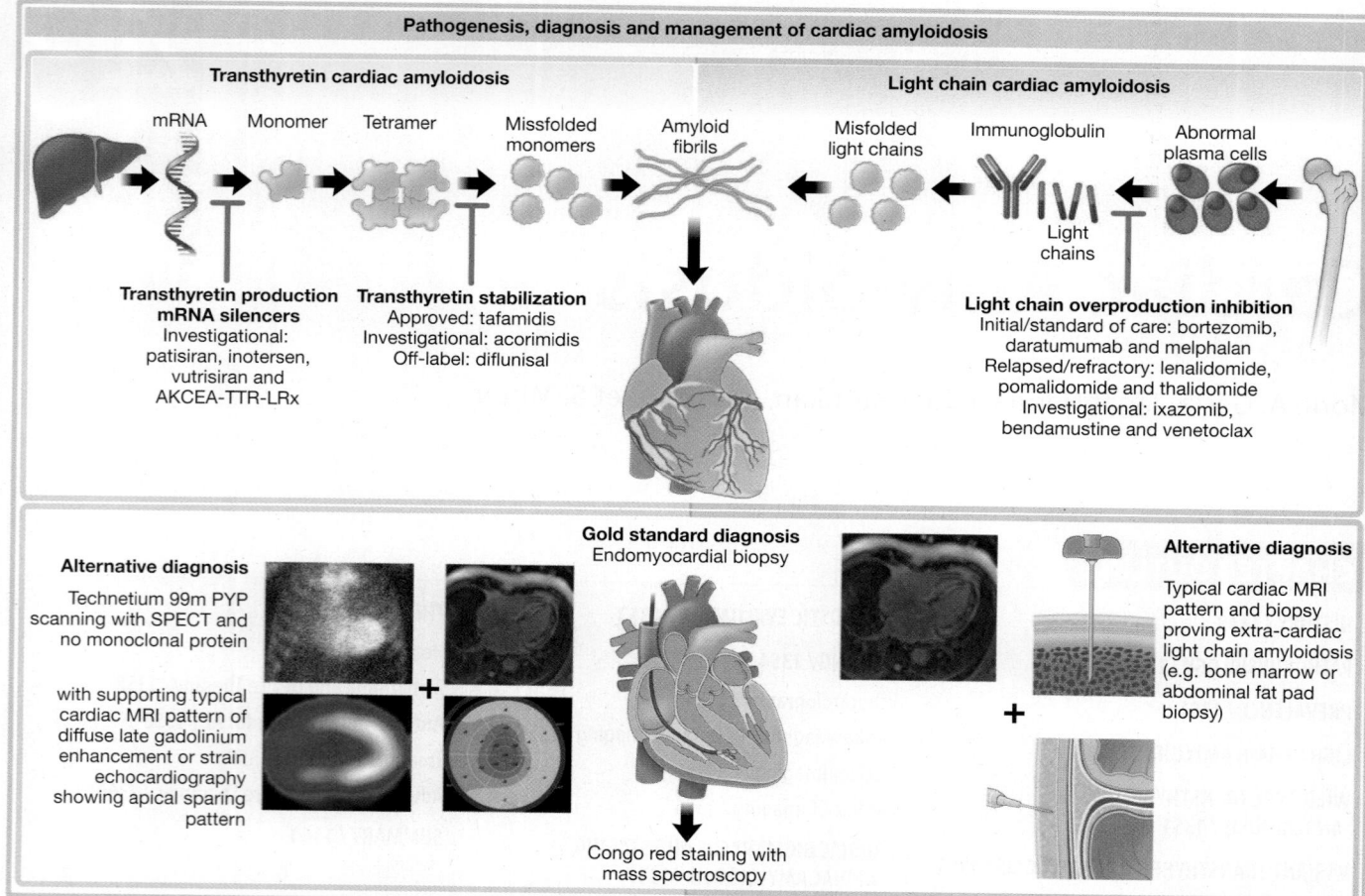

Chapter 43 Fuster and Hurst's Central Illustration. Cardiac amyloidosis leads to left ventricular wall thickening and primarily presents with heart failure with preserved ejection fraction (HFpEF) in early stages of the disease. Pathogenesis and the mechanisms of action of approved, investigational, and off-label therapies for transthyretin cardiac amyloidosis and light chain cardiac amyloidosis are shown in the upper panel. Gold standard and alternative methods of diagnosis are depicted in the lower panel.

CHAPTER SUMMARY

This chapter discusses prevalence, pathophysiology, contemporary invasive and noninvasive diagnosis, and emerging management strategies for cardiac amyloidosis, including both wildtype and variant transthyretin disease as well as light-chain disease (see Fuster and Hurst's Central Illustration). Novel therapies can alter the natural history of cardiac amyloidosis and thus the condition should be considered as a differential diagnosis in any individual with heart failure with preserved ejection fraction, increased left ventricular wall thickness beyond 1.2 cm, and other concerning comorbid conditions including but not limited to atrial fibrillation, carpal tunnel syndrome, and autonomic dysfunction. In variant transthyretin amyloidosis, particularly the V142I pathogenic variant affecting 3% to 4% of Black Americans, facilitating genetic cascade testing in first-degree family members, and subsequent earlier recognition of phenotypic disease and treatment with transthyretin stabilizers, may result in slower disease progression and greater mortality benefit. Ongoing clinical trials using transthyretin silencers may dramatically alter the field if they also show morality benefit and less disease progression for both wildtype and/or variant disease. Additionally, if left untreated, light-chain cardiac amyloidosis is a very fatal disease; however, achieving hematologic response in patients with the condition, either with chemotherapy with bortezomib-based regimens or the anti-CD-38 monoclonal antibody daratumumab, can substantially alter prognosis.

HISTORY

Rudolf Virchow described the reaction of amyloid deposits with iodine and sulfuric acid in 1853. Because this reaction was positive, he assumed that these deposits were starch-like and coined the term *amyloid* (derived from *amylum*, the Latin word for "starch")[1] (**Fig. 43–1**). However, they were later found to be devoid of cellulose by Carl Freidreich and in fact were more albuminoid.[2] In ensuing decades after the introduction of Congo red staining, they were found to have apple-green birefringence under polarized light with a beta pleat structure composing the amyloid fibers.

PATHOPHYSIOLOGY

Today, amyloidosis reflects a localized or systemic process as a result of at least 30 precursor proteins that destabilize, rearranging into such beta-pleated sheets that make up the fibers that can deposit in various organs. Amyloid deposits are all extracellular and appear hyaline-like and amorphous when stained with hematoxylin and eosin (**Fig. 43–2**). As mentioned, under polarized light, amyloid deposits exhibit apple-green birefringence with Congo red staining (Fig. 43–2). This finding in any tissue is the gold standard for diagnosis of amyloidosis. Alternatively, some pathology labs will perform staining with sodium sulphate-Alcian Blue in preference to Congo red.

Cardiac amyloidosis is most often due to misfolded amyloid light-chain (AL) disease and amyloid transthyretin (ATTR) aggregates (**Table 43–1**) that lead to a restrictive cardiomyopathy from amyloid infiltration into the extracellular space of the myocardium.[3] In the former case, AL disease is the result of a monoclonal plasma cell producing immunoglobulins, from which the light chain breaks off and rearranges to form amyloid deposits. The heart is affected in 50% to 75% of AL

disease cases. ATTR disease arises from the breakdown of the tetramer transthyretin protein (or pre-albumin) made primarily in the liver into monomers that destabilize and rearrange into amyloid fibers. Transthyretin functions to transport <5% of the thyroxine as well as retinol-binding protein. Transthyretin is also made in small amounts in the choroid plexus for the cerebrospinal fluid and the retinal pigmented cells for the vitreous of the eye. The encoding gene for transthyretin lies within chromosome 18. A pathologic state can be the result of wild-type ATTR (wtATTR) (formerly senile or age-related ATTR disease) disease that primarily affects the heart or variant ATTR (vATTR) due to more than 130 mutations that lead to varying degrees cardiomyopathy and neuropathy (**Fig. 43–3**). The most common mutation in the United States is Val122Ile (p.V142I), implying valine is substituted by isoleucine at amino acid sequence 122 in the gene and is found in 3.4% of Black American population.[4] The mutation is also common among individuals of African Caribbean descent. Untreated median survival of AL, vATTR, and wtATTR cardiomyopathy is 1.5 years, 2.5 years, and 3.6 years, respectively.[5] Thankfully the natural history of these disease states is rapidly changing with earlier detection and the advent of novel therapies. Rarer forms of cardiac amyloidosis are caused by amyloid acquired (AA) due to rheumatologic or chronic inflammatory/infectious processes, ApoA4 due to apolipoprotein 4, and isolated atrial amyloidosis (IAA) from an overproduction of atrial natriuretic peptide leading to primarily atrial amyloid manifesting often with atrial fibrillation[3,6] (Table 43–1).

Cardiac amyloidosis leads to left ventricular wall thickening and primarily presents with heart failure with preserved ejection fraction (HFpEF) in early stages of the disease. It is often confused with hypertensive heart disease or hypertrophic cardiomyopathy on echocardiography. When recognized late,

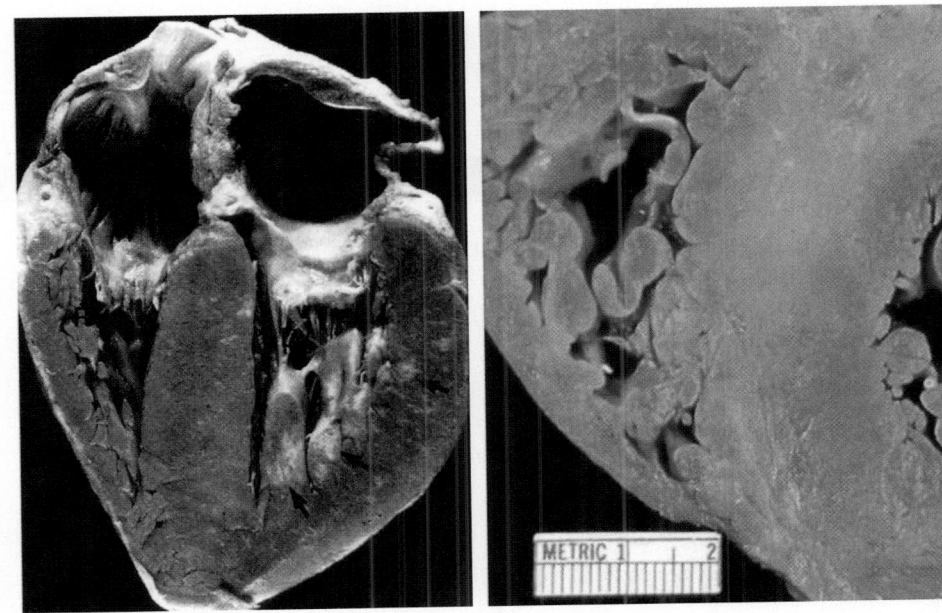

Figure 43–1. **(A)** and **(B)** Cardiac amyloid, note the marked thickening of the right and left ventricular walls. The white deposits of amyloid resulted in the incorrect labeling as "lardaceous degeneration" by Rokitansky in 1842 as "resembling bacon".

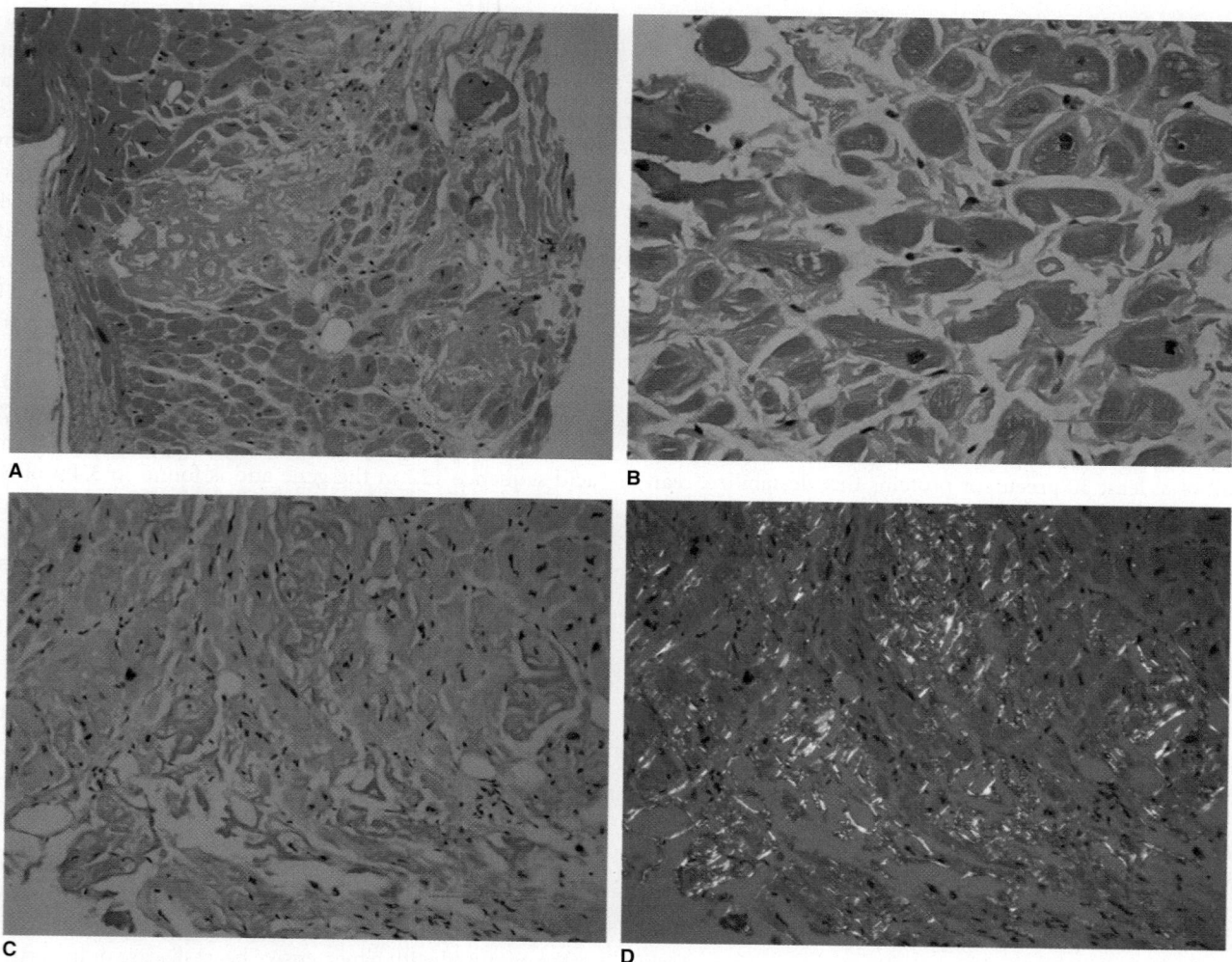

Figure 43–2. Endomyocardial biopsy demonstrating interstitial deposits of amyloid on hematoxylin and eosin staining at **(A)** 200x magnification and **(B)** 400x magnification as well as with Congo red staining at **(C)** 400x magnification and **(D)** under polarized light at 400x magnification showing characteristic apple-green birefringence.

TABLE 43–1. Types of Cardiac Amyloidosis

Precursor Protein	Age of Onset	Other Disease Manifestations	Current Therapies
Light Chain	50 and above	Renal disease, Autonomic dysfunction, Carpal tunnel disease, Pleural effusions, Periorbital purpura	Chemotherapy targeting clonal plasma cell including proteosome inhibitor, daratumumab
Wild-Type Transthyretin	70 and above	Spinal stenosis, Aortic stenosis, Carpal tunnel disease	Tafamidis Acorimidis (in Phase 3 testing) Diflunisal (off label)
Variant Transthyretin	20-70 (varies with pathogenic mutation)	Length-dependent poly sensorimotor neuropathy, Autonomic dysfunction, Carpal tunnel disease	Patisiran and inotersen if concomitant variant ATTR neuropathy
Acquired	Adolescent and above	Liver, kidney (heart rare)	Treat underlying cause
Apolipoprotein A4	Unknown	Unknown	Unknown
Isolated Atrial	Unknown	Atrial fibrillation	None

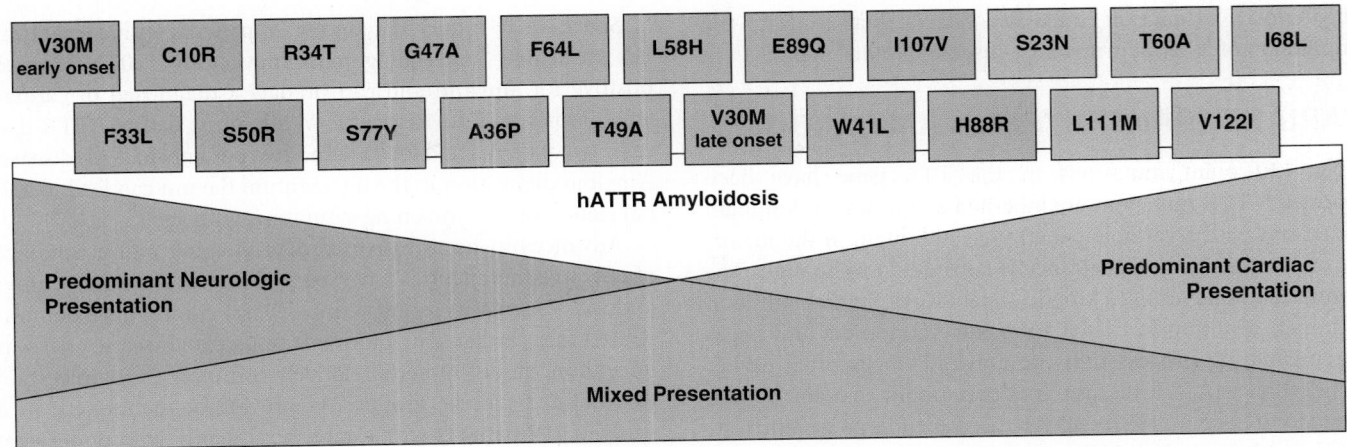

Figure 43–3. Demonstration of cardiac and neurologic phenotypes based on specific vTTR pathogenic mutations.

left ventricular dysfunction may be present and portends to a worse prognosis.

PREVALENCE

The true prevalence of cardiac amyloidosis is not known. Immunoglobulin light-chain amyloidosis has an incidence of 10 patients per million per year, with no evidence of increased frequency over the last 30 years (based on figures from the US, Great Britain, and Europe).[7] Hereditary ATTR prevalence is estimated to be 1 in 100,000 persons in the United States; worldwide prevalence is estimated to be 50,000 persons. Mixed phenotypes with both polyneuropathy and cardiomyopathy can occur in 60% of patients.[8] Wild-type ATTR amyloidosis has an unknown prevalence but can be seen in as many as 25% of autopsies in patients over the age of 80.[9] Today, HFpEF accounts for 50% of hospitalized heart failure.[10] In one recent study of hospitalized HFpEF patients undergoing endomyocardial biopsy to further phenotype disease, 14% had cardiac amyloidosis (including AL, ATTR, and AA disease).[11] Labeling cardiac amyloidosis as a rare disease may actually be a misnomer.

LIGHT-CHAIN AMYLOIDOSIS

Immunoglobulin light-chain amyloidosis represents a clonal plasma cell disorder with an estimated 3500 to 5000 new patients diagnosed annually in the United States. Although this can occur from the misfolding of kappa or lambda immunoglobulin light chains, over 70% of cardiac amyloidosis is lambda-associated, suggesting a unique predisposition for lambda light chains to deposit in the heart when compared to kappa light chains.[12] Occasionally, heavy chains can be found by mass spectroscopic analysis. Progressive build-up of the light-chain amyloid fibers leads to restrictive myopathy and hence a heart failure syndrome due to an elevation in left ventricular filling pressures in the setting of a small left ventricular cavity. Electrical dysfunction with atrial fibrillation and atrial standstill are well reported.

Presentation can be nonspecific and varied and in addition to HFpEF can include nephrotic range proteinuria, carpal tunnel syndrome, periorbital purpura, macroglossia, diarrhea, and autonomic dysfunction. Initial assessment for AL cardiomyopathy when assessing a patient with HFpEF in the absence of hypertension should include serum immunoglobulin-free light-chain assay and serum and urine immunofixation studies. Serum and urine electrophoresis lack significant sensitivity to rule out AL disease and should not be ordered. Should serum and urine markers raise concern for AL disease, a referral to an oncologist should be made at which point fat pad and/or bone marrow biopsy can be performed to obtain tissue needed for diagnostic confirmation. Plasmacytoma with a plasma cell population occupying <20% of the bone marrow is consistent with isolated AL disease, while higher concentrations of plasma cells would indicate multiple myeloma with AL features. The plasma cells in the bone marrow are genetically abnormal, with 50% showing translocations between chromosome 11 and chromosome 14.[12] Occasionally, immunoglobulin light-chain amyloidosis can be seen from nonplasma cell disorders, such as chronic lymphatic leukemia, Waldenström macroglobulinemia, and marginal zone lymphoma.[14] If such biopsy specimens do not detect amyloid, endomyocardial biopsy should be obtained if multimodality imaging raises the index of suspicion for cardiac amyloidosis.

WILD-TYPE TRANSTHYRETIN AMYLOIDOSIS

For unclear reasons in some older individuals, the native tetramer conformation of the TTR protein dissociates into monomers that can misfold into beta sheet–rich fibers that deposit mainly in the heart, but also can lead to biceps tendon rupture and lumbar stenosis.[15,16] Carpal tunnel syndrome is also common and should raise concern for cardiac amyloidosis if elicited in the history of any patient with HFpEF. While peripheral and autonomic neuropathy can occur, it is less common and less severe than that found with vATTR or AL disease.[17,18]

The median age of diagnosis is 74 years. Rarely, disease can be diagnosed as early as age 40.[18] While >90% of cases are found in Caucasian men, some series of hospitalized HFpEF have found equal male and female predominance of ATTR amyloidosis.[19] Hence, it is feasible referral bias leads to the impression of it being primarily a disease of older men.

VARIANT TRANSTHYRETIN AMYLOIDOSIS

Over 130 point mutations in the TTR gene have been reported.[20] TTR mutations are inherited as autosomal-dominant mutations with a variable penetrance; although, in the majority of mutations, the penetrance is considered to be high. The point mutations result in kinetic instability of the transthyretin tetramer, resulting in dissociation into monomers and begin the misfolding process into the amyloid fibrils often earlier in life than wtATTR disease. It is paramount that any patient deemed to have ATTR versus AL disease undergo genetic testing. In addition to Val122Ile, common mutations in the United States include Thr60Ala (p.T80A), and Val30Met (p.V50M).[21] Val122Ile occurs in 3.4% of Black American population and is also found in people of African Caribbean and West African descent and leads to predominantly cardiac involvement with discovery often in a patient's sixties. History of carpal tunnel disease is common and peripheral length dependent sensorimotor neuropathy is rare. The presence of neuropathy however is important because it affects available therapeutic options. Within the Black American population, while the Val122Ile mutation is common, nearly 25% of call cases of ATTR cardiomyopathy will in fact be due to wtATTR disease. Thr60Ala is found in Irish Americans (originating in Donegal) and presents with a mixed cardiac and neuropathy phenotype and also often has antecedent carpal tunnel syndrome. Neuropathy symptoms often appear before HFpEF symptoms. Val30Met is actually the most common mutation worldwide and is endemic in Portugal, Japan, and Sweden leading to vATTR neuropathy. In nonendemic regions of the world, including the United States, Val30Met has a later-onset with a mixed but predominantly cardiac and neuropathic phenotype. Less common but important mutations include Ile68Leu (p.I88L) and Phe64Leu (p.F84L) from Italy, the latter of which has specific considerations during diagnostic workup.

CLINICAL CHARACTERISTICS OF AMYLOID CARDIOMYOPATHIES

AL amyloidosis occurs in approximately 10 patients per million per year with no increase over time (based on reports from the US, Europe, and United Kingdom). Seventy percent of patients have cardiac involvement. The prevalence of variant ATTR cardiac amyloidosis is not known, but there is an estimated worldwide prevalence of 50,000 persons—20% with predominant polyneuropathy and 80% with predominant cardiomyopathy with mixed phenotypes of both in 60% to 70% of patients (Fig. 43–3)—and is likely to be underdiagnosed because the presentation is nonspecific. In AL amyloidosis, extracardiac involvement is very common, with 60% of patients having renal amyloid, 15% having autonomic or peripheral neuropathy, and 15% having hepatomegaly. Dental indentations in the tongue are only seen in AL amyloidosis and are present in approximately 15% of patients.

Sperry et al. found that among 98 patients with carpal tunnel syndrome undergoing tenosynovectomy, 10.2% stained positive for amyloid and can predate a diagnosed of cardiac amyloidosis by 5 to 10 years.[22] While most had wtATTR disease, two patients had vATTR and two patients had AL disease. Amyloid deposition in the ligamentum flavum can lead to spinal stenosis with worsening symptoms with age.[23]

Advances in noninvasive cardiac imaging and emergence of effective therapeutics have sparked interest in cardiac amyloidosis research in recent years. Several studies have demonstrated that cardiac amyloidosis is not a rare disease, as it was once thought, but rather a relatively common entity in certain well-defined patient groups. As previously mentioned, in a study of 108 patients with established HFpEF who underwent endomyocardial biopsy at Johns Hopkins, 15 (14%) patients were diagnosed with cardiac amyloidosis (7 with wtATTR, 4 with vATTR, 3 with AL, and 1 with AA).[11] In another study, of 120 consecutive patients (≥60 years) with hospitalized HFpEF undergoing 99mTc-DPD scintigraphy, 13% had radionuclide evidence of ATTR cardiac amyloidosis (all wild type).[19] Beyond HFpEF, older patients with aortic stenosis may be at high risk for comorbid wtATTR cardiomyopathy. Among 151 patients undergoing transcatheter aortic valve replacement, 24 patients (16%) were positive for TTR cardiac amyloidosis using 99mTc pyrophosphate scintigraphy. Most of these patients had a low-flow, low-gradient aortic stenosis due to decreased cardiac output and restrictive physiology.[24] In another study of 200 aortic stenosis patients aged ≥75 years referred for transcatheter intervention, 26 (13%) were found to have cardiac amyloidosis on a nuclear scan.[25] These studies strongly suggest that cardiac amyloidosis is an underdiagnosed entity, and a strong clinical suspicion is needed in specific patient groups, such as elderly patients with HFpEF and patients with aortic stenosis.

Because of the nonspecific symptomatology associated with cardiac amyloid, there is frequently a delay in diagnosis. Common cardiac misdiagnoses before consideration of ATTR cardiomyopathy include hypertrophic cardiomyopathy, hypertensive heart disease, or changes to the myocardium in patients with advanced/end-stage renal disease based on echo images. The median time from onset of symptoms is 6 to 12 months, but 10% of patients report a >3-year interval between symptoms and diagnosis and, in another 10%, 2 to 3 years between symptoms and diagnosis. Although 70% of patients with amyloidosis have cardiac involvement, only 19% of the diagnosing physicians are cardiologists.[26]

Cardiac amyloidosis should be suspected in a patient with left ventricular hypertrophy and reduced tolerance of antihypertensive medications over time. This reflects an inability to tolerate β-blockers and nondihydropyridine calcium channel blockers due to blunting of cardiac output with lowering of heart rate in patients with restrictive myopathies and a fixed stroke volume. Furthermore, vATTR cardiomyopathy patients often exhibit symptomatic orthostatic hypotension and syncope after taking angiotensin converting enzyme inhibitors or angiotensin receptor blockers due to neurohormonal insufficiency in the presence of autonomic dysfunction. Arrhythmias and conduction disturbances are frequent. Atrial fibrillation is common in AL and ATTR cardiomyopathy with the prevalence of comorbid disease often increasing with advancing age, which can exacerbate heart failure symptoms but may not impact survival.[27,28] In AL amyloidosis, sudden cardiac death represents electrical mechanical dissociation rather than ventricular tachycardia.[29]

DIAGNOSTIC EVALUATION

A schematic on a way to approach patients that carry a suspicion of a diagnosis of cardiac amyloidosis is given in **Fig. 43–4**. An appropriate level of suspicion is the key in timely diagnosis of cardiac amyloidosis. Although the presence of noncardiac manifestations may provide the clue to diagnosis, many patients have symptoms and signs only attributed to cardiac involvement. Classical teaching dictates that patients with cardiac amyloidosis have low-voltage electrocardiograms (ECGs); however, less than 40% of patients have this finding and therefore this is not sensitive in ruling out disease.[30] A discrepancy between left ventricular wall thickening and voltage on ECGs as well as a pseudo-infarct pattern are more reliable ECG findings. Similarly, echocardiographic and magnetic resonance imaging (MRI) features suggestive of amyloid cardiomyopathy should be carefully evaluated.[31] Any patient with

suspicion of cardiac amyloidosis should have serum-free light-chain assay and serum and urine immunofixation studies performed to assess for the presence of monoclonal process. Any lab abnormality should trigger referral to hematology/oncology for evaluation for AL disease. Biopsies to detect amyloid deposits in fat, bone marrow, or lip with Congo red staining and subsequent tissue typing by mass spectroscopy or immunohistochemistry would obviate the need for endomyocardial biopsy in most cases. Regarding AL cardiomyopathy specifically, a bone marrow biopsy is necessary to exclude multiple myeloma and will exhibit positive staining for AL disease in 50% cases. When combined with a subcutaneous fat aspirate, histologic diagnosis of AL disease can be confirmed in 85% of cases after mass spectroscopy or immunofluorescence subtyping. Of note, unfortunately, immunohistochemistry is limited by the size of the antibody panel, and the fact that amyloid proteins are frequently fragmented, having had the epitopes required for antibody recognition deleted.[32] Moreover, the protein misfolding that is characteristic of amyloid will often bury epitopes so that they are not visible to commercially provided antibodies and, as a consequence, immunohistochemistry or immuno-electron gold will be equivocal. Although not widely available and expensive, mass spectroscopic identification of the protein subunit remains the gold standard. In very large

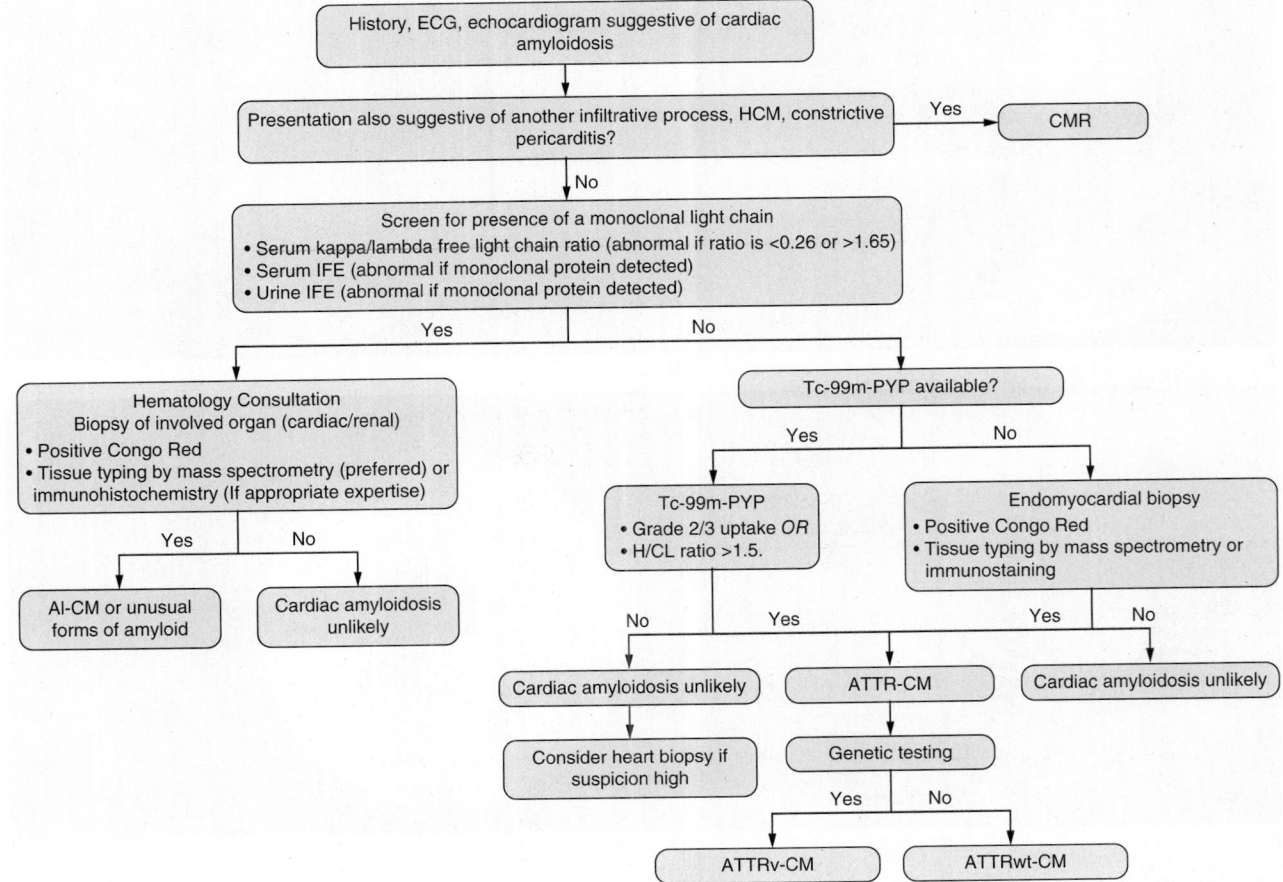

Figure 43–4. Schematic showing a diagnostic workup for cardiac amyloidosis. Reproduced with permission from Kittleson MM, Maurer MS, Ambardekar AV, et al: Cardiac Amyloidosis: Evolving Diagnosis and Management: A Scientific Statement From the American Heart Association, *Circulation*. 2020 Jul 7;142(1):e7-e22.

studies, the technique is capable of identifying the protein sub-unit in 90% of patients and is quite specific.[33]

Endomyocardial biopsy would only be needed if such studies did not exhibit amyloid deposition to confirm AL cardiomyopathy or if despite recognition of a monoclonal process in extracardiac tissue, sufficient suspicion remains for the rare possibility of simultaneous of ATTR cardiomyopathy.[34]

In the absence of a monoclonal protein, nuclear scintigraphy with bone-avid tracers including Technetium-99m (Tc-99m)-pyrophosphate (PYP) in the United States and Tc-99m-3,3-disphosphono-1,2-propandicarboxylic acid (DPD) or Tc-99m-hydroxymethylene diphosphonate (HMDP) in Europe can be obtained to assess for ATTR cardiomyopathy. Should a scan exhibit uptake of the tracer, a diagnosis of ATTR cardiomyopathy can be made, at which point genetic screening should be performed because it has implications for available therapy and familial screening/early detection, regardless of the age of the patient. While fat pad biopsies are commonly performed to assess for systemic amyloidosis, in fact, they offer poor sensitivity to rule out vATTR and wtATTR disease with rates of 45% and 15%, respectively.[35] Nonetheless, gold standard diagnosis of cardiac amyloidosis requires a positive endomyocardial biopsy demonstrating Congo red birefringent deposits (Fig. 43–2) or sodium sulphate-Alcian Blue cardiac staining, with subsequent mass spectroscopic protein subunit typing to discriminate whether AL, wtATTR, vATTR, or other rare forms of amyloidosis are present.

IMAGING

Echocardiography

The standard diagnostic imaging for cardiac amyloidosis includes echocardiography as the first-line test. Most commonly, two-dimensional echocardiography reveals concentric thickening of the left ventricle (1.2 cm or greater) (Fig. 43–5). Occasionally, asymmetric thickening of the septum can be seen, which can phenotypically mimic hypertrophic cardiomyopathy. Abnormal "scintillating" bright echotexture of the left ventricular wall has been described but it is rarely clinically useful in the age of harmonic imaging causing the myocardium can be bright in a number of diagnoses that lead to left ventricular wall thickening including hypertensive heart

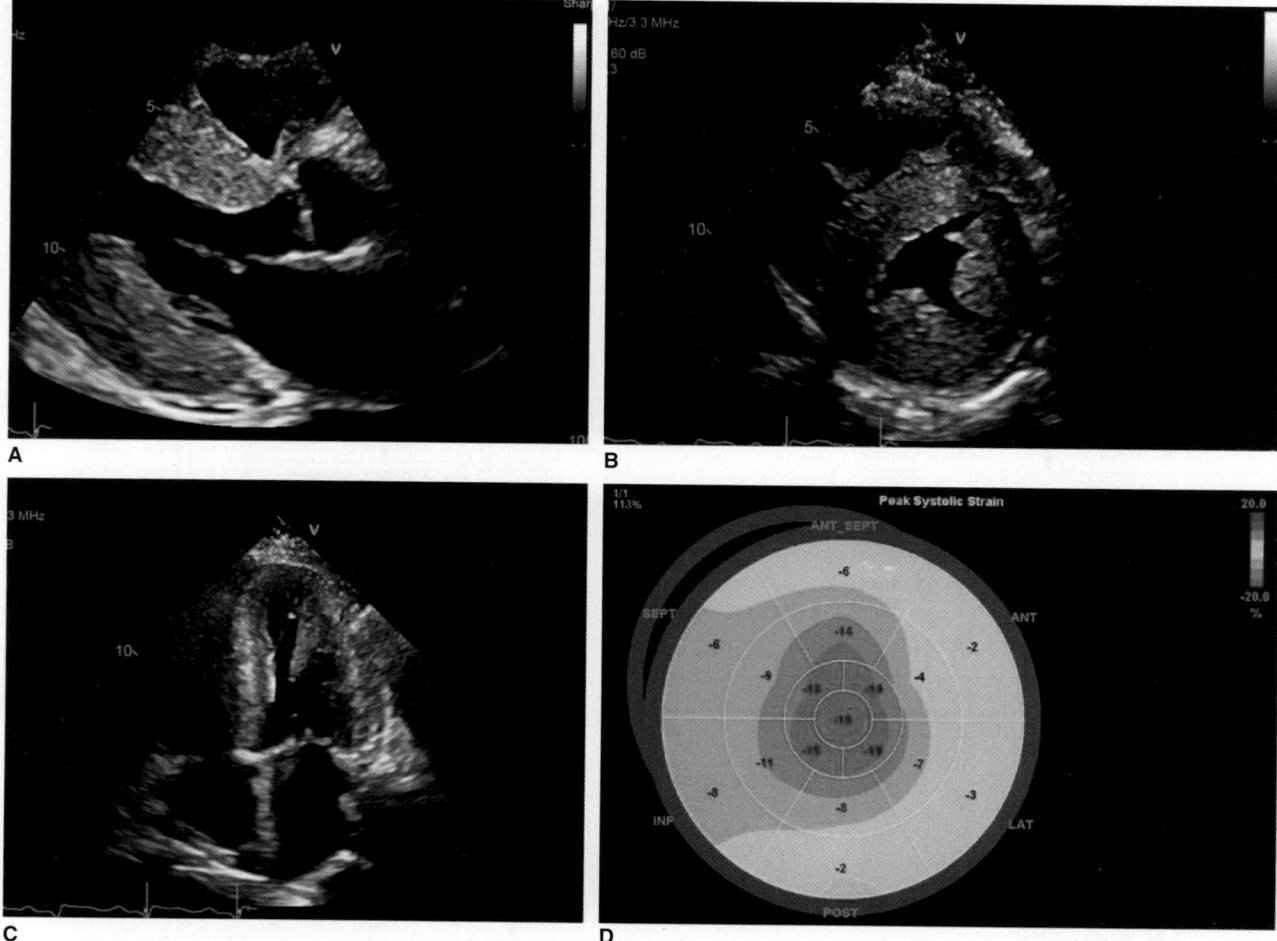

Figure 43–5. Characteristic two-dimensional echocardiographic images of cardiac amyloidosis in **(A)** parasternal long axis, **(B)** parasternal short axis, and **(C)** apical four chamber views notable for concentric left ventricular wall thickening and a "scintillating" myocardium. **(D)** Characteristic strain bull's eye plot showing a relative apical sparing pattern.

disease, advanced/end-stage renal impairment, and lysosomal storage disease. Other echocardiographic findings include valvular thickening, right ventricular hypertrophy, and a small pericardial effusion. Aortic stenosis, specifically low-gradient, has been associated with TTR cardiac amyloidosis, and should raise clinical suspicion especially if the left ventricular cavity appears small. Left ventricular ejection fraction is typically preserved or mildly decreased but stroke volume index is commonly reduced due to concentric remodeling/hypertrophy. In one study, wall thickening and diastolic abnormalities were associated with a low amyloid burden, while left and right ventricular dysfunction as measured by left ventricular ejection fraction and tricuspid annular plane excursion, respectively, with advanced disease.[36]

Diastolic dysfunction is typical for patients with cardiac amyloidosis. Progressive biatrial enlargement is commonly seen. Mitral inflow with impaired relaxation pattern is seen at early stages; however, a restrictive pattern showing grade III diastolic dysfunction is often found at the time of diagnosis with blunted mitral annular tissue Doppler e' velocity resulting in very elevated E/e' values, signifying elevation in left ventricular filling pressures.[37] Pulmonary pressures may be elevated and can be estimated from TR velocities.

Myocardial deformation imaging and evaluation of diastolic function are important echocardiographic measures in these patients. Speckle tracking echocardiography allows reliable evaluation of myocardial function over the cardiac cycle by assessment of global longitudinal strain. Characteristically, patients with cardiac amyloidosis have significantly decreased global longitudinal strain despite preserved left ventricular ejection fraction. Regional deformation heterogeneity with reduction in strain in the base- and mid-myocardial segments and relative preservation of apical longitudinal strain can be seen resulting in relative apical-sparing or "cherry-on-top" pattern on a longitudinal strain bull's eye display[38] (Fig. 43–5). Such a deformation pattern can help differentiate cardiac amyloidosis from hypertrophic cardiomyopathy wherein the latter would show a decrement in strain only in the septum or areas with myocardial fiber disarray.[38] Although this regional deformation pattern has been promoted as characteristic, it may not be sensitive to rule out disease. In one study of patients with aortic stenosis and concomitant cardiac amyloidosis, this pattern was not universally predictive of cardiac amyloidosis.[24] Of note, while echocardiography can raise the index of suspicion for cardiac amyloidosis, it is not a clinically validated tool for diagnosis that can warrant treatment initiation or at this time differentiate between AL and ATTR disease.

Cardiac Magnetic Resonance Imaging

MRI is an important imaging tool in assessing patients with suspected infiltrative cardiomyopathies including sarcoidosis, hemochromatosis, and Fabry's disease in addition to amyloidosis, since it provides structural, physiologic (volumes and flows), and tissue characterization data. MRI-derived chamber volumes and left ventricular mass show a high degree of reproducibility. Gadolinium-based contrast imaging allows detection of abnormal patterns that can be highly suggestive of cardiac amyloidosis, although they again do not discriminate between AL and ATTR disease and cannot at this time be used as a diagnostic tool to warrant treatment initiation by itself. Traditionally, inability to "null" the myocardium (to make it black by the operator) has been described as highly suggestive of cardiac amyloidosis. With phase-sensitive inversion recovery sequence, left ventricular late gadolinium enhancement is very common in these patients, and starts as diffuse subendocardial delayed enhancement but can produce to full thickness delayed enhancement in advanced disease (**Fig. 43–6**). Occasionally, patchy myocardial scar can be seen that is often attributed to cardiac sarcoidosis. Clues to amyloidosis include concomitant right ventricular thickening and delayed enhancement and biatrial enlargement and delayed enhancement. Late gadolinium enhancement has been shown to be a strong predictor of mortality with all typical subtypes of cardiac amyloidosis, especially with transmural enhancement.[39]

Parametric mapping provides unique insights into the disease process in patients with cardiac amyloidosis. Native T1 mapping does not require gadolinium-based contrast. T1 signal is significantly increased with amyloid deposition, which has been demonstrated both in patients with established amyloidosis and vATTR carriers. Postcontrast administration, T1 mapping, and extracellular volume estimation can be performed. Extracellular volume is markedly elevated in cardiac amyloidosis patients (often above 0.5), and it is considered the most reproducible MRI measure of amyloid burden.[40] Similarly, it has stronger prognostic and diagnostic values when compared to native and postcontrast T1 mapping and late gadolinium enhancement.[40,41] Extracellular volume can potentially identify early disease, risk stratify patients, and assess response to therapy in both AL and vATTR disease.[42,43] More studies are needed to define its role in routine patient management.

Obvious limitations of MRI imaging include presence of noncompatible metallic devices, significant renal dysfunction (for contrast administration), poor patient cooperation, and claustrophobia.

Nuclear Imaging

Nuclear medicine techniques have revolutionized the way that patients with ATTR cardiomyopathy are diagnosed in daily practice; obviating the need for biopsy in many patients. Tc-99m PYP is commonly utilized in the United States while Tc-99m DPD and Tc-99m HMDP is used in Europe. On planar imaging, bone tracer uptake is commonly graded qualitatively with visual scores ranging from 0 to 3, where 0 indicates no cardiac uptake, 1 indicates cardiac uptake is less than rib uptake, 2 indicates cardiac uptake is equal to rib uptake, while 3 indicates strong cardiac uptake exceeding rib uptake by intensity (**Fig. 43–7**). A semiquantitative heart to contralateral lung uptake ratio can also be used (>1.5 at 1 hour is diagnostic). Planar imaging must be confirmed by single-photon emission computed tomography (SPECT) in all positive scans to confirm myocardial retention of the tracer as opposed to blood pool signal[44] (Fig. 43–7). There is a >99% sensitivity in cardiac

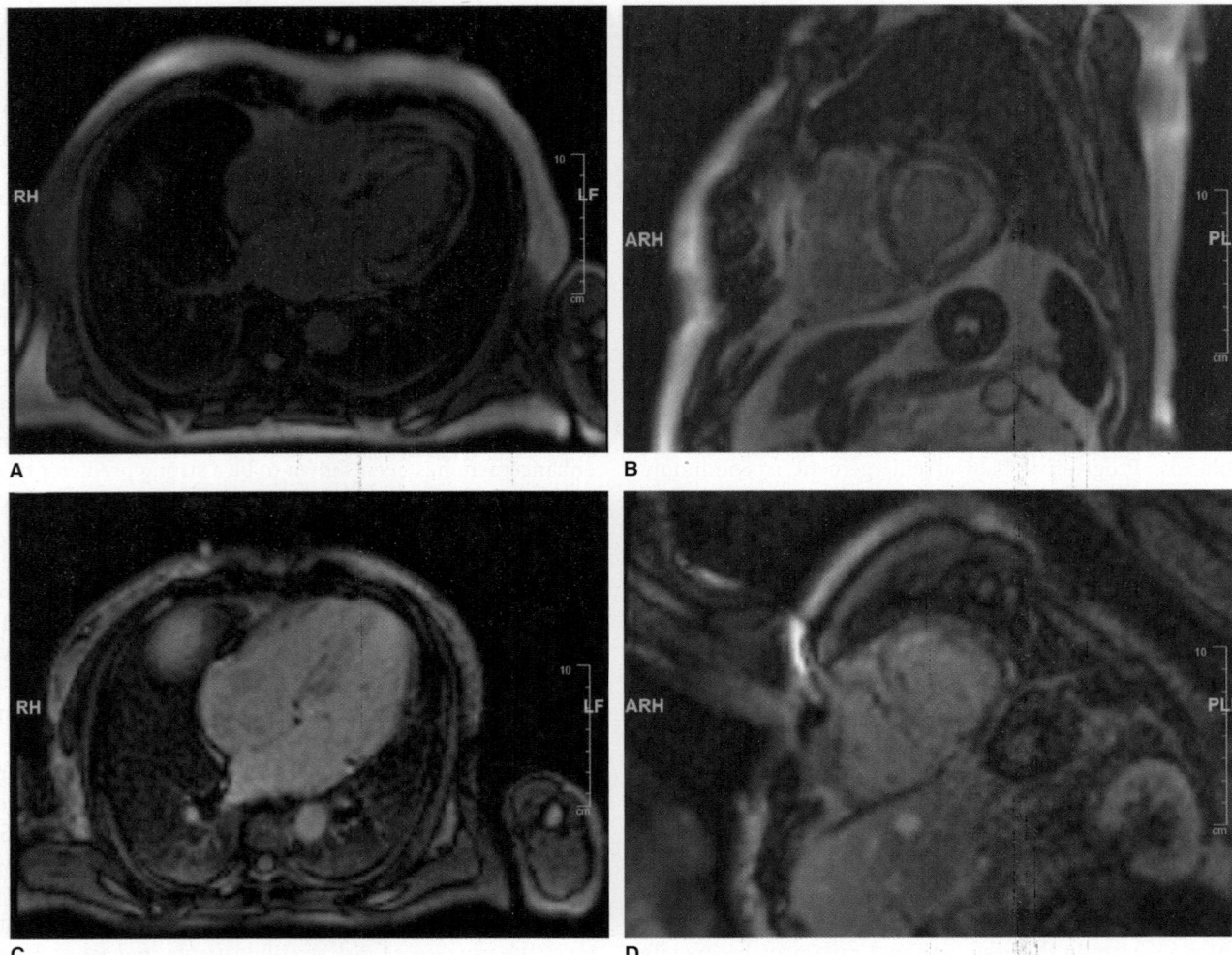

Figure 43–6. Two examples on cardiac MRI of early cardiac amyloidosis with subendocardial delayed enhancement (**A** and **B**) and late-stage disease showing full thickness delayed enhancement (**C** and **D**).

involvement detection in patients with ATTR amyloid, with a specificity of 86%.[45] Ninety-four percent of biopsy-proven cardiac ATTR had moderate-to-high uptake, where only 21% of patients with cardiac AL have this level of uptake, which can lead to false-positive scans. Thus, in the absence of a detectable monoclonal protein, a visual score of 2 or 3 or a heart to contralateral ratio >1.5 confirmed with SPECT is highly predictive of ATTR cardiomyopathy with specificity approaching 100%.[46] After diagnosis by nuclear scintigraphy, genetic testing can discriminate wtATTR versus vATTR cardiomyopathy.

False positives can still occur, however, in the presence of severe renal disease, significant coronary artery disease leading to focal uptake, hydroxychloroquine use in rheumatologic disorders, and ApoA4 cardiomyopathy. Of note, false negatives can occur with the Phe64Leu pathogenic variant for vATTR cardiomyopathy.[47] Thus, if the index of suspicion for cardiac amyloidosis is still high despite negative or equivocal results on nuclear scintigraphy or one is concerned about a false-positive scan, endomyocardial biopsy is needed to confirm a diagnosis.[44]

Investigational areas of nuclear imaging look to quantitate amyloid burden. Early data suggests that quantitative SPECT/

CT imaging correlates well with planar bone avid imaging and may play a future role in assessing disease progression or response to therapy.[48] Amyloid-specific PET tracers (C-11 Pittsburgh-B compound, F-18-florbetapir) allow cardiac and whole-body direct visualization and potential quantification of amyloid fibril deposition.[49,50] While, these compounds are considered investigational and at this time cannot discriminate between amyloid subtypes, some potential PET tracers such as 18F-sodium fluoride may offer the ability to discriminate AL and ATTR amyloidosis when combined with cardiac MRI.[51]

Cardiac CT imaging

Cardiac amyloidosis, specifically TTR subtype, appears to be prevalent in patients with aortic stenosis undergoing transcatheter valve replacement.[24] CT imaging is routinely obtained in patients referred for transcatheter intervention. Studies have shown that CT imaging allows extracellular volume quantification in these patients with minimal increase in acquisition time and radiation dose.[52] Expansion of extracellular volume as seen on CT imaging may allow efficient screening for comorbid cardiac amyloidosis among aortic stenosis patients considered

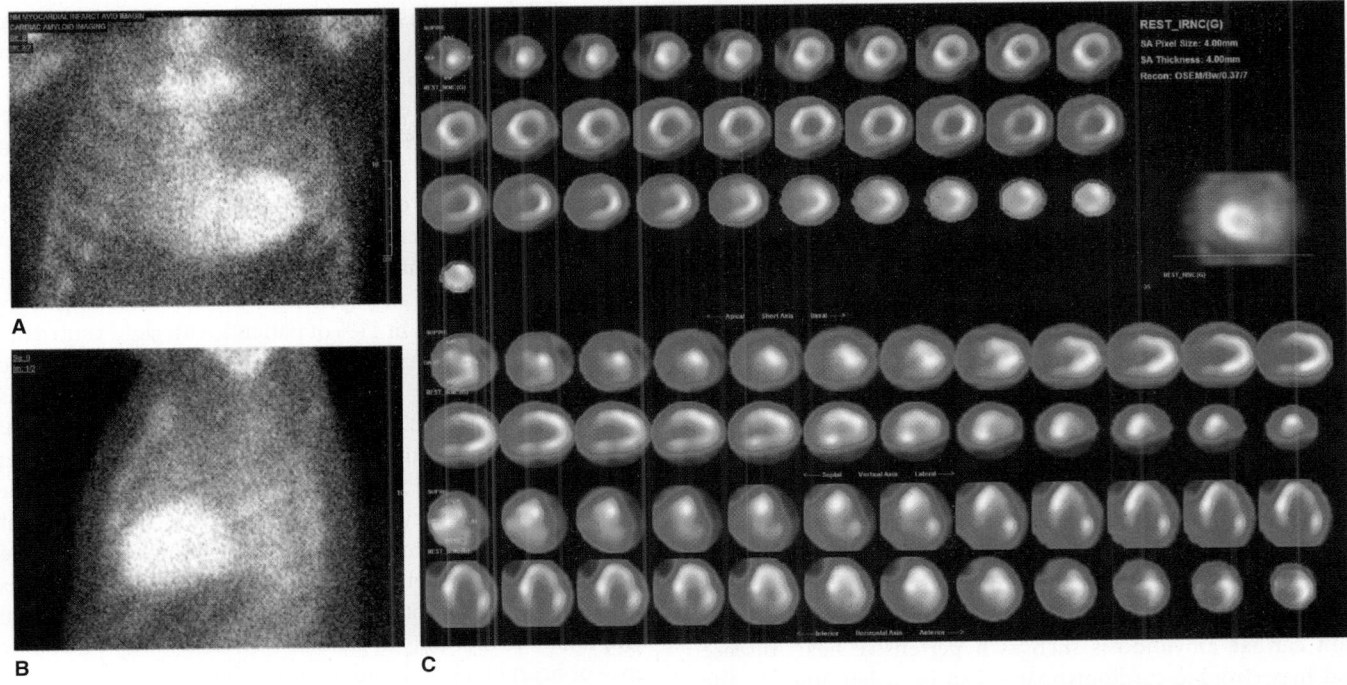

Figure 43–7. Tc-99m PYP scan showing qualitative Grade III uptake on planar images (**A** and **B**) with confirmation of myocardial tracer retention on (**C**) SPECT imaging consistent with a diagnosis of ATTR cardiomyopathy.

for transcatheter intervention. Nonetheless, validation of ATTR cardiomyopathy would still entail either endomyocardial biopsy or positive bone avid Tc-99m scintigraphy in the absence of a monoclonal protein.

CARDIAC BIOMARKERS AND STAGING CARDIAC AMYLOIDOSIS

Once diagnosed, staging helps prognosticate disease. Two scoring systems help prognosticate wtATTR cardiomyopathy: the Mayo wtATTR staging system and the United Kingdom National Amyloidosis Centre staging system (**Table 43–2**). In the Mayo scoring system, one point is assigned for an NT-proBNP >3000 pg/mL and one point is assigned for a troponin T of >0.05 ng/mL (or high-sensitivity cardiac Troponin T >65 ng/L). Stage 1 disease reflects 0 points, Stage 2 reflects

1 point, and Stage 3 reflects 2 points. The median survival of patients with Stage 1, 2, and 3 disease, respectively, is 66, 42, and 20 months.[53] Alternatively, the National Amyloidosis Centre scoring system utilizes eGFR <45 mL/min/1.73 m² in lieu of Troponin T measurements and applies to both wtATTR and vATTR cardiomyopathy and has similar median survivals for Stage 1, 2, and 3 disease at 69.2, 46.7, and 24.1 months, respectively.[54]

In AL amyloidosis, the staging system utilizes 3 classes of biomarkers including NT-proBNP ≥1800 pg/mL (or BNP ≥400 ng/L), cardiac troponin T >0.025 ng/mL (or high-sensitivity cardiac troponin T ≥40 ng/L), and the serum-free light-chain difference between involved and uninvolved light chains of >180 mg/L (Table 43–2). A point is assigned for each factor above the thresholds, resulting in four stages, with median survivals of 73, 35, 15, and 5 months, respectively, which is

TABLE 43–2. Staging of Cardiac Amyloidosis			
	Mayo Staging	**Mayo Staging**	**UK National Amyloidosis Centre**
Population	Light Chain	Wildtype Transthyretin	Wild-Type and Variant Transthyretin
Parameters	NT-proBNP <1800 pg/mL Troponin T ≤0.025 ng/mL Serum Light Chain Difference <180 mg/L	NT-proBNP <3000 pg/mL Troponin T ≤0.05 ng/mL	NT-proBNP <3000 pg/mL eGFR ≥45 mL/min
Median Survival			
Stage 1: all parameters normal	73 months	66 months	69.2 months
Stage 2: 1 parameter abnormal	35 months	40 months	46.7 months
Stage 3: 2 parameters abnormal	15 months	20 months	24.1 months
Stage 4: 3 parameters abnormal	5 months	N/A	N/A

far shorter than TTR amyloidosis.[55] In AL amyloidosis, multiple organ involvement carries an inferior prognosis. Genetic abnormalities in the plasma cells, such as t(11;14), may predict resistance to bortezomib chemotherapy and inferior prognosis, and deletion of 17p, which suggests that chemotherapy drug resistance or short response to chemotherapy are important tests performed on a patient's bone marrow in AL amyloidosis.[56,57]

THERAPY

Heart Failure

Maintaining euvolemia via diet control and loop diuretics remains the cornerstone of congestive symptoms for cardiac amyloidosis. Higher bioavailability of torsemide and bumetanide make them preferable over furosemide and can be used in conjunction with high dose aldosterone antagonists for volume management. There is no current recommended goal-directed medical therapy for cardiac amyloidosis. Common agents used for HFrEF or diagnoses that are often confused with cardiac amyloidosis such as hypertensive heart disease and hypertrophic cardiomyopathy can be deleterious. In the setting of a fixed stroke volume, patients with advanced cardiac amyloidosis often have lower blood pressures from reduce ventricular capacitance and ventricular vascular coupling.[58] Higher heart rates maintain cardiac output and hence patients with cardiac amyloidosis do not feel well when β-blockers are used to excessively blunt heart rate. Relative neurohormonal insufficiency and autonomic dysfunction, especially in AL and vATTR systemic amyloidosis, can lead to symptomatic orthostatic hypotension with the use of angiotensin converting enzyme inhibitors and angiotensin receptor blockers. Furthermore, nondihydropyridine calcium channel blockers are avoided due to older case reports of shock in patients with systemic AL disease.[59] To maintain adequate blood pressure and preload in the setting of advanced disease, compression stockings and midodrine can be helpful. In the subset of patients with comorbid aortic stenosis and ATTR cardiomyopathy that could be exacerbating heart failure, early data shows that transcatheter valve replacement significantly improves one to two year outcomes.[25]

Arrhythmia and Device Therapy

Patients with cardiac amyloidosis often have comorbid and symptomatic atrial fibrillation. Balancing heart rate to control atrial fibrillation without blunting cardiac output can pose challenges. As aforementioned, lowering β-blockers to the lowest acceptable dose to avoid excessive heart rate control is preferable.

Despite literature to the contrary, the use of digoxin, in an effort to control atrial fibrillation rate in carefully selected patients, can be very effective and does not produce excessive toxicity in cardiac amyloidosis.[60] Amiodarone can be used in the treatment of supraventricular arrhythmias in amyloidosis patients.[28,61] Along with cardioversion and ablative therapy, this is more effective earlier in the disease course when trying to restore sinus rhythm.[28] Given propensity to form intracardiac thrombi, even in sinus rhythm, anticoagulation is preferred, either with coumadin or direct oral anticoagulants, at any CHADs-VASc score to attenuate stroke risk.[62]

Heart block due to conduction system should be suspected and investigated with Holter and event monitoring if patients present with syncope. Pacemaker implantation should follow the recommendations of the American College of Cardiology/American Heart Association/Heart Rhythm Society.[53] In a retrospective observational study of 78 patients with ATTR cardiac amyloidosis, with an implantable device, worsening mitral regurgitation was seen in 11% of patients with right ventricular pacing <40%. Furthermore worsening left ventricular ejection fraction and New York Heart Association functional class occurred in 26% and 22% of patients who were right ventricular paced <40% of the time and increased to 89% for both when right ventricular paced >40% of the time.[63] Should patients meet an indication, biventricular pacing can be considered in patients with ATTR cardiac amyloidosis to achieve higher heart rates and theoretically higher cardiac output. Further study is needed to determine if such interventions lead to overall improvement symptoms and mortality in patients with chronotropic incompetence or heart block and cardiac amyloidosis.

At this time, data on the use of primary prevention implantable cardiac defibrillators (ICD) is controversial given lack of survival benefit. Literature, however, may be biased based on prior limited survival without effective therapies or late stage diagnoses of both AL and ATTR cardiomyopathy. Death in patients with AL disease may in fact be due to electromechanical dissociation as well as to a primary arrhythmic etiology.[64] In carefully selected patients with estimated survival >1 year or those who may be awaiting organ transplantation, ICDs can be placed for secondary prevention of sudden cardiac death due to ventricular arrhythmias.[65]

Anti-Amyloid Therapy for AL

Chemotherapy is the mainstay of treatment for AL amyloidosis. The source of the amyloid deposits are clonal plasma cells in the bone marrow, and elimination of these plasma cells using anti-plasma cell chemotherapy has been the standard of care for 50 years. Initially, melphalan and prednisone was used but produced only occasional responses, and the responses were not prolonged. In 1985, myeloablative chemotherapy with autologous stem cell transplantation was introduced for the treatment of amyloidosis and has shown to be an effective technique, capable of very profound responses that were durable, with 15-year survivors being reported. Stem cell transplantation in patients with cardiac amyloidosis, however, carries mortality rates that are reported as high as 10%, which would be unacceptable in the modern era now that there are alternative drugs available.[66] Selection of patients with cardiac amyloidosis for stem cell transplantation is best done at a large center, but typical inclusion criteria include a patient that is ambulatory more than 50% of the day, a systolic blood pressure of >90 mm Hg and serum creatinine <2 mg/dL, and high-sensitivity troponin T <75 ng. With these criteria, transplant-related mortality is approximately 2.5%, with hematologic response rates of 66% and cardiac response rates (30% reduction of NT-proBNP) of

41%. Ten-year survival after stem cell transplant is 25% but is 53% in patients that achieve a complete response.[67]

For nontransplant-eligible patients, the standard of care is bortezomib-based chemotherapy leading to hematologic response in 77% of cases and complete response in 16% of cases. Bortezomib is administered once a week subcutaneously. In a study of 230 AL patients treated with cyclophosphamide, bortezomib, and dexamethasone (CyBorD), the hematologic response rate was 60%, with a cardiac response in 17% of patients, and a renal response in 25% of patients.[68]

The anti CD-38 monoclonal antibody, daratumumab, is highly effective in the treatment of AL amyloidosis. Single center data from the Mayo Clinic using daratumumab-based therapy in 41 patients with relapsed or refractory AL amyloidosis yielded hematologic response in 80% of patients and cardiac response in 33% of patients after a median follow-up of 7.5 months.[69] The ANDROMEDA study showed the completed response rate to be 53.3 vs 18.1% favoring daratumumab. The cardiac response rate in the groups was 41.5 vs 22.2% favoring daratumumab.[70]

Treatment of ATTR

Clinical and investigational therapies for TTR amyloidosis is based on either (1) silencing production of the TTR protein, (2) stabilization of the TTR tetramer, or (3) disruption or extraction of the TTR amyloid fibrils.

The only current approved for therapy ATTR cardiomyopathy in the United States is the TTR tetramer stabilizing compound tafamidis that binds with high affinity to the thyroxine binding site on TTR, largely preventing kinetic destabilization and rearrangement into amyloid fibrils and has virtually no side effect profile. Tafamidis meglumine (20 mg or 80 mg) was tested against placebo in the 2018 randomized controlled ATTR-ACT trial in patients with wtATTR and vATTR cardiomyopathy.[71] The primary hierarchal endpoint of first, all-cause mortality and secondly, rates of cardiovascular hospitalizations using the Finkelstein–Schoenfeld method yielded a "win ratio" of tafamidis over placebo of 1.70 ($P = 0.0006$) for reducing such events.[72] Secondary endpoints of the primary outcomes using Kaplan–Meier time-to-event analysis yielded a 30% reduction in the hazard for all-cause mortality and 32% reduction hazard for cardiovascular hospitalization in patients randomized to tafamidis (pooled 20 mg and 80 mg doses) to placebo. Furthermore, tafamidis resulted in much slower decline in 6-minute walk test distances and Kansas City Cardiomyopathy Questionnaire Scores compared to placebo. While data exists showing that tafamidis can slow the progression of vATTR polyneuropathy,[73] at this time tafamidis only carries an indication for vATTR polyneuropathy outside of the Unites States in Europe and Japan.

AG10 (acoramidis) is a TTR stabilization based on coinheritance of the Thr119Met mutation leading to natural stabilization of the TTR tetramer and is in phase-3 clinical trial testing for wtATTR and vATTR cardiomyopathy (ATTRIBUTE-CM [Efficacy and Safety of AG10 in Subjects with Transthyretin Amyloid Cardiomyopathy]; ClinicalTrials.gov. NCT03860935). It showed a favorable safety profile in Phase 2 testing with near complete TTR stabilization and open label extension data showed that this led to lower mortality and cardiovascular hospitalizations over 15 months.[74]

TTR stabilization can also be achieved with off-label use of the nonsteroidal anti-inflammatory drug diflunisal 250 mg twice a day with only single-center studies showing effectiveness for wtATTR and vATTR cardiomyopathy at this time.[75-77] While rare, diflunisal can result in a small reduction in estimated glomerular filtration rate and slightly increased rates of gastrointestinal complaints, but can be a much more affordable alternative to tafamidis. Notably, response to TTR stabilizers including tafamidis, off-label diflunisal, and under investigation AG10 can be assessed by measurement of serum prealbumin (transthyretin levels), which measures stable transthyretin tetramer conformations as opposed to unstable-dissociated transthyretin monomer subunits.[74]

TTR silencers target hepatic synthesis of the TTR protein. Two currently available silencers are patisiran, an intravenously administered small interfering RNA that targets the TTR mRNA for degradation, and inotersen, a subcutaneously administered antisense oligonucleotide that binds TTR mRNA leading to its degradation. Patisiran and inotersen proved to be efficacious in the randomized APOLLO and NEURO-TTR studies, respectively, assessing for improvements in the Norfolk Quality of Life diabetic neuropathy and mNIS+7 neuropathy scores among patients with vATTR polyneuropathy.[78,79] Prespecified cardiac substudies of patisiran from APOLLO noted that among individuals who had concomitant vATTR cardiomyopathy, treatment with patisiran led to less deterioration of global longitudinal strain, regression of LV wall thickening, and reduction in NT-proBNP.[80,81] Limited data also shows that inotersen may stabilize 6-minute walk test results, global longitudinal strain on echo, and lead to wall regression on cardiac MRI in patients with ATTR cardiomyopathy.[82,83] Of note, inotersen requires frequent monitoring of platelet count and serum creatinine due to rare side effects of fatal thrombocytopenia leading to intracranial hemorrhage and glomerulonephritis. Potential use of silencer therapy for ATTR cardiomyopathy at this time is limited to patients who otherwise have an indication for treatment for vATTR neuropathy. Ongoing clinical studies are assessing the utility of patisiran and inotersen for both wtATTR and vATTR cardiomyopathy and may give insight into the benefit of combination TTR silencer and TTR stabilizer therapy. These include APOLLO-B (A Study to Evaluate Patisiran in Participants with Transthyretin Amyloidosis with Cardiomyopathy; ClinicalTrials.gov. NCT03997383) and 24 Month Open Label Study of the Tolerability and Efficacy of Inotersen in TTR Amyloid Cardiomyopathy Patients (ClinicalTrials.gov. NCT03702829). Furthermore, next generation TTR silencer platforms for ATTR cardiomyopathy with easier administration and potentially less side effects are being tested in phase-3 trials, including HELIOS-B (A Study to Evaluate Vutrisiran in Patients with Transthyretin Amyloidosis with Cardiomyopathy; ClinicalTrials.gov. NCT04153149) and CARDIO-TTRansform (A Study to Evaluate the Efficacy and Safety of AKCEA-TTR-LRx in Participants with Transthyretin Mediated Amyloid Cardiomyopathy; ClinicalTrials.gov.

NCT04136171). If in fact ATTR cardiomyopathy is seen as part of a spectrum of systemic TTR amyloidosis rather than as a distinct disease process by regulatory bodies, such therapies bear clinical weight for a spectrum of disease manifestations.

Lastly, TTR disruptive therapy aims to remove amyloid fibers from organ tissue after deposition. Conflicting evidence exists for the combination of doxycycline and tauroursodeoxycholic acid for TTR disruption.[84,85] The use of monoclonal antibodies targeting portions of deposited ATTR fibers is under investigation.[86]

Advanced Heart Failure Therapies

ACC/AHA Stage D Heart Failure in patients with cardiac amyloidosis poses unique challenges when considering advanced therapies. Given the marked left ventricular hypertrophy, small left ventricular cavity size, and concomitant right ventricular dysfunction, limited data exists for the use of durable univentricular mechanical support with contemporary left ventricular assist devices.[87]

Heart transplantation for cardiac amyloidosis is possible for Stage D cardiac amyloidosis. The updated adult donor allocation system provides a status 4 designation to patients with cardiac amyloidosis given the lack of durable mechanical support options to reduce waiting times on the transplant list. In carefully selected patients, should mechanical support be needed as a bridge to cardiac transplantation, some data supports the use biventricular support either using biventricular extracorporeal devices or a total artificial heart.[88] Such patients would receive a status 2 designation on the transplant waiting list. Recent single-center studies show improving 1-year survival postcardiac transplantation of carefully selected candidates for both AL and ATTR cardiac amyloidosis, with and without biventricular mechanical support, and similar survival rates in patients transplanted for causes other than cardiac amyloidosis.[89,90] However, more data is needed across multiple institutions.

There are special considerations for transplant for both end-stage AL and ATTR cardiomyopathy. In the case of ATTR cardiomyopathy, age is often a limiting factor given the late development of advanced cardiomyopathy in individuals with Stage D heart failure. In the case of vATTR, concomitant neuropathy may affect posttransplant outcomes. Isolated liver transplantation to address vATTR cardiomyopathy and neuropathy, in order to diminish production of a kinetically unstable TTR protein, is not advisable given the possibility of progression of wtATTR deposition on prior sites of vATTR deposition and otherwise would be high risk in the setting of end-stage heart failure.[91,92] The need for combined heart–liver dual organ transplantation to remove mutant TTR from the blood and prevent progression of neuropathy post–heart transplantation has less scope in the new era of TTR silencer therapy, which may have an increasing role post–isolated heart transplantation.

Furthermore, in select patients with end-stage heart failure due to AL cardiomyopathy, cardiac transplantation can be considered if there is evidence of limited extracardiac organ involvement and patients show adequate nutritional status or lack of malabsorption. Standard chemotherapy regimens with proteosome inhibitor therapy and anti-CD-38 monoclonal antibody therapy with daratumumab should be given to target the clonal plasma cell. Once hematologic response is achieved post–heart transplant, there has been a shift in practice paradigms over the last 15 years in some centers in addressing recurrence of light-chain elevation. While some literature supports the use of stem cell transplantation as consolidative therapy when stable post–heart transplant (usually >6 months), use of proteosome inhibitor therapy and/or daratumumab can be achieved to attain hematologic response.[89]

SUMMARY

There is a major educational gap in the diagnosis of cardiac amyloidosis with frequent confusion between amyloid infiltrative cardiomyopathy and hypertensive heart disease or other causes of HFpEF. Failure to incorporate immunoglobulin-free light-chain testing in the workflow of evaluation of patients with thickened heart walls runs the risk of missing the diagnosis of AL amyloidosis. In ATTR amyloidosis, incorporation of the nuclear scan with bone-avid tracers is vital in making a definitive diagnosis. Screening of the TTR gene for mutations helps distinguish wild-type from mutant TTR amyloidosis. Diagnosis is more important than ever since there are now a wide array of effective therapies for AL amyloidosis, two new therapies for the treatment of mutant ATTR amyloidosis, and oral therapy for wtATTR amyloidosis. Key summary differences in TTR

TABLE 43-3. Key Differences in Disease Etiology, Diagnosis, and Management of Transthyretin Cardiac Amyloidosis Between the United States and Europe Based on the Transthyretin Amyloidosis Outcomes Survey and Expert Consensus Statements and Clinical Practice Updates From the American Heart Association and European Society of Cardiology

Parameter	United States	Europe
Percent wild-type	48%	25%
Notable pathogenic vATTR mutations	Val122Ile (p.V142I) Thr60Ala (p.T80A) Val30Met (p.V50M)-late onset	Leu111Met (p.L131M) Ile68Leu (p.I88L) Thr60Ala (p.T80A) Val30Met (p.V50M)-early onset Phe64Leu (p.F84L) Ile107Val (p.I127V)
Tracers for nuclear scintigraphy and non-biopsy diagnosis	Pyrophosphate (PYP)	3,3-disphospho-no-1,2-propandicarboxylic acid (DPD) Hydroxymethylene diphosphonate (HMDP)
Recommended therapy	Tafamidis	Tafamidis
Alternative/adjunct therapies	Diflunisal (off-label) Patisiran (if vATTR with neuropathy) Inotersen (if vATTR with neuropathy)	Diflunisal (off-label)

cardiac amyloidosis disease etiology, diagnosis, and management based on the Transthyretin Amyloidosis Outcomes Survey and recent statements and practice updates from the American Heart Association/European Society of Cardiology are provided for reference in **Table 43–3**.[5,21,93,94]

- Cardiac amyloidosis is a leading cause of HFpEF. It may be confused with hypertrophic cardiomyopathy or hypertensive heart disease.
- Cardiac MRI and strain echocardiography may demonstrate findings that can lead to an early diagnosis.
- Abnormality in the immunoglobulin-free light-chain levels is an important clue to the presence of AL amyloidosis and should be checked in the workup of cardiac amyloidosis.
- Technetium pyrophosphate imaging is highly sensitive and specific in the diagnosis of TTR cardiac amyloidosis provided no monoclonal protein is detected.
- Systemic chemotherapy and stem cell transplantation directed at the plasma cell clone is effective therapy in cardiac AL amyloidosis.
- TTR silencers are currently approved only for vATTR polyneuropathy, with and without concomitant cardiomyopathy. Their use in cardiomyopathy is currently in Phase 3 testing.
- Tafamidis, a TTR stabilizer, improved survival in both wtATTR and vATTR cardiomyopathy and is the only approved therapy in the United States at this time for ATTR cardiomyopathy.

REFERENCES

1. Aterman K. A historical note on the iodine-sulphuric acid reaction of amyloid. *Histochemistry* 1976;49:131-143.
2. Kyle RA. Amyloidosis: a convoluted story. *Br J Haematol.* 2001;114:529-538.
3. Muchtar E, Dispenzieri A, Magen H, et al. Systemic amyloidosis from A (AA) to T (ATTR): a review. *J Intern Med.* 2020;289(3):268-292.
4. Buxbaum JN, Ruberg FL. Transthyretin V122I (pV142I)* cardiac amyloidosis: an age-dependent autosomal dominant cardiomyopathy too common to be overlooked as a cause of significant heart disease in elderly African Americans. *Genet Med.* 2017;19:733-742.
5. Kittleson MM, Maurer MS, Ambardekar AV, et al. Cardiac amyloidosis: evolving diagnosis and management: a scientific statement from the American Heart Association. *Circulation* 2020;142:e7-e22.
6. Sukhacheva TV, Eremeeva MV, Ibragimova AG, Vaskovskii VA, Serov RA, Revishvili A. Isolated atrial amyloidosis in patients with various types of atrial fibrillation. *Bull Exp Biol Med.* 2016;160:844-849.
7. Gertz MA. Immunoglobulin light chain amyloidosis: 2018 Update on diagnosis, prognosis, and treatment. *Am J Hematol.* 2018;93:1169-1180.
8. Schmidt HH, Waddington-Cruz M, Botteman MF, et al. Estimating the global prevalence of transthyretin familial amyloid polyneuropathy. *Muscle Nerve* 2018;57:829-837.
9. Tanskanen M, Peuralinna T, Polvikoski T, et al. Senile systemic amyloidosis affects 25% of the very aged and associates with genetic variation in alpha2-macroglobulin and tau: a population-based autopsy study. *Ann Med.* 2008;40:232-239.
10. Mitter SS, Pinney SP. Advances in the management of acute decompensated heart failure. *Med Clin North Am.* 2020;104:601-614.
11. Hahn VS, Yanek LR, Vaishnav J, et al. Endomyocardial biopsy characterization of heart failure with preserved ejection fraction and prevalence of cardiac amyloidosis. *JACC Heart Fail.* 2020;8:712-724.
12. Sidiqi MH, Aljama MA, Muchtar E, et al. Light chain type predicts organ involvement and survival in AL amyloidosis patients receiving stem cell transplantation. *Blood Adv.* 2018;2:769-776.
13. Keren DF, Schroeder L. Challenges of measuring monoclonal proteins in serum. *Clin Chem Lab Med.* 2016;54:947-961.
14. Basset M, Defrancesco I, Milani P, et al. Nonlymphoplasmacytic lymphomas associated with light-chain amyloidosis. *Blood* 2020;135:293-296.
15. Geller HI, Singh A, Alexander KM, Mirto TM, Falk RH. Association between ruptured distal biceps tendon and wild-type transthyretin cardiac amyloidosis. *JAMA* 2017;318:962-963.
16. Westermark P, Westermark GT, Suhr OB, Berg S. Transthyretin-derived amyloidosis: probably a common cause of lumbar spinal stenosis. *Ups J Med Sci.* 2014;119:223-228.
17. Connors LH, Sam F, Skinner M, et al. Heart failure resulting from age-related cardiac amyloid disease associated with wild-type transthyretin: a prospective, observational cohort study. *Circulation* 2016;133:282-290.
18. Ruberg FL, Grogan M, Hanna M, Kelly JW, Maurer MS. Transthyretin amyloid cardiomyopathy: JACC State-of-the-Art Review. *J Am Coll Cardiol.* 2019;73:2872-2891.
19. Gonzalez-Lopez E, Gallego-Delgado M, Guzzo-Merello G, et al. Wild-type transthyretin amyloidosis as a cause of heart failure with preserved ejection fraction. *Eur Heart J.* 2015;36:2585-2594.
20. Adams D, Koike H, Slama M, Coelho T. Hereditary transthyretin amyloidosis: a model of medical progress for a fatal disease. *Nat Rev Neurol.* 2019;15:387-404.
21. Maurer MS, Hanna M, Grogan M, et al. Genotype and phenotype of transthyretin cardiac amyloidosis: THAOS (Transthyretin Amyloid Outcome Survey). *J Am Coll Cardiol.* 2016;68:161-172.
22. Sperry BW, Reyes BA, Ikram A, et al. Tenosynovial and cardiac amyloidosis in patients undergoing carpal tunnel release. *J Am Coll Cardiol.* 2018;72:2040-2050.
23. Yanagisawa A, Ueda M, Sueyoshi T, et al. Amyloid deposits derived from transthyretin in the ligamentum flavum as related to lumbar spinal canal stenosis. *Mod Pathol.* 2015;28:201-207.
24. Castano A, Narotsky DL, Hamid N, et al. Unveiling transthyretin cardiac amyloidosis and its predictors among elderly patients with severe aortic stenosis undergoing transcatheter aortic valve replacement. *Eur Heart J.* 2017;38:2879-2887.
25. Scully PR, Patel KP, Treibel TA, et al. Prevalence and outcome of dual aortic stenosis and cardiac amyloid pathology in patients referred for transcatheter aortic valve implantation. *Eur Heart J.* 2020;41:2759-2767.
26. McCausland KL, White MK, Guthrie SD, et al. Light chain (AL) amyloidosis: the journey to diagnosis. *Patient* 2018;11:207-216.
27. Longhi S, Quarta CC, Milandri A, et al. Atrial fibrillation in amyloidotic cardiomyopathy: prevalence, incidence, risk factors and prognostic role. *Amyloid* 2015;22:147-155.
28. Donnellan E, Wazni OM, Hanna M, et al. Atrial fibrillation in transthyretin cardiac amyloidosis: predictors, prevalence, and efficacy of rhythm control strategies. *JACC Clin Electrophysiol.* 2020;6:1118-1127.
29. John RM. Arrhythmias in Cardiac Amyloidosis. *J Innov Card Rhythm Manag.* 2018;15;9(3):3051-3057.
30. Rapezzi C, Merlini G, Quarta CC, et al. Systemic cardiac amyloidoses: disease profiles and clinical courses of the 3 main types. *Circulation* 2009;120:1203-1212.
31. Witteles RM, Bokhari S, Damy T, et al. Screening for transthyretin amyloid cardiomyopathy in everyday practice. *JACC Heart Fail.* 2019;7:709-716.
32. Winter M, Tholey A, Kristen A, Rocken C. MALDI mass spectrometry imaging: a novel tool for the identification and classification of amyloidosis. *Proteomics* 2017;17.

33. Abildgaard N, Rojek AM, Moller HE, et al. Immunoelectron microscopy and mass spectrometry for classification of amyloid deposits. *Amyloid* 2020;27:59-66.

34. Fine NM. Challenges and strategies in the diagnosis of cardiac amyloidosis. *Can J Cardiol.* 2020;36:441-443.

35. Quarta CC, Gonzalez-Lopez E, Gilbertson JA, et al. Diagnostic sensitivity of abdominal fat aspiration in cardiac amyloidosis. *Eur Heart J.* 2017;38:1905-1908.

36. Boldrini M, Cappelli F, Chacko L, et al. Multiparametric echocardiography scores for the diagnosis of cardiac amyloidosis. *JACC Cardiovasc Imaging* 2020;13:909-920.

37. Mitter SS, Shah SJ, Thomas JD. A test in context: E/A and E/e' to assess diastolic dysfunction and LV filling pressure. *J Am Coll Cardiol.* 2017;69:1451-1464.

38. Phelan D, Collier P, Thavendiranathan P, et al. Relative apical sparing of longitudinal strain using two-dimensional speckle-tracking echocardiography is both sensitive and specific for the diagnosis of cardiac amyloidosis. *Heart* 2012;98:1442-1448.

39. Fontana M, Pica S, Reant P, et al. Prognostic value of late gadolinium enhancement cardiovascular magnetic resonance in cardiac amyloidosis. *Circulation* 2015;132:1570-1579.

40. Martinez-Naharro A, Kotecha T, Norrington K, et al. Native T1 and extracellular volume in transthyretin amyloidosis. *JACC Cardiovasc Imaging* 2019;12:810-819.

41. Pan JA, Kerwin MJ, Salerno M. Native T1 mapping, extracellular volume mapping, and late gadolinium enhancement in cardiac amyloidosis: a meta-analysis. *JACC Cardiovasc Imaging* 2020;13:1299-1310.

42. Martinez-Naharro A, Abdel-Gadir A, Treibel TA, et al. CMR-verified regression of cardiac AL amyloid after chemotherapy. *JACC Cardiovasc Imaging* 2018;11:152-154.

43. Fontana M, Martinez-Naharro A, Chacko L, et al. Reduction in CMR derived extracellular volume with patisiran indicates cardiac amyloid regression. *JACC Cardiovasc Imaging* 2020.

44. Hanna M, Ruberg FL, Maurer MS, et al. Cardiac scintigraphy with technetium-99m-labeled bone-seeking tracers for suspected amyloidosis: JACC Review Topic of the Week. *J Am Coll Cardiol.* 2020;75:2851-2862.

45. Castano A, Haq M, Narotsky DL, et al. Multicenter study of planar technetium 99m pyrophosphate cardiac imaging: predicting survival for patients with ATTR cardiac amyloidosis. *JAMA Cardiol.* 2016;1:880-889.

46. Gillmore JD, Maurer MS, Falk RH, et al. Nonbiopsy diagnosis of cardiac transthyretin amyloidosis. *Circulation* 2016;133:2404-2412.

47. Musumeci MB, Cappelli F, Russo D, et al. Low sensitivity of bone scintigraphy in detecting Phe64Leu mutation-related transthyretin cardiac amyloidosis. *JACC Cardiovasc Imaging* 2020;13:1314-1321.

48. Scully PR, Morris E, Patel KP, et al. DPD quantification in cardiac amyloidosis: a novel imaging biomarker. *JACC Cardiovasc Imaging* 2020;13:1353-1363.

49. Gallegos C, Miller EJ. Advances in PET-based cardiac amyloid radiotracers. *Curr Cardiol Rep.* 2020;22:40.

50. Manwani R, Page J, Lane T, et al. A pilot study demonstrating cardiac uptake with 18F-florbetapir PET in AL amyloidosis patients with cardiac involvement. *Amyloid* 2018;25:247-252.

51. Trivieri MG, Dweck MR, Abgral R, et al. (18)F-sodium fluoride PET/MR for the assessment of cardiac amyloidosis. *J Am Coll Cardiol.* 2016;68:2712-2714.

52. Scully PR, Patel KP, Saberwal B, et al. Identifying cardiac amyloid in aortic stenosis: ECV quantification by CT in TAVR patients. *JACC Cardiovasc Imaging* 2020;13:2177-2189.

53. Grogan M, Scott CG, Kyle RA, et al. Natural history of wild-type transthyretin cardiac amyloidosis and risk stratification using a novel staging system. *J Am Coll Cardiol.* 2016;68:1014-1020.

54. Gillmore JD, Damy T, Fontana M, et al. A new staging system for cardiac transthyretin amyloidosis. *Eur Heart J.* 2018;39:2799-2806.

55. Kumar SK, Gertz MA, Dispenzieri A. Validation of Mayo Clinic staging system for light chain amyloidosis with high-sensitivity troponin. *J Clin Oncol.* 2019;37:171-173.

56. Dumas B, Yameen H, Sarosiek S, Sloan JM, Sanchorawala V. Presence of t(11;14) in AL amyloidosis as a marker of response when treated with a bortezomib-based regimen. *Amyloid* 2020:1-6.

57. Wong SW, Hegenbart U, Palladini G, et al. Outcome of patients with newly diagnosed systemic light-chain amyloidosis associated with deletion of 17p. *Clin Lymphoma Myeloma Leuk.* 2018;18:e493-e499.

58. Bhuiyan T, Helmke S, Patel AR, et al. Pressure-volume relationships in patients with transthyretin (ATTR) cardiac amyloidosis secondary to V122I mutations and wild-type transthyretin: Transthyretin Cardiac Amyloid Study (TRACS). *Circ Heart Fail.* 2011;4:121-128.

59. Pollak A, Falk RH. Left ventricular systolic dysfunction precipitated by verapamil in cardiac amyloidosis. *Chest* 1993;104:618-620.

60. Donnelly JP, Sperry BW, Gabrovsek A, et al. Digoxin use in cardiac amyloidosis. *Am J Cardiol.* 2020;133:134-138.

61. Mints YY, Doros G, Berk JL, Connors LH, Ruberg FL. Features of atrial fibrillation in wild-type transthyretin cardiac amyloidosis: a systematic review and clinical experience. *ESC Heart Fail.* 2018;5:772-779.

62. Feng D, Syed IS, Martinez M, Oh JK, Jaffe AS, Grogan M, Edwards WD, Gertz MA, Klarich KW. Intracardiac thrombosis and anticoagulation therapy in cardiac amyloidosis. *Circulation.* 2009;12;119(18):2490-2497.

63. Donnellan E, Wazni OM, Saliba WI, et al. Cardiac devices in patients with transthyretin amyloidosis: impact on functional class, left ventricular function, mitral regurgitation, and mortality. *J Cardiovasc Electrophysiol.* 2019;30:2427-2432.

64. Sayed RH, Rogers D, Khan F, et al. A study of implanted cardiac rhythm recorders in advanced cardiac AL amyloidosis. *Eur Heart J.* 2015;36:1098-1105.

65. Varr BC, Zarafshar S, Coakley T, et al. Implantable cardioverter-defibrillator placement in patients with cardiac amyloidosis. *Heart Rhythm* 2014;11:158-162.

66. Sanchorawala V. High-dose melphalan and autologous peripheral blood stem cell transplantation in AL amyloidosis. *Acta Haematol.* 2020;143:381-387.

67. Cordes S, Dispenzieri A, Lacy MQ, et al. Ten-year survival after autologous stem cell transplantation for immunoglobulin light chain amyloidosis. *Cancer* 2012;118:6105-6109.

68. Reece DE, Hegenbart U, Sanchorawala V, et al. Long-term follow-up from a phase 1/2 study of single-agent bortezomib in relapsed systemic AL amyloidosis. *Blood* 2014;124:2498-2506.

69. Abeykoon JP, Zanwar S, Dispenzieri A, et al. Daratumumab-based therapy in patients with heavily-pretreated AL amyloidosis. *Leukemia* 2019;33:531-536.

70. Palladini G, Kastritis E, Maurer MS, et al. Daratumumab plus CyBorD for patients with newly diagnosed AL amyloidosis: safety run-in results of ANDROMEDA. *N Engl J Med.* 2021;385:46-58.

71. Maurer MS, Schwartz JH, Gundapaneni B, et al. Tafamidis treatment for patients with transthyretin amyloid cardiomyopathy. *N Engl J Med.* 2018;379:1007-1016.

72. Finkelstein DM, Schoenfeld DA. Combining mortality and longitudinal measures in clinical trials. *Stat Med.* 1999;18:1341-1354.

73. Coelho T, Maia LF, Martins da Silva A, et al. Tafamidis for transthyretin familial amyloid polyneuropathy: a randomized, controlled trial. *Neurology* 2012;79:785-792.

74. Judge DP, Heitner SB, Falk RH, et al. Transthyretin stabilization by AG10 in symptomatic transthyretin amyloid cardiomyopathy. *J Am Coll Cardiol.* 2019;74:285-295.

75. Castano A, Helmke S, Alvarez J, Delisle S, Maurer MS. Diflunisal for ATTR cardiac amyloidosis. *Congest Heart Fail.* 2012;18:315-319.

76. Ikram A, Donnelly JP, Sperry BW, Samaras C, Valent J, Hanna M. Diflunisal tolerability in transthyretin cardiac amyloidosis: a single center's experience. *Amyloid* 2018;25:197-202.

77. Rosenblum H, Castano A, Alvarez J, Goldsmith J, Helmke S, Maurer MS. TTR (Transthyretin) stabilizers are associated with improved survival in patients with TTR cardiac amyloidosis. *Circ Heart Fail.* 2018;11:e004769.

78. Adams D, Gonzalez-Duarte A, O'Riordan WD, et al. Patisiran, an RNAi therapeutic, for hereditary transthyretin amyloidosis. *N Engl J Med.* 2018;379:11-21.

79. Benson MD, Waddington-Cruz M, Berk JL, et al. Inotersen treatment for patients with hereditary transthyretin amyloidosis. *N Engl J Med.* 2018;379:22-31.

80. Minamisawa M, Claggett B, Adams D, et al. Association of patisiran, an RNA Interference therapeutic, with regional left ventricular myocardial strain in hereditary transthyretin amyloidosis: the APOLLO study. *JAMA Cardiol.* 2019;4:466-472.

81. Solomon SD, Adams D, Kristen A, et al. Effects of patisiran, an RNA interference therapeutic, on cardiac parameters in patients with hereditary transthyretin-mediated amyloidosis. *Circulation* 2019;139:431-443.

82. Benson MD, Dasgupta NR, Rissing SM, Smith J, Feigenbaum H. Safety and efficacy of a TTR specific antisense oligonucleotide in patients with transthyretin amyloid cardiomyopathy. *Amyloid* 2017;24: 219-225.

83. Dasgupta NR, Rissing SM, Smith J, Jung J, Benson MD. Inotersen therapy of transthyretin amyloid cardiomyopathy. *Amyloid* 2020;27:52-58.

84. Obici L, Cortese A, Lozza A, et al. Doxycycline plus tauroursodeoxycholic acid for transthyretin amyloidosis: a phase II study. *Amyloid* 2012;19 Suppl 1: 34-36.

85. Wixner J, Pilebro B, Lundgren HE, Olsson M, Anan I. Effect of doxycycline and ursodeoxycholic acid on transthyretin amyloidosis. *Amyloid* 2017;24:78-79.

86. Higaki JN, Chakrabartty A, Galant NJ, et al. Novel conformation-specific monoclonal antibodies against amyloidogenic forms of transthyretin. *Amyloid* 2016;23:86-97.

87. Swiecicki PL, Edwards BS, Kushwaha SS, Dispenzieri A, Park SJ, Gertz MA. Left ventricular device implantation for advanced cardiac amyloidosis. *J Heart Lung Transplant* 2013;32:563-568.

88. Kittleson MM, Cole RM, Patel J, et al. Mechanical circulatory support for cardiac amyloidosis. *Clin Transplant* 2019;33:e13663.

89. Barrett CD, Alexander KM, Zhao H, et al. Outcomes in patients with cardiac amyloidosis undergoing heart transplantation. *JACC Heart Fail.* 2020;8:461-468.

90. Chen Q, Moriguchi J, Levine R, et al. Outcomes of heart transplantation in cardiac amyloidosis patients: a single center experience. *Transplant Proc.* 2020;53(1):329-334.

91. Carvalho A, Rocha A, Lobato L. Liver transplantation in transthyretin amyloidosis: issues and challenges. *Liver Transpl.* 2015;21:282-292.

92. Nelson LM, Penninga L, Villadsen GE, et al. Outcome in patients treated with isolated liver transplantation for familial transthyretin amyloidosis to prevent cardiomyopathy. *Clin Transplant* 2015;29:1098-1104.

93. Damy T, Kristen AV, Suhr OB, et al. Transthyretin cardiac amyloidosis in continental Western Europe: an insight through the Transthyretin Amyloidosis Outcomes Survey (THAOS). *Eur Heart J.* 2019;1;ehz173.

94. Seferovic PM, Ponikowski P, Anker SD, et al. Clinical practice update on heart failure 2019: pharmacotherapy, procedures, devices and patient management. An expert consensus meeting report of the Heart Failure Association of the European Society of Cardiology. *Eur J Heart Fail.* 2019;21:1169-1186.

44

Restrictive Heart Diseases

Eloisa Arbustini, Alessandro Di Toro, Lorenzo Giuliani,
G. William Dec, and Jagat Narula

CHAPTER OUTLINE

Myo-peri-cardial diseases sharing restrictive physiology

Myocardial diseases: restrictive cardiomyopathy and myocardial phenocopies

- Restrictive ventricular physiology
- Normal or reduced diastolic ventricular volumes
- Normal or reduced systolic volumes
- Normal ventricular wall thickness
- Biatrial enlargement
- Primary genetic (e.g., *TNNI3* or MFM)
- Genetic phenocopies (*HFE*)
- Drug toxicity (chloroquine)

Sarcomeric restrictive cardiomyopathy
Troponinopathies (TNNI3): disarray without hypertrophy

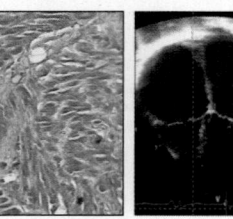
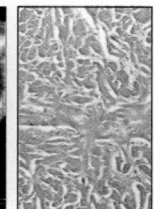

Myofibrillar myopathies (MFM)
Desminopathies (intramyocyte desmin accumulation); other MFM with myofibrillar material (*BAG3, FLNC*)

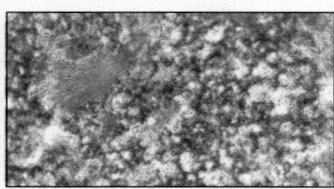

Phenocopies
Acquired: chloroquine toxicity
Genetic: Iron storage

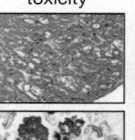
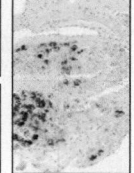

Endo-myo-cardial diseases: endomyocardial fibrosis

Diseases affecting endomyocardial layers may manifest with restrictive physiology and are functional phenocopies of genetic restrictive cardiomyopathy

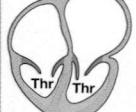

Terms
- Endocardial fibroelastosis
- Endomyocardial fibrosis
- Obliterative cardiomyopathy

Phenocopies:
- Hedinger syndrome
- Right side heart
- Drug toxicity

Acute Febrile phase:
Endo-myo-peri-carditis, thrombosis, thomboembolism

Chronic phase:
Restrictive phenotype, hepatosplenomegaly, ascites

Pathogenetic hypotheses:
Endo-ventricular thrombosis

Possible role:
eosinophils

Possible causes:
parasites

Contributors:
malnutrition, poverty, environmenal and toxic factors, genetic predisposition (?)

Key cells: eosinophils
- Myocyte
- Eosinophilic granulocyte
- Red cell
- Platelets

Surgical Treatment:
Endo(myo)-cardial resection

Myo-peri-cardial diseases

Peri-myocarditis, fibrotic evolution

All diseases affecting pericardium and potentially involving the sub-endocardial myocardium

From epi-pericardial inflammation and fibrosis to constrictive pericarditis

Pericardiectomy
- Epicardial Fat
- Pericardium
- Fibrous layer: Inflammation and fibrosis

Chapter 44 Fuster and Hurst's Central Illustration. Restrictive heart diseases are characterized by diastolic dysfunction in the presence of elevated left ventricular filling pressures and limited increase in volume. Diastolic dysfunction is observed in myocardial, endocardial/endomyocardial, and pericardial/myopericardial diseases.

CHAPTER SUMMARY

This chapter provides an overview of restrictive heart diseases, conditions characterized by diastolic dysfunction in the presence of elevated left ventricular filling pressures and limited increase in volume. The diastolic dysfunction may be observed in myocardial (restrictive cardiomyopathy [RCM] and phenocopies), endocardial/endomyocardial (fibrosis, elastosis), and pericardial (constriction, effusion) diseases (see Fuster and Hurst's Central Illustration). Primary RCMs are rare myocardial diseases and are defined by restrictive ventricular physiology in the presence of normal or reduced diastolic volumes of one or both ventricles, normal or reduced systolic volumes, and normal ventricular wall thickness, with significant atrial dilation. They carry a poor prognosis. Familial RCM are usually caused by mutations in genes encoding for sarcomeric proteins and intermediate filaments. Restrictive endomyocardial diseases include endomyocardial fibrosis of right, left, or both ventricles, frequently with involvement of valves, Hedinger syndrome of the right-sided heart valves in patients with neuroendocrine tumors and carcinoid syndrome, as well as endocardial fibroelastosis associated with congenital heart anomalies.

INTRODUCTION

Restrictive physiology describes a pattern of ventricular filling in which increased myocardial stiffness causes a precipitous elevation of ventricular pressure matched by a limited increase in volume; the resultant diastolic dysfunction is characterized by a pattern of mitral inflow Doppler velocities with an increased ratio of early diastolic filling to atrial filling (greater than or equal to 2), decreased E-deceleration time (<160 ms), and decreased isovolumetric relaxation time.

Diastolic dysfunction occurs in several cardiac diseases with a range of etiologies.[1] Restrictive physiology can be observed in diseases affecting endocardium, myocardium, and epipericardial layers/structures (**Table 44–1**). The recent development of advanced technologies for DNA sequencing, refined imaging techniques, and identification of novel biomarkers have contributed to unraveling the primary causes of many of these different diseases, facilitating more targeted treatments. These dynamic technologies will continue to develop and will transform previous pathology-based nosology of heart diseases into a precise, etiology-based classification of restrictive cardiac diseases (Chapter 40). This chapter illustrates the etiology, phenotypes, and management of these different diseases and separates cardiac and systemic diseases that share similar functional criteria but differ from each other, both etiologically and structurally. The gross inclusion of all myocardial diseases with altered diastolic function, regardless of causes and effects, in fact generates an imprecise nosology. For this reason, amyloid heart disease, for which new epidemiological, diagnostic and therapeutic data are now available, has been deemed worthy of a separate discussion.

RESTRICTIVE CARDIOMYOPATHY

Definition

According to the definition of the European Society of Cardiology (ESC) "Restrictive cardiomyopathies are defined as restrictive ventricular physiology in the presence of normal or reduced diastolic volumes of one or both ventricles, normal or reduced systolic volumes, and normal ventricular wall thickness."[2] According to the definition of the American Heart Association (AHA) "Primary restrictive non-hypertrophied cardiomyopathy is a rare form of heart muscle disease and a cause of heart failure that is characterized by normal or decreased volume of both ventricles associated with biatrial enlargement, normal LV wall thickness and AV valves, impaired ventricular filling with restrictive physiology, and normal (or near normal) systolic function."[3] Both definitions emphasize restrictive ventricular physiology, normal or reduced volume of one or both ventricles, and normal wall thickness. The AHA further stipulates the presence of atrial dilation, normal atrioventricular (AV) valves, and normal systolic function.[3] End-stage hypertrophic cardiomyopathy (HCM) and dilated cardiomyopathy (DCM) may manifest restrictive physiology, but these forms are not assigned to distinct subgroups of cardiomyopathies.[2] Precise epidemiology data are not available, but restrictive cardiomyopathy (RCM) is a less common form of cardiomyopathy. A nationwide epidemiologic survey in Japanese hospitals estimated a prevalence of 0.2 per 100,000 inhabitants.[4]

RCM can be primary/idiopathic or acquired;[5] recent advances in DNA sequencing demonstrated that the former are genetic diseases in both adults and children,[6,7] while the latter are phenocopies of genetic RCM. The criterion common to primary/idiopathic or acquired RCM is the restrictive ventricular physiology. The differentiation between primary/idiopathic RCM from other diseases manifesting restrictive ventricular physiology is essential because the precise diagnosis may determine monitoring, treatment, and prognosis.

"Primary or Idiopathic" Restrictive Cardiomyopathies are Genetic Diseases

RCM is *morphologically* characterized by normal or reduced ventricular size, biatrial dilation, absence of left ventricular hypertrophy (LVH) with LV wall thickness ≤13 mm, and *functionally* defined by diastolic dysfunction with restrictive physiology and preserved systolic function.[1,2,8,9] The early clinical manifestations can be subtle and morphofunctional modifications can be latent. Most RCMs demonstrate familial clustering and genetic origin; the genetic bases are heterogeneous. More than 15 genes have been reported to date in patients and families with RCM.[10] The clinical course is characterized by the development of heart failure (HF) with preserved ejection fraction and late evolution to end-stage biventricular systolic HF when heart transplantation is the most effective treatment option.[8,10–12] Patients with RCM experience long wait

TABLE 44–1. Restrictive Heart Diseases; Myocardial, Pericardial, and Endocardial Diseases

Level	Diseases demonstrating restrictive pathophysiology
Myocardial	Restrictive cardiomyopathy (RCM) Primary RCM Multiorgan genetic diseases with heart involvement and possible restrictive physiology Systemic monogenic diseases • Pseudoxanthoma Elasticum • Cystinosis • Hemochromatosis Phenocopies, acquired • POEMS • Diabetes Mellitus related cardiomyopathy • Cloroquine toxicity (the phenotype may overlap with DCM)
Endocardial/ Endomyo-cardial	Endocardial fibroelastosis Endomyocardial fibrosis Obliterative endocardial disease Carcinoid heart disease with fibrous valvular and endocardial fibrosis, focal (endocardial plaques) or diffuse (valves and endocardium) Iatrogenic diseases (serotonin, methysergide, ergotamine, mercurial agents, busulfan)
Epipericardial	Pericarditis Steatonecrotic, fibrous epicarditis of transplanted hearts Pericardial malignancies Post pericardiectomy

time for heart transplant and high mortality in waitlist. A new heart transplantation allocation system, with increased access to heart transplant without affecting short-term posttransplant survival, has been recently implemented on the basis of data collected from the United Network for Organ Sharing (UNOS) database.[13]

Diagnosis in Probands

Probands (or index patients) are usually diagnosed due to signs and symptoms of HF with preserved ejection fraction.[8,9] The clinical work-up includes physical examination, electrocardiogram (ECG), and two-dimensional (2D) echocardiography. Physical examination reflects the elevated systemic and pulmonary venous pressures, with prominent jugular venous pulse and X and Y descents. In the advanced course of the disease the pulse volume is low, the stroke volume declines, and the heart rate increases. A systolic murmur and filling sound reflect AV valve regurgitation and fast early diastolic filling; a fourth heart sound (S_4) can be present. Hepatomegaly, ascites and peripheral edema are common in decompensated patients. *Echocardiographic criteria* for diagnosing and grading diastolic dysfunction[14] are shown in **Table 44–2**.

In infants, RCM may present with failure to thrive, fatigue, and syncope.[7] Clinical examination usually does not show traits suggesting a specific etiology. ECG may demonstrate increased voltages and signs of atrial enlargement. Two-dimensional echocardiography is the key tool for the diagnosis.[14] In children, the most significant abnormalities are increased left atrial size, increased septal E'/E0, loss of A wave, and presence of mid-diastolic L0-wave; LV compliance may be decreased even with preserved early relaxation properties of the myocardium.[7,14] Interpretation of diastolic dysfunction[14] in children is complicated by the possible absence of key markers such as features of delayed relaxation and scarce contribution of mitral and pulmonary venous Doppler wave patterns.[14,15]

Cardiac magnetic resonance imaging (CMR) contributes to the characterization of different diseases manifesting with the RCM phenotype, to distinguish RCM from constrictive pericarditis, and to evaluate the extent of myocardial fibrosis.[16–18] Certain CMR features characterize RCM with different etiologies (eg, distinguishing metabolic diseases from inflammatory diseases).[19–21]

Endomyocardial biopsy (EMB) is uniquely useful for the diagnosis of desminopathies,[22] iron myocardial overload in both hemochromatosis[23] and Friedriech ataxia with cardiomyopathy,[24] cystinosis,[25,26] pseudoxantoma elasticum,[27] lysosomal storage diseases,[28,29] and cardiac amyloidosis.[30] EMB may show endocardial fibrous thickening,[31] endocardial thrombosis, eosinophilic infiltration,[32] and granulomatous myocardial diseases.[33] EMB may further help distinguish RCM from constrictive pericarditis (specific pathology features can immediately provide a precise diagnosis: eg, restrictive cardiodesminopathy).

Deep phenotyping in probands involves the investigation of cardiac and extracardiac traits that typically occur in etiologically different RCM. Clinical hypothesis on precise etiologies[34] can be obtained by joining information on the clinical phenotype; inheritance pattern; electrocardiographic markers (conduction disease, Wolff-Parkinson-White pattern/short PR interval, QT prolongation, low or high voltages of QRS complex); echocardiographic markers such as LV noncompaction or hypertrabeculation; CMR information such as T2* for iron overload as subsequently discussed;[20] preferential distribution and pattern of late gadolinium enhancement (LGE) on CMR[21] in amyloidosis;[19] and values of biomarkers such as increased creatinine phosphokinase, lactic acid, and N-terminal pro-brain natriuretic peptide (NT-proBNP).[34]

Differential Diagnosis between Restrictive Cardiomyopathy and Constrictive Pericarditis

It is crucial to distinguish between RCM and constrictive pericarditis (CP; Chapter 55) because RCM typically benefits only of medical management and carries a poor prognosis, while CP may be curable by pericardiectomy and represents a potentially reversible cause of HF (**Table 44–3**).[35] The clinical presentation of CP can mimic that of RCM, severe tricuspid regurgitation, and noncardiac conditions such as chronic obstructive airway diseases.[36]

Two-dimensional echocardiography, M-mode, and Doppler blood-flow evaluation including respiratory-related ventricular

TABLE 44–2. Criteria in the American Society of Echocardiography Guidelines Used to Grade Diastolic Function (2014)

IVRT (ms)	Normal	Grade 1 (mild)	Grade 2 (moderate)	Grade 3 (severe)
Mitral E/A ratio	>0.8	≤0.8	0.8–2.0	>2.0
Deceleration time (ms)	140–200	>200	160–200	<160
e' septal (cm/s)	≥8	<8		
e' lateral (cm/s)	≥10	<10		
Average E/e' (cm/s)		<8	9–12	≥13
Left atrial size (mL/m²)	<34	≥34		
Pulmonary vein systolic inflow (S) diastolic inflow (D) ratio (S/D ratio)		>1	<1	
Ar-A (ms)		<0	>30	
Change in E/A ratio with Valsalva		Decrease <50%	Decrease ≥50%	

TABLE 44–3. Major Criteria and Markers for Differential Diagnosis between Restrictive Cardiomyopathy and Constrictive Pericarditis

Items	RCM	Endomyocardial diseases	Constrictive pericarditis	Amyloid heart disease
Ethnic data	none	Epidemics EMF, EFE	none	None* exceptions genetic ATTR
Clinical history	Subtle symptoms	Infections; fatigue,	Possible: pericarditis, cardiac surgery, autoimmune diseases, malignancy	Subtle, fatigue, dyspnea
Family history	Frequently positive	Negative	Negative	Possible positive
Physical examination				
Jugular veins	Large (a) or (v) waves with steep y descent		Short and steep Y descent	Similar to RCM
Paradoxic pulse	Absent	Absent	Possible, 25%	Absent
Murmurs/tones (systole)	Common	Possible	No; friction sound	Common
Murmurs/tones (diastole)	Low pitched S3: 0.12–0.18 s after S2, or a S4	Possible	Pericardial knock: high pitched, usually 0.06–0.12 s after S2	Possible
Electrocardiogram				
P wave	High	High	Low	High
QRS voltage	High	-	Possible, 25%	Low, possible ~50%
Q-wave	Common	Common	no	Possible
LVH	Possible	-	no	no
Atrioventricular block	Possible according to the cause	-	no	Possible, 50%
Arrhythmias, atrial	Possible	Possible	no	Possible, common in advanced phases
Chest x-ray				
Cardiomegaly	Present (atrial dilation)	Possible	no	Possible
Pericardial calcification	No	no	25%	no
Lung congestion	Possible	Possible	no	Possible
2D echocardiography				
Atrial dilation	Present	Present	Possible, mild	Present
Ventricular septal shift	Absent	Absent	Present	Absent
Respiratory variation/valves	Absent	Absent	Present	Absent
TDI e' velocity	< 8 cm/s		>8 cm/s	<8 cm/s
Doppler, color M-mode	Slope > 100 cm/s		Slope <100 cm/s	Slope >100 cm/s
CT Scan				
Pericardial calcification	Absent	Absent	Possible	Absent
Pericardial thickening	Absent	Absent	Present	Absent
CMR				
Pericardial thickening	Absent	Absent	Present	Absent
Respiratory variation/septal	Absent	Absent	Present	Absent
Ventricular morphology, tubular	Absent	Absent	Present	Absent
Tagging: perimyocardium	Systolic breakage		Absent	Systolic breakage
LGE enhancement: pericardium	Absent	Absent	Present	Absent
LGE enhancement: myocardium	Present	Present	Absent	Present
LGE enhancement: endocardium	Present	Present	Absent	Present
Catheterization				
Dip & plateau	Absent	Absent	Present	Absent
Diastolic pressure equalization	Absent	Absent	Present	Absent

(Continued)

TABLE 44–3. Major Criteria and Markers for Differential Diagnosis between Restrictive Cardiomyopathy and Constrictive Pericarditis (Continued)

Items	RCM	Endomyocardial diseases	Constrictive pericarditis	Amyloid heart disease
Respiratory changes of RV and LV systolic pressures	Concordant	Concordant	Discordant	Concordant
RV/LV area, espiration vs inspiration	<1.1	<1.1	>1.1	<1.1
Biomarkers				
Inflammatory	Normal	Increased	Absent	Normal
BNP	Increased	Increased	< normal values	Increased
Pathology: EMB				
Features	Informative	Informative	Useless	Diagnostic

septal shift, preserved or increased medial mitral annular e' velocity, and prominent hepatic vein expiratory diastolic flow reversal are independently associated with the diagnosis of CP.[37–39] The assessment of early diastolic annulus velocity and annulus reversus (reversal of the relationship between lateral and medial e' velocities) by tissue Doppler imaging (TDI) improves the differentiation of constriction from restrictive myocardial disease and can be further facilitated by speckle tracking imaging (STE) as a complementary tool. Three-dimensional (3D) echocardiography precisely evaluates pericardial effusion or pericardial masses because it describes anatomic structures with higher accuracy than does 2D echocardiography.[39]

Computed tomography (CT) and CMR detect global or loculated effusions and measure pericardial thickness, which, in normal conditions, is less than 4 mm and usually around 1 to 2 mm. Cardiac CT demonstrates pericardial thickening and effusions. Delayed gadolinium enhancement CMR detects pericardial and myopericardial inflammation. A multiparametric CMR approach distinguishes among active inflammation, chronic pericarditis with constriction and effusion without inflammation.[40]

Cardiac catheterization is usually planned on an individual basis (eg, in patients with noncalcified or thickened pericardium especially before surgery); CP shows a more pronounced A wave and decline of rapid Y descent, suggesting LV filling abnormalities. However, catheterization may miss up to one-quarter of the cases of CP. Surgical exploration definitely gives an answer in unsolved cases. Finally, *NT-proBNP* levels are significantly higher in RCM than in CP.[41]

Family Studies

Genetic counseling, family history, and evaluation of clinical reports of family members are part of the clinical genetic work-up for patients diagnosed with RCM.[42] Clinical family screening includes physical examination, electrocardiographic, and 2D-echocardiographic evaluations of family members. Further testing such as ambulatory Holter monitoring, treadmill testing, and CMR are performed on an individualized basis. Familial RCM demonstrates autosomal dominant inheritance in the majority of cases; clinically sporadic cases may mask autosomal recessive inheritance or de novo genetic diseases: accordingly, all patients with RCM should receive genetic counseling and testing; relatives should be offered clinical screening.[34,42]

The clinical phenotype in affected members of the same family may vary: HCM or HCM with restrictive physiology or RCM that has progressed through dilation and dysfunction may occur in different family members.[43–47] This phenomenon is confirmed in several families and reflects phenotype heterogeneity: the genetic bases apparently coincide but the end-phenotype may differ. The reasons are still unknown: hypotheses include complex genotypes, modifiers genes, lifestyles (ie, athletes), or epigenetic factors (**Fig. 44–1**).

Family screening studies identify clinically and genetically affected members who may demonstrate borderline LVH. RCM should be distinguished from HCM with a restrictive pattern:[47,48] on echocardiography, a maximum LV thickness less than 13 mm, the absence of LV outflow tract obstruction, and the absence of systolic anterior motion of the mitral valve leaflet favor the diagnosis of RCM. However, long-term follow-up may show progression from RCM to HCM-RCM (**Fig. 44–2**). Cascade genetic testing in families is indicated after identification of the disease-causing mutation in probands.[34,42,49–51]

Genetic Bases

Genes associated with RCM encode sarcomeric structural and regulatory proteins, Z-disc proteins, and intermediate filaments. The *TNNI3* gene that encodes the thin filament Troponin I is the commonest disease gene responsible for RCM;[52] several reports confirm the major role of mutations in *TNNI3* in RCM.[43,45,53–55] Mutations in the Troponin T2 (*TNNT2*) gene are less common in RCM and may also cause HCM and DCM.[56] Other sarcomeric genes involved in RCM include *ACTC1, MYL3, MYH7, TTN, TPM1, MYL3,* and *MYL2*.[47–49,57] Recent reports have described mutations in Z-disc protein-encoding genes, including *MYPN, FLNC,* and *BAG3,* in patients with RCM[58–61] (**Table 44–4**).

Restrictive Troponinopathies: The troponin complex is constituted of three subunits: cardiac troponin I, troponin C, and troponin T. It functions as sensor of the intracellular Ca^{2+} concentration and controls the interaction between the thick and thin filaments during cardiac contraction and relaxation. The inhibitory effect of cardiac troponin I is reversed by troponin C binding to Ca^{2+} resulting in conformational changes of the

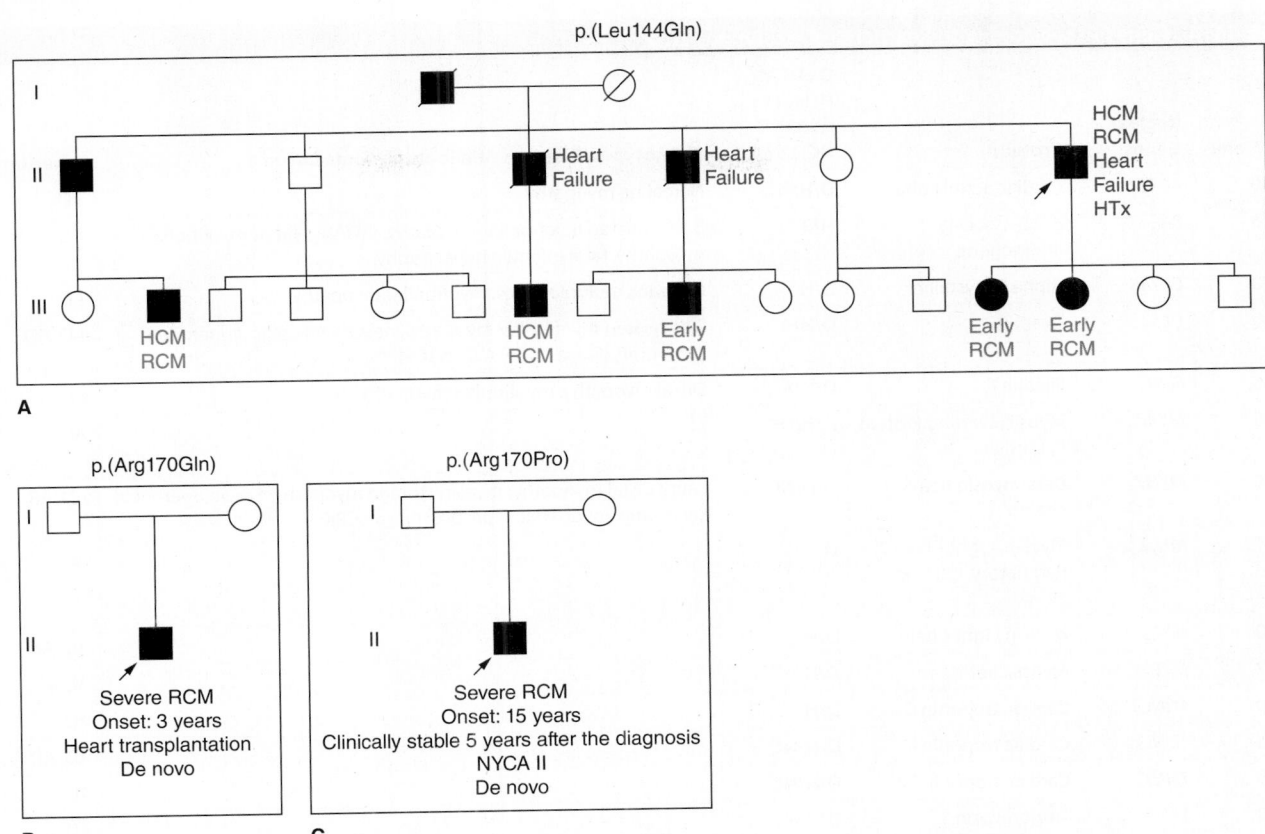

Figure 44–1. The figure shows the pedigrees of two families in which the probands were diagnosed with RCM caused by mutations in the *TNNI3* gene. **(A)** Autosomal dominant RCM in a family in which different affected family members showed HCM (*red bordered symbols*), HCM with restrictive patterns (*blue bordered symbols*), and early RCM with no hypertrophy, mildly dilated left atrium, and NYHA class I. **(B)** De novo RCM in a boy who developed early RCM characterized by severe atrial dilation, absence of LVH, and fast progression to advanced disease. Both parents were clinically and genetically healthy. **(C)** De novo RCM in a boy who developed RCM characterized by severe atrial dilation, absence of LVH, and clinical stability. Both parents were clinically and genetically healthy. HTx, heart transplantation.

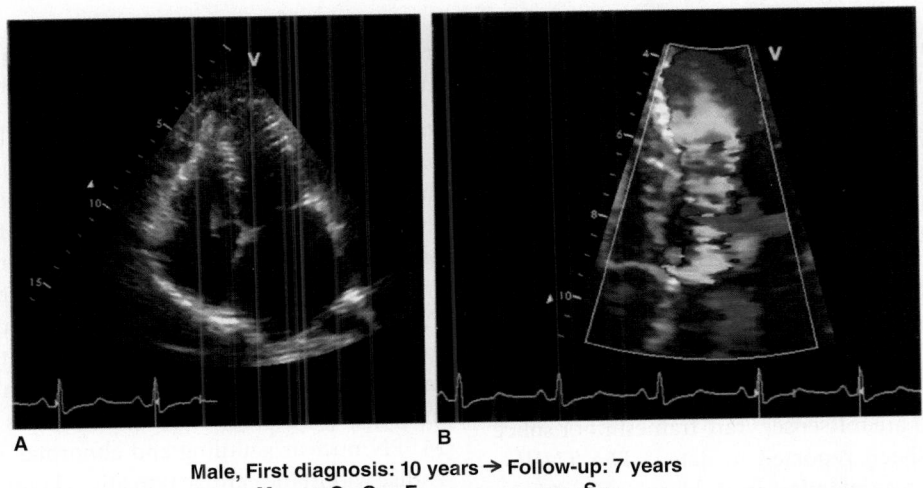

Male, First diagnosis: 10 years → Follow-up: 7 years
$M_{H(Obs)}$ O_H G_{AD} $E_{G\text{-}TNNI3[p.Leu144Gln]}$ $S_{C\text{-}I}$

Figure 44–2. Two-dimensional and color Doppler echocardiography in a 14-year-old boy, who was a member of a family in which mutation in the *TNNI3* gene was associated with RCM, HCM, and overlapping HCM-RCM. **(A)** Apical four-chamber view with biatrial enlargement and a small hyperkinetic left ventricle; an ICD electrode is seen extending into the right ventricle. **(B)** Midventricular obstruction on color Doppler imaging, with evident flow acceleration and turbulent flow, in the same young patient. The young patient was first diagnosed with HCM (mild LVH) at the age of 10 years; the diastolic dysfunction was apparent since the early detection of the disease. In his family, there were three sudden deaths (SDs), one aborted SD, and three heart transplantations. The boy received an ICD at the age of 13 years. Age 9: maximal LV thickness = 8 mm; age 10: maximal LV thickness = 11 mm; age 12: maximal LV thickness = 12 mm; atrial dilation; age 13: ICD; age 14: maximal LV thickness = 14 mm; atrial dilation; age 17: maximal LV thickness = 15 mm; atrial dilation, rest gradient = 22.3 mm Hg; after Valsalva: 40 mm Hg.

TABLE 44–4. Genes Associated with Restrictive Cardiomyopathy

MIM* Gene	Nuclear Genes	Protein	D : DCM H: HCM A: ARVC NC: LVNC	Phenotypes/Diseases Allelic at the Same Locus	Inheritance
102540	ACTC1	Cardiac actin alpha	D/H/NC	Nemaline myopathy	AD
603883	BAG3	BCL2-associated athanogene	H/R	BAG3-related myofibrillar myopathy, CRYAB-related myofibrillar myopathy, fatal infantile hypertrophy,	AD
123590	CRYAB	Alpha B crystallin	D/H	Cataract, multiple types; myofibrillar myopathy,	AD
125660	DES	Desmin	D/H/A	Des-related myofibrillar myopathy, neurogenic scapuloperoneal syndrome, Kaeser type; AVB, > sCPK	AD, AD
102565	FLNC	Filamin C	D/H/A	Distal myopathy, myofibrillar myopathy.	AD
600958	MYBPC3	Myosin-Binding Protein C, Cardiac	D/H/NC		AD
160760	MYH7	Beta-myosin heavy chain 7	D/H/NC	Laing distal myopathy; myosin storage myopathy; Scapuloperoneal syndrome, myopathic type; possible > sCPK	AD, AR
160781	MYL2	Myosin, Light Chain 2, Regulatory, Cardiac, Slow	H		AD
160790	MYL3	Myosin Light Chain 3	D/H		AD, AR
608517	MYPN	Myopalladin	D/H		AD
191040	TNNC1	Cardiac troponin C	D/H		AD
191044	TNNI3	Cardiac troponin I3	D/H/NC		AD, AR
191045	TNNT2	Cardiac troponin T2	D/H/NC		AD
191010	TPM1	Tropomyosin 1	D/H/NC		AD
188840	TTN	Titin	D/H/NC	Limb-girdle muscular dystrophy, early-onset myopathy with fatal CMP, proximal Myopathy with early respiratory muscle involvement, tardive tibial muscular dystrophy	AD

Abbreviations: A, arrhythmogenic cardiomyopathy; D, dilated cardiomyopathy; H, hypertrophic cardiomyopathy; NC, left ventricular noncompaction
This table lists genes, protein and phenotypes, inheritance, as well as nonrestrictive cardiomyopathies that have been reported to be allelic at the same loci of RCM

troponin complex, leading to muscle contraction. Mutations in any one of the components of the troponin complex may modify Ca^{2+} affinity and protein–protein interactions, thus potentially leading to the development of cardiomyopathy.

Founder mutations have been identified in the Netherlands in cardiac troponin I (TNNI3)[46] in families presenting with both RCM and HCM phenotypes in different affected members. Similar data were confirmed in other large families in which different affected members showed different phenotypes: RCM, HCM, and HCM with a restrictive pattern.[47] Intrafamily phenotype variability is not influenced by ethnicity because it is reported in families from different continents.[53] The majority of mutations in TNNI3 are missense;[52] rare frameshift or splice mutations have also been reported to date.[54] The TNNI3-associated phenotype may manifest in children[55] (**Fig. 44–3**). RCM hearts in patients with Troponin I mutations do not show significant loss of protein expression; however, myofibrillar disarray is present even in the absence of significant LVH (**Fig. 44–4**). While TNNI3 should be considered the major candidate gene for RCM, TNNT2 mutations are less commonly responsible.[56] Although the number of published cases and families is low and restrictive troponinopathies are rare, data

from single cases and small series suggest that the clinical evolution is characterized by a poor prognosis.[45,46,53–55]

Restrictive Myopalladinopathies: Recently, mutations in myopalladin (MYPN) and filamin-C (FLNC) have been reported, thus expanding the spectrum of genes potentially causing RCM.[58,60,61] In a large screening study of MYPN, different types of mutations were associated with different cardiac phenotypes: the Q529X-MYPN was found in familial RCM while the Y20C-MYPN variant was associated with HCM or DCM. The mechanism proposed for the development of RCM is disturbed myofibrillogenesis, while the mechanism proposed for DCM or HCM of the Y20C-MYPN variant is perturbation of the MYPN nuclear shuttling and abnormal assembly of terminal Z-disc within the cardiac transitional junction and intercalated disc.[58]

Restrictive Filaminopathies: Mutations in FLNC segregated in two families with autosomal-dominant RCM.[61] FLNC is an actin-crosslinking protein expressed in heart and skeletal muscle. The cardiac myocytes showed cytoplasmic inclusions suggesting protein aggregates, which were FLNC specific for the p.Ser1624Leu by immunohistochemistry. Cytoplasmic

$M_R\ O_H\ G_S\ E_{G\text{-}DN\text{-}TNNI3[p.Arg170Gln]}\ S_{C\text{-}III}$

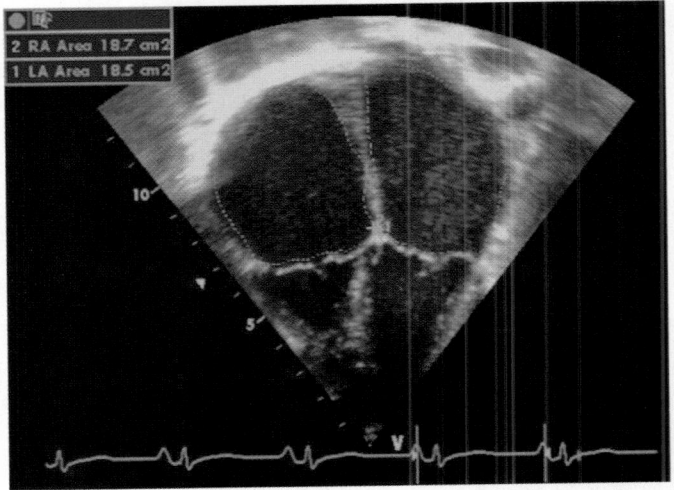

A

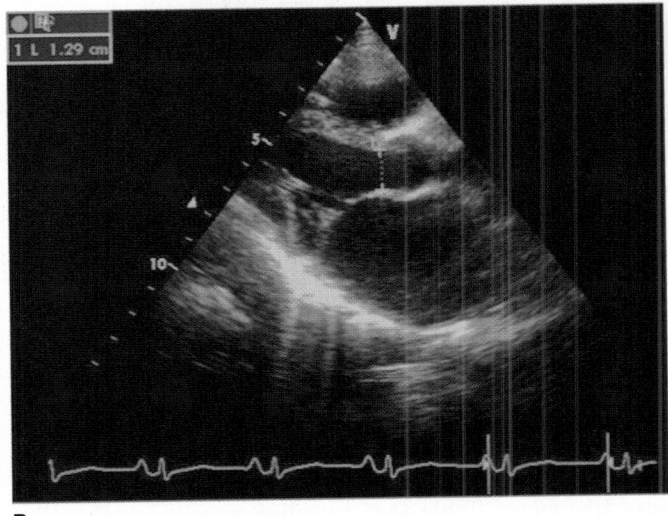

B

Figure 44–3. This figure shows the 2D echocardiographic views in a boy with RCM associated with a de novo mutation in the *TNNI3* gene. The phenotype and the genetic cause are summarized by the MOGES nosology $M_R\ O_H\ G_S\ E_{G\text{-}DN\text{-}TNNI3[p.Arg170Gln]}\ S_{C\text{-}III}$ in which M describes the morphofunctional phenotype (RCM, abbreviated as R); O describes the organs affected in the given patient (in this case, the heart was the only involved organ); G defines whether the cardiomyopathy is genetic or not and includes information on the pattern of inheritance or whether it appeared as sporadic in the family representing a possible de novo disease, which is confirmed after genetic testing; E is the precision diagnostic descriptor and specifies the cause, the disease gene(s), and the mutation(s) (in this patient, the mutation in *TNNI3* was proven de novo); and S is optional and includes NYHA functional class (I–IV) and AHA stage (A–D).

aggregates were also observed in transfected myoblast cell lines expressing this mutant FLNC providing further evidence for its pathogenicity.[61] Due to the rare number of published cases and the very recent association of mutations in these genes, RCM prognostic data are still unavailable.

Restrictive Desminopathies: The desmin intermediate filament network is involved in striated muscle development and maintenance by coordinating cellular components necessary

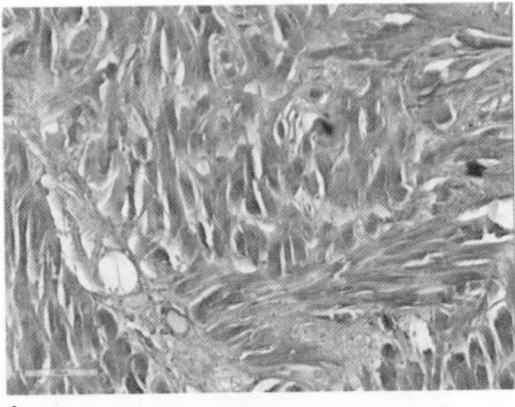

A

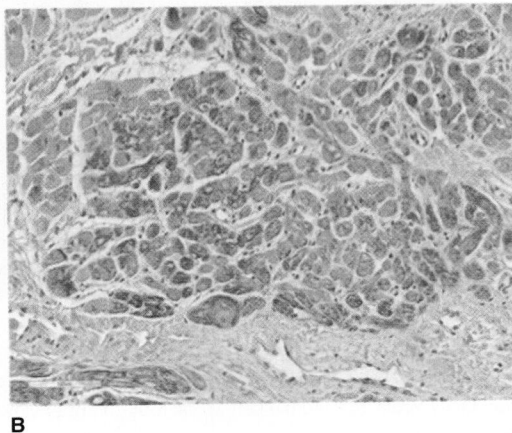

B

Figure 44–4. Anti–troponin I immunostain in myocardial samples from the heart of a patient with restrictive cardiomyopathy associated with the *TNNI3* p.(Leu144Gln) mutation. **(A)** Disarray that typically recurs in cardiomyopathies caused by defects encoding sarcomere proteins. **(B)** Prominent interstitial fibrosis.

for intracellular mechanochemical signaling and trafficking processes.[62] Direct or indirect deregulation of this network causes myopathies and cardiomyopathies.[63–68]

Restrictive desminopathies are autosomal dominant diseases in the majority of cases, and recessive and de novo in the minority of cases. They are clinically characterized by restrictive physiology, mild or absent LVH, absence of LV outflow tract obstruction, atrial dilation, and conduction system disease that may precede the clinical manifestation of RCM[64,65] **(Fig. 44–5).** Subclinical or overt myopathy may occur in these patients.[64] Conduction defect is a typical marker of the disease: it is confirmed in animal models of desminopathy.[66] The course of the disease is characterized by progressive worsening of the cardiac dysfunction to end-stage HF. Heart transplantation is the only therapeutic option.[67] The typical RCM-DES is easily diagnosed by EMB demonstrating desmin immunoreactive granulofilamentous material accumulated within myocytes[64,65,68] **(Fig. 44–6).** Similar findings are observed in skeletal muscle biopsy irrespective of the presence of clinically overt myopathy. Fine-needle biopsy of the skeletal muscle provides diagnostic information when EMB cannot be performed.[64]

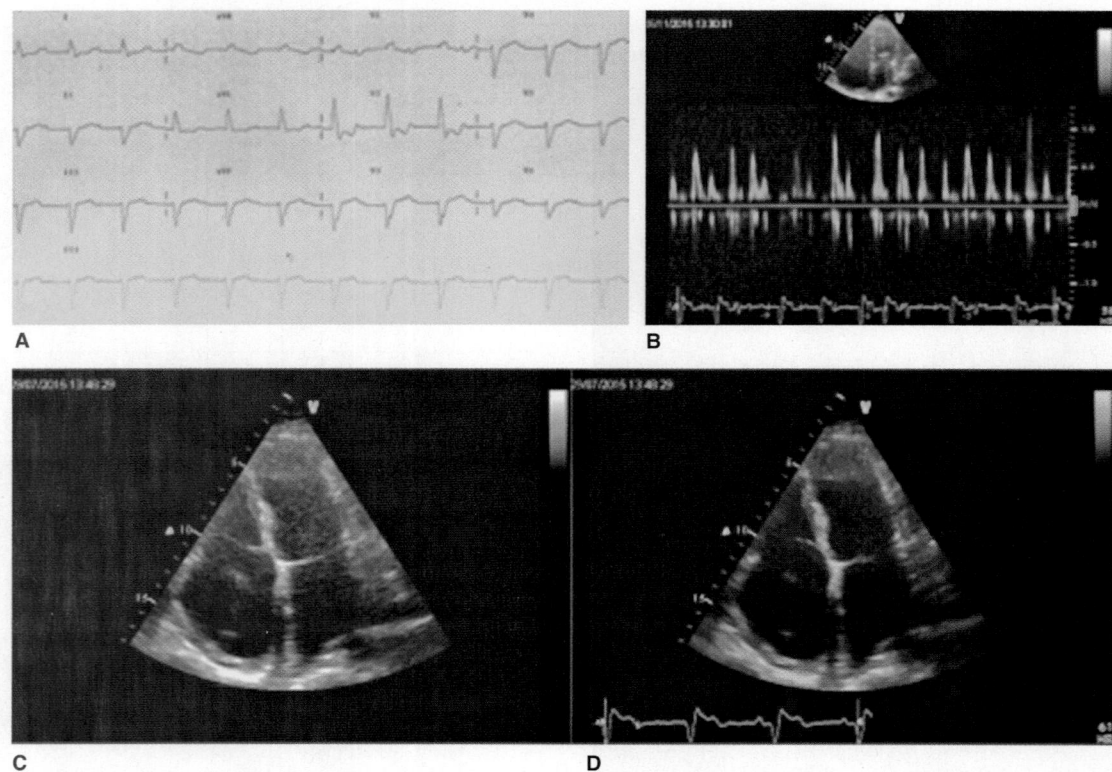

Figure 44–5. Restrictive cardiodesminopathy in a 43-year-old male patient. (**A**) ECG before pacemaker implantation with advanced AV block (PR interval 300 ms). (**B**) Doppler echocardiography with restrictive pattern (E/A wave ratio >3 and shortened deceleration time) at the transmitral flow during an episode of atrial tachycardia. (**C**) and (**D**) Left apical four-chamber view that demonstrates the biatrial enlargement. This patient also had moderate LV systolic dysfunction.

Multiorgan Genetic Diseases with Heart Involvement and Possible Restrictive Physiology

Lysosome storage diseases, cardiac amyloidosis, myocardial iron overload disorders, and collagen diseases may clinically manifest restrictive physiology. The cardiac phenotype is characterized by LV thickening with possible associated diastolic dysfunction, and is therefore similar to HCM. These diseases should be separated from pure RCM to prevent confusion in the nosology of RCM. They are distinct genetic disorders, systemic in the majority of the cases, with disease-specific diagnostic hallmarks and distinct clinical work-up and targeted treatments. **Table 44–5** lists diseases with increased LV thickening and in which restrictive physiology *is systematic* (eg, amyloidosis) or recurrently present in early phases of the

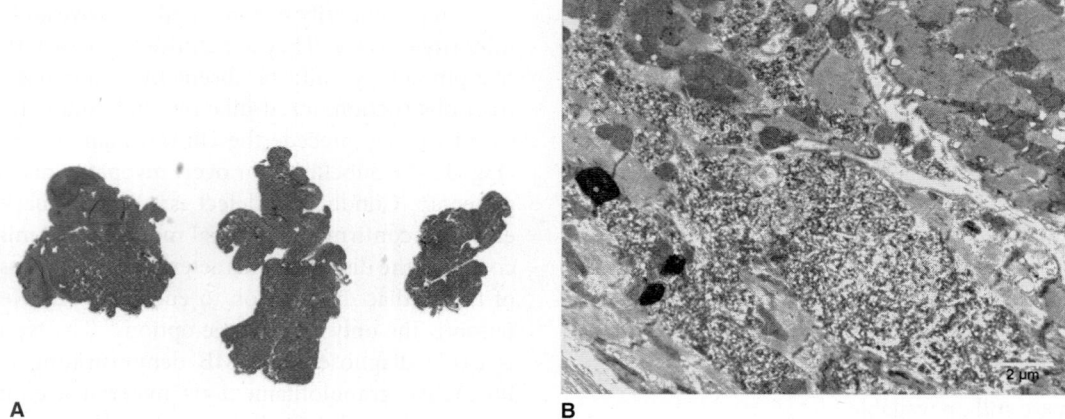

Figure 44–6. Endomyocardial biopsy (EMB), restrictive cardiodesminopathy. (**A**) Low-magnification view of the EMB samples, with prominent endocardial and interstitial fibrosis. (**B**) Electron micrograph demonstrates the typical intramyocyte accumulation of granulofilamentous material that corresponds to the abnormal desmin.

TABLE 44–5. Genes Causing Multiorgan/Systemic Diseases with Cardiac Involvement and Possible Restrictive Physiology

Diseases potentially associated with secondary cardiac restriction

MIM* Gene	Nuclear Genes	Protein	REF	Phenotypes/Diseases Allelic at the Same Locus	Inheritance
603234	ABCC6	ATP-Binding Cassette, Subfamily C, Member 6	69	Pseudoxanthoma elasticum	AR
610860	AGL	Amylo-1,6-Glucosidase, 4-Alpha-Glucanotransferase	70	Glycogen storage disease IIIa, Glycogen storage disease IIIb	AR
107680	APOA1*	Apolipoprotein of High Density Lipoprotein	71	Amyloidosis, hereditary	AD
107670	APOA2*	Apolipoprotein A-II	72	Amyloidosis, hereditary	AD
134820	FGA*	Fibrinogen, A Alpha Polypeptide	73	Amyloidosis, hereditary, familial visceral	AD
606800	GAA	Glucosidase, Alpha, Acid	74	Glycogen storage disease II	AR
606463	GBA	Glucosidase, Beta, Acid	75	Gaucher disease, perinatal lethal, type I, II, III, IIIC	AR
607839	GBE	Glycogen Branching Enzyme	76	Glycogen storage disease IV	AR
300644	GLA	Galactosidase, Alpha	77	Fabry disease	XL
137350	GSN*	Gelsolin	78	Amyloidosis, Finnish type	AD
606464	HAMP	Hepcidin Antimicrobial Peptide	79	Hemochromatosis, type 2B	AR/AD
613609	HFE	HFE Gene	79	Hemochromatosis	AD
608374	HFE2	Hemojuvelin	79	Hemochromatosis	AR/AD
252800	IDUA	Alpha-L-Iduronidase	80	Hurler disease	AR
309060	LAMP2	Lysosome-Associated Membrane Protein 2	81	Danon disease	XLD
610681	PFKM	Phosphofructokinase, Muscle Type	82	Glycogen storage disease VII	AR
172471	PHKG2	Phosphorylase Kinase, Testis/Liver, Gamma-2	83	Glycogen storage disease IXc	AR
602743	PRKAG2	Protein Kinase, AMP-Activated, Noncatalytic, Gamma-2	84	Cardiomyopathy, hypertrophic 6, Glycogen storage disease of heart, lethal congenital, Wolff-Parkinson-White syndrome	AD
613741	PYGL	Glycogen Phosphorylase, Liver	83	Glycogen storage disease VI	AR
604653	SLC40A1	Solute Carrier Family 40 (Iron-Regulated Transporter), Member 1	79	Hemochromatosis, type 4	AR/AD
602671	SLC37A4	Solute Carrier Family 37 (Glucose-6-Phosphate Transporter), Member 4	85	Glycogen storage disease Ib, Ic	AR
604720	TFR2	Transferrin Receptor 2	79	Hemochromatosis, type 3	AR/AD

*Addressed in Chapter 43, "Cardiac Amyloidosis."

disease (iron storage diseases) or *occasionally reported* in single cases (lysosomal storage diseases such as glycogenoses, Anderson–Fabry Disease, Danon Disease, Hurler Disease).[69–85]

Pseudoxanthoma Elasticum

Pseudoxanthoma elasticum (PXE) is a rare autosomal recessive systemic disease of the connective tissue that affects the extracellular matrix of multiple organs[86] with a prevalence that varies from 1 in 70,000 to 1 in 160,000. PXE involves the cutaneous, ocular, cardiovascular, and gastrointestinal systems.[86,87]

The cutaneous lesions (plucked chicken-like appearance) typically occur in flexural areas (**Fig. 44–7B**). The ocular system may show angioid streaks, reticular macular dystrophy, speckled appearance temporal to the macula (peau d'orange, like the dimpled texture of an orange peel), drusen of the optic nerve, and vitelliform-like deposits. Peau d'orange may precede the development of an angioid streak. "Comets," with or without a tail, are seen as solitary subretinal, nodular white bodies

of retinal pigment epithelium (RPE) atrophy, usually present in the mid periphery. The tail points toward the optic disc. Patients sometimes develop choroidal neovascular membrane. Skin changes (plucked chicken-like appearance) occur on the flexure areas, including the neck and axilla, as well as increased skin laxity with excessive skin folding.[87]

The cardiovascular manifestations are characterized by the development of arterial calcifications,[88] premature coronary artery disease, peripheral vascular disease, and RCM.[69,89–91] Sudden death has been occasionally reported.[91,92]

The histopathologic marker of the disease is the mineralization and fragmentation of elastic fibers (**Fig. 44–7**). PXE is caused by homozygous or compound heterozygous mutations in the *ABCC6* (ATP-binding cassette subfamily C member 6) gene that encodes a transmembrane ATP-driven organic anion transporter. Carriers of heterozygous mutations may demonstrate mild and partial traits of the disorder.[93,94] Drugs potentially able to modify the protein conformation, such as sodium

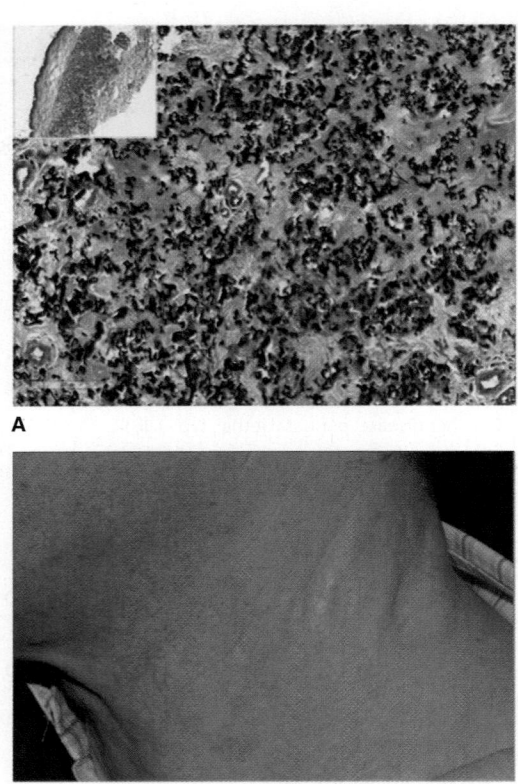

A

B

Figure 44–7. Pseudoxanthoma elasticum. **(A)** Skin biopsy with the typical calcifications that characterize the disease; the inset shows the skin biopsy sample. **(B)** Neck skin of a patient with the typical cutaneous lesions in flexural areas; the patient is carrier of the homozygous p.(Arg1141X) mutation in the *ABCC6* gene.

4-phenylbutyrate, an FDA approved drug for clinical use in urea cycle disorders, seems to be able to restore the plasma membrane localization of mutant *ABCC6*, thus opening the way to target treatment.[95,96] Chronic deficiency of *ABCC6* is also involved in generalized arterial calcification of infancy and PXE phenocopies in thalassemias; it is a susceptibility factor and/or a modifier for myocardial infarction, stroke, cardiac fibrosis, peripheral artery disease, age-related macular degeneration, chronic kidney disease, nephrocalcinosis, and dyslipidemia. A randomized controlled trial tested the oral phosphate binder sevelamer hydrochloride and demonstrated a reduction in both calcification levels and clinical scores.[97]

Cystinosis
Nephropathic cystinosis is a rare lysosomal storage autosomal recessive disease resulting from intracellular accumulation of cystine, leading to multiple organ failure. The incidence is estimated around 0.5 to 1.0 per 100,000 live births. The disease is caused by mutations in the lysosomal cystine/proton symporter termed cystinosin (encoded by *CTNS* gene) and represents the most common cause of inherited renal Fanconi syndrome in the first year of life, which results in end-stage renal disease by the age of 10 years.[98] In the European population, mutations of *CTNS* include a 65-kb deletion-involving marker D17S829 and

11 other small mutations.[99] Other *CTNS* mutations have been confirmed in African American patients with cystinosis.[100]

Early clinical signs commonly include distal myopathy primarily affecting the hands and resulting in intrinsic hand muscles weakness, atrophy, and contractures.[101] Other disease manifestations that occur during disease evolution include dysphagia, hypothyroidism, diabetes mellitus, pancreatic exocrine deficiency, crystalline keratopathy, retinal blindness, hypogonadism, benign intracranial hypertension, and central nervous system involvement. Vascular calcifications affecting coronary arteries,[102] aortic dissection,[103] and cardiomyopathies with restrictive,[104] or dilated[105] phenotype also with increased LV trabeculations[106] have been reported. The pathology of affected tissues is characterized by the tissue deposition of cystine. Cystine crystals have been observed mainly in interstitial cardiac histiocytes, and less commonly in cardiac myocytes.[107] Early administration of cysteamine reduces intracellular levels of cysteine and can delay progression of renal damage.[108] In cases that are diagnosed late, treatment options may be limited to renal transplantation.[109] Pharmacokinetics and safety of ELX-02, a novel eukaryotic ribosomal-specific glycoside, are being investigated in patients with nephropathic cystinosis at earlier stages of renal impairment.[110]

Iron-Overload Cardiomyopathies
Iron-overload cardiomyopathy can result from a primary genetic disease caused by defects in genes coding proteins active in iron metabolism, typically hereditary hemochromatosis, or from secondary causes of iron overload such as acquired hematologic diseases.

Hereditary Hemochromatosis:
Prevalence: Hereditary hemochromatosis (HH) is a heritable disorder of iron metabolism that is characterized by tissue iron overload.[79,111] HF causes approximately one-third of deaths of those with HH. Historically, the average survival was less than 1 year in untreated patients with severe cardiac impairment.[112] In classic HH, about 10% to 15% of affected adults present with cardiac symptoms at diagnosis. HF may develop suddenly in patients with juvenile forms of hemochromatosis. The HH phenotype is clinically heterogeneous and is influenced by gender and complex interactions between genotype and environmental factors (ie, alcohol, other causes of hepatitis). The cardiac phenotype is characterized by early LV diastolic dysfunction with evolution through LV systolic dysfunction and dilation, which is influenced by endocrine dysfunction, neuro-hormonal activation, and inflammatory cytokines.[113]

Genetic Heterogeneity: HH is characterized by genetic heterogeneity (**Table 44–6**).[114–120] The most common HH is HFE1 (or classical HH) that is associated with recurrent mutations [p.(Cys282Tyr) homozygotes or p.(Cys282Tyr)/p.(His63Asp) compound heterozygotes] in the *HFE* gene (**Fig. 44–8**). The most frequent causes of death are complications from cirrhosis, cardiomyopathy, and diabetes, but patients who undergo successful iron depletion before development of cirrhosis or diabetes have normal survival. The diagnosis of HH is established by

TABLE 44-6. Genetic Diseases Causing Iron Overload Potentially Affecting the Heart

MIM* Gene	Nuclear Genes	Protein	HFE	Inheritance	Heart Involvement	Age and Disease Traits
613609	*HFE*	*HFE* related-HH	Hemochromatosis, type1	AR	X[114]	Arthropathy, skin pigmentation, liver damage, diabetes, endocrine dysfunction, hypogonadism
608374	*HJV*	Hemojuvelin	Hemochromatosis, type 2A	AR	X X[115–117]	Earlier onset, <30 years old, hypogonadotrophic hypogonadism, liver damages and endocrine dysfunctions
606464	*HAMP*	Hepcidin Antimicrobial Peptide	Hemochromatosis, type 2B	AR	X[117]	
604720	*TFR2*	Transferrin Receptor 2	Hemochromatosis, type 3	AR	X[118]	Arthropathy, skin pigmentation, liver damage, diabetes, endocrine dysfunction, hypogonadism.
604653	*SLC40A1 (SLC11A3)*	Solute Carrier Family 40 (Iron-Regulated Transporter) Member 1	Hemochromatosis, type 4	AD	X[119]	Lower tolerance to phlebotomies, possible anemia
134770	*FTH1*	Ferritin Heavy Chain 1	Hemochromatosis, type 5	AR	X[120]	Heart involvement (7) by magnetic resonance

genetic testing in patients with elevated serum ferritin (>300 ng/mL) and transferrin saturation values (>55%). Timely diagnosis and treatment prevent iron overload; however, early treatment is limited by the clinically silent or minimally symptomatic manifestations of the disease. Although population screening for HH is controversial, the low cost of genetic tests and the selection of high-risk populations is cost-effective.[121]

The current global prevalence of the different genetic causes of HH can be easily estimated using multigene panels by Next Generation sequencing (NGS); this analysis also provides data on genetic epidemiology of the disease.[122]

Cardiac Involvement: Prevalence. Symptomatic hemochromatosis is estimated to occur in 1 in 500 individuals.[123] Common

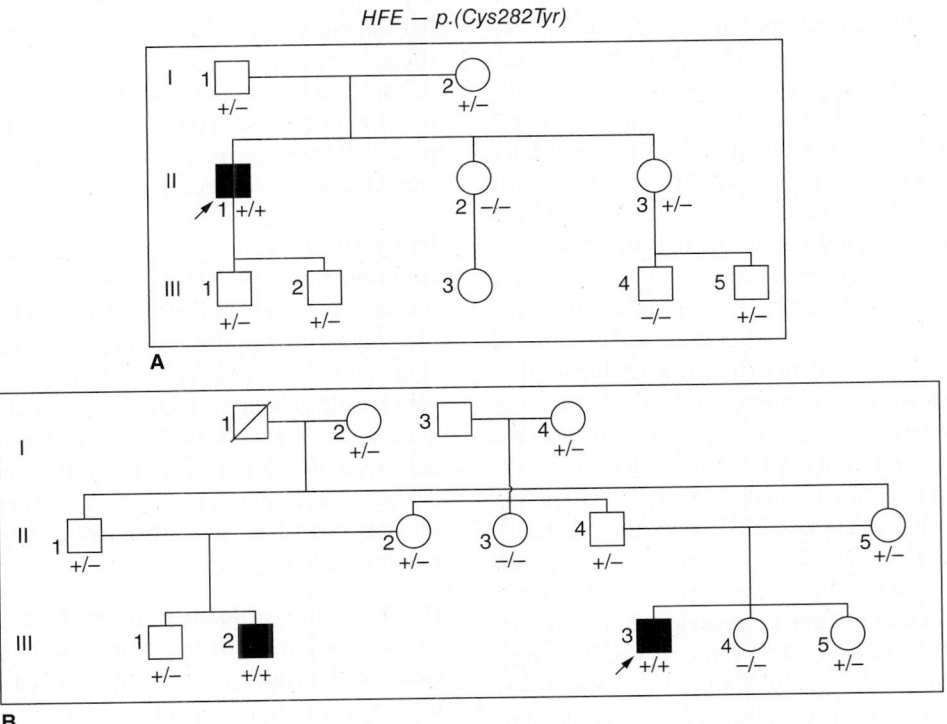

Figure 44-8. Family pedigrees of two patients with autosomal recessive hereditary hemochromatosis caused by homozygous mutation in the *HFE* gene. **(A)** In this family, the disease was apparently sporadic. After the diagnosis in the proband, family screening demonstrated that both parents of the proband are healthy carriers of heterozygous mutations p.(Cys282Tyr) in the *HFE* gene; both sons of the proband are obligate carriers. **(B)** A family in which the genetic diagnosis in the proband led to family screening and identification of a second affected family member.

presenting symptoms such as fatigue, malaise, and arthralgia are nonspecific.[113]

Physical examination. Previously, the clinical diagnosis was typically late and supported by the classic triad of cirrhosis, bronze skin, and diabetes. Today, the diagnosis is established in early phases of the disease when the clinical manifestations are attenuated but cardiac imaging may detect features suggestive of myocardial iron overload.

The electrocardiogram. This is nonspecific and does not significantly contribute to the diagnosis of HH cardiomyopathy; low QRS complex voltage and nonspecific repolarization abnormalities are uncommon in early phases; conduction disease may be present. Atrial fibrillation is the most common arrhythmia while ventricular arrhythmias may occur when the LV dysfunction has manifested.[113]

Echocardiography with TDI, strain imaging, speckle tracking. Two-dimensional echocardiographic evaluation shows early diastolic dysfunction[123] and later evolution through LV dilation and dysfunction. Restrictive physiology may persist in late disease;[124] in patients with asymptomatic cardiac involvement, it maintains stable after conventional phlebotomy treatment, regardless of their treatment history.[123] Echocardiography contributes to early diagnosis of cardiac involvement and provides information on the extent of iron storage and severity of systolic and diastolic dysfunction. In a multivariable analysis, spectral tissue Doppler lower early (E') diastolic velocity was independently associated with hemochromatosis.[125] Midseptal systolic and early diastolic velocities on TDI correlate with myocardial iron content predicted by magnetic resonance imaging.[126] Longer isovolumetric relaxation time and lower E' velocity indicate mildly impaired diastolic function; with aging, filling pressures increase as demonstrated by elevated transmitral early (E) filling velocity, pulmonary venous systolic peak velocity, and higher E/E'-ratio.[127] Real-time 3D echocardiography may contribute to earlier detection of left atrial dysfunction (eg, left atrial active emptying fraction) in asymptomatic patients with cardiac iron overload;[128] exercise stress TDI echocardiography may demonstrates subtle systolic abnormalities that would not have been detected by conventional echocardiography.[129]

CMR imaging:[130] The T2* method is highly sensitive and specific, especially useful for detecting, grading and monitoring iron deposition.[130–132] Patients demonstrating a T2* higher than 20 ms are at low risk for development of HF; T2* between 10 and 20 ms indicates the presence of cardiac iron deposition and an intermediate risk of HF; and a T2* less than 10 ms indicates high risk of HF and need for immediate chelation therapy.[133] The T2* index informs on the risk of HF and arrhythmias.[134] CMR further provides a comprehensive evaluation of myocardial viability, LV ejection fraction, cardiac volume, and mass.[135] The decline in LV ejection fraction correlates with the myocardial iron content measured with T2*.[136] Endomyocardial biopsy shows typical intramyocyte accumulation of iron (**Fig. 44–9**). However, when the diagnosis is established with clinical, imaging, and genetic data, EMB is no longer indicated.

Treatment and Monitoring: Phlebotomy and iron chelators (parenteral deferoxamine, or oral iron chelators, deferiprone and

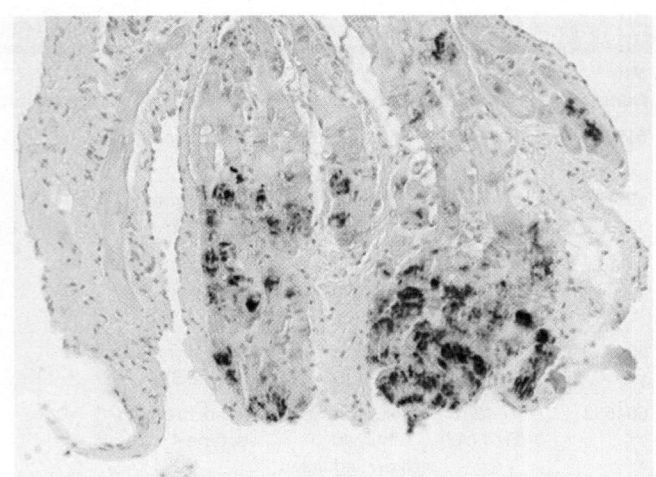

Figure 44–9. Endomyocardial biopsy obtained from a patient presenting with restrictive cardiomyopathy phenotype; the endomyocardial biopsy shows the intramyocyte accumulation of iron (*blue;* Perl's stain). In this patient, genetic testing identified the homozygous p.(Cys282Tyr) mutation in the *HFE* gene.

deferasirox) remain the standard therapy. Adequately treated patients (ie, target ferritin of 50–100 µg/l achieved) demonstrate better prognosis.[137] Chelation improves ventricular function, prevents ventricular arrhythmias and reduces mortality in patients with secondary iron overload. In patients with thalassemia, major and mild-to-moderate cardiac iron loading combination treatment with additional deferiprone reduces myocardial iron and improves ejection fraction and endothelial function.[124] In patients with HF, management is based on the same basic principles as patients with DCM and systolic HF (Chapter 48). Combined heart and liver transplantation should only be considered in severe cases refractory to standard therapies.[124,138] Iron overload–induced cardiomyopathy is reversible when therapy is started before the onset of overt HF.

Family Studies: HH is a genetically heterogeneous disease; common forms of HH are inherited as autosomal recessive diseases; in these families, heterozygous mutation carriers are phenotypically healthy and the illness may appear as sporadic (Fig. 44–8). The diagnosis of HH in a proband should activate family screening including both clinical evaluation and genetic testing. However, at least one of the genetic HH is autosomal dominant: in these families, genetic testing provides a preclinical evidence of the disease. Therefore, family screening may contribute to early diagnosis and should be routinely recommended.

Non-HH Iron Overload: Iron overload potentially involving the heart occurs in hemoglobinopathies (β-thalassemia major, sickle cell disease),[139] sideroblastic anemia,[140,141] myelodysplastic syndromes,[142] aplastic anemia,[143] patients with chronic kidney disease and treated with intravenous iron supplementation,[144] and patients with iron toxicosis (iron poisoning).[145]

Iron overload may occur in *β-thalassemia major,* which is an inherited autosomal recessive hemoglobin disorder causing chronic hemolytic anemia that requires life-long transfusion therapy.[146] Beta-thalassemia is a global health issue: the original geographic prevalence in the Mediterranean area, Southeast Asia, the Middle East, and North India has been modified by population migration to North Europe and North America.[146] Cardiac involvement is due to myocardial iron overload; it constitutes the primary cause of mortality and a major cause of morbidity for HF. The cardiac phenotypes include restrictive beta thalassemia cardiomyopathy and DCM[112] that is usually preceded by diastolic dysfunction (about 80% of cases);[147] in 20% of cases, RV dilation and dysfunction is associated with tricuspid regurgitation, increased pulmonary artery pressure, and restrictive LV filling.[139,148,149] Practice guidelines delineate recommendations for clinical monitoring and treatment (chelation therapy and cardiovascular medications).[150] The precise quantification of myocardial and hepatic iron load by CMR T2* imaging provides useful information on clinical response to iron chelation therapy.[133]

Sideroblastic anemias (SAs) can be either acquired or inherited and are characterized by impaired utilization of iron in the erythroblast, ineffective erythropoiesis, and variable systemic iron overload.[140] Heritable SAs are genetically heterogeneous diseases: heart involvement is occasionally reported. They include the X-linked recessive SA with ataxia caused by mutations in the *ABCB7* gene, the X-linked SA caused by mutations in the *ALAS2* gene; the autosomal recessive SA with myopathy and lactic acidosis (MLASA) caused by mutations in the genes *PUS1* and *YARS2*;[141] the autosomal recessive SA with B-cell immunodeficiency, periodic fevers, and developmental delay caused by mutations in the *TRNT1* gene; and the piridocine-refractory autosomal recessive SA caused by mutations in the *SLC25A38* and *GLRX5* genes. Mutations in *TRNT1* cause the autosomal recessive congenital sideroblastic anemia with immunodeficiency, fevers, and developmental delay (SIFD). In patients diagnosed with MLASA, HF with preserved ejection fraction and pericardial effusion has been reported.[141]

Mitochondrial Iron Overload: Friedreich's Ataxia: Friedreich's ataxia (FRDA) is caused by homozygous GAA trinucleotide repeat expansion that induces a transcriptional defect of the *Frataxin gene (FXN)*.[151] Frataxin is a small mitochondrial protein whose defects are associated with mitochondrial iron overload and are responsible for all phenotypic manifestations of FRDA. The disease affects central and peripheral nervous, cardiovascular, skeletal, and endocrine (particularly pancreatic function) systems. The cardiac involvement in FRDA is characterized by the HCM phenotype (Chapter 42), evolving to LV dysfunction. A restrictive filling pattern is observed in end-stage of Friedreich's cardiomyopathy.[152] Although early studies suggested that global diastolic function was preserved when examined by tissue Doppler,[153] recent studies demonstrate diastolic abnormalities in more than 25% of patients.[154]

Phenocopies of Restrictive Cardiomyopathy

Acquired multiorgan systemic diseases or cardiotoxicity may cause RCM phenotype. This group of diseases includes POEMS, chloroquine toxicity (which may clinically overlap with HCM-DCM), and sarcoidosis. This latter is discussed in the chapter on inflammatory heart diseases (Chapter 46).

POEMS Syndrome

POEMS syndrome (Polyneuropathy, Organomegaly, Endocrinopathy, M protein, and Skin changes) is a paraneoplastic syndrome caused by a plasma cell neoplasm. Diagnoses can be delayed because the clinical manifestations of the syndrome may overlap with other more common neurologic disorders (ie, chronic inflammatory demyelinating polyradiculoneuropathy).[155] Cardiovascular involvement is rare and clinically heterogeneous; it may include heart block,[156] pulmonary hypertension,[157] HF,[158] myocardial infarction,[159] cardiomegaly and cardiomyopathy,[160] and aortic valve fibroma.[161] Although repeatedly mentioned in review articles, RCM is a rare complication.[160]

Diabetes Mellitus-Related Cardiomyopathy

Diabetic cardiomyopathy (DM-CMP) is a clinical condition diagnosed when ventricular dysfunction occurs in the absence of coronary atherosclerosis and hypertension.[162] DM-CMP was originally described as a DCM with eccentric LV remodeling and systolic LV dysfunction. Recent clinical studies outline the prominent restrictive phenotype as one of the major characteristics of the disease. The cardiomyopathy is characterized by both morphologic abnormalities (concentric LVH) and functional abnormalities (diastolic LV dysfunction).[162–164] In DM-CMP, the restrictive phenotypes can progress from HF with preserved LV ejection fraction to HF with reduced LV ejection fraction[165,166] (Chapter 48). A possible hypothesis postulated that "the myocardial remodeling in HF with preserved LV ejection fraction is caused by coronary microvascular endothelial inflammation with cardiomyocytes only exposed to altered paracrine endothelial signaling, while HF with reduced LV ejection fraction is caused by cardiomyocyte cell death due to ischemia, viral infection, or toxic agents."[167] Therapeutic strategies differ between the two phenotypes. Angiotensin-converting enzyme inhibitors, β-blockers, angiotensin II receptor blockers, and mineralocorticoid-receptor antagonists are clearly indicated for diabetics with HF with reduced ejection fraction, while diuretics and lifestyle modifications demonstrated a proven survival benefit in those with HF with preserved ejection fraction.[166]

Microvascular deposition of advanced glycation end products in small myocardial vessels of patients with DM-CMP seems to be the pathologic hallmark of the disease.[168] Several factors have been proposed to play a role in the pathophysiology of the cardiomyopathy: the exposure of cardiac myocytes to hyperglycemia;[169] lipotoxicity and myocardial steatosis;[170] the microvascular deposition of end products of glycation;[171] microvascular dysfunction and rarefaction;[172] "autoimmune myocyte damage" with release of troponins;[173] and insulin resistance/hyperinsulinaemia that could explain myocyte hypertrophy.[168] The combination of the effects of these factors could induce either "restrictive" or "hypertrophic" cardiac phenotypes in patients with diabetes. The diagnostic criteria of the two different phenotypes are reported in the

ESC guidelines on diabetes, prediabetes, and cardiovascular diseases[174] (Chapter 7).

Other Conditions Variably Reported as "Restrictive Heart Diseases"

Cardiotoxic manifestations induced by a variety of drugs or substances (eg, serotonin, methysergide, ergotamine, mercurial agents, busulfan, or heavy metals) have been variably reported. Such substances may cause cardiac toxicity with diastolic dysfunction. However, the maintenance of confounding classifications and nosology delay progression of research, especially when clinical phenotypes are nonspecific, and causes are not proven. Diseases such as cardiac sarcoidosis, or hypereosinophilic diseases, are more appropriately grouped in the chapter on inflammatory heart diseases (Chapter 46). Chloroquine cardiotoxicity, which may manifest with LVH, dilation, and restriction, is revised in Chapter 41.

RESTRICTIVE ENDOMYOCARDIAL DISEASES

Introduction

Diseases affecting both endocardium and endomyocardial layers manifest with restrictive physiology and are functional phenocopies of genetic RCM. The three disorders that can be included in this subgroup of RCM are endocardial fibroelastosis, endomyocardial fibrosis, and "obliterative cardiomyopathy." From early to current classifications of cardiomyopathies, endocardial diseases have been placed in the group of unclassified cardiomyopathies.[2,3] Confusing terms (endocardial fibroelastosis, endomyocardial fibroelastosis, endomyocardial fibrosis, or obliterative cardiomyopathy) and phenotypes reflected the difficult nosology assignment of "pathology-based" diagnoses: the term *endocardial fibroelastosis* described a pathologic feature rather than a precise morphofunctional condition. It represents an endocardial reactive process that may occur in a variety of cardiac diseases (cardiomyopathies and congenital heart diseases, decompensated hearts of different etiology), more the endocardial effect of hemodynamic stressors rather than a primary endocardial disease or endocardium-specific insult[175] (**Fig. 44–10**). In addition, the majority of cases of "endocardial fibroelastosis" have been described in the pregenetic era. Vice versa, *endomyocardial fibrosis (EMF)*, mainly involving the right ventricle, is now recognized as a clinically and pathologically well-defined entity that affects primarily children and adolescents, often in resource-limited regions of sub-Saharan Africa, Latin America, and Asia;[176] it is the most common form of restrictive heart disease worldwide. Although the etiology remains elusive, the clinical profile, and disease course are well established. *Obliterative cardiomyopathy*[177]

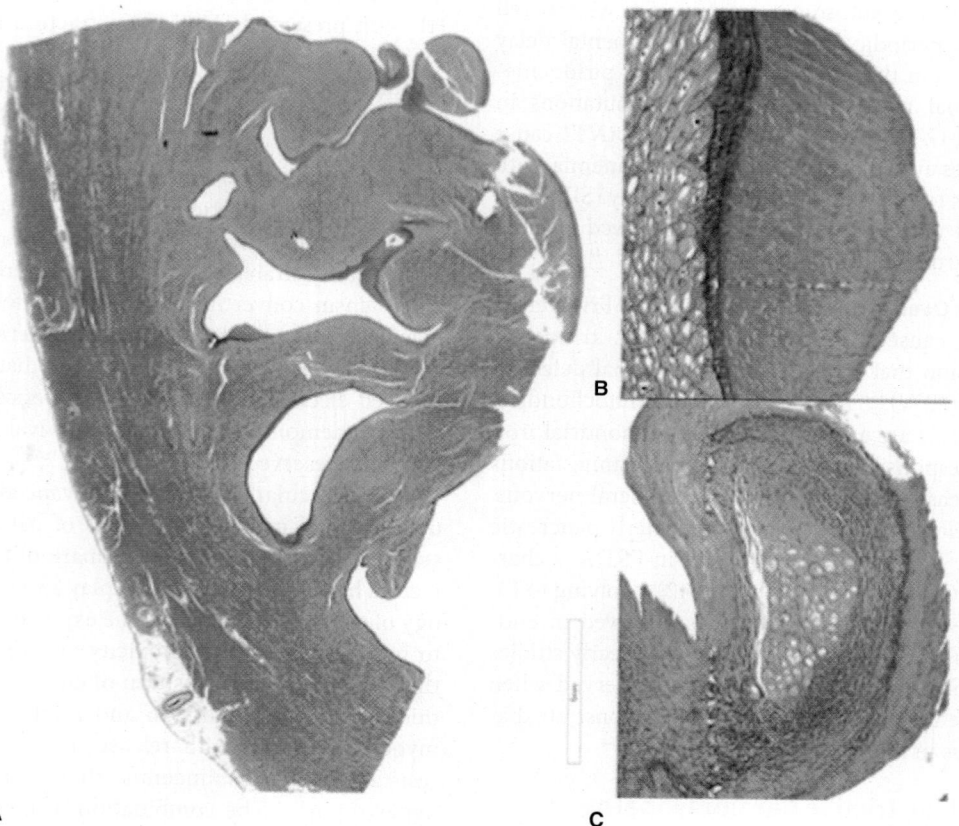

Figure 44–10. (A)–(C) Pathologic characteristics of fibroelastotic endocardial thickening versus fibrous endocardial thickening. The high-magnification views in (B) and (C) show the presence of elastic fibers; the low magnification in (A) gives the proportion of the features. Both findings are common and demonstrate variable extension in decompensated, end-stage hearts.

is a term that confusingly includes either cardiomyopathies with fibrous obliteration of the ventricular apex or the fibrous organization of apical thrombi, typically occurring in hypereosinophilic syndromes (HES) or in other heart diseases where apical thrombi can eventually undergo organization and fibrosis. HES are precisely classified and discussed in the chapter on inflammatory heart diseases (Chapter 46).

Endocardial Fibroelastosis

The term *endocardial fibroelastosis* describes a thickening of the endocardium by layers of collagen and elastic fibers. It corresponds to a right ventricular (RV) endocardial thickness of >10 μm, and an LV endocardial thickness of >20 μm. These microscopic features are commonly observed in several different diseases including congenital heart diseases, cardiomyopathies and decompensated valve disease. The macroscopic appearance shows variable extension of endocardial thickening and is characterized by "white" translucent endocardial ventricular areas versus the normal endocardial aspect.[175] By itself, it does not have a corresponding functional phenotype. Several attempts to identify and confirm a precise etiology have included a viral hypothesis, but mumps and Coxsackie B virus-related mechanisms have proven negative.[175] The possible involvement of lymphatic vessels of the heart has been proposed for both endocardial fibroelastosis and endocardial fibrosis and remains a potential contributor.[178] The term endomyocardial fibroelastosis is also used to describe the same entity.[179] Endocardial fibroelastosis (fibroelastotic thickening of the endocardium) has been repeatedly described in children with hypoplastic heart syndrome but it does not, by itself, demonstrate a causative role: in hypoplastic heart syndrome, the endocardial fibroelastosis is now described as "endocardial fibroelastosis reaction."[180] Its detection in fetal life is a relevant marker for a condition that can now be considered for prenatal interventions aimed at treatment of diastolic dysfunction.[181]

The association of fibroelastosis with endocardial fibroelastosis was originally placed in the group of "unclassified cardiomyopathies" and remains so in the most recent classifications of cardiomyopathies.[2,3] In a critical review article published in 2009, Paul R. Lurie states: "the contemporary author of a report on the endocardial fibroelastosis is confronted by a perplexing literature; most of which was composed when much more was seen, but much less was understood. Confused outdated concepts need to be corrected."[175] We believe that the arguments discussed in this editorial are substantiated by evidence and that this term can be maintained in pathology to describe thickened fibro-elastotic endocardium, which however does not have, by itself, a functional phenotype that justifies its placement in the list of cardiomyopathies. Past "fibroelastosis" cases, especially those that were observed in children with either cardiomyopathy or congenital heart diseases, may represent unrecognized genetic disorders.[182–185]

Endomyocardial Fibrosis

Endomyocardial fibrosis (EMF) is a restrictive endocardiomyopathy that preferentially affects children and adolescents.[186] The variation in geographic distribution supports the hypothesis that common environmental factors in these areas (infectious, nutritional, lifestyles, or climate) play a role in the pathogenesis of the disease.[186–188] However, its occurrence in a range of African, Latin American, and Asian populations does not support the hypothesis that ethnicity factors are associated with the disease.[186–188] The etiology is unknown: research on nutritional deficiencies (cerium, magnesium deficiency, cassava, and malnutrition, in general); infections (parasitic and viral diseases); and autoimmunity and allergic etiology remains unproven.

The RV endocardium is most commonly affected; occasionally, the disease may involve the left ventricle.[186] Patients with right-sided EMF are relatively asymptomatic, despite severe structural and functional abnormalities.[188]

Clinical Presentation and Diagnosis

The diagnosis is based on clinical manifestations and imaging and hemodynamic evaluations. Physical examination may demonstrate hyperpigmentation of the lips and gums, abdominal distension, exophthalmos, jaundice, parotid swelling, asthma-like episodes, finger clubbing, right-sided HF with ascites without lower limb edema even with voluminous ascites, and cyanosis.[189]

Chest x-ray shows cardiomegaly as a result of severe right atrial enlargement and/or pericardial effusion and a possible bulge over the left heart border related to infundibulum dilatation; lung fields are usually hypoperfused.

Electrocardiographic abnormalities include low-voltage QRS complexes, nonspecific ST–T wave changes, and conduction disturbances; in advanced right-sided EMF, the right atrial wave can be prominent and a QR pattern in V3 and V1 can be manifest. Atrial fibrillation is common and ventricular arrhythmias may also occur.[189,190]

Two-dimensional echocardiography demonstrates the thickened ventricular endocardium and provides information on ventricular size and function; obliteration of the RV trabecular portion; abnormal anatomy of both AV valves and subvalvular apparatus, annulus dilatation, and valve regurgitation; right atrial thrombi; pericardial effusion; and dilation of hepatic veins.[190–194] In advanced disease, the right side of the heart may physiologically act as a single functional chamber.[194]

CMR imaging is the ideal tool for both diagnosis of EMF and for monitoring following surgery.[195,196] It provides information on hemodynamics and fibrosis with precise topographic data and characterization of the extent of myocardial fibrosis.[196]

Cardiac catheterization. In advanced right EMF, there is equalization of pressures in the right atrium, right ventricle, and pulmonary artery. The RV angiogram shows loss of the trabeculated pattern, a flattened apex, reduction of ventricular volume, dilated hyper-contractile infundibulum, and free tricuspid reflux, up to severely dilated right atrium and cava veins.[197]

Pathology

EMF typically involves only the heart and spares other organs and tissues. The heart appears enlarged mostly due to atrial dilatation. The endocardium is thickened from fibrosis that is prominent in the right ventricle at the apical level. Endomyocardial fibrosis embeds the RV trabeculae, obliterates the apex of the right ventricle, and fixes the tricuspid valve apparatus.[198] The pulmonary valve leaflets and arteries are not involved. The coronary arteries and small intramural vessels are usually spared. Histologic study shows endocardial fibrous thickening, with myocyte damage with loss of myofibrillar components in the inner portion of the myocardium.[193,199,200] Inflammation is rare, eosinophils are uncommon, and there is no evidence that pathogens such as *Plasmodium falciparum* are causally linked to the disease.[201]

Natural History

The disease seems to evolve through three pathologic stages: endocardial necrosis, thrombosis, and fibrosis. The rate of progression of the three stages is difficult to establish: in fact, the disease is commonly diagnosed in advanced phases, when HF progresses rapidly and causes death within 2 years from onset of clinical manifestations.[186] In some patients, the disease course seems milder showing periods of clinical stability; other patients may experience clinical remission. EMF patients usually die from complications of progressive chronic HF leading to protein-losing enteropathy and hepatic failure. Sudden death can be caused by massive pulmonary embolism, systemic embolic events, or arrhythmias.[202] The thrombogenic and pulmonary embolic risks are high; advanced EMF is associated with chronic thromboembolic pulmonary disease.[198,203,204]

Management

Although there is no specific and effective treatment for EMF, HF therapy is used to control symptoms and reduce the progression of the disease (Chapter 48). Surgery, which resects the endomyocardial fibrosis layer and can include mitral and tricuspid valvuloplasty, constitutes a major advancement in the treatment strategy of EMF and is indicated for symptomatic patients.[205] However, "late presentation and/or lack of expertise and infrastructure for the surgical treatment" are reported as a limitation for the expansion of surgical treatments. Surgery is complicated by high mortality rate especially when the disease requires extensive endocardial resection or tricuspid valve replacement (15% and 30% respectively). Early surgery can prevent the development of pulmonary embolism and hypertension.[202]

The disease carries a poor prognosis: the morbidity and mortality related to refractory HF are high; thromboembolism and arrhythmia further increase the risk of mortality.[206] When possible, heart transplantation can be considered.[207] Innovative surgical approaches to right-sided EMF preventing complete AV block, preserving the native AV valves, releasing the myocardium, and making use of viable myocardium in the obliterated area can improve postoperative mortality and quality of life.[198]

Additional Considerations

EMF remains one of the most neglected cardiovascular diseases with "limited attention from the scientific community."[186,187] Research should concentrate on early diagnosis, treatment, and monitoring; modern imaging could help better elucidate the natural history of the disease and novel biotechnology tools could explore the evolving phenotypes and the cause/s at the molecular level. Indirect evidence that the amelioration of living standards (nutrition, control of infectious diseases) may contribute to control the disease come from India, where the incidence of the disease has declined in the last few decades in areas where the disease was previously endemic.[203] However, EMF remains endemic in many African countries such as Uganda and Mozambique, where it represents a public health problem.

Carcinoid Heart Disease

Introduction

Carcinoid heart disease (Hedinger syndrome) is a rare condition that affects the right side of the heart in up to 60% of patients with neuroendocrine tumors (NETs) and systemic carcinoid syndrome (CS).[208] NETs are rare (2.5 to 5.0 cases per 100,000 of the population per year), slowly progressing, low-grade malignancies with metastatic potential to the liver and possible release of vasoactive amines into the systemic circulation. NETs more commonly associated with carcinoid heart disease originate in the small bowel (72%) followed by those originating in the lung, appendix, large bowel, pancreas, and ovary; the primary site of the tumor remains undetermined in up to 20% of cases.[209] Carcinoid heart disease should be specifically investigated in patients diagnosed with NETs and CS; it carries a poor prognosis and is the major cause of mortality and morbidity.[209,210] Early data reported a mean survival of 1.6 years in patients with NET and cardiac involvement compared with 4.6 years in those with NET and without CS.[211]

CS is caused by vasoactive substances secreted by NET cells. 5-hydroxytryptamine (5-HT, serotonin) is the main peptide, followed by prostaglandins, histamine, bradykinin, tachykinins, and transforming growth factor-β (TGF-β). Both the tachynines and TGF-β display profibrogenic properties inducing fibromixoid plaques that affect the RV endocardium, the ventricular side of the tricuspid valve apparatus (leaflets, chordae and papillary muscles), the ventricular site of the pulmonary valve, and less commonly, the pulmonary artery. Fibromixoid plaques covered by endothelial cells are constituted of fibroblasts, myofibroblasts, smooth muscle cells, collagen, and myxoid material.[209] When the liver is spared by the neoplasm, vasoactive peptides undergo inactivation; however, when hepatic metabolic function is impaired by metastatic dissemination, the vasoactive peptides remain active, thus causing the classical CS.[212] The presence of liver metastases is nonobligate for the development of CS: ovarian NETs may drain into the systemic circulation[213] and patients with retroperitoneal lymphatic metastases may develop CS.

Phenotype and Cardiac Involvement

The clinical phenotype of typical or classic CS is characterized by cutaneous flushing, gut hypermobility with diarrhea, and bronchospasm with wheezing and shortness of breath;[209] the lung variant is characterized by episodes of flushing, headache, and shortness of breath.[214] Depending on the severity of endocardial and tricuspid scarring, the functional effects can be either valve regurgitation or stenosis. The left heart is usually spared but can be involved in patients with patent foramen ovale. Signs and symptoms can be subtle even in patients with cardiac involvement; when present, symptoms include exertional dyspnea and fatigue. As the disease progresses, dyspnea worsens and signs and symptoms of right-sided HF may manifest.[215]

The clinical diagnosis is facilitated by the precise oncologic characterization of the neoplasm; the physical examination may demonstrate elevated jugular venous pressure and a palpable RV impulse; murmurs due to right-sided valve regurgitation are frequent while pulmonary and tricuspid stenosis murmurs are rare.[215]

Imaging. Two-dimensional echocardiography demonstrates tricuspid regurgitation, thickened and hypomobile pulmonary leaflets, and right-side chamber dilation and hypokinesia. In a large series of 252 patients with CS, 52 had carcinoid heart disease. In most severe cases, a 2D transthoracic echocardiogram (TTE) showed thickened, retracted, and noncoapting leaflets; the chordae and papillary muscles were thickened, fused, and shortened; A 3D-TEE showed that all three leaflets were fixed in a semi-open position, thus confirming the noncoaptation. TEE demonstrates thickened RV endocardium with probable deposition of carcinoid plaque.[216] Imaging-based monitoring is recommended by the Guidelines from the Consensus European Neuroendocrine Tumor Society (ENETS): annual echocardiography should be part of the routine surveillance of patients with carcinoid heart disease.[217,218] CMR and CT scans can be variably used to refine, confirm, or implement diagnostic data.[216]

Biomarkers contribute to both diagnosis and monitoring: serum serotonin, platelet serotonin, and urinary 5-hydroxyindoleacetic acid levels are elevated;[219] chromogranin A has also been suggested as a sensitive marker for patients with NETs and carcinoid heart disease.[220] High levels of NT-proBNP are usually measured in patients with remodeled RV chambers;[221] levels of connective tissue growth factor (CTGF) and of TGF-β have been reported as independent predictors of RV dysfunction.[222] Activin A levels can be increased independently of RV dilation;[223] together with impaired myocardial function, levels of Activin A seem to predict mortality in patients with carcinoid intestinal disease.[224]

Management
Once CS is diagnosed, the cardiac involvement should be systematically investigated, monitored, and treated; somatostatin analogues are well-established and well-tolerated antisecretory drugs that have been used as first-line treatment for symptomatic control in hormonally active NETs for three decades. They include depot formulations, long-acting repeatable octreotide, and lanreotide autogel. Treatment has been proven to be associated with significant prolongation of progression-free survival.[225] For patients with symptomatic carcinoid heart disease, tricuspid valve surgery is the only effective treatment option. Without operation, only 10% of patients survive 2 years after the onset of NYHA functional class III or IV symptoms.

A recent study investigated the short-term and long-term outcomes in 195 consecutive patients (70% in NYHA class III and IV) with carcinoid heart disease who underwent tricuspid valve replacement (and further pulmonary valve surgery, n = 157) during a 27-year period (1985–2012) at one institution. Perioperative death was 10% and declined after 2000 (6%). Survival rates (95% confidence intervals) at 1, 5, and 10 years were 69%, 35%, and 24% (18%–32%), respectively. Older age, cytotoxic chemotherapy, and tobacco use were independent predictors of death.[226] The surgical risk also depends on the severity of the RV dysfunction, the involvement of the LV chambers, and on the possible occurrence of carcinoid crises during surgery.[227,228]

SUMMARY

Restrictive heart diseases are a complex group of diseases encompassing a large number of myocardial, endocardial, and pericardial disorders, each of them with different possible etiologies. They all share diastolic dysfunction as a common marker, often without LVH.

Primary Restrictive Cardiomyopathy: The Rarest Genetic Cardiomyopathy
The hallmarks are:

- Impaired ventricular filling with restrictive physiology
- Presence of normal or reduced diastolic volumes of one or both ventricles
- Normal or reduced systolic volumes
- Normal ventricular wall thickness
- Normal AV valves
- Bilateral atrial dilation

The most common disease genes are *TNNI3* and *DES*. Less frequently, *MYPN* and *FLNC* as well as other genes also associated with nonrestrictive cardiomyopathies are involved. The disease course is characterized by progression through end-stage heart failure and the need for substitutive treatment.

Restrictive Cardiomyopathy Phenocopies: Includes Multiorgan Genetic Diseases/Syndromes

- Pseudoxanthoma elasticum, a rare autosomal recessive systemic disease of the connective tissue caused by mutation in the *ACBB6* gene.
- Nephropathic cystinosis, a rare lysosomal storage autosomal recessive disease resulting from intracellular accumulation of cystine caused by cystinosin defects (encoded by *CTNS* gene).
- Other lysosomal storage diseases more typically included in HCM phenocopies with possible restrictive phenotype: glycogenoses, Anderson–Fabry Disease, Danon Disease, and Hurler Disease.
- Iron-overload heart diseases, both hereditary hemochromatosis (HH-HFE1) and the non-HH/non-HFE1 iron overload diseases such as hematological diseases with possible iron accumulation, including iron toxicosis.

Restrictive Endomyocardial Diseases

- Endomyocardial fibrosis (EMF) is now recognized as a clinically and pathologically well-defined entity that primarily affects children and adolescents, often in resource-limited regions of sub-Saharan Africa, Latin America, and Asia; it is the most common form of restrictive heart disease worldwide.

- Hedinger syndrome or carcinoid heart disease is a rare condition that affects the right side of the heart in up to 60% of patients with neuroendocrine tumors (NETs) and systemic carcinoid syndrome.

ACKNOWLEDGMENT

In the previous edition(s), this chapter was contributed to by Alessandra Serio, Valentina Favalli, and Giovanni Palladini, and portions of that chapter have been retained.

REFERENCES

1. Kushwaha SS, Fallon JT, Fuster V. Restrictive cardiomyopathy. *N Engl J Med.* 1997;336:267-276.

2. Elliott P, Andersson B, Arbustini E, et al. Classification of the cardiomyopathies: a position statement from the European Society of Cardiology Working Group on Myocardial and Pericardial Diseases. *Eur Heart J.* 2008;29:270-276.

3. Maron BJ, Towbin JA, Thiene G, et al. Contemporary definitions and classification of the cardiomyopathies: an American Heart Association Scientific Statement from the Council on Clinical Cardiology, Heart Failure and Transplantation Committee; Quality of Care and Outcomes Research and Functional Genomics and Translational Biology Interdisciplinary Working Groups; and Council on Epidemiology and Prevention. *Circulation.* 2006;113:1807-1816.

4. Miura K, Nakagawa H, Morikawa Y, et al. Epidemiology of idiopathic cardiomyopathy in Japan: results from a nationwide survey. *Heart.* 2002;87:126-130.

5. Mogensen J, Arbustini E. Restrictive cardiomyopathy. *Curr Opin Cardiol.* 2009;24:214-220.

6. Teo LY, Moran RT, Tang WH. evolving approaches to genetic evaluation of specific cardiomyopathies. *Curr Heart Fail Rep.* 2015;12:339-349.

7. Kaski JP, Syrris P, Burch et al. Idiopathic restrictive cardiomyopathy in children is caused by mutations in cardiac sarcomere protein genes. *Heart.* 2008;94:1478-1484.

8. Zangwill S, Hamilton R. Restrictive cardiomyopathy. *Pacing Clin Electrophysiol.* 2009;32 Suppl 2:S41-43.

9. Ammash NM, Seward JB, Bailey KR, Edwards WD, Tajik AJ. Clinical profile and outcome of idiopathic restrictive cardiomyopathy. *Circulation.* 2000;101:2490-2496.

10. Cimiotti D, Budde H, Hassoun R, Jaquet K. Genetic restrictive cardiomyopathy: causes and consequences-an integrative approach. *Int J Mol Sci.* 2021;22(2):558.

11. Araki K, Ueno T, Taira M, Kanaya T, Watanabe T, et al. Pediatric patient with restrictive cardiomyopathy on staged biventricular assist device support with Berlin Heart EXCOR® underwent heart transplantation successfully: the first case in Japan. *J Artif Organs.* 2020; Sep 10.

12. Maskatia SA, Decker JA, Spinner JA, et al. Restrictive physiology is associated with poor outcomes in children with hypertrophic cardiomyopathy. *Pediatr Cardiol.* 2012;33:141-149.

13. Raeisi-Giglou P, Rodriguez ER, Blackstone EH, Tan CD, Hsich EM. Verification of heart disease: implications for a new heart transplantation allocation system. *JACC Heart Fail.* 2017;5(12):904-913.

14. Chapman CB, Ewer SM, Kelly AF, Jacobson KM, Leal MA, Rahko PS. Classification of left ventricular diastolic function using American Society of Echocardiography Guidelines: agreement among echocardiographers. *Echocardiography.* 2013;30:1022-1031.

15. Dragulescu A, Mertens L, Friedberg MK. Interpretation of left ventricular diastolic dysfunction in children with cardiomyopathy by echocardiography: problems and limitations. *Circ Cardiovasc Imaging.* 2013;6:254-261.

16. Amaki M, Savino J, Ain DL, et al. Diagnostic concordance of echocardiography and cardiac magnetic resonance-based tissue tracking for differentiating constrictive pericarditis from restrictive cardiomyopathy. *Circ Cardiovasc Imaging.* 2014;7:819-827.

17. Partridge J. The restrictive cardiomyopathies. *Clin Radiol.* 2012;67:1034.

18. Gupta A, Singh Gulati G, Seth S, Sharma S. Cardiac MRI in restrictive cardiomyopathy. *Clin Radiol.* 2012;67:95-105.

19. Mavrogeni S, Markousis-Mavrogenis G, Markussis V, Kolovou G. the emerging role of cardiovascular magnetic resonance imaging in the evaluation of metabolic cardiomyopathies. *Horm Metab Res.* 2015;47:623-632.

20. Mavrogeni S. Evaluation of myocardial iron overload using magnetic resonance imaging. *Blood Transfus.* 2009;7:183-187.

21. Ayoub C, Pena E, Ohira H, Dick A, Leung E, Nery PB, Birnie D, Beanlands RS. Advanced imaging of cardiac sarcoidosis. *Curr Cardiol Rep.* 2015;17:17.

22. Arbustini E, Morbini P, Grasso M, et al. Restrictive cardiomyopathy, atrioventricular block and mild to subclinical myopathy in patients with desmin-immunoreactive material deposits. *J Am Coll Cardiol.* 1998;31:645-653.

23. Arbustini E, Grasso M, Rindi G, et al. H and L ferritins in myocardium in iron overload. *Am J Cardiol.* 1991;68:1233-1236.

24. Koeppen AH, Ramirez RL, Becker AB, et al. The pathogenesis of cardiomyopathy in Friedreich ataxia. *PLoS One.* 2015;10:e0116396.

25. Vicari P, Sthel VM. Images in clinical medicine. Cystine crystals in bone marrow. *N Engl J Med.* 2015;373:e27.

26. Dixit MP, Greifer I. Nephropathic cystinosis associated with cardiomyopathy: a 27-year clinical follow-up. *BMC Nephrol.* 2002;3:8.

27. Giovannoni I, Callea F, Travaglini L, et al. Heart transplant and 2-year follow up in a child with generalized arterial calcification of infancy. *Eur J Pediatr.* 2014;173:1735-1740.

28. Gambarin FI, Disabella E, Narula J, et al. When should cardiologists suspect Anderson-Fabry disease? *Am J Cardiol.* 2010;106:1492-1499.

29. Ben-Ami R, Puglisi J, Haider T, Mehta D. The Mount Sinai Hospital clinical pathological conference: a 45-year-old man with Pompe's disease and dilated cardiomyopathy. *Mt Sinai J Med.* 2001;68:205-212.

30. González-López E, Gallego-Delgado M, Guzzo-Merello G, et al. Wild-type transthyretin amyloidosis as a cause of heart failure with preserved ejection fraction. *Eur Heart J.* 2015;36:2585-2594.

31. Fuchs U, Zittermann A, Schulz U, et al. Unusual case of an 18-year-old heart transplant recipient with endocardial fibroelastosis. *Transplant Proc.* 2006;38:1511-1513.

32. Séguéla PE, Iriart X, Acar P, Montaudon M, Roudaut R, Thambo JB. Eosinophilic cardiac disease: Molecular, clinical and imaging aspects. *Arch Cardiovasc Dis.* 2015;108:258-268.

33. Kusano KF, Satomi K. Diagnosis and treatment of cardiac sarcoidosis. *Heart.* 2016;102:184-190.

34. Rapezzi C, Arbustini E, Caforio AL, et al. Diagnostic work-up in cardiomyopathies: bridging the gap between clinical phenotypes and final diagnosis. A position statement from the ESC Working Group on Myocardial and Pericardial Diseases. *Eur Heart J.* 2013;34:1448-1458.

35. Syed FF, Schaff HV, Oh JK. Constrictive pericarditis-a curable diastolic heart failure. *Nat Rev Cardiol.* 2014;11:530-544.

36. Welch TD, Ling LH, Espinosa RE, et al. Echocardiographic diagnosis of constrictive pericarditis: Mayo Clinic criteria. *Circ Cardiovasc Imaging.* 2014;7:526-534.

37. Klein AL, Abbara S, Agler DA, et al. American Society of Echocardiography clinical recommendations for multimodality cardiovascular imaging of patients with pericardial disease: endorsed by the Society for Cardiovascular Magnetic Resonance and Society of Cardiovascular Computed Tomography. *J Am Soc Echocardiogr*. 2013;26:965-1012.

38. Oh JK, Hatle LK, Seward JB, et al. Diagnostic role of Doppler echocardiography in constrictive pericarditis. *J Am Coll Cardiol*. 1994;23:154-162.

39. Veress G, DaLi Feng, Jae K. Oh. Echocardiography in pericardial diseases: new development. *Heart Fail Rev*. 2013;18:267-275.

40. Aquaro GD, Barison A, Cagnolo A, Todiere G, Lombardi M, Emdin M. Role of tissue characterization by Cardiac Magnetic Resonance in the diagnosis of constrictive pericarditis. *Int J Cardiovasc Imaging*. 2015;31:1021-1031.

41. Parakh N, Mehrotra S, Seth S, et al. NT pro B type natriuretic peptide levels in constrictive pericarditis and restrictive cardiomyopathy. *Indian Heart J*. 2015;67:40-44.

42. Charron P, Arad M, Arbustini E, et al. Genetic counselling and testing in cardiomyopathies: a position statement of the European Society of Cardiology Working Group on Myocardial and Pericardial Diseases. *Eur Heart J*. 2010;31:2715-2726.

43. Mogensen J, Kubo T, Duque M, et al. Idiopathic restrictive cardiomyopathy is part of the clinical expression of cardiac troponin I mutations. *J Clin Invest*. 2003;111:209-216.

44. Arbustini E, Narula N, Tavazzi L, et al. The MOGE(S) classification of cardiomyopathy for clinicians. *J Am Coll Cardiol*. 2014;64:304-318.

45. Gambarin FI, Tagliani M, Arbustini E. Pure restrictive cardiomyopathy associated with cardiac troponin I gene mutation: mismatch between the lack of hypertrophy and the presence of disarray. *Heart*. 2008;94:1257.

46. van den Wijngaard A, Volders P, Van Tintelen JP, et al. Recurrent and founder mutations in the Netherlands: cardiac troponin I (TNNI3) gene mutations as a cause of severe forms of hypertrophic and restrictive cardiomyopathy. *Neth Heart J*. 2011;19:344-351.

47. Kubo T, Gimeno JR, Bahl A, et al. Prevalence, clinical significance, and genetic basis of hypertrophic cardiomyopathy with restrictive phenotype. *J Am Coll Cardiol*. 2007;49:2419-2426.

48. Caleshu C, Sakhuja R, Nussbaum RL, et al. Furthering the link between the sarcomere and primary cardiomyopathies: restrictive cardiomyopathy associated with multiple mutations in genes previously associated with hypertrophic or dilated cardiomyopathy. *Am J Med Genet A*. 2011;155A:2229-2235.

49. Sen-Chowdhry S, Syrris P, McKenna WJ. Genetics of restrictive cardiomyopathy. *Heart Fail Clin*. 2010;6:179-186.

50. Teekakirikul P, Kelly MA, Rehm HL, Lakdawala NK, Funke BH. Inherited cardiomyopathies: molecular genetics and clinical genetic testing in the postgenomic era. *J Mol Diagn*. 2013;15:158-167.

51. Ackerman MJ, Priori SG, Willems S, et al. HRS/EHRA expert consensus statement on the state of genetic testing for the channelopathies and cardiomyopathies: this document was developed as a partnership between the Heart Rhythm Society (HRS) and the European Heart Rhythm Association (EHRA). *Heart Rhythm*. 2011;8:1308-1339.

52. Mogensen J, Hey T, Lambrecht S. A Systematic review of phenotypic features associated with cardiac troponin I mutations in hereditary cardiomyopathies. *Can J Cardiol*. 2015;31:1377-1385.

53. Rai TS, Ahmad S, Ahluwalia TS, et al. Genetic and clinical profile of Indian patients of idiopathic restrictive cardiomyopathy with and without hypertrophy. *Mol Cell Biochem*. 2009;331:187-192.

54. Kostareva A, Gudkova A, Sjoberg G, et al. Deletion in TNNI3 gene is associated with restrictive cardiomyopathy. *Int J Cardiol*. 2009;131:410-412.

55. Chen Y, Yang S, Li J, et al. Pediatric restrictive cardiomyopathy due to a heterozygous mutation of the TNNI3 gene. *J Biomed Res*. 2014;28:59-63.

56. Menon SC, Michels VV, Pellikka PA, et al. Cardiac troponin T mutation in familial cardiomyopathy with variable remodeling and restrictive physiology. *Clin Genet*. 2008;74:445-454.

57. Ware SM, Quinn ME, Ballard ET, Miller E, Uzark K, Spicer RL. Pediatric restrictive cardiomyopathy associated with a mutation in β-myosin heavy chain. *Clin Genet*. 2008;73:165-170.

58. Purevjav E, Arimura T, Augustin S, et al. Molecular basis for clinical heterogeneity in inherited cardiomyopathies due to myopalladin mutations. *Hum Mol Genet*. 2012;21:2039-2053.

59. Kostera-Pruszczyk A, Suszek M, Płoski R, et al. BAG3-related myopathy, polyneuropathy and cardiomyopathy with long QT syndrome. *J Muscle Res Cell Motil*. 2015;36:423-432.

60. Kley RA, Hellenbroich Y, van der Ven PF, et al. Clinical and morphological phenotype of the filamin myopathy: a study of 31 German patients. *Brain*. 2007;130:3250-3264.

61. Brodehl A, Ferrier RA, Hamilton SJ et al. Mutations in FLNC are associated with familial restrictive cardiomyopathy. *Hum Mutat*. 2016;37:269-279.

62. Capetanaki Y, Papathanasiou S, Diokmetzidou A, Vatsellas G, Tsikitis M. Desmin related disease: a matter of cell survival failure. *Curr Opin Cell Biol*. 2015;32:113-120.

63. Ramspacher C, Steed E, Boselli F, et al. developmental alterations in heart biomechanics and skeletal muscle function in desmin mutants suggest an early pathological root for desminopathies. *Cell Rep*. 2015;11:1564-1576.

64. Benvenuti LA, Aiello VD, Falcão BA, Lage SG. Atrioventricular block pathology in cardiomyopathy by desmin deposition. *Arq Bras Cardiol*. 2012;98:e3-e6.

65. Arbustini E, Pasotti M, Pilotto A, et al. Desmin accumulation restrictive cardiomyopathy and atrioventricular block associated with desmin gene defects. *Eur J Heart Fail*. 2006;8:477-483.

66. Clemen CS, Stöckigt F, Strucksberg KH, et al. The toxic effect of R350P mutant desmin in striated muscle of man and mouse. *Acta Neuropathol*. 2015;129:297-315.

67. Arbustini E, Narula N, Dec GW, et al. The MOGE(S) classification for a phenotype-genotype nomenclature of cardiomyopathy: endorsed by the World Heart Federation. *J Am Coll Cardiol*. 2013;62:2046-2072.

68. Bär H, Goudeau B, Wälde S, et al. Conspicuous involvement of desmin tail mutations in diverse cardiac and skeletal myopathies. *Hum Mutat*. 2007;28:374-386.

69. Musumeci MB, Semprini L, Casenghi M, et al. Restrictive cardiomyopathy and pseudoxanthoma elasticum skin lesions. *J Cardiovasc Med (Hagerstown)*. 2014;15.

70. Basit S, Malibari O, Al Balwi AM, Abdusamad F, Abu Ismail F. A founder splice site mutation underlies glycogen storage disease type 3 in consanguineous Saudi families. *Ann Saudi Med*. 2014;34:390-395.

71. Hamidi Asl L, Liepnieks JJ, Hamidi Asl K, Uemichi T, Moulin G, et al. Hereditary amyloid cardiomyopathy caused by a variant apolipoprotein A1. *Am J Pathol*. 1999;154:221-227.

72. Dubrey SW, Comenzo RL. Amyloid diseases of the heart: current and future therapies. *QJM*. 2012;105:617-631.

73. Stangou AJ1, Banner NR, Hendry BM, Hereditary fibrinogen A alphachain amyloidosis: phenotypic characterization of a systemic disease and the role of liver transplantation. *Blood*. 2010;115:2998-3007.

74. Leslie N, Tinkle BT. Glycogen storage disease type II (Pompe disease). In: Pagon RA, Adam MP, Ardinger HH, et al., eds. *GeneReviews®*. Seattle, WA: University of Washington, Seattle; 2007 [updated May 9, 2013].

75. Solanich X, Claver E, Carreras F, et al. Myocardial infiltration in Gaucher's disease detected by cardiac MRI. *Int J Cardiol*. 2012;155:e5-e6.

76. Magoulas PL, El-Hattab AW. Glycogen storage disease type IV. In: Pagon RA, Adam MP, Ardinger HH, et al., eds. *GeneReviews*. Seattle, WA: University of Washington, Seattle; 2013.

77. Weidemann F, Ertl G, Wanner C, Krämer J. The Fabry cardiomyopathy—diagnostic approach and current treatment. *Curr Pharm Des*. 2015;21:473-478.

78. Kiuru S1, Matikainen E, Kupari M, Haltia M, Palo J. Autonomic nervous system and cardiac involvement in familial amyloidosis, Finnish type (FAF). *J Neurol Sci*. 1994;126:40-48.

79. Santos PC1, Krieger JE, Pereira AC. Molecular diagnostic and pathogenesis of hereditary hemochromatosis. *Int J Mol Sci.* 2012;13:1497-1511.

80. Wiseman DH, Mercer J, Tylee K, et al. Management of mucopolysaccharidosis type IH (Hurler's syndrome) presenting in infancy with severe dilated cardiomyopathy: a single institution's experience. *J Inherit Metab Dis.* 2013;36:263-270.

81. Endo Y, Furuta A, Nishino I. Danon disease: a phenotypic expression of LAMP-2 deficiency. *Acta Neuropathol.* 2015;129:391-398.

82. Musumeci O, Bruno C, Mongini T, et al. Clinical features and new molecular findings in muscle phosphofructokinase deficiency (GSD type VII). *Neuromuscul Disord.* 2012;22325-22330.

83. Roscher A, Patel J, Hewson S. et al. The natural history of glycogen storage disease types VI and IX: long-term outcome from the largest metabolic center in Canada. *Mol Genet Metab.* 2014;113:171-176.

84. Porto AG, Brun F, Severini GM, et al. Clinical spectrum of PRKAG2 syndrome. *Circ Arrhythm Electrophysiol.* 2016;9:pii.e003121.

85. Goeppert B, Lindner M, Vogel MN, Noncompaction myocardium in association with type Ib glycogen storage disease. *Pathol Res Pract.* 2012;208:620-622.

86. Uitto J, Pulkkinen L, Ringpfeil F. Molecular genetics of pseudoxanthoma elasticum: a metabolic disorder at the environment-genome interface? *Trends Mol Med.* 2001;7:13-17.

87. Uitto J, Jiang Q. Pseudoxanthoma elasticum-like phenotypes: more diseases than one. *J Invest Dermatol.* 2007;127:507-510.

88. Nitschke Y, Baujat G, Botschen U et al. Generalized arterial calcification of infancy and pseudoxanthoma elasticum can be caused by mutations in either ENPP1 or ABCC6. *Am J Hum Genet.* 2012;90:25-39.

89. Navarro-Lopez F, Llorian A, Ferrer-Roca O, Betriu A, Sanz G. Restrictive cardiomyopathy in pseudoxanthoma elasticum. *Chest.* 1980;78:113-115.

90. Stöllberger C, Finsterer J. Extracardiac medical and neuromuscular implications in restrictive cardiomyopathy. *Clin Cardiol.* 2007;30:375-380.

91. Combrinck M, Gilbert JD, Byard RW. Pseudoxanthoma elasticum and sudden death. *J Forensic Sci.* 2011;56:418-422.

92. Lebwohl M, Halperin J, Phelps RG. Brief report: occult pseudoxanthoma elasticum in patients with premature cardiovascular disease. *N Engl J Med.* 1993;329:1237-1239.

93. De Vilder EY, Hosen MJ, Vanakker OM. The ABCC6 transporter as a paradigm for networking from an orphan disease to complex disorders. *Biomed Res Int.* 2015;2015:648569.

94. Iliás A, Urbán Z, Seidl TL, et al. Loss of ATP-dependent transport activity in pseudoxanthoma elasticum-associated mutants of human ABCC6 (MRP6). *J Biol Chem.* 2002;277:16860-16867.

95. Prulière-Escabasse V, Planès C, Escudier E, Fanen P, Coste A, Clerici C. Modulation of epithelial sodium channel trafficking and function by sodium 4-phenylbutyrate in human nasal epithelial cells. *J Biol Chem.* 2007;282:34048-34057.

96. Uitto J, Váradi A, Bercovitch L, Terry PF, Terry SF. Pseudoxanthoma elasticum: progress in research toward treatment: summary of the, PXE international research meeting. *J Invest Dermatol.* 2012;2013:1444-1449.

97. Yoo JY, Blum RR, Singer GK, A randomized controlled trial of oral phosphate binders in the treatment of pseudoxanthoma elasticum. *J Am Acad Dermatol.* 2011;65:341-348.

98. Gahl WA, Thoene JG, Schneider JA. Cystinosis. *N Engl J Med.* 2002;347:111-121.

99. Town M, Jean G, Cherqui S, Attard M, et al. A novel gene encoding an integral membrane protein is mutated in nephropathic cystinosis. *Nat Genet.* 1998;18:319-324.

100. Kleta R, Anikster Y, Lucero C, et al. *CTNS* mutations in African American patients with cystinosis. *Mol Genet Metab.* 2001;74:332-337.

101. Kushlaf H. Cystinosis myopathy: Searching for optimal clinical outcome measures. *Muscle Nerve.* 2020;62(6):652-653.

102. Ueda M, O'Brien K, Rosing DR, Ling A, Kleta R, et al. Coronary artery and other vascular calcifications in patients with cystinosis after kidney transplantation. *Clin J Am Soc Nephrol.* 2006;1(3):555-562.

103. Tajdini M, Bayati M, Vasheghani-Farahani A. Aortic dissection and cystinosis: is there any relationship? *Cardiol Young.* 2017;27(7):1434-1436.

104. Edelman M, Silverstein D, Strom J, Factor SM. Cardiomyopathy in a male with cystinosis. *Cardiovasc Pathol.* 1997;6(1):43-47.

105. Ramappa AJ, Pyatt JR. Pregnancy-associated cardiomyopathy occurring in a young patient with nephropathic cystinosis. *Cardiol Young.* 2010;20(2):220-222.

106. Ahmed I, Phan TT, Lipkin GW, Frenneaux M. Ventricular noncompaction in a female patient with nephropathic cystinosis: a case report. *J Med Case Rep.* 2009;3:31.

107. Dixit MP, Greifer I. Nephropathic cystinosis associated with cardiomyopathy: a 27-year clinical follow-up. *BMC Nephrol.* 2002;3:8.

108. Ivanova E, De Leo MG, De Matteis MA, Levtchenko E. Cystinosis: clinical presentation, pathogenesis and treatment. *Pediatr Endocrinol Rev.* 2014;176-184.

109. Kashtan CE, McEnery PT, Tejani A, Stablein DM. Renal allograft survival according to primary diagnosis: a report of the North American Pediatric Renal Transplant Cooperative Study. *Pediatr Nephrol.* 1995;9:679-684.

110. Haverty T, Wyatt DJ, Porter KM, Leubitz A, Banks K, et al. Phase 1 renal impairment trial results supports targeted individualized dosing of ELX-02 in patients with nephropathic cystinosis. *J Clin Pharmacol.* 2020;Dec 23.

111. Buja LM, Roberts WC. Iron in the heart. Etiology and clinical significance. *Am J Med.* 1971;51:209-221.

112. Kremastinos DT, Tsetsos GA, Tsiapras DP, Karavolias GK, Ladis VA, Kattamis CA. Heart failure in beta thalassemia: a 5-year follow-up study. *Am J Med.* 2001;111:349-354.

113. Gulati V, Harikrishnan P, Palaniswamy C, Aronow WS, Jain D, Frishman WH. Cardiac involvement in hemochromatosis. *Cardiol Rev.* 2014;22:56-68.

114. Alexander J, Kowdley KV. HFE-associated hereditary hemochromatosis. *Genet Med.* 2009;11:307-313.

115. Nagayoshi Y, Nakayama M, Suzuki S, et al A Q312X mutation in the hemojuvelin gene is associated with cardiomyopathy due to juvenile haemochromatosis. *Eur J Heart Fail.* 2008;10:1001-1006.

116. Militaru MS, Popp RA, Trifa AP. Homozygous G320V mutation in the HJV gene causing juvenile hereditary haemochromatosis type A. A case report. *J Gastrointestin Liver Dis.* 2010;19:191-193.

117. Goldberg YP. Juvenile hereditary hemochromatosis. In: Pagon RA, Adam MP, Ardinger HH, et al., eds. *GeneReviews®.* Seattle, WA: University of Washington, Seattle; 2005.

118. Roetto A, Totaro A, Piperno A, et al. New mutations inactivating transferrin receptor 2 in hemochromatosis type 3. *Blood.* 2001;97:2555-2560.

119. Njajou OT, de Jong G, Berghuis B, et al. Dominant hemochromatosis due to N144H mutation of SLC11A3: clinical and biological characteristics. *Blood Cells Mol Dis.* 2002;29:439-443.

120. Kato J, Fujikawa K, Kanda M, et al. A mutation, in the iron-responsive element of H ferritin mRNA, causing autosomal dominant iron overload. *Am J Hum Genet.* 2001;69:191-197.

121. Barosi G, Salvaneschi L, Grasso M, et al. High prevalence of a screening-detected, HFE-unrelated, mild idiopathic iron overload in Northern Italy. *Haematologica.* 2002;87:472-478.

122. Wallace DF, Subramaniam VN. The global prevalence of HFE and non-HFE hemochromatosis estimated from analysis of next-generation sequencing data. *Genet Med.* 2015. doi:10.1038/gim.2015.140.

123. Shizukuda Y, Tripodi DJ, Sachdev V, et al. Changes in left ventricular diastolic function of asymptomatic hereditary hemochromatosissubjects during five years of follow-up. *Am J Cardiol.* 2011;108:1796-1800.

124. Murphy CJ, Oudit GY. Iron-overload cardiomyopathy: pathophysiology, diagnosis, and treatment. *J Card Fail.* 2010;16:888-900.

125. Davidsen ES, Hervig T, Omvik P, et al. Left ventricular long-axis function in treated haemochromatosis. *Int J Cardiovasc Imaging.* 2009;25:237-247.

126. Aypar E, Alehan D, Hazirolan T, et al. The efficacy of tissue Doppler imaging in predicting myocardial iron load in patients with beta-thalassemia

major: correlation with T2* cardiovascular magnetic resonance. *Int J Cardiovasc Imaging.* 2010;26:413-421.

127. Davidsen ES, Omvik P, Hervig T, et al. Left ventricular diastolic function in patients with treated haemochromatosis. *Scand Cardiovasc J.* 2009;43:32-38.

128. Aggeli C, Felekos I, Poulidakis E, et al. Quantitative analysis of left atrial function in asymptomatic patients with b-thalassemia major using real-time three-dimensional echocardiography. *Cardiovasc Ultrasound.* 2011;9:38.

129. Barbero U, Destefanis P, Pozzi R, et al. Exercise stress echocardiography with tissue doppler imaging (TDI) detects early systolic dysfunction in beta-thalassemia major patients without cardiac iron overload. *Mediterr J Hematol Infect Dis.* 2012;4:e2012037.

130. Wood JC. Use of magnetic resonance imaging to monitor iron overload. *Hematol Oncol Clin North Am.* 2014;28:747-764.

131. Anderson LJ, Holden S, Davis B, et al. Cardiovascular T2-star (T2*) magnetic resonance for the early diagnosis of myocardial iron overload. *Eur Heart J.* 2001;22:2171-2179.

132. Barrera Portillo MC, Uranga M, Sánchez González J, et al. Liver and heart T2* measurement in secondary haemochromatosis. *Radiologia.* 2013;55:331-339.

133. Pepe A, Positano V, Santarelli MF, et al. Multislice multiecho T2* cardiovascular magnetic resonance for detection of the heterogeneous distribution of myocardial iron overload. *J Magn Reson Imaging.* 2006;23:662-668.

134. Kirk P, Roughton M, Porter JB, et al. Cardiac T2* magnetic resonance for prediction of cardiac complications in thalassemia major. *Circulation.* 2009;120:1961-1968.

135. Mavrogeni S, Gotsis E, Verganelakis D, et al. Effect of iron overload on exercise capacity in thalassemic patients with heart failure. *Int J Cardiovasc Imaging.* 2009;25:777-783.

136. Cheong B, Huber S, Muthupillai R, et al. Evaluation of myocardial iron overload by T2* cardiovascular magnetic resonance imaging. *Tex Heart Inst J.* 2005;32:448-449.

137. Zoller H, Henninger B. Pathogenesis, diagnosis and treatment of hemochromatosis. *Dig Dis.* 2016;34:364-373.

138. Ekanayake D, Roddick C, Powell LW. Recent advances in hemochromatosis: a 2015 update: a summary of proceedings of the 2014 conference held under the auspices of Hemochromatosis Australia. *Hepatol Int.* 2015;9:174-182.

139. Kremastinos DT, Farmakis D, Aessopos A, et al. Beta-thalassemia cardiomyopathy: history, present considerations, and future perspectives. *Circ Heart Fail.* 2010;3:451-458.

140. Bottomley SS, Fleming MD. Sideroblastic anemia: diagnosis and management. *Hematol Oncol Clin North Am.* 2014;28:653-670.

141. Shahni R, Wedatilake Y, Cleary MA, Lindley KJ, Sibson KR, Rahman S. A distinct mitochondrial myopathy, lactic acidosis and sideroblastic anemia (MLASA) phenotype associates with YARS2 mutations. *Am J Med Genet A.* 2013;161A:2334-2338.

142. Delea TE, Hagiwara M, Phatak PD. Retrospective study of the association between transfusion frequency and potential complications of iron overload in patients with myelodysplastic syndrome and other acquired hematopoietic disorders. *Curr Med Res Opin.* 2009;25:139-147.

143. Nishio M, Endo T, Nakao S, Sato N, Koike T. Reversible cardiomyopathy due to secondary hemochromatosis with multitransfusions for severe aplastic anemia after successful non-myeloablative stem cell transplantation. *Int J Cardiol.* 2008;127:400-401.

144. Slotki I. Intravenous iron supplementation in the anaemia of renal and cardiac failure–a double-edged sword? *Nephrol Dial Transplant.* 2005;20 Suppl 7:vii16-23.

145. Fraga CG, Oteiza PI. Iron toxicity and antioxidant nutrients. *Toxicology.* 2002;180:23-32.

146. Rund D, Rachmilewitz E. Beta-thalassemia. *N Engl J Med.* 2005;353: 1135-1146.

147. Spirito P, Lupi G, Melevendi C, Vecchio C. Restrictive diastolic abnormalities identified by Doppler echocardiography in patients with thalassemia major. *Circulation.* 1990;82:88-94.

148. Aessopos A, Farmakis D. Pulmonary hypertension in beta-thalassemia. *Ann N Y Acad Sci.* 2005;1054:342-349.

149. Hahalis G, Manolis AS, Gerasimidou I, et al. Right ventricular diastolic function in beta-thalassemia major: echocardiographic and clinical correlates. *Am Heart J.* 2001;141:428-434.

150. Tubman VN, Fung EB, Vogiatzi M, et al. Thalassemia clinical research network. Guidelines for the standard monitoring of patients with thalassemia: report of the thalassemia longitudinal cohort. *J Pediatr Hematol Oncol.* 2015;37:e162-e169.

151. Abrahão A, Pedroso JL, Braga-Neto P, et al. Milestones in Friedreich ataxia: more than a century and still learning. *Neurogenetics.* 2015;16(3): 151-160.

152. Weidemann F, Liu D, Hu K, et al. The cardiomyopathy in Friedreich's ataxia—new biomarker for staging cardiac involvement. *Int J Cardiol.* 2015;194:50-57.

153. Koc F, Akpinar O, Yerdelen D, Demir M, Sarica Y, Kanadasi M. The evaluation of left ventricular systolic and diastolic functions in patients with Friedreich ataxia. A pulse tissue Doppler study. *Int Heart J.* 2005;46: 443-452.

154. Regner SR, Lagedrost SJ, Plappert T, et al. Analysis of echocardiograms in a large heterogeneous cohort of patients with Friedreich ataxia. *Am J Cardiol.* 2012;109:401-405.

155. Dispenzieri A. POEMS syndrome: update on diagnosis, risk-stratification, and management. *Am J Hematol.* 2015;90:951-962.

156. Ashrafi F, Darakhshandeh A, Nematolahy P, Khosravi A. Complete heart block in a patient with POEMS syndrome: a case report. *ARYA Atheroscler.* 2014;10:276-279.

157. Yokokawa T, Nakazato K, Kanno Y, Pulmonary hypertension and refractory heart failure in a patient with Crow-Fukase (POEMS) syndrome. *Intern Med.* 2013;52:1061-1065.

158. Inoue D, Kato A, Tabata S, et al. Successful treatment of POEMS syndrome complicated by severe congestive heart failure with thalidomide. *Intern Med.* 2010;49:461-466.

159. Soullier C, Micolich J, Croisille P. Multiple myocardial infarctions in a 35 year-old woman with POEMS syndrome. *Eur Heart J.* 2010;31:1097.

160. Tanus T, Miller HJ. POEMS syndrome presenting with cardiomegaly and cardiomyopathy. *J Intern Med.* 1992;231:445-448.

161. Huth M, Gordon D, Verrier ED, Otto CM. Aortic valvular fibroma as a source of systemic emboli in POEMS syndrome. *J Am Soc Echocardiogr.* 1991;4:401-404.

162. Marwick TH. Diabetic cardiomyopathy. In: Crawford MH, DiMarco JP, Paulus WJ, eds. *Cardiology,* 3rd ed. Philadelphia, PA: Mosby-Elsevier; 2010;1107-1109.

163. Forbes JM, Cooper ME. Mechanisms of diabetic complications. *Physiol Rev.* 2013;93:137-188.

164. Fang ZY, Prins JB, Marwick TH. Diabetic cardiomyopathy: evidence, mechanisms, and therapeutic implications. *Endocrine Rev.* 2004;25: 543-567.

165. Dunlay SM, Roger VL, Weston SA, Jiang R, Redfield MM. Longitudinal changes in ejection fraction in heart failure patients with preserved and reduced ejection fraction. *Circ Heart Fail.* 2012;5:720-726.

166. Seferović PM, Paulus WJ. Clinical diabetic cardiomyopathy: a two-faced disease with restrictive and dilated phenotypes. *Eur Heart J.* 2015;36:1718-27,1727a-1727c.

167. Paulus WJ, Tschoepe C. A novel paradigm for heart failure with preserved ejection fraction: comorbidities drive myocardial dysfunction and remodeling through coronary microvascular endothelial inflammation. *J Am Coll Cardiol.* 2013;62:263-271.

168. Van Heerebeek L, Hamdani N, Handoko L, et al. Diastolic stiffness of the failing diabetic heart: importance of fibrosis, advanced glycation end-products and myocyte resting tension. *Circulation.* 2008;117:43-51.

169. Montaigne D, Marechal X, Coisne A, et al. Myocardial contractile dysfunction is associated with impaired mitochondrial function and dynamics in type 2 diabetic but not in obese patients. *Circulation.* 2014;130:554-564.

170. Rijzewijk LJ, van der Meer RW, Smit JW, et al. Myocardial steatosis is an independent predictor of diastolic dysfunction in type 2 diabetes mellitus. *J Am Coll Cardiol.* 2008;52:1793-1799.

171. Donaldson C, Taatjes DJ, Zile M, et al. Combined immunoelectron microscopic and computer-assisted image analyses to detect advanced glycation end-products in human myocardium. *Histochem Cell Biol.* 2010;134:23-30.

172. Camici PG, Crea F. Coronary microvascular dysfunction. *N Engl J Med.* 2007;356:830-840.

173. Selvin E, Lazo M, Chen Y, et al. Diabetes mellitus, prediabetes and incidence of subclinical myocardial damage. *Circulation.* 2014;130:1374-1382.

174. Authors/Task Force Members Rydén L, Grant PJ, Anker SD, et al. ESC Committee for Practice Guidelines (CPG), Document Reviewers. ESC Guidelines on diabetes, pre-diabetes, and cardiovascular diseases developed in collaboration with the EASD: the Task Force on diabetes, pre-diabetes, and cardiovascular diseases of the European Society of Cardiology (ESC) and developed in collaboration with the European Association for the Study of Diabetes (EASD). *Eur Heart J.* 2013;34:3035-3087.

175. Lurie PR. Changing concepts of endocardial fibroelastosis. *Cardiol Young.* 2010;20:115-123.

176. Mocumbi AO, Ferreira MB, Sidi D, Yacoub MH. A population study of endomyocardial fibrosis in a rural area of Mozambique. *N Engl J Med.* 2008;359:43-49.

177. Webb-Peploe MM. Obliterative and restrictive cardiomyopathies. *Eur Heart J.* 1988;9(Suppl G):159-167.

178. Miller AJ. Primary endocardial fibroelastosis of the left ventricle. *Tex Heart Inst J.* 2012;39:913-914.

179. Aherrahrou Z, Schlossarek S, Stoelting S, et al. Knock-out of nexilin in mice leads to dilated cardiomyopathy and endomyocardial fibroelastosis. *Basic Res Cardiol.* 2016;111(1):6. doi: 10.1007/s00395-015-0522-5.

180. Cole CR, Eghtesady P. The myocardial and coronary histopathology and pathogenesis of hypoplastic left heart syndrome. *Cardiol Young.* 2016;26:19-29.

181. Emani SM, Marx GR. Operations for improving left ventricular diastolic function. *Curr Opin Cardiol.* 2016;31:101-108.

182. Seki A, Patel S, Ashraf S, Perens G, Fishbein MC. Primary endocardial fibroelastosis: an underappreciated cause of cardiomyopathy in children. *Cardiovasc Pathol.* 2013;22:345-350.

183. Pastor Quirante FA, Pastor-Pérez FJ, Manzano-Fernández S, et al. Unexpected autopsy findings after sudden cardiac death: cardiovascular myxoedema and endocardial fibroelastosis. *Int J Cardiol.* 2015;182:281-283.

184. Arya SO, Karpawich PP, Gupta P, Buddhe S, Singh HR, Hussein Y, Gowda ST. Primary endocardial fibroelastosis presenting in a young child as incessant ventricular tachycardia and dilated cardiomyopathy. *Tex Heart Inst J.* 2012;39:714-718.

185. Steger CM, Antretter H, Moser PL. Endocardial fibroelastosis of the heart. *Lancet.* 2012;379(9819):932.

186. Mocumbi AO, Yacoub S, Yacoub MH. Neglected tropical cardiomyopathies: II. Endomyocardial fibrosis. *Heart.* 2008;94:384-390.

187. Chelo D, Nguefack F, Mbassi Awa HD, Kingue S. Endomyocardial fibrosis in Sub Saharan Africa: the geographical origin, socioeconomic status, and dietary habits of cases reported in Yaounde, Cameroon. *Ann Pediatr Cardiol.* 2015;8:202-209.

188. Kutty VR, Abraham S, Kartha CC. Geographical distribution of endomyocardial fibrosis in south Kerala. *Int J Epidemiol.* 1996;25:1202-1207.

189. Mocumbi AO, Falase AO. Recent advances in the epidemiology, diagnosis and treatment of endomyocardial fibrosis in Africa. *Heart.* 2013;99:1481-1487.

190. Chelo D, Nguefack F, Menanga AP, et al. Endomyocardial fibrosis in Cameroon: Echocardiographic and clinical description of a pediatric series in Yaoundé. *Arch Pediatr.* 2016;23:128-135.

191. Berensztein CS, Pineiro G, Marcotegui M, Brunoldi R, Vazquez Blanco M, Lerman J. Usefulness of echocardiography and Doppler echocardiographiy in endomyocardial fibrosis. *J Am Soc Echocardiogr.* 2000;13: 385-392.

192. Irwin RB, Luckie RB, Luckie M, Khattar RS. Tricuspid regurgitation: contemporary management of a neglected valvular lesion. *Postgrad Med J.* 2010;86:648-655.

193. Mocumbi AO, Carrilho C, Burke MM, Wright G, Yacoub MH. Emergency surgical treatment of advanced endomyocardial fibrosis in Mozambique. *Nat Clin Pract Cardiovasc Med.* 2009;6:210-214.

194. Mocumbi AO, Carrilho C, Sarathchandra P, Ferreira MB, Yacoub M, Burke M. Echocardiography accurately assesses the pathological abnormalities of chronic endomyocardial fibrosis. *Int J Cardiovasc Imaging.* 2011;27:955-964.

195. Cury RĆ, Abbara S, Sandoval LJ, Houser S, Brady TJ, Palacios IF. Visualization of EMF by delayed-enhancement magnetic resonance imaging. *Circulation.* 2005;111:e115-e117.

196. Heredero A, Garcia-Vega M, Tomas M, et al. Combined endocardiectomy and bidirectional Glenn shunt for right ventricular endomyocardial fibrosis. *Ann Thorac Surg.* 2012;93:310-312.

197. Hassan W, Fawzy ME, Al Helaly S, Hegazy H, Malik S. Pitfalls in diagnosis and clinical, echocardiographic, and hemodynamic findings in endomyocardial fibrosis: a 25-year experience. *Chest.* 2005;128:3985-3992.

198. Mocumbi AO, Yacoub MH, Yokohama H, Ferreira MB. Right ventricular endomyocardial fibrosis. *Cardiovasc Pathol.* 2009;18:64-65.

199. Chopra P, Narula J, Talwar KK, Kumar V, Bhatia ML. Histomorphologic characteristics of endomyocardial fibrosis: an endomyocardial biopsy study. *Hum Pathol.* 1990;21:613-616.

200. Seth S, Thatai D, Sharma S, Chopra P, Talwar KK. Clinicopathological evaluation of restrictive cardiomyopathy (endomyocardial fibrosis and idiopathic restrictive cardiomyopathy) in India. *Eur J Heart Fail.* 2004;6:723-729.

201. Mocumbi AO, Songane M, Salomão C, Ulibarri R, Ferreira MB, Yacoub MH. Lack of evidence of myocardial damage in children with Plasmodium falciparum severe and complicated malaria from an endemic area for endomyocardial fibrosis. *J Trop Pediatr.* 2011;57:312-314.

202. Fernandez Vazquez E, Lacarcel Bautista C, Alcazar Navarrete B, Casado Moreno I, Espejo Guerrero A, Ruiz Carazo E. Chronic thromboembolic pulmonary hypertension associated with endomyocardial fibrosis of the right ventricle. *Arch Bronconeumol.* 2003;39:370-372.

203. Vijayaraghavan G, Sivasankaran S. Tropical endomyocardial fibrosis in India: a vanishing disease! *Indian J Med Res.* 2012;136:729-738.

204. Ribeiro PA, Muthusamy R, Duran CM. Right-sided endomyocardial fibrosis with recurrent pulmonary emboli leading to irreversible pulmonary hypertension. *Br Heart J.* 1992;68:326-329.

205. Graham JM, Lawrie GM, Feteih NM, Debakey ME. Management of endomyocardial fibrosis: successful surgical treatment of biventricular involvement and consideration of the superiority of operative intervention. *Am Heart J.* 1981;102:771-775.

206. Mocumbi AO. Recent trends in the epidemiology of endomyocardial fibrosis in Africa. *Pediatr Int Child Health.* 2012;32:63-64.

207. Smedema JP, Winckels SK, Snoep G, Vainer J, Bekkers SC, Crijins HJ. Tropical endomyocardial fibrosis (Davies' disease): case report demonstrating the role of magnetic resonance imaging. *Int J Cardiovasc Imaging.* 2004;20:517-522.

208. Fox DJ, Khattar RS: Carcinoid heart disease: presentation, diagnosis, and management. *Heart.* 2004;90:1224-1228.

209. Patel C, Mathur M, Escarcega RO, Bove AA. Carcinoid heart disease: current understanding and future directions. *Am Heart J.* 2014;167:789-795.

210. Moller JE, Pellikka PA, Bernheim AM, Schaff HV, Rubin J, Connolly HM. Prognosis of carcinoid heart disease: analysis of 200 cases over two decades. *Circulation.* 2005;112:3320-3327.

211. Pellikka PA, Tajik, Khandheria, et al. Carcinoid heart disease. Clinical and echocardiographic spectrum in 74 patients. *Circulation.* 1993;87:1188-1196.

212. Modlin IM, Kidd M, Latich I, Zikusoka MN, Shapiro MD. Current status of gastrointestinal carcinoids. *Gastroenterology.* 2005;128:1717-1751.

213. Daigeler A, Imoberdorf R, Haller A. Carcinoid tumor with carcinoid heart disease: the rare case of Hedinger syndrome without hepatic metastases. *Int J Cardiol.* 2003;92:295-296.

214. Soga J. Carcinoids and their variant endocrinomas. An analysis of 11,842 reported cases. *J Exp Clin Cancer Res.* 2003;22:517-530.

215. Dobson R, Burgess MI, Pritchard DM, Cuthbertson DJ. The clinical presentation and management of carcinoid heart disease. *Int J Cardiol.* 2014;173:29-32.

216. Bhattacharyya S, Toumpanakis C, Burke M, Taylor AM, Caplin ME, Davar J. Features of carcinoid heart disease identified by 2- and 3-dimensional echocardiography and cardiac MRI. *Circ Cardiovasc Imaging.* 2010;3:103-111.

217. Franzen D, Boldt A, Raute-Kreinsen U, Koerfer R, Erdmann E. Magnetic resonance imaging of carcinoid heart disease. *Clin Cardiol.* 2009;32:E92-E93.

218. Caplin M, Sundin A, Nillson O, et al. ENETS Consensus Guidelines for the management of patients with digestive neuroendocrine neoplasms: colorectal neuroendocrine neoplasms. *Neuroendocrinology.* 2012;95: 88-97.

219. Pape UF, Perren A, Niederle B, et al. ENETS Consensus Guidelines for the management of patients with neuroendocrine neoplasms from the jejuno-ileum and the appendix including goblet cell carcinomas. *Neuroendocrinology.* 2012;95:135-156.

220. Korse CM, Taal BG, de Groot CA, Bakker RH, Bonfrer JM. Chromogranin-A and N-terminal pro-brain natriuretic peptide: an excellent pair of biomarkers for diagnostics in patients with neuroendocrine tumor. *J Clin Oncol.* 2009;27:4293-4299.

221. Bhattacharyya S, Toumpanakis C, Caplin ME, Davar J. Usefulness of N-terminal pro-brain natriuretic peptide as a biomarker of the presence of carcinoid heart disease. *Am J Cardiol.* 2008;102:938-942.

222. Bergestuen DS, Gravning J, Haugaa KH, et al. Plasma CCN2/connective tissue growth factor is associated with right ventricular dysfunction in patients with neuroendocrine tumors. *BMC Cancer.* 2010;10:6.

223. Bergestuen DS, Edvardsen T, Aakhus S, et al. Activin A in carcinoid heart disease: a possible role in diagnosis and pathogenesis. *Neuroendocrinology.* 2010;92:168-177.

224. Zahid W, Bergestuen D, Haugaa KH, et al. Myocardial function by two-dimensional speckle tracking echocardiography and activin A may predict mortality in patients with carcinoid intestinal disease. *Cardiology.* 2015;132:81-90.

225. Rinke A, Krug S. Neuroendocrine tumours—medical therapy: biological. *Best Pract Res Clin Endocrinol Metab.* 2016;30:79-91.

226. Connolly HM, Schaff HV, Abel MD, et al. Early and late outcomes of surgical treatment in carcinoid heart disease. *J Am Coll Cardiol.* 2015;66:2189-2196.

227. Jahagirdar V, Kamal A, Steeds R2, Ayuk J. Metastatic small bowel neuroendocrine tumour with bilateral carcinoid heart disease. *BMJ Case Rep.* 2016;2016. pii: bcr2015213693.

228. Ockert DB, White RD. Anesthetic management of patients with carcinoid heart disease undergoing cardiac surgery: two case reports and a review of previous experience. *J Cardiothorac Anesth.* 1988;2:658-665.

45

Left Ventricular Noncompaction

Eloisa Arbustini, Alessandra Serio, Lorenzo Giuliani, Nupoor Narula, and Alessandro Di Toro

Left ventricular noncompaction: definition, pathogenesis, diagnosis and pathology

Definition

The term "Left ventricular noncompaction (LVNC)" does not include descriptors related to the left ventricular function and size, which are essential for the definition of cardiomyopathy.

The definition includes three macro-morphology descriptors:

1. **Thin compact layer**
2. **Prominent trabeculae** (working as mechanical levers that contract in early systole and relax in late diastole)
3. **Deep intertrabecular recesses**

Pathogenic hypotheses

1. **Embryogenic:** arrest of maturation with involvement of multiple molecular pathways (eg, NKx2-5, and NOTCH-1 signaling)
2. **Genetic:** poorly supported by extreme genetic heterogeneity, overlapping with CMP genes, segregation of the mutations with the underlying cardiac disease but not with the noncompaction morphology
3. **Hemodynamic:** supported by the evidence that LVNC can be acquired and reversible

Diagnostic criteria

Imaging-based diagnosis—noncompact/compact layer ratio ≥2; # of affected segments

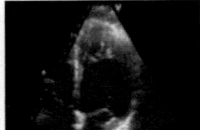
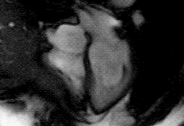
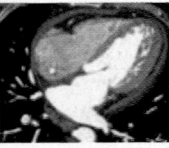

2D-TTE   CMR   MDCT

Many heterogeneous imaging criteria
– No shared, standardized criteria

No functional, electrical or biochemical criteria
No gold standard
No guidelines

Pathology in cardiomyopathies

Hypertrophic cardiomyopathy

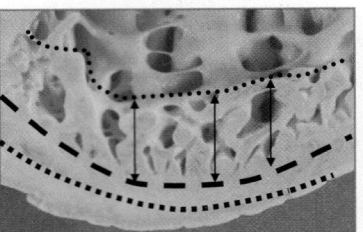

Dilated cardiomyopathy, up to compactless left ventricle

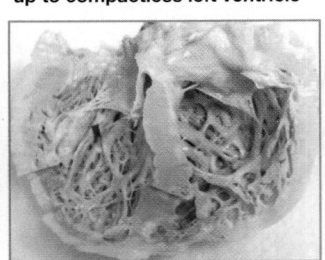

Gene mutations: no segregation with noncompaction

I:1 → M H(N–Obs)+D+NC OH GAD E G-MYH7[p,(Gly716Arg)]SC-IV

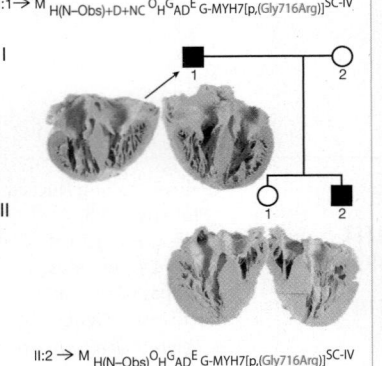

II:2 → M H(N–Obs) OH GAD E G-MYH7[p,(Gly716Arg)]SC-IV

Anticoagulation: dictated by left ventricular dysfunction and dilation

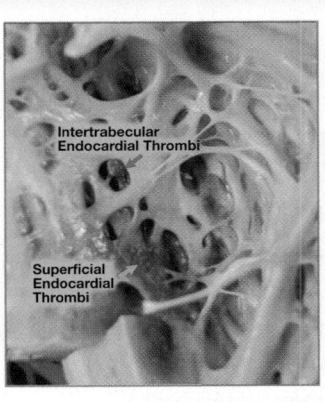

Intertrabecular Endocardial Thrombi

Superficial Endocardial Thrombi

Chapter 45 Fuster and Hurst's Central Illustration. In adults, left ventricular noncompaction (LVNC) can be observed in healthy individuals, athletes, and patients with various diseases. The diagnosis of isolated LVNC does not in itself modify therapy. Similarly, the presence of LVNC does not significantly influence prognosis. Genetic testing cannot replace the role of clinical evaluation and should be carefully prescribed only when a genetic disease is suspected. Upper right image of dilated cardiomyopathy up to compactless left ventricle reproduced with permission from Arbustini E, Favalli V, Narula N, et al. Left Ventricular Noncompaction: A Distinct Genetic Cardiomyopathy? *J Am Coll Cardiol.* 2016 Aug 30;68(9):949-966. Lower right image showing endocardial thrombi reproduced with permission from Arbustini E, Weidemann F, Hall JL. Left ventricular noncompaction: a distinct cardiomyopathy or a trait shared by different cardiac diseases? *J Am Coll Cardiol.* 2014 Oct 28;64(17):1840-1850.

CHAPTER SUMMARY

This chapter reviews left ventricular noncompaction (LVNC). LVNC is an anatomical descriptor that does not inform on left ventricular function and size. The three morphologic features of LVNC are prominent trabeculae, deep intertrabecular recesses, and thin compact myocardial layer (see Fuster and Hurst's Central Illustration). The right ventricle can be involved as isolated right ventricular noncompaction (RVNC) or biventricular noncompaction. LVNC can occur in patients with cardiomyopathies, congenital heart disease, or syndromes with cardiac and multiorgan malformations. Isolated LVNC can also be observed in healthy individuals, including athletes, and in patients with renal failure, and hematological or neuromuscular diseases. LVNC seen in primigravida in the third trimester is reversible and regresses after delivery. Diagnostic criteria are variable for both echocardiography and cardiac magnetic resonance (CMR), and based on the measurement of the ratio of noncompact to compact myocardial layers being ≥2. The presence of LVNC does not influence prognosis nor modify management strategy: both are driven by the underlying cardiac disease. Genetic testing identifies defects associated with the cardiac disease and should be prescribed when a genetic disorder is really suspected. LNVC such as that observed in young athletes with normal left ventricular size and function, unremarkable CMR, and family history for cardiomyopathy should be evaluated with great caution before assigning pathological significance.

INTRODUCTION

In normal hearts, trabeculae undergo continuous and quantifiable geometric changes during the cardiac cycle; their contraction occurs during early systolic ejection while relaxation occurs in late diastole, at larger ventricular volumes. Trabeculae work as small, mechanically active levers during systole and increase perfusion of the subendocardium by expanding the interface between the endocardium and ventricular blood during diastole.[1] Their number and size are highly variable, from few and flat to numerous and prominent, to confer a "spongy" appearance to the endocardial surface of the ventricles. This aspect corresponds to the term *left ventricular noncompaction* (LVNC).

LVNC describes a ventricular wall anatomy characterized by the presence of prominent left ventricular (LV) trabeculae, a thin compacted layer, and deep intertrabecular recesses that are in continuity with the LV cavity and separated from the epicardial coronary arteries.[2] By definition, noncompaction pertains to the LV but may also involve the right ventricle, as either a biventricular[3] or an isolated right ventricular variant.[4] The American Heart Association (AHA) classification defines LVNC as a genetic/congenital cardiomyopathy,[5] whereas the European Society of Cardiology (ESC) classification defines LVNC as a nonclassified entity.[6] The recent MOGE(S) nosology (*M*orphofunctional phenotype, *O*rgan(s) involvement, *G*enetic inheritance pattern, *E*tiologic annotation including genetic defect or underlying disease/substrate, and functional *S*tatus of the disease) proposes a simple description of the trait in individuals with either normal LV size, wall thickness, preserved systolic and diastolic function, or in combination with hypertrophic cardiomyopathy (HCM), dilated cardiomyopathy (DCM), restrictive cardiomyopathy (RCM), or arrhythmogenic cardiomyopathy (ACM).[7] This latter descriptive approach is the expression of the clinical uncertainties regarding the unique interpretation of LVNC as a cardiomyopathy.[8]

In the official guidelines of scientific societies, the requirements for the definition of a cardiomyopathy include "diseases of the myocardium associated with mechanical and/or electrical dysfunction" (AHA)[5] and "myocardial diseases characterized by structurally and functionally abnormal heart muscle and absence of other diseases sufficient to cause the observed myocardial abnormality" (ESC).[6] When isolated and benign, LVNC is not associated with mechanical and/or electrical dysfunction (AHA) and is characterized by hypertrabeculation and normal LV size and function.[8] Therefore, an abnormal ventricular morphology by itself does not meet the structural and functional requirements needed to define a cardiomyopathy. In fact, increasing number of reports that describe LVNC in the normal population questions the definition of LVNC as cardiomyopathy.

This chapter illustrates the current criteria for diagnosing LVNC, available data in normal populations, the association of LVNC with cardiomyopathies and disease genes, congenital heart diseases, rare syndromes affecting or not affecting cardiac function, acquired and possibly reversible LVNC, and diagnostic workup.

CURRENT DIAGNOSTIC CRITERIA FOR LEFT VENTRICULAR NONCOMPACTION

Diagnostic criteria have been established for echocardiography, cardiac magnetic resonance (CMR), and multidetector computed tomography (MDCT). The list of different criteria is by itself evidence that common, standardized, and uniform rules do not exist. This is likely because isolated LVNC represents a spectrum of LV trabecular morphology rather than an independent heart muscle disease. **Table 45–1**[9–21] summarizes current diagnostic criteria that are based on ratios between thickness, mass, or volume or percentages of noncompacted (NC) and compacted LV. The number of NC segments provides information on the extent of LVNC. Alternative methods integrate the count or evaluation of the global trabeculation index. **Figures 45–1** and **45–2** illustrate echocardiographic and CMR features of LVNC, respectively.

MDCT is useful when CMR is contraindicated or when echocardiography and CMR provide discordant data[21,22] and further adds the advantage of noninvasive investigation of the coronary tree. A computed tomography (CT) study that used the AHA 17-segment model and an end-diastolic NC-to-compacted (NC/C) ratio >2.3 distinguished pathologic LVNC with 88% sensitivity and 97% specificity, with positive and negative predictive values of 78% and 99%, respectively.[22]

The independent diagnostic contribution of the maximum thickness of the compacted layer is limited. In the context of using ratios or proportions, the same ratio can result from different absolute values of the two components. In most diagnostic indices, the ratios between compacted and NC thickness, volume, or mass drive the diagnosis. However, reduced thickness of the compacted layer has been proposed as a novel echocardiographic criterion for NC cardiomyopathy; a maximal systolic thickness <8 mm of the compacted layer seems to be specific for LVNC and to differentiate LVNC from normal hearts as well as hearts with myocardial thickening caused by aortic valve stenosis. The addition of this criterion may eventually contribute to preventing the overdiagnosis of LVNC.[23] **Figure 45–3** shows how the criteria for LVNC can be fulfilled either for the prominent trabecular layer but in the presence of the preserved compacted layer (Panels A and B) or for the nearly absent compacted layer (Panel C).

Although CMR is considered the diagnostic gold standard, a unique validated tool and calculation method endorsed by scientific societies are still missing. In fact, the different CMR methods and software do not share the same diagnostic criteria.[13–20]

LEFT VENTRICULAR NONCOMPACTION IN HEALTHY SUBJECTS

LVNC diagnosed according to current criteria may occur in functionally normal hearts. In 2012, the publication of data in 1000 participants (551 women; age, 68.1 ± 8.9 years) of the Multi-Ethnic Study of Atherosclerosis (MESA) cohort suggested the need of reevaluation of CMR criteria for LVNC. The thickness of trabeculated and compact myocardium was measured in

TABLE 45–1. Imaging Criteria for the Diagnosis of Left Ventricular Noncompaction (LVNC)

Echocardiography		Cardiac Phase	Imaging Plan(s)	LVNC	Reference
Echocardiography	X = distance from the epicardial surface to the trough of the trabecular recess; Y = distance from the epicardial surface to peak of trabeculation	End diastole	• Parasternal short axis • Apical 4-chamber • Subcostal	X/Y ≤0.5	9
	Noncompacted/compacted (NC/C) >2	End systole	• Parasternal short axis • Apical 4-chamber	NC/C >2	10
	• >3 trabeculations • Synchronous motion of trabeculae with compacted myocardium • Connection between ventricular cavity and intertrabecular recesses • 2-Layered wall	End diastole	Parasternal short axis		11
	Maximal NC/C planimetered area Ratio of the maximum linear length of noncompacted to compacted myocardium (NC/C) Planimetered area of LVNC on apical 4-chamber view	End systole	Apical 4-chamber Modified apical 2-chamber	*(see sub-table below)*	12

	Linear NC/C (ratio)	Planimeter
	0	0
Mild	>0 and <1	≥0 cm² and <2.5 cm²
Moderate	≥1 and <2	≥2.5 cm² and <5.0 cm²
Severe	2+	≥5.0 cm²

CMR		Cardiac Phase	Imaging Plan(s)	Normal	LVNC Cutoff	Reference
CMR; balanced steady-state free precession	NC/C ratio per segment using horizontal long axis (HLA) and vertical long axis (VLA); apex excluded	End diastole	• Horizontal long axis • Vertical long axis • Left ventricular outflow tract view	1.1 ± 0.1	NC/C 2.3	13
	A. Compacted LV mass subtracted from global LV mass after semiautomated contouring and indexing to BSA B. Ratio of trabeculated LV mass (TLVM) to global LV mass expressed as percentage	End diastole	Short-axis stack	9.0 ± 4.0 g/m² TLVM 12.5 ± 5.0%	Mean TLVM 43 ± 19 g/m² TLVM >20%	14
	17-Segment model excluding apex, evaluated for NC and C wall thickness in ED and ES, taking the peak value for NC per segment	Diastole and systole	Short-axis stack	NC/C ranges: End diastole: 0–0.9 End-systole: 0–0.5	—	15
	A. Software for contouring NC and C; epicardial border manually traced in ES and ED in HLA and registration marks applied	End diastole	• Horizontal long axis • Vertical long axis • Short axis stack	Ai 5.3 ± 2.4g/m² Aii 9.9 ± 4.5g/m²	LV-MMI noncompacted, noncompacted LV myocardial mass index >15 g/m² % LV-MMI noncompacted index >25%	16

	Measurement	Phase	Imaging plane	Criteria	Normal value	
	B. Maximal NC/C from measurements in ED on SAX in 16 of 17 segments		Short axis stack	NC/C ≥3.1	—	16
	Apical SAX 16 to 24 mm from the true apical slice for measurements; papillary muscles excluded; ES NC/C wall thickness ratio	End systole	Short axis stack	ES NC/C ≥2	—	17
	Java-based box-counting fractal analysis to extract the maximal apical fractal dimension (FD) after analyzing all SAX cines (excluding apex)	End diastole	Short axis stack	FD max apical ≥1.30	1.203 ± 0.06	18
	A. Segmental trabeculation index (STI) = NC/C ratio per segment 1-15 in SAX; apical values for segment 16 from HLA and VLA B. Global trabeculation index (GTI) = ratio of the sum of total NC to the sum of total C	End diastole	• Horizontal long axis • Vertical long axis • Short axis stack	STI range in DCM, 0.1–2.2 (apex included) or 0.1–1.5 (apex excluded) Mean GTI in DCM, 0.68 0.32	— —	19
	Epicardial and endocardial contours, paps and trabecular-free LV/RV volumes manually outlined	End diastole	Short axis stack	LV trabecular volume/BSA not defined in LVNC	Males 4.31 ± 8.7 mL/m² Females 38.1 ± 5.9 mL/m²	20
MDCT						
Cardiac Tomography	NC/C ratio >2.2 in at least two segments can be considered diagnostic of LVNC	End diastole	Short axes (basal, mid-ventricular, apical), and long axes (2-, 3-, and 4-chamber views), using the AHA cardiac segmentation model True apex (segment 17) excluded	≥2.2 in the NC/C ratio in ≥2 myocardial segments	—	21

Abbreviations: BSA, body surface area; CMR, cardiac magnetic resonance; CT, computed tomography; DCM, dilated cardiomyopathy; ED, end diastole; ES, end systole; LV, left ventricle; MDCT, multidetector computed tomography; MMI, myocardial mass index; RV, right ventricle; SAX, short axis.

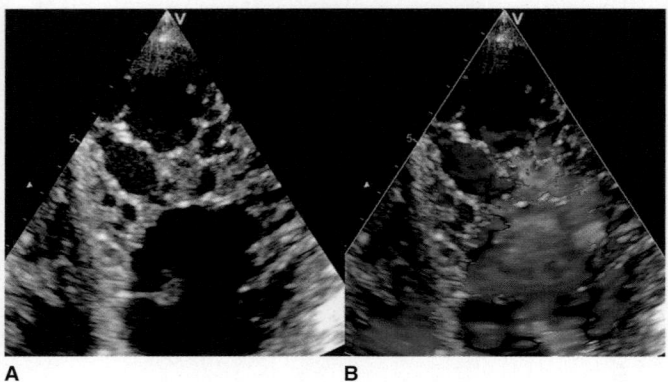

A   **B**

Figure 45–1. Echocardiographic and color Doppler images from a patient with LVNC. (**A**) In the echocardiographic image, an atypical four-chamber view was used to better illustrate the noncompaction in the LV apex. (**B**) The same view with color Doppler imaging. This view highlights perfusion of intertrabecular recesses from the LV cavity. Reproduced with permission from Arbustini E, Weidemann F, Hall JL. Left ventricular noncompaction: a distinct cardiomyopathy or a trait shared by different cardiac diseases? *J Am Coll Cardiol*. 2014 Oct 28;64(17):1840-1850.

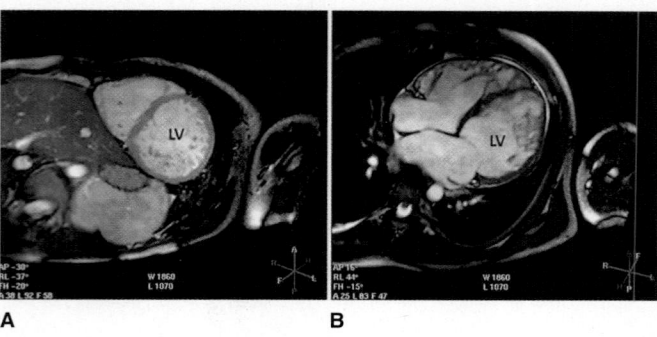

A   **B**

Figure 45–2. Cardiac magnetic resonance image from a patient with LVNC. (**A**) Short-axis view showing the hypertrabeculation in all mid-LV segments apart from the interventricular septum. (**B**) Long-axis view showing the hypertrabeculation mainly in the apical and mid-LV segments. Reproduced with permission from Arbustini E, Weidemann F, Hall JL. Left ventricular non-compaction: a distinct cardiomyopathy or a trait shared by different cardiac diseases? *J Am Coll Cardiol*. 2014 Oct 28;64(17):1840-1850.

eight LV regions on long-axis CMR steady-state free precession cine images. The study demonstrated that (1) 43% of subjects without cardiac disease or hypertension had an NC/C ratio >2.3 in at least one myocardial segment; (2) the NC/C ratio was not associated with age, sex, race/ethnicity, height, or weight; (3) the maximum thickness of trabeculation was positively associated with race/ethnicity (Chinese and Black) and male sex; (4) there was a negative association of LV ejection fraction (LVEF) and a positive association of LV end-diastolic volume and LV end-systolic volume with the maximum NC/C ratio, versus a positive association of LV end-diastolic volume and LV end-systolic volume with maximum trabeculation thickness; and (5) there was technique–related variability in measurement of thickness of trabeculation and compact myocardium as well as NC/C ratio. The study concluded that an NC/C ratio >2.3 is common in a large population-based cohort.[24]

In 2014, long-term follow-up data in 2742 participants in the MESA cohort (mean age, 68.7 years; 52.3% women; 56.4% with hypertension; 16.8% with diabetes) demonstrated that even in subjects with excessive trabeculation, there were no clinically relevant differences in LV volumes and systolic function changes among the quintiles of trabeculation extent. The authors found that 25% of participants exhibited at least one cardiac segment with NC/C ratio >2.3 and that 8% of participants displayed two or more affected segments. Although LV volumes increased and LVEF decreased in the 9.5 years between the first and last examinations, there were no differences across the maximal NC/C ratio quintiles, and patients with greater trabeculation showed even smaller LV end-diastolic volume changes. There were no racial variations in the maximal NC/C ratio. Finally, adverse clinical events were scarce, despite the apparently high proportion of participants with a potential unmasked cardiomyopathy.[25]

CMR studies in normal adult volunteers demonstrated the following sex- and age-related differences: (1) the compacted

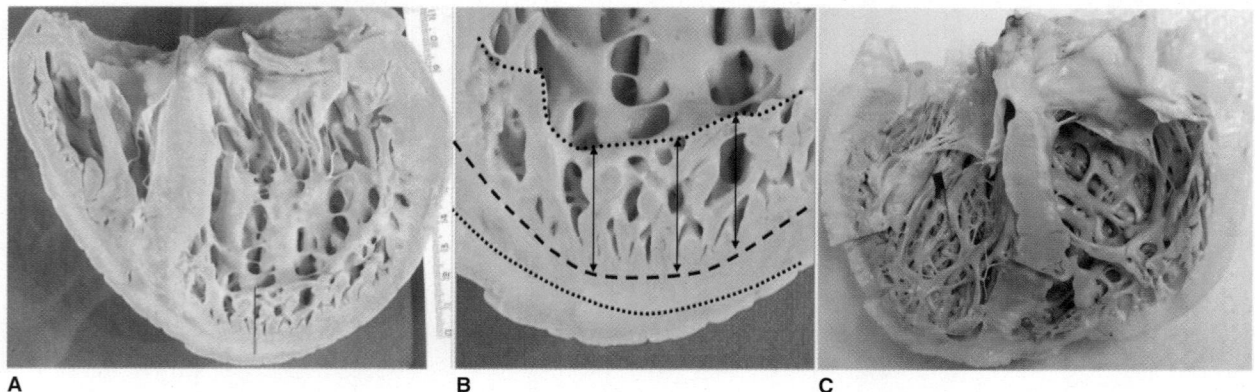

A   **B**   **C**

Figure 45–3. The figure shows two examples of how the anomalous ratio of NC/C can be induced by: (**A**) and (**B**) presence of prominent trabeculae in HCM with preservation of the compact layer or (**C**) by the absence of compacted layer in DCM. (A) Reproduced with permission from Arbustini E, Weidemann F, Hall JL. Left ventricular noncompaction: a distinct cardiomyopathy or a trait shared by different cardiac diseases? *J Am Coll Cardiol*. 2014 Oct 28;64(17):1840-1850. (C) Reproduced with permission from Arbustini E, Favalli V, Narula N, et al. Left Ventricular Noncompaction: A Distinct Genetic Cardiomyopathy? *J Am Coll Cardiol*. 2016 Aug 30;68(9):949-966.

but not the trabeculated layer is thicker in men than in women; (2) the compacted layer thickens whereas the trabeculated layer thins with systole; (3) trabeculated LV segments show increased systolic thinning of trabeculated layers and greater thickening of the compact segments (P <0.05) with age; (4) total wall thickening is neither sex nor age-dependent; (5) there were no sex-specific differences in the trabeculated/compacted ratio at end systole or end diastole; and (6) in end systole, the trabeculated/compacted ratio was lower in older (50–79 years) compared to younger (20–49 years) subjects (P <0.05).[15] Overall, the application of current diagnostic criteria demonstrates that LVNC may occur in a relevant proportion of healthy individuals. In a recent systematic review and meta-analysis of studies reporting LVNC prevalence in 59 eligible studies documenting LVNC in 67 distinct cohorts, the prevalence of LVNC amongst control cohorts of healthy subject ranged between 1.05% when assessed with echocardiography and 15.03% when assessed with CMR (**Fig. 45–4**).

These data call for a consideration on the risk of overdiagnosis, overtreatment, and unnecessary follow-up.[26]

EPIDEMIOLOGY

Epidemiology data reflect the context, methods, and clinical characteristics of the series in which LVNC has been investigated. In sum, the precise proportion of LVNC remains elusive.

Prevalence data demonstrate impressive discrepancies, with LVNC being paradoxically higher in imaging series obtained in normal individuals and in screening studies of volunteers[13,22,23] than in selected clinical series of children and adults. In the aforementioned review and meta-analysis of studies reporting LVNC prevalence in adults,[26] the pooled prevalence estimates for LVNC significantly differed depending on imaging technique, being 12 times higher amongst cohorts diagnosed on CMR versus echocardiography (14.79% and 1.28%, respectively).[26]

Children

Data on annual incidence of LVNC in children report values less than 0.1 per 100,000.[27] Isolated LVNC accounted for 9.2% of all cases in a population-based retrospective cohort study of primary cardiomyopathies in Australian children,[28] with LVNC identified as the third most frequent cardiomyopathy after DCM and HCM. This prevalence was close to that recorded in the Texas Children's Hospital echocardiography database (9.5%).[29] In the Pediatric Cardiomyopathy Registry (1990–2008), 155 (4.8%) of 3219 children had LVNC. This was associated with DCM, HCM, RCM, or indeterminate cardiomyopathies in 120 children and isolated in 35 children. In the latter group, heart failure was not present in any individuals at time of diagnosis. The majority of children with isolated LVNC

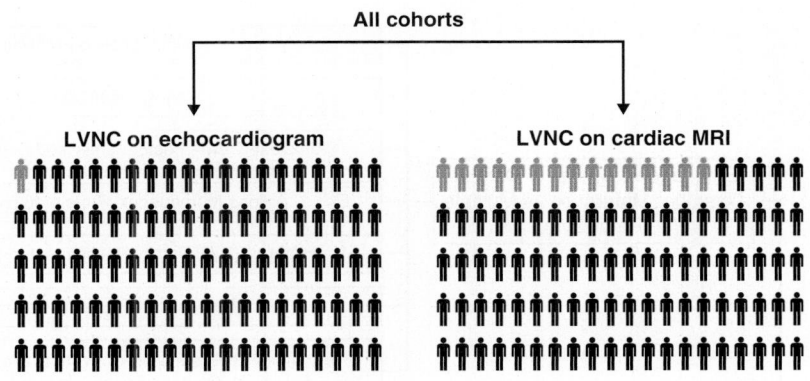

Cohort	Echocardiogram ES (95% CI)	Cardiac MRI ES (95% CI)
Cardiac patient cohorts	0.90 (0.64, 1.20)	9.76 (4.59, 16.56)
Control cohorts	1.05 (0.00, 7.88)	15.03 (8.94, 22.24)
Population representative cohorts	-	19.72 (11.64, 29.28)
Athlete cohorts	3.16 (0.26, 8.48)	27.29 (13.58, 43.27)
Non-cardiac patient cohorts	2.21 (0.24, 5.46)	36.21 (23.64, 49.72)
Primigravida pregnancy cohort	18.63 (11.60, 27.55)	
All cohorts	**1.28 (0.95, 1.64)**	**14.79 (8.85, 21.85)**

Figure 45–4. The difference in prevalence of LVNC depending on the use of either echocardiography or CMR imaging for diagnosis. Reproduced with permission from Ross SB, Jones K, Blanch B, et al. A systematic review and meta-analysis of the prevalence of left ventricular non-compaction in adults. *Eur Heart J.* 2020 Apr 7;41(14):1428-1436.

were referred for reasons such as heart murmurs, chest pain, or family history of cardiomyopathy. Few isolated patients with LVNC developed an associated cardiomyopathy phenotype during the 3.3-year follow-up.[30]

Adults

In adult clinical series, the echocardiographic prevalence ranges from 0.014% to 0.26%.[31-35] As for sex, LVNC is reported to be more common in men (56%–82%) than women.[31,36-38] Ethnic or racial differences have been suggested, with higher prevalence in Blacks than Whites.[24,39,40] Hypertrabeculation may be found as a normal variant in Black Africans. Assessing trabeculation alone may infer isolated LVNC; normal individuals with hypertrabeculation have normal LV function and normal rotation patterns, with no differences in rotational parameters or net twist.[41] In three groups of volunteers including patients diagnosed with LVNC according to criteria by Jenni et al.,[2] the fractal dimension (FD) of the endocardial border was measured as a quantitative parameter distinguishing normal from abnormal trabecular patterns. Among healthy volunteers, Blacks had a higher FD than Whites in the apical third of the LV. Maximal apical FD was higher in individuals with LVNC compared to healthy volunteers.[18] In 38 healthy elite male soccer players (mean age, 23.0; range, 19–34 years; European, n = 28; Black African, n = 10) who underwent CMR and electrocardiography (ECG), hypertrabeculation was assessed using the NC/C ratio on long-axis and short-axis segments; a greater degree of LV hypertrabeculation was seen in healthy Black African athletes, combined with biventricular ejection fraction reduction at rest.[40] Overall, ethnic differences should be taken into consideration when evaluating individuals of different races, including athletes.

PATHOGENETIC HYPOTHESES

The clinical evidence available to date refer to three different pathogenetic hypotheses. The first is the classical embryogenetic one according to which the LVNC would be due to the arrest of maturation of the cardiac chambers. The second hypothesis would relate more to the possibility that LVNC is caused by genetic defects. The third hypothesis is based on increasing evidence that LVNC may be absent at birth, acquired during life in pathological or physiological conditions of overload or hemodynamic stress, and may eventually regress when the load is reduced (**Fig. 45–5**).

Embryogenetic Hypothesis

The most cited pathogenetic hypothesis is the embryogenic arrest of the normal process of trabecular maturation during early intrauterine life[42] when the heart undergoes cardiac chamber maturation. Chamber maturation occurs through the formation of myocardial trabeculae, conduction system, and growth of compact myocardium. Cardiac trabeculation begins after the looping stage when a network of myocardial

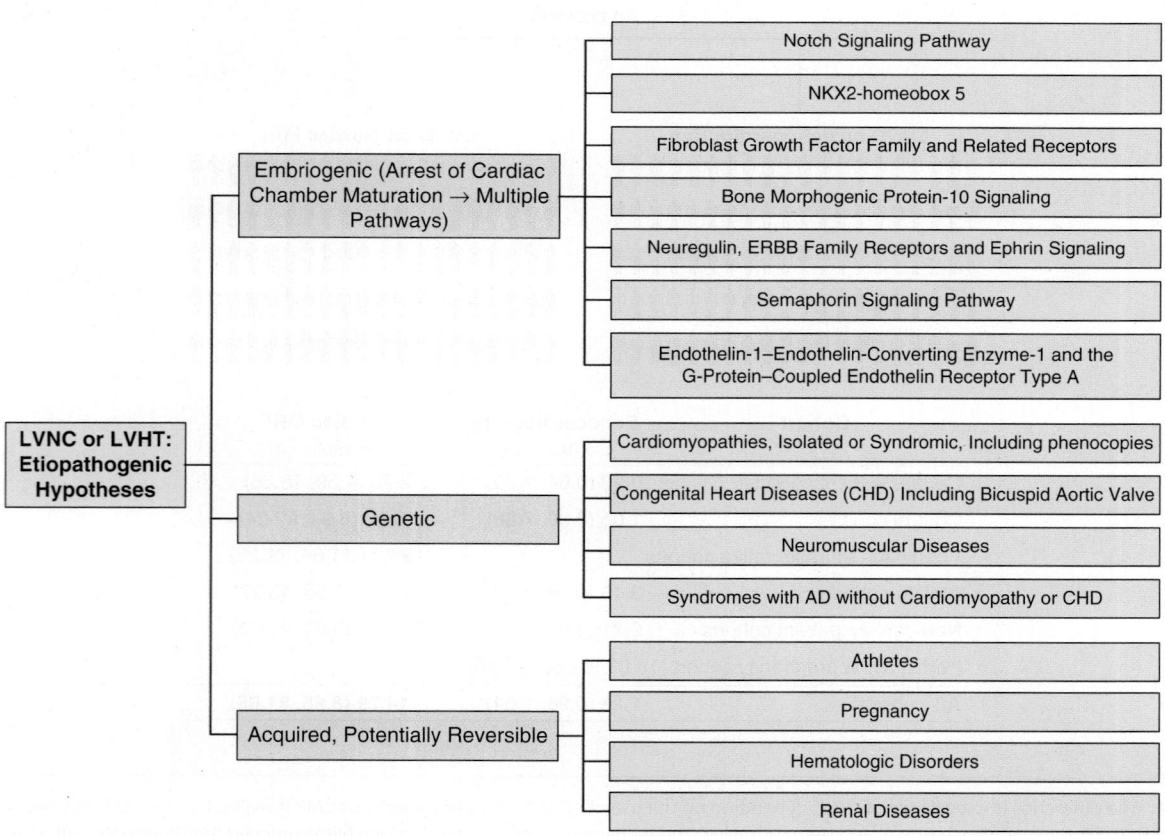

Figure 45–5. The figure summarizes the current pathogenetic hypotheses on LVNC/left ventricular hypertrabeculation.

cells covered by endothelial cells appears and projects in the LV cavity. Projections propagate radially and vertically.[42] Trabeculae then undergo compaction. The epicardial layers enter the myocardial wall and generate the coronary network, which is strictly accompanied by the formation of the compact layer.

The numerous molecular pathways active in cardiac chamber maturation include: (1) the Notch signaling pathway that is involved in the maturation of endocardium and cardiac chambers, with downregulation in the compacted myocardial layer;[43,44] (2) Nkx2-5 gene whose deletion is associated with severe hypertrabeculation and subendocardial fibrosis with Purkinje fiber hypoplasia;[45] (3) the bone morphogenic protein-10 signaling that modulates cardiomyocyte differentiation through activation of transcription factors;[46] (4) the fibroblast growth factor family and related receptors that contribute to the proliferation of the compact myocardium;[47] (5) transmembrane paracrine ligand neuregulin, ERBB family receptors, and ephrin signaling that regulate endothelial cell function and modulate directional migration of cardiomyocytes[48] (ephrin-B2 [EFNB2] and one of its receptors, EPHB4, are expressed in the endothelial cells lining trabeculae);[49] (6) the semaphorin signaling pathway that modulates gene transcription and cardiac patterning;[50] and (7) the endothelin-1–endothelin-converting enzyme-1 and the G-protein–coupled endothelin receptor type A that modulate cardiomyocytes to differentiate into Purkinje cells.[51]

Although all genes involved in pathways active in chamber maturation may potentially influence LV trabecular anatomy, none of the genes active in the above pathways to date has been identified as an LVNC-causing gene. The only exception seems to be the MIB1 gene encoding a ubiquitin ligase that regulates endocytosis of Notch ligands. Endocytosis of Notch ligands in the signal-sending cells is needed for Notch activation.[52] This observation deserves confirmation. To date, mutations in this gene have been reported in individuals with LVNC in two Spanish families.[53] Finally, extracellular matrix (ECM) interacts with cell compartments. ECM contains collagen, versican, and nephronectin;[54,55] it separates endocardial, myocardial, and epicardial layers. ECM–cell interactions are mediated by integrins that modulate cell growth, migration, survival, and differentiation. During cardiac morphogenesis, matrix metalloproteases facilitate cell migration. ECM composition is regulated in part by the matrix metalloprotease ADAMTS1, which is necessary for trabeculation.[56]

According to the embryogenetic hypothesis, the occurrence and extent of LVNC would be conditioned by the stage at which the arrest of the normal embryonic myocardial maturation takes place, considering that during the 5th and 8th week that the myocardium becomes compacted from the basal segments to the apex and from epicardium to endocardium.[57] Causes of interruption of myocardial compaction are unknown.

Genetic Hypothesis

The genetic hypothesis is based on the observation of LVNC in numerous and phenotypically different cardiomyopathies. However, no gene to date has been found to be specifically and causally associated with LVNC; all the variants described in LVNC were in genes associated with cardiomyopathies, congenital heart disease, and syndromes with and without cardiac involvement. This evidence has been recently confirmed by exome sequencing demonstrating that genetic testing is useless in adults with only isolated LVNC without family history.[58] A paradigmatic exception is Barth syndrome, which deserves separate mention because the young boys with Barth syndrome typically present with dilated cardiomyopathy with LVNC at birth.

Barth Syndrome

Barth syndrome is mentioned as a separate entity because it represents the paradigmatic example of LVNC cardiomyopathy. It should be suspected in all male infants with heart failure, DCM, and LVNC, especially when associated with other markers of disease. Barth syndrome is a rare X-linked recessive disorder characterized by cardiomyopathy, neutropenia, skeletal myopathy, prepubertal growth delay, and distinctive facial characteristics. The disease is caused by mutations in the G4.5 gene (TAZ).[59,60] The protein localizes to the mitochondrial membrane and plays a role in mitochondrial structure and function. LVNC and low mitochondrial membrane potential are reported as specific for Barth syndrome.[60] LVNC is commonly associated with LV dilation and dysfunction at onset.[59] Less commonly, Barth cardiomyopathy may present with a hypertrophic or hypertrophic-dilated phenotype. Heart involvement occurs in almost all children before the age of 5 years. Thereafter, the cardiomyopathy may demonstrate an intermittent course during which the heart can undergo remodeling. Improvement can be observed after infancy, with possible stabilization after the toddler years.[61] Heart failure is a major cause of morbidity and mortality. Overall, however, cardiac function varies and tends to decline over time. Arrhythmias, both supraventricular and ventricular, are more commonly reported in adolescents and young adults than in infants.[59,61]

Genes and Left Ventricular Noncompaction in Cardiomyopathies

LVNC can occur in hearts fulfilling the diagnostic criteria for DCM, HCM, RCM, or ARVC. In these cases, cardiomyopathies and LVNC are both present. Family studies may contribute to unraveling whether the two traits (cardiomyopathy and LVNC) can exist as independent entities or are part of the same phenotype in all or some affected family members.

In the current Online Mendelian Inheritance in Man (OMIM) catalogue, 10 genes, one locus with unidentified gene, and one syndrome are formally associated with a Mendelian Inheritance in Man (MIM) phenotype number (**Table 45–2**). The candidacy of the DTNA gene for isolated LVNC is provisionally supported by absence of mutations in cardiomyopathies without LVNC. Alpha-dystrobrevinopathies are caused by mutations in DTNA, which is part of the cytoplasmic complex of the dystrophin-associated proteins.[62] Rare dilated and dysfunctional hearts and LVNC have been associated with mutations in MIB1 that encode Dapk-interacting protein 1

TABLE 45-2. Genes and Loci Formally Included in the OMIM Catalogue as Associated with LVNC*: Ordered by Phenotype OMIM Numbers

Locus	Phenotype	MIM Phenotype No.	Gene	MIM°	Disorders Allelic at the Same Locus	Inheritance
18q12.1	LVNC1	604169	DTNA	601239	With or without congenital heart defects	AD
11p15	LVNC2	609470	None	—	—	—
10q23.2	LVNC3	601493	LDB3	605906	DCM with or without LVNC, HCM, myofibrillar myopathy	AD
15q14	LVNC4	613424	ACTC1	102540	DCM, HCM, atrial septal defects	AD
14q11.2	LVNC5	613426	MYH7	160760	DCM, HCM, Liang distal myopathy, myopathy, myosin storage AD and AR, scapuloperoneal syndrome, myopathic type	AD
1q32.1	LVNC6	611494	TNNT2	191045	DCM, RCM, HCM	AD
18q11.2	LVNC7	615092	MIB1	608677	DCM	AD
1p36.32	LVNC8	615373	PRDM16	605557	DCM	AD
15q22.2	LVNC9	611878	TPM1	191010	DCM, HCM	AD
11p11.2	LVNC10	615396	MYBPC3	600958	DCM, HCM	AD

°Last access, October 09, 2020.
Note: The LVNC phenotypes are numbered from 1 to 10; 9 disease genes are known, while 1 is still unknown (LVNC2). This latter has been mapped at 11p15 locus; No disease-causing mutation identified to date.
Abbreviations: AD, autosomal dominant; AR, autosomal recessive; DCM, dilated cardiomyopathy; HCM, hypertrophic cardiomyopathy; LVNC, left ventricular noncompaction; MIM, Mendelian Inheritance in Man; OMIM, Online Mendelian Inheritance in Man; RCM, restrictive cardiomyopathy; XL, X-linked.
°Indicates the gene.

acting in the Notch pathway.[53] LVNC can be observed in cardiomyopathies with overlapping phenotypes, typically dilated HCM such as in mitochondrial DNA-related cardiomyopathies[63] (**Table 45-3**). The lists of cardiomyopathy genes associated with LVNC demonstrate wide heterogeneity (**Tables 45-2** and **45-4**) and remain incomplete (**Fig. 45-6**). All genes reported to date as associated with LVNC also cause cardiomyopathies. Main groups include genes encoding sarcomere proteins, nuclear envelope components, Z-band proteins, and ion channels.

Sarcomere Genes: Mutations in *ACTC1* (cardiac actin alpha) were first reported in LVNC by Klaassen et al.[64] in 2008, with identification of the p.(Glu101Lys) mutation described previously in apical HCM.[65] LVNC associated with mutations in *ACTC1* gene is labeled in the OMIM catalogue as LVNC4. Mutations in the same gene also cause DCM, RCM, and HCM, as well as congenital heart disease (CHD).[66] Several mutations in the *MYH7* gene were reported in both children and adults with LVNC.[67-69] Nine diseases are allelic at the same locus (LVNC5, HCM, DCM, RCM, familial autosomal dominant Ebstein anomaly with LVNC, autosomal dominant and recessive myosin storage myopathy, Liang distal myopathy, and scapuloperoneal syndrome, myopathic type). Similar, but less complex, is the list of cardiomyopathies allelic at the *MYBPC3* locus (HCM, DCM, and LVNC).[70,71] A relevant clinical observation is the potentially lethal phenotype of cardiomyopathy with LVNC in infants who carry compound heterozygous, double heterozygous, or homozygous truncating mutations.[72] Mutations in *TPM1* (LVNC6)[73] and *TNNT2* (LVNC9)[74] are less commonly associated with LVNC. The

mechanisms by which mutations in sarcomere genes cause LVNC remain to be elucidated. Incomplete genotype is possible. Given the overlapping phenotypes associated with mutations of sarcomeric genes and the number of diseases allelic at the same loci, members of a family with the mutation may show different cardiac profiles, with or without the presence of LVNC (**Fig. 45-7**).

Genes Encoding Nuclear Envelope Proteins: Mutations in genes encoding nuclear envelope proteins (ie, *LMNA*, which typically causes DCM and conduction disease) seem to be less common than those on sarcomere genes. To date, three *LMNA* mutations [p.(Arg644Cys), p.(Arg190W), and p.(Val455Glu)] have been described in patients with DCM and LVNC.[75-77] Given the high arrhythmogenic risk associated with *LMNA* mutations, these patients and families deserve the same monitoring and management strategies currently adopted for cardiolaminopathies without LVNC. Guidelines on the prevention of sudden death recommend that an implantable cardioverter-defibrillator (ICD) should be considered in patients with DCM, a confirmed disease-causing *LMNA* mutation, and clinical risk factors (New York Heart Association [NYHA] class IIa, level of evidence B).[78] Risk factors include nonsustained ventricular tachycardia during ambulatory ECG monitoring, LVEF <45% at first evaluation, male sex, and non-missense mutations (insertion, deletion, truncation, or mutations affecting splicing). These factors correspond to those previously identified in a large European cohort of patients with dilated cardiolaminopathy.[79] LVNC can represent an early marker of cardiolaminopathy and may or may not segregate with DCM in the families (**Fig. 45-8**).

TABLE 45-3. Mitochondrial DNA Mutations Reported at Least Once as Associated with Cardiac Phenotypes Including LVNC

Mitochondrial DNA Genes			Allele	Phenotype
MTTL1	Transfer RNA leucine (UUR)	tRNA^Leu(UUR)	A3243G	MELAS, DCM, HCM
MTTQ	Transfer RNA glutamine	tRNA^Glu	T4373C	DCM, HCM, possibly LVNC-associated
MTRNR1	12S ribosomal RNA	12S rRNA	T721C	Possibly LVNC-associated
MTRNR1	12S ribosomal RNA	12S rRNA	T850C	DCM, possibly LVNC-associated
MTRNR1	12S ribosomal RNA	12S rRNA	T921C	DCM, possibly LVNC-associated
MTRNR1	12S ribosomal RNA	12S rRNA	T961C	DEAF; DCM, possibly LVNC-associated
MTRNR2	16S ribosomal RNA	16S rRNA	T2352C	DCM, possibly LVNC-associated
MTRNR2	16S ribosomal RNA	16S rRNA	G2361A	DCM, possibly LVNC-associated
MTRNR2	16S ribosomal RNA	16S rRNA	A2755G	DCM, HCM, possibly LVNC-associated
MTND1	NADH dehydrogenase subunit 1	ND1	T3308C (M-T)	Possibly LVNC-associated; MELAS, DEAF enhancer; PM[a]
MTND1	NADH dehydrogenase subunit 1	ND1	A3397G (M-V)	ADPD /possibly LVNC cardiomyopathy–associated
MTND1	NADH dehydrogenase subunit 1	ND1	T3398C (M-T)	DMDF+HCM /GDM/possibly LVNC cardiomyopathy–associated
MTND1	NADH dehydrogenase subunit 1	ND1	T4216C (Y-H)	LHON, possibly LVNC-associated
MTATP8	ATP synthase subunit 8	ATP8	A8381G (T-A)	MIDD/LVNC cardiomyopathy–associated
MTATP8/6	ATP synthase subunit 8	ATP8	C8558T (P-S)	Possibly LVNC cardiomyopathy–associated
MTATP6	ATP synthase subunit 6	ATP6	A9058G (T-A)	Possibly LVNC cardiomyopathy–associated
MTCYB	Cytochrome b	CytB	T15693C (M-T)	DCM, HCM, possibly LVNC–associated

Abbreviations: ADPD, Alzheimer disease and Parkinson disease; DCM, dilated cardiomyopathy; DEAF, maternally inherited deafness or aminoglycoside-induced deafness; DMDF, diabetes mellitus and deafness; GDM, gestational diabetes mellitus; HCM, hypertrophic cardiomyopathy; LHON, Leber hereditary optic neuropathy; LVNC, left ventricular noncompaction; MELAS, mitochondrial encephalomyopathy, lactic acidosis, and stroke-like episodes; MIDD, maternally inherited diabetes and deafness; PM, point mutation/polymorphism;
[a]Status indicates that some published reports have determined the variant to be a nonpathogenic polymorphism.

Genes Coding Z-Line Components: Genes coding Z-line components in both skeletal and cardiac muscle include the *CYPHER-ZASP* (*LDB3*) gene, which is a major candidate for LVNC.[80] In fact, carriers of mutations in *LDB3* may demonstrate DCM or LVNC (MIM# LVNC4) and, less commonly, HCM and ARVC.[81,82] Mutations in the same gene also cause myofibrillar myopathy; experimental ablation of Cypher, the PDZ-LIM domain Z-line protein, causes a severe form of congenital myopathy and DCM with premature death.[83] The p.(Asp117Asn) variant in the LIM domain-binding protein 3–encoding Z-band alternatively spliced PDZ motif gene (*ZASP*) has been described in a patient with LVNC and conduction disturbances.[84] Patients with DCM and LVNC/hypertrabeculation carriers of p.(Asp117Asn) commonly carry a second variant in a cardiomyopathy gene.

Genes Causing Muscle Dystrophies and Myopathies: Hypertrabeculation or noncompaction of the LV has been described in several neuromuscular disorders, including Duchenne muscular dystrophy (DMD) and mitochondrial myopathies.[61,63,85–87] In a large CMR study including 96 patients with DMD, 27 patients (28%) fulfilled criteria for the diagnosis of LVNC.[87] LVNC was defined as a diastolic NC/C ratio >2.3 and was measured according to the AHA 16-segment model. In patients with ejection fraction <55%, the median NC/C ratio was 2.46 versus 3.69 for isolated LVNC patients and 1.54 for normal controls. The relevant contribution of this study goes beyond

the prevalence of LVNC in DMD. Serial CMR in 78 boys with DMD demonstrated a mean rate of change in NC/C ratio per year of +0.36 that resulted from the progressive decrease of the compacted layer and relative increase of the NC layer.[87] This information adds a "dynamic view" of NC anatomy in cardiomyopathies and potential prognostic information. LVNC was in fact associated with worsening LV systolic function. The progressive thinning of the compacted layer may result in a relative increased ratio of the two layers. This helps to explain the data reported by Kimura et al.,[88] who found that LVNC is an independent negative prognostic factor in carriers of *DMD* defects.

Ion Channel Genes: Ion channel genes such as the sodium channel, type V, subunit alpha (*SCN5A*), genes encoding calcium-release channels such as the ryanodine receptor 2 (*RYR2*), and genes encoding calcium ion reservoir such as calsequestrin 2 (*CASQ2*, which is part of a protein complex that contains RYR2), typically cause diseases affecting the QT interval and catecholaminergic polymorphic ventricular tachycardia (CPVT; types 1 and 2). Pathogenic variants in *SCN5A* have been reported in Japanese patients with LVNC.[89] Mutations in *RYR2* and *CASQ2* are also associated with LVNC.[90–92] More than 80% of carriers of exon 3 deletion in the *RYR2* gene demonstrated LVNC and malignant arrhythmogenic phenotypes with syncope and CPVT.[90,91] A relevant contribution from *RYR2*-related LVNC is the demonstration that NC can develop

TABLE 45–4. Genes That Have Been Associated with LVNC in at Least One Case/Family but Are Not Listed in the OMIM Catalogue as LVNC Genes

Gene	MIM*	Protein	MIM#	Inheritance	Phenotypes
ABCC9	601439	ATB-binding cassette, subfamily C members	608569 614050 614050 —	AD	DCM Atrial fibrillation Cantu syndrome 1 reported variant in LVNC
ACTN2	102573	Alpha-actinin 2	612158 612158	AD	HCM with/without LVNC DCM with/without LVNC
CASQ2	114251	Calsequestrin 2	611938	AD	Catecholaminergic polymorphic ventricular tachycardia 2
HCN4	605206	Hyperpolarization-activated cyclic nucleotide-gated K channel 4	613123 163800 —	AD	Brugada syndrome 8 Sick sinus syndrome 2 LVNC and bradycardia: 1 report
LMNA	150330	Lamin AC	115200	AD	DCM, ARVC, no isolated LVNC
NNT	607878	Nicotinamide nucleotide transhydrogenase	614736	AR	Glucocorticoid deficiency 4
PLEKHM2	609613	Pleckstrin homology domain containing protein, family M, member 2	—	AD	DCM, LVNC in 1 report
RYR2	180902	Ryanodine receptor 2	604772 600996	AD	Catecholaminergic polymorphic ventricular tachycardia 1 ARVC (LVNC associated with exon 3 deletion)
SCN5A	600163	Sodium channel, voltage gated, type V, alpha subunit	601144 603830 614022 608567 601154 113900 113900 603829 272120	AD	Brugada syndrome 1 Long QT syndrome 3 Familial atrial fibrillation Sick sinus syndrome 1 DCM Heart block nonprogressive Heart block progressive, type IA Familial Ventricular fibrillation,1 Susceptibility to sudden infant death syndrome
TNNI3	191044	Cardiac troponin I 3	611880 613286 613690 115210	AR AD AD AD	DCM DCM HCM RCM

Abbreviations: AD, autosomal dominant; AR, autosomal recessive; ARVC, arrhythmogenic right ventricular cardiomyopathy; DCM, dilated cardiomyopathy; HCM, hypertrophic cardiomyopathy; LVNC, left ventricular noncompaction; MIM, Mendelian Inheritance in Man; RCM, restrictive cardiomyopathy.
*Indicates the gene.
#Indicates the phenotype.

during the evolution of the genetic disease. Specifically, a young patient with *RYR2* deletion of exon 3 showed normal LV function and structure at the age of 14 years when he presented with two episodes of exertional syncope and demonstrated LVNC with normal function 2 years later when he presented with a third episode of syncope.[90]

Descriptors of Cardiomyopathies with Left Ventricular Noncompaction

The nosology description of clinical, imaging, and genetic data does not meet LVNC-specific rules and criteria. Diagnoses such as "dilated LVNC" versus "DCM with LVNC" or "hypertrophic LVNC" versus "HCM with LVNC" are equally used to describe the phenotypes. When LV dilation and dysfunction are present, the diagnosis of LVNC cardiomyopathy is supported more by the DCM phenotype than by the trabecular morphology. When LVNC is observed in hearts with

HCM, the diagnosis of LVNC cardiomyopathy is supported more by the HCM criteria than those of LVNC. Nonetheless, both descriptors (either leading or subordinating the LVNC to the cardiomyopathy diagnosis) give an immediate perception of the phenotype. In comparison, the diagnosis of "LVNC cardiomyopathy" may limit clinical information and, in parallel, automatically assigns a driving role of LVNC in the diagnosis.

Left Ventricular Noncompaction in Congenital Heart Diseases

LVNC can occur in hearts with CHD such as uni- or bicuspid aortic valves, aortic coarctation, diffuse aortic hypoplasia and subaortic stenosis, atrial/ventricular septal defects, Ebstein anomaly,[93–95] tetralogy of Fallot, double outlet right ventricle, hypoplastic left heart syndrome,[96] and 5q34-q35.2 deletion syndrome.[97]

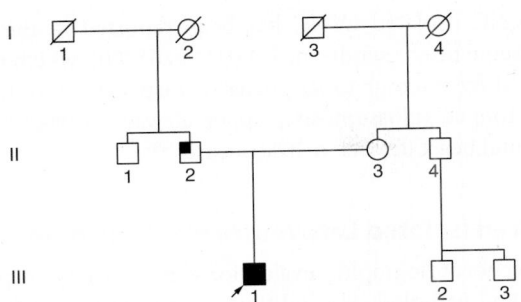

M_{NC} O_H G_{Undet} $E_{G\text{-}DSG2}$ [p.(Ile16Thr)] $S_{C\text{-}I}$

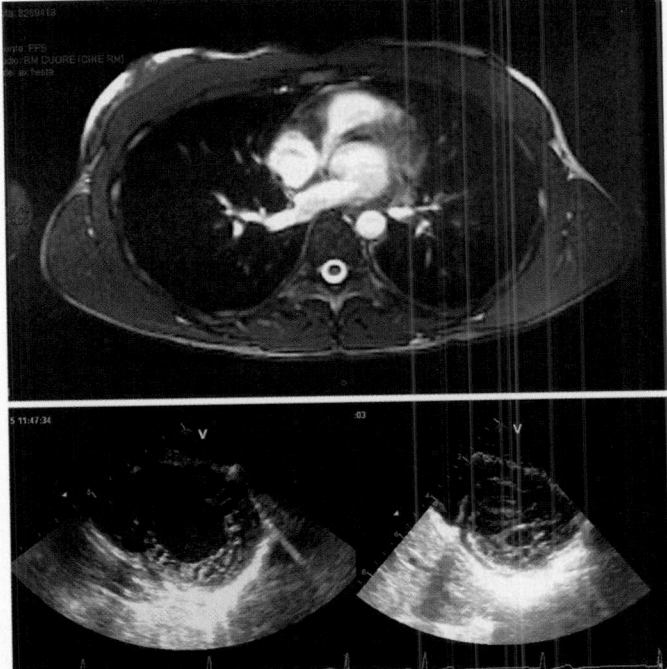

Figure 45–6. The figure shows the pedigree of a family in which the young proband (*arrow*, 23 years) had the first diagnosis of suspected LVNC/hypertrabeculation at the age of 13 years; he had played soccer for about 8 years. The boy suffered growth retardation and was treated with growth hormone (from the age of 5 to 16 years). Over the course of 10 years, he underwent several cardiology evaluations, including three CMR scans and yearly echocardiographic evaluations, treadmill tests, and 24-Holter monitoring, without a conclusive diagnosis. At present, his echocardiographic evaluation showed prominent apical trabeculation with an NC/C ratio of 2.15. Left ventricular dimensions and functions are within normal ranges. Last CMR confirmed the hypertrabeculation, but measurements have been considered as not fulfilling criteria for the diagnosis of LVNC. The right ventricle did not show abnormalities. Clinical family screening was performed before deciding about genetic testing. Multigene panel analysis by next-generation sequencing demonstrated a variant of uncertain significance/likely benign in *DSG2* gene [p.(Ile16Thr)], inherited from the father who does not show LVNC or hypertrabeculation but suffers lone atrial fibrillation. The patient is being monitored. This is a paradigmatic case of nonpathogenic variant and nonsegregation.

A high prevalence of LVNC is reported in patients fulfilling the echocardiographic criteria for bicuspid aortic valve (BAV). Specifically, in one study, 12 (11.0%) of 109 patients with BAV fulfilled the criteria for LVNC, with 9 of the 12 patients being men. Although the pathophysiologic basis of LVNC in patients

with BAV is unclear, special attention should be given to the evaluation of LV trabecular anatomy.[98] However, in a recent CMR study including 79 patients with BAV and 85 controls with tricuspid aortic valve and free of known cardiovascular disease, patients with BAV did not show more LVNC than the controls and did not demonstrate a higher risk of LVNC development.[99]

All of these disorders can be sporadic or familial, with CHD recurring in more than one member of the family.[93–96] The association of CHD and LVNC increases the risk of heart failure.[100]

Syndromic Left Ventricular Noncompaction

Syndromes with LVNC (or syndromic LVNC) are either sporadic or familial. The NC morphology is one of the traits associated with both monogenic defects and chromosomal anomalies.[101,102] Monogenic syndromes mostly include rare diseases. Some of them, such as Anderson–Fabry disease and Danon disease, are well known by cardiologists[103–105] because

I:1 → $M_{H(N\text{-}Obs)+D+NC}$ O_H G_{AD} $E_{G\text{-}MYH7}$[p.(Gly716Arg)] **SC-IV**

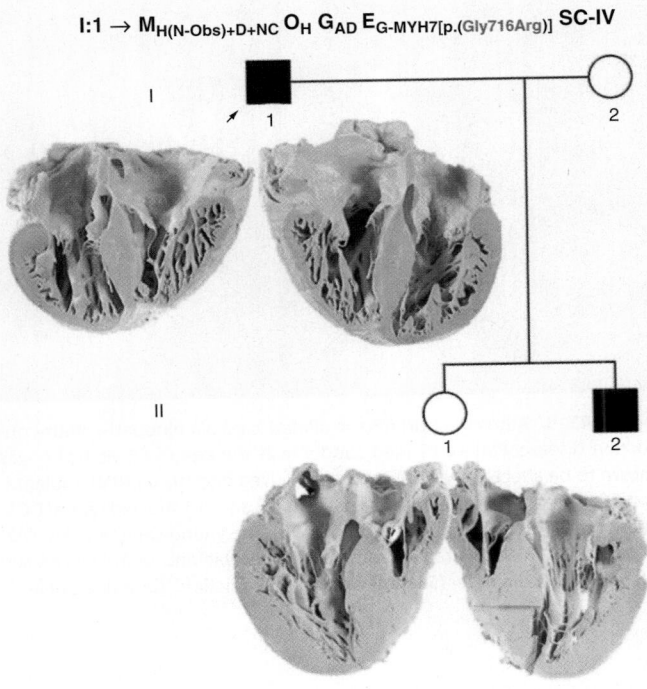

II:2 → $M_{H(N\text{-}Obs)}$ O_H G_{AD} $E_{G\text{-}MYH7}$[p.(Gly716Arg)] **SC-IV**

Figure 45–7. Phenotype heterogeneity in affected members of the same family and lack of segregation of the LVNC with the disease mutation. The figure shows the pedigree and the macroscopic view of the hearts excised at transplantation from I:1 and his son (II:2). The father was first diagnosed at the age of 36 years and underwent heart transplantation 10 years later; the son was first diagnosed with HCM at the age of 20 years and underwent heart transplantation 4 years later. Although father and son carry the same mutation in the *MYH7* gene, the cardiac remodeling in the two hearts differs. In I:1, the heart shows prominent trabeculae in both right and left ventricle; in II:2, the macroscopic phenotype is that of a typical HCM. I:1, MOGE(S) descriptor: the morphofunctional (M) phenotype indicates the hypertrophic cardiomyopathy (H), with dilated evolution (D) and associated noncompaction (NC); O (organ) specifies that the only involved organ was the heart (H); G (genetic) indicates that the disease had genetic basis and the inheritance was autosomal dominant (AD); E (etiology) specification indicates that the disease gene is *MYH7* and the mutation was p.(Gly716Arg); the pathologic mutation is in *red*.

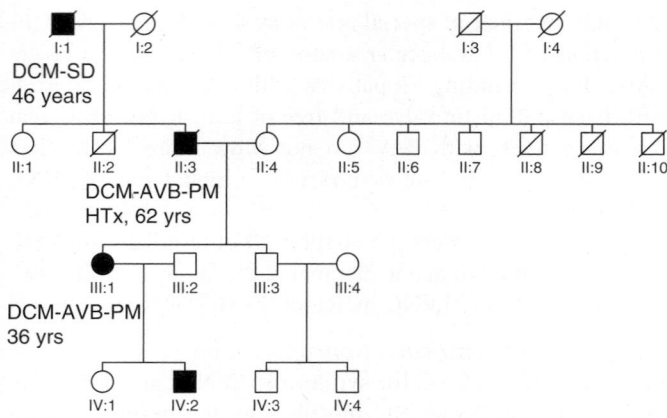

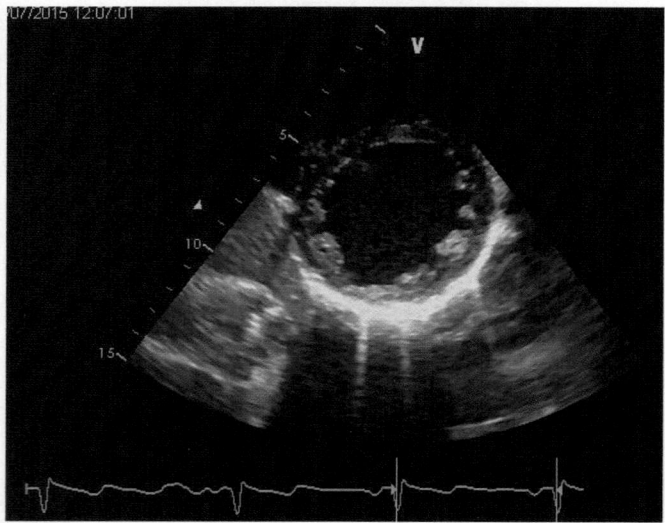

IV:2, 16 yrs M$_{0(LVNC)}$ O$_H$ G$_{AD}$ E $_{G-LMNA[p.(Arg72Cys)]}$ S$_{A-I}$

Figure 45–8. Autosomal dominant dilated cardiolaminopathy with conduction disease. Patient I:1 died suddenly at the age of 46 years; he was known to be affected by DCM and had received pacemaker (PM) implantation a few years before death. Both patients II:3 and III:1 showed typical DCM phenotype with atrioventricular block (AVB). The young son (14 years, IV:2) of patient III:1 demonstrated prominent trabeculae and slightly increased left ventricular diameter (55 mm) with normal function. SD, sudden death.

the HCM phenotype is often the first recognized manifestation. Other monogenic syndromes are less commonly observed in the cardiology setting (**Table 45–5**). Chromosomal anomalies are usually observed in complex syndromes that display several multiorgan defects. Chromosomal abnormalities include deletions, translocations, and trisomy or tetrasomy [1p36 deletion syndrome; interstitial 1q43-q43del; del(1)(q) syndrome; del5q35; 7p14.3-p14.1 deletion; 8p23.1 del syndrome; 18p subtelomeric deletion; 22q11.2 deletion syndrome; 22q11.2 distal deletion syndrome; trisomy 13 and 18; tetrasomy 5q35.2–5q35; Robertsonian translocation 13;14; mosaics such as 45,X/46XX and 45,X/46,X,i(Y)(p11)]. Most chromosomal abnormalities represent isolated cases.[93–95] Reasons for scientific and clinical interest include the possible identification of new disease or modifier genes when abnormal chromosomal regions involve novel candidate genes in patients with the typical syndrome

and LVNC. Isolated LVNC has been reported in the Pierre Robin sequence or syndrome (OMIM #261800), which is characterized by micrognathia, posterior displacement/retraction of the tongue (glossoptosis), upper airway obstruction, and congenital heart defects in 20% of cases.[106]

Acquired Isolated Left Ventricular Noncompaction

Serial echocardiographic evaluations in a variety of physiological and pathological conditions demonstrate that there are forms of LVNC that are acquired and reversible in training athletes,[107] pregnancy,[108] hematologic disorders,[109] and chronic renal diseases.[110]

A trabeculated ventricle can work at lower strain compared to a nontrabeculated ventricle to produce the same stroke volume, which could be a possible explanation why athletes and pregnant women develop reversible signs of LVNC, since the trabeculations may help generate increased cardiac output.[111]

These observations expand the spectrum of pathogenetic hypotheses from arrested embryogenesis maturation of LV trabeculae or genetic hypothesis to acquired pathogenetic mechanisms, including hemodynamics, phenotype-driven trabecular gene expression, or epigenetic factors.

Athletes

The identification of LVNC in preparticipation screening studies had demonstrated that intense physical training may induce increased trabeculation that may fulfill current diagnostic criteria for the diagnosis of LVNC. In a large series including more than 1000 asymptomatic athletes, 18% had increased LV trabeculation and 76 (8%) fulfilled echocardiographic criteria for LVNC.[107] The issue of athletes demonstrating LVNC is emerging from different sources[112,113] and in real life (**Fig. 45–9**). Distinguishing between pathologic LVNC and physiologic hypertrabeculation is a diagnostic challenge, and detection is becoming increasingly common with enhanced echocardiography and magnetic resonance imaging modalities.[26,112] The proportion of athletes who develop LVNC under intensive exercise is relevant (about 10%), but the proportion of those who do not develop LVNC under the same exercise levels is 90%. The impact of LVNC on otherwise normal hearts requires long-term follow-up studies to establish with certainty whether LVNC can be an early marker of myocardial disease or the phenotype of maladaptation of different individuals to strenuous physical effort. Therefore, "healthy" athletes diagnosed with LVNC should undergo deep phenotype examination, advanced imaging, and clinical monitoring as suggested by experts.[114]

Pregnancy

A form of reversible LVNC has been described in pregnancy. In a prospective longitudinal echocardiographic study of 102 primigravida pregnant normotensive women (66 White women and 36 Black women) without family history of cardiomyopathy or premature sudden cardiac death, 25% developed increased LV trabeculations during pregnancy. The finding was more common in Black women than in White women. Furthermore, 10 women (9.8%) fulfilled the Jenni et al.[2] criteria,

TABLE 45–5. Monogenic Syndromes with Cardiac Involvement Including LVNC

Gene	MIM*	Protein	MIM#	Inheritance	Phenotypes
G4.5	300394	Tafazzin	302060	XL	Barth syndrome with DCM-LVNC; rare HCM
ARFGEF2	605371	ADP-ribosylation factor guanine nucleotide-exchange factor 2	608097	AR	Periventricular heterotopia with microcephaly
DNAJC19	608977	DNAJ/HSP40 homolog, subfamily C, member 19	610198	AR	DCM with ataxia (DCMA)
LAMP2	309060	Lysosome-associated membrane protein 2	300257	XL	Danon disease
NNT	607878	Nicotinamide nucleotide transhidrogenase	614736	AR	Glucocorticoid deficiency 4 (GCCD4)
RSK2	300075	Ribosomal S6 kinase 2	303600 300844	XL	Coffin-Lowry syndrome (faciodigital mental retardation syndrome) Mental retardation
YWHAE (14-3-3ε)	605066	Monooxygenase activation protein, epsilon isoform	—	AD	LVNC and hypoplasia of the corpus callosum

Abbreviations: AD, autosomal dominant; AR, autosomal recessive; DCM, dilated cardiomyopathy; HCM, hypertrophic cardiomyopathy; LVNC, left ventricular noncompaction; MIM, Mendelian Inheritance in Man.
*Indicates the gene.
#Indicates the phenotype.

19 (18.6%) fulfilled the Chin et al.[9] criteria, and 8 (7.8%) fulfilled both criteria for LVNC. There was no significant association between increased LV trabeculations and age, body mass index, systolic blood pressure, LV cavity dimension, stroke volume, or LV mass. Ethnicity was the only independent predictor for the presence of increased (three or more) trabeculations during pregnancy, with Black women being almost three times more likely to develop increased LV trabeculations than White women during pregnancy after adjustment for the aforementioned factors. After delivery, 18 women (69.2%) showed complete resolution of LV trabeculations over a mean duration of 8.1 ± 4.2 months, whereas 7 women (27%) continued to display LV trabeculations, without predilection for ethnicity.[108] However, the study[108] adds evidence to the possibility that LVNC can not only be acquired, but also transient and, therefore, does not necessarily represent a primary myocardial disorder but rather an adaptation to physiological needs of higher stoke volume.[115] Further series are necessary to confirm this transient trabecular remodeling and the low risk.[116,117]

Hematologic diseases

LVNC may occur in patients affected by different hematologic disorders such as Congenital dyserythropoietic anemia type 1 (CDA1) (higher prevalence of LVHT/NC than normal individuals),[118] hereditary spherocytosis,[119] essential thrombocytopenia,[120] and β-thalassemia[109,121] with and without myocardial overload. In patients with β-thalassemia, isolated LVNC was identified in 13.3% of patients.[109] The mechanisms by which chronic anemia, hemolysis, or ineffective erythropoiesis may influence the remodeling of the trabecular compartments are not known. In patients with myocardial iron overload and siderosis, a preferential distribution of intramyocyte iron in the compacted or NC layers has not been observed.[122] Myocardial T2*-weighted CMR values should be able to provide more information about intramyocyte iron storage. However, cardiac abnormalities could be triggered by toxic iron species such as non–transferrin-bound iron.[122] Regarding outcome and prognosis, LVNC in 560 patients with thalassemia was not associated with a worsening of LV function and adverse events after a long-term follow-up (5,1 years) based on repeated CMR studies.[123] Whether LVNC represents a physiologic adaptation to the chronic nonprimary cardiac disorders or a disease-related pathologic effect is not clear.[124]

Chronic Renal Disease

LVNC has been reported in two patients with chronic renal failure. In both cases, echocardiography demonstrated a dilated LV with thickened walls and a thin, compacted myocardium on the epicardial side and a thicker noncompacted endocardial layer. Ratio between the NC myocardium and the compaction myocardial layer fulfilled diagnostic criteria in both cases. Clinically relevant is the fact that oral anticoagulation therapy was initiated in both patients after the diagnosis of LVNC. Family screening with echocardiography in first-degree relatives of one of the patients did not show additional affected members. Regular echocardiographic monitoring of patients with chronic renal failure is suggested to diagnose cardiovascular diseases including this rare association.[110]

RIGHT VENTRICULAR NONCOMPACTION

Right ventricular noncompaction (RVNC) can occur as an isolated entity,[4,125–127] in association with LVNC[5] with predominant right ventricular involvement,[128] or in patients with CHD.[129] In rare cases, it may cause right ventricular outflow tract obstruction as a result of hypertrophied spongy muscle at the infundibular region.[130] Given the complex trabecular anatomy of the right ventricle, the diagnosis is difficult but feasible with routine imaging tools and, when necessary, right ventriculography.[130] RVNC may be an occasional finding in family

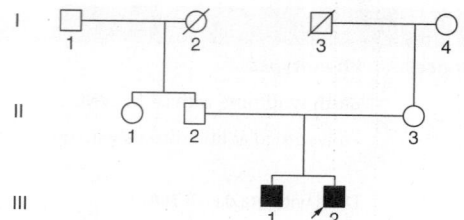

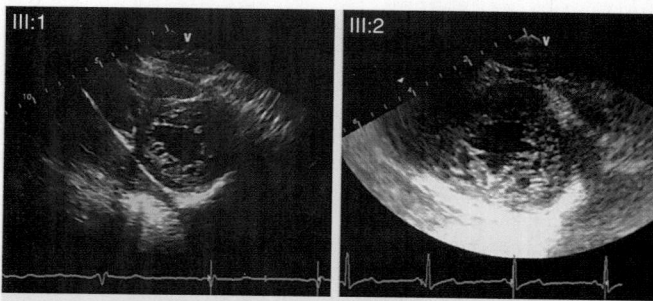

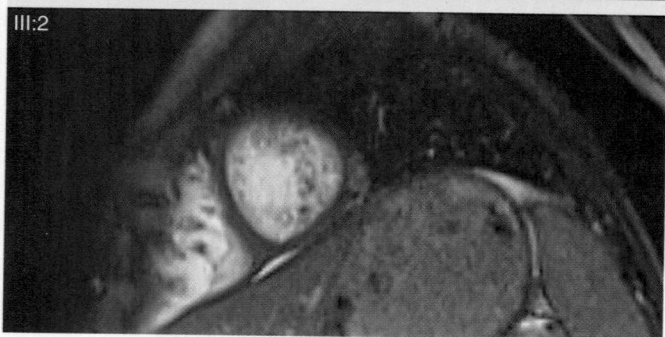

Figure 45–9. The figure shows the pedigree of a small family in which the proband (III:2) is a 12-year-old healthy boy, who plays soccer. He has been incidentally diagnosed with LVNC after identification of nonspecific ECG abnormalities in preparticipation screening (diphasic T waves in V_2-V_3, D_2, aVF). LV function and dimensions were within normal ranges (LVEF, 55%; LV end-diastolic diameter, 52 mm; according to Henry, 104.8; Z-score, 0.50). The echocardiographic evaluation of the brother (III:1; soccer player) showed prominent trabeculation confirmed by CMR, not fulfilling criteria for the diagnosis of LVNC. Both parents are not athletes and had normal echocardiographic evaluation. Extensive genetic testing analysis did not identify pathologic mutations. Both siblings are carriers of a likely benign genetic variant [p.(Lys393Asn)] in the *KCNQ1* gene. The two echocardiographic panels show the trabecular pattern in the two siblings; the CMR panel shows prominent trabeculae in III:2. The variant is inherited from the healthy father. This is another example of nonsegregation and pointless genetic testing.

screening studies (**Fig. 45–10**). Advanced fetal imaging may provide prenatal diagnoses.[131]

LEFT VENTRICULAR NONCOMPACTION: DIAGNOSTIC WORKUP

In patients with LVNC associated with cardiomyopathies, CHDs, or complex syndromes, clinical workup is guided by the primary disease rather than by the LVNC itself. Vice versa, in individuals demonstrating isolated LVNC with normal cardiac function and dimensions, the diagnostic workup should be tailored based on individual characteristics and findings emerging from cardiologic investigations, family history (and eventually

$M_{0(RVHypertrabeculation)}$ O_H G_{Undet} E_{G-N} S_{A-I}

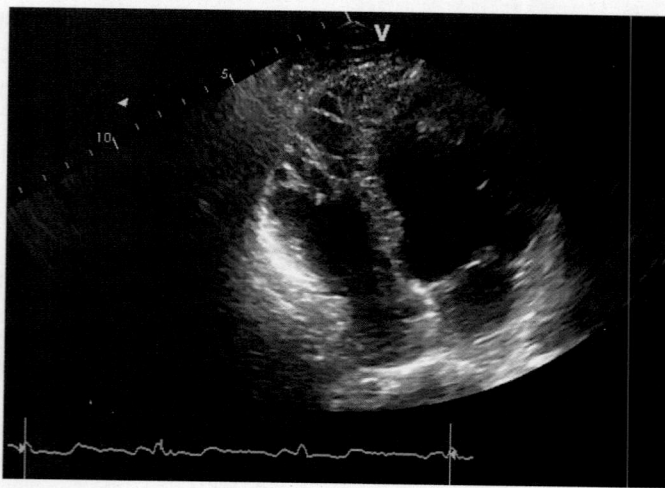

Figure 45–10. Prominent right ventricular trabeculations in a young man (36 years) who was addressed to genetic counseling after the sudden death of his first son (first day of life). The echocardiographic study showed normal LV dimension and morphology; although trabeculae were prominent in the LV apex, criteria for LVNC were not fulfilled. The patient is undergoing regular clinical monitoring.

screening), advanced imaging, and monitoring. Over the last 20 years, LVNC has been repeatedly described as *LVNC cardiomyopathy*. Efforts by several groups of researchers to establish precise diagnostic criteria (Table 45–1) for diagnosing LVNC reflect the lack of gold standards for the diagnosis. The potentially dynamic evolution of LVNC, either progression or regression, and the possibility of controlling abnormal trabecular remodeling with current treatments are matters of investigation. A recent study reported LV mass reduction among patients with LVNC during β-blocker therapy.[132]

Physical Examination

In patients with heart disease and LVNC, physical examination can contribute to the diagnosis. Extracardiac traits recurring in patients with LVNC (and vice versa) can eventually help to generate a diagnostic hypothesis, particularly in genetic cardiomyopathies, syndromes, and congenital heart defects.[133] Deep cardiomyopathy phenotyping can help to generate a clinical hypothesis, especially in patients with LVNC.[133]

Genetics and Family Screening

Genetic evaluation, both counseling and testing, is recommended for patients with cardiomyopathy and LVNC, patients diagnosed with one of the syndromes in which LVNC may recur, and individuals in whom LVNC is incidentally identified during medical screening.[134,135] A key question is whether the trait is familial or sporadic, and the answer may come from clinical family screening. In fact, isolated LVNC in individuals with normal LV size and function and nonthickened LV walls is asymptomatic and only detectable using imaging.

The medical genetic examination explores anthropometric profiles, facies, skin, eyes, hair, and skeletal and nervous systems.[133] Deep phenotyping may identify extracardiac traits that recur in syndromes with LVNC and that can be present in some family members. Data from probands and relatives contribute to generating family pedigrees, which give a "graphic" view of the mode of inheritance of the disease. In the post–genetic test phase, the pedigree shows the segregation of the mutation(s) with the phenotype, thus highlighting the correct interpretation of the genetic results.

Genetic testing should be performed in probands with LVNC and cardiomyopathy, in patients with familial CHD with LVNC, and in patients with syndromes including LVNC.[134] The indication to perform genetic testing in individuals with normal LV function and an incidental diagnosis of LVNC is not regulated by guidelines. Genetic counseling and extensive clinical information are essential.[133,134] Probands should be aware that activation of genetic testing, in particular multigene panels, can demonstrate the presence of genetic variants of unknown significance whose role in the determination of the trait may remain uncertain, and therefore, results can be inconclusive. Athletes are especially exposed to the risk of labeling a potentially reversible trait with the diagnosis of a possible genetic disease, with obvious implications regarding suitability for sport activity and lifestyles.

In families with LVNC and cardiomyopathy, affected members may demonstrate different or combined cardiac phenotypes, with isolated LVNC in some relatives and cardiomyopathy with or without LVNC in others. Therefore, the segregation of LVNC may not coincide with the segregation of a coexisting cardiomyopathy. This explains why segregation studies are major contributors in unraveling the role of mutations, especially in families with complex genetics, when more than one pathologic mutation is identified.[136] Information gathered from large families can be effectively transferred to small families or single patients, especially when evaluating the role of debated genetic variants such as *LDB3* p.(Asp117Asn), which was originally described as causing DCM and LVNC[80] and is now reported as a possible single nucleotide polymorphism.[137]

Electrocardiography

ECG data do not provide LVNC-specific diagnostic information.[138] From available observations, it appears that although a normal ECG finding is rare in LVNC and observed in a minority of patients (from 6% to 13%), there are no changes specific to LVNC.[138-141] However, certain ECG changes, such as negative T waves >1 mm in depth in two or more leads (particularly V_4-V_6, II and aVF, or I and aVL), ST-segment depression ≥0.5 mm in depth in any lead, or pathologic Q waves (>3 mm in depth or >40 milliseconds in duration) in two or more leads (except III and aVR), are more compatible with a cardiomyopathy. A significant number of Black athletes (almost 13%) show negative T waves in the anterior precordial leads that are not associated with structural disease.[142]

Imaging
Echocardiography
Echocardiography is the first-choice imaging tool for suspecting or diagnosing LVNC. It is noninvasive and easy to both perform and repeat. Serial echocardiographic investigations are sustainable and can be offered as both screening studies and in the diagnostic setting. The different diagnostic criteria proposed to date are summarized in Table 45–1. The role of the thickness of the compacted myocardial layer in the diagnosis should be emphasized.[23]

However, echocardiography has limitations. Visualization of the apex, which is commonly affected in LVNC, can be difficult. The profile of a dual-layered myocardium or trabeculations may not be sharp. Indistinct trabeculae may also result in diagnostic difficulty. Interpretation of echocardiographic findings may vary among experts. In a recent study, echocardiographic records from 100 patients with and without LV hypertrabeculation matched for age and systolic function were reviewed by experts according to the following predefined criteria: (1) greater than three prominent trabeculae at end diastole; (2) an NC part of a two-layered myocardial structure formed by these trabeculations; (3) a ratio of >2:1 of the NC/C layer at end systole; and (4) perfusion of the intertrabecular spaces from the ventricular cavity. The observers disagreed over presence or absence of LV hypertrabeculation in 35 cases, and even after mutual review, 11% of cases remained questionable.[143] A possible limitation occurs when the short axis is not perpendicular to the LV long axis, which can give the morphologic appearance of prominent trabeculations mimicking LVNC.[12] The above limitations are those currently listed in most review articles and scientific communications. However, modern echocardiographic instruments are providing high imaging quality. In addition, contrast-enhanced echocardiography can better profile endocardial borders and show trabeculations alternating with the intertrabecular recesses.[144] Finally, three-dimensional echocardiography can further contribute to evaluate the extent of noncompacted myocardium. In 26 Olympic rowing athletes and 49 healthy volunteers, the trabeculated LV volume and its value normalized by LV end-diastolic volume were significantly higher in patients with LVNC as compared to controls and athletes. Given the high spatial resolution and accuracy in volumetric quantification, three-dimensional echocardiography can provide an accurate measurement of the extent of the NC myocardium and identification of patients with LVNC.[145]

Cardiac Magnetic Resonance
CMR is performed in patients with echocardiographic evidence or suspicion of LVNC. The use of balanced steady-state free precession (SSFP) cine imaging instead of simple gradient-echo imaging improves image quality and increases sensitivity for myocardial trabeculae, which are better seen at end diastole[13-19] (Table 45–1). In clinical practice, an NC/C ratio >2.3 is considered diagnostic for LVNC (Petersen criteria). Measures are taken in short axis at the midcavity and basal segments. A four-chamber view may be preferred in hearts with prominent apical LVNC. As a result of the complex right ventricular trabecular anatomy, right ventricular involvement in LVNC or isolated RVNC can be better evaluated with CMR than with echocardiography.[13,146,147] Criteria for the diagnosis of RVNC are not established. From observations in autopsy series, transmural

thickness of the NC right ventricle >75% should correspond to a diagnosis of RVNC.[148] Dilatation of the right ventricle may be a supportive feature for the diagnosis.[149] The three-dimensional view shows the entire volume of the heart independently of the thoracic conformation of patients.[150] CMR further provides information on possible associated CHD, endocardial thrombi, or incidental extracardiac pathologies. In general, CMR performance is superior to echocardiography for characterization of the ventricular trabecular anatomy.[16] Although myocardial fibrosis is not a criterion for the diagnosis of LVNC, late gadolinium enhancement (LGE) is an adjunct value, useful in the general evaluation of the disease context in which LVNC is observed. CMR may have limitations in children because of lack of patient cooperation and small cardiac size.[16] In any case, CMR is superior to two-dimensional echocardiography in assessing the presence and the extent of noncompaction.[26,151] It also provides supplemental morphologic information beyond that obtained with conventional echocardiography.[26,151] However, CMR also has limitations. It may be contraindicated in patients with old intracavitary device implantation and in those suffering from claustrophobia. CMR is more expensive than echocardiography and may be more time consuming. In addition, serial CMR studies can be performed but at reasonably longer intervals than serial echocardiography.

Multidetector Computed Tomography

MDCT offers advantages to both patients and operators. Duration of the test is short, making it especially advantageous for those who suffer from claustrophobia. Newer scanners and dose modulation techniques have decreased the effective radiation exposure. In addition, CT can be used for patients with defibrillators or resynchronizing devices. A major advantage of MDCT is the exclusion of coronary artery disease and coronary anomalies.[23,152–154] With the increase in the number of thoracic and coronary MDCT angiographic studies, LVNC may be incidentally detected during examinations performed for other reasons. Major limitations include the administration of ionizing radiation and lower capability of characterizing myocardial tissue and identifying fibrosis compared with CMR. Cost-related limitations are similar to those of CMR, and serial studies are not routinely feasible.

Biomarkers and Pathology

There are no specific biomarkers for LVNC. Potentially useful markers are either those that provide information on myocardial injury or heart failure, namely troponins and natriuretic peptides. In genetic cardiomyopathies with LVNC, relevant biomarkers may be those that characterize the genetic disease and are equally increased in cardiomyopathy patients independent of LVNC (eg, in dystrophin cardiomyopathy).[87,88] Recently, the up-regulation of miR-21, miR-29a, miR-30d, and miR-133a indicates the presence of LGE in LVNC patients, and therefore these may serve as potential biomarkers for myocardial fibrosis.[155] The possibility that LGE occurs precisely at the level of the trabeculae has not received much attention to date. Trabeculae LGE has been described in 2 of 42 cases with LVNC

diagnosed with both two-dimensional transesophageal echocardiography (2D-TEE) and CMR.[156]

Macroscopic pathology is highly informative. Both autopsy and hearts excised at transplantation may demonstrate typical features of LVNC.[8,148,157] However, microscopic features are nonspecific. Endomyocardial biopsy may show interstitial fibrosis, fibrous endocardial thickening, and nonspecific myocyte changes similar to those seen in cardiomyopathies. In rare cases of cardiac amyloidosis with imaging features of apical hypertrabeculations suggestive of LVNC, endomyocardial biopsy can play a diagnostic role for amyloid heart disease.[158]

LEFT VENTRICULAR NONCOMPACTION MANAGEMENT

In general, the management of patients with LVNC consists of evidence-based treatments for systolic heart failure and arrhythmias as well as oral anticoagulation to prevent mural thrombosis. Indications for ICD placement are similar to those in other patients with DCM.[159]

LVNC specific treatment does not exist. At present, the possible distinct clinical problem is the thrombogenic risk, which is present only in dysfunctional hearts. Therefore, decisions about anticoagulation can eventually be anticipated in patients with LV dilation and impaired systolic function.[160,161] Stroke and embolism are rare in patients with LV hypertrabeculation or LVNC, especially when rhythm and systolic function are normal. When present, atherosclerosis-related causes should be assessed.[160] The $CHADS_2$ (congestive heart failure, hypertension, age ≥75 years, diabetes mellitus, stroke) score may be useful for clinical decision making regarding oral anticoagulation for prevention of stroke and embolism in patients with increased LV trabeculations.[161]

Patients diagnosed with Barth syndrome with heart failure should receive standard medications as per guidelines. Aspirin can eventually be added to decrease the risk of stroke in patients with severe LV dysfunction. The monitoring of arrhythmias and related prevention strategies should be maintained over the course of the patient's life. Disease-specific treatments can include the administration of granulocyte colony-stimulating factor either routinely or in high-risk clinical situations (eg, infections, surgery) along with prophylactic antibiotics. Diets should include administration of uncooked cornstarch to prevent muscle protein loss overnight. Succinylcholine, a nondepolarizing neuromuscular blocker that could have a prolonged effect, should be avoided.[61] As a general rule, patients with Barth syndrome should be cared for by specialized pediatricians in the context of a multidisciplinary setting that guarantees continuity of care from the pediatric setting to adulthood.

In other conditions, such as HCM with LVNC or RCM with LVNC, anticoagulation treatment is driven more by complications of the native disease, such as left atrial dilation with and without arrhythmias.

Pregnant women can be incidentally diagnosed with isolated, de novo LVNC that may regress after delivery, or develop peripartum cardiomyopathy (PPCM; dilated, congestive phenotype) with features of LVNC.[162] The management of LVNC associated with PPCM and of LVNC in pregnant women with normal LV function and dimensions may differ. The former may require management of the PPCM with possible adjunct of anticoagulation (see Chapter 51), whereas the latter may potentially only require clinical monitoring.

The administration of medications such as β-blockers seems to decrease LV mass among patients with LVNC. It is not clear whether the effect is a result of the decrease of the trabeculae or the compacted LV myocardial mass or both. Effects of β-blocker treatment in LVNC require validation in prospective controlled studies.[132]

Left Ventricular Trabeculectomy

In 1985, Oglesby et al. postulated that in mammalian hearts, free-running trabeculae provide tensile support to the left ventricle and minimize diastolic wall stress and that this supportive role can become pathologic, worsening diastolic compliance in LV hypertrophy. Therefore, in an ex vivo experimental study, they set up a novel operation involving cutting trabeculae to acutely increase diastolic compliance in patients presenting with heart failure and diastolic dysfunction with the aim of improving the left ventricle compliance.[163] Since then, there have been no new studies on trabeculectomy procedures in the presence of LVNC. Recently, however, Takamatsu et al. reported the first case of isolated trabeculectomy and postoperative echocardiographic follow-up showing the recovery of the cardiac function for isolated LVNC.[164] This case is unique and remains anecdotal.

PROGNOSTIC STRATIFICATION

Prognosis in LVNC depends on the clinical presentation and on the associated heart disease. The contracted term *LVNC cardiomyopathy* is confusing because it does not specify the type of cardiomyopathy (dilated, hypokinetic, hypertrophic, etc). In general, the lack of specification of the type of cardiomyopathy generates a category of cardiomyopathies defined only by the anatomical characteristics of the LV trabeculae and not by abnormalities of function and size of the left ventricle. In practice, the use of the term *LVNC cardiomyopathy* is often synonymous with "DCM with LVNC." This is particularly manifest in pediatric age. In fact, symptomatic children with LVNC usually present in early infancy with a predominant dilated phenotype. Long-term outcomes are worse than for matched children without dilated cardiomyopathy.[165]

Asymptomatic patients or individuals with LVNC and normal LV function and dimensions have a good prognosis. This is demonstrated by the large group of asymptomatic (26%) first- and second-degree family members of patients with LVNC.[166] Alternatively, patients presenting with heart failure (NYHA class III or IV), sustained ventricular arrhythmias, or left atrial dilation have an unfavorable prognosis.[166,167] Adverse outcomes of isolated LVNC occur in patients with advanced heart failure, dilated left heart with systolic dysfunction, reduced systolic blood pressure, pulmonary hypertension, and right bundle branch block.[166] Survival tracks closely with the presence of symptoms at presentation (69% when present vs 100% when

absent).[144] To further support this observation, in an imaging-based meta-analysis including four prospective studies comparing a total of 574 patients with LVNC and 677 without LVNC, in the group of patients with LVNC, no LGE, and preserved LVEF, no hard cardiac events (ie, cardiac death, sudden cardiac death, appropriate ICD firing, resuscitated cardiac arrest, cardiac transplantation, LV assist device implantation) occurred. When matched for LVEF, patients with LVNC shared the same prognosis compared to those without. Only the presence of LGE was significantly associated with the combined endpoint of the above hard events, heart failure hospitalization, ischemic stroke, and other thromboembolic events.[168]

In subgroups of patients (eg, DMD, Becker muscular dystrophy), the presence of LVNC is significantly associated with rapid deterioration in LV function and higher mortality.[87,88] Therefore, prognosis depends upon the severity of the underlying cardiac disease rather than the trabecular anatomy of the LV. Prognostic stratification is driven by the criteria used for the cardiomyopathy (eg, DCM) in which LVNC is observed. Recent evidence further demonstrates that patients with LVNC carry a similar cardiovascular risk when compared with DCM patients. LVEF—a conventional indicator of heart failure severity, not the extent of trabeculation—appears to be an important determinant of adverse outcomes in LVNC patients.[169]

SUMMARY

LVNC is a morphology-based diagnosis that does not have, by itself, corresponding LV dysfunction. Based on current diagnostic criteria, LVNC can be identified in healthy individuals, or it can be acquired and reversible in pregnant women, athletes, and patients with hematologic disorders, myopathies, chronic renal failure, and bicuspid aortic valve. A trabeculated ventricle can work at lower strain compared to a nontrabeculated ventricle to produce the same stroke volume, which could explain why athletes and pregnant women develop reversible signs of LVNC,[111] since trabeculations allow for an increase in stroke volume with less strain, essentially generating more cardiac output. The observation of reversible LVNC in athletes suggests that it may represent a phenotypic variant of athlete's heart.[170]

When associated with cardiomyopathies, CHDs, or syndromes, LVNC commonly has a genetic cause, which coincides with that of the underlying disease. The proportion of echocardiographic diagnoses is increasing, and this implies cascades of further clinical evaluation, including CMR, family studies, monitoring, and lifestyle modifications and/or restrictions.[171] Genetics may contribute to the overall interpretation of LVNC, either associated with heart disease or isolated in healthy individuals with normally functioning hearts, in whom LVNC may be acquired or reversible. In the former condition, genetic defects will coincide with those that cause the underlying disease. In the latter, genetic testing remains non informative. When present in association with heart disease, the specific role or impact of LVNC on disease manifestations, progression and outcome remains difficult to separate from that of the underlying heart disease. There are no specific treatments that decrease the trabecular burden, which is unique for each individual and acquired in the course of life in the context of different physiological and pathological conditions; anticoagulation plans can be eventually anticipated in dilated and dysfunctional hearts (DCM with LVNC). For isolated LVNC, a precise definition (trabecular anatomy variant, adaptation phenotype, transient/reversible or permanent, or heart muscle disease) based upon consensus diagnostic criteria by scientific bodies is a major missing in clinical practice.

Definition

LVNC describes a ventricular wall anatomy characterized by the presence of a prominent LV trabeculae, a thin compacted layer, and deep intertrabecular recesses that are in continuity with the LV cavity and separated from the epicardial coronary arteries. Isolated LVNC does not fulfill the criteria for cardiomyopathies.

Epidemiology

- In cardiac, control, representative population, athletes, noncardiac, and primigravida cohorts, the prevalence varies from 1.28% with 2D-TTE to 14.89% with CMR—highest in the noncardiac cohort (36.21%).
- Also observed in renal, hematological, and neuromuscular diseases.
- Dynamic, potentially reversible morphologic trait.

Pathogenesis

- Embryogenic hypothesis: arrest of maturation, multiple pathways.
- Genetic hypothesis: extreme genetic heterogeneity, nonspecifically linked with the LVNC. Segregation studies in families demonstrate segregation of the genetic defects with the underlying cardiac disease but not with the LVNC morphology.
- Hemodynamic hypothesis: supported by the evidence of being acquired and reversible (the most plausible hypothesis).

Genetics

- Heterogeneous; genes and defects reported to date as associated with LVNC are mainly those that cause the underlying cardiomyopathy or congenital heart disease, or syndrome in which LVNC is observed.
- The paradigmatic example of LVNC typically associated with hypokinetic dilated phenotype is Barth syndrome that is an X-linked recessive disease caused by defects of the TAZ gene (*G4.5*).

Diagnosis

- The diagnosis is exclusively based upon imaging (2D-TTE and CMR, CT when CMR is not feasible).
- There are no functional, electrical, or biochemical criteria.

Medical Treatment

- Medications are prescribed on the basis of the associated cardiac disease, as per guidelines.
- In hypokinetic dilated cardiomyopathy with LVNC, the anticoagulation is prescribed on the clinical indications dictated by the cardiomyopathy.

Surgical/Interventional Management

- Anecdotal trabeculectomy has been reported in a unique patient.
- Heart transplantation indications are those of the underlying cardiomyopathy.

Guidelines from Scientific Societies

- Unavailable.

REFERENCES

1. Moore B, Prasad Dasi L. Quantifying left ventricular trabeculae function: application of image-based fractal analysis. *Physiol Rep.* 2013;1:e00068.
2. Jenni R, Oechslin EN, van der Loo B. Isolated ventricular non-compaction of the myocardium in adults. *Heart.* 2007;93:11-15.
3. Ulusoy RE, Kucukarslan N, Kirilmaz A, Demiralp E. Noncompaction of ventricular myocardium involving both ventricles. *Eur J Echocardiogr.* 2006;7:457-460.
4. Ranganathan A, Ganesan G, Sangareddi V, Pillai AP, Ramasamy A. Isolated noncompaction of right ventricle-a case report. *Echocardiography.* 2012;29:E169-E172.
5. Maron BJ, Towbin JA, Thiene G, et al. Contemporary definitions and classification of the cardiomyopathies: an American Heart Association Scientific Statement from the Council on Clinical Cardiology, Heart Failure and Transplantation Committee; Quality of Care and Outcomes Research and Functional Genomics and Translational Biology Interdisciplinary Working Groups; and Council on Epidemiology and Prevention. *Circulation.* 2006;113:1807-1816.
6. Elliott P, Andersson B, Arbustini E, et al. Classification of the cardiomyopathies: a position statement from the European Society of Cardiology Working Group on Myocardial and Pericardial Diseases. *Eur Heart J.* 2008;29:270-276.
7. Arbustini E, Narula N, Dec GW, et al. The MOGE(S) classification for a phenotype-genotype nomenclature of cardiomyopathy: endorsed by the World Heart Federation. *J Am Coll Cardiol.* 2013;62:2046-2072.
8. Arbustini E, Weidemann F, Hall JL. Left ventricular noncompaction: a distinct cardiomyopathy or a trait shared by different cardiac diseases? *J Am Coll Cardiol.* 2014;64:1840-1850.
9. Chin TK, Perloff JK, Williams RG, Jue K, Mohrmann R. Isolated noncompaction of left ventricular myocardium. A study of eight cases. *Circulation.* 1990;82:507-513.
10. Jenni R, Oechslin E, Schneider J, Jost CA, Kaufmann PA. Echocardiographic and pathoanatomical characteristics of isolated left ventricular non-compaction: a step towards classification as a distinct cardiomyopathy. *Heart.* 2001;86:666-671.
11. Stöllberger C, Gerecke B, Finsterer J, et al. Refinement of echocardiographic criteria for left ventricular noncompaction. *Int J Cardiol.* 2013;165:463-467.
12. Belanger AR, Miller MA, Donthireddi UR, Najovits AJ, Goldman ME. New classification scheme of left ventricular noncompaction and correlation with ventricular performance. *Am J Cardiol.* 2008;102:92-96.
13. Petersen JB, Selvanayagam F, Wiesmann F, et al. Left ventricular non-compaction: insights from cardiovascular magnetic resonance imaging. *J Am Coll Cardiol.* 2005;46:101-105.
14. Jacquier A, Thuny F, Jop B, et al. Measurement of trabeculated left ventricular mass using cardiac magnetic resonance imaging in the diagnosis of left ventricular non-compaction. *Eur Heart J.* 2010;31:1098-1104.
15. Dawson DK, Maceira AM, Raj VJ, et al. Regional thicknesses and thickening of compacted and trabeculated myocardial layers of the normal left ventricle studied by cardiovascular magnetic resonance. *Circ Cardiovasc Imaging.* 2011;4:139-146.
16. Grothoff M, Pachowsky M, Hoffmann J, et al. Value of cardiovascular MR in diagnosing left ventricular non-compaction cardiomyopathy

and in discriminating between other cardiomyopathies. *Eur Radiol.* 2012;22:2699-2709.

17. Stacey RB, Andersen MM, St Clair M, Hundley WG, Thohan V. Comparison of systolic and diastolic criteria for isolated LV noncompaction in CMR. *JACC Cardiovasc Imaging.* 2013;6:931-940.

18. Captur G, Muthurangu V, Cook C, et al. Quantification of left ventricular trabeculae using fractal analysis. *J Cardiovasc Magn Reson.* 2013;15:36.

19. Marchal P, Lairez O, Cognet T, et al. Relationship between left ventricular sphericity and trabeculation indexes in patients with dilated cardiomyopathy: a cardiac magnetic resonance study. *Eur Heart J Cardiovasc Imaging.* 2013;14:914-920.

20. André F, Burger A, Loβnitzer D, et al. Reference values for left and right ventricular trabeculation and non-compacted myocardium. *Int J Cardiol.* 2015;185:240-247.

21. Melendez-Ramirez G, Castillo-Castellon F, Espinola-Zavaleta N, Meave A, Kimura-Hayama ET. Left ventricular noncompaction: a proposal of new diagnostic criteria by multidetector computed tomography. *J Cardiovasc Comput Tomogr.* 2012;6:346-354.

22. Sidhu MS, Uthamalingam S, Ahmed W, et al. Defining left ventricular noncompaction using cardiac computed tomography. *J Thorac Imaging.* 2014;29:60-66.

23. Gebhard C, Stähli BE, Greutmann M, Biaggi P, Jenni R, Tanner FC. Reduced left ventricular compacta thickness: a novel echocardiographic criterion for non-compaction cardiomyopathy. *J Am Soc Echocardiogr.* 2012;25:1050-1057.

24. Kawel N, Nacif M, Arai AE, et al. Trabeculated (noncompacted) and compact myocardium in adults: the multi-ethnic study of atherosclerosis. *Circ Cardiovasc Imaging.* 2012;5:357-366.

25. Zemrak F, Ahlman MA, Captur G, et al. The relationship of left ventricular trabeculation to ventricular function and structure over a 9.5-year follow-up: the MESA study. *J Am Coll Cardiol.* 2014;64:1971-1980.

26. Ross SB, Jones K, Blanch B, Puranik R, McGeechan K, Barratt A, Semsarian C. A systematic review and meta-analysis of the prevalence of left ventricular non-compaction in adults. *Eur Heart J.* 2020;41(14):1428-1436.

27. Ichida F. Left ventricular noncompaction. *Circ J.* 2009;73:19-26.

28. Nugent AW, Daubeney PE, Chondros P, et al. The epidemiology of childhood cardiomyopathy in Australia. *N Engl J Med.* 2003;348:1639-1646.

29. Pignatelli RH, McMahon CJ, Dreyer WJ, et al. Clinical characterization of left ventricular noncompaction in children: a relatively common form of cardiomyopathy. *Circulation.* 2003;108:2672-2678.

30. Jefferies JL, Wilkinson JD, Sleeper LA, et al. Cardiomyopathy phenotypes and outcomes for children with left ventricular myocardial noncompaction: results from the pediatric cardiomyopathy registry. *J Card Fail.* 2015;21:877-884.

31. Ritter M, Oechslin E, Sütsch G, Attenhofer C, Schneider J, Jenni R. Isolated noncompaction of the myocardium in adults. *Mayo Clin Proc.* 1997;72:26-31.

32. Oechslin EN, Attenhofer Jost CH, Rojas JR, Kaufmann PA, Jenni R. Long-term follow-up of 34 adults with isolated left ventricular noncompaction: a distinct cardiomyopathy with poor prognosis. *J Am Coll Cardiol.* 2000;36:493-500.

33. Aras D, Tufekcioglu O, Ergun K, et al. Clinical features of isolated ventricular noncompaction in adults long-term clinical course, echocardiographic properties, and predictors of left ventricular failure. *J Card Fail.* 2006;12:726-733.

34. Stanton C, Bruce C, Connolly H, et al. Isolated left ventricular noncompaction syndrome. *Am J Cardiol.* 2009;104:1135-1138.

35. Sandhu R, Finkelhor RS, Gunawardena DR, Bahler RC. Prevalence and characteristics of left ventricular noncompaction in a community hospital cohort of patients with systolic dysfunction *Echocardiography.* 2008;25(1):8-12.

36. Oechslin E, Jenni R. Left ventricular non-compaction revisited: a distinct phenotype with genetic heterogeneity? *Eur Heart J.* 2011;32:1446-1456.

37. Zarrouk-Mahjoub S, Finsterer J. Noncompaction with valve abnormalities is rarely associated with neurologic or genetic disease. *Int J Cardiol.* 2016;202:627-628.

38. Ichida F, Hamamichi Y, Miyawaki T, et al. Clinical features of isolated noncompaction of the ventricular myocardium: long-term clinical course, hemodynamic properties, and genetic background. *J Am Coll Cardiol.* 1999;34:233-240.

39. Kohli SK, Pantazis A, Shah JS, et al. Diagnosis of left-ventricular non-compaction in patients with left-ventricular systolic dysfunction: time for a reappraisal of diagnostic criteria? *Eur Heart J.* 2008;29:89-95.

40. Luijkx T, Cramer MJ, Zaidi A, et al. Ethnic differences in ventricular hypertrabeculation on cardiac MRI in elite football players. *Neth Heart J.* 2012;20:389-395.

41. Nel S, Khandheria BK, Libhaber E, et al. Prevalence and significance of isolated left ventricular non-compaction phenotype in normal black Africans using echocardiography. *Int J Cardiol Heart Vasc.* 2020;30:100585.

42. Sedmera D, Thompson RP. Myocyte proliferation in the developing heart. *Dev Dyn.* 2011;240:1322-1334.

43. Yang J, Bucker S, Jungblut B, et al. Inhibition of Notch2 by Numb/Numblike controls myocardial compaction in the heart. *Cardiovasc Res.* 2012;96:276-285.

44. Del Monte-Nieto G, Ramialison M, Adam AAS, et al. Control of cardiac jelly dynamics by NOTCH1 and NRG1 defines the building plan for trabeculation. *Nature.* 2018 May;557(7705):439-445.

45. Choquet C, Nguyen THM, Sicard P, et al. Deletion of Nkx2-5 in trabecular myocardium reveals the developmental origins of pathological heterogeneity associated with ventricular non-compaction cardiomyopathy. *PLoS Genet.* 2018;14(7):e1007502.

46. Lowery JW, de Caestecker MP. BMP signaling in vascular development and disease. *Cytokine Growth Factor Rev.* 2010;21:287-298.

47. Lu SY, Sheikh F, Sheppard PC, et al. FGF-16 is required for embryonic heart development. *Biochem Biophys Res Commun.* 2008;373:270-274.

48. Liu J, Bressan M, Hassel D, et al. A dual role for ErbB2 signaling in cardiac trabeculation. *Development.* 2010;137:3867-3875.

49. Salvucci O, Tosato G. Essential roles of EphB receptors and EphrinB ligands in endothelial cell function and angiogenesis. *Adv Cancer Res.* 2012;114:21-57.

50. Zhou Y, Gunput RF, Pasterkamp RJ. Semaphorin signaling: progress made and promises ahead. *Trends Biochem Sci.* 2008;33:161-170.

51. Hall CE, Hurtado R, Hewett KW, et al. Hemodynamic-dependent patterning of endothelin converting enzyme 1 expression and differentiation of impulse-conducting Purkinje fibers in the embryonic heart. *Development.* 2004;131:581-592.

52. Hansson EM, Lanner F, Das D, et al. Control of Notch-ligand endocytosis by ligand-receptor interaction. *J Cell Sci.* 2010;123(Pt 17):2931-2942.

53. Luxán G, Casanova JC, Martínez-Poveda B, et al. Mutations in the NOTCH pathway regulator MIB1 cause left ventricular noncompaction cardiomyopathy. *Nat Med.* 2013;19:193-201.

54. Cooley MA, Fresco VM, Dorlon ME, et al. Fibulin-1 is required during cardiac ventricular morphogenesis for versican cleavage, suppression of ErbB2 and Erk1/2 activation, and to attenuate trabecular cardiomyocyte proliferation. *Dev Dyn.* 2012;241:303-314.

55. Patra C, Diehl F, Ferrazzi F, et al. Nephronectin regulates atrioventricular canal differentiation via Bmp4-Has2 signaling in zebrafish. *Development.* 2011;138:4499-4509.

56. Stankunas K, Hang CT, Tsun ZY, et al. Endocardial Brg1 represses ADAMTS1 to maintain the microenvironment for myocardial morphogenesis. *Dev Cell.* 2008;14:298-311.

57. Sedmera D, Pexieder T, Vuillemin M, Thompson RP, Anderson RH. Developmental patterning of the myocardium. *Anat Rec.* 2000;258:319-337.

58. Ross SB, Singer ES, Driscoll E, et al. Genetic architecture of left ventricular noncompaction in adults. *Hum Genome Var.* 2020;7:33.

59. Bleyl SB, Mumford BR, Thompson V, et al. Neonatal, lethal noncompaction of the left ventricular myocardium is allelic with Barth syndrome. *Am J Hum Genet.* 1997;61:868-872.

60. Karkucinska-Wieckowska A, Trubicka J, Werner B, et al. Left ventricular noncompaction (LVNC) and low mitochondrial membrane potential are specific for Barth syndrome. *J Inherit Metab Dis.* 2013;36:929-937.

61. Ferreira C, Thompson R, Vernon H. Barth syndrome. In: Pagon RA, Adam MP, Ardinger HH, et al., eds. *GeneReviews(*).* Seattle, WA: University of Washington; 1993. http://www.ncbi.nlm.nih.gov/books/NBK247162/. [Updated July 9, 2020].

62. Ichida F, Tsubata S, Bowles KR, et al. Novel gene mutations in patients with left ventricular noncompaction or Barth syndrome. *Circulation.* 2001;103:1256-1263.

63. Liu S, Bai Y, Huang J, et al. Do mitochondria contribute to left ventricular non-compaction cardiomyopathy? New findings from myocardium of patients with left ventricular non-compaction cardiomyopathy. *Mol Genet Metab.* 2013;109:100-106.

64. Klaassen S, Probst S, Oechslin E, et al. Mutations in sarcomere protein genes in left ventricular noncompaction. *Circulation.* 2008;117:2893-2901.

65. Monserrat L, Hermida-Prieto M, Fernandez X, et al. Mutation in the alpha-cardiac actin gene associated with apical hypertrophic cardiomyopathy, left ventricular non-compaction, and septal defects. *Eur Heart J.* 2007;28:1953-1961.

66. Greenway SC, McLeod R, Hume S, et al. Exome sequencing identifies a novel variant in ACTC1 associated with familial atrial septal defect. *Can J Cardiol.* 2014;30:181-187.

67. Dellefave LM, Pytel P, Mewborn S, et al. Sarcomere mutations in cardiomyopathy with left ventricular hypertrabeculation. *Circ Cardiovasc Genet.* 2009;2:442-449.

68. Hoedemaekers YM, Caliskan K, Majoor-Krakauer D, et al. Cardiac beta-myosin heavy chain defects in two families with non-compaction cardiomyopathy: linking non-compaction to hypertrophic, restrictive, and dilated cardiomyopathies. *Eur Heart J.* 2007;28:2732-2737.

69. Budde BS, Binner P, Waldmüller S, et al. Noncompaction of the ventricular myocardium is associated with a de novo mutation in the beta-myosin heavy chain gene. *PLoS One.* 2007;2:e1362.

70. Probst S, Oechslin E, Schuler P, et al. Sarcomere gene mutations in isolated left ventricular noncompaction cardiomyopathy do not predict clinical phenotype. *Circ Cardiovasc Genet.* 2011;4:367-374.

71. Schaefer E, Helms P, Marcellin L, et al. Next-generation sequencing (NGS) as a fast molecular diagnosis tool for left ventricular noncompaction in an infant with compound mutations in the MYBPC3 gene. *Eur J Med Genet.* 2014;57:129-132.

72. Haberer K, Buffo-Sequeira I, Chudley AE, Spriggs E, Sergi C. A case of an infant with compound heterozygous mutations for hypertrophic cardiomyopathy producing a phenotype of left ventricular noncompaction. *Can J Cardiol.* 2014;30:1249.e1-e3.

73. Chang B, Gorbea C, Lezin G, et al. 14-3-3ε gene variants in a Japanese patient with left ventricular noncompaction and hypoplasia of the corpus callosum. *Gene.* 2013;515:173-180.

74. Luedde M, Ehlermann P, Weichenhan D, et al. Severe familial left ventricular non-compaction cardiomyopathy due to a novel troponin T (TNNT2) mutation. *Cardiovasc Res.* 2010;86:452-460.

75. Rankin J, Auer-Grumbach M, Bagg W, et al. Extreme phenotypic diversity and nonpenetrance in families with the LMNA gene mutation R644C. *Am J Med Genet.* 2008;146A:1530-1542.

76. Hermida-Prieto M, Monserrat L, Castro-Beiras A, et al. Familial dilated cardiomyopathy and isolated left ventricular noncompaction associated with lamin A/C gene mutations. *Am J Cardiol.* 2004;94:50-54.

77. Liu Z, Shan H, Huang J, Li N, Hou C, Pu J. A novel lamin A/C gene missense mutation (445 V > E) in immunoglobulin-like fold associated with left ventricular non-compaction. *Europace.* 2016;18(4):617-622.

78. Priori SG, Blomström-Lundqvist C, Mazzanti A, et al. 2015 ESC Guidelines for the management of patients with ventricular arrhythmias and the prevention of sudden cardiac death: the Task Force for the Management of Patients with Ventricular Arrhythmias and the Prevention of Sudden Cardiac Death of the European Society of Cardiology (ESC) endorsed by: Association for European Paediatric and Congenital Cardiology (AEPC). *Eur Heart J.* 2015:36:2793-2867.

79. van Rijsingen IAW, Arbustini E, Elliott PM, et al. Risk factors for malignant ventricular arrhythmias in lamin a/c mutation carriers a European cohort study. *J Am Coll Cardiol.* 2012;59:493-500.

80. Vatta M, Mohapatra B, Jimenez S, et al. Mutations in Cypher/ZASP in patients with dilated cardiomyopathy and left ventricular non-compaction. *J Am Coll Cardiol.* 2003;42:2014-2027.

81. Theis JL, Bos JM, Bartleson VB, et al. Echocardiographic-determined septal morphology in Z-disc hypertrophic cardiomyopathy. *Biochem Biophys Res Commun.* 2006;351:896-902.

82. Lopez-Ayala JM, Ortiz-Genga M, Gomez-Milanes I, et al. A mutation in the Z-line Cypher/ZASP protein is associated with arrhythmogenic right ventricular cardiomyopathy. *Clin Genet.* 2015;88:172-176.

83. Zhou Q, Chu PH, Huang C, et al. Ablation of Cypher, a PDZ-LIM domain Z-line protein, causes a severe form of congenital myopathy. *J Cell Biol.* 2001;155:605-612.

84. Xi Y, Ai T, De Lange E, et al. Loss of function of hNav1.5 by a ZASP1 mutation associated with intraventricular conduction disturbances in left ventricular noncompaction. *Circ Arrhythm Electrophysiol.* 2012;5:1017-1026.

85. Arbustini E, Di Toro A, Giuliani L, Favalli V, Narula N, Grasso M. Cardiac phenotypes in hereditary muscle disorders: JACC State-of-the-Art Review. *J Am Coll Cardiol.* 2018;72(20):2485-2506.

86. Stöllberger C, Finsterer J, Blazek G. Left ventricular hypertrabeculation/noncompaction and association with additional cardiac abnormalities and neuromuscular disorders. *Am J Cardiol.* 2002;90:899-902.

87. Statile CJ, Taylor MD, Mazur W, et al. Left ventricular noncompaction in Duchenne muscular dystrophy. *J Cardiovasc Magn Reson.* 2013;15:67.

88. Kimura K, Takenaka K, Ebihara A, et al. Prognostic impact of left ventricular noncompaction in patients with Duchenne/Becker muscular dystrophy: prospective multicenter cohort study. *Int J Cardiol.* 2013;168:1900-1904.

89. Shan L, Makita N, Xing Y, et al. SCN5A variants in Japanese patients with left ventricular noncompaction and arrhythmia. *Mol Genet Metab.* 2008;93:468-474.

90. Campbell MJ, Czosek RJ, Hinton RB, Miller EM. Exon 3 deletion of ryanodine receptor causes left ventricular noncompaction, worsening catecholaminergic polymorphic ventricular tachycardia, and sudden cardiac arrest. *Am J Med Genet A.* 2015;167A:2197-2200.

91. Ohno S, Omura M, Kawamura M, et al. Exon 3 deletion of RYR2 encoding cardiac ryanodine receptor is associated with left ventricular non-compaction. *Europace.* 2014;16:1646-1654.

92. Nozaki Y, Kato Y, Uike K, Yamamura K, Kikuchi M, Yasuda M, Ohno S, Horie M, Murayama T, Kurebayashi N, Horigome H. Co-phenotype of left ventricular non-compaction cardiomyopathy and atypical catecholaminergic polymorphic ventricular tachycardia in association with R169Q, a ryanodine receptor type 2 missense mutation. *Circ J.* 2020;84(2):226-234.

93. Stähli BE, Gebhard C, Biaggi P, et al. Left ventricular non-compaction: prevalence in congenital heart disease. *Int J Cardiol.* 2013;167:2477-2481.

94. Attenhofer Jost CH, Connolly HM, Warnes CA, et al. Noncompacted myocardium in Ebstein's anomaly: initial description in three patients. *J Am Soc Echocardiogr.* 2004;17:677-680.

95. Vermeer AM, van Engelen K, Postma AV, et al. Ebstein anomaly associated with left ventricular noncompaction: an autosomal dominant condition that can be caused by mutations in MYH7. *Am J Med Genet Semin Med Genet.* 2013;163:178-184.

96. Digilio MC, Bernardini L, Gagliardi MG, et al. Syndromic non-compaction of the left ventricle: associated chromosomal anomalies. *Clin Genet.* 2013;84:362-367.

97. Arya P, Wilson TE, Parent JJ, et al. An adult female with 5q34-q35.2 deletion: A rare syndromic presentation of left ventricular non-compaction and congenital heart disease. *Eur J Med Genet.* 2020;63(4):103797.

98. Agarwal A, Khandheria BK, Paterick TE, Treiber SC, Bush M, Tajik AJ. Left ventricular noncompaction in patients with bicuspid aortic valve. *J Am Soc Echocardiogr.* 2013;26:1306-1313.

99. Shen M, Capoulade R, Tastet L, et al. Prevalence of left ventricle noncompaction criteria in adult patients with bicuspid aortic valve versus healthy control subjects. *Open Heart.* 2018;5(2):e000869.

100. Hirono K, Hata Y, Miyao N, LVNC Study Collaborators. Left ventricular noncompaction and congenital heart disease increases the risk of congestive heart failure. *J Clin Med.* 2020;9(3):785.

101. Bhatia S, Qasim A, Almasri M, Frank L, Aly AM. Left ventricular noncompaction in a child with Turner syndrome. *Case Rep Pediatr.* 2019;2019:6824321.

102. Sewani M, Nugent K, Blackburn PR, Tarnowski JM, et al. Further delineation of the phenotypic spectrum associated with hemizygous loss-of-function variants in NONO. *Am J Med Genet A.* 2020;182(4):652-658.

103. Azevedo O, Gaspar P, Sá Miranda C, Cunha D, Medeiros R, Lourenço A. Left ventricular noncompaction in a patient with Fabry disease: overdiagnosis, morphological manifestation of Fabry disease or two unrelated rare conditions in the same patient? *Cardiology.* 2011;119:155-159.

104. Stöllberger C, Finsterer J, Voigtländer T, Slany J. Is left ventricular hypertrabeculation/noncompaction a cardiac manifestation of Fabry's disease? *Z Kardiol.* 2003;92:966-969.

105. Van Der Starre P, Deuse T, Pritts C, Brun C, Vogel H, Oyer P. Late profound muscle weakness following heart transplantation due to Danon disease. *Muscle Nerve.* 2013;47:135-137.

106. Aypar E, Sert A, Gokmen Z, Aslan E, Odabas D. Isolated left ventricular noncompaction in a newborn with Pierre-Robin sequence. *Pediatr Cardiol.* 2013;34:452-454.

107. Gati S, Chandra N, Bennett RL, et al. Increased left ventricular trabeculation in highly trained athletes: do we need more stringent criteria for the diagnosis of left ventricular non-compaction in athletes? *Heart.* 2013;99:401-408.

108. Gati S, Papadakis M, Papamichael ND, et al. Reversible de novo left ventricular trabeculations in pregnant women: implications for the diagnosis of left ventricular noncompaction in low-risk populations. *Circulation.* 2014;130:475-483.

109. Piga A, Longo F, Musallam KM, et al. Left ventricular noncompaction in patients with b-thalassemia: uncovering a previously unrecognized abnormality. *Am J Hematol.* 2012;87:1079-1083.

110. Markovic NS, Dimkovic N, Damjanovic T, Loncar G, Dimkovic S. Isolated ventricular noncompaction in patients with chronic renal failure. *Clin Nephrol.* 2008;70:72-76.

111. Paun B, Bijnens B, Butakoff C. Relationship between the left ventricular size and the amount of trabeculations. *Int J Numer Method Biomed Eng.* 2018;34(3).

112. Pitzer ME, Seidenberg PH, Silvis M. Asymptomatic left ventricular noncompaction: implications for athletic participation. *Curr Sports Med Rep.* 2015;14:91-95.

113. Peritz DC, Vaughn A, Ciocca M, Chung EH. Hypertrabeculation vs left ventricular noncompaction on echocardiogram: a reason to restrict athletic participation? *JAMA Intern Med.* 2014;174:1379-1382.

114. D'Ascenzi F, Pelliccia A, Natali BM, Bonifazi M, Mondillo S. Exercise-induced left-ventricular hypertrabeculation in athlete's heart. *Int J Cardiol.* 2015;181:320-322.

115. Gati S, Papadakis M, Papamichael ND, et al. Response to letter regarding article, "Reversible de novo left ventricular trabeculations in pregnant women: implications for the diagnosis of left ventricular noncompaction in low-risk populations." *Circulation.* 2015;131:e426.

116. Stöllberger C, Finsterer J. Letter by Stöllberger and Finsterer regarding article, "Reversible de novo left ventricular trabeculations in pregnant women: implications for the diagnosis of left ventricular noncompaction in low-risk populations." *Circulation.* 2015;131:e425.

117. Reimold SC. Reversible left ventricular trabeculations in pregnancy: is this sufficient to make the diagnosis of left ventricular noncompaction? *Circulation.* 2014;130(6):453-454.

118. Abramovich-Yoffe H, Shalev A, Barrett O, Shalev H, Levitas A. Prevalence of left ventricular hypertrabeculation/noncompaction among patients with congenital dyserythropoietic anemia Type 1 (CDA1). *Int J Cardiol.* 2020;317:96-102.

119. Alter P, Maisch B. Non-compaction cardiomyopathy in an adult with hereditary spherocytosis. *Eur J Heart Fail.* 2007;9:98-99.

120. Celebi AS, Gulel O, Cicekcioglu H, Celebi OO, Ulusoy V. Isolated noncompaction of the left ventricular myocardium complicated by thromboembolic cerebrovascular accident in a patient with essential thrombocythemia. *Int J Cardiol.* 2008;128:e22-e24.

121. Luckie M, Irwin B, Nair S, et al. Left ventricular non-compaction in identical twins with thalassaemia and cardiac iron overload. *Eur J Echocardiogr.* 2009;10:509-512.

122. Wood JC. Cardiac iron across different transfusion-dependent diseases. *Blood Rev.* 2008;22(Suppl 2):S14-S21.

123. Bonamini R, Imazio M, Faletti R, Gatti M, Xhyheri B, Limone M, Longo F, Piga A. Prevalence and prognostic impact of left ventricular non-compaction in patients with thalassemia. *Intern Emerg Med.* 2019;14(8):1299-1306.

124. Gati S, Papadakis M, Van Niekerk N, Reed M, Yeghen T, Sharma S. Increased left ventricular trabeculation in individuals with sickle cell anaemia: physiology or pathology? *Int J Cardiol.* 2013;168:1658-1660.

125. Maheshwari M, Gokroo RK, Kaushik SK. Isolated non compacted right ventricular myocardium. *J Assoc Physicians India.* 2012;60:56-57.

126. Lahmiti S, Aboussad A. Isolated non-compaction of the right ventricular myocardium: two cases report. *Ann Cardiol Angeiol.* 2012;61:299-302.

127. Huo Q, Liang L, Ding X, et al. Isolated right ventricular noncompaction caused ventricular tachycardia and pulmonary embolism. *Ann Noninvasive Electrocardiol.* 2020;25(5):e12731.

128. Said S, Cooper CJ, Quevedo K, Rodriguez E, Hernandez GT. Biventricular non-compaction with predominant right ventricular involvement, reduced left ventricular systolic and diastolic function, and pulmonary hypertension in a Hispanic male. *Am J Case Rep.* 2013;14:539-542.

129. Singh AP, Patra S, Agrawal N, Shankarappa RK. Congenitally corrected transposition of the great vessels associated with morphological right ventricular non-compaction presenting with supraventricular tachycardia. *BMJ Case Rep.* 2013;pii:bcr2013010470.

130. Sirin BH, Kurdal AT, Iskesen I, Cerrahoglu M. Right ventricular outflow obstruction of the patient with biventricular non-compaction. *Thorac Cardiovasc Surg.* 2010;58:364-366.

131. Zhang J, Wang Y, Feng W, Wu Y. Prenatal ultrasound diagnosis of fetal isolated right ventricular noncompaction with pulmonary artery sling: a rare case report. *Echocardiography.* 2019;36(11):2118-2121.

132. Li J, Franke J, Pribe-Wolferts R, et al. Effects of β-blocker therapy on electrocardiographic and echocardiographic characteristics of left ventricular noncompaction. *Clin Res Cardiol.* 2015;104:241-249.

133. Rapezzi C, Arbustini E, Caforio AL, et al. Diagnostic work-up in cardiomyopathies: bridging the gap between clinical phenotypes and final diagnosis. A position statement from the ESC Working Group on Myocardial and Pericardial Diseases. *Eur Heart J.* 2013;34:1448-1458.

134. Charron P, Arad M, Arbustini E, et al. Genetic counselling and testing in cardiomyopathies: a position statement of the European Society of Cardiology Working Group on Myocardial and Pericardial Diseases. *Eur Heart J.* 2010;31:2715-2726.

135. Hoedemaekers YM, Caliskan K, Michels M, et al. The importance of genetic counseling, DNA diagnostics, and cardiologic family screening in left ventricular noncompaction cardiomyopathy. *Circ Cardiovasc Genet.* 2010;3:232-239.

136. Marziliano N, Mannarino S, Nespoli L, et al. Barth syndrome associated with compound hemizygosity and heterozygosity of the TAZ and LDB3 genes. *Am J Med Genet A.* 2007;143A:907-915.

137. Levitas A, Konstantino Y, Muhammad E, et al. D117N in Cypher/ZASP may not be a causative mutation for dilated cardiomyopathy and ventricular arrhythmias. *Eur J Hum Genet.* 2016;24(5):666-671.

138. Steffel J, Kobza R, Oechslin E, Jenni, R, Duru F. Electrocardiographic characteristics at initial diagnosis in patients with isolated left ventricular noncompaction. *Am J Cardiol.* 2009;104:984-989.

139. Murphy RT, Thaman R, Blanes JG, et al. Natural history and familial characteristics of isolated left ventricular non-compaction. *Eur Heart J.* 2005;26:187-192.

140. Lofiego C, Biagini E, Pasquale F, et al. Wide spectrum of presentation and variable outcomes of isolated left ventricular non-compaction. *Heart.* 2007;93:65-71.

141. Brescia ST, Rossano JW, Pignatelli R, et al. Mortality and sudden death in pediatric left ventricular noncompaction in a tertiary referral center. *Circulation.* 2013;127:2202-2208.

142. Papadakis M, Carre F, Kervio G, et al. The prevalence, distribution, and clinical outcomes of electrocardiographic repolarization patterns in male athletes of African/Afro-Caribbean origin. *Eur Heart J.* 2011;32:2304-2313.

143. Stöllberger C, Gerecke B, Engberding R, et al. Interobserver agreement of the echocardiographic diagnosis of LV hypertrabeculation/noncompaction. *JACC Cardiovasc Imaging.* 2015;8:1252-1257.

144. Gianfagna P, Badano LP, Faganello G, Tosoratti E, Fioretti PM. Additive value of contrast echocardiography for the diagnosis of noncompaction of the left ventricular myocardium. *Eur J Echocardiogr.* 2006;7:67-70.

145. Nemes A, Caliskan K, Soliman OII, McGhie JS, Geleijnse ML, Ten Cate FJ. Diagnosis of biventricular non-compaction cardiomyopathy by real-time three-dimensional echocardiography. *Eur J Echocardiogr.* 2009;10:356-357.

146. Gomathi SB, Makadia N, Ajit SM. An unusual case of isolated non-compacted right ventricular myocardium. *Eur J Echocardiogr.* 2008;9:424-425.

147. Tatu-Chitoiu A, Bradisteanu S. A rare case of biventricular non-compaction associated with ventricular septal defect and descendent aortic stenosis in a young man. *Eur J Echocardiogr.* 2008;9:306-308.

148. Burke A, Mont E, Kutys R, Virmani R. Left ventricular noncompaction: a pathological study of 14 cases. *Hum Pathol.* 2005;36:403-411.

149. Fazio G, Lunetta M, Grassedonio E, et al. Noncompaction of the right ventricle. *Pediatr Cardiol.* 2010;31:576-578.

150. Saremi F, Grizzard JD, Kim RJ. Optimizing cardiac MR imaging: practical remedies for artifacts. *RadioGraphics.* 2008;28:1161-1187.

151. Thuny F, Jacquier A, Jop B, et al. Assessment of left ventricular non-compaction in adults: side-by-side comparison of cardiac magnetic resonance imaging with echocardiography. *Arch Cardiovasc Dis.* 2010;103:150-159.

152. Schwartzenberg S, Sherez J, Wexler D, Aviram G, Keren G. Isolated ventricular non-compaction: an underdiagnosed cause of congestive heart failure. *Isr Med Assoc J.* 2009;11:426-429.

153. Zuccarino F, Vollmer I, Sanchez G, Navallas M, Pugliese F, Gayete A. Left ventricular noncompaction: imaging findings and diagnostic criteria. *AJR Am J Roentgenol.* 2015;204(5):W519-W530.4

154. Dodd JD, Ferencik M, Liberthson RR, et al. Congenital anomalies of coronary artery origin in adults: 64-MDCT appearance. *Am J Roentgenol.* 2007;188:W138-W146.

155. Szemraj-Rogucka ZM, Szemraj J, Masiarek K, Majos A. Circulating microRNAs as biomarkers for myocardial fibrosis in patients with left ventricular non-compaction cardiomyopathy. *Arch Med Sci.* 2019;15(2):376-384.

156. Asmakutlu O, Alis D, Topel C, Sahin A. Late gadolinium enhancement on CMRI in patients with LV noncompaction: An overestimated phenomenon? *Clin Imaging.* 2020;66:121-126.

157. Finsterer J, Stollberger C, Feichtinger H. Histological appearance of left ventricular hypertrabeculation/noncompaction. *Cardiology.* 2002;98:162-164.

158. Paterick TE, Tercius AJ, Agarwal A, Treiber SC, Khandheria BK, Tajik AJ. Double jeopardy in the echocardiography laboratory: coexistence of two distinct cardiomyopathies? *Echocardiography.* 2014;31:931-935.

159. Epstein AE, DiMarco JP, Ellenbogen KA, et al. ACC/AHA/HRS 2008 guidelines for device-based therapy of cardiac rhythm abnormalities: a report of the American College of Cardiology/American Heart Association Task Force on Practice Guidelines (Writing Committee to Revise the ACC/AHA/ NASPE 2002 Guideline Update for Implantation of Cardiac Pacemakers and Antiarrhythmia Devices). *J Am Coll Cardiol.* 2008;51:e1-e62.

160. Stollberger C, Blazek G, Dobias C, Hanafin A, Wegner C, Finsterer J. Frequency of stroke and embolism in left ventricular hypertrabeculation/noncompaction. *Am J Cardiol.* 2011;108:1021-1023.

161. Stollberger C, Wegner C, Finsterer J. CHADS2 and CHA2DS2VASc scores and embolic risk in left ventricular hypertrabeculation/noncompaction. *J Stroke Cerebrovasc Dis.* 2013;22:709-712.

162. Sawant RD, Freeman LJ, Stanley KP, McKelvey A. Pregnancy and treatment outcome in a patient with left ventricular non-compaction. *Eur J Heart Fail.* 2013;15:592-595.

163. Oglesby M, Escobedo D, Escobar GP, Fatemifar F, Sako EY, Bailey SR, Han HC, Feldman MD. Trabecular cutting: a novel surgical therapy to increase diastolic compliance. *J Appl Physiol (1985).* 2019;127(2):457-463.

164. Takamatsu M, Kamohara K, Sato M, Koga Y. Effect of noncompacted myocardial resection on isolated left ventricular noncompaction. *Ann Thorac Surg.* 2020;110(5):e387-e389.

165. Shi WY, Moreno-Betancur M, Nugent AW, et al. Long-term outcomes of childhood left ventricular noncompaction cardiomyopathy: results from a national population-based study. *Circulation.* 2018;138(4):367-376.

166. Tian T, Liu Y, Gao L, et al. Isolated left ventricular noncompaction: clinical profile and prognosis in 106 adult patients. *Heart Vessels.* 2014;29:645-652.

167. Caliskan K, Michels M, Geleijnse ML, et al. Frequency of asymptomatic disease among family members with noncompaction cardiomyopathy. *Am J Cardiol.* 2012;110:1512-1517.

168. Grigoratos C, Barison A, Ivanov A, et al. Meta-analysis of the prognostic role of late gadolinium enhancement and global systolic impairment in left ventricular noncompaction. *JACC Cardiovasc Imaging.* 2019;12(11 Pt 1):2141-2151.

169. Aung N, Doimo S, Ricci F, et al. Prognostic significance of left ventricular noncompaction: systematic review and meta-analysis of observational studies. *Circ Cardiovasc Imaging.* 2020;13(1):e009712.

170. Lorca R, Martín M, Gómez J, et al. Diagnostic impact of genetic testing in hypertrophic cardiomyopathy: the story of two families. *Int J Cardiol.* 2016;205:161-162.

171. Captur G, Flett AS, Jacoby DL, Moon JC. Left ventricular noncompaction: the mitral valve prolapse of the 21st century? *Int J Cardiol.* 2013;164:3-6.

46

Myocarditis

Eloisa Arbustini, Alessandro Di Toro, Mario Urtis, Sean Pinney, and Jagat Narula

Causes, presentation, diagnosis, and management of myocarditis

Epidemiology	Clinical presentation	Diagnostic criteria and tools		Evolution	Treatments
Global Burden of Disease Study data from 195 countries indicates 1.80 million cases of myocarditis in 2017 (21)	"Fulminant"/acute Subacute Cardiogenic shock Heart failure Arrhythmias	Clinical (signs, symptoms) Pathology (EMB) Imaging (Echo, CMR) Biomarkers	EMB	Healing/repair Worsening with death or HTx Evolution through DCM, chronic HF	Causes are treated, when identified, and antiinfective medications or other cause-related treatments are available

Types of myocarditis

Acute

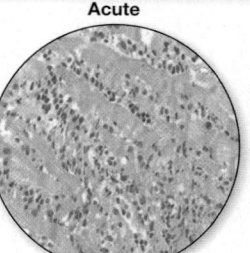

Eosinophilic

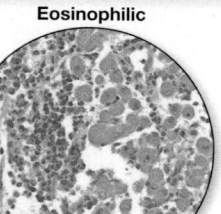

Giant Cell

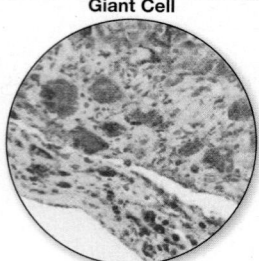

Sarcoidosis

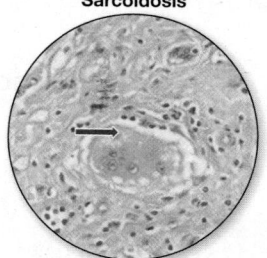

Acute

Heterogeneous causes

Acquired
- Infectious, viral and nonviral
- Immune-mediated
- Toxic: drugs and toxic agents

Genetic
- Twin and families
- Autoinflammatory diseases
- Associated with heritable chromosomally integrated HHV-6 (ciHHV-6)

Eosinophilic

Hypereosinophilic syndromes
Eosinophil count:
- Mild (up to 1,500/mm^3)
- Moderate (1,500–5,000/mm^3)
- Severe (>5,000/mm^3)

Classification
- Hematologic eosinophilia (clonal, Neoplastic, primary, HE$_N$)
- Nonhematologic (secondary or Reactive HE$_R$)
- Eosinophilic diseases of Unknown Significance (HE$_{US}$)
- Familial diseases (HE$_F$)

Giant Cell

GCM: rare, potentially fatal illness of unknown etiology

Hypotheses: autoimmune, infections, drug toxicities, "genetic predisposition"

Common presentation: cardiogenic shock or acute HF

Possible association with myasthenia gravis and thymoma

Sarcoidosis

Noninfectious disease

Hallmark: noncaseating, epithelioid granuloma with asteroid bodies (arrow)

10–40/100,000 persons

In adults: nongenetic but with genetic susceptibility

In children: genetic
- Blau syndrome
- Early onset sarcoidosis (EOS)
- Gene: CARD15 or NOD1 (MIM*605956)

Chapter 46 Fuster and Hurst's Central Illustration. The term myocarditis is the key descriptor of myocardial inflammation; it does not specify the immune phenotype of inflammatory cells or the cause. The most common causes of myocarditis are infectious, in particular, viral. Different forms of myocarditis should be supported by specific diagnostic algorithms. Treatment aims at resolution of the cause, when known, and at the management of cardiac manifestations, regardless of the cause and according to the guidelines addressing clinical phenotype.

CHAPTER SUMMARY

This chapter reviews inflammatory heart diseases; their infectious, autoimmune/immune-mediated, and toxic etiology; diagnostic algorithms; pathologic characteristics; clinical manifestations; and management (see Fuster and Hurst's Central Illustration). The most common etiology of infectious myocarditis is viral; immune-mediated myocarditis is often related to underlying systemic autoimmune diseases, and the most common toxic causes include drugs. The term myocarditis is the key descriptor of myocardial inflammation; it does not specify the immune phenotype of inflammatory cells or the cause. The diagnostic process involves suspicion based on clinical presentation of recent onset of symptoms in previously healthy individuals with exposure to infectious or toxic agents, detection of suggestive imaging abnormalities, and demonstration of the histological evidence of myocardial inflammation with an effort to define etiologic basis. Treatment aims at resolution of the cause, when known, and at the management of cardiac manifestations, regardless of the cause, according to guidelines addressing the clinical phenotype. In most cases, acute myocarditis undergoes spontaneous resolution, but it can evolve toward chronic inflammatory disease with the most common phenotype mimicking dilated-hypokinetic cardiomyopathy. Recent reports have suggested that in some of the viral infections, the viral genome may be chromosomally incorporated and eventually transmitted. Finally, more eventful outcomes are observed when inflammation occurs in patients genetically predisposed to develop dilated cardiomyopathy.

INTRODUCTION

The term *myocarditis* describes the presence of inflammatory cells in the myocardium. This descriptive diagnosis encompasses a wide spectrum of etiologically different diseases that share, as a unique criterion, the pathologically proven evidence of myocardial inflammation.[1] The definition does not specify the inflammatory burden, the immunophenotype of inflammatory cells, and the cause. In clinics, the formulation of a diagnosis of myocarditis implies that the observed cardiac phenotype is attributable to the inflammation of the myocardium.

The Historical Definition

In the 1980s, the World Health Organization and the International Society and Federation of Cardiology defined myocarditis as an inflammatory disease of the myocardium wherein the diagnosis is established by histologic, immunologic, and immunohistochemical criteria. Idiopathic, autoimmune, and infectious forms of inflammatory cardiomyopathy were recognized.[2] Whereas the Dallas criteria[3] insisted on the demonstration of mononuclear cellular infiltration accompanying a demonstrable and ongoing myocyte damage, the definition of myocarditis recently updated by the European Society of Cardiology (ESC) working group on myocardial and pericardial diseases requires the presence of ≥14 lymphocytes/mm[2] including CD3[+] T lymphocytes ≥7 cells/mm[2] but no more than 4 monocytes/mm.[3,4] These descriptive definitions did not include the etiologic basis of myocardial involvement and clinical information.

The Heterogeneous Etiology

Myocarditis can occur in immunocompetent and immunodeficient hosts and be infectious, noninfectious (autoimmune, immune-mediated, or auto-inflammatory), and toxic (**Table 46–1**). The causes of infectious myocarditis include DNA and RNA viruses, bacteria, fungi, protozoa, and helminths. The most common causes of infectious myocarditis in both children and adults are cardiotropic viruses.[1] In immunocompetent individuals residing in endemic areas, major nonviral cardiotropic infections include *Trypanosoma cruzi* (Chagas disease)[5] and *Borrelia burgdorferi* (Lyme disease),[1,6] while in immunocompromised patients, typically heart transplant recipients, the most common opportunistic infections include the human cytomegalovirus (HCMV) and *Toxoplasma gondii*. In this chapter, the epidemiological, diagnostic, therapeutic, and prognostic aspects of infectious and noninfectious myocarditis will be discussed, excluding SARS-CoV-2 infection that is dealt with in Chapter 84.

Requirements for Precise Etiological Diagnosis

Precise rules establish the criteria for the diagnosis of organ infection, including the heart. Myocardial infection is diagnosed when the infectious agent is detected in myocardial tissue by pathologic and pathogen-related genomic studies.[7] The infectious agent's tropism may be either for cardiac myocytes (true specific myocardial tropism often shared with skeletal muscle myocytes) or endothelial cells (endothelial tropism, which can pertain to the endothelial cells of the myocardium as well as other organs/tissues; eg, parvovirus B19). Infectious agents can reach the heart as either free microorganisms or carried by infected circulating-cells. Failure to precisely identify the cause can lead to ignoring endogenous toxic origin (eg, Pheochromocytoma)[8] and familial diseases with similar clinical onset or manifestations, but always bearing in mind that acute infections may cluster in families.[9,10] The precise diagnosis should incorporate both the pathologic evidence of myocardial inflammation and the certainty of causes.[11] Surrogate terms such as *clinically suspected myocarditis* or diagnoses based on *imaging* cannot be equated with the diagnostic certainty of histologically verified disease. However, development of molecular imaging strategies targeting the presence of myocardial inflammation is not beyond the realm of possibility.[12] At present, endomyocardial biopsy (EMB) remains a unique tool for the diagnosis in vivo; surgical samples can be equally informative, such as the left ventricular (LV) apex resected during ventricular assist device implantation. Reasons for not performing EMB include the invasiveness of the procedure and possible complications, such as ventricular wall perforation, pericardial effusion, and tamponade. Although these reasons are repeatedly claimed as the major limitations, EMBs are routinely and frequently performed to monitor allogeneic reaction and opportunistic infections in transplanted patients and have been reported safe both in adults[11] and children.[13] The major reasons why clinical utilization of EMB is discouraged include (1) the lack of evidence-based effective treatment for myocarditis; (2) the nonuniform and nonuniversally agreed upon diagnostic criteria; and (3) the interobserver variability among pathologists interpreting the same biopsy samples. The reports of limitations of Dallas criteria–based interpretation[14] and the results of the National Institutes of Health Myocarditis Treatment Trial[15] have negatively changed the diagnostic work-up for myocarditis as a disease entity. Nonetheless, the need for diagnostic certainty in many acute and chronic clinical settings is refocusing attention on EMB as a diagnostic tool that is currently not replaceable both to explain causes and to provide a rationale for targeted therapeutic choices.[16–19]

EPIDEMIOLOGY

Precise epidemiologic estimates are difficult because of the different diagnostic criteria and clinically heterogeneous manifestations of the disease ranging from nonspecific signs and symptoms to life-threatening arrhythmias and cardiogenic shock. Data can be derived from administrative databases (eg, using International Classification of Diseases [ICD] codes), from clinical and pathological series in adults and children, as well as from prospective surveillance programs during influenza seasons. In the future, large registries, including pancontinental ones, may contribute with greater precision to the epidemic estimates relating to myocarditis.[20]

Data from Global Burden of Disease Study 2017 provide a systematic assessment of health loss due to diseases and injuries in 21 regions, covering 195 countries and territories.[21]

TABLE 46–1. Different Causes of Myocarditis, Including the Most Common and Rare Causes

	Acquired Myocarditis								Heritable Myocarditis
	Infectious				Noninfectious		Autoimmune/Immune-Mediated		
	RNA Viruses	DNA Viruses	Bacteria	Protozoa/Helminths/Fungi	Medicaments	Toxic Agents/Poisons/Physical Agents/Drugs	Autoimmune Diseases	Giant Cell, Granulomatous, Inflammatory Diseases	Heritable Myocarditis
	• **Coxsackieviruses A and B**	• **Adenoviruses**	• **Staphylococcus**	• **Trypanosoma cruzi (Chagas disease)**	• Penicillin	• Lithium	• Systemic lupus erythematosus	• Sarcoidosis	• Heritable autoinflammatory diseases
	• Echoviruses	• **Parvovirus B19**	• **Streptococcus**	• **Toxoplasma gondii**	• Phenylbutazone	• Arsenic	• Rheumatoid arthritis	• Giant cell myocarditis	• Early-onset sarcoidosis
	• Polioviruses	• Human cytomegalovirus	• Pneumococcus	• Entamoeba histolytica	• Methyldopa	• Lead	• Churg-Strauss syndrome	• Tuberculous myocarditis	• Familial hypereosinophilia
	• Influenza A and B viruses	• Human herpesvirus-6	• Meningococcus	• Leishmania	• Thiazide diuretics	• Copper	• Kawasaki disease	• Myocardial involvement in systemic diseases with giant cells	
	• Respiratory syncytial virus	• Epstein-Barr virus	• Gonococcus	• Echinococcus	• Amitriptyline	• Iron	• Inflammatory bowel disease	• Rheumatic heart disease with Aschoff nodules	
	• Mumps virus	• Varicella-zoster virus	• Salmonella	• Trichinella	• Cefaclor	• Phosphorus	• Scleroderma	• Farber disease (lipogranulomatosis)	
	• Measles virus	• Herpes simplex virus	• **Corynebacterium diphtheriae**	• Taenia solium	• Colchicine	• Carbon monoxide	• Polymyositis	• Foreign body reactions	
	• Hepatitis C virus	• Variola virus	• Haemophilus influenzae	• Fungal	• Furosemide	• Ethanol	• Myasthenia gravis		
	• Dengue virus	• Vaccinia virus	• Leptospira (Weil disease)	• Aspergillus,	• Isoniazid	• Poisons by insect stings and bites	• Insulin-dependent diabetes mellitus		
	• Yellow fever virus	• Polyoma virus	• **Borrelia burgdorferi (Lyme disease)**	• Actinomyces	• Lidocaine	• Electric shock	• Thyrotoxicosis		
	• Chikungunya virus	• Trichodysplasia spinulosa-associated polyomavirus[b]	• Neisseria	• Blastomyces	• Tetracycline	• Heat	• Sarcoidosis		
	• Junin virus		• Mycobacterium (tuberculosis)	• Candida	• Phenytoin	• Radiation/radiotherapy	• Wegener granulomatosis		
	• Lassa fever virus		• Mycoplasma pneumoniae	• Coccidioides	• Sulfonamides	• Cocaine			
	• Rabies virus		• Brucella	• Cryptococcus	• Phenylbutazone	• Heroin			
	• Rubella virus		• Tropheryma whipplei	• Histoplasma	• Methyldopa				
	• Human immunodeficiency virus-1			• Mucormycosis	• Thiazide diuretics				
	• Coronavirus[a]			• Nocardia	• Dobutamine				
	• Cardiovirus B (Saffold virus)			• Sporothrix	• Clozapine				
					• Amitriptyline				
					• Interleukin-2				

Note. The most common causes are in bold.

[a]Causing the Middle East respiratory syndrome and COVID-19

[b]Human polyomavirus identified in 2010.

Estimates of myocarditis burden included prevalence, deaths, years lived with disability (YLDs), and years of life lost (YLLs). All estimates were presented as counts, age-standardized rates per 100,000 people, and percentage change, with 95% uncertainty intervals (UIs). Myocarditis was ascertained using the ICD-9 (422–422.9) and ICD-10 (B33.2, I40–I41.9, and I51.4) codes. Worldwide, there were 1.80 million (95% UI, 1.64–1.98) cases of myocarditis, contributing to 46,486 (95% UI, 39,709–51,824) deaths in 2017. Furthermore, there were 131,376 (95% UI, 90,113–183,001) YLDs and 1.26 million (95% UI, 1.10–1.42) YLLs attributable to myocarditis in 2017 (**Fig. 46–1**).[22]

Autopsy studies have provided variable data. In a large autopsy report of 377,841 deceased persons, the prevalence of nonspecific myocarditis and giant cell myocarditis (GCM) was 0.11% and 0.007%, respectively.[23] In another retrospective review of 17,162 postmortem records, myocarditis was histologically confirmed in 91 cases (0.53%; 95% confidence interval [CI], 0.4%–0.7%). However, in a prospectively planned standardized myocardial sampling in 605 autopsies, the prevalence was 5.1%,[24] which is substantially higher than the 2% rate of incidental myocardial infiltrates associated with myocyte necrosis in consecutive noncardiac deaths.[25]

Clinical reports have promulgated myocarditis based on varied phenotypes. A search algorithm based on sentinel reports (using ICD, 9th Revision, codes 420.90, 420.99, 422.90, 422.91, and 429.0) identified 59 cases of suspected myopericarditis among 492,671 US military service personnel who received the smallpox vaccine between 2002 and 2003.[26] In a well-characterized series of competitive athletes, myocarditis was reported as the third leading cause of sudden cardiac death.[27] However, of 672 young Finnish men presenting with myocardial infarction from 1977 to 1996, clinical diagnosis of myocarditis was suggested in 98 (0.17% [95% CI, 0.14%–0.21%]/1000 person-years); Coxsackievirus etiology was confirmed in 4% of the cases.[28] In 3055 patients who underwent EMB, myocardial inflammation was found in 17.2% (n = 525); only 182 of these 525 patients demonstrated decreased ejection fraction (<45%), and viral genome was identified in 11.8%.[29] In a review of 1,698,397 patients aged ≥16 years over 9.5 years from 29 Finnish hospitals, 3198 were discharged as having myocarditis (0.0019%); researchers reported a higher prevalence in affected young men and postmenopausal women.[30] Acute myocarditis has been reported to be more common in hospitalized patients aged 18 to 29 years than acute myocardial infarction.[31]

In children, nationwide surveys, registries, and surveillance programs are contributing to provide estimates of the burden of the disease. A nationwide survey aimed at determining the clinicoepidemiologic features of myocarditis in Japanese children and adolescents demonstrated an incidence of 43.5 cases per year, or 0.24 cases per 100,000 population; pathogens were identified in 37 of 169 subjects, with Coxsackievirus accounting for 60%.[32] Of 62 children with clinical profiles of acute myocarditis and dilated cardiomyopathy (DCM) before diagnosis, 24 (39%) had a final diagnosis of myocarditis.[33] Of the 11 children (median age, 1 year; range 0–9 years) presenting with fulminant myocarditis between 1998 and 2003 in a single center, 5 were confirmed with viral etiology; 10 survivors were asymptomatic with normalized LV ejection fraction (LVEF) at a median follow-up of 58.7 months (range, 33.8–83.1 months).[34] Recent data from the Australian Paediatric Surveillance Unit in children with <15 years of age hospitalized with severe complications of laboratory-confirmed influenza during 10 influenza

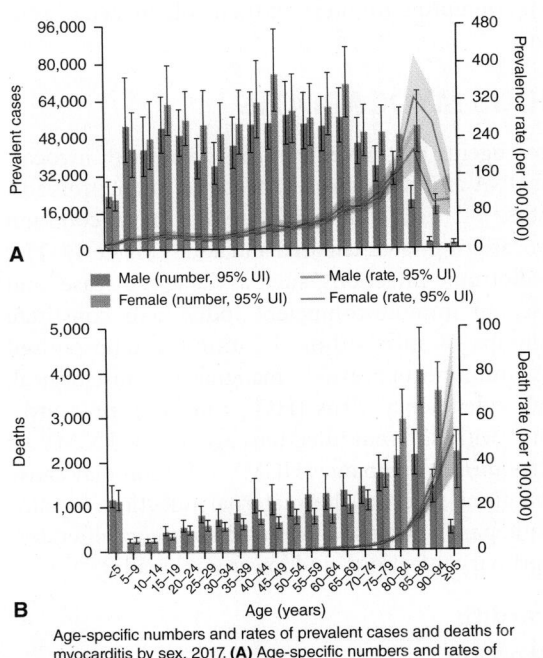

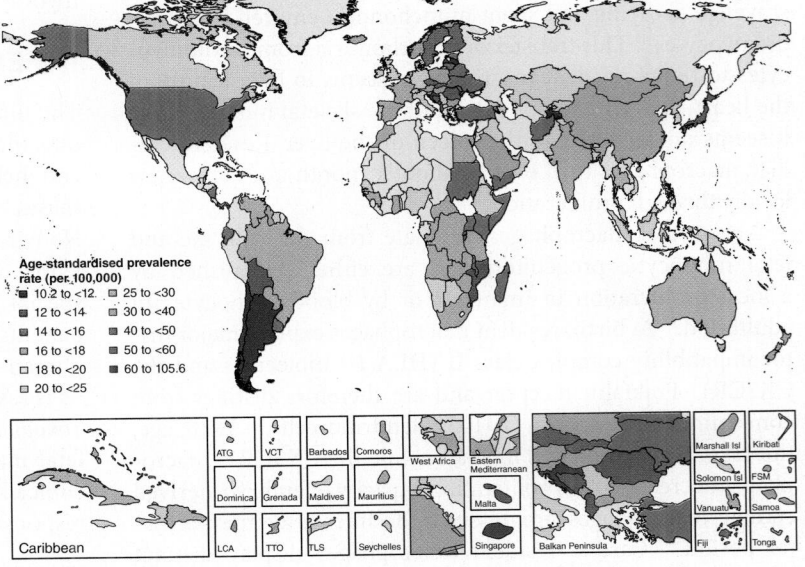

A Male (number, 95% UI) — Male (rate, 95% UI)
Female (number, 95% UI) — Female (rate, 95% UI)

Age-specific numbers and rates of prevalent cases and deaths for myocarditis by sex, 2017. **(A)** Age-specific numbers and rates of myocarditis prevalent cases; **(B)** Age-specific numbers and rates of myocarditis deaths.

Age-standardized prevalence rate (per 100,000)
- 10.2 to <12
- 12 to <14
- 14 to <16
- 16 to <18
- 18 to <20
- 20 to <25
- 25 to <30
- 30 to <40
- 40 to <50
- 50 to <60
- 60 to 105.6

Age-standardized prevalence rates of myocarditis for 195 countries and territories, both sexes, 2017. ATG, Antigua and Barbuda; Isl, Islands; FSM, Federated States of Micronesia; LCA. Saint Lucia; TLS, Timor-Leste; TTO, Trinidad and Tobago; VCT, Saint Vincent and the Grenadines.

Figure 46–1. Data from the global burden of myocarditis between 1990 and 2017 from the Global Burden of Disease study 2017. Reproduced with permission from Dai H, Lotan D, Much AA, et al. Global, Regional, and National Burden of Myocarditis and Cardiomyopathy, 1990-2017. *Front Cardiovasc Med.* 2021 Feb 11;8:610989.

seasons 2008 to 2017, report myocarditis (P = 0.015), pericarditis (P = 0.013), and cardiomyopathy (P = 0.035) in the list of major complications in patients with Influenza B.[35,36] A nationwide epidemiological study investigated acute myocarditis in Korean children using data collected between 2007 and 2016 (n = 1627 children observed during the study period) from the Health Insurance Review and Assessment database. The overall incidence was 1.4 per 100,000 children in 2007 and 2.1 per 100,000 children in 2016 indicating significant increase in the trend over time. The age distribution was bimodal with a larger peak in infancy and a smaller peak in the mid-teenage years. Male preponderance was observed in adolescents aged ≥13 years (482 boys vs 152 girls). Acute fulminant myocarditis occurred in 371 children (22.8%) who needed extracorporeal membrane oxygenation and/or mechanical ventilator support. Of the 371 children with acute fulminant myocarditis, 258 (69.5%) survived. The survival rate of children with acute fulminant myocarditis remained nearly identical over the 10-year study period.[37]

RESIDENT INFLAMMATORY/ IMMUNOCOMPETENT CELLS IN MYOCARDIAL TISSUE

The human myocardium does not host "structured" lymphoid tissue (eg, BALT in lung, MALT in gastrointestinal tract), does not possess resident "reticuloendothelial (RE)" cell systems (eg, liver and spleen), or macrophages as alveolar macrophages in the lung, or glia cell system in the brain, or glomerular-mesangial cells in the kidney. However, a fair amount of resident macrophages are present in steady-state myocardial tissue and participates in supporting normal-tissue homeostasis and immunosurveillance.[38,39] A recent study proposes an additional function of resident cardiac macrophages that would be able to scavenge decaying and spent mitochondria emitted from cardiomyocytes.[40] This transfer of mitochondria from cardiomyocytes to tissue-resident macrophages seems to be a feature of the heart, and, to a minor extent, of the skeletal muscle, while it seems not to occur in the spleen or the liver. Resident cardiac macrophages turn over in about 1 month and self-renew locally through proliferation.[38]

Myocardial macrophages originate from the yolk sac and fetal monocytic progenitors and are either replenished by a local proliferation in infancy,[41] or by blood monocytes in adulthood.[39] At birth, resident macrophages express major histocompatibility complex class II (HLA II) molecules and the CX3CR1+ Fraktalin receptor and are therefore distinct from conventional E integrin CD103+ dendritic cells.[41] With age, the HLA II macrophages increase while the CX3CR1+ macrophages decrease;[42] the proliferation capacity of embryo-derived cardiac macrophages progressively declines after the perinatal period.[42] Cardiac-resident macrophages display distinct functional properties from those of monocyte-derived macrophages in cardiac tissue. Resident macrophages interweave a complex molecular dialogue with cardiomyocytes, likely mediated by cytokines; macrophages can modulate the different signals that originate from the injured cardiac tissue.[43] In cardiac inflammatory diseases, resident macrophages likely participate in attracting circulating monocytes and other inflammatory cells, depending on the local triggers of inflammation.[44] Therefore, even though the myocardial tissue does not lack in resident immune defenses, it does not have a structured lymphoid or RE system like other organs more commonly targeted by infections.

Mast cells are also resident in human hearts.[45] Their number, activation properties, and effects vary in the different myocardial diseases; recently, activation of pericardial mast cells was reported to exacerbate in animal models of Coxsackievirus B3-induced myocarditis.[46] A specific role in human myocarditis remains to be clarified; they have been described in myocarditis caused by immune checkpoint blockade[47] where they could rapidly release cytotoxic mediators.[48]

Myocardial inflammatory cells have been observed in autopsy reports of noncardiac death, wherein the inflammation was a presumptive, but not proven, contributor to the final outcome. In 384 consecutive hearts seen in consultation from a single medical examiner's office, infiltrates were most frequent in natural noncardiac deaths (31%) than in traumatic deaths (12%); eosinophilic infiltrates were especially common in patients on antibiotics (18%). Incidental inflammation with myocyte necrosis in noncardiac deaths was less common (2%).[25] Inflammatory infiltrates have been commonly observed in donor hearts before implantation.[49] Although normal myocardium is expected to be free from pathologic inflammatory infiltrates, lymphocytes in particular, their incidental detection in noncardiac death suggests that, by itself, inflammatory cells may not have clinical significance. The distinction between resident inflammatory cells such as macrophages versus inflammatory cells triggered by local stimuli should be considered when attempting to interpret their role in steady-state myocardium.

INFECTIOUS MYOCARDITIS

The infectious agents that have been associated with myocarditis include DNA and RNA viruses, bacteria, fungi, protozoa, and helminths.[1,50,51] Viral infections are the most common causes of myocarditis in both children and adults (Table 46–1).[50] Nonviral cardiotropic infections, such as Chagas disease[5] and Lyme disease,[6] in immunocompetent individuals constitute special subgroups of myocarditis. In immunocompromised patients (eg, immunosuppressed, malignancy, postsurgical, human immunodeficiency virus [HIV] infected), myocarditis is associated with different infectious agents (eg, HCMV or *Toxoplasma gondii)*. In pregnancy, HCMV infection may cause fetal malformations wherein the maternal infection remains clinically subtle partly because of delayed lymphoproliferative response in primary infection[52] and lower viral load.[53]

Viral Myocarditis

Diagnostic Work-Up

Myocardial infection is diagnosed when the infectious agent is detected in myocardial tissue by pathology and/or genomic studies.[7] The diagnostic work-up of myocardial infection should begin with timely sampling of informative tissue and paired samples of peripheral blood. The diagnostic processes include cell culture, antibody detection, antigen detection, hemagglutination assay, nucleic acid detection, and gene sequencing. Specific antibodies are always produced when the adaptive immune system encounters a virus. As a general rule, immunoglobulin (Ig)Ms are highly effective at neutralizing viruses, are produced only for the initial few weeks, and are indicative of acute infections. IgGs are produced indefinitely and are tested to demonstrate prior infection. Antigens are detected by enzyme-linked immunosorbent assay (ELISA) in biologic fluids with immunofluorescence and immunoperoxidase as the alternative methods. Quantitative assays for measuring the viral genome copy number and nucleic acid sequencing establish the viral presence. In the appropriate diagnostic work-up, the serology is systematically performed, routine inflammatory markers are tested, and markers of myocardial damage are monitored. Neutralizing antibodies in serum can be tested by the neutralization test based on the enzyme-linked immunospot assay.[54] EMB is the gold standard for the confirmation of viral infection.[11,55] Inflammatory cells are detected with routine pathology stains such as hematoxylin and eosin. The immunophenotyping of inflammatory cells for prevalent subtypes of T lymphocytes including CD4+ and CD8+, B lymphocytes, natural killer cells, or macrophages may add information on the presence of effector and regulatory pathogenetic pathways. Immunohistochemical detection of the infective pathogen and molecular transcription signature from the affected myocardium can contribute to the diagnosis of inflammatory heart diseases.[56]

Enteroviruses

Enteroviruses belong to the family of Picornaviridae and are grouped into 12 species: enteroviruses A to H and J and rhinoviruses A to C. The disease in humans is caused by poliovirus, coxsackievirus, rhinovirus, enterovirus, and echovirus serotypes. The clinical presentation may be relatively mild (eg, fever, herpangina, conjunctivitis, hand-foot-mouth disease, tonsillitis, pharyngitis, lower respiratory tract infection, acute gastroenteritis) or, uncommonly, severe (eg, pneumonia, meningitis, encephalitis, myocarditis, pericarditis, hepatic necrosis, coagulopathy).[57] The cardiotropic coxsackievirus B3 (CV-B3) is one of the most common causes of myocarditis.[57] The myocardial infection is mediated by the transmembrane coxsackievirus-adenovirus receptor (CAR); the ablation of CAR blocks viral binding to myocardial cells and inflammation in the myocardium in experimental models.[58] Similarly, increased cardiac expression of CAR may partially explain increased susceptibility to myocarditis.[59] In CV-B3–infected myocytes, the cell damage is induced by direct cytotoxicity and mediated by viral proteinases.[60] CV-B3 replicates on the surface of autophagosomes[61,62] and enhances replication by employing microRNA (miRNA);[63,64] CV-B3–induced differential expression of miRNA modulates expression of both host and viral genes. Patients with defects of dystrophin and dysferlin demonstrate increased susceptibility to myocardial CV-B3 infection by enhancing viral propagation to adjacent cardiomyocytes and disrupting membrane repair function.[65–67] The history of a recent flu episode in patients with X-linked DCM caused by defects of dystrophin could mislead the clinical diagnosis, but the possibility that a viral flu triggers the clinical manifestations of a preexisting asymptomatic disease cannot be excluded. Although myocarditis and viral genome may not be found in the EMB from patients with X-linked DCM,[68] the myocardium with dystrophin defects could suffer greater damage from coxsackievirus proteases known to affect host cell proteins such as dystrophin.[69]

In viral infections, the early innate immune response provides the first defense mechanism and is mediated by cytokines. The virus is recognized by specific receptors (toll-like, retinoic acid inducible gene-I–like, nucleotide-binding oligomerization domain-like, and C-type lectin receptors) through pathogen-specific molecules.[70,71] This interaction induces the production of proinflammatory cytokines (eg, tumor necrosis factor-α and interleukin-1) to recruit T cells (including regulatory T cells and interleukin-17–producing cells) and modulate immune response.[72] The late adaptive immune response contributes to the myocardial lymphocyte infiltration that must clear virus-infected cells, typically cardiac myocytes in CV-B3 myocarditis. Depletion or ablation of T lymphocytes, both CD4+ and CD8+, decreases the mortality and reduces cardiac inflammation and injury after CV-B3 infection.[73] In addition, a molecular mimicry between viral and host antigens has been proposed as a mechanism subsequently responsible for the postinfectious autoimmune-mediated damage of the myocardium.[74] Acute infections are clinically characterized by febrile illness that commonly evolves without complications; when complicated by myocarditis, the febrile illness is commonly reported as having preceded the cardiac symptoms. The cardiac manifestations range from mild, nonspecific symptoms to life-threatening complications such as cardiogenic shock and sudden cardiac death. The pathologic features of CV-B3 myocarditis are T-lymphocyte inflammatory infiltrate and myocyte damage/necrosis (**Fig. 46–2**). Markers of myocardial damage and systemic inflammation can be increased. IgMs are usually missed unless the diagnosis of myocarditis is done close to the onset of the systemic illness. In the acute phase, viral particles can be recognized in infected myocytes.[75,76] Polymerase chain reaction (PCR)–based demonstration of the viral genome in the affected myocardium concludes the diagnostic work-up; molecular assays are paired in blood and myocardial samples.

Human Parvovirus B19 (B19V)

B19V belongs to the genus *Erythroparvovirus* of the Parvoviridae family, which is composed of a group of small DNA viruses with a linear single-stranded DNA genome.[77] B19V usually infects human erythroid progenitor cells (EPC) to cause mild-to-severe hematologic disorders,[78] but may also infect nonerythroid lineage cells such as endothelial cells.[79] B19V infection typically presents clinically with erythema infectiosum, arthralgia, fetal death, transient aplastic crisis, and persistent infection in immunocompromised hosts; less common clinical manifestations include atypical skin rashes, neurologic syndromes, cardiac manifestations, and cytopenias.[77,79]

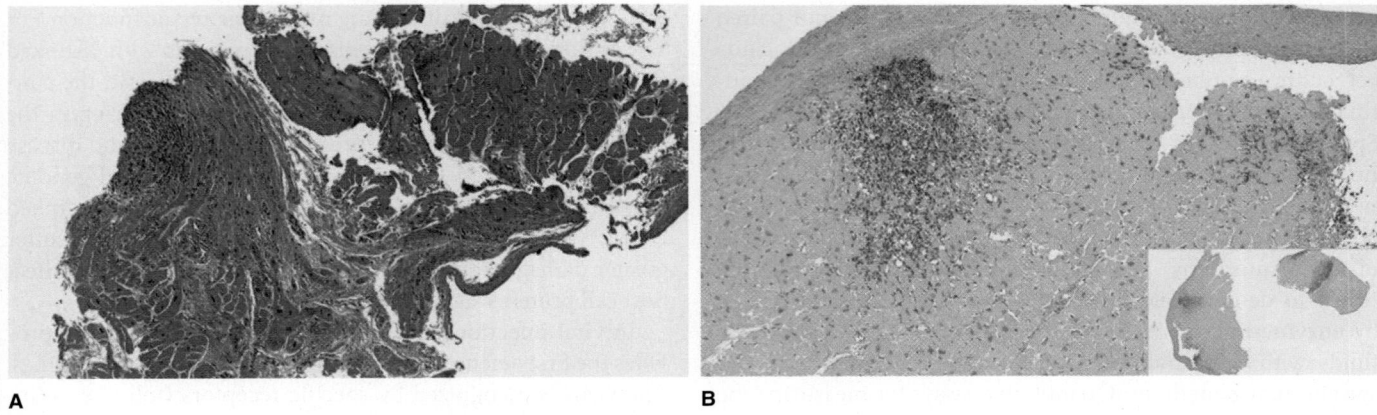

Figure 46–2. (**A**) Active myocarditis, with plurifocal inflammatory infiltrates demonstrating (CD3⁺) immunoreactivity (**B**); the inset shows the very low magnification view of two endomyocardial biopsy (EMB) samples (coxsackievirus B3 positive; onset: 18 days before EMB).

The cardiac manifestations of B19V infection range from mild and nonspecific symptoms (eg, fatigue, arrhythmias) to cardiogenic shock requiring mechanical support. Recently, fatal B19V hemophagocytic syndrome and myocarditis have been reported in two unrelated children who received a shot of AdimFlu-S (A/H1N1) vaccine and of MF59-adjuvanted influenza vaccine; both were supposed to be vaccine-related deaths, on the basis of the temporal relationships between vaccination and lethal outcomes (essentially coincidental).[80] Mechanistically, the B19V-antibody complex enters the cells through an endocytosis process mediated by the direct interaction of antibody-bound complement factor C1q with its receptor CD93 on the cell surface.[81,82] B19V enters myocardial endothelial cells but does not replicate intracellularly.[83] The tropism of B19V for endothelial progenitor cells (EPCs) depends upon the expression of viral receptors and coreceptors on the cell surface and by the viral use of host factors such as RNA binding motif protein 38 (RBM38) for the processing of its pre-mRNA during viral replication.[84] The RBM38 protein (coded by the RBM38 gene, 20q13.31, MIM* 612428) interacts with the intronic splicing enhancer 2 (ISE2) element of B19V pre-mRNA and promotes 11-kDa protein expression that regulates the 11-kDa protein-mediated augmentation of B19V replication.[85]

B19V genome has been identified in the myocardial tissue of patients with myocarditis and DCM, but also in control cases.[86,87] In 72 EMBs from 35 patients with DCM, 17 patients with active myocarditis, and 20 surgical myocardial samples from patients undergoing surgery for valve disease or coronary artery disease, real-time PCR failed to identify enteroviruses, Epstein–Barr virus, or herpes simplex viruses type 1 or 2; only one DCM patient tested positive, but for adenovirus. On the other hand, 20 of 52 patients (38%) with cardiomyopathy and 8 of 20 controls (40%) tested positive for B19V, disproving the hypothesis that persistent myocardial viral infection might be a frequent cause of DCM or myocarditis.[86] A recent review demonstrates that the mean rate of PCR detected B19V genomes in patients presenting with MC/DCM does not differ significantly from the findings in control myocardial tissues. These data imply pathogenetically insignificant latency of B19V genomes

in a proportion of myocardial tissues, both in MC-/DCM-patients and in controls.[88]

A possible hypothesis that could explain the role of B19V in myocarditis and cardiomyopathy is the potential role of trigger of the viral genome for innate immunity, inducing proinflammatory cytokine secretion[83] and myocardial inflammation. EMB typically shows T-lymphocyte inflammatory infiltrates and prominent endothelial cells; myocytes may not show damage or necrosis (**Fig. 46–3**). B19V infection has also been associated with adult and pediatric autoimmune diseases, including systemic diseases that involve the heart, either directly or indirectly.[89–91] Documented mechanisms in B19-associated autoimmunity include molecular mimicry (IgG antibodies to B19 proteins cross-react with human autoantigens), virus-induced apoptosis with presentation of self-antigens to T lymphocytes, and the phospholipase activity of the B19 unique VP1 protein.

Human Herpesviruses

The human herpesviruses (HHV) are currently assigned to three subfamilies: α-, β-, and γ-herpesvirinae. Herpesvirus infections are characterized by their ability to establish lifelong infections with periods of latency followed by reactivation. The diagnosis of HHV myocarditis is based on the demonstration of HHV actively replicating in cardiac cells and by the presence of T-lymphocyte infiltration associated with myocyte injury. In infected cells, HHV typically causes a morphologically manifest cytopathic effect; commercially available antibodies can detect viral antigens expressed in the immediate/early and late phases of viral replication. PCR can selectively detect genes expressed by replicating viruses, and quantitative PCR measures the number of copies of viral genomes in the affected tissues compared to the peripheral blood. HHV6, adenovirus, and Epstein–Barr virus of the herpesvirinae family are associated with myocarditis, which may occur both in immunocompetent and immunocompromised hosts, as well as in children and adults.[92–98] In immunocompromised patients, the HHV6 myocarditis can be fatal.[95–96] Double virus infection may also occur.[99] Myocardial infection with HCMV is more commonly observed in immunocompromised hosts. The myocardial

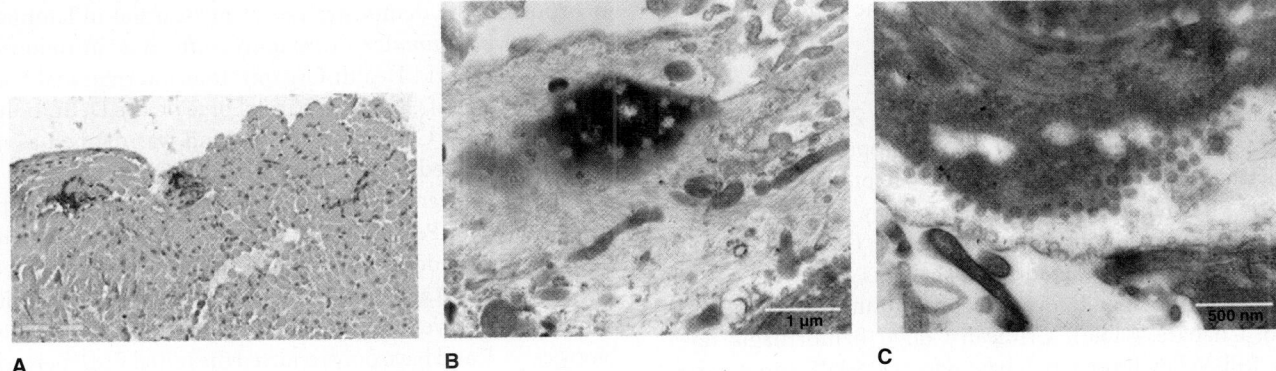

Figure 46–3. Parvovirus B19 (B19V) myocardial infection: cardiogenic shock, female, aged 37 years, ejection fraction = 10%. The patient was admitted to the hospital after 7 days of fever and one episode of syncope the night before; both of her children had suffered febrile flu in the course of the month before the onset of her symptoms. The patient was immediately supported with medical treatment and extracorporeal membrane oxygenation. The endomyocardial biopsy showed mild focal inflammatory infiltrates without significant myocyte damage. Molecular tests gave negative results for enteroviruses (coxsackievirus B3) and Ebstein–Barr virus. B19V was present as 402 copies/10⁶ cells in blood and 109,496 copies/10⁶ cells in myocardium. (**A**) Anti-CD3 immunostain showing focal inflammatory infiltrates. (**B**) and (**C**) Electron micrographs showing virus-like particles in endothelial cells. The patient experienced full recovery of LV function during the next 10 days and was discharged 24 days later with LVEF of 54%.

pathology is characterized by T-cell inflammatory infiltrate and by the presence of typical intranuclear amphophilic inclusion bodies that specifically immune-stain with anti-HCMV antibodies. The virus infects both myocytes and endothelial cells. Seroepidemiologic studies suggest HCMV infection to be widespread and influenced by age, geography, and cultural and socioeconomic status. Children become infected early in life in developing countries. Up to 80% of the adult population is infected in developed nations. The course of primary infection is usually mild or asymptomatic in immunocompetent hosts as HCMV establishes a latent but persistent infection, reflecting the inability of the immune system to clear the virus; immune evasion mechanisms allow infected cells to escape both innate and adaptive effector immunity.[100] In immunosuppressed patients (eg, solid organ or bone marrow transplant recipients), the infection can be reactivated to result in systemic and organ infection; the heart is a possible target for tissue infection.[101] The diagnosis and treatment of viral infections in transplanted patients are managed by preemptive or prophylactic therapy, and antiviral treatment is based on established protocols.[102] Prophylactic therapy is recommended by the Transplantation Society guidelines for high-risk (donor's CMV-IgG antibody positive and recipient's negative) pediatric recipients[103] and in patients who receive allogeneic hematopoietic stem cell transplantation (HSCT).[104] Myocarditis uncommonly complicates infections with herpes simplex virus types 1 and 2 and varicella-zoster virus; recently, an association between myocarditis and HHV7 infection has been described.[105] In the last 50 years, the development of antiviral compounds has substantially contributed to control HHV infections.[106,107] Acyclovir (or its prodrug valacyclovir) and famciclovir have greatly reduced the burden of disease and have demonstrated a remarkable safety record. In the otherwise healthy population, drug resistance has remained below 0.5% after more than 30 years of antiviral use. Vice versa, drug resistance remains more common in immuno-compromised patients, and alternative drugs with good safety

profiles are needed. At present, ganciclovir and valganciclovir are a first-line approach, and foscarnet and cidofovir provide a second-line therapy, mostly limited to treatment of refractory or resistant HCMV infections. Letermovir (LTV), which targets the HCMV DNA terminase complex, was licensed for prophylaxis of HCMV infections in HSCT recipients, preliminarily showing low toxicity and low incidence of resistant infections. Finally, for refractory/resistant HCMV infections by antiviral drugs, HCMV-specific adoptive T-cell immunotherapy should be taken into consideration.[108]

Inherited Chromosomally Integrated HHV-6 (iciHHV-6)

iciHHV-6 has been known for decades to be associated with human diseases,[109] including transplant donors and recipients,[110–112] neonatal sepsis,[113] autoimmune diseases,[114] heart failure,[115] acute myocarditis.[116,117] HHV-6 has been recently classified as HHV-6A and HHV-6B, which share about 90% sequence identity.[118] Whereas HHV-6B is ubiquitous in the population, and primary infection occurs early in childhood as the febrile illness exanthema subitum,[119,120] HHV-6A infection occurs later in life. The prevalence of HHV-6A is less well defined, and the distribution shows geographical variation.[121] Similar to other herpesviruses, HHV6A and HHV-6B demonstrate latency upon primary infection and lifelong viral persistence, possibly in monocytes/macrophages. HHV-6A and HHV-6B integrate their genomes into the chromosomal telomeres of infected cells;[121,122] reported integration sites include both long and short arms of various chromosomes: 1q44; 9q34; 10q26; 11p15.5; 17p13.3; 18p11.3; 18q23; 19qttel; 22q13; Xp. When integration occurs in germ cells,[123] the viral genome can be transmitted from parents to child in a Mendelian manner,[124,125] and therefore be present in every cell of the body. Approximately 1% of the people worldwide carry iciHHV-6, varying from 0.2% to 2.5% in different studies.[109,125,126] Up to 86% of HHV-6 congenital infections seem to be attributable to iciHHV-6, while transplacental transmission of the virus following reactivation or reinfection in the mother accounts only for 14% of them.[12]

Emerging Viral Infections and Myocarditis

Chikungunya (CHIKV), Dengue (DENV), Zika virus (ZIKV), and Mayaro virus (MAYV) are arthropod-borne viruses (arboviruses). Beyond SARS-CoV-2 (Chapter 84), numerous emerging new and reemerging viruses may cause severe and/or lethal diseases in humans: filoviruses (Ebola, Marburg), henipaviruses (Nipah, Hendra), Lassa virus, Lujo virus, South American hemorrhagic fever viruses (Junin, Machupo, Guanarito, Chapare, Sabia), Crimean-Congo hemorrhagic fever virus, Rift Valley fever virus, hantaviruses, SARS coronavirus, MERS coronavirus, and tick-borne encephalitis viruses. Clinical manifestations of these infections include fever, arthralgia, maculopapular rash, chronic polyarthritis, neurological complications, hemorrhage, myocarditis, and even death.[128-131]

The "c" (NET-Heart project) is a recent initiative aimed at systematically reviewing all devastating endemic conditions affecting the heart, to spread knowledge and propose algorithms for early diagnosis and treatment.[132]

Clinical Presentation and Evolution of Viral Myocarditis

Acute myocarditis can have a "fulminant" presentation and course (cardiogenic shock) or present with acute heart failure, a wide spectrum of arrhythmias up to life-threatening arrhythmic storms, or may mimic acute coronary syndromes, or apical ballooning.[1] Then, it can either worsen ending in death, or recover after having required mechanical support or intensive medication, or heal spontaneously (common) or, in a minority of cases, can evolve into a chronic, low-grade inflammatory myocardial disease (**Fig. 46–4**). The diagnosis of chronic myocarditis is ideally established by biopsy-proven evidence of the acute phase and demonstration of the persistent myocardial inflammation. Different terms are currently found in the literature describing the latter pathologic substrate, including chronic myocarditis, subacute myocarditis, inflammatory cardiomyopathy, and myocarditis-induced DCM. Each term

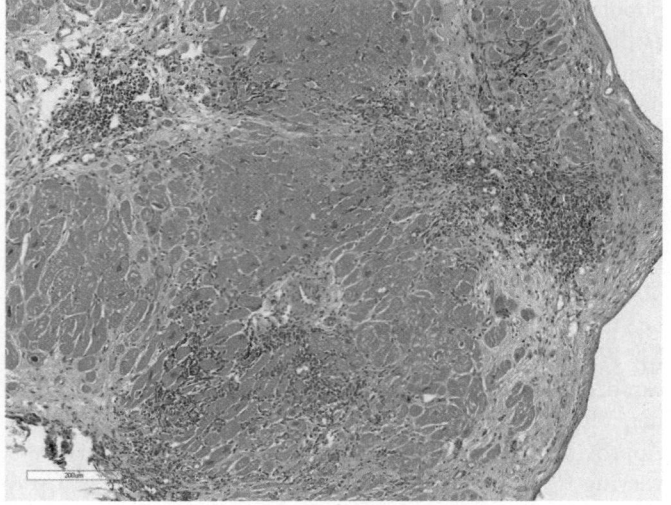

Figure 46–4. Ongoing active inflammation and early granulation tissue in coxsackievirus B3–positive myocarditis.

incorporates the demonstration of myocardial inflammation. The term *inflammatory cardiomyopathy* was introduced in 1995 by the World Health Organization/International Society and Federation of Cardiology Task Force on the Definition and Classification of Cardiomyopathies, and was defined as myocarditis associated with cardiac dysfunction.[2] The term and the definition were adopted by the ESC Working Group for Myocardial and Pericardial Diseases.[4] The term *inflammatory cardiomyopathy* does not describe the phenotype (dilated or arrhythmogenic) and does not specify the cause. Most available clinical series have rarely included both baseline and follow-up biopsies[133-135] and have only reported the initial EMB performed at the onset of symptoms. The non-EMB series inferred the diagnosis of chronic myocarditis on the basis of clinical presentation suggestive of a recent-onset, flu-like syndrome shortly preceding the onset of cardiac symptoms, elevated inflammatory markers, and imaging characterization in patients with angiographically proven normal coronary arteries.[136] Previous studies estimated that 30% of DCM could represent the chronic evolution of a prior myocarditis.[134,135,137,138] In 82 patients with biopsy-proven active myocarditis who were consecutively enrolled and followed-up for 147 ± 107 months, improvement or normalization of LVEF was observed in 53% of patients.[137] In another study including 174 patients with either active or borderline myocarditis, 124 patients were alive without being transplanted, 26 were dead or transplanted, and 24 (14%) were lost at a median follow-up of 23.5 months (interquartile range, 10–54 months).[138] A further series included 181 consecutive patients with clinically suspected viral myocarditis; 69 patients fulfilled Dallas criteria for the diagnosis of myocarditis, 91 showed immunohistologic markers of inflammation, and 79 had a positive PCR-based genome search in the EMB. Twenty-two percent of the patients (n = 40) either died or underwent heart transplantation at a mean age of 59 ± 42 months.[139] In another series of 222 consecutive patients with biopsy-proven viral myocarditis, mortality was 19.2% at a median follow-up of 4.7 years.[140] Overall, about 25% of patients with biopsy-proven myocarditis evolve through worsening of cardiac function and either undergo heart transplantation or die.

Predictors of outcome vary in different myocardial biopsy studies. Persistence of New York Heart Association (NYHA) classes III to IV, left atrium enlargement, and improvement in LVEF at 6 months emerged as independent predictors of long-term outcome in one study.[137] Biventricular dysfunction at diagnosis was the main predictor of death/transplantation in another study.[138] Advanced NYHA functional class, immunohistologic signs of inflammation, and lack of β-blocker therapy (but not histologic characteristics [positive Dallas criteria] or detectability of viral genome) were found to relate to poor outcome.[139] However, poor survival for fulminant myocarditis was associated with the type of inflammatory infiltrates comprising giant cell > eosinophilic > lymphocytic,[141] whereas the high rates of cardiomyocyte apoptosis were associated with functional recovery at 1 year.[142] The presence of late gadolinium enhancement (LGE) emerged as the best independent predictor of all-cause and cardiac mortality, whereas the initial presentation with heart failure was a predictor of incomplete long-term recovery.[140] Similarly, a high LV end-diastolic dimension Z-score on admission in children also was a predictor of worse outcomes, with higher mortality and incomplete recovery.[143] In 203 consecutive patients with an initial cardiac magnetic resonance (CMR)–based diagnosis of acute myocarditis (typical LGE) and a mean follow-up of 18.9 ± 8.2 months, an initial alteration of LVEF was the only independent CMR predictor of adverse clinical outcome.[144] Overall, most studies demonstrate that the most consistent predictors of worse outcomes include NYHA functional class and presence of heart failure or LV dilation and dysfunction, and suggest little prognostic added value to myocarditis or postmyocarditis substrate.

Three pathogenetic hypotheses support the evolution from acute to chronic myocarditis or chronic inflammatory heart disease.

Immunopathogenic Hypothesis: It has been proposed that immunopathogenic or inflammatory reactions could lead to tissue damage uncoupled from the original viral injury.[57] The original myocyte damage induced by the acute inflammation might trigger an abnormal immune response that could subsequently smolder into a subacute and chronic phase of myocardial inflammation and myocyte damage. Few studies have reported the presence of anticardiac autoantibodies and immunoglobulins in blood samples.[145] This hypothesis supports the potential benefit of immunosuppression.

Viral Persistence: It has also been suggested that the infectious agent, or virus in particular, could persist and induce chronic inflammation and myocyte damage.[57] Based on this hypothesis, antiviral agents could help cleanse the infected myocardium from the persistent viral infection. However, the pertinent issues include how to detect viral persistence, demonstrate its virulence, and implicate it as the basis of myocardial dysfunction. Several studies have questioned the validity of PCR-based detection of viral genome in myocardial tissue as the cause of the underlying myocardial disease, because many nonmyocarditis and noncardiomyopathy controls also test positively for the viral genome load.[87,146–148]

Combined Mechanisms: It is reasonable to propose that both mechanisms—viral persistence and the autoimmune reaction—might contribute to the progression of myocardial damage, chronic myocardial remodeling, and dysfunction. Both mechanisms, although biologically plausible, have been variably demonstrated and lend importance to the antiviral and immunosuppressive interventions. However, the major missing link in patients with poor clinical outcome is the systematic evaluation of the family to exclude underlying genetic causes that can either cause or contribute to the eventual phenotype.[149]

Treatment of Viral Myocarditis
Treatment of myocarditis consists of supportive care with heart failure medical therapy and diuretics to relieve congestion, as per guidelines.[150,151] Temporary or implantable mechanical support devices are frequently employed in patients with refractory cardiogenic shock.[152]

Immunosuppressive Therapy: Current clinical guidelines do not support the use of immunosuppressive therapy in the routine management of acute myocarditis.[4] A study of 102 patients with acute-onset DCM classified as either reactive or nonreactive (based on the biopsy or other evidence of inflammation) failed to resolve LVEF after 9 months of prednisone treatment, even after an early transient improvement in reactive patients.[153] The multicenter Myocarditis Treatment Trial randomized 111 patients with biopsy-proven myocarditis of unknown etiology and an LVEF less than 45% to conventional therapy versus immunosuppressive therapy consisting of prednisone together with azathioprine or cyclosporine. Both groups experienced an average LVEF increase of 9% over 28 weeks, but immunosuppressive therapy failed to attenuate clinical disease or improve survival.[15] Reserving immunosuppressive therapy for only those patients with ongoing inflammation has met with mixed success. A randomized study of 84 patients with unexplained DCM and increased human leukocyte antigen expression in biopsy specimens compared guideline-directed medical therapy of heart failure alone or in combination with prednisone and azathioprine.[154] The addition of immunosuppressive therapy was associated with an increase in LVEF and NYHA functional class at 3 and 24 months, but failed to reduce a primary composite end point of death, transplantation, or hospitalization. The favorable response to immunosuppressive therapy has been reported predominantly in virus-negative, autoimmune forms of myocarditis. In a study of 41 patients with active myocarditis and chronic heart failure treated with prednisone and azathioprine,[155] 21 patients were considered responders, experiencing an increase in LVEF from an average of 25.7% at baseline to 47.4% following treatment. Cardiac autoantibodies were present in 91% of these patients and in none of the nonresponders. Interestingly, viral genomes were detectable in 85% of the nonresponders and only 14% of responders. The Tailored Immunosuppression in Inflammatory Cardiomyopathy study was a randomized, placebo-controlled trial of prednisone and azathioprine in virus-negative myocarditis;[156] immunosuppressive therapy of 85 patients was associated with an increase in LVEF, reduction in LV volumes, and improved NYHA functional class.

Immunomodulatory Therapies: High-dose intravenous immunoglobulin (IVIG) has both immunomodulatory and antiviral effects. Clinical trial results of its use in myocarditis have been mixed. In an open-label study, 9 of 10 adult patients with new-onset heart failure treated with IVIG had a significant improvement in LV function.[157] The Intervention in Myocarditis and Acute Cardiomyopathy trial was a randomized, placebo-controlled trial of IVIG that enrolled 62 patients with recent-onset DCM and LVEF <40%.[158] Of these, 15% of patients had biopsy-proven myocarditis. No benefit of immunomodulation was demonstrated in terms of ejection fraction or survival at 6 and 12 months. Direct removal of circulating cardiac autoantibodies through the use of immunoadsorption has also been reported in a small, single-center study of patients with recent-onset cardiomyopathy.[159] In the absence of positive results from randomized controlled trials, it is not possible to make a recommendation for the use of IVIG or immunoadsorption.[4] A recent meta-analysis evaluated the effect of immunosuppression (IS)/immunomodulation (IM); in prospective studies, the difference in mortality between the IS and control groups tended to be lower in the combined IS groups (12.5% vs 18.2%) (95% CI of odds ratio 0.7[0.3, 1.64]) and the pooled difference of the increase of LVEF between the IS and control groups tended to be higher in the combined IS groups (95% CI, 7.26 [−2.29, 16.81]). In retrospective studies, the difference of survival between the IS and control group was in favor of IS (95% CI hazard ratio 0.82[0.69, 0.96]).[160]

Antiviral Therapies: In patients with enterovirus myocarditis and viral persistence, treatment with interferon-β (IFN-β) has been reported to produce hemodynamic and clinical improvement.[135,161] Twenty-two patients with adenoviral or enteroviral genomes from EMBs and heart failure refractory to guideline-directed medical therapy were treated for 6 months with IFN-β. Treatment produced structural and functional LV improvement, and a majority of patients showed an improvement in NYHA functional class; viral genome was successfully eliminated in all patients, and myocardial inflammation was substantially reduced. Long-term follow-up of this cohort and others who spontaneously cleared enterovirus infection showed improved survival as compared to those with viral persistence.[135] Elevated levels of IFN-β, either through spontaneous production or exogenous administration over 6 months, were associated with effective enterovirus clearance and improved outcome. Conversely, the lack of spontaneous IFN-β production was associated with enterovirus persistence and reduced long-term survival. In a recent phase II study, 143 patients with symptoms of heart failure and biopsy-based confirmation of the enterovirus, adenovirus, and/or B19V genomes in their myocardial tissue were randomly assigned to double-blind treatment with either placebo (n = 48) or 4 × 10⁶ IU (n = 49) or 8 × 10⁶ IU (n = 46) of IFN-β-1b for 24 weeks, in addition to standard heart failure treatment. Compared to placebo, virus elimination and/or virus load reduction was higher in the IFN-β-1b groups (odds ratio 2.33, $P = 0.048$; similarly in both IFN groups). IFN-β-1b treatment was associated with favorable effects on NYHA functional class and improvement in quality of life and patient global assessments. The frequency of adverse cardiac events was similar in the IFN-β-1b groups compared to the placebo group.[133] Results of major clinical trials are listed in **Table 46–2.**

Primary Prevention in Viral Myocarditis: Malignant arrhythmias associated with viral myocarditis are potential predictors of future sudden cardiac death in patients not only with a reduced but also with a preserved EF.[16] This observation gives insights into clinical decision-making, despite a lack of clearcut guideline recommendations during (2006)[162] and even after (2015/2018)[163,164] the time of data collection (2002–2015). The implantable cardioverter-defibrillator (ICD) therapy in these patients was not fully covered by guidelines recommendations at the time;[162] the decision was based upon a clinical risk-benefit assessment in patients who survived life-threatening ventricular arrhythmia, as a secondary prevention measure. In 2015, the European guidelines recommended (class IIb) patients with potentially life-threatening arrhythmia resulting from acute viral myocarditis to receive wearable ICD life vests until the resolution of the acute episode.[4,163] ICD implantation can be postponed until the resolution of the acute phase (2–4 weeks) and considered for patients with residual LV dysfunction and/or ventricular electrical instability. Other recent

TABLE 46–2. Randomized Controlled Trials in Myocarditis and Inflammatory Cardiomyopathies

Diagnosis	No. of Patients	Treatments	Primary End Point	Results	Reference
• DCM	102	Prednisone vs placebo	>LVEF at 3 months or <LV end-diastolic dimensions	Mean LVEF >4.3% ± 1.5% in the prednisone vs 2.1% ± 0.8% in the control group ($P = 0.054$)	154
• Biopsy-proven myocarditis (unknown etiology)	111	Prednisone + cyclosporine or azathioprine vs conventional therapy	LVEF at 28 weeks	No difference in LVEF or survival in the two groups ($P = 0.96$)	16
• Inflammatory DCM (unknown etiology, increased HLA expression on EMB)	84	Prednisone plus azathioprine vs placebo	Composite: death, heart transplantation, and hospital readmission over 2 years	No difference in primary end point (22.8% immunosuppression group vs 20.5% placebo group)	155
• Recent-onset unexplained DCM (≤6 months)	62	IVIG vs placebo	LVEF at 6 and 12 months	Similar improvement in LVEF at 6 and 12 months	159
• Inflammatory, virus-negative DCM	85	Prednisone plus azathioprine vs placebo	LVEF at 6 months	Significantly improved LVEF and decreased LV dimensions in immunosuppressive group	157
Symptoms of HF and biopsy-based confirmation of EV, ADV, PVB19 genomes in myocardial tissue	143	4 × 10⁶ (n = 49) and 8 × 10⁶ IU (n = 46) interferon-β-1b vs placebo (n = 48)	Virus elimination and/ or virus load reduction at 24 months	Virus elimination/load reduction: higher in the interferon-β-1b groups (odds ratio, 2.33; $P = 0.048$), similar in both interferon groups and strata	137

Abbreviations: ADV, adenovirus; DCM, dilated cardiomyopathy; EMB, endomyocardial biopsy; EV, enterovirus; HF, heart failure; HLA, human leukocyte antigen; IVIG, intravenous immunoglobulin; LV, left ventricular; LVEF, left ventricular ejection fraction; PVB19, parvovirus B19.

studies showed, after viral myocarditis, mortality rates reaching 20% at 5 years[140] or the need of adequate ICD therapy in 50% of all patients with an indication for ICD implantation.[165] These patients did not have arrhythmias as primary presentation of viral inflammation. The rate of ventricular fibrillation over 5 years was 17.6%, with a further 43.1% having ventricular tachycardia. The aforementioned results highly suggest more frequent implantation of ICDs in such patients.

Nonviral Infectious Myocarditis

Bacterial Myocarditis

Although the list of the causes of infective myocarditis (see Table 46–1) may include several different bacteria, the proportion of bacterial myocarditis in immunocompetent hosts is low. Recent reports suggest a changing epidemiologic scenario of myocarditis-causing bacterial infections (eg, *Corynebacterium diphtheriae* infection is increasing worldwide, particularly in developing countries).[166–168] Uncommon pathogens with atypical clinical presentation such as *Listeria monocytogenes* and *Leptospira* are rare causes of myocarditis, and *Legionella*, typically associated with pneumonia, may occasionally present with fulminant myocarditis.[169–171] Warning messages come from single case reports or small clinical series demonstrating myocarditis in both immunocompetent and immunodeficient patients with multidrug-resistant infectious agents.[172] Typhoid infection from H58 lineage is one of the numerous reports on the re-emergence of typhoid in southern and eastern Africa, particularly in Blantyre, Malawi, since 2011, highlighting the need for identifying the reservoirs and transmission of disease.[172] Recently, nontyphoid *Salmonella*, most commonly *Salmonella enteritidis*, was reported to inflict an overall mortality of 24%, wherein 42% of patients required intensive care and myocarditis affecting young adults was associated with poor prognosis.[172] In immunocompromised hosts, myocarditis can complicate meningococcal infection, with poor prognosis and high mortality.[174–176]

Rare acute nonrheumatic myocarditis mimicking ST-elevation myocardial infarction (STEMI) is a well-documented complication of streptococcal infection. The diagnosis is typically reported in young men with streptococcal pharyngitis or tonsillitis, but should be considered in any acute myocardial presentation associated with active *Streptococcus pyogenes* infection.[177]

Viral infections presenting concurrently with bacterial pneumonia are now known to occur with a frequency of 30% to 50% in both adult and pediatric populations.[178] Bacterial coinfections with prevalent *Staphylococcus aureus* and *Streptococcus pneumoniae* in patients with influenza can cause myocarditis.[179] Immunocompromised children with preexisting neurologic conditions are at increased risk of pH1N1-associated death after intensive care unit admission. Secondary complications of pH1N1, including myocarditis, encephalitis, and clinical diagnosis of methicillin-resistant *Staphylococcus aureus* coinfection of the lung, have been reported as fatal risk factors.[180] Tubercular myocarditis is still known to occur and cause sudden death.[181,182] Finally, myocarditis can follow medical treatments for rare infections such as ehrlichiosis.[183,184]

Fungal Myocarditis

In immunocompetent hosts, fungal myocarditis is rare; Candida and Aspergillus may occasionally cause myocarditis and can represent hospital-acquired infections;[185–187] post influenza aspergillosis, triggered by influenza B virus, can be associated with a fulminant course of respiratory decline and high mortality.[188] Fungal myocarditis can rarely occur in immunocompromised hosts.[189] Fungal infections are more commonly associated with endocarditis (see Chapter 33), in particular in postsurgical patients and in patients receiving implantable devices.

Myocarditis Associated with Parasitic Infections

Protozoal Infections: In immunocompetent hosts, *Trypanosoma cruzi* is the most common parasitic infection known to be associated with myocarditis (see section Endemic Myocarditis).[1,5,50] Between 5 and 18 million people are currently infected, and the infection is estimated to cause more than 10,000 deaths annually.[1,50] *Toxoplasma gondii* causes a disease known as toxoplasmosis.[190] While the parasite is found throughout the world, the prevalence of human *Toxoplasma* infection varies in different parts of the world and has been reported with rates up to 75%.[191,192] Few infected individuals have symptoms. Toxoplasmic myocarditis is a challenging diagnosis that requires evidence of the infection in endomyocardial biopsy.[19]

In pregnant women and individuals who have compromised immune systems, *Toxoplasma* infection can cause severe consequences. The implementation of prophylaxis with trimethoprim-sulfamethoxazole in transplanted patients has significantly contributed to prevent posttransplantation myocarditis.[192]

A rare infection is sarcocystosis, which typically affects muscle but rarely involves the heart;[193] it can be suspected in travelers complaining of myalgia with or without fever, returning ill from high-risk areas. Acute muscular sarcocystosis shows an apparent biphasic course with fever and acute myalgia followed subsequently by elevated creatine phosphokinase, eosinophilia, and possible relapses.[194]

Helminthic Infections: Helminths are multicellular worm-like parasites classified into three taxonomical groups:

1. The nematodes (roundworms) including major intestinal worms (or soil-transmitted helminths) and filarial worms that cause lymphatic Filariasis and onchocerciasis.
2. Cestode (tapeworms), such as Cysticercosis.
3. Trematodes (or flukes) such as the schistosomes. Helminthic infections rarely affect the heart.

Helminthic infections that may affect the myocardium include Trichiniasis, Echinococcosis, Schistosomiasis, Ascariasis, Heterophydiasis, Filariasis, Paragonimiasis, Strongyloidiasis, Cysticercosis, and Visceral larva migrans.

Trichinellosis or Trichinosis: Eosinophilic myocarditis is a possible complication in patients with trichinosis, a zoonosis caused by nematodes of the genus *Trichinella*. The most common species affecting humans is *Trichinella spiralis*, which has a global distribution and is most commonly found worldwide in carnivorous and omnivorous animals.[195,196] The burden of annual infection worldwide is estimated at around 10,000 cases. *Trichinella* is endemic in the areas with unregulated slaughter of pigs and particularly in areas where these are in contact with wild animals.[197] A systematic analysis of six international databases with 494 studies and 65,818 cases reported 42 deaths in 41 countries from 1986 through 2009. The World Health Organization European Region accounted for 87% of cases; 50% of those occurred in Romania from 1990 to 1999.[198] With a prevalence of 1.1 to 8.5 infected cases per 100,000 population,[199] cardiac involvement continues to be a major complication in Romania.[200]

The myocardial involvement occurs in the second phase of the infection cycles, and humans are affected when consuming raw or undercooked meat infected with the *Trichinella* parasite; high temperatures (>77°C) and freezing (−25°C) are known to kill the larvae of the parasite. After exposure to gastric acid, the larvae are released from the cysts (after 1 week of the infection) and invade the small bowel mucosa where they develop into adult worms. Then the larvae migrate through peripheral blood and may reach striated muscles where the encystment is completed in 4 to 5 weeks, and the encysted larvae may remain viable for several years. When informative, muscle biopsy shows inflammatory infiltrates, collagen capsule of the "nurse cell," and intersected muscle larva.[199,200]

The clinical presentation depends on the stage of infection, number of invading larvae, infected tissues, and general physical condition of the patient. The course of the infection can remain asymptomatic. Symptoms of trichinosis occur in two stages. Intestinal infection is the first stage and develops 1 to 2 days after consuming contaminated meat. The most common symptoms are nausea, diarrhea, abdominal cramps, and fever. The second stage corresponds to the larval invasion of muscles and starts after about 7 to 15 days. The most common symptoms are muscle pain and tenderness, weakness, fever, headache, and swelling of the face, particularly periorbital swelling. The pain is pronounced in the respiratory, masticatory, retropharyngeal, and orbicular muscles and tongue. It may be accompanied by skin rash and ocular involvement.[198-201]

Eosinophilic myocarditis may occur in the second stage of the disease; it can be life-threatening and may manifest with heart failure and arrhythmias; right ventricular (RV) outflow tract obstruction is rarely reported.[201] The diagnosis of trichinellosis should be based on clinical findings; pathology findings of muscle and/or EMB detecting larvae; laboratory findings of specific antibody response by indirect immunofluorescence, ELISA, or Western blot; hypereosinophilia (1000 eosinophils/mL) and/or increased total IgE levels; increased levels of muscle enzymes; and investigation of the possible source and origin of infection[195-198] (**Table 46–3**). When the diagnosis is proven, the treatment is based on antihelminthic drugs, such as albendazole or mebendazole, and supportive therapy in patients with heart failure.[198]

Echinococcosis: Echinococcosis is endemic in several geographic areas such as North Africa, South America (Argentina), New Zealand, Greece, and Iceland. In infected patients, cardiac involvement is uncommon (<2%), and even in patients with

TABLE 46–3. European Center for Disease Control: Case Definition for Human Trichinellosis

Case classification:
1. Probable: nonapplicable
1. Possible: any person meeting the clinical criteria and with an epidemiologic link
2. Confirmed: any person meeting the laboratory criteria and with clinical criteria within the past 2 months
3. To be reported: confirmed cases should be reported to European Union level

Criteria Groups	Criteria
Clinical criteria	At least three of the following six: 1. Fever 2. Muscle soreness and pain 3. Gastrointestinal symptoms 4. Facial edema 5. Eosinophilia 6. Subconjunctival, subungual, and retinal hemorrhages
Laboratory criteria	At least one of the following two laboratory tests: 1. Demonstration of *Trichinella* larvae in tissue obtained by muscle biopsy 2. Demonstration of *Trichinella*-specific antibody response by indirect immunofluorescence, ELISA, or Western blot (ie, seroconversion)
Epidemiology criteria	At least one of the following three: 1. Consumption of laboratory-confirmed parasitized meat, 2. Consumption of potentially parasitized products from a laboratory-confirmed infected animal, 3. Epidemiologic link to a laboratory-confirmed human case by exposure to the same common source

Abbreviation: ELISA, enzyme-linked immunosorbent assay.

cardiac involvement, signs and symptoms are rare (<10%). The host of *Echinococcus granulosus* is the dog; humans could serve as the intermediate host if they accidentally ingest ova from contaminated dog feces. Hydatid cysts more commonly affect the liver and lungs and are usually solitary. Combined liver and extraliver cysts are observed in 25% of cases; cardiac cysts comprise 0.5% to 2% of all cases. Within the heart, hydatid cysts are usually located in the left ventricle (up to 60%) or right ventricle (up to 20%) and rarely found in the pericardium (10%–15%).[202] Pericardial cysts usually do not cause symptoms and remain silent until they grow large and result in cardiac compression, atrial fibrillation, and even sudden death. Myocardial cysts localized in the interventricular septum or LV wall remain segregated and undergo calcification or generate daughter cysts and undergo rupture.[203,204]

Depending on the localization, the effects of the ruptured hydatid cysts vary. It could result in pericarditis and may evolve to chronic constrictive pericarditis when ruptured in the pericardium; cardiac tamponade is uncommon.[205,206] When the cyst ruptures in the right cardiac chambers, possible complications include pulmonary embolism and pulmonary hypertension.[207-209] Syncope can occasionally be the first manifestation of the disease.[210] The rupture of the hydatid cysts with the release of the fluid may cause severe anaphylactic reactions. Symptoms may occur in patients with pericardial involvement or with mass-induced right-sided obstruction. Echocardiography and CMR may localize the myocardial cysts.[211] When present, eosinophilia may contribute to the diagnostic suspicion. Serologic tests such as the Casoni test demonstrate false-positive and false-negative results in up to 30% of cases; ELISA test has a sensitivity of 91% and specificity of 82%.[212]

Medical treatment is based on albendazole and mebendazole; surgical resection is the treatment of choice for the prevention of rupture of cysts. Novel application of the cardiac stabilizer (Octopus IV) was reported to safely lift the heart up and excise a hydatid cyst that was firmly adherent to the posterior surface of the heart.[213]

Toxocariasis: Toxocariasis occurs worldwide. The highest prevalence is reported from tropical and subtropical countries.[196] Myocarditis is the most frequent clinical presentation (58%), followed by pericarditis (25%) with or without tamponade. Cardiac involvement in *Toxocara* infection is a potentially life-threatening complication. The cardiac workup is based on electrocardiography (ECG), chest x-ray, echocardiography, and laboratory tests. ECG may show nonspecific abnormalities, including peripheral and thoracic low-voltage and nonspecific ST-T alterations. The chest x-ray shows cardiomegaly and signs of pulmonary congestion. Echocardiography shows wall thickening, hypokinesia, and a reduced LVEF with possible pericardial effusion or endomyocardial fibrosis and restrictive cardiomyopathy.[214] Thrombotic complications may occur. The therapeutic regimens vary widely, especially with regard to the duration of therapy, and the combination of an anthelmintic drug and corticosteroids appears to be a valuable option. Clinical manifestation of the tissue infection by parasites should be considered in cases of nonspecific organ manifestations (ie, heart, lungs, liver) accompanied by fever and eosinophilia, with or without allergic skin rash.[214,215]

Myocardial Transmission of Infections in Heart Transplantation

Organ transplant recipients can develop infections as a result of transmission through the graft, reactivation of silent infection, reinfection in a healthy graft, or de novo infection. Infections can manifest in the posttransplant period as a consequence of immunosuppression.

In 1994, the United Network for Organ Sharing (UNOS) introduced the label of "high-risk donor" to identify donors who meet the Centers for Disease Control and Prevention criteria for high-risk behavior for infection; since then UNOS provides regular recommendations for reducing transmission of HIV, HBV, and HCV through organ transplantation.[216] In a recent single-center series including 55 recipients of heart transplants from high-risk donors, survival was excellent (short-term survival [1 year] 94%; long-term survival [3 years] 80%), and there was no increased incidence of perioperative or postoperative complications; the risk of transmission of infection from donors in this subgroup seemed to be minimal; only 1 of 55 patients (1.9%) had hepatitis C seroconversion at 105 days after receiving the transplant. After antiviral treatment, the patient had undetectable viral loads. All other patients (n = 54) had undetectable plasma viral loads of HIV, hepatitis C, and hepatitis B.[217] These data encourage revision of criteria for declining grafts from high-risk donors. However, UNOS has not modified the requirement regarding consent language around "high risk donors" (https://unos.org/news/policy-changes/new-optn-policies-to-align-with-updated-u-s-public-health-service-guideline/).

Early reports on the use of organs from donors with resolved SARS-CoV-2 infection[218] and arguments against using SARS-CoV-2 positive donors[219] are opening a new unexplored field of priority investigation. To this aim, the organ procurement organizations (OPOs) and transplant centers in the United States began to report potential donor-derived SARS-CoV-2 transmission to the Organ Procurement and Transplantation Network (OPTN) for investigation by the Disease Transmission Advisory Committee (DTAC) (see Chapter 84).[220]

Some infectious diseases, such as Chagas disease, endemic fungal infections, tuberculosis (which could be drug-resistant), leishmaniasis, and other viral and parasitic diseases, should be considered in the differential diagnosis of posttransplant infections in foreign-born recipients.[221]

MYOCARDITIS IN AUTOIMMUNE DISEASES

Involvement of myocardium, endocardium, pericardium, valves, both small intramural vessels, and epicardial coronary arteries is common in autoimmune diseases. The diagnosis is based on the recommendations of scientific societies for the different disorders.[4] The diagnosis of isolated autoimmune myocarditis in patients who do not demonstrate systemic or extracardiac autoimmune disease is difficult and requires demonstration of both myocarditis and autoantibodies mediating myocyte damage or inducing inflammatory autoimmune reaction. This complex diagnostic workup is based on the demonstration of circulating autoantibodies. The significance and role of autoantibodies vary in the different diseases wherein they represent markers of disease, disease-inducing autoantibodies, or both. A paradigmatic example of autoimmune myocarditis is neonatal lupus or autoimmune congenital heart block (atrioventricular block) that is caused by the placental transfer of maternal Ro/La autoantibodies (anti-SSA/Ro and anti-SSB/La antibodies) damaging the conduction tissues during fetal development.[222] Infants may demonstrate transient skin and systemic lesions and permanent atrioventricular block associated with significant morbidity and mortality; pacemakers are implanted in two-thirds of cases. Acute myocarditis may appear in the early phases of the disease and is characterized by lymphocytic infiltrates.[223,224] Serum cardiac autoantibodies may be found in autoimmune myocarditis, DCM, and normal controls[4] and include anti sarcolemmal (ASA), anti fibrillary (AFA), organ-specific and partially organ-specific anti heart (AHA), anti intercalated disk (AIDA), anti adenine nucleotide translocator (anti-ANT), anti myolemmal (AMLA), anti adrenergic receptor (anti-AR), anti interfibrillary (anti-IFA), branched chain α-ketoacid dehydrogenase dihydrolipoyl transacylase (anti-BCKD), anti heat shock protein (HSP), anti myosin heavy chain (MHC), anti myosin light chain 1 ventricular (MLC1v), anti actin, anti tropomyosin, and anti laminin antibodies. The significance of these antibodies is still a matter of research.[4] Recommendation 9 of the recent position statement of the ESC Working Group on Myocardial and Pericardial Diseases suggests testing for cardiac autoantibodies based on the availability of tests and center expertise; unfortunately, no commercially available and standardized cardiac autoantibody tests have been validated.[4] Autoantibodies in postviral cardiomyopathy can be secondary to the effects of primary myocyte damage induced by the viral infection; picornavirus infections (type 1 diabetes, myocarditis, or paralysis) demonstrate a strong association with autoimmunity, with particular evidence in type 1 diabetes and myocarditis.[225,226] The recent demonstration of T cells expressing dual T-cell receptors on a single cell, induced as a natural consequence of Theiler virus infection, which may occasionally cause human myocarditis, could explain the pathogenicity resulting from induction of autoimmunity to organ-specific antigens.[227]

TOXIC MYOCARDITIS

Toxic substances can cause myocardial injury and inflammation (see Table 46–1). The myocardial insult can be transient and reversible or chronic and persistent.

Direct Toxic Substances

Well-known examples are myocarditis forms caused by arsenic and lithium. Historically, arsenic was used in agriculture to control parasites and pests, and exposure in industry is possible during the processing of minerals and coloring of glass. Elimination from the body is easier for organic than for pentavalent or trivalent inorganic arsenic. Trivalent derivatives are 100 times more toxic than pentavalent forms. Injection of arsenic may cause myocarditis characterized by myocyte necrosis, infiltration of leukocytes and lymphocytes, and neutrophilic perivasculitis.[228] Lithium is used in psychiatry as an antimanic and mood stabilizer. It can cause various adverse effects including myocarditis and arrhythmias;[229] sinus node dysfunction can occur with serum lithium levels in the therapeutic range.[230] Zinc phosphide has been used as a rodenticide and is toxic by ingestion; its conversion to phosphine gas that is absorbed into the bloodstream causes metabolic and nonmetabolic toxic effects, including myocarditis, pericarditis, acute pulmonary edema, and congestive heart failure.[231,232] Several other substances may cause toxic myocarditis (see Table 46–1). Their precise diagnosis is based on the identification of the toxic agent.

Drug-Induced Myocarditis

Different drugs may induce similar cardiac toxicity. The clinical manifestations include the entire spectrum of cardiac phenotypes, including cardiomyopathy, conduction disturbances, arrhythmias, hypertension, and coronary artery disease. Each of them is discussed in their corresponding chapter in this text.

Myocarditis is one of the possible complications; it can either regress if the drug is discontinued or persist and evolve through a cardiomyopathy phenotype.

In the acute drug hypersensitivity syndrome, the clinical manifestations occur after a few weeks from initiation of a new drug; less commonly, the syndrome may manifest at any time after drug consumption. Drugs known to potentially cause hypersensitivity syndrome include antibiotics, antiepileptics, allopurinol, and sulfonamide-containing drugs (see Table 46–1). In addition, drugs used for hemodynamic support in patients with cardiogenic shock or acute heart failure, such as dobutamine, may trigger hypereosinophilia and hypersensitivity myocarditis. When present, traits such as cutaneous rash associated with fever, eosinophilia, and multiorgan dysfunction (liver, kidney, and heart) may be indicative of drug toxicity. The cardiac involvement may be extensive and associated with LV dysfunction, hypotension, and thromboembolic risk.

Chemotherapy

5-fluorouracil (5-FU) is one of the most common causes of cardiotoxicity associated with chemotherapy.[233–235] Tyrosine kinase inhibitors targeting human epidermal growth factor receptor (HER)-2, immune checkpoint inhibitors (ICI), and cyclin-dependent kinase (CDK) inhibitors are new targeted breast cancer treatments.[236] Myocarditis, along with colitis and hepatitis, is the most frequent immune-related adverse events.[237] Endomyocardial biopsy can contribute to early diagnosis especially when CMR is negative.[238,239]

Clozapine

Clozapine is an effective antipsychotic drug that is selectively and cautiously used in patients with treatment-resistant schizophrenia because of its hematologic and cardiovascular adverse effects. A recent review describes 250 cases of clozapine-induced myocarditis and highlights the possibility that myocarditis is underdiagnosed in patients receiving clozapine.[240] Warning data potentially useful for suspecting myocarditis in patients treated with clozapine include recent onset of treatment (mean 14 days), the occurrence of fever close to the initial administration of the drug, old age, concomitant treatment with sodium valproate, rapid drug titration, respiratory illness, or pneumonia. The incidence of myocarditis was approximately 3%, and the need of implementing monitoring procedures cannot be overemphasized. More precise data on the prevalence of myocarditis would lead to formal indications for cardiac monitoring. The higher prevalence of clozapine myocarditis reported in Australia likely results from awareness of the complications, as well as from the systematic data collection of the treated patients.[240] Clozapine myocarditis can be fatal and only diagnosed at autopsy.[241] Timely early diagnosis is feasible, and drug removal may reverse signs and symptoms.[242,243]

DIAGNOSTIC WORK-UP IN MYOCARDITIS

Individual Medical History and Physical Examination

Myocarditis is an unexpected, often sudden, and rapidly evolving condition. Patients presenting with acute myocarditis

TABLE 46–4. Acute Myocarditis[a]

Life-threatening events in the absence of CAD and known causes of HF
- Cardiogenic shock
- Aborted sudden death

New-onset HF
- Symptoms include dyspnea and fatigue or arrhythmias
- Signs of HF on physical examination
- ECG signs such as nonspecific ST/T changes, conduction disturbances, and arrhythmias
- Imaging data demonstrating impaired systolic LV and/or RV function, with mildly dilated LV and/or RV

Syndromes simulating ACS with acute chest pain and possible presence of ECG, imaging or biochemical markers, either single or combined
- ECG changes: ST/T-wave changes and T-wave inversions (when available, a prior ECG is useful for comparative evaluation)
- Imaging demonstrating global or regional LV and/or RV impairment
- Increased markers of myocyte injury (increased TnT/TnI) evolving as in AMI or persisting over several weeks or months
- Increased inflammatory markers

Arrhythmias
- Atrial arrhythmias
- Ventricular arrhythmias
- Isolated
- Associated with HF, ACS-like syndrome

Abbreviations: ACS, acute coronary syndrome; AMI, acute myocardial infarction; CAD, coronary artery disease; ECG, electrocardiogram; HF, heart failure; IHD, ischemic heart disease; LV, left ventricle; RV, right ventricle; TnI, troponin I; TnT, troponin T
[a]Clinical scenarios in patients with proven absence of acute IHD/CAD, negative family history, and absence of known cardiac and systemic illness potentially cause of the observed clinical manifestations.

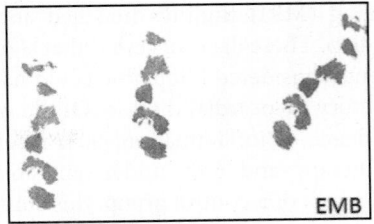

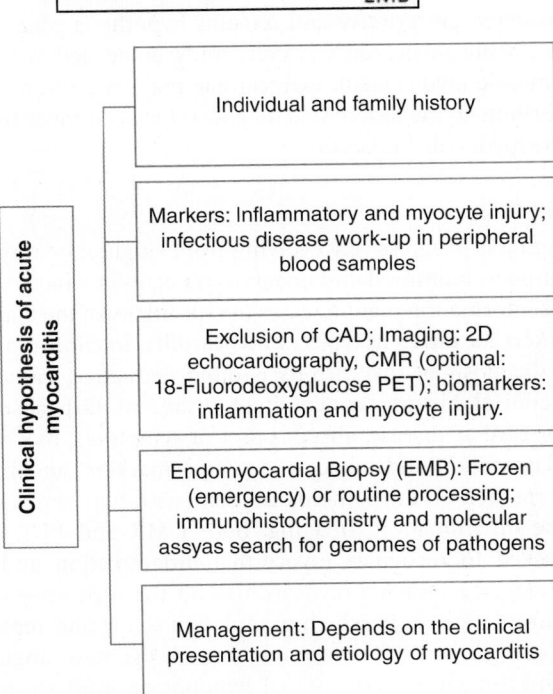

Figure 46–5. Clinical hypothesis of acute myocarditis. 2D, two-dimensional; CAD, coronary artery disease; CMR, cardiac magnetic resonance; EMB, endomyocardial biopsy; PET, positron emission tomography.

frequently describe episodes of recent febrile illness. The clinical manifestations range from severe and life-threatening, to recent onset of heart failure, to mild signs and symptoms such as fatigue and arrhythmias. **Table 46–4** summarizes various scenarios of clinical manifestations. Fulminant myocarditis may present with life-threatening events (in the absence of coronary artery disease and known causes of heart failure), such as cardiogenic shock or aborted sudden death, associated with underlying GCM or acute viral myocarditis. However, patients presenting with aborted sudden death with a history of sudden death in the family should invoke investigation for genetic cardiomyopathy (**Fig. 46–5**).

Myocarditis may present as a new onset of heart failure with symptoms such as dyspnea and fatigue or arrhythmias and signs of heart failure on physical examination. With ECG nonspecific ST-T wave changes, conduction disturbances, and arrhythmias, these patients may demonstrate echocardiographic evidence of impaired systolic LV and/or RV function, with mildly dilated ventricular chambers. The clinical distinction between such presentation of myocarditis and recent-onset DCM is complex and is dependent on pathologic demonstration of myocarditis as the cause of the phenotype. Family history is usually negative. Chronic forms of myocarditis could also be associated with specific myocardial diseases such as sarcoidosis, autoimmune diseases, Chagas disease, or Lyme disease. The differential diagnosis between chronic myocarditis, inflammatory cardiomyopathy, and DCM is essential to prevent misdiagnosis. In clinical practice, a report concluding with the diagnosis of chronic myocarditis is uncommon,

and most patients are diagnosed with DCM. Lack of investigation for genetic cause of the disease in recent-onset DCM may impact not only the management of patients, but also the families.

Uncommonly, acute myocarditis masquerades as an acute coronary event with ST-T wave changes, global or regional LV hypokinesia, and elevated markers of myocyte injury.[244] The ECG alterations and wall motion abnormalities usually extend beyond a single coronary artery territory as expected in a coronary event. Infrequently, myocarditis may also present with unexplained ventricular arrhythmias in a setting of DCM. A recent study evaluated fasting positron emission tomography (PET) scan findings in more than 100 consecutive patients referred with unexplained cardiomyopathy and ventricular arrhythmia for possible ablation.[245] Almost 50% of patients exhibited focal fluorodeoxyglucose (FDG) uptake. The EMB revealed granulomatous inflammation representing sarcoidosis in a small subset of patients and also nongranulomatous inflammation suggestive of myocarditis in another. Correlation between low-voltage regions on electroanatomic mapping and FDG uptake was observed in 75%, and magnetic resonance imaging (MRI) findings matched abnormal PET regions in only 40%. These data suggested that significant proportion of patients considered idiopathic could have harbored occult inflammatory myocardial disease. Of the patients with FDG-based evidence of inflammation, 90% received immunosuppressive therapy and 60% underwent ablation; however, because of a lack of a control group, this study cannot be considered prescriptive and remains hypothesis generating.[245] Since acute myocarditis is commonly associated with skeletal muscle involvement, extracardiac magnetic resonance can contribute to the differential diagnosis between myocardis and acute myocardial infarction.[246]

Imaging

Imaging is progressively evolving from single-modality investigation to multimodality imaging strategies in which each test adds information that increases the specificity of the diagnostic markers for different types of myocarditis. In clinical practice, the diagnosis of myocarditis is often deductive, based more on clinical history (concomitant or recent flu), absence of prior cardiac disease, abrupt onset of symptoms, biochemical (inflammation and myocyte damage) markers, and imaging criteria than on the pathological demonstration of myocardial tissue inflammation. Imaging, both CMR and PET, should be asked to recognize myocardial inflammation and myocyte damage in acute myocarditis and the reparative aspects in chronic forms, in which granulation tissue and repair features are present (therefore ongoing fibrogenesis, angiogenesis, macrophages, and residual lymphocyte infiltrates). CMR informs about edema and fibrosis but not about the presence of inflammatory cells. Functional imaging (PET-based imaging) informs about the presence of metabolically active cells, also targetable with radio-tracers capable of discriminating the different interstitial cells (eg, macrophages), hybrid techniques could integrate the two types of information and add value to the role of imaging in the diagnosis of myocarditis.

Echocardiography

Echocardiography is the initial investigation in patients with suspected myocarditis. Echocardiographic findings are nonspecific and include LV global or regional dysfunction with decreased ejection fraction, LV dilation, RV involvement, and pericardial effusion.[247] Strain and strain rate imaging using speckle tracking may add information on early regional contractility and dysfunction;[248] in patients with biopsy-proven myocarditis, LV fractional shortening, longitudinal strain, and strain rate are reduced and correlate with the burden of myocardial inflammation.[249] In patients with suspected, but non-EMB proven, acute myocarditis, longitudinal strain and circumferential strain have specificities of 93% and 94%, respectively; the degree of strain correlates with the risk of future clinical events.[250] Irrespective of the specific contribution to myocarditis, echocardiography remains the first line of investigation.

Cardiac Magnetic Resonance

CMR is now systematically used for the diagnosis, irrespective of the demonstration of the myocardial inflammation. The first International Consensus Group on Cardiovascular Magnetic Resonance Diagnosis of Myocarditis (the Lake Louse Criteria, LLC) first provided imaging-based "diagnostic" criteria ("two out of three" criteria -T2, LGE, and EGE).[251] According to the Lake Louise CMR criteria, acute myocarditis is associated with (1) increased regional or global myocardial signal intensity in T2-weighted images (indicating myocardial edema); (2) increased global myocardial early gadolinium enhancement (EGE) ratio between myocardium and skeletal muscle in T1-weighted images (supporting hyperemia/capillary leakage); and (3) at least one focal lesion with nonischemic distribution in LGE T1-weighted images (suggestive of cell injury/necrosis).[251] The diagnostic accuracy does not increase with the addition of pericardial effusion.[252]

T2 Mapping for Myocardial Edema: T2-weighted short tau inversion recovery (STIR) imaging can detect and localize epicardial, transmural, or global myocardial edema; T2-STIR high signal intensity identifies areas of tissue edema.[253] When evaluated as an independent measure, T2-STIR has demonstrated variable sensitivity (58%–74%) and specificity (57%–93%).[251] An alternative method for evaluation of myocardial edema is the low b-value diffusion-weighted echo-planar imaging sequence that has offered higher sensitivity (92% vs 54%) and diagnostic accuracy (95% vs 70%) compared with standard STIR-T2 images, but similar specificity, in acute myocarditis.[254,255] T2 mapping is able to quantitatively define the area of edematous myocardium[256] through a 16-LV segment T2-mapping protocol that provides more robust imaging of myocardial edema than standard T2-weighted imaging.[257] Protocols based on gradient spin echo imaging techniques further improve accuracy and reduce acquisition time for T2 mapping.[257]

Early Gadolinium Enhancement: EGE represents an increased distribution into the interstitial space early in the washout phase[12] as a result of hyperemia and capillary leakage.[258] EGE displays a sensitivity of 63% to 85% and specificity of 68% to 100% for the diagnosis of myocarditis in the given clinical context.[251] However, EGE does not describe relative regional distribution of gadolinium uptake and is a time-consuming process. An alternative method, the contrast-enhanced steady-state free precession technique, allows better visualization of hyperintense myocardial regions of gadolinium uptake. In a recent study of 19 patients with myocarditis, hyperemia was observed in 77% of patients and was associated with increased inflammatory markers and greater LGE.[258] CMR with contrast-enhanced steady-state free precession potentially represents a more efficient method for detecting hyperemia, but it should always be compared directly with traditional EGE.

T1 Mapping: T1 prolongation indicates myocardial edema and hyperemia.[259] A T1 value more than 990 ms indicates myocardial injury and is used to create topographic maps representative of the degree of myocardial involvement.[260] In patients with clinically suspected myocarditis,[261] T1 mapping seems to be more sensitive and offers similar diagnostic accuracy as that of dark-blood T2 imaging, bright-blood T2 imaging, and LGE. The performance of T1 mapping has been reported to be similar to LGE and better than the T2-weighted imaging methods. Additional modified protocols showed that longer relaxation times were associated with high diagnostic accuracy.[262] Native T1 relaxation time combined with T2-weighted imaging criteria increase sensitivity (92%), specificity (97%), and diagnostic accuracy (95%). T1 mapping improves the diagnostic confidence in cases in which traditional methods have failed to recognize any disease; incrementally elevated T1 thresholds were associated with enhancement on LGE images, suggesting a role for the absolute T1 value in determining size of myocardial injury.[262]

Late Gadolinium Enhancement: T1-weighted LGE detects irreversible cell injury, myocyte necrosis, and myocardial fibrosis.[264] LGE detects the patchy distribution of the disease, but can also demonstrate transmural patterns.[265] In acute myocarditis, automated calculation of LGE[265,266] correlates with LGE quantified by visual assessment.

The addition of *quantitative markers* such as extracellular volume calculation seemed to improve the diagnostic contribution of CMR in patients with severe myocarditis.[267] In the MyoRacer study performed in patients with acute symptoms, mapping techniques proved useful for confirming or rejecting the diagnosis of myocarditis and superior to the LLC. However, only T2 mapping demonstrated acceptable diagnostic performance in patients with chronic symptoms.[268] Using quantitative CMR, T2 mapping discriminated between acute and healed stages of myocarditis.[269] New parametric mapping techniques further improved the diagnostic accuracy of CMR.[270] A meta-analysis including studies enrolling only biopsy proven cases of acute and chronic myocarditis found that CMR based on LLC does not substantially improve accuracy when compared with the individual components.[271] A further meta-analysis including parametric mapping techniques obtained similar results,[272] even though mapping parameters show excellent agreement between observers in the assessment of myocarditis.[273] Finally, at the end of 2018, updated LLC incorporated experiences with LLC and parametric mapping. The new criteria recommend the use of at least one edema-sensitive technique (T2-weighted sequence or T2 mapping) and at least one T1-based sequence (T1 map, ECV, or T1-weighted LGE). The presence of a signal abnormality on both a T2- and T1-based imaging constitutes a diagnosis, which can be thought of as a "two out of two" approach rather than a "two out of three" as in the original LLC.[274] Overall, LLC has >60% sensitivity and about 90% specificity for acute myocarditis but does not demonstrate the same accuracy for chronic myocarditis. The ambition of diagnosing "chronic" and "borderline" myocarditis is reasonable but these two diagnoses are often questionable even in endomyocardial biopsies, the first difficult to distinguish from DCM, the second with limited clinical impact.

More recently, myocardial perfusion scintigraphy -PET and single-photon emission computed tomography (SPECT), are being implemented in the diagnostic path of myocarditis, adding advantages of functional information.

18F-Fluorodeoxyglucose–Positron Emission Tomography

^{18}F-FDG-PET has played a diagnostic role in myocarditis[275] and in clinically suspected myocarditis, demonstrating a sensitivity of 46% and a specificity of 81%.[276] Although current evidence is not sufficient to support its routine use for the diagnosis of myocarditis, it may add functional information to the currently employed structural imaging. FDG accumulates in inflammatory cells. Sarcoidosis provides an informative example of combined approach of perfusion (eg, ^{13}N-NH$_3$) and inflammation (eg, ^{18}F-FDG) PET imaging in assessing myocardial inflammation. Normal perfusion and intense ^{18}F-FDG uptake indicate active cardiac sarcoidosis, hypoperfusion and high glucose metabolism indicate advanced sarcoidosis, and decreased or absent perfusion and negative FDG uptake indicate end-stage cardiac sarcoidosis.

Hybrid imaging—SPECT and PET/computed tomography (CT), and now PET/MRI—is going to further expand the spectrum of information achievable with simultaneous cardiac FDG–PET/MR for evaluation of myocarditis, compared to PET/CT or MR alone. However, data from well-designed and sized studies in myocarditis are missing. FDG–PET/CT can detect and localize active inflammation in acute myocarditis[277] by providing metabolism information in the absence of relevant myocardial necrosis,[278] a criterion needed for myocarditis in early diagnostic criteria[2] but no longer mentioned in the ESC criteria, that exclusively points on the presence of inflammatory cells irrespective of the morphologically detectable damage related with the inflammation.[4] Overall, any hybrid/combined approach to the in vivo noninvasive diagnosis of myocarditis, either PET/MRI or PET/CT needs to be expanded to add or integrate diagnostic information. An important development will concern the clinical applications of radiotracers for macrophages,[279] as cells that are metabolically active and always present in myocarditis. The development of metabolism-based PET imaging, radiotracers targeting receptors for chemokines, somatostatin, translocator protein and mannose, as well as nanoparticles-based PET is an actively progressing research field. However, it is stimulated more by the clinical needs in malignancies than by those of niche pathologies such as myocarditis. For myocarditis and sarcoidosis, developing radiotracers include 11C-methionine,[280] 68Ga-DOTA-TOC,[281] 68Ga-DOTA-NOC,[282,283] and the 68Ga-NOTE-MSA.[284,285]

Biomarkers

Biomarkers may contribute to the diagnosis of acute myocarditis and its evolution to the chronic state. Beyond serology, antigenemia, viremia, and DNA-emia in infectious myocarditis, biomarkers may inform about inflammatory and myocyte injury processes.

Markers of Myocyte Injury/Damage/Overload

Adults and children myocarditis can be associated with increased levels of markers of myocyte injury such as cardiac troponin (cTn; troponins I and T);[286-287] elevated cTn has been reported predominantly in myocarditis with either fulminant or acute clinical presentation. Previous studies indicated that sensitivity of cTn for the diagnosis of myocarditis is low. Whereas only 34% of patients enrolled in the Myocarditis Treatment Trial had cardiac troponin I elevation,[288] recent studies have demonstrated superior predictive values of high-sensitivity troponin T for acute myocarditis when other causes of increased myocardial necrosis markers, such as myocardial infarction, have been systematically excluded.[289] Cardiac troponin T is routinely used in the clinical work-up for both children[290] and adult patients.[291] In a screening report of 38,197 veterans, 4469 tested positive for influenza virus. Of these, 600 had further cardiac biomarker testing, and 143 (24%) demonstrated an increase in one or more cardiac biomarkers, which was associated with acute congestive heart failure (6%), myocarditis (4%), atrial fibrillation (3%), noncardiac explanations (8%), or no documented explanation (31%).[292]

Although cTn levels have been reported as a prognostic marker in patients with GCM,[293] these data have not been confirmed in other studies, wherein cTn levels predict neither the diagnosis nor severity of disease.[294] cTn may be elevated in myocardial toxicity of known and novel drugs: in patients included in phase I trials of novel targeted therapies for a metastatic solid tumor, cTn was one of the most useful markers for measuring cardiac toxicity. In a series of 90 patients, 2 experienced chest pain and troponin I elevation and 8 revealed asymptomatic elevation of troponin I during follow-up.[295] Markers of myocyte injury can either contribute to the diagnosis or provide information for correlation with other clinical parameters in all forms of myocarditis with myocyte injury.

N-Terminal Pro-B Type (Brain) Natriuretic Peptide

N-terminal pro-B type natriuretic peptide (NT-proBNP) levels increase in myocarditis associated with LV dysfunction, but normal values do not exclude myocarditis;[296] levels rapidly decline with recovery of the LV function.[297] In a pediatric series including 58 children with myocarditis and reduced ejection fraction (<30%), peak BNP >10,000 ng/L and cardiac MRI late enhancement were identified as predictors of poor outcomes.[298] In a series of 70 patients with clinically suspected myocarditis and 42 patients with EMB-confirmed myocarditis, NT-proBNP in the highest quartile (>4225 ng/mL) was predictive for cardiac death or heart transplantation at 7.5 months from the diagnosis.[298] However, newer biomarkers, such as copeptin or midregional pro-adrenomedullin, have not offered additional diagnostic or prognostic information.[298,299]

Serum cardiac autoantibodies (eg, anti fibrillary, organ-specific and partially organ-specific anti heart, anti intercalated disks, anti interfibrillary) in high levels have been described to be useful in the absence of viral genome in EMB, suggesting an immune-mediated myocarditis or inflammatory cardiomyopathy.[3,4]

The role of miRNA profiling is being investigated in acute, chronic, and fulminant myocarditis. miR-208b and miR-499 are upregulated after myocardial damage and can be measured in the plasma of patients with myocarditis. Their simultaneous upregulation seems to characterize fulminant viral myocarditis.[300] Their role as possible positive regulators of toll-like receptor 4 in blood monocyte-derived dendritic cells and macrophages suggests that they can be future diagnostic contributors in patients with suspected myocarditis.[301] Recent studies suggest that miRNA profile provides a new noninvasive tool to identify patients with intramyocardial inflammation and/or viral persistence: the expression of let-7f, miR-197, miR-223, miR-93, and miR-379 seem to differentiate between patients with a virus and/or inflammation and healthy donors (specificity >93%).[300]

Markers of Inflammation

High-sensitivity C-reactive protein and erythrocyte sedimentation rate are routinely measured in patients with suspected myocarditis,[302] but with limited contribution to the diagnosis. As correlation factors, C-reactive protein at admission does not seem to correlate with LGE on CMR in adult patients with myocarditis.[299] Conversely, increased levels of C-reactive protein can be critical early signs of drug toxicity myocarditis (eg, warranting close monitoring and serious consideration for cessation of drugs such as clozapine).[302,303] Experts recommend that C-reactive protein and troponin I levels should be measured at baseline, two times per week for 1 month, then once per week for another 1 month, and then once per month for the remainder of the first year.[304]

Serology

Viral serology can provide information in the acute phases of infectious myocarditis. These phases can be missed unless the clinical onset is cardiogenic shock or acute heart failure and patients are tested shortly after onset of the illness. In chronic myocarditis and in inflammatory cardiomyopathy, the clinical contribution of viral serology is limited; IgG antibodies for cardiotropic virus can be found in the bloodstream of the general population without accompanying cardiac involvement.[305] Serology is routinely performed in parallel with molecular tests seeking genomes of the suspected pathogens. A positive virus PCR in peripheral blood does not prove viral myocarditis. However, when viral genome is present in the EMB, blood viral PCR can exclude or confirm systemic infection.[4] It may also differentiate an acute viral infection from endogenous viral reactivation in which there is higher virus replication.

Endomyocardial Biopsy

EMB is the current gold standard for the diagnosis of myocarditis.[4,55] EMB samples are processed with conventional methods. The frozen samples are processed in case of clinical emergency such as nonischemic cardiogenic shock or resuscitated cardiac arrest, when EMB is performed during implantation of the circulatory support devices. EMB offers immediate information about the basis of cardiogenic shock allowing differentiation between fulminant myocarditis and nonmyocarditic causes. Although frozen sections for histomorphologic studies are not optimal, at least the diagnosis of myocarditis is feasible. In patients presenting with clinically stable heart failure, even of recent onset, EMB samples are routinely processed. The interpretation of pathologic features is based on light microscopic examination of routine stains and immunohistochemistry, and electron microscopy is undertaken when possible and indicated. One or more samples are used for viral investigation, both pathogen isolation and search of replicating pathogens.

Inflammation

The extent of myocardial inflammation and the type of inflammatory cells are major pathologic contributors to the diagnosis; acute myocarditis is characterized by conspicuous focal or diffuse inflammatory infiltrates. Inflammatory cells are routinely recognized on cytomorphology, but immunophenotyping of inflammatory infiltrates allows precise characterization of T-cell CD4+ and CD8+ subsets and identification of the extent of infiltration by the cells of monocyte-macrophage lineage. Neutrophilic and eosinophilic infiltrates, mast cells, and plasma cells are easily detectable using routine stains. Serial sectioning of routine EMB sampling (about 2–3 mm size/sample) usually provides sufficient material for multiple staining and immunohistochemical staining. Immunohistochemical characterization of the inflammatory infiltrate substantially contributes to the diagnosis of rare primary lymphomas of the heart or unusual cardiac involvement in diseases such as Erdheim–Chester disease. The presence of a few scattered inflammatory cells in the myocardium, even when highlighted by immunohistochemical stains, should not be labeled as myocarditis because some inflammatory cells can be present in the normal myocardium[15] and hearts affected by genetic cardiomyopathy.[306]

Eosinophilic inflammatory infiltrates are present in a variety of myocarditides of different origin. Eosinophilic granulocytes may infiltrate in both myocardium and endocardium. EMB can contribute to differentiate neoplastic, reactive, and secondary eosinophilic syndromes and eosinophilic syndromes of unknown significance.

Giant cells are found in GCM, sarcoid granulomas, tubercular myocarditis, rheumatic heart disease, and brucellosis. In GCM, inflammatory cells heavily infiltrate the myocardial tissue. In small EMB samples, giant cells may be missed.

Small intramural vessels occasionally demonstrate vasculitis, with inflammatory infiltrates involving small arteriolar walls. Small thrombi may occur in intramural vessels (**Fig. 46–6**). When both interstitial inflammatory infiltrates and vasculitis are present, patterns of myocarditis and ischemic myocyte damage may coexist.

Endocardium may also show inflammatory cell infiltration, which should always be reported. In addition, the endocardium may occasionally show thrombotic stratification with or without inflammation. The finding may provide the rationale for antiaggregation or anticoagulation treatments (**Fig. 46–7**).

Myocyte Damage

The myocyte injury is typically noncoagulative and ease to distinguish from the coagulative necrosis in small EMB specimens on hematoxylin and eosin stain (**Fig. 46–8**); acid fuchsin orange G stain may further help differentiation. Myocyte injury in myocarditis reflects the cytotoxic effect exerted by T lymphocytes and related cytokines, and is characterized by discontinuity/rupture of sarcolemma, myocyte edema, and loss of intracellular organelles in the interstitium. Nuclei may be prominent and show evident nucleoli. Unless microthrombi occur in small vessels, coagulative necrosis is absent. The

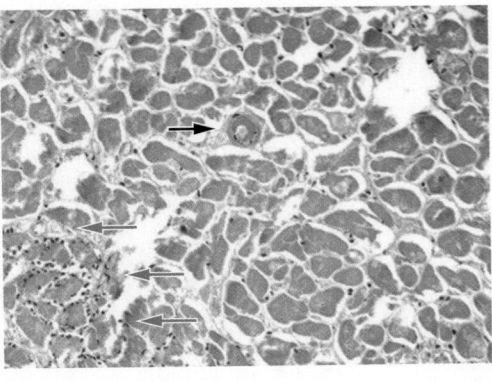

A

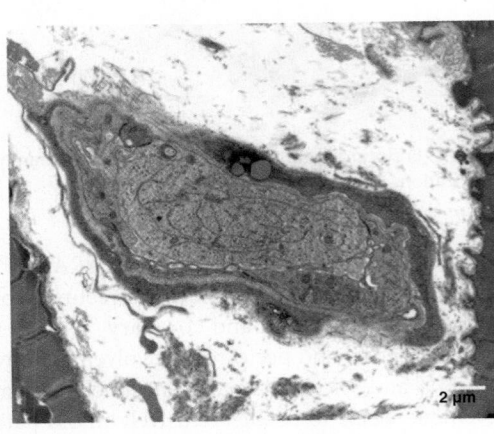

B

Figure 46–6. Small intramural vessels may show thrombi, either fibrin (**A**, *arrow*) or platelets (**B**; degranulated platelets occluding a small vessel).

inflammation-induced myocyte injury also differs from contraction band necrosis that may occur in cardiogenic shock in patients with pheochromocytoma.[307]

Pathologic Evidence of Myocardial Infection

There are pathogens that can be easily seen with routine hematoxylin and eosin stains; parasites, bacteria, and viral infections causing cytopathic effect are unlikely to be missed by routine pathology study. Morphologic evidence of infection is common in transplanted hearts, and HCMV shows a marked endotheliotropic effect usually coincident with increased viremia and DNA-emia. Patients with acute CV-B3 infection with replicating virus in the myocardium may show ultrastructural evidence of viral infection; the confirmation is obtained by molecular analysis with reverse transcriptase PCR, which should be the standard for the etiologic diagnosis. There are viruses or phases of viral infection (and viral replication) that cannot be easily recognized using conventional pathology studies. In these cases, immunohistochemistry for detection of viral antigens is consistent with active viral replication.

MYOCARDITIS WITH GIANT CELLS

Giant cells are the morphologic marker of GCM and sarcoidosis. Touton-like giant cells are also found in diseases such as Erdheim–Chester disease, a rare form of non–Langerhans cell

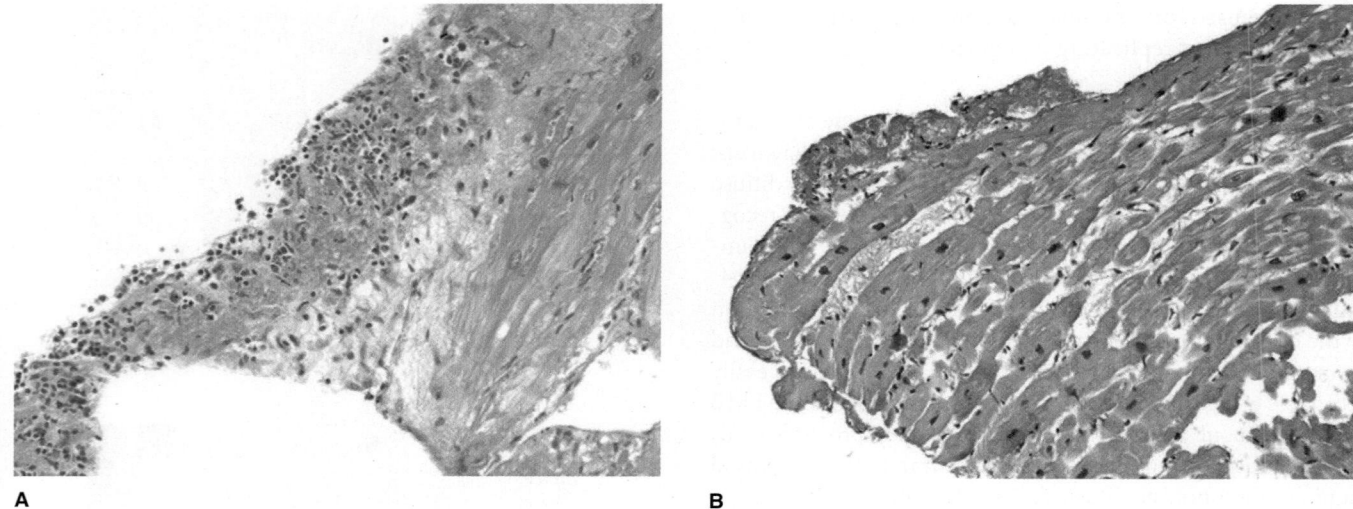

Figure 46–7. (**A**) Endocardial thrombus with prominent inflammatory infiltrates. (**B**) Endocardial thrombus with scattered inflammatory cells and early re-endothelialization.

histiocytosis, associated in more than 50% of *BRAF*[V600E] mutations in early multipotent myelomonocytic precursors or in tissue-resident histiocytes. Heart and coronary "pseudo-tumor" infiltration and pleural and pericardial involvement have been reported in 11% and 9% of patients, respectively. The myocardial involvement seems to occur exclusively in old patients.[308] Tuberculosis is a less common cause of myocarditis. Three distinct forms of myocardial involvement are recognized: nodular tuberculosis of the myocardium characterized by granulomatous disease with central caseation; miliary tuberculosis of the myocardium; and an uncommon diffuse giant cell and lymphocyte infiltrative type associated with tuberculous pericarditis.[309] The myocardium is involved by hematogenous spread, retrograde lymphatic spread from mediastinal lymph nodes, or direct invasion from the pericardium. The confirmatory diagnosis can be made by biopsy of the myocardium or of lymph nodes if clinical suspicion is strong and imaging findings are suggestive.[310–312]

Giant Cell Myocarditis

GCM is a rare disease characterized by myocardial inflammation with giant cells and myocyte necrosis.[313,314] Although the true statistics are unknown, data from autopsy series indicate relatively low prevalence rates of 0.007% to 0.051%.[315]

Etiology and Pathogenesis

GCM is considered a multifactorial disease. Etiologic hypotheses include infectious causes, autoimmune diseases or autoimmune reactions, and genetic predisposition.[313,314,316] Infections reported in GCM include coxsackie B2 virus,[317] B19V,[318] and *Mycobacterium tuberculosis*.[319] In about one-fifth of cases, GCM seems to be associated with autoimmune diseases such as inflammatory bowel disease, cryofibrinogenemia, optic neuritis, fibromyalgia, hyper- or hypothyroidism[313,314] and Hashimoto thyroiditis,[320] rheumatoid arthritis,[313] thymoma,[321] myasthenia gravis,[322] Takayasu arteritis, alopecia totalis, vitiligo, orbital myositis, discoid lupus erythematosus,[320] autoimmune hepatitis,[320] Guillain–Barré syndrome,[323] systemic lupus erythematosus,[320] and Sjögren syndrome.[323] GCM is being reported among novel syndromes such as immune reconstitution inflammatory syndrome that may occur in patients receiving highly active antiretroviral therapy against HIV-1.[324]

The autoimmune or immune-mediated hypothesis is supported by partial remission of GCM in patients treated with immunosuppression,[313,314] as well as by a nonaggressive occurrence (10%–50%) of the disease during immunosuppression treatment in transplanted patients.[325] A recent hypothesis highlights the possibility that GCM is characterized by a chemokine profile related to toll-like receptors and dendritic cells. Distinct

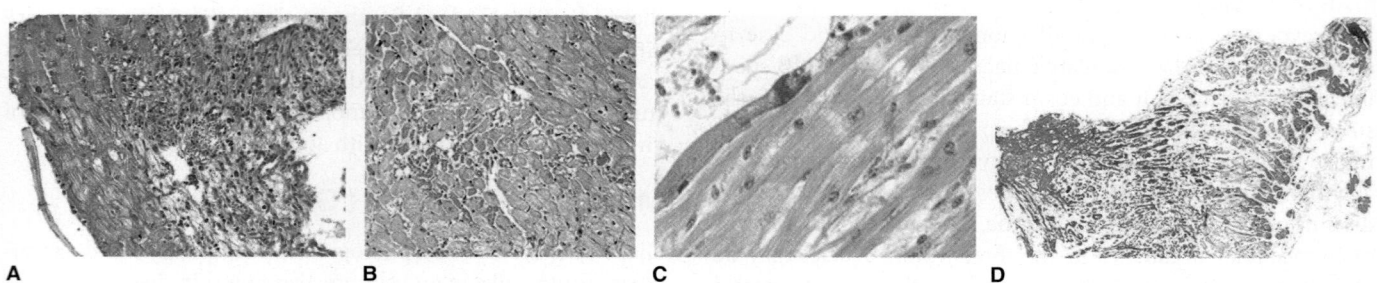

Figure 46–8. (**A**) Typical myocyte damage in myocarditis. (**B–D**) Coagulative necrosis in the absence of inflammatory infiltrates.

differential gene expression profiles seem to discriminate tissues harboring giant cells (GCM and cardiac sarcoidosis) from those with active myocarditis or inflammation-free controls. The expression levels of genes coding for cytokines or chemokines, cellular receptors, and proteins involved in the mitochondrial energy metabolism are deregulated 2- to 300-fold in GCM.[326] Decreased expression of interleukin (IL)-17– and tumor necrosis factor-α–mediated plakoglobin is observed in GCM, cardiac sarcoidosis, and arrhythmogenic RV cardiomyopathy, but not in lymphocytic myocarditis.[327] These data need confirmation.

Clinical Manifestations and Diagnostic Work-Up

Clinical manifestations of GCM are variable. Most patients commonly present with cardiogenic shock requiring mechanical circulatory support, conduction disease such as atrioventricular nodal or infranodal heart block, and atrial or ventricular arrhythmias, which can be the first manifestation of the disease. Occasionally, GCM may mimic an acute myocardial infarction.[315,319] Less common is presentation as an atrial variant with atrial fibrillation, severe atrial dilation, but preserved ventricular function.[328,329]

A precise diagnosis of GCM is established only when typical pathologic features are demonstrated on EMB or surgical samples (**Fig. 46–9**). The inflammatory infiltrate is comprised of CD8+ lymphocytes, eosinophils, and multinucleated giant cells (**Fig. 46–10**); myocytes show damage and necrosis. Sensitivity of RV EMB is 68% to 80%.[314,330] CMR can guide EMB sampling.[331] Differential diagnosis between GCM and cardiac sarcoidosis relies on pathologic features (noncaseating epithelioid granulomas in sarcoidosis) and is supported by the different T-cell subsets (CD4+ in sarcoidosis and CD8+ in GCM). Gene expression profiles vary between the two disorders and can contribute to differential diagnosis.[326,327,332] EMB is recommended by the Heart Failure Society of America in patients presenting with malignant arrhythmias out of proportion to LV dysfunction or in rapidly progressive clinical heart failure or ventricular dysfunction.[333]

Evolution

GCM carries a poor prognosis, with a median survival of 5.5 months from the onset of symptoms; in one report, 89% of patients either died or required cardiac transplantation,[313] and another report showed 1-year survival of 30% to 69%.[314] These data may underestimate the risk of death because some patients may die with undiagnosed disease.[334]

Treatment

Heart failure treatment includes standard regimen with β-blockers, angiotensin-converting enzyme inhibitors, angiotensin receptor blockers, and aldosterone antagonists, as per guidelines.[150,335] The management of GCM has also included the use of muromonab-CD3, pulse steroids, and varying combinations of azathioprine, cyclosporine, and prednisone monitored with surveillance EMB (**Table 46–5**). Cytolytic therapy with other monoclonal or polyclonal antibodies is debated.[313,336] Mechanical circulatory support for bridge to recovery is rare, whereas it is more commonly used as bridge to transplant;[337,338] biventricular support has been frequently required. Patients most commonly end up needing cardiac transplantation despite immunosuppression.[313,314,338,339] Transplantation should be considered even in stable patients.[340]

Posttransplant survival is similar to that of patients who underwent heart transplantation for other diseases;[313,314] however, GCM may recur in 10% to 50% of transplanted hearts,[313,341] with variable response to immunosuppression,[341,342] and may require novel immune-modifiers such as the CD52-binding monoclonal antibody CAMPATH-1 or alemtuzumab.[325,343]

Sarcoidosis

Sarcoidosis is a chronic multisystem inflammatory disease of unknown etiology that carries the pathologic hallmark of

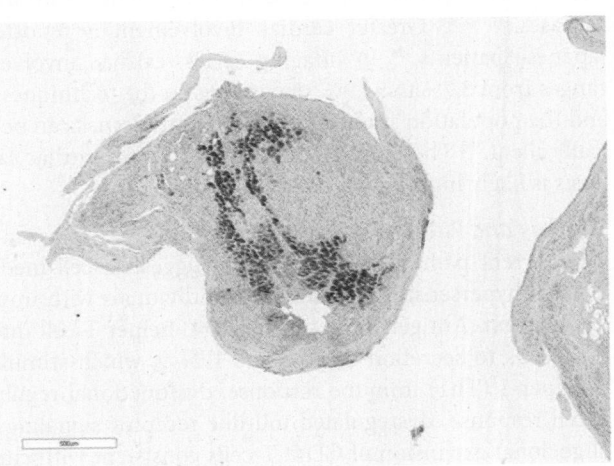

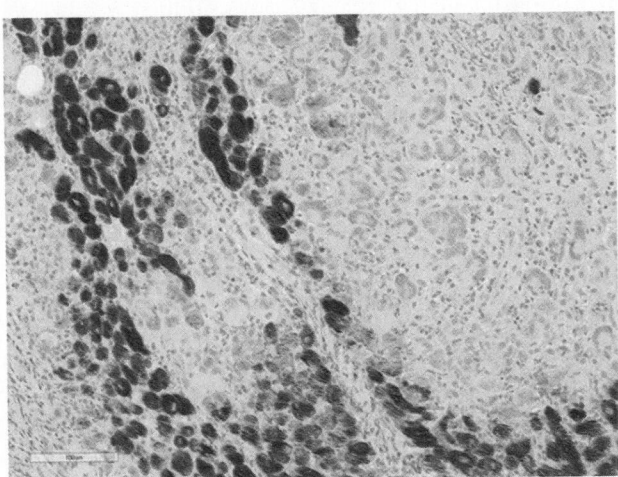

A   **B**

Figure 46–9. (**A**) and (**B**) Antidesmin antibody immunostain demonstrating a few residual layers of myocytes embedded in the context of severe giant cell myocarditis; the giant cells are clearly visible in the higher magnification panel (**B**).

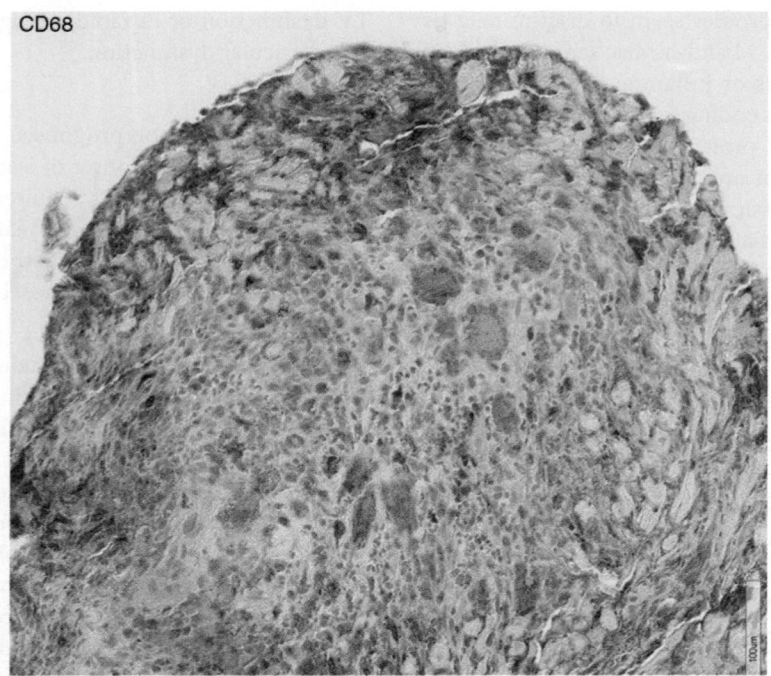

CD68

Figure 46–10. Giant multinucleated cells immunostained with anti-CD68 antibodies in giant cell myocarditis; fulminant onset.

noncaseating epithelioid granulomas in the affected tissues.[344] The incidence varies between 3 to 4 and 35 to 80 per 100,000, reflecting ethnicity, geographic preponderance, and gender bias.[345,346] The prevalence is 10 to 40 per 100,000 persons in the United States and Europe, and is higher in Scandinavians and lower in Turks;[347,348] the ratio between Black and White individuals is 10:1 to 17:1.[349] Women between the age of 20 and 40 years are preferentially affected.[350] Cardiac involvement is influenced by ethnicity but not by gender; cardiac involvement is reported in 58% of Japanese patients, which is the cause of

death in up to 85%.[350] Sarcoidosis typically occurs in adults and is rare in children. In adults, sarcoidosis may manifest with the typical involvement of lungs, lymph nodes, and eyes, or with very early-onset ("early-onset sarcoidosis") in skin, joints, and eyes evolving aggressively to cause blindness, joint destruction, and visceral involvement. The latter aggressive form of sarcoidosis is associated with heterozygous mutations in the *CARD15* gene that cause constitutive nuclear factor-κB activation.[351] When sarcoidosis is suspected in children, the autosomal dominant Blau syndrome/early-onset sarcoidosis has to be considered.[352]

The prevalence of cardiac involvement ranges from 2% to 7% in patients diagnosed with systemic sarcoidosis; autopsy studies have demonstrated cardiac involvement in up to 25% of cases.[344,345,348] Greater cardiac involvement is reported in Japanese patients.[353] In imaging series, cardiac involvement ranges from 3.7% to 54.9%, depending on the techniques used and the population studied.[354] Sarcoid granulomas can be clinically silent.[355] Therefore, the real proportion of cardiac sarcoidosis is likely higher than clinically apparent.

Etiology and Pathogenesis

The current pathogenetic paradigm suggests a cell-mediated delayed hypersensitivity reaction in individuals with immune dysfunction. Antigen and effector CD4+ helper T-cell interaction leads to secretion of IL-2 and IFN-γ, which stimulate a T-helper-1 (Th1) immune response, dysfunctional regulatory T-cell response, dysregulated toll-like receptor signaling, and oligoclonal expansion of CD4+ T cells consistent with chronic antigenic stimulation.[356] Hyperimmune Th1 response to pathogenic microbial and tissue antigens could be associated with the aberrant aggregation of serum amyloid A within granulomas, which in turn promotes progressive chronic granulomatous

TABLE 46–5. Treatment of Giant Cell Myocarditis	
Drug Class	**Drug**
Calcineurin inhibitor	Cyclosporine
	Tacrolimus
Corticosteroids	Methylprednisolone
	Prednisone
Antimetabolite	Imuran
	Mycophenolate mofetil
Cytolytic therapy	ATGAM (antithymocyte globulin)
	Thymoglobulin
Combined treatments	Corticosteroids with cyclosporine
	Corticosteroids with azathioprine
	Corticosteroids, cyclosporine, and azathioprine
	Corticosteroids, cyclosporine, and OKT3
	Corticosteroids, azathioprine, and OKT3

Abbreviation: OKT3, muromonab-CD3.

TABLE 46–6. Family Studies of Genetic Predisposition to Systemic Sarcoidosis

Study	Relatives	Risk Compared with the General Population
Series		
210 twin pairs	Twins, monozygotic	80-fold
	Twins, dizygotic	7-fold
ACCESS (A Case-Control Etiologic Study in Sarcoidosis)	First- or second-degree relative of a patient with sarcoidosis	4- and 7-fold
Genetic Studies		
Genetic association	Chromosome 6, MHC genes	• Acute sarcoidosis: HLA-DRB1*0301 • Remitting disease: HLA-DQB1*0201-DRB1*0301 • Chronic active disease: DQB1*0602-DRB1*150101 • Extrapulmonary manifestations: HLA-DRB1*11
Candidate genes	Case-control studies and family-based studies	• Variation of TNF production: *TNFA1/TNFA2*; rs1800629 • Chronic sarcoidosis: *IL23R*; rs11209026 (Arg381Gln) • Sarcoidosis and uveitis: *IL23R*; rs11209026 (Arg381Gln)
Genome-wide association studies	Susceptibility loci and candidate genes	• Butyrophilin-like 2 (*BTNL2*) gene: *BTNL2* rs2076530 A • Annexin A11 (*ANXA11*) gene: rs1049550 • Ras-related protein Rab-23 (*RAB23*): rs1040461 • Osteosarcoma amplified 9 (*OS9*): rs1050045 • Coiled-coil domain containing 88B (*CCDC88B*) • Peroxiredoxin 5 (*PRDX5*) gene • Neurogenic locus notch homolog protein 4 (*NOTCH4*) gene region: SNP rs715299
Gene-environment interactions	1101 patients with extrapulmonary sarcoidosis and exposed to insecticides, molds, and musty odors	*HLADRB1*

inflammation in the absence of ongoing infection.[356] Mycobacterial ESAT-6 and *Propionibacterium acnes* proteins have been identified by matrix-assisted laser desorption ionization imaging/mass spectrometry in sarcoidosis granulomas, and immune responses to both microbes have been identified in bronchoalveolar lavage of patients with sarcoidosis,[357] which supports the role of infectious agents in the pathogenesis of sarcoidosis. Genetic factors are being investigated in studies of families of probands with sarcoidosis (**Table 46–6**); the co-twin of an affected twin carries a much greater risk of developing sarcoidosis compared to the general population.[358] In the Case-Control Etiologic Sarcoidosis Study (ACCESS), the relative risk for the first- or second-degree relative of a sarcoidosis patient was 4.7 times that of controls.[359] Genetic studies have identified several candidate genes and susceptibility loci; recent epigenetic studies suggest an inverse relationship between methylation and expression of genes involved in T-helper cell type 1 differentiation, chemokines, and chemokine receptors in bronchoalveolar lavage (BAL) cells of patients with pulmonary sarcoidosis.[360] These studies are opening novel avenues in the research of the etiology and pathogenesis of the disease. Sarcoidosis is currently considered as a disease resulting from environmental exposure in genetically susceptible host, to be distinguished from early-onset sarcoidosis/Blau syndrome causally linked with defects of the *CARD15* gene.[361]

Clinical Presentation and Diagnostic Work-Up

The cardiac manifestations are caused by non-necrotizing epithelioid granulomas that preferentially affect the myocardial layer, followed by endocardium, pericardium, and valves. They are most commonly located in the septum, free wall, papillary muscles, and RV free wall in the areas that are not commonly involved by ischemic heart disease. The granulomas heal by fibrosis and evolve to form scars that can be transmural in advanced stages mimicking ischemic disease (**Fig. 46–11**). Clinical manifestations include arrhythmias, conduction disturbances, LV dilation, and systolic or diastolic dysfunction.[344,349] In patients with advanced sarcoidosis, pulmonary hypertension is highly prevalent, may result from both cardiac and pulmonary involvement, and serves as a predictor of poor prognosis.[362] Ventricular aneurysms occur in up to 40% of patients and are also associated with poor prognosis.[363] Involvement of the pericardium and cardiac valves is uncommon.[344,349]

The diagnostic work-up of cardiac involvement is relatively straightforward in patients with established systemic sarcoidosis. However, it is more challenging when cardiac disease presents in isolation (cardiac sarcoidosis) or represents the phenotype of onset, because of the wide spectrum of clinical manifestations, and the possibility that sudden death could be the first clinical manifestation of the disease.[364] The diagnosis of cardiac sarcoidosis is based on EMB, eventually supported by the pathologic evidence of the disease in lung or lymph nodes, and is established on the basis of major and minor criteria recommended by the consensus documents of National Institutes of Health, World Association of Sarcoidosis and Other Granulomatous Disorders, and Heart Rhythm Society (**Table 46–7**).[365–367] The clinical work-up should include a thorough discussion of individual and family medical history,

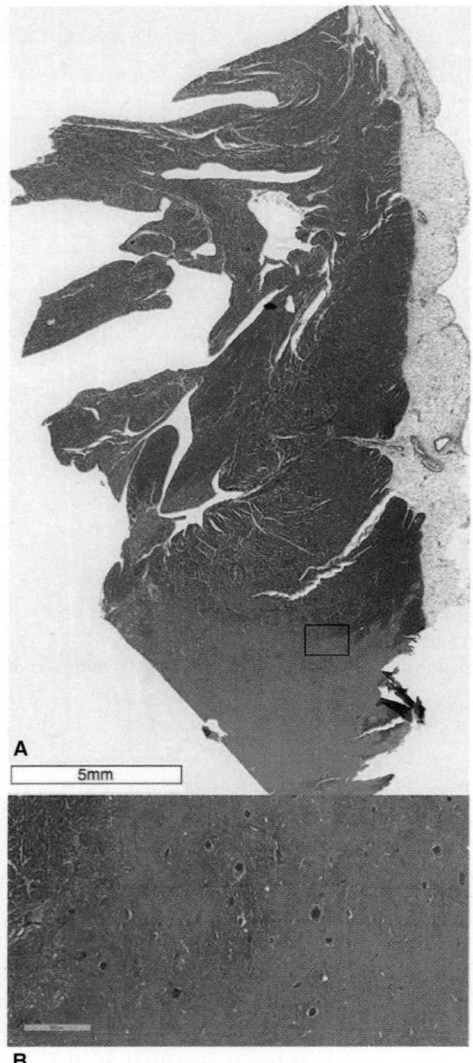

Figure 46–11. End-stage cardiac sarcoidosis. (**A**) A low-magnification view of an LV sample from a heart with end-stage sarcoidosis; note the large transmural scarred area alternated with preserved myocardial tissue and focal thinning of the compacted layer of the left ventricle. (**B**) A scar area with residual giant cells.

physical examination, ECG, 24-hour Holter monitoring, echocardiography, and advanced imaging, as appropriate.

ECG may show conduction disturbances, arrhythmia, or nonspecific ST-segment and T-wave changes. Signal-averaged ECG has a modest diagnostic sensitivity (52%) and reasonable specificity (82%).[368] Holter monitoring is often used as a screening tool for cardiac involvement in patients with systemic sarcoidosis; it predicts cardiac involvement with a sensitivity ranging from 50% to 67% and a specificity of 80% to 97% compared to CMR or PET as a reference standard.[369] Echocardiography remains the most commonly used imaging investigation in suspected sarcoidosis, but detects late stages of the disease (in up to 80% of advanced cases) with regional wall motion abnormalities, LV dilation, LV aneurysms, thinning of the basal septum, and impaired LV or RV systolic function.

Diastolic dysfunction may occur early. The right heart pressures are elevated in patients with lung disease. In early cardiac involvement, when LV function and size are normal, strain and strain rate imaging using speckle tracking are potentially useful for identifying subclinical myocardial involvement.[370]

CMR offers a high sensitivity and specificity for the assessment of cardiac involvement. Whereas T2 hyperenhancement identifies early edema, the LGE in a nonvascular distribution supports myocardial scarring. LGE correlates with cardiac biopsy findings of granulomatous inflammation;[371,372] extensive LGE reliably predicts adverse cardiac outcomes,[373] and major cardiac events in survivors of sudden cardiac death.[374] The LGE features vary during acute inflammation and with scars. CMR-verified cardiac involvement correlates with decreased LVEF, increased diastolic interventricular septal thickness, and diastolic dysfunction.[375] In patients with preserved LVEF and extracardiac sarcoidosis, major adverse cardiac events including death and ventricular tachycardia are associated with a greater LGE and RV involvement; preserved LVEF does not exclude the risk for adverse events.[375] RV involvement and dysfunction are common and are associated with LV involvement, lung disease, or pulmonary hypertension or may even be isolated.[376] However, cardiac PET using ^{18}F-FDG identifies regional inflammatory activity, defines the cause of arrhythmia, and guides treatment.[377] Quantitative imaging assessment can monitor changes in FDG uptake on serial studies. Reduced inflammatory activity with improvement of LVEF and decrease in size and/or intensity of resting perfusion defects (such as by ^{13}N-ammonia imaging) may indicate a favorable response to treatment, but may also indicate progression of scarring processes. Novel indices of FDG uptake allow calculation of the burden of inflammation (cardiac metabolic volume) and the volume-intensity product (cardiac metabolic activity); increased cardiac metabolic activity is associated with adverse clinical events in patients with cardiac sarcoidosis.[378] Using ^{18}F-FDG to assess inflammation after a high-fat/low-carbohydrate diet to suppress normal myocardial glucose uptake, 71 (60%) of 118 consecutive patients with suspected cardiac sarcoidosis demonstrated abnormal cardiac PET findings.[379] The presence of focal perfusion defects (rubidium-82 imaging in this report) and FDG uptake identified higher risk of death or ventricular tachycardia.[380] Overall, PET studies have proved to be clinically useful for diagnostic and prognostic information, especially for the risk of ventricular arrhythmias in patients with cardiac sarcoidosis. The potential translational impact of the serial PET scans could inform about evolution or regression of cardiac granulomas and about active myocardial inflammation or the process of healing. Although gallium-67 scintigraphy has also been employed for the detection of myocardial inflammation in systemic sarcoidosis and relates to response to treatment,[381,382] ^{18}F-FDG PET imaging is preferred both for diagnosis and prognostication because of superior sensitivity and reduced radiation exposure. FDG-PET is now included as a diagnostic criterion in the expert consensus statement on the diagnosis of cardiac sarcoidosis[367] (see Table 46–7).

Biomarkers are not included in the diagnostic criteria for cardiac sarcoidosis. There are no disease-specific markers for

TABLE 46-7. Diagnostic Criteria for Cardiac Sarcoidosis

1999 (revised 2006)	2013[366]	2014[382]
Histologic diagnosis group CS is confirmed when endomyocardial biopsy specimens demonstrate noncaseating epithelioid granulomas with histologic or clinical diagnosis of extracardiac sarcoidosis	**Histologic diagnosis of cardiac sarcoidosis** Endomyocardial biopsy specimens with noncaseating epithelioid granulomas and no alternative cause identified	**1. Histologic diagnosis from myocardial tissue** CS is diagnosed in the presence of noncaseating granuloma on histologic examination of myocardial tissue. Absence of alternative causes. Negative organismal stains.
Clinical diagnosis group Although endomyocardial biopsy specimens do not demonstrate noncaseating epithelioid granulomas, extracardiac sarcoidosis is diagnosed histologically or clinically and satisfies the following conditions and more than 1 of 6 basic diagnostic criteria: I. 2 or more of the 4 major criteria are satisfied II. 1 of 4 of the major criteria and 2 or more of the 5 minor criteria are satisfied **Major criteria** Advanced AV block Basal thinning of the interventricular septum Positive gallium-67 uptake in the heart Depressed LVEF < 50% **Minor criteria** Abnormal ECG findings: ventricular arrhythmias (VT or multifocal or frequent PVCs), complete RBBB, axis deviation, or abnormal Q waves Abnormal echocardiography: wall motion abnormality or morphologic abnormality (aneurysm or wall thickening or ventricular dilation) Perfusion defects on nuclear imaging: thallium-201, technetium-99m SPECT Delayed gadolinium enhancement on CMR Interstitial fibrosis or monocyte infiltration on cardiac biopsy	**Clinical diagnosis of probable cardiac sarcoidosis** Histologic diagnosis of extracardiac sarcoidosis and 1 or more of the following are present while reasonable alternative cardiac causes other than CS have been excluded: Corticosteroid or immunosuppressive therapy responsive cardiomyopathy or heart block Unexplained reduced LVEF (< 40%) Mobitz type II second-degree heart block or third-degree heart block Depressed LVEF < 50% Patchy uptake on cardiac FDG-PET in a pattern consistent with CS LGE on CMR imaging in a pattern consistent with CS Positive gallium uptake in a pattern consistent with CS	**2. Clinical diagnosis from invasive and noninvasive studies** It is probable[a] that there is CS if: A. There is a histologic diagnosis of extracardiac sarcoidosis AND B. One or more of following is present 1. Steroid ± immunosuppressant responsive cardiomyopathy or heart block 2. Unexplained reduced LVEF (< 40%) 3. Unexplained sustained (spontaneous or induced) VT 4. Mobitz type II second-degree heart block or third-degree heart block 5. Patchy uptake on dedicated cardiac PET (in a pattern consistent with CS) 6. LGE on CMR (in a pattern consistent with CS) 7. Positive gallium uptake (in a pattern consistent with CS) AND C. Other causes for the cardiac manifestation(s) have been reasonably excluded

Abbreviations: AV, atrioventricular; CMR, cardiac magnetic resonance; CS, cardiac sarcoidosis; ECG, electrocardiographic; FDG, fluorodeoxyglucose; LGE, late gadolinium enhancement; LVEF, left ventricular ejection fraction; PET, positron emission tomography; PVC, premature ventricular contraction; RBBB, right bundle branch block; SPECT, single-photon emission computed tomography; VT, ventricular tachycardia.

[a]In general, probable involvement is considered adequate to establish a clinical diagnosis of CS.

cardiac sarcoidosis.[383] The circulating level of serum angiotensin-converting enzyme is reported as increased in 60% of patients with systemic sarcoidosis and 21.8% of patients with cardiac sarcoidosis.[384,385] Other biomarkers, including serum soluble IL-2 receptor,[386] IgG, high-sensitivity troponin T,[383,387] and atrial and brain natriuretic peptides,[388] are neither sufficiently sensitive nor specific, and there are no data pertaining to their role in management of cardiac sarcoidosis.[389]

Cardiac sarcoidosis is diagnosed with certainty by EMB demonstrating noncaseating epithelioid granulomas[12,390] (**Fig. 46-12**). Although EMB has low sensitivity (19%-32%) as a result of the inherent sampling limitation for focal epithelioid granulomas, it offers high specificity for the diagnosis.[391] Biopsies are commonly performed in the right ventricle but LV EMB can be performed if necessary.[392] Besides epithelioid granulomas, EMB commonly reveals nonspecific findings including myocardial interstitial fibrosis, myofibrillar disarrangement and fragmentation, and inflammatory mononuclear cell infiltrates.

Treatment

Treatment options largely depend on the symptoms and the phase of the disease evolution, and are summarized in **Table 46-8** based on recommendations of the American College of

Cardiology, American Heart Association,[164] and the Heart Rhythm Society.[365]

ENDEMIC MYOCARDITIS

Chagas Disease

Chagas disease (CD) is caused by the protozoan parasite *Trypanosoma cruzi*,[393] which is transmitted through the feces of an infected triatomine, direct oral contact, contaminated blood transfusion, or bone marrow transplantation; it can also be congenital and transmitted vertically from mother to infant. Triatomines are found in the southern United States, Mexico, Central America, and South America, where CD is endemic.[394] Contamination of food and drink has been reported in northern South America, where transmission cycles may involve wild vector populations and mammalian reservoir hosts.[395] In the acute phase, the disease can manifest with myocarditis, conduction system abnormalities, and pericarditis. In untreated patients, the disease progresses to the chronic phase.[396-398]

Etiology and Pathogenesis

The first description dates back to 1909, when Carlos Chagas isolated *T cruzi* from the blood of a Brazilian patient.[398] Global population epidemiology considers both the local resident

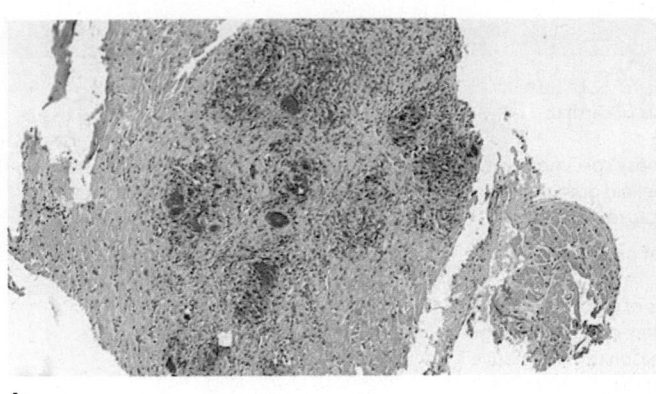
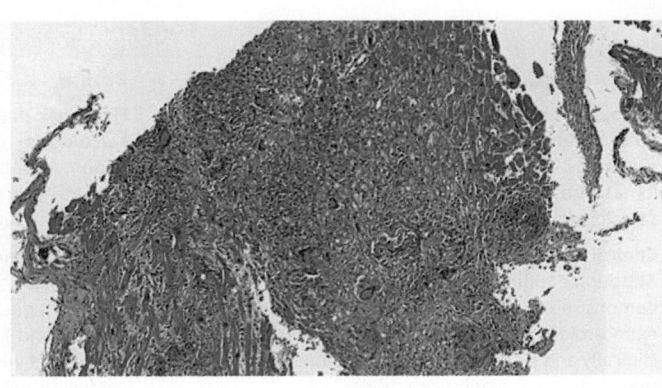

A   **B**

Figure 46–12. Active sarcoidosis. The figure shows the endomyocardial biopsy (EMB) sample of a 46-year-old male patient who presented with dyspnea. He showed conduction disease, LVEF of 50%; LV end-diastolic diameter of 56 mm; and maximum left ventricular thickness of 13 mm. Family history was negative. (**A**) Anti-CD68 immunostain; note positive macrophages and giant cells. (**B**) Hematoxylin and eosin view of the same EMB sample.

TABLE 46–8. Summary of Treatments for Cardiac Sarcoidosis Based on Recommendations of the American College of Cardiology, American Heart Association, and the Heart Rhythm Society

Treatment Type	Treatment	Level of Evidence	Mechanism	Potential Benefit/Class Recommendation
Immunosup-pressive medical therapy	Prednisone	C	Anti inflammatory	^{18}F-FDG PET may guide steroid therapy (LVEF of 3.8% per reduction in SUV volume of 100 cm^3 above a threshold value, $P = 0.022$)
	Methotrexate	C	Antimetabolite and immunomodulator	Steroid-sparing. In a 3-year open-label study steroid + methotrexate had improved LVEF (44.5% ± 13.8% vs 60.7% ± 14.3%, $P = 0.04$)
	Steroid-sparing immunomodulators	C	Variable, depending on the medication	Case reports only have included: infliximab, azathioprine, cyclosporine, antimalarials, pentoxifylline, thalidomide
Heart failure medical therapy	ACE-I/ARB	A	Improves cardiac remodeling	Class I; reduce mortality and morbidity of HFrEF; class IIa for structural heart disease without impaired LVEF or symptoms
	β-Blockers	C	Negative inotrope; delays AV conduction	Class I; reduce mortality and morbidity for HFrEF
	Diuretics and sodium-restricted diet	C	Fluid and sodium excretion	Class I for HFrEF and symptoms
Device therapy	ICD, secondary prevention	C	Defibrillation of potential recurrent VT/VF	Class I; reduce mortality in patients with structural heart disease and syncope, VT/VF, or sustained VT/VF inducible by EP study; class III if life expectancy <1 year
	ICD, primary prevention	C	Defibrillation of potential VT/VF	• Class I; reduce mortality in patients with structural heart disease and EF < 30%–35% despite medical therapy. • Class IIa for patients needing pacemaker, unexplained syncope, or sustained VT/VF inducible by EP study; LGE on CMR may be used to consider EP study. • Class IIb for LVEF 36%–49% or RVEF <40% despite medical therapy. • Class III when life expectancy <1 year
	Pacemaker	C	Prevention of fatal arrhythmia	Class I; reduce mortality and symptoms from complete heart block and bradyarrhythmia
Surgical treatment	Heart and lung transplantation	C	Organ replacement therapy	In patients with end-stage organ dysfunction that may include refractory cardiogenic shock, intravenous inotrope dependence, peak oxygen consumption <10 mL/kg/min with achievement of anaerobic metabolism, refractory VT/VF

Abbreviations: ACE-I, angiotensin-converting enzyme inhibitor; ARB, angiotensin receptor blocker; AV, atrioventricular; CMR, cardiac magnetic resonance; CS, cardiac sarcoidosis; EF, ejection fraction; EP, electrophysiologic; ^{18}F-FDG PET, ^{18}F-fluorodeoxyglucose positron emission tomography; HFrEF, heart failure with reduced ejection fraction; ICD, implantable cardioverter-defibrillator; LGE, late gadolinium enhancement; LVEF, left ventricular ejection fraction; RVEF, right ventricular ejection fraction; SUV, standardized uptake value; VF, ventricular fibrillation; VT, ventricular tachycardia.

population of Latin America and the population of Latin Americans migrating to other countries, particularly the United States. In endemic regions, infected vectors are prevalent in rural houses where people are exposed to the risk of infection for years. The incidence of new infection and transmission though the feces of an infected vector is relatively low and estimated at 1% per year, with a peak of 4% in Bolivian population.[399] The incidence of infected populations and CD cardiomyopathy increases with age. The large-scale migration from rural to urban areas and from Latin America to the United States, Spain, and other countries has been associated with endemic transfer of infected immigrants.[400–402] By systematic serologic screening and screening of congenital disease, the National Health Services in Latin America have significantly contained the infection, with the estimated global prevalence of *T cruzi* infection declining from 18 million in 1991 (when the first regional control initiative began) to 5.7 million in 2010.[400]

Clinical Manifestations and Diagnostic Work-Up

CD evolves in three phases: acute, intermediate, and chronic (**Table 46–9**). After the infected vector transmission, the incubation period is 1 to 2 weeks, and the acute disease lasts 2 to 3 months, comprising the period of parasitemia. In the acute phase, patients present with mild and nonspecific symptoms such as fever, malaise, hepatosplenomegaly, and atypical lymphocytosis. Chagoma (an inflammatory nodule at the site of inoculation) or unilateral painless periorbital swelling (Romana sign) is rarely observed. The majority of infections in the acute phase are not detected. Occasionally, acute CD imposes life-threatening consequences, such as meningoencephalitis and myocarditis.[403] About 30% of infected subjects develop cardiac complications with arrhythmias and transient ECG abnormalities,[404] and develop systolic and diastolic dysfunction and end-stage DCM.[405] This phase is characterized by positive serologic and parasitologic tests.[406] The cardiac manifestations include ECG abnormalities (prolongation of QRS complex and QT interval, right bundle branch block, and/or left anterior fascicular block) and ventricular segmental wall

motion abnormalities;[407] CMR detects cardiac fibrosis and diastolic dysfunction.[406,407] In this phase, illness is severe, with LV dilation and dysfunction, aneurysm, congestive heart failure, thromboembolism, pulmonary hypertension, ventricular arrhythmias, and sudden cardiac death, which is the leading cause of death in patients with Chagas heart disease.[408] Heart transplantation is a possible option. Hearts affected by end-stage CD demonstrate severe dilation and multifocal scars; the histopathology shows persistent chronic inflammation in the context of fibrosis (**Fig. 46–13**). Serial blood PCR testing in transplanted patients is consensually recommended for monitoring CD reactivation. When PCR in blood tests positive with low parasitic load, EMB PCR is useful, with positive test reinforcing the possibility of graft CD.[409] Chagas cardiomyopathy can be complicated by stroke caused by embolization of intracardiac mural thrombi resulting from depressed LV function and/or aneurysm formation.[408]

Although a direct association between parasite burden and CD phase is not clear, parasite persistence remains central to the disease. A serologic test for IgG antibodies to *T cruzi* is the most effective diagnostic tool.[410,411] The mature form of the parasite (trypomastigote) can be detected by microscopy in blood samples during the acute phase, wherein quantitative PCR is the gold standard for quantitation. After the first 90 days, as the *T cruzi* burden is decreasing, the antiparasite serum antibodies show rising titers by serologic tests including indirect hemagglutination, indirect immunofluorescence, and enzyme-linked immunosorbent assays.

Management

Management of cardiac CD must importantly consider the high likelihood of ventricular arrhythmias and sudden death in patients with chronic CD.[412] Ambulatory ECG monitoring has been suggested for patients with an abnormal resting ECG or echocardiographic ventricular wall motion abnormalities. Patients with nonsustained ventricular tachycardia are usually candidates for electrophysiologic studies. Echocardiographic monitoring demonstrates both structural and functional changes in the early stages of cardiac involvement, including regional wall motion abnormalities and diastolic dysfunction; the cardiac phenotype shows LV dilation and severe dysfunction in advance phases.[413]

Two antiparasitic drugs are available for the treatment of CD: benznidazole and nifurtimox.[414] These drugs commonly produce dermatologic side effects that are well controlled by antihistaminic drugs. An ongoing prospective international trial testing antitrypanocidal treatment is evaluating the efficacy of benznidazole in patients with chronic Chagas cardiomyopathy.[415] Heart failure is treated according to current guidelines. Because patients with CD may demonstrate lower blood pressure and higher incidence of bradyarrhythmias than non-CD patients, doses of angiotensin-converting enzyme inhibitors and β-blockers are tailored on individual needs. Cardiac resynchronization therapy in patients with severe systolic dysfunction (LVEF <35%) and prolonged QRS duration[416] has been shown to improve NYHA functional class, increase LVEF, and enhance survival. Patients with end-stage heart failure

TABLE 46–9. Chagas Disease: Three Phases		
Acute Phase (duration: weeks)	**Indeterminate Phase (duration: decades)**	**Chronic Phase (duration: decades)**
• Fever • Malaise • Lymphadenopathy • Chagoma—inflammatory nodule at site of inoculation • Romana's sign—periorbital swelling • ECG abnormalities: sinus tachycardia, first-degree AV block • Myocarditis (rare)	• Asymptomatic (most) • Conduction abnormalities, regional LV wall motion abnormalities, or sudden cardiac death (rare)	• Asymptomatic • Cardiac: LV dilation, congestive heart failure, conduction abnormalities, ventricular arrhythmias, thromboembolic disease, sudden cardiac death

Abbreviations: AV, atrioventricular; ECG, electrocardiogram; LV, left ventricular.

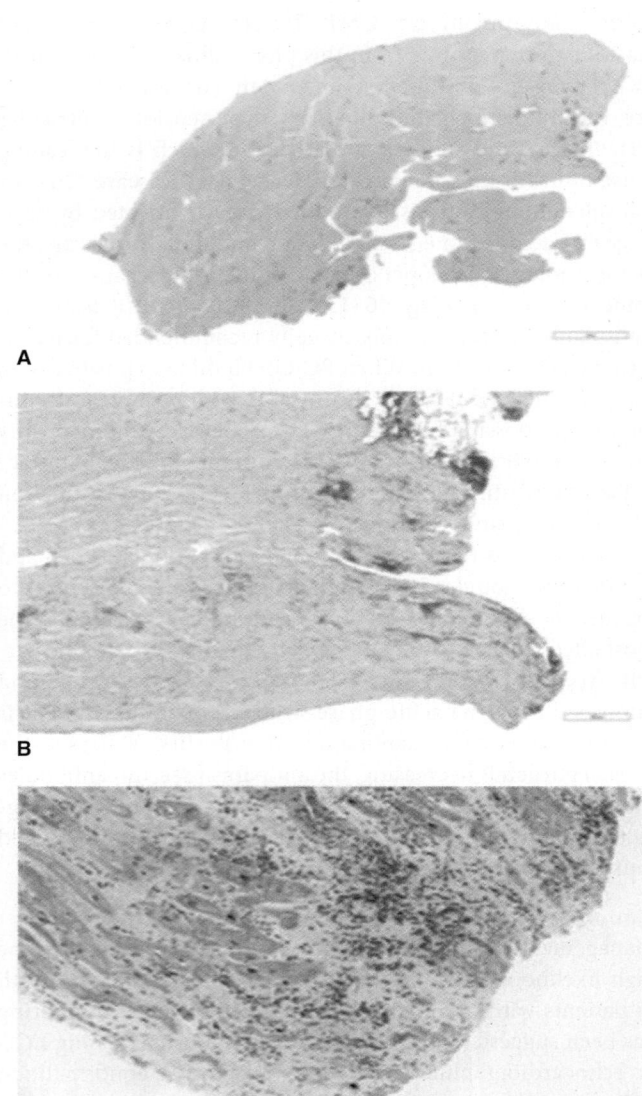

A

B

C

Figure 46–13. Myocardial sections obtained from the left ventricle of a 55-year-old man from South America who was diagnosed with Chagas disease and successfully transplanted for end-stage heart failure, after LV mechanical support. The heart excised at transplantation weighed 360 g and did not show significant LV hypertrophy. After transplantation, he suffered Chagas disease reactivation, with major gastrointestinal clinical manifestations. He is currently doing well 20 months after transplantation (**A**) shows a low-magnification-view section immunostained with anti CD45RO antibodies: spotted clusters of inflammatory infiltrates are variably sparse in the myocardium. (**B**) shows a higher magnification view of the mid part of the right border of (**A**), demonstrating the variable amount of inflammatory infiltrates. (**C**) shows intense inflammatory infiltrates in the context of dense interstitial fibrosis. Cardiac myocyte demonstrates prominent nuclei without significant hypertrophy. (**A**) and (**B**), peroxidase-antiperoxisade, immunostain; magnification bar: low right corner; (**C**) H&E stain, magnification bar: low right corner.

refractory to medical treatment may receive an LV assist device and undergo cardiac transplantation.[417,418] An ICD is effective in both primary and secondary prevention of sudden cardiac death.[419] The combination of ICD and amiodarone seems to be superior for secondary prevention, resulting in a 72% reduction in all-cause mortality and a 95% decrease in sudden cardiac death in the ICD group compared to those receiving amiodarone alone.[419] Permanent cardiac pacing is indicated in patients with high-degree atrioventricular block or with symptomatic bradycardia.[420]

Lyme Disease

Lyme disease is a tick-borne disease caused by *Borrelia burgdorferi*; 60% to 80% of cases demonstrate a characteristic rash (erythema migrans) typically accompanied by fever, headache, and fatigue. Untreated Lyme disease can evolve to chronic arthritis and neurologic and cardiac manifestations.[421] Lyme disease is common in Europe and North America, and may afflict 1 in 1000 persons in some US states and 1 in 300 people in Southern Europe. Cardiac involvement occurs in a minority of patients and predominantly manifests with conduction abnormality, followed by arrhythmias, myocarditis, pericarditis, and DCM; the cardiac involvement is known as *Lyme carditis*.[422] The rates of cardiac involvement in Lyme disease have declined measurably.[423,424] The main vertebrate reservoirs for Lyme *Borrelia* are small mammals, such as mice and voles, and some species of birds. In most tick habitats, deer are essential for the maintenance of tick populations because they are one of the few wild hosts that can feed sufficient numbers of adult ticks, but they are not competent reservoirs for spirochetes.[425] The reservoir hosts and patients can be coinfected with multiple *Borrelia* species or other tick-borne pathogens. Most human infections occur during spring, summer, and early fall months.[424]

Annual incidence of Lyme disease seems to increase from northern to southern parts of central Europe,[425] and ranges from 69 cases per 100,000 population in Sweden to 111 cases per 100,000 in Germany[426] and 155 cases per 100,000 in Slovenia; the lowest incidence in Europe is in the United Kingdom (0.7 per 100,000) and Ireland (0.6 per 100,000).[427] The incidence declines from south to north in Scandinavia and north to south in Italy, Spain, and Greece. In France, the yearly Lyme disease incidence rate averages 42 cases per 100,000 inhabitants.[428] In the United States and Canada, Lyme disease is the major vector-born zoonosis, with approximately 30,000 reported cases and an estimated 300,000 human cases occurring annually in the United States.[429,430] Men are more commonly infected than women. Although the distribution per age is bimodal (children 5–9 years old and adults 45–59 years old), patients of all ages are exposed to the risk of infection.

Etiology and Pathogenesis

The vector deposits Lyme *Borrelia* into the skin of a host that disseminates through blood or soft tissue to other locations. Several days or weeks elapse from the infection to the appearance of erythema migrans, which occurs in 60% to 80% of patients.[431] In the majority of patients, early infection is asymptomatic or presents with influenza-like symptoms, fever, fatigue, muscle or joint pain, and headache.[432] The second phase of involvement of organ systems, such as the cardiac

TABLE 46–10. Clinical Manifestations of Lyme Disease

Organ/System	Signs and Symptoms
Skin	Erythema migrans
Neuromuscular system	Recurrent, brief attacks (weeks or months) of joint swelling in one or a few joints, sometimes followed by chronic arthritis in one or a few joints
Nervous system	Lymphocytic meningitis; cranial neuritis, particularly facial palsy (may be bilateral); radiculoneuropathy; or, rarely, encephalomyelitis. Encephalomyelitis must be confirmed by demonstration of antibody production against *Borrelia burgdorferi* in the cerebrospinal fluid (CSF), evidenced by a higher titer of antibody in CSF than in serum
Cardiovascular system	Acute onset of high-grade (second-degree or third-degree) atrioventricular conduction defects that resolve in days to weeks and are sometimes associated with myocarditis

or neurologic systems, may come to attention among untreated patients as part of early disseminated disease (**Table 46–10**).[433]

Clinical Manifestations and Diagnostic Work-Up

Recent guidelines have addressed prevention, diagnosis, and treatment of Lyme Disease.[434] Lyme carditis is rare and typically manifests 2 to 5 weeks after the erythema migrans. It affects 1% to 5% of diagnosed patients with Lyme disease.[422] Patients who develop Lyme disease may first demonstrate atrioventricular block at 14 days (range, 2–24 days) after the onset; only one-third of patients recall the erythema migrans.[435,436] Myopericarditis can present with chest pain, dyspnea, or syncope,[436] and the signs and symptoms of Lyme myopericarditis can mimic acute coronary syndrome, with ECG ST-segment alterations and elevated peripheral blood cardiac biomarkers. In such cases, echocardiography demonstrates diffuse ventricular hypokinesis rather than the focal wall motion abnormalities expected with an acute coronary syndrome.[435] The mechanism of the development of cardiomyopathy in Lyme disease is debated, and myocardial persistence of *Borrelia* may contribute to the pathophysiology in individuals living in endemic areas;[437] this observation[438] seems to be supported by the finding of 20% of unexplained DCM patients who test positive for *Borrelia*. Diffuse erythema migrans throughout the body indicates dissemination. Subsequently, Lyme disease may present as inflammatory arthritis several months after the initial infection, and has been reported to occur in approximately 11% of patients with untreated erythema migrans.

The history of tick bite combined with erythema migrans (see Table 46–10) should be carefully investigated in patients with suspected Lyme carditis. However, patients may not always recall a tick bite, and 20% to 40% of patients do not develop erythema migrans. The diagnosis is based on *Borrelia* isolation or on a two-step test including a sensitive ELISA screening test for IgM and IgG antibody and then confirmation through Western blot assay for positive or borderline results.[437] In the early stage of the disease, results may be false negative as a result of the delayed immune response. Methods such as immune PCR

assay have been validated for detection of antibodies to the *Borrelia* C6 peptide.[439] Immune PCR exploits the amplification property of PCR to increase the sensitivity of standard ELISAs by 100- to 10,000-fold.[439] Methods based on metabolomics are being tested;[440] they are based on the use of liquid chromatography/mass spectrometry and statistical modeling to define a metabolic profile of biosignatures present in patients with early-stage Lyme disease.[438,440]

Treatment

Lyme disease is treated with a 10- to 21-day course of doxycycline or amoxicillin orally. Intravenous ceftriaxone (2 g every 24 hours for 2–3 weeks) may be indicated when the infection is not detected in the early stages or is refractory to initial treatments.[429,435] Treated patients who do not recover after *Borrelia* infection may experience chronic peripheral and central nervous system manifestations, including depression, fatigue, sleep disorders, and memory loss, for months to years after the initial infection. In pregnant women, doxycycline should be avoided because of the potential adverse effects to both fetus and mother.[441] Since high-degree atrioventricular block is the most common presentation of Lyme carditis, and usually resolves with antibiotic therapy, the precise diagnosis and appropriate treatment prevents unnecessary implantation of permanent pacemakers in otherwise healthy young individuals.[442]

Malaria

Severe malaria remains a leading cause of death worldwide. Although cardiac involvement is not considered as a frequent cause of morbidity and mortality, cardiovascular involvement is clinically heterogeneous, with cardiac involvement manifesting with myocarditis, pericarditis, pericardial effusion, ischemic disease, and heart failure.[443] Myocarditis can be associated with hemorrhagic manifestations induced by the typical haemolysis.[444,445] Pathogenetic mechanisms include an imbalanced proinflammatory cytokine response and/or erythrocyte sequestration by increased cytoadherence to endothelium.[446,447]

The disease is well controlled with specific medications but patients who do not receive antimalarial chemoprophylaxis can get sick and become carriers.[448] Malaria transmission can occur through heart transplantation: screening in organ donors should be considered in endemic regions.[449]

HYPEREOSINOPHILIC SYNDROMES

Eosinophils are the descendants of the granulocytic lineage that differentiate in the bone marrow under the influence of IL-5, IL-3, and granulocyte-macrophage colony-stimulating factor.[450] They produce and store enzymes, basic proteins, cytokines, chemokines, membrane-derived factors, and antifibrinolytic mediators.[450,451] Although their function is not fully clarified, they are involved in host immune response to infection, cancer surveillance, and maintenance of other immune cells.[450,451] In peripheral blood, the normal range of eosinophils is 3% to 5%, which corresponds to an absolute count of 350 to 500/μL.[451,452] Eosinophilia refers to an increased absolute eosinophilic count (AEC) in peripheral blood and is graded as mild

(AEC from upper normal limit to 1500/µL), moderate (AEC 1500–5000/µL), or severe (AEC >5000/µL).[452] The complex groups of eosinophilias encompass a broad range of disorders including hematologic eosinophilias (clonal, neoplastic, primary), nonhematologic (secondary or reactive), eosinophilic diseases of unknown significance, and familial diseases with either known or unknown genetic causes; organ damage may occur in several of these forms (**Table 46–11**).[453] The heart is either potentially involved in the context of systemic diseases or is the major or unique clinically involved organ. During the course of the last 30 years, the progress of knowledge on both causes and markers of hypereosinophilic syndromes (HES) has led to development of diagnostic criteria that were modified in 2006, when the definition of HES was expanded to include other previously distinct disease entities associated with eosinophilia, such as eosinophilic granulomatosis with polyangiitis (EGPA; formerly known as Churg–Strauss syndrome), chronic eosinophilic pneumonia, and eosinophilic gastrointestinal disorders.[454] In 2010, the time limit of a 6-month diagnostic period was substituted with the suggestion of an elevation of the AEC to >1500/µL on at least two occasions.[455] Because tissue eosinophilic infiltration and related end-organ damage may occur in patients with peripheral AEC <1500/µL, it was recommended that the diagnosis can be formulated in patients with "tissue eosinophilia and marked peripheral eosinophilia"; the AEC value is no longer a requirement for the diagnosis. The definition of HES was also expanded to include molecular evidence of end-organ damage.[455]

The age-adjusted prevalence is approximately 0.036 per 100,000 wherein the estimates are based on the International Classification of Diseases for Oncology (Version 3), coding 9964/3 (HES including chronic eosinophilic leukemia) and the Surveillance, Epidemiology, and End Results database from 2001 to 2005. In this estimate, eosinophilias with somatic genetic abnormalities (*PDGFRA/B*, *FGFR1*) account for a minority of cases (median, 23%; range, 3%–56%).[456] In developing countries, the *FIP1L1-PDGFRA* fusion occurs in approximately 10% to 20% of patients with idiopathic hypereosinophilia.[457,458] Idiopathic hypereosinophilia is usually diagnosed between the ages of 20 and 50 years, but also occurs in children and the elderly.[459–463] In 131 incident cases observed between 2001 and 2005, the male-to-female ratio was 1.5, and rates increased with age (peak between 65–74 years).[456] Most patients with *FIP1L1-PDGFRA* or myeloproliferative variants are male,[458,464,465] whereas other eosinophilia subtypes do not show differences between the two genders.

Etiology and Pathogenesis

The causes include malignancies, hypersensitivity myocarditis, autoimmune reactions in the heart (typically related to a drug reaction), parasitic infections, and eosinophilic granulomatosis with polyangiitis (EGPA; also known as Churg–Strauss syndrome).[451,452,454,455] Patients who develop eosinophilic myocarditis often demonstrate fever, rash, ECG abnormalities, and peripheral eosinophilia. The pathologic substrate is myocardial eosinophilic inflammation associated with limited myocyte damage and necrosis. Endomyocardial fibrosis that typically affects the right ventricle is a distinct disease of the endocardium and may not be associated with hypereosinophilia. Eosinophilic myocarditis in its end-fibrotic endocardial stage is also distinct from carcinoid heart disease.

Clinical Manifestations and Diagnostic Work-Up

The clinical presentation is heterogeneous and demonstrates nonspecific signs and symptoms, including weakness, fatigue, dyspnea, myalgias, angioedema, rash, fever, rhinitis, and diarrhea.[465] Patients demonstrate leukocytosis (eg, 20,000–30,000/µ or higher) with peripheral eosinophilia in the range of 30% to 70%, neutrophilia, basophilia, myeloid immaturity, and both mature and immature eosinophils with varying degrees of dysplasia.[465,466] Anemia occurs in more than 50% of patients; thrombocytopenia, bone marrow eosinophilia with Charcot-Leyden crystals, and possible increased blasts and marrow fibrosis can also recur.[452,453]

The most common organ/tissue manifestations occur in skin (about 70% of patients), followed by lung and gastrointestinal manifestations in 40% and 30% of cases, respectively. Cardiac involvement occurs in 20% of patients, in the majority during the course of the disease,[467,468] and affects myocardial layers, endocardium, and valves. Eosinophilic infiltration of the myocardium with release of toxic mediators is associated with heart failure. Endocardial infiltration causes mural thrombi with increased embolic risk. Late phases are characterized by endocardial fibrosis manifesting with restrictive physiology. Valve regurgitation is prominently observed when mural endocardial thrombosis and fibrosis involve leaflets of the mitral or tricuspid valves.[467,468]

Eosinophilic Heart Disease

Cardiac involvement is a major cause of morbidity and mortality in HES.[469] The cardiac pathology is divided into three stages: (1) an acute necrotic stage, (2) a thrombotic stage, and (3) a fibrotic stage (**Table 46–12**).

The early, acute necrotic stage is characterized by eosinophilic and lymphocyte infiltration; in the myocardial interstitium, eosinophils undergo degranulation with release of biologically active factors that cause myocyte injury (**Fig. 46–14**). Clinical presentation may comprise nonspecific manifestations. Patients may infrequently present with acute heart failure or cardiogenic shock at onset.[470] ECG may show tachycardia, nonspecific ST-segment changes, or conduction delays. cTn levels may be increased, mimicking acute myocardial infarction.[471,472] Echocardiography may show increased LV wall thickness caused by interstitial edema, LV systolic dysfunction, and wall motion abnormalities. CMR shows endocardial delayed enhancement, and T2 mapping may demonstrate subendocardial edema.[473] EMB differentiates eosinophilic infiltration of the endocardium and subendocardial spaces. Corticosteroids inhibit the degranulation of eosinophils and are the first-line treatment for eosinophilic myocarditis.[474,475] In case of fulminant heart failure, mechanical support may become necessary.[476]

TABLE 46–11. 2008 World Health Organization Classification of Eosinophilic Disorders

Primary Eosinophilia	Secondary Eosinophilia	Familial Eosinophilia (HE_F)			Eosinophilia, Unknown Significance (HE_US)

Primary Eosinophilia

Myeloid and lymphoid neoplasms with eosinophilia and abnormalities of *PDGFRA*, *PDGFRB*, or *FGR1*
- MPN with eosinophilia associated with *FIP1L1-PDGFRA* fusion gene
- MPN associated with *ETV6-PDGFRB* fusion gene or other rearrangement of *PDGFRB*
- Diagnostic criteria of MPN or acute leukemia associated with *FGFR1* rearrangement,

Chronic eosinophilic leukemia, NOS
1. Eosinophil count >1.5 × 10⁹/L
2. No Ph chromosome or *BCR-ABL* fusion gene or other MPNs or MDS/MPN
3. No t(5;12)(q31–q35;p13) or other rearrangement of *PDGFRB*
4. No *FIP1L1-PDGFRA* fusion gene or other rearrangement of *PDGFRA*
5. No rearrangement of *FGFR1*
6. The blast cell count in the peripheral blood and bone marrow <20% and no inv(16)(p13q22) or t(16;16)(p13;q22) or other feature diagnostic of AML
7. Clonal cytogenetic or molecular genetic abnormality, or blast cells are >2% in peripheral blood or >5% in bone marrow

Idiopathic hypereosinophilic syndrome
Exclusion of the following:
1. Reactive eosinophilia
2. Lymphocyte-variant hypereosinophilia (cytokine-producing, immunophenotypically aberrant T-cell population)
3. Chronic eosinophilic leukemia, NOS
4. WHO-defined myeloid malignancies associated eosinophilia (eg, MDS, MPNs, MDS/MPNs, or AML)
5. Eosinophilia-associated MPNs or AML/ALL with rearrangements of *PDGFRA*, *PDGFRB*, or *FGR1*

Secondary Eosinophilia

Infections
Parasitic: helminths; *Strongyloides stercoralis; Isospora belli; Sarcocystis hominis*; viral: human immunodeficiency virus and human T-cell leukemia virus; fungal: coccidiomycosis, *Aspergillus*

Allergy/atopy
Allergic rhinitis, asthma, atopic dermatitis, allergic bronchopulmonary aspergillosis, allergic gastroenteritis (with associated peripheral eosinophilia)

Drug reactions
Medications causing DIHS
- Anticonvulsants: carbamazepine, phenytoin, phenobarbital, lamotrigine, zonisamide
- Antimicrobials: metronidazole, piperacillin/tazobactam, ceftriaxone, nitrofurantoin, minocycline
- Antiretrovirals: abacavir, nevirapine
- Sulfonamides/sulfones: trimethoprim/sulfamethoxazole, dapsone, sulfasalazine
- Nonsteroidal anti-inflammatories: diclofenac, ibuprofen, naproxen
- Other: allopurinol, amitriptyline, fluoxetine
Medications causing organ-specific eosinophilic dysfunction
- Lung → Pulmonary infiltrates: sulfasalazine, nitrofurantoin, nonsteroidal anti-inflammatories
- Kidney → Acute interstitial nephritis: semisynthetic penicillins, cephalosporins, sulfonamides, phenytoin, cimetidine, nonsteroidal anti-inflammatories, allopurinol
- Gastrointestinal tract → Enterocolitis: nonsteroidal anti-inflammatories
- Hepatitis → Tetracyclines, penicillins
- Vasculitis → Allopurinol
- Asymptomatic eosinophilia → Penicillins, cephalosporins, quinine, fluoroquinolones

Systemic diseases
Churg-Strauss syndrome; granulomatosis with polyangiitis (Wegener); systemic lupus erythematosus; Crohn disease; polyarteritis nodosa; rheumatoid arthritis

Pulmonary eosinophilic diseases
Idiopathic acute or chronic eosinophilia pneumonia, tropical pulmonary eosinophilia; allergic bronchopulmonary aspergillosis, etc

Metabolic conditions such as adrenal insufficiency

Familial Eosinophilia (HE_F)

Hyper IgE syndrome

MIM	Gene	Inheritance
102582	*STAT3*	AD
611432	*DOCK8*	AR

Omenn Syndrome

MIM	Gene	Inheritance
605988	*DCLRE1C*	AR
179615	*RAG1*	AR
179616	*RAG2*	AR

Eosinophilic granulomatosis with polyangiitis (possible familial)

Eosinophilia, Unknown Significance (HE_US)

Eosinophilia-myalgia syndrome
- With giant cell myocarditis
- Associated with tryptophan ingestion,
- Toxic oil syndrome

Eosinophilic gastrointestinal disease
- Eosinophilic esophagitis when the eosinophilia is limited to the esophagus
- Eosinophilic gastritis if it is limited to the gastric tract
- Eosinophilic colitis if it is limited to the colon
- Eosinophilic gastroenteritis if the eosinophilia involves one or more parts of the gastrointestinal tract

Cytokine-associated angioedema syndromes (Gleich syndrome)
- Episodic angioedema with eosinophilia; increased IgM, IgE
- Nonepisodic angioedema with eosinophilia
- NERDS (nodules, eosinophilia, rheumatism, dermatitis, and swelling) syndrome; increased IgE

Abbreviations: AD, autosomal dominant; ALL, acute lymphoblastic leukemia; AML, acute myeloid leukemia; AR, autosomal recessive; DIHS, drug-induced hypersensitivity syndrome; Ig, immunoglobulin; MDS, myelodysplastic syndrome; MIM, Mendelian Inheritance in Man; MPN, myeloproliferative neoplasm; NOS, not otherwise specified; WHO, World Health Organization.

TABLE 46–12. Pathologic Features and Frequency of Symptoms in the Three Stages of Hypereosinophilic Syndrome

Acute Necrotic Stage	Thrombotic Stage	Fibrotic Stage
Myocarditis with eosinophilic and lymphocytic infiltration	Thrombus along damaged endocardium	Thrombi undergo organization, reabsorption and fibrosis, ending in endocardial scarring
Myocyte necrosis and apoptosis	Thrombi localize in the ventricular apex	Endocardial fibrosis involves the base of the heart
Possible rare microembolic phenomena	Thrombi can extend to the base of the heart and subvalvular regions	Fibrosis can involve valve structures with regurgitation
Symptoms: rare	Symptoms: possible embolic complications	Symptoms: the functional phenotype is diastolic dysfunction with restrictive pattern

In the thrombotic stage, mural thrombi develop on the endocardium. Mechanisms potentially explaining the endocardial thrombophilia include the release of antifibrinolytic mediators such as plasminogen activator inhibitor-2 and thrombomodulin-eosinophilic proteins that impair the anticoagulant property of the endocardial cells.[465] Thrombi most commonly involve the ventricular apex and further extend to subvalvular regions and, occasionally, to atria. Both echocardiography and CMR detect mural thrombi.[465,469] Thromboembolic complications occur in up to 30% of patients; oral anticoagulation is appropriate to prevent major embolic events. Antiplatelet therapy has also been proposed to prevent the formation of thrombi at the stage of eosinophilic myocarditis.

In the scarring, fibrotic stage both ventricles and subvalvular structures of the atrioventricular valves are involved. The functional phenotype is typically restrictive as in endomyocardial fibrosis. Echocardiography demonstrates regurgitation of the atrioventricular valves; spectral Doppler flow shows restrictive pattern. The severity of the endomyocardial fibrosis can be graded according to the combination of major and minor echocardiographic criteria.[469] CMR provides better profile of the endocardial diseases and confirms the diastolic dysfunction. The fibrotic state corresponds to an irreversible endomyocardial fibrosis.

Although surgery can be considered for releasing endocardium and subvalvular apparatus from fibrosis (as done in endomyocardial fibrosis), indications should be evaluated on individually tailored programs that consider cause, comorbidity, and complications. Heart transplantation has alternatively been proposed.[477,478]

Churg–Strauss Syndrome or Eosinophilic Granulomatosis with Polyangiitis

Churg-Strauss syndrome, recently renamed as EGPA,[450] is a systemic necrotizing vasculitis that affects small- to medium-sized vessels. The recommendations for the management of small- and medium-sized vessel vasculitides that apply to EGPA have recently been published.[479] Much progress has been made over the last 30 years in understanding, redefining, and treating systemic necrotizing vasculitis. EGPA belongs to the group of antineutrophil cytoplasmic antibody (ANCA)–associated vasculitides (AAV) and is characterized by blood and tissue eosinophilia and asthma, thus differing from granulomatosis with polyangiitis (Wegener) and microscopic polyangiitis. ANCA positivity ranges from 30% to 70% of EGPA patients, but is usually less frequently observed than in other AAV. Diagnostic and management algorithms for EGPA are summarized in **Table 46–13.**[479]

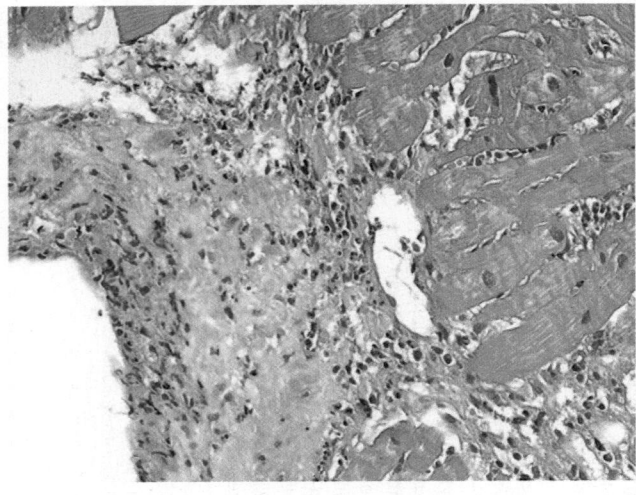

A

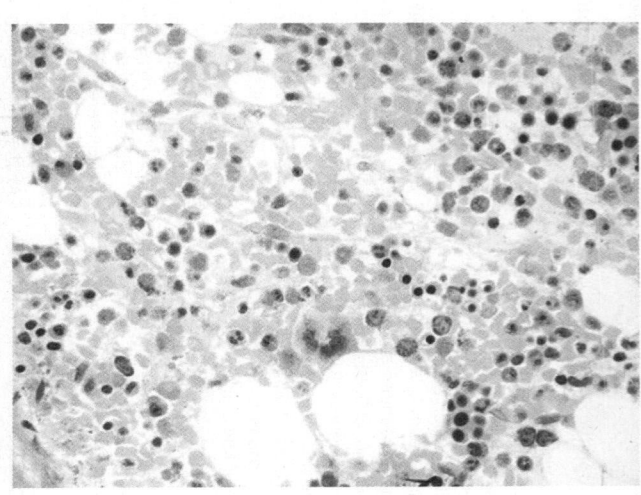

B

Figure 46–14. An endomyocardial biopsy sample (**A**) with interstitial and endocardial inflammatory infiltrates largely constituted of eosinophils. The patient had heart failure at onset and demonstrated hypereosinophilia; the patient was diagnosed with clonal, neoplastic, primary hypereosinophilia (HE_N) (*PDGFRA/B* rearrangement). (**B**) Bone marrow biopsy demonstrating a high number of eosinophilic granulocytes.

TABLE 46–13. Churg-Strauss Syndrome or Eosinophilic Granulomatosis with Polyangiitis

The EGPA Consensus Task Force Recommendations	Level of Evidence
1. EGPA should be managed in collaboration with, or in, centers with established expertise in the management of small and medium-sized vessel vasculitides.	NA
2. Recommended: Serologic testing for toxocariasis and HIV, specific IgE and IgG dosages for *Aspergillus* spp, search for *Aspergillus* spp on a sputum and/or bronchoalveolar lavage fluid, tryptase and vitamin B$_{12}$ dosages, peripheral blood smear (looking for dysplastic eosinophils or blasts), and chest CT scan are the minimal initial differential diagnosis workup; additional investigations should be guided by patient-specific clinical findings, and extensive search for causes of hypereosinophilia should be considered.	NA
3. Obtaining biopsies from patients with suspected EGPA is encouraged.	NA
4. ANCA testing (with indirect immunofluorescence and ELISA) should be done for patients with suspected EGPA.	NA
5. There is currently no reliable biomarker to measure EGPA activity.	NA
6. Once EGPA is diagnosed, evaluating possible lung, kidney, heart, GI, and/or peripheral nerve involvement is recommended.	NA
7. Definition of EGPA remission: The absence of a clinical systemic manifestation (excluding asthma and/or ENT).	NA
8. Definition of EGPA relapse: The new appearance or recurrence or worsening of clinical EGPA manifestation(s) (excluding asthma and/or ENT) requiring the addition, change, or dose increase of glucocorticoids and/or other immunosuppressants.	NA
9. Use of glucocorticoids is appropriate to achieve EGPA remission; the dose prescribed should be ~1 mg/kg/d of prednisone for patients with organ- or life-threatening manifestations.	A
10. Patients with life- and/or organ-threatening disease manifestations (ie, heart, GI, central nervous system, severe peripheral neuropathy, severe ocular disease, alveolar hemorrhage, and/or glomerulonephritis) should be treated with a remission-induction regimen combining glucocorticoids and an additional immunosuppressant (eg, cyclophosphamide).	B
11. Maintenance therapy (with azathioprine or methotrexate) is recommended for patients with life- and/or organ-threatening disease manifestations on a remission-induction therapeutic regimen.	C
12. Glucocorticoids alone may be suitable for patients without life- and/or organ-threatening disease manifestations; additional immunosuppression can be considered for selected patients for whom the prednisone dose cannot be tapered to 7.5 mg/d after 3-4 months of therapy or patients with recurrent disease.	C
13. Plasma exchanges are generally not effective in EGPA, but can be considered for selected patients with ANCA and rapidly progressive glomerulonephritis or pulmonary-renal syndrome.	D
14. Rituximab can be considered for selected ANCA-positive patients with renal involvement or refractory disease.	C
15. IVIG can be considered a second-line therapy for patients on glucocorticoids (and/or other immunosuppressants) with EGPA flares refractory to other treatments or during pregnancy; in the context of drug-induced hypogammaglobulinemia with severe and/or recurrent infections, Ig replacement may be considered.	C
16. Interferon-α may be reserved as a second- or third-line drug for selected patients.	C
17. LRA can be prescribed, if needed, for EGPA patients.	B
18. Vaccinations with inactivated vaccines and against influenza and pneumococci should be encouraged; live-attenuated vaccines are contraindicated in patients taking immunosuppressants and/or ≥ 20 mg/d of prednisone.	D
19. Implementation of patient educational programs is encouraged.	D
20. Patients with peripheral nerve involvement and motor deficit(s) should routinely be referred to a physiotherapist.	D
21. Patients should be advised to avoid tobacco smoke and irritants.	D
22. Venous thromboembolic events and pulmonary embolism should be treated according to general guidelines for the management of thromboembolic disease; it is unknown whether anticoagulation should be prolonged in selected patients with persistent or recurring disease activity.	D

Abbreviations: ANCA, antineutrophil cytoplasm antibody; CT, computed tomography; EGPA, eosinophilic granulomatosis with polyangiitis (Churg-Strauss); ELISA, enzyme-linked immunosorbent assays; ENT, ear, nose, and throat; GI, gastrointestinal; HIV, human immunodeficiency virus; Ig, immunoglobulin; IVIG, intravenous immunoglobulins; LRA, leukotriene receptor antagonists; NA, not applicable.

SUMMARY

The term myocarditis remains fundamental to describe myocardial inflammation, but does not specifically describe phenotype and etiologies. The recent advancements in the identification of the different causes of myocarditis; the novel emerging infectious diseases, and drug-resistant infections; the reclassification of syndromes such as eosinophilic diseases; and the recent discovery of "monogenic" myocarditis and autoinflammatory diseases challenge cardiologists in their diagnostic work-up, when deciding about performing EMB, progressing from echocardiography to advanced molecular imaging, or establishing target treatments. The individual history, family history, imaging, biomarkers, and molecular tests flanking the conventional infectious work-up to identify the genome of the pathogens are now necessary for a complete diagnostic work-up in infectious myocarditis. Different forms of noninfectious myocarditis and autoimmune or toxic diseases with myocarditis need to be supported by specific diagnostic algorithms. The clear distinction of the different forms of myocarditis would help generate reliable epidemiology data and bases for precise nosology and classification.

Diagnosis

- The descriptive diagnosis of myocarditis encompasses a wide spectrum of etiologically different diseases that share, as unique criterion, the pathologically proven evidence of myocardial inflammation.
- The definition does not specify the inflammatory burden, the immunophenotype of inflammatory cells and the cause.
- In clinics, the formulation of a diagnosis of myocarditis implies that the observed cardiac phenotype is attributable to the inflammation of the myocardium.

Pathophysiology

- Myocarditis can occur in immunocompetent and immunodeficient hosts and be infectious, noninfectious (autoimmune, immune-mediated, or auto-inflammatory), and toxic. Infectious causes include DNA and RNA viruses, bacteria, fungi, protozoa, and helminths.
- The most common causes of infectious myocarditis in both children and adults are cardiotropic viruses, such as enteroviruses.
- In immunocompetent individuals residing in endemic areas, major nonviral infections include *Trypanosoma cruzi* (Chagas disease) and *Borrelia burgdorferi* (Lyme disease), while in immunocompromised patients, typically heart transplant recipients, the most common opportunistic infections include the human cytomegalovirus (HCMV) and *Toxoplasma gondii*.

Presentation and Investigations

- The clinically heterogeneous presentation ranges from acute fulminant manifestations to acute heart failure and cardiac rhythm disturbances.
- The diagnostic work-up is based on the clinical presentation, noninvasive imaging, biomarkers of inflammation and myocyte damage, endomyocardial biopsy, serology, and molecular test for the suspected infectious agent.

Treatment and Prognosis

- Treatment depends on the severity of the clinical manifestations, ranging from circulatory support in ICU, to management for acute heart failure and conduction rhythm disturbances, both arrhythmias and conduction defects.
- The target treatments are used for specific infectious agents, when their presence is proven. Steroids, Immunoglobulin, can be administered in noninfectious myocarditis.
- The course of the disease is benign in most cases; fatal evolution or the need for heart transplant is uncommon. Finally, the acute phase can be followed by chronic evolution through a DCM-like phenotype that demonstrates outcome similar to that of DCM.

REFERENCES

1. Fung G, Luo H, Qiu Y, Yang D, McManus B. Myocarditis. *Circ Res.* 2016;118(3):496-514.
2. Aretz HT, Billingham ME, Edwards WD, et al. Myocarditis: a histopathologic definition and classification. *Am J Cardiovasc Pathol.* 1987;1:3-14.
3. Richardson P, McKenna W, Bristow M, et al. Report of the 1995 World Health Organization/International Society and Federation of Cardiology Task Force on the Definition and Classification of cardiomyopathies. *Circulation.* 1996;93:841-842.
4. Caforio AL, Pankuweit S, Arbustini E, et al. European Society of Cardiology Working Group on Myocardial and Pericardial Diseases. Current state of knowledge on aetiology, diagnosis, management, and therapy of myocarditis: a position statement of the European Society of Cardiology Working Group on Myocardial and Pericardial Diseases. *Eur Heart J.* 2013;34:2636-2648.
5. Stanaway JD, Roth G. The burden of Chagas disease: estimates and challenges. *Glob Heart.* 2015;10:139-144.
6. Chomel B. Lyme disease. *Rev Sci Tech.* 2015;34:569-576.
7. Banoo S, Bell D, Bossuyt P, et al. TDR Diagnostics Evaluation Expert Panel. Evaluation of diagnostic tests for infectious diseases: general principles. *Nat Rev Microbiol.* 2010;8:S17-S29.
8. Rostoff P, Nessler B, Pikul P, et al. Fulminant adrenergic myocarditis complicated by pulmonary edema, cardiogenic shock and cardiac arrest. *Am J Emerg Med.* 2018;36(2):344.e1-e344.e4
9. Bissel SJ, Winkler CC, DelTondo J, et al. Coxsackievirus B4 myocarditis and meningoencephalitis in newborn twins. *Neuropathology.* 2014;34(5):429-437.
10. Amdani SM, Kim HS, Orvedahl A, et al. Successful treatment of fulminant neonatal enteroviral myocarditis in monochorionic diamniotic twins with cardiopulmonary support, intravenous immunoglobulin and pocapavir. *BMJ Case Rep.* 2018;2018:bcr2017224133.
11. Leone O, Veinot JP, Angelini A, et al. 2011 consensus statement on endomyocardial biopsy from the Association for European Cardiovascular Pathology and the Society for Cardiovascular Pathology. *Cardiovasc Pathol.* 2012;21:245-274.
12. Temme S, Bönner F, Schrader J, et al. 19F magnetic resonance imaging of endogenous macrophages in inflammation. *Nanomed Nanobiotechnol.* 2012;4:329-343.
13. Zhorne D, Petit CJ, Ing FF, et al. A 25-year experience of endomyocardial biopsy safety in infants. *Catheter Cardiovasc Interv.* 2013;82:797-801.
14. Baughman KL. Diagnosis of myocarditis: death of Dallas criteria. *Circulation.* 2006;113:593-595.
15. Mason JW, O'Connell JB, Herskowitz A, et al. A clinical trial of immunosuppressive therapy for myocarditis. The Myocarditis Treatment Trial Investigators. *N Engl J Med.* 1995;333:269-275.
16. Sasko B, Patschan D, Nordbeck P, et al. Secondary prevention of potentially life-threatening arrhythmia using implantable cardioverter defibrillators in patients with biopsy-proven viral myocarditis and preserved ejection fraction. *Cardiology.* 2021:146(2):213-221.
17. Haanschoten DM, Adiyaman A, 't Hart NA, et al. Value of 3D mapping-guided endomyocardial biopsy in cardiac sarcoidosis: Case series and narrative review on the value of electro-anatomic mapping-guided endomyocardial biopsies. *Eur J Clin Invest.* 2021;51(4):e13497.
18. Bohné M, Chung DU, Tigges E, et al. Short-term use of "ECMELLA" in the context of fulminant eosinophilic myocarditis with cardiogenic shock. *BMC Cardiovasc Disord.* 2020;20(1):519.
19. Zhou Z, Ortiz Lopez HIA, Pérez GE, et al. Toxoplasmosis and the Heart. *Curr Probl Cardiol.* 2021;46(3):100741.
20. Kraus SM, Shaboodien G, Francis V, et al. Rationale and design of the African Cardiomyopathy and Myocarditis Registry Program: The IMHOTEP study. *Int J Cardiol.* 2021:S0167-5273(21)00279-5.
21. GBD 2017 Disease and Injury Incidence and Prevalence Collaborators. Global, regional, and national incidence, prevalence, and years lived with

disability for 354 diseases and injuries for 195 countries and territories, 1990–2017: a systematic analysis for the Global Burden of Disease Study 2017. *Lancet.* 2018;392:1789–1858.

22. Dai H, Lotan D, Much AA, et al. Global, regional, and national burden of myocarditis and cardiomyopathy, 1990-2017. *Front Cardiovasc Med.* 2021;8:610989.

23. Wakafuji S, Okada R. Twenty year autopsy statistics of myocarditis incidence in Japan. *Jpn Circ J.* 1986;50:1288-1293.

24. Passarino G, Burlo P, Ciccone G, et al. Prevalence of myocarditis at autopsy in Turin, Italy. *Arch Pathol Lab Med.* 1997;121:619-622.

25. Zhang M, Tavora F, Zhang Y, et al. The role of focal myocardial inflammation in sudden unexpected cardiac and noncardiac deaths-a clinicopathological study. *Int J Legal Med.* 2013;127:131-138.

26. Arness MK, Eckart RE, Love SS, et al. Myopericarditis following smallpox vaccination. *Am J Epidemiol.* 2004;160:642-651.

27. Maron BJ, Levine BD, Washington RL, et al. American Heart Association Electrocardiography and Arrhythmias Committee of the Council on Clinical Cardiology, Council on Cardiovascular Disease in the Young, Council on Cardiovascular and Stroke Nursing, Council on Functional Genomics and Translational Biology, and the American College of Cardiology. Eligibility and disqualification recommendations for competitive athletes with cardiovascular abnormalities: Task Force 2: preparticipation screening for cardiovascular disease in competitive athletes: a scientific statement from the American Heart Association and American College of Cardiology. *Circulation.* 2015;132:e267-e272.

28. Karjalainen J, Heikkilä J. Incidence of three presentations of acute myocarditis in young men in military service. A 20-year experience. *Eur Heart J.* 1999;20:1120-1125.

29. Hufnagel G, Pankuweit S, Richter A, et al. The European Study of Epidemiology and Treatment of Cardiac Inflammatory Diseases (ESETCID). First epidemiological results. *Herz.* 2000;25:279-285.

30. Kytö V, Sipilä J, Rautava P. Gender differences in myocarditis: a nationwide study in Finland. *Eur Heart J.* 2013;34:3505-3505.

31. Kytö V, Sipilä J, Rautava P. Acute myocardial infarction or acute myocarditis? Discharge registry-based study of likelihood and associated features in hospitalised patients. *BMJ Open.* 2015;5:e007555.

32. Saji T, Matsuura H, Hasegawa K, et al. Comparison of the clinical presentation, treatment, and outcome of fulminant and acute myocarditis in children. *Circ J.* 2012;76:1222-1228.

33. Durani Y, Egan M, Baffa J, et al. Pediatric myocarditis: presenting clinical characteristics. *Am J Emerg Med.* 2009;27:942-947.

34. Amabile N, Fraisse A, Bouvenot J, et al. Outcome of acute fulminant myocarditis in children. *Heart.* 2006;92:1269-1273.

35. Teutsch SM, Zurynski YA, Nunez C, et al. Ten years of national seasonal surveillance for severe complications of influenza in Australian children. *Pediatr Infect Dis J.* 2021;40(3):191-198.

36. Putschoegl A, Auerbach S. Diagnosis, evaluation, and treatment of myocarditis in children. *Pediatr Clin North Am.* 2020;67(5):855-874.

37. Kim J, Cho MJ. Acute Myocarditis in Children: a 10-year Nationwide Study (2007-2016) based on the Health Insurance Review and Assessment Service Database in Korea. *Korean Circ J.* 2020;50(11):1013-1022.

38. Heidt T, Courties G, Dutta P, et al. Differential contribution of monocytes to heart macrophages in steady-state and after myocardial infarction. *Circ Res.* 2014;115(2):284-95.

39. Pinto AR, Paolicelli R, Salimova E, et al. An abundant tissue macrophage population in the adult murine heart with a distinct alternatively-activated macrophage profile. *PLoS One.* 2012;7(5):e36814.

40. Nicolás-Ávila JA, Lechuga-Vieco AV, Esteban-Martínez L, et al. A network of macrophages supports mitochondrial homeostasis in the heart. *Cell.* 2020;183(1):94-109.e23

41. Epelman S, Lavine KJ, Beaudin AE, et al. Embryonic and adult-derived resident cardiac macrophages are maintained through distinct mechanisms at steady state and during inflammation. *Immunity.* 2014;40:91-104.

42. Molawi K, Wolf Y, Kandalla PK, et al. Progressive replacement of embryo-derived cardiac macrophages with age. *J Exp Med.* 2014;211(11):2151-2158.

43. Gomez I, Duval V, Silvestre JS. Cardiomyocytes and macrophages discourse on the method to govern cardiac repair. *Front Cardiovasc Med.* 2018;5:134.

44. Monnerat G, Alarcón ML, Vasconcellos LR, et al. Macrophage-dependent IL-1β production induces cardiac arrhythmias in diabetic mice. *Nat Commun.* 2016;7:13344.

45. Epelman S, Liu PP, Mann DL. Role of innate and adaptive immune mechanisms in cardiac injury and repair. *Nat Rev Immunol.* 2015;15(2):117-129.

46. Bruno KA, Mathews JE, Yang AL, et al. BPA alters estrogen receptor expression in the heart after viral infection activating cardiac mast cells and T cells leading to perimyocarditis and fibrosis. *Front Endocrinol (Lausanne).* 2019;10:598.

47. Johnson DB, Balko JM, Compton ML, et al. Fulminant myocarditis with combination immune checkpoint blockade. *N Engl J Med.* 2016;375(18):1749-1755.

48. Wroblewski M, Bauer R, Cubas Córdova M, et al. Mast cells decrease efficacy of anti-angiogenic therapy by secreting matrix-degrading granzyme B. *Nat Commun.* 2017;8(1):269.

49. Arbustini E, Gavazzi A, Pozzi R, et al. Endomyocardial biopsy of normal donor hearts before cardiac transplantation. A morphological and morphometrical study in 97 cases. *Am J Cardiovasc Pathol.* 1992;4:1-8.

50. Kindermann I, Barth C, Mahfoud F, et al. Update on myocarditis. *J Am Coll Cardiol.* 2012;59:779-792.

51. Klingel K, Sauter M, Bock CT, Szalay G, Schnorr JJ, Kandolf R. Molecular pathology of inflammatory cardiomyopathy. *Med Microbiol Immunol.* 2004;193:101-107.

52. Adams Waldorf KM, McAdams RM. Influence of infection during pregnancy on fetal development. *Reproduction.* 2013;146:R151-162.

53. Fornara C, Furione M, Lilleri D, et al. Primary human cytomegalovirus infections: kinetics of ELISA-IgG and neutralizing antibody in pauci/asymptomatic pregnant women vs symptomatic non-pregnant subjects. *J Clin Virol.* 2015;64:45-51.

54. Yang L, He D, Tang M, et al. Development of an enzyme-linked immunosorbent spot assay to measure serum-neutralizing antibodies against coxsackievirus B3. *Clin Vaccine Immunol.* 2014;21:312-320.

55. Thiene G, Bruneval P, Veinot J, Leone O. Diagnostic use of the endomyocardial biopsy: a consensus statement. *Virchows Arch.* 2013;463:1-5.

56. Heidecker B, Kittleson MM, Kasper EK, et al. Transcriptomic biomarkers for the accurate diagnosis of myocarditis. *Circulation.* 2011;123:1174-1184.

57. Garmaroudi FS, Marchant D, Hendry R, et al. Coxsackievirus B3 replication and pathogenesis. *Future Microbiol.* 2015;10:629-653.

58. Shi Y, Chen C, Lisewski U, et al. Cardiac deletion of the coxsackievirus-adenovirus receptor abolishes coxsackievirus B3 infection and prevents myocarditis in vivo. *J Am Coll Cardiol.* 2009;53:1219-1226.

59. Noutsias M, Fechner H, de Jonge H, et al. Human coxsackie-adenovirus receptor is colocalized with integrins alpha(v)beta(3) and alpha(v)beta(5) on the cardiomyocyte sarcolemma and upregulated in dilated cardiomyopathy: implications for cardiotropic viral infections. *Circulation.* 2001;104:275-280.

60. Jagdeo JM, Dufour A, Fung G, et al. Heterogeneous nuclear ribonucleoprotein M facilitates enterovirus infection. *J Virol.* 2015;89:7064-7078.

61. Alirezaei M, Flynn CT, Wood MR, et al. Coxsackievirus can exploit LC3 in both autophagy-dependent and independent manners in vivo. *Autophagy.* 2015;11:1389-1407.

62. Robinson SM, Tsueng G, Sin J, et al. Coxsackievirus B exits the host cell in shed microvesicles displaying autophagosomal markers. *PLoS Pathog.* 2014;10:e1004045.

63. Hemida MG, Ye X, Zhang HM, et al. MicroRNA-203 enhances coxsackievirus B3 replication through targeting zinc finger protein-148. *Cell Mol Life Sci.* 2013;70:277-291.

64. Corsten MF, Papageorgiou A, Verhesen W, et al. MicroRNA profiling identifies microRNA-155 as an adverse mediator of cardiac injury and dysfunction during acute viral myocarditis. *Circ Res.* 2012;111:415-425.

65. Wang C, Wong J, Fung G, et al. Dysferlin deficiency confers increased susceptibility to coxsackievirus-induced cardiomyopathy. *Cell Microbiol.* 2015;17:1423-1430.

66. Badorff C, Lee GH, Lamphear BJ, et al. Enteroviral protease 2A cleaves dystrophin: evidence of cytoskeletal disruption in an acquired cardiomy-opathy. *Nat Med.* 1999;5:320-326.

67. Xiong D, Lee GH, Badorff C, et al. Dystrophin deficiency markedly increases enterovirus- induced cardiomyopathy: a genetic predisposition to viral heart disease. *Nat Med.* 2002;8:872-877.

68. Diegoli M, Grasso M, Favalli V, et al. Diagnostic work-up and risk strat-ification in X-linked dilated cardiomyopathies caused by dystrophin defects. *J Am Coll Cardiol.* 2011;58:925-934.

69. Knowlton KU. CBV infection and mechanisms of viral cardiomyopathy. *Curr Top Microbiol Immunol.* 2008;323:315-335.

70. Gorbea C, Makar KA, Pauschinger M, et al. A role for toll-like receptor 3 variants in host susceptibility to enteroviral myocarditis and dilated car-diomyopathy. *J Biol Chem.* 2010;285:23208-23223.

71. Abston ED, Coronado MJ, Bucek A, et al. TLR3 deficiency induces chronic inflammatory cardiomyopathy in resistant mice following cox-sackievirus B3 infection: role for IL-4. *Am J Physiol Regul Integr Comp Physiol.* 2013;304:R267-R277.

72. Martinez NE, Sato F, Kawai E, et al. Regulatory T cells and Th17 cells in viral infections: implications for multiple sclerosis and myocarditis. *Future Virol.* 2012;7:593-608.

73. Opavsky MA, Penninger J, Aitken K, et al. Susceptibility to myocarditis is dependent on the response of alphabeta T lymphocytes to coxsackieviral infection. *Circ Res.* 1999;85:551-558.

74. Rose NR. Learning from myocarditis: mimicry, chaos and black holes. *F1000Prime Rep.* 2014;6:25.

75. Arbustini E, Porcu E, Bellini O, et al. Enteroviral infection causing fatal myocarditis and subclinical myopathy. *Heart.* 2000;83:86-90.

76. Arbustini E, Grasso M, Porcu E, et al. Enteroviral RNA and virus-like particles in the skeletal muscle of patients with idiopathic dilated cardio-myopathy. *Am J Cardiol.* 1997;80:1188-1193.

77. Rogo LD, Mokhtari-Azad T, Kabir MH, Rezaei F. Human parvovirus B19: a review. *Acta Virol.* 2014;58:199-213.

78. Kerr JR. A review of blood diseases and cytopenias associated with human parvovirus B19 infection. *Rev Med Virol.* 2015;25:224-240.

79. Adamson-Small LA, Ignatovich IV, Laemmerhirt MG, et al. Persistent parvovirus B19 infection in non-erythroid tissues: possible role in the inflammatory and disease process. *Virus Res.* 2014;190:8-16.

80. Hu HY, Wei SY, Huang WH, Pan CH. Fatal parvovirus B19 infections: a report of two autopsy cases. *Int J Legal Med.* 2019;133(2):553-560.

81. Von Kietzell K, Pozzuto T, Heilbronn R, et al. Antibody-mediated enhancement of parvovirus B19 uptake into endothelial cells mediated by a receptor for complement factor C1q. *J Virol.* 2014;88:8102-8115.

82. Tschope C, Müller I, Xia Y, et al. NOD2 (nucleotide-binding oligomer-ization domain 2) is a major pathogenic mediator of coxsackievirus B3 induced myocarditis. *Circ Heart Fail.* 2017;10(9):e003870

83. Luo Y, Qiu J. Human parvovirus B19: a mechanistic overview of infection and DNA replication. *Future Virol.* 2015;10:155-167.

84. Ganaie SS, Chen AY, Huang C, et al. RNA binding protein RBM38 reg-ulates expression of the 11-kilodalton protein of parvovirus B19, which facilitates viral DNA replication. *J Virol.* 2018;92(8):e02050-17.

85. Lyoo H, van der Schaar HM, Dorobantu CM, et al. ACBD3 Is an essential pan-enterovirus host factor that mediates the interaction between viral 3A protein and cellular protein PI4KB. *mBio.* 2019;10(1):e02742-18.

86. Moimas S, Zacchigna S, Merlo M. Idiopathic dilated cardiomyopathy and persistent viral infection: lack of association in a controlled study using a quantitative assay. *Heart Lung Circ.* 2012;21:787-793.

87. Schenk T, Enders M, Pollak S, et al. High prevalence of human parvovirus B19 DNA in myocardial autopsy samples from subjects without myocar-ditis or dilative cardiomyopathy. *J Clin Microbiol.* 2009;47:106-110.

88. Rigopoulos AG, Klutt B, Matiakis M, et al. Systematic review of PCR proof of parvovirus B19 genomes in endomyocardial biopsies of patients presenting with myocarditis or dilated cardiomyopathy. *Viruses.* 2019;11(6):566.

89. Kerr JR. The role of parvovirus B19 in the pathogenesis of autoimmunity and autoimmune disease. *J Clin Pathol.* 2016;69(4):279-291.

90. Koliou M, Karaoli E, Soteriades ES, et al. Acute hepatitis and myositis associated with erythema infectiosum by parvovirus B19 in an adoles-cent. *BMC Pediatr.* 2014;14:6.

91. Page C, Duverlie G, Sevestre H, et al. Erythrovirus B19 and autoimmune thyroid diseases. Review of the literature and pathophysiological hypoth-eses. *J Med Virol.* 2015;87:162-169.

92. Cavigelli-Brunner A, Schweiger M, Knirsch W, et al. VAD as bridge to recovery in anthracycline-induced cardiomyopathy and HHV6 myocar-ditis. *Pediatrics.* 2014;134:e894-9.

93. Ashrafpoor G, Andréoletti L, Bruneval P, et al. Fulminant human her-pesvirus 6 myocarditis in an immunocompetent adult: role of car-diac magnetic resonance in a multidisciplinary approach. *Circulation.* 2013;128:e445-e447.

94. Leveque N, Boulagnon C, Brasselet C, et al. A fatal case of human herpes-virus 6 chronic myocarditis in an immunocompetent adult. *J Clin Virol.* 2011;52:142-145.

95. Brennan Y, Gottlieb DJ, Baewer D, et al. A fatal case of acute HHV-6 myocarditis following allogeneic haemopoietic stem cell transplantation. *J Clin Virol.* 2015;72:82-84.

96. Stefanski HE, Thibert KA, Pritchett J, et al. Fatal myocarditis associated with HHV-6 following immunosuppression in two children. *Pediatrics.* 2016;137:1-4.

97. Horovitz A, El ZI, Valentino R, et al. How an Ebstein-Barr virus may induce acute fulminant myocarditis in a young immunocompetent adult: a case report. *West Indian Med J.* 2012;61:640-642.

98. Heydari H, Mamishi S, Khotaei GT, et al. Fatal type 7 adenovirus asso-ciated with human bocavirus infection in a healthy child. *J Med Virol.* 2011;83:1762-1763.

99. Yamamoto T, Kenzaka T, Matsumoto M, et al. A case report of myocarditis combined with hepatitis caused by herpes simplex virus. *BMC Cardiovasc Disord.* 2018;18(1):134.

100. Poole E, Sinclair J. Sleepless latency of human cytomegalovirus. *Med Microbiol Immunol.* 2015;204:421-429.

101. Scherger S, Mathur S, Bajrovic V, et al. Cytomegalovirus myocarditis in solid organ transplant recipients: a case series and review of literature. *Transpl Infect Dis.* 2020;22(3):e13282.

102. Perez Romero P, Blanco P, Gimenez E, et al. An update on the manage-ment and prevention of cytomegalovirus infection following allogeneic hematopoietic stem cell transplantation. *Future Virol.* 2015;10:113-134.

103. Kotton CN, Kumar D, Caliendo AM, et al. The third international con-sensus guidelines on the management of cytomegalovirus in solid-organ transplantation. *Transplantation.* 2018;102:900-931.

104. Ljungman P, de la Camara R, Robin C, et al. 2017 European Conference on Infections in Leukaemia group. Guidelines for the management of cytomegalovirus infection in patients with haematological malignancies and after stem cell transplantation from the 2017 European Conference on Infections in Leukaemia (ECIL 7). *Lancet Infect Dis.* 2019;19(8):e260-e272.

105. Ozdemir R, Kucuk M, Dibeklioglu SE. Report of a myocarditis outbreak among pediatric patients: human herpesvirus 7 as a causative agent? *J Trop Pediatr.* 2018;64(6):468-471.

106. Vigant F, Santos NC, Lee B. Broad-spectrum antivirals against viral fusion. *Nat Rev Microbiol.* 2015;13:426-437.

107. Gonçalves BC, Lopes Barbosa MG, Silva Olak AP, et al. Antiviral ther-apies: advances and perspectives. *Fundam Clin Pharmacol.* 2020. doi:10.1111/fcp.12609.

108. Gerna G, Lilleri D, Baldanti F. An overview of letermovir: a cytomegalovirus prophylactic option. *Expert Opin Pharmacother.* 2019;20(12):1429-1438.

109. Komaroff AL, Zerr DM, Flamand L. Summary of the 11th international conference on human herpesviruses-6A, -6B, and -7. *J Med Virol.* 2020;92:4-10.

110. Hill JA. Human herpesvirus 6 in transplant recipients: an update on diagnostic and treatment strategies. *Curr Opin Infect Dis.* 2019;32(6):584-590.

111. Petit V, Bonnafous P, Fages V, et al. Donor-to-recipient transmission and reactivation in a kidney transplant recipient of an inherited chromosomally integrated HHV-6A: Evidence and outcomes. *Am J Transplant.* 2020;20(12):3667-3672.

112. Bonnafous P, Marlet J, Bouvet D, et al. Fatal outcome after reactivation of inherited chromosomally integrated HHV-6A (iciHHV-6A) transmitted through liver transplantation. *Am J Transplant.* 2018;18(6):1548-1551.

113. Pugni L, Pietrasanta C, Ronchi A, et al. Inherited chromosomally integrated human herpesvirus 6: an unexpected finding in a septic neonate. *Pediatr Infect Dis J.* 2021;40(1):74-75.

114. Kawamura Y, Hashimoto T, Miura H, et al. Inherited chromosomally integrated human herpesvirus 6 and autoimmune connective tissue diseases. *J Clin Virol.* 2020;132:104656.

115. Kühl U, Lassner D, Wallaschek N, et al. Chromosomally integrated human herpesvirus 6 in heart failure: prevalence and treatment. *Eur J Heart Fail.* 2015;17(1):9-19.

116. Nguyen AB, Chung BB, Sayer G, et al. Acute Myocarditis Secondary to Reactivated Chromosomally-Integrated Human Herpesvirus 6. *J Card Fail.* 2017;23(7):576-577.

117. Yoshikawa T, Ihira M, Suzuki K, et al. Fatal acute myocarditis in an infant with human herpesvirus 6 infection. *J Clin Pathol.* 2001;54(10):792-5.

118. Ablashi D, Agut H, Alvarez-Lafuente R, et al. Classification of HHV-6A and HHV-6B as distinct viruses. *Arch Virol.* 2014;159(5):863-870.

119. Yamanishi K, Okuno T, Shiraki K, et al. Identification of human herpesvirus-6 as a causal agent for exanthem subitum. *Lancet.* 1988;1(8594):1065-1067.

120. Hall CB, Long CE, Schnabel KC, et al. Human herpesvirus-6 infection in children. A prospective study of complications and reactivation. *N Engl J Med.* 1994;331(7):432-438.

121. Bates M, Monze M, Bima H, et al. Predominant human herpesvirus 6 variant A infant infections in an HIV-1 endemic region of Sub-Saharan Africa. *J Med Virol.* 2009;81(5):779-789.

122. Arbuckle JH, Medveczky MM, Luka J, et al. The latent human herpesvirus-6A genome specifically integrates in telomeres of human chromosomes in vivo and in vitro. *Proc Natl Acad Sci U S A.* 2010;107(12):5563-5568.

123. Osterrieder N, Wallaschek N, Kaufer BB. Herpesvirus genome integration into telomeric repeats of host cell chromosomes. *Annu Rev Virol.* 2014;1(1):215-235.

124. Tanaka-Taya K, Sashihara J, Kurahashi H, et al. Human herpesvirus 6 (HHV-6) is transmitted from parent to child in an integrated form and characterization of cases with chromosomally integrated HHV-6 DNA. *J Med Virol.* 2004;73(3):465-473.

125. Collin V, Flamand L. HHV-6A/B integration and the pathogenesis associated with the reactivation of chromosomally integrated HHV-6A/B. *Viruses.* 2017;9(7):160.

126. Zhang E, Bell AJ, Wilkie GS, et al. Inherited chromosomally integrated human herpesvirus 6 genomes are ancient, intact, and potentially able to reactivate from telomeres. *J Virol.* 2017;91(22):e01137-17.

127. Hall CB, Caserta MT, Schnabel K, et al. Chromosomal integration of human herpesvirus 6 is the major mode of congenital human herpesvirus 6 infection. *Pediatrics.* 2008;122(3):513-520.

128. Vairo F, Haider N, Kock R, et al. Chikungunya: epidemiology, pathogenesis, clinical features, management, and prevention. *Infect Dis Clin North Am.* 2019;33(4):1003-1025.

129. Bai C, Hao J, Li S, et al. Myocarditis and heart function impairment occur in neonatal mice following in utero exposure to the Zika virus. *J Cell Mol Med.* 2021;25(5):2730-2733.

130. Aletti M, Lecoules S, Kanczuga V, et al. Transient myocarditis associated with acute Zika virus infection. *Clin Infect Dis.* 2017;64(5):678-679.

131. Kularatne SAM, Rajapakse MM, Ralapanawa U, et al. Heart and liver are infected in fatal cases of dengue: three PCR based case studies. *BMC Infect Dis.* 2018;18(1):681.

132. Scatularo CE, Ballesteros OA, Saldarriaga C, et al. Neglected tropical diseases and other infectious diseases affecting the heart (NET-Heart project). Zika & heart: a systematic review. *Trends Cardiovasc Med.* 2020:S1050-1738(20)30147-X.

133. Schultheiss HP, Piper C, Sowade O, et al. Betaferon in chronic viral cardiomyopathy (BICC) trial: Effects of interferon-β treatment in patients with chronic viral cardiomyopathy. *Clin Res Cardiol.* 2016;105(9):763-773.

134. Kuhl U, Pauschinger M, Seeberg B, et al. Viral persistence in the myocardium is associated with progressive cardiac dysfunction. *Circulation.* 2005;112:1965-1970.

135. Kuhl U, Lassner D, von Schlippenback J, et al. Interferon-beta improves survival in enterovirus-associated cardiomyopathy. *J Am Coll Cardiol.* 2012;60:1295-1296.

136. Cihakova D, Rose NR. Pathogenesis of myocarditis and dilated cardiomyopathy. *Adv Immunol.* 2008;99:95-114.

137. Anzini M, Merlo M, Sabbadini G, et al. Long-term evolution and prognostic stratification of biopsy-proven active myocarditis. *Circulation.* 2013;128:2384-2394.

138. Caforio AL, Calabrese F, Angelini A, et al. A prospective study of biopsy-proven myocarditis: prognostic relevance of clinical and aetiopathogenetic features at diagnosis. *Eur Heart J.* 2007;28(11):1326-1333.

139. Kindermann I, Kindermann M, Kandolf R, et al. Predictors of outcome in patients with suspected myocarditis. *Circulation.* 2008;118:639-648.

140. Grün S, Schumm J, Greulich S, et al. Long-term follow-up of biopsy-proven viral myocarditis: predictors of mortality and incomplete recovery. *J Am Coll Cardiol.* 2012;59(18):1604-1615.

141. Ammirati E, Veronese G, Brambatti M, et al. Fulminant versus acute non-fulminant myocarditis in patients with left ventricular systolic dysfunction. *J Am Coll Cardiol.* 2019;74(3):299-311.

142. Abbate A, Sinagra G, Bussani R, et al. Apoptosis in patients with acute myocarditis. *Am J Cardiol.* 2009;104:995-1000.

143. Kim G, Ban GH, Lee HD, et al. Left ventricular end-diastolic dimension as a predictive factor of outcomes in children with acute myocarditis. *Cardiol Young.* 2016;26:1-9.

144. Sanguineti F, Garot P, Mana M, et al. Cardiovascular magnetic resonance predictors of clinical outcome in patients with suspected acute myocarditis. *J Cardiovasc Magn Reson.* 2015;17:78.

145. Meier LA, Binstadt BA. The contribution of autoantibodies to inflammatory cardiovascular pathology. *Front Immunol.* 2018;9:911.

146. Donoso Mantke O, Meyer R. High prevalence of cardiotropic viruses in myocardial tissue from explanted hearts of heart transplant recipients and heart donors: a 3-year retrospective study from a German patients' pool. *J Heart Lung Transplant.* 2005;24:1632-1638.

147. Wang X, Zhang G, Liu F, et al. Prevalence of human parvovirus B19 DNA in cardiac tissues of patients with congenital heart diseases indicated by nested PCR and in situ hybridization. *J Clin Virol.* 2004;31:20-24.

148. Stewart GC, Lopez-Molina J, Gottumukkala RV, et al. Myocardial parvovirus B19 persistence: lack of association with clinicopathologic phenotype in adults with heart failure. *Circ Heart Fail.* 2011;4:71-78.

149. Hazebroek MR, Moors S, Dennert R, et al. Prognostic relevance of gene-environment interactions in patients with dilated cardiomyopathy: applying the MOGE(S) classification. *J Am Coll Cardiol.* 2015;66:1313-1323.

150. Yancy CW, Jessup M, Bozkurt B, et al. 2013 ACCF/AHA guideline for the management of heart failure: a report of the American College of Cardiology Foundation/American Heart Association Task Force on Practice Guidelines. *J Am Coll Cardiol.* 2013;62:e147-e239.

151. Yancy CW, Jessup M, Bozkurt B, et al. 2017 ACC/AHA/HFSA Focused Update of the 2013 ACCF/AHA Guideline for the Management of Heart

Failure: A Report of the American College of Cardiology/American Heart Association Task Force on Clinical Practice Guidelines and the Heart Failure Society of America. *J Am Coll Cardiol.* 2017;70(6):776-803.

152. Rihal CS, Naidu SS, Givertz MM, et al. 2015 SCAI/ACC/HFSA/STS Clinical expert consensus statement on the use of percutaneous mechanical circulatory support devices in cardiovascular care. *J Am Coll Cardiol.* 2015;65:2140-2141.

153. Parrillo JE, Cunnion RE, Epstein SE, et al. A prospective, randomized, controlled trial of prednisone for dilated cardiomyopathy. *N Engl J Med.* 1989;321:1061-1068.

154. Wojnicz R, Nowalany-Kozielska E, Wojciechowska C, et al. Randomized, placebo-controlled study for immunosuppressive treatment of inflammatory dilated cardiomyopathy: two-year follow-up results. *Circulation.* 2001;104:39-45.

155. Frustaci A, Chimenti C, Calabrese F, et al. Immunosuppressive therapy for active lymphocytic myocarditis: virological and immunologic profile of responders versus nonresponders. *Circulation.* 2003;107:857-863.

156. Frustaci A, Russo MA, Chimenti C. Randomized study on the efficacy of immunosuppressive therapy in patients with virus-negative inflammatory cardiomyopathy: the TIMIC study. *Eur Heart J.* 2009;30:1995-2002.

157. McNamara DM, Rosenblum WD, Janosko KM, et al. Intravenous immune globulin in the therapy of myocarditis and acute cardiomyopathy. *Circulation.* 1997;95:2476-2478.

158. McNamara DM, Holubkov R, Starling RC, et al. Controlled trial of intravenous immune globulin in recent-onset dilated cardiomyopathy. *Circulation.* 2001;103:2254-2259.

159. Staudt A, Hummel A, Ruppert J, et al. Immunoadsorption in dilated cardiomyopathy: 6-month results from a randomized study. *Am Heart J.* 2006;152:712.e1.

160. Cheng CY, Cheng GY, Shan ZG, et al. Efficacy of immunosuppressive therapy in myocarditis: a 30-year systematic review and meta analysis. *Autoimmun Rev.* 2021;20(1):102710.

161. Kuhl U, Pauschinger M, Schwimmbeck PL, et al. Interferon-beta treatment eliminates cardiotropic viruses and improves left ventricular function in patients with myocardial persistence of viral genomes and left ventricular dysfunction. *Circulation.* 2003;107:2793-2798.

162. Zipes DP, Camm AJ, Borggrefe M, et al. ACC/AHA/ESC 2006 guidelines for management of patients with ventricular arrhythmias and the prevention of sudden cardiac death: a report of the American College of Cardiology/American Heart Association task force and the European Society of Cardiology Committee for practice guidelines (writing committee to develop guidelines for management of patients with ventricular arrhythmias and the prevention of sudden cardiac death). *J Am Coll Cardiol.* 2006;48:e247-e346.

163. Priori SG, Blomstrom-Lundqvist C, Mazzanti A, et al. ESC guidelines for the management of patients with ventricular arrhythmias and the prevention of sudden cardiac death: the task force for the management of patients with ventricular arrhythmias and the prevention of sudden cardiac death of the European Society of Cardiology (ESC). Endorsed by: Association for European Paediatric and Congenital Cardiology (AEPC). *Eur Heart J.* 2015;36:2793-2867.

164. Al-Khatib SM, Stevenson WG, Ackerman MJ, et al. 2017 AHA/ACC/HRS guideline for management of patients with ventricular arrhythmias and the prevention of sudden cardiac death: a report of the American College of Cardiology/American Heart Association task force on clinical practice guidelines and the heart rhythm society. *Circulation.* 2018;138(13):e272-e391.

165. Pavlicek V, Kindermann I, Wintrich J, et al. Ventricular arrhythmias and myocardial inflammation: Long-term follow-up of patients with suspected myocarditis. *Int J Cardiol.* 2019;274:132-137.

166. Washington CH, Issaranggoon na ayuthaya S, Makonkawkeyoon K, et al. 9-year-old boy with severe diphtherial infection and cardiac complications. *BMJ Case Rep.* 2014;2014:bcr2014206085.

167. Meera M, Rajarao M. Diphtheria in Andhra Pradesh: a clinical-epidemiological study. *Int J Infect Dis.* 2014;19:74-78.

168. Sharma NC, Efstratiou A, Mokrousov I, et al. Diphtheria. *Nat Rev Dis Primers.* 2019;5(1):81.

169. Ladani AP, Biswas A, Vaghasia N, et al. Unusual presentation of listerial myocarditis and the diagnostic value of cardiac magnetic resonance. *Tex Heart Inst J.* 2015;42:255-258.

170. Panagopoulos P, Terzi I, Karanikas M, et al. Myocarditis, pancreatitis, polyarthritis, mononeuritis multiplex and vasculitis with symmetrical peripheral gangrene of the lower extremities as a rare presentation of leptospirosis: a case report and review of the literature. *J Med Case Rep.* 2014;8:150.

171. Briceño DF, Fernando RR, Nathan S, et al. Tandem heart as a bridge to recovery in Legionella myocarditis. *Tex Heart Inst J.* 2015;42:357-361.

172. Feasey NA, Gaskell K, Wong V, et al. Rapid emergence of multidrug resistant, H58-lineage *Salmonella typhi* in Blantyre, Malawi. *PLoS Negl Trop Dis.* 2015;9:e0003748.

173. Villablanca P, Mohananey D, Meier G, et al. *Salmonella berta* myocarditis: case report and systematic review of non-typhoid *Salmonella* myocarditis. *World J Cardiol.* 2015;7:931-937.

174. Shrestha P, Shrestha NK, Giri S. Rapid recovery following fulminant meningococcemia complicated by myocarditis in a 15-year-old Nepalese girl: a case report. *Int Med Case Rep J.* 2013;6:33-36.

175. Taldir G, Parize P, Arvis P, et al. Acute right-sided heart failure caused by *Neisseria meningitidis. J Clin Microbiol.* 2013;51:363-365.

176. Razminia M, Salem Y, Elbzour M, et al. Importance of early diagnosis and therapy of acute meningococcal myocarditis: a case report with review of literature. *Am J Ther.* 2005;12:269-271.

177. Fox-Lewis A, Merz TM, Hennessy I. Severe non-rheumatic streptococcal myocarditis requiring extracorporeal membrane oxygenation support. *Lancet Infect Dis.* 2020;20(12):1481. doi: 10.1016/S1473-3099(20)30689-7.

178. Kalil AC, Thomas PG. Influenza virus-related critical illness: pathophysiology and epidemiology. *Crit Care.* 2019;23(1):258. doi: 10.1186/s13054-019-2539-x.

179. Dawood FS, Chaves SS, Pérez A, et al. Complications and associated bacterial coinfections among children hospitalized with seasonal or pandemic influenza, United States, 2003-2010. *J Infect Dis.* 2014;209:686-694.

180. Randolph AG, Vaughn F, Sullivan R, et al. Critically ill children during the 2009-2010 influenza pandemic in the United States. *Pediatrics.* 2011;128:e1450-e1458.

181. Mteirek M, Beuret P, Convert G. Tubercular myocarditis: two case reports and review of the literature. *Ann Cardiol Angeiol.* 2011;60:105-108.

182. Liu A, Hu Y, Coates A. Sudden cardiac death and tuberculosis: how much do we know? *Tuberculosis.* 2012;92:307-313.

183. Nayak SU, Simon GL. Myocarditis after trimethoprim/sulfamethoxazole treatment for ehrlichiosis. *Emerg Infect Dis.* 2013;19:1975-1977.

184. Havens NS, Kinnear BR, Mató S. Fatal ehrlichial myocarditis in a healthy adolescent: a case report and review of the literature. *Clin Infect Dis.* 2012;54:e113-e114.

185. Harris M, Ananth Narayan S, Orchard EA. Fungal myocarditis in a preterm neonate. *BMJ Case Rep.* 2012;2012:bcr-2012-007174.

186. Chatterjee D, Bal A, Singhal M, et al. Fibrosing mediastinitis due to *Aspergillus* with dominant cardiac involvement: report of two autopsy cases with review of literature. *Cardiovasc Pathol.* 2014;23:354-357.

187. Vaideeswar P. *Aspergillus* pancarditis manifesting as hospital-acquired infection: report of two cases and review of literature. *Cardiovasc Pathol.* 2010;19:e253-e257.

188. Nulens EF, Bourgeois MJ, Reynders MB. Post-influenza aspergillosis, do not underestimate influenza B. *Infect Drug Resist.* 2017;10:61-67. doi: 10.2147/IDR.S122390.

189. Bullis SS, Krywanczyk A, Hale AJ. Aspergillosis myocarditis in the immunocompromised host. *IDCases.* 2019;17:e00567. doi: 10.1016/j.idcr.2019.e00567.

190. Liu Q, Wang ZD, Huang SY, Zhu XQ. Diagnosis of toxoplasmosis and typing of *Toxoplasma gondii. Parasit Vectors.* 2015;8:292.

191. Pappas G, Roussos N, Falagas ME. Toxoplasmosis snapshots: global status of *Toxoplasma gondii* seroprevalence and implications for pregnancy and congenital toxoplasmosis. *Int J Parasitol.* 2009;39:1385-1394.

192. Saadatnia G, Golkar M. A review on human toxoplasmosis. *Scand J Infect Dis.* 2012;44:805-814.

193. Harris VC, Van Vugt M, Aronica E, et al. Human extraintestinal sarcocystosis: what we know, and what we don't know. *Curr Infect Dis Rep.* 2015;17:495.

194. Esposito DH, Stich A, Epelboin L, et al. Tioman Island Sarcocystosis Investigation Team. Acute muscular sarcocystosis: an international investigation among ill travelers returning from Tioman Island, Malaysia, 2011-2012. *Clin Infect Dis.* 2014;59:1401-1410.

195. Centers for Disease Control and Prevention. Parasites: trichinellosis (also known as trichinosis). https://www.cdc.gov/parasites/trichinellosis. Accessed March 1, 2021.

196. Okello AL, Burniston S, Conlan JV, et al. Prevalence of endemic pig-associated zoonoses in Southeast Asia: a review of findings from the Lao People's Democratic Republic. *Am J Trop Med Hyg.* 2015;92:1059-1066.

197. Murrell KD, Pozio E. Worldwide occurrence and impact of human trichinellosis, 1986-2009. *Emerg Infect Dis.* 2011;17:2194-2202.

198. Rawla P, Sharma S. Trichinella spiralis. 2020. In: *StatPearls [Internet].* Treasure Island (FL): StatPearls Publishing; 2021.

199. Neghina R, Neghina AM, Marincu I. Reviews on trichinellosis (III): cardiovascular involvement. *Foodborne Pathog Dis.* 2011;8:853-860.

200. Neghina R, Neghina AM, Marincu I, et al. Cardiac involvement in patients with trichinosis hospitalized in western Romania. *Foodborne Pathog Dis.* 2010;7:1235-1238.

201. Bang SH, Park JB, Chee HK, et al. Cardiac parasitic infection in trichinellosis associated with right ventricle outflow tract obstruction. *Korean J Thorac Cardiovasc Surg.* 2014;47:145-148.

202. Yaliniz H, Tokcan A, Salih OK, et al. Surgical treatment of cardiac hydatid disease: a report of 7 cases. *Texas Heart Inst J.* 2006;33:333-339.

203. Shakil U, Rehman AU, Shahid R. Isolated cardiac hydatid cyst. *J Coll Physicians Surg Pak.* 2015;25:374-375.

204. Dasbaksi K, Haldar S, Mukherjee K, et al. A rare combination of hepatic and pericardial hydatid cyst and review of literature. *Int J Surg Case Rep.* 2015;10:52-55.

205. Elkarimi S, Ouldelgadia N, Gacem H, et al. Tamponade reveals an intrapericardial hydatid cyst: a case report. *Ann Cardiol Angeiol.* 2014;63:267-270.

206. Demircan A, Keles A, Kahveci FO, et al. Cardiac tamponade via a fistula to the pericardium from a hydatid cyst: case report and review of the literature. *J Emerg Med.* 2010;38:582-586.

207. Menassa-Moussa L, Braidy C, Riachy M, et al. Hydatid disease diagnosed following a pulmonary embolism. *J Mal Vasc.* 2009;34:354-357.

208. Akgun V, Battal B, Karaman B, et al. Pulmonary artery embolism due to a ruptured hepatic hydatid cyst: clinical and radiologic imaging findings. *Emerg Radiol.* 2011;18:437-439.

209. Bach AG, Restrepo CS, Abbas J, et al. Imaging of nonthrombotic pulmonary embolism: biological materials, nonbiological materials, and foreign bodies. *Eur J Radiol.* 2013;82:e120-e141.

210. Turak O, Ozcan F, Sökmen E, et al. Syncope as the primary manifestation of hydatid cyst. Report of two cases with different etiologies. *Herz.* 2014;39:287-290.

211. Kahlfuß S, Flieger RR, Roepke TK, Yilmaz K. Diagnosis and treatment of cardiac echinococcosis. *Heart.* 2016;102(17):1348-1353.

212. Poretti D, Felleisen E, Grimm F, et al. Differential immunodiagnosis between cystic hydatid disease and other cross-reactive pathologies. *Am J Trop Med Hyg.* 1999;60:193-198.

213. Musleh M, Abuhussein N, Musleh G, et al. Innovative use of the octopus stabilizer in the excision of a cardiac hydatid cyst. *J Surg Case Rep.* 2016;2016:rjw019.

214. Kuenzli E, Neumayr A, Chaney M, Blum J. Toxocariasis-associated cardiac diseases: a systematic review of the literature. *Acta Trop.* 2016;154:107-120.

215. Centers for Disease Control and Prevention. Toxocariasis. http://www.cdc.gov/parasites/toxocariasis/. Accessed March 1, 2021.

216. Jones JM, Kracalik I, Levi ME, et al. Assessing solid organ donors and monitoring transplant recipients for human immunodeficiency virus, hepatitis B virus, and hepatitis C virus infection—U.S. Public Health Service Guideline, 2020. *MMWR Recomm Rep.* 2020;69(4):1-16.

217. Gaffey AC, Doll SL, Thomasson AM, et al. Transplantation of "high-risk" donor hearts: implications for infection. *J Thorac Cardiovasc Surg.* 2016;152(1):213-220.

218. Kates OS, Fisher CE, Rakita RM, et al. Use of SARS-CoV-2-infected deceased organ donors: Should we always "just say no?". *Am J Transplant.* 2020;20:1787-1794.

219. Shah MB, Lynch RJ, El-Haddad H, et al. Utilization of deceased donors during a pandemic: argument against using SARS-CoV-2-positive donors. *Am J Transplant.* 2020;20:1795-1799.

220. Jones JM, Kracalik I, Rana MM, et al. SARS-CoV-2 infections among recent organ recipients, March–May 2020, United States. Center for Disease Control and Prevention. *Dispatch. EID J,* 2021; 27. https://wwwnc.cdc.gov/eid/article/27/2/20-4046_article#r1

221. Miró JM, Blanes M, Norman F, et al. Infections in solid organ transplantation in special situations: HIV-infection and immigration. *Enferm Infecc Microbiol Clin.* 2012;30:76-85.

222. Brito-Zerón P, Izmirly PM, Ramos-Casals M, et al. Autoimmune congenital heart block: complex and unusual situations. *Lupus.* 2016;25:116-128.

223. Eronen M, Heikkilä P, Teramo K. Congenital complete heart block in the fetus: hemodynamic features, antenatal treatment, and outcome in six cases. *Pediatr Cardiol.* 2001;22(5):385-392.

224. Morel N, Georgin-Lavialle S, Levesque K, et al. Neonatal lupus syndrome: literature review. *Rev Med Interne.* 2015;36:159-166.

225. Eringsmark Regnell S, Lernmark A. The environment and the origins of islet autoimmunity and type 1 diabetes. *Diabet Med.* 2013;30:155-160.

226. Massilamany C, Koenig A, Reddy J, et al. Autoimmunity in picornavirus infections. *Curr Opin Virol.* 2016;16:8-14.

227. Cusick MF, Libbey JE, Fujinami RS. Molecular mimicry as a mechanism of autoimmune disease. *Clin Rev Allergy Immunol.* 2012;42:102-111.

228. Tournel G, Houssaye C, Humbert L, et al. Acute arsenic poisoning: clinical, toxicological, histopathological, and forensic features. *J Forensic Sci.* 2011;56(Suppl 1):S275-S279.

229. Hagiwara H, Fukushima A, Iwano H, Anzai T. Refractory cardiac myocarditis associated with drug rash with eosinophilia and systemic symptoms syndrome due to anti-bipolar disorder drugs: a case report. *Eur Heart J Case Rep.* 2018;2(4):yty100.

230. Ataallah B, Al-Zakhari R, Sharma A, et al. A rare but reversible cause of lithium-induced bradycardia. *Cureus.* 2020;12(6):e8600.

231. Doğan E, Güzel A, Ciftçi T, et al. Zinc phosphide poisoning. *Case Rep Crit Care.* 2014;2014:589712.

232. Giacon G, Boon K. Cobalt toxicity: a preventable and treatable cause for possibly life threatening cardiomyopathy. *N Z Med J.* 2021;134(1529):103-108.

233. More LA, Lane S, Asnani A. 5-FU cardiotoxicity: vasospasm, myocarditis, and sudden death. *Curr Cardiol Rep.* 2021;23(3):17.

234. Allison JD, Tanavin T, Yang Y, et al. Various manifestations of 5-fluorouracil cardiotoxicity: a multicenter case series and review of literature. *Cardiovasc Toxicol.* 2020;20(4):437-442.

235. Mishra T, Shokr M, Ahmed A, Afonso L. Acute reversible left ventricular systolic dysfunction associated with 5-fluorouracil therapy: a rare and increasingly recognised cardiotoxicity of a commonly used drug. *BMJ Case Rep.* 2019;12(9):e230499.

236. Chen DH, Tyebally S, Malloupas M, et al. Cardiovascular disease amongst women treated for breast cancer: traditional cytotoxic chemotherapy, targeted therapy, and radiation therapy. *Curr Cardiol Rep.* 2021;23(3):16.

237. Ma R, Wang Q, Meng D et al. Immune checkpoint inhibitors-related myocarditis in patients with cancer: an analysis of international spontaneous reporting systems. *BMC Cancer.* 2021;21(1):38.

238. Ederhy S, Fenioux C, Cholet C, et al. Immune checkpoint inhibitor myocarditis with normal cardiac magnetic resonance imaging: importance of cardiac biopsy and early diagnosis. *Can J Cardiol.* 2020:S0828-282X(20)31189-2.

239. Behravesh S, Shomali N, Danbaran GR, et al. Cardiotoxicity of immune checkpoint inhibitors: an updated review. *Biotechnol Appl Biochem.* 2020.

240. Ronaldson KJ, Fitzgerald PB, McNeil JJ. Clozapine-induced myocarditis, a widely overlooked adverse reaction. *Acta Psychiatr Scand.* 2015;132:231-243.

241. Chopra N, de Leon J. Clozapine-induced myocarditis may be associated with rapid titration: a case report verified with autopsy. *Int J Psychiatry Med.* 2016;51:104-115.

242. Chow V, Feijo I, Trieu J, et al. Successful rechallenge of clozapine therapy following previous clozapine-induced myocarditis confirmed on cardiac MRI. *J Child Adolesc Psychopharmacol.* 2014;24:99-101.

243. Munshi TA, Volochniouk D, Hassan T, et al. Clozapine-induced myocarditis: is mandatory monitoring warranted for its early recognition? *Case Rep Psychiatry.* 2014;2014:513108.

244. Hausvater A, Smilowitz NR, Li B, Redel-Traub G, et al. Myocarditis in relation to angiographic findings in patients with provisional diagnoses of MINOCA. *JACC Cardiovasc Imaging.* 2020;13(9):1906-1913.

245. Tung R, Bauer B, Schelbert H, et al. Incidence of abnormal positron emission tomography in patients with unexplained cardiomyopathy and ventricular arrhythmias: the potential role of occult inflammation in arrhythmogenesis. *Heart Rhythm.* 2015;12:2488-2498.

246. Glenn-Cox S, Foley RW, Pauling JD, Rodrigues JCL. Fulminant immune-mediated necrotising myopathy (IMNM) mimicking myocardial infarction with non-obstructive coronary arteries (MINOCA). *BMJ Case Rep.* 2020;13(11):e236603.

247. Mavrogeni S, Dimitroulas T, Kitas GD. Multimodality imaging and the emerging role of cardiac magnetic resonance in autoimmune myocarditis. *Autoimmun Rev.* 2012;12:305-312.

248. Polat TB, Yalcin Y, Erdem A, et al. Tissue Doppler imaging in rheumatic carditis. *Cardiol Young.* 2014;24:359-365.

249. Escher F, Kasner M, Kuhl U, et al. New echocardiographic findings correlate with intramyocardial inflammation in endomyocardial biopsies of patients with acute myocarditis and inflammatory cardiomyopathy. *Mediators Inflamm.* 2013;2013:875420.

250. Gursu HA, Cetin II, Azak E, et al. The assessment of treatment outcomes in patients with acute viral myocarditis by speckle tracking and tissue Doppler methods. *Echocardiography.* 2019;36(9):1666-1674.

251. Kirkbride RR, Rawal B, Mirsadraee S, et al. Imaging of cardiac infections: a comprehensive review and investigation flowchart for diagnostic workup. *J Thorac Imaging.* 2020.

252. Lurz P, Eitel I, Klieme B, et al. The potential additional diagnostic value of assessing for pericardial effusion on cardiac magnetic resonance imaging in patients with suspected myocarditis. *Eur Heart J Cardiovasc Imaging.* 2014;15:643-650.

253. Friedrich MG, Marcotte F. Cardiac magnetic resonance assessment of myocarditis. *Circ Cardiovasc Imaging.* 2013;6:833-839.

254. Sprinkart AM, Luetkens JA, Traber F, et al. Gradient spin echo (GraSE) imaging for fast myocardial T2 mapping. *J Cardiovasc Magn Reson.* 2015;17:12.

255. Potet J, Rahmouni A, Mayer J, et al. Detection of myocardial edema with low-b-value diffusion-weighted echo-planar imaging sequence in patients with acute myocarditis. *Radiology.* 2013;269(2):362-369.

256. Thavendiranathan P, Walls M, Giri S, et al. Improved detection of myocardial involvement in acute inflammatory cardiomyopathies using T2 mapping. *Circ Cardiovasc Imaging.* 2012;5:102-110.

257. Perfetti M, Malatesta G, Alvarez I, et al. A fast and effective method to assess myocardial hyperemia in acute myocarditis by magnetic resonance. *Int J Cardiovasc Imaging.* 2014;30:629-637.

258. Schumm J, Greulich S, Sechtem U, et al. T1 mapping as new diagnostic technique in a case of acute onset of biopsy-proven viral myocarditis. *Clin Res Cardiol.* 2014;103:405-408.

259. Ferreira VM, Piechnik SK, Dall'Armellina E, et al. Native T1-mapping detects the location, extent and patterns of acute myocarditis without the need for gadolinium contrast agents. *J Cardiovasc Magn Reson.* 2014;16:36.

260. Ferreira VM, Piechnik SK, Dall'Armellina E, et al. T(1) mapping for the diagnosis of acute myocarditis using CMR: comparison to T2-weighted and late gadolinium enhanced imaging. *JACC Cardiovasc Imaging.* 2013;6:1048-1058.

261. Luetkens JA, Doerner J, Thomas DK, et al. Acute myocarditis: multiparametric cardiac MR imaging. *Radiology.* 2014;273:383-392.

262. Roller FC, Harth S, Schneider C, et al. T1, T2 mapping and extracellular volume fraction (ECV): application, value and further perspectives in myocardial inflammation and cardiomyopathies. *Rofo.* 2015;187:760-770.

263. Rottgen R, Christiani R, Freyhardt P, et al. Magnetic resonance imaging findings in acute myocarditis and correlation with immunohistological parameters. *Eur Radiol.* 2011;21:1259-1266.

264. Yilmaz A, Ferreira V, Klingel K, et al. Role of cardiovascular magnetic resonance imaging (CMR) in the diagnosis of acute and chronic myocarditis. *Heart Fail Rev.* 2013;18:747-760.

265. Vermes E, Childs H, Carbone I, et al. Auto-threshold quantification of late gadolinium enhancement in patients with acute heart disease. *J Magn Reson Imaging.* 2013;37:382-390.

266. Mavrogeni S, Bratis K, Markussis V, et al. The diagnostic role of cardiac magnetic resonance imaging in detecting myocardial inflammation in systemic lupus erythematosus. Differentiation from viral myocarditis. *Lupus.* 2013;22:34-43.

267. Radunski UK, Lund GK, Stehning C et al. CMR in patients with severe myocarditis: diagnostic value of quantitative tissue markers including extracellular volume imaging. *JACC Cardiovasc Imaging.* 2014;7(7):667-675.

268. Lurz P, Luecke C, Eitel I, et al. Comprehensive cardiac magnetic resonance imaging in patients with suspected myocarditis: the MyoRacer-Trial. *J Am Coll Cardiol.* 2016;67(15):1800-1811.

269. von Knobelsdorff-Brenkenhoff F, Schüler J, Dogangüzel S, et al. Detection and monitoring of acute myocarditis applying quantitative cardiovascular magnetic resonance. *Circ Cardiovasc Imaging.* 2017;10(2):e005242.

270. Hahn L, Kligerman S. Cardiac MRI evaluation of myocarditis. *Curr Treat Options Cardiovasc Med.* 2019;21(11):69.

271. Wei S, Fu J, Chen L, Yu S. Performance of cardiac magnetic resonance imaging for diagnosis of myocarditis compared with endomyocardial biopsy: a meta-analysis. *Med Sci Monit.* 2017;23:3687-3696.

272. Kotanidis CP, Bazmpani MA, Haidich AB. Diagnostic accuracy of cardiovascular magnetic resonance in acute myocarditis: a systematic review and meta-analysis. *JACC Cardiovasc Imaging.* 2018;11:1583–1590.

273. Wetscherek MTA, Rutschke W, Frank C, et al. High inter- and intra-observer agreement in mapping sequences compared to classical Lake Louise Criteria assessment of myocarditis by inexperienced observers. *Clin Radiol.* 2020;75(10):796.e17-e796.e26.

274. Ferreira VM, Schulz-Menger J, Holmvang G, et al. Cardiovascular magnetic resonance in nonischemic myocardial inflammation: expert recommendations. *J Am Coll Cardiol.* 2018;72:3158–76.

275. Hanneman K, Kadoch M, Guo HH, et al. Initial experience with simultaneous 18F-FDG PET/MRI in the evaluation of cardiac sarcoidosis and myocarditis. *Clin Nucl Med.* 2017;42(7):e328-e334.

276. Ozawa K, Funabashi N, Daimon M, et al. Determination of optimum periods between onset of suspected acute myocarditis and 18F-fluorodeoxyglucose positron emission tomography in the diagnosis of inflammatory left ventricular myocardium. *Int J Cardiol.* 2013;169:196-200.

277. Tanimura M, Dohi K, Imanaka-Yoshida K, et al. Fulminant myocarditis with prolonged active lymphocytic infiltration after hemodynamic recovery. *Int Heart J.* 2017;58:294-297.

278. Nensa F, Kloth J, Tezgah E, Poeppel TD, Heusch P, Goebel J. Feasibility of FDG-PET in myocarditis: comparison to CMR using integrated PET/MRI. *J Nucl Cardiol.* 2018;25:785-794.

279. Li X, Rosenkrans ZT, Wang J, Cai W. PET imaging of macrophages in cardiovascular diseases. *Am J Transl Res*. 2020;12(5):1491-1514.

280. Maya Y, Werner RA, Schütz C, et al. 11C-Methionine PET of myocardial inflammation in a rat model of experimental autoimmune myocarditis. *J Nucl Med*. 2016;57(12):1985-1990.

281. Pizarro C, Kluenker F, Dabir D, et al. Cardiovascular magnetic resonance imaging and clinical performance of somatostatin receptor positron emission tomography in cardiac sarcoidosis. *ESC Heart Fail*. 2018;5:249-261.

282. Bravo PE, Bajaj N, Padera RF, et al. Feasibility of somatostatin receptor-targeted imaging for detection of myocardial inflammation: a pilot study. *J Nucl Cardiol*. 2019.

283. Gormsen LC, Haraldsen A, Kramer S, et al. A dual tracer (68) Ga-DOTANOC PET/CT and (18)F-FDG PET/CT pilot study for detection of cardiac sarcoidosis. *EJNMMI Res*. 2016;6:52.

284. Lee SP, Im HJ, Kang S et al. Noninvasive imaging of myocardial inflammation in myocarditis using (68)Ga-tagged mannosylated human serum albumin positron emission tomography. *Theranostics*. 2017;7:413-424.

285. Rischpler C, Nekolla SG, Kunze KP, et al. PET/MRI of the heart. *Semin Nucl Med*. 2015;45:234-247.

286. Eisenberg M, Hopkins I, Alexander M, et al. Cardiac troponin T as a screening test for myocarditis in children. *Pediatr Emerg Care*. 2012;11:1173-1178.

287. Wildi K, Twerenbold R, Mueller C. How acute changes in cardiac troponin concentrations help to handle the challenges posed by troponin elevations in non-ACS-patients. *Clin Biochem*. 2015;48:218-222.

288. Smith SC, Ladenson JH, Mason JW, et al. Elevations of cardiac troponin I associated with myocarditis. experimental and clinical correlates. *Circulation*. 1997;95:163-168.

289. Ukena C, Kindermann M, Mahfoud F, et al. Diagnostic and prognostic validity of different biomarkers in patients with suspected myocarditis. *Clin Res Cardiol*. 2014;103:743-751.

290. Pettit MA, Koyfman A, Foran M. Myocarditis. *Pediatr Emerg Care*. 2014;30:832-835.

291. Lewandrowski KB. Special topics: cardiac markers in myocarditis: cardiac transplant rejection and conditions other than acute coronary syndrome. *Clin Lab Med*. 2014;34:129-135.

292. Ludwig A, Lucero-Obusan C, Schirmer P, et al. Acute cardiac injury events ≤30 days after laboratory-confirmed influenza virus infection among U.S. veterans, 2010-2012. *BMC Cardiovasc Disord*. 2015;15:109.

293. Freixa Pettit X, Sionis A, Castel A, et al. Low troponin-I levels on admission are associated with worse prognosis in patients with fulminant myocarditis. *Transplant Proc*. 2009;41:2234-2236.

294. Gilotra NA, Minkove N, Bennett MK, et al. Lack of relationship between serum cardiac troponin I level and giant cell myocarditis diagnosis and outcomes. *J Card Fail*. 2016;22(7):583-585.

295. Ederhy S, Massard C, Dufaitre G, et al. Frequency and management of troponin I elevation in patients treated with molecular targeted therapies in phase I trials. *Invest New Drugs*. 2012;30:611-615.

296. Jensen J, Ma LP, Fu ML, et al. Inflammation increases NT-proBNP and the NT-proBNP/ BNP ratio. *Clin Res Cardiol*. 2010;99:445-452.

297. Teele SA, Allan KC, Laussen PC, et al. Management and outcomes in pediatric patients presenting with acute fulminant myocarditis. *J Pediatr*. 2011;158:638-643.

298. Mlczoch E, Darbandi-Mesri F, Luckner D, et al. NT-pro BNP in acute childhood myocarditis. *J Pediatr*. 2012;160:178-179.

299. Sachdeva S, Song X, Dham N, et al. Analysis of clinical parameters and cardiac magnetic resonance imaging as predictors of outcome in pediatric myocarditis. *Am J Cardiol*. 2015;115:499-504.

300. Aleshcheva G, Pietsch H, Escher F, Schultheiss HP. MicroRNA profiling as a novel diagnostic tool for identification of patients with inflammatory and/or virally induced cardiomyopathies. *ESC Heart Fail*. 2021;8(1):408-422.

301. Tserel L, Runnel T, Kisand K, et al. MicroRNA expression profiles of human blood monocyte-derived dendritic cells and macrophages reveal miR-511 as putative positive regulator of Toll-like receptor 4. *J Biol Chem*. 2011;286:26487-26495.

302. Fehily SR, Forlano R, Fitzgerald PB. C-reactive protein: an early critical sign of clozapine-related myocarditis. *Australas Psychiatry*. 2016;24:181-184.

303. Ronaldson KJ, Fitzgerald PB, McNeil JJ. Evolution of troponin, C-reactive protein and eosinophil count with the onset of clozapine induced myocarditis. *Aust N Z J Psychiatry*. 2015;49:486-487.

304. Cook SC, Ferguson BA, Cotes RO, Heinrich TW, Schwartz AC. Clozapine-induced myocarditis: prevention and considerations in rechallenge. *Psychosomatics*. 2015;56:685-690.

305. Kuhl U, Schultheiss HP. Viral myocarditis. *Swiss Med Wkly*. 2014; 144:w14010.

306. Dec GW, Arbustini E. Utilizing the MOGE(S) classification for predicting prognosis in dilated cardiomyopathy. *J Am Coll Cardiol*. 2015;66: 1324-1326.

307. Kodama T, Agozzino M, Pellegrini C, et al. Endomyocardial biopsy in acute cardiogenic shock: diagnosis of pheochromocytoma. *Int J Cardiol*. 2016;202:897-899.

308. Raptis DA, Raptis CA, Jokerst C, et al. Erdheim-Chester disease with interatrial septum involvement. *J Thorac Imaging*. 2012;27:105-107.

309. Michira BN, Alkizim FO, Matheka DM. Patterns and clinical manifestations of tuberculous myocarditis: a systematic review of cases. *Pan Afr Med J*. 2015;21:118.

310. Afzal A, Keohane M, Keeley E, Borzak S, Callender CW, Iannuzzi M. Myocarditis and pericarditis with tamponade associated with disseminated tuberculosis. *Can J Cardiol*. 2000;16:519-521.

311. Khurana R, Shalhoub J, Verma A, et al. Tubercular myocarditis presenting with ventricular tachycardia. *Nat Clin Pract Cardiovasc Med*. 2008;5:169-174.

312. Cowley A, Dobson L, Kurian J, Saunderson C. Acute myocarditis secondary to cardiac tuberculosis: a case report. *Echo Res Pract*. 2017;4(3):K25-K29.

313. Cooper L, Berry G, Shabetai R. Idiopathic giant-cell myocarditis: natural history and treatment. *N Engl J Med*. 1997;336:1860-1866.

314. Kandolin R, Lehtonen J, Salmenkivi K, et al. Diagnosis, treatment, and outcome of giant-cell myocarditis in the era of combined immunosuppression. *Circ Heart Fail*. 2013;6:15-22.

315. Vaideeswar P, Cooper L. Giant cell myocarditis: clinical and pathological disease characteristics in an Indian population. *Cardiovasc Pathol*. 2013;22:70-74.

316. Blauwet LA, Cooper LT. Idiopathic giant cell myocarditis and cardiac sarcoidosis. *Heart Fail Rev*. 2013;18:733-746.

317. Lee M, Kwon GY, Kim JS, et al. Giant cell myocarditis associated with Coxsackievirus infection. *J Am Coll Cardiol*. 2010;56:e19.

318. Dennert R, Schalla S, Suylen RJ, et al. Giant cell myocarditis triggered by a parvovirus B19 infection. *Int J Cardiol*. 2009;134:115-116.

319. Everett RJ, Sheppard MN, Lefroy DC. Chest pain and palpitations: taking a closer look. *Circulation*. 2013;128:271-277.

320. Shariff S, Straatiamn L, Allard M, et al. Novel associations of giant cell myocarditis: tow case reports and a review of the literature. *Can J Cardiol*. 2004;4:557-561.

321. Sasaki H, Yano M, Kawano O, et al. Thymoma associated with fatal myocarditis and polymyositis in a 58-year-old man following treatment with carboplatin and paclitaxel: a case report. *Oncol Lett*. 2012;3:300-302.

322. Joudinaud TM, Fadel E, Thomas-de-Montpreville V, et al. Fatal giant cell myocarditis after thymoma resection in myasthenia gravis. *J Thorac Cardiovasc Surg*. 2006;131:494-495.

323. Schumann C, Faust M, Gerharz M, et al. Autoimmune polyglandular syndrome associated with idiopathic giant cell myocarditis. *Exp Clin Endocrinol Diabetes*. 2005;113:302-307.

324. Ikeda Y, Inomata T, Nishinarita R, et al. Giant cell myocarditis associated with multiple autoimmune disorders following highly active

antiretroviral therapy for human immunodeficiency virus type 1 infection. *Int J Cardiol.* 2016;206:79-81.

325. Evans JD, Pettit SJ, Goddard M, et al. Alemtuzumab as a novel treatment for refractory giant cell myocarditis after heart transplantation. *J Heart Lung Transplant.* 2016;35:256-258.

326. Lassner D, Kühl U, Siegismund CS, et al. Improved diagnosis of idiopathic giant cell myocarditis and cardiac sarcoidosis by myocardial gene expression profiling. *Eur Heart J.* 2014;35:2186-2195.

327. Asimaki A, Tandri H, Duffy E, et al. Altered desmosomal proteins in granulomatous myocarditis and potential pathogenic links to arrhythmogenic right ventricular cardiomyopathy. *Circ Arrhythm Electrophysiol.* 2011;4:743-752.

328. Larsen BT, Maleszewski JJ, Edwards WD, et al. Atrial giant cell myocarditis: a distinctive clinicopathologic entity. *Circulation.* 2013;127:39-47.

329. Bose AK, Bhattacharjee M, Martin V, et al. Giant cell myocarditis of the left atrium. *Cardiovasc Pathol.* 2010;19:e37-e38.

330. Shields RC, Tazelaar HD, Berry GJ, et al. The role of right ventricular endomyocardial biopsy for idiopathic giant cell myocarditis. *J Card Fail.* 2002;8:74-78c.

331. Sujino Y, Kimura F, Tanno J. Cardiac magnetic resonance imaging in giant cell myocarditis: intriguing associations with clinical and pathological features. *Circulation.* 2014;129:e467-e469.

332. Elezkurtaj S, Lassner D, Schultheiss H, et al. Vascular involvement in cardiac giant cell myocarditis: a new pathophysiological aspect. *Clin Res Cardiol.* 2014;103:161-163.

333. Lindenfeld J, Albert NM, Boehmer JP. Heart Failure Society of America, HFSA 2010 comprehensive heart failure practice guideline. *J Card Fail.* 2010;16:e1-e194.

334. Casali MB, Lazzaro A, Gentile G, et al. Forensic grading of myocarditis: an experimental contribution to the distinction between lethal myocarditis and incidental myocarditis. *Forensic Sci Int.* 2012;223:78-86.

335. Cooper LT Jr, Hare JM, Tazelaar HD, et al. Giant cell myocarditis treatment trial investigators. Usefulness of immunosuppression for giant cell myocarditis. *Am J Cardiol.* 2008;102:1535-1539.

336. Steinhaus D, Gelfand E, VanderLaan PA, et al. Recovery of giant cell myocarditis using combined cytolytic immunosuppression and mechanical circulatory support. *J Heart Lung Transplant.* 2014;33:769-771.

337. Murray LK, Gonzalez-Costello J, Jonas SN, et al. Ventricular assist device support as a bridge to heart transplantation in patients with giant cell myocarditis. *Eur J Heart Fail.* 2012;14:312-318.

338. Seeburger J, Doll N, Doll S. Mechanical assist and transplantation for treatment of giant cell myocarditis. *Can J Cardiol.* 2010;26:96-97.

339. Kong G, Madden B, Spyrou N, et al. Response of recurrent giant cell myocarditis in a transplanted heart to intensive immunosuppression. *Eur Heart J.* 1991;12:554-557.

340. Bang V, Ganatra S, Shah SP, et al. Management of patients with giant cell myocarditis: JACC Review Topic of the Week. *J Am Coll Cardiol.* 2021;77(8):1122-1134.

341. Maleszewski JJ, Orellana VM, Hodge DO, et al. Long-term risk of recurrence, morbidity and mortality in giant cell myocarditis. *Am J Cardiol.* 2015;115:1733-1738.

342. Cooper LT Jr, El Amm C. Giant cell myocarditis. Diagnosis and treatment. *Herz.* 2012;37:632-636.

343. Bhowmick M, Auckbarallee F, Edgar P, et al. Humanized monoclonal antibody alemtuzumab treatment in transplant. *Exp Clin Transplant.* 2016;14:17-21.

344. Sekhri V, Sanal S, DeLorenzo LJ, et al. Cardiac sarcoidosis: a comprehensive review. *Arch Med Sci.* 2011;7:546-554.

345. Rybicki BA, Major M, Popovich J Jr, et al. Racial differences in sarcoidosis incidence: a 5-year study in a health maintenance organization. *Am J Epidemiol.* 1997;145:234-241.

346. Iannuzzi MC, Rybicki BA, Teirstein AS. Sarcoidosis. *N Engl J Med.* 2007;357(21):2153-2165.

347. Musellim B, Kumbasar OO, Ongen G, et al. Epidemiological features of Turkish patients with sarcoidosis. *Respir Med.* 2009;103:907-912.

348. Trivieri MG, Spagnolo P, Birnie D, et al. Challenges in cardiac and pulmonary sarcoidosis: JACC State-of-the-Art Review. *J Am Coll Cardiol.* 2020;76:1878-1901.

349. Schatka I, Bengel FM. Advanced imaging of cardiac sarcoidosis. *J Nucl Med.* 2014;55:99-106.

350. Lynch JP, Hwang J, Bradfield J, et al. Cardiac involvement in sarcoidosis: evolving concepts in diagnosis and treatment. *Semin Respir Crit Care Med.* 2014;35:372-390.

351. Kanazawa N, Okafuji I, Kambe N, et al. Early-onset sarcoidosis and CARD15 mutations with constitutive nuclear factor-kappa-B activation: common genetic etiology with Blau syndrome. *Blood.* 2005;105:1195-1197.

352. Ellis JC, Faber BG, Uri IF, Emerson SJ. Early onset sarcoidosis (Blau syndrome): erosive and often misdiagnosed. *Rheumatology (Oxford).* 2020;59(5):1190.

353. Ardehali H, Howard DL, Hariri A, et al. A positive endomyocardial biopsy result for sarcoid is associated with poor prognosis in patients with initially unexplained cardiomyopathy. *Am Heart J.* 2005;150:459-463.

354. Iwai K, Takemura T, Kitaichi M, et al. Pathological studies on sarcoidosis autopsy. II. Early change, mode of progression and death pattern. *Acta Pathol Jpn.* 1993;43:377-385.

355. Burke RR, Stone CH, Havstad S, Rybicki BA. Racial differences in sarcoidosis granuloma density. *Lung.* 2009;187:1-7.

356. Chen ES, Moller DR. Etiologies of sarcoidosis. *Clin Rev Allergy Immunol.* 2015;49:6-18.

357. Oswald-Richter KA, Beachboard DC, Seeley EH, et al. Dual analysis for mycobacteria and propionibacteria in sarcoidosis BAL. *J Clin Immunol.* 2012;32:1129-1140.

358. Sverrild A, Backer V, Kyvik KO, et al. Heredity in sarcoidosis: a registry-based twin study. *Thorax.* 2008;63:894-896.

359. Rybicki BA, Iannuzzi MC, Frederick MM, et al. Familial aggregation of sarcoidosis. A case-control etiologic study of sarcoidosis (ACCESS). *Am J Respir Crit Care Med.* 2001;164:2085-2091.

360. Yang IV, Konigsberg I, MacPhail K et al. DNA methylation changes in lung immune cells are associated with granulomatous lung disease. *Am J Respir Cell Mol Biol.* 2019;60(1):96-105.

361. Kaufman KP, Becker ML. Distinguishing Blau syndrome from systemic sarcoidosis. *Curr Allergy Asthma Rep.* 2021;21(2):10.

362. Baughman RP, Engel PJ, Nathan S. Pulmonary hypertension in sarcoidosis. *Clin Chest Med.* 2015;36:703-714.

363. Miyazawa K, Yoshikawa T, Takamisawa I, et al. Presence of ventricular aneurysm predicts poor clinical outcomes in patients with cardiac sarcoidosis. *Int J Cardiol.* 2014;177:720-722.

364. Ekström K, Lehtonen J, Nordenswan HK, et al. Sudden death in cardiac sarcoidosis: an analysis of nationwide clinical and cause-of-death registries. *Eur Heart J.* 2019;40:3121-3128.

365. Birnie DH, Sauer WH, Bogun F, et al. HRS expert consensus statement on the diagnosis and management of arrhythmias associated with cardiac sarcoidosis. *Heart Rhythm.* 2014;11:1305-1323.

366. Judson MA, Costabel U, Drent M, et al. The WASOG sarcoidosis organ assessment instrument: An update of a previous clinical tool. *Sarcoidosis Vasc Diffuse Lung Dis.* 2014;31:19-27.

367. Birnie DH, Sauer WH, Judson MA. Consensus statement on the diagnosis and management of arrhythmias associated with cardiac sarcoidosis. *Heart.* 2016;102:11-14.

368. Schuller JL, Lowery CM, Zipse M, et al. Diagnostic utility of signal-averaged electrocardiography for detection of cardiac sarcoidosis. *Ann Noninvasive Electrocardiol.* 2011;16:70-76.

369. Bami K, Haddad T, Dick A, et al. Noninvasive imaging in acute myocarditis. *Curr Opin Cardiol.* 2016;31:217-223.

370. Tigen K, Sunbul M, Karaahmet T, et al. Early detection of bi-ventricular and atrial mechanical dysfunction using two-dimensional

speckle tracking echocardiography in patients with sarcoidosis. *Lung.* 2015;193:669-675.

371. Ise T, Hasegawa T, Morita Y, et al. Extensive late gadolinium enhancement on cardiovascular magnetic resonance predicts adverse outcomes and lack of improvement in LV function after steroid therapy in cardiac sarcoidosis. *Heart.* 2014;100:1165-1172.

372. Yoshida H, Ishibashi-Ueda N, Yamada N, et al. Direct comparison of the diagnostic capability of cardiac magnetic resonance and endomyocardial biopsy in patients with heart failure. *Eur J Heart Fail.* 2013;15:166-175.

373. Neilan TG, Farhad H, Mayrhofer T, et al. Late gadolinium enhancement among survivors of sudden cardiac arrest. *JACC Cardiovasc Imaging.* 2015;8:414-423.

374. Pizarro C, Goebel A, Dabir D, et al. Cardiovascular magnetic resonance-guided diagnosis of cardiac affection in a Caucasian sarcoidosis population. *Sarcoidosis Vasc Diffuse Lung Dis.* 2016;32:325-335.

375. Murtagh G, Laffin LJ, Beshai JF, et al. Prognosis of myocardial damage in sarcoidosis patients with preserved left ventricular ejection fraction: risk stratification using cardiovascular magnetic resonance. *Circ Cardiovasc Imaging.* 2016;9:e003738.

376. Patel MB, Mor-Avi V, Murtagh G, et al. Right heart involvement in patients with sarcoidosis. *Echocardiography.* 2016;33:734-741.

377. Paz YE, Bokhari S. The role of F18-fluorodeoxyglucose positron emission tomography in identifying patients at high risk for lethal arrhythmias from cardiac sarcoidosis and the use of serial scanning to guide therapy. *Int J Cardiovasc Imaging.* 2014;30:431-438.

378. Ahmadian A, Brogan A, Berman J, et al. Quantitative interpretation of FDG PET/CT with myocardial perfusion imaging increases diagnostic information in the evaluation of cardiac sarcoidosis. *J Nucl Cardiol.* 2014;21:925-939.

379. Blankstein R, Osborne M, Naya M, et al. Cardiac positron emission tomography enhances prognostic assessments of patients with suspected cardiac sarcoidosis. *J Am Coll Cardiol.* 2014;63:329-336.

380. Mc Ardle BA, Birnie DH, Klein R, et al. Is there an association between clinical presentation and the location and extent of myocardial involvement of cardiac sarcoidosis as assessed by ^{18}F-flurodoexyglucose positron emission tomography? *Circ Cardiovasc Imaging.* 2013;6:617-626.

381. Kouranos V, Wells AU, Sharma R, et al. Advances in radionuclide imaging of cardiac sarcoidosis. *Br Med Bull.* 2015;115:151-163.

382. Isobe M, Tezuka D. Isolated cardiac sarcoidosis: clinical characteristics, diagnosis and treatment. *Int J Cardiol.* 2015;182:132-140.

383. Kandolin R, Lehtonen J, Airaksinen J, et al. Usefulness of cardiac troponins as markers of early treatment response in cardiac sarcoidosis. *Am J Cardiol.* 2015;116:960-964.

384. Kato Y, Morimoto S. Analysis of clinical manifestations of cardiac sarcoidosis: a multicentre study: preliminary report. *Jpn J Sarcoidosis Granulomatous Disord.* 2010;30:73-76.

385. Shijubo N, Ichimura S, Itoh T, et al. Analysis of several examinations in 516 histologically proven sarcoidosis patients. *Jpn J Sarcoidosis Granulomatous Disord.* 2007;27:29-35.

386. Grutters JC, Fellrath JM, Mulder L, et al. Serum soluble interleukin-2 receptor measurement in patient with sarcoidosis. *Chest.* 2003;124:186-195.

387. Baba Y, Kubo T, Kitaoka H, et al. Usefulness of high-sensitive cardiac troponin T for evaluating the activity of cardiac sarcoidosis. *Int Heart J.* 2012;53:287-292.

388. Yasutake H, Seino Y, Kashiwagi M, et al. Detection of cardiac sarcoidosis using cardiac markers and myocardial integrated backscatter. *Int J Cardiol.* 2008;102:259-268.

389. Ipek E, Demirelli S, Ermis E, Inci S. Sarcoidosis and the heart: a review of the literature. *Intractable Rare Dis Res.* 2015;4:170-180.

390. Kandolin R, Lehtonen J, Graner M, et al. Diagnosing isolated cardiac sarcoidosis. *J Intern Med.* 2011;270:461-468.

391. Lagana SM, Parwani AV, Nichols LC. Cardiac sarcoidosis. A pathology-focused review. *Arch Pathol Lab Med.* 2010;134:1039-1046.

392. Sperry BW, Oldan J, Hachamovitch R, et al. Insights into biopsy-proven cardiac sarcoidosis in patients with heart failure. *J Heart Lung Transplant.* 2016;35:392-393.

393. Malik LH, Singh GD, Amsterdam EA. The epidemiology, clinical manifestations, and management of Chagas heart disease. *Clin Cardiol.* 2015;38:565-569.

394. Bern C. Chagas' disease. *N Engl J Med.* 2015;373:456-466.

395. Shikanai-Yasuda MA, Carvalho NB. Oral transmission of Chagas disease. *Clin Infect Dis.* 2012;54:845-852.

396. Garcia MN, Woc-Colburn L, Aguilar D, et al. Historical perspectives on the epidemiology of human Chagas disease in Texas and recommendations for enhanced understanding of clinical Chagas disease in the southern United States. *PLoS Negl Trop Dis.* 2015;9:e0003981.

397. Nouvellet P, Dumonteil E, Gourbière S. The improbable transmission of *Trypanosoma cruzi* to human: the missing link in the dynamics and control of Chagas disease. *PLoS Negl Trop Dis.* 2013;7:e2505-e2505.

398. Samuels AM, Clark EH, Galdos-Cardenas G, et al. Epidemiology of and impact of insecticide spraying on Chagas disease in communities in the Bolivian Chaco. *PLoS Negl Trop Dis.* 2013;7:e2358-e2358.

399. Chagas disease in Latin America: an epidemiological update based on 2010 estimates. *Wkly Epidemiol Rec.* 2015;90:33-43.

400. World Health Organization. Chagas disease (American trypanosomiasis) 2015. Updated March 2015. http://www.who.int/mediacentre/factsheets/fs340/en/. Accessed March 1, 2021.

401. Kapelusznik L, Varela D, Montgomery SP, et al. Chagas disease in Latin American immigrants with dilated cardiomyopathy in New York City. *Clin Infect Dis.* 2013;57:e7.

402. Cantey PT, Stramer SL, Townsend RL, et al. The United States *Trypanosoma cruzi* Infection Study: evidence for vector-borne transmission of the parasite that causes Chagas disease among United States blood donors. *Transfusion.* 2012;52:1922-1930.

403. Bern C, Martin DL, Gilman RH. Acute and congenital Chagas disease. *Adv Parasitol.* 2011;75:19-47.

404. Alvarado-Tapias E, Miranda-Pacheco R, Rodríguez-Bonfante C, et al. Electrocardiography repolarization abnormalities are characteristic signs of acute Chagasic cardiomyopathy. *Invest Clin.* 2012;53:378-394.

405. Ribeiro A, Nunes M, Teixeira M, et al. Diagnosis and management of Chagas disease cardiomyopathy. *Nat Rev Cardiol.* 2012;9:576-589.

406. Marcolino MS, Palhares DM, Ferreira LR, Ribeiro AL. Electrocardiogram and Chagas disease: a large population database of primary care patients. *Glob Heart.* 2015;10:167-172.

407. Regueiro A, Garcia-Alvarez A, Sitges M, et al. Myocardial involvement in Chagas disease: insights from cardiac magnetic resonance. *Int J Cardiol.* 2013;165:107-112.

408. Rassi A Jr, Rassi S, Rassi A. Sudden death in Chagas disease. *Arq Bras Cardiol.* 2001;76:75-96.

409. Benvenuti LA, Freitas VLT, Roggério A, et al. Usefulness of PCR for Trypanosoma cruzi DNA in blood and endomyocardial biopsies for detection of Chagas disease reactivation after heart transplantation: a comparative study. *Transpl Infect Dis.* 2021:e13567.

410. Del Puerto R, Nishizawa JE, Kikuchi M, et al. Lineage analysis of circulating *Trypanosoma cruzi* parasites and their association with clinical forms of Chagas disease in Bolivia. *PLoS Negl Trop Dis.* 2010;4:e687.

411. Haberland A, Saravia SG, Wallukat G, et al. Chronic Chagas disease: from basics to laboratory medicine. *Clin Chem Lab Med.* 2013;51:271-294.

412. Healy C, Viles-Gonzalez JF, Sáenz LC, et al. Arrhythmias in Chagasic cardiomyopathy. *Card Electrophysiol Clin.* 2015;7:251-268.

413. Pereira Júnior Cde B, Markman Filho B. Clinical and echocardiographic predictors of mortality in Chagasic cardiomyopathy: systematic review. *Arq Bras Cardiol.* 2014;102:602-610.

414. Viotti R, Alarcón de Noya B, Araujo-Jorge T, et al. Towards a paradigm shift in the treatment of chronic Chagas disease. *Antimicrob Agents Chemother.* 2014;58:635-639.

415. Molina I, Prat J, Salvador F, et al. Randomized trial of posaconazole and benznidazole for chronic Chagas disease. *N Engl J Med*. 2014;370:1899-1908.

416. Bestetti RB, Cardinalli-Neto A. Device therapy in Chagas disease heart failure. *Expert Rev Cardiovasc Ther*. 2012;10:1307-1317.

417. Kransdorf EP, Zakowski PC, Kobashigawa JA. Chagas disease in solid organ and heart transplantation. *Curr Opin Infect Dis*. 2014;27:418-424.

418. Pereira F, Rocha E, Monteiro Mde P, et al. Long-term follow-up of patients with chronic Chagas disease and implantable cardioverter-defibrillator. *Pacing Clin Electrophysiol*. 2014;37:751-756.

419. Gali W, Sarabanda A, Baggio A, et al. Implantable cardioverter defibrillators for treatment of sustained ventricular arrhythmias in patients with Chagas' heart disease: comparison with a control group treated with amiodarone alone. *Europace*. 2014;16:674-680.

420. Arce M, Van Grieken J, Femenia F, et al. Permanent pacing in patients with Chagas' disease. *Pacing Clin Electrophysiol*. 2012;35:1494-1497.

421. Stanek G, Wormser GP, Gray J, et al. Lyme borreliosis. *Lancet*. 2012;379:461-473.

422. Rivera OJ, Nookala V. Lyme Carditis. 2020. In: *StatPearls [Internet]*. Treasure Island (FL): StatPearls Publishing; 2021.

423. Centers for Disease Control and Prevention. Reported cases of Lyme disease by state or locality, 2004–2013. http://www.cdc.gov/lyme/stats/chartstables/reportedcases_statelocality.html. Accessed March 1, 2021.

424. Lindgren E, Jaenson TG. Lyme borreliosis in Europe: influences of climate and climate change, epidemiology, ecology and adaptation measures, WHO Regional Office for Europe (2006). http://www.euro.who.it/InformationSources/Publications/Catalogue/20061219_1. Accessed March 1, 2021.

425. Kugeler KJ, Jordan RA, Schulze TL, Griffith KS, Mead PS. Will culling white-tailed deer prevent Lyme disease? *Zoonoses Public Health*. 2016;63:337-345.

426. Scheffold N, Herkommer B, Kandolf R, et al. Lyme carditis: diagnosis, treatment and prognosis. *Dtsch Arztebl Int*. 2015;112:202-208.

427. Dubrey SW, Bhatia A, Woodham S, et al. Lyme disease in the United Kingdom. *Postgrad Med J*. 2014;90:33-42.

428. Stanek G, Fingerle V, Hunfeld KP, et al. Lyme borreliosis: clinical case definitions for diagnosis and management in Europe. *Clin Microbiol Infect*. 2011;17:69-79.

429. Hinckley AF, Connally NP, Meek JI, et al. Lyme disease testing by large commercial laboratories in the United States. *Clin Infect Dis*. 2014;59:676-681.

430. Nelson CA, Saha S, Kugeler KJ, et al. Incidence of clinician-diagnosed Lyme disease, United States, 2005-2010. *Emerg Infect Dis*. 2015;21:1625-1631.

431. Franke J, Hildebrandt A, Dorn W. Exploring gaps in our knowledge on Lyme borreliosis spirochaetes: updates on complex heterogeneity, ecology, and pathogenicity. *Ticks Tick Borne Dis*. 2013;4:11-25.

432. Sanchez JL. Clinical manifestations and treatment of Lyme disease. *Clin Lab Med*. 2015;35:765-778.

433. Halperin JJ. Nervous system Lyme disease. *Clin Lab Med*. 2015;35:779-795.

434. Lantos PM, Rumbaugh J, Bockenstedt LK, et al. Clinical Practice Guidelines by the Infectious Diseases Society of America (IDSA), American Academy of Neurology (AAN), and American College of Rheumatology (ACR): 2020 Guidelines for the Prevention, Diagnosis and Treatment of Lyme Disease. *Clin Infect Dis*. 2021;72(1):e1-e48.

435. Robinson ML, Kobayashi T, Higgins Y, et al. Lyme carditis. *Infect Dis Clin North Am*. 2015;29:255-268.

436. Forrester JD, Mead P. Third-degree heart block associated with Lyme carditis: review of published cases. *Clin Infect Dis*. 2014;59:996-1000.

437. Kubánek M, Šramko M, Berenová D, et al. Detection of *Borrelia burgdorferi* sensu lato in endomyocardial biopsy specimens in individuals with recent-onset dilated cardiomyopathy. *Eur J Heart Fail*. 2012;14:588-596.

438. Kuchynka P, Palecek T, Havranek S, et al. Recent-onset dilated cardiomyopathy associated with *Borrelia burgdorferi* infection. *Herz*. 2015;40:892-897.

439. Theel ES. The past, present and (possible) future of serologic testing for Lyme disease. *J Clin Microbiol*. 2016;54:1191-1196.

440. Molins CR, Ashton LV, Wormser GP, et al. Development of a metabolic biosignature for detection of early Lyme disease. *Clin Infect Dis*. 2015;60:1767-1775.

441. Smith GN, Gemmill I, Moore KM. Management of tick bites and lyme disease during pregnancy. *J Obstet Gynaecol Can*. 2012;34(11):1087-1091.

442. Yeung C, Baranchuk A. Diagnosis and treatment of lyme carditis: JACC Review Topic of the Week. *J Am Coll Cardiol*. 2019;73(6):717-726.

443. Wooldridge G, Nandi D, Chimalizeni Y, O'Brien N. Cardiovascular findings in severe malaria: a review. *Glob Heart*. 2020;15(1):75.

444. Ventura AM, Chaves Tdo S, Monteiro JC et al. Myocarditis associated with Plasmodium vivax malaria: a case report. *Rev Soc Bras Med Trop*. 2014;47(6):810-813.

445. Gantait K, Gantait I. Vivax malaria complicated by myocarditis. *J Assoc Physicians India*. 2013;61(12):944-945.

446. Gupta S, Gazendam N, Farina JM et al. Malaria and the heart: JACC State-of-the-Art Review. *J Am Coll Cardiol*. 2021;77(8):1110-1121.

447. Nayak KC, Meena SL, Gupta BK, et al. Cardiovascular involvement in severe vivax and falciparum malaria. *J Vector Borne Dis*. 2013;50:285-291.

448. Khan FY. Imported *Plasmodium vivax* malaria complicated by reversible myocarditis. *J Family Community Med*. 2019;26(3):232-234.

449. Vernaza A, Pinilla-Monsalve G, Cañas F, et al. Malaria and encephalopathy in a heart transplant recipient: a case report in the context of multiorgan donation. *Transpl Infect Dis*. 2021:e13565.

450. Kita H. Eosinophils: multifaceted biological properties and roles in health and disease. *Immunol Rev*. 2011;242:161-177.

451. Valent P, Klion AD, Horny H-P, et al. Contemporary consensus proposal on criteria and classification of eosinophilic disorders and related syndromes. *J Allergy Clin Immunol*. 2012;130:607-612.e9.

452. Gotlib J. World Health Organization-defined eosinophilic disorders: 2011 update on diagnosis, risk stratification, and management. *Am J Hematol*. 2011;86:678-688.

453. Valent P, Gleich GJ, Reiter A, et al. Pathogenesis and classification of eosinophil disorders: a review of recent developments in the field. *Expert Rev Hematol*. 2012;5:157-176.

454. Klion AD, Bochner BS, Gleich GJ, et al. Approaches to the treatment of hypereosinophilic syndromes: a workshop summary report. *J Allergy Clin Immunol*. 2006;117:1292-1302.

455. Simon H-U, Rothenberg ME, Bochner BS, et al. Refining the definition of hypereosinophilic syndrome. *J Allergy Clin Immunol*. 2010;126:45-49.

456. Crane MM, Chang CM, Kobayashi MG, et al. Incidence of myeloproliferative hypereosinophilic syndrome in the United States and an estimate of all hypereosinophilic syndrome incidence. *J Allergy Clin Immunol*. 2010;126:179-181.

457. Pardanani A, Ketterling RP, Li CY, et al. FIP1L1-PDGFRA in eosinophilic disorders: prevalence in routine clinical practice, long-term experience with imatinib therapy, and a critical review of the literature. *Leuk Res*. 2006;30:965-970.

458. Jovanovic JV, Score J, Waghorn K, et al. Low-dose imatinib mesylate leads to rapid induction of major molecular responses and achievement of complete molecular remission in FIP1L1-PDGFRA-positive chronic eosinophilic leukemia. *Blood*. 2007;109:4635-4640.

459. Giovannini-Chami L, Hadchouel A, Nathan N, et al. Idiopathic eosinophilic pneumonia in children: the French experience. *Orphanet J Rare Dis*. 2014;9:28.

460. Tamse T, Rampersad A, Jordan-Villegas A, et al. A case of idiopathic hypereosinophilic syndrome causing mitral valve papillary muscle rupture. *Case Rep Pediatr*. 2015;2015:538762.

461. Tai CP, Chung T, Avasarala K. Endomyocardial fibrosis and mural thrombus in a 4-year-old girl due to idiopathic hypereosinophilia syndrome described with serial cardiac magnetic resonance imaging. *Cardiol Young*. 2016;26:168-171.

462. Cools J, DeAngelo DJ, Gotlib J, et al. A tyrosine kinase created by fusion of the PDGFRA and FIP1L1 genes as a therapeutic target of imatinib in idiopathic hypereosinophilic syndrome. *N Engl J Med.* 2003;348:1201-1214.

463. Kuang FL, Legrand F, Makiya M, et al. Benralizumab for *PDGFRA*-negative hypereosinophilic syndrome. *N Engl J Med.* 2019;380(14):1336-1346.

464. Baccarani M, Cilloni D, Rondoni M, et al. The efficacy of imatinib mesylate in patients with FIP1L1-PDGFRalpha-positive hypereosinophilic syndrome. Results of a multicenter prospective study. *Haematologica.* 2007;92:1173-1179.

465. Ogbogu PU, Bochner BS, Butterfield JH, et al. Hypereosinophilic syndromes: a multicenter, retrospective analysis of clinical characteristics and response to therapy. *J Allergy Clin Immunol.* 2009;124:1319-1325.

466. Riley LK, Rupert J. Evaluation of patients with leukocytosis. *Am Fam Physician.* 2015;92:1004-1011.

467. Mankad R, Bonnichsen C, Mankad S. Hypereosinophilic syndrome: cardiac diagnosis and management. *Heart.* 2016;102:100-106.

468. Séguéla PE, Iriart X, Acar P, et al. Eosinophilic cardiac disease: molecular, clinical and imaging aspects. *Arch Cardiovasc Dis.* 2015;108:258-268.

469. Kleinfeldt T, Nienaber CA, Kische S, et al. Cardiac manifestation of the hypereosinophilic syndrome: new insights. *Clin Res Cardiol.* 2010;99:419-427.

470. Cheung CC, Constantine M, Ahmadi A, et al. Eosinophilic myocarditis. *Am J Med Sci.* 2017 Nov;354(5):486-492.

471. D'Orazio J, Pulliam J. Hypereosinophilic syndrome presenting as acute myocardial infarction in an adolescent. *J Pediatr.* 2011;158:685.

472. Amini R, Nielsen C. Eosinophilic myocarditis mimicking acute coronary syndrome secondary to idiopathic hypereosinophilic syndrome: a case report. *J Med Case Rep.* 2010;4:40.

473. Campbell RT, Jhund PS, Dalzell JR, et al. Diagnosis and resolution of Löeffler endocarditis secondary to eosinophilic granulomatosis with polyangiitis demonstrated by cardiac magnetic resonance-T2 mapping. *Circulation.* 2015;131:114-117.

474. May LJ, Patton DJ, Fruitman DS, et al. The evolving approach to pediatric myocarditis: a review of the current literature. *Cardiol Young.* 2011;21:241-251.

475. Yanagisawa T, Inomata T, Watanabe I, et al. Clinical significance of corticosteroid therapy for eosinophilic myocarditis. *Int Heart J.* 2011;52:110-113.

476. Lo MH, Huang CF, Chang LS, et al. Drug reaction with eosinophilia and systemic symptoms syndrome associated myocarditis: a survival experience after extracorporeal membrane oxygenation support. *J Clin Pharm Ther.* 2013;38:172-174.

477. Fassnacht F, Roumier M, Fouret P, et al. Successful heart transplantation for unreversible endomyocardial fibrosis related to FIP1L1-PDGFRA chronic eosinophilic leukemia. *Transplantation.* 2015;99:e176-e177.

478. Groh M, Masciocco G, Kirchner E, et al. Heart transplantation in patients with eosinophil granulomatosis with polyangiitis (Churg-Strauss syndrome). *J Heart Lung Transplant.* 2014;33:842-850.

479. Groh M, Pagnoux C, Baldini C, et al. Eosinophilic granulomatosis with polyangiitis (Churg-Strauss) (EGPA) Consensus Task Force recommendations for evaluation and management. *Eur J Intern Med.* 2015;26:545-553.

47

Obstructive and Nonobstructive Coronary Disease in Heart Failure

Charlotte Lee and G. William Dec

Obstructive and non-obstructive coronary disease in heart failure

Obstructive disease

Non-obstructive disease

Risk factors for HF in stable CAD

- Older age
- Lower LVEF
- Atrial fibrillation
- Higher body mass index
- Diabetes mellitus
- HTN
- Angina at baseline
- Multivessel CAD

Risk factors

- Similar to those in obstructive disease, and also include HTN, lung disease, obesity, anemia, kidney disease and sleep-disordered breathing

Diagnostic testing

Non-invasive: Myocardial perfusion imaging or stress echo for known CAD and de novo HF

Invasive: Angiography for those with HF and angina, unexplained LV systolic dysfunction

Viability: Assessment of myocardial viability (PET most sensitive) not shown to correlate with improved ventricular function

Diagnostic testing

Non-invasive: PET to assess global myocardial flow reserve, cardiac MRI to assess coronary flow reserve

Separate testing for other risk factors above

Phenotypes

Intermittent episodes of ischemia, fixed myocardial fibrosis and endothelial dysfunction superimposed on progressive nature of HFrEF; ischemic MR is associated with poor prognosis

High incidence of CAD

Presence of CAD associated with increased mortality and greater deterioration in ventricular function; worse prognosis with increasing extent of CAD

| HFrEF: LVEF < 40% |
| HFmrEF: LVEF 41%-49% |
| HFpEF: LVEF ≥50% |

Phenotypes

Non-obstructive disease is associated with an increased risk of death and adverse cardiac events

High incidence of CAD; other clinical characteristics similar to HFpEF (older age, female sex, HTN, COPD, diabetes)

Microvascular endothelial inflammation may play a role in those with angiographically normal coronaries

Treatment

- Coronary revascularization may improve quality of life and outcome in patients with or without symptomatic angina pectoris in HFrEF
- Percutaneous repair in HFrEF? ERO ≥ 0.30 cm^2; no excessive LV dilatation, ongoing HF despite intense GDMT
- Screen/treat for CAD in HFmrEF
- Revascularization improves clinical outcomes in those with symptomatic CAD in HFpEF
- CABG favored for patients with preserved exercise capacity, multivessel CAD, lower LVEF, three-vessel disease and higher LV end-systolic volume index, diabetic patients with LV dysfunction

Treatment

- Ongoing studies on GDMT across phenotypes
- Screen/treat for CAD in HFmrEF, pharmacologic treatment similar to HFpEF
- Treat comorbid conditions

Prompt reperfusion and use of pharmacologic therapies with GDMT may prevent adverse remodeling in **post-MI** heart failure

Chapter 47 Fuster and Hurst's Central Illustration. Coronary artery disease (CAD) is the most common etiology for heart failure, regardless of whether the phenotype is heart failure with reduced ejection fraction (HFrEF; left ventricular ejection fraction [LVEF] <40%), mildly reduced ejection fraction (HFmrEF; LVEF 41%-49%), or preserved ejection fraction (HFpEF; LVEF ≥50%). The extent of CAD has a direct bearing on clinical outcome. CABG, coronary artery bypass grafting; GDMT, guideline-directed medical therapy; HTN, hypertension; LV, left ventricular; MI, myocardial infarction; MR, mitral regurgitation; PET, positron emission tomography; MRI, magnetic resonance imaging; COPD, chronic obstructive pulmonary disease.

CHAPTER SUMMARY

This chapter discusses the epidemiology of heart failure due to coronary atherosclerosis, as well as the pathophysiology and treatment options for promoting reverse remodeling of the left ventricle following myocardial infarction. Coronary artery disease remains the most common etiology for heart failure, regardless of whether the phenotype is heart failure with reduced ejection fraction (left ventricular ejection fraction [LVEF] up to 40%), mildly reduced ejection fraction (LVEF 41% to 49%), or preserved ejection fraction (LVEF of at least 50%) (see Fuster and Hurst's Central Illustration). The extent of coronary artery disease has a direct bearing on clinical outcome. While guideline-directed pharmacotherapy remains a cornerstone for managing heart failure with reduced ejection fraction, coronary revascularization may improve quality of life and outcome in patients with or without symptomatic angina pectoris. Surgical coronary revascularization is more effective than medical therapy alone in the setting of hemodynamically significant multivessel disease, impaired left ventricular function, ventricular enlargement, moderate or severe mitral regurgitation and relatively preserved functional capacity. Coronary bypass grafting is more beneficial than multivessel percutaneous coronary intervention among diabetic patients with ischemic cardiomyopathy. For heart failure with preserved ejection fraction, the role of microvascular dysfunction and intermittent ischemia is summarized and treatment recommendations, including revascularization, are discussed.

EPIDEMIOLOGY OF HEART FAILURE DUE TO ISCHEMIC HEART DISEASE

Common risk factors for heart failure (HF) include increased age, hypertension, diabetes, obesity, valvular heart disease, metabolic syndrome, and coronary artery disease (CAD). HF prevalence is also age-dependent, increasing significantly in the Framingham Heart Study from ~1% for those aged 50 to 59 years to ~10% in those aged 80 to 89 years.[1] The incidence of CAD has been found to vary globally. In the United States, 50% to 70% of all cases of HF are attributed to CAD, compared to only 10% of cases in sub-Saharan Africa and 30% to 40% of all cases in Asia and Latin America.[2] The incidence of HF has also been increasing with the lifetime risk for developing HF ranging from 20% to 45% in those aged 45 to 95 years old.[1] Further, data from community surveillance studies have shown that HF hospitalizations are expected to increase over time, largely driven by increases in heart failure with preserved ejection fraction (HFpEF).[3]

Several large community-based studies have examined the relationship between CAD and incident HF. Major advances in the treatment of acute ST-segment elevation myocardial infarction (STEMI) during the last four decades have resulted in a substantial decline in mortality rates after myocardial infarction (MI). However, HF is now an increasingly common complication among post-MI survivors. Investigators from the Framingham Heart Study evaluated the temporal trends in HF incidence after symptomatic acute MI. While the 30-day mortality rates after MI declined from 12.2% (1970–1979) to 4.1% (1990–1999), the 30-day incidence of HF after MI rose from 10% to 23% during the same time interval.[4] Importantly, the 5-year incidence of HF after MI rose from 27.6% to 32.0% while the 5-year mortality after MI declined from 41.1% to 17.3% during the same timeframe. The extent of CAD (eg, number of diseased vessels, history of revascularization, or MI) has also been found to be an important factor in prognosis[5] (**Fig. 47–1**).

A key question is how often does HF develop in patients with stable CAD? A recent French registry study identified over 4000 unselected outpatients with stable ischemic heart disease (ie, prior MI and/or revascularization >1 year earlier).[6] The 5-year cumulative incidence of new symptomatic HF was 5.7%. Independent predictors of HF hospitalization were older age, lower left ventricular ejection fraction (LVEF), atrial fibrillation, higher body mass index, diabetes mellitus, history of hypertension, angina at baseline, and multivessel CAD. The vast majority (92%) of HF admissions were not preceded by an incident MI. Hospitalization for HF was a powerful independent predictor of mortality (adjusted hazard ratio [HR], 5.97).

Data from a large registry have demonstrated that the presence of symptomatic angina pectoris in patients with ischemic cardiomyopathy and reduced ejection fraction is not associated with increased long-term rates of death, MI, or death/all-cause mortality.[7] Three-vessel coronary disease was present in over 50% of both cohorts and over 60% had undergone prior coronary revascularization. While mortality rates did not differ, patients with symptomatic angina had higher rates of cardiovascular hospitalization.

An earlier study from the Framingham Heart group examined the natural history of asymptomatic left ventricular systolic dysfunction (ALVD) in the community.[8] Routine

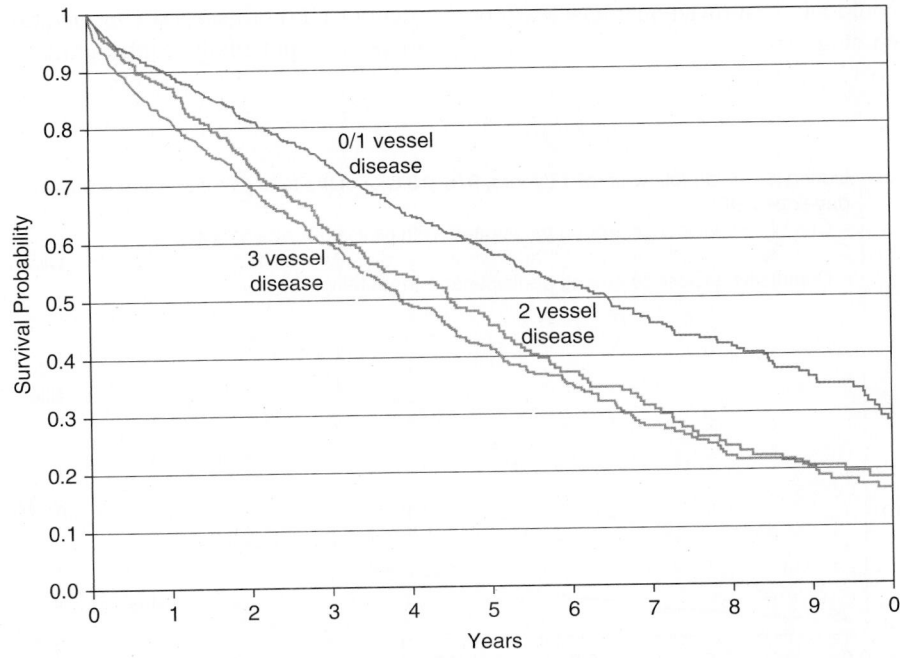

Figure 47–1. Adjusted survival curves via modified number-of-diseased-vessels classification. Adjusted survival curve using modified number-of-diseased-vessels classification to quantify CAD. Curves were adjusted for age, ejection fraction, gender, NYHA functional class, diabetes mellitus, and valvular heart disease. This classification scheme provided the best overall prognostic value. Reproduced with permission from Felker GM, Shaw LK, O'Connor CM. A standardized definition of ischemic cardiomyopathy for use in clinical research. *J Am Coll Cardiol.* 2002 Jan 16;39(2):210-218.

echocardiography identified the prevalence of ALVD (defined as LVEF ≤50% without a history of symptomatic HF) in 6% of men and in 0.8% of women. Overall, prior MI was identified in 49% of the ALVD cohort compared to 2% of patients with normal systolic function. ALVD was associated with a substantially higher risk of developing overt HF (adjusted HR, 4.7) compared to individuals with normal function. Importantly, even individuals with heart failure with midrange ejection fraction (HFmidEF) (LVEF 40%–50%) were at increased risk of developing overt HF over the next decade.

Electrocardiogram (ECG)-defined silent MI (SMI) accounts for 5% to 30% of the total number of all nonfatal MIs. Investigators from the ARIC (Atherosclerosis Risk In Communities) study compared the association with of SMI and clinically manifested MI (CMI) on the subsequent development of HF.[9] All patients were free of known cardiovascular disease at baseline community assessment. The incident rate of HF was higher in both CMI and SMI participants than in those free of MI (**Fig. 47–2**). After adjustment for demographics and known HF risk factors, both SMI (HR, 1.35) and CMI (HR, 2.85) were strongly associated with an increased risk of HF compared to those without MI. Surprisingly, a stronger association with SMI was noted in younger patients (<53 years of age).

The ETICS (Epidemiologie et Thereutique de L'Insuffisance Cardiaque das la Somme) registry examined 10-year outcomes of patients enrolled at the time of initial HF hospitalization.[10] CAD was identified in 39% of the heart failure with reduced ejection fraction (HFrEF) cohort. The 10-year event rate was significantly greater in the CAD group than in the non-CAD cohort (86% vs 67%). Specifically, CAD was associated with an increased risk of HF-related (adjusted has ratio: 2.03) and MI-related fatal events (adjusted HR, 3.84). Whether aggressive revascularization could have improved outcomes was not examined in this epidemiologic study.

DIAGNOSTIC TESTING

Noninvasive testing

CAD is the most common etiology for HF regardless of HFrEF, HFmidEF, or HFpEF phenotype. Thus, an ischemia work-up should be considered for any patient with unexplained HF with more than a low pretest probability of coronary atherosclerosis (eg, males over 40 years of age, diabetics, those with a family history of premature coronary disease, or marked hyperlipidemia). Chronotropic incompetence during exercise testing has been associated with increased likelihood of CAD and higher overall mortality. A meta-analysis comparing exercise to pharmacologic stress perfusion imaging found a comparable ability to risk-stratify patients, although those undergoing a pharmacologic test had an increased risk of subsequent cardiac events likely due to their inability to exercise.[11] In a study of 5183 patients who underwent SPECT imaging, incremental prognostic value was noted for those having at least a moderately severe perfusion defect or several abnormal regions of perfusion for future MI or cardiac death[12] (**Fig. 47–3**). Exercise echocardiography provides additional information including wall motion abnormalities and has an increased predictive value when combined with other exercise test parameters. Noninvasive stress testing (either myocardial perfusion imaging or stress echocardiography) should be considered for all patients who present with de novo HF and have known coronary disease with or without symptomatic angina pectoris, unless the patient is not eligible for revascularization (American College of Cardiology/American Heart Association [ACC/AHA] class IIa recommendation).[13] Of note, although there are differences and similarities between ACC and European Society of Cardiology (ESC) guidelines on diagnosis and management of HF, both suggest consideration of angiography when ischemia is potentially contributing to HF or in patients with

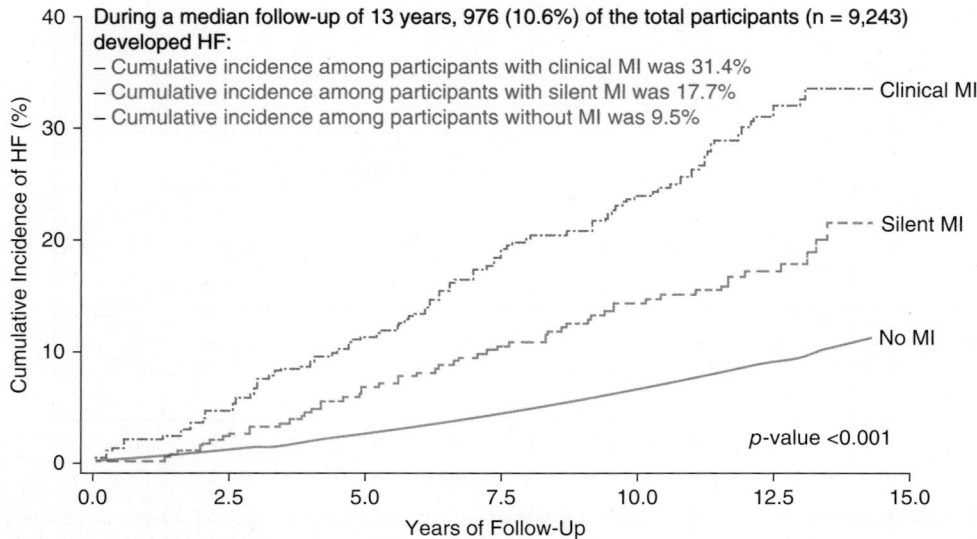

Figure 47–2. Risk of HF associated with different patterns of MI. Cumulative incidence of HF stratified by MI status. Reproduced with permission from Qureshi WT, Zhang ZM, Chang PP, et al. Silent Myocardial Infarction and Long-Term Risk of Heart Failure: The ARIC Study. *J Am Coll Cardiol.* 2018 Jan 2;71(1):1-8.

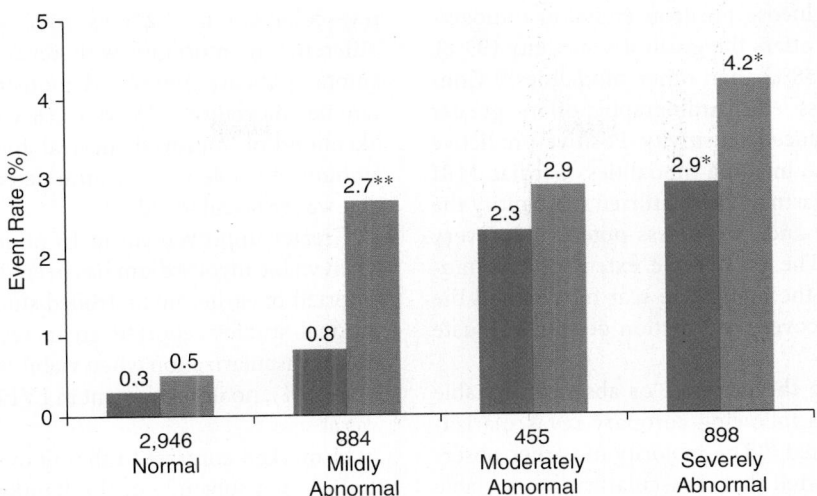

Figure 47–3. **SPECT myocardial perfusion imaging predicts cardiac death and MI.** The frequency of events per year of follow-up as a function of scan result are shown. The presence and severity of an abnormal myocardial perfusion imaging scan during treadmill stress testing was predictive of cardiac death (*open bars*) or MI (*closed bars*) during a 2-year follow-up (n = 5183 patients).

*Statistically significant increase as a function of scan result. **Statistically significant increase in rate of MI versus cardiac death within scan category. Reproduced with permission from Hachamovitch R, Berman DS, Shaw LJ, et al. Incremental prognostic value of myocardial perfusion single photon emission computed tomography for the prediction of cardiac death: differential stratification for risk of cardiac death and myocardial infarction. *Circulation.* 1998 Feb 17; 97(6):535–543.

intermediate-to-high pretest probability of coronary disease with ischemia on noninvasive stress testing (class IIa recommendation).[14] The ESC guidelines do recommend coronary angiography in patients with HF and angina pectoris refractory to medical therapy, or patients with a history of symptomatic ventricular arrhythmia or cardiac arrest,[13] whereas the ACC guidelines recommend coronary angiography for those with HF and angina, those with known CAD and angina, or those with significant ischemia on ECG or noninvasive testing and impaired ventricular function.[15]

Among patients without known CAD and a low pretest probability, coronary computed tomographic angiography (CCTA) has been found to be effective in screening for proximal multivessel coronary disease. Sensitivity, specificity, and negative predictive value for the identification of >50% stenoses in one or more vessel have been reported at 99%, 96%, and 99%, respectively.[16] A Johns Hopkins study of 1230 patients with initially unexplained dilated cardiomyopathy who were felt to have nonischemic cardiomyopathy were subsequently found to have unsuspected coronary disease in 7% of cases.[17] Thus, a low threshold for diagnostic testing is mandatory.

Invasive Testing

Invasive coronary angiography is indicated for patients with HF and angina and may be useful for patients without angina but unexplained left ventricular (LV) systolic dysfunction. Patients with acute pulmonary edema should also be considered for coronary angiography. Further, patients who have significant ischemia diagnosed by ECG or noninvasive testing should undergo coronary angiography (AHA/ACC class I recommendation). Among patients in whom CAD had previously been excluded as a cause for LV dysfunction, coronary angiography

is generally not indicated unless a change in clinical status suggests the interim development of ischemic heart disease.[18]

Viability Assessment

Prior observational studies have found the incidence of viable myocardium in ischemic LV dysfunction to be approximately 50% to 60%.[19] It has been proposed that those with LV systolic dysfunction may have either transient ischemic stunning or hibernation from hypoperfused myocardium from a potentially treatable coronary stenosis. In transient ischemic stunning, an abrupt decrease in blood flow leads to contractile dysfunction with recovery of function over hours to days, whereas hibernating myocardium has undergone an adaptive process with structural changes that require a longer time for recovery.[20] Interestingly, a study by Narula et al. found that different mechanisms—stunning, hibernation, remodeling, and scarring—can exist simultaneously in a given region of myocardium and that approximately 50% of patients in their study had stunned and/or hibernating myocardium.[21] In the CHRISTMAS trial, an association between the extent of hibernating or ischemic myocardium and the degree of LVEF improvement with carvedilol treatment was observed.[22] Studies using PET and SPECT imaging have also found improvement in functional capacity correlated to the extent of viability.[19,23]

The spectrum of viability testing includes conventional myocardial perfusion imaging employing thallium 201 or technetium 99 sestamibi, single-photon admission computed tomography (SPECT), positron emission tomography (PET), dobutamine stress echocardiography, and cardiac magnetic resonance imaging (MRI). Prior studies have reported sensitivity ranging from 80% to 92%, specificity ranging from 54% to 78%, and positive predictive value ranging from 67% to

75%.[24] 18 F-fluorodeoxyglucose positron emission tomography (FDG-PET) imaging offers the greatest sensitivity (93%), with a lower specificity (58%) than other modalities.[25] Conversely, dobutamine stress echocardiography offers greater specificity at a cost of reduced sensitivity. Positive predictive value is similar among the imaging modalities. Cardiac MRI with gadolinium has increasingly been utilized to quantify the extent of myocardial scar and thus assess potential recovery of myocardial function. The greater the extent of transmural LV late enhancement, the higher the scar burden and the lower the likelihood of recovery of function despite adequate revascularization.[26]

The utility of detecting the presence or absence of viable myocardium on outcomes following coronary revascularization continues to be debated.[24] The majority of earlier observational studies have reported that revascularization of viable hibernating myocardium among patients with ischemic cardiomyopathy results in both improved survival and ventricular function compared to continued medical therapy.[24,27] However, important limitations including selection bias among patients who underwent coronary bypass grafting, negative publication bias, and lack of contemporary medical therapies hinder interpretation of these nonrandomized trials. The potential survival benefit of revascularization was best demonstrated in a 2002 meta-analysis that included 24 nonrandomized studies of over 3000 patients with multivessel coronary disease and LV dysfunction.[27] Patients demonstrated to have myocardial viability had an 80% reduction in annual mortality following revascularization (3.2% vs 16% with medical therapy); no difference in mortality with revascularization was observed among patients without demonstrable myocardial viability (annual mortality 7.7% vs 6.2% with medical therapy). The likelihood of improved survival appeared to be related to the amount of viable myocardium detected by FDT-PET imaging that was revascularized.[28]

Greater improvement in LVEF following revascularization when viable myocardium has been demonstrated has also been reported in earlier uncontrolled studies. A review of 29 observational studies reported an increase in global LVEF of 8% after revascularization when viability was demonstrated (LVEF 37%–45%); no improvement in LVEF was noted when viability was absent.[19]

In marked contrast to these nonrandomized observational studies, in a substudy of the Randomized Surgical Treatment for Ischemic Heart failure (STICH) trial, approximately 50% of patient underwent preoperative viability testing. Following adjustment in differences in baseline variables, myocardial viability was not found to predict a benefit following coronary revascularization[29,30] (**Fig. 47–4**). However, myocardial viability was assessed using older less sensitive techniques including stress echocardiography and SPECT myocardial perfusion imaging.

Several clinical scenarios may require greater precision in assessing for potential recovery in areas of prior infarction when surgical morbidity or mortality are high (ie, chronic kidney disease), or outcomes may not be optimal (evidence of

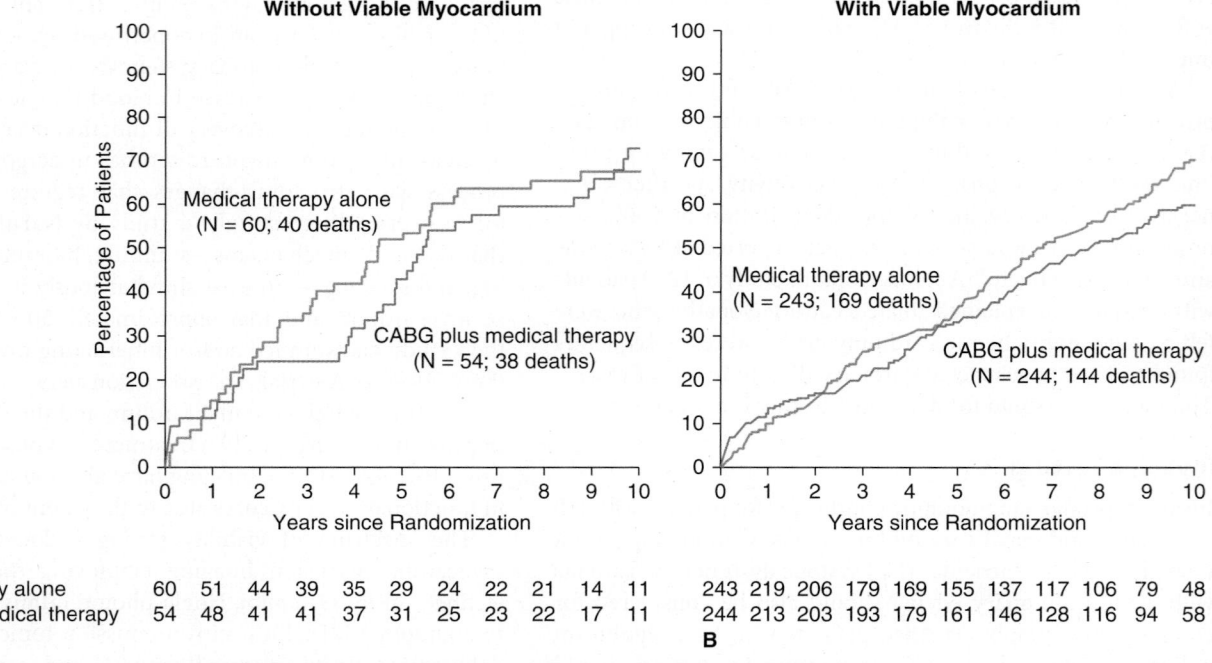

Figure 47–4. Kaplan–Meier analysis of the incidence of death from any cause by CABG versus medical therapy. Kaplan–Meier curves for the incidence of death from any cause among patients without viable myocardium (**A**) and among those with viable myocardium (**B**), according to treatment group. Reproduced with permission from Panza JA, Ellis AM, Al-Khalidi HR, et al. Myocardial Viability and Long-Term Outcomes in Ischemic Cardiomyopathy. *N Engl J Med.* 2019 Aug 22;381(8):739-748.

marked ventricular remodeling, inability to achieve complete revascularization). In these scenarios, myocardial viability assessment utilizing more contemporary techniques such as cardiac MRI or FDG-PET may be considered to further define potential risks and benefits in a high-risk population.[24]

POSTMYOCARDIAL INFARCTION VENTRICULAR REMODELING

Adverse Remodeling

Acute HF is not uncommon in the setting of acute MI. Acute elevation left-sided filling pressures may be due to either systolic dysfunction or decreased LV compliance leading to diastolic dysfunction. The reported incidence of in-hospital HF after MI ranges from 15% to 48%; an additional 3% to 51% will subsequently develop HF following discharge over the course of days to months.[31] The prognostic significance of HF complicating acute MI has been assessed in many studies. Two large registry studies indicated the presence of HF on admission increases the odds of in-hospital mortality by 1.8- to 2.2-fold.[32,33] The risk of HF was similar in patients with STEMI or non-STEMI. Further, this increased mortality rate does not decline over time. In the French registry of Acute ST elevation or non-ST-elevation Myocardial Infarction (FAST-MI), acute MI patients with HF had a significantly increased risk of death 12 months later.[34] It has been found that those who experience late-onset HF post-MI have an over 10-fold increased risk of death compared to other post-MI survivors and that mortality does not decline over time.[31,35] Of note, most of the patients who developed late-onset post-MI HF did not have a recurrent MI, suggesting that remodeling and perhaps residual

myocardial damage plays a significant role.[35] Clinical factors associated with the development of post-MI HF include older age, prior hypertension, female sex, prior MI, diabetes mellitus, increased heart rate, and LVEF.[31]

A sizable percentage of patients who sustained STEMI will be left with impairment in systolic function and increased risk of late chronic HF development. However, prompt myocardial reperfusion and the use of aggressive neurohormonal blockade may promote favorable LV remodeling and delay or prevent the development of HFrEF. Among younger patients who experienced acute MI (≤50 years of age), 29% had impaired LVEF during index hospitalization.[36] Patients with lower LVEF were more likely to have experienced STEMI, had higher troponin values, and had more severe angiographic CAD. In this population, 42% of patients recovered to an LVEF >50%. Over a median of 11.1 years of follow-up, LVEF recovery was associated with an 8-fold reduction in all-cause mortality (**Fig. 47–5**).

Ventricular remodeling may develop in response to pressure overload, volume overload, or myocardial injury. Following acute MI, the extent of LV chamber enlargement, or remodeling, is related, in part, to the size of the infarct. Using cardiac MRI, smaller infarct sizes (<18.5% of LV mass) were associated with a 15% progression and adverse LV remodeling while larger infarct sizes (≥18.5% of LV mass) were associated with an approximately 40% likelihood of progressive LV remodeling.[37] Baseline differences in hypertension, hyperlipidemia, tobacco smoking, or diabetes did not explain differences in the amount of adverse remodeling between groups. During the first few days after a moderate-to-large-sized MI, the LV cavity may enlarge due to infarct expansion (ie, elongation and thinning of the infarcted segment). Once initiated, progressive LV

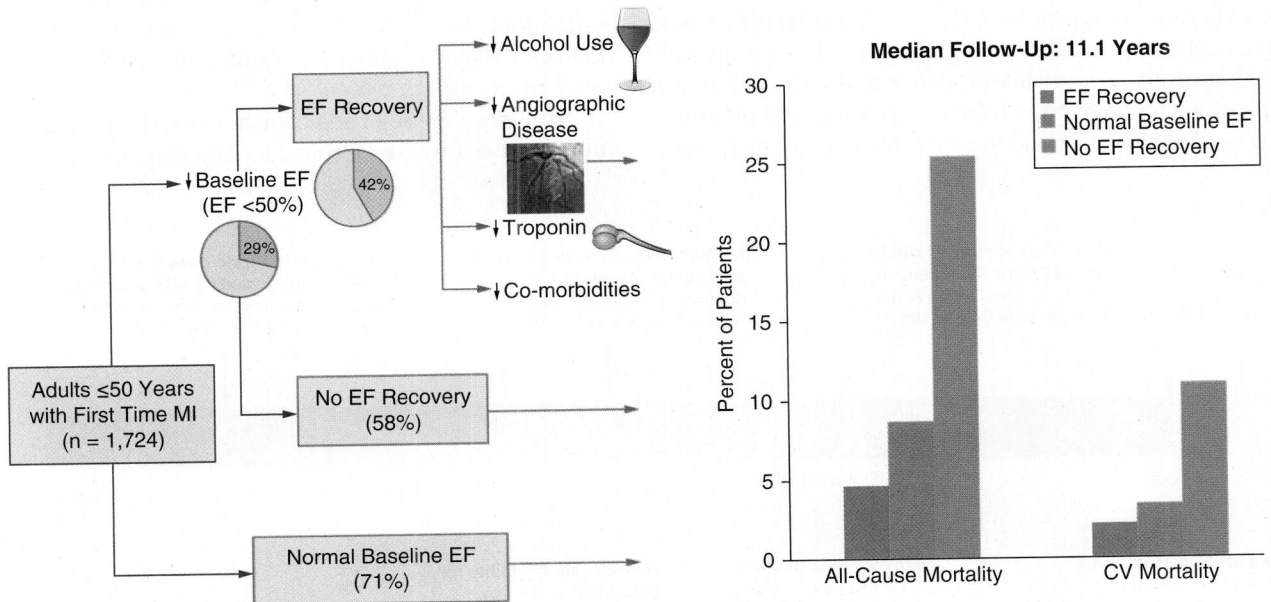

Figure 47–5. Outcomes of young adults after a first MI stratified by baseline ejection fraction and ejection fraction recovery. This shows the proportion of patients who presented with abnormal baseline ejection fraction (n = 503), and among them, the proportion of those who recovered (*green*) (42%) versus those who did not (*red*) (58%). Ejection fraction recovery was associated with decreased alcohol consumption, lower burden of angiographic disease, lower peak troponin values, and a lower burden of comorbidities. Reproduced with permission from Wu WY, Biery DW, Singh A, et al. Recovery of Left Ventricular Systolic Function and Clinical Outcomes in Young Adults With Myocardial Infarction. *J Am Coll Cardiol*. 2020 Jun 9;75(22):2804-2815.

dilatation may continue to occur over months or years. This time-dependent remodeling appears to largely result from elongation and dysfunction of the noninfarcted LV segments. Ventricular remodeling early following acute infarction has short-term benefits because stroke-volume will increase by the Frank–Starling mechanism. However, long-term structural and biochemical adaptations are detrimental to ventricular function and often lead to chronic HF. The transition to failure is related to marked alterations in the expression of multiple genes that regulate the composition of contractile elements, the cytoskeleton, the extracellular matrix, and continued myocyte loss due to apoptosis. Fibroblasts appear to play a major role in adverse remodeling. Both the production and degradation of the complex collagen network are regulated by fibroblast activity. While inflammation is a critical component of tissue healing following infarction, excessive inflammatory response may contribute to adverse remodeling.[37] Finally, over time, the left ventricle acquires a more spherical shape after injury that is associated with increased wall stress, abnormal distribution of fiber shortening, and progressive dilatation of the mitral annulus with functional mitral regurgitation (MR).

The molecular mechanisms responsible for adverse ventricular remodeling continue to be elucidated. Both cardiomyocytes and nonmyocytes are active sensors of pressure overload. In response to biomechanical stress, there is increased release of growth factors and cytokines, including peptides that stimulate G protein-coupled receptors such as endothelin-1 and angiotensin II, interleukin-6-related cytokines, and tumor necrosis factor-α; biomechanical stress also concomitantly activates hypertrophic and apoptotic pathways. Further, activation of the renin-angiotensin system and adrenergic stimulation occur following acute MI. Angiotensin II further stimulates cardiac fibroblasts to increase collagen formation. Finally, a variety of cytokines appear important in regulating the balance between collagen degradation and excess production through regulation of metalloproteinases. Better understanding of the complex interaction of growth factors cytokines and other signaling mechanisms may lead to better therapies in the future.

It should be recognized that remodeling is a dynamic process. Patients may have progressive adverse remodeling over time after acute MI leading to HF or experience favorable reverse remodeling when guideline-directed medical therapy is instituted.[38] Conversely, adverse ventricular remodeling can occur in previously stable patients when guideline-directed medical therapy is withdrawn. Serum biomarkers (B-type natriuretic peptide [BNP], NT-proBNP, and sST2) have been shown to be useful in predicting remodeling and for tailoring pharmacologic therapy. Patients with persistently low concentrations of natriuretic peptides (eg, BNP <100 ng/L and NT-proBNP <1000 ng/L) have a low likelihood of adverse remodeling and favorable long-term prognosis.[39] However, patients with persistently elevated or rising biomarkers are at increased risk of further ventricular enlargement, greater decline in LVEF, and require more aggressive follow-up and treatment.

Neurohormonal blockade has been shown to have a highly favorable effect in ameliorating adverse ventricular remodeling following acute myocardial injury[40] (**Fig. 47–6**). The benefits of long-term β-blockers following MI have been well-established. In a meta-analysis of 31 randomized trials that included approximately 25,000 patients, the long-term use of β-blockers reduced the risk of reinfarction and death by approximately 20% to 25%.[41] The efficacy of carvedilol on morbidity and mortality among patients with LV dysfunction after an MI was assessed in the CAPRICORN (Carvedilol Post-myocardial Infarction Survival Cohort in Left Ventricular Dysfunction study).[42] Among patients with acute MI and LV ejection ≤40% who received carvedilol within 3 to 21 days, all-cause mortality was lower than it was in a placebo group (HR, 0.77). Current ACC/AHA and ESC guidelines continue to recommend the initiation of a β-blocker within the first 24 hours in patients with STEMI who do not have contraindications such as overt HF, low output state, hypotension, or sinus tachycardia (class I). A β-blocker should continue to be administered following hospital discharge (class I).[43]

Similarly, the use of angiotensin-converting enzyme inhibitors has been well-established among patients with impaired

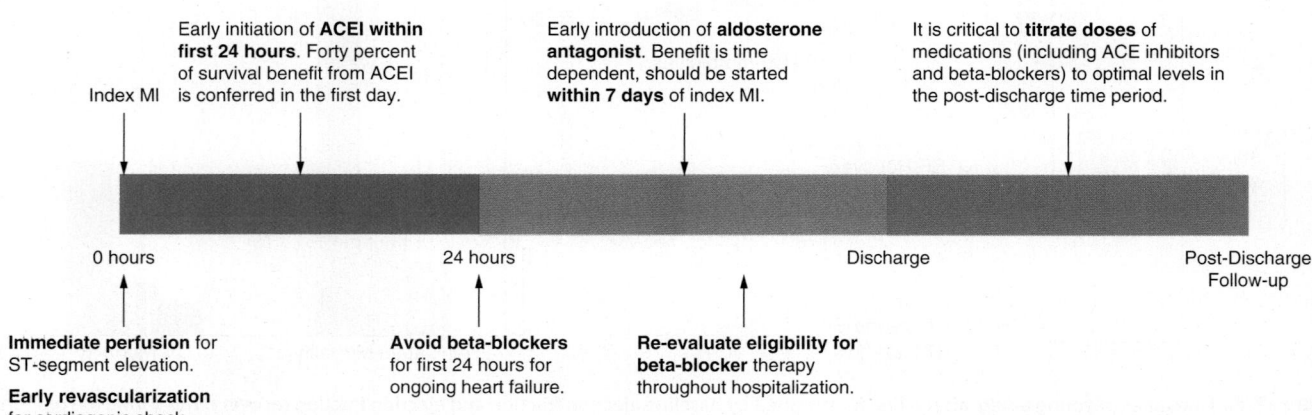

Figure 47–6. **Time-dependent therapies to promote post-MI LV remodeling.** ACE, angiotensin-converting enzyme; ACEI, angiotensin-converting enzyme inhibitor; MI, myocardial infarction. Reproduced with permission from Bahit MC, Kochar A, Granger CB. Post-Myocardial Infarction Heart Failure. *JACC Heart Fail.* 2018 Mar;6(3):179-186.

LVEF following an MI. Systemic overview of four large trials of angiotensin-converting enzyme (ACE) inhibitor therapy initiated within 36 hours of presentation showed a 7% relative reduction in 30-day mortality.[44] Importantly, the absolute benefit was found to be greater in high-risk populations (eg, Killip class II/III, heart rate >100 bpm, or anterior MI). In the three largest post-MI trials, SAVE (Survival And Ventricular Enlargement), AIRE (Acute Reinfarction Ramipril Efficacy), and TRACE (TRAndolapril Cardiac Evaluation), ACE inhibitors demonstrated a 26% relative risk reduction mortality, 27% relative risk reduction in HF readmission rate, and a 20% reduction in reinfarction.[40] Current ACC/AHA and ESC guidelines continue to recommend ACE inhibitor therapy for patients with STEMI with anterior location, HF findings, or LVEF ≤40%, unless contraindicated. Angiotensin receptor blockers (ARBs) have been shown to be equally effective to ACE inhibitors and should be considered for patients who are intolerant of ACE inhibitor therapy (class I).[43]

Aldosterone levels have been demonstrated to be elevated in the peri-infarction period and the beneficial role of aldosterone antagonism has been convincingly demonstrated in the EPHESUS (Eplerenone Post-acute Myocardial Infarction Heart failure Efficacy and Survival) study. Eplerenone initiated between days 3 and 14 after STEMI in patients with LVEF ≤40% or symptomatic HF or diabetes experienced a 15% relative reduction in all-cause mortality.[40] The effect of eplerenone was time dependent and attenuated if the drug was initiated beyond 7 days after index acute MI.[45]

Studies have shown increasing cardiovascular risk with increasing extent of CAD[46,47] (**Fig. 47–7**). In a population-based cohort study performed in Olmstead County, 1922 participants who sustained initial MI were followed for the development of symptomatic HF. During a mean follow-up of 6 years, 30.6% developed HF. The extent of angiographic coronary atherosclerosis determined by angiography demonstrated that more severe coronary disease was associated with a higher cumulative incident rate of post-MI HF. Among patients with 0 or 1, 2, and 3 diseased epicardial vessels, HF incidence rates were 14.7%, 20.6%, and 29% 0.8% at 5 years, respectively.[47] The increased risk with a greater number of diseased vessels was independent of the occurrence of recurrent MI and did not differ appreciably by HF phenotype.

Reverse Remodeling

Reverse ventricular remodeling is observed in 26% to 46% of HFrEF patients. Reverse remodeling typically occurs following intensification of drug or device therapy but the magnitude of ventricular recovery varies considerably among patients (**Table 47–1**).[2] Patients with ischemic cardiomyopathy are less likely to demonstrate extensive reverse remodeling than those with nonischemic etiologies for systolic dysfunction but often will show some favorable improvement.[38] Other variables associated with greater likelihood of reverse remodeling include shorter duration of HF symptoms, female sex, absence of left bundle branch block, and intensity of neurohormonal therapy.[48,49] Cardiac resynchronization therapy (CRT) is less likely to produce substantial reverse remodeling in ischemic cardiomyopathy due to the fixed nature of transmural scar.[50] Marked depression of ventricular systolic function and or greater degrees of ventricular enlargement do not preclude the possibility of reverse remodeling.[48,49,51] Greater contractility on echocardiography-derived strain imaging may predict a more favorable outcome. Less pronounced scar burden by late gadolinium enhancement on cardiac MRI is also a favorable prognostic marker.[52] Finally, improvement in serum biomarkers, particularly NT-proBNP, during intensification of pharmacologic therapy is highly predictive of favorable remodeling.[39,51]

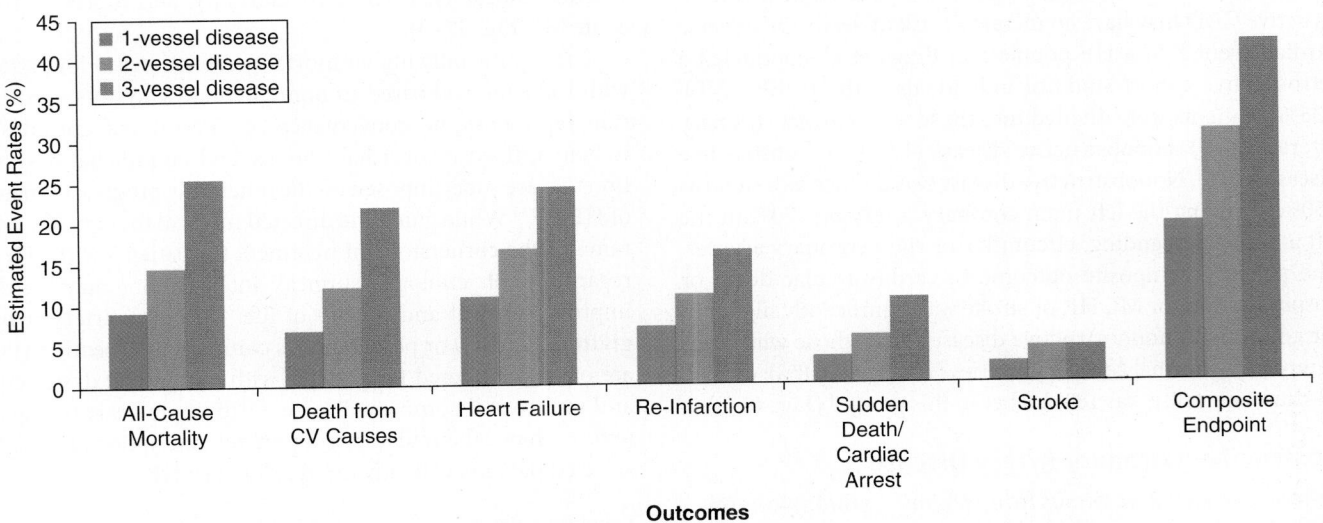

Figure 47–7. **Kaplan-Meier estimates of outcomes (at 3 years) according to the extent of CAD.** The composite end point consisted of cardiovascular death, reinfarction, HF, resuscitated sudden death, and stroke. Reproduced with permission from Janardhanan R, Kenchaiah S, Velazquez EJ, et al. Extent of coronary artery disease as a predictor of outcomes in acute myocardial infarction complicated by heart failure, left ventricular dysfunction, or both. *Am Heart J.* 2006 Jul; 152(1):183-189.

TABLE 47–1. Current Guideline Recommendations for Medical Therapy to Improve Mortality in Heart Failure with Reduced Ejection Fraction

Medication Class	Recommendation	Recommendation Class/Level of Evidence	Guidelines
β-blockers	Recommended for all patients with current or prior symptoms of HFrEF	Class I; LOE: A	2013 ACCF/AHA Heart Failure Guideline 2016 ESC Heart Failure Guideline
ACE inhibitors	Recommended in all patients with HFrEF and current or prior symptoms	Class I; LOE: A	2013 ACCF/AHA Heart Failure Guideline 2017 ACC/AHA/HFSA Heart Failure Focused Update 2016 ESC Heart Failure Guideline
Angiotensin receptor blockers	Recommended in patients with HFrEF with current or prior symptoms who are intolerant to ACE inhibitor	Class I; LOE: A	2013 ACCF/AHA Heart Failure Guideline 2017 ACC/AHA/HFSA Heart Failure Focused Update 2016 ESC Heart Failure Guideline
Mineralocorticoid receptor antagonists	Recommended for all patients with NYHA Class II–IV heart failure with LVEF ≤35%. Patients with NYHA Class II should have a history of prior heart failure hospitalization or elevated BNP before initiation	Class I; LOE: A	2013 ACCF/AHA Heart Failure Guideline 2016 ESC Heart Failure Guideline
Angiotensin receptor neprilysin inhibitor	Recommended in selected patients with chronic HFrEF in conjunction with β-blockers and aldosterone antagonists	Class I; LOE: B	2017 ACC/AHA/HFSA Heart Failure Focused Update

Abbreviations: ACC, American College of Cardiology; ACCF, American College of Cardiology Foundation; ACE, angiotensin-converting enzyme; AHA, American Heart Association; BNP, B-type natriuretic peptide; ESC: European Society of Cardiology; HFrEF, heart failure with reduced ejection fraction; HFSA, Heart Failure Society of America; LOE, Level of Evidence; LVEF, left ventricular ejection fraction; and NYHA, New York Heart Association.
Reproduced with permission from Elgendy IY, Mahtta D, Pepine CJ. Medical Therapy for Heart Failure Caused by Ischemic Heart Disease. *Circ Res*. 2019 May 24;124(11):1520-1535.

HEART FAILURE WITH REDUCED EJECTION FRACTION

Nonobstructive Coronary Artery Disease and Outcome

HF etiology is often classified broadly as ischemic or nonischemic with patients demonstrated to have normal coronary arteries compared to those with nonobstructive CAD. Recent studies, however, have demonstrated that patients with nonobstructive CAD may have an increased risk of death and adverse cardiac event.[53] In a HF population, Braga et al. conducted a retrospective cohort study of individuals with HFrEF (LVEF ≤35%). Patients were divided into those with normal coronary arteries (21%), nonobstructive disease (17%), and obstructive disease (62%). Nonobstructive disease was defined as a stenosis <50% involving the left main coronary artery or <70% in the left anterior descending, circumflex or right coronary arteries. The primary composite outcome of cardiovascular death or hospitalization for MI, HF, or stroke was significantly higher in the cohort with nonobstructive disease versus those with angiographically normal coronary arteries (20.8% vs 16.8%); overall, all-cause mortality was 18% higher in this group[54] (**Fig. 47–8**).

Obstructive Coronary Artery Disease

Outcome in Ischemic versus Nonischemic Cardiomyopathy

Chronic ischemic heart disease is the most common etiology for HFrEF and HFmidEF. While symptomatic angina often coexists with acute or chronic HF symptoms, silent ischemia is also common, particularly in elderly or diabetic patients. Older observational studies have reported worse outcomes in patients with ischemic versus nonischemic cardiomyopathy. Mortality is lower among women with comparable degrees of LV systolic dysfunction.[55] Felker and colleagues evaluated outcomes in 1230 patients with new onset cardiomyopathy and demonstrated higher early and late mortality for those found to have underlying CAD.[17] Indeed, HFrEF patients with underlying CAD had significantly higher rates of all-cause death, cardiovascular mortality, HF-related mortality, and mortality from acute MI (**Fig. 47–9**).

The significantly higher mortality rate observed for patients with ischemic compared to nonischemic LV systolic dysfunction represents the convergence of intermittent episodes of ischemia, fixed myocardial fibrosis, and endothelial dysfunction that are superimposed on the inherently progressive nature of HFrEF.[56] While guideline directed medical therapy (GDMT) remains the cornerstone of treatment for patients with HFrEF, regardless of etiology, surgical intervention may further improve survival and quality of life. Coronary artery bypass grafting (CABG) or percutaneous coronary intervention (PCI) are often considered for patients with LV systolic dysfunction and multivessel coronary disease. Orthotopic heart transplant and mechanical circulatory support remain options for highly selected patients with advanced refractory HF.

Coronary Revascularization and Outcome

Coronary Artery Bypass Grafting: A variety of retrospective observational studies performed in the 1980s and 1990s suggested that CABG improves survival in patients with ischemic

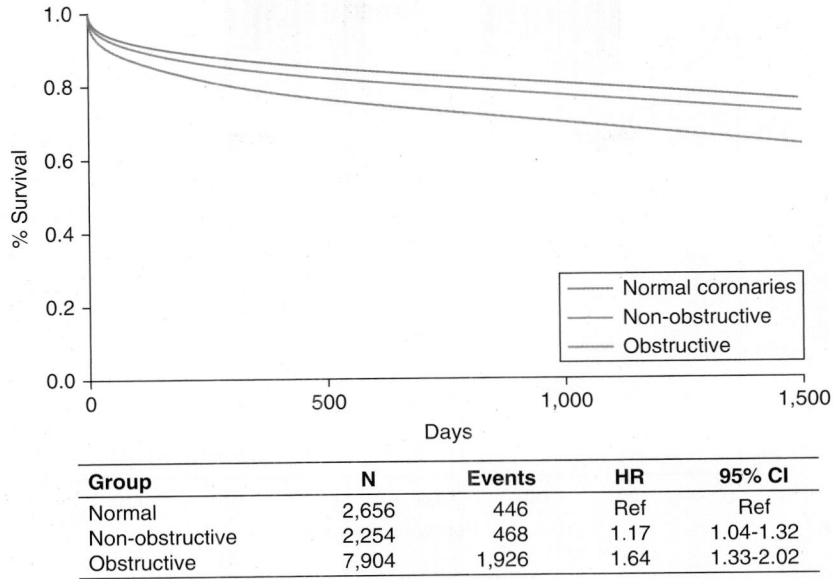

Group	N	Events	HR	95% CI
Normal	2,656	446	Ref	Ref
Non-obstructive	2,254	468	1.17	1.04-1.32
Obstructive	7,904	1,926	1.64	1.33-2.02

Figure 47–8. Adjusted survival curves according to the extent of epicardial CAD. The primary outcome was the composite of cardiovascular death, nonfatal acute MI, nonfatal stroke, or HF hospitalization. Patients with nonobstructive CAD had a higher hazard of experiencing the primary composite outcome compared with no apparent CAD. Reproduced with permission from Braga JR, Austin PC, Ross HJ, et al. Importance of Nonobstructive Coronary Artery Disease in the Prognosis of Patients With Heart Failure. *JACC Heart Fail.* 2019 Jun;7(6):493-501.

cardiomyopathy compared to medical therapy.[57,58] Mortality reductions with CABG compared with medical therapy ranged from 10% to greater than 50%. The single randomized controlled trial of CABG versus medical therapy during that era was the Coronary Artery Surgery Study (CASS).[59] Among patients with three-vessel CAD and a history of HF, sudden cardiac death was significantly lower in the surgical cohort (9% vs 31%, for CABG and medical therapy, respectively). However, all studies were generally performed before the routine use of β-blockers, or renin-angiotensin-aldosterone inhibition and failed to provide sufficient detail on whether medical management had been optimized.

The STICH trial was the first randomized trial to directly compare surgical revascularization with optimal medical therapy among patients with LVEF ≤35%.[60] Overall, 1212 patients were randomized to medical therapy plus CABG or medical therapy alone. All patients underwent coronary angiography to define the extent of CAD; patients with significant left main disease or unstable coronary symptoms were excluded from the trial. The majority of patients (85%) had New York Heart Association (NYHA) functional class II or III HF symptoms. At a median follow-up of 56 months, the CABG cohort demonstrated a nonsignificant trend toward improvement in the primary outcome of all-cause mortality (36% vs 41% for medical therapy alone). Significantly lower cardiovascular mortality and significantly improved quality of life as assessed by the Kansas City Cardiomyopathy Questionnaire were demonstrated.[61]

The STICH Extension Study (STICHES), published in 2016, extended follow-up to almost 10 years.[62] With longer follow-up, the primary outcome of all-cause mortality was significantly lower in the CABG group compared to patients in the medical group (59% vs 66%; HR, 0.84) (**Fig. 47–10**). Further, the CABG group experience significant reductions in prespecified secondary outcomes of cardiovascular mortality (40.5% vs 49.3%) and the combination of all-cause mortality and cardiovascular hospitalizations (76.6% vs 87%). Based upon the observed 7% absolute reduction in long-term mortality and improved quality of life, CABG should be considered for patients with multivessel CAD that is amenable to complete revascularization, LVEF ≤35%, and mild-to-moderate HF symptoms provided that they do not have substantial comorbidities that would substantially increase perioperative mortality or limit their likelihood of achieving long-term survival.

Angina pectoris was present in approximately two-thirds of the entire cohort at baseline. While CABG was associated with a significantly greater improvement in angina compared to medical therapy alone, it did not identify patients who had a greater survival benefit following revascularization.[63]

Several factors have been associated with higher survival rates following multivessel CABG including a better functional status as assessed by the 6-minute walk test (>300 m) and/or the Kansas City Cardiomyopathy Questionnaire prior to surgery,[64] angiographic severity of CAD, severity of LV systolic dysfunction, and severity of LV remodeling (as assessed by end-systolic volume index). Panza et al. specifically investigated the impact of three anatomic variables on survival following revascularization: presence of three-vessel CAD (defined as ≥50% stenoses), baseline LVEF, and baseline LVESVI (end-systolic volume index). They observed a progressive time-dependent benefit from CABG as the risk score increased.[65] Myocardial viability did not predict better outcome following CABG. Similarly, while circulating levels of BNP were strongly related to survival in both surgical and medical cohorts, they did not identify those with a survival advantage following revascularization.[66]

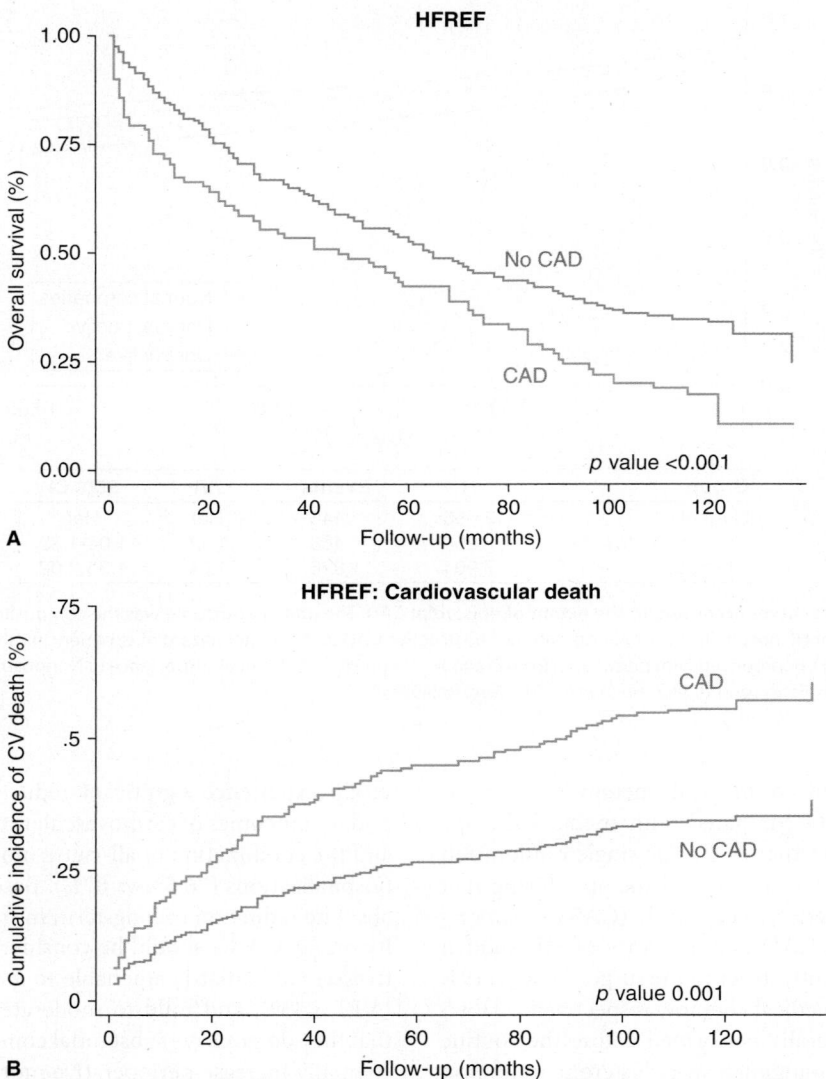

Figure 47–9. Long-term prognostic impact of CAD in HFrEF patients by (A) overall survival and (B) cardiovascular mortality. Reproduced with permission from Rusinaru D, Houpe D, Szymanski C, et al. Coronary artery disease and 10-year outcome after hospital admission for heart failure with preserved and with reduced ejection fraction. *Eur J Heart Fail*. 2014 Sep;16(9):967-976.

Patients with preserved exercise capacity but multivessel CAD, lower LVEF, and higher end-systolic volume index appear most likely to benefit from CABG with respect to long-term survival[56] (**Fig. 47–11**).

The most recent 2018 ESC/European Association for Cardio-Thoracic Surgery (EACTS) guidelines on myocardial revascularization recommends CABG for patients with stable CAD and low predicted surgical mortality who have three-vessel disease with or without diabetes and left main CAD (class I, level of evidence [LOE] A). Furthermore, in patients with chronic HF and systolic LV dysfunction with EF ≤35%, CABG is recommended in those with multivessel disease and acceptable surgical risk (class I, LOE B).[67] In comparison, the ACC/AHA guidelines from 2017 recommend CABG be considered for patients with multivessel disease or proximal LAD disease and LVEF 35% to 50% (class IIa, LOE B).[68] Data are less convincing among patients with LVEF <35%, unless symptomatic angina fails to respond to anti ischemic medical therapy (class IIb, LOE B).

Percutaneous Coronary Intervention: Data remain limited on the relative efficacy of PCI in patients with ischemic cardiomyopathy and no prospective studies have directly compared to PCI to CABG in this population. The best observational data comes from 4616 patients with LVEF <35% enrolled in the New York State registry of PCI and CABG.[69] Using propensity matching, no significant difference in mortality was noted at a median follow-up of 2.9 years between contemporary PCI and CABG. PCI was associated with a greater risk of MI (has a ratio 2.16) and the need for repeat revascularization (HR, 2.54) but a significantly lower risk of stroke compared to CABG (HR, 0.57).[69]

Two relatively large trials included patients with LV systolic dysfunction-BARI (Bypass Angioplasty Revascularization

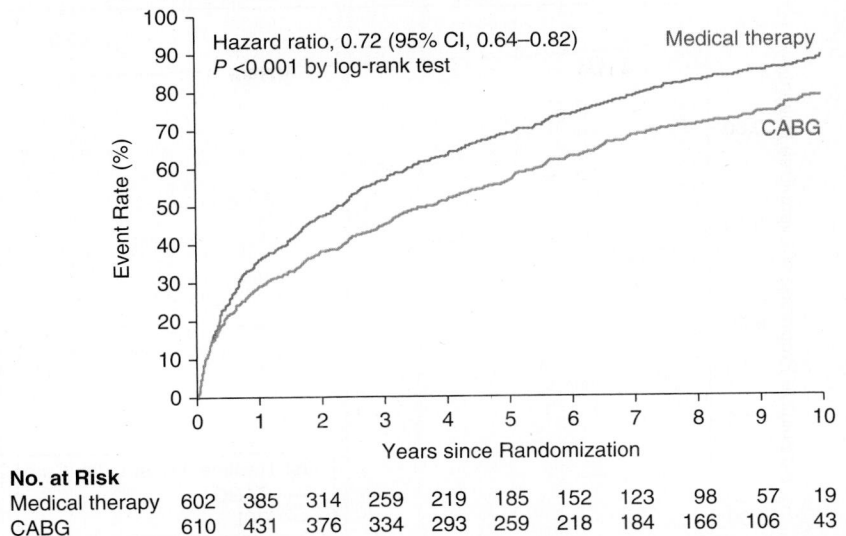

Death from any Cause or Cardiovascular Hospitalization

Hazard ratio, 0.72 (95% CI, 0.64–0.82)
P <0.001 by log-rank test

Medical therapy

CABG

Event Rate (%)

Years since Randomization

No. at Risk

	0	1	2	3	4	5	6	7	8	9	10
Medical therapy	602	385	314	259	219	185	152	123	98	57	19
CABG	610	431	376	334	293	259	218	184	166	106	43

Figure 47–10. Kaplan–Meier estimates of the rates of death from any cause (primary outcome) or hospitalization for cardiovascular causes. Reproduced with permission from Velazquez EJ, Lee KL, Jones RH, et al. Coronary-Artery Bypass Surgery in Patients with Ischemic Cardiomyopathy. *N Engl J Med.* 2016 Apr 21; 374(16):1511-1520.

Investigation) that included 29% of patients with LVEF ≤50%, and AWESOME (Angina With Extremely Serious Operative Mortality Evaluation) that had 21% with LVEF <35%.[70,71] Subgroup analysis in patients with impaired LV function from these trials suggested no difference in outcome between PCI and CABG. In a propensity-matched cohort study of diabetic patients with ischemic LV dysfunction, Canadian investigators found that CABG demonstrated significantly lower rates of revascularization compared to PCI (**Fig. 47–12**). In addition, CABG exhibited a significantly lower incidence of major adverse cardiac and cerebrovascular events and improved long-term survival compared to PCI without an increased risk for stroke.[72] These findings were similar to prior trials among diabetic patients with preserved ventricular function.

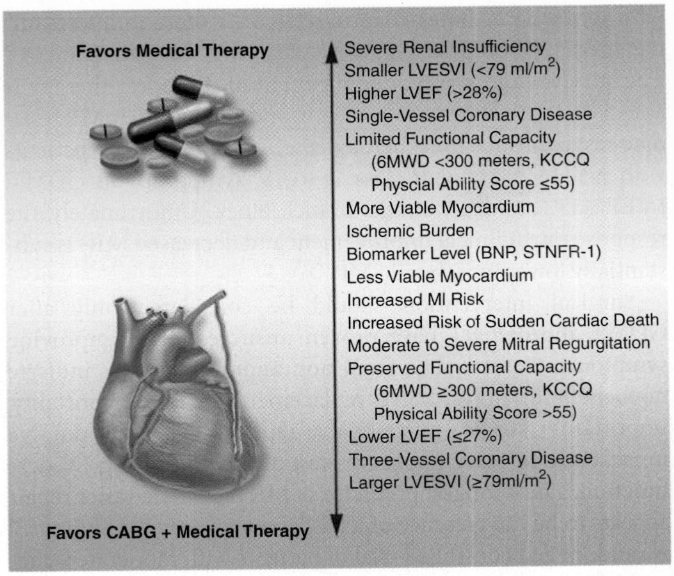

Ischemic Mitral Regurgitation

Restricted leaflet motion in ischemic MR is primarily attributed to LV remodeling with tethering of normal-appearing mitral leaflets from apical and lateral papillary muscle displacement after an infarction and secondarily attributed to inadequate mitral leaflet closure due to LV dysfunction and/or dyssynchrony. As these changes are dependent on loading conditions, secondary forms of MR are dynamic in nature. Conventional two-dimensional (2D) echocardiographic quantification of MR relies on measurement of the MR jet core at its vena contract or proximal convergence zone using methods that assume circular orifice geometry.[73] Ischemic MR may therefore be significantly underestimated when the orifice is elliptical (as is typically observed in secondary forms of MR). Clinically, the degree of MR is often substantially underestimated by auscultation.

Ischemic MR contributes to HF morbidity and is a powerful marker of poor prognosis in patients with CAD and LV dysfunction (**Fig. 47–13**). Bursi et al. demonstrated that among a cohort of 1331 post-MI patients of whom half were found to have MR on echocardiography within 30 days of the MI,

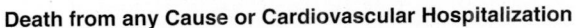

Favors Medical Therapy

Severe Renal Insufficiency
Smaller LVESVI (<79 ml/m²)
Higher LVEF (>28%)
Single-Vessel Coronary Disease
Limited Functional Capacity
  (6MWD <300 meters, KCCQ
  Physcial Ability Score ≤55)
More Viable Myocardium
Ischemic Burden
Biomarker Level (BNP, STNFR-1)
Less Viable Myocardium
Increased MI Risk
Increased Risk of Sudden Cardiac Death
Moderate to Severe Mitral Regurgitation
Preserved Functional Capacity
  (6MWD ≥300 meters, KCCQ
  Physical Ability Score >55)
Lower LVEF (≤27%)
Three-Vessel Coronary Disease
Larger LVESVI (≥79ml/m²)

Favors CABG + Medical Therapy

Figure 47–11. Revascularization in ischemic HF: contributing factors influencing the decision for revascularization in patients with severe LV dysfunction. BNP, B-type natriuretic peptide; CABG, coronary artery bypass graft surgery; KCCQ, Kansas City Cardiomyopathy Questionnaire; LVEF, left ventricular ejection fraction; LVESVI, left ventricular end systolic volume index; MI, myocardial infarction; 6MWD, 6-min walk distance; STNFR-1, soluble tumor necrosis factor receptor 1. Reproduced with permission from Velazquez EJ, Bonow RO. Revascularization in severe left ventricular dysfunction. *J Am Coll Cardiol.* 2015 Feb 17;65(6):615-624.

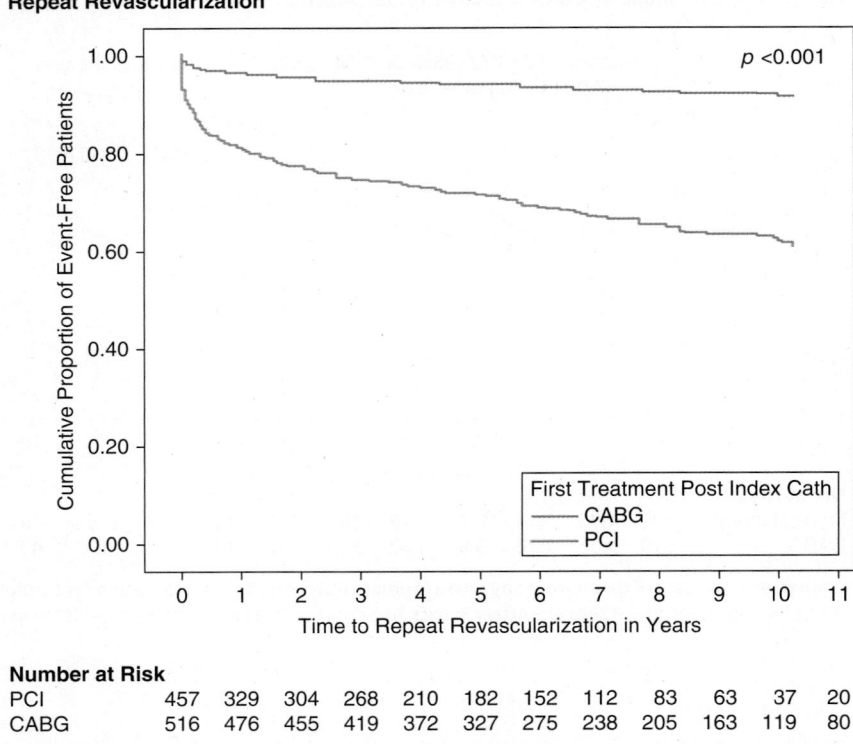

Repeat Revascularization

Figure 47–12. Cumulative risk for repeat revascularization among diabetic patients with ischemic cardiomyopathy by CABG versus PCI in the ejection fraction <35% cohort. Reproduced with permission from Nagendran J, Bozso SJ, Norris CM, et al. Coronary Artery Bypass Surgery Improves Outcomes in Patients With Diabetes and Left Ventricular Dysfunction. *J Am Coll Cardiol.* 2018 Feb 27;71(8):819-827.

12% having moderate-to-severe MR had an increased risk of HF (risk ratio [RR], 3.44) and death (RR, 1.55).[74] Similarly, 4-year cardiac mortality in ischemic cardiomyopathy has been reported in 43% and 45% when MR is moderate or severe compared to only 6% when mild MR is present.[75]

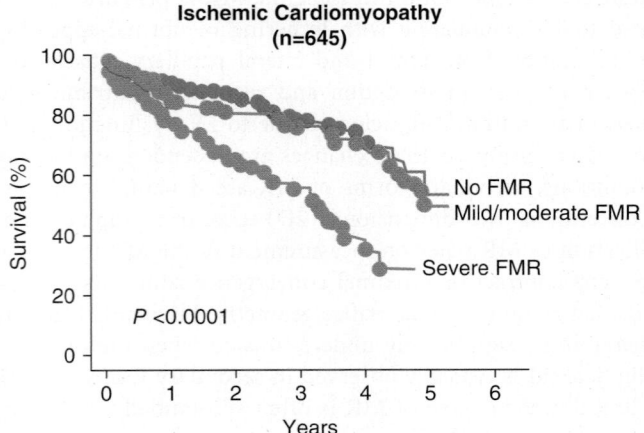

Figure 47–13. Prognosis of quantitatively determined secondary MR in patients with ischemic cardiomyopathy. Freedom from death according to the degree of functional MR in patients with ischemic cardiomyopathy. Reproduced with permission from Asgar AW, Mack MJ, Stone GW. Secondary mitral regurgitation in heart failure: pathophysiology, prognosis, and therapeutic considerations. *J Am Coll Cardiol.* 2015 Mar 31;65(12):1231-1248.

It has proven difficult to ascertain whether ischemic MR is predominantly a marker of the severity of LV dysfunction or directly contributes to progressive LV deterioration. Initial therapy should be GDMT (ACC/AHA MR guidelines).[76] The survival and symptomatic benefit of β-blocker therapy is associated with reverse remodeling and reduction in MR. Cardiac resynchronization therapy is well-established for patients with NYHA functional class II to IV symptoms on GDMT, LVEF ≤35%, and left bundle branch block. Unfortunately, the response rate (clinical improvement and decreased MR) is substantially lower in ischemic MR.[73]

Surgical intervention should be considered only after GDMT and/or CRT have proven unsuccessful in improving symptoms. Current data from nonrandomized trials indicate no benefit of mitral valve replacement/repair on mortality. Importantly, surgical mitral valve repair is often not durable in ischemic MR due to progression of the underlying LV dysfunction. The strongest predictor of MR recurrence after repair appears to be the presence of a basilar aneurysm or dyskinesis.[73] A randomized controlled trial of patients with moderate ischemic MR undergoing CABG did not find an improvement in mortality or higher likelihood of reverse LV remodeling but did note a higher risk of postoperative complications.[77] The most recent ACC/AHA guidelines indicate that mitral valve repair or replacement may be considered for severely symptomatic patients (NYHA class III or IV) with chronic severe secondary MR (stage D) who have persistent symptoms despite optimal GDMT for HF (AHA/ACC class IIb, LOE B).[78]

Percutaneous mitral valve therapies are rapidly evolving in the management of patients at high risk for surgical intervention, including those with secondary MR related to ischemic cardiomyopathy. Percutaneous treatments include annuloplasty, edge-to-edge repair, or prosthesis implantation. Edge-to-edge repair by MitraClip is the most widely studied procedure. The MITRA-FR (Percutaneous Repair with the MitraClip device for Severe Functional/Secondary Mitral Regurgitation) trial randomized patients with symptomatic MR, LVEF of 15% to 40%, and effective regurgitant orifice (ERO) >20 mm^2 to GDMT or GDMT and MitraClip.[79] No benefit in the primary endpoint of all-cause mortality or HF hospitalizations at 1 year was noted (54.6% for MitraClip, 51.3% for GDMT). In contrast, the COAPT trial (Cardiovascular Outcomes Assessment of the MitralClip Percutaneous Therapy for heart failure patients with functional mitral regurgitation) randomized symptomatic patients with LVEF of 20% to 50%, end-systolic dimension ≤69 mm, and MR grade 3 or 4+. At 2 years, HF hospitalization rate (the primary endpoint) was markedly lower in the MitraClip cohort (35.8 vs 67.9 per 100 patient-years).[80] In addition, all secondary endpoints also favored MitraClip: MR severity, quality of life metrics, 6-minute walk test, LV remodeling, hospitalization rate, and 2-year mortality (29.1% vs 46.1%). Much has been written about the marked difference in findings between the two clinical trials. Post hoc analysis suggest that the COAPT trial enrolled patients with more recoverable LV function and more severe functional MR causing more advanced HF, while the MITRAL-HF trial population had less severe MR and larger LV cavity size, possibly with less potential for reverse remodeling.[81] More intense GDMT was also utilized in the COAPT study. Given these contradictory findings, patients most likely to benefit for a percutaneous mitral clip appear to be those with ERO ≥0.30 cm^2, without excessive LV dilatation, and after intense GDMT has been proven unsuccessful in controlling HF symptoms.

HEART FAILURE WITH MIDRANGE EJECTION FRACTION

Initially described in the 2013 AHA/ACC HF guidelines and more recently better characterized in the 2016 ESC HF guidelines is a new HF phenotype: HFmidEF. This describes patients with LVEF of 40% to 49%. Among >40,000 Medicare patients hospitalized with HF in the Get With The Guidelines-Heart Failure program, HFmidEF was detected in 14%.[82] A variety of retrospective studies have documented a high incidence of CAD, ranging from 57% to 79%.[82,83] Overall, this cohort had clinical characteristics that were more similar to HFpEF including older age, female sex, greater comorbidities (hypertension, chronic obstructive pulmonary disease, and diabetes), and elevation in creatinine and NT-proBNP.[84] Mortality rates at 30 days and 12 months have been shown to be intermediate between HFrEF and HFpEF but were more similar to those observed in HFpEF populations.[84] Prospective randomized trials have not specifically examined this population. Current HF guidelines are based upon observational studies and subgroup analyses and suggest pharmacological treatment should be similar to that employed for HFrEF with ACE/ARB, β-blocker, and an aldosterone antagonist. Sacubitral valsartan may be more effective than an ACE-I/ARB in this phenotype than the HFpEF phenotype based upon the results of the recent PARAGON-HF (Prospective Comparison of ARNI [angiotensin receptor-neprilysin inhibitor] and ARB Global Outcomes in HF with Preserved Ejection Fraction) trial.[85] This cohort often demonstrates dynamic variation in LVEF with a significant percentage of patients having improvement in LVEF on treatment and a similar percentage of patients demonstrating deterioration in LV function over time. CAD has been associated with greater declines in LVEF among patients with HFpEF; thus, screening and treatment of CAD is recommended for patients with HFmidEF to help prevent further progression of LV systolic dysfunction and perhaps lead to improvement in LVEF with revascularization.[86]

HEART FAILURE WITH PRESERVED EJECTION FRACTION

CAD and diastolic dysfunction are interrelated because both myocardial ischemia and infarction are major causes of diastolic dysfunction.[87] Tissue Doppler imaging and 2D-speckle tracking techniques have demonstrated in acute MI and ischemic cardiomyopathy that LV twisting and untwisting motion are reduced; further, diastolic dyssynchrony is highly prevalent in CAD patients with or without prior MI.[87] Further, diastolic dysfunction weakly correlates with neurohormonal activation in chronic ischemic cardiomyopathy.

Nonobstructive (Microvascular) Coronary Disease

The prominent association of metabolic risk factors and endothelial inflammatory activation led Paulus and colleagues to propose a new paradigm for the HFpEF phenotype.[88] In their model, metabolic abnormalities lead to LV remodeling and diastolic dysfunction through coronary microvascular endothelial inflammation, which alters signaling of endothelial cells to the surrounding cardiomyocytes. The fall in nitric oxide-cyclic guanosine model phosphate (cyclic GMP)-protein kinase G (PKG) signaling predisposes to cardiomyocyte hypertrophy and increased diastolic resting tension. Microvascular inflammatory endothelial activation, high oxidative stress, eNOS uncoupling, and impaired cyclic GMP-PKG signaling have all been demonstrated in LV myocardial samples from HFpEF patients.[89] Similar changes were confirmed in an obese, leptin-resistant, hypertensive rat model of HFpEF.

Microvascular endothelial inflammation is associated with endothelial dysfunction and microvascular rarefaction. HFpEF has been shown to be associated with reduced microvascular density due to an increase in myocardial fibrosis.[90] Patients with HFpEF and angiographically normal coronary arteries have been shown to demonstrate significant reductions in global myocardial flow reserve as assessed by 82 rubidium PET imaging compared to hypertensive and normal controls.[91] Similarly, coronary flow reserve, measured using phase-contrast cardiac MRI of the coronary sinus at rest and during adenosine stress imaging, showed a significant inverse correlation with serum brain natriuretic peptide levels in HFpEF patients without significant epicardial coronary disease.[92] Patients with microvascular dysfunction generally have a number of other comorbidities including hypertension, diabetes mellitus, obesity, and hyperlipidemia. It is currently unknown whether HFpEF patients with microvascular dysfunction have a different clinical prognosis than those without dysfunction. Unfortunately, therapies aimed at reducing inflammation and/or improving endothelial function (eg, statins, ARBs, and phosphodiesterase-5 inhibitors) have not been shown to be effective in improving patient outcomes in HFpEF.[90]

Obstructive Coronary Disease

Outcomes

Although abnormal relaxation is the first mechanical manifestation of acute myocardial ischemia, acute coronary syndromes seldom precipitate HFpEF decompensation or present as chronic HFpEF.[93] The prevalence of underlying CAD, diagnosed based on history of MI, revascularization, or ECG changes, ranges from 35% to 53% in large community-based registries.[93] Compared with HFpEF patients without CAD, those with CAD are more likely to be male, to have typical atherosclerotic risk factors, and to be treated with anti-ischemic medications.[94] Dyspnea and anginal symptoms are typically similar between groups. Further, noninvasive diagnostic testing fails to detect the presence of significant CAD in at least one-third of HFpEF patients.[94] Among HFpEF patients with CAD who were hospitalized for decompensated HF, Rusinaru et al. found a higher rate of SCD while in-hospital mortality rates did not differ from those without CAD.[10] Further, hospital admissions in HFpEF patients were more likely to be triggered by arrhythmia compared to HFrEF patients in whom an acute coronary syndrome was more likely to precipitate an admission.[10] While earlier studies suggested better outcomes than

HFrEF, more recent studies have shown similar cumulative survival probabilities and readmission rates as those with systolic dysfunction.[82]

CAD has significant clinical implications among HFpEF patients.[95,96] A study by Hwang et al. demonstrated angiographically proven CAD in 68% of 376 patients with chronic HFpEF.[94] The presence of CAD was associated with increased mortality and greater deterioration in ventricular function. A worse prognosis was associated with increasing extent of CAD (**Fig. 47–14**). In a large single institution database, only 40% of patients with significant obstructive CAD had exertional angina pectoris. Those with symptomatic angina were older with more comorbidities and a higher prevalence of prior revascularization.[97] After multivariable adjustment for comorbidities, patients with angina remained at increased risk for MACE (death, MI, revascularization, or stroke). The majority of the increased risk was due to need for revascularization with similar risk of death, MI, or HF hospitalizations.[95] Furthermore, in a recent investigation of the prognostic impact of MI in HFpEF patients, prior MI was independently associated with a greater risk of cardiovascular death with a 31-fold increased risk in the first 30 days after first post enrollment MI. Specifically, Cunningham et al. conducted a pooled analysis of three clinical trials—CHARM Preserved (Candesartan Cilexietil in Heart Failure Assessment of Reduction in Mortality and Morbidity), I-Preserve (Irbesartan in Heart Failure With Preserved Systolic Function), and the Americas region of TOPCAT (Treatment of Preserved Cardiac Function Heart Failure With an Aldosterone Antagonist)—and found that the greater risk of cardiovascular death was driven by excess sudden death (adjusted HR, 1.55) with the risk remaining elevated over time.[98] Of note, this study found that HFpEF patients with prior MI had a higher prevalence of atherosclerotic risk factors and lower prevalence of hypertension, obesity, and atrial fibrillation—risk factors

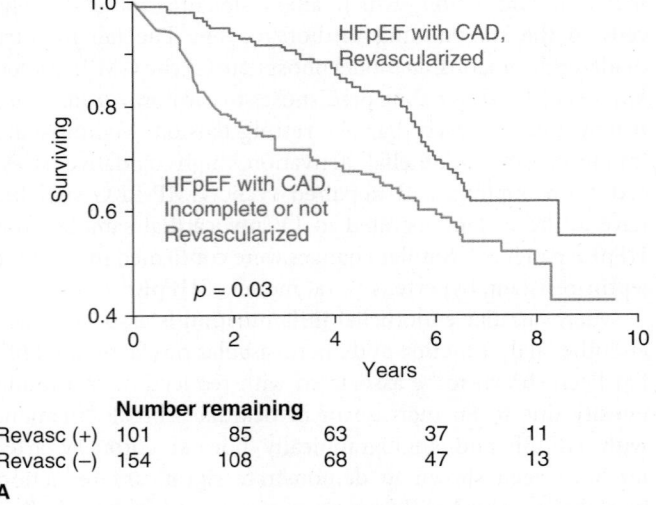

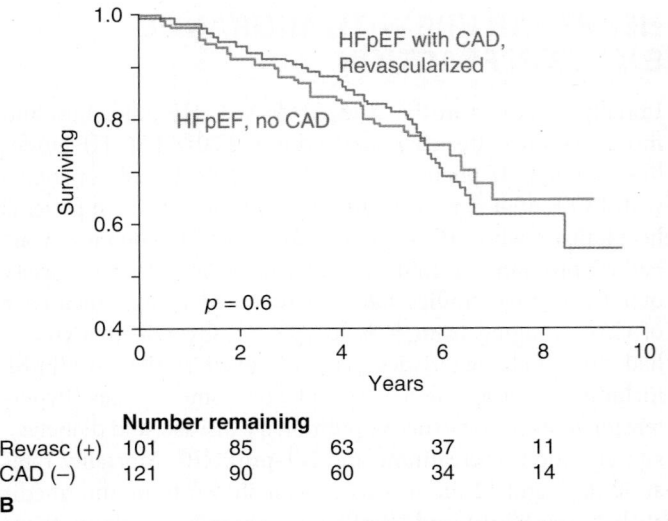

Number remaining				
Revasc (+) 101	85	63	37	11
Revasc (−) 154	108	68	47	13

A

Number remaining				
Revasc (+) 101	85	63	37	11
CAD (−) 121	90	60	34	14

B

Figure 47–14. Impact of revascularization on survival in patients with HFpEF and CAD. Kaplan-Meier plots showing (**A**) greater survival among patients with CAD who were revascularized (revasc) (*green*) compared with patients with CAD who were not completely revascularized (*blue*) and (**B**) similar survival among patients with CAD who were revascularized (*green*) and patients without significant CAD (*black*). CAD, coronary artery disease; HFpEF, heart failure with preserved ejection fraction. Reproduced with permission from Hwang SJ, Melenovsky V, Borlaug BA. Implications of coronary artery disease in heart failure with preserved ejection fraction. *J Am Coll Cardiol.* 2014 Jul 1;63(25 Pt A):2817-2827.

traditionally associated with HFpEF. Although there was no difference in HF hospitalization by prior MI status, there was a 2.4-fold increased risk of first or recurrent HF hospitalization after MI.

Medical Therapy: Unlike HFrEF, therapeutic options remain quite limited. While diuretics can improve symptoms of volume overload, no pharmacological agent has been shown to improve survival. A post hoc analysis of the TOPCAT trial suggested a survival advance for spironolactone, which is now commonly utilized for management (AHA/ACC class IIb).[99] Current treatment strategies focus on improving known risk factors and cardiac and noncardiac comorbidities and conditions that impact the clinical trajectory of HFpEF. These include hypertension, lung disease, atrial fibrillation, obesity, anemia, diabetes, kidney disease, and sleep-disordered sleeping.[95]

Coronary Artery Revascularization: Surgical or percutaneous coronary revascularization improves clinical outcomes in patients with HFpEF and symptomatic CAD.[94] Patients who underwent complete revascularization experienced less deterioration in LVEF and had improved overall survival compared with patients who had incomplete or no revascularization, particularly among patients with more extensive CAD.[94] The failure of anginal-like symptoms and the high false-negative rate of noninvasive diagnostic testing to adequately identify patients with extensive CAD argues for an aggressive approach among patients with risk factors or a high pretest suspicion of coronary atherosclerosis as the cause for their HF.

Sudden onset acute (flash) pulmonary edema is one of the most dramatic HF manifestations and is frequently due to obstructive CAD. It is generally felt to be due to ischemia-induced acute increase in pulmonary capillary wedge pressure due to diastolic dysfunction. Marked hypertension leading to elevation in afterload is also commonly observed. Coronary angiography and revascularization are recommended for treating this potentially life-threatening presentation. Successful coronary revascularization has been shown to decrease the frequency of this clinical manifestation but does not entirely prevent the possibility of relapse.[100] Aggressive control of hypertension may play an important role in preventing repeat occurrence of pulmonary edema as does coronary revascularization.

SUMMARY

- HF is an increasingly common complication among post-MI survivors with the extent of CAD found to be an important prognostic factor; furthermore, both silent MI and clinical MI are associated with subsequent development of HF.

- An ischemia work-up should be considered for any patient with unexplained HF with more than a low pretest probability of coronary atherosclerosis.

- The benefit of myocardial viability testing on outcomes following revascularization continues to be debated and may be suitable for certain scenarios in which surgical morbidity or mortality is high or outcomes may not be optimal; in these cases, more contemporary techniques including cardiac MRI or FDG-PET may be helpful.

- HF complicating acute MI is not uncommon and late-onset HF post-MI has an over 10-fold increased risk of death compared to other post-MI survivors. This occurs via ventricular remodeling in a time-dependent fashion through a series of structural and biochemical adaptations that include altered expression of multiple genes that regulate the contractile elements, cytoskeleton, and extracellular matrix with fibroblasts playing a key role.

- Therapies to ameliorate adverse ventricular remodeling include those aimed at neurohormonal blockade (eg, β-blockers, ACE inhibitors, or ARBs) and aldosterone antagonism.

- Reverse ventricular remodeling is observed in 26% to 46% of patients with HFrEF through pharmacologic and device therapies, although those with ischemic cardiomyopathy are less likely to demonstrate extensive reverse remodeling.

- Recent studies have found that patients with HFrEF with nonobstructive CAD may have an increased risk of death and adverse cardiac events. In HFrEF patients with chronic ischemic heart disease, management strategies include GDMT, CABG, or PCI. Those who appear to benefit from CABG most likely with respect to long-term survival are patients with preserved exercise capacity but multivessel CAD, lower LVEF, and higher end-systolic volume index; further studies are needed for those more likely to benefit from PCI versus CABG.

- Ischemic MR contributes to HF morbidity and is a powerful marker of poor prognosis in patients with CAD and LV dysfunction. Therapies include GDMT and/or CRT and surgical intervention if the prior therapies are unsuccessful in reducing symptoms. A percutaneous mitral clip may be of benefit to patients with certain characteristics (ERO ≥0.3 cm^2, lack marked LV dilation, and have limiting symptoms despite GDMT).

- A high incidence of CAD (57%–79%) has also been reported in patients with HFmidEF who have characteristics similar to patients with HFpEF. Current guidelines recommend similar pharmacologic therapies as with HFrEF.

- Microvascular endothelial inflammation appears to play a prominent role in HFpEF patients and likely microvascular dysfunction plays a large role in those without significant CAD. On the other hand, HFpEF patients with CAD appear to have traditional atherosclerotic risk factors with the presence of CAD associated with increased mortality and greater deterioration in ventricular function. Therapeutic options continue to be limited and no agent has been shown thus far to improve survival. In those with HFpEF and symptomatic CAD, surgical or percutaneous coronary revascularization improves clinical outcomes.

REFERENCES

1. Lloyd-Jones DM, Larson MG, Leip EP, et al. Lifetime risk for developing congestive heart failure: the Framingham Heart Study. *Circulation.* 2002;106(24):3068-3072. doi:10.1161/01.cir.0000039105.49749.6f.

2. Elgendy IY, Mahtta D, Pepine CJ. Medical therapy for heart failure caused by ischemic heart disease. *Circ Res.* 2019;124(11):1520-1535. doi:10.1161/CIRCRESAHA.118.313568.

3. Owan TE, Hodge DO, Herges RM, Jacobsen SJ, Roger VL, Redfield MM. Trends in prevalence and outcome of heart failure with preserved ejection fraction. *N Engl J Med.* 2006;355(3):251-259. doi:10.1056/NEJMoa052256.

4. Velagaleti RS, Pencina MJ, Murabito JM, et al. Long-term trends in the incidence of heart failure after myocardial infarction. *Circulation.* 2008;118(20):2057-2062. doi:10.1161/CIRCULATIONAHA.108.784215.

5. Felker GM, Shaw LK, O'Connor CM. A standardized definition of ischemic cardiomyopathy for use in clinical research. *J Am Coll Cardiol.* 2002;39(2):210-218. doi:10.1016/S0735-1097(01)01738-7.

6. Lamblin N, Meurice T, Tricot O, de Groote P, Lemesle G, Bauters C. First hospitalization for heart failure in outpatients with stable coronary artery disease: determinants, role of incident myocardial infarction, and prognosis. *J Card Fail.* 2018;24(12):815-822. doi:10.1016/j.cardfail.2018.09.013.

7. Mentz RJ, Fiuzat M, Shaw LK, et al. Comparison of Clinical characteristics and long-term outcomes of patients with ischemic cardiomyopathy with versus without angina pectoris (from the Duke Databank for Cardiovascular Disease). *Am J Cardiol.* 2012;109(9):1272-1277. doi:10.1016/j.amjcard.2011.12.021.

8. Wang TJ, Evans JC, Benjamin EJ, Levy D, LeRoy EC, Vasan RS. Natural history of asymptomatic left ventricular systolic dysfunction in the community. *Circulation.* 2003;108(8):977-982. doi:10.1161/01.CIR.0000085166.44904.79.

9. Qureshi WT, Zhang Z-M, Chang PP, et al. Silent myocardial infarction and long-term risk of heart failure: the ARIC study. *J Am Coll Cardiol.* 2018;71(1):1-8. doi:10.1016/j.jacc.2017.10.071.

10. Rusinaru D, Houpe D, Szymanski C, Lévy F, Maréchaux S, Tribouilloy C. Coronary artery disease and 10-year outcome after hospital admission for heart failure with preserved and with reduced ejection fraction. *Eur J Heart Fail.* 2014;16(9):967-976. doi:10.1002/ejhf.142.

11. Navare S, Mather J, Shaw L, Fowler M, Heller G. Comparison of risk stratification with pharmacologic and exercise stress myocardial perfusion imaging: a meta-analysis. *J Nucl Cardiol.* 2004;11(5):551-561. doi:10.1016/j.nuclcard.2004.06.128.

12. Hachamovitch R, Berman DS, Shaw LJ, et al. Incremental prognostic value of myocardial perfusion single photon emission computed tomography for the prediction of cardiac death: differential stratification for risk of cardiac death and myocardial infarction. *Circulation.* 1998;97(6):535-543. doi:10.1161/01.cir.97.6.535.

13. Ponikowski P, Voors AA, Anker SD, et al. 2016 ESC Guidelines for the diagnosis and treatment of acute and chronic heart failure: the Task Force for the diagnosis and treatment of acute and chronic heart failure of the European Society of Cardiology (ESC). Developed with the special contribution of the Heart Failure Association (HFA) of the ESC. *Eur Heart J.* 2016;37(27):2129-2200. doi:10.1093/eurheartj/ehw128.

14. van der Meer P, Gaggin HK, Dec GW. ACC/AHA versus ESC guidelines on heart failure: JACC guideline comparison. *J Am Coll Cardiol.* 2019;73(21):2756-2768. doi:10.1016/j.jacc.2019.03.478.

15. Yancy CW, Jessup M, Bozkurt B, et al. 2013 ACCF/AHA guideline for the management of heart failure: a report of the American College of Cardiology Foundation/American Heart Association Task Force on Practice Guidelines. *J Am Coll Cardiol.* 2013;62(16):e147-e239. doi:10.1016/j.jacc.2013.05.019.

16. Andreini D, Pontone G, Pepi M, et al. Diagnostic accuracy of multidetector computed tomography coronary angiography in patients with dilated cardiomyopathy. *J Am Coll Cardiol.* 2007;49(20):2044-2050. doi:10.1016/j.jacc.2007.01.086.

17. Felker GM, Thompson RE, Hare JM, et al. Underlying causes and long-term survival in patients with initially unexplained cardiomyopathy. *N Engl J Med.* 2000;342(15):1077-1084. doi:10.1056/NEJM200004133421502.

18. Scanlon PJ, Faxon DP, Audet AM, et al. ACC/AHA guidelines for coronary angiography: executive summary and recommendations. A report of the American College of Cardiology/American Heart Association Task Force on Practice Guidelines (Committee on Coronary Angiography) developed in collaboration with the Society for Cardiac Angiography and Interventions. *Circulation.* 1999;99(17):2345-2357. doi:10.1161/01.cir.99.17.2345.

19. Bax JJ, Wall EE van der, Harbinson M. Radionuclide techniques for the assessment of myocardial viability and hibernation. *Heart.* 2004;90(suppl 5):v26-v33. doi:10.1136/hrt.2002.007575.

20. Chareonthaitawee P, Gersh BJ, Araoz PA, Gibbons RJ. Revascularization in severe left ventricular dysfunction: the role of viability testing. *J Am Coll Cardiol.* 2005;46(4):567-574. doi:10.1016/j.jacc.2005.03.072.

21. Narula J, Dawson MS, Singh BK, et al. Noninvasive characterization of stunned, hibernating, remodeled and nonviable myocardium in ischemic cardiomyopathy. *J Am Coll Cardiol.* 2000;36(6):1913-1919. doi:10.1016/S0735-1097(00)00959-1.

22. Cleland J, Pennell D, Ray S, et al. Myocardial viability as a determinant of the ejection fraction response to carvedilol in patients with heart failure (CHRISTMAS trial): randomised controlled trial. *Lancet.* 2003;362(9377):14-21. doi:10.1016/S0140-6736(03)13801-9.

23. Di Carli MF, Asgarzadie F, Schelbert HR, et al. Quantitative relation between myocardial viability and improvement in heart failure symptoms after revascularization in patients with ischemic cardiomyopathy. *Circulation.* 1995;92(12):3436-3444. doi:10.1161/01.CIR.92.12.3436.

24. Anavekar NS, Chareonthaitawee P, Narula J, Gersh BJ. Revascularization in patients with severe left ventricular dysfunction: is the assessment of viability still viable? *J Am Coll Cardiol.* 2016;67(24):2874-2887. doi:10.1016/j.jacc.2016.03.571.

25. Bax JJ, Poldermans D, Elhendy A, Boersma E, Rahimtoola SH. Sensitivity, specificity, and predictive accuracies of various noninvasive techniques for detecting hibernating myocardium. *Curr Probl Cardiol.* 2001;26(2):147-181. doi:10.1067/mcd.2001.109973.

26. Kim RJ, Wu E, Rafael A, et al. The use of contrast-enhanced magnetic resonance imaging to identify reversible myocardial dysfunction. *N Engl J Med.* 2000;343(20):1445-1453. doi:10.1056/NEJM200011163432003.

27. Allman KC, Shaw LJ, Hachamovitch R, Udelson JE. Myocardial viability testing and impact of revascularization on prognosis in patients with coronary artery disease and left ventricular dysfunction: a meta-analysis. *J Am Coll Cardiol.* 2002;39(7):1151-1158. doi:10.1016/s0735-1097(02)01726-6.

28. Desideri A, Cortigiani L, Christen AI, et al. The extent of perfusion-F18-fluorodeoxyglucose positron emission tomography mismatch determines mortality in medically treated patients with chronic ischemic left ventricular dysfunction. *J Am Coll Cardiol.* 2005;46(7):1264-1269. doi:10.1016/j.jacc.2005.06.057.

29. Panza JA, Ellis AM, Al-Khalidi HR, et al. Myocardial viability and long-term outcomes in ischemic cardiomyopathy. *N Engl J Med.* 2019;381(8):739-748. doi:10.1056/NEJMoa1807365.

30. Bonow RO, Maurer G, Lee KL, et al. Myocardial viability and survival in ischemic left ventricular dysfunction. *N Engl J Med.* 2011;364(17):1617-1625. doi:10.1056/NEJMoa1100358.

31. Hellermann JP, Jacobsen SJ, Redfield MM, Reeder GS, Weston SA, Roger VL. Heart failure after myocardial infarction: clinical presentation and survival. *Eur J Heart Fail.* 2005;7(1):119-125. doi:10.1016/j.ejheart.2004.04.011.

32. Segev A, Strauss BH, Tan M, et al. Prognostic significance of admission heart failure in patients with non-ST-elevation acute coronary syndromes (from the Canadian Acute Coronary Syndrome Registries). *Am J Cardiol.* 2006;98(4):470-473. doi:10.1016/j.amjcard.2006.03.023.

33. Steg PG, Dabbous OH, Feldman LJ, et al. Determinants and prognostic impact of heart failure complicating acute coronary syndromes: observations from the Global Registry of Acute Coronary Events (GRACE). *Circulation.* 2004;109(4):494-499. doi:10.1161/01.CIR.0000109691.16944.DA.

34. Bahit MC, Lopes RD, Clare RM, et al. Heart failure complicating non-ST-segment elevation acute coronary syndrome: timing, predictors, and clinical outcomes. *JACC: Heart Fail.* 2013;1(3):223-229. doi:10.1016/j.jchf.2013.02.007.

35. Lewis EF, Moye LA, Rouleau JL, et al. Predictors of late development of heart failure in stable survivors of myocardial infarction: The

CARE study. *J Am Coll Cardiol.* 2003;42(8):1446-1453. doi:10.1016/S0735-1097(03)01057-X.

36. Wu WY, Biery DW, Singh A, et al. Recovery of left ventricular systolic function and clinical outcomes in young adults with myocardial infarction. *J Am Coll Cardiol.* 2020;75(22):2804-2815. doi:10.1016/j.jacc.2020.03.074.

37. Westman PC, Lipinski MJ, Luger D, et al. Inflammation as a driver of adverse left ventricular remodeling after acute myocardial infarction. *J Am Coll Cardiol.* 2016;67(17):2050-2060. doi:10.1016/j.jacc.2016.01.073.

38. Aimo A, Gaggin HK, Barison A, Emdin M, Januzzi JL. Imaging, biomarker, and clinical predictors of cardiac remodeling in heart failure with reduced ejection fraction. *JACC Heart Fail.* 2019;7(9):782-794. doi:10.1016/j.jchf.2019.06.004.

39. Daubert MA, Adams K, Yow E, et al. NT-proBNP goal achievement is associated with significant reverse remodeling and improved clinical outcomes in HFrEF. *JACC Heart Fail.* 2019;7(2):158-168. doi:10.1016/j.jchf.2018.10.014.

40. Bahit MC, Kochar A, Granger CB. Post-myocardial infarction heart failure. *JACC Heart Fail.* 2018;6(3):179-186. doi:10.1016/j.jchf.2017.09.015.

41. Freemantle N, Cleland J, Young P, Mason J, Harrison J. Beta blockade after myocardial infarction: systematic review and meta regression analysis. *BMJ.* 1999;318(7200):1730-1737. doi:10.1136/bmj.318.7200.1730.

42. Dargie HJ. Effect of carvedilol on outcome after myocardial infarction in patients with left-ventricular dysfunction: the CAPRICORN randomised trial. *Lancet.* 2001;357(9266):1385-1390. doi:10.1016/s0140-6736(00)04560-8.

43. Antman EM, Anbe DT, Armstrong PW, et al. ACC/AHA guidelines for the management of patients with ST-elevation myocardial infarction: a report of the American College of Cardiology/American Heart Association Task Force on Practice Guidelines (Committee to Revise the 1999 Guidelines for the Management of Patients with Acute Myocardial Infarction). *Circulation.* 2004;110(9):e82-e292.

44. Indications for ACE inhibitors in the early treatment of acute myocardial infarction: systematic overview of individual data from 100,000 patients in randomized trials. ACE Inhibitor Myocardial Infarction Collaborative Group. *Circulation.* 1998;97(22):2202-2212. doi:10.1161/01.cir.97.22.2202.

45. Adamopoulos C, Ahmed A, Fay R, et al. Timing of eplerenone initiation and outcomes in patients with heart failure after acute myocardial infarction complicated by left ventricular systolic dysfunction: insights from the EPHESUS trial. *Eur J Heart Fail.* 2009;11(11):1099-1105. doi:10.1093/eurjhf/hfp136.

46. Janardhanan R, Kenchaiah S, Velazquez EJ, et al. Extent of coronary artery disease as a predictor of outcomes in acute myocardial infarction complicated by heart failure, left ventricular dysfunction, or both. *Am Heart J.* 2006;152(1):183-189. doi:10.1016/j.ahj.2005.11.013.

47. Gerber Y, Weston SA, Enriquez-Sarano M, et al. Atherosclerotic burden and heart failure after myocardial infarction. *JAMA Cardiol.* 2016;1(2):156-162. doi:10.1001/jamacardio.2016.0074.

48. Aimo A, Vergaro G, Castiglione V, et al. Effect of sex on reverse remodeling in chronic systolic heart failure. *JACC Heart Fail.* 2017;5(10):735-742. doi:10.1016/j.jchf.2017.07.011.

49. Wilcox JE, Fonarow GC, Yancy CW, et al. Factors associated with improvement in ejection fraction in clinical practice among patients with heart failure: findings from IMPROVE HF. *Am Heart J.* 2012;163(1):49-56.e2. doi:10.1016/j.ahj.2011.10.001.

50. Linde C, Abraham WT, Gold MR, Daubert C, REVERSE Study Group. Cardiac resynchronization therapy in asymptomatic or mildly symptomatic heart failure patients in relation to etiology: results from the REVERSE (REsynchronization reVErses Remodeling in Systolic Left vEntricular Dysfunction) study. *J Am Coll Cardiol.* 2010;56(22):1826-1831. doi:10.1016/j.jacc.2010.05.055.

51. Lupón J, Gaggin HK, de Antonio M, et al. Biomarker-assist score for reverse remodeling prediction in heart failure: the ST2-R2 score. *Int J Cardiol.* 2015;184:337-343. doi:10.1016/j.ijcard.2015.02.019.

52. Selvanayagam JB, Kardos A, Francis JM, et al. Value of delayed-enhancement cardiovascular magnetic resonance imaging in predicting myocardial viability after surgical revascularization. *Circulation.* 2004;110(12):1535-1541. doi:10.1161/01.CIR.0000142045.22628.74.

53. Shaw LJ, Arbustini E, Narula J. Heart failure with obstructive, nonobstructive, and no coronary artery disease. *JACC Heart Fail.* 2019;7(6):502-504. doi:10.1016/j.jchf.2019.03.003.

54. Braga JR, Austin PC, Ross HJ, Tu JV, Lee DS. Importance of nonobstructive coronary artery disease in the prognosis of patients with heart failure. *JACC Heart Fail.* 2019;7(6):493-501. doi:10.1016/j.jchf.2019.02.014.

55. Dewan P, Rørth R, Jhund PS, et al. Differential impact of heart failure with reduced ejection fraction on men and women. *J Am Coll Cardiol.* 2019;73(1):29-40. doi:10.1016/j.jacc.2018.09.081.

56. Velazquez EJ, Bonow RO. Revascularization in severe left ventricular dysfunction. *J Am Coll Cardiol.* 2015;65(6):615-624. doi:10.1016/j.jacc.2014.10.070.

57. O'Connor CM, Velazquez EJ, Gardner LH, et al. Comparison of coronary artery bypass grafting versus medical therapy on long-term outcome in patients with ischemic cardiomyopathy (a 25-year experience from the Duke Cardiovascular Disease Databank). *Am J Cardiol.* 2002;90(2):101-107. doi:10.1016/s0002-9149(02)02429-3.

58. Velazquez EJ, Williams JB, Yow E, et al. Long-term survival of patients with ischemic cardiomyopathy treated by coronary artery bypass grafting versus medical therapy. *Ann Thorac Surg.* 2012;93(2):523-530. doi:10.1016/j.athoracsur.2011.10.064.

59. Emond M, Mock MB, Davis KB, et al. Long-term survival of medically treated patients in the Coronary Artery Surgery Study (CASS) Registry. *Circulation.* 1994;90(6):2645-2657. doi:10.1161/01.cir.90.6.2645.

60. Velazquez EJ, Lee KL, Deja MA, et al. Coronary-artery bypass surgery in patients with left ventricular dysfunction. *N Engl J Med.* 2011;364(17):1607-1616. doi:10.1056/NEJMoa1100356.

61. Mark DB, Knight JD, Velazquez EJ, et al. Quality-of-life outcomes in surgical treatment of ischemic heart failure quality-of-life outcomes with coronary artery bypass graft surgery in ischemic left ventricular dysfunction. *Ann Intern Med.* 2014;161(6):392-399. doi:10.7326/M13-1380.

62. Velazquez EJ, Lee KL, Jones RH, et al. Coronary-artery bypass surgery in patients with ischemic cardiomyopathy. *N Engl J Med.* 2016;374(16):1511-1520. doi:10.1056/NEJMoa1602001.

63. Jolicœur EM, Dunning A, Castelvecchio S, et al. Importance of angina in patients with coronary disease, heart failure, and left ventricular systolic dysfunction: insights from STICH. *J Am Coll Cardiol.* 2015;66(19):2092-2100. doi:10.1016/j.jacc.2015.08.882.

64. Stewart RAH, Szalewska D, She L, et al. Exercise capacity and mortality in patients with ischemic left ventricular dysfunction randomized to coronary artery bypass graft surgery or medical therapy: an analysis from the STICH Trial (Surgical Treatment for Ischemic Heart Failure). *JACC: Heart Fail.* 2014;2(4):335-343. doi:10.1016/j.jchf.2014.02.009.

65. Panza JA, Velazquez EJ, She L, et al. Extent of coronary and myocardial disease and benefit from surgical revascularization in LV dysfunction. *J Am Coll Cardiol.* 2014;64(6):553-561. doi:10.1016/j.jacc.2014.04.064.

66. Feldman AM, Mann DL, She L, et al. Prognostic significance of biomarkers in predicting outcome in patients with coronary artery disease and left ventricular dysfunction: results of the biomarker substudy of the Surgical Treatment for Ischemic Heart Failure trials. *Circ Heart Fail.* 2013;6(3):461-472. doi:10.1161/CIRCHEARTFAILURE.112.000185.

67. Neumann F-J, Sousa-Uva M, Ahlsson A, et al. 2018 ESC/EACTS Guidelines on myocardial revascularization. *Eur Heart J.* 2019;40(2):87-165. doi:10.1093/eurheartj/ehy394.

68. Patel MR, Calhoon JH, Dehmer GJ, et al. ACC/AATS/AHA/ASE/ASNC/SCAI/SCCT/STS 2017 appropriate use criteria for coronary revascularization in patients with stable ischemic heart disease: a report of the American College of Cardiology Appropriate Use Criteria Task Force, American Association for Thoracic Surgery, American Heart Association, American Society of Echocardiography, American Society of Nuclear Cardiology, Society for Cardiovascular Angiography and Interventions, Society of Cardiovascular Computed Tomography, and Society of Thoracic Surgeons. *J Am Coll Cardiol.* 2017;69(17):2212-2241. doi:10.1016/j.jacc.2017.02.001.

69. Bangalore S, Guo Y, Samadashvili Z, Blecker S, Hannan EL. Revascularization in patients with multivessel coronary artery disease and severe left ventricular systolic dysfunction: everolimus-eluting stents versus coronary artery bypass graft surgery. *Circulation.* 2016;133(22):2132-2140. doi:10.1161/CIRCULATIONAHA.115.021168.

70. Berger PB, Velianou JL, Aslanidou Vlachos H, et al. Survival following coronary angioplasty versus coronary artery bypass surgery in anatomic subsets in which coronary artery bypass surgery improves survival compared with medical therapy. Results from the Bypass Angioplasty Revascularization Investigation (BARI). *J Am Coll Cardiol.* 2001;38(5):1440-1449. doi:10.1016/s0735-1097(01)01571-6.

71. Sedlis SP, Ramanathan KB, Morrison DA, Sethi G, Sacks J, Henderson W. Outcome of percutaneous coronary intervention versus coronary bypass grafting for patients with low left ventricular ejection fractions, unstable angina pectoris, and risk factors for adverse outcomes with bypass (the AWESOME Randomized Trial and Registry). *Am J Cardiol.* 2004;94(1):118-120. doi:10.1016/j.amjcard.2004.03.041.

72. Nagendran J, Bozso SJ, Norris CM, et al. Coronary artery bypass surgery improves outcomes in patients with diabetes and left ventricular dysfunction. *J Am Coll Cardiol.* 2018;71(8):819-827. doi:10.1016/j.jacc.2017.12.024.

73. Asgar AW, Mack MJ, Stone GW. Secondary mitral regurgitation in heart failure: pathophysiology, prognosis, and therapeutic considerations. *J Am Coll Cardiol.* 2015;65(12):1231-1248. doi:10.1016/j.jacc.2015.02.009.

74. Bursi F, Enriquez-Sarano M, Nkomo VT, et al. Heart failure and death after myocardial infarction in the community: the emerging role of mitral regurgitation. *Circulation.* 2005;111(3):295-301. doi:10.1161/01.CIR.0000151097.30779.04.

75. Agricola E, Ielasi A, Oppizzi M, et al. Long-term prognosis of medically treated patients with functional mitral regurgitation and left ventricular dysfunction. *Eur J Heart Fail.* 2009;11(6):581-587. doi:10.1093/eurjhf/hfp051.

76. Nishimura RA, Otto CM, Bonow RO, et al. 2014 AHA/ACC guideline for the management of patients with valvular heart disease: executive summary: a report of the American College of Cardiology/American Heart Association Task Force on Practice Guidelines. *Circulation.* 2014;129(23):2440-2492. doi:10.1161/CIR.0000000000000029.

77. Smith PK, Puskas JD, Ascheim DD, et al. Surgical treatment of moderate ischemic mitral regurgitation. *N Engl J Med.* 2014;371(23):2178-2188. doi:10.1056/NEJMoa1410490.

78. Nishimura RA, Otto CM, Bonow RO, et al. 2017 AHA/ACC focused update of the 2014 aha/acc guideline for the management of patients with valvular heart disease: a report of the American College of Cardiology/American Heart Association Task Force on Clinical Practice Guidelines. *J Am Coll Cardiol.* 2017;70(2):252-289. doi:10.1016/j.jacc.2017.03.011.

79. Obadia J-F, Messika-Zeitoun D, Leurent G, et al. Percutaneous repair or medical treatment for secondary mitral regurgitation. *N Engl J Med.* 2018;379(24):2297-2306. doi:10.1056/NEJMoa1805374.

80. Stone GW, Lindenfeld J, Abraham WT, et al. Transcatheter mitral-valve repair in patients with heart failure. *N Engl J Med.* 2018;379(24):2307-2318. doi:10.1056/NEJMoa1806640.

81. Enriquez-Sarano M, Michelena HI, Grigioni F. Treatment of functional mitral regurgitation. *Circulation.* 2019;139(20):2289-2291. doi:10.1161/CIRCULATIONAHA.118.038207.

82. Cheng RK, Cox M, Neely ML, et al. Outcomes in patients with heart failure with preserved, borderline, and reduced ejection fraction in the Medicare population. *Am Heart J.* 2014;168(5):721-730. doi:10.1016/j.ahj.2014.07.008.

83. Rickenbacher P, Kaufmann BA, Maeder MT, et al. Heart failure with mid-range ejection fraction: a distinct clinical entity? Insights from the Trial of Intensified versus standard Medical therapy in Elderly patients with Congestive Heart Failure (TIME-CHF). *Eur J Heart Fail.* 2017;19(12):1586-1596. doi:10.1002/ejhf.798.

84. Hsu JJ, Ziaeian B, Fonarow GC. Heart failure with mid-range (borderline) ejection fraction: clinical implications and future directions. *JACC Heart Fail.* 2017;5(11):763-771. doi:10.1016/j.jchf.2017.06.013.

85. Solomon SD, Vaduganathan ML, Claggett B, et al. Sacubitril/valsartan across the spectrum of ejection fraction in heart failure. *Circulation.* 2020;141(5):352-361. doi:10.1161/CIRCULATIONAHA.119.044586.

86. Dunlay SM, Roger VL, Weston SA, Jiang R, Redfield MM. Longitudinal changes in ejection fraction in heart failure patients with preserved and reduced ejection fraction. *Circ Heart Fail.* 2012;5(6):720-726. doi:10.1161/CIRCHEARTFAILURE.111.966366.

87. Ohara T, Little WC. Evolving focus on diastolic dysfunction in patients with coronary artery disease. *Curr Opin Cardiol.* 2010;25(6):613-621. doi:10.1097/HCO.0b013e32833f0438.

88. Paulus WJ, Tschöpe C. A novel paradigm for heart failure with preserved ejection fraction: comorbidities drive myocardial dysfunction and remodeling through coronary microvascular endothelial inflammation. *J Am Coll Cardiol.* 2013;62(4):263-271. doi:10.1016/j.jacc.2013.02.092.

89. Franssen C, Chen S, Unger A, et al. Myocardial microvascular inflammatory endothelial activation in heart failure with preserved ejection fraction. *JACC Heart Fail.* 2016;4(4):312-324. doi:10.1016/j.jchf.2015.10.007.

90. Lewis GA, Schelbert EB, Williams SG, et al. Biological phenotypes of heart failure with preserved ejection fraction. *J Am Coll Cardiol.* 2017;70(17):2186-2200. doi:10.1016/j.jacc.2017.09.006.

91. Srivaratharajah K, Coutinho T, deKemp R, et al. Reduced myocardial flow in heart failure patients with preserved ejection fraction. *Circ Heart Fail.* 2016;9(7). doi:10.1161/CIRCHEARTFAILURE.115.002562.

92. Kato S, Saito N, Kirigaya H, et al. Impairment of coronary flow reserve evaluated by phase contrast cine-magnetic resonance imaging in patients with heart failure with preserved ejection fraction. *J Am Heart Assoc.* 2016;5(2). doi:10.1161/JAHA.115.002649.

93. Samson R, Jaiswal A, Ennezat PV, Cassidy M, Le Jemtel TH. Clinical phenotypes in heart failure with preserved ejection fraction. *J Am Heart Assoc.* 2016;5(1). doi:10.1161/JAHA.115.002477.

94. Hwang S-J, Melenovsky V, Borlaug BA. Implications of coronary artery disease in heart failure with preserved ejection fraction. *J Am Coll Cardiol.* 2014;63(25 Part A):2817-2827. doi:10.1016/j.jacc.2014.03.034.

95. Mentz RJ, Kelly JP, von Lueder TG, et al. Noncardiac comorbidities in heart failure with reduced versus preserved ejection fraction. *J Am Coll Cardiol.* 2014;64(21):2281-2293. doi:10.1016/j.jacc.2014.08.036.

96. Greenberg B. Heart failure preserved ejection fraction with coronary artery disease: time for a new classification? *J Am Coll Cardiol.* 2014;63(25 Pt A):2828-2830. doi:10.1016/j.jacc.2014.03.033.

97. Mentz RJ, Broderick S, Shaw LK, Fiuzat M, O'Connor CM. Heart failure with preserved ejection fraction: comparison of patients with and without angina pectoris (from the Duke Databank for Cardiovascular Disease). *J Am Coll Cardiol.* 2014;63(3):251-258. doi:10.1016/j.jacc.2013.09.039.

98. Cunningham JW, Vaduganathan M, Claggett BL, et al. Myocardial infarction in heart failure with preserved ejection fraction: pooled analysis of 3 clinical trials. *JACC: Heart Fail.* 2020;8(8):618-626. doi:10.1016/j.jchf.2020.02.007.

99. Yancy CW, Jessup M, Bozkurt B, et al. 2017 ACC/AHA/HFSA focused update of the 2013 ACCF/AHA guideline for the management of heart failure: a report of the American College of Cardiology/American Heart Association Task Force on Clinical Practice Guidelines and the Heart Failure Society of America. *Circulation.* 2017;136(6):e137-e161. doi:10.1161/CIR.0000000000000509.

100. Kramer K, Kirkman P, Kitzman D, Little WC. Flash pulmonary edema: association with hypertension and reoccurrence despite coronary revascularization. *Am Heart J.* 2000;140(3):451-455. doi:10.1067/mhj.2000.108828.

Diagnosis and Management of Chronic Heart Failure

Muhammad Shahzeb Khan, Muthiah Vaduganathan, and Javed Butler

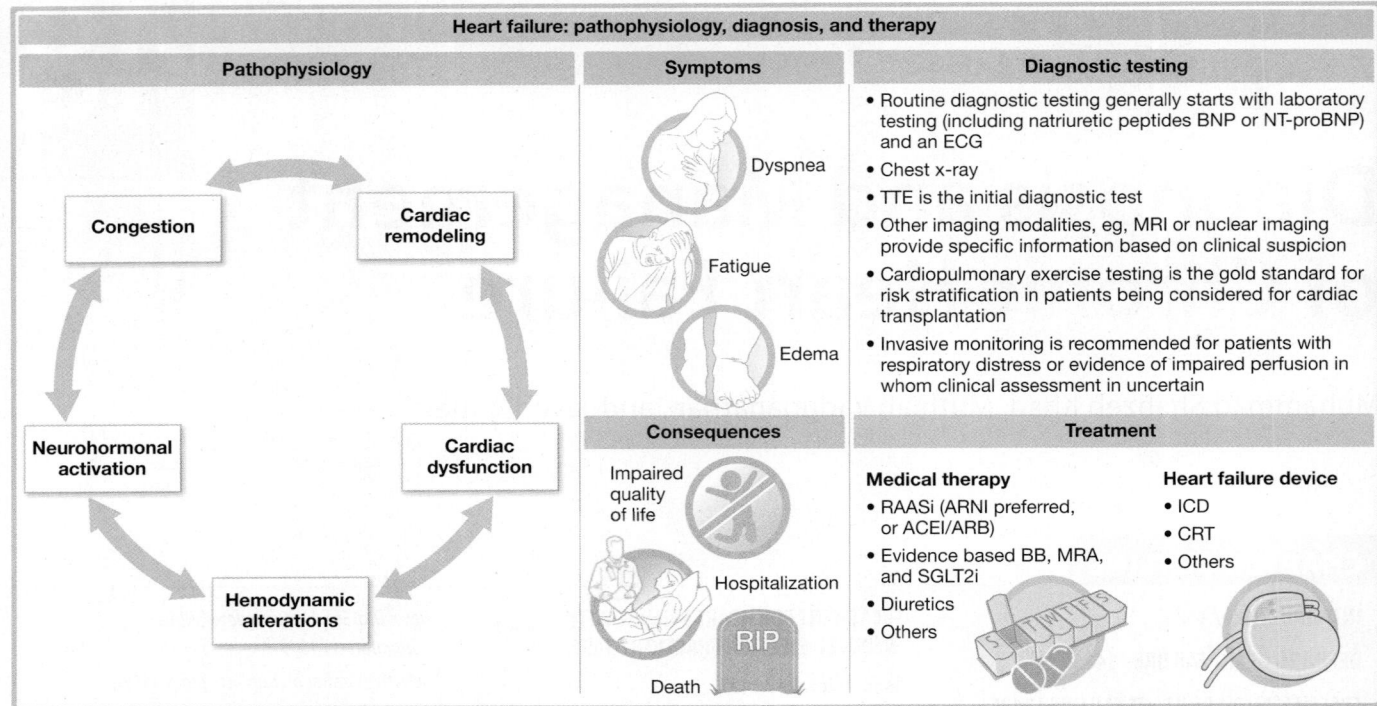

Chapter 48 Fuster and Hurst's Central Illustration. Heart failure is a clinical syndrome that involves a complex interplay between myocardial, vascular, neurohormonal, hemodynamic and comorbid factors. Signs and symptoms of heart failure can be fairly nonspecific and thus diagnosis of heart failure is often challenging. However, early diagnosis and treatment of heart failure can improve quality of life, and reduce risk of hospitalization and/or death. BB, beta blockers; BNP, B-type natriuretic peptide; CRT, cardiac resynchronization therapy; ECG, electrocardiogram; ICD, implantable cardioverter defibrillator; MRA, mineralocorticoid receptor antagonist; NT-proBNP, N-terminal-pro B-type natriuretic peptide; RAASi, renin–angiotensin–aldosterone system inhibitors; SGLT2i, sodium-glucose co-transporter 2 inhibitors; TTE, transthoracic echocardiography.

CHAPTER SUMMARY

This chapter discusses the diagnosis and treatment of heart failure with reduced ejection fraction (HFrEF), mid-range EF (HFmrEF) and recovered EF (HFrecEF), clinical syndromes that involve a complex interplay between myocardial, vascular, hemodynamic neurohormonal, and comorbid factors (see Fuster and Hurst's Central Illustration). Early diagnosis and treatment of heart failure can improve quality of life and reduce rates of hospitalization and death. Cardinal manifestations of heart failure include dyspnea, which may limit exercise tolerance, and fluid retention, which may lead to pulmonary, splanchnic and peripheral edema. Foundational pharmacological therapies for chronic heart failure include diuretics, beta blockers, angiotensin receptor-neprilysin inhibitors, aldosterone receptor antagonists, and sodium glucose co-transporter 2 inhibitors. Certain heart failure patients may benefit from device-based therapies such as implantable cardioverter defibrillators and cardiac resynchronization therapy. Considering the high morbidity and mortality associated with heart failure, it is essential to appropriately diagnose and employ guideline directed medical therapy.

INTRODUCTION

The syndrome of heart failure has existed since humans first began to document disease. Clinical texts attributable to Hippocrates describe patients with shortness of breath, edema, and anasarca, in a manner not too varied from contemporary accounts.[1] It has also long been realized that heart failure is not caused by a single disease; rather, it is an amalgamate of several diseases that have unique etiologies, natural histories, and treatments.[2] The shared feature of this cluster of illnesses is damage to the cardiac issue. Initially, the heart compensates in various manners to a loss in reserve; however, once there is a critical degree of impairment in its structure and function, a final common pathway emerges that shares similarities in symptoms and findings.

Over the last several decades, dramatic improvements in management of valvular and ischemic heart disease have decreased mortality from these illnesses and consequently led to an increase in the incidence and prevalence of heart failure. Coupled with the aging of the global population, there has been a growth of the heart failure prevalence to epidemic proportions. Currently, heart failure affects more than 60 million people globally.[3] Heart failure is a difficult disease to manage and is associated with high rates of morbidity and mortality, and costs associated with it, both in terms of direct financial costs as well as indirect cost of patient and caregiver burden.[4] Therefore, it is imperative to recognize and manage the syndrome using the best currently available information, and to make concerted efforts to find novel ways to further improve its management.

DEFINING HEART FAILURE

According to the 2013 American College of Cardiology/American Heart Association (ACC/AHA) heart failure guidelines, "Heart failure is a complex clinical syndrome that results from any structural or functional impairment of ventricular filling or ejection of blood." The cardinal manifestations of heart failure are dyspnea and fatigue, which may limit exercise tolerance, and fluid retention, which may lead to pulmonary and/or splanchnic congestion and/or peripheral edema. Some patients have exercise intolerance but little evidence of fluid retention, whereas others complain primarily of edema, dyspnea, or fatigue. Because some patients present without signs or symptoms of volume overload, the term *heart failure* is preferred over *congestive heart failure*. There is no single diagnostic test for heart failure because it is largely a clinical diagnosis based on a careful history and physical examination.[5] The definition used by the 2016 European Society of Cardiology (ESC) heart failure guidelines states that "Heart failure is a clinical syndrome characterized by typical symptoms (eg, breathlessness, ankle swelling and fatigue) that may be accompanied by signs (eg, elevated jugular venous pressure, pulmonary crackles and peripheral oedema) caused by a structural and/or functional cardiac abnormality, resulting in a reduced cardiac output and/or elevated intracardiac pressures at rest or during stress."[6]

While previously thought of as simply a syndrome of disordered hemodynamics and fluid balance caused by alterations in the structure of the heart, our understanding of heart failure has progressed to a systemic illness that involves complex interplay between myocardial factors, systemic inflammation, kidney abnormalities, and neurohormonal dysfunction (**Fig. 48–1**).[2,7,8] As a result, there is an evolution in our assessment and treatment from a focus solely on examination findings and improving hemodynamics to measuring and modifying the maladaptive molecular processes that contribute to disease progression.[9] In the absence of universally agreed-upon objective biological descriptors of the syndrome, however, we must rely on an assortment of clinical descriptors to diagnose the syndrome that vary in their ability to adequately phenotype heart failure.[10]

CLASSIFICATION OF HEART FAILURE

Several constructs have been created for the purpose of describing heart failure such that there is greater uniformity in its diagnosis and treatment. The most common of these is the New York Heart Association (NYHA) functional classification that was first introduced in 1928 and still persists due to its ease of use and clinical relevance (**Table 48–1**).[11] Furthermore, currently approved therapies are anchored in this classification because it was used to select patients for almost all randomized clinical trials in heart failure. Patients with NYHA class I have no symptoms attributable for heart disease; those in NYHA classes II, III, or IV have mild, moderate, and severe symptoms, respectively. It is important to note that this classification has numerous limitations: it correlates poorly with objective measures of heart failure, is not a static measure, and there is significant intraobserver variability in assignment of class.[12]

Another classification introduced by the ACC/AHA is the heart failure staging approach that emphasizes the importance of development and progression of disease (Table 48–1).[5] These stages are progressive and associated with prognosis, and interventions can vary based on stage: modifying risk factors (stage A), treating structural heart disease (stage B), and reducing morbidity and mortality (stages C and D).

Another key classifier of heart failure is left ventricular ejection fraction (LVEF), principally because this was a fundamental variable used in clinical trials and there is a belief that it captures distinct phenotypes of heart failure.[13-15] Mathematically, it is LV stroke volume divided by the end-diastolic volume. In patients with reduced contraction and emptying of the LV due to systolic dysfunction, output is maintained by the heart ejecting a smaller percentage of a larger end diastolic volume.[6] As systolic function decreases, this is generally parallel by reduction in ejection fraction and greater end-diastolic and end-systolic volumes. In patients with heart failure symptoms in whom reductions in ejection fraction do not occur, there is generally increase in thickness of the LV suggestive of chronically high filling pressures, as well as increased left atrial size.

A commonly used clinical classification of heart failure relies on bedside physician assessment of perfusion and volume status (see section Signs and Symptoms).[16] Indicators of congestion include history of orthopnea and/or physical exam evidence of jugular venous distention, rales, hepatojugular

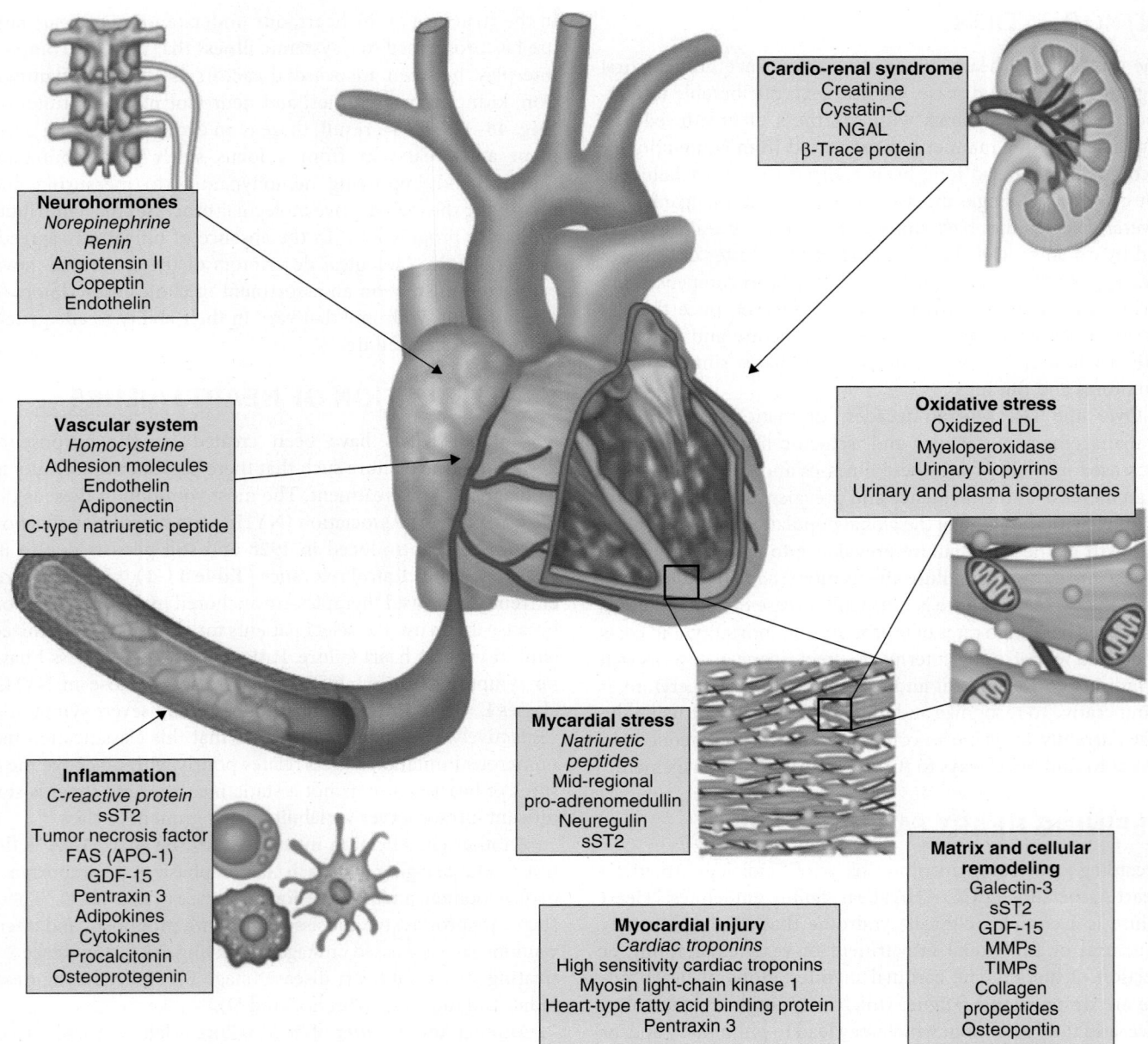

Neurohormones
Norepinephrine
Renin
Angiotensin II
Copeptin
Endothelin

Cardio-renal syndrome
Creatinine
Cystatin-C
NGAL
β-Trace protein

Vascular system
Homocysteine
Adhesion molecules
Endothelin
Adiponectin
C-type natriuretic peptide

Oxidative stress
Oxidized LDL
Myeloperoxidase
Urinary biopyrrins
Urinary and plasma isoprostanes

Inflammation
C-reactive protein
sST2
Tumor necrosis factor
FAS (APO-1)
GDF-15
Pentraxin 3
Adipokines
Cytokines
Procalcitonin
Osteoprotegenin

Mycardial stress
Natriuretic
peptides
Mid-regional
pro-adrenomedullin
Neuregulin
sST2

Matrix and cellular
remodeling
Galectin-3
sST2
GDF-15
MMPs
TIMPs
Collagen
propeptides
Osteopontin

Myocardial injury
Cardiac troponins
High sensitivity cardiac troponins
Myosin light-chain kinase 1
Heart-type fatty acid binding protein
Pentraxin 3

Figure 48–1. Heat failure involves an interplay between myocardial factors, systemic inflammation, renal dysfunction, and neurohormonal activation. Biomarkers can be classified according to broad categories of processes that are involved in the development and progression of heart failure. Several biomarkers have been characterized for each of these processes; these vary greatly in their ease of measurement, cost, turnaround time, and evaluation in the clinical setting. Traditional biomarkers that have been studied fairly rigorously appear in italics. APO, apoptosis antigen; GDF, growth differentiation factor; HF, heart failure; ICAM, intercellular adhesion molecule; LDL, low-density lipoprotein; MMPs, matrix metalloproteinases; NGAL, neutrophil gelatinase-associated lipocalin; TIMPs, matrix metalloproteinase tissue inhibitors. Reproduced with permission from Ahmad T, Fiuzat M, Felker GM, et al. Novel biomarkers in chronic heart failure. *Nat Rev Cardiol.* 2012 Mar 27;9(6):347-359.

reflux, ascites, peripheral edema, leftward radiation of the pulmonic heart sound, or a square wave blood pressure response to the Valsalva maneuver. Compromised perfusion is assessed by the presence of a narrow proportional pulse pressure ([systolic–diastolic blood pressure]/systolic blood pressure <25%), pulsus alternans, symptomatic hypotension (without orthostasis), cool extremities, and/or impaired mentation.[16]

Heart failure itself is not synonymous with a certain degree of LV dysfunction and similar abnormalities can exist across the spectrum of LVEF.[17,18] However, important clinical decisions hinge on a dichotomous classification of ejection fraction because only randomized clinical trials that enrolled patients with LVEF ≤35% to 40% to date have shown efficacious results (**Table 48–2**).[19,20] Therefore, one of the most common ways to describe heart failure is as heart failure with reduced ejection fraction (HFrEF) and heart failure with preserved ejection fraction (HFpEF). The prevalence of HFrEF and HFpEF is approximately 50% each.[21] In addition, patients with LVEF

TABLE 48-1. Comparison of ACCF/AHA Stages of HF and NYHA Functional Classifications

ACCF/AHA Stages of HF		NYHA Functional Classification
A At high risk for HF but without structural heart disease or symptoms of HF	None	
B Structural heart disease but without signs or symptoms of HF	I	No limitation of physical activity. Ordinary physical activity does not cause symptoms of HF.
C Structural heart disease with prior or current symptoms of HF	I	No limitation of physical activity. Ordinary physical activity does not cause symptoms of HF.
	II	Slight limitation of physical activity. Comfortable at rest, but ordinary physical activity results in symptoms of HF.
	III	Marked limitation of physical activity. Comfortable at rest, but less than ordinary activity causes symptoms of HF.
	IV	Unable to carry on any physical activity without symptoms of HF, or symptoms of HF at rest.
D Refractory HF requiring specialized interventions	IV	Unable to carry on any physical activity without symptoms of HF, or symptoms of HF at rest.

Abbreviations: ACCF indicates American College of Cardiology Foundation; AHA, American Heart Association; HF, heart failure; NYHA, New York Heart Association.

between 40% and 50%, referred to as heart failure with mid-range or mildly reduced ejection fraction, share characteristics of both heart failure phenotypes. LVEF is also recognized to be a dynamic measure that may improve with medical therapies; select patients with HFrEF may achieve durable improvements in LVEF above 40% and are called heart failure with recovered ejection fraction. However, studies have shown that many such patients who have recovered their LVEF may relapse following treatment withdrawal.[22] Of note, the descriptors *systolic* and *diastolic* are often used in place of HFrEF and HFpEF, but from a purist's perspective, these are incorrect because systolic and diastolic dysfunction coexists in the majority of patients with heart failure, irrespective of ejection fraction.[15]

Finally, there are a few other terminologies used. Patients who have had heart failure for some time are often said to have *chronic heart failure*. If symptoms in such patient are unchanged for some length of time, they are said to have chronic stable heart failure; however, this terminology may not be entirely accurate because many "stable" patients may still experience high rates of clinical events in practice.[23]

If a chronic heart failure patient declines, they are said to have *worsening heart failure* and in general if this leads to hospitalization, it is referred to as *acute heart failure* or *acutely decompensated heart failure. Congestive heart failure* is an older term and implies the symptoms of excessive volume retention that are frequent but by no means the sine qua non for heart failure.[6] Terms such as *right-sided heart failure* and *left-sided heart failure* attempt to isolate symptoms to a specific ventricle; for example, lower extremity edema and ascites are ascribed to a failing right ventricle (RV), whereas dyspnea and low blood pressure to the LV. These descriptors are less informative because abnormalities of all cardiac chambers have been recognized to exist in patients with heart failure.

DIAGNOSIS AND EVALUATION OF HEART FAILURE

Signs and Symptoms

It is often challenging to diagnose heart failure, especially in its early stages. Its signs and symptoms can be fairly nonspecific, and may not prompt further testing that would lead to a more certain diagnosis.[24-26] In the acute setting, heart failure can be mistaken for disorders such as myocardial ischemia, chronic obstructive pulmonary disease, pulmonary embolism, or infections. In the more chronic setting, heart failure can be mistaken for diseases such as depression, asthma, cirrhosis, or

TABLE 48-2. Definitions of Heart Failure

Classification	EF (%)	Description
I. Heart failure with reduced ejection fraction (HFrEF)	≤40	Also referred to as systolic HF. Randomized controlled trials have mainly enrolled patients with HFrEF, and it is only in these patients that efficacious therapies have been demonstrated to date.
II. Heart failure with preserved ejection fraction (HFpEF)	≥50	Also referred to as diastolic HF. Several different criteria have been used to further define HFpEF. The diagnosis of HFpEF is challenging because it is largely one of excluding other potential noncardiac causes of symptoms suggestive of HF. To date, efficacious therapies have not been identified.
a. HFpEF, borderline	41 to 49	These patients fall into a borderline or intermediate group. Their characteristics, treatment patterns, and outcomes appear similar to those of patients with HFpEF.
b. HFpEF, improved	>40	It has been recognized that a subset of patients with HFpEF previously had HFrEF. These patients with improvement or recovery in EF may be clinically distinct from those with persistently preserved or reduced EF. Further research is needed to better characterize these patients.

Abbreviations: EF indicates ejection fraction; HF, heart failure; HFpEF, heart failure with preserved ejection fraction; and HFrEF, heart failure with reduced ejection fraction.

hypothyroidism. Therefore, a heightened clinical suspicion is required when a clinician encounters a patient with suspected heart failure such that the appropriate set of diagnostic and therapeutic interventions are performed. Once it is confirmed that abnormalities of the heart are driving the patient's symptoms, the diversity of causes for cardiomyopathy should be considered.[27] Another challenge is that criteria for early detection of heart failure in the community have not been well established at this time.

Table 48–3 outlines some of the findings noted in heart failure. As with many medical conditions, key information can be gleaned from a thoughtful history and physical exam.[28,29] Identification of risk factors such as prior myocardial infarction and a family history can provide important clues about etiology.[30] The duration and triggers of symptoms can identify potential drivers of cardiac dysfunction. Other clues might come from comorbid conditions and treatments. Social history might reveal use of cocaine, methamphetamine, or alcohol, which may all contribute to cardiomyopathy.

Physical examination findings are generally ascribed to findings of increased total body volume (edema, anasarca) or decreased cardiac output (fatigue, exercise intolerance, decreased urine output), which are useful for ruling in heart failure, rather than ruling it out.[16,31] Findings such as elevations in jugular venous pressure and third heart sound are strongly specific for heart failure but difficult to detect and suffer from lack of reproducibility.[32,33] Furthermore, they are dependent on the patient's body habitus and can be misleading in the presence of RV dysfunction and/or tricuspid regurgitation. That said, the astute clinician can garner important clues by examination, especially when it is well integrated.[34] A proportional pulse pressure [(systolic−diastolic)/systolic)] of <25% has been correlated with a cardiac index <2.2 L/min/m^2.[25] An elevated jugular venous pressure is among the most important exam findings to identify congestion.[32]

The cardiovascular response to the Valsalva maneuver is a simple and highly sensitive bedside test for estimation of volume status and detection of LV systolic dysfunction. With the blood pressure cuff inflated 15 mm Hg over the systolic pressure, the patient is asked to perform a Valsalva maneuver. A normal response is when Korotkoff sounds are audible only at the onset of straining and at release. In patients with heart failure, Korotkoff sounds can be heard throughout the Valsalva maneuver (the square wave response) or a lack of reappearance of the sounds after release (the absent overshoot response).[31] The third heart sound (or gallop rhythm) is commonly present with tachycardia (but may be challenging to hear) and volume overload and signifies elevated left-sided filling pressures. Even in the absence of complaints, examination should be performed to determine the presence of ascites, hepatosplenomegaly, or a pulsatile liver. It is not uncommon for patients with advanced heart failure to present with severe right upper quadrant pain and to undergo cholecystectomy when the actual culprit is acute hepatic congestion.[35] Peripheral edema is common in heart failure but is nonspecific because it can result from a number of other disease states, including obesity. The finding of cachexia in patients with end-stage heart failure

is associated with a particularly poor prognosis.[36] Finally, it is important to remember that signs of pulmonary congestion such as rales and pulmonary edema are commonly lacking in patients with heart failure, even elevated pulmonary pressures given the development of a collateral lymphatic circulation in the thoracic cavity.[28,29,37]

Routine Diagnostic Testing

Routine diagnostic testing generally starts with laboratory testing and electrocardiogram (ECG) analysis.[38] Assessments of kidney function and potassium can have therapeutic implications. Reversible causes of heart failure such as thyroid disorders, anemia, select vitamin deficiencies, and hypocalcemia should be ruled out. The ECG can provide information about rhythm and conduction[39] and can help select therapies. Chest x-ray is commonly performed in patients with suspected or new-onset heart failure but is limited by low sensitivity and specificity[40] and significant LV dysfunction and volume overload can exist in the presence of a normal chest x-ray.[41]

Biomarkers

Natriuretic peptides, specifically the B-type natriuretic peptide (BNP) and N-terminal-proBNP (NT-proBNP), have revolutionized the diagnosis and prognostication of heart failure.[42] Before its activation, BNP is stored as a 108–amino acid polypeptide precursor, proBNP, in secretory granules in both ventricles and, to a lesser extent, in the atria. After proBNP is secreted in response to volume overload and resulting myocardial stretch, it is cleaved to the 76-peptide, biologically inert N-terminal fragment NT-proBNP and the 32-peptide, biologically active hormone BNP. The two fragments are secreted into the plasma in equimolar amounts, and both have been extensively evaluated for use in the management of heart failure. BNP has diuretic, natriuretic, and antihypertensive effects; furthermore, it may provide a protective effect against the detrimental fibrosis and remodeling that occurs in progressive heart failure. Normal natriuretic peptide level in an untreated patient virtually excludes significant cardiac disease, potentially making further testing unnessary.[38,43] Assays for BNP and NT-proBNP are reasonably correlated and either can be used clinically. Inhibition of neprilysin, which degrades BNP, with sacubitril/valsartan may increase BNP levels; levels may still be interpretable with maintenance therapy and still carry prognostic value.[44] Natriuretic peptides are supported with an ACC/AHA class I recommendation for the diagnosis of acute heart failure and establishment of prognosis in chronic heart failure.[5] Both BNP and NT-proBNP levels can also be elevated from a variety of other causes (**Table 48–4**).[45]

An abundance of biomarkers can provide unique information about various aspects of heart failure pathophysiology but only a few are approved for use in the clinical setting (Fig. 48–1).[9,46] Cardiac troponin[47] elevations in heart failure are associated with more severe disease and prognosis, but management implications of these elevations remain unclear.[48] It is currently reasonable to measure levels in the hospital setting to rule out an ischemic trigger and establish prognosis.

TABLE 48–3. History and Physical Examination in Heart Failure

	Comments
History	
Potential clues suggesting etiology of HF	A careful family history may identify an underlying familial cardiomyopathy in patients with idiopathic DCM. Other etiologies outlined in Section 5 should be considered as well.
Duration of illness	A patient with recent-onset systolic HF may recover time.
Severity and triggers of dyspnea and fatigue, presence of chest pain, exercise capacity, physical activity, sexual activity	To determine NYHA class; identify potential symptoms of coronary ischemia.
Anorexia and early satiety, weight loss	Gastrointestinal symptoms are common in patients with HF. Cardiac cachexia is associated with adverse prognosis.
Weight gain	Rapid weight gain suggests volume overload.
Palpitations, (pre)syncope, ICD shocks	Palpitations may be indications of paroxysmal AF or ventricular tachycardia. ICD shocks are associated with adverse prognosis.
Symptoms suggesting transient ischemic attack or thromboembolism	Affects consideration of the need for anticoagulation.
Development of peripheral edema or ascites	Suggests volume overload.
Disordered breathing at night, sleep problems	Treatment for sleep may improve cardiac function and decrease pulmonary hypertension.
Recent or frequent prior hospitalizations for HF	Associated with adverse prognosis.
History of discontinuation of medications for HF	Determine whether lack of GDMT in patients with HFrEF reflects intolerance, an adverse event, or perceived contraindication to use. Withdrawal of these medications has been associated with adverse prognosis.
Medications that may exacerbate HF	Removal of such medications may represent a therapeutic opportunity.
Diet	Awareness and restriction of sodium and fluid intake should be assessed.
Adherence to medical regimen	Access to medications; family support; access to follow-up; cultural sensitivity
Physical Examination	
BMI and evidence of weight loss	Obesity may be a contributing cause of HF; cachexia may correspond with poor prognosis.
Blood pressure (supine and upright)	Assess for hypertension or hypotension. Width of pulse pressure may reflect adequacy of cardiac output. Response of blood pressure to Valsalva maneuver may reflect LV filling pressure.
Pulse	Manual palpation will reveal strength and regularity of pulse rate.
Examination for orthostatic changes in blood pressure and heart rate	Consistent with volume depletion or excess vasodilation from medications.
Jugular venous pressure at rest and following abdominal compression (http://wn.com/jugular_venous_distension_example)	Most useful finding on physical examination to identify congestion.
Presence of extra heart sounds and murmurs	S_3 is associated with adverse prognosis in HFrEF. Murmurs may be suggestive of valvular heart disease.
Size and location of point of maximal impulse	Enlarged and displaced point of maximal impulse suggests ventricular enlargement.
Presence of right ventricular heave	Suggests significant right ventricular dysfunction and/or pulmonary hypertension.
Pulmonary status: respiratory rate, rales, pleural effusion	In advanced chronic HF, rales are often absent despite major pulmonary congestion.
Hepatomegaly and/or ascites	Usually markers of volume overload.
Peripheral edema	Many patients, particularly those who are young, may be not edematous despite intravascular volume overload. In obese patients and elderly patients, edema may reflect peripheral rather than cardiac causes.
Temperature of lower extremities	Cool lower extremities may reflect inadequate cardiac output.

Abbreviations: AF indicates atrial fibrillation; BMI, body mass index; DCM, dilated cardiomyopathy; GDMT, guideline-directed medical therapy; HF, heart failure; HFrEF, heart failure with reduced ejection fraction; ICD, implantable cardioverter-defibrillator; LV, left ventricular; NYHA, New York Heart Association.

TABLE 48-4. Selected Causes of Elevated Natriuretic Peptide Concentrations

Cardiac
- Heart failure, including RV syndromes
- Acute coronary syndrome
- Heart muscle disease, including LVH
- Valvular heart disease
- Pericardial disease
- Atrial fibrillation
- Myocarditis
- Cardiac surgery
- Cardioversion

Noncardiac
- Advancing age
- Anemia
- Renal failure
- Pulmonary: obstructive sleep apnea, severe pneumonia, pulmonary hypertension
- Critical illness
- Bacterial sepsis
- Severe burns
- Toxic-metabolic insults, including cancer chemotherapy and envenomation

Abbreviations: LVH indicates left ventricular hypertrophy; RV, right ventricular.

Soluble ST2 and galectin-3 are predictive of adverse outcomes in chronic heart failure and are additive in their value to natriuretic peptides.[49] Along with other prognostic factors, they can provide unique and objective information about the patient, and are likely be included in future multimarker approaches to heart failure care.[50] In chronic heart failure, measurement of cardiac troponins, ST2, and galectin-3 has an ACC/AHA Class IIb recommendation for risk stratification.[51]

Transthoracic Echocardiogram

Transthoracic echocardiography is the initial diagnostic test for heart failure assessment (**Table 48-5**).[13,14,52,53] It can be performed at the bedside, is accurate and safe, and provides key information on chamber size and volumes, systolic and diastolic function, wall thickness, and valve function. A two-dimensional echocardiogram with Doppler during an initial assessment of a patient with suspected heart failure, as well as those with changes in symptoms, is a class I recommendation.[5] The LVEF is measured using several different methods, with the recommended technique being the apical biplane method of discs (the modified Simpson's rule). LVEF must be interpreted in its clinical context as it depends on several parameters such as heart rate, preload, afterload, and valvular function, and is not the same as stroke volume. Assessment of diastolic parameters are an important part of the assessment of patients with heart failure. No single echocardiographic parameter can make the diagnosis of diastolic dysfunction in heart failure; a comprehensive inclusion of two-dimensional and Doppler data is required (Table 48-5). Other key echocardiographic measures in heart failure patients are assessments of RV function, presence of pulmonary hypertension, inferior vena cava diameters and collapsibility, which are useful in the estimation of right atrial pressure, and severity of coexisting valvular heart disease.[54]

Other Noninvasive Imaging

Other imaging modalities are available that provide unique information about various aspects of myocardial dysfunction (**Table 48-6 and Fig. 48-2**).[55] Transesophageal echocardiography is useful when chest wall windows are inadequate, in patients with complex valvular or congenital heart disease, and to evaluate the left atrial appendage for thrombus.[6] Stress echocardiography is useful to identify ischemia and to gauge if the dysfunctional myocardium is viable.[54] It is also valuable for the evaluation of aortic stenosis severity or contractile reserve in the setting of reduced LVEF and low transvalvular gradient. Single-photon emission computer tomography (SPECT) or positron emission tomography (PET) may be used to assess ischemia and viability if coronary artery disease is present.

Cardiac magnetic resonance (CMR) can provide almost all the information gleaned from a comprehensive echocardiogram, as well as additional assessments.[56] It is considered the gold standard for assessment of myocardial volumes, mass, and wall motion. CMR can provide key input in regards to whether an inflammatory or infiltrative condition might be present. Furthermore, it is an extremely helpful tool for the understanding of potential sources of arrhythmias, pericardial disease, and anatomy in patients with congenital heart disease.

Cardiopulmonary Exercise Testing

Cardiopulmonary exercise testing (CPX) measures a broader range of variables related to cardiorespiratory function, including expiratory ventilation ($\dot{V}E$) and pulmonary gas exchange (oxygen uptake [$\dot{V}O_2$] and carbon dioxide output [$\dot{V}CO_2$]), and helps quantitatively link metabolic, cardiovascular, and pulmonary responses to exercise.[57] It objectively correlates the subjective findings in heart failure and helps understand the relative contributions of the heart, lungs, and peripheral muscles to symptoms of dyspnea and fatigue.[58] The test uses treadmill and bicycle protocols along with gas exchange analysis, and provides key information that can be used to gauge candidacy for advanced therapies such as a left ventricular assist device (LVAD) and transplantation. Cardiopulmonary exercise testing is the gold standard for risk stratification in patients being considered for cardiac transplantation.[59] Originally, a threshold of peak $\dot{V}O_2$ of ≤14 mL/kg/min had been suggested, but in the current era of improved therapies, a lower threshold of 10 to 12 mL/kg/min has been suggested for consideration of advanced therapies. Some studies have suggested that the $\dot{V}E/\dot{V}CO_2$ slope is a better predictor of outcome than peak $\dot{V}O_2$, LVEF, and NYHA class.[60]

Genetic Testing

Familial syndromes are thought to account to up to 20% to 35% of patients with apparent idiopathic dilated cardiomyopathy. Additionally, genetic testing in now readily available to assess for mutations in several other disease-causing genes that can lead to unexplained cardiomyopathies, or syndromes with cardiac involvement (**Table 48-7**).

TABLE 48–5. Common Echocardiographic Abnormalities in Patients with Heart Failure

Measurement	Abnormality	Clinical implications
Parameters related to systolic function		
LV ejection fraction	Reduced (<50%)	LV global systolic dysfunction
LV fractional shortening	Reduced (<25%)	LV radial systolic dysfunction
LV regional function	Hypokinesis, akinesis, dyskinesis	Myocardial infarction/ischemia Cardiomyopathy, myocarditis
LV end-diastolic size	Increased (diameter ≥60 mm, >32 mm/m², volume >97 mL/m²)	Volume overload HF likely
LV end-systolic size	Increased (diameter >45 mm/>25 mm/m², volume >43 mL/m²)	Volume overload HF likely
LV outflow tract velocity time integral	Reduced (<15 cm)	Reduced LV stroke volume
Parameters related to diastolic function		
LV diastolic dysfunction parameters	Abnormalities of the mitral inflow pattern, tissue velocities (e') or the E/e' ratio	Indicate LV diastolic dysfunction degree and suggest level of filling pressure
Left atrial volume index	Increased (volume >34 mL/m²)	Increased LV filling pressure (past or present) Mitral valve disease
LV mass index	Increased: >95 g/m² in women and >115 g/m² in men	Hypertension, aortic stenosis, hypertrophic cardiomyopathy
Parameters related to valvular function		
Valvular structure and function	Valvular stenosis or regurgitation (especially aortic stenosis and mitral regurgitation)	May be the cause of HF or a complicating factor or the result of HF (secondary mitral regurgitation) Assess dysfunction severity and hemodynamic consequences Consider surgery
Other parameters		
RV function (eg, TAPSE)	Reduced (TAPSE <16 mm)	RV systolic dysfunction
Tricuspid regurgitation peak velocity	Increased (>3.4 m/s)	Increased RV systolic pressure
Systolic pulmonary artery pressure	Increased (>50 mmHg)	Pulmonary hypertension likely
Inferior vena cava	Dilated, with no respiratory collapse	Increased right atrial pressure RV dysfunction, volume overload Pulmonary hypertension possible
Pericardium	Effusion, hemopericardium, calcification	Consider tamponade, malignancy, systemic diseases, acute or chronic pericarditis, constrictive pericarditis
Measurement	**Abnormality**	**Clinical implications**
e'	Decreased (<8 cm/s septal, <10 cm/s lateral, or <9 cm/s average)	Delayed LV relaxation
E/e' ratio[a]	High (>15)	High LV filling pressure
	Low (<8)	Normal LV filling pressure
	Intermediate (8–15)	Grey zone (additional parameters necessary)
Mitral inflow E/A ratio[b]	"Restrictive" (>2)	High LV filling pressure
		Volume overload
	"Impaired relaxation" (<1)	Delayed LV relaxation
		Normal LV filling pressure
	Normal (1–2)	Inconclusive (may be "pseudonormal")
Mitral inflow during Valsalva maneuvre	Change of the "pseudonormal" to the "impaired relaxation" pattern (with a decrease in E/A ratio ≥0.5)	High LV filling pressure (unmasked through Valsalva)
(A pulm—A mitral) duration	>30 ms	High LV filling pressure

TABLE 48–6. Possible Applications of Various Imaging Techniques in the Diagnosis of Heart Failure

		Echo	CMR	Cath	SPECT	MDCT	PET
Remodeling/dysfunction							
LV	EDV	++	+++	++	++	++	++
	ESV	++	+++	++	++	++	++
	EF	++	+++	++	++	++	++
	Mass	++	+++	–	–	++	–
RV	EDV	++	+++	+	–	++	–
	ESV	++	+++	+	–	++	–
	EF	++	+++	+	–	++	–
	Mass	++	+++	–	–	++	–
LV diastolic dysfunction		+++	+	+++	–	–	–
Dyssynchrony		++	+	–	+	–	–
Etiology							
CAD	Ischemia	+++	+++	+++	+++	–	+++
	Hibernation	+++	+++	–	+++	–	+++
	Scar	++	+++	–	++	–	++
	Coronary anatomy	–	–	+++	–	+++	–
Valvular	Stenosis	+++	+	+++	–	++	–
	Regurgitation	+++	++	++	–	–	–
Myocarditis		+	+++	+++	–	–	–
Sarcoidosis		+	+++	++	–	–	++
Hypertrophic CMP	HCM	+++	++	++	–	–	–
	Amyloidosis	++	+++	+++	–	–	–
Dilated CMP	Myocarditis	+	+++	+++	–	–	–
	Eosinophilic syndromes	+	+++	+++	–	–	–
	Iron hemochromatosis	+	+++	–	–	–	–
	Iron thalassemia	+	+++	–	–	–	–
ARVC		++	+++	+++	–	+	–
Restrictive CMP	Pericarditis	++	++	++	–	++	–
	Amyloidosis	++	+++	+++	–	–	–
	Endomyocardial fibrosis	+	+++	+++	–	–	–
	Anderson-Fabry	+	+	–	–	–	-
Unclassified CMP	Takotsubo cardiomyopathy	++	++	+++	–	–	–
Main advantages							
		Wide availability Portability No radiation Relatively low cost	Good-quality images No radiation	Good availability	Good availability	Reasonable availability High-quality images	Limited availability Good-quality images
Main disadvantages							
		Echo window needed	Limited availability Contraindications Functional analysis Image quality limited if arrhythmia	Radiation Invasive	Radiation	Radiation Image quality limited if arrhythmia	Radiation Limited availability

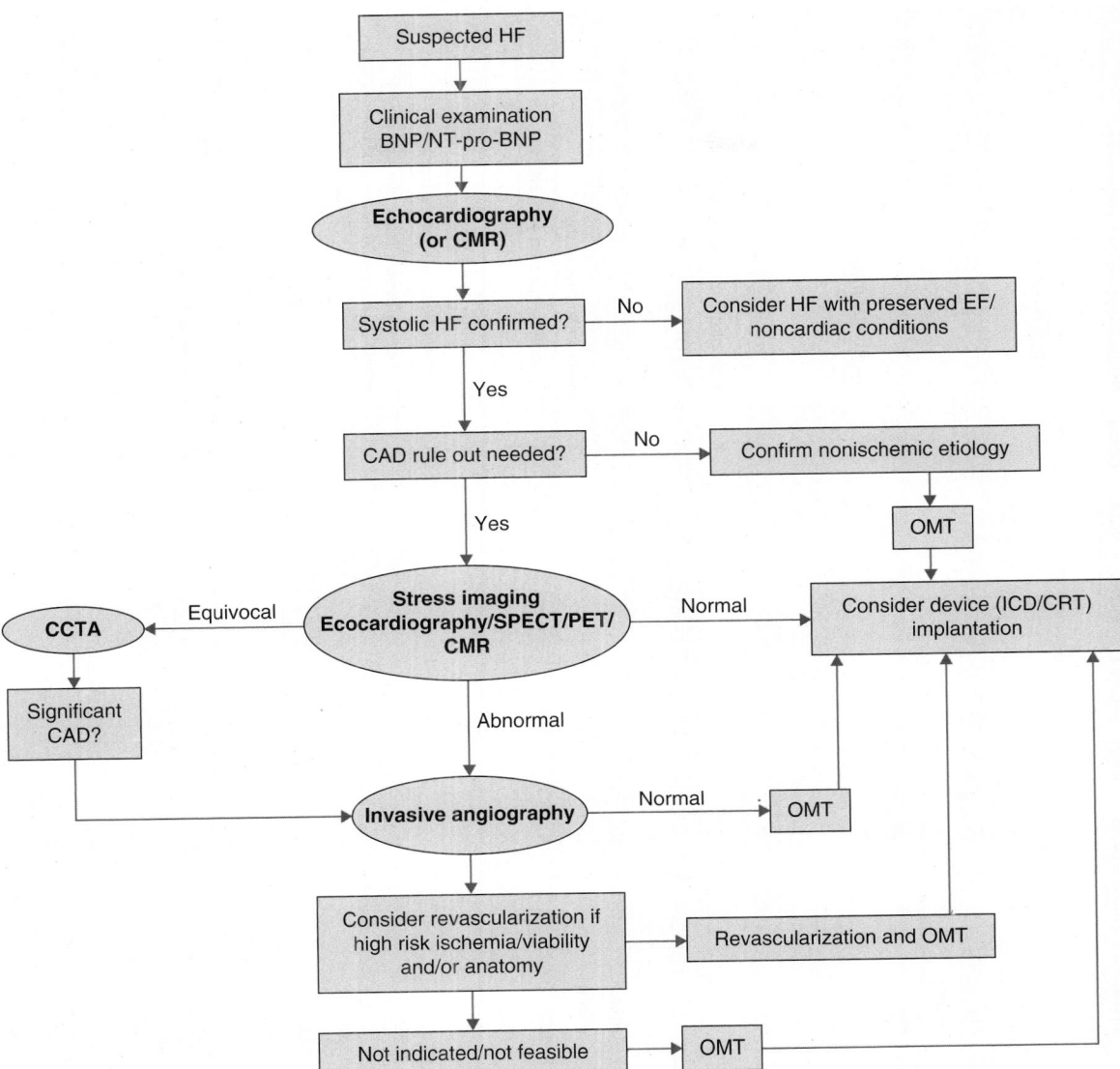

Figure 48–2. Use of cardiac imaging for the management of patients with chronic systolic heart failure (HF). BNP, brain natriuretic peptide; CAD, coronary artery disease; CCTA, cardiac computed tomographic angiography; CMR, cardiac magnetic resonance; CRT, cardiac resynchronization therapy; EF, ejection fraction; ICD, implantable cardioverter-defibrillator; NT-proBNP, N-terminal proBNP; OMT, optimal medical therapy; PET, positron emission tomography; SPECT, single-photon emission computed tomography. Reproduced with permission from Gimelli A, Lancellotti P, Badano LP, et al. Non-invasive cardiac imaging evaluation of patients with chronic systolic heart failure: a report from the European Association of Cardiovascular Imaging (EACVI). *Eur Heart J.* 2014 Dec 21;35(48):3417-3425.

Invasive Testing

Right heart catheterizations are commonly used in the diagnosis or management of heart failure, but there are little data to help guide appropriate settings for when hemodynamic measurements are indicated. Based on expert consensus, invasive monitoring is recommended for patients with respiratory distress or evidence of impaired perfusion in whom clinical assessment falls short. It is also recommended for (1) presumed cardiogenic shock requiring escalating pressor therapy and consideration of mechanical circulatory support, (2) severe clinical decompensation in which therapy is limited by uncertain contributions of elevated filling pressures, hypoperfusion, and vascular tone, (3) apparent dependence on intravenous inotropic infusions, (4) persistent severe symptoms despite adjustment of recommended therapies, or (5) consideration for mechanical circulatory support or transplantation in a patient with advance disease. Routine use of right heart catheterization is not recommended in normotensive patients who are responding appropriately to diuretics and vasodilators.

Based on the premise that providing clinicians with continuous invasive data in heart failure patients could improve outcomes, an implantable device (CardioMEMS) that allows therapeutic adjustment based on continuously measures pulmonary artery (PA) pressures was tested in a randomized trial of 550 high-risk heart failure patients. The CHAMPION (CardioMEMS Heart Sensor Allows Monitoring of Pressure to Improve Outcomes in NYHA Class III Heart Failure Patients) trial showed that the PA pressure-guided treatment arm had

TABLE 48–7. Cardiomyopathy Panels

Gene	Cardiomyopathy Panels — Pan Cardiomyopathy Panel (62 Genes)	HCM Panel (20 Genes)	DCM/Arrythmogenic Cardiomyopathy Panel (53 Genes)	Inher.	HCM	DCM	ARVC	CPVT	LVNC	RCM	Other	Other Diseases or Syndromes
ABBC9	X			AD		X					X	Cantu syndrome
ACTC1	X	X	X	AD	X	X			X	X		
ACTN2	X	X	X	AD	X	X				X		
ANKRD1	X			Unkn	X	X						
BAG3	X		X	AD	X	‥				X	X	Myofibrillar myopathy
CASQ2	X		X	AD				X	X			
CAV3	X			AD	X	X					X	Limb-girdle muscular dystrophy
CHRM2	X		X	AD		X					X	Long QT
CRYAB	X		X	Unkn		X					X	Myofibrillar myopathy
CSRP3	X	X	X	AD/AR	X	‥					X	Myopathy reported with HCM
DES	X		X	AD/AR		X	X			X	X	Myofibrillar myopathy; Limb-girdle muscular dystrophy
DMD	X		X	XL		‥					X	Duchenne/Becker muscular dystrophy; Female carriers may develop isolated DCM
DOLK	X		X	AR		X						
DSC2	X		X	AD		X	X					
DSG2	X		X	AD		X	X					
DSP	X		X	AD		X	X					
DTNA	X		X	AR		‥	‥		X		X	Carvajal syndrome
EMD	X		X	XL		‥			X		X	Emery-Dreifuss muscular dystrophy
FHL2	X			Unkn		X						
GATAD1	X		X	AR		X						
GLA	X	X	X	XL	‥						X	Fabry disease

Gene	1	2	Inheritance	3	4	5	6	7	Disease
ILK	X		Unkn	X	X				
JPH2	X	X	Unkn	X	X				
JUP	X	X	AD	X	X	X		X	Naxos disease
LAMA4*	X		Unkn	X	X				
LAMP2	X	X	XL	⋮	⋮		⋮		Danon disease
LDB3	X	X	AD	X	X	X			Myofibrillar myopathy
LMNA	X		AD	X	X			X	Limb-girdle muscular dystrophy
									Charcot-Marie-Tooth disease
									Malouf syndrome
									Partial lipodystrophy
			AD/AR	⋮	⋮		⋮		Emery-Dreifuss muscular dystrophy
MURC	X	X	AD	X	X	X			
MYBPC3	X	X	AD	X	X	X	X		
MYH6	X	X	AD	X	X	X			CHD
MYH7	X	X	AD	X	X	X	X		Myopathies
								X	Laing distal myopathy
								X	Myosin storage myopathy
MYL2	X	X	AD	X	X	X			
MYL3	X	X	AD	X	X	X	X		
MYLK2	X		Unkn	X	X				
MYOM1	X	X	AD	X	X				
MYOZ2	X	X	AD	X	X				
MYPN	X	X	AD	X	X	X			
NEBL	X	X	Unkn	X	X			X	Endocardial fibroelastosis
NEXN	X	X	Unkn	X	X				
PDLIM3	X		Unkn	X	X				
PKP2	X	X	AD	X	X	X			
PLN	X	X	AD	X	X	X		X	
PRDM16	X	X	Unkn	X	X	X			
PRKAG2	X	X	AD	X	X	⋮		X	Glycogen storage disease (with WPW)
PTPN11	X	X	AD	X	X	⋮		X	Noonan spectrum disorders

(Continued)

TABLE 48–7. Cardiomyopathy Panels (Continued)

Gene	Pan Cardiomyopathy Panel (62 Genes)	HCM Panel (20 Genes)	DCM/Arrythmogenic Cardiomyopathy Panel (53 Genes)	Inher.	HCM	DCM	ARVC	CPVT	LVNC	RCM	Other	Other Diseases or Syndromes
RAF1	X	X		AD	X						X	Noonan spectrum disorders
RBM20	X		X	AD		X						
RYR2	X		X	AD	X			X				Presentation can overlap with ARVC
SCN5A	X		X	AD		X	X				X	Brugada syndrome, Long QT syndrome
SGCD	X		X	AD		X						
				AR	X	X					X	Limb-girdle muscular dystrophy
TAZ	X		X	XL	X	X			X		X	Barth syndrome
TCAP	X		X	Unkn	X							
				AR	X	X					X	Limb-girdle muscular dystrophy
TMEM43	X		X	AD			X					
TNNC1	X	X	X	AD	X	X						
TNNI3	X	X	X	AD	X	X				X		
TNNT2	X	X	X	AD	X	X			X	X		
TPM1	X	X	X	AD	X	X				X		
TRDN	X		X	AR				X				
TTN	X		X	AD	X	X	X					
				AD/AR							X	HMERF
											X	Tibial muscular dystrophy
				AR							X	Centronuclear myopathy
												Limb-girdle muscular dystrophy
TTR	X	X	X	AD	X	X					X	Amyloidosis
VCL	X		X	AD	X	X			X			

a 37% reduction in heart failure hospitalizations compared with the control group.[61] Based on these results, the device is approved by the US Food and Drug Administration (FDA) for use in patients with heart failure and NYHA class III symptoms. The appropriate application of this device in clinical practice is still evolving.[62] Left heart catheterizations or coronary angiography should be performed in patients who are candidates for revascularization in whom it is felt that ischemia is contributing to the development or worsening of heart failure.[63] Endomyocardial biopsy may be considered when seeking a specific diagnosis that would influence therapy, such as suspected giant cell myocarditis or cardiac amyloidosis; however, this must be weighed against the known procedural risks associated with a native heart biopsy.[64]

TREATMENT FOR HEART FAILURE WITH REDUCED EJECTION FRACTION

Sodium Intake

Despite the absence of credible data, dietary sodium restriction for the management of heart failure is widely recommended, and is borne out of historical beliefs, putative mechanistic data, and observational studies.[65,66] No study to date has evaluated the effects of sodium restriction on outcomes in optimally treated patients,[67] and there are data showing that reduction in sodium intake might lead to adverse outcomes in heart failure[68] underscoring the need for a randomized clinical trial in this area.[69]

Exercise

Both the ESC and the ACC/AHA guidelines extend exercise training a class I recommendation for treatment of HFrEF.[5,6] Several studies have showed that exercise has numerous benefits in heart failure.[70,71] The HF-ACTION (Heart Failure: A Controlled Trial Investigating Outcomes of Exercise Training) trial randomized 2331 patients with LVEF ≤35% to exercise training versus usual care[72] and showed improvements in quality of life, depression, physical fitness, and reduction in risk of heart failure hospitalizations. The Center for Medicare and Medicaid Services (CMS) supports cardiac rehabilitation for heart failure.[73]

Pharmacological Treatments

The goal for pharmacological treatment of heart failure is to help patients feel better, live longer, and stay out of the hospital. Until the evaluation of vasodilators in 1980s, no options were available to treat heart failure other than diuretics and digoxin.[74] Subsequently, hydralazine plus isosorbide dinitrate, angiotensin-converting enzyme (ACE) inhibitors,[75,76] β-blockers, and mineralocorticoid receptor antagonists have all been shown to improve outcomes in patients with HFrEF (**Fig. 48–3**). Three novel therapies—sacubitril/valsartan, ivabradine, and sodium-glucose cotransporter 2 inhibitors—were recently approved for use in HFrEF.

Diuretics

Many of the clinical manifestations of heart failure are related to excessive salt and volume retention and several downstream deleterious consequences.[77] Diuretics can restore salt and water homeostasis, relief congestion and symptoms, and improve exercise capacity; however, no long-term studies examining the effects of diuretics on morbidity or mortality have been performed to date.[78] **Figure 48–4** shows the tubular sites of action of commonly used diuretics and **Table 48–8** reviews usual dosage recommendations.

Proximal tubular diuretics act primarily by decreasing proximal tubular sodium reabsorption and include osmotic diuretics such as mannitol and carbonic anhydrase inhibitors such as acetazolamide, and are not very effective when used alone. Although 50% to 70% of the glomerular filtrate is reabsorbed isosmotically in the proximal tubule, the distal nephron (particularly the ascending limb of the loop of Henle) has the capacity to increase its rate of sodium reabsorption substantially. Therefore, an increase in glomerular filtration or decrease in proximal tubular reabsorption alone may not be associated with a significant diuresis. Thus, these agents are infrequently used.

Loop of Henle diuretics include ethacrynic acid, furosemide, bumetanide, and torsemide. Loop diuretics inhibit the $Na^+/2Cl^-/K^+$ cotransporter of the thick ascending loop of Henle, resulting in decreased sodium and chloride reabsorption.[79] The potency of these agents depends on renal blood flow and proximal tubular secretion to deliver these agents to their site of action. Bioavailability of furosemide ranges from 40% to 70% of the oral dose; in contrast, bumetanide and torsemide exceeds 80%.[80] Despite belief that continuous infusions of loop diuretics were superior to bolus dosing and that higher doses might be harmful, the Diuretic Strategies in Patients with Acute Decompensated Heart Failure (DOSE) trial showed that these therapeutic strategy largely made no difference, and it appeared to be beneficial to use of higher doses of diuretics.[81] Loop diuretics also induce prostaglandins synthesis resulting in renal and peripheral vascular smooth muscle relaxation and vasodilatation.

Thiazide diuretics include drugs like chlorthalidone and metolazone.[79] These agents are chemically different. Metolazone is an oral quinazoline that inhibits the Na^+-Cl^- transporter in the cortical portion of the ascending loop of Henle and prevents maximal dilution of the urine and decreasing the kidneys ability to secrete free water. It may contribute to hyponatremia. It increases Ca^{2+} and decreases Mg^{2+} resorption, and may be associated with hypercalcemia and hypomagnesemia. Increased delivery of NaCl and H_2O to the collecting duct can trigger potassium secretion, causing hypokalemia. Metolazone and chlorothiazide can be used in conjunction with loop diuretics to overcome diuretic resistance.

The mineralocorticoid receptor antagonists spironolactone and eplerenone are the most relevant *potassium-sparing diuretics* in heart failure.[79] Spironolactone is a synthetic steroid that competes for the cytoplasmic aldosterone receptor. It increases the secretion of water and sodium, while decreasing the excretion of potassium, by competing for the aldosterone-sensitive Na+/K+ channel in the distal tubule of the nephron. Since sodium exchange in the distal tubule is low, potassium-sparing diuretics are generally relatively weak diuretics. As a nonselective aldosterone receptor antagonist, endocrine-related adverse effects (such as gynecomastia) are

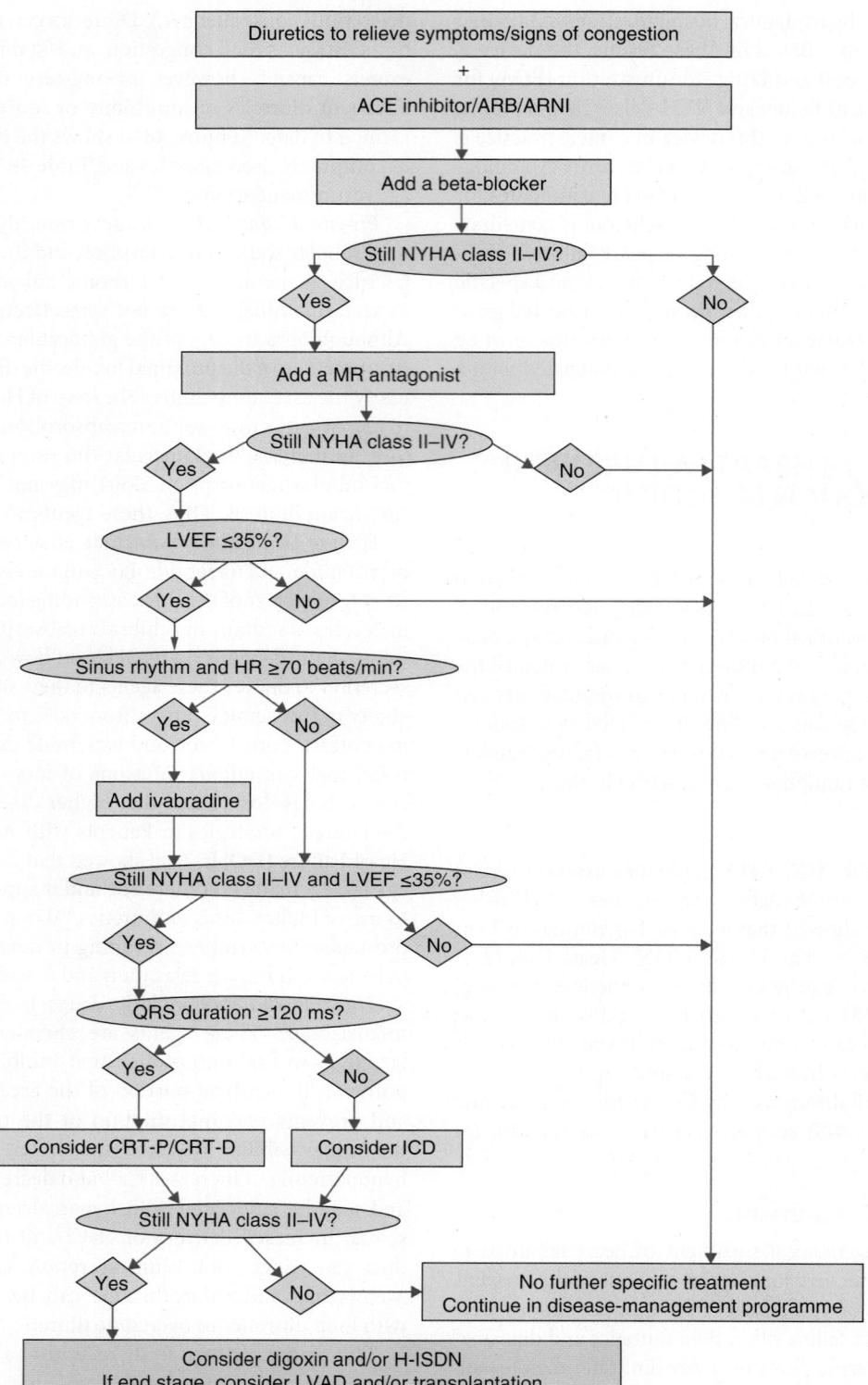

Figure 48–3. Treatment options for patients with chronic symptomatic systolic heart failure (New York Heart Association [NYHA] functional class II–IV). ACE, angiotensin-converting enzyme; ARB, angiotensin-receptor blocker; ARNI, angiotensin receptor-neprilysin inhibitor; CRT-D, cardiac resynchronization therapy defibrillator; CRT-P, cardiac resynchronization therapy pacemaker; H-ISDN, hydralazine–isosorbide dinitrate; HR, heart rate; ICD, implantable cardioverter-defibrillator; LVEF, left ventricular ejection fraction; LVAD, left ventricular assist device; MR, mineralocorticoid receptor. Reproduced with permission from McMurray JJ, Adamopoulos S, Anker SD, et al. ESC Guidelines for the diagnosis and treatment of acute and chronic heart failure 2012: The Task Force for the Diagnosis and Treatment of Acute and Chronic Heart Failure 2012 of the European Society of Cardiology. Developed in collaboration with the Heart Failure Association (HFA) of the ESC. *Eur Heart J.* 2012 Jul;33(14):1787-1847.

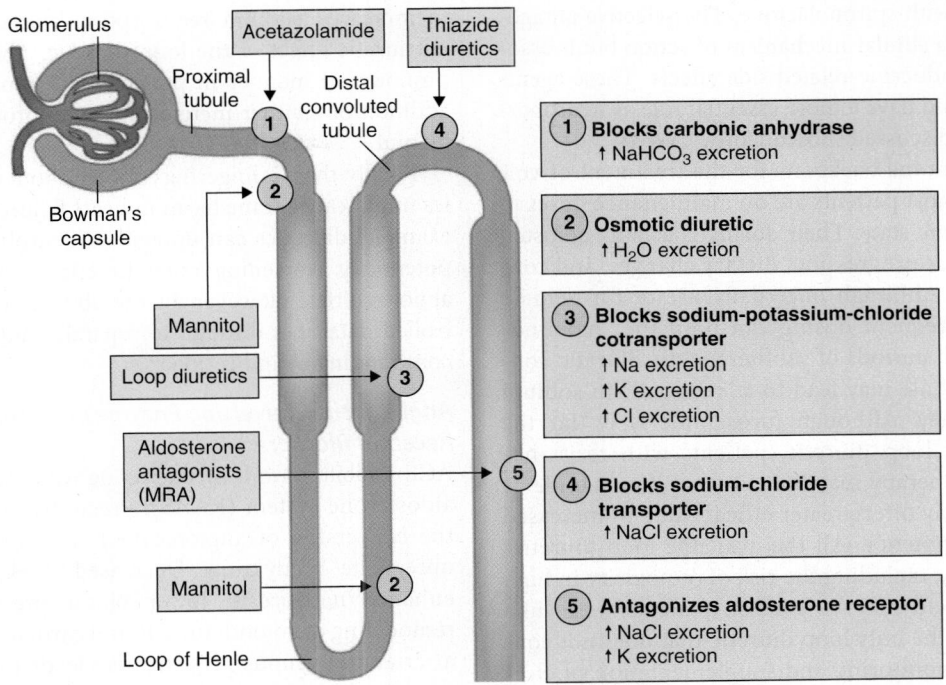

Figure 48–4. (1) Acetazolamide functions in the proximal tubule by blocking carbonic anhydrase and increasing $NaHCO_3$ excretion. (2) Mannitol functions in both the proximal tubule and the loop of Henle by increasing H_2O excretion. (3) Loop diuretics function in thick ascending limb of the loop of Henle by blocking the sodium-chloride-potassium cotransporter and increasing sodium, potassium, and chloride excretion. (4) Thiazide functions in the distal convoluted tubule by blocking the sodium-chloride transporter and increasing sodium chloride excretion. (5) Mineralocorticoid receptor antagonists (MRAs) function in the collecting duct of the distal tubule and antagonize the aldosterone receptor, hence increasing sodium excretion and potassium retention. Reproduced with permission from ter Maaten JM, Valente MAE, Damman K, et al. Diuretic response in acute heart failure—pathophysiology, evaluation, and therapy. *Nat Rev Cardiol*. 2015 Mar;12(3):184-192.

TABLE 48–8. Oral Diuretics Recommended for Use in the Treatment of Chronic Heart Failure

Drug	Initial Daily Dose(s)	Maximum Total Daily Dose	Duration of Action
Loop diuretics			
Bumetanide	0.5 to 1.0 mg once or twice	10 mg	4 to 6 h
Furosemide	20 to 40 mg once or twice	600 mg	6 to 8 h
Torsemide	10 to 20 mg once	200 mg	12 to 16 h
Thiazide diuretics			
Chlorothiazide	250 to 500 mg once or twice	1,000 mg	6 to 12 h
Chlorthalidone	12.5 to 25.0 mg once	100 mg	24 to 72 h
Hydrochlorothiazide	25 mg once or twice	200 mg	6 to 12 h
Indapamide	2.5 mg once	5 mg	36 h
Metolazone	2.5 mg once	20 mg	12 to 24 h
Potassium-sparing diuretics*			
Amiloride	5 mg once	20 mg	24 h
Spironolactone	12.5 to 25.0 mg once	50 mg†	1 to 3 h
Triamterene	50 to 75 mg twice	200 mg	7 to 9 h
Sequential nephron blockade			
Metolazone	2.5 to 10.0 mg once plus loop diuretic	N/A	N/A
Hydrochlorothiazide	25 to 100 mg once or twice plus loop diuretic	N/A	N/A
Chlorothiazide (IV)	500 to 1,000 mg once plus loop diuretic	N/A	N/A

*Eplerenone, although also a diuretic, is primarily used in chronic HF.
†Higher doses may occasionally be used with close monitoring.
HF indicates heart failure; IV, intravenous; and N/A, not applicable.

relatively common with spironolactone. The selective antagonist eplerenone has a similar mechanism of action but is associated with fewer endocrine-related side effects. These agents are weak diuretics and have a more essential role as neurohormonal modulators, discussed subsequently.

Loop diuretics are the backbone for the treatment of volume overload and most patients are on maintenance doses to preserve an euvolemic state. Their dosing is usually adjusted in response to disease progression, dietary changes, and concurrent therapies.[79] Although once-daily use of furosemide is standard, more frequent dosing can limit the "rebound" period during which periods of subtherapeutic diuretic concentration in the tubule may lead to a "rebound" in sodium avidity by the kidney. Although furosemide is by far the most common oral loop diuretic, patients with resistance to oral furosemide therapy may benefit from bumetanide or torsemide, which may offer greater efficacy due to increased bioavailability and potency. All the available loop diuretics share similar toxicity, including the risk of ototoxicity in high doses. Ethacrynic acid may be used in patients with sulfa allergy because it is the only loop diuretic that does not contain sulfa. Careful monitoring and supplementation of electrolytes, particularly potassium and magnesium, are a crucial aspect of loop diuretic therapy.

Over time, some patients develop diuretic resistance. Once issues such as noncompliance and concomitant use of nonsteroidal anti-inflammatory drug use are addressed, it is important to achieve an adequate dose of loop diuretics by requiring a higher dose in order to achieve the same level of sodium excretion (**Fig. 48–5**). This "breaking phenomenon" is felt to be from both hemodynamic changes at the glomerulus, adaptive changes in the distal nephron, and stimulation of the renin-angiotensin and sympathetic nervous systems. Chronically high amounts of sodium delivered to the distal nephron causes hypertrophy of distal convoluted tubule cells, leading

to increased sodium reabsorption and negating the overall natriuretic effect of the loop diuretic. This occurs in a more pronounced manner in patients with renal dysfunction. The addition of a either metolazone or chlorothiazide can also be helpful.

Finally, there is lingering concern about whether loop diuretics might cause some harm in heart failure (**Fig. 48–6**).[82,83] For example, diuretics can upregulate neurohormonal activation, potentially worsening renal function, and cause electrolyte abnormalities. However, in the absence of randomized controlled data, it is difficult to separate causal association from confounding by indication.[84]

Angiotensin-Converting Enzyme Inhibitors/Angiotensin Receptor Blockers

ACE inhibitors work by interfering with the renin-angiotensin-aldosterone system (RAAS). Precisely, ACE inhibitors block the conversion of angiotensin I to angiotensin II and also upregulate bradykinin. Decreased levels of angiotensin II enhance natriuresis, lower blood pressure, and prevent remodeling of smooth muscle and cardiac myocytes. Lowered arterial and venous pressure also leads to decreased preload and afterload.[85] Several trials have shown that ACE inhibitors reduce the risk of death and hospitalization in patients with HFrEF, and are an ACC/AHA class I recommendation for patients with current or prior symptoms of heart failure.[5] **Table 48–9** shows all the major trials conducted on ACE inhibitors and angiotensin receptor blockers (ARBs).[75,76,86–107] Two key randomized trials were Cooperative North Scandinavian Enalapril Survival Study (CONSENSUS) and Studies of Left Ventricular Dysfunction (SOLVD)-Treatment.[75,76] Both trials showed reductions in mortality; a relative risk reduction of 27% in CONSENSUS, and of 16% in SOLVD-Treatment. The Assessment of Treatment with Lisinopril And Survival (ATLAS) trial randomized 3164 patients to with moderate-severe heart failure to low versus high dose lisinopril and showed a 15% relative reduction in risk of death or hospitalization with the latter approach.[108] Furthermore, in 4228 patients with low LVEF but no symptoms of heart failure, enalapril in the SOLVD-Prevention trial showed a 20% reduction in risk of death or heart failure hospitalization.[107]

ACE inhibitors should be used with caution in patients with low systemic blood pressures, markedly elevated creatinine, bilateral renal artery stenosis, or elevated levels of serum potassium.[5] There are no differences among the various ACE inhibitors and there is a class recommendation for their use. Kidney function and potassium should be monitored 1 to 2 weeks after initiation and at periodic timepoints afterward. Up to 20% of patients develop an ACE inhibitor–induced cough. In these patients and others who are intolerant to ACE inhibitors, ARBs may provide an equally efficacious alternative.[5] ARBs are receptor antagonists that block type 1 angiotensin II (AT1) receptors on bloods vessels and other tissues such as the heart. These receptors are coupled to the Gq-protein and IP3 signal transduction pathway that stimulates vascular smooth muscle contraction. Because ARBs do not inhibit ACEs, they do not cause an increase in bradykinin. However, their other

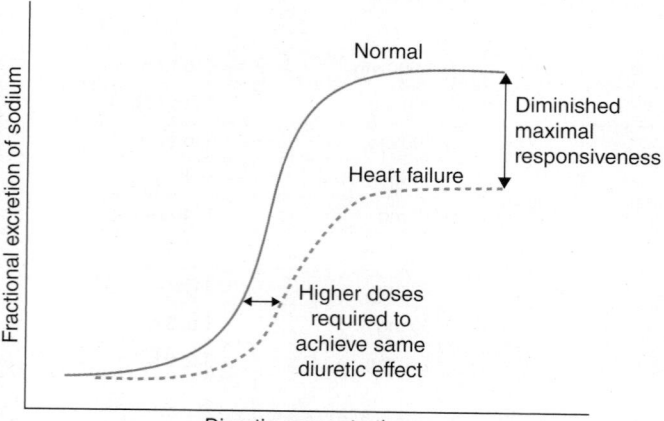

Figure 48–5. Schematic of dose-response curve of loop diuretics in heart failure patients compared with normal controls. In heart failure patients, higher doses are required to achieve a given diuretic effect, and the maximal effect is blunted. Reproduced with permission from Felker GM, Mentz RM. Diuretics and Ultrafiltration in Acute Decompensated Heart Failure. *J Am Coll Cardiol.* 2012;59(24):2145-2153.

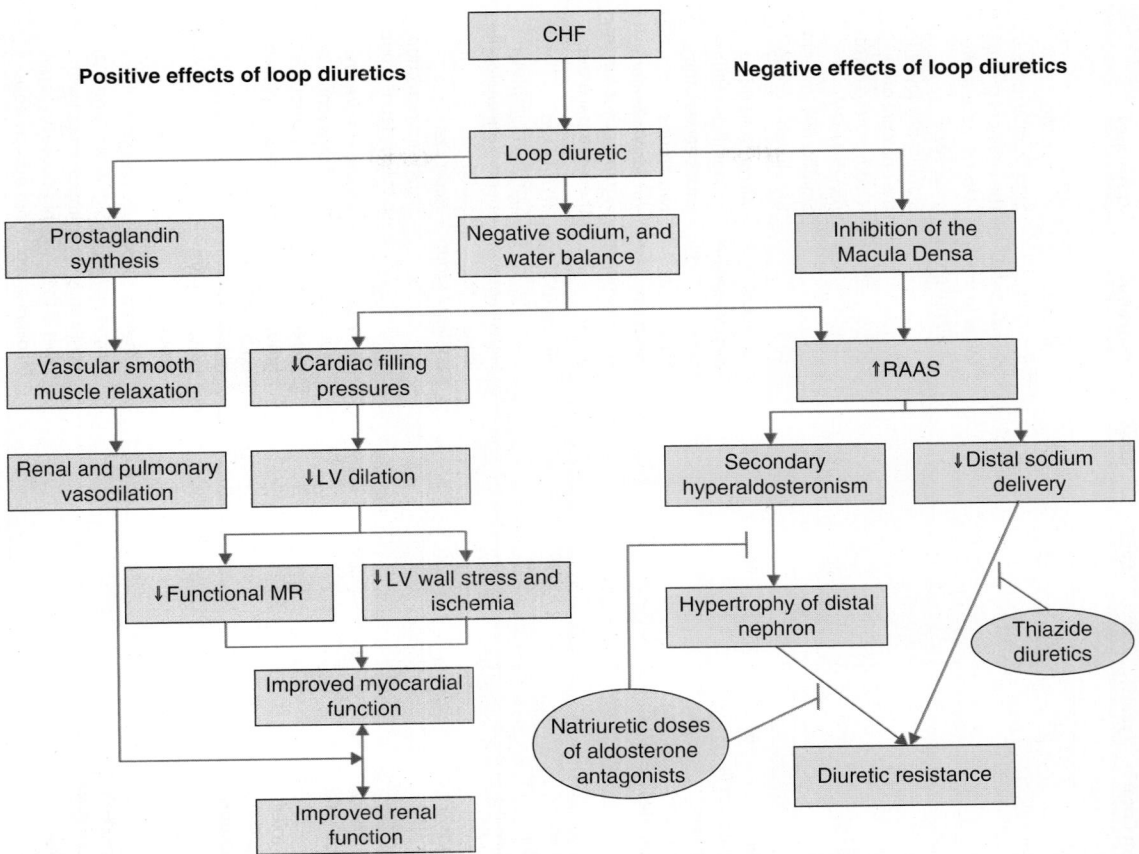

Figure 48–6. Proposed positive and negative effects of loop diuretics as well as sites of action for thiazide diuretics and natriuretic doses of aldosterone antagonists. CHF, congestive heart failure; LV, left ventricular; MR, mitral regurgitation; RAAS, renin-angiotensin-aldosterone system. Reproduced with permission from Felker GM, Mentz RM. Diuretics and Ultrafiltration in Acute Decompensated Heart Failure. *J Am Coll Cardiol.* 2012;59(24):2145-2153.

effects are very similar to ACE inhibitors that include dilatation of arteries and veins and thereby reducing arterial pressure and preload and afterload. These drugs also cause renal excretion of sodium and water (natriuretic and diuretic effects) by blocking the effects of angiotensin II in the kidney and by blocking angiotensin II stimulation of aldosterone secretion.[109] In several placebo-controlled studies, ARBs have been shown to yield similar long-term hemodynamic, neurohormonal, and clinical effects as those of ACE inhibition (Table 48–9). Two key trials were the Valsartan Heart Failure Trial (Val-HeFT) and CHARM-Added that randomized patients with mild to severe heart failure to placebo versus valsartan and candesartan, respectively,[110,111] Treatment with an ARB improved symptoms and quality of life, and reduced the risk of heart failure hospitalization. Further evidence of the benefit of ARBs comes from the CHARM-Alternative trial that randomized ACE inhibitor–intolerant patients to placebo versus candesartan, and showed an relative risk reduction of 23% in risk of cardiovascular death and heart failure hospitalizations.[112] Other trials in acute myocardial infarction have continued to solidify the proposition that ARBs are worthy alternatives to ACE inhibitors in HFrEF.[6] **Table 48–10** displays the recommended and target doses for ARBs in heart failure. Considerations for initiation of ARBs are similar to those of ACE inhibitors.

β-Blockers

While RAAS is the main target of ACE inhibitors and ARBs, the main target for β-blockers is the sympathetic nervous system. Of note, they do also partly affect the RAAS by inhibiting renin release by blocking β-1 receptors in the juxtaglomerular apparatus. Activation of the sympathetic nervous system plays an important role in remodeling, leading to impaired β-adrenergic receptor function, myocyte necrosis, and fibrosis. β-blockers reduce the sympathetic tone and increase vagal tone that may contribute to their beneficial effect. β-blockers also myocardial work/oxygen consumption ratio thereby reducing the risk of subendocardial ischemia. The use of β-blocker therapy was initially considered counterintuitive in heart failure.[74,113] That belief was overturned by three landmark key clinical trials—CIBIS II, COPERNICUS, and MERIT-HF—that randomized more than 9000 patients with mild-to-severe HFrEF to a β-blocker bisoprolol, carvedilol, and metoprolol, respectively, or placebo.[114–116] In these trials, more than 90% of patients were on an ACE inhibitor or ARB. Each of these trials showed a significant reduction in risk of both mortality (including sudden cardiac death) and hospitalization by approximately 30%. Another randomized controlled trial, COMET, showed that carvedilol increased survival compared with short acting metoprolol.[117] It is now felt that β-blockers act

TABLE 48–9. Major Clinical Trials on Angiotensin-Converting Enzyme Inhibitors and Angiotensin Receptor Blockers in Heart Failure

Study, Year	Design	Mean Follow-Up (Months)	Total Participants	Comparators	Essential Concomitant Therapy	Inclusion Criteria	Mean Age (years)	Males (%)	Mean Baseline LVEF	Mean Baseline NYHA Class	Primary Outcome	Other Key Outcomes
ACEIs versus Placebo												
SOLVD-treat, 1991[76,107]	DB, MC	41	2569	-Enalapril (n = 1285) -Placebo (n = 1284)	NA	-EF ≤35% -Symptomatic CHF	61	80	25	2.2	-All-cause mortality: Significantly lower in the enalapril group	-CV mortality: Significantly lower in the enalapril group -Mortality due to progressive HF: Significantly lower in the enalapril group -Death or hospitalization due to HF: Significantly lower in the enalapril group
FEST, 1995[86]	DB, MC	3	307	-Fosinopril (n = 155) -Placebo (n = 153)	NA	-EF ≤30% -NYHA class II or III -Exercise tolerance between 1 and 11 minutes	63	75	26	2.4	-Maximal bicycle exercise time: Significantly greater increase in the fosinopril group	-All cause mortality: No significant difference between the two groups -HF hospitalizations: Significantly lower in the fosinopril group
CONSENSUS, 1987[75]	DB, MC	6	253	-Enalapril (n = 126) -Placebo (n = 127)	NA	-Patients with severe CHF (NYHA class IV) -Reduced EF	70	71	NR	4.0	-All-cause mortality: Significantly lower in the enalapril group	-NYHA Class: Significant improvement in the enalapril group -Heart size: Significant reduction in the enalapril group
CASSIS, 1995[87]	DB, MC	3	248	-Spirapril (n = 152) -Enalapril (n = 48) -Placebo (n = 48)	NA	-EF ≤40% or a cardiothoracic ratio of >0.55 -Exercise tolerance between 2 and 14 minutes	58	83	28%	2.9	-Exercise tolerance: Increase in all groups but no significant difference between any groups	-All-cause mortality: Significant reduction in spirapril group, compared to placebo
van Veldhuisen, 1998[88]	DB, MC	5	244	-Imidapril (n = 182) -Placebo (n = 62)	Digoxin and diuretic therapy	-EF ≤45% -NYHA class II–III -Stable on digoxin and diuretics	61	77	34	2.2	-Development of progressive HF: Significantly lower in the imidapril group	-Exercise tolerance: Significantly greater improvement with high dose imidapril, but not low dose

Study, year	Design	Duration	n	Treatment groups	Background therapy	Inclusion criteria					Outcome	Outcome
Shettigar, 1999[89]	DB, MC	4	206	-Fosinopril (n = 102) -Placebo (n = 104)	Diuretic therapy	-EF ≤35% -NYHA class II–IV -Hospitalized for worsening HF -Maintenance diuretic therapy	62	75	24	3.6	-Exercise tolerance: Significantly greater improvement in the fosinopril group	-Hospitalization for worsening HF: Significantly lower in lisinopril group -NYHA class, dyspnea, fatigue, PND: Significantly greater improvement in lisinopril group
Goldstein, 1988[90]	DB, SC	6.5	204	-Captopril (n = 104) -Placebo (n = 100)	Diuretic therapy	-EF ≤40% -Mild to moderate CHF -Maintenance diuretic therapy	56	82	25	2.1	-Exercise tolerance: Significantly greater improvement in the captopril group	-NYHA class: Significantly greater improvement in the captopril group
Beller, 1995[91]	DB, MC	3	193	-Lisinopril (n = 130) -Placebo (n = 63)	NA	-EF ≤45% or a cardiothoracic ratio >0.5 -Uncontrolled HF despite optimal therapy -Treadmill exercise tolerance between 1 and 12 minutes	60	75	28	2.7	-Treadmill exercise tolerance: Significantly greater improvement in the lisinopril group	-Change in LVEF: Significantly greater increase in the lisinopril group
Colfer, 1992[92]	DB, MC	3	172	-Benazepril (n = 114) -Placebo (n = 58)	NA	-EF ≤35% -NYHA class II–IV -Symptomatic CHF	62	83	25	2.5	-Exercise tolerance: Significantly greater improvement in the benazepril group	-Improvement in clinical status: Significantly greater
MHFT, 1991[93]	DB, MC	32	170	-Captopril (n = 83) -Placebo (n = 87)	NA	-NYHA class I–III -Clinical symptoms of heart failure	62	78	35	2.0	-Progression of HF: Significantly less progression in the captopril group	-Death due to progression of HF: Significantly lower in the captopril group -All-cause death: No significant difference between the groups

(Continued)

TABLE 48-9. Major Clinical Trials on Angiotensin-Converting Enzyme Inhibitors and Angiotensin Receptor Blockers in Heart Failure (Continued)

Study, Year	Design	Mean Follow-Up (Months)	Total Participants	Comparators	Essential Concomitant Therapy	Inclusion Criteria	Mean Age (years)	Males (%)	Mean Baseline LVEF	Mean Baseline NYHA Class	Primary Outcome	Other Key Outcomes
Brown, 1995[94]	DB, MC	6	141	-Fosinopril (n = 116) -Placebo (n = 125)	NA	-EF ≤35% -NYHA class II or III -Exercise tolerance: between 2 and 14 minutes	62	80	25	2.7	-Mean change in exercise tolerance: Significantly greater improvement in fosinopril group -Clinical events indicative of worsening HF: Significantly lower in the fosinopril group	-NYHA class: Significant improvement in the fosinopril group
Chalmers, 1987[95]	DB, MC	3	130	-Lisinopril (n = 87) -Placebo (n = 43)	NA	-EF ≤45% -NYHA class II-IV	58	69	NR	2.9	-Exercise tolerance: Significantly greater improvement in the lisinopril group	-HF related clinical parameters: Significant improvement in all clinical parameters in the lisinopril group, except edema and paroxysmal nocturnal dyspnea
Lewis, 1989[96]	DB, MC	3	130	-Lisinopril (n = 87) -Placebo (n = 43)	NA	-NYHA class II-IV	NR	NR	38	2.9	-Exercise tolerance: Significantly greater improvement in the lisinopril group	-Cardiothoracic ratio, EF, functional and clinical status: Significant improvement in the lisinopril group
CARMEN, 2004[97]	DB, MC	18	572	-Carvedilol + placebo (n = 191) -Enalapril + placebo (n = 190) -Carvedilol + enalapril (n = 191)	NA	-EF ≤40% -Mild HF symptoms -Clinically stable	62	81	30	2.2	-Safety and tolerability: Similar across all three treatment arms	-LVEF: Significant improvement in the combination arm when compared to enalapril alone -All-cause mortality: No significant difference between the groups

ARBs versus Placebo

Study	Design			Treatment groups	ACEIs and beta-blockers	Inclusion criteria						Outcome	
CHARM-added, 2003[98]	DB, MV	41	2548	-Candesartan (n = 1276) -Placebo (n = 1272)	ACEIs and beta-blockers	-EF ≤40% -NYHA class II–IV -On current treatment with ACEIs	64	79	28	2.7	-Composite of CV death or hospitalization for CHF: Significantly lower in the candesartan group	-CV death: Significantly lower in the candesartan group -HF hospitalization: Significantly lower in the candesartan group
STRETCH, 1999[99]	DB, MC	3	844	-Candesartan (n = 633) -Placebo (n = 211)	NA	-EF 30%–45%	62	69	39	2.4	-Exercise time: Significantly greater improvement in the candesartan group	-Dyspnea: Significantly greater improvement in the candesartan group -NYHA class: No significant difference between the two groups
SPICE, 2000[100]	DB, MC	3	270	-Candesartan (n = 179) -Placebo (n = 91)	NA	-EF ≤35% -Symptomatic CHF -ACE inhibitor intolerance	66	69	27	2.6	-Discontinuation rate: No significant difference between the two groups	-Death and morbidity: No significant difference between the two groups
Mitrovic, 2003[101]	DB, MC	12	221	-Candesartan (n = 174) -Placebo (n = 44)	NA	-EF ≤40% -NYHA class II–III -Pulmonary capillary wedge pressure >13 mm	73	67	30	2.4	-Pulmonary capillary wedge pressure and mean pulmonary arterial pressure: Significantly greater reduction in the candesartan group in the short term and long term	-Systemic vascular resistance: No significant difference between the two groups

ACEIs versus ARBs

Study	Design			Treatment groups	ACEIs and beta-blockers	Inclusion criteria						Outcome	
ELITE II, 2000[102]	DB, MC	23	3152	-Losartan (n = 1578) -Captopril (n = 1574)	NA	-EF ≤40% -NYHA class II–IV -Age 60 or more	71	70	31	2.5	-All-cause mortality: No significant difference between the two groups	-Sudden death or resuscitated arrests: No significant difference between the two groups

(Continued)

TABLE 48–9. Major Clinical Trials on Angiotensin-Converting Enzyme Inhibitors and Angiotensin Receptor Blockers in Heart Failure (Continued)

Study, Year	Design	Mean Follow-Up (Months)	Total Participants	Comparators	Essential Concomitant Therapy	Inclusion Criteria	Mean Age (years)	Males (%)	Mean Baseline LVEF	Mean Baseline NYHA Class	Primary Outcome	Other Key Outcomes
ELITE I, 1997[103]	DB, MC	12	722	-Losartan (n = 352) -Captopril (n = 372)	NA	-EF ≤40% -NYHA class II–IV -ACE inhibitor naïve	73	67	30	2.4	*-Persisting increase in serum creatinine:* No significant difference between the two groups	*-Discontinuation due to adverse effects:* Significantly lower in the losartan group *-Death and/or hospitalization for HF:* No significant difference between the two groups *-Death:* Significantly lower in the losartan group *-Hospitalization for HF:* No significant difference between the two groups.
REPLACE, 2001[104]	DB, MC	3	378	-Telmisartan (n = 301) -Enalapril (n = 77)	NA	-EF ≤40% -NYHA class III or IV	64	89	26	2.4	*-Exercise tolerance:* No significant difference between the two groups	*-Change in blood pressure:* Small but significant increase in blood pressure in the telmisartan groups
Dickstein, 1995[105]	DB, MC	2	166	-Losartan (n = 78) -Enalapril (n = 38)	NA	-EF ≤35% -NYHA class III or IV	64	78	23	3.2	*-Exercise capacity:* No significant difference between the two groups	*-Clinical status:* No significant difference between the two groups
HEAVEN, 2002	DB, MC	3	141	-Valsartan (n = 70) -Enalapril (n = 71)	Beta-blockers	-EF ≤40% -Symptomatic HF -Not receiving ACEIs due to previous intolerance	67	53	NR	2.3	*-6MWT distance:* Valsartan was significantly non-inferior to enalapril	*-LV size and function:* Significant improvement only in the valsartan group
Lang, 1997[106]	DB, MC	3	116	-Losartan (n = 78) -Enalapril (n = 38)	NA	-EF ≤45% -NYHA class II–IV	64	78	23	2.6	*-Treadmill exercise time and 6MWT:* No significant difference	*-Dyspnea-fatigue index or LVEF:* No significant difference between the two groups

TABLE 48–10. Drugs Commonly Used for Stage C HFrEF

Drug	Initial Daily Dose(s)	Maximum Dose(s)	Mean Doses Achieved in Clinical Trials
ACE inhibitors			
Captopril	6.25 mg 3 times	50 mg 3 times	122.7 mg/d
Enalapril	2.5 mg twice	10 to 20 mg twice	16.6 mg/d
Fosinopril	5 to 10 mg once	40 mg once	N/A
Lisinopril	2.5 to 5 mg once	20 to 40 mg once	32.5 to 35.0 mg/d
Perindopril	2 mg once	8 to 16 mg once	N/A
Quinapril	5 mg twice	20 mg twice	N/A
Ramipril	1.25 to 2.5 mg once	10 mg once	N/A
Trandolapril	1 mg once	4 mg once	N/A
ARBs			
Candesartan	4 to 8 mg once	32 mg once	24 mg/d
Losartan	25 to 50 mg once	50 to 150 mg once	129 mg/d
Valsartan	20 to 40 mg twice	160 mg twice	254 mg/d
Aldosterone antagonists			
Spironolactone	12.5 to 25.0 mg once	25 mg once or twice	26 mg/d
Eplerenone	25 mg once	50 mg once	42.6 mg/d
Beta blockers			
Bisoprolol	1.25 mg once	10 mg once	8.6 mg/d
Carvedilol	3.125 mg twice	50 mg twice	37 mg/d
Carvedilol CR	10 mg once	80 mg once	N/A
Metoprolol succinate extended release (metoprolol CR/XL)	12.5 to 25 mg once	200 mg once	159 mg/d
Hydralazine and isosorbide dinitrate			
Fixed-dose combination	37.5 mg hydralazine/20 mg isosorbide dinitrate 3 times daily	75 mg hydralazine/40 mg isosorbide dinitrate 3 times daily	~175 mg hydralazine/90 mg isosorbide dinitrate daily
Hydralazine and isosorbide dinitrate	Hydralazine: 25 to 50 mg, 3 or 4 times daily and isosorbide dinitrate: 20 to 30 mg 3 or 4 times daily	Hydralazine: 300 mg daily in divided doses and isosorbide dinitrate: 120 mg daily in divided doses	N/A

by attenuating deleterious long-term effects of sustained sympathetic system activation in heart failure. **Table 48–11** lists all the major randomized controlled trials of β-blockers in heart failure.[97,114,116,118–136]

β-blockers should be initiated in all stable patients with HFrEF except those who have a clear contraindication to their use. Types of β-blockers and target doses are shown in Table 48–10; the ones shown to be efficacious in heart failure are bisoprolol and metoprolol succinate (β-1 antagonists) and carvedilol (α-1, β-1, and β-2 antagonists). They must be used cautiously in those with recent decompensations. If a patient is admitted with acute heart failure, β-blockers can be continued, but in setting of worsening clinical status (such as development of cardiogenic shock), the dose should be lowered or they should be discontinued. Clinicians should attempt to achieve target doses suggested by clinical trials. Abrupt withdrawal can lead to clinical decompensation. Adverse effects such as hypotension and bradycardia might necessitate lowering dose or discontinuation; however, symptoms of fatigue or volume overload can be managed without medication discontinuation.

Mineralocorticoid Receptor Antagonists

Aldosterone is synthesized by the adrenal glands to preserve intravascular sodium, potassium, and water homeostasis. Aldosterone binds to mineralocorticoid receptors in the kidney, colon, and sweat glands and induces sodium reabsorption with concomitant potassium excretion. In heart failure, aldosterone levels increase as a response to perceived reductions in intravascular volume, and cause several unfavorable effects including adverse remodeling of the heart through enhanced collagen deposition.[137]

Two aldosterone receptor antagonists, spironolactone and eplerenone, block these deleterious effects and have been shown to have significant morbidity and mortality benefits in symptomatic heart failure. Aldosterone receptor antagonists significantly reduce LV hypertrophy and blood pressure. These agents have also been shown to have beneficial effects on net fluid balance by promoting diuresis and natriuresis. In addition, they improve heart rate variability and improve cardiac sympathetic nervous system activity in patients with heart failure. Spironolactone has also shown to improve endothelial

TABLE 48–11. Major Clinical Trials of β-Blockers in Heart Failure

Study, Year	Design	Mean Follow-Up (Months)	Total Participants	Comparators	Essential Concomitant Therapy	Inclusion Criteria	Mean Age (years)	Males (%)	Mean Baseline LVEF	Mean Baseline NYHA Class	Primary Outcome	Other Key Outcomes
β-blockers versus Placebo												
MERIT-HF, 1999[116]	DB, MC	12	3991	-Metoprolol (n = 1990) -Placebo (n = 2001)	NA	-EF ≤40% -NYHA class II to IV -Stabilized with optimum standard therapy	64	78	28	2.6	*-Total mortality or all-cause hospitalization:* Significantly lower in the metoprolol group *-Total mortality or hospitalizations due to worsening HF:* Significantly lower in the metoprolol group	*-NYHA class:* Significantly greater improvement in the metoprolol group
BEST, 2001[117]	DB, MC	24	2708	-Bucindolol (n = 1354) -Placebo (n = 1354)	NA	-EF ≤35% -NYHA class III or IV	60	78	23	3.1	*-All-cause mortality:* There was no significant added mortality benefit in the bucindolol group	*-Death from CV causes:* Significantly lower in the bucindolol group
CIBIS II, 1999[118]	DB, MC	16	2647	-Bisoprolol (n = 1327) -Placebo (n = 1320)	ACEIs and diuretics	-EF ≤35% -NYHA class III or IV -Standard therapy with ACEIs and diuretics	61	81	28	3.2	*-All-cause mortality:* Significantly lower in the bisoprolol group	*-Sudden deaths:* Significantly lower in the bisoprolol group
COPERNICUS, 2001[119]	DB, MC	12	2289	-Carvedilol (n = 1156) -Placebo (n = 1133)	NA	-EF ≤25% -Symptoms of HF at rest or minimal exertion -Clinically euvolemic	63	79	20	NR	*-Death:* No significant difference between the two groups *-Hospitalization:* No significant difference between the two groups	*-Permanent withdrawal for adverse events:* No significant difference between the two groups
Packer, 1996[120]	DB, MC	6 (severe HF group) and 12 (mild HF group)	1094	-Carvedilol (n = 696) -Placebo (n = 398)	ACEIs and diuretics	-EF ≤35% -Symptomatic HF -At least 2 months of treatment with diuretics and ACEIs	58	77	23	2.5	*-All-cause mortality:* Significantly lower in the carvedilol group	*-Hospitalization for CV causes:* Significantly lower in the carvedilol group

Study	Design	Duration	N	Treatment arms		Inclusion criteria						
CIBIS, 1994[121]	DB, MC	23	641	-Bisoprolol (n = 320) -Placebo (n = 321)	NA	-EF ≤40% -NYHA class III or IV	60	83	17	3.1	-All-cause mortality: No significant difference between the two groups	-Functional status: Significantly greater improvement in the bisoprolol group -Sudden death rate: No significant difference between the two groups -Ventricular tachycardia or fibrillation: No significant difference between the two groups
CARMEN, 2004[97]	DB, MC	18	572	-Carvedilol + placebo (n = 191) -Enalapril + placebo (n = 190) -Carvedilol + enalapril (n = 191)	NA	-EF ≤40% -Mild HF symptoms -Clinically stable	62	81	30	2.2	-Safety and tolerability: Similar across all three treatment arms	-LVEF: Significant improvement in the combination arm when compared to enalapril alone -All-cause mortality: No significant difference between the groups
Colucci, 1996[122]	DB, MC	12	366	-Carvedilol (n = 232) -Placebo (n = 134)	NA	-EF ≤35% -6MWT distance of 450–550 m -Receiving optimal standard therapy	54	85	23	2.1	-Clinical progression of HF (defined as death due to heart failure, hospitalization for heart failure, or a sustained increase in heart failure medications): Significantly lower in the carvedilol group	-LVEF, HF score, NYHA class, physician and patient global assessments: Significantly greater improvement in the carvedilol group
MOCHA, 1996[123]	DB, MC	6	345	-Carvedilol (n = 261) -Placebo (n = 84)	NA	-EF ≤35% -NYHA class II to IV	60	76	23	2.9	-6MWT: No significant difference between the two groups -9-minute self-powered treadmill test: No significant difference between the two groups	-LVEF: Significant dose-related improvement in the carvedilol group -Survival: Significant dose related benefit in the carvedilol group -Hospitalization: Significantly lower in the carvedilol group

(Continued)

TABLE 48–11. Major Clinical Trials of β-Blockers in Heart Failure (Continued)

Study, Year	Design	Mean Follow-Up (Months)	Total Participants	Comparators	Essential Concomitant Therapy	Inclusion Criteria	Mean Age (years)	Males (%)	Mean Baseline LVEF	Mean Baseline NYHA Class	Primary Outcome	Other Key Outcomes
PRECISE, 1996[124]	DB, MC	6	278	-Carvedilol (n = 133) -Placebo (n = 145)	NA	-6MWT distance: 150–450m -EF ≤35%	60	73	22	2.6	*-NYHA class or global condition:* Greater improvement in the carvedilol group	*-LVEF:* Significantly greater increase in the carvedilol group *-Morbidity and mortality:* Significantly lower in the carvedilol group
ENECA, 2005[125]	DB, MC	8	260	-Nebivolol (n = 134) -Placebo (n = 126)	NA	-EF ≤35% -NYHA class II–IV -Age ≤65	72	73	26	2.6	*-Change in LVEF:* Significantly greater improvement in LVEF in the nebivolol group	*-Clinical status, quality of life, safety:* No significant difference between the two groups
RESOLVD, 2003[126]	DB, MC	43	226	-Metoprolol (n = 214) -Placebo (n = 212)	Candesartan OR Enalapril OR Candesartan + Enalapril	-EF ≤40% -NYHA class II to IV	61	82	28	2.2	*-Cardiac function:* The group receiving metoprolol + candesartan + enalapril had a modest but significant beneficial effect on cardiac function compared to other groups	NA
CELICARD, 2000[127]	DB, MC	12	124	-Celiprolol (n = 62) -Placebo (n = 62)	NA	-EF ≤40% -NYHA class II or III	57	90	26	2.5	*-Functional class:* No significant difference between the two groups	*-CV mortality:* No significant difference between the two groups *-Arrhythmias:* No significant difference between the two groups *-Worsening HF:* No significant difference between the two groups
Sturm, 2000[128]	DB, SC	13	100	-Atenolol (n = 51) -Placebo (n = 49)	High-dose enalapril	-EF ≤25% -NYHA class II or III -Already on high-dose enalapril	52	88	17	2.2	*-Combined worsening HF or death at 2 years:* Significantly lower in the atenolol group	*-Hospitalization for cardiac events:* No significant difference between the two groups

Study											*Quality of life / outcomes*	*Global assessment (assessed by physicians)*
Cohn, 1997[129]	83	6	DB, MC	-Carvedilol (n = 70) -Placebo (n = 35)	NA	-EF ≤35% -NYHA class III or IV	60	58	22	3.1	-Quality of life: Similar improvement in both groups	-Global assessment (assessed by physicians): Significantly favored the carvedilol group -LVEF: Significantly greater improvement in the carvedilol group
Palazzuoli, 2005[130]	58	12	DB	-Carvedilol (n = 33) -Placebo (n = 25)	NA	-EF ≤40% -NYHA class III or IV -Clinically stable	71	66	32	3.4	-Diastolic function: Significantly greater improvement in the carvedilol group	NA
de Milliano, 2002[131]	54	6	DB, MC	-Metoprolol (n = 43) -Placebo (n = 11)	NA	-EF ≤35% -NYHA class II or III	65	67	25	2.5	-Mean myocardial MIBG uptake: Significantly greater increase in the metoprolol group	NA
MIC, 2000[132]	52	6	DB, MC	-Metoprolol (n = 26) -Placebo (n = 26)	NA	-EF ≤40% -NYHA class II or III	54	71	28	2.4	-Maximal exercise: Significantly greater improvement in the metoprolol group	-Heart rate: Significantly lower in the metoprolol group after submaximal and maximal exercise -LVEF, 6MWT: Significantly greater improvement in the metoprolol group at rest, submaximal exercise, and maximal exercise
SYMPOXY-DEX, 2004[133]	50	6	DB, MC	-Carvedilol (n = 28) -Placebo (n = 22)	NA	-EF ≤40%	59	84	26	2.2	-Renin and ACE activity: Activity was significantly lower in the carvedilol group	-LVEF: Significantly greater improvement in the carvedilol group
Krum, 1995[134]	49	2.5	DB	-Carvedilol (n = 33) -Placebo (n = 16)	NA	-Severe CHF	55	78	16	2.8	-LVEF, stroke-volume index: Significantly greater increase in the carvedilol group -Pulmonary capillary wedge pressure, mean right atrial pressure, systemic vascular resistance: Significantly greater decrease in the carvedilol group	-Clinical status, functional status and exercise capacity: Significantly greater improvement in the carvedilol group

(Continued)

TABLE 48–11. Major Clinical Trials of β-Blockers in Heart Failure (Continued)

Study, Year	Design	Mean Follow-Up (Months)	Total Participants	Comparators	Essential Concomitant Therapy	Inclusion Criteria	Mean Age (years)	Males (%)	Mean Baseline LVEF	Mean Baseline NYHA Class	Primary Outcome	Other Key Outcomes
Dubach, 2002[135]	DB	12	28	-Bisorpolol (n = 13) -Placebo (n = 15)	NA	-EF ≤40%	58	NR	26	NR	*Exercise capacity:* Significant improvement in the bisoprolol group	NA
Beta-blockers vs ACEIs												
CIBIS III, 2008[136]	OL, MC	14	1010	-Bisoprolol (n = 505) -Enalapril (n = 505) **Patients received either bisoprolol or enalapril for first 6 months. From 6 months to 24 months, patients received both drugs	NA	-EF ≤35% -NYHA class II or III -Age >65	72	68	29	2.5	-*Death or all-cause hospitalization:* No significant difference between the two groups	*All-cause mortality:* No significant difference between the two groups *All-cause hospitalization:* No significant difference between the two groups
CARMEN, 2004[97]	DB, MC	18	572	-Carvedilol + placebo (n = 191) -Enalapril + placebo (n = 190) -Carvedilol + enalapril (n = 191)	NA	-EF ≤40% -Mild HF symptoms -Clinically stable	62	81	30	2.2	-*Safety and tolerability:* Similar across all three treatment arms	*LVEF:* Significant improvement in the combination arm when compared to enalapril alone *All-cause mortality:* No significant difference between the groups

function, increase nitric oxide bioactivity, inhibit vascular angiotensin I to II conversion, and reduce thrombotic response to injury.[137]

The Randomized Aldactone Evaluation Study (RALES) enrolled 1663 patients with severe heart failure (NYHA class III–IV) and LV systolic dysfunction to receive either spironolactone or placebo in combination with ACE inhibition and diuretics.[138] Only 11% of the patients were on β-blockers. Spironolactone led to a relative risk reduction in death of 30% and in heart failure hospitalization of 35%. The Eplerenone in Patients with Systolic Heart Failure and Mild Symptoms (EMPHASIS-HF) trial randomized 2737 patients with NYHA class II symptoms and LVEF ≤30% (≤35% if QRS ≥130 ms).[139] Treatment with eplerenone led to a relative risk reduction of 37% in cardiovascular death or heart failure hospitalization. EPHESUS trial that enrolled 6632 patients with LV systolic dysfunction (LVEF ≤40%) within 2 weeks following an acute myocardial infarction and showed a 15% reduction in risk of all-cause mortality with eplerenone treatment.[140] Importantly, the majority of patients in both EPHESUS trials were on β-blockers and ACE inhibitors/ARBs. **Table 48–12** shows all the major randomized controlled trials of mineralocorticoid receptor agonists in heart failure.[139,141-144]

It is recommended that spironolactone or eplerenone be used in all patients with HFrEF who are already on an ACE inhibitor (or ARB) and β-blocker.[5,6] Table 48–10 shows the recommended target doses. The biggest concern is hyperkalemia and therefore, these medications should not be used in patients with an estimated glomerular filtration rate (eGFR) <30 mL/min/1.73 m² (serum creatinine ≈ 2.5 mg/dL in men and 2.0 mg/dL in women) and/or potassium greater >5 mEq/L. Even in the absence of these findings, patients on these medications require rigorous monitoring of their kidney function and serum potassium levels. Patients should be advised to eat foods low in potassium; potassium supplementation should be lowered or discontinued upon mineralocorticoid receptor antagonist initiation. Men on spironolactone can experience gynecomastia or breast pain (≈10%), in which case, they should be switched to eplerenone because the major difference between the medications is selectivity of aldosterone receptor antagonism. Eplerenone is more specific for the aldosterone receptor and has a relatively lower affinity for progesterone and androgen receptors compared with spironolactone. Therefore, eplerenone lacks the major endocrine adverse effects that are associated with spironolactone.

Hydralazine and Isosorbide Dinitrate
Hydralazine and isosorbide dinitrate combination pill acts as a vasodilator affecting both arteries and veins that release nitric oxide and thereby activating guanylyl cyclase for vascular smooth muscle activation and endothelial function. Heart failure is closely linked with reactive oxygen species, and is also associated with endothelial dysfunction due to the nitric oxide–reactive oxygen species imbalance. Because hydralazine and isosorbide dinitrate combination pill increases the availability of nitric oxide and enhances productive blood flow, it was believed to be beneficial for heart failure patients.

The effect of long-acting nitrates plus hydralazine on survival was evaluated in the First Veterans Heart Failure Trial (V-HeFT-I),[145] when 642 men with mild-to-moderate heart failure were randomized to receive placebo, or prazosin, or the combination of isosorbide dinitrate plus hydralazine. Compared with placebo, the mortality-risk reduction in the group treated with isosorbide dinitrate plus hydralazine was 36% by 3 years. In contrast, the mortality in the prazosin group was the same as that seen in the placebo-treated patients. The V-HeFT-II trial published in 1991 directly compared the combination of isosorbide dinitrate plus hydralazine with enalapril in patients with predominantly NYHA class II to III heart failure.[146] Overall, 804 men were randomized to one of these two regimens for an average of 2.5 years. The study demonstrated the superiority of the ACE inhibitor in reducing cumulative mortality. The African American Heart Failure Trial (A-HeFT) tested the hypothesis that a fixed-dose combination of isosorbide dinitrate and hydralazine could improve outcomes in African Americans with HFrEF. In A-HeFT, 1050 African American subjects with NYHA class III to IV heart failure were randomized to the fixed-dose combination or placebo. Combination therapy significantly improved the primary endpoint, a composite response including morbidity, mortality, and quality of life. Most impressively, a 43% reduction in all-cause mortality was seen in the treatment group. The results of this study led the FDA to approve fixed-dose combination of isosorbide dinitrate and hydralazine for African American patients with NYHA class III or class IV heart failure and reduced ejection fraction. **Table 48–13** shows the details of the major trials of isosorbide dinitrate and hydralazine in heart failure.[147,148]

Clinicians can use the combination of hydralazine and isosorbide dinitrate for African American patients with HFrEF who remain symptomatic while on ACE inhibitors, β-blockers, and aldosterone antagonists. These therapies are not a substitute for ACE inhibitors or ARBs, but may also be used in non–African American patients who are intolerant of these medications (Table 48–10). These therapies may not be well tolerated due to the need for frequent dosing and numerous adverse reactions such as headache, dizziness, and gastrointestinal complaints.[149]

Digoxin
Digitalis has been used to treat heart failure for more than 200 years. The most commonly used preparation is digoxin.[150] Its mechanism of action is via inhibition of the Na-K-ATPase pump in myocardial cells, augmenting intracellular calcium, thus increasing inotropy. Digitalis also has an antiadrenergic effect and upregulate parasympathetic tone.[151] In the Digitalis Investigation Group (DIG) trial,[152] 6800 patients with LVEF ≤45% and NYHA class II to IV symptoms were randomized to 0.25 mg digoxin versus placebo. The patient population was on concomitant diuretics (82%) and ACE-inhibitors (95%). Treatment with digoxin did not reduce all-cause or heart failure mortality but led to a 28% reduction in heart failure admissions. Digoxin was associated with a trend toward an increased incidence of sudden (presumed arrhythmic) death. A post hoc analysis showed a relationship between mortality and plasma

TABLE 48-12. Major Clinical Trials of Mineralocorticoid Receptor Agonists in Heart Failure

Study, Year	Design	Mean Follow-Up (months)	Total Participants	Comparators	Essential Concomitant Therapy	Inclusion Criteria	Mean Age (years)	Males (%)	Mean Baseline LVEF	Mean Baseline NYHA Class	Primary Outcome	Other Key Outcomes
EMPHA-SIS-HF, 2011[139]	DB, MC	21	2737	-Eplerenone (n = 1364) -Placebo (n = 1373)	ACEIs and beta-blockers	-EF ≤35% -NYHA class II	69	78	26	2.0	-Composite of death from CV causes or hospitalization for HF: Significantly lower in the eplerenone group	-All-cause mortality: Significantly lower in the eplerenone group -CV death: Significantly lower in the eplerenone group -Hospitalization for HF: Significantly lower in the eplerenone group -Hospitalization for any cause: Significantly lower in the eplerenone group
RALES, 1999[141]	DB, MC	24	1663	-Spirono-lactone (n = 822) -Placebo (n = 841)	ACEIs	-EF ≤35% -NYHA class III or IV	65	73	25	3.3	-All-cause mortality: Significantly lower in the spironolactone group	-Death from progressive HF: Significantly lower in the spironolactone group -Sudden cardiac death: Significantly lower in the spironolactone group -Hospitalization for worsening HF: Significantly lower in the spironolactone group
AREA-IN CHF, 2009[142]	DB, MC	12	467	-Canrenone (n = 231) -Placebo (n = 236)	ACEIs and beta-blockers	-EF ≤45% -NYHA class II	63	84	40	2.0	-Left ventricular end diastolic volume: Similar reduction in both groups -LVEF: Significantly greater increase in the canrenone group	-Brain natriuretic peptide: Significantly greater reduction in the can-renone arm -Left atrial dimensions: Significantly greater reductions in the can-renone arm
Vizzardi, 2014[143]	SB, SC	44	130	-Spirono-lactone (n = 65) -Placebo (n = 65)	ACEIs and beta-blockers	-EF ≤40% -NYHA class I or II	63	NR	36	1.8	-Event-free survival for CV death or CV hospitalizations: Significantly greater in the spironolactone group -CV hospitalizations: Significantly lower in the spironolactone group	NA
Cicoira, 2002[144]	OL	12	106	-Spirono-lactone (n = 54) -Placebo (n = 52)	ACEIs and beta-blockers	-EF ≤40%	62	87	33	NR	-LV volumes and function: Significant improvement with spironolactone	-Exercise tolerance: Significantly improved with spironolactone when administered at its highest dose

TABLE 48–13. Major Clinical Trials of Hydralazine/Isosorbide Dinitrate in Heart Failure

Study, Year	Design	Mean Follow-Up (Months)	Total Participants	Comparators	Essential Concomitant Therapy	Inclusion Criteria	Mean Age (years)	Males (%)	Mean Baseline LVEF	Mean Baseline NYHA Class	Primary Outcome	Other Key Outcomes
A-HeFT, 2004[147]	DB, MC	10	1050	-Isosorbide dinitrate/hydralazine (n = 518) -Placebo (n = 532)	NA	-Self-identified as Black (or of African descent) -EF ≤45% -NYHA class III or IV	57	56	24	3	-Composite score derived from following endpoints - all cause death, first HF hospitalization, and change in quality of life: Significant benefit in the isosorbide dinitrate/hydralazine group	-All-cause mortality: Significantly lower in the isosorbide dinitrate/hydralazine arm -First HF hospitalization: Significantly lower in the isosorbide dinitrate/hydralazine group -Quality of life score: Significantly greater improvement in quality of life in the isosorbide dinitrate/hydralazine group
V-HeFT, 1986[148]	DB, MC	28	642	-Isosorbide dinitrate/hydralazine (n = 186) -Prazosin (n = 183) -Placebo (n = 273)	NA	-EF ≤45 or cardiothoracic ratio >0.55 on CXR -Reduced exercise tolerance	58	NR	30	NR	-All-cause mortality (entire study period): Lower in the hydralazine + isosorbide dinitrate group. This result was borderline significant	-All-cause mortality (2-year follow-up): Significantly lower in the hydralazine + isosorbide dinitrate group

digoxin concentration with a serum concentration >1 ng/mL associated with increased risk. Clinical improvement have been supported by smaller trials that suggest a role for digoxin for the improvement or prevention of clinical deterioration.[153,154]

Clinicians can consider adding digoxin if they have persistent symptoms on guideline-recommended therapy. Generally, therapy is started at 0.125 to 0.25 mg a day, with lower or every-other-day dosing in patients with impaired renal function, elderly, or the frail. Serum levels of 0.5 to 0.9 ng/mL should be targeted. The major side effects are arrhythmias (ectopic and reentry rhythms and heart block), gastrointestinal symptoms (anorexia, nausea, and vomiting), and neurological symptoms (visual disturbances, disorientation, and confusion). Toxicity generally occurs at serum levels of >2 ng/mL but may be potentiated at lower levels in the presence of hypokalemia, hypomagnesemia, and hypothyroidism. Several medications interact with digoxin and interactions should be considered prior to initiation.

Sacubitril/Valsartan

A first-in-class of drug that involves dual inhibition of neprilysin and the ATII receptor (ARNI: Angiotensin Receptor Neprilysin Inhibitor) was approved for use in HFrEF and NYHA class II to IV heart failure in the PARADIGM-HF (Prospective Comparison of ARNI With ARB Global Outcomes in Heart Failure With Preserved Ejection Fraction) trial that randomized 8442 patients to sacubitril/valsartan versus enalapril.[155] The trial was stopped early due to significant reductions in the primary endpoint after a median duration of follow-up of 27 months. Sacubitril/valsartan reduced the primary composite endpoint of cardiovascular death or heart failure hospitalization by 20%. Similar results were observed for cardiovascular death, hospitalization, and all-cause mortality. Of note, a 22% decrease in the risk of sudden death (hazard ratio [HR], 0.78; 95% confidence interval [CI], 0.66–0.92; $P = 0.002$) was also observed in HFrEF patients receiving sacubitril/valsartan compared with enalapril. Hypotension was more common in patients receiving sacubitril/valsartan, although discontinuation because of hypotension was similar in both arms of the study. Elevations in serum creatinine and potassium and cough were less frequent in those assigned to sacubitril/valsartan.

Valsartan blocks the angiotensin type I (AT_1) receptor. Sacubitril is converted to the active neprilysin inhibitor LBQ657, which inhibits neprilysin, an enzyme that breaks down atrial natriuretic peptide (ANP), BNP, and C-type natriuretic peptide (CNP), as well as other vasoactive substances (**Fig. 48–7**). NT-proBNP is not a substrate for neprilysin, and more appropriately reflects heart failure condition among patients on this therapy. The combined beneficial effects of ARBs in heart failure along with the natriuretic, vasodilatory, antisympathetic,

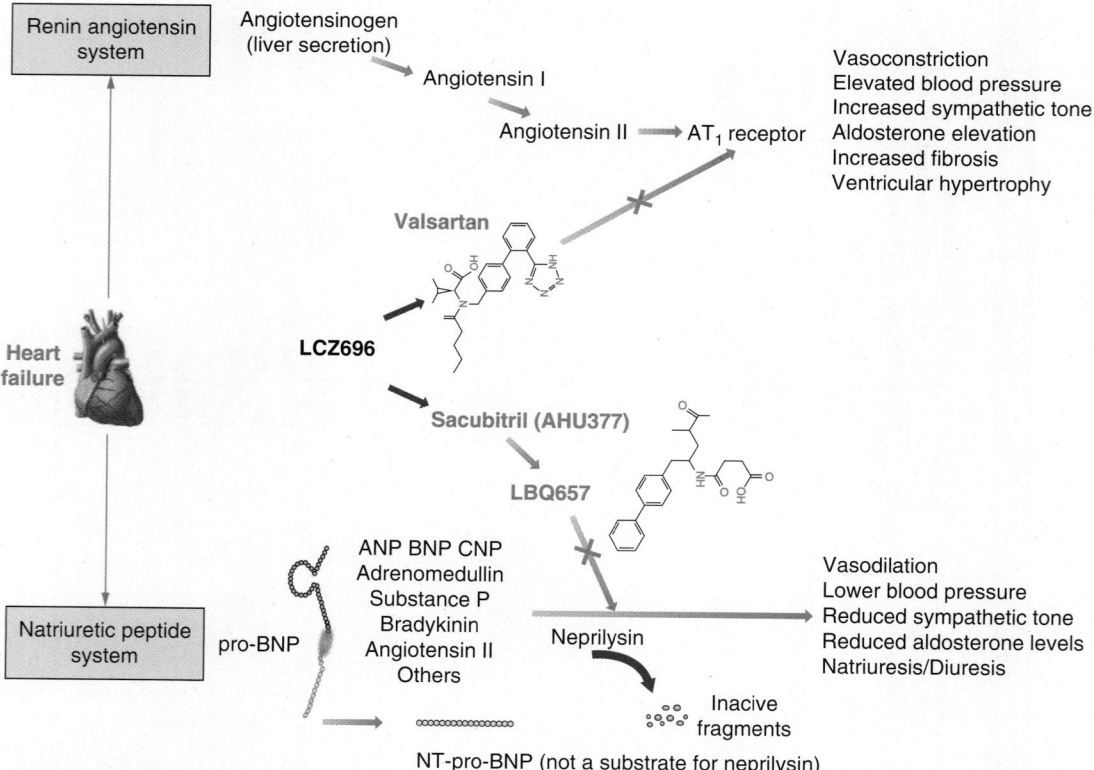

Figure 48–7. Schematic showing the mechanism of action of LCZ696. Heart failure stimulates both the renin-angiotensin system and the natriuretic peptide system. LCZ696 is composed of two molecular moieties, the angiotensin receptor blocker valsartan and the neprilysin inhibitor prodrug sacubitril (AHU377). Valsartan blocks the angiotensin type I (AT₁) receptor. Sacubitril is converted enzymatically to the active neprilysin inhibitor LBQ657, which inhibits neprilysin, an enzyme that breaks down the breakdown of atrial natriuretic peptide (ANP), brain (or B-type) natriuretic peptide (BNP), and C-type natriuretic peptide (CNP), as well as other vasoactive substances. N-terminal pro-BNP (NT-proBNP) is not a substrate for neprilysin. Reproduced with permission from Vardeny O, Miller R, Solomon SD. Combined Neprilysin and Renin-Angiotensin System Inhibition for the Treatment of Heart Failure. *JACC Heart Fail.* 2014 Dec;2(6):663-670.

and antiadverse remodeling effects of natriuretic peptides likely account for the benefit with this agent. The single-arm PROVE-HF (Prospective Study of Biomarkers, Symptom Improvement, and Ventricular Remodeling During Sacubitril/Valsartan Therapy for Heart Failure) study found that reduction in NT-proBNP concentration was significantly correlated with improvements in cardiac volume and function at 12 months in HFrEF patients treated with sacubitril/valsartan suggesting that reverse cardiac remodeling may be a major factor responsible for the clinical benefit observed with sacubitril/valsartan.[156] On the basis of substantial benefit, sacubitril/valsartan has received a class I recommendation with level of evidence B in the European and US Guidelines and a class I level A recommendation in Canadian Guidelines for HFrEF patients with NYHA class II to IV.

Ivabradine

Ivabradine is a heart rate–lowering agent that mainly acts by inhibiting the cardiac pacemaker current (I_f), a mixed sodium/potassium inward current that regulates the spontaneous diastolic depolarization in the sinoatrial node and therefore controls the heart rate. By inhibiting this channel, I_f ion current flow is disrupted, which prolongs diastolic depolarization and thereby slows the firing in the sinus node, which eventually reduces the heart rate. The heart rate reduction is dose dependent with almost linear effect up to 15 mg twice daily. The drug effects are particular to the sinus node, and ivabradine has no major impact on blood pressure, intracardiac conduction, myocardial contractility, or ventricular repolarization.

Ivabradine is approved for stable patients with HFrEF who have a resting heart rate of at least 70 bpm on maximally tolerated β-blockers. The Systolic Heart failure treatment with the I*f* inhibitor ivabradine Trial (SHIFT) enrolled 6588 heart failure patients with NYHA functional class II to IV, sinus rhythm with a rate of ≥70 bpm, and an LVEF ≤35%.[157] Patients were randomized to ivabradine versus placebo, and ivabradine was associated with an 18% reduction in cardiovascular death or heart failure hospitalization (driven by reductions in the latter). Ivabradine also improved LV function and quality of life. The major side effects were symptomatic bradycardia (5%) and visual disturbances (3%). The recommended starting dosage of the drug is 5 mg twice daily, while maximum dosage is 7.5 mg twice daily.

Sodium-Glucose Cotransporter 2 Inhibitors

Sodium-glucose cotransporter 2 (SGLT2) inhibitors selectively inhibit SGLT2 and thus promote decreased renal absorption of glucose in the proximal renal tubule. This mechanism is dependent on blood glucose levels and is completely independent of the actions of insulins compared with other antihyperglycemic agents. Through glycosuria and natriuresis, SGLT2 inhibitors induce osmotic diuresis. These agents also appear to have broader multisystem metabolic benefits including weight loss and reduction in blood pressure.[158] Unlike other antihyperglycemics, SGLT2 inhibitors have consistently shown to reduce heart failure hospitalizations among various at-risk populations with type 2 diabetes in various different trials.[159-161]

In the landmark DAPA-HF trial (Dapagliflozin and Prevention of Adverse Outcomes in Heart Failure), dapagliflozin was shown to reduce the composite endpoint of worsening heart failure events or cardiovascular mortality by 26% compared with placebo in patients with chronic HFrEF, irrespective of type 2 diabetes status.[162] This led to the approval of dapagliflozin by the FDA for use in the treatment of HFrEF with or without type 2 diabetes. Consistent benefit in heart failure hospitalization with SGLT2 inhibitors has been observed in all subgroups including age, race, estimated glomerular filtration rate, baseline ejection fraction, baseline atherosclerotic cardiovascular disease, and baseline medications for heart failure or diabetes. These randomized clinical trial results are further reinforced by evidence from several real-world observational studies.[163,164] Moreover, the EMPEROR-Reduced (Evaluating the effects of Empagliflozin on morbidity and mortality in patients with chronic heart failure and reduced ejection fraction) has met its primary endpoint, demonstrating superiority of empagliflozin compared with standard of care in reducing the risk for the composite of cardiovascular death or heart failure hospitalization (see **Table 48–14**).[165,166]

SGLT2 inhibitors have several unique properties that make them ideal agents to fit in the current heart failure regimen. First, SGLT2 inhibitors are once-daily medications and do not require any dose titration compared with other heart failure medications. Second, SGLT2 inhibitors have minimal drug–drug interactions. Third, SGLT2 inhibitors cause osmotic diuresis and natriuresis, which may be synergistic when used in combination with other diuretics. Importantly, compared with loop diuretics, SGLT2 inhibitors result in less compensatory RAAS activation owing to their preferentially reduction in interstitial volume compared with intravascular volume.[167] Fourth, SGLT2 inhibitors offer substantial kidney-protective benefits that are closely linked with development and progression of heart failure. In the CREDENCE (The Evaluation of the Effects of Canagliflozin on Renal and Cardiovascular Outcomes in Participants with Diabetic Nephropathy) trial, canagliflozin significantly reduced the relative risk of the primary outcome (doubling of serum creatinine, end stage renal disease or mortality due to cardiovascular or renal cause) by 30% compared with placebo (event rates of 43.2 and 61.2 per 1000 patient-years respectively; HR, 0.70; 95% CI, 0.59–0.82).[168] Moreover, DAPA-CKD was terminated prematurely due to overwhelming efficacy of dapagliflozin in reducing the primary composite of worsening renal function defined as eGFR decline of at least 50%, onset of end-stage kidney disease, and death from cardiovascular or renal cause.[169] Finally, for most patients, SGLT2 inhibitors cause minimal blood pressure lowering, and has no effect on potassium levels. This is crucial because one of the main reasons why guideline-directed medical therapy is not started or maintained in heart failure patients is because of concerns around hyperkalemia and low blood pressure.

SGLT2 inhibitors are generally well tolerated and serious adverse events are rarely reported. Common side effects of SGLT2 inhibitors include genital mycotic infections, which generally do not necessitate discontinuation of SGLT2 inhibitors. Heart failure patients should be specifically counselled

TABLE 48–14. Major Clinical Trials of SGLT2 Inhibitors in Heart Failure

Study, Year	Design	Mean Follow-Up (Months)	Total Participants	Comparators	Essential Concomitant Therapy	Inclusion Criteria	Mean Age (years)	Males (%)	Mean Baseline LVEF	Mean Baseline NYHA Class	Primary Outcome	Other Key Outcomes
EMPEROR-Reduced, 2020[66]	DB, MC	16	7220	-Empagliflozin (n = 1863) -Placebo (n = 1867)	NA	-EF ≤40% -NYHA class II to IV -HF hospitalization within 12 months	67	76	27	27	*-CV death or HF hospitalization:* Significantly lower in the empagliflozin group	*-Total hospitalizations:* Significantly lower in the empagliflozin group *-Composite renal outcome (chronic hemodialysis, renal transplantation, profound sustained reduction in eGFR):* Significantly lower in the empagliflozin group *-All cause mortality:* No significant difference between the two groups
DAPA-HF, 2019[62]	DB, MC	18	4744	-Dapagliflozin (n = 2373) -Placebo (n = 2371)	NA	-EF ≤40% -NYHA class II to IV	66	76	31	2.4	*-Worsening HF (hospitalization or urgent visit resulting in IV therapy) or CV mortality:* Significantly lower in the dapagliflozin arm	*-Worsening HF:* Significantly lower in the dapagliflozin group *-CV mortality:* Significantly lower in the dapagliflozin group *-CV death or HF hospitalization:* Significantly lower in the dapagliflozin group *-KCCQ score:* Significantly greater improvement in the dapagliflozin group *-All cause mortality:* Significantly lower in the dapagliflozin arm

about maintenance of perineal hygiene because in 2018, the FDA released a warning related to 12 cases of Fournier's gangrene, a rare, but serious perineal infection associated with SGLT2 inhibitors.[170] Although seldom, diabetic ketoacidosis at relatively normal glucose levels ("euglycemic diabetic ketoacidosis") can also occur with SGLT2 inhibitors.

Novel Oral Soluble Guanylate Cyclase Stimulators

Vericiguat is a novel oral soluble guanylate cyclase (sGC) stimulator that enhances the cyclic guanosine monophosphate (GMP) signaling by directly activating soluble guanylate cyclase through a binding site that is independent of nitric oxide. Patients with heart failure are especially prone to relative deficiency of soluble guanylate cyclase and reduced cyclic GMP generation owing to the reactive oxygen species production and endothelial dysfunction commonly seen in heart failure patients. The elevation of cyclic GMP is associated with vasodilatation, antifibrotic, and antiinflammatory effects. Although there are two main types of oral selective sGC simulators (vericiguat and riociguat), vericiguat is the main drug investigated for heart failure patients. Table 48–10 shows the recommended target doses.

In the phase 3 VICTORIA (Vericiguat Global Study in Subjects with Heart Failure with Reduced Ejection Fraction) trial, 5050 patients with chronic heart failure with an ejection fraction of less than 45% who had recently been hospitalized or had received intravenous diuretic therapy, were randomized to receive vericiguat (10 mg once daily) or placebo.[171] Incidence of cardiovascular mortality or first hospitalization for heart failure was significantly lower in the vericiguat compared with placebo (35.5% vs 38.5%; HR, 0.90; 95% CI, 0.82–0.98). There was no significance difference in the occurrence of adverse events such as syncope and hypotension. These results suggest that vericiguat may offer health benefits in HFrEF patients who had recent decompensation with good tolerance and safety.

Selective Cardiac Myosin Activator

The primary initial pathogenesis in HFrEF is decreased myocardial contractility. Omecamtiv mecarbil is a novel, selective cardiac myosin activator that has been shown to increase contractility and therefore significantly improve cardiac function and decrease heart rate, NT-proBNP, and ventricular volumes in patients with chronic heart failure. The ongoing GALACTIC-HF (Global Approach to Lowering Adverse Cardiac outcomes Through Improving Contractility in Heart Failure) trial, which is a randomized, double-blind, placebo-controlled, event-driven cardiovascular outcomes trial enrolling >8000 patients, will provide further information regarding the clinical benefit achieved with omecamtiv mecarbil.[172]

Intravenous Iron

Iron deficiency is a common comorbidity in heart failure patients. Although exact mechanisms remain unclear, important contributing factors are believed to be decreased iron absorption, increased gastrointestinal losses, and reduced availability of utilizable iron from the reticulo-endothelial system. Iron deficiency, with or without anemia, can substantially decrease functional capacity, quality of life, and survival in heart failure patients.[173] Therefore, targeting iron deficiency has recently gained popularity.

In the FAIR-HF (Ferinject Assessment in Patients with Iron Deficiency and Chronic Heart Failure) trial, treatment with intravenous ferric carboxymaltose resulted in significant improvement in the distance on the 6-minute walk test, self-reported patient global assessment, and quality-of-life in chronic heart failure patients.[174] These beneficial results with IV iron were confirmed in EFFECT-HF (Effect of Ferric Carboxymaltose on Exercise Capacity in Patients With Iron Deficiency and Chronic Heart Failure) and CONFIRM (Ferric CarboxymaltOse evaluatioN on perFormance in patients with IRon deficiency in coMbination with chronic Heart Failure) trials (Table 48–15).[174-176] Moreover, an individual patient level meta-analysis showed that patients on intravenous (IV) iron had lower rates of recurrent cardiovascular hospitalizations and cardiovascular mortality (rate ratio, 0.59; 95% CI, 0.40–0.88).[177]

The current ESC guidelines recommend screening for iron deficiency in heart failure patients (recommendation Class I). Moreover, a recommendation Class IIa has been given to consider using IV iron in symptomatic HFrEF patients with iron deficiency. It is important to emphasize that there is limited benefit achieved with oral iron supplementation. This may be because of poor absorption and tolerability due to gastrointestinal side effects. Four large randomized controlled trials are currently underway that will evaluate the effects of IV iron on all-cause mortality and hospitalizations in various different heart failure populations.

Other Therapies

Anticoagulation

Derangements in the clotting cascade are common in heart failure and the triad of prerequisites for thrombus formation—endothelial dysfunction, hypercoagulopathy, and stasis—commonly coexist in heart failure.[178,179] However, large trials testing vitamin K antagonism in HFrEF without atrial fibrillation yielded mixed results (Table 48–16).[180] The WASH (Warfarin/Aspirin Study in Heart Failure) and HELAS (Heart failure Long-term Anticoagulation Study) trials showed no benefit but noted an increased rate of major bleeding with warfarin.[181,182] The WATCH (Warfarin and Anti-platelet Therapy in Chronic Heart failure) trial (n = 1587) showed no difference in patients randomized to aspirin 162 mg versus clopidogrel 75 mg versus warfarin for the primary endpoint of death, myocardial infarction, or stroke.[183] The WARCEF (Warfarin versus Aspirin in Reduced Cardiac Ejection Fraction) trial enrolled 2305 patients with LVEF ≤35% and sinus rhythm, found no differences in the rates of the primary endpoint of death, ischemic stroke, or intracerebral hemorrhage for warfarin versus aspirin.[184] A reduced risk of ischemic stroke with warfarin was offset by an increased risk of major hemorrhage. Similarly, in the COMMANDER-HF (a study to assess the effectiveness and safety of rivaroxaban in reducing the risk of death, myocardial infarction, or stroke in participants with heart failure and coronary artery disease following an episode of decompensated heart failure), only a modest reduction in stroke events was

TABLE 48–15. Major Clinical Trials of Iron Therapy in Heart Failure

Study, Year	Design	Mean Follow-Up (Months)	Total Participants	Comparators	Essential Concomitant Therapy	Inclusion Criteria	Mean Age (years)	Males (%)	Mean Baseline LVEF	Mean Baseline NYHA Class	Primary Outcome	Other Key Outcomes
FAIR-HF, 2009[174]	DB, MC	6	459	-Ferric car-boxymaltose (n = 344) -Placebo (n = 155)	NA	-EF ≤45% with NYHA class II or III -EF ≤40% with NYHA class II -Elevated natriuretic peptides -Hb 9.5–13.5 g/dL -Iron deficiency	67	55	33	2.8	-Improvement in patient global assessment at week 24: Significantly greater in the group receiving iron therapy -Improvement in NYHA class at week 24: Significantly greater in the group receiving iron therapy	-6MWT distance: Significantly greater improvement in the iron therapy arm -KCCQ questionnaire: Significantly greater improvement in the iron therapy arm -First HF hospitalization: No significant difference between the two groups
CONFIRM-HF, 2014[176]	DB, MC	12	304	-Ferric car-boxymaltose (n = 152) -Placebo (n = 152)	NA	-EF ≤45% -Elevated natriuretic peptides -Iron deficiency	69	47	37	2.4	-6MWT distance: Significantly greater improvement in the iron therapy group	-Patient global assessment, NYHA class, quality of life score: All significantly reduced in the iron therapy group -HF hospitalization: Significantly lower in the iron therapy group -Death: No significant difference between the two groups
EFFECT-HF, 2017[175]	OL, MC	6	174	-Ferric car-boxymaltose (n = 86) -Standard of care (n = 86)	NA	-EF ≤45% -NYHA class II or III -Elevated natriuretic peptides -Iron deficiency	64	75	32	2.3	-Peak VO2: Significantly lower decrease in the iron therapy group	-Patients global assessment, NYHA class: Significantly greater improvement in the iron therapy group

TABLE 48–16. Major Clinical Trials of Anticoagulation in Heart Failure

Study, Year	Design	Mean Follow-Up (Months)	Total Participants	Comparators	Essential Concomitant Therapy	Inclusion Criteria	Mean Age (years)	Males (%)	Mean Baseline LVEF	Mean Baseline NYHA Class	Primary Outcome	Other Key Outcomes
COMMAND-ER-HF, 2018[180]	DB, MC	21	5022	-Rivaroxaban (n = 2507) -Placebo (n = 2515)	NA	-EF ≤40% -CAD -Recent WHF -Elevated natriuretic peptide concentration	66	77	35	2.5	-Composite of death from any cause, myocardial infarction, or stroke: There was no significant difference between the two groups	-All-cause mortality: No significant difference between the two groups -Safety: No significant difference between the two groups -Stroke: Significantly lower in the rivaroxaban group
WARCEF, 2012[184]	DB, MC	42	2305	-Warfarin (n = 1142) -Aspirin (n = 1163)	NA	-EF ≤35% -No clear indication warfarin or aspirin	61	80	25	2.2	-Time to the first event in a composite end point of ischemic stroke, intracerebral hemorrhage or all cause death: No significant difference between the two groups	-All cause death: No significant difference between the two groups -Ischemic stroke: Significantly lower in the aspirin group -Intracerebral hemorrhage: No significant difference between two groups
WATCH, 2009[183]	DB, MC	23	1587	-Aspirin (n = 523) -Clopidogrel (n = 524) -Warfarin (n = 540)	Diuretics and ACEIs (unless not tolerated)	-EF ≤35% -Diuretic +ACEI therapy -Sinus rhythm	63	85	24	2.6	-Composite of all cause death, nonfatal myocardial infarction, and nonfatal stroke: No significant difference between the groups	-Nonfatal strokes: Significantly lower incidence in the warfarin group compared to the aspirin and clopidogrel group -CV hospitalization: Significantly greater in patients randomized to aspirin
WASH, 2004[181]	OL, MC	27	279	-Warfarin (n = 89) -Aspirin (n = 91) -No antiplatelet therapy (n = 99)	Diuretics	-EF ≤35% -HF requiring diuretics	63	74	NA	NA	-Death, nonfatal myocardial infarction, nonfatal stroke: No significant difference between the groups	NA
HELAS, 2006[182]	DB, MC	19	197	Ischemic heart disease group: -Aspirin (n = 61) -Warfarin (n = 54) Dilated cardiomyopathy group: -Warfarin (n = 38) -Placebo (n = 44)	NA	-EF ≤35% -NYHA class II to IV Age 20 to 75 years	59	85	28	NA	-Incidence of myocardial infarction, hospitalization, exacerbation of HF, death and hemorrhage: No significant difference between the groups	NA

observed.[185] Therefore, at this time, in the absence of another indication for anticoagulation, such as atrial fibrillation or flutter, anticoagulation for routine management of HFrEF is not supported.[5,6]

Novel Potassium Binders as Enabling Therapy

Heart failure patients have many risk factors for developing hyperkalemia including old age and high prevalence of chronic kidney disease. Fear of hyperkalemia is often the primary reason for clinicians not to initiate or maximize dosing of renin-angiotensin aldosterone inhibitors. It has been shown that approximately 30% of eligible heart failure patients are not prescribed mineralocorticoid receptor antagonists because of concerns around hyperkalemia.[186] Furthermore, around 80% of heart failure patients are on less than the recommended doses of ACE inhibitors or ARBs because of concerns of side effects such as hyperkalemia.[187] Therefore, to maximize the use of life saving drugs such as renin-angiotensin aldosterone inhibitors without adversely impacting the safety, novel potassium binders may serve as enabling therapy.

The two most commonly used novel potassium binders are patiromer and sodium zirconium cyclosilicate (SZC). Table 48–10 shows the recommended doses. The PEARL-HF (Evaluation of Patiromer in Heart Failure Patients) trial showed that patients receiving patiromer had significantly less hyperkalemia (7% vs 25%; $P = 0.015$) at 4 weeks and were more likely to be up-titrated to spironolactone 50 mg/day from 25 mg/day compared with patients receiving placebo (91% vs 74%, respectively; $P = 0.019$).[188] However, guidelines currently do not recommend the use of novel potassium binders as enabling therapy mainly because of insufficient evidence to show that novel potassium binder enabled optimization of heart failure drugs would result in improved heart failure outcomes. The ongoing DIAMOND (Patiromer for the management of hyperkalemia in subjects receiving RAASi medications for the treatment of heart failure) trial, which is estimated to enroll more than 2000 patients with time to occurrence of cardiovascular death or hospitalization as the primary endpoint, will provide further insights regarding the future role of novel potassium binders in heart failure.

Device-Based Therapies

Three types of device have been shown to reduce morbidity and mortality in select heart failure patients. They include implanted cardiac defibrillators (ICD), cardiac resynchronization therapy (CRT), and LVADs.

Implantable Cardioverter-Defibrillators

Patients with HFrEF are at increased risk for ventricular arrhythmias and sudden cardiac death (SCD). Whereas therapy with neurohormonal blockade can decrease this risk of SCD, an unacceptable degree of residual risk remains. For these patients, an ICD can be lifesaving. The benefits of these therapies have been evaluated in several clinical trials, both for primary and secondary prevention, leading to the current recommendations.

For primary prevention, current recommendations are largely based on three key trials: the Sudden Cardiac Death in Heart Failure Trial (SCD-HeFT), Multicenter Automatic Defibrillator Implantation Trial II (MADIT II), and Defibrillators in Non-ischemic Cardiomyopathy Treatment Evaluation (DEFINITE).[189-191] SCD-HeFT enrolled 2521 patients with NYHA class II to III heart failure from ischemic or nonischemic etiologies and LVEF ≤35%, and randomized them to placebo, amiodarone, or standard medical therapy. Amiodarone did not reduce mortality but ICD was associated with a relative risk reduction of 23% over the follow-up period of ≈5 years. The MADIT-II trial enrolled 1232 patients with ischemic cardiomyopathy and an LVEF ≤30% who were at least 40 days postmyocardial infarction. Follow-up was prematurely discontinued at 20 months due to a significant 31% reduction in all-cause mortality in the ICD group. DEFINITE trial attempted to evaluate the role of primary prevention ICDs in 458 patients with a nonischemic etiology and LVEF ≤35%. A nonsignificant trend toward reduction in mortality was observed. Of note, in the relatively recent DANISH (Defibrillator Implantation in Patients with Non-ischemic Systolic Heart Failure) trial, ICD implantation in patients with symptomatic heart failure with reduced ejection fraction not caused by coronary artery disease was not associated with a lower all-cause mortality compared with usual care.[192] Therefore, in the context of contemporary pharmacotherapy, the role of ICDs should continue to be reassessed given longitudinal declines in SCD rates.[193]

The ACC/AHA 2013 guidelines provide the following class I recommendations for ICD use in primary prevention: (1) for the primary prevention of SCD to reduce mortality in patient with both ischemic and nonischemic cardiomyopathy and LVEF≤35% with NYHA class II to III symptoms on guideline recommended medical therapy for at least 3 months, and (2) for the primary prevention of SCD in patients who are at least 40 days postmyocardial infarction and LVEF ≤30% and NYHA class I symptoms or more while receiving guideline recommended medical therapy. For secondary prevention, ICDs are indicated for survivors of cardiac arrest and in patients with sustained ventricular arrhythmias, irrespective of LVEF. ICD therapy should only be offered to patients who have a reasonable expectation of survival beyond a year and lack of frailty and/or advanced comorbid conditions.

The decision to recommend an ICD is highly complex and should be approached with a high degree of contemplation, because an injudicious insertion can lead to significant suffering. Patients should be advised that the ICD is not a disease modifying therapy, which is a common misconception. ICD shocks, whether appropriate or not, can lead to anxiety and even posttraumatic stress disorder. Patients with multiple comorbid conditions have far higher rates of device complications and competing risks of death from noncardiac issues might blunt benefit from an ICD. There is unclear data on benefit in patients >75 years and those with chronic kidney disease. An ICD should not be implanted in patients with NYHA class IV symptoms who are not candidates for LVAD or cardiac transplantation. Finally, heart failure is a progressive disease and patients with functional ICDs will eventually come to a point where the risk/benefit ratio from the device shifts to increased harm, in which case discussions with the patients and families about deactivation are challenging but obligatory.

Cardiac Resynchronization Therapy

Approximately one-third of patients with HFrEF have prolongation of the QRS interval on ECG, inferring a degree of mechanical dyssynchrony of the failing heart, which is associated with worse clinical outcomes (**Fig. 48–8**).[194] CRT or biventricular pacing is accomplished through simultaneous pacing of both the LV and RV and can lead to improvements in echocardiographic and hemodynamic parameters, functional status (average of 1–2 mL/kg/min increased in peak VO_2), and clinical outcomes (reduction in hospitalizations and all-cause mortality). CRT is recommended for patients in normal sinus rhythm with LVEF ≤35%, and a left bundle branch block (LBBB) with QRS

of ≥120 ms. Less clarity exists for patients with non-LBBB patterns on ECG, those who are not in normal sinus rhythm, or those with wide QRS but ≤150 ms.

Figure 48–9 presents an algorithm for the consideration of CRT in heart failure patients. Key studies to note are the Comparison of Medical Therapy, Pacing, and Defibrillation in Heart Failure (COMPANION) and Cardiac Resynchronization in Heart Failure Study (CARE-HF) that together randomized 2333 patients with NYHA class III to ambulatory IV symptoms, LVEF ≤35%, and QRS ≥120 ms, to CRT versus usual medical care.[195,196] Each of these two trials showed that CRT reduced the risk of death from any cause and hospital admission for worsening heart failure (relative risk reduction for death of 24% with a CRT-pacemaker [CRT-P] and of 36% with CRT-defibrillator [CRT-D] in COMPANION and of 36% with CRT-P in CARE-HF). In CARE-HF, the relative risk reduction

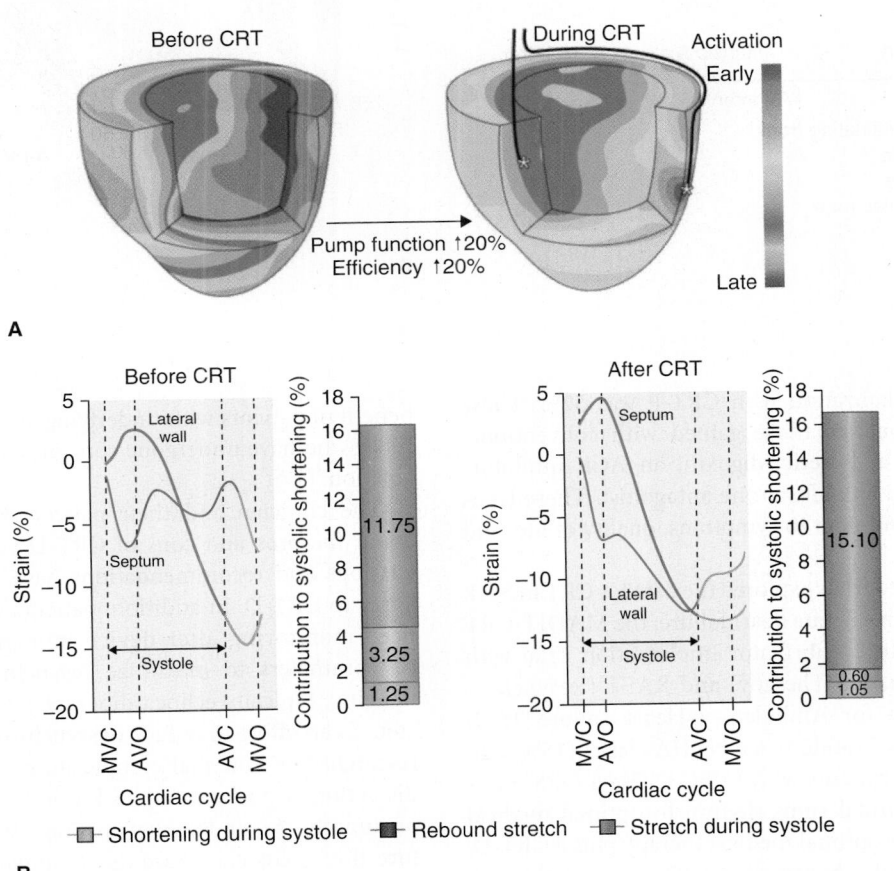

Figure 48–8. **(A)** Three-dimensional representations of electrical activation indicate regions with early (*red*) or late (*blue*) activation. Before pacing, the electrical activation progresses slowly from the right ventricle (RV) to the left ventricle (LV), but resynchronization is seen after biventricular pacing (*asterisks*). **(B)** Myocardial strain curves are also shown (shortening indicated by negative values). Before cardiac resynchronization therapy (CRT), the different strain curves in the septum and lateral wall indicate poor coordination of contraction, quantified by the sum of early systolic stretch (*green*) and rebound stretch (*blue*). After CRT, the contributions of early systolic stretch and rebound stretch to total systolic deformation are substantially reduced, which indicates improved coordination between the various regions. **(C)** Interactions between activation wavefronts originating from the RV and LV pacing electrodes and from the RBB. **(D)** Contour plots of changes in LVdP/dt_max, stroke work (SW), and electric resynchronization during 100 combinations of A-LV and A-RV intervals in two dogs with left bundle branch block, but different PQ interval. The higher the percentage change, the greater the benefit from CRT. AV, atrioventricular; AVC, atrial valve closing; AVO, atrial valve opening; MVC, mitral valve closing; MVO, mitral valve opening; RBB, right bundle branch; (A, B, and C) Reproduced with permission from Vernooy K, van Deursen CJM, Strik M, et al. Strategies to improve cardiac resynchronization therapy. *Nat Rev Cardiol.* 2014 Aug;11(8):481-493 (D) Reproduced with permission from Strik M, van Middendorp LB, Houthuizen P, et al. Interplay of electrical wavefronts as determinant of the response to cardiac resynchronization therapy in dyssynchronous canine hearts. *Circ Arrhythm Electrophysiol.* 2013 Oct;6(5):924-931.

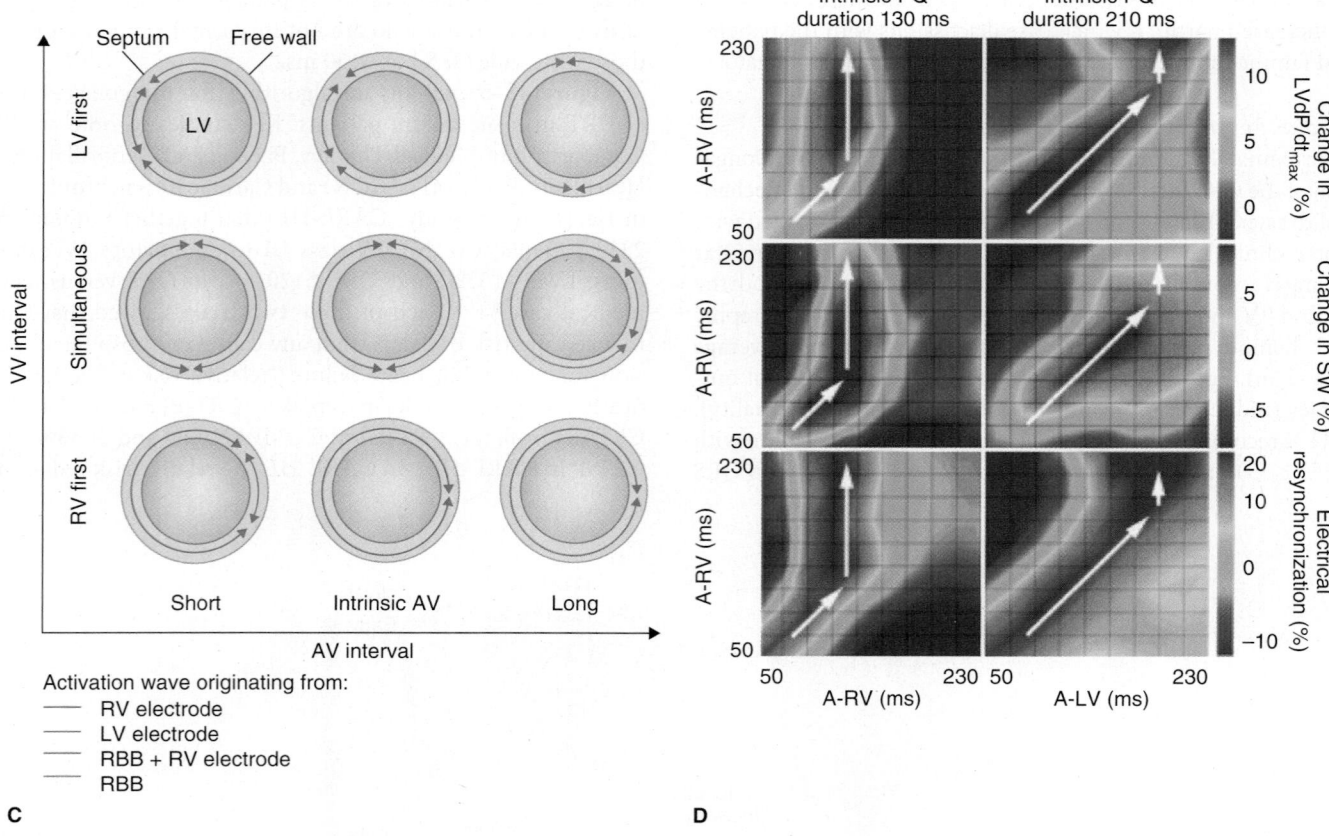

C

D

Figure 48–8. (Continued)

in heart failure hospitalization with CRT-P was 52%. These benefits were additional to those gained with conventional treatment, including a diuretic, digoxin, an ACE inhibitor/ARB, a β-blocker, and an aldosterone antagonist. These trials also showed an improvement in symptoms, quality of life, and ventricular function.

Two key randomized trials explored the data for CRT in 3618 patients with mild-to-moderate heart failure: the MADIT-CRT (Multicenter Automatic Defibrillator Implantation Trial with Cardiac Resynchronization Therapy) and RAFT (Resynchronization/Defibrillation for Ambulatory Heart Failure Trial) trials.[197,198] MADIT-CRT randomized NYHA class I (15%) and NYHA class II (85%) patients with LVEF ≤30%, a QRS duration ≥130 ms, and normal sinus rhythm to optimal medical therapy plus an ICD or optimal medical therapy plus a CRT-D. Each of these two trials showed that CRT reduced the risk of mortality and heart failure hospitalization by 25% to 35%. Only RAFT showed a decrease in all-cause mortality. In either study, there was significant heterogeneity in treatment effect based on baseline QRS duration, diminishing the strength of recommendation of CRT in patients with mild heart failure to those with a QRS ≥150 ms or ≥120 ms plus an LBBB pattern. CRT is also indicated in heart failure patients who have an indication for conventional RV pacing that alters cardiac activation in a manner similar to a native LBBB. Finally, since effective CRT requires high rates of biventricular pacing, the

benefit of patients with underlying atrial fibrillation is most in those who have undergone concomitant atrioventricular node ablation.[199,200]

The clinician and their patient should have discussions about the pros and cons of CRT-D versus CRT. Similar discussions and recommendations have been laid out for ICD apply to CRT-D. In addition, patients with CRT +/− ICD will need monitoring after device implantation for adjustment of parameters to maximize resynchronization. The use of imaging, typically echocardiography, to adjust device parameters in an effort to reduce dyssynchrony is still the subject of research.[201,202] Potential complications include coronary sinus dissection or perforation, lead dislodgement, device infection, pneumothorax, and pocket erosion. High LV lead pacing capture thresholds can cause diaphragmatic pacing from stimulation of the phrenic nerve that runs parallel to the lateral LV free wall.

COMPARISON OF UNITED STATES AND EUROPEAN GUIDELINES

ACC/AHA published guidelines on heart failure in 2013 (with focused updates in 2017) while ESC guidelines were issued in 2016. Both guidelines offer practical evidence-based recommendations for patients with chronic heart failure. While both guidelines have many similarities, they have some subtle

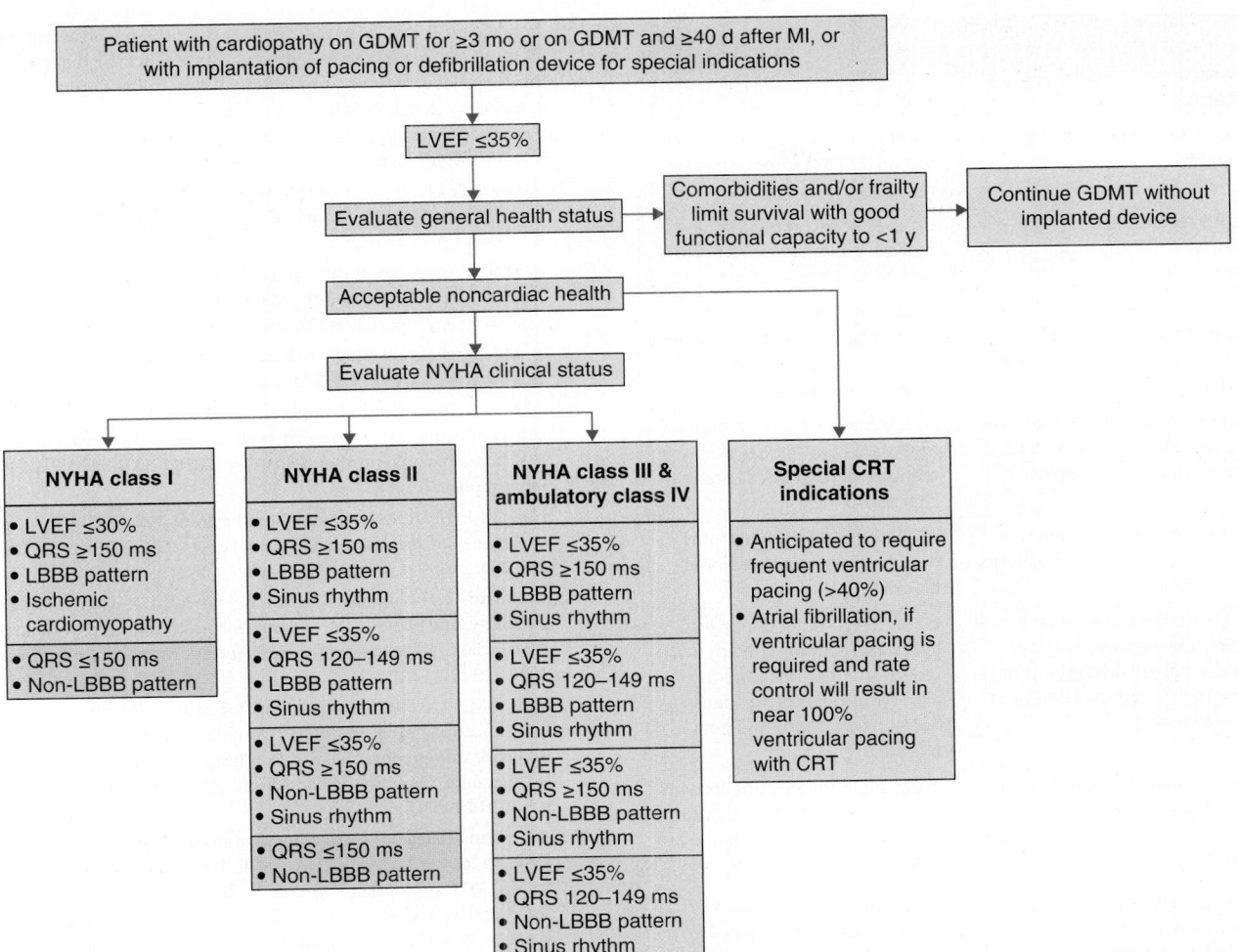

Figure 48–9. Indications for cardiac resynchronization therapy (CRT) algorithm. GDMT, guideline-directed medical therapy; LBBB, left bundle-branch block; LVEF, left ventricular ejection fraction; MI, myocardial infarction; NYHA, New York Heart Association. Please note that the colors in the figure correspond to the class of recommendations in the American College of Cardiology Foundation/American Heart Association guidelines. Reproduced with permission from Yancy CW, Jessup M, Bozkurt B, et al. 2013 ACCF/AHA guideline for the management of heart failure: a report of the American College of Cardiology Foundation/American Heart Association Task Force on Practice Guidelines. *J Am Coll Cardiol*. 2013 Oct 15;62(16):e147-e239.

differences especially regarding the treatment of chronic heart failure patients. These differences may be due to the timing of the guidelines published (2013 vs 2016) and also because of how evidence was weighted by the expert panel. Important differences between the guidelines are summarized in **Table 48–17.** Briefly, ESC gives a class I recommendation for cardiac resynchronization therapy (CRT) in symptomatic heart failure patients with LVEF ≤35% and LBBB with intermediate QRS duration while ACC/AHA gives a class IIb recommendation for such patients. Another major difference is regarding utilization of ARNI. ESC recommends ARNI only for heart failure patients who have persistent symptoms despite triple neurohormonal blockade while ACC/AHA gives a class Ia recommendation of switching ACE inhibitors or ARB to ARNI in all chronic heart failure patients with NYHA functional class II/III symptoms. Moreover, initiation of hydralazine-nitrate therapy in African American patients with NYHA functional class III or IV symptoms despite

optimal therapy with ACE inhibitors, β-blockers, and mineralocorticoid receptor antagonist is a class Ia recommendation in ACC/AHA guidelines while ESC guidelines give it a class IIa recommendation. In terms of diagnostic testing in chronic heart failure patients, both guidelines are pretty similar except two important differences. First, ESC gives a class IIa recommendation for measuring NT-proBNP to assess prognosis and severity in heart failure patients while ACC/AHA gives it a class I recommendation. Similarly, ACC/AHA recommends that biomarkers of myocardial stress or fibrosis such as ST2 and galectin-3 may be considered in heart failure patients (class IIb) while ESC remains silent about the use of these biomarkers. Second, ESC guidelines strongly advocate for CMR in heart failure patients. ESC guidelines give a class Ia recommendation regarding utilization of CMR for tissue characterization (myocarditis, amyloid) while ACC/AHA give a class IIa recommendation for CMR for assessment of myocardial scar or infiltration.

TABLE 48–17. Differences between American and European Guidelines

ACC/AHA	ESC
Cardiac MRI for myocardial scar or infiltration	Cardiac MRI for tissue characterization and to distinguish ischemic versus non-ischemic
Class II b recommendation for biomarkers of fibrosis such as ST-2 or galectin-3	No specific recommendation regarding biomarkers of fibrosis such as ST-2 or galectin-3
Class I recommendation for natriuretic peptide measurement to assess prognosis or disease severity in HF patients	Class IIa recommendation for natriuretic peptide measurement to assess prognosis or disease severity in HF patients
Class IIa recommendation for natriuretic peptide measurement to assess predischarge prognosis	No specific recommendation regarding natriuretic peptide measurement to assess predischarge prognosis
ACE inhibitors or ARBs should be switched to ARNI in HFrEF patients with symptoms	ARNI for persistent symptoms despite triple neurohormonal blockade
Class Ia recommendation for hydralazine-nitrate therapy in African American patients with symptoms despite neurohormonal blockade and beta blockers	Class IIa recommendation for hydralazine-nitrate therapy in African American patients with symptoms despite neurohormonal blockade and beta blockers
In symptomatic HF patients with LVEF <35% and LBBB with intermediate duration, CRT therapy is a class IIb recommendation	In symptomatic HF patients with LVEF <35% and LBBB with intermediate duration, CRT therapy is a class I recommendation

Abbreviations: ACC, American College of Cardiology; AHA, American Heart Association; ESC, European Society of Cardiology; MRI, Magnetic Resonance Imaging; HF, Heart failure; ACE, Angiotensin Converting Enzyme; ARB, Angiotensin Receptor Blocker; ARNI, Angiotensin Receptor Neprilysin Inhibition; CRT, Cardiac Resynchronization Therapy; LVEF, Left Ventricular Ejection Fraction; LBBB, Left Bundle Branch Block.

ACKNOWLEDGMENT

In the previous edition, this chapter was written by Tariq Ahmad, Javed Butler, and Barry Borlaug, and portions of that chapter have been retained.

REFERENCES

1. Katz AM. The "modern" view of heart failure: how did we get here? *Circ Heart Fail.* 2008;1:63-71.

2. Braunwald E. Heart failure. *JACC Heart Fail.* 2013;1:1-20, doi: 10.1016/j.jchf.2012.10.002.

3. Global, regional, and national incidence, prevalence, and years lived with disability for 354 diseases and injuries for 195 countries and territories, 1990-2017: a systematic analysis for the Global Burden of Disease Study 2017. *Lancet.* 2018;392:1789-1858. doi: 10.1016/s0140-6736(18)32279-7.

4. Go AS, et al. Heart disease and stroke statistics–2014 update: a report from the American Heart Association. *Circulation.* 2014;129:e28-e292. doi: 10.1161/01.cir.0000441139.02102.80.

5. Yancy CW, et al. 2013 ACCF/AHA guideline for the management of heart failure: a report of the American College of Cardiology Foundation/American Heart Association Task Force on Practice Guidelines. *J Am Coll Cardiol.* 2013. doi: 10.1016/j.jacc.2013.05.019.

6. Ponikowski P, et al. 2016 ESC Guidelines for the diagnosis and treatment of acute and chronic heart failure: the Task Force for the diagnosis and treatment of acute and chronic heart failure of the European Society of Cardiology (ESC). Developed with the special contribution of the Heart Failure Association (HFA) of the ESC. *Eur Heart J.* 2016;37;2129-2200. doi: 10.1093/eurheartj/ehw128.

7. Ahmad T, Fiuzat M, Felker GM, O'Connor C. Novel biomarkers in chronic heart failure. *Nature reviews. Cardiology.* 2012;9:347-359. doi: 10.1038/nrcardio.2012.37.

8. Ahmad T, et al. Prognostic implications of long-chain acylcarnitines in heart failure and reversibility with mechanical circulatory support. *J Am Coll Cardiol.* 2016;67:291-299. doi: 10.1016/j.jacc.2015.10.079.

9. Ahmad T, et al. Charting a roadmap for heart failure biomarker studies. *JACC Heart Fail.* 2014;2:477-488. doi: 10.1016/j.jchf.2014.02.005.

10. Ahmad T, et al. Clinical Implications of cluster analysis-based classification of acute decompensated heart failure and correlation with bedside hemodynamic profiles. *PLoS One.* 2016;11:e0145881. doi: 10.1371/journal.pone.0145881.

11. New York Heart Association. *Nomenclature and Criteria for Diagnosis of Diseases of the Heart and Great Vessels.* Little, Brown & Co; 1994: 253-256.

12. Goldman L, Hashimoto B, Cook EF, Loscalzo A. Comparative reproducibility and validity of systems for assessing cardiovascular functional class: advantages of a new specific activity scale. *Circulation.* 1981;64:1227-1234.

13. Lang RM, et al. Recommendations for cardiac chamber quantification by echocardiography in adults: an update from the American Society of Echocardiography and the European Association of Cardiovascular Imaging. *J Am Soc Echocardiogr.* 2015;28:1-39 e14. doi: 10.1016/j.echo.2014.10.003.

14. American College of Cardiology Foundation Appropriate Use Criteria Task, et al. ACCF/ASE/AHA/ASNC/HFSA/HRS/SCAI/SCCM/SCCT/SCMR 2011 appropriate use criteria for echocardiography. A report of the American College of Cardiology Foundation Appropriate Use Criteria Task Force, American Society of Echocardiography, American Heart Association, American Society of Nuclear Cardiology, Heart Failure Society of America, Heart Rhythm Society, Society for Cardiovascular Angiography and Interventions, Society of Critical Care Medicine, Society of Cardiovascular Computed Tomography, and Society for Cardiovascular Magnetic Resonance Endorsed by the American College of Chest Physicians. *J Am Coll Cardiol.* 2011;57:1126-1166. doi: 10.1016/j.jacc.2010.11.002.

15. Borlaug BA, Paulus WJ. Heart failure with preserved ejection fraction: pathophysiology, diagnosis, and treatment. *Eur Heart J.* 2011;32:670-679. doi: 10.1093/eurheartj/ehq426.

16. Nohria A, Lewis E, Stevenson LW. Medical management of advanced heart failure. *JAMA.* 2002;287:628-640.

17. Tan YT, et al. The pathophysiology of heart failure with normal ejection fraction: exercise echocardiography reveals complex abnormalities of both systolic and diastolic ventricular function involving torsion, untwist, and longitudinal motion. *J Am Coll Cardiol.* 2009;54:36-46. doi: 10.1016/j.jacc.2009.03.037.

18. Sanderson JE. HFNEF, HFpEF, HF-PEF, or DHF: what is in an acronym? *JACC Heart Fail.* 2014;2:93-94. doi: 10.1016/j.jchf.2013.09.006.

19. McMurray J, Pfeffer MA. New therapeutic options in congestive heart failure: Part II. *Circulation.* 2002;105:2223-2228.

20. McMurray J, Pfeffer MA. New therapeutic options in congestive heart failure: Part I. *Circulation.* 2002;105:2099-2106.

21. Bhatia RS, et al. Outcome of heart failure with preserved ejection fraction in a population-based study. *N Engl J Med* 2006;355:260-269. doi: 10.1056/NEJMoa051530.

22. Halliday BP, et al. Withdrawal of pharmacological treatment for heart failure in patients with recovered dilated cardiomyopathy (TRED-HF): an open-label, pilot, randomised trial. *Lancet.* 2019;393:61-73. doi: 10.1016/s0140-6736(18)32484-x.

23. Solomon SD, et al. Efficacy of sacubitril/valsartan relative to a prior decompensation: the PARADIGM-HF trial. *JACC Heart Fail*. 2016;4: 816-822. doi: 10.1016/j.jchf.2016.05.002.

24. Kelder JC, et al. The diagnostic value of physical examination and additional testing in primary care patients with suspected heart failure. *Circulation*. 2011;124:2865-2873. doi: 10.1161/CIRCULATIONAHA.111.019216.

25. Stevenson LW, Perloff JK. The limited reliability of physical signs for estimating hemodynamics in chronic heart failure. *JAMA*. 1989;261:884-888.

26. Jessup M, Brozena S. Heart failure. *N Engl J Med*. 2003;348:2007-2018. doi: 10.1056/NEJMra021498.

27. Felker GM, et al. Underlying causes and long-term survival in patients with initially unexplained cardiomyopathy. *N Engl J Med*. 2000;342: 1077-1084. doi: 10.1056/NEJM200004133421502.

28. Leier CV, et al. Nuggets, pearls, and vignettes of master heart failure clinicians. Part 2–the physical examination. *Congest Heart Fail*. 2001;7:297-308.

29. Leier CV, Chatterjee K. The physical examination in heart failure–Part I. *Congest Heart Fail*. 2007;13:41-47.

30. Assimes TL. Family history of heart disease: the re-emergence of a traditional risk factor. *J Am Coll Cardiol*. 2011;57:628-629. doi: 10.1016/j.jacc.2010.09.036.

31. Felker GM, Cuculich PS, Gheorghiade M. The Valsalva maneuver: a bedside "biomarker" for heart failure. *Am J Med*. 2006;119:117-122. doi: 10.1016/j.amjmed.2005.06.059.

32. Drazner MH, Rame JE, Stevenson LW, Dries DL. Prognostic importance of elevated jugular venous pressure and a third heart sound in patients with heart failure. *N Engl J Med*. 345;574-581. doi: 10.1056/NEJMoa010641.

33. Ishmail AA, et al. Interobserver agreement by auscultation in the presence of a third heart sound in patients with congestive heart failure. *Chest*. 1987;91;870-873.

34. Ahmad T, Patel CB, Milano CA, Rogers JG. When the heart runs out of heartbeats: treatment options for refractory end-stage heart failure. *Circulation*. 2012;125:2948-2955. doi: 10.1161/CIRCULATIONAHA.112.097337.

35. Samsky MD, et al. Cardiohepatic interactions in heart failure: an overview and clinical implications. *J Am Coll Cardiol*. 2013;61:2397-2405. doi: 10.1016/j.jacc.2013.03.042.

36. Anker SD, Rauchhaus M. Insights into the pathogenesis of chronic heart failure: immune activation and cachexia. *Curr Opin Cardiol*. 1999;14:211-216.

37. Caldentey G, et al. Prognostic value of the physical examination in patients with heart failure and atrial fibrillation: insights from the AF-CHF trial (atrial fibrillation and chronic heart failure). *JACC Heart Fail*. 2014;2:15-23. doi: 10.1016/j.jchf.2013.10.004.

38. Ahmad T, et al. Evaluation of the incremental prognostic utility of increasingly complex testing in chronic heart failure. *Circ Heart Fail*. 2015;8:709-716. doi: 10.1161/CIRCHEARTFAILURE.114.001996.

39. Davie AP, et al. Value of the electrocardiogram in identifying heart failure due to left ventricular systolic dysfunction. *BMJ*. 1996;312:222.

40. Thomas JT, et al. Utility of history, physical examination, electrocardiogram, and chest radiograph for differentiating normal from decreased systolic function in patients with heart failure. *Am J Med*. 2002;112:437-445.

41. Miller WL, Mullan BP. Understanding the heterogeneity in volume overload and fluid distribution in decompensated heart failure is key to optimal volume management: role for blood volume quantitation. *JACC Heart Fail*. 2014;2:298-305. doi: 10.1016/j.jchf.2014.02.007.

42. Januzzi JL Jr. Natriuretic peptides as biomarkers in heart failure. *J Investigat Med*. 2013. doi: 10.231/JIM.0b013e3182946b69.

43. Januzzi JL, Troughton R. Are serial BNP measurements useful in heart failure management? Serial natriuretic peptide measurements are useful in heart failure management. *Circulation*. 2013;127:500-507; discussion 508. doi: 10.1161/CIRCULATIONAHA.112.120485.

44. Vardeny O, Miller R, Solomon SD. Combined neprilysin and renin-angiotensin system inhibition for the treatment of heart failure. *JACC Heart Fail*. 2014;2:663-670. doi: 10.1016/j.jchf.2014.09.001.

45. Felker GM, et al. Rationale and design of the GUIDE-IT study: guiding evidence based therapy using biomarker intensified treatment in heart failure. *JACC Heart Fail*. 2014;2:457-465. doi: 10.1016/j.jchf.2014.05.007.

46. Gandhi PU, Testani JM, Ahmad T. The current and potential clinical relevance of heart failure biomarkers. *Curr Heart Fail Rep*. 2015;12:318-327. doi: 10.1007/s11897-015-0268-2.

47. Januzzi JL Jr, Filippatos G, Nieminen M, Gheorghiade M. Troponin elevation in patients with heart failure: on behalf of the third Universal Definition of Myocardial Infarction Global Task Force: Heart Failure Section. *Eur Heart J*. 2012;33:2265-2271. doi: 10.1093/eurheartj/ehs191.

48. O'Connor CM, et al. Impact of serial troponin release on outcomes in patients with acute heart failure: analysis from the PROTECT pilot study. *Circ Heart Fail*. 2011;4:724-732. doi: 10.1161/CIRCHEARTFAILURE.111.961581.

49. Ahmad T, et al. Biomarkers of myocardial stress and fibrosis as predictors of mode of death in patients with chronic heart failure. *JACC Heart Fail*. 2014;2:260-268. doi: 10.1016/j.jchf.2013.12.004.

50. Ky B, et al. Multiple biomarkers for risk prediction in chronic heart failure. *Circ Heart Fail*. 2012;5:183-190. doi: 10.1161/CIRCHEARTFAILURE.111.965020.

51. Yancy CW, et al. 2013 ACCF/AHA guideline for the management of heart failure: executive summary: a report of the American College of Cardiology Foundation/American Heart Association Task Force on Practice Guidelines. *J Am Coll Cardiol*. 2013. doi: 10.1016/j.jacc.2013.05.020.

52. Gardin JM, et al. M-mode echocardiographic predictors of six- to seven-year incidence of coronary heart disease, stroke, congestive heart failure, and mortality in an elderly cohort (the Cardiovascular Health Study). *Am J Cardiol*. 2001;87:1051-1057.

53. Grayburn PA, et al. Echocardiographic predictors of morbidity and mortality in patients with advanced heart failure: the Beta-blocker Evaluation of Survival Trial (BEST). *J Am Coll Cardiol*. 2005;45:1064-1071. doi: 10.1016/j.jacc.2004.12.069.

54. American College of Cardiology Foundation Appropriate Use Criteria Task, et al. ACCF/ASE/AHA/ASNC/HFSA/HRS/SCAI/SCCM/SCCT/SCMR 2011 appropriate use criteria for echocardiography. A report of the American College of Cardiology Foundation Appropriate Use Criteria Task Force, American Society of Echocardiography, American Heart Association, American Society of Nuclear Cardiology, Heart Failure Society of America, Heart Rhythm Society, Society for Cardiovascular Angiography and Interventions, Society of Critical Care Medicine, Society of Cardiovascular Computed Tomography, Society for Cardiovascular Magnetic Resonance American College of Chest Physicians. *J Am Soc Echocardiogr*. 2011;24:229-267. doi: 10.1016/j.echo.2010.12.008.

55. Gimelli A, et al. Non-invasive cardiac imaging evaluation of patients with chronic systolic heart failure: a report from the European Association of Cardiovascular Imaging (EACVI). *Eur Heart J*. 2014;35:3417-3425. doi: 10.1093/eurheartj/ehu433.

56. Karamitsos TD, Francis JM, Myerson S, Selvanayagam JB, Neubauer S. The role of cardiovascular magnetic resonance imaging in heart failure. *J Am Coll Cardiol*. 2009;54:1407-1424. doi: 10.1016/j.jacc.2009.04.094.

57. Arena R, Sietsema KE. Cardiopulmonary exercise testing in the clinical evaluation of patients with heart and lung disease. *Circulation*. 2011;123:668-680. doi: 10.1161/CIRCULATIONAHA.109.914788.

58. Milani RV, Lavie CJ, Mehra MR. Cardiopulmonary exercise testing: how do we differentiate the cause of dyspnea? *Circulation*. 2004;110:e27-e31. doi: 10.1161/01.CIR.0000136811.45524.2F.

59. Mancini DM, et al. Value of peak exercise oxygen consumption for optimal timing of cardiac transplantation in ambulatory patients with heart failure. *Circulation*. 1991;83:778-786

60. Arena R, et al. Development of a ventilatory classification system in patients with heart failure. *Circulation*. 2007;115:2410-2417. doi: 10.1161/CIRCULATIONAHA.107.686576.

61. Abraham WT, et al. Wireless pulmonary artery haemodynamic monitoring in chronic heart failure: a randomised controlled trial. *Lancet*. 2011;377:658-666. doi: 10.1016/S0140-6736(11)60101-3.

62. Sandhu AT, et al. Cost-effectiveness of implantable pulmonary artery pressure monitoring in chronic heart failure. *JACC Heart Fail.* 2016. doi: 10.1016/j.jchf.2015.12.015.

63. Velazquez EJ, Bonow RO. Revascularization in severe left ventricular dysfunction. *J Am Coll Cardiol.* 2015;65:615-624. doi: 10.1016/j.jacc.2014.10.070.

64. Cooper LT, et al. The role of endomyocardial biopsy in the management of cardiovascular disease: a scientific statement from the American Heart Association, the American College of Cardiology, and the European Society of Cardiology. Endorsed by the Heart Failure Society of America and the Heart Failure Association of the European Society of Cardiology. *J Am Coll Cardiol.* 2007;50:1914-1931. doi: 10.1016/j.jacc.2007.09.008.

65. O'Connor CM, Ahmad T. The role of sodium and chloride in heart failure: does it take two to tango? *J Am Coll Cardiol.* 2015;66:667-669. doi: 10.1016/j.jacc.2015.05.070.

66. Gupta D, et al. Dietary sodium intake in heart failure. *Circulation.* 2012;126:479-485. doi: 10.1161/CIRCULATIONAHA.111.062430.

67. Hummel SL, Konerman MC. Dietary sodium restriction in heart failure: a recommendation worth its salt? *JACC Heart Fail.* 2016;4:36-38. doi: 10.1016/j.jchf.2015.10.003.

68. Doukky R, et al. Impact of dietary sodium restriction on heart failure outcomes. *JACC Heart Fail.* 2016;4:24-35. doi: 10.1016/j.jchf.2015.08.007.

69. Yancy CW. The uncertainty of sodium restriction in heart failure: we can do better than this. *JACC Heart Fail.* 2016;4:39-41. doi: 10.1016/j.jchf.2015.11.005.

70. Whellan DJ, et al. Heart failure and a controlled trial investigating outcomes of exercise training (HF-ACTION): design and rationale. *Am Heart J.* 2007;153:201-211. doi: 10.1016/j.ahj.2006.11.007.

71. O'Connor CM, Ahmad T. Can we prevent heart failure with exercise? *J Am Coll Cardiol.* 2012;60:2548-2549. doi: 10.1016/j.jacc.2012.09.021.

72. O'Connor CM, et al. Efficacy and safety of exercise training in patients with chronic heart failure: HF-ACTION randomized controlled trial. *JAMA.* 2009;301:1439-1450.

73. O'Connor C. It is time to exercise change for heart failure. *JACC Heart Fail.* 2013;1:549-550. doi: 10.1016/j.jchf.2013.10.001.

74. Sacks CA, Jarcho JA, Curfman GD. Paradigm shifts in heart-failure therapy–a timeline. *N Engl J Med.* 2014;371:989-991. doi: 10.1056/NEJMp1410241.

75. Effects of enalapril on mortality in severe congestive heart failure. Results of the Cooperative North Scandinavian Enalapril Survival Study (CONSENSUS). The CONSENSUS Trial Study Group. *N Engl J Med.* 1987;316:1429-1435. doi: 10.1056/NEJM198706043162301.

76. Effect of enalapril on survival in patients with reduced left ventricular ejection fractions and congestive heart failure. The SOLVD Investigators. *N Engl J Med.* 1991;325:293-302. doi: 10.1056/NEJM199108013250501

77. Brater DC. Diuretic therapy. *N Engl J Med.* 1998;339:387-395. doi: 10.1056/NEJM199808063390607.

78. Heart Failure Society of America, et al. HFSA 2010 Comprehensive Heart Failure Practice Guideline. *J Card Fail.* 2010;16:e1-e194. doi: 10.1016/j.cardfail.2010.04.004.

79. Felker GM. Diuretic management in heart failure. *Congest Heart Fail.* 2010;16(Suppl 1):S68-S72. doi: 10.1111/j.1751-7133.2010.00172.x.

80. Testani JM, et al. Loop diuretic efficiency: a metric of diuretic responsiveness with prognostic importance in acute decompensated heart failure. *Circ Heart Fail.* 2014;7:261-270. doi: 10.1161/CIRCHEARTFAILURE.113.000895.

81. Felker GM, et al. Diuretic strategies in patients with acute decompensated heart failure. *N Engl J Med.* 2011;364:797-805. doi: 10.1056/NEJMoa1005419.

82. Felker GM, O'Connor CM, Braunwald E, Heart Failure Clinical Research Network. Loop diuretics in acute decompensated heart failure: necessary? Evil? A necessary evil? *Circ Heart Fail.* 2009;2:56-62. doi: 10.1161/CIRCHEARTFAILURE.108.821785.

83. Butler J, et al. Relationship between heart failure treatment and development of worsening renal function among hospitalized patients. *Am Heart J.* 2004;147:331-338. doi: 10.1016/j.ahj.2003.08.012.

84. Felker GM, Mentz RJ. Diuretics and ultrafiltration in acute decompensated heart failure. *J Am Coll Cardiol.* 2012;59:2145-2153. doi: 10.1016/j.jacc.2011.10.910.

85. Pfeffer MA. ACE inhibitors in acute myocardial infarction: patient selection and timing. *Circulation.* 1998;97:2192-2194.

86. Erhardt L, Maclean A, Ilgenfritz J, et al. Fosinopril attenuates clinical deterioration and improves exercise tolerance in patients with heart failure. *Eur Heart J.* 1995;16(12):1892-1899.

87. Widimský J, Uhlíř O, Kremer HJ, et al. Czech and Slovak spirapril intervention study (CASSIS). *Eur J Clin Pharmacol.* 1995;49(1-2):95-102.

88. van Veldhuisen DJ, Genth-Zotz S, Brouwer J, et al. High- versus low-dose ACE inhibition in chronic heart failure. *J Am Coll Cardiol.* 1998;32(7):1811-1818.

89. Shettigar U, Hare T, Gelperin K, et al. Effects of fosinopril on exercise tolerance, symptoms, and clinical outcomes in patients with decompensated heart failure. *Congest Heart Fail.* 1999;5(1):27-34.

90. Goldstein S, Kennedy HL, Hall C, et al. Metoprolol CR/XL in patients with heart failure: a pilot study examining the tolerability, safety, and effect on left ventricular ejection fraction. *Am Heart J.* 1999;138(6):1158-1165.

91. Beller B, Bulle T, Bourge RC, et al. Lisinopril versus placebo in the treatment of heart failure: the Lisinopril Heart Failure Study Group. *J Clin Pharmacol.* 1995;35(7):673-680.

92. Colfer HT, Ribner HS, Gradman A, et al. Effects of once-daily benazepril therapy on exercise tolerance and manifestations of chronic congestive heart failure. *Am J Cardiol.* 1992;70(3):354-358.

93. Kleber FX, Niemöller L. Long-term survival in the Munich Mild Heart Failure Trial (MHFT). *Am J Cardiol.* 1993;71(13):1237-1239.

94. Brown EJ, Chew PH, MacLean A, et al. Effects of fosinopril on exercise tolerance and clinical deterioration in patients with chronic congestive heart failure not taking digitalis. *Am J Cardiol.* 1995;75(8):596-600.

95. Chalmers JP, West MJ, Cyran J, et al. Placebo-controlled study of lisinopril in congestive heart failure. *J Cardiovasc Pharmacol.* 1987;9:S89-S97.

96. Lewis GR. Comparison of lisinopril versus placebo for congestive heart failure. *Am J Cardiol.* 1989;63(8):D12-D16.

97. Komajda M, Lutiger B, Madeira H, et al. Tolerability of carvedilol and ACE-Inhibition in mild heart failure. Results of CARMEN (Carvedilol ACE-Inhibitor Remodelling Mild CHF EvaluatioN). *Eur J Heart Fail.* 2004;6(4):467-475.

98. McMurray JJV, Östergren J, Swedberg K, et al. Effects of candesartan in patients with chronic heart failure and reduced left-ventricular systolic function taking angiotensin-converting-enzyme inhibitors: the CHARM-Added trial. *Lancet.* 2003;362(9386):767-771.

99. Riegger GAJ, Bouzo H, Petr P, et al. Improvement in exercise tolerance and symptoms of congestive heart failure during treatment with candesartan cilexetil. *Circulation.* 1999;100(22):2224-2230.

100. Granger CB, Ertl G, Kuch J, et al. Randomized trial of candesartan cilexetil in the treatment of patients with congestive heart failure and a history of intolerance to angiotensin-converting enzyme inhibitors. *Am Heart J.* 2000;139(4):609-617.

101. Mitrovic V, Willenbrock R, Miric M, et al. Acute and 3-month treatment effects of candesartan cilexetil on hemodynamics, neurohormones, and clinical symptoms in patients with congestive heart failure. *Am Heart J.* 2003;145(3):E14.

102. Pitt B, Poole-Wilson PA, Segal R, et al. Effect of losartan compared with captopril on mortality in patients with symptomatic heart failure: randomised trial—the Losartan Heart Failure Survival Study ELITE II. *Lancet.* 2000;355(9215):1582-1587.

103. Pitt B, Segal R, Martinez FA, et al. Randomised trial of losartan versus captopril in patients over 65 with heart failure (Evaluation of Losartan in the Elderly Study, ELITE). *Lancet.* 1997;349(9054):747-752.

104. Dunselman PHJM. Effects of the replacement of the angiotensin converting enzyme inhibitor enalapril by the angiotensin II receptor blocker telmisartan in patients with congestive heart failure. *Int J Cardiol.* 2001;77(2-3):131-138.

105. Dickstein K, Chang P, Willenheimer R, et al. Comparison of the effects of losartan and enalapril on clinical status and exercise performance in patients with moderate or severe chronic heart failure. *J Am Coll Cardiol.* 1995;26(2):438-445.

106. Lang RM, Elkayam U, Yellen LG, et al. Comparative effects of losartan and enalapril on exercise capacity and clinical status in patients with heart failure. This study was supported by a grant from Merck Research Laboratories, West Point, Pennsylvania. *J Am Coll Cardiol.* 1997;30(4):983-991.

107. Effect of enalapril on mortality and the development of heart failure in asymptomatic patients with reduced left ventricular ejection fractions. The SOLVD Investigators. *N Engl J Med.* 1992;327:685-691. doi: 10.1056/NEJM199209033271003.

108. Packer M, et al. Comparative effects of low and high doses of the angiotensin-converting enzyme inhibitor, lisinopril, on morbidity and mortality in chronic heart failure. ATLAS Study Group. *Circulation.* 1999;100:2312-2318.

109. Liu YH, et al. Effects of angiotensin-converting enzyme inhibitors and angiotensin II type 1 receptor antagonists in rats with heart failure. Role of kinins and angiotensin II type 2 receptors. *J Clin Invest.* 1997;99: 1926-1935. doi: 10.1172/JCI119360.

110. Cohn JN, Tognoni G, Valsartan Heart Failure Trial. A randomized trial of the angiotensin-receptor blocker valsartan in chronic heart failure. *N Engl J Med.* 2001;345:1667-1675. doi: 10.1056/NEJMoa010713.

111. McMurray JJ, et al. Effects of candesartan in patients with chronic heart failure and reduced left-ventricular systolic function taking angiotensin-converting-enzyme inhibitors: the CHARM-Added trial. *Lancet.* 2003; 362:767-771. doi: 10.1016/S0140-6736(03)14283-3.

112. Granger CB, et al. Effects of candesartan in patients with chronic heart failure and reduced left-ventricular systolic function intolerant to angiotensin-converting-enzyme inhibitors: the CHARM-Alternative trial. *Lancet.* 2003;362:772-776. doi: 10.1016/S0140-6736(03)14284-5.

113. Waagstein F, Hjalmarson A, Varnauskas E, Wallentin, I. Effect of chronic beta-adrenergic receptor blockade in congestive cardiomyopathy. *Br Heart J.* 1975;37:1022-1036.

114. The Cardiac Insufficiency Bisoprolol Study II (CIBIS-II): a randomised trial. *Lancet.* 1999;353:9-13.

115. Packer M, et al. Effect of carvedilol on the morbidity of patients with severe chronic heart failure: results of the carvedilol prospective randomized cumulative survival (COPERNICUS) study. *Circulation.* 2002;106:2194-2199.

116. Effect of metoprolol CR/XL in chronic heart failure: Metoprolol CR/XL Randomised Intervention Trial in Congestive Heart Failure (MERIT-HF). *Lancet* 1999;353:2001-2007.

117. Poole-Wilson PA, et al. Comparison of carvedilol and metoprolol on clinical outcomes in patients with chronic heart failure in the Carvedilol Or Metoprolol European Trial (COMET): randomised controlled trial. *Lancet.* 2003;362:7-13. doi: 10.1016/S0140-6736(03)13800-7.

118. A trial of the beta-blocker bucindolol in patients with advanced chronic heart failure. *N Engl J Med.* 2001;344(22):1659-1667.

119. Krum H, Roecker EB, Mohacsi P, et al. Effects of initiating carvedilol in patients with severe chronic heart failure: results from the COPERNICUS Study. *JAMA.* 2003;289(6):712-718.

120. Packer M, Bristow MR, Cohn JN, et al. The effect of carvedilol on morbidity and mortality in patients with chronic heart failure. *N Engl J Med.* 1996;334(21):1349-1355.

121. A randomized trial of beta-blockade in heart failure. The Cardiac Insufficiency Bisoprolol Study (CIBIS). CIBIS Investigators and Committees. *Circulation.* 1994;90(4):1765-1773.

122. Colucci WS, Packer M, Bristow MR, et al. Carvedilol inhibits clinical progression in patients with mild symptoms of heart failure. *Circulation.* 1996;94(11):2800-2806.

123. Bristow MR, Gilbert EM, Abraham WT, et al. Carvedilol produces dose-related improvements in left ventricular function and survival in subjects with chronic heart failure. *Circulation.* 1996;94(11):2807-2816.

124. Packer M, Colucci WS, Sackner-Bernstein JD, et al. Double-blind, placebo-controlled study of the effects of carvedilol in patients with moderate to severe heart failure. *Circulation.* 1996;94(11):2793-2799.

125. Edes I, Gasior Z, Wita K. Effects of nebivolol on left ventricular function in elderly patients with chronic heart failure: results of the ENECA study. *Eur J Heart Fail.* 2005;7(4):631-639.

126. McKelvie R. Comparative impact of enalapril, candesartan or metoprolol alone or in combination on ventricular remodelling in patients with congestive heart failure. *Eur Heart J.* 2003;24(19):1727-1734.

127. Witchitz S, Cohen-Solal A, Dartois N, et al. Treatment of heart failure with celiprolol, a cardioselective beta blocker with beta-2 agonist vasodilatory properties. *Am J Cardiol.* 2000;85(12):1467-1471.

128. Sturm B, Pacher R, Strametz-Juranek J, et al. Effect of β1 blockade with atenolol on progression of heart failure in patients pretreated with high-dose enalapril. *Eur J Heart Fail.* 2000;2(4):407-412.

129. Cohn JN, Fowler MB, Bristow MR, et al. Safety and efficacy of carvedilol in severe heart failure. *J Cardiac Fail.* 1997;3(3):173-179.

130. Palazzuoli A, Quatrini I, Vecchiato L, et al. Left ventricular diastolic function improvement by carvedilol therapy in advanced heart failure. *J Cardiovasc Pharmacol.* 2005;45(6):563-568.

131. de Milliano PAR, de Groot AC, Tijssen JGP, et al. Beneficial effects of metoprolol on myocardial sympathetic function: Evidence from a randomized, placebo-controlled study in patients with congestive heart failure. *Am Heart J.* 2002;144(2):A14-A22.

132. Genth-Zotz S, Zotz RJ, Sigmund M, et al. MIC trial: metoprolol in patients with mild to moderate heart failure: effects on ventricular function and cardiopulmonary exercise testing. *Eur J Heart Fail.* 2000;2(2):175-181.

133. Solal AC, Jondeau G, Beauvais F, et al. Beneficial effects of carvedilol on angiotensin-converting enzyme activity and renin plasma levels in patients with chronic heart failure. *Eur J Heart Fail.* 2004;6(4): 463-466.

134. Krum H, Sackner-Bernstein JD, Goldsmith RL, et al. Double-blind, placebo-controlled study of the long-term efficacy of carvedilol in patients with severe chronic heart failure. *Circulation.* 1995;92(6):1499-1506.

135. Dubach P, Myers J, Bonetti P, et al. Effects of bisoprolol fumarate on left ventricular size, function, and exercise capacity in patients with heart failure: Analysis with magnetic resonance myocardial tagging. *Am Heart J.* 2002;143(4):676-683.

136. Dobre D, van Veldhuisen DJ, Goulder MA, et al. Clinical effects of initial 6 months monotherapy with bisoprolol versus enalapril in the treatment of patients with mild to moderate chronic heart failure. Data from the CIBIS III Trial. *Cardiovasc Drugs Therapy.* 2008;22(5):399-405.

137. Maron BA, Leopold JA. Aldosterone receptor antagonists: effective but often forgotten. *Circulation.* 2010;121:934-939. doi: 10.1161/CIRCULATIONAHA.109.895235.

138. Pitt B, et al. The effect of spironolactone on morbidity and mortality in patients with severe heart failure. Randomized Aldactone Evaluation Study Investigators. *N Engl J Med.* 1999;341:709-717. doi: 10.1056/NEJM199909023411001.

139. Zannad F, McMurray JJV, Krum H, et al. Eplerenone in patients with systolic heart failure and mild symptoms. *N Engl J Med.* 2011;364:11-21. doi: 10.1056/NEJMoa1009492.

140. Pitt B, et al. Eplerenone, a selective aldosterone blocker, in patients with left ventricular dysfunction after myocardial infarction. *N Engl J Med.* 2003;348:1309-1321. doi: 10.1056/NEJMoa030207.

141. Pitt B, Zannad F, Remme WJ, et al. The effect of spironolactone on morbidity and mortality in patients with severe heart failure. *N Engl J Med.* 1999;341(10):709-717.

142. Boccanelli A, Mureddu GF, Cacciatore G, et al. Anti-remodelling effect of canrenone in patients with mild chronic heart failure (AREA IN-CHF study): final results. *Eur J Heart Fail.* 2009;11(1):68-76.

143. Vizzardi E, Nodari S, Caretta G, et al. Effects of spironolactone on long-term mortality and morbidity in patients with heart failure and mild or no symptoms. *Am J Med Sci.* 2014;347(4):271-276.

144. Cicoira M, Zanolla L, Rossi A, et al. Long-term, dose-dependent effects of spironolactone on left ventricular function and exercise tolerance in patients with chronic heart failure. *J Am Coll Cardiol.* 2002;40(2):304-310.

145. Cohn JN, et al. Effect of vasodilator therapy on mortality in chronic congestive heart failure. Results of a Veterans Administration Cooperative Study. *N Engl J Med.* 1986;314:1547-1552. doi: 10.1056/NEJM198606123142404.

146. Cohn JN, et al. A comparison of enalapril with hydralazine-isosorbide dinitrate in the treatment of chronic congestive heart failure. *N Engl J Med.* 1991;325:303-310. doi: 10.1056/NEJM199108013250502.

147. Taylor AL, Ziesche S, Yancy C, et al. Combination of isosorbide dinitrate and hydralazine in blacks with heart failure. *N Engl J Med.* 2004;351(20):2049-2057.

148. Cohn JN, Archibald DG, Ziesche S, et al. Effect of vasodilator therapy on mortality in chronic congestive heart failure. Results of a Veterans Administration Cooperative Study. *N Engl J Med.* 1986;314(24):1547-1552.

149. Cole RT, et al. Hydralazine and isosorbide dinitrate in heart failure: historical perspective, mechanisms, and future directions. *Circulation.* 2011;123:2414-2422. doi: 10.1161/CIRCULATIONAHA.110.012781.

150. Rahimtoola SH. Digitalis therapy for patients in clinical heart failure. *Circulation.* 2004;109:2942-2946. doi: 10.1161/01.CIR.0000132477.32438.03.

151. Smith TW. Digitalis. Mechanisms of action and clinical use. *N Engl J Med.* 1988;318:358-365. doi: 10.1056/NEJM198802113180606.

152. Digitalis Investigation Group. The effect of digoxin on mortality and morbidity in patients with heart failure. *N Engl J Med.* 1997;336:525-533. doi: 10.1056/NEJM199702203360801.

153. Hood WB Jr, Dans AL, Guyatt GH, Jaeschke R, McMurray JJ. Digitalis for treatment of congestive heart failure in patients in sinus rhythm: a systematic review and meta-analysis. *J Card Fail.* 2004;10:155-164.

154. Packer M, et al. Withdrawal of digoxin from patients with chronic heart failure treated with angiotensin-converting-enzyme inhibitors. RADIANCE Study. *N Engl J Med.* 1993;329:1-7. doi: 10.1056/NEJM199307013290101.

155. McMurray JJ, et al. Angiotensin-neprilysin inhibition versus enalapril in heart failure. *N Engl J Med.* 2014;371:993-1004. doi: 10.1056/NEJMoa1409077.

156. Januzzi JL Jr, et al. Association of change in n-terminal pro-b-type natriuretic peptide following initiation of sacubitril-valsartan treatment with cardiac structure and function in patients with heart failure with reduced ejection fraction. *JAMA.* 2019;322:1-11. doi: 10.1001/jama.2019.12821.

157. Swedberg K, et al. Ivabradine and outcomes in chronic heart failure (SHIFT): a randomised placebo-controlled study. *Lancet.* 2010;376:875-885. doi: 10.1016/S0140-6736(10)61198-1.

158. Vardeny O, Vaduganathan M. Practical guide to prescribing sodium-glucose cotransporter 2 inhibitors for cardiologists. *JACC Heart Fail.* 2019;7:169-172. doi: 10.1016/j.jchf.2018.11.013.

159. Zinman B, et al. Empagliflozin, cardiovascular outcomes, and mortality in type 2 diabetes. *N Engl J Med.* 2015;373:2117-2128. doi: 10.1056/NEJMoa1504720.

160. Neal B, et al. Canagliflozin and cardiovascular and renal events in type 2 diabetes. *N Engl J Med.* 2017;377:644-657. doi: 10.1056/NEJMoa1611925.

161. Wiviott SD, et al. Dapagliflozin and cardiovascular outcomes in type 2 diabetes. *N Engl J Med.* 2019;380:347-357. doi: 10.1056/NEJMoa1812389.

162. McMurray JJV, Solomon SD, Inzucchi SE, et al. Dapagliflozin in patients with heart failure and reduced ejection fraction. *N Engl J Med.* 2019;381:1995-2008. doi: 10.1056/NEJMoa1911303.

163. Cavender MA, et al. SGLT-2 Inhibitors and cardiovascular risk: an analysis of CVD-REAL. *J Am Coll Cardiol.* 2018;71:2497-2506. doi: 10.1016/j.jacc.2018.01.085.

164. Kosiborod M, et al. Cardiovascular events associated with SGLT-2 inhibitors versus other glucose-lowering drugs: the CVD-REAL 2 study. *J Am Coll Cardiol.* 2018;71:2628-2639. doi: 10.1016/j.jacc.2018.03.009.

165. Empagliflozin meets primary endpoint in reducing risk of cardiovascular death or hospitalization for heart failure in Phase III trial in adults with and without diabetes. Boehringer Ingelheim. July 30, 2020. https://www.boehringer-ingelheim.com/press-release/emperor-reduced-heart-failure-toplineresults

166. Packer M, Butler J, Filippatos GS, et al. Evaluation of the effect of sodium-glucose co-transporter 2 inhibition with empagliflozin on morbidity and mortality of patients with chronic heart failure and a reduced ejection fraction: rationale for and design of the EMPEROR-Reduced trial. *Eur J Heart Fail.* 2019;21(10):1270-1278.

167. Griffin M, et al. Empagliflozin in heart failure: diuretic and cardio-renal effects. *Circulation.* 2020. doi: 10.1161/circulationaha.120.045691.

168. Perkovic V, et al. Canagliflozin and renal outcomes in type 2 diabetes and nephropathy. *N Engl J Med.* 2019;380:2295-2306. doi: 10.1056/NEJMoa1811744.

169. Farxiga Phase III DAPA-CKD trial will be stopped early after overwhelming efficacy in patients with chronic kidney disease. Astra Zeneca. 2020. https://www.astrazeneca.com/media-centre/press-releases/2020/farxiga-phase-iii-dapa-ckd-trial-will-be-stopped-early-after-overwhelming-efficacy-in-patients-with-chronic-kidney-disease.html

170. FDA warns about rare occurrences of a serious infection of the genital area with SGLT2 inhibitors for diabetes. US Food and Drugs Administration. 2018. https://www.fda.gov/drugs/drug-safety-and-availability/fda-warns-about-rare-occurrences-serious-infection-genital-area-sglt2-inhibitors-diabetes

171. Armstrong PW, et al. Vericiguat in patients with heart failure and reduced ejection fraction. *N Engl J Med.* 2010;382:1883-1893. doi: 10.1056/NEJMoa1915928.

172. Teerlink JR, et al. Omecamtiv mecarbil in chronic heart failure with reduced ejection fraction: rationale and design of GALACTIC-HF. *JACC Heart Fail.* 2020;8:329-340. doi: 10.1016/j.jchf.2019.12.001

173. Chopra VK, Anker SD. Anaemia, iron deficiency and heart failure in 2020: facts and numbers. *ESC Heart Fail.* 2020. doi: 10.1002/ehf2.12797.

174. Anker SD, Comin Colet J, Filippatos G, et al. Ferric carboxymaltose in patients with heart failure and iron deficiency. *N Engl J Med.* 2009;361:2436-2448. doi: 10.1056/NEJMoa0908355.

175. van Veldhuisen DJ, Ponikowski P, van der Meer P, et al. Effect of ferric carboxymaltose on exercise capacity in patients with chronic heart failure and iron deficiency. *Circulation.* 2017;136:1374-1383. doi: 10.1161/circulationaha.117.027497.

176. Ponikowski P, et al. Beneficial effects of long-term intravenous iron therapy with ferric carboxymaltose in patients with symptomatic heart failure and iron deficiency. *Eur Heart J.* 2015;36:657-668. doi: 10.1093/eurheartj/ehu385.

177. Anker SD, et al. Effects of ferric carboxymaltose on hospitalisations and mortality rates in iron-deficient heart failure patients: an individual patient data meta-analysis. *Eur J Heart Fail.* 2018;20:125-133. doi: 10.1002/ejhf.823.

178. Ahmad T, Butler J. Disrupting Virchow's triad: can factor X inhibition reduce risk of adverse outcomes in patients with ischaemic cardiomyopathy? *Eur J Heart Fail.* 2015;17:647-651. doi: 10.1002/ejhf.296.

179. Gurbel PA, Tantry US. Antiplatelet and anticoagulant agents in heart failure: current status and future perspectives. *JACC Heart Fail.* 2014;2:1-14. doi: 10.1016/j.jchf.2013.07.007.

180. Zannad F, Anker SD, Byra WM, et al. Rivaroxaban in patients with heart failure, sinus rhythm, and coronary disease. *N Engl J Med.* 2018;379(14):1332-1342.

181. Cleland JG, Findlay I, Jafri S, et al. The Warfarin/Aspirin Study in Heart failure (WASH): a randomized trial comparing antithrombotic strategies for patients with heart failure. *Am Heart J.* 2004;148:157-164. doi: 10.1016/j.ahj.2004.03.010.

182. Cokkinos DV, Haralabopoulos GC, Kostis JB, Toutouzas PK. HELAS Investigators Efficacy of antithrombotic therapy in chronic heart failure: the HELAS study. *Eur J Heart Fail.* 2006;8:428-432. doi: 10.1016/j.ejheart.2006.02.012.

183. Massie BM, Collins JF, Ammon SE, et al. Randomized trial of warfarin, aspirin, and clopidogrel in patients with chronic heart

failure: the Warfarin and Antiplatelet Therapy in Chronic Heart Failure (WATCH) trial. *Circulation.* 2009;119:1616-1624. doi: 10.1161/CIRCULATIONAHA.108.801753.

184. Homma S, Thompson JL, Pullicino PM, et al. Warfarin and aspirin in patients with heart failure and sinus rhythm. *N Engl J Med.* 2012;366:1859-1869. doi: 10.1056/NEJMoa1202299.

185. Mehra MR, et al. A comprehensive analysis of the effects of rivaroxaban on stroke or transient ischaemic attack in patients with heart failure, coronary artery disease, and sinus rhythm: the COMMANDER HF trial. *Eur Heart J.* 2019;40:3593-3602. doi: 10.1093/eurheartj/ehz427.

186. Butler J, Khan MS, Anker SD. Novel potassium binders as enabling therapy in heart failure. *Eur J Heart Fail.* 2019;21:550-552, doi:10.1002/ejhf.1474.

187. Khan MS, et al. Dose of angiotensin-converting enzyme inhibitors and angiotensin receptor blockers and outcomes in heart failure: a meta-analysis. *Circ Heart Fail.* 2017;10. doi: 10.1161/circheartfailure.117.003956.

188. Pitt B, et al. Evaluation of the efficacy and safety of RLY5016, a polymeric potassium binder, in a double-blind, placebo-controlled study in patients with chronic heart failure (the PEARL-HF) trial. *Eur Heart J.* 2011;32:820-828. doi: 10.1093/eurheartj/ehq502.

189. Moss AJ, et al. Improved survival with an implanted defibrillator in patients with coronary disease at high risk for ventricular arrhythmia. Multicenter Automatic Defibrillator Implantation Trial Investigators. *N Engl J Med.* 1996;335:1933-1940. doi: 10.1056/NEJM199612263352601.

190. Bardy GH, et al. Amiodarone or an implantable cardioverter-defibrillator for congestive heart failure. *N Engl J Med.* 2005;352:225-237. doi: 10.1056/NEJMoa043399.

191. Kadish A, et al. Prophylactic defibrillator implantation in patients with nonischemic dilated cardiomyopathy. *N Engl J Med.* 2004;350:2151-2158. doi: 10.1056/NEJMoa033088.

192. Køber L, et al. Defibrillator implantation in patients with nonischemic systolic heart failure. *N Engl J Med.* 2016;375:1221-1230. doi: 10.1056/NEJMoa1608029.

193. Shen L, et al. Declining risk of sudden death in heart failure. *N Engl J Med.* 2017;377:41-51. doi: 10.1056/NEJMoa1609758.

194. Saxon LA, Ellenbogen KA. Resynchronization therapy for the treatment of heart failure. *Circulation.* 2003;108:1044-1048. doi: 10.1161/01.CIR.0000085656.57918.B1.

195. Bristow MR, et al. Cardiac-resynchronization therapy with or without an implantable defibrillator in advanced chronic heart failure. *N Engl J Med.* 2004;350:2140-2150. doi: 10.1056/NEJMoa032423.

196. Cleland JG, et al. The effect of cardiac resynchronization on morbidity and mortality in heart failure. *N Engl J Med.* 2005;352:1539-1549. doi: 10.1056/NEJMoa050496.

197. Moss AJ, et al. Cardiac-resynchronization therapy for the prevention of heart-failure events. *N Engl J Med.* 2009;361:1329-1338. doi: 10.1056/NEJMoa0906431.

198. Tang AS, et al. Cardiac-resynchronization therapy for mild-to-moderate heart failure. *N Engl J Med.* 2010;363:2385-2395. doi: 10.1056/NEJMoa1009540.

199. Brignole M, et al. Cardiac resynchronization therapy in patients undergoing atrioventricular junction ablation for permanent atrial fibrillation: a randomized trial. *Eur Heart J.* 2011;32:2420-2429. doi: 10.1093/eurheartj/ehr162.

200. Upadhyay GA, Choudhry NK, Auricchio A, Ruskin J, Singh JP. Cardiac resynchronization in patients with atrial fibrillation: a meta-analysis of prospective cohort studies. *J Am Coll Cardiol.* 2008;52:1239-1246. doi: 10.1016/j.jacc.2008.06.043.

201. Risum N, et al. Identification of typical left bundle branch block contraction by strain echocardiography is additive to electrocardiography in prediction of long-term outcome after cardiac resynchronization therapy. *J Am Coll Cardiol.* 2015;66;631-641: doi: 10.1016/j.jacc.2015.06.020.

202. Risum N, Kisslo J, Wagner G. Cardiac resynchronization therapy: identifying an activation delay by regional strain analysis. *J Electrocardiol.* 2015;48:779-782. doi: 10.1016/j.jelectrocard.2015.07.020.

Diagnosis and Management of Heart Failure with Preserved Ejection Fraction

49

João Pedro Ferreira, Kavita Sharma, and Javed Butler

CHAPTER OUTLINE

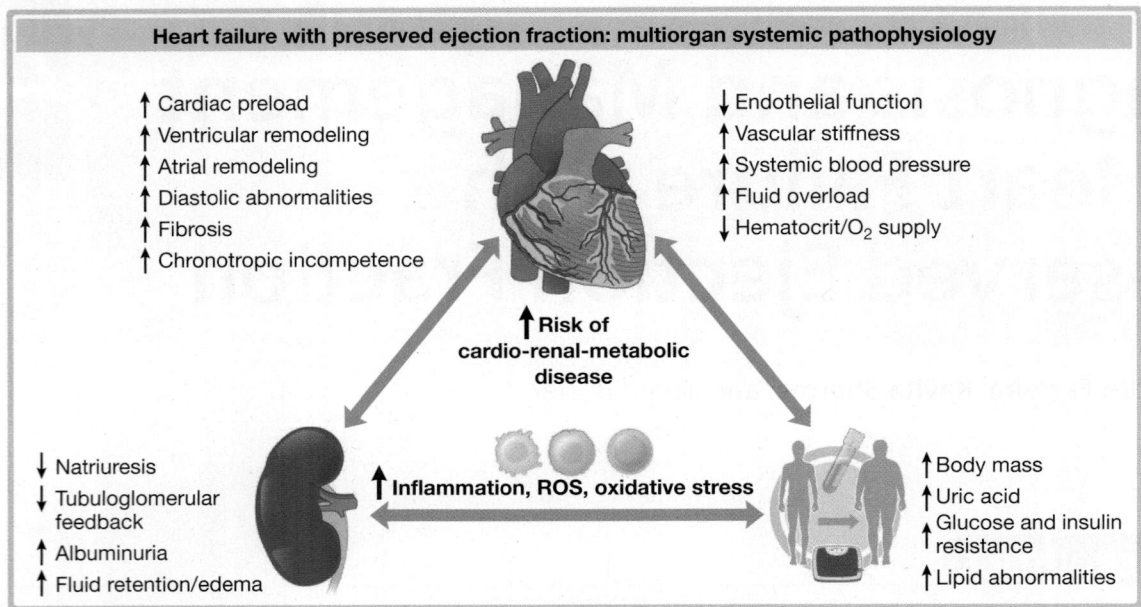

Heart failure with preserved ejection fraction: multiorgan systemic pathophysiology

- ↑ Cardiac preload
- ↑ Ventricular remodeling
- ↑ Atrial remodeling
- ↑ Diastolic abnormalities
- ↑ Fibrosis
- ↑ Chronotropic incompetence

- ↓ Endothelial function
- ↑ Vascular stiffness
- ↑ Systemic blood pressure
- ↑ Fluid overload
- ↓ Hematocrit/O_2 supply

↑ Risk of cardio-renal-metabolic disease

↑ Inflammation, ROS, oxidative stress

- ↓ Natriuresis
- ↓ Tubuloglomerular feedback
- ↑ Albuminuria
- ↑ Fluid retention/edema

- ↑ Body mass
- ↑ Uric acid
- ↑ Glucose and insulin resistance
- ↑ Lipid abnormalities

Chapter 49 Fuster and Hurst's Central Illustration. Patients with heart failure with preserved ejection fraction have increased risk of cardio-renal-metabolic disease. ROS, reactive oxygen species.

CHAPTER SUMMARY

This chapter provides an in-depth description of heart failure with preserved ejection fraction (HFpEF), from pathophysiology to treatment. Patients with HFpEF have a multifaceted constellation of comorbidities and clinical presentations. Numerous pathogenic mechanisms, including diastolic dysfunction, impaired systolic reserve, abnormal ventricular–arterial coupling, inflammation, endothelial dysfunction, chronotropic incompetence, altered myocardial energetics, impaired peripheral skeletal muscle metabolism and perfusion, pulmonary hypertension, atrial fibrillation, coronary artery disease, obesity, and renal insufficiency, contribute to the disease burden of HFpEF (see Fuster and Hurst's Central Illustration). The prognosis of patients with HFpEF remains poor. Many treatments (including angiotensin-converting enzyme inhibitors, angiotensin receptor blockers, mineralocorticoid receptor antagonists, sacubitril/valsartan, and sodium glucose cotransporter-2 inhibitors) have been tested in HFpEF. Candesartan, spironolactone, and sacubitril/valsartan all demonstrated a modest effect to reduce heart failure hospitalizations in patients with HFpEF, at least up to left ventricular ejection fractions in the 50% to 55% range. Empagliflozin showed a more pronounced effect to reduce the composite of heart failure hospitalizations or cardiovascular death across the spectrum of ejection fraction of HFpEF patients.

INTRODUCTION

For a general introduction on heart failure definition, classification, and diagnosis, please see Chapter 48, Diagnosis and Management of Chronic Heart Failure.

Given the multifaceted constellation of comorbidities and clinical presentation that is almost invariably present in patients with heart failure with preserved ejection fraction (HFpEF), its underlying pathophysiology remains subject to debate. Among the leading contenders over the last two decades are diastolic dysfunction, impaired systolic reserve, and perhaps even resting dysfunction, abnormal ventricular-arterial coupling, inflammation and endothelial dysfunction, depressed heart rate response (chronotropic incompetence), altered myocardial energetics and peripheral skeletal muscle metabolism and perfusion, pulmonary hypertension, and renal insufficiency. More recent myocardial tissue studies have revealed distinct transcriptomic profile in HFpEF compared to heart failure with reduced ejection fraction (HFrEF) and nonfailing hearts. A major challenge to the field is that truly representative experimental models of HFpEF do not fully capture the clinical syndrome, and yet human data, particularly direct myocardial analysis, remains very limited. The leading mechanisms of interest in HFpEF are subsequently summarized, and in **Fig. 49–1**.

MYOCARDIAL ABNORMALITIES

Diastolic Relaxation

HFpEF often presents with diastolic abnormalities including delayed early relaxation, myocardial and myocyte stiffening, and associated changes in filling dynamics. Slow relaxation has been documented in patients by means of invasive pressure recordings or echo-Doppler imaging parameters.[1-7] Most of the reported data compares relaxation rates to that of age-matched normotensive subjects or hypertensive patients without left ventricular hypertrophy (LVH); however, the combination of LVH and hypertension without HF generates similar delay.[7] Many of the same abnormalities that result in slowed chamber relaxation in HFrEF are suspected in HFpEF, although direct proof remains limited given the lack of live tissue for human myocardial analysis. In an interesting study of biopsy samples from HFpEF and HFrEF patients, Hamdani et al.[8] found the expression of calcium handling proteins and phosphorylation of myofilament proteins were very similar between the groups. Relaxation is also controlled by passive recoil of elastic elements, notably titin, compressed during systole.[9] Dilated hearts have depressed recoil,[10] because the heart does not contract sufficiently to compress the elastic elements. However, because HFpEF volumes are generally normal, recoil may be less impacted.

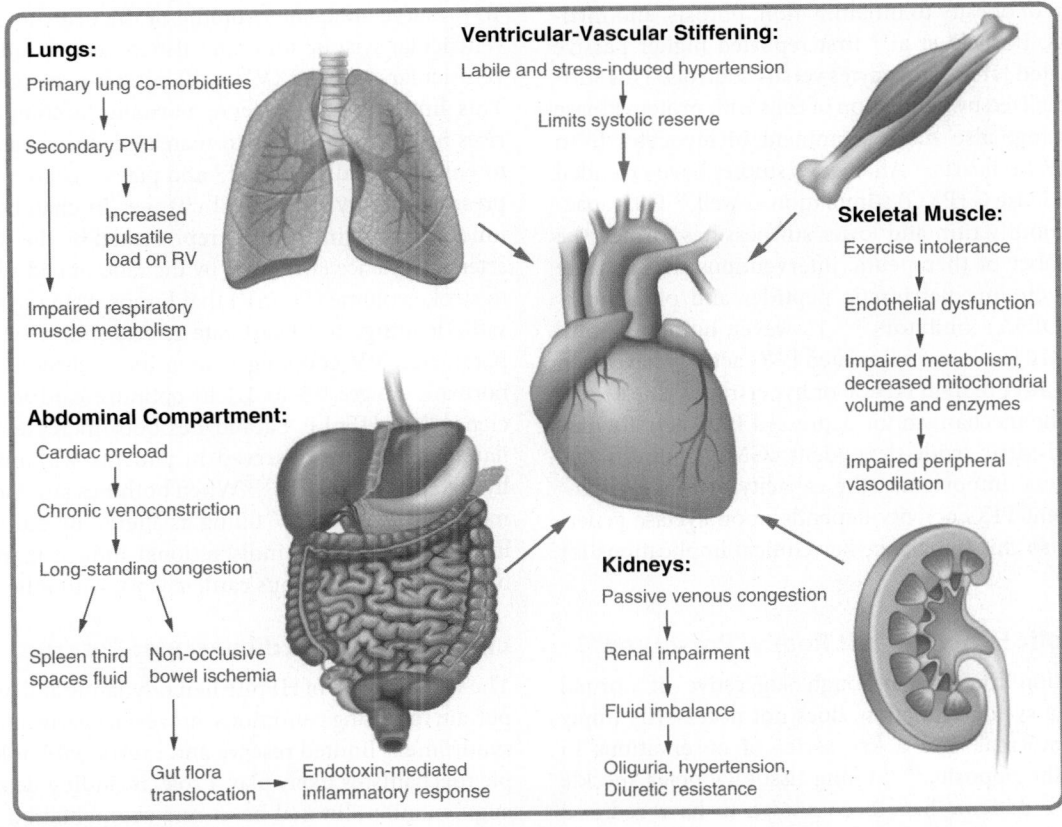

Figure 49–1. Pathophysiology of HFpEF.

Myocardial Stiffness, Fibrosis, and Inflammation

Passive myocardial stiffness is often observed in HFpEF and is considered an important contributor to disease manifestations. Chamber-level analysis has consisted of invasively measured steady-state pressure–volume relations,[2,11] as well as simplified noninvasive estimates.[12] The causes for myocardial stiffening can be divided into factors influencing the extracellular space such as fibrosis and infiltrative processes, and those intrinsic to the myocyte itself. Myocardial fibrosis is a well-established feature of HFrEF and total collagen volume is similarly increased in HFpEF endomyocardial biopsy tissue.[13–16] In 2000, Hahn et al. reported results from a prospective endomyocardial biopsy study in well-characterized HFpEF patients.[16] Myocardial fibrosis was increased in HFpEF compared to donor-controls; however, it was mild in severity in the majority of cases.[16] Both collagen type I and type III expression and tissue staining are elevated in HFpEF and are coupled to reduced collagenase, metalloproteinase-1 (MMP-1), but increased tissue inhibitor of MMP (TIMP-1) expression, which may further enhance fibrosis.[17,18] In addition to altering matrix turnover, cross-linking of collagen including the formation of advanced glycation end products (AGEs) contribute to fibrosis and stiffening.[19,20] Potential mechanisms for the altered matrix structure include inflammation, diabetes, and neurohumoral stimuli such as the renin-angiotensin-aldosterone system (RAAS). Markers of inflammatory cells are found in HFpEF tissue,[16,18] including in the Hahn et al. study, and have been proposed to play an important role in the disease.[21,22] Of increasing interest is the role of obesity, the growing predominant phenotype of HFpEF,[23] and the relationship of obesity to inflammation, fibrosis, and myocardial stiffness. Borbely et al.[13] first reported higher passive stiffness in isolated HFpEF myocytes versus controls. This stiffening was normalized by incubation of cells with protein kinase A (PKA), a change also more prominent in myocytes from HFpEF than HFrEF hearts.[15] Analogous studies have extended this to protein kinase G (PKG) stimulation as well.[24] The capacity of PKG to modify titin and lower stiffness has formed the basis for a number of therapeutic interventions that activate this pathway including natriuretic peptides and phosphodiesterase 5A (PDE5A) inhibitors.[25,26] However, human HFpEF myocardial cGMP levels and associated PKG activity have been observed to be lower than in HFrEF or hypertrophy due to aortic stenosis.[24] The mechanism for depressed PKG activity may involve reduced nitric oxide-dependent cGMP synthesis due to oxidative stress. Importantly, the capacity of PDE5A inhibition to augment PKG activity depends upon cyclase generation of cGMP, so this imbalance has clinical implications for treatments.

Resting Systolic Function: Is It Really "Preserved"?

Preserved ejection fraction, although suggestive of normal contractility and systolic function, does not necessarily imply that systole is normal, and a key series of observations in fact suggested the opposite.[27–30] Using tissue Doppler speckle tracking, HFpEF patients have been shown to have reduced longitudinal and circumferential strain compared to age- and gender-matched hypertensive patients with diastolic dysfunction but without clinical HF.[31] However, studies employing catheterization with imaging or conductance catheter measurements to derive pressure–volume relations find resting load-independent indexes of systolic function are essentially normal in HFpEF.[32–34] Some measures of systole, such as end-systolic elastance (Ees) a measure of systolic stiffening, have been reported as higher in HFpEF,[12,34] although this seems particularly true in urban populations with a high Black population. Rather than implying increased resting contractility, the higher Ees may reflect myocardial hypertrophy, fibrosis, infiltrative disease, and/or titin modifications. Until recently, we had very little data from human myocardial tissue to understand contractility in HFpEF. In a recent study by Aslam et al., right ventricular (RV) sarcomere contractility from endomyocardial biopsy samples was compared between a predominantly hypertensive-LVH phenotype of HFpEF to a predominantly obese phenotype of HFpEF.[35] Strikingly, while RV sarcomere contractility was preserved in the hypertensive-hypertrophied group, it was markedly depressed by ~40% in the obesity group in comparison; body mass index (BMI) strongly and inversely correlating with maximal sarcomere tension.[35]

Ventricular–Arterial Coupling

Systolic ejection involves the interaction of time-varying properties of the ventricular pump and the vascular impedance to which it is connected. Vascular stiffening has long been associated with aging and is exacerbated by comorbidities such as hypertension, obesity, diabetes, and chronic kidney disease. To preserve adequate coupling of the heart to arterial system, ventricular systolic stiffening also increases, and this combined ventricular–vascular (VV) stiffening is a feature of HFpEF.[3,5,36] This limits systolic reserve normally accompanying further rises in Ees, contributes to increased cardiac energy demands to enhance cardiac output,[3] and plays a central role in arterial pressure lability with small changes in chamber preload volume. VV coupling is often represented by the ratio of effective arterial elastance (Ea) given by the ratio of end-systolic pressure to stroke volume (Pes/SV) that lumps systemic resistance, pulsatile loading, and heart rate effects into a single "afterload" parameter. VV coupling is then indexed by Ea/Ees ratio that normally ranges 0.5 to 1.2 to optimize cardiac work and efficiency.[37] In HFpEF, Ea and Ees both increase, although similar increases are observed in patients without HF but with hypertension (±LVH).[3,12] When both Ees and Ea are increased, modest changes in LV filling as altered by diuresis or sodium loading (eg, dietary indiscretions) induce marked swings in blood pressure and thus cardiac work with little change in SV.[3]

Limitations of Cardiovascular Reserve

The vast majority of HFpEF hemodynamic and myocardial data pertain to resting conditions; however, nearly ubiquitous to this syndrome is limited reserve and exertional intolerance. Multiple mechanisms likely play a role, including depressed systolic augmentation, limited heart rate augmentation (chronotropic incompetence), diastolic filling abnormalities, and reduced peripheral vascular dilation. Kitzman et al. reported among the first studies of exercise capacity in HFpEF patients and highlighted failure of these patients to increase end-diastolic volume and thus engage the Frank–Starling mechanism.[38] Borlaug et al. also found reduced exercise capacity and peak oxygen consumption in a HFpEF group related to reduced cardiac output reserve; however, rather than being from impaired diastolic filling, low carbon monoxide augmentation was related to a failure to enhance heart rate and peripherally vasodilate.[39] Chronotropic incompetence has since been reported by multiple investigators[40,41] and found in large trials[42] and impaired peripheral vasodilation has been documented in exercised HFpEF patients using MRI.[43] Borlaug et al. examined cardiac systolic reserve in exercising HFpEF subjects and found that in addition to peripheral dilation and HR limitations, contractility increases were also depressed, resulting in VV mismatching.[32] More recently, obese HFpEF patients have been shown to have worse exercise capacity (peak oxygen consumption), higher biventricular filling pressures with exercise, and depressed pulmonary artery vasodilator reserve than nonobese HFpEF.[23]

Role of Inflammation

Results from LV endomyocardial biopsy[24] and analyses of inflammatory cell markers[18] suggest increased oxidative stress and depressed nitric oxide signaling resulting in inflammation play a key role in this syndrome.[21,22] The aforementioned endomyocardial biopsy study from HFpEF demonstrated increased CD68+ staining macrophages in HFpEF myocardium compared to donor-controls and HFrEF.[35] The multitude of HFpEF comorbidities may contribute to a proinflammatory state,[44] because circulating inflammatory cytokines such as interleukin-6 (IL-6), tumor necrosis factor-α (TNF-α), soluble ST2, and pentraxin 3 are elevated in HFpEF.[45–48] Systemic inflammation has been postulated to lead to endothelial dysfunction supported by higher expression of vascular cell adhesion molecules such as VCAM-1, E-selectin, and reactive oxygen species (ROS),[18] with downstream implications for bioavailable nitric oxide and cGMP/PKG activation.

Myocardial Transcriptomics

In a recent first in human myocardial gene expression analysis study in 41 HFpEF patients, Hahn et al. compared HFpEF to HFrEF (explanted hearts with dilated cardiomyopathy) and to controls (unused donor hearts).[49] Using RNAseq, the group reported strong within-group clustering of these three groups that remained so after adjusting for major differentiating clinical features (sex, age, body mass index, renal function, and diabetes). Interestingly, although there were many gene changes shared by both HFpEF and HFrEF, thousands were uniquely altered in HFpEF. Uniquely upregulated genes were enriched for mitochondrial ATP synthesis and electron transport pathways, whereas HFpEF-specific down-regulated genes were in endoplasmic reticulum stress, angiogenesis, and autophagy. Sex had no impact on the results, and while adjusting for BMI removed most enrichment in up-regulated gene pathways it had no impact on down-regulated gene pathways. Using agnostic

clustering methods (eg, nonnegative matrix factorization), three HFpEF subgroups with distinctive clinical and hemodynamic features were identified, based solely on their transcriptomes, including a group closest to HFrEF with significantly higher mortality.[49] Further study is needed to better understand molecular mechanisms in HFpEF that may help identify therapeutic targets.

COMORBIDITIES IN HFPEF

Pulmonary Hypertension and Right Ventricular Dysfunction

Pulmonary hypertension (PH) defined by a mean pulmonary artery (PA) pressure >25 mm Hg is commonly associated with HFrEF and harbingers a worse outcome. Data on PH in HFpEF are more limited, but studies have reported a fairly high prevalence that importantly predicts increased morbidity and mortality.[50–52] The development of PH in HFpEF has been linked to chronic left atrial (LA) dysfunction, diffuse endothelial dysfunction, and myocardial stiffness leading to advanced disease[53,54] Beyond postcapillary PH attributable to LV volume overload and pulmonary venous hypertension (PVH), subsets of individuals with HFpEF have been shown to have combined postcapillary PH with precapillary pulmonary arterial hypertension (PAH) consistent with underlying pulmonary vascular disease.[55] Pulmonary artery systolic pressure (PASP) has been observed to rise along with pulmonary capillary wedge pressure (PCWP) in patients with both hypertension and HFpEF; however, after adjusting for PCWP, PASP was still higher in HFpEF.[51] Borlaug has demonstrated that many HFpEF patients who have normal PCWP at rest display marked increases with supine exercise associated with PAH.[56] The implications of such data are that many patients with PH may have an underrecognized component of PVH linked to left-sided HF (including HFpEF) that is more manifest under conditions of exertion or volume loading.[57] Finally, RV dysfunction is a well-established predictor of poor outcomes and increased mortality in HFrEF, and is notably worse in obese HFpEF.[23,35,50]

Atrial Fibrillation

Atrial fibrillation (AF) prevalence in HFpEF is approximately 21% to 41% and represents a significant comorbid condition in HFpEF.[29,58,59] Both conditions have been linked to a generalized proinflammatory state, microvascular dysfunction, and myocardial fibrosis. AF may increase risk of incident HFpEF through development of LA remodeling and LV fibrosis, while HFpEF may lead to development AF through LA dilation from elevated LV pressures.[60] The association between the two is complicated by subclinical development and progression of both diseases with overlapping symptomatology; however, studies suggest that one can lead to the other.[61,62] Studies suggest that individuals with concomitant HFpEF and AF have worse outcomes in terms of mortality and event-free survival driven in part by cerebrovascular disease;[63] further study is needed regarding best treatment strategies for AF in HFpEF.

Coronary Artery Disease

Coronary artery disease (CAD) represents a common comorbidity for individuals with HFpEF and mechanistically can contribute to the diastolic and systolic abnormalities involved in HFpEF.[64,65] Although ischemic events are traditionally associated with HFrEF, there is equal likelihood of development of HFpEF or HFrEF from CAD, especially early after diagnosis from an incident event. CAD in HFpEF portends worse overall survival, increased mortality from cardiovascular disease, increased risk of sudden death, and increased risk of development of reduced ejection fraction.[64,65]

Renal Dysfunction

Chronic kidney disease occurs in 26% to 53% of HFpEF and is associated with poor prognosis.[58,66,67] Beyond baseline impairment, worsening renal function during HFpEF hospital admission predicts higher mortality at 6 months, with a 7-year survival of only 9%.[67] The underlying mechanisms of how renal dysfunction (as a complication of other comorbidities) is implicated in myocardial inflammation, fibrosis, and resultant HFpEF are unclear. There are intriguing pathways that may link renal and cardiac disease such as transient receptor potential channel-6 (TRPC6), a Gq-receptor and ROS activated nonselective cation channel that plays an important role in proteinuria and glomerular dysfunction[68] as well as cardiac hypertrophy[69] and fibrosis.[70]

Obesity

Correlating with the obesity epidemic at a population level,[71] the obesity subgroup of HFpEF is increasingly becoming the predominant phenotype in HFpEF.[23,72] Up to 80% of HFpEF patients have been reported to be obese, and this proportion is expected to rise.[71] The obesity subgroup is associated with worse outcomes by survival and burden of symptoms; although, there does appear to be a paradoxical protective effect with mild obesity that is not fully understood. Clinically, obese HFpEF patients demonstrate worse RV function, worse hemodynamic changes during exercise, and demonstrate evidence of pericardial restraint.[23,72] Tissue-based investigations are beginning to reveal distinct pathophysiology and molecular changes that in the obesity subgroup including impaired sarcomere function in obese HFpEF, mitochondrial dysfunction, autophagy, and angiogenesis.[35,49]

TREATMENT FOR HFPEF

Patients with an LVEF below or equal to 40% are usually defined as having HFrEF and those with an LVEF greater than 40% are defined as HFpEF. Based on this definition, the prevalence of HFrEF and HFpEF is approximately 50% each.[73] Patients with an LVEF between 41% and 49% are often referred to as HF with midrange or mildly reduced ejection fraction.[74] Additionally, one should note that LVEF is a dynamic measure that may change with time and medical therapies. For example, some HFrEF patients may transition to HFpEF and vice versa; however, optimal HF treatment should not be stopped in the case of LVEF recovery because many patients who have recovered their LVEF may relapse following treatment withdrawal.[75] Furthermore, it should be noted that an LVEF >40% or even 50% does not exclude a systolic impairment of the LV. Among various limitations of LVEF as a diagnostic tool is the confounding effect of LVH and increased afterload. There is a difference between LV chamber function (ie, fractional shortening or LVEF) and myocardial function (ie, midwall shortening). Because the myocardial contractile element is located in the midwall, the estimation of LV systolic function depends on the distance from the endocardium to the midwall. In the estimation of the LVEF, the wall is assumed to be thin. However, this is not the case in concentric remodeling and hypertrophy, where, a seemingly normal LVEF is accompanied by a depressed midwall shortening, lower cardiac output, and higher peripheral resistance. Additionally, in the context of concentric LVH, the LVEF may appear normal or supranormal despite a substantial reduction in myocardial shortening and stroke volume.[76] Therefore, the myocardial contractile function in the context of hypertrophy (often present in HFpEF) may be depressed despite a "preserved" LVEF. A truly depressed ejection fraction may be better captured by measurements of longitudinal LV strain.[77] As consequence, HFpEF is a heterogeneous condition in terms of pathophysiological triggers and clinical presentation; therefore, assigning patients to clinical subphenotypes may allow the identification and development of more targeted treatment strategies.[78] But for the average HFpEF patient enrolled in randomized controlled outcome trials (RCTs), the optimal treatment strategy is not as well established as the treatment for patients with HFrEF due to the paucity of clearly "positive" outcome trials.[79–81] Importantly, patients with HFpEF often have multiple comorbid conditions (eg, hypertension, diabetes, and chronic kidney disease) that should be targeted with therapy; however, the choice of the "optimal" medical therapy for HFpEF (ie, therapy that can improve outcomes) while also targeting the comorbid conditions requires some in-depth analysis of the available data.

Pharmacological Treatment

Several landmark RCTs provided robust evidence that angiotensin-converting enzyme inhibitors (ACEi), angiotensin receptor blockers (ARBs), β-blockers, mineralocorticoid receptor antagonists (MRAs), sacubitril/valsartan, and the sodium-glucose cotransporter 2 inhibitors (SGLT2i) dapagliflozin and empagliflozin significantly improve mortality and morbidity in HFrEF.[79–83] All of these treatments have been tested in HFpEF but, in many cases, with different results from those found in HFrEF.

Angiotensin Receptor Blockers

In the Candesartan in Heart Failure: Assessment of Reduction in Mortality and Morbidity study (CHARM program), HF patients with an LVEF ≤40% were allocated to the CHARM-Added (candesartan vs placebo added to standard treatment including ACEi) or CHARM-Alternative (if intolerant to ACEi) trials, and patients with LVEF >40% were allocated to the CHARM-Preserved trial.[84] CHARM-Preserved included 3023 patients (65% of the patients had an LVEF ≥50% and 35%

an LVEF >40% and <50%). A 14% relative reduction in the rate of the primary outcome (a composite of cardiovascular death or HF hospitalization) with candesartan versus placebo was seen, but it did not reach statistical significance (unadjusted hazard ratio [HR], 0.86; 95% confidence interval [CI], 0.77–1.03; $P = 0.12$). In the prespecified covariate adjusted analysis, the treatment effect became more pronounced (HR 0.86; 95% CI, 0.74–1.00; $P = 0.051$). Moreover, fewer patients were hospitalized for HF in the candesartan group (230 vs 279; $P = 0.017$). Together, these findings support, at least, a moderate impact of candesartan for preventing HF admissions among patients who have HF and an LVEF >40%.[84]

The I-PRESERVE (Irbesartan in Heart Failure with Preserved Ejection Fraction) trial tested the ARB irbesartan versus placebo in 4133 patients with an LVEF ≥45% who were aged 60 or older.[85] Irbesartan did not reduce mortality nor hospitalizations for cardiovascular causes (HR, 0.95; 95% CI, 0.86–1.05; $P = 0.35$) nor HF hospitalizations (HR, 0.95; 95% CI, 0.81–1.10; $P = 0.50$). A post hoc analysis adjusting for prognostic baseline variables suggested some benefit with irbesartan (HR 0.87; 95% CI, 0.77–0.99; $P = 0.039$) for the composite of cardiovascular death or HF hospitalization.[86]

Angiotensin-Converting Enzyme Inhibitors

In the PEP-CHF (Perindopril in Elderly People with Chronic Heart Failure) study, a total of 850 patients aged 70 years or older with an echocardiogram suggesting diastolic dysfunction and excluding substantial LV systolic dysfunction or valve disease were randomized to receive either perindopril 4 mg or placebo.[87] This trial had a low event rate and a high proportion of treatment withdrawal and open-label ACEi use after the first year of follow-up. The composite endpoint of all-cause mortality or HF hospitalization was not different between groups. By 1 year, treatment with perindopril improved symptoms, exercise capacity, and reduced hospitalizations for HF (HR, 0.63; 95% CI, 0.41–0.97; $P = 0.033$).

β-Blockers and Ivabradine

β-blockers have been postulated as potentially beneficial to HFpEF patients because heart rate lowering could improve early diastolic filling and reduce the myocardial oxygen demand. However, trial data did not show beneficial effects of β-blockers for patients with an LVEF >40%. The ELANDD (Effects of Long-term Administration of Nebivolol on the clinical symptoms, exercise capacity, and left ventricular function of patients with Diastolic Dysfunction) study did not show benefit of nebivolol in symptoms or exercise capacity among 116 patients with an LVEF >45% and evidence of diastolic dysfunction.[88] The Beta-blockers in Heart Failure Collaborative Group recently pooled individual patient-level data from double-blind RCTs in HF in order to examine the effects of β-blockers across the spectrum of LVEF.[89] Among 14,262 patients in sinus rhythm, β-blockers improved LVEF and prognosis for patients with an LVEF <40%, with a similar benefit for patients with an LVEF 40% to 49%, and no benefit seen in patients with an LVEF ≥50% but only 244 patients could be analyzed in this subgroup.

It should also be mentioned that in patients with HFpEF and a heart rate ≥70 bpm, the I(f) channel inhibitor ivabradine did not improve filling pressures, functional capacity, or NT-proBNP levels.[90]

Mineralocorticoid Receptor Antagonists

Mineralocorticoid receptor antagonists can improve endothelial function and cardiac remodeling, and reduced fibrosis and vascular stiffness.[91] In the Aldo-DHF (Aldosterone Receptor Blockade in Diastolic Heart Failure) trial, spironolactone (vs placebo) improved echocardiographic markers of LV diastolic function, and reduced LV mass and the circulating levels of NT-pro BNP.[92] The TOPCAT (Treatment of Preserved Cardiac Function Heart Failure with an Aldosterone Antagonist) trial investigated the prognostic effect of spironolactone versus placebo in 3,445 patients with an LVEF ≥45% randomized in North America, South America, and Canada (ie, the Americas) and Russia/Georgia (ie, Eastern Europe).[93] The primary outcome was a composite endpoint of cardiovascular death or HF hospitalization. Spironolactone did not reduce the primary outcome (HR, 0.89; 95% CI, 0.77–1.04; $P = 0.14$) but did reduced HF hospitalizations (HR, 0.83; 95% CI, 0.69–0.99; $P = 0.04$). However, marked regional variations were seen in the trial, whereby patients from Eastern Europe had event rates similar to the general population of those countries and not compatible with HFpEF, did not experience rises in serum potassium and creatinine while randomized to spironolactone, and the analysis of blood spironolactone metabolites showed a low treatment adherence in Eastern Europe.[94,95] Taking these differences into account, spironolactone did reduce primary outcome events in the Americas (27.3% events in the spironolactone group vs 31.8% events in the placebo group [HR, 0.82; 95% CI, 0.69–0.98; $P = 0.026$]) but not in Eastern Europe (9.3% events in the spironolactone vs 8.4% events in the placebo group [HR, 1.10; 95% CI, 0.79–1.51; $P = 0.58$]). Taken together, these findings show superiority of spironolactone versus placebo in patients with HFpEF.

Angiotensin Receptor Neprilysin Inhibitor

The first-in-class Angiotensin Receptor Neprilysin inhibitor (ARNi) sacubitril/valsartan decreased the risk of HF hospitalization or cardiovascular death versus enalapril by 20% in patients with HFrEF.[96] A phase-II study documented greater reductions in NT-proBNP, LA size, blood pressure, and dyspnea with ARNi compared to valsartan in HF patients with an LVEF >45%.[97] These data served as basis for the PARAGON-HF (Efficacy and Safety of LCZ696 Compared to Valsartan on Morbidity and Mortality in Heart Failure Patients With Preserved Ejection Fraction trial) trial, an RCT examining the efficacy and safety of sacubitril/valsartan versus valsartan. A total of 4822 patients aged 50 years or older with an LVEF ≥45%, structural cardiac alterations, and increased natriuretic peptides were enrolled. The primary outcome was a composite of total hospitalizations for HF or cardiovascular mortality.[98] Compared with valsartan, sacubitril/valsartan narrowly failed statistical significance for the reduction in the event rate of the primary outcome (risk reduction [RR] 0.87; 95% CI, 0.75–1.01;

P = 0.06). Subgroup analyses showed that patients with an LVEF below the median (of 57%), women, and those with a recent HF hospitalization could benefit more from sacubitril/valsartan.[99-101] Additionally, sacubitril/valsartan led to significant improvements in quality-of-life scores and New York Heart Association (NYHA) class, as well as lower rates of renal events and worsening renal function, particularly when combined with a mineralocorticoid receptor antagonist.[102]

It is important to highlight that PARAGON-HF tested sacubitril/valsartan versus valsartan as the active comparator. A putative placebo analysis suggested a clear treatment benefit of sacubitril/valsartan versus putative placebo for HF hospitalization or cardiovascular death across the full range of LVEF up to 60%.[103]

The PARALLAX (Randomized, Double-blind Controlled Study Comparing LCZ696 to Medical Therapy for Comorbidities in HFpEF Patients) trial (NCT number: NCT03066804) studied the effects of sacubitril/valsartan in 2566 NYHA class II to IV patients with an LVEF >40%, structural heart disease, and increased NT-proBNP. The study population was stratified into three groups based on background therapy: enalapril, valsartan, and placebo without ACEi or ARB. Overall, sacubitril/valsartan reduced NT-proBNP, but it did not improve 6-minute walk distance nor health-related quality of life.[104]

Sodium-Glucose Cotransporter 2 Inhibitors

Compared with placebo, SGLT1/2i reduced morbidity and mortality (particularly HF hospitalizations) in patients with type 2 diabetes and a high cardiovascular risk, type 2 diabetes and chronic kidney disease, type 2 diabetes and worsening HF, and HFrEF with and without diabetes.[82,105-108] While some of the patients enrolled in SGLT1/2i trials had HFpEF, a more robust answer was provided by the EMPEROR-Preserved trial (Empagliflozin Outcome trial in Patients with Chronic Heart Failure with Preserved Ejection Fraction), where, compared with placebo, empagliflozin reduced the composite of cardiovascular death or heart failure hospitalizations by 21% (HR, 0.79; 95% CI, 0.69–0.90; *P* <0.001) and recurrent HF hospitalizations by 27% (HR, 0.73; 95% CI, 0.61–0.88; *P* <0.001) with no treatment effect modification by diabetes status or LVEF for the primary outcome.[109] These results may be further confirmed by the DELIVER (Dapagliflozin Evaluation to Improve the Lives of Patients With Preserved Ejection Fraction Heart Failure) trial (NCT03619213). While at the time of the writing of this chapter, the practice guidelines for HFpEF are not updated, based on the results of the EMPEROR-Preserved trial, the use of empagliflozin in patients with HFpEF should be considered in all patients unless there are contraindications or tolerability concerns.

Devices

Currently approved and novel device therapies that are in the pipeline generally allow targeting of a structural or neurohormonal abnormality that is not directly amendable to pharmacologic therapeutic interventions. Given the more invasive nature and inherent risk of device-based therapies, they are primarily developed and approved for patients with persistent symptomatic or progressive disease despite optimal HF therapy. Thus, device-based therapies for HF should be considered complementary to pharmacologic therapy

Several device-based therapies have been recently approved for HF, particularly HFrEF (eg, transcatheter edge-to-edge mitral valve repair, cardiac contractility modulation, baroreflex activation therapy). In patients with HF regardless of ejection fraction, phrenic nerve stimulation may be considered for patients with moderate-to-severe central sleep apnea.

Other Treatment Options

Several other agents were tested for the treatment of HFpEF and did not show benefit or require further investigation. These include (but are not limited to) nitrates, statins, soluble guanylyl cyclase stimulators, phosphodiesterase-5 inhibitors, and cytokine inhibitors. More trials examining novel treatments such as antifibrotic, anti-inflammatory, and antioxidant agents, as well as cell therapies, are underway. A detailed description is beyond the scope of this chapter.

Lifestyle Changes

Even though there is limited evidence of the effect of different lifestyle measures in patients with HFpEF, promotion of lifestyle changes, smoking cessation, and weight control is recommended.

The role of salt in the pathophysiology of fluid overload in HFpEF is unclear, and the evidence for salt restriction even for patients with HFrEF is weak.[110] Until more data are available, the current general recommendation of salt restriction to <5 g per day should be followed in patients with HFpEF, who should also be advised to pursue a balanced diet rich in vegetables, legumes, whole grains, fresh fruits, low-fat dairy products, fish, and unsaturated fatty acids, and low in red meat and saturated fatty acids.

Regular exercise has been shown to improve cardiorespiratory fitness and quality of life in patients with HFpEF.[111]

IMPACT AND MANAGEMENT OF ASSOCIATED COMORBIDITIES

Comorbidities are highly prevalent in HFpEF in population-based studies and registries, and include hypertension, AF, CAD, diabetes mellitus, obesity, and chronic kidney disease. Other conditions, such as sleep apnea or iron deficiency, are also frequent. These comorbidities complicate diagnosis, treatment, and prognosis by reducing quality of life and increasing hospitalization and mortality rates.[112] The treatment of comorbidities should be tailored to each patient, but it should include treatments that have been show to improve outcomes (at least reduce hospitalizations) in HFpEF, and these agents are spironolactone and sacubitril/valsartan. For now, the use of SGLT1/2i in people with a preserved ejection fraction should be restricted to patients with diabetes; ongoing trials in HFpEF patients with and without diabetes will better elucidate the role of these agents for the treatment of HFpEF.

REFERENCES

1. Zile MR, Brutsaert DL. New concepts in diastolic dysfunction and diastolic heart failure: Part I: diagnosis, prognosis, and measurements of diastolic function. *Circulation.* 2002;105(11):1387-1393.

2. Wachter R, Schmidt-Schweda S, Westermann D, et al. Blunted frequency-dependent upregulation of cardiac output is related to impaired relaxation in diastolic heart failure. *Eur Heart J.* 2009;30(24):3027-3036. doi: 10.1093/eurheartj/ehp341.

3. Kawaguchi M, Hay I, Fetics B, Kass DA. Combined ventricular systolic and arterial stiffening in patients with heart failure and preserved ejection fraction: implications for systolic and diastolic reserve limitations. *Circulation.* 2003;107(5):714-720.

4. Lester SJ, Tajik AJ, Nishimura RA, Oh JK, Khandheria BK, Seward JB. Unlocking the mysteries of diastolic function: deciphering the Rosetta Stone 10 years later. *J Am Coll Cardiol.* 2008;51(7):679-689. doi: 10.1016/j.jacc.2007.09.061.

5. Lam CS, Roger VL, Rodeheffer RJ, et al. Cardiac structure and ventricular-vascular function in persons with heart failure and preserved ejection fraction from Olmsted County, Minnesota. *Circulation.* 2007;115(15):1982-1990. doi: 10.1161/CIRCULATIONAHA.106.659763.

6. Yamamoto K, Redfield MM, Nishimura RA. Analysis of left ventricular diastolic function. *Heart.* 1996;75(6 Suppl 2):27-35.

7. Melenovsky V, Borlaug BA, Rosen B, et al. Cardiovascular features of heart failure with preserved ejection fraction versus nonfailing hypertensive left ventricular hypertrophy in the urban Baltimore community: the role of atrial remodeling/dysfunction. *J Am Coll Cardiol.* 2007;49(2):198-207. doi: 10.1016/j.jacc.2006.08.050.

8. Hamdani N, Paulus WJ, van Heerebeek L, et al. Distinct myocardial effects of beta-blocker therapy in heart failure with normal and reduced left ventricular ejection fraction. *Eur Heart J.* 2009;30(15):1863-1872. doi:10.1093/eurheartj/ehp189.

9. Helmes M, Lim CC, Liao R, Bharti A, Cui L, Sawyer DB. Titin determines the Frank-Starling relation in early diastole. *J Gen Physiol.* 2003;121(2):97-110.

10. Bell SP, Nyland L, Tischler MD, McNabb M, Granzier H, LeWinter MM. Alterations in the determinants of diastolic suction during pacing tachycardia. *Circ Res.* 2000;87(3):235-240.

11. Penicka M, Bartunek J, Trakalova H, et al. Heart failure with preserved ejection fraction in outpatients with unexplained dyspnea: a pressure-volume loop analysis. *J Am Coll Cardiol.* 2010;55(16):1701-1710. doi: 10.1016/j.jacc.2009.11.076.

12. Lam CS, Roger VL, Rodeheffer RJ, et al. Cardiac structure and ventricular-vascular function in persons with heart failure and preserved ejection fraction from Olmsted County, Minnesota. *Circulation.* 2007;115(15):1982-1990.

13. Borbely A, van der Velden J, Papp Z, et al. Cardiomyocyte stiffness in diastolic heart failure. *Circulation.* 2005;111(6):774-781. doi: 10.1161/01.CIR.0000155257.33485.6D.

14. Kasner M, Westermann D, Lopez B, et al. Diastolic tissue Doppler indexes correlate with the degree of collagen expression and cross-linking in heart failure and normal ejection fraction. *J Am Coll Cardiol.* 2011;57(8):977-985. doi: 10.1016/j.jacc.2010.10.024.

15. van Heerebeek L, Borbely A, Niessen HW, et al. Myocardial structure and function differ in systolic and diastolic heart failure. *Circulation.* 2006;113(16):1966-1973. doi: 10.1161/CIRCULATIONAHA.105.587519.

16. Hahn VS, Yanek LR, Vaishnav J, et al. Endomyocardial biopsy characterization of heart failure with preserved ejection fraction and prevalence of cardiac amyloidosis. *JACC Heart Fail.* 2020;8(9):712-724. doi: 10.1016/j.jchf.2020.04.007.

17. Gonzalez A, Lopez B, Querejeta R, Zubillaga E, Echeverria T, Diez J. Filling pressures and collagen metabolism in hypertensive patients with heart failure and normal ejection fraction. *Hypertension.* 2010;55(6):1418-1424. doi: 10.1161/Hypertensionaha.109.149112.

18. Westermann D, Lindner D, Kasner M, et al. Cardiac inflammation contributes to changes in the extracellular matrix in patients with heart failure and normal ejection fraction. *Circulation Heart Fail.* 2011;4(1):44-52. doi: 10.1161/CIRCHEARTFAILURE.109.931451.

19. van Heerebeek L, Hamdani N, Handoko ML, et al. Diastolic stiffness of the failing diabetic heart: importance of fibrosis, advanced glycation end products, and myocyte resting tension. *Circulation.* 2008;117(1):43-51. doi: 10.1161/circulationaha.107.728550.

20. Badenhorst D, Maseko M, Tsotetsi OJ, et al. Cross-linking influences the impact of quantitative changes in myocardial collagen on cardiac stiffness and remodelling in hypertension in rats. *Cardiovasc Res.* 2003;57(3):632-641.

21. Glezeva N, Baugh JA. Role of inflammation in the pathogenesis of heart failure with preserved ejection fraction and its potential as a therapeutic target. *Heart Failure Rev.* 2013. doi: 10.1007/s10741-013-9405-8.

22. Paulus WJ, Tschope C. A novel paradigm for heart failure with preserved ejection fraction: comorbidities drive myocardial dysfunction and remodeling through coronary microvascular endothelial inflammation. *J Am Coll Cardiol.* 2013;62(4):263-271. doi: 10.1016/j.jacc.2013.02.092.

23. Obokata M, Reddy YNV, Pislaru SV, Melenovsky V, Borlaug BA. Evidence supporting the existence of a distinct obese phenotype of heart failure with preserved ejection fraction. *Circulation.* 2017;136(1):6-19. doi: 10.1161/CIRCULATIONAHA.116.026807.

24. van Heerebeek L, Hamdani N, Falcao-Pires I, et al. Low myocardial protein kinase G activity in heart failure with preserved ejection fraction. *Circulation.* 2012;126(7):830-839. doi: 10.1161/CIRCULATIONAHA.111.076075.

25. Bishu K, Hamdani N, Mohammed SF, et al. Sildenafil and B-type natriuretic peptide acutely phosphorylate titin and improve diastolic distensibility in vivo. *Circulation.* 2011;124(25):2882-2891. doi: 10.1161/CIRCULATIONAHA.111.048520.

26. Hamdani N, Franssen C, Lourenco A, et al. Myocardial titin hypophosphorylation importantly contributes to heart failure with preserved ejection fraction in a rat metabolic risk model. *Circulation Heart Fail.* 2013;6(6):1239-1249. doi: 10.1161/CIRCHEARTFAILURE.113.000539.

27. Bruch C, Gradaus R, Gunia S, Breithardt G, Wichter T. Doppler tissue analysis of mitral annular velocities: evidence for systolic abnormalities in patients with diastolic heart failure. *J Am Soc Echocardiogr.* 2003;16(10):1031-1036. doi: 10.1016/S0894-7317(03)00634-5.

28. Vinereanu D, Nicolaides E, Tweddel AC, Fraser AG. "Pure" diastolic dysfunction is associated with long-axis systolic dysfunction. Implications for the diagnosis and classification of heart failure. *Eur J Heart Fail.* 2005;7(5):820-828. doi: 10.1016/j.ejheart.2005.02.003.

29. Yip G, Wang M, Zhang Y, Fung JW, Ho PY, Sanderson JE. Left ventricular long axis function in diastolic heart failure is reduced in both diastole and systole: time for a redefinition? *Heart.* 2002;87(2):121-125.

30. Yu CM, Lin H, Yang H, Kong SL, Zhang Q, Lee SW. Progression of systolic abnormalities in patients with "isolated" diastolic heart failure and diastolic dysfunction. *Circulation.* 2002;105(10):1195-1201.

31. Kraigher-Krainer E, Shah AM, Gupta DK, et al. Impaired systolic function by strain imaging in heart failure with preserved ejection fraction. *J Am Coll Cardiol.* 2014;63(5):447-456. doi: 10.1016/j.jacc.2013.09.052.

32. Borlaug BA, Olson TP, Lam CS, et al. Global cardiovascular reserve dysfunction in heart failure with preserved ejection fraction. *J Am Coll Cardiol.* 2010;56(11):845-854. doi: 10.1016/j.jacc.2010.03.077.

33. Baicu CF, Zile MR, Aurigemma GP, Gaasch WH. Left ventricular systolic performance, function, and contractility in patients with diastolic heart failure. *Circulation.* 2005;111(18):2306-2312. doi: 10.1161/01.CIR.0000164273.57823.26.

34. Kawaguchi M, Hay I, Fetics B, Kass DA. Combined ventricular systolic and arterial stiffening in patients with heart failure and preserved ejection fraction: implications for systolic and diastolic reserve limitations. *Circulation.* 2003;107(5):714-720.

35. Aslam MI, Hahn VS, Jani V, Hsu S, Sharma K, Kass DA. Reduced right ventricular sarcomere contractility in heart failure with preserved ejection fraction and severe obesity. *Circulation.* 2021;143(9):965-967. doi: 10.1161/CIRCULATIONAHA.120.052414.

36. Borlaug BA, Kass DA. Ventricular-vascular interaction in heart failure. *Cardiol Clin*. 2011;29(3):447-459. doi: 10.1016/j.ccl.2011.06.004.

37. Kelly RP, Ting CT, Yang TM, et al. Effective arterial elastance as index of arterial vascular load in humans. *Circulation*. 1992;86(2):513-521.

38. Kitzman DW, Higginbotham MB, Cobb FR, Sheikh KH, Sullivan MJ. Exercise intolerance in patients with heart failure and preserved left ventricular systolic function: failure of the Frank-Starling mechanism. *J Am Coll Cardiol*. 1991;17(5):1065-1072.

39. Borlaug BA, Melenovsky V, Russell SD, et al. Impaired chronotropic and vasodilator reserves limit exercise capacity in patients with heart failure and a preserved ejection fraction. *Circulation*. 2006;114(20):2138-2147. doi: 10.1161/CIRCULATIONAHA.106.632745.

40. Brubaker PH, Joo KC, Stewart KP, Fray B, Moore B, Kitzman DW. Chronotropic incompetence and its contribution to exercise intolerance in older heart failure patients. *J Cardiopulm Rehabil*. 2006;26(2):86-89.

41. Phan TT, Shivu GN, Abozguia K, et al. Impaired heart rate recovery and chronotropic incompetence in patients with heart failure with preserved ejection fraction. *Circulation Heart Fail*. 2010;3(1):29-34. doi: 10.1161/CIRCHEARTFAILURE.109.877720.

42. Redfield MM, Chen HH, Borlaug BA, et al. Effect of phosphodiesterase-5 inhibition on exercise capacity and clinical status in heart failure with preserved ejection fraction: a randomized clinical trial. *JAMA*. 2013;309(12):1268-1277. doi: 10.1001/jama.2013.2024.

43. Puntawangkoon C, Kitzman DW, Kritchevsky SB, et al. Reduced peripheral arterial blood flow with preserved cardiac output during submaximal bicycle exercise in elderly heart failure. *J Cardiovasc Magn Reson*. 2009;11:48. doi: 10.1186/1532-429X-11-48.

44. Edelmann F, Stahrenberg R, Gelbrich G, et al. Contribution of comorbidities to functional impairment is higher in heart failure with preserved than with reduced ejection fraction. *Clin Res Cardiol*. 2011;100(9):755-764. doi: 10.1007/s00392-011-0305-4.

45. Kalogeropoulos A, Georgiopoulou V, Psaty BM, et al. Inflammatory markers and incident heart failure risk in older adults: the Health ABC (Health, Aging, and Body Composition) study. *J Am Coll Cardiol*. 2010;55(19):2129-2137. doi: 10.1016/j.jacc.2009.12.045.

46. Collier P, Watson CJ, Voon V, et al. Can emerging biomarkers of myocardial remodelling identify asymptomatic hypertensive patients at risk for diastolic dysfunction and diastolic heart failure? *Eur J Heart Fail*. 2011;13(10):1087-1095. doi: 10.1093/eurjhf/hfr079.

47. Shah KB, Kop WJ, Christenson RH, et al. Prognostic utility of ST2 in patients with acute dyspnea and preserved left ventricular ejection fraction. *Clin Chem*. 2011;57(6):874-882. doi: 10.1373/clinchem.2010.159277.

48. Matsubara J, Sugiyama S, Nozaki T, et al. Pentraxin 3 is a new inflammatory marker correlated with left ventricular diastolic dysfunction and heart failure with normal ejection fraction. *J Am Coll Cardiol*. 2011;57(7):861-869. doi: 10.1016/j.jacc.2010.10.018.

49. Hahn VS, Knutsdottir H, Luo X, et al. Myocardial gene expression signatures in human heart failure with preserved ejection fraction. *Circulation*. 2020. doi: 10.1161/CIRCULATIONAHA.120.050498.

50. Burke MA, Katz DH, Beussink L, et al. Prognostic importance of pathophysiologic markers in patients with heart failure and preserved ejection fraction. *Circ Heart Fail*. 2014;7(2):288-299. doi: 10.1161/CIRCHEARTFAILURE.113.000854.

51. Lam CS, Roger VL, Rodeheffer RJ, Borlaug BA, Enders FT, Redfield MM. Pulmonary hypertension in heart failure with preserved ejection fraction: a community-based study. *J Am Coll Cardiol*. 2009;53(13):1119-1126. doi: 10.1016/j.jacc.2008.11.051.

52. Shah AM, Shah SJ, Anand IS, et al. Cardiac structure and function in heart failure with preserved ejection fraction: baseline findings from the echocardiographic study of the treatment of preserved cardiac function heart failure with an aldosterone antagonist trial. *Circ Heart Fail*. 2013. doi:10.1161/CIRCHEARTFAILURE.113.000887.

53. Guazzi M, Ghio S, Adir Y. Pulmonary Hypertension in HFpEF and HFrEF: JACC Review Topic of the Week. *J Am Coll Cardiol*. 2020;76(9):1102-1111. doi: 10.1016/j.jacc.2020.06.069.

54. Guazzi M. Pulmonary hypertension in heart failure preserved ejection fraction: prevalence, pathophysiology, and clinical perspectives. *Circ Heart Fail*. 2014;7(2):367-377. doi: 10.1161/CIRCHEARTFAILURE.113.000823.

55. Dixon DD, Trivedi A, Shah SJ. Combined post- and pre-capillary pulmonary hypertension in heart failure with preserved ejection fraction. *Heart Fail Rev*. 2016;21(3):285-297. doi: 10.1007/s10741-015-9523-6.

56. Borlaug BA, Nishimura RA, Sorajja P, Lam CS, Redfield MM. Exercise hemodynamics enhance diagnosis of early heart failure with preserved ejection fraction. *Circ Heart Fail*. 2010;3(5):588-595. doi: 10.1161/CIRCHEARTFAILURE.109.930701.

57. Borlaug BA. Invasive assessment of pulmonary hypertension: time for a more fluid approach? *Circ Heart Fail*. 2014;7(1):2-4. doi: 10.1161/CIRCHEARTFAILURE.113.000983.

58. Yancy CW, Lopatin M, Stevenson LW, De Marco T, Fonarow GC. Clinical presentation, management, and in-hospital outcomes of patients admitted with acute decompensated heart failure with preserved systolic function: a report from the Acute Decompensated Heart Failure National Registry (ADHERE) Database. *J Am Coll Cardiol*. 2006;47(1):76-84. doi: 10.1016/j.jacc.2005.09.022.

59. Fonarow GC, Stough WG, Abraham WT, et al. Characteristics, treatments, and outcomes of patients with preserved systolic function hospitalized for heart failure: a report from the OPTIMIZE-HF Registry. *J Am Coll Cardiol*. 2007;50(8):768-777. doi: 10.1016/j.jacc.2007.04.064.

60. Packer M, Lam CSP, Lund LH, Redfield MM. Interdependence of atrial fibrillation and heart failure with a preserved ejection fraction reflects a common underlying atrial and ventricular myopathy. *Circulation*. 2020;141(1):4-6. doi: 10.1161/CIRCULATIONAHA.119.042996.

61. Zakeri R, Chamberlain AM, Roger VL, Redfield MM. Temporal relationship and prognostic significance of atrial fibrillation in heart failure patients with preserved ejection fraction: a community-based study. *Circulation*. 2013;128(10):1085-1093. doi: 10.1161/CIRCULATIONAHA.113.001475.

62. Oluleye OW, Rector TS, Win S, et al. History of atrial fibrillation as a risk factor in patients with heart failure and preserved ejection fraction. *Circ Heart Fail*. Nov 2014;7(6):960-966. doi: 10.1161/CIRCHEARTFAILURE.114.001523.

63. Zafrir B, Lund LH, Laroche C, et al. Prognostic implications of atrial fibrillation in heart failure with reduced, mid-range, and preserved ejection fraction: a report from 14 964 patients in the European Society of Cardiology Heart Failure Long-Term Registry. *Eur Heart J*. 2018;39(48):4277-4284. doi: 10.1093/eurheartj/ehy626.

64. Choudhury L, Gheorghiade M, Bonow RO. Coronary artery disease in patients with heart failure and preserved systolic function. *Am J Cardiol*. 2002;89(6):719-722.

65. Hwang SJ, Melenovsky V, Borlaug BA. Implications of coronary artery disease in heart failure with preserved ejection fraction. *J Am Coll Cardiol*. 2014;63(25 Pt A):2817-2827. doi: 10.1016/j.jacc.2014.03.034.

66. Shah SJ, Heitner JF, Sweitzer NK, et al. Baseline characteristics of patients in the treatment of preserved cardiac function heart failure with an aldosterone antagonist trial. *Circ Heart Fail*. 2013;6(2):184-192. doi: 10.1161/CIRCHEARTFAILURE.112.972794.

67. Rusinaru D, Buiciuc O, Houpe D, Tribouilloy C. Renal function and long-term survival after hospital discharge in heart failure with preserved ejection fraction. *Int J Cardiol*. 2011;147(2):278-282. doi: 10.1016/j.ijcard.2009.09.529.

68. Dryer SE, Reiser J. TRPC6 channels and their binding partners in podocytes: role in glomerular filtration and pathophysiology. *Am J Physiol Renal Physiol*. 2010;299(4):F689-701. doi: 10.1152/ajprenal.00298.2010.

69. Eder P, Molkentin JD. TRPC channels as effectors of cardiac hypertrophy. *CircRes*. 2011;108(2):265-272.

70. Davis J, Burr AR, Davis GF, Birnbaumer L, Molkentin JD. A TRPC6-dependent pathway for myofibroblast transdifferentiation and wound healing in vivo. *Development Cell* 2012;23(4):705-715. doi: 10.1016/j.devcel.2012.08.017.

71. Dunlay SM, Roger VL, Redfield MM. Epidemiology of heart failure with preserved ejection fraction. *Nat Rev Cardiol*. 2017;14(10):591-602. doi: 10.1038/nrcardio.2017.65

72. Reddy YNV, Lewis GD, Shah SJ, et al. Characterization of the obese phenotype of heart failure with preserved ejection fraction: a RELAX trial ancillary study. *Mayo Clin Proc.* 2019;94(7):1199-1209. doi: 10.1016/j.mayocp.2018.11.037.

73. Bhatia RS, Tu JV, Lee DS, et al. Outcome of heart failure with preserved ejection fraction in a population-based study. *N Engl J Med.* 2006;355(3):260-269. doi: 10.1056/NEJMoa051530.

74. Bozkurt B, Coats AJ, Tsutsui H, et al. Universal definition and classification of heart failure: a report of the Heart Failure Society of America, Heart Failure Association of the European Society of Cardiology, Japanese Heart Failure Society and Writing Committee of the Universal Definition of Heart Failure. *J Card Fail.* 2021. doi: 10.1016/j.cardfail.2021.01.022.

75. Halliday BP, Wassall R, Lota AS, et al. Withdrawal of pharmacological treatment for heart failure in patients with recovered dilated cardiomyopathy (TRED-HF): an open-label, pilot, randomised trial. *Lancet.* 2019;393(10166):61-73. doi: 10.1016/s0140-6736(18)32484-x.

76. Aurigemma GP, Silver KH, Priest MA, Gaasch WH. Geometric changes allow normal ejection fraction despite depressed myocardial shortening in hypertensive left ventricular hypertrophy. *J Am Coll Cardiol.* 1995;26(1):195-202. doi: 10.1016/0735-1097(95)00153-q.

77. Stokke TM, Hasselberg NE, Smedsrud MK, et al. Geometry as a confounder when assessing ventricular systolic function: comparison between ejection fraction and strain. *J Am Coll Cardiol.* 2017;70(8):942-954. doi: 10.1016/j.jacc.2017.06.046.

78. Lam CSP, Voors AA, de Boer RA, Solomon SD, van Veldhuisen DJ. Heart failure with preserved ejection fraction: from mechanisms to therapies. *Eur Heart J.* 2018;39(30):2780-2792. doi: 10.1093/eurheartj/ehy301.

79. Ponikowski P, Voors AA, Anker SD, et al. 2016 ESC Guidelines for the diagnosis and treatment of acute and chronic heart failure: the Task Force for the diagnosis and treatment of acute and chronic heart failure of the European Society of Cardiology (ESC). Developed with the special contribution of the Heart Failure Association (HFA) of the ESC. *Eur J Heart Fail.* 2016. doi:10.1002/ejhf.592.

80. Yancy CW, Jessup M, Bozkurt B, et al. 2016 ACC/AHA/HFSA focused update on new pharmacological therapy for heart failure: an update of the 2013 ACCF/AHA guideline for the management of heart failure: a report of the American College of Cardiology/American Heart Association Task Force on Clinical Practice Guidelines and the Heart Failure Society of America. *J Am Coll Cardiol.* 2016. doi: 10.1016/j.jacc.2016.05.011.

81. Yancy CW, Jessup M, Bozkurt B, et al. 2017 ACC/AHA/HFSA focused update of the 2013 ACCF/AHA guideline for the management of heart failure: a report of the American College of Cardiology/American Heart Association Task Force on Clinical Practice Guidelines and the Heart Failure Society of America. *J Am Coll Cardiol.* 2017;70(6):776-803. doi: 10.1016/j.jacc.2017.04.025.

82. Zannad F, Ferreira JP, Pocock SJ, et al. SGLT2 inhibitors in patients with heart failure with reduced ejection fraction: a meta-analysis of the EMPEROR-Reduced and DAPA-HF trials. *Lancet.* 2020. doi: 10.1016/s0140-6736(20)31824-9.

83. Vaduganathan M, Claggett BL, Jhund PS, et al. Estimating lifetime benefits of comprehensive disease-modifying pharmacological therapies in patients with heart failure with reduced ejection fraction: a comparative analysis of three randomised controlled trials. *Lancet.* 2020;396(10244):121-128. doi: 10.1016/s0140-6736(20)30748-0.

84. Yusuf S, Pfeffer MA, Swedberg K, et al. Effects of candesartan in patients with chronic heart failure and preserved left-ventricular ejection fraction: the CHARM-Preserved Trial. *Lancet.* 2003;362(9386):777-781. doi: 10.1016/s0140-6736(03)14285-7.

85. Massie BM, Carson PE, McMurray JJ, et al. Irbesartan in patients with heart failure and preserved ejection fraction. *N Engl J Med.* 2008;359(23):2456-2467. doi: 10.1056/NEJMoa0805450.

86. Ferreira JP, Dewan P, Jhund PS, et al. Covariate adjusted reanalysis of the I-Preserve trial. *Clin Res Cardiol.* 2020. doi: 10.1007/s00392-020-01632-x.

87. Cleland JG, Tendera M, Adamus J, Freemantle N, Polonski L, Taylor J. The perindopril in elderly people with chronic heart failure (PEP-CHF) study. *Eur Heart J.* 2006;27(19):2338-2345. doi: 10.1093/eurheartj/ehl250.

88. Conraads VM, Metra M, Kamp O, et al. Effects of the long-term administration of nebivolol on the clinical symptoms, exercise capacity, and left ventricular function of patients with diastolic dysfunction: results of the ELANDD study. *Eur J Heart Fail.* 2012;14(2):219-225. doi: 10.1093/eurjhf/hfr161.

89. Cleland JGF, Bunting KV, Flather MD, et al. Beta-blockers for heart failure with reduced, mid-range, and preserved ejection fraction: an individual patient-level analysis of double-blind randomized trials. *Eur Heart J.* 2018;39(1):26-35. doi: 10.1093/eurheartj/ehx564.

90. Komajda M, Isnard R, Cohen-Solal A, et al. Effect of ivabradine in patients with heart failure with preserved ejection fraction: the EDIFY randomized placebo-controlled trial. *Eur J Heart Fail.* 2017;19(11):1495-1503. doi: 10.1002/ejhf.876.

91. Cleland JGF, Ferreira JP, Mariottoni B, et al. The effect of spironolactone on cardiovascular function and markers of fibrosis in people at increased risk of developing heart failure: the heart "OMics" in AGEing (HOMAGE) randomized clinical trial. *Eur Heart J.* 2020. doi: 10.1093/eurheartj/ehaa758.

92. Edelmann F, Wachter R, Schmidt AG, et al. Effect of spironolactone on diastolic function and exercise capacity in patients with heart failure with preserved ejection fraction: the Aldo-DHF randomized controlled trial. *JAMA.* 2013;309(8):781-791. doi: 10.1001/jama.2013.905.

93. Pitt B, Pfeffer MA, Assmann SF, et al. Spironolactone for heart failure with preserved ejection fraction. *N Engl J Med.* 2014;370(15):1383-1392. doi: 10.1056/NEJMoa1313731.

94. Pfeffer MA, Claggett B, Assmann SF, et al. Regional Variation in Patients and Outcomes in the Treatment of Preserved Cardiac Function Heart Failure with an Aldosterone Antagonist (TOPCAT) Trial. *Circulation.* 2015;131(1):34-42. doi: 10.1161/circulationaha.114.013255.

95. de Denus S, O'Meara E, Desai AS, et al. Spironolactone Metabolites in TOPCAT—New Insights into Regional Variation. *N Engl J Med.* 2017;376(17):1690-1692. doi: 10.1056/NEJMc1612601.

96. McMurray JJ, Packer M, Desai AS, et al. Angiotensin-neprilysin inhibition versus enalapril in heart failure. *N Engl J Med.* 2014;371(11):993-1004. doi: 10.1056/NEJMoa1409077.

97. Solomon SD, Zile M, Pieske B, et al. The angiotensin receptor neprilysin inhibitor LCZ696 in heart failure with preserved ejection fraction: a phase 2 double-blind randomised controlled trial. *Lancet.* 2012;380(9851):1387-1395. doi: 10.1016/s0140-6736(12)61227-6.

98. Solomon SD, McMurray JJV, Anand IS, et al. Angiotensin-neprilysin inhibition in heart failure with preserved ejection fraction. *N Engl J Med.* 2019. doi: 10.1056/NEJMoa1908655.

99. McMurray JJV, Jackson AM, Lam CSP, et al. Effects of sacubitril-valsartan versus valsartan in women compared with men with heart failure and preserved ejection fraction: insights from PARAGON-HF. *Circulation.* 2020;141(5):338-351. doi: 10.1161/circulationaha.119.044491.

100. Solomon SD, Vaduganathan M, B LC, et al. Sacubitril/valsartan across the spectrum of ejection fraction in heart failure. *Circulation.* 2020;141(5):352-361. doi: 10.1161/circulationaha.119.044586.

101. Vaduganathan M, Claggett BL, Desai AS, et al. Prior heart failure hospitalization, clinical outcomes, and response to sacubitril/valsartan compared with valsartan in HFpEF. *J Am Coll Cardiol.* 2020;75(3):245-254. doi: 10.1016/j.jacc.2019.11.003.

102. Jering KS, Zannad F, Claggett B, et al. Cardiovascular and renal outcomes of mineralocorticoid receptor antagonist use in PARAGON-HF. *JACC Heart Fail.* 2021;9(1):13-24. doi: 10.1016/j.jchf.2020.08.014.

103. Vaduganathan M, Jhund PS, Claggett BL, et al. A putative placebo analysis of the effects of sacubitril/valsartan in heart failure across the full range of ejection fraction. *Eur Heart J.* 2020;41(25):2356-2362. doi: 10.1093/eurheartj/ehaa184.

104. Wachter R, Shah SJ, Cowie MR, et al. Angiotensin receptor neprilysin inhibition versus individualized RAAS blockade: design and rationale of the PARALLAX trial. *ESC Heart Fail.* 2020;7(3):856-864. doi: 10.1002/ehf2.12694.

105. Zelniker TA, Wiviott SD, Raz I, et al. SGLT2 inhibitors for primary and secondary prevention of cardiovascular and renal outcomes in type 2 diabetes: a systematic review and meta-analysis of cardiovascular outcome trials. *Lancet*. 2019;393(10166):31-39. doi: 10.1016/s0140-6736(18)32590-x.

106. Neuen BL, Young T, Heerspink HJL, et al. SGLT2 inhibitors for the prevention of kidney failure in patients with type 2 diabetes: a systematic review and meta-analysis. *Lancet Diabetes Endocrinol*. Nov 2019;7(11):845-854. doi: 10.1016/s2213-8587(19)30256-6.

107. Bhatt DL, Szarek M, Steg PG, et al. Sotagliflozin in patients with diabetes and recent worsening heart failure. *N Engl J Med*. 2020. doi: 10.1056/NEJMoa2030183.

108. Bhatt DL, Szarek M, Pitt B, et al. Sotagliflozin in patients with diabetes and chronic kidney disease. *N Engl J Med*. 2020. doi: 10.1056/NEJMoa2030186.

109. Anker SD, Butler J, Filippatos G, et al. Empagliflozin in heart failure with a preserved ejection fraction. *N Engl J Med*. 2021. doi: 10.1056/NEJMoa2107038.

110. Khan MS, Jones DW, Butler J. Salt, no salt, or less salt for patients with heart failure? *Am J Med*. 2020;133(1):32-38. doi: 10.1016/j.amjmed.2019.07.034.

111. Pandey A, Parashar A, Kumbhani D, et al. Exercise training in patients with heart failure and preserved ejection fraction: meta-analysis of randomized control trials. *Circ Heart Fail*. 2015;8(1):33-40. doi: 10.1161/circheartfailure.114.001615.

112. Mentz RJ, Kelly JP, von Lueder TG, et al. Noncardiac comorbidities in heart failure with reduced versus preserved ejection fraction. *J Am Coll Cardiol*. 2014;64(21):2281-2293. doi: 10.1016/j.jacc.2014.08.036.

Evaluation and Management of Acute Heart Failure

Anuradha Lala, Kiran Mahmood, and Eric J. Velazquez

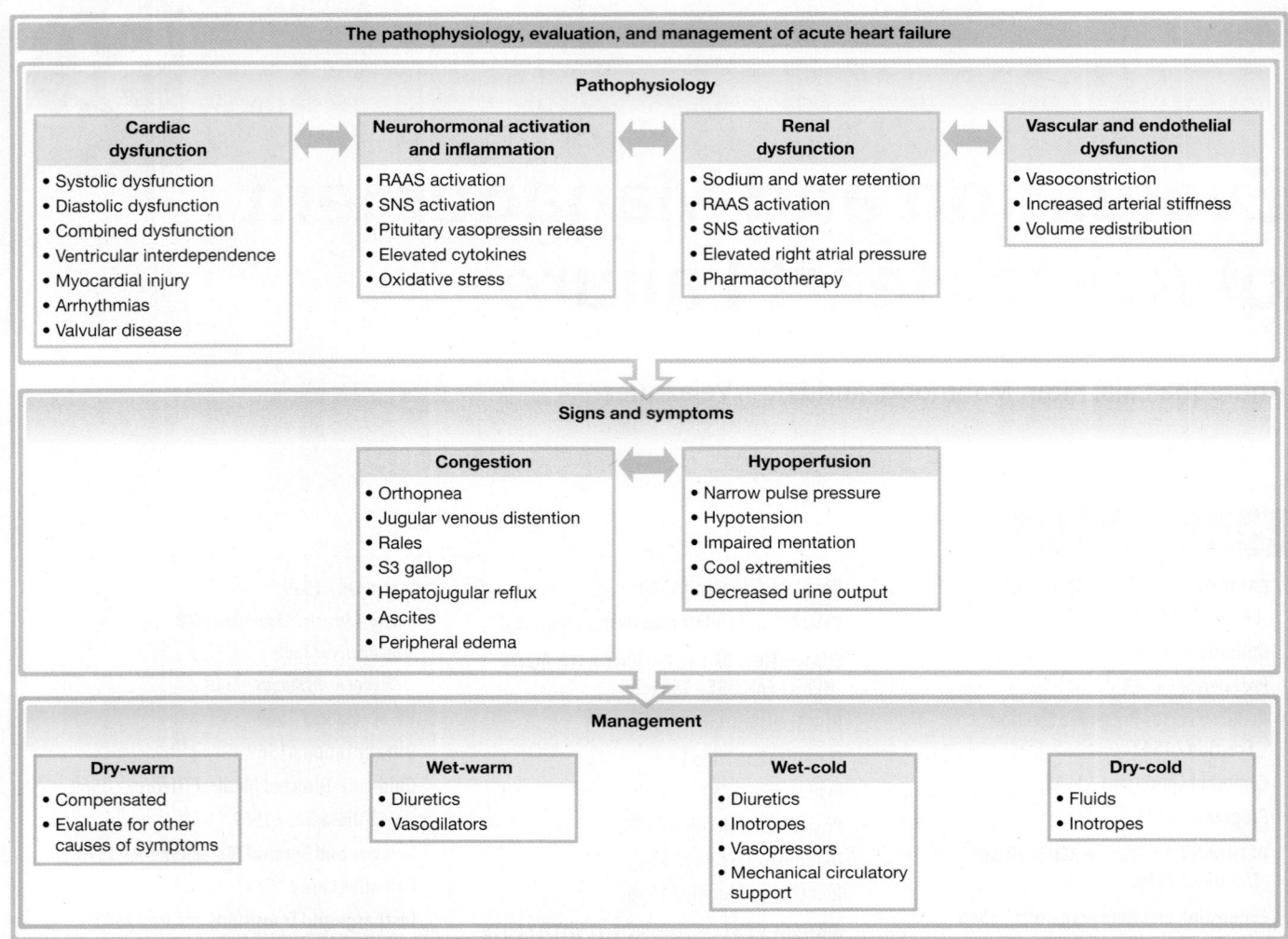

The pathophysiology, evaluation, and management of acute heart failure

Pathophysiology

Cardiac dysfunction
- Systolic dysfunction
- Diastolic dysfunction
- Combined dysfunction
- Ventricular interdependence
- Myocardial injury
- Arrhythmias
- Valvular disease

Neurohormonal activation and inflammation
- RAAS activation
- SNS activation
- Pituitary vasopressin release
- Elevated cytokines
- Oxidative stress

Renal dysfunction
- Sodium and water retention
- RAAS activation
- SNS activation
- Elevated right atrial pressure
- Pharmacotherapy

Vascular and endothelial dysfunction
- Vasoconstriction
- Increased arterial stiffness
- Volume redistribution

Signs and symptoms

Congestion
- Orthopnea
- Jugular venous distention
- Rales
- S3 gallop
- Hepatojugular reflux
- Ascites
- Peripheral edema

Hypoperfusion
- Narrow pulse pressure
- Hypotension
- Impaired mentation
- Cool extremities
- Decreased urine output

Management

Dry-warm
- Compensated
- Evaluate for other causes of symptoms

Wet-warm
- Diuretics
- Vasodilators

Wet-cold
- Diuretics
- Inotropes
- Vasopressors
- Mechanical circulatory support

Dry-cold
- Fluids
- Inotropes

Chapter 50 Fuster and Hurst's Central Illustration. The pathophysiology of acute heart failure incorporates cardiac dysfunction, neurohormonal activation and inflammation, renal dysfunction, and vascular and endothelial dysfunction, leading to signs and symptoms of congestion, hypoperfusion, or both. Determining the hemodynamic profile of the patient allows for appropriate management. RAAS, renin-angiotensin-aldosterone system; SNS, sympathetic nervous system.

CHAPTER SUMMARY

This chapter discusses the epidemiology, pathophysiology, evaluation, and management of acute heart failure (AHF), which is the onset or recurrence of symptoms and signs of heart failure requiring urgent or emergent therapy. The pathophysiology of AHF is complex, incorporating cardiac dysfunction, neurohormonal activation and inflammation, renal dysfunction, and vascular and endothelial dysfunction (see Fuster and Hurst's Central Illustration). The interplay of these systems ultimately leads to signs and symptoms related to congestion, hypoperfusion, or both. The evaluation of the patient with AHF requires rapidly establishing the diagnosis, treating potentially life-threatening presentations such as shock or respiratory failure, identifying triggers or precipitating factors requiring specific treatment such as acute coronary syndrome, risk stratifying to provide the appropriate level of care, and defining the hemodynamic profile to implement appropriate therapy. Management involves relieving congestion and restoring or maintaining perfusion primarily with diuretics and vasodilators. In patients with decreased cardiac output with organ hypoperfusion, inotropes and vasopressors may be needed. Escalation of therapy to mechanical circulatory support may be needed for patients with cardiogenic shock. Transitioning care from the inpatient setting to the outpatient setting is a vulnerable period for patients with AHF and postdischarge follow-up is imperative.

EPIDEMIOLOGY OF ACUTE HEART FAILURE

Definition

The clinical syndrome of heart failure (HF) is defined as current or prior symptoms and/or signs of congestion in the setting of a structural and/or functional cardiac abnormality, corroborated by elevated natriuretic peptide levels or objective evidence by imaging or hemodynamic assessment.[1] Acute heart failure (AHF) therefore relates to the onset or recurrence of symptoms and signs of HF requiring urgent or emergent therapy, and resulting in unscheduled care or hospitalization. Although the word "acute" suggests a sudden onset, many patients have a more subacute course, with gradual worsening of symptoms that ultimately reach a level of severity sufficient to seek unscheduled medical care.

Prevalence

AHF is among the most common causes for hospitalization in patients older than age 65. In the United States, 4 million people are hospitalized each year with a primary (1 million) or secondary diagnosis of HF (3 million), the latter highlighting the prevalence of comorbid conditions in patients with HF.[2]

With an increasing aging population, improvement in medical and device-based therapies resulting in increased survival after myocardial infarction as well as prevention of sudden death, the prevalence of HF is only expected to increase with time. In the United States alone, the costs associated with management of HF approach 40 billion dollars annually, with the majority of expenditures related to the costs of hospitalizations.[3,4] Therefore, in efforts to reduce hospitalizations and associated costs, initiatives such as outpatient diuretic clinics and observation units have evolved wherein less severe HF decompensations can be managed.[5,6]

Additionally, substantial heterogeneity in HF prevalence and mortality across US states and among racial and ethnic groups requires attention to social determinants of health, as well as inequities in access and delivery of care for the optimization of AHF care (**Fig. 50–1**).

Reduced versus Preserved Ejection Fraction

Important epidemiologic differences exist between heart failure with reduced ejection fraction (HFrEF) and heart failure with preserved ejection fraction (HFpEF). Patients with HFpEF are more likely to be older and female. Although they have less coronary artery disease (CAD), there is a higher prevalence of

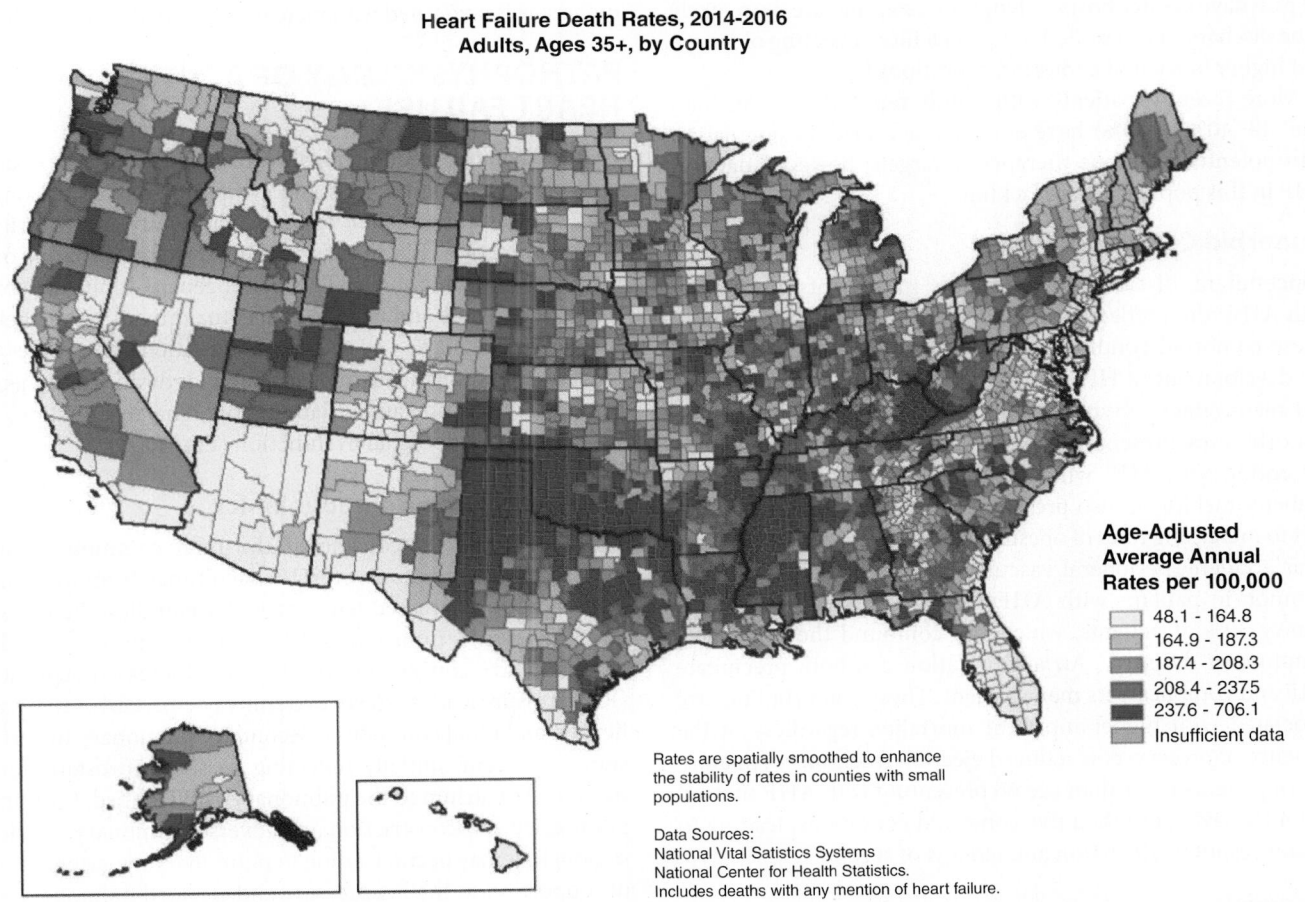

Heart Failure Death Rates, 2014-2016
Adults, Ages 35+, by Country

Age-Adjusted Average Annual Rates per 100,000

- 48.1 - 164.8
- 164.9 - 187.3
- 187.4 - 208.3
- 208.4 - 237.5
- 237.6 - 706.1
- Insufficient data

Rates are spatially smoothed to enhance the stability of rates in counties with small populations.

Data Sources:
National Vital Satistics Systems
National Center for Health Statistics.
Includes deaths with any mention of heart failure.

Figure 50–1. A map of the death rates from heart failure by county during 2014 to 2016 shows that heart failure is more common in some areas of the United States than in others. Reproduced with permission from National Center for Chronic Disease Prevention and Health Promotion , Division for Heart Disease and Stroke Prevention, Heart Disease. https://www.cdc.gov/heartdisease/heart_failure.htm.

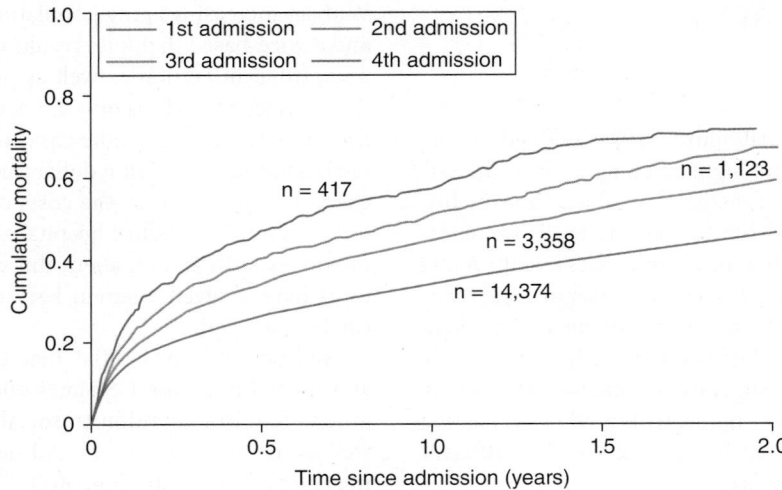

Figure 50–2. Kaplan–Meier survival curves for cumulative mortality after repeated acute decompensated heart failure hospitalizations. Reproduced with permission from Setoguchi S, Stevenson LW, Schneeweiss S. Repeated hospitalizations predict mortality in the community population with heart failure. *Am Heart J.* 2007 Aug;154(2):260-266.

atrial fibrillation, chronic kidney disease (CKD), hypertension, and chronic obstructive pulmonary disease (COPD).[7] Over 50% of AHF admissions occur in patients with HFpEF.[8] The proportion of hospitalizations in those with HFpEF is increasing considerably compared to those with HFrEF. Patients with HFpEF have greater hospital lengths of stay and are more likely to be discharged to a skilled nursing facility, reflecting older age and higher burden of comorbid conditions.[7]

More recently, patients with mildly reduced ejection fraction (EF 40% to 49%) have emerged as a distinct population with potentially unique therapeutic targets; however, data on AHF in this population are lacking.

Comorbid Conditions

Concomitant diseases are common in patients presenting with AHF, often reflective of an increasingly aging population. These comorbid conditions serve not only as risk factors for the development of HF, but may also complicate its diagnosis and management. Hypertension is the most prevalent of the comorbidities, present in approximately two-thirds of patients presenting with AHF, whereas CAD is present in about half. Diabetes mellitus is also present in more than 40%, related in part to increasing rates of obesity.[8] Hyperlipidemia, cerebrovascular accident, peripheral vascular disease, and CKD are also common in patients with AHF. COPD is present in approximately 30% of patients, which can confound the presenting symptom of dyspnea.[8] Atrial fibrillation can both precipitate AHF and complicate its management. These comorbidities are associated with higher inpatient mortality, regardless of the presence of preserved or reduced ejection fraction.[9,10] An analysis of patients older than age 65 presenting with AHF showed that 40% have more than five comorbid conditions, leading to greater resource utilization and lengths of stay.[10]

Prognosis

AHF is associated with an often underrecognized, but significant mortality and morbidity. In-hospital mortality ranges from

2% to 5% and is similar for patients with HFrEF and HFpEF.[7] Postdischarge mortality approaches 10% at 90-day follow-up, and 30% at 1 year.[11,12] Nearly 25% of patients are readmitted within 30 days of discharge, and 50% are readmitted within 6 months.[13,14] Each subsequent hospitalization following the index stay is associated with increasing risk of death (**Fig. 50–2**).

PATHOPHYSIOLOGY OF ACUTE HEART FAILURE

AHF is a heterogeneous clinical syndrome with complex pathophysiology leading to signs and symptoms related to congestion, decreased perfusion, or both. The acuity and severity of presentation of AHF can vary, ranging from mild volume overload to cardiogenic shock. This heterogeneity limits the ability to create a simple and unified conceptual model. Nevertheless, several factors play a key role in the initiation and progression of AHF, including myocardial and valvular dysfunction, neurohormonal activation and inflammation, renal dysfunction, and vascular and endothelial dysfunction (**Fig. 50–3**).

Congestion and Hemodynamics

Congestion can be considered the final common pathway underlying the symptoms of AHF that ultimately prompts medical attention. Increased left ventricular end diastolic pressure (LVEDP) results in increased left atrial (LA) pressure, leading to pulmonary congestion and dyspnea. Increased right atrial (RA) pressure leads to lower extremity edema, early satiety, and hepatic and renal congestion. Secondary pulmonary hypertension may occur, initially reflecting passive hydrostatic forces from the left atrium to the pulmonary capillary bed. Over time, pulmonary vasoconstriction and adverse pulmonary arteriolar remodeling may occur, leading to pulmonary hypertension out of proportion to the LA pressure and elevated pulmonary vascular resistance.[15]

One important concept that has evolved is the distinction between clinical congestion and hemodynamic congestion.

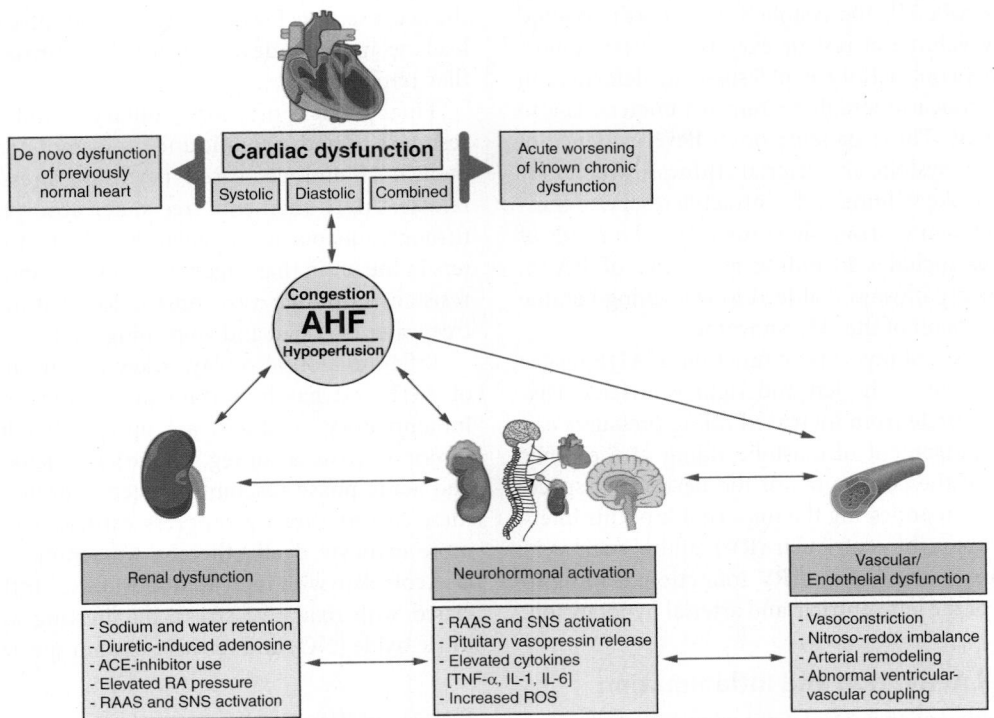

Figure 50–3. The basic pathophysiology of acute heart failure (AHF). ACE, angiotensin-converting enzyme; IL, interleukin; RA, right atrial; RAAS, renin-angiotensin-aldosterone system; ROS, reactive oxygen species; SNS, sympathetic nervous system; TNF-α, tumor necrosis factor-α.

Patients present with signs and symptoms of systemic congestion, including dyspnea, rales, elevated jugular venous pressure, and edema. However, hemodynamic congestion, elevated LVEDP without overt clinical signs or symptoms, often precedes clinical congestion.[16] Studies using implantable hemodynamic monitors suggest that increases in invasively measured LV filling pressures can occur without substantial changes in body weight.[16] These observations have led to an increasing focus on the concept of volume redistribution, where blood is centrally redistributed due to peripheral vasoconstriction, increasing pulmonary venous congestion and edema. Studies with implantable hemodynamic monitors also show that chronically elevated filling pressures are associated with increased risk of future events.[17]

In most cases of AHF, cardiac output (CO) is normal or only mildly reduced, especially when AHF develops from a progressive exacerbation of chronic LV dysfunction. In the case of an acute process, such as myocardial infarction or fulminant myocarditis, CO may decrease significantly, leading to shock characterized by decreased end-organ perfusion requiring inotropic or mechanical circulatory support.

Cardiac Dysfunction

Cardiac dysfunction may manifest as systolic dysfunction with impaired contractility, diastolic dysfunction with impaired relaxation or decreased ventricular compliance, or more often than not, both. AHF in the setting of primarily systolic dysfunction may result from an abrupt insult such as myocardial infarction or myocarditis or, more commonly, a worsening of a chronic, progressive process. The features of acute systolic HF

include elevated LV filling pressures, manifesting as congestion and dyspnea, and decreased arterial filling, manifesting as hypoperfusion or cardiogenic shock in extreme cases. When systolic dysfunction occurs abruptly, CO may be significantly reduced, however when it occurs progressively, CO is usually not impaired until late stages. This is due to a cascade of effects that are adaptive in the short term but maladaptive chronically. These mechanisms, including renin-angiotensin-aldosterone system (RAAS) activation, sympathetic nervous system (SNS) upregulation, and pituitary vasopressin (antidiuretic hormone [ADH]) release, augment circulating blood volume and maintain mean arterial pressure. Although activation of these neurohormonal axes may acutely augment perfusion pressures, they ultimately lead to vasoconstriction, sodium and fluid retention, myocardial damage and fibrosis, and adverse ventricular remodeling.[18]

Although systolic dysfunction is important in the pathophysiology of AHF, epidemiology data previously discussed show that approximately half of patients with AHF have preserved ejection fraction. Importantly, abnormalities in diastolic function are present in HF patients regardless of ejection fraction. Diastolic HF results from the inability of the LV to effectively fill in diastole, related to passive stiffness, abnormal active relaxation, or both. This may occur abruptly, such as in acute onset atrial fibrillation with rapid ventricular response or progressively, such as in worsening hypertensive heart disease. As diastolic dysfunction progresses, LA pressures become increasingly elevated to facilitate ventricular filling. This escalating pressure reflects back to the pulmonary capillary circulation, leading to pulmonary congestion and dyspnea. Although ejection fraction is preserved in diastolic HF, the systolic function as measured by effective stroke volume at rest or exercise is often abnormal and myocardial contractility as measured by deformation imaging, such as echocardiographic strain parameters, is also commonly abnormal. These patients often have evidence of increased ventricular systolic and arterial stiffness, which may manifest as lower stroke volume and contractile reserve.[19] Similar to patients with acute primarily systolic HF, the result of these abnormalities includes including activation of RAAS, SNS, and vasopressin pathways that lead to worsening volume overload and progression of the HF syndrome.

An important aspect of myocardial function in AHF relates to the interdependence of the left and right ventricles. Distention of either ventricle from increased filling pressures can result in direct impingement of diastolic filling of the other ventricle, because of the constraints of the pericardial space. One clinical scenario manifesting the importance of this interdependence is abrupt right ventricular (RV) failure, such as in the case of pulmonary embolism or RV infarction, leading to diminished filling of the left ventricle and arterial hypotension.

Neurohormonal Activation and Inflammation

The primary objective of the circulatory system is the perfusion to vital organs by maintaining mean arterial pressure and blood volume. Organ perfusion is mediated by a variety of processes and feedback loops embedded in the RAAS and SNS, in addition to pituitary vasopressin release. Although acute upregulation of these systems is effective at restoring circulating blood volume and perfusion pressures, chronic activation leads to sodium and fluid retention as well as cardiac fibrosis and adverse remodeling.

When perfusion pressures decrease, the juxtaglomerular cells of the nephron release renin into the circulation. Renin cleaves angiotensinogen to angiotensin I, which is then converted to angiotensin II by angiotensin-converting enzyme (ACE). Angiotensin II has multiple downstream effects, including increased systemic vascular resistance (SVR) through vasoconstriction, volume expansion by promoting sodium reabsorption in the proximal tubule, stimulation of adrenal aldosterone release, and activation of the SNS. Aldosterone release from the adrenal glands leads to additional sodium resorption in the distal tubule and collecting duct, volume expansion, and ultimately myocardial fibrosis. Thus, RAAS activation plays a fundamental role in the precipitation of AHF through fluid retention and vasoconstriction while also contributing to chronic ventricular remodeling.

Reductions in perfusion pressure also lead to activation of the SNS, primarily through the suppression of cardioinhibitory baroreceptor reflexes and the augmentation of excitatory reflexes.[20] SNS activation results in increased CO by increasing myocardial contractility and heart rate, while also increasing blood pressure through norepinephrine-mediated vasoconstriction. Additionally, heightened sympathetic activity leads to renin release from the kidney and the propagation of the RAAS axis, further exacerbating AHF. Like the RAAS axis, the acute effects of SNS activation favorably support organ perfusion in

the acute setting; however, augmented catecholamine exposure leads to myocyte death, myocardial fibrosis, and adverse cardiac remodeling.

Finally, the posterior pituitary gland releases ADH in response to both osmotic and nonosmotic mechanisms. Angiotensin II and decreased perfusion pressure trigger ADH release. ADH augments free water absorption in the kidney through aquaporin upregulation, which stimulates thirst centers in the brain that trigger fluid intake, and increases vascular resistance through vasoconstriction. Ultimately, this leads to free water overload and worsening AHF.

Inflammation also plays a key role in the pathophysiology of AHF and has important prognostic significance. Several inflammatory cytokines are upregulated in AHF, including tumor necrosis factor (eg, TNF-α), interleukins (eg, IL-1, IL-6), and acute-phase reactant C-reactive protein (CRP). Many of these factors directly suppress cardiac contractility and promote myocyte death, thereby worsening AHF. Higher levels also correlate with increased mortality.[21] Inflammation is associated with oxidative stress, manifesting as an imbalance in nitric oxide (NO) and reactive oxygen species (ROS).

Renal Dysfunction

Change in renal function is common in AHF, affecting between 30% and 67% of patients.[22] Specifically, as many as 20% to 40% of patients experience worsening renal function (WRF) while being treated for AHF, a finding associated with worse prognosis.[22-25] Despite the high prevalence of renal dysfunction in AHF, our understanding of the complex interactions between the two organs remains inadequate. The pathophysiology of renal dysfunction in AHF likely incorporates hemodynamic factors, activation of the RAAS and SNS, inflammation and oxidative stress, renovascular congestion and altered fluid distribution, and the iatrogenic effects of pharmacotherapy, among other factors.

The term cardiorenal syndrome has been increasingly used to describe pathologic interactions between the cardiac and renal axes in the setting of HF. In the context of AHF, cardiorenal syndrome describes the clinical scenario of worsening renal function in the setting of persistent congestion. Although previously assumed to be related to low CO, hemodynamic studies have revealed that the strongest predictor of WRF relates to elevated RA pressure, which is reflected back to the renal veins and leads directly to changes in glomerular filtration rate.[26-29]

Neurohormonal activation once again plays a critical role in WRF in the setting of decompensation. The downstream effects of RAAS and SNS activation include angiotensin II and catecholamine-induced renal efferent arteriolar constriction, which increases glomerular filtration at the expense of renal blood flow. Additionally, stimulation of aldosterone secretion increases sodium resorption and exacerbates volume overload and congestion, which in turn promotes WRF. Chronic RAAS and SNS activation may lead to renal interstitial fibrosis and inflammation, resulting in CKD.[30]

Highlighting the complex interplay between cardiac and renal dysfunction in AHF, WRF in the setting of aggressive diuresis in a patient who is clinically improving may represent a delayed equilibration of fluid between the extra- and intra-vascular compartments. This may actually be associated with improved and not worse outcomes.[31–33] This transient WRF at the cost of effective decongestion has been shown to be associated with better outcomes compared to persistent WRF during treatment for AHF.[34]

Vascular and Endothelial Dysfunction

Endothelial dysfunction related to NO-dependent regulation of vascular tone is well described in HF, both in HFrEF and HFpEF.[35–37] Arterial stiffness increases afterload or SVR and impairs cardiac performance. Endothelial dysfunction leads to systemic vasoconstriction leading to greater ventricular wall stress and higher LV filling pressures resulting in pulmonary congestion. Endothelial dysfunction is associated with worse prognosis and higher rate of cardiovascular events.[37]

EVALUATION OF THE PATIENT WITH ACUTE HEART FAILURE

The initial evaluation of the patient with AHF focuses on rapidly establishing the diagnosis, treating potentially life-threatening presentations such as shock or respiratory failure, identifying triggers or precipitating factors requiring specific treatment such as acute coronary syndrome, risk stratifying to provide the appropriate level of care, and defining the hemodynamic profile of the patient to implement appropriate therapy. The European Society of Cardiology (ESC) has proposed an algorithm for the initial evaluation of the patient with AHF (**Fig. 50–4**).

Risk Stratification

Careful patient assessment and recognition of presentation and comorbid conditions may help stratify patients more likely to experience adverse outcomes or who may require closer observation. Specifically, several clinical variables and biomarkers have been identified that may allow for the identification of such, and prediction models and risk scores have been developed to better facilitate stratification of patients with AHF (**Table 50–1**).[38–43]

- The Acute Decompensated Heart Failure National Registry (ADHERE) "risk tree" was derived from an analysis of 39 admission variables in over 60,000 AHF patients. Investigators found that the best predictors of inpatient mortality were markers of renal dysfunction (elevated blood urea nitrogen and creatinine) and lower systolic blood pressure. A risk tree was developed incorporating these variables, enabling clinicians to estimate inpatient mortality ranging from low risk (~2%) to intermediate risk (~6%–13%) to high risk (~20%) (**Fig. 50–5**).[38]

- The Enhanced Feedback for Effective Cardiac Treatment (EFFECT) risk index uses several demographic, laboratory, and clinical variables at the time of admission to determine death risk at 30 days and 1 year. Developed from a retrospective study of over 4000 community-based AHF patients

in Ontario, Canada, the EFFECT risk index can be used to categorize patients into low risk (mortality 0.4% at 30 days and 7.8% at 1 year) and high risk for death during follow-up (mortality 59% at 30 days and 79% at 1 year).[39]

- The Get With the Guidelines–Heart Failure (GWTG-HF) risk score was derived from a cohort of over 39,000 patients admitted with AHF between 2007 and 2009. This score incorporates admission variables associated with risk of death in a multivariable analysis, including age, systolic blood pressure, blood urea nitrogen, heart rate, sodium, COPD, and non-Black race. This model is effective in both HFpEF and HFrEF patients.[42]

- The Multiple Estimation of risk based on the Emergency department Spanish Score In patients with AHF (MEESSI-AHF) score aims to predict morality within 30 days using data available in the emergency department (ED) that can be important to identify patients at lower risk for whom hospitalization may not be required.[43] A systematic review identified 19 scales for risk stratification that have been applied in ED patients with AHF in 28 different studies.[44] However, further research is still needed about the outcomes of risk stratification on decision-making regarding whether to admit or discharge patients with AHF who present to the ED.

Several established and novel biomarkers have also been shown to predict either low or high risk for postdischarge events. In one study of 1653 patients who presented with AHF, 47 biomarkers were serially evaluated. Patients were classified as low risk if postdischarge 30-day risk of death or heart failure rehospitalization was <5% while risk >20% was used to define high risk. Cardiac-specific troponin I was the strongest biomarker for low-risk prediction while endothelin-1 (ET-1) showed better performance for high-risk prediction. Several biomarkers (individually and in combination) provided added predictive value, on top of a clinical model, in both low-risk and high-risk regions.[45]

Classification

The variability of patients who present with AHF makes the development of a classification model difficult and there is no one single classification system that is universally accepted. Previous ESC guidelines proposed six groups based on clinical and hemo-dynamic characteristics, but the most recent guidelines classify patients clinically based on determining their hemodynamic profile at the bedside as described by Nohria et al.[46–48] The most recent American College of Cardiology Foundation/American Heart Association (ACCF/AHA) guidelines also classify patients based on these hemodynamic profiles.[49]

Characterization of hemodynamic profile entails the clinical appraisal of congestion and perfusion. Patients are described as either "wet" or "dry" depending on their volume status and either "cold" or "warm" depending on their perfusion status (**Fig. 50–6**). The presence of congestion is determined by orthopnea, jugular venous distention, rales, hepatojugular reflux, ascites, peripheral edema, leftward radiation of the pulmonic

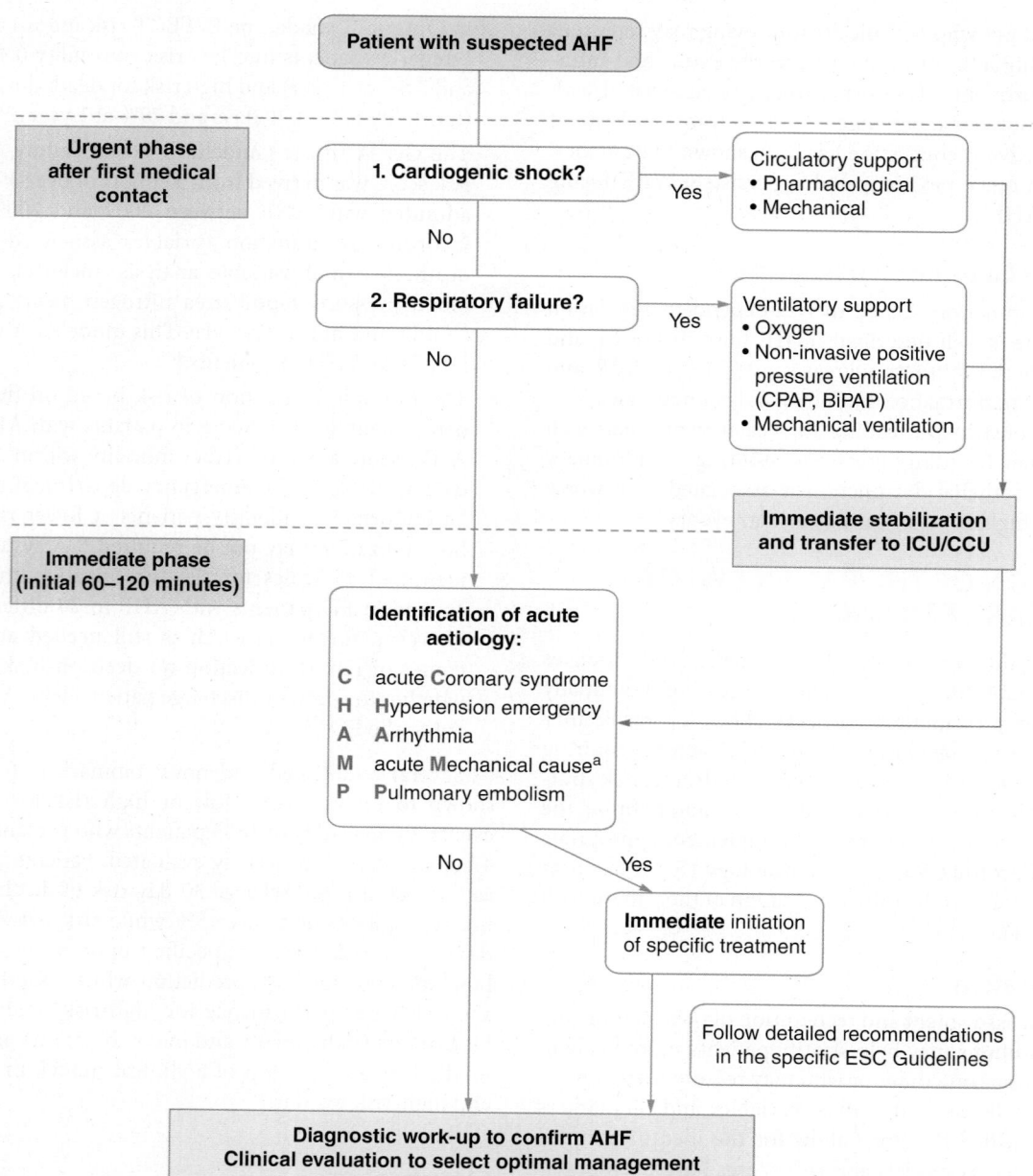

Figure 50–4. Initial management of a patient with acute heart failure. [a]Acute mechanical cause: myocardial rupture complicating acute coronary syndrome (free wall rupture, ventricular septal defect, acute mitral regurgitation), chest trauma or cardiac intervention, acute native or prosthetic valve incompetence secondary to endocarditis, aortic dissection, or thrombosis. Reproduced with permission from Ponikowski P, Voors AA, Anker SD, et al. 2016 ESC Guidelines for the diagnosis and treatment of acute and chronic heart failure: The Task Force for the diagnosis and treatment of acute and chronic heart failure of the European Society of Cardiology (ESC)Developed with the special contribution of the Heart Failure Association (HFA) of the ESC. *Eur Heart J.* 2016 Jul 14; 37(27):2129-2200.

heart sound, or a square wave blood pressure response to the Valsalva maneuver. Hypoperfusion is determined by the presence of narrow pulse pressure, pulsus alternans, hypotension, cool extremities, reduced urine output, and/or impaired mentation.[48]

Profiling patients by congestion and perfusion allows for appropriate therapeutic intervention but also provides prognostic information. Patients in Profile A are without evidence of congestion with adequate perfusion ("dry-warm"). These patients are compensated from a cardiac perspective, and presence of dyspnea in these patients should prompt evaluation for

alternative causes. Patients in Profile B have congestion but adequate perfusion ("wet-warm") and represent the majority of patients encountered with AHF, generally requiring diuresis with or without vasodilation. Patients in Profile C show signs and symptoms of congestion and hypoperfusion ("wet-cold"). These patients are generally a sicker group who may require inotropic support or invasive hemodynamic monitoring, particularly if conventional therapy does not result in clinical improvement. Finally, patients in Profile L are patients without congestion, but have signs of hypoperfusion ("dry-cold"). This profile is less frequently encountered but includes those

TABLE 50-1. Risk Scores for Acutely Decompensated Heart Failure

Risk Score	Population	Outcome	Variables in Model	Utility
ADHERE risk tree	ADHERE registry (AHF admissions at 263 hospitals in the United States); derivation cohort, n = 33,046; validation cohort, n = 32,229	Inpatient mortality	39 variables analyzed; 3 variables strongly associated with risk of death: BUN <43 mg/dL; SBP >115 mm Hg; Cr >2.75 mg/dL	Stratify patients into low risk (~3%), low/intermediate (~6%), intermediate/high risk (~13%), and high risk (~20%) for inpatient death
EFFECT risk index	Over 4000 patients admitted with AHF to 24 hospitals in Ontario, Canada; derivation cohort, n = 2624; validation cohort, n = 1407	All-cause 30-day and 1-year mortality	Age, RR, SBP, BUN, sodium <136 mEq/L, cerebrovascular disease, dementia, COPD, cirrhosis, cancer, hemoglobin <10 g/dL	Categorize patients into low risk (score <60): <1% 30-day and ~8% 1-year mortality; or high risk (score >150): 69% 30-day mortality and ~79% 1-year mortality
PROTECT risk score	2015 AHF patients with complete data enrolled in PROTECT study (AHF patients with renal dysfunction)	Risk of death, worsening HF, or readmission for HF at 7 days	BUN, albumin, SBP, RR, HR, cholesterol, HF hospitalization in last year, DM; incremental points awarded for increasing severity of each	Probability of an event ranges from 4.8% (lowest scores) to 39% (highest scores)
GWTG-HF risk score	GWTG-HF registry (AHF admissions to 198 participating hospitals); derivation cohort, n = 27,850; validation cohort, n = 11,933	Inpatient mortality	BP, BUN, sodium, age, HR, black race, COPD; incremental points awarded for increasing severity/presence of each	Discriminate mortality from <1% in lowest decile of scores to ~10% in the highest decile of scores; valid for both HFpEF and HFrEF
ESCAPE discharge risk score	423 patients with complete data discharged during the ESCAPE study; validated by data from FIRST trial	6-month mortality following discharge	Age >70, BUN >40 or >90 mg/dL, 6MWT <300 ft, sodium <130 mEq/L, CPR/ventilator use, D/C diuretic >240 mg, no BB at D/C, D/C BNP >500 or >1300 pg/mL	D/C risk score discriminates mortality from 5% (score = 0) to 94% (score = 8) at 6 months
MEESSI-AHF risk score	EAHFE registry (AHF patients from 34 EDs in Spain); derivation cohort, n = 4867; validation cohort, n = 3229	30-day mortality	Barthel index, SBP, age, NT-proBNP level, potassium, positive troponin, NYHA IV, RR, low output symptoms, SpO2, ACS, hypertrophy on ECG, Cr	Discriminate mortality from >2% in 2 lowest risk quintiles to 45% in highest risk decile

Abbreviations: 6MWT, 6-minute walk test; ACS, acute coronary syndrome; ADHERE, Acute Decompensated Heart Failure National Registry; AHF, acute heart failure; BB, β-blocker; BNP, B-type natriuretic peptide; BP, blood pressure; BUN, blood urea nitrogen; COPD, chronic obstructive pulmonary disease; CPR, cardiopulmonary resuscitation; Cr, creatinine; D/C, discharge; DM, diabetes mellitus; EAHFE, Epidemiology of Acute Heart Failure in Emergency Departments; ECG, electrocardiogram; ED, emergency department; EFFECT, Enhanced Feedback for Effective Cardiac Treatment; ESCAPE, Evaluation Study of Congestive Heart Failure and Pulmonary Artery Catheterization and Effectiveness; FIRST, Flolan International Randomized Survival Trial; GWTG-HF, Get With the Guidelines–Heart Failure; HF, heart failure; HFpEF, heart failure with preserved ejection fraction; HFrEF, heart failure with reduced ejection fraction; HR, heart rate; MEESSI-AHF, Multiple Estimation of risk based on the Emergency department Spanish Score In patients with AHF; NT-proBNP, N-terminal pro B-type natriuretic peptide; NYHA, New York Heart Association; PROTECT, Pro-BNP Outpatient Tailored Chronic Heart Failure Therapy; RR, respiratory rate; SBP, systolic blood pressure; SpO2, peripheral oxygen saturation.

with severe limitation in cardiovascular reserve. Patients with profiles B and C have an increased risk of death or urgent transplantation.[48]

Symptoms

The presenting symptoms in patients with AHF are primarily due to congestion, but can also be due to hypoperfusion or both. Dyspnea is the most common symptom reported by patients with AHF and can include exertional dyspnea, paroxysmal nocturnal dyspnea, or orthopnea. Peripheral edema, abdominal discomfort or bloating, and early satiety are also seen. Fatigue and changes in mental status can be related to hypoperfusion.

Physical Examination

AHF is a clinical diagnosis and, therefore, the physical examination is pivotal to assessment and subsequent management. The physical examination must focus on vital signs (bradycardia, tachycardia, hypertension, hypotension, narrow pulse pressure, hypoxia), jugular venous pressure (JVP),

cardiac, respiratory, abdominal, and extremity examinations.[49] Although blood pressure is generally related to cardiac output and organ perfusion, hypotension and hypoperfusion are not synonymous. Patients with systemic hypoperfusion may have normal blood pressures, and likewise, patients with advanced HF may have chronically low blood pressures not associated with acute hypoperfusion. In AHF, proportional pulse pressure ([systolic–diastolic blood pressure]/systolic blood pressure) <25% is associated with low cardiac index (<2.2 L/min/m²) with high sensitivity and specificity.[50]

The presence of jugular venous distention suggests elevated right-sided filling pressures, which in 80% of cases (wherein there is no significant isolated right heart dysfunction) suggests elevated left-sided filling pressures.[51] The JVP may not reflect left-sided filling pressures in isolated RV failure and can be difficult to assess with significant tricuspid regurgitation. Cardiac examination may reveal a third heart sound, suggestive of LV dilatation, or fourth heart sound, which may indicate poor LV compliance. The Valsalva maneuver may be used to indicate the presence of altered arterial pressures, suggesting LV systolic dysfunction, but may be more challenging to perform in the

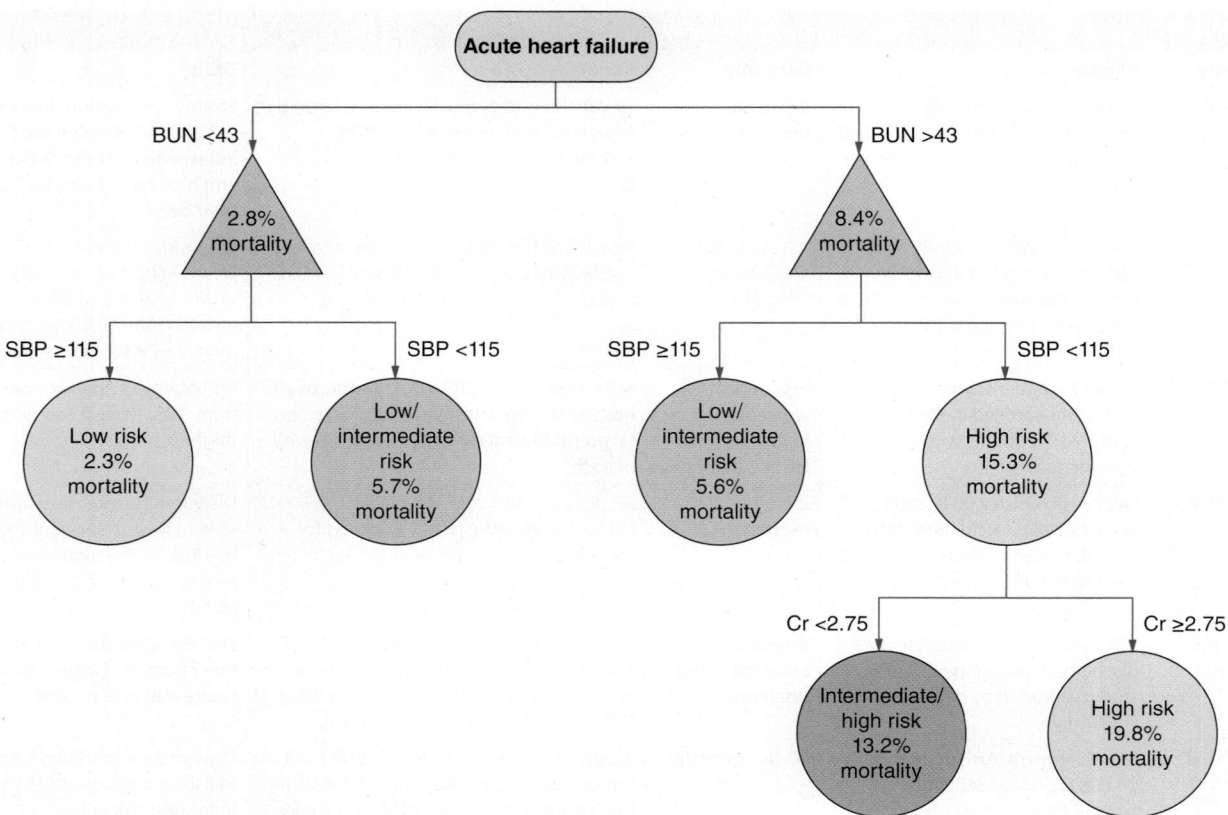

Figure 50–5. The Acute Decompensated Heart Failure National Registry (ADHERE) "risk tree" assessing inpatient mortality in patients admitted with acute decompensated heart failure in the ADHERE registry. Mortality varies based on admission blood urea nitrogen (BUN), systolic blood pressure (SBP), and serum creatinine (Cr).

acute setting.[52] New or worsened murmur may indicate worsened ventricular dilatation or new valvular disease.

In Organized Program to Initiate Lifesaving Treatment in Hospitalized Patients with Heart Failure (OPTIMIZE-HF), 64% of enrolled patients had rales on exam, likely reflecting increased pulmonary capillary wedge pressure (PCWP).[53] However, rales are often not heard in patients with progressive chronic HF because of increased lymphatic drainage, and the absence of rales does not necessarily imply normal LV filling pressures. Abdominal examination may reveal hepatomegaly signifying passive congestion, or ascites. The presence of a hepatojugular reflux can indicate RV dysfunction. An extremity exam can provide insight on both congestion with lower extremity and dependent edema and perfusion with poor capillary refill and cool temperature (**Table 50–2**).[54]

Diagnostic Testing

Several diagnostic tests are essential as part of a work-up for AHF, including laboratory testing, electrocardiogram (ECG), chest radiograph, and echocardiogram. Initial laboratory testing should include complete blood count, serum electrolytes, blood urea nitrogen, serum creatinine, liver function tests, thyroid-stimulating hormone, and urinalysis.[49] Specific attention should be paid to the presence of anemia, hyponatremia, and renal dysfunction. Evidence of hepatic abnormalities may be from passive congestion and RV dysfunction.

Measurement of natriuretic peptides is recommended for patients in whom the diagnosis of AHF is uncertain or for prognostic information.[49] Both atrial natriuretic peptide (ANP) and B-type natriuretic peptide (BNP) have vasodilatory,

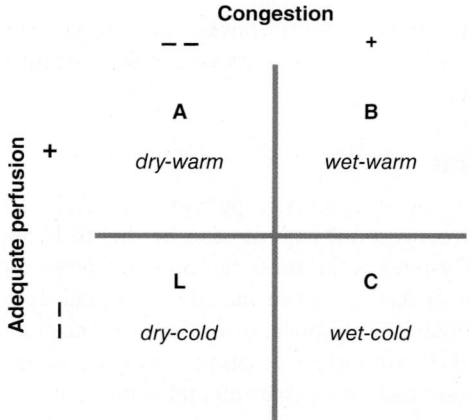

Figure 50–6. Hemodynamic assessment of clinical profiles. Congestion evaluated by orthopnea, jugular venous distention, rales, hepatojugular reflux, ascites, peripheral edema, leftward pulmonic heart sound, or square-wave blood pressure response to Valsalva maneuver. Poor perfusion determined by presence of narrow pulse pressure, pulsus alternans, symptomatic hypotension, cool extremities, and/or decreased mentation. Reproduced with permission from Nohria A, Tsang SW, Fang JC, et al. Reproduced from Clinical assessment identifies hemodynamic profiles that predict outcomes in patients admitted with heart failure. *J Am Coll Cardiol.* 2003 May 21;41(10):1797-1804.

TABLE 50-2. History and Physical Examination in Acute Heart Failure

History	Physical Examination	Clinical/Hemodynamic Significance
Establishment of diagnosis (ie, volume status and assessment of precipitating factors)		
Dyspnea	Rales, dullness to percussion, cardiac wheezing, reduced oxygen saturation, accessory respiratory muscle use, elevated jugular venous pressure, peripheral edema, hepatomegaly, ascites	Pulmonary edema, left heart failure, right heart failure
Confusion, lightheadedness, dizziness	Systolic blood pressure (SBP) <90 mm Hg, orthostatic hypotension, poor peripheral perfusion	Low output state, poor perfusion, possible hypovolemia
Weakness, fatigue	SBP <90 mm Hg, elevated jugular venous pressure, hepatomegaly, peripheral edema, decreased strength and muscle mass	Low output state, right heart failure
Cold periphery	Cool extremities, anuria, oliguria	Low output state, poor perfusion, renal insufficiency, possible cardiogenic shock
Abdominal discomfort	Hepatomegaly, ascites	Right ventricular dysfunction
Palpitations	Tachycardia, bradycardia, irregular rhythm	Atrial fibrillation, heart block
Evaluation of comorbidities		
Hypertension	Blood pressure, fourth heart sound	Stiff left ventricle, impaired relaxation
Dyslipidemia	Xanthomas	Suggestive of coronary artery disease or metabolic syndrome
Coronary artery disease, chest pain	Bruits, diaphoresis, visible discomfort	Acute coronary syndrome
Valvular abnormalities (ie, mitral regurgitation, aortic stenosis, or regurgitation)	Systolic or diastolic murmur	Altered left ventricular geometry; elevated left ventricular diastolic and/or left atrial pressures
Arrhythmias (ie, atrial fibrillation)	Heart rate, irregular rhythm	Risk of stroke or sudden cardiac death

Reproduced with permission from Harinstein ME, Flaherty JD, Fonarow GC, et al. Clinical assessment of acute heart failure syndromes: emergency department through the early post-discharge period. *Heart*. 2011 Oct;97(19):1607-1618.

natriuretic, and diuretic properties.[55] N-terminal pro–B-type natriuretic peptide (NT-proBNP) is part of the precursor peptide BNP and has a longer half-life.[56] BNP and NT-proBNP are similar for diagnosis of AHF, but NT-proBNP is superior in predicting clinical outcome.[57,58] Serial measurement may add to prognostic prediction. The Pro-BNP Outpatient Tailored Chronic Heart Failure Therapy (PROTECT) study showed that a 50% reduction in NT-proBNP correlated with a nearly 50% reduction in event rate.[59] Biomarkers of myocardial injury, such as troponins T and I, are associated with worse clinical outcomes and mortality and should be routinely measured in patients presenting with AHF.[49,60]

Besides natriuretic peptides and troponins, multiple other biomarkers, including those reflecting neurohormonal activation, inflammation, and myocardial remodeling have been studied in AHF. Biomarker utilization may add to risk prediction, although in which combination and in what capacity remain largely undefined. Biomarkers of myocardial fibrosis, soluble suppression of tumorigenesis-2 (sST2) and galectin-3 are predictive of hospitalization and death and additive to natriuretic peptides in their prognostic value.[49] The Multinational Observational Cohort on Acute Heart Failure (MOCA) trial studied the value of adding biomarkers to a clinical prediction model. The strongest biomarkers in this analysis were midregional pro-adrenomedullin (MRproADM), a marker of neurohormonal activation, and sST2.[61] The Biomarkers in Acute Heart Failure (BACH) trial, a prospective multicenter study of patients presenting with dyspnea, showed MRproADM

to be the best predictor of mortality compared with BNP and NT-proBNP.[62] Future research will need to focus on comprehensive biomarker investigations to reveal the clinical potential of novel biomarkers.

All patients presenting with AHF should have an initial ECG to look for changes suggestive of ischemia and arrhythmias, which are common triggers for AHF.[49] Chest radiography should be performed to assess for pulmonary congestion, cardiomegaly, pleural and pericardial effusions, and other pulmonary processes that may be contributing factors, such as infection or pulmonary disease.[54] Other noninvasive testing includes echocardiogram and, in appropriate cases, assessment for the presence of ischemia and myocardial viability. Echocardiography is useful for evaluating the etiology of HF. It allows for the determination of systolic and diastolic function, wall motion abnormalities, valvular function, and hemodynamics including estimates of filling pressures and cardiac output.[63] Although the role of handheld echocardiography is still evolving, this imaging modality may also aid in estimation of filling pressures.[64] There are several modalities that can be used for noninvasive assessment of myocardial ischemia and/or viability in appropriate patients, including stress echocardiography, nuclear imaging, and cardiac magnetic resonance imaging.[49]

Pulmonary artery catheters (PACs) may be useful in the management of some patients with AHF. The Evaluation Study of Congestive Heart Failure and Pulmonary Artery Catheterization and Effectiveness (ESCAPE) trial randomized patients to receive therapy guided by clinical assessment and PAC or

TABLE 50–3. Precipitating Factors Leading to Acute Heart Failure

Medical Factors	Psychosocial Factors
CARDIAC:	Nonadherence to
Changes to cardiac meds (negative inotropes such as BBs or non-DHPs)	Sodium restriction
	Fluid restriction
Accelerated or uncontrolled HTN	Medications
Ischemia/Acute coronary syndrome	Daily weights
Valvular disease	Poor insight into illness
Arrhythmia	Poor access to medications or
NONCARDIAC:	health care as a result of cost or
Endocrine abnormalities	physical condition
Infection	ETOH or illicit drug use
Anemia	OTC drugs such as NSAIDS,
Pregnancy	herbal, dietary
Pulmonary embolus	

Abbreviations: BB, β-blocker; DHP, dihydropyridine; ETOH, alcohol; HTN, hypertension; NSAID, nonsteroidal anti-inflammatory drug; OTC, over the counter.

by clinical assessment alone. In ESCAPE, use of PACs did not significantly affect the days alive and out of hospital during the first 6 months, mortality, or number of days hospitalized compared to clinical assessment alone.[65] It is important to note that the ESCAPE trial excluded patients whom physicians felt clearly required PAC for optimal management and involved physician investigators who were highly experienced in the evaluation and treatment of HF. The ACCF/AHA guidelines state that invasive hemodynamic monitoring with a PAC should be performed to guide therapy in patients who have respiratory distress or clinical evidence of impaired perfusion in whom filling pressures cannot be determined from clinical assessment. Invasive hemodynamic monitoring can also be useful for patients with AHF who have persistent symptoms despite empirically adjusting therapy.[49]

Identifying Triggers

Patients requiring hospitalization for AHF can often be characterized as having a precipitating event (**Table 50–3**). Data from OPTIMIZE-HF represents the most comprehensive identification of precipitants leading to hospitalization for AHF, reporting that of the almost 50,000 patients included, roughly 60% had one or more identified precipitating factors. These precipitants independently predicted clinical outcomes, making early identification and targeted therapy critical. These precipitants included ischemia or acute coronary syndromes, arrhythmia, uncontrolled hypertension, pneumonia, WRF, and nonadherence with diet or medications.[66] Prompt identification and early medical management of precipitating factors in AHF are essential to improve outcomes of these patients.

MANAGEMENT OF THE PATIENT WITH ACUTE HEART FAILURE

Management of AHF involves relieving congestion and restoring or maintaining systemic perfusion. The ESC has proposed an algorithm for the management of patients with AHF based on their hemodynamic profile (**Fig. 50–7**). After initial stabilization, usually in the emergency department, patients admitted with AHF require comprehensive and multidisciplinary care in the hospital with focused and careful discharge planning (**Table 50–4**).[54,67]

Traditionally, two phases of AHF care have been described.[68,69] Phase I is the stabilization phase, often beginning with care in the emergency department, where the main goals include identification and improvement of signs and symptoms, hemodynamics, and volume overload. Phase II continues into the hospitalization and through discharge planning. Primary goals include prevention of disease progression, focus on improvement of cardiac function, and following evidence-based guidelines. Critical to phase I is the early and appropriate identification of precipitating factors and determination of clinical profiles whereby therapies can be targeted. Paramount to phase II is the incorporation of guideline-directed medical therapy (GDMT) to optimize mortality benefit.

More recently, the ACC expert consensus decision pathway emphasizes the importance of assessing the clinical trajectory of HF continuously during admission. Three main in-hospital trajectories have been defined: *improving towards target, stalled after initial response, and not improved/worsening.* These trajectories translate into different management strategies throughout hospitalization and postdischarge (**Fig. 50–8**).[70] The ACCF/AHA guidelines provide recommendations for therapies in the hospitalized patient with AHF (**Table 50–5**).[49] Despite a multitude of clinical trials evaluating therapies to improve outcomes in AHF, few have translated to direct benefit, underscoring the need for multidisciplinary care and ongoing research (**Table 50–6**).

Diuretics

Loop diuretics (furosemide, torsemide, and bumetanide) are the primary treatment to restore euvolemia in patients with volume overload related to salt and water retention. Most patients with AHF will require intravenous diuretics, with the initial dose either equivalent to or exceeding their home dose.[49] Diuretic therapy should be delivered without delay because early intervention has been shown to improve outcome in observational studies.[58,71] The Diuretic Optimization Strategies Evaluation (DOSE) trial randomized AHF patients to low-dose (equal to daily diuretic dose) or high-dose (2.5 times total daily dose) furosemide, administered as either an intravenous bolus every 12 hours or as a continuous infusion. The study found no significant difference between strategies in the patient-reported global assessment of symptoms and no change in serum creatinine from baseline to 72 hours.[72] However, there was a trend toward greater improvement in patients' global assessment of symptoms in the high-dose versus the low-dose group. In addition, the high-dose strategy was associated with more favorable outcomes in some secondary measures, including lower levels of BNP, higher levels of diuresis, and relief of dyspnea.

Patients with refractory volume retention may require higher doses of their current loop diuretic, a switch to an alternative loop diuretic, or addition of a diuretic with a different mechanism of action such as a thiazide diuretic (metolazone

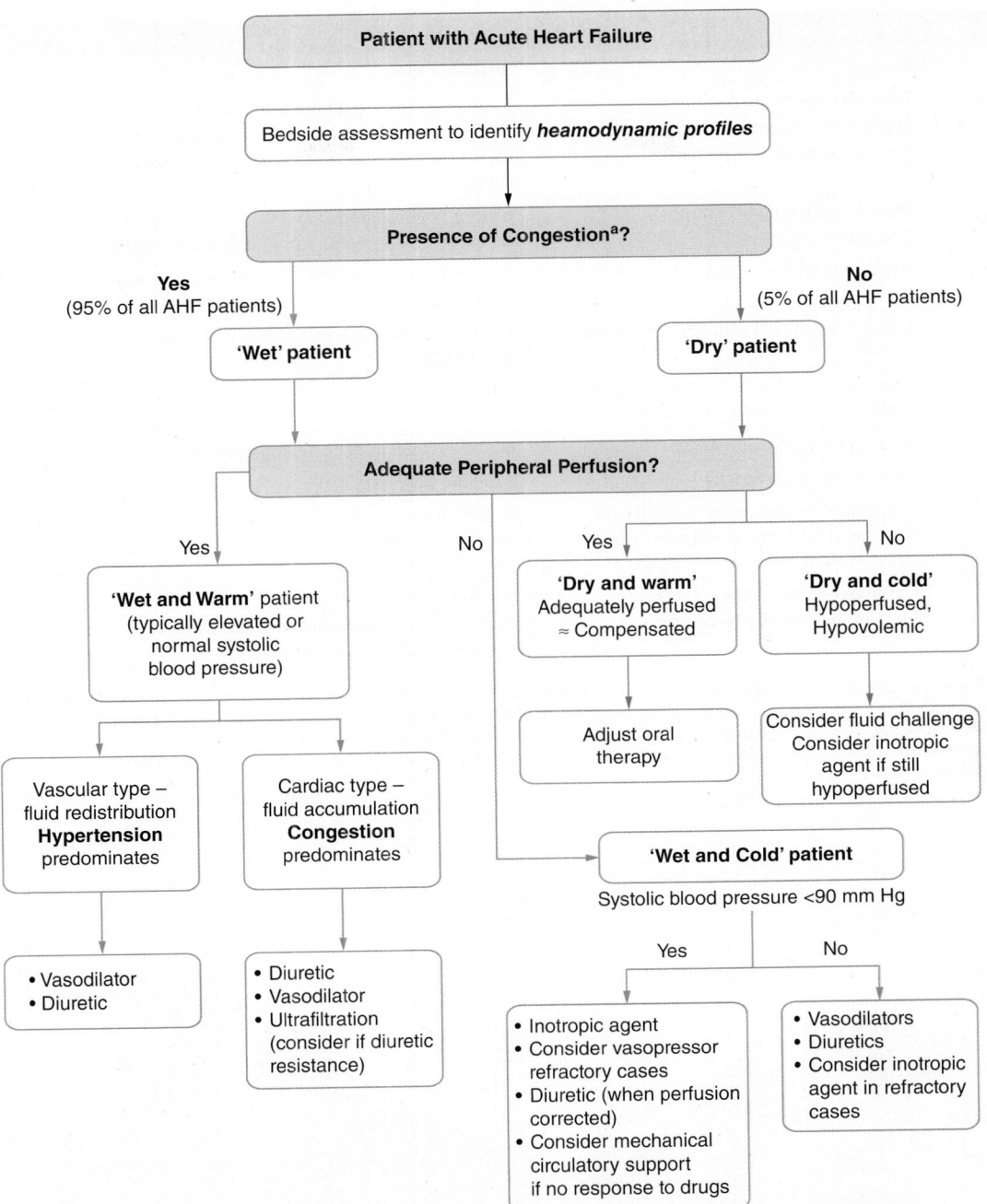

Figure 50–7. Management of patients with acute heart failure based on clinical profile during an early phase. ªSymptoms/signs of congestion: orthopnea, paroxysmal nocturnal dyspnea, breathlessness, bi-basilar rales, an abnormal blood pressure response to the Valsalva maneuver (left-sided); symptoms of gut congestion, jugular venous distension, hepatojugular reflux, hepatomegaly, ascites, and peripheral edema (right-sided). Reproduced with permission from Ponikowski P, Voors AA, Anker SD, et al. 2016 ESC Guidelines for the diagnosis and treatment of acute and chronic heart failure: The Task Force for the diagnosis and treatment of acute and chronic heart failure of the European Society of Cardiology (ESC)Developed with the special contribution of the Heart Failure Association (HFA) of the ESC. *Eur Heart J*. 2016 Jul 14;37(27):2129-2200.

or chlorthiazide). Thiazides may be useful as an addition in patients on chronic loop diuretics because they may overcome loop diuretic resistance, but they should be used with caution because they can cause electrolyte disturbances such as hypokalemia. Mineralocorticoid receptor antagonists (MRAs) such as spironolactone and eplerenone have established mortality benefit in chronic HFrEF patients.[49] They can also augment diuresis by blocking salt-retaining aldosterone receptors.[73]

Mild elevations in blood urea nitrogen and creatinine should be monitored closely, but should not prompt lowering or withholding diuretics in patients with volume overload. In some patients in whom volume overload is accompanied by preexisting renal impairment, response to diuretic therapy may be attenuated. In most cases, adequate diuretic dosing improves renal function as a result of venous decongestion.[74] Patients requiring augmentation of diuretics require frequent

TABLE 50–4. Phases of Acute Heart Failure Management

Phases	Goals	Available Tools
Initial or emergency department phase of management	Treat life threatening conditions Establish the diagnosis Determine the clinical profile	Examples: STEMI → reperfusion therapy History, physical exam, ECG, x-ray, natriuretic peptide level BP, HR, signs (pulmonary edema), ECG, x-ray, laboratory analysis, echocardiography
	Identify and treat precipitant Disposition	History, physical exam No universally accepted risk-stratification method
In-hospital phase	Monitoring and reassessment	Signs/symptoms, HR, SBP, ECG, orthostatic changes, body weight, laboratory analysis (BUN/Cr, electrolytes), potentially BNP
	Assess right and left ventricular pressures	SBP (orthostatic changes, Valsalva maneuver), echocardiography, BNP/NT-pro BNP, PA catheter
	Assess and treat (in the right patient) other cardiac and non-cardiac conditions	Echo-Doppler, cardiac catheterization, electrophysiology testing
	Assess for myocardial viability	MRI, stress testing, echocardiography, radionuclear studies
Discharge phase	Assess functional capacity	6-minute walk test
	Re-evaluate exacerbating factors (eg, non-adherence, infection, anemia, arrhythmias, hypertension) and treat accordingly	Physical therapy, education for diet control and medication, evaluation for sleep apnea
	Optimize pharmacological therapy Establish post-discharge planning	ACCF/AHA and ESC guidelines Discharge instructions including body weight monitoring, smoking cessation, medication adherence, follow-up

Abbreviations: ACCF, American College of Cardiology Foundation; AHA, American Heart Association; BNP, B-type natriuretic peptide; BP, blood pressure; BUN, blood urea nitrogen; Cr, creatinine; ECG, electrocardiogram; ESC, European Society of Cardiology; HR, heart rate; MRI, magnetic resonance imaging; NT-proBNP, N-terminal pro–B-type natriuretic peptide; PA, pulmonary artery; SBP, systolic blood pressure; STEMI, ST-segment elevation myocardial infarction.
Reproduced with permission from Gheorghiade M, Zannad F, Sopko G, et al. Acute heart failure syndromes: current state and framework for future research. *Circulation.* 2005 Dec 20;112(25):3958-3968.

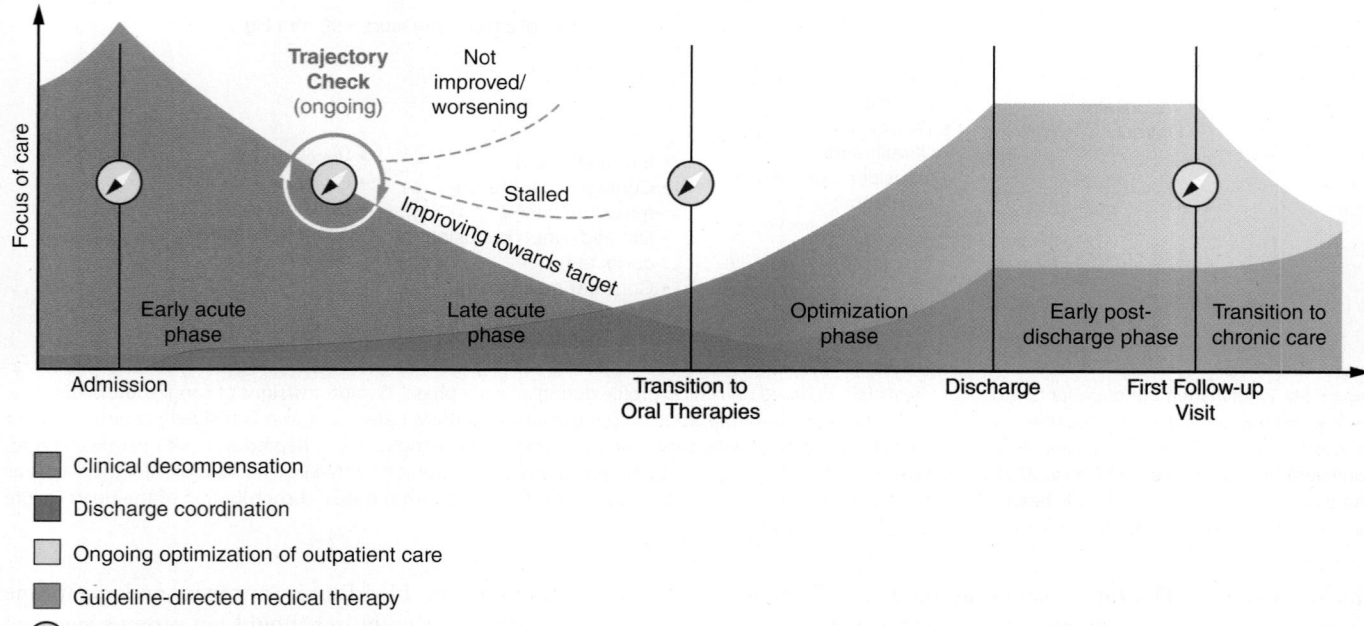

Figure 50–8. Graphic depiction of course of heart failure admission, showing the degree of focus on clinical decompensation (*red*), discharge coordination (*blue*), ongoing coordination of outpatient care (*light blue*), and optimization of guideline-directed medical therapy (*green*), with ongoing assessment of the clinical course (*circle with arrows*), and key time points for review and revision of the long-term disease trajectory for the HF journey (*compass signs*). Reproduced with permission from Hollenberg SM, Warner Stevenson L, Ahmad T, et al. 2019 ACC Expert Consensus Decision Pathway on Risk Assessment, Management, and Clinical Trajectory of Patients Hospitalized With Heart Failure: A Report of the American College of Cardiology Solution Set Oversight Committee. *J Am Coll Cardiol.* 2019 Oct 15;74(15):1966-2011.

TABLE 50–5. American College of Cardiology Foundation/American Heart Association Recommendations for Therapies in the Hospitalized Heart Failure Patient

Recommendations	COR	LOE
HF patients hospitalized with fluid overload should be treated with intravenous diuretics	I	B
HF patients receiving loop diuretic therapy should receive an initial parenteral dose greater than or equal to their chronic oral daily dose; then dose should be serially adjusted	I	B
HFrEF patients requiring HF hospitalization on GDMT should continue GDMT except in cases of hemodynamic instability or where contraindicated	I	B
Initiation of beta-blocker therapy at a low dose is recommended after optimization of volume status and discontinuation of intravenous agents	I	B
Thrombosis/thromboembolism prophylaxis is recommended for patients hospitalized with HF	I	B
Serum electrolytes, urea nitrogen, and creatinine should be measured during titration of HF medications, including diuretics	I	C
When diuresis is inadequate, it is reasonable to	IIa	
a. give higher doses of intravenous loop diuretics; or		B
b. add a second diuretic (eg, thiazide)		B
Low-dose dopamine infusion may be considered with loop diuretics to improve diuresis	IIb	B
Ultrafiltration may be considered for patients with obvious volume overload	IIb	B
Ultrafiltration may be considered for patients with refractory congestion	IIb	C
Intravenous nitroglycerin, nitroprusside, or nesiritide may be considered an adjuvant to diuretic therapy for stable patients with HF	IIb	A
In patients hospitalized with volume overload and severe hyponatremia, vasopressin antagonists may be considered	IIb	B

Abbreviations: COR, class of recommendation; GDMT, guideline-directed medical therapy; HF, heart failure; HFrEF, heart failure with reduced ejection fraction; LOE, level of evidence.
Reproduced with permission from Yancy CW, Jessup M, Bozkurt B, et al. 2013 ACCF/AHA guideline for the management of heart failure: a report of the American College of Cardiology Foundation/American Heart Association Task Force on Practice Guidelines. *J Am Coll Cardiol.* 2013 Oct 15;62(16):e147-e239.

reassessment and monitoring of volume status by measurement of vital signs, physical exam, measurement of daily weight, and daily serum laboratory testing. Hospital discharge should only be considered once euvolemia has been achieved and an appropriate diuretic strategy for maintenance therapy has been established. Roughly 50% of patients are discharged from the hospital with residual congestion after which they are at considerably higher risk of early readmission and poor outcomes.[75]

Vasodilators

In patients with volume overload without systemic hypotension, intravenous vasodilators such as nitroglycerin, nitroprusside, or nesiritide may provide benefit when added to diuretic therapy.[49] Intravenous nitroglycerin, primarily a venodilator, lowers preload, thereby relieving pulmonary congestion. Patients with hypertension, coronary ischemia, or severe mitral regurgitation are considered good candidates for nitroglycerin therapy.[76] Limitations include rapid development of tachyphylaxis, leading to drug resistance even at high doses.

Sodium nitroprusside is a balanced venous and arterial vasodilator that also provides some pulmonary vasodilation. Sodium nitroprusside can be used in markedly congested patients with hypertension or severe mitral regurgitation, although use is often limited by potential for systemic hypotension and potential thiocyanate toxicity, especially in patients with renal insufficiency.[76]

Nesiritide reduces LV filling pressures and relieves dyspnea, but may lead to hypotension. Nesiritide was shown to improve early hemodynamics in the Vasodilation in the Management of Acute Heart Failure (VMAC) trial.[77] However, the subsequent Acute Study of Clinical Effectiveness of Nesiritide in Decompensated Heart Failure (ASCEND-HF) trial failed to reach statistical significance for either relief of dyspnea or HF readmission or death at 30 days compared with placebo.[78] Furthermore, the Renal Optimization Strategies Evaluation in Acute Heart Failure (ROSE-HF) trial, with low-dose nesiritide versus low-dose dopamine in patients with AHF and renal failure, also failed to show improvements in urine output, renal function, rehospitalization, HF symptoms, or mortality, and showed nesiritide to be associated with more symptomatic hypotension than placebo.[79]

Vasodilators should be used with caution in patients who are preload or afterload dependent (severe diastolic dysfunction, aortic stenosis, CAD), since they can cause severe hypotension. As outlined in ACCF/AHA guidelines, there are no data that suggest that intravenous vasodilators improve outcomes in the patient hospitalized with HF. Therefore, use of intravenous vasodilators is limited to the relief of dyspnea in the hospitalized HF patient with intact blood pressure.[49]

Inotropes

Some patients with AHF present with low CO, manifested by low blood pressure (with or without congestion) accompanied by signs of decreased end-organ perfusion. Clinical manifestations may include cool or clammy skin, cool extremities, decreased urine output, and mental status changes. In patients

TABLE 50-6. Major Clinical Trials in Patients with Acute Heart Failure

Study	Year	Total Participants	Design	Inclusion Criteria	Primary outcomes	Results
VMAC	2002	489	Randomized, double-blind IV nesiritide (n = 204), nitroglycerin (n = 143), or placebo (n = 142) for 3 h, followed by nesiritide (n = 278) or nitroglycerin (n = 216) for 24 h	Inpatients with dyspnea at rest from AHF Estimated or measured elevation of cardiac filling pressures (PCWP ≥20 mm Hg in catheterized patients) and ≥2 of following: (1) JVD, (2) PND or 2-pillow orthopnea within 72 h, (3) abdominal discomfort due to mesenteric congestion, or (4) CXR consistent with decompensated HF	Change in PCWP in catheterized patients and patient self-evaluation of dyspnea in all patients at 3 h	3 h: mean (SD) decrease in PCWP −5.8 (6.5) mm Hg for nesiritide (vs placebo, p <0.001; vs nitroglycerin, p = 0.03), −3.8 (5.3) mm Hg for nitroglycerin (vs placebo, p = 0.09), −2 (4.2) mm Hg for placebo 3 h: nesiritide resulted in improvement in dyspnea vs placebo (p = 0.03) No difference in dyspnea or global clinical status with nesiritide vs nitroglycerin
OPTIME-CHF	2002	951	Randomized, double-blind IV milrinone (0.5 μg/kg/min initially) (n = 477) or placebo (n = 472) for 48 h	Inpatients with AHF not requiring IV inotropes LVEF <40%	Cumulative days of hospitalization for CV cause within 60 days	Median number of days hospitalized for CV causes within 60 days did not differ between milrinone vs placebo (6 vs 7 days; p = 0.71) Sustained hypotension requiring intervention (10.7% vs 3.2%; p <0.001) and new atrial arrhythmias (4.6% vs 1.5%; p = 0.004) occurred more with milrinone Groups did not differ in in-hospital mortality, 60-day mortality, or composite incidence of death or readmission
ESCAPE	2005	433	Randomized Therapy guided by clinical assessment and a PAC (n = 215) or clinical assessment alone (n = 218)	Inpatients with severe symptomatic HF despite recommended therapies Severe defined as: (1) hospitalization for HF within past year, (2) urgent visit to ED, or (3) treatment during preceding month with >160 mg furosemide daily (or equivalent) LVEF ≤30% SBP ≤125 mm Hg ≥3 months of symptoms despite ACE inhibitors and diuretics ≥1 sign and 1 symptom of congestion	Days alive out of hospital during first 6 months	Both groups had substantial reduction in symptoms, JVP, and edema Use of PAC did not significantly affect primary end point of days alive and out of hospital during first 6 months (133 vs 135 days; HR 1.00; 95% CI 0.82–1.21; p = 0.99), mortality (p = 0.35), or number of days hospitalized (p = 0.67) In-hospital adverse events more common in PAC group (47 [21.9%] vs 25 [11.5%]; p = 0.04) No deaths related to PAC use, and no difference for in-hospital plus 30-day mortality (p = 0.97)
VERITAS	2007	1435	2 independent, identical, and concurrent randomized, double-blind, parallel-group trials IV tezosentan (5 mg/h for 30 minutes, followed by 1 mg/h for 24 to 72 h) (n = 730) or placebo (n = 718)	Inpatients admitted within 24 h with persisting dyspnea and resp rate ≥24/min and 2 of 4 criteria: (1) elevated BNP or NT-proBNP, (2) clinical pulmonary edema, (3) pulmonary congestion or edema on CXR, or (4) LV systolic dysfunction	Coprimary end points: change in dyspnea using VAS AUC over 24 h in individual trials and incidence of death or worsening HF at 7 days in both trials combined	No change in dyspnea with tezosentan vs placebo in either trial Mean treatment difference of −12 mm × h (p = 0.80) in first trial and −25 mm × h (p = 0.60) in second trial Incidence of death or worsening HF at 7 days in combined trials 26% in each treatment group (p = 0.95)
SURVIVE	2007	1327	Randomized, double-blind IV levosimendan (n = 664) or IV dobutamine (n = 663)	Inpatients with AHF who required inotropic support LVEF ≤30% Insufficient response to IV diuretics and/or vasodilators, and ≥1 of following: (1) dyspnea at rest or mechanical ventilation for HF, (2) oliguria not as result of hypovolemia, or (3) PCWP ≥18 mm Hg and/or cardiac index ≤2.2 L/min/m²	All-cause mortality at 180 days	All-cause mortality at 180 days occurred in 173 (26%) patients in levosimendan group and 185 (28%) patients in dobutamine group (HR 0.91; 95% CI 0.74–1.13; p = 0.40) Levosimendan group had greater decreases in BNP at 24 h that persisted through 5 days (p <0.001) Higher incidences of atrial fibrillation, hypokalemia, and headache in levosimendan group

EVEREST[125]	2007	4133	Randomized, double-blind Oral tolvaptan (30 mg daily) (n = 2072) or placebo (n = 2061) for minimum of 60 days	Inpatients admitted within 48 h for exacerbation of chronic HF LVEF ≤40% NYHA class III/IV Signs of volume expansion	Coprimary end points: all-cause mortality (superiority and noninferiority) and CV death or HFH (superiority only)	During median follow-up of 9.9 months, 537 patients (25.9%) in tolvaptan group and 543 (26.3%) in placebo group died (HR 0.98; 95% CI 0.87-1.11; p = 0.68) Upper confidence limit for mortality difference was within prespecified noninferiority margin of 1.25 (p <0.001) Composite of CV death or HFH occurred in 871 tolvaptan patients (42.0%) and 829 placebo patients (40.2%; HR 1.04; 95% CI 0.95-1.14; p = 0.55)
UNLOAD	2007	200	Randomized UF (n = 100) or IV diuretics (n = 100)	Inpatients admitted within 24 h for AHF ≥2 signs of hypervolemia: (1) peripheral edema ≥2+, (2) JVD ≥7 cm, (3) pulmonary edema or pleural effusion on CXR, (4) enlarged liver or ascites, or (5) pulmonary rales, PND, or orthopnea	Weight loss and dyspnea assessment at 48 h	48 h: weight (5.0 ± 3.1 kg vs 3.1 ± 3.5 kg; p = 0.001) and net fluid loss (4.6 vs 3.3 l; p = 0.001) greater in UF group Dyspnea scores similar 90 days: UF had fewer patients rehospitalized for HF (p = 0.037), HF rehospitalizations (p = 0.022), rehospitalization days per patient (p = 0.022), and unscheduled visits (p = 0.009)
HORIZON-HF	2008	120	Randomized, double-blind IV istaroxime (n = 89) or placebo (n = 31) in 3 sequential, escalating-dose cohorts for 6 h	Inpatients with AHF LVEF ≤35% SBP <150 and >90 mm Hg Heart rate <110 and >60 beats/min	Change in PCWP at 6 h	All doses of istaroxime lowered PCWP (mean ± SD: −3.2 ± 6.8 mm Hg, −3.3 ± 5.5 mm Hg, and −4.7 ± 5.9 mm Hg compared with 0.0 ± 3.6 mm Hg with placebo; p <0.05 for all doses)
3CPO[126]	2008	1069	Randomized Oxygen (n = 367), CPAP (5 to 15 cm of water) (n = 346), or NIPPV (inspiratory pressure, 8 to 20 cm of water; expiratory pressure, 4 to 10 cm of water) (n = 356)	ED patients Clinical acute cardiogenic pulmonary edema Resp rate ≥20/min Pulmonary edema on CXR Arterial pH <7.35	Primary end point between noninvasive ventilation and oxygen: death within 7 days Primary end point between NIPPV and CPAP: death or intubation within 7 days	No difference in 7-day mortality between oxygen (9.8%) and noninvasive ventilation (9.5%, p = 0.87) No difference in combined end point of death or intubation within 7 days between two groups of patients undergoing noninvasive ventilation (11.7% for CPAP and 11.1% for NIPPV, p = 0.81)
DAD-HF	2010	60	Randomized, double-blind IV high-dose furosemide (20 mg/h) or low-dose furosemide (5 mg/h) combined with low-dose dopamine (5 μg/kg/min) for 8 h	Inpatients with AHF History of HF Deterioration of HF symptoms of recent onset (<6 h), namely, dyspnea at rest, orthopnea, and PND accompanied by signs of congestion (S3, JVD, pulmonary rales) Oxygen saturation <90% on admission BNP >400 pg/mL or NT-proBNP >1500 pg/mL eGFR ≥30 mL/min/1.73 m²	Incidence of WRF (rise in serum creatinine of >0.3 mg/dL) at 24 h	WRF more frequent in HDF (n = 9; 30%) than in LDFD group (n = 2; 6.7%; p = 0.042) Length of stay and 60-day mortality or rehospitalization rates (all-cause, CV, and worsening HF) similar in two groups

(Continued)

TABLE 50-6. Major Clinical Trials in Patients with Acute Heart Failure (Continued)

Study	Year	Total Participants	Design	Inclusion Criteria	Primary outcomes	Results
PROTECT[127]	2010	2033	Randomized, double-blind IV rolofylline (30 mg daily) (n = 1356) or placebo (n = 677) for up to 3 days	Inpatients admitted within 24 h with AHF with impaired renal function (estimated CrCl 20–80 ml/min) Persistent dyspnea at rest or with minimal activity BNP ≥500 pg/mL or NT-proBNP ≥2000 pg/mL Ongoing IV loop diuretic therapy	Treatment success, treatment failure, or no change in patient's clinical condition; this end point was defined according to survival, HF status, and changes in renal function	Rolofylline did not provide benefit with respect to primary end point (OR 0.92; 95% CI 0.78 to 1.09; p = 0.35)
DOSE	2011	308	Randomized, double-blind IV furosemide as either bolus every 12 h (n = 156) or continuous infusion (n = 152) and either low dose (equivalent to patient's previous oral dose) (n = 151) or high dose (2.5 times previous oral dose) (n = 157)	Inpatients admitted within 24 h with AHF History of chronic HF >1 symptom (dyspnea, orthopnea, or edema) and >1 sign (rales, peripheral edema, ascites, or pulmonary vascular congestion on CXR) of HF Receipt of oral loop diuretic for >1 month before hospitalization, at dose of 80–240 mg daily of furosemide or an equivalent dose different loop diuretic	Coprimary end points: patients' global assessment of symptoms by VAS AUC over 72 h and change in serum creatinine level at 72 h	With bolus vs continuous infusion, no difference in patients' global assessment of symptoms (mean AUC, 4236 ± 1440 vs 4373 ± 140; p = 0.47) or in mean change in creatinine level (0.05 ± 0.3 mg per deciliter [4.4 ± 26.5 µmol per liter] vs 0.07 ± 0.3 mg per deciliter [6.2 ± 26.5 µmol per liter]; p = 0.45) With high-dose vs low-dose, a nonsignificant trend toward greater improvement in patients' global assessment of symptoms in high-dose group (p = 0.06) With high-dose vs low-dose, no difference in mean change in creatinine level (0.08 ± 0.3 mg per deciliter [7.1 ± 26.5 µmol per liter] vs 0.04 ± 0.3 mg per deciliter [3.5 ± 26.5 µmol per liter]; p = 0.21)
ASCEND-HF	2011	7141	Randomized, double-blind IV nesiritide (n = 3496) or placebo (n = 3511) for 24 to 168 h	Inpatients with AHF within 24 h of first IV treatment for HF Dyspnea at rest or with minimal activity ≥1 sign (resp rate ≥20/min or pulmonary congestion or edema with rales) and ≥1 objective measure of HF (congestion or edema on CXR, BNP ≥400 pg/mL or NT-proBNP ≥1000 pg/mL, PCWP >20 mm Hg, or LVEF <40% in previous 12 months)	Coprimary end points: change in dyspnea at 6 and 24 h by Likert scale and composite end point of HFH or death within 30 days	With nesiritide patients more frequently reported markedly or moderately improved dyspnea at 6 h (44.5% vs 42.1%, p = 0.03) and 24 h (68.2% vs 66.1%, p = 0.007), but prespecified level for significance (p ≤.005 for both assessments or p ≤.0025 for either) was not met Rate of HFH or death from any cause within 30 days was 9.4% in nesiritide group vs 10.1% in placebo group (p = 0.31)
CARRESS-HF	2012	188 (200 planned)	Randomized UF (n = 94) or stepped pharmacologic therapy (n = 94)	Inpatients with AHF and WRF (increase in serum creatinine level of at least 0.3 mg/dL) within 12 weeks before or 10 days after admission ≥2 of following: (1) ≥2+ peripheral edema, (2) jugular venous pressure >10 cm, or (3) pulmonary edema or pleural effusion on CXR	Bivariate change from baseline in serum creatinine level and body weight at 96 h	UF was inferior to pharmacologic therapy with respect to bivariate end point of change in serum creatinine level and body weight at 96 h (p = 0.003), owing primarily to increase in creatinine level in UF group 96 h: mean change in creatinine level −0.04 ± 0.53 mg per deciliter (−3.5 ± 46.9 µmol per liter) in pharmacologic-therapy group vs +0.23 ± 0.70 mg per deciliter (20.3 ± 61.9 µmol per liter) in UF group (p = 0.003) No difference in weight loss at 96 h (loss of 5.5 ± 5.1 kg [12.1 ± 11.3 lb] in pharmacologic-therapy group vs 5.7 ± 3.9 kg [12.6 ± 8.5 lb] in UF group; p = 0.58)

Trial	Year	N	Design	Inclusion Criteria	Primary End Point	Results
RELAX-AHF	2013	1161	Randomized, double-blind IV serelaxin (30 µg/kg/day) (n = 581) or placebo (n = 580) for 48 h	Inpatients admitted within 16 h with AHF Dyspnea at rest or with minimal exertion, congestion on CXR, BNP ≥350 ng/L or NT-proBNP ≥1400 ng/L, eGFR 30–75 mL/min/1.73 m², and SBP >125 mm Hg	Change from baseline in VAS AUC at 5 days and proportion of patients with moderate or marked dyspnea improvement by Likert scale within 24 h	Serelaxin improved VAS AUC primary dyspnea endpoint (448 mm × h, 95% CI 120–775; p = 0.007), but had no effect on other primary endpoint (Likert scale; p = 0.70)
ASTRONAUT	2013	1639	Randomized, double-blind Aliskiren (150 mg increased to 300 mg daily as tolerated) (n = 821) or placebo (n = 818)	Inpatients with AHF after stabilization, defined as SBP ≥110 mm Hg for ≥6 h and no use of IV vasodilators (except nitrates) or IV inotropes LVEF ≤40% BNP ≥400 pg/mL or NT-proBNP ≥1600 pg/mL on admission	First occurrence of CV death or HFH at 6 months	24.9% of patients receiving aliskiren (77 CV deaths, 153 HFH) and 26.5% of patients receiving placebo (85 CV deaths, 166 HFH) experienced primary end point at 6 months (HR 0.92; 95% CI 0.76–1.12; p = 0.41) Rates of hyperkalemia, hypotension, and renal impairment/renal failure higher in aliskiren group
REVIVE-II	2013	600	Randomized, double-blind IV levosimendan (n = 299) or placebo (n = 301) for 24 h	Inpatients with AHF who remained dyspneic at rest despite treatment with IV diuretics LVEF ≤35%	Composite that evaluated changes in clinical status within 5 days	More levosimendan than placebo patients (58 vs 44) improved at all 3 pre-specified time points (6 h, 24 h, and 5 days), whereas fewer levosimendan patients (58 vs 82) experienced clinical worsening (p = 0.015 for difference between groups) Improvements in patient self-assessment and declines in BNP with levosimendan persisted for 5 days and were associated with reduced length of stay (p = 0.009) Levosimendan associated with more frequent hypotension and cardiac arrhythmias during infusion period and numerically higher risk of death across REVIVE-I and REVIVE-II (49/350 on levosimendan vs 40/350 on placebo at 90 days, p = 0.29)
ROSE-HF	2013	360	Randomized, double-blind IV dopamine (n = 22), IV nesiritide (n = 119), or IV pooled placebo (n = 119)	Inpatients admitted within 24 h with AHF and eGFR 15–60 mL/min/1.73 m² ≥1 symptom (dyspnea, orthopnea, or edema) and 1 sign of HF (rales, edema, ascites, or pulmonary vascular congestion on CXR)	Cumulative urine volume (decongestion end point) and change in serum cystatin C (renal function end point) at 72 h	Low-dose dopamine had no effect on 72-h cumulative urine volume (dopamine, 8524 mL; 95% CI 7917-9131 vs placebo, 8296 mL; 95% CI 7762–8830; difference, 229 mL; 95% CI −714 to 1171 mL; p = 0.59) or on change in cystatin C level (dopamine, 0.12 mg/L; 95% CI 0.06–0.18 vs placebo, 0.11 mg/L; 95% CI 0.06–0.16; difference, 0.01; 95% CI −0.08 to 0.10; p = 0.72) Low-dose nesiritide had no effect on 72-h cumulative urine volume (nesiritide, 8574 mL; 95% CI 8014-9134 vs placebo, 8296mL; 95% CI 7762–8830; difference, 279 mL; 95% CI −618 to 1176 mL; p = 0.49) or on change in cystatin C level (nesiritide, 0.07 mg/L; 95% CI 0.01–0.13 vs placebo, 0.11 mg/L; 95% CI 0.06–0.16; difference, −0.04; 95% CI −0.13 to 0.05; p = 0.36)

(Continued)

TABLE 50-6. Major Clinical Trials in Patients with Acute Heart Failure (Continued)

Study	Year	Total Participants	Design	Inclusion Criteria	Primary outcomes	Results
DAD-HF II	2014	161	Randomized, single-blind IV high dose furosemide (20 mg/h) (n = 50), low-dose furosemide and low-dose dopamine (5 mg/h and 5 μg/kg/min) (n = 56), or low-dose furosemide (5 mg/h) (n = 55) for 8 h	Inpatients with AHF Dyspnea at rest or with minimal exertion Oxygen saturation <90% on ABG ≥1 of following: (1) signs of congestion (S3, pulmonary rales, or lower extremity/sacral edema ≥1+), (2) interstitial congestion or pleural effusion on CXR, or (3) BNP >400 pg/mL or NT-proBNP >1500 pg/mL	All-cause mortality and HFH at 60 days and 1 year	Neither all-cause mortality at day 60 (4.0%, 7.1%, and 7.2%; p = 0.74) or at 1 year (38.1%, 33.9% and 32.7%, p = 0.84) nor HFH at day 60 (22.0%, 21.4%, and 14.5%, p = 0.55) or 1 year (60.0%, 50.0%, and 47%, p = 0.40) differed between HDF, LDFD, and LDF groups
AVOID-HF	2016	224 (810 planned)	Randomized Adjustable ultrafiltration (n = 110) or adjustable IV loop diuretics (n = 114)	Inpatients admitted within 24 h with AHF Chronic daily oral loop diuretics Fluid overload by ≥2 of following: (1) pitting edema ≥2+ of lower extremities, (2) JVD >8 cm, (3) pulmonary edema or pleural effusion on CXR, (4) PND or ≥2 pillow orthopnea, or (5) resp rate ≥20/min Received ≤2 IV loop diuretics doses	Time to first HF event (HFH or as unscheduled outpatient or ED treatment with IV loop diuretics or UF) within 90 days	Estimated days to first HF event for AUF and ALD groups were 62 and 34 (p = 0.106) More AUF patients experienced an adverse effect of special interest (p = 0.018) and serious study product–related adverse event (p = 0.026).
ATOMIC-AHF	2016	606	Randomized, double-blind IV omecamtiv mecarbil or placebo in 3 sequential, escalating-dose cohorts (n ~ 200 per cohort) for 48 h	Inpatients with AHF LVEF ≤40% Dyspnea at rest or with minimal exertion BNP ≥400 pg/ml or NT-proBNP ≥1600 pg/ml, BNP ≥600 pg/ml or NT-proBNP ≥2400 pg/ml with atrial fibrillation Within 24 h of initial IV loop diuretic dose	Dyspnea improvement by Likert scale	OM did not improve primary endpoint of dyspnea relief (3 OM dose groups and pooled placebo: placebo, 41%; OM cohort 1, 42%; cohort 2, 47%; cohort 3, 51%; p = 0.33) In supplemental, pre-specified analyses, OM resulted in greater dyspnea relief at 48 h (p = 0.034) and through 5 days (p = 0.038) in high-dose cohort OM exerted plasma concentration–related increases in LV systolic ejection time (p <0.0001) and decreases in end-systolic dimension (p <0.05)
TACTICS-HF[128]	2017	257	Randomized, double-blind Tolvaptan (30 mg daily) (n = 129) or placebo (n = 128) for 3 doses	Inpatients admitted within 24 h with AHF Dyspnea at rest or with minimal exertion BNP >400 pg/ml or NT-proBNP >2000 pg/ml 1 additional sign or symptom of congestion (orthopnea, edema, elevated JVP, rales, or congestion on CXR) Serum Na ≤140 mmol/L	Proportion of patients with at least moderate improvement in dyspnea by Likert scale at both 8 and 24 h without death or need for rescue therapy within 24 h (defined as responders) Rescue therapy: need for additional open-label loop diuretic agents or addition of thiazide diuretic agents, IV vasoactive drug for HF, or mechanical circulatory or respiratory support	Dyspnea relief by Likert scale similar between groups at 8 h (25% moderately or markedly improved with tolvaptan vs. 28% placebo; p = 0.59) and at 24 h (50% tolvaptan vs. 47% placebo; p = 0.80) Need for rescue therapy similar at 24 h (21% tolvaptan, 18% placebo; p = 0.57) Proportion defined as responders at 24 h (primary study endpoint) was 16% for tolvaptan and 20% for placebo (p = 0.32)

Trial	Year	N	Design	Inclusion Criteria	Endpoint	Results
TRUE-AHF	2017	2157	Randomized, double-blind IV ularitide (15 ng/kg/min) (n = 1088) or placebo (n = 1069) for 48 h	Patients with unplanned ED visit or hospitalization for AHF; Possibility of initiating study drug within 12 h after initial clinical evaluation; Dyspnea at rest that had worsened during previous week; Evidence of HF on CXR; BNP >500 pg/mL or NT-proBNP >2000 pg/mL	Coprimary end points: death from CV causes during median follow-up of 15 months and hierarchical composite end point that evaluated initial 48-h clinical course	Death from CV causes in 236 patients in ularitide group and 225 patients in placebo group (21.7% vs 21.0%; HR 1.03; 96% CI 0.85 to 1.25; p = 0.75). No between-group difference with respect to hierarchical composite outcome
BLAST-AHF	2017	621	Randomized, double-blind IV TRV027 1 mg/h (n = 129), 5 mg/h (n = 183), 25 mg/h (n = 126), or placebo (n = 183) for 48 to 96 h	Inpatients with AHF; BNP >400 pg/mL or NT-proBNP >1600 pg/mL (for BMI >30 kg/m², BNP >200 pg/mL or NT-proBNP >800 pg/mL and for atrial fibrillation, BNP >600 pg/mL or NT-proBNP >2400 pg/mL); >2 physical HF signs including congestion on CXR, rales, edema, and/or elevated JVP; SBP ≥120 and ≤200 mm Hg; eGFR 20-75 mL/min/1.73 m²	Composite endpoint of time from baseline to death through day 30, time from baseline to HFH through day 30, first assessment time point following worsening HF through day 5, change in dyspnea VAS AUC from baseline through day 5, and length of initial hospital stay (in days) from baseline	TRV027 did not have any benefit over placebo at any dose with regards to primary composite endpoint or any individual components
ROPA-DOP[29]	2018	90	Randomized, single-blind IV furosemide bolus every 12 h (n = 19), furosemide continuous infusion (n = 23), furosemide bolus with low-dose dopamine (n = 24), furosemide continuous infusion with low-dose dopamine (n = 24)	Inpatients with HFpEF admitted within 24 h with AHF; LVEF ≥50% within 12 months of admission; >1 symptom (dyspnea, orthopnea, or edema) and 1 sign (rales, JVD, positive hepatojugular reflex, peripheral edema, ascites, or pulmonary vascular congestion on CXR); eGFR >15 ml/min/1.73 m²	Percent change in creatinine at 72 h	Compared to intermittent bolus strategy, continuous infusion strategy was associated with higher percent increase in creatinine (continuous infusion: 16.01%; 95% CI 8.58% to 23.45% vs intermittent bolus: 4.62%; 95% CI −1.15% to 10.39%; p = 0.02). Low-dose dopamine had no effect on percent change in creatinine (p = 0.33). No interaction seen between diuretic strategy and low-dose dopamine (p >.10)
PIONEER-HF	2019	881	Randomized, double-blind Sacubitril–valsartan (target dose 97–103 mg twice daily) (n = 440) or enalapril (target dose 10 mg twice daily) (n = 441)	Inpatients with AHF; LVEF ≤40%; NT-proBNP ≥1600 pg/mL or BNP ≥400 pg/mL; Signs and symptoms of fluid overload; Hemodynamically stable, defined by maintenance of SBP ≥100 mm Hg for preceding 6 h with no increase in IV diuretic dose and no use of IV vasodilators during preceding 6 h and no use of IV inotropes during preceding 24 h	Time-averaged proportional change in NT-proBNP concentration from baseline through weeks 4 and 8	Time-averaged reduction in NT-proBNP concentration was greater in sacubitril–valsartan group than in enalapril group; ratio of geometric mean of values obtained at weeks 4 and 8 to baseline value was 0.53 in sacubitril–valsartan group as compared with 0.75 in enalapril group (percent change, −46.7% vs −25.3%; ratio of change with sacubitril–valsartan vs enalapril, 0.71; 95% CI 0.63 to 0.81; p <0.001). Greater reduction in NT-proBNP concentration with sacubitril–valsartan than with enalapril evident as early as week 1 (ratio of change, 0.76; 95% CI 0.69 to 0.85). Rates of WRF, hyperkalemia, symptomatic hypotension, and angioedema did not differ significantly between groups

(Continued)

TABLE 50–6. Major Clinical Trials in Patients with Acute Heart Failure (Continued)

Study	Year	Total Participants	Design	Inclusion Criteria	Primary outcomes	Results
RELAX-AHF-2	2019	6545	Randomized, double-blind IV serelaxin (30 μg/kg/day) (n = 3274) or placebo (n = 3271) for 48 h	Inpatients admitted within 16 h with AHF Dyspnea, vascular congestion on CXR, elevated natriuretic peptides, eGFR 25–75 ml/min/1.73m², and SBP ≥125 mm Hg	Coprimary end points: death from CV causes at 180 days and worsening HF at 5 days	Day 180: death from CV causes in 285 patients (8.7%) in serelaxin group and in 290 patients (8.9%) in placebo group (HR 0.98; 95% CI 0.83 to 1.15; p = 0.77) Day 5: worsening HF in 227 patients (6.9%) in serelaxin group and in 252 (7.7%) in placebo group (HR 0.89; 95% CI 0.75–1.07; p = 0.19)
VICTORIA	2020	5050	Randomized, double-blind Vericiguat (target dose 10 mg daily) (n = 2526) or placebo (n = 2524)	Patients with worsening HF, 3 cohorts based on timing: hospitalized within 3 months, hospitalized within 3 to 6 months, and receiving IV diuretic therapy without hospitalization within 3 months LVEF <45% NYHA class II-IV Elevated natriuretic peptide level	Composite of death from CV causes or first HFH	Over median of 10.8 months, a primary-outcome event occurred in 897 patients (35.5%) in vericiguat group and in 972 patients (38.5%) in placebo group (HR 0.90; 95% [CI 0.82–0.98; p = 0.02) 691 patients (27.4%) in vericiguat group and 747 patients (29.6%) in placebo group were hospitalized for HF (HR 0.90; 95% CI 0.81–1.00) Death from CV causes in 414 patients (16.4%) in vericiguat group and in 441 patients (17.5%) in placebo group (HR 0.93; 95% CI 0.81–1.06).
GALACTIC-HF	2021	8256	Randomized, double-blind Omecamtiv mecarbil (25 mg, 37.5 mg, or 50 mg twice daily) (n = 4120) or placebo (n = 4112)	Inpatients with AHF and outpatients with an urgent visit to ED or HFH within 1 year LVEF ≤35% NYHA II-IV NT-proBNP ≥400 pg/mL or BNP ≥125 pg/mL (for atrial fibrillation or flutter, NT-proBNP ≥1200 pg/mL or BNP ≥375 pg/mL	Composite of a first heart-failure event (hospitalization or urgent visit for HF) or death from CV causes	During median of 21.8 months, a primary-outcome event occurred in 1523 patients (37.0%) in omecamtiv mecarbil group and in 1607 patients (39.1%) in placebo group (HR 0.92; 95% CI 0.86–0.99; p = 0.03) 808 patients (19.6%) vs 798 patients (19.4%), died from CV causes (HR 1.01; 95% CI 0.92–1.11)
SOLO-IST-WHF[30]	2021	1222	Randomized, double-blind Sotagliflozin (200 mg daily with dose increase to 400 mg depending on side effects) (n = 608) or placebo (n = 614)	Patients with type 2 DM who were recently hospitalized for AHF (either before or within 3 days after hospital discharge) Stable defined as no need for oxygen, SBP ≥100 mm Hg, no need for IV inotropes or vasodilators (excluding nitrates), and having transitioned from IV to oral diuretic therapy BNP ≥150 pg/mL or NT-proBNP ≥600 pg/mL (for atrial fibrillation BNP ≥450 pg/mL or NT-proBNP ≥1800 pg/mL)	Total number of deaths from CV causes and hospitalizations and urgent visits for HF (first and subsequent events)	First dose of sotagliflozin or placebo was administered before discharge in 48.8% and median of 2 days after discharge in 51.2% During median of 9.0 months, 600 primary end-point events occurred (245 in sotagliflozin group and 355 in placebo group) Rate (number of events per 100 patient-years) of primary end-point events lower in sotagliflozin group vs placebo group (51.0 vs 76.3; HR 0.67; 95% CI 0.52–0.85; p <0.001)

| STAND-UP AHF | 2021 | Part I 100 Part II 222 | Randomized, double-blind, 2 sequential parts Part I: IV cimlanod (3 µg/kg/min for 4 h, then 6 µg/kg/min for another 4 h, then 12 µg/kg/min for remaining 40 h) (n = 49) or escalating doses of placebo (n = 49) for 48 h Part II: IV cimlanod at 6 µg/kg/min (n = 71), cimlanod at 12 µg/kg/min (n = 72), or placebo (n = 71) for 48 h | Inpatients with AHF LVEF ≤40% Signs and symptoms of congestion that required treatment with IV loop diuretics SBP >105 mm Hg or <160 mm Hg No IV vasodilators or IV inotropes, with exception of IV nitroglycerin at a stable dose NT-proBNP ≥1600 pg/mL or BNP ≥400 pg/mL (for atrial fibrillation, NT pro-BNP ≥,400 pg/mL or BNP ≥600 pg/mL) | Rate of clinically relevant hypotension, defined as either SBP <90 mm Hg or symptoms up to 6 h after end of drug infusion | Part I: clinically relevant hypotension more common with cimlanod than placebo (20% vs 8%; RR 2.45; 95% CI 0.83 to 14.53) Part II: incidence of clinically relevant hypotension 18% for placebo, 21% for cimlanod 6 µg/kg/min (RR 1.15; 95% CI 0.58 to 2.43), and 35% for cimlanod 12 µg/kg/min (RR 1.9; 95% CI 1.04 to 3.59) NT-proBNP and bilirubin decreased during infusion of cimlanod compared with placebo, but these differences did not persist after treatment discontinuation |

Abbreviations: ACE, angiotensin converting enzyme; AHF, acute heart failure; ALD, adjustable loop diuretic; AUC, area under curve; AUF, adjustable ultrafiltration; BNP, B-type natriuretic peptide; CI, confidence interval; CrCl, creatinine clearance; CV, cardiovascular; CXR, chest x-ray; DM, diabetes mellitus; ED, emergency department; eGFR, estimated glomerular filtration rate; h, hour; HDF, high dose furosemide; HF, heart failure; HFH, heart failure hospitalization; HFpEF, heart failure with preserved ejection fraction; HR, hazard ratio; IV, intravenous; JVD, jugular venous distention; JVP, jugular venous pressure; LDF, low dose furosemide; LDFD, low dose furosemide plus dopamine; LVEF, left ventricular ejection fraction; mm Hg, millimeter of mercury; NT-proBNP, N-terminal pro B-type natriuretic peptide; NYHA, New York Heart Association; OM, omecamtiv mecarbil; OR, odds ratio; PAC, pulmonary artery catheter; PCWP, pulmonary capillary wedge pressure; PND, paroxysmal nocturnal dyspnea; Resp, respiratory; RR, relative risk; SBP, systolic blood pressure; SD, standard deviation; UF, ultrafiltration; VAS, visual analogue scale; vs, versus; WRF, worsening renal failure.

TABLE 50–7. Intravenous Inotropic Agents Used in the Management of Heart Failure

Intropic Agent	Dose (mcg/kg)		Drug Kinetics and Metabolism	Effects				Adverse Effects	Special Considerations
	Bolus	Infusion (/min)		CO	HR	SVR	PVR		
Adrenergic agonists									
Dopamine	N/A	5 to 10	$t_{1/2}$: 2 to 20 min	↑	↑	↔	↔	T, HA, N, tissue necrosis	Caution: MAO-I
	N/A	10 to 15	R,H,P	↑	↑	↑	↔		
Dobutamine	N/A	2.5 to 5	$t_{1/2}$: 2 to 3 min	↑	↑	↓	↔	↑/↓BP, HA, T, N, F, hypersensitivity	Caution: MAO-I; CI: sulfite allergy
	N/A	5 to 20	H	↑	↑	↔	↔		
PDE inhibitor									
Milrinone	N/R	0.125 to 0.75	$t_{1/2}$: 2.5 h H	↑	↑	↓	↓	T, ↓BP	Renal dosing, monitor LFTs

Abbreviations: BP, blood pressure; CI, contraindication; CO, cardiac output; F, fever; H, hepatic; HA, headache; HF, heart failure: HR, heart rate; LFT, liver function test; MAO-I, monoamine oxidase inhibitor; N, nausea; N/A, not applicable; N/R, not recommended; P, plasma; PDE, phosphodiesterase; PVR, pulmonary vascular resistance; R, renal; SVR, systemic vascular resistance; T, tachyarrhythmias; $t_{1/2}$, elimination half-life.

Reproduced with permission from Yancy CW, Jessup M, Bozkurt B, et al. 2013 ACCF/AHA guideline for the management of heart failure: a report of the American College of Cardiology Foundation/American Heart Association Task Force on Practice Guidelines. *J Am Coll Cardiol.* 2013 Oct 15;62(16):e147-e239.

considered to be "low output," consideration should be given to use of inotropic agents, such as dopamine, milrinone, and dobutamine (**Table 50–7**).

Beta Adrenergic Agonists

Low-dose dopamine in addition to loop diuretics may improve diuresis and better preserve renal function.[49] The Dopamine in Acute Decompensated Heart Failure (DAD-HF) study of 60 patients admitted for AHF suggested that a combination of low-dose furosemide and low-dose dopamine resulted in comparable urine output and dyspnea relief, but improved renal function and potassium homeostasis, compared to high-dose furosemide.[80] However, the DAD-HF II study of 161 patients found no beneficial effect of the addition of low-dose dopamine to furosemide.[81]

Dobutamine stimulates beta$_1$ receptors and, therefore, its effect may be attenuated in patients who are concurrently taking β-blockers. Dobutamine typically does not affect pulmonary vascular resistance because it does not have direct pulmonary vasodilating properties. Dobutamine has a half-life of 2 minutes with largely hepatic clearance.

Inodilators

Milrinone, a phosphodiesterase-3 inhibitor, decreases the degradation of cyclic adenosine monophosphate, thus increasing protein kinase A, leading to phosphorylation of multiple myocardial targets downstream augmenting contractility. Milrinone is an inodilator because it effects contractility and decreases systemic and pulmonary vascular resistance. Because of its ability to improve pulmonary vascular resistance, milrinone administration may produce reversibility of marked pulmonary hypertension associated with poor CO.[82] The mechanism of action of milrinone is independent of beta receptors and therefore, the effect of the drug is independent of concomitant use of β-blockers. Milrinone has a half-life of roughly 2.4 hours and is renally cleared. Outcomes of a Prospective Trial of Intravenous Milrinone for Exacerbations of Chronic

Heart Failure (OPTIME-CHF) evaluated the use of milrinone (0.5 µg/kg/min) versus placebo within 48 hours of hospital admission in all AHF patients not limited to the low-output group. Milrinone use did not result in decreased duration of hospitalization and was associated with a nonsignificant higher mortality both in hospital and after discharge, as well as higher rates of new-onset atrial arrhythmias and sustained hypotension requiring intervention.[83]

Levosimendan is a calcium sensitizer whose inotropic effect relates to its binding to calcium-saturated troponin C in the myocardial thin filament, which results in prolongation of actin-myosin coupling. In contrast to other inotropic agents, levosimendan does not cause an increase in myocardial oxygen demand. Additionally, levosimendan also has vasodilatory, anti-inflammatory, and antiapoptotic properties.[84] The second Randomized Multicenter Evaluation of Intravenous Levosimendan Efficacy (REVIVE-II) trial and Survival of Patients With Acute Heart Failure in Need of Intravenous Inotrope Support (SURVIVE) trial did not show an overall mortality benefit in levosimendan compared with placebo or dobutamine, respectively, and the drug is currently not approved for use in AHF in the United States.[85,86]

Risks of Arrhythmias

Both milrinone and dobutamine can cause a tachycardic response and are often arrhythmogenic, portending a higher risk of death. Observational analysis from the ADHERE registry suggested increased mortality with inotrope use in patients hospitalized with AHF, mostly in those with normal or elevated blood pressure.[87] ACCF/AHA guidelines suggest that short-term inotropic support may be considered only for patients with hypotension and signs of low CO, and long-term inotrope use may be considered for palliative treatment in stage D patients who are not candidates for advanced therapies. Guidelines also warn of harm in routine use of such parenteral agents and should not be used routinely to augment diuresis as is often clinically encountered.[49] Despite the hypothesis that levosimendan may be less arrhythmogenic, the SURVIVE trial showed more tachycardia and atrial fibrillation in the levosimendan group than in the dobutamine group.[86]

Vasopressors

Vasopressors should be reserved for patients with marked hypotension in whom organ hypoperfusion is evident. Vasopressors will redistribute CO centrally at the expense of peripheral perfusion and increased afterload. Norepinephrine is a potent agonist of $beta_1$ and $alpha_1$ receptors but is a weaker agonist of $beta_2$ receptors, resulting in marked vasoconstriction. In general, norepinephrine is the preferred vasopressor for cardiogenic shock.[47] In the Sepsis Occurrence in Acutely Ill Patients (SOAP) II trial, 1679 patients with shock were randomized to either dopamine or norepinephrine with no statistical difference in mortality but a significant increase in arrhythmias in the dopamine group. In a subgroup analysis including the 280 patients with cardiogenic shock, norepinephrine had improved survival compared to dopamine.[88] Epinephrine, an agonist of adrenergic receptors, should be restricted to patients with persistent hypotension despite adequate cardiac filling pressures and the use of other vasoactive agents.[47]

Ultrafiltration

Patients may require mechanical removal of volume with ultrafiltration (UF) or hemodialysis if marked volume retention persists and more conservative strategies are limited by renal dysfunction.[89,90] UF uses a volume removal strategy of moving water and small- to medium-weight solutes across a semipermeable membrane, using two peripheral venous catheters, thus avoiding complications of central venous access.[91] The Ultrafiltration Versus Intravenous Diuretics for Patients Hospitalized for Acute Decompensated Congestive Heart Failure (UNLOAD) trial was a 200-patient trial demonstrating the UF group to have greater weight loss and volume removal with no differences in dyspnea at 48 hours. By 90 days, the UF group had lower risk of HF hospitalization and fewer unscheduled clinic visits without any difference in renal function or overall mortality.[92] The subsequent Cardiorenal Rescue Study in Acute Decompensated Heart Failure (CARRESS-HF) trial randomized 188 patients with AHF, WRF, and persistent intravascular congestion to receive either UF or high-dose loop diuretics and found no differences in mean weight loss at 96 hours. The UF group had more serious adverse events, mainly bleeding and worsened serum creatinine levels.[93] As a result of uncertainty surrounding the results of these trials, a subsequent 800-patient trial, the Aquapheresis Versus Intravenous Diuretics and Hospitalization for Heart Failure (AVOID-HF) trial, was undertaken but terminated prematurely secondary to slow patient recruitment.[94] The ACCF/AHA guidelines currently state that UF is reasonable in patients with refractory congestion once other strategies have failed.[49]

Guideline-Directed Medical Therapy

Neurohormonal antagonists have dramatically improved outcomes for HFrEF.[49] When possible, continuation of GDMT through hospitalization or initiation before discharge is associated with substantially better outcomes, both due to the benefit of the therapies and to the better prognostic profile of patients who can tolerate them.[95] In patients hospitalized with HFrEF not already being treated with oral therapies known to improve outcomes, such as angiotensin receptor–neprilysin inhibitors (ARNIs)/ACE inhibitors (ACEIs)/angiotensin II receptor blockers (ARBs), β-blockers, and MRAs, these agents should be initiated prior to discharge.[70] Hospitalization for AHF often presents an opportunity to optimize HF medications in a controlled setting with careful attention to blood pressure and renal function. The PIONEER-HF trial studied the use of sacubitril-valsartan in comparison with enalapril upon initial stabilization from AHF and included a diverse patient population. The primary outcome, time-averaged reduction in NT-proBNP, for sacubitril/valsartan versus enalapril was −46.7% versus −25.3% (hazard ratio 0.71; 95% confidence interval 0.63–0.81; $P < 0.001$). Importantly however, this trial showed a reduction in the secondary clinical outcomes of all-cause death, HF rehospitalization, requirement for LV assist device or listing for transplant, with no evidence of safety concerns of hypotension, renal dysfunction, or hyperkalemia.[96]

Novel Therapies

There are a variety of novel molecules with vasodilator or inotropic properties that have been studied as therapeutics for AHF. Relaxin was first identified as a hormone of pregnancy with systemic and renal vascular effects, as well as beneficial effects on cardiac preconditioning and ischemia, inflammation, fibrosis, and apoptosis. Serelaxin (recombinant human relaxin-2) demonstrated encouraging effects in a dose-finding pilot study of 234 patients with AHF and the phase III Efficacy and Safety of Relaxin for the Treatment of Acute Heart (RELAX-AHF) trial.[97,98] Based on the promising results of RELAX-AHF, the RELAX-AHF-2 trial enrolled more than 6500 patients admitted for AHF and evaluated the effects of serelaxin compared to placebo on the independently powered primary endpoints of cardiovascular mortality at 180 days and worsening heart failure at 5 days. In this large study, serelaxin did not improve either primary endpoint compared to placebo.[99] Currently, the data do not support the routine use of serelaxin in patients with AHF.

Multiple different natriuretic peptides continue to be developed and investigated for the treatment of AHF. Urodilatin, a modified version of pro-ANP, is an amino acid hormone synthesized and secreted from the distal tubules of the kidney that regulates renal sodium absorption and water homeostasis. Ularitide, a synthetically produced urodilatin, has demonstrated beneficial effects on hemodynamics and symptom relief in two studies of patients with AHF.[100] The Trial of Ularitide Efficacy and Safety in Acute Heart Failure (TRUE-AHF) enrolled 2157 patients with symptomatic AHF and randomized them to a 48-hour infusion of either ularitide or placebo. Ularitide did not significantly improve a hierarchical clinical composite endpoint or cardiovascular mortality.[101]

Direct renin inhibitors (DRIs) block the first enzymatic step in the RAAS cascade, leading to a suppression of this neurohormonal system. Aliskiren is the first oral DRI on the market and currently approved for the treatment of hypertension. The Aliskiren Trial on Acute Heart Failure Outcomes (ASTRONAUT) enrolled 1639 hemodynamically stable patients at a median 5 days after admission for AHF who were randomized to daily oral aliskiren or placebo. Aliskiren treatment was associated with higher rates of hyperkalemia, hypotension, and renal impairment compared to placebo, but there was no difference in cardiovascular death or HF rehospitalization.[102]

Endothelin receptor antagonists block the actions of ET-1, an endogenous vasoconstrictor produced by the vascular endothelial cells. It exerts its effects by binding to two receptors, ET_A and ET_B, located on the vascular smooth muscle cells, resulting in systemic arterial vasoconstriction. Tezosentan, a nonselective ET_{A-B} antagonist, has been shown to improve hemodynamics in patients with AHF. The Value of Endothelin Receptor Inhibition with Tezosentan in Acute Heart Failure Study (VERITAS) studied more than 1400 patients admitted with AHF in a large international trial. The addition of intravenous tezosentan to standard therapy did not improve symptoms nor decrease worsening HF or mortality at 7 days after randomization.[103]

Another approach to neurohormonal antagonism in AHF includes the angiotensin II type I receptor beta-arrestin–biased ligand TRV027, which stimulates inotropy and antagonizes the angiotensin II–signaling pathways. The Biased Ligand of the Angiotensin Receptor Study in Acute Heart Failure (BLAST-AHF) enrolled 621 patients admitted with AHF in a dose-ranging study of a 48- to 96-hour infusion of TRV027 compared to placebo. TRV027 conferred no benefit over placebo at any dose with regard to the primary composite endpoint or any of the individual components.[104]

Cinaciguat activates the soluble form of guanylate cyclase (sGC) in smooth muscle cells, thus leading to the synthesis of cyclic guanosine monophosphate (cGMP) and subsequent vasodilation. Cinaciguat has been shown to improve hemodynamics in patients with AHF but at high doses, it has been associated with significant hypotension, which resulted in the termination of early clinical studies.[105] Vericiguat is an oral sGC stimulator studied in patients with worsening heart failure. In the Soluble Guanylate Cyclase Stimulator in Heart Failure Patients with Reduced EF (SOCRATES-REDUCED) study of 456 patients, vericiguat did not significantly improve NT-proBNP concentrations compared to placebo, but there was a suggestion of a dose-response effect.[106] In the Vericiguat Global Study in Subjects with Heart Failure with Reduced Ejection Fraction (VICTORIA) of 5050 patients, the incidence of death from cardiovascular causes or hospitalization for HF was lower among those who received vericiguat than among those who received placebo.[107]

Cardiac myosin activators increase myocardial contractility by increasing the transition rate from the weakly bound to the strongly bound state necessary for initiation of a force-generating power stroke. Omecamtiv mecarbil is the first drug of this class to undergo human testing. In the Acute Treatment With Omecamtiv Mecarbil to Increase Contractility in Acute Heart Failure (ATOMIC-AHF) study, a phase IIb dose-finding study

of 606 patients with AHF, intravenous omecamtiv mecarbil did not meet the primary endpoint of dyspnea improvement, but it was generally well tolerated, increased systolic ejection time, and improved dyspnea in the high-dose group.[108] In the Global Approach to Lowering Adverse Cardiac outcomes Through Improving Contractility in Heart Failure (GALACTIC-HF) trial, which enrolled 8256 inpatients and outpatients with HFrEF, those who received omecamtiv mecarbil had a lower incidence of a composite of a HF event or death from cardiovascular causes than those who received placebo.[109]

Istaroxime stimulates the membrane-bound Na^+/K^+-ATPase pathway and enhances the activity of the sarcoendoplasmic reticulum Ca^{2+}-ATPase type 2a (SERCA2a). These two mechanisms result, respectively, in increased cytosolic calcium accumulation during systole, with positive inotropic effects, and in rapid sequestration of cytosolic calcium into the sarcoplasmic reticulum during diastole, leading to an enhanced lusitropic effect. The Hemodynamic, Echocardiographic, and Neurohormonal Effects of Istaroxime (HORIZON-HF) trial evaluated 120 patients admitted with AHF and HFrEF. The addition of istaroxime to standard therapy lowered PCWP and increased systolic blood pressure. There were no changes in neurohormones, renal function, or troponin I levels during the short, 6-hour infusion.[110,111]

Nitroxyl (HNO) donors have vasodilator, inotropic, and lusitropic effects by enhancing myocardial contractility and relaxation, and reducing preload and afterload without increasing heart rate or myocardial oxygen consumption. Cimlanod is an HNO donor developed for AHF. In the Study Assessing Nitorxyl Donor Upon Presentation with Acute Heart Failure (STAND-UP AHF) trial, a phase II, randomized, double-blind, placebo-controlled clinical trial of continuous 48-hour intravenous infusions of cimlanod or placebo in patients hospitalized for AHF, cimlanod at a dose of 6 μg/kg/min was reasonably well-tolerated compared with placebo. Cimlanod reduced markers of congestion, but this did not persist beyond the treatment period.[112]

Invasive and Surgical Management

Cardiogenic shock is defined as systemic tissue hypoperfusion caused by inadequate CO despite adequate circulatory volume and filling pressure. Hemodynamic criteria include systolic blood pressure <90 mm Hg for >30 minutes, a drop in mean arterial pressure >30 mm Hg below baseline with cardiac index <1.8 L/min/m² without hemodynamic support, and a PCWP >15 mm Hg.[113,114] For patients with advanced HF, the Interagency Registry for Mechanically Assisted Circulatory Support has defined seven clinical profiles with respect to acuity of hemodynamic deterioration, where profiles 1 and 2 refer to patients who are failing inotropic therapy.[115] These patients need escalation of therapy to mechanical circulatory support (MCS). The optimal timing for placement of MCS remains a source of debate, but the available options for support have increased.[116] Many factors influence the type of MCS to use, including the degree of hemodynamic instability, acuity of need for implantation, and technical considerations. The options for temporary MCS include intra-aortic balloon pump,

Impella (Abiomed, Danvers, MA), TandemHeart (TandemLife, Pittsburgh, PA), and extracorporeal membrane oxygenation either as veno-veno or veno-arterial support. Bleeding, infection, limb ischemia, and hemolysis can complicate any of the MCS devices.

Palliative Care

Palliative care addresses goals of care, advance care planning, and symptom management for patients with life-threatening conditions or debilitating illness. There is a growing recognition of the importance of palliative care in the management of patients with HF and emerging evidence to support its routine incorporation.[117] Palliative care can coexist with active and even invasive treatments up to the point of transition to hospice care.

Goals of care discussions should play an important part in the care of many patients admitted with AHF.[118] Advance care planning involves identification of a surrogate decision-maker and consideration of the type and degree of care that patients would choose in the event they lose decision-making capacity. Ideally, all patients with HF would have advance care planning discussions as stable outpatients, but sometimes it is necessary to have them as inpatients.

Specialists in palliative care can be useful at several points during the hospitalization. They are particularly skilled at helping patients and families navigate the difficult process of complicated goals of care and advance care planning discussions, particularly in the setting of unrealistic expectations. Palliative care specialists also provide expertise in managing noncardiac symptoms and holistically improving quality of life near the end. Palliative care specialists may also help to facilitate the transition to hospice.[70]

Discharge and Transitions of Care

A critical performance measure set forth for HF hospitalization involves transitions of care, which includes written discharge instructions or educational materials provided to patients explaining discharge medications, activity level, diet, weight monitoring, follow-up visit instructions, and what to do if symptoms worsen.[119] Many registries suggest that patients with AHF are commonly discharged before euvolemia is achieved, without optimal blood pressure control and without optimal use of GDMT.[54] Maintenance diuretic dosing should be planned recognizing that lower doses are required for fluid balance than for net diuresis, but also that fluid balance is usually harder to maintain at home than in the hospital. A rescue dosing plan should be included in the discharge regimen, to specify not only the increased diuretic therapy but also the trigger that should prompt the rescue. Patients should be encouraged to call their clinician if unsure and to avoid delay in starting therapy.[70] Comprehensive discharge planning ensuring compliance with GDMT can reduce readmissions and improve patient outcomes.[120]

Patients admitted with AHF should be evaluated prior to discharge for appropriateness for devices, including cardiac resynchronization therapy and an implantable

TABLE 50–8. Clinical Events and Findings Useful in Identifying Patients with Advanced Heart Failure

Repeated (≥2) hospitalizations or ED visits for HF in the past year
Progressive deterioration in renal function (eg, rise in BUN and creatinine)
Weight loss without other cause (eg, cardiac cachexia)
Intolerance to ACE inhibitors due to hypotension and/or worsening renal function
Intolerance to beta blockers due to worsening HF or hypotension
Frequent systolic blood pressure <90 mm Hg
Persistent dyspnea with dressing or bathing requiring rest
Inability to walk 1 block on the level ground due to dyspnea or fatigue
Recent need to escalate diuretics to maintain volume status, often reaching daily furosemide equivalent dose over 160 mg/d and/or use of supplemental metolazone therapy
Progressive decline in serum sodium, usually to <133 mEq/L
Frequent ICD shocks

Abbreviations: ACE, angiotensin-converting enzyme; BUN, blood urea nitrogen; ED; emergency department; HF, heart failure; and ICD, implantable cardioverter-defibrillator.
Reproduced with permission from Yancy CW, Jessup M, Bozkurt B, et al. 2013 ACCF/AHA guideline for the management of heart failure: a report of the American College of Cardiology Foundation/American Heart Association Task Force on Practice Guidelines. *J Am Coll Cardiol.* 2013 Oct 15;62(16):e147-e239.

cardioverter-defibrillator.[121] Consideration should also be given to candidacy for implantable pressure sensors such as CardioMEMS (St. Jude Medical, St. Paul, MN), which may decrease rehospitalization.[122] Patients with advanced heart failure (**Table 50–8**) should be provided with a referral to tertiary care centers with expertise in implantable left ventricle assist device and/or orthotopic heart transplantation.[49]

The postdischarge follow-up comprises two events: a follow-up phone call within 2 to 3 days of discharge and the clinic visit within 7 to 14 days of hospital discharge. The follow-up phone call should assess clinical signs of congestion, check on availability and affordability of medications, confirm understanding of and adherence with the medical regimen, and ensure that follow-up appointments have been made and that transportation to those appointments is not an issue. The first postdischarge appointment provides the opportunity to reassess clinical status, to provide additional patient education, to review medications and adjust their doses, and to address issues that might lead to readmission or worsening HF, including social determinants of risk such as insurance status.[70] Data suggest that follow-up with a physician within 7 days of discharge and follow-up with a cardiologist can lower 30-day mortality.[123,124]

FUTURE DIRECTIONS

AHF continues to have a high mortality and morbidity, therefore posing a major public health burden. Most patients are treated primarily with intravenous loop diuretics. However, novel therapies targeting the underlying pathophysiology of AHF are actively being studied. AHF is a heterogeneous clinical syndrome and will likely require tailored therapies for specific subgroups to allow for improved outcomes. As we develop and study novel therapies, it is important to recognize and utilize the HF hospitalization as an opportunity to identify reversible causes, ensure GDMT, appropriately manage comorbid conditions, and deliver patient and caregiver education to improve long-term outcomes in patients with HF.

SUMMARY

Definition

- Acute heart failure refers to the clinical syndrome wherein symptoms and/or signs of congestion occur in the setting of a structural and/or functional cardiac abnormality, corroborated by elevated natriuretic peptide levels or other objective evidence of congestion.

Epidemiology

- Acute heart failure is the most common cause of hospitalizations in patients older than age 65, with expected increases in prevalence over time.

- Acute heart failure is associated with significant morbidity and mortality, with high rates of readmission and up to 10% mortality following discharge.

Pathophysiology

- Congestion regardless of ejection fraction is what ultimately prompts clinical attention, wherein hemodynamic congestion precedes clinical congestion by days to weeks.

- The renin-angiotensin-aldosterone and sympathetic nervous systems as well as inflammatory cytokines are upregulated in acute heart failure. Chronic activation leads to cardiac fibrosis, adverse remodeling, and sodium and fluid retention.

- Change in renal function is common in acute heart failure with 20% to 40% experiencing worsening renal function, often labeled "cardiorenal syndrome," and can be transient to allow for effective decongestion.

Diagnosis

- Assessment of hemodynamic profile in acute heart failure based on perfusion and volume status allows for classification of patients as either "wet" or "dry" depending on their volume status and either "cold" or "warm" depending on their perfusion status.

- Measurement of natriuretic peptides is recommended in those patients for whom the diagnosis of acute heart failure is uncertain, and for purposes of prognostication.

- Special attention should be paid to identifying triggers for decompensation and acute heart failure so as to prevent subsequent events.

Management

- Hemodynamic profiles inform management, which can range from diuretic therapy alone to mechanical circulatory support for cardiogenic shock.

- Phases of management of acute heart failure include stabilization, hospitalization, and discharge planning, where focus of therapy is hemodynamic optimization, incorporation of guideline-directed medical therapy, education, and arranging follow-up, respectively.

- The hospitalization for acute heart failure should be considered a vulnerable and ripe setting to appropriately decongest patients, address comorbid conditions, educate and ensure guideline-directed medical therapy, and orchestrate a post-discharge and follow-up plan.

ACKNOWLEDGMENT

In the previous edition(s), this chapter was written by Michelle Weisfelner, Robert T. Cole, and Javed Butler, and portions of that chapter have been retained.

REFERENCES

1. Bozkurt B, Coats AJ, Tsutsui H, et al. Universal definition and classification of heart failure: a report of the Heart Failure Society of America, Heart Failure Association of the European Society of Cardiology, Japanese Heart Failure Society and Writing Committee of the Universal Definition of Heart Failure. *J Card Fail.* 2021:S1071-9164(21)00050-6.

2. Mozaffarian D, Benjamin EJ, Go AS, et al. Heart disease and stroke statistics-2016 update: a report from the American Heart Association. *Circulation.* 2016;133(4):e38-e360.

3. Heidenreich PA, Albert NM, Allen LA, et al. Forecasting the impact of heart failure in the United States: a policy statement from the American Heart Association. *Circ Heart Fail.* 2013;6(3):606-619.

4. Voigt J, Sasha John M, Taylor A, et al. A reevaluation of the costs of heart failure and its implications for allocation of health resources in the United States. *Clin Cardiol.* 2014;37(5):312-321.

5. Butler J, Gheorghiade M, Kelkar A, et al. In-hospital worsening heart failure. *Eur J Heart Fail.* 2015;17(11):1104-1113.

6. Okumura N, Jhund PS, Gong J, et al. Importance of clinical worsening of heart failure treated in the outpatient setting: evidence from the prospective comparison of ARNI with ACEI to determine impact on global mortality and morbidity in heart failure trial (PARADIGM-HF). *Circulation.* 2016;133(23):2254-2262.

7. Steinberg BA, Zhao X, Heidenreich PA, et al. Trends in patients hospitalized with heart failure and preserved left ventricular ejection fraction: prevalence, therapies, and outcomes. *Circulation.* 2012;126(1):65-75.

8. Yancy CW, Lopatin M, Stevenson LW, et al. Clinical presentation, management, and in-hospital outcomes of patients admitted with acute decompensated heart failure with preserved systolic function: a report from the acute decompensated heart failure national registry (ADHERE) database. *J Am Coll Cardiol.* 2006;47(1):76-84.

9. Mentz RJ, Kelly JP, von Lueder TG, et al. Noncardiac comorbidities in heart failure with reduced versus preserved ejection fraction. *J Am Coll Cardiol.* 2014;64(21):2281-2293.

10. Braunstein JB, Anderson GF, Gerstenblith G, et al. Noncardiac comorbidity increases preventable hospitalizations and mortality among Medicare beneficiaries with chronic heart failure. *J Am Coll Cardiol.* 2003;42(7):1226-1233.

11. Fonarow GC, Stough WG, Abraham WT, et al. Characteristics, treatments, and outcomes of patients with preserved systolic function hospitalized for heart failure: a report from the OPTIMIZE-HF Registry. *J Am Coll Cardiol.* 2007;50(8):768-777.

12. Shahar E, Lee S, Kim J, Duval S, Barber C, Luepker RV. Hospitalized heart failure: rates and long-term mortality. *J Card Fail.* 2004;10(5):374-379.

13. Giamouzis G, Kalogeropoulos A, Georgiopoulou V, et al. Hospitalization epidemic in patients with heart failure: risk factors, risk prediction, knowledge gaps, and future directions. *J Card Fail.* 2011;17(1):54-75.

14. Ross JS, Chen J, Lin Z, et al. Recent national trends in readmission rates after heart failure hospitalization. *Circ Heart Fail.* 2010;3(1):97-103.

15. Vachiery JL, Adir Y, Barbera JA, et al. Pulmonary hypertension due to left heart diseases. *J Am Coll Cardiol.* 2013;62(25 Suppl):D100-D108.

16. Zile MR, Bennett TD, St John Sutton M, et al. Transition from chronic compensated to acute decompensated heart failure: pathophysiological insights obtained from continuous monitoring of intracardiac pressures. *Circulation.* 2008;118(14):1433-1441.

17. Stevenson LW, Zile M, Bennett TD, et. al. Chronic ambulatory intracardiac pressures and future heart failure events. *Circ Heart Fail.* 2010;3(5)580-587.

18. Braunwald E. Heart failure. *JACC Heart Fail.* 2013;1(1):1-20.

19. Borlaug BA, Kass DA. Ventricular-vascular interaction in heart failure. *Cardiol Clin.* 2011;29(3):447-459.

20. Kishi T. Heart failure as an autonomic nervous system dysfunction. *J Cardiol.* 2012;59(2):117-122

21. Marti CN, Georgiopoulou VV, Kalogeropoulos AP. Acute heart failure: patient characteristics and pathophysiology. *Curr Heart Fail Rep.* 2013;10(4):427-433.

22. Cole RT, Masoumi A, Triposkiadis F, et al. Renal dysfunction in heart failure. *Med Clin North Am.* 2012;96(5):955-974.

23. Damman K, Navis G, Voors AA, et al. Worsening renal function and prognosis in heart failure: systematic review and meta-analysis. *J Card Fail.* 2007;13(8):599-608.

24. Klein L, Massie BM, Leimberger JD, et al. Admission or changes in renal function during hospitalization for worsening heart failure predict post-discharge survival: results from the Outcomes of a Prospective Trial of Intravenous Milrinone for Exacerbations of Chronic Heart Failure (OPTIME-CHF). *Circ Heart Fail.* 2008;1(1):25-33.

25. Kociol RD, Greiner MA, Hammill BG, et al. Long-term outcomes of Medicare beneficiaries with worsening renal function during hospitalization for heart failure. *Am J Cardiol.* 2010;105(12):1786-1793.

26. Damman K, van Deursen VM, Navis G, Voors AA, van Veldhuisen DJ, Hillege HL. Increased central venous pressure is associated with impaired renal function and mortality in a broad spectrum of patients with cardiovascular disease. *J Am Coll Cardiol.* 2009;53(7):582-588.

27. Guglin M, Rivero A, Matar F, Garcia M. Renal dysfunction in heart failure is due to congestion but not low output. *Clin Cardiol.* 2011;34(2):113-116.

28. Mullens W, Abrahams Z, Francis GS, et al. Importance of venous congestion for worsening of renal function in advanced decompensated heart failure. *J Am Coll Cardiol.* 2009;53(7):589-596.

29. Mullens W, Abrahams Z, Skouri HN, et al. Elevated intra-abdominal pressure in acute decompensated heart failure: a potential contributor to worsening renal function? *J Am Coll Cardiol.* 2008;51(3):300-306.

30. Mezzano SA, Ruiz-Ortega M, Egido J. Angiotensin II and renal fibrosis. *Hypertension.* 2001;38(3 Pt 2):635-638.

31. Felker GM, Lee KL, Bull DA, et al. Diuretic strategies in patients with acute decompensated heart failure. *N Engl J Med.* 2011;364(9):797-805.

32. Testani JM, Chen J, McCauley BD, Kimmel SE, Shannon RP. Potential effects of aggressive decongestion during the treatment of decompensated heart failure on renal function and survival. *Circulation.* 2010;122(3):265-272.

33. Metra M, Davison B, Bettari L, et. al. Is worsening renal function an ominous prognostic sign in patients with acute heart failure? The role of congestion and its interaction with renal function. *Circ Heart Fail.* 2012;5(1)54-62.

34. Aronson D, Burger AJ. The relationship between transient and persistent worsening renal function and mortality in patients with acute decompensated heart failure. *J Card Fail.* 2010;16(7):541-547.

35. Marti CN, Gheorghiade M, Kalogeropoulos AP, et. al. Endothelial dysfunction, arterial stiffness, and heart failure. *J Am Coll Cardiol.* 2012;60(16)1455-1469.

36. Hare JM, Stamler JS. NO/redox disequilibrium in the failing heart and cardiovascular system. *J Clin Invest.* 2005;115(3):509-517.

37. Zuchi C, Tritto I, Carluccio E, et al. Role of endothelial dysfunction in heart failure. *Heart Fail Rev.* 2020;25(1):21-30.

38. Fonarow GC, Adams KF Jr, Abraham WT, et al. Risk stratification for in-hospital mortality in acutely decompensated heart failure: classification and regression tree analysis. *JAMA.* 2005;293(5):572-580.

39. Lee DS, Austin PC, Rouleau JL, Liu PP, Naimark D, Tu JV. Predicting mortality among patients hospitalized for heart failure: derivation and validation of a clinical model. *JAMA.* 2003;290(19):2581-2587.

40. O'Connor CM, Hasselblad V, Mehta RH, et al. Triage after hospitalization with advanced heart failure: the ESCAPE (Evaluation Study of Congestive Heart Failure and Pulmonary Artery Catheterization Effectiveness) risk model and discharge score. *J Am Coll Cardiol.* 2010;55(9):872-878.

41. O'Connor CM, Mentz RJ, Cotter G, et al. The PROTECT in-hospital risk model: 7-day outcome in patients hospitalized with acute heart failure and renal dysfunction. *Eur J Heart Fail.* 2012;14(6):605-612.

42. Peterson PN, Rumsfeld JS, Liang L, et al. A validated risk score for in-hospital mortality in patients with heart failure from the American Heart Association get with the guidelines program. *Circ Cardiovasc Qual Outcomes.* 2010;3(1):25-32.

43. Miro O, Rosello X, Gil V, et al. Predicting 30-day mortality for patients with acute heart failure in the emergency department: a cohort study. *Ann Intern Med.* 2017;167(10):698-705.

44. Miro O, Rossello X, Platz E, et al. Risk stratification scores for patients with acute heart failure in the emergency department: a systematic review. *Eur Heart J Acute Cardiovasc Care.* 2020;9(5):375-398.

45. Demissei BG, Postmus D, Cleland JG, et al. Plasma biomarkers to predict or rule out early post-discharge events after hospitalization for acute heart failure. *Eur J Heart Fail.* 2017;19(6):728-738.

46. Dickstein K, Cohen-Solal A, Filippatos G, et al. ESC guidelines for the diagnosis and treatment of acute and chronic heart failure 2008: the task force for the diagnosis and treatment of acute and chronic heart failure 2008 of the European Society of Cardiology. Developed in collaboration with the Heart Failure Association of the ESC (HFA) and endorsed by the European Society of Intensive Care Medicine (ESICM). *Eur Heart J.* 2008;29(19):2388-2442.

47. Ponikowski P, Voors AA, Anker SD, et al. 2016 ESC guidelines for the diagnosis and treatment of acute and chronic heart failure: the task force for the diagnosis and treatment of acute and chronic heart failure of the European Society of Cardiology (ESC). Developed with the special contribution of the Heart Failure Association (HFA) of the ESC. *Eur Heart J.* 2016;37(27):2129-2200.

48. Nohria A, Tsang SW, Fang JC, et al. Clinical assessment identifies hemodynamic profiles that predict outcomes in patients admitted with heart failure. *J Am Coll Cardiol.* 2003;41(10):1797-1804.

49. Yancy CW, Jessup M, Bozkurt B, et al. 2013 ACCF/AHA guideline for the management of heart failure: a report of the American College of Cardiology Foundation/American Heart Association task force on practice guidelines. *J Am Coll Cardiol.* 2013;62(16):e147-e239.

50. Stevenson LW, Perloff JK. The limited reliability of physical signs for estimating hemodynamics in chronic heart failure. *JAMA.* 1989;261(6):884-888.

51. Drazner MH, Hamilton MA, Fonarow G, Creaser J, Flavell C, Stevenson LW. Relationship between right and left-sided filling pressures in 1000 patients with advanced heart failure. *J Heart Lung Transplant.* 1999;18(11):1126-1132.

52. Felker GM, Cuculich PS, Gheorghiade M. The Valsalva maneuver: a bedside "biomarker" for heart failure. *Am J Med.* 2006;119(2):117-122.

53. Abraham WT, Fonarow GC, Albert NM, et al. Predictors of in-hospital mortality in patients hospitalized for heart failure: insights from the Organized Program to Initiate Lifesaving Treatment in Hospitalized Patients with Heart Failure (OPTIMIZE-HF). *J Am Coll Cardiol.* 2008;52(5):347-356.

54. Harinstein ME, Flaherty JD, Fonarow GC, et al. Clinical assessment of acute heart failure syndromes: emergency department through the early post-discharge period. *Heart (British Cardiac Society).* 2011;97(19):1607-1618.

55. Brunner-La Rocca HP, Kaye DM, Woods RL, Hastings J, Esler MD. Effects of intravenous brain natriuretic peptide on regional sympathetic activity in patients with chronic heart failure as compared with healthy control subjects. *J Am Coll Cardiol.* 2001;37(5):1221-1227.

56. Kimura K, Yamaguchi Y, Horii M, et al. ANP is cleared much faster than BNP in patients with congestive heart failure. *Eur J Clin Pharmacol.* 2007;63(7):699-702.

57. Mueller T, Gegenhuber A, Poelz W, Haltmayer M. Diagnostic accuracy of B type natriuretic peptide and amino terminal proBNP in the emergency diagnosis of heart failure. *Heart (British Cardiac Society).* 2005;91(5):606-612.

58. Maisel AS, Peacock WF, McMullin N, et al. Timing of immunoreactive B-type natriuretic peptide levels and treatment delay in acute decompensated heart failure: an ADHERE (Acute Decompensated Heart Failure National Registry) analysis. *J Am Coll Cardiol.* 2008;52(7):534-540.

59. Januzzi JL Jr, Rehman SU, Mohammed AA, et al. Use of amino-terminal pro-B-type natriuretic peptide to guide outpatient therapy of patients with chronic left ventricular systolic dysfunction. *J Am Coll Cardiol.* 2011;58(18):1881-1889.

60. Peacock WF, De Marco T, Fonarow GC, et al. Cardiac troponin and outcome in acute heart failure. *N Engl J Med.* 2008;358(20):2117-2126.

61. Lassus J, Gayat E, Mueller C, et al. Incremental value of biomarkers to clinical variables for mortality prediction in acutely decompensated heart failure: the Multinational Observational Cohort on Acute Heart Failure (MOCA) study. *Int J Cardiol.* 2013;168(3):2186-2194.

62. Maisel A, Mueller C, Nowak RM, et al. Midregion prohormone adrenomedullin and prognosis in patients presenting with acute dyspnea: results from the BACH (Biomarkers in Acute Heart Failure) trial. *J Am Coll Cardiol.* 2011;58(10):1057-1067.

63. Porter TR, Shillcutt SK, Adams MS, et al. Guidelines for the use of echocardiography as a monitor for therapeutic intervention in adults: a report from the American Society of Echocardiography. *J Am Soc Echocardiogr.* 2015;28(1):40-56.

64. Blair JE, Brennan JM, Goonewardena SN, Shah D, Vasaiwala S, Spencer KT. Usefulness of hand-carried ultrasound to predict elevated left ventricular filling pressure. *Am J Cardiol.* 2009;103(2):246-247.

65. Binanay C, Califf RM, Hasselblad V, et al. Evaluation study of congestive heart failure and pulmonary artery catheterization effectiveness: the ESCAPE trial. *JAMA.* 2005;294(13):1625-1633.

66. Fonarow GC, Abraham WT, Albert NM, et al. Factors identified as precipitating hospital admissions for heart failure and clinical outcomes: findings from OPTIMIZE-HF. *Arch Intern Med.* 2008;168(8):847-854.

67. Greene SJ, Fonarow GC, Vaduganathan M, Khan SS, Butler J, Gheorghiade M. The vulnerable phase after hospitalization for heart failure. *Nat Rev Cardiol.* 2015;12(4):220-229.

68. Pang PS, Komajda M, Gheorghiade M. The current and future management of acute heart failure syndromes. *Eur Heart J.* 2010;31(7):784-793.

69. Gheorghiade M, Braunwald E. A proposed model for initial assessment and management of acute heart failure syndromes. *JAMA.* 2011;305(16):1702-1703.

70. Hollenberg SM, Stevenson LW, Ahmad T, et al. 2019 ACC expert consensus decision pathway on risk assessment, management, and clinical trajectory of patients hospitalized with heart failure: a report of the American College of Cardiology solution set oversight committee. *J Am Coll Cardiol.* 2019;74(15):1966-2011.

71. Peacock WF, Fonarow GC, Emerman CL, Mills RM, Wynne J. Impact of early initiation of intravenous therapy for acute decompensated heart failure on outcomes in ADHERE. *Cardiology.* 2007;107(1):44-51.

72. Felker GM, Lee KL, Bull DA, et al. Diuretic strategies in patients with acute decompensated heart failure. *N Engl J Med.* 2011;364(9):797-805.

73. van Vliet AA, Donker AJ, Nauta JJ, Verheugt FW. Spironolactone in congestive heart failure refractory to high-dose loop diuretic and low-dose angiotensin-converting enzyme inhibitor. *Am J Cardiol.* 1993;71(3):21a-28a.

74. Firth JD, Raine AE, Ledingham JG. Raised venous pressure: a direct cause of renal sodium retention in oedema? *Lancet.* 1988;1(8593):1033-1035.

75. Lala A, McNulty SE, Mentz RJ, et al. Relief and recurrence of congestion during and after hospitalization for acute heart failure: insights From Diuretic Optimization Strategy Evaluation in Acute Decompensated Heart Failure

76. Elkayam U, Janmohamed M, Habib M, Hatamizadeh P. Vasodilators in the management of acute heart failure. *Criti Care Med.* 2008;36(1 Suppl):S95-S105.

77. Intravenous nesiritide vs nitroglycerin for treatment of decompensated congestive heart failure: a randomized controlled trial. *JAMA.* 2002;287(12):1531-1540.

78. O'Connor CM, Starling RC, Hernandez AF, et al. Effect of nesiritide in patients with acute decompensated heart failure. *N Engl J Med.* 2011;365(1):32-43.

79. Chen HH, Anstrom KJ, Givertz MM, et al. Low-dose dopamine or low-dose nesiritide in acute heart failure with renal dysfunction: the ROSE acute heart failure randomized trial. *JAMA.* 2013;310(23):2533-2543.

80. Giamouzis G, Butler J, Starling RC, et. al. Impact of dopamine infusion on renal function in hospitalized heart failure patients: results of the Dopamine in Acute Decompensated Heart Failure (DAD-HF) Trial. *J Card Fail.* 2010;16(12):922-930.

81. Triposkiadis FK, Butler J, Karayannis G, et. al. Efficacy and safety of high dose versus low dose furosemide with or without dopamine infusion: the Dopamine in Acute Decompensated Heart Failure II (DAD-HF II) trial. *Int J Cardiol.* 2014;172(1):115-121.

82. Givertz MM, Hare JM, Loh E, Gauthier DF, Colucci WS. Effect of bolus milrinone on hemodynamic variables and pulmonary vascular resistance in patients with severe left ventricular dysfunction: a rapid test for reversibility of pulmonary hypertension. *J Am Coll Cardiol.* 1996;28(7):1775-1780.

83. Cuffe MS, Califf RM, Adams KF Jr, et al. Short-term intravenous milrinone for acute exacerbation of chronic heart failure: a randomized controlled trial. *JAMA.* 2002;287(12)1541-1547.

84. Pierrakos C, Velissaris D, Franchi F, Muzzi L, Karanikolas M, Scolletta S. Levosimendan in critical illness: a literature review. *J Clin Med Res.* 2014;6(2):75-85.

85. Packer M, Colucci W, Fisher L, et al. Effect of levosimendan on the short-term clinical course of patients with acutely decompensated heart failure. *JACC Heart Fail.* 2013;1(2):103-111.

86. Mebazaa A, Nieminen MS, Filippatos GS, et al. Levosimendan vs. dobutamine: outcomes for acute heart failure patients on beta-blockers in SURVIVE. *Eur J Heart Fail.* 2009;11(3):304-311.

87. Fonarow GC, Heywood JT, Heidenreich PA, Lopatin M, Yancy CW. Temporal trends in clinical characteristics, treatments, and outcomes for heart failure hospitalizations, 2002 to 2004: findings from Acute Decompensated Heart Failure National Registry (ADHERE). *Am Heart J.* 2007;153(6):1021-1028.

88. De Backer D, Biston P, Devriendt J, et. al.: Comparison of dopamine and norepinephrine in the treatment of shock. *N Engl J Med.* 2010;362(9):779-789.

89. Pepi M, Marenzi GC, Agostoni PG, et al. Sustained cardiac diastolic changes elicited by ultrafiltration in patients with moderate congestive heart failure: pathophysiological correlates. *Br Heart J.* 1993;70(2):135-140.

90. Iorio L, Simonelli R, Nacca RG, Saltarelli G, Violi F. The benefits of daily hemofiltration in the management of anuria in patients with severe heart failure (NYHA IV). *Int J Artific Organs.* 1998;21(8):457-459.

91. Dahle TG, Blake D, Ali SS, Olinger CC, Bunte MC, Boyle AJ. Large volume ultrafiltration for acute decompensated heart failure using standard peripheral intravenous catheters. *J Card Fail.* 2006;12(5):349-352.

92. Costanzo MR, Guglin ME, Saltzberg MT, et al. Ultrafiltration versus intravenous diuretics for patients hospitalized for acute decompensated heart failure. *J Am Coll Cardiol.* 2007;49(6):675-683.

93. Bart BA, Goldsmith SR, Lee KL, et al. Ultrafiltration in decompensated heart failure with cardiorenal syndrome. *N Engl J Med.* 2012;367(24):2296-2304.

94. Costanzo MR, Negoianu D, Fonarow GC, et al. Rationale and design of the Aquapheresis Versus Intravenous Diuretics and Hospitalization for Heart Failure (AVOID-HF) trial. *Am Heart J.* 2015;170(3):471-482.

95. Tran RH, Aldemerdash A, Chang P, et al. Guideline-directed medical therapy and survival following hospitalization in patients with heart failure. *Pharmacotherapy.* 2018;38(4):406-416.

(DOSE-AHF) and Cardiorenal Rescue Study in Acute Decompensated Heart Failure (CARESS-HF). *Circ Heart Fail.* 2015;8(4):741-748.

96. Velazquez EJ, Morrow DA, DeVore AD, et al. Angiotensin-neprilysin inhibition in acute decompensated heart failure. *N Engl J Med.* 2019;380(6):539-548.

97. Teerlink JR, Metra M, Felker GM, et. al. Relaxin for the treatment of patients with acute heart failure (Pre-RELAX-AHF): a multicentre, randomised, placebo-controlled, parallel-group, dose-finding phase IIb study. *Lancet.* 2009;373(9673):1429-1439.

98. Teerlink JR, Cotter G, Davison BA, et. al. Serelaxin, recombinant human relaxin-2, for treatment of acute heart failure (RELAX-AHF): a randomised, placebo-controlled trial. *Lancet.* 2013;381(9860):29-39.

99. Metra M, Teerlink JR, Cotter G, et al. Effects of serelaxin in patients with acute heart failure. *N Engl J Med.* 2019;381(8):716-726.

100. Anker SD, Ponikowski P, Mitrovic V, Peacock WF, Filippatos G. Ularitide for the treatment of acute decompensated heart failure: from preclinical to clinical studies. *Eur Heart J.* 2015;36(12):715-723.

101. Packer M, O'Connor C, McMurray JJ, et. al. Effect of ularitide on cardiovascular mortality in acute heart failure. *N Engl J Med.* 2017;376(20):1956-1964.

102. Gheorghiade M, Bohm M, Greene SJ, et. al. Effect of aliskiren on postdischarge mortality and heart failure readmissions among patients hospitalized for heart failure: the ASTRONAUT randomized trial. *JAMA.* 2013;309(11):1125-1135.

103. McMurray JJ, Teerlink JR, Cotter G, et. al. Effects of tezosentan on symptoms and clinical outcomes in patients with acute heart failure: the VERITAS randomized controlled trials. *JAMA.* 2007;298(17):2009-2019.

104. Pang PS, Butler J, Collins SP, et. al. Biased ligand of the angiotensin II type 1 receptor in patients with acute heart failure: a randomized, double-blind, placebo-controlled, phase IIb, dose ranging trial (BLAST-AHF). *Eur Heart J.* 2017;38(30):2364-2373.

105. Erdmann E, Semigran MJ, Nieminen MS, et. al. Cinaciguat, a soluble guanylate cyclase activator, unloads the heart but also causes hypotension in acute decompensated heart failure. *Eur Heart J.* 2013;34(1):57-67.

106. Gheorghiade M, Greene SJ, Butler J, et. al. Effect of vericiguat, a soluble guanylate cyclase stimulator, on natriuretic peptide levels in patients with worsening chronic heart failure and reduced ejection fraction: the SOCRATES-REDUCED randomized trial. *JAMA.* 2015;314(21):2251-2262.

107. Armstrong PW, Pieske B, Anstrom KJ, et al. Vericiguat in patients with heart failure and reduced ejection fraction. *N Engl J Med.* 2020;382(20):1883-1893.

108. Teerlink JR, Felker GM, McMurray JJ, et. al. Acute Treatment with Omecamtiv Mecarbil to Increase Contractility in Acute Heart Failure: the ATOMIC-AHF study. *J Am Coll Cardiol.* 2016;67(12):1444-1455.

109. Teerlink JR, Diaz R, Felker GM, et al. Cardiac myosin activation with omecamtiv mecarbil in systolic heart failure. *N Engl J Med.* 2021;384(2):105-116.

110. Gheorghiade M, Blair JE, Filippatos GS, et. al. Hemodynamic, echocardiographic, and neurohormonal effects of istaroxime, a novel intravenous inotropic and lusitropic agent: a randomized controlled trial in patients hospitalized with heart failure. *J Am Coll Cardiol.* 2008;51(23):2276-2285.

111. Shah SJ, Blair JE, Filippatos GS, et. al. Effects of istaroxime on diastolic stiffness in acute heart failure syndromes: results from the Hemodynamic, Echocardiographic, and Neurohormonal Effects of Istaroxime, a novel intravenous inotropic and lusitropic agent: a randomized controlled trial in patients hospitalized with heart failure (HORIZON-HF) trial. *Am Heart J.* 2009;157(6):1035-1041.

112. Felker GM, McMurray JJV, Cleland JG, et al. Effects of a novel nitroxyl donor in acute heart failure: the STAND-UP AHF study. *JACC Heart Fail.* 2021;9(2):146-147.

113. Antonelli M, Levy M, Andrews PJ, et al. Hemodynamic monitoring in shock and implications for management. International Consensus Conference, Paris, France, 27-28 April 2006. *Intensive Care Med.* 2007;33(4):575-590.

114. Reynolds HR, Hochman JS. Cardiogenic shock: current concepts and improving outcomes. *Circulation.* 2008;117(5):686-697.

115. Stevenson, LW, Pagani FD, Young JB, et al. INTERMACS profiles of advanced heart failure: the current picture. *J Heart Lung Transplant.* 2009;28(6):535-541.

116. Rihal CS, Naidu SS, Givertz MM, et al. 2015 SCAI/ACC/HFSA/STS clinical expert consensus statement on the use of percutaneous mechanical circulatory support devices in cardiovascular care (endorsed by the American Heart Association, the Cardiological Society of India, and Sociedad Latino Americana de Cardiologia Intervencion; Affirmation of Value by the Canadian Association of Interventional Cardiology-Association Canadienne de Cardiologie d'intervention). *J Card Fail.* 2015;21(6):499-518.

117. Kavalieratos D, Gelfman LP, Tycon LE, et al. Palliative care in heart failure: rationale, evidence, and future priorities. *J Am Coll Cardiol.* 2017;70(15):1919-1930.

118. Allen LA, Stevenson LW, Grady KL et al. Decision making in advanced heart failure: a scientific statement from the American Heart Association. *Circulation.* 2012;125(15):1928-1952.

119. Bonow RO, Bennett S, Casey DE Jr, et al. ACC/AHA clinical performance measures for adults with chronic heart failure: a report of the American College of Cardiology/American Heart Association Task Force on Performance Measures (Writing Committee to Develop Heart Failure Clinical Performance Measures) endorsed by the Heart Failure Society of America. *J Am Coll Cardiol.* 2005;46(6):1144-1178.

120. Larsen PM, Teerlink JR. Team-based care for patients hospitalized with heart failure. *Heart Fail Clin.* 2015;11(3):359-370.

121. Epstein AE, DiMarco JP, Ellenbogen KA, et al. ACC/AHA/HRS 2008 guidelines for device-based therapy of cardiac rhythm abnormalities: a report of the American College of Cardiology/American Heart Association task force on practice guidelines (writing committee to revise the ACC/AHA/NASPE 2002 guideline update for implantation of cardiac pacemakers and antiarrhythmia devices) developed in collaboration with the American Association for Thoracic Surgery and Society of Thoracic Surgeons. *J Am Coll Cardiol.* 2008;51(21):e1-e62.

122. Costanzo MR, Stevenson LW, Adamson PB, et al. Interventions linked to decreased heart failure hospitalizations during ambulatory pulmonary artery pressure monitoring. *JACC Heart Fail.* 2016;4(5):333-344.

123. Hernandez AF, Greiner MA, Fonarow GC, et al. Relationship between early physician follow-up and 30-day readmission among Medicare beneficiaries hospitalized for heart failure. *JAMA.* 2010;303(17):1716-1722.

124. Metra M, Gheorghiade M, Bonow RO, Dei Cas L. Postdischarge assessment after a heart failure hospitalization: the next step forward. *Circulation.* 2010;122(18):1782-1785.

125. Konstam MA, Gheorghiade M, Burnett JC Jr, et al. Effects of oral tolvaptan in patients hospitalized for worsening heart failure: the EVEREST outcome trial. *JAMA.* 2007;297(12):1319-1331.

126. Gray A, Goodacre S, Newby DE, et al. Noninvasive ventilation in acute cardiogenic pulmonary edema. *N Engl J Med.* 2008.359(2)142-151.

127. Massie BM, O'Connor CM, Metra M, et al. Rolofylline, an adenosine A1-receptor antagonist, in acute heart failure. *N Engl J Med.* 2010;363(15):1419-1428.

128. Felker GM, Mentz RJ, Cole R, et al. Efficacy and safety of tolvaptan in patients hospitalized with acute heart failure. *J Am Coll Cardiol.* 2017;69(11):1399-1406.

129. Sharma K, Vaishnav J, Kalathiya R, et al. Randomized evaluation of heart failure with preserved ejection fraction patients with acute heart failure and dopamine: the ROPA-DOP trial. *JACC Heart Fail.* 2018;6(10):859-870.

130. Bhatt DL, Szarek M, Steg PG, et al. Sotagliflozin in patients with diabetes and recent worsening heart failure. *N Engl J Med.* 2021;384(2):117-128.

51

Peripartum Cardiomyopathy

Uri Elkayam and Jena Pizula

Peripartum cardiomyopathy

Definition

Idiopathic nonischemic cardiomyopathy with reduced LVEF that usually presents in the first month postpartum but can present towards the end of pregnancy or in the first few months postpartum

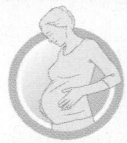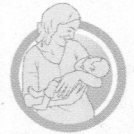

Potential important and lasting complications

- Severe heart failure
- Cardiogenic shock
- Cardiopulmonary arrest secondary to heart failure or arrythmias
- Thromboembolic complications
- Brain injury
- Mechanical circulatory support
- Cardiac transplantation
- Death

Management

During pregnancy
- Diuretics, vasodilators, digoxin, LMWH
- Mechanical circulatory support for severe heart failure/cardiogenic shock
- Consider early delivery if unstable
- Not recommended: ACEi/ARBs, spironolactone, ivabradine

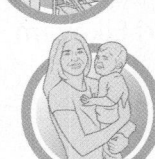

After delivery
- Diuretics, ACEi/ARB, spironolactone
- Mechanical circulatory device for severe heart failure/cardiogenic shock

Long term
- Optimal duration of pharmacotherapy after LV recovery unknown
- In case of stopping medications, wean gradually and observe closely
- Continue surveillance after recovery

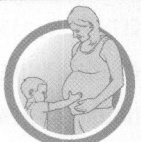

Risk factors

- Age >30 years
- African American race
- Hypertension
- Preeclampsia
- Multigestational pregnancy

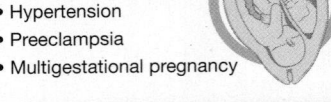

Predictors of poor outcome

- LVEF <30%
- LVEDD >6.0 cm
- African American race
- Late diagnosis
- High levels of NT-proBNP and troponin

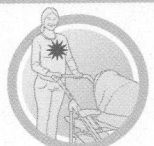

Signs and symptoms

- Shortness of breath
- Orthopnea
- Paroxysmal nocturnal dyspnea
- Chest pain
- Tachycardia
- Leg edema

Risk of subsequent pregnancy

- In women with persistent LV dysfunction (LVEF <50%): high risk of reduced EF and clinical deterioration
- In women with recovered LV function: favorable outcome in most, but modest reduction in EF in 20%, which persists in 10%, and occasional severe EF deterioration

Chapter 51 Fuster and Hurst's Central Illustration. Peripartum cardiomyopathy is an idiopathic cardiomyopathy presenting with heart failure due to severe left ventricular systolic dysfunction towards the end of pregnancy or in the first few months postpartum; it most commonly presents within the first month postpartum. Peripartum cardiomyopathy is a diagnosis of exclusion, and other causes of cardiac dysfunction should be ruled out. Although many patients do improve, peripartum cardiomyopathy can be associated with important and lasting complications. ACEi, angiotensin receptor inhibitors; ARB, angiotensin receptor antagonists; EF, ejection fraction; LMWH, low molecular weight heparin; LV, left ventricular; LVEF, left ventricular ejection fraction; LVEDD, left ventricular end-diastolic diameter; NT-proBNP, N-terminal pro-brain natriuretic protein

CHAPTER SUMMARY

This chapter reviews the epidemiology, pathophysiology, and management of peripartum cardiomyopathy (PPCM), an idiopathic cardiomyopathy presenting with heart failure due to severe left ventricular systolic dysfunction. Presentation is usually during the first month after delivery but can be during the second or third trimester of pregnancy or a few months postpartum (see Fuster and Hurst's Central Illustration). The incidence of PPCM in the United States is approximately 1 in 3000 live births and is significantly higher in Black women than in White women. The incidence worldwide varies and is higher in Africa and Haiti than in Europe and the United States. Risk factors for the condition include advanced age, preeclampsia, Black ethnicity, and multifetal pregnancy. Normalization of left ventricular function occurs in >50% of women in the United States, mostly within 2 to 6 months after diagnosis. Reported recovery rates in other countries vary. Although many patients do improve, PPCM can be associated with important and lasting complications. Moreover, subsequent pregnancy in women with a history of PPCM can be associated with relapse with reduced ejection fraction and worsening of symptoms; this is more likely in women with persistent left ventricular dysfunction prior to their subsequent pregnancy but occasionally occurs in women with recovered left ventricular function.

DEFINITION

Peripartum cardiomyopathy (PPCM) is a pregnancy-associated myocardial disease, reported to occur in different parts of the world.[1-3] PPCM is an idiopathic cardiomyopathy presenting with heart failure (HF) secondary to LV systolic dysfunction toward the end of pregnancy or in the months following delivery, where no other cause of HF is found.[2-4] PPCM is therefore a diagnosis of exclusion, and other causes of cardiac dysfunction should be ruled out. At the same time, however, transient and unexpected depression of LV function typical to PPCM has been described in women with other forms of heart disease.[5]

INCIDENCE AND EPIDEMIOLOGY

The incidence of PPCM varies widely, between ~1:100 and 1:300 in Africa and Haiti, respectively, to an average of 1:20,000 live births in Japan.[2] Incidence of PPCM in the United States has been reported to range from ~1 in 1000 to 1 in 4000 live births[6,7] with a significantly higher incidence in Black women.[8,9] Multiple studies from the United States also reported a more severe disease and worse outcomes in Black women with PPCM, which could be related to racial differences due to genetic predisposition and environmental difference.[10,11] PPCM incidence in the United States is increasing most likely due to older maternal age, an increase in the rate of multifetal pregnancies, and an increased recognition of the disease.[5]

ETIOLOGY AND PATHOPHYSIOLOGY

The etiology of PPCM remains unclear. Mechanisms proposed have included low selenium level, viral infection, stress-activated cytokines, inflammation, autoimmune reactions, and hemodynamic changes of pregnancy.[2] Studies based on animal models of pregnancy-associated cardiomyopathy (PACM) in the last decade have suggested that PPCM may be a vascular disease caused by hormonal changes occurring in late pregnancy[12,13] (**Fig. 51–1**). Experimental support of this suggestion was a

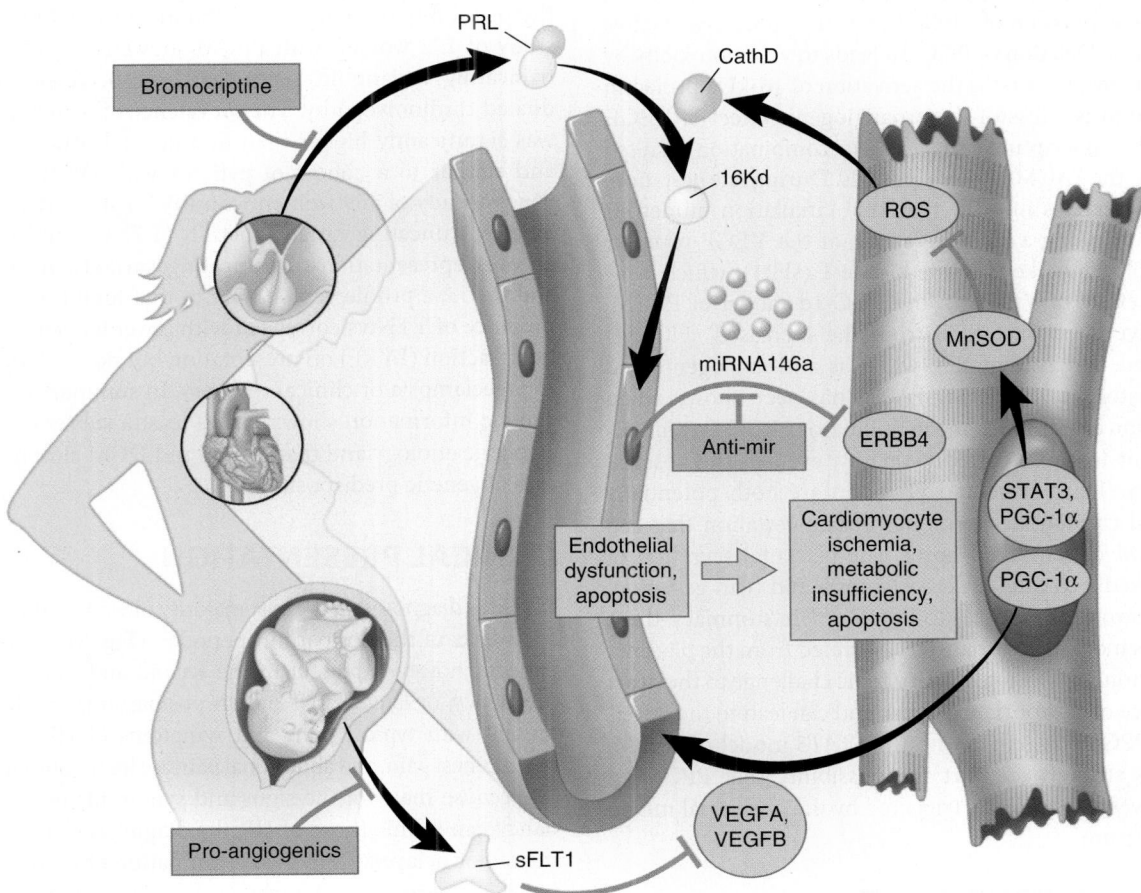

Figure 51–1. Loss of *STAT3* in murine hearts leads to reduced expression of MnSOD, which neutralizes superoxides generated by the robust mitochondrial activity in beating cardiomyocytes. The consequent rise in reactive oxygen species leads to the secretion of the peptidase cathepsin D that cleaves the pregnancy hormone prolactin into a 16-kDa fragment that promotes apoptosis in endothelial cells and the development of pregnancy-associated DCM.[16] Blocking prolactin secretion from the pituitary with bromocriptine reversed the cardiomyopathy. 16-kDa prolactin induces endothelial cells to package miR-146a into exosomes, which are then secreted and taken up by cardiomyocytes. The miR-146a internalized into cardiomyocytes then suppresses the neuregulin/ErbB pathway, thereby promoting cardiomyocyte apoptosis.[46] A different mouse model of PADCM with cardiac-specific deletion of proliferator-activated receptor-gamma coactivator-1α (PGC-1α) was found to promote vasculotoxicity by two pathways: the activation of an antivascular 16-kDa prolactin-mediated pathway (as in the *STAT3* model) and the loss of a provascular VEGF-mediated pathway together with the toxic challenge of sFlt1 secreted from the placenta in late gestation.[17] Reproduced with permission from Arany Z, Elkayam U. Peripartum Cardiomyopathy. *Circulation.* 2016 Apr 5;133(14):1397-409.

mouse model of PPCM with genetically deleted *STAT3* transcription specifically in cardiomyocytes leading to reduced expression of manganese superoxide dismutase (MnSOD), which neutralizes increased level of superoxide generated by increased mitochondrial activity in beating cardiomyocytes during pregnancy.[12] Unopposed high level of reactive oxygen species leads to the expression of cathepsin D, a peptidase that cleaves prolactin into a 16- kDa fragment that promotes the expression of miRNA 146a, which leads to endothelial dysfunction and apoptosis and cardiomyocyte ischemia, metabolic insufficiency, and apoptosis and leads to the development of a dilated cardiomyopathy.[14] Treatment of *STAT3* cardiac knockout mice with bromocriptine that blocks prolactin secretion from the pituitary completely reversed the observed cardiomyopathy. The vasculo-hormonal mechanism of PACM was later supported in a different mouse model with cardiac-specific deletion of proliferator-activated receptor-gamma coactivator-1α (PGC-1α), which is a powerful transcriptional regulator[3,13] (Fig. 51–1). PGC-1α drives the expression of vascular endothelial growth factor (VEGF) and similar to *STAT3*, increases the expression of MnSOD, which suppresses reactive oxygen species. Deletion of PGC-1α leads to vasculotoxicity by two mechanisms: the first is the activation of 16-kDa prolactin and the second is a loss of the proangiogenic effect of VEGF. The use of bromocriptine and VEGF in combination resulted in a rescue of the PACM in these animals. During late gestation, the placenta secretes into the maternal circulation numerous hormones, including a soluble variant of the VEGF receptor 1, and soluble Fms-like tyrosine kinase 1 (sFlt1), which neutralizes the effect of VEGF. In the PGC-1α model of PACM, the protective effect of VEGF from the increased sFlt level is diminished. The role of sFlt, which is anti-angiogenic and proinflammatory, in triggering PACM has been shown when administration of this hormone to nulliparous PGC-1α animals was sufficient to cause cardiomyopathy, even in the absence of pregnancy, Thus, sFlt1 and prolactin are both potentially vasculo- and cardiotoxic hormones of late gestation that can trigger PPCM in sensitized hosts. The placental secretion of sFlt1 is markedly elevated in preeclampsia and twin gestation, which have strong association to PPCM.[15,16] In summary, these observations may suggest that sFlt1, secreted from the placenta in late gestation, is associated with a toxic challenge to the heart in the absence of appropriate defense and can lead to the development of PPCM. Together with the *STAT3* model of PACM, the findings strongly support the possibility that PPCM in women is a vascular disease, triggered by the hormonal milieu of the peripartum.

ASSOCIATED CONDITIONS

The mean age of women with PPCM ranges from 27 to 33 years[1,2] with >50% of patients reported to be >30 years of age.[1,7,17] The incidence of the disease is also considerably higher among Black patients.[8,9] Preeclampsia and hypertension are also strongly associated with PPCM with a 4-fold higher incidence in women with PPCM compared to those without it.[15] Multi-gestational status has been reported in 7% to 14.5% of patients

with PPCM in the United States compared with only 3% of twin pregnancies in the overall population.[2,16] Multiparity has been traditionally considered to be a risk factor for PPCM, although most studies in the United States have reported the development of PPCM in conjunction with the first or second pregnancy in >50% of patients.[5]

GENETICS OF PERIPARTUM CARDIOMYOPATHY

Some evidence has supported the notion that PPCM may have a hereditary or genetic component. The strikingly higher incidence of PPCM in Black women in the United States compared to White women and in African countries and Haiti suggests a possible genetic contribution.[3,11,18] Observations of familial clustering of PPCM, cardiac history of cardiac disease in 15% of-first degree relatives of women included in a German registry of PPCM,[19] as well as approximately co-occurrence with idiopathic dilated cardiomyopathy (DCM), a phenotypically similar disease that is linked to genetic variation,[20] also suggest the possibility of genetic contribution to PPCM.[21,22] A recent study of 172 women with PPCM showed that 15% bore rare truncating variants in genes that have been associated with dilated cardiomyopathy. The prevalence of truncating variants was significantly higher than in a normal control population and similar to a cohort of patients with DCM.[23,24] A recent genetic study of 469 women with PPCM showed a 10% prevalence of truncating variants in TTN (TTNtvs) and additionally an overrepresentation of truncating variants in *FLNC*, *DCP*, and *BAG3*, a profile very similar to that found in DCM.[25] The presence of TTNtvs correlated with lower left ventricular ejection fraction (LVEF) on presentation but not with the presence of preeclampsia or clinical recovery. In summary, the available genetic information shows that at least a subset of PPCM has a genetic etiology and that PPCM and DCM closely share profiles of genetic predispositions.

CLINICAL PRESENTATION

PPCM is diagnosed in the vast majority of women during the first few weeks of the postpartum period[5,26] (**Fig. 51–2**). A subset of patients, however, present in the second and third trimester of pregnancy, or later than 1 month postpartum.[2,5,26] Most patients present with typical signs and symptoms of HF.[5] In addition, cough, chest pain, and abdominal pain are frequently encountered.

Because many of the signs and symptoms of normal pregnancy can mimic those of HF, the diagnosis of PPCM is often missed or delayed.[27] Physical examination often reveals orthopnea, tachycardia and tachypnea, increased jugular venous pressure, right ventricular heave, and displaced apical impulse. A third heart sound and murmurs of mitral and tricuspid regurgitation may be present as well as pulmonary rales and peripheral edema.[2] The most common electrocardiogram (ECG) findings on presentation are sinus tachycardia and T-wave flattening and/or inversion and non-specific ST-segment depression. Left atrial enlargement, left ventricular hypertrophy, and left bundle branch block (LBBB) may be present.[28,29]

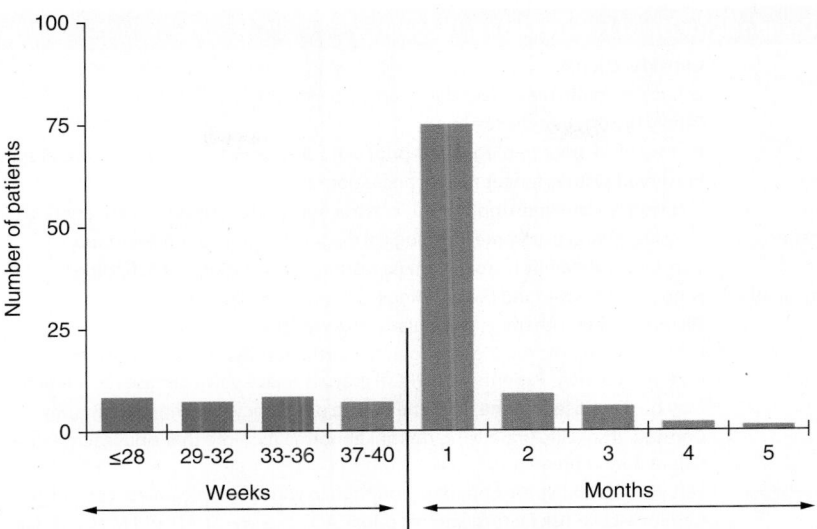

Figure 51–2. Time of diagnosis of cardiomyopathy in 123 patients. *Black bars* represent 23 patients with early PACM; *white bars* represent 100 patients with traditional PPCM. Reproduced with permission from Elkayam U, Akhter MW, Singh H, et al. Pregnancy-associated cardiomyopathy: clinical characteristics and a comparison between early and late presentation. *Circulation*. 2005 Apr 26;111(16):2050-2055.

Chest radiography usually shows cardiomegaly and pulmonary venous congestion. Echocardiographic findings include variable degrees of LV dilatation, with moderate-to-severe depression of systolic function.[2] LV apical thrombi can be seen in those with severely depressed LV function. Right ventricular and biatrial dilatation as well as moderate-to-severe mitral and tricuspid regurgitation are also commonly seen, with increased pulmonary pressures and mild pulmonary regurgitation.[5] Cardiac MRI can be used for accurate assessment of chamber measurements and ejection fraction and for detection of mural thrombi.[30] Brain natriuretic peptide (BNP) levels are usually markedly elevated at the time of presentation.

DIFFERENTIAL DIAGNOSIS

PCCM is a diagnosis of exclusion that needs to be made after exclusion of other possible causes of HF. A list of potential differential diagnoses is shown in **Table 51–1**.

PROGNOSIS

Complications

PPCM can be associated with important and lasting complications, including severe HF, cardiogenic shock, cardiopulmonary arrest secondary to HF or arrythmias, thromboembolic complications, brain injury, mechanical circulatory support, cardiac transplantation, and death.[2,7] Because of delayed diagnosis, preventable complications often preceded the diagnosis.[27] Predictors of complications are LVEF <30%, Black ethnicity, and delay of diagnosis.[17,27]

Mortality

Reported rate of mortality has varied significantly in different racial groups and geographical regions. One-year mortality in the United States ranged between 4% in the prospective IPAC

(Investigation of Pregnancy Associated Cardiomyopathy) study that included 30% Black women[17] and 11% in a population of 96% Black women.[31] A recent publication from the worldwide registry of PPCM reported 6 months mortality of 6%, which was lower in Europe (4%) and highest in the Middle East (10%). Most deaths were due to HF or sudden cardiac death.[32]

Recovery of LV Function

Available information in the United States has demonstrated normalization of LV function in >50% of women with PPCM, mostly occurring within 2 to 6 months after diagnosis.[17,26,33] Later recovery, however, is possible and occurs in some patients. The rate of LV recovery seems to be significantly lower, and the timing longer in Black patients compared with White patients.[10,17,34,35] Reports of recovery rates in other countries are variable with high recovery rates in Germany,[19] Japan, China, Pakistan, and low recovery rates in African countries, Turkey, and Haiti.[35-37]

Predictors of LV Recovery

Factors shown to be associated with failure to recover include low EF (<30%), enlarged LV diastolic dimension (>6.0 cm), and late diagnosis.[17,34] In addition, troponin elevation, high plasma BNP,[2] presence of LV thrombus,[38] and Black ethnicity[272,5] are associated with lower likelihood of recovery.[2,3] Genetic testing showed that women with the *GNB3* TT genotype had significantly less myocardial recovery at 1 year and its impact was particularly evident in Black women with PPCM.[39]

Evidence of Subclinical LV Dysfunction After Recovery

A recent study by Goland et al.[40] demonstrated a significantly lower LV global longitudinal and apical circumferential two-dimensional strain in 29 women with EF >50%

TABLE 51–1. Differential Diagnosis for Heart Failure During Pregnancy

Differential Diagnosis	Considerations
Takotsubo cardiomyopathy	Echocardiogram may show classic apical ballooning
Preexisting cardiomyopathy	Family history, genetic testing
Pre-eclampsia	History of HF prior to pregnancy; prior echo studies with low LVEF before pregnancy
Hypertrophic cardiomyopathy	Preserved systolic function on echocardiogram
Myocarditis	Left ventricular hypertrophy, LVOT obstruction, preserved systolic function, genetic testing
Arrythmogenic RV cardiomyopathy	Consider if viral prodrome, histological diagnosis, fulminant presentation
Left ventricular noncompaction	Consider with family history, genetic testing, echocardiographic findings
Chemotherapy-related cardiomyopathy	Echocardiographic and CMR findings
Valvular heart disease	History of chemotherapy, particularly doxorubicin
Congenital heart disease	Echocardiographic findings; congenital aortic stenosis; mitral stenosis from rheumatic heart disease in endemic country. Patients with PPCM may also have valve disease (ie, mitral regurgitation)
Tachycardia-arrhythmia mediated cardiomyopathy	May be diagnosed for the first time during pregnancy by echocardiography
Hypertensive heart disease	Consider if specific underlying rhythm abnormality. Note that sinus tachycardia may be secondary to heart failure during pregnancy
Ischemic heart disease	Left ventricular hypertrophy; less common in young people unless very long-standing history of hypertension
Cardiomyopathy related to other acute conditions	Cardiovascular risk factors; angina; prior CAD; consider SCAD and MINOCA diagnoses
Pulmonary embolism	May consider if patient has other conditions such as sepsis, postrespiratory arrest
	Dyspnea, tachycardia with preserved LVEF

CAD, coronary artery disease; CMR, cardiac magnetic resonance imaging; HF, heart failure; LVEF, left ventricular ejection fraction; LVOT, left ventricular outflow tract; MINOCA, myocardial infarction in nonobstructive coronary arteries; PPCM, peripartum cardiomyopathy.
Reproduced with permission from Davis MB, Arany Z, McNamara DM, et al. Peripartum Cardiomyopathy: JACC State-of-the-Art Review. *J Am Coll Cardiol.* 2020 Jan 21; 75(2):207-221.

at least 12 months after presentation with PPCM compared to controls. These findings support early echocardiographic study of women with PPCM with recovered LV function that revealed decreased contractile reserve in response to dobutamine challenge, indicating the presence of persistent subclinical dysfunction in women with a history of PPCM even after normalization of LVEF.[2]

MANAGEMENT

The goals of management in PPCM are to improve hemodynamics and symptoms of HF to achieve recovery of cardiac function, to prevent thromboembolic complications, and to prevent sudden arrhythmic death. In general, the pharmacological treatment of HF should follow recent guideline recommendations except during pregnancy and lactation, when drug therapy may need to be altered because of potential risk to the fetus or the breastfed infant[2] (**Fig. 51–3**). Because of the high incidence of thromboembolism associated with PPCM,[38,41–47] anticoagulation from the time of the diagnosis until LV function recovers (LVEF >35%) is advisable.[2,3] Anticoagulation seems particularly important during pregnancy and the first 6 to 8 weeks postpartum because of persistent hypercoagulable state.

Because only limited long-term, prospective data are available, no recommendations can be made about stopping HF medications after normalization of LV function. Patients with persistent LV dysfunction should continue treatment with β-blockers and RAAS inhibitors. Discontinuation of medications in women with complete recovery (LVEF >55%) should only be done gradually with close monitoring of LV function.[2]

Annual assessment of LV function is recommended in all women with history of PPCM after LV recovery for early detection of recurrent cardiomyopathy.

Bromocriptine and the Role of Breastfeeding

The potential benefit of bromocriptine for the treatment of PPCM was initially suggested based on the concept of enhanced oxidative stress–mediated cleavage of the nursing hormone prolactin into an antiangiogenic and proapoptotic 16-kDa form that may be responsible for the development of PPCM.[12] The benefit of bromocriptine has been shown in two small human studies in Africa[48,49] while a small, randomized German study was inconclusive.[50] No information is available in the United States regarding safety and efficacy of bromocriptine and it is not routinely used. The European guidelines include a level IIb recommendation for the use of the drug.[51] Because of the risk of thromboembolic complications, anticoagulation should be prescribed to women taking bromocriptine. While bromocriptine will hinder milk production, breastfeeding does not worsen prognosis and can be allowed in a stable patient.[52]

Devices and Heart Transplantation

Implantable Cardioverter-Defibrillators

About 30% of PPCM-related mortality is due to sudden death and most deaths occur within the first 6 months and in women with LVEF <30%. For these reasons and because recovery of LV function occurs in the majority of patients within 2 to 6 months after the diagnosis, it is reasonable to consider wearable external defibrillators in patients with severe LV dysfunction (EF <35%) as a bridge to recovery or permanent implantable

MEDICATION	DURING PREGNANCY	POTENTIAL ADVERSE EFFECTS	INDICATIONS	DURING LACTATION
HEART FAILURE MEDICATIONS				
Loop diuretics	Yes	Caution for hypovolemia or hypotension that may lead to decreased placental perfusion	For signs and symptoms of congestion and fluid overload.	Yes, but over-diuresis can lead to decreased milk production.
Beta blockers (metoprolol tartrate used most commonly)	Yes	IUGR; fetal bradycardia and hypoglycemia	For standard treatment of HF; consider treatment of women with subsequent pregnancy.	Yes
Hydralazine/nitrates	Yes	Caution with hypotension	Use for afterload reduction during pregnancy (instead of ACE-I/ARB) when needed.	Yes, but ACE-I/ARB typically chosen post-partum
Digoxin	Yes	No associated congenital defects	Can be used with symptomatic heart failure and/or systolic dysfunction during pregnancy, or afterwards per guidelines.	Yes
ACE-I/ARB	No	Anuria, oligohydramnios, fetal limb contractures, craniofacial deformation, pulmonary atresia, fetal hypocalvaria, intra uterine growth restriction, prematurity, patent ductus arteriosus, stillbirth, neonatal hypotension, and death	Cannot use during pregnancy. After delivery, should be used as part of guideline-directed medical therapy for afterload reduction and LV remodeling.	Enalapril and captopril can be used
Aldosterone receptor antagonists	No	Spironolactone has been associated with antiadrenergic activity, feminization of male rat fetuses and permanent changes in reproductive tract in both sexes	As per guideline-directed medical therapy for heart failure.	Spironolactone can be used
Sacubitril-valsartan	No	Same as ACE-I/ARB	As per guideline-directed medical therapy for heart failure.	No information in human, present in rat milk
Ivabradine	Scant data in humans; would avoid due to concerns in animal studies	Scant data in humans, animal data suggest risk	As per guideline-directed medical therapy for heart failure.	No information in human, present in rat milk
ANTICOAGULANTS				
Low molecular weight heparin	Yes	Caution at time of delivery and with neuraxial anesthesia; does not cross placenta; consider the need for monitoring anti-Xa levels	For prevention and treatment of thromboembolic complications during pregnancy and as bridge to warfarin postpartum.	Yes
Warfarin	Avoid	Warfarin embryopathy and fetopathy	For prevention and treatment of thromboembolic complications postpartum.	Yes

Legend:

	Data or experience to support use
	Caution with using this medication
	Data is limited or inconclusive

Figure 51–3. Heart failure and anticoagulant medications: Indications and safety in pregnancy and during lactation. Reproduced with permission from Davis MB, Arany Z, McNamara DM, et al. Peripartum Cardiomyopathy: JACC State-of-the-Art Review. *J Am Coll Cardiol.* 2020 Jan 21;75(2):207-221.

cardioverter-defibrillator (ICD) implantation in women with no recovery of LV function on appropriate medical therapy.[2] In women with LBBB and persistent LVEF <35% in spite of appropriate medical therapy, a cardiac resynchronization therapy defibrillator (CRTD) implantation is recommended.[53]

Mechanical Circulatory Devices

In patients demonstrating rapid hemodynamic deterioration not responding to medical therapy including vasoactive medications, mechanical support (intra-aortic balloon pumps, Impella) can be used.[54] In cases with impaired oxygenation, extracorporeal membrane oxygenation (ECMO) has been successfully used.[55-60] Because the rate of recovery in patients with PPCM is higher than in other forms of DCM, an attempt should be made to use temporary devices as a bridge to recovery before referral for cardiac transplantation.[55,57,61]

Durable Left Ventricular Assist Device

Recent data from INTERMACS reported better survival in women with PPCM receiving durable left ventricular assist device (LVAD) compared with non-PPCM patients, probably because of younger age and fewer comorbidities. At 36 months, LV recovery, however, was found in only 6% of PPCM patients (compared to 2% in non-PPCM women) and almost half of patients ultimately underwent cardiac transplantation.[62]

Cardiac Transplantation

This procedure has been performed successfully in patients with PPCM. A recent review of the UNOS registry of patients receiving a heart transplant between 1987 and 2019 identified 666 with PPCM. These patients were younger and 48% were Black. They required higher frequency of support pretransplant including IABP and VAD but not ECMO. The PPCM patients had fewer days on the wait list and demonstrated a greater incidence of pretransplant panel reactive antibodies. The overall posttransplant survival was slightly lower in the PPCM group.[63]

OUTCOME OF SUBSEQUENT PREGNANCY

Women with a history of PPCM are at risk of relapse with deterioration of LV function and symptoms during subsequent pregnancies.[64] The risk of relapse is higher in women with persistent LV dysfunction compared to those who have normalized LV function. Almost 50% of women with persistent LV dysfunction had significant deterioration of LV function and approximately 1 out of 6 women died during recurrent pregnancy. The recent European practice guidelines for the management of pregnant women with heart disease recommend discouraging subsequent pregnancy when the EF has not recovered to >50% to 55%.[51] Almost 25% of woman with recovered LV function have been reported to have a decrease in LV function with the subsequent pregnancy,[65,66] which persisted in about half them. Isolated cases of severe deterioration of LV function and life-threatening arrythmias have been described;[64] however, there have fortunately been no reported deaths. Patients who decide to become pregnant again should be counseled about the increased risk of complications with subsequent pregnancies. Unintentional pregnancy should be prevented by effective contraception. Recommendations for the follow-up and management of subsequent pregnancy in women with a history of PPCM are shown in **Tables 51-2 and 51-3**. Early termination of an unintentional pregnancy should be considered to prevent worsening of LV function and potential maternal mortality, especially in patients with persistent LV dysfunction.[64] Although a majority of women usually receive reproductive counseling, based on a self-reported national, web-based registry focused of health-related quality assessment in women with PPCM, 25% of patients still reported no discussion of contraceptive strategies to prevent unintended

pregnancy and HF worsening.[67] The recommendations for the use of contraceptives in women with previous PPCM are generally similar to those recommended for women with other forms of heart disease.[68] Women with PPCM and LV dysfunction are at high thromboembolic risk, therefore, contraceptives containing estrogen should be avoided. Progesterone releasing

TABLE 51-2. Suggested Algorithm for Management of Subsequent Pregnancy in Women with a History of PPCM and Persistent LV Dysfunction

Women with persistent LV dysfunction (LVEF <50%) should be informed about the risk of significant morbidity and even mortality associated with subsequent pregnancy and the alternative ways to build a family.
During Pregnancy
- Base line echocardiography and BNP level prior to pregnancy or during the first visit.
- Symptoms are followed monthly for 30 weeks and biweekly thereafter.
- Continue β-blockers, switch ACEi/ARBs/Sacubitril-Valsartan to Hydralazine/Isosorbide dinitrate.
- Diuretics for volume overload.
- Aspirin 81 mg/daily started between 12 to 28 weeks until delivery in women at increased risk of preeclampsia.
- Consider Digoxin for symptoms improvement.
- Therapeutic anti coagulation for LVEF <35%.
- Life Vest for LVEF ≤35%.
- Repeat echocardiography and BNP at the end of 1st and 2nd trimester, 1 month prior to estimated time of delivery, prior to discharge after the delivery, 1-month postpartum and at any time if symptoms worsen.

After Delivery
- Start Enalapril and Spironolactone.
- Continue anticoagulation for 6 weeks if LVEF <35%.
- Continue Life Vest as a bridge to recovery or implantation of implantable cardioverter defibrillator if LVEF <35%.
- Breast feeding can be allowed unless the patient is unstable.
- Close follow-up for 6 months.

Abbreviations: ACEi, angiotensin converting enzyme inhibitors; ARB, angiotensin receptor blockers; BNP, brain natriuretic peptide; LV, left ventricular; LVEF, LV ejection fraction.

TABLE 51-3. Suggested Algorithm for Management of Subsequent Pregnancy in Women with a History of PPCM and Recovered LV function (≥50%)

- Baseline echocardiography and BNP level prior to or at first visit during pregnancy.
- Follow up for symptoms q 1 to 2 months for 30 weeks and q 2 weeks until delivery.
- Discontinue ACEi/ARBs in patients who are on these medications and continue β-blockers.
- Repeat echocardiogram and BNP level 1 to 2 months after discontinuation of RAAS inhibitors medications to reassess LV function.
- No drug therapy in patients who are not on medications.
- ASA 81 mg/d started between 12 and 28 weeks until delivery in women at increased risk of preeclampsia.
- Repeat echocardiogram and BNP at the end of 2nd trimester, 1 month prior to estimated time of delivery, prior to discharge, 1-month postpartum or at any time if symptoms develop.
- Breast feeding can be allowed
- Close follow-up for 6 months.

Abbreviations: ACEi, angiotensin converting enzyme inhibitors; ARB, angiotensin receptor blockers; BNP, brain natriuretic peptide; RAAS, renin angiotensin aldosterone system.

intrauterine device such as Mirena or progesterone subcutaneous implant are preferred. Tubular ligation can be used as well when decided upon by the women. The decision on the type of contraception has to be made after counselling of both a gynecologist and cardiologist to choose the optimal approach.

LABOR AND DELIVERY

The timing and mode of delivery in a patient diagnosed with PPCM during pregnancy should be determined by the clinical status of the mother and the fetus. Termination of pregnancy or early delivery may result in improvement of both symptoms and cardiac function and should be considered in patients with deteriorating symptoms or cardiac function.[65] Continuation of pregnancy can be allowed, with frequent monitoring, to allow fetal maturity in patients who can be stabilized on medical therapy. The mode of delivery in a stable patient with PPCM should be determined jointly by the obstetrician and the cardiologist. Vaginal delivery prevents potential risks associated with anesthesia and surgical delivery that include hemodynamic fluctuations, larger blood loss, pain, infections, respiratory and thromboembolic complications, damage to pelvic organs, and potential unfavorable effects on future reproductive health.[69] At the same time, an elective cesarean section is more rapid and allows better planning of the time of delivery as well as the presence of the most experienced medical team during the delivery. Hemodynamic monitoring for labor and delivery may be desirable in a patient with PPCM who is diagnosed during pregnancy and allows optimization of hemodynamic status before delivery as well as monitoring of changes related to fluid intake and blood loss during delivery and early hemodynamic changes as a result of increased venous return and peripheral vascular resistance after delivery. In case of vaginal delivery, an assisted second stage may be recommended to reduce maternal efforts and shorten labor. Maternal vital signs as well as oxygen saturation, ECG, and fetal heart rate should be continuously monitored.

PSYCHOLOGICAL SEQUENCES AMONG PPCM SURVIVORS

Most research is focused on survival and cardiac complications of PPCM and little is known about psychosocial outcomes of these previously healthy young women. A nationwide, web-based quality of life registry revealed that 32% of 177 PPCM patients (median time since diagnosis of 3.0 ± 4.3 years) had clinically significant symptoms of depression, which was associated with worse record of follow-up visits.[70] Another study showed high anxiety in response to the diagnosis of PPCM and feeling a sense of doom even after recovery. Women had difficulty caring for their newborns during the postpartum period and recommendations to avoid additional pregnancy may have negative influence on their family relationship.[71] Another survey of 116 women showed that more than half (56%) never returned to their previous emotional condition and only 26% were satisfied with the counselling they received from their physician.[72] All of this information emphasizes the need for many survivors of PPCM for ongoing support and education.

SUMMARY

- PPCM is an idiopathic cardiomyopathy presenting with HF secondary to LV systolic dysfunction toward the end of pregnancy or in the months following delivery.

- The incidence varies widely between ~1:100 livebirths in Africa and 1:20,000 in Japan and between 1:1000 and 1:4000 live births in the United States.

- Etiology of PPCM remains unclear; animal models suggest vasculo-hormonal mechanism of PACM.

- Associated conditions to PPCM include Black ethnicity, older age, preeclampsia, and multifetal pregnancies.

- Most patients with PPCM present with typical signs and symptoms of HF. Because many of the signs and symptoms of normal pregnancy can mimic those of HF, the diagnosis of PPCM is often missed or delayed.

- PPCM can be associated with important and lasting complications including severe HF/cardiogenic shock, arrythmias, thromboembolism, and sudden death.

- Genetic studies suggest that at least a subset of women with PPCM has a genetic etiology and that PPCM and nonischemic DCM closely share profiles of genetic predisposition.

- Recovery of cardiac function occurs in >50% of women with PPCM in the United States mostly within 2 to 6 months after diagnosis.

- Factors associated with lower or delayed recovery rate include low EF (<30%), enlarged LV diastolic dimension (>6.0 cm), Black ethnicity, elevated troponin, and BNP levels.

- Goals of management are to improve symptoms of HF, achieve recovery of cardiac function, and prevent thromboembolic complications and sudden cardiac death.

- Choice of drugs used during pregnancy and lactation should take into account drug efficacy but also fetal and newborn safety.

- Discontinuation of cardiac medications after complete recovery should be done gradually with close monitoring of LV function.

- Women with a history of PPCM are at risk of relapse with deterioration of LV function and symptoms during subsequent pregnancies.

- Risk of cardiac deterioration during subsequent pregnancy is higher in women with persistent LV dysfunction.

- Subsequent pregnancy after recovery of LV function (LVEF >50%) can also be associated with important decrease in LV function.

- Timing and mode of delivery in women with PPCM diagnosed during pregnancy should be determined by the clinical status of the mother and the fetus.

- PPCM is associated with important psychological and emotional complications that require ongoing support and education.

REFERENCES

1. Sliwa K, Mebazaa A, Hilfiker-Kleiner D, et al. Clinical characteristics of patients from the worldwide registry on peripartum cardiomyopathy (PPCM): EURObservational Research Programme in conjunction with the Heart Failure Association of the European Society of Cardiology Study Group on PPCM. *Eur J Heart Fail.* 2017;19(9):1131-1141.

2. Davis MB, Arany Z, McNamara DM, Goland S, Elkayam U. Peripartum cardiomyopathy: JACC State-of-the-Art Review. *J Am Coll Cardiol.* 2020;75(2):207-221.

3. Arany Z, Elkayam U. Peripartum cardiomyopathy. *Circulation.* 2016;133(14):1397-1409.

4. Sliwa K, Hilfiker-Kleiner D, Petrie MC, et al. Current state of knowledge on aetiology, diagnosis, management, and therapy of peripartum cardiomyopathy: a position statement from the Heart Failure Association of the European Society of Cardiology Working Group on peripartum cardiomyopathy. *Eur J Heart Fail.* 2010;12(8):767-778.

5. Elkayam U. Clinical characteristics of peripartum cardiomyopathy in the United States: diagnosis, prognosis, and management. *J Am Coll Cardiol.* 2011;58(7):659-670.

6. Gunderson EP, Croen LA, Chiang V, Yoshida CK, Walton D, Go AS. Epidemiology of peripartum cardiomyopathy: incidence, predictors, and outcomes. *Obstet Gynecol.* 2011;118(3):583-591.

7. Kolte D, Khera S, Aronow WS, et al. Temporal trends in incidence and outcomes of peripartum cardiomyopathy in the United States: a nationwide population-based study. *J Am Heart Assoc.* 2014;3(3):e001056.

8. Gentry MB, Dias JK, Luis A, Patel R, Thornton J, Reed GL. African-American women have a higher risk for developing peripartum cardiomyopathy. *J Am Coll Cardiol.* 2010;55(7):654-659.

9. Harper MA, Meyer RE, Berg CJ. Peripartum cardiomyopathy: population-based birth prevalence and 7-year mortality. *Obstet Gynecol.* 2012;120(5):1013-1019.

10. Irizarry OC, Levine LD, Lewey J, et al. Comparison of clinical characteristics and outcomes of peripartum cardiomyopathy between African American and Non–African American women. *JAMA Cardiology.* 2017;2(11):1256-1260.

11. Goland S, Modi K, Hatamizadeh P, Elkayam U. Differences in clinical profile of African-American women with peripartum cardiomyopathy in the United States. *J Card Fail.* 2013;19(4):214-218.

12. Hilfiker-Kleiner D, Kaminski K, Podewski E, et al. A cathepsin D-cleaved 16 kDa form of prolactin mediates postpartum cardiomyopathy. *Cell.* 2007;128(3):589-600.

13. Patten IS, Rana S, Shahul S, et al. Cardiac angiogenic imbalance leads to peripartum cardiomyopathy. *Nature.* 2012;485(7398):333-338.

14. Halkein J, Tabruyn SP, Ricke-Hoch M, et al. MicroRNA-146a is a therapeutic target and biomarker for peripartum cardiomyopathy. *J Clin Invest.* 2013;123(5):2143-2154.

15. Bello N, Rendon ISH, Arany Z. The relationship between pre-eclampsia and peripartum cardiomyopathy: a systematic review and meta-analysis. *J Am Coll Cardiol.* 2013;62(18):1715-1723.

16. Russell RB, Petrini JR, Damus K, Mattison DR, Schwarz RH. The changing epidemiology of multiple births in the United States. *Obstet Gynecol.* 2003;101(1):129-135.

17. McNamara DM, Elkayam U, Alharethi R, et al. Clinical outcomes for peripartum cardiomyopathy in North America: results of the IPAC Study (Investigations of Pregnancy-Associated Cardiomyopathy). *J Am Coll Cardiol.* 2015;66(8):905-914.

18. Karaye KM, Sa'idu H, Balarabe SA, et al. Clinical features and outcomes of peripartum cardiomyopathy in Nigeria. *J Am Coll Cardiol.* 2020;76(20):2352-2364.

19. Haghikia A, Podewski E, Libhaber E, et al. Phenotyping and outcome on contemporary management in a German cohort of patients with peripartum cardiomyopathy. *Basic Res Cardiol.* 2013;108(4):366.

20. Demakis JG, Rahimtoola SH, Sutton GC, et al. Natural course of peripartum cardiomyopathy. *Circulation.* 1971;44(6):1053-1061.

21. van Spaendonck-Zwarts KY, van Tintelen JP, van Veldhuisen DJ, et al. Peripartum cardiomyopathy as a part of familial dilated cardiomyopathy. *Circulation.* 2010;121(20):2169-2175.

22. Morales A, Painter T, Li R, et al. Rare variant mutations in pregnancy-associated or peripartum cardiomyopathy. *Circulation.* 2010;121(20):2176-2182.

23. van Spaendonck-Zwarts KY, Posafalvi A, van den Berg MP, et al. Titin gene mutations are common in families with both peripartum cardiomyopathy and dilated cardiomyopathy. *Eur Heart J.* 2014;35(32):2165-2173.

24. Ware JS, Li J, Mazaika E, et al. Shared genetic predisposition in peripartum and dilated cardiomyopathies. *N Engl J Med.* 2016;374(3):233-241.

25. Goli R, Li J, Brandimarto J. Genetic and phenotypic landscape of peripartum cardiomyopathy. *Circulation.* 2021;143(19):1852-1862.

26. Elkayam U, Akhter MW, Singh H, et al. Pregnancy-associated cardiomyopathy: clinical characteristics and a comparison between early and late presentation. *Circulation.* 2005;111(16):2050-2055.

27. Goland S, Modi K, Bitar F, et al. Clinical profile and predictors of complications in peripartum cardiomyopathy. *J Card Fail.* 2009;15(8):645-650.

28. Tibazarwa K, Lee G, Mayosi B, Carrington M, Stewart S, Sliwa K. The 12-lead ECG in peripartum cardiomyopathy. *Cardiovasc J Afr.* 2012;23(6):322-329.

29. Honigberg M, Elkayam U, McNamara DM, Givertz M. Prognostic value of electrocardiographic findings in peripartum cardiomyopathy. *J Am Coll Cardiol.* 2018;71(11 Supplement):A705.

30. Ntusi NB, Chin A. Characterisation of peripartum cardiomyopathy by cardiac magnetic resonance imaging. *Eur Radiol.* 2009;19(6):1324-1325; author reply 1326-1327.

31. Briasoulis A, Mocanu M, Marinescu K, et al. Longitudinal systolic strain profiles and outcomes in peripartum cardiomyopathy. *Echocardiography.* 2016;33(9):1354-1360.

32. Sliwa K, Petrie MC, van der Meer P, et al. Clinical presentation, management, and 6-month outcomes in women with peripartum cardiomyopathy: an ESC EORP registry. *Eur Heart J.* 2020;41(39):3787-3797.

33. Goland S, Bitar F, Modi K, et al. Evaluation of the clinical relevance of baseline left ventricular ejection fraction as a predictor of recovery or persistence of severe dysfunction in women in the United States with peripartum cardiomyopathy. *J Card Fail.* 2011;17(5):426-430.

34. Rasmusson KD, Budge D, Alharethi R, et al. Long-term outcomes in patients with peripartum cardiomyopathy and no recovery of ventricular function. *J Cardiac Fail.* 2010;16(8, Supplement):S97.

35. Blauwet LA, Libhaber E, Forster O, et al. Predictors of outcome in 176 South African patients with peripartum cardiomyopathy. *Heart.* 2013;99(5):308-313.

36. Biteker M, Ilhan E, Biteker G, Duman D, Bozkurt B. Delayed recovery in peripartum cardiomyopathy: an indication for long-term follow-up and sustained therapy. *Eur J Heart Fail.* 2012;14(8):895-901.

37. Fett JD. Promoting full recovery and improved relapse-free prognosis in the diagnosis and treatment of peripartum cardiomyopathy. *J Am Coll Cardiol.* 2020;76(20):2365-2367.

38. Amos AM, Jaber WA, Russell SD. Improved outcomes in peripartum cardiomyopathy with contemporary. *Am Heart J.* 2006;152(3):509-513.

39. Sheppard R, Hsich E, Damp J, et al. GNB3 C825T polymorphism and myocardial recovery in peripartum cardiomyopathy: results of the Multicenter Investigations of Pregnancy-Associated Cardiomyopathy Study. *Circ Heart Fail.* 2016;9(3):e002683.

40. Goland S, Weinstein JM, Zalik A, et al. Angiogenic imbalance and residual myocardial injury in recovered peripartum cardiomyopathy patients. *Circ Heart Fail.* 2016;9(11).

41. Napporn AG, Kane A, Damorou JM, et al. Intraventricular thrombosis complicating peri-partum idiopathic myocardiopathy. *Ann Cardiol Angeiol (Paris).* 2000;49(5):309-314.

42. Agunanne E. Peripartum cardiomyopathy presenting with pulmonary embolism: an unusual case. *South Med J.* 2008;101(6):646-647.

43. Box LC, Hanak V, Arciniegas JG. Dual coronary emboli in peripartum cardiomyopathy. *Tex Heart Inst J.* 2004;31(4):442-444.

44. Ibebuogu UN, Thornton JW, Reed GL. An unusual case of peripartum cardiomyopathy manifesting with multiple thrombo-embolic phenomena. *Thromb J.* 2007;5:18.

45. Jha P, Jha S, Millane TA. Peripartum cardiomyopathy complicated by pulmonary embolism and pulmonary hypertension. *Eur J Obstet Gynecol Reprod Biol.* 2005;123(1):121-123.

46. Quinn B, Doyle B, McInerney J. Postnatal pre-cordial pain. Pulmonary embolism or peripartum cardiomyopathy. *Emerg Med J.* 2004;21(6): 746-747.

47. Shimamoto T, Marui A, Oda M, et al. A case of peripartum cardiomyopathy with recurrent left ventricular apical thrombus. *Circ J.* 2008;72(5):853-854.

48. Sliwa K, Blauwet L, Tibazarwa K, et al. Evaluation of bromocriptine in the treatment of acute severe peripartum cardiomyopathy: a proof-of-concept pilot study. *Circulation.* 2010;121(13):1465-1473.

49. Yaméogo NV, Kagambèga LJ, Seghda A, Owona A, Kaboré O. Bromocriptine in management of peripartum cardiomyopathy: a randomized study on 96 women in Burkina Faso. *J Cardiol Clin Res.* 2017;5(2):1098.

50. Hilfiker-Kleiner D, Haghikia A, Berliner D, et al. Bromocriptine for the treatment of peripartum cardiomyopathy: a multicentre randomized study. *Eur Heart J.* 2017;38(35):2671-2679.

51. Regitz-Zagrosek V, Roos-Hesselink JW, Bauersachs J, et al. 2018 ESC Guidelines for the management of cardiovascular diseases during pregnancy. *Eur Heart J.* 2018;39(34):3165-3241.

52. Koczo A, Marino A, Jeyabalan A, et al. Breastfeeding, cellular immune activation, and myocardial recovery in peripartum cardiomyopathy. *JACC: Basic Translati Sci.* 2019;4(3):291-300.

53. Ponikowski P, Voors AA, Anker SD, et al. 2016 ESC Guidelines for the diagnosis and treatment of acute and chronic heart failure: the Task Force for the diagnosis and treatment of acute and chronic heart failure of the European Society of Cardiology (ESC). Developed with the special contribution of the Heart Failure Association (HFA) of the ESC. *Eur J Heart Fail.* 2016;18(8):891-975.

54. Elkayam U, Schäfer A, Chieffo A, et al. Use of Impella heart pump for management of women with peripartum cardiogenic shock. *Clin Cardiol.* 2019;42(10):974-981.

55. Zimmerman H, Bose R, Smith R, Copeland JG. Treatment of peripartum cardiomyopathy with mechanical assist devices and cardiac transplantation. *Ann Thorac Surg.* 2010;89(4):1211-1217.

56. Zimmerman H, Coelho-Anderson R, Smith R, Nolan P, Copeland J. Bridge to recovery with a thoratec biventricular assist device for postpartum cardiomyopathy. *Asaio J.* 2010;56(5):479-480.

57. Emmert MY, Prêtre R, Ruschitzka F, Krähenmann F, Falk V, Wilhelm MJ. Peripartum cardiomyopathy with cardiogenic shock: recovery after prolactin inhibition and mechanical support. *Ann Thorac Surg.* 2011;91(1):274-276.

58. Park SH, Chin JY, Choi MS, Choi JH, Choi YJ, Jung KT. Extracorporeal membrane oxygenation saved a mother and her son from fulminant peripartum cardiomyopathy. *J Obstet Gynaecol Res.* 2014;40(7):1940-1943.

59. Bouabdallaoui N, Mastroianni C, Revelli L, Demondion P, Lebreton G. Predelivery extracorporeal membrane oxygenation in a life-threatening peripartum cardiomyopathy: save both mother and child. *Am J Emerg Med.* 2015;33(11):1713.e1711-e1712.

60. Gevaert S, Van Belleghem Y, Bouchez S, et al. Acute and critically ill peripartum cardiomyopathy and "bridge to" therapeutic options: a single center experience with intra-aortic balloon pump, extra corporeal membrane oxygenation and continuous-flow left ventricular assist devices. *Crit Care.* 2011;15(2):R93.

61. Oosterom L, de Jonge N, Kirkels J, Klöpping C, Lahpor J. Left ventricular assist device as a bridge to recovery in a young woman admitted with peripartum cardiomyopathy. *Neth Heart J.* 2008;16(12):426-428.

62. Loyaga-Rendon RY, Pamboukian SV, Tallaj JA, et al. Outcomes of patients with peripartum cardiomyopathy who received mechanical circulatory support. Data from the Interagency Registry for Mechanically Assisted Circulatory Support. *Circ Heart Fail.* 2014;7(2):300-309.

63. Genyk PA, Liu GS, Nattiv J, et al. Heart transplantation outcomes in adults with postpartum cardiomyopathy. *J Heart Lung Transplant.* 2020;39 (4, Supplement):S223-S224.

64. Elkayam U. Risk of subsequent pregnancy in women with a history of peripartum cardiomyopathy. *J Am Coll Cardiol.* 2014;64(15):1629-1636.

65. Elkayam U, Tummala PP, Rao K, et al. Maternal and fetal outcomes of subsequent pregnancies in women with peripartum cardiomyopathy. *N Engl J Med.* 2001;344(21):1567-1571.

66. Codsi E, Rose CH, Blauwet LA. Subsequent pregnancy outcomes in patients with peripartum cardiomyopathy. *Obstet Gynecol.* 2018;131(2):322-327.

67. Rosman L, Salmoirago-Blotcher E, Wuensch KL, Cahill J, Sears SF. Contraception and reproductive counseling in women with peripartum cardiomyopathy. *Contraception.* 2017;96(1):36-40.

68. Roos-Hesselink JW, Cornette J, Sliwa K, Pieper PG, Veldtman GR, Johnson MR. Contraception and cardiovascular disease. *Eur Heart J.* 2015;36(27):1728-1734, 1734a-1734b.

69. Ecker JL, Frigoletto FD, Jr. Cesarean delivery and the risk-benefit calculus. *N Engl J Med.* 2007;356(9):885-888.

70. Rosman L, Salmoirago-Blotcher E, Cahill J, Wuensch KL, Sears SF. Depression and health behaviors in women with peripartum cardiomyopathy. *Heart Lung.* 2017;46(5):363-368.

71. Dekker RL, Morton CH, Singleton P, Lyndon A. Women's experiences being diagnosed with peripartum cardiomyopathy: a qualitative study. *J Midwifery Womens Health.* 2016;61(4):467-473.

72. Koutrolou-Sotiropoulou P, Lima FV, Stergiopoulos K. Quality of life in survivors of peripartum cardiomyopathy. *Am J Cardiol.* 2016;118(2):258-263.

Mechanical Circulatory Support and Heart Transplantation in Severe Heart Failure

Adam D. DeVore, Michelle M. Kittleson, Carmelo A. Milano, Jignesh K. Patel, Joseph G. Rogers, and Jon A. Kobashigawa

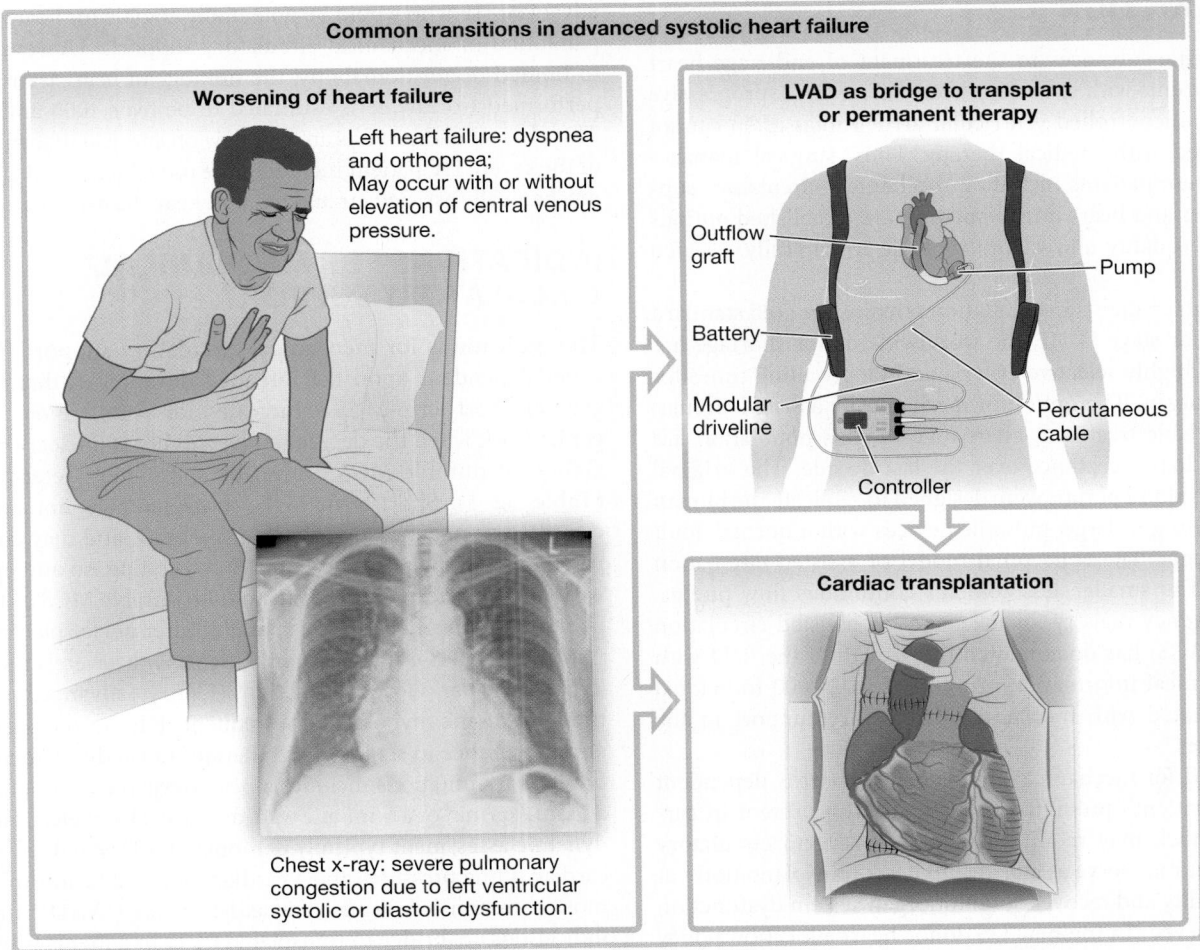

Common transitions in advanced systolic heart failure

Worsening of heart failure

Left heart failure: dyspnea and orthopnea;
May occur with or without elevation of central venous pressure.

Chest x-ray: severe pulmonary congestion due to left ventricular systolic or diastolic dysfunction.

LVAD as bridge to transplant or permanent therapy

Outflow graft
Pump
Battery
Modular driveline
Percutaneous cable
Controller

Cardiac transplantation

Chapter 52 Fuster and Hurst's Central Illustration. In many patients with systolic heart failure will ultimately experience worsening dyspnea, exertional intolerance, frequent hospitalizations, and end-organ dysfunction despite receiving guideline-directed medical therapy. As the disease progresses, a left ventricular assist device (LVAD) may be required to support the patient as a bridge to transplant or as permanent therapy. A subset of those with advanced heart failure will be candidates for cardiac transplantation.

CHAPTER SUMMARY

This chapter explores the current status of mechanically assisted circulation and cardiac transplantation. Since the first successful heart transplant in 1967, refinements to candidate and donor selection and management, manipulating the immune system, and surveillance for acute and chronic complications have been associated with progressively improved outcomes. Contemporary median survival following heart transplant is 12.5 years, extending to 14.8 years in those surviving the first year after the procedure. Similarly, mechanically assisted circulation using left ventricular assist devices (LVADs) has become a standard of care for patients failing medical therapies awaiting transplantation or in those ineligible for transplant (see Fuster and Hurst's Central Illustration). Newer devices are small, continuous flow pumps with enhanced hemocompatibility to minimize bleeding and thrombosis complications. The mean survival after LVAD implantation is nearly 5 years. Patient selection approaches for mechanical and biologic replacement, as well as the roles for palliative care and shared decision-making in supporting the patients with advanced heart failure and their families, are discussed.

INTRODUCTION

Despite major advances in the treatment of end-stage heart disease, patients with refractory heart failure (HF), progressive angina, or uncontrolled ventricular arrhythmias often cannot be stabilized with medical therapy. Thus, surgical management of these patients including mechanical circulatory support devices and heart transplantation are established options to improve quality and quantity of life in carefully selected patients.

Although cardiac transplantation remains the gold standard treatment for stage D HF, the worldwide donor shortage has resulted in highly selective criteria and long waiting times for a suitable organ. The option of mechanically assisted circulation as a viable treatment alternative for this population has gained gradual acceptance over the last decade. The original mechanical blood pumps were designed to replicate the human heart, resulting in large, pulsatile devices with a normal adult stroke volume. The conceptual model of assisted circulation has evolved to smaller, less complex continuous flow pumps. The interagency registry for mechanically assisted circulation (INTERMACS) has documented the growth of the field with detailed clinical information on more than 24,000 individual patients treated with mechanical circulatory support in the United States.[1]

The need for mechanical circulatory support is dependent upon the patient's presentation. Patients who present in cardiogenic shock may require acute or short-term circulatory support that may serve as a bridge to heart transplantation but only if stability and recovery of multiorgan system dysfunction can be achieved. In the new US donor heart allocation policy (October 2018), patients who have met criteria for cardiogenic shock and have stabilized with short-term devices have the highest priority for donor hearts. This change in policy appears to have led to the increased use of short-term mechanical circulatory support for these patients.[2] The criteria for heart transplantation have remained unchanged despite the donor heart allocation policy change.

Heart transplantation has progressed over 50 years since the first human heart transplant was performed in South Africa in December 1967.[4] Shortly thereafter, the first US adult heart transplant was performed by Shumway and colleagues at Stanford in January 1968. A flurry of transplant activity began at many centers, but initial enthusiasm waned as it became evident that postoperative survival was limited by a variety of complex medical problems, including opportunistic infections and graft rejection. Most major centers discontinued their heart transplant programs in the early 1970s. It was not until the introduction of cyclosporine-based immunosuppression in 1980 and the demonstration of the attendant improvement in survival rate that the procedure reemerged as a widely accepted therapy for end-stage heart disease.[4] By the 1990s, many tertiary care and academic centers had established programs for heart transplantation, and most medical care payers in the United States, including the federal government, provided coverage for such care. Currently, there are over 6 million patients in the United States with HF, with an estimated 300,000 with

advanced HF who would be potentially eligible for heart transplantation or mechanical circulatory support.[5] However, due to limited donor availability, the number of heart transplants performed worldwide is estimated to be over 4000 annually.[6] This chapter will serve as an overview on surgical management of the severe HF patient including the use of acute and chronic mechanically assisted circulation and heart transplantation.

INDICATIONS FOR MECHANICAL CIRCULATORY SUPPORT

The indications for mechanical circulatory support (MCS) differ dependent upon the intended duration of therapy. In general, short-term MCS is indicated for acute HF or cardiogenic shock when the degree of reversibility is unclear or suitability for durable MCS cannot be completely determined[7] (**Table 52–1**). Short-term MCS strategies may not provide complete circulatory support, limit mobility, and may confine patients to an intensive care unit (ICU) setting, so attempts to wean these devices, and/or transition to durable MCS or transplant, should begin as soon as possible after device placement.

Durable MCS is indicated for patients with severely reduced left ventricular ejection fraction (LVEF), advanced symptoms, systemic hypotension, frequent HF hospitalizations, and intolerance to standard HF therapy. Objective evidence of functional limitations includes a peak oxygen consumption of ≤14 mL/kg/min or a 6-minute walk distance <300 meters. Hemodynamic assessment typically demonstrates elevated left-sided cardiac filling pressures and a cardiac index <2 L/min/m². The most common left ventricular assist device (LVAD) implant indications are bridge to transplant (BTT) in patients listed for transplantation at high priority who are failing optimal medical therapies or as permanent cardiac replacement in patients currently ineligible for transplant (ie, destination therapy). The latter group have New York Heart Association (NYHA) class IIIb to IV functional limitations on maximally tolerated medical therapy, an LVEF <25%, and a peak oxygen consumption on cardiopulmonary exercise test of <14 mL/kg/min. In less stable patients, treatment with continuous infusion of inotropic medications for at least 14 days or need for short-term MCS for at least 7 days are also indications for durable LVAD therapy.

SPECIFIC DEVICE TYPES AND APPLICATIONS

Short-term MCS devices can be subdivided into percutaneously and peripherally inserted pumps versus those implanted centrally through a thoracic incision. A subset of short-term VADs are designed and applied uniquely for right heart support. Extracorporeal membrane oxygenation (ECMO) is another category of short-term MCS capable of circulatory support and gas exchange.

Percutaneous Short-Term Left Ventricular Assist Devices

The simplest and most commonly applied percutaneous MCS device is the intra-aortic balloon pump (IABP). This is

TABLE 52-1. Anticipated Duration of Support Based on Condition and Likelihood of Reversibility

Condition	Reversibility of Ventricular Dysfunction	Anticipated Duration of Support	Additional Comments
Acute MI with Shock	++	Days to Weeks	Examples: papillary muscle rupture, infarct-related VSD, etc.
Postcardiac Surgery Inability to Wean CPB	++	Days to Weeks	Severe ventricular dysfunction may have preceded the operation and did not recover with the procedure, or unexpected myocardial injury occurred during the procedure
Viral Myocarditis	+++	Weeks	Compared with chronic HF, patients often have normal ventricular diameters and a higher incidence of ventricular functional recovery
Procedure Support for Increased-Risk Patients Including Those with LV Dysfunction	++++	Hours	Increased-risk PCI, ventricular arrhythmia ablation, or catheter valve procedure
Post–Heart Transplant Graft Dysfunction	Early after Transplant ++++	Days	
	Late after Transplant ++++	Days	
RV Failure from Acute PE	++++	Days	
Ventricular Dysfunction from Drug Overdose or Electrolyte Disturbance	++++	Days	
Decompensated Chronic HF Support	+	Weeks	Can be utilized as a bridge to cardiac transplant

Abbreviations: CBP, cardiopulmonary bypass; HF, heart failure; LV, left ventricle; MI, myocardial infarction; PCI, percutaneous coronary intervention; PE, pulmonary embolism; RV, right ventricle; VSD, ventricular septal defect.

a catheter with a pressure transducer and an elongated balloon that is inflated during ventricular diastole and deflated during ventricular systole (**Fig. 52–1**). A lumen within the catheter delivers and removes helium gas from the balloon. IABPs are most commonly inserted percutaneously utilizing a Seldinger technique in a retrograde manner from the femoral artery into the descending aorta. Other approaches may be utilized in special circumstances: direct insertion into the ascending aorta with antegrade delivery into the descending aorta has been described in conditions of severe peripheral vascular disease or insertion into the axillary or subclavian artery enabling ambulation.[8] Axillary insertion may utilize cutdown and attachment of a graft to the axillary artery or percutaneous insertion. Complications from axillary insertion are generally similar to those encountered with femoral insertion. The device is inserted into the arterial system over a wire with fluoroscopy but intraoperative guidance with transesophageal echocardiography is also possible. Optimal balloon position is in the descending thoracic aorta, just distal to the ostium of the left subclavian artery. For adult patients, the balloon volume is typically 40 mL to 50 mL but there are smaller sizes for adult or pediatric patients.

Direct effects of counterpulsation include increased diastolic pressure, improved coronary and cerebral blood flow, and decreased afterload. Indirect benefits may include increased stroke volume (increased cardiac output), reduced LV end diastolic pressure and volume, and reduced wall stress. The effectiveness of IABP support is dependent on the presence of organized native heart rhythm and LV ejection. Relative contraindications to use of the IABP support include significant aortic valve insufficiency, severe atherosclerotic vascular disease between the femoral artery and the aortic arch, and rapid or irregular heart rhythm. Profound shock or cardiac arrest may also be considered relative contraindications to IABP support because this form provides only partial support for the circulation. Complications include arterial bleeding, limb ischemia, dissection, infection, gas embolus, and stroke.

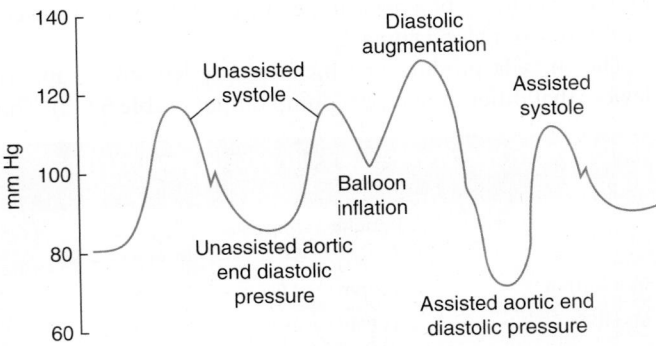

Figure 52–1. Optimal timing of inflation for IABP support. Timing of inflation for the IABP can be determined from the ECG or arterial pressure waveform. Optimal timing consists of initiation of inflation just after closure of the aortic valve and completion of deflation just prior to opening of the aortic valve during the next cardiac cycle. Therefore, the initiation of balloon inflation should occur at the dicrotic pressure notch on the arterial pressure tracing. In this manner, augmentation of the mid-diastolic pressure is achieved with reduction of the end diastolic pressure compared to the non-augmented cycle. Adapted with permission from Trost JC, Hillis LD. Intra-aortic balloon counterpulsation. *Am J Cardiol.* 2006 May 1;97(9):1391-1398.

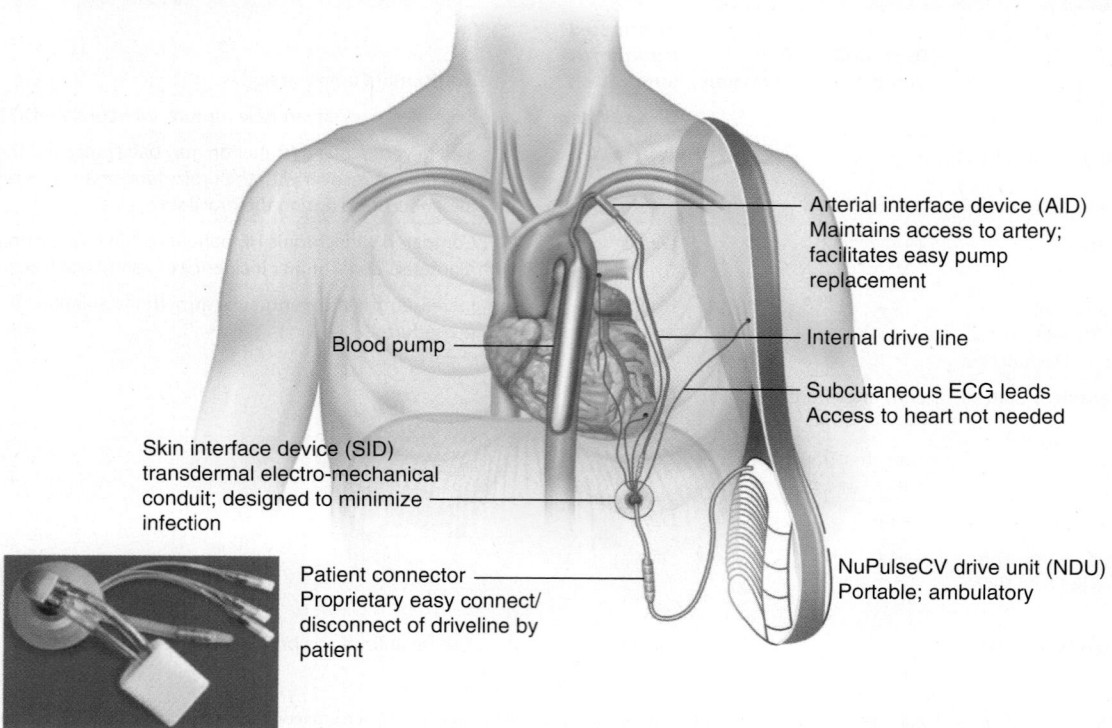

Figure 52–2. **Diagram of iVAS demonstrating components of this ambulatory intra-aortic balloon counterpulsation device.** Insertion is via the axillary artery and tracking utilizes ECG signal acquired from three internal leads that provide input to the skin interface device. Reproduced with permission from Nupulse Inc., Cary, NC.

Given the relatively low rates of adverse events, IABP support is commonly utilized, although randomized clinical trial data supporting its use in cardiogenic shock are lacking.[9] Weaning IABP support is achieved by decreasing the frequency of counterpulsation or reducing the degree of augmentation.

Newer devices are in clinical trials that are designed to provide longer-term counterpulsation. The Nupulse intravascular ventricular assist device (iVAS) (Nupulse, Cary NC) is a 50-mL balloon catheter pump that is inserted via the axillary artery and attached to a subcutaneous skin interface device, which acquires electrocardiographic information from three internal leads. The skin interface device is in turn coupled to an external driver that is portable (battery driven; **Fig. 52–2**). This device has been studied first in man and feasibility clinical trials, during which device modifications were made. Over 100 patients have now been supported with the longest support period being greater than 1 year.[10,11] The hemodynamic effects of iVAS support include a small increase in cardiac output and cardiac power with a small decrease in LV filling pressures. iVAS falls between short-term and durable MCS because some patients have been safely discharged to independent living with this device. The most common indication has been for chronic HF as a BTT. Limitations include inability to insert into small axillary arteries, inability to track irregular heart rhythms (eg, atrial fibrillation), and incomplete hemodynamic support. A planned pivotal trial will help to define indications for this experimental device.

The Impella Device

Impella (Abiomed Inc., Danvers, MA) is a catheter-mounted, axial flow VAD demonstrated to provide greater hemodynamic support relative to IABP. The catheter is inserted into the LV using an over-the-wire technique. The device draws blood from the LV and ejects into the aortic root. In addition to housing the electrical power cord, the catheter also contains a lumen for delivery of a heparin dextrose solution that protects the motor from blood contact.

The Impella product line includes five left-sided support devices that differ in maximal pump output (**Table 52–2**). The

TABLE 52–2. Specifications of Four Impella Products for LV Support

	Impella 2.5	Impella CP	Impella 5.0/LD
Max Output	2.5 lpm	4.0 lpm	5.0 lpm
Max RPM	51,000	46,000	33,000
Guiding Catheter Size	9Fr	9Fr	9Fr
Guide Wire Diameter (in)	.018	.018	.018
Motor Size	12Fr	14Fr	21/22Fr
Introducer Size	13Fr	14Fr	Dacron Graft, 10mm
Access	Perc. Femoral	Perc. Femoral	Surgical

Abbreviations: Fr, French; Lpm, liters per minute; Perc, percutaneous; RPM, rotations per minute.

PROTECT II trial randomized nearly 500 patients to either the Impella 2.5 or IABP during high-risk percutaneous coronary intervention (PCI).[12] There was no difference in major adverse events during the 30 days following the procedure despite the Impella-supported patients receiving more extensive coronary revascularization. The most common application of the Impella 2.5 device remains high-risk PCI, with great variability in rates of utilization between institutions.[13] Concerns over the magnitude of support with the 2.5 device led to the development of the CP device, which is also designed for percutaneous femoral insertion but provides greater output (greater LV unloading) (**Fig. 52–3**).

Another important clinical application of the Impella devices is acute myocardial infarction (MI) complicated by cardiogenic shock. While multiple studies have documented that the Impella CP achieves improved hemodynamics relative to IABP support alone, its impact on survival outcomes for acute MI shock patients has not been shown. The IMPRESS trial randomized patients with acute MI and cardiogenic shock, to support with IABP versus Impella CP. Twenty-four patients were randomized into each arm of the trial and all patients in both arms underwent PCI revascularization. Thirty-day and 6-month mortality were not different between the two groups; 6-month mortality was 50% in both groups.[14] Other registry (nonrandomized) studies have also failed to demonstrate a survival benefit to Impella versus IABP support in acute MI shock.[15] These studies raise the idea that earlier application of

MCS for this condition may be as important as the over magnitude of the hemodynamic support.

The Impella LD, 5.0, and most recently the 5.5 are intended for surgical insertion through a 10-mm Dacron vascular graft that is applied to the ascending aorta or axillary artery (Fig. 52–3). These devices are capable of 5 liters per minute of blood flow under ideal circumstances and may be utilized after cardiac surgery in the setting of inability to wean from cardiopulmonary bypass.[16] In addition, these devices have also been used to bridge patients with left HF to cardiac transplantation.

Impella device malposition may occur over time and requires careful assessment. The inlet is ideally positioned 3.5 cm below the aortic valve (this can be deeper for the 5.5 device that lacks the pigtail design) and the outlet cannula just above the valve. Impella features a position monitoring screen that simultaneously displays aortic and LV pressure and motor current tracings. Proper device positioning is confirmed by a normal aortic and LV pressure tracing and motor current phasic with the native cardiac cycle. Abnormal positioning results in changes in motor current and ventricular pressure tracing that can be used to diagnosis the problem. Echocardiographic or fluoroscopic imaging can also be used to confirm and guide positioning. Device weaning is accomplished by decreasing pump speeds while examining ventricular function on echocardiography and measuring hemodynamics.

Adverse events related to use of the Impella devices include arterial insertion site complications, ventricular perforation,

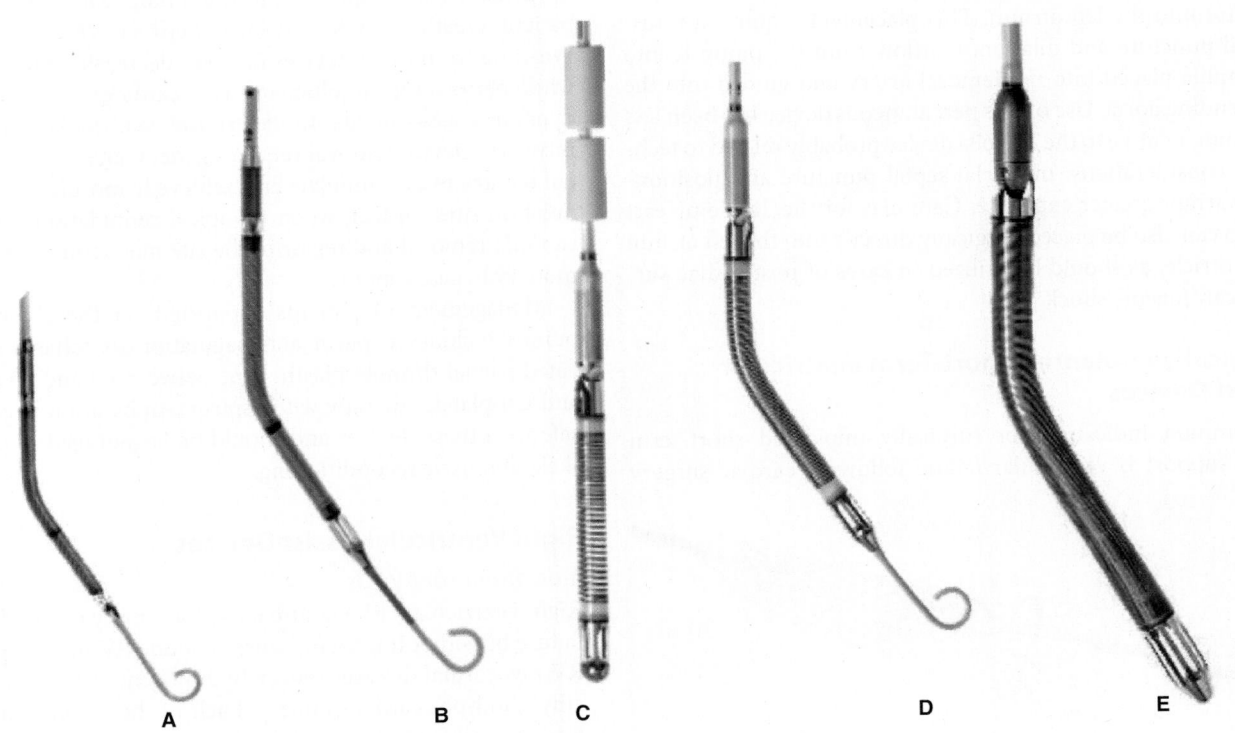

Figure 52–3. Impella products for LV support. Impella 2.5® (**A**) and Impella CP® (**B**) are designed for percutaneous femoral insertion. Impella LD® (**C**) employs direct aortic insertion. Impella 5.0® or Impella 5.5® can be inserted directly in the ascending aorta or wire guided from an axillary arterial site. Reproduced with permission from Abiomed Inc. Danvers, MA.

ventricular arrhythmias, mitral insufficiency related to the device impinging on the anterior mitral valve leaflet or chordal attachments, and hemolysis. In addition, patients with advanced LV failure may not receive adequate flow rates and remain in a low output state, particularly with the smaller devices (Fig. 52–3). The most recent Impella 5.5 design features higher flow rates at lower RPM settings, which may reduce the complication of hemolysis. Furthermore, insertion and fixation at the ascending aorta or axillary artery locations may reduce migration and malposition. The Impella 5.5 also lacks the pigtail design that may become entangled in the mitral apparatus.

The HeartMate PHP Device

HeartMate PHP (Abbott Inc., Chicago, IL) is another electrical axial flow pump mounted on a catheter (**Fig. 52–4**). The ongoing SHIELD II trial in the United States is randomizing patients undergoing high-risk PCI to receive either the HeartMate PHP or an Impella device, with the endpoint being freedom from major adverse events at 90 days. This device has many similarities to the Impella devices including insertion technique. After insertion, the inlet component expands to 24 Fr and the device is capable of 4 liters per minute of blood flow under ideal loading conditions. The adverse event profile for this device is expected to mimic the Impella devices.

TandemHeart™ Pump and Cannula System (LivaNova Inc., London, UK) is another percutaneous device for LV support. This extracorporeal centrifugal pump is attached by blood tubing to two percutaneously inserted cannulas. The left heart drainage cannula (ProtekSolo) is inserted from the femoral vein into the right atrium, then across the intra-atrial septum into the left atrium. This placement requires a transseptal puncture and dilation. Outflow from the pump is into a cannula placed into the femoral artery and guided into the descending aorta. Use of this percutaneous device has been less common relative to the Impella device probably related to technical considerations; the atrial septal puncture and positioning warrant greater expertise. Cannulas for the TandemHeart pump can also be placed surgically directly into the left atrium or ventricle, as should be utilized in cases of postcardiac surgery cardiogenic shock.

Surgically Implanted Short-Term Ventricular Assist Devices

A common indication for surgically implanted short-term VAD support is ventricular failure following cardiac surgery

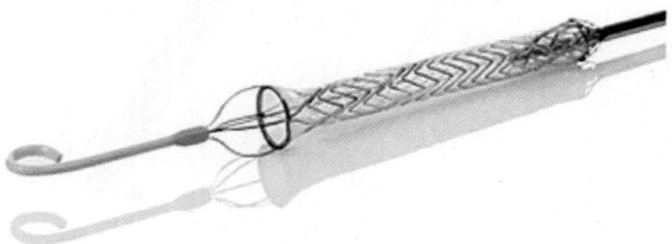

Figure 52–4. The HeartMate PHP device is inserted through a 14 Fr femoral sheath and is positioned across the aortic valve in the LV. After insertion, the cannula inlet area expands to 24 Fr.

including primary graft failure after heart transplant. These devices may also be used for conditions such as viral myocarditis where there is a high likelihood for ventricular recovery and in cases of decompensated chronic HF when suitability for durable LVAD is unclear. Historically, these devices were extracorporeal, pulsatile devices based in part on the theory that pulsatile blood flow was advantageous for end-organ recovery from shock state. This theory has not been supported by clinical observation, and currently the majority of surgically placed short-term VADs are centrifugal flow devices that are set a fixed speed and provide minimal pulsatility. These devices have gained popularity in part due to their simplicity and reliability. Furthermore, the absence of a pump diastole may reduce thrombosis risk for centrifugal versus pulsatile devices.

Centrifugal Extracorporeal Blood Pumps

Two examples of this type of device are the CentriMag (Abbott Inc., Chicago, IL) and the Rotaflow pumps (Maquet Inc., Wayne, NJ). These rotary flow systems provide right heart and/or left heart support and utilize surgically attached cannulas tunneled out of chest onto the upper abdomen. Pump speed can be altered to change output and ventricular unloading and is typically higher for left-sided than right-sided support. Since there is no "pump diastole," pump thrombus is uncommon in the setting of adult pump flows (3–6 L/min). Device blood flow is measured with an ultrasonic flow probe attached to the blood tubing that provides reliable measurement. Total systemic blood flow consists of that provided by the device plus residual flow ejected from the native ventricle. If required, an oxygenator can be spliced into the tubing leading back to the patient, creating a hybrid strategy between VAD and ECMO. Weaning from these devices involves decreasing pump speeds while performing simultaneous echocardiography and hemodynamics assessments to determine ventricular functional recovery. Device removal requires general anesthesia and sternal reentry to de-cannulate and achieve hemostasis at the cannulation sites. In fact, when LV apical cannulation is utilized, cannula removal and repair of the site may require cardiopulmonary bypass support.

Management of patients supported on these centrifugal pumps includes heparin anticoagulation to achieve an activated partial thromboplastin time between 60 and 80 seconds and antiplatelet therapy with aspirin. Ambulation is generally safe with these devices and should be encouraged to promote skeletal muscle reconditioning.

Right Ventricular Assist Devices

Indications for RVADs

Right ventricular (RV) failure most commonly results from LV failure but other important causes include RV infarct, primary RV myocardial diseases (eg, arrhythmogenic RV cardiomyopathy), and postcardiac surgery. Each of these conditions may lead to need for isolated RV mechanical support.

Extracorporeal RVADs

The extracorporeal centrifugal pumps described for short-term LV support can also be surgically implanted for RV support.

Standard cannulas employed in cardiac surgery can be used to cannulate the right atrium and the main pulmonary artery. Potential adverse events include bleeding and device thrombosis that may cause pulmonary embolism. Other pulmonary complications include development of edema and hemoptysis. These events can result from supraphysiologic pulmonary artery pressures or flows, and emphasize the need for caution when increasing the pump speeds particularly when LV performance is not normal. Unlike the percutaneous devices for RV support, the surgically placed devices typically require reopening of a thoracic incision for removal.

Percutaneous RVADs

Recently, percutaneous devices have become available that provide RV mechanical support. An example is the Impella RP (Abiomed, Inc., Danvers, MA) (**Fig. 52–5**). Like the other Impella devices, the right-sided device is an axial flow, electrically driven pump. It is placed through a 23 Fr sheath inserted in the right femoral vein and guided over an 0.025-inch (0.6-mm) wire into the right heart. The inlet is positioned at the junction between the right atrium and the inferior vena cava with the device outlet positioned in the main pulmonary artery. This device was studied clinically in the Recover Right Trial, a single-arm study that enrolled patients with RV failure following LVAD implantation, acute RV infarct, or postcardiac surgery.[17] Patients supported with the Impella RP demonstrated a significantly reduced central venous pressure, increased cardiac output, and reduction in intravenous inotropic or vasopressor support. The primary endpoint was survival to 30 days, hospital discharge, or transition to a durable RVAD; 73% of the patients supported with the Impella RP achieved the primary endpoint compared to a predetermined performance measure of 50%. Adverse events experienced in the trial included device

malposition, hemolysis, and bleeding either at the insertion site or related to lung injury.

Another device utilized for percutaneous RV mechanical support is the TandemHeart™ Centrifugal Pump System and ProtekDuo cannula (LivaNova Inc., London, UK). The Protekduo cannula is a two-lumen catheter that is positioned to draw blood from the right atrium and deliver it to the main pulmonary artery (Fig. 52–5). The catheter interfaces with a Centrifugal TandemHeart" Blood Pump. An oxygenator can be inserted to provide gas exchange creating a venovenous ECMO circuit. One potential advantage of this device is the ability for patients to ambulate (relative to the Impella RP). Potential adverse events include hemolysis, bleeding complications, and inadequate blood flows due to either the cannula size or malposition.

Extracorporeal Membrane Oxygenation

ECMO is another temporary MCS strategy capable of supporting the cardiovascular and respiratory systems. Venovenous (VV) ECMO drains and oxygenates venous blood prior to returning it to the venous system and is primarily utilized for severe pulmonary insufficiency and impaired gas exchange. Veno-arterial (VA) ECMO consists of a circuit in which blood is drawn from the venous circulation, oxygenated, and returned to the arterial system. VA ECMO has been adopted for management of cardiogenic shock and its utilization in the United States is increasing.[13]

VA ECMO deployment requires venous and arterial access and systemic anticoagulation, usually with heparin. There are many potential components to a VA ECMO circuit but most commonly venous blood is drawn out of the body via a cannula into a centrifugal pump and then delivered out of the pump through a membrane oxygenator into an arterial cannula. A

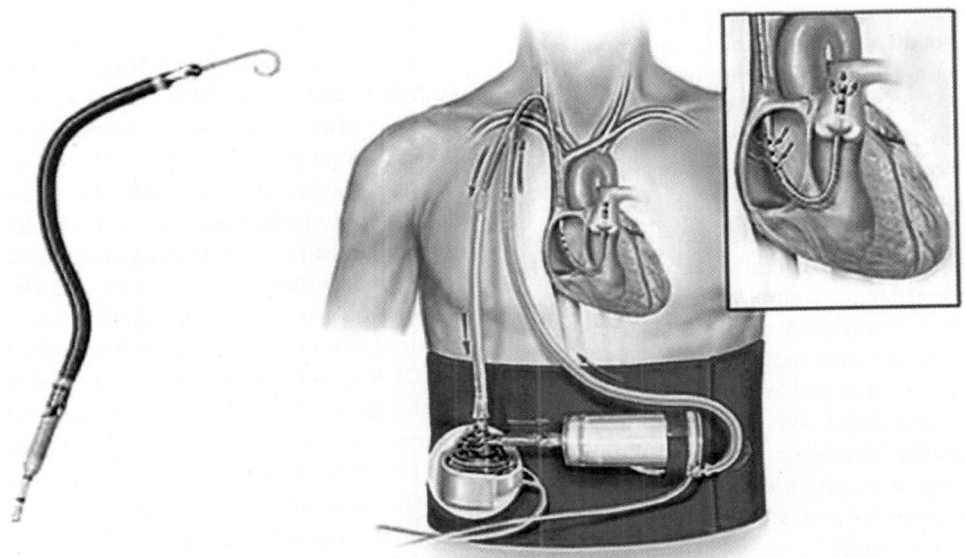

Figure 52–5. Percutaneous devices designed for RV support. The left panel is the Impella RP device. The outlet portion of the device located at the pigtail portion is delivered above the pulmonary valve. The right panel is the PROTEK™ Duo Cannula consisting of an outer proximal lumen that is positioned at the right atrium and an inner distal lumen positioned in the main pulmonary artery. The two independent lumens are attached via blood.

flow probe is attached to the circuit to measure flow and bubble detector locking mechanisms is placed on the circuit as a safeguard against air being introduced into the arterial system.

VA ECMO for management of cardiogenic shock has a number of advantages. First, hospital systems have developed teams for emergency ECMO deployment. While VA ECMO can be established within an operating room or catheterization lab, emergency placement and initiation can also take place in ICU settings, in the emergency department, and in patients experiencing cardiac arrest, undergoing cardiopulmonary resuscitation. VA ECMO provides RV and LV replacement as well as gas exchange support. Therefore, VA ECMO is particularly useful in the setting of profound biventricular dysfunction associated with pulmonary edema or other lung injuries. It has become the most common form of MCS for postcardiac surgery shock and failure to wean from CPB. In fact, existing cannulas used for CPB may be detached from the CPB circuit and attached to an ECMO circuit. A final advantage of this technology is that newer circuits have been miniaturized and are portable. CARDIOHELP (Maquet, Inc., Wayne, NJ) is a highly condensed circuit and allows greater patient mobility within a hospital but also facilitates hospital-to-hospital transfers.

Adverse events associated with VA ECMO are related to the cannulation and artificial blood circuit as well as to the underlying shock state that prompted treatment. Peripheral arterial complications associated with VA ECMO include bleeding, arterial obstruction, and distal extremity ischemia. When femoral arterial cannulation is utilized, ipsilateral lower extremity perfusion must be monitored. Insertion of a small antegrade limb perfusion catheter or surgical cutdown and graft arterial cannulation enables antegrade lower extremity perfusion. Central aortic cannulation for VA ECMO is appropriate when the patient has had recent heart surgery and a previous incision can be reopened to place the arterial aortic cannula. In other instances, cannulas can be inserted into the aorta and right atrium through a small right anterior thoracotomy.

VA ECMO does not directly unload the LV and blood return from an incompetent aortic valve or from pulmonary venous system may cause LV distention and hydrostatic pulmonary circulatory injury. PA pressure monitoring and echocardiography are tools which help define this problem. Placement of an LV vent via the apex or right superior pulmonary vein with return of blood to the ECMO circuit can prevent this complication. For patients who are peripherally cannulated, another common LV venting strategy is employment of an Impella device with VA ECMO. The Impella device is placed on a low setting and serves to decompress the LV while the majority of the systemic blood flow is provided by the ECMO circuit.

ECMO support is associated with hemolysis, platelet activation, and coagulopathy. Hemolysis related to blood contact with the ECMO tubing is usually not clinically significant as long as appropriate cannulas and pump speeds are utilized. Thrombocytopenia may result from platelet consumption or clumping trigger by the foreign surfaces. Exposure of the blood to the artificial surfaces also may trigger inflammatory responses manifested as fever, leukocytosis, or peripheral arterial vasodilation requiring vasopressors.

Durable Circulatory Support Devices

Contemporary durable LVADs have similar conceptual designs. Access to the circulation is obtained via an inflow cannula inserted in the LV apex. The pump housing contains a rotor that draws blood from the LV and delivers it to the ascending aorta via an outflow graft. Devices receive power via a driveline tunneled subcutaneously across the anterior abdomen that attaches to a controller that drives the pump and collects information on device performance. The driver is powered by either battery or alternating current (AC) electric current. Early durable LVADs utilized an axial flow configuration in which the impeller was in line with the direction of blood flow (eg, HeartMate II LVAD, Abbott Inc., Chicago, IL). Contemporary LVADs utilize a centrifugal flow design in which the direction of the blood is perpendicular to the rotor (eg, HeartWare HVAD Medtronic, Minneapolis, MN, and HeartMate 3 LVAD, Abbott Inc., Chicago, IL).

The HeartWare HVAD is implanted in the pericardial space and the rotor is suspended magnetically and on a blood bearing, preventing contact with the interior surface of the pump housing. The HVAD was approval in the United States for both BTT and destination therapy indications. The BTT indication was based on a 140-patient trial that compared outcomes for patients receiving an HVAD to a cohort of patients in INTERMACS that received an FDA-approved LVAD.[18] The outcomes of patients receiving an HVAD were similar to the INTERMACS cohort for the primary endpoint of survival to 180 days on the originally implanted pump, transplantation, or explantation due to myocardial recovery. The destination therapy indication was based on the ENDURANCE trial, a multicenter, randomized, noninferiority trial that compared HVAD to HeartMate II in 446 patients who were ineligible for transplant.[19] The primary endpoint was survival to 24 months on the originally implanted device without a disabling stroke (measured 6 months after any stroke), transplantation, or explantation for LV recovery. The two groups had similar outcomes for the primary endpoint.[13] Quality of life and functional outcomes were also similar between devices. Adverse event analysis demonstrated a higher rate of stroke with HVAD relative to HeartMate II. Secondary analysis demonstrated that mean arterial blood pressure >90 mm Hg was a risk factor for stroke as were aspirin dosing and international normalized ratio.[20] In a follow-up study, the ENDURANCE Supplemental Trial included a blood pressure protocol of frequent monitoring and mean arterial blood pressure targets of ≤85 mm Hg.[21] Patients following the protocol in the ENDURANCE Supplemental Trial had a reduced risk of stroke compared with the HVAD cohort of the ENDURANCE trial. In June, 2021, Medtronic announced discontinuation of HVAD manufacturing and implantation citing excessive numbers of adverse events associated with the potential for serious health consequences for patients.

The HeartMate 3 LVAD is also implanted in the pericardial space and is fully magnetically levitated. In contrast to the HVAD and HeartMate II, the HeartMate 3 has wide gaps for blood flow through the pump, friction-free movement without bearings, and intrinsic pulsatility to reduce shear stress and stasis of blood.[22] In the MOMENTUM 3 trial, patients were randomized to either the HeartMate 3 or HeartMate II, either as a BTT or as destination therapy.[23] Over 2 years of follow-up, the HeartMate 3 was superior to the HeartMate II with respect to survival free of disabling stroke or reoperation to replace or remove a malfunctioning LVAD. The HeartMate 3 also had a lower incidence of either ischemic or hemorrhagic strokes of any severity and fewer bleeding events, including gastrointestinal bleeding. Mucosal bleeding, including gastrointestinal bleeding (25% of patients with HeartMate 3 vs 31% with HeartMate II; relative risk ratio 0.64; 95% confidence interval 0.54–0.75; *P* <0.001) remained common, however. Optimal antithrombotic regimens have not been well-studied in LVADs and will be compared in the currently enrolling ARIES HeartMate 3 randomized controlled trial of vitamin K antagonist plus aspirin 100 mg versus vitamin K antagonist plus placebo.[24] There was no significant different between the HeartMate 3 and HeartMate II LVADs in rates of all-cause mortality or major infections.[23]

SURGICAL TECHNIQUE AND CONSIDERATIONS

The majority of durable LVAD implants use a sternotomy approach, which is the most common thoracic incision for cardiac surgery. However, a sternal sparing approach has been more recently described for the HVAD and HeartMate 3. The sternal sparing approach utilizes a left anterior thoracotomy to expose the LV apex and attach the apical sewing ring; a second incision is required to attach the outflow graft to the ascending aorta, usually either a right anterior thoracotomy or an upper partial sternotomy (**Fig. 52–6**). McGee et al. reported a cohort of 144 patients who underwent implantation via a sternal sparing approach and compared these cases to historical control patients implanted via sternotomy.[24] The primary composite endpoint was survival to 6 months free of stroke or need for device replacement and 88% of the sternal sparing cohort achieved the primary end point versus 78% for the historical sternotomy approach. This report and others have increased enthusiasm for implant techniques which avoid sternotomy. Additional benefits to the nonsternotomy approach may include reduced operative blood loss; however, others have reported greater postoperative pain with the thoracotomy approach.

After the thoracic incision is performed but before heparinization for cardiopulmonary bypass, the tract for the power cord is established with a tunneling device. Most commonly, the cord exits the body either on the right upper abdomen or on the left upper abdomen. Counterincisions may be employed to lengthen the course of the power cord. Too low an exit may interfere with the belt line. The cord typically contains a

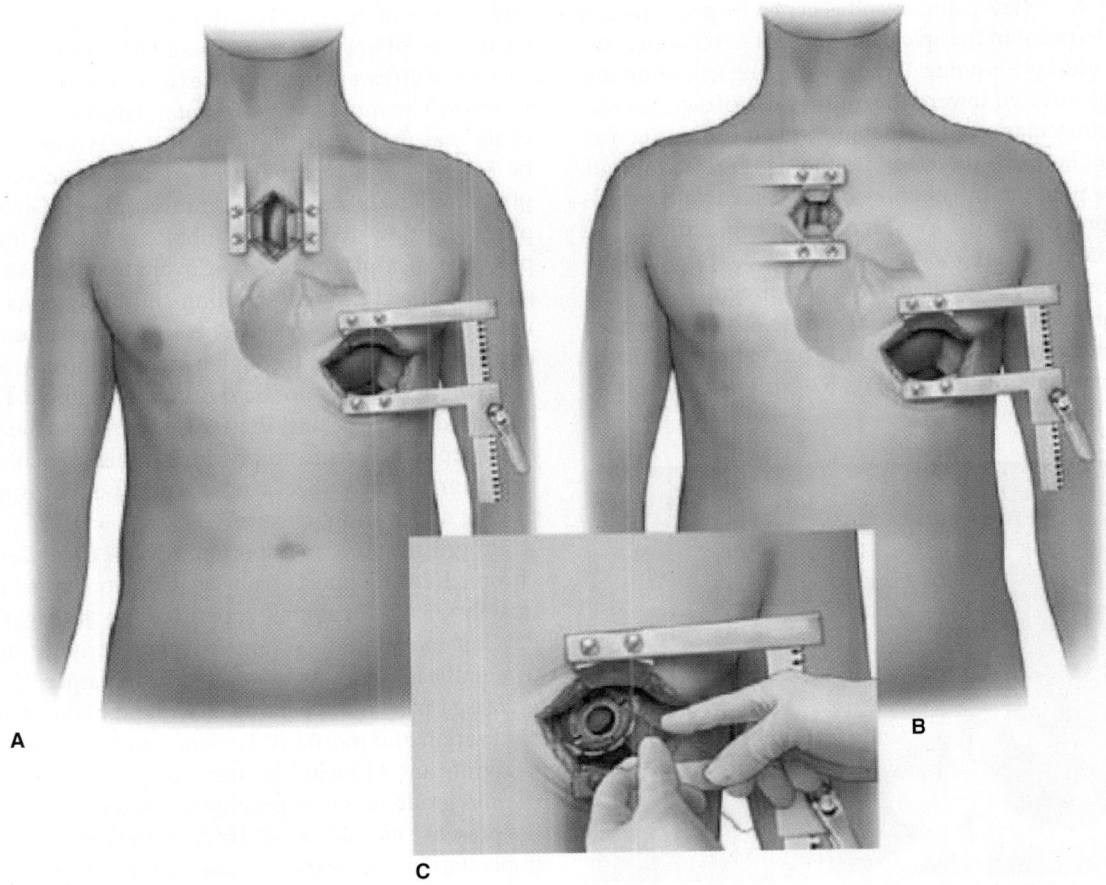

Figure 52–6. Nonsternotomy approaches utilized for implantation of centrifugal durable LVAD. (C) shows application of sewing cuff to the LV apex via a small left anterior thoracotomy. **(A)** and **(B)** show second thoracic incision consisting of either upper partial sternotomy **(A)** or right anterior thoracotomy **(B)** utilized for application of the outflow graft to the ascending aorta. Reproduced with permission from McGee E Jr, Danter M, Strueber M, et al. Evaluation of a lateral thoracotomy implant approach for a centrifugal-flow left ventricular assist device: The LATERAL clinical trial. *J Heart Lung Transplant.* 2019 Apr;38(4):344-351.

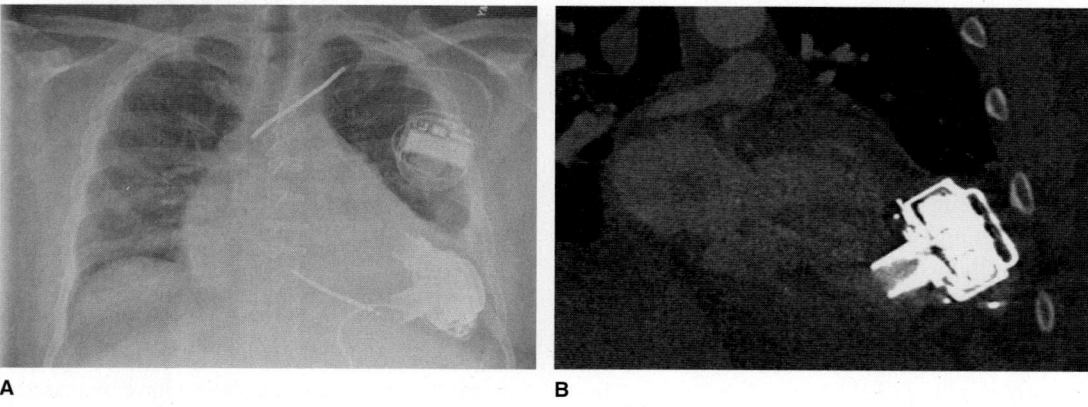

A   **B**

Figure 52–7. Chest x-ray (**A**) and CT scan (**B**) demonstrating malposition of HeartMate 3 apical cannula; anterior sewing cuff placement results in cannula directed into the posterior LV wall and away from the mitral valve inlet.

segment of velour (designed for tissue ingrowth), which should be entirely buried within the chest or abdominal wall; the exit point on the cord should be just distal to the end of the velour.

There are two attachments of the LVAD to the heart: the first is the attachment of the sewing ring to the LV apex and the second is the attachment of the outflow graft to the ascending aorta. Generally, these steps are accomplished while the patient is supported with cardiopulmonary bypass. The apical sewing ring supports the inflow cannula and is generally positioned at the apex just leftward of the apical left anterior descending coronary artery. Ideal positioning of the sewing ring will result in a cannula that is directed toward the mitral valve orifice, parallel to the interventricular septum. Inappropriate positioning may lead to a cannula that is directed into the septum, lateral wall, or posterior wall of the LV and may be associated with suboptimal decompression of the LV (**Fig. 52–7**). The outflow graft is most commonly sutured in an end-to-side configuration to the midportion of the ascending aorta; attachment of the graft to the right lateral aspect of the aorta helps to displace the graft away from the sternal closure, making sternal reentry safer, versus a retrosternal positioning (**Fig. 52–8**). The graft should

meet the aorta at a 30- to 45-degree angle to reduce turbulence in the ascending aorta. Too low a positioning or a less acute angle has been associated with increased turbulence in the root and more rapid progression of aortic valve insufficiency.

In addition to the two attachments to the heart, LVAD implantation may require associated procedures to optimize LVAD support. There are at least three other considerations for concurrent cardiac surgical procedures: (1) assessment for and closure of atrial or ventricular septal defects, (2) surgical correction of aortic insufficiency (AI), and (3) surgical correction of atrioventricular valve (ie, mitral or tricuspid) insufficiency. The most common septal defect is a patent foramen ovale that may occur in up to 20% of patients. This should be assessed with preoperative transthoracic echocardiography as well as intraoperative transesophageal echocardiography; color flow doppler and bubble studies are indicated. The presence of a patent foramen ovale may be associated with significant right to left shunting and hypoxemia after LVAD unloading of the left heart. Therefore, such shunts are generally surgically closed through a right atriotomy. Small patent foramen ovales may not be significant and post-LVAD catheter-based device occlusion has also been described. Iatrogenic atrial septal defects from previous catheter ablations or other procedures that utilize a transseptal puncture may also be present and warrant closure.

Progressive AI is an important adverse event associated with chronic LVAD support. Truby et al. demonstrated that approximately 25% of patients supported on rotary flow LVADs develop moderate-to-severe AI.[25] Furthermore, the presence of significant AI was associated with larger LV diameters, increased natriuretic peptide levels, and higher rates of rehospitalization and mortality. Factors associated with progression to significant AI included older age, female sex, and presence of mild grade of AI on preimplant studies. For these reasons, the presence of mild or greater AI at the time of durable LVAD implantation may warrant a concurrent surgical procedure to reduce or prevent AI progression. Bioprosthetic aortic valve replacement or central aortic valve oversewing are the two most common concurrent strategies to address progression of AI (**Fig. 52–9**).

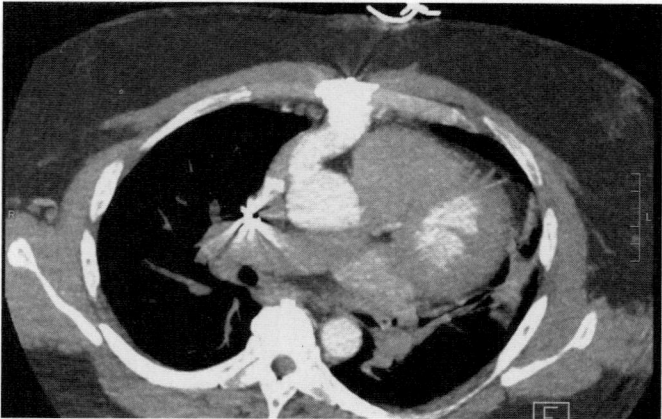

Figure 52–8. Chest CT scan demonstrating malposition of the LVAD outflow graft; the outflow graft is positioned anteriorly and immediate retrosternal. Redo sternotomy for LVAD replacement or transplant is difficult and associated with a high incidence of graft disruption.

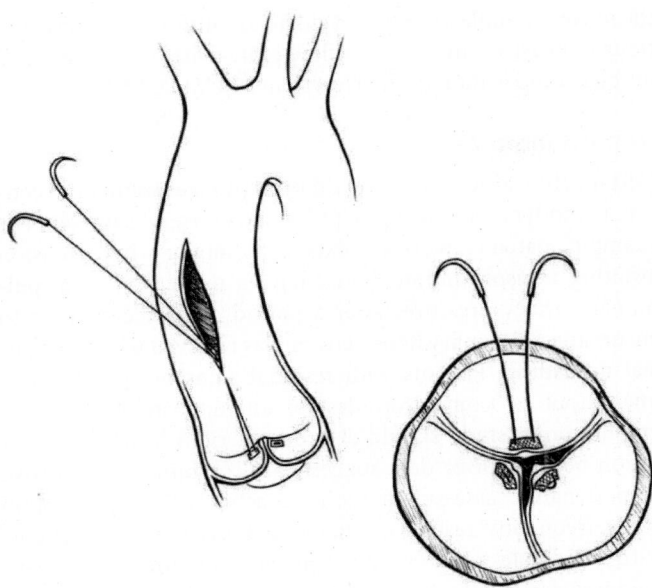

Figure 52–9. Technique for surgical coaptation of the aortic valve cusps to eliminate aortic insufficiency. Pledgeted sutures are applied to approximate the fibrous nodules of Arantius. Reproduced with permission from Park SJ, Liao KK, Segurola R, et al. Management of aortic insufficiency in patients with left ventricular assist devices: a simple coaptation stitch method (Park's stitch). *J Thorac Cardiovasc Surg.* 2004 Jan;127(1):264-266.

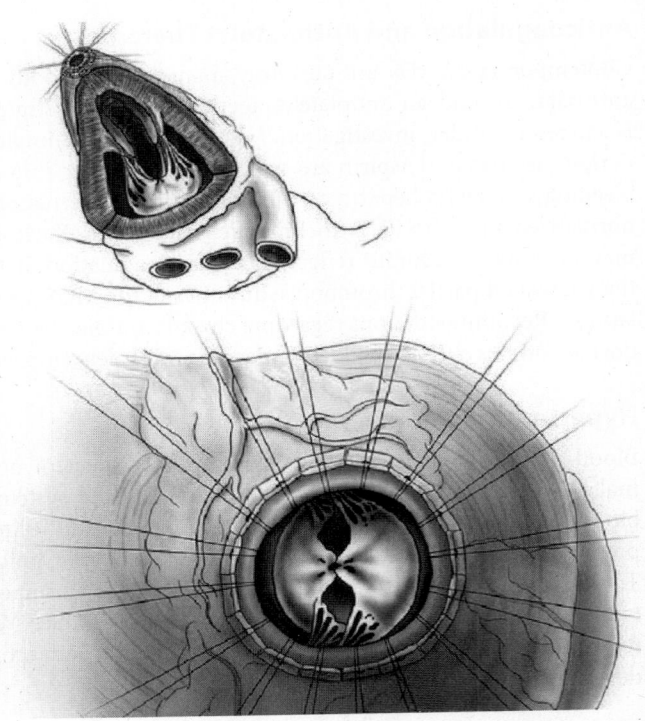

Figure 52–10. Sutures placed in LV apex for attachment of LVAD apical sewing cuff provide exposure to the mitral valve and performance of edge-to-edge repair of functional mitral insufficiency. Reproduced with permission from Russo MJ, Merlo A, Johnson EM, et al. Transapical approach for mitral valve repair during insertion of a left ventricular assist device. *Scientific World Journal.* 2013 Jun 26;2013:925310.

Advanced HF patients who present for LVAD implantation commonly have significant mitral valve regurgitation (MR) and tricuspid valve regurgitation (TR). Generally, the etiology of the MR and TR is secondary to changes in ventricular geometry. As the ventricles dilate, annuli of the atrioventricular valves are stretched or dilated; furthermore, chordal attachments can be apically displaced leading to restriction of the leaflets and central regurgitation. Reverse remodeling after LVAD unloading can lead to reduction of this regurgitation. Some patients, however, fail to resolve MR or TR following LVAD unloading and may experience worse clinical outcomes compared with patients without MR and/or TR.[26] Therefore, a variety of concurrent surgical approaches have been described to reduce or eliminate MR or TR at the time of implantation. The goal of these additional procedures is to reduce right HF, which is an important adverse event following LVAD support. The most common procedure is annuloplasty ring repair of the tricuspid valve, performed via a right atriotomy. Edge-to-edge repair of the mitral valve via the apical cannulation site has also been described as a strategy to address MR (**Fig. 52–10**).[27] Unfortunately, there are no randomized studies that provide guidance on when these procedures are beneficial, and concurrent application with LVAD implantation is often center specific.

Sternotomy closure after LVAD implantation may have detrimental effect on right heart function manifested as elevated central venous pressures or reduced LVAD output. Therefore, some cases may benefit from delay in sternal closure after a period of diuresis and correction of coagulopathy. Final closure may employ a GORE-TEX membrane (WL Gore and Associates, Inc.) or other barrier materials that facilitate redo sternotomy for future transplant, by preventing adhesion formation.

DEVICE MANAGEMENT

Measuring Blood Pressure

The unique physiology of continuous flow LVADs poses interesting challenges in seemingly simple medical tasks such as measuring blood pressure or obtaining peripheral pulse oximetry, both dependent on detection of a peripheral pulse. Use of a Doppler and a peripheral blood pressure cuff is the most effective means to measure blood pressure. When compared to an automated blood pressure, palpation, and auscultation, Doppler was more highly correlated with the blood pressure obtained simultaneously from direct measurement with an arterial catheter.[28] The narrow pulse pressure observed with continuous flow LVADs minimizes the distinction between systolic and diastolic pressure often making them imperceptible. If the peripheral pulse is not detectable, the first sound (ie, the opening sound) detected with a Doppler can be considered the mean arterial pressure. Detection of a palpable pulse should prompt consideration for device malfunction or insufficient pump speed. It is common for the pulse oximeter to provide inaccurate data. The pulse oximeter may not display a clinically accurate value or may read a value that is lower than obtained by blood gas analysis.

Anticoagulation and Antiplatelet Therapies

Contemporary LVADs are currently managed with both an anticoagulant and an antiplatelet agent though that strategy is currently under investigation.[29] During the peri-implant period, heparin and aspirin are typically started after surgical bleeding slows with heparin continuing until the international normalized ratio (INR) is therapeutic. Anti-factor Xa levels may be a more accurate reflection of anticoagulation status than activated partial thromboplastin times in the MCS population.[30] Recommendations regarding chronic antiplatelet drug dosing and target INR are device-specific and largely empiric.

Hypertension Management

Blood pressure management is an important aspect of normal LVAD function and postimplant care. Elevated systemic blood pressure reduces cardiac output and increases LV filling pressures in continuous flow LVADs. The HeartWare Clinical Trials Program identified systemic hypertension as an important contributor to both ischemic and hemorrhagic stroke.[20] To date, it is less clear that the same relationship exists with other devices.

Setting Device Speed

Regardless of the specific LVAD device implanted, there are several general goals of mechanically assisted circulation including reduction of HF symptoms, ventricular unloading, reduction of LV diameter and MR, and maintenance of the interventricular septum in a neutral position. Excessive device speeds with excessive lowering of the LV end diastolic pressure will cause septal shift toward the lateral wall of the LV resulting in secondary TR as well as RV enlargement and dysfunction.

Imaging

The only adjustment that a clinician can make with current durable LVADs is speed alteration, and transthoracic echocardiography plays a key role in optimizing this parameter.[31] Prior to discharge, many programs assess the adequacy of LVAD support using a hemodynamic or echocardiographic ramp study. This technique involves reducing the LVAD speed to a level nominal support and then incrementally increasing the speed with simultaneous assessment of the patient symptoms, ventricular size, septal position, mitral regurgitation, and aortic valve opening. The ramp study has been shown to be beneficial in both setting the most optimal speed and assessing for HeartMate II malfunction.[32] In the case in which speed increases do not reduce ventricular size, consideration should be given to obstruction of flow into or out of the pump.

Other imaging techniques are intermittently used to assess the positioning of the LVAD inflow cannula. Routine chest x-ray is useful to serially evaluate the angulation of the inflow cannula. The cannula should be positioned in the long axis of the LV and directed at the mitral valve. Positioning toward the ventricular septum or lateral wall may lead to suboptimal device function. Gated computed tomography (CT) angiography is another technique that is useful to determine positioning of the inflow cannula as well as evaluate for outflow graft obstructions or twist-occlusions. Outflow graft twist occlusions are a unique complication of the HeartMate 3 LVAD.[33,34]

Hemodynamics

Certain clinical scenarios should prompt measurement of central hemodynamics using a pulmonary artery catheter. For example, patients with secondary pulmonary hypertension awaiting transplantation should have a measurement of pulmonary artery pressures after a period of device support to ensure the pulmonary hypertension has resolved with mechanical unloading. Patients with residual signs or symptoms of low-output or congestion despite attempts an echocardiographic ramp study should also have a right heart catheterization because prior data suggest that combining an invasive hemodynamic assessment with an echocardiographic ramp study frequently results in changing LVAD speed.[35] Patients with moderate-to-severe AI may also require an invasive hemodynamic evaluation to determine LV filling pressures.

COMMON COMPLICATIONS

The most recent INTERMACS report demonstrated that major adverse events remain common within the first year after LVAD implantation.[1] Common complications include bleeding, infections, arrhythmia, stroke, and death.

Systemic Bleeding

Both surgical and nonsurgical bleeding are common adverse events associated with LVAD therapy. Bleeding in LVAD recipients results from hematologic alterations including acquired von Willebrand disease (vWD), impaired platelet aggregation, and the requisite use of antiplatelet agents and anticoagulation.[36,37] Acquired vWD, a consequence of high shear stress generated in the LVAD, exposes enzymatic cleavage sites on the von Willebrand protein with resultant proteolysis to smaller molecular weight fragments that are less effective at platelet binding.[38,39] LVAD patients have measurable reductions of large molecular weight vWF multimers within 30 days after implantation but restoration following heart transplantation suggesting a primary role of the LVAD.[40–42]

Mucosal Bleeding

Nasal and gastrointestinal bleeding occur in 10% to 30% of LVAD patients with 21% to 44% having recurrence often leading to readmission and invasive diagnostic and therapeutic procedures.[43–49] It is postulated that gastrointestinal bleeding is a consequence of continuous blood flow physiology. High shear stress on blood elements causes hematologic alterations in vWF as aforementioned. Reduced pulse pressure leads to alterations in microcirculatory flow promoting proliferation of arteriovenous malformations (AVMs) in the gastrointestinal tract. AVMs have been identified as the bleeding source in up to one-third of GI bleeding events and most commonly identified in the small bowel.[49] The proposed pathophysiological mechanisms by which continuous flow support promotes formation of AVMs are (1) elevated intraluminal pressures and smooth muscle alterations causing arteriovenous dilatation; and (2) decreased pulse pressure causes hypoperfusion, regional hypoxia, and vascular dilatation. Patients with mucosal bleeding require interruption of standard anticoagulation and antiplatelet treatments. In addition to endoscopic evaluation/treatment and modification of anticoagulation targets, novel strategies to reduce the incidence gastrointestinal bleeding are being explored including restoration of pulsatility and novel pharmacological therapies to reduce AVM formation or stabilize vWF multimers. As aforementioned, the HeartMate 3 had fewer bleeding events, including gastrointestinal bleeding, compared with the HeartMate II, although the burden of gastrointestinal remains high.[23]

Infection

Infections, including device-related infections, are common complications after LVAD implantation.[50] Device-related infections may present as a driveline infection, a deep tissue infection, or bacteremia. The importance of driveline infections cannot be underestimated—the majority of LVAD-related infections begin at the driveline and 64% are associated with invasive disease.[51] In addition, in the MOMENTUM 3 trial, approximately 50% of patients with a major infection experienced a recurrence within 2 years of follow-up and had in increased hazard for death.[52] The most common pathogens involved in LVAD-related infections are bacterial, including *Staphylococcus* and *Pseudomonas* species, though other pathogens including *Candida* species can be involved.[51–52] Fungal infections are difficult to eradicate and carry a high risk of mortality.[53] Infections in this population require active microbiologic and imaging diagnoses as well as aggressive antibiotic therapy and possibly surgical treatment. In general, LVAD-related bloodstream infections are difficult to eliminate, frequently requiring pump exchange or transplantation.[54]

Ventricular Arrhythmias

Ventricular tachycardia (VT) and ventricular fibrillation (VF) occur in 30% to 55% of patients supported with LVAD therapy.[55,56] Ventricular arrhythmias are often related to the underlying cardiomyopathy but can be induced by ongoing ischemia or originate from areas of myocardial scarring/fibrosis including the apical cannulation site. Ventricular arrhythmias may also be caused by contact of the LVAD with the myocardium. Preimplant arrhythmias are associated with postimplant VT/VF, suggesting a role for targeted antiarrhythmic therapy, intraoperative surgical ablation, biventricular VAD support, or heart transplantation.[57] Catheter ablation for postimplant refractory VT/VF is often well-tolerated resulting from the hemodynamic stability provided by the LVAD.[58–60] Following LVAD implantation, strategies to reduce ventricular arrhythmias and antitachycardia therapies include careful volume management and LVAD speed adjustment to avoid interaction between the myocardium and LVAD as well as careful reprogramming of implantable cardioverter defibrillator parameters to limit defibrillator therapies.[61]

Neurologic Events

Neurologic complications after LVAD therapy can have devastating consequences for patients and negatively impact survival and transplant candidacy. Ischemic and hemorrhagic strokes have been observed following LVAD implantation with an incidence of 5% to 30%.[19,23,62–65] Ischemic events are likely thromboembolic resulting from complex interactions of blood components with the device. However, concomitant atherosclerotic disease in the intracranial or extracranial head and neck vasculature should be excluded. Hemorrhagic CVAs have been postulated to result from elevated blood pressure in fully anticoagulated patients, higher velocity flow, or hemorrhagic conversion from thromboembolic ischemic strokes.[20]

Durable LVAD Exchange

The transition from pulsatile to continuous flow LVADs was driven in part by improved durability. While this change has resulted in reduced need for LVAD exchange, device replacement is still occasionally required. Indications for LVAD exchange include device thrombosis, driveline electrical fault, and infection. The incidence of pump replacement for all causes in the ENDURANCE trial was 10% per patient-year for the Heartmate II versus 6% per patient-year for the HVAD.[19] In the MOMENTUM 3 trial, pump replacement was less common in the HeartMate 3 than the HeartMate II, 12 patients (2.3%) versus 57 patients (11.3%).[23] In many instances, LVAD exchange can be performed without redo sternotomy, particularly if the outflow graft to the ascending aorta is free of thrombus or malalignment. Therefore, a preoperative contrasted chest CT scan may be helpful in planning the approach to exchange. For the centrifugal LVADs, device replacement can be performed through an anterior thoracotomy.[66] In both instances, peripheral cardiopulmonary bypass is established and the old outflow graft is retained and attached to the new LVAD pump. This strategy may also be appropriate in cases of ascending power cord infections or electrical fault involving the power cord. While short-term survival for replacement procedures approaches 100%, long-term outcomes may be diminished relative to primary implants. The exact reasons for this are unclear but recurring pump thrombosis has been reported and reinfection can occur when replacement is required for infections.

OTHER DEVICES AND SPECIAL POPULATIONS

Syncardia Total Artificial Heart

The Syncardia Total Artificial Heart (Syncardia, Tuscon, AZ) is the only commercially available total artificial heart that has achieved BTT approval in patients with severe biventricular HF. This device is manufactured in 50 cc and 70 cc sizes to accommodate a range of body sizes. The device was approved based upon a prospective study comparing TAH to medical therapy or IABP. Patients supported with TAH had a superior survival to transplantation (79% vs 46%) than the control cohort.[67]

Excor Pediatric Ventricular Assist Device

The Excor Pediatric VAD (Berlin Heart, Woodlands, TX) is a miniaturized, pneumatically-driven, extracorporeal LVAD manufactured with stroke volumes from 10 cc to 60 cc to fulfill the hemodynamic needs of children from newborn through adolescence. The Excor was tested in a single arm trial in pediatric patients ranging in weight from 3 kg to 60 kg using historical outcomes with ECMO as a control group.[68] Children treated with the Excor had a statistically lower likelihood of death, withdrawal of support for stroke with serious neurological injury, or inability to wean from the device than control. Based upon the results of this trial, Excor is approved as a BTT for children in the United States.

Biventricular Heart Failure

At present, there are no LVADs specifically designed for chronic, out-of-hospital treatment of RV failure with the exception of the Syncardia TAH. Post-LVAD RV failure is associated with decreased survival.[69] The use of LVADs in a biventricular configuration has been described including the use of two HeartMate 3 devices as TAH configuration.[70,71]

HEART TRANSPLANTATION

Recipient Selection and Management

Indications

Given the relative scarcity of donor organs, it is essential to determine if advanced HF patients are truly refractory to maximal medical therapy and merit transplant evaluation. The commonly acceptable indications for heart transplantation are shown in **Table 52–3**. Generally, the three major indications for heart transplantation are severe HF symptoms, refractory angina, or uncontrolled ventricular arrhythmias not responsive to maximal medical, electrical, and surgical therapies.[72] The

TABLE 52–3. Commonly Accepted Indications for Cardiac Transplantation

Advanced heart failure with severe functional limitations or refractory symptoms despite optimal medical and device therapy
   NYHA functional class IIIb–IV
Cardiogenic shock not expected to recover
   Acute myocardial infarction
   Acute myocarditis
Ischemic heart disease with intractable angina not amenable to surgical or percutaneous revascularization and refractory to maximal medical therapy
Intractable ventricular arrhythmias, uncontrolled with standard antiarrhythmic, device, or ablative therapy
Congenital heart disease in which severe, fixed pulmonary hypertension is not a complication

Abbreviations: LVEF, left ventricular ejection fraction; NYHA, New York Heart Association.

Low LVEF alone is not an adequate indication for heart transplantation

Abnormal cardiopulmonary exercise testing in the absence of functional limitations is not a sufficient criteria for transplantation

most common indication for heart transplantation is intractable HF. Patients with severe angina in the absence of HF are often not considered, since the survival benefit is unclear. Intractable ventricular arrhythmias, commonly referred to as "VT storm," may merit heart transplant evaluation, and often urgent listing given the associated hemodynamic compromise and mortality.

Although these indications for cardiac transplantation are generally well accepted, identifying the subgroup of patients most likely to derive a benefit from transplantation can be challenging. Prior to consideration of advanced HF therapies such as heart transplantation, it is essential to first optimize guideline-directed medical therapy as detailed in other chapters in Section 7. For patients with ischemic cardiomyopathy, surgical revascularization may also be indicated to improve long-term survival.[73]

Thus, the goal of a heart transplant evaluation is to determine if (1) the patient's cardiac status is limited enough, on optimal medical therapy, to benefit from heart transplantation (ie, "sick enough"); (2) the patient does not have comorbidities that would preclude heart transplantation (ie, "well enough"); and (3) the patient demonstrates compliance and possesses adequate social support ("can adapt to a transplant lifestyle"). At an advanced HF center, patients may undergo right heart and pulmonary arterial catheterization for optimization of filling pressures and cardiac output, revascularization of coronary artery disease (CAD), or ablation of ventricular tachycardia before considering heart transplantation. As a result, most heart transplant centers have evolved into centers for advanced HF management in addition to providing the opportunity for transplantation or mechanical circulatory support.

Role of Exercise Testing

In ambulatory patients, evaluation often includes cardiopulmonary exercise stress testing to determine if a patient is limited enough to merit heart transplant evaluation.[72,74] The cardiopulmonary exercise stress test measures maximal oxygen consumption (VO_2 max), which is proportional to cardiac output. Patients with a peak VO_2 of more than 14 mL/kg/min have 1- and 2-year survival rates that are comparable or better than those achieved with transplantation, and these patients should be managed medically and undergo serial exercise testing.[72]

Patients with a peak VO_2 between 10 and 14 mL/kg/min constitute an intermediate-risk group in which continued medical therapy may offer a survival benefit similar to heart transplantation among selected patients that are able to tolerate β-blockers and have the protection of a defibrillator.[75] In patients tolerating β-blockers, a peak VO_2 of less than 12 mL/kg/min has been suggested as an appropriate threshold to identify individuals who are likely to derive a survival benefit from transplantation.[76] Patients with a peak VO_2 of 10 mL/kg/min or less, regardless of β-blocker use, have significantly reduced survival rates with medical therapy compared with cardiac transplantation, and these patients should be listed for transplantation.[77] Adequate effort is defined as the patient's achievement of anaerobic threshold, at which point CO_2 production exceeds O_2 consumption (indicated by the respiratory exchange ratio [RER] >1.10).[78,79] Other parameters of cardiopulmonary exercise testing that are also associated with increased mortality include a predicted VO_2 max <50%[80] and VE/VCO$_2$ slope >35[81] and may be considered in the evaluation for heart transplantation.

Contraindications

Appropriate candidates for cardiac transplantation should have severe functional limitations, limited life expectancy from their heart disease, and a limited number of established contraindications (**Table 52–4**). Many of these factors are not absolute and need to be considered in the context of the severity of the patient's heart disease and associated comorbidities. The degree to which they are interpreted and applied may vary considerably among transplant programs.

Advanced Age: In general, patients are considered for heart transplantation if they are 70 years of age or less, since advances in posttransplant care have shown that survival in the older age group is comparable to that of younger recipients.[6] Patients

TABLE 52–4. Contraindications to Heart Transplantation

Age	Over 70 is a relative contraindication depending on associated comorbidities
Obesity	BMI <35 kg/m² is recommended
Malignancy	Active neoplasm, except nonmelanoma skin cancer, is an absolute contraindication; cancers that are low-grade or in remission may be acceptable in consultation with an oncologist
Pulmonary hypertension	The inability to achieve PVR <3 Wood units with vasodilator or inotropic therapy is a contraindication; such patients may benefit from unloading with a temporary or durable mechanical circulatory support
Diabetes	Uncontrolled diabetes or that associated with significant end-organ damage is an absolute contraindication; Hgb A1c >7.5% is a relative contraindication
Renal dysfunction	Irreversible renal dysfunction (eGFR <30 mL/min/1.73 m²) is a relative contraindication to heart transplantation and may be an indication for combined heart-kidney transplantation
Cirrhosis	May be secondary to cardiac disease and is an absolute contraindication in most centers (unless combined heart/liver transplant is considered)
Peripheral vascular disease	Severe disease not amenable to revascularization is an absolute contraindication, especially if associated with ischemic ulcers
Infection	Selected HIV-positive candidates may be considered if they have no active or prior opportunistic infections, are stable on combination antiretroviral therapy (cART) for >3 months, have undetectable HIV RNA, and have CD4 counts >200 cells/µL for >3 months
Substance use	6 months of abstinence from smoking, alcohol, and illicit drugs is required; in critically ill patients, consultation with psychiatry and social work is essential
Psychosocial issues	Nonadherence, lack of caregiver support, and dementia are absolute contraindications; mental retardation may be a relative contraindication if the patient lacks the ability to understand and cooperate with medical care

Abbreviations: BMI, body mass index; PVR, pulmonary vascular resistance.

over the age of 70 years may have acceptable outcomes, but careful consideration of associated comorbidities is essential in these cases. At some centers, such patients are offered nonstandard donor hearts, including those with mild CAD, mildly decreased LVEF, LV hypertrophy, or donor age older than 55 years. This practice allows older patients to undergo heart transplantation without denying the scarce resource to younger candidates, with comparable outcomes.[82] Physiologic age may be more important than chronologic age with respect to survival and rehabilitation potential. As a result, many programs focus less on fixed upper age limits and instead assess the patient's functional status, integrity of major organ systems, and the presence of comorbidities that might impact survival, rehabilitation potential, and quality of life.

Pulmonary Hypertension: Pulmonary hypertension from chronic elevation of LV end-diastolic pressure is a common complication of long-standing HF and, if unrecognized and untreated, can result in irreversible changes to the pulmonary vasculature.[83] In the early years of heart transplantation, it was discovered that a normal donor RV is unable to increase its external workload acutely to overcome elevated pulmonary vascular resistance (PVR), resulting in acute RV failure and cardiogenic shock postoperatively.[84] Elevated PVR remains a strong risk factor for RV failure and early postoperative mortality in the modern era. Potential heart transplant candidates must therefore undergo measurements of pulmonary artery pressures and calculation of PVR in the cardiac catheterization laboratory or in the ICU as part of their transplant evaluation.

A pulmonary artery systolic pressure above 60 mm Hg, a PVR value above 5 Wood units, or a transpulmonary gradient above 15 to 20 mm Hg is generally considered prohibitive of successful heart transplantation. A vasodilator challenge should be administered when the pulmonary artery systolic pressure is ≥50 mm Hg and either the transpulmonary gradient (TPG) is ≥15 or the PVR is >3 Wood units.[72]

A vasodilator challenge is considered successful if the PVR can be reduced below 3 with a vasodilator while maintaining a systolic arterial blood pressure over 85 mm Hg. If the PVR cannot be reduced below 3 or if the systolic blood pressure falls below 85 mm Hg with reduction in the PVR, the patient remains at high risk of right HF and mortality after cardiac transplantation. In this situation, hospitalization with continuous hemodynamic monitoring should be performed, because the PVR will often decline after 24 to 48 hours of treatment consisting of diuretics, nitroprusside, prostaglandin E$_1$, milrinone, and dobutamine or inhaled nitric oxide. If pharmacologic measures fail, temporary or durable mechanical circulatory support may be indicated for longer-term unloading.[85,86]

Infections: Patients must be free of active infection before transplantation because the immunosuppression that is required after transplantation to prevent rejection can exacerbate infections. The presence of an active systemic infection or severe localized infection is often considered a temporary contraindication to transplantation. Patients with a history of infection should not be activated or reactivated on the transplant waiting list until there is sufficient evidence that the infection is resolved or controlled, as demonstrated by absence of fever for a minimum of 72 hours on appropriate antibiotics, a normal white blood cell count, negative blood culture results, and resolving signs or symptoms of infection. However, it is important to note that MCS driveline infections are generally not a contraindication to transplantation because definitive treatment involves removal of the driveline at the time of transplant.

Hepatitis B and C are generally no longer considered absolute contraindications to heart transplantation. In particular, the advent of direct-acting antiviral agents with >95% cure rate for hepatitis C after 12 weeks or less of therapy[87,88] has changed practice at many centers.

In addition, HIV infection is no longer considered a contraindication to heart transplantation at some centers as long as the patient has no opportunistic infections, acceptable CD4 count, and an undetectable viral load.[89–91] Chagas disease, while uncommon in the United States, is a common indication for transplantation in South America, and reactivation of disease can occur.[92] The decision to proceed with transplantation in these situations must be made in collaboration with an infectious disease specialist well-versed in transplantation.

Malignancy: Patients with current malignancies, except for nonmelanoma cutaneous cancers, primary cardiac tumors restricted to the heart, and low-grade neoplasms of the prostate, are generally excluded from cardiac transplantation. However, neoplasms are diverse with respect to their response to immunosuppressive therapy and risk of recurrence. Consultation with an oncologist is essential to assess the risk of tumor recurrence. Cardiac transplantation should be considered when the risk of tumor recurrence is low based on the tumor type, response to therapy, and negative metastatic work-up. The specific amount of time to wait before transplantation after neoplasm remission depends on the aforementioned factors, and no arbitrary time period for observation should be used.

Other Comorbidities: Potential cardiac transplant recipients are screened for the existence of other conditions or systemic diseases that may independently limit their survival or rehabilitation potential. Obese patients have a greater risk of poor wound healing, infections, and pulmonary complications after cardiac surgery, although the outcomes in heart transplant recipients are less clear.[93] Nevertheless, it is recommended that patients achieve a body mass index <35 kg/m² before listing.[72]

The presence of preexisting insulin-requiring diabetes mellitus was once considered a relative contraindication to heart transplantation because of concerns regarding diminished survival, increased infection rates, and worsening glycemic control in the context of corticosteroid immunosuppression. However, several reports have demonstrated comparable short- and long-term survival rates in diabetic and nondiabetic heart transplant recipients with similar rates of infection, rejection, renal function, and cardiac allograft vasculopathy.[94–96] Although the safety and efficacy of heart transplantation in these very carefully selected patients has been documented in the literature, most transplant programs continue to consider the presence of diabetes with end-organ damage (proliferative retinopathy, neuropathy, or nephropathy) a relative contraindication to transplantation. Corticosteroid therapy may worsen glycemic control in patients with preexisting diabetes, and thus the presence of poorly controlled diabetes is also considered a relative contraindication. At most centers, patients are expected to achieve control with a hemoglobin A1c under 7.5% before listing;[73] ongoing collaboration with an endocrinologist may be helpful to achieve this goal.

Other comorbid conditions must be considered on an individual basis, but irreversible organ dysfunction such as pulmonary fibrosis, severe emphysema, and hepatic or renal dysfunction are strong relative contraindications, although selected patients with irreversible renal, pulmonary, or hepatic dysfunction may be considered for multiorgan transplantation.[97–100]

Advanced noncardiac vascular disease, including symptomatic cerebrovascular disease or peripheral vascular disease not amenable to revascularization, is considered a relative contraindication to transplantation if the condition is expected to limit survival or impair rehabilitation after transplantation.

Psychosocial Factors

All cardiac transplant candidates should undergo a careful psychosocial assessment with emphasis on current and previous substance abuse history, adherence with medical therapy and follow-up, comprehension of and ability to follow a complex medical regimen, and adequacy of caregiver support. Active cigarette smoking is a contraindication to heart transplantation, and smoking during the 6 months prior transplant is a risk factor for poor outcomes.[72] At most centers, patients must display abstinence from smoking for 6 months, documented by urine nicotine screens, prior to listing. Addiction to alcohol or illicit drugs is an absolute contraindication because it suggests that these patients will have poor adherence after transplantation, and 6 months abstinence with participation in counseling programs is required. This assessment may be difficult to make in the critically ill patient in whom transplantation cannot be delayed for 6 months. In this scenario, consultation with social workers and psychiatrists is essential to gauge the patient's commitment to abstinence.

Medical marijuana poses a specific conundrum and whether heart transplant candidates on medical marijuana or those that obtain it through other legal means should receive organ transplantation is not clear. As abuse is possible and would render potential candidates unsuitable for transplantation, centers generally request abstinence from marijuana whenever possible.[101]

In addition to freedom from dependence on cigarettes, alcohol, and illicit substances, patients must be able to demonstrate the ability to adhere with medications and follow-up after transplantation, which includes the presence of dedicated caregiver support. Mental retardation and dementia are relative contraindications to heart transplantation; the former due to concerns of adherence (which may be overcome with dedicated close caregiver support) and the latter due to overall poor prognosis.

The Role of Antibody Sensitization

Sensitization

The number of heart transplant candidates with antibodies to human leukocyte antigens (HLA), so-called "sensitization," has increased over the last decade.[102] Risk factors for sensitization include pregnancy, transfusions, VADs, or prior transplantation. Such preformed antibodies may cause hyperacute rejection, increase the risk of rejection posttransplantation,[103] and predispose patients to the development of cardiac allograft vasculopathy.[104]

Detection of Anti-HLA Antibodies

The detection of anti-HLA antibodies is most commonly performed using solid phase assays. With these assays, latex beads bound with single HLAs are mixed with patient serum. Antibodies bind to their respective antigen-coated beads, are tagged with an anti-IgG fluorescent carrier, and are then detected by flow cytometry, allowing the identity and quantification of anti-HLA antibodies to be determined. Quantification is important because antibodies of greater binding intensity in vitro are considered to be potentially more cytotoxic in vivo. The presence of anti-HLA antibodies in high binding levels (usually median fluorescent intensity above 5000) are considered potentially cytotoxic.[104]

However, binding intensity of antibodies may not be the best test of potential cytotoxicity because not all antibodies at high binding intensity may be detrimental to graft function; to assess the ability of donor-specific antibodies to fix complement, a functional assay (C1q assay) may be a better marker of their cytotoxicity.[105-107] For centers where the C1q assay is not available, considering only antibodies that are strong binding by mean fluorescence intensity (MFI) after a 1:8 or 1:16 dilution may offer comparable information on potential cytotoxicity.[106]

Approach to the Crossmatch

The detection of anti-HLA antibodies prior to transplantation is important since one would avoid donors who have HLA corresponding to high-binding anti-HLA antibodies in the potential recipient to prevent hyperacute rejection. Previously, the only way to assess for this was with a prospective crossmatch, in which the potential recipient's serum was mixed with donor cells to assess for complement-dependent cytotoxicity. However, this severely geographically restricted the donor pool to hospitals near where the candidate's serum was stored, thus reducing the number of potential donors. The virtual crossmatch has replaced the prospective crossmatch at most centers. With the virtual crossmatch, HLA corresponding to high-binding anti-HLA antibodies in the transplant candidate are listed as "avoids" in the United Network of Organ Sharing database, and, thus, potential donors with such HLA are not considered. This method has proven safe and successful in heart transplantation.[108]

The Calculated PRA

The identity and binding intensity of anti-HLA antibodies is useful not only in safely finding a donor organ for a sensitized recipient, but also in deciding on which sensitized patients require treatment prior to transplantation.[103,104] Centers often use a certain number of the calculated panel reactive antibody (cPRA) to decide on treatment of the sensitized patient. The cPRA is the frequency of unacceptable HLA in the donor population.[109] It is computed based on HLA frequencies of 12,000 kidney donors in the United States between 2003 and 2005. For example, if a heart transplant candidate had antibodies against common HLA, the cPRA might be 90%, and, thus, only 10% of all potential donors would be compatible. On the other hand, if a heart transplant candidate had only antibodies against rare HLA, the cPRA might be 10%, and, thus, 90% of all potential donors would be compatible. The cPRA is very dependent on what the individual program determines the antibody binding threshold to be in order to identify an antibody as being unacceptable. Most centers use an antibody binding threshold of more than 5000 MFI to avoid corresponding antigens in a potential donor. A higher threshold would avoid less antibodies, which would result in a lower cPRA. cPRA highlights the fact that some anti-HLA antibodies will impact the ability to find a suitable donor heart more than others.[110] If the cPRA is above 50% to 70%, therapies to reduce antibody binding prior to transplantation may be used because high cPRA results in longer time on the waiting list with attendant increased mortality.[111]

Approach to Desensitization

Management of the sensitized patient involves protocols to target antibodies by inactivation (intravenous immune globulin [IV Ig][112]), removal (plasmapheresis), and decreased production (rituximab[112] and bortezomib[113]). Production of IV Ig begins with pooled human plasma from several thousand screened volunteer donors, from which highly purified polyvalent IgG is derived. While the mechanisms of action are incompletely understood, intravenous immune globulin suppresses inflammatory and immune-mediated processes. Rituximab is a monoclonal antibody directed against the CD20 antigen on B-lymphocytes. It is most commonly used for B-cell lymphoma but, in conjunction with IV Ig, also reduces HLA antibodies in patients awaiting kidney transplantation.[112]

If the protocol of intravenous immune globulin and rituximab is ineffective in reducing the cPRA below 50%, or if a patient requires rapid desensitization, then bortezomib, a proteasome inhibitor against plasma cells, may be used in conjunction with plasmapheresis. It is most commonly used for the treatment of multiple myeloma but also reduces HLA antibodies in patients awaiting heart transplantation.[113]

Donor Selection and Management

Acceptance of the concept of irreversible brain death, both legally and medically, has been integral to the emergence of organ transplantation in the modern era. Brain death is defined as irreversible cessation of all functions of the entire brain.[114] The heart does not need to stop for a valid declaration of death and this definition has facilitated heart transplantation. Criteria for brain death have been adapted from Harvard Ad Hoc Committee in 1968[115] and codified into law in the Uniform Determination of Death Act in 1981 following the President's

TABLE 52–5. Criteria for Determining Brain Death

Clinical evaluation

Mechanism of brain injury is sufficient to account for irreversible loss of brain function

Absence of reversible causes of CNS depression

   CNS depressant drugs*

   Hypothermia (<32°C)

   Hypotension (MAP <55 mm Hg)

Absence of neuromuscular blocking drugs that may confound the results of the neurologic examination

No spontaneous movements, motor responses, or posturing

No gag or cough reflexes

No corneal or pupillary light reflexes

No oculovestibular reflex (cold calorics)

Confirmatory tests

Apnea test for minimum of 5 min showing

   No respiratory movements

   pCO_2 >55 mm Hg

   pH <7.40

No intracranial blood flow

Abbreviations: CNS, central nervous system; MAP, mean arterial pressure; pCO_2, partial pressure.

*Removal of CNS depressant drugs may take several days to take effect.

TABLE 52–6. More Favorable Donor Characteristics

Age <55 years

Absence of significant cardiac structural abnormalities such as:

   LV hypertrophy (wall thickness >13 mm by echocardiography)*

   Significant valvular dysfunction

   Significant congenital cardiac abnormality

   Significant coronary artery disease

Adequate physiologic function of donor heart

   LVEF ≥45%** or

   Achievement of target hemodynamic criteria after hormonal resuscitation and hemodynamic management

      MAP >60 mm Hg

      PCWP 8–12 mm Hg

      Cardiac index >2.4 L/min·m²

      CVP 4–12 mm Hg

      SVR 800–1200 dyne/s·cm⁵

      No inotrope dependence

      Predicted heart mass donor/recipient ratio >0.86

Negative hepatitis C antibody,*** hepatitis B surface antigen, and HIV serologies. Absence of active malignancy (except nonmelanoma skin cancers and certain primary brain tumors) or overwhelming infection

Abbreviations: CVP, central venous pressure; LV, left ventricular; LVEF, left ventricular ejection fraction; MAP, mean arterial pressure; PCWP, pulmonary capillary wedge pressure; SVR, systemic vascular resistance.

*Echocardiograms are often reviewed by the accepting center to confirm the accuracy of the reported left ventricular dimensions.

**LVEF may be reduced due to catecholamine-induced myocardial stunning and may resolve in a period of days to hours.

***Hepatitis C donors may not be contraindicated at all centers with the advent of antiviral therapy that offers the chance of cure.

Commission Report.[116] Fundamental requirements for brain death are summarized in **Table 52–5.**

The most common causes of brain death include intracranial hemorrhage, blunt traumatic injury to the head, penetrating traumatic injury, and anoxic brain injury. Patients with irreversible brain injury accompanied by the intent to withdraw life support are also considered potential organ donors. The complete absence of brainstem function is not required; many patients who meet all the criteria for brain death do not in fact have irreversible cessation of all functions of the entire brain, because some of the brain stem's homeostatic functions remain, such as temperature control and water and electrolyte balance.[117]

Donor Evaluation

After a potential donor is identified, the procurement process is initiated by contacting the local, or "host," organ procurement organization (OPO). The host OPO is responsible for obtaining consent for organ donation, verifying pronouncement of brain death, evaluating and managing the donor, and equitably allocating the donor organs. The process of donor evaluation begins with a detailed history and physical examination, focusing on cause of death, past medical history, donor height and weight, and clinical course. Basic laboratory studies, including a complete blood count, metabolic panel, ABO blood typing, and viral serologies (hepatitis B and C, HIV, human T-cell leukemia virus, Ebstein-Barr virus [EBV], and cytomegalovirus [CMV]) are ordered; in addition other serologies may be obtained in the presence of outbreaks such as West Nile virus, SARS-CoV-2, or in donors considered high risk for infections such as Chagas disease. Additional studies include chest radiography, 12-lead electrocardiography (ECG), and echocardiography.

To be considered suitable donors for cardiac transplantation, brain-dead individuals must meet certain minimum criteria (**Table 52–6**). Most cardiac donors are younger than age 55 years, although older donors may be used selectively in critically ill or older recipients. There should be no evidence of severe cardiothoracic trauma. An initial echocardiogram is performed to identify significant structural heart disease such as LV hypertrophy or dysfunction, occlusive CAD, valvular dysfunction, and congenital lesions. Donors with these conditions are typically excluded, although selected marginal organs may be allocated to higher-risk recipients. Angiography is performed to exclude significant CAD in male donors older than age 45 years and in female donors older than age 50 years but may also be performed in younger patients with multiple risk factors for CAD. Younger patients with a history of cocaine and methamphetamine abuse may also warrant consideration for angiography. Patients with active malignancy (excluding nonmelanocytic skin cancers and certain isolated brain tumors) or severe systemic infections are typically excluded.

HIV and hepatitis B infections generally preclude organ donation, though there is renewed interest in the use of hearts from hepatitis C donors with the advent of effective cure from direct-acting antiviral agents (DAA).[118] As this is an emerging area of organ transplantation, HCV-specific informed consent of waitlisted patients is recommended before organ offer. There are two possible approaches to the management of donor-derived HCV infection in transplant recipients: (1) prophylactic strategy: DAA is initiated preoperatively or within a few hours following transplantation from an HCV NAT+ donor; or (2) preemptive strategy: After HCV infection acquisition is confirmed by serial posttransplant testing, DAA is started within 90 days of transplantation.

Donor Management

After brain death has been determined and the patient has been identified as a potential organ donor, the main goals of organ donor management are to ensure optimal organ function by providing volume resuscitation; optimizing cardiac output; normalizing systemic vascular resistance; maintaining adequate oxygenation; correcting anemia, acid–base, and electrolyte abnormalities; and correcting hormonal imbalances that occur after brain death and that can impair circulatory function. Standardized algorithms incorporating early use of invasive hemodynamic monitoring along with aggressive hemodynamic management and hormonal resuscitation with insulin, corticosteroids, triiodothyronine, and arginine vasopressin have been proposed to improve cardiac donor management and maximize organ utilization, particularly in patients with a LVEF below 45% on initial echocardiography.[119] In brain death, particularly in cases of subarachnoid hemorrhage, there is a catecholamine surge that can result in LV dysfunction and regional wall motion abnormalities.[120] This dysfunction is often not associated with structural abnormalities and may be reversible, so such donors may ultimately be acceptable for transplantation.[121]

Most donor hearts are currently harvested locally from the donor by an organ procurement team from the transplant center and transported back to the center for implantation. A cold ischemic period of less than 4 to 6 hours in adult hearts is considered optimal. This requirement for short ischemic times leads to the rationale for geographic subdivision in the US into OPOs.

One way to minimize ischemic injury would be to limit cold ischemic time through use of an ex vivo heart perfusion platform that maintains the donor heart in a warm, beating state for transplantation.[122] The PROCEED II study demonstrated that the Organ Care System (OCS™ TransMedics, Andover MA) for ex vivo perfusion of human hearts offered comparable 30-day patient and graft survival rates to standard cold storage in 130 heart transplant recipients.[122] An ongoing Phase 3 clinical trial, the EXPAND trial (International Trial for Preserving and Assessing Expanded Criteria Donor Hearts for Transplantation NCT02323321) will offer further insight into the utility of this platform.

Between 2005 and 2014, only 29% percent of potential organ donors in the United States become heart transplant donors.[123] Despite ongoing efforts to increase the identification of potential donors, increase the consent rate among eligible donors, expand donor selection criteria, and maximize potential donor organ function, heart transplantation will likely remain a donor-limited field for the foreseeable future.[124]

Donation after Cardiac Death

To expand the donor pool, there is interest in donation after circulatory death (DCD) for heart transplantation.[125] DCD applies to donors with devastating brain injury who depend on life support but do not meet the legal criteria for brain death. After the withdrawal of life support, death is declared on the basis of cardiac arrest. Asystole must be confirmed for at least 5 minutes for declaration of death. This practice differs from donation after brain death (DBD), which involves donation of a beating heart. The challenges for heart transplantation using DCD donors include minimization of ischemic injury of the donor organs as well as ethical concerns.

There are a number of techniques for DCD heart procurement: normothermic regional perfusion, ex situ reperfusion, and modified conventional procurement[126] and they differ in the management of the heart after declaration of death on the basis of circulatory arrest. In normothermic regional perfusion, the donor is centrally cannulated, and the heart reanimated on cardiopulmonary bypass and then procured in the usual fashion. In ex situ reperfusion, the explanted heart is reanimated by ex vivo perfusion using the TransMedics Organ Care System device. Finally, in modified conventional procurement, the explanted heart is not reanimated but instead expediently transplanted into a recipient in close proximity.

The practice of restarting circulation after declaration of death according to circulatory criteria for procurement of DCD donors appears to challenge the legal circulatory death definition requiring irreversible cessation. Permanent cessation for life-saving efforts must be achieved and ligating principal vessels to maintain no blood flow to the brain, may be performed to ensure natural progression to cessation of brain function. This practice raises unique concerns about prioritizing life-saving efforts, informed authorization from decision-makers, and the clinician's role in the patient's death. To mitigate these issues, the donation conversation must not take place until after an uncoerced decision to withdraw life-sustaining treatment made in accordance with the patient's treatment goals. The decision-maker must understand DCD procedure well enough to provide genuine authorization and the preservation/procurement teams must be separate from the clinical care team.[127]

Organ Matching and Allocation

Donor–recipient matching is performed based on ABO blood group compatibility and body size. Although the benefit of matching donor organs and recipients with respect to human leukocyte antigen (HLA) has been well established in renal transplantation, HLA matching is not performed in potential heart transplant recipients due to the relatively scarcity of donor organs. However, heart transplant candidates who are sensitized (those with preformed anti-HLA antibodies related to prior pregnancy, transplant, blood transfusions, or MCS), will undergo crossmatching (see section Approach to the Crossmatch) to determine if there are potentially cytotoxic antibodies against the donor HLA.

Predicted Heart Mass

The 2010 International Society of Heart and Lung Transplantation guidelines for the care of heart transplant recipients recommended avoidance of donor–recipient undersizing by more than 30% based on total body weight.[128] Yet undersizing by total body weight is not associated with worse outcomes after transplantation,[129] perhaps because the assumption of a direct correlation between body weight and cardiac size is not valid. However, predicted heart mass (PHM) is derived from magnetic resonance imaging studies and factors in height, weight, age, and sex to account for variations in heart mass not accounted for by total body weight alone, and analyses of the both the United Network for Organ Sharing (UNOS) registry[130] and International Society of Heart and Lung Transplantation (ISHLT) registry[93] indicate that undersizing by PHM is associated with worse posttransplant survival. Thus, in the current era, the optimal metric for donor–recipient size matching is PHM.

Allocation System

UNOS under contract to the Organ Procurement and Transplantation Network (OPTN) implemented an adult organ allocation system in 1988 with periodic updates to optimize fair allocation of donor hearts.[131,132] In an update in 2005, patients listed for cardiac transplantation were stratified into a three-tiered system of escalating urgency for heart transplantation to enhance broader access to donor. By 2015, the sickest patients in the Status 1A tier increased 5-fold and accounted for two-thirds of heart transplantation recipients.[133]

Despite good intentions to optimize organ allocation, there were critiques of the 2005 system,[133] namely that the former Status 1A provided inadequate resolution among the sickest patients: a heterogenous group of unstable heart transplant candidates received the same prioritization despite different waitlist mortality.[70] The OPTN/UNOS Thoracic Organ Transplantation Committee redesigned a six-tiered heart allocation system with a broader geographic sharing policy, implemented on October 18, 2018 (**Table 52–7**). Advantages of the new system include prioritization of more unstable inpatient candidates, such as those with ECMO support (Status 1), over those receiving inotropic support with hemodynamic monitoring (Status 3), as well as prioritization of ambulatory heart transplant candidates with poorer prognosis, those with infiltrative or hypertrophic cardiomyopathy (Status 4), over those with nonischemic dilated cardiomyopathy (Status 6).

Long-term registry data on mortality, as well as single-center analysis of morbidity, will be essential to determine the impact of the new allocation system on waitlist and posttransplant morbidity and mortality.

Surgical Technique

The donor heart is explanted, or "harvested," by a surgical team at a hospital usually remote from the transplant center, and the procedure must be coordinated with the surgical teams procuring other organs for transplantation. The donor heart is first arrested with cardioplegic solution. The original surgical technique for orthotopic heart transplantation, the biatrial technique, was described by Lower and Shumway in 1960.[134] In this procedure, both the donor and recipient hearts are removed by transecting the atria at the midatrial level, leaving the multiple pulmonary venous connections to the left atrium (LA) intact in the posterior wall of the LA, and then transecting the aorta and pulmonary artery just above their respective semilunar valves. The explanted heart is cooled topically by being placed in an iced preservation solution; it is then placed in a secure container and transported expeditiously to the transplant center. Ischemic times average 3 to 4 hours.

TABLE 52–7. United Network of Organ Sharing Heart Transplant Allocation System as of October 2018

Status	Status Description
1	VA-ECMO Nondischargeable surgically implanted Bi-VAD LVAD with life-threatening VT or VF
2	Nondischargeable surgically implanted LVAD IABP Life-threatening VT or VF LVAD with mechanical failure, admitted to the hospital Percutaneous endovascular pump (eg, Impella®) TAH, Bi-VAD, RVAD, or VAD for single ventricle patient
3	LVAD discharged with discretionary 30 days LVAD with device infection, hemolysis, pump thrombosis, right heart failure, mucosal bleeding or aortic regurgitation Multiple inotropes or single high-dose inotrope with PA catheter VA-ECMO, IABP, or percutaneous endovascular pump that downgrades
4	Dischargeable LVAD without discretionary 30 days Multiple inotropes or single high dose inotrope without PA catheter Congenital heart disease, refractory angina, retransplantation Amyloidosis, hypertrophic or restrictive cardiomyopathy
5	Listed for heart transplant and at least one other organ
6	All other adult heart candidates not meeting higher status
7	Inactive

Abbreviations: VA-ECMO, veno-arterial extracorporeal membranous oxygenation; Bi-VAD, biventricular assist device; LVAD, left ventricular assist device; VT, ventricular tachycardia; VF, ventricular fibrillation; IABP, intra-aortic balloon pump; Impella® (Abiomed Inc., Danvers MA); TAH, total artificial heart; RVAD, right ventricular assist device.

Adapted with permission from Organ Procurement and Transplantation Network. US Department of Health & Human Services.

Implantation of the heart in the orthotopic position historically began with re-anastomosis at the midatrial level, beginning with the atrial septum (**Fig. 52–11**). Efforts are made to include a generous cuff of donor right atrium so the sinoatrial node will be included. The great vessels are connected just above the semilunar valves. Commonly seen with the biatrial technique was the presence of two asynchronous P waves on electrocardiography. One P wave emanates from the sinus node of the donor heart and the other from the sinus node in the right atrial remnant of the native heart. Currently, the biatrial technique has been modified by leaving the donor right atrium intact and making anastomoses at the level of the superior and inferior vena cavae and pulmonary veins.[135] This so-called "bicaval technique" (**Fig. 52–12**) results in less distortion of atrioventricular geometry, resulting in improved atrial and ventricular function, less atrioventricular valve regurgitation, decreased incidence of atrial arrhythmias, and decreased incidence of donor sinus node dysfunction and heart block requiring permanent pacemaker implantation.[136–138]

Immediate postoperative care differs little from that after more routine heart surgery except for the institution of

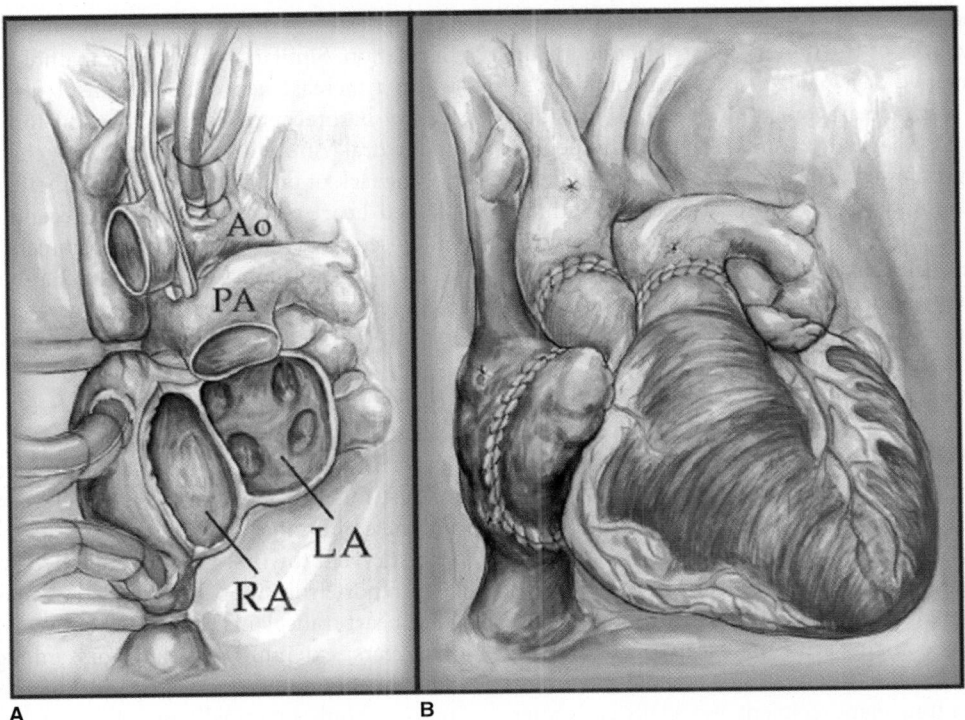

Figure 52–11. Original bilatrial technique for orthotopic heart transplantation. (A) shows the completed recipient cardiectomy with the recipient atria transected at the midatrial level. **(B)** shows the completed re-anastomosis of the donor heart. Ao, aorta; LA, left atrium; PA, pulmonary artery; RA, right atrium. Reproduced with permission from Pahl E, Backer CL, Mavroudis C. Heart transplantation at Children's Memorial. *The Children's Doctor: Journal of Children's Memorial Hospital*, Chicago, IL; Fall 1999.

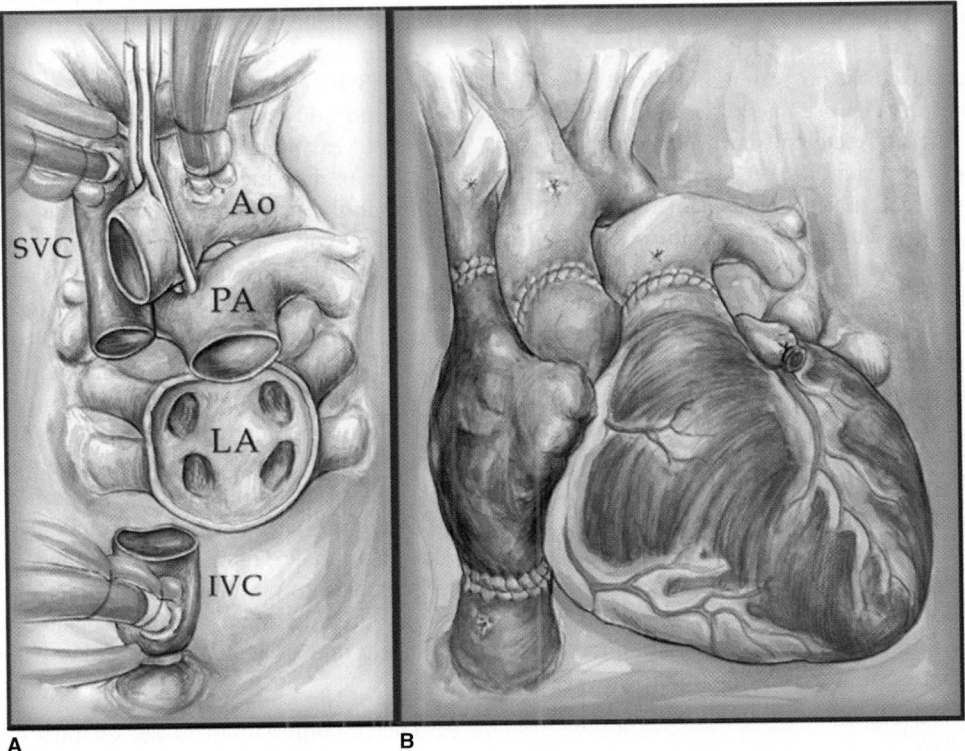

Figure 52–12. Bicaval technique for orthotopic heart transplantation. (A) shows the completed recipient cardiectomy. The recipient atria are completed removed except for except for a cuff of tissue around the pulmonary vein orifices. The superior and inferior vena cavae are transected at their junction with the right atrium. **(B)** shows the completed anastomoses of the donor heart at the level of the superior and inferior venae cavae and pulmonary veins. Ao, aorta; IVC, inferior vena cava; LA, left atrium; PA, pulmonary artery; SVC, superior vena cava. Reproduced with permission from Pahl E, Backer CL, Mavroudis C. Heart transplantation at Children's Memorial. *The Children's Doctor: Journal of Children's Memorial Hospital*, Chicago, IL; Fall 1999.

immunosuppression (subsequently described) and the need for chronotropic support of the donor sinoatrial node for the first 2 to 3 postoperative days, usually with temporary pacemaker support or with beta-agonist intravenous infusions. Postoperative bradycardia usually results from sinus node dysfunction due to surgical trauma, ischemia to the sinus node, or pretransplant use of amiodarone.[139] Most cases resolve within a few weeks to months. The incidence of refractory bradycardia requiring permanent pacemaker implantation is between 10% and 20% with the biatrial technique and less than 10% with the bicaval technique.[137] Patients with uncomplicated postoperative courses are discharged from the hospital as early as 7 to 10 days after heart transplantation.

Physiology of the Transplanted Heart

Lack of Innervation

When the donor heart is placed into the recipient, both afferent (from the heart to the central nervous system) and efferent (from the central nervous system to the heart) nerve supply is lost. The loss of afferent nerve supply means that the recipient will not experience angina with the exception of a small subgroup that may have re-innervation.[140] Therefore, chest discomfort in a heart transplant recipient, especially early after transplant, is likely not caused by coronary ischemia, and coronary ischemia will likely not present with chest discomfort. The standard practice of annual angiograms for surveillance of transplant CAD is a direct consequence of the lack of afferent nerves supplying the transplanted heart and required for early detection of allograft vasculopathy.

The consequences of the loss of efferent nerves are related to the loss of vagal tone and the postganglionic direct release of norepinephrine stores in response to exercise. With the loss of vagal tone, heart transplant recipients have a higher than resting heart rate usually of around 90 to 110 bpm. The lack of efferent nerves also means that the transplant recipient must rely on circulating catecholamines to respond to exercise, so there is a blunting of the heart-rate response to exercise. Similarly, after exercise, the heart rate returns to baseline more slowly because of the gradual decline of circulating catecholamine concentrations to baseline.

Heart transplant recipients lack the baroreceptor reflex, which relies on intact baroreceptors and sympathetic and parasympathetic innervation. Thus, heart transplant recipients are more susceptible to orthostasis and carotid sinus massage will not break a reentrant tachycardia in these patients.

Nevertheless, heart transplant recipients often experience reinnervation of the heart, with possible angina, an improvement in exercise tolerance, and a decrease in resting heart rate. This process is variable among patients, although tends to increase over time. Restoration of sympathetic innervation correlates with improved responses of heart rate and contractile function to exercise.[141]

Response to Medications

Some cardiac drugs are not effective in the denervated heart. Due to the lack of vagal tone, digoxin will have little effect on sinoatrial and atrioventricular conduction velocity and will not achieve rate control if the transplanted heart develops atrial fibrillation. Similarly, the parasympatholytic effect of atropine will not increase heart rate in transplanted hearts. Due to the lack of baroreceptor reflexes, vasodilators such as nifedipine and hydralazine will not cause reflex tachycardia.

The lack of postganglionic sympathetic nerves in the transplanted heart results in increased receptor density, and thus more sensitivity to sympathetic agonists and antagonists.[142] Clinically, this is most often seen with β-blockers; heart transplant recipients will often have exaggerated fatigue in response to β-blockers, especially with exercise.

Posttransplant Outcomes

Survival

Survival after heart transplantation has steadily improved in the last four decades. In the 1980s, 1-year survival was 70% and the conditional half-life, the time at which 50% of patients who survived the first year are still alive, was 9.4 years. In the 2019 report from the ISHLT registry,[93] median survival after adult heart transplants performed between 2002 and 2009 was 12.5 years, extending to 14.8 years among 1-year survivors. Notably, the mortality rate beyond 1 year after transplant has improved only marginally for patients who received allografts after 1992 without significant improvement in the last two decades. This stable annual mortality rate of approximately 3% to 4% is higher than that of the general population, and likely exists because the processes responsible for long-term mortality, including cardiac allograft vasculopathy and malignancy, remain a challenge of detection and treatment.

An in-depth analysis of risk factors for survival is provided in the ISHLT registry report.[93] The strongest risk factors for 1-year mortality, associated with a 50% or more increase in the risk of 1-year mortality, are mainly related to technical issues and the underlying disease responsible for transplantation, including the use of temporary circulatory support, congenital cardiomyopathy versus nonischemic cardiomyopathy, prior transplant, pretransplant ventilatory support, or dialysis. Risk factors for 5- and 10-year mortality, on the other hand, are most referable to immunological issues and toxicity related to immunosuppression, including dialysis or infection after transplant, rejection during the first posttransplant year, and lack of immunosuppression therapy with a combination of at least two of the following classes: cell cycle inhibitors, calcineurin inhibitors (CNIs), and proliferation signal inhibitors (PSIs).

Women also have a somewhat higher risk of death compared with their male counterparts. Younger donor age, younger recipient age, lower allograft ischemic time, and higher center volume are additional factors associated with long-term survival, and these risk factors appear consistent across countries.

Quality of Life

Patients not only gain increased quantity of life after transplantation, but quality of life is improved as well. In the first years after heart transplant, over 70% of recipients report having a normal healthy lifestyle or only few disease symptoms.[93]

In-depth analysis of a smaller cohort of transplant patients indicates that the most frequently reported symptoms long-term after heart transplantation, at moderate rates of 50% to 65%, were fatigue, sexual dysfunction, memory problems, bruising, and cramps.[143] These symptoms are less common in recipients who are married and those with a higher educational level.

Based on information from the ISHLT registry, among recipients aged 25 to 55 years old, less than 40% were employed 5 years after transplantation.[93] On the basis of the functional data reviewed above, it appears that a higher proportion could return to the workplace; however, in the United States, the structure of disability benefits and health insurance considerations may represent a barrier to this process.

Postoperative Management
Primary Graft Dysfunction
Primary graft dysfunction (PGD) occurs when there is dysfunction of the donor heart within 24 hours of completion of the heart transplant surgery. It must be differentiated from secondary graft dysfunction due to surgical issues (tamponade, bleeding, anastomosis injury) or recipient issues (hyperacute rejection, pulmonary hypertension, sepsis). A strict definition was developed at an international consensus conference in 2013[144] (**Table 52–8**). In an international survey of 47 heart transplant centers comprising almost 10,000 patients, a PGD rate of 7.4% was reported with a 30-day mortality of 30%.[144] Treatment is ultimately supportive (**Fig. 52–13**). In severe cases, ECMO may be used with acceptable outcomes, especially if initiated early in the course of decompensation.[145,146]

Hyperacute Rejection: Prevention with Eculizumab
Pretransplant interventions with IV Ig, rituximab, and bortezomib can reduce antibody levels such that it is possible to find an acceptable donor even for highly sensitized patients. However, hyperacute rejection related to preformed cytotoxic anti-HLA antibodies can still occur due to donor-specific antibodies that were considered unlikely to be cytotoxic by virtual crossmatch or that formed after banked blood was collected

for a prospective crossmatch. In this setting, eculizumab offers further insurance and protection against hyperacute rejection.

Eculizumab is a monoclonal antibody that selectively inhibits the terminal portion of the complement cascade. Eculizumab is FDA-approved for use in paroxysmal nocturnal hemoglobunuria and atypical hemolytic-uremic syndrome, two complement-mediated conditions. However, benefit has been seen in sensitized kidney transplant recipients[147] and results of the DUET study (De-novo Use of Eculizumab alongside Conventional Therapy in Presensitized Patients Receiving Cardiac Transplantation: An Open-Label, Investigator-Initiated Pilot [NCT02013037]) are forthcoming.

Immunosuppression
General Principles: Most of the immunosuppressive regimens used in clinical transplantation consist of a combination of several agents used concurrently and use several general principles. The first general principle is that immune reactivity and tendency toward graft rejection are highest early (within the first 3–6 months) after graft implantation. Thus, most regimens target the highest levels of immunosuppression immediately after transplant and decrease those levels over the first year, eventually settling on the lowest maintenance levels of immune suppression required to prevent graft rejection and minimize drug toxicities. The second general principle is to use low doses of several drugs without overlapping toxicities in preference to higher (and more toxic) doses of fewer drugs whenever feasible. The third principle is that excessive immunosuppression is undesirable because it results in susceptibility to infection and malignancy.

Induction Therapy: Currently, about 50% of transplant programs use a strategy of augmented immunosuppression, or "induction" therapy, with antilymphocyte antibodies or interleukin-2 receptor antagonists during the early postoperative period.[93] The goal of induction therapy is to provide intense immunosuppression during a time when the risk of allograft

TABLE 52–8. Definition of Severity Scale for Primary Graft Dysfunction (PGD)

1. PGD–Left ventricle (PGD-LV):	*Mild PGD–LV: One* of the following criteria must be met:	LVEF ≤ 40% by echocardiography, *or* Hemodynamics with RAP >15 mm Hg, PCWP >20 mm Hg, CI <2.0 L/min/m² (lasting more than 1 hour) requiring low-dose inotropes
	Moderate PGD-LV: Must meet one criterion from I *and* another criterion from II:	I. *One* criteria from the following: Left ventricular ejection fraction ≤40%, *or* Hemodynamic compromise with RAP >15 mm Hg, PCWP >20 mm Hg, CI <2.0 L/min/m², hypotension with MAP <70 mm Hg (lasting more than 1 hour)
		II. *One* criteria from the following:
		i. High-dose inotropes—Inotrope score >10[a] *or*
		ii. Newly placed IABP (regardless of inotropes)
	Severe PGD–LV	Dependence on left or biventricular mechanical support including ECMO, LVAD, BiVAD, or percutaneous LVAD. Excludes requirement for IABP.
2. PGD-right ventricle (PGD-RV):	Diagnosis requires either both i and ii, or iii alone:	i. Hemodynamics with RAP >15 mm Hg, PCWP <15 mm Hg, CI <2.0 L/min/m² ii. TPG <15 mm Hg and/or pulmonary artery systolic pressure <50 mm Hg, *or* iii. Need for RVAD

Abbreviations: BiVAD, biventricular assist device; CI, cardiac index; ECMO, extracorporeal membrane oxygenation; IABP, intra-aortic balloon pump; LVAD, left ventricular assist device; PCWP, pulmonary capillary wedge pressure; RAP, right atrial pressure; RVAD, right ventricular assist device; TPG, transpulmonary pressure gradient.

[a]Inotrope score = dopamine (×1) + dobutamine (×1) + amrinone (×1) + milrinone (×15) + epinephrine (×100) + norepinephrine (×100) with each drug dosed in µg/kg/min.

Reproduced with permission from Kobashigawa J, Zuckermann A, Macdonald P, et al. Report from a consensus conference on primary graft dysfunction after cardiac transplantation. *J Heart Lung Transplant.* 2014 Apr;33(4):327-340.

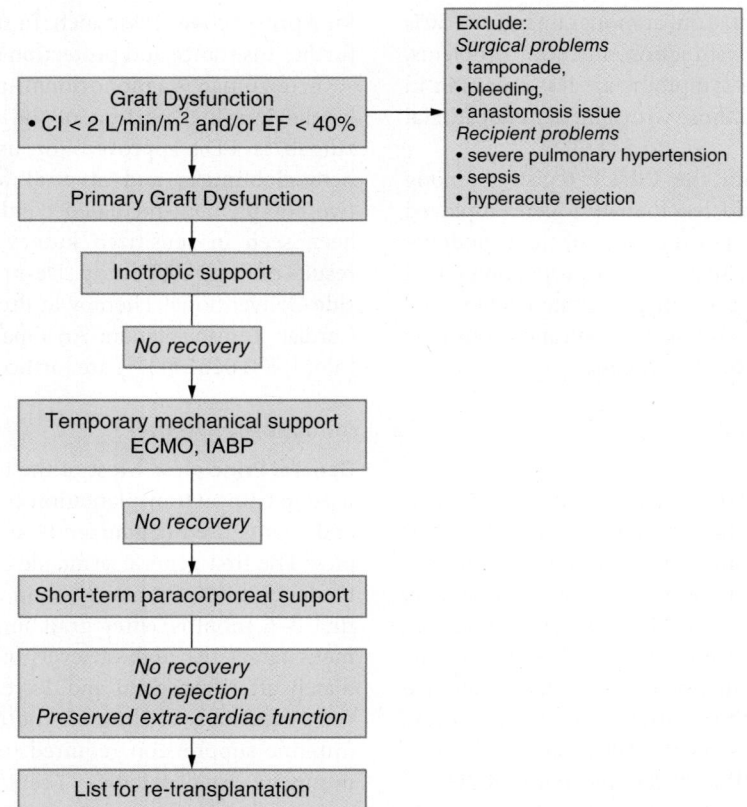

Figure 52–13. Management of primary graft dysfunction (PGD). The first step in the management of PGD is to exclude treatable/reversible causes. Once surgical and recipient factors have been excluded, the treatment is supportive. For select patients with refractory graft dysfunction and preserved end-organ function, urgent listing for retransplantation may be considered, although outcomes are worse. ECMO, extracorporeal membrane oxygenation; EF, ejection fraction; IABP, intraaortic balloon pump. Modified with permission from Kittleson MM. Changing Role of Heart Transplantation. *Heart Fail Clin.* 2016 Jul; 12(3):411-421.

rejection is highest. Additionally, induction therapy allows delayed initiation of nephrotoxic immunosuppressive drugs in patients with compromised renal function. Agents used for induction therapy include polyclonal antithymocyte antibodies derived by immunization of horses (ATGAM) or rabbits (thymoglobulin) with human thymocytes. These agents may reduce the risk of early rejection but have been associated with an increased risk of infection.[148,149]

Anti–interleukin-2 (IL-2) receptor antagonists such as daclizumab result in reduced rates of moderate or severe cellular rejection among heart transplant patients treated with standard immunosuppression (cyclosporine, mycophenolate mofetil [MMF], and corticosteroids) without increasing the incidence of opportunistic infection or cancer at 1 year. However, among patients receiving daclizumab induction, there was an increased risk of fatal infection when cytolytic therapy was concomitantly used.[150] While daclizumab is no longer manufactured, basiliximab is currently available for use as an induction therapy. Although induction therapy is commonly used, there have been no large, randomized trials or registry analyses conclusively demonstrating benefit or harm from induction therapy.

Maintenance Immunosuppression: Most maintenance immunosuppressive protocols use a three-drug regimen consisting

of a CNI (cyclosporine or tacrolimus), an antimetabolite agent (MMF or azathioprine), and tapering doses of corticosteroids over the first year posttransplantation. The commonly used drugs and their toxicities are outlined in **Table 52–9**. Recent trends in the use of these drugs are presented in **Fig. 52–14**.

The CNIs exert their immunosuppressive effects by inhibiting calcineurin, which is responsible for the transcription of IL-2 and several other cytokines, including tumor necrosis factor-α (TNF-α), granulocyte-macrophage colony-stimulating factor, and interferon-β. The result is blunting of T-lymphocyte activation and proliferation in response to alloantigens. The two available agents, cyclosporine and tacrolimus, inhibit calcineurin by forming complexes with different intracellular binding proteins. Since the introduction of cyclosporine in the early 1980s, the CNIs have remained the cornerstone of maintenance immunosuppressive therapy in patients undergoing solid organ transplantation. Tacrolimus is favored over cyclosporine as tacrolimus-based immunosuppression may be associated with decreased risk of acute rejection.[151,152] While nephrotoxicity is seen with both agents, cyclosporine is associated with more hypertension and dyslipidemia and tacrolimus is associated with a higher incidence of new-onset insulin-requiring diabetes.[153,154]

MMF has replaced azathioprine as the preferred antimetabolite agent based on a randomized clinical trial demonstrating

TABLE 52–9. Common Immunosuppressive Agents Used in Heart Transplantation

Drug	Typical Dose	Major Toxicities
Calcineurin inhibitors		
Cyclosporine	3–6 mg/kg/d in two divided doses titrated to keep therapeutic 12-h trough levels*	Renal dysfunction Hypertension Dyslipidemia Hypokalemia and hypomagnesemia Hyperuricemia Neurotoxicity (encephalopathy, seizures, tremors, neuropathy) Gingival hyperplasia Hirsutism
Tacrolimus	0.02–0.04 mg/kg/d in two divided doses titrated to keep therapeutic 12-h trough levels	Renal dysfunction Hypertension Hyperglycemia and diabetes mellitus Dyslipidemia Hyperkalemia Hypomagnesemia Neurotoxicity (tremors, headaches)
Antimetabolite agents		
Azathioprine	1.0–3.5 mg/kg/d, titrated to keep WBC ~3000K	Bone marrow suppression Hepatitis (rare) Pancreatitis Malignancy
Mycophenolate mofetil	2000–3000 mg/d in two divided doses titrated to tolerance	GI disturbances (nausea, diarrhea) Leukopenia
Proliferation signal inhibitors		
Sirolimus	0.5–2 mg daily titrated to keep therapeutic 24-h trough levels	Oral ulcerations Hypercholesterolemia and hypertriglyceridemia Poor wound healing Lower extremity edema Pleural and pericardial effusions Pulmonary toxicities (interstitial pneumonitis, alveolar hemorrhage) Bone marrow suppression (leukopenia, anemia, and thrombocytopenia) Potentiation of calcineurin inhibitor–mediated nephrotoxicity
Everolimus	1.5mg/d in two divided doses	Similar to sirolimus with less marked impairment in wound healing
Prednisone	≤1 mg/kg/d in two divided doses, usually rapidly tapered to 0–0.05 mg/kg/d by 6–12 months	Weight gain Hypertension Hyperlipidemia Osteopenia Hyperglycemia Poor wound healing Salt and water retention Proximal myopathy Cataracts Peptic ulcer disease Growth retardation

Abbreviations: GI, gastrointestinal; WBC, white blood cell.

*Two-hour peak cyclosporine levels are more reliable but are not practical and not routinely performed.

a significant reduction in both mortality and in the incidence of treated rejection at 1 year with MMF versus azathioprine.[155] Mycophenolate sodium is an enteric-coated, delayed-release formulation developed to improve the upper gastrointestinal tolerability of MMF. It is therapeutically similar to MMF with respect to the prevention of biopsy-proven and treated acute rejection episodes, graft loss, and death.[156]

PSIs, or mammalian target of rapamycin (mTOR) inhibitors, are more recent advances in maintenance immunosuppression. The two agents in this class, sirolimus and everolimus, inhibit the proliferation of T cells, B cells, and vascular smooth muscle cells in response to growth factor and cytokine signals. Compared with azathioprine, both sirolimus and everolimus reduce the incidence of acute rejection and prevent the development

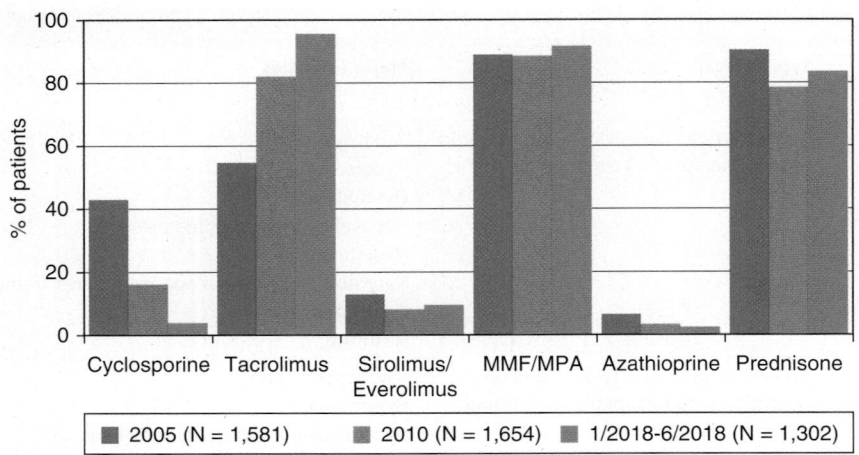

Figure 52–14. Trends in maintenance immunosuppression at 1 year in adult heart transplant recipients. MMF, mycophenolate mofetil. Data from Hayes D Jr, Cherikh WS, Chambers DC, et al. The International Thoracic Organ Transplant Registry of the International Society for Heart and Lung Transplantation: Twenty-second pediatric lung and heart-lung transplantation report-2019; Focus theme: Donor and recipient size match. *J Heart Lung Transplant.* 2019 Oct;38(10):1015-1027.

of cardiac allograft vasculopathy (CAV) when used in conjunction with cyclosporine and prednisone in de novo heart transplant recipients.[157,158] Compared to MMF, everolimus is noninferior with respect to the combined endpoint of rejection, graft loss, and death[159] and demonstrates less CAV progression as measured by intravascular ultrasound (IVUS) at 1 year.[160] Other benefits of sirolimus include slowing of CAV progression reduction in the incidence of clinically significant cardiac events.[161]

Sirolimus and everolimus are generally not initiated de novo post transplantation due to an increased risk of sternal wound dehiscence,[157] and due to exacerbation of the nephrotoxic effects of CNIs. However, based on the benefits observed in clinical trials, the PSIs can be initiated later after transplant for specific indications. The PSIs are often used in place of MMF in patients with rejection, allograft vasculopathy, malignancy, and viral infections such as cytomegalovirus[162] to prevent recurrence or progression. When used in place of the CNI, the PSIs may prevent progression of renal dysfunction.

In the SCHEDULE[163] and MANDELA[164] trials, when the CNI was withdrawn within 3 to 6 months of transplant with conversion to PSI in addition to MMF, patients had improved renal function (and in the SCHEDULE trial, less CAV as measured by intravascular ultrasound) by 1 year compared to those maintained on CNI along with MMF and corticosteroids. However, the renal benefits of the CNI-free regimen came at a cost of more frequent episodes of biopsy-proven rejection. This concern of has limited widespread implementation of CNI-free regimens, which are generally tailored to those patients over 1-year posttransplant with significant renal dysfunction who are also at low risk for rejection.

Corticosteroids are nonspecific anti-inflammatory agents that interrupt multiple steps in immune activation, including antigen presentation, cytokine production, and proliferation of lymphocytes. Although steroids are highly effective for the prevention and treatment of acute rejection, their long-term use is associated with new-onset or worsening diabetes mellitus, hyperlipidemia, hypertension, fluid retention, myopathy, osteoporosis, and a predisposition toward opportunistic infections. Thus, although corticosteroids are used in relatively high doses in the early postoperative period, they are then tapered to low doses or discontinued altogether within the first 6 to 12 months.

Although dual- or triple-drug therapy are the most commonly used strategies for maintenance immunosuppression after heart transplantation, single-drug therapy using tacrolimus following early withdrawal of corticosteroids and MMF has also been shown to be safe and efficacious.[165] However, this strategy required higher tacrolimus trough levels that resulted in higher serum creatinine levels at 1 year.

Drug Interactions

In managing patients on immunosuppressive drug therapy, clinicians should be aware of the potential for drug interactions when other agents are added to or removed from the patient's regimen.[166] A list of the most common and clinically important drug interactions is shown in **Table 52–10**. The CNIs and PSIs are predominantly metabolized by the cytochrome P450 3A4 pathway in the liver. Drugs that induce the P450 3A4 pathway, such as phenytoin, rifampin, and St. John's wort, enhance the metabolism of the CNIs and PSIs, thus lowering their blood levels and clinical effectiveness. Alternatively, drugs that inhibit the enzyme pathway such as calcium channel blockers, antifungal agents, and HIV protease inhibitors, decrease the metabolism of cyclosporine, tacrolimus, or sirolimus, thus increase their drug levels and potentiating their nephrotoxic effects. Finally, the lipid-lowering agents lovastatin, atorvastatin, and simvastatin have decreased clearance and increased drug concentrations when used concurrently with the CNIs. Therefore, the use of higher doses of these statins may lead to an increased risk of myopathy or rhabdomyolysis. When a drug with the potential to interact with the immunosuppressive agents is added to or removed from a patient's regimen, immunosuppressive drug levels and renal function should be carefully monitored.

TABLE 52–10. Important Drug Interactions	
Drugs that increase levels of CNIs and PSIs (inhibitors of cytochrome P450 3A4)	
Calcium channel blockers	Diltiazem Nifedipine Nicardipine Verapamil
Antifungal drugs	Itraconazole Fluconazole Ketoconazole Voriconazole Posaconazole
Macrolide antibiotics	All
Fluoroquinolone antibiotics	Ciprofloxacin
HIV protease inhibitors	All
Antiarrhythmic agents	Amiodarone
Gastrointestinal agents	Metoclopramide
Miscellaneous	Grapefruit juice
Drugs that decrease levels of CNIs and PSIs (inducers of cytochrome P450 3A4)	
Antitubercular drugs	Rifampin
Antiseizure drugs	Phenytoin Phenobarbital
Miscellaneous	St. John's wort
Drugs with synergistic nephrotoxicity when used with CNIs	
Aminoglycoside antibiotics	
Amphotericin B	
Colchicine	
NSAIDs	
Drugs whose concentrations are increased when used with CNIs	
Lovastatin	
Simvastatin	
Atorvastatin	
Ezetimibe	

Abbreviations: GI, gastrointestinal; NSAID, nonsteroidal anti-inflammatory drug, CNI, calcineurin inhibitor, PSI, proliferation signal inhibitor.

Recognition and Treatment of Acute Rejection

Diagnosis

Transplant rejection remains one of the major causes of death after heart transplantation[32] and is classified as hyperacute rejection, acute cellular rejection (ACR), or antibody-mediated rejection (AMR). In the current era, 12.6% of heart transplant recipients experience some form of rejection within the first year posttransplant.[93] The incidence of specific forms of rejection is not further classified in registry analyses, but a survey of 5406 patients from 67 heart transplant centers indicated that AMR occurred in approximately 6% of recipients.[104] Hyperacute rejection is rare but may occur in the setting of circulating preformed antibodies to the ABO blood group (in cases of ABO blood group incompatibility) or to major histocompatability antigens in the donor. Possible risk factors include presensitization following after blood transfusions, multiparity, and previous organ grafts.[167] Hyperacute rejection manifests as severe graft failure within the first few minutes to hours after transplantation. Without inotropic and mechanical circulatory support, plasmapheresis, and intense immunosuppression, the recipient usually does not survive.

While the presentation of hyperacute rejection is dramatic, the signs and symptoms of acute rejection are generally nonspecific and may only manifest in the late stages. Patients may present with fatigue, low-grade fevers, HF symptoms, or hypotension. Occasionally, rejection will manifest as atrial arrhythmias or new pericardial effusions. On examination, patients may have an elevated jugular venous pressure or a new S3 gallop. However, the majority of patients with acute cellular or AMR are asymptomatic without signs of allograft dysfunction.

Because symptoms are often vague, routine testing for rejection is standard practice. Unlike renal or liver transplantation, there are no laboratory markers for rejection in heart transplantation and the endomyocardial biopsy remains the cornerstone of rejection surveillance. It is performed via the right internal jugular vein or femoral vein by introducing a bioptome into the RV and obtaining three to five pieces of endomyocardium, typically from the RV septum (**Fig. 52–15**).

While the timing of biopsies will vary from center to center, in general biopsies are performed frequently early after transplantation and less frequently over time. Most programs perform surveillance biopsies on a weekly basis for the first 4 to 6 postoperative weeks and then with diminishing frequency in a stable patient but at a minimum of every 3 months

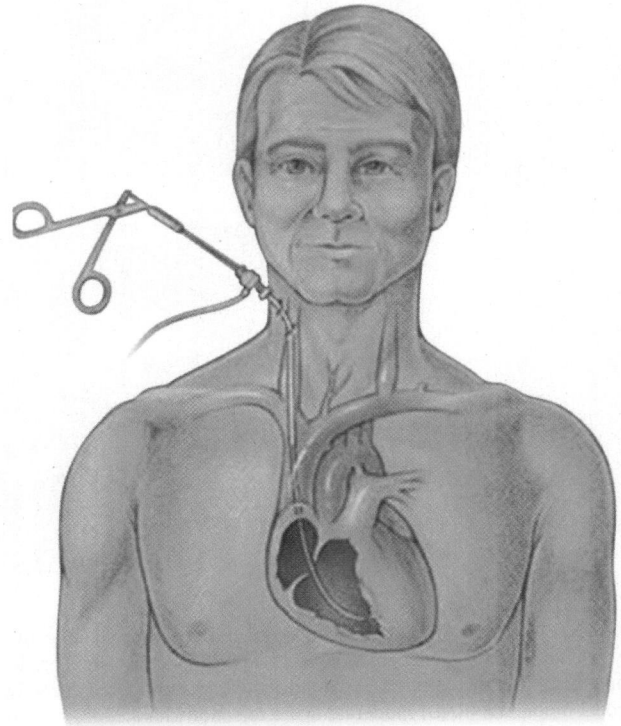

Figure 52–15. Endomyocardial biopsy via the right internal jugular vein.

for the first postoperative year. The need for continued surveillance biopsies after the first year in clinically stable patients has been questioned.[168,169]

The purpose of the endomyocardial biopsy is to assess for myocardial damage in the form of ACR (**Fig. 52–16**) or AMR (**Fig. 52–17**). The ISHLT grading scales for diagnosis of ACR[170] and AMR[171] are shown in **Tables 52–11** and **52–12**, respectively.

While not required for the diagnosis of AMR, many centers also perform screening for antibodies against HLA post-transplantation. Strong-, and especially complement-binding,

donor-specific anti-HLA antibodies (DSA) are considered potentially cytotoxic.[106,172] Their presence may merit a change in treatment, depending on the clinical situation, as subsequently discussed.

While the gold standard for diagnosis of rejection relies on histology for ACR and histology and immunopathology for AMR, there is a significant interobserver variability with only 28% agreement between pathologists when evaluating samples graded ≥2R in one study.[173] There are emerging innovative molecular techniques to improve the accuracy of current endomyocardial biopsy grading methods.

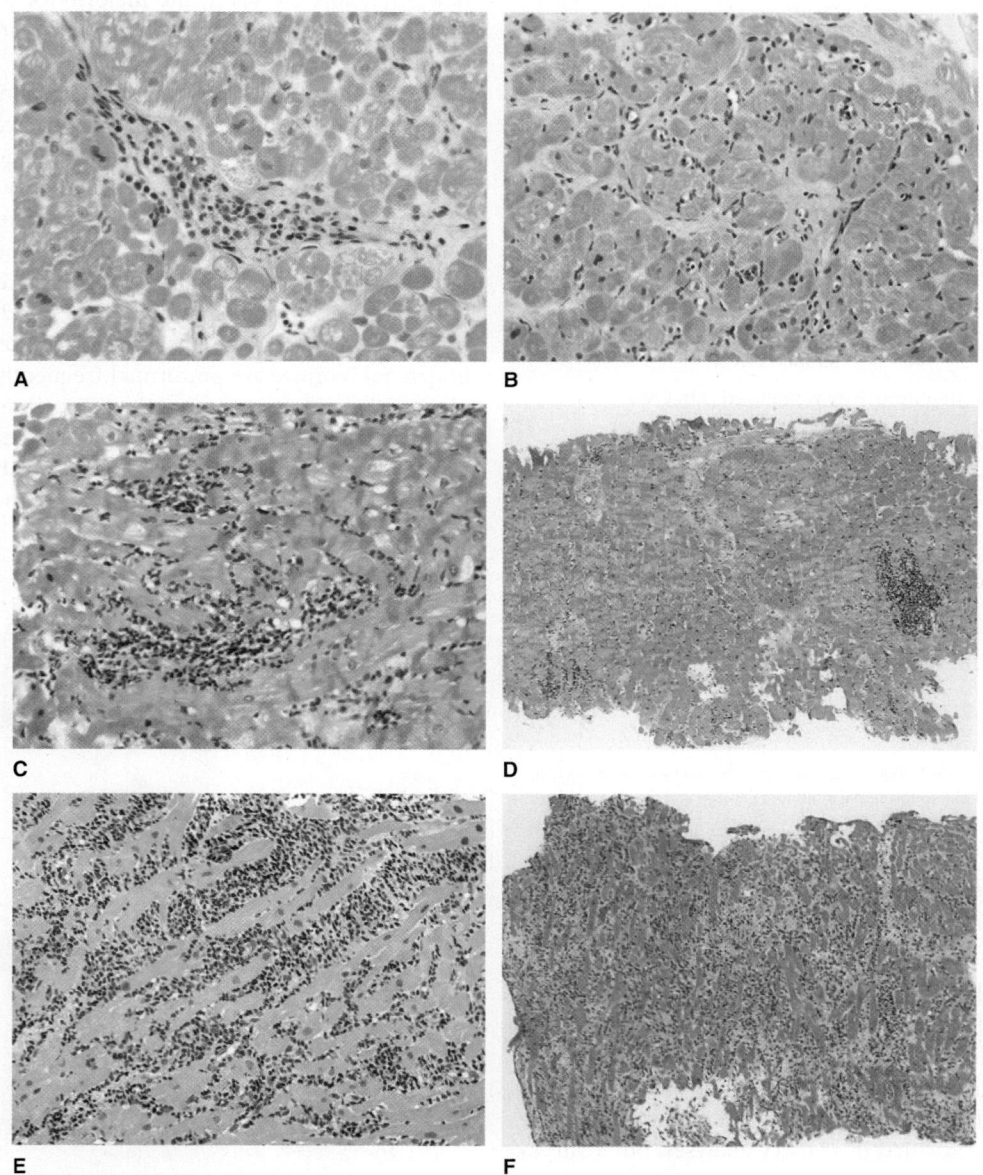

Figure 52–16. 2004 ISHLT acute cellular rejection grading scheme. (A) Mild acute rejection characterized by a perivascular cuff of mononuclear inflammatory cells without myocyte damage. This corresponds to focal mild grade 1R. **(B)** Mild acute rejection characterized by a diffuse interstitial pattern. This corresponds to diffuse mild grade 1R. **(C)** Mild acute rejection characterized by a solitary focus of mononuclear cells with rare myocyte damage. This corresponds to focal moderate 1R. **(D)** Moderate acute rejection characterized by multiple foci of inflammation and myocyte damage. This corresponds to multifocal moderate 2R. **(E)** Severe acute rejection showing dense interstitial infiltrates and myocyte damage. This corresponds to diffuse moderate, borderline severe grade 3R. **(F)** Severe acute rejection corresponding to grade 3R.

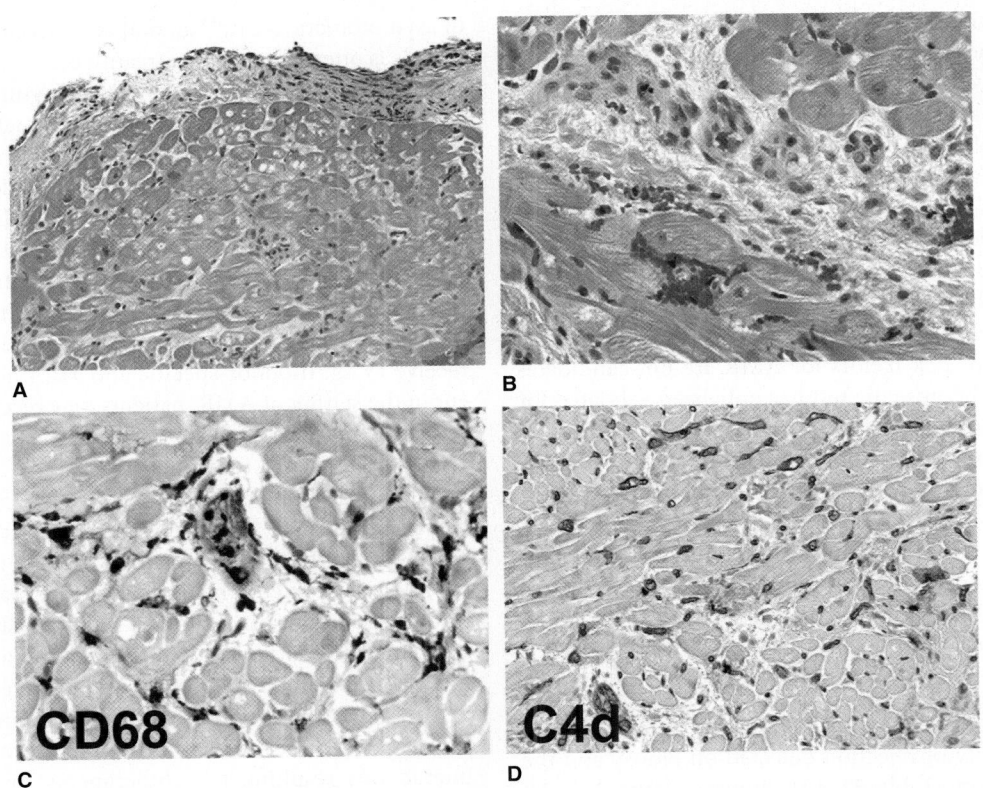

Figure 52–17. Acute antibody-mediated (humoral) rejection. (A) Scanning magnification of endomyocardial biopsy specimen showing a mononuclear cell infiltrate within the endocardium. In the central part of the figure, the small vessel displays prominent endothelial cells. **(B)** High-power magnification showing endothelial cell hyperplasia and perivascular edema. **(C)** CD68 staining of interstitial and intravascular histiocytes. **(D)** Strong, uniform staining of the microvascular for C4d, a marker of complement activation and deposition.

The Molecular Microscope System (MMDx™) is a diagnostic approach initially described in kidney transplant recipients that has been adapted for heart transplantation. The MMDx™ system measures specific mRNA transcripts that represent various immune pathways in the allograft biopsy specimen and is designed to more accurately diagnose both ACR and AMR compared to histology.[174] An ongoing prospective study (the INTERHEART trial [NCT02670408]) will compare the

TABLE 52–11. International Society for Heart and Lung Transplant Standardized Cardiac Biopsy Grading: Acute Cellular Rejection

Grade	Description	Prior classification
0R	No rejection	0
1R, mild	Interstitial and/or perivascular infiltrate with up to one focus of myocyte damage	1A, 1B, 2
2R, moderate	Two or more foci of infiltrate with associated myocyte damage	3A
3R, severe	Diffuse infiltrate with multifocal myocyte damage ± edema ± hemorrhage ± vasculitis	3B, 4

Data from Stewart S, Winters GL, Fishbein MC, et al. Revision of the 1990 working formulation for the standardization of nomenclature in the diagnosis of heart rejection. *J Heart Lung Transplant*. 2005 Nov;24(11):1710-1720.

TABLE 52–12. International Society for Heart and Lung Transplant Standardized Cardiac Biopsy Grading: Acute Antibody-Mediated Rejection

Grade	Definition	Substrates
pAMR 0	Negative for pathologic AMR	Histologic and immunopathologic studies are both negative.
pAMR 1 (H+)	Histopathologic AMR alone	Histologic findings are present and immunopathologic findings are negative.
pAMR 1 (I+)	Immunopathologic AMR alone	Histologic findings are negative and immunopathologic findings are positive (CD68+ and/or C4d+).
pAMR 2	Pathologic AMR	Histologic and immunopathologic findings are both present.
pAMR 3	Severe pathologic AMR	Interstitial hemorrhage, capillary fragmentation, mixed inflammatory infiltrates, endothelial cell pyknosis, and/or karyorrhexis, and marked edema and immunopathologic findings are present. These cases may be associated with profound hemodynamic dysfunction and poor clinical outcomes.

Reproduced with permission from Berry GJ, Burke MM, Andersen C, et al. The 2013 International Society for Heart and Lung Transplantation Working Formulation for the standardization of nomenclature in the pathologic diagnosis of antibody-mediated rejection in heart transplantation. *J Heart Lung Transplant*. 2013 Dec; 32(12):1147-1162.

molecular microscope to the current standard of care in diagnosing cellular and AMR. Although the MMDx™ does not overcome the procedural risk of the endomyocardial biopsy, it may be a more reliable standard to assess noninvasive methods for the diagnosis of rejection.

The gene expression profile (GEP) test (AlloMap®, CareDx Inc., Brisbane, CA), an 11-gene expression signature derived from peripheral blood mononuclear cells, has a high negative predictive value for the presence of ACR,[175] is noninferior to the biopsy in the diagnosis of ACR,[176] and may be useful early posttransplant.[177] However, it must be emphasized that patients with a history of, or risk factors for AMR are not candidates for GEP screening because the test has only been validated for ACR.

Another emerging technology in the noninvasive diagnosis of rejection involves cell-free DNA technology (AlloSure®; CareDx, Inc., Brisbane, CA). Donor-derived cell-free DNA is detectable in both the urine and blood of transplant recipients.[178,179] Increased levels of donor-derived cell-free DNA correlate with ACR and AMR events as determined by endomyocardial biopsy.[180]

Treatment

The management of rejection proceeds in a step-wise fashion based on the severity of rejection detected on biopsy and the patient's presentation (**Table 52–13**). Biopsies with grade 1R or AMR1, in the absence of clinical or hemodynamic compromise, may merit no intervention.

More serious findings on the biopsy, including grade 2R or higher and AMR1h, AMR2, or higher warrant treatment. The intensity of treatment depends on the patient's clinical presentation. If the patient is asymptomatic (no HF symptoms and normal LVEF), treatment options include oral pulse steroids, targeting higher levels of immunosuppressive medications, switching from cyclosporine to tacrolimus,[151,152,181] or switching from MMF to a PSI.[159,182] Given the equivalent success of intravenous and oral corticosteroid therapy for the treatment

of asymptomatic ACR,[183] an outpatient course of oral corticosteroids is often the first-line treatment.

Asymptomatic AMR is more challenging. It may be associated with poor outcomes,[184,186] but it is unclear whether treatment affects outcomes. At some centers, such patients will receive an oral corticosteroid bolus, consideration of intravenous immune globulin, and monitoring of DSA.[104]

For patients with HF symptoms or reduced ejection fraction, treatment is more aggressive, with intravenous corticosteroids and cytolytic therapy with antithymocyte globulin. If there is evidence of AMR2 or higher, patients will also often receive IV Ig. If donor-specific anti-HLA antibodies are present in the setting of AMR, patients may receive more intensive therapy with rituximab or bortezomib. Plasmapheresis may also be used in this setting.

Finally, in patients presenting with cardiogenic shock, empiric aggressive treatment includes intravenous corticosteroids, cytolytic therapy, plasmapheresis, IV Ig, eculizumab (if AMR suspected), heparin (because patients often have thrombotic occlusion of the cardiac microvasculature on postmortem examination),[187,188] and hemodynamic support with intra-aortic balloon counterpulsation or even ECMO.[146]

Any rejection episode should prompt an investigation for precipitating causes such as infection, noncompliance, or drug interactions resulting in subtherapeutic immunosuppressive drug levels. A biopsy should be repeated 2 weeks after completion of treatment to document improvement or resolution of the rejection episode.

Long-Term Management

While ACR is often successfully treated with corticosteroids and cytolytic therapy, resulting in a resolution of HF and normalization of the ejection fraction, management of AMR is often more complicated. Patients may have a persistent reduction in ejection fraction, restrictive physiology with recurrent HF, and accelerated progression of transplant CAD.[185]

TABLE 52–13. Treatment of Acute Cellular and Antibody-Mediated Rejection

	Asymptomatic	Reduced EF	Heart Failure/Shock
Cellular Rejection	• Target higher CNI levels • Oral steroid bolus + taper • MMF → PSI	• Oral steroid bolus/taper or • IV pulse steroids	*Treat based on clinical presentation; do not await biopsy findings* • IV pulse steroids • Cytolytic therapy (ATG) • Plasmapheresis (before ATG dose) • IV immune globulin • Inotropic therapy • IV heparin • IABP or ECMO support
Antibody-Mediated Rejection with no/↓ DSA	• Target higher CNI levels • MMF → PSI	• IV pulse steroids • consider IV immune globulin	
Antibody-Mediated Rejection with ↑DSA	• Oral steroid bolus + taper • MMF → PSI • Consider IV immune globulin and rituximab	• IV pulse steroids • IV immune globulin • consider ATG, rituximab or bortezomib	

Patients receiving augmented immunosuppression with high-dose steroids or ATG should also be given prophylaxis against pneumocystis pneumonia and cytomegalovirus.
Reproduced with permission from Kittleson MM, Kobashigawa JA. Long-term care of the heart transplant recipient. *Curr Opin Organ Transplant.* 2014 Oct;19(5):515-524.

The management of such patients with a persistent drop in ejection fraction after treatment of symptomatic rejection is not well established. Some centers rely on therapies to reduce the levels of DSA, including rituximab and bortezomib, as well as photopheresis to alter the function of T cells.[104] In small case series, such therapies have shown benefit,[189,190] although such patients often go on to require redo heart transplantation.

Cardiac Allograft Vasculopathy

Incidence and Clinical Presentation

The incidence of CAV varies widely due to differences in definition of disease and patient populations, but by various estimates ranges from 42% at 5 years to 50% at 10 years.[93] CAV can occur as early as one year after transplantation and this accelerated form of disease is more aggressive and associated with a worse prognosis.[91] Even in patients without apparent angiographic epicardial disease, microvascular abnormalities may be present and are associated with adverse outcomes.[192] Despite improvements in immunosuppression over the last three decades, the incidence of CAV has not significantly decreased, and its development continues to limit long-term posttransplant survival.

Over time, patients may develop cardiac reinnervation, and chest pain due to ischemia and infarction in transplant patients has been documented.[140,193,194] However, given the denervation of the transplanted heart, patients usually do not experience typical angina and the presentation of CAV differs from that of nontransplant CAD (**Table 52–14**). Thus, routine surveillance angiography is performed in cardiac transplant recipients.

Morphologic Features

In CAV, the major epicardial vessels, their branches, and often the intramyocardial divisions display uniform, diffuse involvement extending along their entire length (**Fig. 52–18**). The asymmetric and calcified plaques or lesions composed of cholesterol that are characteristic of conventional atherosclerosis are not found in uncomplicated lesions of vessels affected by CAV. Histopathologic sections show a concentrically thickened intimal layer composed of modified smooth muscle cells, foamy macrophages, and variable numbers of histiocytes and lymphocytes within a connective tissue matrix that ranges

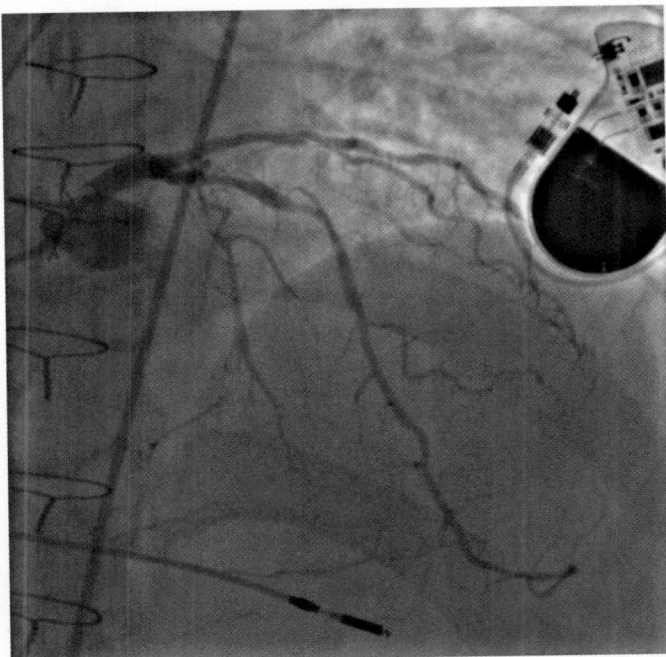

Figure 52–18. Coronary angiogram in a patient with severe cardiac allograft vasculopathy showing diffuse disease of the left anterior descending coronary artery, occlusion of the left circumflex coronary artery, and obliteration of the obtuse marginal branches.

from loose, edematous, and myxoid in early lesions to densely hyalinized and fibrotic in older lesions. Intraluminal thrombosis is uncommon.

Diagnosis

CAV is usually beyond therapeutic intervention by the time symptoms develop, so surveillance is essential to monitor the development of CAV and graded by the ISHLT grading scheme (**Table 52–15**).[195] Coronary angiography remains the mainstay of CAV detection, although it has limitations. Coronary angiography relies upon the ability to compare normal segments of the vessel with diseased segments. The diffuse nature of CAV often results in underestimation of disease because there is no reference segment in which the normal diameter of the vessel can be assessed. Comparison with prior studies may help but requires the use of the same angiographic protocol at each study to avoid confounding by technical factors.

IVUS offers cross-sectional images of the coronary vessel wall comparable to histological sections to detect even early plaque burden (**Fig. 52–19**). IVUS is more sensitive than angiography in detecting CAV[196–199] and has prognostic value: progression of intimal thickening greater than 0.5 mm in the first year after transplantation is associated with an increased risk of death and development of angiographic CAV up to 5 years later.[160]

Optical coherence tomography (OCT) is another intravascular imaging modality that employs long wavelengths of light, typically near-infrared, which penetrate the coronary vessel wall, allowing for a 10-fold increase in spatial resolution over

TABLE 52–14. Cardiac Allograft Vasculopathy versus Coronary Artery Disease in Nontransplant Patients	
Nontransplant Atherosclerosis	**Cardiac Allograft Vasculopathy**
Mainly epicardial disease	Panvascular disease (may include microvasculature)
Slower progression	Rapid progression
Eccentic lesions	Concentric lesions (usually)
Lipid rich	Generally lipid poor
Early calcification	Late calcification

Modified with permission from Kittleson MM, Kobashigawa JA. Management of the ACC/AHA Stage D patient: cardiac transplantation. *Cardiol Clin.* 2014 Feb;32(1):95-112.

TABLE 52–15. Standardized Nomenclature for Cardiac Allograft Vasculopathy

ISHLT CAV$_0$ (Not significant)	No detectable angiographic lesion
ISHLT CAV$_1$ (Mild)	Angiographic left main (LM) <50%, or primary vessel with maximum lesion of <70%, or any branch stenosis <70% (including diffuse narrowing) without allograft dysfunction
ISHLT CAV$_2$ (Moderate)	Angiographic LM <50%; a single primary vessel ≥70%, or isolated branch stenosis ≥70% in branches of 2 systems, without allograft dysfunction
ISHLT CAV$_3$ (Severe)	Angiographic LM ≥50%, or two or more primary vessels ≥70% stenosis, or isolated branch stenosis ≥70% in all 3 systems; or ISHLT CAV1 or CAV2 with allograft dysfunction (defined as LVEF ≤45% usually in the presence of regional wall motion abnormalities) or evidence of significant restrictive physiology (which is common but not specific; see text for definitions)

Definitions

a). A "Primary Vessel" denotes the proximal and middle 33% of the left anterior descending artery, the left circumflex, the ramus and the dominant or codominant right coronary artery with the posterior descending and posterolateral branches.

b). A "Secondary Branch Vessel" includes the distal 33% of the primary vessels or any segment within a large septal perforator, diagonals and obtuse marginal branches or any portion of a nondominant right coronary artery.

c). Restrictive cardiac allograft physiology is defined as symptomatic heart failure with echocardiographic E to A velocity ratio >2 (>1.5 in children), shortened isovolumetric relaxation time (<60 ms), shortened deceleration time (<150 ms), or restrictive hemodynamic values (Right Atrial Pressure >12 mm Hg, Pulmonary Capillary Wedge Pressure >25 mm Hg, Cardiac Index <2 L/min/m^2)

Adapted with permission from Mehra MR, Crespo-Leiro MG, Dipchand A, et al. International Society for Heart and Lung Transplantation working formulation of a standardized nomenclature for cardiac allograft vasculopathy-2010. *J Heart Lung Transplant.* 2010 Jul;29(7):717-727.

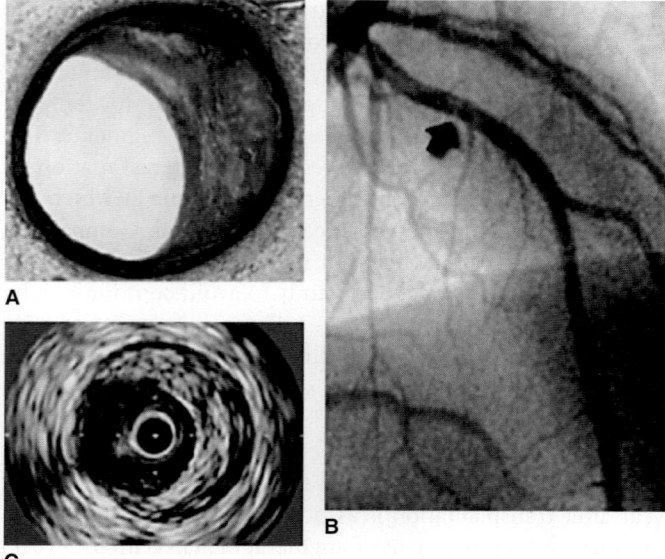

Figure 52–19. Concentric or eccentric subintimal proliferation in CAV seen histologically (A) are underestimated in lesion severity angiographically (B) but are better appreciated by IVUS (C). Reproduced with permission from Ahsan N. *Chronic allograft failure: natural history, pathogenesis, diagnosis and management.* Austin, TX: CRC Press; 2007.

IVUS. Since the normal intimal thickness is below the resolution of IVUS, OCT might in theory also allow the detection of intimal changes earlier in the natural history of CAV. In early studies, demonstrated that markers of plaque vulnerability demonstrated in heart transplant recipients by OCT—lipid pools, a thin fibrous cap, macrophages, and microchannels—observed at 1-year posttransplantation were predictive for CAV progression over time.[200]

Given the variable development of CAV, identification of specific trajectories would allow for more individually tailored CAV surveillance protocols. A prospective observational multicenter international study identified four distinct trajectories associated with distinct prognoses: (1) CAV trajectory 1: no CAV at 1 year and stable over time with 10-year survival 80%; (2) CAV trajectory 2: no CAV at 1 year, with a slight increase starting 4 years after transplantation with 10-year survival 83%; (3) CAV trajectory 3: intermediate CAV grade at 1 year with moderate increase during follow-up and 10-year survival 73%; and (4) CAV trajectory 4: intermediate CAV at 1 year and acceleration over time; 10-year survival 52%.[191] Independent predictive variables of CAV trajectories were donor age, donor sex, donor tobacco consumption, recipient low-density lipoprotein cholesterol (LDL-C) ≥1 g/dL 1 year after transplantation, recipient immunologic profile as defined by the presence of preexisting or de novo circulating class II anti–HLA donor-specific antibodies, and allograft injury defined by acute cellular rejection ≥2R occurring in the first year after transplantation.

Treatment

Clinically apparent CAV is associated with a poor prognosis and therefore prevention is an important strategy. Aspirin is given, due to its established role in nontransplant coronary disease. Control of hypertension and hyperlipidemia is paramount. HMG Co-A reductase inhibitors are particularly important because they also prevent allograft rejection in addition to reducing CAV development.[201] The PSIs also show significant promise in reducing the progression of intimal thickening by IVUS.[158,159,161,182]

Once clinically significant CAV is apparent, PCI is successful for focal disease, although restenosis is common and there is no evidence to date that PCI alters the prognosis of CAV. Drug-eluting stents may help, but restenosis rates continue to be higher than in the nontransplant population.[202-204] Patients with multivessel focal disease with adequate distal target vessels may be candidates for surgical revascularization with coronary artery bypass grafting, although this is rarely performed due to the rapid progression and diffuse nature of this disease.

Retransplantation may be considered for select patients with advanced CAV. After retransplantation, patients have comparable survival and CAV incidence to those patients undergoing a first transplant.[203] The scarcity of donor hearts, however, creates an ethical dilemma. Some argue that it is better to maximally distribute organs, rather than to allocate two organs to the same individual. Others contend that patients needing a second transplant should be considered on the same basis as those being evaluated for a first transplant.

Complications of Immunosuppression

Infection

Infections are the major cause of death during the first postoperative year and remain a threat throughout the life of a chronically immunosuppressed patient. Infections in the first postoperative month are commonly bacterial and typically related to indwelling catheters and wound infections. They involve nosocomial organisms such as *Legionella, Staphylococcus, Pseudomonas, Proteus, Klebsiella,* and *Escherichia coli.* These infections typically present in the form of pneumonias, urinary tract infections, sternal wound infections and mediastinitis, and bacteremia. Late infections (those that occur 2 months to 1 year after transplantation) are more diverse. In additional to typical pathogens, transplant patients are susceptible to viruses (particularly CMV), fungi (*Aspergillus, Candida,* and *Pneumocystis* spp.), *Mycobacterium* spp., *Nocardia* spp., and *Toxoplasma* spp. Effective therapy requires an aggressive approach to diagnosis and experience in recognizing the presentations of CMV, *Aspergillus* spp., and other opportunistic infectious agents.

Balancing the risks of infection and rejection with immunosuppression relies on an understanding of the patient's global immune state. An immune-monitoring assay (ImmuKnow®; Vircor-IBT, Lee's Summit, MO) performed on peripheral blood, which measures adenosine triphosphate (ATP) release from activated lymphocytes, may offer some guidance in profoundly immunosuppressed patients.[205,206] In heart transplant recipients, an immune monitoring score <200 was associated with a higher risk of infection within 1 month.[207] Thus, centers may target lower CNI trough levels or reduce MMF doses in patients with scores less than 200 ng ATP/mL, especially those with recurrent infections or malignancy.

Given the degree of immunosuppression, all transplant recipients receive antimicrobial prophylaxis for oral candidiasis, toxoplasmosis and pneumocystis, and cytomegalovirus over the first posttransplant year. The use of vaccines in heart transplant recipients remains controversial. Live vaccines are definitely contraindicated because of patients' immunosuppressed states. Even dead vaccines may pose a risk because they can promote activation of the immune system and cause rejection.[208] At some centers, dead vaccines such as the influenza or pneumococcal vaccines are recommended only to patients more than 6 months after transplant and with no history of rejection within the previous 6 months.

Malignancy

Incidence: Malignancy is one of the most common causes of late mortality in heart transplant recipients.[93] Malignancies are approximately 2- to 4-fold more common in heart compared with renal transplant recipients.[209–212] The enhanced risk of cancer among heart transplant recipients is thought to reflect the greater degree of immunosuppression in heart transplant recipients, possibly due to inherent immunologic requirements.[213]

All immunosuppressive agents are believed to contribute to the cumulative risk of malignancy, with the possible exception of corticosteroids. However, the PSIs sirolimus and everolimus may have a decreased incidence and progression of malignancy compared with CNIs and antimetabolites.[214–217]

Clinical Presentation: Cancer in solid organ transplant recipients usually presents at least 3 to 5 years posttransplantation. Cutaneous malignancies are the most common, mainly squamous cell and basal cell carcinomas.[218] Risk factors common to the general population for the development of skin cancers include fair skin, previous history of skin cancer, and geographic location (in areas of high sun exposure).[219] Specifically in heart transplant recipients, increased intensity of immunosuppression and long-term voriconazole use for treatment of fungal infections such as aspergillosis are associated with a higher increased risk of developing skin cancer.[220]

Posttransplant lymphoproliferative disorder (PTLD), most commonly a B-cell lymphoma related to Epstein-Barr virus (EBV) infection, may occur after transplantation.[221] More than 50% of patients with PTLD present with extranodal masses involving the gastrointestinal tract, lungs, skin, liver, central nervous system, and the allograft itself. Risk factors for the development of PTLD include the use of cytolytic therapy for induction[222] and EBV serostatus (with EBV-seronegative recipients of EBV-seropositive donors being at the highest risk).[223]

Neoplasms common in the general population also occur in heart transplant recipients, including breast, lung, and prostate. Lung cancer is more common in heart and lung transplant recipients than in recipients of other solid organs, likely because smoking, a strong risk factor for lung cancer, may also contribute to advanced heart and lung disease requiring transplantation.[224]

Prevention and Treatment: The most critical management of malignancies is prevention. Heart transplant recipients should undergo routine health maintenance screenings with their primary care physicians, including mammograms, pap smears, prostate exams, and colonoscopies as indicated for nontransplant patients. In addition, patients are instructed to utilize sun protection and to establish care with a dermatologist for routine skin exams.

The initial approach to malignancy is reduction of immunosuppression, and this may be the only treatment required for some forms of PTLD. Patients with newly diagnosed malignancy are often switched to a PSI such as sirolimus or everolimus, due to its possible beneficial effect in malignancies,[214–217] in place of a CNI or MMF.

General Medical Management

Heart transplant recipients should receive regular care from an internist for routine health maintenance. Such patients require the same general medical surveillance as nontransplant patients, including age-appropriate cancer screening. Internists also manage the long-term complications of heart transplant recipients, including renal dysfunction, hypertension, dyslipidemia, diabetes, osteoporosis, and gout. However, it is essential that patients inform the transplant center of any new medication recommended by another physician, because there may be unforeseen interactions (Table 52–10).

Renal dysfunction occurs in up to one-third of individuals and is related to the direct effects of the CNIs on the kidney tubules and from CNI–mediated vasoconstriction of the afferent arteriole, leading to decreased kidney perfusion. Renal insufficiency is a common adverse effect of the CNIs, and often worsens over time, such that up to 8% of heart transplant recipients will develop end-stage renal disease at 5 or more years posttransplant.[93,225,226] "Renal-sparing" immunosuppressive regimens are often utilized in such patients, including a reduction in CNI dose or substitution of the CNI with a PSI, as previously discussed in detail.

Hypertension after cardiac transplantation is primarily a result of CNI use and occurs in up to 80% of patients.[93] Posttransplant hypertension is often difficult to control and often requires a combination of several antihypertensive agents.[227,228] No agent has proven superior in clinical trials of renal[229–231] or heart transplant recipients.[232] However, β-blockers are less often used because the denervated heart relies on circulating catecholamines to maintain cardiac function during exercise, and thus heart transplant recipients often experience fatigue from β-blockers. Angiotensin-converting enzyme inhibitors and angiotensin receptor blockers may not be tolerated due to renal dysfunction or hyperkalemia. Dihydropyridine calcium channel blockers such as amlodipine and nifedipine are often effective, but may result in troublesome dependent edema and will increase levels of CNIs, which should be monitored after initiation.

Elevated lipid levels are common after heart transplantation, due to the use of steroids, CNIs, and PSIs.[233] Statins are effective in reducing total and LDL-C in heart transplant recipients. Notably, treatment initiated within 2 weeks of transplantation with statins is also associated with a lower frequency of hemodynamically compromising rejection episodes and improved survival over the first transplant year.[201] Pravastatin is the statin of choice, since it hydrophilic and is not metabolized by the cytochrome 3A4 system, reducing the possible interactions with CNIs.[166]

Diabetes is common pretransplantation because it increases the risk of cardiovascular disease. Furthermore, the use of steroids and tacrolimus posttransplant may cause or worsen diabetes; up to one-third of patients are diabetic by 5 years posttransplant.[93] While diabetes is associated with poorer long-term survival,[234] optimal treatment is not clear. Since renal insufficiency is common, metformin is often avoided. Sulfonylureas may be the agents of choice for heart transplant recipients.[166]

Osteoporosis resulting in vertebral compression fractures is a common and debilitating problem after heart transplantation, exacerbated by steroid use. Annual screening bone-density examinations may be useful for heart transplant recipients on chronic steroids. To prevent osteoporosis, patients should receive supplemental calcium and vitamin D, engage in weight-bearing exercises, and receive bisphosphonates as recommended by the primary care physician.

Gout is common after heart transplantation. In these patients, causes of gout include CNI use, diuretic use, and renal insufficiency. Nonsteroidal anti-inflammatory agents are often avoided in heart transplant recipients due to the potential of renal insufficiency. Colchicine may be used to treat acute attacks, although there is a risk of myoneuropathy when colchicine is combined with CNIs. Thus, for acute flares, systemic or intra-articular steroids may be considered. Allopurinol is useful as suppressive therapy as long as the patient is not receiving azathioprine, because the combination may result in severe myelosuppression.

Pediatric Heart Transplantation

Pediatric heart transplantation remains a relatively rare event with only about 700 transplants being reported globally on an annual basis.[235] From the early days, it became apparent that heart transplantation in children is quite different than in adults. The primary indication for transplant varies by age, with congenital heart disease (CHD) being the most common indication in infants (57%) and cardiomyopathy being the most common indication in older children (43% in children aged 1–10 years and 53% in children aged 11–17 years). Outcomes following pediatric transplantation surpass experience in adult transplantation with an overall median survival of more than 18 years. However, median survival varies widely by age at transplant and is highest (22 years) among patients who underwent transplantation in infancy and lowest (13 years) for those who received their transplant at age 11 to 17 years, which is comparable to outcomes in adults. Recipients that survive to 1-year posttransplant have excellent long-term survival, particularly infants, with more than 60% alive 25 years later. Rejection in the first year is associated with increased mortality.

As in adults, MCS as a bridge to heart transplantation is being increasingly utilized in children with about 37% of children supported to transplant on some form of MCS, mostly a durable VAD. Although more ill pretransplant, CHD patients bridged with a VAD appear to have similar posttransplant survival compared with CHD patients without a VAD and with other non-CHD heart transplant patients.[236]

Pediatric heart transplant recipients are at risk for allosensitization from a variety of factors including prior surgeries, blood product exposure, and the use of homografts for the repair of CHD. Allosensitization, (defined as a PRA level ≥ 10%, continues to increase among pediatric heart transplant recipients). In 2007, only 14% of recipients had allosensitization compared with 32% in 2017. Allosensitization is more common in older children than infants and among patients with CHD and retransplant than DCM or other types of heart disease.[235] While the increasing use of a VAD is associated with risk of sensitization, this does not appear to affect risk of posttransplant rejection or survival.[237]

Induction therapy with anti-thymocyte globulin (ATG) or interleukin 2 receptor antagonist (basiliximab) has been utilized in three quarters of pediatric transplants in the most recent era. The use of basiliximab has been associated with increased rejection and late graft loss compared to ATG in a matched registry cohort.[238] Advantages for ATG have been shown in low-risk patients given tacrolimus and MMF in a steroid-free regimen, in sensitized patients with preformed alloantibodies with or without a positive donor-specific crossmatch, and in ABO-incompatible (ABOi) pediatric heart transplantation. There appears to be no indication for increased risk of infection or posttransplant lymphoproliferative disorder in children receiving ATG after heart transplantation.[239]

Maintenance immunosuppression regimen reflects use in adults with the majority receiving tacrolimus with mycophenolate-based anti-proliferative. However, only two-thirds of patients are discharged on prednisone given the concern for its prolonged use on growth. While increased mortality has been associated with those patients developing acute rejection in the first year, overall rates of rejection have declined from 24% to 13% in the last two consecutive decades.[235] Interestingly, use of induction therapy does not appear to affect risk of rejection, although higher rates have been observed with cyclosporine compared to tacrolimus.

Although nearly 50% of all transplant recipients have developed CAV by 15 years posttransplant, freedom from CAV has improved in the recent era. The use of induction therapy may be associated with increased freedom from CAV.

The risk of developing malignancy increases over time posttransplant with 16% of survivors developing a malignancy by 15 years posttransplant.[235] The vast majority of malignancies are lymphomas and, in contrast to adult heart transplant recipients, skin cancers are exceptionally rare. Historically, EBV load and use of azathioprine have been associated of posttransplant lymphoproliferative disease.[240]

Due to even greater constraints of donor availability in pediatric heart transplantation, ABOi transplantation has evolved into a progressively acceptable therapy in young children.[241] ABO-i transplantation has been adapted mainly in the neonatal population because of the immaturity of the immune system in the first year of life. Over the last decade, almost 20% of listed patients reaching transplant were ABOi representing up to 40% of the annual volume. Primary listing for ABOi heart transplant has now become routine for the majority of children less than 2 years of age, with shorter waitlist time, especially in blood group O. Posttransplant survival has been similar despite ABOi-listed children still showing a higher risk profile. ABOi transplantation is achieved with intra-operative antibody removal using blood exchange or plasmapheresis if isohemagglutinin titers are 1:16 or above. It is routinely considered in children up to 2 years of age but in select cases may be considered for older children with additional desensitization strategies.[242]

PALLIATIVE CARE IN ADVANCED HEART DISEASE

Despite advances is therapies, HF is associated with a high symptom burden and decreased quality of life and remains one of the most common causes for hospitalizations, with a 5-year mortality rate up to 50%.[243] Palliative care has been defined by the World Health Organization as an approach that improves the quality of life of patients and their families facing life-threatening illness, through the prevention and relief of suffering by means of early identification and treatment of pain and other problems—physical, psychosocial, and spiritual—using a holistic, interdisciplinary approach. The goals of palliative care include treatment of symptoms, improving quality of life, helping patients maintain a sense of control, reducing the burden on caregivers, and facilitating the dying process. The Palliative Care in Heart Failure Trial (PAL-HF) randomized 150 patients to usual care or usual care with palliative care intervention.[244] Patients receiving palliative care had significantly higher scores for quality of life, functional assessment, improved depression, anxiety, and well-being at 6 months, although rehospitalization or mortality was not affected. However, in a recent integrated review of prior studies on outpatient palliative care in HF, in addition to improvements in symptoms and quality of life, three of four studies reported a decrease in hospitalization rates.[245] Palliative care intervention before temporary or durable MCS implantation or heart transplantation is crucial in empowering patients and caregivers to articulate their goals and health measures that they may find unacceptable in the event of complications. Despite some progress, only a minority of patients with HF are referred for palliative care even in their last month of life.[246] Palliative care should therefore be integrated with conventional medical therapies for HF and can be initiated at any point in the illness trajectory and there is an increasing appreciation that early involvement should be considered to optimize benefits.

SUMMARY

For select patients with severe HF, surgical management including mechanical circulatory support and heart transplantation have emerged as viable options. Mechanically assisted circulation has evolved over the last decade from a niche therapy used for short periods to support unstable patients awaiting transplantation to a viable long-term treatment for advanced HF. Clinical trials have demonstrated that MCS prolongs survival and simultaneously improve functionality and quality of life in carefully selected patients. The therapy remains imperfect with a higher than desirable rate of important adverse events that result in morbidity, mortality, and cost. However, this field has entered a new phase of rapid change in which critical feedback loops between patients, clinicians, and engineers are being leveraged to support devices, peripheral components in adjuvant management. With continued progress, the ultimate goal of the field may be realized—widespread availability of a treatment that rivals heart transplantation.

For now, heart transplantation has become the preferred therapy for select patients with end-stage heart disease. Improvements in immunosuppression, donor procurement, surgical techniques, and posttransplant care have resulted in a substantial decrease in acute allograft rejection that had previously significantly limited survival of transplant recipients. Major impediments to long-term allograft survival exist, including rejection, infection, cardiac allograft vasculopathy, and malignancy. Nevertheless, through careful balance of immunosuppressive therapy and vigilant surveillance for complications, we can expect further advances in the long-term outcomes of heart transplant recipients over the decades to come.

ACKNOWLEDGEMENT

The authors would like to acknowledge Chetan B. Patel. MD who contributed content related to mechanically assisted circulation in the previous edition(s) of this chapter.

REFERENCES

1. Teuteberg JJ, Cleveland JC, Cowger J, et al. The Society of Thoracic Surgeons Intermacs 2019 annual report: the changing landscape of devices and indications. *Ann Thorac Surg.* 2020;109:649-660.

2. Goff RR, Uccellini K, Lindblad K, et al. A change of heart: preliminary results of the US 2018 adult heart allocation revision. *Am J Transplant.* 2020;20:2781-2790.

3. Barnard CN. The operation. A human cardiac transplant: an interim report of a successful operation performed at Groote Schuur Hospital, Cape Town. *S Afr Med J.* 1967;41:1271-1274.

4. Virani SS, Alonso A, Benjamin EJ, et al. Heart disease and stroke statistics-2020 update: a report from the American Heart Association. *Circulation.* 2020;141(9):e139-e596.

5. Khush KK, Cherikh WS, Chambers DC, et al. The International Thoracic Organ Transplant Registry of the International Society for Heart and Lung Transplantation: thirty-sixth adult heart transplantation report - 2019; focus theme: donor and recipient size match. *J Heart Lung Transplant.* 2019;38:1056-1066.

6. Rihal CS, Naidu SS, Givertz MM, et al. 2015 SCAI/ACC/HFSA/STS Clinical Expert Consensus Statement on the use of percutaneous mechanical circulatory support devices in cardiovascular care: Endorsed by the American Heart Association, the Cardiology Society of India and Sociedad Latino Americana de Cardiologia Intervencion; Affirmation of Value by the Canadian Association of Interventinal Cardiology-Association Canadienne de Cardiologie d'intervention. *J Am Coll Cardiol.* 2015;65:e7-e26.

7. Estep JD, Cordero-Reyes AM, Bhimaraj A, et al. Percutaneous placement of an intra-aortic balloon pump in the left axillary/subclavian position provides safe, ambulatory long-term support as bridge to heart transplantation. *J Am Coll Cardiol HF.* 2013;1:382-388.

8. Thiele H, Zeymer U, Neumann FJ, et al. Intraaortic balloon support for myocardial infarction with cardiogenic shock. *N Engl J Med.* 2012;367:1287-1296.

9. Jeevanandam V, Song T, Onsager D, et al. The first-in-human experience with a minimally invasive, ambulatory, counterpulsation heart assist system for advanced congestive heart failure. *J Heart Lung Transplant.* 2018;37:1–6.

10. Uriel N, Jeevanandam V, Imamura T, et al. Clinical outcomes and quality of life with an ambulatory counterpulsation pump in advanced heart failure patients: results of the multicenter feasibility trial. *Circ Heart Fail.* 2020;13:e006666.

11. O'Neill WW, Kleiman BS, Moses J, et al. A prospective randomized clinical trial of hemodynamic support with Impella 2.5 versus intra-aortic balloon pump in patients undergoing high-risk percutaneous coronary intervention. *The PROTECT II Study. Circulation.* 2012;126:1717-1727.

12. Stretch R, Sauer CM, Yuh DD, et al. National trends in the utilization of short-term mechanical circulatory support. Incidence, outcomes and cost analysis. *J Am Coll Cardiol.* 2014;64:1407-1415.

13. Ouweneel DM, Eriksen E, Sjauw KD, et al. Percutaneous mechanical circulatory support versus intra-aortic balloon pump in cardiogenic shock after acute myocardial infarction. *J Am Coll Cardiol.* 2016;69:278-287.

14. Schrage B, Ibrahim K, Loehn T et al. Impella support for acute myocardial infarction complicated by cardiogenic shock. *Circulation.* 2019;139:1249-1258.

15. Griffith BP, Anderson MB, Samuels LE, et al. The RECOVER I: a multicenter prospective study of Impella 5.0/LD for postcardiotomy circulatory support. *J Thorac Cardiovasc Surg.* 2013;145:548-554.

16. Anderson MB, Goldstein J, Milano C, et al. Benefits of a novel percutaneous ventricular assist device for right heart failure: the prospective RECOVER RIGHT study of the Impella RP device. *J Heart Lung Transplant.* 2015;34:1549-1560.

17. Aaronson KD, Slaughter MS, Miller LW, et al. Use of an intrapericardial continuous-flow, centrifugal pump in patients awaiting heart transplantation. *Circulation.* 2012;125:3191-3200.

18. Rogers JG, Pagani, FD, Tatooles AJ, et al. Intrapericardial left ventricular assist device for advanced heart failure. *N Engl J Med.* 2017;376:451-460.

19. Teuteberg JJ, Slaughter MS, Rogers JG, et al. The HVAD left ventricular assist device: risk factors for neurological events and risk mitigation strategies. *JACC Heart Fail.* 2015;3:818-828.

20. Milano CA, Rogers JG, Tatooles AJ, et al. HVAD: The ENDURANCE Supplemental Trial. *JACC Heart Fail.* 2018;6:792-802.

21. Bourque K, Cotter C, Dague C, et al. Design rationale and preclinical evaluation of the HeartMate 3 left ventricular assist system for hemocompatibility. *ASAIO J.* 2016;62:375-383.

22. Mehra MR, Uriel N, Naka Y, et al. A fully magnetically levitated left ventricular assist device—final report. *N Engl J Med.* 2019;380:1618-1627.

23. McGee E, Danter M, Strueber M, et al. Evaluation of a lateral thoracotomy implant approach for a centrifugal-flow left ventricular assist device: the LATERAL clinical trial. *J Heart Lung Transplant.* 2019;38:344-351.

24. Truby LK, Garan AR, Givens RC, et al. Aortic insufficiency during contemporary left ventricular assist device support: analysis of the INTERMACS Registry. *JACC Heart Fail.* 2018;6:951-960.

25. Piacentino V, Troupes C, Ganapathi A et al. Clinical impact of concomitant tricuspid valve procedures during left ventricular assist device implantation. *Ann Thor Surg.* 2011;92:1414-1418.

26. Russo MJ, Merlo A, Johnson EM et al. Transapical approach for mitral valve repair during insertion of a left ventricular assist device. *Scientific World J.* 2013;26:925310.

27. Bennett MK, Roberts CA, Russell SD. Ideal methodology to assess systemic blood pressure in patients with continuous-flow left ventricular assist devices. *J Heart Lung Transplant.* 2010;29:593-594.

28. The ARIES HeartMate 3 Pump IDE Study. https://clinicaltrials.gov/ct2/show/NCT04069156. Accessed October 22, 2020.

29. Adatya S, Uriel N, Yarmohammadi H, et al. Anti-factor Xa and activated partial thromboplastin time measurements for heparin monitoring in mechanical circulatory support. *JACC Heart Fail.* 2015;3:314-322.

30. Stainback RF, Estep JD, Agler DA, et al. Echocardiography in the management of patients with left ventricular assist devices: Recommendations from the American Society of Echocardiography. *J Am Soc Echocardiogr.* 2015;28:853-909.

31. Uriel N, Morrison KA, Gargan AR, et al. Development of a novel echocardiography ramp test for speed optimization and diagnosis of device thrombosis in continuous-flow left ventricular assist devices. *J Am Coll Cardiol.* 2012;60:1764-1775.

32. Duero Posada JG, Moayedi Y, Alhussein M, et al. Outflow graft occlusion of the HeartMate 3 left ventricular assist device. *Circ Heart Fail* 2017; 10:e004275-e004275.

33. Mehra MR, Salerno C, Naka Y, et al. A tale of the twist in the outflow graft: an analysis from the MOMENTUM 3 trial. *J Heart Lung Transplant.* 2018;37:1281-1284.

34. Uriel N, Sayer G, Addetia K, et al. Hemodynamic ramp tests in patients with left ventricular assist devices. *J Am Coll Cardiol HF.* 2016;4:208-217.

35. John R, Boyle A, Pagani F, et al. Physiologic and pathologic changes in patients with continuous-flow ventricular assist devices. *J Cardiovasc Trans Res.* 2009;2:154-158.

36. Suarez J, Patel CB, Felker GM, et al. Mechanisms of bleeding and approach to patients with axial-flow left ventricular assist devices. *Circ Heart Fail*. 2011;4:779-784.

37. Tsai HM, Sussman, II, Nagel RL. Shear stress enhances the proteolysis of von Willebrand factor in normal plasma. *Blood*. 1994;83:2171-2179.

38. Baldauf C, Schneppenheim R, Stacklies W, et al. Shear-induced unfolding activates von Willebrand factor A2 domain for proteolysis. *J Thromb Haemost*. 2009;7:2096-2105.

39. Crow S, Chen D, Milano C, et al. Acquired von Willebrand syndrome in continuous-flow ventricular assist device recipients. *Ann Thorac Surg*. 2010;90:1263-1269.

40. Crow S, Milano C, Joyce L, et al. Comparative analysis of von Willebrand factor profiles in pulsatile and continuous left ventricular assist device recipients. *ASAIO J*. 2010;56:441-445.

41. Uriel N, Pak SW, Jorde UP, et al. Acquired von Willebrand syndrome after continuous-flow mechanical device support contributes to a high prevalence of bleeding during long-term support and at the time of transplantation. *J Am Coll of Cardiol*. 2010;56:1207-1213.

42. Crow S, John R, Boyle A, et al. Gastrointestinal bleeding rates in recipients of nonpulsatile and pulsatile left ventricular assist devices. *J Thorac Cardiovasc Surg*. 2009;137:208-215.

43. Genovese EA, Dew MA, Teuteberg JJ, et al. Incidence and patterns of adverse event onset during the first 60 days after ventricular assist device implantation. *Ann Thorac Surg*. 2009;88:1162-1170.

44. John R, Kamdar F, Eckman P, et al. Lessons learned from experience with over 100 consecutive HeartMate II left ventricular assist devices. *Ann Thorac Surg*. 2011;92:1593-1599.

45. Stern DR, Kazam J, Edwards P, et al. Increased incidence of gastrointestinal bleeding following implantation of the HeartMate II LVAD. *J Card Surg*. 2010;25:352-356.

46. Aggarwal A, Pant R, Kumar S, et al. Incidence and management of gastrointestinal bleeding with continuous flow assist devices. *Ann Thoracic Surg*. 2012;93:1534-1540.

47. Morgan JA, Paone G, Nemeh HW, et al. Gastrointestinal bleeding with the HeartMate II left ventricular assist device. *J Heart Lung Transplant*. 2012;31:715-718.

48. Demirozu ZT, Radovancevic R, Hochman LF, et al. Arteriovenous malformation and gastrointestinal bleeding in patients with the HeartMate II left ventricular assist device. *J Heart Lung Transplant*. 2011;30:849-853.

49. Hannan MM, Xie R, Cowger J, et al. Epidemiology of infection in mechanical circulatory support: a global analysis from the ISHLT mechanically assisted circulatory support registry. *J Heart Lung Transplant*. 2019;38:364-373.

50. Gordon RJ, Weinberg AD, Pagani FD, et al. Prospective, multicenter study of ventricular assist device infections. *Circulation*. 2013;127:691-702.

51. Patel CB, Blue L, Cagliostro B, et al. Left ventricular assist systems and infection-related outcomes: a comprehensive analysis of the MOMENTUM 3 trial. *J Heart Lung Transplant*. 2020;39:774-781.

52. Shoham S, Shaffer R, Sweet L, et al. Candidemia in patients with ventricular assist devices. *Clin Infect Dis*. 2007;44:e9-e12.

53. Moazami N, Milano CA, John R, et al. Pump replacement for left ventricular assist device failure can be done safely and is associated with low mortality. *Ann Thorac Surg*. 2013;95:500-505.

54. Oswald H, Schultz-Wildelau C, Gardiwal A, et al. Implantable defibrillator therapy for ventricular tachyarrhythmia in left ventricular assist device patients. *Eur J Heart Fail*. 2010;12:593-599.

55. Andersen M, Videbaek R, Boesgaard S, et al. Incidence of ventricular arrhythmias in patients on long-term support with a continuous-flow assist device (HeartMate II). *J Heart Lung Transplant*. 2009;28:733-735.

56. Brenyo A, Rao M, Koneru S, et al. Risk of mortality for ventricular arrhythmia in ambulatory LVAD patients. *J Cardiovasc Electrophysiol*. 2012;23:515-520.

57. Cantillon DJ, Tarakji KG, Kumbhani DJ, et al. Improved survival among ventricular assist device recipients with a concomitant implantable cardioverter-defibrillator. *Heart Rhythm*. 2010;7:466-471.

58. Dandamudi G, Ghumman WS, Das MK, et al. Endocardial catheter ablation of ventricular tachycardia in patients with ventricular assist devices. *Heart Rhythm*. 2007;4:1165-1169.

59. Rehorn MR, Koontz J, Barnett AS, et al. Noninvasive electrocardiographic mapping of ventricular tachycardia in a patient with a left ventricular assist device. *Heart Rhythm Case Rep*. 2020;6:398-401.

60. Gopinathannair R, Cornwell WK, Dukes JW, et al. Device therapy and arrhythmia management in left ventricular assist device recipients: a scientific statement from the American Heart Association. *Circulation*. 2019;139:e967-e989.

61. Slaughter MS, Rogers JG, Milano CA, et al. Advanced heart failure treated with continuous-flow left ventricular assist device. *N Engl J Med*. 2009;361:2241-2251.

62. Park SJ, Milano CA, Tatooles AJ, et al. Outcomes in advanced heart failure patients with left ventricular assist devices for destination therapy. *Circ Heart Fail*. 2012;5:241-248.

63. Slaughter MS, Pagani FD, McGee EC, et al. HeartWare ventricular assist system for bridge to transplant: combined results of the bridge to transplant and continued access protocol trial. *J Heart Lung Transplant*. 2013;32:675-683.

64. Lietz K, Long JW, Kfoury AG, et al. Impact of center volume on outcomes of left ventricular assist device implantation as destination therapy: analysis of the Thoratec HeartMate Registry, 1998 to 2005. *Circ Heart Fail*. 2009;2:3-10.

65. Barac YD, Wojnarski CM, Junpaparp P, et al. Early outcomes with durable left ventricular assist device replacement using the HeartMate 3. *J Thorac Cardiovasc Surg*. 2020;160:132-139.

66. Copeland JG, Smith RG, Arabia FA, et al. Cardiac replacement with a total artificial heart as a bridge to transplantation. *N Eng J Med*. 2004;351:859-867.

67. Fraser CD, Jaquiss RD, Rosenthal DN, et al. Prospective trial of a pediatric ventricular assist device. *N Engl J Med*. 2012;367:532-541.

68. Kormos RL, Teuteberg JJ, Pagani FD, et al. Right ventricular failure in patients with the HeartMate II continuous-flow left ventricular assist device: Incidence, risk factors, and effect on outcome. *J Thorac Cardiovasc Surg*. 2010;139:1316-1324.

69. Krabatsch T, Potapov E, Stepaneko A, et al. Biventricular circulatory support with two miniaturized implantable assist devices. *Circulation*. 2011;124:S179-S186.

70. Daneshmand MA, Bishawi M, Milano CA, Schroder JN. The HeartMate 6. *ASAIO J*. 2020;66:e46-e49.

71. Mehra MR, Canter CE, Hannan MM, et al. The 2016 International Society for Heart Lung Transplantation listing criteria for heart transplantation: A 10-year update. *J Heart Lung Transplant*. 2016;35:1-23.

72. Velazquez EJ, Lee KL, Jones RH, et al. Coronary-artery bypass surgery in patients with ischemic cardiomyopathy. *N Engl J Med*. 2016;374:1511-1520.

73. Mancini DM, Eisen H, Kussmaul W, et al. Value of peak exercise oxygen consumption for optimal timing of cardiac transplantation in ambulatory patients with heart failure. *Circulation*. 1991;83:778-786.

74. Butler J, Khadim G, Paul KM, et al. Selection of patients for heart transplantation in the current era of heart failure therapy. *J Am Coll Cardiol*. 2004;43:787-793.

75. Peterson LR, Schechtman KB, Ewald GA, et al. Timing of cardiac transplantation in patients with heart failure receiving beta-adrenergic blockers. *J Heart Lung Transplant*. 2003;22:1141-1148.

76. O'Neill JO, Young JB, Pothier CE, set al. Peak oxygen consumption as a predictor of death in patients with heart failure receiving beta-blockers. *Circulation*. 2005;111:2313-2318.

77. Arena R, Myers J, Abella J, et al. Development of a ventilatory classification system in patients with heart failure. *Circulation*. 2007;115:2410-2417.

78. Corrà U, Mezzani A, Bosimini E, et al. Ventilatory response to exercise improves risk stratification in patients with chronic heart failure and intermediate functional capacity. *Am Heart J*. 2002;143:418-426.

79. Stelken AM, Younis LT, Jennison SH, et al. Prognostic value of cardiopulmonary exercise testing using percent achieved of predicted peak oxygen uptake for patients with ischemic and dilated cardiomyopathy. *J Am Coll Cardiol.* 1996;27:345-52.

80. Poggio R, Arazi HC, Giorgi M, et al. Prediction of severe cardiovascular events by VE/VCO2 slope versus peak VO2 in systolic heart failure: a meta-analysis of the published literature. *Am Heart J.* 2010;1601004-1601014.

81. Laks H, Marelli D, Fonarow GC, et al. Use of two recipient lists for adults requiring heart transplantation. *J Thorac Cardiovasc Surg.* 2003;125:49-59.

82. Delgado JF, Conde E, Sánchez V, et al. Pulmonary vascular remodeling in pulmonary hypertension due to chronic heart failure. *Eur J Heart Fail.* 2005;7:1011-1016.

83. Costard-Jäckle A, Fowler MB. Influence of preoperative pulmonary artery pressure on mortality after heart transplantation: testing of potential reversibility of pulmonary hypertension with nitroprusside is useful in defining a high risk group. *J Am Coll Cardiol.* 1992;19:48-54.

84. Tsukashita M, Takayama H, Takeda K, et al. Effect of pulmonary vascular resistance before left ventricular assist device implantation on short- and long-term post-transplant survival. *J Thorac Cardiovasc Surg.* 2015;150:1352-1360.

85. Kutty RS, Parameshwar J, Lewis C, et al. Use of centrifugal left ventricular assist device as a bridge to candidacy in severe heart failure with secondary pulmonary hypertension. *Eur J Cardiothorac Surg.* 2013;43:1237-1242.

86. Zeuzem S, Foster GR, Wang S, et al. Glecaprevir-Pibrentasvir for 8 or 12 Weeks in HCV genotype 1 or 3 infection. *N Engl J Med.* 2018;378:354-369.

87. Bourlière M, Gordon SC, Flamm SL, et al. Sofosbuvir, Velpatasvir, and Voxilaprevir for previously treated HCV infection. *N Engl J Med.* 2017;376:2134-2146.

88. Agüero F, Castel MA, Cocchi S, et al. An update on heart transplantation in human immunodeficiency virus-infected patients. *Am J Transplant.* 2016;16:21-28.

89. Halpern SD, Ubel PA, Caplan AL. Solid-organ transplantation in HIV-infected patients. *N Engl J Med.* 2002;347:284-287.

90. Uriel N, Jorde UP, Cotarlan V, et al. Heart transplantation in human immunodeficiency virus-positive patients. *J Heart Lung Transplant.* 2009;28:667-669.

91. Morillo CA, Marin-Neto JA, Avezum A, et al. Randomized trial of benznidazole for chronic Chagas' cardiomyopathy. *N Engl J Med.* 2015;373:1295-1306.

92. Khush KK, Cherikh WS, Chambers DC, et al. The International Thoracic Organ Transplant Registry of the International Society for Heart and Lung Transplantation: thirty-sixth adult heart transplantation report—2019; focus theme: Donor and recipient size match. *J Heart Lung Transplant.* 2019;38:1056-1066.

93. Ladowski JS, Kormos RL, Uretsky BF, et al. Heart transplantation in diabetic recipients. *Transplantation.* 1990;49303-49305.

94. Morgan JA, John R, Weinberg AD, et al. Heart transplantation in diabetic recipients: a decade review of 161 patients at Columbia Presbyterian. *J Thorac Cardiovasc Surg.* 2004;127:1486-1492.

95. Munoz E, Lonquist JL, Radovancevic B, et al. Long-term results in diabetic patients undergoing heart transplantation. *J Heart Lung Transplant.* 1992;11:943-949.

96. Raichlin E, Daly RC, Rosen CB, et al. Combined heart and liver transplantation: a single-center experience. *Transplantation.* 2009;88:219-225.

97. Te HS, Anderson AS, Millis JM, et al. Current state of combined heart-liver transplantation in the United States. *J Heart Lung Transplant.* 2008;27:753-759.

98. Vermes E, Grimbert P, Sebbag L, et al. Long-term results of combined heart and kidney transplantation: a French multicenter study. *J Heart Lung Transplant.* 2009;28:440-445.

99. Gill J, Shah T, Hristea I, Chavalitdhamrong D, et al. Outcomes of simultaneous heart-kidney transplant in the US: a retrospective analysis using OPTN/UNOS data. *Am J Transplant.* 2009;9:844-852.

100. Neyer J, Uberoi A, Hamilton M, et al. Marijuana and listing for heart transplant: a survey of transplant providers. *Circ Heart Fail.* 2016;9:e002851.

101. Eckman PM, Hanna M, Taylor DO, et al. Management of the sensitized adult heart transplant candidate. *Clin Transplant.* 2010;24:726-734.

102. Kobashigawa J, Mehra M, West L, et al. Report from a consensus conference on the sensitized patient awaiting heart transplantation. *J Heart Lung Transplant.* 2009;28:213-225.

103. Kobashigawa J, Crespo-Leiro MG, Ensminger SM, et al. Report from a consensus conference on antibody-mediated rejection in heart transplantation. *J Heart Lung Transplant.* 2011;30:252-269.

104. Loupy A, Lefaucheur C, Vernerey D, et al. Complement-binding anti-HLA antibodies and kidney-allograft survival. *N Engl J Med.* 2013;369:1215-1226.

105. Zeevi A, Lunz J, Feingold B, et al. Persistent strong anti-HLA antibody at high titer is complement binding and associated with increased risk of antibody-mediated rejection in heart transplant recipients. *J Heart Lung Transplant.* 2013;32:98-105.

106. Sutherland SM, Chen G, Sequeira FA, et al. Complement-fixing donor-specific antibodies identified by a novel C1q assay are associated with allograft loss. *Pediatric Transplantation.* 2012;16:12-17.

107. Stehlik J, Islam N, Hurst D, et al. Utility of virtual crossmatch in sensitized patients awaiting heart transplantation. *J Heart Lung Transplant.* 2009;28:1129-1134.

108. Cecka JM. Calculated PRA (CPRA): the new measure of sensitization for transplant candidates. *Am J Transplant.* 2010;10:26-29.

109. Cecka JM, Kucheryavaya AY, Reinsmoen NL, et al. Calculated PRA: initial results show benefits for sensitized patients and a reduction in positive crossmatches. *Am J Transplant.* 2011;11:719-724.

110. Kransdorf EP, Kittleson MM, Patel JK, et al. Calculated panel-reactive antibody predicts outcomes on the heart transplant waiting list. *J Heart Lung Transplant.* 2017;36:787-796.

111. Vo AA, Lukovsky M, Toyoda M, et al. Rituximab and intravenous immune globulin for desensitization during renal transplantation. *N Engl J Med.* 2008;359:242-251.

112. Patel J, Everly M, Chang D, et al. Reduction of alloantibodies via proteosome inhibition in cardiac transplantation. *J Heart Lung Transplant.* 2011;30:1320-1326.

113. Wijdicks EF, Varelas PN, Gronseth GS, et al. Evidence-based guideline update: determining brain death in adults: report of the Quality Standards Subcommittee of the American Academy of Neurology. *Neurology.* 2010;74:1911-1918.

114. A definition of irreversible coma. Report of the Ad Hoc Committee of the Harvard Medical School to Examine the Definition of Brain Death. *JAMA.* 1968;205:337-340.

115. Burroughs JT, Terrance G, Furlow MC. Guidelines for the determination of death. Report of the medical consultants on the diagnosis of death to the President's Commission for the Study of Ethical Problems in Medicine and Biomedical and Behavioral Research. *JAMA.* 1981;246(19):2184-2186.

116. Sade RM. Brain death, cardiac death, and the dead donor rule. *J SC Medl Associ.* 2011;107:146-149.

117. Aslam S, Grossi P, Schlendorf KH, et al. Utilization of hepatitis C virus-infected organ donors in cardiothoracic transplantation: an ISHLT expert consensus statement. *J Heart Lung Transplant.* 2020;39:418-432.

118. Zaroff JG, Rosengard BR, Armstrong WF, et al. Consensus conference report: maximizing use of organs recovered from the cadaver donor: cardiac recommendations. *Circulation.* 2002;106:836-841.

119. Zaroff JG, Rordorf GA, Ogilvy CS, et al. Regional patterns of left ventricular systolic dysfunction after subarachnoid hemorrhage: evidence for neurally mediated cardiac injury. *J Am Soc Echocardiogr.* 2000;13:774-779.

120. Chen CW, Sprys MH, Gaffey AC, et al. Low ejection fraction in donor hearts is not directly associated with increased recipient mortality. *J Heart Lung Transplant.* 2017;36:611-615.

121. Ardehali A, Esmailian F, Deng M, et al. Ex-vivo perfusion of donor hearts for human heart transplantation (PROCEED II): a prospective, open-label, multicentre, randomised non-inferiority trial. *Lancet.* 2015;385(9987):2577-2584.

122. Trivedi JR, Cheng A, Gallo M, et al. Predictors of donor heart utilization for transplantation in United States. *Ann Thorac Surg.* 2017;103:1900-1906.

123. Khush KK. Donor selection in the modern era. *Ann Cardiothorac Surg.* 2018;7:126-134.

124. Dhital KK, Iyer A, Connellan M, et al. Adult heart transplantation with distant procurement and ex-vivo preservation of donor hearts after circulatory death: a case series. *Lancet.* 2015;385(9987):2585-2591.

125. Rajab TK, Jaggers J, Campbell DN. Heart transplantation following donation after cardiac death: History, current techniques, and future. *J Thorac Cardiovasc Surg.* 2020;S0022-5223(20)30529-8.

126. Parent B, Moazami N, Wall S, et al. Ethical and logistical concerns for establishing NRP-cDCD heart transplantation in the United States. *Am J Transplant.* 2020;20:1508-1512.

127. Costanzo MR, Dipchand A, Starling R, et al. The International Society of Heart and Lung Transplantation Guidelines for the care of heart transplant recipients. *J Heart Lung Transplant.* 2010;29:914-956.

128. Patel ND, Weiss ES, Nwakanma LU, et al. Impact of donor-to-recipient weight ratio on survival after heart transplantation. *Circulation.* 2008;118(14suppl1):S83-S88.

129. Kransdorf EP, Kittleson MM, Benck LR, et al. Predicted heart mass is the optimal metric for size match in heart transplantation. *J Heart Lung Transplant.* 2019;38:156-165.

130. Meyer DM, Rogers JG, Edwards LB, et al. The future direction of the adult heart allocation system in the United States. *Am J Transplant.* 2015;15:44-54.

131. Van Meter CH. The organ allocation controversy: how did we arrive here? *Ochsner J.* 1999;1:6-11.

132. Committee OUTOT. Proposal to modify the adult heart allocation system. 2016.

133. Reitz BA, Bieber CP, Raney AA, et al. Orthotopic heart and combined heart and lung transplantation with cyclosporin-A immune suppression. *Transplant Proc.* 1981;13(1 Pt 1):393-396.

134. Dreyfus G, Jebara V, Mihaileanu S, et al. Total orthotopic heart transplantation: an alternative to the standard technique. *Ann Thorac Surg.* 1991;52:1181-1184.

135. el-Gamel A, Deiraniya AK, Rahman AN, et al. Orthotopic heart transplantation hemodynamics: does atrial preservation improve cardiac output after transplantation? *J Heart Lung Transplant.* 1996;15:564-571.

136. Meyer SR, Modry DL, Bainey K, et al. Declining need for permanent pacemaker insertion with the bicaval technique of orthotopic heart transplantation. *Can J Cardiol.* 2005;21:159-163.

137. Traversi E, Pozzoli M, Grande A, et al. The bicaval anastomosis technique for orthotopic heart transplantation yields better atrial function than the standard technique: an echocardiographic automatic boundary detection study. *J Heart Lung Transplant.* 1998;17:1065-1074.

138. Goldstein DR, Coffey CS, Benza RL, et al. Relative perioperative bradycardia does not lead to adverse outcomes after cardiac transplantation. *Am J Transplant.* 2003;3:484-491.

139. Stark RP, McGinn AL, Wilson RF. Chest pain in cardiac-transplant recipients. Evidence of sensory reinnervation after cardiac transplantation. *N Engl J Med.* 1991;324:1791-1794.

140. Bengel FM, Ueberfuhr P, Schiepel N, et al. Effect of sympathetic reinnervation on cardiac performance after heart transplantation. *N Engl J Med.* 2001;345:731-738.

141. Farrukh HM, White M, Port JD, et al. Up-regulation of beta 2-adrenergic receptors in previously transplanted, denervated nonfailing human hearts. *J Am Coll Cardiol.* 1993;22:1902-1908.

142. Grady KL, Wang E, Higgins R, et al. Symptom frequency and distress from 5 to 10 years after heart transplantation. *J Heart Lung Transplant.* 2009;28:759-768.

143. Kobashigawa J, Zuckermann A, Macdonald P, et al. Report from a consensus conference on primary graft dysfunction after cardiac transplantation. *J Heart Lung Transplant.* 2014;33:327-340.

144. DeRoo SC, Takayama H, Nemeth S, et al. Extracorporeal membrane oxygenation for primary graft dysfunction after heart transplant. *J Thorac Cardiovasc Surg.* 2019;158:1576-1584.e3.

145. Kittleson MM, Patel JK, Moriguchi JD, et al. Heart transplant recipients supported with extracorporeal membrane oxygenation: outcomes from a single-center experience. *J Heart Lung Transplant.* 2011;30:1250-1256.

146. Stegall MD, Diwan T, Raghavaiah S, et al. Terminal complement inhibition decreases antibody-mediated rejection in sensitized renal transplant recipients. *Am J Transplant.* 2011;11:2405-2413.

147. Smart FW, Naftel DC, Costanzo MR, et al. Risk factors for early, cumulative, and fatal infections after heart transplantation: a multiinstitutional study. *J Heart Lung Transplant.* 1996;15:329-341.

148. Miller LW, Naftel DC, Bourge RC, et al. Infection after heart transplantation: a multiinstitutional study. Cardiac Transplant Research Database Group. *J Heart Lung Transplant.* 1994;13:381-392.

149. Hershberger RE, Starling RC, Eisen HJ, et al. Daclizumab to prevent rejection after cardiac transplantation. *N Engl J Med.* 2005;352:2705-2713.

150. Grimm M, Rinaldi M, Yonan NA, et al. Superior prevention of acute rejection by tacrolimus vs. cyclosporine in heart transplant recipients—a large European trial. *Am J Transplant.* 2006;6:1387-1397.

151. Kobashigawa JA, Miller LW, Russell SD, et al. Tacrolimus with mycophenolate mofetil (MMF) or sirolimus vs. cyclosporine with MMF in cardiac transplant patients: 1-year report. *Am J Transplant.* 2006;6:1377-1386.

152. Taylor DO, Barr ML, Radovancevic B, et al. A randomized, multicenter comparison of tacrolimus and cyclosporine immunosuppressive regimens in cardiac transplantation: decreased hyperlipidemia and hypertension with tacrolimus. *J Heart Lung Transplant.* 1999;18:336-345.

153. Ye F, Ying-Bin X, Yu-Guo W, et al. Tacrolimus versus cyclosporine microemulsion for heart transplant recipients: a meta-analysis. *J Heart Lung Transplant.* 2009;28:58-66.

154. Kobashigawa J, Miller L, Renlund D, et al. A randomized active-controlled trial of mycophenolate mofetil in heart transplant recipients. Mycophenolate Mofetil Investigators. *Transplantation.* 1998;66:507-515.

155. Kobashigawa JA, Renlund DG, Gerosa G, et al. Similar efficacy and safety of enteric-coated mycophenolate sodium (EC-MPS, myfortic) compared with mycophenolate mofetil (MMF) in de novo heart transplant recipients: results of a 12-month, single-blind, randomized, parallel-group, multicenter study. *J Heart Lung Transplant.* 2006;25:935-941.

156. Keogh A, Richardson M, Ruygrok P, et al. Sirolimus in de novo heart transplant recipients reduces acute rejection and prevents coronary artery disease at 2 years. *Circulation.* 2004;110:2694-2700.

157. Eisen HJ, Tuzcu EM, Dorent R, et al. Everolimus for the prevention of allograft rejection and vasculopathy in cardiac-transplant recipients. *N Engl J Med.* 2003;349:847-858.

158. Eisen HJ, Kobashigawa J, Starling RC, et al. Everolimus versus mycophenolate mofetil in heart transplantation: a randomized, multicenter trial. *Am J Transplant.* 2013;13:1203-1216.

159. Kobashigawa JA, Pauly DF, Starling RC, et al. Cardiac allograft vasculopathy by intravascular ultrasound in heart transplant patients: substudy from the Everolimus versus mycophenolate mofetil randomized, multicenter trial. *JACC Heart Fail.* 2013;1:389-399.

160. Mancini D, Pinney S, Burkhoff D, et al. Use of rapamycin slows progression of cardiac transplantation vasculopathy. *Circulation.* 2003;108:48-53.

161. Kobashigawa J, Ross H, Bara C, et al. Everolimus is associated with a reduced incidence of cytomegalovirus infection following de novo cardiac transplantation. *Transpl Infect Dis.* 2013;15:150-162.

162. Andreassen AK, Andersson B, Gustafsson F, et al. Everolimus initiation and early calcineurin inhibitor withdrawal in heart transplant recipients: a randomized trial. *Am J Transplant.* 2014;14:1828-1838.

163. Barten MJ, Hirt SW, Garbade J, et al. Comparing everolimus-based immunosuppression with reduction or withdrawal of calcineurin inhibitor

reduction from six months after heart transplantation: the randomized MANDELA study. *Am J Transplant.* 2019. doi: 10.1111/ajt.15361

164. Baran DA, Zucker MJ, Arroyo LH, et al. Randomized trial of tacrolimus monotherapy: tacrolimus in combination, tacrolimus alone compared (the TICTAC trial). *J Heart Lung Transplant.* 2007;26:992-997.

165. Page RL, 2nd, Miller GG, Lindenfeld J. Drug therapy in the heart transplant recipient: part IV: drug-drug interactions. *Circulation.* 2005;111:230-239.

166. Kemnitz J, Cremer J, Restrepo-Specht I, et al. Hyperacute rejection in heart allografts. Case studies. *Pathol Res Pract.* 1991;187:23-29.

167. Sethi GK, Kosaraju S, Arabia FA, et al. Is it necessary to perform surveillance endomyocardial biopsies in heart transplant recipients? *J Heart Lung Transplant.* 1995;14(6 Pt 1):1047-1051.

168. White JA, Guiraudon C, Pflugfelder PW, et al. Routine surveillance myocardial biopsies are unnecessary beyond one year after heart transplantation. *J Heart Lung Transplant.* 1995;14(6 Pt 1):1052-1056.

169. Stewart S, Winters GL, Fishbein MC, et al. Revision of the 1990 working formulation for the standardization of nomenclature in the diagnosis of heart rejection. *J Heart Lung Transplant.* 2005;24:1710-1720.

170. Berry GJ, Burke MM, Andersen C, et al. The 2013 International Society for Heart and Lung Transplantation Working Formulation for the standardization of nomenclature in the pathologic diagnosis of antibody-mediated rejection in heart transplantation. *J Heart Lung Transplant.* 2013;32:1147-1162.

171. Loupy A, Lefaucheur C, Vernerey D, et al. Complement-binding anti-hla antibodies and kidney-allograft survival. *N Engl J Med.* 2013;369:1215-1226.

172. Crespo-Leiro MG, Zuckermann A, Bara C, et al. Concordance among pathologists in the second Cardiac Allograft Rejection Gene Expression Observational Study (CARGO II). *Transplantation.* 2012;94:1172-1177.

173. Halloran PF, Potena L, Van Huyen JD, et al. Building a tissue-based molecular diagnostic system in heart transplant rejection: The heart Molecular Microscope Diagnostic (MMDx) System. *J Heart Lung Transplant.* 2017;361192-1200.

174. Deng MC, Eisen HJ, Mehra MR, et al. Noninvasive discrimination of rejection in cardiac allograft recipients using gene expression profiling. *Am J Transplant.* 2006;6:150-160.

175. Pham MX, Teuteberg JJ, Kfoury AG, et al. Gene-expression profiling for rejection surveillance after cardiac transplantation. *N Engl J Med.* 2010;362:1890-1900.

176. Kobashigawa J, Patel J, Azarbal B, et al. Randomized pilot trial of gene expression profiling versus heart biopsy in the first year after heart transplant: early invasive monitoring attenuation through gene expression trial. *Circ Heart Fail.* 2015;8(3):557-564.

177. Zhang J, Tong KL, Li PK, et al. Presence of donor- and recipient-derived DNA in cell-free urine samples of renal transplantation recipients: urinary DNA chimerism. *Clin Chem.* 1999;45:1741-1746.

178. Lo YM, Tein MS, Pang CC, et al. Presence of donor-specific DNA in plasma of kidney and liver-transplant recipients. *Lancet.* 1998;351(9112):1329-1330.

179. Khush KK, Patel J, Pinney S, et al. Noninvasive detection of graft injury after heart transplant using donor-derived cell-free DNA: A prospective multicenter study. *Am J Transplant.* 2019;19:2889-2899.

180. Kobashigawa JA, Patel J, Furukawa H, et al. Five-year results of a randomized, single-center study of tacrolimus vs microemulsion cyclosporine in heart transplant patients. *J Heart Lung Transplant.* 2006;25:434-439.

181. Keogh A, Richardson M, Ruygrok P, et al. Sirolimus in de novo heart transplant recipients reduces acute rejection and prevents coronary artery disease at 2 years: a randomized clinical trial. *Circulation.* 2004;110:2694-2700.

182. Kobashigawa JA, Stevenson LW, Moriguchi JD, et al. Is intravenous glucocorticoid therapy better than an oral regimen for asymptomatic cardiac rejection? A randomized trial. *J Am Coll Cardiol.* 1993;21:1142-1144.

183. Kfoury AG, Hammond ME, Snow GL, et al. Cardiovascular mortality among heart transplant recipients with asymptomatic antibody-mediated

184. Wu GW, Kobashigawa JA, Fishbein MC, et al. Asymptomatic antibody-mediated rejection after heart transplantation predicts poor outcomes. *J Heart Lung Transplant.* 2009;28417-28422.

185. Kfoury AG, Stehlik J, Renlund DG, et al. Impact of repetitive episodes of antibody-mediated or cellular rejection on cardiovascular mortality in cardiac transplant recipients: defining rejection patterns. *J Heart Lung Transplant.* 2006;25:1277-1282.

186. Arbustini E, Roberts WC. Morphological observations in the epicardial coronary arteries and their surroundings late after cardiac transplantation (allograft vascular disease). *Am J Cardiol.* 1996;78:814-820.

187. Fishbein MC, Kobashigawa J. Biopsy-negative cardiac transplant rejection: etiology, diagnosis, and therapy. *Curr Opin Cardiol.* 2004;19:166-169.

188. Patel J, Everly M, Chang D, et al. Reduction of alloantibodies via proteasome inhibition in cardiac transplantation. *J Heart Lung Transplant.* 2011;30:1320-1326.

189. Kirklin JK, Brown RN, Huang ST, et al. Rejection with hemodynamic compromise: objective evidence for efficacy of photopheresis. *J Heart Lung Transplant.* 2006;25:283-288.

190. Loupy A, Coutance G, Bonnet G, et al. Identification and characterization of trajectories of cardiac allograft vasculopathy after heart transplantation: a population-based study. *Circulation.* 2020;141:1954-1967.

191. Potluri SP, Mehra MR, Uber PA, et al. Relationship among epicardial coronary disease, tissue myocardial perfusion, and survival in heart transplantation. *J Heart Lung Transplant.* 2005;24:1019-1025.

192. Ramsdale DB, Bellamy CM. Angina and threatened acute myocardial infarction after cardiac transplantation. *Am Heart J.* 1990;119:1195-1197.

193. Schroeder JS, Hunt SA. Chest pain in heart-transplant recipients. *N Engl J Med.* 1991;324:1805-1807.

194. Mehra MR, Crespo-Leiro MG, Dipchand A, et al. International Society for Heart and Lung Transplantation working formulation of a standardized nomenclature for cardiac allograft vasculopathy—2010. *J Heart Lung Transplant.* 2010;29:717-727.

195. Kapadia SR, Nissen SE, Tuzcu EM. Impact of intravascular ultrasound in understanding transplant coronary artery disease. *Curr Opin Cardiol.* 1999;14:140-150.

196. Kapadia SR, Nissen SE, Ziada KM, et al. Development of transplantation vasculopathy and progression of donor-transmitted atherosclerosis: comparison by serial intravascular ultrasound imaging. *Circulation.* 1998;98:2672-2678.

197. König A, Theisen K, Klauss V. Intravascular ultrasound for assessment of coronary allograft vasculopathy. *Z Kardiol.* 2000;89(Suppl 9):Ix/45-49.

198. Rickenbacher P. Role of intravascular ultrasound versus angiography for diagnosis of graft vascular disease. *Transplant Proc.* 1998;30:891-892.

199. Park K-H, Sun T, Liu Z, et al. Relationship between markers of plaque vulnerability in optical coherence tomography and atherosclerotic progression in adult patients with heart transplantation. *J Heart Lung Transplant.* 2017;36:185-192.

200. Kobashigawa JA, Katznelson S, Laks H, et al. Effect of pravastatin on outcomes after cardiac transplantation. *N Engl J Med.* 1995;333:621-627.

201. Azarbal B, Arbit B, Ramaraj R, et al. Clinical and angiographic outcomes with everolimus eluting stents for the treatment of cardiac allograft vasculopathy. *J Interv Cardiol.* 2014;27:73-79.

202. Simpson L, Lee EK, Hott BJ, et al. Long-term results of angioplasty vs stenting in cardiac transplant recipients with allograft vasculopathy. *J Heart Lung Transplant.* 2005;24:1211-1217.

203. Tanaka K, Li H, Curran PJ, et al. Usefulness and safety of percutaneous coronary interventions for cardiac transplant vasculopathy. *Am J Cardiol.* 2006;97:1192-1197.

204. Kowalski R, Post D, Schneider MC, et al. Immune cell function testing: an adjunct to therapeutic drug monitoring in transplant patient management. *Clin Transplant.* 2003;17:77-88.

205. Kowalski RJ, Post DR, Mannon RB, et al. Assessing relative risks of infection and rejection: a meta-analysis using an immune function assay. *Transplantation.* 2006;82:663-668.

206. Kobashigawa JA, Kiyosaki KK, Patel JK, et al. Benefit of immune monitoring in heart transplant patients using ATP production in activated lymphocytes. *J Heart Lung Transplant.* 2010;29:504-508.

207. Schaffer SA, Husain S, Delgado DH, et al. Impact of adjuvanted H1N1 vaccine on cell-mediated rejection in heart transplant recipients. *Am J Transplant.* 2011;11:2751-2754.

208. Mihalov ML, Gattuso P, Abraham K, et al. Incidence of post-transplant malignancy among 674 solid-organ-transplant recipients at a single center. *Clin Transplant.* 1996;10:248-255.

209. Penn I. Incidence and treatment of neoplasia after transplantation. *J Heart Lung Transplant.* 1993;12(6 Pt 2):S328-336.

210. Fortina AB, Caforio AL, Piaserico S, et al. Skin cancer in heart transplant recipients: frequency and risk factor analysis. *J Heart Lung Transplant.* 2000;19:249-255.

211. Jensen P, Hansen S, Møller B, et al. Skin cancer in kidney and heart transplant recipients and different long-term immunosuppressive therapy regimens. *J Am Acad Dermatol.* 1999;40(2 Pt 1):177-186.

212. Dantal J, Soulillou JP. Immunosuppressive drugs and the risk of cancer after organ transplantation. *N Engl J Med.* 2005;352:1371-1373.

213. Euvrard S, Morelon E, Rostaing L, et al. Sirolimus and secondary skin-cancer prevention in kidney transplantation. *N Engl J Med.* 2012;367:329-339.

214. Mathew T, Kreis H, Friend P. Two-year incidence of malignancy in sirolimus-treated renal transplant recipients: results from five multicenter studies. *Clin Transplant.* 2004;18:446-449.

215. Salgo R, Gossmann J, Schöfer H, et al. Switch to a sirolimus-based immunosuppression in long-term renal transplant recipients: reduced rate of (pre-)malignancies and nonmelanoma skin cancer in a prospective, randomized, assessor-blinded, controlled clinical trial. *Am J Transplant.* 2010;10:1385-1393.

216. Campistol JM, Gutierrez-Dalmau A, Torregrosa JV. Conversion to sirolimus: a successful treatment for posttransplantation Kaposi's sarcoma. *Transplantation.* 2004;77:760-762.

217. Vajdic CM, van Leeuwen MT. Cancer incidence and risk factors after solid organ transplantation. *Int J Cancer.* 2009;125:1747-1754.

218. Ramsay HM, Fryer AA, Hawley CM, et al. Factors associated with nonmelanoma skin cancer following renal transplantation in Queensland, Australia. *J Am Acad Dermatol.* 2003;49:397-406.

219. Williams K, Mansh M, Chin-Hong P, et al. Voriconazole-associated cutaneous malignancy: a literature review on photocarcinogenesis in organ transplant recipients. *Clin Infect Dis.* 2014;58:997-1002.

220. Opelz G, Henderson R. Incidence of non-Hodgkin lymphoma in kidney and heart transplant recipients. *Lancet.* 1993;342(8886-8887):1514-1516.

221. Swinnen LJ, Costanzo-Nordin MR, Fisher SG, et al. Increased incidence of lymphoproliferative disorder after immunosuppression with the monoclonal antibody OKT3 in cardiac-transplant recipients. *N Engl J Med.* 1990;323:1723-1728.

222. Walker RC. Pretransplant assessment of the risk for posttransplant lymphoproliferative disorder. *Transplant Proc.* 1995;27(5 Suppl 1):41.

223. Rinaldi M, Pellegrini C, D'Armini AM, et al. Neoplastic disease after heart transplantation: single center experience. *Eur J Cardiothorac Surg.* 2001;19:696-701.

224. Goldstein DJ, Zuech N, Sehgal V, et al. Cyclosporine-associated end-stage nephropathy after cardiac transplantation: incidence and progression. *Transplantation.* 1997;63:664-668.

225. Zietse R, Balk AH, vd Dorpel MA, et al. Time course of the decline in renal function in cyclosporine-treated heart transplant recipients. *Am J Nephrol.* 1994;14:1-5.

226. Frohlich ED, Ventura HO, Ochsner JL. Arterial hypertension after orthotopic cardiac transplantation. *J Am Coll Cardiol.* 1990;15:1102-1103.

227. Starling RC, Cody RJ. Cardiac transplant hypertension. *Am J Cardiol.* 1990;65:106-111.

228. Hausberg M, Barenbrock M, Hohage H, et al. ACE inhibitor versus beta-blocker for the treatment of hypertension in renal allograft recipients. *Hypertension.* 1999;33:862-868.

229. Sennesael J, Lamote J, Violet I, et al. Comparison of perindopril and amlodipine in cyclosporine-treated renal allograft recipients. *Hypertension.* 1995;26:436-444.

230. Midtvedt K, Hartmann A, Holdaas H, et al. Efficacy of nifedipine or lisinopril in the treatment of hypertension after renal transplantation: a double-blind randomised comparative trial. *Clin Transplant.* 2001;15:426-431.

231. Brozena SC, Johnson MR, Ventura H, et al. Effectiveness and safety of diltiazem or lisinopril in treatment of hypertension after heart transplantation. Results of a prospective, randomized multicenter trail. *J Am Coll Cardiol.* 1996;27:1707-1712.

232. Lindenfeld J, Page RL, Zolty R, et al. Drug therapy in the heart transplant recipient: part III: common medical problems. *Circulation.* 2005;111:113-117.

233. Kobashigawa JA, Starling RC, Mehra MR, et al. Multicenter retrospective analysis of cardiovascular risk factors affecting long-term outcome of de novo cardiac transplant recipients. *J Heart Lung Transplant.* 2006;25:1063-1069.

234. Rossano JW, Cherikh WS, Chambers DC, et al. The International Thoracic Organ Transplant Registry of the International Society for Health and Lung Transplantation: twenty-first pediatric heart transplantation report- 2018; Focus theme: multi-organ transplantation. *J Heart Lung Transplant.* 2018;37:1184-1195.

235. Bryant R 3rd, Rizwan R, Villa CR, et al. Transplant outcomes for congenital heart disease patients bridged with a ventricular assist device. *Ann Thorac Surg.* 2018;106:588-594.

236. Castleberry C, Zafar F, Thomas T, et al. Allosensitization does not alter post-transplant outcomes in pediatric patients bridged to transplant with a ventricular assist device. *Pediatr Transplant.* 2016;20(4):559-564.

237. Butts RJ, Dipchand AI, Sutcliffe D, et al. Comparison of basiliximab vs. antithymocyte globulin for induction in pediatric heart transplant recipients: an analysis of the International Society of Heart and Lung Transplantion database. *Pediatr Transplant.* 2018;22(4):e13190. doi:10.1111/petr.13190

238. Schweiger M, Zuckermann A, Beiras-Fernandez A, et al. A review of induction with rabbit antithymocyte globulin in pediatric heart transplant recipients. *Ann Transplant.* 2018;23:322-333.

239. Schubert S, Renner C, Hammer M, et al. Relationship of immunosuppression to Epstein-Barr viral load and lymphoproliferative disease in pediatric heart transplant patients. *J Heart Lung Transplant.* 2008;27:100-105.

240. Urschel S, McCoy M, Cantor RS, et al. A current era analysis of ABO incompatible listing practice and impact on outcomes in young children requiring heart transplantation. *J Heart Lung Transplant.* 2020;39:627-635.

241. Urschel S, West LJ. ABO-incompatible heart transplantation. *Curr Opin Pediatr.* 2016;28(5):613-619. doi: 10.1097/MOP.0000000000000398

242. Yancy CM, Jessup M, Bozkurt B, et al. ACCF/AHA guideline for the management of heart failure: a report of the American College of Cardiology Foundation/American Heart Association Task Force on practice guidelines. *Circulation.* 2013;128:e240-e327.

243. Rogers JG, Patel CB, Mentz RJ, et al. Palliative Care in Heart Failure: the PAL-HF Randomized, Controlled Clinical Trial. *J Am Coll Cardiol.* 2017;70:331-341.

244. DeGroot L, Koirala B, Pavlovic N, et al. Outpatient Palliative Care in Heart Failure: an Integrative Review *J Palliat Med.* 2020;23:1257-1269.

245. Wiskar K, Toma M, Rush B. Palliative care in heart failure. *Trends Cardiovasc Med.* 2018;28:445-450.

SECTION VIII

DISEASES OF THE PERICARDIUM

53

Acute Pericarditis

James W. Lloyd, Sushil Allen Luis, Zi Ye, and Jae K. Oh

CHAPTER OUTLINE

Diagnosis and management of acute pericarditis

Diagnosis

History and physical examination
- Characteristic chest pain (classically, acute, pleuritic, positional)
- Pericardial rub (variably present in 1/3 of idiopathic cases)

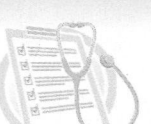

Electrocardiographic changes consistent with pericarditis (diffuse ST-segment elevation/ PR-segment depression, save aVR)

Pericardial effusion (new/worsening)

High sedimentation rate

Assessment by imaging and biopsy

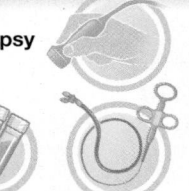

Treatment

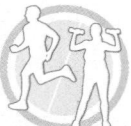

Non-pharmacologic (consideration of exercise modification/restriction)

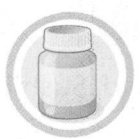

Pharmacologic (NSAID*, colchicine, and, as applicable, disease-specific therapy)

Etiologic evaluation

Laboratory assessment, imaging, biopsy
- Idiopathic (presumed viral)
- Non-idiopathic (non-viral infectious, non-infectious, acute myopericardial syndromes)

Complications

Arrhythmias

Pericardial effusions with/without tamponade

Recurrent pericarditis

Incessant/chronic pericarditis

Constrictive pericarditis

Chapter 53 Fuster and Hurst's Central Illustration. Acute pericarditis is diagnosed on the basis of clinical, electrocardiographic and, as necessary, imaging criteria. Depending on the clinical scenario, additional evaluation may prove necessary to identify causative factors, though the majority of cases are idiopathic and presumed viral in origin. Treatment rests on nonpharmacologic and pharmacologic approaches. While most cases of acute pericarditis have a benign course, resolving spontaneously, pericarditis can recur despite initial resolution, persist without clinical resolution, and give rise to additional complications, including arrhythmias and constrictive pericarditis. *NSAIDs are not used to treat pericarditis associated with acute myopericardial syndromes.

CHAPTER SUMMARY

This chapter outlines the pathophysiology and management of acute pericarditis as well as prognosis and potential complications (see Fuster and Hurst's Central Illustration). Of pericardial diseases, acute pericarditis represents the most commonly encountered entity after pericardial effusions. Diagnosis typically involves combined clinical and electrocardiographic assessment, although further evaluation with laboratory studies and imaging (particularly echocardiography) is often required. Frequently, initial assessment yields no particular etiology, suggesting an idiopathic cause (often presumed viral), and treatment rests on combined therapy with nonsteroidal anti-inflammatory agents and colchicine. Less commonly, however, acute pericarditis may develop secondary to either alternative infectious processes (eg, bacterial) or noninfectious factors, including autoimmune/autoinflammatory disorders, pericardial injury (eg, surgery), metabolic derangements, malignancy, or medications. In such instances, treatment may include nonsteroidal anti-inflammatory agents and colchicine as well as therapy directed toward the underlying cause(s). Following its initial identification and treatment, acute pericarditis may be accompanied by one or more complicating factors, including arrhythmias and pericardial effusions (with/without tamponade). Depending on the response to therapy and the successful treatment of contributing factors, acute pericarditis may recur despite initial clinical resolution and can assume an incessant/chronic form. In such cases, a related, but distinct entity may arise in the form of constrictive pericarditis.

ANATOMY AND PHYSIOLOGY OF THE PERICARDIUM

As a doubled-layered sac surrounding the heart, the pericardium consists of two separate layers: the outer parietal pericardium and the inner visceral pericardium (**Fig. 53–1**). A dense collagenous network chiefly forms this outer parietal pericardium, while the inner visceral pericardium contributes to the epicardium, the outermost contiguous layer of the heart. Together, these layers define the pericardial cavity, which is itself lined by a single-layered columnar mesothelium, the serous pericardium. The serous pericardium arises from two contiguous components: the visceral and parietal. The visceral component extends along the epicardium, contributes to the outer aspect of the visceral pericardium, and reflects onto the inner surface of the parietal pericardium at the base of the heart and proximal great vessels. This reflection gives rise simultaneously to separate recesses within the pericardial cavity, including the oblique and transverse sinuses, and constitutes the inner lining of the parietal pericardium. While the transverse sinus separates the great arteries and veins, the more inferior oblique sinus separates the left atrium and pulmonary veins. Together, they contribute to pericardial reserve volume.

In conjunction with the outer fibrous pericardium, the visceral and parietal components serve several critical physiologic roles beyond their anatomic function, including immunologic, fibrinolytic, and hemodynamic. A shared blood supply arising from branches of neighboring pericardiophrenic arteries and aortic tributaries supports these roles in combination with rich innervation from surrounding phrenic and plexus neurons. In the case of the former, these neurons arise from cervical spinal nerves C4-C6 and fuse to form the phrenic nerves, arching over the anterolateral aspects of the parietal pericardium as they extend inferiorly to the diaphragm and serving as crucial intraoperative landmarks during cardiothoracic surgery, including pericardiectomy. While these supportive structures contribute critically to proper pericardial function, they—in conjunction with the pericardium as a whole—also contribute to the genesis of several important clinicopathologic conditions. These conditions include acute pericarditis and pericardial effusions with and without tamponade.

As enabled by its structure, innervation, and blood supply, the pericardium serves several critical functions under normal conditions (**Table 53–1**). With its fibrous framework, the pericardium modulates cardiac chamber filling and thereby cardiac output, helping define end-diastolic ventricular volumes, preload, and thus stroke volume. These effects become more apparent—and even functionally limiting—in certain scenarios, including exercise and pericardial disease (eg, constrictive pericarditis). Beyond hemodynamic function, the pericardium also displays several mechanical functions. These functions include physical protection of the heart from injury and infection (such as neighboring mediastinitis) and effectively frictionless equalization of external gravitational and related forces

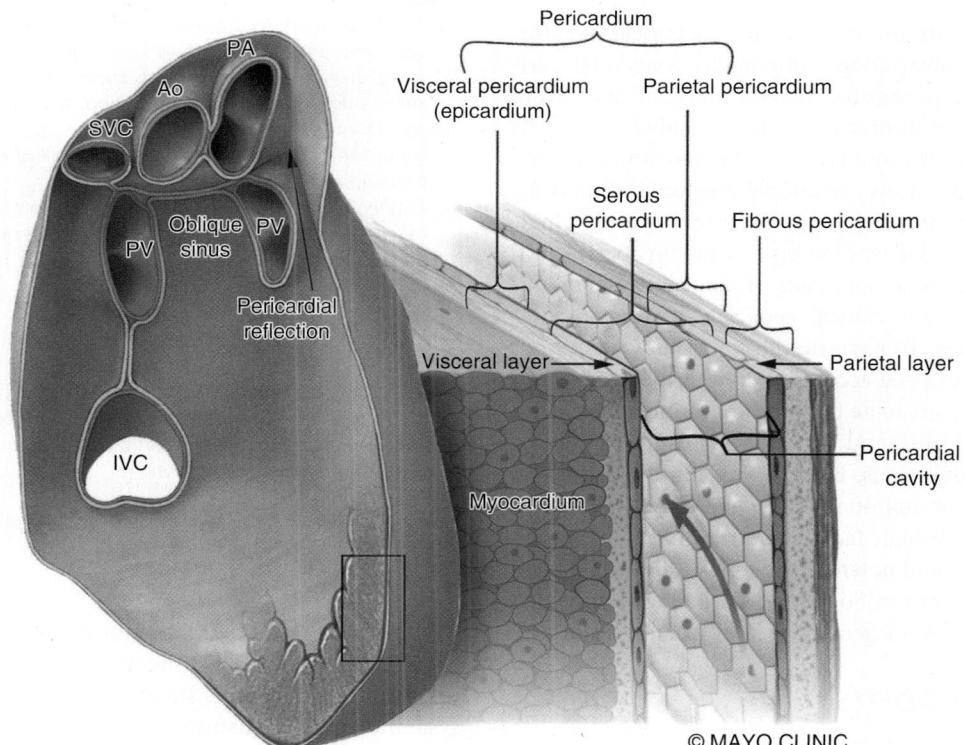

Figure 53–1. Anatomy of the pericardium. External to the myocardium, the pericardium consists of an outer parietal pericardium and an inner visceral pericardium that define the pericardial cavity. The serous pericardium includes a visceral layer, which lines the surface of the visceral pericardium, and a parietal layer, a continuous reflection of the visceral layer that lines the inner aspect of the parietal pericardium. From Melduni RM. Chapter 77: Pericardial Diseases. In: Murphy JG & Lloyd MA, editors. In: *Mayo Clinic Cardiology Concise Textbook*, 4th edition. New York: Oxford University Press, May 2013 used with permission of Mayo Foundation for Medical Education and Research, all rights reserved.

TABLE 53–1. Functions of the Pericardium

Mechanical
  Effects on chambers
    Limits short-term cardiac distention
    Facilitates cardiac chamber coupling and interaction
    Maintains pressure-volume relationship of the cardiac chambers
    and output from them
    Maintains geometry of left ventricle
  Effects on whole heart
    Lubricates, minimizes friction
    Equalizes gravitation and inertial hydrostatic forces
    Mechanical barrier to infection
Immunologic
Vasomotor
Fibrinolytic
Autocrine/paracrine (modulation of myocyte structure and function and gene expression)
Vehicle for drug delivery and gene therapy

TABLE 53–2. Etiology of Pericardial Diseases

Infectious Causes
Viral (common): Enteroviruses (coxsackieviruses, echoviruses), herpesviruses (Epstein-Barr virus, cytomegalovirus, human herpesvirus-6), adenoviruses, parvovirus B19 (possible overlap with etiologic viral agents of myocarditis)
Bacterial: *Mycobacterium tuberculosis* (common, other bacterial causes are rare), *Coxiella burnetii, Borrelia burgdorferi,* rarely: *Pneumococcus* spp., *Meningococcus* spp., *Gonococcus* spp., *Streptococcus* spp., *Staphylococcus* spp., *Haemophilus* spp., *Chlamydia* spp., *Mycoplasma* spp., *Legionella* spp., *Leptospira* spp., *Listeria* spp., *Providencia stuartii*
Fungal (rare): *Histoplasma* spp. (more likely in immunocompetent patients), *Aspergillus* spp., *Blastomyces* spp., *Candida* spp. (more likely in immunocompromised host)
Parasitic (rare): *Echinococcus* spp., *Toxoplasma* spp.
SARS-CoV-2
Noninfectious Causes
Autoimmune (common): Systemic autoimmune and autoinflammatory diseases (systemic lupus erythematosus, Sjögren syndrome, rheumatoid arthritis, scleroderma), systemic vasculitides (eg, eosinophilic granulomatosis with polyangiitis or allergic granulomatosis, previously named Churg-Strauss syndrome, Horton disease, Takayasu disease, Behçet syndrome), sarcoidosis, familial Mediterranean fever, inflammatory bowel diseases, Still disease
Neoplastic: Primary tumors (rare; especially pericardial mesothelioma), secondary metastatic tumors (common; especially lung and breast cancer, lymphoma)
Metabolic: Uremia, myxedema, anorexia nervosa, other rare
Traumatic and iatrogenic:
Early onset (rare):
• Direct injury (penetrating thoracic injury, esophageal perforation)
• Indirect injury (nonpenetrating thoracic injury, radiation injury)
Delayed onset:
• Pericardial injury syndromes (common) postmyocardial infarction syndrome, postpericardiotomy syndrome, posttraumatic, including forms after iatrogenic trauma (eg, coronary percutaneous intervention, pacemaker lead insertion, radiofrequency ablation).
Drug related (rare):
• Lupus-like syndrome (procainamide, hydralazine, methyldopa, isoniazid, phenytoin)
• Antineoplastic drugs (often associated with a cardiomyopathy; may cause a pericardiopathy): doxorubicin and daunorubicin, cytosine arabinoside, 5-fluorouracil, cyclophosphamide, immune checkpoint inhibitors
• Hypersensitivity pericarditis with eosinophilia: penicillins, amiodarone, methysergide, mesalamine, clozapine, minoxidil, dantrolene, phenylbutazone, thiazides, streptomycin, thiouracils, streptokinase, p-aminosalicylic acid, sulfa drugs, cyclosporine, bromocriptine, several vaccines, GM-CSF, anti-TNF agents
Other (common): Amyloidosis, aortic dissection, pulmonary arterial hypertension, chronic heart failure

Abbreviations: GM-CSF, granulocyte-macrophage colony-stimulating hormone; TNF, tumor necrosis factor.

across cardiac chambers through the production of pericardial fluid by the pericardial mesothelium. While performing these mechanical functions, the pericardium also assumes numerous well-defined physiologic roles, releasing autocrine and paracrine signals to influence neurovascular responses and myocyte function. Derangements in these and other functions form the basis of pericardial disease.

DISEASES OF THE PERICARDIUM

Diseases of the pericardium can manifest as pericardial effusions, pericarditis, constriction, tamponade, congenital pericardial disease, and pericardial masses and can arise from either infectious or noninfectious causes (**Table 53–2**). As inflammation of one or more layers of the pericardium, pericarditis represents the most commonly encountered pericardial disease after pericardial effusions and can vary widely in its extent and chronicity. Depending on its etiology, pericarditis can also manifest a broad spectrum of clinical presentations with decidedly different clinical sequelae, treatment paradigms, and prognoses. To navigate this variability, definitions of pericarditis have evolved according to both the time course of disease, ranging from acute to chronic and including incessant and recurrent forms, and suspected etiologies, including infectious and noninfectious. Beyond their utility in classifying pericarditis, these definitions have also evolved to guide research into the pathologic factors contributing to pericarditis, disease diagnosis, and potential therapies. **Table 53–3** summarizes the 2015 European Society of Cardiology Guidelines for the Diagnosis and Management of Pericardial Diseases.[1]

ACUTE PERICARDITIS

Epidemiology of Acute Pericarditis

Acute pericarditis accounts for approximately 5% of emergency department presentations for chest pain without acute coronary syndrome.[2] Among cases of acute pericarditis in developed countries, the majority (variably reported as 55%–86%) arise idiopathically, are of assumed viral origin, and occur more frequently in men.[3-6] Following acute idiopathic pericarditis, pericarditis stemming from systemic disease (eg, systemic lupus erythematosus), pericardial injury syndromes, malignancy-related pericarditis, and tuberculous pericarditis comprise the next most commonly encountered forms of pericarditis. In developing countries, tuberculous pericarditis accounts for the majority of documented cases.[7] The following sections will focus first on acute idiopathic pericarditis

TABLE 53–3. Summary of the 2015 European Society of Cardiology Guidelines on the Diagnosis and Management of Pericardial Diseases[1]

	Indication	Evidence
Acute and recurrent pericarditis		
A triage is recommended to identify high-risk patients who should be admitted to hospital. Low-risk patients can be managed as outpatients.	Class I	Level B
Colchicine is now a first-choice drug to be used as adjunct to aspirin/NSAID or corticosteroids to treat and prevent pericarditis either in acute or recurrent pericarditis (weight-adjusted doses are recommended without a loading dose; eg, 0.5 mg twice a day for 3 months in acute pericarditis and 6 months in recurrent pericarditis; colchicine should be given only as 0.5 mg once for patients <70 kg).	Class I	Level A
Levels of C-reactive protein are useful to guide the treatment duration and assess the response to treatment in acute and recurrent pericarditis; anti-inflammatory therapy should be maintained until symptom resolution and C-reactive protein normalization.	Class IIa	Level C
Corticosteroids should not be prescribed as first choice in patients with acute pericarditis since it may favor disease recurrence.	Class III	Level C
Pericardial effusion		
The essential indications to drain a pericardial effusion include: (1) cardiac tamponade (therapeutic pericardiocentesis), (2) a suspicion of bacterial or neoplastic etiology, and (3) persistent moderate to large pericardial effusion without response to medical therapy.	Class I	Level C
A triage system is proposed also for the management of pericardial effusion and is essentially based on the following: (1) recognize cardiac tamponade and possible bacterial of neoplastic etiologies, (2) exclude concomitant pericarditis or treat as pericarditis, (3) identify associated underlying diseases, and (4) if chronic and large (>20 mm), consider pericardial drainage to prevent cardiac tamponade during follow-up.	Class I	Level C
Treatment of pericardial effusions should be tailored as much as possible to the underlying etiology.	Class I	Level C
Cardiac tamponade		
In a patient with clinical suspicion of cardiac tamponade, echocardiography is recommended as the first imaging technique to evaluate the size, location, and degree of hemodynamic impact of the pericardial effusion.	Class I	Level C
Urgent pericardiocentesis or cardiac surgery is recommended to treat cardiac tamponade.	Class I	Level C
A judicious clinical evaluation including echocardiographic findings is recommended to guide the timing of pericardiocentesis.	Class I	Level C
Vasodilators and diuretics are not recommended in the presence of cardiac tamponade.	Class III	Level C
Constrictive pericarditis		
CT and CMR are indicated for the evaluation of a suspected constrictive pericarditis as second-level imaging techniques after echocardiography.	Class I	Level C
Cardiac catheterization is indicated only in complex cases when noninvasive imaging does not provide a clear-cut diagnosis or provides conflicting results.	Class I	Level C
The mainstay of therapy for chronic constriction is radical pericardiectomy, but it is acknowledged that there is a need to assess the possible presence of pericardial inflammation (eg, elevation of C-reactive protein, pericardial inflammation on CT/CMR) as precipitating cause in new-onset cases in order to treat with empiric anti-inflammatory therapy.	Class I	Level C
Diagnostic workup of pericardial diseases		
First diagnostic evaluation in a patient with a clinical suspicion of pericardial disease should include focused history and physical examination, ECG, chest x-ray, and routine blood tests, including markers of myocardial inflammation and lesion and renal function.	Class I	Level C
Echocardiography is the first essential diagnostic imaging tool, whereas CT and CMR are second-level imaging techniques for specific indications.	Class I	Level C
Additional diagnostic testing should be targeted and clinically guided.	Class I	Level C
Main specific forms _Tuberculosis_		
Empiric antituberculous therapy is only recommended in countries where tuberculosis is endemic and the disease is highly probable in the setting of a patient with pericarditis and pericardial effusion.	Class I	Level C
In cases with an established diagnosis of tuberculous pericarditis, standard antituberculous therapy is recommended for 6 months and prevents the evolution to constrictive pericarditis.	Class I	Level C
In patients with tuberculous pericarditis with features of constriction and not responding to antituberculous therapy, pericardiectomy is recommended after 4–8 weeks of medical therapy.	Class I	Level C

(Continued)

TABLE 53–3. Summary of the 2015 European Society of Cardiology Guidelines on the Diagnosis and Management of Pericardial Diseases[1] (Continued)

	Indication	Evidence
Neoplastic pericardial diseases		
The definite diagnosis of neoplastic pericardial disease relies on the evidence of neoplastic cells on cytology of pericardial fluid.	Class I	Level B
Pericardial biopsy should be considered for the final etiologic diagnosis in selected cases.	Class IIa	Level B
Tumor markers in pericardial fluid may be helpful to differentiate a benign vs a malignant pericardial effusion.	Class IIa	Level B
In cases with a confirmed diagnosis of neoplastic pericardial disease, systemic antineoplastic treatment is indicated.	Class I	Level B
Extended pericardial drainage is recommended to prevent recurrent cardiac tamponade and pericardial effusion and to provide a way for intrapericardial therapy.	Class I	Level B
Intrapericardial therapy with cytostatic agents should be considered to treat neoplastic pericardial disease.	Class IIa	Level B

Abbreviations: CT, computed tomography; CMR, cardiac magnetic resonance; ECG, electrocardiography; NSAID, nonsteroidal anti-inflammatory drugs.

(ie, pericarditis arising from presumed viral origin without other cause) and subsequently on secondary forms.

Evaluation and Diagnosis of Acute Pericarditis

History and Physical Examination

The initial evaluation of acute idiopathic pericarditis rests fundamentally on thorough clinical assessment through careful history taking and physical examination. From this assessment, the initial diagnosis of acute pericarditis can often be made, relying clinically on the presence of at least two of four characteristics features as subsequently described (**Table 53–4, Fig. 53–2**).[1] Of these features, half derive from clinical evaluation alone and include characteristic chest pain and a pericardial friction rub.

The chest pain characteristic of acute idiopathic pericarditis traditionally develops suddenly in a substernal to left-sided location along the anterior thorax. Routinely, it is sharp and pleuritic, worsening with deep inspiration and/or supine positioning and improving with leaning forward. Given the shared innervation of the pericardium by the phrenic nerves, this pain can radiate and be referred to the left and/or right shoulders, interscapular region, and, in particular, the trapezius ridge. In fact, the report of chest pain radiating to the trapezius ridge offers a very specific clinical finding strongly suggestive of acute pericarditis.[2,8] Despite these notable features, the chest pain classically associated with acute pericarditis, while common on presentation in acute idiopathic disease (more than 85%–90% of cases), does not appear uniformly and may be atypical and even absent in other causes of acute pericarditis.[9]

Beyond classic acute-onset, pleuritic chest pain, other symptoms, and historical features contribute to the diagnosis of acute idiopathic pericarditis. Additional symptoms on initial presentation may include atypical chest discomfort (variably described as dull and/or pressure like), dyspnea (either at rest or with exertion), and fatigue. Patients may also report a preceding history of symptoms suggestive of viral illness, including accompanying malaise, myalgias, and upper and/or lower respiratory tract symptoms. The elicitation of such symptoms may support a diagnosis of acute idiopathic pericarditis secondary to an antecedent viral infection. Similarly, review of prior medical diagnoses, procedural and surgical interventions, medications, and environmental exposures may aid further in the diagnosis of acute pericarditis and afford revealing clues to one or more contributing factors.

Apart from clinical history, the physical examination forms a second crucial element of diagnosing acute pericarditis, and descriptions of acute pericarditis have classically included pericardial friction rub as a specific finding. Present in roughly one-third of all patients with acute idiopathic pericarditis,[10] the pericardial friction rub arises from inflammation of the visceral and parietal layers of the serous pericardium and is often transient, requiring careful serial examinations with the patient upright, leaning forward, and holding respirations to maximize detection.[11] As historically described, three separate components on auscultation combine to characterize the classic rub and reflect different portions of the cardiac cycle, including atrial systole, ventricular diastole, and ventricular systole.[12] As these components arise from the cardiac cycle, the pericardial friction rub commonly (though not necessarily) occurs independently of respiration, helping to distinguish it from a pleural rub. In most cases, however, auscultation discloses a three-component rub in only approximately 50% of patients presenting with a rub, and the examiner may appreciate only either a two- or one-component rub in the remaining 33 and 17% of patients, respectively.[12]

TABLE 53–4. Definition and Diagnostic Criteria for Acute Pericarditis

Inflammatory pericardial syndrome to be diagnosed with at least 2 of the 4 following criteria:
(1) pericarditis chest pain (classically sharp, pleuritic, and positional)
(2) pericardial rub
(3) characteristic electrocardiographic change (eg, new widespread ST-segment elevation or PR-segment depression)
(4) pericardial effusion (new or worsening)
Additional supporting findings:
　Elevation of markers of inflammation (ie, elevated C-reactive protein, erythrocyte sedimentation rate, and/or white blood cell count);
　Evidence of pericardial inflammation by cross-sectional imaging (computed tomography and/or cardiac magnetic resonance).

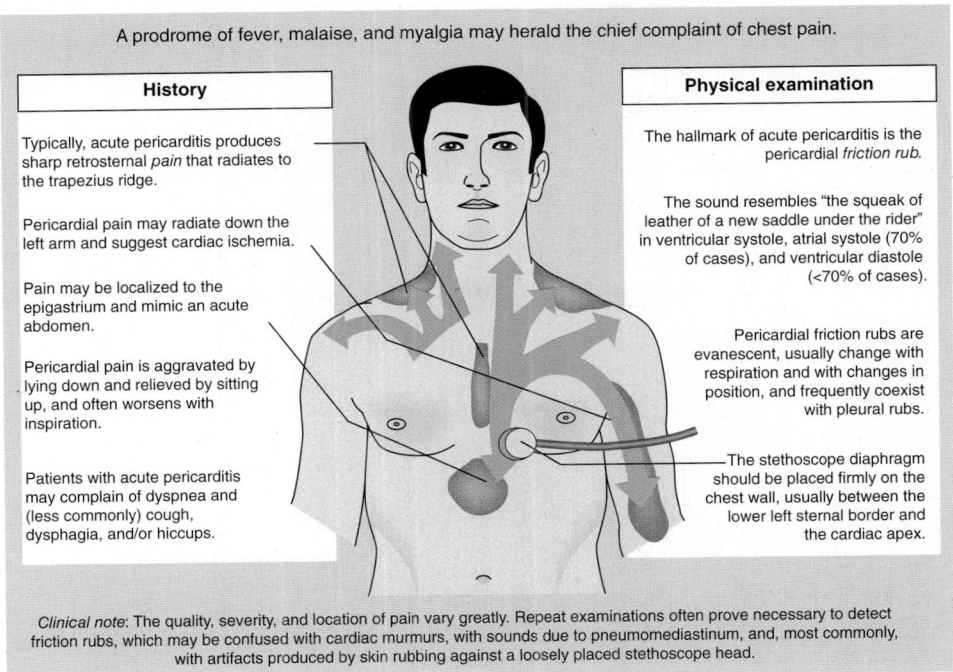

A prodrome of fever, malaise, and myalgia may herald the chief complaint of chest pain.

History

Typically, acute pericarditis produces sharp retrosternal *pain* that radiates to the trapezius ridge.

Pericardial pain may radiate down the left arm and suggest cardiac ischemia.

Pain may be localized to the epigastrium and mimic an acute abdomen.

Pericardial pain is aggravated by lying down and relieved by sitting up, and often worsens with inspiration.

Patients with acute pericarditis may complain of dyspnea and (less commonly) cough, dysphagia, and/or hiccups.

Physical examination

The hallmark of acute pericarditis is the pericardial *friction rub.*

The sound resembles "the squeak of leather of a new saddle under the rider" in ventricular systole, atrial systole (70% of cases), and ventricular diastole (<70% of cases).

Pericardial friction rubs are evanescent, usually change with respiration and with changes in position, and frequently coexist with pleural rubs.

The stethoscope diaphragm should be placed firmly on the chest wall, usually between the lower left sternal border and the cardiac apex.

Clinical note: The quality, severity, and location of pain vary greatly. Repeat examinations often prove necessary to detect friction rubs, which may be confused with cardiac murmurs, with sounds due to pneumomediastinum, and, most commonly, with artifacts produced by skin rubbing against a loosely placed stethoscope head.

Figure 53–2. Diagnostic criteria of acute pericarditis. A diagnosis is made based on the presence of at least two of four of the presented criteria. Reproduced with permission from Hoit BD. Acute pericarditis: diagnosis and differential diagnosis. *Hosp Pract.* 1991;27:23-43.

Other examination findings offer valuable insights and may reflect the simultaneous development of complications. Such findings on assessment could include decreased heart sounds to support the presence of a pericardial effusion; evidence of heart failure (eg, S3, lower extremity edema, rales, and abdominal distension); and elevated jugular venous pressure with pulsus paradoxus, tachycardia, and hypotension to suggest simultaneous tamponade. In uncomplicated acute idiopathic pericarditis, jugular venous pressure remains normal. In addition to findings suggestive of potential complications, physical examination may also reveal one or more causative factors, including, for instance, evidence of an underlying connective tissue disease process and/or manifestations of an evolving malignancy.

Electrocardiographic Assessment

Following clinical evaluation, electrocardiographic assessment with resting 12-lead electrocardiogram (ECG) should be performed as part of the routine evaluation of patients presenting with possible acute pericarditis.[1] This evaluation aids in diagnosis through the identification of characteristic changes associated with acute pericarditis and can provide further insight into etiology and complications.

In patients with acute idiopathic pericarditis, the resting 12-lead ECG has historically been described as evolving through four stages in concert with disease progression and resolution.[13,14] As the pericardium itself is nonconducting, changes on ECG necessarily imply involvement of the subepicardium (ie, the myocardium), and their appreciation depends on the timing of presentation. With pericarditis onset, widespread ST-segment elevation (often less than 5 mm) in a noncoronary distribution with concomitant PR-segment depressions appear secondary to subepicardial inflammation and augmented atrial repolarization (**Fig. 53–3**).[13] Simultaneously, lead aVR may disclose PR-segment elevation, further suggesting acute pericarditis and referred to as the "knuckle sign."[15] These changes form stage 1 of ECG evolution in acute idiopathic pericarditis, can develop within hours of symptom onset, and characterize one of four diagnostic features (beyond the clinical criteria).[16,17] At this stage, the ratio of ST-segment elevation to T-wave amplitude in lead V6 can be assessed, with a value in excess of 0.24 additionally suggestive of underlying acute pericarditis.[16]

Following stage 1 and over the course of hours to days, ST- and PR-segment deviations resolve (stage 2), giving way to diffuse T-wave inversions (stage 3). As the disease subsides, the ECG returns to baseline over weeks to months (stage 4) in most instances, although T-wave inversions may persist in select cases (eg, chronic pericarditis).[16,17] As with classically reported historical and physical examination features, however, patients with acute pericarditis may not uniformly display and/or progress through each of these four separate stages. In fact, while 90% of patients presenting with acute pericarditis will have some kind of ECG abnormality, less than 60% will demonstrate progression through all four stages described.[18] As a result, a normal ECG does not exclude pericarditis. Nonetheless, despite their shortcomings, the specific nature of these changes makes them an essential element of the diagnosis of acute pericarditis and may, with the advent and application of artificial intelligence, contribute even more to the diagnosis of acute idiopathic pericarditis in the future.

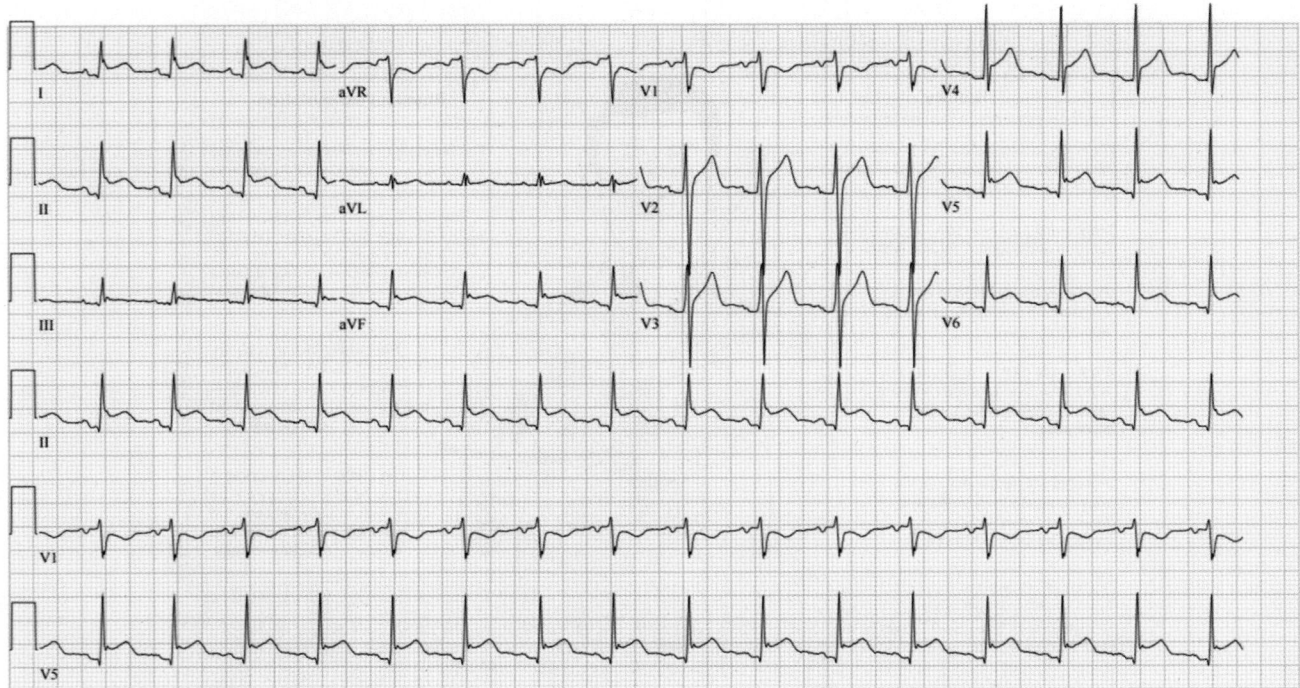

Figure 53–3. Resting 12-lead electrocardiogram revealing for class stage I electrocardiographic changes in patient presenting with acute pericarditis. Key features include diffuse ST-segment elevation with concordant PR-segment depression in a nonterritory-specific distribution. Of note, aVR classically demonstrates simultaneous ST-segment depression with PR-segment elevation.

While the aforementioned pattern of ST-segment elevation has routinely been associated with acute pericarditis, other diagnostic considerations of acute chest pain also display ST-segment elevation. Careful inspection of the presenting ECG and serial ECG assessments can aid in distinguishing acute pericarditis from these other considerations, which notably include benign early repolarization and acute coronary syndrome (**Table 53–5**). In contrast to the ECG features of acute pericarditis, those of acute coronary syndrome, for instance, commonly include more convex and localized ST-segment elevation with reciprocal ST-segment depression (eg, in lead aVL in the setting of an inferior ST-segment myocardial infarction), Q-wave formation with loss of R-wave amplitude to suggest underlying infarction, and simultaneous (as opposed to temporally separate) T-wave inversion reflecting ischemia-related changes in repolarization.[9,16] Additionally, in the case of acute coronary syndrome, PR-segment depression—in the absence of atrial infarction—is decidedly less common.[19] These differences aid in the critical distinction of acute pericarditis from acute coronary syndrome and may guide the often difficult decision to pursue (or not to pursue) invasive assessment, particularly since the latter condition requires urgent coronary angiography.[20]

Laboratory Evaluation

Initial laboratory assessment in acute pericarditis includes serum creatinine, complete blood count (CBC), and markers of inflammation (ie, erythrocyte sedimentation rate [ESR]

TABLE 53–5. Differential Diagnosis of Acute Pericarditis versus Early Repolarization and ST-Segment Elevation Myocardial Infarction (STEMI)

Electrocardiographic Feature	Acute Pericarditis	Early Repolarization	STEMI
PR-segment depression	Possible	No	No
ST-segment elevation	Concave up	Concave up	Usually convex
Localization of ST-segment elevation	Widespread	Usually precordial, inferior leads	Localized
Reciprocal ST-segment changes	No	No	Common
T-wave inversion	Yes, but after ST-segment normalization	No	Yes, before ST-segment normalization
ST/T ratio in lead V$_6$	>0.25	<0.25	Variable
Presence of Q waves	No	No	Possible
QT-interval prolongation	No	No	Possible

and C-reactive protein [CRP]). While elevated creatinine can suggest nephropathy and guide subsequent therapy, CBC may reveal anemia, possibly reflecting a simultaneous systemic process and a secondary form of acute pericarditis. At the same time, CBC may also disclose prominent leukocytosis (greater than 13,000 cells/mm³), supporting, in the appropriate clinical context, a related infection (ie, purulent pericarditis).[2] Increased markers of inflammation, although nonspecific, can provide further evidence of acute pericarditis and guide therapy. For example, approximately 75% to 80% of patients with acute idiopathic pericarditis will have an elevated CRP that peaks around 48 hours after disease onset and often normalizes within approximately 1 to 2 weeks. Persistent elevation despite therapy indicates an increased risk of recurrence and constrictive pericarditis.[21]

In addition to abnormalities on routine laboratory assessment, patients with acute idiopathic pericarditis frequently present with detectable elevations in troponin (variably reported as 30%–50%).[22,23] Such elevation reflects concomitant involvement of the myocardium through contiguous inflammation and/or simultaneous acute myocardial injury. While ST-segment elevation alone does not reliably predict troponin elevation on presentation (specificity 43%), the degree of troponinemia does correlate with the magnitude of ST-segment elevation.[23] In cases of isolated acute pericarditis without significant myocardial involvement, elevated levels will typically normalize within 1 to 2 weeks of diagnosis and treatment initiation. Persistent elevation beyond 2 weeks, however, indicates more prominent inflammation and a likely underlying myopericardial syndrome.[22,23] In contrast to other causes of troponin elevation (in particular, acute coronary syndrome), however, the short- and long-term prognosis in such patients generally remains good (with both clinical heart failure and death uncommon events).[24]

Further laboratory evaluation beyond that already described depends on suspected causes of acute pericarditis. As the majority of cases are idiopathic and presumed viral in etiology, temptation often arises to test for specific viral pathogens, including, for example, with viral serologies and/or nucleic acid amplification testing. Frequently, however, such pathogens are themselves without dedicated treatment options beyond supportive care, and their identification is accordingly of limited clinical utility. Notable exceptions include acute pericarditis related to influenza and severe acute respiratory syndrome coronavirus 2 (SARS-CoV-2). In other cases, initial clinical evaluation may reveal findings that raise the suspicion of nonviral causes and inform crucial additional laboratory assessment. In these instances, targeted assessment to identify bacterial, fungal, and/or parasitic infections; connective tissue disease and other autoimmune phenomena; and specific malignancies can be pursued.

Echocardiography

Transthoracic echocardiography (TTE) is the principal imaging modality in the evaluation of acute pericarditis, both in diagnosis and in the assessment of any associated complications, and carries a class I recommendation.[1] As suggested, the diagnosis of acute pericarditis requires at least two of four features be present, one of which includes the identification of a new and/or worsening pericardial effusion. Although frequently normal in the case of acute idiopathic pericarditis, TTE provides a safe and noninvasive diagnostic modality with excellent sensitivity and specificity to identify pericardial effusions and potential coexistent cardiac tamponade.

When visualized echocardiographically, effusions appear anechoic and are located external to the visualized epicardium and within the surrounding parietal pericardium (**Fig. 53–4**). The greatest effusion depth at end-diastole determines its size; small effusions are those with an anechoic space less than 10 mm in depth at end-diastole, while intermediate and large effusions have depths of 10 to 20 and greater than 20 mm, respectively. Effusions beyond 20 mm in depth more likely reflect a nonidiopathic cause of acute pericarditis and increased risk of subsequent complications (eg, tamponade).[5] Beyond depth, however, distribution (eg, circumferential vs localized) and complexity further distinguish effusions. Simple effusions, for

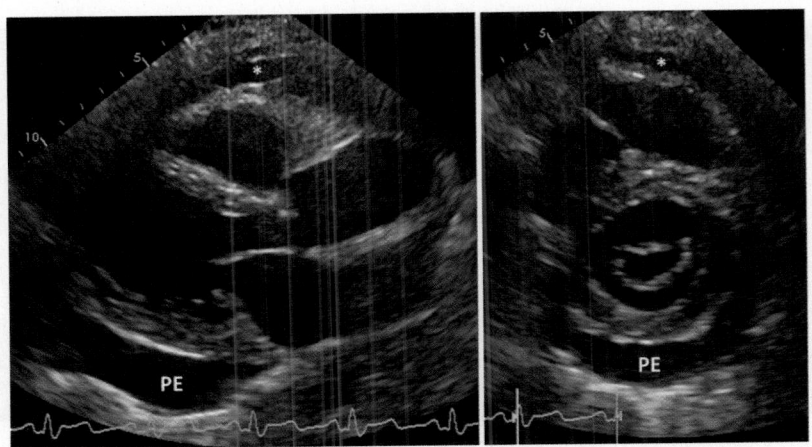

Figure 53–4. Transthoracic echocardiographic assessment of patient with acute pericarditis. Parasternal long-axis (*left*) and mitral valve short-axis (*right*) views reveal a large, circumferential pericardial effusion with anterior (*asterisk*) and posterior (PE) components. Based on its depth at end diastole (>20 mm), this effusion is large.

instance, demonstrate a uniformly anechoic void in the pericardial cavity. In contrast, a heterogeneous appearance of the pericardial space on TTE characterizes complicated effusions, with hemorrhage and coagulum, fibrin exudates and stranding, active infection, and malignant infiltration potentially contributing to this heterogeneity and assisting with the differential diagnosis further (**Fig. 53–5**).

TTE also provides insight into other pericarditis-related complications, including tamponade and constriction. As discussed separately, tamponade refers to a condition in which a pericardial effusion and/or additional space-occupying material within the pericardial cavity exhausts the pericardial reserve volume, increasing intrapericardial pressure (even above intracardiac pressure), augmenting ventricular interdependence, and

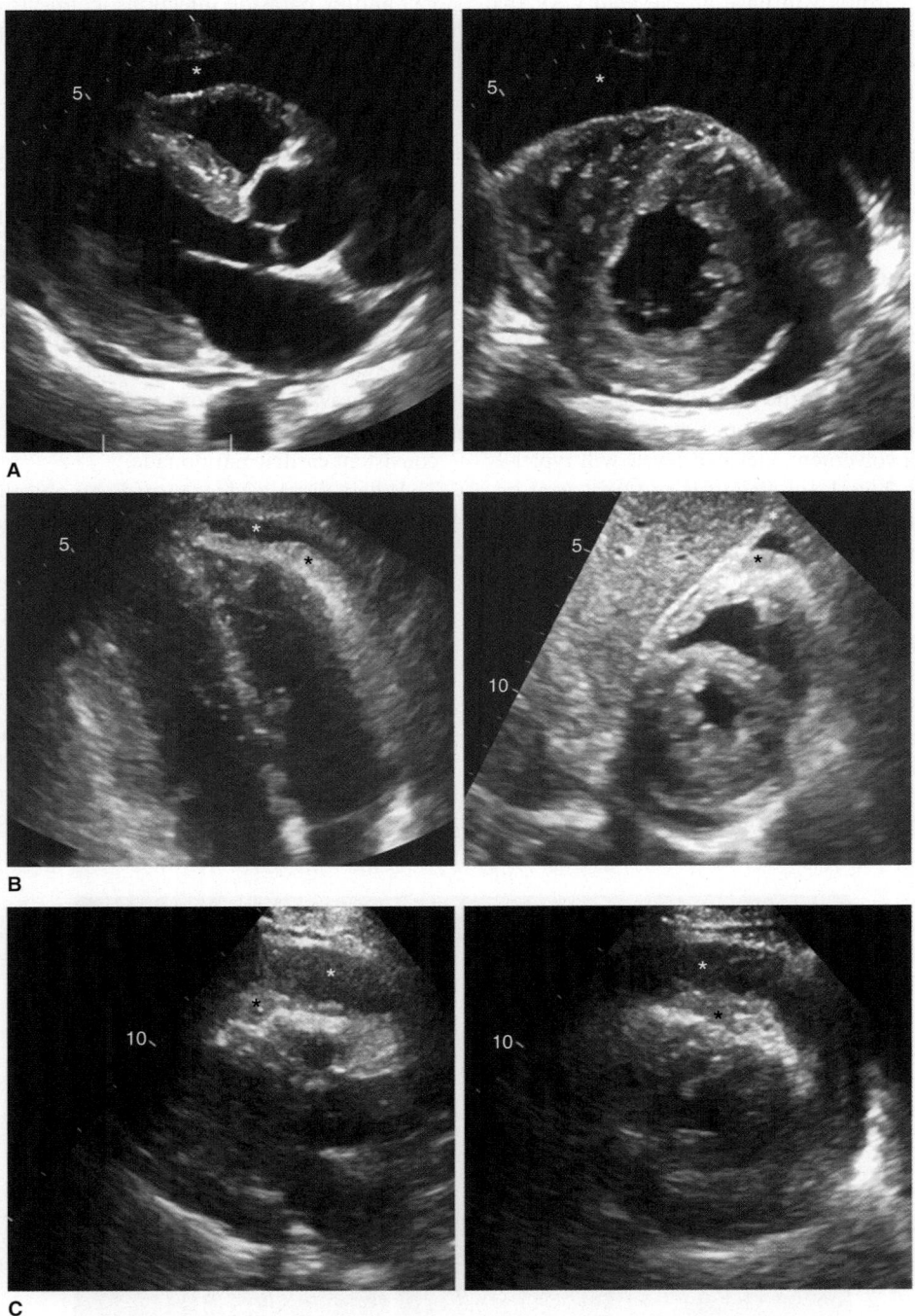

Figure 53–5. Two-dimensional echocardiography with parasternal long-axis views (*left*) and parasternal short-axis views (*right*) revealing pericardial effusions (*white asterisk*) in patients presenting with acute pericarditis, including (**A**) simple transudative, (**B**) exudative with fibrinous echogenic material (*black asterisk*), and (**C**) and hemorrhagic with coagulum (*black asterisk*).

precipitating a clinical syndrome of impaired cardiac output and heart failure. Echocardiographically, several findings can reveal tamponade with high specificity and sensitivity, including right ventricular diastolic collapse, abnormal diastolic ventricular septal wall motion, respirophasic variation in early tricuspid and mitral inflow velocities (to greater than 60% and 30%, respectively), and reduced stroke volume index.[25,26] Tamponade constitutes a medical emergency and requires immediate treatment independent of acute pericarditis. Simultaneously, its presence on initial evaluation should raise the suspicion of a secondary form of acute pericarditis (eg, malignant pericarditis).

Pericardial constriction is a second important complication of pericarditis and may be a presenting feature of acute disease. As with tamponade, constriction reflects a clinical syndrome with notable echocardiographic features. In some cases, constriction may first present as tamponade in the form of effusive-constrictive pericarditis. In such instances, the effusion effects tamponade physiology that persists until removed via pericardiocentesis, unmasking underlying constriction in the process. Echocardiographic findings of constrictive pericarditis are similar to those in tamponade, including important manifestations of heightened ventricular interdependence. Beyond these features, however, several findings distinguish constrictive pericarditis and include characteristic hepatic vein expiratory diastolic flow patterns with notable end-expiratory reversal; annulus and strain reversus; and altered superior vena cava flow patterns.[25,26] Notably, however, in the setting of acute pericarditis, constrictive physiology arising from pericardial inflammation is usually transient and may no longer be present on follow-up assessment after successful treatment. Transient constrictive pericardial physiology, where present, should be treated with aggressive and potentially prolonged anti-inflammatory therapy, with down-titration and withdrawal of therapy guided by normalization of inflammatory markers. Although the natural history of acute pericardial inflammation has not been clearly delineated, it is suspected that inadequately treated pericardial inflammation contributes to fibrosis and scar, potentially resulting in pericardial calcification and/or chronic constrictive pericarditis many years later.

Chest X-Ray

Routine evaluation of acute pericarditis includes chest x-ray with combined posteroanterior and lateral views. Although often normal in most patients with acute idiopathic pericarditis, chest x-ray can suggest the presence of associated complications, including, for instance, an enlarged cardiac silhouette to suggest a pericardial effusion or pericardial calcification indicating recurrent and/or chronic disease concerning for constrictive pericarditis (**Fig. 53–6**). In addition, such evaluation can provide insight into other cardiac and extracardiac processes that may be contributing to the patient's presentation (eg, tuberculosis).

Computed Tomography

Cross-sectional imaging with computed tomography (CT) in acute pericarditis aids in diagnosis, the identification of contributing and causative conditions, and the appreciation of complicating factors. Not infrequently, CT is the imaging modality in patients with chest pain for a "triple rule-out" diagnostic strategy and can detect pericardial effusion, prompting diagnostic consideration of acute pericarditis. It should be reserved, however, for when the initial presentation is atypical; echocardiography is nondiagnostic; or a secondary cause, including trauma, is suspected. In such instances, CT may provide important diagnostic clues to a patient's presentation beyond findings appreciated on clinical evaluation and TTE

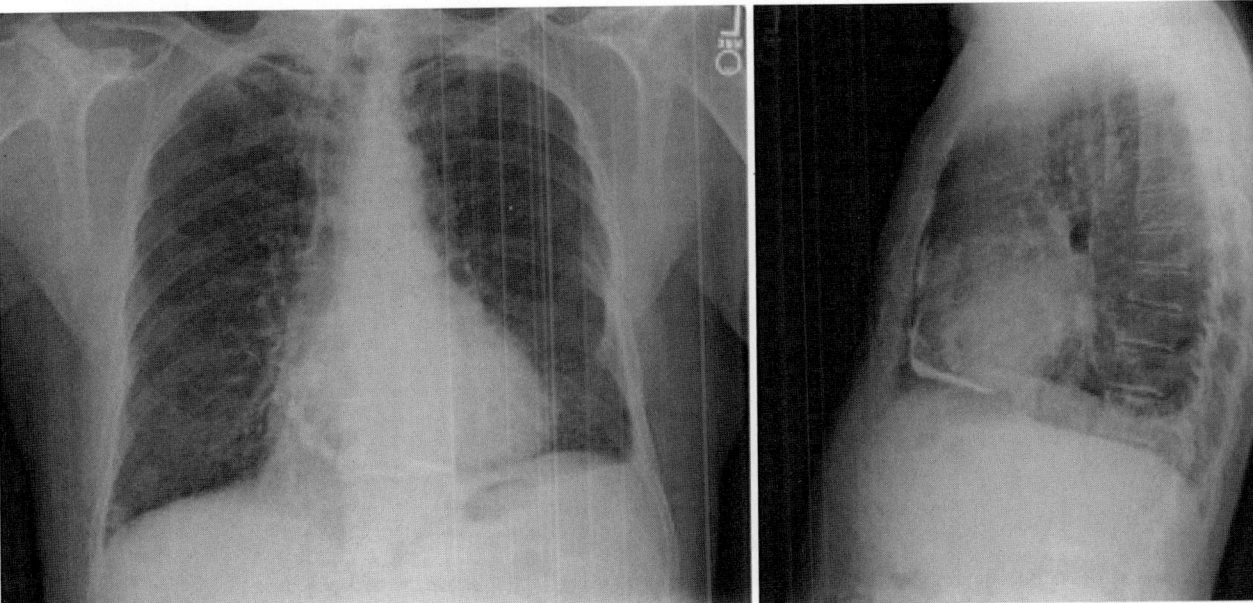

Figure 53–6. Posteroanterior and lateral upright radiograms revealing dense right-sided, anterior, and inferior pericardial calcification in a patient with recurrent constrictive pericarditis following remote partial pericardiectomy. Of note, a retained surgical needle lateral to the right heart border and in the lung parenchyma is also visualized.

alone. Relative to TTE, for instance, CT affords greater sensitivity to detect smaller pericardial effusions and can also reveal pathology both within and external to the pericardium (eg, primary pulmonary malignancy with contiguous lymphatic and/or hematogenous spread to the pericardium).[26] Additionally, in suspected acute pericarditis when the index of suspicion is low for an acute coronary syndrome, but uncertainty exists (eg, elevated troponin), ECG-gated cardiac CT offers the opportunity to exclude flow-limiting coronary artery disease as a cause for presentation and may be an alternative to coronary angiography in this setting.

Cardiac Magnetic Resonance Imaging

Similar to CT, cardiac magnetic resonance imaging (MRI) in patients with suspected acute pericarditis can characterize pericardial and extracardiac pathology in a fashion complementary to and beyond that offered by routine clinical and echocardiographic assessments. In contrast to CT, however, cardiac MRI offers additional important information in patients with possible acute pericarditis—in particular, tissue characterization, hemodynamic assessment, and prognosis.

With cardiac MRI, tissue characterization of the perimyocardium becomes possible. Through the application of particular MRI sequences, for instance, cardiac MRI with T1-weighted black blood and T2-weighted STIR imaging can characterize pericardial effusion and reveal pericardial edema, respectively. Meanwhile, late gadolinium enhancement may suggest pericardial inflammation and/or fibrosis (even in the absence of pericardial effusion) (**Fig. 53–7**).[23] In this fashion, cardiac MRI can clarify the presence/absence of pericardial inflammation in patients with suspected acute pericarditis presenting with atypical symptoms, serving to guide not only diagnosis but also treatment initiation. Through similar techniques, cardiac MRI can reveal concomitant myocardial involvement, expanding diagnostic considerations, clarifying the nature of simultaneous elevations in cardiac biomarkers, and providing useful

prognostic information. Once identified at baseline, findings obtained via cardiac MRI can subsequently guide the duration and modification of dedicated therapies.

In addition to perimyocardial characterization at presentation, cardiac MRI also provides simultaneous hemodynamic assessment and separate prognostic information. Similar to TTE, real-time cine imaging with free-breathing exercises enables cardiac MRI to identify features of tamponade and constriction in patients with suspected pericarditis, providing acute prognostic information in the process. Beyond the acute period, perimyocardial inflammation visualized on cardiac MRI provides separate prognostic information. When present at baseline, for instance, most affected patients have persistent inflammation on follow-up MRI assessment at 3 months, resolving in the majority of individuals, however, by 6 months. Persistence of this inflammation beyond 6 months may reflect a worse clinical prognosis (eg, increased propensity to develop constrictive pericarditis and/or recurrent disease). With these findings in mind, serial cardiac MRI may guide treatment of acute pericarditis, including duration and intensity, particularly in those patients with atypical, recurrent, and diagnostically challenging presentations.

Additional Evaluation and Diagnostic Means

The diagnosis of acute pericarditis rests on clinical evaluation and other noninvasive assessments already described. When presenting with typical acute idiopathic pericarditis, no concern for complication, and prompt response to treatment (see section Treatment, Management, and Prognosis of Acute Pericarditis), such assessments generally suffice. In specific clinical scenarios, however, including, in particular, cases of suspected purulent acute pericarditis, connective tissue disease, or malignancy, further evaluation beyond clinical and noninvasive strategies proves necessary.

Above routine evaluation in acute pericarditis, additional diagnostic tools include pericardiocentesis and pericardial

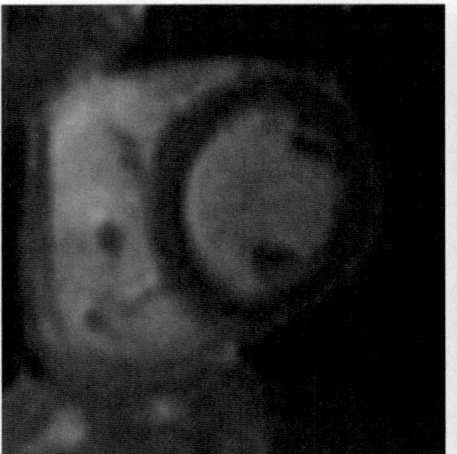 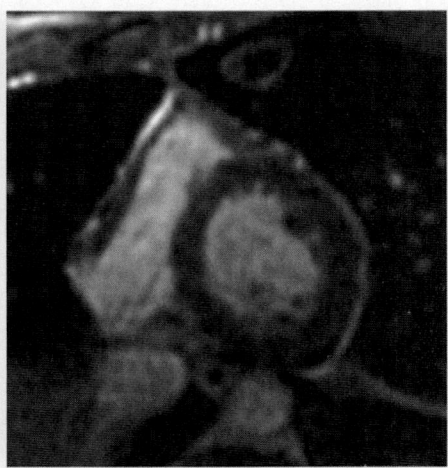 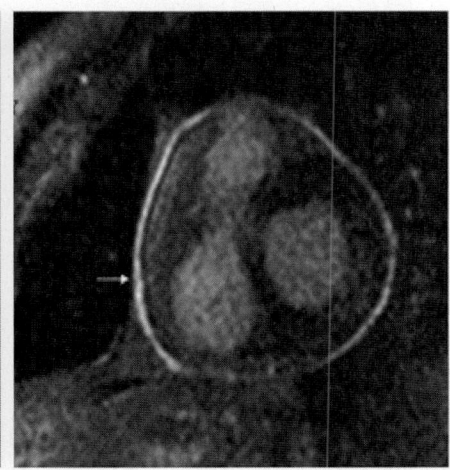

Figure 53–7. Short-axis cardiac magnetic resonance imaging views of the left and right ventricles in patients with acute pericarditis demonstrating progressively more prominent late gadolinium enhancement (*white arrow*) and thus pericardial inflammation. From left to right, increasing enhancement reveals mild, moderate, and severe pericardial inflammation, respectively. Reproduced with permission from Feng D, Glockner J, Kim K, et al. Cardiac magnetic resonance imaging pericardial late gadolinium enhancement and elevated inflammatory markers can predict the reversibility of constrictive pericarditis after antiinflammatory medical therapy: a pilot study. *Circulation*. 2011 Oct 25;124(17):1830-1837.

biopsy. In the case of the former, indications for pericardiocentesis include tamponade, suspected malignancy, or concerns for purulent pericarditis.[27] With pericardiocentesis, the pericardial space is accessed percutaneously, and pericardial fluid aspirated (**Fig. 53–8**). Aspirated fluid is subsequently sent for biochemical, infectious, and cytopathologic evaluation and, in the setting of cardiac tamponade, provides diagnostic findings in roughly 30% of presenting cases.[3] In the case of the latter, traditional means of pericardial biopsy have involved open surgical assessment with direct visualization. Over time, however, minimally invasive approaches have evolved and currently include pericardioscopy. With pericardioscopy, an endoscope is inserted percutaneously into the pericardial cavity, allowing for both visualization of the pericardial surface and guided biopsy of the pericardium. In the diagnosis of specific causes of acute pericarditis, these methods find their greatest utility.[28]

Apart from cases of suspected secondary causes, routine pericardiocentesis and biopsy have also been applied to all-comers with acute pericarditis. In such applications, pericardiocentesis and biopsy improve diagnostic yields, allowing for many patients with previously diagnosed "idiopathic" disease to be reassigned a specific cause for their presentation.[1,27-29] In these instances, however, reassignment for most patients equates to the identification of a particular viral cause of their acute pericarditis and not necessarily the reclassification of their disease, for instance, from an infectious to a noninfectious cause. Considering that most viral pathogens lack dedicated treatment beyond standard acute idiopathic pericarditis care, reassignment does not routinely lead to a change in clinical management, and the routine performance of pericardiocentesis and pericardial biopsy in suspected acute idiopathic pericarditis is not recommended. Instead, pericardiocentesis with/without biopsy demonstrates the greatest diagnostic yield in cases of tamponade; large pericardial effusions; and suspected malignancy, tuberculous pericarditis, or purulent pericarditis.[27,30,31]

TREATMENT, MANAGEMENT, AND PROGNOSIS OF ACUTE PERICARDITIS

Acute Management

The immediate management of acute pericarditis depends on the presence of clinically significant complications, particularly tamponade, and contributing factors (**Fig. 53–9**). When cardiac tamponade is present, prompt pericardiocentesis enables rapid treatment of both symptoms and reversal of underlying cardiovascular impairment. Beyond the management of such immediate complications, however, further treatment of acute pericarditis depends on etiology.

In the case of suspected acute idiopathic pericarditis, hospitalization should be considered for those individuals with either suspected or demonstrated complications and those with higher-risk features associated with worse prognosis (**Table 53–6**). Features that may raise the suspicion for nonidiopathic disease include a subacute-chronic presentation (developing over days to weeks), immunosuppression, related trauma, inadequate response to previous nonsteroidal anti-inflammatory drug (NSAID) therapy (if begun earlier), use of anticoagulant therapy, fever (greater than 38°C), a large pericardial effusion, and/or evidence of concomitant myocarditis.[5] Such findings suggest a nonidiopathic form of acute pericarditis and/or risk of complications, indicating a need for more extensive and urgent evaluation. In cases of uncomplicated idiopathic pericarditis without high-risk features (eg, a previously healthy adult with antecedent viral prodrome and typical symptoms), routine hospitalization is not required, and treatment can commence in the outpatient setting. In both hospitalized and nonhospitalized cases, as subsequently outlined, treatment principally consists of NSAID therapy, colchicine, activity restriction, and close follow-up.

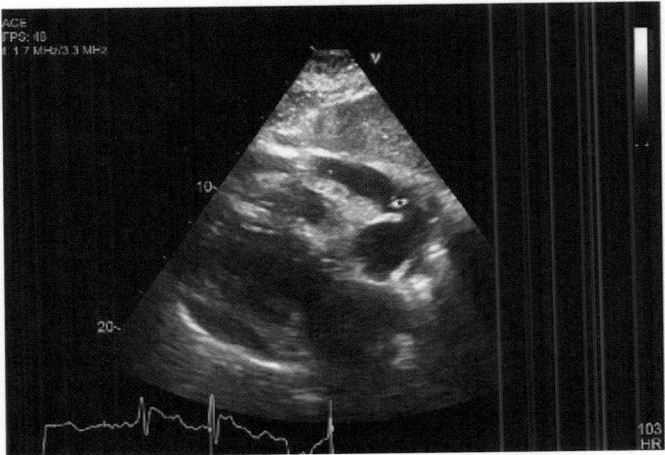

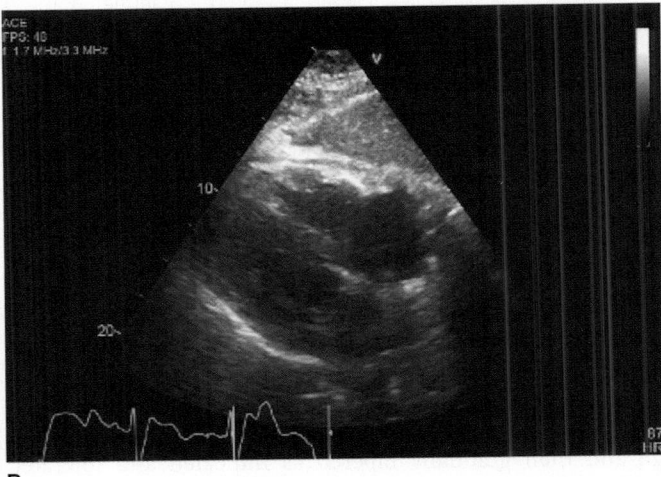

Figure 53–8. Subxiphoid transesophageal echocardiographic evaluation of patient with cardiac tamponade undergoing pericardiocentesis. During pericardiocentesis, the anechoic pericardial space and fluid are accessed (**A**) with a percutaneous drain (*black asterisk*). Follow-up evaluation minutes later (**B**) demonstrates successful drainage with resolution of the pericardial effusion.

NSAID Therapy

NSAID therapy forms the cornerstone of symptomatic management in acute pericarditis, including in both idiopathic and most nonidiopathic forms (note that in acute pericarditis

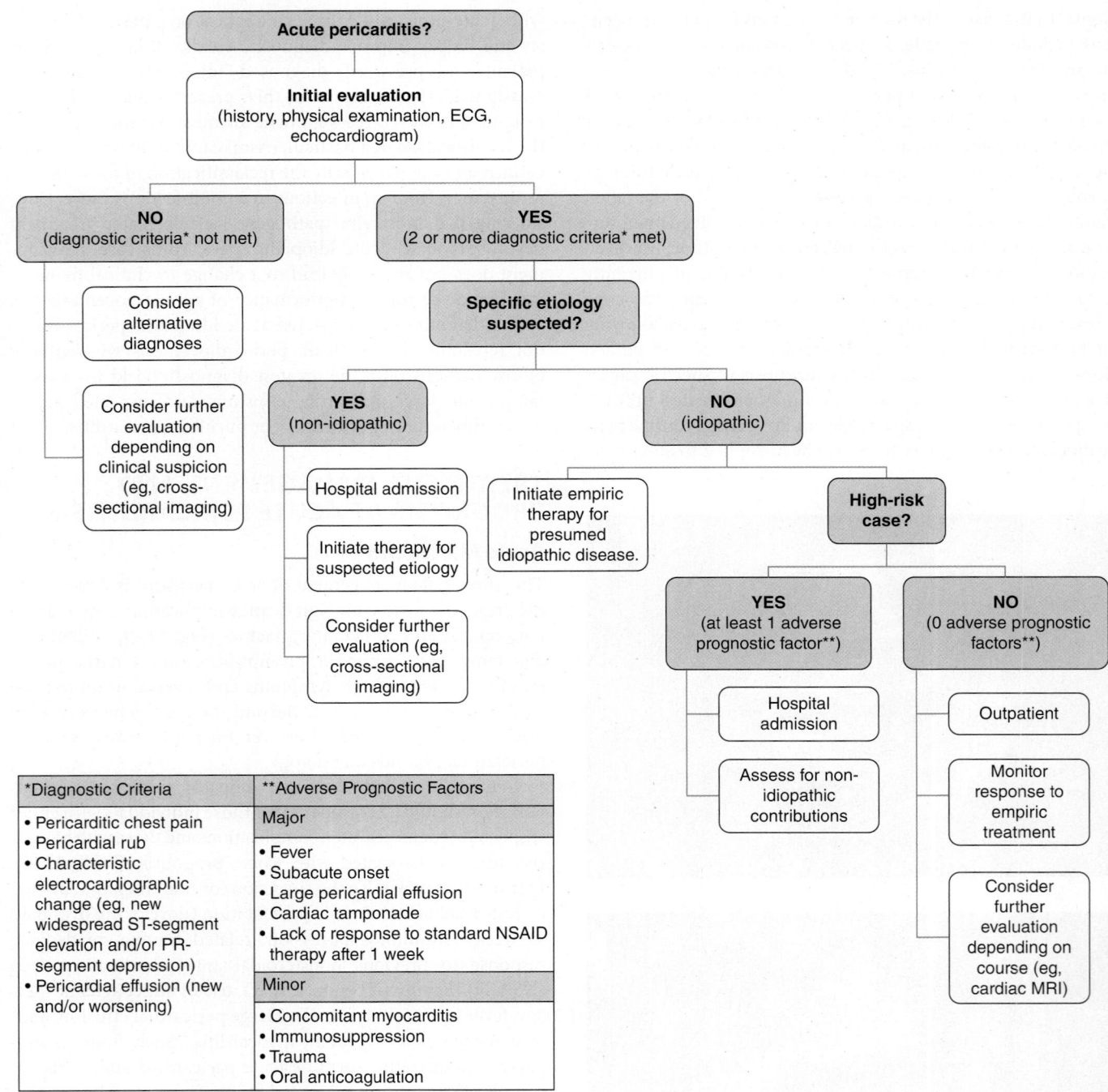

Figure 53–9. Overall approach to the evaluation and triage of acute pericarditis.

related to myocardial infarction, aspirin is recommended over alternative NSAID therapy due to a theoretical risk of impaired scar formation and mechanical complication with the latter).[32] In its capacity to treat pericarditis-related symptoms, particularly chest pain, NSAID therapy modulates the inflammatory milieu through prostaglandin synthesis inhibition. With this modulation, most patients with acute idiopathic pericarditis often experience prompt and sustained relief once initiated on NSAID therapy at appropriate, full-strength doses (**Table 53–7**). Over the course of the ensuing

1 to 2 weeks and predicated on close follow-up evaluation, NSAID therapy is initially maintained at full-strength doses until symptoms resolve and inflammatory markers normalize and then gradually tapered as indicated and tolerated by the patient. If tolerated by the patient and not otherwise contraindicated, the authors would recommend continued NSAID therapy 1 month beyond the resolution of chest pain to minimize pericardial inflammation and the risk of future constrictive pericarditis. Beyond clinical assessment, including a careful review of systems and physical examination,

TABLE 53–6. Indicators of Poor Prognosis and Nonidiopathic Etiology in Acute Pericarditis

Major
- Fever >38°C
- Subacute onset
- Large pericardial effusion (ie, >20 mm end-diastolic depth on echocardiography)
- Cardiac tamponade
- Lack of response to aspirin or NSAID after at least 1 week of therapy

Minor
- Pericarditis associated with myocarditis
- Immunosuppression
- Trauma
- Oral anticoagulant therapy

Abbreviation: NSAID, nonsteroidal anti-inflammatory drug.

additional information gleaned from follow-up laboratory and imaging assessment(s) directs this titration.

Historically, the presence of pericarditis-related symptoms and, for instance, the appreciation of a pericardial friction rub (or lack thereof) on physical examination have guided modifications in NSAID therapy. As suggested by more recent developments, however, follow-up laboratory evaluation and imaging assessment(s) can augment the clinical evaluation and, importantly, tailor NSAID therapy more closely, enabling a reduction in therapy duration and intensity and a corresponding reduction in therapy-related adverse outcomes. For instance, with the use of serial CRP monitoring, NSAID titration can be accelerated in many patients relative to historic timelines, resulting in reduced medication exposure and a curtailing of adverse side effects.[21] Such therapy modification becomes critically important in those patients at heightened risk of adverse outcomes (eg, gastritis), including those with underlying medical comorbidities such as baseline renal dysfunction, prior history of gastrointestinal bleeding and/or

TABLE 53–7. Empiric Anti-inflammatory Therapy for Acute Pericarditis

Drug	Usual Dosing	Duration	Tapering
Aspirin	750–1000 mg every 8 hours	1–2 weeks	Decrease doses every week: eg, 750 mg TID for 1 week, then 500 mg TID for 1 week, then stop
Ibuprofen	600 mg every 8 hours	1–2 weeks	Decrease doses every week: eg, 600 mg plus 400 mg plus 600 mg for 1 week, then 600 mg plus 400 mg plus 400 mg for 1 week, then 400 mg TID for 1 week, then stop
Colchicine	0.6 mg once (<70 kg) or 0.6 mg BID (≥70 kg)	3 months	Not mandatory; alternatively, 0.6 mg every other day (<70 kg) or 0.6 mg once (≥70 kg) in the last weeks

Abbreviations: BID, twice a day; TID, three times a day.

peptic ulcer disease, and simultaneous anticoagulant use. In cases involving patients with these and other risk factors, the routine use of concomitant proton pump inhibitor therapy is recommended.

Colchicine

In addition to NSAID therapy, colchicine forms the second prong of a characteristic and fundamental two-pronged approach to acute idiopathic pericarditis management. Molecularly, colchicine binds to and impairs the cellular cytoskeleton and its function, specifically at the level of the microtubule. In doing so, colchicine inhibits microtubule-dependent neutrophil migration, reduces the activity of cellular inflammasomes and the release of inflammatory mediators, and thus tempers overall inflammation.[33] These effects have established colchicine as an integral therapy in several conditions, including commonplace disorders such as gouty arthritis and acute pericarditis and less frequently encountered autoinflammatory disorders such as familial Mediterranean fever and tumor necrosis factor receptor-associated periodic syndrome.

Beginning in the early 21st century, several pivotal studies established the role of colchicine, a centuries-old medication, in the treatment of acute pericarditis and related complications.[34,35] Utilizing the outlined anti-inflammatory properties, these studies revealed an improvement in the rate of symptom resolution in acute idiopathic pericarditis and a reduction in both the rate of hospitalization and frequency of short- and long-term recurrence with the addition of colchicine to standard NSAID therapy. In response, colchicine has become a mainstay of acute idiopathic pericarditis treatment and, through additional investigation, achieved further prominence in the treatment and prevention of both postpericardiotomy syndrome, an iatrogenic pericarditis syndrome, and recurrent pericarditis. In the setting of an initial episode of acute idiopathic pericarditis, a 3-month course therapy is prescribed (at 0.5 mg–0.6 mg orally twice daily for patients in excess of 70 kg and once daily for those less than 70 kg) in conjunction with at least one month of simultaneous NSAID therapy (Table 53–7). Despite the evidence supporting its use, however, colchicine is not without its shortcomings.

Although supported by several prominent investigations, colchicine—like NSAID therapy itself—has several limitations. Colchicine, as an agent metabolized by the CYP450 and P-glycoprotein systems and dependent on renal function for adequate clearance, has several potentially limiting drug–drug interactions and side effects, including, most notably, gastrointestinal distress.[36,37] Given its mechanism of metabolism and route of elimination, these side effects may become more prominent in the presence of certain medications (eg, antibiotics) and underlying renal dysfunction. In such situations, dose reduction (if not outright cessation of therapy) may be necessary.

Corticosteroids

When added to conventional NSAID and colchicine therapies in the treatment of acute idiopathic pericarditis, patients treated with corticosteroids have demonstrated often rapid symptom resolution but a higher rate of adverse effects and recurrent inflammation or pericarditis.[34] Consequently, corticosteroids are customarily deployed as second-line therapies in the treatment of idiopathic pericarditis refractory to standard treatment. When prescribed for this purpose, low-dose therapy (with starting doses often of 0.2 mg–0.5 mg prednisone per kg) with a slow taper guided by serial clinical evaluation and monitoring of inflammatory markers may minimize recurrence risk and maximize tolerance relative to alternative, higher-dose regimens.[38] Despite rapid symptom resolution, it is imperative to note that rapid withdrawal of steroids is associated with a high risk of pericarditis recurrence. In most cases, initial commencement of prednisone (eg, at 20 mg daily) is sufficient for disease control, and steroids therapy must be tapered over months as suggested by current guidelines (**Table 53–8**).[1] In contrast to acute idiopathic pericarditis, corticosteroids may be first-line therapy in the treatment of acute pericarditis arising secondary to an underlying, corticosteroid-responsive process (eg, systemic lupus erythematosus) and in cases in which contraindications to NSAID and/or colchicine therapies exist (eg, pregnancy, drug–drug interactions, and concurrent anticoagulant use). In these instances, corticosteroids may form the preferred therapy and often effect prompt symptom resolution.

Nonpharmacologic Intervention

Nonpharmacologic interventions for the treatment of acute idiopathic pericarditis include avoidance of contributing factors (if nonidiopathic) and activity modification. Expert opinion recommends activity restriction in both nonathletes and athletes following a diagnosis of acute pericarditis.[1,39,40] In the case of nonathletes, this restriction limits activity to effectively sedentary levels and is encouraged until both associated symptoms and objective findings of pericarditis (eg, elevated inflammatory markers) normalize. In athletes, a minimal period of 3 months of activity restriction, including, importantly, avoidance of competitive athletics, is recommended (irrespective of the clinical resolution of acute pericarditis). These recommendations stem from the theory that increased activity raises average heart rates; results in greater pericardial friction, inflammation, and symptoms; and are supported by expert-level opinion and anecdotal clinical observations. Recent evaluation with serial laboratory assessment and cardiac MRI has supported this theory and expert-guided recommendation by demonstrating at least a correlation between activity restriction and both lower markers of inflammation and reduced pericardial enhancement on MRI in patients with acute idiopathic pericarditis.[41]

Prognosis

The prognosis of acute pericarditis depends fundamentally on its cause. Acute idiopathic pericarditis carries a favorable prognosis, particularly with the prompt deployment of appropriate therapy, and will resolve completely in nearly 90% of affected patients over the course of 2 to 6 weeks.[35] Complications amongst acute idiopathic pericarditis patients include tamponade (<5%), constrictive pericarditis (<2%), and recurrent disease (15%–30%).[34,35,42] As suggested, the initiation of appropriate therapy at the time of diagnosis limits the development of such complications. In nonidiopathic pericarditis, however, prognosis varies prominently with the underlying cause. In tuberculous and purulent pericarditides, for example, the incidence of constrictive pericarditis, as diagnosed clinically and by corroborative imaging findings, may approach approximately 20% to 30%.[43]

Prevention

In acute idiopathic pericarditis, preventive efforts focus on minimizing complications and the risk of recurrence. As suggested, these efforts rest on timely diagnosis and initiation of appropriate therapy. In addition, they depend on the avoidance of potentially exacerbating factors, including high-intensity activity and, in the setting of acute idiopathic pericarditis, steroid-based regimens.[34,44] With such approaches, complications and recurrence are less common but not eliminated, and routine clinical surveillance remains paramount. In the case of secondary causes of acute pericarditis, prevention stems from the thorough treatment of the underlying condition.

RECURRENT PERICARDITIS

Recurrent pericarditis is defined as pericarditis in a patient with a previously documented episode of acute pericarditis that responded to therapy originally and was followed by an intervening asymptomatic period of at least 4 to 6 weeks (and thus after completion of NSAID therapy) (**Table 53–9**).[42] In those with prior acute idiopathic pericarditis, recurrent disease occurs in 20% to 40% of patients and may be less characteristic than the initial episode, including atypical chest pain, an absent pericardial friction rub, and normal inflammatory markers.[35] Risk factors for recurrence include female sex, a limited response to initial therapy, inadequate treatment at onset

TABLE 53–8. Tapering of Corticosteroids in Acute and Recurrent Pericarditis

Prednisone dose[b]	Starting dose 0.2–0.5 mg/kg/d[a]	Tapering[c]
Prednisone daily dose	>50 mg	10 mg/d every 1–2 weeks
	50–25 mg	5–10 mg/d every 1–2 weeks
	25–15 mg	2.5 mg/d every 2–4 weeks
	<15 mg	1.25–2.5 mg/d every 2–6 weeks

[a]Calcium intake (supplement plus oral intake; 1200–1500 mg/d) and vitamin D supplementation (800–1000 IU/d) should be offered to all patients receiving glucocorticoids. Moreover, bisphosphonates are recommended to prevent bone loss in all men ≥50 years old and postmenopausal women in whom long-term treatment with glucocorticoids is initiated at a dose ≥5.0 to 7.5 mg/d of prednisone or equivalent.
[b]Avoid higher doses except for special cases, and only for a few days, with rapid tapering to 25 mg/d. Prednisone 25 mg is equivalent to methylprednisolone 20 mg.
[c]Every decrease in prednisone dose should be done only if the patient is asymptomatic and C-reactive protein is normal, particularly for doses <25 mg/d.

TABLE 53–9. Definitions of Recurrent, Incessant, and Chronic Pericarditis

	Definition
Recurrent	Recurrence of pericarditis after a documented first episode of acute pericarditis and a symptom-free interval of 4–6 weeks or longer[a]
Incessant	Pericarditis lasting for >4–6 weeks but <3 months[b] without remission
Chronic	Pericarditis lasting for >3 months[b]

[a]Usually, recurrences occur within 18 to 24 months of the index episode.
[b]Arbitrary term defined by experts.

(eg, absence of colchicine), prior corticosteroid therapy, persistent elevation in inflammatory markers, large pericardial effusion, and the presence of an underlying causative disorder (eg, malignancy).[42] In fact, previous investigations suggest the recurrence rate is nearly 2-fold higher without concomitant colchicine therapy and even higher when steroid therapy was initially used for treatment of acute pericarditis.[45] Of those with idiopathic disease, most will have one to two recurrences and few (<5%) more than two.[46] In such cases, proposed mechanisms for recurrence include recurrent viral infection and autoimmune- and autoinflammatory-like phenomena (eg, molecular mimicry arising from viral antigen exposure).

The evaluation and diagnosis of recurrent pericarditis are pursued in the same manner as for the index episode. Repeat echocardiography aids in the identification of related complications and should include respirometry to evaluate for features suggestive of constrictive pericarditis and/or tamponade. As presentations with recurrence may be more atypical, including normal inflammatory markers (as reported in 22% of patients), further evaluation with cardiac MRI may afford higher sensitivity to detect recurrent pericardial inflammation and can help navigate unclear situations.[42] The presence of mild late

gadolinium enhancement as a marker for recurrent pericarditis, however, should be interpreted with some caution as such enhancement may persist for a prolonged duration of time (ie, many months) even after the preceding episode has clinically resolved. In the absence of suspected alternative causes (including musculoskeletal chest pain), further assessment for other contributing factors is not generally warranted, and most originally idiopathic cases recur in a similarly idiopathic fashion. In the setting of previous acute idiopathic pericarditis, however, consideration should be given to rare, but nonetheless defined autoinflammatory syndromes such as familial Mediterranean fever. In addition, tuberculosis, Whipple's disease, and IgG-4–related disease should be considered as possible causes depending on the clinical scenario.

Once identified, treatment for recurrent pericarditis rests fundamentally on prompt initiation of combined NSAID and colchicine therapies (extending the latter to 6 months) (**Table 53–10**).[42] As with initial acute idiopathic pericarditis, ample evidence supports the utility of this combination in recurrent pericarditis in promoting symptom resolution, lowering hospitalization rates, and reducing the risk of further recurrence.[45,47,48] At onset, steroid therapy should not be used as it can lessen the response to colchicine therapy.[49] If there is a response to NSAID and colchicine therapies, the overall prognosis is good, and the incidence of tamponade and constriction low (7% and 0%, respectively, in one study of 61 patients).[50] For those unresponsive to this standard therapy, alternatives exist, including corticosteroids. With corticosteroid therapy, lower dosing regimens with slower tapering schedules (eg, initial dose 0.2 mg–0.5 mg/kg daily for 2 weeks followed by a slow taper) (Table 53–8) have proven themselves more efficacious and more tolerable with fewer side effects and less risk of future recurrence than higher-dose regimens.[42] Beyond corticosteroids, however, immunosuppressive agents such as azathioprine (antimetabolite),[51] intravenous

TABLE 53–10. Therapeutic Options for Recurrent Pericarditis

Therapy	Dosing	Duration[a]	Tapering	Monitoring[b]	LOE[c]
Aspirin[d]	750–500 mg 3 times daily	1–2 weeks	Weekly in 3–4 weeks	Needed	A
Ibuprofen[d]	600–800 mg 3 times daily	1–2 weeks	Weekly in 3–4 weeks	Needed	A
Indomethacin	50 mg 3 times daily	1–2 weeks	Weekly in 3–4 weeks	Needed	B
Colchicine	0.5 mg twice daily (reduced to 0.5 once daily if <70 kg, chronic kidney disease, and/or intolerant of higher dosing)	6 months	May be considered	Needed	A
Prednisone	0.2–0.5 mg/kg/d	2–4 weeks	Several months	Needed	B
Azathioprine	Starting with 1 mg/kg/d, then gradually increased to 2–3 mg/kg/d	Several months	Several months	Needed	C
IVIG	400–500 mg IV daily for 5 days	5 days	Not required	Needed	C
Anakinra	1–2 mg/kg/d up to 100 mg/d in adults	Several months	To be determined	Needed	C
Pericardiectomy	NA	NA	NA	Needed	C

Abbreviations: IV, intravenous; IVIG, intravenous immunoglobulin; LOE, level of evidence; NA, not applicable.
[a]Therapy duration as initial dosing
[b]Monitoring is essentially based on the assessment of blood count, creatinine, creatinine kinase, transaminases, C-reactive protein, and echocardiography.
[c]LOE A, data derived from multiple randomized clinical trials or meta-analyses; LOE B, data derived from a single randomized clinical trial or large nonrandomized studies (in this review, a study with at least 100 patients is considered large); LOE C, consensus of opinion of the experts and/or small studies, retrospective studies, or registries.
[d]Aspirin and ibuprofen are common first-level.

immunoglobulin therapy,[52,53] and anakinra (IL-1 receptor antagonist)[54-56] have been trialed, demonstrating success in several case series of refractory recurrent pericarditis due to idiopathic disease (Table 53–10). In such cases, at least 1 year of therapy is frequently required, and significant risk of rebound disease may exist after therapy taper and discontinuation. Phase 3 clinical trial of interleukin-1 trap Rilonacept in recurrent pericarditis was performed in 86 patients. Among a total of 61 patents who were randomized, Rilonacept resulted in rapid resolution of recurrent pericarditis and lower risk of recurrence compared to placebo. This treatment requires an weekly injection and we will need further clinical experience to determine therapeutic strategy in recurrent pericarditis.[57]

In select cases of recurrent (and, as subsequently described, incessant/chronic) pericarditis, radical pericardiectomy has demonstrated superiority over continued medical management alone, and pericardiectomy has yielded greater success and efficacy over partial removal.[58-60] One investigation of 184 patients with recurrent pericarditis, for instance, assigned patients to either medical management alone (126 patients) or medical management with pericardiectomy (58 patients).[58] This study demonstrated an excellent safety profile of pericardiectomy in this patient population (with 0% perioperative mortality) and improved long-term outcomes. Indeed, following pericardiectomy, only 9% of patients treated with pericardiectomy experienced recurrence over a mean follow-up period 5.5 ± 3.5 years (compared with 29% in those treated medically), and 70% required no chronic medical therapy (relative to 57% treated with medical management alone). Similar published experiences have reinforced these findings, underscoring—in experienced centers—the low mortality of pericardiectomy, the superiority of complete over partial removal, and the potential ability to minimize medical therapy as a result.[60]

INCESSANT/CHRONIC PERICARDITIS

Definitions of incessant and chronic pericarditis originate from the standard duration of NSAID therapy used to treat acute pericarditis (approximately 4–6 weeks) and the often predictable time course of acute pericarditis and its response to treatment (Table 53–9).[1] In the case of the former, "incessant pericarditis" is defined as symptomatic pericarditis lasting longer than 4 to 6 weeks without an intervening period of complete symptomatic relief. Should symptoms subsequently persist beyond 3 months, incessant pericarditis becomes "chronic." Apart from more sustained symptoms, patients with either incessant or chronic pericarditis suffer from an increased risk of downstream complications, including constriction. Similar to recurrent pericarditis, aggressive treatment strategies beyond standard combination therapy with NSAID and colchicine treatments are often required and include pericardiectomy. Prevention of incessant/chronic pericarditis, however, begins with appropriate management of acute pericarditis, including both early diagnosis and adequate treatment.

In combination with standard NSAID therapy, colchicine significantly lowers the incidence of both incessant and recurrent pericarditis (by nearly 50%) following an initial episode of acute pericarditis. In the absence of such therapy, the incidence of incessant/recurrent pericarditis following acute idiopathic disease ranges from 15% to 30%. When this is the result of non-idiopathic causes (eg, bacterial/purulent percarditis), however, this incidence of incessant/chronic pericarditis following an acute episode increases further, reaching as high as nearly 60% in patients suffering from nonidiopathic disease.[43] On subsequent serial assessment of patients originally diagnosed with acute disease, clinical, laboratory, and imaging evaluations may indicate evolution to incessant/chronic disease and reveal, for instance, persistent symptoms, sustained elevation in inflammatory markers, and ongoing pericardial enhancement on cross-sectional imaging. Such cross-sectional imaging may reveal further changes suggestive of incessant/chronic pericardial inflammation (eg, pericardial fibrosis, thickening, and nodularity). In such settings, providers must maintain constant vigilance for the emergence of other complications, including, notably, constrictive pericarditis.

SPECIFIC FORMS OF PERICARDITIS

Idiopathic

Acute idiopathic pericarditis constitutes the most commonly encountered form of acute pericarditis in developed countries, accounting for approximately 80% of encountered cases depending on the series. Although labeled "idiopathic," this form of acute pericarditis is believed to arise in the vast majority of cases from an antecedent viral infection. Such cases are diagnosed and treated as already described. In other instances, however, pericarditis may be the result of an underappreciated secondary etiology, effectively being labeled "idiopathic" in the absence of adequate, complete, and/or feasible diagnostic assessment. Beyond idiopathic disease, causes of acute pericarditis can be further divided into infectious (including idiopathic cases assumed to be viral in origin) and noninfectious categories.

Infectious

Viral

Acute viral pericarditis often presents in the form of acute idiopathic pericarditis following a preceding viral upper respiratory tract infection (or alternative viral syndrome). Common viral pathogens associated with acute pericarditis include echovirus, coxsackievirus, and adenovirus, and several mechanisms have been proposed to describe the pathogenesis of such viruses in acute pericarditis.[6,61] These proposed mechanisms range from molecular mimicry, whereby viral antigens with structural similarity to host epitopes activate an autoimmune-like reaction, to genetic variants of the host inflammatory response that create an inappropriate and seemingly self-propagating autoinflammatory cascade. In both cases, the pericardium is targeted, leading to acute pericarditis.

In routine practice, the identification of the causative virus (eg, through polymerase chain reaction [PCR]) in acute viral pericarditis does not influence clinical management and may be misleading. In one series of patients with acute pericarditis, for instance, PCR identified viral genomes in 20% of pericardial fluid samples in all patients presenting with pericarditis, including 16% of those with malignant pericarditis and 13% with postpericardial injury syndromes.[6] These results suggest that certain viruses may be present generally and not necessarily contribute pathogenically. Depending on the clinical scenario, however, specific identification may be warranted, including, for example, in cases of suspected infection with influenza and SARS-CoV-2.[62,63] Overall, however, routine viral testing is not recommended. Instead, in the absence of secondary factors, acute viral pericarditis is synonymous with idiopathic pericarditis, often resolving in a predictable fashion with adjunctive NSAID and colchicine therapy.

Bacterial

Pericarditis may also develop as a consequence of bacterial infection and, in the presence of an accompanying effusion, is known as "purulent pericarditis." Among bacteria, *Mycobacterium tuberculosis* contributes frequently to bacterial pericarditis and, in fact, constitutes the most common overall cause of pericarditis in developing countries.[64] In addition to acute pericarditis, tuberculous involvement of the pericardium may also present as an isolated pericardial effusion, tamponade, or constrictive pericarditis. Apart from *M. tuberculosis*, however, other bacterial causes of pericarditis exist. As with M. tuberculosis, these infections may either develop, as in the case of penetrating trauma, in a primary fashion or evolve secondarily, reaching the pericardium through hematogenous spread, lymphatic transmission, or direct contiguous extension of an adjacent but originally extrapericardial infectious process.

Though accounting for less than 5% of pericarditis cases in developed countries, tuberculous pericarditis occurs with much greater frequency in developing areas and arises from a delayed-type hypersensitivity response to *M. tuberculosis* infection.[64] In contrast to its idiopathic counterpart, tuberculous pericarditis assumes a more subacute-chronic form; presents more commonly with dyspnea, cough, and constitutional symptoms; and is more frequently associated with larger pericardial effusions through an initial effusive phase. Despite therapy, over 30% of affected patients will progress to an adhesive phase of disease marked by constrictive pericarditis.[64,65] Consistent with these differences in presentation, initial electrocardiographic assessment discloses a typical acute idiopathic pericarditis pattern in only approximately 10% of presenting patients. Factors that contribute to the development of tuberculous pericarditis notably include a prior history of extracardiac tuberculosis, occurring, for example, in 1% to 2% of patients with known pulmonary tuberculosis, and immunosuppression, including, in particular, concomitant HIV infection.[64]

The approach to diagnosing and treating tuberculous pericarditis depends on the perceived risk of underlying infection. When presenting from endemic regions, a presumptive diagnosis can stem from a combination of supportive clinical findings, perceived exposure, risk assessment scoring, and even response to already initiated therapy (a so-called *ex juvantibus* diagnosis). Once diagnosed, treatment routinely consists of a four-drug regimen of rifampicin, isoniazid, pyrazinamide, and ethambutol for 2 months and subsequent 4-month course of

isoniazid and rifampicin. In those patients without endemic exposure and consistent clinical picture, however, further evaluation to prove underlying infection is required. As patients with tuberculous pericarditis routinely display neither acute symptoms nor typical electrocardiographic findings, evaluation begins with echocardiography and cross-sectional imaging (either CT or MRI). If these assessments reveal an underlying effusion, pericardiocentesis with/without biopsy is in turn recommended to confirm the diagnosis through the identification of elevated pericardial fluid adenosine deaminase levels, tubercle bacilli, and/or caseating necrosis. In such cases, adenosine deaminase levels greater than 40 U/L have demonstrated particularly good sensitivity and specificity for the diagnosis of tuberculous pericarditis (93% and 97%, respectively).[66] Once confirmed, treatment is pursued as already described and may include pericardiectomy should evidence of constriction arise and response to therapy be limited.[64,67]

Beyond tuberculous pericarditis, purulent pericarditis may also arise from infection with nontuberculous bacteria, particularly *Staphylococcus aureus*, *Streptococcus pneumoniae*, *Haemophilus influenzae*, and other Gram-negative bacteria. Additional considerations include Legionella, a common cause of community-acquired pneumonia, and Lyme disease. Historically, such cases arose from contiguous neighboring infections (eg, pneumonia). Presently, however, with widespread and prompt antibiotic use, purulent pericarditis develops in approximately 70% of cases from the metastatic spread of infection to the pericardium rather than contiguous extension, although pneumonia and, in particular, empyema remain prominent risk factors.[68] Apart from secondary infection of the pericardium, purulent pericarditis arising iatrogenically from procedural intervention has become an increasingly recognized phenomenon as well, including, for example, following gastric band placement.[69]

As expected, patients affected with nontuberculous purulent pericarditis may have a history of underlying immunosuppression, malignancy, other chronic disease (eg, chronic kidney disease), and/or injury. Such patients routinely present in a more fulminant fashion with fever (especially in excess of 38°C). Chest pain is not a uniform feature, and other features of typical acute idiopathic pericarditis are often absent. Evaluation and diagnosis require a dedicated search for concomitant infection(s) and, should effusion be present, pericardiocentesis. Treatment begins with intravenous broad-spectrum antibiotic therapy, often including empiric antifungal treatment, and close observation. In certain cases, intrapericardial fibrinolytic therapy may be required with pursuit of surgical drainage and possible pericardiectomy should medical management alone prove insufficient and complications arise. As with tuberculous pericarditis, long-term complications occur with greater frequency than in idiopathic disease and include constrictive pericarditis, developing in approximately 20% to 30% of survivors; mycotic aneurysms; and pseudoaneurysms.[43,70] Despite therapy, mortality is high (approximately 40%).[68]

Fungal

Fungal pericarditis represents a rare form of pericarditis and is most commonly seen in cases of either injury (particularly traumatic, including surgical) or significant immunosuppression.[6,71] As a result, only infrequent and scattered case reports document the occurrence of fungal pericarditis. Causative organisms have included *Cryptococcus neoformans*, Candida species, Aspergillus, and Blastomyces in immunocompromised hosts and endemic fungi (eg, Histoplasma) in immunocompetent patients.[72,73] Clinical history and examination may raise initial suspicion of acute fungal pericarditis, while echocardiogram may demonstrate a complicated effusion with, for example, echogenic septations and loculations. Ultimately, however, diagnosis requires microbiologic identification, frequently necessitating pericardiocentesis and assessment of aspirated pericardial fluid. Once diagnosed, optimal treatment rests on prompt microbiologic identification, pericardial drainage, and dedicated, often prolonged antifungal therapy. Despite treatment, outcomes remain poor, a likely reflection of the baseline health and intersecting comorbidities of those affected.

Parasitic

Similar to fungal pericarditis, parasitic pericarditis occurs seldomly, although with particularly higher frequency in less-developed countries.[74] To date, a handful of case reports details its presentation, which often resembles that of bacterial and fungal pericarditis, and describes infections with Echinococcus, Leishmania, and Toxoplasma.[74,75] As with other microbial infections, therapy is tailored to the causative organism, and prognosis is dependent on extent of infection and the rapidity of diagnosis and treatment.

Noninfectious

Systemic Autoimmune and Autoinflammatory Diseases

Connective tissue diseases and systemic inflammatory disorders can each present with pericarditis, either at their onset or during their disease course, and account for approximately 10% of cases of acute pericarditis.[6,16] Connective tissue diseases with predominant pericarditis-related associations include systemic lupus erythematosus. Autoinflammatory disorders with similar associations include hereditary periodic fever syndromes with inherited mutations in inflammatory response pathways (eg, familial Mediterranean fever). Routinely, pericarditis related to these and similar conditions presents acutely and in proportion to disease severity. On evaluation, patients may endorse symptoms akin to acute idiopathic pericarditis but also a personal history of autoimmune/autoinflammatory disease, a family history of such disease, and prior episodes of acute pericarditis with limited/refractory response to standard therapies. Laboratory testing, including genetic assessment, can facilitate diagnosis. Following presentation, the subsequent clinical course and treatment depend on the underlying condition and its simultaneous extracardiac activity.

Postpericardial Injury Syndromes

Acute pericarditis arising from pericardial injury, particularly of the pericardial mesothelium, forms the basis of postpericardial injury syndromes and includes postpericardiotomy syndrome, posttraumatic pericarditis, and postmyocardial infarction pericarditis. By arising from pericardial injury, these conditions are believed to result from an autoimmune response to native perimyocardial tissue. First reported in the context of cardiac surgery, postpericardiotomy syndrome, for instance, affects 10% to 40% of patients undergoing cardiac surgery. Risk factors for its development include female gender and further mesothelial injury through simultaneous pleural incision.[76] Affected patients most often present within the first month after surgery (80%) and almost always within 3 months.[77] Affected patients manifest pleuritic chest pain (56%), fever (54%), and elevated inflammatory markers (74%). The majority of patients (over 80%) will have an accompanying pericardial effusion, although few will have typical electrocardiographic changes of acute pericarditis.[77]

Once suspected, treatment of postpericardiotomy syndrome should proceed with combined NSAID and colchicine therapy as circumstances permit and address any identified complications. Generally, the clinical syndrome is self-limiting. In conjunction with NSAID therapy, however, colchicine hastens symptom relief and disease course.[77] In fact, additional investigation suggests that colchicine can also be employed prophylactically in the perioperative period to minimize the risk of development of postpericardiotomy syndrome.[78,79] Following treatment, most patients are without recurrent symptoms, and few develop either tamponade (less than 2% in one series at 20 months) or constriction.[77]

Pericarditis can also develop secondary to percutaneous and other less invasive procedural interventions and mechanical trauma. As with postpericardiotomy syndrome, however, acute pericarditis in these situations arises from injury to the pericardium and ensuing inflammation. Procedures previously associated with acute pericarditis include percutaneous coronary intervention, transcatheter valve replacement, left atrial appendage occlusion, pacemaker implantation, and other electrophysiologic interventions.[76,80,81] As with surgically related postpericardiotomy syndrome, affected patients often present with chest pain, dyspnea, fever, and elevated inflammatory markers. Combined clinical and echocardiographic evaluation remains critical to both the diagnosis of acute pericarditis in affected patients and the identification of any related complications. Analogous to postpericardiotomy syndrome, treatment consists of combined NSAID and colchicine therapies.

Pericardial inflammation can also occur in the context of myocardial infarction and develop either acutely, in the form of postmyocardial infarction pericarditis, or in a subacute-chronic fashion referred to as Dressler's syndrome. In one study of acute myocardial infarction, acute pericarditis developed in approximately 20% of patients as defined by the emergence of consistent symptoms and pericardial rub.[82] Affected patients were more likely to have sustained a transmural infarction and display evidence of greater myocardial injury, including higher average troponin elevation and lower average ejection fraction on echocardiographic assessment. Apart from symptomatic myocardial infarction, however, acute pericarditis may also arise secondary to an otherwise clinically silent infarction as well. Such instances of acute pericarditis are treated with a combination of high-dose aspirin (eg, 650 mg three times daily) and colchicine, foregoing alternative NSAIDs given known associations of nonaspirin NSAID therapy with increased risk of mechanical and other complications in the acute postinfarction period.

Following an acute myocardial infarction, related inflammation can reveal neoantigens in the perimyocardium that in turn stimulate a systemic response and give rise to Dressler's syndrome (or postmyocardial infarction syndrome). In these circumstances, patients present most commonly 2 to 4 weeks after their acute myocardial infarction with features of pericarditis, including pleuritic chest pain, and often additional symptoms of dyspnea, malaise, and fever. As with acute idiopathic pericarditis, treatment is supportive and consists of a combination of high-dose aspirin and colchicine therapies.

Metabolic

Metabolic causes of acute pericarditis include hypothyroidism (myxedema) and end-stage renal disease. In cases of significant hypothyroidism, pericardial effusions may develop in 37% of affected patients and are believed to form from several proposed mechanisms, including increased permeability of epicardial vessels in the hypothyroid state that leads to often large, slowly expanding effusions with low incidence of tamponade.[83] In addition, concomitant heart failure, also a consequence of untreated and significant hypothyroidism, may further complicate the patient's clinical presentation. Rarely, acute pericarditis may occur concurrently, although a direct association is lacking. While treatment of hypothyroidism is mandatory, further symptomatic management related to accompanying acute pericarditis may mirror that of acute idiopathic pericarditis.

Another more well-known metabolic cause of acute pericarditis is end-stage renal disease. Historically, acute pericarditis related to underlying renal dysfunction arose from untreated, effectively end-stage renal disease at a time of limited (if any) dialysis access. In such cases, acute pericarditis would arise secondary to untreated uremia, occurring either before or within 8 weeks of dialysis onset and affecting approximately 20% of patients.[84,85] In such cases, affected patients would often present atypically, manifesting a more subacute process with atypical chest discomfort and very infrequently fever. Physical examination would disclose a pericardial friction rub in the majority of patients and subsequent evaluation tended to reveal more routinely an underlying pericardial effusion with tamponade-like physiology. Interestingly, blood urea nitrogen levels on presentation did not correlate with the incidence of uremic pericarditis, suggesting a multifactorial process behind acute pericarditis in affected patients.[86] Regardless, such patients were treated with intensive dialysis therapy.

With the advent and more widespread utilization of dialysis, acute pericarditis related to untreated end-stage renal disease has become less frequent but has not disappeared. Instead, acute pericarditis previously related to untreated end-stage renal disease has been replaced with acute pericarditis related to inadequate dialysis (classically, 8 weeks or longer after dialysis onset), including, for instance, complications arising from arteriovenous fistula malfunction. As with its predecessor, however, treatment rests on intensive dialysis therapy and can be further enhanced with dose-adjusted NSAID and colchicine therapies

as tolerated. With this approach, most patients improve within 2 weeks of intensive therapy, although long-term consequences include a higher incidence of constrictive pericarditis.[85]

Malignant

Malignant involvement of the pericardium can occur as a result of either de novo development of a primary pericardial malignancy (eg, pericardial mesothelioma) or, more commonly, secondary spread of an originally extrapericardial malignancy. In the case of the latter, spread can occur hematogenously, lymphatically, or through contiguous extension of an adjacent malignancy. Breast, hematologic, pulmonary, and gastrointestinal malignancies are principally involved. Most commonly, malignant involvement of the pericardium presents as a pericardial effusion but may occasionally manifest as acute pericarditis. Indeed, among patients presenting with acute pericarditis and no preceding history of malignancy, approximately 5% will have malignant pericarditis.[87] At the same time, however, in patients with known malignancy presenting with acute pericarditis, two-thirds will have pericardial disease from a nonmalignant cause (eg, infection).[88]

When presenting as acute pericarditis, initial signs and symptoms of malignant pericarditis may differ from those classically associated with idiopathic disease, although diagnostic criteria for acute pericarditis otherwise remain identical. Certain features on clinical evaluation, including a history of known malignancy and a large pericardial effusion with/without tamponade, increase the suspicion of malignancy.[88] When presenting with tamponade, for example, approximately one-third of patients with acute pericarditis will ultimately be diagnosed with malignancy.[88] In such instances, diagnostic evaluation should consist of image-guided pericardiocentesis. A densely hemorrhagic effusion raises the likelihood of underlying malignancy, and cytologic and biomarker assessment (eg, carcinoembryonic antigen) of aspirated fluid aids in further diagnosis.[30] History and physical examination guide further assessment (eg, colonoscopy). In certain clinical scenarios, assessment with FDG-PET/CT may afford a useful noninvasive intermediary by helping confirm underlying pericarditis, reveal pericardial and/or extracardiac malignancy, and provide suitable alternative biopsy sites.

Following identification, treatment involves directed therapies for acute pericarditis and for the underlying malignancy. Prognosis is inherently worse than that of acute idiopathic pericarditis and worse than that of comparable malignancy without pericardial involvement. Consequently, it is recommended that malignancy-directed treatment be continued as clinically tolerated and permitted. The type of underlying malignancy subsequently dictates clinical course and prognosis. On the whole, however, approximately 4% of patients with acute malignancy-related pericarditis will ultimately develop constriction.[43]

Medication-Induced/Immunotherapy

Though less commonly encountered, certain medications have demonstrated associations with acute pericarditis. Traditionally, medication-related pericarditis fell under the umbrella of "lupus-like" reactions, denoting the tendency of particular medications to generate a form of drug-induced lupus characterized by serosal inflammation, including inflammation of the pericardium. Medications with such potential included hydralazine, phenytoin, isoniazid, and procainamide.[1] Apart from these medications, however, chemotherapeutic agents have gained increasing attention as causes of acute pericarditis, particularly with the introduction of immune checkpoint inhibitors.

Prior to the advent and increased application of immune checkpoint inhibitors, scattered case reports documented associations between chemotherapeutic agents and acute pericarditis.[89] In such instances, various mechanisms for pericardial injury were proposed, including direct cellular toxicity. In contrast, immune checkpoint inhibitors result in unique modulation of the immune system, altering T-cell-mediated activity and contributing to a variety of now well-documented autoimmune phenomena. Included among these phenomena is acute pericarditis. Distinct from direct toxicity related to traditional chemotherapy, acute pericarditis in such cases appears variably following treatment and arises in general from an idiosyncratic autoimmune reaction.[90]

Radiation-Induced

Historically, radiation-induced acute pericarditis occurred following direct irradiation of the heart and surrounding mediastinum. In such cases, radiation injury would precipitate acute pericarditis within days to weeks of exposure and would, apart from its antecedent clinical history, mirror acute idiopathic pericarditis.[91-93] With the introduction of newer techniques aimed at focusing and minimizing radiation, however, the incidence of acute radiation-induced pericarditis has fallen substantially (from 20% previously to 2.5% of acute pericarditis cases currently).[91] Nonetheless, acute radiation pericarditis remains an important source of morbidity and mortality in patients receiving radiation therapy, and the pericardium itself represents the most commonly affected component of the heart in thoracic radiation treatment. In fact, in one series of 27 patients examined on autopsy with a history of malignancy and previous radiation therapy, 70% showed evidence of pericardial injury/inflammation, including pericardial effusion, acute radiation pericarditis, and constrictive pericarditis.[92]

Factors that contribute to the occurrence of acute radiation pericarditis include the location irradiated, the extent of radiation, and the concomitant use of any medication that could function as a radiosensitizing agent (eg, certain chemotherapeutic agents, including 5-fluoruacil).[91] As with acute idiopathic pericarditis, diagnosis rests on combined clinical, electrocardiographic, and/or echocardiographic assessment, with patients frequently presenting with nonspecific symptoms akin to acute idiopathic pericarditis. Treatment involves a combination of minimizing/avoiding further radiation and the use of NSAID- and colchicine-based therapies, which may, however, be limited based on the possible simultaneous use of agents with potentially significant drug–drug interactions (eg, select chemotherapies). Prognosis is heavily dependent on the type and extent of radiation exposure, the nature of the underlying malignancy, and the development of any associated complications (eg, constrictive pericarditis). Overall, however, acute radiation pericarditis often has a self-limiting course.[93]

Acute Myopericardial Syndromes

As the visceral layer of the serous pericardium contributes to the epicardium and is thus contiguous with the underlying myocardium, myocarditis of varying degrees often accompanies pericardial inflammation. Generally, myocardial involvement should be suspected when the patient manifests electrocardiographic changes, arrhythmias, plasma troponin elevation, and/or left ventricular dysfunction. Depending on the degree of concomitant myocarditis, the presenting clinical syndrome is described as "myopericarditis" when, based on available evidence, the predominant layer involved is the pericardium and as "perimyocarditis" when the myocardium is principally affected. The integration of findings on clinical presentation, subsequent laboratory evaluation, and additional imaging assessment aids in distinguishing these two entities. This distinction has decided diagnostic, therapeutic, and clinical implications.

Myopericarditis reflects extension of pericardial inflammation to the underlying myocardium. In such instances, the clinical syndrome resembles isolated pericarditis (rather than myocarditis). Laboratory evaluation may reveal evidence of direct underlying myocardial inflammation (eg, elevated cardiac troponin), while further imaging assessment with cardiac MRI, for example, may disclose contiguous myopericardial inflammation and an accompanying pericardial effusion. Given the principal pericardial involvement in these patients, treatment is supportive and resembles treatment deployed in isolated acute pericarditis. Additionally, similar to acute pericarditis, prognosis is often good, and complication rates low. As there is a greater risk of arrhythmia, however, secondary to myocardial involvement, such patients require close immediate observation with hospitalization. Following resolution of the acute episode, the risk of recurrence is relatively low (approximately 11% after median follow-up of 3 years).[24] Because of a concern for possible increased risk of sudden cardiac death secondary to myocardial involvement, guidelines suggest activity restriction for 6 months from initial diagnosis.[1]

In contrast to myopericarditis, predominant myocardial involvement characterizes perimyocarditis. The clinical syndrome of perimyocarditis resembles that of isolated myocarditis, although features of pericarditis (eg, pleuritic chest discomfort) may appear superimposed. Clinical presentation, laboratory evaluation, and imaging assessment identify this condition and reveal findings of underlying myocardial injury, including possible signs and symptoms of heart failure, significant elevations in troponin, and cardiac dysfunction. Because of this direct and often significant myocardial involvement, patients tend to display a relatively worse prognosis than in myopericarditis and uniformly require closer observation with inpatient admission. Depending on course, further evaluation with coronary angiogram and/or cardiac MRI and treatment for heart failure, cardiogenic shock, and other complications may prove necessary.[1] With resolution of the acute episode, however, prognosis, as with acute myopericarditis, is generally good, and a recurrence rate of approximately 12% has been cited.[24] Similarly, a 6-month period of activity restriction is recommended.[1]

COMPLICATIONS

Arrhythmias

Inflammation related to acute pericarditis can involve varying degrees of underlying myocardium and thus the conduction system. Involvement of the conduction system in this fashion can infrequently precipitate any one of several arrhythmias, whereby atrial fibrillation is most common and may be present in 5% of patients on presentation.[94] Depending on the degree of concomitant myocarditis and presence of baseline structural heart disease, ventricular arrhythmias ranging from asymptomatic and infrequent ventricular ectopy to malignant ventricular tachycardia can develop. Although such arrhythmias arise uncommonly, their potential development mandates inpatient observation of patients with acute perimyocarditis/myopericarditis.

Pericardial Effusions

Pericardial effusions form in roughly 67% of all cases of acute pericarditis.[11] Generally, such effusions are usually small and develop without complication (ie, without either tamponade or constriction). Given the gravity of possible complications, however, and their distinct treatment, echocardiography is mandatory, enabling both the identification of an effusion and any accompanying complications. With respect to effusion size, larger effusions (ie, those defined echocardiographically as deeper than 20 mm) more commonly form in the setting of acute pericarditis secondary to a specific underlying factor, including malignancy and infection (particularly tuberculosis).[5] With further evaluation using other imaging modalities, additional features of identified pericardial effusions may become apparent. In the case of CT, for instance, the Hounsfield units of pericardial fluid can suggest whether the fluid is transudative, exudative, or hemorrhagic in nature.[42]

Although the identification of a pericardial effusion and the presence of any related complications forms a critical aspect of patient evaluation in acute pericarditis, most patients will present with uncomplicated effusions that are tiny or smaller in size. In these cases, pericardiocentesis is not indicated. In select other patients, however, further evaluation with pericardiocentesis becomes a critical part of their evaluation. These patients include those with clinical evidence of tamponade, features suggestive of purulent pericarditis, or findings concerning for underlying malignancy. In the case of the latter, such findings include a known history of previous/current malignancy and large effusion on echocardiography and/or cross-sectional imaging. In these cases, image-guided pericardiocentesis affords indispensable diagnostic information that can also prove pivotal to treatment.

Tamponade

Cardiac tamponade reflects a situation of impaired early diastolic filling and exaggerated ventricular interdependence due to exhaustion of the pericardial reserve volume and reduced pericardial compliance. Frequently, as in the case of acute pericarditis, tamponade arises from an accumulating pericardial effusion, occupying the pericardial cavity and precipitating this clinical syndrome. The incidence of tamponade in acute pericarditis varies by etiology, ranging from 15% in acute idiopathic pericarditis to as high as 60% in cases of malignant and purulent acute pericarditides.[30] Because of its clinical implications and relatively straightforward treatment—pericardiocentesis—echocardiographic evaluation in acute pericarditis is mandatory.

Constrictive Pericarditis

Constrictive pericarditis constitutes a clinical heart failure syndrome arising from either reversible or permanent reductions in pericardial compliance, reserve volume, and thus late diastolic filling. On gross visual and radiographic assessment, the involved pericardium often appears thickened and calcified and can be affected either focally or diffusely. Histopathologically, affected areas demonstrate nonspecific inflammation and evidence of chronic remodeling with fibrosis characteristic of constrictive pericarditis. These changes limit late diastolic filling, enhance ventricular interdependence, and effect a right heart failure state as appreciated on history, physical examination, and noninvasive studies. Although an infrequent complication of acute idiopathic pericarditis (less than 1% of cases), the incidence is much higher in secondary causes of acute pericarditis.[43] Evaluation should involve assessment for evidence of acute pericardial inflammation, suggesting potential reversibility, which may successfully be treated with aggressive anti-inflammatory therapy; however, when irreversible pericardial fibrosis has ensued, definitive treatment may necessitate surgical complete pericardiectomy.[60]

REFERENCES

1. Adler Y, Charron P, Imazio M, et al. 2015 ESC Guidelines for the diagnosis and management of pericardial diseases. *Eur Heart J*. 2015;36(42):2921-2964. doi:10.1093/eurheartj/ehv318
2. Lewinter MM. Acute pericarditis. *N Engl J Med*. 2014;371(25):2410-2416. doi:10.1056/NEJMcp1404070
3. Permanyer-Miralda G, Sagristá-Sauleda J, Soler-Soler J. Primary acute pericardial disease: a prospective series of 231 consecutive patients. *Am J Cardiol*. 1985;56(10):623-630. doi:10.1016/0002-9149(85)91023-9
4. Zayas R, Anguita M, Torres F, et al. Incidence of specific etiology and role of methods for specific etiologic diagnosis of primary acute pericarditis. *Am J Cardiol*. 1995;75(5-6):378-382. doi:10.1016/S0002-9149(99)80558-X
5. Imazio M, Cecchi E, Demichelis B, et al. Indicators of poor prognosis of acute pericarditis. *Circulation*. 2007;115(21):2739-2744. doi:10.1161/CIRCULATIONAHA.106.662114
6. Gouriet F, Levy PY, Casalta JP, et al. Etiology of pericarditis in a prospective cohort of 1162 cases. *Am J Med*. 2015;128(7):784.e1-784.e8. doi:10.1016/j.amjmed.2015.01.040
7. Mayosi BM. Contemporary trends in the epidemiology and management of cardiomyopathy and pericarditis in sub-Saharan Africa. *Heart*. 2007;93(10):1176-1183. doi:10.1136/hrt.2007.127746
8. Shabetai R. *The Pericardium*. Norwell, MA: Kluwer; 2003.
9. Farzad A, Schussler JM. Acute myopericardial syndromes. *Cardiol Clin*. 2018;36(1):103-114. doi:10.1016/j.ccl.2017.09.004
10. Imazio M, Demichelis B, Parrini I, et al. Day-hospital treatment of acute pericarditis: a management program for outpatient therapy. *J Am Coll Cardiol*. 2004;43(6):1042-1046. doi:10.1016/j.jacc.2003.09.055

11. Lange RA, Hillis LD. Clinical practice. Acute pericarditis. *N Engl J Med.* 2005;351(21):2195-2202. doi:10.1056/NEJMcp041997

12. Spodick DH. Pericardial rub: prospective, multiple observer investigation of pericardial friction in 100 patients. *Am J Cardiol.* 1975;35(March):357-362. doi:10.32388/cqko7h

13. Spodick DH. Diagnostic electrocardiographic sequences in acute pericarditis. *Circulation.* 1973;48(3):575-580. doi:10.1161/01.cir.48.3.575

14. Surawicz B, Lasseter KC. Electrocardiogram in pericarditis. *Am J Cardiol.* 1970;26(5):471-474. doi:10.1016/0002-9149(70)90704-6

15. George A, Arumugham PS, Figueredo VM. aVR—The forgotten lead. *Exp Clin Cardiol.* 2010;15(2).

16. Imazio M, Brucato A, DeRosa FG, et al. Aetiological diagnosis in acute and recurrent pericarditis: when and how. *J Cardiovasc Med.* 2009;10(3):217-230. doi:10.2459/JCM.0b013e328322f9b1

17. Yusuf SW, Hassan SA, Mouhayar E, Negi SI, Banchs J, Ogara PT. Pericardial disease: a clinical review. *Expert Rev Cardiovasc Ther.* 2016;14(4):525-539. doi:10.1586/14779072.2016.1134317

18. Chetrit M, Xu B, Verma BR, Klein AL. Multimodality imaging for the assessment of pericardial diseases. *Curr Cardiol Rep.* 2019;21(5):41. doi:10.4250/jcvi.2019.27.e48

19. Nagahama Y, Sugiura T, Takehana K, Tarumi N, Iwasaka T, Inada M. PQ segment depression in acute Q wave inferior wall myocardial infarction. *Circulation.* 1995;91(3):641-644. doi:10.1161/01.cir.91.3.641

20. Salisbury AC, Olalla-Gómez C, Rihal CS, et al. Frequency and predictors of urgent coronary angiography in patients with acute pericarditis. *Mayo Clin Proc.* 2009;84(1):11-15. doi:10.4065/84.1.11

21. Imazio M, Brucato A, Maestroni S, et al. Prevalence of C-reactive protein elevation and time course of normalization in acute pericarditis: implications for the diagnosis, therapy, and prognosis of pericarditis. *Circulation.* 2011;123(10):1092-1097. doi:10.1161/CIRCULATIONAHA.110.986372

22. Imazio M, Demichelis B, Cecchi E, et al. Cardiac troponin I in acute pericarditis. *J Am Coll Cardiol.* 2003;42(12):2144-2148. doi:10.1016/j.jacc.2003.02.001

23. Bonnefoy E, Godon P, Kirkorian G, Fatemi M, Chevalier P, Touboul P. Serum cardiac troponin I and ST-segment elevation in patients with acute pericarditis. *Eur Heart J.* 2000;21(10):832-836. doi:10.1053/euhj.1999.1907

24. Imazio M, Brucato A, Barbieri A, et al. Good prognosis for pericarditis with and without myocardial involvement: results from a multicenter, prospective cohort study. *Circulation.* 2013;128(1):42-49. doi:10.1161/CIRCULATIONAHA.113.001531

25. Cosyns B, Plein S, Nihoyanopoulos P, et al. European Association of Cardiovascular Imaging (EACVI) position paper: multimodality imaging in pericardial disease. *Eur Heart J Cardiovasc Imaging.* 2015;16(1):12-31. doi:10.1093/ehjci/jeu128

26. Klein AL, Abbara S, Agler DA, et al. American society of echocardiography clinical recommendations for multimodality cardiovascular imaging of patients with pericardial disease: endorsed by the society for cardiovascular magnetic resonance and society of cardiovascular computed tomography. *J Am Soc Echocardiogr.* 2013;26(9):965-1012.e15. doi:10.1016/j.echo.2013.06.023

27. Imazio M, Spodick DH, Brucato A, Trinchero R, Adler Y. Controversial issues in the management of pericardial diseases. *Circulation.* 2010;121(7):916-928. doi:10.1161/CIRCULATIONAHA.108.844753

28. Maisch B, Rupp H, Ristic A, Pankuweit S. Pericardioscopy and epi- and pericardial biopsy—A new window to the heart improving etiological diagnoses and permitting targeted intrapericardial therapy. *Heart Fail Rev.* 2013;18(3):317-328. doi:10.1007/s10741-013-9382-y

29. Seferović PM, Ristić AD, Maksimović R, Tatić V, Ostojić M, Kanjuh V. Diagnostic value of pericardial biopsy: improvement with extensive sampling enabled by pericardioscopy. *Circulation.* 2003;107(7):978-983. doi:10.1161/01.CIR.0000051366.97361.EA

30. Permanyer-Miralda G. Acute pericardial disease: approach to the aetiologic diagnosis. *Heart.* 2004;90(3):252-254. doi:10.1136/hrt.2003.024802

31. Mercé J, Sagristà-Sauleda J, Permanyer-Miralda G, Soler-Soler J. Should pericardial drainage be performed routinely in patients who have a large pericardial effusion without tamponade? *Am J Med.* 1998;105(2):106-109. doi:10.1016/S0002-9343(98)00192-2

32. Hammerman H, Alker KJ, Schoen FJ KR. Morphologic and functional effects of piroxicam on myocardial scar formation after coronary occlusion in dogs. *Am J Cardiol.* 1984;53(4):604-607.

33. Leung YY, Yao Hui LL, Kraus VB. Colchicine—update on mechanisms of action and therapeutic uses. *Semin Arthritis Rheum.* 2015;45(3):341-350. doi:10.1016/j.semarthrit.2015.06.013

34. Imazio M, Bobbio M, Cecchi E, et al. Colchicine in addition to conventional therapy for acute pericarditis: results of the COlchicine for acute PEricarditis (COPE) trial. *Circulation.* 2005;112(13):2012-2016. doi:10.1161/CIRCULATIONAHA.105.542738

35. Imazio M, Brucato A, Cemin R, et al. A randomized trial of colchicine for acute pericarditis. *N Engl J Med.* 2013;369(16):1522-1528. doi:10.1056/NEJMoa1208536

36. Tong DC, Wilson AM, Layland J. Colchicine in cardiovascular disease: an ancient drug with modern tricks. *Heart.* 2016;102(13):995-1002. doi:10.1136/heartjnl-2015-309211

37. Schenone AL, Menon V. Colchicine in pericardial disease: from the underlying biology and clinical benefits to the drug-drug interactions in cardiovascular medicine. *Curr Cardiol Rep.* 2018;20(8). doi:10.1007/s11886-018-1008-5

38. Lotrionte M, Biondi-Zoccai G, Imazio M, et al. International collaborative systematic review of controlled clinical trials on pharmacologic treatments for acute pericarditis and its recurrences. *Am Heart J.* 2010;160(4):662-670. doi:10.1016/j.ahj.2010.06.015

39. Maron BJ, Udelson JE, Bonow RO, et al. Eligibility and disqualification recommendations for competitive athletes with cardiovascular abnormalities: task force 3: hypertrophic cardiomyopathy, arrhythmogenic right ventricular cardiomyopathy and other cardiomyopathies, and myocarditis: a scientific statement from the American Heart Association and American College of Cardiology. *Circulation.* 2015;132(22):e273-e280. doi:10.1161/CIR.0000000000000239

40. Pelliccia A, Solberg EE, Papadakis M, et al. Recommendations for participation in competitive and leisure time sport in athletes with cardiomyopathies, myocarditis, and pericarditis: position statement of the Sport Cardiology Section of the European Association of Preventive Cardiology (EAPC). *Eur Heart J.* 2019;40(1):19-33. doi:10.1093/eurheartj/ehy730

41. Shah NP, Verma BR, Ala CK, et al. Exercise is good for the heart but not for the inflamed pericardium? *JACC Cardiovasc Imaging.* 2019;12(9):1880-1881. doi:10.1016/j.jcmg.2019.01.022

42. Andreis A, Imazio M, de Ferrari GM. Contemporary diagnosis and treatment of recurrent pericarditis. *Expert Rev Cardiovasc Ther.* 2019;17(11):817-826. doi:10.1080/14779072.2019.1691916

43. Imazio M, Brucato A, Maestroni S, et al. Risk of constrictive pericarditis after acute pericarditis. *Circulation.* 2011;124(11):1270-1275. doi:10.1161/CIRCULATIONAHA.111.018580

44. Seidenberg PH, Haynes J. Pericarditis: diagnosis, management, and return to play. *Curr Sport Med Rep.* 2006;5(2):74-79. doi:10.1007/s11932-006-0034-z'

45. Imazio M, Bobbio M, Cecchi E, et al. Colchicine as first-choice therapy for recurrent pericarditis results of the CORE (COlchicine for REcurrent pericarditis) trial. *Arch Intern Med.* 2005;165(17):1987-1991.

46. Imazio M, Brucato A, Adler Y, et al. Prognosis of idiopathic recurrent pericarditis as determined from previously published reports. *Am J Cardiol.* 2007;100(6):1026-1028. doi:10.1016/j.amjcard.2007.04.047

47. Guindo J, De la Serna AR, Gusi G, De Miguel MA, Cosin J, De Luna AB. Recurrent pericarditis: relief with colchicine. *Primary Cardiol.* 1992;18(8):1117-1120.

48. Millaire A, De Groote P, Decoulx E, Goullard L, Ducloux G. Treatment of recurrent pericarditis with colchicine. *Eur Heart J.* 1994;15(1):120-124. doi:10.1093/oxfordjournals.eurheartj.a060363

49. Artom G, Koren-Morag N, Spodick DH, et al. Pretreatment with corticosteroids attenuates the efficacy of colchicine in preventing recurrent pericarditis: a multi-centre all-case analysis. *Eur Heart J.* 2005;26(7):723-727. doi:10.1093/eurheartj/ehi197

50. Brucato A, Brambilla G, Moreo A, et al. Long-term outcomes in difficult-to-treat patients with recurrent pericarditis. *Am J Cardiol.* 2006;98(2):267-271. doi:10.1016/j.amjcard.2006.01.086

51. Vianello F, Cinetto F, Cavraro M, et al. Azathioprine in isolated recurrent pericarditis: a single centre experience. *Int J Cardiol.* 2011;147(3):477-478. doi:10.1016/j.ijcard.2011.01.027

52. Moretti M, Buiatti A, Merlo M, et al. Usefulness of high-dose intravenous human immunoglobulins treatment for refractory recurrent pericarditis. *Am J Cardiol.* 2013;112(9):1493-1498. doi:10.1016/j.amjcard.2013.06.036

53. Imazio M, Lazaros G, Picardi E, et al. Intravenous human immunoglobulins for refractory recurrent pericarditis: a systematic review of all published cases. *J Cardiovasc Med.* 2016;17(4):263-269. doi:10.2459/JCM.0000000000000260

54. Brucato A, Imazio M, Gattorno M, et al. Effect of anakinra on recurrent pericarditis among patients with colchicine resistance and corticosteroid dependence: the AIRTRIP randomized clinical trial. *JAMA* 2016;316(18):1906-1912. doi:10.1001/jama.2016.15826

55. Lazaros G, Imazio M, Brucato A, et al. Anakinra: an emerging option for refractory idiopathic recurrent pericarditis: a systematic review of published evidence. *J Cardiovasc Med.* 2016;17(4):256-262. doi:10.2459/JCM.0000000000000266

56. Dagan A, Langevitz P, Shoenfeld Y, Shovman O. Anakinra in idiopathic recurrent pericarditis refractory to immunosuppressive therapy; a preliminary experience in seven patients. *Autoimmun Rev.* 2019;18(6):627-631. doi:10.1016/j.autrev.2019.01.005

57. Klein AL, Imazio M, and Cremer P. RHAPSODY Investigators. Phase 3 Trial of Interleukin-1 Trap Rilonacept in Recurrent Pericarditis. *N Engl J Med.* 2021 Jan 7;384(1):31-41.

58. Khandaker MH, Schaff H V, Greason KL, et al. Pericardiectomy vs medical management in patients with relapsing pericarditis. *Mayo Clin Proc.* 2012;87(11):1062-1070. doi:10.1016/j.mayocp.2012.05.024

59. Gillaspie E, Stulak J, Daly R, et al. A 20-year experience with isolated pericardiectomy: analysis of indications and outcomes. *J Thorac Cardiovasc Surg.* 2016;152(2):448-458. doi:10.1016/j.jtcvs.2016.03.098

60. Unai S, Johnston DR. Radical pericardiectomy for pericardial diseases. *Curr Cardiol Rep.* 2019;21(2):1-6. doi:10.1007/s11886-019-1092-1

61. Hammer Y, Bishara J, Eisen A, Iakobishvili Z, Kornowski R, Mager A. Seasonal patterns of acute and recurrent idiopathic pericarditis. *Clin Cardiol.* 2017;40(11):1152-1155. doi:10.1002/clc.22804

62. Fried JA, Ramasubbu K, Bhatt R, et al. The variety of cardiovascular presentations of COVID-19. *Circulation.* 2020;141(23):1930-1936. doi:10.1161/CIRCULATIONAHA.120.047164

63. Hua A, O'Gallagher K, Sado D, Byrne J. Life-threatening cardiac tamponade complicating myo-pericarditis in COVID-19. *Eur Heart J.* 2020;41(22):2130. doi:10.1093/eurheartj/ehaa253

64. Mayosi BM, Burgess LJ, Doubell AF. Tuberculous pericarditis. *Circulation.* 2005;112(23):3608-3616. doi:10.1161/CIRCULATIONAHA.105.543066

65. Sagristà-Sauleda J, Permanyer-Miralda G, Soler-Soler J. Tuberculous pericarditis: ten year experience with a prospective protocol for diagnosis and treatment. *J Am Coll Cardiol.* 1988;11(4):724-728. doi:10.1016/0735-1097(88)90203-3

66. Koh KK, Kim EJ, Cho CH, et al. Adenosine deaminase and carcinoembryonic antigen in pericardial effusion diagnosis, especially in suspected tuberculous pericarditis. *Circulation.* 1994;89(6):2728-2735. doi:10.1161/01.CIR.89.6.2728

67. Tirilomis T, Unverdorben S, von der Emde J. Pericardiectomy for chronic constrictive pericarditis: risks and outcome. *Eur J Cardiothorac Surg.* 1994;8(9):487-492. doi:10.1016/1010-7940(94)90020-5

68. Sagristà-Sauleda J, A. Barrabés J, Permanyer-Miralda G, Soler-Soler J. Purulent pericarditis: Review of a 20-year experience in a general hospital. *J Am Coll Cardiol.* 1993;22(6):1661-1665. doi:10.1016/0735-1097(93)90592-O

69. De Jong Y, Van Loenhout RB, Swank DJ, Jansen CL, Sorgdrager BJ. Polymicrobial bacterial pericarditis and cardiac tamponade caused by pericardial penetration of an adjustable gastric band. *BMJ Case Rep.* 2018;2018. doi:10.1136/bcr-2017-221589

70. Parikh SV, Memon N, Echols M, Shah J, McGuire DK, Keeley EC. Purulent pericarditis report of 2 cases and review of the literature. *Medicine (Baltimore).* 2009;88(1):52-65. doi:10.1097/MD.0b013e318194432b

71. Rubin RH, Moellering RC. Clinical, microbiologic and therapeutic aspects of purulent pericarditis. *Am J Med.* 1975;59(1):68-78. doi:10.1016/0002-9343(75)90323-X

72. Chang SA. Tuberculous and infectious pericarditis. *Cardiol Clin.* 2017;35(4):615-622. doi:10.1016/j.ccl.2017.07.013

73. El Helou G, Hellinger W. Cryptococcus neoformans pericarditis in a lung transplant recipient: case report, literature review and pearls. *Transpl Infect Dis.* 2019;21(5):e13137. doi:10.1111/tid.13137

74. Hidron A, Vogenthaler N, Santos-Preciado JI, Rodriguez-Morales AJ, Franco-Paredes C, Rassi A. Cardiac involvement with parasitic infections. *Clin Microbiol Rev.* 2010;23(2):324-349. doi:10.1128/CMR.00054-09

75. Nunes MCP, Guimarães MH, Diamantino AC, Gelape CL, Ferrari TCA. Cardiac manifestations of parasitic diseases. *Heart.* 2017;103(9):651-658. doi:10.1136/heartjnl-2016-309870

76. Imazio M, Hoit BD. Review: Post-cardiac injury syndromes. An emerging cause of pericardial diseases. *Int J Cardiol.* 2013;168(2):648-652. doi:10.1016/j.ijcard.2012.09.052

77. Imazio M, Brucato A, Rovere ME, et al. Contemporary features, risk factors, and prognosis of the post-pericardiotomy syndrome. *Am J Cardiol.* 2011;108(8):1183-1187. doi:10.1016/j.amjcard.2011.06.025

78. Finkelstein Y, Shemesh J, Mahlab K, et al. Colchicine for the prevention of postpericardiotomy syndrome. *Herz.* 2002;27(8):791-794. doi:10.1007/s00059-002-2376-5

79. Imazio M, Trinchero R, Brucato A, et al. COlchicine for the Prevention of the Post-pericardiotomy Syndrome (COPPS): a multicentre, randomized, double-blind, placebo-controlled trial. *Eur Heart J.* 2010;31(22):2749-2754. doi:10.1093/eurheartj/ehq319

80. Gunda S, Reddy M, Nath J, et al. Impact of periprocedural colchicine on postprocedural management in patients undergoing a left atrial appendage ligation using LARIAT. *J Cardiovasc Electrophysiol.* 2016;27(1):60-64. doi:10.1111/jce.12869

81. Llubani R, Böhm M, Imazio M, Fries P, Khreish F, Kindermann I. The first post-cardiac injury syndrome reported following transcatheter aortic valve implantation: a case report. *Eur Hear J— Case Reports.* 2018;2(4):1-6. doi:10.1093/ehjcr/yty107

82. Tofler GH, Muller JE, Stone PH, et al. Pericarditis in acute myocardial infarction: characterization and clinical significance. *Am Heart J.* 1989;117(1):86-92. doi:10.1016/0002-8703(89)90660-1

83. Chahine J, Ala CK, Gentry JL, Pantalone KM, Klein AL. Pericardial diseases in patients with hypothyroidism. *Heart.* 2019;105(13):1027-1033. doi:10.1136/heartjnl-2018-314528

84. Renfrew R, Buselmeier TJ, Kjellstrand CM. Pericarditis and renal failure. *Annu Rev Med.* 1980;31(1):345-360. doi:10.1146/annurev.me.31.020180.002021

85. Rehman KA, Betancor J, Xu B, et al. Uremic pericarditis, pericardial effusion, and constrictive pericarditis in end-stage renal disease: insights and pathophysiology. *Clin Cardiol.* 2017;40(10):839-846. doi:10.1002/clc.22770

86. Dad T, Sarnak MJ. Pericarditis and pericardial effusions in end-stage renal disease. *Semin Dial.* 2016;29(5):366-373. doi:10.1111/sdi.12517

87. Imazio M, Demichelis B, Parrini I, et al. Relation of acute pericardial disease to malignancy. *Am J Cardiol.* 2005;95(11):1393-1394. doi:10.1016/j.amjcard.2005.01.094

88. Imazio M, Colopi M, De Ferrari GM. Pericardial diseases in patients with cancer: contemporary prevalence, management and outcomes. *Heart.* 2020;106(8):569-574. doi:10.1136/heartjnl-2019-315852

89. Yeh ETH, Tong AT, Lenihan DJ, et al. Cardiovascular complications of cancer therapy: diagnosis, pathogenesis, and management. *Circulation.* 2004;109(25):3122-3131. doi:10.1161/01.CIR.0000133187.74800.B9

90. Altan M, Toki MI, Gettinger SN, et al. Immune checkpoint inhibitor–associated pericarditis. *J Thorac Oncol.* 2019;14(6):1102-1108. doi:10.1016/j.jtho.2019.02.026

91. Stewart JR, Fajardo LF, Gillette SM, Constine LS. Radiation injury to the heart. *Int J Radiat Oncol Biol Phys.* 1995;31(5):1205-1211. doi:10.1016/0360-3016(94)00656-6

92. Veinot JP, Edwards WD. Pathology of radiation-induced heart disease: a surgical and autopsy study of 27 cases. *Hum Pathol.* 1996;27(8):766-773. doi:10.1016/S0046-8177(96)90447-5

93. Yusuf SW, Sami S, Daher IN. Radiation-induced heart disease: a clinical update. *Cardiol Res Pract.* 2011;1(1). doi:10.4061/2011/317659

94. Imazio M, Lazaros G, Picardi E, et al. Incidence and prognostic significance of new onset atrial fibrillation/flutter in acute pericarditis. *Heart.* 2015;101(18):1463-1467. doi:10.1136/heartjnl-2014-307398

54

Pericardial Effusion and Tamponade

Darryl J. Burstow, Sushil Allen Luis, Garvan C. Kane, and Jae K. Oh

Etiology, evaluation and management of pericardial effusions and cardiac tamponade

Etiology

Pericardial effusion:

Idiopathic (most common etiology in developed countries)

Inflammatory

Tuberculosis (most common etiology in developing countries)

Other infectious

Iatrogenic
• Post-surgery
• Post-catheter or device intervention

Connective tissue disease

Malignant

Post-myocardial infarction

Type A ascending aortic dissection

Uremic

See Table 54-1 for a comprehensive list of etiologies

Cardiac tamponade:
Results when intrapericardial pressure elevation impairs cardiac filling with resulting hemodynamic derangements

Evaluation

History and Clinical Examination
• Pulsus paradoxus (inspiratory decrease in systolic BP > 10mmHg)
• Jugular venous pressure elevation

ECG
• Electrical alternans

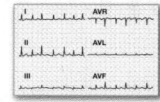

Chest X-Ray
• Globular cardiomegaly

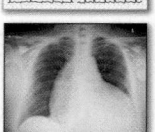

Echocardiography
• RV and RA chamber collapse
• IVC plethora
• Abnormal respiratory variation in ventricular filling
• Progressive loss of diastolic forward flow in central venous flow

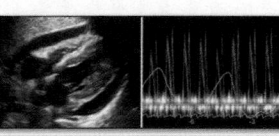

Computed Tomography
• Pericardial mass
• Pericardial thickness
• Cardiac anatomy

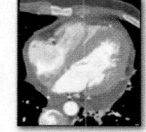

Magnetic Resonance Imaging
• Pericardial inflammation

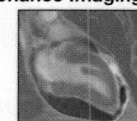

Management

Small and Moderate Asymptomatic Effusions
• Anti-inflammatories and colchicine if inflammatory
• Periodic observation

Acute Tamponade
• Pericardiocentesis
• Pericardial window

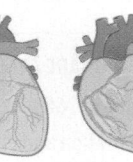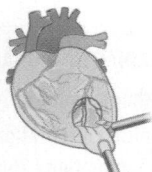

Large Asymptomatic Effusion
• Anti-inflammatories and colchicine if inflammatory
• Periodic observation versus pericardiocentesis due to potential risk of progressing to tamponade

Management After Pericardiocentesis
• NSAID and colchicine for 1 month following pericardiocentesis unless contraindications

Chapter 54 Fuster and Hurst's Central Illustration. Clinical evaluation of patients with pericardial effusions should assess for features of cardiac tamponade. Transthoracic echocardiography is the key diagnostic test in the evaluation of pericardial effusions and assessment of cardiac tamponade. Management of pericardial effusions should target the underlying etiology. BP, blood pressure, ECG, electrocardiography; IVC, inferior vena cava; NSAID, nonsteroidal anti-inflammatory drug; RA, right atrium; RV, right ventricle. Chest x-ray, echocardiogram, CT and MR images used with permission from the Mayo Foundation for Medical Education and Research.

CHAPTER SUMMARY

This chapter outlines the etiology, clinical presentation, investigation, and management of pericardial effusions and cardiac tamponade (see Fuster and Hurst's Central Illustration). Pericardial effusions are most commonly idiopathic in etiology in developed countries, while tuberculous pericarditis is the predominant etiology in developing countries. Cardiac tamponade results when intrapericardial pressure elevation impairs cardiac filling with resulting hemodynamic derangements. The rate of pericardial fluid accumulation is a key factor in the development of cardiac tamponade, whereby small volume rapidly accumulating pericardial effusions can result in cardiac tamponade. Clinical evaluation of patients with pericardial effusions should assess for features of cardiac tamponade, including symptoms, tachycardia, hypotension, pulsus paradoxus, and jugular venous pressure elevation. Transthoracic echocardiography is the key diagnostic test in the evaluation of pericardial effusions and assessment of cardiac tamponade, and should be performed in patients with suspected cardiac tamponade. Management of pericardial effusions should target the underlying etiology, with utilization of anti-inflammatory therapy in those with evidence of active pericardial inflammation. Amongst patients with cardiac tamponade, pericardiocentesis is the intervention of choice and should ideally be performed under imaging guidance.

PERICARDIAL PHYSIOLOGY

The pericardial cavity arises between the visceral and parietal layers of the serous pericardium (see Fig. 53.1, Chapter 53), typically containing 15 mL to 35 mL of physiologic pericardial fluid. Pericardial fluid, which is produced through ultrafiltration of plasma, provides lubrication between the actively contracting heart beneath it and adjacent surrounding structures. The serous pericardial surface comprises of a single layer of mesothelial cells with numerous microvilli and occasional cilia that protrude into the pericardial space. Tight intracellular junctions between these mesothelial cells, comprising of zona occludens and desomsomal junctions, form a barrier allowing filtration of plasma to create pericardial fluid.[1] Pericardial fluid production is a balance between hydrostatic pressure pushing fluid into the pericardial space and osmotic pressure drawing fluid back into the intravascular space, and so alterations in these can result in increases in pericardial fluid volumes. Increased hydrostatic pressures resulting from intravascular volume expansion such as in patients with heart failure; or decreased plasma osmotic pressure resulting from hypoproteinemia in conditions such as cirrhosis and nephrotic syndrome can result in increased pericardial fluid volumes. Pericardial inflammation can result in increased vascular permeability, which also results in pericardial fluid accumulation. Pericardial fluid drainage occurs via the lymphatic system. Distinctive connective tissue structures, with a macroscopic milky spot-like appearance protruding into

the pericardial cavity, allow direct communication between the pericardial cavity and lymphatic capillaries allowing drainage of the pericardial fluid via lymphatic vessels.[2] Hence damage to lymphatic structures, including particularly the thoracic duct, can result in the formation of chylous pericardial effusions (**Fig. 54–1**).

ETIOLOGIES

Any disease or traumatic process that causes injury to the pericardium and the subsequent development of pericarditis can cause pericardial effusion due to inflammation of the visceral and parietal layers with increased production of pericardial fluid (typically an exudate on biochemical analysis). Less commonly, accumulation of pericardial fluid can occur due to decreased reabsorption secondary to a general increase in systemic venous pressure as seen in congestive heart failure or pulmonary hypertension (transudate or hydropericardium). Rarely, a transudative pericardial effusion may also be seen in advanced hypoalbuminemia secondary to cirrhosis or nephrotic syndrome. Hemopericardium is a unique form of pericardial effusion caused by blood directly entering the pericardial space from an aortic or cardiac rupture that can occur secondary to thoracic trauma, aortic dissection, myocardial infarction, or iatrogenic causes. A more comprehensive list of known etiologies of pericardial effusion is presented in **Table 54–1**. Their relative frequency varies with patient demographics.

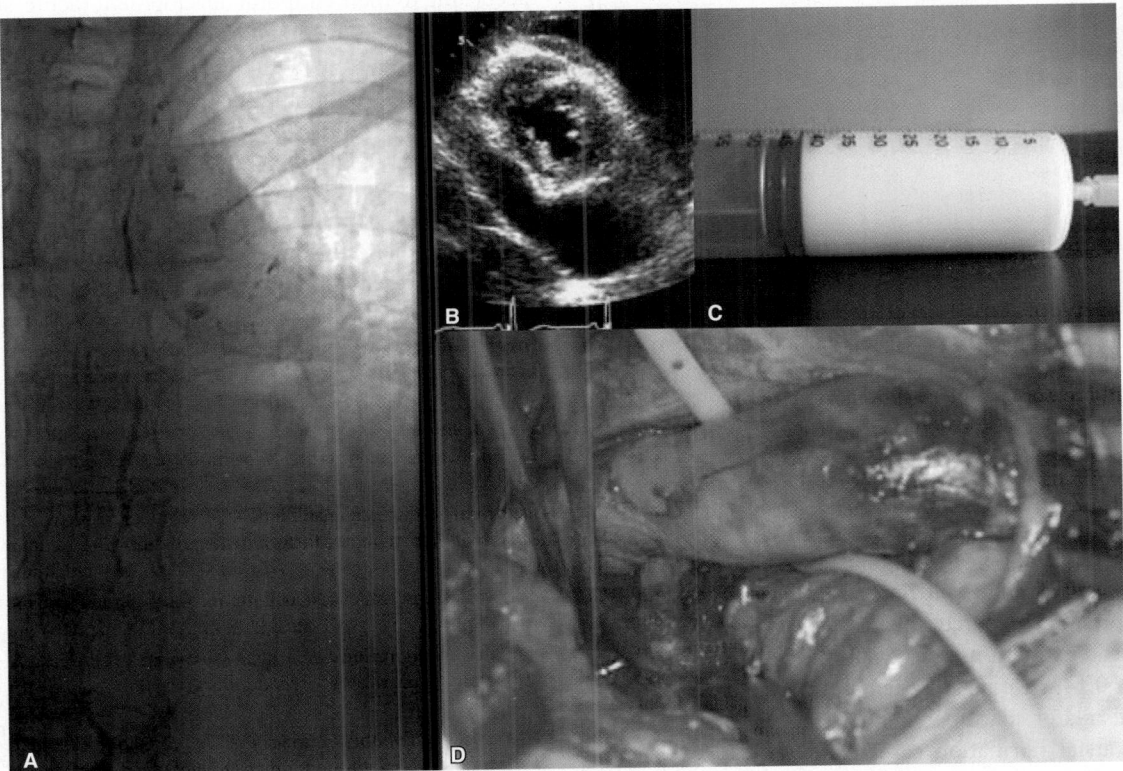

Figure 54–1. A composite of lymphangiogram (**A**) showing obstruction of thoracic duct, transthoracic echocardiogram (**B**) showing large pericardial effusion, and chylous fluid drained by pericardiocentesis (**C**), and intraoperative photo demonstrating anastomosis between the thoracic duct and subclavian vein to cure recurrent collection of pericardial effusion (**D**).

TABLE 54–1. Etiology of Pericardial Effusions

Idiopathic

Infectious

  Viral (enteroviruses: echovirus, coxsackievirus, herpes viruses: EBV, cytomegalovirus, adenovirus, parvovirus B19, HIV)

  Bacterial (Mycobacterium TB, *Coxiella burnetii, Borrelia burgdorferi,* rarely: *Pneumococcus* spp., *Meningococcus* spp., *Gonococcus* spp., *Streptococcus* spp., *Staphylococcus* spp., *Haemophilus* spp., *Chlamydia* spp., *Mycoplasma* spp., *Legionella* spp., *Leptospira* spp., *Listeria* spp., *Providencia stuartii*)

  Fungal Histoplasma spp., *Aspergillus* spp., *Blastomyces* spp., *Candida* spp.

  Protozoal (*Echinococcus* spp. and *Toxoplasma* spp.)

Inflammatory

  Connective tissue disease (systemic lupus erythematosus, rheumatoid arthritis, or scleroderma)

  Vasculitis (polyarteritis nodosa, temporal arteritis, or Churg–Strauss disease)

Drug induced (procainamide, hydralazine, or isoniazid)

Postcardiotomy/thoracotomy

Miscellaneous (sarcoidosis, familial Mediterranean fever, or inflammatory bowel disease)

Postmyocardial infarction

  Early

  Late (Dressler syndrome)

Hemopericardium

  Trauma

  Post–myocardial infarction complications (free wall rupture)

  Dissecting aortic aneurysm (Type A)

  Iatrogenic (endomyocardial biopsy, post–percutaneous coronary intervention, post insertion of cardiac devices, transcatheter valve implants, postcardiac surgery)

  Anticoagulants

Malignancy

Miscellaneous

  Metabolic: Chronic renal failure, Hypothyrodisim

  Radiation therapy

  Chylopericardium

  Hydropericardium: Heart failure, pulmonary hypertension, cirrhosis, nephrotic syndrome

---

Data from multiple studies[3–6] suggest that in developed countries, the etiology of pericardial effusion remains undiagnosed despite investigation in up to 50% of cases and are labeled idiopathic although many of these are presumed to have an infectious cause. Other common causes are confirmed infectious agents (15%–30%), cancer (10%–25%), and connective tissue disorders (5%–15%). In patients requiring pericardiocentesis, malignancy and iatrogenic causes (postsurgery, postcatheter intervention) become more common and accounted for nearly 70% of cases in one large series with over 1000 patients.[7] Iatrogenic cardiac perforation can complicate numerous percutaneous procedures including electronic cardiac device placements, arrhythmia ablations, percutaneous coronary interventions, and device lead extractions. Large national registries report an incidence of 0.14% amongst patients undergoing implantable cardiac defibrillator placement and 0.61% amongst patients undergoing atrial fibrillation catheter ablation.[8,9] Case complexity, procedure and device type, and proceduralist volumes and experience contribute to the risk of cardiac perforation. Proceduralists should maintain a high index of suspicion

particularly in instances of unexplained hemodynamic instability. Tuberculosis continues to be the predominant etiology in developing countries, accounting for 50% to 60% of the cases.[6] The characteristics of the intrapericardial contents may aid in determining the etiology of the effusion (**Figs. 54–2** and **54–3**). Hemopericardium is typically an echodense effusion due to its high cellularity and formation of intrapericardial hematoma may be seen. Fibrinous strands with associated pericardial thickening or phlegmon suggest a chronic inflammatory process[10] and may identify patients at risk of developing an effusive-constrictive form of pericardial disease. In cases of malignant effusion, tumor masses within the pericardial space can sometimes be demonstrated. In end-stage renal failure, pericardial effusions may arise due to a combination of uremic pericarditis and volume overload. Uremic pericarditis results from the accumulation of toxic metabolites that promote pericardial inflammation, and is associated with pericardial effusions in the majority of cases. Uremic pericarditis should be treated by institution of dialysis, although caution should be taken in patients with evidence of tamponade physiology because intravascular fluid shifts during dialysis can exacerbate cardiac tamponade and result in marked hemodynamic instability. In such uremic patients with evidence of cardiac tamponade, drainage of pericardial effusions as subsequently detailed should be considered to allow institution of dialysis.

CLINICAL PRESENTATION

In addition to etiology, pericardial effusions can be classified according to their temporal development (acute, subacute, and chronic), effusion volume (small, moderate, large), and the presence of hemodynamic effect (cardiac tamponade). Transthoracic echocardiography is the standard imaging modality used for detection and assessment of pericardial effusion and its utility will be described in more detail later in this chapter. Clinical presentation is variable being influenced by the underlying etiology as well as the size and speed of accumulation of the pericardial effusion. For example, if the etiology is infectious, the presentation is often acute and dominated by clinical features of acute pericarditis. The effusion size is frequently small and may not result in any features of hemodynamic compromise. Conversely, conditions resulting in a rapid accumulation of pericardial effusion, as in thoracic trauma, cardiac perforation, or aortic dissection, present with a clinical picture of rapid hemodynamic deterioration and shock despite relatively small pericardial effusions. Patients with slowly accumulating pericardial effusions, usually due to a noninfectious etiology (eg, malignancy), might be entirely asymptomatic with the detection of the effusion, often moderate or large, being an incidental finding during thoracic imaging or transthoracic echocardiography.

Classic symptoms may include pleuritic chest pain, atypical chest pain or fullness, exertional dyspnea, orthopnea (rarely), or other less specific findings such as cough, malaise, or fatigue. Compression of local contiguous anatomic structures by the pericardial effusion can lead to dysphagia (esophagus), hoarseness (recurrent laryngeal nerve), or hiccups (phrenic nerve).

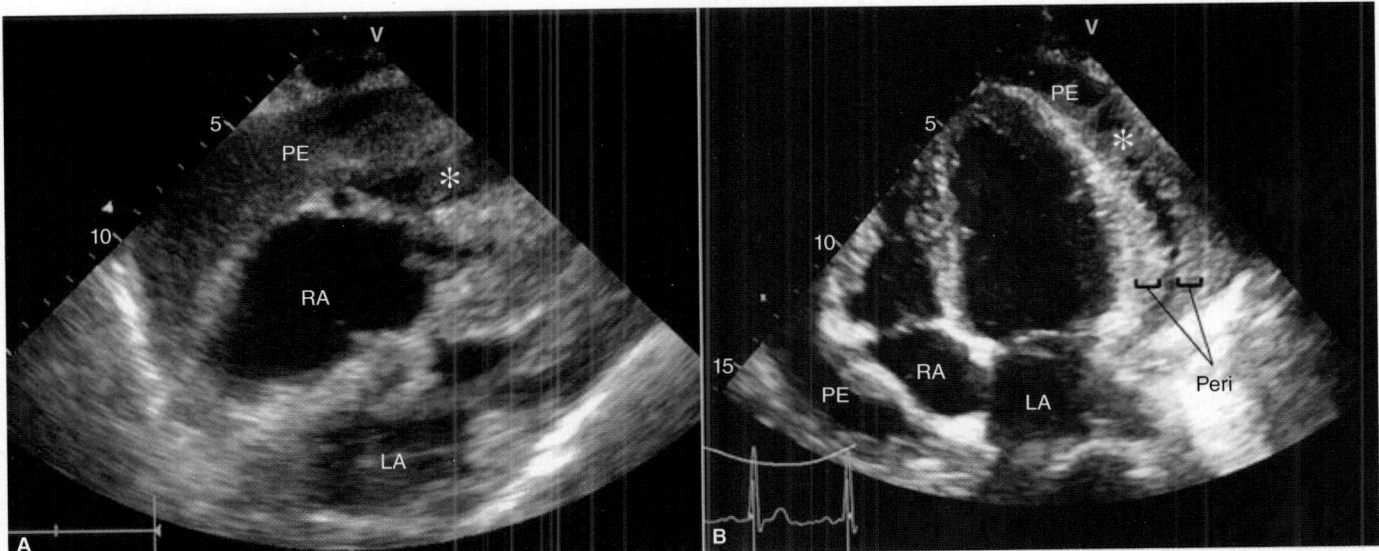

Figure 54–2. (**A**) demonstrates transthoracic echocardiography (subcostal view) in a patient with hemopericardium secondary to Type A aortic dissection. The pericardial effusion (PE) is echodense and contains semi-solid material consistent with hematoma (*asterisk*). (**B**) demonstrates the apical four chamber view of a transthoracic echo in a patient with a pericardial effusion secondary to a severe inflammatory pericarditis. The pericardial effusion (PE) contains fibrinous strands (*asterisk*) and the pericardium (Peri) is markedly thickened (*brackets*). LA, left atrium, RA, right atrium.

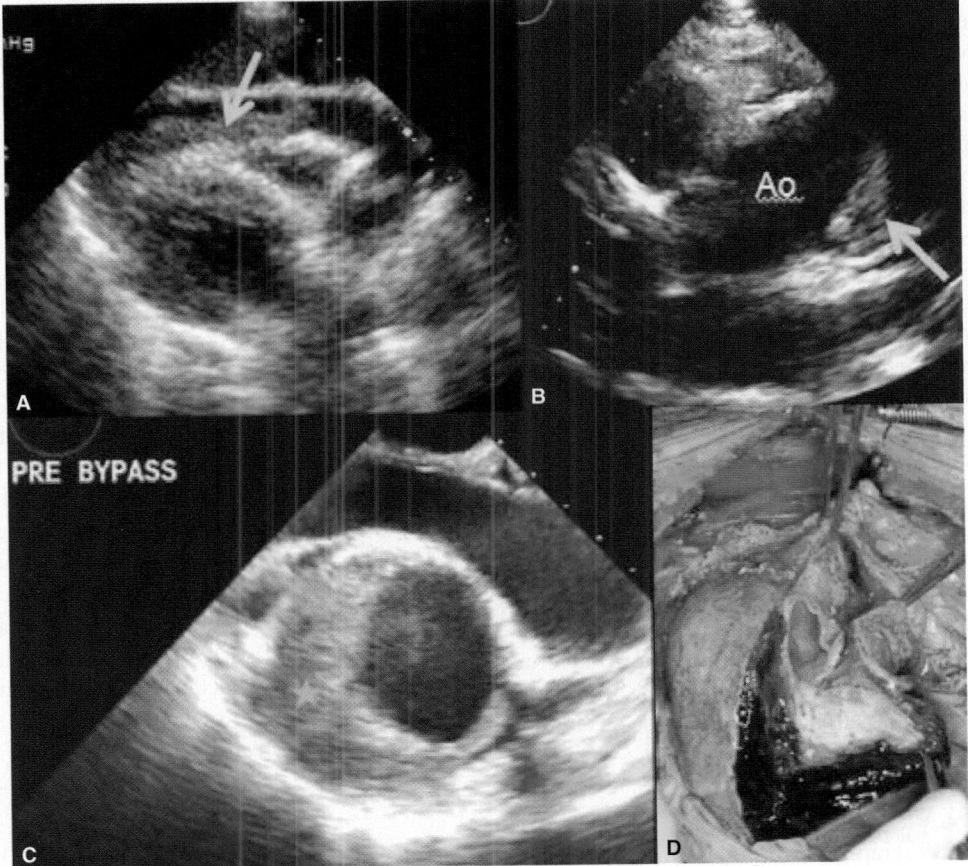

Figure 54–3. Characteristic appearance of hemopericardium (*arrow* in **A**) from a patient with intramural hematoma shown in the parasternal long-axis view (*arrow* in **B**) by transthoracic echocardiogram. It was confirmed by intraoperative transesophageal echocardiogram (*star* in **C**) and surgery (**D**).

Physical Examination

The diagnosis of pericardial effusion at the bedside can be challenging and usually echocardiography or sometimes cardiac computed tomography (CT) provides a definite diagnosis of pericardial effusion. In patients with a known pericardial effusion, the role of the physical examination is, firstly, to assess the hemodynamic consequences of the pericardial effusion looking for features of cardiac tamponade and, secondly, to identify signs of an underlying etiology (such as infection, pericardial trauma, systemic inflammatory disorder, malignancy, etc). Heart rate and blood pressure should be manually recorded, and the presence of pulsus paradoxus should be sought. A thorough examination of the jugular veins is mandatory to determine whether systemic venous pressure is elevated. In patients with larger but uncomplicated pericardial effusions, distant heart sounds might be present, but cardiac examination can be otherwise unremarkable. A pericardial friction rub may be auscultated in patients with concomitant pericarditis. The pathophysiology and clinical features of cardiac tamponade are discussed in more detail later in this chapter.

INVESTIGATIONS

Laboratory Investigations

Investigations should be chosen to assess potential causative etiologies based on clinical history and physical examination. Baseline assessment of renal function is reasonable both as a potential causative etiology and as new acute renal impairment may be a marker of cardiac tamponade. Inflammatory markers, including C-reactive protein (CRP) and erythrocyte sedimentation rate (ESR), can be useful markers of pericardial inflammation. Thyroid function testing may be considered because thyroid dysfunction, most commonly hypothyroidism, is associated with pericardial effusion.

Where rheumatologic etiologies are suspected, autoimmune antibody testing should be considered. This includes assessment of antinuclear antibodies (ANA) and extractable nuclear antigen (ENA) antibodies for suspected systemic lupus erythematosus and systemic sclerosis; rheumatoid factor and anticyclic citrullinated peptide (anti-CCP) antibodies for suspected rheumatoid arthritis; and antineutrophil cytoplasmic antibodies (ANCA) for suspected eosinophilic granulomatosis with polyangiitis (Churg–Strauss syndrome).

Chest X-Ray

Although not diagnostic or specific, a globular or flask shape of the heart on chest x-ray suggests pericardial effusion. Unless there is a component of effusive-constriction, pericardial effusion does not cause pulmonary venous congestion. In certain clinical situation, pericardial effusion should be suspected by increasing size of cardiac shadow (**Fig. 54–4**).

Echocardiography

Transthoracic echocardiography is routinely utilized for the assessment of pericardial effusions, and provides a high sensitivity and specificity for the diagnosis. It offers advantages of being widely available, portable, and of lower cost than cross-sectional imaging techniques. Circumferential pericardial effusions lie anterior to the descending thoracic aorta in the parasternal long axis view, allowing them to be distinguished from pleural effusions which lie posterior to this structure (**Fig. 54–5**). Pericardial effusion size can be assessed semi-quantitatively by echocardiography based on the end-diastolic linear dimension between parietal and visceral layers of the serous pericardium. Pericardial effusions are described as small if measured as <10 mm at end-diastole, moderate if 10 mm to 20 mm, and large if >20 mm.[11] A major strength of echocardiography is its ability to diagnose the hemodynamic consequences of the pericardial effusion, as described in detail in the section Cardiac Tamponade. If transthoracic echocardiographic imaging windows are nondiagnostic, consideration could be given to further echocardiographic evaluation using transesophageal echocardiography, cardiac CT, or cardiac magnetic resonance (CMR) imaging.

Cardiac Computed Tomography and Cardiac Magnetic Resonance

Cardiac CT and CMR provide alternatives to echocardiography in the minority of patients in whom pericardial effusions cannot be adequately imaged using echocardiography. Such instances include nondiagnostic echocardiographic acoustic windows, posterior or superior loculated effusions, and pneumopericardium. Discrepancies are frequently reported between cross-sectional imaging, with cardiac CT and CMR, and echocardiography in terms of pericardial effusion size such that cross-sectional imaging reported effusion sizes are typically reported as being larger than those by echocardiography. These differences in reported pericardial effusion size are due to differences in grading criteria between modalities, rather than discrepancies in pericardial effusion visualization or actual differences in effusion size.

Pericardial effusions are often incidentally discovered on cardiac CT. Cardiac CT also provides valuable extracardiac imaging where aortic dissection or malignant invasion of the pericardium is suspected as the etiology for pericardial effusions. Cardiac CT can also be useful to differentiate epicardial fat from pericardial fluid where uncertainty exists by echocardiography. Additionally, CT attenuation coefficients can be useful to distinguish effusion etiologies including simple transudates, hemorrhage, chyle, and purulent fluid.[11]

In addition to being able to visualize small effusions, CMR offers particular strengths in tissue characterization, including being able to distinguish epicardial fat and define pericardial fluid characteristics, including transudates, exudates, and hemorrhage. Pericardial delayed gadolinium enhancement and edema-sensitive triple inversion recovery sequences may suggest coexistent pericardial inflammation.

GENERAL MANAGEMENT

Pericardial effusion management should be tailored to the underlying etiology. Anti-inflammatory therapy including non-steroidal anti-inflammatory drugs (NSAIDS) and colchicine

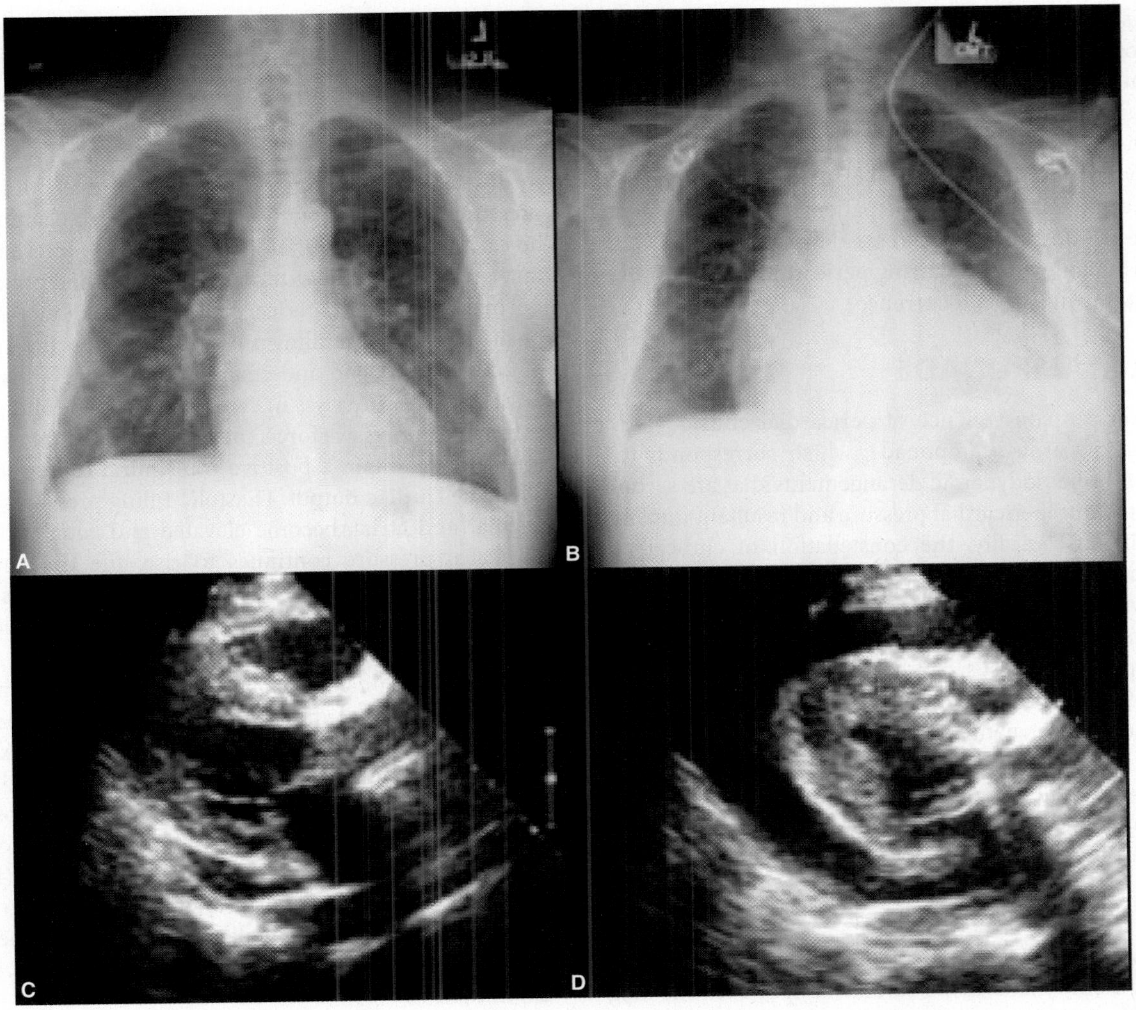

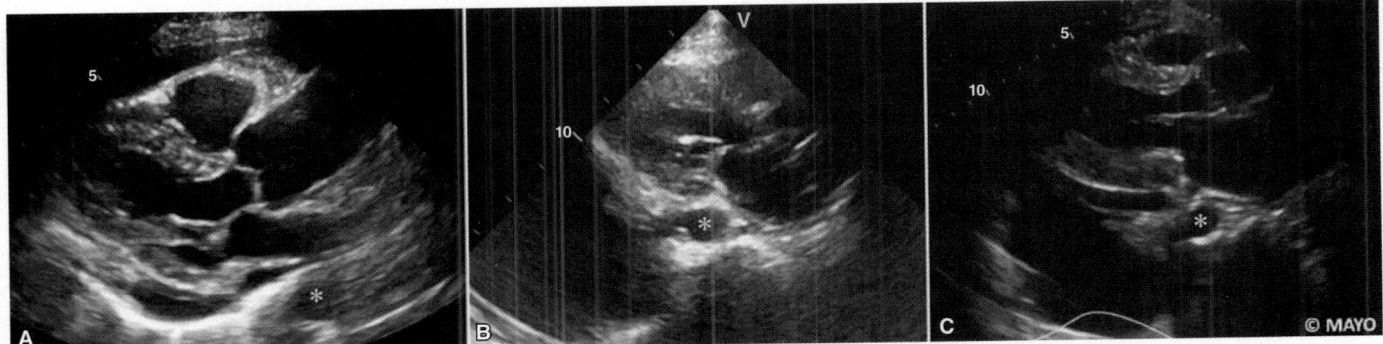

Figure 54–4. Cardiac silhouette increased from soon after aortic valve replacement (**A**) to 2 weeks later when the patient presented with increasing dyspnea (**B**). Echocardiogram showed large pericardial effusion (**D**) that was not present when he was dismissed after surgery (**C**).

should be considered among patients with evidence of active pericardial inflammation. Rheumatologic etiologies should be treated with the usual disease-modifying antirheumatic drugs with input from a rheumatologist. Routine diagnostic pericardiocentesis and/or pericardial biopsy are not indicated and should only be considered where diagnostic evaluation will alter management. Such instances include where there is a high index of suspicion for a bacterial, fungal, or protozoal infectious etiology. Similarly, pericardiocentesis and/or pericardial biopsy may be considered where a malignant pericardial

Figure 54–5. Distinction of pericardial effusion from pleural effusion in parasternal long-axis view of transthoracic echocardiography. Pericardial effusion (**A** and **C**) is located anterior to the descending thoracic aorta (*asterisk*) and pleural effusion posterior to it (**B** and **C**).

effusion is suspected, and where a definitive diagnosis would alter oncologic therapy. Therapeutic pericardiocentesis should be performed if there is evidence of cardiac tamponade or in selected patients with large pericardial effusions, as described in the section Cardiac Tamponade. Although not common, chronic asymptomatic pericardial effusion (ie, longer than 6 months) can be present in some patients without an identifiable cause. Almost 30% of patients developed cardiac tamponade during follow-up, requiring pericardiocentesis or even pericardiectomy due to its recurrence.

CARDIAC TAMPONADE

The most serious consequence of pericardial effusion is the development of cardiac tamponade, which corresponds to a constellation of hemodynamic derangements that are secondary to elevated intrapericardial pressure and resultant impaired cardiac filling. Classically, the constellation of clinical and hemodynamic findings that we recognize as cardiac tamponade include elevation of systemic and pulmonary venous pressure, equalization of diastolic pressures within the heart, reduced cardiac output, and pulsus paradoxus. However, it has been recognized for some time that cardiac tamponade represents a continuum of hemodynamic compromise,[12,13] which limits the accuracy of clinical diagnosis. Thus, echocardiography plays an important adjunctive role in confirming the presence of cardiac tamponade with characteristic cardiac hemodynamic compromise often before overt clinical signs have developed.

Pathophysiology

Elevated intrapericardial pressure is the fundamental hemodynamic abnormality that leads to cardiac tamponade. The magnitude of the rise in intrapericardial pressure is determined by the rate at which the effusion develops, and the pericardial compliance as illustrated in pericardial pressure-volume curves (**Fig. 54–6**). Thus, effusion size and the degree of clinical decompensation often correlate poorly. When the pericardial volume increases rapidly (eg, following iatrogenic cardiac perforation or as a result of aortic rupture from dissection), a small amount (as little as 150 mL) of fluid in the pericardial space results in a significant, abrupt elevation in intrapericardial

pressure and can lead to sudden hemodynamic decompensation. Conversely, in the setting of chronic pericardial effusions, the pericardium "stretches out" and is sometimes able to accommodate liters of fluid without major hemodynamic consequences.

Transmural filling pressure[14-16] is the distending or filling pressure across the free wall of any cardiac chamber and can be calculated as the difference between the internal intracavitary pressure and the external intrapericardial pressure. In the normal setting, intrapericardial pressure is low resulting in a positive transmural filling pressure that favors the maintenance of adequate preload and chamber geometry. Thus, as intrapericardial pressure rises in cardiac tamponade and provides an external compressive force, intracardiac pressure will also need to rise to maintain a positive transmural filling pressure and adequate cardiac output. Diastolic filling pressures, both ventricular and atrial, become elevated and equalized. If intrapericardial pressure continues to rise, the transmural filling pressure will continue to fall, further impeding diastolic filling of the heart and, ultimately, becomes negative allowing diastolic compression of the cardiac chambers.[16]

Ventricular interdependence is seen in all forms of compressive pericardial disease. In cardiac tamponade, the total intrapericardial volume is operating at or near maximum levels preventing any significant increase in total cardiac volume. Thus, when the filling and subsequent volume of one ventricular chamber increases, the filling of the other ventricle is impeded.[12,17,18] As a result, when right ventricular (RV) stroke volume increases with inspiration (secondary to increased venous return), left ventricular (LV) stroke volume decreases (the origin of pulsus paradoxus); the opposite occurs during expiration.

Also, the presence of pericardial effusion *attenuates the transmission of normal intrathoracic pressure changes to the left ventricle*. Therefore, when intrathoracic pressure falls with inspiration, pulmonary venous pressure falls more than does intracardiac pressure resulting in a reduction in the diastolic filling gradient between the pulmonary veins and left ventricle.[12,19] The opposite changes are noted during expiration resulting in an increase in diastolic filling gradient. This mechanism likely plays a secondary but contributing role to the

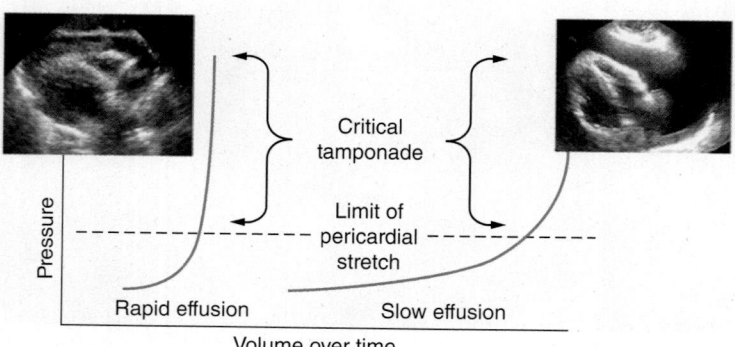

Figure 54–6. Pressure–volume relationship depends on the rate of pericardial fluid accumulation.

abnormal respiratory variation in LV filling and stroke volume seen in cardiac tamponade.

As the severity of tamponade worsens, RV diastolic filling is further compromised resulting in less inspiratory augmentation in RV filling, progressive underfilling of both ventricles, and reduction in cardiac output. Tachycardia and increased peripheral vascular resistance initially compensate for the reduction in stroke volume, but as pericardial pressures increase further, the reduction in cardiac output leads to hypotension, shock, and ultimately death, unless the pericardial effusion is drained.

Clinical Presentation and Physical Examination

Cardiac tamponade should always be considered in patients presenting with shock in the clinical context of recent intracardiac procedures, chest trauma, or cardiothoracic surgery. However, its diagnosis can be more challenging if cardiac tamponade has developed slowly resulting in less dramatic presenting symptoms such as dyspnea or fatigue. Thus, any clinical decompensation in the context of a known or possible pericardial effusion should trigger further clinical evaluation and testing to exclude cardiac tamponade.

Although described as the classic diagnostic criteria for cardiac tamponade, *Beck's triad*— the constellation of hypotension, distended neck veins, and distant heart sounds—is present in less than a half of the patients with tamponade and, therefore, its absence does not exclude the diagnosis.[20] Based on pooled data from eight studies where clinical examination was compared to a reference standard for the diagnosis of cardiac tamponade, the clinical features that occurred in the majority of patients were tachycardia, pulsus paradoxus, and elevated jugular venous pressure (together with dyspnea and cardiomegaly on chest radiography).[21]

Tachycardia (heart rate >100 bpm) develops secondary to increased adrenergic stimulation to maintain cardiac output. Hypotension is an ominous sign of falling cardiac output and advanced tamponade. However, blood pressure may initially be normal due to increased adrenergic tone and should always be assessed in the context of the patient's baseline blood pressure as a "normal" blood pressure level may represent hypotension in patients with chronic hypertension. Blood pressure should be manually measured with special attention to the presence of pulsus paradoxus, which is defined as an inspiratory drop in systolic blood pressure >10 mm Hg. Although a useful clinical sign in the context of a patient with suspected tamponade, it should be remembered that in severe tamponade, blood pressure and stroke volume may be so low that pulsus paradoxus becomes undetectable. Also, there are other conditions without pericardial effusion that have been associated with pulsus paradoxus where pericardial constraint and increased ventricular interaction play a role such as in acute respiratory failure, RV infarction, and acute pulmonary embolism. Inspection of the jugular veins will show elevation in central venous pressure and analysis of the venous pressure waveform may be valuable. As cardiac tamponade results in a progressive impairment in diastolic filling, the contour of the venous waveform will reveal absence or blunting of the y descent, which corresponds

to the period of ventricular diastolic filling. In patients with significant tachycardia, analysis of the timing of the venous waveform descents is usually not feasible. Following pericardiocentesis, with restoration of normal diastolic filling, the jugular venous pressure should fall with restoration of the y descent. In some cases, elevation in central venous pressure persists despite adequate drainage and this scenario suggests the presence of effusive-constrictive pericarditis (see Chapter 55) where ventricular filling is now limited by a noncompliant pericardium rather than pericardial effusion.[22] In this scenario, careful inspection of the jugular venous pressure may reveal rapid and deep y descents reflecting the rapid and abbreviated ventricular filling seen in constrictive pericarditis. Cardiac auscultation might reveal distant heart sounds. Because early diastolic filling is progressively impaired in tamponade, a third heart sound will not be present; its occurrence suggests an alternative diagnosis. For unclear reasons, tamponade does not lead to pulmonary edema; the lungs are usually clear on auscultation in patients with isolated cardiac tamponade. Right upper quadrant pain may be a presenting symptom of chronic pericardial effusion and tamponade due to hepatic congestion. Hepatomegaly along with increased jugular venous pressure strongly suggests this situation, which needs to be confirmed by cardiac imaging.

Evaluation and Testing

Patients with suspected cardiac tamponade should undergo urgent echocardiography, particularly in hemodynamically unstable cases with tachycardia and hypotension. In other clinical scenarios, ECG and chest radiography may also have been performed and can provide diagnostic clues. The ECG classically shows sinus tachycardia, electrical alternans (**Fig. 54–7**), and low QRS voltages. Electrical alternans is characterized by beat-to-beat variation in the QRS complex because of the swinging motion of the heart in the large effusion; changes in P and QRS axes might also be present. Chest radiography might reveal an enlarged cardiac silhouette in the setting of a large pericardial effusion but might be entirely normal. In isolated cardiac tamponade, pulmonary parenchymal abnormalities should not be seen; although pleural effusions might be found in the case of a pleuro-pericarditic process.

Diagnostic Role of Echocardiography

Two-dimensional (2D) and Doppler transthoracic echocardiography is the key diagnostic tool in the evaluation and management of patients with cardiac tamponade (Class I recommendation; level of evidence: C).[23] Firstly, echocardiography confirms the presence of pericardial fluid and also demonstrates certain characteristics of the effusion that may in some cases be helpful in pointing to a specific etiology (Fig. 54–1). Although the size and location of an effusion are important for planning and feasibility of pericardiocentesis, the size of the effusion does not favor or exclude the presence of cardiac tamponade as previously discussed. Secondly, both the 2D echo and Doppler components of the echocardiographic examination can provide important additional information

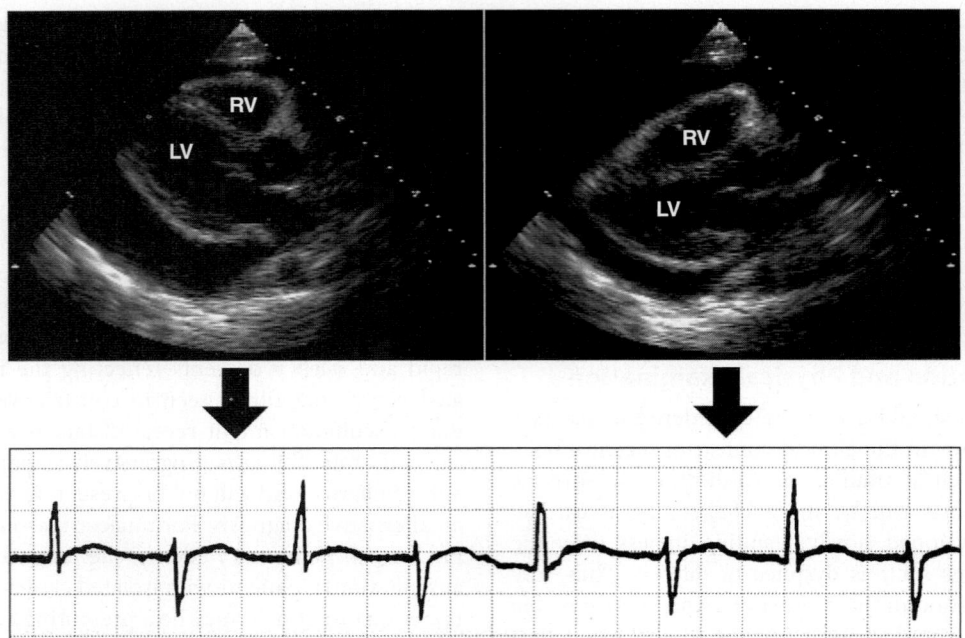

Figure 54–7. Electrical alternans (lower panel) due to swinging motion of the heart (upper panel) within a large amount of pericardial fluid. The magnitude and the direction of "QRS" voltage alternate as shown.

about the likely presence and severity of cardiac tamponade. The pathophysiology and hemodynamic sequelae of cardiac tamponade outlined earlier in this chapter are reflected in various 2D and Doppler echocardiographic abnormalities.

Chamber Compression

Chamber compression occurs when intrapericardial pressure exceeds intracardiac pressure (negative transmural filling pressure) and so is more commonly seen in diastole and affecting the lower pressure right heart chambers (**Fig. 54–8**). The most widely applied signs of chamber compression detected by 2D echocardiography are right atrial (RA) inversion[24,25] and RV diastolic collapse.[25,26] RV compression occurs when RV pressure is lowest and RA inversion typically begins in late diastole and continues into ventricular systole for a variable period. The sensitivity and specificity of this sign appears to increase if the duration of inversion is greater than one-third of the cardiac cycle.[24] RV diastolic collapse is characterized by an abnormal inward motion of the RV free wall during early diastole. A 2D-directed M-mode examination of the abnormal wall motion is often useful in clarifying the timing of these events. It should be remembered that the predictive value of these echocardiographic signs will vary with the patient's pretest likelihood of having cardiac tamponade[27] and they are most accurate in patients who also have a high clinical probability of tamponade. Conversely, in low probability patients, the positive predictive value is significantly reduced but the negative predictive value is high. Thus, in a patient with a low clinical probability of cardiac tamponade, the absence of 2D echocardiographic signs confidently excludes this entity. The sensitivity of both RA diastolic inversion and RV diastolic collapse can be affected by coexistent pathologies (eg, RV hypertrophy, pulmonary

hypertension, and pericardial adhesions). In the presence of these conditions, diastolic collapse may not be observed despite significant elevation in intrapericardial pressure.

IVC Plethora

In cardiac tamponade, central venous pressure becomes elevated and thus the inferior vena cava (IVC) typically becomes dilated with visible blood stasis (plethora)[28] and shows diminished (<50%) or absent collapse with "sniffing maneuver" (Fig. 54–4). An entirely normal inferior vena cava makes tamponade unlikely.

Ventricular Interdependence

Ventricular interdependence is manifested as respirophasic changes in the interventricular septal motion on M-mode and 2D echocardiographic assessment[18] (Fig. 54–8) as well as abnormal respirophasic variation in the Doppler assessment of LV and RV filling (mitral and tricuspid inflow respectively) (**Fig. 54–9**), LV stroke volume and central venous flow profiles (hepatic venous and superior vena cava flow)[12,17] (**Fig. 54–10**). Importantly, the abnormal ventricular filling is reciprocal, being seen maximally and in the opposite direction on the first beats of inspiration and expiration. The published diagnostic thresholds for tamponade physiology are a 30% change in mitral E velocity and a 60% change in tricuspid E velocity when defining velocity change relative to the velocity in expiration.[11] The abnormal respiratory changes in mitral and tricuspid inflow are also reflected in the pulmonary and hepatic venous flow profiles as follows: an inspiratory decrease and expiratory increase in pulmonary venous diastolic forward flow and an expiratory decrease in hepatic venous diastolic forward flow and expiratory increase in reversal flow (Figs. 54–9 and 54–10).

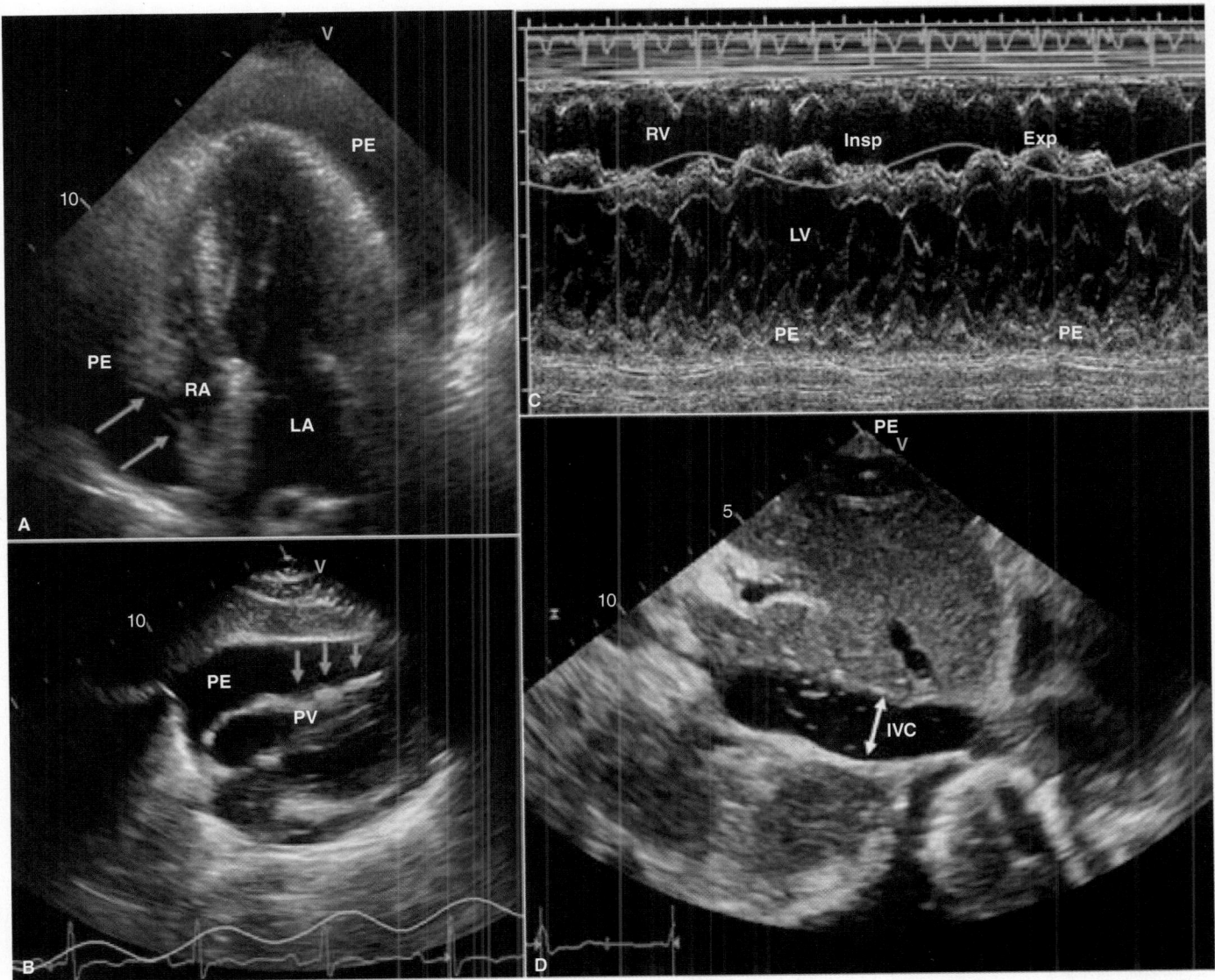

Figure 54–8. M-mode and 2D echocardiographic signs of cardiac tamponade. (A) is a transthoracic echocardiogram (four chamber view) demonstrating a large pericardial effusion (PE) and right atrial (RA) inversion (*blue arrows*). **(B)** is a transthoracic echocardiogram (subcostal view) demonstrating a large pericardial effusion (PE) with right ventricular (RV) diastolic inversion. **(C)** is an M-mode tracing through left ventricle (LV) and RV demonstrating ventricular interaction in a patient with a relatively small pericardial effusion (PE). Note the respirophasic variation in LV and RV diameters which are reciprocal in nature; RV increases with inspiration (upward deflection of the respirometer trace) while LV decreases with the opposite changes noted during expiration. **(D)** is a transthoracic echocardiogram (subcostal view) demonstrating a plethoric inferior vena cava (IVC) with visible stasis of blood flow. Exp, expiration; Insp, inspiration; LA, left atrium.

The most specific finding, however, is the presence of expiratory diastolic flow reversals in the hepatic veins.[12,17,29] The use of a respirometer facilitates the accurate timing of inspiratory and expiration, and should always be used in the evaluation of patients suspected of having tamponade.

Ventricular Filling Profiles

Increased intrapericardial pressure provides a constant external resistance to filling of the cardiac chambers. Thus, as intrapericardial pressures rises, transmural filling pressure falls resulting in impairment in LV filling throughout diastole, particularly early diastole, resulting in a low E velocity and E/A <0.8 (Fig. 54–9). As aforementioned, the presence of

pericardial effusion limits the transmission of normal intrathoracic pressure changes to the left ventricle resulting in respiratory variation in the filling gradient from the pulmonary veins to left ventricle. In addition to respiratory changes in mitral E velocity, the variation in filling gradient results in later or earlier opening of the mitral valve reflected in respiratory variation in the interval from aortic valve closure to mitral valve opening (isovolumic relaxation time [IVRT]) (Fig. 54–9). This finding is also useful for confirming that the variation in mitral inflow reflects genuine variation in LV filling. In case of effusive-constrictive pericarditis, mitral inflow and hepatic vein Doppler velocities resemble those of constriction. This is further discussed in Chapter 55.

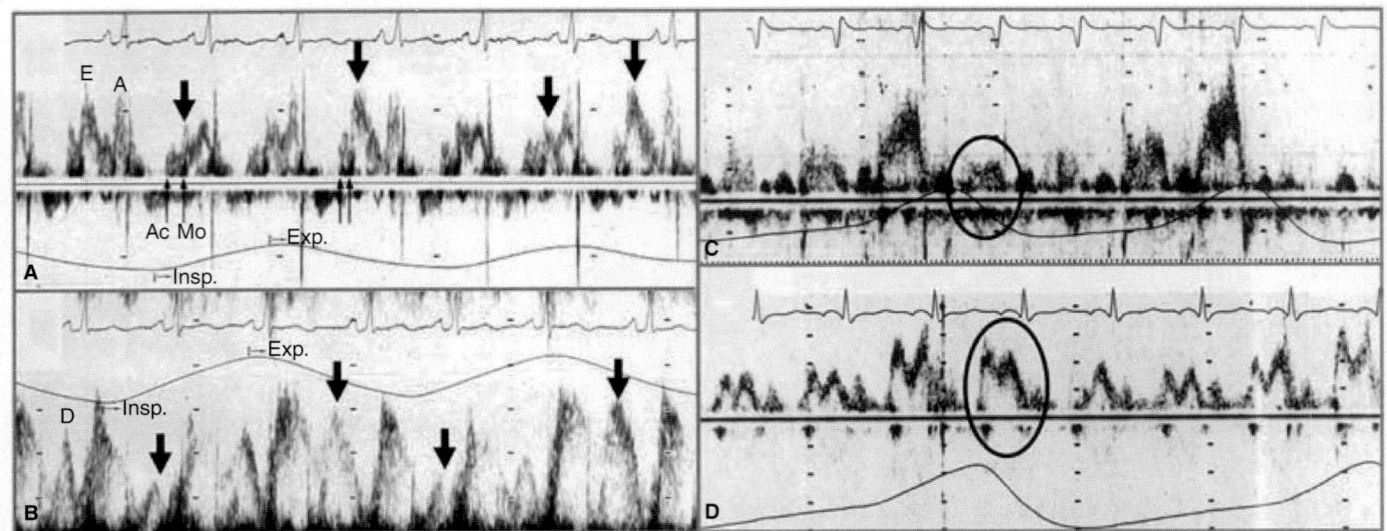

Figure 54–9. (**A**) represents the mitral inflow trace in a patient with cardiac tamponade. There is abnormal respiratory variation (*bold arrows*) with a marked reduction in the early diastolic (E) wave on inspiration, consistent with impairment in left ventricular filling, particularly in early diastole. Also note the variation in isovolumic relaxation time (IVRT), which lengthens in inspiration and shortens during expiration due to later or earlier opening of the mitral valve respectively. (**B**) is the pulmonary venous flow trace from the same patient as (**A**). Pulmonary venous diastolic (D) velocity (*bold arrows*) parallels the changes seen in the mitral E velocity. (**C**) is the tricuspid inflow trace in a patient with tamponade. Note the increased respiratory variation with the most marked reduction in flow on the first beat of expiration (*circled*), which is opposite in timing to changes seen in mitral inflow, a sign of increased ventricular interaction. (**D**) is the same trace post pericardiocentesis. Respiratory variation is still present but the sign of ventricular interaction (loss of filling on the first beat of expiration) is absent (*circled*). A, atrial flow; AC, aortic valve closure; exp, expiration; insp, inspiration.

Tamponade Severity

Cardiac tamponade represents a "continuum" of hemodynamic compromise depending on the level of intrapericardial pressure elevation. Respirophasic variation in LV and RV filling have been shown to occur with only mild elevations in intrapericardial pressure, often precede the development of chamber compression, and thus correlate poorly with the severity of tamponade.[30] As intrapericardial pressure rises, right heart filling and subsequently cardiac output is progressively compromised. Central venous flow velocities (hepatic venous and SVC) demonstrate the degree to which diastolic filling of the right heart is compromised. This is seen as a progressive loss of diastolic forward flow and, ultimately, with severe tamponade, right heart filling is only seen when total cardiac volume is decreasing during ventricular systole (Fig. 54–10). When a reduction in cardiac output is present, this can be seen as a fall in all intracardiac flow velocities (tricuspid, mitral, and RV and LV outflow tract [RVOT/LVOT]). LVOT flow velocity is the easiest to formally measure allowing calculation of LVOT stroke volume and thus cardiac output.

Specific Scenarios

Low-Pressure Tamponade: Low pressure tamponade is a condition where a pericardial effusion, typically small, exerts hemodynamic effects in the presence of an intrapericardial pressure that is only minimally elevated. The patient is typically hypovolemic. Right sided chamber compression and abnormal respirophasic variation in ventricular filling suggest the presence of cardiac tamponade. However, clinical signs of elevated central venous pressure are absent. Depending on the clinical scenario, careful volume replacement may improve haemodynamics and/or further delineate the significance of the effusion.

Regional Tamponade: Regional tamponade occurs when a pericardial effusion causes selective compression of a cardiac chamber, most commonly behind the right atrium. This is most commonly seen in the postoperative cardiac surgical patient where hematoma is collecting within loculated pericardial spaces. In this situation, the patient is hypotensive due to severe underfilling of one cardiac chamber and may not have typical features of cardiac tamponade. In addition, transthoracic echocardiography may also be technically difficult due to limited acoustic windows. A low threshold for performing transesophageal echocardiography is appropriate in this clinical setting (**Fig. 54–11**).

Role of Invasive Hemodynamics

Cardiac catheterization is rarely used for the initial diagnosis of cardiac tamponade. More typically, a patient in intensive care with a pericardial effusion will have invasive hemodynamic monitoring and thus several hemodynamic variables will be available for the assessment of tamponade severity. An arterial line can confirm pulsus paradoxus. If a Swan-Ganz catheter is in place, this will classically show elevation in right- and left-sided filling pressures, equalization of end-diastolic pressures and a falling cardiac index by thermodilution technique. However, in some cases, left-sided filling pressures might be lower than those on the right as a result of significant underfilling of the left ventricle. An additional diagnostic feature of cardiac tamponade is seen in the contour of the right atrial or central

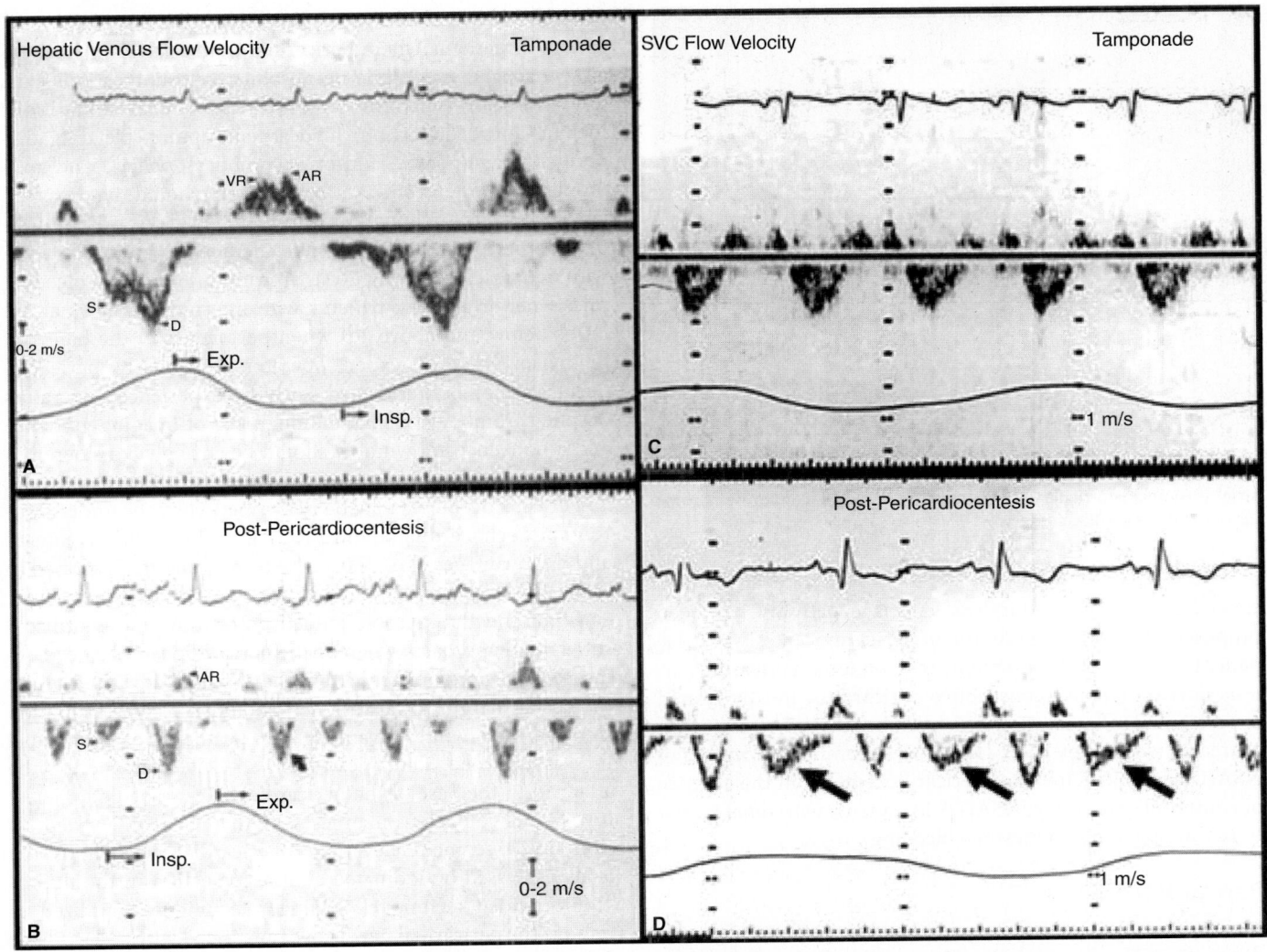

Figure 54–10. (**A**) demonstrates pulsed wave Doppler hepatic venous flow tracing from a patient with cardiac tamponade. (**B**) demonstrates a tracing of the same patient postpericardiocentesis. In (**A**), on expiration, there is a marked reduction in right ventricular diastolic filling as indicated by minimal diastolic forward flow (D) with increased atrial flow reversal (AR), a sign of increased ventricular interaction, paralleling the changes seen in tricuspid inflow depicted in **Fig. 54–9C**. In panel (**B**), post pericardiocentesis, diastolic forward flow is restored with expiration (*arrow*). (**C**) demonstrates pulsed wave Doppler through the superior vena cava in a patient with cardiac tamponade. (**D**) demonstrates a tracing of the same patient postpericardiocentesis. In (**C**), there is complete loss of diastolic flow and minimal inspiratory increase in flow velocity consistent with severe tamponade. In (**D**), diastolic flow has been restored consistent with relief of tamponade (*arrows*). Exp, expiration; Insp, inspiration; S, systolic flow; VR, ventricular flow reversal. Reproduced with permission from Burstow DJ, Oh JK, Bailey KR, et al. Cardiac tamponade: characteristic Doppler observations. *Mayo Clin Proc.* 1989 Mar;64(3):312-324.

venous pressure wave forms with blunting or absence of *y* descents as a result of impaired early RV diastolic filling[31] consistent with changes of the jugular venous pressure waveforms on physical examination and the SVC flow on Doppler assessment (Fig. 54–10).

MANAGEMENT OF CARDIAC TAMPONADE

Classical teaching states that cardiac tamponade is a clinical diagnosis and thus should be based on a constellation of clinical findings and confirmatory testing results. Once the clinical diagnosis is made, patients should in most cases undergo urgent pericardiocentesis. If cardiac tamponade is related to hemopericardium from cardiac perforation, recent cardiac surgery or aortic dissection, an emergency surgical approach with open drainage is recommended when available (Class I recommendation; level of evidence: C).[23] In most other clinical scenarios, a percutaneous approach is recommended with needle puncture usually guided by echocardiography or CT depending on institutional experience and expertise (see section Pericardiocentesis). As cardiac tamponade is part of continuum and not an all-or-none phenomenon; some patients in present at earlier stages and may have "tamponade physiology" (typically by echocardiography) on complementary testing before overt (decompensated) clinical signs develop. The management of those patients should be individualized, and intervention should be based on clinical status, risks of the pericardiocentesis (location and size of the effusion), and

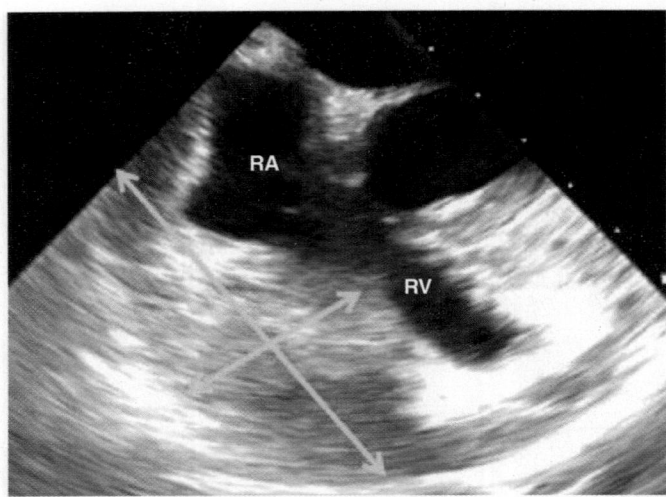

Figure 54–11. Treansesophageal echocardiographic finding of right atrial (RA) and ventricular (RV) compression by pericardial hematoma (*arrows*) after a cardiac surgery.

expertise of the proceduralists. A triage pathway has been proposed to guide in the timing of pericardiocentesis in these patients.[23] About 20% of patients who undergo pericardiocentesis develop effusive-constrictive pericarditis, mostly related to pericardial inflammation which can be progress to scar if left untreated (see Chapter 56). Hence, we recommend 1 month of NSAID and colchicine after pericardiocentesis, in the absence of contraindications (eg, NSAIDS in patients with renal failure or recent upper gastrointestinal bleeding).

Pericardiocentesis

Pericardiocentesis should be performed in patients with evidence of cardiac tamponade. It may also be considered in selected patients with large chronic pericardial effusions without evidence of tamponade due to the long-term risk of progression to cardiac tamponade, and as a diagnostic procedure in patients where pericardial fluid analysis is likely to alter management. While no absolute contraindications exist to performing pericardiocentesis, relative contraindications include aortic dissection, myocardial rupture, bleeding disorders (coagulopathy and/or thrombocytopenia), and pulmonary hypertension. Anticoagulation should be reversed where feasible, although imaging-guided pericardiocentesis may be performed safely despite therapeutic anticoagulation with one series reporting no significant differences in bleeding rates when evaluating patients with international normalized ratios below and above 1.5 when performed in the hands of highly experienced, expert operators.[32] Similarly, pericardiocentesis may be performed safely by experienced operators despite thrombocytopenia, although use of imaging guidance and a nonsubcostal window should be strongly considered in patients with platelet counts <50 x 10⁹/L.[32,33]

Pericardiocenteses may be performed blind, or under fluoroscopic, echocardiographic, or CT guidance. The advantages and disadvantages of each of these techniques are described in **Table 54–2**.

Blind and fluoroscopic-guided pericardiocentesis utilize a subxiphoid approach, whereby the pericardiocentesis needle is inserted at approximately 30° to the skin and advanced under the costal margin toward the left shoulder. Needle aspiration is performed while advancing the needle until pericardial fluid is aspirated. The V-lead from an ECG machine may be attached to the base of the pericardiocentesis needle to detect myocardial contact, as manifest by either PR-segment depression or ST-segment elevation.[34] Pericardial needle position is also assessed by iodinated contrast injection in the fluoroscopic guided technique. Seldinger technique is utilized to remove the pericardial needle over a J-tipped wire and a dilator sheath inserted over the J-tipped guide wire to secure pericardial access, with subsequent removal of the dilator leaving the sheath in place. If fluoroscopic-guidance is used, the J-tipped

TABLE 54–2. Pericardiocentesis				
	Blind pericardiocentesis	**Fluroscopic guided pericardiocentesis**	**Echocardiography-guided pericardiocentesis**	**CT-guided pericardiocentesis**
Advantages	Widely available Portable allowing bedside performance No imaging equipment required	Widely available Ability to confirm pericardial catheter position	Widely available Highly feasible Ability to confirm pericardial catheter position Multiple access site options limited only by available acoustic windows Portable allowing bedside performance Excellent visualization of adjacent structures	Highly feasible Ability to confirm pericardial catheter position Unlimited access site options Excellent visualization of adjacent structures
Limitations	Unable to confirm pericardial catheter position and exclude myocardial puncture Subxiphoid access only Inability to visualize adjacent structures Loculated pericardial effusions	Cannot be performed at bedside Subxiphoid access only Inability to visualize adjacent structures Radiation use Iodinated contrast use Loculated pericardial effusions	Nondiagnostic acoustic windows (eg, pneumopericardium) Loculated posterior pericardial effusions	Availability and operator experience Cannot be performed at bedside Radiation use Iodinated contrast use (in some cases)

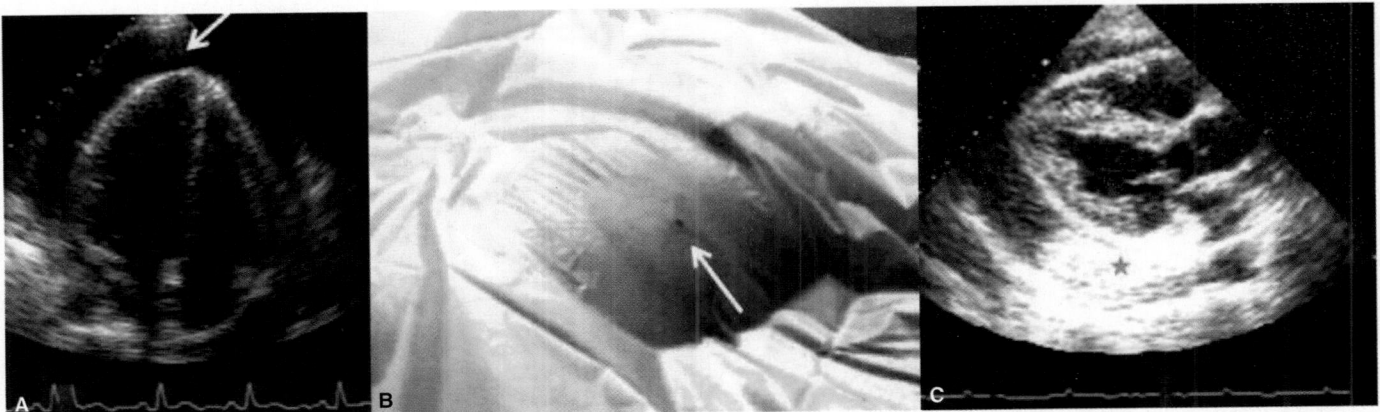

Figure 54–12. Echocardiography-guided pericardiocentesis. The most common location for pericardiocentesis is the apex shown by the apical four chamber view demonstrating a large pericardial effusion located very close to the apex (*arrow* in **A**). An ultrasound probe can guide the location and the direction of pericardiocentesis needle (*arrow* in **B**). When in doubt about the location of the needle, agitated saline is administered to confirm its position in the pericardium (*asterisk* in **C**).

guide wire position should be assessed in orthogonal planes to confirm an intrapericardial rather than intravascular course, prior to insertion of the dilator sheath.

Imaging-guided pericardiocentesis offers an improved margin of safety over blind and fluoroscopic techniques by allowing visualization of adjacent structures, offering multiple potential access sites, and potentially avoiding subxiphoid access. Given its widespread availability, high feasibility, portability and increased margin of safety, echocardiographic-guided pericardiocentesis should be considered the standard of care in contemporary practice. A step-by-step description of the echocardiographic-guided pericardiocentesis procedure is presented in **Fig. 54–12**, with typical access sites illustrated in **Fig. 54–13**. CT-guided pericardiocentesis should be considered second-line and reserved for those patients where echocardiographic-guided pericardiocentesis is not feasible. By offering numerous potential access sites (**Fig. 54–14**) with excellent visualization of adjacent structures unbounded by acoustic windows, CT-guided pericardiocentesis offers high procedural success even in the face of failed echocardiographic-guidance, providing an excellent alternative to surgical drainage.[35,36]

Regardless of the pericardiocentesis technique used, prolonged pericardial catheter drainage is recommended over simple pericardial aspiration in all patients undergoing pericardiocentesis, due to a significant reduction recurrence risk.[7,37] To facilitate this pericardial catheters should be secured and left in place at the conclusion of the procedure. Every 6 hours, the pericardial catheter should be flushed using 5 mL of sterile 0.9% saline, the entire pericardial fluid volume removed by aspirated, followed by injection of 3 mL of sterile 0.9% saline to lock the pericardial catheter. Pericardial catheter related pain may be managed by administering 10 mL of 1% lidocaine (without epinephrine) after each aspiration and as required up to every 2 hours. Repeat echocardiographic imaging should be performed once net pericardial fluid drainage decreases to <50 mL/24 hours to ensure that no residual pericardial effusion is present, with subsequent removal of the pericardial catheter.

Pericardial Window and Pericardiectomy

Surgical pericardial windows, performed via a subxiphoid or transpleural approach, may be considered as an alternative to pericardiocentesis, especially where the pericardial effusion is inaccessible via pericardiocentesis. Such windows typically involve excision of an approximately 2.5-cm square of pericardium. Subxiphoid pericardial windows are performed via a midline vertical incision over the xiphoid, incision of the linea alba and dissection to allow access to the retrosternal space and pericardium, without entry into the peritoneal cavity. Transpleural pericardial windows are typically performed using video-assisted thorascopic surgery and involve pericardial access via the pleural space to allow pericardial fluid evacuation and persistent drainage of pericardial fluid into the adjoining pleural space. Surgical pericardial windows create a larger postprocedural pericardial defect than pericardiocentesis, and hence are associated with lower 30-day reaccumulation rates.[38] Hence, surgical pericardial windows may be considered in patients where symptomatic pericardial effusions recur despite multiple prior pericardiocenteses.[23] Pericardial effusions can recur at medium and long-term follow up despite pericardial window creation, due either to healing or adhesion of the pericardial window margin to the underlying myocardium.[39,40] Transpleural pericardial window creation with insertion of the tip of a tunneled long-term pleural catheter system into the pericardial space may provide a durable therapeutic option in recurrent malignant pericardial effusions.[41]

Where definitive therapy for symptomatic recurrent pericardial effusions is desired, surgical complete pericardiectomy should be considered, especially in symptomatic patients with nonmalignant pericardial effusions.[23,42]

Pericardial Fluid Analysis

Clinical history and macroscopic pericardial fluid appearance should guide pericardial fluid analysis. Routine evaluation of pericardial fluid for cell counts, hemoglobin, aerobic and

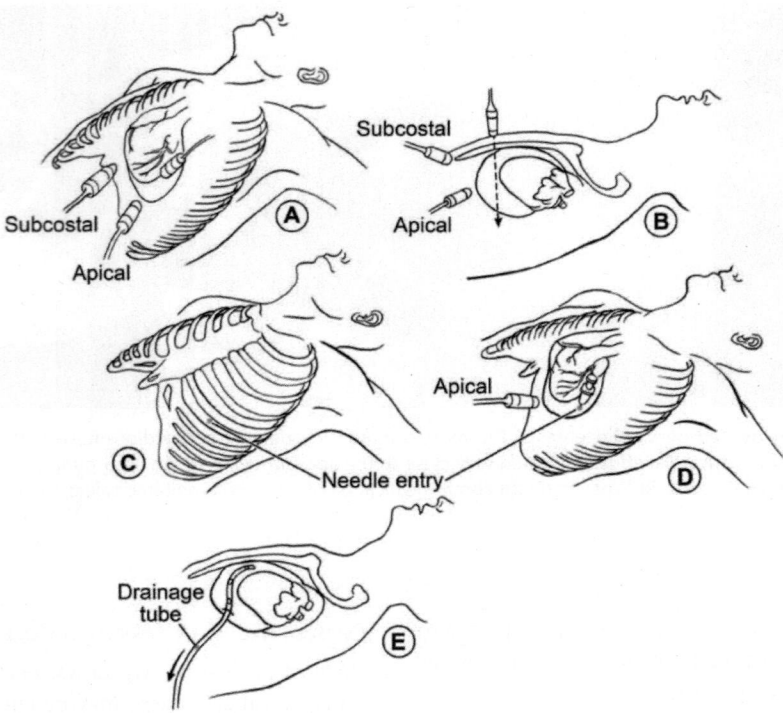

Figure 54–13. Echocardiographically guided pericardiocentesis.

Step 1. Locate an area on the chest or subcostal region from which the largest amount of pericardial effusion can be visualized, and mark it (**A–C**).

Step 2. Determine the depth of effusion from the marked position and the optimal angulation.

Step 3. After sterile preparation and local anesthesia, perform pericardiocentesis (**D**).

Step 4. To assess and confirm the location of the needle, inject agitated saline solution through the needle and image to visualize bubbles and confirm insertion into the pericardial space.

Step 5. Monitor the withdrawal of pericardial fluid with repeat echocardiography.

Step 6. Place a 6F or 7F pigtail catheter in the pericardial space to minimize reaccumulation of fluid (**E**).

Step 7. Drain any residual fluid or fluid that has reaccumulated via the pigtail catheter every 4 to 6 hours. If after 2 to 3 days, pericardial fluid has not reaccumulated, as seen echocardiographically, the pigtail catheter may be removed. Always have the pericardial fluid analyzed: cell counts, glucose and protein measurements, culture, and cytology.

Reproduced with permission from Callahan JA, Seward JB, Tajik AJ, et al. Pericardiocentesis assisted by two-dimensional echocardiography. *J Thorac Cardiovasc Surg.* 1983 Jun;85(6):877-879.

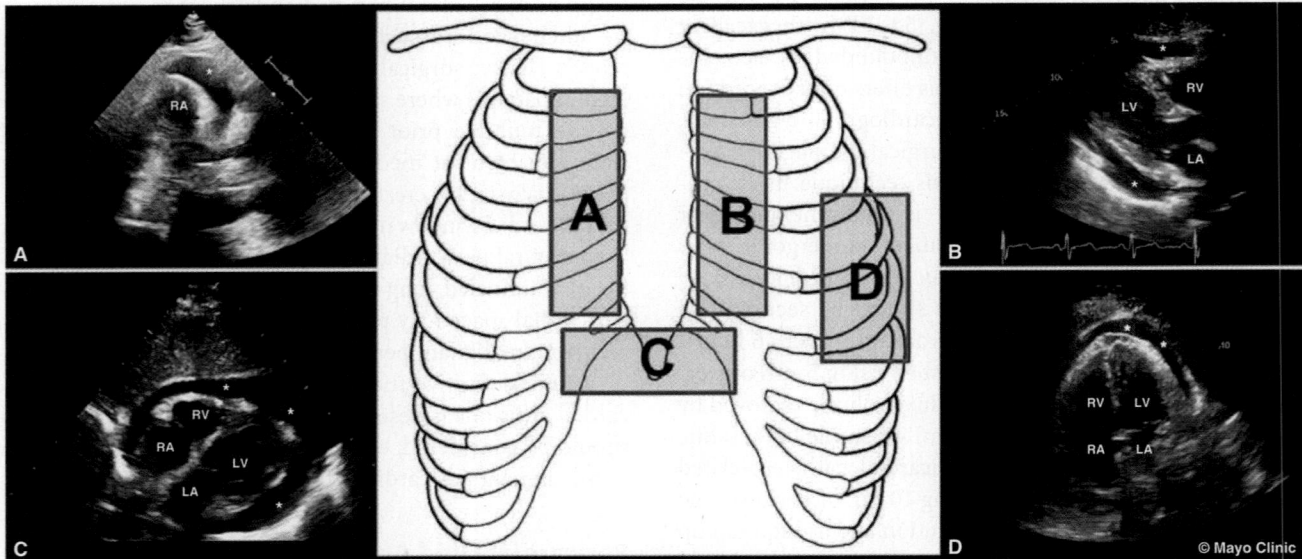

Figure 54–14. Echocardiographic-guided pericardiocentesis access sites. (**A**) Right parasternal window. (**B**) Left parasternal window. (**C**) Apical and para-apical window. (**D**) Subcostal window. LA, left atrium; LV, left ventricle; RA, right atrium; RV, right ventricle; asterisk, pericardial effusion. Reproduced with permission from Luis SA, Kane GC, Luis CR, et al. Overview of Optimal Techniques for Pericardiocentesis in Contemporary Practice. *Curr Cardiol Rep.* 2020 Jun 19;22(8):60.

anerobic cultures, and cytology may be considered, although detection of malignancy and infection is unlikely. Pericardial fluid electrolytes are not of clinical value. Unlike pleural effusions, Light's criteria cannot be used to distinguish transudative from exudative pericardial effusions.[43] Pericardial fluid lactate dehydrogenase (LDH), protein, albumin, and glucose are hence of limited value and should not be routinely assessed.[44,45] Straw-colored fluid is consistent with inflammatory pericarditis; while bloody fluid suggests trauma, postoperative states, and malignancy. However, sanguineous and serosanguineous effusions can be difficult to differentiate visually, and pericardial fluid hemoglobin or hematocrit levels approximately 50% of peripheral blood suggest cardiac chamber or great vessel rupture or perforation.[41] It should be noted that pericardial fluid cytology carries a low diagnostic yield,[46,47] even amongst those patients with known malignancy,[48] and so care must be taken to submit the entire volume of aspirated pericardial fluid in order to maximize diagnostic yield.[49] Pericardial fluid triglycerides should be evaluated if the fluid has a milky appearance, because such appearance would be consistent with a chylous pericardial effusion due to lymphatic injury (eg, thoracic duct injury). Uremic pericarditis is typically diagnosed clinically, but pericardial fluid urea and uric acid levels may be evaluated noting that normal mean values are reported to be at the upper limit of normal for serum.[44]

REFERENCES

1. Ishihara T, Ferrans VJ, Jones M, Boyce SW, Kawanami O, Roberts WC. Histologic and ultrastructural features of normal human parietal pericardium. *Am J Cardiol.* 1980;46:744-753.

2. Takada K, Otsuki Y, Magari S. Lymphatics and pre-lymphatics of the rabbit pericardium and epicardium with special emphasis on particulate absorption and milky spot-like structures. *Lymphology.* 1991;24:116-124.

3. Corey GR, Campbell PT, Van Trigt P, et al. Etiology of large pericardial effusions. *Am J Med.* 1993;95:209-213.

4. Levy PY, Corey R, Berger P, et al. Etiologic diagnosis of 204 pericardial effusions. *Medicine (Baltimore).* 2003;82:385-391.

5. Sagrista-Sauleda J, Merce J, Permanyer-Miralda G, Soler-Soler J. Clinical clues to the causes of large pericardial effusions. *Am J Med.* 2000;109:95-101.

6. Syed FF, Ntsekhe M, Mayosi BM. Tailoring diagnosis and management of pericardial disease to the epidemiological setting. *Mayo Clin Proc.* 2010;85:866; author reply 866.

7. Tsang TS, Enriquez-Sarano M, Freeman WK, et al. Consecutive 1127 therapeutic echocardiographically guided pericardiocenteses: clinical profile, practice patterns, and outcomes spanning 21 years. *Mayo Clin Proc.* 2002;77:429-436.

8. Hsu JC, Varosy PD, Bao H, Dewland TA, Curtis JP, Marcus GM. Cardiac perforation from implantable cardioverter-defibrillator lead placement: insights from the national cardiovascular data registry. *Circ Cardiovasc Qual Outcomes.* 2013;6:582-590.

9. Friedman DJ, Pokorney SD, Ghanem A, et al. Predictors of cardiac perforation with catheter ablation of atrial fibrillation. *JACC Clin Electrophysiol.* 2020;6:636-645.

10. Martin RP, Bowden R, Filly K, Popp RL. Intrapericardial abnormalities in patients with pericardial effusion. Findings by two-dimensional echocardiography. *Circulation.* 1980;61:568-572.

11. Klein AL, Abbara S, Agler DA, et al. American Society of Echocardiography clinical recommendations for multimodality cardiovascular imaging of patients with pericardial disease: endorsed by the Society for

12. Cardiovascular Magnetic Resonance and Society of Cardiovascular Computed Tomography. *J Am Soc Echocardiogr.* 2013;26:965-1012 e15.

12. Appleton CP, Hatle LK, Popp RL. Cardiac tamponade and pericardial effusion: respiratory variation in transvalvular flow velocities studied by Doppler echocardiography. *J Am Coll Cardiol.* 1988;11:1020-1030.

13. Levine MJ, Lorell BH, Diver DJ, Come PC. Implications of echocardiographically assisted diagnosis of pericardial tamponade in contemporary medical patients: detection before hemodynamic embarrassment. *J Am Coll Cardiol.* 1991;17:59-65.

14. Boltwood CM, Jr. Ventricular performance related to transmural filling pressure in clinical cardiac tamponade. *Circulation.* 1987;75:941-955.

15. Fowler NO, Shabetai R, Braunstein JR. Transmural ventricular pressures in experimental cardiac tamponade. *Circ Res.* 1959;7:733-739.

16. Gaffney FA, Keller AM, Peshock RM, Lin JC, Firth BG. Pathophysiologic mechanisms of cardiac tamponade and pulsus alternans shown by echocardiography. *Am J Cardiol.* 1984;53:1662-1666.

17. Burstow DJ, Oh JK, Bailey KR, Seward JB, Tajik AJ. Cardiac tamponade: characteristic Doppler observations. *Mayo Clin Proc.* 1989;64:312-324.

18. Settle HP, Adolph RJ, Fowler NO, Engel P, Agruss NS, Levenson NI. Echocardiographic study of cardiac tamponade. *Circulation.* 1977;56:951-959.

19. Reddy PS, Curtiss EI, O'Toole JD, Shaver JA. Cardiac tamponade: hemodynamic observations in man. *Circulation.* 1978;58:265-272.

20. Guberman BA, Fowler NO, Engel PJ, Gueron M, Allen JM. Cardiac tamponade in medical patients. *Circulation.* 1981;64:633-640.

21. Roy CL, Minor MA, Brookhart MA, Choudhry NK. Does this patient with a pericardial effusion have cardiac tamponade? *JAMA.* 2007;297:1810-1818.

22. Syed FF, Ntsekhe M, Mayosi BM, Oh JK. Effusive-constrictive pericarditis. *Heart Fail Rev.* 2013;18:277-287.

23. Adler Y, Charron P, Imazio M, et al. 2015 ESC Guidelines for the diagnosis and management of pericardial diseases: the Task Force for the Diagnosis and Management of Pericardial Diseases of the European Society of Cardiology (ESC). Endorsed by: The European Association for Cardio-Thoracic Surgery (EACTS). *Eur Heart J.* 2015;36:2921-2964.

24. Gillam LD, Guyer DE, Gibson TC, King ME, Marshall JE, Weyman AE. Hydrodynamic compression of the right atrium: a new echocardiographic sign of cardiac tamponade. *Circulation.* 1983;68:294-301.

25. Singh S, Wann LS, Schuchard GH, et al. Right ventricular and right atrial collapse in patients with cardiac tamponade—a combined echocardiographic and hemodynamic study. *Circulation.* 1984;70:966-971.

26. Singh S, Wann LS, Klopfenstein HS, Hartz A, Brooks HL. Usefulness of right ventricular diastolic collapse in diagnosing cardiac tamponade and comparison to pulsus paradoxus. *Am J Cardiol.* 1986;57:652-656.

27. Eisenberg MJ, Schiller NB. Bayes' theorem and the echocardiographic diagnosis of cardiac tamponade. *Am J Cardiol.* 1991;68:1242-1244.

28. Himelman RB, Kircher B, Rockey DC, Schiller NB. Inferior vena cava plethora with blunted respiratory response: a sensitive echocardiographic sign of cardiac tamponade. *J Am Coll Cardiol.* 1988;12:1470-1477.

29. Tsang TS, Oh JK, Seward JB. Diagnosis and management of cardiac tamponade in the era of echocardiography. *Clin Cardiol.* 1999;22:446-452.

30. Gonzalez MS, Basnight MA, Appleton CP. Experimental pericardial effusion: relation of abnormal respiratory variation in mitral flow velocity to hemodynamics and diastolic right heart collapse. *J Am Coll Cardiol.* 1991;17:239-248.

31. Holmes DR, Jr., Nishimura R, Fountain R, Turi ZG. Iatrogenic pericardial effusion and tamponade in the percutaneous intracardiac intervention era. *JACC Cardiovasc Interv.* 2009;2:705-717.

32. Ryu AJ, Kane GC, Pislaru SV, et al. Bleeding complications of ultrasound-guided pericardiocentesis in the presence of coagulopathy or thrombocytopenia. *J Am Soc Echocardiogr.* 2020;33:399-401.

33. Iliescu C, Khair T, Marmagkiolis K, Iliescu G, Durand JB. Echocardiography and fluoroscopy-guided pericardiocentesis for cancer patients with cardiac tamponade and thrombocytopenia. *J Am Coll Cardiol.* 2016;68:771-773.

34. Bishop LH, Jr., Estes EH, Jr., McIntosh HD. The electrocardiogram as a safeguard in pericardiocentesis. *J Am Med Assoc.* 1956;162:264-265.

35. Eichler K, Zangos S, Thalhammer A, et al. CT-guided pericardiocenteses: clinical profile, practice patterns and clinical outcome. *Eur J Radiol.* 2010;75:28-31.

36. Palmer SL, Kelly PD, Schenkel FA, Barr ML. CT-guided tube pericardiostomy: a safe and effective technique in the management of postsurgical pericardial effusion. *AJR Am J Roentgenol.* 2009;193:W314-320.

37. Rafique AM, Patel N, Biner S, et al. Frequency of recurrence of pericardial tamponade in patients with extended versus nonextended pericardial catheter drainage. *Am J Cardiol.* 2011;108:1820-1825.

38. Horr SE, Mentias A, Houghtaling PL, et al. Comparison of outcomes of pericardiocentesis versus surgical pericardial window in patients requiring drainage of pericardial effusions. *Am J Cardiol.* 2017;120:883-890.

39. Balla S, Zea-Vera R, Kaplan RA, Rosengart TK, Wall MJ, Jr., Ghanta RK. Mid-term efficacy of subxiphoid versus transpleural pericardial window for pericardial effusion. *J Surg Res.* 2020;252:9-15.

40. Lazaros G, Antonopoulos AS, Lazarou E, et al. Long-term outcome of pericardial drainage in cases of chronic, large, hemodynamically insignificant, c-reactive protein negative, idiopathic pericardial effusions. *Am J Cardiol.* 2020.

41. Luis SA, Kane GC, Luis CR, Oh JK, Sinak LJ. Overview of optimal techniques for pericardiocentesis in contemporary practice. *Curr Cardiol Rep.* 2020;22:60.

42. Sagrista-Sauleda J, Angel J, Permanyer-Miralda G, Soler-Soler J. Long-term follow-up of idiopathic chronic pericardial effusion. *N Engl J Med.* 1999;341:2054-2059.

43. Ben-Horin S, Bank I, Shinfeld A, Kachel E, Guetta V, Livneh A. Diagnostic value of the biochemical composition of pericardial effusions in patients undergoing pericardiocentesis. *Am J Cardiol.* 2007;99:1294-1297.

44. Xiang F, Guo X, Chen W, et al. Proteomics analysis of human pericardial fluid. *Proteomics.* 2013;13:2692-2695.

45. Hutchin P, Nino HV, Suberman R. Electrolyte and acid-base composition of pericardial fluid in man. *Arch Surg.* 1971;102:28-30.

46. Lane CE, Diaz Soto JC, Padang R, Luis SA. Contained right atrial rupture: an unusual presentation of a rare primary cardiac tumour. *Eur Heart J.* 2018;39:1574-1575.

47. Monte SA, Ehya H, Lang WR. Positive effusion cytology as the initial presentation of malignancy. *Acta Cytol.* 1987;31:448-52.

48. Lekhakul A, Assawakawintip C, Fenstad ER, et al. Safety and outcome of percutaneous drainage of pericardial effusions in patients with cancer. *Am J Cardiol.* 2018;122:1091-1094.

49. Rooper LM, Ali SZ, Olson MT. A minimum volume of more than 60 mL is necessary for adequate cytologic diagnosis of malignant pericardial effusions. *Am J Clin Pathol.* 2016;145:101-106.

55

Constrictive Pericarditis

William R. Miranda, Kevin L. Greason, John M. Stulak, and Jae K. Oh

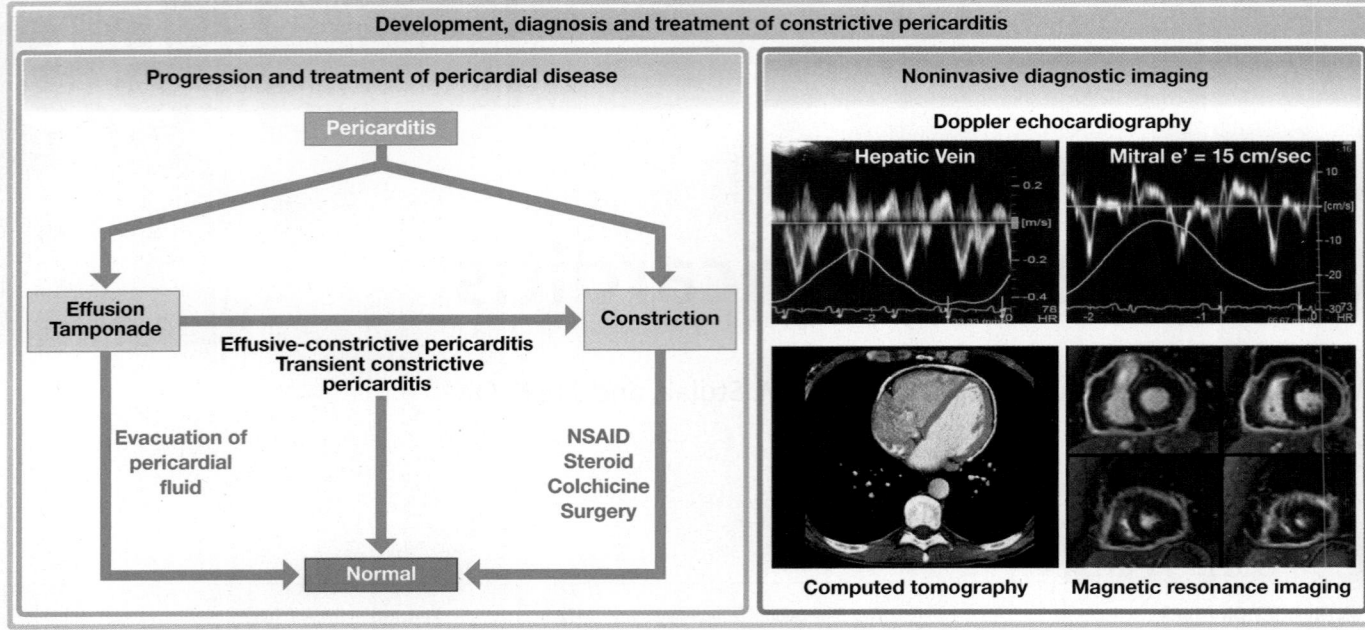

Chapter 55 Fuster and Hurst's Central Illustration. One stage of pericardial disease can transition into another stage. Patients with pericardial constriction have a very poor prognosis if left untreated, but appropriate treatment (shown in red) can potentially cure pericardial conditions. Traditionally, cardiac catheterization has been the gold standard for diagnosing constrictive pericarditis, but advances in cardiac imaging have enabled noninvasive diagnostic hemodynamic assessment by echocardiography, delineation of pericardial and cardiac anatomy by computed tomography, and detection of pericardial inflammation by cardiac magnetic resonance imaging. Transthoracic echocardiography is now the main diagnostic tool in the evaluation of constrictive pericarditis. NSAID, nonsteroidal anti-inflammatory drug.

CHAPTER SUMMARY

This chapter discusses the etiology, presentation, diagnosis and treatment of constrictive pericarditis, a potentially curable form of diastolic heart failure due to inflamed, scarred, or even calcified pericardium limiting diastolic filling of the heart. Effusive or chronic constrictive pericarditis can result from progression of acute pericarditis with pericardial inflammation or pericardial effusion (see Fuster and Hurst's Central Illustration). Traditionally, cardiac catheterization has been the gold standard for diagnosing constrictive pericarditis, but advances in cardiac imaging have allowed diagnostic hemodynamic assessment by echocardiography, delineation of pericardial and cardiac anatomy by computed tomography, and detection of pericardial inflammation by cardiac magnetic resonance imaging. A subset of the patients with constrictive pericarditis predominantly due to pericardial inflammation, as seen in effusive or transient constrictive pericarditis, can be managed medically. Cardiac imaging can identify this subset of the patients. However, therapeutic pericardiectomy is the recommended treatment for symptomatic patients with constrictive pericarditis. Surgical pericardiectomy can cure chronic constrictive pericarditis unless it is mixed with myocardial diseases from radiation, ischemia, or fibrosis. Constriction can recur if pericardiectomy is incomplete.

INTRODUCTION

Constrictive pericarditis (CP) occurs in the setting of inflammation and/or scarring of the pericardium, resulting in impaired cardiac filling.[1] Therefore, CP is a form of diastolic heart failure. The importance of its recognition lies in the fact that pericardial constriction is a potentially curable disease and it is still underdiagnosed, carrying a very poor prognosis if left untreated.[2]

PATHOPHYSIOLOGY AND CLINICAL PRESENTATION

CP develops after an injury to the pericardium triggers ongoing pericardial inflammation and ultimately fibrosis. This process might be acute (over the course of days), subacute, or chronic; in acute cases, inflammation prevails whereas fibrosis tends to be predominant in chronic forms of the disease. Pericardial inflammation may resolve spontaneously or with anti-inflammatory therapy, but the pericardium typically becomes fibrotic or scarred if the inflammatory process is not resolved within 3 months. The reason for which some patients will evolve into CP after an acute event is unclear; however, certain etiologies (for example, tuberculous pericarditis) are associated with higher risk of developing CP.[3,4] The disease also appears to favor men (2:1 ratio).[1] Although, CP is primarily a pericardial disease, subepicardial myocardial atrophy might be present[5] (particularly in long-standing cases), leading to concomitant myocardial systolic and diastolic dysfunction. A mixed pattern with coexistent myocardial disease is also the norm in patients who develop constriction after cardiac surgery or in those with a history of mediastinal irradiation therapy.

Given the abnormal pericardial compliance, diastolic filling is significantly impaired in patients with CP (ie, steeper increase in pressure per change in volume in the pressure–volume curve). As a consequence, cardiac filling pressures increase and cardiac output falls as stroke volume decreases. The thickened pericardium has limited expansion and the cardiac chambers "compete" for pericardial space during diastolic filling. With respiration, an increase in preload in one ventricle occurs at the expense of filling in the other (*ventricular interdependence*). In addition, the abnormal pericardium insulates the heart from respirophasic changes in intrathoracic pressures and, therefore, negative intrathoracic pressures generated by inspiration are not transmitted to cardiac chambers. This phenomenon—the so-called *dissociation of intrathoracic and intracardiac pressures*—contributes to decreased filling of the left atrium and ventricle upon inspiration (due to decreased pressure gradient between pulmonary veins and the left atrium as the pulmonary veins are located outside the pericardium). These two physiologic/hemodynamics characteristics constitute the hallmarks of CP and are the basis of most noninvasive and cardiac catheterization criteria for the diagnosis of CP.

Patients with CP typically show features of right-sided heart failure, presenting with elevated venous pressure, ascites, and leg edema. Exertional dyspnea is a common complaint, particularly in those with concomitant myocardial disease. It should be highlighted that pericardial constriction must always be considered when right heart failure is disproportional to degree of pulmonary congestion or in patients presenting with heart failure following cardiac surgery. For unknown reasons, patients with CP are more prone to the development of ascites than are patients with other forms of right heart failure, with ascites often being more striking than the degree of lower extremity edema. Additional common complaints are fatigue, decreased functional capacity, and head fullness. Orthopnea and paroxysmal nocturnal dyspnea are rare and suggest another etiology. In more advanced stages, liver and renal dysfunction might be present.

ETIOLOGIES

Causes of CP are illustrated in **Table 55–1**. The epidemiology of the disease has substantially changed over the last 50 to 60 years, paralleling the advances and wide use of cardiac surgery. Data from the Mayo Clinic showed that 72% of cases of CP seen between 1936 and 1982 were idiopathic, whereas only 2% involved patients with prior cardiac surgery.[6] Between 1985 and 2006, postoperative cases accounted for 29% while the prevalence of idiopathic cases decreased to 22%.[7] This shift in epidemiology has also been shown by others in the United States and in European centers.[8-10] CP occurs in 0.2% to 0.4% of patients undergoing cardiac surgery and on average occurs 2 years after the surgical procedure.[11,12] Although data on the incidence of CP following an episode of idiopathic and postviral pericarditis are still limited, this has been reported in less than 1% of cases.[3]

In areas where tuberculosis is still prevalent (such as in some parts of Africa and Asia), tuberculous pericarditis continues to be most common cause of pericardial constriction.[13,14] Thus, a thorough travel and social history should be obtained in the evaluation of patients with CP. A history of radiation therapy is also of great importance, given the risk of concomitant myocardial and valvular disease, which has diagnostic and therapeutic implications.

PHYSICAL EXAMINATION

General examination will typically reveal muscle wasting, increased abnormal girth, and leg edema, with patients generally appearing chronically ill. In patients with a subacute

TABLE 55–1. Etiologies of Constrictive Pericarditis

Idiopathic
Postcardiac surgery
Connective tissue disorders
Radiation-induced
Tuberculous
Neoplastic
Purulent
Uremia
Other (rare)
Trauma, sarcoid, parasites, drugs-induced (procainamide, methylsergide), asbestos

course, these findings can be absent and the complaints will appear out of proportion to the patient's "healthy" appearance. Abdominal exam will show signs of liver enlargement and often ascites; signs of cirrhosis should be noted since the presence of liver failure has implications regarding surgical risk. Pleural effusions are not infrequently present but rales should not be expected.

Detailed assessment of jugular venous pressure is mandatory in the evaluation of CP. Elevated central venous pressure is essentially always present, unless the patient has been aggressively diuresed; in contrast, a normal venous pressure in an individual off diuretic therapy strongly argues against clinically significant pericardial constriction. If the venous pulse cannot be seen with the patient sitting, they should be asked to stand; failure to do this will preclude proper analysis of venous pressure and contour in patients with very elevated filling pressures. The *Kussmaul sign* corresponds to an increase in venous pressure associated with inspiration; this, however, is not pathognomonic of constriction and can be seen in other situations where severe elevation in right atrial pressure is present. Jugular venous waveforms will show prominent *y* descents or sometimes prominent *x* and *y* descents (if sinus rhythm is present and there is absence of significant concomitant myocardial disease)—the *W* or *M* pattern. It should be noted that if CP is present, the predominant waves are the descents (down strokes), which is the opposite of normal. In severe tricuspid regurgitation, although a deep *y* descent will be present, the predominant wave is a positive one, the large *v* wave. Restrictive cardiomyopathy can be associated with deep *y* descents and the distinction between restriction and constriction at the bedside can be extremely challenging.

Auscultation might reveal the presence of a low-pitched third heart sound, sometimes only heard during inspiration or expiration. The presence of a high-pitched early diastolic sound (slightly earlier than a typical third heart sound)—the *pericardial knock*—is very specific, but not a sensitive sign of CP. A loud pulmonary component of the second heart sound would be an unusual finding and should suggest the presence of a concomitant myocardial process (resulting in significant elevation in pulmonary pressures).

EVALUATION AND TESTING

Electrocardiogram, Chest Radiography, and Laboratory Testing

Electrocardiography usually shows nonspecific ST-T wave abnormalities; atrial fibrillation occurs commonly in patients with CP. *P mitrales* (broad, notched P waves in lead II) in the absence of mitral disease has also been described as a sign of CP.[15] Chest radiography may reveal pericardial calcification (**Fig. 55-1**), although this is not a sensitive nor specific sign and it is seen in only 25% to 30% of cases.[16] Pleural effusions are frequently present. Plasma brain natriuretic peptide levels appear to be lower in patients with CP compared to patients with myocardial restrictive disease,[17] particularly among patients with idiopathic CP.

Echocardiography

Transthoracic echocardiography is now the main diagnostic tool in the evaluation of CP. In addition, it allows for the diagnosis of other pathologies that might mimic CP clinically. Guidelines recommend transthoracic echocardiography to be performed in all patients with suspected CP (class of recommendation [COR] I, level of evidence [LOE] C).[18] In our practice, transthoracic echocardiography will suffice for the diagnosis of CP in 75% of cases,[7] foregoing the need for invasive hemodynamic assesment. The echocardiographic evaluation of constrictive physiology should include thorough two-dimensional (ventricular septal motion, inferior vena cava size/collapsibility) and Doppler (mitral inflow, mitral annulus tissue Doppler and hepatic vein) assessments. Speckle tracking echocardiography has also been suggested to have incremental diagnostic value, particularly in discriminating CP from restrictive cardiomyopathy.[19,20]

Two-Dimensional Echocardiography

The evaluation of ventricular septal motion in patients with suspected CP is a pivotal component of the echocardiography evaluation. Two distinct septal motion abnormalities can be present: The septal "bounce" or "shudder" occurs in early diastole and reflects instantaneous differences in right and left

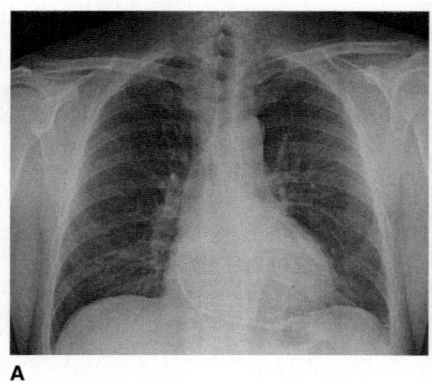
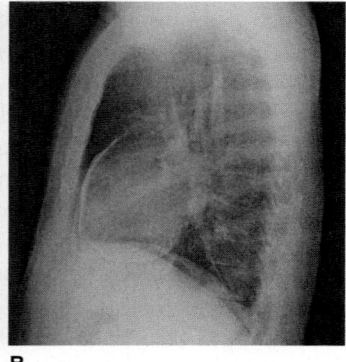

A   **B**

Figure 55-1. **Chest radiograph demonstrating pericardial calcification. (A)** Posteroanterior and **(B)** lateral chest radiography in patient with calcific constrictive pericarditis.

ventricular pressures during early diastolic filling,[21] resulting in a brief oscillation of the ventricular septum. It is a sensitive but less specific finding since it might be hard to differentiate this "shudder" from septal motion abnormalities seen in patients with prior cardiac surgery or due to conduction disease. A more specific feature of constrictive physiology is the presence of the respirophasic septal shift. With this phenomenon, the ventricular septum moves toward the left ventricle during inspiration as systemic venous return increases. During expiration, the opposite occurs, with the ventricular septum bulging toward the right. This respiratory variation in septal position is the echocardiographic marker of ventricular interdependence as it reflects the reciprocal respiratory changes in right and left ventricular preload in the setting of a noncompliant pericardium. Due to its better special resolution, this respirophasic shift is better appreciated on M-mode echocardiography; in addition, if CP is suspected 10-beats clips should be acquired in order to avoid underappreciation of this finding.

Since increased right-sided filling pressure should be universal in individuals of CP, the assessment of the inferior cava size and inspiratory collapsibility also provide important diagnostic information. Although the presence of dilated or poorly collapsible inferior vena cava does not aid in the differentiation from other causes of right-sided heart failure (such as tricuspid regurgitation or myocardial disease), the identification of a normal-sized inferior vena cava or >50% inspiratory caval collapse was present in <5% of patients in our series,[22] thus strongly arguing against constrictive physiology.

Echo-Doppler

Assessment of mitral annular tissue Doppler velocities is now one of the pillars of the echocardiographic diagnosis of CP. As highlighted in the guidelines for the assessment of diastolic function,[23] the early diastolic mitral annular (e') velocity is a marker of left ventricular relaxation, and therefore, reflective of underlying myocardial disease. Accordingly, reduced mitral e' velocities are to be expected in those with heart failure secondary to myocardial pathology. In contrast, in CP, as the lateral mitral annulus is tethered to adjacent pericardium, medial mitral e' velocities are augmented. Thus, most patients with CP will demonstrate medial mitral e' velocities ≥9 cm/s; the presence of increased mitral e' velocities in patients with overt heart failure should be one of the first clues that CP is present. It should be noted that, as it parallels the degree of concomitant myocardial disease, individuals with CP following cardiac surgery therapy will have lower medial e' velocities than those with idiopathic CP (11.1 ± 3.5 cm/s vs 14.5 ± 3.7 cm/s in our series). Those patients with radiation-induced CP have the lowest values (9.5 ± 3.7 cm/s) of all. Moreover, increased medial e' velocities not only provide diagnostic information in CP but were found to be independent predictors of more favorable outcomes postpericardiectomy.[24] Lastly, due to myocardial tethering, mitral annular lateral e' velocity might be lower than its medial counterpart—the so-called annulus reversus (**Fig. 55-2**).

Reflecting the increased left atrial pressures, mitral inflow Doppler profile will show grade II or grade III patterns; accordingly, a mitral E/A ratio <0.8 would be exceptional in CP.[25]

Similar to ventricular septal position, inspiratory changes in left ventricular preload can be appreciated on mitral inflow pulse-wave Doppler (**Fig. 55-3**). Although a >25% decrease in mitral early diastolic (E) velocity has been classically suggested as the cutoff for diagnosis of CP, this degree of variation is insensitive because most patients with CP show lesser degrees of mitral inflow variation.

Interrogation of the hepatic veins by pulse-wave Doppler is a mandatory step in the echo-Doppler evaluation of pericardial disorders. Patients with CP will show increased expiratory diastolic flow reversals, with this being the most specific criteria for the presence of CP.[22,25] As subsequently outlined, hepatic vein Doppler also aids in the differentiation of CP and other pathologies that also manifest themselves as right-sided failure.

Mimickers of CP

Severe tricuspid regurgitation and restrictive cardiomyopathy have been the classic mimickers of CP. Given the advances in echocardiography, the distinction between the two diseases and CP can now be made without difficulties in the vast majority cases. Echo-Doppler features of restrictive cardiomyopathy include severe biatrial enlargement, normal-sized ventricles, and restrictive mitral inflow pattern with significantly reduced mitral e' velocities (consistent with markedly abnormal ventricular relaxation/underlying myocardial disease). Those with severe tricuspid regurgitation show significant right ventricular enlargement, right atrial enlargement, and malcoaption of tricuspid leaflets with tricuspid insufficiency being easily apparent on color-flow Doppler. It is important to note, however, the at least moderate tricuspid regurgitation coexists in approximately 20% of patients with CP undergoing pericardiectomy[26,27] and is associated with worse outcomes in this population.[28]

Hepatic vein Doppler also provides important diagnostic information in these two entities. In contrast to the expiratory flow reversals seen in CP, individuals with restrictive cardiomyopathy will show increased inspiratory hepatic flow reversals[29] due to inability of the noncompliant right ventricle to accommodate the augmentation in venous return. In severe tricuspid regurgitation, systolic flow reversals (commonly holosystolic in the most severe cases) will be seen on hepatic vein Doppler, analogous to the large v-waves seen in the jugular venous pulsations.

Diagnostic Algorithm for the Diagnosis of CP on Echocardiography

Given the multitude of echocardiographic findings described in CP[15,68,83] our group proposed the use of three echocardiographic criteria to simplify its diagnosis (Mayo Clinic Echocardiographic Diagnostic Criteria[22]; Fig. 55-3): diastolic respirophasic shift of the ventricular septum, medial mitral annulus e' ≥9 cm/s, and diastolic expiratory hepatic vein flow ratio >0.8, as well as plethoric inferior vena cava and restrictive mitral inflow velocities. If septal shift is present in conjunction with one of the other two criteria, sensitivity and specificity approach 90%. If all three are present, specificity increased to 97% but sensitivity decreased to 67%. A proposed algorithm of the echocardiographic diagnosis of CP is illustrated in **Fig. 55-4**.

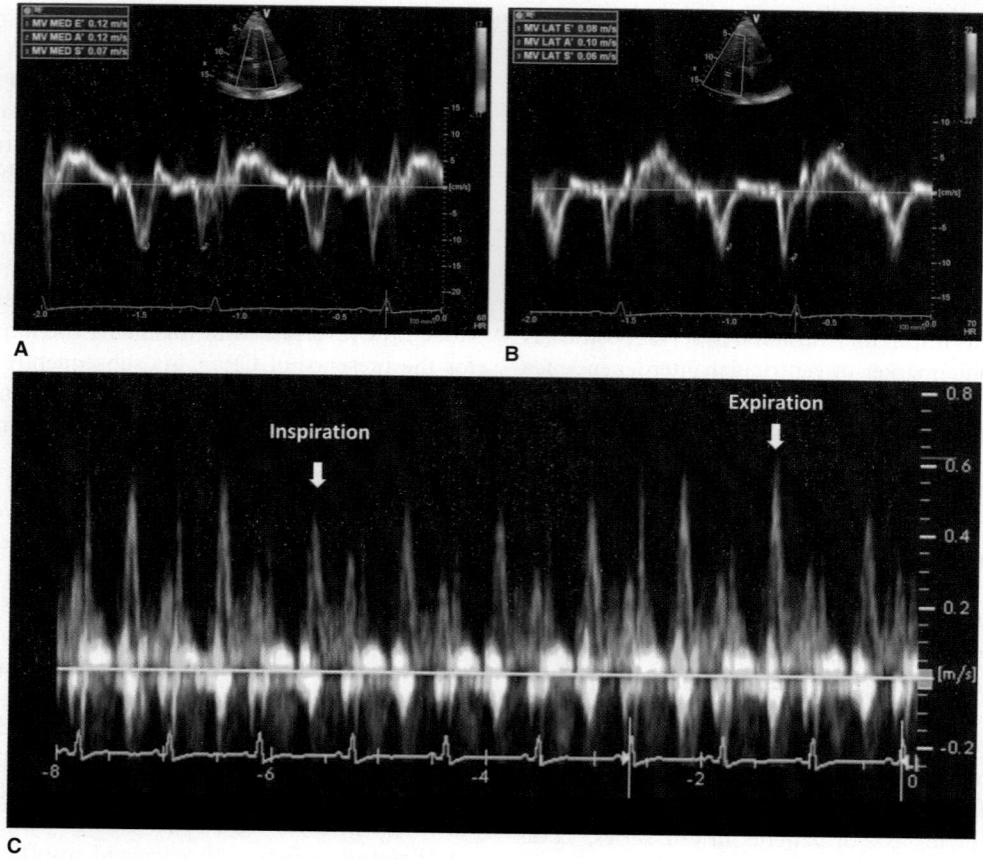

Figure 55–2. Echo-Doppler findings in a patient with constrictive pericarditis. Tissue Doppler shows (**A**) medial e′ greater than (**B**) lateral e′ velocities—the so-called annulus reversus. (**C**) Mitral inflow pulse-wave Doppler revealed marked respirophasic changes in E velocity; note reduction in mitral E velocity during inspiration.

Cardiac Catheterization

Classic cardiac catheterization findings[30,31] (**Fig. 55–5**) of CP include elevation of biventricular filling pressures with equalization of end diastolic pressures (within 5 mm Hg), presence of rapid ventricular filling waves (≥5 mm Hg; so-called square root sign), right ventricular systolic pressures <55 mm Hg with right ventricular end-diastolic pressures greater than a third of right ventricular systolic pressures, and right atrial pressures showing prominent x and y descents with no drop in mean right atrial pressure with inspiration (Kussmaul sign). However, there is a large overlap of these hemodynamic criteria between constriction and restrictive myocardial diseases. A normal cardiac output argues against the presence of clinically significant CP.

More specific, two "dynamic criteria" have been introduced to the diagnostic armamentarium. With inspiration, there is a significant decrease in the gradient between the pulmonary artery wedge pressure and left ventricular diastolic pressures, owing to dissociation of intrathoracic and intracardiac pressures. In addition, discordance between right and left ventricular tracings during inspiration marks the presence of ventricular interdependence. This finding is of great diagnostic importance given its sensitivity and specificity for diagnosis of CP,[32,33] especially when differentiating it from restrictive cardiomyopathy (when ventricular concordance will be seen). If atrial fibrillation is present, temporary pacing might be necessary during the catheterization procedure in order to appreciate respirophasic changes. Since most of the invasive features of CP are load dependent and might not be present if filling pressures are normal or only mildly elevated, fluid challenge (rapid infusion of 1 liter of fluid) should be considered in patients with right atrial pressures <15 mm Hg.

Noteworthy, concomitant pulmonary hypertension (at least mild to moderate) during cardiac catheterization is traditionally felt to argue against the diagnosis of CP. Although this is still true for most cases of idiopathic constriction, more significant elevations in pulmonary pressures were prevalent in a current cohort of patients with surgically proven CP undergoing cardiac catheterization at our institution. In this population, combined pre- and postcapillary pulmonary hypertension occurred in approximately 12% of patients and was an independent predictor of survival postpericardiectomy.[34]

Cross-Sectional Imaging

Additional imaging with cardiac computed tomography or magnetic resonance imaging might be performed to assess pericardial thickness (**Fig. 55–6**) because pericardial thickening is present in 80% of patients with surgically proven CP.[35]

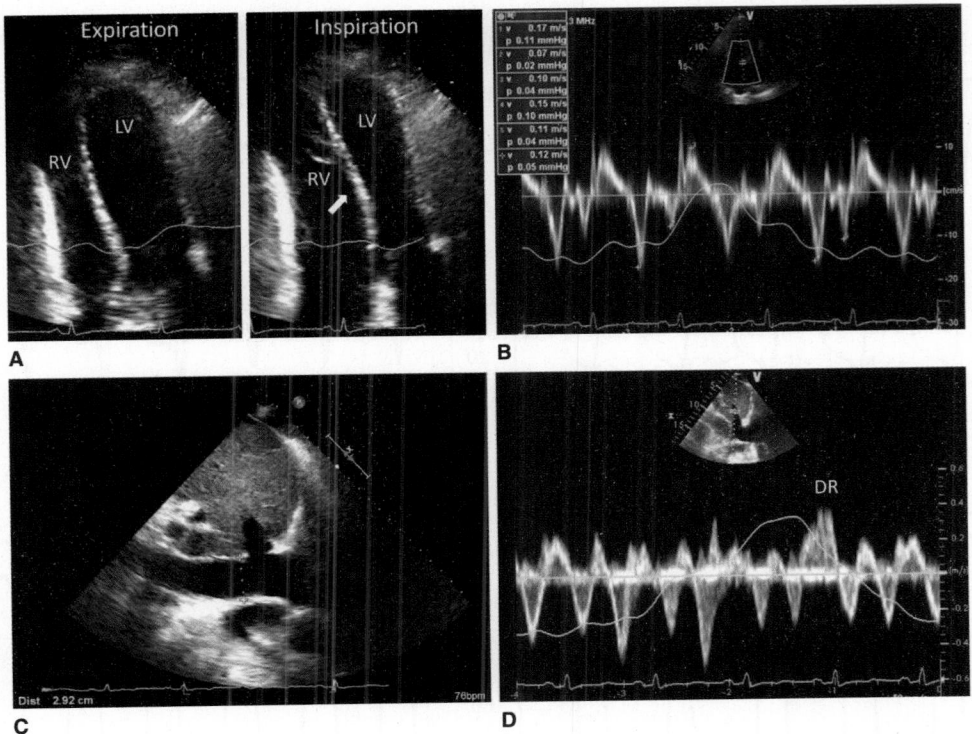

Figure 55–3. Two-dimensional and Doppler echocardiographic findings illustrating the Mayo Clinic constrictive pericarditis criteria:

1. respirophasic interventricular septal shift (*arrow*) (**A**)
2. medial e' velocity ≥9 cm/s on tissue Doppler (**B**)
3. dilated inferior vena cava (**C**)
4. hepatic vein expiratory end-diastolic reversal (DR)/forward flow ≥0.8 (**D**)

(LV, left ventricle; RV, right ventricle)

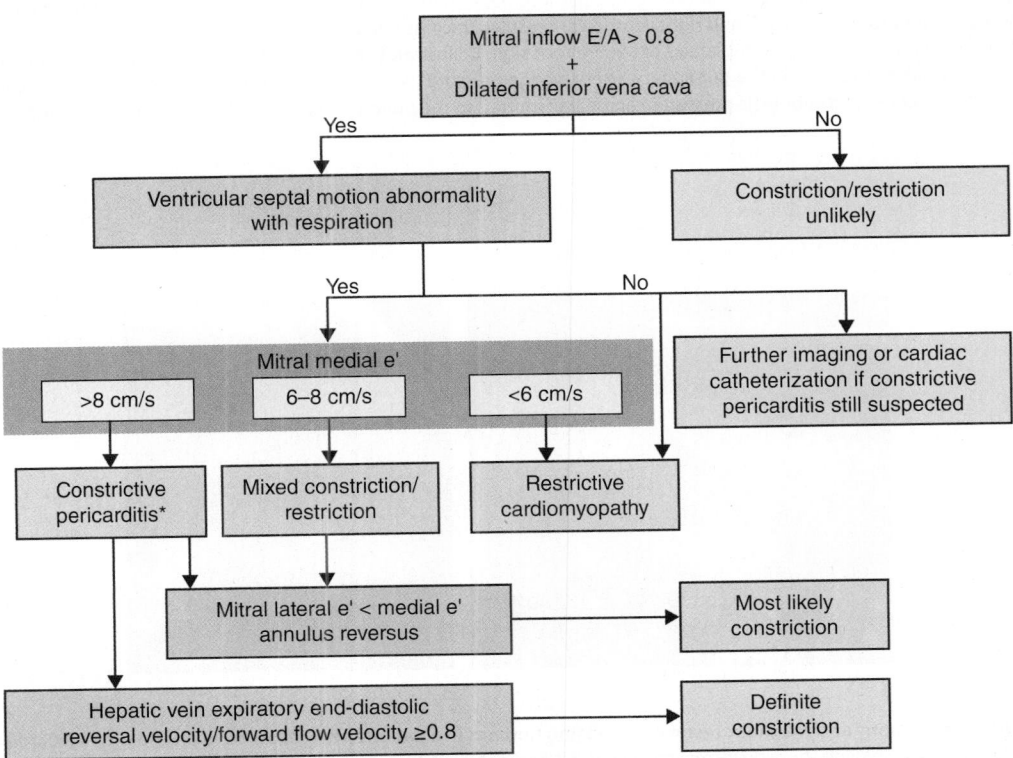

Figure 55–4. Algorithm for the evaluation of patients with constrictive pericarditis based on echocardiographic findings.

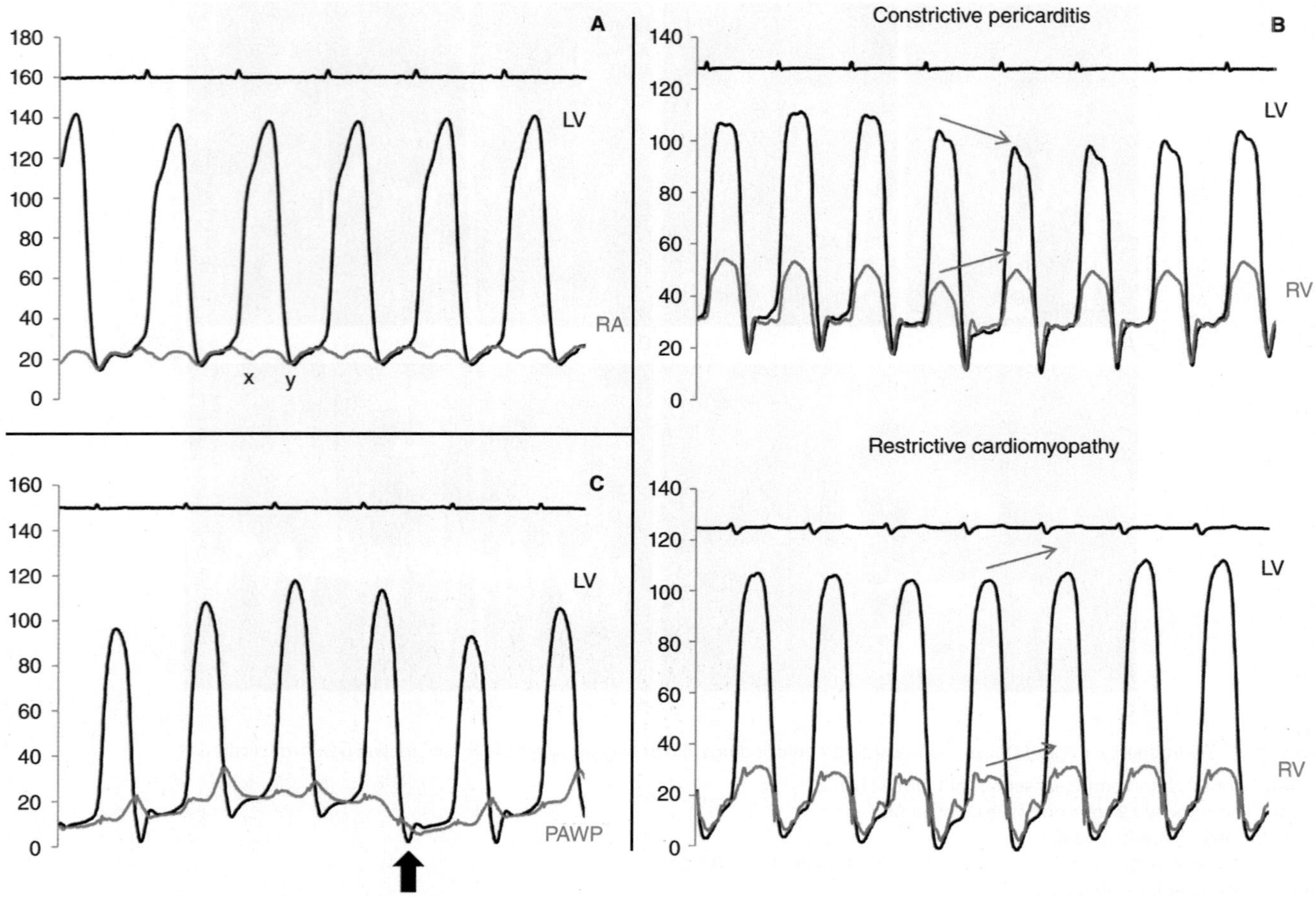

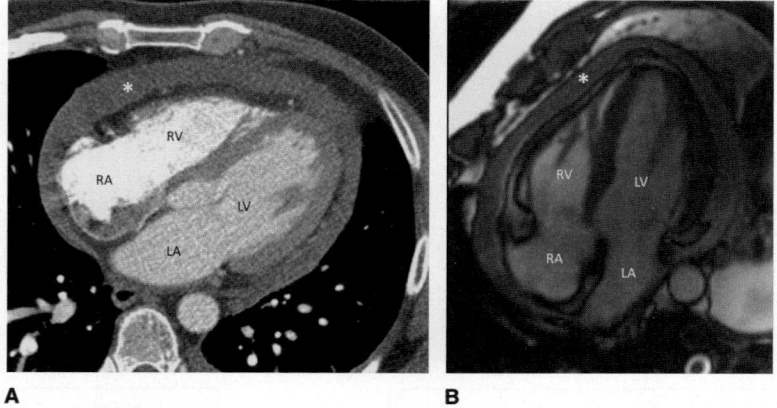

Figure 55–5. Cardiac catheterization findings in constrictive pericarditis. (A) Right atrial (RA, *red*) pressure tracings show prominent *x* and *y* descents; elevation in filling pressures is also present; **B** shows discordance (*converging blue arrows*) between left ventricular (LV, *black*) and right ventricular (RV, *red*) pressure tracings upon inspiration, representing enhanced ventricular interdependence; this finding is compared to findings in a patient with restrictive cardiomyopathy, where concordance between left and right ventricular pressure tracings (*parallel blue arrows*) is present (lower panel). Please note the rapid filling waves in both ventricular tracings—dip-and-plateau or square root sign. **C** illustrates the dissociation of intrathoracic and intracardiac pressures; on inspiration (*arrow*), there is marked decrease in the pulmonary artery wedge pressure (PAWP) to left ventricular diastolic pressure gradient. Due to scarred pericardium, respirophasic changes in intrathoracic pressures can be transmitted to the pulmonary veins (PAWP) but not to the cardiac chambers.

Figure 55–6. Computed tomography and magnetic resonance imaging findings in a patient with constrictive physiology. (A) Cardiac computed tomography and **(B)** magnetic resonance imaging showing increased pericardial thickness with the pericardial space being occupied by semisolid material (*asterisk*); (LA, left atrium; LV, left ventricle; RA, right atrium; RV, right ventricle).

Normal pericardial thickness on cross-sectional imaging (≤2 mm[36]) makes the diagnosis of CP less likely but does not rule it out (particularly in those with a history of prior cardiac surgery where normal pericardial thickness tends to more prevalent). In contrast, a pericardial thickness >4 mm has been associated with a >90% diagnostic accuracy when differentiating constriction from restrictive cardiomyopathy.[37]

Other diagnostic findings of CP on computed tomography include calcification of the pericardium, distortion of the cardiac chambers, and abnormal septal motion on gated cine studies. Computed tomography can also provide valuable preoperative information, such as assessment of the coronaries arteries (thus, potentially avoiding coronary angiography in younger individuals or those with at lower risk for atherosclerosis), outlining residual pericardial tissue in those with prior pericardiectomy, and delineating the thoracic anatomy prior to chest reentry in those with previous cardiac operations.

Currently, cardiac magnetic resonance imaging is a widely used tool in the evaluation of pericardial disorders.[38,39] Similar to computed tomography, cardiac magnetic resonance allows for the identification of pericardial thickening and the presence of ventricular interdependence (based on septal motion on free breathing series). However, cardiac magnetic resonance imaging has the advantage of offering incremental information regarding associated pericardial inflammation according to the presence of pericardial gadolinium enhancement and pericardial edema, which has important therapeutic implications for patients with CP.

Diagnostic Algorithm

The evaluation of patients with CP can be rather complex, in particular in patients with previous cardiac surgery, severe concomitant myocardial/valvular disease, or radiation heart disease. The work-up should be individualized and the threshold to intervene (most times with therapeutic pericardiectomy) will depend on concordant/discordant test results. If the history, physical exam, and echocardiogram findings are typical for the disease, no additional testing will typically be required. This, however, requires familiarity with bedside and echocardiographic assessment of CP. If necessary, additional imaging (computed tomography and magnetic resonance) and/or cardiac catheterization are the next steps (COR I, LOE C). In our practice, cardiac catheterization is only performed in one-third of the patients undergoing pericardiectomy, generally for more complex cases. If the diagnosis is still unclear despite extensive evaluation, exploratory surgery and surgical inspection of the pericardium ("gold standard" in the hands of an experienced surgeon) can be performed; the need for diagnostic thoracotomy current practice is very rare nowadays.

TREATMENT

Although patients presenting with CP and evidence of active pericardial inflammation (either by cardiac magnetic resonance or elevated inflammatory markers) might respond to anti-inflammatory therapy (COR IIb, LOE C),[18] therapeutic pericardiectomy is the recommended treatment for symptomatic patients with CP (COR I, LOE C).[18]

Pericardiectomy

Pericardiectomy is the surgical removal of the pericardium, and the procedure is applicable to all variants of pericardial disease.[10,40–47] Successful operation is predecated on two fundamental caveats: obtain adequate operative exposure and remove the appropriate amount of pericardium. Although median sternotomy and thoractomy both allow for safe removal of the pericardium, thoracotomy exposure may require extension across the midline into the right chest to allow for resection of all right-sided pericardium (**Fig. 55–7**).[40,42,48] The Mayo Clinic Rochester experience includes 513 patients operated with isolated pericardiectomy from 1993 through 2013. During that time period, the majority (n = 412; 80%) of operations were performed through a median sternotomy.[49]

From a surgical perspective, pericardiectomy can be classified as either radical or complete (also referred to as total). The nomenclature is controversial and can be confusing.[48] It is probably best to frame the discussion about amount of pericardial resection in the context of the underlying disease process. For example, effusive and replapsing pericariditis represent inflammatory pathologies that can involve the entire pericardium.[42] Therefore when operation is undertaken, total or complete pericardiectomy is indicated.[40] CP, on the other hand, is a disease of the ventricles.[1,40] Operation in that setting mandates resection of the pericardium overling the the venticles (ie, radical pericardiectomy).[40]

The key procedure-related elements of pericardiectomy are to remove the pericardium and to preserve phrenic nerve function. From the median sternotomy approach, the pericardial resection typically begins up near the great vessels, where the pericardium is usually less inflamed and less scarred to the underlying cardiac structures (Fig. 55–7). The "anterior" pericardium is resected from the great vessels, to the diaphragm, and from the left phrenic nerve to the atrioventricular groove (at a minimum for constriction) or right phrenic nerve (for inflammatory etiologies), as needed or allowed (Fig. 55–7). To prevent injury to the phrenic nerves, a 1- to 2-cm pedicled strip of pericardium should be left undisturbed along the course of the nerves.

Resection of the anterior pericardium is also referred to as a "phrenic-to-phrenic" pericardiectomy. Specific attention is brought to this nomenclature to make the point that such limited resection (Fig. 55–7) is inadequate surgical therapy for essentially all pericardial disease processes; furthermore, it puts the patient at risk of treatment failure and disease recurerrence.[40,48,50] As such, it is imperative that the pericardium be removed off the diaphragm and posterior to the left phrenic nerve (Fig. 55–7). Exposure to facilitate removal of that pericardium may require cardiopulmonary bypass support and sometimes even aortic occlusion (ie, aortic cross-clamp).[10,47,50] In the Mayo Clinic Rochester exerience, 207 patients (40%) received cardiopulmonary bypass support during pericardiectomy, but only 4 patients (0.8%) received aortic occlusion.[49]

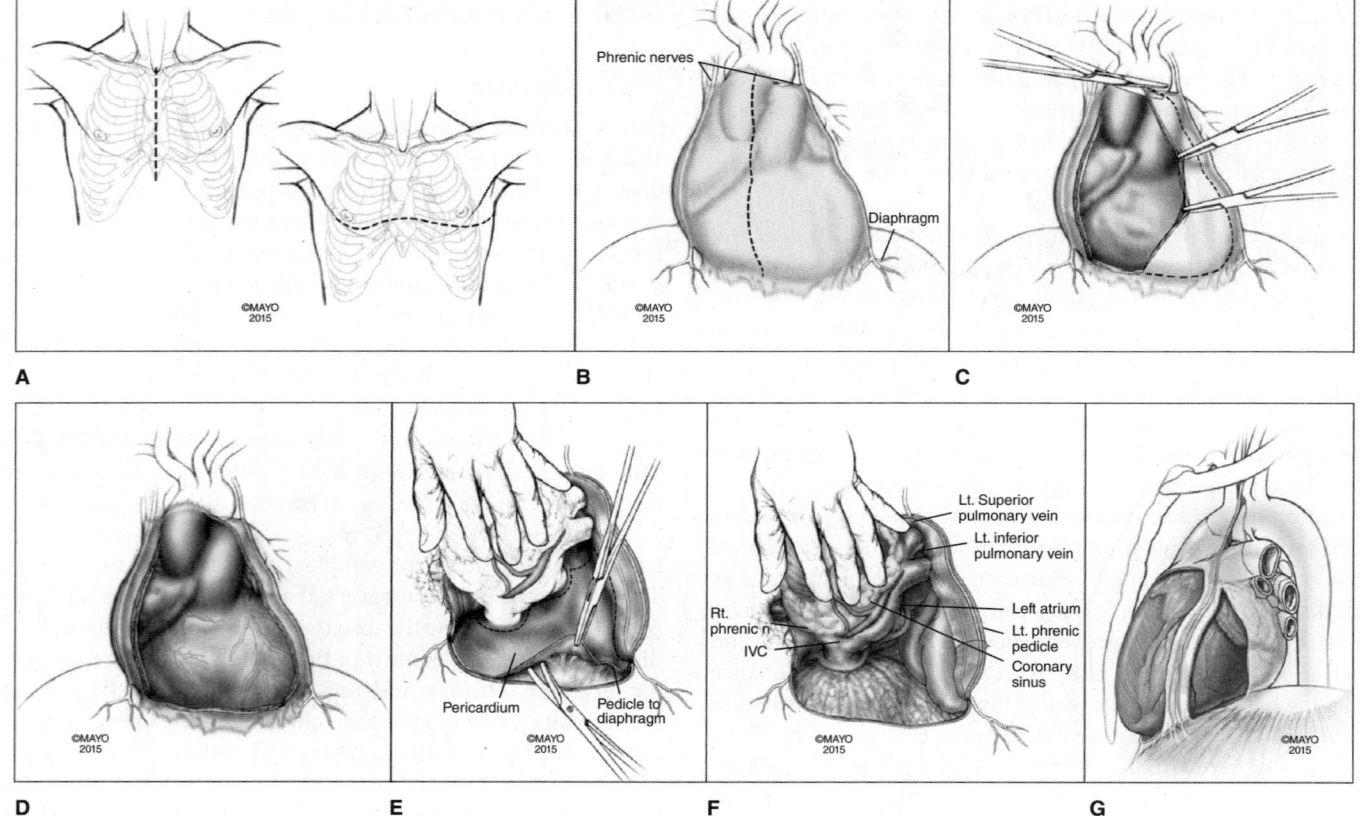

Figure 55–7. **Schematic of surgical pericardiectomy.** (A) Surgical approaches to pericardiectomy; (B) exposure of anterior pericardium; (C) resection of anterior pericardium; (D) completed anterior or "phrenic-to-phrenic" pericardiectomy; (E) removal pericardium off diaphragm; (F) completed diaphragm and posterior pericardiectomy; and (G) left lateral view of completed pericardiectomy showing pedicle along left phrenic nerve.

CP is a surgical disease that is best treated with pericardiectomy.[1,18] For this condition, the European Society of Cardiology recommends removal of as much of the pericardium as possible.[1,18] This is ideally and theoretically correct, but in practice it can be misguided thinking because the constricting peel often is densely fibrosed to the heart and calcification may even penetrate into the myocardium. This is especially true in the area of the atria, inferior vena cava, and atrioventricular groove. Attempts to resect the densely adhered pericardium can be dangerous, and injury to the thin-walled structures can even prove fatal. The pathophysiology requires release of the ventricles (Fig. 55-7), which must include the visceral pericardium.[48,51] Tricuspid valve regurgitation can be a confounding condition and should be addressed prior to the completion of the operation.[27]

Pericardiectomy can be performed with an associated low operative morbidity and mortality, and results in significant improvement in quality of life up to 10 years.[49] In the Mayo Clinic Rochester experience, overall mortality was 2.3%; for the CP group, mortality was 2.5%. Variables associated with an increased operative mortality have been well described by several investigators and commonly include a delay in treatment, advanced heart failure (eg, increased New York Heart Association class or reduced ejection fraction), and need of completion pericardiectomy (ie, for inadequate first operation

or recurrence of disease).[10,46,47,50,52,53] The take-home message is that early and adequate pericacardiectomy is both life-changing and life-saving. Referral for operation should not be denied.

PROGNOSIS

As previously stated, if left untreated, CP is associated with very high morbidity and mortality.[2] The survival 5 and 10 years postpericardiectomy have been reported to be 78% and 57%, respectively.[16] Postpericardiectomy outcomes are directly related to the underyling etiology, with patients with idopathic CP having very good long-term prognosis (>85% survival at 7 years) when compared to those with CP following cardiac surgery and particularly to those with radiation-related CP.[54,55] Other proposed indicators of unfavorable prognosis in patients with CP are shown in **Table 55–2**.

EFFUSIVE–CONSTRICTIVE PERICARDITIS

Most patients with CP present with the classic, chronic form of the disease. However, other "uncommon" presentations have been recognized.[56] Although typically described as two separate entities,[57,58] transient and effusive–constrictive pericarditis are most likely part of a clinical spectrum and distinction between the two might be academic.

TABLE 55–2. Clinical Predictors of Worse Prognosis in Patients with Constrictive Pericarditis

Age[16,52]
Etiology[16,52]
   Postcardiac surgery
   Radiation-induced
New York Heart Association functional class III–IV[16,52]
Renal dysfunction[52]
Hyponatremia[52]
Atrial fibrillation[66]
Echocardiography
   Left ventricular systolic dysfunction[52]
   Reduced medial mitral e' velocity[67]
   Degree of tricuspid valve regurgitation[25,68]
Cardiac catheterization[69]
   Low right atrial pressure: pulmonary artery wedge pressure ratio
   Increased pulmonary artery mean pressure

Some patients presenting with cardiac tamponade demonstrate features of CP immediately after pericardiocentesis is performed and tamponade relieved[59,60] (**Fig. 55–8**). This is felt to be secondary to decreased pericardial compliance in the setting of acute inflammation. The reported incidence of effusive–constrictive pericarditis has varied according to the population analyzed, chosen methodology (echocardiography vs. right heart catheterization), and most common etiologies, ranging from 8% in developed countries to more than 50% in African patients with tuberculous pericarditis.[57,61] In a recent publication, we observed typical echo-Doppler features of CP in 16% of patients undergoing pericardiocentesis at our institution,[62] showing that effusive–constrictive pericarditis is common in those undergoing percutaneous pericardial drainage. In addition, our data also suggest that effusive–constrictive

pericarditis can be suspected even prior to pericardiocentesis, with these patients demonstrating echo-Doppler findings that are a combination of those of cardiac tamponade and CP.[63] Therapy should be focused on treating active inflammation;[59] our results suggest that in the current era, the number of individuals evolving into chronic CP and requiring pericardiectomy is small. However, they might be at an increased risk of rehospitalization due to heart failure; therefore, we suggest close follow-up of patients with effusive–constrictive pericarditis.

TRANSIENT CONSTRICTIVE PERICARDITIS

The definition of transient CP has been variable in the literature. Initially described by Sagrista-Sauleda,[58] this group included patients initially presenting with acute pericarditis (not necessarily tamponade), subsequently developing constrictive features when the acute process was resolving and the pericardial effusion was either small or absent. The long-term prognosis for affected patients was good with none of them requiring surgical treatment. Others have defined transient constriction as CP that resolved with corticosteroids or anti-inflammatory therapy;[64] currently, the latter is the most widely used definition.

Pericardial effusions are common in patients with transient constriction, reported in two-thirds of cases. Affected patients tend to have signs of inflammation with elevated inflammatory markers and pericardial gadolinium enhancement on magnetic resonance imaging at the time of the diagnosis of CP (**Fig. 55–9**).[65] Cardiac magnetic resonance results are of critical importance in these individuals as both qualitative[65] and quantitative[66] analysis of pericardial late gadolinium enhancement have been shown to predict response to anti-inflammatory agents in those with transient CP.

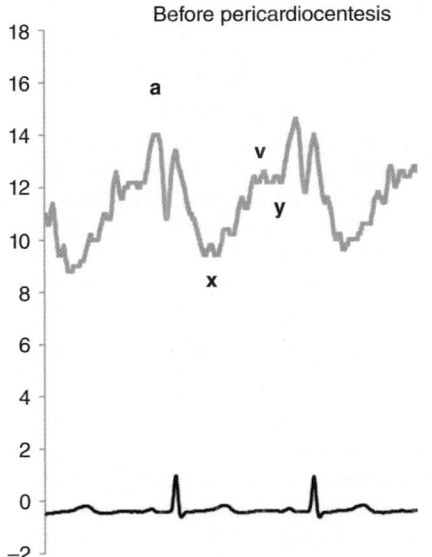
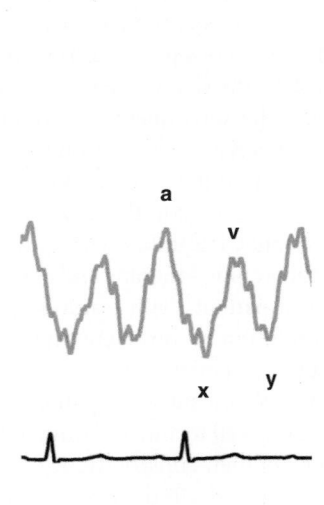

Figure 55–8. Hemodynamic pressure tracings in effusive–constrictive pericarditis. Right atrial pressure tracings before and after pericardiocentesis—prior to the pericardiocentesis, there is blunting of the *y* with a prominent *x* descent in the setting of elevated right atrial pressures, findings consistent with cardiac tamponade. After pericardiocentesis, although mean right atrial pressures drop, it remains slightly elevated with the development of deep *x* and *y* descents; this finding is diagnostic of effusive–constrictive pericarditis.

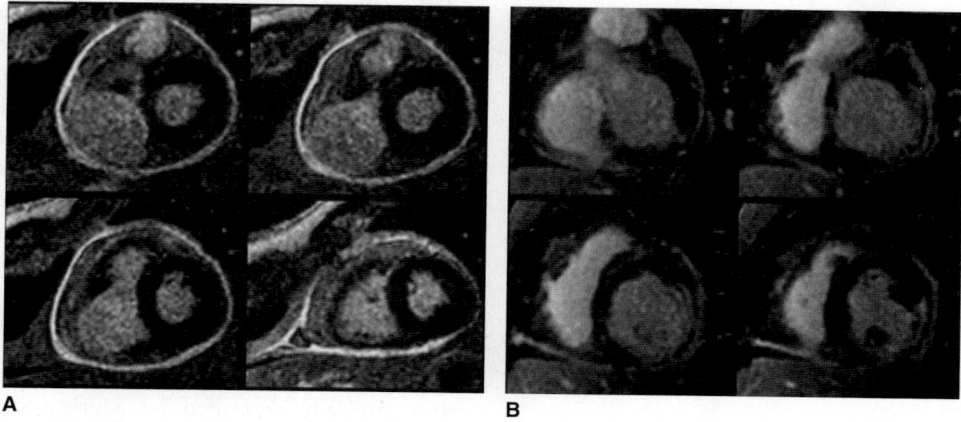

Figure 55–9. Cardiac magnetic resonance findings in a patient with transient constrictive pericarditis before and after anti-inflammatory therapy. Severe pericardial delayed enhancement is present before therapy **(A)**. With anti-inflammatory therapy, there was clinical and echocardiographic resolution of constrictive pericarditis. Posttreatment images show improvement in the degree of pericardial delayed enhancement **(B)**.

Optimal type and duration of nonsteroidal anti-inflammatory versus corticosteroids ± colchicine for transient CP is yet to be determined. However, in our experience, clinical response to medical therapy is relatively quick (less than a week), particularly when corticosteroids are used. Lack of immediate response to therapy typically indicates that the constrictive process will not be amenable to medical therapy. At least 3 months of medical therapy is required for a complete or clinically satisfactory response. Currently, the role and yield of steroid-sparing agents (including anakinra) for the treatment of transient CP is still unknown.

Similar to uncomplicated pericarditis associated with rheumatologic disorders (such as systemic lupus erythematosus), medical therapy for transient CP secondary to these diseases should be directed to treating the underlying process. Therefore, the management of these patients requires a multidisciplinary approach, including a cardiologist and rheumatologist. Data on the preferred medical regimen in these individuals are lacking, but in our experience, corticosteroids are frequently needed in those presenting with symptomatic CP.

The management of tuberculous pericarditis is complex and it involves a multidrug anti-tuberculous regimen.[67] The use of corticosteroids to prevent the subsequent development of CP have been recommended as a reasonable option for those without concomitant human immunodeficiency virus infection[66] but the optimal medical therapy for those with established tuberculosis-related transient CP is unknown.[69] In a series of 50 patients receiving anti-tuberculosis therapy and corticosteroids (88% of the cohort), most patients with features of CP at the time of diagnosis had resolution of constrictive hemodynamics during follow-up (18 out of 22 patients after 6 months).[70]

It should be mentioned that a subset of patients with transient CP initially responding well to anti-inflammatory therapy will experience worsening of their constrictive features as medication dosages are decreased or will demonstrate an inability to be weaned off steroids. Most of these patients will require surgical pericardiectomy and, thus, close follow-up is required even in patients that might have an initial favorable response to medial therapy.

OCCULT CONSTRICTIVE PERICARDITIS

Occult CP was described in a group of patients where constrictive features were only noticeable after fluid challenge.[71] Although we do use rapid saline infusion in the catheterization laboratory for patients with suspected CP and low filling pressures related to overdiuresis, we do not use fluid challenge routinely to identify occult CP. Given the lack of data, we would not recommend the diagnosis or treatment of CP solely based on post–saline infusion changes for patients who do not otherwise have diagnostic features of the CP.

ACKNOWLEDGMENT

In the previous edition, this chapter was contributed to by Massimo Imazio, and portions of that chapter have been retained.

REFERENCES

1. Syed FF, Schaff HV, Oh JK. Constrictive pericarditis—a curable diastolic heart failure. *Nat Rev Cardiol.* 2015;12(12):682.
2. Wood P. Chronic constrictive pericarditis. *Am J Cardiol.* 1961;7(1):48-61.
3. Imazio M, Brucato A, Maestroni S, et al. Risk of constrictive pericarditis after acute pericarditis. *Circulation.* 2011;124(11):1270-1275.
4. Sagrista-Sauleda J, Permanyer-Miralda G, Soler-Soler J. Tuberculous pericarditis: ten year experience with a prospective protocol for diagnosis and treatment. *J Am Coll Cardiol.* 1988;11(4):724-728.
5. Dines DE, Edwards JE, Burchell HB. Myocardial atrophy in constrictive pericarditis. *Proc Staff Meet Mayo Clin.* 1958;33(4):93-99.
6. McCaughan BC, Schaff HV, Piehler JM, et al. Early and late results of pericardiectomy for constrictive pericarditis. *J Thorac Cardiovasc Surg.* 1985;89(3):340-350.
7. Ling LH, Schaff HV, dal-Bianco J, et al. Detection of constrictive pericarditis: a single-centre experience of 523 surgically confirmed cases [abstract]. *J Am Coll Cardiol.* 2009;53(Supp 1):A176.
8. George TJ, Arnaoutakis GJ, Beaty CA, Kilic A, Baumgartner WA, Conte JV. Contemporary etiologies, risk factors, and outcomes after pericardiectomy. *Ann Thorac Surg.* 2012;94(2):445-451.
9. Oreto L, Mayer A, Todaro MC, et al. Contemporary clinical spectrum of constrictive pericarditis: a 10-year experience. *Int J Cardiol.* 2013;163(3):339-341.

10. Szabo G, Schmack B, Bulut C, et al. Constrictive pericarditis: risks, aetiologies and outcomes after total pericardiectomy: 24 years of experience. *Eur J Cardiothorac Surg*. 2013;44(6):1023-1028; discussion 1028.

11. Im E, Shim CY, Hong GR, et al. The incidence and clinical outcome of constrictive physiology after coronary artery bypass graft surgery. *J Am Coll Cardiol*. 2013;61(20):2110-2112.

12. Matsuyama K, Matsumoto M, Sugita T, et al. Clinical characteristics of patients with constrictive pericarditis after coronary bypass surgery. *Jpn Circ J*. 2001;65(6):480-482.

13. Lin Y, Zhou M, Xiao J, Wang B, Wang Z. Treating constrictive pericarditis in a Chinese single-center study: a five-year experience. *Ann Thorac Surg*. 2012;94(4):1235-1240.

14. Yetkin U, Kestelli M, Yilik L, et al. Recent surgical experience in chronic constrictive pericarditis. *Tex Heart Inst J*. 2003;30(1):27-30.

15. Avgoustakis D, Lazarides D, Athanasiades D, Michaelides G. The electrocardiogram in constrictive pericarditis before and after radical pericardectomy. *Chest*. 1970;57(5):460-467.

16. Ling LH, Oh JK, Schaff HV, et al. Constrictive pericarditis in the modern era: evolving clinical spectrum and impact on outcome after pericardiectomy. *Circulation*. 1999;100(13):1380-1386.

17. Babuin L, Alegria JR, Oh JK, Nishimura RA, Jaffe AS. Brain natriuretic peptide levels in constrictive pericarditis and restrictive cardiomyopathy. *J Am Coll Cardiol*. 2006;47(7):1489-1491.

18. Adler Y, Charron P, Imazio M, et al. 2015 ESC Guidelines for the diagnosis and management of pericardial diseases: The Task Force for the Diagnosis and Management of Pericardial Diseases of the European Society of Cardiology (ESC) Endorsed by: The European Association for Cardio-Thoracic Surgery (EACTS). *Eur Heart J*. 2015;36(42):2921-2964.

19. Madeira M, Teixeira R, Costa M, Goncalves L, Klein AL. Two-dimensional speckle tracking cardiac mechanics and constrictive pericarditis: systematic review. *Echocardiography*. 2016;33(10):1589-1599.

20. Sengupta PP, Krishnamoorthy VK, Abhayaratna WP, et al. Disparate patterns of left ventricular mechanics differentiate constrictive pericarditis from restrictive cardiomyopathy. *JACC Cardiovasc Imaging*. 2008;1(1):29-38.

21. Coylewright M, Welch TD, Nishimura RA. Mechanism of septal bounce in constrictive pericarditis: a simultaneous cardiac catheterisation and echocardiographic study. *Heart*. 2013;99(18):1376.

22. Welch TD, Ling LH, Espinosa RE, et al. Echocardiographic diagnosis of constrictive pericarditis: Mayo Clinic criteria. *Circ Cardiovasc Imaging*. 2014;7(3):526-534.

23. Nagueh SF, Smiseth OA, Appleton CP, et al. Recommendations for the evaluation of left ventricular diastolic function by echocardiography: an update from the American Society of Echocardiography and the European Association of Cardiovascular Imaging. *J Am Soc Echocardiogr*. 2016;29(4):277-314.

24. Yang JH, Miranda WR, Nishimura RA, Greason KL, Schaff HV, Oh JK. Prognostic importance of mitral e' velocity in constrictive pericarditis. *Eur Heart J Cardiovasc Imaging*. 2021;22(3):357-364.

25. Oh JK, Hatle LK, Seward JB, et al. Diagnostic role of Doppler echocardiography in constrictive pericarditis. *J Am Coll Cardiol*. 1994;23(1):154-162.

26. Choi MS, Jeong DS, Oh JK, Chang SA, Park SJ, Chung S. Long-term results of radical pericardiectomy for constrictive pericarditis in Korean population. *J Cardiothorac Surg*. 2019;14(1):32.

27. Gongora E, Dearani JA, Orszulak TA, Schaff HV, Li Z, Sundt TM, 3rd. Tricuspid regurgitation in patients undergoing pericardiectomy for constrictive pericarditis. *Ann Thorac Surg*. 2008;85(1):163-170; discussion 170-161.

28. Calderon-Rojas R, Greason KL, King KS, et al. Tricuspid valve regurgitation in patients undergoing pericardiectomy for constrictive pericarditis. *Semin Thorac Cardiovasc Surg*. 2020;32(4):721-728.

29. Asher CR, Klein AL. Diastolic heart failure: restrictive cardiomyopathy, constrictive pericarditis, and cardiac tamponade: clinical and echocardiographic evaluation. *Cardiol Rev*. 2002;10(4):218-229.

30. Nishimura RA. Constrictive pericarditis in the modern era: a diagnostic dilemma. *Heart*. 2001;86(6):619-623.

31. Nishimura RA, Carabello BA. Hemodynamics in the cardiac catheterization laboratory of the 21st century. *Circulation*. 2012;125(17):2138-2150.

32. Hurrell DG, Nishimura RA, Higano ST, et al. Value of dynamic respiratory changes in left and right ventricular pressures for the diagnosis of constrictive pericarditis. *Circulation*. 1996;93(11):2007-2013.

33. Talreja DR, Nishimura RA, Oh JK, Holmes DR. Constrictive pericarditis in the modern era: novel criteria for diagnosis in the cardiac catheterization laboratory. *J Am Coll Cardiol*. 2008;51(3):315-319.

34. Kyunghee L, Jeong HY, William RM, et al. Clinical significance of pulmonary hypertension in patients with constrictive pericarditis. *Heart*. 2021 Oct;107(20):1651-1656.

35. Talreja DR, Edwards WD, Danielson GK, et al. Constrictive pericarditis in 26 patients with histologically normal pericardial thickness. *Circulation*. 2003;108(15):1852-1857.

36. Bull RK, Edwards PD, Dixon AK. CT dimensions of the normal pericardium. *Br J Radiol*. 1998;71(849):923-925.

37. Masui T, Finck S, Higgins CB. Constrictive pericarditis and restrictive cardiomyopathy: evaluation with MR imaging. *Radiology*. 1992;182(2):369-373.

38. Alajaji W, Xu B, Sripariwuth A, et al. Noninvasive multimodality imaging for the diagnosis of constrictive pericarditis. *Circ Cardiovasc Imaging*. 2018;11(11):e007878.

39. Klein AL, Abbara S, Agler DA, et al. American Society of Echocardiography clinical recommendations for multimodality cardiovascular imaging of patients with pericardial disease: endorsed by the Society for Cardiovascular Magnetic Resonance and Society of Cardiovascular Computed Tomography. *J Am Soc Echocardiogr*. 2013;26(9):965-1012.e1015.

40. Villavicencio MA, Dearani JA, pericarditis TMSPfcori. Pericardiectomy for constrictive or recurrent inflammatory pericarditis. *Oper Tech Thorac Cardiovasc Surg*. 2008;18:2-13.

41. Ali-Hassan-Sayegh S, Mirhosseini SJ, Liakopoulos O, et al. Posterior pericardiotomy in cardiac surgery: systematic review and meta-analysis. *Asian Cardiovasc Thorac Ann*. 2015;23(3):354-362.

42. Chowdhury UK, Subramaniam GK, Kumar AS, et al. Pericardiectomy for constrictive pericarditis: a clinical, echocardiographic, and hemodynamic evaluation of two surgical techniques. *Ann Thorac Surg*. 2006;81(2):522-529.

43. Khandaker MH, Espinosa RE, Nishimura RA, et al. Pericardial disease: diagnosis and management. *Mayo Clin Proc*. 2010;85(6):572-593.

44. Patel N, Rafique AM, Eshaghian S, et al. Retrospective comparison of outcomes, diagnostic value, and complications of percutaneous prolonged drainage versus surgical pericardiotomy of pericardial effusion associated with malignancy. *Am J Cardiol*. 2013;112(8):1235-1239.

45. Piehler JM, Pluth JR, Schaff HV, Danielson GK, Orszulak TA, Puga FJ. Surgical management of effusive pericardial disease. Influence of extent of pericardial resection on clinical course. *J Thorac Cardiovasc Surg*. 1985;90(4):506-516.

46. Porta-Sanchez A, Sagrista-Sauleda J, Ferreira-Gonzalez I, Torrents-Fernandez A, Roca-Luque I, Garcia-Dorado D. Constrictive pericarditis: etiologic spectrum, patterns of clinical presentation, prognostic factors, and long-term follow-up. *Rev Esp Cardiol (Engl Ed)*. 2015;68(12):1092-1100.

47. Vistarini N, Chen C, Mazine A, et al. Pericardiectomy for constrictive pericarditis: 20 years of experience at the Montreal Heart Institute. *Ann Thorac Surg*. 2015;100(1):107-113.

48. Chowdhury UK, S SS, Reddy SM. Pericardiectomy for chronic constrictive pericarditis via left anterolateral thoracotomy. *Oper Tech Thorac Cardiovasc Surg 2008*. 2008;18:14-25.

49. EA G. A 20-year experience with isolated pericardiectomy: analysis of indications and outcomes. *J Thorac Cardiovasc Surg*. 2016;152(2):448-458.

50. Busch C, Penov K, Amorim PA, et al. Risk factors for mortality after pericardiectomy for chronic constrictive pericarditis in a large single-centre cohort. *Eur J Cardiothorac Surg*. 2015;48(6):e110-e116.

51. Matsuura K, Mogi K, Takahara Y. Off-pump waffle procedure using an ultrasonic scalpel for constrictive pericarditis. *Eur J Cardiothorac Surg.* 2015;47(5):e220-e222.

52. Cho YH, Schaff HV, Dearani JA, et al. Completion pericardiectomy for recurrent constrictive pericarditis: importance of timing of recurrence on late clinical outcome of operation. *Ann Thorac Surg.* 2012;93(4):1236-1240.

53. Komoda T, Frumkin A, Knosalla C, Hetzer R. Child-Pugh score predicts survival after radical pericardiectomy for constrictive pericarditis. *Ann Thorac Surg.* 2013;96(5):1679-1685.

54. Bertog SC, Thambidorai SK, Parakh K, et al. Constrictive pericarditis: etiology and cause-specific survival after pericardiectomy. *J Am Coll Cardiol.* 2004;43(8):1445-1452.

55. Siddharth P, Juan C, William M, et al. Annalisa Bernabei, Andreas Polycarpou, Hartzell Schaff, Joseph Dearani, John Stulak, Alberto Pochettino, Richard Daly, Brian Lahr, Jason Viehman, Kevin Greason. Outcomes of pericardiectomy for constrictive pericarditis following mediastinal irradiation. *J Card Surg.* 2021 Dec;36(12):4636-4642.

56. Sagrista-Sauleda J. Pericardial constriction: uncommon patterns. *Heart.* 2004;90(3):257-258.

57. Sagrista-Sauleda J, Angel J, Sanchez A, Permanyer-Miralda G, Soler-Soler J. Effusive-constrictive pericarditis. *N Engl J Med.* 2004;350(5):469-475.

58. Sagrista-Sauleda J, Permanyer-Miralda G, Candell-Riera J, Angel J, Soler-Soler J. Transient cardiac constriction: an unrecognized pattern of evolution in effusive acute idiopathic pericarditis. *Am J Cardiol.* 1987;59(9):961-966.

59. Syed FF, Ntsekhe M, Mayosi BM, Oh JK. Effusive-constrictive pericarditis. *Heart Fail Rev.* 2013;18(3):277-287.

60. Miranda WR, Oh JK. Effusive-Constrictive Pericarditis. *Cardiol Clin.* 2017;35(4):551-558.

61. Ntsekhe M, Matthews K, Syed FF, et al. Prevalence, hemodynamics, and cytokine profile of effusive-constrictive pericarditis in patients with tuberculous pericardial effusion. *PLoS One.* 2013;8(10):e77532.

62. Kim KH, Miranda WR, Sinak LJ, et al. Effusive-constrictive pericarditis after pericardiocentesis: incidence, associated findings, and natural history. *JACC Cardiovasc Imaging.* 2018;11(4):534-541.

63. Miranda WR, Newman DB, Sinak LJ, et al. Pre- and post-pericardiocentesis echo-Doppler features of effusive-constrictive pericarditis compared with cardiac tamponade and constrictive pericarditis. *Eur Heart J Cardiovasc Imaging.* 2019;20(3):298-306.

64. Haley JH, Tajik AJ, Danielson GK, Schaff HV, Mulvagh SL, Oh JK. Transient constrictive pericarditis: causes and natural history. *J Am Coll Cardiol.* 2004;43(2):271-275.

65. Feng D, Glockner J, Kim K, et al. Cardiac magnetic resonance imaging pericardial late gadolinium enhancement and elevated inflammatory markers can predict the reversibility of constrictive pericarditis after antiinflammatory medical therapy: a pilot study. *Circulation.* 2011;124(17):1830-1837.

66. Cremer PC, Tariq MU, Karwa A, et al. Quantitative assessment of pericardial delayed hyperenhancement predicts clinical improvement in patients with constrictive pericarditis treated with anti-inflammatory therapy. *Circ Cardiovasc Imaging.* 2015;8(5).

67. Isiguzo G, Du Bruyn E, Howlett P, Ntsekhe M. Diagnosis and management of tuberculous pericarditis: what is new? *Curr Cardiol Rep.* 2020;22(1):2.

68. Adler Y, Charron P, Imazio M, et al. 2015 ESC Guidelines for the diagnosis and management of pericardial diseases: The Task Force for the Diagnosis and Management of Pericardial Diseases of the European Society of Cardiology (ESC)Endorsed by: The European Association for Cardio-Thoracic Surgery (EACTS). *Eur Heart J.* 2015;36(42):2921-2964.

69. Ntsekhe M, Shey Wiysonge C, Commerford PJ, Mayosi BM. The prevalence and outcome of effusive constrictive pericarditis: a systematic review of the literature. *Cardiovasc J Afr.* 2012;23(5):281-285.

70. Kim MS, Chang SA, Kim EK, et al. The clinical course of tuberculous pericarditis in immunocompetent hosts based on serial echocardiography. *Korean Circ J.* 2020;50(7):599-609.

71. Bush CA, Stang JM, Wooley CF, Kilman JW. Occult constrictive pericardial disease. Diagnosis by rapid volume expansion and correction by pericardiectomy. *Circulation.* 1977;56(6):924-930.

SECTION IX

CARDIOPULMONARY DISEASE

Diagnosis and Management of Diseases of the Peripheral Venous System

Daniella Kadian-Dodov, Hillary Johnston-Cox, and Jeffrey W. Olin

Risk factors, diagnosis and management of acute and chronic peripheral venous diseases

Upper extremity

Axillary vein
Subclavian vein
Brachial veins

Lower extremity

Profunda femoral vein
Femoral vein
Tibial veins

External iliac vein
Common femoral vein
*Great saphenous vein**
Popliteal vein
Small saphenous vein
Gastrocnemius veins (muscular)
Soleal veins (muscular)
Peroneal vein

Acute venous disease

Deep vein thrombosis, calf vein thrombosis, superficial vein thrombosis

Risk Factors

Intrinsic: cancer, thrombophilia, obesity, anatomic variants (e.g. May Thurner)

Extrinsic: injury, surgery, exogenous hormones, SARS-CoV2

Diagnosis

Duplex ultrasound: dilated, non-compressible vein; echolucent thrombus; altered flow dynamics

CT or MR Venogram: useful for pelvic veins, outflow obstruction

Venography: limited to planned treatment

Medical Treatment

Anticoagulation (treatment & extended therapy)
• Duration dependent on reversible/nonreversible risk factors, and thrombus burden, location (i.e. deep veins, calf veins, superficial veins)
• Agent dependent on renal function, oral absorption (i.e. bariatric patients), malignancy e.g. GI, uro cancers), high risk thrombophilias (i.e. antiphospholipid antibody syndrome)

Intervention

IVC filter typically if anticoagulation is contraindicated

Thrombolysis, thrombectomy: typically IVC and iliac vein occlusive disease within 14 days of acute event

Chronic venous disease

Venous insufficiency, venous ulcers

Risk Factors

Primary: autosomal dominant with incomplete penetrance

Secondary: prior VTE, female sex, obesity, multiparity, age

Diagnosis

Clinical: swelling, lipodermatosclerosis hyperpigmentation.

Venous duplex: measured reflux with Valsalva, dilated veins, varicose veins

Treatment

Compression therapy:
• Wraps (edema control), stockings or garment (edema maintenance)
• Varicose veins (20-30 mm Hg), healed venous ulcer (30-40 mm Hg)

Endovenous ablation:
• GSV or SSV only, if failed conservative therapy (i.e. compression)

Vein stripping or phlebectomy
• Very superficial or large superficial veins

Venous Ulcers (Tenets of Healing)
• **Compression, i.e. edema control**
• **Skin Care**
• **Infection control**
• **Arterial perfusion**

Chapter 56 Fuster and Hurst's Central Illustration. Peripheral vein anatomy is shown in the left panel; bolded words are deep veins, italic words (not bolded) are superficial veins, and non-bolded, non-italic words are calf veins. *The great saphenous vein runs along the medial side of the leg from the groin to the lower calf.

CHAPTER SUMMARY

This chapter reviews the pathophysiology and treatment of peripheral venous disease. The anatomy of the venous system is central to the diagnosis and management of acute and chronic venous disease (see Fuster and Hurst's Central Illustration). Both intrinsic and extrinsic risk factors may contribute to venous thrombosis in the deep veins, calf veins, or superficial veins. Duplex ultrasonography is useful for diagnosis in most cases; computed tomography or magnetic resonance venography may be considered to evaluate pelvic vein thrombosis or outflow obstruction. Catheter-based venography is reserved for planned treatment. The cornerstone of medical therapy for venous thrombosis is anticoagulation. Advanced therapies such as inferior vena cava filter or catheter-directed thrombolysis and thrombectomy may be considered in specialized cases. Prior venous thrombosis is a risk factor for chronic venous disease, as well as family history, age, sex, parity, and obesity. Candidacy for advanced therapies may be assessed by duplex ultrasonography to quantify the extent of insufficiency and anatomy. Compression therapy is central to management of chronic venous disease; in refractory cases, endovenous ablation, vein stripping, or other surgical techniques may be considered. Venous ulcers require additional attention beyond compression to skin care, infection control, and assessment of arterial perfusion, which may be compromised in up to 26% of patients.

INTRODUCTION

The lower extremity venous system includes the deep, superficial, and perforating veins that work in concert to return blood to the heart (**Fig. 56–1**).[1] Unlike the arterial system, the venous system is low resistant and must overcome gravitational and hydrostatic pressure forces to achieve blood return to the heart. The venules and veins have very thin walls and low resting basal tone, which allows for enormous distensibility. As a result, small changes in hydrostatic forces, central pressure, and/or external forces result in changes of the vein diameter. Venous blood flow is reliant upon muscular leg contraction, historically referred to as "the peripheral heart,"[2] as well as bicuspid venous valves that open and close to prevent backflow; together, muscular leg contraction and venous valves help to overcome hydrostatic forces within the vein itself. Venous disease results due to degeneration and dysfunction of the veins and/or valves, which may occur following an obstruction such as deep vein thrombosis (DVT) or in the setting of increased central pressures as in heart failure. Venous disease is associated with a wide array of clinical manifestations due to complex hemodynamic and anatomic failures. A basic understanding of these complexities is essential in the evaluation, diagnosis, and appropriate treatment of venous disease.

ANATOMY

The veins of the lower extremities are divided into three main subgroups that are interconnected and together ultimately drain into the external and common iliac veins to the inferior vena cava: (1) perforator veins, (2) superficial veins, and (3) deep veins. The *fascia muscularis* divides the deep and superficial vein compartments; the perforator veins cross the fascial plane to connect the deep and superficial venous systems. A network of bicuspid venous valves exists in the deep and superficial veins to assist in venous return and prevent backflow. In the lower extremity, the deep veins accompany the corresponding arteries and their branches.[3] The popliteal vein is formed by the confluence of the calf veins, which include the gastrocnemius vein draining into the popliteal vein and the soleal veins emptying into the tibial and then popliteal veins. Subsequently, the popliteal vein empties into the femoral, common femoral, and iliac veins. The common femoral and external iliac vein each have one venous valve approximately 63% of the time; in 37% of patients, there is no valve present in this location.[4]

The largest of the superficial veins, the great saphenous vein (GSV), is also the longest vein in the human body. It courses from the ankle medially up the calf and into the thigh to ultimately confluence with the common femoral vein at the saphenofemoral junction (Fig. 56–1). Normal GSV caliber ranges from 3 mm to 4 mm in diameter and 10 to 20 valves scattered along its course aide in venous outflow.[4] Almost all patients have a "terminal valve" located at the saphenofemoral junction. The second largest superficial vein is the small saphenous vein (SSV), which courses along the lateral calf and typically drains into the popliteal vein at the saphenopopliteal junction. The SSV contains 7 to 13 venous valves and is typically 3 mm in diameter. Notably, anatomic variants of the venous system are common and alternative drainage routes can be seen

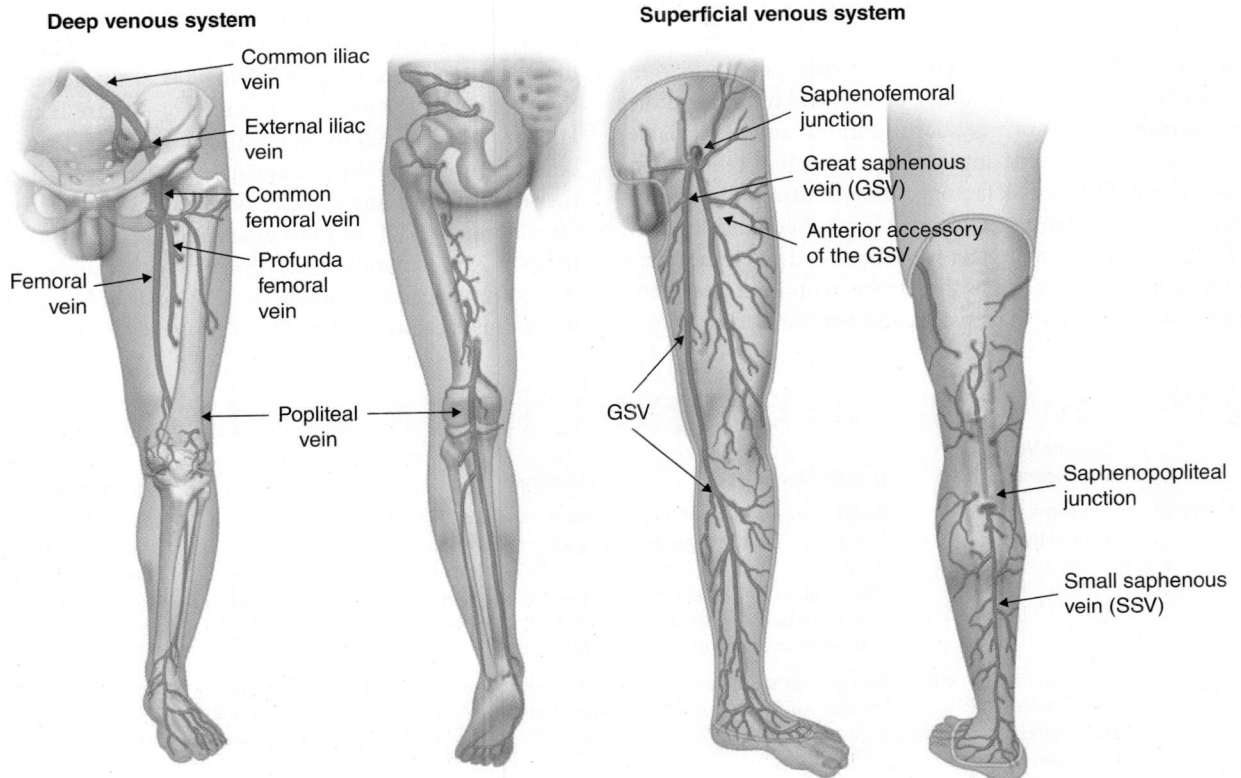

Figure 56–1. Peripheral venous anatomy.

TABLE 56–1. Categorization of Risk Factors for Venous Thromboembolism Based on the Risk of Recurrence Over the Long-Term

Estimated risk for long-term recurrence*	Risk factor category for index VTE	Examples
Low (<3% per year)	Major transient or reversible factors associated with >10-fold increased risk for the index VTE event (compared to patients without the risk factor)	• Surgery with general anesthesia for >30 min • Confined to hospital bed (eg, bathroom privileges only) for ≥3 days due to acute illness or acute exacerbation of chronic illness
Intermediate (3%–8% per year)	Transient of reversible factors associated with ≤10-fold increased risk for first (index) VTE	• Minor surgery (general anesthesia <30 min) • Admission to hospital for <3 days with an acute illness • Estrogen therapy/contraception • Confined to bed out of hospital for ≥3 days with an acute illness • Leg injury (without fracture) associated with reduced mobility for ≥3 days • Long-haul flight
	Nonmalignant persistent risk factors	• Inflammatory bowel disease • Active autoimmune disease
	No identifiable risk factor	
High (>8% per year)		• Active cancer • One or more previous episodes of VTE in the absence of a major transient or reversible risk factor • Antiphospholipid antibody syndrome

*If anticoagulation is discontinued after the first 3 months
Reproduced with permission from Konstantinides SV, Meyer G, Becattini C, et al. 2019 ESC Guidelines for the diagnosis and management of acute pulmonary embolism developed in collaboration with the European Respiratory Society (ERS). *Eur Heart J.* 2020 Jan 21;41(4):543-603.

in as many as 50% of patients.[4] Rich networks of subcutaneous and dermal vein plexuses exist as embryologic remnants of the venous system, which are spread across the lateral thigh and calf. In some conditions, abnormal development of the superficial veins may result in large varices across these networks, as seen in Klippel–Trénaunay or Parkes–Weber syndromes.

VENOUS THROMBOSIS

Venous thrombosis may occur due to the risks as identified in Virchow's Triad—circulatory stasis, endothelial injury, and the hypercoagulable state—or may occur without any identifiable risk factors. The treatment approach and duration relies upon the patient's modifiable risk factors, extent of thrombus, and/or affected venous segments.[5,6] The terms "provoked" and "unprovoked" thrombosis are no longer recommended given the oversimplification of these terms as they relate to optimal treatment strategies for patients with transient and persistent risk factors

for venous thromboembolism (VTE) (**Table 56–1**).[6,7] We will consider venous thrombosis in the superficial and deep venous systems separately.

Superficial Thrombophlebitis

Superficial thrombophlebitis (STP) classically presents as a tender, red, and indurated cord that follows the line of the affected superficial vein. Most often, the GSV is involved. The disease is reported in up to 3% to 11% of the general population, although the annual incidence of disease is not known. Higher rates are seen in malignancy, women over age 60 years, obesity, thrombophilia, pregnancy or estrogen use, sclerotherapy, autoimmune disease, and those with varicose veins.[8,9] Overlap with DVT or pulmonary embolism (PE) is reported in up to 25% of patients with STP.[10] Duplex ultrasonography is recommended to confirm the diagnosis of STP and exclude other causes of the swollen limb (**Table 56–2**), as well as screen

TABLE 56–2. Causes of the Swollen Limb

	Chronic Venous Insufficiency	Lymphedema	Lipedema	Cellulitis	Deep Venous Thrombosis
Distribution of Edema	Below the knee Around the ankle	Distal; involves the foot "buffalo hump" and toes "sausage toes" "Stemmer's sign" – inability to pinch skin between the base of the first and second toe	Always bilateral Spares the foot: "ankle cut-off sign"; concentrated edema over the malleolus: "fat pad sign"	Often unilateral and well demarcated. Skip areas of involved and uninvolved skin	Often unilateral, limited to the affected limb and distal to the obstructed vein. Many patients with DVT may have no symptoms or signs
Skin Findings	Telangiectasia, reticular veins, varicose veins, skin pigmentation and/or eczema, atrophie blanche, lipodermatosclerosis, ulcerations	Skin pigmentation and/or fibrosis; verrucous changes	Disproportionate fat distribution below the waist; tender to palpation	Well-demarcated erythema, tender to palpation, warm	Erythema, warmth, tenderness to palpation. Dilated superficial veins, suffusion of leg

for the presence of a concomitant DVT or extension of the clot into the deep venous system that would warrant treatment with anticoagulation.[9,11] First-line management of STP typically includes warm compresses and nonsteroidal anti-inflammatory agents for a period of 7 to 10 days. Most cases of STP are self-limited; however, anticoagulation should be considered in cases that do not respond to conservative management, or if the STP is in close proximity to the deep veins at the sapheno-popliteal (5 cm) or sapheno-femoral junction (10 cm).[11,12] Both low-molecular-weight heparin (LMWH) and fondaparinux at prophylactic or therapeutic doses are acceptable therapies for the prevention of DVT or PE in patients deemed to be high risk.[11,13] In cases of recurrent STP, testing for thrombophilias, search for systemic diseases (ie, thromboangiitis obliterans, Behcet's syndrome), and investigation for underlying malignancy may be appropriate.[9]

Deep Vein Thrombosis

Presentation, Risk Factors, and Diagnosis

The classic clinical description of DVT includes unilateral pain, limb swelling, skin erythema, and warmth with symptoms acute to subacute in onset. However, diagnostic testing is necessary to confirm the diagnosis as the signs and symptoms of DVT are not reliable and cases may be clinically subtle or entirely absent in some patients.[14] The use of clinical prediction scores, such as the Wells' score (**Table 56–3**), may be helpful in the initial evaluation of outpatients with possible DVT to guide healthcare providers in deciding who may warrant additional testing with D-dimer and duplex ultrasound.[15–17] If DVT is suspected, an evaluation to confirm and define the extent of DVT should be pursued.[17] Findings that support the diagnosis of DVT on duplex ultrasonography include a dilated noncompressible vein due to the presence of thrombus, direct visualization of thrombus, as well as altered venous flow dynamics with a lack of respiratory variation resulting from outflow obstruction or a lack of flow augmentation with calf muscle compression, indicating distal obstruction between the calf muscle and ultrasound

transducer.[18] Duplex ultrasound has a reported sensitivity of 96.5% for symptomatic proximal DVT, 71.2% for distal DVT, and 94% specificity.[19] There is controversy with regard to proximal vein duplex ultrasound (popliteal and more proximal) versus whole leg ultrasound in the evaluation of patients with DVT because not all patients with isolated distal calf vein thrombosis will require anticoagulation. All calf vein thromboses require a follow-up plan as subsequently addressed in the treatment section. Catheter-based venography, magnetic-resonance (MR), and computed-tomographic (CT) venography may have a role in specific situations (ie, evaluation of the pelvic veins, assessing for extrinsic vein compression), although duplex ultrasonography is the standard method for detection of acute DVT in most cases.[18,20] Challenges with CT venography surround appropriate contrast timing of the target vein and subsequent difficulty in obtaining a diagnostic study; MR venography, on the other hand, shows promise in overcoming the contrast issue seen with CT, although its use is limited in patients with metallic implants.[20] Catheter-based venography is the gold standard for the direct visualization of venous flow and collaterals, and allows for intraluminal pressure gradient measurements and the use of intravascular ultrasound to detect a significant stenosis within the venous segment.[20] The use of catheter-based venography is generally limited to the evaluation of cases with possible stenosis or venous compression, and patients in whom a therapeutic intervention to relieve the obstruction is considered.[18,20]

The morbidity and mortality associated with DVT is related to the proximal extent of the thrombus and risk for pulmonary embolism (PE).[21] Upper extremity DVT, at the level of the axillary veins or more proximal, carries risk for PE estimated as high as ~12%.[21,22] Up to 30% of patients with VTE suffer a mortal event within 30 days,[23] most often due to PE of which 25% to 30% present with hemodynamic compromise and higher risk of associated sudden death.[24] The number of people who experience VTE per year in the United States is not known. However, it is estimated that as many as 900,000 could be affected (1–2 per 100,000).[23,25] It is estimated that 60,000 to 100,000 people per year die from VTE in the United States. In general, VTE, including DVT and PE, without identifiable risk factors tends to recur with a cumulative incidence of 10% at 1 year and 30% at 8 years after the first event.[26] Risk factors for DVT and PE are many, and may include both intrinsic and extrinsic factors such as sex, ethnicity, inherited or acquired thrombophilia, obesity, malignancy, pregnancy, exogenous estrogen hormones, chronic disease with prolonged bedrest, stroke, recent surgery, or injury (Table 56–1). Anatomic variants leading to extrinsic vein compression, such as in May–Thurner Syndrome (**Fig. 56–2**), are found in up to 20% to 24% of the general population[27,28] and may account for the left-sided predominance of DVT described in the lower extremity.[29] In the upper extremity, venous thoracic outlet syndrome also known as "Paget–Schroetter" syndrome or effort related thrombosis and the use of central venous catheters and pacemakers account for most cases.[30] Inherited thrombophilias such as Factor V Leiden, Prothrombin (G20210A) gene mutation, Plasminogen-Activator-Inhibitor 1 (PAI-1) levels, abnormal PAI-1 gene

TABLE 56–3. Wells Score for Assessing Probability of Deep Vein Thrombosis[14,15]

+1 Point Each:
Active Malignancy
Paralysis, paresis, or recent plaster immobilization of lower limb
Recently bedridden >3 days and/or major surgery within 4 weeks
Localized tenderness along distribution of lower extremity deep veins
Entire lower limb swollen
Calf swelling >3 cm compared with the asymptomatic leg
Strong family history of DVT (≥2 first degree relatives with history of DVT)
–2 Points if alternative diagnosis to DVT is at least as likely

Probability:	
High	≥3 points
Moderate	1–2 points
Low	≤0 points

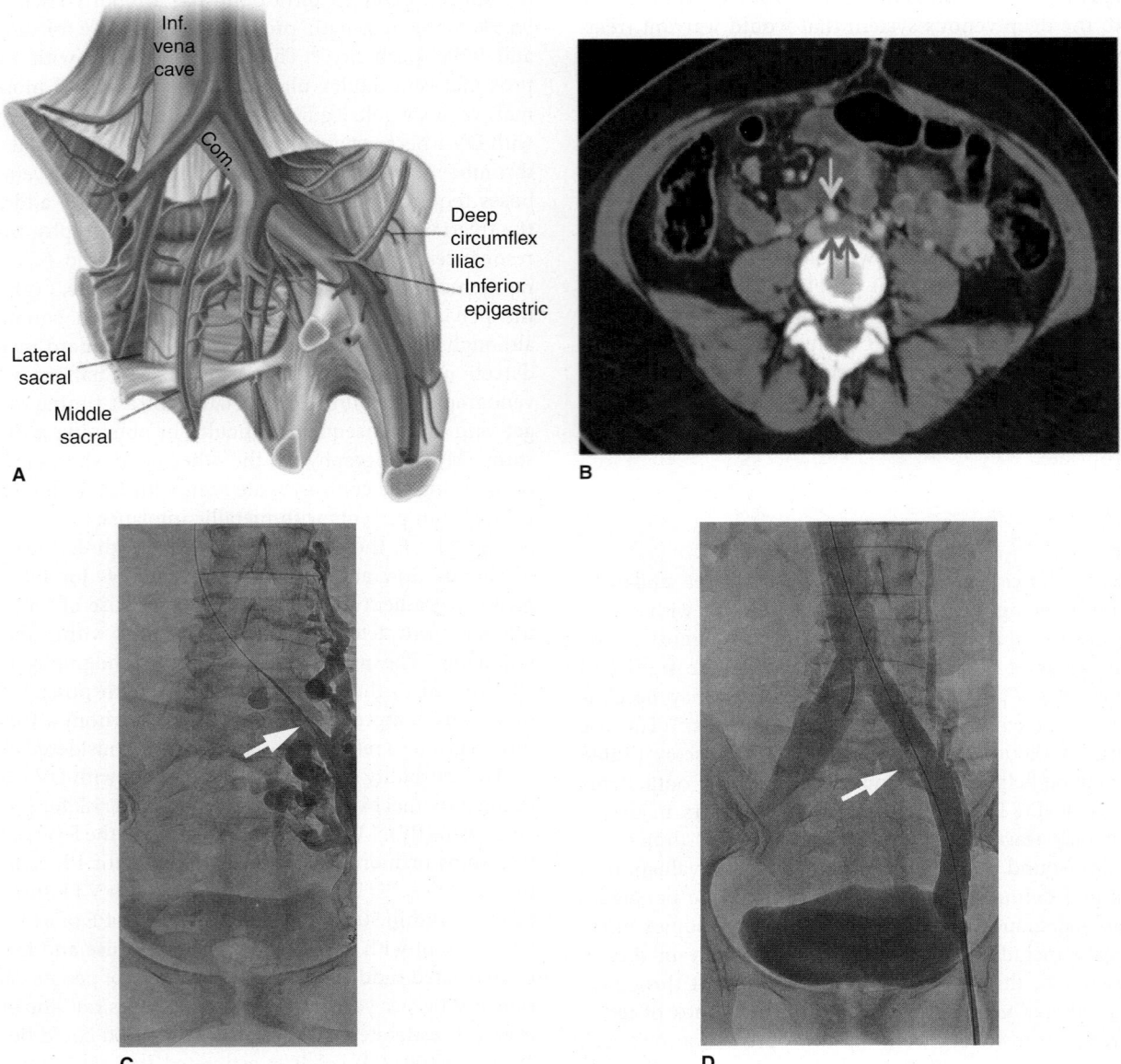

Figure 56–2. **May–Thurner anatomy and syndrome. (A)** Anatomic variant causing compression of the left common iliac vein by the overlying right common iliac artery, which results in an outflow obstruction that may result in DVT; **(B)** May–Thurner Syndrome diagnosed by CT venogram: filling defect seen in the left common iliac vein (*red arrows*) consistent with DVT due to compression of the overlying right common iliac artery (*yellow arrow*); **(C)** catheter-based venogram demonstrating occlusion of the left common iliac vein (*white arrow*) with collateral flow in the pelvis; **(D)** status-post thrombectomy, thrombolysis, venoplasty, and left common iliac stent placement with restored flow through the left common iliac vein (*white arrow*).

polymorphism, Antithrombin, and Protein C/S deficiency are present in approximately 30% of patients presenting with VTE and may confer up to a 5-fold increased risk of DVT or PE in their heterozygous state.[31,32] Despite these rates, routine testing for thrombophilia is not recommended because the presence of an abnormal allele only rarely affects the management of a patient with DVT or PE. Of note, in 25% to 50% of all DVT and PE, no underlying cause or risk factor is identified.[25]

Treatment

In the case of distal calf vein DVT, it is estimated that approximately 15% to 25% will propagate to the popliteal vein and/or

result in a pulmonary embolus.[33] For this reason, it is recommended that patients be treated with anticoagulation if symptomatic and no contraindication to anticoagulation. If the patient is asymptomatic (ie, DVT identified on screening in a stroke unit, or postoperative in a high-risk surgical procedure such as post total hip or knee replacement), one may still choose to treat with anticoagulation if the bleeding risk is not high. However, if there is a high risk of bleeding, an ultrasound surveillance program (ie, duplex ultrasound weekly for 3 to 4 weeks is perfectly acceptable to assess for thrombus propagation).[21]

Treatment of DVT involving the popliteal veins, or subclavian-axillary veins in the upper extremity, and more proximal segments is dictated by the presence of reversible or modifiable risk factors (ie, surgery or exogenous hormone use), persistent risk factors (ie, cancer, obesity, nephrotic syndrome, inflammatory bowel disease, immobility), the extent of thrombus (ie, DVT vs. PE), the patient's risk of bleeding with anticoagulation therapy, and patient preference. The guidelines for anticoagulation recommend that patients with an identifiable and reversible risk factor be treated with anticoagulation for at least 3 months prior to discontinuation.[6,21,34] In contrast, those without modifiable or identifiable risk factors should be considered for longer treatment duration if the risks of anticoagulation do not outweigh the perceived benefit.[6,21,34] Newer guidelines recognize direct oral anticoagulants (DOACs) as first-line alternatives to warfarin therapy for the treatment of acute DVT and PE.[6,21] DOACs include one direct thrombin inhibitor, dabigatran, as well as the factor Xa inhibitors rivaroxaban, apixaban, and edoxaban (**Table 56–4**).[35-47] There is variability in the recommended dosing regimens, use of heparin versus oral run-in to therapy, cost of drug, and recommended use in the setting of renal insufficiency. All have demonstrated noninferiority in comparison to warfarin for the acute treatment of venous thromboembolic disease.[37-39,41,48] Apixaban was superior compared to warfarin with regard to rates of major bleeding.[48] Since the recurrence rate of DVT/PE is so high (10% at 1 year and 30% at 8 years, as mentioned), it is now recommended that most patients be treated with lower doses of a DOAC after completing their planned treatment course. In the AMPLIFY EXT trial, low-dose apixaban (2.5 mg twice daily) and in the EINSTEIN CHOICE trial, low-dose rivaroxaban (10 mg daily) demonstrated a safety profile equal to placebo or aspirin, respectively, and was as effective as full-dose therapy (apixaban 5 mg twice daily; rivaroxaban 20 mg) for the prevention of recurrent VTE.[40,47] Total treatment duration must be individualized to accommodate the patient's specific risks and benefits with continued anticoagulation.

Early meta-analysis of the DOAC phase III trials, which included 3% to 9% of patients with concomitant malignancy, evaluated the efficacy of these new agents in cancer-related thrombosis and suggested that DOACs may be an acceptable alternative to LMWH or warfarin.[49] Recent randomized trials of rivaroxaban and edoxaban have shown a significant decrease in the rates of recurrent VTE as compared to LMWH, although higher rates of bleeding were noted, particularly in patients with gastric cancer.[43,44] The most recent guideline iterations advocate for direct oral anticoagulants as alternatives to LMWH to treat cancer-related VTE in patients with low bleeding risk and the absence of gastric cancer (**Fig. 56–3**).[6,50,51] The multicenter, international Caravaggio study published in 2020, additionally demonstrated similar decreased rates of recurrent VTE compared to LMWH in patients with cancer receiving treatment-dose apixaban (5 mg twice a day) with no difference in bleeding outcomes.[42]

In the setting of chronic kidney disease (CKD) or end-stage kidney disease (ESKD), DOACs have been increasingly used in clinical practice and observational data suggest that these agents have comparable efficacy with reduced bleeding in this setting.[52-54] It is important to note that the US and European prescribing information, which provides dosing guidance for rivaroxaban, apixaban, and edoxaban, is based on pharmacodynamic data without any clinical outcome data.[55] Data remains limited for other special populations, such as those with morbid obesity (body mass index >40 kg/m² or weight >120 kg), and available guidelines recommend against the use of DOACs in the absence of randomized trials for this population.[56]

Advanced therapies including thrombolysis and inferior vena cava filter (IVC filter) placement may be considered in specific scenarios, although in general these treatments are recommended only on a case-by-case assessment. For patients with a contraindication to anticoagulation, IVC filter placement may be considered for the prevention of PE.[6,21] However, a recent randomized trial failed to demonstrate any benefit for the use of retrievable IVC filters in patients receiving concomitant treatment with anticoagulation or thrombolysis,[57] and the most recent guidelines do not recommend routine use in this setting.[6,21] Catheter-directed thrombolysis (CDT) and mechanical thrombectomy are typically reserved for patients with occlusive ilio-femoral DVT and symptoms ≤14 days duration. CDT is used in this setting to correct the outflow obstruction, rapidly relieve patient symptoms, and prevent the complication of the post thrombotic syndrome (PTS).[21] However, the data for use of CDT to prevent PTS is limited to small and/or nonrandomized studies.[58-61] A large randomized trial entitled "Acute Venous Thrombosis: Thrombus Removal With Adjunctive Catheter-Directed Thrombolysis (ATTRACT)" demonstrated no difference in PTS in patients with iliac, femoral, and/or popliteal DVT receiving CDT in addition to anticoagulation, but higher rates of bleeding.[62] A subgroup analysis of this trial evaluated 391 patients with acute iliofemoral DVT (56% of the original trial population), and confirmed no difference in rates of PTS; however, pain severity and severity of PTS was reduced acutely within 30 days, as well as out to 24 months follow-up in patients that underwent CDT.[63]

Phlegmasia Cerulea Dolens

Phlegmasia cerulea dolens (PCD) is the most severe manifestation of DVT and occurs when there is near-total venous outflow obstruction of the lower extremity, resulting in limb ischemia.[64] In most patients with ileofemoral DVT, the superficial veins remain open and collaterals develop so that venous outflow is sufficient to allow arterial perfusion to be unaffected. However, in PCD, not only are the main veins thrombosed but the superficial and collateral veins are thrombosed as well. This leads to massive leg swelling resulting in tissue interstitial pressure and venous pressure that is higher than arterial pressure. This may result in venous gangrene in up to 50% of cases.[64] Most patients who develop PCD have an underlying malignancy or heparin-induced thrombocytopenia with thrombosis. Although literature is scarce, associated mortality rates of 25% to 40% are reported and up to 15% to 25% of survivors will require amputation.[64,65] The clinical triad of PCD includes acute limb pain, massive swelling, and cyanosis, which herald a reversible phase of venous occlusion before gangrene sets in (**Fig. 56–4A**). Urgent management is imperative at this phase and may include systemic or catheter-directed thrombolysis,

TABLE 56–4. Various Options for Oral Anticoagulation in the Treatment of VTE

	Warfarin	Dabigatran	Rivaroxaban	Apixaban	Edoxaban
Mechanism of Action	Vitamin K Antagonist	Direct Thrombin Inhibitor	Factor Xa Inhibitor	Factor Xa Inhibitor	Factor Xa Inhibitor
Half-Life	40 h (mean)	12–17 h	5–9h	8–15 h	8–10 h
Cost (30d)	$	$$$	$$$	$$$	$$$
VTE Treatment					
Trial	[35,36][4,5]	RE-COVER[37]	EINSTEIN[38, 39]	AMPLIFY[48]	HOKUSAI-VTE[49]
Heparin Run-in	Yes	Yes	No	No	Yes
Dosing Regimen	2–10 mg/d (INR 2–3)	150 mg BID	Acute VTE: initiate at 15 mg BID × 3 weeks, then 20mg daily for treatment duration	Acute VTE: initiate at 10 mg BID × 7 days, then 5 mg BID for treatment duration	60 mg daily or 30 mg daily[a]
Recurrent VTE (DOAC vs warfarin)		2.4% vs 2.1% $P < 0.001$ (noninferiority)	2.1% vs 3.0% $P < 0.001$[38] 2.1% vs 1.8% $P = 0.003$[39] (noninferiority)	2.3% vs 2.7% RR 0.84 CI 0.6–1.18 $P < 0.001$ (noninferiority)	3.2% vs 3.5% HR 0.89, CI 0.7–1.13, $P < 0.001$ (noninferiority)
Major Bleeding (DOAC vs warfarin)		1.6% vs 1.9% HR 0.82, CI 0.45–1.48	0.8% vs 1.2% $P = 0.21$[38]; 1.1% vs 2.2% $P = 0.003$[39,8]	0.6% vs 1.8% RR 0.31 CI 0.17–0.55 $P < 0.001$ (superiority)	1.4% vs 1.6% HR 0.84, CI 0.59–1.21
Special Populations					
CrCl <30 ml/min	No dose adjustment	Not recommended	No dose adjustment[c]	No dose adjustment	30 mg daily
Recurrent VTE vs LMWH in Cancer-related Thrombosis[42–44]	4 % (dalteparin) vs 11% (warfarin); $P = 0.002$		4% (rivaroxaban) vs 11% (dalteparin); HR 0.43, 95% CI 0.19–0.99, pilot trial	5.6% (apixaban) vs 7.9% (dalteparin), $P < 0.001$ (noninferiority)	12.8% (edoxaban) vs 13.5% (dalteparin), $P < 0.006$ (noninferiority)
Major Bleeding vs LMWH in Cancer-related Thrombosis[42–44]	6% (dalteparin) vs 4% (warfarin), $P = 0.27$		4% (rivaroxaban) vs 13% (dalteparin); HR 3.76, 95% CI 1.63–8.69, pilot trial	3.8% (apixaban) vs 4% (dalteparin) $P = 0.6$	6.9% (edoxaban) vs 4% (dalteparin), $P = 0.04$
Extended Treatment of VTE[b]					
Trial	PREVENT[45]	RE-SONATE and RE-MEDY[46]	EINSTEIN-CHOICE[47]	AMPLIFY-EXT[40]	NA
Dosing Regimen	2–10 mg/day (INR 1.5–2) vs placebo	Dabigatran 150 mg BID vs warfarin or placebo	Rivaroxaban (10 mg daily or 20 mg daily) vs aspirin	Apixaban (2.5 mg BID or 5 mg BID) vs placebo	
Recurrent VTE (OAC vs control)	2.6 vs 7.2 (per 100 person-yr) HR 0.36 CI 0.19–0.67 $P < 0.001$	0.4% vs 5.6% and 1.8% vs 1.3% $P = 0.03$	1.2% (10 mg) and 1.5% (20 mg) vs 4.4% $P < 0.001$ (superiority)	1.7% (2.5 mg) and 1.7% (5 mg) vs 8.8% $P < 0.001$ (superiority)	
Major Bleeding (OAC vs control)	0.4 vs 0.9 (per 100 person-yr) HR 2.53 CI 0.49–13.03 $P = 0.25$	0.3% vs 0.0% and 0.9% vs 1.8% $P = 0.06$	0.4% (10 mg) and 0.5% (20 mg) vs 0.3% $P = 0.32$	0.2% (2.5 mg) and 0.1% (5 mg) vs 0.5% RR (2.5 mg vs control) 0.49, CI 0.09–2.64 RR (5 mg vs control) 0.25, CI 0.03–2.24	

Abbreviations: BID, twice daily; CI, confidence interval; HR, hazard ratio; LMWH, low-molecular-weight heparin; RR, risk ratio; VTE, venous thromboembolism.

[a]Patients with body weight below 60 kg or a creatinine clearance of 30–50 mL per minute, as well as patients who were receiving P-glycoprotein inhibitors (ie, verapamil, quinidine) received 30 mg edoxaban instead of 60 mg daily.

[b]Patients with VTE completed at least 3 months of planned anticoagulation prior to study enrollment.

[c]European guidelines suggest dose adjustment to rivaroxaban 15 mg daily for CrCl 15–29 ml/min.

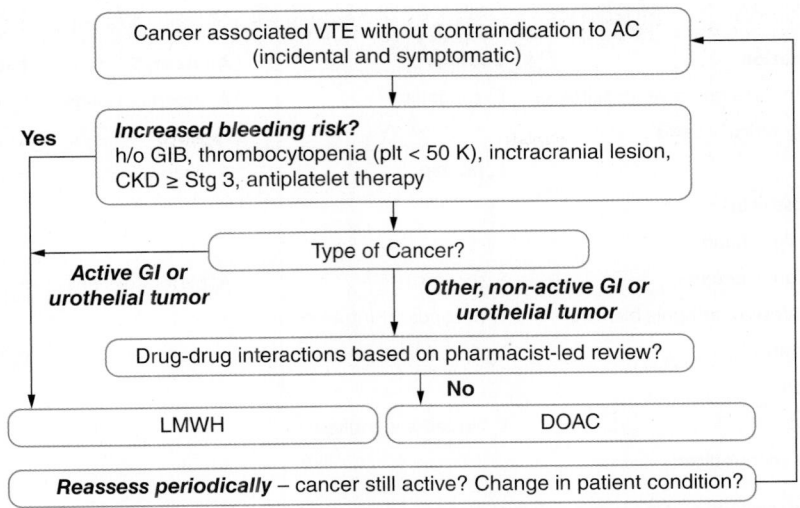

Figure 56–3. Treatment algorithm for cancer-associated venous thromboembolism. Adapted with permission from Carrier M, Blais N, Crowther M, et al. Treatment algorithm in cancer-associated thrombosis: Canadian expert consensus. *Curr Oncol.* 2018 Oct;25(5):329-337.

mechanical or surgical thrombectomy with or without fasciotomy, or a combination of these modalities in addition to systemic anticoagulation.[65–67] The characteristic changes of gangrene begin distally and move proximal as ischemia progresses (**Fig. 56–4B**).

SARS-CoV2 and Venous Thrombosis

SARS-CoV2 is a novel coronavirus that originated in Wuhan, China, in the fall of 2019. It was first reported to the World Health Organization (WHO) on December 31, 2019.[68] In February 2020, the WHO named the disease COVID-19. The understanding of the distinct pathophysiology, natural history,

and treatment of this viral pandemic is a rapidly evolving field, but the current understanding is that the SARS-CoV2 virus binds angiotensin converting enzyme-2 receptors throughout the body. In the majority of patients, a mild-to-moderate respiratory illness results, but some patients experience a systemic inflammatory illness characterized by multiorgan failure with profound cytokinemia.[69] The hypoxia related to the respiratory syndrome, and the massive inflammatory response, create an environment ripe for coagulopathy and thrombosis.[70,71] Series from China, Europe, and the United States have demonstrated high rates of VTE in patients hospitalized with COVID-19 and support a role for aggressive anticoagulation.[72–80] At present,

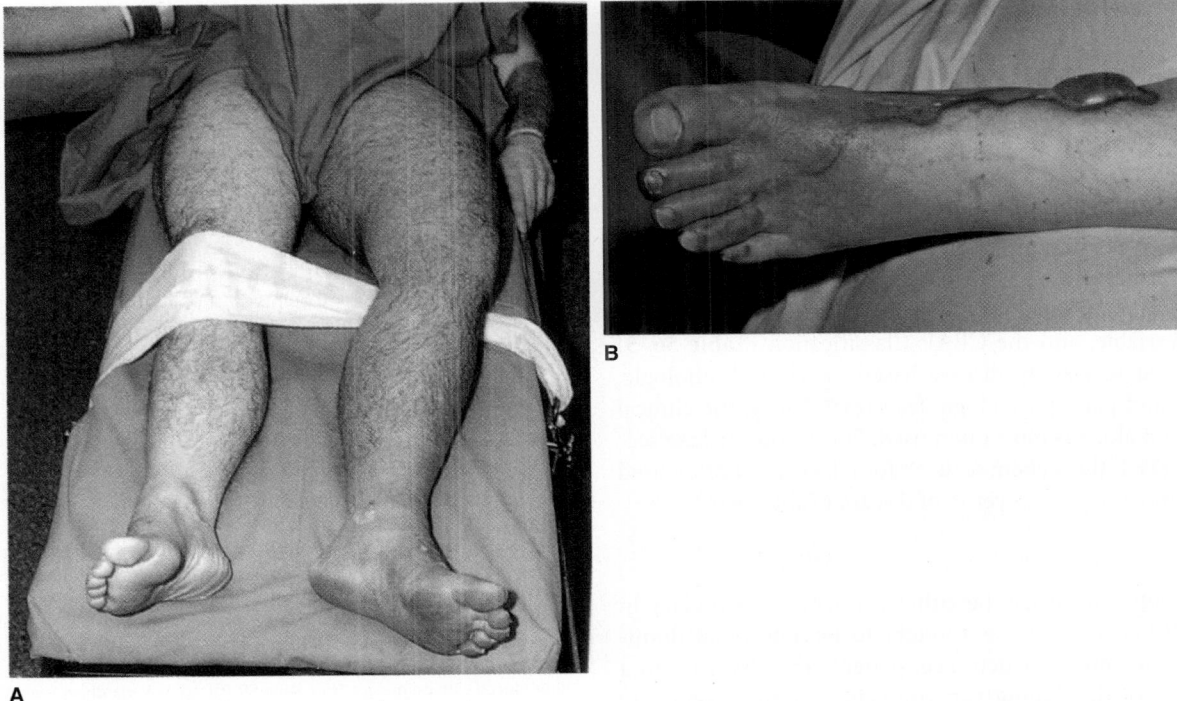

Figure 56–4. Phlegmasia cerulea dolens (A), a life and limb-threatening emergency that heralds venous gangrene (B).

TABLE 56–5. The 2020 Revision of CEAP[a]

	Clinical Presentation	Etiology	Anatomy[b]	Pathophysiology
C_0	No visible of palpable signs of venous disease	E_c congenital	A_s superficial veins	P_r reflux
C_1	Telangiectasia, or reticular veins			
C_2	Varicose veins	E_p primary	A_d deep veins	P_o obstruction
C_{2r}	Recurrent varicose veins			
C_3	Edema without skin changes			
C_{4a}	Skin pigmentation or eczema	E_s secondary	A_p perforator veins	$P_{r,O}$ reflux and obstruction
C_{4b}	Lipodermatosclerosis or atrophie blanche	E_{si} Secondary - intravenous		
C_{4C}	Corona phlebectatica	E_{se} Secondary – extravenous		P_n No pathophysiology identified
C_5	Healed ulceration			
C_6	Active ulceration	E_n No cause identified		
C_{6r}	Recurrent active venous ulcer			

[a]Each category is scored independently of the others. For example, with this scheme, a patient with postphlebitic syndrome, an active venous ulcer, and hemodynamic evidence of reflux but no obstruction is scored as $C_6 E_s A_D P_R$. A patient with telangiectasias and no other symptoms or findings is $C_2 E_P A_S$.
[b]The complete anatomy classification also identifies the venous segment(s) involved.
CEAP, clinical manifestation, etiologic factor, anatomic involvement, and pathophysiology feature.
Adapted with permission from Lurie F, Passman M, Meisner M, et al. The 2020 update of the CEAP classification system and reporting standards. *J Vasc Surg Venous Lymphat Disord.* 2020 May;8(3):342-352.

expert consensus and guidelines recommend weight-adjusted or intermediate dose thromboprophylaxis with enoxaparin in patients admitted with COVID-19; however, some advocate for full dose anticoagulation in the sickest patients.[81–83] Additionally, the massive inflammatory response to SARS-CoV2 suggests there may be a role for immune modulator therapy such as interleukin-6 inhibitors or complement inhibition.[71,84] A number of ongoing clinical trials will hopefully provide clarity on best practice for patients with COVID-19 (NCT04406389, NCT04412291, NCT04345848, NCT04367831, NCT04373707, NCT04366960, NCT04416048, NCT04372589, NCT04391179, NCT04368377, NCT04408235, NCT04356833, NCT04412304, NCT04394000, NCT04359277).

VENOUS INSUFFICIENCY

Venous insufficiency occurs as a result of inadequate venous outflow due to incompetent venous valves or obstruction. It is estimated that up 25% of the adult population in the United States and Western Europe have varicose veins, and cross-sectional studies demonstrate that >50% of the population have some clinical manifestations of venous disease.[85–87] The presentation is variable, and the CEAP Classification (**Table 56–5**) is often used to classify disease based on clinical, etiologic, anatomic, and pathophysiologic features.[88] Today, the clinical classification alone is most often used. For venous disease secondary to DVT, the Villalta scale[89,90] for PTS is most often used to define and grade the severity of disease (**Table 56–6**).[89,91,92]

Etiology, Risk Factors, and Presentation

Venous insufficiency may be either primary or secondary in etiology. Primary disease is thought to be autosomal dominant with incomplete penetrance; patients may have up to a 90% chance of developing varicose veins if both parents are affected.[93] No candidate genes have been identified; however,

familial studies in twins confirm a heritable influence on the development of disease.[94] Additional risk factors include female sex, obesity, prolonged standing, multiparity, and age.[95,96] Secondary causes of venous insufficiency include the PTS related to DVT or increased hydrostatic pressure as in heart failure. The clinical signs and symptoms are widely varied and may range

TABLE 56–6. Villalta Post-Thrombotic Syndrome Scale

Symptoms and Clinical Signs	None	Mild	Moderate	Severe
Symptoms				
Pain	0 points	1 point	2 points	3 points
Cramps	0 points	1 point	2 points	3 points
Heaviness	0 points	1 point	2 points	3 points
Paresthesia	0 points	1 point	2 points	3 points
Pruritis	0 points	1 point	2 points	3 points
Clinical Signs				
Pretibial Edema	0 points	1 point	2 points	3 points
Skin Induration	0 points	1 point	2 points	3 points
Hyperpigmentation/ Erythema	0 points	1 point	2 points	3 points
Venous Ectasia	0 points	1 point	2 points	3 points
Pain on Calf Compression	0 points	1 point	2 points	3 points
Venous Ulcer	Absent	Present		

Points are summed into a total (range 0–33). PTS is defined as a score ≥5 or the presence of a venous ulcer. PTS is classified as *mild* if score is 5–9, *moderate* if score is 9–14, and *severe* if the score is ≥15 or a venous ulcer is present. To use the Villalta score as a continuous measure, it is recommended that those with severe PTS based solely on the presence of a venous ulcer (ie, total Villalta score <15) should be assigned a score of 15.[19]
Reproduced with permission from Kahn SR, Partsch H, Vedantham S, et al. Definition of post-thrombotic syndrome of the leg for use in clinical investigations: a recommendation for standardization. *J Thromb Haemost.* 2009 May;7(5):879-883.

from cosmetic complaints such as spider veins and asymptomatic varicose veins to painful varicosities, edema, skin hyperpigmentation, lipodermatosclerosis, and ulceration.[1,95] A large proportion of patients may live indefinitely without symptoms related to their venous disease; however, the more severe manifestations like ulceration have a poor overall prognosis when present, with frequently delayed healing times and a high risk of recurrent ulceration.[97] Medical costs related to the management of venous disease in the United States are estimated to be upward of $1 billion annually.[1,95] Additional indirect costs may be incurred due to missed workdays related to leg symptoms of chronic venous insufficiency often described as bursting, leg

fullness and heaviness, burning, cramping, pruritis, and restlessness.[98,99] Symptoms are exacerbated by prolonged standing and dependency, as well as during pregnancy or other volume overload states. Leg elevation typically relieves the symptoms.

Diagnosis and Treatment

The diagnosis of chronic venous insufficiency is often clinical because the characteristic skin changes and symptoms readily expose the disease. Skin hyperpigmentation is due to hemosiderin deposition resulting from long-standing venous hypertension (**Figs. 56–5A** and **56–5B**). Venous hypertension

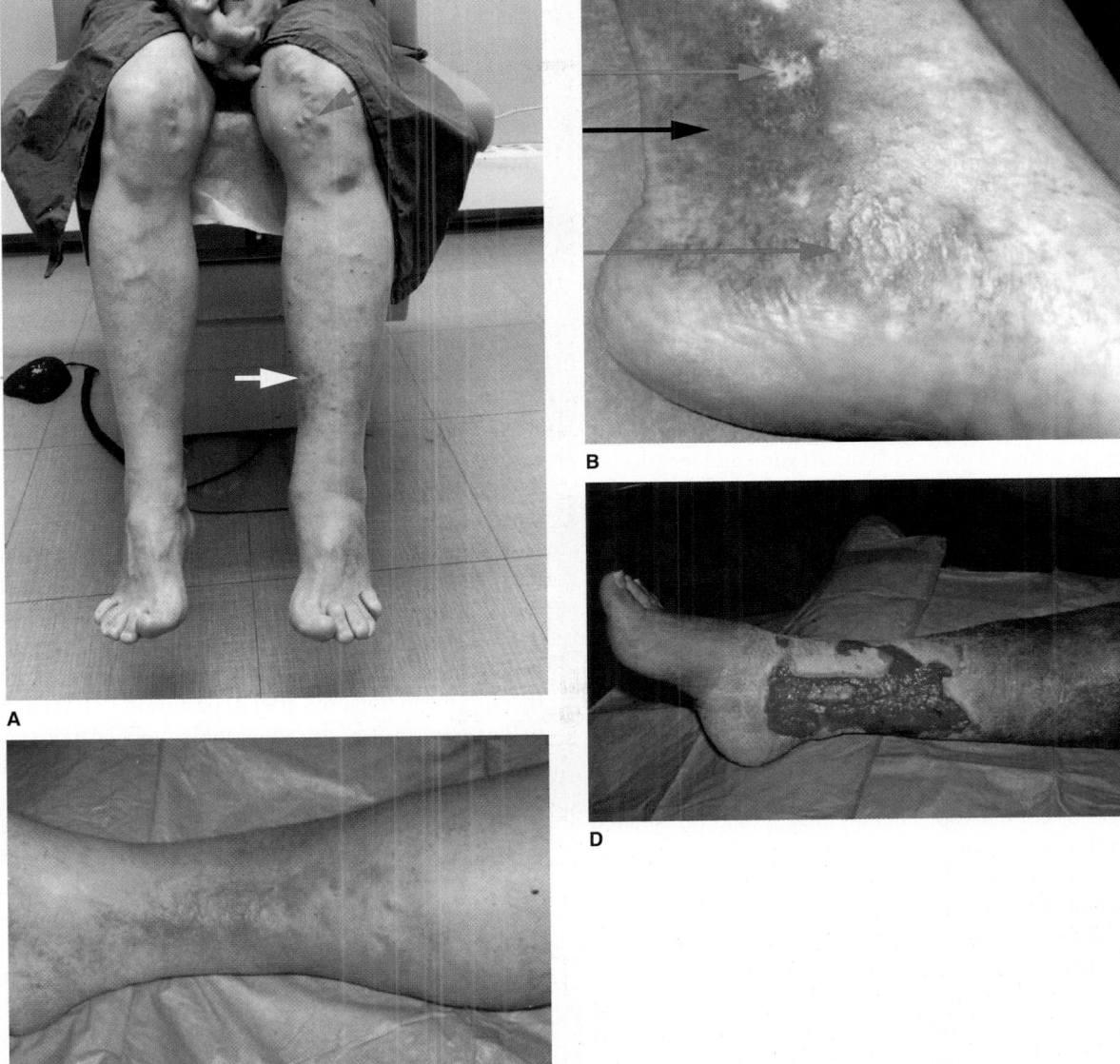

Figure 56–5. Chronic venous insufficiency and venous ulcerations. (A) The legs are swollen with visible large varicose veins (*red arrow*). There is stasis pigmentation (*white arrow*) present. **(B)** This patient has three findings often present in patients with venous insufficiency: stasis pigmentation (*black arrow*), atrophie blanche (*red arrow*), corona phlebectatica (*blue arrow*). **(C)** Lipodermatosclerosis, stasis associated panniculitis. **(D)** Typical venous ulcer located on the medial aspect of the leg. The ulcer bed is beefy red with healthy granulation tissue; these ulcers are typically wet and drain serous fluid. Edema control is the most important measure to heal these ulcerations. B, Reproduced with permission from Steven Dean, D.O., Ohio State School of Medicine.

causes edema that leads to transudation of interstitial fluid and hemosiderin in the skin and subcutaneous space. The swelling may occur in any part of the leg below the knee while stasis pigmentation and stasis dermatitis usually is present on and above the medial malleolus. If this remains untreated (lack of compression), lipodermatosclerosis and venous ulceration may occur (**Figs. 56–5C** and **56–5D**). In lipodermatosclerosis, the skin is indurated and fibrotic with more extensive pigmentation and erythema. Lipodermatosclerosis is a stasis-associated panniculitis that may mimic acute bacterial cellulitis. In its most severe form, the leg has the appearance of a "bowling pin" or "inverted champagne bottle." For most patients with venous insufficiency, conservative management including compression therapy and good skin care are mainstay. We advise that our patients keep the feet clean, dry, and well moisturized to prevent any skin breakdown or seeding of a potential infectious nidus that may complicate the disease. Control of edema is also imperative, because the excess fluid in the legs is a setup for poor wound healing in the case of venous ulceration. Compression therapy has been used for over 2000 years as treatment of chronic venous insufficiency.[100] The goals of compression therapy include (1) reduction of limb size by alteration of the venous pressure gradient and improved effectiveness of the muscle pump, (2) maintaining the limb at the smallest possible size, and (3) prevention of the complications of venous insufficiency.[100] Initially, compression wraps are recommended to achieve a reduction in limb size because the wraps may be adjusted to the ever-decreasing limb girth, day to day. Once edema control is achieved, a compression garment or stocking may be used to maintain edema control. Compression garments come in different grades of compression and lengths (ie, knee-thigh, thigh-high, pantyhose). The most important area of compression is below the knee, where the standing venous pressure is greatest.[1] Most patients with varicose veins and venous insufficiency will require compression of 20 to 30 mm Hg, and some 30 to 40 mm Hg, for control. For those with an ulcer related to venous insufficiency, 30 to 40 mm Hg compression is usually needed. In patients with more severe disease related to lymphedema, compression therapy in the 40 to 50 mm Hg grade is recommended.[1,100] For patients who are morbidly obese, they may need custom-made stockings in which the compression can be specified (ie, 40 mm Hg). There is one aspect of compression therapy that should be adhered to: never put a compression garment on a swollen leg. These stockings do not reduce the amount of edema present, they merely prevent it from worsening. Thus, wraps as described above should first be used. When the edema is improved, the patient should be measured by a certified fitter for a stocking. The patient should be instructed to put the stocking on in the morning and take it off at night. Four to five pairs of stockings usually last 1 year before they lose their compression.

Venous Ulcers

Venous ulcers are the most common leg ulceration and the most severe manifestation of venous disease (Fig. 56–5D). Up to 10% of patients in the United States living with venous insufficiency have a healed or active venous ulcer (CEAP Class 5–6 disease).[87,101] Despite the fact that most patients are treated in the outpatient setting, the per-patient cost of venous ulcer management is estimated to be $2500 per month.[102,103] This reflects the high intensity of care needed to manage these ulcerations, including wound care supplies, medications, patient education, facility costs, vascular testing, and provider reimbursements. For patients with a healed venous ulcer, up to 50% will experience a recurrence in their lifetime, primarily due to noncompliance with compression garments.

The evaluation of a venous ulcer should include a thorough medical history and physical assessment, including area and depth measurements of the ulcer. A number of medical conditions are associated with leg ulcers, and these should be excluded.[103] Venous ulcers are generally wet, with good granulation tissue and localize to the gaiter area of the leg with a predilection for the medial and malleoli (Fig. 56–5D). In contrast, arterial (ischemic) ulcers are extremely painful and often located distally (tip of toes, over pressure points). Unlike venous ulcers, they are dry and have a dark eschar because of lack of blood supply. Treatment involves revascularization and wound care. Neurotrophic ulcers (often referred to as diabetic ulcers) occur over pressure points on the foot (metatarsal area, toes, heel) and have the appearance of an open ulcer surrounded by callous. This type of ulcer occurs in patients with a peripheral neuropathy (most often from diabetes) because the patient cannot feel that they are putting abnormal pressure over a specific area. This ulcer is the most common ulcer to lead to osteomyelitis and amputation of the toe, foot, or leg. Treatment of this type of ulcer involves investigation (and treatment) for osteomyelitis, debriding the abnormal callous that is present and fitting for a shoe that will unload this area of abnormal weight bearing.

Once venous disease is confirmed, compression therapy with wound care is the foundation of venous ulcer treatment. However, four cardinal tenets (**Table 56–7**) promote wound healing, and in the setting of an active ulcer each should be considered and optimized. Notably, up to 26% of patients with a lower extremity ulcer have both peripheral artery (PAD) and venous disease, which may limit their tolerance of compression therapy due to impaired arterial perfusion.[104] PAD is diagnosed in the presence of an abnormal ankle-brachial index (ABI <0.9), and PAD may be severe with an ABI <0.5.[105] Above this threshold (ABI >0.5), or absolute ankle pressure >60 mm Hg, inelastic compression may be tolerated up 40 mm Hg without impaired arterial perfusion.[103,104,106] Below this threshold, modified compression and/or revascularization may be necessary to achieve wound healing. We favor adjustable compression devices (ie, ACE wraps, Profore® 4-layer wrap, Unna boot, etc.) over compression garments (ie, stockings) when treating an active ulcer in order to optimize edema control, as well as to allow for a clean wound care supplies that are regularly turned over. Multilayer compression is superior to single-layer compression for the promotion of ulcer healing.[103,107] There is limited evidence regarding the use of intermittent pneumatic compression as an alternative to compression therapy, and in general this modality is not preferred. Once ulcer healing is achieved, continued edema control with compression garments and good skin care should be optimized to minimize the risk of recurrence.

TABLE 56-7. The Cardinal Tenets of Venous Ulcer Healing

1. Edema control: this is the most important aspect of care. Without adequate control of edema, the ulcer will not heal
2. Assure adequate arterial perfusion
3. Good skin care in the nonulcerated areas of the leg
4. Put a nonirritating dressing (ie, saline wet to dry, Profore 4-layer wrap, Unna Boot) on the ulcer itself.

The main body of evidence surrounding the pharmacology of venous disease and venous ulcers includes pentoxifylline and the saposides (horse chestnut seed extracts). Horse chestnut seed (*Aesculus hippocastanum L.*) is thought to inhibit enzymes, such as hyaluronidase, which are activated by accumulated leukocytes in limbs affected by chronic venous disease, thereby reducing associated leg edema and pain although long-term safety and efficacy has not been established.[108] In a Cochrane review examining the use of horse chestnut seed extract for the prevention of PTS, no improvement in symptoms of PTS was observed.[109] Pentoxifylline has been studied in the treatment of advanced venous disease and may promote venous ulcer healing via its anti inflammatory properties and rheolytic activities.[110] Several trials suggest modestly improved healing rates with pentoxifylline, although the magnitude of effect is small and its role in the treatment of venous disease is unclear.[111-114] Diuretics are not useful to control limb swelling related to venous insufficiency in the absence of another cause of systemic edema (ie, heart failure, nephrotic syndrome, advanced liver disease).

Duplex Ultrasonography in Chronic Venous Insufficiency

For patients in whom therapies beyond conservative measures may be considered, such as recurrent venous ulceration or painful varicosities despite a trial of compression therapy, duplex ultrasonography is standard for evaluation. The goal of the exam is to define the anatomy and malfunctioning veins, as well as the extent of insufficiency. By consensus standards, evaluation should include the vein diameters, location and competence of all saphenous junctions, perforating veins, and source veins of superficial varices.[115,116] The deep veins are also evaluated for competence, anatomy, and the presence of an obstructive lesion.[115] In addition to the maneuvers discussed in the evaluation for obstruction or DVT, the duplex exam for venous insufficiency includes provocative maneuvers to unmask abnormal reversal of flow in the vein. Normal valve mechanics include a period of proximal antegrade flow with calf muscle contraction followed by flow reversal, which leads to a reversal of the transvalvular gradient and allows for vein valve closure. Clinically relevant reflux can be measured as prolonged flow reversal. The vein is interrogated with color-Doppler and spectral waveform analysis; incompetence is demonstrated as retrograde flow occurring above the baseline (**Fig. 56-6A**).[116] The Valsalva maneuver is performed by asking the patient to bear down, thereby increasing intrathoracic pressure and potentially reversing the transvalvular gradient. The Parana maneuver is more widely used outside of the United States, and works to initiate calf compression by having the patient stand and lean slightly forward and backward.[116] Compression of the proximal limb and release of the distal limb, either manually or with standardized pressure cuffs, also work to disturb and test the normal resting pressure gradient across the valves. All maneuvers may be performed with the patient supine and standing to reveal otherwise subtle reflux disease. The majority of normal valves will close within 0.5 seconds of a maneuver, although the defined normal duration is shorter in perforating veins (<0.35 seconds) and longer in the deeper venous segments (>1 second).[117] While flow may also be detected by color-flow Doppler analysis, the duration of reflux may be underestimated as compared to measurement of flow via the spectral waveform.[118]

Other Noninvasive Testing

Physiologic testing with plethysmography relies on volume change in the limb due to venous outflow or reflux disease. The most common techniques are strain gauge plethysmography, air plethysmography, and impedance plethysmography (IPG). IPG is the best-studied technique, and useful for the evaluation of venous outflow obstruction (ie, DVT) as well as venous insufficiency.[119,120] To evaluate for venous insufficiency, the legs are raised to empty the veins followed by rapid lowering of the legs. If there is incompetence, blood rushes retrograde from the proximal veins into the calves resulting in volume increase.[121] If in the superficial veins only, application of a light tourniquet around the legs will normalize the refilling time. Exercise plethysmography assesses ejection of blood by the calf pump as well as the subsequent refilling of the lower extremities. Unlike the duplex ultrasound assessment, these modalities do not precisely localize the level of disease and most vascular laboratories do not perform these physiologic tests.

Advanced Treatments

For patients with lifestyle limiting symptoms or complications related to venous insufficiency, advanced therapies to ablate the offending veins may be considered.[122] There is variability in insurance requirements for these procedures, although most plans will consider advanced therapies for those patients that have failed a period of conservative therapy. The techniques to treat venous insufficiency depend upon the size and location of the veins, patient preference, and etiology of their disease. To date, endovenous procedures such as laser therapy or radiofrequency ablation are most often used for treatment of reflux in the GSV and SSV.[1,123-125] Both modalities use a thermal source to cause injury to the vein wall, which leads to vein occlusion. The procedures are performed under ultrasound guidance, and often in the outpatient setting, with only local anesthesia and instillation of perivenous tumescent anesthesia, which serves to encase the vein and protect adjacent structures from the heat source. During the procedure, a mixture of normal saline with lidocaine is infiltrated into the saphenous sheath under ultrasound guidance to create tumescence. Distal access is obtained (**Fig. 56-6B**) and the catheter is tip is positioned ~2 cm from the sapheno-femoral junction. The vein is then ablated in a retrograde fashion with withdrawal of the active

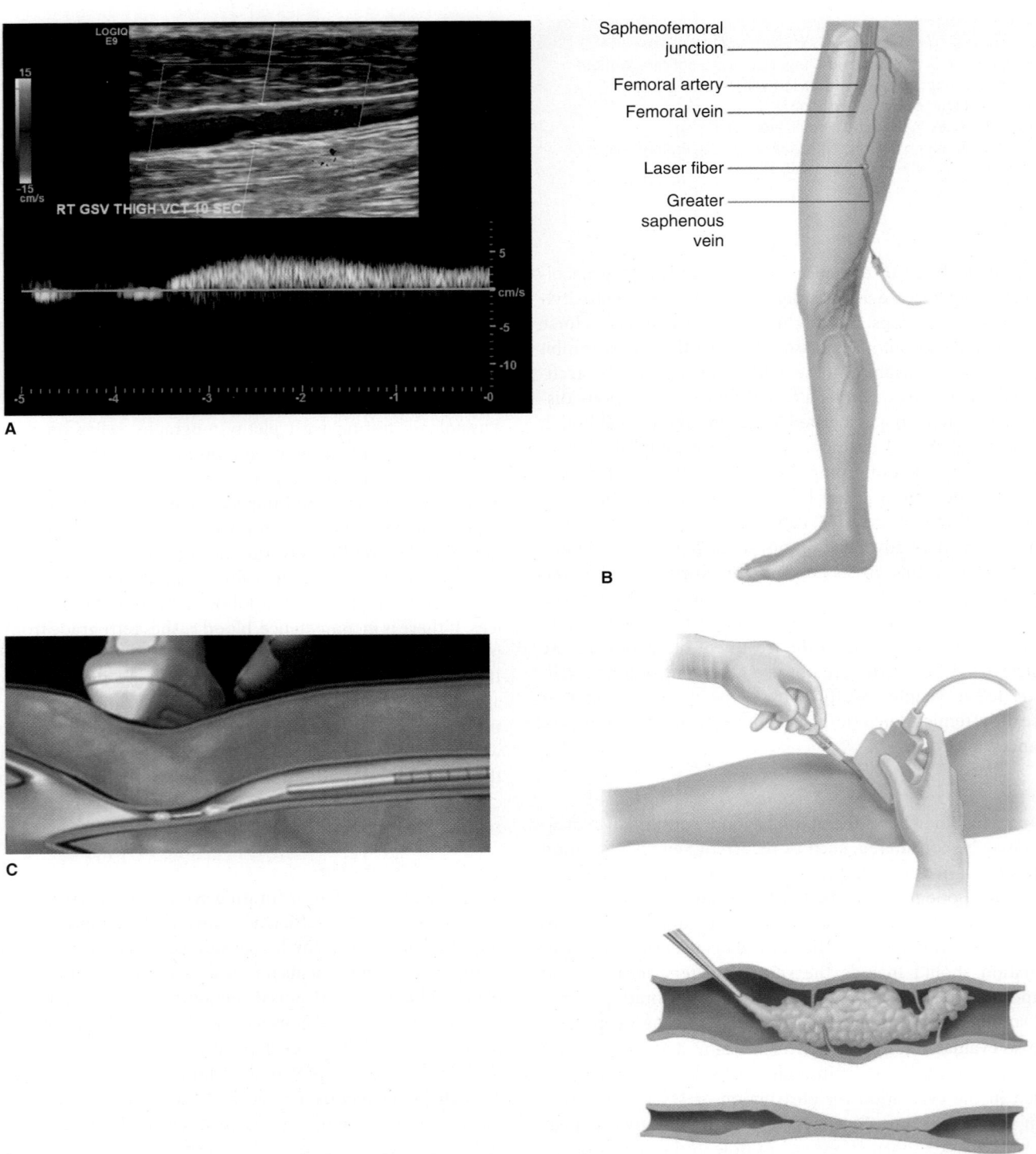

Figure 56–6. Invasive treatments for varicose veins and chronic venous insufficiency. (A) Spectral waveform analysis demonstrating retrograde flow with a valve closure time of 10 seconds at the sapheno-femoral junction consistent with venous insufficiency. **(B)** Endovenous ablation involves treatment of the GSV with a laser fiber that is introduced via the distal GSV. The entire segment is treated from 2 cm distal to the saphenofemoral junction to the distal puncture site. **(C)** Endovenous cyanoacrylate glue application in the GSV with external manual compression to facilitate closure. **(D)** Sclerotherapy of varicose veins under ultrasound guidance. Sclerosing agent is directly injected into the varicose vein resulting in vein occlusion and obliteration.

laser fiber. The patient is placed in graduated compression wraps or stockings for at least 2 weeks. Postprocedure, all patients should return within a 48- to 72-hour period for an office clinical assessment and a duplex ultrasound exam to evaluate the result and exclude the complication of DVT. Additional potential complications may include paresthesia, skin burns, thrombophlebitis, and transient pain or bruising.[126] Recently, mechanochemical endovenous ablation techniques have emerged in lieu of thermal therapies of the GSV and SSV, and this therapy does not require infiltration with perivenous tumescence.[127] The technique uses a rotational wire that induces vein spasm while infusing a chemical sclerosing agent to ablate the vein. The studies available to date report high short-term occlusion rates with lower reported pain scores in patients receiving mechanochemical endovenous therapies as compared to thermal ablation, although the long-term outcomes are not yet known.[128,129] Endovenous cyanoacrylate glue has also been compared to thermal ablation with noninferior efficacy of long-term vein closure at 36 months follow-up and similar safety profile.[130] The benefit of this therapy is it is a nonthermal and

nontumescent proprietary microfoam that does not require a sclerosant (**Fig. 56–6C**).

Chemical ablation with sclerosing agents is an alternative to thermal therapies, without the mechanical counterpart described above, most often for the treatment of varicose veins and larger spider veins. A variety of agents are available including hypertonic saline, glycerin, polidocanol, and sodium tetradecyl sulfate, which cause endothelial damage and subsequent thrombosis and fibrosis of the treated veins (**Fig. 56–6D**).[1,122] Complications may include hyperpigmentation or staining, due to extravasation of the agent with hemosiderin deposition into the surrounding skin, as well as allergic reactions, matting and rarely cutaneous ulceration. Most patients achieve a cosmetic improvement initially, although with a high risk of recurrence in their lifetime.[1]

Vein stripping and phlebectomy or microphlebectomy procedures are less often used today due to the prolific availability of less invasive procedures with lower pain rates and good success. However, surgery may still be preferred in patients with very superficial veins (which carry a higher potential for

TABLE 56–8. Comparison of Available Guidelines for the Management of Venous Thromboembolism

	Categorizing VTE to Guide Anticoagulation	Anticoagulation Duration and Extended Therapy	Treatment of Cancer-Related VTE	DOACs in Obesity (BMI >40 kg/m² or weight >120 kg)
American College of Chest Physicians (2016)	VTE classified as provoked vs unprovoked[21]	Favor ≥6 months anticoagulation in unprovoked iliofemoral DVT or PE Favor >3 months anticoagulation in unprovoked proximal DVT or PE if low-moderate bleeding risk[21]	LMWH favored over warfarin and DOACs[21]	NA
International Society of Thrombosis and Haemostasis	VTE classified as provoked with transient risk factor, provoked with persistent risk factor vs unprovoked[34]	Favor extended therapy regimens >3 months for patients without identifiable risk factors or high bleeding risk[34]	Rivaroxaban or edoxaban may be an alternative to LMWH in patients with low bleeding risk[50]	Should not be used in obese patients; if used, recommend checking drug-specific peak and trough levels[56]
Thrombosis Canada Expert Consensus (2018)			DOACs favored in patients with low bleeding risk, depending on type of cancer and pharmacist-led review of drug-drug interactions[51]	
European Society of Cardiology, European Respiratory Society (2020)[6]	Risk factors for VTE recurrence are classified as low, intermediate or high risk (Table 56–1)	Favor extended therapy regimens >3 months for patients without identifiable risk factors or persistent risk factors	Rivaroxaban or edoxaban may be an alternative to LMWH in patients with low bleeding risk	NA

US labeling for DOACs VTE Treatment			European labeling for DOACs for VTE Treatment	
	CrCl 15–29 mL/min	CrCl 30–50 mL/min	CrCl 15–29 mL/min	CrCl 30–50 mL/min
Dabigatran	Not recommended	150 mg twice a day	Not recommended	150 mg or 110 mg twice a day
Rivaroxaban	15 mg twice a day × 3 weeks, then 20 mg daily	15 mg twice a day × 3 weeks, then 20 mg daily	15 mg twice a day × 3 weeks, then 20 mg daily	15 mg twice a day × 3 weeks, then 20 mg daily
Apixaban	10 mg twice a day × 1 week, then 5 mg twice a day	10 mg twice a day × 1 week, then 5 mg twice a day	10 mg twice a day × 1 week, then 5 mg twice a day	10 mg twice a day × 1 week, then 5 mg twice a day
Edoxaban	30 mg daily	30 mg daily	30 mg daily	30 mg daily

[a]Consider dose adjustment to 15 mg once daily.
[b]Data from Derebail VK, Rheault MN, Kerlin BA. Role of direct oral anticoagulants in patients with kidney disease. *Kidney Int.* 2020 Apr;97(4):664-675.

skin thermal injury), extremely tortuous veins (which may not allow for passage of a catheter), previous failure of endovenous therapy, or the presence of thrombus.[131]

ACKNOWLEDGMENTS

We would like to thank Dr. Paul W. Wennberg and Dr. Thom W. Rooke, who contributed to a previous version of this chapter in the 13th edition.

REFERENCES

1. Hamdan A. Management of varicose veins and venous insufficiency. *JAMA.* 2012;308(24):2612-2621.

2. Bauer G. Patho-physiology and treatment of the lower leg stasis syndrome. *Angiology.* 1950;1(1):1-8.

3. Kachlik D, Pechacek V, Musil V, Baca V. The deep venous system of the lower extremity: new nomenclature. *Phlebology.* 2012;27(2):48-58.

4. Golviczki P, Mozes G. Development and anatomy of the venous system. In: Golviczki P, ed. *Handbook of Venous Disorders.* 3rd ed. Hodder Arnold; 2009:12-24.

5. Albertsen IE, Piazza G, Goldhaber SZ. Let's stop dichotomizing venous thromboembolism as provoked or unprovoked. *Circulation.* 2018;138(23):2591-2593.

6. Konstantinides SV, Meyer G, Becattini C, et al. 2019 ESC guidelines for the diagnosis and management of acute pulmonary embolism developed in collaboration with the European Respiratory Society (ERS). *Eur Heart J.* 2020;41(4):543-603.

7. Kearon C, Ageno W, Cannegieter SC, et al. Categorization of patients as having provoked or unprovoked venous thromboembolism: guidance from the SSC of ISTH. *J Thromb Haemost.* 2016;14(7):1480-1483.

8. Leon L, Giannoukas AD, Dodd D, Chan P, Labropoulos N. Clinical significance of superficial vein thrombosis. *Eur J Vasc Endovasc Surg.* 2005;29(1):10-17.

9. Marchiori A, Mosena L, Prandoni P. Superficial vein thrombosis: risk factors, diagnosis, and treatment. *Sem Thromb Hemost.* 2006;32(7):737-743.

10. Di Minno MN, Ambrosino P, Ambrosini F, Tremoli E, Minno GD, Dentali F. Prevalence of deep vein thrombosis and pulmonary embolism in patients with superficial vein thrombosis: a systematic review and meta-analysis. *J Thromb Haemost.* 2016.

11. Kearon C, Akl EA, Comerota AJ, et al. Antithrombotic therapy for VTE disease: *Antithrombotic Therapy and Prevention of Thrombosis,* 9th ed: American College of Chest Physicians Evidence-Based Clinical Practice Guidelines. *Chest.* 2012;141(2 Suppl):e419S-e494S.

12. Di Nisio M, Wichers IM, Middeldorp S. Treatment for superficial thrombophlebitis of the leg. *Cochrane Database Syst Rev.* 2013;4:CD004982.

13. Di Nisio M, Middeldorp S. Treatment of lower extremity superficial thrombophlebitis. *JAMA.* 2014;311(7):729-730.

14. Wells PS, Hirsh J, Anderson DR, et al. Accuracy of clinical assessment of deep-vein thrombosis. *Lancet.* 1995;345(8961):1326-1330.

15. Wells PS, Anderson DR, Rodger M, et al. Evaluation of D-dimer in the diagnosis of suspected deep-vein thrombosis. *N Engl J Med.* 2003;349(13):1227-1235.

16. Silveira PC, Ip IK, Goldhaber SZ, Piazza G, Benson CB, Khorasani R. Performance of Wells score for deep vein thrombosis in the inpatient setting. *JAMA Intern Med.* 2015;175(7):1112-1117.

17. Needleman L, Cronan JJ, Lilly MP, et al. Ultrasound for lower extremity deep venous thrombosis: multidisciplinary recommendations from the society of radiologists in ultrasound consensus conference. *Circulation.* 2018;137(14):1505-1515.

18. Dawson DL, Beals H. Acute lower extremity deep vein thrombosis. In: Zierler RE, ed. *Strandness's Duplex Scanning in Vascular Disorders.* 4th ed. Philadelphia, PA: Lippincott Williams & Wilkins, a Wolter Kluwer business; 2010:179-199.

19. Goodacre S, Sampson F, Thomas S, van Beek E, Sutton A. Systematic review and meta-analysis of the diagnostic accuracy of ultrasonography for deep vein thrombosis. *BMC Med Imaging.* 2005;5:6.

20. Birn J, Vedantham S. May-Thurner syndrome and other obstructive iliac vein lesions: meaning, myth, and mystery. *Vasc Med.* 2015;20(1):74-83.

21. Kearon C, Akl EA, Ornelas J, et al. Antithrombotic therapy for VTE disease: CHEST guideline. *Chest.* 2016. doi: 10.1016/j.chest.2015.11.026.

22. Grant JD, Stevens SM, Woller SC, et al. Diagnosis and management of upper extremity deep-vein thrombosis in adults. *Thromb Haemost.* 2012;108(6):1097-1108.

23. Beckman MG, Hooper WC, Critchley SE, Ortel TL. Venous thromboembolism: a public health concern. *Am J Prevent Med.* 2010;38(4 Suppl):S495-S501.

24. Goldhaber SZ, Visani L, De Rosa M. Acute pulmonary embolism: clinical outcomes in the International Cooperative Pulmonary Embolism Registry (ICOPER). *Lancet.* 1999;353(9162):1386-1389.

25. White RH. The epidemiology of venous thromboembolism. *Circulation.* 2003;107(23 Suppl 1):I4-I8.

26. Prandoni P, Lensing AW, Cogo A, et al. The long-term clinical course of acute deep venous thrombosis. *Ann Intern Med.* 1996;125(1):1-7.

27. May R, Thurner J. The cause of the predominantly sinistral occurrence of thrombosis of the pelvic veins. *Angiology.* 1957;8(5):419-427.

28. Kibbe MR, Ujiki M, Goodwin AL, Eskandari M, Yao J, Matsumura J. Iliac vein compression in an asymptomatic patient population. *J Vasc Surg.* 2004;39(5):937-943.

29. Thijs W, Rabe KF, Rosendaal FR, Middeldorp S. Predominance of left-sided deep vein thrombosis and body weight. *J Thromb Haemost.* 2010;8(9):2083-2084.

30. Kucher N. Clinical practice. Deep-vein thrombosis of the upper extremities. *N Engl J Med.* 2011;364(9):861-869.

31. Sundquist K, Wang X, Svensson PJ, et al. Plasminogen activator inhibitor-1 4G/5G polymorphism, factor V Leiden, prothrombin mutations and the risk of VTE recurrence. *Thromb Haemost.* 2015;114(6):1156-1164.

32. Stevens SM, Woller SC, Bauer KA, et al. Guidance for the evaluation and treatment of hereditary and acquired thrombophilia. *J Thromb Thrombolysis.* 2016;41(1):154-164.

33. Hughes MJ, Stein PD, Matta F. Silent pulmonary embolism in patients with distal deep venous thrombosis: systematic review. *Thromb Res.* 2014;134(6):1182-1185.

34. Baglin T, Bauer K, Douketis J, et al. Duration of anticoagulant therapy after a first episode of an unprovoked pulmonary embolus or deep vein thrombosis: guidance from the SSC of the ISTH. *J Thromb Haemost.* 2012;10(4):698-702.

35. Duxbury BM, Poller L. The oral anticoagulant saga: past, present, and future. *Clin App Thromb/Hemost.* 2001;7(4):269-275.

36. Wardrop D, Keeling D. The story of the discovery of heparin and warfarin. *Br J Haematol.* 2008;141(6):757-63.

37. Schulman S, Kearon C, Kakkar AK, et al. Dabigatran versus warfarin in the treatment of acute venous thromboembolism. *N Engl J Med.* 2009;361(24):2342-2352.

38. Investigators E, Bauersachs R, Berkowitz SD, et al. Oral rivaroxaban for symptomatic venous thromboembolism. *N Engl J Med.* 2010;363(26):2499-2510.

39. Investigators E-P, Buller HR, Prins MH, et al. Oral rivaroxaban for the treatment of symptomatic pulmonary embolism. *N Engl J Med.* 2012;366(14):1287-1297.

40. Agnelli G, Buller HR, Cohen A, et al. Apixaban for extended treatment of venous thromboembolism. *N Engl J Med.* 2013;368(8):699-708.

41. Hokusai VTEI, Buller HR, Decousus H, et al. Edoxaban versus warfarin for the treatment of symptomatic venous thromboembolism. *N Engl J Med.* 2013;369(15):1406-1415.

42. Agnelli G, Becattini C, Meyer G, et al. Apixaban for the treatment of venous thromboembolism associated with cancer. *N Engl J Med.* 2020;382(17):1599-1607.

43. Raskob GE, van Es N, Verhamme P, et al. Edoxaban for the treatment of cancer-associated venous thromboembolism. *N Engl J Med.* 2018;378(7):615-624.

44. Young AM, Marshall A, Thirlwall J, et al. Comparison of an oral factor Xa inhibitor with low molecular weight heparin in patients with cancer with venous thromboembolism: results of a randomized trial (SELECT-D). *J Clin Oncol.* 2018;36(20):2017-2023.

45. Ridker PM, Goldhaber SZ, Danielson E, et al. Long-term, low-intensity warfarin therapy for the prevention of recurrent venous thromboembolism. *N Engl J Med.* 2003;348(15):1425-1434.

46. Schulman S, Kearon C, Kakkar AK, et al. Extended use of dabigatran, warfarin, or placebo in venous thromboembolism. *N Engl J Med.* 2013;368(8):709-718.

47. Weitz JI, Lensing AWA, Prins MH, et al. Rivaroxaban or aspirin for extended treatment of venous thromboembolism. *N Engl J Med.* 2017;376(13):1211-1222.

48. Agnelli G, Buller HR, Cohen A, et al. Oral apixaban for the treatment of acute venous thromboembolism. *N Engl J Med.* 2013;369(9):799-808.

49. Posch F, Konigsbrugge O, Zielinski C, Pabinger I, Ay C. Treatment of venous thromboembolism in patients with cancer: a network meta-analysis comparing efficacy and safety of anticoagulants. *Thromb Res.* 2015;136(3):582-589.

50. Khorana AA, Noble S, Lee AYY, et al. Role of direct oral anticoagulants in the treatment of cancer-associated venous thromboembolism: guidance from the SSC of the ISTH. *J Thromb Haemost.* 2018;16(9):1891-1894.

51. Carrier M, Blais N, Crowther M, et al. Treatment algorithm in cancer-associated thrombosis: Canadian expert consensus. *Curr Oncol.* 2018;25(5):329-337.

52. Schafer JH, Casey AL, Dupre KA, Staubes BA. Safety and efficacy of apixaban versus warfarin in patients with advanced chronic kidney disease. *Ann Pharmacother.* 2018;52(11):1078-1084.

53. Siontis KC, Zhang X, Eckard A, et al. Outcomes associated with apixaban use in patients with end-stage kidney disease and atrial fibrillation in the United States. *Circulation.* 2018;138(15):1519-1529.

54. Ha JT, Neuen BL, Cheng LP, et al. Benefits and harms of oral anticoagulant therapy in chronic kidney disease: a systematic review and meta-analysis. *Ann Intern Med.* 2019;171(3):181-189.

55. Derebail VK, Rheault MN, Kerlin BA. Role of direct oral anticoagulants in patients with kidney disease. *Kidney Int.* 2020;97(4):664-675.

56. Martin K, Beyer-Westendorf J, Davidson BL, Huisman MV, Sandset PM, Moll S. Use of the direct oral anticoagulants in obese patients: guidance from the SSC of the ISTH. *J Thromb Haemost.* 2016;14(6):1308-1313.

57. Mismetti P, Laporte S, Pellerin O, et al. Effect of a retrievable inferior vena cava filter plus anticoagulation vs anticoagulation alone on risk of recurrent pulmonary embolism: a randomized clinical trial. *JAMA.* 2015;313(16):1627-1635.

58. Watson LI, Armon MP. Thrombolysis for acute deep vein thrombosis. *Cochrane Database Syst Rev.* 2004;(4):CD002783.

59. Enden T, Klow NE, Sandvik L, et al. Catheter-directed thrombolysis vs. anticoagulant therapy alone in deep vein thrombosis: results of an open randomized, controlled trial reporting on short-term patency. *J Thromb Haemost.* 2009;7(8):1268-1275.

60. Enden T, Haig Y, Klow NE, et al. Long-term outcome after additional catheter-directed thrombolysis versus standard treatment for acute iliofemoral deep vein thrombosis (the CaVenT study): a randomised controlled trial. *Lancet.* 2012;379(9810):31-38.

61. Haig Y, Enden T, Slagsvold CE, Sandvik L, Sandset PM, Klow NE. Determinants of early and long-term efficacy of catheter-directed thrombolysis in proximal deep vein thrombosis. *J Vasc Intervent Radiol.* 2013;24(1):17-24;quiz 6.

62. Vedantham S, Goldhaber SZ, Julian JA, et al. Pharmacomechanical catheter-directed thrombolysis for deep-vein thrombosis. *N Engl J Med.* 2017;377(23):2240-2252.

63. Comerota AJ, Kearon C, Gu CS, et al. Endovascular thrombus removal for acute iliofemoral deep vein thrombosis. *Circulation.* 2019;139(9):1162-1173.

64. Perkins JM, Magee TR, Galland RB. Phlegmasia caerulea dolens and venous gangrene. *Br J Surg.* 1996;83(1):19-23.

65. Chinsakchai K, Ten Duis K, Moll FL, de Borst GJ. Trends in management of phlegmasia cerulea dolens. *Vasc Endovasc Surg.* 2011;45(1):5-14.

66. Dayal R, Bernheim J, Clair DG, et al. Multimodal percutaneous intervention for critical venous occlusive disease. *Ann Vasc Surg.* 2005;19(2):235-240.

67. Klok FA, Huisman MV. Seeking optimal treatment for phlegmasia cerulea dolens. *Thromb Res.* 2013;131(4):372-373.

68. World Health Organization. Coronavirus disease (COVID-19) outbreak situation. https://www.who.int/emergencies/diseases/novel-coronavirus-2019. Accessed on June 5, 2020.

69. Zhou F, Yu T, Du R, et al. Clinical course and risk factors for mortality of adult inpatients with COVID-19 in Wuhan, China: a retrospective cohort study. *Lancet.* 2020;395(10229):1054-1062.

70. Gupta N, Zhao YY, Evans CE. The stimulation of thrombosis by hypoxia. *Thromb Res.* 2019;181:77-83.

71. Magro C, Mulvey JJ, Berlin D, et al. Complement associated microvascular injury and thrombosis in the pathogenesis of severe COVID-19 infection: a report of five cases. *Transl Res.* 2020.

72. Klok FA, Kruip M, van der Meer NJM, et al. Incidence of thrombotic complications in critically ill ICU patients with COVID-19. *Thromb Res.* 2020;191:145-147.

73. Llitjos JF, Leclerc M, Chochois C, et al. High incidence of venous thromboembolic events in anticoagulated severe COVID-19 patients. *J Thromb Haemost.* 2020.

74. Artifoni M, Danic G, Gautier G, et al. Systematic assessment of venous thromboembolism in COVID-19 patients receiving thromboprophylaxis: incidence and role of D-dimer as predictive factors. *J Thromb Thrombolysis.* 2020.

75. Demelo-Rodriguez P, Cervilla-Munoz E, Ordieres-Ortega L, et al. Incidence of asymptomatic deep vein thrombosis in patients with COVID-19 pneumonia and elevated D-dimer levels. *Thrombosis Res.* 2020;192:23-26.

76. Zhang L, Feng X, Zhang D, et al. Deep vein thrombosis in hospitalized patients with coronavirus disease 2019 (COVID-19) in Wuhan, China: prevalence, risk factors, and outcome. *Circulation.* 2020.

77. Wichmann D, Sperhake JP, Lutgehetmann M, et al. Autopsy findings and venous thromboembolism in patients with COVID-19. *Ann Intern Med.* 2020.

78. Lax SF, Skok K, Zechner P, et al. Pulmonary arterial thrombosis in COVID-19 with fatal outcome: results from a prospective, single-center, clinicopathologic case series. *Ann Intern Med.* 2020.

79. Tang N, Bai H, Chen X, Gong J, Li D, Sun Z. Anticoagulant treatment is associated with decreased mortality in severe coronavirus disease 2019 patients with coagulopathy. *J Thromb Haemost.* 2020;18(5):1094-1099.

80. Middeldorp S, Coppens M, van Haaps TF, et al. Incidence of venous thromboembolism in hospitalized patients with COVID-19. *J Thromb Haemost.* 2020.

81. Bikdeli B, Madhavan MV, Jimenez D, et al. COVID-19 and thrombotic or thromboembolic disease: implications for prevention, antithrombotic therapy, and follow-up. *J Am Coll Cardiol.* 2020.

82. Thachil J, Tang N, Gando S, et al. ISTH interim guidance on recognition and management of coagulopathy in COVID-19. *J Thromb Haemost.* 2020;18(5):1023-1026.

83. Spyropoulos AC, Levy JH, Ageno W, et al. Scientific and standardization committee communication: clinical guidance on the diagnosis, prevention and treatment of venous thromboembolism in hospitalized patients with COVID-19. *J Thromb Haemost.* 2020.

84. Campbell CM, Kahwash R. Will complement inhibition be the new target in treating COVID-19-related systemic thrombosis? *Circulation.* 2020;141(22):1739-1741.

85. Callam MJ. Epidemiology of varicose veins. *Br J Surg.* 1994;81(2):167-173.

86. Allan PL, Bradbury AW, Evans CJ, Lee AJ, Vaughan Ruckley C, Fowkes FG. Patterns of reflux and severity of varicose veins in the general population–Edinburgh Vein Study. *Eur J Vasc Endovasc Surg.* 2000;20(5):470-477.

87. Criqui MH, Jamosmos M, Fronek A, et al. Chronic venous disease in an ethnically diverse population: the San Diego Population Study. *Am J Epidemiol.* 2003;158(5):448-456.

88. Lurie F, Passman M, Meisner M, et al. The 2020 update of the CEAP classification system and reporting standards. *J Vasc Surg Venous Lymphat Disord.* 2020;8(3):342-352.

89. Villalta S, Bagatella P, Piccioli A, Lensing A, Prins M, Prandoni P. Assessment of validity and reproducibility of a clinical scale for the post-thrombotic syndrome (abstract). *Haemostasis.* 1994;24:158a.

90. Kahn SR. Measurement properties of the Villalta scale to define and classify the severity of the post-thrombotic syndrome. *J Thromb Haemost.* 2009;7(5):884-888.

91. Kahn SR, Partsch H, Vedantham S, et al. Definition of post-thrombotic syndrome of the leg for use in clinical investigations: a recommendation for standardization. *J Thromb Haemost.* 2009;7(5):879-883.

92. Jayaraj A, Meissner MH. A comparison of Villalta-Prandoni scale and venous clinical severity score in the assessment of post thrombotic syndrome. *Ann Vasc Surg.* 2014;28(2):313-317.

93. Cornu-Thenard A, Boivin P, Baud JM, De Vincenzi I, Carpentier PH. Importance of the familial factor in varicose disease. Clinical study of 134 families. *J Dermatol Surg Oncol.* 1994;20(5):318-326.

94. Brinsuk M, Tank J, Luft FC, Busjahn A, Jordan J. Heritability of venous function in humans. *Arterioscler Thromb Vasc Biol.* 2004;24(1):207-211.

95. Eberhardt RT, Raffetto JD. Chronic venous insufficiency. *Circulation.* 2005;111(18):2398-2409.

96. Criqui MH, Denenberg JO, Bergan J, Langer RD, Fronek A. Risk factors for chronic venous disease: the San Diego Population Study. *J Vasc Surg.* 2007;46(2):331-337.

97. Callam MJ, Harper DR, Dale JJ, Ruckley CV. Chronic ulcer of the leg: clinical history. *Br Med J.* 1987;294(6584):1389-1391.

98. Da Silva A, Navarro MF, Batalheiro J. The importance of chronic venous insufficiency. Various preliminary data on its medico-social consequences. *Phlebologie.* 1992;45(4):439-443.

99. Rabe E, Pannier F. Societal costs of chronic venous disease in CEAP C4, C5, C6 disease. *Phlebology.* 2010;25(Suppl 1):64-67.

100. Felty CL, Rooke TW. Compression therapy for chronic venous insufficiency. *Sem Vasc Surg.* 2005;18(1):36-40.

101. Chiesa R, Marone EM, Limoni C, Volonte M, Schaefer E, Petrini O. Chronic venous insufficiency in Italy: the 24-cities cohort study. *Eur J Vasc Endovasc Surg.* 2005;30(4):422-429.

102. Olin JW, Beusterien KM, Childs MB, Seavey C, McHugh L, Griffiths RI. Medical costs of treating venous stasis ulcers: evidence from a retrospective cohort study. *Vasc Med.* 1999;4(1):1-7.

103. O'Donnell TF, Jr., Passman MA. Clinical practice guidelines of the Society for Vascular Surgery (SVS) and the American Venous Forum (AVF)–Management of venous leg ulcers. Introduction. *J Vasc Surg.* 2014;60 (2 Suppl):1S-2S.

104. Hedayati N, Carson JG, Chi YW, Link D. Management of mixed arterial venous lower extremity ulceration: a review. *Vasc Med.* 2015;20(5):479-486.

105. Aboyans V, Criqui MH, Abraham P, et al. Measurement and interpretation of the ankle-brachial index: a scientific statement from the American Heart Association. *Circulation.* 2012;126(24):2890-2909.

106. Mosti G, Iabichella ML, Partsch H. Compression therapy in mixed ulcers increases venous output and arterial perfusion. *J Vasc Surg.* 2012;55(1):122-128.

107. O'Meara S, Cullum N, Nelson EA, Dumville JC. Compression for venous leg ulcers. *Cochrane Database Syst Rev.* 2012;11:CD000265.

108. Pittler MH, Ernst E. Horse chestnut seed extract for chronic venous insufficiency. *Cochrane Database Syst Rev.* 2012;11:CD003230.

109. Morling JR, Yeoh SE, Kolbach DN. Rutosides for treatment of post-thrombotic syndrome. *Cochrane Database Syst Rev.* 2015;9:CD005625.

110. Pascarella L, Shortell CK. Medical management of venous ulcers. *Sem Vasc Surg.* 2015;28(1):21-28.

111. Jull A, Arroll B, Parag V, Waters J. Pentoxifylline for treating venous leg ulcers. *Cochrane Database Syst Rev.* 2007;(3):CD001733.

112. Nelson EA, Prescott RJ, Harper DR, Gibson B, Brown D, Ruckley CV. A factorial, randomized trial of pentoxifylline or placebo, four-layer or single-layer compression, and knitted viscose or hydrocolloid dressings for venous ulcers. *J Vasc Surg.* 2007;45(1):134-141.

113. Dale JJ, Ruckley CV, Harper DR, Gibson B, Nelson EA, Prescott RJ. Randomised, double blind placebo controlled trial of pentoxifylline in the treatment of venous leg ulcers. *BMJ.* 1999;319(7214):875-878.

114. Jull A, Waters J, Arroll B. Pentoxifylline for treatment of venous leg ulcers: a systematic review. *Lancet.* 2002;359(9317):1550-1554.

115. Coleridge-Smith P, Labropoulos N, Partsch H, Myers K, Nicolaides A, Cavezzi A. Duplex ultrasound investigation of the veins in chronic venous disease of the lower limbs–UIP consensus document. Part I. Basic principles. *Eur J Vasc Endovasc Surg.* 2006;31(1):83-92.

116. Meissner MH. Chronic Venous Disorders. In: Zierler RE, ed. *Strandness's Duplex Scanning in Vascular Disorders.* 4th ed. Philadelphia, PA: Lippincott Williams & Wilkins, a Wolter Kluwer business; 2010:223-229.

117. Labropoulos N, Tiongson J, Pryor L, et al. Definition of venous reflux in lower-extremity veins. *J Vasc Surg.* 2003;38(4):793-798.

118. Araki CT, Back TL, Padberg FT, Jr., Thompson PN, Duran WN, Hobson RW, 2nd. Refinements in the ultrasonic detection of popliteal vein reflux. *J Vasc Surg.* 1993;18(5):742-748.

119. Robinson BJ, Kesteven PJ, Elliott ST. The role of strain gauge plethysmography in the assessment of patients with suspected deep vein thrombosis. *Br J Haematol.* 2002;118(2):600-603.

120. Kahn SR, Joseph L, Grover SA, Leclerc JR. A randomized management study of impedance plethysmography vs. contrast venography in patients with a first episode of clinically suspected deep vein thrombosis. *Thromb Res.* 2001;102(1):15-24.

121. Persson LM, Arnhjort T, Larfars G, Rosfors S. Hemodynamic and morphologic evaluation of sequelae of primary upper extremity deep venous thromboses treated with anticoagulation. *J Vasc Surg.* 2006; 43(6):1230-1235;discussion 5.

122. Masuda E, Ozsvath K, Vossler J, et al. The 2020 appropriate use criteria for chronic lower extremity venous disease of the American Venous Forum, the Society for Vascular Surgery, the American Vein and Lymphatic Society, and the Society of Interventional Radiology. *J Vasc Surg Venous Lymphat Disord.* 2020;8(4):505-525.e4.

123. Puggioni A, Kalra M, Carmo M, Mozes G, Gloviczki P. Endovenous laser therapy and radiofrequency ablation of the great saphenous vein: analysis of early efficacy and complications. *J Vasc Surg.* 2005;42(3): 488-493.

124. Nordon IM, Hinchliffe RJ, Brar R, et al. A prospective double-blind randomized controlled trial of radiofrequency versus laser treatment of the great saphenous vein in patients with varicose veins. *Ann Surg.* 2011;254(6):876-881.

125. Shepherd AC, Gohel MS, Brown LC, Metcalfe MJ, Hamish M, Davies AH. Randomized clinical trial of VNUS ClosureFAST radiofrequency ablation versus laser for varicose veins. *Br J Surg.* 2010;97(6):810-818.

126. Dexter D, Kabnick L, Berland T, et al. Complications of endovenous lasers. *Phlebology.* 2012;27(Suppl 1):40-45.

127. Elias S, Raines JK. Mechanochemical tumescentless endovenous ablation: final results of the initial clinical trial. *Phlebology.* 2012;27(2):67-72.

128. Kim PS, Bishawi M, Draughn D, et al. Mechanochemical ablation for symptomatic great saphenous vein reflux: a two-year follow-up. *Phlebology.* 2016.

129. Bishawi M, Bernstein R, Boter M, et al. Mechanochemical ablation in patients with chronic venous disease: a prospective multicenter report. *Phlebology.* 2014;29(6):397-400.

130. Morrison N, Kolluri R, Vasquez M, Madsen M, Jones A, Gibson K. Comparison of cyanoacrylate closure and radiofrequency ablation for the treatment of incompetent great saphenous veins: 36-Month outcomes of the VeClose randomized controlled trial. *Phlebology.* 2019;34(6):380-390.

131. Theivacumar NS, Dellagrammaticas D, Beale RJ, Mavor AI, Gough MJ. Factors influencing the effectiveness of endovenous laser ablation (EVLA) in the treatment of great saphenous vein reflux. *Eur J Vasc Endovasc Surg.* 2008;35(1):119-123.

57

Pulmonary Hypertension

Yogesh N. V. Reddy and Barry A. Borlaug

Clinical classification and management of various forms of pulmonary hypertension

Group 1: Pulmonary arterial hypertension

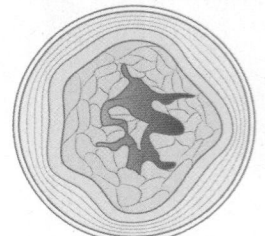

- Pulmonary arterial remodeling

- Frequently idiopathic

- Therapies focused on targeting endothelin, nitric oxide and prostaglandin pathways to promote pulmonary vasodilation and improve right heart functional reserve

Group 2: Left heart disease

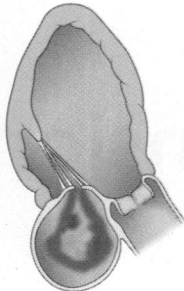

Group 3: Lung disease

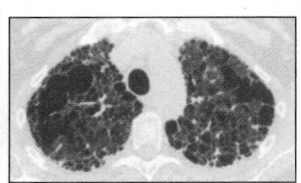

- Pulmonary hypertension develops secondary to left heart or lung insults

- Therapy primarily directed towards underlying cause

- No role for routine use of pulmonary vasodilator therapy

Group 4: Chronic thromboembolic pulmonary hypertension

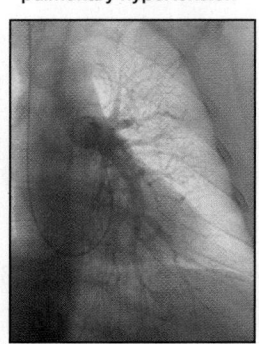

- First line therapy: mechanical relief of chronic thromboembolic obstruction

- Vasodilator therapy may be helpful in inoperable disease

Chapter 57 Fuster and Hurst's Central Illustration. Group 1, pulmonary arterial hypertension, is the classic precapillary form of pulmonary hypertension that is often idiopathic and is treated with pharmacological vasodilator therapy. Group 2, pulmonary hypertension from left heart disease, and Group 3, pulmonary hypertension from lung disease, have therapy directed primarily towards the underlying pathology. Group 4, chronic thromboembolic pulmonary hypertension, arises from chronic pulmonary emboli and requires mechanical relief of obstruction when feasible, with pharmacological vasodilator therapy reserved for inoperable disease.

CHAPTER SUMMARY

This chapter summarizes the diagnosis, pathophysiology, and treatment of various forms of pulmonary hypertension. Pulmonary hypertension is defined by a mean pulmonary artery pressure >20 mm Hg, and it can arise from primary pulmonary vascular pathology (WHO group 1), left heart disease (WHO group 2), lung disease (WHO group 3), or chronic thromboembolic disease (WHO group 4) (see Fuster and Hurst's Central Illustration). The diagnosis of pulmonary hypertension can be suspected from noninvasive testing, but it requires confirmation with invasive right heart catheterization. Group 1 pulmonary hypertension is frequently idiopathic and associated with poor outcomes, but multiple pharmacological treatment options are now available to improve symptoms and prognosis. Group 4 pulmonary hypertension requires treatment directed toward mechanical relief of thromboembolic obstruction with pharmacological therapy reserved for inoperable or residual disease. Pulmonary hypertension for groups 2 and 3 primarily involves treatment directed toward the underlying pathology. Regardless of etiology, worsening pulmonary hypertension and associated right heart dysfunction are associated with poor outcomes. The diagnostic and therapeutic approach to pulmonary hypertension requires careful clinical phenotyping and thoughtful consideration of the multiple treatment options available.

DEFINITION OF PULMONARY HYPERTENSION

Pulmonary hypertension (PH) refers to a pathologic elevation of pressure in the pulmonary artery (PA). In contrast to systemic hypertension where etiologic evaluation is rarely undertaken, it is important to determine the underlying cause of PH because there are specific treatments directed for some of the specific etiologies. The presence of PH was traditionally defined by a mean PA pressure ≥25 mm Hg, but this has recently been revised to include patients with a mean PA pressure >20 mm Hg.[1] The term pulmonary arterial hypertension (PAH) is typically used to connote patients with PH that is caused by an elevation in the pulmonary vascular resistance (PVR) that is not secondary to other disorders such as heart disease or hypoxemic lung disease. There is a paucity of evidence to guide treatment decisions in patients with a mean PA pressure between 21 and 25 mm Hg, and most of the literature to date has primarily evaluated patients with a mean PA pressure ≥25 mm Hg.

EPIDEMIOLOGY AND CLASSIFICATION OF PULMONARY HYPERTENSION

Regardless of etiology, the presence of an elevated PA pressure is consistently associated with poor prognosis.[2,3,4] PH affects approximately 1% of the world's population, and increases with aging.[5] PH is categorized as being "postcapillary" when the cause is distal to the alveolar-pulmonary capillary interface (predominantly in the left heart), or "precapillary" when the pathologic process affecting the pulmonary arterial vessels. The prevalence of PH is higher in developing countries where previously important causes of PH such as rheumatic heart disease, unrepaired congenital heart disease, schistosomiasis, and human immunodeficiency virus infection remain problematic[5,6] (**Fig. 57–1**).

There are five categories of PH grouped by major etiology or underlying pathophysiological mechanisms (**Table 57–1**). Four of the five categories are caused by precapillary mechanisms and one (left heart [LH] disease, World Symposium on Pulmonary Hypertension [WSPH] Group 2) is postcapillary. Left heart (LH) disease and lung disease are the most common causes of PH in developed countries.[5,7] In a large cohort of patients undergoing right heart catheterization (RHC), 16% displayed precapillary PAH whereas nearly three times as many patients (46%) had PH from LH disease.[3] The most common causes of LH disease are heart failure with preserved ejection fraction (HFpEF) and heart failure with reduced ejection fraction (HFrEF), with HFpEF increasingly becoming the leading cause for Group 2 PH.[3]

WSPH Group 1 PAH is the prototypical form of isolated pulmonary vascular pathology. This is a rare condition with an estimated prevalence of around 15 cases per million adults,[8] but frequently impacts young otherwise healthy individuals (disproportionately young women). PAH may be idiopathic, heritable, associated with infectious or inflammatory disorders, or caused by toxin exposures (Table 57–1).[5] In more developed countries, patients with Group 1 PAH are increasingly older-aged and have multiple risk factors for LH disease, creating overlap between Group 1 PAH and HFpEF.[9]

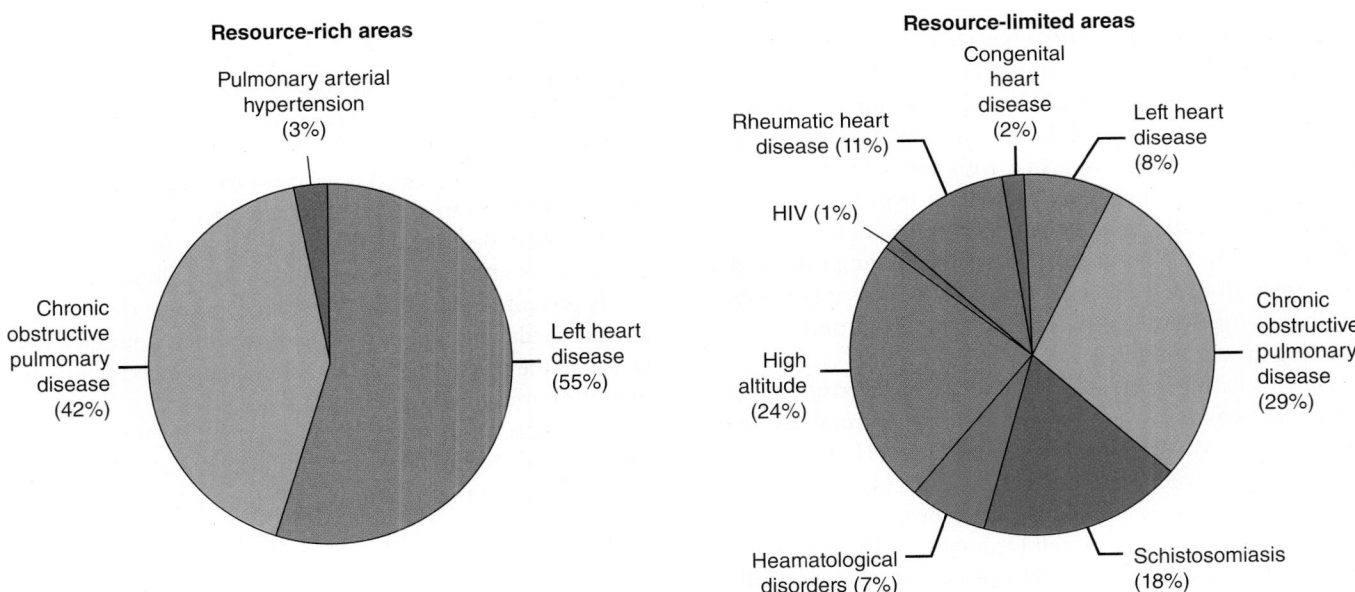

Pulmonary vascular disease

Resource-rich areas

- Pulmonary arterial hypertension (3%)
- Chronic obstructive pulmonary disease (42%)
- Left heart disease (55%)

Resource-limited areas

- Congenital heart disease (2%)
- Rheumatic heart disease (11%)
- Left heart disease (8%)
- HIV (1%)
- Chronic obstructive pulmonary disease (29%)
- High altitude (24%)
- Schistosomiasis (18%)
- Heamatological disorders (7%)

Figure 57–1. **The different causes of pulmonary vascular disease in resource-rich and research-limited areas of the world.** Heart and lung disease represent the vast majority of causes in resource rich regions whereas infectious and inflammatory disorders are a greater problem in the developing world. Pulmonary arterial hypertension, the only group for whom there are clearly effective treatments, represents a minority of patients. Modified with permission from Gidwani S, Nair A. The burden of pulmonary hypertension in resource-limited settings. *Glob Heart.* 2014 Sep;9(3):297-310.

TABLE 57–1. Clinical Classification of Pulmonary Hypertension (PH) per 6th World Symposium on Pulmonary Hypertension

Group 1: Pulmonary Arterial Hypertension (PAH)
1.1 Idiopathic PAH
1.2 Heritable PAH
1.3 Drug- and toxin-induced PAH
1.4 PAH associated with
   1.4.1 Connective tissue disease
   1.4.2 Human immunodeficiency virus infection
   1.4.3 Portal hypertension
   1.4.4 Congenital heart disease
   1.4.5 Schistosomiasis
1.5 PAH long-term responders to calcium channel blockers
1.6 PAH with overt features of venous/capillaries (PVOD/PCH) involvement
1.7 Persistent PH of the newborn syndrome

Group 2: PH due to left heart disease
2.1 PH due to heart failure with preserved ejection fraction
2.2 PH due to heart failure with reduced ejection fraction
2.3 Valvular heart disease
2.4 Congenital/acquired cardiovascular conditions leading to post-capillary PH

Group 3: PH due to lung diseases and/or hypoxia
3.1 Obstructive lung disease
3.2 Restrictive lung disease
3.3 Other lung diseases with mixed obstructive/restrictive pattern
3.4 Hypoxia without lung disease
3.5 Developmental lung disorders

Group 4: PH due to pulmonary artery obstructions
4.1 Chronic thromboembolic PH
4.2 Other pulmonary artery obstructions

Group 5: PH due to unclear and/or multifactorial mechanisms
5.1 Hematologic disorders
5.2 Systemic and metabolic disorders
5.3 Others
5.4 Complex congenital heart disease

Lung disease (World Health Organization [WHO] Group 3) represents the second most common cause of PH in developed countries (Fig. 57–1).[5,6] Approximately one-third of end-stage COPD patients referred for lung transplantation display evidence of PH, which is associated with parenchymal and pulmonary vascular remodeling as well as hypoxic pulmonary arterial vasoconstriction. Patients may also develop WSPH Group 3 PH in the absence of parenchymal lung disease due to hypoxic disorders such as obstructive sleep apnea (OSA) or obesity-hypoventilation (Pickwickian) syndrome, usually resulting in only mild PH.

Patients with persistent PH despite adequate treatment of a pulmonary embolic event represent chronic thromboembolic PH (CTEPH, WSPH Group 4), where the PH is caused by mechanical obstruction and secondary vascular responses to this obstruction. This represents a small proportion of patients with pulmonary emboli overall (around 3%–4% of all known pulmonary emboli).[10–12] CTEPH can be virtually identical in presentation to idiopathic PAH, but involves different treatments, so it is essential to distinguish between these two forms of PH.[10] Only a quarter of patients with CTEPH present with no known history of an acute pulmonary embolism[13] which

contributes to underdetection,[14] and one study suggested that CTEPH may represent up to 9% of cases of PAH.[7]

PHYSIOLOGY OF THE PULMONARY CIRCULATION

The high compliance, low-resistance pulmonary circulation operates at a pressure that is 8-fold lower than the systemic circulation. Maintaining low PA pressures therefore is dependent on the compliance of the pulmonary vascular bed to ensure that PA pressures remain within normal limits. The primary level of resistance in the PA vasculature is at the level of the smaller pulmonary arterioles.[15] The pulmonary vasculature has ample distensibility reserve, such that during the augmented blood flow during exercise, PVR decreases substantially through vascular recruitment and distention.[16] This helps to maintain optimal right ventricular (RV) performance during exercise when blood flow demands increase.[17] Because of the enormous vascular reserve of the lungs, substantial disease must develop before resting PH is present.

Contributors to Mean Pulmonary Artery Pressure

Blood flow through the lungs is driven by the pressure difference between the mean PA pressure and the downstream left atrial pressure (LAP). Mean PA pressure increases proportionally to the resistance across the pulmonary circulation through which blood must travel (PVR) and the amount of pulmonary blood flow (cardiac output, CO). Expressing this in algebraic form:

$$\text{mean PAP} = \text{LAP} + (\text{PVR} * \text{CO})$$

While a myriad of specific diseases can result in elevated mean PAP, this equation demonstrates that there are fundamentally only these three hemodynamic mechanisms (increase in LAP, PVR, and/or CO), that can lead to PH, although more than one may coexist in an individual patient.

Pulmonary Vascular Load

The resistance that the pulmonary vasculature imparts is a critical component of the afterload on the RV. In contrast to the systemic circulation where downstream venous pressure (ie, right atrial pressure [RAP]) is very low relative to mean arterial pressure, downstream pressure from the LA is an important contributor to the load that the RV faces.[18] Steady-state load reflects resistance assuming continuous, nonpulsatile blood flow, which is only present in patients with certain congenital disorders (eg, Fontan circulation) and in patients with a mechanical RV assist device. In the normal circulation, pulmonary blood flow is pulsatile and varies throughout the cardiac cycle.

Quantification of nonpulsatile afterload on the RV is performed using transpulmonary gradient (TPG), which forms the numerator of the equation for PVR:

$$\text{PVR} = (\text{mean PA} - \text{PCWP})/\text{CO} = \text{TPG}/\text{CO}$$

A PVR >3 Wood units is considered to reflect significant precapillary disease. Other indices reflecting precapillary pathology include an elevated pressure gradient between the PA and the pulmonary capillary wedge pressure (PCWP) at end diastole (diastolic pressure gradient, DPG >7 mm Hg).[19]

Pulsatile load to the RV can be evaluated by PA compliance (usually estimated by quotient of stroke volume/PA pulse pressure) or PA elastance (PA systolic pressure/stroke volume).[20] These pulsatile variables are more prognostic when compared to PVR in both LH disease[20] and PAH.[21]

Right Ventricular Function and Coupling to the Pulmonary Circulation

Clinical outcomes in PH are determined predominantly by the RV response to PH, rather than the severity of PH itself.[22-25] Patients with PH and severe RV dysfunction display a 1-year mortality of ~40%.[23] The interaction between RV function and pulmonary vascular afterload is referred to RV–PA coupling.[22,26] Impaired RV–PA coupling is associated with impairments in the ability to augment CO with exertion,[17,27] alterations in pulmonary ventilation,[28] abnormal metabolic profiling, RV dilation, development of lung congestion,[29] and enhanced ventricular interaction.[27,30] In research studies, RV–PA coupling requires sophisticated assessments of pressure and volume simultaneously. In clinical practice, indexing echocardiographic indices of systolic function such as tricuspid annular plane systolic excursion (TAPSE) to PA systolic pressure has been validated as an estimate of end-systolic elastance to effective arterial elastance (Ees/Ea) in PAH[22] and is related to abnormal hemodynamics and outcomes.[26,31]

Impact of Ventricular Interaction and Pericardial Restraint

The pressure measured in the left heart (left ventricular end diastolic pressure [LVEDP] or PCWP) is related to the distending pressure within the chamber (left atrium or ventricle) summed with the external contact pressure mediated across the interventricular septum from the RV and across the lateral wall by the pericardium.[30] This external pericardial pressure is best reflected by the RAP[32] and is substantially elevated in the presence of right-sided heart failure due to PH, especially when the right heart chamber dilates to increase pericardial constraint. In these patients, there may be a greater portion of PCWP elevation that is not primarily due to left ventricular (LV) disease, but rather reflects enhanced diastolic ventricular interaction with relative pericardial restraint[27] (**Fig. 57–2**).

If the left heart pressure is elevated simply because of pericardial restraint, this could lead to misdiagnosis of LH disease when in fact precapillary etiologies are predominant and have caused right heart failure. This possibility should be entertained when RAP equals or even exceeds PCWP, particularly when the PA pressure is elevated greatly out of proportion to PCWP. Pericardial restraint and diastolic ventricular interaction also contribute to limitations in LV filling and stroke volume response during rest[33] and exercise,[34] since the diseased and enlarged RV competes within the limited space of the pericardium with the LV during diastolic filling.

Determinants of Pulmonary Vascular Resistance

Autopsy series from patients with precapillary PH revealed a characteristic spectrum of histopathologic changes (**Fig. 57–3**),

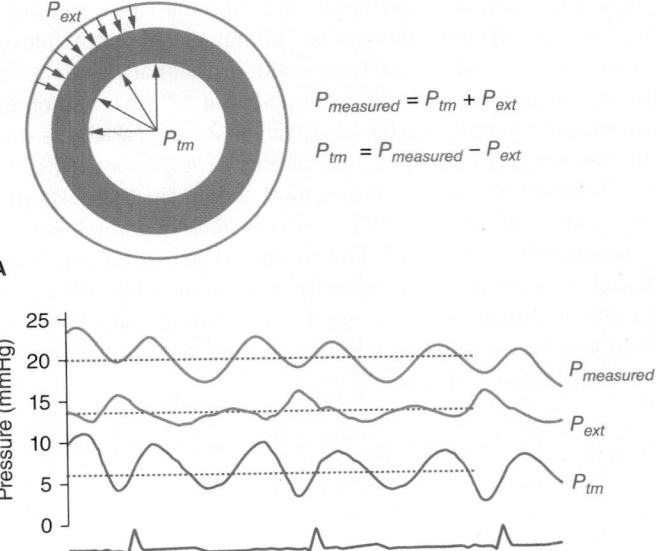

Figure 57–2. Differences between measure intraluminal pressure (P_measured) and transmural pressure (P_tm). (A) The intravascular pressure measured in the pulmonary artery reflects the sum of the net distending pressure within the vessel, defined as the P_tm, plus the external pressure (P_ext), which is related to pressures in the lung, thorax, and pericardium. During inspiration, the intrathoracic pressure decreases, reducing P_ext, such that P_measured decreases even as P_tm remains unchanged. For this reason, pulmonary vascular pressures are measured at end expiration, where P_ext is closest to zero. (B) The top pressure in *red* represents pulmonary capillary wedge pressure in a patient with pulmonary hypertension due to heart failure. The pressure is elevated (20 mm Hg) due to both an increase in P_tm and P_ext. The external pressure applied on the left atrium and ventricle is that measured in the pericardium. Pericardial pressure is most closely approximated by right atrial pressure (*green*). Thus, the true distending P_tm (*blue*) that determines left ventricular preload is much lower than P_measured. In patients with severe right heart failure due to various causes of PH, there is greater elevation in right atrial pressure and thus P_ext, representing an important contributor to elevations in measured pressure. Reproduced with permission from Borlaug BA, Reddy YNV. The Role of the Pericardium in Heart Failure: Implications for Pathophysiology and Treatment. *JACC Heart Fail.* 2019 Jul;7(7):574-585.

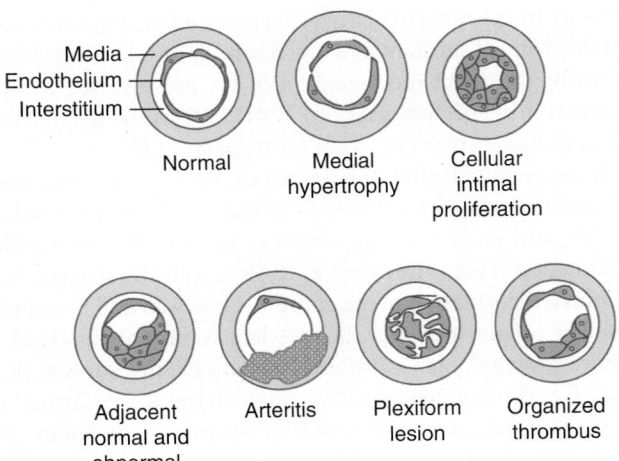

Figure 57–3. Vascular lesions observed in patients with pulmonary arterial hypertension.

including intimal hyperplasia and fibroelastosis, muscular medial hypertrophy, obliterative intimal vasculopathy, plexogenic lesions in advanced disease, and occasionally evidence of in situ thrombosis and venous remodeling.[35,36] Such pathological vascular remodeling has also been observed in patients with LH disease and a significant precapillary component of PH.[37]

However, numerous studies have shown that a substantial component of elevated PVR in PH is acutely reversible with pulmonary vasodilators.[38] The combined structural and functional vasoconstriction typically determine high PVR.[39] A minority patients with Group 1 PAH demonstrate favorable response to vasodilators administered acutely, and outcomes are excellent in this cohort.[40]

EVALUATION OF SUSPECTED PULMONARY HYPERTENSION

Physical Examination

Patients with PH present with symptoms of dyspnea and fatigue on activity. If there is coexisting right heart failure, they also display elevation in jugular venous pressure, often with a prominent "a" wave due to abnormal RV compliance, and a prominent "c-v" wave due to severe tricuspid regurgitation from RV remodeling. Chronic elevations in RA pressure may result in other signs of systemic congestion including tender hepatomegaly, ascites, and peripheral edema. Auscultation may disclose a right-sided S3 or parasternal heave from RV enlargement, and a loud P2 or pulmonary ejection click from PH. Severe tricuspid regurgitation may result in a holosystolic murmur that augments with inspiration, but in torrential TR with advanced RV failure, the murmur may be soft due to rapid equalization between the RV and RA pressures.

Echocardiography

PA systolic pressure can be estimated using Doppler interrogation of the tricuspid regurgitant velocity jet summed with estimated RA pressure. Although this approach is useful for population screening and has prognostic value, there are inaccuracies to this methodology, including underestimation of RA pressure by echo, particularly when assessed during exercise or in the setting of substantial RA pressure elevation[41] (**Fig. 57–4**). Accordingly, direct measurement of PA pressures by RHC is essential in suspected cases of PH to confirm the diagnosis of PH and differentiate pre- from postcapillary PH.

In patients with PH, the degree of RV dysfunction cannot be solely explained on the basis of the increased afterload on the RV, and there is a component of intrinsic RV myocardial dysfunction.[42] Measures such as RV free wall strain assess longitudinal deformation of the entire RV free wall and have independent prognostic value, but are less commonly assessed in echocardiography laboratories.[43] In contrast, measures such as TAPSE and tissue Doppler RVs reflect basal RV deformation, and are important measures of RVs' velocity performance. RV fractional area change provides a monoplane assessment of RV ejection fraction (RVEF) but may be limited by the complex geometry of the RV.

Cardiac Magnetic Resonance Imaging

Echocardiographic assessment of volume is limited owing to the complex shape of the RV, and magnetic resonance imaging (MRI) provides much more accurate volumetric assessments that have prognostic relevance. This is particularly true if the RVEF is low[24] or in the presence of RV dilation.[44] MRI also provides accurate estimates of LV volumes and septal configuration, which will favorably increase with effective PAH therapy from relief of pericardial restraint resulting in better LV diastolic filling. Cardiac MRI is most frequently used in the longitudinal evaluation of patients with PH and not part of routine initial diagnostic workup.

Cardiac Catheterization

An invasive RHC is essential for confirmation of PH given the limited accuracy of echocardiography. The presence of LH disease is inferred from an abnormal PCWP ≥15 mm Hg, although even normal PCWP does not exclude LH disease in patients with risk factors.[45] Measurement of pressures is performed at passive, end expiration, where intrathoracic pressure equals atmospheric pressure (Fig. 57–2). The practice of averaging pressures throughout the respiratory cycle introduces error and underestimates true intracardiac pressures due to confounding influence of inspiratory declines in intrathoracic and intracardiac pressures.

Patients with PAH often display intrinsic RV myocardial changes due to hypertrophy, fibrosis, and myocyte stiffening, resulting in elevation in RA pressure and systemic congestion.[46] As the RV becomes stiffer during diastole, this increases right atrial afterload, resulting in prominent RA "a" wave. Many patients will also display a prominent "v" wave reflecting poor operating atrial compliance as well as the common coexistence of significant tricuspid regurgitation.

An elevated LVEDP localizes pathology to the level of the left ventricle and provides a measure of preload, but it is important to recognize that the LVEDP (and LA pressure) provide complementary but not interchangeable information. It is the mean LA pressure (and not the LVEDP) that more accurately reflects the downstream pulmonary venous pressure that is "seen" by the pulmonary capillary bed and right ventricle, and therefore best reflects whether the PH is pre- or postcapillary (**Fig. 57–5**). In the presence of a diseased and myopathic left atrium, the LA pressure may be elevated out of proportion to the degree of LV pathology or LVEDP, and therefore the LA pressure best reflects the postcapillary contribution to PA pressure. These patients typically display an LA "v" wave that may be dramatically increased above the LVEDP.

The pulmonary arterial wedge pressure (PAWP) provides a convenient method to estimate LA pressure without transseptal access and the mean PAWP and LA pressure should be equal and used for the PVR calculation. By convention, LA (and RA) pressure are measured at the midpoint of the mid "a" wave (or "c" wave in atrial fibrillation), which is closest in timing to end diastole and provides the best estimate of LVEDP. The "v" wave in contrast begins shortly after ventricular systole and represents filling of the atrium, thereby reflecting left atrial

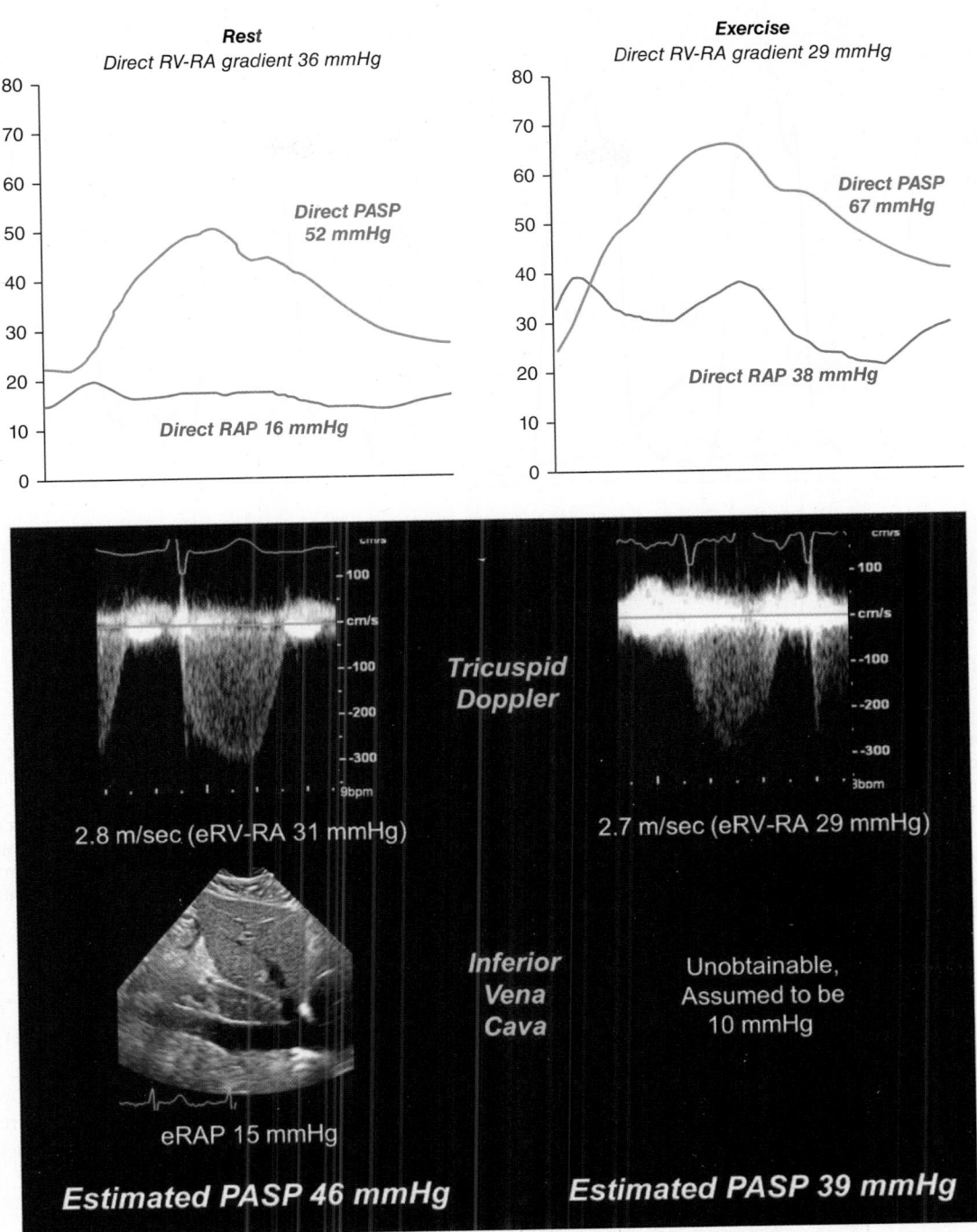

Figure 57–4. Estimation of pulmonary artery systolic pressure (PASP) from Doppler echocardiography. The PASP is estimated by echocardiography based upon the velocity of regurgitant blood flow across the tricuspid valve during systole (*bottom panels*), which reflects the pressure gradient between the right ventricle (RV, *red*) and right atrium (RA, *blue*). Because this reflects a pressure gradient, it is necessary to accurately estimate RA pressure (eRAP). This is done by echocardiography based upon the size, respiratory variation, and collapsibility of the inferior vena cava (*bottom*). When eRAP cannot be obtained, or if it deviates from invasively-measured values, as commonly occurs during exercise or in patients with severe right-sided heart failure, the accuracy of the PASP estimate decreases. Reproduced with permission from Obokata M, Kane GC, Sorimachi H, et al: Noninvasive evaluation of pulmonary artery pressure during exercise: the importance of right atrial hypertension. *Eur Respir J.* 2020 Feb 12;55(2):1901617.

operating compliance. A large "v" wave can reflect either reduced operating compliance of the LA or increased filling of the LA, as with mitral regurgitation or other volume overload states.

Cardiac Output Determination

In addition to direct pressure measurements, cardiac catheterization allows calculation of the cardiac output and forward flow to the body through either the thermodilution or Fick method, which is essential for calculation of PVR. The thermodilution method involves injection of saline through the proximal port of a Swan-Ganz catheter, with measurement of the area under the curve of temperature change over time in the distal catheter tip. The thermodilution method is less accurate in low output states or when there is severe tricuspid regurgitation.

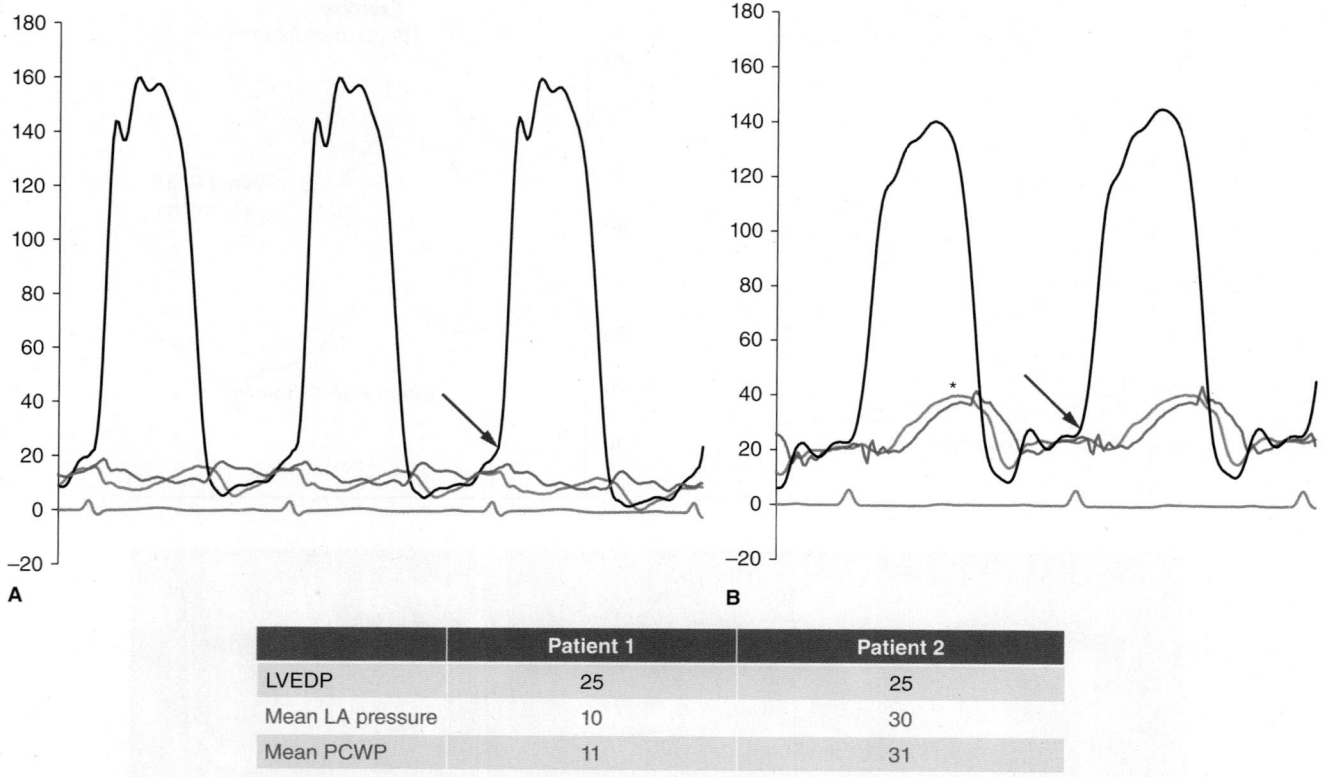

	Patient 1	Patient 2
LVEDP	25	25
Mean LA pressure	10	30
Mean PCWP	11	31

Figure 57–5. Discordant measures of left heart filling pressure. Pressure tracings from the left ventricle (LV, *black*), left atrium (LA, *red*), and pulmonary capillary wedge pressure (PCWP, *blue*) in two patients with pulmonary hypertension. Patient 1 (**A**) has normal LA pressure and PCWP, but markedly elevated LV pressure at end diastole. The increase in LV pressure at end-diastole (LVEDP, *arrow*) does not reflect the mean LA diastolic pressure during diastole, which is the more relevant downstream pressure that increases load in the pulmonary artery (PA). This pattern is common in patients with LV diastolic dysfunction and an increase in viscoelastic chamber stiffness. Patient 2 (**B**) displays the same degree of elevation in LVEDP, but LV pressure is higher throughout the entirety of diastole. In addition, there is a prominent V wave (*asterisk*), which is most commonly related to increased LA stiffness or mitral regurgitation. In this case, the mean LA pressure downstream of the PA is higher than the LVEDP, even as LA pressure at end diastole is equal to LVEDP. In both patients, the most relevant downstream pressure that is "seen" by the PA is that in the LA (which is also reflected by the PCWP).

The direct Fick method is considered the gold standard method to measure cardiac output, and is performed by measuring total body oxygen consumption (VO_2, which can be directly measured at the mouth using a metabolic cart) and systemic arterial and PA O_2 contents. Cardiac output is then calculated using the Fick equation:

$$CO \text{ (L/min)} = VO_2/[\text{arterial} - \text{venous } O_2 \text{ content difference}]*10$$

Although nomograms are available to provide estimates of VO_2 (indirect Fick method), this introduces error particularly when patients are obese[47] or deviate from normal physiological states.[48] In patients with PAH, in particular, the direct Fick method has been shown to be superior to thermodilution and indirect Fick methods that are all associated with decreased precision which can misclassify risk in at least one-third of patients.[49]

Vasodilator Testing

Acute vasodilator testing is performed in PAH to identify the subset of patients where there is a reversible component of active pulmonary vasoconstriction. Vasodilator testing can be performed using adenosine, intravenous prostaglandin, or most commonly using inhaled nitric oxide. A "responder" is defined by a patient with a 10 mm Hg or greater reduction in mean PA pressure to values less than 40 mm Hg, with a stable or increased CO. Patients with PAH and this favorable acute response have a better prognosis and often respond more favorably to treatment with calcium channel blockers.

Exercise Testing

In many patients with borderline or normal hemodynamics at rest and risk factors for LH disease, exercise testing may provide diagnostic clarification.[50] Patients with pulmonary vascular disease will demonstrate abnormal PA pressure flow relationships during exercise (>3 mm Hg of mean PA pressure rise per 1 L/min of cardiac output), which is associated with adverse prognosis.[51] Simultaneous measures of ventilation and gas exchange may also quantify the degree of ventilatory inefficiency, which is related to abnormal RV–PA coupling and ventilation–perfusion mismatch during exercise. Fluid challenge is a less sensitive and less physiological stress, but may also unmask occult LH disease in patients at risk and may be predictive of a rise in PCWP and lack of symptom response following PAH therapy.[52]

PULMONARY ARTERIAL HYPERTENSION (GROUP I)

Clinical Features

The clinical presentation of Group 1 PAH typically involves exercise intolerance in the early stages, which progresses to symptoms and signs reflective of systemic venous congestion and reduced cardiac output. Patients typically present with dyspnea, fatigue, and in severe cases positional or exertional syncope. Patients may experience exertional angina even in the absence of coronary artery disease reflecting a form of RV supply-demand mismatch. In a notable subset, this reflects compression of the left main coronary artery by an enlarged PA, in whom percutaneous stenting may alleviate symptoms.[53] Patients with advanced PAH frequently display evidence of systemic venous congestion along with pericardial effusion or pleural effusions.

Pathobiology

The pathology of Group 1 PAH is characterized by a combination of intimal hyperplasia and fibroelastosis, muscular medial hypertrophy, obliterative intimal vasculopathy, plexogenic lesions in advanced disease, and occasionally evidence of thrombosis (Fig. 57–3).[54] While most patients display idiopathic disease, others display a heritable component, with the most notable including abnormalities in BMPR2 (Bone Morphogenetic Protein Receptor Type 2) signaling pathways.[55] Even in patients with idiopathic PAH without BMPR2 mutations, the level of BMPR2 may be low in the lungs, suggesting an important causal role for this molecular pathway in the pathogenesis.[56] Inflammation and fibroproliferative signaling pathways become altered and activate transcription pathways that result in vascular smooth muscle proliferation.[57] Accumulated DNA damage and alterations in DNA repair mechanisms, insulin resistance, autonomic imbalance, neurohormonal activation, and pulmonary arterial endothelial dysfunction have all been variably implicated in the pathogenesis of PAH. Many of these sporadic, environmental, and genetic factors synergize in complex ways to produce pulmonary vascular disease (**Fig. 57–6**).

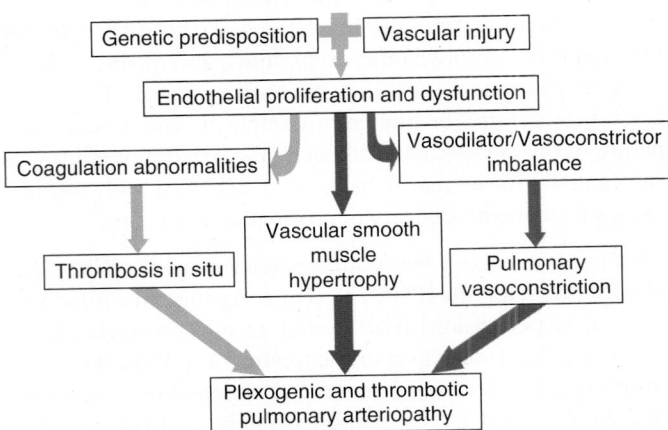

Figure 57–6. Summary of the pathobiology of Group 1 pulmonary hypertension (PAH).

Environmental Basis

Drug and toxin exposures remain the most easily identifiable culprit in specific cases of PAH in a minority of cases. A number of prescription drugs including appetite suppressants, the chemotherapeutic agent dasatinib (a tyrosine kinase inhibitor), and recreational drugs such as methamphetamines are associated with PAH. Among individuals exposed to these drugs, only a minority actually develop clinical PAH, suggesting a role for host susceptibility. Indeed, a subset of patients (~8%) with anorexigen-associated PAH will demonstrate BMPR2 mutations suggesting a combined genetic and environmental insult resulting in the clinical phenotype.[58] Recent data suggest that acquired somatic mutations in bone marrow-derived stem cells accumulated throughout life (clonal hematopoiesis of indeterminate potential), may increase the risk of systemic inflammation and pulmonary vascular remodeling seen in patients with PAH.[59]

Genetic Basis

Mutations in BMPR2 account for approximately 15% of all cases of otherwise idiopathic Group 1 PAH, with a higher prevalence in familial cases (around 75%).[58,60] There are some unique pathophysiological associations in BMPR2 mutation associated with PAH including a greater histological involvement of the bronchial circulation and pulmonary veins with a greater risk for hemoptysis and younger age at presentation with worse hemodynamics and prognosis.[61] The BMPR2 mutation, however, is associated with incomplete penetrance, which varies with sex. Disease penetrance in men with the genotype is around 14% compared to approximately 42% in females.[62] A number of rarer additional genes apart from BMPR2 have been identified [TBX4, ACVRL1, ENG, SMAD9, KCNK3, ATP13A3, SOX17, AQP1, and GDF2], which individually each account for 1% or less of otherwise "idiopathic" PAH cases.[58]

Other Common Etiologies of Group 1 PAH

Congenital Heart Disease

Chronic high-flow states as a result of intracardiac shunts result in increased pulmonary blood flow that can induce pulmonary vascular remodeling, increasing PA pressure. Pulmonary vascular changes in congenital shunt-related PH resemble those of Group 1 patients but may reverse remodel in response to shunt closure. Therefore, evaluation for shunt closure must always be considered in congenital heart disease-associated PH. Once substantial pulmonary vascular remodeling and RV failure has emerged, patients may develop right to left shunting (Eisenmenger syndrome). Secundum atrial septal defects represent the most common cause of left to right shunting presenting with PH in adults in the current era.

Connective Tissue Disease

Patients with systemic sclerosis frequently develop Group 1 PAH, even in the absence of interstitial lung disease, which is associated with poorer prognosis when compared to idiopathic PAH.[63] This is partly related to greater degree of RV dysfunction in systemic sclerosis PAH as well as other contributors such as LV diastolic dysfunction, venous involvement, or interstitial lung disease. Patients with limited systemic sclerosis (formerly known as CREST syndrome) may also develop PAH, and this form is notable for a lower prevalence of interstitial lung disease. Some patients with limited systemic sclerosis may also develop a high output heart failure state with associated PH.[64] Other connective tissue diseases may also cause the clinical syndrome.

Portal Hypertension

The presence of hepatic cirrhosis is associated with a unique pathophysiology of splanchnic vasodilation, decreased systemic vascular resistance, and a high-flow state resulting in high-output heart failure.[64] Cirrhosis can also be associated with a rare complication of pulmonary vascular remodeling called porto-pulmonary hypertension, which is associated with poorer outcomes. Pulmonary vasodilator therapy may afford some benefit in carefully selected patients, but great caution in follow-up must be undertaken to avoid an iatrogenic high output state from the systemic vasodilation that occurs with PAH drugs.[65] In patients who are candidates for liver transplantation, there may be reversibility in PAH with transplantation and vasodilator therapy that may serve as a bridge to liver transplant in appropriate patients.

Treatment for Group 1 PAH

General Measures

There is currently not an established role for neurohormonal or β-blocker therapy in patients with PAH. Even though digoxin has favorable acute hemodynamic effects,[66] it has not been studied in a randomized trial in PAH, and therefore its long-term use is of uncertain utility. In patients with overt right-sided congestion, diuretics are necessary to improve symptoms, and this may be associated with improved forward CO through reduction in relative pericardial restraint and functional tricuspid regurgitation.[30] Exercise training exerts beneficial effects on exercise performance and quality of life and appears safe in patients with PH.[67]

Role of Empiric Anticoagulation

The demonstration of intravascular thrombosis in pathology specimens of the PA circulation led to the hypothesis that in situ thrombosis may contribute to the progression of idiopathic PAH.[35] This was further supported by observational studies suggesting a survival advantage with anticoagulation,[36,40] but these data are confounded by the observational nature of treatment assignment, as well as the inclusion of patients with CTEPH (who are known to benefit from anticoagulation). Recent registry results have also been conflicting, with some signals of increased mortality in PAH associated with systemic sclerosis.[68] Therefore, currently anticoagulation is recommended only for those with an alternate indication such as CTEPH or atrial fibrillation.

Supplemental Oxygen

In many patients with PAH, there is a low PA saturation coupled with modest V/Q mismatch (ventilation/perfusion mismatch).[69] This results in hypoxic vasoconstriction that exacerbates V/Q mismatch promoting arterial hypoxemia.[69] Treatment with PAH vasodilator therapies (subsequently discussed) improves systemic blood flow, with a higher PA O_2 saturation, contributing to an improvement in systemic arterial saturation.[70] Although no randomized trials are available, persistent hypoxia despite PAH therapy is generally treated with chronic supplemental oxygen therapy.

PAH-Specific Pharmacological Therapy

The pharmacological approach to treatment for PAH involves the therapeutic modulation of three relatively unique pathways: (1) prostaglandin, (2) endothelin, and (3) the nitric oxide-guanylate cyclase-cyclic GMP pathways (**Fig. 57–7; Table 57–2**). Drugs targeting these pathways in general promote pulmonary vasodilation with favorable effects on RV performance. Changes in hemodynamics measured at steady state are often modest and it is unknown whether favorable effects are mediated by vasodilation or other disease-modifying effects on the pulmonary vasculature.[71] Pulmonary vasodilators improve exercise capacity in PAH and reduce clinical worsening, but to date only intravenous (IV) prostaglandin therapy has demonstrated a clear mortality advantage.[72]

Prostaglandin Pathway:

Parenteral Prostacyclin: Intravenous epoprostenol (prostaglandin I2) reduces PVR leading to improved symptoms, hemodynamics, and right heart structure and survival in patients with PAH.[70,72] Treprostinil is a more chemically stable form of prostaglandin I2 with a half-life around 4 hours (compared to 6 minutes for epoprostenol) that can be used either intravenously or subcutaneously. Like epoprostenol, intravenous treprostinil improves exercise capacity and symptoms in PAH.[73] Treprostinil is also available in a subcutaneous formulation that cannot achieve as high doses as intravenous formulations but improves functional capacity.[74,75] The hemodynamic effects of parenteral prostaglandins are not limited only to the pulmonary circulation, with nearly 50% reduction in systemic vascular resistance commonly observed, which may limit dose escalation.[70]

Inhaled Prostaglandins: Inhaled prostaglandin therapy (inhaled iloprost or treprostinil) avoids the risks of an intravenous catheter, but requires multiple inhalations a day. Although this may improve hemodynamics, symptoms, and quality of life,[76] there are pharmacological troughs in such periodic drug delivery, inhalation may be limited by complexity and burdensome nature of the devices, and ultimately the maximum efficacy is substantially lower than what can be achieved with intravenous/subcutaneous delivery of prostaglandin therapy,

Oral Prostaglandin and Prostaglandin Receptor Agonist: The GRIPHON (Prostacyclin [PGI2] Receptor Agonist In Pulmonary Arterial Hypertension) trial[77] tested an oral prostaglandin I2 receptor agonist, selexipag in the treatment of PAH. The most common side effect was headache affecting about two-thirds of patients, but diarrhea, nausea, myalgia, and jaw pain also occurred similar to other prostaglandin therapies. There was no mortality or symptom benefit with selexipag but it did

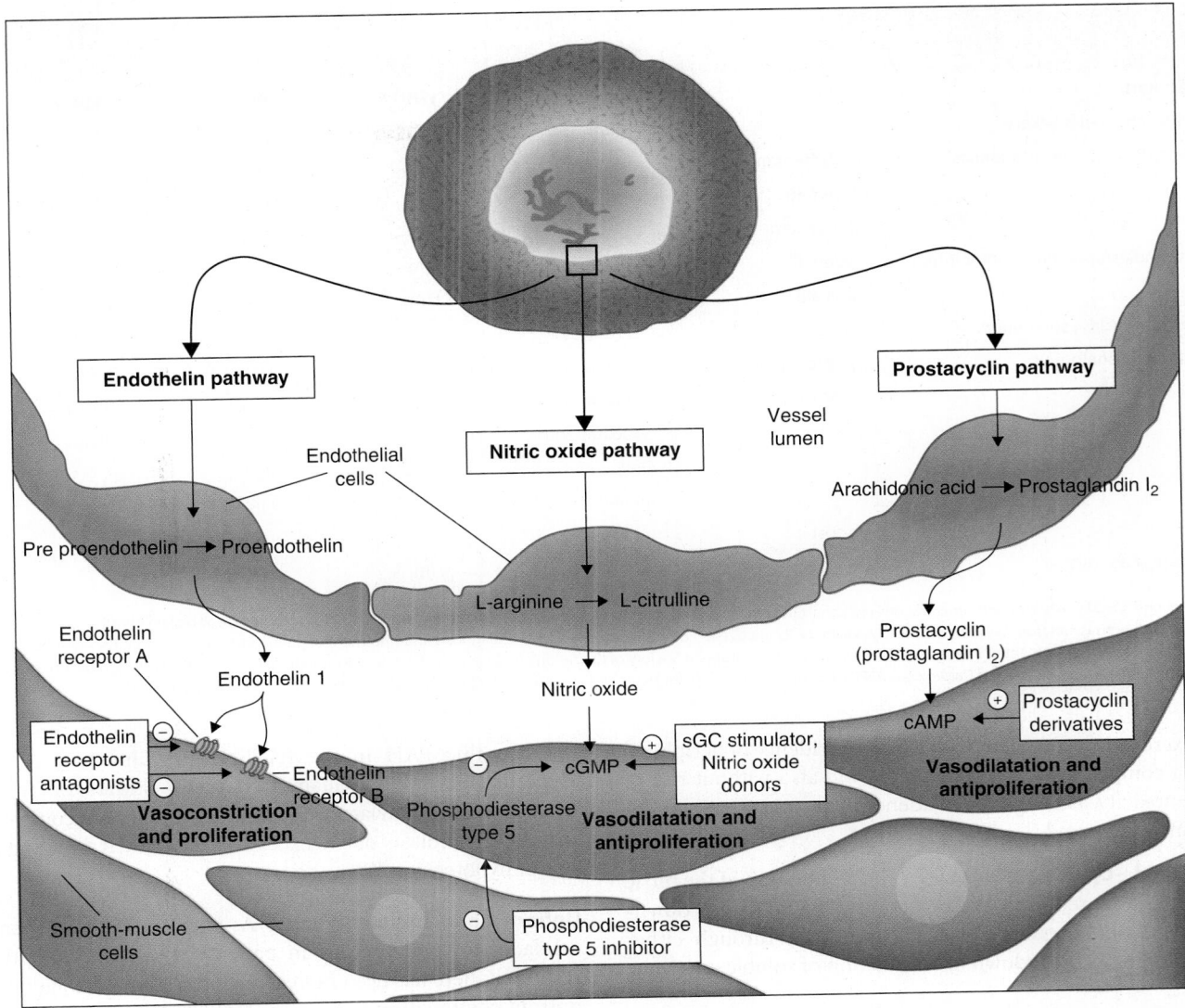

Figure 57–7. Pathways involved in the pathophysiology of PAH. Endothelin is released from vascular endothelium where it binds to receptors in vascular smooth muscle cells promoting vasoconstriction and proliferation. ERAs work by inhibiting this response. Nitric oxide is also synthesized in vascular endothelium and diffuses out of the endothelial cell and into the vascular smooth muscle cell, where it activates soluble guanylate cyclase, increasing levels of cyclic guanosine monophosphate (cGMP) and activation of downstream signaling pathways that promote vasodilation and have antiproliferative effects. Cellular cGMP levels may be augmented through agonists such soluble guanylate cyclase stimulators (sGC) or exogenous nitric oxide donors, or through inhibition of PDE-5. Finally, the prostacyclin derivatives act through the prostacyclin I2 receptor to increase intracellular cyclic adenosine monophosphate (cAMP), resulting in vasodilation and antiproliferative effects through mechanisms that complement but are distinct from cGMP-dependent signaling pathways.

appear to prevent clinical worsening with a small effect on 6-minute walking distance in both treatment naive patients as well as those already on other oral therapies (sildenafil, endothelin antagonists, or both).[77] An oral version of treprostinil is now also available and appears to modestly improve symptoms, exercise capacity, and mitigate clinical worsening when added to PAH monotherapy in the randomized FREEDOM-EV trial.[78] Side effects were also typical for prostaglandin stimulation including headache, flushing, and gastrointestinal symptoms.[78]

Endothelin Pathway: Bosentan is a nonselective endothelin antagonist that has demonstrated symptom and hemodynamic benefit in PAH with a reduced time to clinical worsening.[79] Hepatotoxicity is a notable side effect with bosentan, with up

to 17% developing aminotransferase elevations, and monthly liver enzyme monitoring is required. Ambrisentan is a selective endothelin A antagonist with less hepatotoxicity risk that favorably improves symptoms.[80] Endothelin antagonists in general and ambrisentan in particular have been associated with a risk of renal fluid retention, which can exacerbate peripheral edema in patients with PAH, and this may also contribute to the increased prevalence of anemia associated with these agents. Nasopharyngitis is another notable complication of the endothelin antagonists. More recently, macitentan, which is also a dual endothelin receptor antagonist (ERA), was studied in the SERAPHIN (Study with an Endothelin Receptor Antagonist in Pulmonary Arterial Hypertension to Improve Clinical Outcome) trial and demonstrated favorable symptom

TABLE 57–2. European Society of Cardiology Recommendations for Drug Monotherapy in Group 1 Pulmonary Arterial Hypertension According to WHO Functional Class

Treatment	Drug	Route**	WHO FC II	WHO FC III	WHO FC IV
Calcium channel blockers			I (C)*	I (C)*	-
Endothelin receptor antagonists	Ambrisentan		I (A)	I (A)	IIb (C)
	Bosentan		I (A)	I (A)	IIb (C)
	Macitentan		I (B)	I (B)	IIb (C)
Phosphodiesterase type 5 inhibitors	Sildenafil		I (A)	I (A)	IIb (C)
	Tadalafil		I (B)	I (B)	IIb (C)
Guanylate cyclase stimulators	Riociguat		I (B)	I (B)	IIb (C)
Prostacyclin analogues	Epoprostenol	Intravenous	-	I (A)	I (A)
	Treprostinil	Intravenous	-	IIa (C)	IIb (C)
		Subcutaneous	-	I (B)	IIb (C)
		Oral	-	IIb (B)	
		Inhaled	-	I (B)	IIb (C)
	Ilopost	Inhaled	-	I (B)	IIb (C)
IP receptor agonist	Selexipag		I (B)	I (B)	-

Abbreviations: WHO FC, World Health Organization Functional Class, *only in responders to acute vasoreactivity testing with group 1 PAH **drugs are all oral unless otherwise specified.
Modified with permission from Galiè N, Humbert M, Vachiery JL, et al: 2015 ESC/ERS Guidelines for the diagnosis and treatment of pulmonary hypertension: The Joint Task Force for the Diagnosis and Treatment of Pulmonary Hypertension of the European Society of Cardiology (ESC) and the European Respiratory Society (ERS): Endorsed by: Association for European Paediatric and Congenital Cardiology (AEPC), International Society for Heart and Lung Transplantation (ISHLT). *Eur Respir J.* 2015 Oct;46(4):903-975.

and exercise improvement with a lower incidence of peripheral edema compared to the other agents and also without risk of hepatotoxicity, although the incidence of anemia remained significantly increased.[81]

Nitric Oxide-Cyclic GMP Pathway: The stimulation of the nitric oxide pathway relies on augmentation of nitric oxide's downstream second messenger (ie, cyclic GMP), through either inhibition of its breakdown or stimulation of soluble guanylate cyclase.

Phosphodiesterase Inhibitors: Phosphodiesterase (PDE)-5 inhibitors augments nitric oxide (NO) signaling by preventing the breakdown of its second messenger cyclic GMP. PDE-5 has been identified in human PA vascular smooth muscle cells, and PDE-5 inhibitors such as sildenafil lead to significant pulmonary vasodilation.[82] In the SUPER (Sildenafil Use in Pulmonary Arterial Hypertension) trial, sildenafil demonstrated favorable effects on both symptoms and exercise capacity.[83] A Cochrane meta-analysis suggested that PDE inhibitors may even reduce mortality in PAH.[84] Tadalafil has advantages over sildenafil because a once-a-day drug has also demonstrated favorable symptom benefits and may be an easier to use alternative in some patients.[80,85] Headache, flushing, myalgia, and dyspepsia are common side effects of the PDE5 inhibitors.[83,85]

Soluble Guanylate Cyclase Stimulator: Riociguat is a soluble guanylate cyclase stimulator that increases sensitivity of guanylate cyclase to existing NO. This drug is associated with substantial peripheral vasodilation through cyclic GMP mechanisms resulting in an average drop in mean arterial pressure of approximately 7 to 9 mm Hg.[86,87] Riociguat has demonstrated symptom and exercise benefits with delay in clinical worsening

in idiopathic PAH in the PATENT-1 (Pulmonary Arterial Hypertension Soluble Guanylate Cyclase–Stimulator Trial 1) trial.[86] Soluble guanylate cyclase stimulators are not compatible with PDE inhibitors due to excessive cyclic GMP signaling and risk of hypotension.[88]

Upfront Combination Therapy: As opposed to a sequential escalation of oral therapy in patients who have suboptimal response, there has been increasing interest in more aggressive upfront combination therapy in PAH. The largest randomized trial testing this strategy was the AMBITION (Ambrisentan and Tadalafil in Patients with Pulmonary Arterial Hypertension) trial that tested the combination of ambrisentan and tadalafil compared to monotherapy in Group 1 PAH. This study showed that upfront combination therapy reduced clinical worsening and improved 6-minute walking distance, but there was no difference in mortality.[80] Given the available evidence base, the combination of ambrisentan and tadalafil is generally favored, but other combinations are often utilized in practice including sildenafil with macitentan, riociguat with an ERA, and selexipag with an ERA and/or PDE-5 inhibitor.

Ca Channel Blockers: There are a small subset of Group 1 patients who have a more prominent vasoconstrictive component. Observational studies have suggested improved survival of such patients treated with calcium channel blockers,[40] but there are no randomized trials of this therapy. Identification of potential candidates for calcium channel blockade is based on a positive vasoreactivity test with reduction in mean PA pressure by at least 10 mm Hg to reach an absolute value below 40 mm Hg, without a drop in cardiac output.[1] Even among this subset with acute vasodilatory response (12.6% in one study), only half of these patients have a satisfactory long-term clinical response to calcium channel blockade.[89]

Atrial Septostomy: In patients with advanced and end-stage right heart failure, palliative atrial septostomy can be utilized as a means to offload the right heart through right to left atrial shunting. This decreases right-sided congestion and RAP and increases systemic cardiac output albeit at the expense of systemic desaturation.

Heart–Lung or Lung Transplant: In patients with advanced PH with persistent heart failure despite therapy, lung transplantation is the only meaningful therapy to improve survival. If RV function remains adequate, then isolated lung transplantation may be sufficient, and the right heart failure will improve with the removal of abnormal pulmonary vascular load from transplantation of normal pulmonary vascular bed into the recipient. However, in patients with severe right heart failure or those with Eisenmenger syndrome, combined heart–lung transplantation is often necessary.

Special Considerations for Patients with Congenital Heart Disease

The management of PAH due to congenital heart disease is complex as summarized in the AHA (American Heart Association) and ESC (European Society of Cardiology).[90,91] Patients with Eisenmenger syndrome generally benefit from treatment with parenteral therapy for advanced symptoms (subcutaneous or inhaled therapy preferred over intravenous when feasible due to the risk for paradoxical embolism); and oral therapy with an ERA or PDA inhibitor when symptoms are less severe.

The other common clinical scenario relates to closure of left to right shunts in the setting of PH. In general, a substantial left to right shunt (Qp/Qs ≥1.5) in the absence of very severe PVR elevation or Eisenenger-related right to left shunting suggests increasing likelihood of benefit with shunt closure. The benefits of closure relate to reverse chamber remodeling, pulmonary vascular reverse remodeling, and acute PA pressure reduction from decreased pulmonary blood flow. The ACC and ESC guidelines differ slightly in their recommendations for degree of PVR that precludes shunt closure. The ACC recommends against routine closure for a significant left to right shunt if the PVR is more than one-third of the SVR or if the PA systolic pressure is >50% of systemic systolic pressure, but this can be reconsidered depending on the response to chronic PAH therapy.[91] In contrast, the ESC provides different recommendations for pretricuspid shunt (ASD) compared to post tricuspid shunts (Ventricular Septal Defects [VSD] or Patent Ductus Arteriosus [PDA]). For patients with a significant ASD (Qp/Qs >1.5), the ESC recommends against closure with a PVR ≥5 Wood units, unless the PVR can be reduced below 5 Wood units, in which case fenestrated closure can then be considered. For patients with a significant VSD or PDA (Qp/Qs >1.5), closure with a PVR ≥5 Wood units can still be considered for closure, but a careful rule out of Eisenmenger physiology with rest or exercise (arterial saturation <90%) must be performed first.[90]

Clinical Follow-Up and Risk Stratification

Figure 57–8 shows an evidence-based treatment algorithm for patients with Group 1 PAH, both the newly diagnosed patient and also patients with known disease that are being followed in clinic. A number of noninvasive and invasive measures can help guide treatment decisions and provide risk stratification for patients with PAH. Functional class should be assessed with each clinical visit. The 6-minute walk test is prognostic, easy to perform during clinic visits, and can be used to objectively monitor therapeutic response. NTproBNP levels are secreted in response to increases in cardiac wall stress and are related to abnormal hemodynamics and prognosis in PAH. The ESC guidelines recommend that patients with NTproBNP below 300 ng/L can be considered as low risk, while patients with values >1400 ng/L are high risk.[92] Echocardiography after therapy can identify favorable changes in RV size and function with improved LV filling.

Although many patients who achieve low-risk clinical status after treatment can be followed without repeat invasive assessment, there is an important role for cardiac catheterization in patients with persistent or worsening symptoms, or a poor therapeutic response. In a large French registry of idiopathic PAH patients, low stroke volume index and high RA pressure on follow-up catheterization after treatment were highly predictive of prognosis, while baseline hemodynamics were not.[93] Invasive cardiopulmonary exercise testing with determination of peak exercise capacity and pressure flow relationships may further help risk stratify patients, although this is not yet widely used for this purpose.[51]

Patients with Group 1 PAH have a very poor prognosis if untreated, with a median survival of 2.8 years, and 1- and 5-year survival rates of 68% and 34%, respectively.[94] Even with IV prostaglandin therapy, hemodynamic and symptom improvement is not complete,[95,96] and a 5-year survival of 55% on treatment remains suboptimal for the typical young patient affected by idiopathic PAH. In a more modern cohort of idiopathic, heritable, and drug-induced Group 1 PAH, the demographics have shifted to an older age at diagnosis, with much lower upfront use of IV prostaglandin therapy and more oral therapy use.[93] But despite the older average age and less IV prostaglandin use, survival did compare favorably to prior eras, with survival rates at 1, 2, and 3 years from diagnosis being 90%, 81%, and 73%, respectively, although reductions in PA pressure are in fact quite modest.[93] Survival decreases with more adverse hemodynamics, and given the incomplete improvement afforded by current treatments, early transplant referral should be considered in appropriate candidates with high-risk features.

PULMONARY VENO-OCCLUSIVE DISEASE AND PULMONARY CAPILLARY HEMANGIOMATOSIS

Clinical Features

Pulmonary veno-occlusive disease (PVOD) and Pulmonary Capillary Hemangiomatosis (PCH) are less common causes of

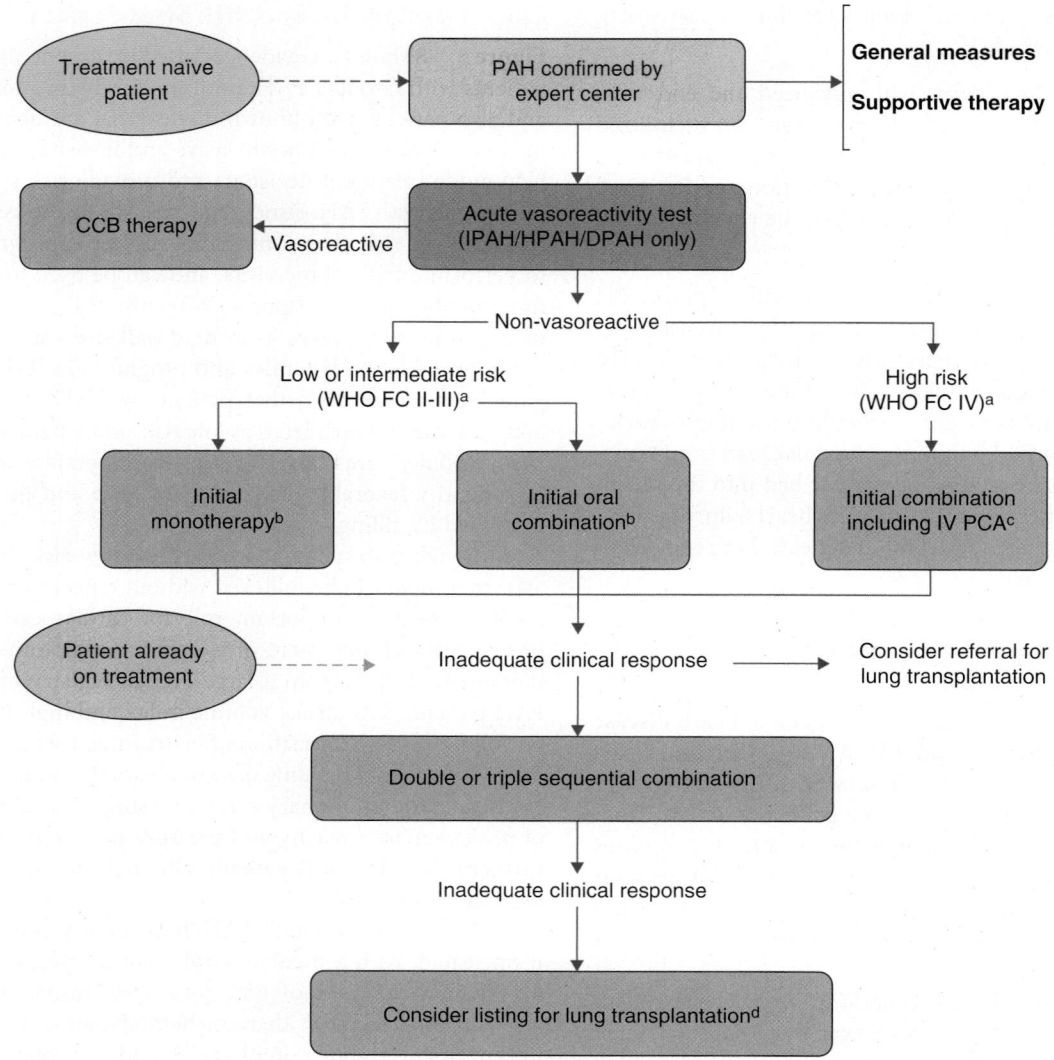

CCB = calcium channel blockers; DPAH = drug-induced PAH; HPAH = heritable PAH; IPAH = idiopathic PAH; IV = intravenous; PAH = pulmonary arterial hypertension; PCA = prostacyclin analogues; WHO-FC = World Health Organization functional class.
aSome WHO-FC III patients may be considered high risk
bInitial combination with ambrisentan plus tadalafil has proven to be superior to initial monotherapy with ambrisentan or tadalafil in delaying clinical failure.
cIntravenous epoprostenol should be prioritised as it has reduced the 3 month mortality in high risk PAH patients also as monotherapy.
dConsider also balloon atrial septostomy.

Figure 57–8. Evidence-based treatment algorithm for patients with Group 1 PAH.

PAH characterized by greater pulmonary venous and capillary remodeling.[97] PCH is associated with infiltrative proliferation of thin-walled microvessels in the alveolar wall. The distinction between PCH and PVOD is often challenging, but in clear cut cases there is venous obliteration from proliferating capillaries in PCH as opposed to intimal fibrosis in PVOD.

These patients display very high pulmonary capillary pressures that may lead to pulmonary edema with vasodilator therapy due to downstream obstruction, emphasizing the importance of accurate phenotyping. Patients with PVOD typically display normal PCWP despite small vessel venous obstruction, because the PCWP in the static column of blood more closely reflects the normal LA pressure in these patients. A number of radiographic computed tomography (CT) features have been associated with PVOD, including poorly defined nodular or ground glass opacities, septal lines, and lymphadenopathy.[98] The presence of underlying PVOD can be suspected by a very low diffusion capacity (DLCO), severe hypoxia and ventilatory inefficiency during exertion, or the appearance of pulmonary edema with vasodilator therapy,[98] but can only be truly confirmed by lung biopsy.

Pathogenesis

Genetic mutations in eukaryotic translation initiation factor 2 α kinase 4 (*EIF2AK4*) have been recognized in around one-third of cases with clinical PVOD.[60,99] A notable minority of patients with clinically idiopathic Group 1 PAH (around 1%) may also have the typical biallelic *EIF2AK4* mutation, supporting a missed diagnosis of PVOD, and suggests the potential for misclassification in clinical practice based only on the clinical phenotype.[60] *BMPR2* mutations have also been described in PVOD[100] and the delineation between PVOD and idiopathic PAH is often unclear.[61,97] Recent studies in PH due to LH disease have also revealed remodeling at the level of the small pulmonary veins.[101]

Treatment

Patients with PVOD/PCH may have a poor response to pulmonary arterial vasodilator therapy, with pulmonary edema developing in 30% to 40% of patients, while others have a poor clinical and symptomatic response.[98] As a result of the high proportion of poor response to traditional PH therapy, early referral for lung transplantation is recommended in the case of confirmed or suspected PVOD.

PULMONARY HYPERTENSION ASSOCIATED WITH LEFT HEART DISEASE (GROUP 2)

In a large institutional database of 4621 patients with Group 2 PH undergoing RHC, 39% of cases were a result of HFrEF and 61% were from HFpEF.[3] Less common etiologies of LH disease such as valvular heart disease, amyloid, and hypertrophic cardiomyopathy are also associated with a reasonably high prevalence of PH but are proportionally less common than HFpEF or HFrEF on a population level.

PH in LH disease has been universally recognized as a marker of not only poor prognosis but also impaired exercise tolerance and risk for progressive HF.[3,25,27,31,51,102] Furthermore, when the PH is "out of proportion" to the degree of LH filling pressure elevation, outcomes are substantially poorer.[3,4] Such patients have been defined as combined pre- and postcapillary PH (CpC-PH), differing from patients with isolated LA hypertension as the cause of PH (isolated postcapillary PH [IpC-PH]) (**Table 57–3**). The frequency of superimposed precapillary PH in LH disease varies depending on way that it is defined[4,103] and based upon the adequacy of decongestion prior to assessment,[104] but the best estimate is that roughly ~10% to 15% of patients with Group 2 PH have coexisting precapillary disease, defined by an elevated PVR.[3,31,103]

Pulmonary Hypertension in HFrEF

HFrEF is characterized by LV dilatation and systolic dysfunction that leads to progressive LA hypertension, although PA

TABLE 57–3. Hemodynamic Definitions of Pulmonary Hypertension (PH)

Definition	Mean PA pressure	PCW pressure*	PVR
Precapillary PH (Groups 1, 3, 4)	>20 mm Hg	≤15 mm Hg	>3 Wood units
Isolated post capillary PH (IpC PH)	>20 mm Hg	>15 mm Hg	<3 Wood units
Combined pre and post capillary PH (CpC PH)	>20 mm Hg	>15 mm Hg	≥3 Wood units
High output HF**	>20 mm Hg	>15 mm Hg	<3 Wood units

Abbreviations: PA, pulmonary artery; PCW, pulmonary capillary wedge; PVR, pulmonary vascular resistance.
*Some guidelines use values of 15 or greater to indicate Group 2.
**Also requires a cardiac index >4.0 L/min/m² differentiating from IpC PH.

pressures often improve through use of guideline-directed medical therapy.[105] The presence of PH after medical therapy optimization is a poor prognostic sign. If LA pressures remain elevated for a prolonged period of time, this can result in pulmonary vascular remodeling, with an associated decrease in lung diffusion capacity (Fig. 57–8).[101]

Patients with HFrEF may become accustomed to elevated PCWP over sustained durations of time due to enhancement of pulmonary lymphatic drainage and thickening of the capillary basement membrane, which limits transudation of fluid into the alveolar interstitium.[106] While these changes may be adaptive to reduce lung congestion, they also impair gas exchange and worsen RV afterload by increasing PVR even further (**Fig. 57–9**).

The presence of CpC-PH is important in the evaluation of patients for heart transplantation. Exposing a normal "virgin" heart to a diseased pulmonary vasculature may lead to RV dysfunction and primary graft failure. However, if the PVR elevation is reversible, outcomes following transplantation are acceptable. This importantly indicates that not all "precapillary" PH in LH disease is from irreversible histological remodeling.[107] Sustained reduction in PCWP through LVAD support has demonstrated reversibility of the precapillary components of PH in HFrEF, followed by successful transplantation.[108]

Pulmonary Hypertension in HFpEF

Although IpC-PH is the most common form of PH in HFpEF, pulmonary vascular reserve limitations during exercise are present even in the earliest stages of HFpEF where filling pressures and PH are normal at rest.[17,109] Impairments in pulmonary vascular function constrain cardiac output reserve during exercise, even when PVR is not extremely high. All efforts should be made to reduce LA pressures in patients with Group 2 PH. Experimental interventions such as atrial septostomy that reduce LA pressure reduction and increases in pulmonary blood flow may improve pulmonary vascular function in patients with IpC PH HFpEF,[110] but LA pressure reduction is most commonly achieved using diuretics in this cohort.

Patients with CpC-PH HFpEF display similar patterns of pulmonary vascular remodeling as patients with PH due to HFrEF (Fig. 57–9). These patients also display prominent abnormalities in RV–PA coupling culminating in marked increases in RA pressure during exercise, increasing ventricular interaction, and limiting cardiac output responses to stress.[27] Recent data suggest overlap between PAH and CpC-PH HFpEF, implying a spectrum of disease expression.[103] Obesity and metabolic syndrome play important roles in Group 2 PH. Patients with the obese phenotype of HFpEF display even more deranged RV–PA coupling and pulmonary vascular remodeling compared to nonobese HFpEF,[111] and weight loss may be associated with reduced PA pressures.[112]

High-Output Heart Failure

High-output heart failure is an uncommon disorder that may lead to PH and be confused with HFpEF. The pathogenesis involves excessive increases in whole-body oxygen

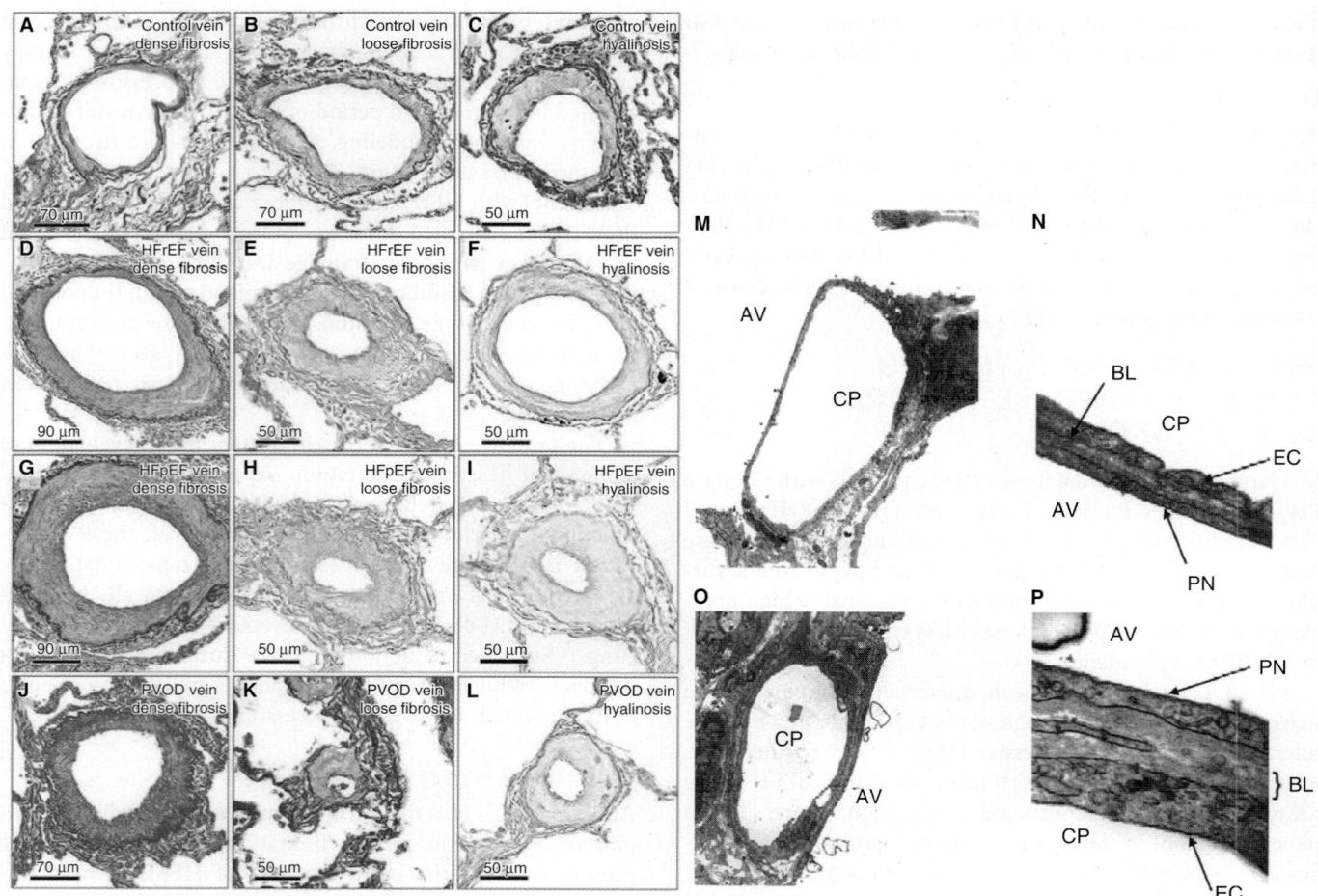

Figure 57–9. Pulmonary vascular remodeling in chronic Group 2 PH. (A–L) show small vessel venous remodeling in autopsy samples from human controls (**A–C**), heart failure with reduced ejection fraction (HFrEF, **D–F**), heart failure with preserved ejection fraction (HFpEF, **G–I**), and patients with pulmonary veno-occlusive disease (PVOD, **J–L**). Extensive intimal thickening is noted with fibrosis and hyalinosis that develops in the setting of chronic pulmonary venous and arterial hypertension. **(M and N)** show normal alveolus (AV) and pulmonary capillary (CP) interface, with thin alveolar-capillary interface and basal lamina (BL). **(O and P)** show changes with chronic heart failure, with thickening of the interstitial space and the BL. A–L, Reproduced with permissions from Fayyaz AU, Edwards WD, Maleszewski JJ, et al: Global Pulmonary Vascular Remodeling in Pulmonary Hypertension Associated With Heart Failure and Preserved or Reduced Ejection Fraction. *Circulation.* 2018 Apr 24;137(17):1796-1810. M–P, Reproduced with permission from Huang W, Kingsbury MP, Turner MA, et al: Capillary filtration is reduced in lungs adapted to chronic heart failure: morphological and haemodynamic correlates. *Cardiovasc Res.* 2001 Jan;49(1):207-217.

consumption and/or peripheral vasodilation that cause arterial underfilling, with impaired renal perfusion. This promotes salt and water retention with resultant volume overload and increase in filling pressures. Obesity, arteriovenous fistulas, cirrhosis, lung disease, and myeloproliferative disorders are the most common causes in the modern era.[64]

Treatment of Pulmonary Hypertension in Left Heart Disease

In patients with Group 2 PH, normalization of LA pressure through decongestion is the most important treatment intervention. This is most often accomplished using diuretics and vasodilators. Neurohormonal antagonists may also directly reduce PA pressures through vasoactive or anti-remodeling effects, but this possibility remains little studied. Mechanical unloading may also be effective when sustained chronically to improve pulmonary vascular properties.[107,108] Some patients with high-output heart failure–related PH may respond to treatments targeting the inciting problem, for example, closure of an arteriovenous fistula. There is currently no evidence-based role for therapies used in patients with Group 1 PAH in patients with Group 2 PH, although a number of patients are prescribed these therapies in current practice.[7]

PULMONARY HYPERTENSION ASSOCIATED WITH LUNG DISEASE (GROUP 3)

Although any form of chronic hypoxic lung disease can lead to PH, the most common forms of lung disease that result in PH are chronic obstructive pulmonary disease (COPD), interstitial fibrosis, and obesity hypoventilation syndrome/sleep apnea. In general, the treatment for these forms of PH involves addressing the underlying cause and no specific PAH directed therapy has shown benefit with some potential for harm with inappropriate use of these therapies. Many of these patients also display an element of PH due to LH disease (usually HFpEF).

Chronic Obstructive Airway Disease

Most patients with COPD who develop PH display only mild elevations in PVR and PA pressure but a notable subset may develop severe PH out of proportion to their lung disease.[113] This leads to reduced cardiac output during exercise through abnormal RV–PA coupling greatly limiting functional capacity.[114] A subset of COPD patients may also develop hypoxia and hypercapnia mediated peripheral vasodilation resulting in renal hypoperfusion and secondary salt and water retention[115] representing a form of high-output heart failure with associated PH.[64] Patients with COPD frequently display multiple risk factors for HFpEF and careful evaluation for coexisting LH disease is essential.[116]

Interstitial Lung Disease

The most common form of interstitial fibrosis is idiopathic pulmonary fibrosis (IPF). In a series of patients with mild to moderate IPF undergoing invasive hemodynamic evaluation, 14% of patients displayed Group 3 PH, and notably another 4% displayed Group 2 PH due to HFpEF.[117] The prevalence of PH is higher among more severe IPF, approaching 50%, with a higher prevalence of elevated left-sided filling pressures and HFpEF.[118] In patients with combined emphysema and interstitial fibrosis (emphysema in the upper lobes and fibrosis in the lower lobes), the prevalence of PH is particularly high and associated with abysmal outcomes.[119] Clinical trials testing therapies effective in PAH have decidedly failed in IPF-associated PH, with no benefit and a potential for harm, with worsening oxygenation and increased rates of disease progression, hospitalization, and mortality with PAH-specific therapy.[120,121] Therefore, lung transplantation remains the treatment of choice in the presence of substantial PH and IPF.

Obesity Hypoventilation and Sleep Apnea

Obesity hypoventilation syndrome is characterized by obesity associated with resting daytime hypercapnia and hypoventilation, and in most cases is associated with underlying OSA, both of which can be associated with PH. Patients with OSA are frequently obese and have risk factors for left-sided heart disease such as HFpEF. PH in isolated OSA without obesity hypoventilation syndrome is frequently mild and present in only a minority of patients. The PH in OSA is in fact most strongly associated with the degree of PCWP elevation, but also associated with the degree of nocturnal hypoxia.[122] Since these original studies, there has been a greater appreciation of the detrimental impact of obesity in directly contributing to global cardiac reserve abnormalities that leads to obesity-related HFpEF.[25,50,111,123]

Although nocturnal noninvasive positive pressure ventilation can alleviate the degree of intermittent nocturnal hypoxia in OSAs, there are no large randomized trials demonstrating a benefit of continuous positive airway pressure (CPAP) therapy on outcomes in PH. For patients with OSA coupled with obesity hypoventilation syndrome, nocturnal noninvasive ventilation or CPAP helps alleviate chronic resting hypercapnia and hypoxia,[124] and this may have potential benefits for long term pulmonary vascular function and PH.[125] Weight loss has substantial impacts on reversing sleep apnea,[126] but may also have beneficial impacts on central pulmonary and left heart hemodynamic impairments that can result in PH.[112]

PULMONARY HYPERTENSION ASSOCIATED WITH PULMONARY EMBOLI (GROUP 4)

Definitions

Most patients with pulmonary embolism respond well to chronic anticoagulation with resolution of symptoms. In a small percentage of patients (around 3%–4%), there can be persistence of symptoms with evidence of PH from organization and incomplete resolution of the thrombus.[10] Even more patients may suffer from persistent exercise intolerance in the absence of resting PH, which is associated with increased dead space and deranged exercise hemodynamics—a condition termed *chronic thromboembolic disease.*

Pathophysiology and Therapeutic Implications

There is great variability in clinical phenotype depending on whether the afterload on the RV is primarily related to large proximal clot burden, more distal embolic disease, small vessel remodeling, or a combination of these. In highly experienced centers, surgical pulmonary endarterectomy affords substantial improvements in hemodynamics and quality of life and may be associated with improved survival.[127] In patients who are not surgical candidates, peripheral segmental and subsegmental disease may be approachable by percutaneous balloon angioplasty with symptom and hemodynamic improvement, although again this intervention is only available at select centers.[128] A subset of patients with CTEPH develop pulmonary arteriolar remodeling with intimal hyperplasia and medial hypertrophy resulting in pathophysiologic changes similar to those in Group 1 PAH.[129] The small vessel changes with intimal thickening in arterial segments can be seen even in nonobstructed lung territory and contributes to persistent PH, symptoms, and increased mortality despite successful pulmonary endarterectomy.[129]

Treatment

A ventilation-perfusion scan is the screening test of choice should be done in all suspected patients with PH, since around 20% to 25% of CTEPH patients may have had clinically unrecognized pulmonary embolism in the past.[130] Invasive pulmonary angiography can provide further anatomic details and allow assessment for the feasibility of percutaneous pulmonary balloon angioplasty in appropriate candidates. This has demonstrated symptom and hemodynamic improvement in observational studies[128] and is an increasingly viable alternative for patients with more distal disease that cannot be easily approached surgically, or in patients who are not candidates for surgical endarterectomy. Although there is substantial upfront risk (5% in-hospital mortality), surgery remains the standard of care in the approximately 60% of CTEPH patients who are appropriate candidates given the potentially curative nature of the operation, particularly in patients with more proximal disease.[130] A notable subset of patients may have persistent PAH after surgery or catheter-based therapy reflective of small vessel disease, with approximately 20% to 50% of patients after surgical embolectomy continuing to have residual (but improved) PH. These patients may benefit from medical therapy, and riociguat has been specifically studied in CTEPH with modest benefit on exercise capacity, symptoms, and hemodynamics[87] in patients with persistent PH after surgery or with inoperable disease.

PULMONARY HYPERTENSION WITH UNCLEAR AND MULTIFACTORIAL DISORDERS (GROUP 5)

This is by far the smallest group of patients and includes a widely heterogenous assortment of disorders. Treatments are highly individualized and directed at the underlying disease processes, and little prospective data is available to guide treatment decisions. The evolution of classification of the various groups of PH over time is depicted in **Table 57–4**.

FUTURE DIRECTIONS

Remarkable advances have been made in the treatment of patients with Group 1 PAH in the last two decades, but outcomes remain suboptimal in this population, and treatment options are even more limited for the substantially larger number of individuals worldwide afflicted with other types of PH. Future research into targeting novel pathways to target the underlying processes driving pulmonary vascular remodeling

and right heart dysfunction to change the natural history are needed, because it is likely that many patients with non-Group 1 PAH display pathophysiologic features that are more typical of PAH, and might accordingly respond to existing treatments. With advances in molecular diagnostics and more detailed hemodynamic profiling, more refined diagnostic phenotyping of the various forms of PH will allow more targeted and personalized management in the near future.

REFERENCES

1. Simonneau G, Montani D, Celermajer DS, et al. Haemodynamic definitions and updated clinical classification of pulmonary hypertension. *Eur Respir J.* 2019;53.
2. Rich S, Dantzker DR, Ayres SM, et al. Primary pulmonary hypertension. A national prospective study. *Ann Intern Med.* 1987;107:216-223.
3. Vanderpool RR, Saul M, Nouraie M, Gladwin MT, Simon MA. Association between hemodynamic markers of pulmonary hypertension and outcomes in heart failure with preserved ejection fraction. *JAMA Cardiol.* 2018;3:298-306.
4. Miller WL, Grill DE, Borlaug BA. Clinical features, hemodynamics, and outcomes of pulmonary hypertension due to chronic heart failure with reduced ejection fraction: pulmonary hypertension and heart failure. *JACC Heart Fail.* 2013;1:290-299.
5. Hoeper MM, Humbert M, Souza R, et al. A global view of pulmonary hypertension. *Lancet Respir Med.* 2016;4:306-322.
6. Hasan B, Hansmann G, Budts W, et al. Challenges and special aspects of pulmonary hypertension in middle- to low-income regions: JACC State-of-the-Art Review. *J Am Coll Cardiol.* 2020;75:2463-2477.
7. Wijeratne DT, Lajkosz K, Brogly SB, et al. Increasing incidence and prevalence of World Health Organization Groups 1 to 4 Pulmonary Hypertension: a population-based cohort study in Ontario, Canada. *Circ Cardiovasc Qual Outcomes.* 2018;11:e003973.
8. Humbert M, Sitbon O, Chaouat A, et al. Pulmonary arterial hypertension in France: results from a national registry. *Am J Respir Crit Care Med.* 2006;173:1023-1030.
9. Opitz CF, Hoeper MM, Gibbs JS, et al. Pre-capillary, combined, and post-capillary pulmonary hypertension: a pathophysiological continuum. *J Am Coll Cardiol.* 2016;68:368-378.
10. Pengo V, Lensing AW, Prins MH, et al. Incidence of chronic thromboembolic pulmonary hypertension after pulmonary embolism. *N Engl J Med.* 2004;350:2257-2264.
11. Zhang M, Wang N, Zhai Z, et al. Incidence and risk factors of chronic thromboembolic pulmonary hypertension after acute pulmonary embolism: a systematic review and meta-analysis of cohort studies. *J Thorac Dis.* 2018;10:4751-4763.
12. Ende-Verhaar YM, Cannegieter SC, Vonk Noordegraaf A, et al. Incidence of chronic thromboembolic pulmonary hypertension after acute pulmonary embolism: a contemporary view of the published literature. *Eur Respir J.* 2017;49.
13. Pepke-Zaba J, Delcroix M, Lang I, et al. Chronic thromboembolic pulmonary hypertension (CTEPH): results from an international prospective registry. *Circulation.* 2011;124:1973-1981.
14. Gall H, Hoeper MM, Richter MJ, Cacheris W, Hinzmann B, Mayer E. An epidemiological analysis of the burden of chronic thromboembolic pulmonary hypertension in the USA, Europe and Japan. *Eur Respir Rev.* 2017;26.
15. Vonk Noordegraaf A, Westerhof BE, Westerhof N. The relationship between the right ventricle and its load in pulmonary hypertension. *J Am Coll Cardiol.* 2017;69:236-243.
16. Lewis GD, Bossone E, Naeije R, et al. Pulmonary vascular hemodynamic response to exercise in cardiopulmonary diseases. *Circulation.* 2013;128:1470-1479.

TABLE 57–4. Key Changes in Clinical Classification from the 5th to 6th World Society of Pulmonary Hypertension (WSPH) Classification

	6th WSPH
Group 1	• Group 1.3 Drug and toxin-induced PAH was simplified to two subgroups: "Definite association" and "Possible association." PAH due to methamphetamine and dasatinib now considered a definite association • Group 1.5 created to represent PAH patients who are long-term responders to calcium channel blockers • Group 1.6 created to represent PAH with overt features of venous/capillaries (PVOD/PCH) involvement
Group 2	No change
Group 3	• Sleep disordered breathing, alveolar hypoventilation disorders, and chronic exposure to high altitude combined under Group 3.4 Hypoxia without lung disease
Group 4	• Creation of two groups 4.1 Chronic thromboembolic PH and 4.2 Other pulmonary artery obstructions
Group 5	• PH in lymphangioleiomyomatosis classified together with parenchymal lung diseases in Group 3 and removed from Group 5 • Thyroid disorders removed from Group 5 • Tumoral obstructions moved to Group 4.2 under other pulmonary artery obstruction

17. Borlaug BA, Kane GC, Melenovsky V, Olson TP. Abnormal right ventricular-pulmonary artery coupling with exercise in heart failure with preserved ejection fraction. *Eur Heart J.* 2016;37:3293-3302.

18. Tedford RJ, Hassoun PM, Mathai SC, et al. Pulmonary capillary wedge pressure augments right ventricular pulsatile loading. *Circulation.* 2012;125:289-297.

19. Gerges C, Gerges M, Lang MB, et al. Diastolic pulmonary vascular pressure gradient: a predictor of prognosis in "out-of-proportion" pulmonary hypertension. *Chest.* 2013;143:758-766.

20. Tampakakis E, Shah SJ, Borlaug BA, et al. Pulmonary effective arterial elastance as a measure of right ventricular afterload and its prognostic value in pulmonary hypertension due to left heart disease. *Circ Heart Fail.* 2018;11:e004436.

21. Mahapatra S, Nishimura RA, Sorajja P, Cha S, McGoon MD. Relationship of pulmonary arterial capacitance and mortality in idiopathic pulmonary arterial hypertension. *J Am Coll Cardiol.* 2006;47:799-803.

22. Tello K, Wan J, Dalmer A, et al. Validation of the tricuspid annular plane systolic excursion/systolic pulmonary artery pressure ratio for the assessment of right ventricular-arterial coupling in severe pulmonary hypertension. *Circ Cardiovasc Imaging.* 2019;12:e009047.

23. Padang R, Chandrashekar N, Indrabhinduwat M, et al. Aetiology and outcomes of severe right ventricular dysfunction. *Eur Heart J.* 2020;41:1273-1282.

24. van de Veerdonk MC, Kind T, Marcus JT, et al. Progressive right ventricular dysfunction in patients with pulmonary arterial hypertension responding to therapy. *J Am Coll Cardiol.* 2011;58:2511-2519.

25. Obokata M, Reddy YNV, Melenovsky V, Pislaru S, Borlaug BA. Deterioration in right ventricular structure and function over time in patients with heart failure and preserved ejection fraction. *Eur Heart J.* 2019;40:689-697.

26. Guazzi M, Bandera F, Pelissero G, et al. Tricuspid annular plane systolic excursion and pulmonary arterial systolic pressure relationship in heart failure: an index of right ventricular contractile function and prognosis. *Am J Physiol Heart Circ Physiol.* 2013;305:H1373-H1381.

27. Gorter TM, Obokata M, Reddy YNV, Melenovsky V, Borlaug BA. Exercise unmasks distinct pathophysiologic features in heart failure with preserved ejection fraction and pulmonary vascular disease. *Eur Heart J.* 2018;39:2825-2835.

28. Obokata M, Olson TP, Reddy YNV, Melenovsky V, Kane GC, Borlaug BA. Haemodynamics, dyspnoea, and pulmonary reserve in heart failure with preserved ejection fraction. *Eur Heart J.* 2018;39:2810-2821.

29. Reddy YNV, Obokata M, Wiley B, et al. The haemodynamic basis of lung congestion during exercise in heart failure with preserved ejection fraction. *Eur Heart J.* 2019;40:3721-3730.

30. Borlaug BA, Reddy YNV. The role of the pericardium in heart failure: implications for pathophysiology and treatment. *JACC Heart Fail.* 2019;7:574-585.

31. Gerges M, Gerges C, Pistritto AM, et al. Pulmonary hypertension in heart failure. epidemiology, right ventricular function, and survival. *Am J Respir Crit Care Med.* 2015;192:1234-1246.

32. Tyberg JV, Taichman GC, Smith ER, Douglas NW, Smiseth OA, Keon WJ. The relationship between pericardial pressure and right atrial pressure: an intraoperative study. *Circulation.* 1986;73:428-432.

33. Kasner M, Westermann D, Steendijk P, et al. Left ventricular dysfunction induced by nonsevere idiopathic pulmonary arterial hypertension: a pressure-volume relationship study. *Am J Respir Crit Care Med.* 2012;186:181-189.

34. Holverda S, Gan CT, Marcus JT, Postmus PE, Boonstra A, Vonk-Noordegraaf A. Impaired stroke volume response to exercise in pulmonary arterial hypertension. *J Am Coll Cardiol.* 2006;47:1732-1733.

35. Pietra GG, Edwards WD, Kay JM, et al. Histopathology of primary pulmonary hypertension. A qualitative and quantitative study of pulmonary blood vessels from 58 patients in the National Heart, Lung, and Blood Institute, Primary Pulmonary Hypertension Registry. *Circulation.* 1989;80:1198-1206.

36. Fuster V, Steele PM, Edwards WD, Gersh BJ, McGoon MD, Frye RL. Primary pulmonary hypertension: natural history and the importance of thrombosis. *Circulation.* 1984;70:580-587.

37. Goodale F, Jr., Sanchez G, Friedlich AL, Scannell JG, Myers GS. Correlation of pulmonary arteriolar resistance with pulmonary vascular changes in patients with mitral stenosis before and after valvulotomy. *N Engl J Med.* 1955;252:979-983.

38. Weir EK, Rubin LJ, Ayres SM, et al. The acute administration of vasodilators in primary pulmonary hypertension. Experience from the National Institutes of Health Registry on Primary Pulmonary Hypertension. *Am Rev Respir Dis.* 1989;140:1623-1630.

39. Curti PC, Cohen G, Castleman B, Scannell JG, Friedlich AL, Myers GS. Respiratory and circulatory studies of patients with mitral stenosis. *Circulation.* 1953;8:893-904.

40. Rich S, Kaufmann E, Levy PS. The effect of high doses of calcium-channel blockers on survival in primary pulmonary hypertension. *N Engl J Med.* 1992;327:76-81.

41. Obokata M, Kane GC, Sorimachi H, et al. Noninvasive evaluation of pulmonary artery pressure during exercise: the importance of right atrial hypertension. *Eur Respir J.* 2020;55.

42. Bogaard HJ, Natarajan R, Henderson SC, et al. Chronic pulmonary artery pressure elevation is insufficient to explain right heart failure. *Circulation.* 2009;120:1951-1960.

43. Wright L, Dwyer N, Wahi S, Marwick TH. Relative importance of baseline and longitudinal evaluation in the follow-up of vasodilator therapy in pulmonary arterial hypertension. *JACC Cardiovasc Imaging.* 2019;12:2103-2111.

44. Lewis RA, Johns CS, Cogliano M, et al. Identification of cardiac magnetic resonance imaging thresholds for risk stratification in pulmonary arterial hypertension. *Am J Respir Crit Care Med.* 2020;201:458-468.

45. Maor E, Grossman Y, Balmor RG, et al. Exercise haemodynamics may unmask the diagnosis of diastolic dysfunction among patients with pulmonary hypertension. *Eur J Heart Fail.* 2015;17:151-158.

46. Rain S, Handoko ML, Trip P, et al. Right ventricular diastolic impairment in patients with pulmonary arterial hypertension. *Circulation.* 2013;128:2016-2025.

47. Narang N, Thibodeau JT, Levine BD, et al. Inaccuracy of estimated resting oxygen uptake in the clinical setting. *Circulation.* 2014;129:203-210.

48. Opotowsky AR, Hess E, Maron BA, et al. Thermodilution vs estimated fick cardiac output measurement in clinical practice: an analysis of mortality from the veterans affairs clinical assessment, reporting, and tracking (VA CART) program and Vanderbilt University. *JAMA Cardiol.* 2017;2:1090-1099.

49. Khirfan G, Ahmed MK, Almaaitah S, et al. Comparison of different methods to estimate cardiac index in pulmonary arterial hypertension. *Circulation.* 2019;140:705-707.

50. Reddy YNV, Carter RE, Obokata M, Redfield MM, Borlaug BA. A simple, evidence-based approach to help guide diagnosis of heart failure with preserved ejection fraction. *Circulation.* 2018;138:861-870.

51. Ho JE, Zern EK, Lau ES, et al. Exercise pulmonary hypertension predicts clinical outcomes in patients with dyspnea on effort. *J Am Coll Cardiol.* 2020;75:17-26.

52. Huis In't Veld AE, Oosterveer FPT, et al. Hemodynamic effects of pulmonary arterial hypertension-specific therapy in patients with heart failure with preserved ejection fraction and with combined post- and precapillay pulmonary hypertension. *J Card Fail.* 2020;26:26-34.

53. Galie N, Saia F, Palazzini M, et al. Left main coronary artery compression in patients with pulmonary arterial hypertension and angina. *J Am Coll Cardiol.* 2017;69:2808-2817.

54. Humbert M, Guignabert C, Bonnet S, et al. Pathology and pathobiology of pulmonary hypertension: state of the art and research perspectives. *Eur Respir J.* 2019;53.

55. Morrell NW, Aldred MA, Chung WK, et al. Genetics and genomics of pulmonary arterial hypertension. *Eur Respir J.* 2019;53.

56. Atkinson C, Stewart S, Upton PD, et al. Primary pulmonary hypertension is associated with reduced pulmonary vascular expression of type II bone morphogenetic protein receptor. *Circulation*. 2002;105:1672-1678.

57. Savai R, Al-Tamari HM, Sedding D, et al. Pro-proliferative and inflammatory signaling converge on FoxO1 transcription factor in pulmonary hypertension. *Nat Med*. 2014;20:1289-1300.

58. Graf S, Haimel M, Bleda M, et al. Identification of rare sequence variation underlying heritable pulmonary arterial hypertension. *Nat Commun*. 2018;9:1416.

59. Potus F, Pauciulo MW, Cook EK, et al. Novel mutations and decreased expression of the epigenetic regulator TET2 in pulmonary arterial hypertension. *Circulation*. 2020;141:1986-2000.

60. Hadinnapola C, Bleda M, Haimel M, et al. Phenotypic characterization of EIF2AK4 mutation carriers in a large cohort of patients diagnosed clinically with pulmonary arterial hypertension. *Circulation*. 2017;136:2022-2033.

61. Ghigna MR, Guignabert C, Montani D, et al. BMPR2 mutation status influences bronchial vascular changes in pulmonary arterial hypertension. *Eur Respir J*. 2016;48:1668-1681.

62. Larkin EK, Newman JH, Austin ED, et al. Longitudinal analysis casts doubt on the presence of genetic anticipation in heritable pulmonary arterial hypertension. *Am J Respir Crit Care Med*. 2012;186:892-896.

63. Tedford RJ, Mudd JO, Girgis RE, et al. Right ventricular dysfunction in systemic sclerosis-associated pulmonary arterial hypertension. *Circ Heart Fail*. 2013;6:953-963.

64. Reddy YNV, Melenovsky V, Redfield MM, Nishimura RA, Borlaug BA. High-output heart failure: a 15-year experience. *J Am Coll Cardiol*. 2016;68:473-482.

65. Rich S, McLaughlin VV. The effects of chronic prostacyclin therapy on cardiac output and symptoms in primary pulmonary hypertension. *J Am Coll Cardiol*. 1999;34:1184-1187.

66. Rich S, Seidlitz M, Dodin E, et al. The short-term effects of digoxin in patients with right ventricular dysfunction from pulmonary hypertension. *Chest*. 1998;114:787-792.

67. Pandey A, Garg S, Khunger M, et al. Efficacy and safety of exercise training in chronic pulmonary hypertension: systematic review and meta-analysis. *Circ Heart Fail*. 2015;8:1032-1043.

68. Khan MS, Usman MS, Siddiqi TJ, et al. Is anticoagulation beneficial in pulmonary arterial hypertension? *Circ Cardiovasc Qual Outcomes*. 2018;11:e004757.

69. Dantzker DR, Bower JS. Mechanisms of gas exchange abnormality in patients with chronic obliterative pulmonary vascular disease. *J Clin Invest*. 1979;64:1050-1055.

70. McLaughlin VV, Genthner DE, Panella MM, Rich S. Reduction in pulmonary vascular resistance with long-term epoprostenol (prostacyclin) therapy in primary pulmonary hypertension. *N Engl J Med*. 1998;338:273-277.

71. Ventetuolo CE, Gabler NB, Fritz JS, et al. Are hemodynamics surrogate end points in pulmonary arterial hypertension? *Circulation*. 2014;130:768-775.

72. Barst RJ, Rubin LJ, Long WA, et al. A comparison of continuous intravenous epoprostenol (prostacyclin) with conventional therapy for primary pulmonary hypertension. *N Engl J Med*. 1996;334:296-301.

73. Hiremath J, Thanikachalam S, Parikh K, et al. Exercise improvement and plasma biomarker changes with intravenous treprostinil therapy for pulmonary arterial hypertension: a placebo-controlled trial. *J Heart Lung Transplant*. 2010;29:137-149.

74. Simonneau G, Barst RJ, Galie N, et al. Continuous subcutaneous infusion of treprostinil, a prostacyclin analogue, in patients with pulmonary arterial hypertension: a double-blind, randomized, placebo-controlled trial. *Am J Respir Crit Care Med*. 2002;165:800-804.

75. Sadushi-Kolici R, Jansa P, Kopec G, et al. Subcutaneous treprostinil for the treatment of severe non-operable chronic thromboembolic pulmonary hypertension (CTREPH): a double-blind, phase 3, randomised controlled trial. *Lancet Respir Med*. 2019;7:239-248.

76. Olschewski H, Simonneau G, Galie N, et al. Inhaled iloprost for severe pulmonary hypertension. *N Engl J Med*. 2002;347:322-329.

77. Sitbon O, Channick R, Chin KM, et al. Selexipag for the treatment of pulmonary arterial hypertension. *N Engl J Med*. 2015;373:2522-2533.

78. White RJ, Jerjes-Sanchez C, Bohns Meyer GM, et al. Combination therapy with oral treprostinil for pulmonary arterial hypertension. A double-blind placebo-controlled clinical trial. *Am J Respir Crit Care Med*. 2020;201:707-717.

79. Galie N, Rubin L, Hoeper M, et al. Treatment of patients with mildly symptomatic pulmonary arterial hypertension with bosentan (EARLY study): a double-blind, randomised controlled trial. *Lancet*. 2008;371:2093-2100.

80. Galie N, Barbera JA, Frost AE, et al. Initial use of ambrisentan plus tadalafil in pulmonary arterial hypertension. *N Engl J Med*. 2015;373:834-844.

81. Pulido T, Adzerikho I, Channick RN, et al. Macitentan and morbidity and mortality in pulmonary arterial hypertension. *N Engl J Med*. 2013;369:809-818.

82. Michelakis ED, Tymchak W, Noga M, et al. Long-term treatment with oral sildenafil is safe and improves functional capacity and hemodynamics in patients with pulmonary arterial hypertension. *Circulation*. 2003;108:2066-2069.

83. Galie N, Ghofrani HA, Torbicki A, et al. Sildenafil citrate therapy for pulmonary arterial hypertension. *N Engl J Med*. 2005;353:2148-2157.

84. Barnes H, Brown Z, Burns A, Williams T. Phosphodiesterase 5 inhibitors for pulmonary hypertension. *Cochrane Database Syst Rev*. 2019;1:CD012621.

85. Galie N, Brundage BH, Ghofrani HA, et al. Tadalafil therapy for pulmonary arterial hypertension. *Circulation*. 2009;119:2894-2903.

86. Ghofrani HA, Galie N, Grimminger F, et al. Riociguat for the treatment of pulmonary arterial hypertension. *N Engl J Med*. 2013;369:330-340.

87. Ghofrani HA, D'Armini AM, Grimminger F, et al. Riociguat for the treatment of chronic thromboembolic pulmonary hypertension. *N Engl J Med*. 2013;369:319-329.

88. Galie N, Muller K, Scalise AV, Grunig E. PATENT PLUS: a blinded, randomised and extension study of riociguat plus sildenafil in pulmonary arterial hypertension. *Eur Respir J*. 2015;45:1314-1322.

89. Sitbon O, Humbert M, Jais X, et al. Long-term response to calcium channel blockers in idiopathic pulmonary arterial hypertension. *Circulation*. 2005;111:3105-3111.

90. Brugada J, Katritsis DG, Arbelo E, et al. 2019 ESC Guidelines for the management of patients with supraventricular tachycardia The Task Force for the management of patients with supraventricular tachycardia of the European Society of Cardiology (ESC). *Eur Heart J*. 2020;41:655-720.

91. Stout KK, Daniels CJ, Aboulhosn JA, et al. 2018 AHA/ACC guideline for the management of adults with congenital heart disease: a report of the American College of Cardiology/American Heart Association Task Force on Clinical Practice Guidelines. *J Am Coll Cardiol*. 2019;73:e81-e192.

92. Galie N, Humbert M, Vachiery JL, et al. 2015 ESC/ERS Guidelines for the diagnosis and treatment of pulmonary hypertension: The Joint Task Force for the Diagnosis and Treatment of Pulmonary Hypertension of the European Society of Cardiology (ESC) and the European Respiratory Society (ERS): endorsed by: Association for European Paediatric and Congenital Cardiology (AEPC), International Society for Heart and Lung Transplantation (ISHLT). *Eur Heart J*. 2016;37:67-119.

93. Weatherald J, Boucly A, Chemla D, et al. Prognostic value of follow-up hemodynamic variables after initial management in pulmonary arterial hypertension. *Circulation*. 2018;137:693-704.

94. D'Alonzo GE, Barst RJ, Ayres SM, et al. Survival in patients with primary pulmonary hypertension. Results from a national prospective registry. *Ann Intern Med*. 1991;115:343-349.

95. Barst RJ, Rubin LJ, McGoon MD, Caldwell EJ, Long WA, Levy PS. Survival in primary pulmonary hypertension with long-term continuous intravenous prostacyclin. *Ann Intern Med*. 1994;121:409-415.

96. Sitbon O, Humbert M, Nunes H, et al. Long-term intravenous epoprostenol infusion in primary pulmonary hypertension: prognostic factors and survival. *J Am Coll Cardiol*. 2002;40:780-788.

97. Nossent EJ, Antigny F, Montani D, et al. Pulmonary vascular remodeling patterns and expression of general control nonderepressible 2 (GCN2) in pulmonary veno-occlusive disease. *J Heart Lung Transplant.* 2018;37:647-655.

98. Montani D, Achouh L, Dorfmuller P, et al. Pulmonary veno-occlusive disease: clinical, functional, radiologic, and hemodynamic characteristics and outcome of 24 cases confirmed by histology. *Medicine (Baltimore).* 2008;87:220-233.

99. Montani D, Girerd B, Jais X, et al. Clinical phenotypes and outcomes of heritable and sporadic pulmonary veno-occlusive disease: a population-based study. *Lancet Respir Med.* 2017;5:125-134.

100. Runo JR, Vnencak-Jones CL, Prince M, et al. Pulmonary veno-occlusive disease caused by an inherited mutation in bone morphogenetic protein receptor II. *Am J Respir Crit Care Med.* 2003;167:889-894.

101. Fayyaz AU, Edwards WD, Maleszewski JJ, et al. Global pulmonary vascular remodeling in pulmonary hypertension associated with heart failure and preserved or reduced ejection fraction. *Circulation.* 2018;137:1796-1810.

102. Malhotra R, Dhakal BP, Eisman AS, et al. Pulmonary vascular distensibility predicts pulmonary hypertension severity, exercise capacity, and survival in heart failure. *Circ Heart Fail.* 2016;9.

103. Assad TR, Hemnes AR, Larkin EK, et al. Clinical and biological insights into combined post- and pre-capillary pulmonary hypertension. *J Am Coll Cardiol.* 2016;68:2525-2536.

104. Aronson D, Eitan A, Dragu R, Burger AJ. Relationship between reactive pulmonary hypertension and mortality in patients with acute decompensated heart failure. *Circ Heart Fail.* 2011;4:644-650.

105. Stevenson LW, Tillisch JH. Maintenance of cardiac output with normal filling pressures in patients with dilated heart failure. *Circulation.* 1986;74:1303-1308.

106. Hoeper MM, Meyer K, Rademacher J, Fuge J, Welte T, Olsson KM. Diffusion capacity and mortality in patients with pulmonary hypertension due to heart failure with preserved ejection fraction. *JACC Heart Fail.* 2016;4:441-449.

107. Costard-Jackle A, Fowler MB. Influence of preoperative pulmonary artery pressure on mortality after heart transplantation: testing of potential reversibility of pulmonary hypertension with nitroprusside is useful in defining a high risk group. *J Am Coll Cardiol.* 1992;19:48-54.

108. Mikus E, Stepanenko A, Krabatsch T, et al. Reversibility of fixed pulmonary hypertension in left ventricular assist device support recipients. *Eur J Cardiothorac Surg.* 2011;40:971-977.

109. Obokata M, Kane GC, Reddy YNV, et al. The neurohormonal basis of pulmonary hypertension in heart failure with preserved ejection fraction. *Eur Heart J.* 2019;40:3707-3717.

110. Obokata M, Reddy YNV, Shah SJ, et al. Effects of interatrial shunt on pulmonary vascular function in heart failure with preserved ejection fraction. *J Am Coll Cardiol.* 2019;74:2539-2550.

111. Obokata M, Reddy YNV, Pislaru SV, Melenovsky V, Borlaug BA. Evidence supporting the existence of a distinct obese phenotype of heart failure with preserved ejection fraction. *Circulation.* 2017;136:6-19.

112. Reddy YNV, Anantha-Narayanan M, Obokata M, et al. Hemodynamic effects of weight loss in obesity: a systematic review and meta-analysis. *JACC Heart Fail.* 2019;7:678-687.

113. Chaouat A, Bugnet AS, Kadaoui N, et al. Severe pulmonary hypertension and chronic obstructive pulmonary disease. *Am J Respir Crit Care Med.* 2005;172:189-194.

114. Boerrigter BG, Bogaard HJ, Trip P, et al. Ventilatory and cardiocirculatory exercise profiles in COPD: the role of pulmonary hypertension. *Chest.* 2012;142:1166-1174.

115. Anand IS, Chandrashekhar Y, Ferrari R, et al. Pathogenesis of congestive state in chronic obstructive pulmonary disease. Studies of body water and sodium, renal function, hemodynamics, and plasma hormones during edema and after recovery. *Circulation.* 1992;86:12-21.

116. Mentz RJ, Kelly JP, von Lueder TG, et al. Noncardiac comorbidities in heart failure with reduced versus preserved ejection fraction. *J Am Coll Cardiol.* 2014;64:2281-2293.

117. Raghu G, Nathan SD, Behr J, et al. Pulmonary hypertension in idiopathic pulmonary fibrosis with mild-to-moderate restriction. *Eur Respir J.* 2015;46:1370-1377.

118. Shorr AF, Wainright JL, Cors CS, Lettieri CJ, Nathan SD. Pulmonary hypertension in patients with pulmonary fibrosis awaiting lung transplant. *Eur Respir J.* 2007;30:715-721.

119. Cottin V, Le Pavec J, Prevot G, et al. Pulmonary hypertension in patients with combined pulmonary fibrosis and emphysema syndrome. *Eur Respir J.* 2010;35:105-111.

120. Nathan SD, Behr J, Collard HR, et al. Riociguat for idiopathic interstitial pneumonia-associated pulmonary hypertension (RISE-IIP): a randomised, placebo-controlled phase 2b study. *Lancet Respir Med.* 2019;7:780-790.

121. Raghu G, Behr J, Brown KK, et al. Treatment of idiopathic pulmonary fibrosis with ambrisentan: a parallel, randomized trial. *Ann Intern Med.* 2013;158:641-649.

122. Sanner BM, Doberauer C, Konermann M, Sturm A, Zidek W. Pulmonary hypertension in patients with obstructive sleep apnea syndrome. *Arch Intern Med.* 1997;157:2483-2487.

123. Reddy YNV, Rikhi A, Obokata M, et al. Quality of life in heart failure with preserved ejection fraction: importance of obesity, functional capacity, and physical inactivity. *Eur J Heart Fail.* 2020.

124. Masa JF, Mokhlesi B, Benitez I, et al. Long-term clinical effectiveness of continuous positive airway pressure therapy versus non-invasive ventilation therapy in patients with obesity hypoventilation syndrome: a multicentre, open-label, randomised controlled trial. *Lancet.* 2019;393: 1721-1732.

125. Masa JF, Mokhlesi B, Benitez I, et al. Echocardiographic changes with positive airway pressure therapy in obesity hypoventilation syndrome. long-term Pickwick randomized controlled clinical trial. *Am J Respir Crit Care Med.* 2020;201:586-597.

126. Foster GD, Borradaile KE, Sanders MH, et al. A randomized study on the effect of weight loss on obstructive sleep apnea among obese patients with type 2 diabetes: the Sleep AHEAD study. *Arch Intern Med.* 2009;169:1619-1626.

127. Archibald CJ, Auger WR, Fedullo PF, et al. Long-term outcome after pulmonary thromboendarterectomy. *Am J Respir Crit Care Med.* 1999;160: 523-528.

128. Kalra R, Duval S, Thenappan T, et al. Comparison of balloon pulmonary angioplasty and pulmonary vasodilators for inoperable chronic thromboembolic pulmonary hypertension: a systematic review and meta-analysis. *Sci Rep.* 2020;10:8870.

129. Gerges C, Gerges M, Friewald R, et al. Microvascular disease in chronic thromboembolic pulmonary hypertension: hemodynamic phenotyping and histomorphometric assessment. *Circulation.* 2020;141:376-386.

130. Delcroix M, Lang I, Pepke-Zaba J, et al. Long-term outcome of patients with chronic thromboembolic pulmonary hypertension: results from an international prospective registry. *Circulation.* 2016;133:859-871.

58

Pulmonary Embolism

Victor F. Tapson

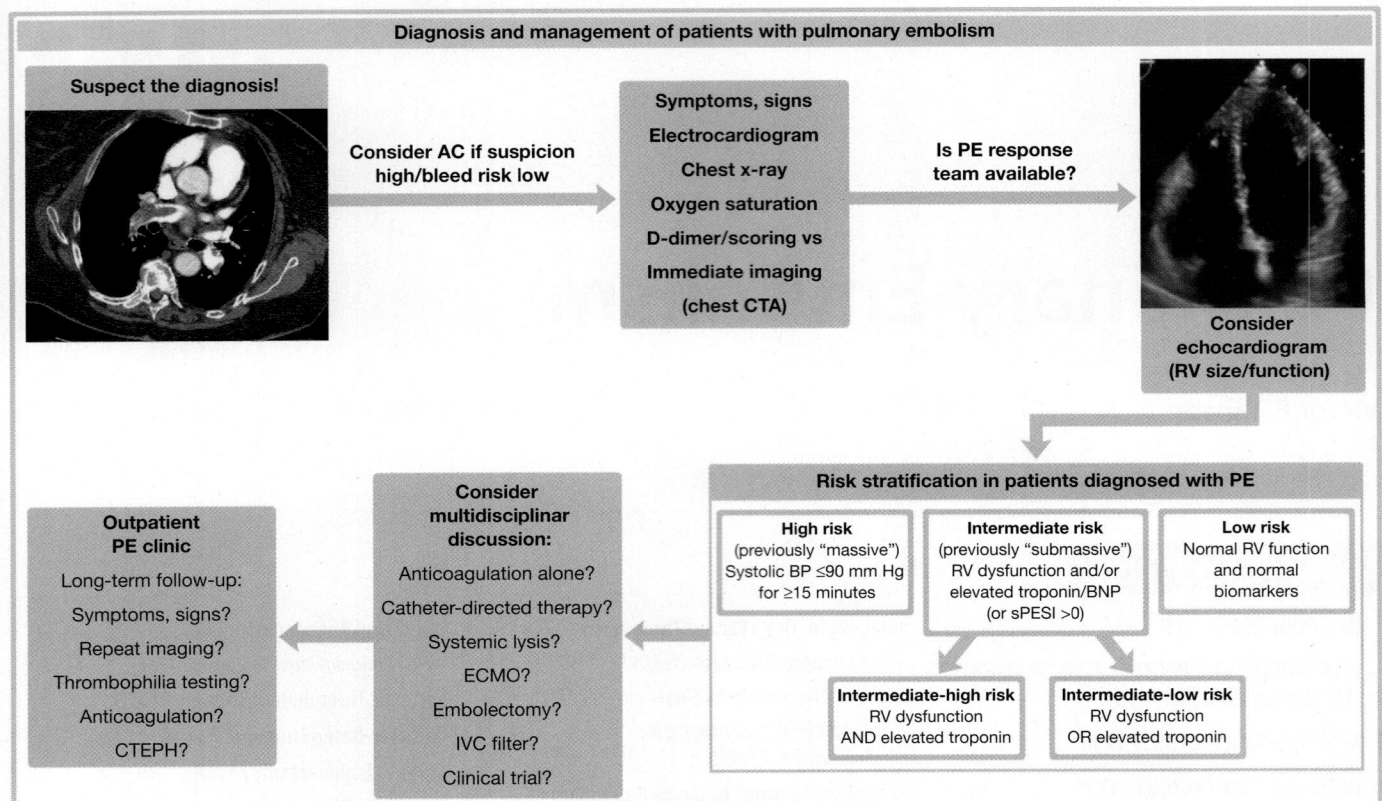

Diagnosis and management of patients with pulmonary embolism

Suspect the diagnosis!

Consider AC if suspicion high/bleed risk low

Symptoms, signs
Electrocardiogram
Chest x-ray
Oxygen saturation
D-dimer/scoring vs
Immediate imaging
(chest CTA)

Is PE response team available?

Consider echocardiogram (RV size/function)

Outpatient PE clinic
Long-term follow-up:
Symptoms, signs?
Repeat imaging?
Thrombophilia testing?
Anticoagulation?
CTEPH?

Consider multidisciplinar discussion:
Anticoagulation alone?
Catheter-directed therapy?
Systemic lysis?
ECMO?
Embolectomy?
IVC filter?
Clinical trial?

Risk stratification in patients diagnosed with PE

High risk
(previously "massive")
Systolic BP ≤90 mm Hg
for ≥15 minutes

Intermediate risk
(previously "submassive")
RV dysfunction and/or
elevated troponin/BNP
(or sPESI >0)

Low risk
Normal RV function
and normal
biomarkers

Intermediate-high risk
RV dysfunction
AND elevated troponin

Intermediate-low risk
RV dysfunction
OR elevated troponin

Chapter 58 Fuster and Hurst's Central Illustration. Once pulmonary embolism (PE) is diagnosed, risk stratification is critical. Consider anticoagulation even before diagnosis confirmed, if suspicion high and bleeding risk low. Risk stratification is critical in selecting the optimal management strategy and to potentially improve patient outcome. While this form of risk stratification has proven helpful in decision making, each of these PE risk groups remain heterogeneous and so clear decisions cannot always be made based solely on this stratification. AC, anticoagulation; CTA, computed tomographic angiography; CTEPH, chronic thromboembolic pulmonary hypertension; ECMO, extracorporeal membrane oxygenation; IVC, inferior vena cava; PE, pulmonary embolism; RV, right ventricle; sPESI, simplified pulmonary embolism severity index.

CHAPTER SUMMARY

This chapter discusses the pathogenesis, diagnosis, and management of acute pulmonary embolism (PE). Approximately one-third of patients die from PE within the first hours of presentation, often before the diagnosis can be confirmed and therapy initiated, or because the diagnosis was simply missed. When acute PE is suspected, if the bleeding risk is deemed acceptable, anticoagulation should be initiated because this is the one approach that has proven to reduce mortality. Once PE is diagnosed, risk stratification is critical and should involve consideration of clot burden, heart rate, respiratory rate, blood pressure, oxygenation, right ventricular size and function, and biomarkers. The risk-stratification terminology has evolved (see Fuster and Hurst's Central Illustration) and the term "high-risk" (rather than "massive") is suggested, while "intermediate-risk" is now used more commonly than "submassive." Carefully selected low-risk patients can be considered for outpatient anticoagulation therapy. Therapy more aggressive than anticoagulation alone is indicated when patients are hemodynamically compromised—hypotension caused by PE is the clearest indication. Various potential aggressive therapeutic options are available, including systemic thrombolysis, catheter-directed therapy, surgical embolectomy, and extracorporeal membrane oxygenation (ECMO). Following an acute PE episode, resolution may be incomplete despite optimal anticoagulant therapy, which in approximately 1% of cases may lead to chronic thromboembolic pulmonary hypertension.

INTRODUCTION

Venous thromboembolism (VTE) comprises deep vein thrombosis (DVT) and pulmonary embolism (PE). It is the third most frequent cardiovascular disease with an overall annual incidence of between 75 and 270 cases per 100,000 inhabitants.[1] The risk of VTE approximately doubles with each subsequent decade after the age of 40, therefore a larger number of patients are expected to be diagnosed with VTE in aging societies in the coming future.[1] PE is the most serious clinical presentation of VTE with 1-month and 3-month mortality between 9% and 11%, and up to 17%, respectively.[2,3] Undiagnosed or late diagnosed cases impact the mortality; anticoagulation therapy reduces the mortality substantially.[2,3] Although a number of patients die from comorbidities that predispose them to the thromboembolic event, approximately one-third of patients die from PE within the first hours of presentation, often before the diagnosis can be confirmed and therapy initiated, or because the diagnosis was overlooked.[4] Despite advances in diagnostic imaging tests and therapeutic interventions, PE remains underdiagnosed and prophylaxis continues to be underused. Following the acute PE episode, resolution is maybe incomplete despite optimal anticoagulant therapy,[5] which in approximately 1% of cases may lead to chronic thromboembolic pulmonary hypertension (CTEPH).[6]

Over the last few decades, a number of valuable insights into the natural history of venous thrombosis and PE have enhanced our diagnostic and therapeutic approaches. One such insight is the awareness that patients hospitalized for medical problems face a thromboembolic risk similar to that of their surgical counterparts. Another is an understanding of the substantial thromboembolic recurrence risk among patients with idiopathic or unprovoked venous thrombosis.[7] We have also learned that the presence of right ventricular (RV) dysfunction and increased levels of troponin and/or natriuretic peptides in the setting of acute PE may be associated with an increased risk of adverse consequences, including subsequent cardiovascular collapse and death.[8] Risk stratification is thus, critically important in acute PE. In view of this, terminology has evolved and patients are more commonly classified as high-risk (rather than massive), intermediate-risk (rather than submassive), and low-risk PE.

Parenteral anticoagulation with low-molecular-weight heparin (LMWH) or standard heparin as a "bridge" to oral anticoagulation is still considered the standard treatment for acute PE, except in the case of carefully screened low-risk PE patients who may be initiated directly on an oral direct oral anticoagulant (DOAC). Many new studies evaluating more advanced therapies such as catheter-directed PE approaches and extracorporeal membrane oxygenation (ECMO) have been conducted, although precise indications are frequently debated.[9] Finally, the SARS-CoV-2 virus causing COVID-19 infection has been shown to be a prothrombotic entity and emphasizes the link between severe inflammation and thrombosis.[10]

RISK FACTORS AND PATHOGENESIS OF VENOUS THROMBOEMBOLISM

In 1856, Virchow proposed a triad of factors leading to intravascular coagulation, including stasis, vessel wall injury, and hypercoagulability. Risk factors for VTE are based on these processes (**Table 58–1**). VTE is considered to be provoked in the presence of a temporary or reversible—usually acquired—risk factor (ie, surgery, trauma, immobilization, pregnancy) within the 3 months before the diagnosis, and unprovoked in the absence of such risks.[11] The presence of a persistent—usually inherited—risk factor may affect the decision of the duration of anticoagulation therapy after a first episode of VTE. The overwhelming majority of emboli originate from the deep veins of the lower extremities, although any venous bed can be involved. Although thrombi may form at any point along the vein wall, most originate in valve pockets. The veins of the calf are the most common site of origin, with subsequent extension of the clot prior to embolization.[12] Eventually, the thrombus

TABLE 58–1. Risk Factors for Venous Thromboembolism*†
Hereditary factors
Antithrombin deficiency
Factor V Leiden
Activated protein C resistance without factor V Leiden
Prothrombin gene mutation
Protein C deficiency
Protein S deficiency
Plasminogen deficiency
Dysfibrinogenemia
Acquired factors
Advanced age
Decreased mobility
Cancer
Acute medical illness
Major surgery
Trauma/spinal cord injury
Pregnancy and the postpartum period
Oral contraceptives
Hormone replacement therapy
Polycythemia vera
Antiphospholipid antibody syndrome
Heparins (heparin-induced thrombocytopenia)
Cancer chemotherapy
Obesity
Central venous lines
Limb immobilizer or cast
Probable factors†
Elevated homocysteine
Elevated factors VIII, IX, XI
Elevated fibrinogen
Elevated thrombin-activated fibrinolysis inhibitor
Low levels of tissue factor pathway inhibitor

*In a compatible clinical setting, acute DVT and/or PE should be considered even without potential risk factors.
†It remains unclear whether certain disorders listed above are hereditary, acquired, or both.

may expand to fill the vessel entirely, with both retrograde and proximal extension. If embolization does not occur, the thrombosis can partially or completely resolve via three mechanisms: recanalization, organization, and lysis. Postthrombotic syndrome occurs in 20% to 50% of patients and involves chronic pain, swelling, edema, and skin changes, which can substantially impact quality of life and incur significant healthcare costs.[13]

ACQUIRED RISK FACTORS

Frequently, more than one risk factor for venous thrombosis is present; knowledge of these risk factors provides the rationale for both prophylaxis and clinical suspicion. Comorbidities enhance the risk of VTE. In the DVT FREE prospective registry of 5451 patients with ultrasound-confirmed DVT, the most common comorbidities were systemic hypertension (50%), surgery within the prior 3 months (38%), immobility within 30 days (34%), cancer (32%), and obesity (27%).[14]

Although studies to date have yielded inconsistent results, long automobile or airplane trips appear to be risk factors for VTE. Thromboembolic events developing during or after air travel are often associated with other thrombotic risk factors, such as the presence of a thrombophilia or the use of oral contraceptive agents, and correlates with flight distance. In 2019, the number of scheduled passengers boarded by the global airline industry reached over 4.5 billion people.[15] The risk of PE significantly increases with a flight distance of greater than 5000 km or a duration longer than 8 hours.[16]

Clinical studies have implicated obesity as a risk factor for VTE for decades, particularly in developed countries, where obesity represents a major health issue.[17,18] The Nurses' Health Study explored risk factors for PE in women and found that a body mass index of 29 kg/m^2 or greater was an independent risk factor.[19] The Framingham Study confirmed that obesity is a risk factor for PE, particularly in women.[20] In addition to increased venous stasis, obesity may also increase the risk for VTE as a consequence of elevated plasma levels of certain clotting factors, such as fibrinogen, factor VII, and plasminogen activator inhibitor-1, and as a result of platelet activation caused by enhanced lipid peroxidation.[21]

An abundance of literature documents that the risk of VTE and its mortality increases with age, with a relative risk for those 70 years of age approximately 25-fold greater than the risk for those 20 to 29 years of age.[22] Prior VTE substantially increases the risk of subsequent events. Surgical patients with a previous history of VTE who do not receive prophylaxis are at particularly high risk for DVT. Surgery itself significantly enhances the risk. The risk of VTE is highest during the first 2 postoperative weeks but may remain elevated for 2 to 3 months. Spinal surgery, pelvic surgery (and joint replacement in general), and neurosurgery place patients at a particularly high risk for VTE.[23] Prophylactic anticoagulation may be initiated either before surgery or shortly thereafter to prevent the development of intraoperative and early postoperative thrombosis. The incidence of VTE is reduced with increasing duration of thromboprophylaxis after major orthopedic surgery and cancer surgery,

whereas this association has not been observed for general surgery.[24] Trauma, particularly major trauma, and of the lower extremities and pelvis, heightens the risk of DVT.[23]

Upper extremity DVT has become more important because of an increasing use of pacemakers; implantable defibrillators; and long-term, indwelling, central venous catheters.[25] Symptomatic PE may originate from upper extremity thrombi, although this appears much less common than embolization from lower extremity DVT. Upper extremity DVT poses the risk of superior vena cava syndrome and loss of vascular access.[26] Effort-related, upper extremity axillary-subclavian thrombosis (Paget–Schroetter syndrome) may occur spontaneously or be associated with an underlying thrombophilic tendency, and may result in significant, long-term functional impairment; fortunately, it is commonly surgically correctable.[25]

Epidemiologic analyses suggest that patients with cardiac disease are predisposed to VTE. Myocardial infarction (MI) and heart failure increase the risk of PE;[27] conversely, patients with VTE are at increased risk of subsequent MI and stroke.[28] Cancer clearly augments the risk of VTE, although the precise pathogenesis of thromboembolism in cancer is not well understood. Numerous mechanisms, including intrinsic tumor procoagulant activity and extrinsic factors such as chemotherapeutic agents and indwelling access catheters, contribute to this process. The thrombophilic tendency associated with cancer is often amplified by clinical factors such as patient weakness and immobility.[29] An analysis based on data from PIOPED (Prospective Investigation of Pulmonary Embolism Diagnosis) found that of 399 patients with PE, 73 (18.3%) had cancer.[30] The risk of VTE varies with different types of cancer.[31] Hematological malignancies, lung cancer, gastric and pancreatic malignancies, brain cancer, genitourinary tract, and breast malignancies are associated with a particularly high risk of DVT and PE.[32] About half of all cancer patients and approximately 90% of those with metastases exhibit abnormalities of one or more coagulation parameters.[33] After the administration of various chemotherapeutic agents, changes in the levels of coagulation factors, suppression of anticoagulant and fibrinolytic activity, and direct endothelial damage have been documented clinically and experimentally.[34] Hormonal therapy, particularly tamoxifen in breast cancer adjuvant therapy, is also associated with an increased risk of thromboembolism, particularly when combined with chemotherapy.[35] Neutropenia and sepsis, which often accompany chemotherapeutic regimens, often necessitate hospitalization and bedrest, which contribute further to the risk of VTE. A subsequent malignancy has been reported to occur within 2 to 3 years in approximately 5% to 10% of patients presenting with idiopathic venous thrombosis.[36] Although an aggressive search for cancer does not appear to be warranted in patients presenting with idiopathic DVT, recent data suggest that a limited approach in selected patients (age-appropriate testing, eg, carcinoembryonic antigen and prostatic specific antigen as well as mammography and colonoscopy) may be cost-effective[37] while abdominal/pelvic computed tomography (CT) scanning does not appear routinely indicated in unprovoked VTE.[38]

Oral contraception, pregnancy, and the postpartum period are the most common settings in which women younger than age 40 years acquire thromboembolic disease. Venous thrombosis develops in these settings 3 to 6 times more often than in age-matched women not on oral contraceptives.[39] When occurring during pregnancy, VTE is a major cause of maternal mortality.[40] The risk is highest in the third trimester of pregnancy and over the 6 weeks of the postpartum period;[40] still, the risk is considerable throughout pregnancy.[41] Cesarean section further augments the risk. In vitro fertilization also increases the risk of pregnancy-associated VTE, particularly during the first trimester of pregnancy.[42] Oral contraceptives are associated with an increased relative risk of VTE, although the absolute risk (~1 to 3 cases per 10,000 woman-years) remains small.[39] The VTE risk is higher in agents containing third-generation progestins such as drospirenone or cyproterone acetate, compared with earlier generations. Oral contraceptive use should be avoided when possible by women with protein C, protein S, and antithrombin deficiency, as well as in homozygous carriers of the factor V Leiden mutation. Results from a clinical trial evaluating hormone replacement therapy indicated that such therapy increased the incidence of VTE in women 45 to 64 years of age. The best available evidence suggests a 2- to 4-fold increased relative risk of VTE among oral hormone replacement therapy users compared with nonusers.[39,43] The risk of VTE also appears to be highest during the first year of exposure to hormone replacement.[43] Although such therapy is associated with quality-of-life benefits in women who require postmenopausal symptom control, physicians must balance this benefit against the risk of VTE, cardiovascular disease, and breast cancer before prescribing hormone replacement therapy.[44] Whether routine screening should be performed before the initiation of oral contraceptive agents or hormone replacement therapy remains controversial. Given the low absolute risk, especially among users of oral contraceptive agents, the general consensus is that such an approach would not be cost-effective.[45]

Antiphospholipid antibodies represent a diverse family of immunoglobulins that bind to cardiolipin or to phospholipid-associated plasma proteins such as β 2-glycoprotein I, and prothrombin or annexin A5. Antiphospholipid antibody syndrome (APLS) is associated with both arterial and venous thrombi,[46] and in rare settings a variant known as catastrophic APLS may cause life-threatening thromboembolic events.[47]

INHERITED RISK FACTORS

Inherited thrombophilias result in variable degrees of VTE risk.[48] Antithrombin deficiency was first described in 1965 and was the first inherited trait associated with thrombophilia. Functional and quantitative abnormalities of protein C and protein S were subsequently described. The factor V Leiden mutation, a single base mutation (substitution of A for G at position 506), is a far more common genetic polymorphism associated with activated protein C resistance. It is present in approximately 4% to 6% of European populations and is less common among those of Asian or African descent.[49,50] The relative risk of a first idiopathic DVT among men heterozygous for the mutation is 3- to 7-fold higher than that of those not

affected.[49] This genetic mutation is also a risk factor for recurrent pregnancy loss, probably because of placental thrombosis.[51] Oral contraceptive use in patients with heterozygous factor V Leiden mutation is associated with a 10-fold higher risk of VTE, although the absolute risk still remains low.[52]

Another less frequent thrombophilic mutation has been identified in the 3 untranslated region of the prothrombin gene (substitution of A for G at position 20210).[53] This mutant allele is present in 2% to 4% of the general population and causes increased levels of prothrombin. This prothrombin gene defect increases the risk of DVT by a factor of 2.7 to 3.8.[53,54] It appears that carriers of both factor V Leiden and the prothrombin G20210A defect have an increased risk of recurrent DVT after a first episode and are candidates for lifelong anticoagulation.[55]

Homocysteine has potential thrombogenic effects, including injury to vascular endothelium and antagonism of the synthesis and function of nitric oxide.[56] Coexisting hyperhomocysteinemia has been shown to increase the risk for thrombosis in patients with factor V Leiden.[57] However, the thermolabile methylenetetrahydrofolate reductase gene variant is not independently associated with thrombosis, emphasizing that the precise role of homocysteine in venous thrombosis is unclear. Thus, interactions between the genetic factors (defects in enzymes) that control homocysteine metabolism and nutritional factors (folate, vitamin B_6, and vitamin B_{12} deficiencies) that affect homocysteine metabolism warrant additional investigation with regard to VTE.[58]

Elevated factor VIII levels have been demonstrated to be a strong and independent risk factor for both acute and recurrent venous thrombosis; elevated levels of other clotting factors including VII, IX, XI, and XII have also been associated with an increased risk.[59,60] The real dilemma is determining who to test. Clearly, testing does not change the treatment plan in many cases.

PATHOPHYSIOLOGY OF ACUTE PULMONARY EMBOLISM

Gas-Exchange Abnormalities

The effect of PE on oxygenation and hemodynamics depends on the extent of obstruction of the pulmonary vascular bed and the severity of underlying cardiopulmonary disease.[8] Hypoxemia develops in the preponderance of patients with PE and has been attributed to various mechanisms, including intrapulmonary or intracardiac right-to-left shunting, elevated alveolar dead space, ventilation–perfusion (V/Q) inequality, and decreases in the mixed venous O_2 level, thereby magnifying the effect of the normal venous admixture. The two latter mechanisms are proposed to account for the majority of hypoxemia and hypocarbia associated with acute embolism. Shunt may occur as a consequence of atelectasis related to loss of surfactant, alveolar hemorrhage, or bronchoconstriction related to regional areas of hypocarbia. Hypoxemia leads to an increase in sympathetic tone with systemic vasoconstriction and may actually increase venous return with augmentation of stroke volume at least initially, if there is no significant underlying cardiac or pulmonary disease already present.

Hemodynamic Alterations

The hemodynamic effects of embolism are related to three factors: the degree of reduction of the cross-sectional area of the pulmonary vascular bed, the preexisting status of the cardiopulmonary system, and the physiologic consequences of both hypoxic and neurohumorally mediated vasoconstriction.[8] Obstruction of the pulmonary vascular bed by embolism acutely increases the workload on the RV, a chamber ill-equipped to deal with a high-pressure load. In patients without preexisting cardiopulmonary disease, obstruction of less than 20% of the pulmonary vascular bed results in a number of compensatory events that minimize adverse hemodynamic consequences. Recruitment and distension of pulmonary vessels occur, resulting in a normal or near-normal pulmonary artery pressure and pulmonary vascular resistance; cardiac output is maintained by increases in the RV stroke volume and increases in the heart rate. As the degree of pulmonary vascular obstruction exceeds 30% to 40%, increases in pulmonary artery pressure and modest increases in right atrial pressure occur. The Frank–Starling mechanism maintains RV stroke work and cardiac output. When the degree of pulmonary artery obstruction exceeds 50% to 60%, compensatory mechanisms are overcome, cardiac output begins to decrease, and right atrial pressure increases dramatically. With acute obstruction beyond this amount, the right heart dilates, RV wall tension increases, RV ischemia may develop, the cardiac output decreases, and systemic hypotension develops. In patients without prior cardiopulmonary disease, the maximal mean pulmonary artery pressure capable of being generated by the RV appears to be 40 mm Hg. The correlation between the extent of pulmonary vascular obstruction and the pulmonary vascular resistance appears to be hyperbolic, reflecting at its lower end the expansible nature of the pulmonary vascular bed, and at its upper end, the precipitous decline in cardiac output that may occur as the RV fails.[61]

The hemodynamic response to acute PE in patients with preexisting cardiopulmonary disease may be considerably different.[62] Such patients may demonstrate degrees of pulmonary hypertension that are disproportionate to the degree of pulmonary vascular obstruction. As a result, severe pulmonary hypertension may develop in response to a relatively small reduction in pulmonary artery cross-sectional area. Thus, evidence of RV hypertrophy (rather than RV dilation) associated with a mean pulmonary artery pressure in excess of 40 mm Hg should suggest an element of chronic pulmonary hypertension resulting from a potentially diverse group of etiologic possibilities, including chronic thromboembolic pulmonary hypertension (CTEPH), left ventricular (LV) failure, valvular disease, right-to-left cardiac shunts, or chronic lung disease.

DIAGNOSIS OF DEEP VENOUS THROMBOSIS AND PULMONARY EMBOLISM

History and Physical Examination

Erythema, warmth, pain, swelling, and tenderness are not specific for DVT but suggest the need for further evaluation.

PE must always be considered when unexplained dyspnea is present. Pleuritic chest pain and hemoptysis are also common in patients with PE. Coughing may be present, and although it is sometimes caused by PE, it more commonly occurs with bronchitis or pneumonia. Anxiety and lightheadedness are symptoms that may be caused by PE but may also be caused by a number of other entities that result in hypoxemia or hypotension. Severe dyspnea and syncope are the principal symptoms that may suggest massive, life-threatening PE.[63-65] Tachypnea and tachycardia are the most common signs of PE, but they are also nonspecific.[64] A pleural rub or accentuated pulmonic component of the second heart sound may suggest PE but can also be explained by other disorders. With embolism of sufficient magnitude to cause RV dysfunction, a murmur of tricuspid regurgitation, systemic hypotension, or jugular venous distension might be present. Clinical symptoms and signs of acute PE are listed in **Table 58–2**.

Differential Diagnosis

PE may mimic a large spectrum of diseases. The most common differential diagnoses are pneumonia, musculoskeletal

---

TABLE 58–2. Symptoms and Signs in Patients Presenting with Acute Pulmonary Embolism[†*]

Common Symptoms (>50%)[‡]
Dyspnea
Sudden onset dyspnea
Pleuritic chest pain
Less Common Symptoms (16%–49%)
Cough[‡]
Lightheadedness/presyncope
Syncope
Leg pain/swelling
Rare Symptoms (<15%)
Gradual onset of dyspnea
Orthopnea
Hemoptysis
Angina-like chest pain
Palpitations
Wheezing
Signs
Visible anxiety
Fever
Tachycardia
Tachypnea
Hypotension
Chest wall tenderness (with pulmonary infarction)
Leg swelling/tenderness
Wheezing
Signs of overt right ventricular failure (eg, neck vein distension, right ventricular S3)

[†]Symptoms can vary based upon the pulmonary embolic burden and physiologic response to the clot, as well as based on the presence/absence of underlying cardiopulmonary disease.
[‡]Note that these % values are estimates and not based on a specific clinical study.
[*]Data from Stein PD, Terrin ML, Hales CA, et al. Clinical, laboratory, roentgenographic, and electrocardiographic findings in patients with acute pulmonary embolism and no pre-existing cardiac or pulmonary disease. *Chest.* 1991 Sep;100(3):598-603.

pain/costochondritis, pneumothorax, congestive heart failure, chronic lung disease, asthma, acute MI, aortic dissection, pericarditis, and anxiety states. Importantly, patients with pulmonary infarction may not only have pain but may also have chest wall tenderness mimicking musculoskeletal disease.

Clinical Probability, Lab Testing, and Imaging

Clinical Probability Models and D-Dimer Testing

A major advance in the diagnostic approach to both venous thrombosis and PE has been a transition from a technique-oriented approach to one that uses Bayesian analysis. In doing so, the pretest probability of the disease, calculated independently of a particular test result through either empiric means or through a standardized prediction rule, is calculated. This pretest probability aids in the selection and interpretation of further diagnostic tests to create a posttest probability of the disease. The posttest probability can then be used as a basis for clinical decision-making.

For PE, three such scores have been developed and validated. Wells and coworkers[66] prospectively tested a rapid seven-item bedside assessment to estimate the clinical pretest probability for PE. An alternative scoring system, the Geneva score, involved seven variables and required gas exchange and radiographic information.[67] More recently, a revised Geneva score requiring eight clinical variables without gas exchange or radiographic information was validated and published.[68] Although such scoring systems have not proven to be more accurate than implicit assessment, they have been adequately validated[69-71] and do provide a means of standardization that compensates for variability in physician experience and judgment. Both the Wells and the revised Geneva rule were simplified in an attempt to increase their adoption into clinical practice;[72,73] and these simplified versions have been adequately validated as well.[70,72] The simplified Geneva score attributes 1 point per variable (except heart rate >95/min = 2 points) and was prospectively validated in outpatients in the ADJUST-PE management outcome study, facilitating its effective use in the management of suspected PE.[74]

D-dimer is a specific derivative of cross-linked fibrin and this test has been incorporated into clinical decision-making, particularly in outpatients presenting to the emergency department. It is important to recognize that the usefulness of D-dimer testing in inpatients is more limited as a result of comorbidities in hospitalized patients that elevate D-dimer levels. However, the negative predictive value of a (negative) D-dimer test remains high in these situations. Measurement of circulating plasma D-dimer has been comprehensively evaluated as a diagnostic test for acute VTE.[75] A normal enzyme-linked immunosorbent assay (ELISA) or ELISA-derived assay result is highly sensitive in excluding PE and DVT. When an ELISA D-dimer level is below an established cutoff level, the sensitivity and negative predictive value for VTE are 95% or above.[75] Therefore, it can be used to exclude PE in patients with either a low or a moderate pretest probability. An increased D-dimer level is nonspecific for PE and may be seen with advancing age and in patients with various conditions, including infections and

other inflammatory states, cancer, MI, the postoperative state, and the second and third trimesters of pregnancy. Thus, the specificity of D-dimer in suspected PE decreases steadily with age, to almost 10% in patients older than 80 years.[74]

The Pulmonary Embolism Rule-out Criteria (PERC) rule was developed to exclude PE and to minimize unnecessary diagnostic testing.[76,77] When a patient is deemed to *have low gestalt clinical suspicion for PE* and the eight criteria are absent (age <50 years, pulse <100/min, SaO2 >94%, no unilateral leg swelling, no hemoptysis, no recent trauma or surgery, no history of VTE, no estrogen use), it is suggested that the diagnosis of PE should not be pursued.[76,77] Inclusion criteria for a prospective validation of the PERC rule in the United States were new-onset or worsening of shortness of breath or chest pain and a low clinical probability of PE. It was found that of the 24% of patients excluded by the PERC rule, 1.3% were found to have PE.[76] Naturally, "low gestalt clinical probability" is subjective. The PERC rule was validated in the European PROPER trial;[77] however, the low overall prevalence of PE in these studies warrants caution regarding the generalizability of the results and lessens its utility. The YEARS clinical decision rule (diagnosed DVT, hemoptysis, clinician feels PE is the most likely diagnosis) also appears to be a promising, relatively easy to implement algorithm; Van der Hulle and colleagues, reported a 14% decrease in computed tomography angiography (CTA) exams required to rule out suspected PE when YEARS was paired with D-dimer level testing.[78] Furthermore, in the ADJUST-PE study, the use of an age-adjusted D-dimer (rather than a fixed D-dimer cutoff of 500 µg/L), combined with a pretest clinical probability assessment was associated with a larger number of patients in whom PE could be considered ruled out with a low likelihood of subsequent clinical VTE.[75] It should be noted that recent data suggest the utility of a low clinical pretest probability combined with D-dimer <1000, as well as moderate clinical pretest probability combined with D-dimer <500, in excluding PE and avoiding the need for chest imaging.[79]

Finally, clinical gestalt is crucial and would be expected to increase with clinical experience. It has been suggested that gestalt can outperform clinical probability scoring models in suspected acute PE although understandably this depends on the experience and knowledge base of the clinician.[80] Clinical probability tables are shown in **Table 58–3**.

Oxygen Saturation and Arterial Blood Gas Analysis

Although hypoxemia is common in acute PE, some patients, particularly young individuals without underlying cardiopulmonary disease, may have a normal PaO_2 (arterial oxygen partial pressure). In a retrospective study of hospitalized patients with PE, the PaO_2 was greater than 80 mm Hg in 29% of patients who were younger than 40 years compared with 3% in the older group.[64] However, the alveolar–arterial (A–a) difference was elevated in all patients. An important tenet should be that unexplained hypoxemia, particularly in the setting of risk factors for DVT, suggests the possibility of PE. O_2 saturations should be interpreted cautiously. A "normal" or "adequate" O_2 saturation in a patient having breathing difficulty may be associated with a very low pCO_2 by blood gas analysis indicating

TABLE 58–3. Clinical Prediction Rules for Acute Pulmonary Embolism

The Wells Score*

PE is most likely diagnosis	Yes = 3 points
Symptoms and signs of DVT present	Yes = 3 points
Heart rate >100/minute	Yes = 1.5 points
Immobilization at least 3 days, or surgery in prior 4 weeks	Yes = 1.5 points
Previous, objectively diagnosed DVT or PE	Yes = 1 point
Hemoptysis	Yes = 1 point
Malignancy with treatment within 6 months	Yes = 1 point

*In the validation cohort, a score <4.0 (PE unlikely) combined with a negative Simpli-Red D-dimer assay (not an ELISA-based assay), accurately excluded acute PE in 98% of patients. Based on the first 3-point item in the score "PE most likely," gestalt is part of the method that introduces subjectivity.[66]

The Simplified Revised Geneva Score*

Variable	Score
Age ≥65 years	1
Previous DVT or PE	3
Surgery or fracture within 1 month	2
Active malignancy	2
Hemoptysis	2
Heart rate 75 to 94/minute	3
Heart rate >95/minute	5
Unilateral lower limb pain	3
Pain on deep palpation of lower limb and unilateral edema	4

*The Geneva score was originally designed as a somewhat complex clinical prediction rule which required arterial blood gas analysis. It was revised, and ultimately, simplified. The simplified Geneva score includes the same parameters as the revised score but the score for each parameter is uniformly 1 point, and if heart rate is >95/minute an addition point was added. It is suggested that the likelihood of patients having PE with a simplified Geneva score <2 and a normal D-dimer is 3%.[68,73]

The PERC Score*

Pulmonary embolism is ruled out if no criteria are present and pretest probability is ≤15%:

Age <50 years

Pulse <100/minute

Oxygen saturation >94%

Absence of:
    Unilateral leg swelling
    Hemoptysis
    Recent surgery/trauma
    Prior DVT/PE
    Oral contraceptive use

*The PERC rule was designed to rule out acute PE in patients presenting to the emergency room without additional testing. The eight variables are listed above. As a diagnostic test, low gestalt clinical suspicion for PE and PERC negative status has been shown to have a sensitivity of 97.4% (CI, 95.8%–98.5%) and specificity of 21.9% (CI, 21.0%–22.9%).[76,77]

The YEARS Score*

Clinical signs of DVT

Hemoptysis

PE most likely diagnosis

D-dimer ≥500 ng/mL or ≥1000 ng/mL

*In patients without YEARS items and D-dimer <1000 ng/mL, or in patients with ≥1 YEARS items and D-dimer <500 ng/mL, PE was considered excluded. All others had chest CTA.

The primary outcome was number of VTE events during 3-month follow up. Of 3465 patients, PE was excluded and CTA withheld in 1651 patients with either: no YEARS items and D-dimer level <1000 ng/mL; or ≥1 YEARS items and D-dimer level <500 ng/mL. VTE occurred in 0.43% of patients with PE excluded based on YEARS algorithm alone and 0.84% of patients with PE excluded based on CTA.[78]

that the patient is working very hard to achieve that "normal" O$_2$ saturation.

Electrocardiography

Electrocardiography (ECG) findings in acute PE are generally nonspecific and include T-wave changes, ST-segment abnormalities, incomplete or complete right bundle-branch block, right axis deviation in the extremity leads, and clockwise rotation of the QRS vector in the precordial leads. The changes that do occur are likely caused by right-heart dilatation. In milder cases, the only anomaly may be sinus tachycardia, present in around 40% of patients. Atrial arrhythmias, most frequently atrial fibrillation, may be associated with acute PE. Approximately 20% of patients with PE have no ECG changes. Therefore, ECG cannot be relied upon to rule in or rule out PE, although ECG proof of a clear alternative diagnosis, such as MI, is useful when PE is among the possible diagnoses. The "classic" S$_1$Q$_3$T$_3$ pattern described by McGinn and White[81] in 1935 in seven patients with acute cor pulmonale secondary to PE was subsequently demonstrated to be present in approximately 10% of PE cases.[82] In patients without underlying cardiac or pulmonary disease from the UPET (Urokinase Pulmonary Embolism Trial), ECG abnormalities were documented in 87% of patients with proven PE.[83] These findings were not specific for PE, however. In this clinical trial, 26% of patients with high-risk (massive) or intermediate-risk (submassive) PE and 32% of those with high-risk PE had manifestations of acute cor pulmonale, such as the S$_1$Q$_3$T$_3$ pattern, right bundle-branch block, a P-wave pulmonale, or right axis deviation. The low frequency of specific ECG changes associated with PE was confirmed

in the PIOPED study.[64] It clearly correlates with degree of RV enlargement.

Despite its lack of diagnostic accuracy, ECG may be helpful in predicting adverse clinical outcomes in patients with PE. It was recently suggested that a T-wave inversion in V$_2$ or V$_3$ is the most frequent ECG sign of high-risk PE.[84] In another PE study, both the pseudoinfarction pattern (Qr in V$_1$) (**Fig. 58–1**) and T-wave inversion in V$_2$ were closely related to the presence of RV dysfunction and were independent predictors of adverse clinical outcome.[85] In a recent trial, an abnormal ECG at presentation proved to be an independent predictor of an adverse outcome, although no individual abnormality appeared capable of predicting such an outcome after being adjusted for the patients' clinical symptoms and findings on admission and for the presence of preexisting cardiac or pulmonary disease.[86]

Imaging Studies for Pulmonary Embolism

Chest Radiography

The chest radiograph is abnormal in the majority of patients with PE, but the findings are nonspecific and often subtle. Atelectasis, cardiomegaly, pulmonary infiltrates, small pleural effusions, and mild elevation of a hemidiaphragm may be present.[64,87] Classic radiographic evidence of pulmonary infarction (Hampton's hump) or proximal dilation of the pulmonary artery with decreased peripheral vascularity (Westermark sign) are suggestive but uncommon. A normal or near-normal chest radiograph in the presence of significant dyspnea and hypoxemia without evidence of bronchospasm or anatomic cardiac shunt is strongly suggestive of PE. In most situations, however,

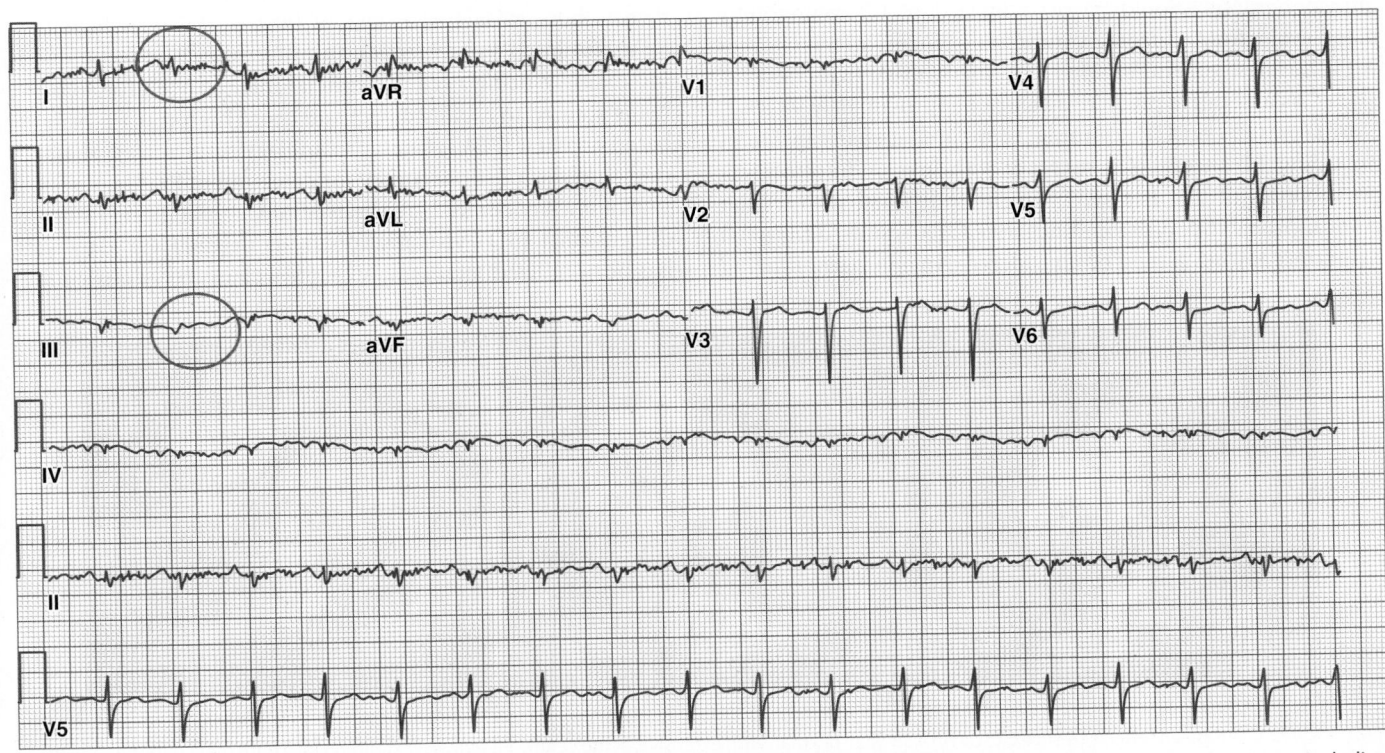

Figure 58–1. **Twelve-lead ECG from a 60-year-old man with high-risk (massive) PE and cardiogenic shock.** Several signs of RV strain are present, including sinus tachycardia with a heart rate of 116 bpm, right axis deviation, classic S1Q3T3, and flattened T-wave in V$_2$.

the chest radiograph cannot be used to definitively diagnose or exclude PE. Although exclusion of other processes such as pneumonia, congestive heart failure, pneumothorax, or rib fracture (which may cause symptoms similar to acute PE) is important, it is important to recognize that PE often coexists with other underlying lung diseases.

Computed Tomographic Angiography of the Chest

Since the introduction of multidetector CTA, contrast-enhanced CT of the chest has become the most useful imaging test in patients with clinically suspected acute PE. It allows adequate visualization of the pulmonary arteries—often down to the subsegmental level. The latest generation of CT scanners (**Fig. 58–2**) permits image acquisition of the entire chest with 1-mm or submillimeter resolution with a breathhold of less than 10 seconds.[88] Today, it is generally accepted that a chest CTA, either refuting the presence of acute PE or diagnosing it, can serve as a stand-alone test.[89] On the basis of a meta-analysis of observational and randomized studies, a normal chest CTA is associated with a pooled incidence of VTE at 3 months of 1.2% (0.8% to 1.8%) and negative predictive value of 98.8% (98.2% to 99.2%).[90]

In PIOPED II, combining CT venography with CT angiography increased sensitivity for PE from 83% to 90% and had a similar specificity (around 95%).[91,92] However, the corresponding increase in negative predictive value was not deemed clinically significant and this practice is generally not undertaken nowadays. CT venography adds a significant amount of irradiation, which may be a concern, especially in younger women.[93] As CT venography and ultrasonography yielded similar results in patients with signs or symptoms of DVT in PIOPED II, ultrasonography should be used instead of CT venography if leg evaluation is deemed indicated. Finally, newer studies with the latest generation of CT scanners reveal that chest CT alone has a negative predictive value of approximately 98.8%.[90] Normal results on CT scanning, therefore, appear capable of excluding PE in embolic suspects with low or intermediate probabilities of the disease.[90,94] In the individual with a high clinical probability of PE and negative CTA results, additional diagnostic testing should be considered. An approach utilizing

clinical probability and imaging has recently been published.[95] As demonstrated in the original PIOPED trial, a negative V/Q scan or contrast pulmonary angiogram would achieve this end.[96] Sequential, noninvasive, lower extremity examinations in patients with adequate cardiopulmonary reserve, although not confirming that PE did not occur, would render the probability of recurrence unlikely. Alternatively, additional testing should be considered in patients with a low clinical probability of embolism and a CTA that is suggestive but not clearly diagnostic of embolism because the positive predictive value of chest CTA scanning under this circumstance in PIOPED II was only 58%.[92,95]

The use of chest CTA to evaluate RV size and the presence of contrast reflux into the IVC and liver may be helpful in determining the impact of PE on the RV.[97] Furthermore, an important advantage of chest CT is the concomitant ability to define nonvascular and vascular structures such as airway, parenchymal, and pleural abnormalities; lymphadenopathy; and cardiac and pericardial disease. This is very important for rapid detection of alternative diagnoses (eg, aortic dissection, pneumonia, pericardial tamponade) in patients with acute "chest syndromes" in the emergency setting. Intravenous (IV) contrast agents may precipitate renal failure in patients with renal insufficiency. Patients with a history of allergy to contrast agents should receive preprocedure treatment with steroids administered at least 6 hours before the procedure if possible. H1 and H2 histamine blockers may be used in addition to corticosteroids. Imaging for acute PE in pregnancy is discussed in the section Pulmonary Embolism in Pregnancy.

Newer technology, including *dual-energy* CTA offers the opportunity to examine not only pulmonary arterial filling defects but also actual extent of lung perfusion which may be useful in risk stratification in proven PE. The technique is increasingly being used.[98] Artificial intelligence protocols are being studied to rapidly detect and triage high-risk PE patients based on chest CTA images; preliminary studies suggest a high degree of diagnostic accuracy for detection of PE.[99]

Volume-rendered reconstruction, obtaining three-dimensional (3D) visualization from original CT data sets, has been utilized increasingly by physicians in various clinical

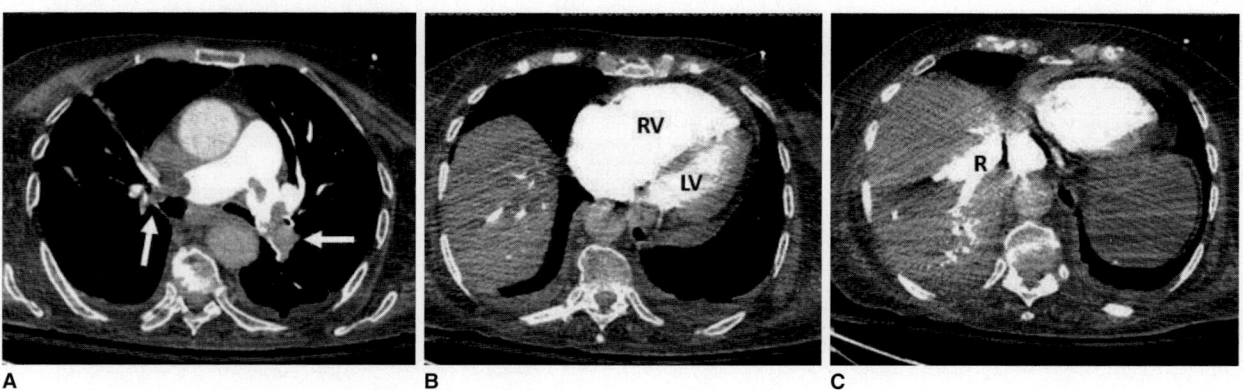

Figure 58–2. Contrast-enhanced 16-slice CT scan in a 58-year-old man with extensive, acute central PE (*arrows*) extending into both main pulmonary arteries (**A**). The center image (**B**) shows the dilated right ventricle (RV) compressing the left ventricle (LV). The image in (**C**) demonstrates the reflux of intravenous contrast (R) into the inferior vena cava and hepatic veins due to the increased pulmonary artery/RV pressure.

and educational scenarios. *Cinematic rendering* is a novel 3D rendering technique that simulates the propagation and inter-action of light rays as they pass through the volumetric data, showing a more photorealistic representation of 3D images than can be achieved with standard volume rendering.[100] While the images can be spectacular, it has not been proven that they actually add to diagnostic accuracy.

Ventilation–Perfusion Scanning

V/Q scanning has been the pivotal diagnostic test for suspected PE for many years. Although clinical indications for the study remain (contrast allergy, renal insufficiency, pregnancy), chest CT has now virtually replaced lung scanning.

The test is based on the intravenous injection of techne-tium (Tc)-99m-labeled albumin particles, which block a small fraction of the pulmonary capillaries and thereby enable scin-tigraphy assessment of lung perfusion. Perfusion scans are combined with ventilation studies, for which multiple tracers can be used. The purpose of the ventilation scan is to increase specificity: in acute PE, ventilation is expected to be normal in hypoperfused segments (mismatch).

V/Q scanning is nondiagnostic in up to 70% of patients with suspected PE, which has been a cause for criticism, because they indicate the necessity for further diagnostic testing. Normal and high-probability scans (**Fig. 58–3**) are considered diagnostic. A normal perfusion scan excludes the diagnosis of PE with enough certainty that further diagnostic testing is unnecessary.

In the PIOPED study, the usefulness of lung scanning combined with clinical assessment of patients with suspected PE was prospectively evaluated.[96] Patients with PE had scans that were of high, intermediate, or low probability, but so did most individuals without PE. Although the specificity of high-probability scans was 97%, the sensitivity was only 41%. Of interest, 33% of patients with intermediate-probability scans and 12% of those with low-probability scans were diagnosed definitively with PE by pulmonary arteriography. Forty percent of low-probability scans in the presence of high clinical sus-picion were followed by documentation of PE at angiography. When the clinical suspicion of PE was considered very high, the positive predictive value of high-probability scans for PE was 96%. In patients with nondiagnostic lung scans, further diagnostic testing for PE should be undertaken. Finally, por-table V/Q scanning may be used in patients too ill to easily move to the CT scanner and may be diagnostically useful even if there are other radiographic abnormalities.[101]

Pulmonary Angiography

Standard contrast pulmonary arteriography (**Fig. 58–4**) has long been considered the established "gold standard" imaging test for the diagnosis of PE. However, it is rarely performed now for diagnosis because less invasive chest CTA offers almost similar diagnostic accuracy; it is, however, more often used to guide percutaneous catheter-directed treatment of acute PE during the actual procedure.

Magnetic Resonance Imaging

Gadolinium-enhanced magnetic resonance (MR) angiography is also being used to evaluate clinically suspected PE. Earlier studies demonstrated that when MR was performed under opti-mal conditions, it appeared to be highly sensitive and specific

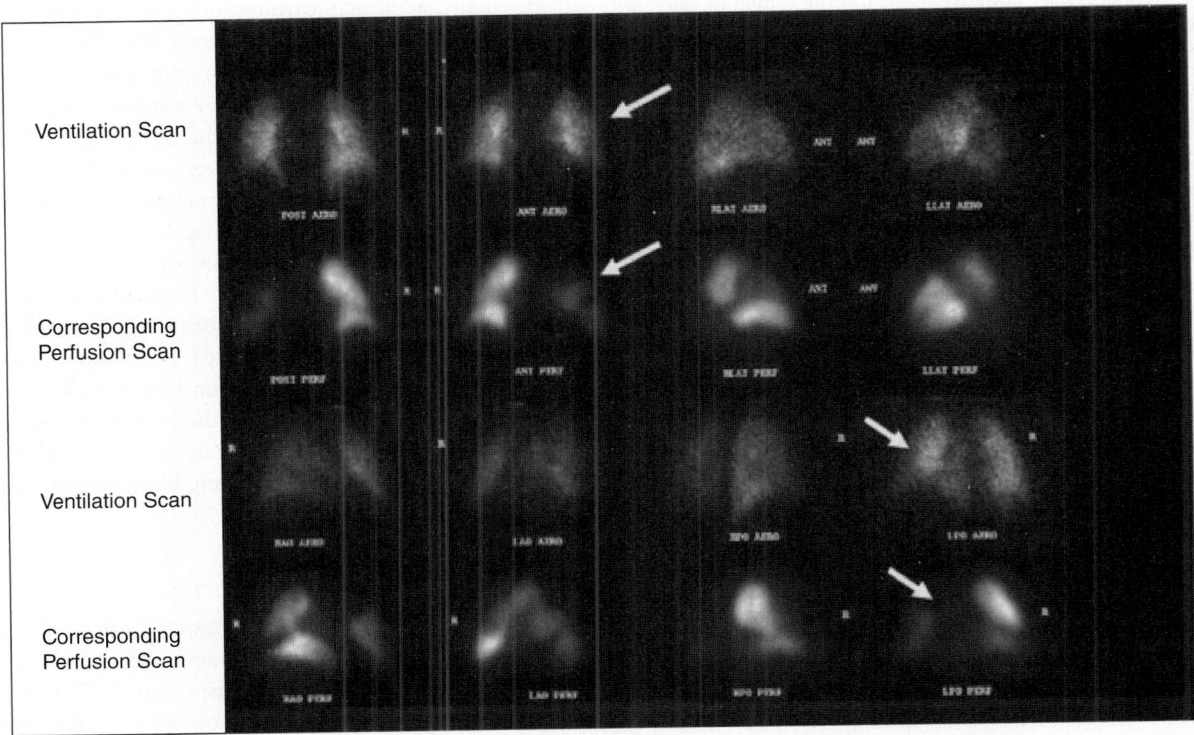

Figure 58–3. **Ventilation-perfusion scan in a 46-year-old woman with colon cancer and acute PE.** The scan demonstrates large perfusion defects that are not matched on the ventilation scan (*arrows*).

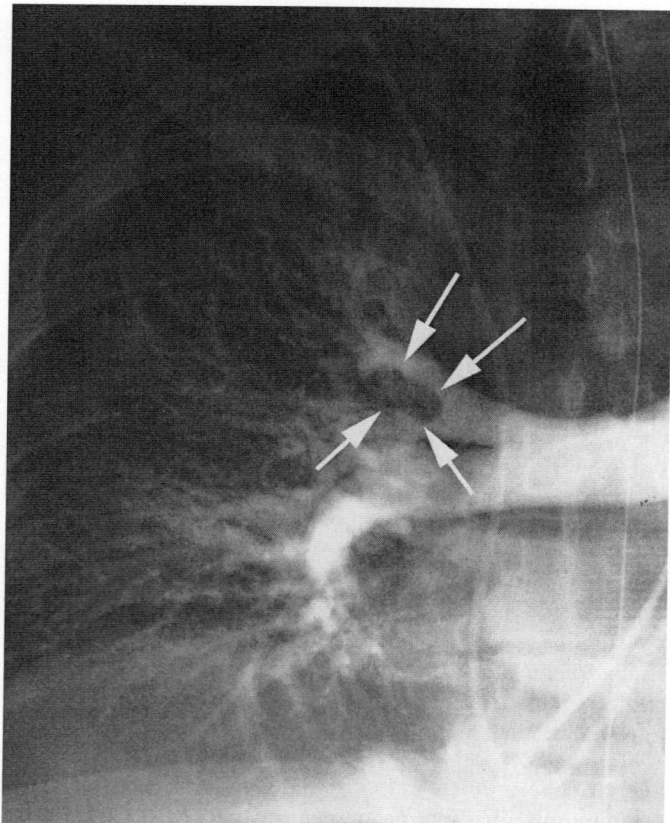

Figure 58–4. Selective conventional angiography of the right pulmonary artery in a 67-year-old woman with pneumonia and the new acute onset of dyspnea and chest pain, and a nondiagnostic V/Q scan. The right upper lobe artery is obstructed with visualization of the tail of the embolus in the proximal right upper lobe artery (*arrows*). Standard pulmonary angiography is rarely necessary nowadays except in the setting of catheter-directed therapy for PE.

even for segmental PE compared with pulmonary angiography.[102,103] Large-scale studies have shown that MR, although promising, is not yet ready for clinical practice in suspected PE due to its low sensitivity, high proportion of nondiagnostic scans, and low availability in most emergency settings.[104] MR has several attractive advantages over chest CT, including no requirement of ionizing radiation or iodinated contrast agents. Furthermore, MR technology also allows assessment of RV and RV size and function—potentially important for the risk stratification of PE patients. Use of the technique has been hampered by the cost, required scanning time in relationship to CT, and availability of scanners.

Echocardiography

Transthoracic echocardiography (**Figs. 58–5B to 58–5D**) has emerged as a potentially important tool for risk assessment and treatment guidance in patients with acute PE, complementing the findings on chest CTA (**Fig. 58–5A**). Acute PE may lead to RV pressure overload and dysfunction, which can be detected by echocardiography. While a negative result of course cannot exclude PE, in the setting of severe hypotension and shock, a normal right ventricle effectively rules out PE as the cause.[105] Importantly, signs of RV overload or dysfunction may also be

found in the absence of acute PE and be due to concomitant cardiac or respiratory disease. The presence of RV dysfunction on a baseline echocardiogram in normotensive patients appears to represent an independent predictor of an adverse outcome or early death.[106] Patients with severe RV dysfunction may show regional wall motion abnormalities of the RV known as the *McConnell sign* (ie, evidence of severe hypokinesia of the RV free wall combined with preserved/increased systolic contraction of the RV apex).[107] Patients with only mild RV dysfunction do not need more aggressive therapy in the absence of other concerning findings.

Echocardiographic examination is not recommended as part of the diagnostic work-up in hemodynamically stable, normotensive patients with low-risk PE.[104,105] This is in contrast to suspected high-risk PE, in which the absence of echocardiographic signs of RV overload or dysfunction practically excludes PE as the cause of hemodynamic instability. In the latter case, echocardiography may be of further help in the differential diagnosis of the cause of shock, by detecting pericardial tamponade, acute valve dysfunction, severe global or regional LV dysfunction, aortic dissection, or hypovolemia. Conversely, in a hemodynamically compromised patient with suspected PE, unequivocal signs of RV pressure overload and dysfunction may justify emergency reperfusion treatment for PE if immediate CTA is not feasible.

Echocardiography is also useful to diagnose a patent foramen ovale (PFO) in patients with suspected paradoxical embolism, directly visualizing thrombi in the main pulmonary artery (**Fig. 58–5D**), right heart chambers, and vena cava.[108] It has long been known that presence of a PFO can worsen the prognosis in acute PE, based on the risk of paradoxical embolism. Finally, while echocardiography can document clot in the heart "clot-in-transit" more accurately than chest CTA, data do not support ordering echocardiography specifically to look for clot-in-transit. A comparison of 57 patients who had clot-in-transit with 608 PE patients who did not have this feature suggested that presence of heart failure, a central venous catheter, and hypotension should alert physicians to patients who may require an echocardiogram to diagnose clot-in-transit. The mortality of PE with clot-in-transit appears high even relative to a population with severe PE.[109] Nonetheless, that does not allow for clear recommendations for management of this entity and it remains a frequent topic of discussion. The decision regarding whether these patients undergo simply anticoagulation, systemic thrombolysis, a catheter-directed approach, or direct surgical approach requires careful individualization. The size of the clot-in-transit, PE burden, bleeding risk, and overall clinical status must be considered.

Imaging for Deep Venous Thrombosis

In the majority of cases, PE originates from DVT in the leg or pelvic veins. A number of diagnostic techniques can be used to evaluate patients with suspected DVT. Compression ultrasonography (duplex ultrasonography) is the most common technique used in the United States and in many other areas of the world. Impedance plethysmography is rarely used

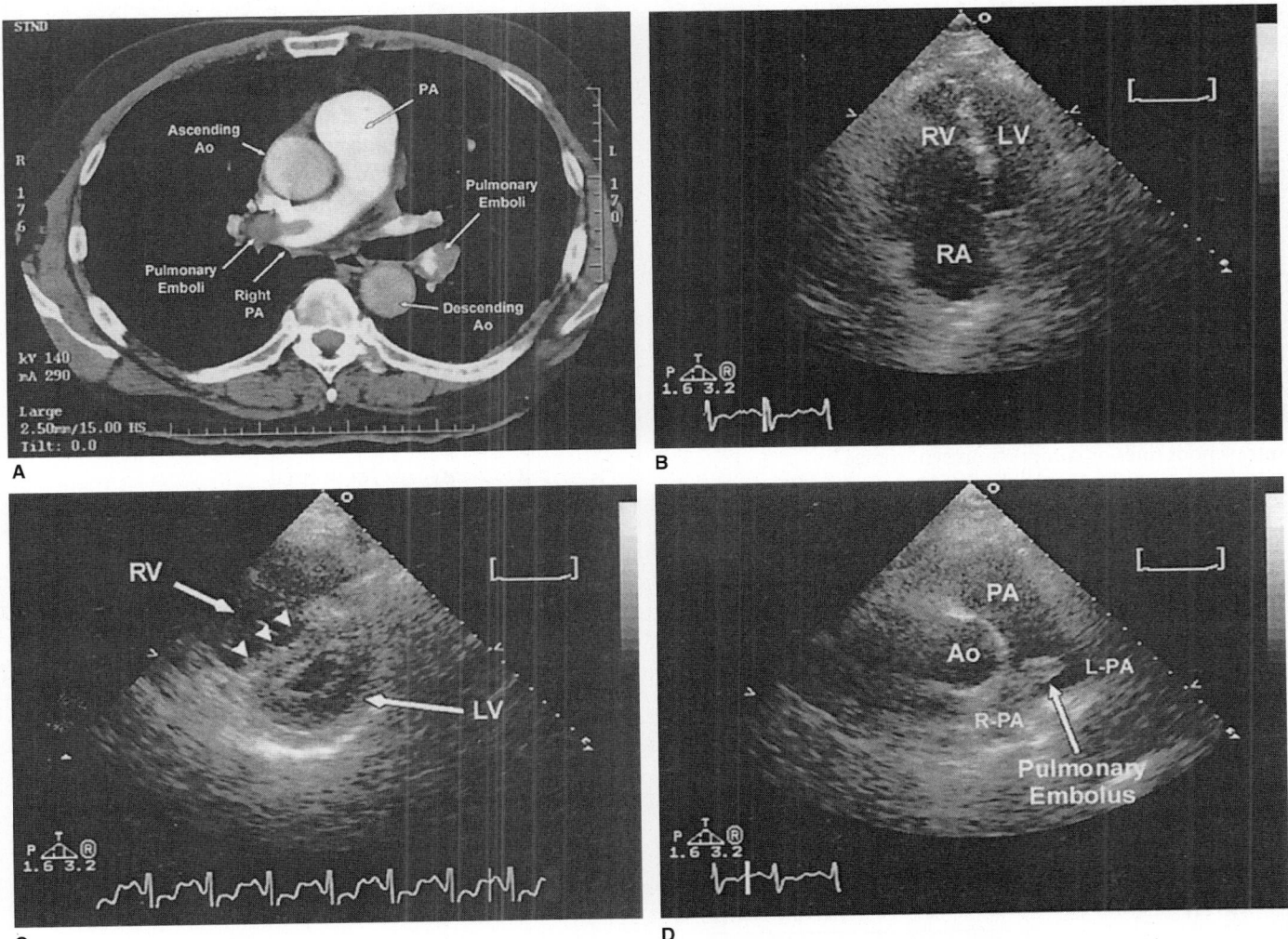

Figure 58–5. Chest CT and echocardiographic findings in a 55-year-old man with intermediate-risk (submassive) PE. (A) Chest CT scan demonstrating extensive proximal emboli, including a central embolus in main pulmonary artery and extending into right pulmonary artery (R-PA). **(B)** Transthoracic apical four-chamber view with severe right ventricular (RV) dilation. **(C)** Transthoracic parasternal short-axis view showing flattening of the interventricular septum (*arrowheads*) with "D-shaped" left ventricle (LV). **(D)** Transthoracic short-axis view demonstrating the central clot in the main and R-PAs. Ao, aorta; L-PA, left pulmonary artery; PA, pulmonary artery; RA, right atrium; R-PA, right pulmonary artery. Reproduced with permission from Garg RK, Bednarz J, Spencer KT, Lang RM. Acute pulmonary embolism. *Circulation.* 2000 Nov 7;102(19):2441-2442.

nowadays. Magnetic resonance imaging (MRI) appears to have some important advantages, but it has not generally been used as a first-line test because of cost and convenience. CT venography appears to have a sensitivity and specificity equivalent to that of duplex ultrasonography but exposes the patient to additional radiation. Contrast venography remains the gold standard, but it is almost never needed except as guidance for catheter-directed procedures. Each diagnostic technique has advantages and limitations. Although diagnostic algorithms may be suggested for suspected DVT, these are institution specific, depending on resources and available expertise with certain techniques.

Ultrasonography for Suspected DVT

Compression ultrasonography with venous imaging is a portable, accurate, and widely available diagnostic technique for DVT.[110] The primary criterion to diagnose DVT by ultrasonography is the noncompressibility of the vein. Combined with a Doppler

reading, this technique is referred to as *duplex ultrasonography*. Ultrasound technology has been further improved by the development of color duplex instrumentation that displays Doppler frequency shifts as color superimposed on the grayscale image. The color duplex images display both mean blood-flow *velocity*, expressed as a change in hue or saturation, and *direction* of blood flow, displayed as red or blue. Ultrasound imaging techniques can also identify or suggest the presence of pathology other than DVT such as Baker cysts, hematomas, lymphadenopathy, arterial aneurysms, superficial thrombophlebitis, and abscesses.[111] The sensitivity and specificity of ultrasonography for symptomatic proximal DVT has been well above 90% in most clinical trials.[112,113] There are limitations, including lower sensitivity for asymptomatic DVT, operator dependence, the inability to accurately distinguish acute from chronic DVT in symptomatic patients, and insensitivity for calf vein thrombosis. Compared with other technologies, ultrasonography is relatively inexpensive and is the preferred diagnostic modality for symptomatic suspected proximal DVT.

Ultrasonography is considered diagnostic for PE if it confirms DVT in patients with PE symptoms. However, approximately 50% of patients with CT-confirmed PE have no imaging evidence of lower extremity venous thrombosis.[112,113] Thus, PE cannot safely be *ruled out* in patients with suspected PE on the basis of a negative lower extremity duplex ultrasonography. In patients with suspected PE and a negative chest CTA, the addition of duplex ultrasonography appears to only minimally increase diagnostic yield.[113] Recent evidence suggests that multiorgan ultrasonography might increase the accuracy of PE diagnosis and reduce the CT pulmonary angiography burden.[114] Finally, upper extremity ultrasound is also accurate for axillary-subclavian or jugular vein thrombosis that may occur due to intravenous lines or compression syndromes.[115]

Contrast Venography for Suspected DVT

Contrast venography is a costly and invasive procedure that may result in superficial phlebitis or hypersensitivity reactions, but it is generally safe and accurate. Although it is the gold standard for DVT diagnosis, it is now rarely performed. Venography is performed whenever noninvasive testing is nondiagnostic or impossible to perform or during interventional procedures such as catheter-directed thrombolysis, catheter embolectomy, percutaneous angioplasty, or insertion of an inferior vena cava (IVC) filter. Compression or Doppler ultrasonography is widely available, noninvasive, and accurate, and thus favored in most settings. Alternative diagnostic approaches are contrast CT and MRI.

Magnetic Resonance Imaging for Suspected DVT

MRI has clear advantages as a diagnostic test for suspected DVT and appears to be an accurate, noninvasive alternative to venography.[116] A major feature of this technique is excellent resolution of the IVC and pelvic veins. Preliminary experience with MRI suggests that it is at least as accurate as contrast venography or ultrasound imaging and more sensitive than ultrasonography for pelvic vein and calf-limited thrombosis.[117] Simultaneous bilateral lower extremity imaging can be accomplished, and MRI appears to accurately distinguish acute from chronic DVT. This technique is also useful in differentiating other entities such as cellulitis or a Baker cyst from acute DVT. As with many other diagnostic techniques, its usefulness depends to a certain degree on the experience of the reader.

Diagnostic Strategy for Acute Pulmonary Embolism

Diagnostic testing for acute suspected PE should be undertaken as expediently as feasible. The overall diagnostic approach depends on the hemodynamic presentation of the patient. Rapid diagnosis and therapeutic intervention are required in patients with shock and suspected high-risk PE. Higher clinical suspicion and lower bleed risk suggests considering initiation of anticoagulation therapy even before PE is proven. It is critical to divide PE patients into those who are hemodynamically unstable (ie, high-risk [massive] PE) and those who are hemodynamically stable (ie, either intermediate-risk [submassive] PE or low-risk PE). The specific definitions for these categories are outlined in **Fig. 58–6.**

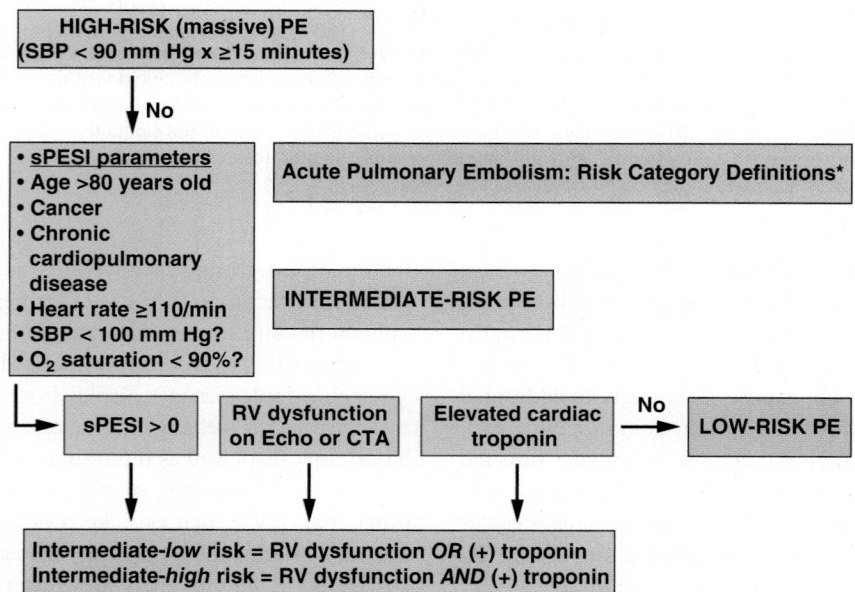

*Modified from [89] PE = pulmonary embolism; SBP = systolic blood pressure; sPESI= simplified pulmonary embolism scoring index; min = minute; Echo = echocardiogram; CTA = computed tomographic angiography; RV = right ventricular

Figure 58–6. Classification of acute PE. High-risk and low-risk PE definitions are more straightforward. Intermediate-risk (submassive) PE can be defined by either a sPESI of >0, or abnormal RV function, defined either as an elevated biomarker (troponin) or abnormal RV function by echocardiography. The 2019 ESC guidelines[89] have focused only on troponin as the key biomarker, but data support the use of BNP as also important in characterizing RV function. Each of these categories is heterogeneous and thus, denoting a specific category does not necessarily clearly define the therapeutic approach. Low-risk PE, however, is nearly always treated by anticoagulation alone.

Patients with Suspected Pulmonary Embolism and Shock or Hypotension

Patients with acute PE are generally classified as high-risk (massive), intermediate-risk (submassive), or low-risk, PE (see section Risk Stratification).[89] In patients with hypotension or cardiogenic shock associated with suspected high-risk (massive) PE, rapid initiation of therapy is potentially lifesaving. The definition of high-risk PE should be based on hemodynamic considerations rather than purely anatomic considerations and the generally accepted definition is a systolic blood pressure of 90 mm Hg or less for at least 15 minutes.[9] Occasionally, patients may present with large clot burdens with disproportionately severe hypoxemia, rather than hypotension; such patients should also be considered for aggressive therapy. Irrespective of the degree of vascular obstruction, patients with PE who present with shock have a mortality rate that approaches 30%, but those with cardiopulmonary arrest have a mortality rate of approximately 70%. Time-consuming imaging tests often can be avoided when emergency bedside echocardiography is available. In patients with suspected high-risk PE and evidence of severe acute RV dysfunction on the echocardiogram, thrombolysis or embolectomy may be considered. A caveat to this general recommendation exists in patients presenting with decompensated right-heart failure caused by nonembolic forms of pulmonary hypertension or other disorders in which there is disproportionate RV dysfunction. Clues to chronic RV dysfunction include a history of chronic rather than acute dyspnea, the presence of RV hypertrophy rather than simple dilation, or estimated pulmonary artery systolic pressures by echocardiography that are greater than approximately 70 mm Hg. As with other risk categories of acute PE, the high-risk PE category is heterogeneous and can range from, for example, a mildly hypotensive patient on a very low dose of vasopressor therapy, to a "catastrophic PE" patient on very high-dose vasopressors who is still not achieving an adequate blood pressure or has already arrested; such variability often requires differing treatment approaches in spite of both being classified as high-risk PE.

The PE response team (PERT) concept represents a multidisciplinary approach to management of acute PE and has permeated the field of acute PE management.[118,119] The PERT concept is not limited to addressing patients with proven PE but also difficult cases of suspected PE. Recent data suggest that following PERT implementation, patients with intermediate- and high-risk acute PE received more aggressive and advanced treatment modalities and received more efficient patient care, with a trend toward decreased mortality compared to before the development of a PERT.[118]

Patients with Suspected Pulmonary Embolism without Shock or Hypotension

PE cannot be excluded without objective testing. The history, physical examination, and diagnostic studies (eg, chest radiography, ECG, arterial blood gas analysis) can raise or lower the clinical suspicion of embolism but are incapable of excluding or confirming it unless a clearly identifiable condition (eg, pneumothorax) is identified to account for the patient's complaints. Noninvasive strategies have been investigated and algorithms constructed that are capable of confirming or excluding the diagnosis of embolism under most circumstances. A diagnostic algorithm is presented in **Fig. 58–7**. In all emergency department patients and other outpatients, the clinical pretest probability for PE should be calculated by implicit assessment or, through a standardized technique.[66–73,80,89] PE can be excluded by a highly sensitive D-dimer result below the assay-specific cutoff level except in patients with a high pretest clinical probability. In patients with elevated D-dimer levels or a high clinical probability of PE, chest CTA should be obtained (Fig. 58–7). In patients with significant impairment of renal function, pregnancy, or allergy to contrast agents, V/Q perfusion scanning can be the primary imaging test (see aforementioned details in section Imaging Studies for Pulmonary Embolism).

A V/Q scan can also be performed in patients with a nondiagnostic or negative chest CT when the clinical suspicion of PE persists. A normal V/Q is capable of excluding the diagnosis, and a high-probability scan is capable of confirming the diagnosis in patients with a high or intermediate probability of disease.[96] If a high clinical suspicion for PE persists after nondiagnostic chest imaging, venous compression ultrasonography and standard pulmonary angiography can be performed, although the latter is rarely necessary.[89]

The approach to a *hospitalized* patient with suspected PE is often different. At the present time, the safe exclusion of PE in inpatients using a clinical prediction rule and D-dimer in a hospitalized patient with either surgical or medical illness is less well established because of its reduced specificity.[69,71] Clinical findings suggestive of PE may be misleading due to comorbid conditions. A negative chest CTA result excludes PE under most circumstances. In renal insufficiency, a strategy using V/Q scanning with or without lower extremity ultrasound is often the most prudent approach. Under this circumstance, clinical judgment must come into play with the potential need for empiric anticoagulation at least temporarily.[80,89] When available, there should be a low threshold to consult the PERT service.[118,119]

RISK STRATIFICATION

An important advance in the therapeutic approach to PE has been the development of predictive models capable of stratifying patient by mortality risk. In-hospital mortality associated with PE depends on clinical features at admission and increases significantly when RV dysfunction is present. Accurate risk stratification in patients with PE is important in selecting the optimal management strategy for each individual patient and to potentially improve patient outcome.

Patients should be stratified as high-risk (massive) PE, low-risk, or intermediate-risk PE with the latter subdivided into intermediate-low risk, and intermediate-high risk. As already described, the generally accepted definition of high-risk PE is a systolic blood pressure of 90 mm Hg or less for at least 15 minutes.[9] Intermediate-risk (submassive) PE refers to patients with RV dysfunction by echocardiography or an elevated biomarker—generally troponin and brain natriuretic peptide (BNP). This category is further broken down into

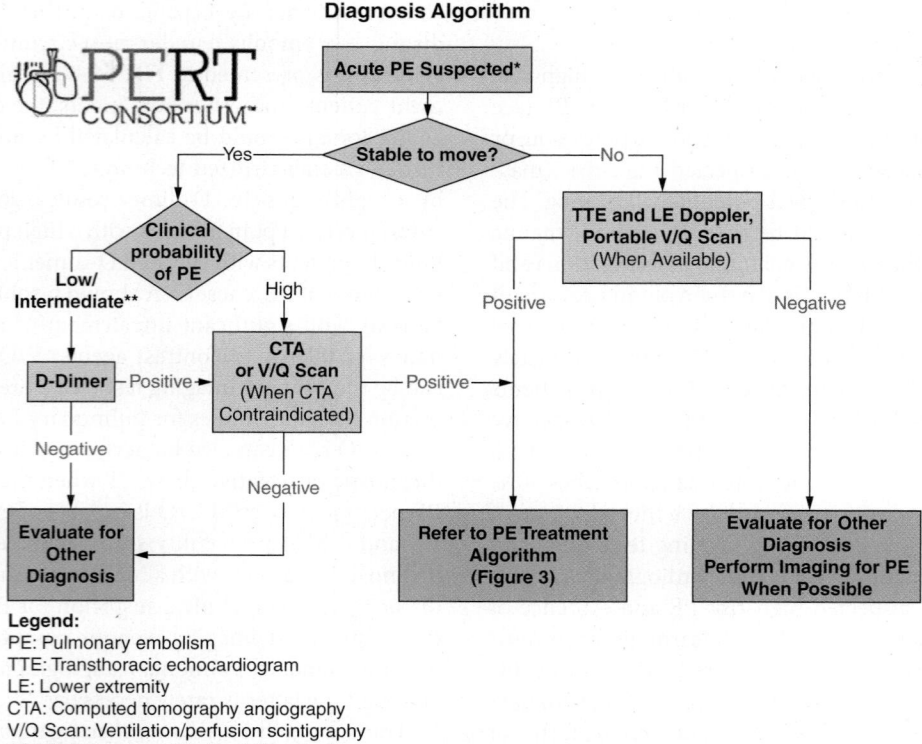

Figure 58–7. This diagnostic algorithm demonstrates the approach to suspected acute PE. Scoring systems such as PERC can be carefully used to avoid the need for imaging in some patients. Reproduced with permission from Rivera-Lebron B, McDaniel M, Ahrar K, et al. Diagnosis, Treatment and Follow Up of Acute Pulmonary Embolism: Consensus Practice from the PERT Consortium. *Clin Appl Thromb Hemost.* 2019 Jan-Dec;25:1076029619853037.

intermediate-low risk (abnormal RV function by echocardiogram *or* elevated biomarker) and intermediate-high risk (both abnormal RV function by echocardiogram *and* elevated biomarker). Intermediate-risk PE can also be identified using the pulmonary embolism severity index (PESI) bedside prediction rule (based on 11 simple patient characteristics), which has been simplified (Fig. 58–6).[120–122] An sPESI >0 also identifies an intermediate-risk PE patient. Finally, low-risk PE is the case when these parameters are all normal. While this form of classification has proven helpful in decision-making, each of these PE risk groups still remain heterogeneous and so clear decisions cannot always be made based solely on this stratification.[89] The diagnostic imaging used in risk stratification has been described above, but it is briefly outlined below in this context.

Use of Imaging in Risk Stratification

As outlined above, transthoracic echocardiography is the most important tool for risk stratification in PE because RV dysfunction on the echocardiogram is a powerful and independent predictor of mortality[123] and is the basis for determining low- versus intermediate-risk PE. Problems include the occasional poor imaging quality of the RV, particularly in obese patients and those with chronic lung disease.

While chest CTA is not generally used for risk stratification solely based upon clot burden, it is logical that the more clots present, the higher the mortality (total occlusion of the vasculature would lead to death) and there are data that support this concept.[124] Thus, assessing clot burden is included in our approach to therapy, but does not solely guide as vital signs, and RV function are deemed more critical. A number of methods have been proposed to quantify the extent of vascular obstruction and RV enlargement/dysfunction by CT scanning. Following a number of early retrospective studies with divergent results,[125,126] the prognostic value of an enlarged RV on chest CTA (RV to LV ratio ≥0.9) was confirmed by a prospective multicenter cohort study.[127] In this study, RV enlargement was an independent predictor for and adverse in-hospital outcome, both in the overall population and in hemodynamically stable patients. Interventricular septal bowing on CT was also shown to have the same prognostic value.

Use of Biomarkers in Risk Stratification

Troponins and natriuretic peptides are useful in prognosticating (**Figs. 58–8** and **58–9**).[128] RV pressure overload is associated with increased myocardial stretch, which leads to the release of BNP or N-terminal (NT)-proBNP. Thus, the plasma levels of

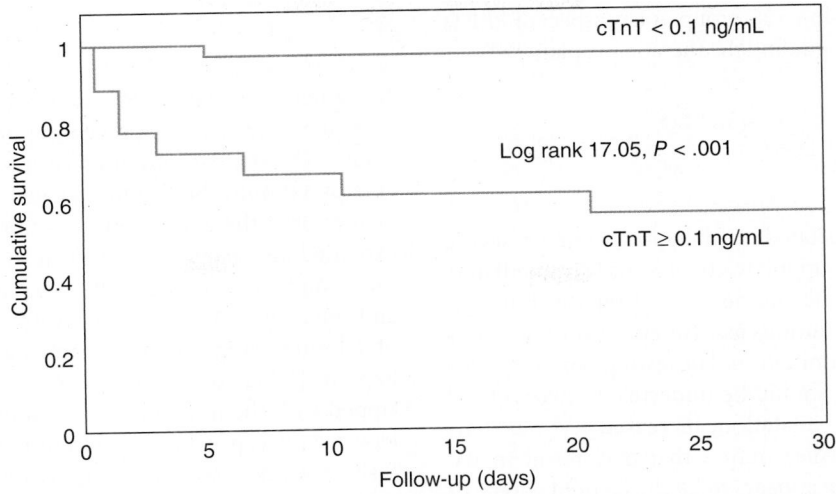

Figure 58–8. Cumulative survival rate at 30 days in patients with acute PE according to the level of cardiac troponin T (cTNT). A level above 0.1 ng/mL identifies patients at high risk for adverse clinical outcomes. Reproduced with permission from Giannitsis E, Muller-Bardorff M, Kurowski V, et al. Independent prognostic value of cardiac troponin T in patients with confirmed pulmonary embolism. *Circulation.* 2000 Jul 11;102(2):211-217.

natriuretic peptides reflect the severity of hemodynamic compromise and RV dysfunction in acute PE.[129,130] The positive predictive value of elevated BNP or NT-proBNP concentration for early mortality is low. Conversely, low levels can identify patients with a favorable short-term clinical outcome based on their high negative predictive value.[129,130]

Similar findings have been reported with troponins.[130,131] Thus, elevated plasma troponin concentrations at admission in acute PE patients have been associated with poor prognosis. Similarly, the reported positive predictive value of troponin elevation for PE-related early mortality is low, while the negative predictive value of normal levels is high. The cutoff levels for troponins are the lower detection limits for myocardial ischemia reported by the manufacturer. Recently developed high-sensitivity assays have further improved the prognostic performance of this biomarker, particularly with regard to normal values of troponin and the exclusion of patients with and adverse short-term outcome.[131,132]

Summary: Classification of Pulmonary Embolism Patients for Consideration of Therapy

At present, the patient should be classified as either high, intermediate-low, intermediate-high, or low-risk and other parameters and comorbidities should be taken into consideration for prediction of early (in-hospital or 30-day) outcome in patients with acute PE.[89] Hemodynamically unstable patients with shock or persistent hypotension should immediately be identified as high-risk patients; they require an emergency diagnosis and, if PE confirmed, pharmacological (or alternatively, surgical or interventional) reperfusion therapy.[89,133]

Patients without shock or hypotension are not at high risk of adverse early outcomes, and further risk stratification should be considered after diagnosis of PE has been confirmed, because this may influence the therapeutic strategy and the duration of hospitalization. In these patients, risk assessment should begin with the evaluation of the PESI or sPESI clinical prognostic score to distinguish between intermediate and low-risk patients. Accordingly, normotensive patients in sPESI >0 or PESI class ≥III are considered in the intermediate-risk group. In these patients, further risk assessment should be considered, focusing on vital signs, oxygenation, the status of the RV (by echocardiography or CT) and cardiac biomarkers level. Patients who display evidence of *both* RV dysfunction and elevated cardiac biomarker levels (particularly cardiac troponin) should be classified into an intermediate-high-risk category. These patients should be closely monitored to permit early detection of hemodynamic decompensation and the need of rescue reperfusion therapy.[132] On the other hand, patients in whom the RV is normal *or* cardiac biomarker levels are normal,

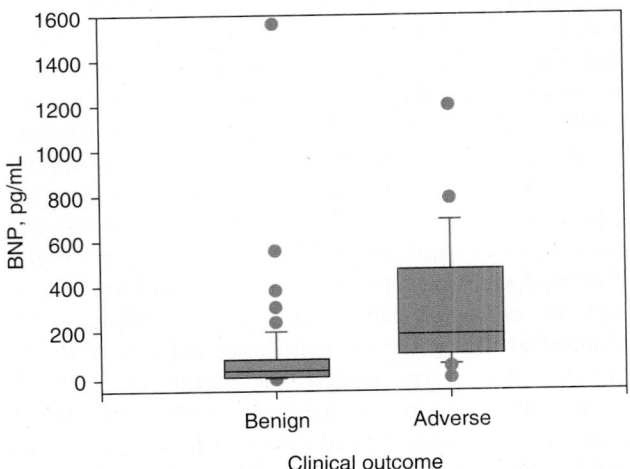

Figure 58–9. BNP levels (median, confidence interval, and outliers) in patients with acute PE according to clinical outcome. Although BNP levels between patients with benign and adverse outcome overlap, the negative predictive value for the absence of adverse outcomes for BNP triage levels below 50 pg/mL was 97%. Data from Kucher N, Printzen G, Doernhoefer T, et al. Low pro-brain natriuretic peptide levels predict benign clinical outcome in acute pulmonary embolism. *Circulation.* 2003 Apr 1;107(12):1576-1578.

belong to an intermediate-low-risk group. A key aspect of PERTs is in risk stratification and guiding the therapeutic plan.[118,119]

THERAPEUTIC APPROACHES

Supportive Measures

Volume Replacement and Vasopressor Therapy

When high-risk PE associated with hypotension or severe hypoxemia is suspected, supportive treatment is immediately initiated. Intravenous saline can be infused rapidly, but caution is recommended. A cautious assessment of volume status using history, clinical examination, lab testing, and echocardiography (IVC collapse) should be undertaken. Excess fluid may result in further RV dilatation, increased RV wall tension, and a decreased cardiac output that may result in RV ischemia.[9] Norepinephrine appears to be the favored choice of vasoactive therapy in massive PE and should be administered if the blood pressure is not rapidly restored.[89,134] Death from high-risk PE results from RV failure, and dobutamine may augment RV output.[89,134] A vasopressor, such as norepinephrine combined with dobutamine, might offer optimal results.[89] Caution with dobutamine is advised based on its inodilator properties.

Oxygenation and Mechanical Ventilation

Hypoxemia and hypocapnia are frequently encountered in patients with PE, in most cases of moderate severity, which usually reversed with administration of oxygen. Mechanical ventilation may be instituted to decrease systemic oxygen demands or manage respiratory failure. Intubation in the setting of a decompensated RV, however, is fraught with risk. Premedications may cause systemic vasodilatation, and positive-pressure ventilation may abruptly reduce preload and cardiac output. Therefore, positive end-expiratory pressure should be applied with caution, and low tidal volumes (approximately 6 mL/kg lean body weight) should be used in an attempt to keep the end-inspiratory plateau pressure <30 cm H_2O.

Extracorporeal Membrane Oxygenation

Randomized controlled human trials of ECMO in acute PE have not been done, but its role is becoming increasingly defined. The European Society of Cardiology (ESC) 2019 acute PE guidelines states that ECMO can be used for high-risk PE as a method for hemodynamic support and as an adjunct to surgical embolectomy.[89] The 2016 CHEST Antithrombotic Therapy guidelines do not mention ECMO in the management of massive PE. However, multiple case reports and small series cited benefit with ECMO for massive PE.[135] Further, ECMO may facilitate stabilization for surgical embolectomy. Unfortunately, ECMO requires full anticoagulation to maintain the functionality of the system; hence, significant bleeding complicates its use in 35% of patients. Contraindications to ECMO include high bleeding risk, recent surgery or hemorrhagic stroke, poor baseline functional status, advanced age, neurologic dysfunction, morbid obesity, unrecoverable condition, renal failure, and prolonged cardiopulmonary resuscitation without adequate perfusion of end organs.[135]

Anticoagulation

General Principles

In patients with acute PE, anticoagulation is recommended with the objectives of preventing early death and recurrent VTE.[89] The standard duration of anticoagulation should cover at least 3 months but is often longer if there are persisting risk factors or if the VTE event was unprovoked. In some cases, extended anticoagulation even indefinitely, may be necessary for secondary prevention, after weighing the risk of recurrence and bleeding. Acute-phase treatment previously consisted of administering parenteral anticoagulation (unfractionated heparin [UFH] or LMWH) over the first 5 to 10 days overlapped with the initiation of a vitamin K antagonist (VKA).[136] However, except when the bleeding risk is deemed high and a short acting parenteral anticoagulant is preferred, the initial use of LMWH offers a more bioavailable and predictable approach, with a generally guaranteed therapeutic level in 3 to 4 hours without monitoring in most cases.[137] Alternatively, in selected stable patients, oral anticoagulation can be initiated with a DOAC (ie, rivaroxaban or apixaban) alone instead of the standard parenteral/VKA regimen.[89] When DOACs are contraindicated, a VKA can be used and must be overlapped with parenteral anticoagulation for at least 5 days with monitoring (in the case of standard UFH). This initial anticoagulation approach applies to both acute DVT and PE.[136] Finally, when the dabigatran or edoxaban are utilized, they must be preceded by upfront parenteral anticoagulation as for VKAs based on how the clinical trials leading to drug approval were designed. Parenteral anticoagulation should be initiated while awaiting the results of diagnostic tests in patients with intermediate or high clinical probability for PE, and low perceived bleeding risk.[89]

Standard Unfractionated Heparin

Anticoagulation has been shown to reduce mortality in acute PE.[138] Standard UFH is still used very widely although LMWH has distinct advantages. A clear advantage of UFH, however, is that it is short acting and reversible with protamine, but it is less bioavailable, and requires monitoring. It is favored when the risk of bleeding is higher, but the clinical team still feels that anticoagulation can be undertaken. A weight-based approach substantially enhances the chances of attaining the therapeutic range quickly.[136] A widely utilized UFH and very effective regimen consists of a bolus of 80 U/kg followed by 18 U/kg/h.[136] Subsequent adjusting of the heparin dose should also be weight based. It is critical to realize that despite the efficacy of UFH in controlled clinical trials it may not be as predictable in the real world. Recent data suggest that the majority of patients with acute PE spend most of their first 48 hours outside of the therapeutic range when treated with guideline standard dosing of UFH.[139] Thus, when possible, LMWH is favored as subsequently described.

The two most common methods for monitoring UFH infusions are the activated partial thromboplastin time (aPTT) and the antifactor Xa heparin assay (anti-Xa). When IV UFH is instituted, monitoring at 6-hour intervals until it is consistently in the therapeutic range is critical. The peak anti-Xa level is particularly useful for monitoring heparin therapy under the following circumstances: (1) a baseline elevated aPTT because of antiphospholipid antibodies or other circulating anticoagulants in patients being treated with UFH, (2) extremes of body weight (<40 kg and ≥150 kg), (3) renal failure or insufficiency (creatinine clearance <30 mL/min), (4) pregnancy, and (5) the occurrence of an unexpected bleeding or clotting event during therapy.[140]

Bleeding is the primary concern with anticoagulation. This is minimized with heparin based on its short half-life and reversibility. Heparin-induced thrombocytopenia (HIT) typically develops 5 or more days after the initiation of heparin therapy and occurs in 5% to 10% of patients.[141] If a patient is placed on heparin for VTE and the platelet count progressively decreases either by 50% or to 100,000/mm³ or less, heparin therapy should be discontinued. Although the risk of HIT appears to be lower with LMWH, it is important for clinicians to realize that HIT can occur with the use of either form of heparin. Prolonged administration of UFH may cause asymptomatic osteopenia, osteoporosis, and (rarely) pathologic bone fractures. After discontinuation of heparin, bone metabolism by densitometry usually improves within 1 year.

Low-Molecular-Weight Heparin

These agents differ in a number of respects from standard UFH. Except when the bleeding risk is deemed high and a short acting parenteral anticoagulant is preferred, the initial use of LMWH offers a more bioavailable and predictable approach, with a generally guaranteed therapeutic level in 3 to 4 hours without monitoring in most cases.

Numerous clinical trials have demonstrated the efficacy and safety of LMWHs for the treatment of patients with acute proximal DVT and PE, using recurrent symptomatic VTE as the primary outcome measure.[137,142] Treatment with LMWHs is more convenient for the patient and the nursing staff for several reasons. A continuous IV line is not required because these agents can be administered once or twice per day subcutaneously at fixed therapeutic doses, usually without laboratory monitoring. When necessary, LMWH therapy can be monitored by measuring anti-Xa levels. The therapeutic target peak anti-Xa level drawn 4 hours after administration should be in the range of 0.6 to 1 IU/mL for twice-daily administration, and 1 to 2 IU/mL for once-daily administration. LMWH must be dose adjusted for those with creatinine clearance <30 mL/min or UFH should be used.

Unlike regimens for prophylaxis, in which fixed dosing is used, a weight-based dosing regimen is used for the treatment of patients with established VTE with these agents. In addition to being more convenient, the LMWH preparations appear to be cost-effective, particularly when outpatient therapy is used. Particular caution should be used with LMWHs and spinal/epidural anesthesia based on the risk of epidural or spinal hematoma, which can cause permanent paraplegia.[143] A comparison between standard UFH and LMWH as well as potential advantages of LMWH are shown in **Tables 58–4** and **58–5**, respectively.

TABLE 58–4. A Comparison of Low Molecular Weight Heparin with Unfractionated Heparin

Characteristic	UFH	LMWH
Mean molecular weight	12,000–15,000	4000–6000
Protein binding	Substantial	Minimal
Anti-Xa activity	Substantial	Substantial
Anti-IIa activity	Substantial	Minimal
Platelet inhibition	Substantial	Minimal
Vascular permeability	Moderate	None
Microvascular permeability	Substantial	Minimal
Elimination (predominant)	Hepatic/macrophages	Renal

Abbreviations: LMWH, low-molecular-weight heparin; UFH, unfractionated heparin.

Fondaparinux

Fondaparinux is a synthetic pentasaccharide that selectively inhibits factor Xa. It has been approved by the FDA and Europe for the initial treatment of VTE, including PE. In hemodynamically stable patients with acute symptomatic PE, fondaparinux is as safe and effective as IV UFH.[144] Fondaparinux is administered subcutaneously on a once-daily basis in fixed doses of 5 mg for body weight below 50 kg, 7.5 mg for body weight of 50 to 100 kg, and 10 mg for body weight greater than 100 kg. Unlike IV UFH, fondaparinux is administered in a fixed dose and does not require dose adjustment with laboratory coagulation tests. As is the case with LMWH, fondaparinux is cleared through the renal route and is contraindicated in patients with severe renal disease (creatinine clearance <30 mL/min). In patients with clearance, a 30 to 50 mL/min dose should be reduced by 50%.[145] In contrast to heparin compounds, fondaparinux does not cause HIT and has proven safe and effective for use in that setting.[145]

Vitamin K Antagonists

VKA therapy is rarely used for acute VTE nowadays. It is used in certain settings where DOACs are not proven or contraindicated such as during breastfeeding, or with supermorbid obesity. The convenience of DOACs have rendered warfarin almost (but not quite) obsolete. Warfarin must be initiated with concomitant UFH or LMWH; otherwise, the first few days of

TABLE 58–5. Potential Advantages of LMWH Over Unfractionated Heparin

Efficacy: Comparable or superior[a]
Safety: Comparable or superior[b]
No laboratory monitoring[c]
Less phlebotomy
Earlier ambulation
Home therapy in certain patient subsets

Abbreviation: LMWH, low-molecular-weight heparin.
[a]Based on objectively documented recurrence rates in clinical trials.
[b]Based on rates of major and minor bleeding in clinical trials.
[c]In certain patient populations (significant obesity, renal insufficiency), monitoring is suggested.

VKA administration may lead to a prothrombotic state because of rapid depletion of proteins C and S. The procoagulant effect of VKA can be inhibited by overlapping with a heparin compound for at least 5 days.

Ordinarily, the initial dose of warfarin should be 10 mg for 2 days, with monitoring performed daily. A dose of 5 mg for 2 days is recommended for older (>60 years of age), debilitated, or malnourished patients.[142,146] A standardized nomogram has long been available and can be used to make dose adjustments based on international normalized ratio (INR) values obtained on days 3 and 5.[146] A few patients have extremely low daily warfarin dose requirements of 1 to 2 mg, with an increased bleeding risk because of CYP2C9 and VKORC1 variant alleles. At the present time, however, data indicate that pharmacogenetic-based dosing, used on top of clinical parameters, does not improve the quality of anticoagulation (more effective and/or less risky than empiric, clinically based dosing).[146,148] In selected patients, self-management of VKA therapy using INR measurement with "point of care" devices may be effective and safe.[149]

Risk factors for VKA-related bleeding include hepatic disease, renal dysfunction, alcoholism, drug interactions, trauma, cancer, and a history of gastrointestinal bleeding. The risk of bleeding is greatest in the first month after initiation of anticoagulation.[150] Depending on the extent and site, patients with major bleeding can routinely be treated with fresh-frozen plasma or prothrombin complex concentrates. Although vitamin K should be administered, it can take many hours to take effect. In patients with excessive INR values without bleeding, withholding one or two doses of warfarin with elective administration of oral vitamin K 2.5 mg is an effective strategy.

Rare complications of VKAs are skin necrosis and cholesterol microembolization, causing the "purple toes" syndrome by enhancing crystal release from ulcerated plaques.[151] Reliable contraception and patient education are mandatory in women of childbearing potential because VKAs are teratogenic, particularly during weeks 6 to 12 of gestation (see subsequent section Pulmonary Embolism in Pregnancy).

Direct Oral Anticoagulants

Phase III clinical trials on the acute-phase treatment and duration of anticoagulation after VTE (DVT or PE) with parenteral therapy followed by non–vitamin K-dependent direct oral anticoagulants DOACs have led to the approval of four DOACs in the United States and Europe.[152-157] The overall results of these trials indicate that these agents are noninferior (in terms of efficacy) and safer with regard to major bleeding, than the standard parenteral/VKA regimen.[158] These DOACs include rivaroxaban, apixaban, edoxaban, and dabigatran. Rivaroxaban and apixaban allow for single drug therapy, eliminating the need for initial parenteral anticoagulation, while dabigatran and edoxaban are initiated after a short course of parenteral anticoagulation regimen. Practical recommendations for dosing and bleeding complications are summarized in **Table 58–6**.

Importantly, reversal agents for DOACs are now available. The monoclonal antibody idarucizumab that binds dabigatran

is effective in emergency situations;[159] as is andexanet for reversing oral factor Xa inhibitors (rivaroxaban, apixaban, and edoxaban).[160] Both of these drugs are reserved for critical bleeding emergencies such as intracranial hemorrhage. The DOACs have simplified the treatment of acute VTE, shortened hospitalization, and facilitated out of hospital management because these anticoagulants can be administered safely in fixed doses without the need for laboratory monitoring and have far fewer food and drug interactions than the VKAs.[161,162]

Consequently, clinical guidelines now recommend DOACs as first-line VTE treatment for most patients, although notable exclusions are patients with severe renal or liver impairment, triple-positive antiphospholipid syndrome, or women who are pregnant.[163]

While the LMWHs have been the therapy of choice for cancer-related VTE, recent data strongly support the use of DOACs for this indication, since LMWH has been demonstrated to be superior to VKAs in reducing the rate of recurrent VTE in this setting.[164] Patients with cancer-associated VTE have a both higher risk of VTE recurrence and of bleeding and were underrepresented in the early pivotal DOAC trials. Recent trials evaluating DOACs in the treatment of cancer-associated VTE now provide evidence that the DOACs are at least as effective and safe as LMWH. The four trials representing each DOAC—the Hokusai VTE Cancer Trial comparing edoxaban with LMWH, SELECT-D comparing rivaroxaban and LMWH, and the ADAM-VTE and Caravaggio trials comparing apixaban with LMWH—have proven that DOACs are at least as effective as LMWH.[165-168] However, caution is recommended in certain luminal cancers such as active gastrointestinal malignancies based upon increased bleeding. Notably, Hokusai VTE Cancer, SELECT-D, and ADAM-VTE each included patients with intracerebral metastases, and in spite of this, there was no reported increase in intracranial bleeding hemorrhage.[165-167]

The few drug interactions involving the two DOACs most commonly used in the United States (rivaroxaban and apixaban) involve strong cytochrome P (CYP) 3A and P-glycoprotein (P-gp) inhibitors or inducers.[169] For example, some of the earlier human immunodeficiency virus (HIV) drugs (ie, the protease inhibitors as well as older antifungals such as ketoconazole) are strong CYP3A/P-gp inhibitors and can result in ineffectively low levels of the DOAC, placing patients at higher risk of bleeding. Conversely, strong inducers such as rifampin, certain anticonvulsants (diphenylhydantoin, phenobarbital, and carbamazepine), as well as St. John's wort can result in very low DOAC levels resulting in high risk of recurrent VTE.[169]

New Anticoagulation Strategies

Several evolving strategies for novel anticoagulant development are on the horizon. Recent data have suggested that the contact activation pathway appears critical for thrombus growth and stability while having minimal role in mediating hemostasis. Recent preclinical and preliminary clinical data suggest reducing factor XI or XII levels might be a potential strategy to achieve thrombosis prevention and/or treatment without a significant increase in bleeding risk.[170,171] Several trials have

TABLE 58–6. Direct Oral Anticoagulants: A Comparison

| Compound | Dosage | | Contraindicated or Caution | Handling of Bleeding Complications |
	Initial phase	Long-term phase		Common for all DOACs
Dabigatran exilate	Parenteral anti-coagulation for 5–10 days before initiation	150 mg bid 110 mg bid*	CrCl <30 mL/min Concomitant treatment with P-glycoprotein inhibitors/inducers	Supportive measures (local hemostatic, fluid replacement PRBC transfusion if necessary) Platelet transfusion for thrombocytopenia (≤60 x 10^9/L) FFP as plasma expander (not useful as reversal agent) Tranexamic acid For life-threatening bleeding: Idarucizumab (dabigatran-related bleeding) Andexanet (for edoxaban, rivaroxaban, and apixaban-related bleeding) PCC 25 U/kg; activated PCC 50 IE/kg; activated factor VII (90 μg/kg);
Edoxaban	Parenteral anti-coagulation for 5–10 days before initiation	60 mg qd 30 mg qd†	CrCl <15 mL/min Moderate/severe hepatic impairment Concomitant treatment with P-glycoprotein and strong CYP3A4 inhibitors/inducers	
Rivaroxaban	15 mg bid for 21 days	20 mg qd	CrCl <15 mL/min Moderate/severe hepatic impairment Concomitant treatment with P-glycoprotein and strong CYP3A4 inhibitors/inducers	
Apixaban	10 mg bid for 7 days	5 mg bid	CrCl <15 mL/min Severe hepatic impairment Concomitant treatment with strong dual inhibitors or inducers of P-glycoprotein/CYP3A4	

Abbreviations: PRBC, packed red blood cells; FFP, fresh frozen plasma; PCC, prothrombin complex concentrate.
*Dabigatran 110 mg bid may be considered in elderly patients (≥80y); those under concomitant treatment with moderate P-glycoprotein inhibitors (ie, amiodarone, verapamil, quinidine); at higher risk of bleeding; or with CrCl 30–50 mL/min.
†Edoxaban 30 mg qd may be considered in patients with at least 1 of the following factors: CrCl 15–50 mL/min; concomitant use with strong P-glycoprotein inhibitors; body weight ≤60 kg.
Apart from the specific conditions listed above, all DOACs are contraindicated in patients: (1) expected to be treated with thrombolysis or embolectomy; (2) receiving concomitant treatment with another anticoagulant; (3) with active bleeding or at very high risk of bleeding; (4) pregnant women or during breast feeding.
In general, all DOACs should be administered with caution in patients with an increased risk of bleeding, including those receiving concomitant treatment with nonsteroidal anti-inflammatory drugs and antiplatelet agents.
A full updated list of drug interactions and tables of drug interactions can be found at: https://www.fda.gov/drugs/drug-interactions-labeling/drug-development-and-drug-interactions-table-substrates-inhibitors-and-inducers#potency

evaluated the role of FXI and FXII inhibition in prevention and treatment of VTE; currently several phase-2 clinical trials evaluating these coagulation factors are completed or underway. In addition, targeting platelets, leukocyte recruitment, or the fibrinolysis pathway may offer potential antithrombotic options.[172]

Systemic Thrombolytic Therapy

Thrombolytic therapy of acute PE restores pulmonary perfusion more rapidly than anticoagulation with UFH alone, which leads to a prompt reduction in clot burden and thus, pulmonary vascular resistance with improvement in RV function.[173] Thrombolytic therapy may reduce total mortality, PE recurrence, and PE-related mortality in *selected* patients with acute PE, particularly in hemodynamically unstable patients or massive PE. However, a decrease in mortality has not been proven overall in hemodynamically stable patients with acute PE.[174] In the absence of hemodynamic compromise, the clinical

benefits of thrombolysis have remained controversial for many years. Recent evidence suggest that hemodynamically stable patients *with evidence of RV enlargement/dysfunction and elevated troponins* and no contraindications may benefit from thrombolytic therapy,[133] possibly at a cost of higher rates of major hemorrhage.[133] Systematic review data even suggest the possibility of lower mortality in this population.[175]

Chatterjee et al.[175] evaluated 16 trials performed over the last 45 years including 2115 patients and conducted subset analyses in the 1775 patients with intermediate risk. In summary, thrombolysis was associated with lower mortality risk compared with standard anticoagulation (3.89% vs 2.17%, relative reduction of 47%). However, it was also associated with increased major bleeding (9.24% vs 3.42%) and intracranial hemorrhage (1.46% vs 0.19%) compared with anticoagulation. In the subset of patients 65 years or older, thrombolysis was associated with increased major bleeding while this was not the case in patients 65 years or younger.[175] It is feasible that a more enriched population (eg, more tachycardic or hypox-emic, or with more severely abnormal biomarkers) but without hypotension might more convincingly benefit from systemic thrombolysis. Future studies may be revealing.

FDA- and European-approved thrombolytic agents include recombinant tissue-type plasminogen activator (tPA), strep-tokinase, and urokinase; the latter two drugs are essentially not used anymore. Tenecteplase was used in the PEITHO trial;[133] an advantage of this drug is that is delivered by bolus, rather than over 2 hours as with tPA; this drug, however, is not cur-rently FDA-approved for treatment of acute PE.

In practice, in severely hypotensive patients, it may be pru-dent to deliver tPA over a shorter period of time instead of 2 hours, although randomized controlled trial data are lack-ing in this realm. The primary concern regarding thrombolytic therapy is increased risk of bleeding, particularly an increase in major and fatal or intracranial hemorrhage.[133,175] Abso-lute and relative contraindications for thrombolytic therapy include conditions that increase the possible risk of bleeding complications, such as recent bleeding, surgery, stroke, or gas-trointestinal hemorrhage (**Table 58–7**). In general, heparin is withheld until the thrombolytic infusion is completed, and the aPTT is then determined, and heparin is initiated without a loading dose if this value is less than twice the upper limit of normal. If the aPTT exceeds this value, the test is repeated every 4 hours until it is safe to proceed with heparin. If heparin levels are being utilized, then heparin should not be restarted if the level is in the supratherapeutic therapeutic range. While there are no data proving an increased risk of bleeding when heparin is continued during tPA infusion, holding it appears prudent. Anticoagulation with UFH is generally restarted and continued for 24 hours after completion of thrombolytic ther-apy before switching to LMWH or a DOAC. In patients receiv-ing LMWH at the time thrombolytics are infused, initiation of UFH should be delayed until 12 hours after the last LMWH injection if given twice daily, or until 24 hours after the last LMWH if given once daily.

Some of these trials, including the landmark PEITHO trial, studied tenecteplase as the thrombolytic agent.[133] While the primary endpoint was met in the PEITHO trial, tenecteplase was associated with an increased risk of intracranial hemor-rhage and is not currently approved for the treatment of PE. At present, systemic thrombolysis is not routinely recommended as primary treatment for patients with intermediate-high risk PE, but should be considered if clinical signs of hemodynamic decompensation appear.[89] The efficacy of half-dose systemic thrombolysis has been recently explored in small trials with preliminary modest positive results and acceptable safety;[176,177] but level 1A data are lacking. If bleeding risk is deemed high, half-dose systemic thrombolysis, surgical pulmonary embolec-tomy, or percutaneous catheter-directed treatment should be considered.[89] No comparative trials have been conducted. Alternative approaches to systemic thrombolysis are catheter-directed therapies (ie, either thrombolysis or clot extraction without thrombolysis).[9]

Catheter-Based Therapies

Percutaneous catheter-directed therapy (CDT) can be consid-ered as an alternative to surgical pulmonary embolectomy for patients in whom full-dose systemic thrombolysis is contrain-dicated or has failed, if appropriate expertise and resources are available on-site;[9,89] early studies suggested potential ben-efit utilizing lower doses of thrombolytics.[178–181] Interventional options include more than simply thrombolysis and include: thrombus fragmentation with a pigtail or balloon catheter, rheolytic thrombectomy with hydrodynamic catheter devices, suction thrombectomy with aspiration catheters, rotational thrombectomy, and low-dose catheter-directed thrombolysis.[9] Of these, ultrasound-facilitated catheter-directed thrombolysis (UCDT) has offered more clinical data than other tech-niques.[181–183] The ULTIMA trial of 59 patients showed a clear benefit with regard to improvement in RV/LV ratio at 24 hours compared to standard UFH alone.[181] Subsequent UCDT stud-ies suggested that this technique is effective at reducing RV/LV ratio and with a low rate of intracranial hemorrhage (ICH). In the three aforementioned UCDT studies, there was only 1 ICH event out of 277 patients that was attributed to the pro-cedure.[181–183] Catheter-directed clot extraction without throm-bolysis has also been studied in prospective, nonrandomized trials.[9,184,185] Finally, the larger AngioVac suction device utilizes veno-veno bypass in order to minimize blood removal from circulation has proven effective in extracting IVC and right atrial thrombi as well as clot-in-transit.[186] Overall, most cath-eter-directed devices appear to be effective and safe, although randomized controlled trial data are very few—the ULTIMA trial is one example.[181]

Surgical Embolectomy

Urgent surgical embolectomy should be considered in patients with hemodynamically massive PE or right-heart thrombus who have an absolute contraindication to anticoagulant or

---

TABLE 58–7. Absolute and Relative Contraindications to Thrombolysis in Pulmonary Embolism

Absolute contraindications
Hemorrhagic stroke or stroke of unknown cause at any time
Ischemic stroke in preceding 6 months
CNS damage or neoplasm
Recent major trauma, surgery, or head injury (within preceding 3 weeks)
GI bleed within the past month
Known bleeding

Relative contraindications
Transient ischemic attacks in the preceding 6 months
Oral anticoagulant therapy
Pregnancy or within 1 week postpartum
Noncompressible punctures
Traumatic resuscitation
Refractory hypertension (systolic blood pressure ≥180 mm Hg)
Advanced liver disease
Infective endocarditis
Active peptic ulcer

Abbreviations: CNS, central nervous system; GI, gastrointestinal

thrombolytic therapy; in patients with impending paradoxical embolism; and in patients in whom aggressive medical therapy, including the use of thrombolysis, has proven ineffective. Aortic cross-clamping and cardioplegic cardiac arrest should be avoided. Current surgical embolectomy mortality rates with a rapid multidisciplinary approach, including the use of peripheral extracorporeal membrane oxygenators[187] and individualized indications before hemodynamic collapse, have been reported to be lower than 10%.[188] Preoperative thrombolysis increases the risk of bleeding, but it is not an absolute contraindication to surgical embolectomy (ECMO is discussed in the section Supportive Measures).

Vena Cava Filters

Routine use of IVC filters in patients with PE is not recommended. The essential indications for filter placement include contraindications to anticoagulation/significant bleeding complications during anticoagulation in the acute phase, or recurrent embolism while on adequate therapy. A frequent consideration for IVC filters is in patients with recent VTE or those on indefinite anticoagulation in whom surgery or an invasive procedure is necessary. In such patients, anticoagulation can sometimes be transiently held and resumed (generally safer when acute VTE is not recent), especially if there is not extensive, fresh, proximal DVT. In higher risk patients, especially when anticoagulation must be held for more than a few hours, a filter may be considered. Another option when holding anticoagulation is to do serial ultrasounds every 24 to 48 hours. The latter may entail a high risk of recurrence and there are no prospective, randomized trial data or guidelines suggesting the optimal approach. Such decisions must be carefully risk-assessed and individualized, with a very low threshold for filter placement when therapeutic anticoagulation is indicated but cannot be given.

Although IVC filters can be potentially lifesaving by preventing early recurrence of PE, patients with filters appear to be at higher mid- and long-term risk for recurrent VTE.[189] Consequently, anticoagulation is generally continued when a filter is placed unless it is contraindicated. These devices can be inserted via the jugular or femoral vein and are usually placed in the infrarenal portion of the IVC. Complications associated with IVC filters are common, although rarely fatal.[190,191] Possible mechanisms of IVC filter failure include filter migration; improper filter positioning, allowing thrombi to bypass the filter; and formation of thrombosis proximal to the filter or on the proximal tip of the filter with subsequent embolization. Rare complications include clinically significant perforation of the IVC, migration to the heart, and displacement of the filter during insertion. Occasionally, these devices may erode through the wall of the IVC, or IVC obstruction caused by thrombosis at the filter site may occur. Filters placed now are always retrievable but may be left in place. Depending on the filter type, retrievable filters should be removed within weeks to months when possible but can remain permanently if necessary, because of persistent contraindication to anticoagulation. Although some works have suggested that IVC filters could be associated with significant lower rates of mortality in patients with PE who were hemodynamically unstable whether or not treated with fibrinolysis,[192,193] recent studies have investigated the use of retrievable filters with no convincing data suggesting improved mortality.[194] Therefore, the use of filters beyond these indications listed is not supported by evidence at present.

CHRONIC THROMBOEMBOLIC PULMONARY HYPERTENSION

In a few patients with acute PE, the residual thromboembolic burden is sufficiently extensive to cause thromboembolic pulmonary hypertension.[195] Estimates of the incidence of CTEPH range from 0.5% to 3.8% after an initial episode of embolism and 13.4% after recurrent episodes of VTE, with an estimated incidence of 5 individuals per million population per year.[195] Approximately 30% of patients who develop CTEPH have no documented history of acute DVT or PE, and this feature greatly impedes the diagnosis. Antiphospholipid antibodies have been detected in approximately 10% of patients, and elevated factor VIII levels have been detected in 40%.[196] Apart from major pulmonary vascular obstruction, the pathophysiology of CTEPH included pulmonary microvascular disease, pulmonary vascular remodeling, immune phenomena, and inflammation.[196,197]

The median age of patients at diagnosis of CTEPH is 63 years, and both genders are equally affected.[198] Clinical symptoms and signs are nonspecific or absent in early CTEPH, with signs of right heart failure only becoming evident in advanced disease. As in other forms of pulmonary hypertension, progressive exertional dyspnea and exercise intolerance are characteristic. Later in the course of the disease, exertional chest pain, presyncope, or syncope may occur. Diagnostic delay, particularly in the absence of a history of acute VTE, occurs commonly.[198]

The chest radiograph usually reveals RV enlargement and enlarged main pulmonary arteries. ECG changes are consistent with RV hypertrophy. Arterial blood gases generally reveal hypoxemia with a widened A–a gradient, although some patients may demonstrate only exercise-induced hypoxemia. Echocardiography documents the presence of pulmonary hypertension, as well as RV hypertrophy.

V/Q lung scanning represents a simple, noninvasive means of differentiating disorders of the peripheral pulmonary vascular bed from those of the central vascular bed, and remains the first-line imaging modality for CTEPH. In chronic thromboembolic disease, at least one segmental or larger mismatched perfusion defect is present. In disorders of the distal pulmonary vascular bed, perfusion scans either are normal or exhibit a "mottled" appearance characterized by subsegmental defects. Mismatched segmental or larger defects in patients with pulmonary hypertension may also arise from other processes that result in obstruction of the central pulmonary arteries or veins, such as pulmonary artery sarcoma, large vessel pulmonary vasculitides, extrinsic vascular compression by mediastinal adenopathy or fibrosis, and pulmonary veno-occlusive disease.[199] Multidetector CT angiography has become an established imaging technique diagnostic algorithms for CTEPH after intermediate or high probability V/Q scan. A variety of CT abnormalities have been described in patients with chronic thromboembolic disease, including right-sided cardiac enlargement, enlargement of the pulmonary arteries, a mosaic perfusion pattern, intraluminal thrombi, subpleural densities, and dilated bronchial arteries.[199] The absence of these findings, however, cannot absolutely exclude the diagnosis; therefore, CT alone cannot rule out the disease. Right heart catheterization is an essential diagnostic tool since provide important diagnostic and prognostic information. Finally, contrast pulmonary arteriography can be performed to establish the diagnosis with certainty and to determine operability. The angiographic findings in CTEPH are distinct from those encountered in acute embolism and considerable experience is required for accurate angiographic interpretation (**Fig. 58–10**).

Thus, the diagnosis of CTEPH is based on the following findings obtained after at least 3 months of anticoagulation: mean pulmonary arterial pressure ≥25 mm Hg with pulmonary arterial wedge pressure ≤15 mm Hg plus at least one segmental or large-sized defect detected by V/Q or chest CTA scan; generally, bilateral defects are present.

Pulmonary endarterectomy is the treatment of choice for CTEPH. General criteria for the operability of patients include NYHA functional class II to IV and the surgical accessibility of the thrombi up to the segmental level. There are no particular age, pulmonary vascular resistance, or RV dysfunction thresholds that absolutely preclude pulmonary endarterectomy, since patients who do not undergo surgery or suffer from persistent residual pulmonary hypertension after surgery face a very poor prognosis. However, all these parameters constitute important prognostic factors after surgery. Pulmonary endarterectomy is performed via median sternotomy on cardiopulmonary bypass with periods of deep hypothermic circulatory arrest and is technically quite distinct from pulmonary embolectomy for acute embolic disease. The procedure is a true endarterectomy, which requires careful dissection of chronic endothelialized material from the native intima to restore pulmonary arterial patency (**Fig. 58–11**). Balloon pulmonary angioplasty seems promising as a therapeutic alternative for selected patients with nonoperable CTEPH or rescue therapy after surgery.[200–202]

Optimal medical treatment for CTEPH consists of anticoagulants, diuretics, and oxygen.[203] Lifelong anticoagulation is recommended, even after pulmonary endarterectomy. Riociguat, a soluble oral stimulator of guanylate cyclase, is FDA-approved for use in CTEPH and should be considered in symptomatic patients who have been classified as having inoperable CTEPH by an experienced group/center or have persistent/recurrent CTEPH after surgical treatment.[204] The use of other drugs approved for pulmonary arterial hypertension may be justified in inoperable patients or in patients with persistent or residual pulmonary hypertension after surgery if riociguat failed or was not tolerated. However, off-label use of drugs approved for pulmonary arterial hypertension as a therapeutic bridge to endarterectomy in patients considered to be at high risk due to poor hemodynamics, is

Figure 58–10. Representative right-sided pulmonary angiogram in a patient with CTEPH demonstrating classic "pouch" defect with absent flow to the right middle and lower lobes.

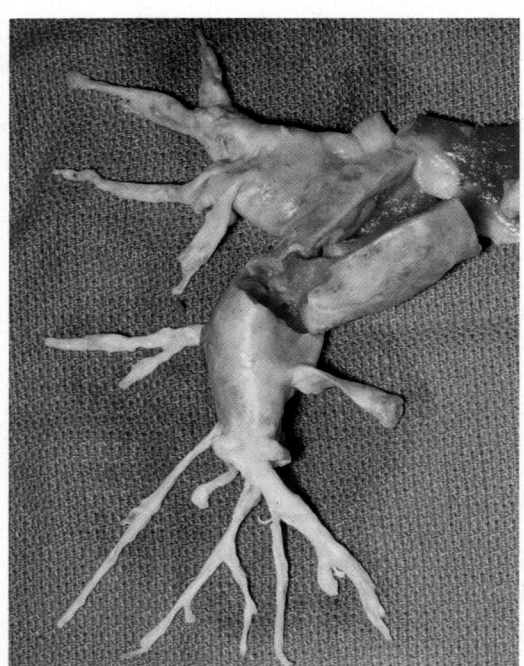

Figure 58–11. Example of chronic thromboembolic material obtained from the right pulmonary artery at the time of pulmonary thromboendarterectomy. Note the chronic fibrotic material that must be meticulously dissected from the native intima to achieve an optimal outcome.

currently not justified. It is worthwhile reiterating that pulmonary endarterectomy remains the first-line intervention for Chronic thromboembolic pulmonary hypertension (CTEPH), although Balloon pulmonary angioplasty (BPA) is evolving as experience increases. At present, the hemodynamic and symptomatic benefits to be accrued from medical therapy, although often positive, are modest compared with those resulting from surgery.

PREVENTION OF VENOUS THROMBOEMBOLISM

Background

Prophylaxis for DVT is effective. Evidence-based clinical guidelines for the prevention of thromboembolism in a wide range of patient populations have been published by the American College of Chest Physicians.[205-208]

A substantial reduction in the incidence of DVT can be accomplished when individuals at risk receive appropriate preventive care; however, such measures appear to be grossly underused. Data support that prophylaxis can be administered safely with major bleeding complications occurring in only 0.2% of surgical patients.[207,209]

Prophylaxis can be pharmacologic or nonpharmacologic. Pharmacologic prophylaxis options include low-dose UFH, LMWH, fondaparinux, warfarin, and new oral anticoagulants.[205-208] Aspirin has a slight benefit but not enough to be used as a standard therapy to prevent VTE. LMWHs are increasingly used in clinical practice for both the prevention and treatment of established VTE. The LMWH preparations are advantageous in that they produce a more predictable dose response and are administered subcutaneously only once or twice daily (without monitoring), depending on the preparation. Early ambulation whenever possible is always recommended in postoperative patients.

General Medical Patients

Prophylactic measures to prevent VTE has not traditionally been widely implemented among patients with medical illnesses. In the DVT FREE Registry of 5451 DVT patients, 59% of those who did not receive prophylaxis were medical patients.[14] Completed trials have demonstrated that medical patients have a thrombosis risk equivalent to that of moderate-risk surgical patients and that the use of prophylaxis can significantly reduce the rate of venous thromboembolic events with an acceptable rate of bleeding.[208] Rates of prophylaxis in hospitalized medically ill patients is now nearly universal based on a number of influential trials.[210]

Patients should be stratified according to DVT risk, and certain prophylactic measures are more appropriate for some patients than for others. The intensity of a prophylactic regimen should take into account the relative risk for thrombosis. Generally, low-dose anticoagulation with standard UFH, LMWH, or fondaparinux is indicated in medical patients who are deemed to be at risk for DVT. In patients who are bleeding or are at high risk of major bleeding, it is recommended to use mechanical thromboprophylaxis with graduated compression stockings or intermittent pneumatic compression if indicated.

Hospitalized patients with cancer are at high risk for VTE and are at risk for complications associated with full-dose anticoagulation. Prophylaxis for cancer patients should follow the recommendations outlines for medical patients.[208,210] Recent data in outpatients with cancer and no additional risk factors for VTE, suggest potential benefit from routine thromboprophylaxis, but it appears to be outweighed by the risk of bleeding and is not currently recommended.[211] Anticoagulation together with mechanical prophylaxis is appropriate in patients who are deemed to be at exceptionally high risk and for those who have multiple risk factors for DVT.[206]

Extensive evidence-based recommendations for prevention of VTE in general medical patients (including hospitalized medical patients, outpatients with cancer, the chronically immobilized, long-distance travelers, and those with asymptomatic thrombophilia) can be found elsewhere.[208,210] Increasing data now support prophylactic initiation of a DOAC (rivaroxaban) in medically ill inpatients, with extension for approximately a month postdischarge.[210]

General Surgical Patients

In general surgical patients, a number of prophylactic strategies have been used.[207] Approximately one-third of the 150,000 to 200,000 VTE-related deaths per year in the United States occur following surgery.[212] The high incidence of postoperative VTE and the availability of effective methods of prevention mandate that thromboprophylaxis should be considered in every surgical patient. Thus, an overview of the results of randomized trials in surgical patients demonstrated the substantial benefit of DVT prophylaxis.[207] For patients undergoing minor operations who are younger than age 40 years and who have no additional risk factors for DVT, no prophylaxis other than early ambulation is recommended. Older patients who are undergoing major operations without additional risk factors should receive standard low-dose UFH two or three times daily, LMWH, fondaparinux, or intermittent pneumatic compression. For patients with a high risk of bleeding, mechanical prophylaxis in the form of graduated compression stockings or intermittent pneumatic compression should be substituted for pharmacologic prophylaxis. Extensive evidence-based recommendations for prevention of VTE in general nonorthopedic surgical patients can be found elsewhere.[207]

Other High-Risk Patients

Total hip arthroplasty and total knee arthroplasty are performed with increasing frequency. The risk for VTE in major orthopedic surgery, in particular total hip arthroplasty and hip fracture surgery, is among the highest for all surgical specialties. For patients undergoing elective total hip or knee arthroplasty, approved regimens include fondaparinux initiated 6 to 8 hours after surgery, LMWH initiated 12 hours before or 12 to 24 hours after surgery, adjusted-dose VKA initiated on the evening of the surgical day, low-dose UFH, aspirin, dabigatran, apixaban, or rivaroxaban (total hip arthroplasty or total knee arthroplasty but not hip fracture surgery). The duration of prophylaxis depends on whether the patient is ambulatory and on additional risk factors, although at least 12 days and as many as 35 days of therapy are recommended.[205,213]

The DOACs, including direct thrombin inhibitors (dabigatran exilate) and factor Xa inhibitors (rivaroxaban, apixaban), appear as effective as enoxaparin in reducing the risk of VTE in patients undergoing total hip or total knee arthroplasty with a similar safety profile, although some studies suggest a trend to increase in major bleeding when compared to LMWH.[213] The introduction of oral, once-daily forms of thromboprophylaxis that do not require monitoring represents a substantial advance in both pre- and potentially postembolic prophylaxis. In summary, given the effective options available, few patients at risk for venous thrombosis cannot be protected. Prophylaxis must occur if a substantial impact is to be made on the considerable and often unnecessary morbidity and mortality associated with PE. Not only must prophylaxis be applied; it must also be applied in a manner proportionate to the patient's risk of thromboembolism.

SPECIAL CIRCUMSTANCES IN ACUTE PULMONARY EMBOLISM

Early Discharge and Outpatient Pulmonary Embolism Treatment

Early discharge and outpatient treatment in patients with acute PE are a matter of debate. The crucial issue with regard to early discharge and outpatient treatment in patients with acute PE is to select those patients who are at low risk of adverse early outcome. A number of risk-prediction models have been developed.[214] Among them, the PESI is the most extensively validated score to date. The value of the simplified form of the PESI score (sPESI) for selecting candidates for early discharge and home treatment has not yet been directly evaluated. Several recent multicenter clinical trials (randomized and nonrandomized) have investigated the 3-month clinical outcome of patients with PE, who were discharge early or treated entirely at home using different prediction rules with divergent results.[215–221] Meta-analytic data suggest that pooled incidences of recurrent VTE, major bleeding, and total mortality did not significantly differ between early discharge patients and those treated as inpatients.[220] Real-world data support these meta-analytic data.[222]

Current clinical guidelines recommend that early discharge (within first 24 hours) and outpatient treatment should be considered in patients with DVT; and those with PE and low risk of an adverse early outcomes (PESI class I or II, and probably those with sPESI of 0) plus low bleeding risk, if it appears feasible based on the patient's anticipated compliance and family/social background.[89]

Follow-Up and Optimal Duration of Anticoagulation

The duration of outpatient anticoagulation for patients with VTE remains controversial, but it is generally agreed upon in patients with a first episode of acute unprovoked VTE (ie, occurring in the absence of reversible risk factors such as surgery, trauma, immobilization, or contraception/hormonal therapy).[89,222,223] The incidence of recurrent VTE does not appear depend on the clinical manifestation of the first event (ie, it is similar after PE than after DVT); however, in patients who have suffered PE, VTE more frequently recurs as symptomatic PE, while in patients who have suffered DVT, it tends to recur more frequently as DVT.[224]

Patients with a clearly defined initial predisposition whose initial thromboembolic risk factors have resolved ("provoked" PE, in the presence of a temporary or reversible risk factor) should receive at least 3 months of anticoagulation. Consideration should be given to a longer course of therapy in those with persistent V/Q/CT scan defects or abnormal lower extremity test results if performed. Treatment beyond this initial period with VKA reduces the risk of recurrent VTE up to 90%, but this benefit is partially offset by at least 1% higher risk of major bleeding.[225,226] Therefore, in patients who receive extended anticoagulation, the risk–benefit ratio of continuing such treatment should be reassessed at a regular basis.

Patients without a clearly defined initial predisposition to thromboembolism (unprovoked PE) should be treated for at least 3 months, although extended oral anticoagulation should always be provided unless the bleeding risk is prohibitive. Certain patients, such as those with recurrent spontaneous or unprovoked episodes of VTE (≥2 episodes), an irreversible clinical risk factor, combined thrombophilic tendencies, antithrombin III deficiency, deficit of protein C or protein S, homozygous factor V Leiden or homozygous prothrombin G20210A, or the presence of a lupus anticoagulant, should also be treated with an indefinite period of anticoagulation. In previous trials, such a strategy has been associated with an increased risk of bleeding complications. It has been proposed that D-dimer testing might, alone[227] or integrated in recurrence risk scores,[228–230] identify patients in whom anticoagulation can be or not safely discontinued after a first unprovoked VTE. However, a recent prospective study has questioned the utility of this strategy.[231]

Recent trials have evaluated DOACs at reduced doses. This has altered the paradigm of long-term therapy. Reduced-dose rivaroxaban and apixaban have been evaluated for the extended treatment of patients with VTE with the hopes of proving that lower doses could be protective but safer long term. The efficacy and safety of extended therapy beyond 6 to 12 months of half-dose DOACs (ie, prophylactic dose) compared with therapeutic doses has been evaluated in two clinical trials. The Apixaban after the Initial Management of Pulmonary Embolism and Deep Vein Thrombosis with First-Line Therapy–Extended Treatment (AMPLIFY-EXT)[232] and Reduced-dosed Rivaroxaban in the Long-term Prevention of Recurrent Symptomatic Venous Thromboembolism (EINSTEIN CHOICE) trials[233] have evaluated low-dose apixaban and rivaroxaban, respectively. AMPLIFY-EXT assessed therapeutic dose apixaban (5 mg every 12 hours), low-dose apixaban (2.5 mg every 12 hours), and placebo, and found that both doses of apixaban were effective at preventing recurrent VTE and were superior to placebo. Additionally, both therapeutic and low-dose apixaban had no significant difference in combined rates of major and nonmajor bleeding between apixaban and placebo. EINSTEIN CHOICE demonstrated that reduced dose rivaroxaban (10 mg daily) and treatment dose rivaroxaban (20 mg daily) were similarly effective and safe compared with aspirin.[233] A meta-analysis of these studies found low-dose DOACs to be as effective as therapeutic dose, with a trend toward reduced bleeding with the use of low-dose DOACs.[234] These findings to date have led to several clinical guidelines recommending either therapeutic dose or low-dose DOACs for secondary prevention of VTE and suggesting aspirin in patients who are unable to receive a DOAC.

Small (Subsegmental) Acute Pulmonary Emboli

The diagnostic value and clinical significance of subsegmental defects on chest CTA have been debated.[235] One analysis showed similar outcomes (3-month recurrence and mortality rates) between patients with subsegmental and more proximal PE; but outcomes were largely determined by comorbidities.[236] Perhaps compression ultrasound of the lower limbs may be helpful, because the exclusion of proximal DVT in a patient with isolated subsegmental PE might support anticoagulation discontinuation. However, this decision should be made on an individual basis, evaluating both current risk of VTE recurrence and bleeding risk. The critical point is that while a new subsegmental PE, in and of itself, may be of no prognostic significance, the fact that the patient *developed* acute PE means that there *is or recently was* ongoing risk and treatment should be very strongly considered. For example, a small PE discovered incidentally during a screening CT in a cancer patient may not cause current or future clinical symptoms, but in the presence of active cancer, the recurrence rate would be expected to be high, justifying consideration of anticoagulation. Even without active cancer, incidental PE developed for a reason so that there should be a very low threshold to consider at least 3 months of anticoagulation.

Treatment of Isolated Distal Deep Vein Thrombosis and Upper Limb Thrombosis

Although posing a substantially lower embolic risk than proximal vein thrombosis, calf-limited thrombi may extend into the proximal veins. Furthermore, the symptomatic outcome may be worse in the absence of therapy.[206,237] If a contraindication to anticoagulation exists, noninvasive testing over 10 to 14 days should be performed to detect possible proximal extension. Again, the fact that the clot occurred implies the presence of one or more VTE risk factors, and unless the risk resolves, treatment should be strongly considered.[206]

The spectrum of upper extremity venous thrombosis is variable and includes patients with peripherally and centrally placed IV catheters, as well as those with underlying malignancy. Patients with documented upper extremity DVT should be anticoagulated.[238] Cautious line removal should be undertaken whenever possible. Prophylactic anticoagulation in patients with long-term indwelling catheters is

controversial. Effort-related upper extremity venous thrombosis (Paget–Schroetter syndrome) usually affects young, active individuals and is related to extrinsic compression of the subclavian vein at the thoracic inlet.[25,26] A multidisciplinary approach to management is often required to avoid long-term consequences, including recurrence, embolism, and symptomatic sequelae.

Pulmonary Embolism in Pregnancy

PE is a leading cause of pregnancy-related maternal death in developed countries; the risk of PE is higher in the postpartum period, particularly after a cesarean section.[239,240] Symptoms should be interpreted with caution since pregnant women often complain of breathlessness, and data on clinical prediction rules for PE in pregnancy is scarce. Suspicion of PE in pregnancy warrants formal diagnostic assessment with validated methods. A normal D-dimer value has the same exclusion value for PE in pregnant women as for other patients with suspected PE but is found more rarely, because plasma D-dimer levels physiologically increase throughout pregnancy.[241] Imaging of the lungs in pregnant patients with suspected PE is outlined in the Diagnosis of DVT and PE section.

In pregnancy, elective chest imaging should be minimized, but utilized when needed. Radiation exposure in utero can potentially lead to oncogenicity and teratogenicity. Studies have demonstrated equivalent fetal radiation exposure from V/Q and current generation CT scanners.[242] However, available data suggest that the danger of fetal irradiation during standard maternal diagnostic testing for PE is likely overstated. Radiation doses of 5 rad (50 mSv) or less do not appear to be associated with an increased risk of pregnancy loss and the risk of fetal malformation doesn't increase until background levels of radiation reach doses greater than 15 rad (150 mSv).[243,244] Overall, based on the low baseline rate of childhood cancer, this represents a very low absolute risk increase.

Weight-adjusted LMWH is the preferred treatment for acute VTE in pregnancy, given its safety profile.[239,246] Adaptation according to anti-Xa monitoring may be considered in women at extremes of body weight or with renal disease, but routine monitoring is generally not justified.[246] Fondaparinux should not be used in pregnancy due to the lack of data. VKAs should not be administered as well throughout pregnancy, especially during the first and third trimesters. DOACs are contraindicated in pregnant patients and during breast feeding. Thrombolytic treatment during pregnancy and the peripartum period should be used only in life-threatening situations.[239]

The management of labor and delivery require particular attention. Epidural analgesia cannot be used unless LMWH has been discontinued at least 12 hours before delivery. Treatment can be resumed 12 to 24 hours after removal of the epidural catheter if the catheter placement was uncomplicated. After delivery, heparin treatment may be replaced by VKAs, including in breast-feeding mothers, which should be continued for at least 3 months. A recent treatise on acute PE in pregnancy is recommended for a detailed review.[247]

Pulmonary Embolism in Cancer Patients

The overall risk of VTE in cancer patients is four times greater than in the general population. The risk of VTE varies with different types of cancer.[248] Hematological malignancies, lung cancer, gastric and pancreatic malignancies, brain cancer, genitourinary tract, and breast malignancies are associated with a particularly high risk of DVT and PE.[31-34] The risk is higher in patients receiving chemotherapy; nevertheless, prophylactic anticoagulation is not routinely recommended during ambulatory anticancer chemotherapy, with the exception of thalidomide- or lenalidomide-based regimens in multiple myeloma.[249] The risk is particularly increased after cancer surgery, especially in the first 4 to 6 weeks, although it may remain elevated beyond the third month after surgery.[250] Continued vigilance is therefore necessary, as currently recommended prophylactic anticoagulation regimen only covers the first 1 month after surgery.

Malignancy is taken into account in the estimation of clinical probability of PE. A negative D-dimer test has the same diagnostic value as in noncancer patients; therefore, a normal value excludes the diagnosis of VTE in patients with low or intermediate clinical probability of PE. However, D-dimer levels are increased in many patients with cancer but are nonspecific. Thus, as in any patient with suspected PE and elevated D-dimer or those with high clinical probability of PE, further imaging tests should be performed. Cancer is a risk for adverse outcome in PE, which is mainly due to the increased bleeding risk during anticoagulation therapy and to the high rate of recurrence of VTE. Previously, LMWH was recommended in the acute phase (except for high-risk PE) and continued over the first 3 to 6 months as first-line therapy.[250,251] DOAC trials in cancer patients with VTE are discussed in the section Direct Oral Anticoagulants; these drugs have proven effective in this setting.[165-168]

Finally, up to 10% of patients with VTE may be diagnosed with cancer within 1 year following the "unprovoked" index event.[36] However, an extended occult cancer screening does not seem superior to a limited-screening, age-appropriate strategy based on clinical, exploratory, and laboratory parameters.[37,38]

COVID and Thromboembolism

COVID-19 is a multisystem disease caused by the SARS-CoV-2 virus and may be associated with severe thrombotic manifestations. The association between viral respiratory infection and thrombosis, including coronavirus severe acute respiratory syndrome and Middle Eastern respiratory syndrome is not new, but the scope of the COVID-19 pandemic has brought this concern to the forefront of clinical practice.[253,254] Despite extensive research in this area, the direct effects of activation of coagulation on inflammatory pathways and perpetuation of lung injury are not yet well understood but seem to be related to major disturbances to the endothelium, abnormal levels of clotting factors, and platelet activation. The concept of microvascular thrombosis involving the lung and other organs appears to be important in the pathophysiology of the COVID-19 disease. A number of randomized trials are underway that will offer guidance in selecting prophylaxis and treatment approaches.[255]

SUMMARY

- Acute PE continues to cause death frequently and is a worldwide problem.
- Undiagnosed and late diagnosed patients contribute substantially to the death rate.
- Clinicians should maintain a high suspicion for the disease.
- Risk stratification should be undertaken when PE is diagnosed.
- Anticoagulation unequivocally improves mortality.
- More aggressive therapy is indicated in patients with high-risk (massive) PE and may be considered in certain patients with intermediate-risk PE.
- CTEPH occurs in a small percentage of patients and should be addressed with pulmonary endarterectomy when possible.

REFERENCES

1. Raskob GE, Angchaisuksiri P, Blanco AN, et al. Thrombosis: a major contributor to global disease burden. *Arteriosclerosis Thrombos and Vasc Biol.* 2014;34:2363-2371.
2. Aujesky D, Obrosky DS, Stone RA, et al. A prediction rule to identify low-risk patients with pulmonary embolism. *Arch Intern Med.* 2006;166:169-175.
3. Goldhaber SZ, Visani L, De Rosa M. Acute pulmonary embolism: clinical outcomes in the International Cooperative Pulmonary Embolism Registry (ICOPER). *Lancet.* 1999;353:1386-1389.
4. Cohen AT, Agnelli G, Anderson FA, et al. Venous thromboembolism (VTE) in Europe. The number of VTE events and associated morbidity and mortality. *Thromb Haemost.* 2007;98:756-764.
5. Cosmi B, Nijkeuter M, Valentino M, Huisman MV, Barozzi L, Palareti G. Residual emboli on lung perfusion scan or multidetector computed tomography after a first episode of acute pulmonary embolism. *Intern Emerg Med.* 2011;6:521-528.
6. Pengo V, Lensing AW, Prins MH, et al. Incidence of chronic thromboembolic pulmonary hypertension after pulmonary embolism. *New Engl J Med.* 2004;350:2257-2264.
7. Goldhaber SZ. Prevention of recurrent idiopathic venous thromboembolism. *Circulation.* 2004;110:IV20-IV24.
8. Wood KE. Major pulmonary embolism: review of a pathophysiologic approach to the golden hour of hemodynamically significant pulmonary embolism. *Chest.* 2002;121:877-905.
9. Tapson VF, Jimenez D. Catheter-based approaches to acute pulmonary embolism. *Semin Respir Crit Care Med.* 2017;38:73-83.
10. Berkman SA, Tapson VF. Methodological issues and controversies in COVID-19 coagulopathy: a tale of two storms. *Clin Appl Thrombosis/Hemost.* Sept 3, 2020. doi: 10.1177/1076029620945398
11. Kearon C, Akl EA. Duration of anticoagulant therapy for deep vein thrombosis and pulmonary embolism. *Blood.* 2014;123:1794-1801.
12. Cotton LT, Clark C. Anatomical localization of venous thrombosis. *Ann R Coll Surg Engl.* 1965;36:214-224.
13. Kahn SR, Comerota AJ, Cushman M et al. The postthrombotic syndrome: evidence-based prevention, diagnosis, and treatment strategies: a scientific statement from the American Heart Association. *Circulation.* 2014;130:1636-1661.
14. Goldhaber SZ, Tapson VF, Committee DFS. A prospective registry of 5,451 patients with ultrasound-confirmed deep vein thrombosis. *Am J Cardiol.* 2004;93:259-262.
15. Mazareanu E. Global air traffic—scheduled passengers 2004-2021. *Statista.* Jun 10, 2020. https://www.statista.com/statistics/564717/airline-industry-passenger-traffic-globally/

16. Aryal KR, Al-Khaffaf H. Venous thromboembolic complications following air travel: what's the quantitative risk? A literature review. *Eur J Vasc Endovasc Surg.* 2006;31:187-199.

17. Go AS, Mozaffarian D, Roger VL et al. Heart disease and stroke statistics–2014 update: a report from the American Heart Association. *Circulation.* 2014;129:e28-e292.

18. Ogden CL, Carroll MD, Kit BK, Flegal KM. Prevalence of childhood and adult obesity in the United States, 2011-2012. *JAMA.* 2014;311:806-814.

19. Goldhaber SZ, Grodstein F, Stampfer MJ et al. A prospective study of risk factors for pulmonary embolism in women. *JAMA.* 1997;277:642-645.

20. Goldhaber SZ, Savage DD, Garrison RJ et al. Risk factors for pulmonary embolism. The Framingham Study. *Am J Med.* 1983;74:1023-1028.

21. Davi G, Guagnano MT, Ciabattoni G et al. Platelet activation in obese women: role of inflammation and oxidant stress. *JAMA.* 2002;288:2008-2014.

22. Stein PD, Hull RD, Kayali F, Ghali WA, Alshab AK, Olson RE. Venous thromboembolism according to age: the impact of an aging population. *Arch Intern Med.* 2004;164:2260-2265.

23. Rogers MA, Levine DA, Blumberg N, Flanders SA, Chopra V, Langa KM. Triggers of hospitalization for venous thromboembolism. *Circulation.* 2012;125:2092-2099.

24. Kearon C. Natural history of venous thromboembolism. *Circulation.* 2003;107:I22-30.

25. Engelberger RP, Kucher N. Management of deep vein thrombosis of the upper extremity. *Circulation.* 2012;126:768-773.

26. Joffe HV, Goldhaber SZ. Upper-extremity deep vein thrombosis. *Circulation.* 2002;106:1874-1880.

27. Sorensen HT, Horvath-Puho E, Lash TL et al. Heart disease may be a risk factor for pulmonary embolism without peripheral deep venous thrombosis. *Circulation.* 2011;124:1435-1441.

28. Sorensen HT, Horvath-Puho E, Pedersen L, Baron JA, Prandoni P. Venous thromboembolism and subsequent hospitalisation due to acute arterial cardiovascular events: a 20-year cohort study. *Lancet.* 2007;370:1773-1779.

29. Fernandes CJ, Luciana TK, Morinaga J, et al. Cancer-associated thrombosis: the when, how and why. *Eur Respir Rev.* 2019;28:180119. doi: 10.1183/16000617.0119-2018

30. Carson JL, Kelley MA, Duff A et al. The clinical course of pulmonary embolism. *N Engl J Med.* 1992;326:1240-1245.31.

31. Chew HK, Wun T, Harvey D, Zhou H, White RH. Incidence of venous thromboembolism and its effect on survival among patients with common cancers. *Arch Intern Med.* 2006;166:458-464.

32. Timp JF, Braekkan SK, Versteeg HH, Cannegieter SC. Epidemiology of cancer-associated venous thrombosis. *Blood.* 2013;122:1712-1723.

33. Rickles FR, Levine M, Edwards RL. Hemostatic alterations in cancer patients. *Cancer Metastasis Rev.* 1992;11:237-248.

34. Lee AY, Levine MN. The thrombophilic state induced by therapeutic agents in the cancer patient. *Semin Thromb Hemost.* 1999;25:137-145.

35. Decensi A, Maisonneuve P, Rotmensz N et al. Effect of tamoxifen on venous thromboembolic events in a breast cancer prevention trial. *Circulation.* 2005;111:650-656.

36. Sorensen HT, Mellemkjaer L, Steffensen FH, Olsen JH, Nielsen GL. The risk of a diagnosis of cancer after primary deep venous thrombosis or pulmonary embolism. *N Engl J Med.* 1998;338:1169-1173.

37. Di Nisio M, Otten HM, Piccioli A et al. Decision analysis for cancer screening in idiopathic venous thromboembolism. *J Thromb Haemost.* 2005;3:2391-2396.

38. Carrier M, Lazo-Langner A, Shivakumar S, et al. Screening for occult cancer in unprovoked venous thromboembolism. *N Engl J Med.* 2015;373:697-704. doi: 10.1056/NEJMoa1506623

39. Gomes MP, Deitcher SR. Risk of venous thromboembolic disease associated with hormonal contraceptives and hormone replacement therapy: a clinical review. *Arch Intern Med.* 2004;164:1965-1967.

40. Pomp ER, Lenselink AM, Rosendaal FR, Doggen CJ. Pregnancy, the postpartum period and prothrombotic defects: risk of venous thrombosis in the MEGA study. *J Thromb Haemost.* 2008;6:632-637.

41. Toglia MR, Weg JG. Venous thromboembolism during pregnancy. *N Engl J Med.* 1996;335:108-114.

42. Henriksson P, Westerlund E, Wallen H, Brandt L, Hovatta O, Ekbom A. Incidence of pulmonary and venous thromboembolism in pregnancies after in vitro fertilisation: cross sectional study. *BMJ.* 2013;346:e8632.

43. Wu O, Robertson L, Langhorne P et al. Oral contraceptives, hormone replacement therapy, thrombophilias and risk of venous thromboembolism: a systematic review. The Thrombosis: Risk and Economic Assessment of Thrombophilia Screening (TREATS) Study. *Thromb Haemost.* 2005;94:17-25.

44. Sweetland S, Beral V, Balkwill A et al. Venous thromboembolism risk in relation to use of different types of postmenopausal hormone therapy in a large prospective study. *J Thromb Haemost.* 2012;10:2277-2286.

45. Wu O, Robertson L, Twaddle S et al. Screening for thrombophilia in high-risk situations: a meta-analysis and cost-effectiveness analysis. *Br J Haematol.* 2005;131:80-90.

46. Galli M, Luciani D, Bertolini G, Barbui T. Lupus anticoagulants are stronger risk factors for thrombosis than anticardiolipin antibodies in the antiphospholipid syndrome: a systematic review of the literature. *Blood.* 2003;101:1827-1832.

47. Ortel TL, Erkan D, Kitchens CS. How I treat catastrophic thrombotic syndromes. *Blood.* 2015;126(11):1285-1293.

48. Simioni P, Tormene D, Spiezia L et al. Inherited thrombophilia and venous thromboembolism. *Semin Thromb Hemost.* 2006;32:700-708.

49. Ridker PM, Hennekens CH, Lindpaintner K, Stampfer MJ, Eisenberg PR, Miletich JP. Mutation in the gene coding for coagulation factor V and the risk of myocardial infarction, stroke, and venous thrombosis in apparently healthy men. *N Engl J Med.* 1995;332:912-917.

50. Ridker PM, Miletich JP, Hennekens CH, Buring JE. Ethnic distribution of factor V Leiden in 4047 men and women. Implications for venous thromboembolism screening. *JAMA.* 1997;277:1305-1307.

51. Kujovich JL. Thrombophilia and pregnancy complications. *Am J Obstet Gynecol.* 2004;191:412-424.

52. Vandenbroucke JP, Rosing J, Bloemenkamp KW et al. Oral contraceptives and the risk of venous thrombosis. *N Engl J Med.* 2001;344:1527-1535.

53. Poort SR, Rosendaal FR, Reitsma PH, Bertina RM. A common genetic variation in the 3′-untranslated region of the prothrombin gene is associated with elevated plasma prothrombin levels and an increase in venous thrombosis. *Blood.* 1996;88:3698-3703.

54. Hillarp A, Zoller B, Svensson PJ, Dahlback B. The 20210 A allele of the prothrombin gene is a common risk factor among Swedish outpatients with verified deep venous thrombosis. *Thromb Haemost.* 1997;78:990-992.

55. De Stefano V, Martinelli I, Mannucci PM et al. The risk of recurrent deep venous thrombosis among heterozygous carriers of both factor V Leiden and the G20210A prothrombin mutation. *N Engl J Med.* 1999;341:801-806.

56. D'Angelo A, Selhub J. Homocysteine and thrombotic disease. *Blood.* 1997;90:1-11.

57. Ridker PM, Hennekens CH, Selhub J, Miletich JP, Malinow MR, Stampfer MJ. Interrelation of hyperhomocyst(e)inemia, factor V Leiden, and risk of future venous thromboembolism. *Circulation.* 1997;95:1777-1782.

58. Undas A, Brozek J, Szczeklik A. Homocysteine and thrombosis: from basic science to clinical evidence. *Thromb Haemost.* 2005;94:907-915.

59. Kraaijenhagen RA, in't Anker PS, Koopman MM et al. High plasma concentration of factor VIIIc is a major risk factor for venous thromboembolism. *Thromb Haemost.* 2000;83:5-9.

60. Kyrle PA, Minar E, Hirschl M et al. High plasma levels of factor VIII and the risk of recurrent venous thromboembolism. *N Engl J Med.* 2000;343:457-462.

61. Azarian R, Wartski M, Collignon MA et al. Lung perfusion scans and hemodynamics in acute and chronic pulmonary embolism. *J Nucl Med.* 1997;38:980-983.

62. McIntyre KM, Sasahara AA. The hemodynamic response to pulmonary embolism in patients without prior cardiopulmonary disease. *Am J Cardiol.* 1971;28:288-294.

63. Stein PD, Henry JW. Clinical characteristics of patients with acute pulmonary embolism stratified according to their presenting syndromes. *Chest.* 1997;112:974-979.

64. Stein PD, Terrin ML, Hales CA et al. Clinical, laboratory, roentgenographic, and electrocardiographic findings in patients with acute pulmonary embolism and no pre-existing cardiac or pulmonary disease. *Chest.* 1991;100:598-603.

65. Pollack CV, Schreiber D, Goldhaber SZ et al. Clinical characteristics, management, and outcomes of patients diagnosed with acute pulmonary embolism in the emergency department: initial report of EMPEROR (Multicenter Emergency Medicine Pulmonary Embolism in the Real World Registry). *J Am Coll Cardiol.* 2011;57:700-706.

66. Wells PS, Anderson DR, Rodger M et al. Derivation of a simple clinical model to categorize patients probability of pulmonary embolism: increasing the models utility with the SimpliRED D-dimer. *Thromb Haemost.* 2000;83:416-420.

67. Wicki J, Perneger TV, Junod AF, Bounameaux H, Perrier A. Assessing clinical probability of pulmonary embolism in the emergency ward: a simple score. *Arch Intern Med.* 2001;161:92-97.

68. Le Gal G, Righini M, Roy PM et al. Prediction of pulmonary embolism in the emergency department: the revised Geneva score. *Ann Intern Med.* 2006;144:165-171.

69. Ceriani E, Combescure C, Le Gal G et al. Clinical prediction rules for pulmonary embolism: a systematic review and meta-analysis. *J Thromb Haemost.* 2010;8:957-970.

70. Douma RA, Mos IC, Erkens PM et al. Performance of 4 clinical decision rules in the diagnostic management of acute pulmonary embolism: a prospective cohort study. *Ann Intern Med.* 2011;154:709-718.

71. Lucassen W, Geersing GJ, Erkens PM et al. Clinical decision rules for excluding pulmonary embolism: a meta-analysis. *Ann Intern Med.* 2011;155:448-460.

72. Gibson NS, Sohne M, Kruip MJ et al. Further validation and simplification of the Wells clinical decision rule in pulmonary embolism. *Thromb Haemost.* 2008;99:229-234.

73. Klok FA, Mos IC, Nijkeuter M et al. Simplification of the revised Geneva score for assessing clinical probability of pulmonary embolism. *Arch Intern Med.* 2008;168:2131-2136.

74. Righini M, et al. Age-adjusted D-dimer cutoff levels to rule out pulmonary embolism: the ADJUST-PE study. *JAMA.* 2014.311(11):1117-1124.

75. Adam SS, Key NS, Greenberg CS. D-dimer antigen: current concepts and future prospects. *Blood.* 2009;113:2878-2887.

76. Penaloza A, Soulié C, Moumneh T, et al. Pulmonary embolism rule-out criteria (PERC) rule in European patients with low implicit clinical probability (PERCEPIC): a multicentre, prospective, observational study. *Lancet Haematol.* 2017;4(12):e615-e621.

77. Freund Y, Cachanado M, Aubry A, et al. Effect of the pulmonary embolism rule-out criteria on subsequent thromboembolic events among low-risk emergency department patients: The PROPER randomized clinical trial. *JAMA.* 2018;319(6):559-566.

78. van der Hulle T, Cheung WY, Kooij S, et al. Simplified diagnostic management of suspected pulmonary embolism (the YEARS study): a prospective, multicentre, cohort study. *Lancet.* 2017;390(10091):289-297.

79. Righini M, Le Gal G, Perrier A, Bounameaux H. More on: clinical criteria to prevent unnecessary diagnostic testing in emergency department patients with suspected pulmonary embolism. *J Thromb Haemost.* 2005;3: 188-189.

80. Penaloza A, et al. Comparison of the unstructured clinician gestalt, the Wells Score, and the Revised Geneva score to estimate pretest probability for suspected PE. *Ann Emerg Med.* 2013;62(2):117-124.e2. doi: 10.1016/j. annemergmed.2012.11.002

81. McGinn S, White P. Acute cor pulmonale resulting from pulmonary embolism. *JAMA.* 1935;104:1473-1480.

82. Sokolow M, Katz L, Muscovitz A. The electrocardiogram in acute pulmonary embolism. *Am Heart J.* 1940;19:166-184.

83. The urokinase pulmonary embolism trial. A national cooperative study. *Circulation.* 1973;47:II1-108.

84. Ferrari E, Imbert A, Chevalier T, Mihoubi A, Morand P, Baudouy M. The ECG in pulmonary embolism. Predictive value of negative T waves in precordial leads–80 case reports. *Chest.* 1997;111:537-543.

85. Kucher N, Walpoth N, Wustmann K, Noveanu M, Gertsch M. QR in V1–an ECG sign associated with right ventricular strain and adverse clinical outcome in pulmonary embolism. *Eur Heart J.* 2003;24:1113-1119.

86. Geibel A, Zehender M, Kasper W, Olschewski M, Klima C, Konstantinides SV. Prognostic value of the ECG on admission in patients with acute major pulmonary embolism. *Eur Respir.* 2005;25:843-848.

87. Elliott CG, Goldhaber SZ, Visani L, DeRosa M. Chest radiographs in acute pulmonary embolism. Results from the International Cooperative Pulmonary Embolism Registry. *Chest.* 2000;118:33-38.

88. Schoepf UJ, Goldhaber SZ, Costello P. Spiral computed tomography for acute pulmonary embolism. *Circulation.* 2004;109:2160-2167.

89. 2019 ESC Guidelines for the diagnosis and management of acute pulmonary embolism developed in collaboration with the European Respiratory Society (ERS): the Task Force for the diagnosis and management of acute pulmonary embolism of the European Society of Cardiology (ESC). *Eur Heart J.* 2019;41:543-603. doi: 10.1093/eurheartj/ehz405

90. Mos IC, Klok FA, Kroft LJ, et al. Safety of ruling out acute pulmonary embolism by normal computed tomography pulmonary angiography in patients with an indication for computed tomography: systematic review and meta-analysis. *J Thromb Haemost.* 2009;7:1491-1498. doi:10.1111/j.1538- 7836.2009.03518.x

91. Goodman LR, Stein PD, Matta F et al. CT venography and compression sonography are diagnostically equivalent: data from PIOPED II. *AJR Am J Roentgenol.* 2007;189:1071-1076.

92. Stein PD, Fowler SE, Goodman LR et al. Multidetector computed tomography for acute pulmonary embolism. *N Engl J Med.* 2006;354: 2317-2327.

93. Brenner DJ, Hall EJ. Computed tomography—an increasing source of radiation exposure. *N Engl J Med.* 2007;357:2277-2284.

94. Quiroz R, Kucher N, Zou KH et al. Clinical validity of a negative computed tomography scan in patients with suspected pulmonary embolism: a systematic review. *JAMA.* 2005;293:2012-2017.

95. Duffett L, Castellucci LA, Forgie MA. Pulmonary embolism: update on management and controversies. *BMJ.* 2020;370:m2177 doi: https://doi. org/10.1136/bmj.m2177

96. PIOPED Investigators. Value of the ventilation/perfusion scan in acute pulmonary embolism. Results of the prospective investigation of pulmonary embolism diagnosis (PIOPED). *JAMA.* 1990;263:2753-2759.

97. Kang DK, Thilo C, Schoepf UJ, et al. CT signs of right ventricular dysfunction: prognostic role in acute pulmonary embolism. *JACC: Cardiovasc Imaging.* 2011;4(8):841-849. doi:10.1016/j.jcmg.2011.04.013

98. Elster, Allen D. Introduction to dual-energy computed tomography. *J Comput Assist Tomog.* 2018;42:823.

99. Weikert TJ, Winkel DJ, Bremerich J, et al. Automated detection of pulmonary embolism in CT pulmonary angiograms using an AI-powered algorithm. *Eur Radiol.* 2020;30:6545-6553.

100. Eid M, De Cecco CN, Nance, Jr. JW, et al. Cinematic rendering in CT: a novel, lifelike 3D visualization technique. *Med Phys Informatics.* 2017;209:370-379.

101. Weinberg AS, Dohad S, Ramzy D, Madyoon H, Tapson VF. Clot extraction with the FlowTriever device in acute massive pulmonary embolism. *J Intensive Care Med.* 2016;31;676.

102. Sostman HD, Layish DT, Tapson VF, et al. Prospective comparison of helical CT and MR imaging in clinically suspected acute pulmonary embolism. *JMRI.* 1996;6:275-281.

103. Oudkerk M, van Beek EJ, Wielopolski P et al. Comparison of contrast-enhanced magnetic resonance angiography and conventional pulmonary angiography for the diagnosis of pulmonary embolism: a prospective study. *Lancet.* 2002;359:1643-1647.

104. Stein PD, Chenevert TL, Fowler SE et al. Gadolinium-enhanced magnetic resonance angiography for pulmonary embolism: a multicenter prospective study (PIOPED III). *Ann Intern Med.* 2010;152:434-443, W142-W143.

105. Grifoni S, Olivotto I, Cecchini P et al. Short-term clinical outcome of patients with acute pulmonary embolism, normal blood pressure, and echocardiographic right ventricular dysfunction. *Circulation.* 2000;101:2817-2822.

106. Bova C, Greco F, Misuraca G et al. Diagnostic utility of echocardiography in patients with suspected pulmonary embolism. *Am J Emerg Med.* 2003;21:180-183.

107. McConnell MV, Solomon SD, Rayan ME, Come PC, Goldhaber SZ, Lee RT. Regional right ventricular dysfunction detected by echocardiography in acute pulmonary embolism. *Am J Cardiol.* 1996;78:469-473.

108. Konstantinides S, Geibel A, Olschewski M, et al. Patent foramen ovale is an important predictor of adverse outcome in patients with major pulmonary embolism. *Circulation.* 1998;97(19):1946-1951. doi: 10.1161/01.cir.97.19.1946

109. Garvey S, Dudzinski DM, Giordano N, et al. Pulmonary embolism with clot in transit: an analysis of risk factors and outcomes. *Thromb Res.* 2020;187:139-147. doi: 10.1016/j.thromres.2020.01.006.

110. Zierler BK. Ultrasonography and diagnosis of venous thromboembolism. *Circulation.* 2004;109:I9-14.

111. Borgstede JP, Clagett GE. Types, frequency, and significance of alternative diagnoses found during duplex Doppler venous examinations of the lower extremities. *J Ultrasound Med.* 1992;11:85-89.

112. Kearon C, Ginsberg JS, Hirsh J. The role of venous ultrasonography in the diagnosis of suspected deep venous thrombosis and pulmonary embolism. *Ann Intern Med.* 1998;129:1044-1049.

113. Turkstra F, Kuijer PM, van Beek EJ, Brandjes DP, ten Cate JW, Buller HR. Diagnostic utility of ultrasonography of leg veins in patients suspected of having pulmonary embolism. *Ann Intern Med.* 1997;126:775-781.

114. Nazerian P, Vanni S, Volpicelli G et al. Accuracy of point-of-care multiorgan ultrasonography for the diagnosis of pulmonary embolism. *Chest.* 2014;145:950-957.

115. Chin EE, Zimmerman PT, Grant EG. Sonographic evaluation of upper extremity deep venous thrombosis. *J Ultrasound Med.* 2005;24:829-838. doi: 10.7863/jum.2005.24.6.829

116. Fraser DG, Moody AR, Morgan PS, Martel AL, Davidson I. Diagnosis of lower-limb deep venous thrombosis: a prospective blinded study of magnetic resonance direct thrombus imaging. *Ann Intern Med.* 2002;136:89-98.

117. Abdalla G, Fawzi Matuk R, Venugopal V et al. The diagnostic accuracy of magnetic resonance venography in the detection of deep venous thrombosis: a systematic review and meta-analysis. *Clin Radiol.* 2015;70:858-871.

118. Wright C, Elbadawi A, Chen, YL, et al. Initiation of a pulmonary embolism response team: a quality assurance initiative in the emergency department. *J Am Coll Cardiol.* 2019;73(9_Supplement_1):1923.

119. Rivera-Lebron B, McDaniel M, Ahrar K, et al. Diagnosis, treatment and follow up of acute pulmonary embolism: consensus practice from the PERT consortium. *Clin Appl Thromb Hemost.* 2019;25:1-16. doi: 10.1177/1076029619853037

120. Aujesky D, Obrosky DS, Stone RA et al. Derivation and validation of a prognostic model for pulmonary embolism. *Am J Respir Crit Care Med.* 2005;172:1041-1046.

121. Jimenez D, Aujesky D, Moores L et al. Simplification of the pulmonary embolism severity index for prognostication in patients with acute symptomatic pulmonary embolism. *Arch Intern Med.* 2010;170:1383-1389.

122. Righini M, Roy PM, Meyer G, Verschuren F, Aujesky D, Le Gal G. The simplified pulmonary embolism severity index (PESI): validation of a clinical prognostic model for pulmonary embolism. *J Thromb Haemost.* 2011;9:2115-2117.

123. Kucher N, Rossi E, De Rosa M, Goldhaber SZ. Prognostic role of echocardiography among patients with acute pulmonary embolism and a systolic arterial pressure of 90 mm Hg or higher. *Arch Intern Med.* 2005;165:1777-1781.

124. Wu AS, Pezzullo JA, Cronan JJ, et al. CT pulmonary angiography: quantification of pulmonary embolus as a predictor of patient outcome—initial experience. *Home Radiol.* 2004;230. doi: 10.1148/radiol.2303030083

125. Sanchez O, Trinquart L, Colombet I et al. Prognostic value of right ventricular dysfunction in patients with haemodynamically stable pulmonary embolism: a systematic review. *Eur Heart J.* 2008;29:1569-1577.

126. Becattini C, Agnelli G, Germini F, Vedovati MC. Computed tomography to assess risk of death in acute pulmonary embolism: a meta-analysis. *Eur Respir J.* 2014;43:1678-1690.

127. Trujillo-Santos J, den Exter PL, Gomez V et al. Computed tomography-assessed right ventricular dysfunction and risk stratification of patients with acute nonmassive pulmonary embolism: systematic review and meta-analysis. *J Thromb Haemost.* 2013;11:1823-1832.

128. Vuilleumier N, Le Gal G, Verschuren F et al. Cardiac biomarkers for risk stratification in non-massive pulmonary embolism: a multicenter prospective study. *J Thromb Haemost.* 2009;7:391-398.

129. Klok FA, Mos IC, Huisman MV. Brain-type natriuretic peptide levels in the prediction of adverse outcome in patients with pulmonary embolism: a systematic review and meta-analysis. *Am J Respir Crit Care Med.* 2008;178:425-430.

130. Lankeit M, Jimenez D, Kostrubiec M et al. Validation of N-terminal pro-brain natriuretic peptide cut-off values for risk stratification of pulmonary embolism. *Eur Respirat J.* 2014;43:1669-1677.

131. Hakemi EU, Alyousef T, Dang G, Hakmei J, Doukky R. The prognostic value of undetectable highly sensitive cardiac troponin I in patients with acute pulmonary embolism. *Chest.* 2015;147:685-694.

132. Lankeit M, Jimenez D, Kostrubiec M et al. Predictive value of the high-sensitivity troponin T assay and the simplified Pulmonary Embolism Severity Index in hemodynamically stable patients with acute pulmonary embolism: a prospective validation study. *Circulation.* 2011;124:2716-2724.

133. Meyer G, Vicaut E, Danays T et al. Fibrinolysis for patients with intermediate-risk pulmonary embolism. *N Engl J Med.* 2014;370:1402-1411.

134. Layish DT, Tapson VF. Pharmacologic hemodynamic support in massive pulmonary embolism. *Chest.* 1997;111:218-224.

135. Weinberg A, Tapson VF, Ramzy D. Massive pulmonary embolism: Extracorporeal membrane oxygenation and surgical pulmonary embolectomy. *Semin Respir Crit Care Med.* 2017;38:66-72.

136. Raschke RA, Reilly BM, Guidry JR, Fontana JR, Srinivas S. The weight-based heparin dosing nomogram compared with a "standard care" nomogram. A randomized controlled trial. *Ann Intern Med.* 1993;119:874-881.

137. Erkens PM, Prins MH. Fixed dose subcutaneous low molecular weight heparins versus adjusted dose unfractionated heparin for venous thromboembolism. *Cochrane Database Syst Rev.* 2010:CD001100.

138. Smith SB, Geske JB, Maguire JM, et al. Early anticoagulation is associated with reduced mortality for acute pulmonary embolism. *Chest.* 2010;137(6):1382-1390. doi: 10.1378/chest.09-0959.

139. Prucnal CK, Jansson PS, Deadmon E, et al. Analysis of partial thromboplastin times in patients with pulmonary embolism during the first 48 hours of anticoagulation with unfractionated heparin. *Acad Emerg Med.* 2020;27:117-127. doi: 10.1111/acem.13872

140. Duplaga BA, Rivers CW, Nutescu E. Dosing and monitoring of low-molecular-weight heparins in special populations. *Pharmacotherapy.* 2001;21:218-234.

141. Greinacher A. Clinical Practice. Heparin-induced thrombocytopenia. *N Engl J Med*. 2015;373:252-261.

142. Kovacs MJ, Rodger M, Anderson DR et al. Comparison of 10-mg and 5-mg warfarin initiation nomograms together with low-molecular-weight heparin for outpatient treatment of acute venous thromboembolism. A randomized, double-blind, controlled trial. *Ann Intern Med*. 2003; 138:714-719.

143. Horlocker T, Vandermeulen E, Kopp S, et al. Regional anesthesia in the patient receiving antithrombotic or thrombolytic therapy: American Society of Regional Anesthesia and Pain Medicine evidence-based guidelines (fourth edition). *Regional Anesthes Pain Med*. 2018;43:263-309. doi: 10.1097/AAP.0000000000000763

144. Buller HR, Davidson BL, Decousus H et al. Subcutaneous fondaparinux versus intravenous unfractionated heparin in the initial treatment of pulmonary embolism. *N Engl J Med*. 2003;349:1695-1702.

145. Schindewolf M, Steindl J, Beyer-Westendorf J, et al. Use of fondaparinux off-label or approved anticoagulants for management of heparin-induced thrombocytopenia. *J Am Coll Cardiol*. 2017;70:2636-2648.

146. Jonas DE, McLeod HL. Genetic and clinical factors relating to warfarin dosing. *Trends Pharmacol Sci*. 2009;30:375-386.

147. Kimmel SE, French B, Kasner SE et al. A pharmacogenetic versus a clinical algorithm for warfarin dosing. *N Engl J Med*. 2013;369:2283-2293.

148. Pirmohamed M, Burnside G, Eriksson N et al. A randomized trial of genotype-guided dosing of warfarin. *N Engl J Med*. 2013;369: 2294-2303.

149. Heneghan C, Ward A, Perera R et al. Self-monitoring of oral anticoagulation: systematic review and meta-analysis of individual patient data. *Lancet*. 2012;379:322-334.

150. White RH, Beyth RJ, Zhou H, Romano PS. Major bleeding after hospitalization for deep-venous thrombosis. *Am J Med*. 1999;107:414-424.

151. Egred M, Rodrigues E. Purple digit syndrome and warfarin-induced skin necrosis. *Eur J Intern Med*. 2005;16:294-295.

152. Agnelli G, Buller HR, Cohen A et al. Oral apixaban for the treatment of acute venous thromboembolism. *N Engl J Med*. 2013;369:799-808.

153. Hokusai VTEI, Buller HR, Decousus H et al. Edoxaban versus warfarin for the treatment of symptomatic venous thromboembolism. *N Engl J Med*. 2013;369:1406-1415.

154. Investigators E, Bauersachs R, Berkowitz SD et al. Oral rivaroxaban for symptomatic venous thromboembolism. *N Engl J Med*. 2010;363:2499-2510.

155. Investigators E-P, Buller HR, Prins MH et al. Oral rivaroxaban for the treatment of symptomatic pulmonary embolism. *N Engl J Med*. 2012;366:1287-1297.

156. Schulman S, Kakkar AK, Goldhaber SZ et al. Treatment of acute venous thromboembolism with dabigatran or warfarin and pooled analysis. *Circulation*. 2014;129:764-772.

157. Schulman S, Kearon C, Kakkar AK et al. Dabigatran versus warfarin in the treatment of acute venous thromboembolism. *N Engl J Med*. 2009;361:2342-2352.

158. van der Hulle T, Kooiman J, den Exter PL, Dekkers OM, Klok FA, Huisman MV. Effectiveness and safety of novel oral anticoagulants as compared with vitamin K antagonists in the treatment of acute symptomatic venous thromboembolism: a systematic review and meta-analysis. *J Thromb Haemost*. 2014;12:320-328.

159. Pollack CV, Jr., Reilly PA, Eikelboom J et al. Idarucizumab for dabigatran reversal. *N Engl J Med*. 2015;373:511-520.

160. Lu G, DeGuzman FR, Hollenbach SJ et al. A specific antidote for reversal of anticoagulation by direct and indirect inhibitors of coagulation factor Xa. *Nat Med*. 2013;19:446-451.

161. Tran H, Joseph J, Young L, et al. New oral anticoagulants: a practical guide on prescription, laboratory testing and peri-procedural/bleeding management. *Intern Med J*. 2014;44:525-536.

162. van Es N, Coppens M, Schulman S, Middeldorp S, Buller HR. Direct oral anticoagulants compared with vitamin K antagonists for acute venous thromboembolism: evidence from phase 3 trials. *Blood*. 2014;124:1968-1975.

163. Ortel TL, Neumann I, Ageno W, et al. American Society of Hematology 2020 guidelines for management of venous thromboembolism: treatment of deep vein thrombosis and pulmonary embolism. *Blood Adv*. 2020;4:4693-4738.

164. Lee AY, Levine MN, Baker RI, et al. Low-molecular-weight heparin versus a coumarin for the prevention of recurrent venous thromboembolism in patients with cancer. *N Engl J Med*. 2003;349:146-153.

165. Young AM, Marshall A, Thirlwall J, et al. Comparison of an oral factor Xa Inhibitor with low molecular weight heparin in patients with cancer with venous thromboembolism: results of a randomized trial (SELECT-D). *J Clin Oncol*. 2018:JCO2018788034.

166. Raskob GE, van Es N, Verhamme P, et al. Edoxaban for the treatment of cancer-associated venous thromboembolism. *N Engl J Med*. 2018;378:615-624.

167. McBane RD, 2nd, Wysokinski WE, Le-Rademacher JG, et al. Apixaban and dalteparin in active malignancy-associated venous thromboembolism: the ADAM VTE trial. *J Thromb Haemost*. 2020;18:411-421.

168. Agnelli G, Becattini C, Meyer G, et al. Apixaban for the treatment of venous thromboembolism associated with cancer. *N Engl J Med*. 2020;382:1599-1607.

169. Wiggins BS, Dixon DL, Neyens RR, et a. Select drug-drug interactions with direct oral anticoagulants. *JACC*. 2020;75:1341-1350.

170. Crosby JR, Marzec U, Revenko AS et al. Antithrombotic effect of antisense factor XI oligonucleotide treatment in primates. *Arterioscl Thromb Vascular Biol*. 2013;33:1670-1678.

171. Renne T, Schmaier AH, Nickel KF, Blomback M, Maas C. In vivo roles of factor XII. *Blood*. 2012;120:4296-4303.

172. McFadyen JD, Peter K. Novel antithrombotic drugs on the horizon: the ultimate promise to prevent clotting while avoiding bleeding. *Circ Res*. 2017;121:1133-1135.

173. Goldhaber SZ, Haire WD, Feldstein ML et al. Alteplase versus heparin in acute pulmonary embolism: randomised trial assessing right-ventricular function and pulmonary perfusion. *Lancet*. 1993;341:507-511.

174. Marti C, John G, Konstantinides S et al. Systemic thrombolytic therapy for acute pulmonary embolism: a systematic review and meta-analysis. *Eur Heart J*. 2015;36:605-614.

175. Chatterjee S, Chakraborty A, Weinberg I, et al. Thrombolysis for pulmonary embolism and risk of all-cause mortality, major bleeding, and intracranial hemorrhage: a meta-analysis. *JAMA*. doi:10.1001/jama.2014.5990.

176. Sharifi M, Bay C, Skrocki L, Rahimi F, Mehdipour M, Investigators M. Moderate pulmonary embolism treated with thrombolysis (from the "MOPETT" Trial). *Am J Cardiol*. 2013;111:273-277.

177. Wang C, Zhai Z, Yang Y et al. Efficacy and safety of low dose recombinant tissue-type plasminogen activator for the treatment of acute pulmonary thromboembolism: a randomized, multicenter, controlled trial. *Chest*. 2010;137:254-262.

178. Tapson VF, Gurbel PA and Stack RS. Pharmacomechanical thrombolysis of experimental pulmonary emboli: rapid low-dose intraembolic therapy. *Chest*. 1994;106:1558-1562.

179. Engelberger RP, Kucher N. Catheter-based reperfusion treatment of pulmonary embolism. *Circulation*. 2011;124:2139-2144.

180. Kuo WT, Banerjee A, Kim PS et al. Pulmonary Embolism Response to Fragmentation, Embolectomy, and Catheter Thrombolysis (PERFECT): initial results from a prospective multicenter registry. *Chest*. 2015;148:667-673.

181. Kucher N, Boekstegers P, Muller OJ et al. Randomized, controlled trial of ultrasound-assisted catheter-directed thrombolysis for acute intermediate-risk pulmonary embolism. *Circulation*. 2014;129:479-486.

182. Piazza G, Hohlfelder B, Jaff MR et al. A prospective, single-arm, multicenter trial of ultrasound-facilitated, catheter-directed, low-dose fibrinolysis for acute massive and submassive pulmonary embolism: The SEATTLE II Study. *JACC Cardiovasc Interv*. 2015;8:1382-1392.

183. Tapson VF, Sterling K, Jones N, et al. The OPTALYSE PE Trial. A randomized trial of the optimum duration of acoustic pulse thrombolysis procedure in acute intermediate-risk pulmonary embolism. *JACC: Cardiovasc Intervent.* 2018:11;1401-1410.

184. Tu, T, Toma C, Tapson VF, et al, and the FLARE Investigators. A prospective, single-arm, multicenter trial of catheter-directed mechanical thrombectomy for intermediate-risk acute pulmonary embolism. The FLARE Study. *JACC: Cardiovasc Intervent.* 2019;12. http://creativecommons.org/licenses/by-nc-nd/4.0

185. Weinberg AS, Dohad S, Ramzy D, Madyoon H, Tapson VF. Clot extraction with the FlowTriever device in acute massive pulmonary embolism. *J Intensive Care Med.* 2016;31;676-679.

186. Rajput FA, Du L, Woods M, Jacobson K. Percutaneous vacuum-assisted thrombectomy using angiovac aspiration system. *Cardiovasc Revasc Med.* 2020;21(4):489-493. doi: 10.1016/j.carrev.2019.12.020.

187. Aymard T, Kadner A, Widmer A et al. Massive pulmonary embolism: surgical embolectomy versus thrombolytic therapy–should surgical indications be revisited? *Eur J Cardiothor Surg.* 2013;43:90-94; discussion 94.

188. Fukuda I, Taniguchi S, Fukui K, Minakawa M, Daitoku K, Suzuki Y. Improved outcome of surgical pulmonary embolectomy by aggressive intervention for critically ill patients. *Ann Thorac Surg.* 2011;91:728-732.

189. Muriel A, Jimenez D, Aujesky D et al. Survival effects of inferior vena cava filter in patients with acute symptomatic venous thromboembolism and a significant bleeding risk. *J Am Coll Cardiol.* 2014;63:1675-1683.

190. Rajasekhar A, Streiff MB. Vena cava filters for management of venous thromboembolism: a clinical review. *Blood Rev.* 2013;27:225-241.

191. Jia Z, Wu A, Tam M, Spain J, McKinney JM, Wang W. Caval penetration by inferior vena cava filters: a systematic literature review of clinical significance and management. *Circulation.* 2015;132:944-952.

192. Isogai T, Yasunaga H, Matsui H, Tanaka H, Horiguchi H, Fushimi K. Effectiveness of inferior vena cava filters on mortality as an adjuvant to antithrombotic therapy. *Am J Med.* 2015;128:312.e23-e31.

193. Stein PD, Matta F, Keyes DC, Willyerd GL. Impact of vena cava filters on in-hospital case fatality rate from pulmonary embolism. *Am J Med.* 2012;125:478-484.

194. Mismetti P, Laporte S, Pellerin O, et al. Effect of a retrievable inferior vena cava filter plus anticoagulation vs anticoagulation alone on risk of recurrent pulmonary embolism: a randomized clinical trial. *JAMA.* 2015;313:1627-1635.

195. Kim NH, Delcroix M, Jenkins DP et al. Chronic thromboembolic pulmonary hypertension. *J Am Coll Cardiol.* 2013;62:D92-D99.

196. Kim NH, Lang IM. Risk factors for chronic thromboembolic pulmonary hypertension. *Eur Respir Rev.* 2012;21:27-31.

197. Lang IM, Pesavento R, Bonderman D, Yuan JX. Risk factors and basic mechanisms of chronic thromboembolic pulmonary hypertension: a current understanding. *Eur Respir J.* 2013;41:462-468.

198. Pepke-Zaba J, Delcroix M, Lang I et al. Chronic thromboembolic pulmonary hypertension (CTEPH): results from an international prospective registry. *Circulation.* 2011;124:1973-1981.

199. Heinrich M, Uder M, Tscholl D, Grgic A, Kramann B, Schafers HJ. CT scan findings in chronic thromboembolic pulmonary hypertension: predictors of hemodynamic improvement after pulmonary thromboendarterectomy. *Chest.* 2005;127:1606-1613.

200. Andreassen AK, Ragnarsson A, Gude E, Geiran O, Andersen R. Balloon pulmonary angioplasty in patients with inoperable chronic thromboembolic pulmonary hypertension. *Heart.* 2013;99:1415-1420.

201. Inami T, Kataoka M, Shimura N et al. Pulmonary edema predictive scoring index (PEPSI), a new index to predict risk of reperfusion pulmonary edema and improvement of hemodynamics in percutaneous transluminal pulmonary angioplasty. *JACC Cardiovasc Interv.* 2013;6:725-736.

202. Mizoguchi H, Ogawa A, Munemasa M, Mikouchi H, Ito H, Matsubara H. Refined balloon pulmonary angioplasty for inoperable patients with chronic thromboembolic pulmonary hypertension. *Circulation Cardiovasc Intervent.* 2012;5:748-755.

203. Pepke-Zaba J, Jansa P, Kim NH, Naeije R, Simonneau G. Chronic thromboembolic pulmonary hypertension: role of medical therapy. *The Eur Respir J.* 2013;41:985-90.

204. Ghofrani HA, D'Armini AM, Grimminger F et al. Riociguat for the treatment of chronic thromboembolic pulmonary hypertension. *New Engl J Med.* 2013;369:319-329.

205. Falck-Ytter Y, Francis CW, Johanson NA et al. Prevention of VTE in orthopedic surgery patients: Antithrombotic Therapy and Prevention of Thrombosis, 9th ed: American College of Chest Physicians Evidence-Based Clinical Practice Guidelines. *Chest.* 2012;141:e278S-325S.

206. Kearon C, Akl EA, Ornelas J, et al. Antithrombotic therapy for VTE disease. CHEST guideline and expert panel report. *Chest.* 2016;149(2): 315-352.

207. Gould MK, Garcia DA, Wren SM et al. Prevention of VTE in nonorthopedic surgical patients: Antithrombotic Therapy and Prevention of Thrombosis, 9th ed: American College of Chest Physicians Evidence-Based Clinical Practice Guidelines. *Chest.* 2012;141:e227S-e277S.

208. Kahn SR, Lim W, Dunn AS et al. Prevention of VTE in nonsurgical patients: Antithrombotic Therapy and Prevention of Thrombosis, 9th ed: American College of Chest Physicians Evidence-Based Clinical Practice Guidelines. *Chest.* 2012;141:e195S-e226S.

209. Leonardi MJ, McGory ML, Ko CY. The rate of bleeding complications after pharmacologic deep venous thrombosis prophylaxis: a systematic review of 33 randomized controlled trials. *Arch Surg.* 2006;141:790-797; discussion 797-799.

210. Spyropoulos AC, Ageno W, Cohen AT, et al. Prevention of venous thromboembolism in hospitalized medically ill patients: a U.S. perspective. *Thromb Haemost.* 2020;120(6):924-936. doi: 10.1055/s-0040-1710326

211. Carrier M, Abou-Nassar K, Mallick R, et al. Apixaban to prevent venous thromboembolism in patients with cancer. *N Engl J Med.* 380:711-719. doi: 10.1056/NEJMoa1814468

212. Horlander KT, Mannino DM, Leeper KV. Pulmonary embolism mortality in the United States, 1979-1998: an analysis using multiple-cause mortality data. *Arch Intern Med.* 2003;163:1711-1717.

213. Adam SS, McDuffie JR, Lachiewicz PF, Ortel TL, Williams JW, Jr. Comparative effectiveness of new oral anticoagulants and standard thromboprophylaxis in patients having total hip or knee replacement: a systematic review. *Ann Intern Med.* 2013;159:275-284.

214. Squizzato A, Donadini MP, Galli L, Dentali F, Aujesky D, Ageno W. Prognostic clinical prediction rules to identify a low-risk pulmonary embolism: a systematic review and meta-analysis. *J Thromb Haemost.* 2012;10:1276-1290.

215. Agterof MJ, Schutgens RE, Snijder RJ et al. Out of hospital treatment of acute pulmonary embolism in patients with a low NT-proBNP level. *J Thromb Haemost.* 2010;8:1235-1241.

216. Aujesky D, Roy PM, Verschuren F et al. Outpatient versus inpatient treatment for patients with acute pulmonary embolism: an international, open-label, randomised, noninferiority trial. *Lancet.* 2011;378:41-48.

217. Tapson VF, Huisman M. Early discharge for acute pulmonary embolism. Home at last? *Eur Respir J.* 2007;30:613-615.

218. Otero R, Uresandi F, Jimenez D et al. Home treatment in pulmonary embolism. *Thromb Res.* 2010;126:e1-e5.

219. Zondag W, Mos IC, Creemers-Schild D et al. Outpatient treatment in patients with acute pulmonary embolism: the Hestia Study. *J Thromb Haemost.* 2011;9:1500-1507.

220. Zondag W, Kooiman J, Klok FA, Dekkers OM, Huisman MV. Outpatient versus inpatient treatment in patients with pulmonary embolism: a meta-analysis. *Eur Respir J.* 2013;42:134-144.

221. Yoo HH, Queluz TH, El Dib R. Outpatient versus inpatient treatment for acute pulmonary embolism. *Cochrane Database Syst Rev.* 2014;11:CD010019.

222. Dentali F, Di Micco G, Giorgi Pierfranceschi M et al. Rate and duration of hospitalization for deep vein thrombosis and pulmonary embolism in real-world clinical practice. *Annals Med.* 2015;47:546-554.

223. Agnelli G, Becattini C. Treatment of DVT: how long is enough and how do you predict recurrence. *J Thromb Thrombolysis*. 2008;25:37-44.

224. Murin S, Romano PS, White RH. Comparison of outcomes after hospitalization for deep venous thrombosis or pulmonary embolism. *Thromb Haemost*. 2002;88:407-414.

225. Douketis JD, Gu CS, Schulman S, Ghirarduzzi A, Pengo V, Prandoni P. The risk for fatal pulmonary embolism after discontinuing anticoagulant therapy for venous thromboembolism. *Ann Intern Med*. 2007;147:766-774.

226. Schulman S, Rhedin AS, Lindmarker P et al. A comparison of six weeks with six months of oral anticoagulant therapy after a first episode of venous thromboembolism. Duration of Anticoagulation Trial Study Group. *N Engl J Med*. 1995;332:1661-1665.

227. Palareti G, Cosmi B, Legnani C et al. D-dimer to guide the duration of anticoagulation in patients with venous thromboembolism: a management study. *Blood*. 2014;124:196-203.

228. Eichinger S, Heinze G, Jandeck LM, Kyrle PA. Risk assessment of recurrence in patients with unprovoked deep vein thrombosis or pulmonary embolism: the Vienna prediction model. *Circulation*. 2010;121:1630-1636.

229. Rodger MA, Kahn SR, Wells PS et al. Identifying unprovoked thromboembolism patients at low risk for recurrence who can discontinue anticoagulant therapy. *Canadian Medical Association J*. 2008;179:417-426.

230. Tosetto A, Iorio A, Marcucci M et al. Predicting disease recurrence in patients with previous unprovoked venous thromboembolism: a proposed prediction score (DASH). *J Thromb Haemost*. 2012;10:1019-1025.

231. Kearon C, Spencer FA, O'Keeffe D et al. D-dimer testing to select patients with a first unprovoked venous thromboembolism who can stop anticoagulant therapy: a cohort study. *Ann Intern Med*. 2015;162:27-34.

232. Agnelli G, Buller HR, Cohen A et al. Apixaban for extended treatment of venous thromboembolism. *New Engl J Med*. 2013;368:699-708.

233. Weitz JI, Lensing AWA, Prins MH, et al. Rivaroxaban or aspirin for extended treatment of venous thromboembolism. *N Engl J Med*. 2017;376:1211-1222.

234. Vasanthamohan L, Boonyawat K, Chai-Adisaksopha C, Crowther M. Reduced-dose direct oral anticoagulants in the extended treatment of venous thromboembolism: a systematic review and meta-analysis. *J Thromb Haemost*. 2018;16:1288-1295.

235. Stein PD, Goodman LR, Hull RD, Dalen JE, Matta F. Diagnosis and management of isolated subsegmental pulmonary embolism: review and assessment of the options. *Clin Appl Thrombosis/Hemost*. 2012;18:20-26.

236. den Exter PL, van Es J, Klok FA et al. Risk profile and clinical outcome of symptomatic subsegmental acute pulmonary embolism. *Blood*. 2013;122:1144-1149; quiz 1329.

237. Horner D, Hogg K, Body R. Should we be looking for and treating isolated calf vein thrombosis? *Emerg Med J*. 2015;33(6):

238. Fallouh N, McGuirk HM, Flanders SA, Chopra V. Peripherally inserted central catheter-associated deep vein thrombosis: a narrative review. *Am J Med*. 2015;128:722-738.

239. Bates SM, Greer IA, Middeldorp S et al. VTE, thrombophilia, antithrombotic therapy, and pregnancy: Antithrombotic Therapy and Prevention of Thrombosis, 9th ed: American College of Chest Physicians Evidence-Based Clinical Practice Guidelines. *Chest*. 2012;141:e691S-736S.

240. European Society of G, Association for European Paediatric C, German Society for Gender M et al. ESC Guidelines on the management of cardiovascular diseases during pregnancy: the Task Force on the Management of Cardiovascular Diseases during Pregnancy of the European Society of Cardiology (ESC). *Eur Heart J*. 2011;32:3147-3197.

241. Chan WS, Chunilal S, Lee A, Crowther M, Rodger M, Ginsberg JS. A red blood cell agglutination D-dimer test to exclude deep venous thrombosis in pregnancy. *Ann Intern Med*. 2007;147:165-170.

242. Hurwitz LM, Yoshizumi T, Reiman RE et al. Radiation dose to the fetus from body MDCT during early gestation. *AJR Am J Roentgenol*. 2006;186:871-876.

243. Ratnapalan S, Bentur Y, Koren G. Doctor, will that x-ray harm my unborn child? *CMAJ*. 2008;179:1293-1296, 2008.

244. Doll R, Wakeford R: Risk of childhood cancer from fetal irradiation. *Br Radiol*. 1997;70:130-139.

245. Romualdi E, Dentali F, Rancan E et al. Anticoagulant therapy for venous thromboembolism during pregnancy: a systematic review and a meta-analysis of the literature. *J Thromb Haemost*. 2013;11:270-281.

246. Bates SM. Pulmonary embolism in pregnancy. *Semin Respir Crit Care Med*. 2021;42(2):284-298.

247. Palumbo A, Cavo M, Bringhen S et al. Aspirin, warfarin, or enoxaparin thromboprophylaxis in patients with multiple myeloma treated with thalidomide: a phase III, open-label, randomized trial. *J Clin Oncol*. 2011;29:986-993.

248. Louzada ML, Carrier M, Lazo-Langner A et al. Development of a clinical prediction rule for risk stratification of recurrent venous thromboembolism in patients with cancer-associated venous thromboembolism. *Circulation*. 2012;126:448-454.

249. Trujillo-Santos J, Nieto JA, Tiberio G et al. Predicting recurrences or major bleeding in cancer patients with venous thromboembolism. Findings from the RIETE Registry. *Thromb Haemost*. 2008;100:435-439.

250. Carrier M, Cameron C, Delluc A, Castellucci L, Khorana AA, Lee AY. Efficacy and safety of anticoagulant therapy for the treatment of acute cancer-associated thrombosis: a systematic review and meta-analysis. *Thromb Res*. 2014;134:1214-1219.

251. Carrier M, Lazo-Langner A, Shivakumar S et al. Screening for occult cancer in unprovoked venous thromboembolism. *N Engl J Med*. 2015;373:697-704.

252. Bunce PE, High SM, Nadjafi M, et al. Pandemic H1N1 influenza infection and vascular thrombosis. *Clin Infect Dis*. 2011;52:e14-e17.

253. Chong PY, Chui P, Ling AE et al. Analysis of deaths during the severe acute respiratory syndrome (SARS) epidemic in Singapore: challenges in determining a SARS diagnosis. *Arch Pathol Lab Med*. 2004;128:195-204.

254. Tritschler T, Mathieu M-E, Skeith L, et al. Anticoagulant interventions in hospitalized patients with COVID-19: a scoping review of randomized controlled trials and call for international collaboration. *J Thrombos Haemost*. 2020;18:2958-2967. doi: 10.1111/jth.15094

Cor Pulmonale: The Heart in Structural Lung Disease

Lewis J. Rubin

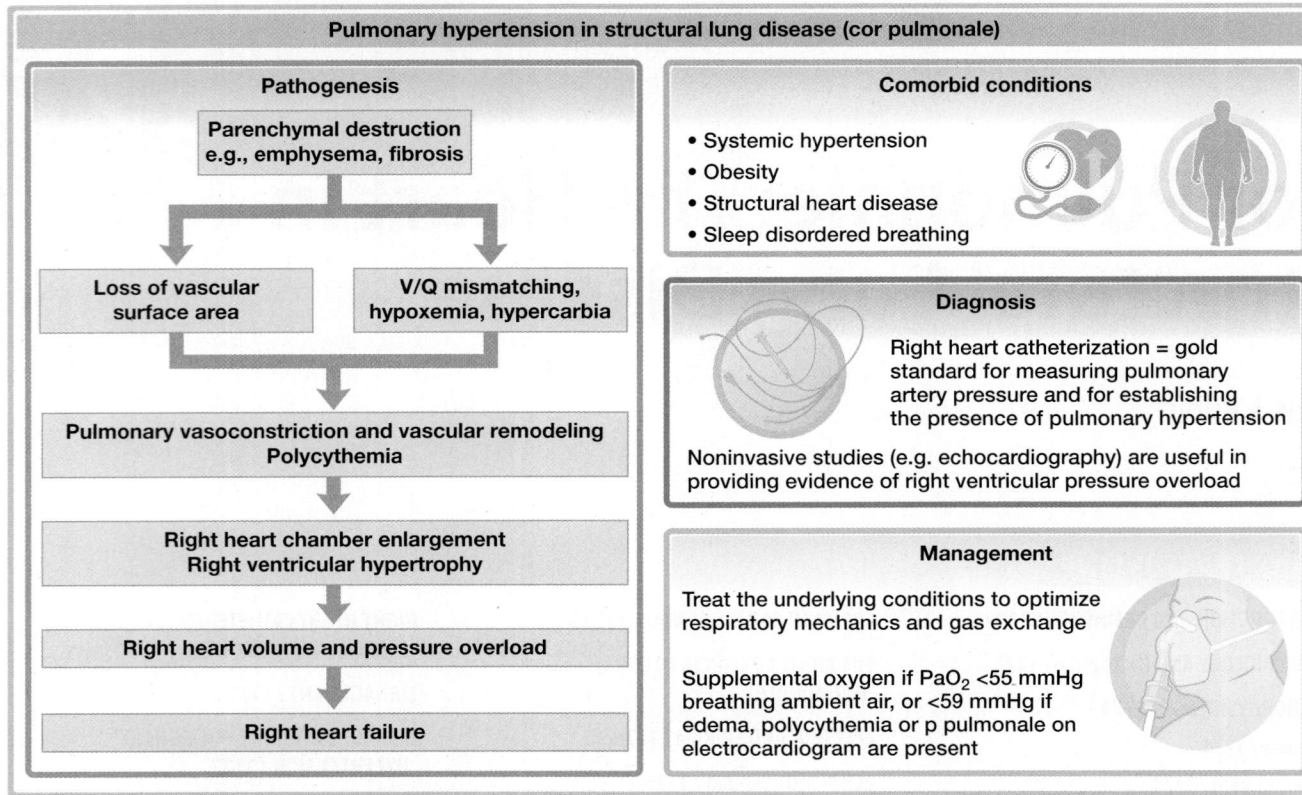

Chapter 59 Fuster and Hurst's Central Illustration. Airway obstruction, lung fibrosis with restriction, or a combination of both factors cause a loss of pulmonary vascular surface area and impairment in intrapulmonary gas exchange, leading to hypoxemia with or without hypercarbia, which are potent stimuli for pulmonary vasoconstriction and vascular remodeling. Polycythemia with increased blood viscosity, resulting from hypoxia-induced increased red blood cell production, may further increase pulmonary vascular resistance. The resultant elevations in pulmonary artery pressure lead to right ventricular pressure and volume overload. Definitive diagnosis requires direct measurement of pulmonary hemodynamics. The mainstay of management is to optimize respiratory mechanics and gas exchange by treating the underlying conditions.

CHAPTER SUMMARY

This chapter addresses the pathogenesis, pathophysiology, and management of pulmonary hypertension (PH) in the setting of structural lung disease, commonly referred to as cor pulmonale. Airway obstruction, lung fibrosis with restriction, or a combination of both factors causes a loss of pulmonary vascular surface area and impairment in intrapulmonary gas exchange, leading to hypoxemia with or without hypercarbia, which are potent stimuli for pulmonary vasoconstriction and vascular remodeling. Polycythemia with increased blood viscosity, resulting from hypoxia-induced increased red blood cell production, may further increase pulmonary vascular resistance. The subsequent elevations in pulmonary artery pressure result in right ventricular pressure and volume overload that may ultimately lead to right heart failure and death (see Fuster and Hurst's Central Figure). The presence of cor pulmonale may be inferred from echocardiographic signs of right ventricular enlargement and hypertrophy, along with measurement of an increased tricuspid regurgitant jet velocity, but the definitive diagnosis requires the direct measurement of pulmonary hemodynamics. Management of cor pulmonale is primarily directed at optimizing lung function and gas exchange with conventional medical therapies (ie, bronchodilators, corticosteroids, and other anti-inflammatory agents), minimizing hypoxemia with supplemental oxygen, and identifying and treating comorbid conditions. The role of pulmonary arterial hypertension–targeted therapies in cor pulmonale is controversial and can result in worsening V/Q mismatching and clinical deterioration.

INTRODUCTION AND DEFINITIONS

The term *cor pulmonale* was coined by Paul Dudley White nearly a century ago and has long been used as a surrogate for right ventricular failure.[1] The development of sophisticated invasive and noninvasive techniques has facilitated the study of right heart and pulmonary circulatory structure and function, yielding a greater understanding of the unique properties of the cardiopulmonary circuit in normal and disease states.

The normal mean pulmonary artery pressure is less than 20 mm Hg at rest.[2] The pulmonary circulation is a high-flow, low-resistance system capable of accepting the entire cardiac output at a pressure one-fifth that of the systemic circulation. Even with maximal exercise, when pulmonary blood flow may increase 5-fold, pulmonary artery pressure changes little, owing to pulmonary vasodilation and recruitment of unused vasculature. This remarkable capacity of the pulmonary circulation to adapt is further demonstrated by the fact that the loss of 50% of the vascular surface area, for example due to pneumonectomy or widespread parenchymal destruction in the setting of advanced lung disease, results in little change in resting pulmonary artery pressures. Pulmonary hypertension (PH), defined as a mean pulmonary artery pressure greater than 25 mm Hg at rest measured by right heart catheterization,[2] may be due to a variety of conditions, as summarized in **Table 59–1**.

In his state-of-the art review, Fishman defined cor pulmonale as "a synonym for pulmonary heart disease … used to signify right ventricular enlargement from disorders that affect either the structure or function of the lungs."[3] He defined the elements of cor pulmonale as (1) the etiology of the heart disease may be either intrinsic pulmonary disease, including abnormalities in the pulmonary vessels, or inadequate function of the chest bellows or inadequate ventilatory drive from the respiratory centers; (2) the cardiomegaly is confined predominantly, if not exclusively, to the right ventricle and may take the form of dilatation, hypertrophy, or both; (3) pulmonary arterial hypertension (PAH) is the sine qua non, and whether dilatation or hypertrophy contributes more depends on the degree and duration of the PH; and (4) neither congenital heart disease nor acquired disease of the left side of the heart can be implicated as initiating mechanisms for the PAH. Using the current World Health Organization classification of PH,[2] conditions associated with cor pulmonale would include some, but not all, of those conditions under the headings of Groups 1 (Pulmonary Artery Hypertension [PAH]), 3 (Pulmonary Hypertension Resulting from Chronic Respiratory Disease and/or Hypoxia), 4 (Chronic Thromboembolic Pulmonary Hypertension [CTEPH]), and 5 (Miscellaneous Causes). Excluded would be Group 2, in which PH is the result of left-sided heart disease, and congenital heart disease (listed under Group 1).

EPIDEMIOLOGY AND INCIDENCE

Chronic cor pulmonale occurs in the setting of advanced structural or functional lung diseases (**Table 59–2**). Examples of the former include chronic obstructive lung disease (COPD) such

TABLE 59–1. Updated Clinical Classification of Pulmonary Hypertension (PH)

1 PAH
1.1 Idiopathic PAH
1.2 Heritable PAH
1.3 Drug- and toxin-induced PAH
1.4 PAH associated with:
    1.4.1 Connective tissue disease
    1.4.2 HIV infection
    1.4.3 Portal hypertension
    1.4.4 Congenital heart disease
    1.4.5 Schistosomiasis
1.5 PAH long-term responders to calcium channel blockers
1.6 PAH with overt features of venous/capillaries (PVOD/PCH) involvement
1.7 Persistent PH of the newborn syndrome
2 PH due to left heart disease
2.1 PH due to heart failure with preserved LVEF
2.2 PH due to heart failure with reduced LVEF
2.3 Valvular heart disease
2.4 Congenital/acquired cardiovascular conditions leading to post capillary PH
3 PH due to lung diseases and/or hypoxia
    3.1 Obstructive lung disease
3.2 Restrictive lung disease
3.3 Other lung disease with mixed restrictive/obstructive pattern
3.4 Hypoxia without lung disease
3.5 Developmental lung disorders
4 PH due to pulmonary artery obstructions
4.1 Chronic thromboembolic PH
4.2 Other pulmonary artery obstructions
5 PH with unclear and/or multifactorial mechanisms
5.1 Hematological disorders
5.2 Systemic and metabolic disorders
5.3 Others
5.4 Complex congenital heart disease

Reproduced with permission from Simonneau G, Montani D, Celermajer DS, et al. Haemodynamic definitions and updated clinical classification of pulmonary hypertension. *Eur Respir J.* 2019 Jan 24;53(1):1801913.

as chronic bronchitis, bronchiolitis, or emphysema; fibrotic lung diseases; and mixed obstructive and restrictive lung diseases such as cystic fibrosis and combined pulmonary fibrosis and emphysema (CPFE). Examples of functional lung diseases than can cause cor pulmonale include hypoventilation syndromes such as sleep disordered breathing, and neuromuscular and mechanical disorders (eg, kyphoscoliosis).

Smoking remains widespread, particularly in less developed parts of the world, and is the most common cause of COPD, which is the most common form of lung disease associated with cor pulmonale.[4] Smoking may cause pulmonary vascular disease even in the absence of severe structural or functional lung disease, and it has been suggested that smoke-induced pulmonary endothelial injury may be the cause. Other risk factors for COPD, including outdoor, indoor, and occupational air pollution, account for approximately 20% of moderate or severe COPD. Burning of wood or other biofuels is a common cause of COPD in undeveloped regions. COPD is among the five leading causes of death worldwide.[5]

The true prevalence of cor pulmonale is unknown, owing to underdiagnosis of advanced lung diseases and the infrequency

TABLE 59-2. Respiratory Diseases Associated with Pulmonary Hypertension

Obstructive lung diseases
Chronic obstructive pulmonary disease (chronic bronchitis, emphysema)
Asthma (with irreversible airway obstruction)
Cystic fibrosis
Bronchiectasis
Bronchiolitis obliterans

Restrictive lung diseases
Neuromuscular diseases
Kyphoscoliosis
Sequelae of pulmonary tuberculosis
Sarcoïdosis
Pneumoconiosis
Drug related lung diseases
Extrinsic allergic alveolitis
Connective tissue diseases
Idiopathic interstitial pulmonary fibrosis
Interstitial pulmonary fibrosis of known origin
Combined pulmonary fibrosis and emphysema

Mixed obstructive and restrictive diseases
Chronic pulmonary fibrosis and emphysema (CPFE)

Respiratory insufficiency of "central" origin
Central alveolar hypoventilation
Obesity-hypoventilation syndrome
Sleep apnea syndrome

of definitive, invasive testing such as right heart catheterization in this population. In studies of candidates for lung transplantation for advanced pulmonary diseases, approximately 30% to 50% had some degree of PH, which is typically mild.[6-8] In a large hemodynamic study of nearly 1000 COPD patients, the prevalence of cor pulmonale was estimated to be ~1%; the highest prevalence was correlated with the severity of lung disease assessed by an FEV_1 <50%, PaO_2 <55 mm Hg, and a low DLCO (diffusing capacity for carbon monoxide). Of patients with Global Initiative for Chronic Lung Disease (GOLD) stage IV disease, up to 5% have moderate PH, with a mean pulmonary artery pressure >35 mm Hg.[9,10]

PATHOPHYSIOLOGY

A variety of mechanisms contribute to the increased pulmonary artery pressure and pulmonary vascular resistance (PVR) in cor pulmonale (**Fig. 59–1; Table 59–3**). These include (1) loss of cross-sectional vascular surface area due to destruction of lung parenchyma, as in emphysema and fibrotic lung disease; (2) alveolar hypoxia, a potent pulmonary vasoconstrictor that normally facilitates ventilation-perfusion matching by diverting blood flow away from poorly ventilated lung units to well ventilated ones. Chronic hypoxia also induces vascular remodeling; (3) inflammation; and (4) endothelial dysfunction.[11]

Hypoxia

Alveolar hypoxia was first demonstrated to be a potent constrictor of pulmonary arteries by von Euler and Liljestrand in the 1940s and is considered a major element of PH in chronic lung diseases.[3,11-12] While acute hypoxia produces constriction of the small, muscular pulmonary arteries (50–100 μm in diameter), chronic hypoxia produces pulmonary vascular stiffness and remodeling, albeit less severe than that observed in idiopathic pulmonary artery hypertension, connective tissue diseases, and Eisenmenger's syndrome, among others. Hypercapnia, which frequently accompanies hypoxia in severe COPD and hypoventilation syndromes, potentiates hypoxic vasoconstriction.

Inflammation

Changes in the structure and function of pulmonary arteries has been demonstrated in smokers and patients with even mild COPD.[13] The severity of vascular remodeling correlates with the degree of inflammation and is characterized by intimal thickening, smooth muscle cell migration and proliferation, and increased extracellular matrix. The inflammatory response in COPD is largely the result of activated lymphocytes and correlates with the extent of airflow obstruction, but even smokers with preserved lung function have increased $CD8^+$ T cells residing within the pulmonary arterial walls.[13]

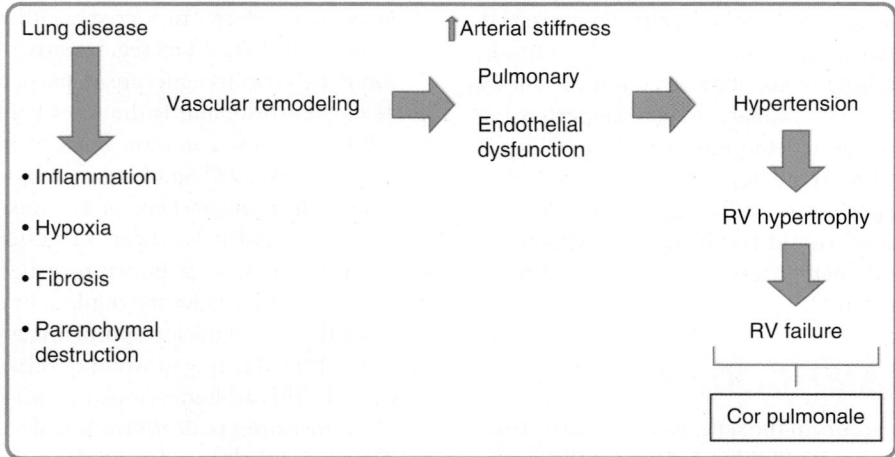

Figure 59–1. The pathophysiology of cor pulmonale. Abbreviation: RV, right ventricular.

TABLE 59–3. Factors Contributing to Increased Pulmonary Vascular Resistance in Chronic Respiratory Diseases

- Reduction in the cross-sectional surface area of the pulmonary vascular bed due to destruction/obliteration (eg, fibrosis or emphysema).
- Thromboembolism
- Functional factors:
  - Acute and chronic alveolar hypoxia (vasoconstriction and remodeling of the pulmonary vascular bed)
  - Acidosis, hypercapnia
  - Hyperviscosity (polycythemia)
  - Hypervolemia
- Mechanical factors

Endothelial Dysfunction

The pulmonary vascular endothelium produces a number of substances that contribute to control of vasomotor tone in both the pulmonary and systemic circulations. These include nitric oxide, prostacyclin, and endothelin, which predominantly affect pulmonary vasomotor tone and proliferation, and angiotensin-converting enzyme, which is an important systemic vascular regulator. In the setting of intimal thickening and proliferation, an imbalance in these local mediators results in a milieu promoting pulmonary vasculopathy. These include reduced nitric oxide and prostacyclin production (potent pulmonary vasodilators and antiproliferative substances) and increased endothelin production (a pulmonary vasoconstrictor and promotor of vascular remodeling). Pulmonary endothelial dysfunction has been observed in patients with mild-to-moderate COPD.[14]

CLINICAL MANIFESTATIONS

The clinical manifestations of chronic cor pulmonale are generally nonspecific and are overshadowed by the signs and symptoms of underlying severe chronic lung disease. Similarly, in acute cor pulmonale, which occurs in the setting of exacerbations of chronic lung disease or massive pulmonary thromboembolism, the clinical features of the underlying lung disorder predominate (severe dyspnea, productive or nonproductive cough, cyanosis, labored breathing).

Physical findings may include jugular venous distention with a prominent *v* wave indicative of tricuspid regurgitation, right ventricular heave, and an accentuated P_2. As the degree of pulmonary disease and PH progresses, a murmur of pulmonic regurgitation (Graham Steell murmur) may be audible. Late in the course of illness as overt right heart failure ensues, signs of right ventricular volume overload, such as hepatomegaly, ascites, and edema may occur.

EDEMA IN COR PULMONALE

Lower extremity edema is frequently observed in patients with moderate or severe COPD. Since cardiac output is well maintained in cor pulmonale until very late in the course of the disease,[11] edema formation is not explained by pump dysfunction as occurs in classic congestive heart failure. Several physiologic alterations, both renal and extra renal, have been proposed to explain this phenomenon:[15]

1. Effective renal plasma flow is reduced in chronic respiratory failure, resulting in reduced renal urinary sodium excretion. Additionally, hypercapnia, which is an almost universal feature of chronic respiratory failure with edema, leads to glomerular sodium reabsorption as the kidneys compensate for the chronic respiratory acidosis by increased reabsorption of bicarbonate and urinary elimination of hydrogen ions.

2. While cardiac output may be preserved, systemic oxygen tissue delivery may be impaired owing to the pumping of poorly oxygenated arterial blood. This may cause some degree of altered cellular metabolism in the kidney as well as other organs, resulting in impaired salt and water handling. Intracellular acidosis, resulting from increased intracellular hydrogen ion concentrations to buffer chronic respiratory acidosis, would augment dysfunction of intracellular processes.

THE RIGHT VENTRICLE IN COR PULMONALE

Cournand and colleagues first characterized several clinical phenotypes of cor pulmonale, particularly focusing on acute and chronic cor pulmonale resulting from chronic lung disease.[16,17] They showed that the clinical features of acute cor pulmonale, typically the result of acute exacerbations of chronic lung disease, may be reversible with time and general treatment measures for the underlying cause. They also noted that, while left-sided heart failure is associated with a reduced cardiac output, cor pulmonale is characterized by a normal or even increased cardiac output, owing to the increased myocardial fiber stretch resulting from increased intravascular volume. Only late in the course of chronic cor pulmonale does overt right heart failure with decreased cardiac output ensue. The COPD cohort in the Multi-Ethnic Study of Atherosclerosis (MESA), which was heavily represented by those with emphysema ("pink puffer"), had lower resting right ventricular end diastolic volumes and similar right ventricular mass compared with controls,[18] likely indicative of decreased venous return due to lung hyperinflation. In contrast, the "blue bloater" phenotype, characterized by chronic airways disease with hypoxemia and hypercapnia, is more likely to have more overt pulmonary vascular disease. Recent studies have emphasized the importance of right ventricular stiffness, increased afterload, ventriculo-arterial uncoupling, and right ventricular dyssynchrony as the key features of right heart failure due to advanced pulmonary artery hypertension.[19-26] The latter mechanism is also thought to contribute to altered left ventricular systolic and diastolic function due to ventricular interdependence that occurs in the setting of right ventricular pressure overload.[26]

At the cellular level, fatty deposits have been found in the right ventricular myocardium of patients with right ventricular pressure overload,[27] although their meaningfulness is unknown, since even a "failing" right ventricle can return to normal function if afterload is normalized, such as after lung transplantation for PH or pulmonary endarterectomy for CTEPH. Studies using uptake of radiolabeled fluorodeoxyglucose (FDG) as an index of efficiency of myocardial metabolism have shown impaired uptake in the right ventricular myocardium of patients with PH.[28] Thus, therapies that target the imbalance between energy substrate supply and demand or efficiency of substrate utilization may be novel approaches to the treatment of conditions associated with right ventricular pressure overload.

ELECTROCARDIOGRAM

Electrocardiographic findings in cor pulmonale include evidence of right axis deviation, right ventricular hypertrophy and strain, and P pulmonale due to right atrial hypertrophy and dilation. Supraventricular tachycardias (atrial flutter and fibrillation and multifocal atrial tachycardia), along with premature atrial and ventricular contractions occur commonly, particularly during acute exacerbations, when worsening hypoxemia and hypercapnia may occur.[29]

ECHOCARDIOGRAM

Owing to the anterior location of the right ventricle, echocardiography is useful for the noninvasive assessment of right heart structure and function. However, the assessment of right ventricular function differs from assessment of left ventricular function as a result of the complex crescent-like shape of the right ventricle, different fiber orientation, and contraction (the septum normally moves with the left ventricle but moves "paradoxically" with the right ventricle with severe right ventricular pressure overload). The salient features on transthoracic echocardiography include right ventricular enlargement and hypertrophy, increased tricuspid regurgitant velocity indicative of an increased pressure gradient between the right ventricle and atrium, increased right ventricular/left ventricular ratio and eccentricity index, and increased tricuspid annular plane systolic excursion (TAPSE). TAPSE reflects the longitudinal myocardial shortening of the right ventricle and reflects right ventricular function. TAPSE is assessed with M-mode in the apical four-chamber view, with a normal value being at least 16 mm and severe RV dysfunction is present when TAPSE is less than 10 mm.

While right heart catheterization remains the gold standard for measuring pulmonary artery pressure and for establishing the presence of PH, noninvasive studies such as echocardiography are useful in providing evidence of right ventricular pressure overload. When tricuspid regurgitation is present, as in almost all patients with PH, the pressure gradient between the two right heart chambers can be estimated by measuring the peak tricuspid regurgitation velocity by Doppler and adding the estimated right atrial pressure, which can be obtained by physical examination of the jugular venous pressure or by echocardiographic-based parameters. While this approach has become widely used to estimate pulmonary artery pressures noninvasively,[30] a wide range of correlations with directly measured pressures have been reported.[8,31] Accordingly, rather than taking the estimated pressure by echocardiogram as the sole determinant of the presence or degree of elevated pulmonary

artery pressure, a complete assessment including right ventricular size, thickness, eccentricity, septal motion, TAPSE, and tricuspid regurgitant velocity will provide a more accurate picture of the state of the right heart. In the absence of technical limitations to echocardiographic imaging (COPD patients often have hyperinflation that makes imaging difficult), the absence of a tricuspid regurgitant jet makes PH unlikely.

RADIOGRAPHY, NUCLEAR SCAN, COMPUTED TOMOGRAPHY, AND MAGNETIC RESONANCE IMAGING

Conventional chest radiography remains a simple tool to evaluate the lung parenchyma for the presence of acute and chronic diseases such as COPD, interstitial lung disease, bronchiolitis, and bronchiectasis, while computed tomography (CT) provides greater detail and assessment of severity. Right ventricular enlargement can be visualized with both forms of imaging, with increased retrosternal density on lateral chest radiograph suggesting right ventricular abnormality. PH may also be suspected when there is enlargement of the descending pulmonary arteries (>16 mm in the right pulmonary artery and >18 mm in the left pulmonary artery). Ventilation perfusion lung scanning remains the imaging technique of choice to screen for the possibility of CTEPH, while CT imaging is more sensitive for identifying specific areas of vascular occlusion in both acute pulmonary embolism and CTEPH, along with other vascular features of CTEPH such as intravascular webs and bands.[32] Computerized imaging may also demonstrate unusual conditions that may mimic CTEPH, such as pulmonary artery sarcoma or mediastinal fibrosis.

Magnetic resonance imaging (MRI) provides useful information regarding the right heart and pulmonary circulation. MRI can be used to assess pulmonary arterial stiffness and compliance, which become altered early in the course of PH and may play a role in the progression of cor pulmonale.[33-34]

RIGHT HEART CATHETERIZATION AND EXERCISE TESTING

As stated previously, right heart catheterization remains the most reliable technique to accurately measure pulmonary artery pressure; when performed with a balloon-tipped catheter it also allows for the measurement of pulmonary artery wedge pressure, with which the assessment of any contribution of left-sided heart disease may be determined.

The impact of PH in chronic lung disease remains controversial. Particularly in COPD, but in interstitial lung disease as well, the elevations in PA pressure are modest compared to pulmonary arterial hypertension (PAH, Group 1), and cardiac output is preserved until late in the course of the disease.[11] Exertional dyspnea is largely driven by the altered respiratory mechanics and impaired gas exchange and oxygen delivery.[35] Nevertheless, exercise capacity appears to be affected by the presence of cor pulmonale. In a study of 42 patients with moderate to very severe COPD, Vonbank et al.[36] identified a cohort of 32 subjects with resting PH (mean Pap = 26.8 +/− 5.9 mm Hg), while the remaining 10 subjects had normal pulmonary artery pressures (mean PAp 16.8 +/− 2 mm Hg). Exercise capacity, assessed by maximal oxygen uptake (VO_2 max) during cardiopulmonary exercise testing (CPET) and was significantly lower in those with PH (785 +/− 244 mL/min) compared with those with normal resting pressures (1052 +/− 207 mL/min, $P = 0.004$). Using the 6-minute walk test as an evaluation of exercise capacity, Sims et al.[37] found that the 6-minute walk decreased by 11 m for every 5 mm Hg elevation in mean PAp in a cohort of severe COPD patients undergoing invasive and noninvasive evaluation for lung transplantation.

MANAGEMENT

The mainstay of management of cor pulmonale is to optimize respiratory mechanics and gas exchange by treating the underlying conditions (eg, bronchodilators for COPD and antifibrotic agents or corticosteroids for interstitial lung diseases). Continuous supplemental oxygen therapy via nasal cannula has been shown to improve survival in patients with hypoxemic COPD[38] and functional capacity, but not dyspnea, in patients with fibrotic lung disease.[39] Generally accepted guidelines for the use of supplemental oxygen are a PaO_2 less than 55 mm Hg breathing ambient air, or 59 mm Hg if edema, polycythemia, or P pulmonale on electrocardiogram are present.[38]

It is tempting to administer diuretics for those patients with edema, but they should be used with caution in cor pulmonale since they can significantly reduce intravascular volume and deleteriously affect the renal contribution to the complex acid-base status typical of chronic respiratory failure.

Efforts using therapies that target pathogenic pathways in PAH to treat cor pulmonale have generally been disappointing.[40] As noted previously, PH and the vascular remodeling are less severe and the cardiac output is generally maintained in cor pulmonale compared with PAH. While survival in chronic lung disease correlates with the presence and severity of PH, it is not clear whether this is due to the vasculopathy or it is simply a marker of lung disease severity. Furthermore, drugs that affect pulmonary vasomotor tone and regional blood flow can worsen ventilation-perfusion matching by increasing blood flow to poorly ventilated lung units, further impairing intrapulmonary gas exchange and resulting in worsening arterial hypoxemia. Studies using sildenafil in COPD have shown worsening gas exchange with no improvement in pulmonary hemodynamics or exercise capacity.[41] A recent trial of riociguat, a guanylate cyclase activator that increases nitric oxide activity, was discontinued due to excess mortality in the active treatment arm compared with placebo,[42] and a study of ambrisentan, an Endothelin Receptor Antagonist (ERA) approved for the treatment of PAH, showed no benefit in a population of patients with interstitial lung disease of various etiologies.[43] At present, PAH-targeted therapies should be considered in cor pulmonale only when the degree of PH is more severe and right heart function is more impaired than typically seen in this population (ie, a phenotype that is more characteristic of PAH).[44]

DISPROPORTIONATE PULMONARY HYPERTENSION

The concept of "disproportionate" PH relates primarily to COPD patients but can be extended to other causes of chronic respiratory disease. While PH is typically mild to moderate from a hemodynamic standpoint, some patients exhibit more severe degrees of PH, often exceeding a resting mean PA pressure >35 to 40 mm Hg. This level of PH is considered as "disproportionate" to the extent and severity of the underlying pulmonary disease. Recently, several studies have aimed to evaluate the frequency of "disproportionate" PH and to clarify its pathogenesis. Chaouat et al.[44] reported that out of 998 patients undergoing right heart catheterization during a period of disease stability, only 27 had a resting mean PAP >40 mm Hg. Of these 27 patients, 16 had a comorbid condition that could cause or contribute to pulmonary vascular disease, such as severe obesity with obstructive sleep apnea. Only 11 patients (1.1%) had COPD as the only identifiable cause of PH. These COPD patients with severe PH tend to have less severe bronchial obstruction, but have severe hypoxemia, hypocapnia, and a severely reduced DLCO. Thabut et al.[45] identified a similar subgroup of 16 out of a total cohort of 263 COPD subjects in whom pulmonary vascular disease was severe. Whether this represents an atypical phenotype of cor pulmonale, the presence of identified or undiagnosed comorbid conditions, or the coexistence of a common disease (COPD) with an uncommon one (idiopathic pulmonary artery hypertension [IPAH]), is unclear.

SUMMARY

Cor pulmonale, defined as PH in the setting of advanced lung disease, is the result of disturbances in a variety of pathophysiological factors that normally maintain the pulmonary circulation as a high-flow, low-resistance circuit. These include hypoxic vasoconstriction and vascular remodeling, hypercapnia, and loss of cross-sectional vascular surface area as a result of destruction or obliteration of lung parenchyma. In contrast to classical left-sided heart failure, right heart function is preserved until late in the course of the disease, when overt right heart failure may ensue. Since edema may develop even in the absence of right heart failure, diuretics should be used cautiously since aggressive diuresis can lead to reduced intravascular volume and worsening acid-base status. Management consists of optimizing lung function with disease-specific therapies and supplemental oxygen. Cardiopulmonary rehabilitation may improve symptoms and quality of life in some patients. Survival is poor, however. Other than continuous oxygen therapy, it remains unclear whether other PH-targeted therapies have a beneficial effect on physical activity, quality of life, or survival and these drugs should be used with extreme caution since they can worsen oxygenation and survival.

- Cor pulmonale is defined as right ventricular enlargement that is due to abnormalities in the structure or function of the lungs, and may occur in the absence of overt right heart failure.

- Edema is common in patients with chronic lung disease and may be due to a variety of causes; accordingly, it is not necessarily indicative of the presence of right heart failure.
- Cor pulmonale is typically characterized hemodynamically by mild-to-moderate PAH with a normal or increased cardiac output. Only late in the course of the disease or during acute respiratory decompensation does cardiac output decrease.
- Management consists of optimizing respiratory function and oxygenation.
- PAH-targeted therapy should be used with caution in the absence of evidence demonstrating beneficial effects; furthermore, these drugs can worsen intrapulmonary gas exchange, thereby causing cardiorespiratory decompensation.

ACKNOWLEDGMENT

In the previous edition, this chapter was written by Ori Ben-Yehuda, and portions of that chapter have been retained.

REFERENCES

1. Chronic cor pulmonale. Report of an expert committee. *Circulation.* 1963;27:594–615.
2. Simonneau G, Montani D, Celermajer DS, et al. Haemodynamic definitions and updated clinical classification of pulmonary hypertension. *Eur Respir J.* 2019;53:1801913.
3. Fishman AP. Chronic cor pulmonale. State of the art. *Am Rev Respir Dis.* 1976;114:775-794.
4. Weitzenblum E, Chaouat A, Canuet M, Kessler R. Pulmonary hypertension in chronic obstructive pulmonary disease and interstitial lung diseases. *Semin Respir Crit Care Med.* 2009;30:458-470.
5. World Health Organization. The top 10 causes of death. December 9, 2020. https://www.who.int/news-room/fact-sheets/detail/the-top-10-causes-of-death. Accessed August 4, 2021.
6. Shorr AF, Wainright JL, Cors CS, Lettieri CJ, Nathan SD. Pulmonary hypertension in patients with pulmonary fibrosis awaiting lung transplant. *Eur Respir J.* 2007;30:715-721.
7. Balcı MK, Arı E, Vayvada M, et al. assessment of pulmonary hypertension in lung transplantation candidates: correlation of doppler echocardiography with right heart catheterization. *Transplant Proc.* 2016;48(8):2797-2802.
8. Arcasoy SM, Christie JD, Ferrari VA, et al. Echocardiographic assessment of pulmonary hypertension in patients with advanced lung disease. *Am J Respir Crit Care Med.* 2003;167(5):735-740.
9. Chen X, Tang S, Liu K et al. Therapy in stable chronic obstructive lung disease patients with pulmonary hypertension: a systematic review and meta-analysis. *J Thorac Dis.* 2015;7:309-319.
10. Anderson KH, Iverson M, Kjaergaard J, et al. Prevalence, predictors and survival in pulmonary hypertension related to end-stage chronic obstructive pulmonary disease. *J Heart Lung Transpl.* 2012;31:373-380.
11. MacNee W. Pathophysiology of cor pulmonale in chronic obstructive pulmonary disease. *Am J Resp Crit Care Med.* 1994;150:833-852.
12. Rowan SC, Keane MP, Gaine S, McLaughlin P. Hypoxic pulmonary hypertension in chronic lung diseases: novel vasoconstrictor pathways. *Lancet Respir Med.* 2016;4:225-236.
13. Peinado V, Pizzaro S, Barbera JA, Abate P. Inflammatory reaction in pulmonary muscular arteries of patients with mild chronic obstructive pulmonary disease. *Am J Respir Crit Care Med.* 1999;159:1605-1611.
14. Paenado VI, Barbera JA, Ramirez J et al. Endothelial dysfunction in pulmonary arteries of patients with mild COPD. *Am J Physiol.* 1998;274:L908-L913.
15. Baudouin SV. Oedema and cor pulmonale revisited. *Thorax.* 1997;52:401-402.
16. Ferrer MI, Harvey RM, Cathcart RT, Webster CA, Richards DW, Cournand A. Some effects of digoxin upon the heart and circulation in man: digoxin in chronic cor pulmonale. *Circulation.* 1950;1:161-186.
17. Harvey RM, Ferrer MI, Cournand A. The treatment of chronic cor pulmonale. *Circulation.* 1953;7:932-940.
18. Kawut SM, Poor HD, Parikh MA, et al. Cor pulmonale parvus in chronic obstructive pulmonary disease and emphysema: the MESA COPD study. *J Am Coll Cardiol.* 2014:64:2000-2009.
19. Hagger D, Condliffe R, Woodhouse N, et al. Ventricular mass index correlates with pulmonary artery pressure and predicts survival in suspected systemic sclerosis-associated pulmonary arterial hypertension. *Rheumatology (Oxford).* 2009;48:1137-1142.
20. van Wolferen SA, Marcus JT, Boonstra A, et al. Prognostic value of right ventricular mass, volume, and function in idiopathic pulmonary arterial hypertension. *Eur Heart J.* 2007;28:1250-1257.
21. Rain S, Handoko ML, Trip P, et al. Right ventricular diastolic impairment in patients with pulmonary arterial hypertension. *Circulation.* 2013;128:2016-2025.
22. Guihaire J, Haddad F, Boulate D, et al. Non-invasive indices of right ventricular function are markers of ventricular-arterial coupling rather than ventricular contractility: insights from a porcine model of chronic pressure overload. *Eur Heart J Cardiovasc Imaging* 2013;14:1140-1149.
23. Vonk-Noordegraaf A, Haddad F, Chin KM, et al. Right heart adaptation to pulmonary arterial hypertension: physiology and pathobiology. *J Am Coll Cardiol.* 2013;62:D22-D33.
24. Vonk Noordegraaf A, Westerhof BE, Westerhof N. The relationship between the right ventricle and its load in pulmonary hypertension. *J Am Coll Cardiol.* 2017;69:236-243.
25. van de Veerdonk MC, Kind T, Marcus JT, et al. Progressive right ventricular dysfunction in patients with pulmonary arterial hypertension responding to therapy. *J Am Coll Cardiol.* 2011;24:2511–2519.
26. Gan C, Lankhaar JW, Marcus JT, et al. Impaired left ventricular filling due to right-to-left ventricular interaction in patients with pulmonary arterial hypertension. *Am J Physiol Heart Circ Physiol.* 2006;290(4):H1528-H1533.
27. Brittain EL, Talati M, Fessel JP, et al. fatty acid metabolic defects and right ventricular lipotoxicity in human pulmonary arterial hypertension. *Circulation.* 2016;133(20):1936-1944.
28. Oikawa M, Kagaya Y, Otani H, et al. Increased [18F]fluorodeoxyglucose accumulation in right ventricular free wall in patients with pulmonary hypertension and the effect of epoprostenol. *J Am Coll Cardiol.* 2005;45(11):1849-1855.
29. Goudis CA, Konstantinides AK, Ntalas IV, Korantzopoulos P. Electrocardiographic abnormalities and cardiac arrhythmias in chronic obstructive pulmonary disease. *Int J Cardiol.* 2015;199:264-273.
30. Yock PG, Popp RL. Noninvasive estimation of right ventricular systolic pressure by Doppler ultrasound in patients with tricuspid regurgitation. *Circulation.* 1984;70:657-662.
31. Fisher MR, Criner GJ, Fishman AP, et al. Estimating pulmonary artery pressures by echocardiography in patients with emphysema. *Eur Respir J.* 2007;30:914-921.
32. Kim NH, Delcroix M, Jais X, et al. Chronic thromboembolic pulmonary hypertension. *Eur Respir J.* 2019;53:1801915.
33. Kuehne T, Yilmaz S, Steendijk P, et al. Magnetic resonance imaging analysis of right ventricular pressure-volume loops: In vivo validation and clinical application in patients with pulmonary hypertension. *Circulation.* 2004;110:2010-2016.
34. Peacock AJ, Crawley S, McLure L, et al. Changes in right ventricular function measured by cardiac magnetic resonance imaging in patients receiving pulmonary arterial hypertension-targeted therapy: the EURO-MR study. *Circ Cardiovasc Imaging.* 2014;7(1):107-114.
35. Hilde JM, Skjorten I, Hansteen V, et al. Haemodynamic responses to exercise in patients with COPD. *Eur Respir J.* 2013;41:1031-1041.

36. Vonbank E, Funk GC, Marzluf B, et al. Abnormal pulmonary arterial pressure limits exercise capacity in patients with COPD. *Wien Klin Wochenschr.* 2008;120:749-755.

37. Sims MW, Margolis DJ, Localio AR, Panettieri RA, Kawut SM, Christie JD. Impact of pulmonary artery pressure on exercise function in severe COPD. *Chest.* 2009;136:412-419.

38. Nocturnal Oxygen Therapy Trial Group. Continuous or nocturnal oxygen therapy in hypoxemic chronic obstructive lung disease. *Ann Intern Med.* 1980;93:391-398.

39. Bell EC, Cox NS, Goh N, et al. Oxygen therapy for interstitial lung disease: a systematic review. *Eur Respir Rev.* 2017;26:160080.

40. Vonk-Noordegraaf A, Boerrtiger BG. Sildenafil: a definitive NO in COPD. *Eur Respir J.* 2013;42:893-894.

41. Rietema H, Holverda S, Bongaard HJ. Sildenafil treatment in COPD does not affect stroke volume or exercise capacity. *Eur Respir J.* 2008;31:759-764.

42. Nathan SD, Behr J, Collard HR, et al. Riociguat for idiopathic interstitial pneumonia-associated pulmonary hypertension (RISE-IIP): a randomised, placebo-controlled phase 2b study. *Lancet Respir Med.* 2019;7: 780-790.

43. Raghu G, Nathan SD, Behr J, et al. Pulmonary hypertension in idiopathic pulmonary fibrosis with mild-to-moderate restriction. *Eur Respir J.* 2015; 46(5):1370-1377.

44. Chaouat A, Bugnet AS, Kadaoui N, et al. Severe pulmonary hypertension and chronic obstructive pulmonary disease. *Am J Resp Crit Care Med.* 2005;172:189-194.

45. Thabut G, Dauriat G, Stern JB, Logeart D, Levy A, Marrash-Chahla R, et al. Pulmonary hemodynamics in advanced COPD candidates for lung volume reduction surgery or lung transplantation. *Chest* 2005;127:1531–1536.

Sleep-Disordered Breathing

Shahrokh Javaheri, Dirk Pevernagie, and Ali Javaheri

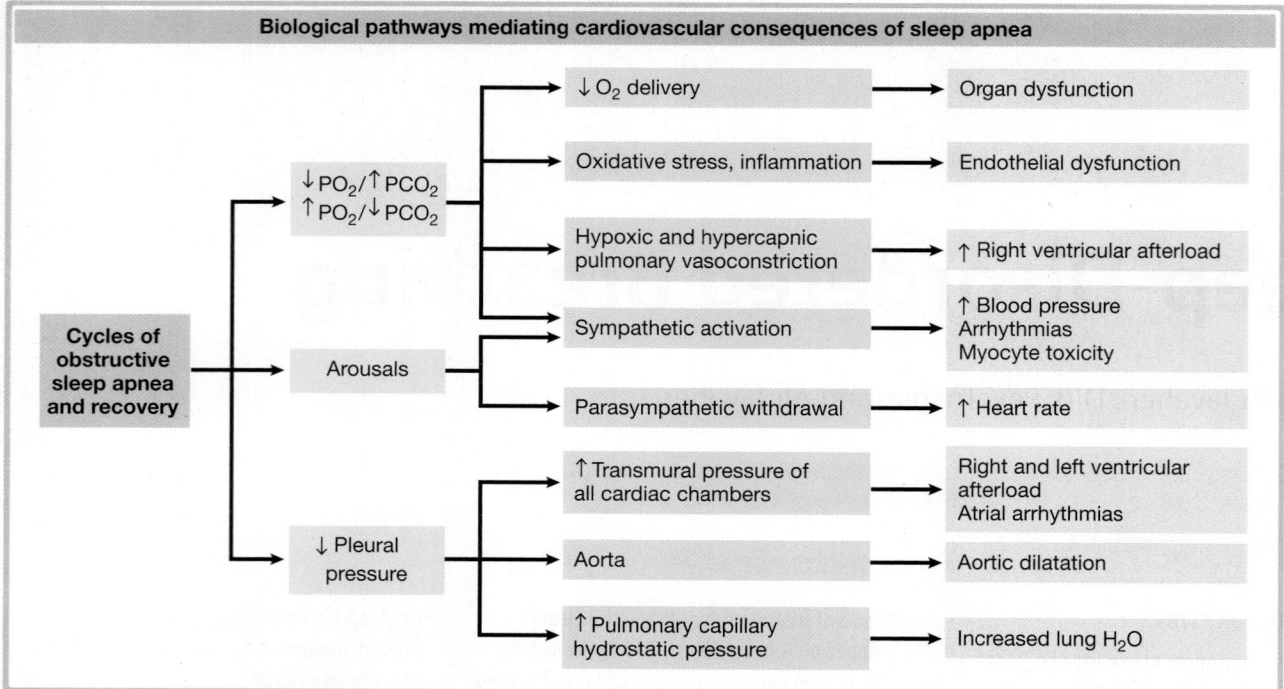

Chapter 60 Fuster and Hurst's Central Illustration. Sleep apnea involves cyclic asphyxia, microarousals from sleep, and negative swings in intrathoracic pressure, which induce adverse systemic effects that disrupt normal cardiovascular physiology and function. The pathways are qualitatively similar in obstructive and central sleep apnea, though most pronounced in obstructive sleep apnea.

CHAPTER SUMMARY

This chapter explores the pathophysiology of obstructive and central sleep apnea, as well as the purported causal relationship between these and hypertension, atherosclerosis, cardiac rhythm disorders, and cardiac failure. Obstructive sleep apnea (OSA)—involving cyclic asphyxia, microarousals from sleep, and negative swings in intrathoracic pressure—induces adverse systemic effects that disrupt normal cardiovascular physiology and function (see Fuster and Hurst's Central Illustration). Notably, however, central sleep apnea of the Hunter-Cheyne-Stokes type is a consequence of cardiac failure rather than a cause. Treatment of sleep-disordered breathing with positive airway pressure devices and other therapeutic regimens has been shown to improve cardiovascular outcomes in patients with OSA. Randomized controlled trials have failed to show any mortality benefit, but this is likely related to methodological issues with the trials. Treatment of central sleep apnea remains difficult. Two randomized, controlled trials are ongoing: one with low-flow nocturnal oxygen and another with improved adaptive servo-ventilation. Phrenic nerve stimulation has shown benefits in a randomized, controlled trial. Finally, cardiac transplant recipients have been of particular interest because it was anticipated that preexisting central sleep apnea might be cured; however, OSA is prevalent in this patient population due to weight gain, potentially contributing to hypertension, poor quality of life, and even cardiac rejection.

INTRODUCTION

Normal sleep is associated with favorable autonomic nervous system activity, and a reduced blood pressure (BP), heart rate, and metabolic rate[1] (**Fig. 60–1**). However, in the presence of sleep-disordered breathing (SDB), sleep is disrupted with adverse consequences. SDB encompasses apneas, hypopneas, and hypoventilation syndromes. Hypoventilation syndromes have been reviewed elsewhere[2,3] and are beyond the scope of this chapter.

There are two main types of respiratory events, namely apneas and hypopneas (apnea implying complete cessation of ventilation and hypopnea diminished ventilation). For each of these events the pathophysiological mechanism can be either obstructive, central or mixed central/obstructive. Obstructive sleep apnea/hypopnea (hitherto referred to as OSA) is quite common in the general population and in subjects with cardiovascular disease (CVD), and is rising in prevalence, primarily linked to the obesity epidemic. Central sleep apnea/hypopnea (hitherto referred to as CSA) is rare in the general population but is common in patients with left ventricular (LV) systolic dysfunction with or without overt clinical heart failure (HF), and is also observed in subjects with atrial fibrillation (AF) and stroke.[3] Another main cause of CSA is opioid use.[4]

The most common symptom of OSA for which subjects are referred to a sleep physician is excessive daytime sleepiness. In addition, OSA is associated with various forms of CVD, such as hypertension, systolic and diastolic LV dysfunction, and AF, and cardiologists frequently refer such individuals for clinical evaluation in the absence of daytime sleepiness, which is often the case in such subjects. In contrast to OSA, which is a known cause of incident CVD, CSA is rather a consequence of HF and AF. Therefore, there is a bidirectional relationship between SDB and CVD.

POLYSOMNOGRAPHY, SLEEP STAGES, SLEEP APNEA, AND HYPOPNEA

Polysomnography (related to Somnus, the ancient Roman god of sleep) consists of electrophysiological recording of brain waves through an electroencephalogram (EEG), eye movements, chin electromyogram, electrocardiogram (ECG), naso-oral airflow (measured by a thermocouple and a pressure sensor), thoracoabdominal excursions (measured by strain gauges, inductive plethysmography, or impedance pneumography), arterial oxyhemoglobin saturation (measured by pulse oximetry), and leg movements. These recordings serve several purposes. First, the combination of EEG, eye movements, and chin electromyogram allow differentiation of state of wakefulness from state of sleep, and recognition of various stages of sleep. Second, the combination of probes allows the classification of sleep-related breathing disorders into apneas, hypopneas, and subclassification into OSA and CSA.

Monitoring of the ECG and the anterior tibialis muscles electromyogram allows detection of nocturnal arrhythmias and a sleep disorder called periodic limb movements, respectively. There are standard criteria for sleep staging, arousal from sleep, and classification of SDB.[5]

Sleep Stages

Sleep is not a homogeneous single state. Sleep consists of two neurophysiologically distinct states of non-rapid-eye-movement (NREM) and rapid-eye-movement (REM) sleep. NREM sleep consists of stages 1 to 3 (N1, N2, and N3) and accounts for about 80% of adult total sleep time. REM sleep is neurophysiologically distinct from NREM sleep and accounts for 20% of total adult sleep time. In REM sleep, there are rapid eye movements (hence the name), which occur intermittently (phasic REM, in contrast to tonic REM), skeletal muscle atonia (characterized by a decrease in the amplitude of chin electromyogram), and dreaming. REM sleep, therefore, is a state of an active brain in an atonic body. Due to the atonia, the dream is not enacted, otherwise, a potentially dangerous sleep disorder referred to as REM sleep behavior disorder ensues when the subject inappropriately acts out the dream. Normally, several sleep cycles occur each night. For a total dark time of 8 hours and a total sleep time of 7.5 hours (sleep efficiency of 94%), there will be five cycles with NREM sleep accounting for about 6 hours and REM sleep accounting for about 1.5 hours of total sleep time.

Sleep-Disordered Breathing

An apnea is defined as the absence of inspiratory airflow for 10 seconds or more recorded by a naso-oral pressure probe and a thermocouple. Apneas are of three kinds: central (**Fig. 60-2**), obstructive (**Fig. 60-3**), and mixed. In central apnea, the absence of airflow is due to the absence of activation of inspiratory pump muscles including the diaphragm. Central apneas are characterized by the simultaneous absence of naso-oral airflow and thoracoabdominal excursions (Fig. 60-2). In contrast, in obstructive apnea, the activity of inspiratory thoracic pump muscles, such as the diaphragm, are present. The absence of airflow is due to upper airway occlusion. This is secondary to inward collapse of the relaxed dilator muscles of the oropharynx that cannot resist the negative intra-airway pressure during inspiration. Polysomnographically, an obstructive apnea is characterized by the absence of naso-oral airflow in spite of

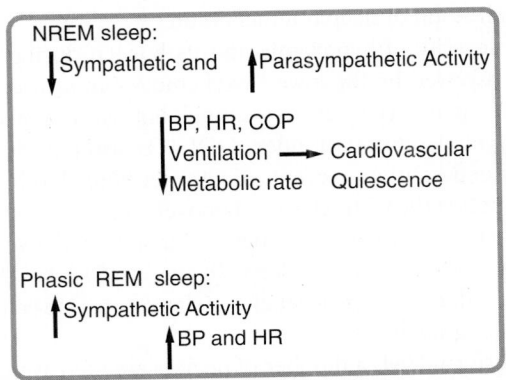

Figure 60–1. Normal cardiovascular changes in non-rapid-eye-movement (NREM) and REM sleep.

REM, rapid eye movement; NREM, non-rapid eye movement; BP, blood pressure; HR, heart rate; COP, cardiac output.

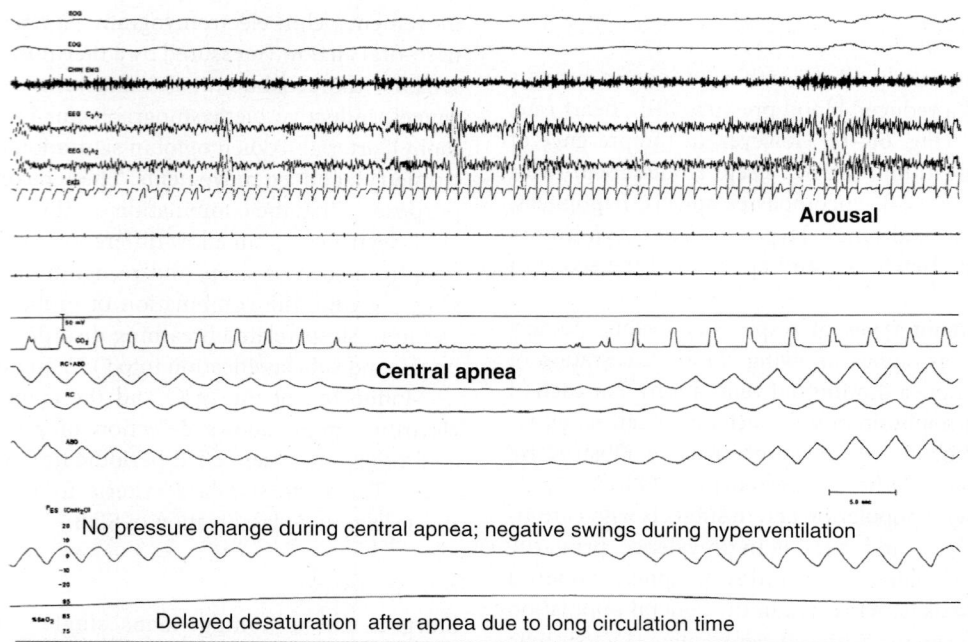

Figure 60–2. Polysomnographic example of OSA. Tracings are: electro-oculogram (EOG, 1st and 2nd); chin electromyogram (EMG, 3rd); electroencephalogram (EEG, 4th and 5th); ECG (7th); airflow measured by thermocouple (8th) and CO_2 (9th); combined (10th) rib cage (RC) and abdominal (ABD); RC (11th) and ABD (12th) excursions; time in seconds (13th); and esophageal pressure (14th). Airflow is absent in the face of effort observed on rib cage, abdominal, and esophageal pressure tracings. Breathing resumes with the onset of arousal (increase in chin EMG and EEG α waves) and opening of upper airway.

continual thoracoabdominal excursions (Fig. 60–3). A mixed apnea has an initial central component followed by an obstructive component.

Hypopnea is a reduction in breathing. It may be defined as reduced naso-oral airflow or thoracoabdominal excursions of 10 seconds or more in duration, resulting in either a 3% or 4%

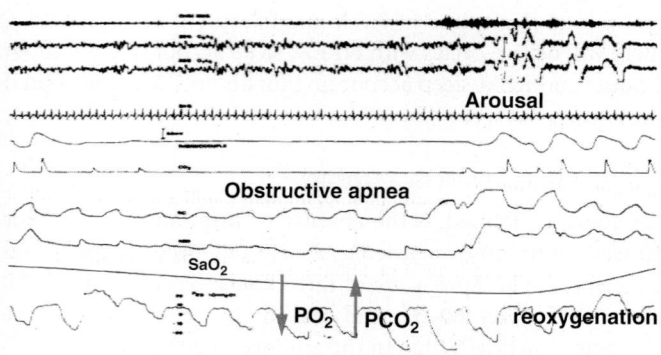

Figure 60–3. Polysomnographic example of CSA. Tracings are: electro-oculogram (EOG, 1st and 2nd); chin electromyogram (EMG, 3rd); electroencephalogram (EEG, 4th and 5th); ECG (7th); airflow measured by thermocouple (8th) and CO_2 (9th); combined (10th) rib cage (RC) and abdominal (ABD); RC (11th) and ABD (12th) excursions; time in seconds (13th); and esophageal pressure (14th). Airflow is absent in the effort channels observed on rib cage, abdominal, and esophageal pressure tracings. Note the smooth and gradual changes in the thoracoabdominal excursions and esophageal pressure in the crescendo and decrescendo arms of the cycle. The arousal occurs at the peak of hyperventilation.

(the Medicare criterion) drop in arterial oxyhemoglobin saturation and/or an electroencephalographic arousal.[6] Similar to apneas, hypopneas may be either obstructive or central, but this distinction is very difficult; for which reason, these two kinds of hypopneas are frequently not reported separately.

To determine the severity of sleep-related breathing disorders, an Apnea–Hypopnea Index (AHI) is calculated as the number of apneas and hypopneas per hour of sleep. Traditionally, an AHI of 5 or greater is considered abnormal and has been used as the criterion for polysomnographic diagnosis. When an obstructive AHI of ≥5 is associated with excessive daytime sleepiness, the combination is referred to as OSA (hypopnea) syndrome. The number of electroencephalographic arousals per hour of sleep is referred to as an arousal index, and is used as an indication of sleep fragmentation.

The severity of hypoxemia and its burden during sleep is usually assessed by the lowest oxyhemoglobin saturation and the time spent below an oxyhemoglobin saturation of 90%. The oxygen desaturation index (ODI 4) is also reported as the number of desaturation events of ≥4% per hour. The biological implication of the ODI relates to hypoxemia reoxygenation episodes that are thought to be a determinant of oxidative stress.

Most recently, Home Sleep Testing (HST) has become popular, due to cost-benefit relative to in-laboratory polysomnography.

To perform HST, a number of devices are increasingly used with important limitations. These devices measure air flow, respiratory effort, and oxygen saturation, but without recording electroencephalography. Therefore, sleep time and arousals are not captured. With HST, an AHI is estimated as the number of apneas and hypopneas (that occur only during sleep time) divided by the total recording time, which is invariably of longer duration than the total sleep time. Depending on the difference between the two denominators, HST underestimates the severity of sleep apnea and could be false negative, particularly in those with insomnia and low-level AHI values (mild OSA). In addition, hypopneas associated with arousals are not captured, further underestimating the severity of OSA. Another limitation is the potential difficulty in distinguishing obstructive from central disordered breathing depending on the number of channels available for monitoring SDB events. For this reason, in diseases in which CSA is common, such as HF, HST is inferior to in-laboratory polysomnography.

Normal Sleep and Cardiovascular Hemodynamics

As previously mentioned, sleep is not a homogeneous state; it consists of both NREM and REM sleep. NREM sleep is characterized by autonomic stability due to a simultaneous decrease in sympathetic nervous system activity and elevated parasympathetic neural tone (Fig. 60–1), which progressively increases with the deepening of sleep stages from N1 to N3.[7] Consequently, arterial BP and heart rate decrease progressively throughout NREM sleep, decreasing cardiac workload, and metabolic rate (Fig. 60–1). Based on these autonomic alterations and hemodynamic changes, NREM sleep is generally considered "peaceful" for the cardiovascular system.[8] However, in NREM sleep, particularly in N3 when sympathetic activity is at its nadir,[7] the normal physiological drop in diastolic BP, one of the main determinants of coronary blood flow, could precipitate myocardial ischemia.[9] Another determinant of coronary blood flow, coronary artery resistance, is increased in the presence of coronary artery disease. Because of the combined drop in diastolic BP and presence of coronary artery stenosis, ischemia becomes more likely even though the heart rate is low.[9] In this regard, it is well known that low diastolic BP, both in the senior population[8] and in patients with HF and sleep apnea[10] is associated with increased mortality, which is at least in part based on the same pathophysiology.

In contrast to NREM sleep, REM sleep is associated with dreaming, is emotional, and provokes increased sympathetic activity with consequent increased heart rate and BP. The increase in BP increases LV afterload and myocardial oxygen consumption, which is further augmented by an increase in heart rate, another determinant of myocardial oxygen consumption. These changes could result in myocardial supply–demand mismatch, precipitated by the increased demand.[9] Also, REM sleep could impose an additional respiratory burden due to decreased activity of both upper airway dilator and intercostal muscles. In particular, in subjects with established OSA, apneas may become more prevalent and lengthen further, contributing to hypoxemia/hypercapnia leading to adverse cardiovascular consequences. The REM-related AHI, not NREM AHI, has been proposed to be the main underlying factor contributing to hypertension.[11] Therefore, REM-related increases in metabolic demand, potentially combined with diminished oxygen delivery, could precipitate myocardial demand ischemia in the vulnerable heart.[9]

Overnight Acute Consequences of Sleep Apnea and Recovery Cycles

Episodes of apneas and hypopneas are followed by compensatory hyperpnea, a period of increased ventilation. These cycles repeat themselves many times across the night. Apnea-recovery cycles are associated with four acute adverse cardiovascular consequences (**Fig. 60–4**): (1) arterial blood gas abnormalities, of longer duration and fluctuations in partial pressure of carbon dioxide (PCO_2); (2) increased number of microarousals (defined as the appearance of alpha waves on EEG for between 3 and 14 seconds); (3) decreased parasympathetic and increased sympathetic activity; and (4) large negative intrathoracic pressure swings (Fig. 60–4).

These consequences are qualitatively similar for OSA and CSA, but more pronounced in OSA.

Fig. 60–5 depicts the multietiological risk factors for OSA and its downstream consequences. Globally, obesity remains the most important risk factor for OSA, because excess fat is deposited in the tongue and the parapharyngeal areas, narrowing the pharyngeal airway. Subjects with a narrow upper airway are most vulnerable to upper airway closure when during sleep, the genioglossus muscle relaxes and falls backward. Meanwhile, roughly 20% to 40% of subjects with OSA are not obese. In these individuals, nonanatomic factors may account for OSA.[1] In particular, a large number of elderly people (65 years and older) with CVD are not necessarily obese and may not snore much or complaining of daytime sleepiness, yet suffer from OSA or CSA, which frequently could be severe.

The downstream consequences of OSA (Fig. 60–5) include increased sympathetic nerve activity, both at night and daytime, inflammation, oxidative stress, metabolic dysregulation, and vascular endothelial dysfunction. These mechanistic pathways are critically involved in the pathogenesis of hypertension, coronary heart disease, left and right ventricular dysfunction, and AF, all of which are etiological risk factors for end-stage CVD. A recent study[12] investigating serum proteomic biomarkers profiling 1300 proteins in serum samples of 713 individuals undergoing polysomnography reported that obstructive AHI was associated with upregulation of 65 proteins, predominantly involved in pathways of complement, coagulation, cytokine signaling, and hemostasis, all of which could be involved in various pathways of OSA-related CVD and hypercoagulopathy.

In contrast to OSA, where obesity is the major risk factor, increased chemosensitivity to hypoxemia and hypercapnia (increased loop gain), the underlying mechanism of CSA, is associated with LV dysfunction and HF with reduced ejection fraction (HFrEF).[1,13]

Diagnostic Aspects of Sleep-Disordered Breathing

Sleep-related respiratory disorders are catalogued and comprehensively explained in the third edition of the *International Classification of Sleep Disorders (ICSD-3)* published by the American Academy of Sleep Medicine (AASM).[14] The nosology of these disorders comprises OSA, CSA, hypoventilation

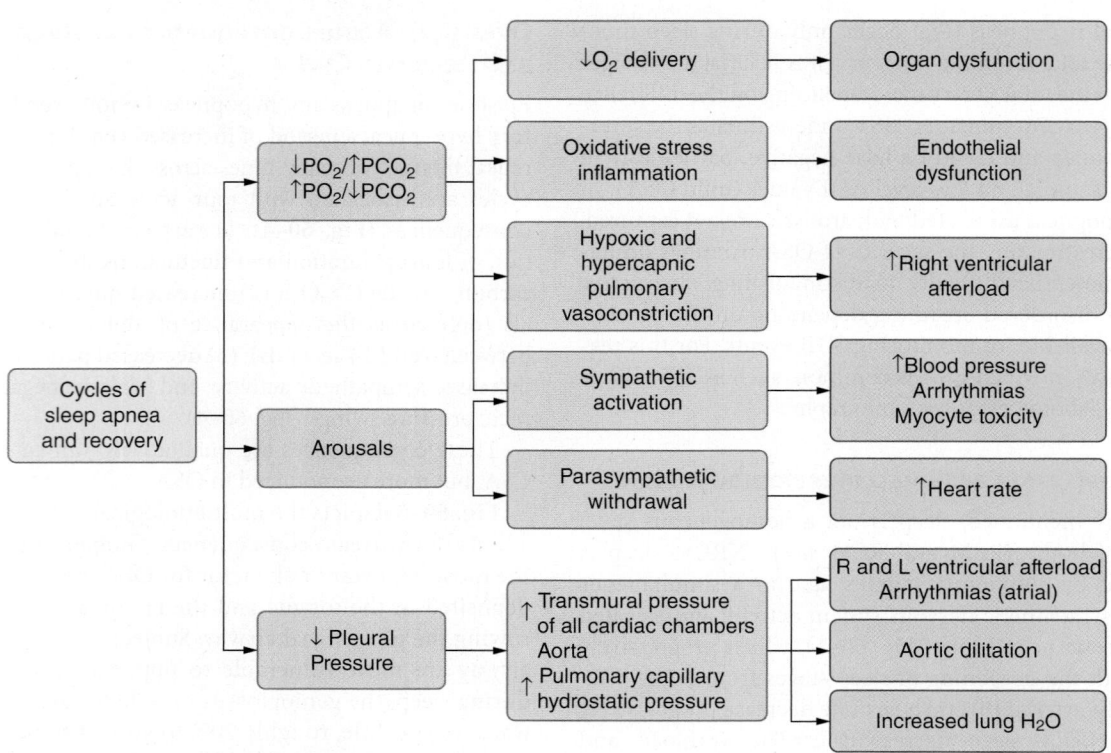

Figure 60–4. **Pathophysiological consequences of sleep apnea and hypopnea.** Pleural pressure (Ppl) is a surrogate of the pressure surrounding the heart and other vascular structures. ↑ increased; ↓ decreased.

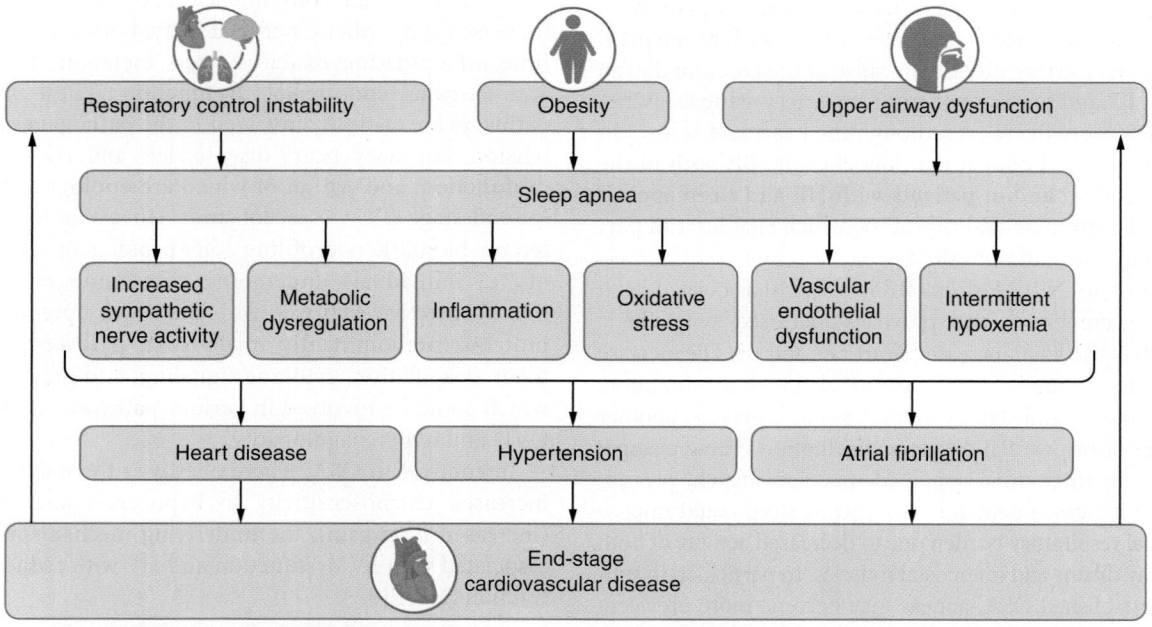

Figure 60–5. **The multietiological risk factors for sleep apnea and its downstream consequences.** These risk factors include increased sympathetic nerve activity (SNA), metabolic dysregulation, inflammation, oxidative stress, vascular endothelial dysfunction (VED), and intermittent hypoxemia (IH). These mechanistic pathways are critical for the pathogenesis coronary heart disease (CHD), hypertension (HTN), and atrial fibrillation (AFIB); all of which are etiological risk factors for end-stage cardiovascular disease (CVD). Reproduced with permission from Javaheri S, Barbe F, Campos-Rodriguez F, et al. Sleep Apnea: Types, Mechanisms, and Clinical Cardiovascular Consequences. *J Am Coll Cardiol.* 2017 Feb 21;69(7):841-858.

syndromes, isolated symptoms, and normal variants. Features of disease severity have only been described for OSA and are differentiated into mild (AHI 5 to 14), moderate (AHI 15 to 29), and severe (AHI 3 and more). OSA is defined as a combination of nocturnal or diurnal symptoms in combination with an AHI ≥ 5 (which is above threshold) or an AHI ≥ 15, even in the absence of relevant symptoms. While this classification is commonly accepted, only weak correlations can be demonstrated between AHI and clinical symptom scores.[15] Subjects in the "severe" range may be asymptomatic. While the clinical significance of OSA without symptoms and objective signs remains equivocal, the US Preventive Services Task Force recommends not to screen for OSA in subjects without suggestive complaints.[16]

The AASM recently published clinical practice recommendations for the diagnosis of OSA, in line with other AASM guidelines on the evaluation and treatment of SDB in adults.[17] Based on the quality of evidence, the balance of benefits and harms, patient values and preferences, and use of resources, good practice statements were issued regarding diagnostic testing for OSA with either polysomnography or HST as described above. Such testing should always be performed in conjunction with a comprehensive sleep evaluation and adequate follow-up.

Obstructive Sleep Apnea, Clinical Manifestations, and Cardiovascular Disease

Obstructive Sleep Apnea

OSA is a highly prevalent disorder and has been on the rise due to the obesity epidemic, the major risk factor for OSA (as aforementioned, obesity has a direct mechanical effect on the respiratory system). Based on the updated Wisconsin Sleep cohort study,[18] it is estimated that in the United States, 34% of men and 17% of women aged between 30 and 70 have mild to severe OSA (ie, at least AHI ≥5/hour of sleep); respective estimations for moderate to severe polysomnographic OSA (AHI of ≥15/hour) are 13% for men and 6% for women. The prevalence of OSA increased by approximately 30% between 1990 and 2010, with an absolute increase of about 4% in women and 8% in men. Based on these data, OSA is approximately twice as common in men as in women. The prevalence of OSA increases with age, but importantly, the association with obesity decreases while the association with CVD increases. Also, the association of OSA with the male gender diminishes with age, while the prevalence of OSA increases in postmenopausal women.

OSA is associated with diurnal symptomtomatology.[19] Nocturnally disruptive snoring affects the sleep of both the patient and the spouse, because snoring goes away with apnea when ventilation ceases. However, apnea is frequently terminated by microarousals with resumption of ventilation and a sudden deep breath associated with snorts. The microarousals are also associated with leg movements and kicking, frequently noticed by the spouse. While there is upper airway closure, the inspiratory muscles are contracting, creating large negative swings in intrathoracic pressure (analogous to the Muller maneuver).

This causes atrial dilatation with the release of atrial natriuretic peptide causing nocturia, an important symptom of OSA. Similarly, during OSA, increased transdiaphragmatic pressure (positive intra-abdominal pressure minus negative intrathoracic pressure, both due to contraction of the diaphragm against a closed airway) facilitates the flux of acid from the stomach into the esophagus. Not surprisingly, nocturnal gastroesophageal reflux is approximately twice as common in patients with OSA as in the general population.[20] Treatment with continuous positive airway pressure (CPAP), which eliminates OSA and increases intrathoracic pressure, invariably eliminates nocturnal reflux.

Another consequence of OSA is frequent morning headaches, which are reported almost twice more commonly in subjects with OSA than in the general population.[21] If cerebral hypoxemia and hypercapnia occur, morning headaches may ensue, resolving shortly after awakening and resumption of normal breathing. Also, similar to nocturnal reflux, treatment of OSA with CPAP eliminates the related morning headache. Finally, waking up with dry mouth or a sore throat is commonly reported by patients with OSA related to mouth breathing.

Due to microarousals (which subjects are not necessarily aware of) and sleep fragmentation, sleep is not restful, is nonrestorative, and subjects may complain of morning grogginess and daytime fatigue and sleepiness.[6,22] Other manifestations of poor sleep quality include irritability and poor productivity, with falling asleep driving (with major public health consequences) or operating heavy machinery being the extreme consequences.[22]

When an AHI of ≥5 per hour is associated with the subject's complaint of daytime sleepiness, the disorder is called OSA syndrome. Most commonly, subjective daytime sleepiness is validated by a metric referred to as the Epworth sleepiness scale (ESS). This metric consists of 8 items evaluating propensity to fall asleep under different circumstances and above 10 is suggestive of sleepiness, and the maximum is 24.[23] This is a useful metric when positive (ESS ≥10), easy to use, but has low sensitivity and a negative scale could be misleading because a large number of subjects could be observed as dozing and snoring by the spouse, yet the subjects dispute snoring and claim that they are awake.

Regarding physical examination, although there are no specific findings, some upper airway anatomical findings such as enlarged tonsils (particularly in children), macroglossia (a subjective observation), and retrognathia may be present. Neck circumference (17 inches or larger in men and 16 or larger in women) could be suggestive; however, OSA needs to be confirmed.

Finally, presence of CVD should increase suspicion for presence of SDB. The prevalence of OSA is much higher in this population than in the general population (**Fig. 60–6**). As will be discussed next, the prevalence of OSA is particularly high in those with HF, stroke, atrial fibrillation, and resistant hypertension.[1,19] Yet, many of these subjects do not complain of daytime sleepiness, which is the most common symptom of

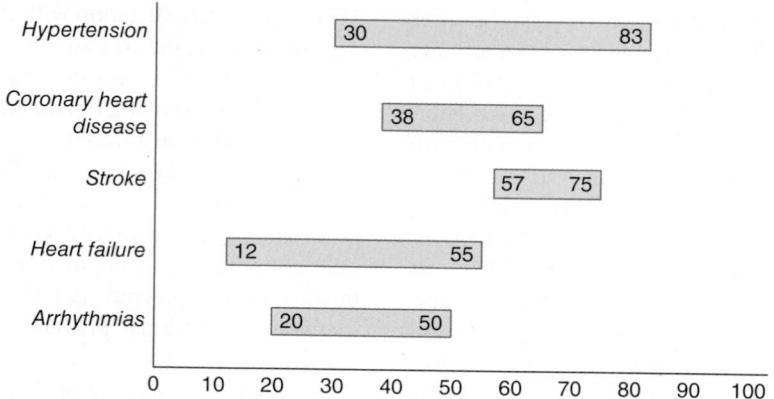

Figure 60–6. Prevalence (%) of OSA in cardiovascular diseases. The lower limit is invariably using an AHI of ≥15 per hour, indicating presence of moderate to severe OSA. The upper part of the range relates to a lower threshold of ≥5 per hour.

OSA in the general population referred to a sleep laboratory for evaluation.

Cardiovascular Consequences of Obstructive Sleep Apnea

OSA is a disorder associated with oxidative stress, up-regulation of redox-sensitive genes, and inflammatory cascade and endothelial dysfunction (Fig. 60–5). Apnea causes hypoxemia, and desaturation and resumption of breathing at the end of apneas/hypopneas leads to rapid reoxygenation and production of free radicals resulting in oxidative stress and upregulation of nuclear factor-kappa B. OSA-related hypoxemia, hypercapnia, and arousals cause perturbations in the autonomic nervous system with increased catecholamines, and increased sympathetic activity occurring during sleep and extending into daytime. Importantly, these intermediary mechanisms are the molecular signatures of OSA that in the long run lead to a variety of CVD[1,25,26] if left untreated. With effective treatment, these CVD-related biomarkers have been shown to change,[1,24,25] catecholamine levels decline and rise again, if treatment is withdrawn.[26]

Last but not least, evidence is accumulating, both from animal studies mimicking OSA and human studies, that OSA-related hypoxemia/reoxygenation and sleep fragmentation/arousals promote specific alterations in microbiota, and the acquired dysbiosis could contribute to adverse cardiometabolic consequences of OSA such as hypertension, insulin resistance, and atherosclerosis.[27–29] Similarly, studies suggest that altered microbiome could influence sleep physiology via the microbiome-gut-brain axis.[30–32] Based on these studies, we[22] speculate that OSA could promote specific alterations in gut microbiota producing cytokines and inflammatory markers that could contribute to adverse outcomes.

To summarize, OSA, particularly when severe, could lead to a variety of CVD, including systemic hypertension, resistant hypertension, pulmonary hypertension (PH), AF, patent foramen ovale, HF, coronary heart disease, myocardial ischemia, myocardial infarction, and sudden death. Cerebral consequences include transient ischemic attack (TIA) and stroke, sometimes at night (wake-up stroke). These downstream consequences of OSA are briefly reviewed in the following subsections.

Obstructive Sleep Apnea and Systemic Hypertension

Increasing acute and chronic sympathetic activity and resetting of the baroreceptors[1,8,33] are the most significant mechanistic, causal links between OSA and hypertension. Intermittent hypoxemia, a hallmark of OSA, stimulates peripheral arterial chemoreceptors, the carotid bodies, leading to a reflex increase in sympathetic activity, resulting in peripheral vasoconstriction and increased BP. In the long-term, persistently increased sympathetic activity along with baroreceptor resetting could induce vascular remodeling, leading to persistent elevation of BP, not only during sleep, but also during waking time.[1,8,33] Once remodeling has occurred, treatment of OSA may not lower elevated BP. The implication is that the earlier the diagnosis of OSA is made and therapy instituted, the better chance of reversing the elevated BP and its adverse cardiovascular consequences.[33]

Meanwhile, fluid retention and leg edema due to increased renal- and aldosterone-mediated sodium retention could further augment OSA. The recumbent position of sleep is associated with the cephalad movement of fluid from the legs to the neck causing vascular congestion and peri-pharyngeal edema, narrowing the upper airway and therefore worsening OSA severity.[34]

It is estimated that about 30% of patients suffering from hypertension have OSA, and conversely, 50% of OSA patients have hypertension.[33] Therefore, the presence of hypertension should signal the presence of OSA, particularly in nonobese subjects,[35] as in obese subjects, obesity itself could be the cause of hypertension and not necessarily OSA. This was demonstrated in the Sleep Heart Health Study (SHHS)[35] concluding that in subjects with a body mass index below 27 kg/m², OSA was independently associated with systemic hypertension. Therefore, presence of hypertension in a nonobese subject should herald presence of OSA as the likely cause needing confirmation with a sleep study.

Prevalence of OSA is higher in subjects with resistant than those without resistant hypertension. Multiple studies have reported a prevalence ranging from 60% to 90% among patients with resistant hypertension.[33] Notably, considering all identifiable causes of resistant hypertension, OSA appears to be the most common cause.[1,33,36]

The aforementioned evidence has led the international guidelines to acknowledge OSA as a cause of systemic hypertension and an important contributing factor to resistant hypertension.

Effects of Treatment for Obstructive Sleep Apnea on Hypertension

The causal association of OSA with hypertension and resistant hypertension is confirmed from a randomized controlled trial (RCT) of treatment of OSA with a CPAP device and using 24-hour ambulatory pressure recording[1,33] demonstrating a reduction in BP (**Figs. 60–7** and **60–8**). As depicted in Fig. 60–7, in systemic hypertension, the overall average drop in BP is modest, although there are individuals with a large drop in BP. Specifically, compared with subtherapeutic or conservative treatment, systolic and diastolic BP decrease by about 2 to 2.5 mm Hg and 1.5 to 2 mm Hg, respectively.

CPAP also restores the normal dipping of the nocturnal BP pattern in OSA patients, and reduction in BP is usually greater for nocturnal than for diurnal measures.[33,37]

Similar to systemic hypertension, the causal association of OSA with resistant hypertension is also confirmed from an RCT of treatment of OSA with a CPAP device and using 24-hour ambulatory pressure recording[1,33] (Figs 60–8). The results of these RCTs reviewed previously[1,33] and a meta-analysis[38] identified a significant reduction in systolic BP of about 5 to 7 mm Hg and diastolic BP ranging from 3 to 5 mm Hg (Fig. 60–8), with the largest reductions achieved in those most adherent to CPAP therapy.[39]

Because, in the long-run, even small reductions in BP have important consequences in preventing downstream cardiocerebrovascular consequences of hypertension, subjects with OSA should be counselled regarding the critical importance of using a CPAP device while asleep.

Obstructive Sleep Apnea, Atherosclerosis, Coronary Heart Disease, and Sudden Death

Mechanistically, OSA induces cyclic patterns of apnea-induced hypoxemia and reoxygenation, resulting in oxidative stress with immediate and sustained sympathetic activation, inflammation, and endothelial dysfunction, all of which could cause atherosclerosis and CAD. Vibration from snoring could also be a cause of damage to carotid arteries, which has been implicated in carotid stenosis.[40]

In addition, OSA induces a state of increased cardiac oxygen demand (due to tachycardia and increased BP related to increased sympathetic activity), which occurs simultaneously with reductions in oxygen delivery due to lack of ventilation. At the same time, because of negative swings in intrathoracic and juxtacardiac pressure (diaphragmatic contraction against closed pharyngeal airway), LV wall tension and afterload increase, further increasing LV work and oxygen consumption (**Fig. 60–9**). Collectively, these adverse consequences of OSA serve as a substrate for experiencing nocturnal angina pectoris, acute coronary syndrome, myocardial infarction, or sudden cardiac death during sleep or in the early morning hours soon after awakening.[41–42]

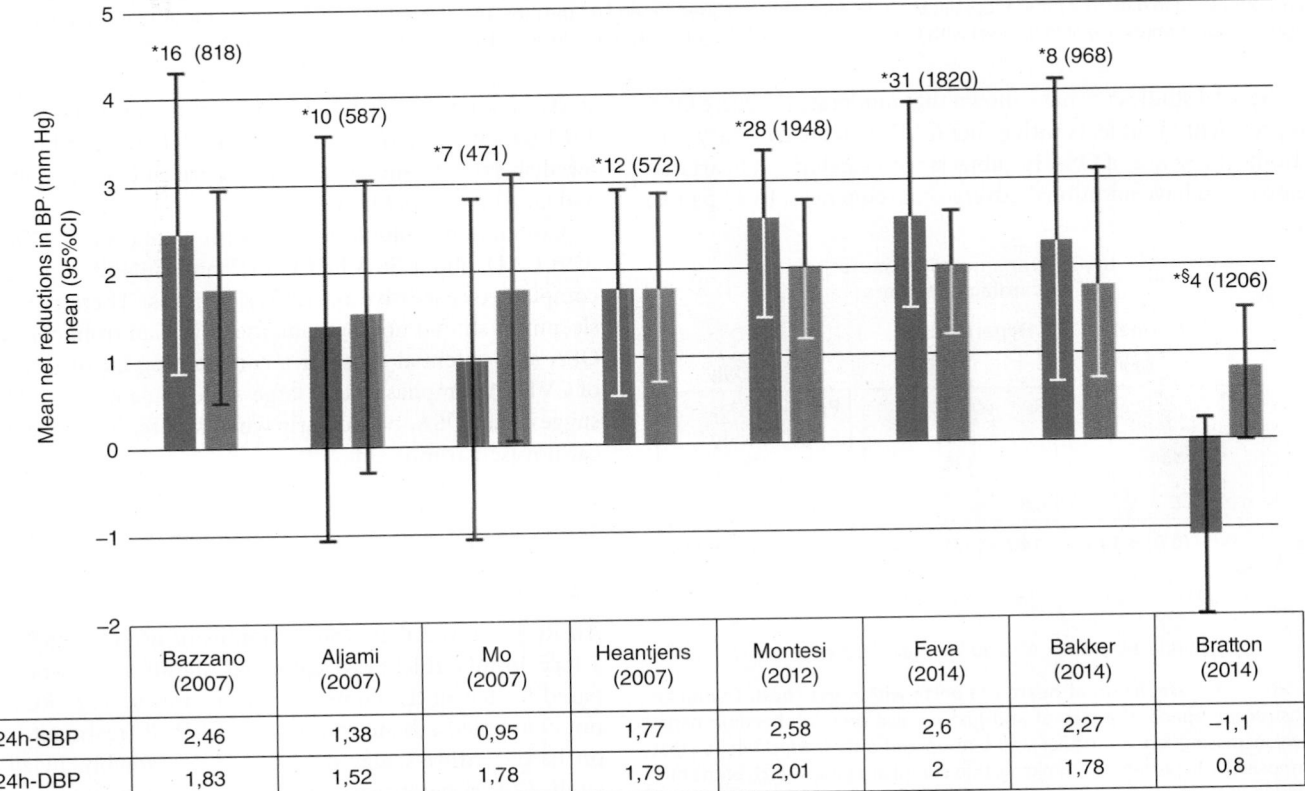

	Bazzano (2007)	Aljami (2007)	Mo (2007)	Heantjens (2007)	Montesi (2012)	Fava (2014)	Bakker (2014)	Bratton (2014)
■ 24h-SBP	2,46	1,38	0,95	1,77	2,58	2,6	2,27	−1,1
■ 24h-DBP	1,83	1,52	1,78	1,79	2,01	2	1,78	0,8

Figure 60–7. **Effect of CPAP therapy on BP in patients with hypertension.** Summary of different meta-analyses of RCTs. Positive figures mean improvement in BP level with CPAP (net changes). *Number of studies included (number of patients included). §Patients without daytime hypersomnia.

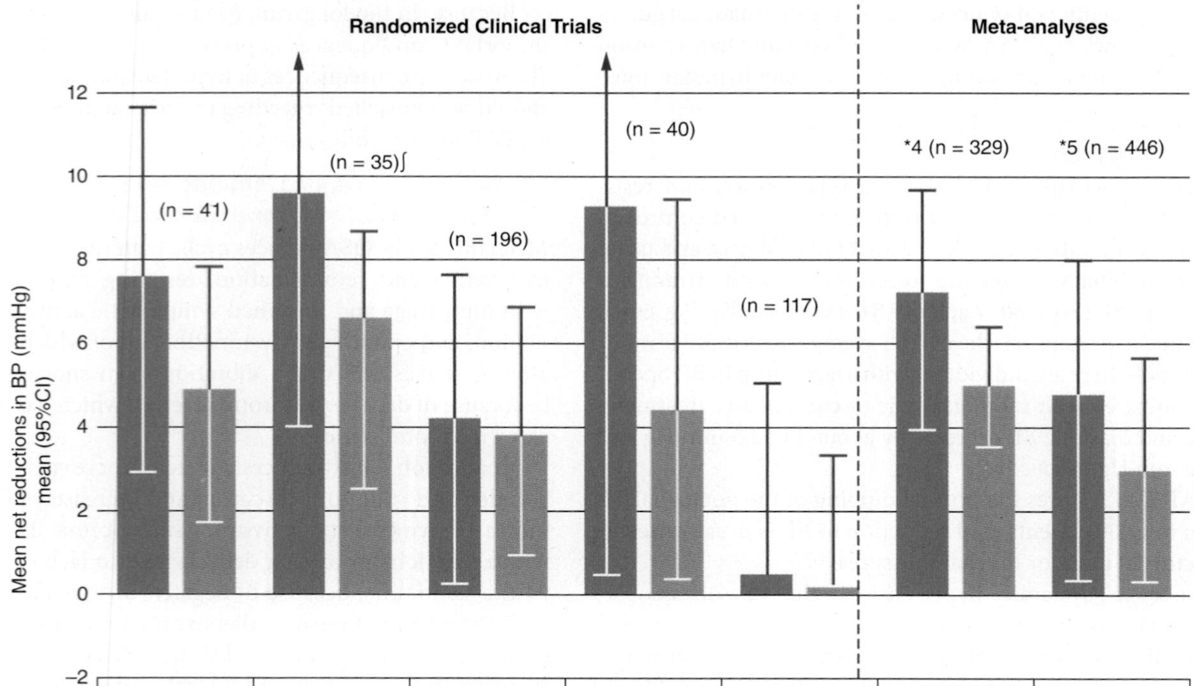

Randomized Clinical Trials

Meta-analyses

Mean net reductions in BP (mmHg) mean (95%CI)

(n = 41)
(n = 35)∫
(n = 40)
(n = 196)
(n = 117)
*4 (n = 329)
*5 (n = 446)

	Lozano (2010)	Pedrosa (2013)	Martinez-Garcia (2014)	De Oliveira (2014)	Muxfeldt (2015)	Iftikhar (2014)	Liu (2015)
■ 24h-SBP	7,6	9,6	4,2	9,3	0,5	7,21	4,78
■ 24h-DBP	4,9	6,6	3,8	4,4	0,2	4,99	2,95

Figure 60–8. Effect of CPAP therapy on BP in patients with resistant hypertension. The figure includes the results of the five RCTs as well as two meta-analyses published to date. The differences between the two meta-analyses depend on the most updated references included in the 2015 meta-analysis. Positive figures mean improvement in BP level with CPAP (net changes). *Number of studies included (number of patients included). ∫Daytime Blood pressure values.

Several studies[43-45] have shown that moderate to severe OSA is prevalent in subjects with either CAD or acute coronary syndrome. Presence of OSA in subjects with established heart disease could have additional adverse consequences. In a Spanish

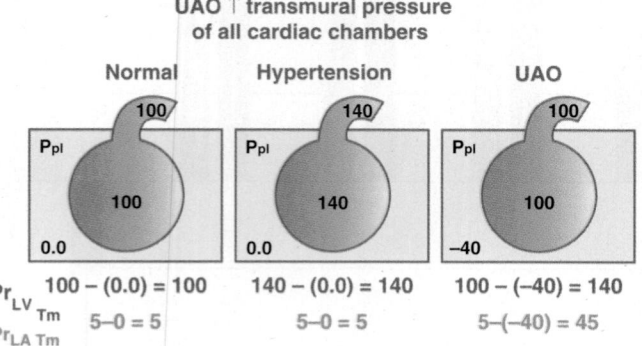

Figure 60–9. Depiction of heart and aorta within the chest. During an obstructive apnea, the pleural and juxtacardiac pressure become negative, increasing left ventricular wall tension and after load, similar to that imposed by hypertension. Similarly, thin compliant atria stretch with stimulation of mechanoreceptors, predisposing to atrial fibrillation. At the same time, atrial natriuretic peptide is released causing nocturia. AF, atrial fibrillation; LV, left ventricular; UAO, upper airway obstruction.

study, among 2551 patients with acute coronary syndrome, 1264 patients (almost 50%) had an AHI ≥15 per hour.[45] In a Swedish study,[44] among 662 revascularized CAD patients, 64% had an AHI ≥15 per hour.

Combining multiple studies with a total of 6672 subjects with CAD, about 56% had OSA,[46] and notably most did not complain of excessive daytime sleepiness. Therefore, lack of sleepiness should not dissuade the physician from considering OSA as a potential cause or a contributing factor to a variety of CVD. We emphasize that large-scale epidemiological studies suggest that OSA, particularly when severe, is associated with cardiovascular mortality.[47-49]

Effects of Treatment for Obstructive Sleep Apnea on Atherosclerosis and Cardiovascular Disease in Randomized Controlled Trials

An RCT showed that after 3 months of use of CPAP, carotid artery intima thickness decreased significantly when compared to that in the control arm.[50] However, large RCTs have not confirmed a beneficial effect of CPAP treatment of OSA on hard cardiovascular outcomes.[43-45,51] Notably, in all these studies, the adherence with CPAP was low, potentially accounting for the absence of benefits,[52-54] and multiple RCTs indicate that only adherent subjects see any benefits in improvement in hypertension, resistant hypertension (noted earlier), and insulin resistance.[55]

In the aforementioned RCTs, the average use of the device was about 3 hours.[52–54] In this regard, analysis of several RCTs (which included the aforementioned trials) subjects with adequate CPAP use, defined as 4 hours or more per night, were selected and were compared to the control group. The only beneficial effect of CPAP was reflected in the cerebrovascular, not cardiac outcomes[52] (**Fig. 60–10**). Lessons learned from these RCTs provide clues for designing future trials.[54,56] These data do not necessarily mean that treatment of OSA has no impact on cardiac outcomes; more long-term and higher powered RCTs than the current ones are needed when cardiac outcomes are the endpoints.

Obstructive Sleep Apnea and Arrhythmias

The neurocardiac axis of the autonomic nervous system plays an important role in controlling the heart rhythm, and the imbalance in sympathovagal activity underlies cardiac arrhythmogenesis.[57,58] In concert with favorable changes in autonomic nervous system activity during NREM sleep,[7] incident ventricular arrhythmias are usually suppressed,[59] evidence which is supported by reduced discharges of implantable

cardioverter–defibrillators in ischemic heart disease.[60] However, surges in cardiac sympathetic nerve activity during REM sleep could cause nocturnal myocardial ischemia and arrhythmias, even in the absence of coronary heart disease.[61] Yet, overall, sleep provides cardioprotection because 80% of total sleep time is occupied by NREM sleep. However, this cardioprotection is removed in subjects with OSA promoting both atrial and ventricular arrhythmias,[62] potentially contributing to sudden death during sleep.[42]

OSA has multiple adverse effects on cardiac electrophysiology[62–69] encompassing abnormal automaticity, triggered automaticity, shortening of the atrial effective refractory period (ERP), QT interval prolongation, and reentrant mechanisms, promoting abnormal cardiac impulse formation, which has been reviewed extensively elsewhere.[68]

A common pattern of heart rate changes is a relative brady-tachyarrhythmia, with the heart rate decreasing during apnea, and increasing with resumption of breathing. The mechanism of these decelerations and accelerations is similar to that of diving reflex and in the case of OSA, enhanced parasympathetic activation during apnea and sympathetic surges subsequent to resumption of breathing,[62] and when observed with Holter monitoring should alert the presence of OSA.

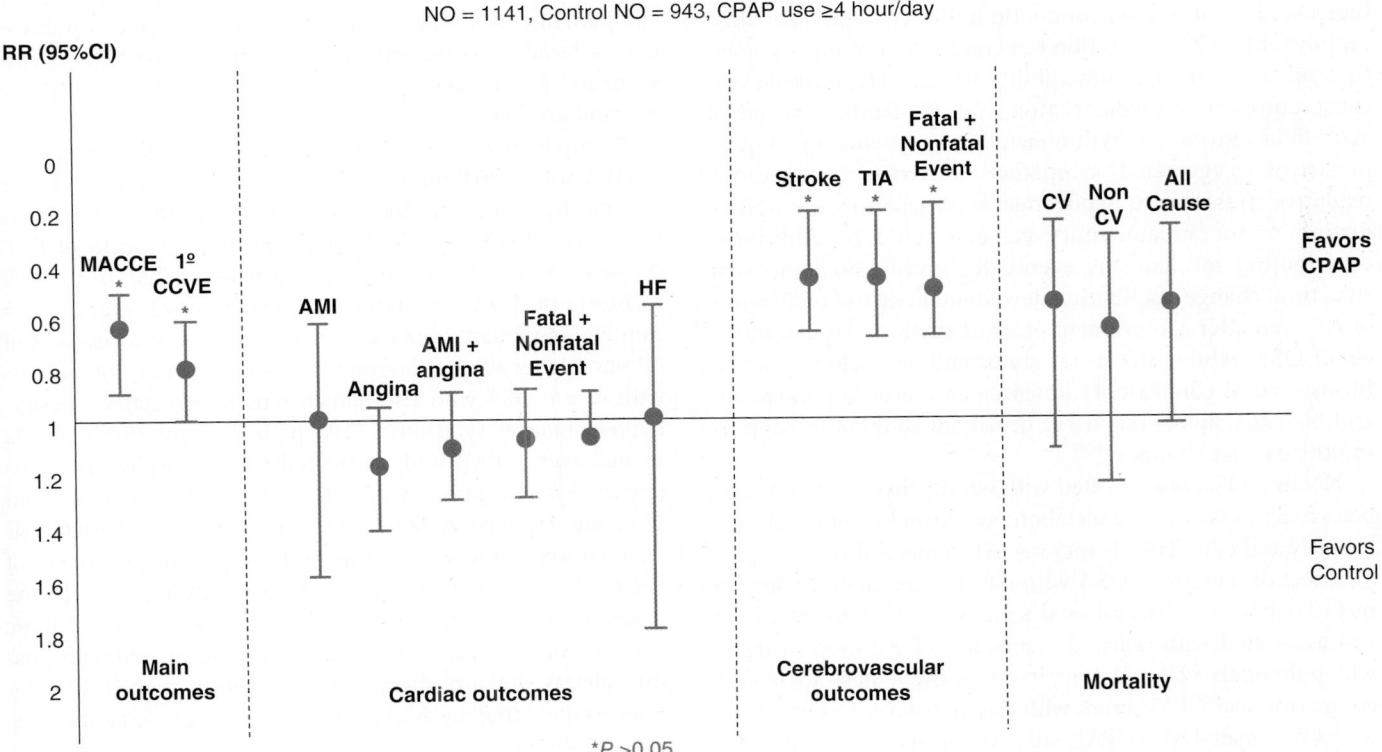

Figure 60–10. Summary of the main results regarding the effects of CPAP treatment on single or composite cardiovascular or cerebrovascular events. Risk ratios with 95% confidence intervals are shown on the y-axis. The x-axis shows the different types of individual and composite cardiovascular events divided into groups corresponding to (from left to right) the primary outcome of the study, the secondary outcome of the study, cerebrovascular outcomes, cardiac outcomes, and mortality outcomes. AMI, acute myocardial infarction; CCVE, cardiovascular and cerebrovascular events; CPAP, continuous positive airway pressure; CV, cardiovascular; HF, heart failure; MACCE, Major adverse cerebrovascular and cardiovascular events; RR, risk ratio; TIA, transient ischemic attack.

Atrial Fibrillation and Sleep-Disordered Breathing

Atrial fibrillation (AF) is the most common chronic sustained cardiac rhythm disorder, affecting millions of individuals worldwide. It is associated with an increased risk of cardiovascular complications, including cerebral and systemic embolization, HF, hospitalization, increased healthcare costs excess, and premature mortality.

Observational polysomnographic studies show that presence of OSA significantly increases the risk of AF and other arrhythmias during sleep.[63–69] In the SHHS cohort,[63] there was a strong association between nocturnal cardiac arrhythmias and SDB with point estimates in the 2 to 4-fold increased risk range, after confounding factors such as obesity and self-reported CVD were accounted for.

There are multiple features of OSA that collectively contribute to inducing and recurrence of AF. These include acute overnight hemodynamic, blood gas alterations, and altered autonomic nervous system activity, intermediate mechanisms encompassing oxidative stress and inflammatory pathways, and long-term structural changes.

Hemodynamically, negative swings in intrathoracic and juxtacardiac pressure distend the compliant thin wall atria (Fig. 60–9), and at the same time cause volume overload of the right atrium, stimulating stretch-mechanoreceptors. In addition, OSA-related cardiomyocyte hypoxemia, hypercapnia/acidosis, and hypocapnia after recovery collectively could facilitate arrhythmogenesis. In regards to PCO_2, hypercapnia increases ERP and slows conduction; ERP changes normalize rapidly with PCO_2 correction but conduction changes persist to result in increased vulnerability to AF.[65] Hypocapnia can cause coronary vasoconstriction and alkalemia. The other acute and chronic arrhythmogenic consequence of OSA is persistent exaggerated sympathetic activity. Conceivably, oxidative stress due to hypoxemia/reoxygenation and upregulation of the inflammatory cascade could be additional contributing mechanisms eventually leading to long-term structural changes facilitating development of and recurrence of AF even after achievement of sinus rhythm. Animal models of OSA exhibit structural abnormalities including atrial fibrosis, atrial connexin 43 downregulation or lateralization, and increased autonomic nerve density in addition to AF-promoting electric changes.[66–69]

Notably, OSA is associated with obesity, hypertension, diabetes mellitus type 2, and metabolic syndrome, all of which collectively and cumulatively increase AF vulnerability.[69]

Effect of therapy of OSA with CPAP were analyzed in two meta-analyses of observational studies.[70,71] The use of CPAP was associated with reduced recurrence of AF even in those with pulmonary vein isolation. In one of these meta-analyses,[70] comparing 698 CPAP users with 549 non-CPAP users, those with OSA treated with CPAP, after AF intervention, had a 44% reduced risk of relapse; younger, more obese, and male patients benefited the most.

For all of the aforementioned reasons, expert consensus supports the presence of OSA as a risk factor for AF recurrence after surgical and catheter ablation, and recommends its treatment.[72] However, in spite of overwhelming pathophysiological evidence

linking OSA to AF, so far, no systematic RCT has been performed to determine if treatment of OSA has any impact in eliminating or reducing the incidence rates of recurrent AF.

So far, we have concentrated on OSA as a cause of AF. However, AF could be a cause of CSA, and epidemiologic data implicate the possible role of CSA in the development of AF, which will be discussed under the CSA section.

Pulmonary Hypertension

Pulmonary hypertension (PH) secondary to OSA falls into the third group of the World Health Organization (WHO) classification, which also includes chronic obstructive pulmonary disease (COPD), interstitial lung diseases, and PH related to chronic exposure to high altitude. The primary pathophysiologic mechanism underlying PH in this group of disorders is hypoxemia.

PH due to OSA is invariably mild, unless another cause of PH from the third group, or left HF, is comorbid.[73] Notably, when OSA is quite severe and associated with hypercapnia, hypoxemia, and obesity, PH is severe, eventually leading to symptomatic right ventricular dysfunction. This is called Pickwickian syndrome, named after Joe, an obese character from the 1836 Charles Dickens novel, *The Pickwick Papers*, who constantly falls asleep in the daytime.

Combining the results of the multiple studies,[33] using polysomnography and right heart catheterization to define PH (and with exclusion of lung and left heart diseases), 29 of 105 patients (28%) satisfy the current criteria (mean pulmonary arterial pressure [mPAP] of 20 mm Hg or higher with a normal pulmonary artery occlusion pressure [PAOP]) for precapillary PH.

Multiple observational studies demonstrate that treatment of OSA with CPAP improves PH.[33,73] But large-scale RCTs are lacking. In a small randomized crossover study,[74] 23 patients with severe OSA (AHI ≥44/hour) and PH, 12 weeks of PAP therapy compared to sham CPAP, decreased mPAP from 29±9 to 24±6 mm Hg (P <0.0001). The reduction was greatest (8.5 mm Hg) in patients with pulmonary artery systolic pressure of 30 mm Hg by echocardiography. In a recent trial[75] of patients with severe OSA who also had chronic hypercapnia (obesity-hypoventilation syndrome), 196 patients were enrolled, 102 treated with CPAP, and 94 treated with a respiratory assist device. Systolic pulmonary artery pressure decreased from 41±2 mm Hg at baseline to 35±1 mm Hg at 3 years with CPAP. Positive airway pressure treatment decreased the prevalence of PH by 37% in the CPAP group on echocardiography. In the study, a large number of participants had echocardiographic evidence of LV diastolic dysfunction that improved with positive airway pressure therapy. It is therefore conceivable that improvement in PH was a consequence of improvement in diastolic dysfunction.

The American College of Cardiology (ACC)/American Heart Association (AHA) expert consensus document recommends polysomnography to rule out OSA for all patients with PH.[76] The recommendation is based on the idea that targeted therapy of OSA could either improve or prevent further deterioration in central hemodynamics.

Obstructive Sleep Apnea and Stroke

In the United States, ischemic stroke is the leading cause of long-term disability in adults, affecting 700,000 individuals annually. There is a bidirectional relationship between OSA and stroke. It is plausible that stroke-related motor impairment of the pharyngeal dilator muscles, as a result of involvement of cranial nerves, predispose to upper airway collapsibility and the development of OSA. On the other hand, OSA is an established risk factor for stroke and epidemiological studies suggest that stroke is the most common downstream consequence of untreated OSA, being associated with an almost 3-fold increased risk for incident stroke. Notably, OSA is found in 50% to 70% of patients with stroke.[40,77-81]

There are several pathophysiological reasons linking OSA to stroke. Because of repetitive cycles of OSA, surges in systolic and diastolic BP, and hypoxemia and hypercapnia have profound effects on cerebral circulation when autoregulation is not operative in non-steady-state conditions dictated by cycles of OSA.[82,83] Furthermore, OSA may cause embolic stroke by way of multiple mechanisms. As noted earlier, OSA is a potential cause of carotid artery atherosclerosis, a source of embolic stroke. Another important pathway is OSA-related cardioembolic stroke,[84] due to AF (paroxysmal during sleep as well as awake or permanent). Lastly, patent foramen ovale is more prevalent in OSA and could be because of paradoxical cerebral embolism.[84,85]

The main question is if treatment of OSA has any effect in subjects with stroke, or incident stroke. As noted earlier, several RCTs failed to show any treatment effect of CPAP on cerebrocardiovascular diseases. In all of these trials, only some subjects used CPAP effectively. Using data from these RCTs, we compared individuals who used CPAP effectively to the control group. We reported that effective use of CPAP was associated with improvement in cerebrovascular, but not cardiac, outcomes[52] (Fig. 60-10).

The Guideline for Healthcare Professionals from the AHA/ American Stroke Association has made the following statements: "A sleep study might be considered for patients with an ischemic stroke or TIA on the basis of the very high prevalence of sleep apnea in this population and the strength of the evidence that the treatment of sleep apnea improves outcomes in the general population."[86]

THE LANDSCAPE OF TREATMENT FOR OBSTRUCTIVE SLEEP APNEA

Therapeutic approaches for treatment of OSA are depicted in **Table 60-1**. Although CPAP is the most effective therapy and therefore the treatment of choice, particularly in the presence of CVD, adherence is low, and as emphasized elsewhere, it is most probably the reason for negative results of the RCTs.[52] Other therapeutic options are oral appliances and hypoglossal nerve stimulation for individuals who refuse or are intolerant to CPAP therapy. Furthermore, combination therapy (eg, CPAP with weight loss, when applicable, or exercise) have shown beneficial effects. Positional therapy is appropriate for

TABLE 60-1. Treatment of OSA

- Promote sleep hygiene
- Avoid alcohol, opioids, benzodiazepines, and phosphodiesterase inhibitors at bedtime
- Weight loss, when applicable
- Exercise
- Continuous positive airway pressure (CPAP) devices
- Mandibular advancement devices (MAD)
- Hypoglossal nerve stimulation
- Upper airway procedures
- Nocturnal use of supplemental oxygen

supine OSA. Phenotypic-guided therapy of OSA is currently in embryonic stages and could prove helpful once long-term RCTs are performed with beneficial outcomes.[87]

Oral Appliances

Oral appliances are mandibular advancement devices (MAD) fabricated using impressions of the patient's teeth/oral anatomy structures and are intended to advance the mandible to which the tongue is inserted. This increases pharyngeal volume and decreases its collapsibility, therefore maintaining a patent's airway during sleep.[88] Oral appliances could be recommended for individuals with mild to moderate OSA, and for those with severe OSA (AHI ≥30/hour) who refuse or are intolerant to CPAP.[89]

There are more than 100 different oral appliances. Custom-made oral appliances are preferable as the mandible is advanced gradually to find the "sweet spot" where OSA is best controlled. Side effects include temporomandibular joint discomfort, jaw misalignment, and hypersalivation. There are no data on hard CV outcomes. A meta-analysis of 34 randomized clinical trials found that these devices were associated with a mean reduction in AHI of 14 (95% confidence interval [CI], 12-15) events per hour.[89] Systematic analyses conclude that oral appliances are nearly equivalent to CPAP in reducing BP.[90] In contrast, in a large RCT, in which 150 subjects were randomized to effective MAD or sham device for 2 months, effective use of MADs for an average of 6.6 hours/night (objective assessment of adherence) improved OSA severity and related symptoms, without a significant change in endothelial function or 24-hour ambulatory BP monitoring, compared to sham MAD.[91]

Hypoglossal Nerve Stimulation

A main reason for OSA is a reduction in drive to the upper airway muscles, and upper airway patency is strongly correlated with the activation of the genioglossus muscle.[92] Like oral appliances, hypoglossal nerve stimulation may be suggested for the treatment of moderate and severe OSA in adults who refuse or are intolerant to CPAP.

Two devices have been approved by the US Food and Drug Administration (FDA). These devices stimulate genioglossus muscle to enhance tongue protrusion with the aim to prevent upper airway collapse. After neck dissection under general anesthesia, the stimulator electrode is placed on the medial branch of the hypoglossal nerve. In addition, a pressure sensor is also implanted inside the chest wall, between the internal and external intercostal muscles to detect inspiratory effort, communicating with the hypoglossal electrode in response to inspiratory effort. In a multicenter, prospective, single-group cohort design, involving 126 patients who had difficulty either accepting or adhering to CPAP therapy, at 12 months, hypoglossal nerve stimulation resulted in a 68% reduction in median AHI score from 29 to 9 events per hour (P <0.001), with improvement in subjective daytime sleepiness and quality of life.[93] In a study on outcomes of 116 out of 126 enrolled individuals with OSA who completed a 36-month follow-up evaluation,[94] lasting improvements were reported regarding objective respiratory and subjective quality-of-life outcome measures. It is unfortunate that 24-hour BP monitoring was not assessed in any the studies. More data are being accumulated for the other device, equally effective, using bilateral hypoglossal nerve stimulation transcutaneously.[95,96] Future trials measuring biomarkers, 24-hour BP monitoring, and other relevant outcomes are needed. Adverse events are similar to those observed with other implantable devices, but are uncommon.

Positional Therapy

Positional OSA is a subtype of OSA when SDB events occur predominantly in the supine position and are minimal in other positions. Although there are no accepted criteria for AHI values in various sleep positions, at its best, nonsupine AHI should be less than 5 events per hour (a threshold indicating lack of clinically significant SDB). This phenotype of OSA is prevalent, particularly in patients with mild and moderate OSA.[97] Different devices such as tennis balls, vests, positional alarms, and pillows are used to avoid sleeping supine.[98]

In 25 subjects with supine OSA (average supine AHI = 31 and a nonsupine AHI = 2 events per hour), Permut and colleagues used the Zzoma Positional Device, which is FDA approved, and reported that positional therapy was equivalent to CPAP at normalizing the AHI with similar effects on sleep quality and nocturnal oxygenation.[99] Therefore, restriction of supine position to sleep on the side or prone position may be sufficient treatment.[100] Other devices are also available.[101]

Exercise

Exercise training and physical activity attenuate OSA. In a meta-analysis enrolling 129 participants, the pooled estimate of mean pre- to postexercise reduction in AHI was −6.3 events/h (95% CI, −8.5 to −4; P <0.001) (about 32 % reduction), without significant changes in body weight.[102] This improvement in severity of OSA with exercise goes along with attenuation of other sequalae of OSA, including hypertension, and impaired glucose tolerance,[103] improved cardiac structure and function,[104] and AF.[105] In an RCT, we found similar results in patients with OSA comorbid with HF.[106]

The proposed mechanisms by which physical activity and exercise may reduce severity of OSA include weight loss,[107] stabilization of chemoreceptor sensitivity,[108] improved strength of pharyngeal dilator muscles,[109] decreased nasal resistance,

and increased sleep quality with consequent respiratory stabilization. Another mechanism involves decreased rostral fluid redistribution. In a small study, 45 minutes of exercise twice weekly resulted in decreased rostral fluid shift during sleep with a consequent increase in pharyngeal volume and a 30% reduction in AHI from 58 to 40 per hour of sleep, without weight change.[110] Exercise also activates the musculovenous pump, which counteracts fluid accumulation in the legs during daytime, and therefore its redistribution into the pharyngeal area in the supine position. Last but not least, there is a possibility of fat redistribution induced by exercise, in analogy with the use of CPAP, which was shown to decrease visceral fat, even in the absence of a change in weight.[111]

Weight Loss

It is well known that weight loss improves OSA and cardiometabolic consequences associated with OSA.[112] In a two-arm 12-month RCT, 264 subjects with OSA and type 2 diabetes mellitus who were overweight and obese were randomized to a control group receiving diabetes education versus the active arm undergoing lifestyle intervention. Comparing the two groups, with weight loss and exercise, AHI and weight decreased by about 10 events per hour and 10 kg, respectively.[113] In another RCT, 181 patients with obesity and moderate-to-severe OSA were allocated to treatment with CPAP, a weight-loss intervention, or CPAP plus a weight-loss intervention for 24 weeks.[114] Reductions in insulin resistance and serum triglyceride levels were greater in the combined-intervention group than in the group receiving CPAP only, but there were no significant differences in these values between the combined-intervention group and the weight-loss group. However, in the 90 participants who met prespecified criteria for adherence, the combined interventions resulted in a larger reduction in systolic BP and mean arterial pressure than did either CPAP or weight loss.[114] The results of this study provide strong evidence that weight reduction and CPAP adherence should be the core element in the treatment of OSA.

Weight loss is associated with the loss of upper body fat, including from the tongue and the throat, and remodeling of the upper airway,[115] all of which should improve OSA.[19,116–119]

A commonly held misperception is that CPAP causes weight loss; however, use of CPAP alone may result in a small amount of weight gain,[120] which may be partly related to reduced respiratory work of breathing.[121] Therefore, lifestyle changes, exercise, and weight loss, when applicable, should be the cornerstone of long-term therapy of OSA.

Avoidance of Alcohol, Smoking, Phosphodiesterase-5 Inhibitors, and Opioids

It is well known that alcohol relaxes the genioglossus muscle, augmenting snoring and promoting the likelihood of upper airway occlusion. We recommend avoidance of alcohol before sleep. Smoking, via mechanisms mediated by nicotine, the active chemical in tobacco, increases efferent sympathetic activity (at least, in part, due to stimulating peripheral chemoreceptors in the carotid bodies, which contain excitatory nicotinic receptors) and plasma catecholamine resulting in increases in BP, heart rate, and myocardial oxygen consumption.[122] In addition, nicotine decreases oxygen availability and causes coronary vasospasm, all promoting ventricular tachyarrhythmia. Because excessive adrenergic overactivity is the underlying mechanism of arrhythmias and HF, sleep apnea in combination with smoking may predispose to these conditions.

Phosphodiesterase inhibitors used to treat erectile dysfunction (eg, sildenafil [Viagra], vardenafil [Levitra], and tadalafil [Cialis]) have been shown to worsen OSA. In a randomized double-blind placebo-controlled study, the use of 50 mg of sildenafil before sleep significantly increased the severity of OSA and desaturation in a group of patients with OSA.[123] This could be related to the vasodilating effect of nitrogen oxide in the upper airway, nasal, and pharyngeal vascular bed.

The emphasis on effectively treating chronic pain syndromes has led to a large increase in the number of patients on opioid medications chronically. A major potentially fatal side effect of chronic opioid use is SDB, including obstructive and central sleep apnea.[4,124-126] These medications are best avoided, in particular, in patients at high risk for sleep apnea (ie, patients with various cardiovascular disorders).

Notably, detoxification and withdrawal of opioids eliminates CSA, and may also improve OSA.[4]

Treatment of Edema

As noted earlier, in the supine position, fluid from the lower extremities is absorbed and moves intravascularly cephalad, causing vascular congestion and pharyngeal narrowing, therefore facilitating upper airway occlusion.[34,127] Patients with OSA, obesity, and hypertension, and those with HF, frequently have salt retention and lower extremity edema. In patients with HF and biventricular dysfunction, elevated right atrial and central venous pressure additionally contribute to pharyngeal vascular congestion and edema. Therefore, an appropriate therapeutic approach to decrease the lower extremity edema and venous congestion is advisable, although care must be taken to avoid volume depletion, hypotension, and renal failure.

HEART FAILURE AND SLEEP-DISORDERED BREATHING

There is a bidirectional relationship between SDB and HF. The results from the SHHS, a large cohort of subjects from the general population, suggests that OSA is linked to incident HF, and that this association is stronger in men than women.[128] On the other hand, both OSA and CSA are common in subjects with HFrEF or HF preserved ejection fraction (HFpEF), patients hospitalized for HF, and even asymptomatic subjects with LV systolic and diastolic dysfunction (**Fig. 60–11**). SDB could contribute to worsening of HF.

For a variety of reasons, patients with HF, even in the absence of SDB, have poor sleep architecture characterized by excessive light sleep, insomnia, and excessive arousals. To this end, in a 2-night sleep laboratory study—the first night for habituation with a sleep-related electrode attached and the second night with polysomnographic recording—sleep architecture was abnormal. Stage N1, the lightest stage of sleep, accounted for 34% of total sleep time (normally about 5%), and N3 (deep sleep) was virtually absent.[129-131] Subjects suffered from mild insomnia with a sleep efficiency of about 72% (normally more than 85%).[129] There were excessive microarousals (15 per hour). Importantly, upon awakening after the second night stay in the laboratory, when asked, the patients noted that their

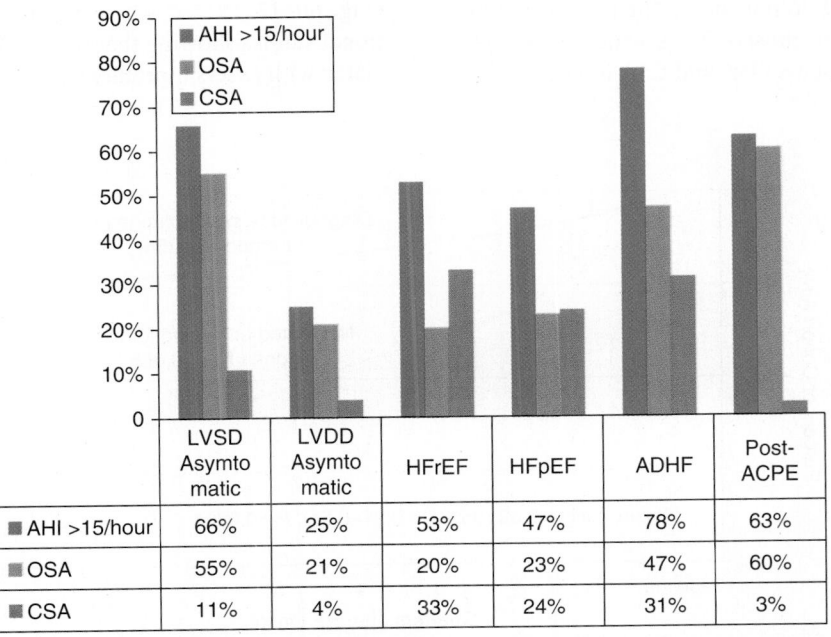

	LVSD Asymtomatic	LVDD Asymtomatic	HFrEF	HFpEF	ADHF	Post-ACPE
AHI >15/hour	66%	25%	53%	47%	78%	63%
OSA	55%	21%	20%	23%	47%	60%
CSA	11%	4%	33%	24%	31%	3%

Figure 60–11. Prevalence (%) of sleep apnea in conditions associated with left ventricular dysfunction. Data show prevalence of moderate-to-severe sleep apnea (AHI ≥15) in asymptomatic left ventricular systolic (LVSD) and diastolic dysfunction (LVDD), heart failure with preserved (HFpEF) and reduced ejection fraction (HFrEF), and acutely decompensated heart failure (ADHF).

sleep quantity and quality was the same as they experienced at home. Symptoms of HF such as cough, paroxysmal nocturnal dyspnea, orthopnea and nocturia, as well as medications used for treatment of HF, and other associated comorbidities such as depression could account for poor sleep. Depression, a common cause of insomnia, is frequently comorbid with HF and carries a poor prognosis if left untreated.[132] Also, the synthesis and secretion of melatonin in the pineal gland is primarily regulated through the β-adrenergic signal transduction system and could be impaired by administration of some β-blockers used for treatment of HF.[133]

Why Sleep-Disordered Breathing Is Underdiagnosed in Patients with Heart Failure

There are many shared diurnal symptoms between SDB and HF chronic comorbid disorders. Shared nocturnal symptoms include paroxysmal nocturnal dyspnea (which could be the hyperventilation following an apnea), cough, nocturia, insomnia, and poor quality of sleep. Shared daytime symptoms include waking up not refreshed (unrestorative sleep) and fatigue.

Lack of subjective daytime sleepiness is typical and we contend that this is due to overlapping symptoms of two chronic disorders: HF and sleep apnea comorbid together. Yet, when an objective test that analyses brain waves to determine sleepiness (multiple sleep latency test) is used, sleepiness is present. In one study of patients with HFrEF and OSA, many subjects exhibited pathological objective sleepiness, in spite of ESS <10.[134] Other investigators have shown the same dissociation in patients with HFrEF and CSA.[135,136]

Clinical differences between patients with HF and OSA versus CSA are the presence of obesity and snoring in the former subtype and the lack thereof in the latter. Subjects with CSA are commonly not obese and do not snore. The lack of symptoms may contribute to underdiagnosis of CSA, which we referred to as "occult."[131] Next, we discuss OSA and CSA in HF.

Heart Failure and Obstructive Sleep Apnea

Although multiple factors play a role in the pathogenesis of OSA,[3,137] obesity remains a major risk factor for OSA, both in the general population and in those with HF. Notably, the prevalence of obesity and morbid obesity is on the rise.

OSA is quite common in subjects with LV systolic and diastolic dysfunction, both asymptomatic and symptomatic subjects (Fig. 60–11). Similarly, sleep apnea is quite common in patients admitted to the hospital with acute decompensated HF[106,138] and cardiogenic pulmonary edema[106] (Fig. 60–11).

In the presence of HF, in addition to OSA-related nocturnal hypoxemia/hypercapnia and increased sympathetic activity, the presence of OSA imposes additional adverse consequences. For example, the large negative swings in juxtacardiac pressure could impair LV stroke volume considerably, by at least two mechanisms, by increasing venous return to the heart leading to right ventricular septal deviation to the left, decreasing LV volume on one hand, and increasing LV afterload, on the other hand (Fig. 60–9). The combined consequences could result in diminished cardiac output and hypotension, particularly during sleep. Meanwhile, although the venous return to the heart increases, apnea-related hypoxemia and hypercapnia cause pulmonary vasoconstriction impeding right ventricular stroke volume. In the long run, overnight consequences of OSA should adversely affect the already impaired cardiac structure and function.

In observational longitudinal studies, OSA has been independently associated with higher rates of readmission, recurrence of acute cardiogenic pulmonary edema, and both fatal and nonfatal cardiovascular events.[106]

A large observational study involving Medicare beneficiaries showed that OSA was associated with increased hospital readmission, excess healthcare costs, and mortality (**Fig. 60–12**),[106,138,139] which is consistent with other observational studies showing that in HF, OSA is independently associated with excess mortality.[106,138–141]

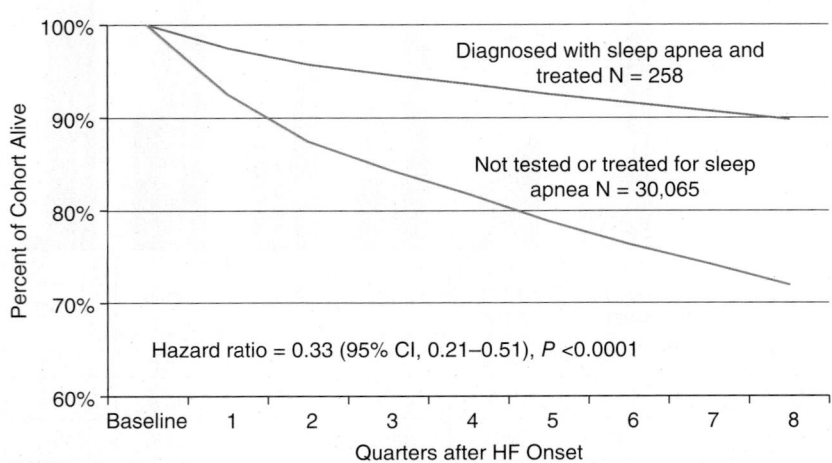

Figure 60–12. Survival of the 258 heart failure patients treated for sleep apnea compared to survival of the 30,000 patients who were not tested for sleep apnea. (Adjusted for age, gender, and Charleston comorbidity index. Reproduced with permission from Javaheri S, Caref EB, Chen E, Tet al. Sleep apnea testing and outcomes in a large cohort of Medicare beneficiaries with newly diagnosed heart failure. *Am J Respir Crit Care Med*. 2011 Feb 15;183(4):539-546.

Treatment of Obstructive Sleep Apnea in Heart Failure

Treatment of OSA, as discussed, also applies to patients with OSA and HF. However, improving cardiopulmonary function by guideline-based therapy of HF is the first-line approach.

As in the general population, the treatment of choice for OSA is the use of CPAP. In the observational study of the Medicare beneficiaries, treatment of OSA with CPAP reduced hospital readmission, health-related costs, and mortality in those treated with CPAP, compared with untreated subjects (Fig. 60–12).[139] Expectedly, mortality is lowest in those who are adherent to CPAP.[140,141] Notably, no RCTs are available using any therapeutic options for treatment of OSA in HF and are increasingly needed.

Treatment of edema in HF is of importance given the state of extracellular volume overload, salt, and fluid retention and presence of lower extremity edema. As aforementioned, in the supine position, fluid from the lower extremities is absorbed and transported intravascularly cephalad causing pharyngeal vascular congestion and narrowing, facilitating upper airway occlusion during sleep.[34,127] Furthermore, in some subjects, the presence of right ventricular dysfunction and elevated right atrial and central venous pressure additionally contributes to pharyngeal vascular congestion and edema. Therefore, an appropriate therapeutic approach to decrease lower extremity edema and venous congestion is advisable.

Multiple studies have shown regular supervised exercise improves snoring and OSA via multiple mechanisms reviewed elsewhere.[3,34] This is the case for OSA the general population[102] and OSA associated with HF.[142] In a four-arm RCT involving patients with OSA and comorbid HF, comparing the baseline versus 3 months, the AHI did not change much in the control group, but decreased significantly in the exercise group from an average of 28 to 18 events per hour of sleep ($P < 0.03$) with minimal change in body weight.[143] Furthermore, compared with the control group, improvements in the quality-of-life scores were significant only in the exercise and exercise with CPAP groups ($P < 0.05$). The postulated mechanisms of the therapeutic effects of exercise include decreased rostral fluid redistribution, stabilization of chemoreceptor sensitivity, improved nasal resistance and strength of pharyngeal dilator muscles, weight loss, and improved sleep quality.[3] Obviously, multimodal therapeutic regimens may have advantages over single point targeted treatment and, therefore, such combined interventions should be routinely recommended to subjects with OSA. Phenotype-guided therapy of OSA is a topic of great interest, but no large systematic trial has been reported.[87]

Heart Failure and Central Sleep Apnea

In the general population, CSA is rare, except in those with HFrEF, AF, stroke, and in patients taking opioids. In HFrEF, CSA occurs in the context of periodic breathing characterized by a repetitive pattern of crescendo-decrescendo ventilation (Fig. 60–13). This pattern is commonly referred to as Cheyne–Stokes breathing (CSB), while the term Hunter–Cheyne–Stokes breathing (HCSB) would be more appropriate, because Hunter

published a case with this breathing pattern almost 37 years before Cheyne's description.[3,144] This unique pattern is a manifestation of instability in breathing during NREM sleep[137] and in prolonged effective circulation time that increases the cycle of periodic breathing.

As aforementioned, both OSA and CSA are common comorbidities with HF, and both subtypes of sleep apnea frequently occur simultaneously when polysomnography is performed. There are some similarities and dissimilarities between the two apneas. As with OSA, CSA is associated with intermittent arousals, hypoxemia/reoxygenation, changes in PCO_2, and negative swings in intrathoracic/juxtacardiac pressure (Fig. 60–2). However, the latter two consequences are less severe with CSA than with OSA. In CSA, the negative swings occur at the peak of hyperventilation, and these swings are relatively large, proportional to the severity of congestion of the respiratory system. In OSA, the large negative swings occur during the apnea itself, as the inspiratory muscles contract in the face of pharyngeal closure.

Another important difference between CSA and OSA is that CSA is primarily a NREM sleep disorder, being rare in REM sleep, in sharp contrast to OSA, which is more permanent and frequently longer in duration in REM sleep. Another difference between the two disorders is the timing of the microarousals that occur at the peak of hyperventilation in CSA, and just at the termination of OSA when the upper airway opens and ventilation resumes.

Important similarities shared by both OSA and CSA are that both apnea subtypes lead to sustained sympathetic overactivity, creating a hyperadrenergic state (Fig. 60–14). In disorders in which sympathetic overactivity already exists, this additional challenge has been shown to carry a poor prognosis. Similar to OSA, CSA is associated with hospital readmissions[138] and premature mortality in observational studies of patients with HFrEF.[10,145] In one of these studies,[10] CSA independently increased the risk of premature death by 150%, compared to those without CSA. In the largest study, in which more than 900 patients with HFrEF were followed for up to 10 years, among a few variables, oxyhemoglobin desaturation was independently associated with premature death.[145] Time with oxygen saturation <90% (T90) predicted the risk of death in a dose-dependent manner, namely an increase of 16% per hour of time below 90%. A similar correlation has been reported in patients with acute decompensated HF.[146]

Atrial Fibrillation and Central Sleep Apnea

SDB and AF also exhibit a bidirectional relationship, with OSA as a cause of AF, and AF as a cause of CSA. In HFrEF, AF is the most common comorbidity heralding presence of CSA.[129] CSA is also observed in polysomnography in subjects with AF without presence of LV dysfunction. In a study of 150 patients with AF and normal LVEF, CSA was observed in 31% of the patients.[147] Further, the presence of polysomnographic CSA heralds incident AF.[148,149] In these individuals, CSA presumably reflects early structural heart disease, which is asymptomatic when polysomnography was performed.

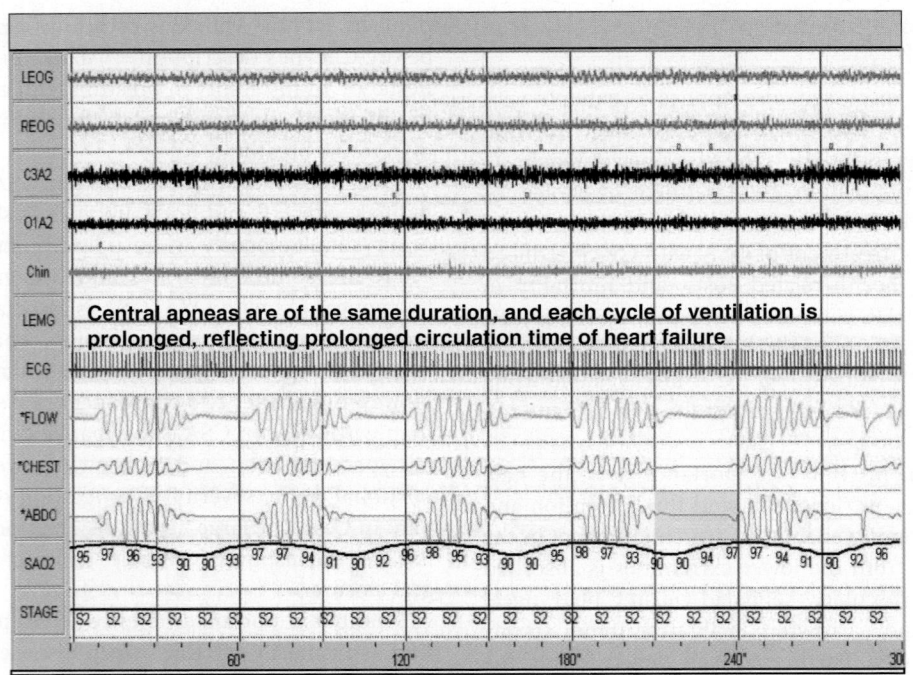

Figure 60–13. **Polysomnographic example of Hunter–Cheyne–Stokes breathing.** Tracings are: electro-oculogram (EOG, 1st and 2nd); chin electromyogram (EMG, 3rd); electroencephalogram (EEG, 4th and 5th); ECG (7th); airflow measured by thermocouple (8th) and CO_2 (9th); combined (10th) rib cage (RC) and abdominal (ABD); RC (11th) and ABD (12th) excursions; time in seconds (13th); and esophageal pressure (14th). Note the smooth and gradual changes in the thoracoabdominal excursions and esophageal pressure in the crescendo and decrescendo arms of the cycle. There is an intervening central apnea, absence of naso-oral airflow and excursions in pleural pressure, thorax, and abdomen. The arousal occurs at the peak of hyperventilation. Desaturation is delayed because of long circulation time in heart failure.

Importantly, in a small study in a subset of participants of the SERVE-HF RCT,[150] the change in the AF burden from baseline to follow-up was –16% with ASV versus +24% with usual care ($P = 0.03$),[58] suggesting that treatment of sleep apnea could improve AF burden.

The mechanism underlying AF causing CSA is probably related to increased left atrial pressure and pulmonary capillary pressure increasing the propensity to periodic breathing. This premise is based on experiments in naturally sleeping dogs in which an elevated atrial pressure (via a balloon in the left atrium) resulted in narrowing the PCO_2 reserve thus facilitating the development of CSA.[151]

In summary, OSA is a potential cause of AF, whereas CSA is present in subjects with AF, and also when observed polysomnographically in individuals without AF or known HF, may herald future AF.

Sleep-Disordered Breathing in Heart Failure with Preserved Ejection Fraction

So far, we have presented data on SDB in HFrEF, because HFrEF has been the most intensely studied. However, SDB are also common in subjects with LV dysfunction with and without the HF syndrome (Fig. 60–11). There are two studies in HFpEF involving a total of 263 consecutive patients that showed that 47% had sleep apnea (AHI ≥15): 24% OSA and 23% CSA.[147,152] There are no large systematic studies on HFpEF in the US population, and in our experience, OSA, rather than CSA, is most common.

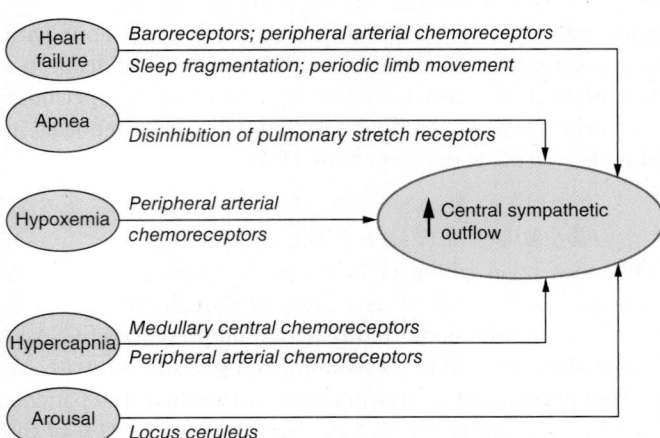

Figure 60–14. **Effects of heart failure and sleep apnea on central sympathetic outflow.** Heart failure is a hyperadrenergic state. Sleep apnea further contributes to increased central sympathetic outflow. Locus ceruleus is the brain stem arousal network, and norepinephrine is the neurotransmitter.

Treatment of Central Sleep Apnea in Heart Failure

LV dysfunction is the most common cause of CSA, and CSA is frequently observed on polysomnography of subjects with symptomatic or asymptomatic LV dysfunction, both with reduced and preserved ejection fraction, although most commonly in HFrEF.

The modalities of therapy of CSA in HF are depicted in **Table 60–2** and have been discussed in detail.[137] Optimization

TABLE 60-2. Treatment of Central Sleep Apnea in Heart Failure with Reduced Ejection Function

- Maximize medical therapy
- Pharmacotherapy of heart failure
- Cardiac resynchronization therapy (CRT)
- Adaptive servo ventilation (ASV) (SERVE-HF trial; ADVENT-HF trial)
- Continuous positive airway pressure (CPAP) devices
- Cardiac transplantation
- Phrenic nerve stimulation
- Nocturnal oxygen
- Acetazolamide
- Theophylline

of cardiopulmonary function has been shown to improve CSA, therefore optimization of guideline-directed HF therapy is the gold-standard therapy for CSA at this point.

Cardiac Resynchronization Therapy

When indicated, cardiac resynchronization therapy (CRT) could improve cardiac function and with that CSA improves. A meta-analysis[88] of CRT trials in patients with HFrEF demonstrated improvement in CSA, but not OSA.[153] CSA improves in those in whom CRT improves cardiac function suggesting HFrEF is causative.

Continuous Positive Airway Pressure Devices

CPAP therapy improves CSA in about 40% to 50% of subjects with HFrEF. In one study, overnight treatment with CPAP improved CSA in about 40% of the subjects and this was associated with reduced ventricular arrhythmias during sleep, a finding in contrast to those in whom CPAP did not suppress CSA.[154] It was suggested that improvement of CSA was associated with reduced sympathetic activity mediating improvement in arrhythmias. This is supported by a randomized trial demonstrating that attenuation of CSA by CPAP was associated with decreases of plasma and urinary norepinephrine.[155]

In the largest RCT with two arms, enrolling subjects with severe HFrEF, comparing subjects with severe CSA using CPAP to the usual care, the control group, treatment with CPAP did not improve survival.[156] However, CPAP therapy was not effective in 53% of the patients, consistent with the results of the acute study. In the post hoc analysis, significant improvement in survival was observed in patients whose AHI was suppressed AHI decreasing to below 15/hour) by CPAP,[157] presumably in part due to improvement in ventricular arrhythmias.[155] In view of uniform lack of efficacy of CPAP, adaptive servo-ventilation (ASV) was invented and clinically assessed as described next.

Adaptive Servo-Ventilation

Adaptive servo-ventilation (ASV) is a positive airway pressure device controlled by a dedicated electronic algorithm to provide varying inspiratory pressure support (IPS = inspiratory pressure minus expiratory pressure), anticyclic (ie, out of phase) to the periodic breathing seen in HF patients. The ASV algorithm is different from CPAP, which provides constant pressure all the time. Aside from the anticyclic variable IPS, current ASV devices have two other virtues, an automatic expiratory positive airway pressure (EPAP) algorithm capable of stabilizing

the upper airway to eliminate obstructive events when they occur, and a mandatory timed back-up mode to abort impending central apneas.[158] Many observational and some small RCTs showed efficacy of ASV in treating CSA.[137] Surprisingly, in the SERVE-HF study—the largest RCT trial so far—not only did ASV fail to show efficacy across the board, it significantly increased CV mortality.[150] Investigators hypothesized that either CSA is adaptive and therefore should not be treated, or the increased intrathoracic pressure imposed by ASV resulted in harmful hemodynamic consequences eventually leading to premature mortality.

Based on adverse cardiovascular consequences of CSA (hypoxemia, arousals, and increased sympathetic activity previously discussed), it has been emphasized that CSA is maladaptive rather than adaptive.[159] Multiple factors[160] including inappropriate pressure delivery with the use of an outdated algorithm of the ASV apparatus, residual SDB, and hypoxemia could have contributed to premature deaths reported in the SERVE-HF trial.

There is an ongoing study (the ADVENT-HF trial) using an ASV device with an improved algorithm.[161] The results of this study will be published after 2021. Thus far, no signs of premature mortality have become apparent with this device.

Phrenic Nerve Stimulation

Unilateral phrenic nerve stimulation has been approved by the FDA for treatment of CSA. In an RCT, 151 patients with predominant CSA of various etiologies were implanted and randomized to phrenic nerve stimulation or sham (device was implanted but not turned on) for 6 months.[162] In patients in whom the device was active, AHI, central apnea index, arousal index, and oxygen desaturation index improved significantly. Along with improvement in sleep metrics, quality of life and daytime sleepiness also significantly improved. The most common side effect was therapy-related discomfort that was resolved with reprogramming in most. Local side effects, such as infection and dislodgment occurred in 13 of 151 implanted patients. Sustained effects have been observed for up to 36 months.[163] However, long-term trials with mortality as an endpoint are not available as yet.

Drug Therapy for Central Sleep Apnea

Oxygen, acetazolamide, and theophylline have been used to treat CSA in observational and RCTs of subjects with HFrEF. Two small RCTs have been performed, one with acetazolamide[164,165] and one with theophylline.[166] In these two crossover trials, both of short duration, CSA improved.[164–166] However, no data from long-term studies are available.

Nocturnal low-flow oxygen has been used extensively. Two early RCTs, using low-flow nocturnal oxygen versus room air showed significant improvement in CSA and oxyhemoglobin desaturation.[167,168] One RCT showed that treatment with oxygen, compared to room air also decreased overnight urinary catecholamine secretion.[168] Two unblended RCTs have shown that compared to placebo, treatment of CSA with oxygen improves quality of life of HF patients.[169,170] Other effects of treating CSA with nocturnal oxygen include decreased muscle sympathetic activity, and improved maximum oxygen consumption during exercise (reviewed elsewhere).[171] Based on these results and the failure of positive airway pressure devices, a phase 3 long-term RCT with O_2 therapy versus room air has been funded by the National Institutes of Health in the United States (LOFT-HF trial). The composite endpoint of the study is rehospitalization and mortality. The study is ongoing and results of this 5-year trial will be available after 2023.

SLEEP DISORDERS IN CARDIAC TRANSPLANT RECIPIENTS

It may be anticipated that cardiac transplantation improves sleep and SDB noted in subjects with HFrEF. Surprisingly, for multiple reasons, sleep is quite disturbed in cardiac transplant recipients (**Fig. 60–15**). In the largest prospective and most systematic study so far reported,[172] 45 of 60 consecutive patients agreed to undergo polysomnography. Subjects were at least 5 months posttransplant, receiving a maintenance dose of prednisone (5 to 10 mg daily), and antirejection medications including cyclosporine. As previously discussed, sleep is compromised in patients with HFrEF, and it was anticipated that with transplantation, quality of sleep should improve. In contrast, polysomnography showed that disturbed sleep architecture reduced sleep efficiency of about 72%, with a large amount of N1 and presence of OSA; 36% of participants had moderate-to-severe OSA with an obstructive AHI of 15 or more per hour.[172] Consistent with obesity being the major risk factor for OSA, patients who had gained the most weight were found to have OSA. These subjects snored habitually, complained of unrefreshing sleep, impaired quality of life (based on the SF-36 questionnaire), and excessive daytime sleepiness. Systemic

hypertension was prevalent in OSA subjects and at the time of the study, one patient had developed LV systolic dysfunction, potentially related to rejection and the impact of SDB. Meanwhile, a small retrospective study involving 29 consecutive cardiac transplant recipients,[173] 20% with untreated OSA, had a three times higher risk of developing late graft dysfunction than those with treated or no OSA.

Cardiac transplant recipients should be checked for development of OSA, particularly those who gain weight, snore, and develop hypertension and rejection, and be treated accordingly.

SUMMARY

Sleep has profound effects on the cardiovascular system. Normally, as sleep deepens from N1 to N3, both systolic and diastolic BP, heart rate, and metabolic rate decrease. Sleep decreases cardiac workload allowing restoration of myocytes while asleep. The phasic REM sleep, however, could cause hemodynamic instability and nondemand myocardial ischemia. However, at the same time, loss of wakefulness input places a healthy ventilatory control system in jeopardy with increased upper airway collapsibility predisposing subjects with anatomically small pharyngeal airways to OSA. Simultaneously, sleep unmasks a very sensitive apneic threshold PCO_2. Therefore, if the prevailing PCO_2 decreases below the apneic threshold PCO_2, ventilation ceases and apnea ensues. These obstructive and central sleep apneas not only adversely affect quality of life but also have adverse consequences on cardiocerebrovascular systems.

OSA is a common cause of CVD including hypertension, HF, coronary artery disease, arrhythmias, and stroke. Whereas OSA can be a cause of HF, HF by itself, and particularly HFrEF,

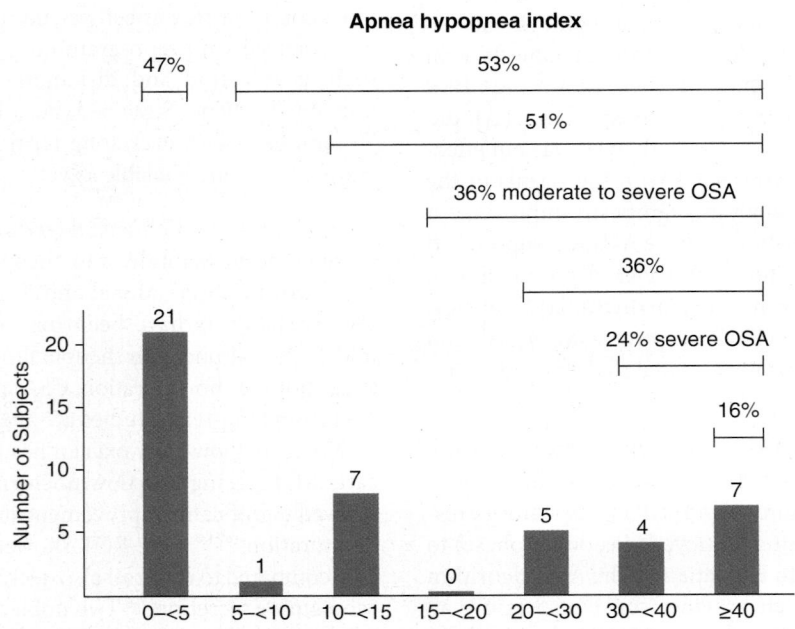

Figure 60–15. Prevalence of obstructive sleep apnea in 45 out of 60 consecutive cardiac transplant recipients. Those who developed sleep apnea had gained the most weight after transplantation. Reproduced with permission from Javaheri S, Abraham WT, Brown C, et al. Prevalence of obstructive sleep apnoea and periodic limb movement in 45 subjects with heart transplantation. *Eur Heart J*. 2004 Feb;25(3):260-266..

causes CSA. Expectedly, cardiac transplantation virtually eliminates CSA, but recipients are prone to gain weight and develop OSA.

RCTs have failed to show beneficial effects of treating OSA with CPAP on hard cardiovascular outcomes. However, in all these studies, the adherence with CPAP was low, potentially accounting for neutral results. And multiple RCT studies have shown that only adequate use of CPAP decreases BP and insulin resistance.

CSA is quite common in LV dysfunction, particularly in HFrEF. Treatment of CSA remains a challenge. Multiple therapeutic options including use of oxygen, acetazolamide, theophylline, CPAP, ASV, and phrenic nerve stimulation have demonstrated efficacy. However, both RCTs using CPAP and ASV failed to show efficacy on hard outcomes. The ASV used in the SERVE-HF trial had deficiencies, which may have contributed to premature death. An RCT with an improved ASV is ongoing.

Phrenic nerve stimulation is a promising treatment option that has been approved by the FDA for treatment of CSA. Also, renewed interest in oxygen therapy for the treatment of CSA has been materialized into a long-term, FDA-approved RCT.

- OSA is quite common in the general population and in subjects with various CVDs including hypertension, resistant hypertension, arrhythmias, coronary heart disease, systolic and diastolic HF, and stroke.
- CPAP devices are the treatment of choice for OSA, particularly for those with established CVD.
- RCTs using ambulatory BP monitoring have consistently demonstrated that treatment of OSA with CPAP lowers BP.
- The drop in BP is most pronounced in those with severe OSA, with resistant hypertension, and those who are most adherent to therapy.
- However, RCTs have failed to show that therapy with CPAP improves cardiovascular outcomes, perhaps in part due to poor adherence with CPAP.
- CSA, a rare polysomnographic finding in the general population, is highly prevalent in patients with HF, particularly in those with reduced ejection fraction. A large RCT using an outdated ASV device was neutral. A second large trial with improved ASV algorithm is in progress. Another phase 3 large trial with use of oxygen has begun.
- Unilateral phrenic nerve stimulation has been approved by the FDA, and has shown promising results for treatment of CSA of various causes.

REFERENCES

1. Javaheri S, Barbe F, Campos-Rodriguez F, et al. Sleep apnea: types, mechanisms, and clinical cardiovascular consequences. *J Am Coll Cardiol.* 2017;69(7):841–858. doi: 10.1016/j.jacc.2016.11.069.

2. Egea-Santaolalla C, Javaheri S. Obesity hypoventilation syndrome. *Cur Sleep Med Rep.* 2016;2:12–19. doi: 10.1007/s40675-016-0035-2.

3. Piper AJ, BaHammam AS, Javaheri S. Obesity hypoventilation syndrome: choosing the appropriate treatment for a heterogeneous disorder. *Sleep Med Clin.* 2017;12:587-596.

4. Javaheri S, Patel S. Opioids cause central and complex sleep apnea in humans: reversal with discontinuation. *J Clin Sleep Med.* 2017;13(6):829-833.

5. Berry RB, Budhiraja R, Gottlieb DJ, et al. Rules for scoring respiratory events in sleep: update of the 2007 AASM Manual for the Scoring of Sleep and Associated Events. Deliberations of the Sleep Apnea Definitions Task Force of the American Academy of Sleep Medicine. *J Clin Sleep Med.* 2012;8(5):597-619.

6. Javaheri S, Gay PC. To die, to sleep—to sleep, perchance to dream...without hypertension: dreams of the visionary Christian Guilleminault revisited. *J Clin Sleep Med.* 2019;15(9):1189-1190. doi:10.5664/jcsm.7952.

7. Somers VK, Dyken ME, Mark AL, Abboud FM. Sympathetic-nerve activity during sleep in normal subjects. *N Engl J Med.* 1993;328(5):303-307. doi:10.1056/NEJM199302043280502.

8. Floras JS. Hypertension and sleep apnea. *Can J Cardiol.* 2015;31(7):889-897. doi:10.1016/j.cjca.2015.05.003.

9. Mehra R, Mittleman MA, Verrier RL. Sleep-related cardiac risk. In: Kryger MH, Roth T, Dement WC, eds. *Principles and Practices of Sleep Medicine.* 7th ed. Philadelphia, PA: WB Saunders; 2021.

10. Javaheri S, Shukla R, Zeigler H, Wexler L. Central sleep apnea, right ventricular dysfunction, and low diastolic blood pressure are predictors of mortality in systolic heart failure. *J Am Coll Cardiol.* 2007;49(20):2028-2034. doi:10.1016/j.jacc.2007.01.084.

11. Mokhlesi B, Finn LA, Hagen EW, et al. Obstructive sleep apnea during REM sleep and hypertension. Results of the Wisconsin Sleep Cohort. *Am J Respir Crit Care Med.* 2014;190(10): 1158-1167. doi:10.1164/rccm.201406-1136OC.

12. Ambati A, Ju YE, Lin L, et al. Proteomic biomarkers of sleep apnea. *Sleep J.* 2020;43:1-12.

13. Javaheri S. A mechanism of central sleep apnea in patients with heart failure. *N Eng J Med.* 1999;341:949-954.

14. AASM. Sleep-related breathing disorders. In: Sateia M, ed. *The International Classification of Sleep Disorders.* 3rd ed. Darien, IL, USA: American Academy of Sleep Medicine; 2014:49-141.

15. Pevernagie DA, Gnidovec-Strazisar B, Grote L, et al. On the rise and fall of the apnea-hypopnea index: a historical review and critical appraisal. *J Sleep Res.* 2020;29(4):e13066.

16. Bibbins-Domingo K, Grossman DC, Curry SJ, et al. Screening for obstructive sleep apnea in adults: US Preventive Services Task Force recommendation statement. *JAMA.* 2017;317(4):407-414.

17. Kapur VK, Auckley DH, Chowdhuri S, et al. Clinical practice guideline for diagnostic testing for adult obstructive sleep apnea: an American Academy of Sleep Medicine clinical practice guideline. *J Clin Sleep Med.* 2017;13(3):479-504.

18. Peppard PE, Young T, Barnet JH, et al. Increased prevalence of sleep-disordered breathing in adults. *Am J Epidemiol.* 2013;177:1006-1014.

19. Gottlieb DJ, Punjabi NM. Diagnosis and management of obstructive sleep apnea: a review. *JAMA.* 2020;323(14):1389-1400. doi:10.1001/jama.2020.3514.

20. Lim KG, Morgenthaler TI, Katzka DA. Sleep and nocturnal gastroesophageal reflux: an update. *Chest.* 2018;154(4):963-971. doi:10.1016/j.chest.2018.05.030.

21. Russell MB, Kristiansen HA, Kværner KJ. Headache in sleep apnea syndrome: epidemiology and pathophysiology. *Cephalalgia.* 2014;34(10):752-755. doi:10.1177/0333102414538551.

22. Javaheri S, Javaheri S. Update on persistent excessive daytime sleepiness in OSA. *Chest.* 2020;158(2):776-786.

23. Johns MW. A new method for measuring daytime sleepiness: the Epworth Sleepiness Scale. *Sleep.* 1991;14(6):540-545. doi:10.1093/sleep/14.6.540.

24. Bauters F, Rietzschel ER, Hertegonne KB, et al. The link between obstructive sleep apnea and cardiovascular disease. *Curr Atheroscler Rep.* 2016;18:1.

25. Baltzis D, Bakker JP, Patel SR, et al. Obstructive sleep apnea and vascular diseases. *Compr Physiol.* 2016;6:1519-1528.

26. Kohler M, Stoewhas AC, Ayers L, et al. Effects of continuous positive airway pressure therapy withdrawal in patients with obstructive sleep apnea: a randomized controlled trial. *Am J Respir Crit Care Med.* 2011;184:1192-1199.

27. Moreno-Indias I, Torres M, Sanchez-Alcoholado L, et al. Normoxic recovery mimicking treatment of sleep apnea does not reverse intermittent hypoxia-induced bacterial dysbiosis and low-grade endotoxemia in mice. *Sleep.* 2016;39(10):1891-1897.

28. Yang W, Shao L, Heizhati M, et al. Oropharyngeal microbiome in obstructive sleep apnea: decreased diversity and abundance. *J Clin Sleep Med.* 2019;15(12):1777-1788.

29. Wu BG, Sulaiman I, Wang J, et al. Severe obstructive sleep apnea is associated with alterations in the nasal microbiome and an increase in inflammation. *Am J Respir Crit Care Med.* 2019;199:99-109.

30. Kim Y-M, Snijders AM, Brislawn CJ, et al. Light-stress influences the composition of the murine gut microbiome, memory function, and plasma metabolome. *Front Mol Biosci.* 2019;6:108.

31. Lin A, Shih C-T, Huang C-L, Wu C-C, Lin C-T, Tsai Y-C. Hypnotic effects of PS150 on pentobarbital-induced sleep in mice. *Nutrients.* 2019;11(10):2409.

32. Smith RP, Easson C, Lyle SM, et al. Gut microbiome diversity is associated with sleep physiology in humans. *PLoS One.* 2019;14(10):e0222394.

33. Campos-Rodriguez F, Martínez-García MA, Mohsenin V, Javaheri S. Systemic and pulmonary hypertension in obstructive sleep apnea. In: Principles and Practices of Sleep Medicine, 7/e. Edited by Kryger MH; WB Saunders, Philadelphia.2021.

34. Lyon OD, Bradley TD. Heart failure and sleep apnea. *Can J Cardiol.* 2015;31(7):898-908. doi:10.1016/j.cjca.2015.04.017.

35. O'Connor GT, Caffo B, Newman AB, et al. Prospective study of sleep-disordered breathing and hypertension: the Sleep Heart Health Study. *Am J Respir Crit Care Med.* 2019; 179(12):1159-1164. doi:10.1164/rccm.200712-1809OC.

36. Pedrosa RP, Drager LF, Gonzaga CC, et al. Obstructive sleep apnea: the most common secondary cause of hypertension associated with resistant hypertension. *Hypertension.* 2011;58:811-817.

37. Hu X, Fan J, Chen S, Yin Y, Zrenner B. The role of continuous positive airway pressure in blood pressure control for patients with obstructive sleep apnea and hypertension: a meta-analysis of randomized controlled trials. *J Clin Hypertens.* 2015;17:215-222.

38. Iftikhar IH, Valentine CW, Bittencourt LRA, et al. Effects of continuous positive airway pressure on blood pressure in patients with resistant hypertension and obstructive sleep apnea: a meta-analysis. *J Hypertens.* 2014;32:2341-2350.

39. Campos-Rodriguez F, Navarro-Soriano C, Reyes-Nuñez N, et al. Good long-term adherence to continuous positive airway pressure therapy in patients with resistant hypertension and sleep apnea. *J Sleep Res.* 2019;28(5):e12805.

40. Bassetti CLA. Sleep disordered breathing and stroke. In: Kryger MH, Roth T, Dement WC, eds. *Principles and Practices of Sleep Medicine.* 7th ed. Philadelphia, PA: WB Saunders; 2021.

41. Gami AS, Howard DE, Olson EJ, Somers VK. Day-night pattern of sudden death in obstructive sleep apnea. *N Engl J Med.* 2015;352(12): 1206-1214. doi:10.1056/NEJMoa041832.

42. Gami AS, Olson EJ, Shen WK, et al. Obstructive sleep apnea and the risk of sudden cardiac death: a longitudinal study of 10,701 adults. *J Am Coll Cardiol.* 2013;62(7):610-616.

43. McEvoy RD, Antic NA, Heeley E, et al. CPAP for prevention of cardiovascular events in obstructive sleep apnea. *N Engl J Med.* 2016;375(10): 919-931. doi:10.1056/NEJMoa1606599.

44. Peker Y, Glantz H, Eulenburg C, Wegscheider K, Herlitz J, Thunstrom E. Effect of positive airway pressure on cardiovascular outcomes in coronary artery disease patients with nonsleepy obstructive sleep apnea. The RICCADSA randomized controlled trial. *Am J Respir Crit Care Med.* 2016;194(5):613-620. doi:10.1164/rccm.201601-0088OC.

45. Sanchez-de-la-Torre M, Sanchez-de-la-Torre A, Bertran S, et al. Effect of obstructive sleep apnoea and its treatment with continuous positive airway pressure on the prevalence of cardiovascular events in patients with acute coronary syndrome (ISAACC study): a randomised controlled trial. *Lancet Respir Med.* 2020;8(4):359-367. doi:10.1016/S2213-2600(19)30271-1.

46. Peker Y, Karl A, Franklin KA, Hedner J. coronary artery disease and obstructive sleep apnea. In: Kryger MH, Roth T, Dement WC, eds. *Principles and Practices of Sleep Medicine.* 7th ed. Philadelphia, PA: WB Saunders; 2021.

47. Young T, Finn L, Peppard PE, et al. Sleep disordered breathing and mortality: eighteen-year follow-up of the Wisconsin Sleep Cohort. *Sleep.* 2018;31(8):1071-1078.

48. Punjabi NM, Caffo BS, Goodwin JL, et al. Sleep-disordered breathing and mortality: a prospective cohort study. *PLoS Med.* 2019;6(8):e1000132. doi:10.1371/journal.pmed.1000132.

49. Campos-Rodriguez F, Martinez-Garcia MA, de la Cruz-Moron I, et al. Cardiovascular mortality in women with obstructive sleep apnea with or without continuous positive airway pressure treatment: a cohort study. *Ann Intern Med.* 2012;156(2):115-122.

50. Drager LF, Bortolotto LA, Figueiredo AC, Krieger EM, Lorenzi GF. Effects of continuous positive airway pressure on early signs of atherosclerosis in obstructive sleep apnea. *Am J Respir Crit Care Med.* 2017;176(7):706-712.

51. Yu J, Zhou Z, McEvoy RD, et al. Association of positive airway pressure with cardiovascular events and death in adults with sleep apnea: a systematic review and meta-analysis. *JAMA.* 2017;318:156-166.

52. Javaheri S, Martinez-Garcia MA, Campos-Rodriguez F, Muriel A, Peker Y. Continuous positive airway pressure adherence for prevention of major adverse cerebrovascular and cardiovascular events in obstructive sleep apnea. *Am J Respir Crit Care Med.* 2020;201(5): 607-610. doi:10.1164/rccm.201908-1593LE.

53. Martinez-García MA, Campos-Rodriguez F, Javaheri S, Gozal, D. Pro: continuous positive airway pressure and cardiovascular prevention. *Eur Respir J.* 2018;51:1702400. doi: 10.1183/13993003.02400-2017.

54. Javaheri S, Martinez-Garcia MA, Campos-Rodriguez F. CPAP treatment and cardiovascular prevention: we need to change the design and implementation of our trials. *Chest.* 2019;156(3):431-437. doi:10.1016/j.chest.2019.04.092.

55. Pamidi S, Wroblewski K, Stepien M, et al. Eight hours of nightly continuous positive airway pressure treatment of obstructive sleep apnea improves glucose metabolism in patients with prediabetes. A randomized controlled trial. *Am J Respir Crit Care Med.* 2015;192:96-105.

56. Martinez-Garcia MA, Campos-Rodriguez F, Gozal D. Obstructive sleep apnoea in acute coronary syndrome. *Lancet Respir Med.* 2020,:8(4):e15. doi:10.1016/S2213-2600(20)30040-0.

57. Waldron NH, Fudim M, Mathew JP, Piccini JP. Neuromodulation for the treatment of heart rhythm disorders. *JACC Basic Transl Sci.* 2019;4(4):546-562. doi:10.1016/j.jacbts.2019.02.009.

58. Piccini JP, Pokorney SD, Anstrom KJ, et al. Adaptive servo-ventilation reduces atrial fibrillation burden in patients with heart failure and sleep apnea. *Heart Rhythm.* 2019;16(1):91-97. doi:10.1016/j.hrthm.2018.07.027.

59. Verrier RL, Josephson ME. Impact of sleep on arrhythmogenesis. *Circ Arrhythm Electrophysiol.* 2019;2(4):450-459. doi:10.1161/CIRCEP.109.867028.

60. Bitter T, Fox H, Gaddam S, Horstkotte D, Oldenburg O. Sleep-disordered breathing and cardiac arrhythmias. *Can J Cardiol.* 2015;31(7):928-934. doi:10.1016/j.cjca.2015.04.022.

61. Nowlin JB, Troyer WG Jr, Collins WS, et al. The association of nocturnal angina pectoris with dreaming. *Ann Intern Med.* 1965;63(6):1040-1046. doi:10.7326/0003-4819-63-6-1040.

62. Somers VK, Javaheri SM. Cardiovascular effects of sleep-related breathing disorders. In: Kryger MH, Roth T, Dement WC, eds. *Principles and Practices of Sleep Medicine.* 7th ed. Philadelphia, PA: WB Saunders; 2021.

63. Mehra R, Benjamin EJ, Shahar E, et al. Association of nocturnal arrhythmias with sleep-disordered breathing: The Sleep Heart Health

Study. *Am J Respir Crit Care Med.* 2006;173(8): 910-916. doi:10.1164/rccm.200509-1442OC.

64. Monahan K, Storfer-Isser A, Mehra R, et al. Triggering of nocturnal arrhythmias by sleep-disordered breathing events. *J Am Coll Cardiol.* 2019; 54(19):1797-1804. doi:10.1016/j.jacc.2009.06.038.

65. Lau, DH, Nattel, S, Kalman, JM, Sanders, P. Modifiable riskfactors and atrialfibrillation. *Circulation.* 2017;136:583-596. doi: 10.1161/CIRCULATIONAHA.116.023163.

66. Iwasaki YK, Kato T, Xiong F, et al. Atrial fibrillation promotion with long-term repetitive obstructive sleep apnea in a rat model. *J Am Coll Cardiol.* 2014;64:2013-2023. doi: 10.1016/j.jacc.2014.05.077.

67. Zhao J, Xu W, Yun F, et al. Chronic obstructive sleep apnea causes atrial remodeling in canines: mechanisms and implications. *Basic Res Cardiol.* 2014;109:427. doi: 10.1007/s00395-014-0427-8.

68. May AM, Van Wagoner DR, Mehra R. OSA and cardiac arrhythmogenesis mechanistic insights. *Chest.* 2017;151(1):225-241.

69. Chamberlain AM, Agarwal SK, Ambrose M, Folsom AR, Soliman EZ, Alonso A. Metabolic syndrome and incidence of atrial fibrillation among blacks and whites in the Atherosclerosis Risk in Communities (ARIC) Study. *Am Heart J.* 2010;159:850-856. doi: 10.1016/j.ahj.2010.02.005.

70. Qureshi WT, Nasir UB, Alqalyoobi S, et al. Analysis of continuous positive airway pressure as a therapy of atrial fibrillation in obstructive sleep apnea. *Am J Cardiol.* 2015;116(11): 1767-1773. doi:10.1016/j.amjcard.2015.08.046.

71. Shukla A, Aizer A, Holmes D, Fowler, et al. Effect of obstructive sleep apnea treatment on atrial fibrillation recurrence: a meta-analysis. *JACC Clin Electrophysiol.* 2015;1(1-2):41-51. doi:10.1016/j.jacep.2015.02.014.

72. Calkins H, Kuck KH, Cappato R, et al. 2012 HRS/EHRA/ECAS expert consensus statement on catheter and surgical ablation of atrial fibrillation: recommendations for patient selection, procedural techniques, patient management and follow-up, definitions, endpoints, and research trial design: a report of the Heart Rhythm Society (HRS) Task Force on Catheter and Surgical Ablation of Atrial Fibrillation. Developed in partnership with the European Heart Rhythm Association (EHRA), a registered branch of the European Society of Cardiology (ESC) and the European Cardiac Arrhythmia Society (ECAS); and in collaboration with the American College of Cardiology (ACC), American Heart Association (AHA), the Asia Pacific Heart Rhythm Society (APHRS), and the Society of Thoracic Surgeons (STS). Endorsed by the governing bodies of the American College of Cardiology Foundation, the American Heart Association, the European Cardiac Arrhythmia Society, the European Heart Rhythm Association, the Society of Thoracic Surgeons, the Asia Pacific Heart Rhythm Society, and the Heart Rhythm Society. *Heart Rhythm.* 2012;9(4):632-696.e621. doi:10.1016/j.hrthm.2011.12.016.

73. Javaheri S, Javaheri S, Javaheri A. Sleep apnea, heart failure and pulmonary hypertension. *Curr Heart Fail Rep.* 2013;10:315-320.

74. Arias MA, Garcia-Rio F, Alonso-Fernandez A, Martinez I, Villamor J. Pulmonary hypertension in obstructive sleep apnoea: effects of continuous positive airway pressure: a randomized, controlled cross-over study. *Eur Heart J.* 2006;27(9):1106-1113.

75. Masa JF, Mokhlesi B, Benitez I, et al. echocardiographic changes with positive airway pressure therapy in obesity hypoventilation syndrome. Long-term Pickwick randomized controlled clinical trial. *Am J Respir Crit Care Med.* 2020;201(5):586-597.

76. McLaughlin VV, Archer SL, Badesch DB, et al. ACCF/AHA 2009 expert consensus document on pulmonary hypertension: a report of the American College of Cardiology Foundation Task Force on Expert Consensus Documents and the American Heart Association: developed in collaboration with the American College of Chest Physicians, American Thoracic Society, Inc., and the Pulmonary Hypertension Association. *Circulation.* 2009;119(16):2250-2294.

77. Redline S, Yenokyan G, Gottlieb DJ, et al. Obstructive sleep apnea-hypopnea and incident stroke: the sleep heart health study. *Am J Respir Crit Care Med.* 2010;182(2):269-277. doi:10.1164/rccm.200911-1746OC.

78. Yaggi H, Mohsenin V. Obstructive sleep apnoea and stroke. *Lancet Neurol.* 2004;3(6):333-342.

79. Yaggi HK, Concato J, Kernan WN, Lichtman JH, Brass LM, Mohsenin V. Obstructive sleep apnea as a risk factor for stroke and death. *N Engl J Med.* 2005;353(19):2034-2041.

80. Lyons OW, Ryan CM. Sleep apnea and stroke. *Can J Cardiol.* 2015;31:918-927.

81. Parra O, Sánchez-Armengol Á, Capote F, et al. Efficacy of continuous positive airway pressure treatment on 5-year survival in patients with ischaemic stroke and obstructive sleep apnea: a randomized controlled trial. *J Sleep Res.* 2015;24:7-53.

82. Catalan-Serra P, Campos-Rodriguez F, Reyes-Nunez N, et al. Increased incidence of stroke, but not coronary heart disease, in elderly patients with sleep apnea. *Stroke.* 2019;50(2):491-494. doi:10.1161/STROKEAHA.118.023353.

83. Balfors EM, Franklin KA. Impairment of cerebral perfusion during obstructive sleep apneas. *Am J Respir Crit Care Med.* 1994;150:1587-1591.

84. Lipford MC, Flemming KD, Calvin AD, et al. Associations between cardioembolic stroke and obstructive sleep apnea. *Sleep.* 2015;38:1699-1705.

85. Ciccone A, Proserpio P, Roccatagliata DV, et al. Wake-up stroke and TIA due to paradoxical embolism during long obstructive sleep apnoeas: a cross-sectional study. *Thorax.* 2013;68(1):97-104.

86. Kernan WN, Ovbiagele B, Black HR, et al. for the American Heart Association Stroke Council, Council on Cardiovascular and Stroke Nursing, Council on Clinical Cardiology, and Council on Peripheral Vascular Disease. Guidelines for the prevention of stroke in patients with stroke and transient ischemic attack: a guideline for healthcare professionals from the American Heart Association/American Stroke Association. *Stroke.* 2014;45:2160-2236.

87. Javaheri S, Brown LK, Abraham WT, Khayat R. Apneas of heart failure and phenotype-guided treatments: part one: OSA. *Chest.* 2020;157(2):394-402. doi:10.1016/j.chest.2019.02.407.

88. Edwards BA, Andara C, Landry S, et al. Upper-airway collapsibility and loop gain predict the response to oral appliance therapy in patients with obstructive sleep apnea. *Am J Respir Crit Care Med.* 2016;194(11):1413-1422. doi:10.1164/rccm. 201601-0099OC.

89. Ramar K, Dort LC, Katz SG, et al. Clinical practice guideline for the treatment of obstructive sleep apnea and snoring with oral appliance therapy: an up-date for 2015. *J Clin Sleep Med.* 2015; 11:773-827.

90. Bratton DJ, Gaisl T, Wons AM. CPAP vs mandibular advancement devices and blood pressure in patients with obstructive sleep apnea a systematic review and meta-analysis. *JAMA.* 2015; 314:2280-2293.

91. Gagnadoux F, Pépin J-L, Vielle B, et al. Impact of mandibular advancement therapy on endothelial function in severe obstructive sleep apnea. *Am J Respir Crit Care Med.* 2017;195:1244-1252.

92. Schwartz AR, Bennett ML, Smith PL, et al. Therapeutic electrical stimulation of the hypoglossal nerve in obstructive sleep apnea. *Arch Otolaryngol Head Neck Surg.* 2001;127:1216-1223.

93. Strollo PJ Jr, Soose RJ, Maurer JT, et al. Upper-airway stimulation for obstructive sleep apnea. *N Engl J Med.* 2014;370(2):139-149. doi:10.1056/NEJMoa1308659.

94. Woodson T, Soose RJ, Gillespie, MB, et al. Three-year outcomes of cranial nerve stimulation for obstructive sleep apnea: the star trial. *Otolaryngol Head Neck Surg.* 2015;154:1-8.

95. Eastwood PR, Barnes M, MacKay SG, et al. Bilateral hypoglossal nerve stimulation for treatment of adult obstructive sleep apnoea. *Eur Respir J.* 2020;55(1):1901320. doi:10.1183/ 13993003.01320-2019.

96. He B, Al-Sherif M, Nido M, et al. Domiciliary use of transcutaneous electrical stimulation for patients with obstructive sleep apnoea: a conceptual framework for the TESLA home programme. *J Thorac Dis.* 2019;11(5):2153-2164. doi:10.21037/jtd. 2019.05.04.

97. Mador MJ, Kufel TJ, Magalang UJ, et al. Prevalence of positional sleep apnea in patients undergoing polysomnography. *Chest.* 2005;128:2130-2137.

98. Randerath WJ, Verbraecken J, Andreas S, et al. Non-CPAP therapies in obstructive sleep apnea. *Eur Respir J.* 2011;37:1000-1028.

99. Permut I, Diaz-Abad M, Chatila W, et al. Comparison of positional therapy to CPAP in patients with positional obstructive sleep apnea. *J Clin Sleep Med.* 2010;6(3):238-243.

100. Srijithesh PR, Aghoram R, Goel A, Dhanya J. Positional therapy for obstructive sleep apnoea. *Cochrane Database Syst Rev.* 2019; 5(5):CD010990.

101. van Maanen JP, de Vries N. Long-term effectiveness and compliance of positional therapy with the Sleep Position Trainer in the treatment of positional obstructive sleep apnea syndrome. *Sleep.* 2014;37:1209-1215.

102. Iftikhar IH, Kline CE, Youngstedt SD. Effects of exercise training on sleep apnea: a meta-analysis. *Lung.* 2014;192(1):175-184. doi:10.1007/s00408-013-9511-3.

103. Cornelissen VA, Fagard RH. Effects of endurance training on blood pressure, blood pressure-regulating mechanisms, and cardiovascular risk factors. *Hypertension.* 2005;46:667-675.

104. Bhella PS, Hastings JL, Fujimoto N, et al. Impact of lifelong exercise "dose" on left ventricular compliance and distensibility. *J Am Coll Cardiol.* 2014;64:1257-1266.

105. Malmo V, Nes BM, Amundsen BH, et al. Aerobic interval training reduces the burden of atrial fibrillation in the short term: a randomized trial. *Circulation.* 2016; 133:466-473.

106. Uchoa CHG, Pedrosa RP, Javaheri S, et al. OSA and prognosis after acute cardiogenic pulmonary edema: the OSA-CARE Study. *Chest.* 2017;152(6):1230-1238. doi:10.1016/j.chest.2017.08.003.

107. Awad KM, Malhotra A, Barnet JH, Quan SF, Peppard PE. Exercise is associated with a reduced incidence of sleep-disordered breathing. *Am J Med.* 2012;125:485-490.

108. Li YL, Ding Y, Agnew C, Schultz HD. Exercise training improves peripheral chemoreflex function in heart failure rabbits. *J Appl Physiol.* 2008;105:782-790.

109. O'Donnell DE, McGuire M, Samis L, et al. General exercise training improves ventilatory and peripheral muscle strength and endurance in chronic airflow limitation. *Am J Respir Crit Care Med.* 1998;157:1489-1497.

110. Taranto-Montemurro L, Arnulf I, Similowski T, et al. Attenuation of obstructive sleep apnea and overnight rostral fluid shift by physical activity. *Am J Respir Crit Care Med.* 2015;191:85-858.

111. Chin K, Shimizu K, Nakamura T, et al. Changes in intra-abdominal visceral fat and serum leptin levels in patients with obstructive sleep apnea syndrome following nasal continuous positive airway pressure therapy. *Circulation.* 1999;100:706-712.

112. Hudgel DW, Patel SR, Ahasic AM, et al; American Thoracic Society Assembly on Sleep and Respiratory Neurobiology. The role of weight management in the treatment of adult obstructive sleep apnea: an official American Thoracic Society clinical practice guideline. *Am J Respir Crit Care Med.* 2018;198(6):e70-e87. doi:10.1164/rccm.201807-1326ST.

113. Foster GD, Borradaile KE, Sanders MH, et al; Sleep AHEAD Research Group of Look AHEAD Research Group. A randomized study on the effect of weight loss on obstructive sleep apnea among obese patients with type 2 diabetes: the Sleep AHEAD study. *Arch Intern Med.* 2009;169(17):1619-1626. doi:10.1001/archinternmed.2009.266.

114. Chirinos JA, Gurubhagavatula I, Teff K, et al. CPAP, weight loss, or both for obstructive sleep apnea. *N Engl J Med.* 2014;370(24):2265-2275. doi:10.1056/NEJMoa1306187.

115. Lin H, Xiong H, Ji C. Upper airway lengthening caused by weight increase in obstructive sleep apnea patients. *Respir Res.* 2020;21(1):272. doi: 10.1186/s12931-020-01532-8.

116. Tuomilehto H, Seppä J, Uusitupa M. Obesity and obstructive sleep apnea—clinical significance of weight loss. *Sleep Med Rev.* 2013 17(5):321-329.

117. Johansson K, Neovius M, Lagerros YT, et al. Effect of a very low energy diet on moderate and severe obstructive sleep apnoea in obese men: a randomized controlled trial. *BMJ.* 2009; 339:4609.

118. Grunstein RR, Stenlof K, Hedner JA, et al. Two-year reduction in sleep apnea symptoms and associated diabetes incidence after weight loss in severe obesity. *Sleep.* 2007;30:703-710.

119. Ng SSS, Chan RSM, Woo J, et al. A randomized controlled study to examine the effect of a lifestyle modification program in OSA. *Chest.* 2015;148:1193-1203.

120. Drager LF, Brunoni AR, Jenner R, Lorenzi-Filho G, Bensenor IM, Lotufo PA. Effects of CPAP on body weight in patients with obstructive sleep apnoea: a meta-analysis of randomised trials. *Thorax.* 2015;70(3):258-264. doi:10.1136/thoraxjnl-2014-205361.

121. Tachikawa R, Ikeda K, Minami T, et al. Changes in energy metabolism after continuous positive airway pressure for obstructive sleep apnea. *Am J Respir Crit Care Med.* 2016;194(6):729-738. doi:10.1164/rccm.201511-2314OC.

122. Javaheri S, Shukla R, Wexler L. Association of smoking, sleep apnea and plasma alkalosis with nocturnal ventricular arrhythmias in men with systolic heart failure. *Chest.* 2012;141:1449-1456.

123. Roizenblatt S, Guilleminault C, Poyares D, Cintra F, Kauati A, Tufik S. A double-blind, placebo-controlled, crossover study of sildenafil in obstructive sleep apnea. *Arch Intern Med.* 2006;166(16):1763-1767.

124. Javaheri S, Randerath WJ. Opioids-induced central sleep apnea: mechanisms therapies. *Sleep Med Clin.* 2014;9:49-56.

125. Cao M, Javaheri S. Chronic opioid use: Effects on respiration and sleep. In: Tvildiani D, Gegechkori K, eds. *Opioids Pharmacology, Clinical Uses and Adverse Effects.* New York: Nova Science Publishers; 2012:1-13.

126. Arora N, Cao M, Javaheri S. Opioids, sedatives, and sleep hypoventilation. *Sleep Med Clin.* 2014;9:391-398.

127. Shepard JW Jr, Pevernagie DA, Stanson AW, Daniels BK, Sheedy PF. Effects of changes in central venous pressure on upper airway size in patients with obstructive sleep apnea. *Am J Respir Crit Care Med.* 1996;153(1):250-254. doi:10.1164/ajrccm.153.1.8542124.

128. Gottlieb DJ, Yenokyan G, Newman AB, et al. Prospective study of obstructive sleep apnea and incident coronary heart disease and heart failure: the sleep heart health study. *Circulation.* 2010;122(4):352-360. doi:10.1161/CIRCULATIONAHA.109.901801.

129. Javaheri S. Sleep disorders in systolic heart failure: a prospective study of 100 male patients. The final report. *Int J Cardiol.* 2006;106(1):21-28. doi:10.1016/j.ijcard.2004.12.068.

130. Javaheri S, Parker TJ, Liming JD, et al. Sleep apnea in 81 ambulatory male patients with stable heart failure. Types and their prevalences, consequences, and presentations. *Circulation.* 1998;97(21):2154-2159. doi:10.1161/01.cir.97.21.2154.

131. Javaheri S, Parker TJ, Wexler L, et al. Occult sleep-disordered breathing in stable congestive heart failure. *Ann Intern Med.* 1995;122(7):487-492. doi:10.7326/0003-4819-122-7-199504010-00002.

132. Kato N, Kinugawa K, Shiga T, et al. Depressive symptoms are common and associated with adverse clinical outcomes in heart failure with reduced and preserved ejection fraction. *J Cardiol.* 2012;60(1):23-30. doi:10.1016/j.jjcc.2012.01.010.

133. Arendt J, Bojkowski C, Franey C, Wright J, Marks V. Immunoassay of 6-hydroxymelatonin sulfate in human plasma and urine: abolition of the urinary 24-hour rhythm with atenolol. *J Clin Endocrinol Metab.* 1985;60(6):1166-1173. doi:10.1210/jcem-60-6-1166.

134. Mehra R, Wang L, Andrews N, et al. dissociation of objective and subjective daytime sleepiness and biomarkers of systemic inflammation in sleep-disordered breathing and systolic heart failure. *J Clin Sleep Med.* 2017;13(12):1411-1422. doi:10.5664/jcsm.6836.

135. Hanly P, Zuberi-Khokhar N. Daytime sleepiness in patients with congestive heart failure and Cheyne-Stokes respiration. *Chest.* 1995;107(4):952-958. doi:10.1378/chest.107.4.952.

136. Pepperell JC, Maskell NA, Jones DR, et al. A randomized controlled trial of adaptive ventilation for Cheyne-Stokes breathing in heart failure. *Am J Respir Crit Care Med.* 2003;168(9):1109-1114. doi:10.1164/rccm.200212-1476OC.

137. Javaheri S, Brown LK, Khayat RN. Update on apneas of heart failure with reduced ejection fraction: emphasis on the physiology of treatment: part 2: central sleep apnea. *Chest.* 2020. doi:10.1016/j.chest.2019.12.020.

138. Khayat R, Jarjoura D, Porter K, et al. Sleep disordered breathing and post-discharge mortality in patients with acute heart failure. *Eur Heart J.* 2015;36(23):1463-1469. doi:10.1093/eurheartj/ehu522.

139. Javaheri S, Caref EB, Chen E, Tong KB, Abraham WT. Sleep apnea testing and outcomes in a large cohort of Medicare beneficiaries with newly diagnosed heart failure. *Am J Respir Crit Care Med.* 2011;183(4):539-546. doi:10.1164/rccm.201003-0406OC.

140. Kasai T, Narui K, Dohi T. Prognosis of patients with heart failure and obstructive sleep apnea treated with continuous positive airway pressure. *Chest.* 2008;133(3):690-696. doi:10.1378/chest.07-1901.

141. Wang H, Parker JD, Newton GE, et al. Influence of obstructive sleep apnea on mortality in patients with heart failure. *J Am Coll Cardiol.* 2007;49(15):1625-1631. doi:10.1016/j.jacc.2006.12.046.

142. Ueno LM, Drager LF, Rodrigues AC, et al. Effects of exercise training in patients with chronic heart failure and sleep apnea. *Sleep.* 2007;32(5):637-647. doi:10.1093/sleep/32.5.637.

143. Servantes DM, Javaheri S, Kravchychyn ACP, et al. Effects of exercise training and cpap in patients with heart failure and OSA: a preliminary study. *Chest.* 2018;154(4):808-817. doi:10.1016/j.chest.2018.05.011.

144. Javaheri, S. Heart failure. In: M Kryger, T Roth, WC Dement, eds. *Principles and Practices of Sleep Medicine.* 6th ed. Philadelphia, PA: Elsevier; 2017:1271-1285.

145. Oldenburg O, Wellmann B, Buchholz A, et al. Nocturnal hypoxaemia is associated with increased mortality in stable heart failure patients. *Eur Heart J.* 2016;7(21):1695-1703. doi:10.1093/eurheartj/ehv624.

146. Huang Y, Wang Y, Huang Y, et al. Prognostic value of sleep apnea and nocturnal hypoxemia in patients with decompensated heart failure. *Clin Cardiol.* 2020;43(4):329-337. doi:10.1002/clc.23319.

147. Bitter T, Faber L, Hering D, Langer C, Horstkotte D, Oldenburg O. Sleep-disordered breathing in heart failure with normal left ventricular ejection fraction. *Eur J Heart Fail.* 2009;11(6):602-608. doi:10.1093/eurjhf/hfp057.

148. Javaheri S, Blackwell T, Ancoli-Israel S, et al. Sleep-disordered breathing and incident heart failure in older men. *Am J Respir Crit Care Med.* 2016;193(5):561-568. doi:10.1164/rccm.201503-0536OC.

149. May AM, Blackwell T, Stone PH, et al. Central sleep-disordered breathing predicts incident atrial fibrillation in older men. *Am J Respir Crit Care Med.* 2016;193(7):783-791. doi:10.1164/rccm.201508-1523OC.

150. Cowie MR, Woehrle H, Wegscheider K, et al. adaptive servo-ventilation for central sleep apnea in systolic heart failure. *N Engl J Med.* 2015;373(12):1095-1105. doi:10.1056/NEJMoa1506459.

151. Chenuel BJ, Smith CA, Skatrud JB, Henderson KS, Dempsey JA. Increased propensity for apnea in response to acute elevations in left atrial pressure during sleep in the dog. *J Appl Physiol.* 2006;101(1):76-83. doi:10.1152/japplphysiol.01617.2005.

152. Herrscher TE, Akre H, Overland B, Sandvik L, Westheim AS. High prevalence of sleep apnea in heart failure outpatients: even in patients with preserved systolic function. *J Card Fail.* 2011;17(5):420-425. doi:10.1016/j.cardfail.2011.01.013.

153. Oldenburg O, Faber L, Vogt J, et al. Influence of cardiac resynchronisation therapy on different types of sleep disordered breathing. *Eur J Heart Fail.* 2007;9(8):820-826.

154. Javaheri S. Effects of continuous positive airway pressure on sleep apnea and ventricular irritability in patients with heart failure. *Circulation.* 2000;101(4):392-397.

155. Naughton MT, Benard DC, Liu PP, et al. Effects of nasal CPAP on sympathetic activity in patients with heart failure and central sleep apnea. *Am J Respir Crit Care Med.* 1995;152:473-479.

156. Bradley TD, Logan AG, Kimoff RJ, et al. Continuous positive airway pressure for central sleep apnea and heart failure. *N Engl J Med.* 2005;353;19:2025-2033.

157. Arzt M, Floras JS, Logan AG, et al. Suppression of central sleep apnea by continuous positive airway pressure and transplant-free survival in heart failure: a post hoc analysis of the Canadian Continuous Positive Airway Pressure for Patients with Central Sleep Apnea and Heart Failure Trial (CANPAP). *Circulation.* 2017;115(25):3173-3180. doi:10.1161/CIRCULATIONAHA.106.683482.

158. Javaheri S, Brown LK, Randerath WJ. Positive airway pressure therapy with adaptive servoventilation: part 1: operational algorithms. *Chest.* 2014;146(2):514-523. doi:10.1378/chest.13-1776.

159. Javaheri S, Brown LK, Khayat R. Rebuttal to Naughton. *J Clin Sleep Med.* 2018;14(6):923-925. doi:10.5664/jcsm.7150.

160. Javaheri S, Brown LK, Randerath W, Khayat R. SERVE-HF: More questions than answers. *Chest.* 2016;149(4):900-904. doi:10.1016/j.chest.2015.12.021.

161. Lyons OD, Floras JS, Logan AG, et al. Design of the effect of adaptive servo-ventilation on survival and cardiovascular hospital admissions in patients with heart failure and sleep apnoea: the ADVENT-HF trial. *Eur J Heart Fail.* 2017;19(4):579-587. doi:10.1002/ejhf.790.

162. Costanzo MR, Ponikowski P, Javaheri S, et al. Transvenous neurostimulation for central sleep apnoea: a randomised controlled trial. *Lancet.* 2017;388(10048):974-982. doi:10.1016/S0140-6736(16)30961-8.

163. Fox H, Oldenburg O, Javaheri S, et al. Long-term efficacy and safety of phrenic nerve stimulation for the treatment of central sleep apnea. *Sleep.* 2019;42(11). doi:10.1093/sleep/zsz158.

164. Javaheri S. Acetazolamide improves central sleep apnea in heart failure: a double-blind, prospective study. *Am J Respir Crit Care Med.* 2006;173(2):234-237.

165. Javaheri S, Sands SA, Edwards BA. Acetazolamide attenuates Hunter-Cheyne-Stokes breathing but augments the hypercapnic ventilatory response in patients with heart failure. *Ann Am Thorac Soc.* 2014;11(1):80-86.

166. Javaheri S, Parker TJ, Wexler L, Liming JD, Lindower P, Roselle GA. Effect of theophylline on sleep-disordered breathing in heart failure. *N Engl J Med.* 1996;335(8):562-567.

167. Hanly PJ, Millar TW, Steljes DG, Baert R, Frais MA, Kryger MH. The effect of oxygen on respiration and sleep in patients with congestive heart failure. *Ann Intern Med.* 1989;111(10):777-782.

168. Staniforth AD, Kinnear WJ, Starling R, Hetmanski DJ, Cowley AJ. Effect of oxygen on sleep quality, cognitive function and sympathetic activity in patients with chronic heart failure and Cheyne-Stokes respiration. *Eur Heart J.* 1998;19(6):922-928.

169. Sasayama S, Izumi T, Matsuzaki M, et al. Improvement of quality of life with nocturnal oxygen therapy in heart failure patients with central sleep apnea. *Circ J.* 2009;73(7):1255-1262.

170. Sasayama S, Izumi T, Seino Y, Ueshima K, Asanoi H, Group C-HS. Effects of nocturnal oxygen therapy on outcome measures in patients with chronic heart failure and Cheyne-Stokes respiration. *Circ J.* 2006;70(1):1-7.

171. Javaheri S. Pembrey's dream: the time has come for a long-term trial of nocturnal supplemental nasal oxygen to treat central sleep apnea in congestive heart failure. *Chest.* 2003;123(2):322-325.

172. Javaheri S, Abraham WT, Brown C, Nishiyama H, Giesting R, Wagoner LE. Prevalence of obstructive sleep apnoea and periodic limb movement in 45 subjects with heart transplantation. *Eur Heart J.* 2004;25(3):260-266. doi:10.1016/j.ehj.2003.10.032.

173. Afzal A, Tecson KM, Jamil AK, et al. The effect of obstructive sleep apnea on 3-year outcomes in patients who underwent orthotopic heart transplantation. *Am J Cardiol.* 2019;124(1):51-54. doi:10.1016/j.amjcard.2019.04.005.

CRITICAL CARDIOVASCULAR CARE

61. Evaluation of Cardiac Critical Care
62. Circulatory and Cardiogenic Shock
63. Sudden Cardiac Death And Resuscitation
64. Perioperative and Postprocedural Care in the Cardiac Intensive Care Unit

Evolution of Cardiac Critical Care

Venu Menon and Penelope Rampersad

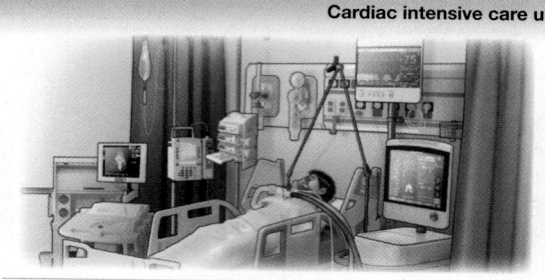

Evolution of the coronary care unit into a cardiac intensive care unit

Coronary care unit

Original concept

In 1961, Dr. Desmond Julian proposed a central unit to cluster patients following acute myocardial infarction, with ready access to electrocardiographic monitoring and trained medical staff

The unit led to an immediate increase in survival following acute myocardial infarction and was adopted worldwide

Became a clinical and research laboratory for the treatment and advancement of cardiac care predominantly in patients following an acute myocardial infarction

Patient population

Mostly acute myocardial infarction and post-reperfusion care

Cardiac intensive care unit

Hub and spoke model

Rapid triage of patients often from regional centers to hubs focused on:
STEMI
Shock
Acute aortic syndromes
Pulmonary embolism
Cardiac arrest

Evolving patient population	Design	Workforce
Elderly	Open versus closed models	Based on local needs
Pre-existing cardiac disease	Quality indicators	Training pathways
Chronic multisystem disease		Critical care cardiology

Unique populations	Critical care needs	Team-based care
Temporary mechanical circulatory support	Neurologic emergencies	Physicians/consultants
Out-of-hospital cardiac arrest	Sedation and delirium	Nurses
Structural heart disease	Mechanical ventilation	Respiratory therapists
Endocarditis	Infection/sepsis	Physical and occupational therapists
Periprocedural management	Coagulopathy	Dietician
VT storm	Nutrition	Social workers
	Early mobilization	Palliative care
	End of life care/ethics	

Chapter 61 Fuster and Hurst's Central Illustration. While the traditional coronary care unit consisted mostly of patients with acute myocardial infarction and post reperfusion care, the contemporary cardiac intensive care unit serves a more complex demographic of patients. STEMI, ST-segment elevation myocardial infarction; VT, ventricular tachycardia.

CHAPTER SUMMARY

This chapter discusses the evolution of the coronary care unit (CCU) into the modern day cardiac intensive care unit (CICU). While the traditional CCU consisted mostly of patients with acute myocardial infarction (MI) and postreperfusion care, the contemporary CICU serves a more complex demographic of patients with acute and chronic cardiac disease, multiple comorbidities, and advanced age. Operationalization requires rapid triage of patients often from regional centers to hubs focused on ST-segment elevation myocardial infarction (STEMI), shock, acute aortic emergencies, pulmonary embolism, and out-of-hospital cardiac arrest. Other unique populations include patients requiring management of structural heart disease, temporary mechanical circulatory support, endocarditis, and periprocedural management. Ensuring appropriate systems of care, infrastructure, and workforce capable of caring for these patients has led to the emerging field of critical care cardiology. The CICU has truly become an intensive care unit requiring knowledge of critical care medicine with guidance largely extrapolated from the general intensive care unit literature, but with a recognized need to develop CICU-specific evidence-based patterns of care.

HISTORY OF THE CORONARY CARE UNIT: 1960 TO 2000

Eugene Braunwald has described the creation of the coronary care unit (CCU) as the "single most important advancement in the treatment of (acute myocardial Infarction)." The concept of the CCU was conceived in 1961 by Dr. Desmond Julian, a young cardiologist at the Edinburgh Royal Infirmary. Aware of the significant incidence of early arrhythmia related mortality following acute myocardial infarction and influenced by the introduction of external defibrillation by Zoll[1] and advances in closed chest cardiopulmonary resuscitation by Kouwenhoven,[2] he proposed a central unit to cluster patients following acute myocardial infarction with ready access to electrocardiographic monitoring and trained medical staff.[3,4] This organizational action led to an immediate 7% absolute increase in survival following acute myocardial infarction and was promptly adopted worldwide. Subsequently, the first unit in the United States was created in 1963 by Dr. Hughes Day at Bethany Medical Center in Kansas City who is also credited with coining the term CCU.[5]

Over the next three decades, the CCU became a clinical and research laboratory for the treatment and advancement of cardiac care predominantly in patients following an acute myocardial infarction (AMI). In 1967, Killip and Kimball risk stratified 250 patients with AMI admitted to the four-bed New York Hospital–Cornell Medical Center CCU and established the profound impact of acute heart failure and cardiogenic shock in this setting.[6] (**Table 61–1**). Shortly thereafter, the design of the balloon tipped catheter by Swan and Ganz enabled continuous direct bedside hemodynamic monitoring that resulted in the recognition of the hemodynamic subsets of myocardial infarction and correlates of cardiogenic shock by Forrester and colleagues (**Fig. 61–1**).[7,8] The invention of the intra-aortic balloon pump (IABP) by Kantrowitz and colleagues provided the CCU access to temporary circulatory support that enabled supportive management of patients presenting with ongoing myocardial ischemia, hemodynamic instability, and mechanical complications of myocardial infarction. Scheidt and colleagues established the hemodynamic benefits of IABP counterpulsation support in improving circulatory and biochemical parameters of ineffective perfusion, but were unable to establish mortality benefit with temporary support alone.[9] Advances in reperfusion therapy utilizing fibrinolytic

agents and percutaneous coronary balloon angioplasty in the 1980s maintained the clinical and research focus on the CCU. By the turn of the century, the superiority of primary percutaneous coronary intervention (PCI) over fibrinolytic therapy had become established and the SHOCK trial had proven the benefits of an early revascularization strategy in patients with cardiogenic shock complicating AMI.[10,11]

THE CHANGING PARADIGM

Success at restoring coronary flow and limiting myocardial infarction size with effective reperfusion therapy, aborting sudden cardiac death with an implantable cardioverter defibrillator (ICD), as well as the development of proven pharmacotherapy (ACE inhibitors and β-blockers) to attenuate and prevent the deleterious consequences of adverse ventricular modeling, along with statin utilization in secondary prevention, transformed the outcome of patients with AMI and heart failure. Having survived their initial cardiac insult, survivors of myocardial infarction and heart failure were now more likely to present later in the disease state with increased comorbidities affecting multiple organ systems and advanced age. This transformation led to the metamorphosis of the CCU to the modern cardiac intensive care unit (CICU) as patients with acute or chronic consequences of myocardial diseases became the dominant population.[12]

CONTINUED EVOLUTION

The changing landscape of patients in the CICU with regards to demographic, etiology of presentation, underlying comorbidities, as well as complexity has resulted in the development and evolution of a new subspecialty of cardiology: cardiac critical care. Recent registry data from a critical care network suggests that CICU admissions were primarily for a heterogeneous spectrum of acute cardiac presentations, followed by combined cardiac and general diagnoses, overflow from general intensive care units (ICUs), and periprocedural monitoring (**Fig. 61–2**).[13] While the severity of illness of patients varied between CICUs around the nation, patients were generally elderly and comorbid with a median age of 65 years, with one-third of patients greater than 70 years of age. Common cardiac conditions such as ischemic heart disease and heart failure with reduced ejection fraction were accompanied by

TABLE 61–1. Clinical Presentation and Outcome in 250 Patients Admitted with Acute Myocardial Infarction to the New York Hospital Coronary Care Unit

Clinical Presentation	Number (%)	Average Age (Years)	Life-Threatening Arrhythmia (%)	Cardiac Arrest (%)	Hospital Mortality (%)
No Heart Failure	33	58	36	5	6
Heart Failure	38	65	46	15	17
Pulmonary Edema	10	69	73	46	38
Cardiogenic Shock	19	67	94	77	81

Adapted with permission from Killip T 3rd, Kimball JT. Treatment of myocardial infarction in a coronary care unit. A two year experience with 250 patients. *Am J Cardiol.* 1967 Oct;20(4):457-464.

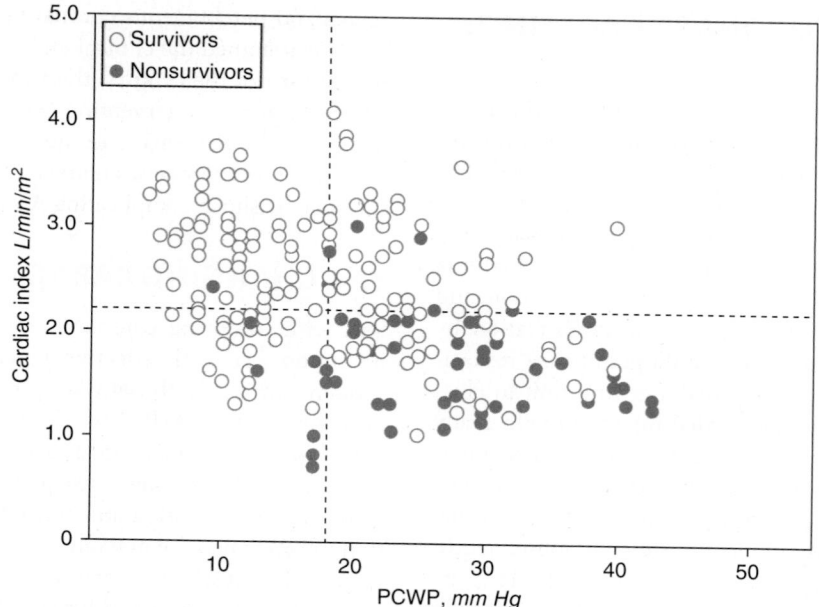

Figure 61–1. **Serial hemodynamics in patients admitted to the CCU at Cedars Sinai with AMI.** Utilizing a wedge pressure of 18 mm Hg and a cardiac index of 2.2 L/min/m², four quadrants are noted. Most of the deaths (*filled arrows*) occur in the bottom right defined as cardiogenic shock. The bottom left quadrant characterized by hypoperfusion and low wedge pressure defines the subset of hemodynamically significant right ventricular infarction.

comorbid illnesses such as diabetes, chronic kidney disease, chronic pulmonary disease, and active malignancy. While the most common causes for admission remains acute coronary syndromes and decompensated heart failure, the indication for ICU level care was warranted by respiratory insufficiency, unstable arrhythmias, shock, and cardiac arrest.[13] Intensive

care therapies necessitating CICU admission included the need for intravenous therapies including vasopressors, inotropes, or vasodilator therapies, followed by invasive mechanical ventilation and need for temporary mechanical circulatory support. However, a substantial proportion of patients admitted to the CICU had no identified need for any of the aforementioned

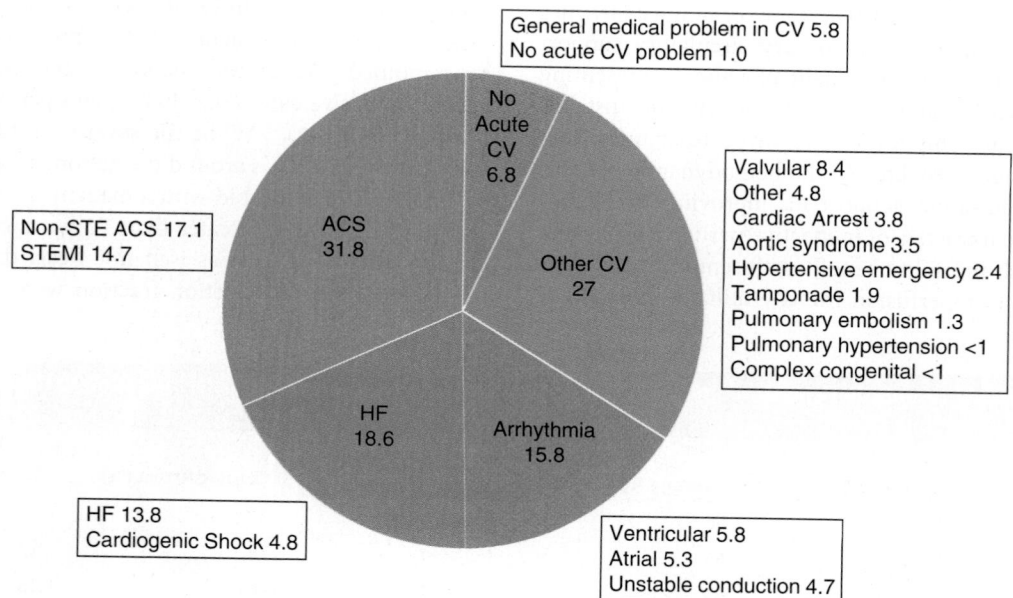

Percentage of patients admitted to CICU by reason for hospitalization

Figure 61–2. **Reason for hospitalization to the CICU in the Cardiac Critical Care Trials Network.** Abbreviations: ACS, acute coronary syndrome. HF, heart failure. CV, cardiovascular. Non-STE ACS, Non-ST elevation-acute coronary syndrome. STEMI, ST elevation myocardial infarction.

therapies or invasive hemodynamic monitoring. Creation of evidence-based criteria to guide and standardize admission criteria to the CICU appears warranted.

A number of other developments have also contributed to the changing patient profile of the CICU; some of which are subsequently outlined.

Creation of Systems of Care

The superiority of primary PCI over fibrinolytic therapy led to the development of systems of care with a hub and spoke model at the national and local community level both in the United States and in many regions around the world. While intended to provide increased access to timely reperfusion, these systems have enabled and facilitated early recognition, triage, and transfer of critically ill patients from the field to CICUs that can provide definitive treatment. Transfer from smaller community hospitals to tertiary institutions has also been facilitated by this process. Consequently, patients with a number of other acute time sensitive cardiac emergencies like out of hospital cardiac arrest (OOHCA), cardiogenic shock, acute aortic dissection, and acute pulmonary embolism now have rapid and seamless access to the CICU.[14–16] Similarly, improved organization of rapid response and acute response teams within hospitals has also led to the improved triage and transfer of critically ill patients to the CICU. The ongoing development of a multidisciplinary "SHOCK Team" is an example of this evolution in the delivery of cardiac critical care. In an observational study, activation of the SHOCK team utilizing a standardized team-based approach was associated with improved survival for cardiogenic shock compared to historical controls.[17]

Availability of Temporary Mechanical Support

Advances in temporary percutaneous mechanical support has transformed our ability to deliver ventricle specific or biventricular support in the CICU. These devices have been shown to effectively support the circulation by improving hemodynamics and preventing the adverse consequences of end organ hypoperfusion. Although not yet proven to improve outcomes with cardiogenic shock in randomized clinical trials, there has been an explosive growth in their utilization. Use of temporary circulatory support has enabled the clinician in the CICU to stabilize patients with circulatory collapse or refractory heart failure as they bridge to a decision of either weaning and recovery, withdrawal and palliation, or consideration of durable mechanical support/transplantation. Adoption of this strategy is associated with increased ICU length of stay with subsequent decrease in ICU throughput, complications of vascular access and nosocomial infection, and extreme demands on multidisciplinary physician and nursing teams.

Out of Hospital Cardiac Arrest and Advances in Postarrest Care

Although prognosis for patients with OOHCA remains dismal with large observed regional variations, public education with bystander cardiopulmonary resuscitation (CPR), availability of an automated external defibrillator (AED), regionalization of arrest care, acute revascularization in patients with manifest ST-elevation myocardial infarction (STEMI), and benefits of targeted temperature management have all resulted in improved survival.[15] Survivors of OOHCA warrant extensive postarrest care and neurological prognostication when admitted to the ICU with multiorgan dysfunction being common and prolonged CICU length of stay.

Advances in Structural Heart Disease Intervention

The revolutionary advances in this area, although originally evaluated in patients with a chronic anatomical substrate, are rapidly being considered on an emergent basis in patients with acute hemodynamic instability. The availability of transcatheter treatment options to treat hemodynamic instability due to native valve disease (especially aortic stenosis and mitral regurgitation) or unexpected bioprosthetic valve failure has expanded our therapeutic armamentarium in the CICU.

Endocarditis

The aging of the population, increased utilization of intravascular devices like pacemakers and ICDs, use of long-term vascular access techniques, frequent use of renal replacement therapy, and the epidemic of intravenous drug abuse in the United States have all led to increasing hospitalizations for infective endocarditis. A number of these patients with adverse hemodynamic or embolic sequelae of endocarditis now populate the CICU.

Procedural Complications

Advances in coronary and structural interventions and frequent electrophysiology procedures now enable us to successfully expand our therapies to more complex patient subsets. These interventions while markedly improving longevity and quality of life can be associated with vascular and nonvascular complications due to their inherent invasive nature and contribute to a proportion of patient admissions to the CICU.

DESIGN OF THE CARDIAC INTENSIVE CARE UNIT

The location for the care of critical cardiac patients can vary. The majority of CICU patients, especially in smaller community hospitals and less developed healthcare systems, will be admitted to a mixed ICU alongside patients with other medical and even surgical conditions. Based on the available capabilities and the supervisory personnel, the American Heart Association (AHA) scientific statement classifies CICU as level 1 to 3.[18] Although most CICU remain open, with individual physicians responsible for individual patients, a closed model with dedicated physician and nursing leadership is recommended. The CICU should not operate in isolation and should harmonize common ICU protocols dealing with common ICU-related issues with other units in the hospital/system. Continuous education and certification processes should be set in place to train, maintain, and ensure maintenance of specific procedure and management competencies amongst physician, advanced practice providers, and nursing personnel. The accepted common ICU quality metrics like rates of central line–associated bloodstream infection (CLABSI), catheter-induced urinary tract infection, and ventilator-associated pneumonia should be measured, monitored, and followed as part of a continuing quality improvement process. Specific unit cardiac metrics should also be identified, measured, analyzed, and followed. Processes for morbidity and mortality review as well as root cause analyses for complications or therapy failures should be in place. In addition to appropriate subspecialty consultation when warranted, the unit should also involve multispecialty input from a number of ancillary areas including bioethics, palliative care, social work, respiratory and physiotherapy, and nutrition. The presence of a cardiac pharmacist on rounds aids in adequate antibiotic stewardship, evaluation of cost considerations, appropriate pharmacotherapy, and avoidance of serious drug interactions.[19]

CREATING THE IDEAL WORKFORCE

The changing patient landscape supports the development of a unique cardiology workforce dedicated to the care and research of patients admitted to the CICU.[18] The ideal physician in this environment would complement the skills of a cardiologist with mastery in more generalizable critical care skills such as management of respiratory failure and renal replacement therapy. Initial investigations into CICU staffing suggest that these patients, similar to other ICUs, benefit from improved outcomes when cared for by dedicated dual-trained cardiology and critical care medicine physicians.[20] However, this may not be practical in all settings and should be determined by available local or community resources. Multiple training and staffing pathways have been proposed for the CICU physician, which should reflect the severity of illness of patients in secondary, tertiary, or quaternary centers.[18,21–23] For the cardiologist pursuing clinical and academic leadership of a tertiary CICU, completion of a dedicated critical care fellowship following completion of a general cardiology fellowship appears warranted. Currently, most dedicated cardiac critical care fellowships involve a dedicated additional year of critical care medicine training to equip cardiologists with skills in acute critical care management. Surveyed dual certified critical care cardiologists cite that their most frequently utilized critical care medicine skills in the CICU include management of ventilators and multiorgan dysfunction, end-of-life care, sedation, multidisciplinary team processes, and airway management.[21] Individual cardiologists may complement their critical care training by considering dedicated additional training in advanced heart failure, mechanical circulatory support, cardiac hemodynamics, heart transplantation, interventional techniques, or cardiac imaging.

System-based care is a frequently used method of organization and prioritization in the management of complex critically ill patients. The CICU staff should have mastery over commonly encountered ICU domains and should readily seek consultation if and when required to improve patient outcomes. Some of the general critical care issues commonly encountered in the CICU include neurologic emergencies and outcome prognostication, sedation and delirium management, sepsis, acute respiratory failure, management of coagulopathies, renal and hepatic failure, nutrition, critical illness myopathy, and end-of-life care. The bulk of literature to support care protocols and bundled care packages are limited to the general critical care population but may be appropriately applied to those with underlying cardiac conditions. Given the paucity of data specific to CICU populations, best clinical practice protocols are usually extrapolated with some specific considerations for cardiac patients (**Table 61–2**).[24]

SPECIFIC CRITICAL CARE ISSUES

Neurologic Emergencies, Sedation, and Delirium

Postcardiac arrest care and temperature-targeted management has moved to the forefront of CICU management with OOHCA being a common clinical presentation. Unique features in management include need for intensive sedation, prevention of shivering and electrolyte disorders, ongoing neurologic monitoring for seizure activity, and assessment of neurologic prognostication for meaningful recovery. Collaboration with neurology intensive care specialists and/or neurologists should be performed, but in their absence; knowledge of continuous neurologic monitors, including electroencephalogram interpretation and intracranial pressure monitoring, may be useful at the bedside along with the ability to accurately evaluate brain function viability. The recognition and initial management of acute neurologic illnesses including seizures, ischemic and hemorrhagic stroke, and elevated intracranial pressure is warranted. Additionally, in all patients, close attention should be paid toward basic critical care principles including sedation strategies and recognition and management of delirium given its deleterious impact on increasing morbidity including ventilator days and length of stay in both general ICU and CICU populations.[25,26] The pharmacologic properties of sedative agents need to be considered in the context of limited cardiac reserve with preexisting evidence of myocardial depression, which can be worsened by agents like propofol, and more recently, with dexmedetomidine that can cause bradycardia, hypotension, increasing vasopressor/inotrope requirements, and asystole in a CICU setting. Delirium, also a culprit of increased morbidity and mortality in the general ICU setting had a prevalence rate of 18% to 20% in two single center CICU studies.[27–29] Again, drug interactions of atypical antipsychotics often used to manage delirium in the ICU setting can cause profound harm in the cardiac patient with underlying conduction disease and prolonged QT interval. The optimal use and abuse of sedative agents in the CICU emphasizes the importance of specialized pharmacists in this setting.[30–32]

Infection

Concomitant infections, both community-acquired and nosocomial, may manifest as acute decompensation of chronic cardiac illness. Governing principles include prompt recognition of sepsis, adequate fluid resuscitation, prompt antimicrobial

TABLE 61–2. Critical Care Complication Prevention Tips for the Coronary Intensive Care Unit Population

Complication	Cardiac Disease	Tip	Rationale
Ventilator-associated pneumonia	Intra-aortic balloon pump and cannulas	Adjust bed to maximum reverse Trendelenburg position and limit head of bed elevation to 10%	Head of bed elevation >10% has risk of kinking catheter or tearing femoral artery
Sedation	Cardiac arrest	RASS and SAS scores not validated	Scales use of motor function in their assessments are not valid in brain injuries
	Cardiogenic shock	Avoid propofol in hemodynamically unstable patients	Propofol has negative inotropic effect
	Bradycardias	Avoid dexmedetomidine	Dexmedetomidine has a negative chronotropic effect
	Significant alcohol consumption	Consider benzodiazepine for alcohol withdrawal symptoms	Benzodiazepines can reduce alcohol withdrawal symptoms and seizures
Central line infections	Multiple antiplatelet agents, anticoagulants or post-thrombolytics	Consider avoiding subclavian insertion sites	The safety of noncompressible venous site insertion in this population unknown
Delirium	Unrevascularized coronary ischemia	Mobility goals should be set below threshold of inducible ischemia prior to revascularization	Mobilization can induce ischemia
Malnutrition	Therapeutic hypothermia	Consider trophic feeding until normothermic (>36.5°C)	Hypothermia causes gastroparesis
Stress ulcers	Dual antiplatelet therapy	Consider continuing stress ulcer prophylaxis after initiating of enteral nutrition	Proton pump inhibitors have been shown to reduce long term bleeding in this population
Medication errors	Nitroglycerine use	Inquire about recent erectile dysfunction medication use prior to initiation	Risk of life-threatening hypotension with recent phosphodiesterase type 5 use
	β-blocker initiation	Inquire about recent cocaine and/or stimulate use	Theoretical risk of unopposed α-vasoconstriction

administration, and source control. Prescriptive fluid resuscitation as suggested in the surviving sepsis campaign in patients with combined reduced cardiac function and septic shock can be detrimental and cause further decompensation.[33] Furthermore, myocardial depression in sepsis can make hemodynamic optimization challenging. Adequacy of fluid resuscitation can be difficult to gauge without supportive guidance utilizing invasive hemodynamic monitoring, mixed or central venous saturation, or echo guidance. ICU-acquired infections secondary to central venous catheters, catheter-associated urinary tract infections, ventilator associated pneumonias, as well as nosocomial infections from MRSA, resistant organism, and *Clostridium difficile* are also thought to be common in the CICU population and should be followed as part of a continuous quality improvement process. CLABSIs have impact not just on patient outcomes, but also on hospital reimbursements in some health systems. The general ICU literature supports subclavian central venous catheters whenever possible and jugular in preference to femoral venous catheters that have increased risks of catheter-related bloodstream infections.[34] Challenges in a CICU population to comply with such recommendations include increased bleeding risks with subclavian access in patients receiving dual antiplatelet agents and frequent anticoagulant therapies. Femoral cannulation is also frequently encountered in cardiac patients who frequently may have postprocedural femoral central venous catheters or

femoral arterial access for IABP or other mechanical circulatory support devices. Ventilator-associated pneumonia precautions recommending elevated head of the bed above 45 degrees can be problematic in patients with femoral access catheters, which can be temporized with reverse Trendelenberg positioning to allow for some head elevation.[24] Overall vigilance and daily reassessment to justify need for all large bore access catheters on multidisciplinary rounds is paramount to decrease the risk of infection. Moreover, bundling of components for central venous access allows for greater compliance with sterile technique at the time of insertion and reduces overall CLABSI rates.[35]

Respiratory Status

The proportion of patients requiring advanced respiratory support including high-flow oxygen therapy, noninvasive mechanical ventilation, or mechanical ventilation was approximately 26.7% in a multicenter North American prospective study, with roughly 21.4% of patients requiring invasive mechanical ventilation.[13] Indications may range from airway protection in the postarrest patient to acute respiratory distress syndrome in patients with underlying cardiac pathology. Data supporting noninvasive mechanical ventilation in acute cardiogenic pulmonary edema with either continuous positive airway pressure (CPAP) or bilevel positive airway pressure ventilation show that both therapies reduced the need for subsequent invasive mechanical ventilation. Additionally, compared to standard therapy, CPAP reduced mortality. Reasons for improved outcomes with noninvasive positive ventilation may be associated with the reduced work of breathing that is achieved. Respiratory distress may require as much as 16% of overall cardiac output, and mechanical ventilation may unload the work of breathing by up to 30% in some studies.[36] Additionally, the positive effects of positive end–expiratory pressure (PEEP) either by invasive or noninvasive mechanical ventilation are many. Positive pressure is known to decrease cardiac preload by decreasing venous return, increasing pulmonary vascular resistance, and perhaps decreasing hypoxemic pulmonary vasoconstriction. It is also thought to decrease the work of breathing by unloading respiratory muscles and thereby cardiac output, as well as decrease pulmonary edema. At the level of the left heart, PEEP may decrease oxygen demand by decreasing the work of breathing, increase oxygen delivery to the myocardium, and decrease cardiac afterload by increasing intrathoracic pressure and thereby decreasing transmural pressure. Depending on the indication for invasive mechanical ventilation, best practices to prevent ventilator-induced lung injury (VILI) are based on the pulmonary critical care literature and management of acute respiratory distress syndrome (ARDS).[37] VILI is thought to be a result of repetitive atelectrauma, volutrauma, and barotrauma that typically occurs in the injured lung on mechanical ventilation. The ARDS literature has produced a number of defining trials that govern lung protective ventilation that consists of low tidal volumes, limiting mean airway pressures, and setting PEEPs.[38–41] However, cardiac patients at the time of initiation of mechanical ventilation may not have parenchymal lung disease and indications for mechanical ventilation may be largely to offset the work of breathing. In these instances, settings for mechanical ventilation to limit VILI have limited data to guide clinical decisions. The most recent trial to examine low versus intermediate tidal volume ventilation at 6-to 8-cc/kg versus 10-cc/kg predicted body weight in patients without ARDS, did not result in a significant difference in ventilator-free days or 28-day mortality.[42] Based on best available data, recommendations are a tidal volume of 6- to 8-cc/kg predicted body weight in those patients at risk for VILI, targeting a plateau pressure of less than 30 cm water and a driving pressure of less than 15 cm water. Weaning and liberation from mechanical ventilation is challenging in the patient with ineffective cardiac reserve. The most common reason for extubation failures, or reintubation, remains decompensated heart failure. As stated, PEEP contributes significantly to decreasing myocardial oxygen demand with the most pronounced benefit in patients with marginal hemodynamics. Aggressive optimization of fluid status and hemodynamics should be established prior to an attempt at liberation from mechanical ventilation in patients with severely reduced ejection fraction. Additionally, discussion over the best predictors of weaning failure should be evaluated individually. The removal of positive pressure may cause acute decompensation. In such cases a T-piece trial may be considered in addition to aggressive avoidance of hypertension at the time of liberation.

Nutrition and Early Mobilization

ICU patients suffer the consequences of prolonged bed rest and underfeeding causing rapidly progressive cachexia that may result in profound debility and critical illness myopathy. CICU patients may be at additional risk for such complications due to the degree of immobility caused by prolonged bed rest. Initiatives for early mobilization with involvement of occupational and physical therapists should be adopted.

End-of-Life Care and Ethical Considerations

Death both unexpected and expected is frequently encountered in the CICU. In a recent registry, the overall observed mortality rate was 8% with up to 38% mortality observed in cardiac arrest patients.[13] Consequently, end-of-life care discussions play an increasingly important role in the CICU. In a retrospective study of CICU patients who died during index admission, there were planned end-of-life discussions in 72.6% (n = 85/117) of patients.[43] Of the patients who died, those having undergone goals of care discussions were more likely to redirect their care toward either no escalation of care or comfort care prior to death. The degree of palliative or hospice care team involvement was noted to be only modest with the majority of discussions being led by the CICU team.

FUTURE DIRECTIONS

There is an important need to standardize admission and practice patterns in the CICU. Creation of registry data highlighting current practices, variations, and deficiencies will help facilitate this goal. Design of high-quality studies specific to ICU care in cardiac patients remains lacking. Randomized clinical trials to generate high-quality evidence, although challenging to perform in a CICU setting on specific patient groups, are sorely needed. The increased patient demands and complexity of care should encourage cardiologists to pursue this area of subspecialization. Currently, training pathways to pursue cardiac critical care appear heterogeneous and standardization of goals and objectives for this training pathway should be a major objective in the future.

REFERENCES

1. Zoll PM, Linenthal AJ, Gibson W, Paul MH, Norman LR. Termination of ventricular fibrillation in man by externally applied electric countershock. *N Engl J Med.* 1956;254:727-732.
2. Kouwenhoven WB, Jude JR, Knickerbocker GG. Closed-chest cardiac massage. *JAMA.* 1960;173:1064-1067.
3. Julian DG. Treatment of cardiac arrest in acute myocardial ischaemia and infarction. *Lancet.* 1961;2:840-844.
4. Julian DG. The evolution of the coronary care unit. *Cardiovasc Res.* 2001;51:621-624.
5. Day HW. A cardiac resuscitation program. *J Lancet.* 1962;82:153-156.
6. Killip T 3rd, Kimball JT. Treatment of myocardial infarction in a coronary care unit. A two year experience with 250 patients. *Am J Cardiol.* 1967;20:457-464.
7. Forrester JS, Diamond G, Chatterjee K, Swan HJ. Medical therapy of acute myocardial infarction by application of hemodynamic subsets (second of two parts). *N Engl J Med.* 1976;295:1404-1413.

8. Forrester JS, Diamond G, Chatterjee K, Swan HJ. Medical therapy of acute myocardial infarction by application of hemodynamic subsets (first of two parts). *N Engl J Med.* 1976;295:1356-1362.

9. Scheidt S, Wilner G, Mueller H, et al. Intra-aortic balloon counterpulsation in cardiogenic shock. Report of a co-operative clinical trial. *N Engl J Med.* 1973;288:979-984.

10. Hochman JS, Sleeper LA, Webb JG, Sanborn TA, White HD, Talley JD, Buller CE, Jacobs AK, Slater JN, Col J, McKinlay SM, LeJemtel TH. Early revascularization in acute myocardial infarction complicated by cardiogenic shock. SHOCK Investigators. Should we emergently revascularize occluded coronaries for cardiogenic shock. *N Engl J Med.* 1999;341: 625-634.

11. Keeley EC, Boura JA, Grines CL. Primary angioplasty versus intravenous thrombolytic therapy for acute myocardial infarction: a quantitative review of 23 randomised trials. *Lancet.* 2003;361:13-20.

12. Katz JN, Shah BR, Volz EM, Horton JR, Shaw LK, Newby LK, Granger CB, Mark DB, Califf RM, Becker RC. Evolution of the coronary care unit: clinical characteristics and temporal trends in healthcare delivery and outcomes. *Crit Care Med.* 2010;38:375-381.

13. Bohula EA, Katz JN, van Diepen S, et al. Demographics, care patterns, and outcomes of patients admitted to cardiac intensive care units: the Critical Care Cardiology Trials Network Prospective North American Multicenter Registry of Cardiac Critical Illness. *JAMA Cardiol.* 2019;4:928-935.

14. Aggarwal B, Raymond CE, Randhawa MS, et al. Transfer metrics in patients with suspected acute aortic syndrome. *Circ Cardiovasc Qual Outcomes.* 2014;7:780-782.

15. Nichol G, Aufderheide TP, Eigel B, et al. Regional systems of care for out-of-hospital cardiac arrest: A policy statement from the American Heart Association. *Circulation.* 2010;121:709-729.

16. van Diepen S, Katz JN, Albert NM, et al. Contemporary management of cardiogenic shock: a scientific statement from the American Heart Association. *Circulation.* 2017;136:e232-e268.

17. Tehrani BN, Truesdell AG, Sherwood MW, et al. Standardized team-based care for cardiogenic shock. *J Am Coll Cardiol.* 2019;73:1659-1669.

18. Morrow DA, Fang JC, Fintel DJ, et al. Evolution of critical care cardiology: transformation of the cardiovascular intensive care unit and the emerging need for new medical staffing and training models: a scientific statement from the American Heart Association. *Circulation.* 2012;126:1408-1428.

19. Dunn SP, Birtcher KK, Beavers CJ, et al. The role of the clinical pharmacist in the care of patients with cardiovascular disease. *J Am Coll Cardiol.* 2015;66:2129-2139.

20. Na SJ, Chung CR, Jeon K, et al. Association between presence of a cardiac intensivist and mortality in an adult cardiac care unit. *J Am Coll Cardiol.* 2016;68:2637-2648.

21. Brusca SB, Barnett C, Barnhart BJ, et al. Role of critical care medicine training in the cardiovascular intensive care unit: survey responses from dual certified critical care cardiologists. *J Am Heart Assoc.* 2019;8:e011721.

22. Geller BJ, Fleitman J, Sinha SS. Critical care cardiology: implementing a training paradigm. *J Am Coll Cardiol.* 2018;72:1171-1175.

23. Miller PE, Kenigsberg BB, Wiley BM. Cardiac critical care: training pathways and transition to early career. *J Am Coll Cardiol.* 2019;73:1726-1730.

24. van Diepen S, Sligl WI, Washam JB, Gilchrist IC, Arora RC, Katz JN. Prevention of critical care complications in the coronary intensive care unit: protocols, bundles, and insights from intensive care studies. *Can J Cardiol.* 2017;33:101-109.

25. Aday AW, Dell'orfano H, Hirning BA, et al. Evaluation of a clinical pathway for sedation and analgesia of mechanically ventilated patients in a cardiac intensive care unit (CICU): the Brigham and Women's Hospital Levine CICU sedation pathways. *Eur Heart J Acute Cardiovasc Care.* 2013;2:299-305.

26. Kress JP, Pohlman AS, O'Connor MF, Hall JB. Daily interruption of sedative infusions in critically ill patients undergoing mechanical ventilation. *N Engl J Med.* 2000;342:1471-1477.

27. Ely EW, Shintani A, Truman B, et al. Delirium as a predictor of mortality in mechanically ventilated patients in the intensive care unit. *JAMA.* 2004;291:1753-1762.

28. Lahariya S, Grover S, Bagga S, Sharma A. Delirium in patients admitted to a cardiac intensive care unit with cardiac emergencies in a developing country: incidence, prevalence, risk factor and outcome. *Gen Hosp Psychiatry.* 2014;36:156-164.

29. Pauley E, Lishmanov A, Schumann S, Gala GJ, van Diepen S, Katz JN. Delirium is a robust predictor of morbidity and mortality among critically ill patients treated in the cardiac intensive care unit. *Am Heart J.* 2015;170:79-86, 86.e1.

30. Barr J, Fraser GL, Puntillo K, et al. Clinical practice guidelines for the management of pain, agitation, and delirium in adult patients in the intensive care unit. *Crit Care Med.* 2013;41:263-306.

31. Devi P, Kamath DY, Anthony N, Santosh S, Dias B. Patterns, predictors and preventability of adverse drug reactions in the coronary care unit of a tertiary care hospital. *Eur J Clin Pharmacol.* 2012;68:427-433.

32. Girard TD, Exline MC, Carson SS, et al. Haloperidol and ziprasidone for treatment of delirium in critical illness. *N Engl J Med.* 2018;379:2506-2516.

33. Rhodes A, Evans LE, Alhazzani W, et al. Surviving sepsis campaign: international guidelines for management of sepsis and septic shock: 2016. *Crit Care Med.* 2017;45:486-552.

34. Timsit JF, Bouadma L, Mimoz O, et al. Jugular versus femoral short-term catheterization and risk of infection in intensive care unit patients. Causal analysis of two randomized trials. *Am J Respir Crit Care Med.* 2013;188:1232-1239.

35. Furuya EY, Dick A, Perencevich EN, Pogorzelska M, Goldmann D, Stone PW. Central line bundle implementation in US intensive care units and impact on bloodstream infections. *PLoS One.* 2011;6:e15452.

36. Kuhn BT, Bradley LA, Dempsey TM, Puro AC, Adams JY. Management of mechanical ventilation in decompensated heart failure. *J Cardiovasc Dev Dis.* 2016;3.

37. Slutsky AS, Ranieri VM. Ventilator-induced lung injury. *N Engl J Med.* 2013;369:2126-2136.

38. Acute Respiratory Distress Syndrome N, Brower RG, Matthay MA, et al. Ventilation with lower tidal volumes as compared with traditional tidal volumes for acute lung injury and the acute respiratory distress syndrome. *N Engl J Med.* 2000;342:1301-1308.

39. Amato MB, Meade MO, Slutsky AS, et al. Driving pressure and survival in the acute respiratory distress syndrome. *N Engl J Med.* 2015;372:747-755.

40. Brower RG, Lanken PN, MacIntyre N, et al. Higher versus lower positive end-expiratory pressures in patients with the acute respiratory distress syndrome. *N Engl J Med.* 2004;351:327-336.

41. Meade MO, Cook DJ, Guyatt GH, et al. Ventilation strategy using low tidal volumes, recruitment maneuvers, and high positive end-expiratory pressure for acute lung injury and acute respiratory distress syndrome: a randomized controlled trial. *JAMA.* 2008;299:637-645.

42. Writing Group for the PI, Simonis FD, Serpa Neto A, et al. Effect of a low vs intermediate tidal volume strategy on ventilator-free days in intensive care unit patients without ARDS: a randomized clinical trial. *JAMA.* 2018;320:1872-1880.

43. Naib T, Lahewala S, Arora S, Gidwani U. Palliative care in the cardiac intensive care unit. *Am J Cardiol.* 2015;115:687-690.

62

Circulatory and Cardiogenic Shock

Gregory Serrao, Benjamin Bier, and Umesh Gidwani

The pathophysiology, assessment, classification and management of cardiogenic shock		
Pathophysiology	**Classification**	**Management**
Maladaptive compensatory cycle triggered by acute reduction in cardiac output All etiologies initiate a physiologic cascade rooted in three main pathways: 1) Increase in left ventricular end diastolic pressure 2) Reduction of blood pressure 3) Triggering of inflammatory responses If left uninterrupted, the compensatory cycle will lead to progressive cardiac dysfunction and ultimately death	Cardiogenic shock with predominant left ventricular failure • More common than isolated right ventricular failure and most often precipitated by coronary ischemia • Etiology categorized as primary, obstructive, or valvular	Management strategies depend on etiology Key clinical goals: • Reduction of ventricular afterload, • Optimization of preload, • Augmentation of cardiac contractility, • Maintenance of adequate mean arterial pressure to ensure perfusion to vital organs Vasopressors and inotropes are the backbone of medical therapy for cardiogenic shock
Assessment • Physical exam • Ultrasonography • Laboratory studies (lactic acid) • Invasive hemodynamics • Coronary angiography, as appropriate	Cardiogenic shock with predominant right ventricular failure • Less common than predominant left ventricular failure but similar overall mortality • Etiology usually primary or obstructive, as from massive or submassive acute pulmonary embolism Cardiogenic shock with biventricular failure • Etiology is primary, obstructive, electrical, or structural	Where cardiogenic shock is driven by acute myocardial infarction, re-establishing and maintaining perfusion to the affected myocardial territory is of high importance; both coronary revascularization and antithrombotic therapies are essential The role of mechanical circulatory support in cardiogenic shock is a growing area of research and clinical interest (refer to Chapter 52)

Chapter 62 Fuster and Hurst's Central Illustration. Cardiogenic shock is diminished cardiac function resulting in life-threatening end-organ hypoperfusion and hypoxemia, and is associated with significant morbidity and mortality. A thorough assessment of the patient with suspected cardiogenic shock is necessary to confirm the diagnosis and inform treatment decisions.

CHAPTER SUMMARY

This chapter describes the pathophysiology, assessment, classification, and management of cardiogenic shock (see Fuster and Hurst's Central Illustration). The pathophysiology of cardiogenic shock involves a maladaptive compensatory cycle triggered by acute reduction in cardiac output. All etiologies initiate a physiologic cascade rooted in three main pathways: (1) increase in left ventricular end diastolic pressure, (2) reduction of blood pressure, and (3) triggering of inflammatory responses. If left uninterrupted, the compensatory cycle will lead to progressive cardiac dysfunction and ultimately death. A thorough assessment of the patient with suspected cardiogenic shock is necessary to confirm diagnosis and inform treatment decisions, and involves physical examination, ultrasonography, laboratory studies, invasive hemodynamics, and coronary angiography, as appropriate. Cardiogenic shock with predominant left ventricular failure is more common than isolated right ventricular failure, and etiology can be categorized as primary, obstructive, or valvular. Etiology of cardiogenic shock with predominant right ventricular failure is usually primary or obstructive, often related to acute pulmonary embolism of hemodynamic significance. Concurrent left ventricular failure and right ventricular failure is relatively common among causes of cardiogenic shock and the underlying etiology is primary, obstructive, electrical, or structural. Treatment for cardiogenic shock depends on etiology, and may involve a combination of vasoactive agents (pressors and inotropes), treatment of myocardial ischemia and revascularization as appropriate, and mechanical circulatory support (e.g. intra-aortic balloon pump counterpulsation, percutaneous left ventricular assist device, and/or extracorporal membrane oxygenation) as needed.

INTRODUCTION

Cardiogenic shock is diminished cardiac function resulting in life-threatening end-organ hypoperfusion and hypoxemia[1] and is associated with major morbidity and frequent mortality.

DEFINITIONS

There are varied definitions of cardiogenic shock. The most widely used are the entry criteria used in the SHOCK trial[2] that highlight three hallmarks of cardiogenic shock: (1) a systolic blood pressure of <90 mm Hg for >30 minutes or vasopressor support to maintain a systolic blood pressure of >90 mm Hg, (2) evidence of end organ hypoperfusion, and (3) a measured cardiac index of <2.2 L/m/m² and pulmonary capillary wedge pressure of >15 mm Hg. Since that time, there have been a number of randomized trials that used similar but slightly varied definitions of cardiogenic shock, many not requiring the measurement of invasive hemodynamic data to meet criteria.[3-5]

Most recently, the Society for Cardiovascular Angiography and Intervention (SCAI) proposed a new classification system.[6] This system describes five stages of cardiogenic shock, from A to E, with A being "at risk," B "beginning," C "classic," D "deteriorating," and E "extremis" (**Fig. 62–1**). Cardiogenic shock begins at Stage C, which is defined by organ hypoperfusion. Stage D is defined by the failure of at least 30 minutes of initial interventions. Stage E is when the patient is highly unstable and often with complete cardiovascular collapse. This classification method was developed with the aim of establishing a common language to support communication across institutions and subspecialties such as interventional cardiology and cardiothoracic surgery. It is also meant to help with interpreting the results of clinical trials, which is often difficult to do because of the varied definitions of cardiogenic shock. This system has already been proven to help predict mortality in this patient subgroup.[7]

PATHOPHYSIOLOGY

The pathophysiology of cardiogenic shock is rooted in a maladaptive compensatory cycle that is triggered by acute reduction in cardiac output. While a number of different etiologies can cause this acute reduction, all initiate the same physiologic cascade rooted in three main pathways (**Fig. 62–2**): (1) increase in left ventricular end diastolic pressure, (2) reduction of blood pressure, and (3) triggering of inflammatory responses. First, acute myocardial dysfunction raises left ventricular end diastolic pressure. This can directly precipitate further coronary ischemia by reducing coronary perfusion pressure (defined as the difference between aortic diastolic pressure and the left ventricular end diastolic pressure) and indirectly by leading to the development of pulmonary edema that may cause systemic hypoxia and result in decreased oxygen delivery to the myocardium. Second, there is an acute reduction in blood pressure.

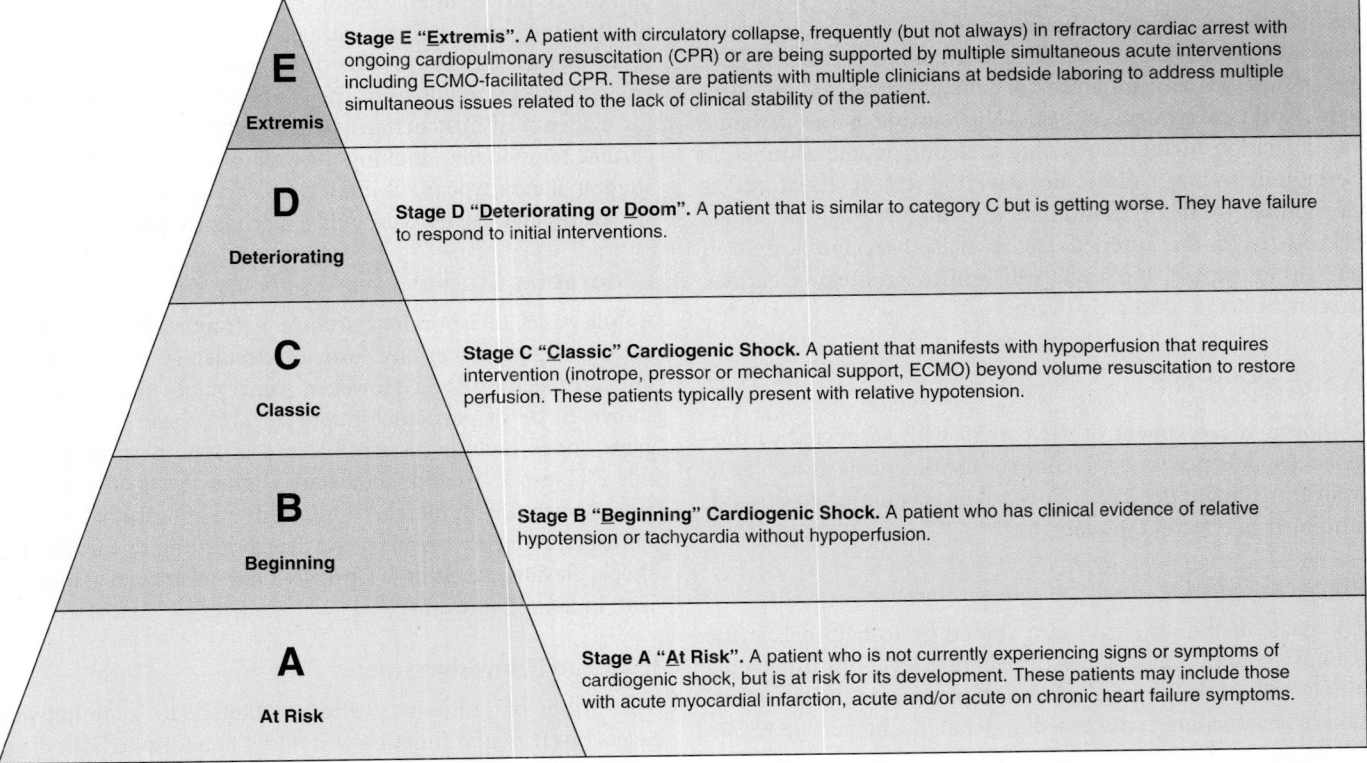

Figure 62–1. SCAI clinical expert consensus statement on the classification of cardiogenic shock. Reproduced with permission from Baran DA, Grines CL, Bailey S, et al. SCAI clinical expert consensus statement on the classification of cardiogenic shock: This document was endorsed by the American College of Cardiology (ACC), the American Heart Association (AHA), the Society of Critical Care Medicine (SCCM), and the Society of Thoracic Surgeons (STS) in April 2019. *Catheter Cardiovasc Interv.* 2019 Jul 1;94(1):29-37.

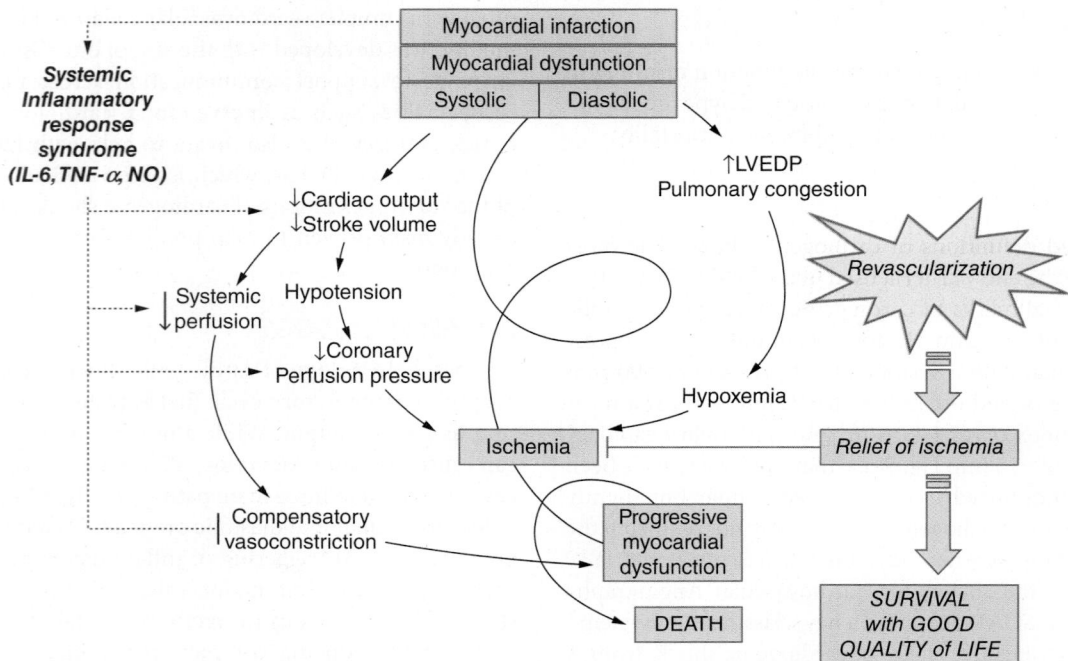

Figure 62–2. Current concept of cardiogenic shock pathophysiology. Reproduced with permission from Reynolds HR, Hochman JS. Cardiogenic shock: current concepts and improving outcomes. *Circulation.* 2008 Feb 5;117(5):686-697.

This directly decreases coronary perfusion pressure (due to reduction in aortic diastolic blood pressure). Furthermore, this reduction in blood pressure induces compensatory peripheral vasoconstriction in an attempt to maintain tissue perfusion; this increases ventricular afterload and further reduces cardiac output. Third, tissue necrosis due to impaired perfusions generates the release of inflammatory mediators including nitric oxide and peroxynitrite radicals. Nitric oxide causes systemic vasodilatation further worsening systemic hypotension while peroxynitrite has a direct negative ionotropic effect and is cardiotoxic.[8] Other inflammatory mediators such as tumor necrosis factor and interleukins have also been implicated.[9] If left uninterrupted, this cycle will lead to progressive cardiac dysfunction and ultimately death.

ASSESSMENT

A thorough assessment of the patient with suspected cardiogenic shock is necessary to confirm the diagnosis as well as to inform treatment decisions. This can be accomplished through a number of different modalities.

Physical Exam

The goals of the physical exam should be to help define the patient's volume status and estimate their level of cardiac output. Details of the physical exam as it pertains to the classification of heart failure is discussed in detail in Chapters 48 to 50.

Ultrasonography

Ultrasound has emerged as an essential tool in the efficient treatment and diagnosis of patients presenting in circulatory

shock, and is of particular importance in patients at risk for cardiogenic shock. Performing an informative point of care ultrasound has been shown to take an average of 6 minutes[10] and can improve patient outcomes. In patients presenting with cardiogenic shock, point of care ultrasound can rapidly determine the involvement of one or both ventricles and can help to diagnose the etiology of the cardiogenic shock by looking for evidence of obstruction (such as pulmonary embolism or cardiac tamponade), looking for wall motion abnormalities to suggest acute myocardial infarction, and assessing the cardiac structures and valves to exclude a mechanical issue.

Laboratory Studies

A full panel of laboratory studies is important in the evaluation of patients in any form of circulatory shock, including cardiogenic shock. However, some values that have been shown to be of particular importance in those with cardiogenic shock include N-terminal pro–B-type natriuretic peptide (NT-proBNP) and lactic acid. Higher levels of lactic acid are associated with increased mortality[11] and, especially in the setting of an acute coronary syndrome leading to cardiogenic shock, elevated levels of NT-proBNP have also been associated with increased mortality.[12]

Invasive Hemodynamics

The utility of pulmonary artery catheters to quantitatively assess biventricular function and filling pressures to both diagnose and guide management in the treatment of cardiogenic shock has been a topic of vigorous debate for years. Several trials have shown no benefit from the routine use of pulmonary artery catheters in managing critically ill patients[13] or patients with decompensated heart failure.[14,15] However, these trials notably excluded patients with cardiogenic shock from their analyses. More recently, several trials have shown benefit in using pulmonary artery catheter data in treating patients in cardiogenic shock,[16,17] particularly in those requiring mechanical circulatory support,[18] and have demonstrated improved survival rates when using a pulmonary artery catheter to completely characterize cardiogenic shock in order to inform treatment decisions.[19]

Cardiac Catheterization

Acute coronary occlusion is one of the most common etiologies of cardiogenic shock[20] and coronary angiography is essential for both the diagnosis and treatment in this scenario. Moreover, treatment and stabilization in a cardiac catheterization laboratory enables rapid invasive hemodynamic assessment and the ability to assess the vasculature and to place mechanical circulatory support devices under continuous fluoroscopic guidance if needed. As such, many cardiogenic shock protocols suggest immediate activation of the cardiac catheterization laboratory for treatment of cardiogenic shock[21] if there are any signs of ischemia on electrocardiogram or by serum biomarkers, such as troponin.

ETIOLOGY, CLASSIFICATION, AND TREATMENT

The clinical trials and guidelines for classification of cardiogenic shock have evolved and become more complex.[22] The modern cardiogenic shock characterizations have increased in nuance and compose a more complete picture of the various phenotypes associated with the disease process.[23] The classical depiction of "Warm-Wet," "Cold-Wet," "Cold-Dry," and "Warm-Dry" has gone through multiple transformations, including the most recent SCAI 5 tiered criteria that have been validated against hospital mortality outcomes.[6] However, there is significant room for further characterizations of clinical presentations of cardiogenic or low-cardiac output shock.

The management of cardiogenic shock secondary to acute myocardial infarction, which can present as right ventricular failure, left ventricular failure, or biventricular failure in the setting of cardiogenic shock, is subsequently discussed.[1] We have classified cardiogenic shock within its anatomical and physiological etiology.

Cardiogenic Shock with Predominant Left Ventricular Failure

Cardiogenic shock with predominant left ventricular failure is more common than isolated right ventricular failure and most often is precipitated by myocardial infarction or coronary ischemia.[24] However, the etiology of predominant left ventricular failure is variable and can be broken into three distinct categories: *primary, obstructive, and valvular.* The reason for further subclassification for predominant left ventricular failure is to distinguish specific management strategies for these variable physiologic presentations.

Primary left ventricular failure corresponds to an abnormality/injury to the myocardium itself. Often caused by ischemia, inflammation, or infiltration, primary left ventricular failure causing cardiogenic shock is diagnosed by exam, echocardiogram, cardiac magnetic resonance imaging, and by characteristic right heart catheterization findings (**Table 62–1**). Management of these patients focuses on treatment of the underlying cause while providing supportive management with inotropes and/or mechanical support to preserve end-organ function.[23] Mechanical support types are varied and the options range from intra aortic balloon pump (IABP), to percutaneous left ventricular assist devices (LVAD-Impella), to venoarterial extracorporeal membrane oxygenation (VA-ECMO).[1]

Obstructive left ventricular failure is often associated with complications from hypertrophic cardiomyopathy or postaortic valve intervention, and favors higher afterload with increased volume resuscitation and vasopressors, in order to decrease the obstructive gradient.[25] Evaluation with echocardiography is recommended to assess specific etiologies and individualized treatment strategies. In addition, negative chronotropic agents (β-blockade), will often increase diastolic filling time and lessen the outflow gradient. Definitive mechanical support with devices that do not cross the aortic valve are preferred as rescue options (TandemHeart LA-FA or VA-ECMO).[23]

Valvular left ventricular failure leading to cardiogenic shock is difficult to manage without procedural or surgical intervention. The mechanical etiology is varied based on the specific valve involved. In addition, the acuity of the complication often complicates the management strategy (Table 62–1). Overall, for definitive treatment of valvular left ventricular failure, procedural interventions are needed.[26]

Cardiogenic Shock with Predominant Right Ventricular Failure

Cardiogenic shock with predominant right ventricular failure is less common than predominant left ventricular failure; however, the overall mortality is similar.[23] In addition, the treatment strategies are less well defined. It is also common to have concurrent left ventricular failure with right ventricular failure that can sometimes be underrepresented on initial work-up.[23] Similar to its counterpart, treatments are based on the various etiologies of right ventricular failure, which we divide in two categories: *primary and obstructive.* Valvular complications affecting the right ventricle are rarely the etiology for underlying shock; however, they do present in patients with a history of congenital abnormalities.[27]

Primary right ventricular failure rarely presents in isolation; however, similar to primary left ventricular failure, it can be due to ischemia, inflammation, or infiltration. Pharmacological treatment is focused on augmentation of contractility while maintaining low-normal pulmonary vascular resistance.[28] In addition, management of these patients favors normal-to-high preload/central venous pressure. Mechanical support options for isolated right ventricular failure include Impella (RP), TandemHeart RA-PA, and VA-ECMO. However, when upgrading management to mechanical support the right ventricular

TABLE 62–1. Cardiogenic Shock Anatomic/Physiologic Stratification

Designation	Etiology	Physiology	Assessment	Treatment
Right Heart				
RH—Primary	AMI	Acute Ischemic infarct affecting RV > LV	**Exam:** peripheral edema, increased JVP; cool extremities **Echo:** RV dysfunction, normal/low RVSP **Coronary Angiography:** RCA disease if ischemic **Swan Ganz:** CPO <0.6W PAPi <1.0; elevated CVP; CVP:PCWP >0.63	**Preload:** favors high CVP **Contractility:** augmentation with selective inotropes favored (milrinone, dobutamine) **Afterload:** favors lower PVR and normal SVR (inhaled nitric oxide) **Mechanical Support:** Impella (RP), TandemHeart—RA/PA; Protec Duo; VA-ECMO
RH—Primary	Myocarditis	Acute myocardial non-ischemic inflammatory process affecting RV > LV		
RH—Primary	Cardiomyopathy-Progressive	Primary progressive deterioration of underlying disease process affecting the RV myocardium		
RH—Obstructive	Pulmonary Embolism	Acute thromboembolism of the pulmonary arteries causing acute increase in RV afterload	**Exam:** peripheral edema, increased JVP; SEM present; cool extremities **Echo:** RV dysfunction, +/− RVSP increase, outflow tract obstructions, pulmonary and tricuspid valve disease **Cardiac CT:** pulmonary embolism; outflow tract obstructions **Right Heart Catheterization:** elevated CVP; CVP:PCWP >0.63;	**Preload:** favors high CVP **Contractility:** augmentation with selective inotropes favored (milrinone, dobutamine) **Afterload:** favors lower PVR and normal SVR (inhaled nitric oxide) **Procedures:** Suction embolectomy; thrombolysis should be considered **Mechanical Support:** Impella (RP), TandemHeart—RA/PA; Protec Duo; VA-ECMO
RH—Obstructive	RVOT Obstruction/ Pulmonic Valve Obstruction	Progressive fixed obstruction of the RVOT or pulmonic valve causing progressive increase in RV afterload		**Preload:** favors high CVP **Contractility:** augmentation with selective inotropes favored (milrinone, dobutamine) **Afterload:** favors normal PVR and normal SVR (inhaled nitric oxide) **Procedures:** Invasive or minimally invasive procedures should be considered **Mechanical Support:** VA-ECMO
RH—Obstructive	Pulmonary Hypertension	Progressive disease of the pulmonary vascular system causing increased afterload of the RV		**Preload:** favors High CVP **Contractility:** augmentation with selective inotropes favored (milrinone, dobutamine) **Afterload:** favors lower PVR and normal SVR (inhaled nitric oxide, advanced pulmonary HTN mngt) **Mechanical Support:** VA-ECMO
Left Heart				
LH—Primary	AMI	Acute Ischemic Infarct affecting LV > RV	**Exam:** pulmonary edema, hypoxemia, S3+, tachycardia, decreased pulse pressure, pulsus alternans; cool extremities **Echo:** LV dysfunction without significant valvular dysfunction **Coronary Angiography:** variable presentation of disease if ischemic **Swan Ganz:** CPO <0.6 W; PAPi >1.0; normal CVP; PCWP elevated	**Preload:** favors low-normal CVP (diuretics, nitroglycerin) **Contractility:** augmentation with selective inotropes favored (milrinone, dobutamine) **Afterload:** favors lower afterload and lower SVR (nipride, nicardipine, nitroglycerin) **Mechanical Support:** balloon pump; Impella (CP, 5.0), TandemHeart—LA/VA; VA-ECMO
LH—Primary	Myocarditis	Acute myocardial non-ischemic inflammatory process affecting LV > RV		

(Continued)

TABLE 62-1. Cardiogenic Shock Anatomic/Physiologic Stratification (Continued)

Designation	Etiology	Physiology	Assessment	Treatment
LH—Primary	Progressive Cardiomyopathy	Progressive worsening of underlying LV cardiomyopathy		
LH—Primary	Peripartum Cardiomyopathy	Acute LV myocardial dysfunction in the peripartum period		
LH—Primary	Stress Cardiomyopathy	Acute LV myocardial dysfunction in the absence of ischemia or inflammation, related to underlying physical or emotional stress		
LH—Obstruction	Ventricular Outflow Obstruction	Progressive (ie, HOCM) or acute (ie, post TAVR) obstruction of the LVOT causing significant increase in gradient from LV cavity to LVOT.	**Exam:** pulmonary edema, hypoxemia, S4+, SEM increasing with valsalva, tachycardia; cool extremities **Echo:** hyperdynamic LV; elevated LVOT or mid-LV cavity gradient without significant Aortic Valve Disease; +/− systolic anterior motion of the mitral valve; +/− mitral regurgitation 2/2 to SAM **Left Heart Catheterization:** elevated LV:Ao gradient without significant aortic valve disease; elevated LVEDP **Swan Ganz:** CPO <0.6 W; PAPi >1.0; normal CVP; PCWP elevated	**Preload:** favors higher CVP, PCWP **Contractility:** favors decrease in contractility and chronotropy (β-blockade) **Afterload:** favors higher afterload and use of pure vasopressors (phenylephrine, vasopressin) **Procedures:** ETOH septal ablation and septal myomectomy can be considered **Mechanical Support:** ECMO available for intractable cases
LH—Valvular	Aortic Regurgitation—Acute	Acute regurgitation 2/2 to mechanical or infective injury of the aortic valve.	**Exam:** pulmonary edema, hypoxemia, diastolic murmur; tachycardia; cool extremities **Echo:** hyperdynamic LV; significant aortic regurgitation seen with short pressure half-time; +/− appearance of valvular abscess/mass **Swan Ganz:** CPO <0.6 W; PAPi >1.0; normal CVP; PCWP elevated	**Preload:** favors low-normal CVP/PCWP **Contractility:** augmentation with inotropes and chronotropes favored (milrinone, dobutamine, norepi, epi, dopamine) **Afterload:** favors lower afterload and SVR (nipride, nicardipine, nitroglycerin) **Procedural:** urgent surgical repair/replacement is recommended **Mechanical:** can consider TandemHeart-LA/FA
LH—Valvular	Aortic Stenosis Progressive[26]	Progressive narrowing of the aortic valve leading to increased fixed afterload of the LV	**Exam:** pulmonary edema, hypoxemia, soft SEM with loss of 2/2 heart sound; +/− S4; cool extremities **Echo:** normal to low normal LVEF; significant aortic stenosis with gradient **Swan Ganz:** CPO <0.6 W; PAPi >1.0; normal CVP; PCWP elevated	**Preload:** favors normal CVP status **Contractility:** augmentation with inopresors favored (norepi; epi) **Afterload:** favors higher afterload to maintain coronary perfusion pressure (phenylephrine, vasopressin) **Procedural:** BAV; TAVR; Surgical AVR can be considered[26] **Mechanical:** balloon pump; TandemHeart—LA/VA; ECMO
LH—Valvular	Mitral Regurgitation-Acute	Acute regurgitation 2/2 to mechanical or infective injury of the mitral valve	**Exam:** pulmonary edema (+/−asymmetry), hypoxemia, holosystolic murmur; cool extremities **Echo:** normal to hyperdynamic LVEF; significant mitral regurgitation (+/− eccentric); +/− left atrial dilation **Swan Ganz:** CPO <0.6 W; PAPi >1.0; normal CVP; PCWP elevated with prominent V-waves	**Preload:** favors low-normal CVP/PCWP **Contractility:** augmentation with inotropes and chronotropes favored (milrinone, dobutamine, norepi, epi, dopamine) **Afterload:** favors lower afterload and SVR (nipride, nicardipine, nitroglycerin) **Procedural:** urgent surgical repair/replacement is recommended **Mechanical:** can consider balloon pump, Impella CP/5.0, TandemHeart LA-FA, VA-ECMO

(Continued)

TABLE 62–1. Cardiogenic Shock Anatomic/Physiologic Stratification (Continued)

Designation	Etiology	Physiology	Assessment	Treatment
LH—Valvular	Mitral Stenosis / Mitral In-Flow Obstruction-Progressive	Progressive narrowing of the mitral valve leading to decreased filling of the LV	**Exam:** pulmonary edema, hypoxemia, soft diastolic murmur; cool extremities **Echo:** normal to hyperdynamic LVEF; significant mitral valve stenosis; +/− mitral regurgitation; +/− significant mitral annular calcification **Swan Ganz:** CPO <0.6 W; PAPi >1.0; normal CVP; PCWP significantly elevated	**Preload:** favors low-normal CVP/PCWP **Contractility:** favors increased diastolic filling time with decreased chronotropy; favor normal Atrial rhythm (SInus) **Afterload:** favors normal—higher afterload and SVR **Procedural:** can consider balloon valvuloplasty for urgent intervention **Mechanical:** can consider TandemHeart—LA/FA; VA-ECMO
Biventricular				
Primary	AMI	Acute ischemic infarct resulting in biventricular failure	**Exam:** increased JVP, pulmonary edema, hypoxemia, S3+, tachycardia, decreased pulse pressure, pulsus alternans; cool extremities **Echo:** biventricular dysfunction w/wo ventricular dilation **Coronary Angiography:** variable presentation of disease if ischemic **Swan Ganz:** CPO <0.6 W; PAPi <1.0; elevated CVP; PCWP elevated	**Preload:** favors low- normal CVP (diuretics, nitroglycerin) **Contractility:** augmentation with selective inotropes favored (milrinone, dobutamine) **Afterload:** favors lower afterload and lower SVR, PVR (inhaled NO, nipride, nicardipine, nitroglycerin) **Mechanical Support:** balloon pump; Impella (RP, CP, 5.0); VA-ECMO
Primary	Acute Myocarditis	Acute myocardial nonischemic inflammatory process affecting both ventricles		
Primary	Toxic, Metabolic, Iatrogenic	A direct myocardial toxic effect by pharmaceuticals, recreational drugs, toxins, electrolyte abnormalities, or underlying physiologic processes		
Electrical	Ventricular Tachycardia	Biventricular decrease in diastolic filling time with severe decreased and dyssynchronous myocardial contraction	**Exam:** increased JVP, pulmonary edema, hypoxemia, S3+, variable pulse rate pending arrhythmia, decreased pulse pressure, cool extremities **ECG:** variable based on diagnosis **Coronary Angiography:** variable based on underlying disease process **Swan Ganz:** CPO <0.6 W; PAPi <1.0; elevated CVP; PCWP elevated	**Preload:** favors low- normal CVP (diuretics, nitroglycerin) **Contractility:** bradycardia arrhythmias favor chronotropic agents (dopamine, dobutamin) **Rhythm:** favors rhythm control strategy with cardioversion or antiarrhythmic medication **Afterload:** favors lower afterload and lower SVR **Mechanical Support:** balloon pump; Impella (RP, CP, 5.0); VA-ECMO
Electrical	Bradycardia	Decreased cardiac output secondary to a low heart rate		
Electrical	Atrial Tachyarrhythmia	Biventricular decrease in diastolic filling time often coupled with decreased myocardial contraction		
Obstructive	Tamponade	External compression of biventricular expansion resulting from fluid accumulation in the pericardial space, leading to limited ventricular filling and respiratory variation in cardiac output	**Exam:** increased JVP, decreased heart sounds, tachycardia, pulsus paradoxus; cool extremities **Echo:** evidence of cardiac tamponade per established criteria; ventricular interdependence **Coronary Angiography:** variable presentation of disease if ischemic **Swan Ganz:** CPO <0.6 W; elevated CVP; PCWP elevated; blunted y-descent	**Preload:** favors normal—high CVP (IVF) **Procedures:** pericardiocentesis indicated for definitive treatment **Mechanical Support:** VA-ECMO

(Continued)

TABLE 62–1. Cardiogenic Shock Anatomic/Physiologic Stratification (Continued)

Designation	Etiology	Physiology	Assessment	Treatment
Obstructive	Pericardial Constriction	Progressive external compression of biventricular expansion leading to a fixed biventricular diastolic volume and lower cardiac output	**Exam:** increased JVP, tachycardia, cool extremities **Echo:** evidence of pericardial constriction by established criteria; ventricular interdependence **Right/Left Heart Catheterization:** CPO <0.6 W; elevated CVP; PCWP elevated; RV/LV pressure discordance	**Preload:** favors normal—high CVP (IVF) **Procedures:** pericardiectomy indicated if available **Mechanical Support:** VA-ECMO
Structural	Postcardiotomy	Acute myocardial dysfunction following cardiac surgery resulting in congestive heart failure and cardiogenic shock	**Exam:** increased JVP, pulmonary edema, hypoxemia, S3+, decreased pulse pressure, cool extremities **Echo:** biventricular failure with +/− myocardial edema **Coronary Angiography:** variable based on underlying disease process **Swan Ganz:** CPO <0.6 W; PAPi <1.0; elevated CVP; PCWP elevated	**Preload:** favors low-normal CVP (diuretics, nitroglycerin) **Contractility:** augmentation with inotropes and chronotropes favored (milrinone, dobutamine, norepi, epi, dopamine) **Rhythm:** favors rhythm control strategy with cardioversion or antiarrhythmic medication **Afterload:** favors lower afterload and lower SVR **Mechanical Support:** balloon pump; Impella (RP, CP, 5.0); VA-ECMO
Structural	Myocardial Wall Rupture	Secondary to acute ischemia, inflammation, or infection, resulting in atypical blood flow patterns and with various hemodynamic complications	**Exam:** increased JVP, pulmonary edema, hypoxemia, S3+, variable pulse rate pending arrhythmia, decreased pulse pressure, cool extremities **Echo:** various presentations based on structural complication **Coronary Angiography:** variable based on underlying disease process **Swan Ganz:** CPO: <0.6 W; variable based on underlying disease process	**Preload:** variable pending structural abnormality **Contractility:** augmentation with inotropes and chronotropes favored (milrinone, dobutamine, norepi, epi, dopamine) **Afterload:** favors lower afterload and lower SVR **Procedures:** urgent surgical intervention indicated pending structural abnormality **Mechanical Support:** balloon pump; VA-ECMO

cardiac output will drastically increase.[29] Since left ventricular failure can go undetected on initial evaluation, isolated right ventricular augmentation can lead to left ventricular failure. Therefore, close monitoring and quick escalation to left ventricular support should be initiated.

Obstructive right ventricular failure most often presents following a massive or submassive pulmonary embolism, leading to an acute increase in pulmonary vascular resistance.[30] Management of acute pulmonary embolism is discussed elsewhere; however, support of the right ventricle is vital while relief of the obstruction with definitive therapy is provided. Antithrombotics and thrombolytics also play an important role; however, they can limit the support options based on overall bleeding risk. In addition to acute pulmonary embolism, obstructive right ventricular failure secondary to worsening pulmonary hypertension or outflow tract obstruction require specialized care focused on reducing the obstructive burden seen by the right ventricle.[30]

Cardiogenic Shock with Biventricular Failure

As with most aspects of cardiology, cardiogenic shock usually involves some degree of dysfunction from both ventricles.[23]

As aforementioned, in situations where one ventricle is the primary culprit, isolated treatments can be implemented. Similar to this, the treatments for biventricular failure leading to cardiogenic shock are managed based on the underlying etiology: *Primary, Obstructive, Electrical, Structural.* For this section, we focus on the etiologies that affect both ventricles simultaneously, leading to biventricular failure.

Primary biventricular failure, predictably, can be caused by ischemia, inflammation, or infiltration. Biventricular failure causing cardiogenic shock is diagnosed by exam, echocardiogram, and by characteristic right heart catheterization findings (Table 62–1). Management of these patients focuses on treatment of the underlying cause while providing supportive management with inotropes and/or mechanical support to preserve end-organ function.[23] There are limited biventricular support options, and if more than one device is used, the cardiac outputs by both the right and left heart must be balanced. Biventricular Impella devices and VA-ECMO are often the salvage mechanical support devices used for stabilization as a bridge to definitive therapy.[31]

Obstructive biventricular failure is characterized by increased external pressure either by fluid (tamponade) or constriction.[23]

The presence of pericardial fluid causing ventricular interdependence and decreased cardiac output leading to shock is known as tamponade.[32] Higher central venous pressure achieved with intravenous fluid resuscitation can temporize the progression to shock; however, definitive treatment is achieved through percutaneous or invasive procedural techniques. Severe pericardial constriction often presents more insidiously and may require extensive surgical procedures for definitive management.[33] Temporization with biventricular mechanical support can be considered for specific cases if definitive management cannot be achieved acutely.[31]

Electrical biventricular failure is characterized by decreased cardiac output stemming from an underlying arrhythmia leading to cardiogenic shock. Most often, this shock is associated with ventricular arrhythmias.[34] Definitive treatment involves correction of the underlying cardiac arrhythmia and a return to normal sinus rhythm. Often, these arrhythmias are combined with underlying structural and valvular abnormalities that also must be considered when treating the patient.[34]

Structural biventricular failure is characterized by a malfunction of anatomical structures or rupture of the myocardium. Postcardiotomy failure can occur postcardiac surgery from various etiologies including graft failure. Treatment requires supportive care with full mechanical support and often primary surgical correction.[24] Myocardial rupture as a result of ischemia, inflammation, or infection presents with varying degrees of ventricular failure. Support often utilizes extracardiac temporary mechanical devices (IABP, Impella-LVAD, VA-ECMO) and definitive procedural correction.[31] The pharmacologic management of myocardial rupture is limited and variable based on the individual defect.[24]

Interdisciplinary Shock Teams

With the introduction of interdisciplinary teams for various diagnoses (pulmonary embolism, stroke, ST-elevation myocardial infarction, etc.), the addition of an interdisciplinary shock team for advanced referral centers is becoming a meaningful strategy.[35] The complexity of assessment and treatment for patients presenting with cardiogenic shock is extensive and time sensitive (as aforementioned). There is growing evidence in the literature that SHOCK Teams decrease the time to definitive therapy and increase the utilization of correct therapies to reverse specific shock etiologies. A team comprising Interventional Cardiology, Cardiac Surgery, Heart Failure, and Cardiac Intensivists allows for high level noninvasive and invasive assessment of the patient.[36] Further decisions including type of temporary mechanical support can be discussed in the context of candidacy for long-term ventricular support (ie, LVAD, BiVAD, total artificial heart, or transplant).

Treatment

Pharmacotherapy

Vasopressors and inotropes are the backbone of medical therapy for cardiogenic shock. In order to interrupt the cascade of cardiogenic shock, one must focus on several key clinical goals: (1) reduction of ventricular afterload, (2) optimization of preload, (3) augmentation of cardiac contractility, and (4) maintenance of adequate mean arterial pressure to ensure that key organs, such as the brain and kidney, remain perfused. This is most often accomplished with a combination of multiple vasoactive agents, each which may serve a different or combined role in reaching these goals based on the clinical situation. Recent data supports the approach of using norepinephrine as a first-line agent for cardiogenic shock, specifically when compared to drugs that have more mixed alpha and beta activity, such as dopamine[37] and epinephrine.[38] Despite the excitement around the novel drug levosimendan, recent data has suggested that it does not confer clear benefit in either a surgical[39] or nonsurgical[40] patient population. **Table 62–2** gives a summary of available pharmacotherapy for cardiogenic shock.

Coronary Revascularization

In situations where cardiogenic shock is driven by acute myocardial infarction, reestablishing perfusion to the affected

---

TABLE 62–2. Summary of Pharmacology Used in Cardiogenic Shock

Agent	Mechanism	Effects	Clinical Importance
Phenylephrine	Pure alpha agonist	Vasoconstriction	Useful in cardiogenic shock related to hypertrophic cardiomyopathy
Norepinephrine	Alpha > Beta Agonist	Vasoconstriction with some ionotropy/chronotropy	Best first-line agent for cardiogenic shock
Epinephrine	Alpha = Beta Agonist	Ionotropy/chronotropy and vasoconstriction	Best reserved for salvage situations of extreme cardiogenic shock
Dopamine	Dose Dependent	Iontropy/chronotropy and vasoconstriction	Best for situations in which chronotropy is desired most
Vasopressin	V1 agonist	Vasoconstriction	Can help to offset vasodilatation which may accompany ionodilators
Dobutamine	Beta Agonist	Iotropy with mild vasodilitation	Good first-line ionotrope but may have blunted response in those on β-blockers
Milrinone	Phosphodiesterase 3 inhibitor	Ionotropy with strong vasodilatation	Caution as may cause hypotension
Nitric Oxide	cGMP Agonist	Pulmonary vasodilator	Best for cardiogenic shock related to right ventricular failure
Levosimendan	Calcium Sensitizer	Ionotropy and mild vasodilatation	Unclear role given recent data

myocardial territory is of high importance. This is most often accomplished by percutaneous coronary intervention.[41] While all agree that revascularization of the culprit artery is essential, the role for revascularization of nonculprit arteries remain controversial. A recent trial, CULPRIT-SHOCK, demonstrated that culprit-only revascularization is associated with reduced rates of 30-day death or renal replacement therapy,[42] although data from the National Cardiogenic Shock Initiative showed similar outcomes in complete versus culprit-only revascularization in the setting of mechanical circulatory support.[43]

Antithrombotic Therapy

In addition to mechanical reperfusion in situations of acute myocardial infarction, pharmacologic therapy to help reperfuse and maintain reperfusion is essential. The optimal use of aspirin and an anticoagulant, usually unfractionated heparin, is the backbone of such medical management. The use of a second antiplatelet agent is of high importance, but selecting the ideal second agent in this setting is controversial. In general, ticagrelor is thought to provide strong and safe antiplatelet activity, and has been shown to be superior to clopidogrel.[44] More recent data has suggested that prasugrel may also be a good choice in selected patients.[45] The newest antiplatelet is cangrelor, and serves a niche role in the management of cardiogenic shock. Cangrelor is delivered intravenously, and because gut absorption may be impaired in shock states, this route of administration ensures that it will lead to adequate platelet inhibition. Moreover, cangrelor has a short half-life, and if cardiothoracic surgery is required to help treat cardiogenic shock, it is more easily accomplished in the setting of cangrelor, because potent oral antiplatelet agents can lead to significant bleeding during surgery and sometimes may delay or prohibit needed urgent surgical intervention.[46]

Mechanical Circulatory Support

The role of mechanical circulatory support in cardiogenic shock is a growing area of research and clinical interest, and is more thoroughly discussed in Chapter 52.

REFERENCES

1. van Diepen S, Katz JN, Albert NM, et al. Contemporary management of cardiogenic shock: a scientific statement from the American Heart Association. *Circulation.* 2017;136:e232-e268.

2. Hochman JS, Sleeper LA, Webb JG, et al. Early revascularization in acute myocardial infarction complicated by cardiogenic shock. SHOCK Investigators. Should we emergently revascularize occluded coronaries for cardiogenic shock. *N Engl J Med.* 1999;341:625-634.

3. Thiele H, Zeymer U, Thelemann N, et al. Intraaortic balloon pump in cardiogenic shock complicating acute myocardial infarction: long-term 6-year outcome of the randomized IABP-SHOCK II trial. *Circulation.* 2019;139:395-403.

4. Bauer T, Zeymer U, Hochadel M, et al. Use and outcomes of multivessel percutaneous coronary intervention in patients with acute myocardial infarction complicated by cardiogenic shock (from the EHS-PCI Registry). *Am J Cardiol.* 2012;109:941-946.

5. Ahn SG, Lee JW, Kang DR, et al. Immediate multivessel intervention versus culprit-vessel intervention only in patients with ST-elevation myocardial infarction and multivessel coronary disease: data from the prospective KAMIR-NIH registry. *Coron Artery Dis.* 2019;30:95-102.

6. Pareek N, Dworakowski R, Webb I, et al. SCAI cardiogenic shock classification after out of hospital cardiac arrest and association with outcome. *Catheter Cardiovasc Interv.* 2021;96(3):E288-E297.

7. Jentzer JC, van Diepen S, Barsness GW, et al. Cardiogenic shock classification to predict mortality in the cardiac intensive care unit. *J Am Coll Cardiol.* 2019;74:2117-2128.

8. Hochman JS. Cardiogenic shock complicating acute myocardial infarction: expanding the paradigm. *Circulation.* 2003;107:2998-3002.

9. Prondzinsky R, Unverzagt S, Lemm H, et al. Interleukin-6, -7, -8 and -10 predict outcome in acute myocardial infarction complicated by cardiogenic shock. *Clin Res Cardiol.* 2012;101:375-384.

10. Jones AE, Tayal VS, Sullivan DM, Kline JA. Randomized, controlled trial of immediate versus delayed goal-directed ultrasound to identify the cause of nontraumatic hypotension in emergency department patients. *Crit Care Med.* 2004;32:1703-1708.

11. Attana P, Lazzeri C, Chiostri M, Picariello C, Gensini GF, Valente S. Strong-ion gap approach in patients with cardiogenic shock following ST-elevation myocardial infarction. *Acute Card Care.* 2013;15:58-62.

12. Shah NR, Bieniarz MC, Basra SS, et al. Serum biomarkers in severe refractory cardiogenic shock. *JACC Heart Fail.* 2013;1:200-206.

13. Marik PE. Obituary: pulmonary artery catheter 1970 to 2013. *Ann Intensive Care* 2013;3:38.

14. Binanay C, Califf RM, Hasselblad V, et al. Evaluation study of congestive heart failure and pulmonary artery catheterization effectiveness: the ESCAPE trial. *JAMA.* 2005;294:1625-1633.

15. Shah MR, Hasselblad V, Stevenson LW, et al. Impact of the pulmonary artery catheter in critically ill patients: meta-analysis of randomized clinical trials. *JAMA.* 2005;294:1664-1670.

16. Hernandez GA, Lemor A, Blumer V, et al. Trends in utilization and outcomes of pulmonary artery catheterization in heart failure with and without cardiogenic shock. *J Card Fail.* 2019;25:364-371.

17. Rossello X, Vila M, Rivas-Lasarte M, et al. Impact of pulmonary artery catheter use on short- and long-term mortality in patients with cardiogenic shock. *Cardiology.* 2017;136:61-69.

18. O'Neill WW, Grines C, Schreiber T, et al. Analysis of outcomes for 15,259 US patients with acute myocardial infarction cardiogenic shock (AMICS) supported with the Impella device. *Am Heart J.* 2018;202:33-38.

19. Garan AR, Kanwar M, Thayer KL, et al. Complete hemodynamic profiling with pulmonary artery catheters in cardiogenic shock is associated with lower in-hospital mortality. *JACC Heart Fail.* 2020;8:903-913.

20. Harjola VP, Lassus J, Sionis A, et al. Clinical picture and risk prediction of short-term mortality in cardiogenic shock. *Eur J Heart Fail.* 2015;17:501-509.

21. Basir MB, Kapur NK, Patel K, et al. Improved outcomes associated with the use of shock protocols: updates from the national cardiogenic shock initiative. *Catheter Cardiovasc Interv.* 2019;93:1173-1183.

22. Josiassen J, Helgestad OKL, Udesen NLJ, et al. Unloading using Impella CP during profound cardiogenic shock caused by left ventricular failure in a large animal model: impact on the right ventricle. *Intensive Care Med Exp.* 2020;8:41.

23. Tehrani BN, Truesdell AG, Psotka MA, et al. A standardized and comprehensive approach to the management of cardiogenic shock. *JACC Heart Fail.* 2020;8:879-891.

24. Mebazaa A, Combes A, van Diepen S, et al. Management of cardiogenic shock complicating myocardial infarction. *Intensive Care Med.* 2018;44:760-773.

25. Suh WM, Witzke CF, Palacios IF. Suicide left ventricle following transcatheter aortic valve implantation. *Catheter Cardiovasc Interv.* 2010;76:616-620.

26. Urena M, Himbert D. Cardiogenic shock in aortic stenosis: is it the time for "Primary" TAVR? *JACC Cardiovasc Interv.* 2020;13:1326-1328.

27. Engelfriet P, Tijssen J, Kaemmerer H, et al. Adherence to guidelines in the clinical care for adults with congenital heart disease: the Euro Heart Survey on adult congenital heart disease. *Eur Heart J.* 2006;27:737-745.

28. Kapur NK, Esposito ML, Bader Y, et al. Mechanical circulatory support devices for acute right ventricular failure. *Circulation*. 2017;136:314-326.

29. Baran DA, Grines CL, Bailey S, et al. SCAI clinical expert consensus statement on the classification of cardiogenic shock: this document was endorsed by the American College of Cardiology (ACC), the American Heart Association (AHA), the Society of Critical Care Medicine (SCCM), and the Society of Thoracic Surgeons (STS) in April 2019. *Catheter Cardiovasc Interv*. 2019;94:29-37.

30. Kucher N, Goldhaber SZ. Management of massive pulmonary embolism. *Circulation*. 2005;112:e28-e32.

31. Kuchibhotla S, Esposito ML, Breton C, et al. Acute biventricular mechanical circulatory support for cardiogenic shock. *J Am Heart Assoc*. 2017;6.

32. Ball JB, Morrison WL. Cardiac tamponade. *Postgrad Med J*. 1997;73:141-145.

33. Spodick DH. The normal and diseased pericardium: current concepts of pericardial physiology, diagnosis and treatment. *J Am Coll Cardiol*. 1983;1:240-251.

34. Saidi A, Akoum N, Bader F. Management of unstable arrhythmias in cardiogenic shock. *Curr Treat Options Cardiovasc Med*. 2011;13:354-360.

35. Hernandez-Perez FJ, Alvarez-Avello JM, Forteza A, et al. Initial outcomes of a multidisciplinary network for the care of patients with cardiogenic shock. *Rev Esp Cardiol (Engl Ed)*. 2021;74(1):33-43.

36. Gibbs D, Eusebio C, Sanders J, et al. Clinician perceptions of the impact of a shock team approach in the management of cardiogenic shock: a qualitative study. *Cardiovasc Revasc Med*. 2021;22:78-83.

37. De Backer D, Biston P, Devriendt J, et al. Comparison of dopamine and norepinephrine in the treatment of shock. *N Engl J Med*. 2010;362:779-789.

38. Levy B, Clere-Jehl R, Legras A, et al. Epinephrine versus norepinephrine for cardiogenic shock after acute myocardial infarction. *J Am Coll Cardiol*. 2018;72:173-182.

39. Mehta RH, Leimberger JD, van Diepen S, et al. Levosimendan in patients with left ventricular dysfunction undergoing cardiac surgery. *N Engl J Med*. 2017;376:2032-2042.

40. Mebazaa A, Nieminen MS, Packer M, et al. Levosimendan vs dobutamine for patients with acute decompensated heart failure: the SURVIVE Randomized Trial. *JAMA*. 2007;297:1883-1891.

41. Thiele H, Zeymer U, Neumann FJ, et al. Intraaortic balloon support for myocardial infarction with cardiogenic shock. *N Engl J Med*. 2012;367:1287-1296.

42. Thiele H, Akin I, Sandri M, et al. PCI strategies in patients with acute myocardial infarction and cardiogenic shock. *N Engl J Med*. 2017;377:2419-2432.

43. Lemor A, Basir MB, Patel K, et al. Multivessel versus culprit-vessel percutaneous coronary intervention in cardiogenic shock. *JACC Cardiovasc Interv*. 2020;13:1171-1178.

44. Wallentin L, Becker RC, Budaj A, et al. Ticagrelor versus clopidogrel in patients with acute coronary syndromes. *N Engl J Med*. 2009;361:1045-1057.

45. Schupke S, Neumann FJ, Menichelli M, et al. Ticagrelor or prasugrel in patients with acute coronary syndromes. *N Engl J Med*. 2019;381:1524-1534.

46. Droppa M, Vaduganathan M, Venkateswaran RV, et al. Cangrelor in cardiogenic shock and after cardiopulmonary resuscitation: a global, multicenter, matched pair analysis with oral P2Y12 inhibition from the IABP-SHOCK II trial. *Resuscitation*. 2019;137:205-212.

Sudden Cardiac Death and Resuscitation

Sanjiv M. Narayan and James P. Daubert

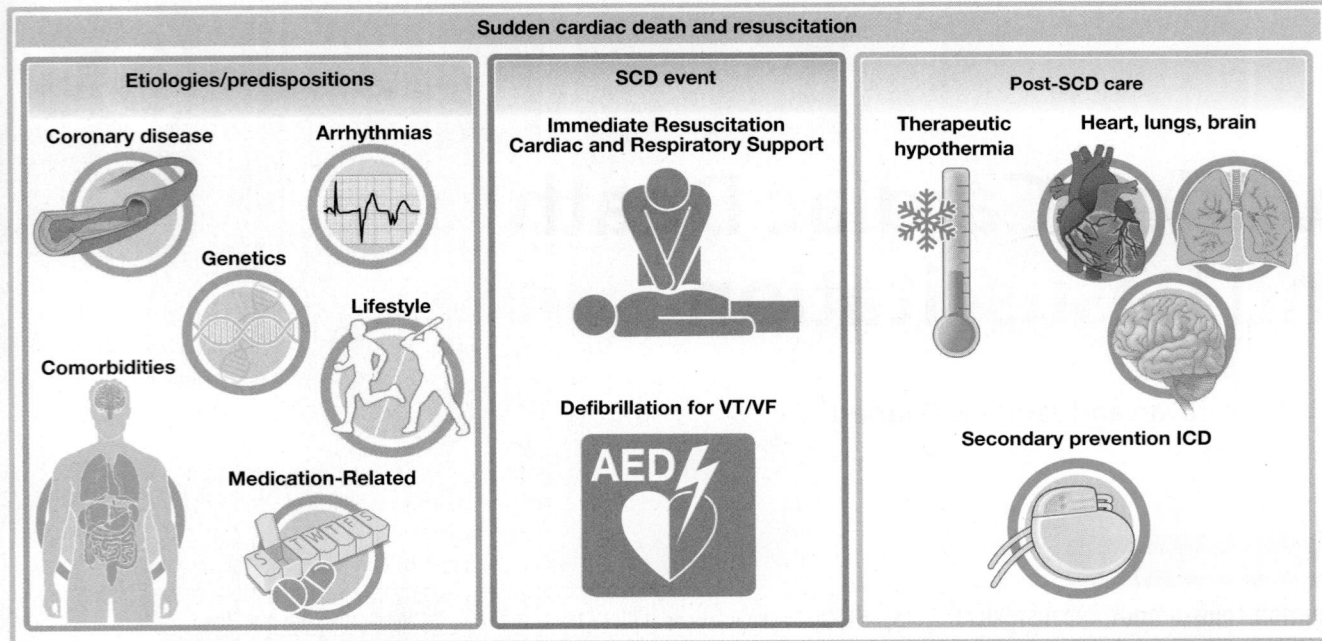

Chapter 63 Fuster and Hurst's Central Illustration. Sudden cardiac death (SCD) can result from various causes. Effective early response is critical in SCD. Post-resuscitation care focuses on preserving the brain, neurological recovery, and cardiopulmonary management. AED, automated external defibrillator; ICD, implantable cardioverter defibrillator; VF, ventricular fibrillation; VT, ventricular tachycardia.

CHAPTER SUMMARY

This chapter provides a structural and practical discussion of sudden cardiac death (SCD), acute resuscitation, and post-resuscitation care. The various etiologies of SCD include arrhythmias, coronary disease, genetic electrical syndromes, and structural causes. SCD can strike individuals in the broad population, as well as special populations at risk, including women, underrepresented minorities, and athletes. Paradoxically, a substantial minority of cases classified as SCD are non-cardiac and span neurological, respiratory, and other causes. Currently, risk stratification for SCD is suboptimal and future avenues for improved mechanism-based prediction are highlighted. Notably, in-hospital SCD is associated with better prognosis than out-of-hospital SCD. Effective early response is critical and shares similarities for both types of arrest. The chapter details basic and cardiopulmonary resuscitation, including current emergency pharmacological management and coronary catheterization. Postresuscitation care focuses on preserving the brain—including via therapeutic temperature management (induced hypothermia)—neurological recovery, as well as cardiopulmonary management. The ethics of end-of-life management and withdrawal of resuscitation are also emphasized.

DEFINITION, EPIDEMIOLOGY, AND HISTORICAL CONSIDERATIONS

Sudden cardiac arrest (SCA) is defined by the World Health Organization (WHO) as a sudden unexpected death either within 1 hour of symptom onset if witnessed, or within 24 hours of having been observed alive and symptom free if unwitnessed.[1] If not successfully resuscitated, individuals with SCA progress rapidly to sudden cardiac death (SCD).

The first successful resuscitation from out-of-hospital SCA was reported in 1956, in a male physician with indigestion who was diagnosed with myocardial infarction and discharged but then collapsed outside the hospital.[2] He was resuscitated by using emergency thoracotomy, cardiac massage, and defibrillation. At about that time, Gurvich in the Soviet Union reported external defibrillation in animal studies and Zoll et al. in the United States reported defibrillation in patients. These studies occurred at a time in history when society was beginning to experience electrocution accidents related to electrification.[2] The subsequent success of external defibrillation for ventricular fibrillation ushered in the era of coronary care units and the model of rapid defibrillation for SCA.

SCD is a leading cause of death worldwide and accounts for 180,000 to 450,000 deaths annually in the United States.[3] SCD may be a patient's first clinical presentation, but is also common in patients with known cardiac disease. The incidence of SCD has risen during crises such as the 9/11 attacks,[4] and during the COVID-19 pandemic[5] in parallel with a drop in admissions for acute coronary syndrome.[6] SCD is less common in women than men (42% vs 58% of victims),[3] but in Black populations its incidence is double that in White populations[7] and it occurs at a younger age[8] (**Fig. 63–1A**). The prevalence of SCD exhibits strong age-dependence, with a rate of 2.28 per 100,000 in those under 35 years, 100 per 100,000 in those 50 to 74 years of age, and 600 per 100,000 in those over 75. While the overall burden of cardiovascular deaths is falling, the burden of SCD is falling more slowly.[3] Only 10% to 12% of victims of out-of-hospital SCA survive to hospital discharge[9] (**Fig. 63–1B**).

CLINICAL AND MECHANISTIC SUBTYPES

SCD is not a single disease but a terminal disturbance of rhythm or hemodynamics from diverse pathological processes (see **Figs. 63–2A** and **63–2B**). Much of our understanding comes from data collected at the scene of an arrest. Historically, two-thirds of cases identified by WHO criteria were due to ventricular tachycardia (VT) or fibrillation (VF).[1] However, the proportion of cases presenting as VF from 1980 to 2000 have fallen in relation to cases presenting at pulseless electrical activity (PEA) or asystole.[3] It is debated whether this reflects increasing use of medications that slow heart rate, such as β-blockers, improved treatment of coronary disease,[10] or factors such as delayed arrival of emergency medical services enabling the rhythm to degenerate to PEA by the time of the first ECG. Patients with SCD without detected VF have lower survival than victims with VF,[10] so this trend has profound implications for risk prediction, therapy, and outcomes.

SCD may result from multiple and diverse causes, which are also age dependent. This is summarized in Figs. 63–2A and 63–2B. Patients with SCD early in life often have inherited causes including defined genetic syndromes. Patients who develop SCD from ages 20 to 40 have a mix of etiologies including genetic syndromes and structural heart disease, while those developing SCD at older ages typically have coronary or

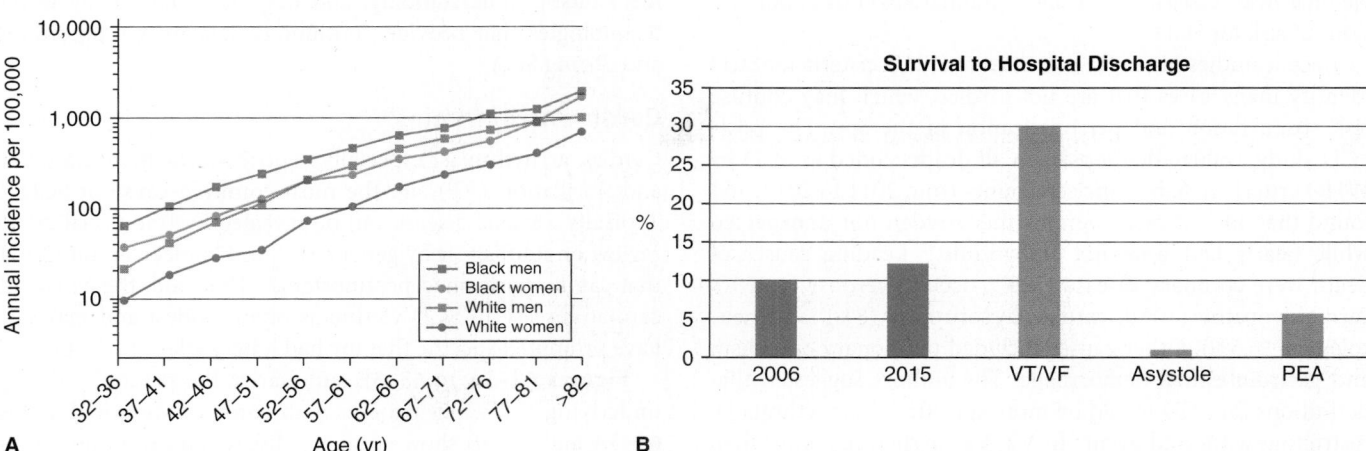

Figure 63–1. Epidemiology of SCD. (A) Age, race, and sex-related annual incidence of SCD in the United States. Incidence rises exponentially with age (note logarithmic scale), and is higher for men versus women and for Black versus White populations across age groups. **(B)** Survival to hospital discharge for selected categories. There has been only a modest increase in survival in 2015 compared to 2006 using data from Resuscitation Outcomes Consortium (ROC) whereas survival in 2015 per the Cardiac Arrest Registry to Enhance Survival (CARES) registry was 10.6% and essentially flat from 2011. Survival rates vary dramatically with presenting rhythm, being lower for the nonshockable rhythms of asystole and PEA than for the shockable rhythms of VT or VF. (A) Reproduced with permission from Becker LB, Han BH, Meyer PM, et al. Racial differences in the incidence of cardiac arrest and subsequent survival. The CPR Chicago Project. *N Engl J Med.* 1993 Aug 26;329(9):600-606. (B) Data from Benjamin EJ, Virani SS, Callaway CW, et al. Heart Disease and Stroke Statistics-2018 Update: A Report From the American Heart Association. *Circulation.* 2018 Mar 20;137(12):e67-e492 and Andrew E, Nehme Z, Lijovic M, et al. Outcomes following out-of-hospital cardiac arrest with an initial cardiac rhythm of asystole or pulseless electrical activity in Victoria, Australia. *Resuscitation.* 2014 Nov;85(11):1633-1639.

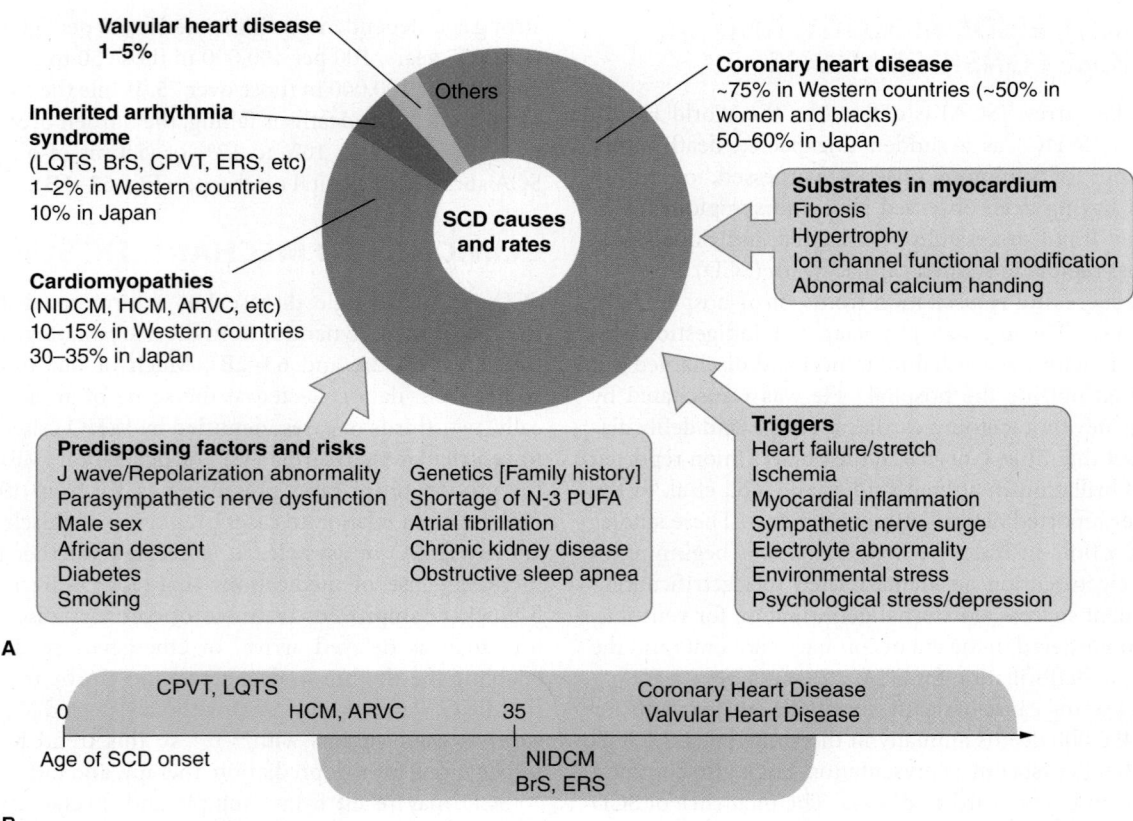

Figure 63–2. The spectrum of epidemiology underlying SCD. Causes of SCD and rates **(A)** and age of SCD onset in each disease **(B)**. (A) Coronary heart disease is the leading cause of SCD, but the rates of baseline heart disease differ between Western countries and Japan. (B) SCDs occur in elderly populations in coronary heart disease and valvular disease, whereas most SCDs in CPVT and LQTS develop at age <35 years. ARVC, arrhythmogenic right ventricular cardiomyopathy; BrS, Brugada syndrome; ERS, early repolarization syndrome; HCM, hypertrophic cardiomyopathy; NIDCM, nonischemic dilated cardiomyopathy; and PUFA, polyunsaturated fatty acids. Reproduced with permission from Hayashi M, Shimizu W, Albert CM. The spectrum of epidemiology underlying sudden cardiac death. *Circ Res.* 2015 Jun 5;116(12):1887-1906.

valvular heart disease. **Table 63–1** summarizes clinical populations at risk for SCD.

Recent studies highlight that current WHO criteria for SCD identify many cases that are not cardiac, which may confuse risk stratification and personalization of therapy. The post-SCD study evaluated autopsies in all deaths coded as SCD by WHO criteria in San Francisco county from 2011 to 2014, and found that 40% of cases were neither sudden nor unexpected while nearly half were not arrhythmic.[11] Leading causes of death were coronary disease (32%), occult overdose (13.5%), cardiomyopathy (10%), cardiac hypertrophy (8%), and neurological (5.5%). Other causes included pulmonary embolism and gastrointestinal hemorrhage. The authors suggested that definitions for SCD would be more specific for arrhythmia by restricting witnessed events to VT/VF or rhythms other than PEA, and restricting unwitnessed cases to <1 hour since the last normal state of health.[1] However, this would also reduce the sensitivity of definitions, and its impact on the prediction, therapy, and outcomes for SCD remain undefined.

The relative frequency of etiologies for SCD is muddied by case ascertainment. Unlike countries such as Finland,[12] there are no mandatory reporting requirements for SCD in the United States. Systematic case reporting would improve

mechanistic understanding, and may be facilitated by novel technologies that provide continuous datastreams preceding and during SCA.[13]

Cardiac Arrhythmias

Cardiac arrhythmias, especially ventricular tachycardia (VT) and fibrillation (VF), are the most common cause of SCD.[10] Typically, cardiac disease can be revealed by traditional chart review or autopsy, or by genetic studies ("molecular autopsy") that can be performed postmortem.[14] That said, the extent of cardiac disease in SCD victims is often modest and may not have prompted specific therapy had it been identified a priori.

Figures 63–3A to **63–3E** summarize the pathophysiology underlying VT/VF in patients with coronary disease. Figures 63–3A and 63–3B show coronary disease and resulting myocardial scar shown on cardiac magnetic resonance (CMR) imaging. Myocardial fibrosis or scar (so-called anatomical "substrates") may result in sustained or nonsustained VT (Fig. 63–3C). Scar causes nonuniform repolarization and regions of slowed conduction (Fig. 63–3D). Premature ventricular complexes (PVCs) can block in refractory tissue but propagate through channels of relatively preserved tissue. If conduction is sufficiently slowed within these channels, the propagating

TABLE 63-1. Patient Groups at Risk for Sudden Cardiac Death

Clinical Phenotype	Clinical Course: Potential Mechanisms
Coronary artery disease	
Acute coronary ischemia	
Acute coronary occlusion (STEMI or NSTEMI) with VT/VF	Size of ischemic zone; genetic determinants. Molecular mechanisms described.[124]
Acute coronary occlusion (STEMI, NSTEMI) without VT/VF	ICD in low LVEF patients 0–40 days after MI not shown to improve long-term outcomes (DINAMIT).[125]
Coronary artery spasm	Diagnosis may be occult. Vasodilator therapy. ICD need unclear. Prognosis worse if atherosclerotic CAD too.
Coronary artery dissection[19]	Female predominance. Arteritis and connective tissue disease (eg, fibromuscular dysplasia). Diagnosis challenging; IVUS, OCT may help.*
Prior myocardial infarction, no acute ischemia	Prior infarct may be clinically apparent or silent. ICD may be beneficial. CABG reduces SCA risk in chronic ischemic cardiomyopathy.
HFrEF (ischemic cardiomyopathy)	For EF ≤35 an ICD is indicated after 40 days; further risk stratification may be warranted however. β-blockers, ACE-I, statins, and other drugs.
HFmEF (ischemic)	SCA cases may outnumber HFrEF, although the risk per patient is lower. [126] β-blockers, ACE-I, statins, and other drugs.
HFpEF (ischemic)	Statins; most pharmacologic trials have been neutral.[127]
Nonischemic cardiomyopathy	
HFrEF (nonischemic)	For EF ≤35, ICD indicated after 90 days;[128] additional risk stratification may be needed. β-blockers, ACE-I, statins, and other drugs.
HFmEF (nonischemic)	ICD not indicated for primary prevention but SCA risk is high; scar may predict events.[44]
HFpEF (nonischemic)	Statins; most pharmacologic trials have been neutral.
Other cardiac	
Inherited channelopathy	Sudden arrhythmic death syndrome; congenital long QT syndrome (15 types); Brugada syndrome; CPVT; short QT syndrome.
Drug-induced QT prolongation	Torsade de pointes and VF. (See text for common drugs and https://crediblemeds.org)
Hypertrophic cardiomyopathy	Risk factors include severe hypertrophy (3.0 cm), unexplained syncope, NSVT, family history of SCD; and to lesser degree: blood pressure fall during exercise, LVOT obstruction, LV aneurysm, substantial fibrosis (>15%) on late gadolinium enhanced MRI.[40]
Arrhythmogenic cardiomyopathy (ACM)	Group of inherited cardiomyopathies including desmosomal proteins (ARVC/ALVC/AC); lamin A/C; others.
Congenital heart disease	Triggered by VT, VF but also AT/AFL with rapid ventricular response; bradyarrhythmias. Common yanotic lesions, tetralogy of Fallot, transposition of great vessels, univentricular hearts and Ebstein's anomaly.[129]
Sarcoidosis[130]	May cause AV block, monomorphic or polymorphic VT, atrial arrhythmias, right and/or left ventricular dysfunction. MRI or PET for diagnosis.
Mitral valve prolapse	Bileaflet prolapse; MR need not be severe;[131] outflow and fascicular or papillary muscle ectopics; localized fibrosis near mitral annulus.
Aortic disease	Aortic Dissection
Subsets at risk for non-VF arrests	
At-risk for PEA	PEA more common in women, Black populations, older patients, pulmonary disease, antipsychotic drug use, prior syncope; OHT recipients. Seizure patients with sudden unexpected death in epilepsy (SUDEP) may present with PEA without antecedent seizure. Survival rates higher than asystole but lower than VF. Women have a higher survival from PEA than men.[132]
At-risk for primary asystole	Nonischemic causes of SCA; dialysis patients; OHT recipients; laryngospasm in SUDEP; pulmonary disease; Asians.[133]
Other	
Obstructive sleep apnea	Nocturnal predominance of SCA; role of stretch, ischemia, autonomic changes, hypoxia.
Neuromuscular disorders	Myotonic dystrophy; Emery-Dreifuss; limb-girdle; facio-scapulo-humeral; mitochondrial; dystrophinopathies (Duchene, Becker, other)
Schizophrenia[134]	Antipsychotic drugs, coronary risk factors, DVT/PE, other.
Hypercoagulable states	Pulmonary embolism

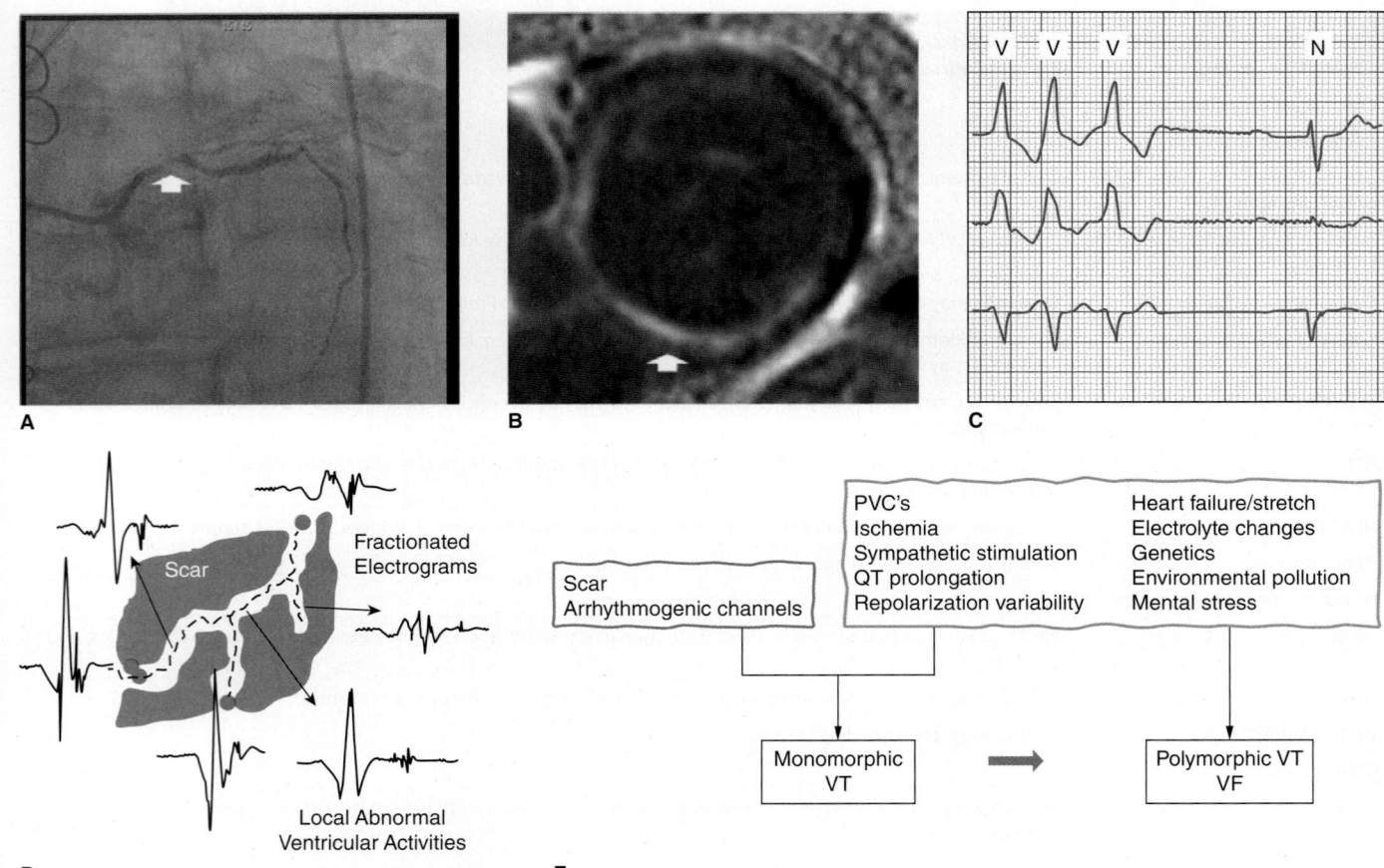

Figure 63–3. Mechanisms underlying VT and VF in the setting of coronary artery disease in a patient with coronary disease and prior coronary artery bypass grafting. (A) Coronary angiogram showing 99% left main stenosis (*arrowhead*) giving rise to occluded left anterior descending artery and diseased circumflex artery. **(B)** Scar on CMR imaging, indicated by delayed gadolinium enhancement in multiple distributions, especially the inferior wall (*arrowhead*). **(C)** Nonsustained VT on ECG telemetry (sustained VT was also recorded at other times). **(D)** Schematic of mechanisms for scar related VT, involving electrical reentry through conducting channels in the dense scar. Characteristic electrograms are shown with delayed components marking the entrance to conducting channels (*red dots*) and internal portions including blind loops. Electrogram signatures such as fractionated electrograms and local abnormal ventricular activities can be targets for catheter ablation to close these channels and eliminate VT. **(E)** Mechanistic contributors to clinical VT or VF include fixed anatomical substrate such as scar and arrhythmogenic channels, the basis for monomorphic VT. Additional contributory factors may be nonmodifiable (eg, genetics) or modifiable. PVCs can trigger VT or VF. Ischemia and global repolarization variability (with QT prolongation) predispose to VF. (D) Reproduced with permission from Berruezo A, Fernández-Armenta J, Andreu D, et al. Scar dechanneling: new method for scar-related left ventricular tachycardia substrate ablation. *Circ Arrhythm Electrophysiol.* 2015 Apr;8(2):326-336.

wavefront can return to sites that were initially blocked but have now recovered, and initiate reentrant VT or VF.[15] The conducting channels may exhibit fractionated or local abnormal ventricular activity electrograms that can be targeted by ablation therapy to close channels and eliminate VT. The heterogeneities required for VT or VF can be exacerbated by nonmodifiable factors such as genetic predisposition, but also by dynamic factors (Fig. 63–3E). Dynamic factors include sympathetic innervation, fluid overload, ventricular stretch, electrolyte abnormalities, or the use of drugs. Thus, VT and VF typically arise in patients with structural heart disease, but can also occur in patients with structurally normal hearts but electrical abnormalities as subsequently discussed.

PEA is a condition in which an organized rhythm that should produce a pulse, which excludes VF but includes sinus rhythm, fails to produce spontaneous circulation. Previously termed electromechanical dissociation, PEA results from myriad causes including myocardial infarction, metabolic derangements such as hypoxia, pharmacological agents, and mechanical compression of the heart from cardiac tamponade or tension pneumothorax.[16,17] Treatment of PEA thus requires identification and reversal of underlying causes, in parallel with treatment of underlying arrhythmias.

Bradycardia can also cause SCD, via asystole, stemming from either sinus pauses or from atrioventricular conduction block. Asystole may reflect degeneration of rhythms including VF, in part due to cases in whom emergency services were delayed. Asystole and bradycardia are treated by resuscitation and removal of any identifiable primary causes, followed by interventions such as pacemaker implantation. Bradycardic causes and PEA are collectively termed nonshockable rhythms, and are associated with the use of medications such as β-blockers, hypoxic respiratory states, and other comorbidities (Table 63–1).[10] SCD due to nonshockable rhythms has a significantly worse prognosis than that associated with shockable rhythms (VT and VF)[3] (Fig. 63–1B).

Coronary Artery Disease

Acute coronary syndromes may present with VF or VT in up to one-third of patients, and this combination exhibits a familial tendency.[18] Acute myocardial ischemia can cause triggered ectopy from delayed afterdepolarizations, exaggerate repolarization heterogeneity, and slow conduction, culminating in reentry. However, implantable cardioverter defibrillators (ICDs) are not of benefit within 40 days after myocardial infarction.[19] In the chronic phase, the development of myocardial infarct scar exacerbates these mechanisms. Less common coronary causes of SCD include vasospasm and dissection,[20] acute pump failure, and myocardial rupture from infarction. Patients are risk stratified based on the presence of reduced left ventricular ejection fraction (LVEF) and other factors discussed above (Table 63–1). Recreational use of agents such as

cocaine may cause acute coronary syndromes and SCD,[21] but ICDs are not typically indicated unless the patient has established LV systolic dysfunction.

Genetic Etiologies for SCD

One-third of SCD victims under 35 years exhibit little or no structural heart disease despite detailed histopathologic studies; these events are termed sudden arrhythmic death syndrome (SADS). Some cases reflect inherited syndromes (Figs. 63–2A and 63–2B), the most common of which are the long QT syndrome, hypertrophic cardiomyopathy, and Brugada syndrome.[22,23] Nevertheless, only a minority of SADS cases can be assigned a definitive diagnosis, and less than half of these have an identifiable genetic abnormality[14,24] suggesting undiscovered genomic variants or other pathology. Genetic etiologies for SCD are discussed in detail in other chapters in this book. Some syndromes have stereotypical electrocardiogram (ECG) appearances, as illustrated in **Figs. 63–4A** to **63–4G**.

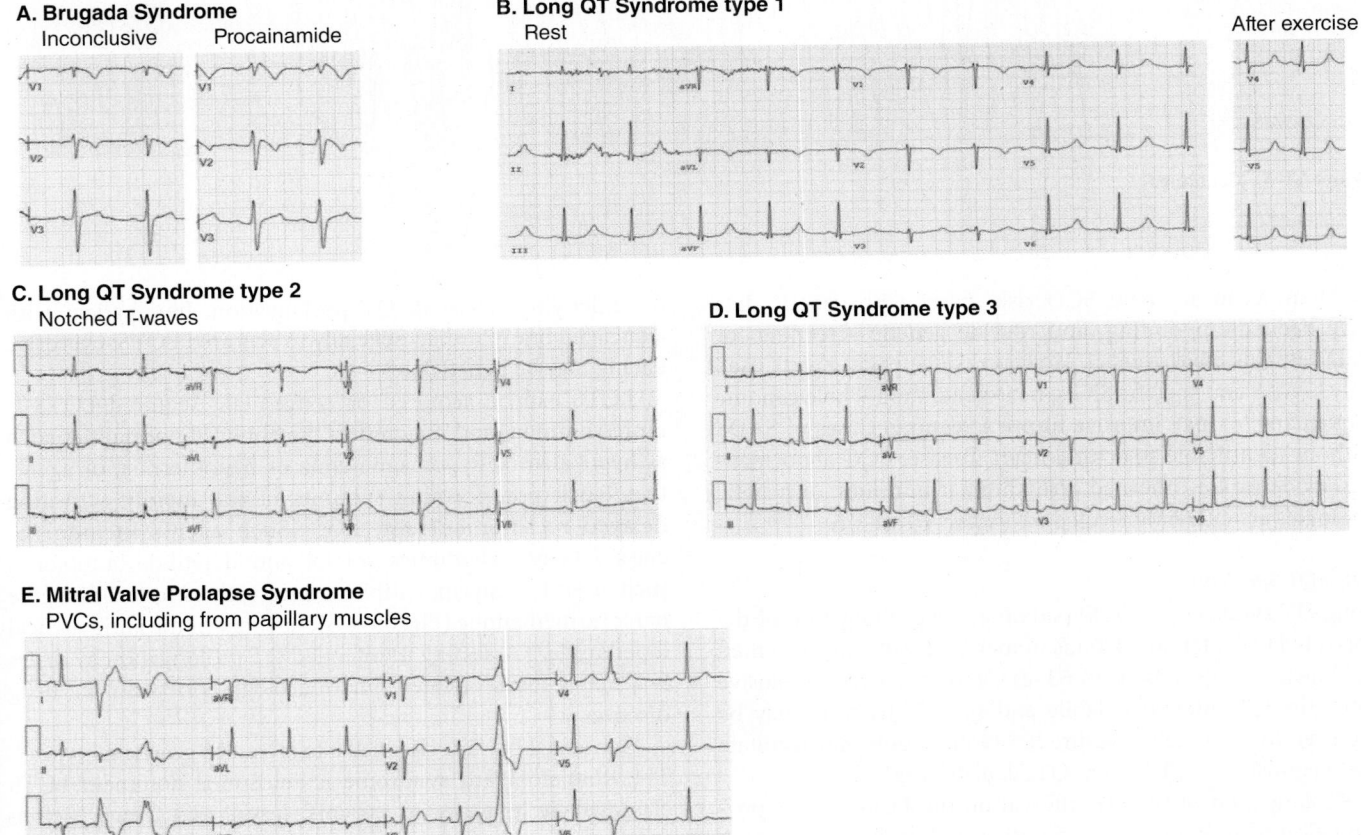

Figure 63–4. Electrocardiographic appearances of SCD syndromes. (A) Brugada syndrome. Right precordial ECG leads are inconclusive at baseline (type III, left panel) but, after procainamide infusion (right panel), are diagnostic of Type I Brugada pattern with 2-mm ST elevation with concave downward (coved) ST elevation in V2 and inverted T-waves in V1-2. **(B)** LQT1, with ECG at rest (left panel) showing QT of 580 ms and QTc 580 ms, and in recovery after stress test (right panel) showing continued QT prolongation of 520 ms and QTc 610 ms illustrating the diminished I$_{KS}$ current with KCNQ1 mutation. **(C)** LQT2 in a patient presenting with syncope after verbal stimuli. ECG shows subtle notching in T-waves with QT 530 ms and QTc 490 ms. **(D)** Long QT Type 3 in a patient with a SCN5A mutation, showing QT 460 ms and QTc 520 ms with relatively delayed T-waves. **(E)** Arrhythmogenic MVP syndrome in a patient presenting with syncope whose brother had SCD with MVP. ECG shows multifocal PVCs including some from the papillary muscles, and abnormal repolarization. **(F)** ARVC in a patient with prolonged terminal QRS in V1-3 (>55 ms from S-wave nadir to end of QRS), epsilon waves (*blue arrows* in double amplified panel on right) and T-wave inversion in V1-5. **(G)** Acquired LQT due to methadone with QT 700 ms and QTC 750 ms, leading to a run of PMVT with alternation of axis known as torsades de pointes.

F. Arrhythmogenic Right Ventricular Cardiomyopathy (ARVC)   Epsilon waves (magnified)

G. Acquired LQT, due to Methadone, and torsades de pointes

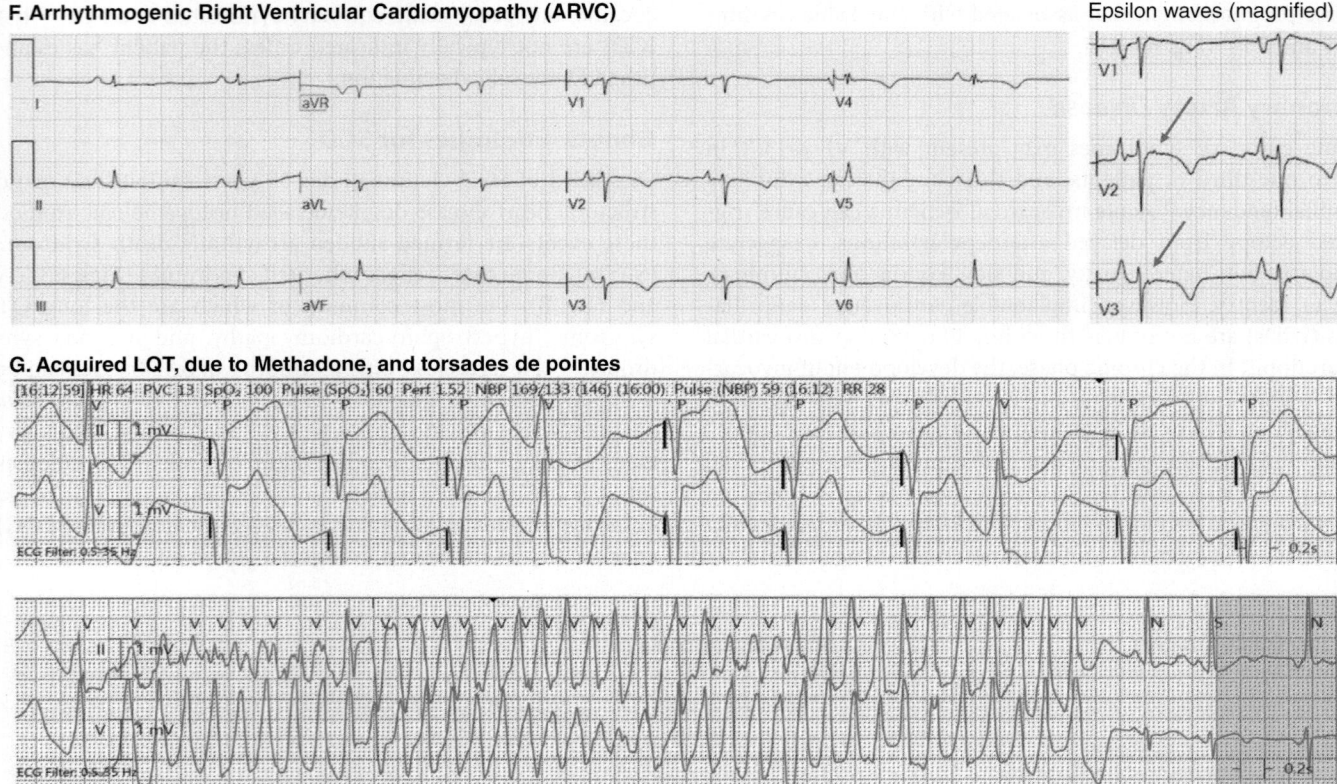

Figure 63–4. (Continued)

Attempts to augment SCD risk scores with genetic data have been disappointing, and routine genetic screening for SCD remains controversial. However, since prior efforts used only GWAS and specific SNPs, next-generation whole genome sequencing[14,24] may improve future screening. Cases of SADS without identifiable structural heart disease, ECG abnormalities, evidence for inherited arrhythmia syndromes, or genetic etiologies are currently termed *idiopathic* VT or VF.

Long QT Syndrome
Long QT syndrome (LQTS) is defined by prolongation of the corrected QT interval >470 ms in men and >480 ms in women as shown in Figs. 63–4B to 63–4D. Diagnosis can be elusive since the QT interval is labile and specific training may be required to accurately measure it.[25] Online tools may facilitate the diagnosis of LQTS (www.QTcalculator.org).

Prolongation of the QT interval on the ECG reflects prolongation of action potential duration within the heart, which may directly cause early after depolarizations and extra systoles via the mechanism of triggered activity.[26] This sets the stage for a form of polymorphic VT known as torsades des pointes, in which the QRS axis appears to twist about its points, in the setting of prior QT prolongation (Fig. 63–4G). Torsades is typically preceded by premature ventricular complexes that follow a beat with prolonged QT interval (Fig. 63–4G).[27] Torsades or VF must be treated by immediate cardioversion. Acute therapy includes intravenous magnesium sulphate (2 g) and correction

of underlying causes of QT prolongation. In a patient with associated bradycardia, especially in acquired LQTS, overdrive pacing may be beneficial.[28]

LQTS can be acquired or congenital. Acquired LQTS is more common, and may reflect metabolic abnormalities such as hypokalemia, hypomagnesemia or hypothermia, or agents that block pore-forming subunits of the rapidly activating delayed rectifier current, IKr.[27] Such agents include the class III antiarrhythmics sotalol and dofetilide, antibiotics such as erythromycin, antihistamines such as terfenadine, the narcotic methadone (Fig. 63–4G), or abuse of the antidiarrheal loperamide.[29] Assessing unintended QT prolongation by drugs is a major focus of safety pharmacology efforts during drug discovery.

Congenital LQTS is classified into at least 15 genetic subtypes.[30] The Romano-Ward syndrome is autosomal dominant LQTS classified by its genomic variants. Jervell and Lange-Nielsen syndrome is associated with nerve deafness and transmitted in autosomal recessive form, and represents either LQT1 or LQT5. Acquired and congenital LQTS can interact, and first-degree relatives of patients with congenital LQTS have an increased risk for drug-induced QT prolongation.[27]

LQT1 to LQT3 account for about a half of all congenital LQT cases (and 90% of those which can be genetically characterized) and have stereotypical ECGs (Figs. 63–4A to 63–4G). LQT1 is the most common form of LQTS representing >35% of cases, caused by abnormalities in the slow component of the delayed rectifier current, I_{Ks}, and usually results in a broad T-wave on the ECG (Fig. 63–4B). The QT fails to shorten appropriately with increasing heart rate, and events are triggered by stress or exercise such as swimming.[30,31] LQT2 is caused by abnormalities in I_{Kr}, the rapid component of the delayed rectifier current and exhibits notched and/or low amplitude ECG T-waves (Fig. 63–4C). LQT2 patients are sensitive to sudden auditory stimuli.[30,31] LQT3 represents 5% to 10% of cases, and is caused by abnormalities resulting in a gain of function in the sodium current I_{Na}. The ECG in LQT3 shows a long delay from the J-point to the T-wave (Fig. 63–4D). LQT3 patients are prone to events during sleep.[30,31]

Therapy for LQTS involves careful assessment of syncope, precipitating causes, and family history.[32] It is first treated by β-blockers, particularly nadolol. β-blockers are most effective in LQT1 and least effective in LQT3. Left-sided sympathectomy can be used in patients with recurrent syncope despite β-blocker use. ICD implantation is recommended in those with prior aborted SCA, prior syncope despite β-blockers, and very high-risk patients (such as those with Jervell and Lange-Nielsen syndrome). Patients with LQT3 may benefit from medications such as mexiletine, flecainide, or ranolazine that block the late sodium current.

Short QT Syndrome
Short QT syndrome (SQTS) is a very rare malignant cause of ventricular arrhythmias that affects young people including infants.[33] SQTS patients display a QTc <340 ms, and minimal variation with heart rate. However, this numerical cutoff lacks specificity. A family history of SQTS, prior aborted SCA, atrial fibrillation at a young age, and/or a genetic mutation may help confirm the diagnosis. Variants in seven genes including *KCNH2, KCNH2* and *KCNQ1* account for 20% to 30% of families. Some genotype positive patients have normal QT intervals. ICD implantation is the optimal therapy for definite cases, although quinidine or sotalol may be effective in some patients.

Catecholaminergic Polymorphic Ventricular Tachycardia
Catecholaminergic polymorphic ventricular tachycardia (CPVT) is a malignant arrhythmia syndrome with a normal resting ECG, in which adrenergic stress may lead to polymorphic VT, syncope, and SCD.[34] The majority of cases are transmitted in autosomal dominant fashion, caused by mutations in the cardiac ryanodine receptor (RyR2). A minority are transmitted in autosomal recessive manner by mutations in genes for the sarcoplasmic reticulum protein calsequestrin 2 (CASQ2). Adrenergic stress results in myocyte calcium loading, triggered activity, and VT with alternating axes ("bidirectional VT"). First-line therapy is β-blockade. Flecainide may be useful by modulating the ryanodine receptor and sodium-channel. Left cardiac sympathetic denervation at experienced centers may be effective.[35] ICD therapy has been used but is not first line, because CPVT patients may experience multiple ICD shocks from triggered VT leading to sympathetic surges, incessant arrhythmia, and death.[36]

Brugada Syndrome
Brugada syndrome (BrS) is an inherited cause of VF.[37] Diagnosis is made from the ECG by coved ST-segment elevation >2 mm followed by a negative T-wave of >1 mm in ECG leads V1 to V2 (the so-called type I Brugada pattern), spontaneously or after administering a sodium-channel blocker drug (Fig. 63–4A). Other ECG patterns, including a "saddleback" J-point elevation or patterns with <2 mm J-point elevation, are not diagnostic.

BrS shows male predominance, and its prevalence varies geographically and ethnically. Variants in the sodium channel gene SCN5A are found in less than half of patients. BrS was initially thought to occur without structural abnormalities, but is increasingly associated with fibrosis in the right ventricular outflow tract that may slow conduction and cause arrhythmias.[38] Recent studies report an autoantibody signature, invoking inflammatory mechanisms.[39] VF can be triggered by medications such as anesthetics and fever. ICD implantation is the main therapy. Patients with one or more shocks can be considered for epicardial RV outflow tract catheter ablation and/or oral quinidine.[37]

Hypertrophic Cardiomyopathy
Hypertrophic cardiomyopathy (HCM) is a structural abnormality that represents the most commonly identified genetic cause of SCD, causing up to 15% of cases overall and up to 30% of cases in athletes <35 years of age.[40] HCM is a structural disorder characterized by unexplained hypertrophy (≥15 mm). The hypertrophy may occur anywhere in the LV but characteristically is asymmetrical and involves the interventricular septum. Septal hypertrophy, combined with systolic anterior movement of the mitral valve, may dynamically obstruct the left ventricular outflow tract. HCM may result from over a dozen mutations in genes for sarcomere-associated proteins, the most common being β-myosin heavy chain and myosin-binding protein C, but causal genes cannot be identified in 40% of patients. Histological features of HCM include myocyte hypertrophy, disarray, and interstitial fibrosis. HCM is often clinically benign, but may cause atypical chest pain, effort dyspnea, palpitations, or syncope from outflow tract obstruction or sustained VT or VF. Atrial fibrillation and stroke commonly occur. Therapy for obstructive physiology includes β-blockade to slow heart rate, reduce cardiac contractility, and increase left ventricular end systolic volume. When these measures are inadequate, surgical myectomy or catheter-based alcohol septal ablation can relieve outflow tract obstruction but do not reduce risk of SCD. A scoring system has been developed to assess the risk of adverse events in patients with HCM.[40] HCM patients with aborted SCA should receive an ICD, as should most HCM patients with strong risk factors, namely, a family history of SCD due to HCM at age ≤50 years, recent syncope deemed likely arrhythmic, extreme septal thickness ≥30 mm, LV apical aneurysm, and/or reduced LVEF (<50%). Extensive myocardial scarring (>15%) detected on MRI, and NSVT, also influence the risk of SCD.[41]

Arrhythmogenic Cardiomyopathy
Arrhythmogenic cardiomyopathy (ACM) refers to a group of genetically determined structural cardiomyopathies with a prominent arrhythmic presentation.[42] The original and best characterized is Arrhythmogenic RV cardiomyopathy (ARVC),

which predisposes to SCA in young patients and may cause up to 22% of SCA in athletes. It is now appreciated that patients may exhibit biventricular or LV only pathology (ALVC). Diagnosis requires fulfilling Task Force criteria that include structural or functional alterations of right or less commonly left ventricles, cellular evidence of myocyte loss, and fibrosis or fibrofatty infiltration into the ventricular wall and ECG abnormalities. ECG depolarization criteria include a prolonged terminal QRS in V1 to V3 (>55 ms from S-wave nadir to end of QRS) distinct from typical right bundle branch block, and small high-frequency epsilon waves after the end of the S-wave. ECG repolarization criteria include T-wave inversions in V1 to V3 and beyond (Fig. 63–4F). Arrhythmias include ventricular tachycardias not arising from the right ventricular outflow tract (major criteria) or minor criteria of premature ventricular contractions or VT from the right ventricular outflow tract. Genetic mutations typically involve desmosomal proteins, causing derangements in cell-to-cell communication, conduction, and arrhythmias. Nondesmosomal mutations include lamin, desmoplakin, and others.[42] Naxos disease is a rare autosomal recessive ARVC syndrome first described on the Greek island of Naxos, that manifests with woolly hair and plantar keratoses. Management of ACM in general involves avoidance of strenuous endurance-type exertion, that may stimulate or exacerbate disease progression. β-blockers and other antiarrhythmic medications (sotalol, amiodarone, or flecainide) are often used. ICD implantation is indicated for prior SCA or sustained VT, as well as LVEF ≤35. Additional primary prevention ICD indications are based on the presence of one or more major risk factors such as nonsustained VT, inducible VT, or LVEF ≤50%, and/or minor risk factors namely ≥1000 PVCs/ 24 hours, significant RV dysfunction, male sex, proband status, or more than one desmosomal mutations. Patients with intractable arrhythmias may require ablation.[19,42]

Finally, genetics may modulate SCA in older victims. In a case control study of individuals at the time of a first ST-segment elevation myocardial infarction (STEMI) aged approximately 55 years, the only factors that associated with SCA from acute VF were a family history of SCA and a larger infarct.[18] This suggests that less clear heritable factors for SCA also exist at least in certain individuals.

Structural Etiologies for SCD

Common Structural Causes

Structural causes for SCD include ventricular hypertrophy (particularly if eccentric),[43] fibrosis, and scar[44,45] (Table 63–1; Figs. 63–2A and 63–2B). Delayed gadolinium enhancement on CMR imaging, that represents myocardial scar, has been shown to predict VT.[46] Stretch can cause extra systoles via the mechanism of mechano-electric feedback,[47] which may explain premature beats, VT, atrial fibrillation, or other arrhythmias in patients with decompensated heart failure.[48] Rarely, SCD is associated with a malignant form of mitral valve prolapse syndrome characterized by inverted or biphasic T waves, and PVCs from the left ventricular outflow and papillary muscles, associated with morphological abnormalities of the mitral apparatus and ventricular fibrosis on CMR imaging[49] (Fig. 63–4E).

Patients with valvular aortic stenosis are also at increased risk of SCD. Causes include tachyarrhythmias related to left ventricular hypertrophy or concomitant coronary disease, bradycardia from atrioventricular block, and/or heart failure. Historically, the risk of SCD in patients with severe stenosis was reported as <1% per year.[50] Some contemporary registries still report a low rate of SCD. In a registry of 1873 patients with mild-to-moderate aortic stenosis, the SCD rate was 0.39% per year and related to the left ventricular hypertrophy but not the severity of stenosis.[51] Conversely, in a registry of 3815 patients with severe aortic stenosis, the cumulative 5-year incidence of SCD was 9.2% in symptomatic patients and 7.2% (1.4% per year) in asymptomatic patients (P <0.001). In this registry, independent risk factors for SCD were hemodialysis, prior myocardial infarction, body mass index <22, peak aortic jet velocity ≥5 m/s, and LVEF <60%.[52] In patients with severe aortic stenosis, aortic valve replacement is associated with reduced all-cause mortality compared with watchful waiting, but it is unclear if this reduces SCD.[53] Aortic valve replacement may also worsen or provoke atrioventricular block. Among 3726 patients undergoing transcutaneous aortic valve replacement, 5.6% of all deaths were due to SCD during follow-up of 22 months. Independent predictors were reduced LVEF, new onset left bundle branch block, and QRS duration >160 ms.[54] In a small pilot study, a restricted approach to pacemaker implantation after transcatheter aortic valve replacement was associated with an increased rate of SCD of 3.4% at 1 year, versus 1.3% for a conservative implantation approach, but with no difference in overall mortality.[55] Clearly, better approaches to risk stratify SCD and heart block after transcutaneous aortic valve replacement are needed.

SCA can also be rarely associated with left bundle branch block in which slow and dys-synchronous conduction may induce regional ventricular stretch and predispose to arrhythmias.

Congenital Heart Disease

Congenital heart disease (CHD) has seen dramatic progress in its noninvasive, interventional, and surgical management,[56] and more adults than children are now living with CHD. Unfortunately, SCD accounts for 7% of mortality in these patients, trailing heart failure (42%), and pneumonia (10%).[57] Most cases of SCD occur in patients with repaired transposition of the great (TGA), univentricular hearts, coarctation, and tetralogy of Fallot (TOF).[58] Repaired TGA contributes 5% of CHD, with a rate of SCA of 1:100 patient years. TOF accounts for 7.5% of CHD and, after surgical repair, regions critical to VT occur near surgical patch repair, at the pulmonic valve, and at scar tissue. Predictors of SCD include near-syncope, nonsustained VT, older age at repair, a transannular patch, QRS duration >180 ms, PVCs, low LVEF, elevated right ventricular systolic pressure, and severe pulmonary regurgitation.[57] Ebstein's disease is strongly associated with SCD, with an 8% rate of SCD by age 50 years.[59] Predictors of SCD proposed in patients with CHD include coexisting supraventricular tachycardia, ventricular systolic dysfunction, subpulmonic ventricular dysfunction, QRS duration, and other ECG parameters including QT dispersion.[60]

Inflammatory Causes of SCD

Several studies report inflammation as a trigger for SCD (Table 63–1; Figs. 63–2A and 63–2B). Inflammation may cause arteritis and precipitate acute coronary syndromes, modulate the autonomic nervous system,[61] or alter cellular electrophysiology[62] to precipitate arrhythmias. An intriguing recent study reported a possible autoantibody signature for SCD.[63] An inflammatory etiology for SCD is supported by the fact that statins, which have anti-inflammatory effects,[64] are associated with lower mortality in patients with nonischemic cardiomyopathy.[65] On the other hand, a trial in which patients with heart failure were randomized to statins did not reveal a reduced incidence of SCD.[64]

Idiopathic Ventricular Fibrillation

This category of SCA comprises patients with VF without clear iatrogenic, congenital, electrical, or structural cause. As such, it is heterogeneous and likely to be subdivided in the future as our mechanistic understanding advances.

One subpopulation of idiopathic VF includes patients with short-coupled premature ventricular complexes from the Purkinje system, yet structurally normal hearts.[66] In general, short-coupled PVCs are an uncommon risk for SCA unless they occur in patients with conditions such as Brugada syndrome, LQTS, SQTS, CPVT. Haissaguerre and colleagues found that idiopathic VF was triggered by PVCs from Purkinje fibers or the right ventricular outflow tract. Elimination of such PVCs by ablation may eliminate recurrent VF in many patients, but an ICD is still indicated even after ablation.[66] Other rare genetic causes of PVC-triggered VF have been described.[67]

Another subpopulation comprises "malignant" early repolarization syndrome (ERS), also termed *J-wave syndromes*, first reported in patients resuscitated from VF with no clear arrhythmic predisposition.[68] These patients have a high risk of recurrent VF, and are distinct from benign ECG J-point elevation. A consensus document defined ERS by Jp >0.1 mV in amplitude, where Jp represents either the peak of an end-QRS notch and/or the onset of an end-QRS slur in the inferior or lateral precordial leads. ST-segment elevation is not a required criterion.[69] This pattern may exaggerate prior to VF. A recent study suggested two forms of ERS. The first shows depolarization abnormalities in the right ventricular outflow tract and inferolateral epicardium, which can be treated by catheter ablation. The second may be associated with VF triggers near Purkinje sites,[70] which can also serve as ablation targets. All patients are candidates for ICD implantation. Notably, asymptomatic individuals with benign ECG early repolarization (in the anterior precordial leads) are common and have a good prognosis. However, clear identification of high-risk ERS individuals remains problematic.[71]

Special Clinical Populations at Risk

Women are less likely than men to experience SCD. In those women with SCA, structural heart disease is found less often than in men (42% vs 58% of victims).[3] Black populations have twice the risk for SCD as White populations, and often experience SCA at a younger age. The excess mortality is not fully explained by socioeconomic status or first response access.[7]

The risk of SCD in patients with Wolff-Parkinson-White (WPW) syndrome is <1 per 1000 patient-years of follow-up,[72] yet it is preventable and such patients are typically otherwise healthy. The predominant mechanism is preexcited AF that may degenerate into VF. The best predictor for SCD risk is a shortest interval between preexcited QRS complexes of <250 ms in AF. Abrupt (not gradual) loss of ECG preexcitation during exercise indicates low risk. At invasive electrophysiological study, ablation of the accessory pathway is indicated in high-risk individuals to prevent SCD, prevent supraventricular tachycardia related to the accessory pathway and to prevent recurrence of AF. Ablation for asymptomatic patients with preexcitation may also be advised in patients with high-risk occupations such as pilots. Whether to observe asymptomatic patients at low risk has been debated, and referral to arrhythmia specialists is warranted.[72]

Patients with end-stage renal disease (ESRD) have a high incidence of SCD, which increases with age and in patients on dialysis, whose estimated risk of SCD is ~50 per 1000 person-years.[73] Chronic kidney disease is an independent risk factor for cardiovascular disease, likely due to factors beyond worse coronary disease. Shifts in electrolytes and the dialysis procedure itself may also contribute to SCD risk. ESRD patients, and even those with severe renal dysfunction, have been excluded from ICD trials, which obscures optimal therapy in these patients. Present evidence suggests that such patients derive less overall benefit from ICD implantation.[74]

Competitive athletes may have dramatic and highly publicized SCD events, yet these are in reality rare with a reported incidence of 0.11 to 33.3 per 100,000.[75,76] US guidelines for preparticipation screening of athletes for cardiac conditions focus on detailed personal and family history and physical examination, but do not emphasize a routine ECG. This differs in some respects from guidelines in Italy and other countries.[77] Causes for SCA in athletes include those in younger individuals as detailed above including HCM, BrS, CPVT, and inherited arrhythmia syndromes. Commotio cordis typically affects young males experiencing nonpenetrating anterior chest trauma from hard sports objects (eg, a baseball or hockey puck), occurring during the T-wave upstroke, leading to VF.[78] Cardiac contusion is an uncommon sequela in these events, and recovery after prompt defibrillation is good. Commotio may be preventable by appropriate protective chest equipment.

Sleep apnea is associated with SCD and may operate via autonomic modulation, blood gas abnormalities, or cardiac stretch from swings in intrathoracic pressure.[79,80] Mortality is higher at night, unlike coronary artery disease–related events. Diabetes mellitus is an important associated risk and may operate via protean mechanisms including fibrosis, inflammation, ventricular hypertrophy, dysautonomia, or modulation of the renin-angiotensin system.[81]

RISK STRATIFICATION FOR SCD

Risk stratification for SCD in the general population is well studied, yet challenging. Myerburg[82] emphasized that individuals at highest risk for SCD are the sickest and easiest to identify, yet contribute far fewer cases than those at lower risk.

Thus, risk stratification in the general population, who contribute a large proportion of total SCD cases but exhibit only 0.1% annual incidence, is difficult.

The highest risk group for future SCD comprises victims who have been resuscitated from SCA. Such individuals have a subsequent VT/VF event rate of nearly 20% at 1 year[83] and a mortality rate of 18% at 2 years, even if potentially "reversible" causes are treated.[84] This may indicate a predisposition to SCA beyond the reversible cause, or an inability to fully reverse that cause. In the largest secondary prevention study of SCA to date, the only "reversible" etiology, which if corrected normalized future risk, was removal of proarrhythmic medications.[84] Secondary prevention ICD therapy is indicated in most SCA survivors.

The next highest at-risk group comprises individuals with reduced LVEF without prior SCD. Several randomized clinical trials have established that patients both with ischemic or nonischemic cardiomyopathy qualify for primary prevention ICDs.[19] However, the rate of appropriate ICD therapy at 1 year in this population using modern programming is now <5%. Several strategies have been attempted to further risk stratify such patients including Signal Averaged ECG, T-wave alternans, heart rate variability, and abnormal gadolinium enhancement on CMR imaging. Recent work has used machine learning of intracardiac signals that link cellular mechanisms to clinical outcomes.[85] At this point, however, none is sufficiently robust to guide ICD therapy.[86]

Individuals with coronary disease, relatively preserved systolic function but without prior SCD, contribute the next largest number of events. However, the actual incidence of SCA is low in this group and it has been difficult to stratify risk.[87] In a meta-analysis of 48,286 patients with prior non-STEMI and preserved or mildly reduced LVEF, SCD represented one-third of all cardiovascular deaths yet still had a rate of only 2.37% over 30 months.[88]

The next largest group of patients are those with coronary disease, in whom risk stratification is again challenging. In patients with coronary disease without severe systolic dysfunction, SCA is associated with moderately reduced LVEF, age, and NYHA class. Invasive electrophysiological study predicts events only modestly in patients with ICDs and LVEF ≤40%, and is less useful in patients with more advanced systolic dysfunction (LVEF ≤30%).[87,89] Several noninvasive risk factors exist, but poorly separate arrhythmic from nonarrhythmic death and are insufficient to guide ICD implantation.[90]

CLINICAL PRESENTATION AND ACUTE MANAGEMENT OF THE SCD VICTIM

Out-of-Hospital Cardiac Arrest

Victims of out-of-hospital cardiac arrest (OHCA) have poor prognosis, with return of spontaneous circulation (ROSC) in fewer than one-fifth and survival to discharge in 10% to 12%.[3] Survival to discharge with good-to-moderate neurological status is even lower, at ~8%.[9] These individuals require systems-of-care that differ from those who experience in-hospital SCA (IHCA).[17]

Effective early response is critical and shares similarities for both types of arrest, which reflect mostly cardiac causes and present with nonshockable rhythms in ~80% of cases.[17] The burden of early response often falls to the community and is arduous: including recognizing the arrest, calling for help, and initiating cardiopulmonary resuscitation (CPR) with public-access defibrillation (PAD) until emergency medical services arrive. Strategies to accelerate resuscitation could thus have a great impact on outcomes.

It is increasingly recognized that SCD may have warning signs. In a prospective study of OHCA survivors and witnesses, three-quarters of victims had preceding symptoms including angina pectoris or dyspnea. These symptoms lasted for over 1 hour in two-thirds of victims, for a median of 50 minutes prior to asystole, 20 minutes prior to PEA, and 30 minutes prior to VF.[91] Recognizing these warning symptoms can improve outcomes. Half of the victims in the Oregon Sudden Unexpected Death Study had premonitory symptoms, and the 21% who contacted emergency services preemptively were more likely to have witnessed arrest, received CPR, had a shockable rhythm, and survived (32.1% vs 6.0%).[92]

The effectiveness of early resuscitation varies greatly. Survival from OHCA to hospital admission varies within the United States from ~19.9% in Seattle and King County, WA to ~3.3% in Detroit,[93] and also by socioeconomic factor and race.[7] Although SCA is often witnessed, less than 1 in 7 witnesses perform resuscitation, which may reflect lack of training and the psychological anguish of performing CPR.[94]

Training and education are top priorities, and should be combined with improved access to emergency services. Smartphone apps that transmit location data can shorten the time to first response.[95] Accessibility of automated external defibrillators (AEDs) must be improved, since many are unavailable at the time of need.[96] A European community volunteer network was used to deliver AEDs to the scene of SCA,[97] while others used drones to fly AEDs to sites of SCA with remote audio and video instructions.[98]

In-Hospital Cardiac Arrest

IHCA affects 209,000 people annually in the United States.[99] Causes include 50% to 60% from cardiac disease such as myocardial infarction, heart failure, and arrhythmias, and 15% to 20% from respiratory insufficiency that is higher than for OHCA.[17] Neurological causes are rare. Notably, IHCA has a higher survival than OHCA,[17] and in a UK National Cardiac Arrest Audit, the survival to hospital discharge varied from 49% when the initial rhythm was shockable to 10.5% when it was not yielding an overall unadjusted rate 18.4%.[100] Survival from IHCA varies between hospitals and is lower in patients with comorbidities such as diabetes.[101] Preventing and treating IHCA requires vigilant surveillance to provide early warning or rapid response. IHCA typically follows an in-patient median admission of 1 to 2 days, which is longer for those suffering respiratory insufficiency than for other causes. Postresuscitation care of IHCA requires a smooth interaction between Institutional code teams, the intensive care unit (ICU), anesthesiology, physicians, nurses, and respiratory therapists.

Ethical Issues in Cardiopulmonary Resuscitation

Cardiopulmonary resuscitation is an invasive and highly aggressive intervention intended to restore life to a subject who could already be classified as deceased. Accordingly, ethical considerations are central considerations regarding the use and the discontinuation of resuscitation. Like anyone else, SCA victims theoretically have ethical and legal rights to make autonomous decisions regarding care, including the right to decline resuscitation. However, the time sensitivity of resuscitation has led to lay and professional rescuers being trained to assume that a victim wishes to receive resuscitation unless information to the contrary is available.[102]

Ascertaining pertinent information on an individual's wishes for resuscitation can be difficult. Living wills, durable power of attorney, advanced directives including "Do Not Attempt Resuscitation (DNAR)" orders, and surrogate decisions are accepted approaches. DNAR status can be documented by a form, an identification bracelet, or other written format. In the absence of written documentation of DNAR, the role of verbal information from family members is gaining traction but is a gray area. The opposite problem is equally challenging—whether to offer treatment that is likely futile.[102] Physicians can reasonably withhold treatment that is likely to be futile, even if requested by patients or their families. In practice, commencing resuscitation is often the default because of difficulty in predicting outcomes.

Resuscitation can and should be withheld, however, in the setting of (1) irreversible death (rigor mortis, decapitation, transection, dependent lividity), (2) when a valid DNAR order is in place and available, or (3) if the rescue scene threatens the rescuer's immediate health or life. Termination of resuscitation is more challenging, and depends on the phase to which resuscitation has progressed, clinical judgment, and sometimes family discussions.

Basic Life Support

Basic life support (BLS) describes the initial aspects of resuscitation for SCA victims by lay or trained individuals. When encountering an unconscious individual, it is critical to maintain a high index of suspicion to minimize delay. Initial assessment includes verifying an arrest via nonresponsiveness, checking for pulse and organized breathing versus agonal gasping, identifying environmental threats like electrical wires, calling for help at the scene, and contacting emergency medical services (911 in the United States, 999 in the United Kingdom, or other appropriate local numbers[103]).

Upon confirming cardiac arrest, an AED is retrieved and applied if nearby. For each minute that a shock is delayed, survival from SCA falls by 10% to 12%.[104] If no AED is available, CPR should commence. Guidelines now recommend that lay rescuers who encounter an unresponsive and nonbreathing victim should assume that cardiac arrest has occurred and initiate CPR, rather than attempting to identify a pulse (as falsely identifying a pulse is possible). If a second responder is available, the AED should be retrieved while the first responder starts CPR. CPR should be continued except at times when the AED is checking rhythm or delivering a shock, after which time CPR should be immediately resumed. There is a need for AED analytical systems that analyze ECG waveforms during CPR artifacts, to eliminate the need to interrupt CPR to analyze rhythm, which may reduce the per-minute fall-off in survival to 3% to 4%.[104] For lay rescuers, compression-only CPR is advised. For healthcare workers, 30 compressions should be delivered followed by 2 breaths, then repeated. **Figure 63–5** shows an algorithm.

Adequacy of BLS

The goal of BLS is ROSC, which is more likely with adequate frequency and intensity of chest compressions. A compression frequency of 100 and 120 per minute is optimal, at a depth of about 5 cm (2 inches) in adults but not more than ~6 cm (2.5 inches). It is essential that the chest recoils completely after a compression, and so rescuers should not lean on the chest between compressions. When a second rescuer is present, it is advisable to quickly and efficiently switch every 2 minutes to avoid fatigue.[105]

Unfortunately, CPR is often not performed optimally. This has motivated the development of systems to monitor progress and provide feedback for training. Automated devices exist to provide CPR at optimal rate and compression depth, but they have not been shown to improve clinical efficacy.[106] However, such devices may offer practical advantages in the setting of infectious concerns during a pandemic, or during ambulance transportation when CPR is difficult to perform.

If AED is Available, Its Use Should Precede CPR

It is no longer recommended to perform CPR prior to applying an AED. In unmonitored or unwitnessed arrests, the rhythm should first be evaluated and a shock delivered if indicated. In monitored arrests due to VT/VF, immediate shock is indicated. While some guidelines advise checking the rhythm before resuming CPR, others advise immediate resumption of CPR. Immediate resumption of CPR improves hemodynamics, but is associated with earlier VF recurrence in some studies.[107] The risk-to-benefit ratio of each approach is debated. Immediate resumption of CPR after a shock for VF did not improve survival in a randomized trial compared to taking up to 30 seconds to recheck the rhythm.[108] Immediately resuming CPR postshock, rather than first waiting to check the rhythm, thus has a class IIb indication.

While initial efforts should focus on restoring circulatory flow, ventilation is also critical. With either a solo or a second trained rescuer, 2 breaths should be interposed between every 30 compressions. The 2 breaths should only interrupt CPR by about 3 to 4 seconds. Ventilation is discussed more fully in the section Advanced Cardiac Life Support.

Discontinuation of BLS

At some point, resuscitation may become futile. It has been suggested that this could be defined as the time point when survival rate falls to <1%, and ethical considerations are very pertinent. In Ontario, Canada, BLS is terminated guided by a rule based on three elements: (1) unwitnessed arrest, (2) three rounds of CPR with AED analysis without return of ROSC,

BLS Healthcare Provider
Adult Cardiac Arrest Algorithm—2015 Update

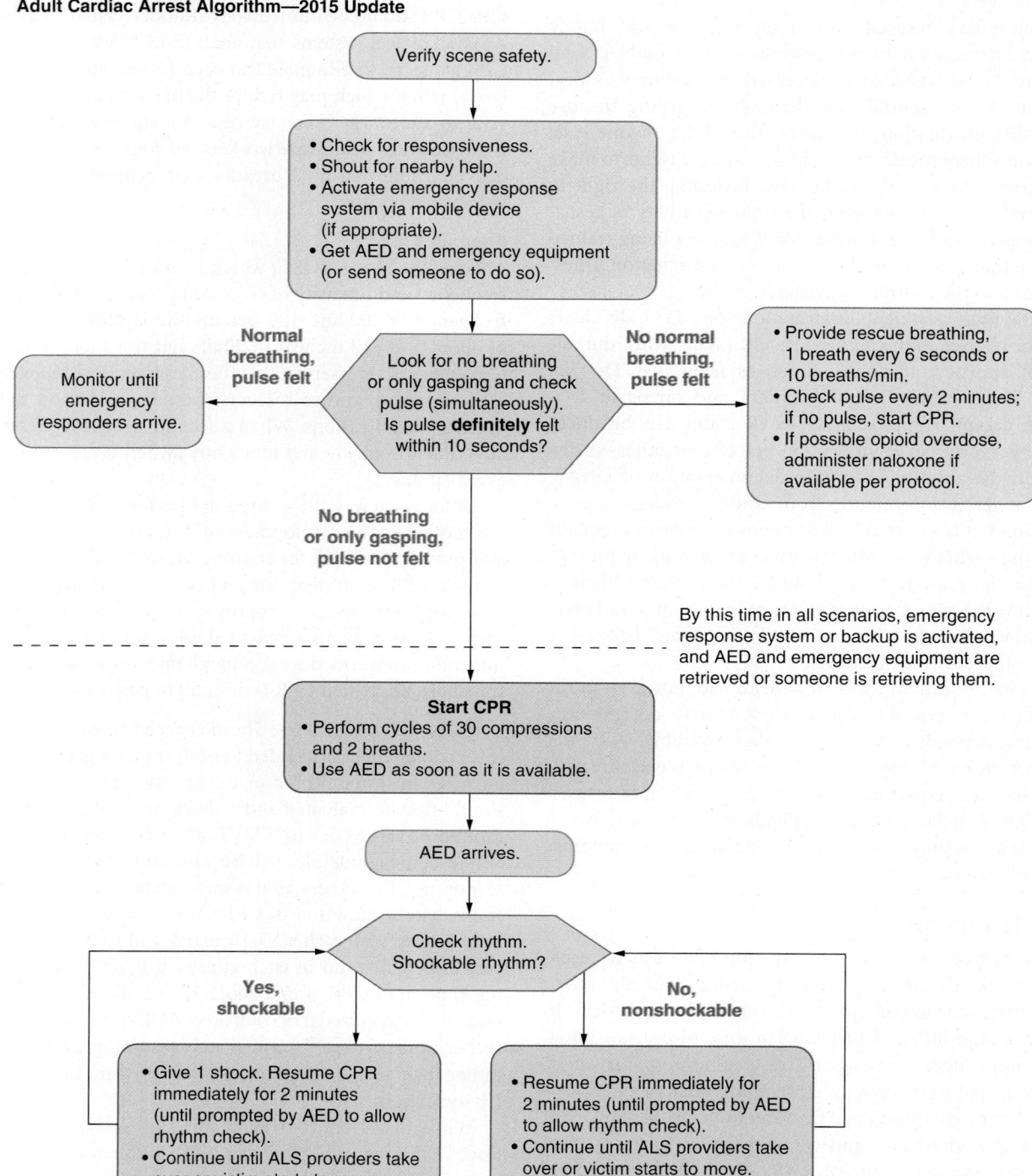

© 2020 American Heart Association

Figure 63–5. BLS for cardiac arrest algorithm in adults. Reproduced with permission from Kleinman ME, Brennan EE, Goldberger ZD, et al. Part 5: Adult Basic Life Support and Cardiopulmonary Resuscitation Quality: 2015 American Heart Association Guidelines Update for Cardiopulmonary Resuscitation and Emergency Cardiovascular Care. *Circulation*. 2015 Nov 3;132(18 Suppl 2):S414-S435.

and (3) absence of any observed shockable rhythms.[109] A trial showed that these BLS termination rules significantly reduced the rate of transporting SCA patients with negligible survival potential to hospital.[110] Any attempt at termination of resuscitation requires detailed discussions with the hospital system, and proper communication with the family and local caregivers.

Advanced Cardiac Life Support

Advanced cardiac life support (ACLS) extends BLS by incorporating airway management, intravenous or intraosseous access and delivery of pressor medications and/or antiarrhythmic drugs, and more advanced physiologic monitoring. ACLS also involves accurate diagnosis and acute management of brady or tachyarrhythmias beyond asystole or PEA and pulseless VT/VF, as detailed in current resuscitation guidelines (see algorithm in **Fig. 63-6**).[28,111]

Airway Management

Airway management in ACLS is not based on the demonstrated benefits of any specific modality, since circulatory support and correction of rhythm disturbances are of primary importance early in resuscitation. The 2019 guidelines support either bag mask ventilation (BMV) or an advanced airway such as endotracheal tube intubation (ETI) or a supraglottic airway (SGA).[111] When BMV is used, breaths should consist of about 600 mL delivered over 1 second using a tight seal with the face. When an advanced airway is used, ventilation should provide one breath every 6 compressions or 10 per minute. While BMV is not always optimal, it may be difficult to place an advanced airway during active resuscitation without interrupting CPR. A randomized study in 2040 subjects with OHCA showed no difference in survival between BMV and ETI despite highly successful (97.9%) utilization of ETI.[112] ETI did, however, show advantages for the secondary endpoints of avoiding difficult airway management ($P = 0.004$), failure of airway management ($P < 0.001$), and regurgitation of gastric contents ($P < 0.001$). Some randomized controlled trials comparing advanced airways have reported superiority of SGA over ETI, but this may reflect a lower rate of successful ETI (50%–70%) in those studies. Accordingly, the 2019 American Heart Association/American College of Cardiology (AHA/ACC) guidelines state that when an advanced airway is used, SGA should be favored over ETI if operator experience in ETI is more limited or when individual clinical circumstances would predict lower ETI success.[111]

Monitoring and Exclusion of Reversible Causes

Reversible causes may explain some presentations of SCA. Patients with PEA require a thorough evaluation and treatment of reversible causes including tension pneumothorax, cardiac tamponade, pulmonary embolus, toxins, hypovolemia, sepsis, massive myocardial infarction, and acidosis. Electrolyte disorders and hypothermia can be implicated. Echocardiography can shed a light on some of these etiologies, if available acutely.

Various forms of monitoring are possible during ACLS. Arterial blood pressure (BP), oximetry, end tidal CO_2 (ET CO_2), and ultrasound are commonly used. ET CO_2 during optimal CPR is usually 15 to 20 mm Hg (normal is 35–45 mm Hg, equivalent to 5%–6% CO_2). When ROSC develops, it is typical for ET CO_2 to jump to >35 mm Hg. End tidal CO_2 has prognostic importance in patients with ETI, in whom an ET CO_2 <10 mm Hg despite >20 minutes of resuscitation is a marker for futility of further efforts.[111]

Adjuvant Pharmacological or Circulatory Therapy

Vasoactive Agents: Vasoactive agents such as epinephrine are used during ACLS to raise diastolic pressure and improve coronary perfusion. However, epinephrine may impair cerebral blood flow via alpha-adrenergically mediated vasoconstriction, and increase myocardial oxygen demand by β-adrenergically mediated inotropy and chronotropy. A randomized trial of epinephrine versus placebo in 8014 patients with cardiac arrest (~20% shockable) showed a slightly but significantly higher 30-day survival for epinephrine (3.2% vs 2.4%, $P = 0.02$) although with no difference in the endpoint of survival with favorable neurologic outcome (2.2% vs 1.9%).[113] When trials are pooled, cardiac arrest victims with nonshockable rhythms may benefit from epinephrine. High-dose epinephrine has not been found superior to standard doses. Vasopressin is another vasoactive agent used in cardiac arrest. Like epinephrine, it increases systemic vascular resistance, but operates by stimulating the V1 receptor to activate Gq proteins and the IP3 pathway. Vasopressin has not been found to be superior to epinephrine, alone or in combination. Neither atropine nor calcium have proven useful for asystolic cardiac arrest. Even emergency pacing is ineffective in the setting of ongoing cardiac arrest is not recommended, although witnessed and acute bradycardia may respond to pacing. In summary, epinephrine should be used early during resuscitation of cardiac arrest in patients with the nonshockable rhythms of PEA/asystole. Conversely, in cardiac arrest due to shockable rhythms, epinephrine is best reserved until after shocks are found to be unsuccessful.

Antiarrhythmic Drugs: Antiarrhythmic drugs are often used for cardiac arrest due to VT/VF. At present, three randomized trials provide supporting evidence (**Table 63–2**). Intravenous amiodarone was first studied in two small randomized clinical trials during 1999 to 2002, and found superior to placebo[114] or lidocaine[115] for the endpoint of survival to hospital admission. This endpoint excludes patients who died in the emergency department, but is a surrogate of the key endpoint of survival to hospital discharge or survival with favorable neurologic status.

More recently, amiodarone or lidocaine were compared to placebo in a three-arm randomized clinical trial for the primary endpoint of survival to hospital discharge or the secondary endpoint of survival to hospital discharge with favorable neurological status.[116] Surprisingly, neither the primary nor secondary endpoints were superior in patients treated with amiodarone or lidocaine compared to placebo, although some surrogate endpoints were superior for lidocaine and/or amiodarone. In the subgroup of patients with witnessed cardiac arrest, survival to hospital discharge was achieved more often for either active drug with borderline significance ($P = 0.05$). The authors speculated that relatively late administration of

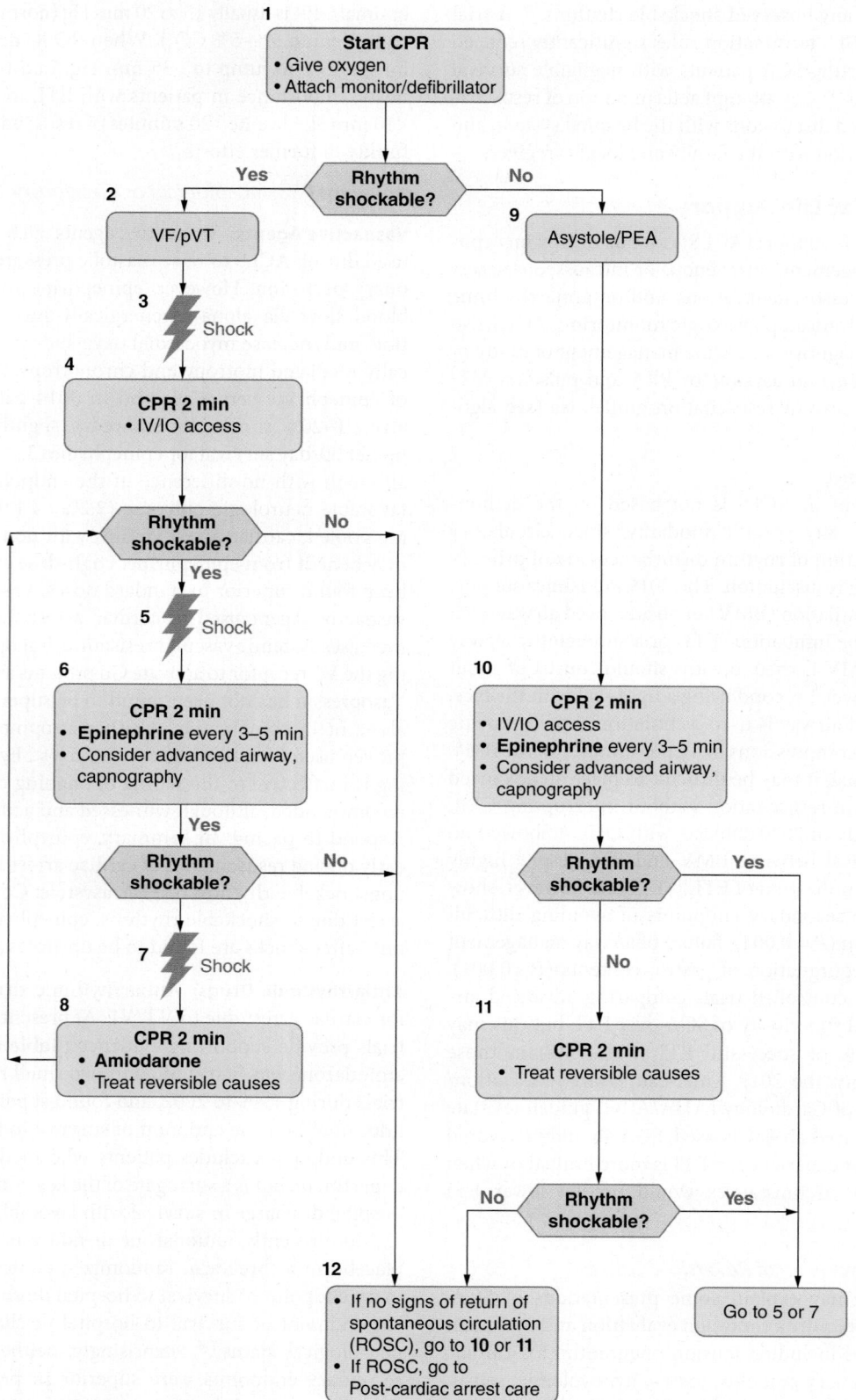

Figure 63–6. ACLS for cardiac arrest algorithm in adults. Treatable or reversible causes in box 11 include *Hypovolemia, Hypoxia, Hydrogen* ion abnormalities (acidosis), *Hypo* or hyperkalemia, *Hypothermia, Tension* pneumothorax, *Tamponade, Toxins,* pulmonary *Thrombosis,* and coronary *Thrombosis* (H^5T^5). Abbreviations: CPR, cardiopulmonary resuscitation; ET, endotracheal; IO, intraosseous; IV, intravenous; PEA, pulseless electrical activity; pVT, pulseless ventricular tachycardia; and VF, ventricular fibrillation. Refer to Guideline document for detailed management steps including ventilation and drug dosages. Reproduced with permission from Panchal AR, Berg KM, Kudenchuk PJ, et al. 2018 American Heart Association Focused Update on Advanced Cardiovascular Life Support Use of Antiarrhythmic Drugs During and Immediately After Cardiac Arrest: An Update to the American Heart Association Guidelines for Cardiopulmonary Resuscitation and Emergency Cardiovascular Care. *Circulation.* 2018 Dec 4;138(23):e740-e749.

TABLE 63–2. Antiarrhythmic Drug Trials for VT/VF Arrest

Trial	Population	Comparator	Primary Outcome
ARREST[106]	OHCA with VF or pulseless VT initially or during resuscitation, despite 3 shocks (n = 504 total)	Amiodarone 300 mg IV vs placebo.	Survival to hospital admission with a stable rhythm: 44% vs 34% ($P = 0.03$); better with amiodarone.
ALIVE[107]	OHCA with recurrent VF or VF resistant to 4 shocks plus epinephrine (n = 347 total)	Amiodarone 5 mg/kg IV vs lidocaine 1.5 mg/kg IV	Survival to hospital admission 22.8% vs 12.0% ($P = 0.009$) better with amiodarone.
ROC-ALPS[108]	OHCA with recurrent or resistant (>1 shock) VF/pulseless VT (n = 3026 total)	Amiodarone (A) vs lidocaine (L) vs placebo (P)	Discharged alive: 24.4%, 23.7%, and 21.0%, respectively; A vs P ($P = 0.08$); L vs P ($P = 0.16$). *Secondary outcome survival with good neurologic status: 18.8%, 17.5%, and 16.6% ($P = NS$). Exploratory outcomes: ROSC: 35.9%, 39.9%, and 34.6%; A vs P ($P = NS$), L vs P ($P = 0.01$); survival to hospital admission 45.7%, 47.0%, and 39.7% (A vs P ($P = 0.01$); L vs P ($P <0.001$).

*ROC-ALPS: in patients with witnessed arrests (n = 1934), a prespecified subgroup, survival to hospital discharge was significantly higher with amiodarone (27.7%) or lidocaine (27.8%) than for placebo (22.7%).

either drug (mean of ~19 minutes after EMS notification) may explain this neutral result. The 2018 AHA guidelines currently assign a class IIb indication for IV amiodarone or lidocaine for shock-refractory VF or pulseless VT and emphasize the likelihood for benefit in those with witnessed arrests.[28]

Intravenous Magnesium: Intravenous magnesium as an adjunct in OHCA was studied in four small randomized controlled trials, and resulted in no improvement in the rate of ROSC or survival. Magnesium retains a class IIb indication for torsades de pointes (polymorphic VT in the setting of long QT), where it appears to prevent the arrhythmia but may not terminate it.[28]

Extracorporeal Membrane Oxygenation: ECMO, also known as extracorporeal CPR (ECPR), has garnered attention given the poor survival from traditional resuscitation. At this time, studies have been small with highly selected patients, without the benefit of randomized data, and thus far, the evidence is not convincing for the presence of benefit.

Discontinuation of ACLS

This is controversial and has substantial ethical implications. Some guidance from Societal guidelines is available, including an algorithm that can be adapted to local situation (**Fig. 63–7**).

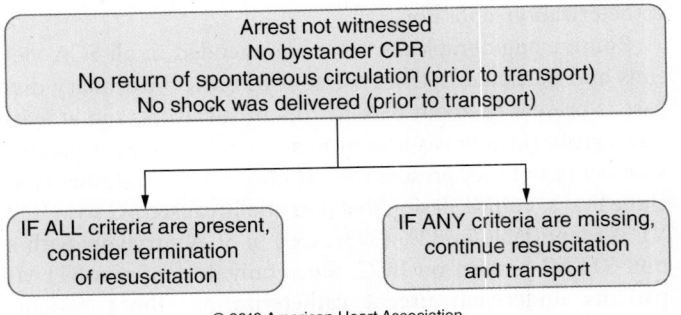

Arrest not witnessed
No bystander CPR
No return of spontaneous circulation (prior to transport)
No shock was delivered (prior to transport)

IF ALL criteria are present, consider termination of resuscitation

IF ANY criteria are missing, continue resuscitation and transport

© 2010 American Heart Association

Figure 63–7. Decision tree for termination of ACLS. Reproduced with permission from Morrison LJ, Kierzek G, Diekema DS, et al. Part 3: ethics: 2010 American Heart Association Guidelines for Cardiopulmonary Resuscitation and Emergency Cardiovascular Care. *Circulation.* 2010 Nov 2;122(18 Suppl 3): S665-S675.

As for BLS, a combination of poor prognostic factors identifies situations where termination may be appropriate.[117]

POSTARREST CARE

Postarrest care commences at the point of ROSC, and represents the transition from restoring circulation to optimizing the chance for meaningful neurologic and optimal cardiac function. Much of this occurs in the ICU. It includes consideration of emergent cardiac catheterization and revascularization for suspected coronary occlusion, tailored ventilation and hemodynamic support, and targeted temperature management. **Figure 63–8** shows a guideline-based algorithm that provides an overview of postarrest care.

Cardiocerebral Resuscitation

This term emphasizes the need to treat the brain and the heart in SCA victims. Cardiac arrest is more fully stated as a multisystem problem that must address ventilation, hemodynamics, cardiac perfusion and cardiac rhythm management, neurological care, metabolic monitoring (eg, potassium, lactate), and subsequently renal and neuropsychiatric care. **Figure 63–9** provides a focused algorithm for cardiovascular and intensive unit care for the postarrest patient. **Figure 63–10** provides a flowchart for neurological care of the postarrest patient that includes targeted temperature management.

Respiratory Management

Endotracheal intubation should be established in patients with impaired consciousness or neurological status. Adequate oxygenation must be confirmed, but excessive FiO_2 should be avoided to maintain a target SpO_2 of 94% and a PaO_2 of 100%. Normal pCO_2 (35–35 mmHg) should be established. Imaging is appropriate to confirm tube placement, to look for evidence of aspiration or possible respiratory causes of arrest such as pneumonia.

Hemodynamic Targets

Targets are a mean BP of 65 mm Hg or SBP of 90 mm Hg. Fluids and pressors should be given as appropriate, including

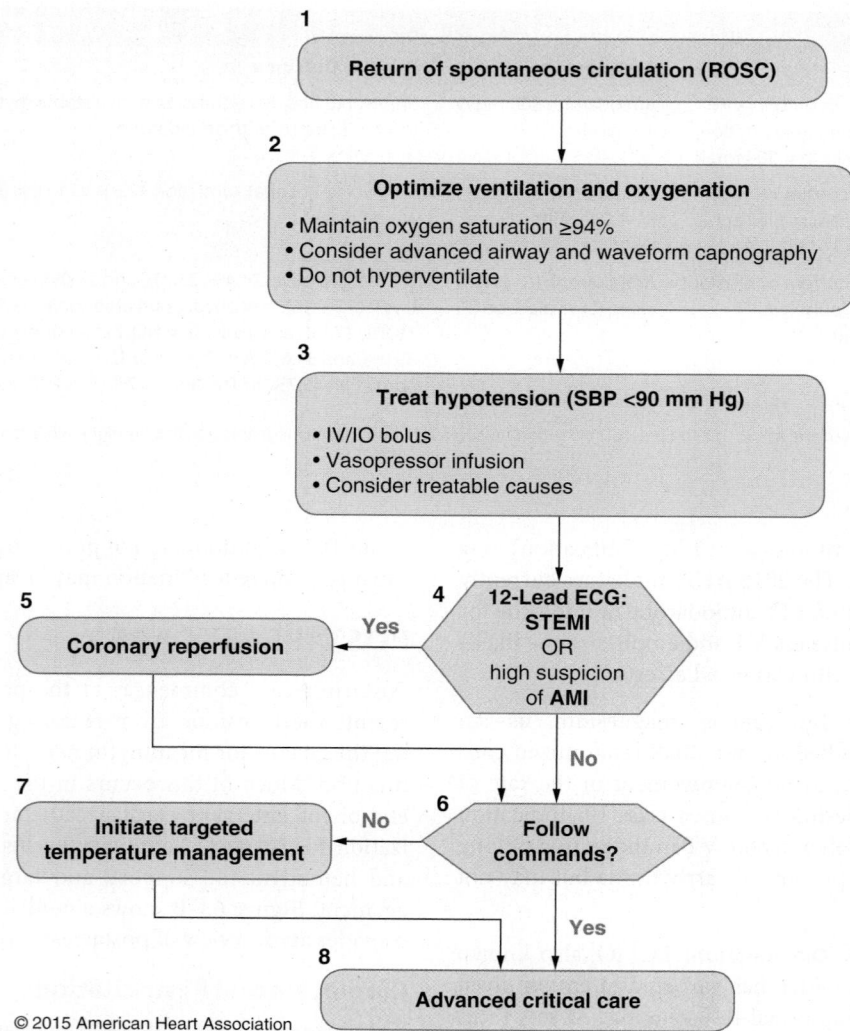

1

Return of spontaneous circulation (ROSC)

2

Optimize ventilation and oxygenation

• Maintain oxygen saturation ≥94%
• Consider advanced airway and waveform capnography
• Do not hyperventilate

3

Treat hypotension (SBP <90 mm Hg)

• IV/IO bolus
• Vasopressor infusion
• Consider treatable causes

4 12-Lead ECG: STEMI OR high suspicion of AMI

5 Coronary reperfusion — Yes

No

6 Follow commands?

7 Initiate targeted temperature management — No

Yes

8 Advanced critical care

© 2015 American Heart Association

Figure 63–8. Algorithm overview for immediate postcardiac arrest care in adults. Treatable or reversible causes in box 3 include *Hypovolemia, Hypoxia, Hydrogen* ion abnormalities (acidosis), *Hypo* or hyperkalemia, *Hypothermia, Tension* pneumothorax, *Tamponade, Toxins,* pulmonary *Thrombosis,* and coronary *Thrombosis* (H⁵T⁵). Reproduced with permission from Peberdy MA, Callaway CW, Neumar RW, et al. Part 9: post-cardiac arrest care: 2010 American Heart Association Guidelines for Cardiopulmonary Resuscitation and Emergency Cardiovascular Care. *Circulation.* 2010 Nov 2;122(18 Suppl 3):S768-S786.

dopamine, norepinephrine, and/or epinephrine. Nonpharmacologic hemodynamic support using an intra-aortic balloon pump may be considered. Echocardiography to evaluate left ventricular function and look for other relevant acute or chronic pathology is advisable. Core temperature should be measured; active temperature interventions are subsequently described. Continuous ECG monitoring should continue and arrhythmias treated, but empirical prophylactic neuro-antiarrhythmic drugs have not yet been proven beneficial.

Investigating Coronary Pathology

Clinicians should maintain a high index of suspicion for acute coronary pathology in cardiac arrest survivors (Figs. 63–8 and 63–9). In patients with cardiac arrest and STEMI, acute percutaneous coronary intervention (PCI) to enable acute reperfusion provides best outcomes (just as it does for STEMI in the absence of cardiac arrest).[118] One study identified STEMI in 31% of 545 patients who had ROSC after cardiac arrest without

an obvious noncardiac cause.[119] Early identification of acute coronary syndromes, using prehospital ECG and with computer-assisted or nonphysician reads, may expedite activation of the catheterization laboratory.

Routine angiography is not recommended in all SCA victims and particularly those without STEMI.[120] Coronary disease is present in about 65% to 70% of survivors, and at least one significant stenosis is seen in about a half of SCA victims whether or not they present with STEMI.[119] Pooled studies conclude that a "culprit" lesion that potentially caused SCA via VT/VF is identifiable in 32% (373/1159) of SCA survivors with a non-STEMI pattern on ECG. Since only 41% of non-STEMI patients underwent urgent catheterization, those patients likely represented a select group enriched for coronary pathology by clinical judgment. Data are conflicting in this area. A meta-analysis of predominantly observational data suggested a survival benefit for early coronary angiography in non-STEMI arrest survivors.[121] Conversely, a trial that randomized 552 SCA

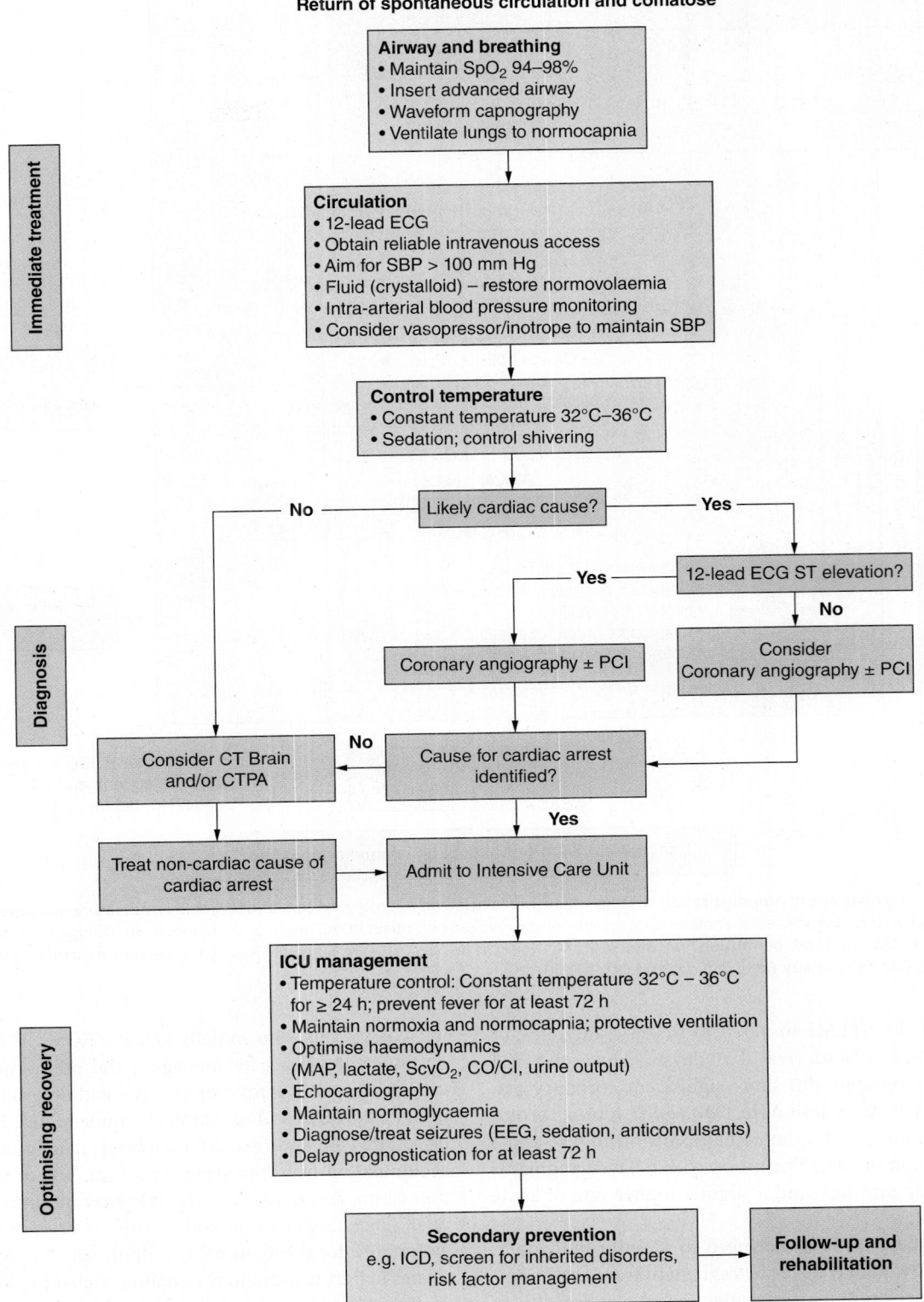

Figure 63–9. Post resuscitation care algorithm focused on cardiac and intensive care. SBP, systolic blood pressure; PCI, percutaneous coronary intervention; CTPA, computed tomography pulmonary angiogram; ICU, intensive care unit; MAP, mean arterial pressure; ScvO2, central venous oxygenation; CO/CI, cardiac output/cardiac index; EEG, electroencephalography; ICD, implanted cardioverter defibrillator. Reproduced with permission from Monsieurs KG, Nolan JP, Bossaert LL, et al. European Resuscitation Council Guidelines for Resuscitation 2015: Section 1. Executive summary. *Resuscitation.* 2015 Oct;95:1-80.

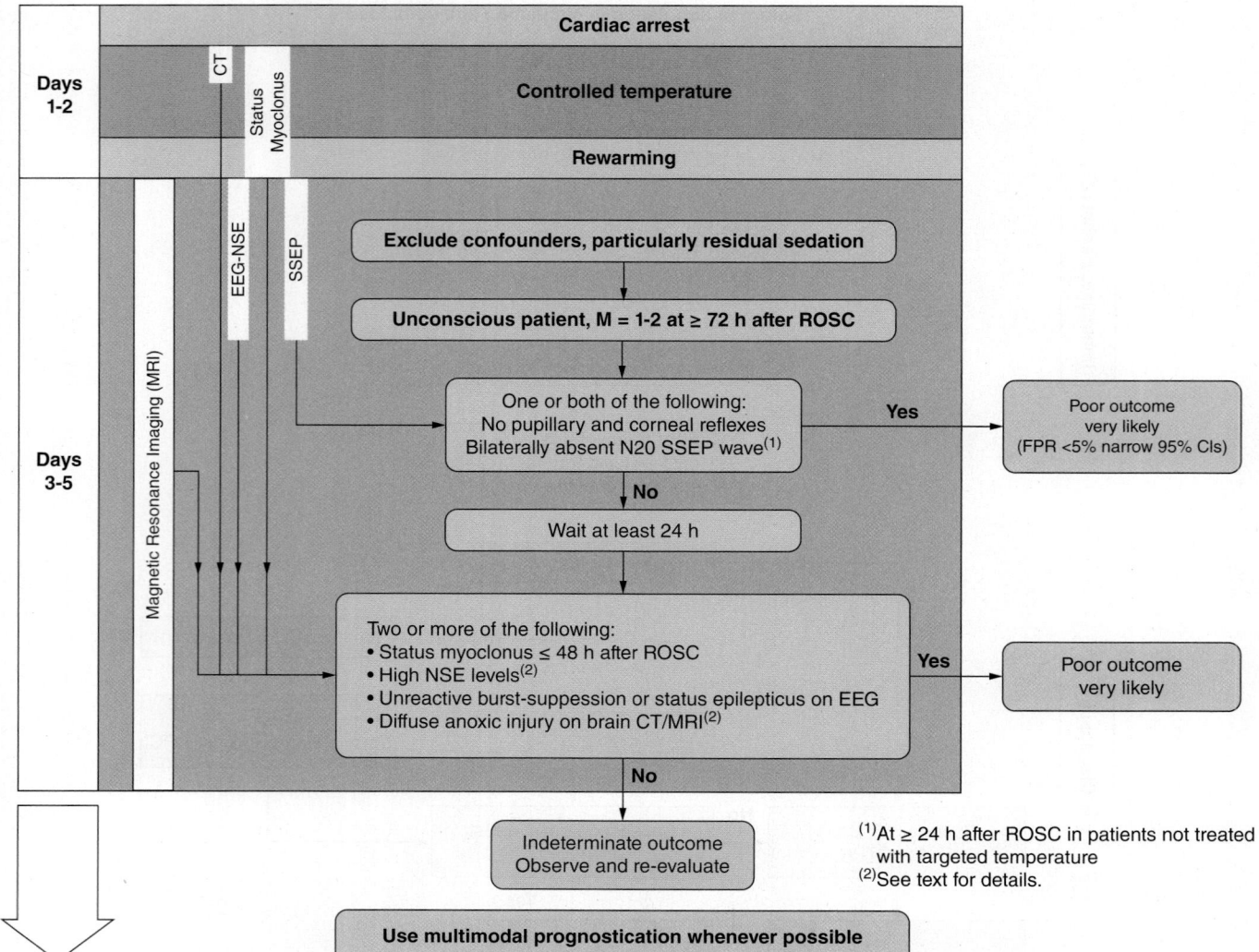

Figure 63–10. Postcardiac arrest, prognostication strategy algorithm focused on neurological care and targeted temperature management. EEG, electroencephalography; NSE, neuron specific enolase; SSEP, somatosensory evoked potentials; ROSC, return of spontaneous circulation; M, Motor score of Glasgow Coma Scale. Reproduced with permission from Monsieurs KG, Nolan JP, Bossaert LL, et al. European Resuscitation Council Guidelines for Resuscitation 2015: Section 1. Executive summary. *Resuscitation.* 2015 Oct;95:1-80.

survivors without STEMI to early versus late angiography reported a similar 65% survival at 90 days.[122] The group with immediate angiography did show significant coronary disease in 65%, an unstable lesion (ie, plaque disruption, thrombus, or dissection) in 14%, an acute occlusion in 4%, and a chronic occlusion in 14%. The group with delayed angiography had similar findings, and a slightly higher rate of acute occlusion (8%).

Therefore, there is an unmet need to identify individuals without STEMI who may nevertheless benefit from acute angiography,[123] since troponin measurements can be nonspecific in the setting of cardiac arrest, CPR, and shocks. One small study reported emergency angiography supported by ECMO in 62 refractory VF patients with encouraging preliminary results.[124]

Assessing Neurological Outcomes

Neurologic management is critical in cardiac arrest survivors, because brain injury is the dominant ultimate cause of death

in SCA victims who initially achieve ROSC.[125] Figure 63–10 outlines a flowchart for managing and preserving neurological function after cardiac arrest. The pathophysiology of brain injury is diverse and incompletely understood. Brain pathology starts with neuronal cell membrane damage and abnormal accumulation of intraneuronal calcium, loss of intraneuronal potassium, and release of cytotoxic enzymes into the extracellular space. Reperfusion adds insult, as does microglial activation and local inflammation. Brain-specific hypoxic injury relates in part to excitatory signaling related to glutamate.

Patients who are comatose or with impairment of consciousness or neurological status should be examined serially.[16] Electro-encephalography (EEG) is indicated to exclude ongoing seizure. A noncontrast CT is indicated to exclude intracranial hemorrhage or other acute process.

Memory abnormalities are often seen after ischemic injury, and evidence suggests parallels to an Alzheimer dementia-type processes. Regions of the brain important to encoding memory such as the hippocampus and thalamus are especially vulnerable to hypoxia, due to high metabolic demand, arterial supply, and density of glutaminergic neurons. Abnormalities in executive functions of the frontal lobe, and neuropsychiatric abnormalities such as anxiety are also frequently seen.

Neurologic outcome after cardiac arrest is often graded by the modified Rankin scale with lower score being more favorable as follows: (1) coma, (2) vegetative state, (3) severe disability, (4) moderate disability (independent but not functioning at level prior to arrest), and (5) good recovery with function similar to prior to arrest. Predictors of worse neurologic outcome after cardiac arrest include the initial rhythm (nonshockable), the time lapse before CPR, the duration of CPR needed, location of cardiac arrest (public site, or home), and severity of hemodynamic insult after ROSC (as indicated by the BP, lactate, creatinine, and need for pressors).[16]

Therapy to Mitigate Neurological Injury

In an effort to mitigate CNS injury, a number of medications including corticosteroids, calcium blockers, and others have been studied but have failed to help. Conversely, systemic hypothermia has emerged as a modality to mitigate ischemic neurologic injury, and is implemented via targeted temperature management (TTM). **Table 63-3** summarizes clinical trials that focused on the use of TTM in cardiac arrest victims.

In preclinical models, hypothermia improves outcomes from cardiac arrest possibly due to decreased cerebral oxygen demand, reduction in free radicals, reduction in intracranial pressure, and/or decreased glutamate levels.[126]

Early and small clinical trials in 2002 reported improved outcomes in VF survivors using hypothermia leading to its incorporation in the guidelines in 2010.[127,128] However, a larger study in 2013 failed to show a benefit of hypothermia compared to a control group in whom temperatures were maintained at low normal (36°C) simply to prevent *hyper*thermia. Criticisms of this study included delays in onset of hypothermia, because the mean temperature in the intervention group did not approach 33°C until 8 hours after randomization, and possible excessive rapid rewarming. In addition, this trial included nonshockable rhythms. A recent trial enrolled only patients with a nonshockable rhythm and found that 90-day survival with favorable neurologic outcome was more likely with hypothermia (33°C, 10.2%) compared to the control group (37°C, 5.7%)[126] (Table 63-3). Guidelines currently recommend temperature between 32°C and 36°C for 24 hours, and strongly emphasize an active prevention of fever during the subsequent several days.[16]

Hypothermia (or targeted temperature management) requires special ICU management protocols. During TTM, sedation and neuromuscular blockade should be administered to prevent shivering. Consequently, EEG surveillance is critical in order to exclude occult seizures. $PaCO_2$ may be artifactually higher during hypothermia, and QT intervals may also be longer.[129] QT prolonging drugs should be avoided. This observation is consistent with the risk of VF in accidental hypothermia. Hypothermia is known to have procoagulation effects raising concern especially in patients receiving acute PCI after OHCA. The actual risk that TTM adds for stent thrombosis is controversial in these already high-risk patients, although at least one study favored the use of ticagrelor over clopidogrel.[130] Beyond hypothermia, several other interventions have been evaluated in preclinical or clinical studies and show promise, including inhaled xenon, as well as nitric oxide.[125]

LONG-TERM SURVIVAL FROM CARDIAC ARREST

After restoring circulation from cardiac arrest, long-term prognosis is the preeminent concern. Unfortunately, sedation, neuromuscular blockade, and hypothermia limit its determination early in the ICU (<72 hours from resuscitation). The recommended time for evaluation is 4 to 5 days after ROSC for most patients.[131]

TABLE 63–3. Trials Evaluating Temperature Management Postcardiac Arrest

Study and Year	Population	Intervention and Control Treatment	Primary End Points	Outcome	Comment
Hypothermia after Cardiac Arrest Study Group[135] 2002	273 post-VF arrest survivors	32–34°C versus normothermia	1°C favorable neurologic outcome at 6 months; 2°C ACM at 6 months and complications	Good neurologic outcome (55% vs 39%) significantly higher; mortality (39% vs 55%) significantly lower with hypothermia	Hypothermia improved neurologic outcome and survival without increasing complications
Bernard[136] 2002	77 post-VF arrest survivors	33°C versus normothermia	1°C survival to discharge to home or rehabilitation (but not to long-term nursing facility)	Better survival with good neurologic status (49% vs 26%)	Moderate hypothermia improved outcomes
Nielsen[137] 2013	950 unconscious postarrest survivors (80% from shockable rhythm)	33°C versus 36°C	1°C ACM; 2°C Poor neurologic function or death	Equivalent 1°C and 2°C outcomes	Hypothermia not superior to targeted temperature management (prevention of hyperthermia)
Lascarrou[117] 2019	584 survivors of PEA/asystolic arrest	33°C versus 37°C	1°C survival with good neurologic function (day 90)	Higher survival with good neurologic function (10.2% vs 5.7%). Mortality at 90-days equivalent (>80%).	Survival poor after PEA/asystole but neurologic outcome better with hypothermia

In the tragic case when postarrest survivors exhibit brain death in the short term, organ donation becomes a valid and important concern. Organs have been found to exhibit appropriate function in these individuals. Thus, patients who do not achieve ROSC who would otherwise have had termination of resuscitation efforts could be considered as potential kidney or liver donors if local conditions allow. Organs transplanted from these donors have success rates comparable to organs recovered from similar donors with other conditions.

Conversely, for cardiac arrest survivors who achieve hospital discharge, contemporary data are encouraging with 73% living independently at 1-year postarrest and a similar percentage at work if they had been working prior to the arrest.[132] Another study found that 90% of cardiac arrest survivors return home rather than residing in an institution, and that less than 20% needed help with everyday activities. Conversely, on deeper investigation, relatives of the SCA victim may report cognitive decline in more than 50% of survivors despite intact cognitive testing in many.[125]

SUMMARY

Definition, Epidemiology, and Historical Considerations

- SCD is defined as occurring within 1 hour of symptom onset if witnessed, or within 24 hours of having been observed alive and symptom free if unwitnessed.
- The term SCA can be used to indicate those successfully resuscitated.
- Incidence is about 350,000 people per year in the United States.
- SCA incidence increases markedly with age and is more common in Black than White populations, and in men than women.

Clinical and Mechanistic Subtypes

- Initial presentations of SCA are VT or VF. Asystole or PEA also present as SCA and are increasing in relative incidence.
- The underlying cause of SCA is typically coronary disease in older individuals.
- Genetic causes (HCM, LQTS, BrS, arrhythmogenic cardiomyopathies) are often identified in younger SCA victims.
- SCA in athletes is rare but highly visible, and usually results from genetic causes, anomalous coronary arteries or a mechanical event called commotio cordis.
- Arrests classified clinically as SCA are noncardiac in up to 40% and include neurological events, pulmonary embolism, gastrointestinal hemorrhage, and occult overdoses.
- Mechanistically, structural causes of SCA are ventricular scar, hypertrophy, and congenital heart disease. Dynamic causes are autonomic changes, volume overload and stretch, premature beats, electrolyte changes, acute ischemia, and repolarization abnormalities.

Risk Stratification for SCD

- Patients with prior SCA are at the highest identifiable risk for future SCA.

- Myocardial infarction survivors with markedly depressed LVEF below 35% have improved survival with an implantable defibrillator.
- Patients with nonischemic cardiomyopathy and heart failure with reduced ejection fraction may have improved survival with an implantable defibrillator.
- Genetic factors may operate in inherited syndromes and even in SCA related to coronary disease.
- Risk stratification is difficult in other patients.
- Other risk factors include extent of ventricular scar, triggering arrhythmias such as premature ventricular complexes, abnormal repolarization patterns (prolonged QT or microvolt alternans), arrhythmia inducibility, and autonomic markers such as heart rate variability.

Clinical Presentation and Acute Management of the SCD Victim

- Survival from OHCA averages 10% to 12% overall, with 8% surviving with a relatively good neurologic status.
- Survival varies dramatically by geography and with respect to race and socioeconomic regions.
- SCA survival is higher for witnessed arrests, when a shockable rhythm is identified, when bystander CPR is performed, and when an AED is used quickly.
- IHCA has a higher overall higher survival rate is higher at ~18% overall and 49% for shockable events.
- BLS describes the immediate and early response to SCA including contacting emergency services, locating and implementing an AED if available, and performing CPR.
- Compression-only CPR, foregoing ventilation, has been proven to be at least as successful as CPR with ventilation and is now recommended for lay responders.
- Survival is correlated to better CPR technique.
- ACLS extends BLS by incorporating airway management, intravenous or intraosseous access and delivery of pressor medications and/or antiarrhythmic drugs, and more advanced physiologic monitoring.
- PEA may be due to a reversible cause that must be identified and corrected, such as tension pneumothorax, cardiac tamponade, pulmonary embolus, toxins, hypovolemia, sepsis, massive myocardial infarction, and/or acidosis.
- Various forms of monitoring are possible during ACLS, including arterial BP, oximetry, ET CO_2, and ultrasound.
- Ventilation is critical during ACLS, unlike lay responder BLS, with early use of a bag valve mask or more definitively via either an endotracheal tube or supraglottic airway.
- Epinephrine increases diastolic BP and coronary perfusion during resuscitation, and has shown modest improvement in 30-day survival.
- Epinephrine has a greater role for nonshockable causes of SCA. Vasopressin has not been found to be preferable or additive to epinephrine.
- Amiodarone and lidocaine may modestly improve survival to hospital admission, but not overall survival in cases of

recurrent or refractory VT/VF. Their early use during refractory SCA events, particularly if witnessed, may be better than that seen overall in randomized trials.

Postarrest Care

- After achieving ROSC, the goals of postarrest care are to optimize long-term neurologic and cardiac function.
- Goals for monitoring, hemodynamics including BP, oxygenation, and electrolyte management have been identified.
- Some SCA, especially VT/VF events, are due to STEMI and acute PCI to enable acute reperfusion provides the best outcomes.
- Some SCA stem from occult acute coronary occlusion without ECG evidence for STEMI; nevertheless, acute catheterization of all SCA survivors has not improved outcomes.
- Hypothermia (32–34°C) has been shown to improve neurologic outcomes over standard care.
- Modest hypothermia (36°C) essentially to prevent hyperthermia may yield similar outcomes to hypothermia (32–34°C), although frank hypothermia appears better for nonshockable SCA.
- Many patients remain comatose after ROSC, and neurological prognostication is not feasible until at least 72 hours after SCA especially in the setting of hypothermia, which necessitates sedation and control of shivering usually with paralytic agents.
- Postarrest survivors who exhibit brain death constitute appropriate organ donor candidates.

Long-Term Survival from Cardiac Arrest

- Although survival from SCA is low, 73% of survivors to hospital discharge achieve independent living status. Those who were working prior to SCA usually are able to return to work.
- Relatives of SCA survivors report cognitive decline in more than 50% of survivors, and a high burden of psychological distress (anxiety and depression) is found in many survivors.

REFERENCES

1. Tseng ZH, Salazar JW, Olgin JE, et al. Refining the World Health Organization definition: predicting autopsy-defined sudden arrhythmic deaths among presumed sudden cardiac deaths in the POST SCD study. *Circ Arrhythm Electrophysiol.* 2019;12:e007171.

2. Daubert JP. Sudden Cardiac Arrest. In: E. Prystowsky, G. Klein and J. P. Daubert, eds. *Cardiac Arrhythmias: Interpretation, Diagnosis and Treatment*: McGraw-Hill; 2020.

3. Hayashi M, Shimizu W, Albert CM. The spectrum of epidemiology underlying sudden cardiac death. *Circ Res.* 2015;116:1887-1906.

4. Shedd OL, Sears J, Samuel F, et al. The World Trade Center attack: increased frequency of defibrillator shocks for ventricular arrhythmias in patients living remotely from New York City. *J Am Coll Cardiol.* 2004;44:1265-1267.

5. Lai PH, Lancet EA, Weiden MD, et al. Characteristics associated with out-of-hospital cardiac arrests and resuscitations during the novel coronavirus disease 2019 pandemic in New York City. *JAMA Cardiol.* 2020.

6. Mountantonakis SE, Saleh M, Coleman K, et al. Out-of-hospital cardiac arrest and acute coronary syndrome hospitalizations during the COVID-19 surge. *J Am Coll Cardiol.* 2020;76:1271-1273.

7. Benjamin EJ, Blaha MJ, Chiuve SE, et al. Heart disease and stroke statistics-2017 update: a report from the American Heart Association. *Circulation.* 2017;135:e146-e603.

8. Reinier K, Nichols GA, Huertas-Vazquez A, et al. Distinctive clinical profile of blacks versus whites presenting with sudden cardiac arrest. *Circulation.* 2015;132:380-387.

9. CARES. CARES Summary Report. Demographic and survival characteristics of OHCA. 2020:2014 cardiac arrest registry to enhance survival (CARES) national summary report. 2014.

10. Niemeijer MN, van den Berg ME, Leening MJ, et al. Declining incidence of sudden cardiac death from 1990-2010 in a general middle-aged and elderly population: the Rotterdam Study. *Heart Rhythm.* 2015;12:123-129.

11. Tseng ZH, Olgin JE, Vittinghoff E, et al. Prospective countywide surveillance and autopsy characterization of sudden cardiac death: POST SCD study. *Circulation.* 2018;137:2689-2700.

12. Junttila MJ, Hookana E, Kaikkonen KS, Kortelainen ML, Myerburg RJ, Huikuri HV. Temporal trends in the clinical and pathological characteristics of victims of sudden cardiac death in the absence of previously identified heart disease. *Circ Arrhythm Electrophysiol.* 2016;9.

13. Narayan SM, Wang PJ, Daubert JP. New concepts in sudden cardiac arrest to address an intractable epidemic: JACC State-of-the-Art Review. *J Am Coll Cardiol.* 2019;73:70-88.

14. Lahrouchi N, Raju H, Lodder EM, et al. Utility of post-mortem genetic testing in cases of sudden arrhythmic death syndrome. *J Am Coll Cardiol.* 2017;69:2134-2145.

15. Berruezo A, Fernandez-Armenta J, Andreu D, et al. Scar dechanneling: new method for scar-related left ventricular tachycardia substrate ablation. *Circ Arrhythm Electrophysiol.* 2015;8:326-336.

16. Monsieurs KG, Nolan JP, Bossaert LL, et al. European Resuscitation Council Guidelines for Resuscitation 2015: Section 1. Executive summary. *Resuscitation.* 2015;95:1-80.

17. Andersen LW, Holmberg MJ, Berg KM, Donnino MW and Granfeldt A. In-hospital cardiac arrest: a review. *JAMA.* 2019;321:1200-1210.

18. Dekker L, Bezzina C, Henriques J, et al. Familial sudden death is an important risk factor for primary ventricular fibrillation: a case-control study in acute myocardial infarction patients. *Circulation.* 2006;114:1140-1145.

19. Al-Khatib SM, Stevenson WG, Ackerman MJ, et al. 2017 AHA/ACC/HRS guideline for management of patients with ventricular arrhythmias and the prevention of sudden cardiac death: a report of the American College of Cardiology/American Heart Association Task Force on Clinical Practice Guidelines and the Heart Rhythm Society. *J Am Coll Cardiol.* 2018;72:e91-e220.

20. Sharma S, Rozen G, Duran J, Mela T, Wood MJ. Sudden cardiac death in patients with spontaneous coronary artery dissection. *J Am Coll Cardiol.* 2017;70:114-115.

21. Havakuk O, Rezkalla SH, Kloner RA. The cardiovascular effects of cocaine. *J Am Coll Cardiol.* 2017;70:101-113.

22. Bagnall RD, Weintraub RG, Ingles J, et al. A prospective study of sudden cardiac death among children and young adults. *N Engl J Med.* 2016;374:2441-2452.

23. Semsarian C, Ingles J, Wilde AA. Sudden cardiac death in the young: the molecular autopsy and a practical approach to surviving relatives. *Eur Heart J.* 2015;36:1290-1296.

24. Rucinski C, Winbo A, Marcondes L, et al. A population-based registry of patients with inherited cardiac conditions and resuscitated cardiac arrest. *J Am Coll Cardiol.* 2020;75:2698-2707.

25. Viskin S, Rosovski U, Sands A, et al. Inaccurate electrocardiographic interpretation of long QT: the majority of physicians cannot recognize a long QT when they see one. *Heart Rhythm.* 2005;2:569-574.

26. Vink AS, Neumann B, Lieve KVV, et al. Determination and Interpretation of the QT Interval. *Circulation.* 2018;138:2345-2358.

27. El-Sherif N, Turitto G, Boutjdir M. Acquired long QT syndrome and electrophysiology of Torsade de Pointes. *Arrhythm Electrophysiol Rev.* 2019;8:122-130.

28. Panchal AR, Berg KM, Kudenchuk PJ, et al. 2018 American Heart Association focused update on advanced cardiovascular life support use of antiarrhythmic drugs during and immediately after cardiac arrest: an update to the American Heart Association Guidelines for Cardiopulmonary Resuscitation and Emergency Cardiovascular Care. *Circulation.* 2018;138:e740-e749.

29. Nattel S. An emerging malignant arrhythmia epidemic due to loperamide abuse underlying mechanisms and clinical relevance. *JACC: Clin Electrophysiol.* 2016;2.

30. Bohnen MS, Peng G, Robey SH, et al. Molecular pathophysiology of congenital long QT syndrome. *Physiol Rev.* 2017;97:89-134.

31. Baskar S, Aziz PF. Genotype-phenotype correlation in long QT syndrome. *Glob Cardiol Sci Pract.* 2015;2015:26.

32. Rohatgi RK, Sugrue A, Bos JM, et al. Contemporary outcomes in patients with long QT syndrome. *J Am Coll Cardiol.* 2017;70:453-462.

33. Campuzano O, Sarquella-Brugada G, Cesar S, Arbelo E, Brugada J, Brugada R. Recent advances in short QT syndrome. *Front Cardiovasc Med.* 2018;5:149.

34. Baltogiannis GG, Lysitsas DN, di Giovanni G, et al. CPVT: arrhythmogenesis, therapeutic management, and future perspectives. a brief review of the literature. *Front Cardiovasc Med.* 2019;6:92.

35. Dusi V, De Ferrari GM, Pugliese L, Schwartz PJ. Cardiac sympathetic denervation in channelopathies. *Front Cardiovasc Med.* 2019;6:27.

36. Roses-Noguer F, Jarman JW, Clague JR, Till J. Outcomes of defibrillator therapy in catecholaminergic polymorphic ventricular tachycardia. *Heart Rhythm.* 2014;11:58-66.

37. Brugada J, Campuzano O, Arbelo E, Sarquella-Brugada G, Brugada R. Present status of Brugada syndrome: JACC State-of-the-Art Review. *J Am Coll Cardiol.* 2018;72:1046-1059.

38. Nademanee K, Raju H, de Noronha SV, et al. Fibrosis, Connexin-43, and conduction abnormalities in the Brugada syndrome. *J Am Coll Cardiol.* 2015;66:1976-1986.

39. Chatterjee D, Pieroni M, Fatah M, et al. An autoantibody profile detects Brugada syndrome and identifies abnormally expressed myocardial proteins. *Eur Heart J.* 2020;41:2878-2890.

40. Marian AJ, Braunwald E. Hypertrophic cardiomyopathy: genetics, pathogenesis, clinical manifestations, diagnosis, and therapy. *Circ Res.* 2017;121:749-770.

41. Ommen SR, Mital S, Burke MA, et al. 2020 AHA/ACC guideline for the diagnosis and treatment of patients with hypertrophic cardiomyopathy: a report of the American College of Cardiology/American Heart Association Joint Committee on Clinical Practice Guidelines. *J Am Coll Cardiol.* 2020;76:e159-e240.

42. Towbin JA, McKenna WJ, Abrams DJ, et al. 2019 HRS expert consensus statement on evaluation, risk stratification, and management of arrhythmogenic cardiomyopathy. *Heart Rhythm.* 2019;16:e301-e372.

43. Aro AL, Reinier K, Phan D, et al. Left-ventricular geometry and risk of sudden cardiac arrest in patients with preserved or moderately reduced left-ventricular ejection fraction. *Europace.* 2017;19:1146-1152.

44. Klem I, Weinsaft JW, Bahnson TD, et al. Assessment of myocardial scarring improves risk stratification in patients evaluated for cardiac defibrillator implantation. *J Am Coll Cardiol.* 2012;60:408-420.

45. Halliday BP, Gulati A, Ali A, et al. Association between midwall late gadolinium enhancement and sudden cardiac death in patients with dilated cardiomyopathy and mild and moderate left ventricular systolic dysfunction. *Circulation.* 2017;135:2106-2115.

46. Piers SR, Everaerts K, van der Geest RJ, et al. Myocardial scar predicts monomorphic ventricular tachycardia but not polymorphic ventricular tachycardia or ventricular fibrillation in nonischemic dilated cardiomyopathy. *Heart Rhythm.* 2015;12:2106-2114.

47. Franz MR, Cima R, Wang D, Profitt D, Kurz R. Electrophysiological effects of myocardial stretch and mechanical determinants of stretch-activated arrhythmias. *Circulation.* 1992;86:968-978.

48. Sutherland GR. Sudden cardiac death: the pro-arrhythmic interaction of an acute loading with an underlying substrate. *Eur Heart J.* 2017;38:2986-2994.

49. Muthukumar L, Jahangir A, Jan MF, Perez Moreno AC, Khandheria BK, Tajik AJ. Association between malignant mitral valve prolapse and sudden cardiac death: a review. *JAMA Cardiol.* 2020;5:1053-1061.

50. Pellikka PA, Nishimura RA, Bailey KR, Tajik AJ. The natural history of adults with asymptomatic, hemodynamically significant aortic stenosis. *J Am Coll Cardiol.* 1990;15:1012-1017.

51. Minners J, Rossebo A, Chambers JB, et al. Sudden cardiac death in asymptomatic patients with aortic stenosis. *Heart.* 2020;106:1646-1650.

52. Taniguchi T, Morimoto T, Shiomi H, et al. Sudden death in patients with severe aortic stenosis: observations from the CURRENT AS registry. *J Am Heart Assoc.* 2018;7.

53. Kumar A, Majmundar M, Doshi R, et al. Meta-analysis of early intervention versus conservative management for asymptomatic severe aortic stenosis. *Am J Cardiol.* 2021;138:85-91.

54. Urena M, Webb J, Eltchaninoff H, et al. Late cardiac death in patients undergoing transcatheter aortic valve replacement: incidence and predictors of advanced heart failure and sudden cardiac death. *J Am Coll Cardiol.* 2015;65:437-448.

55. Schoechlin S, Minners J, Jadidi A, et al. Effect of a restrictive pacemaker implantation strategy on mortality after transcatheter aortic valve implantation. *PACE.* 2020.

56. Neidenbach R, Niwa K, Oto O, et al. Improving medical care and prevention in adults with congenital heart disease-reflections on a global problem-part I: development of congenital cardiology, epidemiology, clinical aspects, heart failure, cardiac arrhythmia. *Cardiovasc Diagn Ther.* 2018;8:705-715.

57. Moore JP, Khairy P. Adults with congenital heart disease and arrhythmia management. *Cardiol Clin.* 2020;38:417-434.

58. Gallego P, Gonzalez AE, Sanchez-Recalde A, et al. Incidence and predictors of sudden cardiac arrest in adults with congenital heart defects repaired before adult life. *Am J Cardiol.* 2012;110:109-117.

59. Attenhofer Jost CH, Tan NY, Hassan A, et al. Sudden death in patients with Ebstein anomaly. *Eur Heart J.* 2018;39:1970-1977a.

60. Koyak Z, Harris L, de Groot JR, et al. Sudden cardiac death in adult congenital heart disease. *Circulation.* 2012;126:1944-1954.

61. Masoud S, Lim PB, Kitas GD, Panoulas V. Sudden cardiac death in patients with rheumatoid arthritis. *World J Cardiol.* 2017;9:562-573.

62. Lazzerini PE, Capecchi PL, Bertolozzi I, et al. Marked QTc prolongation and Torsades de pointes in patients with chronic inflammatory arthritis. *Front Cardiovasc Med.* 2016;3:31.

63. Maguy A, Tardif JC, Busseuil D, Ribi C, Li J. Autoantibody signature in cardiac arrest. *Circulation.* 2020;141:1764-1774.

64. Kjekshus J, Apetrei E, Barrios V, et al. Rosuvastatin in older patients with systolic heart failure. *N Engl J Med.* 2007;357:2248-2261.

65. Goldberger JJ, Subacius H, Schaechter A, et al. Effects of statin therapy on arrhythmic events and survival in patients with nonischemic dilated cardiomyopathy. *J Am Coll Cardiol.* 2006;48:1228-1233.

66. Knecht S, Sacher F, Wright M, et al. Long term follow-up of idiopathic ventricular fibrillation ablation: a multicenter study. *J Am Coll Cardiol.* 2009;54:552-528.

67. Wilde AAM, Garan H, Boyden PA. Role of the Purkinje system in heritable arrhythmias. *Heart Rhythm.* 2019;16:1121-1126.

68. Antzelevitch C, Yan GX, Ackerman MJ, et al. J-Wave syndromes expert consensus conference report: emerging concepts and gaps in knowledge. *Heart Rhythm.* 2016;13:e295-e324.

69. Macfarlane PW, Antzelevitch C, Haissaguerre M, et al. The early repolarization pattern: a consensus paper. *J Am Coll Cardiol.* 2015;66:470-477.

70. Nademanee K, Haissaguerre M, Hocini M, et al. Mapping and ablation of ventricular fibrillation associated with early repolarization syndrome. *Circulation.* 2019;140:1477-1490.

71. Adler A, Gollob MH. A practical guide to early repolarization. *Curr Opin Cardiol.* 2015;30:8-16.

72. Kim SS, Knight BP. Long term risk of Wolff-Parkinson-White pattern and syndrome. *Trends Cardiovasc Med*. 2017;27:260-268.

73. Data USR. System 2015 reference tables. http://www.usrds.org/reference. aspx. 2015; 2020.

74. Goldenberg I, Vyas AK, Hall WJ, et al. Risk stratification for primary implantation of a cardioverter-defibrillator in patients with ischemic left ventricular dysfunction. *J Am Coll Cardiol*. 2008;51:288-296.

75. Harmon KG, Drezner JA, Wilson MG, Sharma S. Incidence of sudden cardiac death in athletes: a state-of-the-art review. *Br J Sports Med*. 2014;48:1185-1192.

76. Landry CH, Allan KS, Connelly KA, et al. Sudden cardiac arrest during participation in competitive sports. *N Engl J Med*. 2017;377:1943-1953.

77. Mont L, Pelliccia A, Sharma S, et al. Pre-participation cardiovascular evaluation for athletic participants to prevent sudden death: Position paper from the EHRA and the EACPR, branches of the ESC. Endorsed by APHRS, HRS, and SOLAECE. *Eur J Prev Cardiol*. 2017;24:41-69.

78. Link MS, Estes NA 3rd, Maron BJ, et al. Eligibility and disqualification recommendations for competitive athletes with cardiovascular abnormalities: Task Force 13: Commotio Cordis: a scientific statement from the American Heart Association and American College of Cardiology. *Circulation*. 2015;132:e339-e342.

79. Kwon Y, Koene RJ, Kwon O, Kealhofer JV, Adabag S, Duval S. Effect of sleep-disordered breathing on appropriate implantable cardioverter-defibrillator therapy in patients with heart failure: a systematic review and meta-analysis. *Circ Arrhythm Electrophysiol*. 2017;10:e004609.

80. May AM, Van Wagoner DR, Mehra R. OSA and cardiac arrhythmogenesis: mechanistic insights. *Chest*. 2017;151:225-241.

81. Marwick TH, Ritchie R, Shaw JE, Kaye D. Implications of underlying mechanisms for the recognition and management of diabetic cardiomyopathy. *J Am Coll Cardiol*. 2018;71:339-351.

82. Myerburg RJ, Kessler KM, Castellanos A. Sudden cardiac death. Structure, function, and time-dependence of risk. *Circulation*. 1992;85:I2-I10.

83. Kloppe A, Proclemer A, Arenal A, et al. Efficacy of long detection interval implantable cardioverter-defibrillator settings in secondary prevention population: data from the Avoid Delivering Therapies for Nonsustained Arrhythmias in ICD Patients III (ADVANCE III) trial. *Circulation*. 2014;130:308-314.

84. Wyse DG, Friedman PL, Brodsky MA, et al. Life-threatening ventricular arrhythmias due to transient or correctable causes: high risk for death in follow-up. *J Am Coll Cardiol*. 2001;38:1718-1724.

85. Rogers AJ, Selvalingam A, Alhusseini MI, et al. Machine learned cellular phenotypes in cardiomyopathy predict sudden death. *Circ Res*. 2020.

86. Goldberger JJ, Basu A, Boineau R, et al. Risk stratification for sudden cardiac death: a plan for the future. *Circulation*. 2014;129:516-526.

87. Al-Khatib SM, Stevenson WG, Ackerman MJ, et al. 2017 AHA/ACC/HRS guideline for management of patients with ventricular arrhythmias and the prevention of sudden cardiac death: a report of the American College of Cardiology/American Heart Association Task Force on Clinical Practice Guidelines and the Heart Rhythm Society. *J Am Coll Cardiol*. 2018;72:e91-e220.

88. Hess PL, Wojdyla DM, Al-Khatib SM, et al. Sudden cardiac death after non-ST-segment elevation acute coronary syndrome. *JAMA Cardiol*. 2016;1:73-79.

89. Daubert JP, Zareba W, Hall WJ, et al. Predictive value of ventricular arrhythmia inducibility for subsequent ventricular tachycardia or ventricular fibrillation in multicenter automatic defibrillator implantation trial (MADIT) II patients. *J Am Coll Cardiol*. 2006;47:98-107.

90. Chatterjee NA, Moorthy MV, Pester J, et al. Sudden death in patients with coronary heart disease without severe systolic dysfunction. *JAMA Cardiol*. 2018;3:591-600.

91. Müller D, Agrawal R, Arntz H-R. How sudden is sudden cardiac death? *Circulation*. 2006;114:1146-1150.

92. Marijon E, Uy-Evanado A, Dumas F, et al. Warning symptoms are associated with survival from sudden cardiac arrest. *Ann Intern Med*. 2016;164: 23-29.

93. Kira Peikoff, NYT. CPR Survival Rates Can Differ Greatly By City. *New York Times*. New York, NYC, NYT Press.

94. Bardy GH, Lee KL, Mark DB, et al. Home use of automated external defibrillators for sudden cardiac arrest. *N Engl J Med*. 2008;358:1793-1804.

95. Berglund E, Claesson A, Nordberg P, et al. A smartphone application for dispatch of lay responders to out-of-hospital cardiac arrests. *Resuscitation*. 2018.

96. Sun CL, Demirtas D, Brooks SC, Morrison LJ, Chan TC. Overcoming spatial and temporal barriers to public access defibrillators via optimization. *J Am Coll Cardiol*. 2016;68:836-845.

97. Capucci A, Aschieri D, Guerra F, et al. Community-based automated external defibrillator only resuscitation for out-of-hospital cardiac arrest patients. *Am Heart J*. 2016;172:192-200.

98. Claesson A, Backman A, Ringh M, et al. Time to delivery of an automated external defibrillator using a drone for simulated out-of-hospital cardiac arrests vs emergency medical services. *JAMA*. 2017;317:2332-2334.

99. Merchant R, Yang L, Becker L and al e. Incidence of treated cardiac arrest in hospitalized patients in the United States. *Crit Care Med*. 2011;39:2401-2406.

100. Nolan J, Soar J, Smith G, et al. Incidence and outcome of in-hospital cardiac arrest in the United Kingdom National Cardiac Arrest Audit. *Resuscitation*. 2014;85:987-992.

101. Petursson P, Gudbjornsdottir S, Aune S, et al. Patients with a history of diabetes have a lower survival rate after in-hospital cardiac arrest. *Resuscitation*. 2008;76:37-42.

102. American Heart Association. Ethical issues in CPR. 2020. https://eccguidelines.heart.org/circulation/cpr-ecc-guidelines/part-3-ethical-issues/.

103. USGovernment. 911 Abroad: Numbers Website Resource. 2020, from https://travel.state.gov/content/dam/students-abroad/pdfs/911_ABROAD. pdf.

104. Waalewijn R, Nijpels M, Tijssen J, Koster R. Prevention of deterioration of ventricular fibrillation by basic life support during out-of-hospital cardiac arrest. *Resuscitation*. 2002;54:31–36.

105. Kleinman ME, Brennan EE, Goldberger ZD, et al. Part 5: adult basic life support and cardiopulmonary resuscitation quality. *Circulation*. 2015;132:S414–S435.

106. Travers AH, Perkins GD, Berg RA, et al. Part 3: adult basic life support and automated external defibrillation: 2015 International Consensus on Cardiopulmonary Resuscitation and Emergency Cardiovascular Care Science With Treatment Recommendations. *Circulation*. 2015;132: S51-S83.

107. Berdowski J, Tijssen JG, Koster RW. Chest compressions cause recurrence of ventricular fibrillation after the first successful conversion by defibrillation in out-of-hospital cardiac arrest. *Circ Arrhythm Electrophysiol*. 2010;3:72-78.

108. Jost D, Degrange H, Verret C, et al. DEFI 2005: a randomized controlled trial of the effect of automated external defibrillator cardiopulmonary resuscitation protocol on outcome from out-of-hospital cardiac arrest. *Circulation*. 2010;121:1614-1622.

109. AHA. Ethical Issues in CPR. 2020, from https://eccguidelines.heart.org/circulation/cpr-ecc-guidelines/part-3-ethical-issues/.

110. Morrison LJ, Eby D, Veigas PV, Implementation trial of the basic life support termination of resuscitation rule: reducing the transport of futile out-of-hospital cardiac arrests. *Resuscitation*. 2014;85:486-91.

111. Panchal AR, Berg KM, Hirsch KG, et al. 2019 American Heart Association focused update on advanced cardiovascular life support: use of advanced airways, vasopressors, and extracorporeal cardiopulmonary resuscitation during cardiac arrest: an update to the American Heart Association Guidelines for Cardiopulmonary Resuscitation and Emergency Cardiovascular Care. *Circulation*. 2019;140:e881-e894.

112. Jabre P, Penaloza A, Pinero D, et al. Effect of bag-mask ventilation vs endotracheal intubation during cardiopulmonary resuscitation on neurological outcome after out-of-hospital cardiorespiratory arrest: a randomized clinical trial. *JAMA*. 2018;319:779-787.

113. Perkins GD, Ji C, Deakin CD, et al. A randomized trial of epinephrine in out-of-hospital cardiac arrest. *N Engl J Med.* 2018;379:711-721.

114. Kudenchuk PJ, Cobb LA, Copass MK, et al. Amiodarone for resuscitation after out-of-hospital cardiac arrest due to ventricular fibrillation. *N Engl J Med.* 1999;341:871-878.

115. Dorian P, Cass D, Schwartz B, Cooper R, Gelaznikas R, Barr A. Amiodarone as compared with lidocaine for shock-resistant ventricular fibrillation (ALIVE Study). *N Engl J Med.* 2002;346:884.

116. Kudenchuk PJ, Brown SP, Daya M, et al. Amiodarone, lidocaine, or placebo in out-of-hospital cardiac arrest. *N Engl J Med.* 2016;374:1711-1722.

117. Morrison LJ, Kierzek G, Diekema DS, et al. Part 3: ethics: 2010 American Heart Association guidelines for cardiopulmonary resuscitation and emergency cardiovascular care. *Circulation.* 2010;122:S665-S675.

118. Welsford M, Nikolaou NI, Beygui F, et al. Part 5: Acute coronary syndromes: 2015 international consensus on cardiopulmonary resuscitation and emergency cardiovascular care science with treatment recommendations. *Circulation.* 2015;132:S146-S176.

119. Dumas F, Cariou A, Manzo-Silberman S, et al. Immediate percutaneous coronary intervention is associated with better survival after out-of-hospital cardiac arrest: insights from the PROCAT (Parisian Region Out of hospital Cardiac ArresT) registry. *Circ Cardiovasc Interv.* 2010;3:200-207.

120. American Heart Association Part 9: Acute coronary syndromes. 2020. https://eccguidelines.heart.org/circulation/cpr-ecc-guidelines/part-9-acute-coronary-syndromes/.

121. Millin MG, Comer AC, Nable JV, et al. Patients without ST elevation after return of spontaneous circulation may benefit from emergent percutaneous intervention: a systematic review and meta-analysis. *Resuscitation.* 2016;108:54-60.

122. Lemkes JS, Janssens GN, van der Hoeven NW, et al. Coronary angiography after cardiac arrest without ST-segment elevation. *N Engl J Med.* 2019;380:1397-1407.

123. Daubert JP, Lee JS, Narayan SM. Role of cardiac angiography in sudden cardiac arrest. *JACC.* 2021;77(4).

124. Yannopoulos D, Bartos JA, Raveendran G, et al. Coronary artery disease in patients with out-of-hospital refractory ventricular fibrillation cardiac arrest. *J Am Coll Cardiol.* 2017;70:1109-1117.

125. Perez CA, Samudra N, Aiyagari V. Cognitive and functional consequence of cardiac arrest. *Curr Neurol Neurosci Rep.* 2016;16:70.

126. Lascarrou JB, Merdji H, Le Gouge A, et al. Targeted temperature management for cardiac arrest with nonshockable rhythm. *N Engl J Med.* 2019;381:2327-2337.

127. Kalra R, Arora G, Patel N, et al. Targeted temperature management after cardiac arrest: systematic review and meta-analyses. *Anesth Analg.* 2018;126:867-875.

128. Polderman KH, Varon J. Confusion around therapeutic temperature management hypothermia after in-hospital cardiac arrest? *Circulation.* 2018;137:219-221.

129. Dietrichs ES, Tveita T, Smith G. Hypothermia and cardiac electrophysiology: a systematic review of clinical and experimental data. *Cardiovasc Res.* 2019;115:501-509.

130. Jimenez-Britez G, Freixa X, Flores-Umanzor E, et al. Out-of-hospital cardiac arrest and stent thrombosis: ticagrelor versus clopidogrel in patients with primary percutaneous coronary intervention under mild therapeutic hypothermia. *Resuscitation.* 2017;114:141-145.

131. American Heart Association. Part 8. Post cardiac arrest care. 2020. https://eccguidelines.heart.org/circulation/cpr-ecc-guidelines/part-8-post-cardiac-arrest-care/.

132. Smith K, Andrew E, Lijovic M, Nehme Z, Bernard S. Quality of life and functional outcomes 12 months after out-of-hospital cardiac arrest. *Circulation.* 2015;131:174-181.

Postoperative and Postprocedural Care in the Cardiac Intensive Care Unit

Venu Menon

Delivering post-operative and post-procedural care in the cardiac intensive care unit

Organization of the cardiac intensive care unit

An organized leadership structure is central to the delivery of optimal care in the CICU

Physician leadership:
- Expertise/special interest in cardiac critical care and familiarity in the management of the heterogeneous group of cardiac disorders that may populate this unit
- Leads a diverse group of medical professionals, including but not limited to: nursing, advanced nurse practitioners, respiratory therapy, pharmacy, occupational and physical therapy, social services and nutritional services, palliative care and bioethics
- Liaise with intensive care unit leadership in other areas across the enterprise

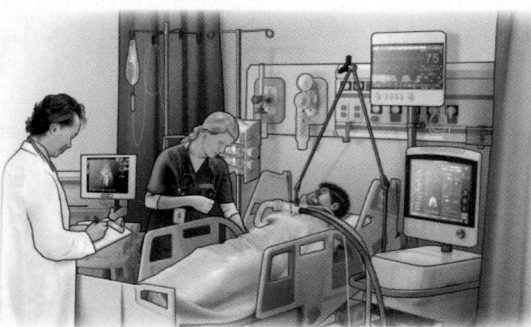

Nursing leadership:
- The CICU nurse is a constant by the bedside and continually interacts with all members of the critical care team, the patient, and family
- Nurses should report to a nursing director for the unit, who ensures adequate staffing, prevention of burnout and implementation of standard operating procedures
- Continuing education and maintenance of proficiency regarding new monitoring and supportive devices, procedural issues and their anticipated complications
- Encouraged to raise issues of concern related to patient care without fear of recrimination

Standard operating procedures

Utilization of standard protocols and implementation bundles guided by best available evidence, and modified for the local environment, can anticipate and prevent most clinical issues. Checklists should be utilized, and ongoing evaluation and critical review are crucial.

Analgesia	Delirium	Sedation	Glycemic control	Infection avoidance	Prevention of DVT	Bleeding
Protocols minimizing utilization of opioid agents with use, as appropriate, of alternative agents (e.g. acetaminophen, tramadol, dexmedetomidine, or gabapentin).	Up to 1 in 5 patients may experience delirium, which has been associated with adverse outcome such as prolonged length of stay and increased in-hospital mortality; screening should be performed in all patients.	Light sedation protocols with adequate pain control, and early extubation after cardiac surgery, are desirable. **Mobilization** Early goal-directed mobilization should be initiated in the absence of contraindications.	Uncontrolled hyperglycemia and/or hypoglycemia associated with adverse outcomes. Conservative management with target glucose of 180 mg/dL preferred.	Prevention of primary CLABSI should be a major focus in the CICU. Minimizing the likelihood of vascular access site infection is also important. Procedures to prevent VAP and CAUTI should additionally be in place.	Individualized risk for developing DVT should be assessed in all patients. Following surgery, patients should receive mechanical thromboprophylaxis utilizing compression stockings with or without intermittent pneumatic compression.	Bleeding is a common complication to be anticipated following most cardiovascular procedures. **Vascular compromise** Baseline and frequent reassessment ensure early recognition of a compromised circulation.

Chapter 64 Fuster and Hurst's Central Illustration. Most patients admitted to the cardiac intensive care unit (CICU) undergo multiple diagnostic and therapeutic procedures. CAUTI, catheter associated urinary tract infection; CLABSI, central line associated blood stream infection; DVT, deep vein thrombosis; VAP, ventilator associated pneumonia.

CHAPTER SUMMARY

This chapter describes broad principles that ensure optimal and consistent postoperative and postprocedural care in the cardiac intensive care unit (CICU). Most patients admitted to the CICU undergo multiple diagnostic and therapeutic procedures. An organized physician and nursing leadership structure is central to the delivery of optimal multidisciplinary care in the CICU (see Fuster and Hurst's Central Illustration). Most clinical issues to be addressed in postprocedural and postoperative settings are well described and can be easily anticipated and prevented by the adoption of evidence-based standard operating protocols and implantation bundles, which ensure consistency and optimal outcomes. Protocol creation should involve a multidisciplinary team including physicians, nurses, and other relevant ancillary medical personnel. Some common clinical areas addressed include provision of analgesia, prevention of infection, screening for and treatment of delirium, sedation for mechanical ventilation, early mobilization and prevention of deep venous thrombosis, and adequate glycemic control. The utilization of checklists and the ability to promptly recognize and treat complications is crucial.

INTRODUCTION

Although only 10% to 15% of patients are admitted to the cardiac intensive care unit (CICU) solely for postprocedural observation, most patients admitted to the unit undergo multiple diagnostic and therapeutic procedures.[1] Procedural advances in cardiology have dramatically improved outcome amongst significant clinical subsets admitted to the CICU. This is best exemplified by the routine utilization of primary percutaneous coronary intervention (PCI) in patients presenting with ST-elevation myocardial infarction (STEMI). Adoption of this strategy, has dramatically lowered mortality while markedly reducing the likelihood of electrical and hemodynamic complications to such a profound degree that a significant proportion of STEMI subjects may now be considered for direct admission to a regular nursing floor, bypassing the CICU itself.[2] While the decision to monitor specific patients following a procedure or cardiac surgery in the CICU will be guided in large part by local circumstance and policies, the broad principles to ensure optimal and consistent postoperative and postprocedural care will be highlighted in this chapter. The management of procedure specific issues to be anticipated/encountered in the postoperative and postprocedural environment will be detailed in the individual chapters addressing these topics.

ORGANIZATION OF THE CARDIAC INTENSIVE CARE UNIT

Having an organized leadership structure is central to the delivery of optimal care in the CICU.

Physician Leadership

The CICU should ideally be led by a physician leader with expertise/special interest in cardiac critical care and with familiarity in the management of the heterogeneous group of cardiac disorders that may populate this unit. The physician leader should lead a diverse group of medical professionals including but not limited to nursing, advanced nurse practitioners, respiratory therapy, pharmacy, occupational and physical therapy, social services and nutritional services, palliative care, and bioethics. The physician leader should be tasked with day-to-day administration of the unit and plays a central role in building consensus and policy across physicians, nurses, and ancillary medical personal on various patient management issues. The physician leader will also serve as the liaison with intensive care unit (ICU) leadership in other areas across the enterprise. This interaction ensures consistency of care across units for common patient-related intensive care issues. Depending on the size and scope of the unit, the physician leader or an appointee should also be directly responsible for setting processes to measuring outcomes and implementing quality improvement projects in the unit. Studies suggest that a closed unit in which the ICU physician assumes complete responsibility for the patients admitted is associated with superior outcomes over an open unit where individual nonintensivist physicians direct patient care.[3]

Nursing Leadership

As the constant by the bedside, the nurse in the CICU is undoubtedly the most valuable team member. The nurse constantly interacts with all members of the critical care team, the patient, and family and is crucial for the implementation of protocols in the postprocedural and postoperative setting. Nurses should report to a nursing director for the unit, who ensures adequate staffing, prevention of burnout, and implementation of standard operating procedures. Similar to physicians, processes should be in place for continuing education and maintenance of proficiency regarding new monitoring and supportive devices, procedural issues, and their anticipated complications. A culture of inquiry should be created and nurses should be encouraged to raise issues of concern related to patient care without fear of recrimination. This ensures prompt identification of errors and reports of shortcomings that should be addressed promptly on an ongoing basis.

Standard Operating Procedures

The majority of clinical issues to be addressed in postprocedural and postoperative settings are well described and can be easily anticipated and prevented by utilizing standard protocols and implementation bundles that should be guided by best available evidence and modified for the local environment. Creation of these protocols should have universal acceptance and should involve a multidisciplinary team involving physicians, nurses, and other relevant ancillary medical personnel. Some but not all of the common salient issues to be addressed in the postoperative and postprocedural setting are subsequently discussed.

Analgesia

Patients should be educated prior to surgery/procedure so that pain is not unexpected.[4] Historically, in postsurgical patients, opioid agents were the mainstay of therapy but the side effects including sedation, respiratory depression, ileus, nausea, and vomiting are now well recognized.[5] As a result, protocols minimizing utilizations of these agents with enhanced introduction of agents like acetaminophen, tramadol, dexmedetomidine, and gabapentin should be implemented.[6] The pharmacological approach should take both the procedure and patient-related characteristics into consideration. In nonverbal patients who can otherwise communicate, a validated instrument like the Numeric Rating Scale (0–10) may be utilized. In those who are intubated and cannot communicate, the Behavioral Pain Scale and the Critical Care Pain Observation Tool to assess pain may be utilized. Similarly, the Behavior Pain Scale-Nonintubated may be utilized in that specific group of patients.[7]

Delirium

Up to 1 in 5 patients admitted to the CICU may experience delirium, which is defined as an acute and dynamic condition characterized by alterations in attention, perception, and cognition. The occurrence of delirium in the CICU has been associated with adverse outcomes including prolonged length of stay and increased in-hospital mortality.[8,9] Screening for delirium utilizing the Intensive Care Delirium Screening Checklist or the Confusion Assessment Method-Intensive Care Unit should be performed in all patients.[10] The American Heart Association (AHA) scientific statement encourages minimizing benzodiazepine utilization and adoption of early ambulation protocols to decrease the risk of this common complication.[11] A single pharmacological agent or intervention is unlikely to impact on the incidence of delirium[12] and a multipronged approach is recommended.[13] Antipsychotic agents that prolong the QTc interval should be utilized with caution in CICU patients with monitoring of the QTc interval and should be considered only in the setting of a hyperactive delirium when the benefits outweigh the risks.

Sedation in Mechanically Ventilated Patients

Adoption of light sedation protocols utilizing the Richmond Agitation–Sedation Scale (RASS) or other validated scales has been shown to significantly decrease the period of ventilator dependence and a RASS target of –1 to 0 is recommended for most patients in the CICU. This should be performed in the background of ensuring adequate pain control that can minimize sedation needs. When deeper sedation goals are warranted, daily interruption of sedation should be performed to prevent drug accumulation, assess neurological status, and consider weaning.

Following cardiac surgery, prolonged intubation has been associated with complications like ventilator associated pneumonia and dysphagia[14] along with observed increased length of stay, expense, and even mortality.[15] Early extubation within 6 hours has been shown to decrease ICU and hospital length of stay without favorably impacting morbidity and mortality.[16]

Avoidance of Infections

Prevention of primary central line–associated bloodstream infection (CLABSI) should be a major focus in the CICU because it is associated with significant morbidity and mortality. The need for a central line, its location, and duration should be continuously assessed so as to minimize risk of infection. **Table 64-1**, incorporated from the AHA scientific statement on prevention of complications in the CICU, outlines a number of strategies to decrease the likelihood of CLABSI.[11] The Center for Disease Control and Prevention recommends washing of hands with soap and water before line placement and manipulation, training and experience in placement of access catheters with use of full barrier precautions, utilization of 2% chlorhexidine for skin preparation, avoidance of femoral access, and limiting duration of catheter use as critical interventions in avoiding CLABSI.[17] These proven recommendations should be incorporated into a central line bundle and compliance should be monitored on an ongoing basis.[18]

Patients receiving temporary mechanical circulatory support with extracorporeal membrane oxygen support (ECMO), Impella, or intra-aortic balloon pump (IABP) support are especially vulnerable to vascular access site infection due to the emergent nature of implementation, accompanying hemodynamic instability, need for prolonged duration of support, femoral access site, and presence of multiple comorbidities. Observed rates of infection range from about 1% with an IABP to one-third of patients requiring ECMO support for over 2 weeks.[19,20] Meticulous and sterile technique, use of alternate

TABLE 64-1. Strategies to Reduce Central Venous Catheter (CVC)–Associated Bloodstream Infection Outlined in the AHA Scientific Statement to Decrease Complications in the Cardiac Intensive Care Unit

Prior to CVC insertion	During CVC insertion	After CVC insertion
Use CVC only when necessary for established indications	Checklist to ensure compliance with CVC bundle	Remove CVC as soon as no longer indicated
Consider alternatives to CVCs when indicated	Perform hand hygiene before and after CVC insertion	Disinfect hubs and injection ports before accessing CVC
Bathe daily with 2% chlorhexidine	Clean skin using alcoholic >0.5% chlorhexidine solution and let dry	Use antiseptic-containing hub/connector caps
Consider appropriate CVC site	Use aseptic technique and sterile equipment for catheter insertion	Change dressing and perform site care with chlorhexidine every 5-7 days or if dressing is compromised
Avoid routine use of guidewire exchanges, especially if infected	Avoid femoral vein site for routine CVC placement	Use antimicrobial ointments for dialysis catheter insertion sites
Ensure proper education regarding CLABSI prevention among providers placing CVCs	Use ultrasound guidance for cannulation when indicated	Perform hand hygiene before and after CVC manipulation
	Use smallest CVC with minimum number of lumens necessary	Properly secure CVC to avoid skin trauma (sutureless device)
	Consider antimicrobial-coated CVCs if infection rates remain high	Do not routinely replace CVC
	Use chlorhexidine-containing dressings	Consider antimicrobial locks for patients with prior CLABSI
	Avoid systemic antibiotic prophylaxis	Use lower nurse-to-patient ratios
		Do not submerge CVC in water, showering only if protected by impermeable barrier

access sites like the axilla, access site care, and limiting duration of support are warranted to minimize the likelihood of this complication.

Similarly, procedures to prevent ventilator-associated pneumonia (VAP) and catheter-associated urinary tract infection (CAUTI) should be in place and are summarized in **Tables 64-2** and **64-3**, respectively, adopted from the AHA scientific statement on prevention of complications in the CICU.[11]

Glycemic Control

Uncontrolled hyperglycemia in the ICU and postoperative setting is associated with adverse clinical outcomes

TABLE 64-2. Strategies to Reduce Ventilator-Associated Pneumonia Outlined in the AHA Scientific Statement to Decrease Complications in the Cardiac Intensive Care Unit

Best practices	
Benefits likely outweigh risks	Use of NI-PPV in selected populations
	Have sedation protocols with targeted light sedation
	Interrupt sedation daily if appropriate
	Assess readiness to extubate daily
	Perform SBT off sedation
	Early mobilization
	Place ETT with subglottic suction (if >48–72 h IMV)
	Change MV only when soiled
	Position head of bed >30°
Special approaches	
Proven efficacy but uncertain risks	Selective oral or digestive decontamination
Uncertain effects on clinical outcomes	Regular oral care with chlorhexidine
	Prophylactic probiotics in selected patients
	Ultrathin polyurethane ETT cuffs
	Automated control of ETT pressure
	Saline instillation during endotracheal suctioning
	Mechanical toothbrushing
Generally not recommended	
Does not lower VAP rates or improve outcomes	Silver-coated ETTs
	Kinetic beds
	Prone positioning
	Stress ulcer prophylaxis
	Early tracheostomy
	Monitoring gastric, residual volumes
	Early parenteral nutrition
	Closed/in-line endotracheal suctioning

Reproduced with permission from Fordyce CB, Katz JN, Alviar CL, et al. Prevention of Complications in the Cardiac Intensive Care Unit: A Scientific Statement From the American Heart Association. *Circulation*. 2020 Dec;142(22):e379-e406.

TABLE 64-3. Strategies for Prevention of Catheter-Associated Bacteriuria and Catheter-Associated Urinary Tract Infection

Before Urinary Catheter Insertion	During Urinary Catheter Insertion	After Urinary Catheter Insertion
Use urinary catheters only when necessary for established indications	Use only trained, dedicated personnel to insert catheters	Remove urinary catheters as soon as no longer indicated
Avoid routine use of urinary catheters for management of incontinence	Perform hand hygiene before and after urinary catheter insertion	Maintain drainage bag and connecting tubing below the level of the bladder
Use portable bladder scanners to assess need for catheterization	Clean urethral meatus with antiseptic solution	Maintain unobstructed urine flow in collecting system
Consider condom catheterization for men without urinary retention	Use aseptic technique and sterile equipment for catheter insertion	Avoid routine catheter irrigation or daily meatal cleansing
Consider intermittent catheterization	Consider use of a preconnected catheter and tubing system	Perform hand hygiene before and after catheter manipulation
	Consider use of antimicrobial-coated urinary catheters	Properly secure catheters to avoid meatal trauma
		Avoid systemic antibiotic prophylaxis
		Replace catheter and collecting system only for breaks in aseptic technique, disconnection, or leakage

Reproduced with permission from Fordyce CB, Katz JN, Alviar CL, et al. Prevention of Complications in the Cardiac Intensive Care Unit: A Scientific Statement From the American Heart Association. *Circulation*. 2020 Dec;142(22):e379-e406.

and hypoglycemia should be avoided. Intensive blood glucose targets utilizing goal blood sugar levels between 80 and 110 mg/dL have been associated with an increased hypoglycemic response and mortality in medical ICU populations. Conservative insulin protocols targeting blood glucose levels of 180 mg/dL should be preferentially utilized.[21] There is limited data in the postcardiac surgery population and a similar strategy has been extrapolated.[4]

Early Mobilization

Prolonged bed rest following surgery or prolonged CICU admission can result in marked neuropathic effects and muscle weakness that is associated with prolonged length of stay and worsening clinical outcomes.[22] The best preventive measure is early goal-directed mobilization that should be initiated in the absence of contraindications in CICU patents who are stable from a hemodynamic, neurological, and respiratory standpoint with no evidence of decompensated heart failure, active ischemia, or electrical instability.

Prevention of Deep Vein Thrombosis

Half of all venous thromboembolic events occur in the background of an acute medical illness or admission to a hospital.[23] Consequently, all patients admitted to the CICU including those that are postprocedure should have their individualized risk for developing deep vein thrombosis assessed. Several risk assessment models have been developed including the Padua and IMPROVE scores[24,25] and in the absence of contraindications, those identified to be at risk should be considered for prophylactic therapy. In critically ill patients, the American Society of Hematology favors pharmacoprophylaxis over mechanical venous thromboembolism (VTE) prophylaxis and suggests utilizing low-molecular-weight heparin over unfractionated heparin for this indication. When mechanical prophylaxis is warranted due to the presence of contraindications, either pneumatic compression devices or graduated compression devices may be utilized.[26]

Cardiothoracic surgery is associated with heightened risk for VTE in the postoperative period.[27] All patients following surgery should receive mechanical thromboprophylaxis utilizing compression stockings with or without intermittent pneumatic compression.[28] Prophylactic anticoagulation should be initiated on the first operative day as soon as hemostasis is achieved and reduces VTE without adverse outcomes of increased bleeding or cardiac tamponade.[29]

Specific Postprocedural Issues

The nature of the underlying procedure performed will guide the focus of care during the observation period. Some of the common procedures encountered in the CICU and their potential complications are outlined in **Table 64–4**. However, the basic principles of postprocedural care remain universal. The nurse by the bedside should have comprehensive understanding of the procedure performed, potential complications,

TABLE 64–4. Common Procedures Encountered in the CICU and Their Potential Complications

Procedure	Checklist on Arrival to CICU Bed	Potential Complications in the Observation Period
Temporary Transvenous Pacing	Confirm lead placement on chest x-ray Confirm pacing and sensing threshold Line Maintenance	Lead dislodgement with failure to capture, undersensing or oversensing, Lead migration with perforation of interventricular septum Right ventricular perforation with tamponade Hemothorax Pneumothorax Pericarditis
Right Heart Catheter	Line Maintenance Chest x-ray to confirm position Zero and obtain pressures	Pulmonary artery rupture from migration during balloon inflation Pneumothorax
Postcatheterization or PCI	Evaluate access site; check for overt bleeding/hematoma Check distal and bilateral pulses Follow immobilization protocol Baseline neurological evaluation	Access site and nonaccess site bleeding Loss of pulses with distal limb ischemia Stroke Neurological injury Acute renal failure Recurrent ischemia, stent thrombosis Tamponade from unrecognized coronary perforation Infection at access site
ECMO (VA)	Check vascular access site integrity Check presence and position of reperfusion cannula Check all distal pulses Baseline neurological evaluation Ensure presence and adequacy of right radial artery oxygenation Ensure adequate cerebral oxygenation utilizing sensors	Major access and nonaccess site bleeding, catheter dislodgement, ischemic distal limb, compartment syndrome, intravascular hemolysis, air/clot in the circuit, stroke, neurological complications, acute kidney injury, infection
Pericardiocentesis	Catheter position if left in situ Care of the access site	Pneumothorax Occult Bleeding Hemothorax Hemopericardium/pneumopericardium Tamponade Arrhythmia Liver laceration
Targeted Temperature Management following Cardiac Arrest	Ensure goal temperature is met and maintained Ensure sedation to RASS of –3 to –5 Ensure OG/NG tube position for decompression: do not initiate tube feeding Monitor for shivering and treat as needed Care of the access site if intravascular cooling catheters are utilized Active rewarming when indicated should be performed at a control rate of 0.25–0.5 degrees Celsius per hour	Access site and nonaccess site bleeding Monitor for electrolytes. Blood glucose and coagulopathy on labs Hypotension due to post arrest vasodilatation and hypothermia induced diuresis

and should have documented proficiency in following the standard procedure-specific operating procedure. A detailed handover should be performed and the receiving team in the CICU should receive details of the procedure, potential challenges, and complications encountered. The nurse-to-patient ratio should be adequate so that necessary monitoring can be performed without compromise. Adequate equipment for monitoring vitals and electrical and hemodynamic stability should be present with suitable alarms. Appropriate physician supervision should be present to address concerns by the bedside and to immediately initiate supportive, diagnostic, or therapeutic interventions when warranted. There should be the ability to perform immediate defibrillation if indicated.

Bleeding is a common complication to be anticipated following most cardiovascular procedures. While overt vascular access bleeding is readily apparent, occult blood loss should be suspected and addressed in the setting of unexplained hypotension or tachycardia. Common sites of occult bleeding include the retroperitoneum and the gastrointestinal tract. Another common complication in the postprocedure cardiovascular setting is ischemic and hemorrhagic stroke. Prompt recognition of this complication entails performing a detailed documented baseline and follow-up neurological examination at regular intervals. Vascular compromise is also commonly encountered in patients with severe peripheral vascular disease and with the use of large bore arterial access. Evaluating the distal limb for ischemia, establishing adequate distal pulses and capillary circulation at baseline, and frequent reassessment will ensure early recognition of a compromised circulation. Decompensation of heart failure, supraventricular and ventricular arrhythmias, bradyarrhythmia, and renal failure are also frequently encountered in this setting.

SUMMARY

Postprocedural and postsurgical care in CICU patients while focused on the unique needs of the individual and the specific procedure can be significantly enhanced by the utilization of established treatment protocols and bundles. Care under a multidisciplinary team can ensure consistency, timeliness, and reliability that will result in superior outcomes and optimized length of care. Measuring and benchmarking observed clinical outcomes is imperative as part of a continuous quality improvement process.

REFERENCES

1. Bohula EA, Katz JN, van Diepen S, et al. Demographics, care patterns, and outcomes of patients admitted to cardiac intensive care units: the Critical Care Cardiology Trials Network Prospective North American Multicenter Registry of Cardiac Critical Illness. *JAMA Cardiol.* 2019;4:928-935.
2. Shavadia JS, Chen AY, Fanaroff AC, de Lemos JA, Kontos MC, Wang TY. Intensive care utilization in stable patients with ST-segment elevation myocardial infarction treated with rapid reperfusion. *JACC Cardiovasc Interv.* 2019;12:709-717.
3. Pronovost PJ, Angus DC, Dorman T, Robinson KA, Dremsizov TT, Young TL. Physician staffing patterns and clinical outcomes in critically ill patients: a systematic review. *JAMA.* 2002;288:2151-2162.
4. Engelman DT, Ben Ali W, Williams JB, et al. Guidelines for perioperative care in cardiac surgery: enhanced recovery after surgery society recommendations. *JAMA Surg.* 2019;154:755-766.
5. White PF, Kehlet H, Neal JM, et al. The role of the anesthesiologist in fast-track surgery: from multimodal analgesia to perioperative medical care. *Anesth Analg.* 2007;104:1380-1396, table of contents.
6. Wick EC, Grant MC, Wu CL. Postoperative multimodal analgesia pain management with nonopioid analgesics and techniques: a review. *JAMA Surg.* 2017;152:691-697.
7. Devlin JW, Skrobik Y, Gelinas C, et al. Clinical practice guidelines for the prevention and management of pain, agitation/sedation, delirium, immobility, and sleep disruption in adult patients in the ICU. *Crit Care Med.* 2018;46:e825-e873.
8. Naksuk N, Thongprayoon C, Park JY, et al. Editor's choice-clinical impact of delirium and antipsychotic therapy: 10-year experience from a referral coronary care unit. *Eur Heart J Acute Cardiovasc Care* 2017;6: 560-568.
9. Pauley E, Lishmanov A, Schumann S, Gala GJ, van Diepen S, Katz JN. Delirium is a robust predictor of morbidity and mortality among critically ill patients treated in the cardiac intensive care unit. *Am Heart J.* 2015;170:79-86, 86.e71.
10. Neto AS, Nassar AP Jr., Cardoso SO, et al. Delirium screening in critically ill patients: a systematic review and meta-analysis. *Crit Care Med.* 2012;40:1946-1951.
11. Fordyce CB, Katz JN, Alviar CL, et al. Prevention of complications in the cardiac intensive care unit: a scientific statement from the American Heart Association. *Circulation.* 2020;142:e379-e406.
12. Maldonado JR. Neuropathogenesis of delirium: review of current etiologic theories and common pathways. *Am J Geriatr Psychiatry* 2013;21:1190-1222.
13. Young J, Murthy L, Westby M, Akunne A, O'Mahony R, Guideline Development G. Diagnosis, prevention, and management of delirium: summary of NICE guidance. *BMJ.* 2010;341:c3704.
14. Barker J, Martino R, Reichardt B, Hickey EJ, Ralph-Edwards A. Incidence and impact of dysphagia in patients receiving prolonged endotracheal intubation after cardiac surgery. *Can J Surg.* 2009;52: 119-124.
15. Rajakaruna C, Rogers CA, Angelini GD, Ascione R. Risk factors for and economic implications of prolonged ventilation after cardiac surgery. *J Thorac Cardiovasc Surg.* 2005;130:1270-1277.
16. Meade MO, Guyatt G, Butler R, et al. Trials comparing early vs late extubation following cardiovascular surgery. *Chest.* 2001;120:445S-453S.
17. Bell T, O'Grady NP. Prevention of central line-associated bloodstream infections. *Infect Dis Clin North Am.* 2017;31:551-559.
18. Pronovost P, Needham D, Berenholtz S, et al. An intervention to decrease catheter-related bloodstream infections in the ICU. *N Engl J Med.* 2006;355:2725-2732.
19. Bizzarro MJ, Conrad SA, Kaufman DA, Rycus P, Extracorporeal Life Support Organization Task Force on Infections EMO. Infections acquired during extracorporeal membrane oxygenation in neonates, children, and adults. *Pediatr Crit Care Med.* 2011;12:277-281.
20. Ternus BW, Jentzer JC, El Sabbagh A, et al. Percutaneous mechanical circulatory support for cardiac disease: temporal trends in use and complications between 2009 and 2015. *J Invasive Cardiol.* 2017;29: 309-313.
21. Griesdale DE, de Souza RJ, van Dam RM, et al. Intensive insulin therapy and mortality among critically ill patients: a meta-analysis including NICE-SUGAR study data. *CMAJ.* 2009;180:821-827.
22. Appleton RT, Kinsella J, Quasim T. The incidence of intensive care unit-acquired weakness syndromes: a systematic review. *J Intensive Care Soc.* 2015;16:126-136.
23. Heit JA, O'Fallon WM, Petterson TM, et al. Relative impact of risk factors for deep vein thrombosis and pulmonary embolism: a population-based study. *Arch Intern Med.* 2002;162:1245-1248.

24. Barbar S, Noventa F, Rossetto V, et al. A risk assessment model for the identification of hospitalized medical patients at risk for venous thromboembolism: the Padua Prediction Score. *J Thromb Haemost.* 2010;8:2450-2457.

25. Spyropoulos AC, Anderson FA Jr., FitzGerald G, et al. Predictive and associative models to identify hospitalized medical patients at risk for VTE. *Chest.* 2011;140:706-714.

26. Schunemann HJ, Cushman M, Burnett AE, et al. American Society of Hematology 2018 guidelines for management of venous thromboembolism: prophylaxis for hospitalized and nonhospitalized medical patients. *Blood Adv.* 2018;2:3198-3225.

27. Parolari A, Mussoni L, Frigerio M, et al. Increased prothrombotic state lasting as long as one month after on-pump and off-pump coronary surgery. *J Thorac Cardiovasc Surg.* 2005;130:303-308.

28. Kakkos SK, Caprini JA, Geroulakos G, et al. Combined intermittent pneumatic leg compression and pharmacological prophylaxis for prevention of venous thromboembolism. *Cochrane Database Syst Rev.* 2016;9:CD005258.

29. Dunning J, Versteegh M, Fabbri A, et al. Guideline on antiplatelet and anticoagulation management in cardiac surgery. *Eur J Cardiothorac Surg.* 2008;34:73-92.

SECTION XI

ADULT CONGENITAL HEART DISEASE

Anatomical and Physiological Classification of Adult Congenital Heart Disease

65

Jasmine Grewal and Alexander R. Opotowsky

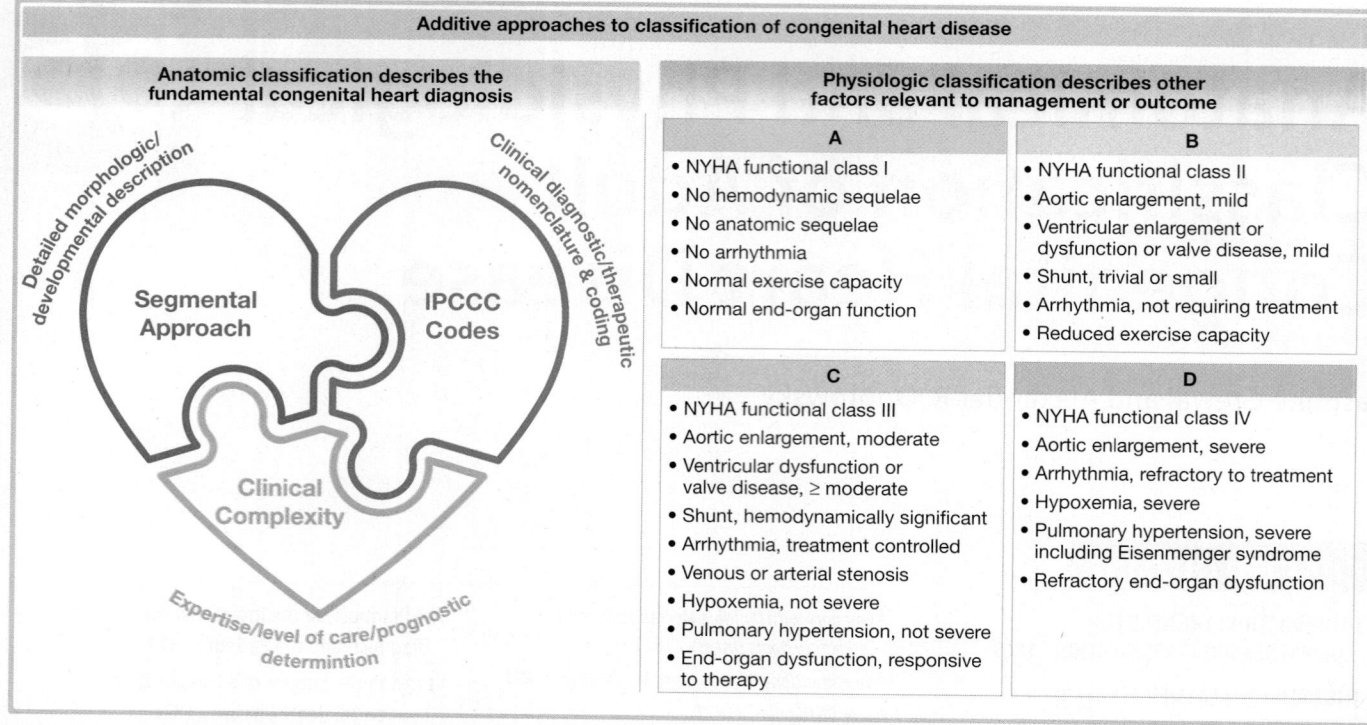

Chapter 65 Fuster and Hurst's Central Illustration. A universally accepted nomenclature is critical to health care providers directly involved in managing the patient with congenital heart disease (CHD), but has remained an unrealized aspiration. Recently developed classification systems have explored involving multiple dimensions to characterize CHD. The overall goal is to standardize and streamline communication and thereby improve patient outcomes. IPCCC, International Pediatric and Congenital Cardiac Code; NYHA, New York Heart Association.

CHAPTER SUMMARY

This chapter describes a brief history of classification of the numerous types of congenital heart disease (CHD) lesions and the additive value of approaches (see Fuster and Hurst's Central Illustration), focusing on recent developments including the anatomic and physiologic (AP) classification and International Pediatric and Congenital Cardiac Code (IPCCC), the basis for ICD-11 codes. Historically, classification has focused on anatomy based on pathology investigations. With the advent of surgical options for CHD management in the 20th century, attention focused on distinctions relevant to available therapeutic decisions. These surgeries, and later catheter-based treatments, modify the initial CHD, often transforming the pathophysiology and long-term consequences. As more individuals survive longer with CHD, so does the need for a common language that comprehensively and concisely describes not only the underlying congenital heart lesion, but also prior medical interventions repairs and cumulative physiologic burden. Recent classifications have explored multiple dimensions to characterizing CHD. The recently proposed AP classification aims to represent CHD anatomy, along with pertinent interventions and current physiologic status. This provides useful nuance, but also adds complexity and associated challenges. Evolving clinical phenotype requires ongoing modification, but these classification efforts share a goal: to standardize and streamline communication and thereby improve outcomes.

INTRODUCTION: THE NEED FOR COMPREHENSIVE CLASSIFICATION

As the number of individuals surviving with congenital heart disease (CHD) grows, so does the need for a common language that describes any given congenital heart lesion and its sequelae. Equally important is the ability to express information comprehensively and concisely. CHD encompasses a wide spectrum of cardiac malformations, ranging from simple to great complexity. This complexity relates not only to the native anatomy, but also to subsequent surgical repairs and long-term cumulative physiologic burden. As such, the same CHD diagnosis may be associated with heterogeneous implications for different patients. For example, take two patients with congenitally corrected transposition of the great arteries (TGA). The first is a 65-year-old patient with mild systemic ventricular dysfunction, no symptoms, and good exercise tolerance. The second is a 28-year-old with severe systemic ventricular dysfunction, prior mechanical systemic atrioventricular valve replacement, secondary prevention implantable defibrillator, and refractory clinical heart failure awaiting heart transplantation. The diagnosis of congenitally corrected transposition of the great arteries alone does not provide substantive insight into the patient's clinical scenario.

In concept, a combined anatomic and physiologic (AP) classification system would allow healthcare providers to communicate the details around a CHD lesion in a standardized way, which is essential to both clinical practice and research. Such a system should represent the principal underlying anatomy as well as pertinent subsequent interventions and current clinical status. Key variables may include surgical and catheter interventions, current hemodynamics, symptoms, exercise tolerance, cardiac and noncardiac comorbidities, and complications. In this way, the classification accounts for factors that may be prognostically important, impact quality of life, and dictate frequency/type of monitoring. A patient's clinical status can change over time, and this becomes especially apparent when using an AP classification, and draws attention to the fact that follow-up and/or management need to be altered accordingly and may become more or less intensive. Ultimately, the AP classification becomes a tool that not only improves communication but also standardizes patient care. All of this is critical to improving patient care and, in some cases, improving outcomes.

THE NEED FOR CLASSIFICATION

Identifies the "Primary Diagnosis"

Intuitively, it seems obvious that each patient has a primary anatomic CHD diagnosis. We believe that the "primary" diagnosis is the one that has the most relevance to a patient's prognosis as related to mortality and/or intensity of required treatment. The list of diagnoses generally follows a hierarchy of severity as reflected by prognosis. One might consider directly ranking diagnoses by their associated life expectancy when encountered in isolation.

When a patient has multiple diagnoses of variable severity, identifying a primary diagnosis can be relatively straightforward. Examples include hypoplastic heart syndrome and aortic coarctation, or Tetralogy of Fallot (TOF) with a secundum atrial septal defect (ASD). Even in such cases, ambiguity may arise. On average, TOF is associated with worse prognosis than ASD. However, if a patient with TOF and ASD develops Eisenmenger syndrome, one might argue that the sequelae of the ASD is more likely to govern appropriate therapy and dominate prognosis. More commonly, patients have multiple diagnoses of similar severity, such as pulmonary stenosis with an ASD, or TOF with a complete atrioventricular septal defect, or tricuspid atresia with TGA. Only by considering clinical characteristics beyond the anatomic diagnosis itself can one make a reasonable decision about primacy. Indeed, each classification of "anatomic" CHD includes some reference to physiologic impacts, such as pulmonary vascular disease or cardiac chamber dilation. This highlights the potential value of a complementary physiologic classification system.

There are a few additional caveats to consider when establishing the primary diagnosis. The same set of diagnoses may lead to a different "primary" diagnosis depending on when a patient is born. For example, take tricuspid atresia with TGA and pulmonary stenosis. In 1950, isolated TGA with a ventricular septal defect (VSD) may have been the diagnosis associated with worse prognosis. In 1960, after development of the atrial switch, tricuspid atresia would presumably now be the primary diagnosis. We have made the assumption that the "primary" diagnosis is the one that has most relevance to a patient's prognosis. But there may be another relevant "primary" diagnosis, depending on the goals of the classification. TGA, for example, may be associated with specific neurodevelopmental impacts independent of its association with mortality. In practice, it is difficult to present a consistent, broadly applicable set of rules that achieves the goal of identifying a primary diagnosis, even when what is meant by "primary" is clear.

Historical Perspective: From Autopsy Case Reports to Segmental Approach and Beyond

The classification of causes of death and disease dates back as far as the early 17th century. Numerous publications described various congenital cardiac lesions through the late 19th century. However, the pioneering systematic classification of congenital cardiac lesions was published by Canadian physician Maude Abbot in 1936 in the *Atlas of Congenital Cardiac Disease*.[1] Over the last several decades, there have been a few notable anatomic classification approaches with which the most complex cardiac malformations can be described in a simple and accurate way. The Van Praagh's introduced a systematic segmental approach to analyzing cardiac morphology, facilitating great improvements in our understanding of cardiac malformations (**Fig. 65–1**).[2,3] This approach focuses on three major segments—visceroatrial situs, ventricular loop, and great artery position and relation. Once segments and intersegmental alignments have been determined, individual chamber, valve, and vessel diagnoses are made. Anderson proposed a modified segmental approach describing connections of cardiac segments in addition to their relations and morphology.[4–6] These classifications described

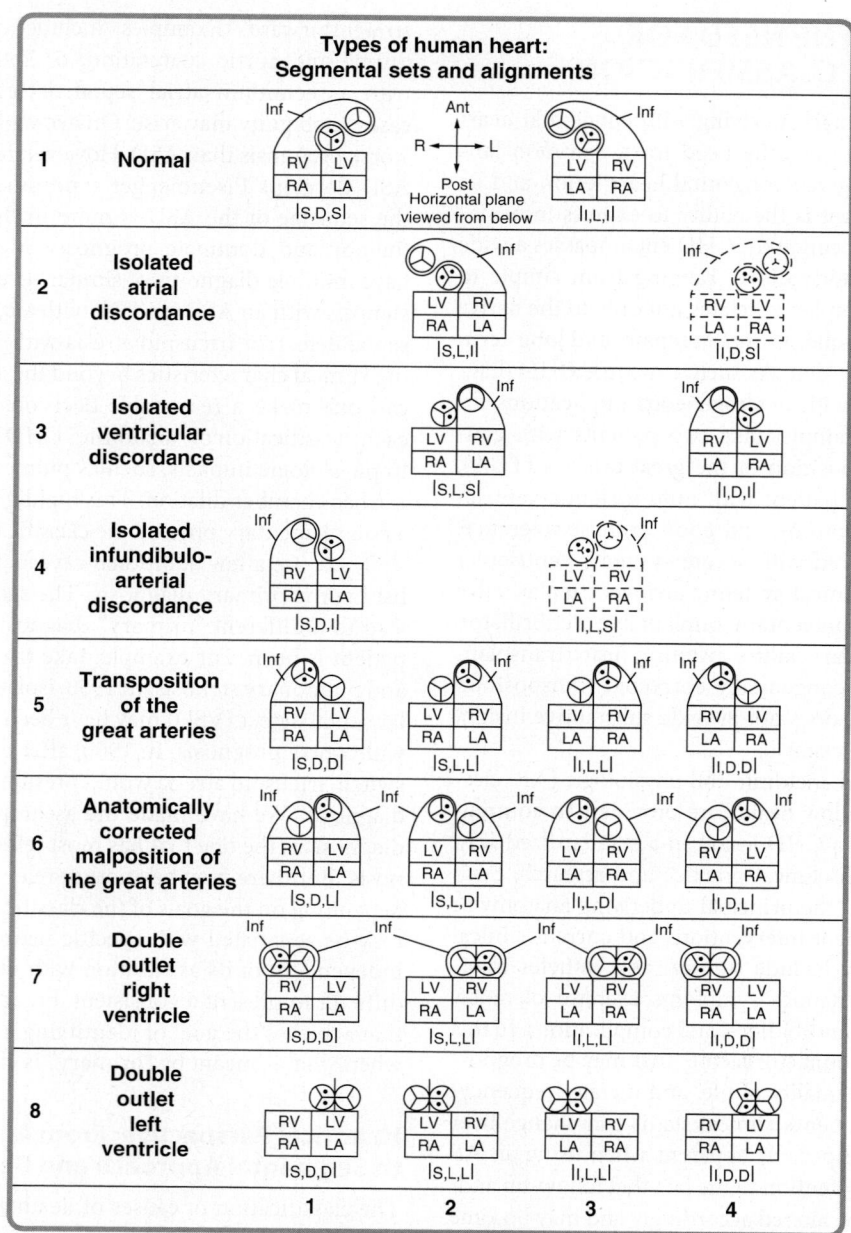

Figure 65–1. Types of human heart in terms of segmental sets (combinations) and segmental alignments. Heart diagrams are viewed from below, as would be achieved with a subxiphoid two-dimensional echocardiogram. Cardiotypes depicted in broken lines had not been documented when this diagram was made. The aortic valve is indicated by the coronary ostia. The pulmonary valve is indicated by the absence of coronary ostia. Braces {} mean "the set of." The columns (1 to 4) are arranged in terms of atrioventricular (AV) concordance or discordance. Column 1 (ie, {S,D,-}) has AV concordance in visceroatrial situs solitus. Column 2 (ie, {S,L,-}) has AV discordance in visceroatrial situs solitus. Column 3 (ie, {I,L,-}) has AV concordance in visceroatrial situs inversus. Column 4 (ie, {I,D,-}) has AV discordance in visceroatrial situs inversus. Situs ambiguus of the viscera and atria in the heterotaxy syndromes, particularly with asplenia (ie, {A,D,-} and {A,L,-}) is omitted; the concepts of AV concordance and AV discordance do not apply in visceroatrial situs ambiguus because the frame of reference, the type of visceroatrial situs, is uncertain or unknown. The rows (1 to 8) are organized in terms of the types of ventriculoarterial (VA) alignment. Normal concordant VA alignments are depicted in rows 1 to 4. Abnormal concordant VA alignments are shown in row 6 and concern anatomically corrected malposition of the great arteries. Discordant VA alignments are depicted in row 5 and concern transposition of the great arteries. Double outlets are shown in rows 7 and 8, double-outlet right ventricle in row 7, and double-outlet left ventricle in row 8. All associated malformations are omitted for diagrammatic simplicity and clarity. Ant, anterior; Inf, infundibulum; LA, morphologically left atrium; L, left; LV, morphologically left ventricle; Post, posterior; R, right; RA, morphologically right atrium; RV, morphologically right ventricle.

Reproduced with permission from Foran RB, Belcourt C, Nanton MA, et la. Isolated infundibuloarterial inversion (S,D,I): a newly recognized form of congenital heart disease. *Am Heart J.* 1988 Nov;116(5 Pt 1):1337-1350.

were intended to describe fundamental definitions and precisely describe underlying developmental and morphologic features. These approaches provide a detailed and reproducible description of the underlying CHD, rather than relying solely on a named diagnosis, which can be an oversimplification, however unlikely to impact clinical practice. This approach is key to determining and understanding the underlying anatomy with foundational importance for clinically focused anatomic diagnosis. However, some of these distinctions important for developmental or morphological purposes have a limited role in clinical practice.

In the 1960s, Donald Fyler developed an extensive, systematic set of numbered codes for CHD and associated procedures as part of work on The New England Regional Infant Cardiac Program, among the earliest attempts to comprehensively classify the range of CHD and associated clinical characteristics. Introduced in an era of punch cards, the Fyler Coding System continues to be used at Boston Children's Hospital, and served as one of the foundational guides in the development of the International Pediatric and Congenital Cardiac Code (IPCCC) (see section IPCCC/ICD-11) along with several other clinical coding systems developed for CHD with particular uses in mind. These include the Society of Thoracic Surgery's Congenital Heart Surgery Nomenclature and Database Project Codes and the European Pediatric Cardiology Codes.[7,8]

Unappreciated Ambiguity

To be useful and avoid misunderstanding, diagnostic names and other systematic categorization must be precise. A term should refer clearly to a specific concept or entity. Perhaps most problematic are terms that seem well-defined but are used and interpreted differently in different contexts. Several examples of pitfalls in classification are provided below.

A Category with Multiple Meanings: Cyanotic Congenital Heart Disease

The term "cyanotic congenital heart disease" is commonly used, and presumably the meaning is clear to those who refer to it. However, cyanotic CHD may be used to refer to a number of different concepts:

1. CHD *usually* associated with hypoxemia at birth or early in life.
   TOF, TGA, total anomalous pulmonary venous connection, truncus arteriosus, tricuspid atresia
2. CHD *that for a given patient at birth or early in life* is associated with hypoxemia.
   Many diagnoses may present this way, such as Ebstein anomaly, pulmonary atresia, left-sided obstructive lesions, hypoplastic left heart syndrome, patent ductus arteriosus
3. CHD *that for a given patient who currently* has related hypoxemia.
   Eisenmenger syndrome, other causes of right-to-left shunting, single ventricle Fontan with venovenous collaterals or pulmonary arteriovenous malformations.

4. A patient who has CHD and *currently* has hypoxemia due to *any* cause.
   This would be invalid, while uses 1 to 3 may be considered incorrect in some situations, but not universally invalid. Nevertheless, providers less familiar with CHD may incorrectly interpret the term to apply to patients with hypoxemia due to parenchymal lung disease unrelated to their existing CHD.

The classic definitions (1 and 2) relate to a set of diagnoses most strongly associated with cyanosis at or soon after birth, when initial identification of one of these diagnoses may be critically important. Beyond the neonatal period, referring to a patient as having "cyanotic congenital heart disease" without further explanation does not indicate a particular diagnosis or severity, or the current presence or absence of cyanosis. Almost always, it is preferable to describe the underlying diagnosis, duration of early life cyanosis (if pertinent), and current saturation or presence of other markers of chronic cyanosis such as hemoglobin concentration.

Other Situations Where Names May Mislead

TOF with pulmonary atresia is alternatively referred to as pulmonary atresia with ventricular septal defect. Most of the time, these terms refer to the same diagnosis, but there are possible exceptions. Another case of ambiguity related to the enormous variety in diagnostic names referring to ventricular septal defects. A VSD can occur in isolation or in the context of more complex disease and there is great morphologic heterogeneity complicating its description. The historical lack of consensus has resulted from differing thoughts on the intrinsic anatomy, but more frequently different nomenclature for the same intrinsic anatomy or same nomenclature applied to different anatomic entities. There has been a huge effort over the course of years to streamline the divergent approaches to describe VSDs, which has been included in the World Health Organization (WHO) 11th iteration of the International Classification of Diseases (ICD-11).[9]

Minor Distinctions

Not uncommonly, groups of clinicians or scientists differ in their strong preference for a particular way to refer to a diagnosis, often because it is "more correct." For example, "sinus venosus defect" might be considered preferable to "sinus venosus atrial septal defect." It is hard to argue: a sinus venosus defect is not a defect in the atrial septum. Likewise, there are minor differences over terms such as bicuspid versus bicommissural; or "physiologically corrected" instead of "congenitally corrected" transposition of the great arteries.

These examples seem trivial, and in most respects they are. However, even minor differences in usage and categorization can have a real impact on searching the literature. One example of a seemingly important distinction is whether or not to use the possessive form of eponyms: Ebstein's versus Ebstein, Eisenmenger's versus Eisenmenger, and so on. Eponyms provide a single, short name for often complex constellations of lesions. There remains debate over whether we should label a diagnosis

subsets of patients or programs. Take the example of bicuspid aortic valve, affecting perhaps 1% of people. The 32nd Bethesda classification includes this as "Simple," while the more recent 2018 American College of Cardiology/American Heart Association (ACC/AHA) guidelines classify this diagnosis as "Moderately Complex." Although debatable, this may suggest that this large patient cohort should be followed by adult congenital heart disease (ACHD) specialists, a minor distinction with enormous consequences for ACHD programs and patients. Some ACHD programs with relatively uncomplicated patient cohorts including a large number of bicuspid aortic valve patients may appear to be caring for more complex patients because bicuspid valve is now equated in terms of complexity with TOF. It is certainly not unreasonable to hypothesize that care by an ACHD specialist or another aortic/valve disease specialist clinic may be associated with better care for many patients with bicuspid aortic valve, but the implications of such a shift needs to be carefully considered.

Additionally, limiting the scale to three broad categories that focus almost entirely on only the "most complex" lesion does not support accurate diagnostic coding across a spectrum of diagnoses in any given patient. Furthermore, the anatomic complexity of a lesion does not fully capture how complicated a given patient may be, as discussed in more detail later in this chapter. In common use, the word "complexity" refers to the number of components in a system and the intricacy of their interaction; a complex problem, therefore, is one with many components. Being complex does not necessarily imply difficulty, whereas the term "complicated" refers to a high level of difficulty. Including a complementary physiologic classification may be helpful to indicate how complicated or difficult it may be to provide care (or avoid adverse outcomes) for a given patient.

IPCCC/ICD-11

In isolation, the aforementioned descriptive approaches to anatomic classification, however, do not address the need of a common diagnostic and therapeutic nomenclature and coding system with which to classify patients with congenital malformations. This is key to easily recording accurate and validated data on the diagnoses, treatment, and outcome of these patients supporting clinical and research related queries across different practice models. In an effort to address this, the International Society for the Nomenclature of Pediatric and Congenital Heart Disease was founded, and in the early 2000s established the IPCCC.[10] The WHO International Classification of Diseases 9th and 10th Revisions (ICD-9 and ICD-10) have been applied for research purposes, but have not been readily used by clinicians as they have lacked detail, accuracy, and clinical relevance. These limitations also apply to research.[14] While ICD-10 has some advantages compared with ICD-9, there remain major shortcomings such as the grouping of ostium secundum ASDs with ostium primum, sinus venosus, coronary sinus defects, and patient foramen ovale under code Q21.1 "Atrial Septal Defect." With these shortcomings in mind, clinicians and other experts in congenital cardiology

nomenclature were invited to contribute to the 11th Revision of this classification scheme (ICD-11) to develop the list of CHD terms. Eventually, a relatively concise list of names for CHD anatomic lesions and repairs derived from the more expansive IPCCC (ipccc.net) were incorporated into ICD-11.[10] Enormous efforts involved have brought the field closer to consensus on an accepted nomenclature and coding system for CHD diagnoses and interventions. **Table 65-2** illustrates how nomenclature/coding would look like using different classification systems.

The CHD terms, definitions, and synonyms can be found in the subsection "Structural developmental anomaly of the heart and great vessels," under the main Developmental Anomalies section that is one of the foundation components of ICD-11. The International Nomenclature Society submitted a list of diagnostic terms presented in a hierarchical manner to the WHO for ICD-11 (**Table 65-3**). Separately, another list of the same diagnostic terms was submitted with the corresponding definitions, comments, synonyms, and 6-digit IPCCC number for each term to minimize nomenclature ambiguity (**Table 65-4**). The coding incorporates the segmental sequential approach describing position and connections with 10 "level 1" items. Each of the 10 "level 1" items can be subdivided further to a maximum of 7 levels of detail, as needed. A separate set of extension codes in ICD-11 can be linked to any stem diagnostic code to describe different characteristics such as severity and time in life.

The Diagnosis or the Interaction Between the Diagnosis and the Patient

Some of these clinical nomenclatures include modifiers representing severity or cause, and additional codes can be used to indicate symptomatology or other clinical characteristics. These are not a requisite part of describing the CHD and there are no requirements that additional codes be recorded to represent the patient's status. These systems categorize CHD, with some allowance to describe relevant pathophysiology (or other clinical characteristics); pathophysiology is not considered integral to describing the diagnosis.

The 2018 ACC/AHA Adult Congenital Heart Disease Guideline document took a remarkably different perspective.[12] The classical simple/moderate/severe complexity remained, with relatively minor modifications (referred to as Anatomic Class I/II/III). In addition, the guideline proposed a new physiologic classification to complement the lesion complexity classification (**Table 65-5**). This classification grades physiologic severity from A to D, with D being the most advanced physiologic stage. The major categories/complications driving the physiologic grade, include aortopathy, arrhythmia, concomitant valvular disease, end organ dysfunction, exercise capacity, hypoxemia/hypoxia/cyanosis, NYHA functional class, pulmonary hypertension, shunting, and venous/arterial stenoses. Any patient at a given moment in time is described by these two dimensions: anatomic class and physiologic stage. This implicitly recognizes not only that these are distinct dimensions, but also that current pathophysiology is equally relevant to clinical

CHAPTER 65 • Anatomical and Physiological Classification of Adult Congenital Heart Disease

TABLE 65–2. Coding Using Different Classification Systems.

	32nd Bethesda & 2008 ACC/AHA ACHD Guidelines	2018 ACC/AHA ACHD guidelines	2020 ESC ACHD guidelines	ICD-9	ICD-10	ICD-11	IPCCC	Van Praagh segmental anatomy	Fyler
Tetralogy of Fallot with pulmonary atresia, repaired with conduit, maximal aortic dimension 5.2 cm, normal exercise capacity	Great Complexity	Moderate complexity (Anatomic Class II), Physiologic Stage D	Severe	745.2 (Tetralogy of Fallot)	Q21.3 (Tetralogy of Fallot) OR Q22.0 (pulmonary valve atresia + Q21.0 (ventricular septal defect)?	165 (Tetralogy of Fallot with pulmonary atresia)	01.01.26 (Tetralogy of Fallot, Pulmonary atresia);	{S,D,S} Tetralogy of Fallot	1050 (Tetralogy of Fallot)
Tetralogy of Fallot with pulmonary stenosis, atrioventricular septal defect, s/p repair	Moderate complexity	Moderate complexity (Anatomic Class II), Physiologic Stage?	Moderate	745.2 (Tetralogy of Fallot)	Q21.3 (Tetralogy of Fallot) + Q21.2 (Atrioventricular septal defect)	143 (Atrioventricular septal defect and Tetralogy of Fallot [atrioventricular canal and Tetralogy of Fallot])	01.01.20 (Tetralogy of Fallot, Common atrioventricular canal [AVSD])	{S,D,S} Tetralogy of Fallot and complete atrioventricular septal defect	1051 (Tetralogy of Fallot with complete atrioventricular canal)
Bicuspid aortic valve, well functioning, normal ventricular function, aortic dimension 5.0 cm unchanged for 8 years	Simple	Moderate complexity (Anatomic Class II), Physiologic Stage D	Simple	746.4 (Congenital insufficiency of aortic valve)	Q23.0 (Congenital stenosis of the aortic valve) or Q23.1 (Congenital insufficiency of the aortic valve)	234 (Bicuspid aortic valve)	09.15.22 (Bicuspid aortic valve)	{S,D,S} bicuspid (or bicommissural) aortic valve	1401 (bicommissural aortic valve)
Bicuspid aortic valve (right-non fusion), severe aortic regurgitation, LV dilation and dysfunction.	Simple	Moderate complexity (Anatomic Class II), Physiologic Stage D	Simple	746.4 (Congenital insufficiency of aortic valve)	Q23.0 (Congenital stenosis of the aortic valve) or Q23.1 (Congenital insufficiency of the aortic valve)	234 (Bicuspid aortic valve)	09.15.22 (Bicuspid aortic valve)	{S,D,S} bicuspid (or bicommissural) aortic valve with fusion of the right and noncoronary cusps	1413 (bicommissural aortic valve [right-non])
Aorto-left ventricular tunnel/fistula	Moderate complexity	Anatomic Class II, Physiologic Stage?	Not mentioned	746.9 (Unspecified congenital anomaly of heart)	Q20.8 (Other congenital malformations of cardiac chambers and connections)	245 (Aortoventricular tunnel)	09.17.01 (Aortoventricular tunnel)	{S,D,S} aorto-left ventricular tunnel	1460 (aortic-left ventricular tunnel)
Moderate size, unrepaired secundum atrial septal defect with Eisenmenger syndrome, NYHA FC IV	Great complexity	Moderate complexity (Anatomic Class II), Physiologic Stage D	Severe	745.5 (Ostium secundum type atrial septal defect)	Q21.1 (atrial septal defect)	98 (Atrial septal defect within oval fossa (secundum atrial septal defect)	05.04.02 (Atrial septal defect within oval fossa (secundum atrial septal defect)	{S,D,S} secundum atrial septal defect	2000 (Atrial septal defect, secundum)

(Continued)

TABLE 65–2. Coding Using Different Classification Systems. (Continued)

	32nd Bethesda & 2008 ACC/AHA ACHD Guidelines	2018 ACC/AHA ACHD guidelines	2020 ESC ACHD guidelines	ICD-9	ICD-10	ICD-11	IPCCC	Van Praagh segmental anatomy	Fyler
Patent foramen ovale	Not included	Not included	Not included	745.5 (Ostium secundum type atrial septal defect)	Q21.1 (atrial septal defect)	97 (Patent oval foramen (patent foramen ovale))	05.03.01 (Patent oval foramen [patent foramen ovale])	{S,D,S} patent foramen ovale	2020 (Patent foramen ovale)
Complete transposition of the great arteries, intact ventricular septum, prior arterial switch operation, neoaorta 3.8cm, otherwise well	Great complexity	Great complexity (Anatomic Class III), Physiologic Stage B	Moderate	745.10 (Complete transposition of great vessels)	Q20.3 (Discordant ventriculoarterial connection)	39 (Transposition of the great arteries (discordant ventriculoarterial connections)	01.05.01 (Transposition of the great arteries (discordant ventriculoarterial connections)	{S,D,D} transposition of the great arteries with intact ventricular septum	710 (D-loop transposition of the great arteries with an intact ventricular septum)

Abbreviations: ACC/AHA American College of Cardiology/American heart Association; ACHD Adult Congenital Heart Disease; ESC European Society of Cardiology; IPCCC International Paediatric and Congenital Cardiac Code

TABLE 65–3. Systematic Hierarchical List of Congenital Cardiology Terms Submitted to the World Health Organization for Inclusion in the Foundation Component of ICD-11—VSD (Outlet VSD Without Malalignment) Classification Example

Level 1	Level 2	Level 3	Level 4	Level 5	Level 6	Level 7
Congenital anomaly of a ventricle or the ventricular septum	Congenital anomaly of the ventricular septum	Ventricular septal defect	Outlet ventricular septal defect	Outlet ventricular septal defect without malalignment	Outlet muscular ventricular septal defect without malalignment Doubly committed juxta-arterial ventricular septal defect without malalignment	Doubly committed juxtaarterial ventricular septal defect without malalignment and with muscular posteroinferior rim Doubly committed juxtaarterial ventricular septal defect without malalignment and with perimembranous extension

care for adults with CHD as CHD anatomy. While the physiologic classification suggested can be problematic in terms of consistent use and interpretation, it nevertheless represents a pioneering leap forward in our attempts to provide a concise description of ACHD patients.

The major challenge facing a physiologic classification is combining factors that are unrelated to simplify the overall grading system and communication. This results in combining factors that variably impact prognosis, and have different follow-up protocols and management strategies. As shown in Table 65–5, an otherwise well patient with a bicuspid aortic valve and an aortic dimension of 5 cm is classified the same as a patient with an unrepaired ASD, Eisenmenger Syndrome, and NYHA IV symptoms. A moderately dilated aorta will not have the same symptom presentation, prognostic importance, follow-up, or management as a moderately dilated systemic ventricle. Classifying cyanosis, Eisenmenger syndrome, and NYHA IV heart failure together satisfies similar symptom status and prognostic importance but not management. Moreover, communicating a severity grade does not lend insight into the specific potential complications that one should be concerned about.

Studying the Success of a Classification in Congenital Heart Disease

No matter how thoughtful and nuanced a classification may be, in order to be effective, it must also be reproducible across contexts and users; what one cardiologist calls TOF should be the same thing as what another cardiologist calls TOF. To be used in clinical practice, a classification is limited to information available to clinicians. In order for a classification to be considered a success, a classification must be able to perform

TABLE 65–4. Systematic List of Congenital Cardiology Terms Submitted to WHO for Inclusion in the Foundation Component of ICD-11 with Their Definitions and Acceptable Synonyms and Their IPCCC Six-Digit Numbers—Ebstein Malformation Example

ICD-11 Congenital Cardiology Term	IPCCC Code	Definition with Commentary	Synonyms
Ebstein malformation of the tricuspid valve	06.01.34	A congenital cardiac malformation of the tricuspid valve and right ventricle that is characterized by downward (apical) displacement of the functional annulus, usually involving the septal and inferior (posterior) leaflets. *Ebstein anomaly is a malformation of the tricuspid valve and right ventricle that is characterised by a spectrum of several features: (1) incomplete delamination of septal and inferior (posterior) tricuspid valve leaflets from the myocardium of the right ventricle; (2) downward (apical) displacement of the functional annulus; (3) dilation of the "atrialized" portion of the right ventricle with variable degrees of hypertrophy and thinning of the wall; (4) redundancy, fenestrations, and tethering of the anterosuperior leaflet; and (5) dilation of the right atrioventricular junction (the true tricuspid annulus). These anatomical and functional abnormalities cause tricuspid regurgitation (and rarely tricuspid stenosis) that results in right atrial and right ventricular dilation and atrial and ventricular arrhythmias. Associated cardiac anomalies include an interatrial communication, the presence of accessory conduction pathways and dilation of the right atrium and right ventricle. Varying degrees of right ventricular outflow tract obstruction may be present, including pulmonary atresia. Some patients with discordant atrioventricular and ventriculo-arterial connections [congenitally corrected transposition] have an Ebstein-like deformity of the left sided morphologically tricuspid valve*	Ebstein syndrome; Ebstein anomaly; Ebstein disease; Ebstein anomaly of tricuspid valve; Congenital Ebstein deformity of tricuspid valve

TABLE 65–5. AHA/ACC Physiological Stage Classification

Physiological Stage

A
- NYHA FC I symptoms
- No hemodynamic or anatomic sequelae
- No arrhythmias
- Normal exercise capacity
- Normal renal/hepatic/pulmonary function

B
- NYHA FC II symptoms
- Mild hemodynamic sequelae (mild aortic enlargement mild ventricular enlargement, mild ventricular dysfunction)
- Mild valvular disease
- Trivial or small shunt (not hemodynamically significant)
- Arrhythmia not requiring treatment
- Abnormal objective cardiac limitation to exercise

C
- NYHA FC III symptoms
- Significant (moderate or greater) valvular disease: moderate or greater ventricular dysfunction (systemic, pulmonic, or both)
- Moderate aortic enlargement
- Venous or arterial stenosis
- Mild or moderate hypoxemia/cyansis
- Hemodynamically significant shunt
- Arrhythmias controlled with treatment
- Pulmonary hypertension (less than severe)
- End-organ dysfunction responsive to therapy

D
- NYHA FC IV symptoms
- Severe aortic enlargement
- Arrhythmias refractory to treatment
- Severe hypoxemia (almost always associated with cyanosis)
- Severe pulmonary hypertension
- Eisenmenger syndrome
- Refractory end-organ dysfunction

the task needed, whatever that may be (eg, selecting a clearly defined group for a research study or predicting survival).

Surprisingly, little empirical research has been done to measure the performance of ACHD classification. Some studies have considered the association between classifications and survival or other outcomes, although there has generally been little consideration to whether the codes were consistently assigned or reliable.[15] To our knowledge, only one study has studied interobserver agreement for CHD classification, focusing on the 2018 ACC/AHA ACHD guideline AP classification.[16] This study reported on agreement between sets of expert ACHD providers and between experts and trained research assistants. On a positive note, Anatomic Class was assigned with good reliability (agreement in 92.7% of cases for experts; however, agreement on Physiologic Stage occurred in 59.5% of cases). Importantly, testing this in a research context exposed substantial ambiguity in many of the Physiologic Class definitions, such as a lack of clarity on what constituted a "refractory" arrhythmia (eg, would persistent symptomatic nonsustained runs of atrial tachycardia on antiarrhythmic medication be considered refractory arrhythmia?). There has been no similar assessment of earlier classifications or of the more recent IPCCC. There has, however, been some research on how well administratively recorded ICD-9 and ICD-10 codes indicative of CHD capture true diagnosis.[17,18] The results have been quite variable and far from consistently reassuring, although in some cases it does appear such codes are accurate enough to provide big picture understanding of CHD epidemiology.

Is There an Ideal Physiologic Classification in Congenital Heart Disease?

A physiologic classification needs to accurately represent a patient's clinical status, which is often independent of the underlying anatomic diagnosis, and therefore the two are complementary. Ideally the physiologic classification would group complicating factors according to clinical similarities, prognostic importance, and management considerations. However, with all of this in mind, no classification will be optimal for all uses, and CHD is a particularly challenging classification problem. Given the heterogeneous nature of the anatomic lesions, interventions, and hence complications, it may be too much to ask for a classification to comprehensively describe anatomy, current physiologic status, prognosis, and particular management considerations.

The main goal of physiologic classification should be to clearly communicate the current complicating factors as per the primary goals of classification (organization, economy, accuracy, precision, and quantification). The clinician can then determine the prognostic importance, follow-up plan, and management based on the communication. Similar to the IPCCC, there could be broad "Level 1" items that are then further subdivided, guided by specifics and severity.

FUTURE AVENUES

There is a remarkable absence of mechanistic criteria to historical or current classifications. Recent advances in understanding the developmental molecular basis of CHD, as well as early forays into understanding genetic, epigenetic, and environmental modifiers of disease course in CHD may pave the way for a more nuanced ability to personalize clinical assessment and therapy. Likewise, advances in computational power and statistical methods to integrate data and learn from it may eventually revolutionize how we view CHD, possibly creating different categories or even viewing diagnosis along a continuous spectrum rather than as distinct categories at all. Integrating these advances in knowledge and technology may provide enormous benefits, but will require equally immense flexibility in our approach to thinking about classification.

SUMMARY

In the end, each decision on how to name a particular diagnosis and each classification algorithm is associated with its own pitfalls and exceptions. While we often view these classifications as "the truth" or a reference framework for defining reality, they are no more than tools to frame our experience and communicate consistently. They do not guarantee effective communication or understanding, and the use of these tools does not allow us to abdicate our ultimate responsibility for conveying our thoughts accurately.

The field of ACHD continues to witness dramatic advances in understanding underlying disease mechanisms, discovery of effective treatments associated with lower risk, and enhanced technologies to measure underlying pathophysiology and patient status. This will require flexibility and ongoing revision to current classification schemes.

Potential Goals of Classification

Primary

- Organization: clear definitions, systematic approach, and consistent coding
- Economy: save time and space
- Accuracy: each diagnosis means the same thing to each user
- Precision: ability to distinguish distinct phenotypes
- Quantification: indicate severity to a specific diagnosis

Secondary

- Maximize understanding of similarities and differences
- Improve communication between providers
- Facilitate reproducible and accurate risk assessment, generalized able to other contexts
- Support risk adjustment for quality measurement, reimbursement, and research
- Guide appropriate follow-up care, other decision support
- Identify similar disease pathophysiology for a specific purpose (eg, research, therapies)
- Public health surveillance

REFERENCES

1. Abbott ME. *Atlas of Congenital Cardiac Disease.* New York: The American Heart Association; 1936.

2. Vanpraagh R, Vanpraagh S, Vlad P, Keith JD. Anatomic types of congenital dextrocardia: diagnostic and embryologic implications. *Am J Cardiol.* 1964;13:510-531.

3. Vanpraagh R, Ongley PA, Swan HJ. Anatomic types of single or common ventricle in man. morphologic and geometric aspects of 60 necropsied cases. *Am J Cardiol.* 1964;13:367-386.

4. Tynan MJ, Becker AE, Macartney FJ, Jimenez MQ, Shinebourne EA, Anderson RH. Nomenclature and classification of congenital heart disease. *Br Heart J.* 1979;41:544-553.

5. Shinebourne EA, Macartney FJ, Anderson RH. Sequential chamber localization–logical approach to diagnosis in congenital heart disease. *Br Heart J.* 1976;38:327-340.

6. Anderson RH, Becker AE, Freedom RM, et al. Sequential segmental analysis of congenital heart disease. *Pediatr Cardiol.* 1984;5:281-287.

7. Mavroudis C, Jacobs JP. Congenital heart surgery nomenclature and database project: overview and minimum dataset. *Ann Thorac Surg.* 2000;69:S2-S17.

8. Franklin RC. The European Paediatric Cardiac Code Long List: structure and function. *Cardiol Young.* 2000;10 Suppl 1:27-146.

9. Lopez L, Houyel L, Colan SD, et al. Classification of ventricular septal defects for the eleventh iteration of the International Classification of Diseases-striving for consensus: a report from the International Society for Nomenclature of Paediatric and Congenital Heart Disease. *Ann Thorac Surg.* 2018;106:1578-1589.

10. Franklin RCG, Beland MJ, Colan SD, et al. Nomenclature for congenital and paediatric cardiac disease: the International Paediatric and Congenital Cardiac Code (IPCCC) and the Eleventh Iteration of the International Classification of Diseases (ICD-11). *Cardiol Young.* 2017;27:1872-1938.

11. Warnes CA, Liberthson R, Danielson GK, et al. Task force 1: the changing profile of congenital heart disease in adult life. *J Am Coll Cardiol.* 2001;37:1170-1175.

12. Stout KK, Daniels CJ, Aboulhosn JA, et al. 2018 AHA/ACC guideline for the management of adults with congenital heart disease: executive summary: a report of the American College of Cardiology/American Heart Association Task Force on clinical practice guidelines. *J Am Coll Cardiol.* 2019;73:1494-1563.

13. Baumgartner H, De Backer J, Babu-Narayan SV, et al. 2020 ESC guidelines for the management of adult congenital heart disease. *Eur Heart J.* 2020.

14. Rodriguez FH, 3rd, Ephrem G, Gerardin JF, Raskind-Hood C, Hogue C, Book W. The 745.5 issue in code-based, adult congenital heart disease population studies: relevance to current and future ICD-9-CM and ICD-10-CM studies. *Congenit Heart Dis.* 2018;13:59-64.

15. Ombelet F, Goossens E, Van De Bruaene A, Budts W, Moons P. Newly developed adult congenital heart disease anatomic and physiological classification: first predictive validity evaluation. *J Am Heart Assoc.* 2020;9:e014988.

16. Lachtrupp CL, Valente AM, Gurvitz M, Landzberg MJ, Brainard SB, Opotowsky AR. Interobserver agreement of the anatomic and physiological classification system for adult congenital heart disease. *Am Heart J.* 2020;229:92-99.

17. Broberg C, McLarry J, Mitchell J, et al. Accuracy of administrative data for detection and categorization of adult congenital heart disease patients from an electronic medical record. *Pediatr Cardiol.* 2015;36:719-725.

18. Cohen S, Jannot AS, Iserin L, Bonnet D, Burgun A, Escudie JB. Accuracy of claim data in the identification and classification of adults with congenital heart diseases in electronic medical records. *Arch Cardiovasc Dis.* 2019;112:31-43.

Shunt Lesions

Ari M. Cedars, Shelby Kutty, and Ashish Doshi

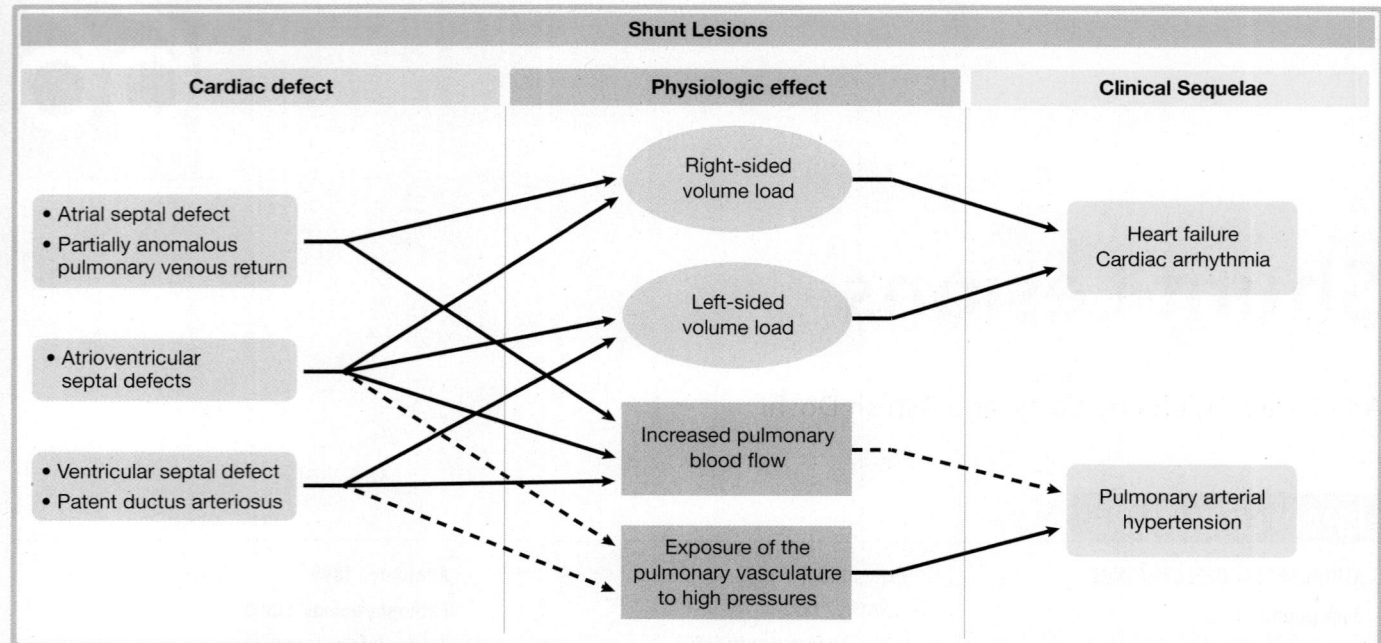

Chapter 66 Fuster and Hurst's Central Illustration. Shunt lesions result in both cardiac chamber volume loading and pulmonary vascular stress. Cardiac chamber volume overload may lead to cardiac arrhythmia and heart failure of the affected side of the heart. Pulmonary stressors include pulmonary over circulation and exposure of the pulmonary vascular bed to elevated pressures (in certain cases). In susceptible individuals, prolonged exposure of the pulmonary vasculature to over circulation may lead to pulmonary arterial hypertension, while exposure to elevated pressures invariably leads to pulmonary hypertension.

CHAPTER SUMMARY

This chapter discusses the various types of congenital cardiac shunt lesions, their anatomy, physiologic impact, epidemiology, clinical presentation, work-up, and management. In congenital shunt lesions, a fundamentally important link exists between anatomy and physiology, such that the location of a shunt dictates its physiologic impact and likely sequelae. As a general rule, shunts upstream of the tricuspid valve (including atrial septal defects and accompanying partially anomalous pulmonary venous return) lead to volume overloading of the right atrium and right ventricle with consequences related to right-sided chamber dilatation and dysfunction. By contrast, shunts downstream of the tricuspid valve (including ventricular septal defects and patent ductus arteriosus) result in volume loading of the left atrium and left ventricle with accompanying consequences. Each lesion has unique associations with other cardiac abnormalities and genetic syndromes. Fundamentally important to all cardiac shunts is the downstream impact of pulmonary overcirculation on the pulmonary vascular bed. Changes in pulmonary vascular physiology, including the development of pulmonary arterial hypertension, play a major role in dictating prognosis and therapeutic decision-making.

ATRIAL SEPTAL DEFECTS

Background

Atrial septal defects (ASDs) are a group of lesions characterized by an abnormal communication between the right and left atria. There are several different types of ASDs[1] that, while etiologically and anatomically distinct, are physiologically similar to one another. In patients with ASDs, the physiologic impact of lesion-related shunting on the myocardium and pulmonary vascular tissues largely drives management decisions. Due to the heterogeneity in anatomy and physiologic sequelae, individualized decision-making is necessary to determine the timing, appropriateness, and technique employed for ASD closure.

Anatomy

Secundum ASDs

Secundum ASDs occur in the region of the fossa ovalis (**Fig. 66–1**). Embryologically, secundum ASDs are the result of either an excessively large ostium secundum, or diminished growth of the septum secundum. Either or a combination of both processes lead to the presence of a defect in the midportion of the interatrial septum, which may be multiple (**Figs. 66–2 and 66–3**).

Primum ASDs

Primum ASDs occur in the region of the posterior crux cordis with variable extension toward the anterior crux cordis (Fig. 66–1). Embryologically, primum ASDs are the result of inadequate fusion between the septum primum and the endocardial cushions (Fig. 66–1). Primum ASDs are thus a physiologically mild or incomplete form of atrioventricular canal defect, the complete form of which will be addressed later in this chapter (**Figs. 66–4 and 66–5**).

Sinus Venosus ASDs with PAPVR

Sinus venosus ASDs occur in one of two locations. Superior sinus venosus ASDs occur in the superior and posterior region of the interatrial septum, adjacent to the ostium of the superior vena cava (SVC) (Fig. 66–1).[2] Inferior sinus venosus ASDs occur in the inferior and posterior region of the interatrial septum, adjacent to the ostium of the inferior vena cava (IVC) (Fig. 66–1). Embryologically, sinus venosus defects are the result of excessive fusion between the pulmonary venous confluence and the posterior atrial wall of the developing atria. Sinus venosus ASDs are commonly associated with partially anomalous pulmonary venous return (PAPVR). The specific veins involved depend on the location of the defect. Superior sinus venosus ASDs are associated with PAPVR of the right superior pulmonary vein to the SVC, while inferior sinus venosus ASDs are associated with PAPVR of the right inferior pulmonary vein to the IVC (**Figs. 66–6, 66–7**, and **66–8**).

Unroofed Coronary Sinus ASDs

Unroofed coronary sinus (CS)–related ASDs occur in the inferior and posterior region of the interatrial septum, slightly anterior to the ostium of the IVC. Embryologically, unroofed CS-related ASDs are the result of excessive fusion between the left horn of the sinus venosus and the posterior wall of the developing atria. Unroofed CS ASDs are commonly associated with a persistent left SVC that drains into the CS and is known as the Raghib syndrome.[3]

Pathophysiology of Shunting in ASDs

Long-term sequelae from ASDs is directly related to the consequences of intracardiac shunting of blood. The primary direction of shunting is from left to right. This is because under normal circumstances, the compliance of the right atrium

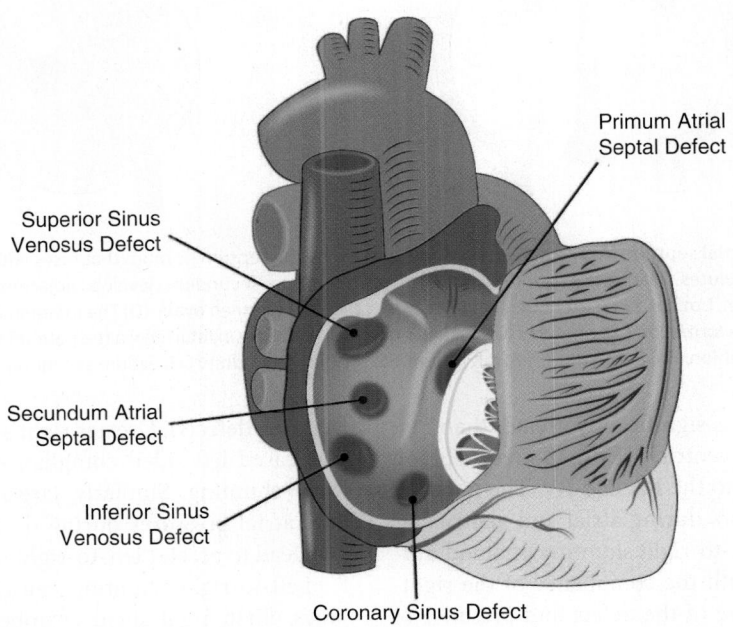

Figure 66–1. The different types of atrial septal defects.

Transection Through
Embryonic Atrial Septum

En Face View of Embryonic
Atrial Septum from Right Atrium

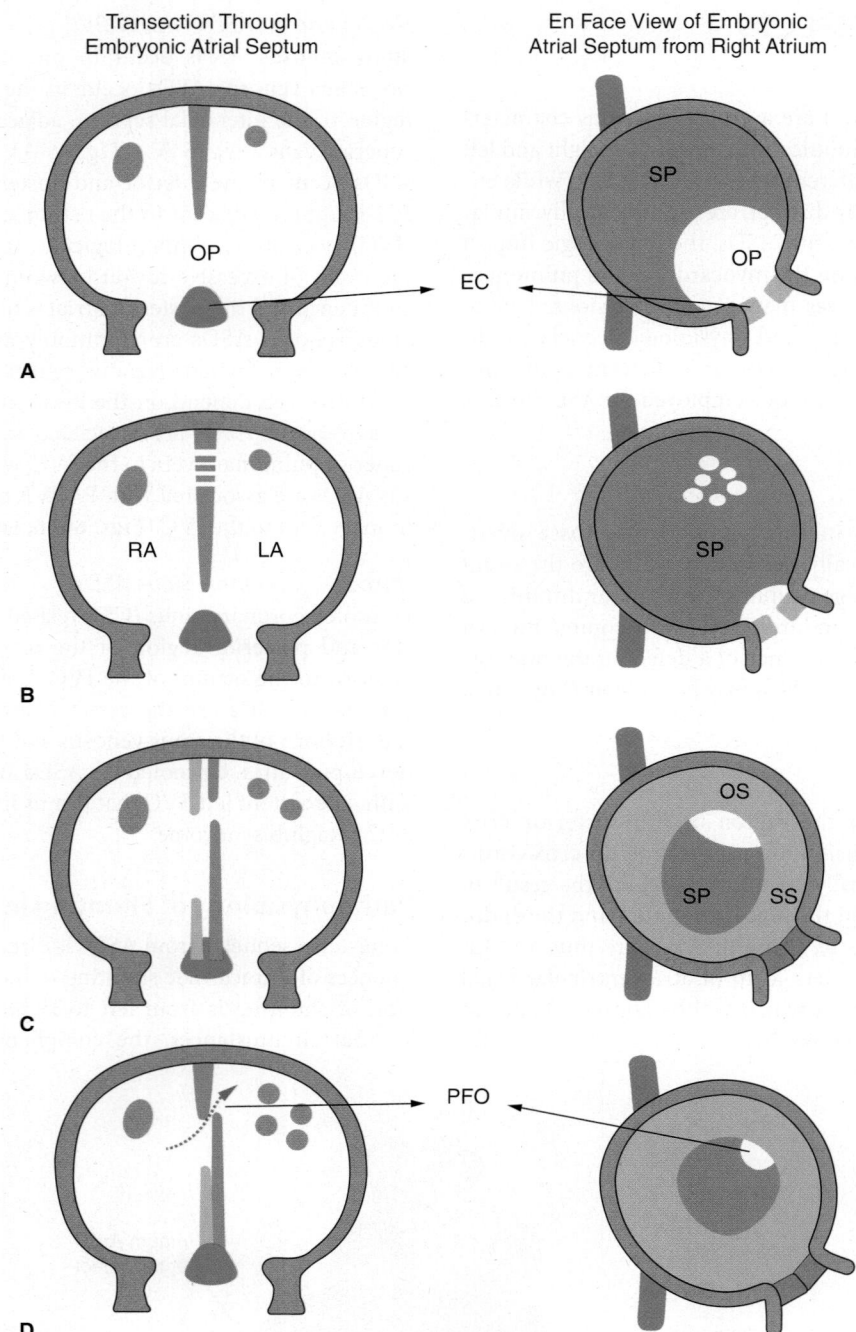

Figure 66–2. Embryology of the atrial septum. (A) The ostium primum is closed by the septum primum that fuses with the endocardial cushion. **(B)** A portion of the septum primum then involutes creating the ostium secundum. **(C)** The septum secundum develops adjacent to the septum primum. This septum does not form an uninterrupted sheet, but has a persistent defect in its center called the foramen ovale. **(D)** The foramen ovale normally does not overlap with the ostium secundum, leading to the formation of a one-way valve allowing right-to-left flow in fetal life via the patent foramen ovale. OP, ostium primum; SP, septum primum; EC, endocardial cushion; RA, right atrium; LA, left atrium; SS, septum secundum; OS, ostium secundum; PFO, patent foramen ovale.

(RA) and right ventricle (RV) is significantly greater than that of the left atrium (LA) and left ventricle (LV). As a result, blood from the LA crosses the ASD to the RA and RV. The majority of ASD-related shunting occurs during atrial and ventricular diastole. The degree of this left-to-right shunting of blood during diastole is governed by both the compliance of the right-sided chambers and by the size of the defect and presence of other sources of shunting (such as PAPVR in the case of sinus venosus defects). Greater right sided diastolic compliance, and decreased left sided compliance both lead to greater left-to-right shunting. Similarly, larger defects with equalization of interatrial pressures during diastole and presence of PAPVR will lead to greater left-to-right shunting.

Left-to-right shunting causes pathology in two primary ways. First, right-sided chambers will distend to accommodate the increased volume with which they are presented. This

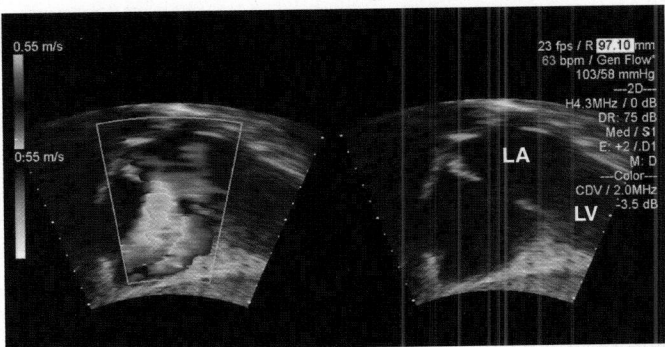

Figure 66–3. Secundum ASD. Color Doppler and 2D echocardiogram images obtained in the subcostal long-axis view from a 35-year-old woman presenting with murmur, demonstrating septum secundum ASD with a left-to-right shunt.

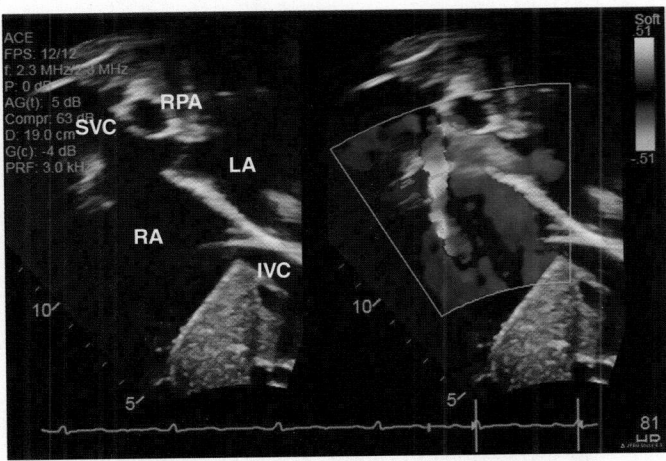

Figure 66–6. Superior Sinus Venosus ASD with PAPVR. 2D and color Doppler echocardiogram images obtained in the subcostal short-axis ("bicaval") view from a 13-year-old young woman presenting with murmur, demonstrating sinus venous ASD with a left-to-right shunt.

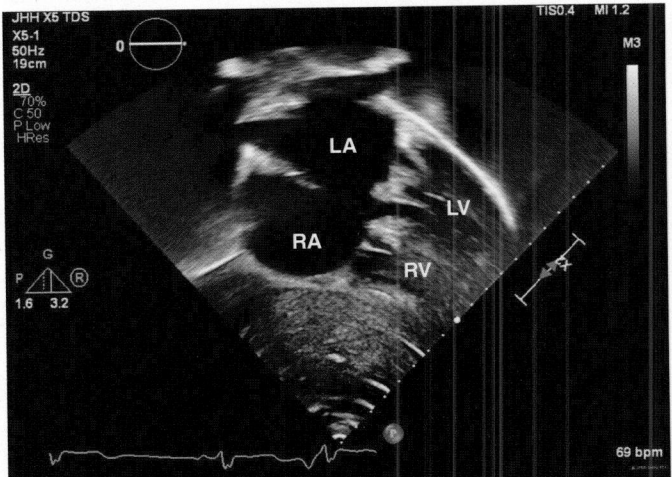

Figure 66–4. Primum ASD. 2D echocardiogram image obtained in the subcostal long-axis view from a 27-year-old woman presenting with murmur, demonstrating septum primum ASD.

process has several consequences. Progressive RA distension leads to electrical remodeling, resulting in a predisposition to atrial arrhythmias.[4] At the same time, progressive RV distension may lead to a predisposition RV dysfunction and then RV failure. This process is attributable in part to increased RV wall tension and therefore increased energy demand. The eventual onset of right-sided atrioventricular valve regurgitation imposes both a further volume load on the right-sided chambers and compromised RV pump efficiency.[5]

Second, left-to-right shunting exposes the pulmonary vascular bed to excessive blood flow. In certain susceptible

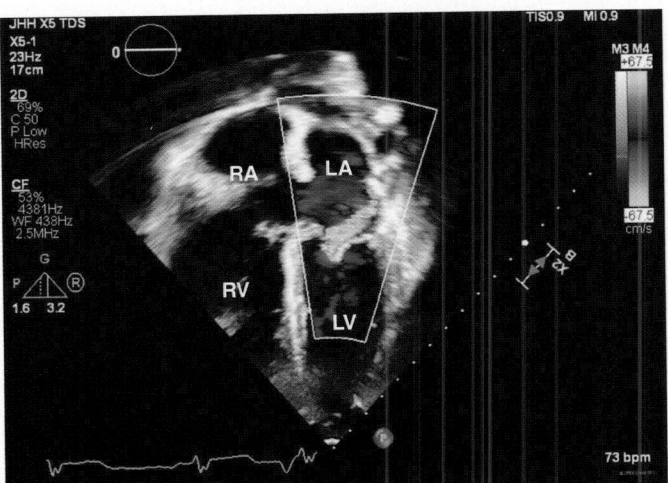

Figure 66–5. Primum ASD. Color Doppler echocardiogram obtained in the apical four-chamber view image, demonstrating septum primum ASD and mitral regurgitation from cleft mitral valve.

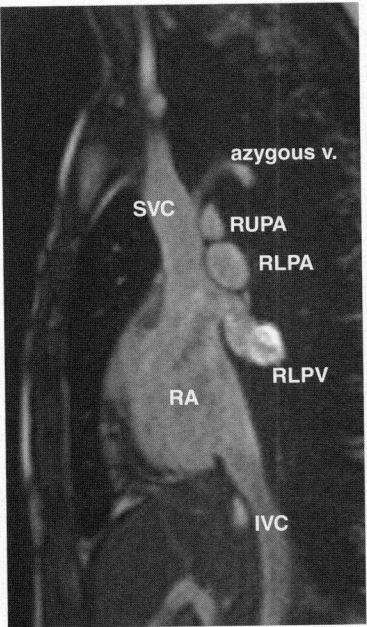

Figure 66–7. Superior Sinus Venosus ASD with PAPVR. Steady-state free procession CMR image demonstrating sinus venous ASD. Of note, the right upper pulmonary vein is not seen.

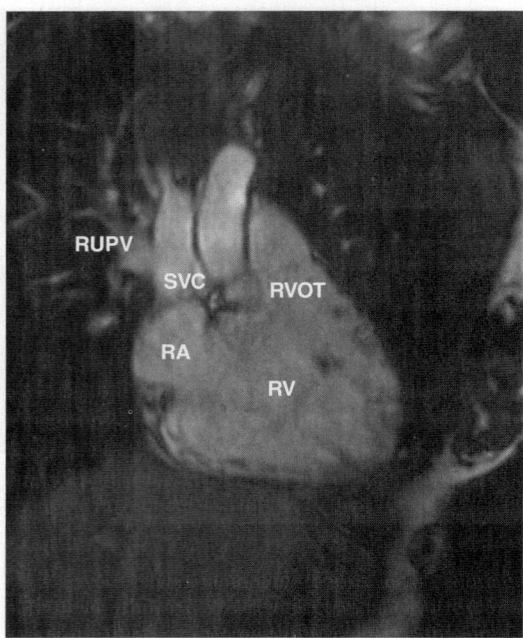

Figure 66–8. Sinus Venosus ASD with PAPVR. Steady-state free procession CMR image from the same patient demonstrate anomalous drainage of the right upper pulmonary vein (RUPV) to the SVC.

individuals, this may result in secondary pulmonary vascular remodeling and the development of World Health Organization Group 1 Pulmonary Arterial Hypertension (PAH).[6,7] The onset of PAH further increases RV wall tension and probability of chronic RV failure.

In rare circumstances, ASDs may also cause right-to-left shunting of blood. This phenomenon occurs transiently during periods of acute shifts in ventricular loading such as during rapid infusion of fluid or Valsalva. It may also occur in the setting of severe right-sided atrioventricular valve regurgitation or severe RV dysfunction and/or RV failure that reflects changing RV compliance. Right-to-left shunting predisposes patients to paradoxical embolization of intravascular thrombi and to systemic embolization of air bubbles or particulate material infused intravenously. In the setting of severe RV dysfunction and/or RV failure, chronic right-to-left shunting results in cyanosis with its accompanying sequelae (addressed in the Eisenmenger Syndrome section).

Epidemiology

The cumulative incidence of ASDs is estimated to be 56 to 88 per 100,000 live births representing between 8% and 10% of congenital heart defects.[8,9] Given the frequently benign clinical course of ASDs, many defects may remain unrecognized and prevalence may in fact be higher. Advances in imaging technology and have led to increases in recent prevalence estimates as asymptomatic cases are incidentally detected.[10] Secundum ASDs are twice as common in females compared to males; however, other types of ASD have equal gender distribution. Secundum ASDs are the most common form of defect, representing approximately 80% of all ASDs, followed by primum

ASDs (10%) and sinus venosus ASDs (5%).[1] CS ASDs are extremely rare (<1%).

Genetics/Inheritance

The majority of ASDs are sporadic. Nevertheless, certain genetic mutations have known associations with ASD. These include mutations in the *NKX2.5/CSX*,[11] *TBX5* (causing Holt-Oram syndrome),[12] and others. Moreover, ASDs commonly are found in association with congenital syndromes including Downs, Williams, Goldenhar, Noonan, Klinefelter, Kabuki, and Ellis–van Creveld.

Incidence of ASD in offspring of affected mothers is estimated to be 8% to 10%. In addition, there is an association between intrauterine environment and ASD. Maternal pregestational diabetes, phenylketonuria, and influenza may increase risk of ASD in the fetus. Similarly, existing data suggest an association between maternal exposure to retinoids, nonsteroidal anti-inflammatory drugs, anticonvulsants, thalidomide, smoking, antihypertensive medications, and alcohol and incident fetal ASD.[13]

Presentation

History

Early in life, the majority of patients with ASDs are asymptomatic. In such patients, the defect may be detected due to abnormal findings on routine physical exam or diagnostic studies obtained for unrelated reasons. With aging and the onset of increased RV wall tension, symptoms of mild fatigue and exertional dyspnea may develop. RA distention may lead to atrial arrhythmias, experienced as palpitations or tachycardia. In cases where RV dilatation progresses, leading to tricuspid valve regurgitation and contractile dysfunction, or when pulmonary vascular disease occurs, patients may develop symptoms typical of RV failure such as dependent edema and poor exercise tolerance. In this setting, patients may develop intermittent cyanosis due to right-to-left shunting across the ASD.

Physical Examination

Classical ASD physical exam findings include a fixed widely split S2 due to atrial pressure equalization through the respiratory cycle and a systolic pulmonary valve murmur due to excessive flow. With progressive ventricular dilatation, the RV may become palpable in the subxiphoid area. With RV failure, jugular venous pressure may be elevated and in the setting of significant tricuspid regurgitation there may be a jugular v-wave. RV failure may also be accompanied by dependent edema (without pulmonary edema) and by cyanosis that may be worse with physical exertion. When pulmonary vascular disease occurs, P2 will become louder and a Graham Steell murmur may be auscultable.

Work-Up/Investigations

Electrocardiography

The electrocardiogram (ECG) in the setting of a significant ASD will typically reveal evidence of delayed RV conduction with an rsR[1] and frequently a right bundle branch block. There will also be evidence of RA enlargement with high peaked P waves in lead II. Depending on the degree of shunting and presence of pulmonary hypertension, there may also be right axis deviation (RAD) and evidence of RV hypertrophy (RVH) with persistent large S waves in the left-sided precordial leads. The exception to this is in individuals with an atrioventricular canal defect that leads to left axis deviation (LAD) due to displacement of the conduction system in the interventricular septum.

Chest Radiography

In the setting of a significant ASD, the cardiac silhouette will be enlarged with RA and RV dilatation. There may be prominent main and branch pulmonary arteries and pulmonary vascular plethora in both lung fields due to pulmonary vascular over-circulation. The LA and LV are normal sized. With the onset of PAH, the right-sided chamber enlargement may decrease and pulmonary vascular plethora will regress, while proximal pulmonary arteries will become more prominent. Should the RV fail in this setting, the RA and RV will again increase in size.

Echocardiography

Transthoracic echocardiography (TTE) is the most widely available modality for assessing ASDs, and yields abundant anatomic and physiologic information.[1,14] TTE may reveal the location and presence of an ASD; however, due to difficulty in visualizing the interatrial septum, more commonly TTE in adults with ASDs will reveal the anatomic and physiologic sequelae of an ASD. Saline contrast may provide evidence of intracardiac shunting. In cases of suspected unroofed CS with a persistent left SVC, the defect's presence may be identified through injection of saline contrast in the left upper extremity.

TTE is most useful in providing evidence of the sequelae of left-to-right shunting associated with an ASD. This may include RA and RV enlargement, flattening of the interventricular septum, and elevated pulmonary blood flow as detected by RV outflow tract (RVOT) Doppler assessment. In cases of PAH, TTE reveals evidence of elevated RV systolic pressures including increased TV peak regurgitant velocity, abbreviated or notched RVOT Doppler envelope, and systolic flattening of the interventricular septum. In cases of RV failure, TTE will reveal evidence of IVC plethora and may reveal the presence of significant tricuspid valve regurgitation.

Transesophageal echocardiography (TEE) is used for evaluating the size and location of ASDs. The esophageal location of insonation permits superior definition of defect anatomy compared to TTE given its comparative proximity to the atria. TEE is also commonly used to guide both surgical and percutaneous ASD closure.

The advent of newer echocardiographic modalities have further expanded the use of the technology in diagnosis and treatment of ASDs. Intracardiac echocardiography (ICE) may be used to facilitate percutaneous closure of ASDs to guide device placement. Three-dimensional echocardiography (3DE) may provide superior anatomic definition and may be uniquely useful in cases of complex defects.

CCT and CMR

Cardiac computed tomography (CCT) and cardiac magnetic resonance (CMR) imaging are not typically part of the work-up for isolated uncomplicated ASDs in which echocardiographic imaging is adequate.[1] Nevertheless, they are important tools for ASD evaluation in specific cases. Gated CCT imaging provides superior anatomic resolution of the intrathoracic structures.[15] In patients with difficult echocardiographic windows, CCT permits accurate anatomical characterization of ASDs. Moreover, CCT will easily delineate associated anatomical abnormalities, most notably PAPVR in the setting of sinus venosus ASDs.

CMR imaging lacks the spatial resolution of CCT,[15,16] and does not permit the accuracy regarding defect sizing that CCT allows. Nevertheless, CMR imaging has the advantage of providing physiologic information specifically by permitting calculation of the ratio of pulmonary (Qp) to systemic (Qs) blood flow, which is a measure of shunting.[17]

3D Printing and Virtual Reality

3D printing and virtual reality (VR) technology use CCT or CMR images to direct the construction of 3D models of the heart and intracardiac structures. 3D printing and VR have evolving roles in procedural planning, permitting practitioners to delineate surgical or catheter-based approach and optimal closure technique. Currently, 3D technology is in use at only a few specialized centers and is not routinely used as part of the work-up for ASDs.

Cardiac Catheterization

Today, cardiac catheterization is an adjunctive procedure after a diagnosis of ASD is made. While angiography can delineate anatomy, the imaging modalities outlined above are currently much more frequently used for this purpose. Cardiac catheterization nevertheless plays an important role in the work-up of ASDs by providing hemodynamic information for decision-making regarding closure in cases where imaging data is insufficient. In this setting, cardiac catheterization delineates Qp:Qs ratio, and is the gold standard for assessment of intracardiac pressures to evaluate RV and LV filling pressures, pulmonary vascular resistance (PVR), and the degree of PAH.

Stress Testing

Stress testing is useful to evaluate limitations in exercise capacity attributable to ASDs. In addition, stress testing with continuous pulse oximetry assessment provides information regarding the physiologic reserve of the RV, and thus the safety of ASD closure (subsequently outlined).

Management

Decision-making regarding closure of ASDs is a complex process involving multiple considerations.[1] (**Table 66–1**). The primary indication for ASD closure is evidence of RV enlargement attributable to left-to-right shunting. In general, a Qp:Qs of >1.5 is required for RV enlargement to develop over time. While there are no data to suggest mortality benefits of ASD closure,[18] the weight of evidence suggests likely clinical benefit to ASD closure in the absence of pulmonary vascular disease in preventing recurrent pneumonias[19] and preserving long-term functional status.[20-22] Moreover, surgical and percutaneous closure are safe[23-27] and lead to regression of right-sided chamber enlargement.[28,29] There are, however, other important considerations that must be included in the decision-making process.

In patients with evidence of pulmonary vascular disease, the evaluation process for ASD closure is more complicated. In this setting, ASD closure may lead to exercise intolerance and hypotension due to RV failure and inadequate LV filling. The mechanism for this physiologic phenomenon is that venous return, which in the setting of a patent ASD may fill the LV either through the pulmonary vascular bed or through right-to-left shunting across the ASD, now must obligatorily traverse the pulmonary vascular bed. If the RV is failing or pulmonary vascular resistance is prohibitively high, the RV pump is unable to overcome the resistance of the pulmonary vascular bed and the LV is left under filled, leading to compromised cardiac

TABLE 66-1. Guideline Comparison for ASD Treatment

COR	LOE	Diagnostic	Therapeutic
Atrial Septal Defects: 2018 AHA/ACC Guidelines for ACHD			
I	C-EO	1. Pulse oximetry at rest and during exercise is recommended for evaluation of adults with unrepaired or repaired ASD with residual shunt to determine the direction and magnitude of the shunt.	
I	B-NR	1. CMR, CCT, and/or TEE are useful to evaluate pulmonary venous connections in adults with ASD 2. Echocardiographic imaging is recommended to guide percutaneous ASD closure	1. In adults with isolated secundum ASD causing impaired functional capacity, right atrial and/or RV enlargement, and net left-to-right shunt sufficiently large to cause physiological sequelae (e.g., pulmonary– systemic blood flow ratio [Qp:Qs] ≥1.5:1) without cyanosis at rest or during exercise, transcatheter or surgical closure to reduce RV volume and improve exercise tolerance is recommended, provided that systolic PA pressure is less than 50% of systolic systemic pressure and pulmonary vascular resistance is less than one third of the systemic vascular resistance 2. Adults with primum ASD, sinus venosus defect or coronary sinus defect causing impaired functional capacity, right atrial and/or RV enlargement and net left-to-right shunt sufficiently large to cause physiological sequelae (e.g., Qp:Qs ≥1.5:1) without cyanosis at rest or during exercise, should be surgically repaired unless precluded by comorbidities, provided that systolic PA pressure is less than 50% of systemic pressure and pulmonary vascular resistance is less than one third of the systemic vascular resistance
IIa	C-LD		1. In asymptomatic adults with isolated secundum ASD, right atrial and RV enlargement, and net left-to-right shunt sufficiently large to cause physiological sequelae (e.g., Qp:Qs 1.5:1 or greater), without cyanosis at rest or during exercise, transcatheter or surgical closure is reasonable to reduce RV volume and/or improve functional capacity, provided that systolic PA pressure is less than 50% of systemic pressure and pulmonary vascular resistance is less than one third systemic resistance 2. Surgical closure of a secundum ASD in adults is reasonable when a concomitant surgical procedure is being performed and there is a net left-to-right shunt sufficiently large to cause physiological sequelae (e.g., Qp:Qs 1.5:1 or greater) and right atrial and RV enlargement without cyanosis at rest or during exercise
IIb	B-NR		1. Percutaneous or surgical closure may be considered for adults with ASD when net left-to-right shunt (Qp:Qs) is 1.5:1 or greater, PA systolic pressure is 50% or more of systemic arterial systolic pressure, and/or pulmonary vascular resistance is greater than one third of the systemic resistance
III	C-LD		1. ASD closure should not be performed in adults with PA systolic pressure greater than two thirds systemic, pulmonary vascular resistance greater than two thirds systemic, and/or a net right-to-left shunt

(Continued)

TABLE 66-1. Guideline Comparison for ASD Treatment (Continued)

Atrial Septal Defects: 2020 ESC Guidelines for ACHD

COR	LOE	Diagnostic	Therapeutic
I	B	1. In patients with evidence of RV volume overload and no PAH (no non-invasive signs of PAP elevation or invasive confirmation of PVR <3 WU in case of such signs) or LV disease, ASD closure is recommended regardless of symptoms.	
I	C	1. In elderly patients not suitable for device closure, it is recommended to carefully weigh the surgical risk against the potential benefit of ASD closure. 2. In patients with non-invasive signs of PAP elevation, invasive measurement of PVR is mandatory. 3. In patients with LV disease, it is recommended to perform balloon testing and carefully weigh the benefit of eliminating L-R 4. shunt against the potential negative impact of ASD closure on outcome due to an increase in filling pressure (taking closure, 5. fenestrated closure, and no closure into consideration).	1. Device closure is recommended as the method of choice for secundum ASD closure when technically suitable.
IIa	C	1. In patients with suspicion of paradoxical embolism (exclusion of other causes), ASD closure should be considered regardless of size providing there is absence of PAH and LV disease. 2. In patients with PVR 3-5 WU, ASD closure should be considered when significant L-R shunt is present (Qp:Qs >1.5)	
IIb	C	1. In patients with PVR ≥ 5 WU, fenestrated ASD closure may be considered when PVR falls below 5WU after targeted PAH treatment and significant L_R shunt is present (Qp:Qs >1.5).	
III	C	1. ASD closure is not recommended in patients with Eisenmenger physiology, patients with PAH and PVR ≥ 5 WU despite targeted PAH treatment, or desaturation on exercise.	

Abbreviations: ASD, atrial septal defect; L–R, left-to-right; LV, left ventricle/ventricular; PAH, pulmonary arterial hypertension; PAP, pulmonary artery pressure; PVR, pulmonary vascular resistance; Qp:Qs, pulmonary to systemic flow ratio; RV, right ventricle/ventricular; WU, Wood units.

output. The degree of PVR or RV failure at which this physiologic event becomes a reality is the subject of debate. Current guidelines suggest that if the ratio of pulmonary (Rp) to systemic vascular resistance (Rs) exceeds 2/3 and if RV systolic pressure is >2/3 systemic systolic pressure, ASD closure is not safe, while if Rp:Rs is <1/3 and RV systolic pressure is <50% systemic systolic pressure then closure is likely to be safe.[1] In between these two values remains a debatable gray zone. For any patient undergoing evaluation for ASD closure, exercise pulse oximetry is recommended to document that there is no significant right-to-left shunting that occurs in the setting of stress that might suggest stress-induced RV dysfunction and/or RV failure due to comprised RV compliance. In patients who either have evidence of right-to-left shunting at rest or with exercise, or in whom Rp:Rs is >2/3 and RV systolic pressure is >2/3 systemic, some have proposed a "treat to close" strategy whereby a multidisciplinary team of congenital heart disease and pulmonary hypertension specialists treat patients with pulmonary vasodilator medications and repeat cardiac catheterizations and exercise tests serially until physiologic numbers improve and the ASD can be safely closed.[30–33] The threshold that should be used after treatment to indicate closure may be safely pursued in this setting remains unclear although the

possibility of fenestrated ASD closure may broaden the window for this strategy.[34,35] Similarly, the need to continue therapy after closure, the probability of continued disease progression versus regression after closure, and the need for fenestration at the time of closure in this setting all remain fundamentally important unanswered questions.

Just as ASD closure in the setting of RV failure may precipitate decompensation, ASD closure in the setting of LV failure may lead to acute decompensated left heart failure and pulmonary edema. Just as an ASD will "offload" the failing RV, in the setting of elevated LV filling pressures, the ASD may offload the LV preventing LA hypertension and pulmonary edema. The idealized example of this phenomenon is Lutembacher syndrome (ASD with mitral stenosis) in which left-to-right shunting is increased due to LA hypertension and ASD closure leads to pulmonary edema. In patients with LV systolic dysfunction and in older patients with diastolic dysfunction, left-to-right shunting may similarly increase and uncover a previously clinically silent ASD.[36] In this setting, it is difficult to predict which individuals will benefit and which will be harmed by ASD closure. Some have advocated test-occlusion of the defect at the time of diagnostic cardiac catheterization prior to closure to assess impact of acute occlusion on LA pressures;

however, this has not been demonstrated to predict success or failure of closure and likely provides little indication of how physiology will respond during periods of physical exertion when LA pressure increases. Moreover, even older individuals generally have good outcomes after ASD closure.[37]

Finally, in individuals with a stroke thought to be thromboembolic in origin, ASD closure is indicated barring contraindications.

ASD Closure

ASDs may be closed either surgically or percutaneously. Currently, the great majority of ASDs are closed using percutaneous devices.[25,38] These devices, however, are suitable only for secundum ASDs with a sufficient rim of atrial septal tissue for device anchoring and in a minority of sinus venosus defects.[39,40] All other defect types must be closed surgically. There are a number of percutaneous closure devices currently available and this will likely continue to expand in the future. Available data suggest that percutaneous devices are nearly as efficacious and are safer than surgical closure.[41] One limitation of earlier generation devices is restriction of access to the interatrial septum, which is significant as patients age and may require pulmonary vein isolation or other therapeutic procedures. Newer generation devices have addressed this limitation by employing newer designs that permit puncture through the device itself.

Surgery for ASD closure is currently the only option for most sinus venosus defects, coronary sinus defects, and primum defects. Given the comparative rarity of these lesions, guidelines recommend that surgical closure of ASDs be undertaken by physicians with experience in congenital cardiac surgery.

Long-Term Outcomes and Prognosis

Long-term outcomes in patients with ASDs are variable depending on if and when the defect is closed, as well as on the degree of left-to-right shunting. There are limited data available on untreated physiologically significant ASDs because the majority of lesions discovered in the current era with significant shunting are closed either surgically or percutaneously. Similarly, data on ASDs that are too small to produce RA and RV enlargement remains limited. With the advent of modern imaging technology, more and more ASDs, including many that are small and of questionable physiologic relevance, are being detected.[42] As a result, recent-era data are likely more accurate than historical reports and suggest a slightly decreased life expectancy and modestly compromised outcomes in the setting of patent ASDs.[43,44] The majority of this liability is in individuals with associated with RA and RV enlargement. Such individuals have a higher probability of atrial arrhythmias and heart failure that may be improved by closure. Prognosis is significantly worse in cases of pulmonary hypertension that may occur in up to 15% of ASDs.

Among patients who undergo ASD closure, outcomes appear to be improved. In addition to preventing the possibility of paradoxical embolization, ASD closure may decrease the probability deteriorating functional status, and rates of pneumonia and atrial arrhythmias. Nevertheless, even after ASD closure, population-based data suggest that life expectancy

remains compromised.[44] The degree of benefit offered by ASD closure appears to be greatest in individuals repaired early in life,[19,21] presumably prior to the advent of irreversible changes in the electrical or mechanical function of myocardial tissue.

VENTRICULAR SEPTAL DEFECTS

Background

Ventricular septal defects (VSDs) are the most common form of congenital heart defects.[45] VSDs are frequently associated with complex anomalies of the heart and great arteries such as transposition of the great arteries (TGA) (both complete and congenitally corrected), tetralogy of Fallot, and pulmonary atresia. The present section will focus on isolated VSDs. Although the most common form of congenital heart disease (CHD) in children, VSDs are the second most common anomaly in adults because up to 80% of VSDs spontaneously close in childhood.[1,46] The pathophysiologic significance of VSDs depends on both the size and location of the lesion.

Anatomy

VSDs are the result of either defective development of embryologic tissue planes, or defective fusion of adjacent tissue planes (**Fig. 66–9**). The interventricular septum forms as part of a complex process through which four primary tissues planes coalesce (**Fig. 66–10**).[47] The location of a particular VSD depends on which of the tissue planes was impacted during development.[48,49]

Perimembranous VSD

Perimembranous VSDs are the most common form of VSDs accounting for between 75% and 80% of defects. These defects are named for their location in or adjacent to the membranous portion of the interventricular septum.

Muscular VSD

Muscular VSDs are the second most common form of VSDs accounting for between 5% and 20% of defects. These VSDs are located in the muscular portion of the interventricular septum between the inlet interventricular septum beneath the atrioventricular valves and the outlet septum above the crista supraventricularis. They are frequently multiple and may be associated with double-chambered RV, even after spontaneous closure in childhood.

Inlet VSD

Inlet VSDs account for approximately 8% of total VSDs. These defects are located in the inlet portion of the interventricular septum or that portion of the septum beneath the septal leaflet of the tricuspid valve. These defects are most commonly associated with atrioventricular canal defects that will be discussed in a later section.

Supracristal VSD

Supracristal VSDs are the least common form of VSDs accounting for 5% to 7% of defects, although in Asian populations it may be more common. These VSDs are located in the infundibular portion of the interventricular septum, above the crista supraventricularis, just beneath the semilunar valves.

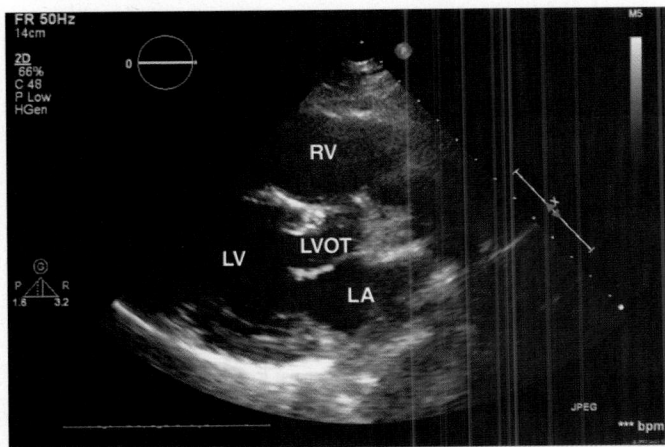

A

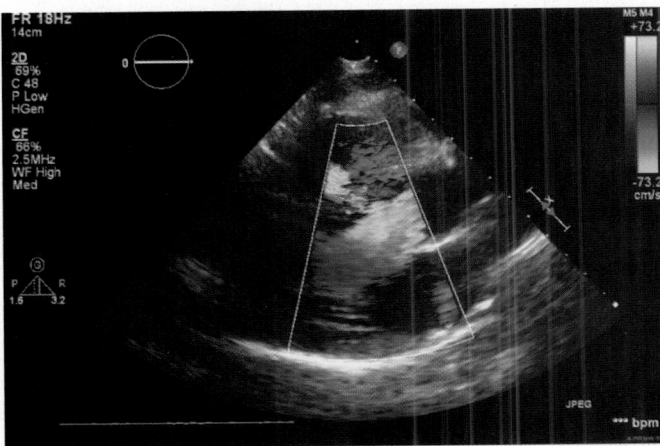

B

Figure 66–9. VSD echocardiogram. (A) 2D and **(B)** color Doppler echocardiogram images obtained in the parasternal long-axis view from a 17-year-old young woman presenting with murmur. On 2D imaging, disruption of normal tissue structure is seen in a membranous septum, consistent with a membranous VSD, with a left-to-right shunt apparent on color Doppler imaging.

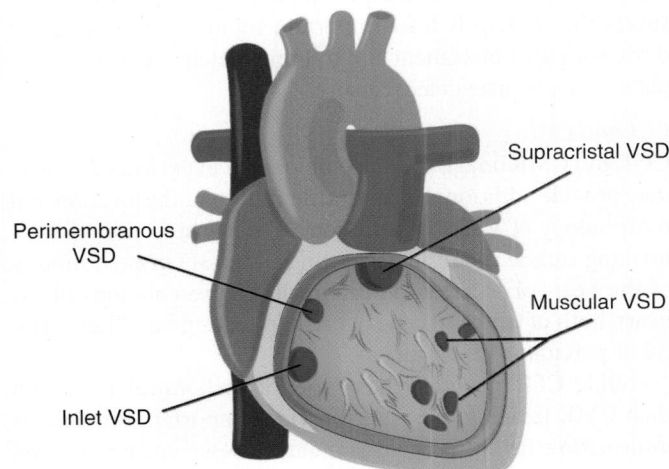

Figure 66–10. **The different types of ventricular septal defects.**

Pathophysiology of VSDs

VSDs cause pathology through two primary mechanisms: shunting with resultant pulmonary overcirculation and associated sequelae, and damage to nearby valvular structures caused by high velocity shunt flow. The degree of shunting across a VSD is dictated by a combination of resistance to flow of the defect itself and impedance to flow through the pulmonary versus the systemic circulation.

Outside of cases of severe pulmonary vascular disease or RVOT stenosis, shunting in VSDs is from left to right and occurs predominantly during ventricular systole. The amount of shunting is dependent on the size of the defect relative to the size of the aortic valve. Classically, defects that are <30% of the size of the aortic annulus do not lead to significant shunting, those between 30% to 65% of aortic annulus size will lead to LA and LV volume overload and may lead to pulmonary hypertension,[50] while those >65% of aortic annulus size will invariably lead to LA and LV volume overload and pulmonary hypertension unless closed early in life. In childhood, with decline in pulmonary vascular resistance shortly after birth, pulmonary overcirculation may be associated with frequent pneumonias and signs left heart failure due to high demands for cardiac output.[51] Over time, pulmonary overcirculation and (in cases of large defects) exposure to high systolic pressures may lead to irreversible pulmonary vascular damage[52] and Eisenmenger syndrome (ES), which will be addressed later in this chapter.[53] With the onset of increasing pulmonary vascular impedance the degree of shunting will decrease and, in cases of ES, may reverse.

Supracristal and perimembranous VSDs may cause damage to the aortic valve.[54] This damage is the result of high velocity flow from the left ventricular outflow tract (LVOT) to the RVOT. The high velocity of flow pulls the leaflets of the aortic valve toward the defect through the Venturi effect, due to imbalance of potential (pressure) and kinetic (flow velocity) energy adjacent to the defect.[55] Over time, the aortic valve leaflets may be damaged leading to aortic insufficiency, imposing a further volume load on the LV.

Small, restrictive VSDs are associated with a high velocity jet from the LV into the RV due to a significant pressure difference between the two chambers throughout ventricular systole. This jet may strike the RV or valvular endocardium, disrupt the endothelium, and result in a nidus for bacterial deposition and the development of endocarditis.[56] This same process may in certain individuals lead to hypertrophy of RV muscle bundles and to the development of a double chambered RV, classically in patients with muscular VSDs.[57]

Epidemiology

VSDs are the most common form of congenital heart disease[58,59] (excluding bicuspid aortic valve), and are present in approximately 50% of individuals affected with congenital heart disease. Most commonly, a VSD is associated with other lesions as part of a complex. In the present section, we will discuss only isolated VSDs, which are still very common and represent approximately 20% of all congenital heart disease.[60]

The prevalence of isolated VSDs is estimated variously to be 1.5 to 53 per 1000 live births, with prevalence increasing as imaging technology has permitted detection in larger numbers of patients who previously would have been unrecognized.[61,62] A large proportion of defects close spontaneously in childhood, and many large defects come to clinical attention in childhood and are surgically closed such that the prevalence in the adult population is significantly lower, although difficult to estimate.

Genetics

The majority of individuals with VSDs do not have an identifiable genetic abnormality. Nevertheless, there are some genetic syndromes that have been linked to VSDs. Down syndrome (trisomy 21), DiGeorge syndrome (22q11 deletion), and Turner syndrome (45X) are all associated with VSDs.[63,64] In addition, Holt Oram syndrome (caused by defects in the *TBX5* gene), defects the *Nkx 2.5* gene, and defects in multiple genes known to share a developmental pathway with these two genes in the developing heart may be associated with VSDs.[65] As more genetic information becomes available, more genetic factors predisposing to VSDs are being identified and likely any gene involved in cardiac development (in particular those involved in cardiac septation) may in some cases lead to VSDs. Currently, the majority of cases are considered polygenic or sporadic and are likely the result of a combination of genetic susceptibility and environment. Recurrence rates in offspring of affected individuals are estimated to be between 2% and 10%.[1]

Presentation

History

The presentation of VSD is largely dependent on the size of the defect. Large defects will frequently present in childhood with recurrent episodes of heart failure or pneumonia. In cases where these symptoms are ignored or missed in childhood, pulmonary overcirculation will eventually lead to severe pulmonary hypertension and ES with unique features as will be discussed in a following section. Individuals with defects that are medium sized may present with symptoms of exertional dyspnea due to increased demand for LV output. Small defects are clinically silent unless they lead to aortic valve damage or endocarditis, in which case symptoms of aortic insufficiency and systemic infection respectively may characterize presentation.

Physical Examination

As with most other aspects of VSDs, there is a size dependence in the physical exam manifestations of the lesions. Early in life, large VSDs may present with a harsh systolic murmur at the left sternal border with rales in the setting of LV failure and pulmonary edema. As pulmonary vascular resistance rises, the flow across the defect will decrease resulting in diminution and eventual disappearance of the murmur with the eventual onset of symptoms of ES. Medium and small defects result in similar harsh holosystolic murmurs dependent on turbulent LV to RV shunt flow. The velocity and hence degree of turbulence and grade of the murmur will depend on the pressure difference between the LV and RV as well as the size of the defect. In the case of medium sized defects, there may be a diastolic rumble at the ventricular apex due to increased flow across an otherwise normal mitral valve. In cases where a perimembranous or supracristal VSD has resulted in aortic valve insufficiency, patients may have physical exam findings attributable to that lesion as well.

Work-Up/Investigations

Electrocardiography

In small defects, there will typically be no ECG findings attributable to the VSD. With medium- and large-sized defects (prior to the development of pulmonary hypertension) there may be evidence of left atrial enlargement or LV hypertrophy as well as intraventricular conduction delay. With the onset of pulmonary vascular disease, signs of RV hypertrophy may appear.

Chest Radiography

In small defects, there are typically no findings. With medium- and large-sized defects, there may be evidence of pulmonary vascular plethora attributable to pulmonary overcirculation and vascular congestion or pulmonary edema due to LV failure. There also may be evidence of cardiomegaly attributable to LA and LV enlargement. With the onset of PAH, the central pulmonary arteries may enlarge with pruning of vascular markings in the peripheral lung fields. In the setting, LA and LV enlargement may regress and RA and RV enlargement may occur.

Echocardiography

Echocardiography (echo) (including both 2D and 3D techniques) is the single most useful tool to assess VSDs. Echocardiographic evaluation permits both identification and localization of VSDs and evaluation of their sequelae including quantification of LA and LV size, identification of shunt direction and velocity, and the presence and degree of pulmonary hypertension. In addition, echo permits identification of VSD-associated lesions and concomitant congenital heart defects, presence and degree of aortic insufficiency, and evidence of endocarditis. In cases where image quality is suboptimal or endocarditis is suspected, TEE can provide additional clarity. At the time of either percutaneous or surgical VSD closure, either TEE or ICE are important adjunctive tools to guide device or patch placement and to immediately identify incomplete or inadequate defect closure.

CCT and CMR

CCT and CMR imaging when employed at experienced centers may provide additional anatomic definition of the location and morphology of VSDs. In addition, 3D reconstruction of CCT imaging can be useful in generating either 3D printed models of the heart or to create virtual reality representations of the heart, both of which may be of use in planning for either surgical or percutaneous closure.

While CCT generally has superior anatomical definition than CMR imaging, the latter provides important physiologic information being the gold standard assessment for RV and LV volumetric assessment and function. More importantly, CMR permits accurate noninvasive assessment of pulmonary and systemic blood flow, which is fundamentally important in assessing overall physiology and candidacy for VSD closure.

Cardiac Catheterization

Catheterization remains the best source for essential information on VSDs including evaluation of pulmonary and systemic blood flow, intracardiac and pulmonary arterial pressures, and systemic and pulmonary vascular resistances. Although invasive angiography may provide anatomical information suggesting the location of VSDs and the presence of aortic insufficiency, the various other modalities already described are likely superior. Catheterization has the advantage of being both diagnostic and potentially therapeutic given the existence of percutaneous devices specifically designed for closure of both emerging muscular and perimembranous VSDs.

Management

Decision-making regarding closure of VSDs is similar to that of ASDs[1] (**Table 66–2**). In general, a Qp:Qs of >1.5 is required for LA or LV enlargement. It is unusual for adult patients with unrepaired VSDs that allow LA or LV enlargement to have avoided developing secondary pulmonary vascular disease and PAH. In cases of younger children, there are clear data indicating that VSDs that cause left heart enlargement have a poor prognosis if left unrepaired. In patients with evidence of pulmonary vascular disease, the approach to and liabilities associated with VSD closure are also similar to those in ASDs. As in the case of ASDs, closure of VSDs in the setting of significant pulmonary vascular disease may lead to exercise intolerance and hypotension attributable to RV failure and inadequate LV filling. Current guidelines recommend that if the ratio of pulmonary (Rp) to systemic vascular resistance (Rs) exceeds 2/3 and if RV systolic pressure is >2/3 systemic systolic pressure, VSD closure is not safe, while if Rp:Rs is <1/3 and RV systolic pressure is <50% systemic systolic pressure then closure is likely to be safe. Between these two lies a group of individuals in whom more complex decision-making is required involving input from both congenital heart disease and pulmonary hypertension specialists.

TABLE 66–2. Guideline Comparison for VSD Treatment

Ventricular Septal Defects: 2018 AHA/ACC Guidelines for ACHD			
COR	**LOE**	**Diagnostic**	**Therapeutic**
I	B-NR		1. Adults with a VSD and evidence of left ventricular volume overload and hemodynamically significant shunts (Qp:Qs ≥1.5:1) should undergo VSD closure, if PA systolic pressure is less than 50% systemic and pulmonary vascular resistance is less than one third systemic
IIa	C-LD		1. Surgical closure of perimembranous or supracristal VSD is reasonable in adults when there is worsening aortic regurgitation (AR) caused by VSD
IIb	C-LD		1. Surgical closure of a VSD may be reasonable in adults with a history of IE caused by VSD if not otherwise contraindicated 2. Closure of a VSD may be considered in the presence of a net left-to-right shunt (Qp:Qs ≥1.5:1) when PA systolic pressure is 50% or more than systemic and/or pulmonary vascular resistance is greater than one third systemic
III	C-LD		1. VSD closure should not be performed in adults with severe PAH with PA systolic pressure greater than two thirds systemic, pulmonary vascular resistance greater than two thirds systemic and/or a net right-to-left shunt
Ventricular Septal Defects: 2020 ESC Guidelines for ACHD			
COR	**LOE**	**Diagnostic**	**Therapeutic**
I	C		1. In patients with evidence of LV volume overload and no PAH (no non-invasive signs of PAP elevation or invasive confirmation of PVR <3 WU in case of such signs), VSD closure is recommended regardless of symptoms.
IIa	C	1. In patients who have developed PAH with PVR 3-5 WU, VSD closure should be considered when there is still significant L-R shunt (Qp:Qp >1.5).	1. In patients with no significant L_R shunt, but a history of repeated episodes of IE, VSD closure should be considered. 2. In patients with VSD-associated prolapse of an aortic valve cusp causing progressive AR, surgery should be considered.
IIb	C	1. In patients who have developed PAH with PVR >_5 WU, VSD closure may be considered when there is still significant L_R shunt (Qp:Qs >1.5), but careful individual decision in expert centers is required	
III	C		1. VSD closure is not recommended in patients with Eisenmenger physiology and patients with severe PAH (PVR ≥5 WU) presenting with desaturation on exercise.

Abbreviations: AR, aortic regurgitation; IE, infective endocarditis; L–R, left-to-right; LV, left ventricle/ventricular; PAH, pulmonary arterial hypertension; PAP, pulmonary artery pressure; PVR, pulmonary vascular resistance; Qp:Qs, pulmonary to systemic flow ratio; VSD, ventricular septal defect; WU, Wood units.

Any patient in whom VSD closure is planned should be evaluated with exercise pulse oximetry to document that right-to-left shunting does not occur in the setting of stress which might suggest a limitation in the capacity of the RV to overcome pulmonary vascular resistance in times of increased demand. In patients who either have evidence of right-to-left shunting at rest or with exercise, or in whom Rp:Rs is >2/3 and RV systolic pressure is >2/3 systemic, treatment with pulmonary vasodilator therapy under the direction of a multidisciplinary team of congenital heart disease and pulmonary hypertension specialists in some cases may permit safe VSD closure. The threshold at which closure is safe and the probability of continued disease progression versus regression after closure remain unanswered questions.

Small restrictive VSDs are not thought to be associated with significantly compromised prognosis and generally are followed without intervention. However, in patients with either a small supracristal or perimembranous VSD and associated aortic insufficiency, closure may be indicated to prevent further valvular deterioration if there is evidence of a progressive increase in aortic insufficiency without other identifiable cause. Similarly, in individuals with small VSDs and infective endocarditis without other identifiable cause, closure may be indicated to prevent recurrence.

Method of VSD Closure

VSD closure is typically performed surgically in centers with expertise in congenital heart surgery and perioperative care. Techniques vary but typically include placing a pericardial or synthetic patch over the defect with sutures placed at some distance from the defect itself to avoid dehiscence. For supracristal and inlet VSDs, surgical closure is the only option because no percutaneous closure device exists. For muscular and perimembranous VSDs, there are now percutaneous devices that may permit closure. The utility of these devices is limited in patients with long or tortuous defects and multiple defects (in particular in the case of muscular VSDs). In addition, perimembranous VSD closure device deployment has been associated with a significant risk of heart block and these devices are therefore only available for use in certain countries.[41,66]

Long-Term Outcomes and Prognosis

Early prognostic studies were hampered by many biases, not the least of which was that individuals who presented to medical attention and were therefore enrolled in these studies were more likely to have had complications related to their defect that led them to medical attention in the first place.[67,68] Moreover, the field of congenital heart disease has advanced significantly over recent decades and an individual born 50 years ago with a VSD was much less likely to be identified and treated than one born today. As a result of this time-dependent bias in prognosis, it is difficult to accurately assess long-term prognosis in VSD.

In general, long-term outcomes of patients with VSDs depends on three major factors: the size of the defect, location of the defect, and whether the defect has been closed. There are recent data to suggest that even in individuals with early closure or with small, restrictive defects, exercise capacity and myocardial function may be compromised.[69,70] In patients with small defects that typically are not closed, there is an increased incidence of bacterial endocarditis over time.[71] Patients with perimembranous or supracristal VSDs may have a higher probability of developing aortic insufficiency and may require aortic valve surgery. Nevertheless, life expectancy in individuals with unrepaired small VSDs is not thought to be significantly different than in the general population.

In individuals with moderate-to-large VSDs, prognosis is poor without repair. Patients with large defects will typically come to medical attention early after birth, because pulmonary vascular resistance declines in the neonatal period. As the impedance of the pulmonary vascular bed decreases, the degree of left-to-right shunting will increase imposing a volume load on the LV with accompanying large demands on the LV for cardiac output. As a result, these children develop pulmonary vascular congestion, pulmonary edema, and evidence of hypoperfusion of systemic organs characteristic of heart failure. With judicious medical therapy, these symptoms of heart failure may be managed to permit closure. Left unattended to, large and moderate sized defects will eventually lead to secondary pulmonary vascular disease and thereafter to ES. Pulmonary vascular disease without ES is associated with a significantly increased risk for heart failure, arrhythmia, and sudden death.[72,73]

In individuals with moderate to large VSDs who have undergone surgical repair prior to the development of significant pulmonary vascular disease, life expectancy is likely similar to the general population. Nevertheless, recent data suggests that such individuals may have a higher risk of aortic valvular disease, arrhythmia, and RV and LV systolic dysfunction and therefore should continue to be monitored throughout life.[60,69]

ATRIOVENTRICULAR SEPTAL DEFECTS

Background

Atrioventricular septal defects (AVSDs) are a relatively rare form of congenital heart disease encompassing a spectrum of pathology from an isolated ASD to the combination of an ASD, VSD, and single atrioventricular valve. Pathophysiology varies depending on anatomy. In the modern era, AVSDs are typically repaired in childhood.

Anatomy

AVSDs are the result of defective fusion of the septum primum with the endocardial cushion or defects with the endocardial cushion itself.[74] Depending on the degree to which this fusion or the endocardial cushion are defective, AVSDs represent a spectrum of disease that is generally divided into the following broad categories[75] (**Fig. 66–11**).

Partial AVSD

Partial AVSDs are synonymous with primum ASDs as addressed in an earlier section.

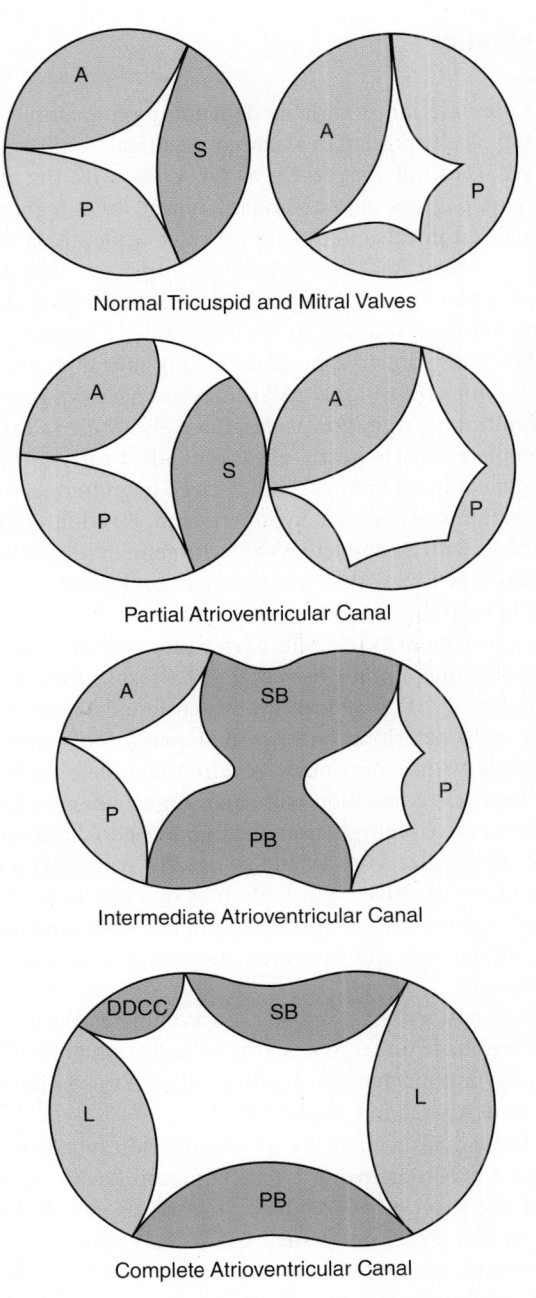

Figure 66–11. Categories of atrioventricular canal defects. A, anterior leaflet; P, posterior leaflet; S, septal leaflet; SB, superior bridging leaflet; PB, posterior bridging leaflet; DDCC, dextrodorsal conus cushion.

Transitional AVSD

Transitional AVSDs are midway between partial and complete AVSDs. They are characterized by a primum ASD in combination with a common atrioventricular valve annulus and bridging atrioventricular valve leaflets without a VSD or with a small restrictive VSD.

Complete AVSD

Complete AVSDs include a primum ASD, a common atrioventricular valve with superior and inferior bridging leaflets, and an inlet VSD. Complete AVSDs are further defined depending on the position of the interventricular septum relative to the

common atrioventricular valve, and the location of superior bridging leaflet attachments. Complete AVSDs in which the crest of the interventricular septum (IVS) does not divide the common atrioventricular valve evenly into two sides are called unbalanced AVSDs while those in which the IVS crest divides the atrioventricular valve evenly are said to be balanced. This has clinical relevance as unbalanced complete AVSDs may lead to unilateral ventricular hypoplasia, precluding two-ventricle repair. Patients falling into this single ventricular physiology are often palliated with a series of surgical procedures leading to a Fontan. Finally, complete AVSDs are defined based on the chordal attachments of the superior bridging leaflet using the Rastelli classification system[76] (**Fig. 66–12**). This classification has clinical relevance as it it impacts the ease and efficacy of surgical repair.

Associated Abnormalities

Due to abnormalities in atrial and ventricular septation, the LVOT is displaced anteriorly and abnormally shaped, in what is called a "gooseneck deformity" based on its angiographic appearance. The gooseneck deformity may lead to varying degrees of LVOT stenosis.[77] This stenosis may be discrete or tunnel-like.

Pathophysiology

The pathophysiology of AVSDs depends largely on the anatomical type of AVSD present. Partial AVSDs are physiologically identical to ASDs as previously described. Transitional AVSDs

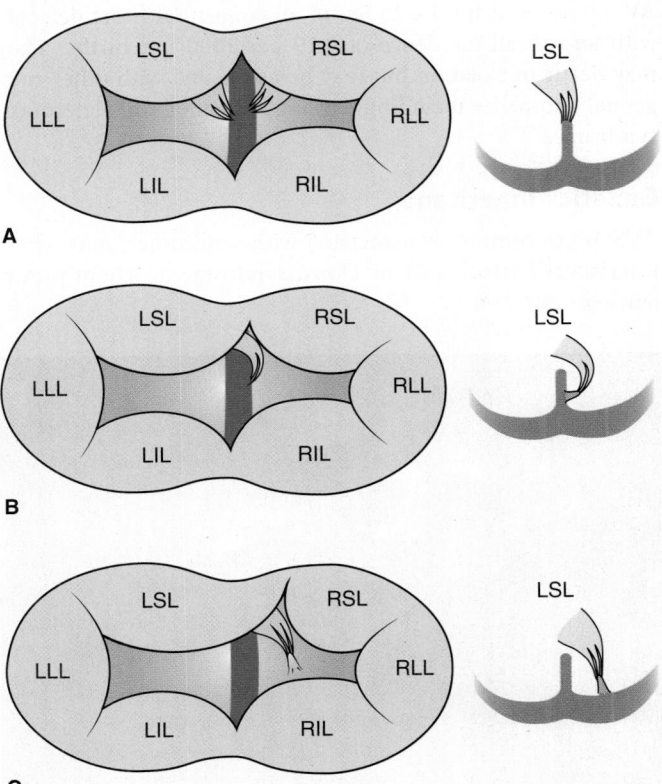

Figure 66–12. Rastelli classification of atrioventricular canal defects (Types A, B, and C). LSL, left superior leaflet; LLL, left lateral leaflet; LIL, left inferior leaflet; RSL, right superior leaflet; RLL, right lateral leaflet; RIL, right inferior leaflet.

are physiologically similar to primum AVSDs superimposed with varying degrees of mitral valve regurgitation due to a cleft in the anterior leaflet of the mitral valve. Complete AVSDs are physiologically characterized by the simultaneous presence of a large ASD and VSD. In the unrepaired state, AVSDs therefore produce a volume load on both the RV and LV, and in the absence of RVOT stenosis expose the pulmonary vasculature to systemic pressures. As a result, unrepaired complete AVSDs may lead to heart failure as pulmonary vascular resistance declines in early postnatal life and invariably cause irreversible pulmonary vascular disease if left unrepaired.

In adulthood, the majority of patients born with complete AVSDs will have been previously repaired[78,79] (**Fig. 66–13**). In this scenario, physiology depends on the presence of a residual ASD, VSD, or associated defects. Patients with repaired AVSDs may have a residual cleft in the anterior mitral valve leaflet, which in combination with other abnormalities[80] commonly leaves patients with some degree of mitral valve regurgitation.[81] The gooseneck deformity that characterizes AVSDs may lead to nondynamic subvalvular aortic stenosis[77] with pathophysiology characteristic of excessive LV afterload as described in other sections. In addition, impairment caused by longstanding high-velocity blood flow produced by the subaortic stenosis striking the underside of the aortic valve may cause aortic valve insufficiency.

Epidemiology

AVSDs account for 4% to 5% of all congenital heart defects[82] with an overall incidence of 0.19 per 1000 live births. They may occur in isolation but may be associated with other congenital anomalies including tetralogy of Fallot and Heterotaxy syndromes.[83,84]

Genetics/Inheritance

AVSDs are commonly associated with syndromes, most characteristically trisomy 21 or Down syndrome in whom prevalence is ~20%.[85,86]

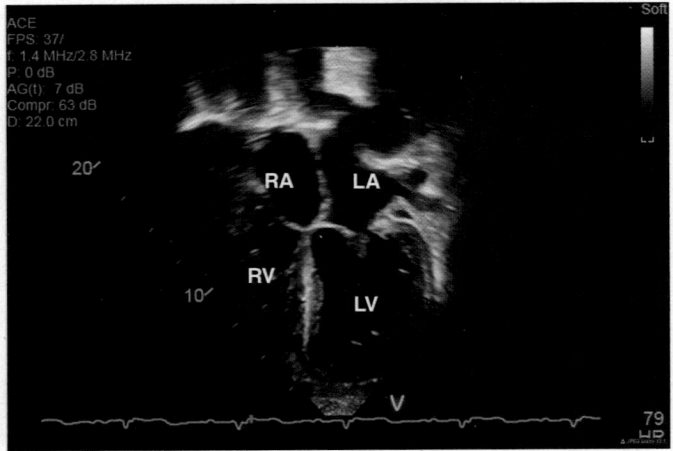

Figure 66–13. Repaired AVCD. 2D echocardiogram image obtained in the apical four-chamber view from a 34-year-old man with complete atrioventricular canal defect repaired in infancy. Of note, the left and right atrioventricular valves are at the same level at the crux of the heart.

Presentation

History

AVSD presentation is variable depending on anatomy. Partial AVSDs typically present in a manner identical to ASDs. Incomplete AVSDs similarly present as do ASDs, with the addition of varying degrees of concomitant mitral valve regurgitation due to a cleft in the anterior mitral valve leaflet. As a result of the concomitant ASD, the physiologic impact of mitral regurgitation is blunted as LA hypertension and left-sided chamber volume load are shunted to the right-sided chambers across the ASD. Therefore, in spite of significant mitral regurgitation, patients with a transitional AVSD may not have symptoms typical of mitral regurgitation as described elsewhere in this text.

Complete AVSDs nearly always manifest early in life with symptoms of heart failure, characterized by pulmonary edema and symptoms of systemic hypoperfusion. By adulthood, most individuals with a complete AVSD who remain unrepaired will have developed ES with associated signs and symptoms as discussed later in this chapter.

The great majority of adults born with a complete AVSD will have undergone a previous repair. As a result, the symptoms of complete AVSD in adults are related to either concomitant defects or to deterioration of prior repairs. Most commonly, individuals with a previously repaired complete AVSD with a two-ventricle circulation will have some evidence of persistent mitral valve regurgitation due to the residual cleft anterior mitral valve leaflet. History and symptoms will depend on the degree of mitral valve regurgitation as described elsewhere in this text. Briefly, this may include symptoms of exertional dyspnea, palpitations, and in severe cases peripheral and pulmonary edema.

Individuals with an unbalanced complete AVSD will in many cases have undergone a Fontan palliation and will present with symptoms typical of individual with this unique physiology as described in Chapter 70.

All individuals with an AVSD may develop subaortic stenosis. This LVOT narrowing typically presents with symptoms characteristic of valvular aortic stenosis as described elsewhere in this text. Briefly, such individuals may present with symptoms of dyspnea with exertion, angina, or in severe cases syncope most commonly associated with exertion. Such individuals may also present with symptoms suggestive of progressive aortic valve regurgitation also as described elsewhere in this text, most commonly dyspnea with exertion.

Physical Examination

Individuals with an incomplete AVSD will have physical exam findings identical to those in ASD with the exception of the ECG that characteristically has left axis deviation due to posterior displacement of the atrioventricular node and inferior displacement of the His-Purkinje system. Other ECG findings generally correlate with the physiologic sequelae of AVSD when present including RV hypertrophy, biatrial, or biventricular enlargement.

Individuals with a transitional AVSD will have physical exam findings similar to those with an incomplete AVSD except that they may have an additional murmur of mitral valve regurgitation. Due to the concomitant presence of an ASD, it is unusual for mitral regurgitation to result in left-sided chamber enlargement on ECG or chest x-ray and findings characteristic of right-sided volume overload predominate.

In children, the unrepaired complete AVSD prior to the development of irreversible pulmonary vascular disease, there will be flow murmurs across the ventricular septal defect, and a murmur of increased flow through the RVOT. The precordium will be hyperdynamic due to increased pulmonary blood flow and cardiomegaly. Chest x-ray findings will reveal pulmonary vascular plethora due to increased pulmonary blood flow but may not be consistent with pulmonary edema as the ASD prevents in part the development of LA hypertension. These findings will progressively fade with the onset of pulmonary vascular disease and accompanying increases in pulmonary vascular impedance and decreased pulmonary blood flow.

In adults with an unrepaired complete AVSD, physical exam findings are those of ES (see section Eisenmenger Syndrome). In those with a repaired complete AVSD with two ventricles and significant mitral regurgitation, physical exam findings will be typical of mitral regurgitation. In those with a Fontan-palliated complete unbalanced AVSD physical exam findings will be characteristic of the Fontan circulation as described in Chapter 70 (Fontan).

Individuals with AVSD who have significant subaortic stenosis may have a systolic murmur at the right upper sternal border on physical exam that is nondynamic and increases with squatting or increased stroke volume. The murmur may radiate to the carotids. They may also have a diastolic murmur of aortic valve insufficiency at the right upper sternal border, also auscultable to the left midsternal border. Individuals with significant aortic insufficiency may also have findings characteristic of that lesion as described elsewhere in this text. Chest x-ray and ECG findings in the setting of significant subaortic stenosis or aortic valve regurgitation will be similar to those of aortic stenosis and regurgitation.

Work-Up/Investigations

Echocardiography

Echocardiography is the modality of choice for diagnosis of AVSD due to its wide availability and the fact that it provides both anatomic and physiologic information. The typical features of unrepaired or repaired AVSD are easily visualized and include tricuspid and mitral valve annuli at the same level relative to the ventricular apex, cleft anterior mitral valve leaflet, and Doppler evidence of both atrial and ventricular septal defects. Echo also permits the facile identification of other congenital heart lesions associated with AVSD as well as sequelae of AVSD including LVOT obstruction, pulmonary hypertension, or ES. TEE may provide additional anatomic information in cases where transthoracic windows are suboptimal and in the intraoperative setting. 3D echocardiography can provide additional anatomic detail, in particular of the mitral valve structure, in cases where surgery is being planned for progressive mitral regurgitation (attributable to a cleft anterior leaflet)

or mitral stenosis (due to a double orifice mitral valve which occurs rarely in association with AVSD).

CCT and CMR

CCT and CMR imaging may help to define anatomy in individuals with difficult echocardiographic visualization. CMR imaging can yield useful information on the quantification of ventricular function and the degree of shunting in individuals who are unrepaired or who have residual ASDs or VSDs.

Cardiac Catheterization

Cardiac catheterization plays little role in the diagnosis and work-up of AVSD in the unrepaired or repaired state. In cases of individuals with overlying pulmonary vascular disease, cardiac catheterization plays an important role in defining intracardiac and pulmonary pressures as well as in assessing the degree of shunting present in unrepaired AVSD or in cases with residual ASDs or VSDs.

Management

AVSDs of all types can only be treated surgically. Treatment of partial or transitional AVSDs is similar to that for ASD, mitral regurgitation, or both as addressed in other sections of this text. The great majority of complete AVSDs are repaired in childhood with excellent success.[87] Adults with unrepaired complete AVSDs typically have some degree of pulmonary vascular disease that may preclude repair. In individuals with a complete AVSD without significant pulmonary hypertension, repair is generally recommended (**Table 66-3**).

In individuals with repaired AVSD with a residual ASD or VSD or in individuals with unrepaired AVSD who also have pulmonary hypertension, pulmonary vasodilator therapy is generally recommended, although the evidence in favor of this approach is retrospective.[88,89] In certain cases with prohibitively high pulmonary vascular resistance prior to therapy, pulmonary vasodilator therapy to facilitate surgical closure may be possible with an associated improvement in prognosis.

In the pediatric population, symptoms of right-sided (in the case of partial or transitional AVSD) or left-sided (in the case of complete AVSD) high-output heart failure may be present. In these cases, diuretic therapy for symptomatic improvement may be helpful. The efficacy of neurohumoral modulation in the setting of AVSD is unproven.

Surgical Repair

Surgical repair for unrepaired AVSD or for residual ASDs or VSDs after childhood repair is recommended in cases with significant shunting without significant pulmonary hypertension. In individuals with a Qp:Qs of >1.5 with a ratio of pulmonary (Rp) to systemic vascular resistance (Rs) <1/3 and RV systolic pressure is <50% systemic systolic pressure then closure is recommended. In cases where Rp/Rs exceeds 2/3 and if RV systolic pressure is >2/3 systemic systolic pressure or in whom shunting is left to right, AVSD closure is not safe. Between these two lies a group of individuals in whom more complex decision-making is required involving input from both congenital heart disease and pulmonary hypertension specialists and in whom there

TABLE 66–3. Guideline Comparison for AVSD Treatment

		Atrioventricular Septal Defects: 2018 AHA/ACC Guidelines for ACHD	
COR	**LOE**	**Diagnostic**	**Therapeutic**
I	C-LD	1. Surgery for severe left atrioventricular valve regurgitation is recommended per GDMT indications for mitral regurgitation	
I	C-EO	1. Surgery for primary repair of atrioventricular septal defect or closure of residual shunts in adults with repaired atrioventricular septal defect is recommended when there is a net left-to-right shunt (Qp:Qs ≥1.5:1), PA systolic pressure less than 50% systemic and pulmonary vascular resistance less than one third systemic.	
IIa	C-EO	1. Cardiac catheterization can be useful in adults with atrioventricular septal defect when pulmonary hypertension is suspected 2. Operation for discrete LVOT obstruction in adults with atrioventricular septal defect is reasonable with a maximum gradient of 50 mm Hg or greater, a lesser gradient if HF symptoms are present, or if concomitant moderate-to-severe mitral or AR are present.	
IIb	C-EO	1. Surgery for primary repair of atrioventricular septal defect or closure of residual shunts in adults with repaired atrioventricular septal defect may be considered in the presence of a net left-to-right shunt (Qp:Qs ≥1.5:1), if PA systolic pressure is 50% or more systemic, and/or pulmonary vascular resistance is greater than one third systemic	
III	C-LD	1. Surgery for primary repair of atrioventricular septal defect or closure of residual shunts in adults with repaired atrioventricular septal defect should not be performed with PA systolic pressure greater than two thirds systemic, pulmonary vascular resistance greater than two thirds systemic, or a net right-to-left shunt	
		Atrioventricular Septal Defects: 2020 ESC Guidelines for ACHD	
COR	**LOE**	**Diagnostic**	**Therapeutic**
I	C		1. Surgical closure is recommended in patients a partial AVSD (primum ASD) with significant RV volume overload and should only be performed by a congenital cardiac surgeon. 2. Valve surgery, preferably AV valve repair, is recommended in symptomatic patients with moderate to severe AV valve regurgitation and should be performed by a congenital cardiac surgeon. 3. In asymptomatic patients with severe left sided AV valve regurgitation, valve surgery is 4. recommended when LVESD ≥ 45 mmd and/or LVEF ≤ 60% provided other causes of LV dysfunction are excluded.
IIa	C		1. In asymptomatic patients with severe left-sided AV valve regurgitation, preserved LV function (LVESD < 45 mmd and/or LVEF > 60%), high likelihood of successful valve repair, and low surgical risk, intervention should be considered when atrial fibrillation or systolic PAP > 50 mmHg is present.
III	C		1. Surgical repair is not recommended in patients with Eisenmenger physiology, and patients with PAH (PVR ≥ 5 WU) presenting with desaturation on exercise.

Abbreviations: ASD, atrial septal defect; AV, atrioventricular; AVSD, atrioventricular septal defect; LV, left ventricle/ventricular; LVEF, left ventricular ejection fraction; LVESD, left ventricular end systolic diameter; LVOTO, left ventricular outflow tract obstruction; PAH, pulmonary artery hypertension; PAP, pulmonary artery pressure; PVR, pulmonary vascular resistance; RV, right ventricle/ventricular; SubAS, subaortic stenosis; VSD, ventricular septal defect; WU, Wood units.

may be a role for pulmonary vasodilator therapy to improve hemodynamics and permit future closure.[1]

Surgical repair of the mitral valve should adhere to guidelines proposed for mitral valve disease as reported elsewhere in this text.

Surgical repair of subaortic stenosis is recommended when there is a maximum gradient of >50 mm Hg, symptoms of stenosis without other identifiable cause, or in cases of moderate-to-severe aortic regurgitation.[1]

Long-Term Outcomes and Prognosis

There are few data available on prognosis given the heterogeneity of AVSD as a lesion, repair status, age at repair, and susceptibility to the development of pulmonary vascular disease. As with all congenital heart disease, individuals with significant pulmonary vascular disease have a significantly worse prognosis.

Prognosis after early repair (prior to the onset of significant pulmonary vascular disease) is excellent with 3% perioperative mortality and 20-year survival as high as 95%.[78,81,87] However, individuals with prior repairs frequently require repeat surgery. The impact of subsequent surgery for long-term deterioration of initial repairs or for mitral or LVOT lesions on prognosis is not defined.

PATENT DUCTUS ARTERIOSUS

Background

The ductus arteriosus is a normal part of the fetal circulation. It is formed by the 6th branchial arch and forms a connection between the pulmonary artery and the descending thoracic aorta. This is necessary to ensure poorly oxygenated blood returning from the developing fetal head returns to the placenta. Normally in early postnatal life, the ductus arteriosus involutes due to a combination of increased blood oxygen concentrations[90–94] and a drop in the prostaglandin PGE_1[94–97] to form the ligamentum arteriosum. In the great majority of cases, the ductus arteriosus closes by 72 hours after birth.[98] In cases where the ductus arteriosus fails to close completely, patients are left with a patent ductus arteriosus (PDA).

Anatomy

PDAs connect the aortic isthmus (just past the left subclavian artery) to the branch point between the left pulmonary artery and the main pulmonary artery. The morphology and size of the PDA itself are variable. Persistence of the right 6th branchial arch may lead to a right-sided PDA. In the setting of aortic arch anomalies, the ductus arteriosus may form one side of a vascular ring (**Fig. 66–14**).

Pathophysiology

Pathophysiologically, a PDA may be considered as similar to a VSD. Shunting in PDAs is from left to right and is continuous throughout the cardiac cycle. The degree of shunting is governed by a combination of resistance to flow through the PDA and impedance to flow in the pulmonary versus the systemic circulation. In the early postnatal period, with the decline in

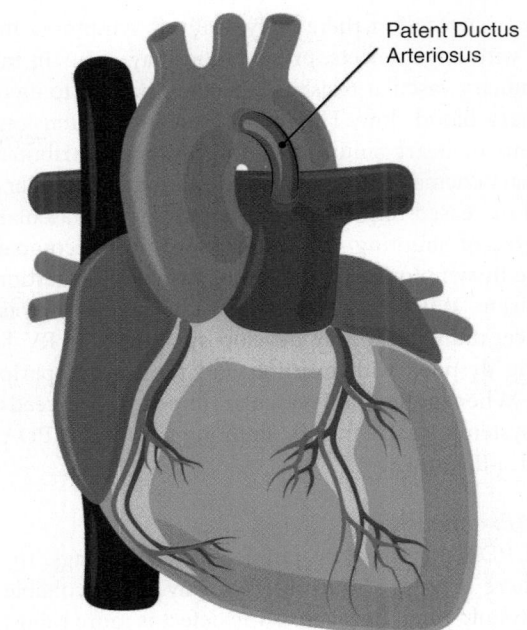

Patent Ductus Arteriosus

Figure 66–14. Location of a typical patent ductus arteriosus.

pulmonary vascular resistance shortly after birth, a PDA that offers little resistance to flow may lead to pulmonary overcirculation and signs LV volume overload or high output heart failure; depending on the size of the defect and the degree of shunting. Over time, pulmonary overcirculation and exposure to high systolic pressures (in the setting of large PDAs) may lead to irreversible pulmonary vascular damage and ES. With the onset of increasing pulmonary vascular impedance the degree of shunting will decrease and, in cases of ES, reverse.

In cases of small PDAs without significant shunting, pathology is related exclusively to high-velocity flow across the defect. This may damage the endothelium and lead to a predisposition to endarteritis typically near the pulmonary arterial ostium of the ductus.

Epidemiology

Isolated PDAs represent 5% to 10% of congenital heart defects,[99,100] although this may be underestimated because the ductus arteriosus is a normal anatomical finding and cases in which shunting is clinically silent may pass unnoticed. Females are more commonly affected than males.[101] PDAs are more common in premature infants (possibly related to immaturity of ductal tissue and suboptimal gas exchange in the premature neonatal lungs[92]) and in infants affected by congenital rubella.[102,103] They are also commonly associated with more complex cyanotic forms of congenital heart disease, possibly as a result of lower oxygen concentrations that may lead to failure of ductal constriction.

Presentation

History

The presentation of PDAs depends largely on the degree of restriction to flow offered by the PDA. In individuals with a small restrictive lesion, there are typically no symptoms. In individuals with large defects, presentation may occur in infancy as pulmonary vascular resistance declines leading to increased pulmonary blood flow. This may result in hypotension, and symptoms of heart failure including dyspnea attributable to pulmonary edema. With progressive pulmonary vascular damage and increased impedance in the pulmonary vascular bed, the degree of shunting will decrease with an accompanying decrease in symptoms of pulmonary vascular congestion and hypotension. With continued increase in pulmonary vascular resistance, individuals may develop symptoms of RV failure including dyspnea with exertion and progressive peripheral edema. When pulmonary vascular impedance exceeds that of the systemic vascular bed, shunting across the PDA may reverse leading to ES.

Physical Examination

A small PDA may have no physical exam findings. In some cases, there may be a murmur that may be auscultable only during systole when flow across the defect is more robust. The classic physical exam findings of a large PDA are a low blood pressure with a widened pulse pressure due to diastolic runoff from the aorta into the pulmonary vascular bed. Because flow across the PDA is continuous, a PDA murmur is classically described as "machine-like" with a louder component during systole and quieter component during diastole. With the advent of pulmonary vascular disease and increased pulmonary impedance to flow, this murmur will decrease in intensity and eventually cease as flow across the defect declines. Pulse pressure will similarly begin to narrow as pulmonary vascular resistance increases.

Work-Up/Investigations

Electrocardiography and Chest Radiography

Chest radiography and electrocardiographic findings are not specific for PDA. Both may reveal evidence of LA or LV enlargement in the setting of large PDAs with significant aortopulmonary shunting. In this setting, a chest x-ray may reveal evidence of pulmonary vascular congestion. With progressive pulmonary vascular disease, there may be ECG evidence of RV hypertrophy with accompanying chest x-ray evidence of enlarged proximal pulmonary arteries and pruning of pulmonary vascular markings in the peripheral lung fields.

Echocardiography

Echocardiography is the primary modality used in the initial diagnosis of PDAs. Echo permits identification of the presence of a PDA, classically appreciated as Doppler flow visualized entering the proximal left pulmonary artery from the aorta on parasternal views (**Fig. 66–15**). Echo also facilitates definition of a PDA's physiologic significance, revealing evidence of LA and LV volume overload as well as evidence of pulmonary hypertension in individuals with a large degree of shunting and with pulmonary vascular disease respectively.[104,105] While in infants and children, echo may permit anatomical definition of the PDA, in adults,

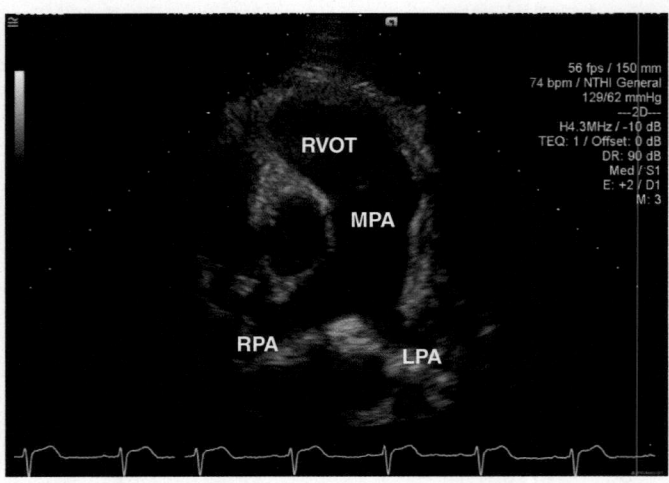

A

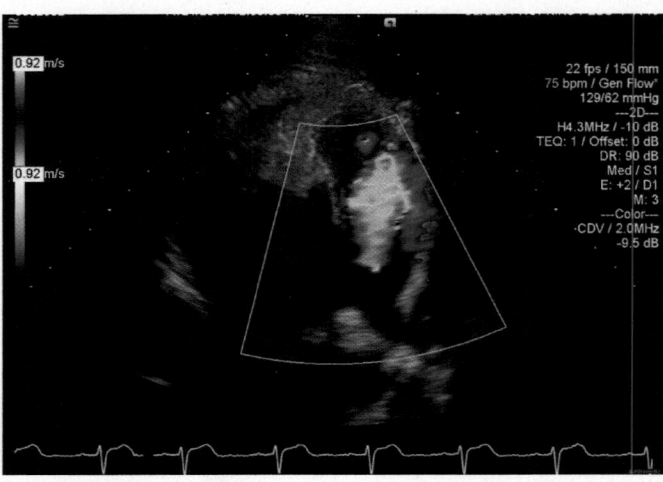

B

Figure 66–15. PDA by echocardiogram. (A) 2D and **(B)** color Doppler echocardiogram images obtained in the parasternal short-axis view from a 21-year-old man presenting with murmur. The small patent ductus arteriosus is not seen on 2D imaging but color Doppler reveals a jet of continuous left-to-right flow in the main pulmonary artery.

echocardiographic windows typically limit accurate anatomic definition of the lesion. TEE and 3D echo contribute little to the diagnosis and work-up of PDAs.

CCT and CMR

CCT and CMR imaging permits excellent anatomical definition including the location, course, size, and morphology of PDAs. This information is very important to guide procedural planning for surgical or catheter-based closure. CCT may also be particularly useful in cases of abnormal aortic anatomy or vascular rings caused by the PDA.

CMR imaging offers good anatomic definition of the PDA. Use of phase contrast imaging also permits objective evaluation of the degree of shunting and accurate assessment of Qp:Qs.

Cardiac Catheterization

Although historically, catheterization was the primary diagnostic modality employed in diagnosis and evaluation of PDAs, today, noninvasive modalities predominate and catheterization is used only in cases where there is concern for elevated pulmonary vascular resistance that is not assessable by noninvasive measures, or when catheter-based PDA closure is considered. Catheterization permits anatomical definition of the PDA using angiography, and evaluation of physiologic significance based on hemodynamic findings. Due to the location of the PDA in which there is no "mixing" chamber upstream of the site of blood sampling, calculation of Qp:Qs is typically more accurate using MRI.

Management

In infants with a PDA, medications that inhibit cyclooxygenase enzymes and therefore decrease the availability of PGE_2 will induce ductal closure in many circumstances. For this indication, ibuprofen or acetaminophen are preferable to indomethacin as a result of a more favorable side effect profile.[106,107]

Decision-making regarding closure of PDAs is similar to that of VSDs[1] (**Table 66–4**). In general, significant shunting is indicated by the presence of LA or LV enlargement without an alternative explanation. Current guidelines recommend that in the presence of a PDA causing left-sided chamber enlargement, if Rp:Rs is <1/3 and RV systolic pressure is <50% systemic systolic pressure then closure is likely to be safe. In contrast, if the ratio of pulmonary (Rp) to systemic vascular resistance (Rs) exceeds 2/3 and if RV systolic pressure is >2/3 systemic systolic pressure, PDA closure is not safe. As is the case with VSD, between these two lies a group of individuals in whom more complex decision-making is required involving input from both congenital heart disease and pulmonary hypertension specialists. It is vitally important in decision-making that oxygen saturations be taken in the lower extremities not just the upper extremities as right-to-left shunting will in most cases only be evident based on lower extremity cyanosis. Such shunting would be a contraindication to closure.

TABLE 66–4. Guideline Comparison for PDA Treatment

COR	LOE	Diagnostic	Therapeutic
Patent Ductus Arteriosus: 2018 AHA/ACC Guidelines for ACHD			
I	C-EO	1. Measurement of oxygen saturation should be performed in feet and both hands in adults with a PDA to assess for the presence of right-to-left shunting	
I	C-LD		1. PDA closure in adults is recommended if left atrial or LV enlargement is present and attributable to PDA with net left-to-right shunt, PA systolic pressure less than 50% systemic and pulmonary vascular resistance less than one third systemic
IIa	C-EO	1. In addition to the standard diagnostic tools, cardiac catheterization can be useful in patients with PDA and suspected pulmonary hypertension	
IIb	B-NR		1. PDA closure in adults may be considered in the presence of a net left-to-right shunt if PA systolic pressure is 50% or greater systemic, and/or pulmonary vascular resistance is greater than one third systemic
III	C-LD		1. PDA closure should not be performed in adults with a net right-to-left shunt and PA systolic pressure greater than two thirds systemic or pulmonary vascular resistance greater than two thirds systemic

COR	LOE	Diagnostic	Therapeutic
Patent Ductus Arteriosus: 2020 ESC Guidelines for ACHD			
I	C		1. In patients with evidence of LV volume overload and no PAH (no non-invasive signs of PAP elevation or invasive confirmation of PVR <3 WU in case of such signs), PDA closure is recommended regardless of symptoms. 2. Device closure is recommended as the method of choice when technically suitable.
IIa	C		1. In patients who have developed PAH with PVR 3-5 WU, PDA closure should be considered when there is still significant L-R shunt (Qp:Qs >1.5).
IIb	C		1. In patients who have developed PAH with PVR ≥ 5 WU, PDA closure may be considered when there is still significant L-R shunt (Qp:Qs >1.5) but careful individual decision in expert centers is required.
III	C		1. PDA closure is not recommended in patients with Eisenmenger physiology and patients with lower limb desaturation on exercise.

Abbreviations: L–R, left-to-right; LV, left ventricle/ventricular; PAH, pulmonary arterial hypertension; PAP, pulmonary artery pressure; PDA, patent ductus arteriosus; PVR, pulmonary vascular.

In adults with a large PDA and evidence of pulmonary hypertension, the use of pulmonary vasodilator medications may be of benefit in altering pulmonary vascular physiology to permit eventual closure, analogous to what has been presented in the sections on ASDs and VSDs with pulmonary hypertension. These medications may also improve outcomes in patients with a PDA and ES.

Methods of PDA Closure

Currently, transcatheter PDA closure is the standard of care using one of multiple devices available and specifically designed for this purpose.[108–110] Surgical closure is reserved only for infants, or in patients with anatomy that precludes transcatheter closure. Surgical closure involves a lateral thoracotomy and ligation. Both transcatheter and surgical closure have very low rates of mortality;[109,11,112] however, surgical closure may rarely be associated with a risk of unilateral vocal cord paralysis due to the location of the recurrent laryngeal nerve adjacent to the PDA.[113]

Long-Term Outcomes and Prognosis

There is a paucity of information on the long-term outcomes with an unrepaired PDA. Data from earlier eras had samples biased by individuals with clinically significant or auscultable shunts who presented for medical attention.[114] The majority of lesions discovered in the current era with significant shunting are closed during childhood. In contrast, data on PDAs which are too small to produce a murmur, LA or LV enlargement are limited by unknown numbers of undiagnosed individuals who die for reasons unrelated to the defect.

Individuals with a PDA are prone to endarteritis; however, the actual incidence is unknown for the reasons outlined above. It is not currently recommended that otherwise clinically silent PDAs be closed to prevent endarteritis, or that patients with a PDA receive endocarditis prophylaxis. Incident endarteritis appears to have been decreasing in the PDA population; however, the degree to which this is attributable to protection offered by PDA closure or dilution of incident cases by greater numbers of individuals identified with PDAs is unknown.[115,116]

In individuals with large PDAs, prognosis is likely poor without repair. Patients with large PDAs will typically come to medical attention early after birth, because pulmonary vascular resistance declines in the neonatal period. As the impedance of the pulmonary vascular bed decreases, the degree of left-to-right shunting will increase imposing a volume load on the LV with accompanying large demands on the LV for cardiac output. As a result, these infants develop pulmonary vascular congestion, pulmonary edema, and evidence of hypoperfusion of systemic organs characteristic of heart failure. With judicious medical therapy, these symptoms of heart failure may be managed to permit closure. As in the case of VSDs, unrepaired moderate and large sized PDAs will eventually lead to secondary pulmonary vascular disease and eventually to ES. Pulmonary vascular disease without ES is associated with a significantly increased risk for heart failure, arrhythmia, and sudden death.

EISENMENGER SYNDROME

Background

ES is a condition that occurs when there has been severe and irreversible pulmonary vascular damage as a result of exposure of the pulmonary vascular bed to chronic left-to-right shunting.[53] The probability of ES developing depends on the degree of shunting, whether the pulmonary vascular bed was exposed to elevated pressures as a result of left to right shunting and underlying genetic susceptibility.[117] In ES, pulmonary vascular damage has progressed to the point at which impedance to flow through the pulmonary vascular bed exceeds that of the systemic vascular bed, resulting in reversal of shunt direction and associated systemic cyanosis.[118]

Pathophysiology

When pulmonary vascular damage occurs as a result of chronic exposure to shunt lesions, histologic changes similar to those seen in primary pulmonary hypertension, resulting eventually in plexiform lesions characteristic of irreversible pulmonary vascular disease.[119] The probability of developing ES is not equal for all shunt lesions. Individuals with a larger degree of left-to-right shunting are more likely to develop ES.[117] The combination of high levels of shunting with exposure of the pulmonary vascular bed to systemic pressure further increases the probability of developing irreversible pulmonary vascular damage. For this reason, individuals with large VSDs and PDAs are more likely to develop ES than are individuals with ASDs or partially anomalous pulmonary venous return. Overlying these hemodynamic risk factors, individual patients may have a genetic susceptibility to the development of pulmonary hypertension that may lead to earlier development of ES, or the development of ES at lower levels of shunting. Likely genetic susceptibility is responsible for ES development in the majority of cases caused by pre-tricuspid shunting. This underlying susceptibility is also thought to be responsible for the earlier development of ES in Down syndrome patients with shunts.[73]

Once ES has developed, pathophysiology is attributable to two primary factors: exposure of the RV to a systemic load and chronic systemic cyanosis. The RV is ill-equipped to handle severely increased afterload. Over time, exposure of the RV to severely elevated pulmonary vascular impedance leads to RV failure.[120] The probability and timing of RV failure is variable and likely depends on factors outside of simple increases in pulmonary vascular resistance. Nevertheless, heart failure, arrhythmia, and sudden death (attributable to one or both of the preceding) are the most common causes for mortality in ES.[117] In rare cases, significant pulmonary artery enlargement may lead to extrinsic compression of the left main coronary artery and induce cardiac ischemia.[121]

Chronic systemic cyanosis predisposes patients with ES to additional pathological risk. In addition to increasing the risk for end-organ dysfunction due purely to inadequate oxygen delivery, chronic cyanosis results in polycythemia. Increased red blood cell mass increases blood viscosity, further increasing the load on the ventricle and probability of heart failure.

In addition, it may lead to systemic symptoms of hyperviscosity. Hypoxemia and hyperviscosity with an associated decrease in platelet count lead to a predisposition to both thrombosis, including in situ thrombosis and hemorrhage.[122] Increased red blood cell turnover leads to a predisposition to cholelithiasis due to pigment stones, as well as hyperuricemia with associated gouty arthritis. Increased red blood cell production and destruction can also lead to iron deficiency that may be further exacerbated by regular phlebotomy and is itself associated with a worse prognosis.[123]

Finally, chronic right-to-left shunting predisposes patients with ES to systemic embolization of venous material. This may include paradoxical embolization of venous thrombi, air embolism in the setting of intravenous catheter placement, and a predisposition to bacteremia with associated endocarditis and systemic abscesses.

Epidemiology

The prevalence of ES is low and is decreasing in the developed world as a result of early detection and repair of shunting lesions. Epidemiologic studies suggest between 1% and 5% of congenital heart disease patients have ES.[124,125] Prevalence is undoubtedly higher in less developed countries where access to medical care is more limited.

Presentation

History

Without complications, ES patients may be asymptomatic and identifiable only based on presence of visible cyanosis that may be a presenting complaint. Although ES patients universally have compromised exercise tolerance, the insidious onset of symptoms may lead to self-limitation and may not be recognized in many cases.[126] Patients may also have chest pain attributable either to the presence of significant pulmonary hypertension or to compromised blood flow in the left-main coronary artery in the setting of compression by a dilated main pulmonary artery.[121] In the great majority of cases, however, the symptoms with which ES patients present will depend on which complication of ES they may be experiencing. In the presence of heart failure, ES patients may present with exertional dyspnea and peripheral edema. In the setting of arrhythmia, ES patients may complain of palpitations, syncope, or presyncope.

In the setting of polycythemia, patients may present with symptoms of cholelithiasis including right upper quadrant pain with fatty meal consumption, gouty arthritic pain, or symptoms of hyperviscosity including fatigue, vertigo, visual disturbances, or disrupted consciousness. In situ thrombosis may lead to local pain at the site of thrombus formation, while bleeding may lead to easy bruisability or pulmonary hemorrhage. In the setting of endocarditis or systemic abscess, patients may present with fevers and sepsis.

Physical Examination

In the great majority of cases, findings typical of chronic cyanosis and lung disease on physical exam confirm a diagnosis of ES. These include peripheral or central cyanosis and digital clubbing. In the unique situation of a large PDA with ES, these findings may be present only in the lower extremities. As net shunting is modest, a shunt murmur that may previously have been present will be diminished or absent. Due to pulmonary hypertension, there may be an accentuation of P2, and patients may exhibit a Graham Steell murmur.

Work-Up/Investigations

Electrocardiography

The ECG will typically reveal evidence for RV hypertrophy including right axis deviation (except in cases of primum ASD that will have left axis deviation), disturbed RV conduction, and persistence of large S waves into the left-sided precordial leads.

Chest Radiography

There may be large central pulmonary arteries, with a paucity of pulmonary vascular markings in the peripheral lung fields. In cases where previously cardiomegaly was present due to shunting, this may have resolved and the cardiac silhouette may be normal sized. There may be evidence of RV or RA enlargement, in particular in cases of RV failure.

Laboratory Studies

ES is a multisystem disease. Regular work-up and longitudinal management require monitoring of the common complications related to ES. These include regular complete blood counts, assessment of iron stores with ferritin and transferrin saturation,[123] evaluation of renal function, electrolytes and liver function with a comprehensive metabolic panel, assessment of uric acid levels, and assessment of B-type natriuretic peptide and potentially C-reactive protein that have been demonstrated to be of prognostic significance.[127,128]

Echocardiography

Echocardiography is a central component of the work-up and long-term management of ES. Echo permits rapid and accurate assessment of biventricular function, in the majority of cases will reveal the shunt lesion responsible for ES and the direction of shunting, and can provide an indirect assessment of RV systolic pressures. Echocardiographic parameters of RV function including tricuspid annular plane systolic excursion and evidence of RV remodeling and failure correlate with prognosis in ES.[129,130] TEE is used primarily as an adjunct in cases where TTE windows are inadequate.

CCT and CMR

Gated contrast-enhanced CCT permits delineation of the shunt lesion responsible for ES. In addition, CCT angiography reveals the size of the pulmonary artery and may uncover evidence of left main coronary artery compression by the dilated main pulmonary artery when present.

In addition to the anatomical definition provided by CCT, CMR imaging will reveal the degree and direction of shunting. This is particularly important in cases of PDA in which catheterization-based assessment of shunting is not reliable.

Cardiac Catheterization

Cardiac catheterization is the definitive test to establish a diagnosis of ES. In general, after the diagnosis has been made,

TABLE 66–5. Pulmonary Arterial Hypertension associated with Congenital Heart Disease and Eisenmenger Syndrome: 2018 AHA/ACC Guidelines for ACHD

COR	LOE	Diagnostic	Therapeutic
I	C-EO	1. When evaluating adults with presumed Eisenmenger syndrome, clinicians should confirm diagnostic imaging and cardiac catheterization data accuracy and exclude other potential contributors to right-to-left shunting or pulmonary hypertension.	
I	A		1. Bosentan is beneficial in symptomatic adults with Eisenmenger syndrome with ASD or VSD
IIa	B-R		1. In symptomatic adults with Eisenmenger syndrome, bosentan and PDE-5 inhibitors are reasonable in combination if symptomatic improvement does not occur with either medication alone
IIa	B-NR		1. Bosentan is a reasonable therapy to treat symptomatic adults with Eisenmenger syndrome with 1 of the following: shunts other than ASD/VSD (e.g., PDA, aortopulmonary window) (Level of Evidence C-EO), or complex congenital heart lesions or Down syndrome
IIa	B-NR		1. It is reasonable to use PDE-5 inhibitors (e.g., sildenafil, tadalafil) to treat symptomatic adults with Eisenmenger syndrome with ASD, VSD, or great artery shunt

Pulmonary Arterial Hypertension associated with Congenital Heart Disease and Eisenmenger Syndrome: 2020 ESC Guidelines for ACHD

COR	LOE	Recommendations
I	C	1. It is recommended that patients with CHD and confirmed pre-capillary PH are counselled against pregnancy. 2. Risk assessment is recommended in all patients with PAH-CHD.
I	A	1. In low- and intermediate-risk patients with repaired simple lesions and pre-capillary PH, initial oral combination therapy or sequential combination therapy is recommended and high-risk patients should be treated with initial combination therapy including parenteral prostanoids.
IIa	B	1. In Eisenmenger patients with reduced exercise capacity (6MWT distance <450 m), a treatment strategy with initial endothelin receptor antagonist monotherapy should be considered followed by combination therapy if patients fail to improve.

Abbreviations: 6MWT, 6-minute walk test; CHD, congenital heart disease; PAH-CHD, pulmonary arterial hypertension associated with congenital heart disease; PH, pulmonary hypertension.

clinical assessments and degree of oxygen desaturation may be followed as surrogates for the health of the pulmonary vascular bed.[131] Pulmonary vasoreactivity testing has no real role in the management of ES.[132]

6-Minute Walk Testing

Adopted from practice in patients with isolated pulmonary vascular disease, 6-minute walk testing (6MWT) provides prognostic information and can be regularly assessed as an objective measure of treatment response. The degree of systemic desaturation with exertion on 6MWT provides useful physiologic information in assessing the interaction between the pulmonary and systemic vascular beds during exertion.[132]

Management [Table 66-5]

In ES, definitive surgical repair of shunt lesions is no longer possible. Treatment therefore focuses on optimizing physiology and preventing sequelae of chronic right-to-left shunting and cyanosis (**Table 66-5**).

Medical Therapy

The overall goal of disease-targeted medical management in ES is to decrease RV afterload (and thus probability of RV failure)

without inducing excessive right-to-left shunting that may result in further clinical deterioration. Due to the comparative rarity of ES, there are few clinical trials investigating therapy in this unique group of patients. Pulmonary vasodilator therapy, in particular endothelin receptor antagonism (ERA) with Bosentan was proven to improve 6MWT and hemodynamics in the BREATHE-5 clinical trial.[133-135] The fact that a trial with a newer ERA Macitentan failed to demonstrate similar findings may temper enthusiasm, and suggests that the benefits of ERA therapy may be heterogeneous.[88] Other small studies and retrospective studies suggest that type 5 phosphodiesterase inhibition (PDE5i) alone or in combination with ERAs may improve clinical outcomes,[136,137] and there are limited data in favor of prostaglandin therapy in ES.[138,139] Angiotensin-converting enzyme inhibitors and angiotensin receptor blockers may increase the degree of right-to-left shunting and induce hypotension, which may preclude therapy with pulmonary vasodilators. These agents may still be used in cases of systemic hypertension; however, they are of unclear benefit in the natural history of ES. β-blockers have been shown to decrease mortality (likely through prevention of sudden death) while digoxin use may be associated with increased mortality.[125]

Mineralocorticoid blockade has not been investigated in ES; however, it has few side effects and may be of benefit based on extrapolation from preclinical and limited clinical data in the pulmonary hypertension literature.[140,141] There is little evidence of benefit from chronic oxygen therapy.

An essential component of ES management is prevention of adverse sequelae related to ES. Patients with ES require antibiotic prophylaxis prior to dental procedures as well as fastidious management of intravenous lines to avoid injection of air or particulate material. While ES patients have been demonstrated to experience in situ thrombosis, regular anticoagulation may increase risk of pulmonary hemorrhage and is not routinely recommended unless there is an unrelated reason for anticoagulation such as atrial arrhythmia or presence of a mechanical valve prosthesis. When anticoagulation is necessary, vitamin K antagonism is recommended to ensure reversibility in case of bleeding. Maintenance of replete iron stores is associated with improved outcomes in ES, which in some cases may require regular oral iron supplementation. Finally, given the acute balance between pulmonary and systemic vascular resistance in ES, patients may be uniquely susceptible to severe sequelae in the setting of pulmonary infections. Regular immunization against influenza and pneumococcus are therefore recommended.

As in other forms of severe, irreversible pulmonary hypertension, pregnancy is contraindicated. Nonestrogen-containing, durable forms of contraception are recommended in ES patients to avoid both pregnancy and the risk of thrombophilia associated with estrogen use.

Phlebotomy

ES patients are prone to hyperviscosity attributable to polycythemia. As a result, it is essential that ES patients avoid dehydration. Nevertheless, regular phlebotomy with associated iron deficiency is associated with adverse events.[123] Therefore, phlebotomy should be avoided outside of individuals with symptomatic hyperviscosity. In these individuals, removed volume should be immediately replaced with saline to dilute polycythemia, and iron stores should be assiduously monitored.

Surgical Therapy

In rare cases, aggressive therapy with pulmonary vasodilator medication may improve pulmonary vascular resistance to the point where closure or partial closure of defects may be an option, as outlined in the preceding sections of this chapter. In general, however, the only surgical option for ES patients is either a lung transplant or heart–lung transplant. Decision-making regarding timing and need for lung alone versus heart–lung transplant require individualized evaluation in specialized care centers.

Outcomes and Prognosis

Interestingly, patients with ES have a generally better prognosis than those with primary pulmonary hypertension or those who develop pulmonary hypertension after shunt closure.[142] The reasons for this are unclear but may have to do with RV adaptation during postnatal development and underlying genetic susceptibility to disease progression. In addition, the presence of a patent shunt allows for maintenance of LV filling in the setting of RV failure, preventing catastrophic hypotension. Individuals with ES attributable to either a VSD or PDA have a better prognosis than those with pre-tricuspid valve shunting, possibly due to earlier acclimatization of the ventricle to increased afterload, or due to as yet undetermined genetic susceptibility responsible for the development of ES in patients with pre-tricuspid shunts.[117] Given small numbers and the heterogeneous nature of the ES population, prognosis is difficult to objectively evaluate but appears to be poor. Five-year survival rates are estimated to be between 74% and 81% with 10-year survival of only 57%.[125,130,142] Increased age and evidence of physiologic decompensation including decreased exercise tolerance, decreased functional class, evidence of RV dysfunction on echo, and elevated B-type natriuretic peptide are associated with worse prognosis.[131]

REFERENCES

1. Stout KK, et al. 2018 AHA/ACC guideline for the management of adults with congenital heart disease: executive summary. *J Am Coll Cardiol.* 2019;73(12):1494-1563. doi: 10.1016/j.jacc.2018.08.1028

2. Van Praagh S, Carrera ME, Sanders SP, Mayer JE, Van Praagh R. Sinus venosus defects: unroofing of the right pulmonary veins-Anatomic and echocardiographic findings and surgical treatment. *Am Heart J.* 1994; 128(2):365-379.

3. Raghib G, et al. Termination of left superior vena cava in left atrium, atrial septal defect, and absence of coronary sinus; a developmental complex. *Circulation.* 1965;31:906-918.

4. Kamphuis VP, et al. Electrical remodeling after percutaneous atrial septal defect closure in pediatric and adult patients. *Int J Cardiol.* 2019;285:32-39.

5. Sugimoto M, et al. Volume overload and pressure overload due to left-to-right shunt-induced myocardial injury: evaluation using a highly sensitive cardiac troponin-I assay in children with congenital heart disease. *Circ J.* 2011;75(9):2213-2219.

6. Steele PM, Fuster V, Cohen M, Ritter DG, McGoon DC. Isolated atrial septal defect with pulmonary vascular obstructive disease—long-term follow-up and prediction of outcome after surgical correction. *Circulation.* 1987;76(5):1037-1042.

7. Gabriels C, et al. A different view on predictors of pulmonary hypertension in secundum atrial septal defect. *Int J Cardiol.* 2014;176(3):833-840.

8. Hoffman JIE, Kaplan S, Liberthson RR. Prevalence of congenital heart disease. *Am Heart J.* 2004;147(3):425-439.

9. Marelli AJ, et al. Lifetime prevalence of congenital heart disease in the general population from 2000 to 2010. *Circulation.* 2014;130(9):749-56.

10. Liu Y, et al. Global birth prevalence of congenital heart defects 1970-2017: updated systematic review and meta-analysis of 260 studies. *Int J Epidemiol.* 2019;48(2):455-463.

11. Stallmeyer B, Fenge H, Nowak-Göttl U, Schulze-Bahr E. Mutational spectrum in the cardiac transcription factor gene NKX2.5 (CSX) associated with congenital heart disease. *Clin Genet.* 2010;78(6):533-540.

12. Basson CT, et al. Different TBX5 interactions in heart and limb defined by Holt-Oram syndrome mutations. *Proc Natl Acad Sci USA.* 1999;96(6):2919-2924.

13. Jenkins KJ, et al. Noninherited risk factors and congenital cardiovascular defects: current knowledge—A scientific statement from the American Heart Association Council on Cardiovascular Disease in the Young. *Circulation.* 2007;115(23):2995-3014.

14. Silvestry FE, et al. Guidelines for the echocardiographic assessment of atrial septal defect and patent foramen ovale: from the American Society

of Echocardiography and Society for Cardiac Angiography and Intervention. *J Am Soc Echocardiogr.* 2015;28(8):910-958.

15. Kim H, et al. Partially unroofed coronary sinus: MDCT and MRI findings. *Am J Roentgenol.* 2010;195(5). doi: 10.2214/AJR.09.3689

16. Teo K, et al. Assessment of atrial septal defects in adults comparing cardiovascular magnetic resonance with transoesophageal echocardiography. *J Cardiovasc Magn Reson.* 2010;12(1). doi: 10.1186/1532-429X-12-44

17. Powell AJ, Tsai-Goodman B, Prakash A, Greil GF, Geva T. Comparison between phase-velocity cine magnetic resonance imaging and invasive oximetry for quantification of atrial shunts. *Am J Cardiol.* 2003; 91(12):1523-1525.

18. Oster M, Bhatt AB, Zaragoza-Macias E, Dendukuri N, Marelli A. Interventional therapy versus medical therapy for secundum atrial septal defect: a systematic review (part 2) for the 2018 AHA/ACC guideline for the management of adults with congenital heart disease: a report of the American College of Cardiology/American Heart Association Task Force on Clinical Practice Guidelines. *Circulation.* 2019;139(14):E814-E830.

19. Attie F, et al. Surgical treatment for secundum atrial septal defects in patients >40 years old: a randomized clinical trial. *J Am Coll Cardiol.* 2001;38(7):2035-2042.

20. Konstantinides S, et al. A comparison of surgical and medical therapy for atrial septal defect in adults. *N Engl J Med.* 1995;333(8):469-473.

21. Murphy JG, et al. Long-term outcome after surgical repair of isolated atrial septal defect: follow-up at 27 to 32 years. *N Engl J Med.* 1990;323(24):1645-1650.

22. Brochu MC, et al. Improvement in exercise capacity in asymptomatic and mildly symptomatic adults after atrial septal defect percutaneous closure. *Circulation.* 2002;106(14):1821-1826.

23. Roos-Hesselink JW, et al. Excellent survival and low incidence of arrhythmias, stroke and heart failure long-term after surgical ASD closure at young age: a prospective follow-up study of 21-33 years. *Eur Heart J.* 2003;24(2):190-197.

24. Dave KS, Pakrashi BC, Wooler GH, Ionescu MI. Atrial septal defect in adults. Clinical and hemodynamic results of surgery. *Am J Cardiol.* 1973;31(1):7-13.

25. Fischer G, Smevik B, Kramer HH, Björnstad PG. Catheter-based closure of atrial septal defects in the oval fossa with the Amplatzer® device in patients in their first or second year of life. *Catheter Cardiovasc Interv.* 2009;73(7):949-955.

26. Moore J, et al. Transcatheter device closure of atrial septal defects: a safety review. *JACC Cardiovasc Interv.* 2013;6(5):433-442.

27. Du ZD, Hijazi ZM, Kleinman CS, Silverman NH, Larntz K. Comparison between transcatheter and surgical closure of secundum atrial septal defect in children and adults: results of a multicenter nonrandomized trial. *J Am Coll Cardiol.* 2002;39(11):1836-1844.

28. Veldtman GR, et al. Right ventricular form and function after percutaneous atrial septal defect device closure. *J Am Coll Cardiol.* 2001;37(8):2108-2113.

29. Kort HW, Balzer DT, Johnson MC. Resolution of right heart enlargement after closure of secundum atrial septal defect with transcatheter technique. *J Am Coll Cardiol.* 2001;38(5):1528-1532.

30. Fujino T, et al. Targeted therapy is required for management of pulmonary arterial hypertension after defect closure in adult patients with atrial septal defect and associated pulmonary arterial hypertension. *Int Heart J.* 2015;56(1):86-93.

31. Bradley EA, et al. "Treat-to-close": Non-repairable ASD-PAH in the adult: results from the North American ASD-PAH (NAAP) Multicenter Registry. *Int J Cardiol.* 2019;291:127-133.

32. Bradley EA, Chakinala M, Billadello JJ. Usefulness of medical therapy for pulmonary hypertension and delayed atrial septal defect closure. *Am J Cardiol.* 2013;112(9):1471-1476.

33. Kijima Y, et al. Treat and repair strategy in patients with atrial septal defect and significant pulmonary arterial hypertension. *Circ J.* 2016;80(1):227-234.

34. Yan C, et al. Combination of F-ASO and targeted medical therapy in patients with secundum ASD and severe PAH. *JACC Cardiovasc Interv.* 2020;13(17):2024-2034.

35. Song J, et al. Hemodynamic follow-up in adult patients with pulmonary hypertension associated with atrial septal defect after partial closure. *Yonsei Med J.* 2016;57(2):306.

36. Masutani S, Senzaki H. Left ventricular function in adult patients with atrial septal defect: implication for development of heart failure after transcatheter closure. *J Card Fail.* 2011;17(11):957-963.

37. Takaya Y, et al. Long-term outcome after transcatheter closure of atrial septal defect in older patients: impact of age at procedure. *JACC Cardiovasc Interv.* 2015;8(4):600-606.

38. Kenny D, et al. A randomized, controlled, multi-center trial of the efficacy and safety of the Occlutech Figulla Flex-II Occluder compared to the Amplatzer Septal Occluder for transcatheter closure of secundum atrial septal defects. *Catheter Cardiovasc Interv.* 2019;93(2):316-321.

39. Batteux C, Meliani A, Brenot P, Hascoet S. Multimodality fusion imaging to guide percutaneous sinus venosus atrial septal defect closure. *Eur Heart J.* 2020;41(46):4444-4445. doi: 10.1093/eurheartj/ehaa292

40. Gertz ZM, Strife BJ, Shah PR, Parris K, Grizzard JD. CT angiography for planning of percutaneous closure of a sinus venosus atrial septal defect using a covered stent. *J Cardiovasc Comput Tomogr.* 2018;12(2):174-175.

41. Butera G, et al. Percutaneous versus surgical closure of secundum atrial septal defects: a systematic review and meta-analysis of currently available clinical evidence. *EuroIntervention.* 2011;7(3):377-385.

42. Udholm S, et al. Lifelong burden of small unrepaired atrial septal defect: results from the Danish National Patient Registry. *Int J Cardiol.* 2019;283:101-106.

43. Campbell M. Natural history of atrial septal defect. *Br Heart J.* 1970;32(6): 820-826.

44. Nyboe C, Karunanithi Z, Nielsen-Kudsk JE, Hjortdal VE. Long-term mortality in patients with atrial septal defect: a nationwide cohort-study. *Eur Heart J.* 2018;39(12):993-998.

45. Penny DJ, Vick GW. Ventricular septal defect. *Lancet.* 2011;377(9771): 1103-1112.

46. Li X, Ren W, Song G, Zhang X. Prediction of spontaneous closure of ventricular septal defect and guidance for clinical follow-up. *Clin Cardiol.* 2019;42(5):536-541.

47. Lamers WH, et al. New findings concerning ventricular septation in the human heart: Implications for maldevelopment. *Circulation.* 1992; 86(4):1194-1205.

48. Van Praagh R, Geva T, Kreutzer J. Ventricular septal defects: how shall we describe, name and classify them? *J Am Coll Cardiol.* 1989;14(5):1298-1299.

49. Jacobs JP, Burke RP, Quintessenza JA, Mavroudis C. Congenital heart surgery nomenclature and database project: ventricular septal defect. *Ann Thoracic Surg.* 2000;69:S25-S35.

50. Magee AG, Fenn L, Vellekoop J, Godman MJ. Left ventricular function in adolescents and adults with restrictive ventricular septal defect and moderate left-to-right shunting. *Cardiol Young.* 2000;10(2):126-129.

51. Stanger P, Lucas RV Jr, Edwards JE. Anatomic factors causing respiratory distress in acyanotic congenital heart diseases. *Pediatrics.* 1969;43:760-9.

52. Neutze JM, et al. Assessment and follow-up of patients with ventricular septal defect and elevated pulmonary vascular resistance. *Am J Cardiol.* 1989;63(5):327-331.

53. Wood P. The Eisenmenger syndrome or pulmonary hypertension with reversed central shunt. *Br Med J.* 1958;2(5099):755.

54. Van Praagh R, McNamara JJ. Anatomic types of ventricular septal defect with aortic insufficiency. Diagnostic and surgical considerations. *Am Heart J.* 1968;75(5):604-619.

55. Tatsuno K, Konno S, Ando M, Sakakibara S. Pathogenic mechanisms of prolapsing aortic valve and aortic regurgitation associated with ventricular septal defect. Anatomical, angiographic and surgical considerations. *Circulation.* 1973;48(5):1028-1037.

56. Gersony WM, et al. Bacterial endocarditis in patients with aortic stenosis, pulmonary stenosis, or ventricular septal defect. *Circulation.* 1993; 87(2 Suppl):I121-I126.

57. Karonis T, et al. Clinical course and potential complications of small ventricular septal defects in adulthood: late development of left ventricular dysfunction justifies lifelong care. *Int J Cardiol.* 2016;208:102-106.

58. Moller JH, Moodie DS, Blees M, Norton JB, Nouri S. Symptomatic heart disease in infants: comparison of three studies performed during 1969-1987. *Pediatr Cardiol.* 1995;16(5):216-222.

59. Hoffman JIE, Kaplan S. The incidence of congenital heart disease. *J Am Coll Cardiol.* 2002;39(12):1890-1900.

60. Ammash NM, Wames CA. Ventricular septal defects in adults. *Ann Intern Med.* 2001;135(9):812-824.

61. Ooshima A, Fukmhige J, Ueda K. Incidence of structural cardiac disorders in neonates: an evaluation by color doppler echocardiography and the results of a 1-year follow-up. *Cardiology.* 1995;86(5):402-406.

62. Roguin N, et al. High prevalence of muscular ventricular septal defect in neonates. *J Am Coll Cardiol.* 1995;26(6):1545-1548.

63. Musewe NN, Hecht BM, Hesslein PS, Rose V, Williams WG. Tricuspid valve endocarditis in two children with normal hearts: diagnosis and therapy of an unusual clinical entity. *J Pediatr.* 1987;110(5):735-738.

64. Marino B, et al. Ventricular septal defect in down syndrome: anatomic types and associated malformations. *Am J Dis Child.* 1990;144(5):544-545.

65. Vaughan CJ, Basson CT. Molecular determinants of atrial and ventricular septal defects and patent ductus arteriosus. *Am J Med Genet.* 2000;97(4):304-309.

66. Walsh MA, et al. Atrioventricular block after transcatheter closure of perimembranous ventricular septal defects. *Heart.* 2006;92(9):1295-1297.

67. Bloomfield DK. The natural history of ventricular septal defect in patients surviving infancy. *Circulation.* 1964;29:914-955.

68. Campbell M. Natural history of ventricular septal defect. *Br Heart J.* 1971;33(2):246-257.

69. Maagaard M, Eckerström F, Redington A, Hjortdal V. Comparison of outcomes in adults with ventricular septal defect closed earlier in life versus those in whom the defect was never closed. *Am J Cardiol.* 2020;133:139-147.

70. Maagaard M, Eckerström F, Boutrup N, Hjortdal VE. Functional capacity past age 40 in patients with congenital ventricular septal defects. *J Am Heart Assoc.* 2020;9(19). doi: 10.1161/JAHA.120.015956

71. Gersony WM, Hayes CJ. Bacterial endocarditis in patients with pulmonary stenosis, aortic stenosis, or ventricular septal defect. *Circulation.* 1977;56(1 Suppl):I84-I87.

72. Clarkson PM, et al. Prognosis for patients with ventricular septal defect and severe pulmonary vascular obstructive disease. *Circulation.* 1968;38(1):129-135.

73. Diller G-P, et al. Survival prospects and circumstances of death in contemporary adult congenital heart disease patients under follow-up at a large tertiary centre. *Circulation.* 2015;132(22):2118-2125.

74. Gutgesell HP, Huhta JC. Cardiac septation in atrioventricular canal defect. *J Am Coll Cardiol.* 1986;8(6):1421-1424.

75. Calkoen EE, et al. Atrioventricular septal defect: from embryonic development to long-term follow-up. *Int J Cardiol.* 2016;202:784-795.

76. Malik M, Khalid Nuri M. Surgical considerations in atrioventricular canal defects. *Semin Cardiothorac Vasc Anesth.* 2017;21(3):229-234.

77. Reeder GS, Danielson GK, Seward JB, Driscoll DJ, Tajik AJ. Fixed subaortic stenosis in atrioventricular canal defect: a Doppler echocardiographic study. *J Am Coll Cardiol.* 1992;20(2):386-394.

78. Minich LLA, et al. Partial and transitional atrioventricular septal defect outcomes. *Ann Thorac Surg.* 2010;89(2):530-536.

79. Ramgren JJ, et al. Long-term outcome after early repair of complete atrioventricular septal defect in young infants. *J Thorac Cardiovasc Surg.* 2021;161(6):2145-2153. doi: 10.1016/j.jtcvs.2020.08.015

80. Colen TM, Khoo NS, Ross DB, Smallhorn JF. Partial zone of apposition closure in atrioventricular septal defect: are papillary muscles the clue? *Ann Thorac Surg.* 2013;96(2):637-643.

81. Atz AM, et al. Surgical management of complete atrioventricular septal defect: associations with surgical technique, age, and trisomy 21. *J Thorac Cardiovasc Surg.* 2011;141(6):1371-1379.

82. Samaának M. Prevalence at birth, "natural" risk and survival with atrioventricular septal defect. *Cardiol Young.* 1991;1(4):285-289.

83. Phoon CK, Neill CA. Asplenia syndrome: insight into embryology through an analysis of cardiac and extracardiac anomalies. *Am J Cardiol.* 1994;73(8):581-587.

84. Peoples WM, Moller JH, Edwards JE. Polysplenia: a review of 146 cases. *Pediatr Cardiol.* 1983;4(2):129-137.

85. Freeman SB, et al. Ethnicity, sex, and the incidence of congenital heart defects: a report from the National Down Syndrome Project. *Genet Med.* 2008;10(3):173-180.

86. Freeman SB et al. Population-based study of congenital heart defects in Down syndrome. *Am J Med Genet.* 1998;80(3):213-217.

87. St. Louis JD, et al. Contemporary outcomes of complete atrioventricular septal defect repair: analysis of the Society of Thoracic Surgeons Congenital Heart Surgery Database. *J Thorac Cardiovasc Surg.* 2014;148(6):2526-2531.

88. Gatzoulis MA, et al. Evaluation of macitentan in patients with Eisenmenger syndrome: results from the randomized, controlled MAESTRO study. *Circulation.* 2019;139(1):51-63.

89. Ren R, He F, Xiao X. Bosentan treatment for pulmonary arterial hypertension due to complete atrioventricular septal defect in an infant with Down's syndrome. *Int J Cardiol.* 2014;177(3):1054-1055.

90. Thébaud B, et al. Oxygen-sensitive Kv channel gene transfer confers oxygen responsiveness to preterm rabbit and remodeled human ductus arteriosus: implications for infants with patent ductus arteriosus. *Circulation.* 2004;110(11):1372-1379.

91. Kajimoto H, et al. Oxygen activates the rho/rho-kinase pathway and induces RhoB and ROCK-1 expression in human and rabbit ductus arteriosus by increasing mitochondria-derived reactive oxygen species: a newly recognized mechanism for sustaining ductal constriction. *Circulation.* 2007;115(13):1777-1788.

92. Thébaud B, et al. Developmental absence of the O2 sensitivity of L-type calcium channels in preterm ductus arteriosus smooth muscle cells impairs O2 constriction contributing to patent ductus arteriosus. *Pediatr Res.* 2008;63(2):176-181.

93. Hong Z, et al. Role of dynamin-related protein 1 (Drp1)-mediated mitochondrial fission in oxygen sensing and constriction of the ductus arteriosus. *Circ Res.* 2013;112(5):802-815.

94. Bouayad A, et al. Characterization of PGE2 receptors in fetal and newborn lamb ductus arteriosus. *Am J Physiol: Hear Circ Physiol.* 2001;280(5). doi: 10.1152/ajpheart.2001.280.5.h2342

95. Freed MD, Heymann MA, Lewis AB. Prostaglandin E1 in infants with ductus arteriosus dependent congenital heart disease. *Circulation.* 1981;64(5):899-905.

96. Waleh N, et al. Prostaglandin E2-mediated relaxation of the ductus arteriosus: effects of gestational age on G protein-coupled receptor expression, signaling, and vasomotor control. *Circulation.* 2004;110(16):2326-2332.

97. Clyman RI, et al. Cyclooxygenase-2 plays a significant role in regulating the tone of the fetal lamb ductus arteriosus. *Am J Physiol: Regul Integr Comp Physiol.* 1999;276(3). doi: 10.1152/ajpregu.1999.276.3.r913

98. Shiraishi H, Yanagisawa M. Bidirectional flow through the ductus arteriosus in normal newborns: evaluation by Doppler color flow imaging. *Pediatr Cardiol.* 1991;12(4):201-205.

99. Mitchell SC, Korones SB, Berendes HW. Congenital heart disease in 56,109 births. Incidence and natural history. *Circulation.* 1971;43(3):323-332.

100. Dickinson DF, Arnold R, Wilkinson JL. Congenital heart disease among 160,480 liveborn children in Liverpool 1960 to 1969. Implications for surgical treatment. *Br Heart J.* 1981;46(1):55-62.

101. Schneider DJ, Moore JW. Patent ductus arteriosus. *Circulation.* 2006;114(17):1873-1882.

102. Gittenberger-De Groot AC, Moulaert AJM, Hitchcock JF. Histology of the persistent ductus arteriosus in cases of congenital rubella. *Circulation.* 1980;62(1):183-186.

103. Webster WS. Teratogen update: Congenital rubella. *Teratology.* 1998; 58(1):13-23.

104. Hiraishi S, et al. Noninvasive Doppler echocardiographic evaluation of shunt flow dynamics of the ductus arteriosus. *Circulation.* 1987;75(6): 1146-1153.

105. Liao PK, Su WJ, Hung JS. Doppler echocardiographic flow characteristics of isolated patent ductus arteriosus: better delineation by Doppler color flow mapping. *J Am Coll Cardiol.* 1988;12(5):1285-1291.

106. Ohlsson A, Walia R, Shah SS. Ibuprofen for the treatment of patent ductus arteriosus in preterm or low birth weight (or both) infants. *Cochrane Database Syst Rev.* 2020;2020(2). doi: 10.1002/14651858.CD003481.pub8

107. Oncel MY, et al. Oral paracetamol versus oral ibuprofen in the management of patent ductus arteriosus in preterm infants: a randomized controlled trial. *J Pediatr.* 2014;164(3). doi: 10.1016/j.jpeds.2013.11.008

108. Francis E, Singhi AK, Lakshmivenkateshaiah S, Kumar RK. Transcatheter occlusion of patent ductus arteriosus in pre-term infants. *JACC Cardiovasc Interv.* 2010;3(5):550-555.

109. El-Said HG, et al. Safety of percutaneous patent ductus arteriosus closure: an unselected multicenter population experience. *J Am Heart Assoc.* 2013;2(6). doi: 10.1161/JAHA.113.000424

110. Rashkind WJ, Mullins CE, Hellenbrand WE, Tait MA. Nonsurgical closure of patent ductus arteriosus: clinical application of the Rashkind PDA Occluder System. *Circulation.* 1987;75(3):583-592.

111. Mavroudis C, et al. Forty-six years of patent ductus arteriosus division at Children's Memorial Hospital of Chicago: standards for comparison. *Ann Surg.* 1994:402-410.

112. Hutchings K, et al. Outcomes following neonatal patent ductus arteriosus ligation done by pediatric surgeons: a retrospective cohort analysis. *J. Pediatr Surg.* 2013:915-918.

113. Strychowsky JE, Rukholm G, Gupta MK, Reid D. Unilateral vocal fold paralysis after congenital cardiothoracic surgery: a meta-analysis. *Pediatrics.* 2014;133(6). doi: 10.1542/peds.2013-3939

114. Coggin CJ, Parker KR, Keith JD. Natural history of isolated patent ductus arteriosus and the effect of surgical correction: twenty years' experience at The Hospital for Sick Children, Toronto. *Can Med Assoc J.* 1970; 102(7):718-720.

115. Sadiq M, Latif F, Ur-Rehman A. Analysis of infective endarteritis in patent ductus arteriosus. *Am J Cardiol.* 2004;93(4):513-515.

116. Fortescue EB, Lock JE, Galvin T, McElhinney DB. To close or not to close: the very small patent ductus arteriosus. *Congenit Heart Dis.* 2010; 5(4):354-365.

117. Kempny A, et al. Predictors of death in contemporary adult patients with Eisenmenger syndrome: a multicenter study. *Circulation.* 2017;135(15): 1432-1440.

118. Beghetti M, Galiè N. Eisenmenger syndrome. a clinical perspective in a new therapeutic era of pulmonary arterial hypertension. *J Am Coll Cardiol.* 2009;53(9):733-740.

119. Heath D, Edwards JE. The pathology of hypertensive pulmonary vascular disease; a description of six grades of structural changes in the pulmonary arteries with special reference to congenital cardiac septal defects. *Circulation.* 1958;18(4 Part 1):533-547.

120. Jensen AS, et al. Impaired right, left, or biventricular function and resting oxygen saturation are associated with mortality in Eisenmenger syndrome: a clinical and cardiovascular magnetic resonance study. *Circ Cardiovasc Imaging.* 2015;8(12). doi: 10.1161/CIRCIMAGING.115.003596

121. Dubois CL, Dymarkowski S, Van Cleemput J. Compression of the left main coronary artery by the pulmonary artery in a patient with the Eisenmenger syndrome. *Eur Heart J.* 2007;28(16):1945.

122. Martin-Garcia AC, et al. Platelet count and mean platelet volume predict outcome in adults with Eisenmenger syndrome. *Heart.* 2018;104(1):45-50.

123. Van De Bruaene A, et al. Iron deficiency is associated with adverse outcome in Eisenmenger patients. *Eur Heart J.* 2011;32(22):2790-2799.

124. Engelfriet P, et al. The spectrum of adult congenital heart disease in Europe: morbidity and mortality in a 5 year follow-up period. The Euro Heart Survey on adult congenital heart disease. *Eur Heart J.* 2005;26(21): 2325-2333.

125. Diller GP, et al. Current therapy and outcome of Eisenmenger syndrome: data of the German National Register for congenital heart defects. *Eur Heart J.* 2016;37(18):1449-1455.

126. Kempny A, et al. Reference values for exercise limitations among adults with congenital heart disease. Relation to activities of daily life–single centre experience and review of published data. *Eur Heart J.* 2012; 33(11):1386-1396.

127. Scognamiglio G, et al. C-reactive protein in adults with pulmonary arterial hypertension associated with congenital heart disease and its prognostic value. *Heart.* 2014;100(17):1335-1341.

128. Schuuring MJ, et al. New predictors of mortality in adults with congenital heart disease and pulmonary hypertension: midterm outcome of a prospective study. *Int J Cardiol.* 2015;181:270-276.

129. Moceri P, et al. Echocardiographic predictors of outcome in Eisenmenger syndrome. *Circulation.* 2012;126(12):1461-1468.

130. Moceri P, et al. Cardiac remodelling amongst adults with various aetiologies of pulmonary arterial hypertension including Eisenmenger syndrome—Implications on survival and the role of right ventricular transverse strain. *Eur Heart J Cardiovasc Imaging.* 2017;18(11):1262-1270.

131. Van De Bruaene A, et al. Worsening in oxygen saturation and exercise capacity predict adverse outcome in patients with Eisenmenger syndrome. *Int J Cardiol.* 2013;168(2):1386-1392.

132. Galiè N, et al. 2015 ESC/ERS Guidelines for the diagnosis and treatment of pulmonary hypertension. *Eur Respirat J.* 2015:903-975.

133. Galie N, et al. Bosentan therapy in patients with Eisenmenger syndrome: a multicenter, double-blind, randomized, placebo-controlled study. *Circulation.* 2006;114(1):48-54.

134. Dimopoulos K, et al. Improved survival among patients with Eisenmenger syndrome receiving advanced therapy for pulmonary arterial hypertension. *Circulation.* 2010;121(1):20-25.

135. Hascoët S, et al. Long-term outcomes of pulmonary arterial hypertension under specific drug therapy in Eisenmenger syndrome. *J Heart Lung Transplant.* 2017;36(4):386-398.

136. Iversen K, Jensen AS, Jensen T V., Vejlstrup NG, Søndergaard L. Combination therapy with bosentan and sildenafil in Eisenmenger syndrome: a randomized, placebo-controlled, double-blinded trial. *Eur Heart J.* 2010;31(9):1124-1131.

137. D'Alto M, et al. Bosentan-sildenafil association in patients with congenital heart disease-related pulmonary arterial hypertension and Eisenmenger physiology. *Int J Cardiol.* 2012;155(3):378-382.

138. D'Alto M, et al. The effects of parenteral prostacyclin therapy as add-on treatment to oral compounds in Eisenmenger syndrome. *Eur Respir J.* 2019;54(5). doi: 10.1183/13993003.01401-2019

139. Thomas IC, Glassner-Kolmin C, Gomberg-Maitland M. Long-term effects of continuous prostacyclin therapy in adults with pulmonary hypertension associated with congenital heart disease. *Int J Cardiol.* 2013;168(4):4117-4121.

140. Aghamohammadzadeh R, et al. Up-regulation of the mammalian target of rapamycin complex 1 subunit Raptor by aldosterone induces abnormal pulmonary artery smooth muscle cell survival patterns to promote pulmonary arterial hypertension. *FASEB J.* 2016;30(7):2511-2527.

141. Maron BA, et al. Effectiveness of spironolactone plus ambrisentan for treatment of pulmonary arterial hypertension (from the [ARIES] Study 1 and 2 Trials). *Am J Cardiol.* 2013;112(5):720-725.

142. Barst RJ, Ivy DD, Foreman AJ, McGoon MD, Rosenzweig EB. Four- and seven-year outcomes of patients with congenital heart disease-associated pulmonary arterial hypertension (from the REVEAL Registry). *Am J Cardiol.* 2014;113(1):147-155.

67

Right-Sided Lesions

Konstantinos Dimopoulos and Andrew Constantine

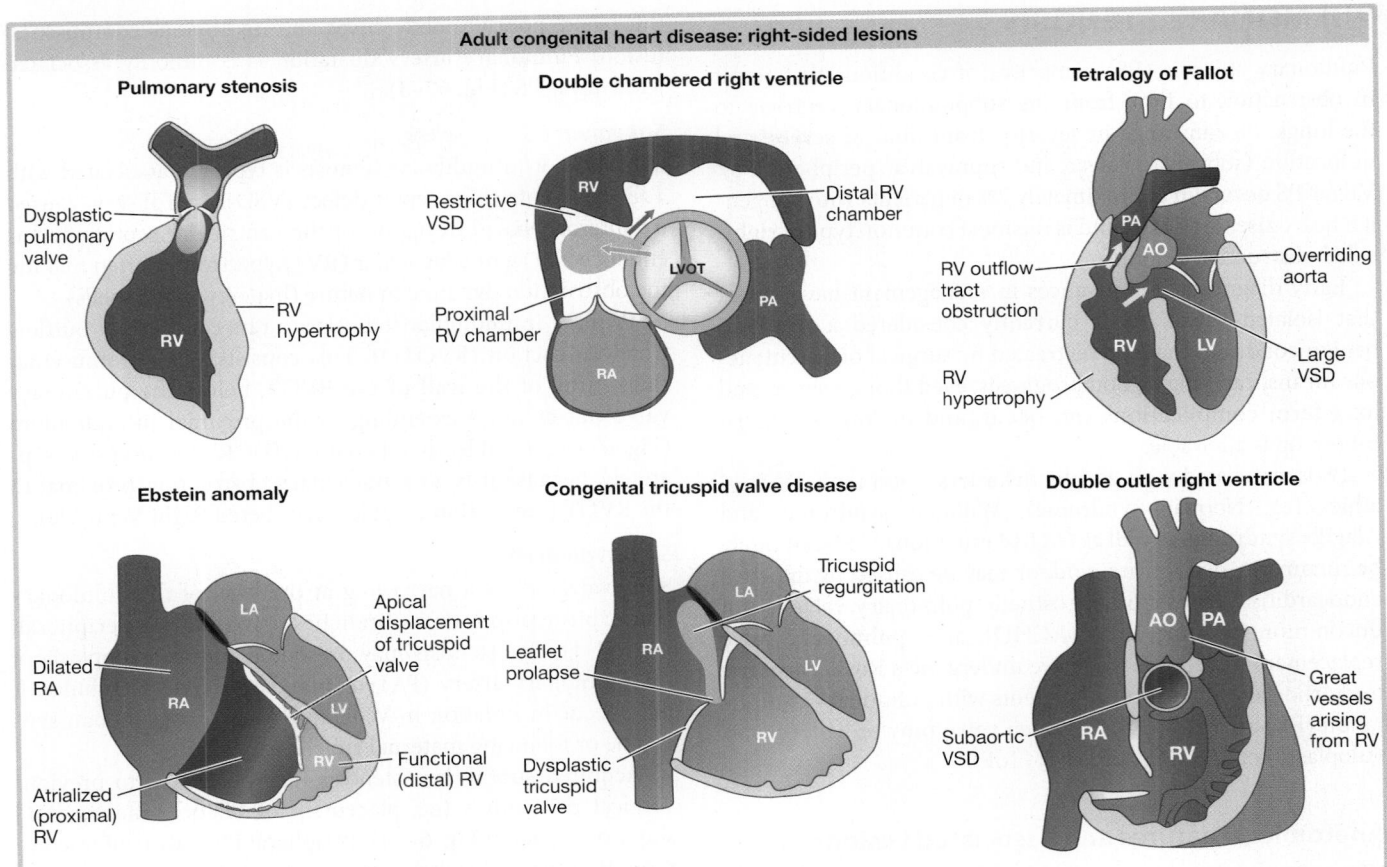

Chapter 67 Fuster and Hurst's Central Illustration. Unlike acquired heart disease, congenital heart disease is frequently a condition of right-sided structures. The anatomical features of each lesion vary in severity between individuals and drive the pathophysiology, clinical presentation and management strategy. AO, aorta; LV, left ventricle; LVOT, left ventricular outflow tract; PA, pulmonary artery; RA, right atrium; RV, right ventricle.

CHAPTER SUMMARY

This chapter provides an overview of the foremost right-sided lesions affecting adults with congenital heart disease (see Fuster and Hurst's Central Illustration), focusing on pathophysiology and clinical management. Right-sided cardiac lesions are typically congenital and include a wide spectrum of conditions of differing complexity. Even "simple" right-sided heart lesions can cause significant right ventricular pressure or volume overload, obstruction of flow to the lungs, and systemic venous congestion. More complex lesions, such as Tetralogy of Fallot, also consist of predominantly right-sided anatomic features and long-term residual right-sided lesions may be present after repair (eg, pulmonary regurgitation). Advances in diagnosis and timely surgical intervention have considerably improved the outlook of these lesions and have minimized long-term complications. However, adults with congenital heart disease remain at risk of long-term sequelae, such as exercise intolerance, right-sided heart failure, and arrhythmias. Long-term specialist care is, therefore, essential, even after successful surgical repair. Expert input and individualized advice are also required in special situations, including pregnancy, noncardiac surgery, and when determining the type and intensity of exercise or sports that patients can practice.

PULMONARY STENOSIS

Pulmonary stenosis (PS) comprises of conditions that result in obstruction to flow from the subpulmonary ventricle to the lungs. PS can range in severity, from mild to severe, and in location (subvalvar, valvar, and supravalvar/peripheral PS). Valvar PS occurs in approximately 7% of patients with congenital heart disease (CHD) and is the most common type of right-sided obstructive lesion.

Early diagnosis and advances in management have meant that isolated valvar PS is currently considered a relatively benign condition that can be treated by surgical or percutaneous means, carrying a good prognosis, even though short- and long-term complications can occur, and lifelong specialist follow-up is advisable.

PS is associated with genetic disorders, commonly RASopathies (eg, Noonan syndrome), Williams syndrome, and Alagille syndrome, as well as *GATA4* mutations.[1,2] PS can rarely be rheumatic, due to carcinoid, or may be caused by infective endocarditis. Stenosis of a prosthetic pulmonary valve is not uncommon in adult CHD (ACHD), after pulmonary valve replacement in patients who have undergone a Ross procedure for aortic valve disease, or in patients with pulmonary regurgitation (PR) after repair of PS (open valvotomy or balloon valvuloplasty) or Tetralogy of Fallot (ToF).

Anatomical Features and Associated Lesions

Valvar PS

Valvar PS (**Fig. 67–1**) is usually an isolated lesion and typically consists of fusion of the commissures of adjacent cusps of the pulmonary valve, leaving a central opening of varying degrees depending on the severity of the stenosis (**Fig. 67–2**). The valve may appear dome-shaped and, in adult patients, thickened and calcific. The number of cusps in a stenotic pulmonary valve may vary between 1 and 4. A "dysplastic" pulmonary valve is often observed in patients with Noonan syndrome, with thickened, poorly mobile cusps and no obvious commissural fusion. Pulmonary artery dilatation is commonly associated with valvar PS (**Fig. 67–3**).

Subvalvar PS

Subvalvar or infundibular stenosis is typically associated with ToF or a ventricular septal defect (VSD). In ToF it is caused by anterocephalad deviation of the ventricular septum and is enhanced by right ventricular (RV) hypertrophy, often making the obstruction dynamic in nature (hypercyanotic spells).

Primary infundibular stenosis is a rare cause of RV outflow tract obstruction (RVOTO). This consists of a fibromuscular thickening of the wall of the RVOT, below the pulmonary valve but at times extending to the proximal infundibulum (Fig. 67–1).[3] Double-chambered RV (DCRV) is discussed separately, because it is an intracavitary obstruction proximal to the RVOT (see section Double-Chambered Right Ventricle).

Supravalvar PS

Supravalvar PS is a narrowing at the level of the pulmonary truck, bifurcation, or its branches (proximal or peripheral, Fig. 67–1). The stenosis may present as diffuse hypoplasia of the pulmonary artery (PA), or may be discrete or tubular. It may occur in isolation in Williams, Alagille, or Noonan syndrome or following maternal rubella exposure.

Acquired supravalvar stenosis may be related to previous surgical procedures (eg, placement of Blalock–Taussig [BT] shunt or PA band; **Fig. 67–4**). Peripheral PS is also not uncommon after arterial switch repair for complete or dextrotransposition of the great arteries (d-TGA), when the Lecompte procedure is used or after surgical pulmonary valve replacement (stenosis at the level of the distal anastomosis; **Fig. 67–5**). In such cases, the main PA is positioned anterior to the aorta, with the branch PAs on either side.

Pulmonary Atresia with Intact Ventricular Septum

Pulmonary atresia is the absence of communication between the subpulmonary ventricle and the pulmonary circulation.

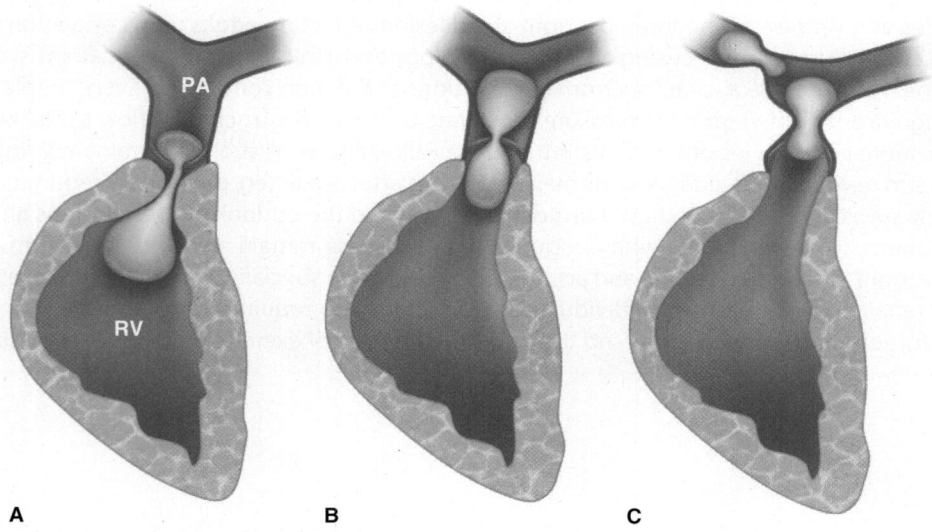

Figure 67–1. Types of pulmonary stenosis. Diagram of the types of pulmonary stenosis: (**A**) Subvalvar, (**B**) valvar, and (**C**) supravalvar/branch pulmonary artery stenosis.

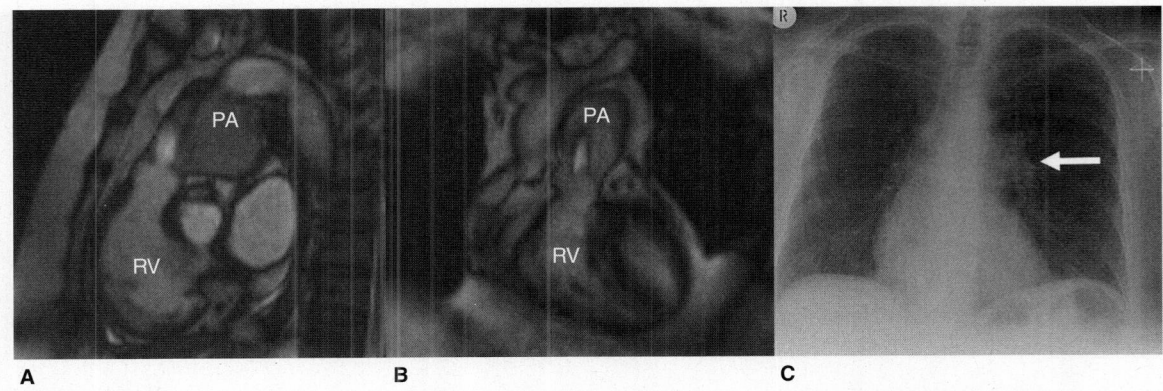

Figure 67–2. Valvar pulmonary stenosis. In (**A**), severe valvar pulmonary stenosis with poststenotic dilatation of the pulmonary artery (PA). Right ventricular (RV) hypertrophy is seen in (**B**). On chest radiography (**C**), the prominent PA is visible (*arrow*).

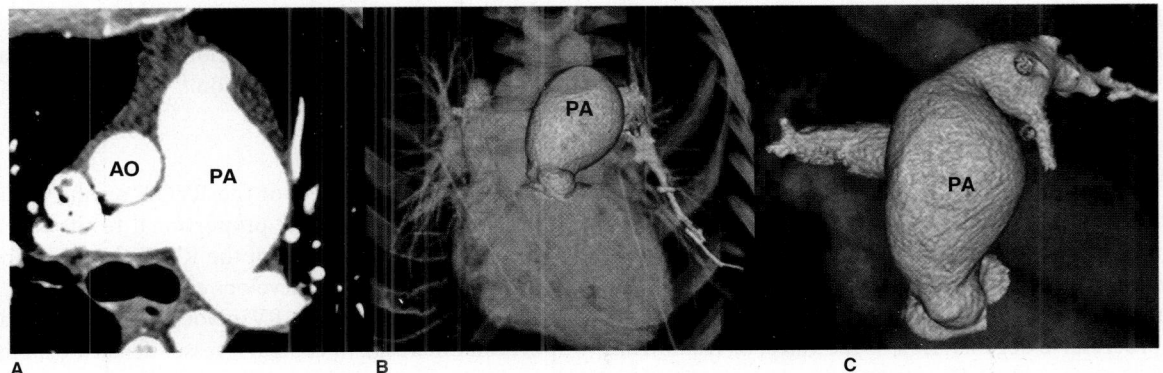

Figure 67–3. Pulmonary artery dilatation after repair of pulmonary stenosis. (**A**) to (**C**) Aneurysmal dilatation of the pulmonary artery (PA) decades after surgical repair of pulmonary stenosis, with residual, severe, long-standing pulmonary regurgitation and mild stenosis. Note the disproportion (in **A**) of the PA compared to the ascending aorta (AO).

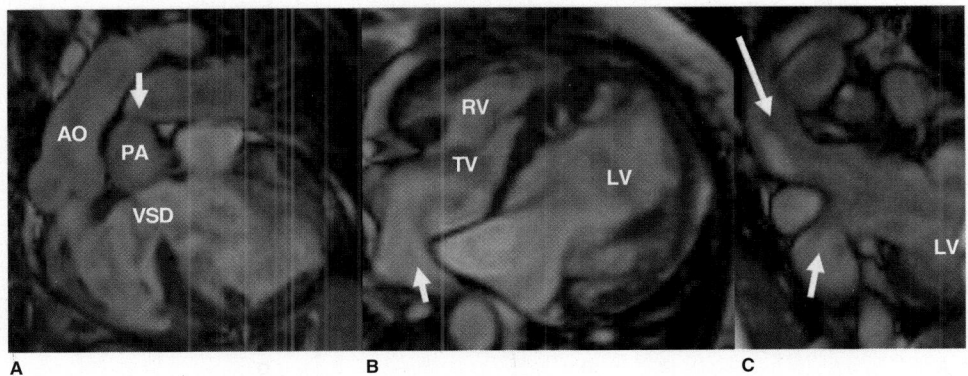

Figure 67–4. Pulmonary artery band causing suprapulmonary stenosis. Patient with TGA and a large VSD who has undergone pulmonary artery (PA) banding (*arrow*) and Mustard (atrial switch) procedure. The PA band (**A**) is causing sufficient suprapulmonary stenosis to protect the pulmonary circulation from developing pulmonary vascular disease. The palliative Mustard procedure allows the VSD to remain open, but redirects pulmonary venous blood (**B**, *arrow*) through the tricuspid valve (TV) into the systemic right ventricle (RV) and the systemic venous blood from the superior and inferior vena cavae (**C**, *long and short arrows*) to the subpulmonary morphologically left ventricle (LV), in an attempt to improve systemic oxygen saturation. AO, aorta.

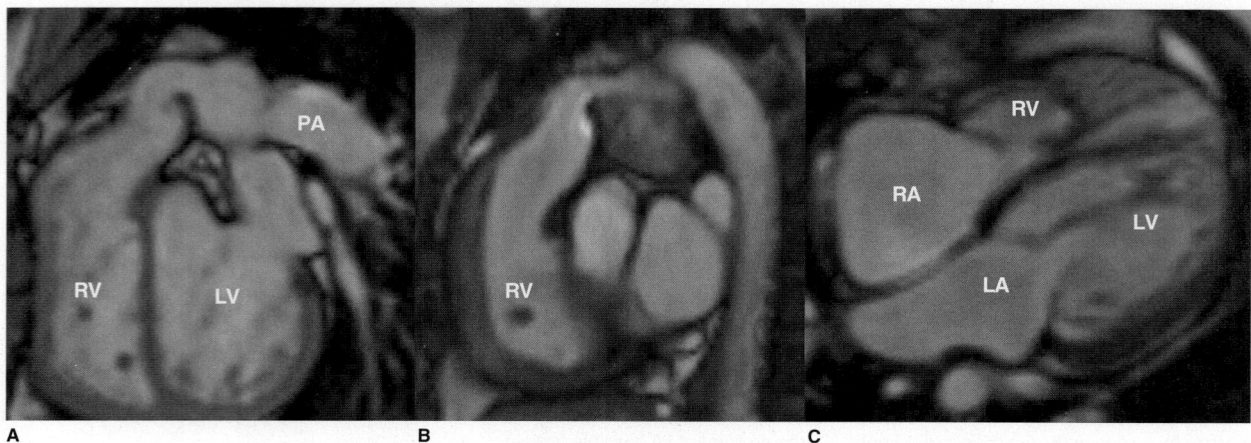

Figure 67–5. Suprapulmonary stenosis after surgical pulmonary valve replacement. Suprapulmonary stenosis after pulmonary valve replacement with homograft. The tortuous stenotic supravalvar segment is visible in (**A**), with flow acceleration in systole (**B**) and evidence of right ventricular hypertrophy (**C**).

Pulmonary atresia may also coexist with other types of CHD (eg, patients with univentricular hearts). Pulmonary atresia with a VSD is described in the section on ToF.

Pulmonary atresia with intact ventricular septum is rare. It is associated with a hypoplastic and restrictive RV, hypoplastic tricuspid valve, and an abnormal coronary artery circulation (RV-dependent coronary circulation, with sinusoids in the RV myocardium that communicate with the coronary arteries).

Prosthetic Pulmonary Valve Stenosis

PS and/or regurgitation may be encountered after pulmonary valve replacement for pulmonary valve disease or as part of the Ross procedure for aortic valve disease (**Fig. 67–6**). PS may be due to progressive degeneration of the valve, or result from thrombosis or endocarditis. Prosthetic valve degeneration may advance rapidly and close monitoring of patients with evidence of progressive stenosis is required.

PS is also common in RV-PA conduits used in the repair of pulmonary atresia, truncus arteriosus, and TGA (Rastelli operation). Infective endocarditis should always be suspected in patients with an RVOT prosthesis and may cause stenosis

or regurgitation of the bioprosthetic pulmonary valve. Percutaneous pulmonary valve prostheses appear to be particularly prone to developing "obstructive endocarditis," at times with rapidly progressive RV dysfunction and decline in cardiac output, requiring urgent intervention.[4]

Pathophysiology

Obstruction at the level of the RVOT results in an increase in RV pressures, typically proportional to the severity of the obstruction. The response of the RV to this pressure overload depends on whether PS develops early or later in life. PS in neonates is accompanied by RV myocyte hyperplasia and a proportional increase in capillary vessel density, enabling the RV to adapt well to the load. When PS develops later in life, RV hypertrophy is associated with a reduction in capillary density and reduced tolerance to severe long-standing PS. On the other hand, severe PS in the neonate may adversely affect the development of the RV cavity and pulmonary arteries and presents with cyanosis (right–left shunting through a patent foramen ovale [PFO]), requiring balloon pulmonary valvuloplasty early

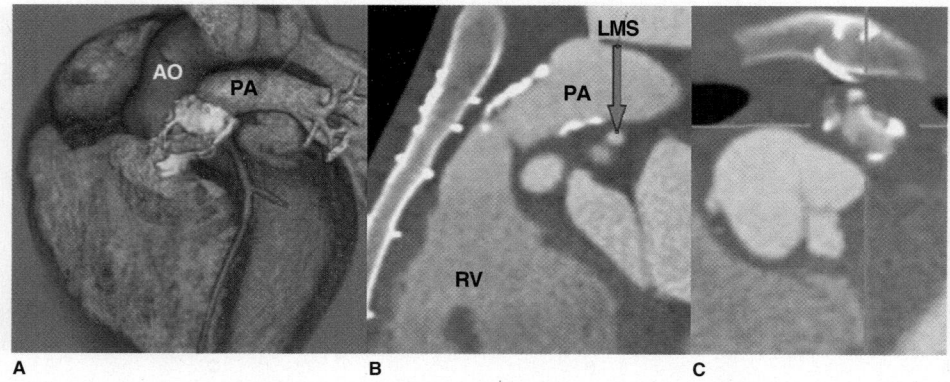

Figure 67–6. Bioprosthetic pulmonary valve stenosis. Computed tomography images of severe bioprosthetic valve stenosis in the pulmonary position after Ross procedure (aortic autograft and pulmonary valve replacement with a bioprosthetic valve), considered for percutaneous valve replacement. Note in (**A**) that the calcification of the RVOT and valve and its proximity to the left coronary artery. In (**B**), the proximity of the left main stem (LMS) of the coronary artery to the pulmonary artery (PA) is shown, raising concerns that this may become compressed at the time of stenting and deployment of the percutaneous valve prosthesis. In (**C**), cross section of the stenosed prosthetic pulmonary valve. AO, aorta; RV, right ventricle.

in life (once the RV is sufficiently developed) or a surgical shunt to augment pulmonary blood flow.

Hence the effects of PS depend on the severity, onset, and duration of the obstruction. In adults:

- Severe PS (peak gradient > 64 mm Hg on echocardiography) causes significant pressure overload of the RV, which adapts by becoming hypertrophic. RV hypertrophy increases the myocardial oxygen requirement, and when long-standing is associated with myocardial fibrosis and diastolic dysfunction. The resultant rise in RV filling pressures and right atrial dilatation, in the presence of an atrial communication, can cause cyanosis by right–left shunting and associated secondary erythrocytosis.

- Extremely severe, long-standing PS can ultimately cause RV dilatation and systolic dysfunction, which is a marker of end-stage disease and is associated with heart failure, arrhythmias, syncope, and death (**Fig. 67–7**).

- Mild PS, with a peak gradient <36 mm Hg, is benign, does not significantly overload the RV, and typically causes no symptoms. It is often diagnosed incidentally (murmur detected on auscultation) or when associated with other lesions. Rapid progression of even mild PS has been described in young children, but progress is much slower in older children and adults.[5]

Significant PS may be beneficial in patients with a large VSD or univentricular heart, protecting the pulmonary circulation from excessive pulmonary blood flow and the development of pulmonary vascular disease. It may also be beneficial for patients with a systemic RV (**Fig. 67–8, Tables 67–1** and **67–2**).

PS in Cyanotic CHD

PS associated with lesions such as ToF or single ventricle physiology are described elsewhere (see section Tetralogy of Fallot and chapter 69). In brief, PS in ToF may be subvalvar and/or involves the valve and pulmonary arteries. The severity of PS dictates the clinical presentation of ToF patients: severe PS is associated with cyanosis and if very severe, may require a palliative shunt to improve oxygen saturation and allow the pulmonary vascular tree to grow; it can also be dynamic, causing cyanotic spells; less severe PS in ToF allows greater pulmonary blood flow, with less cyanosis but greater load on the systemic ventricle and the risk of pulmonary vascular disease if not repaired in a timely fashion.

In patients with single ventricle physiology (eg, tricuspid atresia or double inlet left ventricle [LV]) and a large VSD or transposed great arteries, PS dictates the amount pulmonary blood flow and, when severe, can protect the patient from developing pulmonary vascular disease and protect the systemic ventricle from overload, which is essential when planning

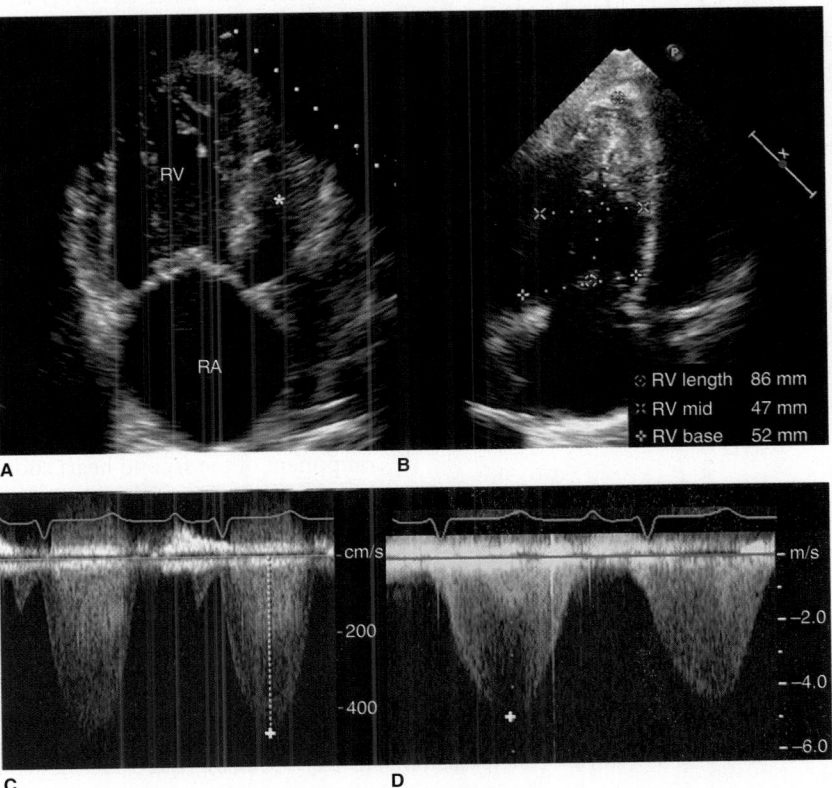

Figure 67–7. Advanced pulmonary stenosis. Severe bioprosthetic pulmonary stenosis in an uncooperative patient with poor parasternal windows. The effect on the right ventricle (RV) is visualized in the apical four-chamber views (**A** and **B**), severely dilated, hypertrophied, and dysfunctional. The left ventricle (left, *star*) is slit-like due to the deviation of the ventricular septum and reduced preload. The RA is also severely dilated and the atrial septum bows to the left, almost obliterating the left atrium. In (**C**) and (**D**), continuous wave Doppler imaging across the pulmonary valve from the parasternal short axis view and the tricuspid view from the apical four-chamber view. There is evidence of severe pulmonary stenosis, especially considering there is severe RV dysfunction. The raised tricuspid regurgitation Doppler velocity reflects RV systolic pressure proximal to the stenosis, rather than pulmonary artery pressure.

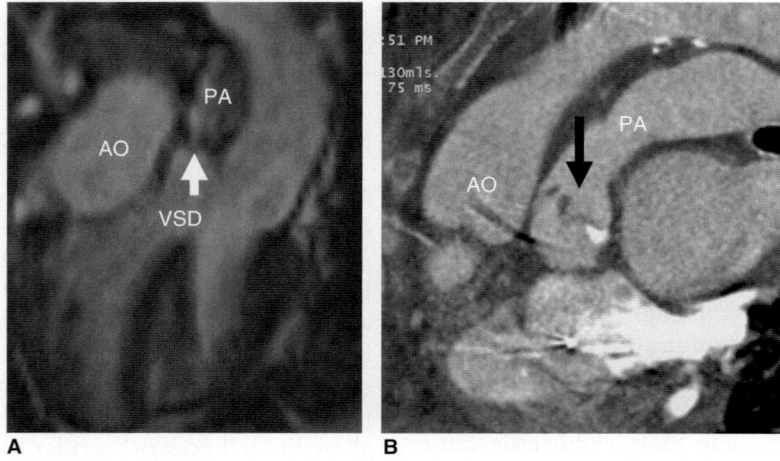

Figure 67–8. Pulmonary stenosis in cc-TGA. cc-TGA with a large VSD and severe pulmonary stenosis (*arrow*). In cc-TGA, there is a systemic RV that typically becomes dilated and hypertrophied, with associated tricuspid regurgitation. The pulmonary stenosis protects the pulmonary circulation from developing pulmonary vascular disease, whilst also minimizing deviation of the ventricular septum toward the subpulmonary LV, thus reducing the likelihood of severe tricuspid regurgitation as the RV dilates. Note the aorta (AO) positioned anterior to the pulmonary artery (PA).

a Fontan-type operation (nowadays, total cavopulmonary connection [TCPC]). However, if PS is very severe, it may significantly restrict pulmonary blood flow (causing severe cyanosis) and the growth of the PAs in patients with univentricular hearts, which is necessary for establishing a working Fontan circulation, the ultimate target for all patients with univentricular circulation. In such cases, pulmonary blood flow can be augmented with a surgical shunt (eg, BT shunt; see Fig. 67–19), at the risk of overloading the ventricle.

PR After Repair of PS
Most children with isolated valvar PS are expected to reach adult life, often after previous surgical or percutaneous intervention to relieve the stenosis, and have a normal life-expectancy with little or no exercise limitation. PR is common after surgical or percutaneous repair of PS. Similar to repaired ToF, PR is well tolerated for years after PS repair, but causes volume overload to the RV and progressive RV dilatation. If left unrepaired, it can lead to significant RV dilatation and systolic RV dysfunction. Pulmonary valve replacement is often required in the long term in patients after previously repaired PS (**Table 67–3**).

Clinical Presentation and Assessment
The clinical presentation of PS depends on the severity of the obstruction and age of the patient. Critical PS of the neonate is a life-threatening condition requiring urgent intervention. In the adult, PS is often a childhood diagnosis (isolated or in association with other CHD). Alternatively, it may be detected incidentally during physical examination, or can present with symptoms and signs of exercise intolerance, fatigue, presyncope, syncope, or heart failure, depending on the severity of the obstruction. Chest pain may be reported, secondary to subendocardial ischemia, in severely hypertensive and hypertrophied RVs. Cyanosis may also be present when RV filling pressures exceed those of the LV in the presence of an atrial septal defect (ASD) or PFO.

On examination, signs of Noonan or Williams syndrome should be noted. In severe PS with RV hypertrophy, a prominent a wave in the jugular venous pressure waveform and an RV heave may be present. A precordial thrill may also be present.

On auscultation, valvar PS causes a systolic crescendo decrescendo murmur, which is longer and prolonged (past the aortic component of the second heart sound [S2]) in severe PS due to

COR	LOE	Diagnostic	Therapeutic
TABLE 67–1. Pulmonary Stenosis: 2018 AHA/ACC Guidelines for ACHD			
I	B-NR	1. For adults with peripheral or branch PS, ongoing surveillance is recommended.	1. In adults with moderate or severe valvular pulmonary stenosis and otherwise unexplained symptoms of HF, cyanosis from interatrial right-to-left communication, and/or exercise intolerance, balloon valvuloplasty is recommended
I	B-NR		1. In adults with moderate or severe valvular pulmonary stenosis and otherwise unexplained symptoms of HF, cyanosis, and/or exercise intolerance who are ineligible for or who failed balloon valvuloplasty, surgical repair is recommended
IIa	C-EO		1. In asymptomatic adults with severe valvular pulmonary stenosis, intervention is reasonable. 2. In adults with peripheral or branch PA stenosis, PA dilation and stenting can be useful.

Abbreviations: ACHD, adult congenital heart disease; AHA/ACC, American Heart Association/American College of Cardiology; COR, class of recommendation; EO, expert opinion; HF, heart failure; LOE, level of evidence; NR, nonrandomized; PA, pulmonary artery; PS, pulmonary stenosis.

TABLE 67-2. Pulmonary Stenosis: 2020 ESC Guidelines for ACHD

COR	LOE	Diagnostic	Therapeutic

I	C		1. In valvular PS, balloon valvuloplasty is the intervention of choice, if anatomically suitable.
			2. Provided that no valve replacement is required, RVOT outflow intervention at any level is recommended regardless of symptoms when the stenosis is severe (Doppler peak gradient is >64 mmHg).
			3. If surgical valve replacement is the only option, it is indicated in patients with severe stenosis who are symptomatic.
			4. If surgical valve replacement is the only option in patients with severe stenosis who are asymptomatic, it is indicated in the presence of one or more of the following:
			• Objective decrease in exercise capacity;
			• Decreasing RV function and/or progression of TR to at least moderate;
			  • RVSP >80 mmHg;
			  • R-L shunting via an ASD or VSD.

IIa	C	1. In patients who have developed PAH with PVR 3-5 WU, VSD closure should be considered when there is still significant L-R shunt (Qp:Qs >1.5).	1. Intervention in patients with a Doppler peak gradient <64 mmHg should be considered in the presence of one or more of the following: • Symptoms related to PS • Decreasing RV function and/or progressive TR to at least moderate; • R-L shunting via an ASD or VSD 2. Peripheral PS, regardless of symptoms, should be considered for catheter interventional treatment if • >50% diameter narrowing, and RVSP >50 mmHg, and/or • related reduced lung perfusion is present.

Abbreviations: ACHD, adult congenital heart disease; ASD, atrial septal defect; COR, class of recommendation; HF, Heart failure; LOE, level of evidence; PA: pulmonary artery; PAH, pulmonary arterial hypertension; PR, pulmonary regurgitation; PS, pulmonary stenosis; PVR, pulmonary vascular resistance; Qp:Qs, ratio of pulmonary to systemic blood flow; R-L, right-to-left; RV, right ventricle; RVOT: right ventricular outflow tract; RVSP, right ventricular systolic pressure; TR, tricuspid regurgitation; VSD, ventricular septal defect.

prolonged RV ejection. For the same reason, the S2 widens and the pulmonary component of the S2 may be absent in severe PS. A systolic ejection click (caused by rapid deceleration of the opening valve/cusps) should precede the murmur and is most likely to be present in mild–moderate rather than severe PS.

Supravalvar PS at the level of the main PA presents with similar findings, with the exception of the ejection click. Peripheral PS (of the branch PAs) causes long systolic murmurs over the lung fields.

The findings in patients with significant PR after previous repair of PS include an RV heave, single S2, ejection systolic murmur over the upper left sternal border, and an early diastolic murmur, which becomes shorter as the PR becomes more severe (even though the length of the murmur is influenced by RV end-diastolic and PA pressure).

ECG and Chest Radiography

Typical findings on ECG include signs of RV hypertrophy and right atrial enlargement observed in severe/long-standing PS. On chest radiography, RV hypertrophy can be seen as an upturned cardiac apex. PA dilation is also typically present in adults with significant PS. Right atrial dilatation may also be observed as a prominent right lower heart border.

Echocardiography

Nowadays, echocardiography is the mainstay of diagnosis of PS for prenatal, neonatal, pediatric, and adult patients. Echocardiography provides the location and severity of the obstruction, anatomical characteristics of a valve, and aggravating features (eg, endocarditis).

The pulmonary valve can be examined from a modified (anterior) parasternal long-axis, short-axis great vessels, apical modified (anterior) 5 chamber, and subcostal short-axis view (**Fig. 67–9**). The RVOT can also be examined on the standard parasternal long-axis view, while the branch PAs can be assessed from the suprasternal window.

The pressure gradient across the pulmonary valve can be assessed by continuous wave Doppler using the modified

TABLE 67-3. Pulmonary Regurgitation: 2018 AHA/ACC Guidelines for ACHD

COR	LOE	Diagnostic	Therapeutic
I	B-NR	1. For asymptomatic patients with residual PR resulting from treatment of isolated pulmonary stenosis with a dilated RV, serial follow-up is recommended.	1. In symptomatic patients with moderate or greater PR resulting from treated isolated pulmonary stenosis, with RV dilation or RV dysfunction, pulmonary valve replacement is recommended.
I	B-NR		1. In adults with moderate or severe valvular pulmonary stenosis and otherwise unexplained symptoms of HF, cyanosis, and/or exercise intolerance who are ineligible for or who failed balloon valvuloplasty, surgical repair is recommended
IIb	C-EO		1. In asymptomatic patients with moderate or greater PR resulting from treatment of isolated pulmonary stenosis with progressive RV dilation and/or RV dysfunction, pulmonary valve replacement may be reasonable.

Abbreviations: ACHD, adult congenital heart disease; COR, class of recommendation; EO, expert opinion; HF, heart failure; LOE, level of evidence; NR, nonrandomized; PR, pulmonary regurgitation; R-L, right-to-left.

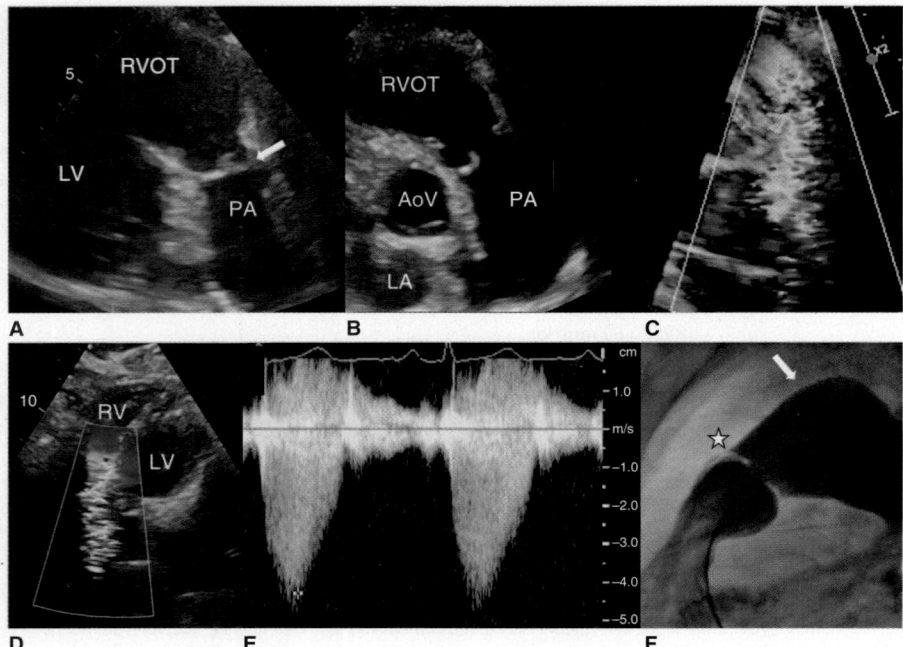

Figure 67–9. Severe valvar pulmonary stenosis. Initial echocardiographic assessment of a patient with valvar pulmonary stenosis (A–E). In (A), parasternal long-axis RVOT view showing a thickened pulmonary valve (*arrow*). The parasternal short-axis (PSAX) view at the level of the great vessels focusing on the pulmonary valve in (B) shows incomplete opening with doming of the valve in systole (note the open aortic valve, AoV) and pulmonary artery dilatation. In (C) and (D), color Doppler demonstrating turbulent flow across the stenotic pulmonary valve in the PSAX and modified five-chamber subcostal (anterior) views, respectively. In (E), the continuous wave Doppler demonstrates severe pulmonary stenosis with a peak gradient of 77 mm Hg. Following referral for balloon pulmonary valvuloplasty, the fluoroscopic image in (F) (left lateral) clearly demonstrates stenosis at the level of the pulmonary valve. The valve leaflets are thickened, calcific, and doming (*star*). Poststenotic dilatation of the main pulmonary artery is visualized (*arrow*).

Bernoulli equation (**Fig. 67–10**), accounting for RV function and the presence of pulmonary hypertension, both of which can result in a reduced pressure gradient across a severely stenotic valve. It is, thus, important to carefully assess RV function and highlight any disproportionate increase in tricuspid regurgitation (TR) gradient, beyond what would be expected from the gradient across the pulmonary valve. The RV systolic pressure should also be estimated using the TR Doppler, which can help quantify the RVOTO (in the absence of pulmonary hypertension), especially when the RVOT Doppler is suboptimal.

Other features of PS on echocardiography include right atrial (RA) dilatation, PA dilatation, and the signs of RV pressure overload (eg, reversal of the ventricular septum, RV hypertrophy). Stenosis at multiple levels (eg, valvar and sub- or supravalvar) and long tubular stenoses may be difficult to quantify on echocardiography.

CMR and CT
Cardiac magnetic resonance (CMR) imaging provides valuable complementary information to echocardiography regarding the anatomical features of the stenosis, especially peripheral or subvalvar PS, the degree of PR, anatomic and functional assessment of the RV, including RV mass, the size and shape of the PAs, and RV fibrosis.

Computed tomography (CT) provides precise imaging of the valve in relation to adjacent structures (eg, coronary

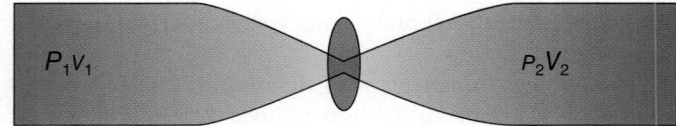

$$P_1 - P_2 = \frac{1}{2}\,p(V_2^2 - V_1^2) + \underbrace{p\int_1^2 \frac{d\bar{V}}{dt}\,\overline{ds}}_{\text{Flow acceleration}} + \underbrace{R(\bar{V})}_{\text{Viscous friction}}$$

$$P_1 - P_2 = \frac{1}{2}\,p(V_2^2 - V_1^2) \approx 4\,(V_2^2 - V_1^2) \approx 4\,(V_2^2)$$

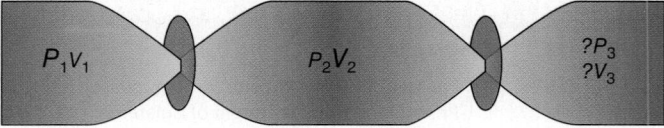

Figure 67–10. Bernoulli's equation. Derivation of the simplified Bernoulli equation. The Bernoulli principle states that, for steady flow, the total mechanical energy per unit volume at locations 1 and 2 is the same but can take different forms. A reduction in pressure across locations may be balanced by an increase in fluid velocity without loss of energy. Bernoulli's initial equation (*top*) can be simplified, making the following assumptions: the flow acceleration and viscous friction terms are negligible, the density of blood p/2 approximates a constant of 4, and V_1 (the velocity in the RVOT) is <1 m/s and therefore contributes minimally to the overall equation. The equation does not hold for multilevel or tandem stenoses as V_2, the velocity of blood approaching the second stenosis is no longer negligible.[24]

arteries), the size of the PAs, and is particularly helpful in delineating peripheral PS in large and smaller PA branches.

Cardiac Catheterization

Cardiac catheterization for solely diagnostic purposes is seldom required in valvar PS, but may be performed to confirm the severity of the stenosis, for RV and PA angiography, and to exclude or quantify shunts or pulmonary hypertension. A diagnostic run is typically performed at the time of percutaneous intervention.

The severity of the PS is assessed during cardiac catheterization by measuring the peak-to-peak gradient between the RV and main PA (or more peripherally, depending on the site of stenosis). The gradient may be affected by general anesthesia and should account for RV dysfunction, when present.

Surgical and Percutaneous Repair

Indications

Relevant American Heart Association (AHA)/American College of Cardiology (ACC) and European Society of Cardiology (ESC) recommendations are shown in Tables 67–1 and 67–2.[6,7] The first-line treatment for (native) valvar PS is balloon pulmonary valvuloplasty for both the ESC and AHA/ACC guidelines. When balloon valvuloplasty is feasible, this is recommended for all patients with severe PS. Surgery or percutaneous valve replacement (which carries an increased long-term risk of endocarditis and need for reintervention) is recommended for symptomatic patients or asymptomatic patients with reduced exercise capacity, decreasing RV function, progressive TR (at least moderate), or cyanosis (right–left shunting through an atrial communication).

In patients with less than severe PS with related symptoms, or progressive RV dysfunction or TR, intervention is recommended.

Peripheral PS should be monitored and intervened upon if there is significant (>50%) stenosis, a raised RV systolic pressure (>50 mm Hg on echocardiography), reduced pulmonary perfusion, or symptoms.

Pulmonary atresia with intact ventricular septum may be amenable to biventricular repair (reestablishing the connection between the adequately sized RV and the pulmonary circulation), a "one-and-a-half" ventricular repair (where only systemic venous return from the inferior vena cava reaches the hypoplastic RV, which is connected to the pulmonary circulation, whereas the superior vena cava [SVC] is connected to the right pulmonary artery via a Glenn shunt), a Fontan-type procedure (nowadays, TCPC, with no ventricle supplying the pulmonary circulation), transplantation, or simple palliation (eg, with an arterial shunt supplying the pulmonary circulation). Long-term complications (eg, arrhythmia, heart failure) and need for reintervention (eg, replacement of an RV-PA conduit) are common.

Technique: Repair versus Replacement

Balloon pulmonary valvuloplasty is the preferred treatment for patients with PS and complications are rare (mortality 0.2%, major complication rate 0.6%). Potential complications include catheter-related injury to vessels or the tricuspid valve, vagal reaction, arrhythmias, and atrioventricular block.[8] A severe but transient RVOTO after relief of valvar PS has been reported and is treated with volume infusion and β-blockers ("suicidal RV").[9]

Balloon pulmonary valvuloplasty may, however, not be suitable for valves with PS and more than mild PR (that is likely to be aggravated by balloon dilatation). Indeed, the aim of balloon pulmonary valvuloplasty is to achieve adequate relief of the severe PS without causing significant PR. Moreover, balloon valvuloplasty may not be suitable patients with very dysplastic valves, a hypoplastic valve annulus, or for subvalvar or supravalvar PS in close proximity to the valve. Prosthetic valve stenosis usually requires surgery or percutaneous pulmonary valve implantation, rather than balloon valvuloplasty alone.

Surgical valvotomy is performed in patients with valvar or supravalvar PS not amenable to percutaneous intervention, and in patients with subvalvar PS in whom muscular resection and/or a surgical patch is required to relieve the subvalvar or supravalvar stenosis. Surgery can be performed via median sternotomy with cardiopulmonary bypass or a closed transventricular approach.

Long-Term Outcome and Management of Complications after PS Repair

Nowadays, the outcomes following percutaneous balloon pulmonary valvuloplasty or surgical valvotomy for PS are excellent. Optimal results have also been reported in adult cohorts of PS patients undergoing balloon valvuloplasty.[10] However, reintervention is frequently needed, most commonly for restenosis or PR, with up to a quarter of patients requiring reintervention at 15 years of follow-up.[11] One half of patients after surgical repair required reintervention at a mean follow-up of 33 years in one study.[12] Another study on 90 patients operated between 1968 and 1980 reported a 93% survival at 25 years and a 15% reoperation rate, but with 37% of patients having moderate to severe PR at last follow-up.[13] They also reported supraventricular arrhythmias in patients with severe PR but no ventricular arrhythmias. Voet et al.[14] reported on 79 patients treated surgically: after a median 22.5 years, 20.3% had needed reintervention, the vast majority of whom for severe PR. Of 139 patients treated percutaneously, 9.4% needed reintervention after a median of 6 years, mainly for PS.[14] Freedom from reintervention at 30 years after surgery was 70.9%, while this was 84.4% at 20 years after percutaneous repair.[14]

The AHA/ACC ACHD guidelines recommend pulmonary valve replacement for symptomatic patients with at least moderate PR after repair of isolated PS when RV dilation or RV dysfunction is present (Table 67–3).

Asymptomatic patients with progressive RV dilation or dysfunction may also be offered pulmonary valve replacement. Progressive PA dilatation is not uncommon in patients with PS, but its management remains unclear, because the risk of dissection or rupture in patients without pulmonary hypertension is deemed small.

Heart failure can occur in patients with severe PS, on a native lesion or degenerating prosthetic valve. Symptoms include dyspnea and fatigue or congestion. The first step toward the management of HF in PS is the identification and treatment of the hemodynamic lesion (ie, relief of PS and/or PR, pulmonary valve replacement for degenerating valve). Additional factors should be excluded (eg, endocarditis or arrhythmia).

Optimal results have also been reported for peripheral PA stenting in adults.[15] In-stent restenosis has been reported in up to 25% of patients who underwent pulmonary angioplasty and stenting.[16] The highest incidence was in patients with ToF and pulmonary atresia, and patients with Williams or Alagille syndrome. The need for reintervention after bilateral PA stenting is high (12 of 26 patients after a mean 41 months).[17]

Patients after repair of pulmonary atresia with intact septum are also at risk of long-term complications and reintervention, depending on the type of repair.[18] This includes PR in patients with patch repair of the outflow tract, degeneration of an RV-PA conduit, heart failure in patients with hypoplastic RV, and a Fontan-type surgery or one-and-a-half repair. In a study of 60 patients with various degrees of RV hypoplasia, 59 of whom received an operation, there were 7 early postprocedure deaths and 1 late death. Survival at 10 years was 86.5% overall but 79.4% for those with severe RV hypoplasia, in whom biventricular repair was not possible.[19]

Infective Endocarditis

All patients with PS are at increased risk of endocarditis compared to the general population. Particular care is warranted for PS patients with a previous pulmonary valve replacement, especially percutaneous valves that are associated with an increased risk of infective endocarditis, which is often obstructive and the source of septic emboli in the lungs, warranting early surgery.[20] Patients should be educated on the merits of adequate dental and skin hygiene, the signs and symptoms of infective endocarditis, and the importance of early diagnosis and treatment. However, antibiotic prophylaxis is not required for the vast majority of patients with PS, unless there is a history of infective endocarditis or they have undergone pulmonary valve replacement.[21]

Pregnancy in Patients with PS

Mild PS is well-tolerated in pregnancy and belongs to the lowest group of the modified World Health Organization (mWHO) classification, according to ESC guidelines on pregnancy in heart disease.[22] Severe PS is less tolerated and should be addressed prior to conception, because it can result in RV failure and manifest as increasing exercise intolerance, edema, arrhythmias, or even (pre-)syncope. Pregnancy may also accelerate the degeneration of mild or moderately stenotic pulmonary biological prostheses. Patients presenting during pregnancy with severe PS and symptoms refractory to medical treatment may benefit form pulmonary balloon valvuloplasty.

TABLE 67–4. Variables Used in the ACHD Anatomic and Physiological Classification

Physiological Variables in ACHD Anatomic and Physiological Classification of the AHA/ACC ACHD Practice Guidelines[6]
Aortopathy, severe ≥5 cm maximum diameter
Arrhythmia, categorized according to presence and response to treatment
Concomitant valvular heart disease, severity defined according to the 2014 AHA/ACC valvular heart disease guidelines (151)
End-organ dysfunction, including renal, hepatic, and pulmonary
Exercise capacity (objective, cardiopulmonary exercise testing)
Hypoxemia/hypoxia/cyanosis: resting oxygen saturation ≤90%, severe if <85%
NYHA functional classification
Pulmonary hypertension
Significant shunt with chamber enlargement (volume overload) and/or Qp:Qs ≥1.5
Venous and arterial stenosis, eg, aortic recoarctation, venous pathway obstruction after atrial switch procedure for transposition of the great arteries, stenosis of cavopulmonary connection, supravalvar or branch pulmonary artery stenosis, pulmonary vein stenosis, or supravalvar aortic stenosis

Abbreviations: ACHD: adult congenital heart disease; Qp:Qs: pulmonary-systemic blood flow ratio.

Routine Follow-Up

All adult patients with PS should be referred to and followed in specialist ACHD services, monitoring for progression of their lesion (PS or PR after repair), and complications such as RV hypertrophy and/or dysfunction, heart failure, or arrhythmia. The frequency of follow-up depends on their physiological state: the AHA/ACC guidelines define physiological stages for ACHD patients (Stages A to D), requiring follow-up and investigations at increasing frequency (**Table 67–4**). Patients in the best physiological state (A) require follow-up every 2 to 3 years with electrocardiogram (ECG), echocardiography, and CMR (as needed). Moreover, exercise testing is recommended every 3 years.

DOUBLE-CHAMBERED RIGHT VENTRICLE

DCRV is an intracavitary obstruction of flow. It was first described over 150 years ago by Thomas Peacock as a constriction of the first portion of the RV infundibulum. Over time, it has been given different names, including "divided right ventricle" or "anomalous right ventricular muscle band," suggesting more than one mechanism/variation for the division of the RV.[23] It is typically associated with restrictive or larger VSD and, when severe, can cause significant intracavitary obstruction limiting cardiac output. It may not be straightforward to diagnose and may be missed on routine echocardiography unless its presence is suspected and investigated.

Anatomical Features and Associated Lesions

To understand the anatomical features of the DCRV, one should remember the three components of the normal RV: the inlet,

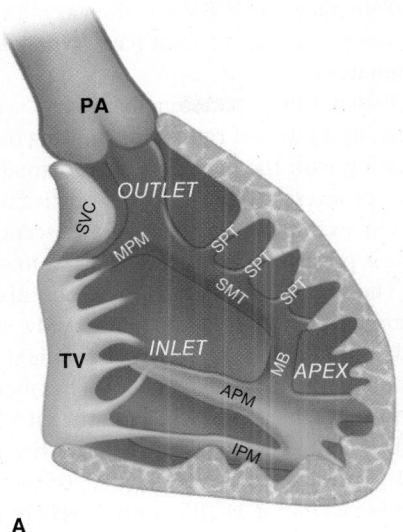
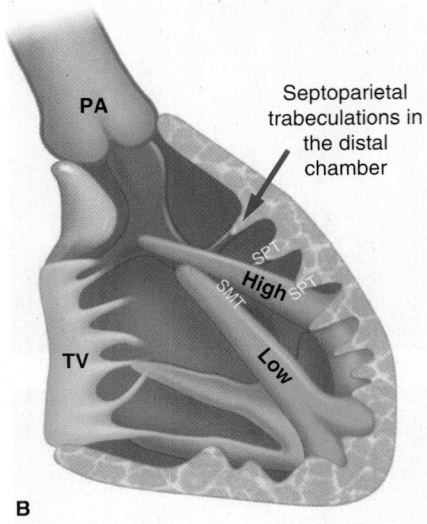

Figure 67–11. The types of double-chambered right ventricle. In (**A**), normal right ventricular anatomy. In (**B**), the two types of double-chambered right ventricle ("high" and "low") according to Restivo et al. and Alva et al.[23,27] (see text for explanation). APM, anterior papillary muscle; IPM, inferior papillary muscle; MB, moderator band; MPM: medial papillary muscle; PA, pulmonary artery; SMT, septomarginal trabeculation; SPT, septoparietal trabeculation; SVC, supraventricular crest; TV, tricuspid valve.

outlet, and apical trabecular portion (**Fig. 67–11**). The latter contains coarse trabeculations, one of which is particularly prominent: the "septomarginal trabeculation." It diverges into two limbs at its base to clasp the supraventricular crest (that separates the pulmonary and tricuspid valves at the roof of the RV).[23] From the posterior limb of this trabeculation arises the medial papillary muscle. The anterior limb expands superiorly to support the pulmonary valve. Therefore, the basal portion of the septomarginal trabeculation lies over the junction of the three portions of the RV.

The apical portion of the septomarginal trabeculation is part of the trabecular component of the RV apex and from its anterior surface several septoparietal bands cross from the septal to the parietal ventricular surface. One of these bands is particularly prominent (the "moderator band") and fuses with the base of the anterolateral papillary muscle. There is significant variability in the anatomy of the septoparietal bands, at times taking off high from the ventricular septum.

Restivo et al. reviewed several DCRV cases and found that the anomaly that was most frequently reported as an "anomalous muscle bundle" is not a unique entity.[23] It can be part of a shelf that divides the apical portion of the RV into two chambers, or it can be a bundle that divides the entrance of the RV outflow.

Alva et al. subsequently described two basic forms of DCRV, caused by muscular division by an obstructive muscular shelf between the body of the septomarginal trabeculation and the ventricular apex, which is either positioned "low" and diagonally across the RV apex, or "high" and horizontal.[27] In the surgical series by Kahr et al., 64% of patients had a "high" and 36% a "low" obstruction intraoperatively.[25]

A high "take-off" of the moderator band from the RV septum has been suggested as potential cause of DCRV.[26] However, according to Alva et al., the muscle bundle is most likely composed of accentuated septoparietal trabeculations (less likely to be the moderator band) and the two parts of the RV on either side of this obstruction each possess part of the apical RV (ie, the distal chamber is never confined to the smooth RV infundibulum).

The majority of patients with DCRV have a VSD (72% in the series by Alva et al., 96% in the series by Kahr et al.), which can be small or large.[25,27] It has been suggested that DCRV may be an acquired lesion in the presence of abnormal ventricular septation.[26] Moreover, it is thought that a DCRV may develop as a result of the VSD jet lesion to the RV endothelium[7,28] caused by the high velocity VSD jet. However, cases of severe DCRV with an intact ventricular septum have been described and a DCRV occurs in a small minority of patients with a VSD.[27] It is felt that a combination of factors are likely to contribute to the development of a DCRV, including the presence of the VSD and abnormally located septoparietal trabeculations.

An association of DCRV with ToF, double-outlet RV (DORV), ASD, aortic or TR, rupture of sinus of Valsalva and subaortic stenosis, pulmonary and mitral stenosis, aortic coarctation, atrioventricular septal defect, and bicuspid aortic valve has been described.[25,27,29] Moreover, an association between DCRV and Down syndrome exists: 11% of patients in the cohort by Kahr et al.[25]

Pathophysiology of Unrepaired DCRV

The implications of a DCRV depend mainly on the severity of the obstruction within the RV and impact of associated lesions (usually a VSD). The severity of obstruction may vary, but when severe, it results in a hypertensive proximal RV chamber and a normotensive distal chamber (**Fig. 67–12**). This results in an increase in right atrial pressure, as filling pressures within the proximal hypertrophied, hypertensive RV chamber rise.

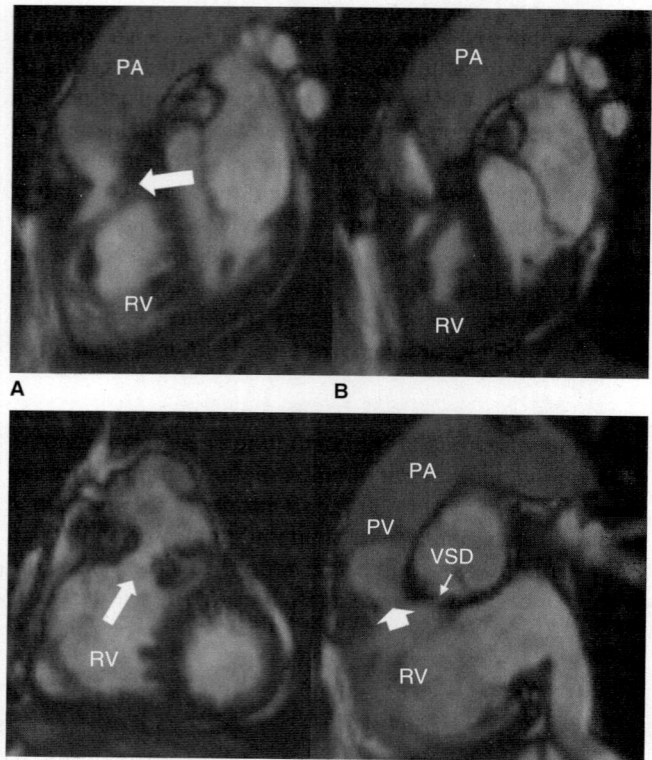

A **B**

C **D**

Figure 67–12. Double-chambered right ventricle. CMR imaging of patients with a restrictive VSD and intracavitary RV obstruction. In (**A**) and (**C**), the obstruction is well below the pulmonary valve (*arrow*), causing significant flow acceleration within the RV. In (**B**) and (**D**), the obstruction is in proximity to the restrictive VSD, which in this case, is in communication with the high pressure (proximal) RV chamber.

Moreover, the obstruction to flow does not permit an adequate increase in cardiac output on efforts, which may cause syncope or presyncope. The obstruction can be dynamic, becoming more severe when RV contractility is enhanced. The remodeling of the RV and, possibly, RV ischemia may also be responsible for cases of sustained ventricular tachycardia described in unrepaired DCRVs, resolving after surgery.

In DCRV, both the severity of the obstruction and the hemodynamic burden from associated lesions need to be considered. In most DCRV cases, a VSD is present, which is most commonly in communication with the proximal (high-pressure), or less commonly with the distal (low-pressure) RV chamber. Knowing the location of the VSD is important for understanding the direction of the shunt through this defect, the VSD, DCRV, and TR pressure gradients, and the findings on auscultation (murmurs) and echocardiography (**Fig. 67–13**). Indeed, depending on the DCRV gradients the shunt across the VSD can be left–right or right–left (or bidirectional). DCRV can be a progressive lesion and long-term monitoring is important.[7,29,30]

Clinical Presentation and Assessment

DCRV is typically diagnosed and, when significant, repaired in childhood or adolescence; however, it may present and require repair in later life.[29,31]

Patients with DCRV are often asymptomatic or complain of exercise intolerance, chest pain, syncope, light-headedness, or palpitations.[6,25]

Patients may occasionally present with cyanosis, which is typically a result of right–left shunting through a VSD communicating with the hypertensive proximal chamber in the presence of severe intracavitary RV obstruction.

On examination, a systolic crescendo–decrescendo murmur is present, typically over the left lower sternal border.

The DCRV murmur may be obscured by the harsh holosystolic murmur of a restrictive VSD. For the VSD murmur to be audible/loud, a pressure gradient should be present in systole between the LV and RV chamber to which the VSD is connected: there will be no significant VSD murmur when the VSD is connected to a very hypertensive proximal RV chamber in the presence of severe DCRV; or the VSD murmur will be audible when the DCRV is not severe or the VSD is communicating with the distal low-pressure chamber of the RV.

The 12-lead ECG may be normal or have a rightward QRS axis, signs of RV hypertrophy or right atrial enlargement (P pulmonale). Right bundle branch block (RBBB) is rare in unrepaired or preoperative DCRV, but is encountered commonly following surgical repair.[25,32,33] The presenting rhythm is sinus in the vast majority of case, although patients may rarely present with atrial arrhythmias (atrial fibrillation or atrial tachycardia). There are few reported cases of sustained

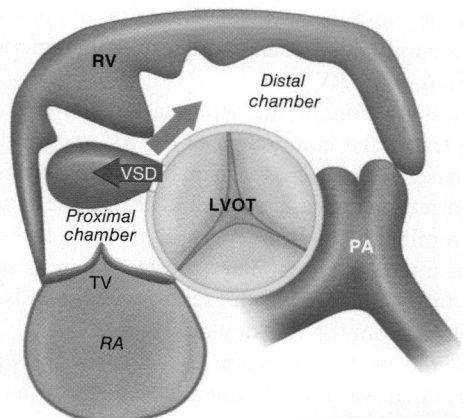

	DCRV Severe	DCRV Mild
DCRV gradient	▲▲▲	▲
Proximal Chamber Pressure	▲▲▲	▲
TR gradient	▲▲▲	▲
Proximal RV chamber-to-LV pressure gradient	~	▲▲▲
VSD gradient (when VSD proximal to obstruction)	0	▲▲▲

Figure 67–13. Mild versus severe DCRV. When a restrictive VSD is in communication with the proximal RV chamber (ie, the VSD is proximal to the obstruction), severe intracavitary obstruction results in a low pressure gradient between the LV and proximal RV chamber, and a low Doppler velocity across the VSD on echocardiography. The tricuspid valve (TV) regurgitation gradient, however, is raised, reflecting the pressures in the proximal RV chamber. In practice, it may be difficult to obtain clear Doppler traces from the VSD, TV, and DCRV due to their proximity to each other. LVOT, left ventricular outflow tract; PA, pulmonary artery; RA, right atrium.

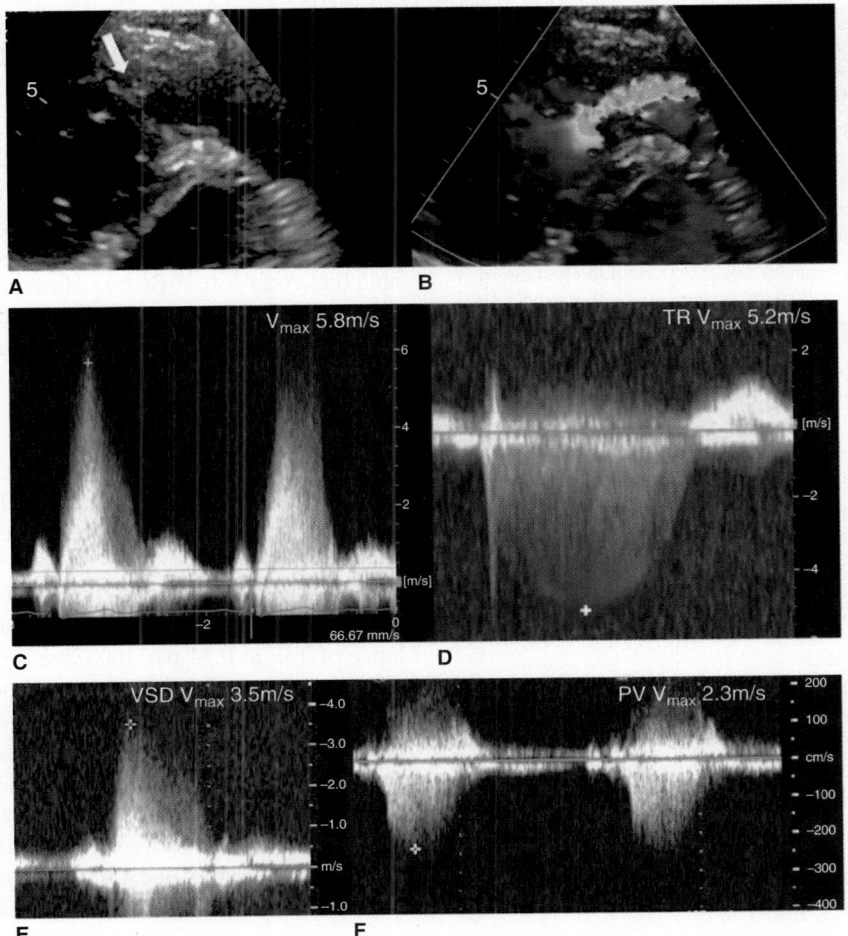

Figure 67–14. Transthoracic echocardiography in DCRV. Echocardiographic assessment of DCRV, displaying the importance of adequate alignment of the Doppler beam when measuring flow across the obstruction, tricuspid, and pulmonary valves and VSD. (**A**) parasternal short-axis view showing intracavitary stenosis (*arrow*). In (**B**), turbulent flow is shown using color Doppler. Continuous wave Doppler interrogation of the stenosis in (**C**) reveals severe obstruction with peak velocity (Vmax) 5.8 m/s. In (**D**), the elevated tricuspid regurgitation (TR) Vmax reflects the hypertensive proximal segment of the right ventricle. In (**E**), the peak pressure gradient across the associated small perimembranous VSD is estimated at 50 mm Hg, although the trace is contaminated by the DCRV flow. Using a noninvasive systolic arterial pressure reading of 125 mm Hg, the RV systolic pressure proximal to the obstruction can be estimated at 75 mm Hg. In (**F**), Doppler interrogation of the pulmonary valve (PV) displays an absence of significant valvar pulmonary stenosis.

ventricular tachycardia in patients with unrepaired DCRV, likely due to a reentry mechanism.[34]

Echocardiography is essential for detecting DCRV, which should be excluded in all VSD patients (**Fig. 67–14**). An index of suspicion is required, because DCRV can be missed on routine echocardiography.[6] The parasternal short-axis great vessels view is best for detecting a DCRV: on two-dimensional (2D) imaging, the anomalous muscle bundles causing stenosis within the RV may be detected in the proximity of a VSD. The presence of septoparietal trabeculations beyond the obstruction distinguishes DCRV from subpulmonary stenosis.[25,27]

On Doppler, turbulent flow across the stenosis is seen and the severity of the intracavitary gradient should be detected and measured on continuous wave Doppler, provided there is adequate alignment of the beam to the flow across the obstruction. However, turbulent flow and a high velocity Doppler trace may be indicative of severe DCRV stenosis or a restrictive VSD without significant DCRV. A "clean" TR trace (eg, from the

apical four-chamber view) may help distinguish between the two (high TR gradient in the presence of severe DCRV), even though "contamination" from the VSD jet may also occur.[25] The size, location, and hemodynamic significance of the VSD should be assessed, as well as the presence of other associated lesions.

CMR imaging can assist in confirming the diagnosis and provides additional information on the anatomy of the obstruction and location of the VSD.[35] Moreover, it can provide information on the hemodynamic significance of the VSD.

Cardiopulmonary exercise testing is important to detect objective limitation in patients with moderate or severe DCRV who are asymptomatic.[6,25]

Cardiac catheterization can be instrumental in establishing the diagnosis, even though in most cases the diagnosis can be established by noninvasive means.[25] Careful collection of pressure tracings is able to detect the gradient within the RV: the main PA and RVOT pressures are similar whereas pullback to

TABLE 67–5. Double-Chambered Right Ventricle: 2018 AHA/ACC Guidelines for ACHD

COR	LOE	Therapeutic
I	C-LD	1. Surgical repair for adults with double-chambered right ventricle and moderate or greater outflow obstruction is recommended in patients with otherwise unexplained symptoms of HF, cyanosis, or exercise limitation
IIb	C-LD	2. Surgical repair for adults with double-chambered right ventricle with a severe gradient may be considered in asymptomatic patients

Abbreviations: ACHD, adult congenital heart disease; COR, class of recommendation; LD, limited data; LOE, level of evidence.

the proximal RV can reveal a significant gradient a hypertensive proximal RV. Angiography in the proximal RV chamber can visualize the stenosis (ie, a dividing muscular shelf and RV trabeculations appearing as filling defects across the RV cavity resulting in an obstruction to flow).

Surgical Repair of DCRV

Indications
The timing of DCRV repair has long been debated. The AHA/ACC ACHD guidelines (**Table 67–5**) recommend surgical repair for adults with DCRV and:[9]

- at least moderate outflow obstruction with otherwise unexplained symptoms of heart failure, cyanosis, or exercise limitation (strong indication, grade I);
- severe obstruction in asymptomatic patients (mild indication, grade IIb).

The progressive nature of DCRV has urged other experts to recommend that repair is considered in all patients with DCRV, even if the gradient is not severe (<64 mm Hg, indication grade IIa).[28]

The 2020 ESC ACHD guidelines include DCRV with RVOTO and provide no DCRV-specific recommendations.[7]

Technique and Outcomes
Previously, repair of DCRV was mainly performed through a ventriculotomy. It is currently performed mainly via a transatrial approach or combined right atriotomy and pulmonary arteriotomy, unless transventricular resection of obstructing muscle bundles and patch enlargement of the RVOT is necessary to relieve the obstruction.[6,29,36,37] The anomalous muscle bundles are transected, avoiding damage to the tricuspid valve. The VSD is also closed. Perioperative risk is low and long-term outcomes are optimal with an extremely low risk of recurrence of DCRV.[25,29] A (residual) VSD may persist and one patient in the series by Khar et al. required permanent pacing postoperatively. RV hypertrophy may also persist long term.[25]

Reoperation for residual VSDs, subaortic stenosis, or aortic valve replacement has been described, but not for recurrence of DCRV.[25,36] Tricuspid valve surgery may also be required.

The risk of endocarditis is also low and most likely related to the presence of residual lesions other than the DCRV. Atrial

arrhythmias (including atrial fibrillation) have been described in patients after repair of DCRV in adult life.[25]

Rarely, ventricular arrhythmia has been reported in patients following right ventriculotomy.[32]

Routine Follow-Up

Despite the low risk of recurrence of DCRV, long-term complications can occur and infrequent specialist follow-up is advisable (eg, every 2 to 3 years).[6] However, in unrepaired patients and repaired patients with residual lesions or other complications, such as arrhythmias and heart failure, more frequent specialist follow-up is required.

TETRALOGY OF FALLOT

ToF is the most common cyanotic CHD. In 1988, Etienne-Louis Arthur Fallot first used the term "tetralogy" to describe the anatomical features of ToF, even though others before him, such as Niels Stensen, had described this condition since the 1600s. A recent meta-analysis has estimated the birth prevalence of ToF at 0.34 per 1000 live births, even though conditions that involved RVOTO (ie, pulmonary stenosis and ToF) were more common in Asia compared to Europe and North America.[38] ToF accounts for approximately 10% of all CHD, and ToF patients are one of the CHD cohorts that have benefited the most from cardiac surgery in the last six decades. Indeed, the vast majority of ToF patients born in developed countries undergo surgical repair, radically transforming their quality of life and long-term prognosis.

Anatomical Features and Pathophysiology of Native ToF

Anatomy
The anatomic features that define ToF are:

1. Stenosis of pulmonary valve/RVOTO
2. Interventricular communication (large VSD)
3. Deviation of the origin of the aorta to the right (overriding aorta)
4. Hypertrophy, almost always concentric, of the RV

All of these anatomical features are the result of a single morphogenetic abnormality: anterocephalad deviation (or malalignment) of the infundibular ventricular septum, with hypertrophy of septoparietal trabeculations (**Fig. 67–15**). The malalignment of the septum involves the perimembranous portion of the septum, with extension to its infundibular part. The VSD is almost always nonrestrictive and perimembranous. Various degrees of aortic override may be encountered, ranging from 5% to a majority of the aortic valve arising from the RV; in the latter case, when >50% of the aortic valve is arising from the RV, this falls into the definition of DORV.

The degree of RVOTO depends on:

- The degree of septal malalignment.
- The severity of hypertrophy of the septoparietal trabeculations, trabecula septomarginalis, and infundibular septum.

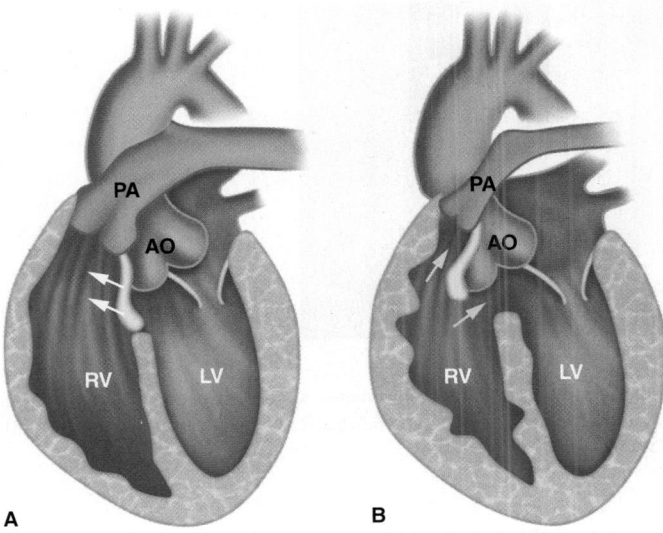

Figure 67–15. Anterocephalad deviation of the septum in ToF. Diagram of a normal heart (**A**) and ToF (**B**). The infundibular ventricular septum is depicted in *yellow*. An anterocephalad deviation of the infundibular septum (**B**) results in a large VSD, RVOTO, and rightward deviation of the aorta (Ao), which overrides the septum. There is RV hypertrophy and right–left shunting (when there is significant RVOTO), causing cyanosis. The pulmonary valve and pulmonary artery (PA) are often hypoplastic and stenosed. LV, left ventricle.

- The presence and severity of pulmonary valve stenosis (which is often a bicuspid or monocusp valve). Acquired pulmonary atresia can occur.
- The size and morphology of the PAs. The PAs are hypoplastic in up to 50% of cases (**Fig. 67–16**).

Associated conditions include:

- Right aortic arch
- Aortic dilatation and aortic valve regurgitation
- Coronary artery anomalies (5%): important for the surgeon, especially if left anterior descending (LAD) from

right coronary artery (RCA), or single coronary artery (**Fig. 67–17**).

- ASD (pentalogy of Fallot) (10%).
- Atrioventricular septal defect (typically in Down syndrome).
- Left SVC.
- DiGeorge syndrome (22q11.2 deletion, in 15% of ToF patients), with implications in term of transmission of this syndrome to offspring (50% vs. 3% in the remainder).
- Down syndrome (7%), CHARGE and Alagille syndrome.

Pathophysiology

ToF comprises a wide anatomical and pathophysiological spectrum, depending on the severity of the RVOTO and anatomy of the PAs (**Fig. 67–18**).

1. Patients with severe RVOTO and/or hypoplastic PAs are typically cyanotic, due to right–left shunting and limited pulmonary blood flow. "Blue" ToF becomes more manifest after the patent ductus arteriosus closes. The RVOTO can be dynamic and hypercyanotic spells in tetralogy can be triggered by an increase in RVOTO or pulmonary vascular resistance, or a drop in systemic vascular resistance, exacerbating right–left shunting across the VSD. Depending on the severity of the RVOTO and cyanosis, a palliative shunt may be required in when direct repair is not feasible (see section Palliative Procedures and ToF Repair).

2. The term "pink tetralogy" is used to describe patients with mild–moderate RVOTO and good-sized PAs, in whom there is normal (at times even excessive) pulmonary blood flow. There is no significant right–left shunting through the ventricular septum, hence no or little cyanosis at rest, but there may be a significant left–right shunt. As the infant grows, RV hypertrophy may cause RVOTO may become more severe, causing more cyanosis. Hypercyanotic spells may also happen in patients with "pink tetralogy."

3. At the extreme end of the ToF spectrum sits pulmonary atresia, in which there is no communication between the

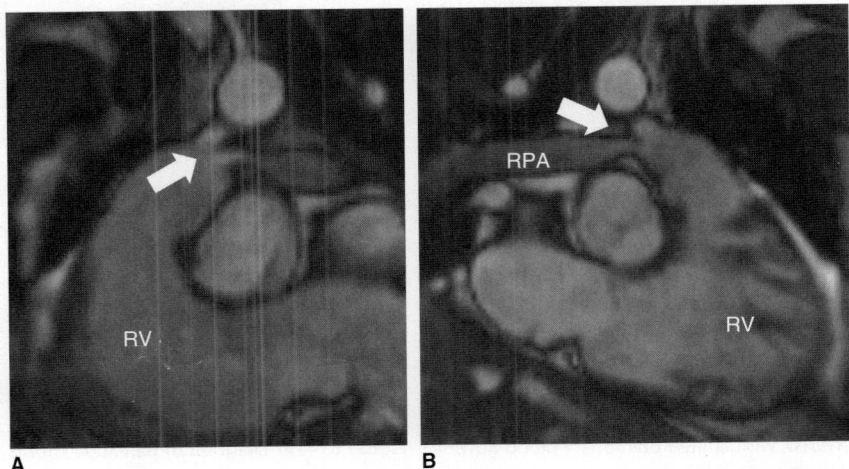

Figure 67–16. Branch pulmonary artery stenosis. Stenosis of the origin of the branch pulmonary arteries that appear somewhat hypoplastic. The right ventricle (RV) is hypertrophied. RPA, right pulmonary artery.

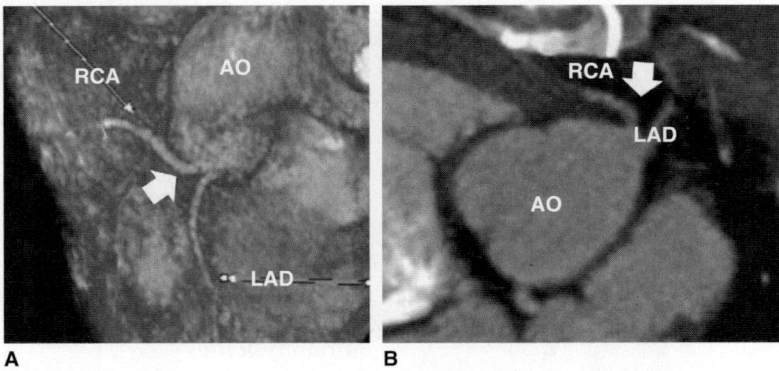

Figure 67–17. Left anterior descending from the right sinus of Valsalva. Multidetector computed tomography images: 3D reconstruction of aortic root (**A**) and double axial oblique view (**B**) showing that both the right coronary artery (RCA) and left anterior descending (LAD) artery originate from the same (right) sinus (*arrow*). The LAD crosses the RVOT and can be damaged with right ventriculotomy.

RV and pulmonary circulation. Within this group, there is again a wide spectrum of anatomies, depending on the level and type of the obstruction (valvar obstruction vs partial or complete absence of PAs) with collateral circulation to the lungs of differing degrees and origin (major aortopulmonary collateral arteries [MAPCAs]).

Palliative Procedures and ToF Repair

Palliative Surgery

Palliative surgery in ToF is usually aimed at augmenting pulmonary blood flow in infants with severe pulmonary stenosis or pulmonary atresia. As surgical techniques and perioperative care evolved, direct repair at a young age (not preceded by a palliative procedure) is the current approach of choice. However, palliative surgery is still performed in:

- Small symptomatic infants who cannot undergo repair
- Infants with hypoplastic PAs, with the aim of augmenting pulmonary blood flow and allowing the PAs to grow in size before repair
- Infants with abnormal coronary arteries, in whom repair is not yet technically feasible

The current palliative procedure of choice is the modified BT shunt, which consists of a small tube graft connecting the subclavian artery to the ipsilateral PA (**Fig. 67–19**). This allows systemic arterial blood (which is partially saturated in a cyanotic child) to shunt into the PA and improves oxygenation, while allowing the PAs to develop. The original BT shunt was achieved by anastomosing the subclavian artery to the PA

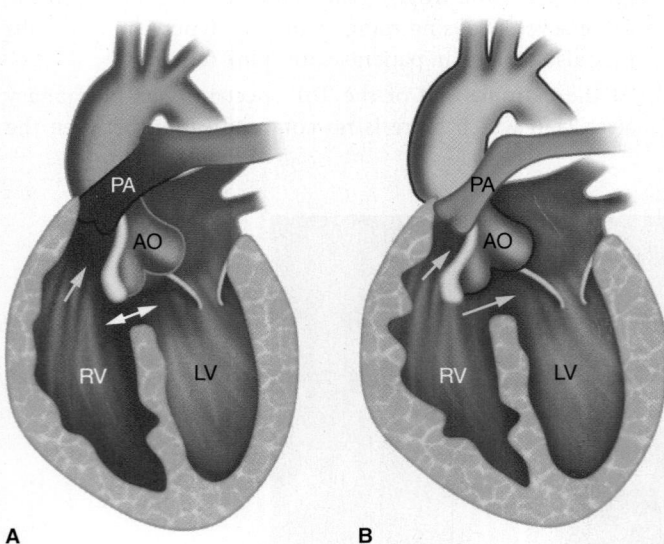

Figure 67–18. Diagram depicting the effect of the severity of the RVOTO on clinical presentation in ToF. In (**A**), "pink tetralogy," in patients with mild–moderate RVOTO, with normal or excessive pulmonary blood flow and no cyanosis at rest. In (**B**), severe RVOTO, with limited pulmonary blood flow, often hypoplastic pulmonary arteries and right–left shunting across the ventricular septal defect causing cyanosis. Dynamic increase in the severity of RVOTO can cause "cyanotic spells."

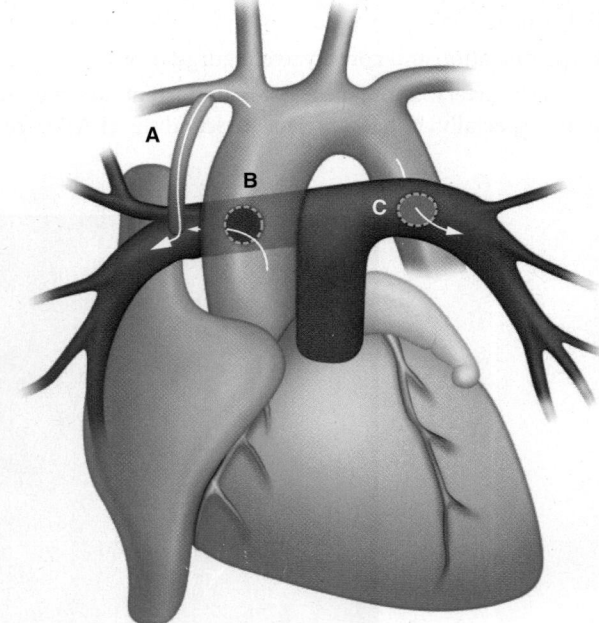

Figure 67–19. Diagram of palliative shunts. (**A**) Modified right BT shunt, between the right subclavian artery and right pulmonary artery. (**B**) Waterston shunt, between the ascending aorta and right pulmonary artery. (**C**) Potts shunt, between the descending aorta and left pulmonary artery.

(end-to-side) hence depriving the arm from direct blood perfusion, relying on collaterals.

Alternatives to the BT shunt included the Waterston shunt (direct anastomosis of the ascending aorta to the right PA) and the Potts shunt (direct anastomosis of the descending aorta to the left PA, physiologically similar to a patent ductus arteriosus). The Waterston and Potts shunt have largely been abandoned for this indication, because the defect created may be under- or oversized, either being ineffective or causing excessive flow to the lungs, triggering pulmonary vascular disease. The modified BT shunt can be easily sized by choosing the correct size for the tube graft.

There are risks associated with a palliative shunt, such as the modified BT. The shunt can volume load the LV (similar to the large patent ductus arteriosus), causing congestive heart failure and long-term LV dysfunction. In the perioperative period, it can cause pulmonary oedema or hemorrhage and, if oversized, and trigger pulmonary vascular disease. Finally, it may be prone to infection and may distort the anatomy of the PA causing stenosis or occlusion.

Surgical Repair

Technique: Surgery for repairing ToF consists of closing the VSD and relieving the RVOTO. The surgical approach to ToF repair has evolved since the first description by Lillehei et al. in 1955.[39] The original procedure involved rather extensive ventriculotomy and patch augmentation of the RVOT and PAs. A transannular patch was used in the presence of a hypoplastic and/or stenotic pulmonary valve. The aim was to relieve most RVOTO at the expense of PR, which was common, especially when a transannular patch was required and when this was thought to be a benign intervention.[40,41] Moreover, extensive

surgery led to a significantly scarred, aneurysmal, and dyskinetic RVOT, which is the substrate for malignant arrhythmias.

As evidence accumulated showing that long-standing significant PR was associated with long-term complications, including heart failure, arrhythmia and sudden death, the surgical approach evolved. Ventriculotomies became small and, eventually, a transatrial approach to repair ToF was introduced and is currently used in most expert centers (**Fig. 67–20**). Moreover, surgical techniques aimed at preserving pulmonary valve function were introduced, mainly pulmonary valvuloplasty, while pulmonary valve replacement (PVR) in young children at the time of ToF repair is avoided.[42-44]

Implantation of an RV-PA conduit becomes necessary when there is ToF with pulmonary atresia. In such cases, extensive multistage surgery to the pulmonary arterial tree is often necessary: in patients with hypoplastic or absent PAs, "unifocalization" of the vessels feeding each lung is performed (ie, reconstruction of the PAs using existing hypoplastic PAs and MAPCAs), connecting each lung to a modified BT shunt; thereafter the reconstructed PAs are connected to an RV-PA conduit and the VSD is closed (providing RV pressures are not significantly raised due to pulmonary vascular disease or significant peripheral pulmonary stenoses).

An RV-PA conduit may also be required in the presence of an anomalous coronary circulation (eg, left anterior descending from the RCA), which could be endangered by surgery to the native RVOT.

Timing of Repair: "Late repair" of ToF (eg, beyond the age of 10 years) is now avoided, due to the detrimental effects of long-standing cyanosis and pressure load to the RV, even though an agreed definition of "late repair" is lacking. Neonatal repair is

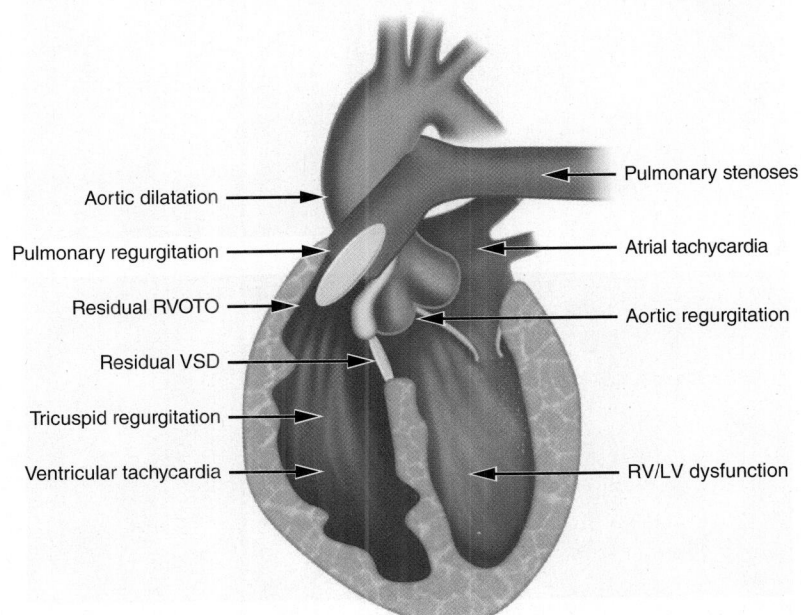

Figure 67–20. Surgical repair of ToF and its long-term sequelae. Diagram depicting a heart repaired ToF. Surgical repair consists of closure of the VSD with a patch and augmentation of the RVOT (and pulmonary artery if the pulmonary valve and pulmonary artery are stenotic) using a patch. The long-term sequalae of tetralogy repair are depicted.

often feasible but does not provide any benefits compared to primary repair at 3 to 6 months of age. Infants who are symptomatic due to severe RVOTO and cyanosis can benefit from duct stenting or palliative surgery (see section Palliative Surgery) early in life to increase pulmonary blood flow and allow the PAs to grow, even though such a procedure does carry risks.[45–47] Balloon dilatation of the pulmonary valve annulus or RVOT stenting has also been proposed for selected patients.[48]

Pathophysiology and Long-Term Outcome after Repair of ToF

The natural history of repaired ToF differs significantly from that of the native lesion. Indeed, ToF patients have benefitted significantly from surgery, with a low perioperative mortality (<3%), and optimal long-term survival.[49–51] This is especially true for the last three to four decades, the so-called "infant era" when primary ToF repair became possible thanks to early diagnosis, the use of prostaglandins for duct-dependent cases (eg, pulmonary atresia) and advances is surgical technique and perioperative care.

Predictors of perioperative mortality include the preoperative size of the PAs and pulmonary valve annulus, severity of cyanosis, and need for transannular patch. Additional risk factors included coronary anomalies or additional CHD (associated) lesions and small or premature infants.[49,52] The same factors dictate many of the long-term complications encountered. For example, patients with more severe RVOTO, a small pulmonary valve annulus, and hypoplastic PAs are more likely to require a transannular patch and will present with either residual stenosis or more commonly PR, depending on the surgical technique used. Patients requiring ventriculotomy are more likely to develop a substrate for ventricular arrhythmias. Patients requiring implantation of an RV-PA conduit are likely to develop stenosis and/or regurgitation of the conduit and may be more prone to infective endocarditis.

While data on the very-long-term survival of ToF patients repaired in the modern era are still lacking, long-term survival is excellent. Most patients with repaired ToF are expected to reach adult life with little everyday limitation, albeit with the risk of long-term complications and need for repeat intervention.[53–55] Indeed, reoperation rates are estimated at 44% at 35 years after the initial repair and are highest in patients after transannular patch.[53–57]

Long-term complications after ToF repair include:

- PR, which is the most common indication for reintervention (**Figs. 67–21** and **67–22**)[58]
- Pulmonary stenosis, which may be valvar, but more commonly subvalvar or supravalvar/ peripheral
- Degeneration of an RV-PA conduit, causing RVOT stenosis and/or regurgitation

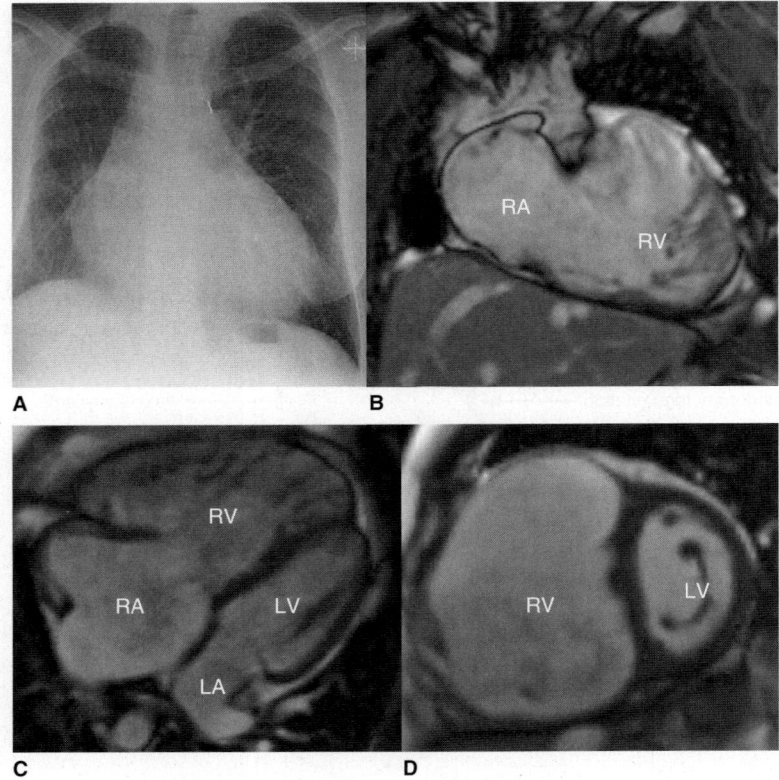

Figure 67–21. Severe pulmonary regurgitation. In (**A**), chest radiograph of an adult patient with severe pulmonary regurgitation after repair of ToF showing significant cardiomegaly. In (**B**) and (**C**), CMR images showing severe right ventricle (RV) and right atrial (RA) dilatation. In D, short axis slice demonstrating the disproportion between the dilated RV and small LV, with flattening of the ventricular septum in diastole due to volume overload of the RV.

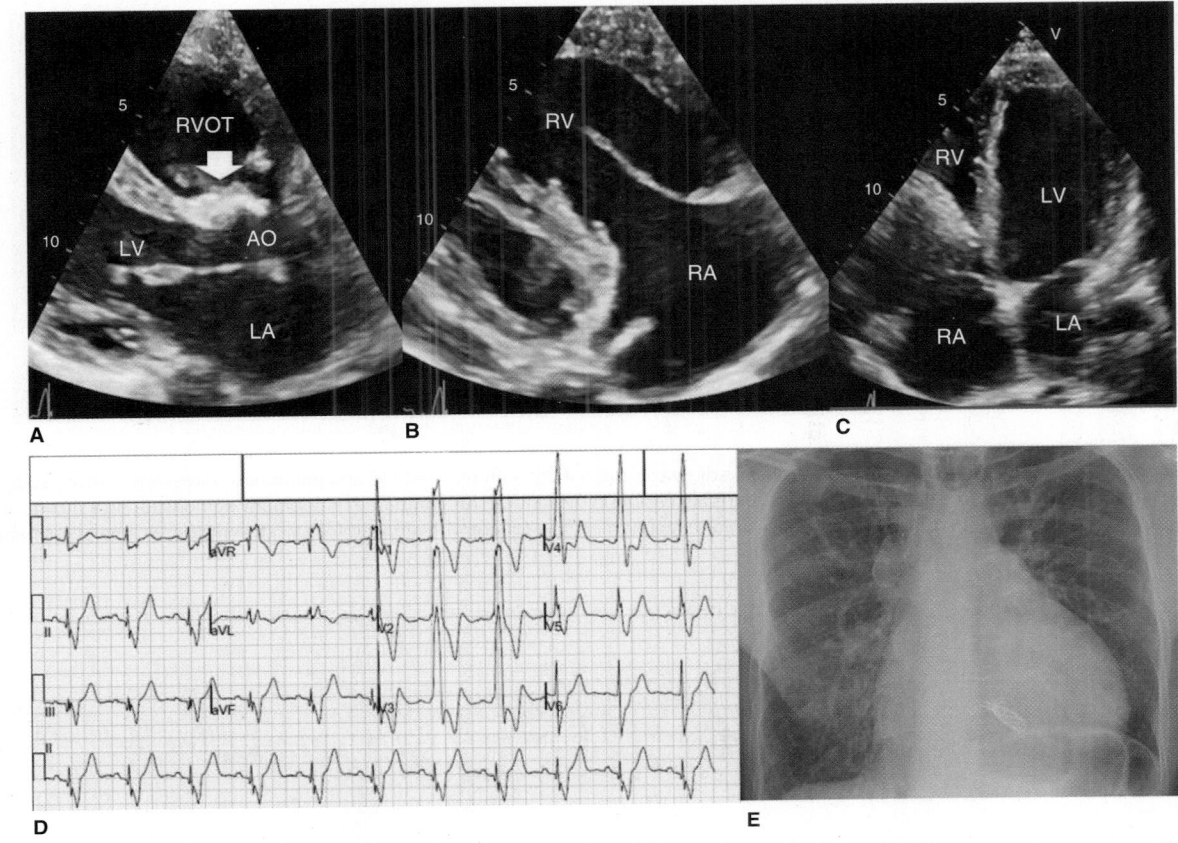

Figure 67–22. Severe pulmonary regurgitation after repair of ToF. In (**A**) to (**C**), echocardiographic images in a patient with repaired ToF and severe RV dilatation due to severe pulmonary regurgitation. A calcified patch closing the VSD is seen in (**A**) (*arrow*). In (**B**), RV and right atrial dilatation is present. In (**D**), ECG showing a RBBB with significantly prolonged QRS duration. In (**E**), chest radiograph showing cardiomegaly with signs of RV dilatation, calcification of a RV-to-pulmonary artery homograft, right pulmonary artery stent, and a dislodged stent in the RV, also visible in (**C**).

- Degeneration of prosthetic valves (commonly a bioprosthetic pulmonary valve), the second most common indication for reoperation/intervention in repaired ToF[58]

- Residual VSD or ASD

- Aortic root dilatation and aortic regurgitation (**Fig. 67–23**)

- Arrhythmias, both supraventricular but also ventricular in origin, with a small but significant (in the young population of patients) risk of sudden cardiac death (SCD; **Fig. 67–24**)

- Late RV dysfunction, resulting from a combination of a residual/ongoing hemodynamic lesion (most commonly PR, but also TR or RVOTO) and the effects of previous surgery (especially when an RV-PA conduit was implanted). RV "restriction" is also common

- LV dysfunction is present in a small but substantial number of patients

- Exercise intolerance and heart failure are more common in older patients repaired in the early surgical era (who may present with ventricular dysfunction and long-standing residual hemodynamic lesions)

- Endocarditis is a risk for all ToF patients, especially those with RV-PA conduits, residual lesions (VSD, PR, or TR), and patients with prosthetic valves (particularly percutaneously implanted pulmonary valves).

Expert lifelong care is, therefore, warranted for all ToF patients who should be followed by physicians and surgeons who are experts in detecting and managing long-term complications.

Long-Term Sequelae and Complications

PR and RVOTO (Including TR and VSD): PR is extremely common in patients with repaired ToF, present in approximately 70% of adults. The severity of the PR after ToF repair depends the original anatomy and type of repair performed. In patients with a small pulmonary valve annulus and PA involvement, who received a transannular patch, PR after repair is inevitable. Modern surgical techniques aiming at achieving a competent pulmonary valve (eg, valve sparing techniques and/or valve repair at the time of surgery) appear promising, but very long-term data are awaited.[43,59]

Severe PR is a volume-loading lesion, leading to progressive remodeling of the RV (ie, dilatation and eccentric hypertrophy). It is typically well-tolerated for several years, but is not a benign lesion in the long term (Figs. 67–21 and 67–22). PR can lead to severe RV dilatation, RV fibrosis, and progressive RV systolic dysfunction, which should be avoided by intervening on the pulmonary valve in a timely fashion. Functional TR is also commonly encountered in patients with significantly

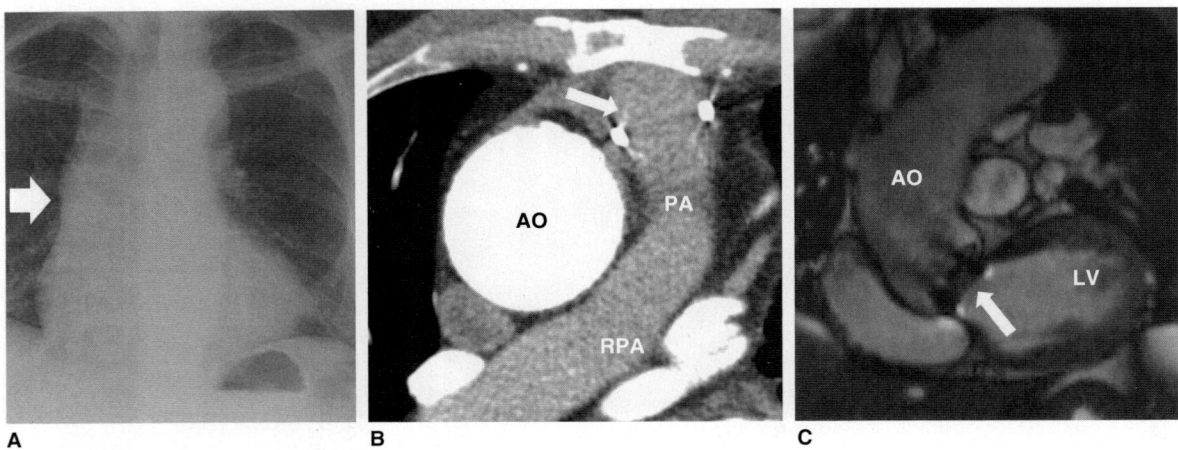

Figure 67–23. Aortic dilatation in repaired ToF. In (**A**), chest radiograph of a patient with repaired ToF and pulmonary valve replacement, suggestive of a dilated ascending aorta (AO, *arrow*); the bioprosthetic valve ring is also visible in the RVOT. In (**B**), computed tomography demonstrating a significantly dilated ascending aorta and the pulmonary bioprosthesis. In (**C**), aortic valve replacement in a patient with repaired ToF. LV, left ventricle; PA, (main) pulmonary artery; RPA, right pulmonary artery.

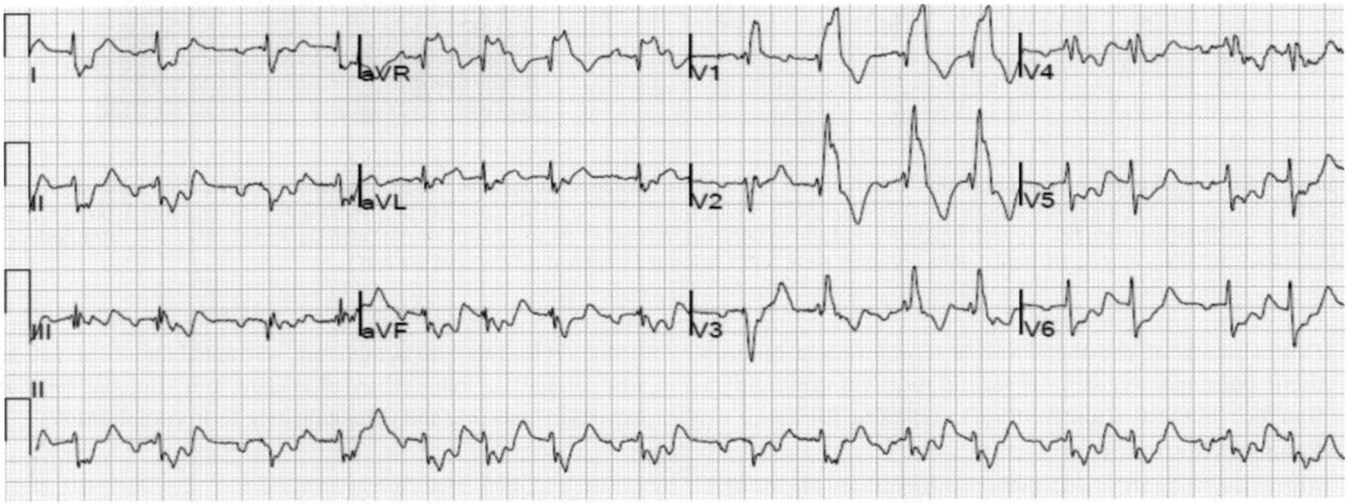

Figure 67–24. Ventricular tachycardia in ToF. In (**A**), ECG of a patient with repaired ToF. Note the atrial tachycardia and RBBB with significantly prolonged QRS duration (~200 ms). In (**B**), CMR image showing late gadolinium enhancement of the RVOT (*arrow*), suggestive of extensive scarring at the area of previous ventriculotomy and the potential for ventricular tachycardia. In (**C**), sustained monomorphic ventricular tachycardia. In (**D**), chest radiograph late after ToF repair showing significant cardiomegaly with signs of right atrial and ventricular dilatation and presence of an ICD.

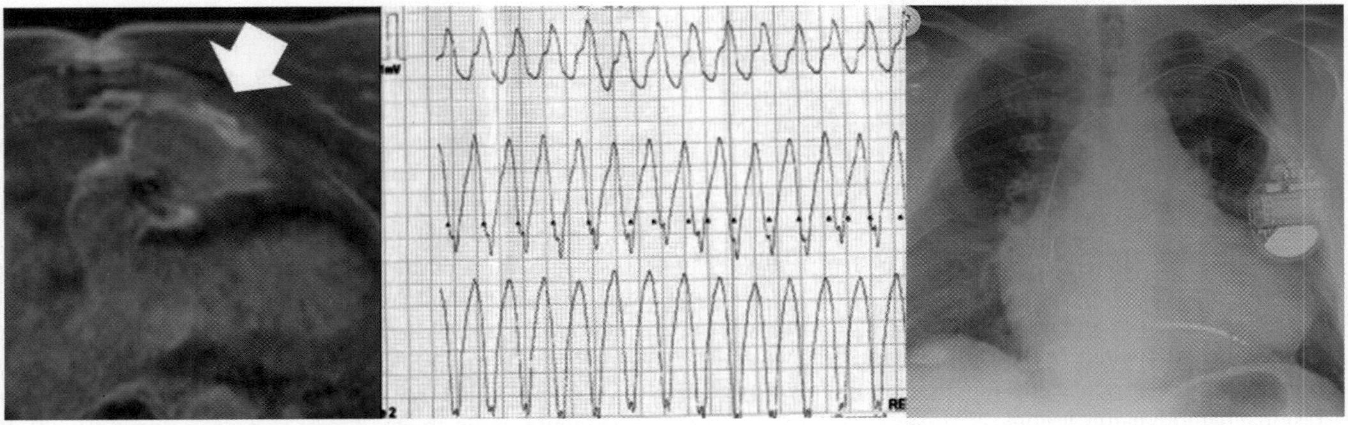

dilated RVs and further aggravates the volume load to the RV.[60] Severe progressive RV dilatation and fibrosis may also increase the risk of malignant tachyarrhythmia and SCD.

Severe PR in combination with "diastolic dysfunction" of the RV ("restrictive RV," not uncommon after ToF repair), causes a rise in RV filling pressures and RA dilatation, and can predispose patients to supraventricular arrhythmias or central venous congestion.

RV fibrosis detected on CMR by late gadolinium enhancement is related to ventricular dysfunction, exercise intolerance, and neurohormonal activation. Moreover, increased RV fibrosis in associated with the risk of clinically relevant arrhythmia.[61]

Symptoms relating to severe PR often present late, for several reasons. Patients are more likely to notice a decline in exercise capacity or signs of heart failure late in the disease course, when RV dysfunction and a reduction in cardiac output occurs. Moreover, as this is a condition present since infancy and progresses over several years, even decades, it may be more difficult for patients to notice a decline until late. PVR should ideally be performed before significant RV dysfunction and symptoms occur, hence regular monitoring with imaging and exercise testing is warranted.

PVR results in significant reverse remodeling, with an improvement in systolic function, especially if this is performed when the RV end-systolic volume does not exceed 82 mL/m².[62] A small but significant improvement in LV ejection fraction is also observed, reflecting the significant ventricular–ventricular interaction in this condition. An improvement in exercise capacity and relief of symptoms in previously symptomatic patients is also observed and related to RV reverse remodeling. However, the effect of PVR on symptoms is more prominent in patients with a combination of RVOTO and PR.[6] Indications for PVR according to AHA/ACC and ESC guidelines are shown in **Tables 67–6** and **67–7**.

Arrhythmias: The potential for malignant tachycardias and SCD is well recognized in patients with repaired ToF and has become integral to the management and risk stratification of these patients (Fig. 67–24).[63] The incidence of SCD reported in various studies is approximately 2% per decade.[53,63,64] Ventricular tachycardia (VT) typically originates from the outflow tract, around areas of scarring from previous ventriculotomy, or the VSD repair. While sustained monomorphic VT is relatively uncommon, nonsustained VT on Holter monitoring or pacing checks is common, but its prognostic implications are still debated.

The study that has provided the most widely used risk stratifiers for SCD in ToF included 121 patients, each with an implantable cardioverter defibrillator (ICD) from 11 specialist centers. After a median of 3.7 years from ICD implantation, 30% of patients received ≥1 appropriate shocks: 7.7%/year in patients with ICD implanted as primary prevention and 9.8%/year for those as secondary prevention.[65]

TABLE 67–6. Tetralogy of Fallot: 2018 AHA/ACC Guidelines for ACHD

COR	LOE	Diagnostic	Therapeutic
I	B-NR	1. CMR is useful to quantify ventricular size and function, pulmonary valve function, pulmonary artery anatomy, and left heart abnormalities in patients with repaired TOF	1. Pulmonary valve replacement (surgical or percutaneous) for relief of symptoms is recommended for patients with repaired TOF and moderate or greater PR with cardiovascular symptoms not otherwise explained
I	B-NR	1. Coronary artery compression testing is indicated before RV to PA conduit stenting or transcatheter valve placement in repaired TOF	
IIa	B-NR	1. Programmed ventricular stimulation can be useful to risk-stratify adults with TOF and additional risk factors for SCD	1. Pulmonary valve replacement (surgical or percutaneous) is reasonable for preservation of ventricular size and function in asymptomatic patients with repaired TOF and ventricular enlargement or dysfunction and moderate or greater PR
IIa	B-NR	1. In patients with repaired TOF, cardiac catheterization with angiography, if indicated, is reasonable to assess hemodynamics when adequate data cannot be obtained noninvasively in the setting of an arrhythmia, HF, unexplained ventricular dysfunction, suspected pulmonary hypertension or cyanosis	1. Primary prevention ICD therapy is reasonable in adults with TOF and multiple risk factors for SCD
IIb	C-EO		1. Surgical pulmonary valve replacement may be reasonable for adults with repaired TOF and moderate or greater PR with other lesions requiring surgical interventions
IIb	C-EO		1. Pulmonary valve replacement, in addition to arrhythmia management, may be considered for adults with repaired TOF and moderate or greater PR and ventricular tachyarrhythmia

Abbreviations: ACHD, adult congenital heart disease; CMR, cardiac magnetic resonance; COR, class of recommendation; EO, expert opinion; HF, heart failure; ICD, implantable cardioverter defibrillator; LD, limited data; LOE, level of evidence; NR, nonrandomized; PA, pulmonary artery; PR, pulmonary regurgitation; RV, right ventricle; SCD, sudden cardiac death; TOF, tetralogy of Fallot.

TABLE 67–7. Tetralogy of Fallot: 2020 ESC Guidelines for ACHD

COR	LOE	Therapeutic
I	C	1. PVR is recommended in symptomatic patients with severe PR and/or at least moderate RVOTO. 2. In patients with no native outflow tract, catheter intervention (TPVI) should be preferred if anatomically feasible.

IIa	C	1. PVR should be considered in asymptomatic patients with severe PR and/or RVOTO when one of the following criteria is present.
		  • Decrease in objective exercise capacity.
		  • Progressive RV dilation to RVESVi $\geq$ 80 mL/m^2, and/or RVEDVi $\geq$160 mL/m^2, and/or progression of TR to at least moderate.
		  • Progressive RV systolic dysfunction.
		  • RVOTO with RVSP > 80 mmHg.

IIa	C	1. In patients with sustained VT who are undergoing surgical PVR or transcutaneous valve insertion, pre-operative catheter mapping and transsection of VT-related anatomical isthmuses before or during the intervention should be considered. 2. Electrophysiologic evaluation, including programmed electrical stimulation, should be considered for risk stratification for SCD in patients with additional risk factors (LV/RV dysfunction; non-sustained, symptomatic VT; QRS duration $\geq$ 180 ms, extensive RV scarring on CMR). 3. ICD implantation should be considered in selected TOF patients with multiple risk factors for SCD, including LV dysfunction, non-sustained, symptomatic VT, QRS duration $\geq$ 180 ms, extensive RV scarring on CMR, or inducible VT at programmed electrical stimulation.
IIb	C	1. Catheter ablation or concomitant surgical ablation for symptomatic monomorphic sustained VT may be considered in those with a preserved biventricular function as an alternative to ICD therapy, provided that the procedure is performed in highly experienced centers and that established ablation endpoints have been reached (e.g. non-inducibility, conduction block across ablation lines).

Abbreviations: ACHD, adult congenital heart disease, CMR, cardiovascular magnetic resonance; COR, class of recommendation; ICD, implantable cardioverter defibrillator; LOE, level of evidence; LV, left ventricle/ventricular; PR, pulmonary regurgitation; PVR, pulmonary valve replacement; RV, right ventricle/ventricular; RVEDVi, right ventricular end diastolic volume indexed; RVESVi, right ventricular end systolic volume indexed; RVOT, right ventricular outflow tract; RVOTO, right ventricular outflow tract obstruction; RVSP, right ventricular systolic pressure; SCD, sudden cardiac death; TOF, Tetralogy of Fallot; TPVI, transcatheter pulmonary valve implantation; TR, tricuspid regurgitation; VSD, ventricular septal defect; VT, ventricular tachycardia.

The AHA/ACC ACHD guidelines include the following as risk factors for SCD in ToF:

• LV systolic or diastolic dysfunction

• Nonsustained VT

• QRS duration $\geq$180 ms

• Extensive RV scarring by CMR

• Inducible sustained VT at electrophysiological study; this is most useful for patients deemed at intermediate risk of SCD and is less likely to influence the decision to implant an ICD in low- or high-risk patients.

The decision to implant an ICD should be weighed against the risk of inappropriate shocks (~5% per year),[6,66,67] other ICD-related complications, and the overall psychological impact on young patients with ToF. Ablation of VT may be useful in reducing arrhythmia burden but does not replace ICD implantation in patients at increased risk of SCD or previous symptomatic VT. Optimization of hemodynamics is also recommended (eg, PVR in a patient with severe PR and severely enlarged RV) as a means of reducing the risk of malignant arrhythmias.

Supraventricular arrhythmias are also common after ToF repair and are incisional (intra atrial tachycardias), atrial flutter, or more rarely atrial fibrillation (in older patients). Long-standing hemodynamic lesions, later repair or repair in the early surgical era and ventricular dysfunction (including "restrictive" RV physiology), are likely to contribute to right atrial dilatation and the incidence of supraventricular arrhythmias.[54] An overlap between supraventricular and ventricular arrhythmias has been described in the presence of PR causing RV overload.

Heart Failure: The number of ACHD patients requiring recurrent admissions for heart failure is rapidly increasing and those admitted with heart failure are at significant risk of mortality.[68,69] While most patients with repaired ToF remain asymptomatic for decades after repair, a small but significant proportion present with symptoms and signs of heart failure, including exercise intolerance and congestion. The potential mechanisms behind the development of heart failure in ToF are multiple.[70] Older patients with later repair or repair during the early surgical era may present with heart failure due to RV or LV systolic and/or diastolic dysfunction. This may be attributed to the prolonged cyanosis and RV overload, suboptimal myocardial preservation around surgery, ventricular overload due to previous palliative shunts, and a large aneurysmal RVOT. Addition causes of heart failure include associated or residual lesions (eg, aortic regurgitation, VSDs, peripheral pulmonary stenosis, or pulmonary hypertension), medication (eg, large doses of β-blockers used to control arrhythmia), long-standing ventricular pacing, detraining, and obesity. A reduction in lung volumes is not uncommon and affects exercise capacity, especially in patients with significant cardiomegaly, previous thoracotomies, and associated skeletal abnormalities.

Endocarditis: All ACHD patients, including those with repaired ToF, are considered at increased risk of developing infective endocarditis. Education on the merits of dental and skin hygiene, and the early recognition of signs and symptoms suggestive of endocarditis, are key and are the responsibility of the CHD specialist who provides lifelong care for these patients. Education of the patient and family start in early infancy, and is reinforced during the transition to ACHD services when patients are prepared for adult life and are empowered to take responsibility for their health.[71]

Current American and European guidelines do not recommend antibiotics for endocarditis prophylaxis for all patients with repaired ToF.[6,21,72] However, patients with prosthetic valves or prosthetic material used for valve repair, cyanotic CHD (uncorrected), or prosthetic material or device implanted within the last 6 months (while endothelialization is ongoing), residual shunts in proximity of prosthetic material/device, and those with previous endocarditis should be offered antibiotic prophylaxis for dental treatment that involves manipulation of the gums or the periapical region of teeth or cause perforation of the oral mucosa/bleeding. Prophylaxis is not recommended for gastrointestinal, genitourinary, or other procedures.

Aortic Dilatation and Aortic Regurgitation: Aortic dilatation is common in ToF, observed in up to 25% of patients.[73,74] It is most commonly seen in patients with ToF and pulmonary atresia and is often associated with aortic regurgitation. It relates to previous increase blood flow to the aorta, due to a longer time from palliative shunt to repair, pulmonary atresia (where both the systemic venous and pulmonary venous flow is ejected to the aorta), aortic regurgitation, and increased LV size.[73] Tan et al. have also demonstrated marked histological abnormalities in the aortic root and ascending aorta of ToF patients from an early age, with changes such as medionecrosis, fibrosis, and elastic fragmentation related to aortic dimensions likely contributing to the aortic dilatation observed in ToF.[74]

However, the risk of major complications, such as aortic dissection or rupture, is low in ToF patients.[75-77] Indeed, there are very few such reports in literature, mostly affecting patients with extremely large aortas.

Assessment of Adults with Repaired ToF

History
When assessing a patient with repaired ToF, one should be aware of their mode of presentation and surgical history. Surgical notes are particularly helpful for providing insight into the anatomy and surgical techniques used by the surgeon. Important information includes:

- Type and timing of palliative shunts
- Type and timing of repair
- Prosthetic material used to augment the RVOT and PA
- Ventriculotomy performed, versus transatrial approach
- Surgery to reconstruct the pulmonary valve
- Additional surgery at the time of repair
- Perioperative complications
- Type and timing of subsequent surgery or interventions to the pulmonary valve, tricuspid valve, PAs, residual VSDs, aortic valve, and so on
- Implantation of pacemaker or ICD

Other important elements of the history focus on complications including arrhythmias, heart failure, and endocarditis, among others. Obstetric history should also be noted.

Regarding recent history, patients should be interrogated with regards to exercise intolerance, congestion/edema, palpitations, syncope or near-syncope, and chest pain.

Physical Examination
Typical findings in an adult with repaired ToF that should be noted include:

- Surgical scars: median sternotomy (from the repair) and thoracotomy scars (from palliative shunts or associated lesions, eg, coarctation of the aorta)
- Facial or other features of DiGeorge syndrome
  In the presence of severe PR, one can appreciate:
- An RV heave
- Single S2
- An ejection systolic murmur over the upper left sternal border, of intensity that depends on the pressure gradient across the RVOT (residual stenosis, prosthetic pulmonary valve or conduit, and/or increased stroke volume due to PR)
- An early diastolic murmur that becomes shorter as the PR becomes more severe. However, the length of the murmur is also influence by RV end-diastolic pressures (the presence of a "restrictive" RV) and PA pressures.
  Other findings on auscultation include:
- A harsh pansystolic murmur, in the presence of a residual VSD
- Ejection systolic murmurs throughout the chest, suggestive of peripheral pulmonary stenosis
- A soft pansystolic murmur of TR, varying with respiration
- A long diastolic murmur of aortic regurgitation
- Extra heart sounds (S3 and S4) in patients with advanced/decompensated heart failure
- Continuous murmurs in the presence of residual surgical shunts or MAPCAs.

ECG and Chest Radiography
The typical feature of the ECG in patients with repaired ToF is an RBBB, with a wide QRS duration, that can progress over time and relates to a previous ventriculotomy, extensive muscle resection in RVOT, transannular pulmonary patch repair, and RV volume overload (Figs. 67–22 and 67–24).[78,79] The ECG took a prominent position in the assessment of ToF patients when Gatzoulis et al. demonstrated a relation between QRS duration and the risk of syncope or SCD.[80] A QRS duration >180 ms (Fig. 67–24) has since been used in the risk stratification of ToF patients for sudden death, even though recent data suggest that the ECG is not as strong a predictor of outcome in more modern cohorts.

Chest radiography can also provide valuable information of cardiac size, dilatation of the PAs or aorta, previous sternotomy or thoracotomy, the presence of a right-sided aortic arch, calcification of surgical patches of conduits, and signs of lung congestion or pulmonary edema. Patients with unrepaired ToF with pulmonary atresia have a characteristic boot-shaped heart, with absence of the RVOT/main PA (**Fig. 67–25**).

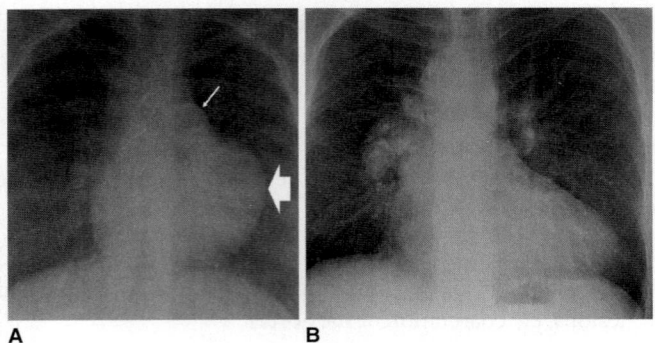

Figure 67–25. Chest radiograms in ToF patients. In (**A**), a patient with repaired ToF and pulmonary valve replacement. The *small arrow* points to the prosthetic pulmonary valve. There is a raised cardiac apex suggestive of RV dilatation (large *arrow*). There is also evidence of previous sternotomy and a prominent RVOT and right pulmonary artery. In (**B**), a patient with unrepaired ToF and pulmonary atresia with a "boot-shaped" heart and prominent right pulmonary artery. There is also a right aortic arch (note the deviation of the trachea to the left).

Imaging

Echocardiography: The echocardiographic assessment of adults with repaired ToF should focus on potential sequelae or residual lesions. The latter includes residual VSDs and RVOTO. Long-term sequelae include PR, ventricular dysfunction (systolic or diastolic), aortic regurgitation or aortic dilatation, and TR. Moreover, echocardiography (transthoracic and transesophageal) is instrumental in the diagnosis of infective endocarditis, typically affecting the pulmonary valve, RV-PA conduit, residual VSDs and adjacent tricuspid valve, and prosthetic material (patches, pacemaker wires, prosthetic valves).

The severity of PR may be assessed by the width of the regurgitant jet and duration of the regurgitation Doppler relative to the duration of diastole (Doppler PR index): in severe PR, RV pressures become equal to PA pressure before the end of diastole, hence the duration of the PR Doppler is short (**Fig. 67–26**). However, when the RV is "restrictive," RV pressure rises rapidly in diastole and may become equal to PA pressure before the end of diastole (providing there is no pulmonary hypertension) in the absence of severe PR. "Restrictive" RV physiology is identified as forward flow in late diastole on the pulmonary Doppler. The presence of pulmonary hypertension or restrictive RV function and the degree of PR need to be taken into consideration when interpreting the characteristics of the Doppler (and 2D) echocardiographic findings (**Fig. 67–27**).

RV-PA conduits (eg, for pulmonary atresia) may be particularly difficult to visualize because they are retrosternal (requiring modified views) and are often heavily calcified. Peripheral pulmonary stenosis may also be difficult to characterize on transthoracic echocardiography (TTE).

Transesophageal echocardiography (TEE) is rarely required in repaired ToF, with the exception of cases of suspected endocarditis, even though this is often right-sided affecting the pulmonary valve or an RV-PA conduit, which is an anterior structure, and which may therefore be visualized better by TTE.

Particular attention is required in repaired pulmonary atresia, peripheral pulmonary stenosis, and RV-PA conduit stenosis that are reflected in the TR gradient. Pulmonary hypertension should also be excluded in patients with "pink tetralogy," previous palliative shunts, and those with complex pulmonary atresia (segmental pulmonary hypertension).[81,82]

CMR Imaging: CMR has become the gold-standard investigation for assessing the RV (including the presence and severity of fibrosis with late gadolinium enhancement) and quantifying PR in repaired ToF (Fig. 67–21). The AHA/ACC ACHD guidelines strongly recommend the use of CMR in patients with repaired ToF to quantify ventricular size and function, pulmonary valve function, PA anatomy, and left heart abnormalities (Tables 67–6 and 67–7).

Three-dimensional (3D) magnetic resonance angiography allows for detailed assessment of peripheral PAs, collateral

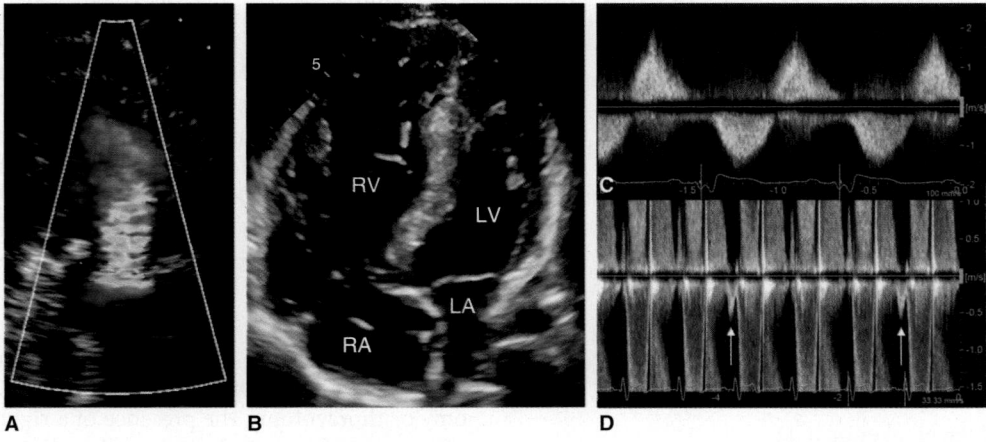

Figure 67–26. Severe pulmonary regurgitation with restrictive RV physiology. In (**A**), there is a broad jet of severe pulmonary regurgitation (PR). In (**B**), a severely dilated RV is displayed that is apex forming. In (**C**), continuous wave Doppler just below the pulmonary valve, showing a rapid descent of the PR velocity in keeping with severe PR. In (**D**), forward atrial flow on the pulmonary Doppler signal varying with respiration (A wave, *arrows*) suggests markedly elevated filling pressures.

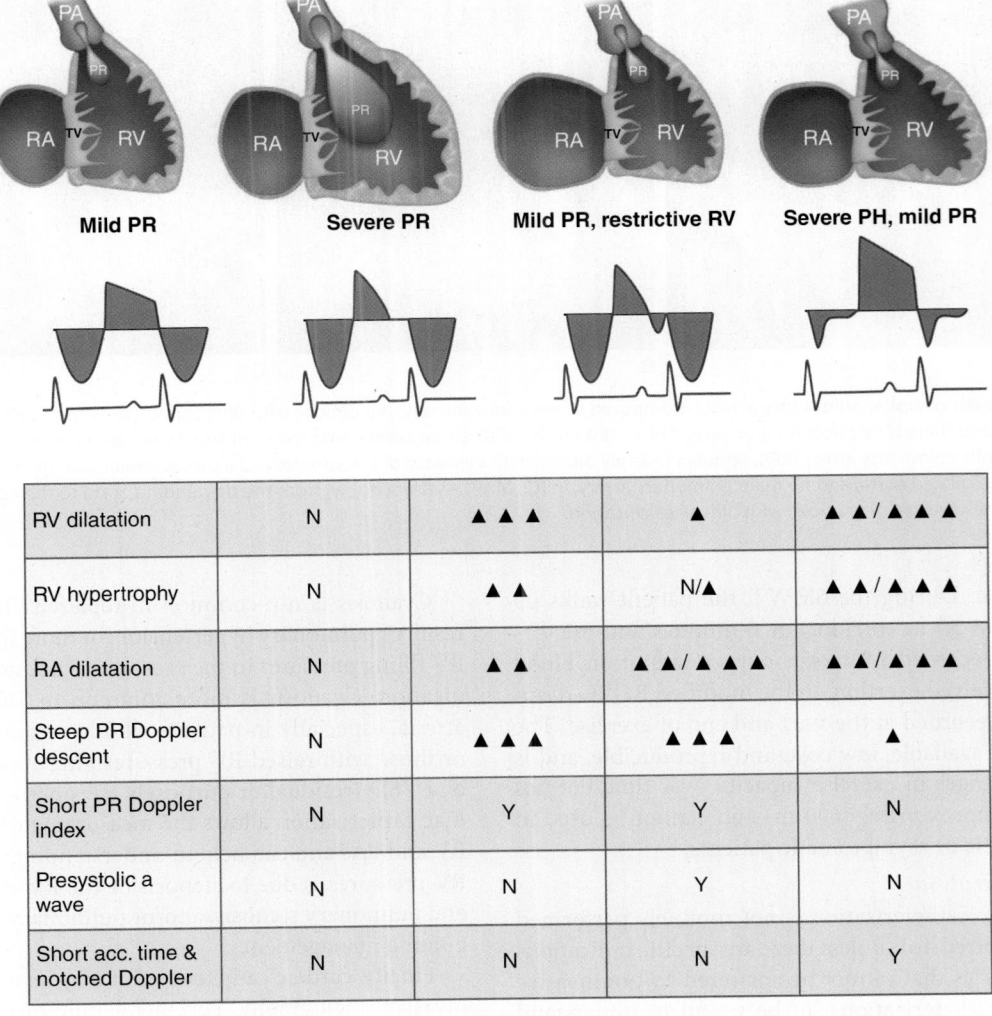

	Mild PR	Severe PR	Mild PR, restrictive RV	Severe PH, mild PR
RV dilatation	N	▲▲▲	▲	▲▲/▲▲▲
RV hypertrophy	N	▲▲	N/▲	▲▲/▲▲▲
RA dilatation	N	▲▲	▲▲/▲▲▲	▲▲/▲▲▲
Steep PR Doppler descent	N	▲▲▲	▲▲▲	▲
Short PR Doppler index	N	Y	Y	N
Presystolic a wave	N	N	Y	N
Short acc. time & notched Doppler	N	N	N	Y

Figure 67–27. Anatomic and continuous wave Doppler characteristics in different pathophysiological states involving pulmonary regurgitation.

arteries (eg, MAPCAs), and in the assessment prior to percutaneous pulmonary valve implantation.

Its accuracy and lack of radiation has allowed CMR to become part of the routine follow-up of ToF patients in specialist centers, monitoring residual hemodynamic lesions, assessing the effect of interventions (eg, PVR), and aiding in the risk stratification of SCD.[6]

Cardiac CT: CT has a complementary role to echocardiography and CMR. It has become standard for the assessment of the coronary artery circulation prior to percutaneous pulmonary valve implantation (assessing the proximity to the RVOT and risk of extrinsic compression at the time of valve implantation), in older patients undergoing cardiac surgery and patients with unexplained LV dysfunction. CT is also useful in delineating the anatomy of the pulmonary circulation, especially in patients with hypoplastic PAs, peripheral PS, and those with complex pulmonary atresia and MAPCAs (**Fig. 67–28**). Finally, CT is useful in identifying calcification in the RV myocardium (eg, at the site of previous ventriculotomy), RV-PA conduits, and ventricular septum.

Exercise Testing

Exercise testing should be used together with functional class and other invasive and noninvasive investigations to risk stratify patients and decide on treatment.[54,83] The cardiopulmonary exercise test (CPET) is routinely used in ToF patients as a tool for assessing baseline exercise physiology and changes over time. It provides objective information on functional capacity and potential mechanisms of exercise intolerance, guiding management. Important parameters, such as the peak oxygen consumption, ventilatory efficiency (VE/VCO$_2$ slope), anaerobic threshold, and chronotropic response to exercise provide a detailed description of the severity of exercise limitation, mechanisms responsible and changes over time or after intervention. In the ACHD population, including ToF patients, the peak VO$_2$, VE/VCO$_2$ slope and heart rate reserve are predictors of mortality. Quality control is extremely important to ensure accuracy and reproducibility, especially for detecting changes over time and around interventions (eg, PVR).

The 6-minute walk test (6MWT) can also be used in patients with advanced disease with moderate or severe

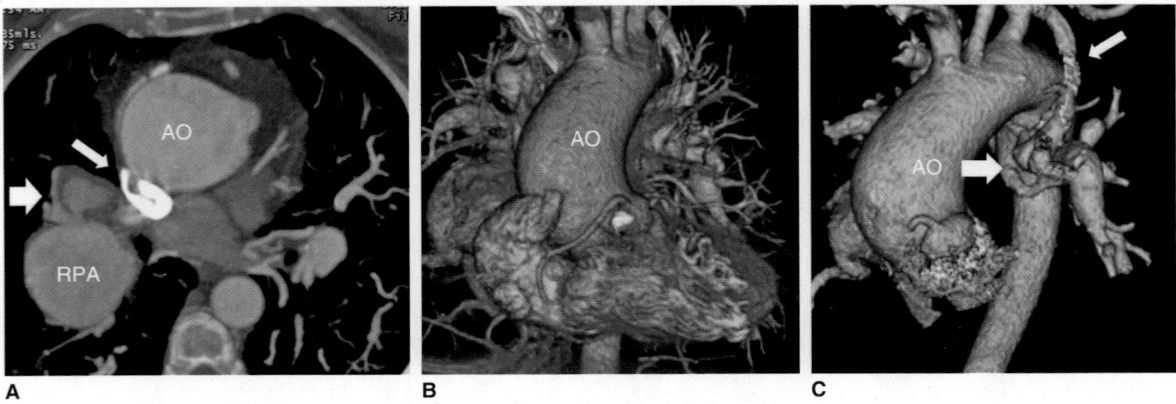

Figure 67–28. ToF with complex pulmonary atresia. Computed tomography images of a patient with unrepaired ToF with pulmonary atresia. In (**A**), the aorta (AO) is dilated and there is calcification (*thin arrow*) of a right modified BT shunt connecting the right subclavian artery to pulmonary artery vessels in the right lung. The right pulmonary artery (RPA) appears severely dilated with evidence of thrombosis and a pseudoaneurysm (*thick arrow*). In (**B**), 3D reconstruction showing the dilated aorta, and no main pulmonary artery. In (**C**), MAPCAs (*thick arrow*) from the descending aorta to the right and left lung. A left modified BT shunt is also visible (*thin arrow*) with diffuse calcification.

exercise limitation. During the 6MWT, the patient walks up and down a 10- to 30-m corridor for 6 minutes and the distance achieved is recorded. Moreover, oxygen saturation, blood pressure, and perceived exertion on the modified BORG dyspnea scale can be recorded at the start and end of exercise. The 6MWT is readily available, low cost, and reproducible, and is able to detect changes in exercise capacity over time but has a ceiling effect (approximately 600 m) and cannot be used in mildly symptomatic or asymptomatic patients.

Cardiac Catheterization

Diagnostic cardiac catheterization is not routinely performed in adults with repaired ToF, unless there are specific indications or diagnostic queries that cannot be answered by noninvasive means. Cardiac catheterization can be useful to understand cardiovascular physiology in patients presenting with restrictive physiology of the RV and/or LV constrictive pericarditis (**Fig. 67–29**), unexplained systolic ventricular dysfunction, or severe heart failure refractory to treatment (see section Heart Failure). Nowadays, invasive coronary angiography has been replaced by CT coronary angiography, but may be performed at the time of cardiac catheterization and can provide additional anatomical or functional information (eg, to interrogate coronary fistulae, extrinsic coronary artery compression).

Cardiac catherization is helpful in diagnosing pulmonary hypertension, either precapillary or postcapillary relating to raised left-sided filling pressures.[81] Precapillary pulmonary hypertension is not common in ToF, especially patients born with severe RVOTO protecting the pulmonary circulation from the effects of the large VSD. However, patients with mild–moderate RVOTO repaired beyond the first year of life may develop pulmonary vascular disease. This is, however, more common in patients who received "oversized" palliative shunts, especially Waterston or Potts shunts (see section Palliative Shunts). Moreover, patients with ToF and pulmonary atresia may develop pulmonary vascular disease in segments of the pulmonary vascular tree that received blood from a large MAPCA or arterial duct (segmental pulmonary hypertension).[82]

Cyanosis is not common in repaired ToF and may be the result of pulmonary hypertension, or more likely severely raised RV filling pressures in the presence of a residual atrial communication. Cyanosis is more common in ToF with pulmonary atresia, especially in patients who have not undergone repair, or those with raised RV pressures after repair in the presence of a VSD (residual or purposely left open). In such cases, cardiac catherization allows the measurement of pressures in the RV and PAs and can help in understanding whether the rise in RV pressures is due to stenosis or the RV-PA conduit, peripheral pulmonary stenosis, and/or pulmonary hypertension, thus guiding management.

Finally, cardiac catheterization may be used for performing invasive angiography. Peripheral pulmonary stenosis is best assessed by a combination of noninvasive imaging, and invasive pulmonary angiography and pressure assessment of the affected areas. Invasive angiography of the RVOT and PAs is also useful in preparation for percutaneous intervention on the pulmonary valve, to quantify PR and assess the anatomy.

Cardiac catherization is not routinely performed in patients with ToF undergoing pulmonary valve implantation. It may, however, be useful to exclude coronary artery disease and pulmonary hypertension, perform pulmonary angiography to quantify PR, and assess the anatomy of the pulmonary circulation, detect and quantify residual shunts (serial oximetry), assess filling pressures, and diagnose diastolic dysfunction or constrictive pericarditis. In patients with repaired pulmonary atresia (after unifocalization and implantation of an RV-PA conduit), cardiac catheterization may be required to determine the cause of RV pressure overload (conduit stenosis vs. peripheral PA stenosis vs. pulmonary vascular disease).

At the time of percutaneous pulmonary valve implantation, detailed characterization of intracardiac pressures and RVOT/PA anatomy is performed. Simultaneous coronary and RVOT angiography is often used to identify patients at risk of coronary compression at the rime of balloon dilatation and stenting of the RVOT (**Fig. 67–30**).[6]

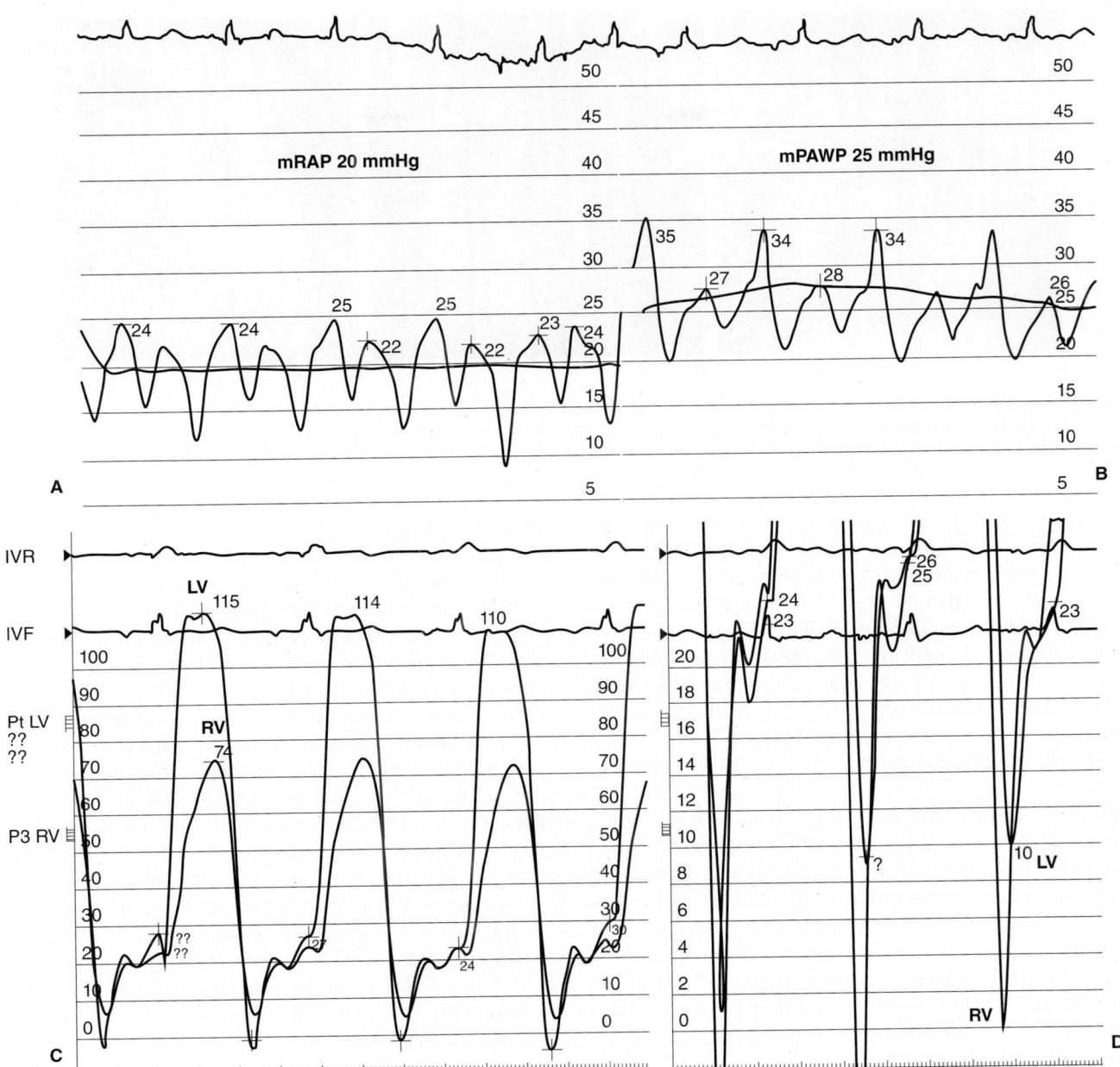

Figure 67–29. Constrictive pericarditis after ToF repair and pulmonary valve replacement. Significantly raised right- and left-sided filling pressures (**A** and **B**) with the square root signs on ventricular pressure waveforms (**C** and **D**). Extremely dense pericardial adhesions were described during surgery, with definite evidence of constriction.

Management of Adults with Repaired ToF

Medical

Patients with repaired ToF are not routinely prescribed medication, unless there is an additional indication. Angiotensin-converting enzyme (ACE) inhibitors or angiotensin receptor blockers are not routinely prescribed and have not shown to be of significant benefit in patients with significant PR.[83] β-blockers have also not proved to be of benefit in this setting and are occasionally used to suppress arrhythmias.[84]

The medical management of heart failure in repaired ToF aims at relieving congestion with the use of diuretics, including aldosterone receptor antagonists (eg, spironolactone).

However, while there is no definitive evidence in this cohort, many specialists use ACE inhibitors or angiotensin receptor blockers in patients with LV dysfunction. Moreover, β-blockade did not confer benefits to asymptomatic or mildly symptomatic repaired ToF patients, but are considered in patients with LV dysfunction.[84]

Surgical

The most common reason of repeat surgery in patients with repaired ToF is PR. Severe PR is typically tolerated well for several years before PVR is needed. The clinical parameters that determine the ideal timing for such a surgery are still debated. PVR is generally performed when RV dilatation is severe, with

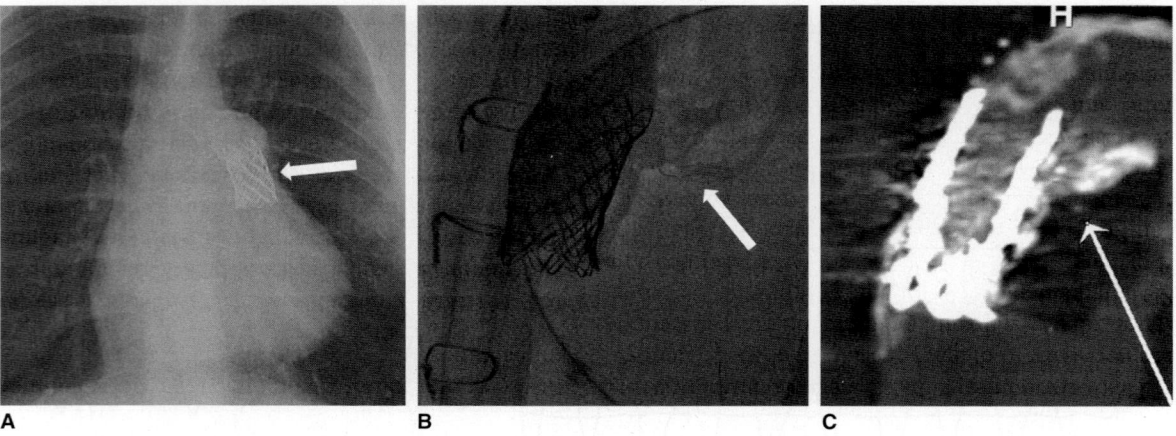

Figure 67–30. Melody transcatheter pulmonary valve implantation. In (**A**), chest radiograph demonstrating a percutaneous bioprosthesis in the RVOT (*arrow*). In (**B**), coronary catheter and guidewire (*arrow*) positioned prior to balloon inflation and deployment of the percutaneous pulmonary valve in case of coronary compression. In (**C**), note the proximity of the left coronary artery (*arrow*) to the pulmonary valve, with extensive calcification of the RVOT.

the scope to preserve ventricular function and achieve a reduction in both end-diastolic and end-systolic dimensions.[85,86] A meta-analysis and meta-regression of 48 studies on PVR showed that 30-day mortality after surgery was low (0.87%), with a pooled 5-year mortality of 2.3% and a repeat PVR rate at 5 years of 4.9%. They also demonstrated improvement in biventricular size and function, QRS duration, and NYHA functional class.[87] A correlation was also observed between the decrease in both end-systolic and end-diastolic RV volume and preoperative end-systolic RV volumes.

When considering PVR for a ToF patient with severe PR, a balance should be achieved between the potential benefits of the PVR (including relief of symptoms and improvement in exercise capacity, preservation of RV and tricuspid valve function, a reduction in the arrhythmia risk or burden, repair of concomitant lesions) versus the perioperative risks and the need for recurrent interventions/operations over a patient's lifetime. Both AHA/ACC and ESC guidelines recommend surgery in patients with significant PR and symptoms attributable to this (**Tables 67–8** and **67–9**).

In asymptomatic patients with significant PR, the decision hinges mainly on the presence of significant RV dilatation or dysfunction, severe coexisting RVOTO, and exercise intolerance. Additional indications include patients with VT in addition to electrophysiological management (as a means of "offloading" the RV and reducing the incidence of VT). In patients with sustained VT undergoing surgery, preoperative electrophysiological mapping and intraoperative transection of the anatomical areas involved in the arrhythmia may be considered. At the time of PVR, residual VSD with evidence of LV volume overload should also be addressed.

Bioprostheses are most commonly used for PVR, in view of the risk of thrombosis and need for anticoagulation of metallic valves. Bioprosthetic valves tend to degenerate less rapidly in the pulmonary position compared to the aortic position and allow percutaneous pulmonary valve (valve-in-valve) implantation when required.

Interventional

Percutaneous interventions are integral to the management of all CHD, including ToF. Examples include balloon pulmonary angioplasty that is useful for relief of aortic or pulmonary valve stenosis, stenting of a patent ductus arteriosus in infants with a duct-dependent circulation (eg, patient with ToF-pulmonary atresia), and balloon angioplasty and stenting of peripheral pulmonary stenoses. Percutaneous valve replacement techniques were introduced less than two decades ago and have further revolutionized the care of ToF patients. Nowadays, percutaneous pulmonary valve implantation is routinely performed in patients with an RV-PA conduit or previous bioprosthetic PVR, in whom there is a rigid structure of contained dimensions that allows stable positioning of the percutaneous valve. Recently, percutaneous PVRs have been implanted in patients with native RVOTs and severe PR or pulmonary stenosis (preceded by stenting of the RVOT to create a rigid landing zone for the valve). Detailed characterization of the RVOT and neighboring coronary arteries is strongly recommended to avoid extrinsic coronary artery compression at the time of stenting and valve implantation.[6]

Finally, balloon dilatation of stenosed MAPCAs may be performed in patients with unrepaired pulmonary atresia and reduced pulmonary blood flow to optimize oxygen saturations. Conversely, residual MAPCAs after repair may be coil-embolized to avoid competitive flow and pulmonary vascular disease and minimize the risk of hemoptysis.

Transplantation

Transplantation should be considered for all ACHD patients with advanced heart failure, refractory to medical management, and deemed unsuitable for conventional surgery due to high perioperative risks or absence of suitable target. ACHD patients tend to have a higher perioperative mortality compared to non-CHD patients but better late survival.[68,88] This is likely due to obstacles to listing in repaired ToF include recurrent operations causing alloimmunization and difficult surgical access, lack of ACHD-specific criteria for eligibility

TABLE 67–8. Repaired TOF: Indications for PVR: 2018 AHA/ACC Guidelines for ACHD

COR	LOE	Diagnostic	Therapeutic
I	B-NR	1. Coronary artery compression testing with simultaneous coronary angiography and high-pressure balloon dilation in the conduit is indicated before RV-PA conduit stenting or transcatheter valve placement.	1. PVR (percutaneous or surgical) for relief of symptoms in patients with at least moderate PR with cardiovascular symptoms not otherwise explained.

IIa	B-NR		1. RV-PA conduit intervention is reasonable for adults with at least moderate PR or stenosis with reduced functional capacity or arrhythmia.
			2. PVR (percutaneous or surgical) in asymptomatic patients with ventricular enlargement or dysfunction and at least moderate PR, with the aim of preserving ventricular size and function (recommendation level IIa): Any 2 of the following criteria:
			  1. Mild or moderate RV or LV systolic dysfunction
			  2. Severe RV dilatation: RVEDV I≥160ml/m² or RVESVI ≥80ml/m² or RVEDV ≥2xLVEDV)
			  3. RVSP (due to RVOT obstruction) ≥2/3 systemic pressure
			  4. Progressive reduction in objective exercise intolerance.

IIb	C-EO		1. Surgical PVR in patients with at least moderate PR and ventricular tachyarrhythmia (in addition to arrhythmia management). 2. Surgical PVR in patients with at least moderate PR undergoing surgery for other lesions. 3. Intervention may be reasonable for asymptomatic adults with severe RV-PA conduit stenosis or regurgitation with reduced RV ejection fraction or RV dilation.

Abbreviations: ACHD, adult congenital heart disease; CMR, cardiac magnetic resonance; COR, class of recommendation; EO, expert opinion; LOE, level of evidence; LVEDV, LV end-diastolic volume; NR, nonrandomized; PA, pulmonary artery; PR, pulmonary regurgitation; PS, pulmonary stenosis; PVR, pulmonary valve replacement; RL, recommendation level; RV, right ventricle; RVEDVi, RV end-diastolic volume indexed; RVESVi, RV end-systolic volume indexed; RVEDV, RV end-diastolic volume; RVSP, RV systolic pressure; RVOT, RV outflow tract; TOF, Tetralogy of Fallot; TR, tricuspid regurgitation; VSD, ventricular septal defect.

delaying transplantation and resulting in multiorgan involvement, reluctance of transplant centers without ACHD expertise to undertake transplantation in an ACHD patient, and limited expertise in VADs for ACHD patients.

Electrophysiological Evaluation, Ablation, and Devices

Electrophysiological evaluation is integral to the management of patients with repaired ToF, for both supraventricular and ventricular arrhythmias. Electrophysiological study with

TABLE 67–9. Repaired TOF: Indications for PVR: 2020 ESC Guidelines for ACHD

COR	LOE	Diagnostic	Therapeutic
I	C		1. PVR in symptomatic patients (dyspnea, chest pain, and/or exercise intolerance referable to PR or otherwise unexplained) with severe PR (defined as a regurgitant fraction by CMR >30%) and/or at least moderate RVOTO. 2. Transcatheter pulmonary valve implantation in patients without a native RVOT and previous surgery using homografts, bovine jugular vein grafts, or bioprostheses/conduits.

IIa	C		1. PVR in asymptomatic patients with:
			  • Objective evidence of exercise intolerance
			  • Progressive RV dilatation to RVESVi ≥80 mL/m², and/or RVEDVi ≥160 mL/m², and/or progression of TR to at least moderate.
			  • Progressive RV systolic dysfunction.
			  • Severe RVOTO with RVSP >80 mmHg.
			2. In patients with sustained VT who are undergoing surgical or percutaneous PVR, pre-operative catheter mapping and transection of VT-related anatomical isthmuses before or during the intervention should be considered.
			3. RV-PA conduit intervention is reasonable for adults with at least moderate PR or PS with reduced functional capacity or arrhythmia.
			4. VSD closure should be considered in patients with residual VSD and significant LV volume overload or if the patient is undergoing pulmonary valve surgery.

IIb	C		1. RV-PA conduit intervention may be reasonable for asymptomatic adults with RV-PA conduit and severe stenosis or severe regurgitation with reduced RV ejection fraction or RV dilation.

Abbreviations: ACHD, adult congenital heart disease; CMR, cardiac magnetic resonance; COR, class of recommendation; EO, expert opinion; LOE, level of evidence; LVEDV, LV end-diastolic volume; NR, nonrandomized; PA, pulmonary artery; PR, pulmonary regurgitation; PS, pulmonary stenosis; PVR, pulmonary valve replacement; RL, recommendation level; RV, right ventricle; RVEDVi, RV end-diastolic volume indexed; RVESVi, RV end-systolic volume indexed; RVEDV, RV end-diastolic volume; RVSP, RV systolic pressure; RVOT, RV outflow tract; TOF, Tetralogy of Fallot; TR, tricuspid regurgitation; VSD, ventricular septal defect.

TABLE 67–10. Arrhythmias in Repaired TOF: 2018 AHA/ACC Guidelines for ACHD

COR	LOE	Diagnostic	Therapeutic
IIa	B-NR	1. Programmed ventricular stimulation can be useful to risk stratify adults with TOF and additional risk factors for SCD 2. In patients with repaired TOF, cardiac catheterization with angiography, if indicated, is reasonable to assess hemodynamics when adequate data cannot be obtained noninvasively in the setting of an arrhythmia, heart failure, unexplained ventricular dysfunction, suspected pulmonary hypertension or cyanosis.	1. Primary prevention ICD therapy is reasonable in adults with TOF and multiple risk factors for SCD.
IIb	C-EO		1. PVR, in addition to arrhythmia management, may be considered for adults with repaired TOF and moderate or greater PR and ventricular tachyarrhythmia.

Abbreviations: COR, class of recommendation; EO, expert opinion; LOE, level of evidence; NR, nonrandomized.

programmed ventricular stimulation may be useful in patients at intermediate risk of malignant tachycardias, when deciding on ICD implantation for primary prevention.[6] In patients with previous sustained VT, ablation may be used to reduce the risk of recurrent arrhythmia, but does not replace the need for an ICD, while also addressing hemodynamic lesions (eg, PR). Surgical VT ablation may be performed at the time of PVR, targeting areas identified on preoperative EP study. Primary prevention ICD should also be considered in patients with "standard" criteria (eg, a reduced LV ejection fraction). Arrhythmia-related recommendations from the AHA/ACC and ESC guidelines are shown in **Tables 67–10** and **67–11**.

ICD implantation should be offered to ToF patients with multiple risk factors, while programmed ventricular stimulation is most helpful in patients at intermediate risk, when the indication for an ICD based on risk factors is not very strong. In patients with arrhythmia, hemodynamic lesions or other

potentially causes should be sought and addressed (including coronary artery disease in adults). There is still debate on whether ablation performed in expert centers should be offered to patients with symptomatic monomorphic sustained VT instead of ICD implantation (providing this is successful). Ablation may be performed around device implantation to minimize the need for ICD discharges.[7]

Routine Follow-Up of Patients with Repaired ToF

Lifelong specialist follow-up is recommended for all patients with repaired ToF. An ACHD cardiologist should review these patients at 12- to 24-month intervals, unless there are additional indications for closer follow-up. The AHA/ACC guidelines define various physiological stages for repaired ToF patients (Stages A–D), requiring follow-up and investigations at increasing frequency. Such stages are defined throughout ACHD and depend on the following (but not exclusively):

TABLE 67–11. Arrhythmias in Repaired TOF: 2020 ESC Guidelines for ACHD

COR	LOE	Diagnostic	Therapeutic
IIa	C	1. In patients with sustained VT who are undergoing surgical PVR or percutaneous valve insertion, pre-operative catheter mapping and transsection of VT-related anatomical isthmuses before or during the intervention should be considered. 2. Electrophysiologic evaluation, including programmed electrical stimulation, should be considered for risk stratification for SCD in patients with additional risk factors (LV/RV dysfunction; non-sustained, symptomatic VT; QRS duration ≥180 ms, extensive RV scarring on CMR).	1. ICD implantation should be considered in selected ToF patients with multiple risk factors for SCD, including LV dysfunction, non-sustained, symptomatic VT, QRS duration ≥180 ms, extensive RV scarring on CMR, or inducible VT at programmed electrical stimulation.
IIb	C		1. Catheter ablation or concomitant surgical ablation for symptomatic monomorphic sustained VT may be considered in those with a preserved biventricular function as an alternative to ICD therapy, provided that the procedure is performed in highly experienced centers and that established ablation endpoints have been reached (e.g. non-inducibility, conduction block across ablation lines).

Abbreviations: ACHD, adult congenital heart disease; CMR, cardiac magnetic resonance; COR, class of recommendation; ICD, implantable cardioverter defibrillator; LOE, level of evidence; LV, left ventricle; PVR, pulmonary valve replacement; RL, recommendation level; RV, right ventricle; SCD, sudden cardiac death; TOF, Tetralogy of Fallot; VT, ventricular tachycardia.

- NYHA functional class
- The presence and severity of hemodynamic or anatomic sequelae, (eg, ventricular dilatation or dysfunction, valve disease, obstructive lesions, aortic enlargement, or residual/palliative shunts)
- Presence of arrhythmias and response to therapy
- Exercise capacity
- Presence of cyanosis and/or pulmonary hypertension
- End-organ dysfunction (kidney, liver, lung function) and response to therapy

Patients with more severe symptoms or comorbidity warrant close follow-up, depending on stability and response to treatment.

Pregnancy in Women with Repaired ToF

Women after repair of ToF generally tolerate pregnancy well and are classified as class II (out of 4) under the mWHO classification in the 2018 ESC guidelines for the management of cardiovascular diseases during pregnancy.[22] The risk of cardiac complications is reported at 8%, affecting mostly patients on cardiac medication prior to becoming pregnant, those with RV dysfunction and/or significant PR, significant RVOTO, or aortic dilatation (especially if aortic dimeter exceeds 50 mm, mWHO risk category IV). There is also an increased risk of fetal growth restriction. Maternal screening for 22q11 deletion should be performed prior to pregnancy.

The guidelines recommend follow-up every trimester in most patients, unless severe PR is present in which case monthly or bimonthly cardiac follow-up is warranted. Diuretic therapy and bed rest is indicated in case of RV failure. If patients do not respond to therapy, early delivery or transcatheter valve implantation may rarely be considered.

Management of Adults with Unrepaired ToF

A quarter of patients with unrepaired ToF die early in life without surgery, with only 30% expected to survive at 10 years of age.[50] The effects of chronic cyanosis and complications such as arrhythmia, infection, and heart failure contribute to the high morbidity and mortality. There are very few patients with ToF who have not undergone repair in developed countries, often those with pulmonary atresia in whom repair could not

be achieved. Adults with unrepaired ToF are more likely those with "balanced" circulation, adequate blood flow, and chronic adaptation to cyanosis of mild or moderate severity, typically exacerbated by efforts.

All adult patients with unrepaired ToF should be considered for repair, balancing the risks of a late operation against the benefits of abolishing cyanosis and improving pulmonary blood flow.

Patients with complex pulmonary atresia may have undergone palliative surgery (**Fig. 67–31**) or partial unifocalization. In others, despite unifocalization and implantation of an RV-PA conduit, the VSD may have been left open to support the RV in the presence of a significant afterload, often due to segmental pulmonary hypertension or peripheral pulmonary stenoses that result in a significant raised RV systolic pressure. In such patients, all effort should be made to optimize oxygenation by means of relief of peripheral pulmonary stenosis, or stenoses, closure of nonessential MAPCAs and, possibly, pulmonary arterial hypertension therapies, even though there is extremely limited evidence for the latter in segmental pulmonary hypertension.[82,89] Moreover, associated lesions, such as aortic or TR, or aortic dilatation, should be detected and monitored, even though surgical repair of valve disease or extreme progressive aortic dilatation in unrepaired pulmonary atresia carries a very high perioperative risk. Other complications, such as heart failure, arrhythmias, or hemoptysis (often triggered by a lower respiratory tract infection), are managed conservatively.

EBSTEIN ANOMALY OF THE TRICUSPID VALVE

Ebstein anomaly (EA) is a rare form of CHD involving the tricuspid valve, with a clinical presentation that varies widely depending on the severity of the defect and associated lesions. It is the most common congenital cause of TR.

In 1866, Wilhelm Ebstein published the case of a 19-year-old man with cyanosis, dyspnea, palpitations, jugular venous distension, and cardiomegaly, who was found to have a markedly dysplastic tricuspid valve at autopsy.[90] More than 150 years since Ebstein's first description, and almost 60 years since Christiaan Barnard performed the first tricuspid valve replacement using

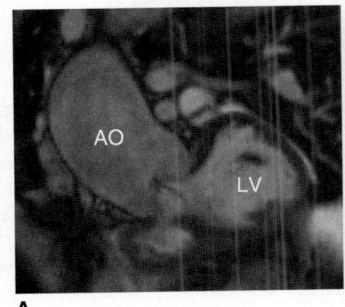
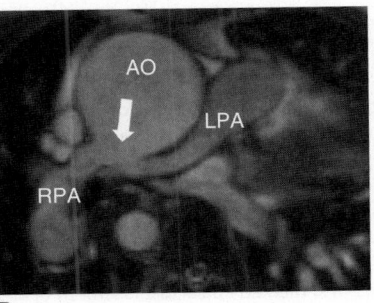

Figure 67–31. Pulmonary atresia with a Waterston shunt. In (**A**), aortic (AO) dilatation with mild aortic regurgitation. In (**B**), the Waterston shunt (*arrow*) between the ascending aorta (AO) and the pulmonary arteries. LPA, left pulmonary artery; RPA, right pulmonary artery.

a bioprosthesis in a patient with EA, remarkable progress has been made in its diagnosis, evaluation, and repair.[91] The birth prevalence has been estimated at between 0.02 and 0.07 per 1,000 live births,[92,93] equating to 90 neonates with EA born in the United States each year. It constitutes less than 1% of all CHD cases, with no sex difference.

EA is associated with genetic syndromes, that include trisomy 21, 18, and 13, CHARGE, VACTERL, and deletions in chromosomes 1p36 and 8p23.1.[94,95] Associated birth defects include cleft lip and palate, congenital diaphragmatic hernia, duodenal atresia, sacrococcygeal teratoma, and fetal hydrops. There is a small increased risk of EA resulting from maternal lithium use, especially with exposures >900 mg/day.[96]

Anatomical Features, Pathophysiology, and Repair of Native EA

Anatomy

EA is defined by the following core anatomic characteristics involving the tricuspid valve and RV (**Fig. 67–32, left**):[97]

- Failure of delamination of the septal and often the posterior tricuspid valve leaflet from the underlying myocardium causing them to appear "adherent" to the RV wall

- Apical displacement of the functional tricuspid valve hinge points (the septal tricuspid valve leaflet is the most commonly affected, followed by the posterior and then the anterior leaflets)

- Division of the RV into a "atrialized" proximal/inlet portion and a "functional" distal portion. There is dilatation of the atrialized RV with a variable degree of myocardial thinning or (less commonly) hypertrophy

- Anterior leaflet redundancy, fenestrations and tethering due to abnormally formed chordae tendineae

- Right atrioventricular junction dilatation.

The anatomic spectrum in EA is broad. In the least severe cases, there is merely an exaggerated "offsetting" of the tricuspid in relation to the anterior mitral valve leaflet, with greater than normal (≥ 8 mm/m^2) apical displacement of the septal and posterior tricuspid valve leaflets. In severe cases, the proximal and distal RV are separated by an imperforate membrane or muscular shelf. The anterior tricuspid valve leaflet is not adherent to the RV wall but is malformed and is commonly displaced into the RVOT. Redundant leaflet tissue leads to a sail-like appearance with tethered chordae which, together with the displacement, can cause intracavitary obstruction (**Figs. 67–32A to 67–32D**).

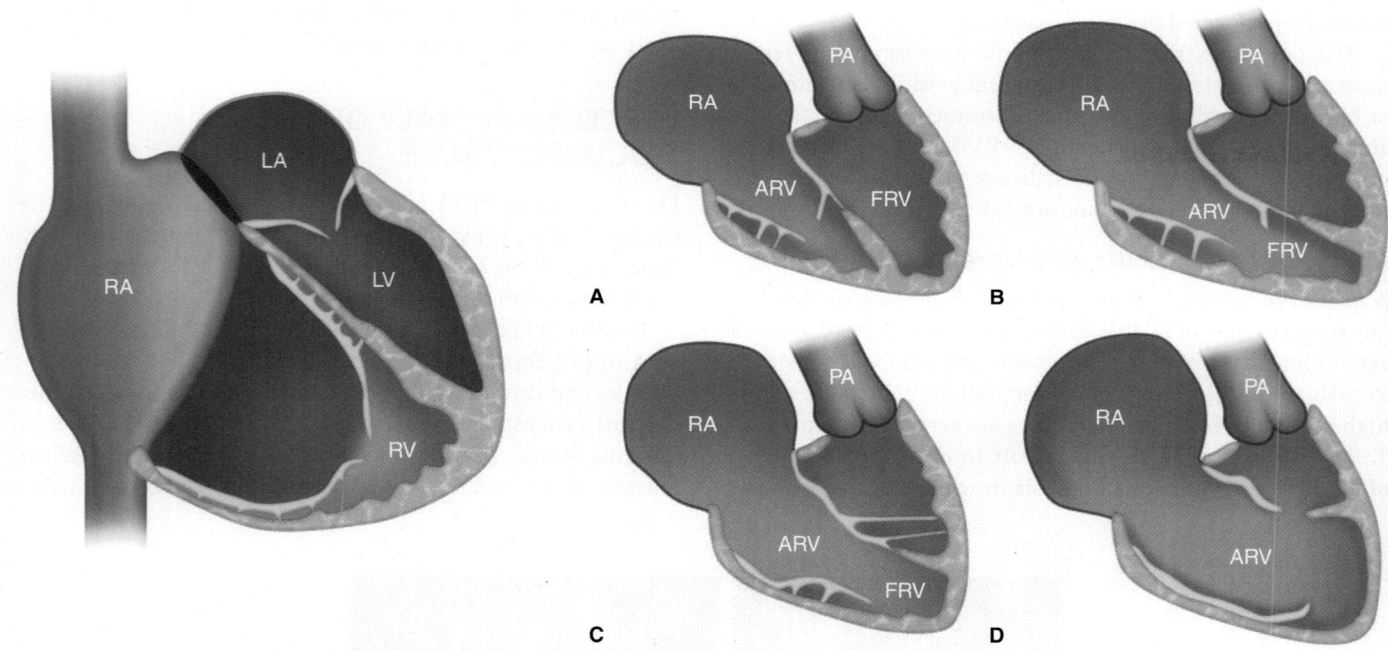

Figure 67–32. **Anatomic characteristics and Carpentier classification of Ebstein anomaly.** *Left*: Ebstein anomaly of the tricuspid valve, resulting in division of the right ventricle (RV) into a proximal "atrialized" portion and a distal "functional" portion. The effective volume of the functional RV is reduced, while the right atrium (RA) is dilated. *Right*: Carpentier classification types A to D by anatomic findings at surgery.[119] In type A, there is moderate displacement of the septal and posterior leaflets, while the anterior leaflet is spared. There is a small contractile atrialized portion of the right ventricle (ARV) and an adequately sized functional right ventricle (FRV). Type B describes marked displacement of the septal and posterior leaflets, with a hypoplastic adherent septal leaflet and a normal anterior leaflet. The ARV is large and noncontractile and the FRV is small. In type C, marked displacement, hypoplasia and adherence of septal and posterior leaflets are accompanied by restricted anterior leaflet motion. There is a large noncontractile ARV with a very small FRV. In type D disease, the tricuspid anatomy is grossly dysplastic, with marked apical displacement of all tricuspid valve leaflets. The septal and posterior leaflets are hypoplastic and adherent, and the anterior leaflet is adherent to the ventricular wall. Almost the entire RV, except for a variable portion of the infundibulum, is atrialized and noncontractile. LA, left atrium; LV, left ventricle; PA, pulmonary artery; RA, right atrium.

The atrialized RV extends from the true position of the tricuspid valve annulus at the right atrioventricular junction, to the tricuspid valve hinge points, thus containing the inlet portion of the RV. The atrialized RV is usually thin, dilated, and lacks ventricular trabeculations. The true annulus is also characteristically dilated and contributes to the development of TR, while the lack of a complete fibrous ring at this location allows for direct muscular connections between the right atrium (RA) and RV, providing the substrate for ventricular preexcitation.[97] The functional RV encompasses the remainder of the RV, namely the trabecular and outlet portions, which is typically dilated but is often small in size compared to a normal RV.

Associated conditions include:

- ASD/PFO; in up to 95%
- Accessory pathways (and Wolff-Parkinson-White syndrome)
- Pulmonary stenosis
- VSDs
- Patent ductus arteriosus
- Coarctation of the aorta
- Mitral valve abnormalities
- LV myocardial changes resembling noncompaction.[98]

In addition, complex CHD can have associated Ebstein-like malformation of the tricuspid valve, including congenitally corrected transposition of the great arteries (cc-TGA, also known as l-TGA): 15% to 50% of ccTGA patients fulfil criteria for EA.[99,100] In ccTGA, the "Ebsteinoid" tricuspid valve is in the systemic position, and impacts significantly on symptoms and prognosis.[101]

Anatomical Classification

Multiple classification systems exist for EA, aimed at providing prognostic information and risk stratification with regards to the surgical strategy (tricuspid valve repair vs replacement). Classification systems either focus on the individual anatomical characteristics of the tricuspid valve and RV, or the functional consequences of this anatomy. The 1988 Carpentier classification takes the former approach, and is aimed at identifying cases that are amenable to tricuspid valve repair versus replacement (Fig. 67-32A to 67-32D).[102] By contrast, the Celermajer index, also referred to as the Great Ormond Street Echocardiography (GOSE) score, takes the ratio of the sum of RA and atrialized RV areas, to that of the areas of the functional RV visible on four-chamber apical view plus the left atrial and LV areas.[103] Ratios of <0.5, 0.5 to 0.99, 1 to 1.49 and ≥1.5 indicate mild, moderate, severe, and very severe disease, respectively. This index was initially developed in 1992 for the risk stratification of neonatal disease, and has also been used in adult EA patients, in whom a higher CMR-derived Celermejer index relates to greater functional impairment.[104]

Pathophysiology

The pathophysiological spectrum of EA is broad and is determined by the following:

- The severity of TR, related to the amount of apical displacement and dysplasia of the valve leaflets

- The extent of the atrialization of the RV, and the size of the functional RV (that usually includes the RV apex and outflow tract)
- The contractility of the functional RV and LV
- The presence of an atrial communication, allowing right–left shunting and cyanosis
- The degree of RVOT and LVOT obstruction
- The presence and type of arrhythmias
- The type and severity of associated lesions.

In its most severe form, EA can present antenatally with massive fetal cardiomegaly ("wall-to-wall" heart), LV compression, and pulmonary hypoplasia, often leading to intrauterine death. At the other end of the spectrum, EA has been diagnosed in asymptomatic adults entering their seventh or eighth decade. In addition to these listed variables, the pathophysiology of pediatric and especially neonatal disease is dependent on postnatal changes in pulmonary vascular resistance, patency of the ductus arteriosus, presence of subvalvar or valvar pulmonary stenosis or pulmonary regurgitation, and adequacy of the RV to generate forward flow across the pulmonary valve, among others.

In the adult patient, the pathophysiology is mainly driven by the TR, causing right-sided volume overload with associated dilatation of the atrialized RV and RA (**Fig. 67–33**). LV dysfunction can be the result of ventricular–ventricular interaction (ventricular interdependence), especially in patients with a large atrialized portion of the RV and/or longstanding severe TR with diastolic shift of the ventricular septum.[70] In severe cases, the geometric distortion of the ventricular septum can contribute to mitral valve prolapse or LVOT obstruction.

In the presence of an atrial communication, the shunt can be left–right or right–left depending the severity of TR and rise of RA pressure. Cyanosis may be apparent from childhood in severe cases, especially in the presence of obstruction caused by the tricuspid valve or a very small functional RV. Cyanosis may only be present on exercise in less severe cases. The presence of a right–left shunt is, at times, deemed beneficial in terms of offloading the RV, but at the expense of cyanosis and its complications.[105]

Palliative Surgery

In EA, palliative procedures aim to offload the RV and augment pulmonary blood flow in infants in whom the tricuspid valve is not amenable to repair and/or the functional RV is not large enough to sustain the entire stroke volume. In such cases during infancy, an aortopulmonary shunt may be recommended (see section Palliative Surgery). The Starnes procedure combines an aortopulmonary shunt, nowadays in the form of a modified BT shunt, RV exclusion with a fenestrated tricuspid valve patch, right atrioplasty, and right ventriculoplasty (to decompress the LV).[106] Biventricular repair may thereafter be possible, otherwise a single-ventricle strategy (Fontan-type operation) is pursued.

A bidirectional superior cavopulmonary (Glenn) shunt (connecting the SVC to the right pulmonary artery) is usually reserved for infants >6 months with massive RV dilatation or

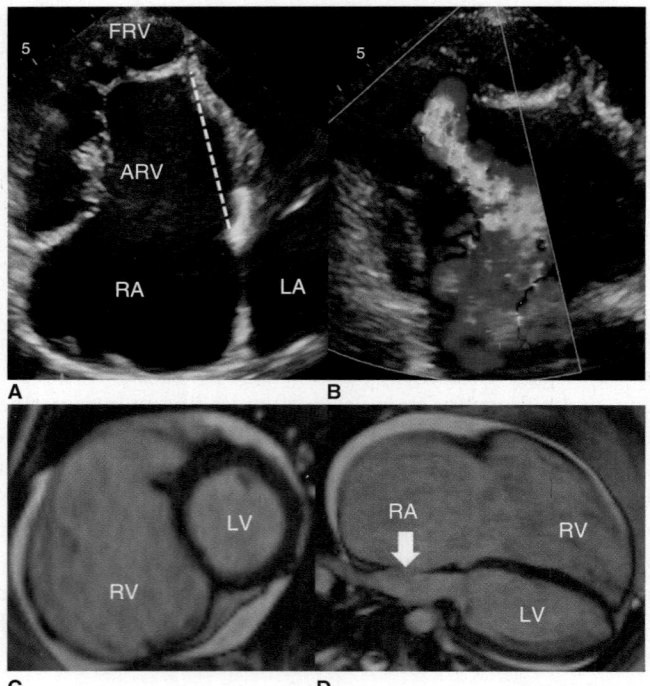

Figure 67–33. Imaging findings in Ebstein anomaly. A 24-year-old patient with Carpentier type III Ebstein anomaly. In (**A**), apical four-chamber showing a septal tricuspid valve leaflet that is displaced toward the apex by 7 cm (*dashed line*) creating a large atrialized portion of the right ventricle (ARV) and a smaller functional right ventricle (FRV). The right atrium (RA) is severely dilated. In (**B**), a modified four-chamber view displaying the tricuspid regurgitation jet, which originates close to the apex of the heart. CMR imaging ventricular short axis and axial four-chamber images are shown in (**C**) and (**D**), displaying the grossly dilated RA and right ventricle (RV) with diminutive left atrium and left ventricle (LV). The associated secundum atrial septal defect is highlighted (*arrow*).

severe RV dysfunction, with inadequate reverse remodeling following initial palliation; the final surgical destination for these patients is a Fontan-type procedure, nowadays through completion of a total cavopulmonary connection (routing inferior vena cava flow to the right pulmonary artery through an extracardiac conduit or lateral tunnel). A Glenn shunt is at times performed in adult patients with severe RV dysfunction in whom there is concern that the RV cannot tolerate the entire stroke volume.[107] The result is that part (approximately half) of the systemic venous return bypasses the RV while augmenting LV preload ("1.5 ventricle repair"). Careful, preoperative assessment of hemodynamics is necessary to ensure that there is adequate LV function, and a normal left atrial and LV end-diastolic pressure that will allow passive flow into the lungs, especially in older patients.

Surgical Repair

Technique: There are numerous variations on the surgical management of EA. Most approaches consist of some form of tricuspid valve repair (or replacement if repair is not feasible), with or without the addition of plication of the RA and atrialized RV, and closure of an atrial communication.[108]

The anatomic cone repair of the Ebstein tricuspid valve and its modifications have emerged as the preferred surgical approach for adults with EA, with low early mortality and excellent durability.[109,110] They aim to restore the valve to its anatomic position and improve valve competency using the native leaflets. The contemporary modified cone procedure involves a series of steps (da Silva technique, **Fig. 67–34**): Delamination of the tricuspid valve leaflets, creation of a cone-shaped valve using tissue from the anterior leaflet and the remnants of the septal and inferior leaflets, a reduction posterior commissuroplasty, with or without limited RV plication over its diaphragmatic surface, a partial ring or de Vega annuloplasty for greater structural support of the valve, and direct suture closure of an ASD or PFO. The most common complications of this procedure include dehiscence requiring reoperation, heart block, and compromise of the right coronary artery by the plication or annular reduction maneuvers. Dehiscence is a major concern, especially in inexperienced hands and is, in part, responsible for the steep learning curve. This, combined with the low median annual institutional case volumes (one case per center per year in the United States, but considerably higher numbers in specialist referral centers),[11] has led to the ACC/AHA and ESC ACHD guidelines recommending that this procedure is performed by a congenital surgeon with experience in Ebstein surgery (**Tables 67–12 and 67–13**).[6,7]

Contraindications to the cone repair include LV dysfunction, either secondary to RV dysfunction or LV noncompaction, a symptomatic neonate with complex anatomic features, and pulmonary hypertension in the older patient. Valve repair may also not be feasible in severe cases of EA when the elongated anterior leaflet of the tricuspid valve is adherent to the RV endocardium and there is almost complete atrialization of the RV. Tricuspid valve replacement is a good alternative in this subset of patients. Some centers have a lower threshold for tricuspid valve replacement in older patients, especially if there is severe RV or tricuspid annular dilatation or pulmonary hypertension, because these findings have been correlated with poor durability of the tricuspid valve repair.[112] Mechanical valves are rarely used nowadays, and should be avoided in the presence of significant RV dysfunction that increases the risk of valve thrombosis.[113]

Timing of Repair: The severity of the condition dictates the need for Ebstein repair. Surgery in the neonatal period is usually necessary in the presence of anatomic pulmonary atresia, congestive cardiac failure, ventilator-dependency, failed medical therapy, or persistent cyanosis. In older children and adults, delaying surgery until the onset of heart failure or severe RV systolic dysfunction has been associated with poor outcomes,[107,114,115] therefore, both the AHA/ACC and ESC guidelines recommend surgical repair at an earlier stage.[6,7] Indications for EA surgery include cyanosis (in the presence of an atrial communication), reduced exercise tolerance, and the onset of atrial arrhythmias.

In addition, the guidelines state that surgical repair should be considered in the absence of symptoms, when there is progressive right heart dilatation or reduction of RV systolic function (Tables 67–12 and 67–13).

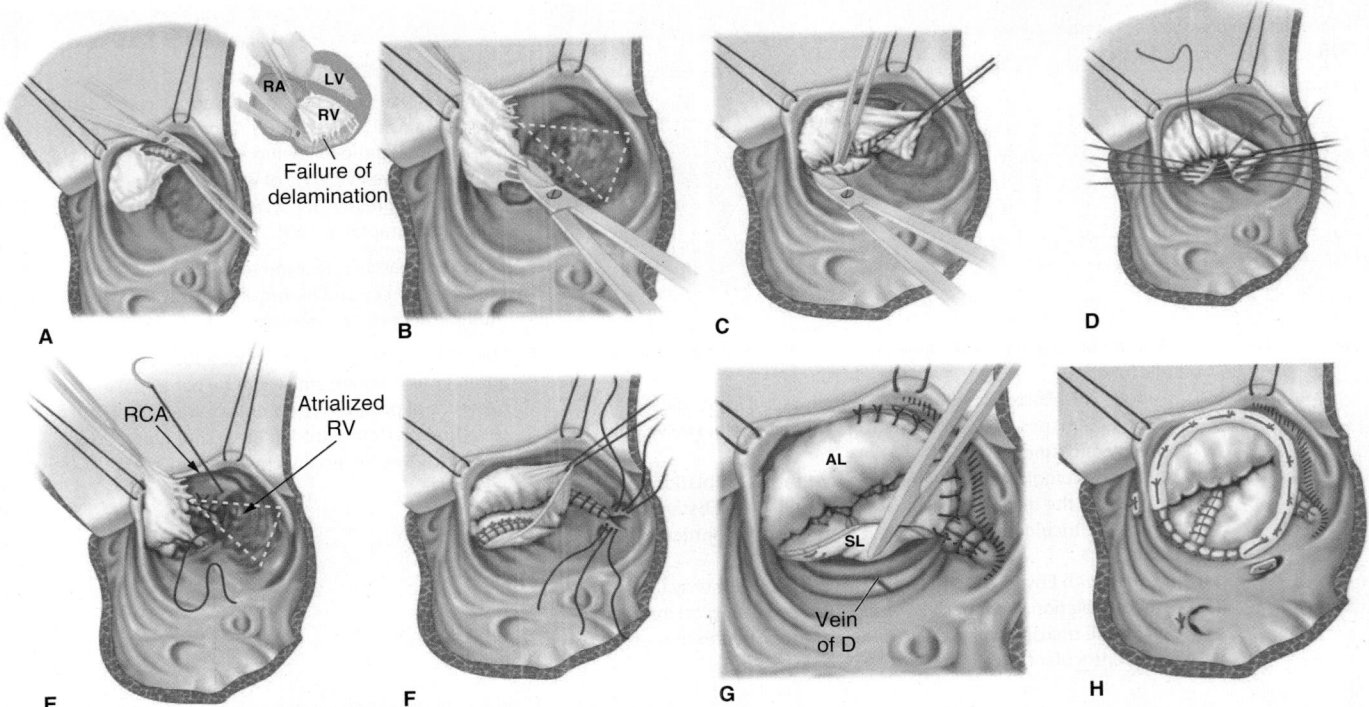

Figure 67–34. The modified cone (da Silva technique) for Ebstein anomaly repair.[215] **(A)** to **(H)**: The operative steps for the da Silva technique for Ebstein anomaly repair. In **(A)**, dissection and surgical delamination of much of the distal anterior and a portion of the posterior leaflet tissue, while maintaining intact all fibrous and muscular attachments of the leading edge of the leaflets to the RV myocardium. In **(B)** and **(C)**, surgical delamination is continued to completely mobilize the anterior, posterior, and septal tricuspid valve (TV) leaflets. In **(D)**, the cone reconstruction, bringing together the inferior and septal leaflet edges resulting in 360° of leaflet tissue that will compose the new TV orifice. In **(E)**, RV plication may or may not be necessary, taking care to avoid the right coronary artery within the true TV annulus. In **(F)**, exclusion of the atrialized RV (*blue dotted triangle* in **B** and **E**) as the suture line is advanced toward the atrioventricular groove, and in some cases crosses the groove to reduce the size of the annulus. In **(G)**, the TV is then reattached at the level of the true annulus, usually with plication of the inferior annulus. Reattachment of the septal leaflet (SL) should be done to the ventricular septum and the ventricular side of the conduction tissue (the vein of D is its anatomical landmark). In **(H)**, the addition of a flexible annuloplasty ring is used in adult patients for further support.

EA affects both the tricuspid valve and RV myocardium, hence a lower threshold for surgical repair compared to other RV-loading conditions is reasonable, especially if a good tricuspid valve repair is likely.[114]

Pathophysiology and Long-Term Outcome after Repair of EA

Outcomes in EA are closely related to age at diagnosis and surgical repair, which reflects the severity of the anatomic lesion and physiological disturbance. Adults with EA are often survivors of pediatric disease, and perceived outcomes following adult intervention must take into account events in earlier life.

In those diagnosed prenatally, early series from the 1990s reported that up to 85% died prior to birth or in the neonatal period;[116,117] even recent reported early mortality in the neonatal period varies from 7% to 65%.[95,118,119] Markers of poor prognosis include diagnosis before 32 weeks of gestation, absence of antegrade flow across the pulmonary valve, pulmonary valve regurgitation, cardiothoracic ratio on chest radiography >0.48, LV dysfunction, or severe tricuspid annular dilatation.[120] In an analysis of the Society of Thoracic Surgeons Congenital Heart Surgery database, neonatal surgery for EA (at a median 7 days of age), had a mortality of 27% and a composite morbidity-mortality of 50%.[121] Over half of the neonates (63%) required reoperation for revision of systemic-to-pulmonary artery shunts. Three-quarters of neonates undergoing surgery for EA required perioperative extracorporeal membrane oxygenation (ECMO) support. When surgery is performed in older infants (median age of 6 months), the mortality is 9%, with a composite morbidity-mortality score of 25% and a reoperation rate of 28%. In older children and adults, perioperative outcomes are vastly better, with an early mortality of 2% to 5%.[114]

Late surgical outcomes are good overall, with 5-, 10-, and 20-year survival of 94%, 90%, and 76%, respectively (mean age at operation 24 years, ranging from 8 days to 79 years). Preoperative multivariate predictors of late mortality include RVOT dilatation or enlargement of the branch pulmonary arteries, raised hematocrit (indicative of cyanosis), prolonged QRS duration, and mitral regurgitation requiring intervention. The presence of sinus rhythm on a preoperative ECG and intraoperative ablation of accessory pathways are associated with improved long-term survival.

Most patients who have undergone Ebstein repair have a good functional status, although survival free from operation

TABLE 67–12. Ebstein Anomaly: 2018 AHA/ACC Guidelines for ACHD

COR	LOE	Diagnostic	Therapeutic
I	B-NR		1. Surgical repair or reoperation for adults with Ebstein anomaly and significant TR is recommended when one or more of the following are present: HF symptoms, objective evidence of worsening exercise capacity, progressive RV systolic dysfunction by echocardiography or CMR
I	C-LD		2. Catheter ablation is recommended for adults with Ebstein anomaly and high-risk pathway conduction or multiple accessory pathways
IIa	B-NR	1. CMR can be useful to determine anatomy, RV dimensions, and systolic function 2. In adults with Ebstein anomaly, TEE can be useful for surgical planning if TTE images are inadequate to evaluate tricuspid valve morphology and function 3. Electrophysiological study with or without catheter ablation can be useful in the diagnostic evaluation of adults with Ebstein anomaly and ventricular preexcitation but without supraventricular tachycardia 4. In adults with Ebstein anomaly, electrophysiological study (and catheter ablation, if needed) is reasonable before surgical intervention on the tricuspid valve even in the absence of preexcitation or supraventricular tachycardia	1. Surgical repair or reoperation for adults with Ebstein anomaly and significant TR can be beneficial in the presence of progressive RV enlargement, systemic desaturation from right-left atrial shunt, paradoxical embolism, and/or atrial tachyarrhythmias
IIb	B-NR		1. Bidirectional superior cavopulmonary (Glenn) anastomosis at time of Ebstein anomaly repair may be considered for adults when severe RV dilation or severe RV systolic dysfunction is present, LV function is preserved, and left atrial pressure and LV end-diastolic pressure are not elevated

Abbreviations: ACHD, adult congenital heart disease, CMR, cardiac magnetic resonance; COR, class of recommendation; HF, heart failure; LD, limited data; LOE, level of evidence; LV, left ventricle/ventricular; NR, nonrandomized; RA, right atrium/atrial; RV, right ventricle/ventricular; TEE, transesophageal echocardiography; TTE, transthoracic echocardiography; TR, tricuspid regurgitation; TV, tricuspid valve.

TABLE 67–13. Ebstein Anomaly: 2020 ESC Guidelines for ACHD

COR	LOE	Indications for Catheter Interventions	Indications for Surgical Interventions
I	C	1. In patients with symptomatic arrhythmias, or pre-excitation on the ECG, electrophysiologic testing followed by ablation therapy, if feasible, or surgical treatment of the arrhythmias in the case of planned heart surgery is recommended.	1. Surgical repair is recommended in patients with severe TR and symptoms or objective deterioration of exercise capacity.
I	C		1. It is recommended that surgical repair is performed by a congenital surgeon with specific experience in Ebstein surgery.
I	C		1. If there is an indication for TV surgery, ASD/PFO closure is recommended at the time of valve repair if it is expected to be hemodynamically tolerated.
IIa	C	1. In the case of documented systemic embolism, probably caused by paradoxical embolism, isolated device closure of ASD/PFO should be considered but requires careful evaluation before intervention to exclude induction of RA pressure increase or fall in cardiac output.	1. Surgical repair should be considered regardless of symptoms in patients with progressive right heart dilation or reduction of RV systolic function.
IIb	C	1. If cyanosis (oxygen saturation at rest <90%) is the leading problem, isolated device closure of ASD/PFO may be considered but requires careful evaluation before intervention to exclude induction of RA pressure increase or fall in cardiac output.	

Abbreviations: ACHD, adult congenital heart disease; ASD, atrial septal defect; COR, class of recommendation; LOE, level of evidence; PFO, patent foramen ovale; RA, right atrium/atrial; RV, right ventricle/ventricular; TR, tricuspid regurgitation; TV, tricuspid valve.

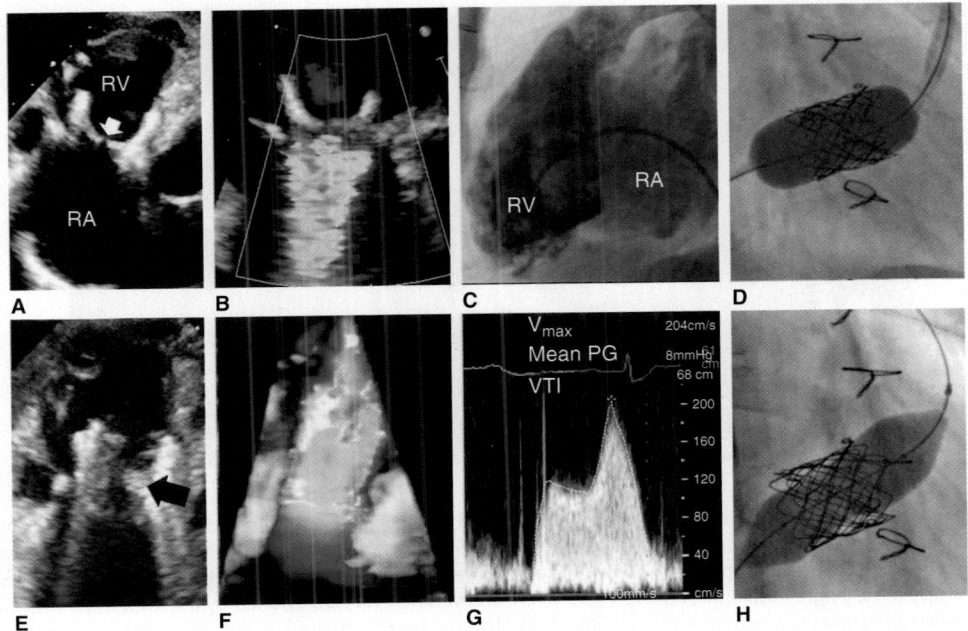

Figure 67–35. Tricuspid regurgitation and tricuspid stenosis following valve replacement. Patient with Carpentier type D Ebstein anomaly and Ebstein surgery involving tricuspid valve replacement 6 months prior to assessment (A–D). (**A**) the valve leaflets of the bioprosthesis are thickened and retracted with noncoaptation (*arrow*) causing, in (**B**), a broad jet of severe tricuspid regurgitation. (**C**) At angiography, contrast in the right ventricle (RV) is seen refluxing into the severely dilated right atrium (RA). (**D**) Melody valve-in-valve placement. Re-assessment (**E–H**) reveals early failure of the new valve. In (**E**), thickened, restricted valve leaflets (*black arrow*) are shown within the stent. In (**F**) and (**G**), there is severe tricuspid stenosis by 3D color and continuous wave Doppler. In (**H**), a third valve is placed percutaneously along with referral for transplantation assessment.

is 82% and 56% at 10- and 20-year follow-up, reflecting an ongoing risk of long-term complications. Approximately one-third of patients require rehospitalization within a decade from surgery. Long-term complications after surgery for EA include:

- Tricuspid valve dysfunction (TR most commonly, or tricuspid stenosis [TS]), causing ventricular dilatation, fibrosis, and dysfunction, requiring late reintervention
- Degeneration of prosthetic valves (bioprosthetic valve is the most common choice) (**Fig. 67–35**)
- Residual atrial communication, which can contribute to the development of cyanosis, exercise intolerance, or paradoxical emboli
- Accessory pathways and arrhythmias, which can be both supraventricular and ventricular. In all age groups, there is an increasing risk of arrhythmias over time and a persistent risk of late hemodynamic decline and SCD
- RV dysfunction, especially affecting the previously atrialized portion of the RV
- LV dysfunction due to ventricular–ventricular interaction, left-sided valve disease, or associated abnormalities (eg, LV noncompaction, mitral valve pathology)
- Exercise intolerance and heart failure
- Endocarditis, especially in patients with residual hemodynamic lesions, prosthetic material used for tricuspid valve repair, or prosthetic valves (especially percutaneously implanted tricuspid valves).

Specialist lifelong follow-up is warranted in patients with EA, as in other forms of CHD, to allow early detection and management of long-term sequelae.

Long-Term Sequelae and Complications

Tricuspid Regurgitation

Significant TR is seen in unoperated patients, as an early or late consequence of Ebstein repair, and as part of prosthetic valve failure in those who have undergone tricuspid valve replacement. It is the most common indication for reintervention. Long-standing severe TR can be well tolerated for many years before symptoms develop, but the lesion is not benign in the longer term (**Fig. 67–36**). Without timely intervention, further RA dilatation and rising RV filling pressures increase the risk of supraventricular arrhythmias and heart failure.

Arrhythmias

Both atrial and ventricular arrhythmias are prevalent in EA patients, likely as a consequence of a combination of significant, longstanding TR, ventricular dilatation, fibrosis and dysfunction, and surgical scarring. Indeed, in adolescent and adult patients, palpitations secondary to atrial arrhythmia are the most common clinical presentation.[122] SCD is not uncommon in EA, accounting for 5% of deaths in unrepaired patients, and representing an ongoing risk following surgical repair.[122,123]

The most common type of atrial arrhythmia encountered is atrial flutter, followed by focal atrial tachycardia and atrial fibrillation; multiple tachycardia substrates are present in over

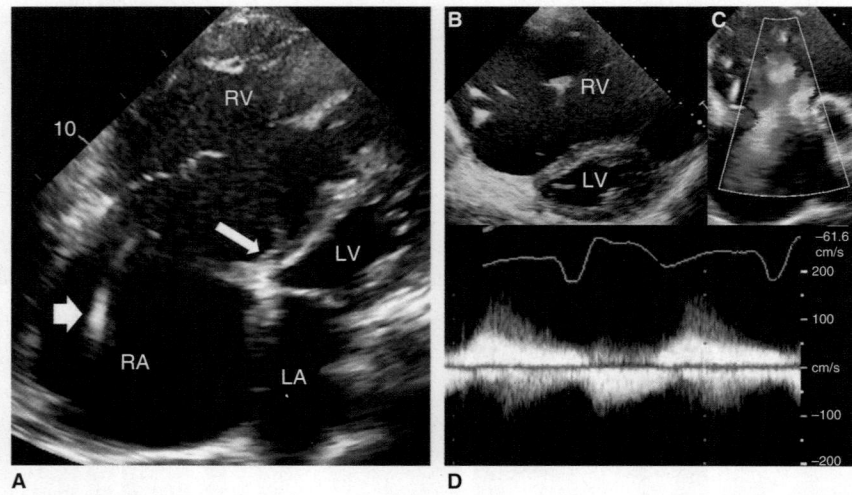

Figure 67–36. Sequelae of long-standing TR in Ebstein anomaly. A 58-year-old patient with Ebstein anomaly presenting with right heart failure and cardiac cirrhosis. In (**A**), apical four-chamber view displaying a severely dilated, apex-forming right ventricle (RV). The septal tricuspid valve leaflet is adherent to the ventricular septum and displaced toward the apex (*long arrow*). The anterior leaflet is elongated and sail-like. A permanent pacemaker lead (*short arrow*) is visualized within the grossly dilated right atrium (RA). The left atrium (LA) and ventricle (LV) are dwarfed by the right heart structures, and the atrial and ventricular septa bow leftward reflecting the pressure and volume overload, also on the parasternal short-axis view in (**B**). In (**C**), there is leaflet malcoaptation and free tricuspid regurgitation, and in (**D**), a low velocity triangular-shaped continuous wave Doppler signal, which cannot be used to estimate the right ventricular systolic pressure.

half of patients undergoing electrophysiological study. Cavotricuspid isthmus-dependent atrial flutter is the most common arrhythmia in patients who had previously undergone atrial Maze, present in >50%. The frequency of this arrhythmia is partly explained by the grossly abnormal anatomy of the isthmus in EA patients (due to the apical displacement of the tricuspid valve tissue and annular dilatation), and in part by the fact that most modern variations of the right-sided Maze procedure do not address this portion of the RA.[124] Incisional intra-atrial reentrant tachycardia is also encountered in this group. Left-sided atrial arrhythmias are rare.

Accessory pathways are commonly encountered in EA, seen in as many as 44% of patients. Direct muscular connections across the atrioventricular junction are due to the downward displacement of the septal tricuspid valve leaflet with discontinuity of the central fibrous body and septal atrioventricular ring. The majority of accessory pathways in EA are right-sided, and approximately one-third of adults with EA and ventricular preexcitation have more than one accessory pathway.[125,126] Concealed accessory pathways may coexist with manifest pathways, including atriofascicular pathways involving Mahaim fibers that can serve as the antegrade limb of macroreentrant supraventricular tachycardia (with the retrograde limb involving the atrioventricular node). The increased risk of both atrial arrhythmias and accessory pathways in patients with EA places these patients at potentially higher risk of lethal ventricular arrhythmia,[127] and proactive screening and ablation is important in reducing the risk of SCD in this patient group (see section Electrophysiological Evaluation, Ablation, and Devices).

Despite the fact that SCD is an important clinical concern in EA patients, risk stratification in EA is not as well established as in other forms of CHD (eg, ToF). The most informative study of sudden death in EA to date was conducted by Attenhofer

Jost et al. on 968 patients over a 40-year evaluation period.[123] There was a 0.2% risk of sudden death per annum, with a significant increase in mortality after the age of 40 years, but also following tricuspid valve surgery, reaching 2% in the first postoperative year. Variables related to mortality included a history of ventricular tachycardia, heart failure, tricuspid valve surgery, syncope, pulmonary stenosis, and a hemoglobin >150 g/L, supporting a role of ventricular tachyarrhythmia in sudden death in EA. However, recommendations for ICDs in primary prevention are still lacking in EA.

Clinically important bradyarrhythmias requiring permanent pacing are mainly encountered perioperatively but are otherwise rare. Conduction delays are, however, common in EA due to dilatation of the right heart and structural abnormalities of the atrioventricular conduction system: first-degree heart block is present in 42% of patients with EA.[128] The right bundle is commonly abnormal, often with marked fibrosis, and RBBB is seen in all but the least severe of cases.[129,130]

Heart Failure

Heart failure is an important complication both in repaired and unrepaired EA. In studies of the natural history of EA, 40% of unrepaired adults over the age of 25 years were in NYHA functional class III or IV.[131] The mechanisms of heart failure in EA are multiple and often include:

- Reduced contractility of the RV, especially the atrialized portion (even after repair)
- Impaired RA reservoir function and contractility, decreasing ventricular filling
- Chronic volume load caused by severe TR
- Ventricular–ventricular interaction, and biventricular dysfunction

- Atrial or ventricular arrhythmias
- Acquired cardiovascular disease and systemic effects in older patients (eg, hypertension, coronary artery disease, renal or liver dysfunction).

Ebstein repair significantly improves indices of RV function,[108] exercise capacity and functional class, but severe RV and LV dysfunction are predictors of early and late mortality, and reoperation following Ebstein surgery.[114] Residual RV dysfunction is common even after optimal surgical repair, particularly affecting the RV inlet.

Residual Shunts
Small atrial communications in EA can act as a relief valve for the right heart, both at rest and especially during periods of increased loading (eg, exercise or arrhythmias). Right–left shunting may also be due to "streaming" of the TR jet toward the ASD/PFO. Cyanosis is associated with the risk of paradoxical embolism and affects exercise capacity through an increase in physiological dead space. Larger atrial communications may allow significant with left–right shunting can contribute to the volume overload of the right heart. When an ASD/PFO is contributing significantly to symptoms, closure may be indicated (see section Transcatheter ASD/PFO Closure).

Endocarditis
Antibiotic prophylaxis around high-risk dental procedures (ie, those involving manipulation of the gingival or periapical region of the teeth or perforation of the oral mucosa, including scaling and root canal procedures), is recommended for EA patients at the highest risk of infective endocarditis. This includes patients with cyanosis, a residual shunt in proximity to prosthetic material, a prosthetic valve, or valve repair with prosthetic material and valve regurgitation.[7,21] Patients should be educated on the importance of maintaining excellent dental hygiene and avoiding piercings, tattoos, and nail biting.

Assessment of Adults with EA

At presentation to adult CHD services, patients with EA either have an established diagnosis, with or without repair in childhood, or milder forms of the disease diagnosed during adult life.

History
When assessing a patient with EA, it is important to gather information about the mode of presentation and past interventions, both surgical and percutaneous: an antenatal diagnosis and neonatal surgery represent the worse end of the spectrum. Important information to glean from medical and surgical notes includes:

- Management during the neonatal period
- Timing of palliative strategy (eg, Starnes procedure, bidirectional Glenn)
- Type and timing of repair
- Additional surgery at the time of repair (surgical ablation, repair of the ASD/PFO, and so on)
- Perioperative complications

- Type and timing of subsequent surgery or interventions on the tricuspid valve, ASD/PFO, and pulmonary or mitral valve
- Long-term complications, including heart failure, endocarditis, and cyanosis
- Device implantation and arrhythmias: arrhythmias account for 40% of presentations in adulthood,[122] and information about previous arrhythmia management should be gathered (eg, antiarrhythmic medication, direct current cardioversion, catheter, and surgical ablation procedures).

Physical Examination
Previous repair is indicated by a median sternotomy scar, or more rarely a thoracotomy scar (from repair of an associated lesion, eg, coarctation of the aorta, or a palliative shunt). Central cyanosis at rest and digital clubbing should be noted.

The presence of severe TR in EA (in contrast to many other causes of TR) is associated with the following:

- Lack of jugular venous distension, rarely displaying large V waves (due to the severely dilated, compliant RA)
- Pansystolic murmur heard over a wide area of the precordium, accentuated during inspiration, and of variable intensity
- Loss of the pansystolic murmur in the setting of severe RV dysfunction and free TR, due to complete failure of tricuspid leaflet coaptation

Other findings on palpation and auscultation may include:

- Displacement of the LV apex toward the axilla
- A low intensity presystolic murmur of anatomic or functional TS
- Wide splitting of S1 and S2
- Presence of a gallop rhythm, the extra sound being an RV S3
- Hepatomegaly, ascites, or peripheral edema.

ECG and Chest Radiography
ECG findings typical to EA include RBBB, which is often atypical, multiphasic with low-amplitude R-waves in leads V1 to V2 (**Fig. 67–37A**). The QRS axis is normal or leftward. This is frequently accompanied by peaked (sometimes "Himalayan") P-waves of RA dilatation, first-degree heart block, or a low atrial rhythm. The presence of an accessory pathway may result in a shortened PR interval with or without delta waves (**Fig. 67–37B**). Arrhythmias are common (see section Long-Term Sequelae and Complications), and periodic screening for silent/asymptomatic arrhythmias with ambulatory ECG monitoring is advised in the AHA/ACC guidelines.

Chest radiography varies in relation to disease severity (**Figs. 67–37C and 67–37D**). In mild forms of EA, the chest radiograph may be normal or bear subtle evidence of right atrial dilatation. In severe cases, there can be massive cardiomegaly, with a bulging right heart border (RA enlargement), raised cardiac apex (RV enlargement) creating a globular cardiac silhouette, which resembles that of a pericardial effusion. Classically, an elevated cardiothoracic ratio >0.6 is related to a worse prognosis and increased risk of reoperation.[115] Incidental

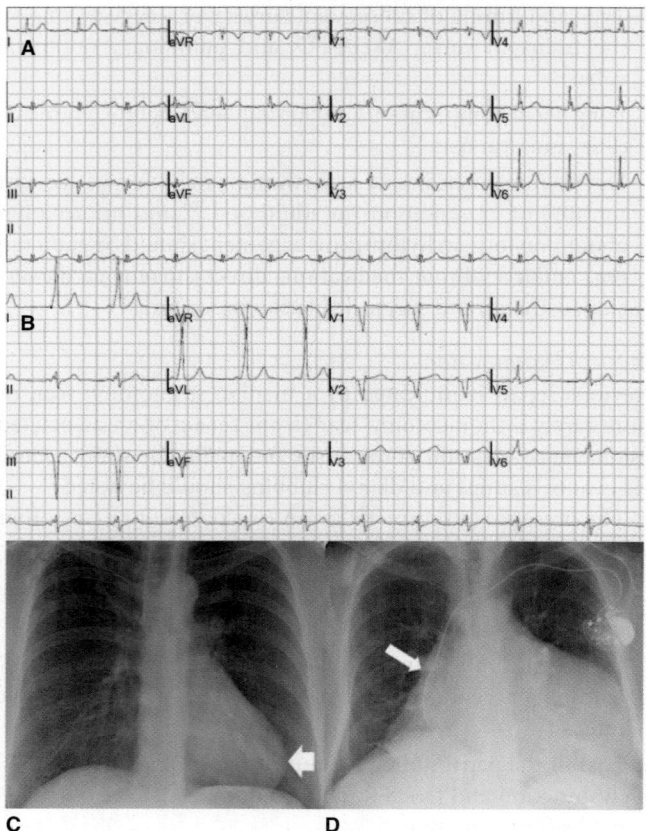

Figure 67–37. ECGs and chest radiographs in Ebstein anomaly. In (**A**), ECG of a patient with Ebstein anomaly and severe tricuspid regurgitation showing many of the typical features, including a first-degree heart block (PR interval 220 ms), peaked P waves, RBBB with low-amplitude R waves in leads V1–V2, and "bizarre" configuration of QRS complexes. In (**B**), ECG of a patient with ventricular preexcitation and manifest accessory pathway (short PR interval, delta waves). The past history of orthodromic atrioventricular reentrant tachycardia indicated Wolff-Parkinson-White syndrome. The patient underwent catheter ablation of a midseptal accessory pathway. In (**C**), a patient with Ebstein anomaly at the mild end of the spectrum, albeit with severe tricuspid regurgitation. There is a raised cardiac apex suggestive of RV dilatation (*arrow*). The cardiothoracic ratio is borderline at 0.49. In (**D**), a patient with advanced disease with severe right atrial (*arrow*) and RV enlargement, cardiothoracic ratio 0.78. Note the displacement of the carina to the right and presence of a permanent pacemaker with single ventricular lead (showing the extent of the RV), implanted for complete heart block at the time of supraventricular tachycardia ablation.

cardiomegaly is the presenting feature in a minority of asymptomatic adults.

Imaging

A multimodality assessment of EA is favored by the AHA/ACC and ESC guidelines.[6,7]

Echocardiography: Transthoracic echocardiography remains the primary imaging modality for the diagnosis and prognostication, in both neonatal disease (eg, using the GOSE score) and adults. It provides valuable information for the assessment of operability, and the noninvasive evaluation of hemodynamics, RV physiology, and associated lesions. Following surgical repair, echocardiography focuses on postoperative sequelae and complications, including TR or stenosis (including prosthetic

valve degeneration), RVOTO, shunt assessment, and other valvular abnormalities. TTE and TEE are also essential in the assessment of infective endocarditis.

The diagnosis of EA on echocardiography is made by measuring the degree of apical displacement of the septal leaflet of the tricuspid valve (ie, the distance between the septal insertions of the anterior mitral valve leaflet and the septal tricuspid valve leaflet) in the apical four-chamber view. Tethering and displacement of the posteroinferior leaflet is best visualized in the subcostal coronal and sagittal views, or parasternal long-axis view with medial angulation of the probe toward the RV. The anterior leaflet is visualized in several planes; in the apical four-chamber view its proximal segment can usually be seen attached to the atrioventricular groove. The parasternal short-axis and subcostal sagittal views allow imaging of the entire RV, from inflow to outflow, and demonstrates the anterior rotation of the tricuspid valve orifice into the RVOT.

Echocardiographic features that predict a poor surgical repair include:

- Small, tethered anterior leaflet with multiple muscular attachments
- Severely hypoplastic septal leaflet
- Severe dilatation of the (true) tricuspid valve annulus or RV
- Severe LV systolic dysfunction
- Pulmonary hypertension.

The presence of severe TR is indicated by a broad TR jet on color Doppler, originating near the RV apex and filling the atrialized RV and true RA. Aliasing of flow may not occur due to the low flow velocities across the tricuspid valve. Multiple valve orifices may be identified on color Doppler. Failure of coaptation on 2D imaging also points to the presence of severe TR. The continuous wave Doppler confirms severe TR with a high-density triangular signal, which peaks early, and a low retrograde velocity; this signal represents early near-equalization of RV and RA pressures, and underestimates RV systolic pressure (**Fig. 67–36D**). Pulsed wave Doppler of superior and inferior caval flow demonstrate flow reversal and dominant early diastolic filling of the RA in the setting of severe TR.[132]

RV dilatation and dysfunction should be assessed, along with sequelae of severe dilatation (ie, paradoxical septal motion and, rarely, obstruction of the LV outflow). The presence of severe TR can lead to overestimation of RV function on echocardiography when using parameters such as tricuspid valve lateral systolic excursion and annular velocity.[133] The use of volumetric quantification of size and function by 3D echocardiography is limited by the massive size of the RV, falling outside the edges of the detection zone.

Echocardiographic assessment following tricuspid valve replacement focuses on the assessment of prosthetic valve function (Fig. 67–35). Mixed tricuspid valve disease is common, and additional challenges in this setting include acoustic shadowing and reflections, low flow rates across the valve limiting accurate evaluation of valve performance by pressure drop and Doppler gradient, and hemodynamic differences between prostheses. Cardiac catheterization should be considered in these cases.

CMR and CT: CMR is the gold standard for the quantitative assessment of the RA and RV, and detailed information about tricuspid valve anatomy,[134] which is useful for surgical planning. For example, a greater tricuspid valve rotation angle and a smaller functional RV end-diastolic volume index have been associated with early surgical breakdown of the Cone reconstruction, and identified cases requiring technical modification or valve replacement.[135] CMR-derived RV ejection fraction has been shown to be predictive of major adverse cardiovascular events and new-onset atrial tachycardia in EA.[136] Myocardial fibrosis, assessed with late gadolinium enhancement, is observed in adult patients with EA and relates to worse LV function and clinical status, although its prognostic value is not established like in ToF (Tables 67–12 and 67–13).[137]

Cardiac CT angiography has replaced invasive coronary for the assessment of the coronary arteries in preoperative planning of EA. It can also be used for chamber quantification when CMR is not feasible, but the frequency of assessment needs to be weighed against radiation exposure.

Exercise Testing
The CPET provides a wealth of data on exercise physiology and can help to determine the mechanisms of exercise limitation, risk stratification, and the impact of time and therapeutic interventions on exercise capacity. Exercise limitation is common in adult EA patients, who have a mean peak oxygen uptake (pVO_2) of 64 ± 19% of predicted.[138,139] A lower pVO_2 is found in those with more severe disease on echocardiography, higher cardiothoracic ratio, and an interatrial shunt, but is not influenced by the degree of TR. Impairment of RV systolic and diastolic function also correlates to poorer exercise capacity.[140] Moreover, many EA patients have evidence of inefficient ventilation (a raised VE/VCO_2 slope) and chronotropic incompetence.[139,141] A lower pVO_2 is predictive of the composite clinical endpoint of death, nonelective hospital admission, and surgical repair.[138]

The 6MWT is a simple alternative, reserved for patients who have advanced disease and cannot undergo a full CPET, or in the presence of pulmonary hypertension with moderate–severe exercise limitation, where the 6-minute walk distance is an established prognostic variable (see Exercise Testing in section Tetralogy of Fallot).

Catheterization
Noninvasive assessment using echocardiography and CMR is usually adequate for the diagnosis and preoperative assessment of EA, avoiding the need for cardiac catheterization in the majority of cases. Catheterization is limited to selected indications (eg, in suspected pulmonary hypertension, raised LV end-diastolic pressure, or to assess candidacy for a superior cavopulmonary [Glenn] shunt or heart transplantation).

Management of Adults with Ebstein Anomaly
Medical
Medical management of EA is aimed at treating specific sequelae and complications of the disease, including arrhythmia, heart failure, and paradoxical embolism.

The pharmacological management of arrhythmia should be concurrent to planning an electrophysiological study and/or catheter ablation. In a series of 285 operated patients with EA, digoxin was the most commonly prescribed medication, used in 22%.[142] In patients with an accessory pathway and atrial fibrillation (preexcited atrial fibrillation), agents that preferentially slow atrioventricular conduction, including digoxin, calcium channel blockers, and β-blockers, are contraindicated and can precipitate rapid conduction down the accessory pathway and SCD.

The medical management of heart failure in EA is aimed at treating congestive symptoms with diuretics. Evidence is lacking to support the use of neurohormonal blockade (eg, using ACE inhibitors, angiotensin receptor blockers, β-blockers, mineralocorticoid receptor antagonists, or neprilysin inhibitors) in right heart failure associated with EA. Specialists reserved these therapies for cases involving biventricular (mainly left) ventricular dysfunction.

The 2020 ESC guidelines recommend oral anticoagulation for EA patients with a history of atrial fibrillation or paradoxical embolism through an atrial communication (see section Transcatheter ASD/PFO Closure).[7] Anticoagulation may also be considered when there is an increased thromboembolic risk or in the presence of a right–left shunt.

Surgical Reintervention
Reintervention in patients with EA and significant tricuspid valve dysfunction or prosthetic valve failure remains an important, long-term issue for patients with repaired EA. In one series, the reoperation rate at 20-years was 30%, with multivariate predictors being younger age at first operation and associated abnormal pulmonary artery architecture.[114,142] Significant TR can be tolerated for years before reintervention is required. The AHA/ACC guideline recommendations for reoperation are identical to those for initial surgical repair.[6] Reoperation involves tricuspid valve replacement more commonly than valve repair (Tables 67–12 and 67–13).

Interventional
Catheter-based interventions employed in EA include catheter ablation (see subsequent section), closure of an atrial communication, and transcatheter tricuspid valve replacement.

Transcatheter ASD/PFO Closure: The indications and timing of isolated ASD/PFO closure are still debated, and practices vary widely between centers. At the Mayo Clinic in Rochester, only 1% of 968 patients under follow-up had undergone isolated ASD/PFO closure at initial evaluation at the tertiary center, and 17% had this closed prior to tricuspid valve surgery.[123] In selected patients, ASD/PFO closure can alleviate cyanosis, prevent paradoxical emboli, and improve exercise capacity.[143] The 2020 ESC ACHD guidelines recommend that isolated device closure of ASD/PFO should be considered in case of documented systemic embolism attributed to paradoxical emboli, or when cyanosis is a leading cause of symptoms (Tables 67–12 and 67–13).

Prior to undertaking this, however, patients need to be carefully evaluated (test balloon occlusion of the atrial communication) to ensure that defect closure will not cause a significant rise in RA pressure or a fall in systemic cardiac output. This is more likely to occur in EA patients with severe TR, congestive cardiac failure, or pulmonary stenosis.

Percutaneous Tricuspid Valve Implantation: Transcatheter tricuspid valve-in-valve implantation in patients with a dysfunctional tricuspid valve prosthesis is a minimally invasive alternative to surgical reoperation. Transcatheter valve-in-ring implantation, following repair using a tricuspid valve annuloplasty ring, has also been performed.[144] A percutaneous approach may be appealing for patients with multiple previous sternotomies or other perioperative risk factors. Immediate procedural success rate is high with effective restoration of tricuspid valve function, and clinical improvement in the majority of patients.[145] The main short- to medium-term complications are valve thrombosis (up to 5%), infective endocarditis (annualized incidence of 1.5% per patient-year), and valve dysfunction (10% reintervention within 3 years).[145,146] Longer-term outcome data are awaited. The approach to postprocedural anticoagulation varies, but almost all patients are discharged on antiplatelet therapy, with over half also on anticoagulation in the largest series of cases.[146]

Transplantation

Heart transplantation is a vital management strategy for eligible ACHD patients with severe advanced heart failure (see Transplantation in section Tetralogy of Fallot).[88] In EA, transplant referral is sought mainly in two groups of patients: in younger children, including neonates with critical EA, who are either unoperated or following palliative procedures EA (accounts for 4% of CHD transplants), or in adults following multiple interventions, when conventional surgical or transcatheter options have been exhausted.[147] Transplant referral should be considered in patients with severe biventricular dysfunction or severe LV dilatation and dysfunction.

Electrophysiological Evaluation, Ablation, and Devices

Electrophysiological evaluation, with proactive identification and treatment of arrhythmia, is an essential component of EA management (Tables 67–12 and 67–13). There is consensus that patients with EA and symptoms of arrhythmia, or preexcitation on ECG, should undergo electrophysiological study and catheter ablation as required (ESC class I; AHA/ACC class IIa recommendation). In the AHA/ACC guidance, this recommendation is strengthened to class I in patients with high-risk pathway conduction or multiple accessory pathways. A preoperative electrophysiological study should be considered in all patients referred for surgery. In a study evaluating this strategy in patients referred for the cone procedure, Shivapour et al.[148] documented significant findings in 69% of the 42 electrophysiological studies, guiding ablation therapy. Furthermore, transcatheter access to right-sided accessory pathways and the slow pathway in atrioventricular node reentry may be obstructed following tricuspid valve surgery, supporting a strategy of electrophysiological study and ablation prior to tricuspid valve surgery.[148]

Surgical ablation of accessory pathways is largely reserved for patients in whom catheter ablation is not feasible or has failed to control the arrhythmia (AHA/ACC ACHD guidelines). European guidelines, however, state that surgical treatment of arrhythmias is recommended in the case of planned heart surgery. Surgical ablation in the presence of atrial arrhythmias is nowadays limited to a modified right atrial Maze procedure unless there are additional indications. In the presence of atrial flutter, the RA isthmus is ablated as well. In cases of atrial fibrillation, additional left atrial Cox Maze III procedure is employed by some surgeons to reduce the risk of arrhythmia recurrence.[123,149]

The indications for pacing and device therapy are the same in EA as for other cardiac conditions. The strongest indications exist for patients with prior symptomatic ventricular tachycardia or aborted SCD (secondary prevention). Data on primary prevention ICD implantation is limited, with a high rate of inappropriate shocks.[123] When a permanent pacemaker is indicated, epicardial LV pacing is preferred.

Routine Follow-Up of Patients with Ebstein Anomaly

All patients with EA require regular, lifelong, specialist follow-up at intervals appropriate for their ACHD anatomic and physiological classification (A–D, see Table 67–4).[6] According to this classification system, patients who suffer a clinical deterioration move up the classification, requiring more frequent follow-up with additional investigations, while patients who undergo successful intervention associated with an improvement in status (eg, Ebstein repair or control of arrhythmia) move down the classification. In uncomplicated EA, patients should undergo outpatient review with ECG and echocardiographic surveillance every 12 to 24 months.

Pregnancy in Women with Ebstein Anomaly

Women with EA without complicated disease normally tolerate pregnancy well, being classified as modified WHO class II in the 2018 ESC guidelines,[22] which reflects a 5.7% to 10.5% risk of maternal cardiac events including arrhythmia and heart failure. There is also an increased risk of preterm delivery.[150] Prepregnancy assessment and counselling, at a minimum including an ECG, echocardiography, and an exercise test, is recommended for all women with EA, and repair should be considered prior to pregnancy in those with severe, symptomatic TR. Women with EA and either cyanosis (resting oxygen saturation <85%) or heart failure are at higher risk of adverse cardiac, obstetric, and fetal outcomes and should be advised against pregnancy.

The guidelines recommend follow-up visits at least once every trimester for women with EA who are otherwise well without complications, with closer monthly or bimonthly follow-up in an expert center for pregnancy and heart disease if cyanosis is present. Clinical review should include assessment for symptoms and signs of paradoxical embolism, which are a risk in women with cyanosis and right–left shunting.

ISOLATED CONGENITAL TRICUSPID VALVE DISEASE

Isolated congenital tricuspid valve (TV) disease describes a rare group of CHDs involving the valvar and/or subvalvar TV apparatus, leading to TR and, much less frequently, TS. Non-EA congenital TR can be due to a range of conditions that culminate in failure of effective valve closure, the most common of which is TV dysplasia. Differentiating a congenital cause of TR or TS from acquired organic TV disease may be difficult, especially in adult patients, and relies on identifying certain features (**Table 67–14**). It is of the utmost importance to distinguish primary disease from functional (secondary) TR, which is far more common and is often associated with left-sided valve disease and/or pulmonary hypertension, both of which dictate the management and prognosis.

The rarity of congenital TV disease has meant that the natural history and genetic associations are not well-defined; indeed, there is no specific mention of isolated congenital TR or TS disease in international ACHD guidelines.[6,7] However, TV disease features in the AHA/ACC or ESC valvular heart disease guidelines.[151,152]

Anatomical Features and Associated Lesions

Tricuspid Stenosis

Congenital TS is caused by TV dysplasia (ie, developmental abnormalities in any of the components of the TV), causing obstruction at the level of the valve or subvalvar apparatus. This can include hypoplasia of the annulus and leaflets, fused commissures, shortened or abnormally arranged chordae (eg, arising from a single papillary muscle causing a parachute-type deformity or double-orifice TV. Supravalvar stenosis rarely arises from a supravalvar ring or persistence of the right venous valve, resulting in a variably perforated partition of the RA into a proximal chamber, that receives the venous return, and a distal chamber; this is known as a double-chambered RA or cor triatriatum dexter. In cases of severe TV hypoplasia or tricuspid atresia (most severe end of the spectrum), there is a variable degree of RV hypoplasia, resulting in a functionally univentricular heart. Per the ACC and ECS guidelines, surgery is recommended for patients with severe tricuspid valve stenosis in symptomatic patients or when being considered for left-sided valvular disease (**Tables 67–15** and **67–16**).

TABLE 67–14. Classification and Features of Non-Ebstein Primary Tricuspid Valve Disease

TV Disease	Hemodynamic Lesion	Additional Valve Involvement	Features on Imaging
Congenital			
TV dysplasia; Unguarded tricuspid orifice	Any or mixed	Pulmonary valve stenosis	Hypoplastic or absent TV leaflets; spectrum of hypoplasia of tricuspid orifice (toward tricuspid atresia); small papillary muscles with shortened, tethered chordae
TV prolapse	TR	Mitral valve (prolapse)	Myxomatous degeneration with leaflet prolapse; elongated, redundant chordae; large leaflets; annular dilatation
RV dysplasia Uhl's anomaly	TR	–	RV free wall aneurysm, focal RV thinning and dysfunction, abnormal septal motion. Almost complete absence of RV myocardium
Acquired			
Tricuspid annular dilatation*	TR	–	Dilated TV annulus, RV +/– LV dilatation, biatrial dilatation
Rheumatic TV disease	Any or mixed	Mitral valve, aortic valve (left-sided valve involvement in ~ all cases affecting TV)	Diffuse marginal or leaflet thickening and calcification, focal chordal thickening, retraction and fusion, commissural fusion
TV endocarditis Infective NBTE	Any or mixed	Any	Vegetations, valvular indentation, ruptured chordae Small, irregular vegetations usual
Traumatic TR	TR	–	Ruptured TV subvalvar apparatus, leaflet perforation
Carcinoid heart disease	Any or mixed	Pulmonary valve, (left-sided valve involvement in 5%–10%, extensive liver metastases, bronchial carcinoid or PFO)	Thickened leaflet margins and/or chordae; retracted, tethered leaflets, carcinoid plaques on TV or RV endocardium
Radiation-associated cardiac disease	Any or mixed	Depends on radiation field	Prominent calcification (valvar, annular, pericardial, aorto-mitral curtain, aortic), biventricular dysfunction, pericardial constriction
Drug-related (ergotamine, anorexogens)	TR	Aortic, mitral valve	Leaflet contraction, thickening with shortened chordae

*Tricuspid annular dilatation caused by pulmonary hypertension, long-standing permanent atrial fibrillation, right ventricular myocardial infarction, or cardiomyopathy.
Abbreviations: NBTE, nonbacterial thrombotic endocarditis; RV, right ventricle; TR, tricuspid regurgitation; TS, tricuspid stenosis; TV, tricuspid valve.

TABLE 67–15. Primary Tricuspid Valve Stenosis: 2018 AHA/ACC Guidelines for ACHD

COR	LOE	Diagnostic	Therapeutic
I	B-NR		1. Surgery is recommended for patients with severe TS at the time of operation for left-sided valve disease. 2. Surgery is recommended for patients with isolated, symptomatic severe TS.
IIb			1. Percutaneous balloon tricuspid commissurotomy might be considered in patients with isolated, symptomatic severe TS without accompanying TR.

Unless otherwise stated, tricuspid valve surgery connotes tricuspid valve repair or replacement, decided on individual assessment.

Abbreviations: ACHD, adult congenital heart disease; COR, class of recommendation; LOE, level of evidence; NR, nonrandomized; TR, tricuspid regurgitation; TS: tricuspid stenosis.

Tricuspid Regurgitation

The most common cause of congenital TR is EA (see section Ebstein Anomaly of the Tricuspid Valve), characterized by a failure of delamination of the TV sufficient to cause apical displacement of the septal tricuspid leaflet by ≥ 8 mm/m^2. The most common cause of non-EA TR is TV dysplasia, characterized by hypoplastic, small or absent leaflets (the latter is referred to as an "unguarded tricuspid orifice"), and an abnormal TV tensor apparatus, including underdeveloped papillary muscles or shortened chordae.[53] Other congenital anomalies causing TR include right-sided congenital partial absence of the pericardium, TV leaflet cleft(s), or Uhl anomaly (an exceptionally rare abnormality with severe hypoplasia of the RV myocardium).

Primary TR caused by TV dysplasia is seen in association with other CHD, including pulmonary stenosis or atresia. In patients with cc-TGA, TV dysplasia is common, and is a major contributing factor to tricuspid (systemic atrioventricular valve) regurgitation requiring surgery. In atrioventricular canal defects (atrioventricular septal defects), abnormal and incomplete development of the right atrioventricular valve is commonly associated with right atrioventricular valve regurgitation, even though this is not a morphologically tricuspid valve.

TABLE 67–16. Primary Tricuspid Valve Stenosis: 2020 ESC Guidelines for ACHD

COR	LOE	Diagnostic	Therapeutic
I			1. Surgery is indicated in symptomatic patients with severe TS. 2. Surgery is indicated in patients with severe TS undergoing left-sided valve surgery.

Unless otherwise stated, tricuspid valve surgery connotes tricuspid valve repair or replacement, decided on individual assessment.

Abbreviations: ACHD, adult congenital heart disease; COR, class of recommendation; LOE, level of evidence; TS: tricuspid stenosis.

TV prolapse caused by myxomatous degeneration is increasingly appreciated in association with mitral valve prolapse in the setting of Marfan syndrome, affecting 12% of patients of all ages and >50% of children diagnosed with Marfan and mitral valve prolapse.[154,155]

Pathophysiology of Congenital Tricuspid Valve Disease

The clinical implications of congenital TS depend primarily on the degree of obstruction to RV inflow. When severe, congenital TS usually manifests in early life. The obstruction to flow causes an elevation in RA pressure and limits the ability of the heart to augment cardiac output on efforts, which may cause syncope.

Unlike TS, TR can be tolerated for a prolonged period with few or no symptoms, even when severe. Over time, however, the right-sided volume load causes RV and RA dilatation, with a rise in central venous pressure. RV remodeling, over time, leads to RV dysfunction and a decrease in exercise capacity.[156] Diastolic ventricular–ventricular interaction can impair LV relaxation and raise its filling pressures.[157]

In severe long-standing TS or TR, there is also a significant risk of atrial arrhythmias, which can precipitate clinical decompensation, commonly manifesting as right-sided heart failure (peripheral edema or ascites). Ventricular arrhythmias may also occur as a result of congenital RV dysplasia or remodeling. In the presence of an atrial communication, TS or TR can cause right–left shunting and cyanosis at rest or on efforts.

Clinical Presentation and Assessment

Isolated congenital TS usually presents and is often repaired in infancy or early childhood. The vast majority of TS identified in adulthood is due to acquired disease (eg, rheumatic valve disease). By contrast, most cases of congenital TV disease causing TR are diagnosed in adolescence or adult life.

Patients with TV disease are often asymptomatic, or complain of exercise intolerance, fatigue, and later as a result of right-sided heart failure, peripheral edema, ascites, progressive exertional breathlessness, and cool peripheries.

Patients with severe TR may occasionally present with cyanosis, the result of "streaming" of the regurgitant jet toward an ASD or PFO and/or rise in RA pressure.

The history and physical examination aim to characterize the severity of the hemodynamic lesion and identify any signs and symptoms of more common acquired tricuspid valve disease, for example, rheumatoid arthritis (joint involvement), systemic lupus erythematosus (SLE) (Raynaud's phenomenon, butterfly rash and mucocutaneous ulcers), carcinoid syndrome (flushing or bronchospasm), current or previous endocarditis (vascular lesions of infective endocarditis in the fingers or toes), drug abuse, history of chest radiotherapy, left-sided heart disease, and pulmonary hypertension.

Features of severe TR include:

- Raised jugular venous pulse with giant *v* waves, which may be absent in instances of severe right atriomegaly
- RV heave due to RV overload (not seen in Uhl anomaly)

- The S1 is appreciably normal, unlike in EA where there is splitting of S1
- The S2 may be normal or have fixed splitting
- An additional, S3 may be present as a result of RV dysfunction
- A holosystolic murmur at the left lower sternal border, which increases in intensity on inspiration (Carvallo's sign). The murmur becomes longer with increasing TR severity, but with torrential TR, early near-equalization of RA and RV pressures causes the murmur to shorten or disappear, along with a diastolic rumble indicating increased flow across the TV
- In TV prolapse, a midsystolic click may be appreciated, accompanied by a mid- to late-systolic murmur
- Pulsatile hepatomegaly.

TTE is the main imaging modality used to diagnose and characterize primary tricuspid valve disease. EA is excluded by measuring the apical displacement of the septal TV leaflet (normal <8 mm/m²) on the apical four-chamber view. Features suggestive of an underlying cause for the TV disease can also be identified on echocardiography (Table 67–14).

TS is often overlooked on echocardiography, and requires clinical suspicion and careful evaluation. Characterization of the valve and subvalvar apparatus is an important for deciding on reparability, with insufficient pliable valve tissue usually precluding repair. TS is frequently associated with TR, hence the continuity equation is rarely applicable, and other quantitative methods that are validated in left-sided disease (eg, pressure half-time) are less accurate. A mean gradient of ≥5 mm Hg in

the absence of tachycardia is indicative of severe TS. Three-dimensional echocardiography and TEE allow better visualization of the valve.

TR severity is graded based on the integration of multiple variables from 2D and Doppler measurements (**Fig. 67–38**), complemented by quantitative Doppler assessment when feasible using the proximal isovelocity surface area (PISA) method with angle correction, and indirect signs from the hepatic veins and inferior vena cava (**Fig. 67–39**). Eccentric TR can be underestimated using the TR jet size and requires modified views and relies more heavily on indirect evidence to grade (**Fig. 67–40**). Estimation of pulmonary artery systolic pressure using the modified Bernoulli equation can be undertaken, but this may be underestimated in very severe TR. When the severity of the TR remains "indeterminate" on transthoracic echo, further testing with TEE or CMR may be indicated.

CMR can provide quantitative assessment of regurgitant volume and fraction, but the assessment of TR is less well-established than with other regurgitant valvular lesions, and TR-specific thresholds (eg, regurgitant volume) have not been validated. The strength of CMR is its ability to accurately assess RA and RV remodeling due to TV disease.

Cardiac catheterization for isolated TR is rarely needed. In contemporary practice, diagnostic catheterization is undertaken for TV disease:

- When there is clinical concern about pulmonary hypertension as a cause/contributing factor of TR[151]
- When the severity of TS cannot be determined by noninvasive means: in this case, two catheters should ideally be used (one in the RV and one in the RA) to measure the tricuspid

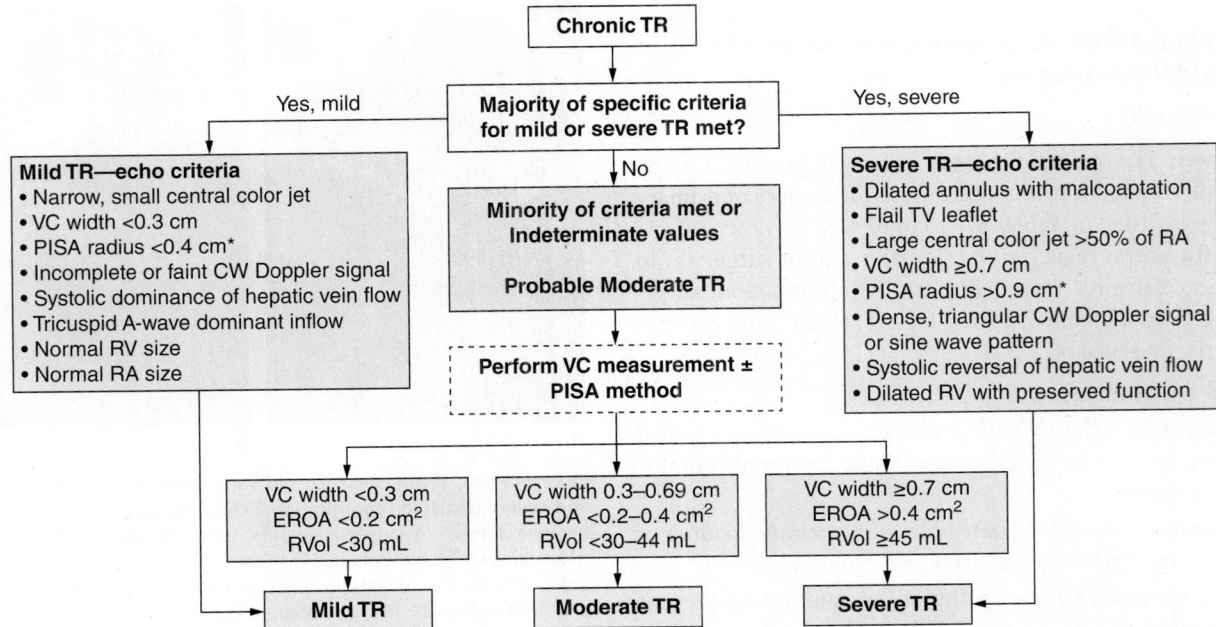

Figure 67–38. Algorithm for the echocardiographic assessment of TR severity. Algorithm for the integration of multiple parameters of TR severity, modified from the ASE Recommendations for Noninvasive Evaluation of Native Valvular Regurgitation.[216] CW, continuous wave; EROA, effective regurgitant orifice area; PISA, proximal isovelocity surface area; RVol, regurgitant volume; VC, vena contracta. *PISA measurement using a Nyquist limit of 28–40 cm/s.

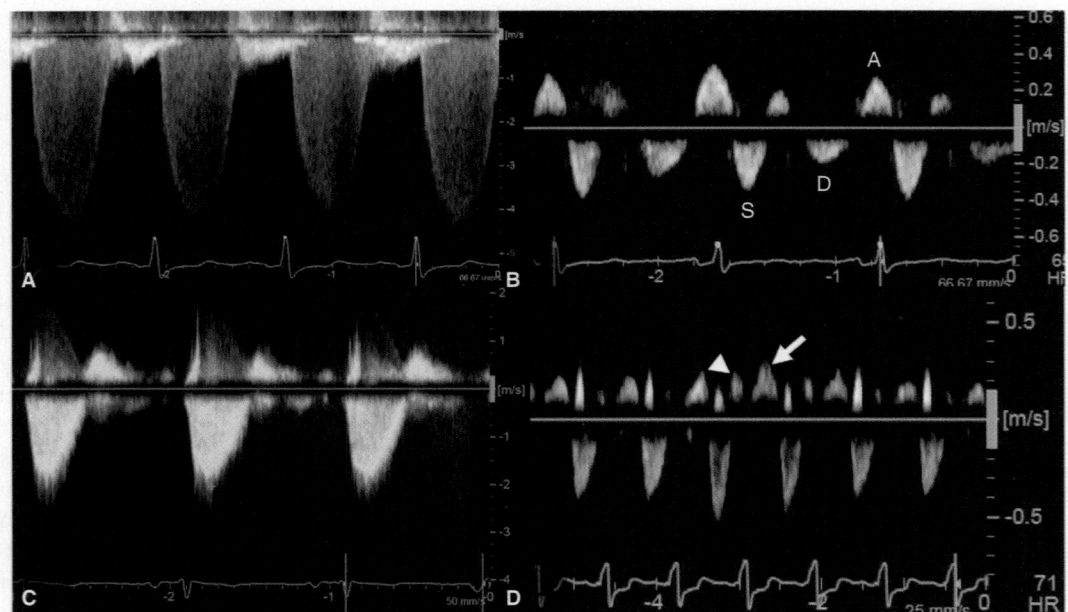

Figure 67-39. Doppler findings in mild and severe tricuspid regurgitation. In (**A**), continuous wave Doppler signal across the tricuspid valve (from apical four-chamber view) in a patient with pulmonary hypertension. There is a symmetrical, low density jet in keeping with mild tricuspid regurgitation (TR). Note that the raised TR peak velocity of above 4 m/s indicates elevated right ventricular systolic pressure (64 mm Hg using the modified Bernoulli equation), but this does not provide information on the severity of the TR. In (**B**), hepatic vein pulsed wave Doppler signal (from a subcostal view) in a patient with mild TR showing a normal pattern of forward systolic (S) and diastolic (D) flow, and atrial reversal (A) flow from normal reflux of blood toward the hepatic vein from atrial contraction. (**C**) and (**D**), by contrast, show Doppler findings in severe TR. (**C**) shows the continuous wave Doppler signal across the tricuspid valve in a patient with torrential TR, showing a dense, triangular signal with early systolic peaking of the jet, representing early equilibration of pressures between the right atrium and right ventricle. In (**D**), the hepatic vein flow signal in a patient in sinus rhythm showing systolic (*arrow*) as well as atrial (*arrowhead*) reversed flow, representing elevated right atrial pressure as a result of severe TR.

valve gradient; the catheters should thereafter be exchanged and measurements repeated to ensure that any gradient detected is not artificial (ie, related to inappropriate calibration of the transducers)

- At the time of transcatheter intervention

Surgical and Transcutaneous Interventions in Tricuspid Valve Disease

Surgical Repair

Indications: The optimal timing of surgery in primary TV disease is still debated. Current indications for surgery of primary TS or TR are listed in **Tables 67-15 to 67-18**.

As with mitral regurgitation, a major aim of surgery is to prevent excessive RV remodeling and RV dysfunction, affecting long-term outcome. Other factors taken into account include the presence of:

- Atrial arrhythmias
- Endocarditis of the TV with inadequate response to medical therapy, or embolic complications, most commonly pulmonary embolism
- Associated lesions that contribute to the volume loading of the RV (eg, ASDs or pulmonary regurgitation)
- Severe congestive hepatopathy, in an attempt to prevent liver cirrhosis

Technique and Outcomes: The surgical approach to TV disease is individualized, focusing on the mechanism responsible.

In TS, reparability of the valve is limited by the availability of pliable tricuspid valve tissue. Hence, replacement using a bioprosthetic is routine practice, while mechanical valves are used less commonly due to the increased risk of thrombosis.

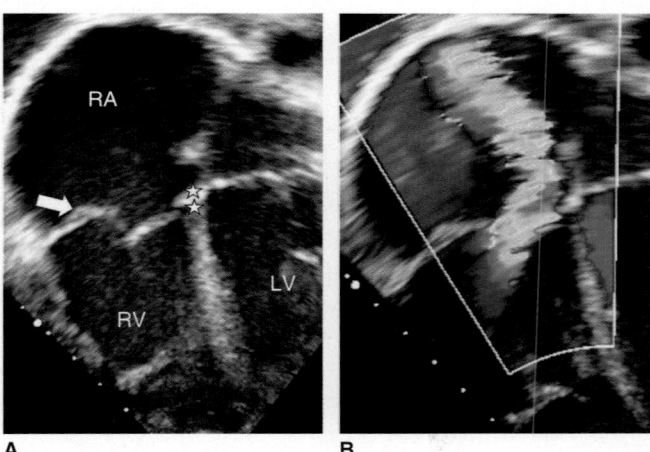

Figure 67-40. Dysplastic tricuspid valve with anterior leaflet prolapse and severe tricuspid regurgitation. Echocardiography (apical four-chamber views) on a 17-year-old male presenting with atypical chest pain, with tricuspid valve (TV) dysplasia. (**A**) There is thickening and tethering of the anterior TV leaflet with anterior leaflet prolapse (*arrow*), with right atrial (RA) and right ventricular (RV) dilatation. Offsetting of the tricuspid and mitral septal attachments is within normal limits, with an apical displacement index of the septal leaflet of the TV of 6 mm or 4 mm/m², indicating this is not Ebstein anomaly. (**B**) There is associated moderate to severe eccentric tricuspid regurgitation, directed toward the atrial septum. LV, left ventricle.

TABLE 67–17. Primary Tricuspid Valve Regurgitation: 2014 AHA/ACC Guidelines for Valvular Heart Disease

COR	LOE	Diagnostic	Therapeutic
I	B-NR		1. Surgery is recommended for patients with severe TR undergoing left-sided valve surgery.
IIa	C-EO		1. Surgery can be beneficial in symptomatic severe TR unresponsive to medical therapy (diuretics).
IIb			1. Surgery can be beneficial in symptomatic or minimally symptomatic patients with severe TR with ≥1 of: • Progressive moderate or greater RV dilatation; • RV systolic dysfunction.

Unless otherwise stated, tricuspid valve surgery connotes tricuspid valve repair or replacement, decided on individual assessment.
Abbreviations: ACHD, adult congenital heart disease; COR, class of recommendation; EO, expert opinion; LOE, level of evidence; NR, nonrandomized; RV, right ventricle; TR, tricuspid regurgitation.

Percutaneous balloon tricuspid valvuloplasty is rarely considered in cases of isolated TS with suitable anatomy, but is associated with a significant risk of postprocedural TR.[158] In patients with primary TR, either TV repair and replacement is chosen based on the extent of the disease, presence of a flail leaflet, involvement of the subvalvar apparatus, and underlying cause of the dysfunction. In general, repair is favored when TV integrity can be achieved and maintained.

Techniques for TV repair are broadly classified into two groups: annuloplasty (by direct suture or ring) and coaptation enhancement. Direct suture annuloplasty procedures include the de Vega annuloplasty, which employs purse-string sutures along the anterior and posterior aspects of the annulus, and the Kay plication, which involves plication of the posterior leaflet, forming a functionally bileaflet valve. Repair using an annuloplasty ring can be complete or incomplete, using either rigid or flexible devices; it has been shown to improve long-term outcome in patients undergoing TV repair and is currently the preferred reconstructive technique.[159] Coaptation enhancement techniques, such as the clover technique, involve stitching together the central part of each leaflet, usually in combination with ring annuloplasty. In patients with isolated congenital TR, degenerative changes of the leaflets and lack of chordae make direct repair challenging, hence additional procedures are required to improve the function of the subvalvar apparatus, including chordal implantation, transposition, or extension.[160]

TV replacement (TVR) is indicated when the TV disease affects all three leaflets and/or the tensor apparatus, where there is concern about the durability of a repair, or in the presence of a disease process that favors replacement (eg, carcinoid syndrome). The decision to use a bioprosthetic versus a mechanical valve should take into account valve anatomy, systemic features (eg, coagulopathy), patient demographics, and choice. The risk of valve thrombosis was prohibitively high (up to 20%)[161] with the older ball-and-cage valves, but the newer, low-profile bileaflet mechanical valves have an improved hemodynamic profile and a lower thrombosis rate. Preoperative RV dysfunction greatly increases the risk of thrombosis, and bioprostheses are favored in this setting.

Early complications are related to the location of the tricuspid annulus, with the base of the septal tricuspid leaflet (forming the triangle of Koch along with the coronary sinus orifice and tendon of Todaro) in proximity to the atrioventricular node, and the right coronary artery running within the right atrioventricular groove. Complete heart block occurs in up to 28% of patients following TVR in adults, increased further in those who undergo combined tricuspid and mitral valve intervention.[162,163] Reoperation is usually the result of bioprosthetic valve failure or valve thrombosis.

Transcatheter Interventions

Early pioneering procedures were performed over 30 years ago in the form of balloon dilatation of both native and bioprosthetic TVs.[164] Balloon valvotomy of the TV is nowadays limited to stenosed rheumatic valves with favorable anatomy, but is associated with a substantial risk of significant postprocedural TR. Recently, transcatheter valve implantation has become established in the management of aortic and pulmonary valve disease. The more complex 3D annular structure of the atrioventricular valves has meant that percutaneous valve implantation has primarily focused on valve-in-valve or valve-in-ring strategies, when there is a stable landing zone for the valve. The

TABLE 67–18. Primary Tricuspid Valve Regurgitation: 2017 ESC/EACTS for the Management of Valvular Heart Disease

COR	LOE	Diagnostic	Therapeutic
I			1. Surgery is indicated in patients with severe TR undergoing left-sided valve surgery.
IIa	C		1. Surgery is indicated in symptomatic patients with severe isolated TR without severe RV dysfunction. 2. Surgery should be considered in asymptomatic or mildly symptomatic patients with severe isolated TR and: RV dilatation, or; Deterioration of RV function.
IIb	C		1. Surgery should be considered in patients with moderate TR undergoing left sided-valve surgery.

*Unless otherwise stated, tricuspid valve surgery connotes tricuspid valve repair or replacement, decided on individual assessment.
Abbreviations: ACHD, adult congenital heart disease, COR, class of recommendation; LOE, level of evidence; RV: right ventricle; TR: tricuspid regurgitation.

main experience to date with transcatheter TVs has been in the treatment of patients with bioprosthetic degenerative TVs. Midterm results in 306 patients with both primary and secondary TR have been acceptable, considering the significant baseline functional limitation in this population (71% in NYHA functional class III or IV):[165] There was a procedural success rate of 99%, with a freedom from reoperation of 85% at 1 year, and freedom from death, TV reintervention, or other valve-related complications of 64% at 3 years. A range of transcatheter devices are being developed, from annuloplasty to coaptation enhancement, which may provide new management options for patients with advanced TV disease.[166]

Outcomes and Management of Complications Following Tricuspid Valve Surgery

The majority of patients undergoing TV surgery for congenital TV disease show sustained improvement in functional capacity and exercise tolerance. However, studies reporting long-term outcomes following TV surgery for primary TV disease are scarce and the few that exist are historical and often do not differentiate between the types of TV disease. In 1998, Rizzoli et al.[167] reported poorer outcomes in patients undergoing TV replacement for congenital TV disease compared to other causes, with a 5-year mortality of 78% in the congenital group.

Earlier intervention and the growing experience over the last two decades are likely to have improved outcomes.[167] Historically, patients were referred for TV surgery late in the disease course, once right-heart failure was established, often with signs of hepatic and renal dysfunction. Long-term outcomes are closely related to RV dysfunction, which has been identified as a marker of poor prognosis in several studies.[168,169] Therefore, surgical intervention should ideally be performed prior to the development of RV failure.

Few studies have compared TV repair to TVR, and results are likely to reflect case selection for repair versus replacement. The initial Cleveland Clinic experience showed a higher mortality following TVR compared to repair.[170] Outcomes with bioprosthetic versus contemporary mechanical valves appear to be similar.[168,171] With bioprostheses, the lower risk of thrombosis and need for lifelong anticoagulation is set against the significant rate of valve dysfunction requiring reoperation.

Late complications after surgery for TS or TR include:

- Prosthetic valve dysfunction
- Recurrent TR following repair. There is a paucity of evidence regarding the rate of late reoperation after valve repair for congenital TR
- RV dysfunction, which may be present preoperatively and is often exacerbated by bypass surgery (especially in patients operated during the early surgical era), causing exercise intolerance, right-sided heart failure and representing a major predictor of late mortality
- Atrial arrhythmias caused by RA dilatation and surgical scarring. Ventricular arrhythmias are uncommon, and usually relate to RV dysfunction or dysplasia
- Valve thrombosis

- Thromboembolism, resulting in pulmonary embolism or systemic embolization in the presence of an atrial communication
- Endocarditis.

Late reintervention is not uncommon in patients who have undergone TV surgery, reported in one series at 34% over 10 years:[167] Valve dysfunction requiring reoperation occurred at a rate of 2.2% per patient-year in the mechanical valve group, and 4.7% in the bioprosthetic valve group. Reoperation for valve thrombosis has been reported at 2.8% per patient-year in patients with St. Jude bileaflet valves, with a mean interval to reoperation of 9.5 years.[172]

Endocarditis is an ongoing risk for all patients with CHD. In the absence of preexisting TV disease, intravenous drug use is strongly associated with right-sided endocarditis. In CHD, pacing leads, previous surgery (eg, VSD repair in patients with a straddling TV) and indwelling catheters are responsible for TV disease.[173] Antibiotic prophylaxis is now limited to patients at the highest risk of infective endocarditis undergoing high-risk dental procedures. This includes patients with a past history of infective endocarditis, presence of cyanosis (eg, where TV disease is a feature of complex CHD), prosthetic TV replacement or transcatheter valve implantation, or TV repair using prosthetic material (eg, annuloplasty), up to 6 months after the procedure or lifelong in the presence of residual TR.[21] Antibiotics are not recommended prior to nondental procedures, and universal advice should be given for meticulous dental and skin hygiene.

Routine Follow-Up

Despite good long-term outcomes in adults with congenital TV disease who have undergone valve repair or replacement, late complications do occur and warrant life-long specialist follow-up at intervals appropriate for the physiological status of the patient.[6]

Pregnancy and Exercise

Pregnancy outcomes specific to women with primary TV disease are lacking, but the principles used for other types of CHD may be applied. Maternal and neonatal risk is increased in the presence of high-risk features, including functional limitation (NYHA functional class III/IV), left-heart disease, pulmonary hypertension, RV dysfunction, cyanosis, or mechanical valve prostheses. As in other valve disease, regurgitant lesions are usually better tolerated than stenotic ones. The maternal risk of arrhythmias and heart failure is increased in severe, symptomatic TR, significant TS, and in women with RV dysfunction.[174] In cases of severe, symptomatic TR or moderate-severe TS, valve intervention should be considered prior to pregnancy. When surgery for left-sided lesions is required prior to pregnancy, additional tricuspid valve repair is indicated in severe TR, and should be considered in moderate TR with an annulus size ≥40 mm. Fetal echocardiography should be offered as standard practice.

Individualized exercise prescription is based on assessment of 5 specific risk modifiers: ventricular function, pulmonary artery pressure, aortic size, presence and severity of arrhythmia, and assessment of oxygen saturation at rest and during exercise. In general, asymptomatic patients with TR without RV dilatation or dysfunction, pulmonary hypertension or complex arrhythmias may partake in high-intensity exercise, including competitive and recreational sports.[175]

DOUBLE-OUTLET RIGHT VENTRICLE

Background

DORV is used to describe a broad family of complex congenital heart lesions where the aorta and pulmonary trunk arise completely or predominantly from the morphologic RV, almost always in association with an interventricular connection. Initial descriptions of autopsy specimens date back to the 18th century,[176,177] and until the introduction of the "double-outlet" right ventricle label in the 1950s, instances of DORV were classified as partial variants of TGA.[178,179]

The clinical presentation and surgical management are wide-ranging, depending on the anatomic subtype and associated lesions (eg, coarctation of aorta). In contemporary practice, biventricular repair is achievable in most cases with adequately sized ventricles, improving the long-term prognosis of this condition, although complications and the need for reintervention are not uncommon, and lifelong specialist follow-up is recommended.

DORV is associated with genetic syndromes in up to 50% of cases, including trisomy 13, trisomy 18, CHARGE, and 22q11 microdeletion. Sporadic cases have been associated with mutations of the *CFC1* and *CSX* genes, and environmental factors such as maternal diabetes and exposure to alcohol, theophylline, retinoids, and valproate.[180]

Embryology and Epidemiology

As with other conotruncal heart defects, the cause of the DORV may be of neural crest origin.[181] The neural crest is involved in the development of the cardiac septum. Deletions of lesser parts of the cardiac neural crest result in deformities such as DORV, VSD, and ToF. Most changes in heart morphology occur while the heart is still in the looped tube stage. In addition to formation of cardiac structures, this area of neural crest cells participates in formation of the thymus, thyroid, and parathyroid glands, serving as the basis for association of congenital heart defects with DiGeorge Syndrome.[177] DORV accounts for 1% to 1.5% of all CHD with an incidence of 1 per 10,000 live births. Most cases of DORV are diagnosed in the first month of life. The long-term (≥10-year) survival of children who undergo repair for DORV is ~80% to 95%.

Anatomical Features and Pathophysiology of DORV

Anatomy

The morphologic definition of DORV has long been debated, with some investigators setting a requirement for the presence of bilateral infundibular muscle (or conus) encompassing the circumference of both arterial valves.[182] This would exclude,

amongst others, all variants of ToF from a DORV label. In contrast, the most widely accepted, contemporary definition refers to a single feature of anatomy, namely a specific type of ventriculoarterial connection in which both great vessels arise either entirely (so-called "200%") or predominantly from the RV. This definition recognizes the fact that DORV is not a discrete phenotypic entity but includes various phenotypes that share this single trait. The term allows for wide variability in morphology, including different types of atrioventricular connection, relation between the great arteries, and the presence or absence of inflow or outflow tract obstruction. DORV describes a number of phenotypes that border and sometimes overlap with other related forms of CHD, and nomenclature can become controversial. These may include:

1. DORV with a subaortic VSD and pulmonary or subpulmonary/infundibular stenosis (ToF-type) are considered a subtype of DORV providing that >50% of the aorta arises from the RV, otherwise they fall within the spectrum of ToF (see section Tetralogy of Fallot).

2. DORV and a subpulmonary VSD, where there is malposition of the great arteries, is considered a subtype of DORV (**Fig. 67–41A**), unless >50% of the pulmonary artery arises from the LV, when they are considered a subtype of TGA with VSD (**Fig. 6–41B**).

3. DORV associated with univentricular atrioventricular connections, atrioventricular valve atresia, or atrial isomerism are usually included in the functionally univentricular hearts and include:

   • single ventricle with double inlet LV and DORV
   • single ventricle with double inlet RV and DORV
   • single ventricle with mitral atresia and DORV
   • single ventricle with heterotaxy syndrome and DORV

Classification systems of DORV prioritize the anatomic features, which will determine the optimal strategy for surgical repair, namely:

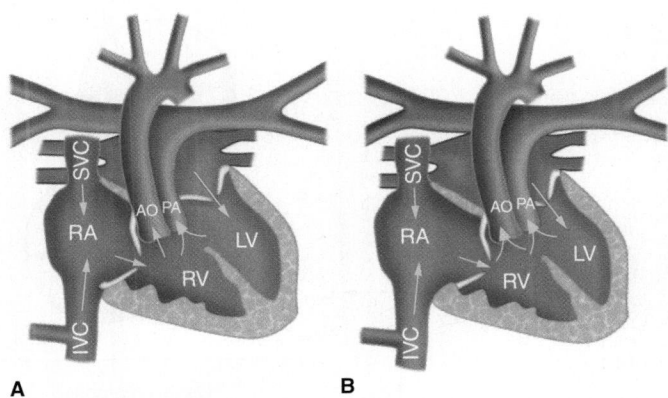

A   **B**

Figure 67–41. The Taussig–Bing anomaly versus TGA. In the Taussig–Bing anomaly (**A**), the great vessels are transposed and >50% of the PA arises from the RV; a subpulmonary VSD coexists with side-by-side great vessels in the absence of pulmonary stenosis. When the PA arises >50% from the LV, this condition is classified as TGA (**B**). AO, aorta; IVC, inferior vena cava.

1. The location and type of interventricular communication, which can be subaortic, subpulmonary, doubly committed, or noncommitted.

2. Presence or absence of valvar or infundibular PS, or varying degrees of hypoplasia of the pulmonary trunk (pulmonary atresia is considered a separate lesion).

3. Relation of the great arteries to each other, which may have a normal arrangement (in a minority of cases) or can be abnormally related in a number of different ways (**Fig. 67–42**). In the normal arrangement, or in mirror-image of normal as is seen in situs inversus, the great arteries take on a spiral arrangement. In other cases, they have a parallel arrangement, with variable degrees of anteroposterior variation of the aorta around the pulmonary artery, from

side-to-side to anterior. The uncommon circumstance where the aorta is leftward and anterior to the pulmonary artery is termed L-malposition; this arrangement resembles cc-TGA, but usually has concordant atrioventricular connections and a subaortic interventricular communication, which simplifies surgical repair.

On the basis of these features, the following subtypes are distinguished in the widely used classification proposed in the Society of Thoracic Surgeons-European Association for Cardio-Thoracic Surgery (STS-EACTS) Congenital Heart Surgery Nomenclature and Database Project (**Fig. 67–43**):[183]

1. VSD type, consisting of a subaortic or doubly committed VSD *without* pulmonary or subpulmonary stenosis (25% of cases)

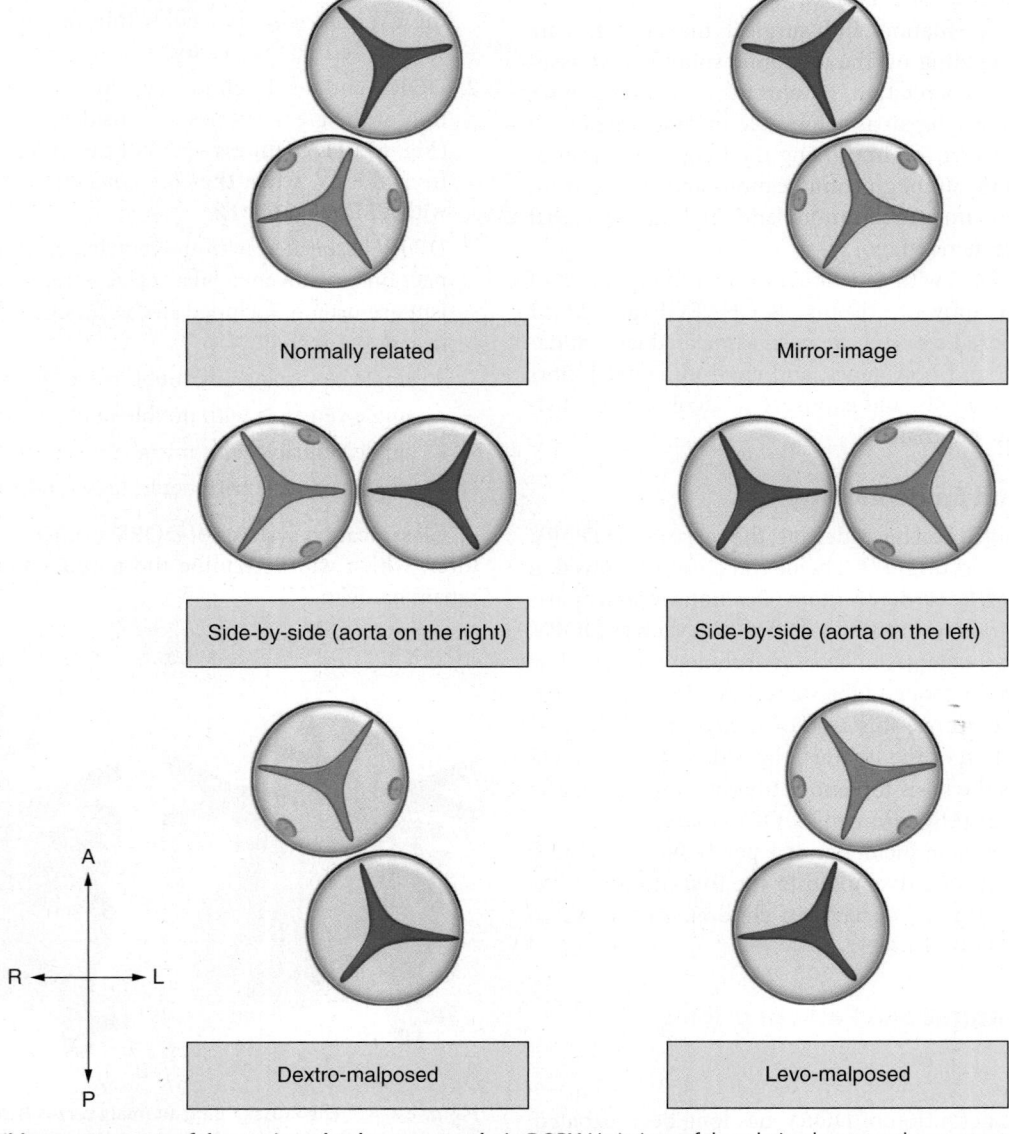

Figure 67–42. Possible arrangements of the aortic and pulmonary trunks in DORV. Variations of the relation between the great arteries arising from the ventricular outflow in DORV, from the perspective of transaxial imaging. The great arteries are normally related in a small minority of cases. Other possible arrangements include mirror-image of normal as is seen in situs inversus, side-by-side great arteries with the aorta to the left or to the right of the pulmonary artery, and dextro- or levo-malposed great arteries, reflecting the arrangement seen in d-TGA and cc-TGA.

2. ToF type, consisting of a subaortic or doubly committed VSD *with* PS (35%, see section Tetralogy of Fallot).

3. TGA type with a subpulmonary VSD. The vast majority of TGA type DORV occur without PS (20%). The term *Taussig–Bing* anomaly or heart is applied in the instance of a subpulmonary VSD, subaortic and subpulmonary coni with absence of the pulmonary-mitral continuity, and side-by-side great arteries (Fig. 67–41A).[184]

4. Remote type, involving a noncommitted VSD (ie, where the interventricular communication is remote from both semilunar valves), with or without PS (20%). To meet the criteria for DORV with noncommitted VSD, some have suggested that the distance between the VSD and the aortic and pulmonary outflow tracts should be at least equal to the aortic valve diameter.

5. DORV with intact interventricular septum is rarely encountered, and most likely represent spontaneous closure of a preexisting defect.

Earlier classifications proposed by Neufeld et al. in 1962[185] and Lev et al.[186] are also based on the VSD position, relation of the great arteries, and presence or absence of PS. Additional important modifiers, which may affect the disease course and surgical strategy, need to be taken into account.[187,188] These include the size and number of VSDs, and the relationship of the VSD margin to the membranous septum (ie, perimembranous VSD, muscular VSD, or atrioventricular septal defect [AVSD]). In the case of a perimembranous VSD, the His bundle runs along the defect's posteroinferior margin whereas it is more distant to the margin of a nonperimembranous VSD. It is key to identify the orientation of the outlet septum relative to the VSD margin. The outlet septum is most frequently perpendicular to the plane of the VSD and fused to either its left (committed to the right-sided arterial trunk, usually the aorta) or right margin (committed to the left-sided arterial trunk, most commonly the pulmonary artery). Less commonly, the outlet septum runs parallel to the plane of the VSD without

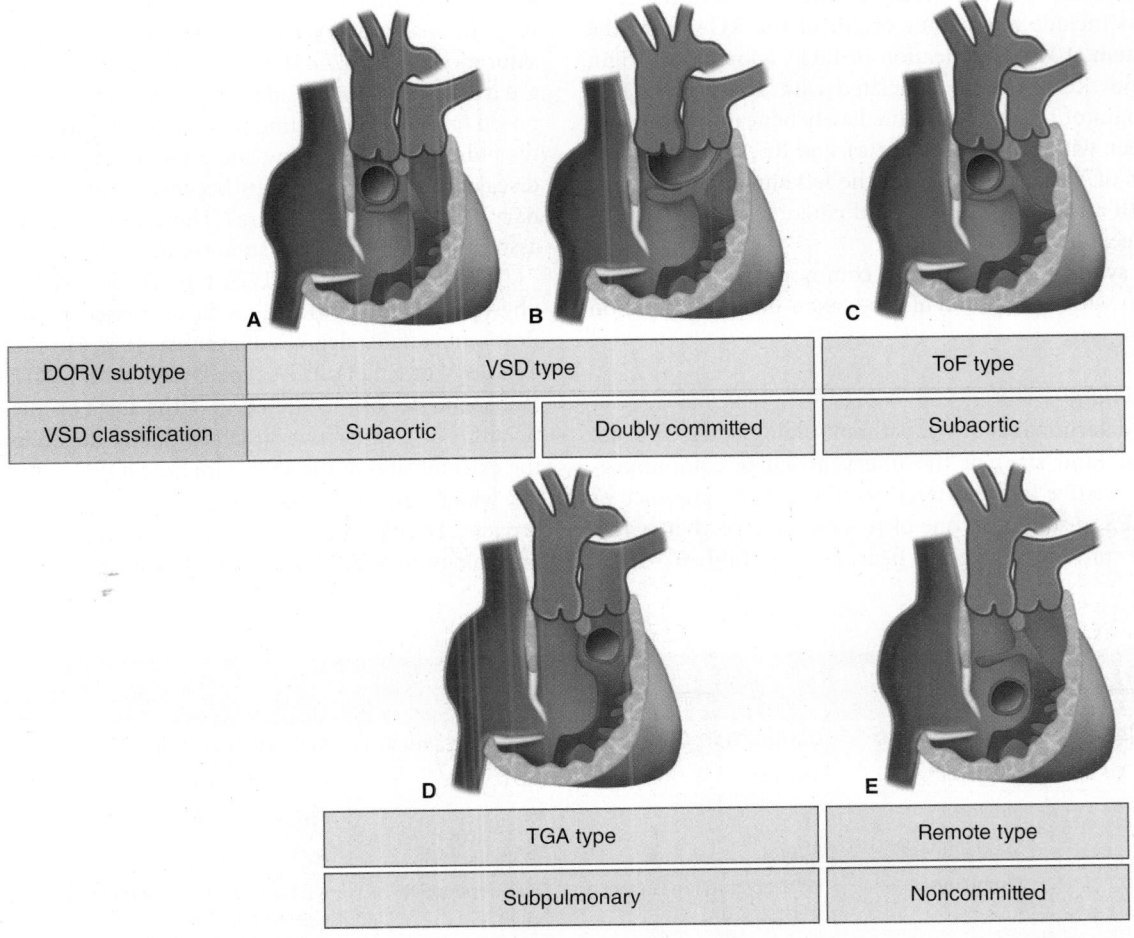

DORV subtype	VSD type		ToF type
VSD classification	Subaortic	Doubly committed	Subaortic

TGA type	Remote type
Subpulmonary	Noncommitted

Figure 67–43. Anatomical Classification of DORV. The clinical classification proposed by the STS-EACTS Congenital Heart Surgery Nomenclature and Database Project.[7] In the upper-left panels, VSD type DORV is shown with either a subaortic (**A**) or doubly committed (**B**) VSD. In (**C**), ToF type DORV is displayed, identified by a subaortic VSD coexisting with infundibular and/or valvar pulmonary stenosis. In the presence of a subaortic VSD, blood flow from the LV is preferentially streamed toward the aorta. In (**D**), TGA type DORV is shown with a subpulmonary VSD; in this arrangement, blood shunting left–right through the VSD preferentially enters the pulmonary arteries, mimicking the physiology of TGA. (**E**) displays the anatomy of remote type DORV. Unlike in the other DORV types, the noncommitted VSD of remote type DORV may not positioned between the limbs of the septomarginal trabeculation.

attachment to the left or right VSD margin. The extent of the septal leaflet of the tricuspid valve in proximity to the VSD margin and the extent of the muscular infundibulum, which determines the distance between the VSD and the semilunar valves, needs to be identified. The distance or remoteness of the VSD from the arterial or semi-lunar valves, the LV and RV volumes, and the coronary anatomy needs to be described for biventricular repair to be undertaken.

Associated congenital heart defects are common in patients with DORV. There may be obstructive lesions that vary according to VSD type. PS and subpulmonary stenosis are more common in patients with a subaortic VSD (66%) than those with a subpulmonary (16%) or noncommitted VSD (32%). Subaortic stenosis is most commonly encountered among those with a doubly committed VSD (14%) and is rare in those with a subaortic VSD. Aortic arch obstruction has been described and occurs most commonly in those with subpulmonary VSD (30%), followed by those with a noncommitted VSD (10%) and doubly committed VSD (9%). Rarely, AVSD has also been described, which is commonly unbalanced and should raise suspicion of heterotaxy. Coronary artery anomalies are common (50%). These vary depending on the relation of the great arteries and include anomalous origin of the RCA from the left main stem (LMS), duplication of LAD, anomalous origin of LAD from RCA usually associated with ToF-type DORV, anterior origin of LAD, RCA immediately beneath pulmonary annulus (seen with L-malposed aorta), and RCA from the posterior sinus of Valsalva/LMS from the left sinus in TGA-type DORV. Both atrial septal defects and patent ductus arteriosus have also been described.

Genetic syndromes that are less commonly associated with DORV than with ToF should also be taken into consideration in DORV.

Pathophysiology
The major determinants of the pathophysiology of DORV are the position (and size) of the interventricular communication (VSD) relative to the arterial trunks and the presence or absence of PS, resulting in one of several patterns that mimic other, more common congenital heart defects (**Table 67–19**).

Patients with VSD type DORV typically present with signs of excessive pulmonary blood flow, resembling the pathophysiology of a large, isolated VSD. The aortic orifice is usually posterior and to the right of the pulmonary orifice, with a spiral arterial relationship. Because the great arteries are normally related, the LV outflow is directed toward the aorta, resulting in aortic oxygen saturations that exceed pulmonary saturations (Figs. 67–43A and 67–43B). The systolic pressures are invariably equal in both ventricles and in the aorta. The ratio of pulmonary-to-systemic blood flow is determined by the pulmonary vascular resistance in the absence of PS. Systemic and pulmonary saturations are also affected by the degree of mixing in the RV. This anatomy may result in congestive heart failure and pulmonary vascular disease. DORV with noncommitted or remote VSD also has a pathophysiology similar to that of an isolated VSD or AVSD (Fig. 67–43E).

In patients with Taussig–Bing anomaly, the pathophysiology is comparable to that seen in TGA with associated VSD, usually with systemic desaturation and pulmonary overcirculation. The LV outflow is directed toward the pulmonary artery leading to preferential streaming of desaturated blood to the aorta and saturated blood to the pulmonary arteries, resulting in pulmonary artery oxygen saturations greater than aortic saturations (Fig. 67–43D). The aortic and pulmonary orifices are usually positioned side-by-side but are described as transposed or malposed. Pulmonary vascular resistance determines the pulmonary blood flow, and early-onset pulmonary vascular disease commonly develops because of the increased pulmonary blood flow and pressures. This type of DORV is frequently associated with subaortic stenosis and arch obstruction.

ToF type DORV and TGA type DORV with PS result in a physiology similar to ToF, with decreased pulmonary blood flow and variable degrees of cyanosis (Fig. 67–43C, see section Tetralogy of Fallot). TGA type DORV with LVOT obstruction (subaortic stenosis, coarctation of the aorta or interrupted aortic arch) or a restrictive VSD is a ductal-dependent lesion. At the extreme end of the spectrum are DORV with LV hypoplasia, which display a single ventricle-type physiology. Like the broader DORV cohort, this group is heterogenous and its physiology may be further complicated by the presence of an

TABLE 67–19. Relation of VSD Location, Presence of Outflow Tract Obstruction, Clinical Presentation, and Preferred Surgical Approach

DORV Classification	Location of VSD	Outflow Tract Obstruction	Physiology (mimic)	Surgical Approach
VSD type	Subaortic	Absent	VSD	Patch baffle or tunnel repair
ToF type	Subaortic	PS	ToF	ToF-type repair
TGA type	Subpulmonary	Absent	TGA	ASO
	Subpulmonary	LVOT obstruction (subaortic stenosis, CoA)	Duct-dependent lesion	ASO with VSD enlargement/infundibular resection/CoA repair
Remote type	Noncommitted	Absent	VSD	Univentricular (Fontan-type) repair. Biventricular repair possible in selected cases
	Noncommitted	PS	ToF	

Abbreviations: ASO, arterial switch operation; CoA, coarctation of the aorta; LVOTO, left ventricular outflow tract obstruction; POT, pulmonary outflow tract obstruction; TGA, transposition of the great arteries; ToF, Tetralogy of Fallot; VSD, ventricular septal defect.

imbalanced AVSD, atrioventricular valve tissue straddling the interventricular connection, criss-cross atrioventricular connections, heterotaxy syndromes, superior-inferior ventricular arrangement, or anomalous pulmonary venous drainage.

Clinical Presentation

This section focuses on the adult patient with DORV, and the remainder of this section will focus on the management of the adult patient with repaired and unrepaired DORV. Briefly, the clinical presentation in patients with DORV prior to surgical repair, which varies based on the location of the VSD and degree of outflow tract obstruction, is summarized below (Table 67–19).

Subaortic or Subpulmonary VSD with PS

Clinical presentation is similar to ToF. If pulmonary oligemia is present, severe cyanosis is seen in the newborn period, and the condition is recognized early. Beyond the newborn period, cyanosis may be accompanied by hypercyanotic spells, polycythemia, and failure to thrive. These children are less likely to develop pulmonary vascular disease due to limitation of blood flow in the setting of PS.

Subaortic VSD without PS

Clinical presentation is similar to patients with a large VSD and pulmonary hypertension. Oxygenation is relatively normal, and patients usually present with congestive heart failure and failure to thrive. These children may have associated chromosomal abnormalities such as trisomy 13 or 18. These children are likely to acquire pulmonary vascular disease without surgical repair, especially if the VSD is large.

Subpulmonary VSD without PS

Clinical presentation is similar to TGA. Cyanosis varies, with oxygen saturations ranging from 40% to 80%. If associated coarctation or interruption of the aorta is present, earlier onset of congestive heart failure can be expected.

Work-Up/Investigations

Most patients with DORV present in early infancy, although there are rare cases of patients with "balanced" circulations presenting in adulthood (see section Management of Adults with Unrepaired DORV)[189] The diagnosis of DORV is a sufficient indication for surgery, unless presenting late with severe pulmonary vascular disease and Eisenmenger physiology.

Electrocardiography

Abnormalities are often present on ECG but are not pathognomic for DORV. In an infant with unrepaired DORV, ECG reveals RV hypertrophy. LV hypertrophy may develop in the presence of a restrictive VSD that leads to LV pressure overload or an increased pulmonary venous return that leads to LV volume overload. Right atrial enlargement is common. Left atrial enlargement may be present if pulmonary venous return or mitral stenosis/atresia is increased. Usually, left axis deviation of the frontal plane QRS is present because of displacement of the bundle of His posterior to VSD.

Chest Radiography

Prior to surgical repair, chest radiography findings usually correlate with clinical presentation, but do not differentiate DORV from other forms of CHD. The presence or absence of PS and pulmonary vascular resistance determines if cardiomegaly and increased pulmonary vascularity are present. Patients with subaortic VSD and severe PS demonstrate diminished pulmonary vascularity and concave left heart border (similar to appearance associated with ToF). If pulmonary vascular disease is present, peripheral pulmonary vascularity may be reduced and proximal pulmonary arteries may be dilated. The appearance of a chest radiograph in patients with subpulmonary VSD is similar to that in patients with TGA, revealing increased pulmonary vascularity and cardiomegaly. In patients in whom the aorta is anterior and to the left, radiography may reveal the leftward position of the aorta.

Echocardiography, CT Angiography, and CMR

Echocardiography is the primary investigation used to diagnose DORV and describe the surgical anatomy and associated features.[190] The spatial relation between the arterial trunks is easily identified in the parasternal long-axis view, but diagnosing DORV requires the integration of information from multiple planes (**Fig. 67–44**). In the presence of complex anatomy, further imaging by TEE, CMR imaging, or dual-source CT

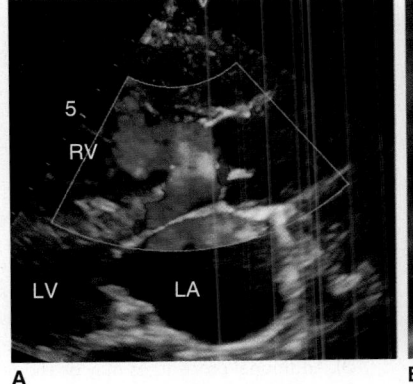 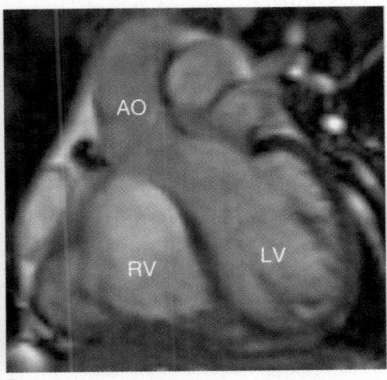

Figure 67–44. DORV with subaortic VSD. In (**A**), parasternal long-axis view showing a subaortic VSD with >50% of the aorta arising from the RV. In (**B**), CMR image of the same patient, showing the aorta arising >50% from the RV. AO, aorta.

provides important complementary information on RV and LV volumes and function, the outflow tracts and aortic arch, morphology of the pulmonary arteries, and the 3D relation of the chambers and the great vessels. Contrast-enhanced CMR imaging or CT angiography also allows for 3D rendering and printing of physical models for anatomic assessment, individualized surgical planning, and education.[187]

Cardiac Catheterization

Cardiac catheterization with angiography is no longer routinely used with modern cross-sectional imaging techniques, but is still required in late presentations to assess for pulmonary vascular disease and, in select cases where CT or CMR imaging are not feasible, to evaluate coronary and aortic arch anatomy, identify a restrictive interventricular communication, and plan the intraventricular baffle by left ventriculography.

Management

Per the ACC/AHA Guidelines for ACHD from 2018, recommendations for the management of the adult patient with DORV can generally be inferred in the recommendations for the lesion with the most similar anatomy and physiology (eg, follow recommendations for patients with lesions similar to repaired ToF or repaired TGA S/P Rastelli procedure or an ASO), recognizing that a patient with DORV is more likely to have residual LVOT obstruction.[6,7] This section highlights the surgical approaches, palliative and complete repair, and long-term management for adult patients with DORV.

Palliative Surgery

In previous decades, palliative procedures were commonly performed in DORV to control (augment or limit) pulmonary blood flow. Advances in neonatal surgery have meant that early direct repair is achievable and is the preferred surgical strategy in most cases, hence palliative procedures in the form of aortopulmonary shunts or PA banding are rarely performed nowadays. Balloon atrial septostomy is still commonly performed for TGA type DORV with restrictive systemic flow. Procedures to regulate pulmonary blood flow are also still used in circumstances where surgery is not feasible in early infancy, such as in the presence of hypoplastic pulmonary arteries. An understanding of palliative procedures is still required when assessing adults with repaired DORV, many of whom have undergone one of the following:

- Modified BT shunt to augment pulmonary blood flow (see Palliative Surgery in section Tetralogy of Fallot).
- Pulmonary artery banding, used to limit excessive pulmonary blood flow in DORV variants without PS, severe subaortic obstruction, restrictive VSD, or aortic arch obstruction.

The main limitation of PA banding is the difficulty in assessing the optimal tightness of the band, with minimal changes in diameter having large effects on pulmonary blood flow. Band adjustment, either tightening or loosening, is frequently required and usually entails an additional invasive procedure, unless an adjustable band is used. Band migration

is not uncommon and can cause suprapulmonary stenosis or band loosening with consequent pulmonary vascular disease. Band erosion is a rare but disastrous complication. Debanding is usually performed at the time of definitive repair, and may require reconstruction of the PA, or may be initially performed percutaneously ("catheter debanding").[191]

Complete Surgical Repair

The main objectives of surgical correction of DORV are to establish continuity of the LV to the aorta and of the RV to the PA. The surgical approach is tailored to the location of the VSD, the location of the coronary arteries, and the size of the LV. Surgical repair usually requires cardiopulmonary bypass with moderate hypothermia and circulatory arrest.

Intraventricular Repair of VSD Type DORV: Repair in patients with this type of DORV is generally achieved (as with the first case of DORV repair performed by Kirklin in 1957) by placing a synthetic baffle around the VSD, connecting the LV outflow to the aorta (**Fig. 67–45**).[192] Adaptation of this technique is needed if there is an inadequate subaortic space, in which case a tunnel-shaped baffle is constructed from a partial tube graft, or when there is a restrictive VSD requiring enlargement at the time of repair.

Intraventricular Repair of ToF Type DORV: DORV associated with subpulmonary stenosis requires a ToF-type repair, usually by preforming an infundibulotomy and establishing RV to pulmonary artery continuity; in DORV, this requires the use of a tunnel rather than a patch to ensure sufficient subaortic space. An RV-PA conduit may be necessary in cases of anomalous coronary arteries crossing the pulmonary outflow tract, or when there is severe hypoplasia of the PA (see section Tetralogy of Fallot).

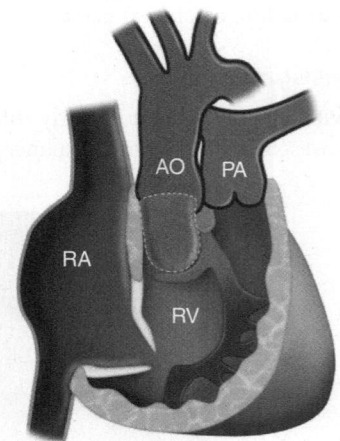

Figure 67–45. Intraventricular tunnel repair of DORV with subaortic VSD. Intraventricular tunnel repair uses a synthetic (usually GORE-TEX) baffle of variable length fashioned on an individual patient basis from a partial tube graft, which redirects blood from the LV, through the VSD to the aorta (AO). Additional procedures may be required during intraventricular repair, such as enlargement of a restrictive VSD, resection of the conal septum, aortic arch/coarctation repair, or ligation of previous palliative shunt(s). PA, pulmonary artery; RA, right atrium; RV, right ventricle.

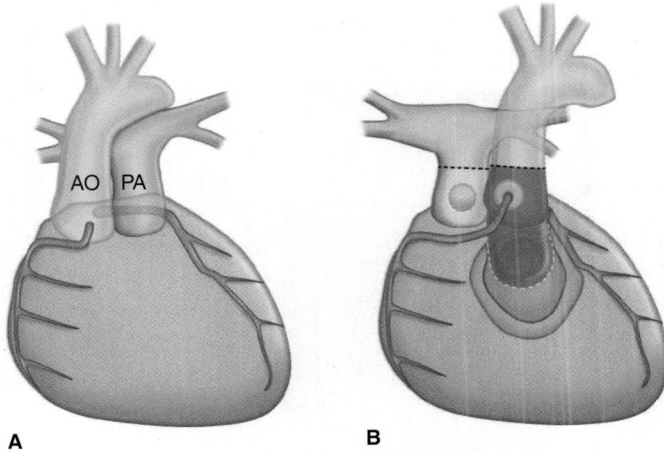

Figure 67–46. Surgical repair of TGA-type DORV. The arterial switch operation with intraventricular tunnel repair of the VSD in TGA-type DORV without subpulmonary or pulmonary stenosis (PS) or coarctation of the aorta. **(A)** Preoperative anatomy. **(B)** Intraventricular tunnel repair of the VSD is performed transatrially or transventricularly. The distal arterial trunks are then transected: the neoaortic root (*right*, below suture line) is sutured to the distal transected ascending aorta (AO), and the neopulmonary root (*yellow*, below suture line) is sewn to the distal main pulmonary artery (PA). Coronary artery transfer to the neoaorta is achieved by dissecting left main and right coronary artery buttons with careful mobilization of the proximal coronary arteries and local wall resection, followed by anastomosis to the appropriate position on the proximal neoaorta (button in *yellow*). Great care is taken to achieve alignment of the proximal and distal neoaortic anastomosis to avoid coronary artery kinking and neoaortic regurgitation. Neopulmonary artery reconstructed is completed using a pericardial patch to fill the defect left by the dissected sinuses of Valsalva (in *gray*).

Repair of TGA Type DORV: Surgical repair of the Taussig–Bing anomaly nowadays involves construction of an LV-to-subpulmonary outflow tract tunnel, with a subsequent arterial switch operation (**Fig. 67–46**). This is technically simpler when the aorta is malposed anteriorly. This is preferred to the alternative operation of a longer intraventricular tunnel rerouting blood through the VSD to the aorta (Kawashima repair).[193]

Without modification, these procedures cannot be applied when there is a significant degree of PS; such cases of TGA-type DORV with PS have imported techniques initially developed for different but related forms of CHD. The Rastelli procedure was first used in TGA, VSD, and PS and has remained in use for over 50 years.[194] It is designed to reestablish the morphologic LV as the systemic ventricle, achieved through the construction of an intraventricular tunnel to establish continuity between the LV and the aorta. An extracardiac (usually) valved conduit connects the RV to the main PA. In-hospital mortality is low and has improved over time, but the need for reintervention is the rule following a Rastelli procedure, and late postrepair survival is lower following Rastelli than other forms of repair for DORV.[195] For coexisting subaortic stenosis, this can be combined with a Damus–Kaye–Stansel procedure (**Fig. 67–47A**), bypassing the obstruction by connecting the proximal pulmonary artery trunk to the ascending aorta and placing the extracardiac conduit between the RV and distal PA (Damus–Rastelli).

Newer alternatives to the Rastelli procedure may be necessary in patients with challenging anatomy, including cases of small or remote interventricular connection, multiple interventricular connections, a small RV, or straddling atrioventricular valve. They offer advantages such as "straighter" LV-to-aorta connections, for example, infundibular resection with an arterial switch operation (as in the REV [réparation à l'étage ventriculaire] procedure) posterior aortic translocation (Nikaidoh–Bex operation), and "en bloc rotation" techniques.[196]

Repair of Remote Type DORV: Biventricular repair, when feasible, usually involves the creation of a longer baffle from the LV to the aorta, or less commonly rerouting blood flow through the interventricular communication to the pulmonary artery, followed by arterial switch operation.[197] Superoanterior enlargement of the interventricular connection is almost invariably necessary, and the ability to perform a biventricular repair may be limited by tricuspid valve chordal attachments to this aspect of the interventricular connection. Use of multiple patches for biventricular repair of DORV with noncommitted VSD, to construct an intraventricular tunnel connecting the LV to the aorta (the double-patch technique), can allow biventricular repair of lesions where single-patch repair would have been impossible and reduces the risk of subaortic stenosis.[198]

Cavopulmonary Connections and Univentricular Repair: Certain anatomies present a surgical challenge for biventricular repair: straddling or abnormal distribution of chordae tendineae of atrioventricular valves and/or severe underdevelopment of LV, complete atrioventricular septal defect, or heterotaxy. These anatomic features, which may be additive, increase the complexity of repair and traditionally favor diversion to a univentricular approach, usually via a Fontan-type operation with redirection of systemic venous blood into the pulmonary artery without traversing a ventricle. In cases with significant overriding of the right atrioventricular valve, biventricular repair may create an RV inlet that is too small to handle the entire systemic venous return. A 1.5 ventricle repair, where the superior caval flow is redirected to the pulmonary arteries via a bidirectional cavopulmonary (Glenn) shunt, is sometimes used (**Fig. 67–47B**).

High-Risk Biventricular versus Univentricular Repair for Complex Anatomy: Patients with remote type DORV and additional anatomical characteristics that increase the complexity of biventricular repair require careful surgical planning. Decision-making includes whether to pursue a univentricular or a complex biventricular repair, either as a primary or staged procedure.[199] The high rate of subaortic stenosis, reintervention, and long-term ventricular dysfunction after complex baffles has to be set against the late consequences of a Fontan circulation. When primary biventricular repair is not easily achievable, a staged approach or a straightforward univentricular repair may allow better preservation of ventricular function with a lower risk of reoperation, at least in the medium term.

Timing of Repair: Adverse consequences of "late repair" of DORV are not as well established as in ToF, although the

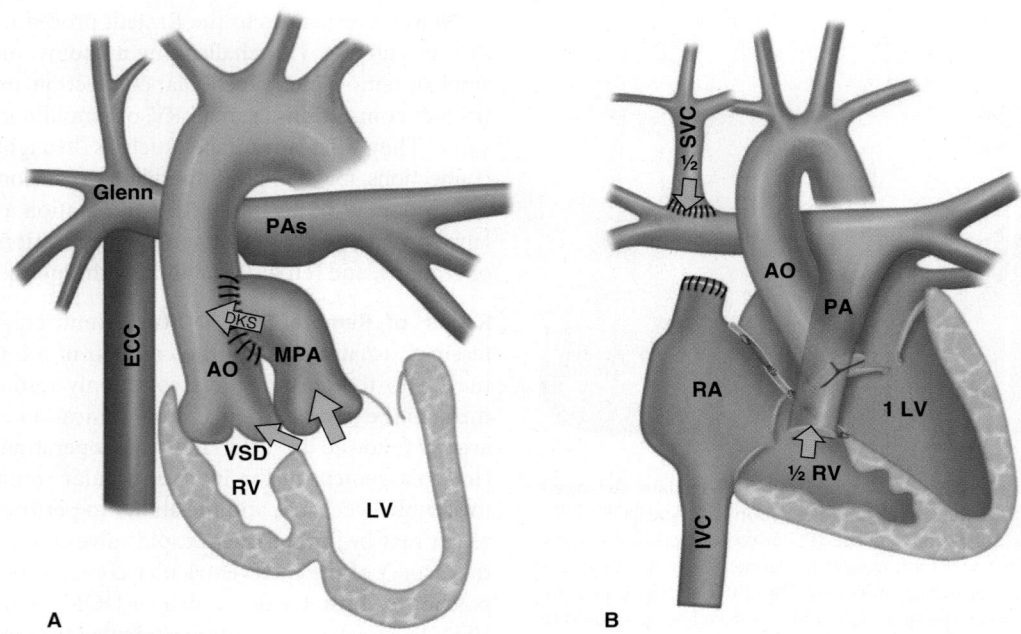

A   **B**

Figure 67–47. **Damus–Kaye–Stansel procedure and the 1.5 ventricle repair. (A)** The Damus–Kaye–Stansel (DKS) procedure is illustrated as part of a Fontan-type repair. An end-to-side DKS anastomosis is formed between the main pulmonary artery (MPA) and ascending aorta (AO) to augment the systemic outflow in this patient with TGA with a restrictive VSD, creating functional subaortic stenosis, and hypoplastic right ventricle (RV). This has been followed by a staged total cavopulmonary anastomosis with a bidirectional Glenn shunt (superior vena cava to right pulmonary artery end-to-side anastomosis in the setting of confluent pulmonary arteries [PAs]) and extracardiac conduit (ECC) redirecting blood from the inferior vena cava to the PAs. **(B)** The concept of a 1.5 ventricle repair is shown. Biventricular repair has restored ventriculoarterial concordance, with the adequately sized LV supporting the entire systemic circulation (1 LV). In this patient, the RV is too small to handle the entire systemic venous return. Therefore, a bidirectional Glenn shunt is fashioned so that around half of the superior vena caval flow (1/2 SVC) is rerouted to the pulmonary artery, leaving the RV to receive systemic venous blood from the inferior vena cava (IVC), hence supporting around half of the venous return to the heart (1/2 RV).

management of DORV is invariably surgical and late repair risks the development of pulmonary vascular disease, which was identified as the only preoperative risk factor associated with early mortality in one large series of cases.[200] Early, single-stage biventricular repair is now feasible in most cases; however, a staged approach with initial palliative procedure is mainly reserved for patients with ToF type DORV (aortopulmonary shunt) or remote type DORV (pulmonary artery banding). The DORV subtype affects surgical timing: TGA type DORV usually requires complete repair in the neonatal period, whereas in asymptomatic neonates with ToF type or VSD type DORV, a one-stage biventricular repair within the first few months of life is preferred.[201]

Long-Term Outcomes

Cardiac surgery has greatly improved outcomes in DORV and has transformed this from a cyanotic condition with a high mortality in infancy and early childhood, to one where survival to adulthood is expected and the majority of patients under follow-up have no or little exercise limitation. Surgical outcomes are, however, still not optimal and depend greatly on the underlying anatomy. The overall perioperative surgical mortality is 4% to 7.5%, while survival at 10 years is estimated at around 86%.[201–203] The reoperation rate is significant, with reintervention required in around 40% of patients at 10 years in the overall DORV group, and more frequently after Rastelli operation

or complex intracardiac repair. Reintervention is least common in patients with ToF type DORV who have undergone simple patch VSD closure.[195]

Long-term sequelae after DORV repair are common, requiring frequent follow-up by an ACHD specialist, ideally in a comprehensive center given the frequency of reintervention. The specific complications depend, at least in part, on the type of operation performed and include:

- LVOT obstruction/subaortic stenosis
- Subpulmonary stenosis
- Baffle stenosis or degeneration
- Extra-cardiac (RV-PA) conduit degeneration and dysfunction
- VSD patch leaks or dehiscence
- Recurrence of coarctation of the aorta (recoarctation)
- Conduction abnormalities, which are more common in the early postoperative period, but may also occur late postoperatively
- Tachyarrhythmias, both supraventricular and ventricular, and the associated risk for SCD
- Neoaortic root dilatation and aortic regurgitation in patients who have undergone an arterial switch procedure as part of their repair
- Infective endocarditis

Ventricular Outflow Tract Obstruction: LVOT obstruction can occur early or late after initial DORV repair and is a major cause of reoperation depending on the underlying anatomy and type of surgery undertaken. The risk of subaortic stenosis is higher among patients who have undergone intraventricular tunnel repair, especially Rastelli repair for TGA type DORV (due to stenosis of the LV-to-aorta internal baffle), with death or reintervention at 15 years reported as high as 79%.[204]

Early subaortic stenosis can occur due to inadequate enlargement of a restrictive VSD or poor baffle configuration with a tortuous course or insufficient subaortic space. Following the Rastelli procedure, functional subaortic stenosis may result from LV-to-aorta internal baffle stenosis. Intraoperative TEE is often necessary to diagnose residual subaortic stenosis and guide surgical management, including muscular resection, further VSD enlargement, or refashioning of the pathway when obstructed or narrowed. Subaortic stenosis may also develop over time and require reoperation several years following initial repair. At reoperation for late subaortic stenosis, obstruction is often due to protrusion of the inferior rim of the VSD into the LVOT associated with a prominent subaortic muscle or membrane, and can be treated by fibromuscular resection or extended septoplasty.[205] RVOTO is managed as for ToF (see section Tetralogy of Fallot).

Conduit Dysfunction: Extracardiac, RV-PA conduits, such as those used in the Rastelli operation and its modifications for DORV with subpulmonary and pulmonary stenosis, are usually implanted in young children (<5 years) but cannot grow with the patient. Most conduits used for this purpose are valved, although nonvalved synthetic tube grafts have also been used. Early conduit dysfunction occurs in a minority of patients due to kinking or aneurysmal dilatation. Late conduit stenosis is more common and is caused by calcification and degeneration, leading to stenosis within conduit or valve stenosis,

regurgitation, or both. This causes pressure and/or volume overload of the RV, with eventual ventricular dysfunction and progressive exercise intolerance if left untreated (**Fig. 67–48**, see also section Tetralogy of Fallot). Acute conduit dysfunction can also result from infective endocarditis.

Reintervention, including conduit revision, is frequent following the Rastelli operation, estimated between 37% and 79% at 15 years, and patients may have undergone multiple conduit revisions as they enter young adulthood.[204,206,207] In children, smaller conduits and non-Dacron grafts have been associated with earlier reoperation, although data from adult cohorts are lacking. Options include surgical conduit revision or transcatheter procedures, including percutaneous pulmonary valve implantation.[6,208,209]

VSD Patch Leak or Dehiscence: Early case series on the outcome of biventricular repair of DORV identified patch leak or dehiscence as one of the main indications for reintervention, affecting more than 25% of patients in some reports.[210] More recent reports on long-term postoperative outcomes have not identified many cases of patch dehiscence, possibly thanks to greater surgical experience and modification of the surgical techniques,[200–202] including the use of interrupted, pledgeted rather than continuous sutures for complex patches.

Patch leaks can result in large residual (usually left–right) shunts, which impose a hemodynamic burden and can lead to progressive exercise intolerance, atrial arrhythmias, and pulmonary hypertension over time. Patients should undergo careful hemodynamic assessment to quantify the shunt and identify established pulmonary vascular disease, followed by interventional or surgical repair when indicated (**Fig. 67–49**). Large, nonrestrictive defects in cyanotic patients, with a right–left (reversed) or bidirectional shunt, cyanosis, and systemic or supra-systemic pulmonary hypertension (ie, Eisenmenger physiology) should not be closed and require specialist

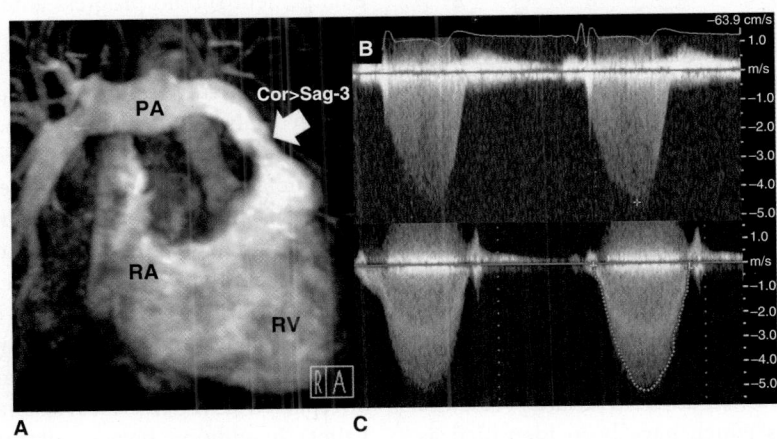

Figure 67–48. Conduit dysfunction following Rastelli repair of DORV. RV-PA conduit dysfunction following Rastelli-type repair with severe pulmonary stenosis. (**A**) The conduit stenosis is visualized on magnetic resonance angiography. (**B**) Continuous wave Doppler across the conduit displays a peak velocity across the conduit of 4.5 m/s equating to a peak gradient of 81 mm Hg. This obstruction to the outflow from the right ventricle (RV) means that the peak TR Doppler velocity no longer reflects pulmonary artery pressure. The peak TR velocity is 5 m/s, giving a peak TR gradient of 100 mm Hg. The pulmonary artery (PA) systolic pressure can be derived by subtracting the RV outflow tract from the TR gradient (PA systolic pressure estimated at 100 – 81 = 19 mm Hg). RA, right atrium.

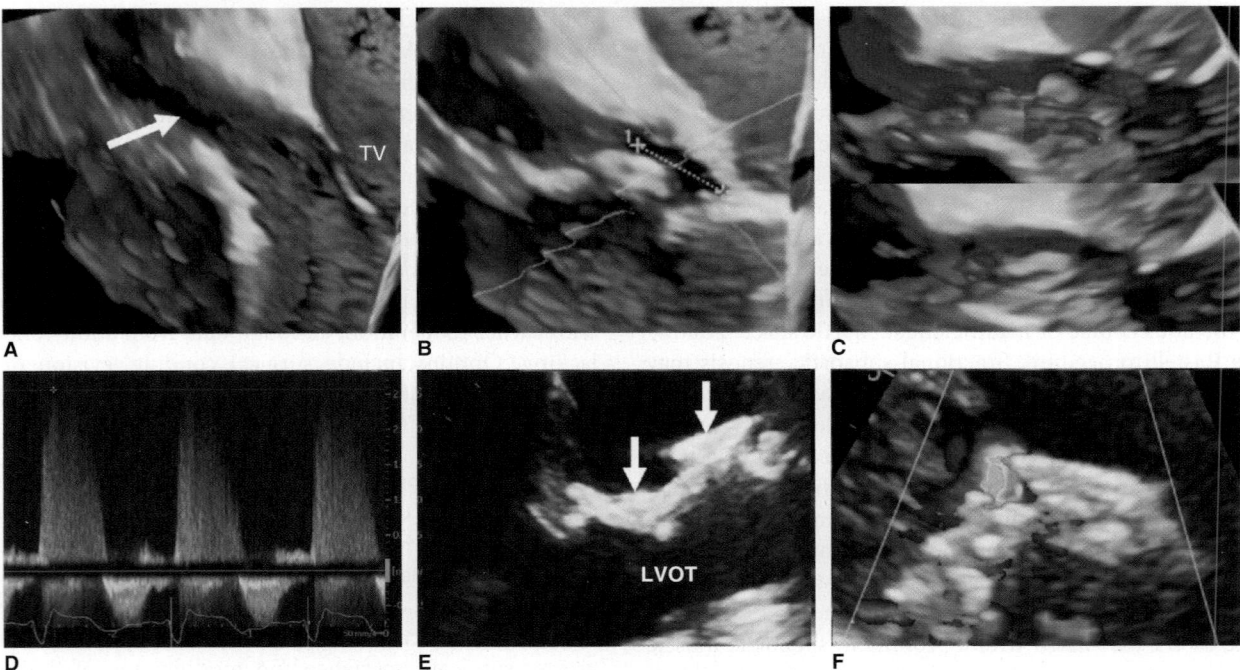

Figure 67–49. Residual VSD requiring transcatheter device closure following DORV repair. This 49-year-old patient presented with peripheral oedema and ascites 28 years after repair of DORV (ToF type) with a subannular Dacron patch with intraventricular tunnel directing blood from the LV, through the VSD to the aorta and an RV to pulmonary artery conduit. On TEE, a crescent-shaped VSD is identified (A and B, *arrow*) due to patch dehiscence. Its RV aspect is located in close proximity to the septal tricuspid valve (TV) leaflet. In (C), there is bidirectional, but predominantly left–right shunting across the defect and, in (D), the peak Doppler velocity is measured at 2.6 m/s. (E) and (F) display the appearances on parasternal long- and short-axis views on TTE following interventional closure of the defect with two Amplatzer occluders (E, *arrows*). There is tiny residual flow between the occluders. LVOT, left ventricular outflow tract.

assessment and management (see section Eisenmenger Syndrome in Chapter 66).

Arrhythmias and Risk for Sudden Cardiac Death: Patients with DORV are at risk of both atrial and ventricular arrhythmias; this remains the case following surgical repair. The pathophysiologic basis for electrical instability in these patients, similar to patients with related forms of CHD, is attributable to multiple factors. This includes myocardial scarring during surgery, especially for repairs that necessitate ventriculotomy, such as the Rastelli procedure or complex intraventricular repairs. This may be compounded by mechanical remodeling of the ventricles in the peri- and postoperative period.

New onset of arrhythmias in repaired DORV should prompt a full clinical evaluation to detect residual hemodynamic lesions, which may contribute to RV or LV overload and progressive ventricular dysfunction, followed by invasive hemodynamic and electrophysiological study. SCD contributes to over one half of late deaths in early repaired cohorts, with older age at repair, the presence of complete heart block, and occurrence of ventricular tachycardia in the perioperative period having been identified as multivariate predictors of SCD.[211] Clinical variables which have been identified as risk factors in ToF, such as QRS prolongation >180 ms, may be relevant in patients with ToF type DORV, but interactions between underlying anatomy, type of repair, and SCD risk in DORV remain unclear and robust risk scores for SCD in DORV patients do not exist.

Bradyarrhythmia and heart block necessitating pacemaker implantation are more common in the early or perioperative period. The atrioventricular node and bundle of His are close to the margin of the VSD and are at risk during VSD enlargement and suture placement. In the presence of a perimembranous VSD, the conduction tissue is positioned at the margin between the tricuspid annulus and the VSD. In the case of a restrictive, noncommitted muscular trabecular defect, defect enlargement should progress anterior and inferiorly, to avoid the conduction system positioned supero-posteriorly.

Congestive Heart Failure: Most patients post-DORV repair remain in NYHA functional class I for several years.[200] A minority of patients with repaired DORV, however, develop systemic and/or subpulmonary ventricular dysfunction, with symptoms and signs of heart failure. This is likely to become more common as the population of postrepair patients grows and patients that have undergone biventricular repair in the 1970s and 1980s reach the fifth decade of life and beyond. Ventricular dysfunction can occur for a variety of reasons in DORV patients, many of which are shared with other forms of repaired CHD (see Heart Failure in section Tetralogy of Fallot). In addition, biventricular repair in patients with small, stiff ventricles may contribute to long-term systolic and/or diastolic dysfunction, while baffle dysfunction is an added source of ventricular pressure or volume overload that contributes to heart failure. Diuretics are used to treat congestive symptoms, and conventional heart failure therapies are prescribed by many specialists to patients with LV dysfunction. In patients with debilitating symptoms, or clinical and biochemical markers indicating a poor prognosis, timely referral for advanced heart failure therapy assessment (including transplantation) is recommended.[6,7]

Valvular Aortic Regurgitation and Neoaortic Dilatation: Patients with TGA type DORV who have undergone repair including an arterial switch procedure develop mild–moderate aortic regurgitation with or without progressive neoaortic dilatation more frequently than "simple" TGA patients.[212] Neoaortic regurgitation is more common in TGA patients following arterial switch operation with associated coronary anomalies requiring complex reconstruction that may cause commissural asymmetry, or those with previous PA banding. In patients with severe aortic regurgitation and neoaortic dilatation, valve-sparing surgery is occasionally possible; otherwise, a Bentall procedure is required, usually with a mechanical valve conduit necessitating lifelong anticoagulation. The alternative for patients in whom anticoagulation is contraindicated (eg, women contemplating pregnancy) is a modified Bentall procedure using a bioprosthetic valve conduit.

Endocarditis: As with other forms of CHD, patients with DORV are at increased risk of infective endocarditis and require consistent education about prevention through good dental and skin hygiene, and early recognition of signs and symptoms that should prompt further evaluation by a specialist. Current guidelines only recommend prophylactic antibiotics prior to high-risk dental procedures (see section Tetralogy of Fallot) for patients with unrepaired cyanotic CHD, which includes those with unrepaired DORV, or those who have received palliative shunts, or conduits.[6,7] Antibiotic prophylaxis is also advised for patients with repaired CHD with residual defects at or adjacent to the site of a prosthetic material (eg, VSD patch or occluder device), those with prosthetic cardiac valves, or those with a personal history of endocarditis.

Follow-Up

Repaired DORV

Lifelong follow-up is recommended for all DORV patients with an ACHD specialist. Recommendations on the interval of follow-up, which can be applied universally in DORV are lacking but can be inferred from lesions with similar anatomies and surgical repair strategies. In general, well patients following biventricular repair require follow-up every 12 to 24 months with ECG and echocardiography. CMR surveillance and exercise testing are recommended every 36 to 60 months or sooner if clinically indicated. As with other CHD, patients at more advanced physiological stages require intensified monitoring.[6]

Adults with Unrepaired DORV

Unoperated DORV is associated with a high morbidity and mortality in adult life, hence surgical repair in early life is desirable in all cases. Unoperated adults with DORV have variable physiology depending on the underlying anatomy (location and size of the VSD, degree of pulmonary or subpulmonary stenosis, arrangement of the arterial trunks, presence of ventricular imbalance, and so on). There will be a variable degree of pulmonary vascular disease determined by the degree of pulmonary or subpulmonary stenosis. Adults without significant PS and, thus, an "unprotected" pulmonary circulation, will invariably have severe pulmonary hypertension with Eisenmenger physiology and should be treated in line with current recommendations, including pulmonary arterial hypertension therapies. Patients with severe PS and severely reduced pulmonary blood flow are unlikely to survive beyond childhood without a palliative shunt to augment pulmonary blood flow; a few of these patients with complex anatomy may have only received palliative surgery (**Fig. 67–50**). Occasionally, an adult may present with a "balanced" circulation (ie, PS that allows sufficient yet not excessive pulmonary blood flow) and mild–moderate cyanosis. Adult patients born in resource-poor countries may also present late to specialist services.

Adult primary presentations of DORV without severe, irreversible pulmonary vascular disease should be evaluated for late repair, balancing the perioperative risks of late intervention against the benefits of abolishing cyanosis, improving exercise tolerance, and controlling pulmonary blood flow. In such cases, rarely, repair with a Fontan-type operation may be performed, but requires a low/normal pulmonary vascular resistance, which is rarely encountered in patients assessed for Fontan surgery as adults. Multimodality imaging along with careful invasive hemodynamic assessment is necessary in all cases. Lifelong dedicated follow-up of unrepaired patients with DORV with an ACHD cardiologist or in an ACHD comprehensive care center is essential to identify and treat progressive associated lesions like atrioventricular valve regurgitation or coarctation, arrhythmias, heart failure, endocarditis and manage the long-term sequelae of Eisenmenger syndrome.

Pregnancy in Women with DORV

Women who have undergone biventricular repair for DORV and are clinically stable are not specifically mentioned under the mWHO classification in the 2018 ESC guidelines for the management of cardiovascular diseases during pregnancy.[213] Successful pregnancies and deliveries have been reported in this cohort, with an increased rate of noncardiac complications, including spontaneous miscarriage, premature labor and small for gestational age infants, and a relatively low risk of cardiac complications.[214] In patients following a biventricular repair of a ToF type DORV, the risk may be similar to the repaired ToF cohort who are in mWHO group II (ie, 5.7%–10.5% maternal cardiac event rate). All DORV patients should undergo assessment prior to pregnancy for the presence of additional risk factors (eg, significant residual hemodynamic lesions, biventricular dysfunction, cyanosis, or pulmonary hypertension). Patients who have had a univentricular repair (ie, Fontan-type operation) and women with unrepaired DORV who have cyanotic CHD are at a significantly increased maternal cardiovascular risk (mWHO III), and require expert counseling prior

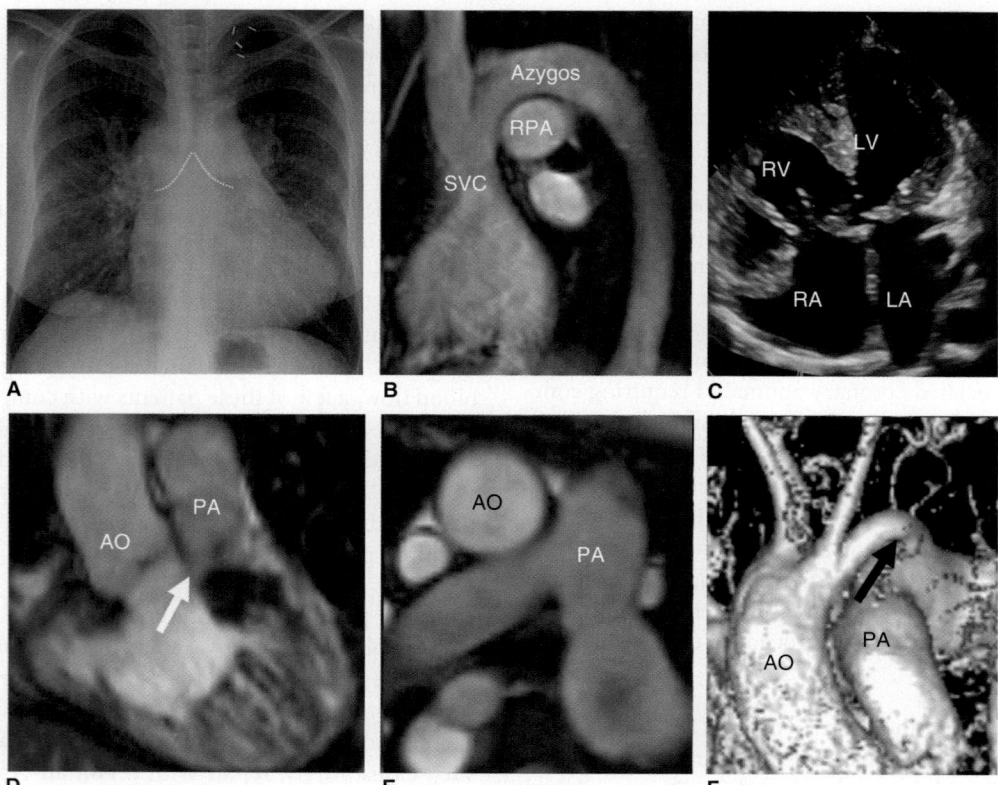

Figure 67–50. Unrepaired DORV with left atrial isomerism, AVSD, and TGA with side-by-side great arteries. An adult patient with unrepaired DORV and functionally univentricular physiology. (**A**) Chest radiography displays left bronchial isomerism with symmetrical, long main bronchi (broken lines) and the stomach "bubble" on the left, suggesting abdominal situs solitus. (**B**) Azygos continuation of the inferior vena cava is shown, the dilated azygos draining into the right-sided left atrium via a right-sided superior vena cava (SVC). (**C**) Normal atrioventricular arrangement is shown with an AVSD without offsetting of the left and right atrioventricular valves. The left ventricle (LV) and right ventricle (RV) are not hypoplastic. (**D**) Subpulmonary stenosis is shown in relation to the subpulmonary, inlet VSD (*white arrow*) and parallel great arteries. (**E**) The aorta (AO) is positioned to the left of the pulmonary artery (PA). (**F**) A left-sided BT shunt (*black arrow*) has been placed, connecting the left subclavian end-to-side to the left pulmonary artery. LA, left atrium; RA, right atrium; RPA, right pulmonary artery.

to pregnancy and close follow-up in an expert pregnancy and heart disease center. Pregnancy is contraindicated in women with coexistence of moderate or severe systemic ventricular dysfunction, severe left heart obstruction, or pulmonary arterial hypertension who are at an extremely high risk (mWHO IV, ≥40% risk of a maternal cardiac event).

REFERENCES

1. LaHaye S, Lincoln J, Garg V. Genetics of valvular heart disease. *Curr Cardiol Rep.* 2014;16(6):487.

2. Xiang R, Fan L-L, Huang H, et al. A novel mutation of GATA4 (K319E) is responsible for familial atrial septal defect and pulmonary valve stenosis. *Gene.* 2014;534(2):320-323.

3. Karamichalis JM, Darst JR, Mitchell MB, Clarke DR. Isolated right ventricular outflow tract obstruction. In: *Pediatric Cardiac Surgery* [Internet]. John Wiley & Sons, Ltd; 2013 [cited 2020 Oct 28]:385-409. doi: 10.1002/9781118320754.ch21.

4. Abdelghani M, Nassif M, Blom NA, et al. Infective endocarditis after melody valve implantation in the pulmonary position: a systematic review. *J Am Heart Assoc.* 2018;7(13):e008163.

5. Rowland DG, Hammill WW, Allen HD, Gutgesell HP. Natural course of isolated pulmonary valve stenosis in infants and children utilizing Doppler echocardiography. *Am J Cardiol.* 1997;79(3):344-349.

6. Stout KK, Daniels CJ, Aboulhosn JA, et al. 2018 AHA/ACC Guideline for the management of adults with congenital heart disease: a Report of the American College of Cardiology/American Heart Association Task Force on Clinical Practice Guidelines. *J Am Coll Cardiol.* 2019;73(12):1494-1563.

7. Baumgartner H, De Backer J, Babu-Narayan SV, et al. 2020 European Society of Cardiology (ESC) Guidelines for the management of adult congenital heart disease. The Task Force for the management of adult congenital heart disease of the ESC. *Eur Heart J.* 2020 Aug 29 [cited 2020 Nov 14];ehaa554. doi: 10.1093/eurheartj/ehaa554/5898606.

8. Stanger P, Cassidy SC, Girod DA, Kan JS, Lababidi Z, Shapiro SR. Balloon pulmonary valvuloplasty: results of the Valvuloplasty and Angioplasty of Congenital Anomalies Registry. *Am J Cardiol.* 1990;65(11):775-783.

9. Ben-Shachar G, Cohen MH, Sivakoff MC, Portman MA, Riemenschneider TA, Van Heeckeren DW. Development of infundibular obstruction after percutaneous pulmonary balloon valvuloplasty. *J Am Coll Cardiol.* 1985;5(3):754-756.

10. Taggart NW, Cetta F, Cabalka AK, Hagler DJ. Outcomes for balloon pulmonary valvuloplasty in adults: comparison with a concurrent pediatric cohort. *Catheter Cardiovasc Interv.* 2013;82(5):811-815.

11. Tabatabaei H, Boutin C, Nykanen DG, Freedom RM, Benson LN. Morphologic and hemodynamic consequences after percutaneous balloon valvotomy for neonatal pulmonary stenosis: medium-term follow-up. *J Am Coll Cardiol.* 1996;27(2):473-478.

12. Earing MG, Connolly HM, Dearani JA, Ammash NM, Grogan M, Warnes CA. Long-term follow-up of patients after surgical treatment for isolated pulmonary valve stenosis. *Mayo Clin Proc.* 2005;80(7):871-876.

13. Roos-Hesselink JW, Meijboom FJ, Spitaels SEC, et al. Long-term outcome after surgery for pulmonary stenosis (a longitudinal study of 22-33 years). *Eur Heart J.* 2006;27(4):482-488.

14. Voet A, Rega F, Bruaene AV de, et al. Long-term outcome after treatment of isolated pulmonary valve stenosis. *Int J Cardiol.* 2012;156(1):11-15.

15. Kenny D, Amin Z, Slyder S, Hijazi ZM. Medium-term outcomes for peripheral pulmonary artery stenting in adults with congenital heart disease. *J Intervent Cardiol.* 2011;24(4):373-377.

16. Hallbergson A, Lock JE, Marshall AC. Frequency and risk of in-stent stenosis following pulmonary artery stenting. *Am J Cardiol.* 2014;113(3):541-545.

17. Gonzalez I, Kenny D, Slyder S, Hijazi ZM. Medium and long-term outcomes after bilateral pulmonary artery stenting in children and adults with congenital heart disease. *Pediatr Cardiol.* 2013;34(1):179-184.

18. Montanaro C, Merola A, Kempny A, et al. The outcome of adults born with pulmonary atresia: high morbidity and mortality irrespective of repair. *Int J Cardiol.* 2018 Nov 7.

19. Schneider AW, Blom NA, Bruggemans EF, Hazekamp MG. More than 25 years of experience in managing pulmonary atresia with intact ventricular septum. *Ann Thorac Surg.* 2014;98(5):1680-1686.

20. McElhinney DB, Sondergaard L, Armstrong AK, et al. Endocarditis after transcatheter pulmonary valve replacement. *J Am Coll Cardiol.* 2018;72(22):2717-2728.

21. Habib G, Lancellotti P, Antunes MJ, et al. 2015 ESC Guidelines for the management of infective endocarditis. The Task Force for the Management of Infective Endocarditis of the European Society of Cardiology (ESC). Endorsed by: European Association for Cardio-Thoracic Surgery (EACTS), the European Association of Nuclear Medicine (EANM). *Eur Heart J.* 2015;36(44):3075-3128.

22. Regitz-Zagrosek V, Roos-Hesselink JW, Bauersachs J, et al. 2018 ESC Guidelines for the management of cardiovascular diseases during pregnancy. *Eur Heart J.* 2018;39(34):3165-3241.

23. Restivo A, Cameron AH, Anderson RH, Allwork SP. Divided right ventricle: a review of its anatomical varieties. *Pediatr Cardiol.* 1984;5(3):197-204.

24. Scantlebury DC, Geske JB, Nishimura RA. Limitations of Doppler Echocardiography in the Evaluation of Serial Stenoses. *Circ Cardiovasc Imaging.* 2013;6:850-852.

25. Kahr PC, Alonso-Gonzalez R, Kempny A, et al. Long-term natural history and postoperative outcome of double-chambered right ventricle—Experience from two tertiary adult congenital heart centres and review of the literature. *Int J Cardiol.* 2014;174(3):662-668.

26. Wong PC, Sanders SP, Jonas RA, et al. Pulmonary valve-moderator band distance and association with development of double-chambered right ventricle. *Am J Cardiol.* 1991;68(17):1681-1686.

27. Alva C, Ho SY, Lincoln CR, Rigby ML, Wright A, Anderson RH. The nature of the obstructive muscular bundles in double-chambered right ventricle. *J Thorac Cardiovasc Surg.* 1999;117(6):1180-1189.

28. Baumgartner H, Bonhoeffer P, De Groot NMS, et al. ESC Guidelines for the management of grown-up congenital heart disease (new version 2010). *Eur Heart J.* 2010;31(23):2915-2957.

29. Hachiro Y, Takagi N, Koyanagi T, Morikawa M, Abe T. Repair of double-chambered right ventricle: surgical results and long-term follow-up. *Ann Thorac Surg.* 2001;72(5):1520-1522.

30. Oliver JM, Garrido A, González A, et al. Rapid progression of midventricular obstruction in adults with double-chambered right ventricle. *J Thorac Cardiovasc Surg.* 2003;126(3):711-717.

31. McElhinney DB, Chatterjee KM, Reddy VM. Double-chambered right ventricle presenting in adulthood. *Ann Thorac Surg.* 2000;70(1):124-127.

32. Lascano ME, Schaad M, Moodie D, Murphy D. Difficulty in diagnosing double-chambered right ventricle in adults. *Am J Cardiol.* 2001.

33. Telagh R, Alexi-Meskishvili V, Hetzer R, Lange PE, Berger F, Abdul-Khaliq H. Initial clinical manifestations and mid- and long-term results after surgical repair of double-chambered right ventricle in children and adults. *Cardiol Young.* 2008;18(3):268-274.

34. Álvarez M, Tercedor L, Lozano JM, Azpitarte J. Sustained monomorphic ventricular tachycardia associated with unrepaired double-chambered right ventricle. *EP Eur.* 2006;8(10):901-903.

35. Ibrahim T, Dennig K, Schwaiger M, Schömig A. Images in cardiovascular medicine. Assessment of double chamber right ventricle by magnetic resonance imaging. *Circulation.* 2002;105(22):2692-2693.

36. Kveselis D, Rosenthal A, Ferguson P, Behrendt D, Sloan H. Long-term prognosis after repair of double-chamber right ventricle with ventricular septal defect. *Am J Cardiol.* 1984;54(10):1292-1295.

37. Penkoske PA, Duncan N, Collins-Nakai RL. Surgical repair of double-chambered right ventricle with or without ventriculotomy. *J Thorac Cardiovasc Surg.* 1987;93(3):385-393.

38. van der Linde D, Konings EEM, Slager MA, et al. Birth prevalence of congenital heart disease worldwide: a systematic review and meta-analysis. *J Am Coll Cardiol.* 2011;58(21):2241-2247.

39. Lillehei CW, Cohen M, Warden HE, et al. Direct vision intracardiac surgical correction of the tetralogy of Fallot, pentalogy of Fallot, and pulmonary atresia defects; report of first ten cases. *Ann Surg.* 1955;142(3):418-442.

40. Wolf MD, Landtman B, Neill CA, Taussig HB. Total correction of tetralogy of Fallot. I. Follow-up study of 104 cases. *Circulation.* 1965;31:385-393.

41. Kirklin JW, Blackstone EH, Pacifico AD, Kirklin JK, Bargeron LM. Risk factors for early and late failure after repair of tetralogy of Fallot, and their neutralization. *Thorac Cardiovasc Surg.* 1984;32(4):208-214.

42. Mavroudis CD, Frost J, Mavroudis C. Pulmonary valve preservation and restoration strategies for repair of tetralogy of Fallot. *Cardiol Young.* 2014;24(6):1088-1094.

43. Padalino MA, Cavalli G, Albanese SB, et al. Long-term outcomes following transatrial versus transventricular repair on right ventricular function in tetralogy of Fallot. *J Card Surg.* 2017;32(11):712-720.

44. Karl TR, Sano S, Pornviliwan S, Mee RB. Tetralogy of Fallot: favorable outcome of nonneonatal transatrial, transpulmonary repair. *Ann Thorac Surg.* 1992;54(5):903-907.

45. van der Ven JPG, van den Bosch E, Bogers AJCC, Helbing WA. Current outcomes and treatment of tetralogy of Fallot. F1000Research [Internet]. 2019 Aug 29 [cited 2020 Jul 28];8. https://www.ncbi.nlm.nih.gov/pmc/articles/PMC6719677/

46. Bentham JR, Zava NK, Harrison WJ, et al. Duct stenting versus modified Blalock-Taussig shunt in neonates with duct-dependent pulmonary blood flow: associations with clinical outcomes in a multicenter national study. *Circulation.* 2018 06;137(6):581-588.

47. Glatz AC, Petit CJ, Goldstein BH, et al. Comparison between patent ductus arteriosus stent and modified Blalock-Taussig Shunt as palliation for infants with ductal-dependent pulmonary blood flow: insights from the Congenital Catheterization Research Collaborative. *Circulation.* 2018;137(6):589-601.

48. Quandt D, Ramchandani B, Penford G, et al. Right ventricular outflow tract stent versus BT shunt palliation in Tetralogy of Fallot. *Heart Br Card Soc.* 2017;103(24):1985-1991.

49. Jacobs JP, Mayer JE, Pasquali SK, et al. The Society of Thoracic Surgeons Congenital Heart Surgery Database: 2018 update on outcomes and quality. *Ann Thorac Surg.* 2018;105(3):680-689.

50. Bertranou EG, Blackstone EH, Hazelrig JB, Turner ME, Kirklin JW. Life expectancy without surgery in tetralogy of Fallot. *Am J Cardiol.* 1978;42(3):458-466.

51. Karamlou T, McCrindle BW, Williams WG. Surgery insight: late complications following repair of tetralogy of Fallot and related surgical strategies for management. *Nat Clin Pract Cardiovasc Med.* 2006;3(11):611-622.

52. Saygi M, Ergul Y, Tola HT, Ozyilmaz I, Ozturk E, Onan IS, et al. Factors affecting perioperative mortality in tetralogy of Fallot. *Pediatr Int Off J Jpn Pediatr Soc.* 2015;57(5):832-839.

53. Nollert G, Fischlein T, Bouterwek S, Böhmer C, Klinner W, Reichart B. Long-term survival in patients with repair of tetralogy of Fallot: 36-year follow-up of 490 survivors of the first year after surgical repair. *J Am Coll Cardiol.* 1997;30(5):1374-1383.

54. Bonello B, Kempny A, Uebing A, et al. Right atrial area and right ventricular outflow tract akinetic length predict sustained tachyarrhythmia in repaired tetralogy of Fallot. *Int J Cardiol.* 2013;168(4):3280-3286.

55. Diller G-P, Kempny A, Alonso-Gonzalez R, et al. Survival prospects and circumstances of death in contemporary adult congenital heart disease patients under follow-up at a large tertiary centre. *Circulation.* 2015 Sep 14.

56. Cuypers JAAE, Menting ME, Konings EEM, et al. Unnatural history of tetralogy of Fallot: prospective follow-up of 40 years after surgical correction. *Circulation.* 2014;130(22):1944-1953.

57. d'Udekem Y, Galati JC, Rolley GJ, et al. Low risk of pulmonary valve implantation after a policy of transatrial repair of tetralogy of Fallot delayed beyond the neonatal period: the Melbourne experience over 25 years. *J Am Coll Cardiol.* 2014;63(6):563-568.

58. Oechslin EN, Harrison DA, Harris L, et al. Reoperation in adults with repair of tetralogy of fallot: indications and outcomes. *J Thorac Cardiovasc Surg.* 1999;118(2):245-2451.

59. Stewart RD, Backer CL, Young L, Mavroudis C. Tetralogy of Fallot: results of a pulmonary valve-sparing strategy. *Ann Thorac Surg.* 2005;80(4):1431-1439.

60. Martin-Garcia AC, Dimopoulos K, Boutsikou M, et al. Tricuspid regurgitation severity after atrial septal defect closure or pulmonic valve replacement. *Heart Br Card Soc.* 2020;106(6):455-461.

61. Babu-Narayan SV, Kilner PJ, Li W, et al. Ventricular fibrosis suggested by cardiovascular magnetic resonance in adults with repaired tetralogy of fallot and its relationship to adverse markers of clinical outcome. *Circulation.* 2006;113(3):405-413.

62. Heng EL, Gatzoulis MA, Uebing A, et al. Immediate and midterm cardiac remodeling after surgical pulmonary valve replacement in adults with repaired tetralogy of Fallot: a prospective cardiovascular magnetic resonance and clinical study. *Circulation.* 2017;136(18):1703-1713.

63. Gatzoulis MA, Balaji S, Webber SA, et al. Risk factors for arrhythmia and sudden cardiac death late after repair of tetralogy of Fallot: a multicentre study. *Lancet Lond Engl.* 2000;356(9234):975-981.

64. Silka MJ, Bar-Cohen Y. A contemporary assessment of the risk for sudden cardiac death in patients with congenital heart disease. *Pediatr Cardiol.* 2012;33(3):452-460.

65. Khairy P, Harris L, Landzberg MJ, et al. Implantable cardioverter-defibrillators in tetralogy of Fallot. *Circulation.* 2008;117(3):363-370.

66. Cook SC, Valente AM, Maul TM, et al. Shock-related anxiety and sexual function in adults with congenital heart disease and implantable cardioverter-defibrillators. *Heart Rhythm.* 2013;10(6):805-810.

67. Bedair R, Babu-Narayan SV, et al. Acceptance and psychological impact of implantable defibrillators amongst adults with congenital heart disease. *Int J Cardiol.* 2015;181:218-224.

68. Dimopoulos K, Muthiah K, Alonso-Gonzalez R, et al. Heart or heart-lung transplantation for patients with congenital heart disease in England. *Heart.* 2019 Jan 10. doi: 10.1136/heartjnl-2018-313984.

69. Zomer AC, Vaartjes I, van der Velde ET, et al. Heart failure admissions in adults with congenital heart disease; risk factors and prognosis. *Int J Cardiol.* 2013;168(3):2487-2493.

70. Stout KK, Broberg CS, Book WM, et al. Chronic heart failure in congenital heart disease a scientific statement from the American Heart Association. *Circulation.* 2016;133(8):770-801.

71. Constantine A, Barradas-Pires A, Dimopoulos K. Modifiable risk factors in congenital heart disease: education, transition, digital health and choice architecture. *Eur J Prev Cardiol.* 2019 Sep 3;2047487319874146.

72. Baddour Larry M, Wilson Walter R, Bayer Arnold S, et al. Infective endocarditis in adults: diagnosis, antimicrobial therapy, and management of complications. *Circulation.* 2015;132(15):1435-1486.

73. Niwa K. Aortic root dilatation in tetralogy of Fallot long-term after repair–histology of the aorta in tetralogy of Fallot: evidence of intrinsic aortopathy. *Int J Cardiol.* 2005;103(2):117-119.

74. Tan JL, Davlouros PA, McCarthy KP, Gatzoulis MA, Ho SY. Intrinsic histological abnormalities of aortic root and ascending aorta in tetralogy of Fallot. *Circulation.* 2005;112(7):961-968.

75. Frischhertz BP, Shamszad P, Pedroza C, Milewicz DM, Morris SA. Thoracic aortic dissection and rupture in conotruncal cardiac defects: a population-based study. *Int J Cardiol.* 2015;184:521-527.

76. Takei K, Murakami T, Takeda A. Implication of aortic root dilation and stiffening in patients with tetralogy of Fallot. *Pediatr Cardiol.* 2018;39(7):1462-1467.

77. Dimopoulos K, Alonso-Gonzalez R, Wort SJ, et al. The incidence of aortic dissection in tetralogy of Fallot. *Eur Heart J* [Internet]. 2017 Aug 1 [cited 2020 Aug 7];38(suppl 1). https://academic.oup.com/eurheartj/article/38/suppl_1/ehx501.329/4087631

78. Davlouros PA, Kilner PJ, Hornung TS, et al. Right ventricular function in adults with repaired tetralogy of Fallot assessed with cardiovascular magnetic resonance imaging: detrimental role of right ventricular outflow aneurysms or akinesia and adverse right-to-left ventricular interaction. *J Am Coll Cardiol.* 2002;40(11):2044-2052.

79. Uebing A, Gibson DG, Babu-Narayan SV, et al. Right ventricular mechanics and QRS duration in patients with repaired tetralogy of Fallot: implications of infundibular disease. *Circulation.* 2007;116(14):1532-1539.

80. Gatzoulis MA, Till JA, Somerville J, Redington AN. Mechanoelectrical interaction in tetralogy of Fallot. QRS prolongation relates to right ventricular size and predicts malignant ventricular arrhythmias and sudden death. *Circulation.* 1995;92(2):231-237.

81. Dimopoulos K, Condliffe R, Tulloh RMR, et al. Echocardiographic screening for pulmonary hypertension in congenital heart disease: JACC Review Topic of the Week. *J Am Coll Cardiol.* 2018;72(22):2778-2788.

82. Dimopoulos K, Diller G-P, Opotowsky AR, et al. Definition and management of segmental pulmonary hypertension. *J Am Heart Assoc.* 2018;7(14).

83. Babu-Narayan SV, Uebing A, Davlouros PA, et al. Randomised trial of ramipril in repaired tetralogy of Fallot and pulmonary regurgitation: The APPROPRIATE study (Ace inhibitors for Potential PRevention Of the deleterious effects of Pulmonary Regurgitation In Adults with repaired TEtralogy of Fallot). *Int J Cardiol.* 2012;154(3):299-305.

84. Norozi K, Bahlmann J, Raab B, et al. A prospective, randomized, double-blind, placebo controlled trial of beta-blockade in patients who have undergone surgical correction of tetralogy of Fallot. *Cardiol Young.* 2007;17(4):372-379.

85. Ghez O, Tsang VT, Frigiola A, et al. Right ventricular outflow tract reconstruction for pulmonary regurgitation after repair of tetralogy of Fallot. Preliminary results. *Eur J Cardiothorac Surg.* 2007;31(4):654-658.

86. Therrien J, Provost Y, Merchant N, Williams W, Colman J, Webb G. Optimal timing for pulmonary valve replacement in adults after tetralogy of Fallot repair. *Am J Cardiol.* 2005;95(6):779–782.

87. Cavalcanti PEF, Sá MPBO, Santos CA, et al. Pulmonary valve replacement after operative repair of tetralogy of Fallot: meta-analysis and meta-regression of 3,118 patients from 48 studies. *J Am Coll Cardiol.* 2013;62(23):2227-2243.

88. Ross HJ, Law Y, Book WM, et al. Transplantation and mechanical circulatory support in congenital heart disease a scientific statement from the American Heart Association. *Circulation.* 2016;133(8):802-820.

89. Schuuring MJ, Bouma BJ, Cordina R, et al. Treatment of segmental pulmonary artery hypertension in adults with congenital heart disease. *Int J Cardiol.* 2013;164(1):106-110.

90. Ebstein W. Ueber einen sehr seltenen Fall von Insufficienz der Valvula tricuspidalis, bedingt durch eine angeborene hochgradige Missbildung derselben. Veit; 1866.

91. Barnard CN, Schrire V. Surgical correction of Ebstein's malformation with prosthetic tricuspid valve. *Surgery.* 1963;54:302-308.

92. Pradat P, Francannet C, Harris JA, Robert E. The epidemiology of cardiovascular defects, part I: a study based on data from three large registries of congenital malformations. *Pediatr Cardiol.* 2003;24(3):195-221.

93. Boyle B, Garne E, Loane M, et al. The changing epidemiology of Ebstein's anomaly and its relationship with maternal mental health conditions: a European registry-based study. *Cardiol Young.* 2017;27(4):677-685.

94. Digilio MC, Bernardini L, Lepri F, et al. Ebstein anomaly: Genetic heterogeneity and association with microdeletions 1p36 and 8p23.1. *Am J Med Genet A.* 2011;155A(9):2196-2202.

95. Freud LR, Escobar-Diaz MC, Kalish BT, et al. Outcomes and predictors of perinatal mortality in fetuses with Ebstein anomaly or tricuspid valve dysplasia in the current era: a multicenter study. *Circulation.* 2015;132(6):481-489.

96. Patorno E, Huybrechts KF, Bateman BT, et al. Lithium use in pregnancy and the risk of cardiac malformations. *N Engl J Med.* 2017;376(23):2245-2254.

97. Edwards WD. Embryology and pathologic features of Ebstein's anomaly. *Prog Pediatr Cardiol.* 1993;2(1):5-15.

98. Jost CHA, Connolly HM, O'Leary PW, Warnes CA, Tajik AJ, Seward JB. Left heart lesions in patients with Ebstein anomaly. *Mayo Clin Proc.* 2005;80(3):361-368.

99. van Son JAM, Danielson GK, Huhta JC, et al. Late results of systemic atrioventricular valve replacement in corrected transposition. *J Thorac Cardiovasc Surg.* 1995;109(4):642-653.

100. Celermajer DS, Cullen S, Deanfield JE, Sullivan ID. Congenitally corrected transposition and Ebstein's anomaly of the systemic atrioventricular valve: Association with aortic arch obstruction. *J Am Coll Cardiol.* 1991;18(4):1056-1058.

101. Silverman NH, Gerlis LM, Horowitz ES, Ho SY, Neches WH, Anderson RH. Pathologic elucidation of the echocardiographic features of Ebstein's malformation of the morphologically tricuspid valve in discordant atrioventricular connections. *Am J Cardiol.* 1995;76(17):1277-1283.

102. Carpentier A, Chauvaud S, Macé L, et al. A new reconstructive operation for Ebstein's anomaly of the tricuspid valve. *J Thorac Cardiovasc Surg.* 1988;96(1):92-101.

103. Celermajer DS, Cullen S, Sullivan ID, Spiegelhalter DJ, Wyse RKH, Deanfield JE. Outcome in neonates with Ebstein's anomaly. *J Am Coll Cardiol.* 1992;19(5):1041-1046.

104. Cieplucha A, Trojnarska O, Bartczak-Rutkowska A, et al. Severity scores for Ebstein anomaly: credibility and usefulness of echocardiographic vs magnetic resonance assessments of the Celermajer Index. *Can J Cardiol.* 2019;35(12):1834-1841.

105. Rudolph AM. Ebstein malformation of the tricuspid valve. In: *Congenital Diseases of the Heart* [Internet]. John Wiley & Sons, Ltd; 2009 [cited 2020 Nov 21]:451-64. doi: 10.1002/9781444311822.ch17

106. Starnes VA, Pitlick PT, Bernstein D, Griffin ML, Choy M, Shumway NE. Ebstein's anomaly appearing in the neonate. A new surgical approach. *J Thorac Cardiovasc Surg.* 1991;101(6):1082-1087.

107. Raju V, Dearani JA, Burkhart HM, et al. Right ventricular unloading for heart failure related to Ebstein malformation. *Ann Thorac Surg.* 2014;98(1):167-174.

108. Hetzer R, Hacke P, Javier M, et al. The long-term impact of various techniques for tricuspid repair in Ebstein's anomaly. *J Thorac Cardiovasc Surg.* 2015;150(5):1212-1219.

109. Silva JP da, Silva L da F da, Moreira LFP, et al. Cone reconstruction in Ebstein's anomaly repair: early and long-term results. *Arq Bras Cardiol.* 2011;97(3):199-208.

110. Ibrahim M, Tsang VT, Caruana M, et al. Cone reconstruction for Ebstein's anomaly: patient outcomes, biventricular function, and cardiopulmonary exercise capacity. *J Thorac Cardiovasc Surg.* 2015;149(4):1144-1150.

111. Davies RR, Pasquali SK, Jacobs ML, Jacobs JJ, Wallace AS, Pizarro C. Current spectrum of surgical procedures performed for Ebstein's malformation: an analysis of the Society of Thoracic Surgeons Congenital Heart Surgery Database. *Ann Thorac Surg.* 2013;96(5):1703-1709; discussion 1709-1710.

112. Attenhofer Jost CH, Connolly HM, Scott CG, Burkhart HM, Warnes CA, Dearani JA. Outcome of cardiac surgery in patients 50 years of age or older with Ebstein anomaly. *J Am Coll Cardiol.* 2012;59(23):2101-2106.

113. Dearani JA, Mora BN, Nelson TJ, Haile DT, O'Leary PW. Ebstein anomaly review: what's now, what's next? *Expert Rev Cardiovasc Ther.* 2015;13(10):1101-1109.

114. Brown ML, Dearani JA, Danielson GK, et al. The outcomes of operations for 539 patients with Ebstein anomaly. *J Thorac Cardiovasc Surg.* 2008;135(5):1120-1136,e1-e7.

115. Badiu CC, Schreiber C, Hörer J, et al. Early timing of surgical intervention in patients with Ebstein's anomaly predicts superior long-term outcome. *Eur J Cardiothorac Surg.* 2010;37(1):186-192.

116. Sharland GK, Chita SK, Allan LD. Tricuspid valve dysplasia or displacement in intrauterine life. *J Am Coll Cardiol.* 1991;17(4):944-949.

117. Hornberger LK, Sahn DJ, Kleinman CS, Copel JA, Reed KL. Tricuspid valve disease with significant tricuspid insufficiency in the fetus: diagnosis and outcome. *J Am Coll Cardiol.* 1991;17(1):167-173.

118. Wertaschnigg D, Manlhiot C, Jaeggi M, et al. Contemporary outcomes and factors associated with mortality after a fetal or neonatal diagnosis of Ebstein anomaly and tricuspid valve disease. *Can J Cardiol.* 2016;32(12):1500-1506.

119. Gottschalk I, Gottschalk L, Stressig R, Ritgen J, Herberg U, Breuer J, et al. Ebstein's anomaly of the tricuspid valve in the fetus—a multicenter experience. *Ultraschall Med Stuttg Ger 1980.* 2017;38(4):427-436.

120. Selamet Tierney ES, McElhinney DB, Freud LR, et al. Assessment of progressive pathophysiology after early prenatal diagnosis of the Ebstein anomaly or tricuspid valve dysplasia. *Am J Cardiol.* 2017;119(1):106-111.

121. Holst KA, Dearani JA, Said SM, et al. Surgical management and outcomes of Ebstein anomaly in neonates and infants: a Society of Thoracic Surgeons Congenital Heart Surgery Database Analysis. *Ann Thorac Surg.* 2018;106(3):785-791.

122. Celermajer DS, Bull C, Till JA, et al. Ebstein's anomaly: presentation and outcome from fetus to adult. *J Am Coll Cardiol.* 1994;23(1):170-176.

123. Attenhofer Jost CH, Tan NY, Hassan A, et al. Sudden death in patients with Ebstein anomaly. *Eur Heart J.* 2018;39(21):1970-1977a.

124. Hassan A, Tan NY, Aung H, et al. Outcomes of atrial arrhythmia radiofrequency catheter ablation in patients with Ebstein's anomaly. *EP Eur.* 2018;20(3):535-540.

125. Pressley JC, Wharton JM, Tang AS, Lowe JE, Gallagher JJ, Prystowsky EN. Effect of Ebstein's anomaly on short- and long-term outcome of surgically treated patients with Wolff-Parkinson-White syndrome. *Circulation.* 1992;86(4):1147-1155.

126. Levine JC, Walsh EP, Saul JP. Radiofrequency ablation of accessory pathways associated with congenital heart disease including heterotaxy syndrome. *Am J Cardiol.* 1993;72(9):689-693.

127. Pediatric and Congenital Electrophysiology Society (PACES), Heart Rhythm Society (HRS), American College of Cardiology Foundation (ACCF), et al. PACES/HRS expert consensus statement on the management of the asymptomatic young patient with a Wolff-Parkinson-White (WPW, ventricular preexcitation) electrocardiographic pattern: developed in partnership between the Pediatric and Congenital Electrophysiology Society (PACES) and the Heart Rhythm Society (HRS). Endorsed by the governing bodies of PACES, HRS, the American College of Cardiology Foundation (ACCF), the American Heart Association (AHA), the American Academy of Pediatrics (AAP), and the Canadian Heart Rhythm Society (CHRS). *Heart Rhythm.* 2012;9(6):1006-1024.

128. Ho SY, Goltz D, McCarthy K, et al. The atrioventricular junctions in Ebstein malformation. *Heart Br Card Soc.* 2000;83(4):444-449.

129. Lev M, Liberthson RR, Joseph RH, et al. The pathologic anatomy of Ebstein's disease. *Arch Pathol.* 1970;90(4):334-343.

130. Anderson KR, Zuberbuhler JR, Anderson RH, Becker AE, Lie JT. Morphologic spectrum of Ebstein's anomaly of the heart: a review. *Mayo Clin Proc.* 1979;54(3):174-180.

131. Watson H. Natural history of Ebstein's anomaly of tricuspid valve in childhood and adolescence. An international co-operative study of 505 cases. *Br Heart J*. 1974;36(5):417-427.

132. Li W, Henein M, Gatzoulis MA. Echocardiography in adult congenital heart disease [Internet]. London: Springer-Verlag; 2007 [cited 2020 Nov 21]. https://www.springer.com/gp/book/9781846288159.

133. Hsiao S-H, Lin S-K, Wang W-C, et al. Severe tricuspid regurgitation shows significant impact in the relationship among peak systolic tricuspid annular velocity, tricuspid annular plane systolic excursion, and right ventricular ejection fraction. *JASE*. 2006;19(7):902-910.

134. Attenhofer Jost CH, Edmister WD, Julsrud PR, et al. Prospective comparison of echocardiography versus cardiac magnetic resonance imaging in patients with Ebstein's anomaly. *Int J Cardiovasc Imaging*. 2012;28(5):1147-1159.

135. Hughes ML, Bonello B, Choudhary P, Marek J, Tsang V. A simple measure of the extent of Ebstein valve rotation with cardiovascular magnetic resonance gives a practical guide to feasibility of surgical cone reconstruction. *J Cardiovasc Magn Reson*. 2019;21(1):34.

136. Rydman R, Shiina Y, Diller G-P, et al. Major adverse events and atrial tachycardia in Ebstein's anomaly predicted by cardiovascular magnetic resonance. *Heart Br Card Soc*. 2018;104(1):37-44.

137. Yang D, Li X, Sun J-Y, et al. Cardiovascular magnetic resonance evidence of myocardial fibrosis and its clinical significance in adolescent and adult patients with Ebstein's anomaly. *J Cardiovasc Magn Reson*. 2018;20(1):69.

138. Radojevic J, Inuzuka R, Alonso-Gonzalez R, et al. Peak oxygen uptake correlates with disease severity and predicts outcome in adult patients with Ebstein's anomaly of the tricuspid valve. *Int J Cardiol*. 2013;163(3):305-308.

139. Chen SSM, Dimopoulos K, Sheehan FH, Gatzoulis MA, Kilner PJ. Physiologic determinants of exercise capacity in patients with different types of right-sided regurgitant lesions: Ebstein's malformation with tricuspid regurgitation and repaired tetralogy of Fallot with pulmonary regurgitation. *Int J Cardiol*. 2016;205:1-5.

140. Akazawa Y, Fujioka T, Kühn A, et al. Right ventricular diastolic function and right atrial function and their relation with exercise capacity in Ebstein anomaly. *Can J Cardiol*. 2019;35(12):1824-1833.

141. Trojnarska O, Szyszka A, Gwizdała A, et al. Adults with Ebstein's anomaly—Cardiopulmonary exercise testing and BNP levels exercise capacity and BNP in adults with Ebstein's anomaly. *Int J Cardiol*. 2006;111(1):92-97.

142. Brown ML, Dearani JA, Danielson GK, et al. Functional status after operation for Ebstein anomaly: the Mayo Clinic experience. *J Am Coll Cardiol*. 2008;52(6):460-466.

143. Silva M, Teixeira A, Menezes I, et al. Percutaneous closure of atrial right-to-left shunt in patients with Ebstein's anomaly of the tricuspid valve. *EuroIntervention J Eur Collab Work Group Interv Cardiol Eur Soc Cardiol*. 2012;8(1):94-97.

144. Aboulhosn J, Cabalka AK, Levi DS, et al. Transcatheter valve-in-ring implantation for the treatment of residual or recurrent tricuspid valve dysfunction after prior surgical repair. *JACC Cardiovasc Interv*. 2017;10(1):53-63.

145. Taggart NW, Cabalka AK, Eicken A, et al. Outcomes of transcatheter tricuspid valve-in-valve implantation in patients with Ebstein anomaly. *Am J Cardiol*. 2018;121(2):262-268.

146. McElhinney DB, Aboulhosn JA, Dvir D, et al. Mid-term valve-related outcomes after transcatheter tricuspid valve-in-valve or valve-in-ring replacement. *J Am Coll Cardiol*. 2019;73(2):148-157.

147. Lambert AN, Weiner J, Hall M, et al. Heart transplant outcomes in children with Ebstein's anomaly. *j heart lung transplant*. 2020;39(4, Supplement):S455-S456.

148. Shivapour JKL, Sherwin ED, Alexander ME, et al. Utility of preoperative electrophysiologic studies in patients with Ebstein's anomaly undergoing the Cone procedure. *Heart Rhythm*. 2014;11(2):182-186.

149. Stulak JM, Sharma V, Cannon BC, Ammash N, Schaff HV, Dearani JA. Optimal surgical ablation of atrial tachyarrhythmias during correction of Ebstein anomaly. *Ann Thorac Surg*. 2015;99(5):1700-1705; discussion 1705.

150. Lima FV, Koutrolou-Sotiropoulou P, Yen TYM, Stergiopoulos K. Clinical characteristics and outcomes in pregnant women with Ebstein anomaly at the time of delivery in the USA: 2003-2012. *Arch Cardiovasc Dis*. 2016;109(6–7):390-398.

151. Nishimura RA, Otto CM, Bonow RO, et al. 2014 AHA/ACC guideline for the management of patients with valvular heart disease: a report of the American College of Cardiology/American Heart Association Task Force on Practice Guidelines. *J Am Coll Cardiol*. 2014;63(22):e57-e185.

152. Baumgartner H, Falk V, Bax JJ, et al. 2017 ESC/EACTS Guidelines for the management of valvular heart disease. *Eur Heart J*. 2017;38(36):2739-2791.

153. Dearani JA, Danielson GK. Congenital heart surgery nomenclature and database project: Ebstein's anomaly and tricuspid valve disease. *Ann Thorac Surg*. 2000;69(3, Supplement 1):106-117.

154. Ozdemir O, Olgunturk R, Kula S, Tunaoglu FS. Echocardiographic findings in children with Marfan syndrome. *Cardiovasc J Afr*. 2011;22(5):245-248.

155. Gu X, He Y, Li Z, Han J, Chen J, Nixon JV (Ian). Echocardiographic versus histologic findings in Marfan syndrome. *Tex Heart Inst J*. 2015;42(1):30-34.

156. Groves PH, Lewis NP, Ikram S, Maire R, Hall RJ. Reduced exercise capacity in patients with tricuspid regurgitation after successful mitral valve replacement for rheumatic mitral valve disease. *Br Heart J*. 1991;66(4):295-301.

157. Andersen MJ, Nishimura RA, Borlaug BA. The hemodynamic basis of exercise intolerance in tricuspid regurgitation. *Circ Heart Fail*. 2014;7(6):911-917.

158. Pande S, Agarwal SK, Majumdar G, Kapoor A, Kale N, Kundu A. Valvuloplasty in the treatment of rheumatic tricuspid disease. *Asian Cardiovasc Thorac Ann*. 2008;16(2):107-111.

159. Tang GHL, David TE, Singh SK, Maganti MD, Armstrong S, Borger MA. Tricuspid valve repair with an annuloplasty ring results in improved long-term outcomes. *Circulation*. 2006;114(1 supplement):I-577.

160. Belluschi I, Del Forno B, Lapenna E, et al. Surgical Techniques for Tricuspid Valve Disease. *Front Cardiovasc Med*. 2018;5:118.

161. Vander Veer JB, Rhyneer GS, Hodam RP, Kloster FE. Obstruction of tricuspid ball-valve prostheses. *Circulation*. 1971;43(5s1):I-62.

162. Koplan BA, Stevenson WG, Epstein LM, Aranki SF, Maisel WH. Development and validation of a simple risk score to predict the need for permanent pacing after cardiac valve surgery. *J Am Coll Cardiol*. 2003;41(5):795-801.

163. Jokinen JJ, Turpeinen AK, Pitkänen O, Hippeläinen MJ, Hartikainen JEK. Pacemaker therapy after tricuspid valve operations: implications on mortality, morbidity, and quality of life. *Ann Thorac Surg*. 2009;87(6):1806-1814.

164. Shrivastava S, Radhakrishnan S, Dev V. Concurrent balloon dilatation of tricuspid and calcific mitral valve in a patient of rheumatic heart disease. *Int J Cardiol*. 1988;20(1):133-137.

165. McElhinney DB, Cabalka AK, Aboulhosn JA, et al. Transcatheter tricuspid valve-in-valve implantation for the treatment of dysfunctional surgical bioprosthetic valves. *Circulation*. 2016;133(16):1582-1593.

166. Giannini F, Colombo A. Percutaneous treatment of tricuspid valve in refractory right heart failure. *Eur Heart J Suppl J Eur Soc Cardiol*. 2019;21(Suppl B):B43-B47.

167. Rizzoli G, Perini LD, Bottio T, Minutolo G, Thiene G, Casarotto D. Prosthetic replacement of the tricuspid valve: biological or mechanical? *Ann Thorac Surg*. 1998;66(6):S62-S67.

168. Van Nooten GJ, Caes F, Taeymans Y, et al. Tricuspid valve replacement: postoperative and long-term results. *J Thorac Cardiovasc Surg*. 1995;110(3):672-679.

169. Nagel E, Stuber M, Hess OM. Importance of the right ventricle in valvular heart disease. *Eur Heart J.* 1996;17(6):829-836.

170. Bajzer CT, Stewart WJ, Cosgrove DM, Azzam SJ, Arheart KL, Klein AL. Tricuspid valve surgery and intraoperative echocardiography. *J Am Coll Cardiol.* 1998;32(4):1023-1031.

171. Scully HE, Armstrong CS. Tricuspid valve replacement: fifteen years of experience with mechanical prostheses and bioprostheses. *J Thorac Cardiovasc Surg.* 1995;109(6):1035-1041.

172. Kawano H, Oda T, Fukunaga S, et al. Tricuspid valve replacement with the St. Jude Medical valve: 19 years of experience. *Eur J Cardio-Thorac Surg Off J Eur Assoc Cardio-Thorac Surg.* 2000;18(5):565-569.

173. Cahill T, Jewell P, Denne L, et al. Contemporary epidemiology of infective endocarditis in patients with congenital heart disease: a UK prospective study. *Am Heart J.* 2019;215:70-77.

174. Khairy P, Ouyang DW, Fernandes SM, Lee-Parritz A, Economy KE, Landzberg MJ. Pregnancy outcomes in women with congenital heart disease. *Circulation.* 2006;113(4):517-524.

175. Pelliccia A, Sharma S, Gati S, et al. 2020 ESC Guidelines on sports cardiology and exercise in patients with cardiovascular diseaseThe Task Force on sports cardiology and exercise in patients with cardiovascular disease of the European Society of Cardiology (ESC). *Eur Heart J.* 2020:1-80.

176. Abernethy J. Surgical and physiological essays. Part 2. 1793 [cited 2021 Feb 7]. https://archive.hshsl.umaryland.edu/handle/10713/2043

177. VanPraagh S, Davidoff A, Chin A, Shiel F, Reynolds J, VanPraagh R. Double outlet right ventricle—anatomic types and developmental implications based on a study of 101 autopsied cases. *Coeur.* 1982;13(4):389-440.

178. Braun K, De Vries A, Feingold DS, Ehrenfeld NE, Feldman J, Schorr S. Complete dextroposition of the aorta, pulmonary stenosis, interventricular septal defect, and patent foramen ovale. *Am Heart J.* 1952;43(5):773-780.

179. Witham AC. Double outlet right ventricle; a partial transposition complex. *Am Heart J.* 1957;53(6):928-939.

180. Obler D, Juraszek AL, Smoot LB, Natowicz MR. Double outlet right ventricle: aetiologies and associations. *J Med Genet.* 2008;45(8):481-497.

181. Bradshaw L, et al. Dual role for neural crest cells during outflow tract septation in the neural crest-deficient mutant Splotch2H. *J Anat.* (2009) 214: 245-257. doi: 10.1111/j.1469-7580.2008.01028.x.

182. Sridaromont S, Ritter D, Feldt R, Davis G, Edwards J. Double-outlet right ventricle. Anatomic and angiocardiographic correlations. *Mayo Clin Proc.* 1978;53(9):555-577.

183. Walters HL, Mavroudis C, Tchervenkov CI, Jacobs JP, Lacour-Gayet F, Jacobs ML. Congenital Heart Surgery Nomenclature and Database Project: double outlet right ventricle. *Ann Thorac Surg.* 2000;69(4 Suppl):S249-S263.

184. Van Praagh R. What is the Taussig-Bing malformation? *Circulation.* 1968;38(3):445-449.

185. Neufeld HN, Lucas RV, Lester RG, Adams P, Anderson RC, Edwards JE. Origin of both great vessels from the right ventricle without pulmonary stenosis. *Br Heart J.* 1962;24(4):393-408.

186. Lev M, Bharati S, Meng CC, Liberthson RR, Paul MH, Idriss F. A concept of double-outlet right ventricle. *J Thorac Cardiovasc Surg.* 1972;64(2):271-281.

187. Yim D, Dragulescu A, Ide H, et al. Essential modifiers of double outlet right ventricle. *Circ Cardiovasc Imaging.* 2018;11(3):e006891.

188. Lecompte Y, Batisse A, Di Carlo D. Double-outlet right ventricle: a surgical synthesis. *Adv Card Surg.* 1993;4:109-136.

189. Ettinger PO, Weisse AB, Khan MI, Levinson GE. Double-outlet right ventricle in an adult with aortic regurgitation. *Am J Med.* 1969;47(5):818-824.

190. Mahle WT, Martinez R, Silverman N, Cohen MS, Anderson RH. Anatomy, echocardiography, and surgical approach to double outlet right ventricle. *Cardiol Young.* 2008;18 (Suppl 3):39-51.

191. Holmström H, Bjørnstad PG, Smevik B, Lindberg H. Balloon dilatation of pulmonary artery banding: Norwegian experience over more than 20 years. *Eur Heart J.* 2012;33(1):61-66.

192. Kirklin JW, Harp RA, McGoon DC. Surgical treatment of origin of both vessels from right ventricle, including cases of pulmonary stenosis. *J Thorac Cardiovasc Surg.* 1964;48(6):1026-1036.

193. Kawashima Y, Fujita T, Miyamoto T, Manabe H. Intraventricular rerouting of blood for the correction of Taussig-Bing malformation. *J Thorac Cardiovasc Surg.* 1971;62(5):825-829.

194. Rastelli GC. A new approach to "anatomic" repair of transposition of the great arteries. *Mayo Clin Proc.* 1969;44(1):1-12.

195. Bradley TJ, Karamlou T, Kulik A, et al. Determinants of repair type, reintervention, and mortality in 393 children with double-outlet right ventricle. *J Thorac Cardiovasc Surg.* 2007;134(4):967-973.e6.

196. Hazekamp MG, Nevvazhay T, Sojak V. Nikaidoh vs Réparation à l'Etage Ventriculaire vs Rastelli. *Sem Thorac Cardiovasc Surg.* 2018;21:58-63.

197. Lacour-Gayet F, Haun C, Ntalakoura K, et al. Biventricular repair of double outlet right ventricle with non-committed ventricular septal defect (VSD) by VSD rerouting to the pulmonary artery and arterial switch. *Eur J Cardiothorac Surg.* 2002;21(6):1042-1048.

198. Barbero-Marcial M, Tanamati C, Atik E, Ebaid M. Intraventricular repair of double-outlet right ventricle with noncommitted ventricular septal defect: advantages of multiple patches. *J Thorac Cardiovasc Surg.* 1999;118(6):1056-1067.

199. Oladunjoye O, Piekarski B, Baird C, et al. Repair of double outlet right ventricle: Midterm outcomes. *J Thorac Cardiovasc Surg.* 2020;159(1):254-264.

200. Li S, Ma K, Hu S, et al. Surgical outcomes of 380 patients with double outlet right ventricle who underwent biventricular repair. *J Thorac Cardiovasc Surg.* 2014;148(3):817-824.

201. Artrip JH, Sauer H, Campbell DN, et al. Biventricular repair in double outlet right ventricle: surgical results based on the STS-EACTS International Nomenclature classification. *Eur J Cardio-Thorac Surg.* 2006;29(4):545-550.

202. Brown JW, Ruzmetov M, Okada Y, Vijay P, Turrentine MW. Surgical results in patients with double outlet right ventricle: a 20-year experience. *Ann Thorac Surg.* 2001;72(5):1630-1635.

203. Villemain O, Belli E, Ladouceur M, et al. Impact of anatomic characteristics and initial biventricular surgical strategy on outcomes in various forms of double-outlet right ventricle. *J Thorac Cardiovasc Surg.* 2016;152(3):698-706.e3.

204. Kreutzer C, De Vive J, Oppido G, et al. Twenty-five-year experience with Rastelli repair for transposition of the great arteries. *J Thorac Cardiovasc Surg.* 2000;120(2):211-223.

205. Belli E, Serraf A, Lacour-Gayet F, et al. Surgical treatment of subaortic stenosis after biventricular repair of double-outlet right ventricle. *J Thorac Cardiovasc Surg.* 1996;112(6):1570-1578; discussion 1578-1580.

206. Hörer J, Schreiber C, Dworak E, et al. Long-term results after the Rastelli repair for transposition of the great arteries. *Ann Thorac Surg.* 2007;83(6):2169-2175.

207. Brown JW, Ruzmetov M, Huynh D, Rodefeld MD, Turrentine MW, Fiore AC. Rastelli operation for transposition of the great arteries with ventricular septal defect and pulmonary stenosis. *Ann Thorac Surg.* 2011;91(1):188-193; discussion 193-194.

208. Ong K, Boone R, Gao M, et al. Right ventricle to pulmonary artery conduit reoperations in patients with tetralogy of fallot or pulmonary atresia associated with ventricular septal defect. *Am J Cardiol.* 2013;111(11):1638-1643.

209. Mainwaring RD, Patrick WL, Punn R, Palmon M, Reddy VM, Hanley FL. Fate of right ventricle to pulmonary artery conduits after complete repair of pulmonary atresia and major aortopulmonary collaterals. *Ann Thorac Surg.* 2015;99(5):1685-1691.

210. Vogt P, Carrel T, Pasic M, Arbenz U, Vonsegesser L, Turina M. Early and late results after correction for double-outlet right ventricle: uni- and multivariate analysis of risk factors. *Eur J Cardio-Thorac Surg.* 1994;8(6):301-307.

211. Shen WK, Holmes DR, Porter CJ, McGoon DC, Ilstrup DM. Sudden death after repair of double-outlet right ventricle. *Circulation.* 1990;81(1):128-136.

212. Haas F, Wottke M, Poppert H, Meisner H. Long-term survival and functional follow-up in patients after the arterial switch operation. *Ann Thorac Surg.* 1999;68(5):1692-1697.

213. Regitz-Zagrosek V, Roos-Hesselink JW, Bauersachs J, Blomström-Lundqvist C, Cífková R, De Bonis M, et al. 2018 ESC Guidelines for the management of cardiovascular diseases during pregnancy. *Eur Heart J.* 2018;39(34):3165-3241.

214. Drenthen W, Pieper PG, van der Tuuk K, et al. Fertility, pregnancy and delivery in women after biventricular repair for double outlet right ventricle. *Cardiology.* 2008;109(2):105-109.

68

Left Heart Obstructive Lesions

Jennifer Cohen, David Ezon, Kenan Stern, and Ali N. Zaidi

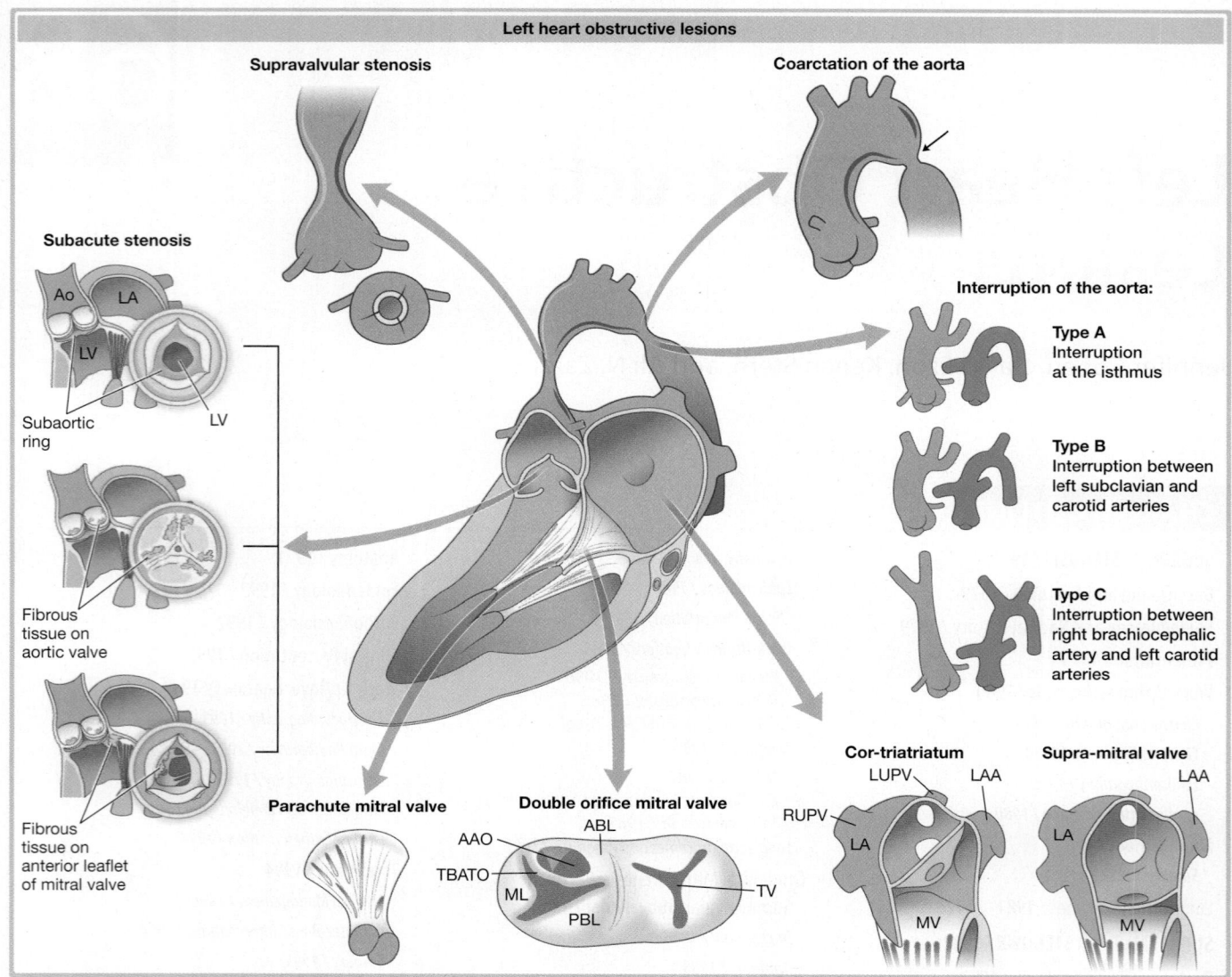

Chapter 68 Fuster and Hurst's Central Illustration. Congenital left heart obstructive lesions are a series of anatomic stenotic lesions from the left atrium extending to the descending portion of the aortic arch. AAO, anterior accessory orifice; ABL, anterior bridging leaflet; Ao, aorta; LA, left atrium; LAA, left atrial appendage; LUPV, left upper pulmonary vein; ML, mural leaflet; MV, mitral valve; PBL, posterior bridging leaflet; RUPV, right upper pulmonary vein; TBATO, tissue bridge between accessory and true orifices; TV, tricuspid valve.

CHAPTER SUMMARY

This chapter describes the presentation, diagnosis, and management of congenital left heart obstructive lesions, a series of anatomic stenotic lesions from the left atrium extending to the descending thoracic aorta (see Fuster and Hurst's Central Illustration). Obstruction may be in the left atrium, at the level of the aortic or mitral valve (subvalvar, valvar, or supravalvar), in the ascending aorta, transverse aortic arch, or in the descending thoracic aorta. These left heart obstructive lesions may present either in isolation or in association with other left-sided lesions. Based on their location, these lesions may cause impairment in valvular function (either aortic or mitral) or may impose increased afterload on the left ventricle and, if severe and untreated, may result in hypertrophy and dysfunction of the left ventricle. Cardiac imaging is essential for diagnosis, management, and long-term follow-up, and it increasingly plays a role in understanding the physiologic changes of left-sided obstructive lesions and the timing for intervention. Treatment is based on the underlying left heart obstructive lesion and may involve either transcatheter or directed surgical repair.

SUBAORTIC STENOSIS

Background and Anatomy

Subaortic stenosis is defined as narrowing of the left ventricular outflow tract. It results in 8% to 20% of left ventricular outflow obstruction.[1,2] It is discrete in 90% of cases. In the remainder, the left ventricular outflow tract is diffusely hypoplastic and tunnel-shaped.[3] In discrete forms, the membrane can be circular or crescent-shaped, and usually made of a nondistensible fibromuscular shelf. The membrane may encroach onto the underside of the aortic valve or the ventricular aspect of the anterior mitral valve leaflet, causing leaflet distortion and secondary regurgitation[4] (**Figs. 68–1** and **68–2**).

The etiology of subaortic stenosis is uncertain. Some have proposed that it is related to incomplete absorption of the subaortic infundibulum,[5] but this is less likely given that it is usually not present in infants. There may be an underlying genetic association given that it can cluster in families.[6] Most likely, the cause is related to change in the flow dynamics of the left ventricular outflow tract. Subaortic membranes are associated with steeper aorto-septal angles, the angle between the plane of the interventricular septum, and midline of the aortic valve. Kleinert et al. found that 68% of patients with subaortic stenosis had an aorto-septal angle less than 135 degrees, compared to 11% in normal controls.[7,8] The angle may cause turbulence in the outflow tract that causes reactive changes in the myocardium due to altered septal shear stress, which in turn causes local cell proliferation that results in the subaortic membrane.

Histologic analysis has found signs of inflammation consistent with this.[7] Subaortic membranes are associated with history of membranous ventricular septal defects (VSDs),[8,9] which may be due to slight malalignments associated with the VSD.[10] Common atrioventricular canal is also associated with left ventricular outflow obstruction, attributed to the gooseneck deformity (elongation of the outflow tract), caused by anterior deviation of the aortic valve that occurs in common atrioventricular canals.[11]

Epidemiology and Natural History

Subvalvular aortic stenosis (SAS) is a rare disorder seen in infants and newborns but is the second most common type of aortic stenosis. It is responsible for approximately 1% of all congenital heart defects (8 in 10,000 births) and 15% to 20% of all fixed left ventricular outflow tract obstructive lesions. Ten percent to 14% of subvalvar AS is observed amongst children with congenital aortic stenosis.[10,12] It is more common in males and is responsible for 65% to 75% of cases,[12] with a male to female ratio of 2:1. The prevalence of SAS is 6.5% of all the adult congenital heart diseases. The course of SAS is gradual. It is rarely an isolated presentation. Subaortic stenosis is associated with congenital heart defects including a VSD, patent ductus arteriosus, coarctation of the aorta, bicuspid aortic valve, abnormal left ventricular papillary muscle, atrioventricular septal defect (AVSD), among others. In the majority of the patients, SAS is incidentally found when evaluating patients for other congenital heart defects.

Presentation

Subaortic stenosis is usually detected at birth while working up the infant for another congenital heart disorder. Most infants are asymptomatic at birth or may have a murmur during evaluation. Among infants who are symptomatic, dyspnea on exertion, angina, effort syncope and presyncope, orthopnea, and sudden cardiac death are commonly observed. Heart failure may be seen in infants with severe obstruction of the left ventricular outflow tract. Exertional dyspnea is the most common symptom seen in 40% of symptomatic patients, and it reflects pulmonary venous hypertension that is induced by an increase in left ventricular filling pressure caused by the impaired diastolic compliance of the hypertrophied left ventricle.

Most patients present by 10 years of age, although it is rare in the newborn period.[4,13] Most patients are initially asymptomatic. However, in one study of patients at a mean of 13 years of age, 54% had New York Heart Association (NYHA) class II or III heart failure symptoms, with symptoms including dyspnea, chest pain, syncope, and palpitations.[14] On exam, patients may have a systolic ejection murmur at the left mid-sternal border that radiates to the upper sternal border and supraclavicular notch, as well as a hyperdynamic left ventricular impulse. A diastolic murmur may indicate the presence of aortic or mitral regurgitation, while a systolic click may indicate valvar aortic stenosis. Patients are at significant risk for infective endocarditis, affecting up to 14% of patients, with higher pressure gradient and worse aortic regurgitation likely risk factors.[15]

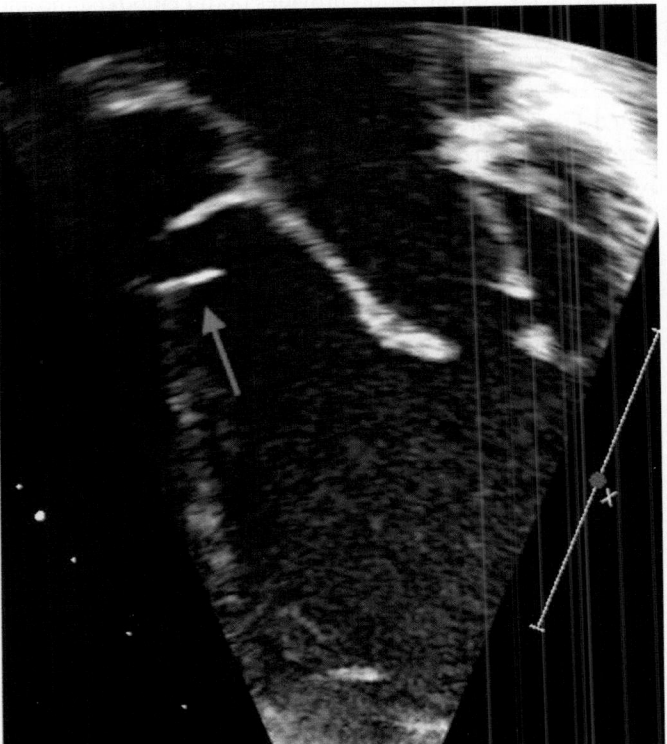

Figure 68–1. Transthoracic echocardiography: apical five chamber image. Discrete subaortic membrane noted in the left ventricular outflow tract (*see arrow*).

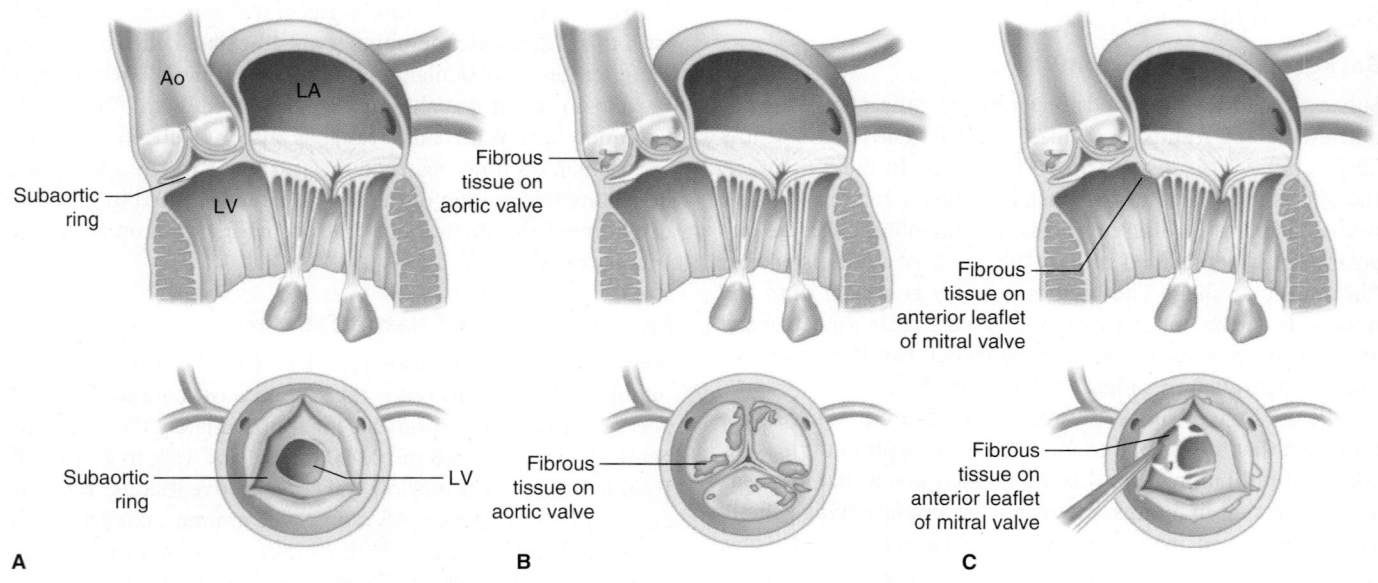

Figure 68–2. Subaortic stenosis: different presentations. (**A**) Isolated geometry. (**B**) Involvement with the aortic valve. (**C**) Involvement with the mitral valve.

Work-Up/Investigations

Electrocardiography

An electrocardiogram (ECG) reveals a varying degree of left ventricular hypertrophy in 50% to 80% of patients. The presence of a prominent Q wave in the left precordial leads may indicate septal hypertrophy. ECG findings may be normal in patients with severe SAS.

Chest Radiography

The chest radiograph is often normal. Some patients, including those with mild stenosis, have mild cardiomegaly or left ventricular prominence.

Echocardiography

Echocardiography is important for assessing the nature of the obstruction as well as associated anomalies, including bicuspid aortic valve, coarctation of the aorta, and a patent ductus arteriosus.[16,17] A distance between the membrane and the aortic valve of ≥8 mm/m², indexed to body surface area, may be associated with increased risk of mitral regurgitation.[5] This may be due to the subaortic membrane tethering the anterior mitral valve leaflet, causing a tenting distortion (**Fig. 68–3**). The distance of the membrane from the aortic valve is also important to assess the risk of significant obstruction to flow and significant aortic valve regurgitation. In one study, a membrane greater than 12 mm from the aortic valve was associated with more than moderate regurgitation, as opposed to those less than 6 mm from the valve.[18] Membranes that are closer to the aortic valve may be associated with greater risk of progressive obstruction.[13] The pressure gradient at diagnosis is important. In one study, a higher left ventricular outflow tract gradient was associated with an increased risk of aortic regurgitation, faster progression of aortic regurgitation, and faster progression of outflow tract obstruction.[13] A peak gradient of greater than 50 mm Hg at age >17 years at diagnosis predicted development of moderate or greater aortic regurgitation.[18]

Cardiac Catheterization

Cardiac catheterization is not routinely indicated in isolated SAS. If multiple levels of obstruction are suspected, it is frequently performed to interpret the degree of subaortic obstruction further. Catheterization provides both hemodynamic and anatomic data, such as the measurement of cardiac output, the gradient across the left ventricular outflow tract, the aortic valve, and estimates of the degree of aortic regurgitation. Associated lesions, such as aortic coarctation, may be evaluated. Cardiac catheterization is often used as part of a preoperative workup to rule out significant coronary artery disease in adult patients who are being evaluated for surgical repair.

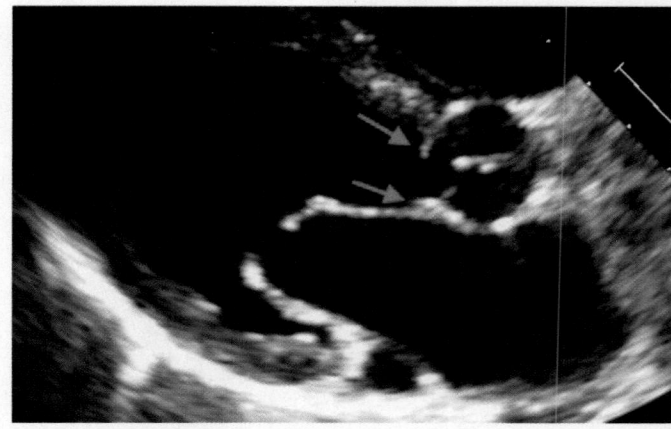

Figure 68–3. Transthoracic echocardiography: parasternal long axis view. Circumferential discrete subaortic membrane noted (*see arrow*). Note the membrane is attached to both the anterior left ventricular outflow tract and the mitral valve.

Management

Surgery

Since most pediatric patients are asymptomatic, medical therapy has no role in the treatment of SAS. As it is progressive, intervention is needed at some point to relieve the left ventricular outflow tract obstruction. Surgical correction of the obstruction is the definitive therapy for SAS. This may range from simple removal of the membrane to extensive ring resection, with or without myectomy. However, if the patient develops heart failure or clinically significant left ventricular dysfunction, the patient is started on medical treatment until the surgery can be performed (**Table 68–1**).

One of the most difficult aspects of caring for persons with subaortic stenosis is predicting whether the degree of stenosis will progress. There is some data that prognosis is worse for children than adults.[17] True indications for surgery based on pressure gradient are unclear. It is also unclear if early repair prevents aortic regurgitation.[17] Higher mean pressure gradient at diagnosis, faster rate of change in pressure gradient, longer left ventricular ejection time, larger aortic valve annulus z-score, smaller mitral valve annulus z-score, and smaller body surface area are some reasons to consider repair.[19] Mean left ventricular outflow tract gradient progressed more quickly if the initial gradient was >30 mm Hg, there was associated aortic valve thickening, or there was membrane attachment to the mitral valve, while those with a gradient of <30 mm Hg

remained low at a mean of 9 years follow up. Bezold et al. created a prediction score to determine the risk of intervention.[20] Shorter distance between the membrane and the valve, indexed to body surface area, was associated with progression. Most nonprogressive membranes were circumferential, thin, mobile folds, or flat, fibrous ridges near the lower margin of a VSD. Most progressive membranes were thicker, less mobile, and protruded further into the outflow tract.

Surgical approach for discrete subaortic membranes usually occurs via an aortotomy extending into the noncoronary sinus. The membrane is then resected, avoiding the conduction system. One open question remains whether to perform a myomectomy concurrently.[21] The risk of a myomectomy includes complete heart block and creation of a VSD.

Long-Term Outcomes

Overall outcomes for subaortic membrane resection are good, although data is limited. Operative mortality is low.[13] In one study, at 15 years postoperation, survival was 95% and freedom from reoperation was 85%, which is similar to other reports.[22] Surgery can adequately reduce the left ventricular outflow tract gradient and symptoms over the short term.[23-25] In one study, 66% of patients had a recurrent gradient at a mean of 3.5 years follow-up.[16] Twenty-three percent of patients required reoperation at a mean of 12 years follow-up. Also, 72% of patients had at least mild aortic regurgitation at a mean of 17 years follow-up.

TABLE 68–1. Guideline Comparison Table for Subaortic Stenosis

			Subaortic Stenosis: 2018 AHA/ACC Guidelines for ACHD	
COR	**LOE**	**Diagnostic**	**Therapeutic**	
I	C-EO		1. Surgical intervention is recommended for adults with subAS, a maximum gradient 50 mm Hg or more and symptoms attributable to the subAS.	
I	C-LD		1. Surgical intervention is recommended for adults with subAS and less than 50 mm Hg maximum gradient and HF or ischemic symptoms, and/or LV systolic dysfunction attributable to subAS	
IIb	C-LD	1. Stress testing for adults with LVOT obstruction to determine exercise capacity, symptoms, electrocardiographic changes, or arrhythmias may be reasonable in the presence of otherwise equivocal indications for intervention	1. To prevent the progression of AR, surgical intervention may be considered for asymptomatic adults with subAS and at least mild AR and a maximum gradient of 50 mm Hg or more	
		Subaortic Stenosis: 2020 ESC Guidelines for ACHD		
COR	**LOE**	**Therapeutic**		
I	C	In symptomatic patients (spontaneous or on exercise test) with a mean Doppler gradient ≥40 mmHg or severe AR, surgery is recommended.		
IIa	C	Asymptomatic patients should be considered for surgery when one or more of the following findings are present: • Mean gradient <40 mm Hg but LVEF <50%. • AR is severe and LVESD >50 mm (or 25 mm/m² BSA) and/or EF <50%d. • Mean Doppler gradient is ≥40 mm Hg and marked LVH present. • Mean Doppler gradient is ≥40 mm Hg and there is a fall in blood pressure below baseline on exercise.		
IIb	C	Asymptomatic patients may be considered for surgery when one or more of the following findings are present: • Mean Doppler gradient is ≥40 mm Hg, LV is normal (EF >50% and no LVH), exercise testing is normal, and surgical risk is low. • Progression of AR is documented and AR becomes more than mild (to prevent further progression).		

Abbreviations: AR, aortic regurgitation; BSA, body surface area; EF, ejection fraction; LV, left ventricle/ventricular; LVEF, left ventricular ejection fraction; LVESD, left ventricular end systolic diameter; LVH, left ventricular hypertrophy.

There is mixed data on whether myomectomy reduces the risk of needing a reoperation, although recent studies have not found a difference.[26-28] Risk for reoperation include a membrane that was less than 7 mm from the aortic valve, a peak gradient at surgery of greater than 60 mm Hg, involvement of the mitral valve, and younger age at resection.[23] Most of these surgeries occurred within 10 years of the initial intervention.[29] In one large meta-analysis, higher pressure gradient and the presence of aortic regurgitation were the strongest predictors of worse outcome.[13]

SUPRAVALVULAR STENOSIS

Background and Anatomy

Supravalvar aortic stenosis (AS) is narrowing of the aortic sinotubular junction, at times extending into the ascending aorta and aortic arch branches.[30] It is usually discrete, forming an hourglass at the sinotubular junction, but by some reports, it is diffuse in up to one-third of patients.[31] It can be congenital, naturally acquired, or iatrogenic. It is considered the rarest form of left ventricular outflow obstruction. Among children with congenital AS, supravalvar AS has accounted for 8% to 14% of cases.[12,32] There are at least two anatomic forms of supravalvar AS, with the majority of patients having an hourglass deformity, consisting of a discrete constriction of a thickened ascending aorta at the superior aspect of the sinuses of Valsalva.[33] The second variation of supravalvular AS is the more diffuse narrowing over a variable distance along the ascending aorta, which is seen in 25% to 40% (**Fig. 68–4**). There are also reports of a discrete membrane, which may be a variant of the hourglass deformity, but is extremely rare. The major histologic feature of the ascending aorta in supravalvar AS is a thickened and dysplastic media with an increased number of hypertrophied smooth muscle cells, increased collagen content, and a paucity

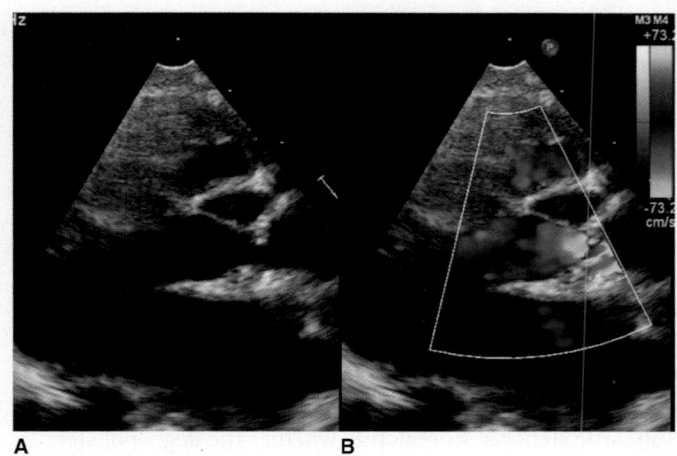

Figure 68–5. Transthoracic echocardiography: parasternal long axis view. **(A)** Supravlavar aortic stenosis with associated tethering of the aortic valve leaflet to the sinotubular junction. **(B)** Same image with color flow Doppler with aliasing at the site of the supravalvular stenosis.

of elastic tissue with disorganized elastin fibers.[30] The aortic valve leaflets may be thickened, redundant, and have reduced mobility. Rarely, the aortic valve leaflets were partially adherent to the stenosing supravalvar ridge in more than one-half of patients (**Fig. 68–5**). Coronary artery stenosis has also been described due to focal or diffuse coronary narrowing or due to obstruction by redundant, dysplastic aortic valve leaflets.[34] Rarely, coarctation of the aorta and ostial stenoses of the carotid, renal, iliac, and other peripheral arteries are seen in some patients. In patients who have supravalvular AS, concomitant pulmonary artery stenoses, either of the main pulmonary artery or of branch pulmonary arteries, has also been described and occurs in approximately one-half of patients, which tends to decrease over time.[35]

Etiology

Congenital supravalvar AS has been associated with several genetic mutations in the *ELN* gene that codes for Elastin synthesis at chromosome 7q11.23. The mutation is usually due to a point mutation or microdeletion, and can occur sporadically or may be inherited in an autosomal dominant manner.[36] It can occur in isolation, but frequently occurs as part of Williams syndrome, which is associated with developmental delay, elfin facies, and short stature, among other findings.[37] Studies report between 45% and 70% of Williams syndrome patients have supravalvar AS.[7,38] The phenotype can vary considerably in patients with *ELN* mutations, from asymptomatic to infantile mortality.[39] These patients with Williams syndrome can have supravalvar AS as the most common lesion, followed by pulmonary stenosis and then coarctation or aortic arch hypoplasia.[39] Supravalvular AS can also be present in a familial form without features of Williams syndrome, inherited in an autosomal dominant pattern.[39] Rarely, sporadic patients can have supravalvular AS without a family history. In adults, homozygous familial hypercholesterolemia (FH), a rare autosomal dominant disorder, has been described with supravalvar

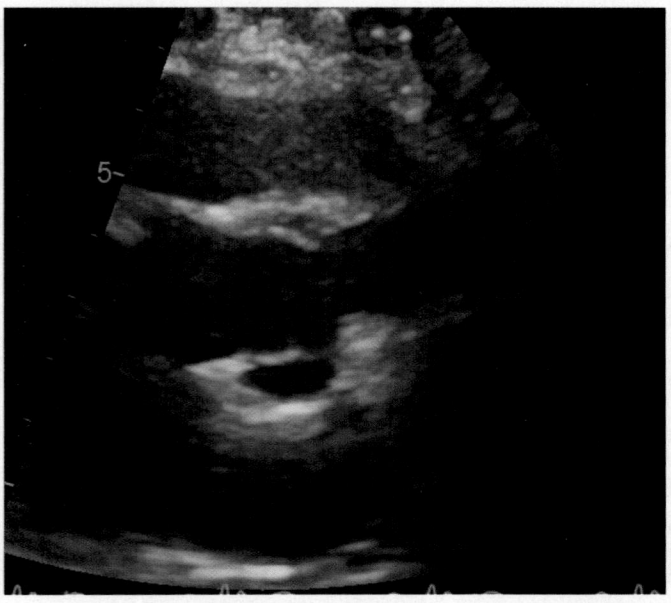

Figure 68–4. Transthoracic echocardiography: parasternal long axis view: Note the hourglass narrowing at the sinotubular junction.

AS.[40] It is not clear whether the lesion is solely a manifestation of aortic atherosclerosis or whether an underlying structural abnormality is present. Iatrogenic supravalvar AS can occur after any surgery involving the aortic root or ascending aorta, including heart transplantation, arterial switch for repair of transposition of the great arteries, aortic dissection repair, and cannulation of the aorta for cardiopulmonary bypass, although these are uncommon.[41,42]

Pathophysiology

The natural history of supravalvar AS is progressive obstruction.[43] Diffuse hypoplasia and multifocal stenosis are associated with worse outcome.[44] The physiology of supravalvar AS is similar to that of valvar and subvalvar stenosis. Significant obstruction is associated with a hyperdynamic, hypertrophied left ventricle. There is also raised systolic pressure in the aortic root that may be responsible for the associated coronary artery enlargement and dilatation of the sinuses of Valsalva.[45] As noted, coronary artery stenosis can occur, and subendocardial ischemic changes may be seen even without coronary narrowing. In some patients, the supravalvar AS creates a systolic jet that hugs the aortic wall and transfers kinetic energy into the right innominate artery. This phenomenon, known as the Coanda effect, is the mechanism that explains higher blood pressure in the right than left arm in most patients with this disorder. Congenital supravalvar AS should be considered a generalized disorder, not simply a disorder of the aorta, because it is associated with stenoses throughout the body, including the main and peripheral pulmonary arteries. Coronary artery anomalies may occur in more than 25% of patients,[10] and include ostial obstruction by aortic valve leaflet and sinotubular junction tissue, ostial stenosis, and fibrodysplasia of the coronary artery. Aortic valve leaflet abnormalities have been reported in up to one-half of affected patients by surgical inspection, and may adhere to the sinotubular junction.[46] It has been proposed that valvar disease may occur as a result of poor distention of the aortic root during systole. In normal hearts, systolic expansion of the root and sinotubular junction allow the aortic valve leaflets to fully straighten, evenly distributing strain across the leaflet. This is reduced in the setting of supravalvar stenosis, leading to early degeneration of the leaflets.[30] Persons with Williams syndrome have associated abnormalities in the vertebral circulation, descending aorta, and renal arteries as well. Strokes related to intracranial coronary artery stenosis have been reported.[46] Systemic hypertension may be seen in patients with supravalvar AS. This is attributed to poor distensibility of the systemic vascular bed, but may also be due to renal artery stenosis.[36]

Clinical Presentation

The clinical features of patients with supravalvar AS vary depending on whether or not the child also has Williams syndrome. Patients with Williams syndrome may have a number of abnormalities in addition to supravalvar AS including intellectual disability, hypercalcemia, renovascular hypertension, facial abnormalities, and short stature. Patients with Williams syndrome have an increased risk of sudden cardiac death, particularly those with biventricular outflow tract obstruction, although sudden cardiac death may occur even in the absence of outflow tract obstruction. Some deaths have been attributed to undiagnosed coronary artery ostial obstruction. Cardiac repolarization abnormalities with prolongation of the QT interval has also been described in a small percentage of patients with Williams syndrome.[47] In patients with familial or sporadic disease, supravalvar AS is usually the only abnormality. Prolonged QTc does not appear to occur in those with nonsyndromic supravalvar AS.[48] Persons with Williams syndrome have a risk of sudden death that is 1 per 1000 patient years, 100 times the risk of the general population.[49] This is attributed to the combination of left ventricular hypertrophy and coronary artery obstruction caused by exposure to high pressure in the sinus of Valsalva. In light of this, early surgical repair should be considered if there is significant obstruction. Regardless, administration of drugs that may decrease systemic vascular resistance including those for moderate sedation or general anesthesia should be given with caution given the risk of coronary insufficiency and sudden death in this patient population.[50]

Work-Up/Investigations

Electrocardiography

The ECG shows left ventricular hypertrophy, which may be accompanied by a strain pattern. Occasionally, the ECG may show right ventricular hypertrophy in patients with significant pulmonary artery obstruction due to peripheral pulmonary artery stenosis.

Echocardiography

The mainstay for the diagnosis of supravalvular AS is echocardiography, which also is able to assess the ventricle function, degree of left ventricular hypertrophy, estimate the pressure gradient across the obstruction, and the status of the aortic valve.[51] Magnetic resonance imaging (MRI) with angiography also provides excellent anatomic detail of supravalvular aortic obstruction, together with associated aortic branch vessel disease, if present. MRI is often utilized in adult patients with concerns for supravalvular AS, when the acoustic windows are poor, or when physical examination or other findings suggest associated lesions of the great vessels. The chest radiograph typically is normal, although some patients have mild-to-moderate cardiomegaly.

Cardiac Catheterization

Cardiac catheterization provides precise hemodynamic and angiographic evaluation but is not routinely necessary due to the advancements with echocardiography and cross-sectional imaging. Cardiac magnetic resonance (CMR) can also be used in assessing the coronary ostia. Electrocardiographic-gated coronary computed tomography angiography (CTA) or invasive selective coronary angiography on cardiac catheterization provides excellent visualization of the coronary arterial anatomy if needed.[52]

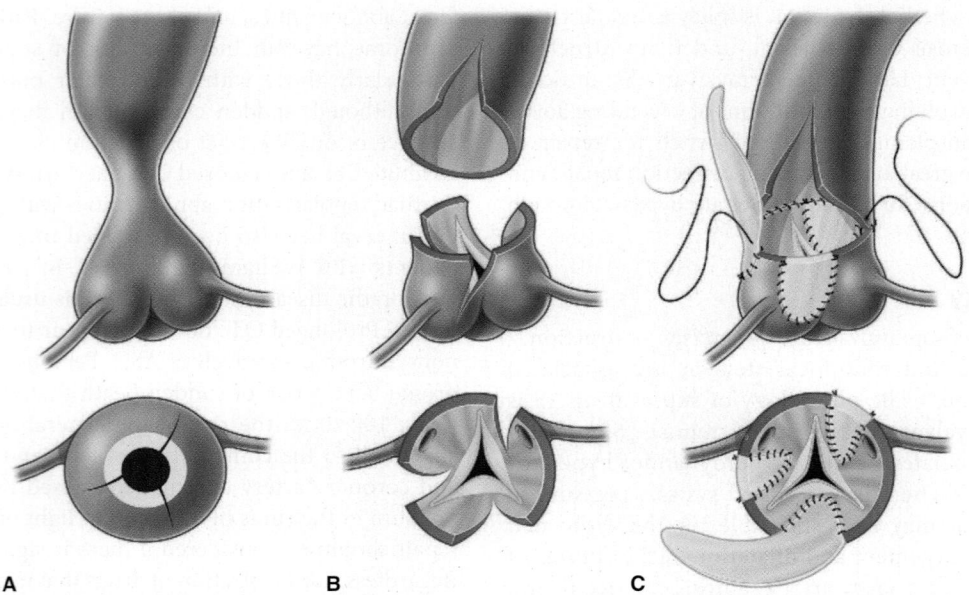

Figure 68–6. Supravalvular stenosis: extended three-patch supravalvular aortic stenosis repair. (**A and B**) The ascending aorta is transected at its narrowest point, and three incisions are extended into the sinuses of Valsalva. (**C**) The sinuses are enlarged with three pericardial patches, and the patch from the non-coronary sinus is extended into the ascending aorta to ensure symmetrical enlargement of the narrow segment.

Management

Surgery

The definitive management for supravalvar AS, whether discrete or diffuse, consists of surgical correction of the obstruction (**Fig. 68–6**). Stent placement has been reported in a few patients, with mixed results and is not routinely utilized (**Table 68–2**). Specific indications to operate for less than moderate obstruction are lacking. However, the association of coronary artery obstruction and sudden death should be considered when weighing the benefits of intervention. The primary goals of surgical correction are enlarging the sinotubular junction, along with any downstream obstruction if diffuse hypoplasia is present, and addressing any coronary narrowing. Originally, it was repaired with a single-patch technique using a diamond shaped patch inserted at the noncoronary sinus of Valsalva. Subsequent approaches include the Doty patch, which consists of inserting an inverted Y-shaped patch across the sinotubular junction near the noncoronary and right coronary sinuses of

TABLE 68–2. Guideline Comparison Table for Supravalvular Aortic Stenosis			
Supravalvular Aortic Stenosis: 2018 AHA/ACC Guidelines for ACHD			
COR	**LOE**	**Diagnostic**	**Therapeutic**
I	C-LD	1. Aortic imaging using TTE, TEE, CMR, or CTA is recommended in adults with Williams syndrome or patients suspected of having supravalvular aortic stenosis 2. Coronary imaging is recommended in patients with Williams syndrome and supravalvular aortic stenosis presenting with symptoms of coronary ischemia	1. Surgical repair is recommended for adults with supravalvular aortic stenosis (discrete or diffuse) and symptoms or decreased LV systolic function deemed secondary to aortic obstruction 2. Coronary artery revascularization is recommended in symptomatic adults with supravalvular aortic stenosis and coronary ostial stenosis
Supravalvular Aortic Stenosis: 2020 ESC Guidelines for ACHD			
COR	**LOE**	**Therapeutic**	
I	C	1. In patients with symptoms (spontaneous or on exercise test) and mean Doppler gradient ≥40 mm Hg, surgery is recommended. 2. In patients with mean Doppler gradient <40 mm Hg, surgery is recommended when one or more of the following findings are present: • Symptoms attributable to obstruction (exertional dyspnea, angina, syncope). • LV systolic dysfunction (EF <50% without other explanation). • Surgery required for significant CAD or valvular disease.	
IIb	C	1. Patients with ≥40 mm Hg but without symptoms, LV systolic dysfunction, LVH, or abnormal exercise test may be considered for repair when the surgical risk is low.	

Abbreviations: CAD, coronary artery disease; EF, ejection fraction; LV, left ventricle/ventricular; LVH, left ventricular hypertrophy.

Valsalva to achieve symmetric enlargement of the root. Other approaches include augmenting each of the three sinuses of Valsalva.[53] In the Brom technique, the aorta is transected above the sinotubular junction, and then each of the sinuses are incised longitudinally, and a patch placed in each of the incisions before the aorta is re-anastomosed. In a similar technique, the aorta is cut to create three flaps that are inserted into each sinus of Valsalva to enlarge them.[54] Surgery in supravalvar AS usually is performed at gradient levels that are lower than in valvar AS to avoid the progressive obstruction that occurs in some patients.[55] The likelihood of progression varies with the initial gradient. Since surgery is usually curative for the discrete form, surgery is often recommended for symptomatic disease and for patients with a measured gradient at catheterization of more than 30 mm Hg. Flap plasty techniques usually are successful in alleviating the discrete type of stenosis, which, as already noted, accounts most of the cases. Other techniques include simple single patch enlargement into the sinotubular junction just above the aortic root, bifurcated patches extended into two sinuses, and separate three sinus patch enlargement methods.[56] Relief of diffuse obstruction is more complex; surgical options include extensive endarterectomy with patch aortoplasty or resection of the stenotic segment with end-to-end anastomosis to the distal ascending aorta, with or without insertion of a pulmonary autograft (the Ross procedure).

Long-Term Outcomes and Prognosis

Overall outcomes are excellent. Early mortality is low, likely between 3% and 5%.[57,58] A postoperative mean pressure gradient of greater than 40 mm Hg is considered significant, and may occur more frequently with a single-patch technique as compared to a Brom repair.[37] Several studies report good long-term outcomes, with 5-year survival of 94% to 98%, and 20-year survival of 61% to 97%.[58,59] Freedom from reoperation ranged from 0% to 32% depending on the study. Data on whether a single patch technique to one sinus of Valsalva, versus augmenting two or three sinuses is superior is mixed. There are reports of late sudden death after repair. Risk factors for poor outcome include diffuse obstruction, valvar obstruction, higher preoperative gradient, and presence of associated coronary artery anomalies.[59]

MITRAL VALVE DISORDERS

Cor Triatriatum

Background

Cor triatriatum sinister (CTS) is a rare form of congenital heart disease that was first described in 1868 by Church and later named in 1905 by Borst.[60,61] It is a congenital malformation in which a septum divides the left atrium into two chambers: a posterior and superior chamber that drains the pulmonary veins, and an anterior and inferior chamber that is adjacent to the mitral valve (**Fig. 68–7**). Cor triatriatum dexter is persistence of the right valve of the sinus venosus and is even more rare than CTS. It is associated with right-sided heart disease, because blood is redirected from the right ventricle into the

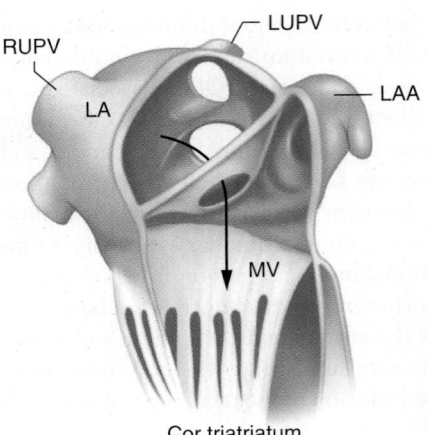

Figure 68–7. Cor triatriatum in relation to the left atrial appendage (LAA).

left atrium by the right valve of the sinus venosus. This chapter section will focus on CTS.

Anatomy

CTS is an abnormal septation in the left atrium. This membrane may be complete, incomplete, or with fenestrations. It divides the left atrium into a posterior pulmonary venous chamber, and an anterior anatomic true left atrial chamber that contains the left atrial appendage (LAA). This anterior chamber also contains the true atrial septum that bears the fossa ovalis. The membrane can vary significantly in shape, ranging from funnel-shaped to bandlike. In most cases, the two chambers communicate through one or more small perforations in the cor triatriatum membrane. Cor triatriatum is distinguished from a supramitral ring (**Fig. 68–8**) in that the LAA is located distal to the membrane (while in a supramitral ring, the LAA is located proximal to the membrane).[62] Atrial septal defects (ASDs) are commonly associated with CTS, with ~50% to 70% of patients having a patent foramen ovale or ASD. The atrial communication can communicate between the right atrium and either the pulmonary venous chamber or true left atrial chamber.[63] Other associated defects include partial or total

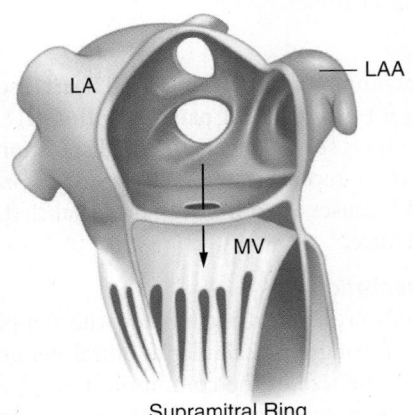

Figure 68–8. Supramitral valve ring in relation to the left atrial appendage (LAA).

anomalous pulmonary venous drainage, found in up to 27% of patients.[64] Cor triatriatum can involve pulmonary veins from only one lung in some cases. Other associated cardiac defects include a patent ductus arteriosus, VSD, persistent left superior vena cava (LSVC) to coronary sinus, and coarctation of the aorta.[63] There are several debated embryonic theories regarding the development of CTS. These include malincorporation, in which the common pulmonary vein fails to fuse normally with the left atrium, malseptation in which abnormal growth of septum primum causes abnormal septation within the left atrium, and the entrapment theory that suggests the left horn of the sinus venosus entraps the common pulmonary vein, which prevents fusion of the common pulmonary vein into the left atrium.[65]

Pathophysiology

The physiology of cor triatriatum depends on the degree of obstruction to flow from the posterior pulmonary venous chamber to the anterior chamber that communicates with the mitral valve. Associated cardiac defects including atrial communications and anomalous pulmonary venous drainage will also impact physiology. Significant obstruction will result in pulmonary venous hypertension with physiology similar to mitral stenosis. Restriction in blood flow from the proximal chamber to the distal chamber results in high pressure in the proximal chamber which is transmitted as high pulmonary venous pressure and manifests as pulmonary edema. High pulmonary venous pressure will then be transmitted through the pulmonary vascular bed resulting in pulmonary capillary and arterial hypertension. This will increase afterload to the right heart that will eventually result in compensatory right ventricular hypertrophy and eventual contractile dysfunction.[66] Initially, this elevated pulmonary pressure is reversible if the inflow restriction is removed, but long-standing increased pressure may lead to irreversible pulmonary vascular changes.[67] CTS can also result in low cardiac output if there is reduced return to the left ventricle due to obstruction through the membrane without an atrial communication to the more anterior chamber. In addition, cyanosis may result from right to left shunting if there is significant obstruction across the membrane with an atrial communication to the more anterior chamber.[68]

Epidemiology

CTS is an uncommon form of congenital heart disease (CHD), representing 0.1% to 0.4% of patients with CHD. It is found equally in either sex. No genetic predisposition had been ascribed until a recent study that described mutations in *HYAL2*, which causes a syndrome of orofacial cleft and CTS in humans and mice.[69]

Clinical Presentation

CTS commonly presents during infancy with symptoms of pulmonary venous congestion, similar to mitral stenosis; however, depending on the size of the communication, it may present later and has been diagnosed at all ages, ranging from infancy to late adulthood.[62] The timing of presentation will depend on the size of the communication between the pulmonary venous

chamber and true atrial chamber, as well as the presence of an ASD and other associated cardiac lesions.

Symptoms of pulmonary edema may be present on history and in younger children often manifest as shortness of breath, feeding intolerance, failure to thrive, and frequent respiratory infections. Patients can also present with cyanosis depending on the presence of atrial communications and degree of obstruction. Clinical symptoms in adults may include exertional dyspnea, orthopnea, and hemoptysis. Adult patients may also present with palpitations, presyncope, syncope, or transient ischemic attacks in the setting of associated atrial arrhythmias.[69,70] Symptoms may be exaggerated during pregnancy and in the postpartum period.[71] If pulmonary hypertension is present, this may manifest as a loud pulmonary component of the second heart sound, right ventricular heave, and pulmonary systolic ejection click. Right heart failure may present with hepatomegaly and jugular venous distention (particularly in adult patients). A diastolic murmur may be detected in the mitral area. Reduced return to the left ventricle may give rise to signs of low cardiac output. Cyanosis may be present depending on exact anatomy.

Work-Up/Investigations

Electrocardiography: ECG findings are nonspecific in cor triatriatum. These can range from atrial fibrillation and no specific P-wave changes to right axis deviation due to pulmonary congestion and right ventricular hypertrophy.

Echocardiography: Echocardiogram is often the modality used for diagnosis of cor triatriatum. Diagnosis on two-dimensional (2D) transthoracic echocardiography (TTE) is often best demonstrated in apical views in which a curvilinear membrane in the midportion of the left atrium is seen (**Fig. 68–9**). The membrane is often thin and may move in response to changes in atrial pressures. The membrane is also well seen in parasternal long-axis views as a vertical linear structure within the left atrium, perpendicular to the ascending aorta. Color Doppler imaging will demonstrate the flow across any opening in the membranes which will be turbulent diastolic flow. Continuous wave Doppler mean gradient is used for grading the severity of the obstruction. It is important to assess the relationship of the LAA to the membrane, which is often most easily seen in parasternal short-axis views. The presence and location of atrial communications should be carefully examined, in addition to assessment of connections of all four pulmonary veins. Associated lesions should be assessed, in particular assessment for a left-sided superior vena cava and examination of the aortic arch. Careful assessment of right ventricular pressure is also necessary, in addition to an assessment of right ventricular function and presence of tricuspid regurgitation. In CTS, the mitral valve is typically normal, in contrast to a supramitral ring in which the membrane is often adherent to the mitral valve.[72] In patients with suboptimal TTE windows, transesophageal echocardiography (TEE) may be needed to better assess the anatomy of the membrane, atrial septum, and pulmonary venous connections.[73] Three-dimensional (3D) echocardiography can improve assessment of the membrane, detection of

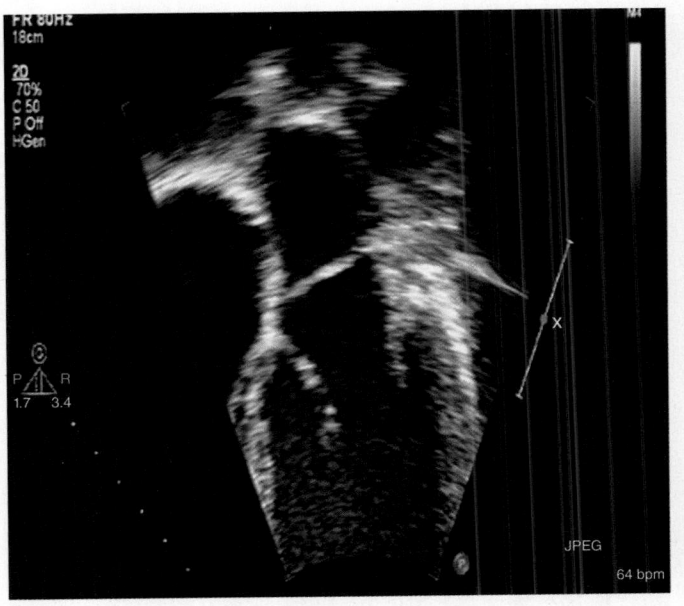
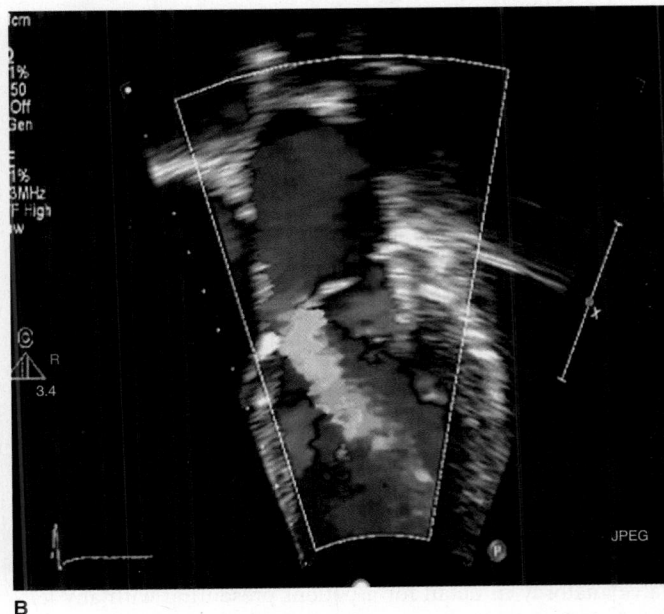

Figure 68–9. Cor triatriatum on transthoracic echocardiography. **(A)** This apical four-chamber view demonstrates a membrane (*arrow*) bisecting the left atrium, separating the pulmonary venous atrium from the mitral inflow portion of the atrium. **(B)** Color Doppler across the membrane demonstrating aliasing consistent with color flow acceleration.

fenestrations, and relationship of the membrane to surrounding structures.[70]

Cardiac CTA and CMR Imaging: CMR or cardiac CTA are often not needed for diagnosis; however, when echocardiography is not diagnostic, they may be helping in further definition of anatomy, or in defining the cause of pulmonary hypertension.[74] Cardiac catheterization is rarely used for diagnosis of cor triatriatum. It may be used to assess pulmonary pressures and pulmonary vascular resistance in adults diagnosed with cor triatriatum. It can be useful to test pulmonary artery pressures and resistance with oxygen to assess for reversibility prior to cardiac surgery.

Treatment

Medical: Typically, when the diagnosis of cor triatriatum is made, if there is significant obstruction or elevated pulmonary artery pressure then membrane resection is indicated. Medical management is not effective. Diuresis could be attempted to alleviate symptoms prior to surgical repair, as well as treatment of arrhythmias if present. Pulmonary vasodilators would

make symptoms worse causing increasing pulmonary edema in this case of a left-sided obstruction and would therefore be contraindicated (**Table 68–3**).[64]

Cardiac Catheterization: Treatment of cor triatriatum with balloon dilation via cardiac catheterization has been reported with some temporary success, but only as a bridge to definitive treatment with surgical excision. This may provide symptomatic relief at times in which cardiac surgery is high risk such as during pregnancy or decompensated heart failure.

Surgical Repair: Surgical correction has excellent results, particularly when diagnosed early and when not complicated by other severe cardiac defects. In a large case series of 25 patients from Mayo Clinic, the median age at time of surgery was 19 years and 10-year survival was 83%. No early mortality was reported and all patients that were alive were in NYHA class I and II at a mean follow-up of 12.8 years.[75]

Long-Term Outcomes and Prognosis

Although earlier surgical series had reported hospital mortality, most reported deaths occurred in children who presented in a

TABLE 68–3. Guideline Synopsis Table for Cor Triatriatum			
Cor Triatriatum: 2018 AHA/ACC Guidelines for ACHD			
COR	**LOE**	**Diagnostic**	**Therapeutic**
I	B-NR	1. Adults presenting with cor triatriatum sinister should be evaluated for other congenital abnormalities, particularly ASD, VSD, and anomalous pulmonary venous connection	1. Surgical repair is indicated for adults with cor triatriatum sinister for symptoms attributable to the obstruction or a substantial gradient across the membrane
IIa	B-NR	1. In adults with prior repair of cor triatriatum sinister and recurrent symptoms, it is reasonable to evaluate for pulmonary vein stenosis	

critically ill condition. In the current era, reported long-term results of surgery are excellent and patient's life expectancy can be expected to approximate that of the general population.

Congenital Mitral Stenosis: Valvular, Supravalvular, Subvalvular

Background

Congenital mitral stenosis is defined as a developmental abnormality at any level of the mitral valve apparatus that results in diastolic filling restriction. Stenosis can occur at the valvular, supravalvular or subvalvar levels. Congenital mitral valve abnormalities may also result in mitral valve regurgitation. They can occur in isolation, although commonly there are other associated left-sided obstructive lesions. Congenital mitral valve abnormalities may be a part of Shone's complex, which is classically defined as the association of supravalvular mitral ring (Fig. 68–8), parachute mitral valve, subvalvar AS, and coarctation of the aorta.[76] It is important to evaluate mitral valve anatomy in detail for a patient presenting with any left-sided obstruction lesion, and conversely to assess all left-sided structures in detail when a patient has a congenital mitral valve abnormality.

Anatomy

The normal mitral valve has two leaflets: the anterior (or aortic) and the posterior (or mural) leaflet. In the normal heart, the anterior mitral valve leaflet is in fibrous continuity with the noncoronary cusp of the aortic valve. Each mitral valve leaflet is attached to chordae tendinae, which attach to two well-spaced papillary muscles: the posteromedial and anterolateral.[77] The anatomy of congenital mitral valve stenosis is often quite complex. Valvular mitral stenosis occurs when there is stenosis at the level of the mitral valve annulus and leaflets. This can occur in cases of a hypoplastic mitral valve annulus, fusion of a mitral valve commissure, or dysplastic leaflets that can be thickened and/or with rolled edges. Hypoplastic mitral valve annulus, in particular, is often associated with other small left-sided structures. Leaflets may be restricted in opening due to abnormal or short chordae tendinae. In rare cases, there can be muscularization of the chordal apparatus in which case the leaflets appear to directly insert into the papillary muscles. This variant is known as a mitral arcade.[78] There can also be abnormal papillary muscle architecture with asymmetric chordal attachments. A parachute mitral valve occurs when all chordae insert into a single papillary muscle (**Fig. 68–10**), while a parachute-like

mitral valve occurs when chordae are unequally distributed between two papillary muscles, with most attachments to a dominant papillary muscle. This often results in restriction to inflow due to restricted leaflet motion and restriction at the level of the chordal apparatus. Parachute mitral valve is a component of Shone's complex and strongly associated with other small left-sided structures. In these cases, the dominant papillary muscle tends to be the posteromedial papillary muscle (**Fig. 68–11A**). This is in contrast to parachute mitral valve in the setting of AVSDs, in which attachments tend to be to the anterolateral papillary muscle.[76,79]

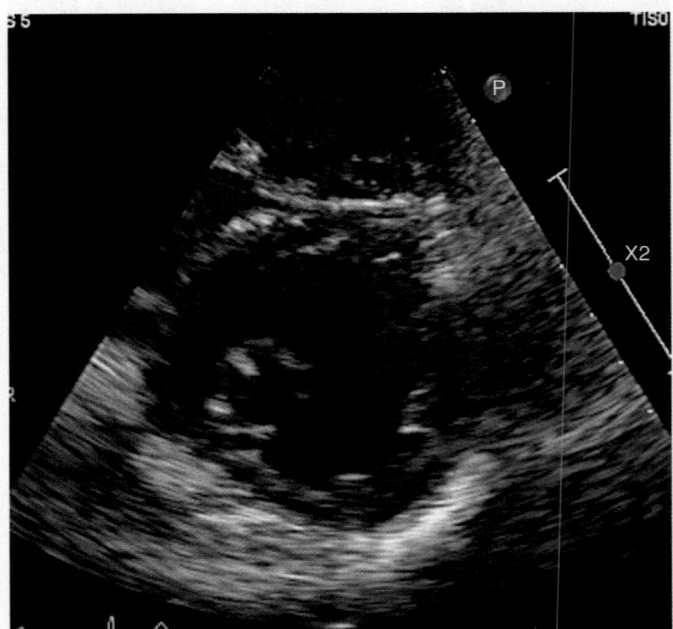

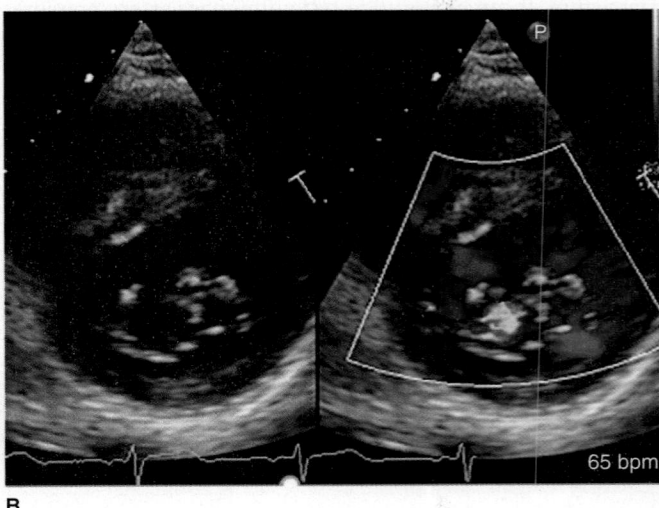

Figure 68–11. (**A**) Transthoracic echocardiography: parasternal short-axis view demonstrating a parachute mitral valve with all attachments to the posteromedial papillary muscle. (**B**) Transthoracic echocardiography: parasternal short-axis color compare view demonstrating a double orifice mitral valve.

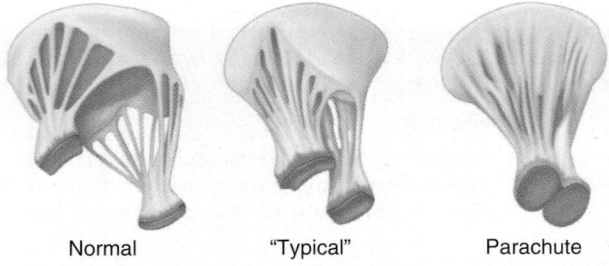

Normal   "Typical"   Parachute

Figure 68–10. Parachute mitral valve in relation to normal mitral valve architecture.

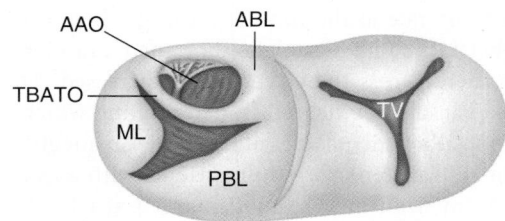

Figure 68–12. Double orifice mitral valve. Eccentric variety of double-orifice left atrioventricular valve (DOLAVV) with accessory orifice near anterior bridging leaflet (ABL). AAO, anterior accessory orifice; ML, mural leaflet; PBL, posterior bridging leaflet; TBATO, tissue bridge between accessory and true orifices; TV, tricuspid valve.

A double orifice mitral valve (DOMV) is another anatomical variant that is defined as two separate mitral valve orifices (**Figs. 68–11B and 68–12**), each supported by its own subvalvar apparatus including chordae and papillary muscles. The two orifices may be equal in size, or one may be significantly smaller than the other. It is more common among patients with AVSDs, but can also be seen in isolation. DOMV in isolation is rare (7% of all DOMV cases). When present in isolation, the valve often functions well and is not clinically significantly. When associated with AVSD, most typically it is complicated by regurgitation rather than stenosis.[80]

A cleft mitral valve occurs when the anterior leaflet is "split" into two separate leaflet components, each of which is attached to a separate papillary muscle group (**Fig. 68–13**). Cleft mitral valve is often associated with an atrioventricular canal defect/primum ASD. An isolated cleft mitral valve is defined as a cleft not associated with an ostium primum ASD. It does, however, frequently occur with other types of congenital heart disease. Isolated clefts are typically oriented toward the left ventricular outflow tract. This is in contrast to in AVSDs in which they

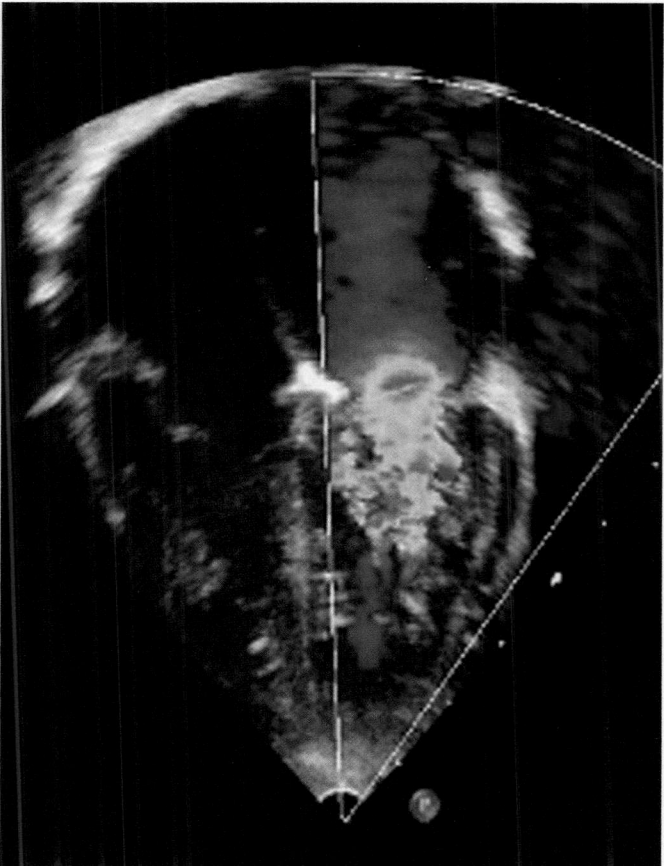

Figure 68–14. Transthoracic echocardiography: 3D apical four-chamber color-compare view demonstrating a supramitral membrane with aliasing starting above the mitral valve annulus. There are also abnormal and short mitral valve chordal attachments.

are oriented toward the ventricular septum. Cleft mitral valves tend to be regurgitant.[81] A supra mitral ring is characterized by a membranous tissue on the left atrial valve of the mitral valve leaflets, which can result in obstruction to inflow (**Fig. 68–14**). It is located beneath the left atrial appendage, distinguishing it from CTS. This membrane may also adhere to mitral valve leaflets and restrict their opening.[82]

Pathophysiology
Congenital mitral valve abnormalities can result in mitral stenosis, regurgitation, or both. Mitral stenosis will result in elevated left atrial pressure, which in turn will result in left atrial dilation and elevated pulmonary venous pressure. In cases of moderate or severe mitral stenosis, this elevated left atrial pressure can be transmitted across the pulmonary vascular bed and result in pulmonary arterial hypertension. Severe pulmonary hypertension can lead to right heart dysfunction and tricuspid regurgitation. Mitral regurgitation will result in a dilated left atrium and left ventricle, and may eventually lead to left ventricular dysfunction. Left atrial dilation in either case significantly increases the risk for atrial arrhythmias including atrial fibrillation, which in turn increases the risk of thrombotic events.[83]

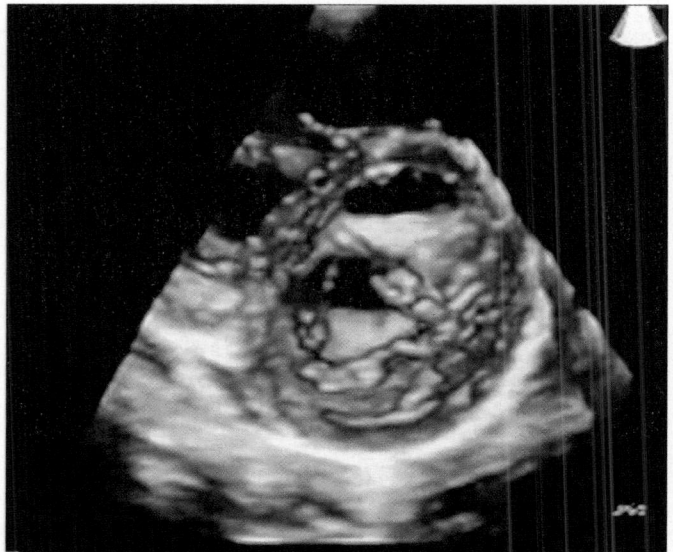

Figure 68–13. Transthoracic echocardiography: 3D echocardiography demonstrating a cleft in the anterior mitral valve leaflet.

Epidemiology

Congenital mitral stenosis is quite rare, and has been found to occur in 0.4% to 0.6% of CHD autopsied patients, and 0.2% to 0.4% in clinical series. It tends to occur more commonly in males, with a male-to-female ratio of 1.5:1.[84]

Clinical Presentation

Symptoms of mitral stenosis are most often secondary to increased pulmonary venous pressure resulting in pulmonary edema and pulmonary hypertension. This can manifest as poor weight gain in children or weight loss in adults, exertional dyspnea, wheezing, and recurrent pulmonary infections. Patients may also present with symptoms of atrial arrhythmias such as palpitations or dizziness.[84] Physical exam findings of mitral stenosis include a low-pitched mid-diastolic rumble and/or a late diastolic murmur during atrial systole. These are better appreciated with the bell of the stethoscope, and are often heard best at the apex. These murmurs are often quiet and can be easily missed. If pulmonary hypertension is present than the pulmonary component of the second heart sound may be loud. There can be respiratory symptoms such as tachypnea and increased work of breathing and if there is right ventricular failure from pulmonary hypertension than hepatomegaly or jugular venous distention may be present. Mitral regurgitation results in a high-pitched pansystolic murmur that can overlap with the first or second heart sound. This murmur is heard best at the left lower sternal border and apex, and may radiate to the left axilla and back. There may also be a diastolic rumble due to increased flow across the mitral valve.[85]

Work-Up/Investigations

Electrocardiography: On the ECG, the P-wave changes suggest left atrial enlargement. A presence of right axis deviation and right ventricular hypertrophy suggest severe pulmonary hypertension. ECG frequently detects atrial arrhythmias such as atrial fibrillation.

Echocardiography: Echocardiography is the primary diagnostic modality used to diagnose and follow mitral valve pathology over time. A 3D echocardiogram provides additional anatomical and function details beyond 2D echocardiography. An echocardiogram can assess the anatomic details of the valve, including the annulus size, leaflet morphology, and assessment of the subvalvar apparatus including the chordae tendinae and papillary muscle architecture. The degree of mitral stenosis and regurgitation can be assessed with the aid of color flow Doppler in combination with pulse-wave Doppler and continuous wave Doppler. It is important to assess left atrial size as well as left ventricular size and function. Presence and degree of pulmonary hypertension should be evaluated based on ventricular septal position, tricuspid valve regurgitation jet velocity, or pulmonary insufficiency end diastolic jet velocity, if present. Right ventricular function and degree of tricuspid regurgitation should also be assessed. Mean gradient is often reported on echocardiogram to assess the severity of mitral stenosis, because this measurement has been found to best correlate with cardiac catheterization transmitral gradient.[86] It is important to

note the heart rate at the time of mean gradient assessment. At a higher heart rate diastole is shortened and therefore the mean gradient across the valve will be increased. The mitral valve area can also be helpful in determining which stage of mitral stenosis a patient is classified. Stage A patients are those at risk for mitral stenosis. Adult patients with a mitral valve area >1.5 cm^2 with mild-to-moderate left atrial enlargement and normal pulmonary pressure would be classified as Stage B, while those with a mitral valve area <1.5 cm^2, severe LA dilation, and elevated pulmonary pressures would be classified as Stage C. Stage D refers to severe symptomatic mitral stenosis.[87]

It is important to assess for associated lesions, particularly any left-sided obstructive lesions including a subaortic membrane, bicuspid aortic valve, and coarctation of the aorta. There may also be an ASD, which would serve as a "pop-off" for the high-pressure left atrium, and in this setting a transmitral gradient would underestimate the true degree of stenosis. All patients require lifelong monitoring for progression of mitral stenosis, assessment of mitral regurgitation, and monitoring of any associated lesions. Three-dimensional echocardiography may allow for a more detailed anatomic diagnosis and add to 2D echocardiographic data. Volumetric 3D echocardiographic data can be displayed in a surgical view from the left atrium, which may aid in planning surgical repair.[88]

CMR Imaging: CMR imaging is typically not used in the diagnosis of mitral stenosis, but may be useful in the setting of mitral regurgitation to obtain accurate left atrial and ventricular volumes. Mitral regurgitant fraction can also be obtained (by subtracting aortic forward flow volume from left ventricular stroke volume).[89]

Cardiac Catheterization: Diagnostic cardiac catheterization is not routinely indicated for assessment of congenital mitral valve pathology. It may be helpful in cases in which there is a discrepancy between clinical and echocardiographic findings or to better assess for pulmonary hypertension.

Management

Management is overall influenced by the severity and mechanism of stenosis and/or regurgitation. Some mitral valve pathology may be more amenable to repair, while others may be more likely to require valve replacement. Associated lesions also play an important role in management and timing of intervention (**Table 68–4**).

Medical Management: Medical management may include diuretic therapy for symptomatic relief of pulmonary edema.

TABLE 68–4. Guideline Synopsis Table for Congenital Mitral Stenosis

Congenital Mitral Stenosis: 2018 AHA/ACC Guidelines for ACHD			
COR	**LOE**	**Diagnostic**	**Therapeutic**
I	B-NR	1. Adults with congenital mitral stenosis or a parachute mitral valve should be evaluated for other left-sided obstructive lesions	

There is controversial data about the use of afterload reduction in the setting of significant mitral regurgitation.[90] Atrial arrhythmias can be treated medically or with catheter ablation, and respiratory infections should be aggressively treated.

Interventional Cardiac Catheterization: Balloon mitral valvuloplasty (BMVP) has been performed in children with congenital mitral stenosis. BMVP did decrease peak and mean mitral stenosis gradients but was often complicated by significant mitral regurgitation and re-intervention rates were high.[91] Given these complications, BMVP is not typically the standard of care in congenital mitral stenosis, unless used as a temporizing measure in a patient who has a contraindication to surgery, or in a patient where mitral valve repair seems unlikely and would benefit from growth prior to mitral valve replacement.

Surgery: Mitral valve surgery is indicated in patients with severe mitral stenosis and/or in those that have significant symptoms (NYHA class III to IV). Mitral valve repair should always be attempted; however, it many cases, mitral valve replacement may be needed.[92] Surgical technique to improve mitral stenosis include chordal fenestration, splitting of a solitary papillary muscle, or resection of subannular or supraannular accessory tissue.[93] Surgical techniques to improve mitral regurgitation include mitral annuloplasty, chordal shortening, commissuroplasty, and accessory orifice closure.[94] Patients who had mitral valve replacement as a small child may have had the valve placed in the supra-annular position, given the lack of pediatric-sized artificial mitral valves. Supra-annular placement has been shown to reduce the likelihood of needing a pacemaker, but in some studies is associated with worse survival.[95] Mitral valve replacement options include bioprosthetic and mechanical valves. Bioprosthetic valves have more rapid degeneration than mechanical valves. There is high rate of reoperation with bioprosthetic valves but it is possible that a new valve could be placed percutaneously.[96] Mechanical valves are more durable; however, they require anticoagulation with warfarin, which is important to consider in reproductive-age women.

Mitral valve clefts can often be successfully repaired, although the degree of mitral valve plasty is a trade-off between improving coaptation, thereby minimizing mitral regurgitation and allowing for an adequate flow orifice to minimize mitral stenosis. Repair of mitral valve clefts have overall good midterm outcomes.[97] Supramitral rings in the absence of other anomalies of the mitral valve have an excellent prognosis, with only 10% having significant postoperative mitral regurgitation. These patients commonly do not need any re-intervention.[98]

Long-Term Outcomes and Prognosis
The management of severe congenital mitral valve stenosis is difficult and associated with a high re-intervention rate and significant mortality. Prognosis is much better in the setting of mild to moderate stenosis. Long-term outcome and prognosis depend on the exact anatomy of the mitral valve abnormality and severity of obstruction or regurgitation, as well as any associated lesions. With regard to intervention during childhood for congenital mitral stenosis, retrospective studies by large centers demonstrate that surgical intervention results in a 60% to 70% decrease in transmitral Doppler gradients. In-hospital mortality in these studies was 10% or less. Repeat surgical intervention at midterm follow-up was necessary in 10% to 25% of patients.[91,93] Long-term follow-up of these patients has not been well described.

COARCTATION OF THE AORTA

Background

Coarctation of the aorta is a congenital narrowing or stricture of the aortic isthmus or proximal descending thoracic aorta, typically at or near the site of ductal insertion and distal to the left subclavian artery (**Fig. 68–15**). The term coarctation is also used to describe narrowing at other sites of the aorta such as the abdomen,[99] although this discussion will focus on the more common aforementioned type. Given the high association of coarctation with other arterial pathologies, systemic hypertension, histopathologic aortic changes,[100] persistent impairment of aortic elasticity even after successful repair,[101] and risk of recoarctation and complications after repair, it is considered part of a generalized arteriopathy that requires life-long management.[102]

Anatomy

Aortic coarctation is thought to result from involution of abnormal ductal tissue that has extended into the aorta[103] or from failure of aortic growth secondary to decreased flow at the isthmus from decreased left ventricular output in comparison with ductal flow.[104] Familial association and higher prevalence in conditions such as Turner syndrome suggest an underlying genetic etiology.[105] Several genes have been identified in its pathogenesis including *VEGF*[106] and *NOTCH1*[107]; however, inheritance is likely complex and multifactorial. Aortic wall pathology includes cystic medial necrosis[108] and has been found distal to the coarctation site, suggesting a more generalized arteriopathy.[100]

There is typically infolding of posterior aortic wall opposite, before, or after the site of ductal insertion, hence the term *juxtaductal*. The narrowed aortic segment may be long segment, or discrete, and there can be associated hypoplasia of the aortic arch. In severe obstruction, circulation to the body distal to the narrowing is maintained by a network of collateral arteries (**Fig. 68–16**). These vessels arise from enlargement of normal parascapular, intrathoracic, and intercostal arteries.[109] Several associated lesions may coexist with aortic coarctation, most commonly other left-sided obstructive lesions. A bicuspid aortic valve is the most frequent association, present in 46% in one series.[110] Other lesions may include tubular hypoplasia of the aortic arch, VSD, subaortic stenosis, and mitral stenosis.110 Intracranial aneurysms are the most common extracardiac association, found in approximately 10% of adults with coarctation, a rate about four to five times that of the general population, and are found more frequently in older patients.[111-113] Given their increasing prevalence with age and association with hypertension, it is thought they may represent

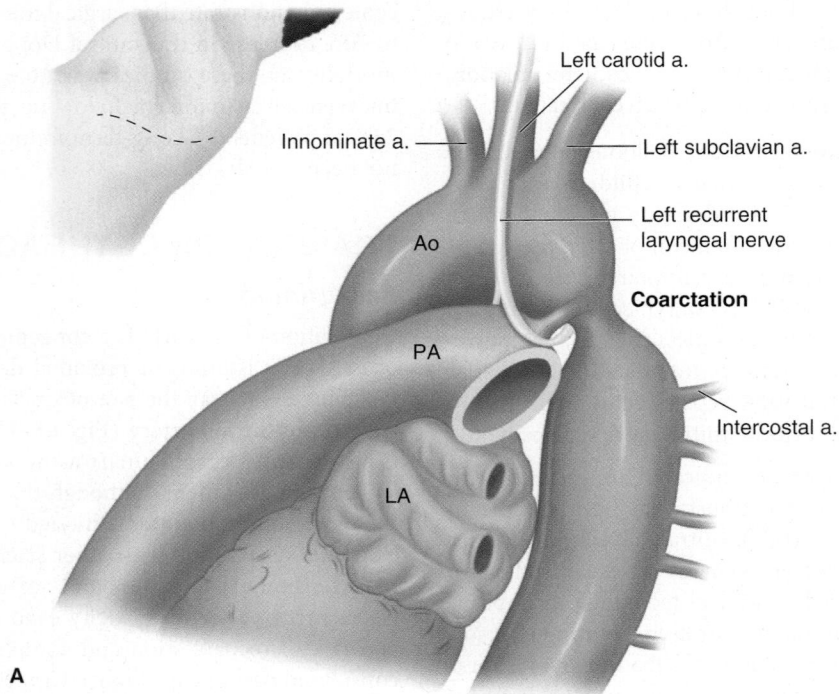

Left carotid a.

Innominate a.

Left subclavian a.

Left recurrent
laryngeal nerve

Ao

Coarctation

PA

Intercostal a.

LA

A

Figure 68–15. Coarctation of the aorta. Ao, aorta; LA, left atrium; PA, pulmonary artery.

and acquired lesion that may be able to be prevented with adequate treatment and blood pressure control.[114] However, their increased prevalence in other aortopathies without the same hemodynamic perturbations associated with aortic coarctation suggests there may be an underlying intrinsic abnormality of the vascular wall.[111]

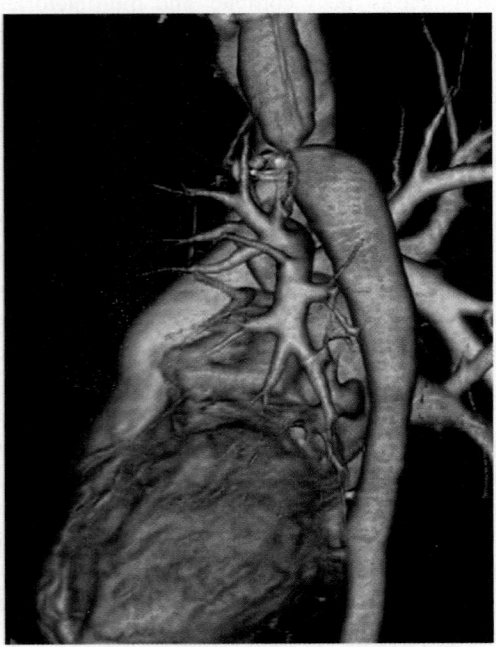

Figure 68–16. 3D reconstruction of CT of unrepaired coarctation of the aorta with aortic collaterals.

Epidemiology

Coarctation of the aorta occurs in approximately 4 per 10,000 live births and accounts for approximately 6% of congenital heart disease.[115,116] There is a male predominance of 1.7 to 1.[117] Patients with Turner syndrome (XO) have an increased risk of left-sided obstructed heart disease that includes isolated coarctation, and karyotype screening is recommended for females with the diagnosis of coarctation. Bicuspid aortic valve is commonly associated with coarctation of the aorta. Offspring and other first-degree relatives diagnosed with an obstructive left-sided cardiac lesion are at 10 times the risk of coarctation and other cardiac lesions.[5]

Pathophysiology

The pathologic sequelae of aortic coarctation result in large part from the complications of severe systemic arterial hypertension. The mechanisms of this hypertension are multifactorial and include hyperactivation of the renin-angiotensin system, impaired vascular elasticity,[101,118] and an attenuation of the baroreceptor reflex.[118] Resultant end-organ manifestations include left ventricular hypertrophy with associated diastolic dysfunction and congestive heart failure,[119] as well as premature atherosclerosis and myocardial infarction.[120] Dissection or rupture of ascending aortic aneurysms as well as the descending aorta distal to the coarctation may occur.[121] Subarachnoid hemorrhage from ruptured intracranial aneurysms and infective endocarditis (more so with associated bicuspid aortic valve) or aortitis can also occur. In a review of 304 autopsies from two series in 1928 and 1947, causes of death related to coarctation were congestive heart failure (25%), rupture of the aorta (21%), bacterial endocarditis or aortitis (28%), and intracranial lesions (11%). The life expectancy without intervention is significantly reduced, reported at 34 years.

Clinical Presentation

Critical coarctation with systemic perfusion dependent on blood flow through a patent ductus arteriosus will present in the neonatal period with cardiovascular collapse with ductal closure. Prenatal detection, while notoriously difficult for this lesion, can sometimes identify fetal cases, allowing for prompt postnatal management.[122] This discussion will focus on the adult presentation of heretofore undiagnosed coarctation, which may often be asymptomatic. In one series, upward of 40% of diagnoses were made in adulthood.[123] Symptoms, when present, may include exertional fatigue or lower extremity claudication. If severe hypertension is present, symptoms may include related headaches and epistaxis. Upper extremity systemic hypertension is quite common,[123] and the initial evaluation of the patient with hypertension should include palpation of femoral pulses and lower extremity blood pressure measurement. Femoral pulses will be weakened and delayed in comparison to the upper extremity pulses. A systolic murmur may be present, particularly in the left interscapular region. If collateral circulation is robust, a continuous murmur may also be noted. Other signs, symptoms, and physical findings depend on the presence of associated anomalies, such as a bicuspid aortic valve or a VSD.

Work-Up/Investigations

Electrocardiography
An ECG may show evidence of increased voltages consistent with left ventricular hypertrophy.

Chest Radiography
On chest x-ray, cardiac enlargement may be present, as well as rib notching caused by erosion of the inferior margin of the third to eighth ribs by collateral arteries. The left posterolateral indentation of the aorta in the area of coarctation may be visualized as a "3" sign.

Echocardiography
Transthoracic echocardiography is often the initial imaging study performed for suspected coarctation. While echocardiography often has limited ability to directly visualize the coarctation in its entirety, it can readily assess for left ventricular hypertrophy, cardiac function, and associated intracardiac lesions. Echocardiographic findings of coarctation include arch hypoplasia (if present), best seen from suprasternal notch views. The isthmus may be difficult to image, especially in adults, although may sometimes be assessed in a left parasagittal view (**Fig. 68–17**). Color flow Doppler will demonstrate turbulent accelerated flow across the area of narrowing and spectral Doppler flow profile will show an increased velocity and continued antegrade flow in diastole, akin to a "sawtooth" pattern (**Fig. 68–18**). The peak velocity as measured by echocardiography typically often overestimates the peak-to-peak

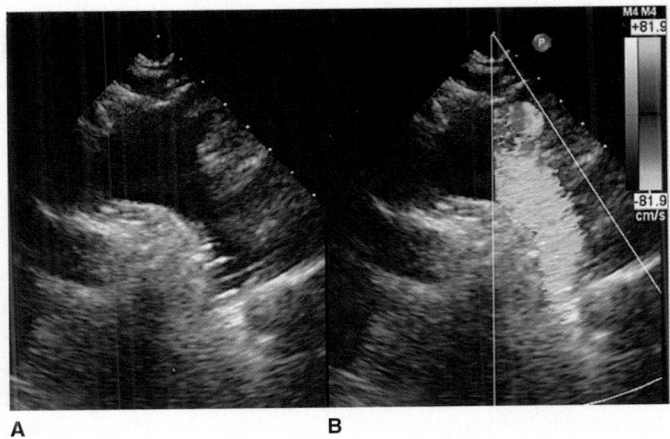

Figure 68–17. (A) Transthoracic echocardiography: suprasternal 2D images of the aortic arch. **(B)** Transthoracic echocardiography with color flow profile in the aortic arch.

catheter-derived pressure gradients. This correlation can be improved by correcting for proximal velocity or using the mean Doppler gradient.[124] Relying on the Doppler gradient may also underestimate the severity of coarctation, particularly in cases where are robust collateral circulation increases the aortic pressure distal to the obstruction.[125] Diminished pulsatility in the abdominal aorta with a flattened tracing indicates a significant coarctation.[126] Abnormalities in myocardial deformation have been noted, including decreased longitudinal strain in adults with unrepaired coarctation.[127] Even after successful repair, however, strain abnormalities may persist.[128]

Cardiac CTA and CMR Imaging
For comprehensive anatomic evaluation of the coarctation and collateral circulation, cross-sectional imaging with cardiac CTA or CMR imaging is needed.[129] CTA offers excellent special resolution and short acquisition times.[130] However, drawbacks of CTA include use of ionizing radiation[131] and intravenous iodinated contrast. Radiation exposure is of concern, especially in

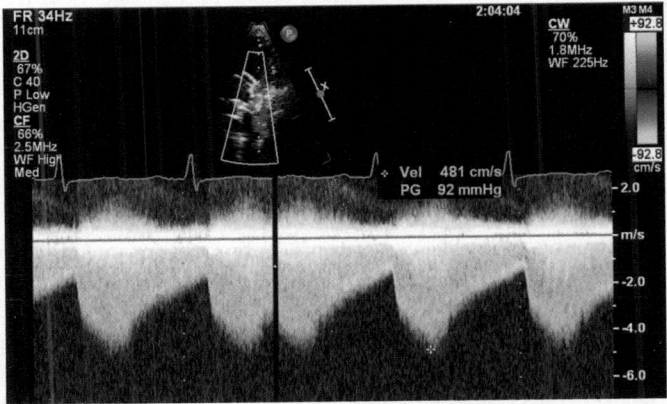

Figure 68–18. Doppler profile of the proximal descending aorta with significant turbulence and a peak velocity of 4.4 m/s consistent with severe aortic coarctation. There is delay in return to baseline and blunting of the abdominal aortic Doppler pattern consistent with significant aortic coarctation.

younger patients, because they are more susceptible to stochastic effects such as cancer, which are increased with repeated exposures.[132] However, radiation dose reduction techniques do continue to evolve, lowering the exposure.[133]

CMR imaging also provides excellent anatomic evaluation of arch anatomy and collateral circulation, while avoiding ionizing radiation. Additional advantages of CMR imaging include functional and anatomic cardiac evaluation, and hemodynamic assessment of coarctation severity and collateral circulation. Phase contrast imaging techniques for flow quantification have allowed for estimation for collateral flow.[134] The combination of anatomic and flow data has been demonstrated to be able to predict catheterization peak-to-peak gradients of ≥20 mm Hg.[135] Emerging work in four-dimensional flow data sets has also demonstrated good correlation with catheter-derived pressure gradients.[136,137] Patients with aortic coarctation have been demonstrated to have increased diffuse myocardial fibrosis by MR T1 mapping techniques, a finding that has been correlated with impaired ventricular function.[138] Disadvantages of CMR imaging include relatively long scanning times, which can complicate scans in anxious or claustrophobic patients. Implanted devices may create significant artifacts, degrading imaging quality, or be contraindications for CMR imaging. Also, intravenous gadolinium-based contrast agents are often administered, which are contraindicated in those with renal insufficiency and have been demonstrated to accumulate in the deep nuclei of the brain, although the clinical significance of this finding remains unclear.[139] Noncontrast angiographic techniques have been demonstrated to accurately define the aortic anatomy, however, thus making contrast unnecessary in some cases.[140] For both CTA and CMR, 3D data sets may be created to assist in visualization for interventional planning and follow-up assessments. These data sets may be viewed virtually or physically printed, which has been shown to be a useful tool for surgical training.[141]

Cardiac Catheterization

While considered the gold standard for assessment of coarctation severity by pressure gradient, it is typically not employed for routine diagnostic assessment unless an invasive measurement of coarctation gradient is required or catheter-based intervention is being considered. In older patients undergoing repair, selective coronary angiography can be performed by catheterization, although CT can also assess for coronary artery lesions.

Treatment

According to guidelines documents, indications for intervention are a resting gradient of ≥20 mm Hg, typically assessed by noninvasive upper/lower extremity blood pressure or peak-to-peak measurement by catheterization.[102,129] In the presence of decreased left ventricular systolic function or significant collateral arterial flow, this threshold may be reduced to 10 mm Hg.[129] The evidence for these specific thresholds is lacking, however. Often, the decision to proceed with intervention is made on the basis of systemic arterial hypertension and anatomic evidence of coarctation. Various surgical and catheter-based interventions

are undertaken to relieve the anatomic obstruction and help reduce systemic arterial hypertension (**Table 68-5**).

Medical Management

While treatment of aortic coarctation requires intervention to relieve anatomic obstruction, systemic hypertension often persists and requires medical management. Reports of prevalence of hypertension after repair range from 25% to 68%, even with an anatomically successful result.[142] The strongest risk factors for late systemic hypertension is older age at repair,[143,144] although it remains common in patients repaired early in life. The prevalence of hypertension increases with age.[145] Guidelines documents from the American College of Cardiology and American Heart Association advise goal-directed medical therapy for management of coarctation-associated hypertension.[129] Ambulatory blood pressure monitoring is useful in identifying patients with masked hypertension and has been associated with markers of arterial load and left ventricular remodeling.[146] Exercise stress testing will also reveal patients with exercise-induced hypertension, which is common after coarctation repair, even in patients without significant residual obstruction.[147]

No specific antihypertensive agent is preferred in management of coarctation-associated hypertension. Commonly used categories include angiotensin-converting enzyme (ACE) inhibitors and β-blockers, although limited treatment data specific to this patient population exist. One group reported better blood pressure control with candesartan, an angiotensin II receptor blocker, than atenolol in an observational study.[148] However, another small study found that Metoprolol was more effective at reducing the mean arterial pressure compared to Candesartan.[149] In a large series late after coarctation repair of patients on one hypertensive agent, most were on a β-blocker (62%), while 27% were on an ACE inhibitor.[145]

Catheter-Based Interventions

Balloon angioplasty for native coarctation was first described in the 1983 by Lock.[150] This technique, however, has a higher rates of recurrence and aneurysm formation than surgical techniques, and is more often reserved for use in infants in whom surgical repair is deemed too risky.[151,152] However, balloon angioplasty is often the technique of choice when treating recurrent coarctation after surgical repair. Stent implantation has also been reported as a bridge to surgical repair in critically ill infants or with comorbidities that preclude immediate surgical repair, including initial reports of a bioresorbable stent that would not need to be resected.[153]

In older children and adult-sized patients, stent implantation has emerged as an alternative to surgery for native coarctation (**Fig. 68-19**). The Coarctation of the Aorta Stent Trial (COAST) reported a high success rate without need for surgical re-interventions on intermediate term follow-up.[154] Patients with aneurysms of aortic wall injury can be treated with covered stents.[155] One strategy that can be employed in the nonadult-sized patient is staged stent re-dilation over time as the patient grows.[156] The decision to operate versus place a stent is multifactorial, and depends on a patient's size, anticipated growth, presence of associated lesions, and anatomic

TABLE 68–5. Guideline Comparison Table for Coarctation of the Aorta

COR	LOE	Diagnostic	Therapeutic
		Coarctation of the Aorta: 2018 AHA/ACC Guidelines for ACHD	
I	B-NR	1. Initial and follow-up aortic imaging using CMR or CTA is recommended in adults with coarctation of the aorta, including those who have had surgical or catheter intervention	1. Surgical repair or catheter-based stenting is recommended for adults with hypertension and significant native or recurrent coarctation of the aorta
I	C-EO	1. Resting blood pressure should be measured in upper and lower extremities in all adults with coarctation of the aorta.	1. GDMT is recommended for treatment of hypertension in patients with coarctation of the aorta
IIa	C-LD	1. Ambulatory blood pressure monitoring in adults with coarctation of the aorta can be useful for diagnosis and management of hypertension	
IIb	B-NR	1. Screening for intracranial aneurysms by magnetic resonance angiography or CTA may be reasonable in adults with coarctation of the aorta	1. Balloon angioplasty for adults with native and recurrent coarctation of the aorta may be considered if stent placement is not feasible and surgical intervention is not an option
IIb	C-LD	1. Exercise testing to evaluate for exercise-induced hypertension may be reasonable in adults with coarctation of the aorta who exercise	

COR	LOE	Therapeutic
		Coarctation of the Aorta: 2020 ESC Guidelines for ACHD
I	C	Repair of coarctation or re-coarctation (surgically or catheter based) is indicated in hypertensive patients with an increased non-invasive gradient between upper and lower limbs confirmed with invasive measurement (peak-to peak ≥20 mmHg) with preference for catheter treatment (stenting), when technically feasible
IIa	C	Catheter treatment (stenting) should be considered in hypertensive patients with ≥50% narrowing relative to the aortic diameter at the diaphragm, even if the invasive peak-to-peak gradient is <20 mm Hg, when technically feasible.
IIa	C	Catheter treatment (stenting) should be considered in normotensive patients with an increased noninvasive gradient confirmed with invasive measurement (peak-to-peak ≥20 mm Hg), when technically feasible.
IIb	C	Catheter treatment (stenting) may be considered in normotensive patients with ≥50% narrowing relative to the aortic diameter at the diaphragm, even if the invasive peak-to-peak gradient is <20 mm Hg, when technically feasible.

complexity of the coarctation (length of segment, relationship to head and neck vessels).

Surgery

The first surgical correction of coarctation was performed in 1944 by Crafoord through excision of the coarctation segment with end-to-end anastomosis.[157] Other surgical techniques include patch aortoplasty, subclavian flap aortoplasty, interposition grafts, extra-anatomic conduits, and a modification of the original technique, an extended end-to-end anastomosis (**Fig. 68–20**). While certain techniques are employed more often in infants and small children, and others in adults, it is important to be familiar with them all since the adult practitioner will likely encounter patients who have such procedures performed.

The extended end-to-end anastomosis, first described in 1977, modifies the traditional end-to-end anastomosis by incising open the inner curvature of the aortic arch and anastomosing it to the descending aorta in a beveled fashion. This enlarges the distal aortic arch and has been found to reduce rates of re-coarctation, which are reported to range from 3% to 5%.[158] This is the technique most commonly preferred today

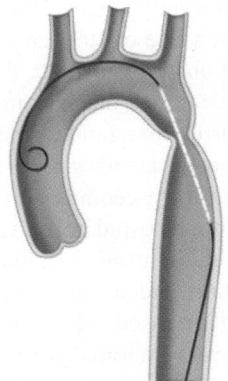
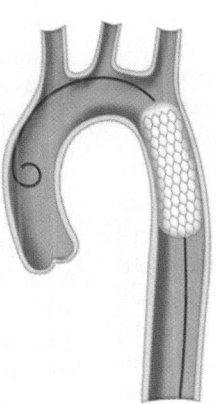
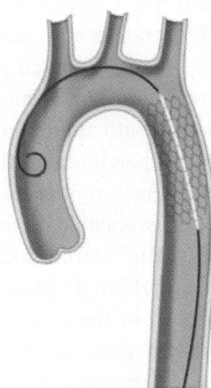

Figure 68–19. Stent implantation following angioplasty for coarctation of the aorta.

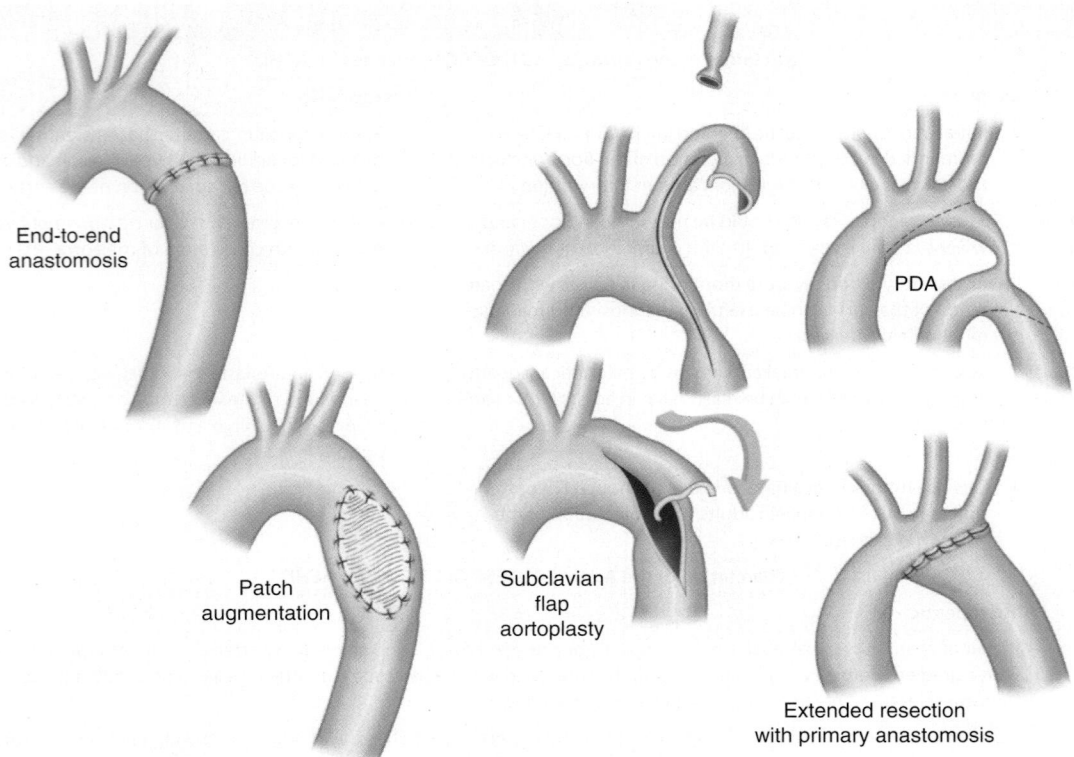

End-to-end
anastomosis

PDA

Patch
augmentation

Subclavian
flap
aortoplasty

Extended resection
with primary anastomosis

Figure 68–20. Surgical techniques to repair coarctation of the aorta. PDA, patent ductus arteriosus.

in infants in small children, where the aorta can be more easily mobilized. In larger adult patients and those with complex or long-segment obstruction, however, this technique is less applicable. The aortic interposition graft is a technique used in adult patients, where the coarctation segment is resected and a prosthetic conduit is placed to connect the proximal and distal aortic segments. This method was first described by Gross in 1951[159] It is not generally used in small children because the graft (typically a Dacron or homograft conduit) does not allow for growth.

In the subclavian flap aortoplasty, which is more commonly used in infants, the subclavian artery is transected and its proximal aspect is turned down onto the aorta and used to patch open the area of narrowing.[160] This can be used in long-segment obstruction; however, it may sometimes lead to subclavian steal and left-arm claudication and has a higher reported rate of recoarctation that the extended end-to-end anastomosis.[161] The patch aortoplasty employs a prosthetic patch placed across the coarctation segment. This technique has generally been abandoned due to its high association with aneurysm formation, particularly when Dacron is used as patch material.[162]

An extra-anatomic conduit is sometimes employed when an anatomic repair is not readily feasible or deemed too complex or risky. In this strategy, the coarctation segment is left untouched, and a prosthetic conduit is placed to bypass the obstruction, most commonly from the ascending to descending aorta. This approach is sometimes used when concomitant intracardiac repairs are needed, because the entire operation can be performed in one stage via a median sternotomy.[163]

Long-Term Outcomes and Prognosis

Long-term management of the patient after coarctation repair requires careful monitoring for several potential sequelae including recoarctation, systemic hypertension and associated cardiovascular disease, and other vascular complications including aneurysms. Although great strides have been made in the surgical and interventional management of this disease, life expectancy is not normal. Two large series found 69% and 80% of patients alive 40 and 50 years after repair, respectively.[144,164]

Recurrent coarctation should be assessed for at follow-up visits through combination of imaging, palpation of lower extremity pulses, and determination of upper and lower extremity blood pressures. In one series, recoarctation was found in 16% of patients and more common in those repaired <1 year of age and with operations prior to 1960.[144] In another, recoarctation was only noted in those operated on as children, not as adults, at a rate of 10%, and was also more common in those operated on prior to 1980.[165] As already discussed, systemic hypertension is a major contributor to morbidity associated with aortic coarctation, and is common after repair. Additionally, aortic aneurysms may still occur after repair, usually either in the ascending aorta, which is more common in patients with a bicuspid aortic valve or associated with the repair site,[166] although they may be found elsewhere.[167] Older age at coarctation and use of the patch repair technique are associated with increased risk of aneurysm.[166] Rupture of intracranial aneurysms also remains a risk.

Guidelines recommend periodic CMR and CTA imaging after aortic coarctation surgery to assess the repair and monitor for aneurysm, the frequency of which depends on the clinical status of the patient, but are generally between every 3 and 5 years. Residual obstruction, defined similarly to native coarctation, warrants treatment, and hypertension should be managed according to goal-directed guidelines.[102,129] A thorough evaluation, including exercise testing, transthoracic echocardiography, and either MRI or CT should be performed prior to making recommendations regarding physical activity. Guidelines allow for participation in competitive athletics as long as there is no significant aortic dilation or aneurysm, no recurrent obstruction, no significant aortic valve disease, and reassuring exercise testing, although high-intensity static activities and those with high risk of bodily collision are discouraged.[168] Given the well-documented cardiovascular benefits of exercise, however, careful consideration should be given to balancing the risks and benefits of restriction from sports participation, and most nonhighly competitive athletes without significant residual lesions or aortic aneurysms will usually be able to participate in most activities.[102]

Pregnant women with coarctation are at increased risk of complications including systemic hypertension.[169,170] While major complications such as aortic dissection are rare, they can occur.[171] Repaired coarctation places women in a modified World Health Organization classification of maternal cardiovascular risk at II to III (depending on patient specifics), which is a small to significant increased risk of maternal morbidity or mortality. Native severe coarctation is in category IV, in which pregnancy is contraindicated. Women should have a complete anatomic and hemodynamic evaluation prior to contemplating pregnancy and should be monitored closely for complications during pregnancy.[172]

INTERRUPTED AORTIC ARCH

Background

Interrupted aortic arch (IAA) is a rare congenital malformation of the aortic arch that is defined as a loss of luminal continuity and complete absence of flow between the ascending and descending portions of the aorta, and entails a very poor prognosis without surgical treatment.[173] IAA is a relatively rare genetic disorder that usually occurs in association with a nonrestrictive VSD and a patent ductus arteriosus (PDA) or, less commonly, with a large aortopulmonary window or truncus arteriosus (TA). Although most cases occur in normally connected great arteries, IAA can coexist with any ventriculoarterial alignment and also with severe underdevelopment of one ventricle.[174] Approximately 50% of patients with IAA have DiGeorge syndrome; in these cases, the IAA is usually type B, although cases of type A or type C have also been reported (**Fig. 68–21**).[175]

Anatomy

According to the Celoria and Patton anatomic classification, IAA can be grouped into three types (Fig. 68–21), depending on the site of the disruption:[176,177]

- Type A: The disruption is located distal to the left subclavian artery; this is the second most common disruption represents approximately 13% of the cases.

- Type B: The disruption is located between the left carotid artery and the left subclavian artery; this is the most common anomaly, representing approximately 84% of the cases.

- Type C: The disruption is located between the innominate artery and the left carotid artery; this is a rare type representing approximately 3% of all cases.

These three types of IAA can be subclassified according to the origin of the right subclavian artery (RSCA):

- Type 1: Normal origin of the RSCA.

- Type 2: Aberrant RSCA, found distal to the left subclavian artery.

- Type 3: Isolated RSCA; found originating from a right patent ductus arteriosus.

Type B interruptions account for about two-thirds of cases, type A occurs in about one-third of cases, and type C is present in less than 1% of cases.[178]

Epidemiology

IAA is an extremely rare type of CHD that affects approximately 1.5% of CHD patients and occurs in 3 per 1 million live births.[179]

Clinical Presentation

During fetal development, left ventricular output supplies the arterial circulation proximal to the interruption whereas right ventricular output supplies arterial circulation distal to the interruption via the (left) ductus arteriosus. Postnatally, this arrangement continues, with the addition of the pulmonary blood flow to the load of the left ventricle. With naturally occurring ductal closure and/or fall in pulmonary vascular resistance after birth, the circulation to the lower part of the body is compromised, resulting in a shock like state. In infants, the clinical presentation involves severe congestive heart failure if the condition is left untreated. Almost 90% of infants with IAA who do not receive surgical repair die at a median age of 4 days. There are only a few documented cases in adults with unrepaired IAA, where the presentation ranges from a lack of symptoms to limb swelling with differential blood pressures in all extremities. Substantial collateral circulation must be present to maintain flow and enable survival. However, collateral vessels are subject to atrophy and atherosclerosis, which can lead to other challenging problems. Most adults who have had surgical repair with IAA are followed for all the usual complications similar to adult patients with repaired coarctation of the aorta.

Work-Up/Investigations

Laboratory Work-Up

A serum calcium measurement is occasionally informative because many patients with interrupted aortic arch have DiGeorge syndrome, including the hypoparathyroidism phenotype. Fluorescent in situ hybridization (FISH) can reveal the typical 22q11.2 deletion seen in 8% to 90% of patients with DiGeorge syndrome.[180]

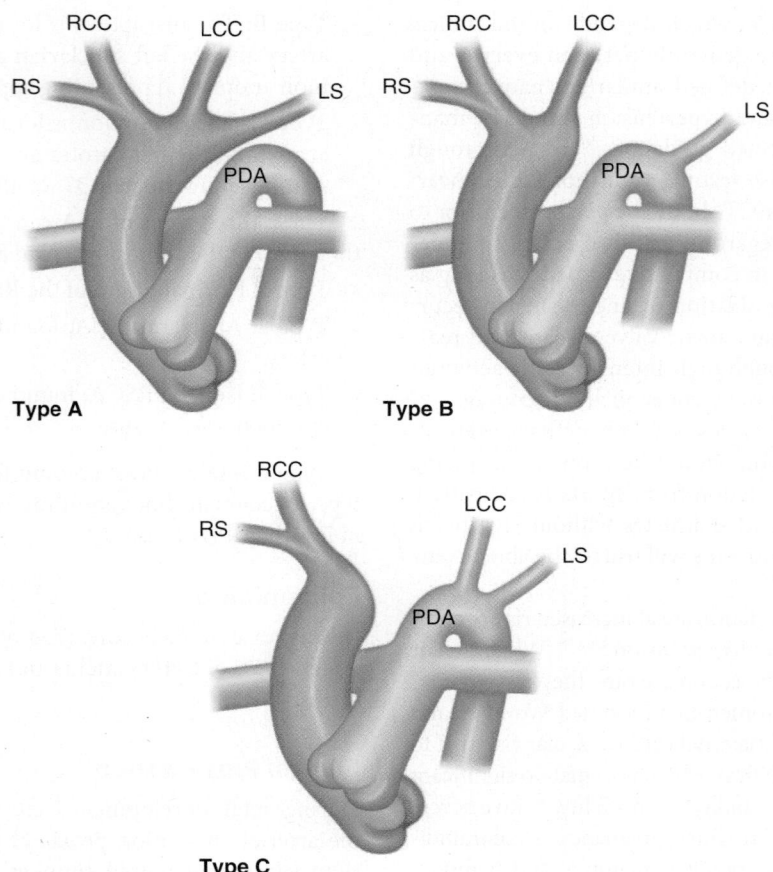

Figure 68–21. Interruption of the aorta: anatomic classification—Type A, Type B, Type C. RS, right subclavian; RCC, right common carotid; LCC, left common carotid; LS, left subclavian; PDA, patent ductus arteriosus.

Echocardiography

Two-dimensional echocardiography is diagnostic for IAA. In addition, it can usually provide at least indirect evidence for the presence or absence of aberrant RSCA artery. Occasionally, the presence of an isolated RSCA can be detected. A suprasternal frontal sweep followed by left oblique and sagittal cuts is recommended. Color-flow Doppler analysis may assist in the ultrasonographic tracing of such vessels by rapidly distinguishing them from venous structures. Furthermore, in the patient whose ductus arteriosus has markedly reduced in size, 2D and Doppler analysis can be used to monitor the effect of exogenous prostaglandin E1 on this structure. The size and anatomic type of the VSD can also be identified. In the setting of a large VSD, additional small VSDs can be missed, just as with cardiac catheterization. The most important contribution of 2D echocardiography to the preoperative characterization of patients with interrupted aortic arch is the display of the aortic outflow region. Echocardiography also demonstrates the site of arch interruption, the size and anatomic type of the VSD, the morphology of the aortic valve, and the anatomic severity of subaortic hypoplasia. Aortic valve and subaortic abnormalities are present in 50% to 80% of patients with IAA.[181]

Cardiac CTA and CMR Imaging

For comprehensive anatomic evaluation of the adult with IAA, cross-sectional imaging with CTA or CMR imaging is needed.[129] CTA offers excellent special resolution and short acquisition times;[130] however, drawbacks include use of ionizing radiation[131] and intravenous iodinated contrast. CMR imaging also provides excellent anatomic evaluation of arch anatomy and collateral circulation, while avoiding ionizing radiation. Additional advantages of CMR imaging include functional and anatomic cardiac evaluation, and hemodynamic assessment of coarctation severity and collateral circulation.

Cardiac Catheterization

Cardiac catheterization is now rarely used due to the advent of cross-sectional CT and CMR imaging. When needed, cardiac catheterization may reveal the site of arch interruption, the size and anatomic type of VSD, and the anatomic severity of subaortic hypoplasia. Cardiac catheterization also reveals whether the RSCA is aberrant as outlined above.

Treatment

Surgical Repair

The objective of the surgery is to form unobstructed continuity between the ascending and descending aorta and to repair associated defects with the most common ASVD or ASD. The repair is done using either native arterial tissue, a homograft, or autograft vascular patch. For VSD, repairs are closed with a synthetic patch that is often made of polyester or polytetrafluoroethylene (ePTFE). An alternative route to a definitive single-operation repair of the arch is to implement a two-stage approach. This approach consists of the reconstruction and placement of a pulmonary artery band in stage 1, postponing the VSD closure to a later time. For the second stage procedure of the procedure, the pulmonary band is removed.[182,183] In cases of significant outflow tract obstruction, it may be necessary to perform a complex combination of the Norwood and Rastelli procedures.[183] The arch interruption itself is usually treated with side-to-side anastomosis, rather than with conduit interposition. If the subaortic region is of good size, the VSD is usually closed with a patch at the same occasion. Whereas the aortic arch interruption is usually treated with side-to-side or end-to-end anastomosis, some surgeons have used the subclavian artery to create an arch-shaped aorta and reported good results.

When a malalignment-type VSD is present, the infundibular septum is not only misplaced but is also frequently hypoplastic. Hence, significant subaortic narrowing is frequently difficult to ameliorate with mere resection of infundibular septal muscle. Two alternative approaches have been adopted: the Ross-Konno procedure and the Norwood-Rastelli procedure.[184,185]

- In the Ross-Konno procedure, the aortic outflow region is directly enlarged (Konno) and the aortic valve is replaced with a pulmonary valve autograft (Ross). The coronary arterial ostia must be relocated to the autograft, and some sort of right ventricle-to-main pulmonary artery conduit is interposed (Ross). One relative contraindication to the Ross-Konno procedure is an unfavorable coronary artery pattern because this may well limit the efficacy of the Konno procedure.

- In the Norwood-Rastelli procedure, an interventricular baffle allows left ventricular blood to reach not only the aortic outflow but also the pulmonary annulus (Rastelli), and the main pulmonary artery is transected. The proximal portion is anastomosed to the ascending aorta (Norwood) while the distal portion is connected to the right ventricle via a conduit (Rastelli).

Long-Term Outcomes and Prognosis

Long-term management of the patient after IAA repair requires careful monitoring for several potential sequelae that are similar to coarctation of the aorta repair (see section Coarctation of the Aorta), including restenosis at the site of prior repair, systemic hypertension, associated cardiovascular disease, and other vascular complications including aneurysms or pseudoaneurysms as outlined in Coarctation of the Aorta.

REFERENCES

1. Braunwald E, et al. Congenital aortic stenosis. I Clinical and hemodynamic findings in 100 patients. II Surgical treatment and the results of operation. *Circulation.* 1963;27:426-462.
2. Katz NM, Buckley MJ, Liberthson RR. Discrete membranous subaortic stenosis. Report of 31 patients, review of the literature, and delineation of management. *Circulation.* 1977;56(6):1034-1038.
3. Aboulhosn J. Child JS. Left ventricular outflow obstruction: subaortic stenosis, bicuspid aortic valve, supravalvar aortic stenosis, and coarctation of the aorta. *Circulation.* 2006;114(22):2412-2422.
4. Somerville J. Stone S, Ross D. Fate of patients with fixed subaortic stenosis after surgical removal. *Br Heart J.* 1980;43(6):629-647.
5. Paul JJ, et al. Relation of the discrete subaortic stenosis position to mitral valve function. *Am J Cardiol.* 2002;90(12):1414-1416.
6. Piacentini G, Marino B, Digilio MC. Familial recurrence of discrete membranous subaortic stenosis. *J Thorac Cardiovasc Surg.* 2007;134(3):818-819; author reply 819.
7. Butany J, Vaideeswar P, David TE. Discrete subaortic membranes in adults—a clinicopathological analysis. *Cardiovasc Pathol.* 2009;18(4):236-242.
8. Kalfa D, et al. Secondary subaortic stenosis in heart defects without any initial subaortic obstruction: a multifactorial postoperative event. *Eur J Cardiothorac Surg.* 2007;32(4):582-587.
9. Roughneen PT, et al. Modified Konno-Rastan procedure for subaortic stenosis: indications, operative techniques, and results. *Ann Thorac Surg.* 1998;65(5):1368-1375; discussion 1375-1376.
10. Kitchiner D, et al. Morphology of left ventricular outflow tract structures in patients with subaortic stenosis and a ventricular septal defect. *Br Heart J.* 1994;72(3):251-260.
11. De Mey N, et al. Subaortic stenosis after atrioventricular septal defect repair. *Anesth Analg.* 2011;113(2):236-238.
12. Liu CW, et al. Aortic stenosis in children: 19-year experience. *Zhonghua Yi Xue Za Zhi (Taipei),* 1997;59(2):107-13.
13. Etnel JR, et al. Paediatric subvalvular aortic stenosis: a systematic review and meta-analysis of natural history and surgical outcome. *Eur J Cardiothorac Surg.* 2015;48(2):212-220.
14. Freedom RM, et al. The progressive nature of subaortic stenosis in congenital heart disease. *Int J Cardiol.* 1985;8(2):137-148.
15. Wright GB et al. Fixed subaortic stenosis in the young: medical and surgical course in 83 patients. *Am J Cardiol.* 1983;52(7):830-835.
16. Lopes R, et al. The natural history of congenital subaortic stenosis. *Congenit Heart Dis.* 2011;6(5):417-423.
17. Oliver JM, et al. Discrete subaortic stenosis in adults: increased prevalence and slow rate of progression of the obstruction and aortic regurgitation. *J Am Coll Cardiol.* 2001;38(3):835-842.
18. Babaoglu K, et al. Echocardiographic follow-up of children with isolated discrete subaortic stenosis. *Pediatr Cardiol.* 2006;27(6):699-706.
19. Karamlou T, et al. Prevalence and associated risk factors for intervention in 313 children with subaortic stenosis. *Ann Thorac Surg.* 2007;84(3):900-906; discussion 906.
20. Bezold LI, et al. Development and validation of an echocardiographic model for predicting progression of discrete subaortic stenosis in children. *Am J Cardiol.* 1998;81(3):314-320.
21. Stassano P, et al. Discrete subaortic stenosis: long-term prognosis on the progression of the obstruction and of the aortic insufficiency. *Thorac Cardiovasc Surg.* 2005;53(1):23-27.
22. Serraf A, et al. Surgical treatment of subaortic stenosis: a seventeen-year experience. *J Thorac Cardiovasc Surg.* 1999;117(4):669-678.
23. Mukadam S, et al. Subaortic stenosis resection in children: emphasis on recurrence and the fate of the aortic valve. *World J Pediatr Congenit Heart Surg.* 2018;9(5):522-528.
24. Talwar S, et al. Resection of subaortic membrane for discrete subaortic stenosis. *J Card Surg.* 2017;32(7):430-435.
25. Donald JS, et al. Outcomes of subaortic obstruction resection in children. *Heart Lung Circ.* 2017;26(2):179-186.
26. Mazurek AA, et al. Routine septal myectomy during subaortic stenosis membrane resection: effect on recurrence rates. *Pediatr Cardiol.* 2018;39(8):1627-1634.
27. Binsalamah ZM, et al. Reoperation after isolated subaortic membrane resection. *Cardiol Young.* 2019;29(11):1391-1396.
28. Tefera E, et al. Outcome in children operated for membranous subaortic stenosis: membrane resection plus aggressive septal myectomy versus membrane resection alone. *World J Pediatr Congenit Heart Surg.* 2015;6(3):424-428.

29. Pickard SS, et al. Long-term outcomes and risk factors for aortic regurgitation after discrete subvalvular aortic stenosis resection in children. *Heart*. 2015;101(19):1547-1553.

30. Stamm C, et al. Congenital supravalvar aortic stenosis: a simple lesion? *Eur J Cardiothorac Surg*. 2001;19(2):195-202.

31. Deo SV, et al. Supravalvar aortic stenosis: current surgical approaches and outcomes. *Expert Rev Cardiovasc Ther*. 2013;11(7):879-890.

32. Kitchiner D, et al. Incidence and prognosis of obstruction of the left ventricular outflow tract in Liverpool (1960-91): a study of 313 patients. *Br Heart J*. 1994;71(6):588-595.

33. Flaker G, et al. Supravalvular aortic stenosis. A 20-year clinical perspective and experience with patch aortoplasty. *Am J Cardiol*. 1983;51(2):256-260.

34. McElhinney DB, et al. Issues and outcomes in the management of supravalvar aortic stenosis. *Ann Thorac Surg*. 2000;69(2):562-567.

35. Eronen M, et al. Cardiovascular manifestations in 75 patients with Williams syndrome. *J Med Genet*. 2002;39(8):554-558.

36. Merla G, et al. Supravalvular aortic stenosis: elastin arteriopathy. *Circ Cardiovasc Genet*. 2012;5(6):692-696.

37. Micale L, et al. Identification and characterization of seven novel mutations of elastin gene in a cohort of patients affected by supravalvular aortic stenosis. *Eur J Hum Genet*. 2010;18(3):317-323.

38. Collins RT 2nd, et al. Long-term outcomes of patients with cardiovascular abnormalities and Williams syndrome. *Am J Cardiol*. 2010;105(6):874-878.

39. Pham PP, et al. Cardiac catheterization and operative outcomes from a multicenter consortium for children with Williams syndrome. *Pediatr Cardiol*. 2009;30(1):9-14.

40. Rallidis L, et al. Extent and severity of atherosclerotic involvement of the aortic valve and root in familial hypercholesterolaemia. *Heart*. 1998;80(6):583-590.

41. Bosco P, Ferrara A, Nashef SAM. Iatrogenic supravalvular aortic stenosis. *Aorta (Stamford)*. 2016;4(5):172-174.

42. Lee JH, et al. Iatrogenic supravalvular aortic stenosis detected by transesophageal echocardiography in a pediatric patient undergoing cardiac surgery. *Anesth Analg*. 2015;120(1):26-29.

43. Pober BR, Johnson M, Urban Z. Mechanisms and treatment of cardiovascular disease in Williams-Beuren syndrome. *J Clin Invest*. 2008;118(5):1606-1615.

44. Mitchell MB, Goldberg SP. Supravalvar aortic stenosis in infancy. *Semin Thorac Cardiovasc Surg Pediatr Card Surg Annu*. 2011;14(1):85-91.

45. Stamm C, et al. The aortic root in supravalvular aortic stenosis: the potential surgical relevance of morphologic findings. *J Thorac Cardiovasc Surg*. 1997;114(1):16-24.

46. Blanc F, et al. Late onset stroke and myocardial infarction in Williams syndrome. *Eur J Neurol*. 2006;13(12):e3-4.

47. Keating MT. Genetic approaches to cardiovascular disease. Supravalvular aortic stenosis, Williams syndrome, and long-QT syndrome. *Circulation*. 1995;92(1):142-147.

48. McCarty HM, et al. Comparison of electrocardiographic QTc duration in patients with supravalvar aortic stenosis with versus without Williams syndrome. *Am J Cardiol*. 2013;111(10):1501-1504.

49. Wessel A, et al. Three decades of follow-up of aortic and pulmonary vascular lesions in the Williams-Beuren syndrome. *Am J Med Genet*. 1994;52(3):297-301.

50. Brown ML, et al. Williams syndrome and anesthesia for non-cardiac surgery: high risk can be mitigated with appropriate planning. *Pediatr Cardiol*. 2018;39(6):1123-1128.

51. Tani LY, et al. Usefulness of doppler echocardiography to determine the timing of surgery for supravalvar aortic stenosis. *Am J Cardiol*. 2000;86(1):114-116.

52. Stout KK, et al. 2018 AHA/ACC guideline for the management of adults with congenital heart disease: a report of the American College of Cardiology/American Heart Association Task Force on clinical practice guidelines. *Circulation*. 2019;139(14):e698-e800.

53. Steinberg JB, Delius RE, Behrendt DM. Supravalvular aortic stenosis: a modification of extended aortoplasty. *Ann Thorac Surg*. 1998;65(1):277-279.

54. Myers JL, et al. Results of surgical repair of congenital supravalvular aortic stenosis. *J Thorac Cardiovasc Surg*. 1993;105(2):281-287; discussion 287-288.

55. Stamm C, et al. Forty-one years of surgical experience with congenital supravalvular aortic stenosis. *J Thorac Cardiovasc Surg*. 1999;118(5):874-885.

56. Arnaiz E, et al. Surgery for supravalvular aortic stenosis—the three-patch technique. *Multimed Man Cardiothorac Surg*. 2008;2008(915):mmcts 2006.002329.

57. Padalino MA, et al. Early and late outcomes after surgical repair of congenital supravalvular aortic stenosis: a European Congenital Heart Surgeons Association multicentric study. *Eur J Cardiothorac Surg*. 2017;52(4):789-797.

58. Liu H, et al. Surgical strategies and outcomes of congenital supravalvular aortic stenosis. *J Card Surg*. 2017;32(10):652-658.

59. Wu FY, et al. Long-term surgical prognosis of primary supravalvular aortic stenosis repair. *Ann Thorac Surg*. 2019;108(4):1202-1209.

60. Church, WS. Congenital malformation of heart; abnormal septum in left auricle. *Trans Path Soc Lond*. 1868;19:188-190.

61. Borst, H. Ein cor triatriatum. *Zentralble Allg Pathol*. 1905;16:812-815.

62. Jha, AK, Makhija N. Cor Triatriatum: a Review. *Sem Cardiothorac Vasc Anesthes*. 2017;21(2):178-185.

63. Marín-García J, et al. Cor triatriatum: study of 20 cases. *Am J Cardiol*. 1975;35(1):59-66.

64. Humpl T, et al. Cor triatriatum sinistrum in childhood. A single institution's experience. *Can J Cardiol*. 2010;26(7):371-376.

65. Van Praagh R, Corsini I. Cor triatriatum: pathologic anatomy and a consideration of morphogenesis based on 13 postmortem cases and a study of normal development of the pulmonary vein and atrial septum in 83 human embryos. *Am Heart J*. 1969;78(3):379-405.

66. İlhan E, et al. Severe right heart failure and pulmonary hypertension because of cor triatriatum sinister in a 54 year-old patient. *Int J Cardiol*. 2011;151(1):e29-e31.

67. Howe MJ, et al. Cor triatriatum: a reversible cause of severe pulmonary hypertension. *Can J Cardiol*. 2015;31(4):548.e1-e3.

68. Alphonso N, et al. Cor triatriatum: presentation, diagnosis and long-term surgical results. *Ann Thoracic Surg*. 2005;80(5):1666-1671.

69. Avari M, et al. Cor triatriatum sinistrum: presentation of syncope and atrial tachycardia. *BMJ Case Rep*. 2017;2017:bcr2016218395.

70. Narayanapillai J., Cor triatriatum sinister with severe obstruction: a rare presentation in an adult. *BMJ Case Rep*. 2016;2016:bcr2016215718.

71. Bojanić K, et al. Isolated cor triatriatum sinistrum and pregnancy: case report and review of the literature. *Can J Anesthes*. 2013;60(6):577-583.

72. Canedo MI, et al. Echocardiographic features of cor triatriatum. *Am J Cardiol*. 1977;40(4):615-619.

73. Schlüter M, et al. Transesophageal two-dimensional echocardiography in the diagnosis of cor triatriatum in the adult. *J Am Coll Cardiol*. 1983;2(5):1011-1015.

74. Gahide G, Barde S, Francis-Sicre N. Cor triatriatum sinister. *J Am Coll Cardiol*. 2009;54(5):487-487.

75. Saxena P, et al. Surgical repair of cor triatriatum sinister: the Mayo Clinic 50-year experience. *Ann Thoracic Surg*. 2014;97(5):1659-1663.

76. Shone JD, et al. The developmental complex of "parachute mitral valve," supravalvular ring of left atrium, subaortic stenosis, and coarctation of aorta. *J Am Coll Cardiol*. 1963;11(6):714-725.

77. van Rijk-Zwikker GL, Delemarre BJ, Huysmans HA. Mitral valve anatomy and morphology: relevance to mitral valve replacement and valve reconstruction. *J Cardiac Surg*. 1994;9:255-261.

78. Parr GV, et al. Anomalous mitral arcade: echocardiographic and angiographic recognition. *Pediat Cardiol*. 1983;4(2):163-165.

79. Oosthoek PW, et al. The parachute-like asymmetric mitral valve and its two papillary muscles. *J Thoracic Cardiovasc Surg*. 1997;114(1):9-15.

80. Zalzstein E, et al. Presentation, natural history, and outcome in children and adolescents with double orifice mitral valve. *Am J Cardiol*. 2004;93(8):1067-1069.

81. Van Praagh S., et al. Cleft mitral valve without ostium primum defect: anatomic data and surgical considerations based on 41 cases. *Ann Thoracic Surg.* 2003;75(6):1752-1762.

82. Vaideeswar P, Baldi MM, Warghade S. An analysis of 24 autopsied cases with supramitral rings. *Cardiol Young.* 2009;19(1):70.

83. Silverman ME, Hurst JW. The mitral complex: interaction of the anatomy, physiology, and pathology of the mitral annulus, mitral valve leaflets, chordae tendineae, and papillary muscles. *Am Heart J.* 1968;76(3):399-418.

84. Collins-Nakai RL, et al. Congenital mitral stenosis. A review of 20 years' experience. *Circulation.* 1977;56(6):1039-1047.

85. Ferencz C, Johnson AL, Wiglesworth F. Congenital mitral stenosis. *Circulation.* 1954;9(2):161-179.

86. Nishimura RA, et al. Accurate measurement of the transmitral gradient in patients with mitral stenosis: a simultaneous catheterization and Doppler echocardiographic study. *J Am Coll Cardiol.* 1994;24(1):152-158.

87. Stout KK, et al. 2018 AHA/ACC guideline for the management of adults with congenital heart disease: executive summary: a report of the American College of Cardiology/American Heart Association Task Force on Clinical Practice Guidelines. *J Am Coll Cardiol.* 2018.

88. Kutty S, Colen TM, Smallhorn JF. Three-dimensional echocardiography in the assessment of congenital mitral valve disease. *J Am Soc Echocardiogr.* 2014;27(2):142-154.

89. Uretsky S, et al. Use of cardiac magnetic resonance imaging in assessing mitral regurgitation: current evidence. *J Am Coll Cardiol.* 2018;71(5):547-563.

90. Baumgartner H, et al. 2017 ESC/EACTS guidelines for the management of valvular heart disease. *Eur Heart J.* 2017;38(36):2739-2791.

91. McElhinney DB, et al. Current management of severe congenital mitral stenosis: outcomes of transcatheter and surgical therapy in 108 infants and children. *Circulation.* 2005;112(5):707-714.

92. Nishimura RA, et al. 2014 AHA/ACC guideline for the management of patients with valvular heart disease: executive summary: a report of the American College of Cardiology/American Heart Association Task Force on Practice Guidelines. *Circulation.* 2014;129(23):2440-2492.

93. Pedro J, Baird C. Congenital mitral valve stenosis: anatomic variants and surgical reconstruction. In: *Seminars in Thoracic and Cardiovascular Surgery: Pediatric Cardiac Surgery Annual.* Elsevier; 2012.

94. Carpentier A, et al. Congenital malformations of the mitral valve in children: pathology and surgical treatment. *J Thoracic Cardiovasc Surg.* 1976;72(6):854-866.

95. Tierney ESS, et al. Echocardiographic predictors of mitral stenosis-related death or intervention in infants. *Am Heart J.* 2008;156(2):384-390.

96. Cullen MW, et al. Transvenous, antegrade Melody valve-in-valve implantation for bioprosthetic mitral and tricuspid valve dysfunction: a case series in children and adults. *JACC: Cardiovasc Intervent.* 2013;6(6):598-605.

97. Tamura M, Menahem S, Brizard C. Clinical features and management of isolated cleft mitral valve in childhood. *J Am Coll Cardiol.* 2000;35(3):764-770.

98. Toscano A, et al. Congenital supravalvar mitral ring: an underestimated anomaly. *J Thoracic Cardiovasc Surg.* 2009;137(3):538-542.

99. Connolly JE, et al. Middle aortic syndrome: distal thoracic and abdominal coarctation, a disorder with multiple etiologies. *J Am Coll Surg.* 2002;194(6):774-781.

100. Niwa K, et al. Structural abnormalities of great arterial walls in congenital heart disease: light and electron microscopic analyses. *Circulation.* 2001;103(3):393-400.

101. Vogt M, et al. Impaired elastic properties of the ascending aorta in newborns before and early after successful coarctation repair: proof of a systemic vascular disease of the prestenotic arteries? *Circulation.* 2005;111(24):3269-3273.

102. Baumgartner H, et al. 2020 ESC Guidelines for the management of adult congenital heart disease. *Eur Heart J.* 2020.

103. Ho SY, Anderson RH. Coarctation, tubular hypoplasia, and the ductus arteriosus. Histological study of 35 specimens. *Br Heart J.* 1979;41(3):268-274.

104. Rudolph AM, Heymann MA, Spitznas U. Hemodynamic considerations in the development of narrowing of the aorta. *Am J Cardiol.* 1972;30(5):514-525.

105. Wessels MW, et al. Autosomal dominant inheritance of left ventricular outflow tract obstruction. *Am J Med Genet A.* 2005;134A(2):171-179.

106. Carmeliet P, et al. Abnormal blood vessel development and lethality in embryos lacking a single VEGF allele. *Nature.* 1996;380(6573):435-439.

107. McBride KL, et al. Linkage analysis of left ventricular outflow tract malformations (aortic valve stenosis, coarctation of the aorta, and hypoplastic left heart syndrome). *Eur J Hum Genet.* 2009;17(6):811-819.

108. Isner JM, et al. Cystic medial necrosis in coarctation of the aorta: a potential factor contributing to adverse consequences observed after percutaneous balloon angioplasty of coarctation sites. *Circulation.* 1987;75(4):689-695.

109. Kirks DR, Currarino G, Chen JT. Mediastinal collateral arteries: important vessels in coarctation of the aorta. *AJR Am J Roentgenol.* 1986;146(4):757-762.

110. Becker, AE, Becker MJ, Edwards JE. Anomalies associated with coarctation of aorta: particular reference to infancy. *Circulation.* 1970;41(6):1067-1075.

111. Yu X, et al. Prevalence of intracranial aneurysm in patients with aortopathy: a systematic review with meta-analyses. *J Stroke.* 2020;22(1):76-86.

112. Curtis SL, et al. Results of screening for intracranial aneurysms in patients with coarctation of the aorta. *AJNR Am J Neuroradiol.* 2012;33(6):1182-1186.

113. Connolly HM, et al. Intracranial aneurysms in patients with coarctation of the aorta: a prospective magnetic resonance angiographic study of 100 patients. *Mayo Clin Proc.* 2003;78(12):1491-1499.

114. Donti A, et al. Frequency of intracranial aneurysms determined by magnetic resonance angiography in children (mean age 16) having operative or endovascular treatment of coarctation of the aorta (mean age 3). *Am J Cardiol.* 2015;116(4):630-633.

115. Hoffman JI, Kaplan S. The incidence of congenital heart disease. *J Am Coll Cardiol.* 2002;39(12):1890-1900.

116. Reller MD, et al. Prevalence of congenital heart defects in metropolitan Atlanta, 1998-2005. *J Pediatr.* 2008;153(6):807-813.

117. Campbell M, Polani PE. The aetiology of coarctation of the aorta. *Lancet.* 1961;1(7175):463-468.

118. Kenny, D, et al. Relationship of aortic pulse wave velocity and baroreceptor reflex sensitivity to blood pressure control in patients with repaired coarctation of the aorta. *Am Heart J.* 2011;162(2):398-404.

119. Egbe, AC, Qureshi MY, Connolly HM. Determinants of left ventricular diastolic function and exertional symptoms in adults with coarctation of aorta. *Circ Heart Fail.* 2020;13(2):e006651.

120. Roifman I, et al. Coarctation of the aorta and coronary artery disease: fact or fiction? *Circulation.* 2012;126(1):16-21.

121. Cohen M, et al. Coarctation of the aorta. Long-term follow-up and prediction of outcome after surgical correction. *Circulation.* 1989;80(4):840-845.

122. Familiari A, et al. Risk factors for coarctation of the aorta on prenatal ultrasound: a systematic review and meta-analysis. *Circulation.* 2017;135(8):772-785.

123. Liberthson RR, et al. Coarctation of the aorta: review of 234 patients and clarification of management problems. *Am J Cardiol.* 1979;43(4):835-840.

124. Aldousany AW, et al. Significance of the Doppler-derived gradient across a residual aortic coarctation. *Pediatr Cardiol.* 1990;11(1):8-14.

125. Scott PJ, Wharton GA, Gibbs JL. Failure of Doppler ultrasound to detect coarctation of the aorta. *Int J Cardiol.* 1990;28(3):379-381.

126. Silvilairat S, et al. Abdominal aortic pulsed wave Doppler patterns reliably reflect clinical severity in patients with coarctation of the aorta. *Congenit Heart Dis.* 2008;3(6):422-430.

127. Avendano-Perez L, et al. Mechanical deformation in adult patients with unrepaired aortic coarctation. *Int J Cardiovasc Imaging* 2018;34(5):735-741.

128. Kowalik E, et al. Global area strain is a sensitive marker of subendocardial damage in adults after optimal repair of aortic coarctation: three-dimensional speckle-tracking echocardiography data. *Heart Vessels* 2016;31(11):1790-1797.

129. Stout KK, et al. 2018 AHA/ACC guideline for the management of adults with congenital heart disease: a report of the American College of Cardiology/American Heart Association Task Force on Clinical Practice Guidelines. *J Am Coll Cardiol.* 2019;73(12):e81-e192.

130. Krupinski M, et al. Morphometric evaluation of aortic coarctation and collateral circulation using computed tomography in the adult population. *Acta Radiol.* 2020;61(5):605-612.

131. Lesser AM, et al. Radiation dose and image quality of 70 kVp functional cardiovascular computed tomography imaging in congenital heart disease. *J Cardiovasc Comput Tomogr.* 2016;10(2):173-178.

132. Johnson JN, et al. Cumulative radiation exposure and cancer risk estimation in children with heart disease. *Circulation.* 2014;130(2):161-167.

133. Hedgire SS, et al. Recent advances in cardiac computed tomography dose reduction strategies: a review of scientific evidence and technical developments. *J Med Imaging (Bellingham)* 2017;4(3):031211.

134. Holmqvist C, et al. Collateral flow in coarctation of the aorta with magnetic resonance velocity mapping: correlation to morphological imaging of collateral vessels. *J Magn Reson Imaging.* 2002;15(1):39-46.

135. Nielsen JC, et al. Magnetic resonance imaging predictors of coarctation severity. *Circulation.* 2005;111(5):622-628.

136. Riesenkampff E, et al. Pressure fields by flow-sensitive, 4D, velocity-encoded CMR in patients with aortic coarctation. *JACC Cardiovasc Imaging.* 2014;7(9):920-926.

137. Goubergrits L, et al. Patient-specific requirements and clinical validation of MRI-based pressure mapping: a two-center study in patients with aortic coarctation. *J Magn Reson Imaging.* 2019;49(1):81-89.

138. Broberg CS, et al. Quantification of diffuse myocardial fibrosis and its association with myocardial dysfunction in congenital heart disease. *Circ Cardiovasc Imaging.* 2010;3(6):727-734.

139. Gulani V, et al. Gadolinium deposition in the brain: summary of evidence and recommendations. *Lancet Neurol.* 2017;16(7):564-570.

140. Potthast S, et al. Measuring aortic diameter with different MR techniques: comparison of three-dimensional (3D) navigated steady-state free-precession (SSFP), 3D contrast-enhanced magnetic resonance angiography (CE-MRA), 2D T2 black blood, and 2D cine SSFP. *J Magn Reson Imaging.* 2010;31(1):177-184.

141. Kleszcz J, et al. Assessing a new coarctation repair simulator based on real patient's anatomy. *Cardiol Young.* 2019;29(12):1517-1521.

142. Canniffe C, et al. Hypertension after repair of aortic coarctation–a systematic review. *Int J Cardiol.* 2013;167(6):2456-2461.

143. Sendzikaite S, et al. Prevalence of arterial hypertension, hemodynamic phenotypes, and left ventricular hypertrophy in children after coarctation repair: a multicenter cross-sectional study. *Pediatr Nephrol.* 2020.

144. Toro-Salazar OH, et al. Long-term follow-up of patients after coarctation of the aorta repair. *Am J Cardiol.* 2002;89(5):541-547.

145. Hager A, et al. Coarctation Long-term Assessment (COALA): significance of arterial hypertension in a cohort of 404 patients up to 27 years after surgical repair of isolated coarctation of the aorta, even in the absence of restenosis and prosthetic material. *J Thorac Cardiovasc Surg.* 2007;134(3):738-745.

146. Egbe AC, et al. Potential benefits of ambulatory blood pressure monitoring in coarctation of aorta. *J Am Coll Cardiol.* 2020;75(16):2089-2090.

147. Egbe AC, Allison TG, Ammash NM. Mild coarctation of aorta is an independent risk factor for exercise-induced hypertension. *Hypertension.* 2019;74(6):1484-1489.

148. Giordano U, et al. Mid-term results, and therapeutic management, for patients suffering hypertension after surgical repair of aortic coarctation. *Cardiol Young.* 2009;19(5):451-455.

149. Moltzer E, et al. Comparison of Candesartan versus Metoprolol for treatment of systemic hypertension after repaired aortic coarctation. *Am J Cardiol.* 2010;105(2):217-222.

150. Lock JE, et al. Balloon dilation angioplasty of aortic coarctations in infants and children. *Circulation.* 1983;68(1):109-116.

151. Hu ZP, et al. Outcomes of surgical versus balloon angioplasty treatment for native coarctation of the aorta: a meta-analysis. *Ann Vasc Surg.* 2014;28(2):394-403.

152. Wu Y, et al. Is balloon angioplasty superior to surgery in the treatment of paediatric native coarctation of the aorta: a systematic review and meta-analysis. *Interact Cardiovasc Thorac Surg.* 2019;28(2):291-300.

153. Sallmon H, et al. First use and limitations of Magmaris(R) bioresorbable stenting in a low birth weight infant with native aortic coarctation. *Catheter Cardiovasc Interv.* 2019;93(7):1340-1343.

154. Meadows J, et al. Intermediate outcomes in the prospective, multicenter Coarctation of the Aorta Stent Trial (COAST). *Circulation.* 2015;131(19):1656-1664.

155. Taggart NW, et al. Immediate outcomes of covered stent placement for treatment or prevention of aortic wall injury associated with coarctation of the aorta (COAST II). *JACC Cardiovasc Interv.* 2016;9(5):484-493.

156. Promphan W, et al. Feasibility and early outcomes of aortic coarctation treatments with BeGraft Aortic stent. *Catheter Cardiovasc Interv.* 2020.

157. Crafoord C, The surgical treatment of coarctation of the aorta. *Surgery.* 1947;21(1):146.

158. Kaushal S, et al. Coarctation of the aorta: midterm outcomes of resection with extended end-to-end anastomosis. *Ann Thorac Surg.* 2009;88(6):1932-1938.

159. Gross RE, Treatment of certain aortic coarctations by homologous grafts; a report of nineteen cases. *Ann Surg.* 1951;134(4):753-768.

160. Waldhausen JA, Nahrwold DL. Repair of coarctation of the aorta with a subclavian flap. *J Thorac Cardiovasc Surg.* 1966;51(4):532-533.

161. Barreiro CJ, et al. Subclavian flap aortoplasty: still a safe, reproducible, and effective treatment for infant coarctation. *Eur J Cardiothorac Surg.* 2007;31(4):649-653.

162. Cramer JW, et al. Aortic aneurysms remain a significant source of morbidity and mortality after use of Dacron(®) patch aortoplasty to repair coarctation of the aorta: results from a single center. *Pediatr Cardiol.* 2013;34(2):296-301.

163. Wang R, et al. Treatment of complex coarctation and coarctation with cardiac lesions using extra-anatomic aortic bypass. *J Vasc Surg.* 2010;51(5):1203-1208.

164. Hoimyr H, et al. Surgical repair of coarctation of the aorta: up to 40 years of follow-up. *Eur J Cardiothorac Surg.* 2006;30(6):910-916.

165. Corno AF, et al. Surgery for aortic coarctation: a 30 years experience. *Eur J Cardiothorac Surg.* 2001;20(6):1202-1206.

166. von Kodolitsch Y, et al. Predictors of aneurysmal formation after surgical correction of aortic coarctation. *J Am Coll Cardiol.* 2002;39(4):617-624.

167. Preventza O, et al. Coarctation-associated aneurysms: a localized disease or diffuse aortopathy. *Ann Thorac Surg.* 2013;95(6):1961-1967; discussion 1967.

168. Van Hare GF, et al. Eligibility and disqualification recommendations for competitive athletes with cardiovascular abnormalities: Task Force 4: congenital heart disease: a scientific statement from the American Heart Association and American College of Cardiology. *J Am Coll Cardiol.* 2015;66(21):2372-2384.

169. Siegmund AS, et al. Pregnancy in women with corrected aortic coarctation: uteroplacental Doppler flow and pregnancy outcome. *Int J Cardiol.* 2017;249:145-150.

170. Siu SC, et al. Prospective multicenter study of pregnancy outcomes in women with heart disease. *Circulation.* 2001;104(5):515-521.

171. Beauchesne LM, et al. Coarctation of the aorta: outcome of pregnancy. *J Am Coll Cardiol.* 2001;38(6):1728-1733.

172. Regitz-Zagrosek V, et al. 2018 ESC Guidelines for the management of cardiovascular diseases during pregnancy. *Eur Heart J.* 2018;39(34):3165-3241.

173. Collins-Nakai RL, et al. Interrupted aortic arch in infancy. *J Pediatr.* 1976;88(6):959-962.

174. Gruber PJ, Epstein JA. Development gone awry: congenital heart disease. *Circ Res.* 2004;94(3):273-283.

175. Marino B, et al. Deletion 22q11 in patients with interrupted aortic arch. *Am J Cardiol.* 1999;84(3):360-361, A9.

176. Celoria GC, Patton RB. Congenital absence of the aortic arch. *Am Heart J.* 1959;58:407-413.

177. Schreiber C, et al. The interrupted aortic arch: an overview after 20 years of surgical treatment. *Eur J Cardiothorac Surg.* 1997;12(3):466-469; discussion 469-470.

178. Hammon JW Jr, et al. Repair of interrupted aortic arch and associated malformations in infancy: indications for complete or partial repair. *Ann Thorac Surg.* 1986;42(1):17-21.

179. Varghese R, et al. Surgical repair of interrupted aortic arch and interrupted pulmonary artery. *Ann Thorac Surg.* 2015;100(6):e139-e140.

180. Belangero SI, et al. Interrupted aortic arch type B in A patient with cat eye syndrome. *Arq Bras Cardiol.* 2009;92(5):e29-31, e56-e58.

181. Apfel HD, et al. Usefulness of preoperative echocardiography in predicting left ventricular outflow obstruction after primary repair of interrupted aortic arch with ventricular septal defect. *Am J Cardiol.* 1998;82(4):470-473.

182. Serraf A, et al. Repair of interrupted aortic arch: a ten-year experience. *J Thorac Cardiovasc Surg.* 1996.;112(5):1150-1160.

183. Alsoufi B, et al. Selective management strategy of interrupted aortic arch mitigates left ventricular outflow tract obstruction risk. *J Thorac Cardiovasc Surg.* 2016;151(2):412-420.

184. Hirooka K, Fraser CD Jr. Ross-Konno procedure with interrupted aortic arch repair in a premature neonate. *Ann Thorac Surg.* 1997;64(1):249-251.

185. Steger V, et al. Combined Norwood and Rastelli procedure for repair of interrupted aortic arch with subaortic stenosis. *Thorac Cardiovasc Surg.* 1998;46(3):156-158.

Single Ventricle Post Fontan Palliation: Tricuspid Atresia, Pulmonary Atresia, and Hypoplastic Left Heart Syndrome

69

Marie-A. Chaix and Paul Khairy

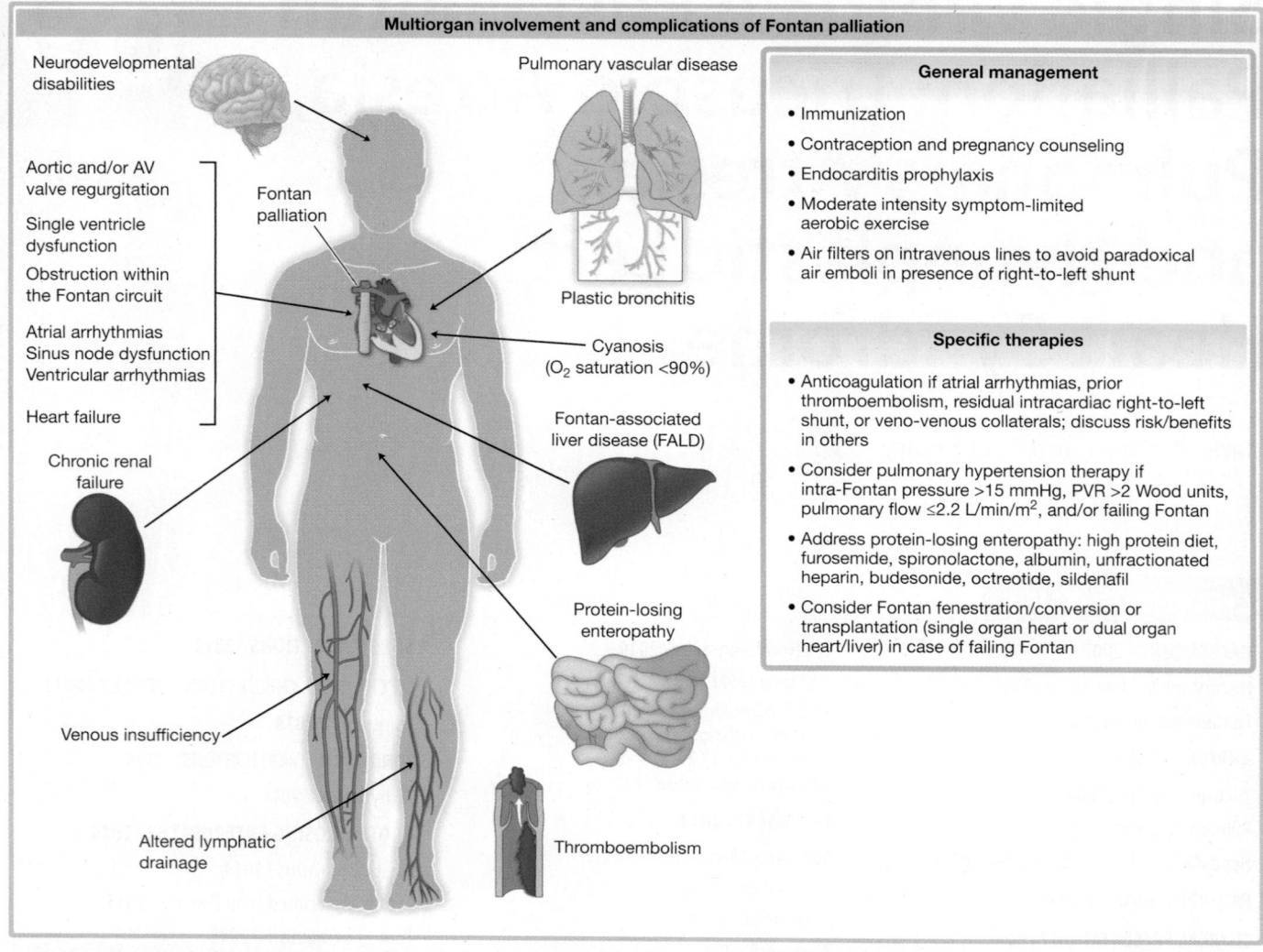

Multiorgan involvement and complications of Fontan palliation

Neurodevelopmental disabilities

Pulmonary vascular disease

Aortic and/or AV valve regurgitation

Single ventricle dysfunction

Obstruction within the Fontan circuit

Atrial arrhythmias
Sinus node dysfunction
Ventricular arrhythmias

Heart failure

Chronic renal failure

Venous insufficiency

Altered lymphatic drainage

Fontan palliation

Plastic bronchitis

Cyanosis
(O_2 saturation <90%)

Fontan-associated liver disease (FALD)

Protein-losing enteropathy

Thromboembolism

General management

• Immunization
• Contraception and pregnancy counseling
• Endocarditis prophylaxis
• Moderate intensity symptom-limited aerobic exercise
• Air filters on intravenous lines to avoid paradoxical air emboli in presence of right-to-left shunt

Specific therapies

• Anticoagulation if atrial arrhythmias, prior thromboembolism, residual intracardiac right-to-left shunt, or veno-venous collaterals; discuss risk/benefits in others
• Consider pulmonary hypertension therapy if intra-Fontan pressure >15 mmHg, PVR >2 Wood units, pulmonary flow ≤2.2 L/min/m^2, and/or failing Fontan
• Address protein-losing enteropathy: high protein diet, furosemide, spironolactone, albumin, unfractionated heparin, budesonide, octreotide, sildenafil
• Consider Fontan fenestration/conversion or transplantation (single organ heart or dual organ heart/liver) in case of failing Fontan

Chapter 69 Fuster and Hurst's Central Illustration. A relatively uneventful clinical course during the first 10–15 years after Fontan surgery may be followed by the onset of complications. Therapeutic management is dictated by the type of complication encountered. AV, atrioventricular; PVR, pulmonary vascular resistance.

CHAPTER SUMMARY

This chapter describes management of the single ventricle post–Fontan palliation. The Fontan procedure has been used to palliate a broad spectrum of univentricular physiologies when biventricular repair is not feasible. Although Fontan physiology represents a hemodynamic compromise between systemic venous hypertension and pulmonary hypotension, it is generally considered successful if venous congestion is mild, along with the reduction in cardiac output. Failing Fontan is characterized by marked venous congestion and low cardiac output with multiorgan manifestations. A relatively uneventful clinical course during the first 10 to 15 years after Fontan surgery may be followed by the onset of complications such as arrhythmias, heart failure, increased pulmonary vascular resistance, protein losing enteropathy, thromboembolism, and liver disease (see Fuster and Hurst's Central Illustration). As a result of considerable morbidity in adulthood, regular screening and surveillance with laboratory tests, imaging studies, arrhythmia monitoring, and objective assessment of functional capacity is required by caregivers with expertise in congenital heart disease. The threshold for cardiac catheterization should generally be low in the setting of new-onset or progressive symptoms. Therapeutic management is dictated by the type of complication encountered. In patients refractory to medical therapy and/or percutaneous interventions, surgical options (including Fontan conversion and transplantation) should be discussed by a multidisciplinary team.

BACKGROUND

History and Epidemiology

The univentricular heart is a rare and complex form of congenital heart disease, with an overall prevalence of approximately 2 per 10,000 live births. The single functional ventricle could be morphologically right (RV) or left (LV), with the second ventricle usually hypoplastic and/or insufficiently functional for a biventricular correction. The different subtypes of univentricular heart include those associated with an absent or atretic atrioventricular (AV) valve (eg, tricuspid atresia, hypoplastic RV in the setting of pulmonary atresia, and hypoplastic left heart syndrome [HLHS]), a common AV valve with only one well-developed ventricle, and heterotaxy syndromes (ie, disorders of lateralization).

Fontan palliation was first introduced by Drs. Francis Fontan and Eugène Beaudet in Bordeaux (France) in 1968. In 1971, they reported three patients with tricuspid atresia palliated by a Fontan procedure, two of whom survived.[1] The Fontan procedure expanded on the work by Dr. William Glenn from Yale University, first described in 1954 and then in 1958, consisting of a cavopulmonary anastomosis of the superior vena cava to the right pulmonary artery. This approach had been used to palliate a broad spectrum of univentricular physiologies, when biventricular repair was not possible. By 2018, it was estimated that 50,000 to 80,000 patients across the world lived with a Fontan procedure.[2] Importantly, the Fontan procedure is likewise palliative because the surgery maintains a univentricular system with no ventricular pump for the pulmonary circulation.

Fontan Procedure

Objectives of Fontan palliation are to provide adequate systemic outflow, controlled pulmonary blood flow, and unobstructed systemic and pulmonary venous return. Patients are managed by a staged surgical approach. For those with severe pulmonary obstruction, initial palliation may consist of an aortopulmonary shunt, such as the Blalock-Taussig (BT) shunt. The classic BT shunt consists of redirecting the subclavian artery to the ipsilateral pulmonary artery with an end-to-side anastomosis. The version used today (ie, the modified BT shunt), consists of a Gore-Tex conduit between the subclavian and pulmonary artery. In contrast, in patients with unrestrictive pulmonary blood flow, pulmonary artery banding, or division may afford initial protection against elevation of pulmonary pressures.

Fontan procedures are typically completed between 2 and 4 years of age and consist of directing systemic venous return to the pulmonary artery without an interposed ventricle. To achieve lower morbidity and mortality, prior to performing the Fontan procedure, patients should ideally have a low pulmonary vascular resistance (PVR) and pulmonary artery pressure, preserved ventricular function, adequate pulmonary artery size, no significant AV valve regurgitation, and a normal rhythm. However, some characteristics are considered modifiable and do not necessarily contraindicate Fontan surgery.[2] For example, moderate-to-severe AV valve regurgitation may require valve repair or replacement, and branch pulmonary artery stenosis or hypoplasia can be addressed surgically or by stenting.

Several modifications and adaptations of the Fontan procedure have been proposed. The atriopulmonary connection consists of a direct anastomosis of the right atrium to a divided pulmonary artery (**Fig. 69–1**), with the RV excluded from the pulmonary circulation. This approach has been supplanted by the total cavopulmonary connection Fontan, which has been associated with improved flow dynamics, lesser risk of thrombus formation, reduced incidence of atrial arrhythmias, and elimination of complications such as pulmonary venous obstruction by a massively enlarged atrium. The first type of total cavopulmonary connection was proposed by De Leval. It consists of anastomosing the superior vena cava to the undivided right pulmonary artery, in association with an intra-atrial tunnel to connect the inferior vena cava to the undivided right pulmonary artery (Fig. 69–1).[3] The more recent modification uses an extracardiac conduit to direct flow from the inferior vena cava to the pulmonary artery (Fig. 69–1).

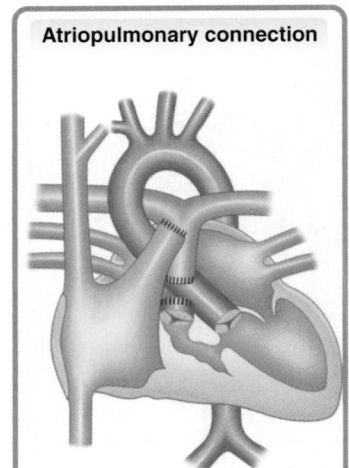
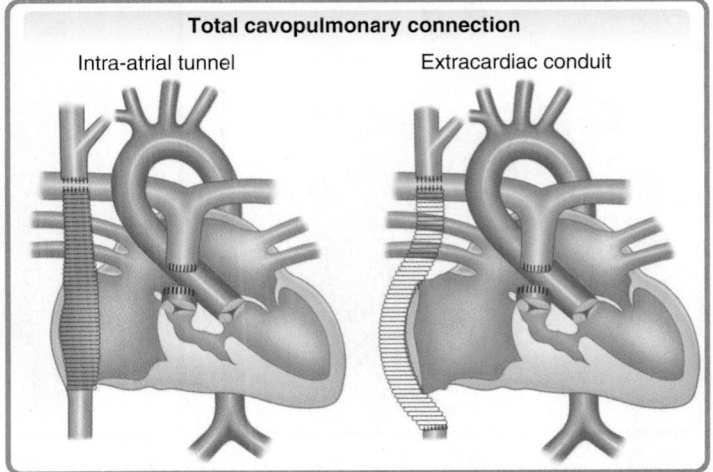

Figure 69–1. Fontan procedures: the atriopulmonary anastomosis and the total cavopulmonary connection with an intra-atrial tunnel or the extracardiac conduit.

Fontan pathways may be "fenestrated" by creating a shunt between the pulmonary circulation and the systemic circulation (ie, between the right and left atrium with an atriopulmonary connection, or between the intra-atrial-tunnel or extracardiac conduit with the pulmonary venous atrium). The objective is to provide an escape valve for blood flow in case of an increase in pulmonary pressure. Some centers perform fenestrations as standard of care to facilitate the postoperative course, whereas others remain skeptical of its benefits. Regardless, fenestrations may subsequently be closed by a percutaneous intervention in case of favorable hemodynamic conditions.

ANATOMY

Tricuspid Atresia

Tricuspid atresia (**Fig. 69–2**) was first described in 1817. It is a rare defect that accounts for 1% to 3% of all forms of congenital heart disease. It is characterized by an absent right AV or tricuspid valve, with no direct communication between the right atrium and RV. Blood flow directed from superior and inferior vena cava to the right atrium and enters the left atrium via an atrial septal defect. There is, therefore, mixing of systemic and pulmonary blood, which results in cyanosis. The LV is dominant with a rudimentary morphologic RV. A large ventricular septal defect connects the two ventricles. The great vessels could be concordant (ie, aorta arising from the LV), or discordant (ie, aorta arising from the RV). Pulmonary or subpulmonary stenosis is commonly associated. The pulmonary circulation is dependent on the ductus arteriosus being kept open at birth by medication.

Pulmonary Atresia

Pulmonary atresia is defined by the absence of a communication between the RV and main pulmonary artery. A ventricular septal defect may be present or the septum may be intact. Patients with pulmonary atresia in association with a ventricular septal defect (Fig. 69–2) usually have good biventricular development and are born with a functional RV. In contrast, the RV is hypoplastic (and the tricuspid valve often atretic) in the setting of pulmonary atresia with an intact septum. The pulmonary arteries could be developed or completely atretic with aorto-pulmonary collaterals. Patients will typically have had a palliative systemic to pulmonary arterial shunt procedure (eg, modified BT shunt) early in life to improve pulmonary blood flow. If possible, it is preferable to conserve biventricular physiology with a valved RV to pulmonary conduit, concomitant closure of the ventricular septal defect, and unifocalization of the pulmonary arteries in cases where they are severely atretic. However, if biventricular physiology cannot realistically be achieved owing to a hypoplastic RV, univentricular Fontan palliation is indicated.

Hypoplastic Left Heart Syndrome

Hypoplastic left heart syndrome is the most extreme form of univentricular physiology (**Fig. 69–3**). It consists of a spectrum of underdevelopment of the left side of the heart (ie, mitral valve, LV cavity, LV outflow tract, aortic valve, ascending aorta, and aortic arch). Systemic venous return is normal (ie, from the vena cava to right atrium and RV). However, pulmonary venous return to the left atrium bypasses the LV through an atrial septal defect. The RV perfuses both systemic and pulmonary circulations by ejecting blood to the pulmonary artery and, via a patent ductus arteriosus, to the aorta with backward cerebral perfusion. The hypoplastic aorta arises from the hypoplastic LV.

Typically, patients with HLHS undergo a variation of Norwood stages of palliation culminating in a Fontan-type circulation. The *Norwood stage 1* procedure, performed within the first 2 weeks of life, consists of reconstructing the hypoplastic aortic arch with a homograft patch and the proximal portion of the main pulmonary trunk (so-called Damus–Kaye–Stansel procedure). The distal pulmonary artery trunk is closed and

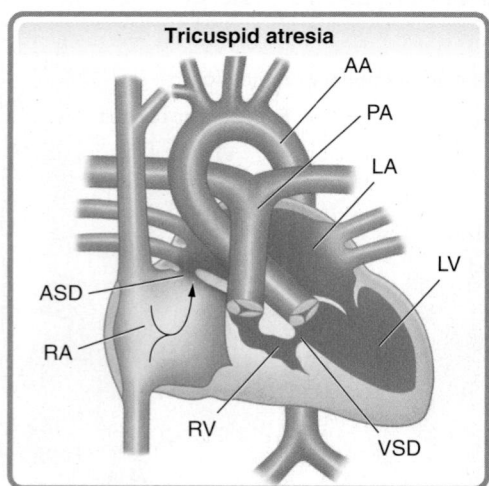

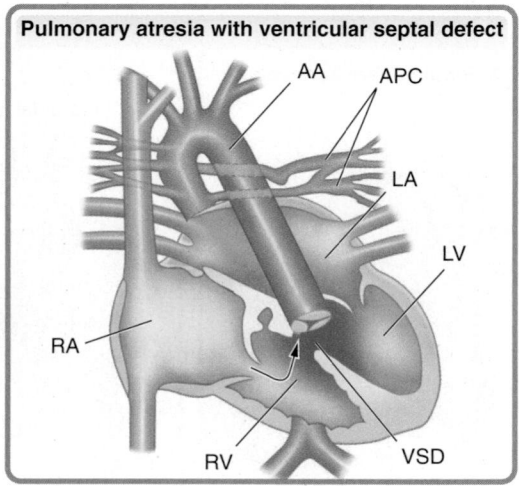

Figure 69–2. Tricuspid atresia and pulmonary atresia with a ventricular septal defect.

AA, ascending aorta; APC, aortopulmonary collaterals: A SD, atrial septal defect; LA, left atrium; LV, left ventricle; PA, pulmonary artery; RA, right atrium; RV, right ventricle; VSD, ventricular septal defect.

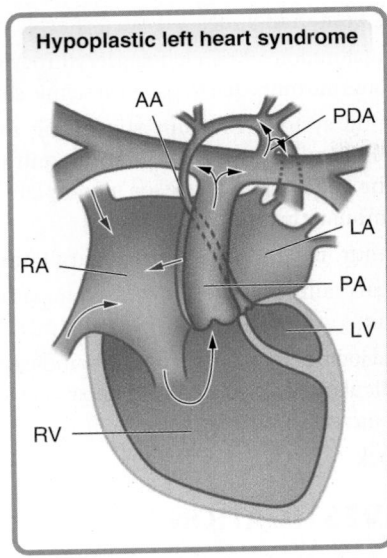
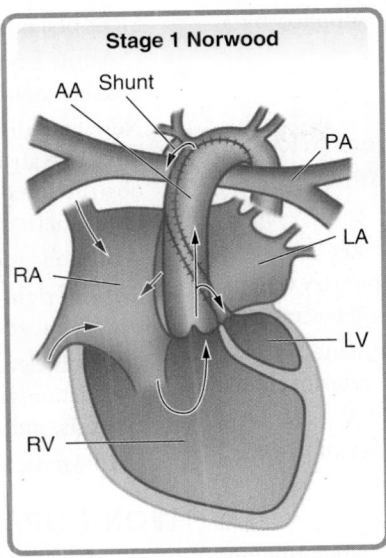
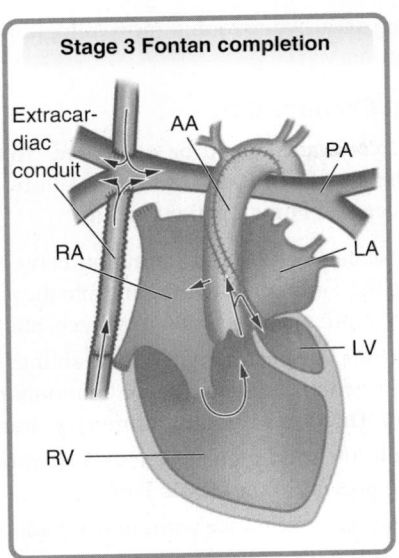

Figure 69–3. Hypoplastic left heart syndrome and the surgical stages. AA, ascending aorta; LA, left atrium; LV, left ventricle; PA, pulmonary artery; RA, right atrium; RV, right ventricle

Adapted with permission from Gatzoulis MA, Webb GD, Daubeney PEF. *Diagnosis and Management of Adult Congenital Heart Disease, 3rd ed*. Philadelphia, PA: Elsevier; 2018.

separated from right and left pulmonary arteries. The RV ejects blood to the systemic circulation. Pulmonary flow is maintained by a modified BT shunt (Fig. 69–3). The *Norwood stage II* procedure, performed prior to 6 months of age (usually between 3 and 6 months), consists of a bidirectional Glenn shunt (connection of the superior vena cava to the right pulmonary artery) or hemi-Fontan (connection of the superior vena cava to the right pulmonary artery without disconnecting it from the atrium, along with a patch to prevent superior vena cava flow from entering the right atrium), and closure of the BT shunt. The *stage III* procedure, performed between 18 months and 3 years of age, completes the total cavopulmonary Fontan by connecting the inferior vena cava to the pulmonary artery (Fig. 69–3). Survival of patients with HLHS has improved during the last three decades. Nevertheless, patients with HLHS remain prone to more complications than other forms of univentricular hearts with Fontan palliation.[4]

PATHOPHYSIOLOGY

In a Fontan circulation, the pulmonary circulation is not supported by a ventricle. Blood flows from vena cava to the right and left pulmonary arteries in a continuous nonpulsatile fashion, with equal pressure throughout the Fontan circulation. Due to the absence of a ventricular pump to propel blood into the pulmonary arteries, there is an obligatory upstream elevation of central venous pressure and a downstream reduction in cardiac output. The cardiac output generated by the systemic (subaortic) ventricle is dependent on blood flow permitted by the Fontan circuit such that the single ventricle is chronically preload-deprived. A Fontan fenestration increases cardiac output but at the expense of a decrease in arterial oxygen saturation.

A Fontan is considered successful if venous congestion is mild, along with the reduction in cardiac output. In contrast,

a failing Fontan is characterized by marked venous congestion and a substantial reduction in cardiac output. The definition of heart failure in a patient with a Fontan differs from other cardiovascular conditions. There are four common categories of Fontan failure, with overlapping hemodynamic problems: (1) systolic and diastolic dysfunction of the single ventricle, especially when it is a morphologic RV; (2) marked atrioventricular or aortic valve regurgitation; (3) systemic complications of the Fontan circuit, such as severe cyanosis (oxygen saturation <90%) secondary to a right-to-left shunt (fenestration, intracardiac, or veno-venous collaterals), hepatic cirrhosis, protein losing enteropathy, plastic bronchitis, and/or atrial arrhythmias; and (4) an increase in pulmonary vascular resistance secondary to pulmonary artery remodeling or thromboemboli.

CLINICAL PRESENTATION

Medical History

During childhood and adolescence, the majority of patients have a favorable clinical course, albeit with a reduction in objective measurements of physical capacity.[5] Reported symptoms are rare until marked deterioration owing to the fact that patients are accustomed to living with a reduced cardiac output since childhood. There is an important distinction between functional class and ability index. Patients with self-reported New York Heart Association (NYHA) class I symptoms may have a low peak VO_2 and a preserved ability index.[5] At each follow-up visit patients should be questioned about changes in functional capacity and activities of daily living. Atrial arrhythmias may be asymptomatic but are more commonly poorly tolerated and often prompt emergency room visits. Chest pain is a relatively rare symptom but coronary thromboemboli have been reported. Moreover, as the Fontan population ages, myocardial ischemia may occur, especially functional ischemia in the setting of a hypertrophic morphologic RV supplied by a single coronary artery.

Physical Examination

The physical exam should be compared from one follow-up visit to the next for any sign of Fontan failure. Typical findings in the successful Fontan patient include:

- A transcutaneous oxygen saturation between 90% and 95% (due to the coronary sinus draining into the pulmonary venous atrium, ventilation-perfusion mismatch, and/or fenestration)
  - If <90%, suspect a right-to-left shunt (eg, fenestration, veno-venous collaterals, or pulmonary-arteriovenous malformation with intrapulmonary shunting)
- Nonpulsatile mild jugular venous distention; giant a-waves may be present in the classic Fontan
- A congested appearance without overt edema
- Single second heart sound that may be loud, depending on the position of the aorta
- No systolic or diastolic murmur or soft systolic murmur (ie, mild atrioventricular valve regurgitation)
- Absent brachial pulses in the case of a classic Blalock-Taussig shunt
  - In this case, blood pressure should be measured on the contralateral side
- Hepatomegaly without overt ascites
- Varicose veins, particularly in the lower limbs; and possibly on the trunk

Signs of a failing Fontan include:

- Cyanosis: oxygen saturation <90%, clubbing, erythrocytosis, and possible continuous murmurs due to patent systemic shunts
- New or worsening systolic murmur suggesting moderate or severe atrioventricular valve regurgitation, outflow tract obstruction of the systemic ventricle, or incomplete ligation of the main pulmonary artery
- A diastolic murmur may indicate aortic regurgitation
- Signs of right heart failure: ascites, increased hepatomegaly, peripheral edema
- Markedly elevated jugular venous pressures may indicate Fontan obstruction, particularly if associated with hepatomegaly, mild cyanosis, and/or increased varicose veins
- Cardiogenic shock

WORK-UP/INVESTIGATIONS

Frequency of Follow-Up

American and European guidelines[6,7] recommend at least yearly follow-up. Frequency of visits should be adapted according to clinical scenario as defined by the NYHA functional class, cyanosis, exercise capacity, hemodynamic sequelae, and specific complications.[6] **Table 69–1** provides recommendations regarding follow-up according to the physiological stage.

Electrocardiography

Electrocardiogram (ECG) profiles depend on the type of congenital heart disease. Typically, the pattern of ventricular

TABLE 69–1. Frequency of Follow-Up

	First Adult Congenital Assessment	Follow-up
Clinical assessment + pulse oximetry + ECG	X	Every 6 months to 1 year
Laboratory: CBC, electrolytes, kidney and liver function tests, albumin, NT-proBNP, INR	X	Every year
Chest x-ray	X	If needed
Transthoracic echocardiography (TTE)	X	An imaging assessment by TTE or CMR is recommended every year and in the event of complications[b]
Cardiac magnetic resonance imaging (CMR)		After the first clinical visit in absence of a contra-indication, then every 3 years and in event of complications depending on the TTE[b]; A CT scan could be considered when CMR is not feasible
Holter monitoring	X	Every 1 to 2 years
Exercise test[a]	X	Every 1 to 2 years
Cardiac catheterization		In the event of complications[b] And prior to cardiac surgery
Hepatic assessment	Hepatic consultation	Every year
Stool alpha-1-antitrypsin (spot stool sample or 24-hour collection) and nutritional evaluation		If needed in case of suspected protein losing enteropathy
Gynecology assessment		If needed for contraception and pregnancy

[a]Exercise test: 6-minute-walk test or cardiopulmonary exercise testing depending on the physiological status of the patient.
[b]New or worsening arrythmias, hepatic failure or cirrhosis, protein-losing enteropathy, cyanosis, reduction in exercise tolerance, unexplained edema, suspected thrombosis, hemoptysis.
Data from Rychik J, Atz AM, Celermajer DS, et al. Evaluation and Management of the Child and Adult With Fontan Circulation: A Scientific Statement From the American Heart Association. *Circulation.* 2019 Jul 1:CIR0000000000000696 and Baumgartner H, De Backer J. The ESC Clinical Practice Guidelines for the Management of Adult Congenital Heart Disease 2020. *Eur Heart J.* 2020 Nov 14;41(43):4153-4154.

hypertrophy parallels the morphology of the systemic ventricle (ie, right or left). Junctional and atrial ectopic rhythms may be present and atrial arrhythmias, including intra-atrial reentrant tachycardia (IART) and atrial fibrillation (AF) are common.

Imaging

Echocardiography: Serial imaging is essential to assess hemodynamics and screen for complications. Transthoracic echocardiography (TTE) can evaluate atrioventricular valve and aortic valve regurgitation or stenosis, outflow tract obstruction of the systemic ventricle, systemic ventricle ejection fraction, and continuous inspiro-phasic flow in the Fontan circulation from the vena cava to the pulmonary arteries.[8] Echogenicity is a major limitation in some patients, particularly those with nonstandard views (eg, meso- or dextrocardia).

CMR Imaging and CCT: Cardiac magnetic resonance (CMR) can provide useful information to complement the TTE, especially in those with limited studies, and is helpful in quantifying ventricular volumes, assessing Fontan pathway patency and flow, characterizing myocardial fibrosis, detecting thrombus, and supplementing the analysis of aortic and atrioventricular valves. Cardiac computed tomographic (CCT) angiography is more challenging in Fontan patients and requires experience to ensure contrast dispersal through the pulmonary vasculature because of the streaming of venous return to the pulmonary arteries from superior vena cava, inferior vena cava, right atrium, and collaterals. An incomplete evaluation could lead to misdiagnosis of thrombus.[9] Using CCT when CMR is not feasible should be weighed against the risks of radiation exposure in this young population.

3D Printing: Three-dimensional (3D) printing is a promising technology based on CMR, CCT, or 3D TTE. Multiple applications have been reported including education of patients and caregivers.[10] It has also been used to plan catheter interventions and surgery.[11-13]

Cardiac Catheterization

Cardiac catheterization allows accurate assessment of intra-Fontan pressures, which should be the same from the vena cava to the pulmonary arteries (usually <12 mm Hg), pulmonary vascular resistance (PVR; typically, <2 Wood Units), systolic and end diastolic pressures of the single ventricle, cardiac output, obstructive lesions, and anomalous vascular connections. In general, the threshold for cardiac catheterization should be low in the setting of clinical deterioration such as new or worsening arrythmias, hepatic failure or cirrhosis, protein-losing enteropathy, cyanosis, decreased exercise tolerance, unexplained edema, suspected thrombosis, or hemoptysis, as well as prior to cardiac surgery.

TREATMENT

Additional Management

Immunizations

All Fontan patients should be advised to be vaccinated against the flu every year. Fontan patients are also considered among the highest risk categories for complications related to COVID-19, such that they should be prioritized for vaccination (**Table 69-2**).

TABLE 69-2. American and European Guidelines for Single-Ventricle Status Post Fontan Palliation

COR	LOE	Diagnostic	Therapeutic
Fontan Palliation of Single Ventricle/Univentricular Heart Physiology: 2018 AHA/ACC Guidelines for ACHD			
I	C-LD	1. New presentation of an atrial tachyarrhythmia in adults with Fontan palliation should be managed promptly and include prevention of thromboembolic events and consultation with an electrophysiologist with CHD expertise	
I	C-EO	1. Adults after Fontan palliation should be evaluated annually with either echocardiography or CMR	1. Anticoagulation with a vitamin K antagonist is recommended for adults with Fontan palliation with known or suspected thrombus, thromboembolic events, or prior atrial arrhythmia, and no contraindications to anticoagulation
I	C-EO	1. Cardiac catheterization should be performed in adults before initial Fontan surgery or revision of a prior Fontan connection to assess suitability of preintervention hemodynamics for Fontan physiology or revision of a prior Fontan connection	
I	C-EO	1. New onset or worsening atrial tachyarrhythmias in adults with single ventricle after Fontan palliation should prompt a search for potential hemodynamic abnormalities, which may necessitate imaging and/or cardiac catheterization.	
IIa	B-R	1. In adults with Fontan palliation, it is reasonable to encourage a regular exercise program appropriate to their abilities	1. Pulmonary vasoactive medications can be beneficial to improve exercise capacity in adults with Fontan repair
IIa	B-NR		1. Antiplatelet therapy or anticoagulation with a vitamin K antagonist may be considered in adults after Fontan palliation without known or suspected thrombus, thromboembolic events, or prior arrhythmia

(Continued)

TABLE 69–2. American and European Guidelines for Single-Ventricle Status Post Fontan Palliation (Continued)

IIa	C-LD	1. Imaging of the liver (ultrasonography, CMR, CT) and laboratory evaluation of liver function for fibrosis, cirrhosis, and/or hepatocellular carcinoma are reasonable in adults after Fontan palliation	1. Catheter ablation can be useful in adults after Fontan palliation with intra-atrial reentrant tachycardia or focal atrial tachycardia
IIa	C-LD		1. Fontan revision surgery, including arrhythmia surgery as indicated, is reasonable for adults with atriopulmonary Fontan connections with recurrent atrial tachyarrhythmias refractory to pharmacological therapy and catheter ablation who have preserved systolic ventricular function and severe atrial dilation
IIa	C-EO	1. In adults after Fontan palliation, it is reasonable to perform biochemical and hematological testing on an annual basis especially for liver and renal function	
IIa	C-LD	1. Cardiac catheterization can be useful to evaluate a symptomatic adult after Fontan palliation when noninvasive testing is insufficient to guide therapy	
IIa	C-LD	1. Evaluation for cardiac transplantation is reasonable in adults with Fontan palliation and signs and symptoms of protein-losing enteropathy	
IIa	C-EO	1. It may be reasonable to perform catheterization in asymptomatic adults after Fontan palliation to evaluate hemodynamics, oxygenation, and cardiac function to guide optimal medical, interventional and/or surgical therapy	
IIa	C-LD		1. Reoperation or intervention for structural/anatomic abnormalities in a Fontan palliated patient with symptoms or with failure of the Fontan circulation may be considered

Fontan Palliation of Single Ventricle/Univentricular Heart Physiology: 2020 ESC Guidelines for ACHD			
COR	**LOE**	**Diagnostic**	**Therapeutic**
I	C	1. It is recommended that adults with unoperated or palliated UVHs undergo careful evaluation in specialized centers, including multimodality imaging as well as invasive work-up to decide whether they may benefit from surgical or interventional procedures. 2. It is recommended that women with a Fontan circulation and any complication are counselled against pregnancy. 3. Cardiac catheterization is recommended at a low threshold in cases of unexplained oedema, exercise deterioration, new-onset arrhythmia, cyanosis, and hemoptysis.	1. Sustained atrial arrhythmia with rapid AV conduction is a medical emergency and should be promptly treated with electrical cardioversion. 2. Anticoagulation is indicated in the presence, or with a history, of atrial thrombus, atrial arrhythmias, or thromboembolic events.
IIa	C	1. Only well-selected symptomatic cyanotic patients, after careful evaluation (low pulmonary vascular resistances, adequate function of the AV valve(s), preserved ventricular function), should be considered candidates for a Fontan circulation. 2. Regular liver imaging (ultrasound, computed tomography, magnetic resonance) should be considered.	1. In patients with arrhythmias, a proactive approach of electrophysiologic evaluation and ablation (where appropriate) should be considered. 2. Patients with increased pulmonary blood flow—unlikely at adult age—should be considered for PA banding or tightening of a previously placed band. 3. Patients with severe cyanosis and decreased pulmonary blood flow, but without elevated PVR or PAP, should be considered for a bidirectional Glenn shunt. 4. Heart transplantation and heart-lung transplantation should be considered when there is no conventional surgical option in patients with poor clinical status.
IIb	C	1. Endothelin receptor antagonists and phosphodiesterase-5 inhibitors may be considered in selected patients with elevated pulmonary pressure/resistance in the absence of elevated ventricular end diastolic pressure.	1. Patients with severe cyanosis and decreased pulmonary blood flow not suitable for a Glenn shunt may be considered for a systemic-to-PA shunt. 2. In selected patients with significant cyanosis, device closure of a fenestration may be considered but requires careful evaluation before intervention to exclude induction of systemic venous pressure increase or fall in cardiac output.

Abbreviations: ACHD, adult congenital heart disease; AV, atrioventricular; PA, pulmonary artery; PAP, pulmonary artery pressure; PVR, pulmonary vascular resistance; UVH, univentricular heart.

Contraception

Estrogen-containing contraceptives must be avoided because of the risk of thromboembolism. Progestogen-only pills and progestogen-eluting intrauterine devices provide safe contraception with smaller cardiovascular risk.

Pregnancy

Patients with complications from a Fontan circulation should be advised against pregnancy. Successful pregnancy is possible in selected patients without complications, albeit at increased risk with 19% to 27% incidence of maternal (common antenatal and peripartum bleeding) and cardiac complications (arrythmias, heart failure, thromboembolic complications), along with a high risk of miscarriage, prematurity, intrauterine growth restriction, and neonatal death. The future mother should receive precounseling with a comprehensive cardiac assessment before pregnancy and careful monitoring on a monthly or bimonthly basis in an expert center during pregnancy and the first weeks/months after delivery.

Endocarditis Prophylaxis

Prophylactic antibiotics are only recommended in patients with a recent redo Fontan procedure (<6 months), cyanosis, prosthetic valve, residual patch leak, or prior endocarditis.

Physical Activity

Fontan patients should be encouraged to exercise regularly with moderate symptom-limited aerobic exercises to target skeletal muscular strength and improve Fontan hemodynamics.

Noncardiac Perioperative Care

Anesthesia can lead to changes in preload and/or pulmonary vascular resistance that could trigger rapid hemodynamic deterioration such that the anesthesia management team should be experienced in congenital heart disease. Pulmonary blood flow is dependent on systemic venous pressures and may be highly sensitive to minor variations in PVR modulated by anesthetics, hypoxemia, and postoperative complications (eg, atelectasis, thromboembolism, and pneumonia). Desaturation commonly occurs upon induction of anesthesia in case of right-to-left shunting (fenestration or collaterals). Regional anesthesia is usually preferable to general anesthesia, although general anesthesia is preferred over epidural anesthesia.

PERCUTANEOUS OPTIONS

A fenestration could be performed percutaneously by creating a shunt between the pulmonary and systemic circulation. It has been proposed in selected candidates with high intra-Fontan pressure for treatment of protein-losing enteropathy (PLE) or plastic bronchitis but with uncertain benefit. It is contraindicated in patients with low arterial oxygen saturation before the intervention. Conversely, in selected adult patients, it may be appropriate to consider device closure of a fenestration if there is symptomatic cyanosis and closure would be tolerated hemodynamically. Catheter interventions may also be required to close anomalous vascular connections, such as systemic venous-to-pulmonary venous (or left atrial) collateral connections associated with cyanosis.

SURGICAL OPTIONS

Surgical options should be contemplated in patients with a failing Fontan. While most patients will be considered for heart transplantation, in the context of donor shortages and high-risk features, selected patients could be candidates for Fontan conversion surgery. This refers to converting an atriopulmonary anastomosis to a total cavo-pulmonary connection. Indications are not straightforward. Objectives include improving flow dynamics, reducing right atrial size, relieving obstructions (eg, thrombus obstructing systemic venous return or severe right atrial dilation compressing the right pulmonary veins), and performing arrhythmia Maze surgery. Conversion should be performed before the onset of irreversible ventricular failure.[14] Patients with elevated intra-Fontan or ventricular end-diastolic pressures, or renal or hepatic dysfunction may not be suitable for Fontan conversion. The reported multicenter in-hospital mortality rate is approximately 10% and morbidities during follow-up remain substantial, including the need for later transplantation. Other surgical revisions in Fontan patients include repair or replacement of the atrioventricular valve due to severe regurgitation. Risks are higher in patients with systemic ventricular systolic dysfunction.

MECHANICAL CIRCULATORY SUPPORT

MCS therapy is limited in the end-stage failing Fontan to patients with univentricular heart dysfunction as a bridge to transplantation. It has not been reported as destination therapy.

Transplant

A growing number of patients with Fontan failure are considered for transplantation. Indications, contraindications, and the timing of transplantation remain controversial. Knowledge is currently too rudimentary to establish uniform criteria. The most common scenarios leading to heart transplantation are PLE (40%), ventricular dysfunction (50%), and other diagnoses such as plastic bronchitis and arrhythmias (10%).[2] However, with heightened awareness about Fontan-associated liver disease (FALD), hepatic dysfunction is increasingly influencing decisions regarding transplantation, which largely remain center-dependent. The survival rate of children transplanted after a Fontan has significantly improved to 89% at 1 year.[15] For adults, the largest single-center experience includes 26 patients over 26 years, with a 1-year survival rate of 65%.[16]

Combined heart and liver transplantations are increasingly discussed because of the concern that deterioration in liver function early after heart transplant increases mortality. Criteria for dual organ transplantation remain uncertain, in part due to the unclear correlation between extent of fibrosis and risk of progression to decompensated cirrhosis with need for liver transplantation.[17] An algorithm has been proposed to determine if a heart transplant alone or a combined heart and liver transplant is indicated in patients with a failing Fontan and advanced liver disease including bridging fibrosis, cirrhosis, hepatocellular carcinoma, or nodular mild-to-moderate fibrosis.[17] There may be immunological benefits to dual organ transplantation, with fewer episodes of acute cellular and humoral rejection.[18] Single organ hepatic transplantation for FALD is not advisable, even in the setting of favorable Fontan hemodynamics.

LONG-TERM COMPLICATIONS

Arrhythmias

Atrial arrhythmias are common in Fontan patients and have been reported in up to 60% by 20 years after Fontan completion. These arrhythmias are facilitated by suture lines and scars, severe atrial dilation, and elevated atrial pressures. The most frequent arrhythmia is IART, although nonautomatic atrial tachycardias and AF are also highly prevalent. Factors associated with the development of arrhythmias include older age at the time of Fontan surgery, a right atrium to pulmonary artery anastomosis, preoperative and early postoperative tachycardia, and atrioventricular valve regurgitation. Right atrial isomerism and sick sinus syndrome have also been proposed as risks factors by some studies. Atrial arrhythmias are associated with a poorer prognosis, including atrial thrombus, heart failure, increased mortality, and transplantation.[2] Atrial arrhythmias with rapid atrioventricular conduction are usually not well tolerated and should be considered a medical emergency. Patients with slower sustained arrhythmias may present with a more insidious history of increased dyspnea and worsening heart failure. New onset or worsening of atrial tachyarrhythmias should be managed and investigated promptly.[6] Arrhythmias may reflect hemodynamic problems such that cardiac catheterization should be considered to assess the integrity of the Fontan circulation. Imaging studies should be performed to rule-out thrombus, ventricular dysfunction, and atrioventricular valve regurgitation.

Anticoagulation is indicated in the setting of sustained atrial arrhythmias. Vitamin K antagonists (international normalized ratio [INR] between 2 and 3) remain the gold standard, pending more definitive safety and efficacy studies on non–vitamin K antagonist oral anticoagulants (NOAC).[19] Given that atrial arrhythmias are often poorly tolerated by the single ventricle, rhythm control is the favored initial approach. It is important to rule-out thrombus prior to cardioversion considering the high baseline risk of thromboembolic complications.[7] Antiarrhythmic agents can be helpful, although recurrences remain common. Patients are at a higher risk of side-effects such as thyrotoxicosis with amiodarone. There should be a low threshold for referral to catheter ablation at a center with expertise in this patient population. It is common for patients to have multiple inducible arrhythmias. Moreover, total cavopulmonary connections complicate catheter access to arrhythmogenic substrates. Patients with uncontrollable arrhythmias may be considered for Fontan conversion or heart transplantation.[6,7]

Sinus node dysfunction is common in patients who have had Fontan surgery that involves a superior vena cava to pulmonary artery connection. Sinus node dysfunction has been associated with a reduction in preload to the single ventricle, increased pulmonary venous pressure, reduced cardiac output,

and atrial arrhythmias.[2] Even if transvenous atrial pacing is feasible in patients with atriopulmonary connections and in some with intracardiac tunnels, an epicardial approach may be preferred due to associated thrombotic complications. Although sudden cardiac death due to ventricular arrhythmias is not the most common cause of mortality, a defibrillator for secondary prevention is required in 1.4% to 2% of the Fontan population.[20,21] In light of access issues, the subcutaneous defibrillator is the preferred option in suitable candidates.

PROTEIN LOSING ENTEROPATHY

PLE occurs in 5% to 10% of Fontan patients and is one of the most challenging complications to manage.[22] It is defined by a reduction in serum albumin to <30 g/dL, with no other identifiable source of protein loss other than the gastrointestinal tract. It is confirmed by an increased clearance of stool alpha-1-antitrypsin. Typical clinical manifestations include chronic diarrhea, abdominal pain, ascites, pleural effusions, and peripheral edema but hypoalbuminemia could be the only initial manifestation. Patients can develop growth failure, decreased bone density, coagulation abnormalities, and lymphopenia. The pathogenesis of PLE is multifactorial and not totally understood, although is thought to implicate chronic venous hypertension, low cardiac output, and abnormal gut lymphatics. A 50% 5-year mortality rate with PLE was initially described, although a more recent study noted 88% survival at 5 years and 72% at 10 years, linked in part to earlier diagnosis.[23] Higher mortality was associated with high Fontan pressure (mean >15 mm Hg), decreased ventricular function (ejection fraction <55%), NYHA functional class above II, higher pulmonary vascular resistance, lower cardiac index, and lower mixed venous saturation.[23]

A diagnosis of PLE requires an extensive assessment to rule-out obstruction in the Fontan circulation, arrhythmias leading to Fontan failure, elevated intra-Fontan pressure, and decreased cardiac output. Renal function and nutritional intake should also be assessed. Other gastrointestinal and nephrotic causes of protein loss should be excluded. Proposed therapies have included combining nutritional support (high-protein diet) with furosemide, spironolactone, albumin, unfractionated heparin, budesonide, octreotide, sildenafil, dopamine, and more recently midodrine.[24] Results have been modest and inconsistent. Treating precipitating factors such as obstructions or arrythmias is essential. Fenestration could benefit patients with high intra-Fontan pressures but is associated with a reduction in systemic oxygen saturation. Evaluation for heart transplant is warranted in acceptable candidates, because PLE may resolve thereafter. However, the survival of transplanted Fontan patients with PLE has not been formally compared to those who do not undergo transplantation.[6,7]

Plastic Bronchitis

Plastic bronchitis is a rare complication (<1%–2% overall). It is characterized by the production of large pale bronchial casts that obstruct the tracheobronchial tree and can result in airway obstruction and asphyxiation. The pathophysiology remains largely unknown but, similar to PLE, plastic bronchitis is considered related to lymphatic system abnormalities associated with high central venous pressures. Decompression of lymph into the airway lumen has been proposed to cause plastic bronchitis. Life-threatening airway obstruction requires aggressive management with combined therapy including inhaled steroids, albuterol, pulmonary physiotherapy, and acetylcysteine. Mechanical clearance of obstructed airways by bronchoscopy could be effective. A few studies reported a benefit of Fontan fenestration and cardiac transplantation.

Fontan-Associated Liver Disease

FALD includes fibrosis, cirrhosis, and hepatic neoplasm. It is secondary to increased central venous pressure, with a chronic increase in hepatic venous congestion, decreased cardiac output, and cyanosis.[17] In Fontan patients, histological evidence of some degree of liver fibrosis is pervasive.[17] Bridging fibrosis to cirrhosis and liver neoplasms are highly prevalent. The relation between poor hemodynamics and progression of bridging fibrosis to cirrhosis remains unclear, with extensive fibrosis described in some patients with ideal Fontan hemodynamics.[25,26]

Annual surveillance of hepatic function is recommended in all patients 10 to 15 years after Fontan surgery.[6] The diagnosis of FALD is challenging due to the absence of symptoms in most and the noncorrelation of serum biomarkers (liver enzymes, MELD-Na, and MELD-XI score) with degree of fibrosis. In one series, the only parameter associated with extensive fibrosis was an elevated INR.[27] Ultrasound imaging, CT scan, and magnetic resonance imaging (MRI) are helpful in detecting nodularity and signs of portal hypertension. Elastography is a noninvasive approach to measure stiffness of the liver but the correlation with cirrhosis remains unclear since it cannot distinguish between passive congestion and fibrosis. Serial measurements showing increased stiffness could be an indicator of a failing Fontan. Esophageal varices have been reported in approximately 20% to 50% of older Fontan patients.[17] Surveillance endoscopy may be useful in patients with evidence of liver fibrosis. Liver biopsy is the gold standard to diagnose cirrhosis. The test is limited by hemorrhagic complications reported in 7.4% of patients and the patchy pattern of fibrosis.[28] Measuring hepatic venous pressure gradients by catheterization comparing the wedged hepatic sinusoidal pressure with the unwedged free hepatic venous pressure could be useful in diagnosing portal hypertension (normal gradient 1–5 mm Hg).

Medical interventions to prevent obesity and avoidance of hepatotoxic medications and alcohol should be considered in all patients with bridging fibrosis to cirrhosis. Screening for hepatocellular carcinoma is challenging, but serial ultrasounds and α-fetoprotein measurements seem reasonable pending the development of FALD-specific approaches. If intra-Fontan pressures and venous pressures are high, a fenestration and/or pulmonary hypertension therapy could be considered. Transplant candidates with progressive FALD should be carefully assessed regarding the need for single (heart) versus combined (heart and liver) organ transplant.

Thromboembolism

The incidence of clinical and silent thromboembolism (TE) in Fontan patients has been reported to be 10% to 35%.[29–33] Most patients can be treated successfully with warfarin alone but recurrence of thrombus is common in the setting of inadequate anticoagulation or discontinuation because of bleeding.[34] The most common site of thrombus is the Fontan circuit, especially in asymptomatic patients.[35] The incidence of thrombus is higher in patients with an atriopulmonary anastomosis compared to total cavopulmonary connections. Thrombus has been associated with mortality, ventricular dysfunction, valvular regurgitation, heart failure, arrhythmias, and cardiac transplantation.[34,35] Even if clinically silent, thrombus in the Fontan circuit contributes to the overall presentation of a failing Fontan.

If thrombus is suspected clinically or by TTE, complementary imaging by CMR or CCT is recommended. Ruling-out thrombus is an important part of annual imaging surveillance even in the absence of symptoms. Anticoagulation with a vitamin K antagonist (INR between 2 and 3) is indicated upon diagnosis of TE. There is no consensus regarding an optimal strategy to prevent TE. Prophylaxis with antiplatelet or anticoagulation therapy has been associated with a lower incidence of thromboembolic events, with no convincing data showing superiority of anticoagulation over antiplatelet therapy. The potential for subclinical, recurrent nonsystemic TE (eventually leading to an increase in PVR) and systemic TE have prompted some centers to recommend routine lifelong anticoagulation or antiplatelet agent in adults with a Fontan circuit. Others reserve anticoagulation for patients with risk factors such as atrial arrhythmia, prior TE, residual intracardiac right-to-left shunt, or veno-veno collaterals.[6,7] There is some emerging data for using one of the novel oral anticoagulants, but these have not made it to guideline-based care as yet.

Pulmonary Vascular Disease

Fontan patients could develop pulmonary vascular disease without meeting the criterion for pulmonary hypertension. A mean pulmonary pressure >20 mm Hg is not compatible with life in a Fontan circulation. But any small increase in pulmonary vascular resistance will decrease pulmonary and systemic outflow and increase central venous pressure, leading to potential complications such as right heart failure, cirrhosis, and PLE.

Pulmonary vascular disease in Fontan patients could be categorized in two groups: (1) residual pulmonary vascular disease from pre-Fontan high pulmonary pressures, leading to early Fontan failure; and (2) pulmonary vascular disease that is a consequence of nonpulsatile continuous flow with low velocity and low shear stress, which leads to a unique pattern of pulmonary artery remodeling that is responsible for a late failing Fontan.[36] Pulmonary hypertension therapies such as endothelin receptor antagonists and phosphodiesterases-5 inhibitors could be considered if the intra-Fontan pressure is >15 mm Hg, PVR >2 Wood units, pulmonary flow is low (≤2.2 L/min/m^2), and/or the Fontan is failing. Routine use of these medications in Fontan patients remains controversial with limited data.[6,7,37-39]

OTHER COMPLICATIONS

Patients with a Fontan circulation present mild renal dysfunction in 40% of cases, with altered renal function being associated with increased mortality. Due to the unique hemodynamics of the Fontan circulation, venous insufficiency is very common. The lymphatic system is profoundly altered in Fontan patients as a result of venous congestion and is believed to underlie complications such as PLE and plastic bronchitis. Patients with Fontan physiology could also have neurodevelopemental disabilities that require early assessment for targeted interventions.

PROGNOSIS

In the modern area, early survival after Fontan surgery approaches 90% at 10 years. This reflects improved surgical techniques, postoperative care, and patient selection. Long-term mortality remains high with 61% to 85% survival at 20 years.[2,40] It has been estimated that a 35-year-old patient with a Fontan has a remaining life expectancy equivalent to a 72-year-old.[41] The principal causes of death are heart failure, thrombosis, perioperative and periprocedural complications, and sudden cardiac death.[41] Outcomes appear to be superior with the total cavopulmonary connections. Nevertheless, a large spectrum of univentricular heart defects culminate in Fontan palliation and survival differs among the various subtypes, with HLHS having the lowest overall long-term survival rate.

SUMMARY

Fontan patients should have regular follow-up by a dedicated multidisciplinary team. Multiorgan involvement and complications are common and merit routine screening, including laboratory tests, imaging studies, arrhythmia monitoring, and objective assessment of functional capacity. The threshold for cardiac catheterization should be low, particularly in the setting of increasing symptoms, new-onset or worsening arrhythmias, PLE, or plastic bronchitis. Routine joint follow-up by a hepatologist is recommended beginning 10 to 15 years after Fontan surgery given that virtually 100% of patients develop silent hepatic fibrosis by adolescence. Surgical options should be considered in patients with complications who fail medical therapy and/or percutaneous interventions. In the absence of standardized criteria, decisions regarding indications and timing of transplantation, along with the need for combined heart–liver transplantation, should be made by a multidisciplinary team at an expert congenital heart disease center.

REFERENCES

1. Fontan F, Baudet E. Surgical repair of tricuspid atresia. *Thorax.* 1971;26:240-248.
2. Rychik J, Atz AM, Celermajer DS, et al. Evaluation and management of the child and adult with Fontan circulation: a scientific statement from the American Heart Association. *Circulation.* 2019:CIR0000000000000696.
3. de Leval MR, Kilner P, Gewillig M, Bull C. Total cavopulmonary connection: a logical alternative to atriopulmonary connection for complex Fontan operations. Experimental studies and early clinical experience. *J Thorac Cardiovasc Surg.* 1988;96:682-695.
4. Iyengar AJ, Winlaw DS, Galati JC, et al. The extracardiac conduit Fontan procedure in Australia and New Zealand: hypoplastic left heart syndrome predicts worse early and late outcomes. *Eur J Cardiothorac Surg.* 2014;46:465-473; discussion 473.
5. Diller GP, Dimopoulos K, Okonko D, et al. Exercise intolerance in adult congenital heart disease: comparative severity, correlates, and prognostic implication. *Circulation.* 2005;112:828-835.
6. Stout KK, Daniels CJ, Aboulhosn JA, et al. 2018 AHA/ACC guideline for the management of adults with congenital heart disease: a report of the American College of Cardiology/American Heart Association Task Force on Clinical Practice Guidelines. *J Am Coll Cardiol.* 2019;73:e81-e192.
7. Baumgartner H, De Backer J, Babu-Narayan SV, et al. 2020 ESC guidelines for the management of adult congenital heart disease. *Eur Heart J.* 2020.
8. Li W, West C, McGhie J, et al. Consensus recommendations for echocardiography in adults with congenital heart defects from the International Society of Adult Congenital Heart Disease (ISACHD). *Int J Cardiol.* 2018;272:77-83.
9. Prabhu SP, Mahmood S, Sena L, Lee EY. MDCT evaluation of pulmonary embolism in children and young adults following a lateral tunnel Fontan procedure: optimizing contrast-enhancement techniques. *Pediatr Radiol.* 2009;39:938-944.
10. Biglino G, Koniordou D, Gasparini M et al. Piloting the use of patient-specific cardiac models as a novel tool to facilitate communication during cinical consultations. *Pediatr Cardiol.* 2017;38:813-818.
11. Bhatla P, Tretter JT, Ludomirsky A, et al. Utility and scope of rapid prototyping in patients with complex muscular ventricular septal defects or double-outlet right ventricle: does it alter management decisions? *Pediatr Cardiol.* 2017;38:103-114.
12. Olivieri L, Krieger A, Chen MY, Kim P, Kanter JP. 3D heart model guides complex stent angioplasty of pulmonary venous baffle obstruction in a Mustard repair of D-TGA. *Int J Cardiol.* 2014;172:e297-e298.
13. Valverde I, Gomez-Ciriza G, Hussain T, et al. Three-dimensional printed models for surgical planning of complex congenital heart defects: an international multicentre study. *Eur J Cardiothorac Surg.* 2017;52:1139-1148.
14. van Melle JP, Wolff D, Horer J, et al. Surgical options after Fontan failure. *Heart.* 2016;102:1127-1133.
15. Simpson KE, Pruitt E, Kirklin JK, et al. Fontan patient survival after pediatric heart transplantation has improved in the current era. *Ann Thorac Surg.* 2017;103:1315-1320.
16. Murtuza B, Hermuzi A, Crossland DS, et al. Impact of mode of failure and end-organ dysfunction on the survival of adult Fontan patients undergoing cardiac transplantation. *Eur J Cardiothorac Surg.* 2017;51:135-141.
17. Emamaullee J, Zaidi AN, Schiano T, et al. Fontan-associated liver disease: screening, management, and transplant considerations. *Circulation.* 2020;142:591-604.
18. Wong TW, Gandhi MJ, Daly RC, et al. Liver allograft provides immunoprotection for the cardiac allograft in combined heart-liver transplantation. *Am J Transplant.* 2016;16:3522-3531.
19. Yang H, Bouma BJ, Mulder BJM. Non vitamin KaOafTpiachdi. Is initiating NOACs for atrial arrhythmias safe in adults with congenital heart disease? *Cardiovasc Drugs Ther.* 2017;31:413-417.
20. Atz AM, Zak V, Mahony L, et al. Longitudinal outcomes of patients with single ventricle after the Fontan procedure. *J Am Coll Cardiol.* 2017;69:2735-2744.
21. Pundi KN, Pundi KN, Johnson JN, et al. Sudden cardiac death and late arrhythmias after the Fontan operation. *Congenit Heart Dis.* 2017;12:17-23.
22. Mertens L, Hagler DJ, Sauer U, Somerville J, Gewillig M. Protein-losing enteropathy after the Fontan operation: an international multicenter study. PLE study group. *J Thorac Cardiovasc Surg.* 1998;115:1063-1073.

23. John AS, Johnson JA, Khan M, Driscoll DJ, Warnes CA, Cetta F. Clinical outcomes and improved survival in patients with protein-losing enteropathy after the Fontan operation. *J Am Coll Cardiol.* 2014;64:54-62.

24. Weingarten AJ, Menachem JN, Smith CA, Frischhertz BP, Book WM. Usefulness of midodrine in protein-losing enteropathy. *J Heart Lung Transplant.* 2019;38:784-787.

25. Trusty PM, Wei Z, Rychik J, et al. Impact of hemodynamics and fluid energetics on liver fibrosis after Fontan operation. *J Thorac Cardiovasc Surg.* 2018;156:267-275.

26. Silva-Sepulveda JA, Fonseca Y, Vodkin I, et al. Evaluation of Fontan liver disease: Correlation of transjugular liver biopsy with magnetic resonance and hemodynamics. *Congenit Heart Dis.* 2019;14:600-608.

27. Surrey LF, Russo P, Rychik J, et al. Prevalence and characterization of fibrosis in surveillance liver biopsies of patients with Fontan circulation. *Hum Pathol.* 2016;57:106-115.

28. Munsterman ID, Duijnhouwer AL, Kendall TJ, et al. The clinical spectrum of Fontan-associated liver disease: results from a prospective multimodality screening cohort. *Eur Heart J.* 2019;40:1057-1068.

29. Grewal J, Al Hussein M, Feldstein J, et al. Evaluation of silent thrombus after the Fontan operation. *Congenit Heart Dis.* 2013;8:40-47.

30. Sughimoto K, Okauchi K, Zannino D et al. Total cavopulmonary connection is superior to atriopulmonary connection fontan in preventing thrombus formation: computer simulation of flow-related blood coagulation. *Pediatr Cardiol.* 2015;36:1436-1441.

31. Tsang W, Johansson B, Salehian O, et al. Intracardiac thrombus in adults with the Fontan circulation. *Cardiol Young.* 2007;17:646-651.

32. Coon PD, Rychik J, Novello RT, Ro PS, Gaynor JW, Spray TL. Thrombus formation after the Fontan operation. *Ann Thorac Surg.* 2001;71:1990-1994.

33. Balling G, Vogt M, Kaemmerer H, Eicken A, Meisner H, Hess J. Intracardiac thrombus formation after the Fontan operation. *J Thorac Cardiovasc Surg.* 2000;119:745-752.

34. Egbe AC, Connolly HM, Niaz T, et al. Prevalence and outcome of thrombotic and embolic complications in adults after Fontan operation. *Am Heart J.* 2017;183:10-17.

35. Sathananthan G, Johal N, Verma T, et al. Clinical importance of fontan circuit thrombus in the adult population: significant association with increased risk of cardiovascular events. *Can J Cardiol.* 2019;35:1807-1814.

36. Ridderbos FJ, Wolff D, Timmer A, et al. Adverse pulmonary vascular remodeling in the Fontan circulation. *J Heart Lung Transplant.* 2015;34:404-413.

37. Wang W, Hu X, Liao W, et al. The efficacy and safety of pulmonary vasodilators in patients with Fontan circulation: a meta-analysis of randomized controlled trials. *Pulm Circ.* 2019;9:2045894018790450.

38. Hebert A, Jensen AS, Idorn L, Sorensen KE, Sondergaard L. The effect of bosentan on exercise capacity in Fontan patients; rationale and design for the TEMPO study. *BMC Cardiovasc Disord.* 2013;13:36.

39. Goldberg DJ, Zak V, Goldstein BH et al. Results of the FUEL Trial. *Circulation.* 2020;141:641-651.

40. Downing TE, Allen KY, Glatz AC, et al. Long-term survival after the Fontan operation: twenty years of experience at a single center. *J Thorac Cardiovasc Surg.* 2017;154:243-253.e2.

41. Diller GP, Kempny A, Alonso-Gonzalez R, et al. Survival prospects and circumstances of death in contemporary adult congenital heart disease patients under follow-up at a large tertiary centre. *Circulation.* 2015;132:2118-2125.

42. Thorne SA. Atrioventricular valve atresia. In: MA Gatzoulis, GD Webb, PEF Daubeney, eds. *Diagnosis and Management of Adult Congenital Heart Disease,* 3rd ed. Philadelphia, PA: Elsevier; 2018:570-577.

70

Complex Cyanotic Congenital Heart Disease: The "Mixing" Lesions

Rafael Alonso-Gonzalez and Danielle Massarella

CHAPTER OUTLINE

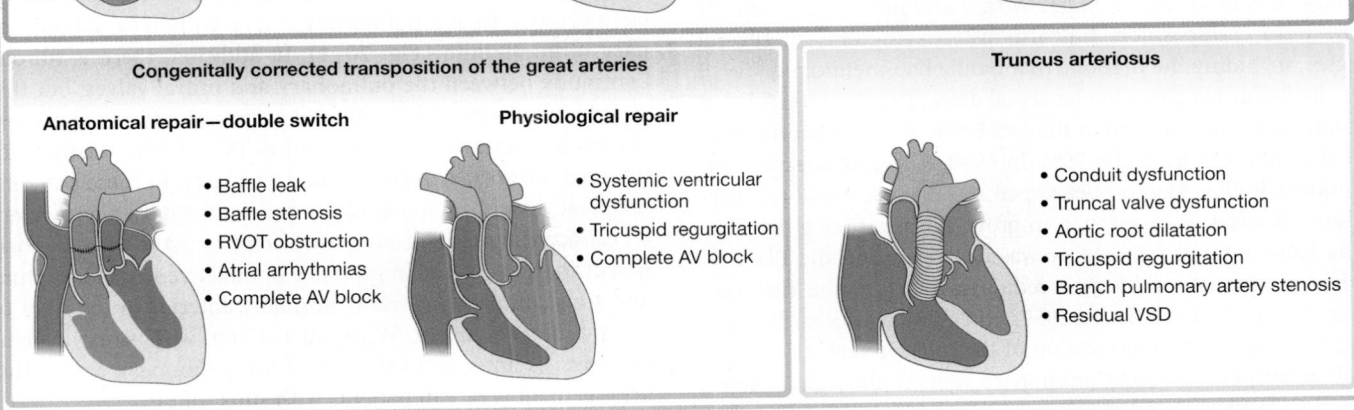

Repair and sequelae of cyanotic congenital cardiac lesions

Transposition of the great arteries

Atrial switch (Mustard/Senning)
- Baffle leak
- Baffle stenosis
- Systemic ventricular dysfunction
- Tricuspid regurgitation
- Atrial arrhythmias
- Pulmonary hypertension

Rastelli procedure
- Conduit dysfunction
- Right/left outflow tract obstruction
- Baffle leak
- Restrictive right ventricle
- Atrial/ventricular arrhythmias

Arterial switch
- RVOT obstruction
- Neo-aortic valve regurgitation
- Neo-aortic root dilatation
- Coronary obstruction

Congenitally corrected transposition of the great arteries

Anatomical repair—double switch
- Baffle leak
- Baffle stenosis
- RVOT obstruction
- Atrial arrhythmias
- Complete AV block

Physiological repair
- Systemic ventricular dysfunction
- Tricuspid regurgitation
- Complete AV block

Truncus arteriosus
- Conduit dysfunction
- Truncal valve dysfunction
- Aortic root dilatation
- Tricuspid regurgitation
- Branch pulmonary artery stenosis
- Residual VSD

Chapter 70 Fuster and Hurst's Central Illustration. Each of these lesions, while resulting from vastly different aberrations of embryonic cardiac development, culminates in mixed pulmonary and systemic venous return to the heart. Surgery assuages the immediacy of these threats to survival; however, residual lesions are nearly universal and determine the future course and outcomes over an individual's lifespan. AV, aortic valve; RVOT, right ventricular outflow tract; VSD, ventricular septal defect.

CHAPTER SUMMARY

This chapter describes the anatomy, physiology, medical and surgical therapies, and outcomes of some of the congenital heart diseases that result in cyanosis at presentation. Lesions discussed in detail include transposition of the great arteries (d-TGA) as well as congenitally corrected d-TGA, anomalies of pulmonary venous return, and truncus arteriosus (see Fuster and Hurst's Central Illustration). Each of these lesions, while resulting from vastly different aberrations of embryonic cardiac development, culminates in mixed pulmonary and systemic venous return to the heart. Depending on associated cardiac lesions, these forms of cardiac disease may be incompatible with life in the neonatal period or, at best, severely life-limiting in their unrepaired form. Advances in the field of cardiothoracic surgery have allowed the immediacy of these threats to survival to be assuaged. However, residual lesions are nearly universal and determine the future course and outcomes over an individual's lifespan. The population of adults born with cyanotic congenital heart disease is increasing, and knowledge of the sequelae of residual lesions is necessary in order to anticipate and mitigate complications.

TRANSPOSITION OF THE GREAT ARTERIES

Background

Transposition of the great arteries (d-TGA) is a congenital cardiac malformation characterized by atrioventricular (AV) concordance and ventriculoarterial (VA) discordance. The malformation was first described by Matthew Baillie in 1788.[1] Baillie reported the findings of an infant's autopsy with d-TGA in his book *The Morbid Anatomy of some of the Most Important Parts of the Human Body*. However, it was John Richard Farre, in 1814, who used for the first time the term *transposition of the great arteries* in his book *Pathological Researches on Malformations of the Human Heart*.[2] Farre mentioned not only the term *transposition*, but also listed symptoms of several cases, including the first one that Baillie had mentioned.

In absence of a ventricular septal defect (VSD), d-TGA is not compatible with life and in the 1950s, the neonatal mortality of this condition was nearly 90%. In 1948, Alfred Blalock and his resident Rollins Hanlon developed the Blalock–Hanlon procedure, an atrial septectomy to improve cardiac mixing. In 1966, the balloon atrial septostomy was described and the Blalock–Hanlon septectomy became redundant. Before the first successful repair of d-TGA in 1957, other procedures such as the Baffes procedure (translocation of the inferior vena cava to the left atrium and the right pulmonary veins to the right atrium), were successfully used to palliate patients with d-TGA.[3] In 1957, Ake Senning performed the first successful atrial switch procedure using flaps from the right atrial tissue and the interatrial septum.[4] Some years later, in 1964, William Mustard described the Mustard procedure,[5] an alternative technique in which the atrial septum is excised and the atrial baffle is created using a shaped patch of pericardial tissue. The Mustard procedure was technically less demanding than the Senning procedure and

became the technique of choice to repair the majority of patients with d-TGA between 1964 and 1975. In 1967, Giancarlo Rastelli developed the Rastelli procedure[6] to correct patients with VSD and obstruction of the subpulmonary outflow tract, leaving the left ventricle in the systemic position. Finally in 1975, Adib Jatene described the first successful arterial switch[7] and since the late 1970s early 1980s, this is the technique of choice to repair patients with d-TGA.

Anatomy

In patients with d-TGA, the right ventricle gives rise to the aorta via a subaortic infundibulum, whereas the left ventricle gives rise to the pulmonary artery without a subpulmonary infundibulum (**Fig. 70–1**). In addition, there is fibrous continuity between the pulmonary and mitral valves, but this is absent between the aorta and tricuspid valves. The most common external abnormality in d-TGA is the relationship between the aorta and the pulmonary artery. In these patients, the great vessels run in parallel instead of the normal crossover, an echocardiographic feature that helps to make the diagnosis in a cyanotic neonate. In presence of intact ventricular septum and situs solitus, the aorta is normally anterior to the right of the pulmonary artery. While in patients with situs inversus the aorta is anterior to the left of the pulmonary artery, this arrangement is rare in patients with situs solitus.

Coronary Arteries

The coronary arteries in patients with d-TGA normally arise from the two sinuses adjacent to the pulmonary artery that are described as facing sinuses. The coronary sinuses are classified according to their orientation, a leftward/anterior and rightward/posterior being the most common pattern.[8] There are several classification schemes for the coronary arteries with the

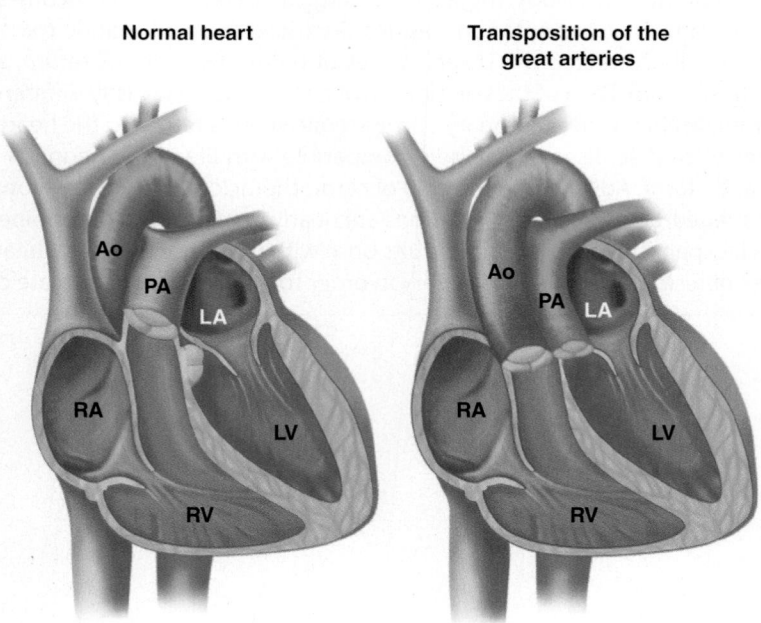

Figure 70–1. Normal heart and transposition of the great arteries. Ao, Aorta; LA, left atrium; LV, left ventricle; PA, pulmonary artery; RA, right atrium; RV, right ventricle.

most commonly used being the Leiden classification, where the left anterior sinus is numbered 1 and the right posterior sinus is numbered 2. The left anterior descending (LAD), circumflex, and right coronary arteries (RCA) are denoted as LAD, LCx, and R. The most common coronary artery pattern in patients with d-TGA is the left main arising from the leftward/anterior sinus (sinus 1) and bifurcating to give rise the LAD and the LCx arteries, and the RCA arising from the rightward/posterior sinus (sinus 2). Using the Leiden classification, this pattern is denoted as the usual pattern or 1LCx; 2R. There are many possible variations of the coronary artery anatomy including the circumflex artery arising from the right sinus, an inverted pattern or a single coronary artery arising from the anterior or posterior sinus and giving rise to the three branches[9] (**Fig. 70–2**). In 3% of cases, one of the coronary arteries can have an intramural course usually associated with an interarterial course between the aorta and pulmonary artery. This confers a risk of early sudden cardiac death (SCD) and increases the surgical mortality of the arterial switch procedure.[10]

Associated Defects

In 50% of the cases, the VA discordance is an isolated finding. This condition is designated as simple transposition. By contrast, complex transposition includes all the cases with coexisting malformations, such as VSDs, left ventricular outflow tract obstruction, or aortic arch anomalies.[11]

Ventricular Septal Defect: The most common associated lesion in d-TGA is a VSD present in 40% to 45% of cases.[12] As in any other VSD, the defect may be small, large, or multiple and can be located in any part of the interventricular septum. The outlet muscular septum in often malaligned relative to the rest of the ventricular septum and located in the right ventricle. A subpulmonary VSD is the most characteristic defect and may extend to the perimembranous area. Other types of defects are rare but also can be found, such as multiple muscular defects, solitary apical muscular defects, or doubly committed defects. The latter is usually associated with left-sided aorta and abnormal coronary artery pattern.

Left Ventricular Outflow Tract Obstruction: This is the second most common associated anomaly in patients with d-TGA and it is present in up to 33% of cases.[11] It is more frequent in patients with VSD but can also be present in those with intact ventricular septum. Isolated valvular obstruction is rare and is commonly associated with muscular subvalvular stenosis. An isolated subvalvular fibrous membrane can also be present mainly in patients with a more directly anteroposterior

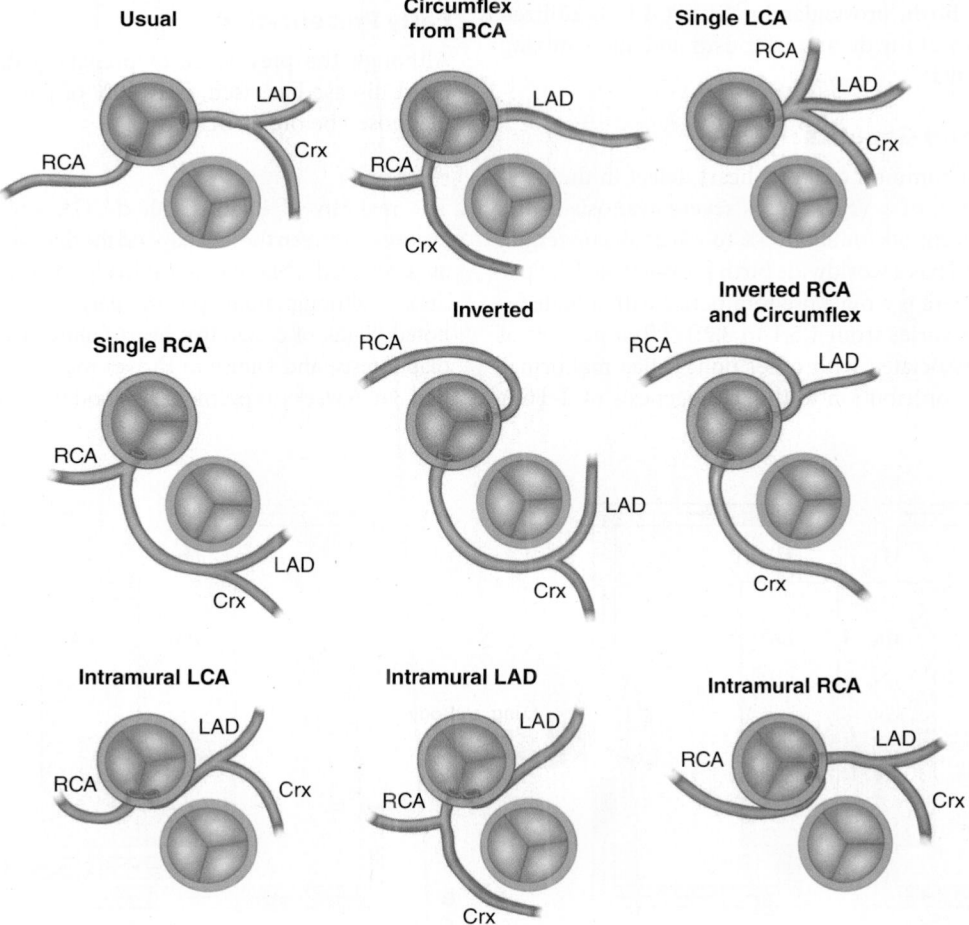

Figure 70–2. Different coronary artery pattens in patients with d-TGA. Cx, circumflex; LAD, left anterior descending; RCA, right coronary artery. Used with permission of Mayo Foundation for Medical Education and Research, all rights reserved.

relationship of the great arteries than when the arteries are side by side.[13] Other rare forms of left ventricular outflow obstruction can be caused by abnormal mitral valve chords attached to the interventricular septum or by aneurysms of fibrous tissue tags bulging into the outflow tract. If an anterior and rightward deviation of the outlet septum is present, concomitant pulmonary overriding and subaortic stenosis can be expected. In these cases, aortic hypoplasia, coarctation, or even interruption of the aortic arch may be encountered.

Coarctation of the Aorta: Coarctation of the aorta can be present in ~5% of patients with d-TGA and can be a discrete lesion or associated with a hypoplastic aortic arch.

Pathophysiology

The anatomical arrangements of d-TGA lead to two separated parallel blood flow circuits rather than the normal single series circuit (**Fig. 70–3**). This causes few problems, if any, in the fetus but it is a major problem after birth with the systemic arteries receiving deoxygenated blood, causing severe cyanosis at birth. The degree of cyanosis will depend on the amount of blood mixing between the two circulation sides and relates to the size of foramen ovale, the patency of the ductus arteriosus, as well as the presence of coexisting pulmonic stenosis. Patients with an associated unrestrictive VSD will be less cyanotic at birth. Immediately after birth, prostaglandin E1 (PGE1) is utilized to maintain patency of the ductus arteriosus and allow mixing between both circuits.

Epidemiology and Genetics

d-TGA is the most common cyanotic heart defect in the newborn and, in absence of a VSD, causes severe cyanosis in the first day of life. It accounts for about 5% to 7% of all congenital cardiac diseases and has a worldwide birth prevalence of 0.3 per 1000 live births. There is a male predominance with a male:female sex ratio that varies from 1.5:1 to 3.2:1.[11] Ten percent of the cases will be associated with other noncardiac malformations. The genetic contribution to the pathogenesis of d-TGA

is not considered to be strong given that very few familial cases have been described and that genetic syndromes or extracardiac malformations are uncommonly associated with d-TGA. Maternal diabetes has been reported as a risk factor for fetal d-TGA and recurrence in offspring is rare, approximately 1% to 2%.

d-TGA might be sporadically associated with trisomy 8 and 18, VACTERL, and CHARGE syndromes.[14] Although d-TGA may be present in patients with 22q11 deletion, it is not considered a characteristic cardiac defect in this population, unlike tetralogy of Fallot, truncus arteriosus, or interrupted aortic arch.[14] However, d-TGA is common in patients with lateralization defects (heterotaxy or isomerisms), and is frequently associated with an AV septal defect in patients with right atrial isomerism. In some patients with isolated d-TGA mutations, genes involved in establishing left–right axis have been identified, such as *ZIC3*, *CFC1*, and *NODAL*.[14]

Some animal studies have obtained d-TGA by treating pregnant mice with retinoic acid competitive antagonist, suggesting that critical levels of retinoic acid must be present for normal heart and conotruncal development.[15] Teratogenic development of d-TGA might be explained due to Hif1α down-regulation in response to blocking retinoic acid[16] and the administration of folic acid during pregnancy might reduce the risk of severe and most common congenital heart disease in offspring.[17]

Early Presentation

Although the prevalence of prenatally diagnosed congenital heart disease has risen, only 10% of patients with d-TGA get diagnosed before birth.[18]

History

The majority of infants with d-TGA will present with severe cyanosis between the first day and the first week of life. Patients with an associated VSD may not initially manifest symptoms of heart disease, although mild cyanosis, particularly when crying, is often noted. Signs of congestive heart failure (tachypnea, tachycardia, diaphoresis, and failure to thrive) may become evident over the first 3 to 6 weeks as pulmonary blood flow increases.

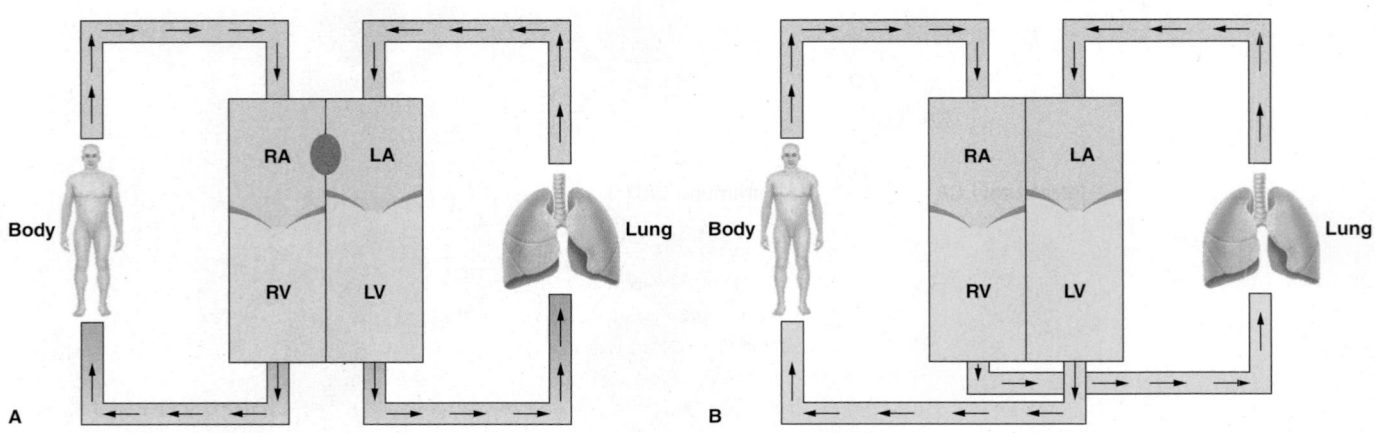

Figure 70–3. (A) Parallel circulation in patients with transposition of the great arteries. **(B)** Normal circulation. LA, left atrium; LV, left ventricle; RA, right atrium; RV, right ventricle.

Physical Examination

Patients with intact ventricular septum will present with progressive central cyanosis. On palpation, there will be a prominent right ventricular impulse and a systolic thrill may be felt when a VSD or severe left ventricular outflow tract obstruction are present. The peripheral pulses are normally bounding and equal. Weak femoral pulses with normal arm pulses should raise the suspicion of an associated coarctation of the aorta. At auscultation, a loud second heart sound is noticed and normally no murmurs are detected, although occasionally a midsystolic murmur might be heard. In patients with severe left ventricular outflow tract obstruction, a loud ejection systolic murmur at the upper sternal edge may be present. When a VSD without no left ventricular outflow tract obstruction is present, a loud pansystolic murmur at the lower left sternal edge can be detected.

Work-Up/Investigations

This section will focus on the investigation prior to surgical repair. Investigations after each type of repair will be discussed in other sections of this chapter.

The most important initial investigation is an arterial blood gas to demonstrate the presence of systemic hypoxemia. In patients with d-TGA, a hyperoxia test may be indicated. Pulmonary disease is suspected if the partial pressure of oxygen increases more than 150 to 180 mm Hg with oxygen. Patients with inadequate mixing might develop acidosis, with values of pH of 6.9 to 7.1 mm Hg not being uncommon.

Chest Radiography

The chest radiograph may appear normal in newborns with d-TGA and intact ventricular septum with adequate atrial level mixing. The specific radiologic features are determined by the extent to which the great arteries are superimposed in the plane of imaging, the size of the communication between the pulmonary and the systemic circulation, and the presence and severity of obstruction to pulmonary flow. The superior mediastinum is normally narrow, and the cardiac silhouette varies from normal to enlarged and globular, with the classic appearance described as an "egg on a string."

Echocardiography

A transthoracic echocardiogram is the technique of choice to diagnose d-TGA in a cyanotic newborn. The diagnosis is based on the sequential segmental analysis to demonstrate the presence of AV concordance and VA discordance. In patients with d-TGA, the aorta is usually anterior and right-sided but since this relationship is not present in all patients and also can be found in other conditions, it should not be used as hallmark for the diagnosis. The feature of particular value in demonstrating the discordant ventriculo-arterial connections is the branching pattern of the posterior pulmonary artery trunk arising from the left ventricle. The parallel alignment of the great arteries, best seen in the parasternal long axis view, can also be seen with other AV connections such as double outlet right ventricle.

Determining the adequacy of cardiac mixing is one of the most important components of the initial evaluation in the neonate with d-TGA. The atrial communication and the patency of the ductus arteriosus must be assessed. Although the size of the atrial communication in 2D is important, an evaluation of the mean pressure gradient across the interatrial septum should be performed to rule out a restrictive atrial septal defect.

A transthoracic echocardiogram will also allow for the characterization of associated lesions such as VSDs, left ventricular outflow tract obstruction, or aortic coarctation. The entire interventricular septum must be assessed to determine the location and size of the defect. Small VSDs may be hemodynamically insignificant or may close spontaneously. With inlet VSDs, imaging must include assessment for a straddling tricuspid valve. Doubly committed subarterial defects have fibrous continuity between the aortic and pulmonary valves and closure of these defects may result in distortion of semilunar valve leaflets and valve regurgitation.[19] Malalignment of the interventricular septum is associated with outflow tract obstruction. Posterior and leftward deviation of the interventricular septum results in left ventricular outflow tract obstruction (subpulmonary obstruction), increasing the risk of associated abnormalities of the pulmonary artery branches; whereas anterior and rightward deviation of the interventricular septum will result in right ventricular outflow obstruction (subaortic obstruction), which may cause hypoplastic aortic arch and/or coarctation of the aorta.

Coronary artery anatomy in patients with d-TGA is highly variable. Although 1LCx; 2R is the most common pattern, multiple patterns have been described (Fig. 70–2). Assessment of coronary artery anatomy is a fundamental component of the echocardiographic evaluation of neonates with d-TGA. Characterization of each coronary ostium and its proximal course is important to identify anomalies, such as an intramural course. Features suggestive of an intramural course include, a coronary artery originating from the opposite sinus of Valsalva that travels between the semilunar valves; a juxtacommissural origin at an acute angle from the aortic root; or a high take-off from the sinotubular junction. The presence of an intramural course increases the risk of coronary translocation in patients suitable for an ASO.

A preoperative transthoracic echocardiogram should include evaluation of the biventricular size and function. Assessment of the left ventricle suitability to support the systemic circulation is paramount before an ASO. The following echocardiographic parameters are examined to ensure the likelihood a good outcome after the ASO: left ventricular muscle mass, posterior wall thickness, shape of the interventricular septum, and the presence of coexisting anomalies such as a patent ductus arteriosus and left ventricular outflow tract obstruction.[20] The left ventricle is considered prepared for an arterial switch when the chamber displays a circular configuration with convexity of the interventricular septum toward the right ventricle on short axis view. Indications for ventricular retraining would include a septum that bulges right to left or has a banana-shape configuration. Aside from echocardiographic criteria, other signs of left ventricle preparedness might be considered.

Cardiac Magnetic Resonance

CMR imaging is seldom requested for preoperative evaluation of infants with d-TGA, because echocardiography usually provides all the necessary diagnostic information for surgical decision-making.[19] The only potential role of CMR in this setting is to accurately quantify left ventricular mass, volume, and systolic function in those patients who have undergone a pulmonary artery banding procedure to prepare a deconditioned left ventricle prior ASO.

Cardiac Computed Tomography

Cardiac computed tomography (CCT) is rarely needed before surgical intervention for patients with d-TGA. The exception is for the definition of complex vascular anatomy in patients with heterotaxy syndrome or patients with extracardiac anomalies.[19]

Cardiac Catheterization

Neonatal diagnostic cardiac catheterization is usually reserved for the subgroup of patients for whom echocardiography does not adequately delineate the coronary artery anatomy. It also might be needed to maintain adequate systemic arterial oxygen saturations prior to the surgical repair (see section Rashkind Procedure).

Treatment

Medical Therapy

There is no medical therapy to treat the physiological problem caused by parallel circulations, hence supportive measures should not delay the balloon atrial septostomy when needed. Cyanotic patients might benefit from a PGE_1 infusion to maintain patency of the ductus arteriosus. This normally improves oxygenation increasing left-to-right shunt but should be used with caution in patients with small patent foramen ovale because PGE_1 might be harmful in this setting. Patients that develop pulmonary edema and respiratory failure may require mechanical ventilatory support.

Balloon Atrial Septostomy (Rashkind Procedure)

Severely cyanotic patients at birth will benefit from early balloon atrial septostomy prior undergoing complete repair. This procedure, described by Rashkind and Miller in 1966, disrupts the foramen flap and creates a larger atrial communication allowing better mixing at the atrial level, leading to better oxygenation. The procedure may be performed in the cardiac catheterization laboratory guided by fluoroscopy or at the bedside guided by echocardiography. The intervention is considered successful when there is a 10% increase in arterial oxygen saturation, a very minimal pressure gradient between the two atria, or an increase in the diameter of the atrial septal defect of more than a third of its original size.[20] Once adequate mixing is obtained, discontinuation of PGE_1 is often possible but patients should be weaned from PGE_1 rather than stopped because of the risk of hypoxemia after abrupt discontinuation.

Surgical Management

Atrial Switch Operation (Mustard and Senning): The atrial switch procedures redirect the venous return at the atrial level streaming the systemic venous flow to the left ventricle and the pulmonary venous flow to the right ventricle. This leaves the right ventricle in systemic position. The atrial switch procedure was first successfully performed in Sweden by Dr. Aka Senning[4] in 1957. In 1963, Dr. William Mustard in Toronto, Canada, described the Mustard procedure that was technically less demanding and became the technique of choice to repair patients with d-TGA in the 1960s. The difference between both procedures is that in the Senning operation, the baffle is created from the right atrial wall and interatrial septum without any prosthetic material, whereas in the Mustard operation, the baffle is created from pericardium or prosthetic material (**Fig. 70–4**). The Senning operation, with its avoidance of foreign material, seemed to provide better growth and less venous obstruction in smaller children. The atrial switch is performed within the first year of life with a low early mortality but significant long-term morbidity (**Table 70–1**).

Arterial Switch Operation: The arterial switch operation (ASO) is the procedure of choice in the current surgical era used to achieve complete physiological and anatomical repair (Fig 70–4). It was first described by Adib Jatene, a Brazilian surgeon, in 1975.[7] In this operation, the aorta and pulmonary

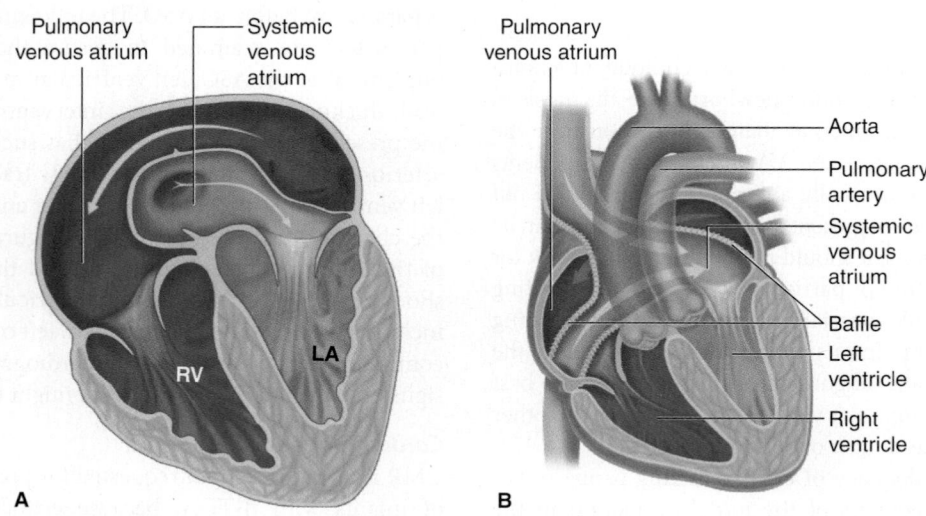

Figure 70–4. (A) Senning procedure. **(B)** Mustard procedure. LA, left atrium; LV, left ventricle; RA, right atrium; RV, right ventricle.

TABLE 70–1. Complication of the Different Surgical Techniques to Correct d-TGA

Arterial switch operation (Mustard and Senning)
- Baffle leak
- Baffle stenosis
- Atrial arrhythmias
- Sinus node dysfunction
- Systemic right ventricle dysfunction
- Tricuspid regurgitation
- Pulmonary hypertension

Arterial switch operation
- Right ventricular outflow tract obstruction
- Branch pulmonary artery stenosis
- Neoaortic root dilatation
- Neoaortic valve regurgitation
- Coronary artery stenosis

Rastelli procedure
- RV-PA conduit stenosis
- RV-PA conduit regurgitation
- LVOT obstruction
- Residual ventricular septal defect
- Left/right ventricular dysfunction
- Restrictive right ventricle
- Atrial arrhythmias
- Sudden cardiac death

Abbreviations: LVOT, left ventricular outflow tract obstruction; PA, pulmonary artery; RV, right ventricle; d-TGA, transposition of the great arteries.

trunks are transected, and their distal ends are transposed and anastomosed; coronary arteries are then translocated to the neoaorta. Initially a conduit was used between the neopulmonary artery and the pulmonary trunk, increasing the risk of right ventricular tract obstruction. In 1981, Lecompte described a maneuver that liberated the posteriorly positioned bifurcation of the pulmonary trunk and threaded the aorta through it, allowing a direct anastomosis of the neopulmonary root and the pulmonary trunk, avoiding the use of a conduit (**Table 70–3**).

The ASO should be performed, ideally, in the first 2 weeks of life and no later than the first month to avoid a significant regression of the left ventricular muscle mass. This would increase the surgical risk and the potential for the left ventricle to fail after the arterial switch. Special consideration should be given to patients with d-TGA that present later than the first month of life. In these patients, mainly in those with intact ventricular septum, the left ventricular muscle mass might have regressed significantly, and the left ventricle might no longer be able to support the systemic circulation. In this scenario, a two-stage repair should be considered.

A majority of patients with d-TGA are suitable for arterial switch. However, patients with left ventricular outflow tract obstruction might need a Rastelli or a Réparation a l'Etage Ventriculaire (REV) operation (subsequently discussed) if the subvalvular stenosis cannot be resected and/or the pulmonary valve is hypoplastic or atretic. The presence of an intramural course of the left coronary artery arising from the right sinus, increases the risk of the ASO and may require individualized techniques for coronary transfer but it is not an absolute contraindication in the current era.

Rastelli, REV, and Nikaidoh Procedures: The Rastelli procedure was developed by Giancarlo Rastelli in 1967[6] for patients with d-TGA, VSD, and left ventricular outflow tract obstruction. The procedure involves patching the VSD to the aorta, ligating and dividing the native pulmonary artery, and inserting a conduit between the right ventricle and the divided pulmonary artery. For a patient to be suitable for a Rastelli procedure, the VSD must extend to the subaortic infundibulum. This normally occurs in patients with subpulmonary stenosis where the outlet septum is deviated toward the left ventricular outflow tract and the aorta overrides the interventricular septum.

The timing to perform the Rastelli procedure remains unclear. Some groups believe that the procedure should be performed in early infancy, whereas others prefer to do a palliative procedure as a first intervention and perform the complete repair between 4 and 6 years when an adult-sized conduit can be implanted. The Rastelli procedure has the advantage of leaving the left ventricle in systemic position but late morbidity and mortality are significant due to recurrent left ventricular outflow tract obstruction, early conduit stenosis or regurgitation, arrhythmias, and SCD (Table 70–1).

The REV procedure[21] consists of resection of the muscular outlet septum, patching the VSD to the aorta and reconstruction of the right ventricular outflow tract by direct implantation of the pulmonary artery to the ventriculotomy. In most cases, the pulmonary artery bifurcation is translocated anteriorly (Lecompte maneuvre).[22]

The Nikaidoh procedure is also an option to repair patients with d-TGA and left ventricular outflow tract obstruction, especially if inadequate anatomy for an REV or Rastelli is present.[23] The repair is achieved by removing the aortic root with its coronaries attached, and translocating them to the prior pulmonary position. The obstruction in the left ventricular outflow tract is relieved through outlet septum dissection and resection of the pulmonary valve. The outflow of the right ventricle is then reconstructed with either a right ventricle to pulmonary artery conduit or patch made of bovine pericardium.[11] The major disadvantages of this approach are that it is technically difficult and has a high reoperation rate. Despite all these disadvantages, Hu et al. suggest that the Nikhaidoh approach obtains better hemodynamics than the REV or the Rastelli.[24] Further studies are needed to establish the role of this surgical approach in d-TGA.

Long-Term Outcome and Prognosis

Before the surgical repair was available, almost half of children born with d-TGA died in the first month of life and 90% within the first year of life.[25] Patients with intact ventricular septum had the worst prognosis and only half of the patients with a VSD survived the first year of life.[26] Patients with VSD and left ventricular outflow tract obstruction have the best prognosis with 50% surviving to 3 years of age.[12] The prognosis of patients after repair will depend significantly on the type of repair.

Atrial Switch Operation (Mustard and Senning)

Early and Long-Term Prognosis: The overall surgical mortality of the Mustard and Senning procedure is low when it is

TABLE 70–2. dTGA S/P Atrial Switch Operation: 2018 AHA/ACC Guidelines for ACHD

COR	LOE	Diagnostic	Therapeutic
I	B-NR		1. GDMT with appropriate attention to the need for anticoagulation is recommended to promptly restore sinus rhythm for adults with d-TGA with atrial switch repair presenting with atrial arrhythmia.
I	C-EO	1. Ambulatory monitoring for bradycardia or sinus node dysfunction is recommended for adults with d-TGA with atrial switch, especially if treated with beta blockers or other rate-slowing agents.	
I	C-EO	1. Adults with d-TGA with atrial switch repair should undergo annual imaging with either echocardiography or CMR to evaluate for common long-term complications of the atrial switch.	
IIa	C-LD	1. Assessment for a communication through the interatrial baffle or venous stenosis is reasonable for adults with d-TGA with atrial switch, particularly if transvenous pacemaker/ICD implantation is considered or leads are already present.	

d-TGA S/P Atrial Switch Operation: 2020 ESC Guidelines for ACHD

COR	LOE	Indications for Catheter Interventions	Indications for Surgical Interventions
I	C	1. In symptomatic patients with baffle stenosis, stenting is recommended when technically feasible. 2. In symptomatic patients with baffle leaks and cyanosis at rest or during exercise, or with strong suspicion of paradoxical emboli, stenting (covered) or device closure is recommended when technically feasible. 3. In patients with baffle leaks and symptoms due to L–R shunt, stenting (covered) or device closure is recommended when technically feasible.	1. In symptomatic patients with pulmonary venous atrium obstruction, surgical repair (catheter intervention rarely possible) is recommended. 2. In symptomatic patients with baffle stenosis not amenable to catheter intervention, surgical repair is recommended. 3. In symptomatic patients with baffle leaks not amenable to catheter-based closure, surgical repair is recommended.
IIa	C	1. In asymptomatic patients with baffle leaks with substantial left ventricular volume overload due to L-R shunt, stenting (covered) or device closure should be considered when technically feasible. 2. In patients with a baffle leak who require a PM/ICD, closure of the baffle leak with a covered stent should be considered, when technically feasible, prior to insertion of transvenous leads.	1. In patients with severe tricuspid valve regurgitation, without significant ventricular systolic dysfunction (EF >40%), valve repair or replacement should be considered, regardless of symptoms.
IIb	C	1. In asymptomatic patients with baffle stenosis, stenting may be considered when technically feasible.	
III	C		1. PA banding in adults, as LV training with subsequent arterial switch procedure, is not recommended.

Abbreviations: AV, atrioventricular; EF, ejection fraction; ICD, implantable cardioverter defibrillator; L-R, left-to-right; LV, left ventricle/ventricular; PA, pulmonary artery; PM, pacemaker.

performed in high-volume centers. Data from the Toronto cohort showed a significant improvement in operative mortality in the late era, 1974 to 1985, when compared to the early era, 1963 to 1973, 0.9% versus 10.1%.[27] Patients with complex d-TGA, associated VSD, and/or left ventricular outflow tract obstruction, have a higher perioperative mortality,[28] which seems be higher with the Senning than the Mustard procedure.[29]

Although the atrial switch operation was replaced in the mid-1980's with the arterial switch operation (which became the procedure of choice), these older patients with the atrial switch operation remain an important cohort in ACHD units. The long-term survival of patients with atrial switch repair will be mainly determined by the progressive deterioration of the systemic right ventricular function and the degree of tricuspid regurgitation that will lead to development of heart failure and SCD. A recent meta-analysis of 29 observational studies comprising 5035 patients with a minimum follow-up of 10 years showed an average survival of 91% at 10 years, 86% at 20 years, 76% at 30 years, and 65% at 40 years, with SCD accounting for 45% of all reported deaths.[30] Congestive heart failure from systemic right ventricular dysfunction was the second most common cause of mortality, responsible for 21% of deaths.[30] Different studies have identified several risk factors for late mortality, such as history of supraventricular tachycardia,[30,31] Mustard procedure compared with Senning,[30,32] and complex d-TGA compared with simple d-TGA.[29,30,32]

After atrial switch repair, patients have initially a good functional capacity, with 75% of them being in New York Heart Association (NYHA) functional class I at the time of transfer to adult care.[33] However, functional class deteriorates over time and approximately half of the patients will be in functional class II by the end of their twenties.[33] Systemic right ventricular function also deteriorates over time with 65% of patients having moderate-to-severe systemic right ventricle dysfunction by the age of 25.[33] Peak oxygen consumption and heart rate reserve are reduced in this population with 44% of the patients having chronotropic incompetence.[34,35] Interestingly, patients with atrial switch have limited ability to increase stroke volume to exercise, probably due to the stiffness of the atrial baffles, hence their aerobic capacity will rely on heart rate response. This should be taken into account when prescribing rate control medications.

Baffle Stenosis and Baffle Leak: Obstruction of the systemic venous baffles is more common after the Mustard (15.3%) than Senning procedure (1.4%).[36] The incidence can be as high as 44%[37] and frequently affects the superior baffle with only 1% to 2% of cases involving the inferior baffle.[38] Systemic venous baffle stenosis is normally asymptomatic due to an effective bypass circulation provided by the azygos or hemiazygos veins, but hepatomegaly and liver cirrhosis might occur with severe obstruction of the inferior baffle. Surgical or percutaneous intervention is not recommended in asymptomatic patients,[39] although might be considered in patients with severe stenosis of the inferior baffle and signs of liver congestion, to avoid further progression to liver cirrhosis. Patency of the superior systemic venous baffle must be assessed prior to pacemaker implantation and baffle limb stenting should be considered if moderate or severe stenosis is present (**Table 70–2**).

Pulmonary venous baffle obstruction is extremely rare, accounting only for 2% of the baffle obstructions.[12] The stenosis is normally produced at the junction between the patch and the left atrial tissue. Severe obstruction of the pulmonary venous baffle will cause pulmonary venous congestion and subsequently pulmonary hypertension. The latter, if not reversible, will be a contraindication for an isolated heart transplant. Mild stenosis can be treated conservatively but significant stenosis may need percutaneous balloon and stent placement or even surgical intervention.[38] It is the authors' preference to stent patients with severe pulmonary venous baffle obstruction and significant pulmonary hypertension to avoid further development of pulmonary vascular disease.

TABLE 70–3. Comparison Table for Transposition of the Great Arteries S/P Arterial Switch Operation: 2018 AHA/ACC Guidelines for ACHD

COR	LOE	Diagnostic	Therapeutic
I	C-LD	1. Baseline and serial imaging with either echocardiography or CMR should be performed in adults with d-TGA with arterial switch who have neoaortic dilation, valve dysfunction or PA or branch PA stenosis or ventricular dysfunction	
I	C-EO	1. Coronary revascularization for adults with d-TGA with arterial switch should be planned by surgeons or interventional cardiologists with expertise in revascularization in collaboration with ACHD providers to ensure coronary and pulmonary artery anatomy are understood	
IIa	B-NR	1. It is reasonable to perform anatomic evaluation of coronary artery patency (catheter angiography, or CT or MR angiography) in asymptomatic adults with d-TGA with arterial switch	
IIa	C-EO	1. Physiological tests of myocardial perfusion for adults with d-TGA after arterial switch can be beneficial for assessing symptoms suggestive of myocardial ischemia	1. GDMT is reasonable to determine indications for aortic valve replacement in adults with d-TGA after arterial switch with severe neoaortic valve regurgitation
IIa	C-EO	1. GDMT is reasonable to determine the need for coronary revascularization for adults with d-TGA after arterial switch	2. Catheter or surgical intervention for PS is reasonable in adults with d-TGA after arterial switch with symptoms of HF or decreased exercise capacity attributable to PS

Transposition of the Great Arteries S/P Arterial Switch Operation: 2020 ESC Guidelines for ACHD

COR	LOE	Indications for Catheter Interventions	Indications for Surgical Interventions
I	C	1. Stenting (depending on substrate) is recommended for coronary artery stenosis causing ischemia	1. Surgery (depending on substrate) is recommended for coronary artery stenosis causing ischemia
IIa	C	1. Stenting should be considered for PA branch stenosis, regardless of symptoms, if >50% diameter narrowing and RVSP >50 mm Hg and/or related reduced lung perfusion are present	1. Neo-aortic root surgery should be considered when the neo-aortic root is >55 mm, providing average adult stature 2. For neoaortic valve replacement or severe neoaortic AR, valvular heart disease guidelines with special considerations apply

Abbreviations: AR, aortic regurgitation; PA, pulmonary artery; RVSP, right ventricular systolic pressure.

Baffle leaks are more common than obstructions. They are present in 25% of patients,[12] are generally small,[38] and frequently located in the distal end of the inferior venous baffle. Shunting can be either left-to-right (systemic-to-pulmonary circulation) or right-to-left (pulmonary-to-systemic circulation). The latter can cause cyanosis and/or paradoxical embolism, whereas the former, if hemodynamically significant, can cause subpulmonary left ventricular volume overload. Baffle leak closure is only needed in 1% to 2% of cases and should be considered in the presence of subpulmonary left ventricular volume overload or prior to pacemaker implantation to reduce the risk of paradoxical embolism.

Assessment of the systemic and pulmonary venous baffles can be accomplished by transthoracic or transesophageal echocardiography, CMR, CCT, or angiography. Echocardiography with agitated saline might be useful to diagnose baffle leaks, although small leaks might only be visualized with a transesophageal echocardiogram. CMR is useful to assess patency of the baffles but also to quantify shunt-related baffle leak (Qp:Qs).

Right Ventricular Function and Tricuspid Valve Regurgitation: After the atrial switch, the right ventricle is in systemic position and at risk of deteriorating over time. Almost all patients with systemic right ventricle will have some degree of systolic dysfunction after 40 years from the atrial switch procedure,[40] with almost two-thirds of them having moderate-to-severe systolic dysfunction already in the third decade of life.[33]

In this population, long-term survival appears to be primarily determined by how well the right ventricle and the tricuspid valve tolerate systemic afterload. To adapt to a high-pressure circulation, the right ventricle geometry becomes more similar to a systemic left ventricle and contraction patterns of the right ventricle free wall change to increased circumferential and reduced longitudinal shortening.[41,42] In addition, the septal curvature on the right ventricle side reverses from convex to concave causing septal dysfunction, contributing to failure of the systemic right ventricle in this population.[42]

The mechanisms of right ventricular failure in these patients are not completely understood. Myocardial perfusion studies and stress echocardiography have demonstrated impaired ventricular function and perfusion defects during exercise suggestive of coronary insufficiency.[43,44] Myocardial fibrosis is common in the systemic right ventricle and is associated with a higher brain natriuretic peptide (BNP) and adverse clinical outcome.[45] A recent study including 48 patients with d-TGA showed that there is a significant correlation between systemic right ventricular function, collagen deposition, and fibrosis,[46] suggesting that myocardial fibrosis plays a role in the deterioration of the systemic right ventricle.

Mild-to-moderate tricuspid regurgitation is very common after atrial switch and tends to progressively worsen. The tricuspid regurgitation is secondary to annular dilatation in the majority of cases, although occasionally the tricuspid valve apparatus may be intrinsically abnormal or may have been damaged at the time of prior VSD repair. The right ventricle in systemic position changes its morphology to a more rounded shape. Progressive deterioration of the systemic right

ventricular function will lead to further annular dilation and ultimately to worsening of the tricuspid regurgitation. Patients with severe tricuspid regurgitation and intrinsic abnormalities of the tricuspid valve might benefit from elective tricuspid valve replacement when the right ventricle ejection fraction is >40%. However, tricuspid valve repair/replacement should be carefully considered in those with functional tricuspid regurgitation and/or more than moderately impaired right ventricular function.

Two-dimensional echocardiography is highly effective in visualizing heart walls, chamber configuration, valve anatomy, intracardiac shunts, and in revealing complex spatial morphologic information. In addition, echocardiography is also reliable and reproducible to assess the left ventricle; however, assessing the right ventricle can be challenging. The assessment of the right ventricle is even more difficult when the right ventricle is in systemic position. Accurate measure of right ventricular size and function drives many clinical decisions in this population, hence CMR is often used to more accurately measure right ventricle volumes and systolic function.

Arrhythmias: Rhythm issues in atrial switch patients range from sinus node dysfunction to atrial and ventricular tachyarrhythmias. Sinus node dysfunction, atrial tachyarrhythmias, and the risk of sudden death have been recognized as important sequelae in this population.[47]

Bradyarrhythmias: Sinus node dysfunction is highly prevalent in the atrial switch population being less common after the Senning procedure.[48] Although 50% of patients will have a sinus node dysfunction 20 years after the atrial switch repair,[49] only 10% of them will need a pacemaker.[50] After atrial switch, patients can present with junctional rhythm and this is associated with a 2.1-fold increased risk of developing supraventricular tachycardia, that can lead to ventricular tachycardia (VT) due to rapid AV conduction.[51] Pacemaker implantation should be consider after atrial switch and junctional rhythm if the resting heart rate is <40 bpm, even if the patient is asymptomatic.

Tachyarrhythmias: Atrial tachyarrhythmias are frequently observed in this population with the incidence increasing over time. Atrial tachyarrhythmias are an important cause of morbidity and mortality and may become life-threatening.[52] Both intra-atrial re-entry tachycardia (IART) and atrial fibrillation (AFib) are predictors of SCD in this population.[53] Cavotricuspid isthmus (CTI) dependent re-entry tachycardia, atrial flutter, is the most common arrhythmia in these patients with a cumulative incidence of up to 25% after 20 years.[50] Cumulative patient-level data from 2143 patients showed a supraventricular tachycardia (SVT) incidence of 14%, with atrial flutter accounting for 83% of SVT.[30] After ASO, the circuit of a CTI dependent reentry tachycardia differs from that of patients without congenital heart disease because of the transection of the CTI by the baffle, various scars, and/or suture lines. Successful ablation of a CTI dependent re-entry tachycardia involves placement of ablative lesions across the CTI in both, the systemic venous atrium and the pulmonary venous atrium in the majority of cases (Fig. 70–4).[54] Other arrhythmias, such as atrioventricular nodal reentry tachycardia (AVNRT), and focal atrial tachycardia have been described but are rare in this population.

Sinus rhythm is favored in patients with systemic right ventricle. Sustained atrial tachyarrhythmias should be urgently controlled and early direct current cardioversion is recommended.[55] Although antiarrhythmic drugs might be considered to maintain sinus rhythm, radiofrequency catheter ablation is a better long-term solution. The ablation of CTI dependent reentry tachycardia often requires baffle puncture to achieve isthmus block. Alternatively, remote magnetic navigation can be used for retrograde access to the pulmonary venous atrium allowing ablation of the CTI without baffle puncture. Conventional retrograde transaortic route access in adults is usually not successful to achieve successful isthmus block.[39]

Sudden Cardiac Death: SCD of presumed arrhythmic etiology is the leading cause of mortality in patients with atrial switch[30] with an estimated incidence of 4 to 5 per 1000 patient-years.[56] In a recent meta-analysis, median annual incidence of SCD in this population was 0.2% with cumulative cohort incidence ranging between 2% and 13%. There are studies suggesting that the late development of spontaneous VT or ventricular fibrillation might be more prevalent in this patient population than has been reported.[56,57]

Over 80% of SCDs after the atrial switch procedure occur during exercise.[53] Risk factors for VT and SCD include a QRS duration ≥140 ms,[57] older age at surgical repair,[58] systemic ventricular dysfunction,[30,57,58] severe tricuspid regurgitation,[55] history of atrial arrhythmias[53,59] and complex d-TGA.[57] Although the pathophysiology linking exercise to sudden death in this population remains unknown, an abnormal stroke volume response to rapid heart rates might increase the vulnerability to ischemia in a chronically pressure overloaded hypertrophied systemic right ventricle, leading to VT and ultimately SCD.

Implantable cardioverter defibrillators (ICDs) are indicated for secondary prevention.[39] However, selecting candidates for primary prevention ICDs remains a major challenge in this population. In addition, there is an increased risk of inappropriate shocks in this setting. In a recent meta-analysis, out of a total 124 ICD discharges over 330 patient-years in patients with ICDs for primary prevention, only 8% were appropriate.[30] In patients with ICDs for primary and secondary prevention treatment with β-blockers should be considered to reduce the risk of appropriate and inappropriate shocks.[59] Cardiac resynchronization therapy (CRT) might be considered in selected cases but frequently the location of the coronary sinus on top of the subpulmonary ventricle precludes intravascular resynchronization in these patients.

Congestive Heart Failure and Systemic Right Ventricle: Despite a high prevalence of moderate to severely impaired right ventricular systolic function 25 years after the atrial switch repair, only a quarter of patients will have clinical signs of heart failure.[33,60] In the atrial switch population, heart failure symptoms are associated with a 4.4-fold increase in the risk of sudden death.[53] Elevated BNP correlates with exercise capacity,

systemic ventricular function, and worsening tricuspid regurgitation; however, prognostic markers for development of heart failure in this population are sparse.[61,62]

The usefulness of conventional heart failure treatment in the setting of a systemic right ventricle is unknown. In fact, the inability to increase stroke volume to exercise in patients with atrial switch might lead to reduction of cardiac output when taking afterload reduction therapy. In addition, altering venous capacitance may decrease ventricular filling rather than increase cardiac output.

A majority of the studies assessing the effect of angiotensin-converting enzyme inhibitors (ACEi) or angiotensin II receptor blockers (ARBs) in patients with systemic right ventricle are small and showed neither benefit nor harm (**Table 70-4**). A small, prospective, randomized/crossover study with losartan in patients with d-TGA demonstrated improvement of ejection fraction and exercise duration in an adolescent/young adult population.[63] Unfortunately, this was not subsequently confirmed in two randomized, placebo-controlled studies with ARBs in this population. Van de Bom et al. showed that patients treated with valsartan had less systemic right ventricular dilatation and mass increase during follow-up. In the same study, a subgroup analysis showed improvement of right ventricular ejection fraction in symptomatic patients treated with valsartan compared to the placebo group.[64] A long-term follow-up study of the same cohort showed that treatment with valsartan does not reduce mortality after 8.3 years of follow-up. However, it showed a significant reduction in the composite endpoint of arrhythmias, worsening heart failure, need for tricuspid valve surgery, and death in symptomatic patients.[65] Data on β-blockers in this population are even more scarce (Table 70-4). Small observational studies with β-blockers have shown improvement in heart failure symptoms in patients with systemic right ventricle. However, β-blockers should be used carefully in this population because they can be detrimental in patients with Mustard repair who rely on heart rate to increase cardiac output.[39]

The available evidence does not support treating asymptomatic patients with systemic right ventricular dysfunction after atrial switch, but treatment with conventional heart failure therapy should be considered in symptomatic patients.[39] Some patients with systemic right ventricle may also benefit from treatment with ICD or CRT-D (see section Arrhythmias).

Ultimately, patients with atrial switch will need to be assessed for heart transplant at some point during follow-up. Early referral to an adult congenital heart disease heart function clinic is recommended (**Table 70-5**). Advanced heart failure therapies, including ventricular assist devices, are now widely available and might need to be considered in selected cases.

Pulmonary Hypertension: Pulmonary hypertension might develop over time in patients with a systemic right ventricle. A study from Toronto, including 141 patients with systemic right ventricle, showed a prevalence of 55% of pulmonary hypertension in this population.[66] A majority of patients had either isolated postcapillary pulmonary hypertension or

TABLE 70–4. Studies with ACEis, ARBs, Mineralocorticoids, and β-Blockers in Patients with Systemic Right Ventricle

	Study Type	Intervention	Sample (N) T/P	Population	Baseline RVEF	NYHA II-IV	Follow-up	Primary End Point/Outcomes
RCT								
Dos et al.[178]	Randomized	Eplerenone	14/12	TGA—100%	55%	3 (11%)	1 year	Change in systemic right ventricular mass (neutral)
Therrien et al.[179]	Randomized	Ramipril	8/9	TGA—100%	44%	1 (6%)	1 year	Change in RVEF and RVEDV (neutral)
van der Bom et al.[64]	Randomized	Valsartan	44/44	TGA—72% ccTGA—28%	36%	28 (32%)	3 years	Change in RVEF (neutral)
van Dissel et al.[65]	Randomized	Valsartan	44/44	TGA—72% ccTGA—28%	36%	28 (32%)	8.3 years	Mortality and MACE (arrhythmias, worsening heart failure, tricuspid valve surgery and death)—no effect in mortality but reduction of MACE
Non-RCT								
Dore et al.[63]	Randomized/ Crossover	Losartan	29	TGA—70% ccTGA—27%	42%	7 (2%)	15 weeks	Improvement in exercise capacity and reduction of NT-Pro-BNP
Hechter et al.[180]	Observational	ACEi	14	TGA—100%	47%	NA	6 months	Change in exercise capacity, RVEF, RVEDV (neutral)
Lester et al.[181]	Randomized/ Crossover	Losartan	7	TGA—100%	48%	NA	8 weeks	Improvement in exercise capacity reduction of tricuspid regurgitation
Giardini et al[182]	Prospective	Carvedilol	8	TGA—75% ccTGA—25%	34%	83 (88%)	1 year	Improvement of RVEF, RVEDV, LVEF and exercise capacity
Doughan et al.[183]	Retrospective	Carvedilol/ Metoprolol XL	31/29	TGA—100%	34%	18 (58%)	10 months	Improved exercise capacity in patients with pacemaker. No change in RVEF, RVED area or degree of tricuspid regurgitation
Tutarel et al.[184]	Prospective– open label	Enalapril	14	TGA—100%	44%	14 (100%)	13 months	No change in exercise capacity but significant reduction in NT-proBNP

Abbreviations: ACEi, angiotensin converting enzyme inhibitors; ARBs, angiotensin II receptor blockers; MACE, major cardiovascular events; NA, Not available; RCT, randomized control trial; RVEDV, right ventricular end-diastolic volume; RVEF, right ventricular ejection fraction; T/P, treatment/placebo

combined pre- and postcapillary pulmonary hypertension, with only 5% of patients having pulmonary arterial hypertension. Pulmonary hypertension was a predictor of outcome and it was uncommon in patients with normal BNP values (BNP <100 pg/mL), regardless of their systemic ventricular function. Treatment with diuretics and afterload reduction medication might be considered in these patients to avoid developing irreversible pulmonary hypertension.[66]

TABLE 70–5. Indications for Referring Patients with Systemic Right Ventricle to an ACHD-HF Clinic

- Patients with heart failure symptoms regardless of the systemic RV function
- Asymptomatic patients with severely impaired systemic RV function
- Severe TR and ≥ moderately impaired systemic RV function
- Patients with ≥ moderately impaired systemic RV function and cardiorenal syndrome
- Patients with pulmonary hypertension, regardless of the systemic RV function or degree of TR
- Symptomatic patients with irreparable baffle obstruction
- Recurrent untreatable atrial arrhythmias
- Recurrent ventricular arrhythmias

Abbreviations: ACHD-HF, adult congenital heart function; RV, right ventricle; TR, tricuspid regurgitation

Arterial Switch Operation

Early and Long-Term Prognosis: The early mortality of patients undergoing arterial switch has reduced significantly since the description of the technique in 1975, with a contemporary surgical mortality rate between 1% and 5% in high-volume centers.[67-69] The surgical mortality is slightly higher in patients with complex d-TGA. A recent study from Belgium reported a long-term survival rate of 89.6% 30 years after the arterial switch with a 3.9% late mortality rate at 20 years follow-up.[70]

Long-term complications are not uncommon after arterial switch. In one of the largest studies to date, where 1200 patients with d-TGA were followed after an ASO, freedom from reintervention was 82% at 10 and 15 years.[71] Mild-to-moderate dilatation of the neoaortic root is the most common long-term complication but right ventricular outflow tract obstruction is the most common cause for reintervention.[71,72] Functional status is normal in the majority of patients with a normal or mildly impaired aerobic exercise capacity.[35]

Neoaortic Root Dilatation and Neoaortic Valve Regurgitation: Dilatation of the neoaortic root is common in patients after arterial switch. Some studies report that up to 70% of patients have dilated aortic root after 20 years follow-up,[73] but in less than 1% of patients it will be larger than 45 mm.[72] To date, we do not have data about the risk of dissection or rupture in this population but close follow-up of patients with severe aortic root dilatation is recommended.[12] The need for elective intervention for aortic root replacement is rare in this population.

Neoaortic valve regurgitation can be present in up 25% of patients 10 years after arterial switch[74] and can progress over time. In our adult cohort, few patients have needed elective neoaortic replacement. In our experience, patients with severe aortic regurgitation after atrial switch might develop left ventricular systolic dysfunction with mildly dilated left ventricle, suggesting the presence of an underlying cardiomyopathy in this population. Risk factors for the development of significant neoaortic valve regurgitation are discrepancy between the size of the great arteries, bicuspid neoaortic (pulmonary) valve, left ventricular outflow obstruction, and progressive dilatation of the neoaortic root.[74–76]

Right Ventricular Outflow Tract Obstruction: Supravalvular pulmonary stenosis or branch pulmonary artery stenosis are frequent complications after an ASO with reintervention needed in up to 40% of patients in some series. Contemporary data suggest a significant improvement in the surgical technique with patients needing less interventions during follow-up.[70,72] The stenosis normally occurs at the level of the distal anastomosis of the pulmonary trunk. Stenosis of the branches of the pulmonary arteries, often as a result of "stretching" produced by the Lecompte maneuvre and in a lesser degree by the compression of the ascending aorta when this dilates, is also a concern. Echocardiography is the technique of choice to diagnose right ventricular outflow tract obstruction; however, it is suboptimal to assess the pulmonary artery branches in adults. Baseline CMR or CCT should be considered in all patients with arterial switch at the time of transfer to the adult department to rule out asymptomatic stenosis of the pulmonary artery branches. Surgical or percutaneous interventions to address right ventricular outflow tract obstruction is required in a minority of patients in the contemporary cohorts.[70]

Coronary Artery Complications: One of the major concerns after arterial switch is late coronary artery complications. Mobilization and reimplantation of the coronary arteries has been one of the major concerns in this population, with survival free of coronary events reported as 92.7%, 91.0%, and 88.2% at 1, 10, and 15 years, respectively.[77] However, 90% of coronary artery events occur in the 3 months postrepair with few cases presenting in adulthood.[77] The best means for assessing the coronary circulation after arterial switch remain controversial but the reported low incidence of coronary-related problems makes it questionable whether routine screening for coronary artery pathologies (with whatever modality) can be justified.[39]

Neurological Outcomes: Long-term studies have shown encouraging overall neurodevelopmental outcomes in patients after arterial switch. However, neurologic impairment appears to be more frequent than in the general population. A study including 60 unselected patients with a mean age of 17 years showed that these patients have above-average scores for analytical thinking, but reduced orthography testing.[78] Magnetic resonance imaging (MRI) demonstrated moderate or severe structural brain abnormalities in 32% of the patients with periventricular leukomalacia being detected in >50%. Preoperative acidosis and hypoxia were the only independent patient-related risk factors for neurologic dysfunction, reduced intelligence, periventricular leukomalacia, and reduced brain volume.[78]

Rastelli Operation

Early and Long-Term Prognosis: The initial experiences with the Rastelli procedure reported an early mortality rate as high as 30%; however, recent series show a significant improvement with an operative mortality rate <5%.[26] Despite of leaving the left ventricle in the systemic position, there is a significant incidence of late mortality after Rastelli repair. Kreutzer et al. reported in large series a survival rate of 82%, 80%, 68%, and 52% at 5, 10, 15, and 20 years of follow-up, respectively. In this study, the most common causes of death were left ventricular failure and SCD. Freedom from death or reintervention (catheterization or surgical) was 53%, 24%, and 21% at 5, 10, and 15 years of follow-up, respectively, with almost 80% of them being to address right ventricular outflow tract obstruction.[79]

Arrhythmias and Sudden Cardiac Death: SCD is the second most common cause of late death in patients with Rastelli.[79] A recent study looking at predictors of SCD in adults with congenital heart disease showed that Rastelli patients are the group with the highest risk of SCD at 20 years of follow-up, ahead of patients with systemic right ventricle or tetralogy of Fallot.[80] Unfortunately, there are no specific indications for primary prevention ICD in this population.

Atrial arrhythmias are prevalent in patients with Rastelli procedure, mainly in those with significant conduit stenosis or regurgitation. The presence of a large VSD patch to reroute the left ventricle to the aorta, reduces the size of the right ventricle and increases the risk of developing restrictive right ventricle. Patients with a restrictive right ventricle rely on AV synchrony to maintain cardiac output. Atrial arrhythmias are not very well tolerated in this setting and prompt restoration of sinus rhythm is recommended. Exercise capacity is mildly to substantially diminished.

Left Ventricular Function and Restrictive Right Ventricle: Left ventricular dysfunction is present in 25% of Rastelli patients at late follow-up.[26] Right ventricular dysfunction is also common, often secondary to conduit stenosis or regurgitation. However, regardless of the functional status of the conduit, diastolic dysfunction of the right ventricle is also common in these patients and should be considered when they present with symptoms of right heart failure.

Right Ventricular Outflow Tract Obstruction: Degeneration of the right ventricle to the pulmonary artery conduit is the most common cause for reintervention in this population. Kreutzer et al. reported that almost one-half of the patients will need conduit replacement within 5 years of the intervention with less than one-quarter being free from reintervention at 15 years follow-up.[79] The use of percutaneous pulmonary implantable valves is the technique of choice if anatomically feasible. Intervention in the right ventricular outflow tract should be considered in symptomatic patients with right ventricular systolic pressure (RVSP) >60 mm Hg and/or severe pulmonary regurgitation. In asymptomatic patients with severe right ventricular outflow tract obstruction, conduit replacement should be considered when RVSP >80 mm Hg or there is objective decreases in exercise capacity.

TOTAL ANOMALOUS PULMONARY VENOUS CONNECTION

Background

Total anomalous pulmonary venous connection is a form of cyanotic congenital heart disease in which pulmonary venous connections to the left atrium are lacking. Rather, all pulmonary veins ultimately return to the heart via the systemic venous system, resulting in complete admixture of systemic and pulmonary venous return in the right atrium. This anomaly was first described in the 18th century; however, prior to the advent of pediatric cardiac surgery, no definitive therapy was available.[81,82] As subsequently discussed in further detail, the typical natural course of this disease is characterized by early cyanosis and cardiac failure. As such, total anomalous pulmonary venous connection is a predominantly pediatric disease requiring surgical repair in infancy. Rare cases have been diagnosed in adult patients.[83,84]

An important distinction is to be made between the terms *anomalous pulmonary venous connection*, and *anomalous pulmonary venous drainage*. Total anomalous pulmonary venous connection will result in total anomalous pulmonary venous drainage, but it is also possible to have normal pulmonary venous connections without normal drainage.[85] While the term *connection* describes the anatomical position of the veins, the term *drainage* is used to the describe the course of pulmonary venous return. For example, in the cases of common atrium or malposition of the primum septum, despite normal connection of the pulmonary veins to the left atrium there is anomalous pulmonary venous drainage.

Forms of anomalous pulmonary venous drainage not associated with anomalous connection are beyond the scope of this chapter. The following sections will focus on the details of anatomy, presentation, and management of total anomalous pulmonary venous drainage secondary to total anomalous pulmonary venous connection.

Anatomy

There are four anatomic variations of total anomalous pulmonary venous connection, as described by Craig et al.[86] Anomalous pulmonary venous connections may be supracardiac, cardiac or infracardiac. In the supracardiac form, all pulmonary veins drain to one or more systemic venous structures above the diaphragm. In the cardiac form, the veins drain to the coronary sinus and in the infracardiac form the

veins will drain into the inferior vena cava (IVC) or hepatic veins. There is a mixed form in which the veins drain to the right heart via some combination of supracardiac, cardiac, and/or infracardiac venous structures (**Fig. 70–5**). Small autopsy series[87-89] as well as larger cohort studies[90,91] demonstrate that the majority of cases are of the supracardiac type, pulmonary venous drainage to the left innominate (or brachiocephalic) vein, with the mixed forms being the least commonly found comprising approximately 10% of cases.[90,91]

Pathophysiology

In fetal life, the pulmonary venous system is derived from the splanchnic plexus, which drains into the systemic venous system until establishing its connection to the left atrium via the common pulmonary vein. Ultimately by the 4th to 5th week gestation, the involution of the common pulmonary vein leaves all of the pulmonary veins directly connected to the left atrium.[92,93] It is hypothesized that total anomalous pulmonary venous connection is the result of early atresia of the common pulmonary vein while the other connections to the systemic venous system are still functional. The most dominant systemic venous connection or connections dictate the specific type of total anomalous pulmonary venous connection that will result.[93]

With all pulmonary venous return delivering fully saturated blood to the right atrium, the postnatal physiology of total anomalous pulmonary venous connection is dependent on the distribution of this mixed venous blood between the systemic and pulmonary circulations. An obligatory intracardiac shunt of sufficient size will support systemic blood flow and cardiac output. In the absence of pulmonary venous obstruction, either at the level of the veins themselves or the intracardiac shunt, systemic oxygen saturations may exceed 90% in older children or adults.[93]

Epidemiology

Among patients with congenital heart disease, the incidence of total anomalous pulmonary venous connection is 0.7% to 1.5%.[94,95] Overall, the incidence of this anomaly is 0.6 to 1.2 per 10,000 live births.[94-96] While there is a male preponderance for the infracardiac type of total anomalous pulmonary venous connection, the remaining types occur equally frequently in males and females.[85,89]

Presentation

Early Presentation

The vast majority of cases of total anomalous pulmonary venous connection present early in life, during the neonatal period or infancy. The timing and specific features of the presentation are dependent on the degree of pulmonary venous obstruction, arising either from the venous channels themselves or restriction of the intracardiac shunt over time.

Obstruction to Pulmonary Venous Return

In the immediate postnatal period, hypoxia will be present due to complete mixing at the right atrium, but it may not be so

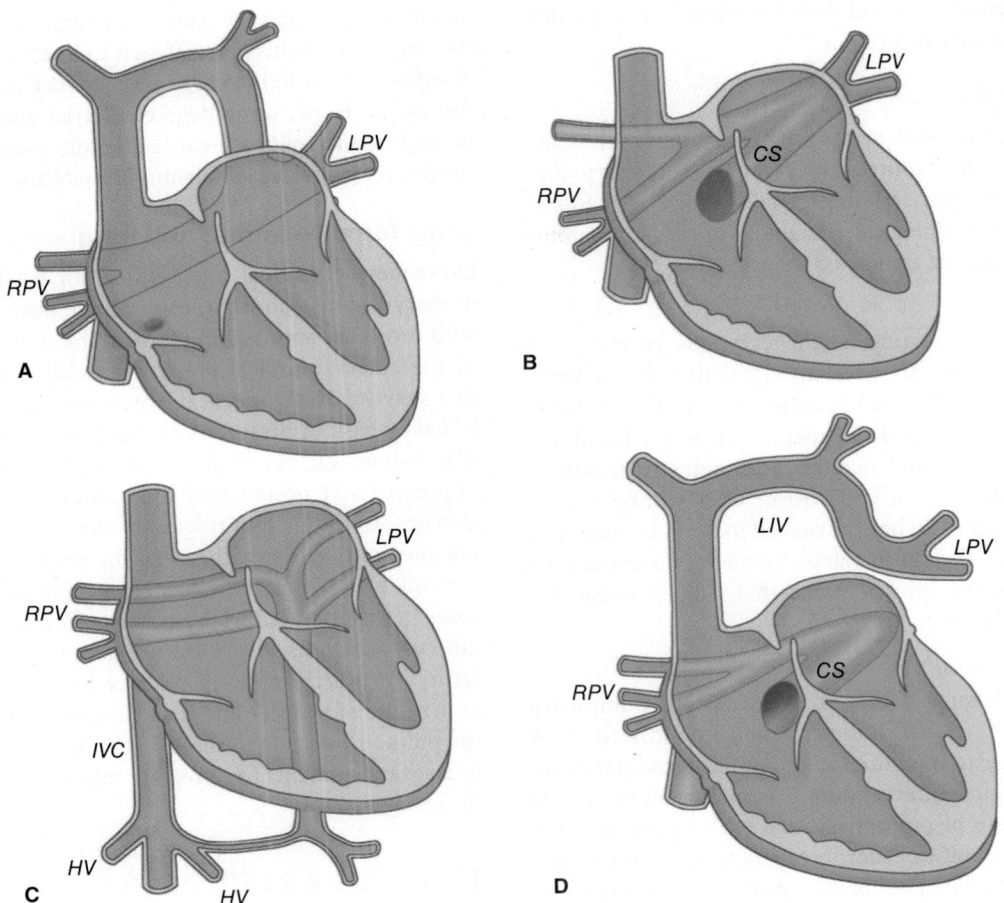

Figure 70–5. **Total anomalous pulmonary venous connection.** (**A**) Supracardiac form. All pulmonary veins join to a common pulmonary venous confluence behind the heart that drains via a vertical vein to the left innominate vein. (**B**) Cardiac form. The pulmonary venous confluence connects to the coronary sinus. (**C**) Infracardiac form. The pulmonary venous confluence drains inferiorly via a vertical vein to the hepatic veins. (**D**) Mixed form. In this example, the left pulmonary veins drain superiorly to the innominate vein, and the right pulmonary veins drain to the coronary sinus. CS, coronary sinus, HV, hepatic vein, IVC, inferior vena cava, LIV, left innominate vein, LPV, left pulmonary veins, RPV, right pulmonary veins. Reproduced with permission from Allen H, Shaddy R, Penny D, et al. *Moss and Adams' Heart Disease in Infants, Children and Adolescents*, 9th ed. Philadelphia, PA: Wolters Kluwer; 2016.

severe to cause clinical cyanosis.[85] Obstruction to pulmonary venous return is rare at birth; however, it will occur over time as the patent foramen ovale becomes restrictive or closes completely.[85,93,97] Over a period of days to weeks, the patient will become more cyanosed and might also display signs of inadequate cardiac output when the obstruction to pulmonary venous flow is severe. The abnormal venous channel by which pulmonary venous blood returns to the right atrium may become stenotic over time, this being most common in the infracardiac form. In this setting, in addition to cyanosis, patients might develop pulmonary edema and ventilatory issues due to increased pulmonary venous pressure.

Unobstructed Pulmonary Venous Return

In the case of unrestricted pulmonary venous return, there may be minimal clinical evidence of this abnormality. As pulmonary vascular resistance falls to its nadir in the first weeks and months of life, pulmonary blood flow increases progressively, resulting frequently in congestive heart failure.[85,93,97]

Late Presentation

Late presentation of total anomalous pulmonary venous return is uncommon, although rare cases have been diagnosed in adulthood.[83,98] Anomalous pulmonary venous return has been described in adults as incidental finding in patients investigated for embolic phenomena or symptoms of right heart failure.[83,84,98] Patients surviving infancy may display clubbing and polycythemia.

Physical Examination

Aside from that of mild hypoxia, physical findings of unrepaired total anomalous pulmonary venous return in those who reach adulthood will vary according to their clinical history and presentation. A parasternal heave is indicative of right ventricular enlargement. The first heart sound may be normal, or of increased intensity due to relative tricuspid stenosis. The second heart sound is widely split without respiratory variation ("fixed"). There may be a systolic ejection murmur of relative pulmonary stenosis at the left upper sternal border, owing to the increased pulmonary blood flow. In isolated cases, pulmonary hypertension may be present.[84,85,93]

Work-Up/Investigations

The goals of the initial work up for total anomalous pulmonary venous return include identifying at least four pulmonary veins and describing their connections in detail, evaluating their size and patency, and describing the remainder of cardiac anatomy in its entirety to rule out associated lesions.

Imaging

In infants, echocardiography is the technique of choice to make the initial diagnosis with a high degree of sensitivity and specificity.[99] Advanced imaging such as MRI is rarely required.[85] In adults, however, elucidating the detailed anatomy of pulmonary venous return is often challenging by transthoracic echocardiography. Cardiac MRI or CCT will be needed to confirm the diagnosis. These advanced modalities also show the relationship of the pulmonary channels to surrounding noncardiac structures, an advantage that can be invaluable with respect to surgical planning.

Cardiac Catheterization

In adults newly diagnosed with total anomalous pulmonary venous connection, cardiac catheterization might need to be considered in order to measure the pulmonary vascular resistance prior to surgical intervention. It is important to sample proximal to the site of pulmonary venous drainage into the systemic venous circuit in order to calculate accurate shunt.[85] Depending on the type of anomalous pulmonary venous connection, even more distal systemic venous saturations could be contaminated by pulmonary venous blood. Pulmonary venous blood saturation, if possible, should be measured rather than assumed. Obstruction can be ruled out by measuring the simultaneous gradients between bilateral pulmonary wedge and right atrial pressures.[97] When total anomalous pulmonary venous connection is diagnosed in infancy, cardiac catheterization is rarely necessary prior to surgical repair.[85,93,97]

Treatment

Definitive treatment of total anomalous pulmonary venous connection is surgical, whereby the pulmonary venous drainage is re-routed to the left atrium, and any intracardiac shunt is closed. Obstructed total anomalous pulmonary venous connection is a surgical emergency in children.[85,97]

Medical Management

In the case of obstructed total anomalous pulmonary venous connection, medical management is limited to intubation, administration of 100% FiO_2, and correction of metabolic acidosis. Emergent surgical correction should be undertaken as soon as possible. Standard decongestive measures can be applied to infants in heart failure secondary to unobstructed total anomalous pulmonary venous connection, however definitive repair should still be done electively in early infancy.[85,97]

Surgical Options

The specific surgical approach to correction of total anomalous pulmonary venous connection is dependent on the type of underlying anomaly.[85,97] Direct manipulation and suturing of the pulmonary veins themselves is to be avoided due to the risk of ostial stenosis following surgery.[93] Once pulmonary vascular disease develops, some degree of atrial communication may be required to maintain cardiac output even after pulmonary venous return to the left atrium is established.

Long-Term Outcomes and Prognosis

Outcomes of surgical intervention for total anomalous pulmonary venous connection were quite poor in the early days, with mortality approaching 90% in the first year.[82,93] However, in the current surgical era this has fallen dramatically such that survival exceeds 95% at experienced surgical centers.[100,101] Mortality risk at present is dictated largely by associated cardiac lesions, such as single ventricle physiology. The presence of preoperative obstruction and pulmonary arterial hypertension are also significant risk factors for mortality.[85,91,100] Following successful surgery, the need for reintervention to address stenosis of the repair site has been reported in up to 20% of cases.[93,102] However, when patients reach adulthood without complications, these are unlikely to develop in the long term.[103,104] It is the authors' practice to perform a cardiac MRI at the time of transfer and if there is wide open connection of the pulmonary veins to the left atrium and no residual lesion, to discharge patients from regular follow-up unless clinical status changes.

TRUNCUS ARTERIOSUS

Background

Truncus arteriosus is a congenital malformation of the heart characterized by a single ventricular outlet. One arterial vessel arising at the base of the heart gives rise to the aorta, coronary, and pulmonary arteries. This form of cardiac disease presents nearly universally in infancy and requires prompt intervention to avoid morbidity and mortality related to heart failure and pulmonary vascular disease.

Anatomy

Some sources refer to this congenital anomaly as *persistent* truncus arteriosus, in acknowledgment of the fact that the truncus arteriosus is a normal component of the human embryologic heart tube. Developmental events, including septation of the truncus and fusion with the conal (infundibular) septum, fail to occur in the embryo resulting in this malformation, which is inevitably associated with a large outlet VSD. It should be noted that errors in this stage of development may result in any conotruncal malformation, such as tetralogy of Fallot or double outlet right ventricle.[105] The truncal valve forms the roof of the VSD and most commonly is trileaflet but may have as many as six leaflets.[105–107] Anomalies of the aortic arch and coronary arteries are commonly associated with truncus arteriosus.

A right aortic arch is seen in approximately 25% of patients, whereas an interrupted aortic arch is seen in up to 20% of patients.[105,106] The latter is particularly common in patients with 22q11 deletion syndrome.[105,106,108] Aberrant subclavian artery can be seen in up to 10% of cases.[108] Left coronary dominance is up to 3-times more common in truncus arteriosus than in the general population.[105] While coronary ostial origins are frequently anomalous, the left coronary tends to arise from the left posterolateral truncal surface and the right coronary tends to arise from the right anterolateral surface.[106,108,109]

Multiple anatomic variations of truncus arteriosus have been described, each with implications for surgical repair. Two main classification systems have been proposed, based on the origins of the branch pulmonary arteries (Collett and Edwards) and commonly associated arterial anomalies (Van Praagh and Van Praagh).[107,110]

Collett and Edwards Classification

This classification, first described in 1949, recognized four types of truncus arteriosus based on the anatomic origins of the branch pulmonary arteries (**Fig. 70–6**). In type I, a rightward vestigial pulmonary arterial trunk gives rise to the branch pulmonary arteries. In types II and III, there is no main pulmonary arterial vestige and the branch pulmonary arteries arise directly from the truncus, either in proximity to each other from the leftward and posterior aspect of the truncus (II), or with origins on opposite sides of it (III). In type IV, the branch pulmonary arteries arise from the thoracic aorta. This type is now considered a discrete entity from truncus arteriosus, namely pulmonary atresia with VSD and major aortopulmonary collaterals.

Van Praagh Classification

The Van Praagh classification was first described in 1965 in a necroscopy study.[107] The main distinctions between Van Praagh and the Collett and Edwards classification are (**Fig. 70–7**): (1) Van Praagh does not distinguish between adjacent and distant truncal origins of the branch pulmonary arteries, such that

type 2 includes both types II and III under Collett and Edwards; (2) Van Praagh expanded their classification to include commonly associated anomalies of the great arteries, as such, type 3 describes a single branch pulmonary arterial origin off the truncus, with the contralateral lung supply originating from the thoracic aorta or ductus arteriosus and type 4 encompasses aortic arch anomalies including hypoplasia, coarctation, or complete interruption.

Associated Anomalies

Aside from VSD and arch anomalies as previously described, commonly associated anomalies include atrial septal defect (9%–20%), persistent left superior vena cava (4%–9%), and tricuspid stenosis (6%). The latter is typically mild.[105,108]

Pathophysiology

Intracardiac anatomy comprising an unrestrictive VSD and single outlet results in complete mixing of systemic and pulmonary venous return. In early infancy, a relatively increased pulmonary vascular resistance may contribute to mild cyanosis that will improve as the resistance falls in the subsequent months. Then, patients will be more normally saturated but the volume of pulmonary blood flow increases, contributing to congestive heart failure.[105] Abnormal function of the truncal valve is present in one-quarter of patients with insufficiency being more common than stenosis.[105,106] Important insufficiency exacerbates ventricular volume overload and hastens clinical decompensation. Truncal stenosis increases ventricular afterload and limits the combined ventricular output, potentially compromising systemic perfusion significantly.[111] Coronary perfusion in truncus arteriosus is suboptimal due not only to desaturated blood supply, but also to competitive flow in diastole between the coronary and pulmonary beds.[106,111] Consequently, the myocardium is chronically underperfused.

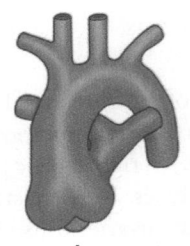 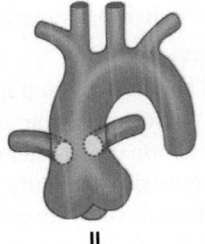 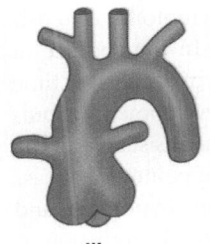 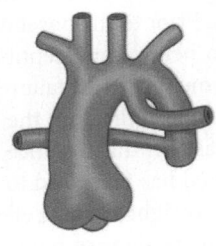

I	II	III	IV
Type I: A short main pulmonary artery gives rise to the branch pulmonary arteries.	**Type II:** The right and left branch pulmonary arteries arise directly from the aorta in close proximity to each other.	**Type III:** The right and left branch pulmonary arteries arise directly from the aorta, distant from each other.	**Type IV:** Absence of the branch pulmonary arteries. The lungs are supplied by collateral vessels arising from the descending aorta. This type is now considered to be a form of pulmonary atresia and is no longer a part of the truncus arteriosus spectrum.

Figure 70–6. The Collett and Edwards classification of truncus arteriosus. Reproduced with permission from Allen H, Shaddy R, Penny D, et al. *Moss and Adams' Heart Disease in Infants, Children and Adolescents*, 9th ed. Philadelphia, PA: Wolters Kluwer; 2016.

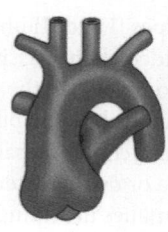 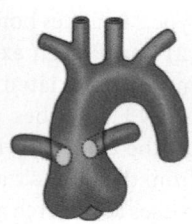 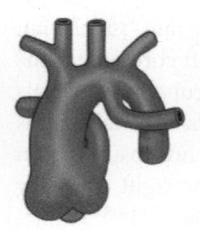 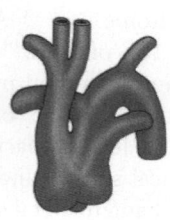

1

Type 1: Partial septation of the truncus results in a short main pulmonary artery, giving rise to the branch pulmonary arteries.

2

Type 2: The truncus fails to septate completely, thus there is no main pulmonary artery, and the branch pulmonary arteries arise directly from the ascending aorta.

3

Type 3: Only one branch pulmonary artery arises from the ascending aorta; the other arises either from the ductus arteriosus or descending aorta.

4

Type 4: The aortic arch is hypoplastic or interrupted, with ductal continuation to the descending aorta.

Figure 70–7. **The Van Praagh classification of truncus arteriosus.** Reproduced with permission from Allen H, Shaddy R, Penny D, et al. *Moss and Adams' Heart Disease in Infants, Children and Adolescents*, 9th ed. Philadelphia, PA: Wolters Kluwer; 2016.

Most patients will succumb to heart failure in the first year of life if left unrepaired[105,106,108]; however, irreversible pulmonary vascular disease is an important sequela, with the tendency to develop early,[105,106,108] and it is the main cause of death in childhood.

Epidemiology

Truncus arteriosus comprises 2% of congenital cardiac anomalies, affecting 0.6 to 1.4 per 10,000 live births.[107,111,112] There is no gender difference in frequency.[105]

Presentation

History

Congestive heart failure in infancy is characterized by poor feeding, tachypnea, diaphoresis, and failure to thrive. Infants with truncus arteriosus typically present within the first weeks to months of life, depending on the pulmonary vascular resistance (magnitude of the left-to-right shunt) and degree of truncal valve insufficiency. Prior to the onset of symptoms, cyanosis may be so mild as to being imperceptible. In the absence of intervention, improvement in heart failure symptoms over time is a poor prognostic sign, indicating the development of pulmonary vascular disease. In this instance, the resistance in the pulmonary capillary bed has increased to the point of decreasing the degree of left to right shunt. Lethargy, hypotonia, and decreased urine output are signs of poor systemic perfusion or cardiogenic shock and might be seen in patients with severe truncal valve stenosis, aortic coarctation, or arch interruption (following ductal closure). Given the dismal prognosis of this lesion if left unrepaired, it is exceedingly rare for patients to present in adulthood.[108,113] Those surviving beyond infancy may report cyanosis, exercise intolerance, dizziness, and/or syncope owing either to Eisenmenger syndrome, or progressive branch pulmonary arterial stenosis.[105,108,113,114] Aortic dissection has been reported in unrepaired patients with truncus arteriosus.[115]

Physical Examination

Physical signs of congestive heart failure secondary to significant left-to-right shunt in infancy include poor weight gain,

tachypnea and tachycardia for age, and hepatomegaly. The precordium is dynamic. Specific findings by auscultation in truncus arteriosus include normal S1 that may be followed by an ejection click, and a single S2. Splitting of S2 may be appreciable in cases where the closure of one or more leaflets of the abnormal truncal valve is delayed. A loud (often associated with a thrill) pansystolic murmur best heard at the left sternal border and radiating throughout the precordium is typical.[105] Murmurs of truncal stenosis or regurgitation may be apparent, as may be a diastolic rumble of relative mitral stenosis owing to increased flow. Peripheral pulses are typically bounding and the pulse pressure is wide, as runoff from the aorta into the pulmonary arteries continues through diastole even in the absence of important truncal valve insufficiency.[105] As pulmonary blood flow is increased early in the unrepaired course, there may be only very mild cyanosis. As the disease progresses, cyanosis and digital clubbing may develop.[105]

Work-Up/Investigations

Imaging

The chest radiograph of an unrepaired patient with truncus arteriosus is characterized by cardiomegaly and increased pulmonary vascularity. A right aortic arch will be seen in approximately 30% of cases. This constellation of findings is strongly suggestive of truncus arteriosus.[105,111] Echocardiography is the technique of choice to establish the primary diagnosis and associated anomalies. Particularly important aspects include ruling out arch anomalies and defining the anatomy of branch pulmonary and coronary arteries.[105,111,116] Advanced imaging is rarely required for surgical planning of initial repair. In adulthood, advanced imaging such as cardiac MRI or CTA may be considered to assess ventricular size and function as well as residual lesions, because echocardiographic windows may be limited.

Cardiac Catheterization

Cardiac catheterization is rarely required preoperatively for the evaluation of truncus arteriosus. In the instance of a late repair (beyond early infancy), it may be necessary to formally assess pulmonary vascular resistance prior to surgery. Pulmonary vascular resistance greater than 8 Wood units/m^2 confers high risk of postoperative mortality, and is considered prohibitive to primary repair in many centers.[105] Following primary repair, typical indications for catheterization include evaluation of acquired cardiac disease and evaluation of conduit dysfunction. Pulmonary valve replacement may be undertaken percutaneously depending on the size of the conduit in situ.

Treatment

Medical Management

At present, no medical therapy is considered to confer acceptable improvement in the morbidity or mortality of patients with truncus arteriosus. Deferral of surgery is in fact associated with higher morbidity and higher risk of poor operative outcome at the time of repair.[106,117] Medical therapies targeting congestive heart failure in the ICU setting may be temporizing to optimize clinical stability preoperatively.

Surgical Options

Complete surgical repair of truncus arteriosus should be undertaken within the first weeks of life. The approach to repair was first described in the 1960s.[105,106] The truncal valve is dedicated to the left ventricle as the VSD is closed, becoming the systemic AV valve. A conduit, an aortic homograft or a heterograft, is placed between the right ventricle and branch pulmonary arteries or main pulmonary artery. The truncal valve, where regurgitant, is usually amenable to repair. Aortic valve replacement is rarely if ever required at the time of surgery.[106] In the early operative era, surgical mortality was high. However, data over the subsequent decades demonstrated a significantly higher mortality rate in patients repaired after 6 months of age.[106,117] At present, early mortality following surgical repair has fallen to approximately 10%.[118-122] The need for late reintervention following initial repair of truncus arteriosus is common, owing to several factors. Conduit sizes appropriate for neonatal repair range between 9 mm and 11 mm internal diameter. As somatic growth progresses, the conduit becomes relatively stenotic. Furthermore, the conduit material itself has limited longevity and is disposed to regurgitation and stenosis over time. Multiple studies have demonstrated significant reintervention rates within the first 3 to 10 years following primary repair.[105,106,123-125]

Long-Term Outcomes and Prognosis

Surviving adults born with truncus arteriosus are likely to have undergone surgical repair in childhood. While long-term survival beyond the first year of life exceeds 90% at 20 years in the current era, the need for conduit replacement is an eventuality.[108,118,120,126-128] Regular follow-up at a congenital cardiac center is necessary throughout adulthood. Primary issues requiring periodic monitoring include biventricular systolic and diastolic function, truncal valvular and conduit function, and progressive aortic root dilation. Tricuspid regurgitation and branch pulmonary artery abnormalities as well as residual lesions associated with comorbid intracardiac anomalies may also represent long-term sequelae in this patient population.[105] To date, long-term follow-up studies have not suggested a significant arrhythmia burden in this population.[127,129] Prophylaxis against bacterial endocarditis is also indicated for life.[130]

CONGENITALLY CORRECTED TRANSPOSITION OF THE GREAT ARTERIES

Background

Congenitally corrected transposition of the great arteries (ccTGA), is a rare structural heart disease constituting less than 1% of all congenital heart disease.[131] The malformation was first described by von Rokitansky in 1875 and it is characterized by AV discordance and VA discordance. In this setting, the morphologic right ventricle receives pulmonary venous blood and gives rise to the aorta, thus supporting the systemic circulation. In contrast, the morphologic left ventricle receives systemic venous blood and connects to the pulmonary artery, supporting the pulmonary circulation. This defect occurs due to abnormal cardiac development during the third gestational week where left looping (L-loop) of the heart tube occurs, rather than right looping, leading to abnormal positioning of the ventricles and abnormal connections between the atrial, ventricular, and arterial segments of the heart. Most cases of ccTGA have normal situs, but situs abnormalities have been reported in 19% to 34% of patients in pediatric series.[132] The majority of patients have one or more associated lesions which will determine the management and outcome of the condition. Patients with either mild or no associated lesions will present later in life with symptoms of heart failure and/or AV conduction abnormalities. However, patients with associated cardiac lesions, including VSD and/or pulmonary stenosis, will present early in life with features of heart failure or cyanosis. This section focuses on ccTGA with two functional ventricles. Patients with ccTGA may be present with criss-cross AV connections, and rarely with single ventricle physiology.

Anatomy

Situs and Origin of the Great Arteries

In most of the patients with ccTGA, the heart is left-sided, although dextrocardia is present in 20% of patients.[133] Situs solitus is the most common atrial arrangement and, as previously outlined, the right atrium connects to the morphologic left ventricle that gives rise to the aorta, and the left atrium connects to the morphologic right ventricle that gives rise to the pulmonary artery (**Fig. 70–8**). As a result of the discordant ventriculo-arterial connections, the pulmonary trunk is wedged between the two AV valves and there is fibrous continuity between the pulmonary and the mitral valves. The aorta arises from the right ventricle usually in an anterior and leftward position, relative to the pulmonary trunk. The outflow into the aorta has the typical configuration of a morphologically right ventricle, with a muscular infundibulum (ventricular conus) separating the aortic and tricuspid valves. Both outflow tracts are parallel to each other and the ventricles tend to be side by side, but other relationships do exist.

Normal heart

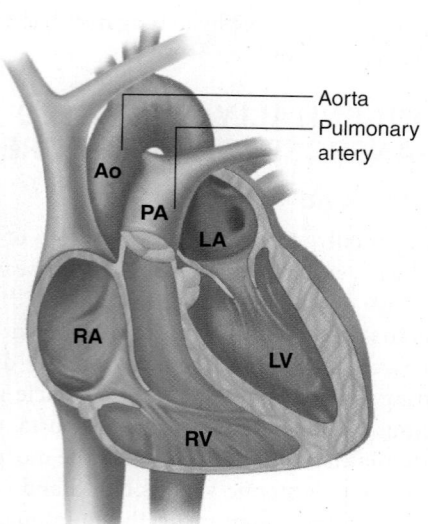

Congenitally corrected transposition of the great arteries

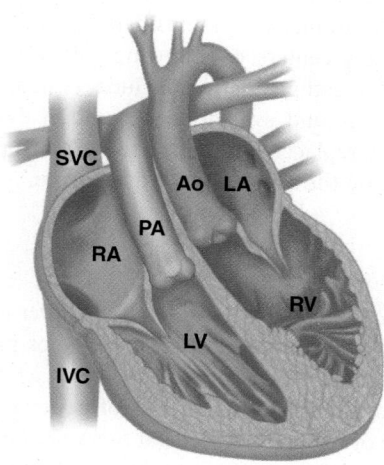

Figure 70–8. Normal heart and congenitally corrected transposition of the great arteries. Ao, Aorta; IVC, inferior vena cava; LA, left atrium; LV, left ventricle; PA, pulmonary artery; RA, right atrium; RV, right ventricle; SVC, superior vena cava.

Coronary Arteries

The coronary arteries arise from the aortic sinuses adjacent to the pulmonary trunk with fairly constant distribution. Generally speaking, in patients with normal atrial arrangement, the right-sided coronary artery is morphologically left and supplies the subpulmonary left ventricle. The left-sided coronary artery is morphologically right and supplies the systemic right ventricle. A solitary coronary artery is the most common anomaly.

Conduction System

While the sinus node is in its normal position in patients with ccTGA, the anatomical distribution of the cardiac conduction system will depend on the situs and the degree of malalignment of the AV septum. In patients with situs solitus, the AV node is placed at the apex of the triangle of Koch and does not penetrate to the ventricular tissue. A secondary node, which is located beneath the opening of the right atrial appendage, in the area of the pulmonary valve to mitral valve fibrous continuity, gives rise to the penetrating bundle of His that courses superficially underneath the pulmonary valve leaflets and then traverses the anterior wall of the morphological left ventricular outflow tract, just caudal to the pulmonary valve annulus. It then dives into the interventricular septum lying subendocardially on the right side of the septum.[134] The bundle lies in relation to the anterosuperior border of the VSD when present.[135] In patients with less malalignment, the regular AV node may be able to make contact with the interventricular septum and both the regular and the anterior nodes may give rise to the penetrating bundles.[136] In patients with situs inversus, the atrial and ventricular septa are better aligned, allowing a regularly located AV node to continue in normal fashion to an AV bundle that passes in a posteroinferior relationship to the margin of a VSD, if there is one[134,137,138] (**Fig. 70–9**). The position of the AV node and the penetrating bundle will determine the risk of complete

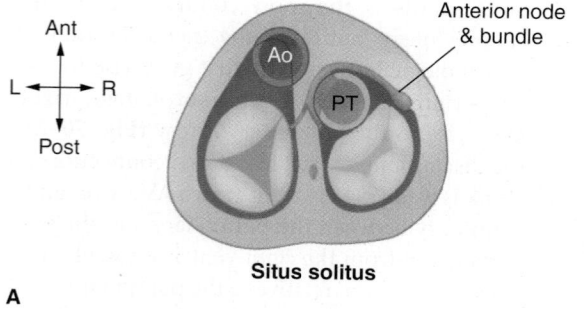

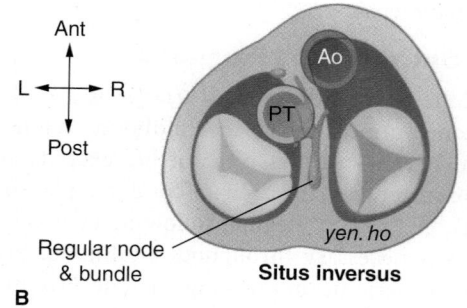

Figure 70–9. Conduction system in patients with ccTGA. Atrial and ventricular septum malalignment in ccTGA with situs solitus (**A**). AV node does not penetrate to ventricular tissue. Thus, a secondary node, located in area of pulmonary valve (PA) to mitral valve fibrous continuity, has a penetrating bundle that courses on anterior segment of septum. In situs inversus (**B**), alignment of atrial and ventricular septum is good, and His bundle branch has its origin in normal AV node. Ao, aortic valve; PT, Pulmonary trunk. Adapted with permission from Baruteau AE, Abrams DJ, Ho SY, et al. Cardiac Conduction System in Congenitally Corrected Transposition of the Great Arteries and Its Clinical Relevance. *J Am Heart Assoc.* 2017 Dec 21;6(12):e007759.

heart block in these patients and has surgical implications when an associated VSD is present.

Associated Defects

The majority of cases with ccTGA have one or more coexisting congenital malformations with an interventricular septal defect being the most common, followed by left ventricular outflow tract obstruction and abnormalities of the tricuspid valve.

Ventricular Septal Defect

VSD occurs in 70% to 80% of patients with ccTGA.[135] The most common VSDs are outlet (38%) and perimembranous (37%).[133] The latter has the feature of having fibrous continuity between the pulmonary valve and the left-sided tricuspid valve.[139] An inlet VSD is present in 13% of the cases and only 4% of patients have a muscular VSD.[133]

Left Ventricular Outflow Tract Obstruction

Left ventricular outflow tract obstruction occurs in 25% to 30% of patients with ccTGA.[5] The obstruction can be valvular (51%) or subvalvular (42%), with a minority of patients presenting with pulmonary atresia (6%).[140] The primary mechanisms of left ventricular outflow tract obstruction include septal muscular hypertrophy, accessory AV valvular tissue, or aneurysmal dilatation of the membranous ventricular septum.[139] The presence of left ventricular outflow tract obstruction in patients with ccTGA may be protective against the development of tricuspid valve regurgitation, systemic right ventricular dysfunction, and ultimately heart failure.[141]

Abnormalities of the Tricuspid Valve

Abnormalities of the tricuspid valve are found in up to 70% of patients with ccTGA. Ebstein-like anomaly is the most common malformation and is recognized by the apical displacement of the septal and posterior leaflets. However, a "sail-like" anterior tricuspid valve leaflet is rare and the atrialization of the right ventricle is minimal in this setting.[142] The degree of tricuspid regurgitation will depend on the severity of the malformation. In the absence of an Ebstein-like anomaly, the tricuspid valve can be dysplastic with thickened leaflets and short chordae. Straddling of the tricuspid valve may preclude biventricular repair.

Epidemiology and Genetics

ccTGA is a rare condition accounting for approximately 0.05% of congenital heart malformations.[139] It is more common in males with a male:female ratio of 1.6:1.[143,144] The etiology is unknown and some studies suggest a familial recurrence rate of up to 5.2%.[145]

Presentation

Patients with associated lesions will present early in life and, depending on the predominant lesion, they can present with heart failure and/or cyanosis. Heart failure and failure to thrive will be the predominant symptoms in patients with VSD due to pulmonary overcirculation, and in patients with severe tricuspid regurgitation due to pulmonary congestion; whereas patients with VSD and significant left ventricular outflow tract obstruction will present with differing degrees of cyanosis.[131] Arrhythmias are the first symptom in approximately 30% of patients.[133] Patients with no lesions or mild associated lesions will be diagnosed in adulthood, either incidentally or after developing symptoms. Whereas an abnormal chest x-ray or electrocardiogram might lead to the diagnosis in asymptomatic patients, most patients diagnosed in adulthood will present with heart failure symptoms due to severe tricuspid valve regurgitation and systemic right ventricular dysfunction.[146] AV block occurs at a rate of 2% per year in patients with ccTGA[147] and can also be the first symptom in adulthood.

Physical Examination

When presenting in adulthood, physical examination might reveal right parasternal lift, loud second heart sound (due to anterior position of the aortic valve), holosystolic murmur (in patients with tricuspid regurgitation) best heard at the apex, and an ejection systolic murmur at the upper sternal border if there is pulmonary stenosis or a left ventricle to pulmonary artery conduit. Diastolic murmurs will be present in patients with pulmonary or, less commonly, aortic regurgitation.

Work-Up/Investigations

Although clinical suspicion for ccTGA can be established by clinical history, physical examination, chest x-ray, and electrocardiogram, definitive diagnosis requires cardiac imaging.

Echocardiography

Transthoracic echocardiogram is the technique of choice to diagnose ccTGA. It will allow for definitive diagnosis and identification of associated abnormalities. As in any other patients with congenital heart disease, echocardiographic examination should begin in the subcostal view to determine the situs and the position of the heart. In the parasternal long axis, mitro-pulmonary continuity will be appreciable and if the great vessels are parallel, both may be seen in this view. Parasternal short axis is helpful to see the anterior and leftward position of the aortic valve and to assess subjectively the systolic function of the systemic right ventricle. In the four-chamber view, the right ventricle is on the left, and the degree of tricuspid regurgitation and/or outflow tract obstruction are best assessed in this plane. This view also allows for appreciation of the tricuspid valve anatomy. In patients with VSD, it is important to rule out a straddling AV valve that would preclude biventricular repair. Objective assessment of the right ventricular function is challenging, and visual assessment is regularly used but requires a high degree of expertise. Tricuspid annular plane systolic excursion (TAPSE) and systolic excursion velocity of the tricuspid annulus (S') can be helpful to monitor deterioration of the systemic right ventricular systolic function overtime. Fractional area change of the right ventricle is widely used to assess the systolic function of the right ventricle in the subpulmonary position; however, references of normal values in patients with systemic right ventricle are lacking. Strain rate echocardiography has been used in a relatively small number of studies to investigate right and left ventricular myocardial deformation and mechanics in patients with a systemic right ventricle.[148,149] These studies have confirmed that global right ventricular peak systolic longitudinal strain is significantly reduced in patients with a systemic right ventricle.

Cardiac Magnetic Resonance Imaging

CMR imaging has emerged over the last few decades as a complementary imaging modality for the investigation of anatomy and function of patients with congenital heart disease. This modality is generally not restricted by body size or poor acoustic windows, and it has many advantages over other imaging modalities. It does not require the use of iodinated contrast agents and does not involve exposure to ionizing radiation. The various CMR techniques, such as steady-state free-precession CMR and phase-velocity imaging allow the accurate assessment of cardiac anatomy, dimensions, and the velocity and volume of blood flow without geometrical assumptions. The administration of contrast agents allows three-dimensional evaluation of contrasted structures, scar tissue, and fibrosis within the myocardium. The main limitations of this technique are the long examination time required and the artifacts caused by stent or cardiac devices.

The unusual shape of the right ventricular cavity and the unpredictable manner in which it dilates make accurate quantitative analysis by echocardiography challenging, and this problem is not unique to ccTGA. CMR is the gold-standard technique to assess right ventricular volumes and systolic function in patients with ccTGA. (**Fig. 70–10**). Stress perfusion CMR and late gadolinium enhancement might be used to detect coronary artery stenosis in patients following a double switch operation and coronary artery reimplantation.[131] CMR should be performed at the time of transfer from pediatric care, and when there is discordance between the clinical and echocardiographic findings. In those with severe tricuspid regurgitation, it may be considered every 2 to 3 years to monitor the systolic function of the systemic right ventricle, or earlier if new symptoms develop.

Cardiac Computed Tomographic Angiography

As a result of improved temporal resolution, several studies have explored the role of computerized cardiac tomographic angiography (CTA) in providing biventricular functional parameters.[150-152] In ccTGA patients with poor echocardiographic windows and contraindications to CMR, such as patients with epicardial pacing wires or intravascular pacemakers, cardiac CTA is a reliable alternative to assess ventricular function. CTA has some drawbacks in comparison to echocardiography and CMR, such as radiation dose and intravenous contrast administration, thus it might be contraindicated in patients with significant renal dysfunction.

Cardiac Catheterization

Diagnostic cardiac catheterization is not regularly used in patients with ccTGA. However, it might be considered in the assessment of pulmonary artery pressures if needed. In patients with a left ventricle to pulmonary artery conduit, cardiac catheterization allows for evaluation of conduit function and may be therapeutic as it provides the possibility of transcatheter valve replacement. A preoperative coronary angiogram is required prior to cardiac surgery in patients over 40 years of age.

Cardiopulmonary Exercise Test

Patients with ccTGA have reduced exercise capacity, even when they are asymptomatic.

A cardiopulmonary exercise test is an excellent tool to monitor objective functional capacity. Peak oxygen consumption is reduced in these patients compared to the general population[153]

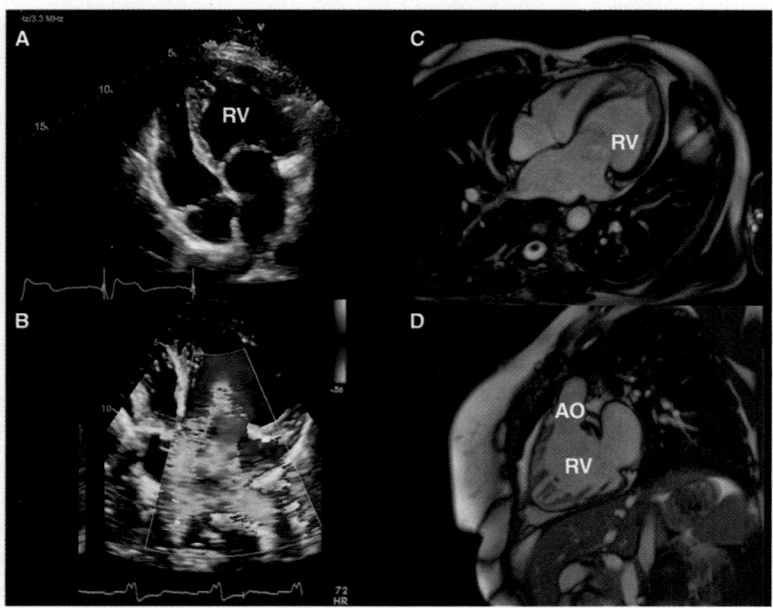

Figure 70–10. **(A)** Four-chamber view (echocardiogram) of a patient with ccTGA showing the Ebstein-like tricuspid valve and the systemic right ventricle on the left side; **(B)** Four-chamber view (echocardiogram) showing a patient with ccTGA with severe tricuspid regurgitation; **(C)** CMR showing a four-chamber view in a ccTGA; **(D)** Sagittal CMR view showing the systemic right ventricle connected to an anterior aorta. RV, right ventricle; Ao, Aorta.

and periodic cardiopulmonary exercise testing is recommended to detect subtle functional decline.

Biomarkers

In patients with systemic right ventricle, blood biomarkers carry significant prognostic value. Geenen et al. showed in a cohort of 86 patients with systemic right ventricle, 21 (~25%) with ccTGA, that patients with elevated BNP, red cell distribution width, factor-15, high-sensitive C-reactive protein, and high-sensitive troponin T have a higher risk of death or of developing heart failure.[154] BNP should be checked yearly in patients with ccTGA and severe tricuspid regurgitation and/or systemic right ventricular dysfunction.

Treatment

Medical Therapy

The natural history of patients with ccTGA depends on the presence and nature of the associated defects.[131] Some degree of systemic right ventricular dysfunction and tricuspid regurgitation are present in the majority of patients. The prevalence of tricuspid regurgitation is similar in patients with or without associated lesions (82% vs 84%); however, systemic right ventricular dysfunction is more common in patients with associated defects (70% vs 55%).[155] Right ventricular dysfunction usually remains subclinical for decades and typically manifests during the fourth and fifth decades of life. Graham et al. reported that 56% of patients with associated lesions and 32% of patients without significant associated lesions will have ventricular dysfunction by the age of 45 years[155] and many of these patients will develop heart failure.

Current evidence regarding the use of conventional heart failure therapy in patients with systemic right ventricle is limited and has been extensively discussed earlier in this chapter. The 2020 European Society of Cardiology (ESC) Adult Congenital Heart Disease Guidelines recommend using conventional heart failure medication in symptomatic patients with systemic right ventricle.[156] It is the authors' practice to start afterload reduction medication in all patients with ccTGA and systemic ventricular ejection fraction under 40% regardless of symptoms. Afterload reduction therapy can paradoxically reduce cardiac output in patients with d-TGA and atrial switch repair due to their inability to augment stroke volume. However, this does not occur in patients with ccTGA, where decreasing afterload will significantly enhance ventricular stroke volume, leading to preload reduction and ultimately improving ejection fraction. Data are lacking to support the use of β-blockers to improve ventricular function in ccTGA. In addition, there are concerns about the propensity for heart block in this population; however, in our experience, β-blockers are generally well tolerated in most adults with ccTGA. Decline in systemic ventricular function in patients with ccTGA should prompt a careful search for treatable causes such as arrhythmias and systemic AV valve regurgitation.[131]

Surgical Management

In patients with ccTGA, surgical intervention is reserved for those who are symptomatic, and those with evidence of declining systemic right ventricular function and worsening tricuspid regurgitation regardless of symptomatology. In the absence of concomitant defects, intervention on asymptomatic patients with preserved systemic right ventricular and tricuspid valve function is controversial. Considering that some patients with ccTGA tend to have a favorable prognosis and surgical intervention is associated with additional risks and long-term issues, the risks in this instance may outweigh potential benefit.[135] Surgical management denotes one of two different strategies, physiological repair (or "classic repair") or anatomical repair.

Physiological Repair

This strategy was introduced in the early 1960s and focuses on repairing the associated defects to complete a biventricular circulation, leaving the right ventricle in systemic position. In the physiological repair, the VSD is closed with special attention to the position of the conduction system to avoid iatrogenic complete heart block. In patients with associated left ventricular outflow tract obstruction, the muscle of septal hypertrophy can be resected at the time of closure of the VSD if the heart is situs inversus; however, muscular resection is discouraged in the setting of situs solitus due to the presence of the conduction system in the subpulmonary left ventricular outflow tract.[157] In this setting, a Rastelli-type procedure with a left ventricle to pulmonary artery conduit should be considered to relieve the left ventricular outflow tract obstruction. Reoperation is frequent following physiological repair, the most common indications being conduit replacement[157] and tricuspid valve repair or replacement.[158] A small study including 32 patients with ccTGA with and without Rastelli-type repair showed that Rastelli patients had better 20-year survival (67% vs 62%) but higher reintervention rate (79% vs 53%)[159] than non-Rastelli patients. The incidence of postoperative complete heart block following physiological repair is high, ranging from 16% to 28%. Tricuspid valve insufficiency and progressive right ventricular dysfunction, common following physiologic repair, are both predictors of poor outcome.[168]

Anatomical Repair

The anatomical repair was described by Ilbawi in 1990[160] with the goal of positioning the left ventricle in systemic position. The anatomical repair can be achieved using different techniques and should not be considered as primary intervention when ccTGA is diagnosed in adulthood.[156] The most common technique is the double switch, a combination of the atrial switch (Mustard or Senning) and arterial switch, but this is contraindicated in patients with pulmonary stenosis. In this setting, the arterial switch is replaced by a Rastelli procedure, a Nikaidoh procedure, or an REV procedure.[161] In patients with hypoplastic right ventricle, a Glenn shunt might need to be considered.[157]

The double switch with arterial switch is indicated in children with no more than mild left ventricular outflow obstruction and a normal pulmonary valve, a minority of ccTGA patients.[158] In patients with unrestrictive VSD, primary double switch is usually performed between 3 and 6 months of age or between 6 and 18 months of age if a pulmonary artery banding is necessary to control congestive heart failure.[162] In absence of a VSD and severe left ventricular outflow tract obstruction, an anatomic repair usually requires staged left ventricular preparation to gain muscle mass before the left ventricle can support the systemic circulation[163] Unfortunately, older adults have limited ability to increase left ventricular mass without inducing fibrosis. They respond to pulmonary artery banding by hypertrophy rather than hyperplasia; as a consequence, they are at risk of developing rapid left ventricular diastolic dysfunction. Impaired systolic and diastolic function of the left ventricle as a result of hypertrophy significantly compromises outcomes in this group, especially if patients are banded for a long period of time.[164] Some groups suggest that successful preparation of the left ventricle is only possible in infants less than 2 years old and should not be considered in patients older than 15 years.[163]

Anatomic repair became the surgery of choice for management of ccTGA in the early 1990s in most centers. Therefore, large, multicenter, clinical trials describing long-term outcomes have not been published yet. A recent meta-analysis including 895 patients who underwent anatomic repair follow-up for 5457.2 patient-years showed an estimated operative mortality of 8.3%. Less than 1% of patients required mechanical support and 1.7% developed postoperative AV block requiring a pacemaker. Patients surviving initial surgery had a transplant free survival of 92.5% per 100 patient-years and a low rate of need for pacemaker, 0.3 per 100 patient-years. After 100 patient-years follow-up, 87.5% of patients were in NYHA functional class I or II and the total reintervention rate was 5.3 per 100 patient-years.[165] In addition, some data suggest that anatomic repair has superior results in higher-risk groups (ie, patients with significant tricuspid valve regurgitation) compared with physiological repair.[166] Tricuspid valve function

significantly improves after anatomic repair and reintervention on the tricuspid valve is usually not necessary.[163] The predictors of outcome after anatomic repair are late left ventricular dysfunction, occurrence of complete or high-degree heart block and pacemaker implantation, neoaortic valve regurgitation, obstruction of Senning/Mustard pathways, and the need for regular reinterventions if conduits have been used.[163,167]

Tricuspid Valve Repair or Replacement

Tricuspid valve abnormalities are present in 70% of patients with ccTGA and progressive tricuspid valve regurgitation is one of the most common complications during follow-up. Timely intervention on the tricuspid valve can interrupt this process and thus improve long-term outcomes.[163]

Early deterioration of systemic ventricular function without tricuspid regurgitation is uncommon in patients with ccTGA, hence, when it occurs, detailed clinical evaluation should be performed to rule out significant tricuspid valve regurgitation.[131] Tricuspid valve replacement is likely to stabilize the systemic right ventricle systolic function when the ejection fraction is preserved, suggesting that the volume overload of the right ventricle secondary to the valve regurgitation is more likely to be the cause of the ventricular dysfunction than a primary cardiomyopathy.[131] Based on this concept, the 2020 ESC Adult Congenital Heart Disease Guidelines recommend tricuspid valve repair or replacement in patients with severe tricuspid valve regurgitation and a right ventricular systolic function >40%, regardless of symptoms (**Table 70-6**).[156] Although the guideline recommendation is tricuspid valve repair or replacement, the former should be avoided due to reduced durability in this population.[168] Risk factors for late mortality or transplantation after tricuspid valve replacement include atrial fibrillation, systemic right ventricular ejection fraction <40%,

TABLE 70-6. ccTGA: 2018 AHA/ACC Guidelines

COR	LOE	Diagnostic	Therapeutic
I	B-NR		1. Tricuspid valve replacement is recommended for symptomatic adults with ccTGA and severe TR, and preserved or mildly depressed systemic ventricular function.
IIa	C-LD	1. CMR is reasonable in adults with ccTGA to determine systemic RV dimensions and systolic function.	1. Tricuspid valve replacement is reasonable for asymptomatic adults with ccTGA and severe TR with dilation or mild dysfunction of the systemic ventricle.
IIb	B-NR		1. Conduit intervention/replacement may be considered for adults with ccTGA and symptomatic sub-pulmonary left ventricle–to-PA conduit dysfunction, recognizing that unloading the subpulmonary ventricle may have a detrimental impact on systemic atrioventricular valve function.

ccTGA: 2020 ESC Guidelines for ACHD

COR	LOE	Therapeutic
I	C	1. In symptomatic patients with severe TR and preserved or mildly impaired systemic RV systolic function (EF >40%), TV replacement is indicated.
IIa	C	1. In asymptomatic patients with severe TR and progressive systemic RV dilatation and/or mildly impaired systemic RV systolic function (EF >40%), TV replacement should be considered. 2. Biventricular pacing should be considered in case of complete AV block or >40% ventricular pacing requirement.
IIb	C	1. In symptomatic patients with severe TR and more than mildly reduced systemic RV systolic function (EF ≤40%), TV replacement may be considered.

Abbreviations: AV, atrioventricular; EF, ejection fraction; RV, right ventricle/ventricular; TR, tricuspid regurgitation; TV, tricuspid valve.

and subpulmonary left ventricle systolic pressure >50 mm Hg.[125,163] The choice of valve prosthesis should be individualized, but a mechanical prosthesis is often preferable to try and avoid re-operation, particularly when ventricular function is already impaired.[131]

Pulmonary Artery Banding

Pulmonary artery banding in adults as left ventricular training for subsequent arterial switch procedure is not recommended.[156] However, it might be considered as a palliative procedure in children not suitable for anatomical repair, or in young patients with severe tricuspid regurgitation and severely impaired systemic right ventricular ejection fraction, with the view of reducing the degree of tricuspid regurgitation and improving the systolic function of the systemic right ventricle. The mechanism of the pulmonary artery banding in this setting is thought be due to the fact that the pulmonary artery banding elevates the left ventricular pressure, reduces leftward septal shift, and prevents further tricuspid annular dilation, thus improving tricuspid regurgitation and the stage of heart failure.[170] The role of pulmonary artery banding in adult patients is not well established.

Nonpharmacological Management of Systemic Right Ventricular Dysfunction

Cardiac Resynchronization Therapy: End-stage heart failure will be inevitable in patients with systemic right ventricle and progressive right ventricular dysfunction. Although we recommend conventional heart failure medication in this population, there is no evidence supporting survival improvement and heart transplantation will be the only lifesaving option. CRT improves survival in patients with acquired heart disease and severely impaired left ventricular function and has been shown to be a potential option in patients with severe systemic right ventricular dysfunction.[171–173] CRT implantation can be challenging in ccTGA patients but, in our experience, it is technically feasible in majority of the cases. Neither the American College of Cardiology/American Heart Association (ACC/AHA) nor the ESC Adult Congenital Heart Disease Guidelines CRT therapy in patients with systemic right ventricle (Table 70–6). Only the PACES/HRS Expert Consensus Statement on the Recognition and Management of Arrhythmias in Adult Congenital Heart Disease gives some clinical guidance, recommending CRT in patients with systemic right ventricle with reduced ejection fraction (≤35%), NYHA function class ≥II, and QRS duration >150 ms with a complete right bundle branch block morphology (spontaneous or paced).[174]

Chronic left ventricular pacing has shown to deteriorate systemic right ventricular function and NYHA functional class in patients with ccTGA[175]; hence, CRT should be considered in patients with AV block and systemic right ventricular ejection fraction <50% who are expected to require ventricular pacing >40% of the time.[176] In this setting, direct His bundle pacing can be also considered, although this requires a high level of expertise.[177]

ICDs are indicated for secondary prevention in patients with ccTGA.[156] However, selecting candidates for primary prevention ICDs remains a major challenge in this population.

Ventricular Assist Devices: Ventricular assist devices (VADs) provide circulatory support to assist damaged ventricles in patients with end-stage heart failure and are widely used in patients with systemic left ventricle. First-generation VADs were large and used pulsatile pumps to mimic the natural pulsing action of the heart, whereas second-generation VADs use a rapidly spinning rotor to produce a continuous flow of blood into the systemic arterial system and are much smaller in size. In patients with systemic right ventricle, VADs should be part of the therapeutic armamentarium and might be considered as a bridge to transplant in severely symptomatic patients with end-stage heart failure or in patients with severe systemic right ventricular dysfunction and pulmonary hypertension. Implantation of a VAD into a morphological right ventricle might be challenging. The inflow cannula should be placed more posteriorly to avoid its obstruction by the moderator band.[163] A close collaboration between the Adult Congenital Heart Disease Unit and the Transplant Unit is needed to manage these patients.

Long-Term Outcomes

The majority of patients with ccTGA will develop symptoms during follow-up due to severe tricuspid regurgitation, systemic right ventricular systolic dysfunction complete heart block, and/or tachyarrhythmias with only a minority reaching advanced age paucisymptomatic. Heart failure and systemic right ventricular dysfunction will develop in the fifth decade of life in two-thirds of patients with associated lesions, whereas they will be present in only 25% of patients without associated lesions.[155] The predictors of congestive heart failure and systemic ventricular dysfunction in this population are age, the presence of significant associated cardiac lesions, history of arrhythmia, pacemaker implantation, and prior surgery of any type, mainly if it involves the tricuspid valve.[155]

Patients with ccTGA require long-life follow-up in a center with expertise in congenital heart disease. They should be followed at least once a year with a comprehensive assessment including echocardiographic evaluation of the systemic right ventricle and tricuspid valve function. When there is discordance between the clinical and echocardiographic findings, advanced imaging with a CMR or CCT should be considered. A cardiopulmonary exercise test should be performed biannually in patients with severe systemic right ventricular dysfunction and in those with severe tricuspid regurgitation to monitor subclinical decline in exercise capacity.

REFERENCES

1. Baillie M. An account of a remarkable transposition of the viscera. *Letter to John Hunter, Esq FRS.* 1788 XXI;78:350-363.
2. Farre J. *Pathological Researches: Essay 1. On Malformations of the Human Heart.* London: Logman, Hurst, Rees, Orme & Brown; 1814.
3. Baffes TG. A new method for surgical correction of transposition of the aorta and pulmonary artery. *Surg Gynecol Obstet.* 1956;102:227-233.
4. Senning A. Surgical correction of transposition of the great vessels. *Surgery.* 1959;45:966-980.
5. Mustard WT. Successful two-stage correction of transposition of the great vessels. *Surgery.* 1964;55:469-472.

6. Rastelli GC. A new approach to "anatomic" repair of transposition of the great arteries. *Mayo Clin Proc.* 1969;44:1-12.

7. Jatene AD, Fontes VF, Paulista PP, et al. Successful anatomic correction of transposition of the great vessels. A preliminary report. *Arq Bras Cardiol.* 1975;28:461-464.

8. Swanson SK, Sayyouh MM, Bardo DME, et al. Interpretation and reporting of coronary arteries in transposition of the great arteries: cross-sectional imaging perspective. *J Thorac Imaging.* 2018;33:W14-W21.

9. Wernovsky G, Sanders SP. Coronary artery anatomy and transposition of the great arteries. *Coron Artery Dis.* 1993;4:148-157.

10. Pasquali SK, Hasselblad V, Li JS, Kong DF, Sanders SP. Coronary artery pattern and outcome of arterial switch operation for transposition of the great arteries: a meta-analysis. *Circulation.* 2002;106:2575-2580.

11. Martins P, Castela E. Transposition of the great arteries. *Orphanet J Rare Dis.* 2008;3:27.

12. Hornung TS, Derrick GP, Deanfield JE, Redington AN. Transposition complexes in the adult: a changing perspective. *Cardiol Clin.* 2002;20:405-420.

13. Chiu IS, Anderson RH, Macartney FJ, de Leval MR, Stark J. Morphologic features of an intact ventricular septum susceptible to subpulmonary obstruction in complete transposition. *Am J Cardiol.* 1984;53:1633-1638.

14. Unolt M, Putotto C, Silvestri LM, et al. Transposition of great arteries: new insights into the pathogenesis. *Front Pediatr.* 2013;1:11.

15. Cipollone D, Amati F, Carsetti R, et al. A multiple retinoic acid antagonist induces conotruncal anomalies, including transposition of the great arteries, in mice. *Cardiovasc Pathol.* 2006;15:194-202.

16. Amati F, Diano L, Campagnolo L, et al. Hif1alpha down-regulation is associated with transposition of great arteries in mice treated with a retinoic acid antagonist. *BMC Genomics.* 2010;11:497.

17. Qu Y, Lin S, Zhuang J, Bloom MS, et al. First-trimester maternal folic acid supplementation reduced risks of severe and most congenital heart diseases in offspring: a large case-control study. *J Am Heart Assoc.* 2020;9:e015652.

18. Landis BJ, Levey A, Levasseur SM, et al. Prenatal diagnosis of congenital heart disease and birth outcomes. *Pediatr Cardiol.* 2013;34:597-605.

19. Cohen MS, Eidem BW, Cetta F, et al. Multimodality imaging guidelines of patients with transposition of the great arteries: a report from the American Society of Echocardiography Developed in Collaboration with the Society for Cardiovascular Magnetic Resonance and the Society of Cardiovascular Computed Tomography. *J Am Soc Echocardiogr.* 2016; 29:571-621.

20. Caplan L, Miller-Hance W. Echocardiographic evaluation of transposition of the great arteries. Congenital Cardiac Anesthesia Society. 2020. https://www.ccasociety.org/education/echoimage/echocardiographic-evaluation-of-transposition-of-the-great-arteries.

21. Rubay J, Lecompte Y, Batisse A, et al. Anatomic repair of anomalies of ventriculo-arterial connection (REV). Results of a new technique in cases associated with pulmonary outflow tract obstruction. *Eur J Cardiothorac Surg.* 1988;2:305-311.

22. Lecompte Y, Vouhe P. Réparation à l'Etage Ventriculaire (REV Procedure): not a rastelli procedure without conduit. *Oper Tech Thorac Cardiovasc Surg.* 2003;8:150-159.

23. Morell VO, Jacobs JP, Quintessenza JA. Aortic translocation in the management of transposition of the great arteries with ventricular septal defect and pulmonary stenosis: results and follow-up. *Ann Thorac Surg.* 2005;79:2089-2092; discussion 2092-2093.

24. Hu SS, Liu ZG, Li SJ, Shen XD, et al. Strategy for biventricular outflow tract reconstruction: Rastelli, REV, or Nikaidoh procedure? *J Thorac Cardiovasc Surg.* 2008;135:331-338.

25. Liebman J, Cullum L, Belloc NB. Natural history of transpositon of the great arteries. Anatomy and birth and death characteristics. *Circulation.* 1969;40:237-262.

26. Hornung T, O'Donnell C. Transposition of the great arteries. In: M Gatzoulis, G Webb, P Daubeney, eds. *Diagnosis and Management of Adult Congenital Heart Disease.* 3rd ed. Philadelphia: Elsevier; 2018.

27. Trusler GA, Williams WG, Duncan KF, et al. Results with the Mustard operation in simple transposition of the great arteries 1963-1985. *Ann Surg.* 1987;206:251-260.

28. Vejlstrup N, Sorensen K, Mattsson E, et al. Long-term outcome of Mustard/Senning correction for transposition of the great arteries in Sweden and Denmark. *Circulation.* 2015;132:633-638.

29. Raissadati A, Nieminen H, Sairanen H, Jokinen E. Outcomes after the Mustard, Senning and arterial switch operation for treatment of transposition of the great arteries in Finland: a nationwide 4-decade perspective. *Eur J Cardiothorac Surg.* 2017;52:573-580.

30. Venkatesh P, Evans AT, Maw AM, et al. Predictors of late mortality in D-transposition of the great arteries after atrial switch repair: systematic review and meta-analysis. *J Am Heart Assoc.* 2019;8:e012932.

31. Wilson NJ, Clarkson PM, Barratt-Boyes BG, et al. Long-term outcome after the mustard repair for simple transposition of the great arteries. 28-year follow-up. *J Am Coll Cardiol.* 1998;32:758-765.

32. Lange R, Horer J, Kostolny M, et al. Presence of a ventricular septal defect and the Mustard operation are risk factors for late mortality after the atrial switch operation: thirty years of follow-up in 417 patients at a single center. *Circulation.* 2006;114:1905-1913.

33. Roos-Hesselink JW, Meijboom FJ, Spitaels SE, et al. Decline in ventricular function and clinical condition after Mustard repair for transposition of the great arteries (a prospective study of 22-29 years). *Eur Heart J.* 2004;25:1264-1270.

34. Diller GP, Okonko DO, Uebing A, et al. Impaired heart rate response to exercise in adult patients with a systemic right ventricle or univentricular circulation: prevalence, relation to exercise, and potential therapeutic implications. *Int J Cardiol.* 2009;134:59-66.

35. Kempny A, Dimopoulos K, Uebing A, et al. Reference values for exercise limitations among adults with congenital heart disease. Relation to activities of daily life–single centre experience and review of published data. *Eur Heart J.* 2012;33:1386-1396.

36. Moons P, Gewillig M, Sluysmans T, et al. Long term outcome up to 30 years after the Mustard or Senning operation: a nationwide multicentre study in Belgium. *Heart.* 2004;90:307-313.

37. Haeffele C, Lui GK. Dextro-transposition of the great arteries: long-term sequelae of atrial and arterial switch. *Cardiol Clin.* 2015;33:543-558, viii.

38. Warnes CA. Transposition of the great arteries. *Circulation.* 2006;114: 2699-2709.

39. Baumgartner H, De Backer J, Babu-Narayan SV, et al. 2020 ESC guidelines for the management of adult congenital heart disease. *Eur Heart J.* 2020.

40. Cuypers JA, Eindhoven JA, Slager MA, et al. The natural and unnatural history of the Mustard procedure: long-term outcome up to 40 years. *Eur Heart J.* 2014;35:1666-1674.

41. Burkhardt BEU, Kellenberger CJ, Franzoso FD, Geiger J, Oxenius A, Valsangiacomo Buechel ER. Right and left ventricular strain patterns after the atrial switch operation for D-transposition of the great arteries–a magnetic resonance feature tracking study. *Front Cardiovasc Med.* 2019;6:39.

42. Storsten P, Eriksen M, Remme EW, et al. Dysfunction of the systemic right ventricle after atrial switch: physiological implications of altered septal geometry and load. *J Appl Physiol (1985).* 2018;125:1482-1489.

43. Li W, Hornung TS, Francis DP, et al. Relation of biventricular function quantified by stress echocardiography to cardiopulmonary exercise capacity in adults with Mustard (atrial switch) procedure for transposition of the great arteries. *Circulation.* 2004;110:1380-1386.

44. Lubiszewska B, Gosiewska E, Hoffman P, et al. Myocardial perfusion and function of the systemic right ventricle in patients after atrial switch procedure for complete transposition: long-term follow-up. *J Am Coll Cardiol.* 2000;36:1365-1370.

45. Broberg CS, Valente AM, Huang J, et al. Myocardial fibrosis and its relation to adverse outcome in transposition of the great arteries with a systemic right ventricle. *Int J Cardiol.* 2018;271:60-65.

46. Ladouceur M, Baron S, Nivet-Antoine V, et al. Role of myocardial collagen degradation and fibrosis in right ventricle dysfunction in transposition of the great arteries after atrial switch. *Int J Cardiol.* 2018;258:76-82.

47. Baysa SJ, Olen M, Kanter RJ. Arrhythmias following the Mustard and Senning operations for dextro-transposition of the great arteries: clinical aspects and catheter ablation. *Card Electrophysiol Clin.* 2017;9:255-271.

48. Love BA, Mehta D, Fuster VF. Evaluation and management of the adult patient with transposition of the great arteries following atrial-level (Senning or Mustard) repair. *Nat Clin Pract Cardiovasc Med.* 2008;5:454-467.

49. Dos L, Teruel L, Ferreira IJ, et al. Late outcome of Senning and Mustard procedures for correction of transposition of the great arteries. *Heart.* 2005;91:652-656.

50. Gelatt M, Hamilton RM, McCrindle BW, et al. Arrhythmia and mortality after the Mustard procedure: a 30-year single-center experience. *J Am Coll Cardiol.* 1997;29:194-201.

51. Gewillig M, Cullen S, Mertens B, Lesaffre E, Deanfield J. Risk factors for arrhythmia and death after Mustard operation for simple transposition of the great arteries. *Circulation.* 1991;84:III187-192.

52. Kirsh JA, Walsh EP, Triedman JK. Prevalence of and risk factors for atrial fibrillation and intra-atrial reentrant tachycardia among patients with congenital heart disease. *Am J Cardiol.* 2002;90:338-340.

53. Kammeraad JA, van Deurzen CH, Sreeram N, et al. Predictors of sudden cardiac death after Mustard or Senning repair for transposition of the great arteries. *J Am Coll Cardiol.* 2004;44:1095-1102.

54. Houck CA, Teuwen CP, Bogers AJ, de Groot NM. Atrial tachyarrhythmias after atrial switch operation for transposition of the great arteries: treating old surgery with new catheters. *Heart Rhythm.* 2016;13:1731-1738.

55. Khairy P. Sudden cardiac death in transposition of the great arteries with a Mustard or Senning baffle: the myocardial ischemia hypothesis. *Curr Opin Cardiol.* 2017;32:101-107.

56. Silka MJ, Hardy BG, Menashe VD, Morris CD. A population-based prospective evaluation of risk of sudden cardiac death after operation for common congenital heart defects. *J Am Coll Cardiol.* 1998;32:245-251.

57. Schwerzmann M, Salehian O, Harris L, et al. Ventricular arrhythmias and sudden death in adults after a Mustard operation for transposition of the great arteries. *Eur Heart J.* 2009;30:1873-1879.

58. Wheeler M, Grigg L, Zentner D. Can we predict sudden cardiac death in long-term survivors of atrial switch surgery for transposition of the great arteries? *Congenit Heart Dis.* 2014;9:326-332.

59. Khairy P, Harris L, Landzberg MJ, et al. Sudden death and defibrillators in transposition of the great arteries with intra-atrial baffles: a multicenter study. *Circ Arrhythm Electrophysiol.* 2008;1:250-257.

60. Verheugt CL, Uiterwaal CS, van der Velde ET, et al. Mortality in adult congenital heart disease. *Eur Heart J.* 2010;31:1220-1229.

61. Chow PC, Cheung EW, Chong CY, et al. Brain natriuretic peptide as a biomarker of systemic right ventricular function in patients with transposition of great arteries after atrial switch operation. *Int J Cardiol.* 2008;127:192-197.

62. Koch AM, Zink S, Singer H. B-type natriuretic peptide in patients with systemic right ventricle. *Cardiology.* 2008;110:1-7.

63. Dore A, Houde C, Chan KL, et al. Angiotensin receptor blockade and exercise capacity in adults with systemic right ventricles: a multicenter, randomized, placebo-controlled clinical trial. *Circulation.* 2005;112:2411-2416.

64. van der Bom T, Winter MM, Bouma BJ, et al. Effect of valsartan on systemic right ventricular function: a double-blind, randomized, placebo-controlled pilot trial. *Circulation.* 2013;127:322-330.

65. van Dissel AC, Winter MM, van der Bom T, et al. Long-term clinical outcomes of valsartan in patients with a systemic right ventricle: follow-up of a multicenter randomized controlled trial. *Int J Cardiol.* 2019;278:84-87.

66. Van De Bruaene A, Norihisa T, Hickey EJ, et al. Pulmonary hypertension in patients with subaortic right ventricle: prevalence, impact and management. *Heart.* 2019;105:1471-1478.

67. Karamlou T, Jacobs ML, Pasquali S, et al. Surgeon and center volume influence on outcomes after arterial switch operation: analysis of the STS Congenital Heart Surgery Database. *Ann Thorac Surg.* 2014;98:904-911.

68. Khairy P, Clair M, Fernandes SM, et al. Cardiovascular outcomes after the arterial switch operation for D-transposition of the great arteries. *Circulation.* 2013;127:331-339.

69. Sarris GE, Chatzis AC, Giannopoulos NM, et al. The arterial switch operation in Europe for transposition of the great arteries: a multi-institutional study from the European Congenital Heart Surgeons Association. *J Thorac Cardiovasc Surg.* 2006;132:633-639.

70. Santens B, Van De Bruaene A, De Meester P, et al. Outcome of arterial switch operation for transposition of the great arteries. A 35-year follow-up study. *Int J Cardiol.* 2020.

71. Losay J, Touchot A, Serraf A, et al. Late outcome after arterial switch operation for transposition of the great arteries. *Circulation.* 2001;104:I121-126.

72. Kempny A, Wustmann K, Borgia F, et al. Outcome in adult patients after arterial switch operation for transposition of the great arteries. *Int J Cardiol.* 2013;167:2588-2593.

73. Co-Vu JG, Ginde S, Bartz PJ, Frommelt PC, Tweddell JS, Earing MG. Long-term outcomes of the neoaorta after arterial switch operation for transposition of the great arteries. *Ann Thorac Surg.* 2013;95:1654-1659.

74. Fricke TA, d'Udekem Y, Richardson M, et al. Outcomes of the arterial switch operation for transposition of the great arteries: 25 years of experience. *Ann Thorac Surg.* 2012;94:139-145.

75. Lim HG, Kim WH, Lee JR, Kim YJ. Long-term results of the arterial switch operation for ventriculo-arterial discordance. *Eur J Cardiothorac Surg.* 2013;43:325-334.

76. Oda S, Nakano T, Sugiura J, Fusazaki N, Ishikawa S, Kado H. Twenty-eight years' experience of arterial switch operation for transposition of the great arteries in a single institution. *Eur J Cardiothorac Surg.* 2012;42:674-679.

77. Legendre A, Losay J, Touchot-Kone A, et al. Coronary events after arterial switch operation for transposition of the great arteries. *Circulation.* 2003;108(Suppl 1):II186-II190.

78. Heinrichs AK, Holschen A, Krings T, et al. Neurologic and psychointellectual outcome related to structural brain imaging in adolescents and young adults after neonatal arterial switch operation for transposition of the great arteries. *J Thorac Cardiovasc Surg.* 2014;148:2190-2199.

79. Kreutzer C, De Vive J, Oppido G, et al. Twenty-five-year experience with rastelli repair for transposition of the great arteries. *J Thorac Cardiovasc Surg.* 2000;120:211-223.

80. Oliver JM, Gallego P, Gonzalez AE, et al. Predicting sudden cardiac death in adults with congenital heart disease. *Heart.* 2020.

81. Wilson J. A description of a very unusual formation of the human heart. *Philos Trans R Soc.* 1798:13,[1]p.,plate.

82. Engle MA. Total anomalous pulmonary venous drainage. Success story at last. *Circulation.* 1972;46:209-211.

83. Ogawa M, Nakagawa M, Hara M, et al. Total anomalous pulmonary venous connection in a 64-year-old man: a case report. *Ann Thorac Cardiovasc Surg.* 2013;19:46-48.

84. Wu FM, Emani SM, Landzberg MJ, Valente AM. Rare case of undiagnosed supracardiac total anomalous pulmonary venous return in an adult. *Circulation.* 2014;130:1205-1207.

85. Brown D, Geva T. Anomalies of the pulmonary veins. In: H Allen, R Shaddy, D Penny, T Feltes, F Cetta, eds. *Moss and Adam's Heart Disease In Infants, Children and Adolescents,* 9th ed. Philadelphia: Wolters Kluwer; 2016.

86. Craig JM, Darling RC, Rothney WB. Total pulmonary venous drainage into the right side of the heart; report of 17 autopsied cases not associated with other major cardiovascular anomalies. *Lab Invest.* 1957;6:44-64.

87. Burroughs JT, Edwards JE. Total anomalous pulmonary venous connection. *Am Heart J.* 1960;59:913-931.

88. Delisle G, Ando M, Calder AL, et al. Total anomalous pulmonary venous connection: Report of 93 autopsied cases with emphasis on diagnostic and surgical considerations. *Am Heart J.* 1976;91:99-122.

89. Lucas RV, Jr., Adams P, Jr., Anderson RC, Varco RL, Edwards JE, Lester RG. Total anomalous pulmonary venous connection to the portal venous system: a cause of pulmonary venous obstruction. *Am J Roentgenol Radium Ther Nucl Med.* 1961;86:561-575.

90. Seale AN, Uemura H, Webber SA, et al. Total anomalous pulmonary venous connection: morphology and outcome from an international population-based study. *Circulation.* 2010;122:2718-2726.

91. Harada T, Nakano T, Oda S, Kado H. Surgical results of total anomalous pulmonary venous connection repair in 256 patients. *Interact Cardiovasc Thorac Surg.* 2019;28:421-426.

92. Yamagishi C, Yamagishi H. Embryology. In: F. Saremi, ed. *Cardiac CT and MR for Adult Congenital Heart Disease.* New York: Springer Science+ Business Media; 2014.

93. Rudolph AM. Total anomalous pulmonary venous connection. In: *Congenital Diseases of the Heart: Clinical-Physiological Considerations,* 3rd ed. West Sussex: Wiley-Blackwell; 2009:320-344.

94. Reller MD, Strickland MJ, Riehle-Colarusso T, Mahle WT, Correa A. Prevalence of congenital heart defects in metropolitan Atlanta, 1998-2005. *J Pediatr.* 2008;153:807-813.

95. Hoffman JI, Kaplan S. The incidence of congenital heart disease. *J Am Coll Cardiol.* 2002;39:1890-1900.

96. Mai CT, Isenburg JL, Canfield MA. National population-based estimates for major birth defects, 2010-2014. *Birth Defects Res.* 2019;111:1420-1435.

97. Jonas R. Total anomalous pulmonary venous connection and other anomalies of the pulmonary veins. In: *Comprehensive Surgical Management of Congenital Heart Disease,* 2nd ed, Boca Raton, FL: CRC Press; 2014.

98. Naha KVG, Shetty RK, Nayak K. Late presentation of TAPVC with multiple cerebral abscesses. *BMJ Case Rep.* 2013.

99. Huhta JC, Gutgesell HP, Nihill MR. Cross sectional echocardiographic diagnosis of total anomalous pulmonary venous connection. *Br Heart J.* 1985;53:525-534.

100. Karamlou T, Gurofsky R, Al Sukhni E, et al. Factors associated with mortality and reoperation in 377 children with total anomalous pulmonary venous connection. *Circulation.* 2007;115:1591-1598.

101. Yong MS, Zhu MZL, Konstantinov IE. Total anomalous pulmonary venous drainage repair: redefining the long-term expectations. *J Thorac Dis.* 2018;10:S3207-S3210.

102. Hyde JA, Stumper O, Barth MJ, et al. Total anomalous pulmonary venous connection: outcome of surgical correction and management of recurrent venous obstruction. *Eur J Cardiothorac Surg.* 1999;15:735-740; discussion 740-741.

103. Yong MS, Yaftian N, Griffiths S, et al. Long-term outcomes of total anomalous pulmonary venous drainage repair in neonates and infants. *Ann Thorac Surg.* 2018;105:1232-1238.

104. St Louis JD, McCracken CE, Turk EM, et al. Long-term transplant-free survival after repair of total anomalous pulmonary venous connection. *Ann Thorac Surg.* 2018;105:186-192.

105. Calbalka A, Edwards WD, Dearani J. Truncus arteriosus. In: H Allen, R Shaddy, D Penny, T Feltes, F Cetta, eds. *Moss and Adams' Heart Disease in Infants, Children and Adolescents* Philadelphia: Wolters Kluwer; 2016.

106. Jonas R. Truncus arteriosus. In: *Comprehensive Surgical Management of Congenital Heart Disease,* 2nd ed. Boca Raton, FL: Taylor & Francis Group; 2014.

107. Van Praagh R, Van Praagh S. The anatomy of common aorticopulmonary trunk (truncus arteriosus communis) and its embryologic implications. A study of 57 necropsy cases. *Am J Cardiol.* 1965;16:406-425.

108. Baggen VJM, Connelly MS, Roos-Hesselink JW. Truncus arteriosus. In: MA Gatzoulis, GD Webb, PE Daubeney, eds. *Diagnosis and Management of Adult Congenital Heart Disease,* 3rd ed. Philadelphia: Elsevier; 2018.

109. Shrivastava S, Edwards JE. Coronary arterial origin in persistent truncus arteriosus. *Circulation.* 1977;55:551-554.

110. Collett RW, Edwards JE. Persistent truncus arteriosus; a classification according to anatomic types. *Surg Clin North Am.* 1949;29:1245-1270.

111. Rudolph AM. Truncus Arteriosus Communis *Congenital Diseases of the Heart: Clinical-Physiological Considerations,* 3rd ed. West Sussex: Wiley-Blackwell; 2009:506-521.

112. Hoffman JI, Kaplan S. The incidence of congenital heart disease. *J Am Coll Cardiol.* 2002;39:1890-1900.

113. Nabati M. An unusual and rare form of truncus arteriosus in an asymptomatic woman. *Ultrasound.* 2017;25:251-254.

114. Kim HS, Kim YH. Persistent truncus arteriosus with aortic dominance in female adult patient. *J Cardiovasc Ultrasound.* 2015;23:32-35.

115. Gutierrez PS, Binotto MA, Aiello VD, Mansur AJ. Chest pain in an adult with truncus arteriosus communis. *Am J Cardiol.* 2004;93:272-273.

116. Lewin MB, Salerno JC. Truncus arteriosus. In: WW Lai, LL Mertens, MS Cohen, T Geva, eds. *Echocardiography in Pediatric and Congenital Heart Disease.* West Sussex: Blackwell; 2009.

117. Ebert PA, Turley K, Stanger P, Hoffman JI, Heymann MA, Rudolph AM. Surgical treatment of truncus arteriosus in the first 6 months of life. *Ann Surg.* 1984;200:451-456.

118. Naimo PS, Bell D, Fricke TA, d'Udekem Y, Brizard CP, Alphonso N, Konstantinov IE. Truncus arteriosus repair: a 40-year multicenter perspective. *J Thorac Cardiovasc Surg.* 2020.

119. Jacobs JP, Mayer JE, Jr., Mavroudis C, et al. The Society of Thoracic Surgeons Congenital Heart Surgery Database: 2016 update on outcomes and quality. *Ann Thorac Surg.* 2016;101:850-862.

120. Chen Q, Gao H, Hua Z, et al. Outcomes of surgical repair for persistent truncus arteriosus from neonates to adults: a single center's experience. *PLoS One.* 2016;11:e0146800.

121. Mastropietro CW, Amula V, Sassalos P, et al. Characteristics and operative outcomes for children undergoing repair of truncus arteriosus: a contemporary multicenter analysis. *J Thorac Cardiovasc Surg.* 2019;157:2386-2398 e4.

122. Buckley JR, Amula V, Sassalos P, et al. Multicenter analysis of early childhood outcomes after repair of truncus arteriosus. *Ann Thorac Surg.* 2019;107:553-559.

123. Thompson LD, McElhinney DB, Reddy M, Petrossian E, Silverman NH, Hanley FL. Neonatal repair of truncus arteriosus: continuing improvement in outcomes. *Ann Thorac Surg.* 2001;72:391-395.

124. Brown JW, Ruzmetov M, Okada Y, Vijay P, Turrentine MW. Truncus arteriosus repair: outcomes, risk factors, reoperation and management. *Eur J Cardiothorac Surg.* 2001;20:221-227.

125. Alamri RM, Dohain AM, Arafat AA, et al. Surgical repair for persistent truncus arteriosus in neonates and older children. *J Cardiothorac Surg.* 2020;15:83.

126. Williams JM, de Leeuw M, Black MD, Freedom RM, Williams WG, McCrindle BW. Factors associated with outcomes of persistent truncus arteriosus. *J Am Coll Cardiol.* 1999;34:545-553.

127. Rajasinghe HA, McElhinney DB, Reddy VM, Mora BN, Hanley FL. Long-term follow-up of truncus arteriosus repaired in infancy: a twenty-year experience. *J Thorac Cardiovasc Surg.* 1997;113:869-878; discussion 878-879.

128. Vohra HA, Whistance RN, Chia AX, et al. Long-term follow-up after primary complete repair of common arterial trunk with homograft: a 40-year experience. *J Thorac Cardiovasc Surg.* 2010;140:325-329.

129. Tlaskal T, Chaloupecky V, Hucin B, et al. Long-term results after correction of persistent truncus arteriosus in 83 patients. *Eur J Cardiothorac Surg.* 2010;37:1278-1284.

130. Nishimura RA, Otto CM, Bonow RO, et al. 2017 AHA/ACC focused update of the 2014 AHA/ACC guideline for the management of patients with valvular heart disease: a report of the American College of Cardiology/ American Heart Association Task Force on Clinical Practice Guidelines. *J Am Coll Cardiol.* 2017;70:252-289.

131. Connolly HM, Miranda WR, Egbe AC, Warnes CA. Management of the adult patient with congenitally corrected transposition: challenges and uncertainties. *Semin Thorac Cardiovasc Surg Pediatr Card Surg Annu.* 2019;22:61-65.

132. Kasar T, Ozturk E, Ayyildiz P, Ergul Y, Guzeltas A. The assessment of patients with situs inversus and corrected transposition of the great arteries. *Rev Port Cardiol.* 2020;39:391-396.

133. Mongeon F-P. Congenitally corrected tranposition of the great arteries. In: M Gatzoulis, G Webb, P Daubeney, eds. *Diagnosis and Management of Adult Congenital Heart Disease,* 3rd ed. Philadelphia: Elsevier; 2018: 545-552.

134. Baruteau AE, Abrams DJ, Ho SY, Thambo JB, McLeod CJ, Shah MJ. Cardiac conduction system in congenitally corrected transposition of the great arteries and its clinical relevance. *J Am Heart Assoc.* 2017;6.

135. Kumar TKS. Congenitally corrected transposition of the great arteries. *J Thorac Dis.* 2020;12:1213-1218.

136. Dick M, 2nd, Van Praagh R, Rudd M, Folkerth T, Castaneda AR. Electrophysiologic delineation of the specialized atrioventricular conduction system in two patients with corrected transposition of the great arteries in situs inversus (I,D,D). *Circulation.* 1977;55:896-900.

137. Oliver JM, Gallego P, Gonzalez AE, et al. Comparison of outcomes in adults with congenitally corrected transposition with situs inversus versus situs solitus. *Am J Cardiol.* 2012;110:1687-1691.

138. Thiene G, Nava A, Rossi L. The conduction system in corrected transposition with situs inversus. *Eur J Cardiol.* 1977;6:57-70.

139. Wallis GA, Debich-Spicer D, Anderson RH. Congenitally corrected transposition. *Orphanet J Rare Dis.* 2011;6:22.

140. Lundstrom U, Bull C, Wyse RK, Somerville J. The natural and "unnatural" history of congenitally corrected transposition. *Am J Cardiol.* 1990;65:1222-1229.

141. Helsen F, De Meester P, Van Keer J, et al. Pulmonary outflow obstruction protects against heart failure in adults with congenitally corrected transposition of the great arteries. *Int J Cardiol.* 2015;196:1-6.

142. Anderson KR, Danielson GK, McGoon DC, Lie JT. Ebstein's anomaly of the left-sided tricuspid valve: pathological anatomy of the valvular malformation. *Circulation.* 1978;58:I87-91.

143. Ferencz C, Rubin JD, McCarter RJ, et al. Congenital heart disease: prevalence at livebirth. The Baltimore-Washington Infant Study. *Am J Epidemiol.* 1985;121:31-36.

144. Samanek M, Voriskova M. Congenital heart disease among 815,569 children born between 1980 and 1990 and their 15-year survival: a prospective Bohemia survival study. *Pediatr Cardiol.* 1999;20:411-417.

145. Piacentini G, Digilio MC, Capolino R, et al. Familial recurrence of heart defects in subjects with congenitally corrected transposition of the great arteries. *Am J Med Genet A.* 2005;137:176-180.

146. Presbitero P, Somerville J, Rabajoli F, Stone S, Conte MR. Corrected transposition of the great arteries without associated defects in adult patients: clinical profile and follow up. *Br Heart J.* 1995;74: 57-59.

147. Huhta JC, Maloney JD, Ritter DG, Ilstrup DM, Feldt RH. Complete atrioventricular block in patients with atrioventricular discordance. *Circulation.* 1983;67:1374-1347.

148. Diller GP, Radojevic J, Kempny A, et al. Systemic right ventricular longitudinal strain is reduced in adults with transposition of the great arteries, relates to subpulmonary ventricular function, and predicts adverse clinical outcome. *Am Heart J.* 2012;163:859-866.

149. Kalogeropoulos AP, Deka A, Border W, et al. Right ventricular function with standard and speckle-tracking echocardiography and clinical events in adults with D-transposition of the great arteries post atrial switch. *J Am Soc Echocardiogr.* 2012;25:304-312.

150. Guo YK, Gao HL, Zhang XC, Wang QL, Yang ZG, Ma ES. Accuracy and reproducibility of assessing right ventricular function with 64-section multi-detector row CT: comparison with magnetic resonance imaging. *Int J Cardiol.* 2010;139:254-262.

151. Muller M, Teige F, Schnapauff D, Hamm B, Dewey M. Evaluation of right ventricular function with multidetector computed tomography: comparison with magnetic resonance imaging and analysis of inter- and intraobserver variability. *Eur Radiol.* 2009;19:278-289.

152. Plumhans C, Muhlenbruch G, Rapaee A, et al. Assessment of global right ventricular function on 64-MDCT compared with MRI. *AJR Am J Roentgenol.* 2008;190:1358-1361.

153. Kempny A, Dimopoulos K, Uebing A, et al. Reference values for exercise limitations among adults with congenital heart disease. Relation to activities of daily life–single centre experience and review of published data. *Eur Heart J.* 2012;33:1386-1396.

154. Geenen LW, van Grootel RWJ, Akman K, et al. Exploring the prognostic value of novel markers in adults with a systemic right ventricle. *J Am Heart Assoc.* 2019;8:e013745.

155. Graham TP, Jr, Bernard YD, Mellen BG, et al. Long-term outcome in congenitally corrected transposition of the great arteries: a multi-institutional study. *J Am Coll Cardiol.* 2000;36:255-261.

156. Baumgartner H, De Backer J, Babu-Narayan SV, et al. 2020 ESC guidelines for the management of adult congenital heart disease. *Eur Heart J.* 2020.

157. Spigel Z, Binsalamah ZM, Caldarone C. Congenitally corrected transposition of the great arteries: anatomic, physiologic repair, and palliation. *Semin Thorac Cardiovasc Surg Pediatr Card Surg Annu.* 2019;22: 32-42.

158. Dyer K, Graham TP. Congenitally corrected transposition of the great arteries: current treatment options. *Curr Treat Options Cardiovasc Med.* 2003;5:399-407.

159. Bogers AJ, Head SJ, de Jong PL, Witsenburg M, Kappetein AP. Long term follow up after surgery in congenitally corrected transposition of the great arteries with a right ventricle in the systemic circulation. *J Cardiothorac Surg.* 2010;5:74.

160. Ilbawi MN, DeLeon SY, Backer CL, et al. An alternative approach to the surgical management of physiologically corrected transposition with ventricular septal defect and pulmonary stenosis or atresia. *J Thorac Cardiovasc Surg.* 1990;100:410-415.

161. Hazekamp MG, Nevvzhay T, Sojak V. Nikaidoh vs Reparation a l'Etage Ventriculaire vs Rastelli. *Semin Thorac Cardiovasc Surg Pediatr Card Surg Annu.* 2018;21:58-63.

162. Hraska V, Woods RK. Anatomic repair of corrected transposition of the great arteries: the double switch. *Semin Thorac Cardiovasc Surg Pediatr Card Surg Annu.* 2019;22:57-60.

163. Filippov AA, Del Nido PJ, Vasilyev NV. Management of systemic right ventricular failure in patients with congenitally corrected transposition of the great arteries. *Circulation.* 2016;134:1293-1302.

164. Winlaw DS, McGuirk SP, Balmer C, et al. Intention-to-treat analysis of pulmonary artery banding in conditions with a morphological right ventricle in the systemic circulation with a view to anatomic biventricular repair. *Circulation.* 2005;111:405-411.

165. Chatterjee A, Miller NJ, Cribbs MG, Mukherjee A, Law MA. Systematic review and meta-analysis of outcomes of anatomic repair in congenitally corrected transposition of great arteries. *World J Cardiol.* 2020;12:427-436.

166. Lim HG, Lee JR, Kim YJ, et al. Outcomes of biventricular repair for congenitally corrected transposition of the great arteries. *Ann Thorac Surg.* 2010;89:159-167.

167. Bautista-Hernandez V, Myers PO, Cecchin F, Marx GR, Del Nido PJ. Late left ventricular dysfunction after anatomic repair of congenitally corrected transposition of the great arteries. *J Thorac Cardiovasc Surg.* 2014;148:254-258.

168. Koolbergen DR, Ahmed Y, Bouma BJ, et al. Follow-up after tricuspid valve surgery in adult patients with systemic right ventricles. *Eur J Cardiothorac Surg.* 2016;50:456-463.

169. Mongeon FP, Connolly HM, Dearani JA, Li Z, Warnes CA. Congenitally corrected transposition of the great arteries ventricular function at the

time of systemic atrioventricular valve replacement predicts long-term ventricular function. *J Am Coll Cardiol.* 2011;57:2008-2017.

170. Kral Kollars CA, Gelehrter S, Bove EL, Ensing G. Effects of morphologic left ventricular pressure on right ventricular geometry and tricuspid valve regurgitation in patients with congenitally corrected transposition of the great arteries. *Am J Cardiol.* 2010;105:735-739.

171. Diller GP, Okonko D, Uebing A, Ho SY, Gatzoulis MA. Cardiac resynchronization therapy for adult congenital heart disease patients with a systemic right ventricle: analysis of feasibility and review of early experience. *Europace.* 2006;8:267-272.

172. Jauvert G, Rousseau-Paziaud J, Villain E, et al. Effects of cardiac resynchronization therapy on echocardiographic indices, functional capacity, and clinical outcomes of patients with a systemic right ventricle. *Europace.* 2009;11:184-190.

173. Moore JP, Cho D, Lin JP, et al. Implantation techniques and outcomes after cardiac resynchronization therapy for congenitally corrected transposition of the great arteries. *Heart Rhythm.* 2018;15:1808-1815.

174. Khairy P, Van Hare GF, Balaji S, et al. PACES/HRS expert consensus statement on the recognition and management of arrhythmias in adult congenital heart disease: developed in partnership between the Pediatric and Congenital Electrophysiology Society (PACES) and the Heart Rhythm Society (HRS). Endorsed by the governing bodies of PACES, HRS, the American College of Cardiology (ACC), the American Heart Association (AHA), the European Heart Rhythm Association (EHRA), the Canadian Heart Rhythm Society (CHRS), and the International Society for Adult Congenital Heart Disease (ISACHD). *Heart Rhythm.* 2014;11:e102-e165.

175. Yeo WT, Jarman JW, Li W, Gatzoulis MA, Wong T. Adverse impact of chronic subpulmonary left ventricular pacing on systemic right ventricular function in patients with congenitally corrected transposition of the great arteries. *Int J Cardiol.* 2014;171:184-191.

176. Kusumoto FM, Schoenfeld MH, Barrett C, et al. 2018 ACC/AHA/HRS guideline on the evaluation and management of patients with bradycardia and cardiac conduction delay: executive summary: a report of the American College of Cardiology/American Heart Association Task Force on Clinical Practice Guidelines, and the Heart Rhythm Society. *J Am Coll Cardiol.* 2019;74:932-987.

177. Mahata I, Macicek SL, Morin DP. Direct His bundle pacing using retrograde mapping in complete heart block and L-transposition of the great arteries. *HeartRhythm Case Rep.* 2019;5:291-293.

178. Dos L, Pujadas S, Estruch M, et al. Eplerenone in systemic right ventricle: double blind randomized clinical trial. The evedes study. *Int J Cardiol.* 2013;168:5167-5173.

179. Therrien J, Provost Y, Harrison J, Connelly M, Kaemmerer H, Webb GD. Effect of angiotensin receptor blockade on systemic right ventricular function and size: a small, randomized, placebo-controlled study. *Int J Cardiol.* 2008;129:187-192.

180. Hechter SJ, Fredriksen PM, Liu P, et al. Angiotensin-converting enzyme inhibitors in adults after the Mustard procedure. *Am J Cardiol.* 2001;87:660-663, A11.

181. Lester SJ, McElhinney DB, Viloria E, et al. Effects of losartan in patients with a systemically functioning morphologic right ventricle after atrial repair of transposition of the great arteries. *Am J Cardiol.* 2001;88:1314-1316.

182. Giardini A, Lovato L, Donti A, et al. A pilot study on the effects of carvedilol on right ventricular remodelling and exercise tolerance in patients with systemic right ventricle. *Int J Cardiol.* 2007;114:241-246.

183. Doughan AR, McConnell ME, Book WM. Effect of beta blockers (carvedilol or metoprolol XL) in patients with transposition of great arteries and dysfunction of the systemic right ventricle. *Am J Cardiol.* 2007;99:704-706.

184. Tutarel O, Meyer GP, Bertram H, et al. Safety and efficiency of chronic ACE inhibition in symptomatic heart failure patients with a systemic right ventricle. *Int J Cardiol.* 2012;154:14-16.

Psychosocial Profiles in Adult Congenital Heart Disease and Transition to Adulthood

71

Philip Moons

CHAPTER OUTLINE

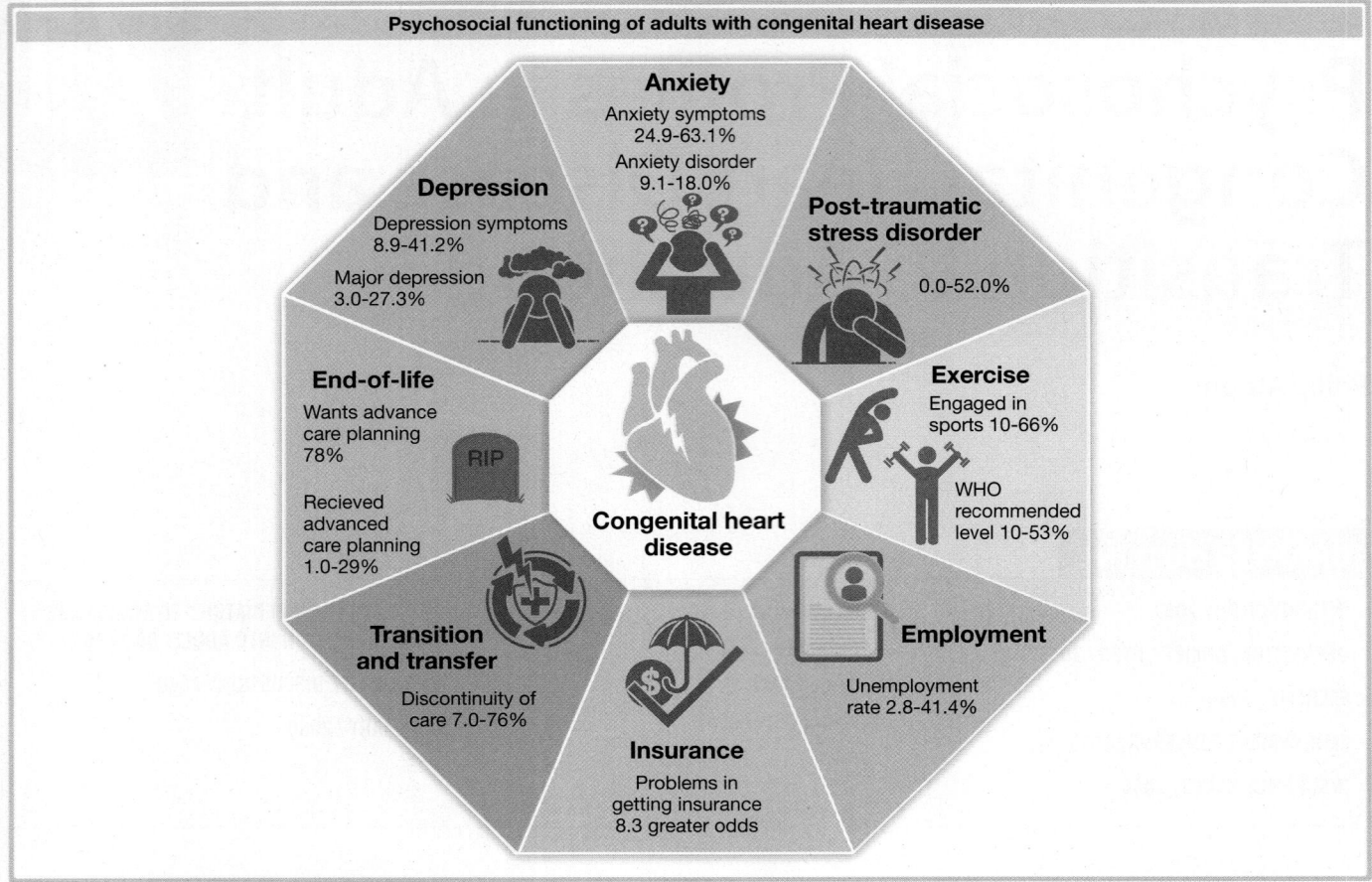

Chapter 71 Fuster and Hurst's Central Illustration. Mental health issues are common in adults with congenital heart disease. Engagement in physical activities improves exercise capacity and psychological functioning. Employability and insurability are jeopardized in adults with congenital heart disease. Discontinuity of care is prevalent as young persons with congenital heart disease transition into adulthood. End-of-life discussions are important: even when in good health, patients prefer to have discussions about advance care planning and advance directives.

CHAPTER SUMMARY

This chapter discusses different aspects of psychosocial functioning of adults with congenital heart disease (ACHD). Mental health issues, such as depression, anxiety, and posttraumatic stress disorder are common in ACHD (see Fuster and Hurst's Central Illustration). Intercountry variations have been found, with higher levels in Asia compared to North America or Europe. Patients generally have higher levels of depression, and equal levels of anxiety than people from the general population. Hence, adequate mental health care is pivotal in ACHD. Another important aspect in the counseling of ACHD patients is physical exercise. Exercise capacity is reduced and skeletal muscle function is compromised in patients with congenital heart disease (CHD) compared to healthy individuals. Nonetheless, it is strongly advised that ACHD engage in physical activities, because it yields significant improvements in exercise capacity and psychological functioning. Social areas of concern are employability and insurability, both of which are jeopardized in ACHD. Because CHD is a lifelong disease, young persons with CHD who are transitioning into adulthood are assumed to transfer from pediatric to adult-focused care. Yet, discontinuity of care is prevalent. End-of-life discussions should be part of standard practice in ACHD. Indeed, even when in good health, patients prefer to have discussions about advance care planning and advance directives.

INTRODUCTION

Congenital heart disease (CHD) represents a heterogeneous group of simple, moderate, and complex structural heart defects. Globally, it is estimated to occur in 9.3 per 1000 newborns,[1] and more than 90% of the children born with CHD now reach adulthood.[2,3] Irrespective of the relatively good life expectancy, afflicted patients remain vulnerable for developing medical and psychosocial problems.

Indeed, psychosocial functioning of persons with CHD is an area of concern. Living with CHD and the required invasive treatments may impact on the psychological and social health of afflicted individuals. Psychosocial functioning is an umbrella term encompassing a range of psychological and social issues, as well as their interplay. Psychological factors include depression, anxiety, and posttraumatic stress disorder (PTSD). Social factors include concerns about employability and insurance. Specific topics that are of particular interest for adults with CHD (ACHD) are physical exercise, transition from pediatric to adult care, and end-of-life discussions. The present chapter addresses these aspects in detail.

DEPRESSION, ANXIETY, PTSD

Mental health issues are common in ACHD. Depression is a serious mood disorder that causes severe symptoms that affect how one feels, thinks, and handles daily activities. In the assessment of depression, it is important to distinguish between the "presence of depressive symptoms" and the diagnosis of "clinical depression." Numerous studies have been conducted to determine the prevalence of depressive symptoms in ACHD patients. A commonly used instrument for this purpose is the Hospital Anxiety and Depression Scale (HADS). HADS scores of ≥8 suggest a possible depression; scores of ≥11 suggest a probable depression.[4] Possible depression was found in 8.9% to 41.2% of the ACHD population (**Table 71–1**). Probable depression occurred in 0.0% to 17.9%. Intercountry variations in depressive symptomatology has been found.[5,6] Indeed, the prevalence of possible depression in Asia (19.3%–41.2%) is higher than in North America (12.3%–16.8%) or Europe (6.4%–17.2%). When looking at ACHD patients with complex conditions, the proportion of possible depression can go up to 68.6% in Fontan patients (Table 71–1).

The diagnosis of major depressive disorder (clinical depression) can only be made by a structured clinical interview, employing diagnostic criteria. Regarding clinical depression, there is less variability across the continents, with depression rates of 19.5% in Asia, 13.8% to 27.3% in North America, and 24.7% to 25.7% in Europe (**Table 71–2**). This suggests that the point prevalence of depressive disorders in ACHD around the globe is around 205 to 25%. The lifetime prevalence of depression, however, is estimated to range from 32.8% to 43.3%.[7,8]

When ACHD patients are compared to the general population, 6 out of 12 studies found a higher rate of depression in patients,[9–14] 1 study found a lower rate,[15] and 5 studies yielded nonsignificant results.[8,16–19] The precise reasons for the higher depression rates are not fully understood yet.

TABLE 71–1. Prevalence of Depressive Symptoms in ACHD as Measured Using the Hospital Anxiety and Depression Scale (HADS)

Author, Year	Country	Possible Depression (HADS score ≥8)	Probable Depression (HADS score ≥11)
North America			
Gleason, 2019[100]	United States	12.3%	
Leslie, 2020[101]	United States	16.8%	
Europe			
Bedair, 2015[102]	United Kingdom	6.4%	
Berg, 2017[103]	Denmark	16.5%	
Martinez-Quintana, 2020[104]	Spain	8.9%	2.4%
Riley, 2012[105]	United Kingdom	17.2%	5.1%
Asia			
Cohen, 2010[19]	Israel	29.6%	0.0%
Enomoto, 2015[a,18]	Japan	19.3%	2.3%
Enomoto, 2015[b,18]	Japan	35.6%	11.1%
Eslami, 2013[16]	Iran	41.2%	17.9%
Global			
Ko, 2019[6]	15 countries	11.9%	3.7%
Special groups			
Bedair, 2015[102]	ACHD + ICD	25.4%	
Amedro, 2016[106]	PAH	9.1%	
Bordin, 2015[107]	Fontan	68.6%	14.3%

Abbreviations: ACHD, adult congenital heart disease; HADS, Hospital Anxiety and Depression Scale; ICD, implanted cardioverter defibrillator; PAH, pulmonary arterial hypertension.
[a]age group 20–29 years; [b]age group 30–39 years.

Disease complexity and the presence of comorbidities seem to make ACHD patients more vulnerable for developing depression.[13,20–23] Depression has significant consequences for afflicted patients. ACHD patients who have been diagnosed with depression have a higher risk for mortality than nondepressed patients.[21,22]

Most studies are cross-sectional, giving a point prevalence of depressive symptoms or clinical depression. However, a longitudinal study demonstrated the importance of assessing persistent or chronic depressive symptoms.[24] Indeed, patients with persisting or recurring depressive symptoms do worse in terms of quality of life and patient-reported health than patients who are experiencing one or no depressive episode.[24] This reminds us of the need for regular and longitudinal assessments of depression throughout clinical follow-up.

Another mood disturbance is anxiety disorders, which are characterized by excessive anxiety or worries in the absence of, or out of proportion to, situational factors. Symptoms of anxiety, as can be measured with the HADS, are even more prevalent in ACHD patients than depressive symptoms. Indeed, possible anxiety ranges from 24.9% to 63.1%, and probable anxiety varies from 3.7% to 40.0% (**Table 71–3**). Intercountry variations in

TABLE 71–2. Prevalence of Major Depressive Disorder in ACHD Based on Clinical Interview

Author, Year	Country	Diagnostic Criteria	Clinical Diagnosis of Depression
North America			
Bromberg, 2003[20]	US	DSM-IV	27.3%
Horner, 2000[108]	US	DSM-III-R	13.8%
Kovacs, 2009[7]	Canada/US	DSM-IV	15.5%
Europe			
Westhoff-Bleck, 2016[9]	Germany	DSM-IV	24.7%
Westhoff-Bleck, 2020[109]	Germany	DSM-IV	25.7%
Asia			
Moon, 2017[110]	South Korea	MINI criteria	19.5%
Special groups			
Kasmi, 2018[8]	ASO for TGA	DSM-IV	3.0%

Abbreviations: MINI, Mini International Neuropsychiatric Interview; ASO, arterial switch operation; TGA, transposition of the great arteries.

TABLE 71–4. Prevalence of Anxiety Disorder in ACHD Based on Clinical Interview

Author, Year	Country	Diagnostic Criteria	Clinical Diagnosis of Depression
North America			
Bromberg, 2003[20]	US	DSM-IV	9.1%
Kovacs, 2009[7]	Canada/US	DSM-IV	17.2%
Europe			
Westhoff-Bleck, 2016[9]	Germany	DSM-IV	9.3%
Asia			
Moon, 2017[110]	South Korea	MINI criteria	18.0%
Special groups			
Kasmi, 2018[8]	ASO for TGA	DSM-IV	35.8%

Abbreviations: DSM, Diagnostic and Statistical Manual of Mental Disorders; MINI, Mini International Neuropsychiatric Interview; ASO, arterial switch operation; TGA, transposition of the great arteries.

TABLE 71–3. Prevalence of Anxiety in ACHD as Measured Using the Hospital Anxiety and Depression Scale (HADS)

Author, Year	Country	Possible Anxiety Disorder (HADS score ≥8)	Probable Anxiety Disorder (HADS score ≥11)
North America			
Gleason, 2019[100]	United States	42.3%	
Leslie, 2020[101]	United States	35.2%	
Europe			
Bedair, 2015[102]	United Kingdom	38.3%	
Berg, 2017[103]	Denmark	27.8%	
Martinez-Quintana, 2020[104]	Spain	24.9%	10.1%
Riley, 2012[105]	United Kingdom	38.4%	13.1%
Asia			
Cohen, 2010[19]	Israel	40.7%	3.7%
Enomoto, 2015[a,8]	Japan	44.3%	19.3%
Enomoto, 2015[b,8]	Japan	57.8%	40.0%
Eslami, 2013[16]	Iran	63.1%	38.3%
Special groups			
Bedair, 2015[102]	ACHD+ICD	42.4%	
Amedro, 2016[106]	PAH	30.8%	
Bordin, 2015[107]	Fontan	88.6%	65.7%

Abbreviations: HADS, Hospital Anxiety and Depression Scale; ACHD, adult congenital heart disease; ICD, implanted cardioverter defibrillator; PAH, pulmonary arterial hypertension.
[a]age group 20–29 years; [b]age group 30–39 years

anxiety symptoms is also documented.[5] However, the disparity across continents is less pronounced for possible anxiety (Asia 40.7%–63.1%; North America 35.2%–42.3%; Europe 24.9%–38.4%) than for probable anxiety (Asia 3.7%–40.0%; Europe 10.1%–13.1%) (Table 71–3). In Fontan patients, possible anxiety occurred in 88.6% and probable anxiety in 65.7%. These data show that anxiety symptoms are very prevalent in ACHD.

Anxiety disorders, diagnosed by a structured clinical interview, are substantially less prevalent than anxiety symptoms. In the ACHD population, anxiety disorders occur in 9.1% to 18% of the patients (**Table 71–4**). However, in patients following an arterial switch operation for transposition of the great arteries, anxiety disorders were diagnosed in 35.8%. The lifetime prevalence of anxiety disorders is found to range between 25.9% and 53.7%.[7,8]

Anxiety rates in ACHD patients have been compared with healthy controls in 12 studies, 4 of which showed higher rates in patients.[9,12,14,16] The other 8 studies showed no differences between the groups.[8,17–19,25–28] The consequences of anxiety and anxiety disorders are less studied.

Early in life, persons with CHD may encounter traumatic experiences due to invasive procedures and prolonged intensive care treatments. Growing up with CHD also may trigger existential questions since patients can be confronted with a potentially reduced life expectancy. From this perspective, it is understandable that some ACHD patients are developing PTSD. The proportion of PTSD in ACHD ranges from 0% to 52% (**Table 71–5**).

EXERCISE

Physical activity is an important determinant for cardiorespiratory fitness, which in turn is a marker for health.[29] This is also true for ACHD patients. In the past, patients were often advised against sport participation by their cardiologists, because the impact of physical activities on CHD were poorly understood and safety was queried.[30] In the meantime, evidence on the benefits of exercise in ACHD is mounting.

TABLE 71–5. Prevalence of Posttraumatic Stress Disorder in ACHD

Author, Year	Country	Prevalence
North America		
Carazo, 2020[21]	United States	1.1%
Deng, 2016[111]	United States	21.3%
Moreland, 2018[112]	United States	24.0%
Europe		
Kasmi, 2018[8]	France	0.0%
Westhoff-Bleck, 2016[9]	Germany	2.7%
Asia		
Eslami, 2013[16]	Iran	52.0%

Admittedly, exercise capacity is reduced in children, adolescents, and adults with CHD in comparison with healthy controls.[31,32] A meta-analysis showed that children and adolescents with CHD have a decrease of 9.31 mL/kg/min in VO_2 max and a lower anaerobic threshold of 4.27 mL/kg/min than controls.[31] The maximum heart rate reached during cardiopulmonary exercise test and stress testing was 15.14 bpm lower as compared with the control group.[31] Obviously, there is also a large variability in exercise capacity across different types of heart defects.[32] In patients with arterial switch operation for transposition of the great arteries, valvular lesions, and coarctation of the aorta, the exercise capacity in half of the patients is normal to mildly impaired.[32] Oppositely, a significant part of the patients with Fontan or Eisenmenger have a severely impaired exercise capacity.[32] This reflects in the perceived physical functioning of patients, where it was found that patients with coarctation of the aorta reported the best physical functioning, and patients with cyanotic heart disease or Eisenmenger syndrome the worst.[33] Not only the cardiac reserve is reduced in ACHD patients, also the skeletal muscle function is compromised. It has been found that patients with complex CHD have an impaired isotonic limb muscle function compared with patients with simple lesions as well as with controls.[34] The underlying mechanism is slower skeletal muscle oxygenation kinetics.[35] Exercise training, both in clinic and home-based interventions, have shown to be safe and suggest to be effective in improving the cardiorespiratory fitness of afflicted patients.[36,37] However, the rather low quality of the studies prevents us from drawing firm conclusions and adherence to the intervention is rather low.[36,37]

Irrespective of the impaired exercise capacity and skeletal muscle function, it is strongly advised that ACHD patients are engaged in physical activities. Participation in sport activities yield significant improvements in exercise capacity[38] and psychological functioning.[6] Almost all patients with CHD can safely perform regular moderate-intensity activities, unless specific contraindications are present.[39] It is important that the prescription of physical activities for recreational purposes is performed on an individual basis. Such individualized exercise prescription has to take the following aspects into consideration: the underlying heart defect; the electrical and hemodynamic stability; the static component of exercise; the degree of intensity; and the control and feedback.[40] A decision matrix has been developed that can guide clinicians in providing advice on recreational physical exercise (**Fig. 71–1**).[40]

Some ACHD patients want to engage in competitive sports, which is not per se contraindicated. The most renowned example is Shaun White, who was born with tetralogy of Fallot and won three Olympic gold medals on the snowboarding halfpipe. An accurate assessment and appropriate advice are warranted. The assessment in preparation of competitive sports include the underlying heart defect, the electrical and hemodynamic stability, the physical fitness, the type of exercise (skills, power, mixed, or endurance), and the control and feedback.[41] Also for this purpose, a decision matrix has been developed (**Fig. 71–2**).[41]

Although it is recommended that clinicians should assess activity levels at regular intervals and counsel patients with ACHD about the types and intensity of exercise appropriate to their clinical status,[42] the levels of physical activity are still relatively low. A large-scale study including over 4000 ACHD patients from 15 countries found that 43% of the patients endorsed sport participation.[43] However, geographic variability was substantial, ranging from 10% in India to 66% in Norway (**Table 71–6**).[43] In terms of levels of activity, the World Health Organization (WHO) recommends 2.5 hours per week of physical activity of three metabolic equivalents (METS) or more in order to have health benefits.[44] Overall, 31% of patients with ACHD indicate to reach this WHO recommended level.[45] Also here, geographic variability was observed, ranging from 10% of patients in India reaching the recommended level to 53% in Norway (Table 71–6).[45] In the interpretation of these data, it is important to note that self-reported physical activities generally yield an overestimation of the true activity level.[46]

EMPLOYMENT CONCERNS

Employment is important for the well-being of an individual. In adults with CHD, it has been found that higher employment rates were associated with better quality of life or less depression.[47–52] A significant proportion of ACHD patients, however, experience problems with employability.[53] Unemployment rates in ACHD patient range from 2.8% to 41.4%, with large geographic differences (**Table 71–7**). Seven studies compared the unemployment rate of ACHD patients with that of the general population,[18,51,54–58] five of which found a higher unemployment rate in ACHD.[18,51,55,57,58] Importantly, the employment rates have increased over the last few decades, yielding more persons with ACHD being successful in obtaining a job.[59]

The level of education is an important predictor for successful employment.[53,54] However, even patients with high academic achievements may have poor job prospects. In particular, patients with complex lesions, poor functional status, or a history of heart failure may find themselves at a disadvantage in obtaining employment.[52–54,57,60] Also, female patients appear to have more difficulties in finding employment.[53,60] Education and career counseling that matches the patient's interests

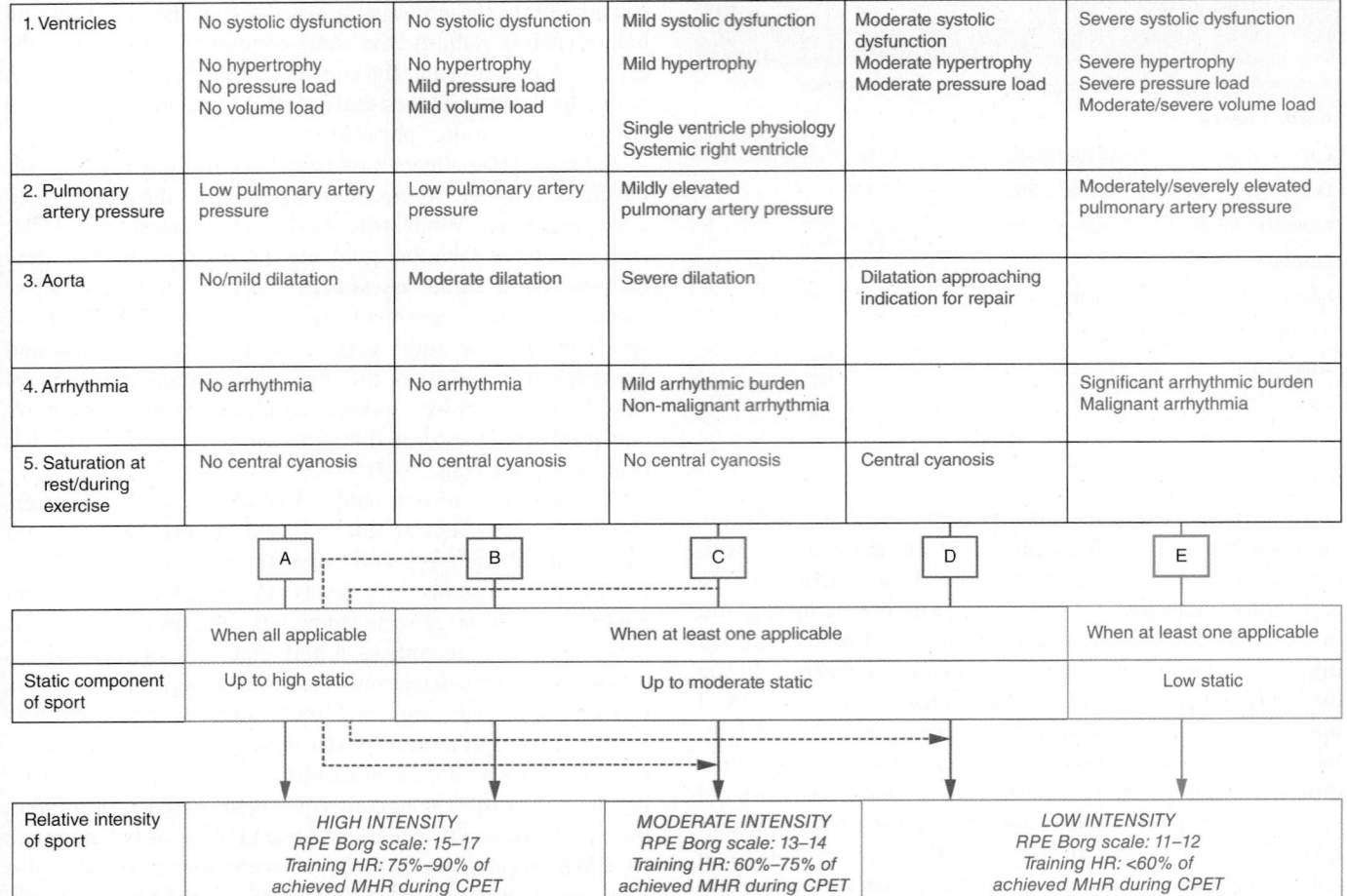

1. Ventricles	No systolic dysfunction No hypertrophy No pressure load No volume load	No systolic dysfunction No hypertrophy Mild pressure load Mild volume load	Mild systolic dysfunction Mild hypertrophy Single ventricle physiology Systemic right ventricle	Moderate systolic dysfunction Moderate hypertrophy Moderate pressure load	Severe systolic dysfunction Severe hypertrophy Severe pressure load Moderate/severe volume load
2. Pulmonary artery pressure	Low pulmonary artery pressure	Low pulmonary artery pressure	Mildly elevated pulmonary artery pressure		Moderately/severely elevated pulmonary artery pressure
3. Aorta	No/mild dilatation	Moderate dilatation	Severe dilatation	Dilatation approaching indication for repair	
4. Arrhythmia	No arrhythmia	No arrhythmia	Mild arrhythmic burden Non-malignant arrhythmia		Significant arrhythmic burden Malignant arrhythmia
5. Saturation at rest/during exercise	No central cyanosis	No central cyanosis	No central cyanosis	Central cyanosis	

	A	B	C	D	E
	When all applicable	When at least one applicable			When at least one applicable
Static component of sport	Up to high static	Up to moderate static			Low static
Relative intensity of sport	*HIGH INTENSITY* *RPE Borg scale: 15–17* *Training HR: 75%–90% of* *achieved MHR during CPET*	*MODERATE INTENSITY* *RPE Borg scale: 13–14* *Training HR: 60%–75% of* *achieved MHR during CPET*			*LOW INTENSITY* *RPE Borg scale: 11–12* *Training HR: <60% of* *achieved MHR during CPET*

Solid lines indicate recommendation; if option for sports with high static component, reduce intensity (dotted lines)

Figure 71–1. Decision matrix for individualized exercise prescription for ACHD patients. Modified with permission from Budts W, Börjesson M, Chessa M, et al. Physical activity in adolescents and adults with congenital heart defects: individualized exercise prescription. *Eur Heart J.* 2013 Dec;34(47):3669-3674.

with their physical abilities may be instrumental to prevent or reduce job-related problems.

INSURANCE ISSUES

Obtaining insurances is essential for many individuals to build up an independent life and reduce financial risks in case of adversity. Having CHD can hinder individuals from obtaining coverage. Some decades ago, insurability of ACHD patients was problematic because a large majority of the patients were refused insurance,[61,62] even for patients whose health status was rated as "excellent" or "good" by a cardiologist. The situation has improved over time. However, the odds of having problems in obtaining insurances in ACHD patients is still 8.3 times greater that in people from the general population.[63]

Health Insurance

Since the Affordable Care Act, ACHD patients in the United States are a well-insured population.[64] People with ACHD seem to be less likely to have Health Maintenance Organization (HMO) and more likely to have Preferred Provider Organization

(PPO) as primary coverage.[64] These patients also were more likely to have Medicare and less likely to have Medicaid.[64] The complexity of the CHD did not play a role in obtaining insurance, neither did the parental plan in patients younger than 26 years.[64] Although the basic healthcare needs are now well insured in most countries, obtaining additional health insurance may still be more difficult for ACHD patients.[63]

Life Insurance

Obtaining life insurance seems to be the most difficult for patients with ACHD.[63] A study in the Netherlands showed that 45% of ACHD patients experienced problems in obtaining life insurance.[63] The odds for having problems obtaining life insurance was 48 times greater in ACHD patients than in the general population.[63] The complexity of the CHD was a determinant for successfully obtaining life insurance, with people having complex heart defects having more problems.[63] More than half of the patients with complex CHD had to pay a higher premium.[63] In a UK study, 34% of the patients were declined for life insurance and 37% had to pay extra.[65] Compared to healthy controls, the odds were 6 and 5.75 times

1. Ventricles	No systolic dysfunction No/mild hypertrophy No/mild pressure load No volume load	Mild systolic dysfunction Volume load without remodelling	Moderate systolic dysfunction Moderate hypertrophy Moderate pressure load Volume load with mild remodelling Single ventricle physiology Systemic right ventricle	Severe systolic dysfunction Severe hypertrophy Severe pressure load Volume load with severe remodelling
2. Pulmonary artery pressure	Low probability of pulmonary hypertension	PH without RV dilatation or dysfunction		PH with RV dilatation or dysfunction
3. Aorta	No/mild dilatation	Moderate dilatation	Severe dilatation	Dilatation approaching indication for repair
4. Arrhythmia at rest/during exercise	No arrhythmia	Mild arrhythmia burden Non-malignant arrhythmia		Significant arrhythmic burden Malignant arrhythmia
5. Saturation at rest/during exercise	No central cyanosis		Mild central cyanosis	Severe central cyanosis
	A	B	C	D
	When all applicable	When ≥1 parameters applicable AND no parameter falls within columns C or D	When ≥1 parameters applicable AND no parameter falls within column D	When ≥1 parameters applicable
Choice of competitive sport	All sports	Skill, power, or mixed sports	Skill sports only	NO COMPETITIVE SPORT

Figure 71–2. Decision matrix for competitive sports in ACHD patients. Modified with permission from Budts W, Pieles GE, Roos-Hesselink JW, et al. Recommendations for participation in competitive sport in adolescent and adult athletes with Congenital Heart Disease (CHD): position statement of the Sports Cardiology & Exercise Section of the European Association of Preventive Cardiology (EAPC), the European Society of Cardiology (ESC) Working Group on Adult Congenital Heart Disease and the Sports Cardiology, Physical Activity and Prevention Working Group of the Association for European Paediatric and Congenital Cardiology (AEPC). *Eur Heart J.* 2020 Nov 14;41(43):4191-4199.

higher, respectively, in ACHD patients.[65] Irrespective of the difficulties that ACHD patients may experience in obtaining life insurance, about one-third of the patients with complex CHD who applied for life insurance were covered at standard rates.[65]

Mortgage

In the Netherlands, 20% of ACHD patients experienced restrictions in obtaining a mortgage.[63] In the United Kingdom, 23% of patients were refused a mortgage.[65] Compared to healthy controls, the odds of having difficulties in obtaining a mortgage is 6 to 8.4 times higher in ACHD patients.[63,65]

Travel Insurance

A survey among ACHD patients in the United Kingdom showed that 9% of patients have been rejected when applying for travel insurance during their lifetime.[66] Unsurprisingly, one-quarter of patients do not declare a preexisting heart condition when applying for travel insurance.[66] In those patients that did declare their condition, 32% reported that their disclosure had incurred a premium charge.[66]

Given that persons with ACHD may experience difficulties in contracting insurance, clinicians need to counsel their patients in this matter. For people who have been declined or those who were offered higher premiums, they should be advised to shop around.[67] Preferably, they shop around before they have been declined, because most insurance companies systematically ask if insurance has been previously declined. An important avenue for obtaining insurance is through group insurance policies from employers or professional organizations, since such applications do not require an individual evaluation.[67] Decline of insurance is often based on the risk for mortality at a certain age. When new treatments and management options have emerged, mortality rates may decrease as well. Consequently, when compared to the general population, the estimated risk difference for mortality may be smaller at the age of 50 years than two decades before, at the age of 30 years. The life expectancy can be further enhanced when ACHD patients are adopting a healthy lifestyle.[43] Therefore, it could be that patients who were uninsurable at the age of 30 years could be able to obtain insurance after the age of 50 years.[67]

TRANSFER FROM PEDIATRICS TO ADULT CARE AND TRANSITION INTO ADULTHOOD

Since more than 90% of children born with heart defects can reach adulthood,[2,3] CHD has to be seen as a life-cycle condition. Therefore, expert care throughout the life cycle has to be

TABLE 71–6. Sports Participation in Patients With ACHD From 15 Countries

Sports Participation	Percentage	Reaching the WHO Recommended Level	Percentage
Norway	66%	Norway	53%
Switzerland	65%	Switzerland	47%
Sweden	59%	Sweden	46%
Netherlands	56%	Netherlands	40%
France	47%	Italy	40%
Italy	47%	Australia	39%
Belgium	46%	Canada	31%
Canada	45%	Belgium	29%
Australia	44%	Malta	26%
Argentina	38%	United States	26%
Taiwan	34%	Argentina	26%
United States	34%	Taiwan	21%
Malta	31%	France	19%
Japan	24%	Japan	11%
India	10%	India	10%
Total	**43%**		**31%**

Data from Holbein CE, Peugh J, Veldtman GR, et al. Health behaviours reported by adults with congenital heart disease across 15 countries. *Eur J Prev Cardiol.* 2020 Jul; 27(10):1077-1087 and Larsson L, Johansson B, Sandberg C, et al. Geographical variation and predictors of physical activity level in adults with congenital heart disease. *Int J Cardiol Heart Vasc.* 2018 Nov 22;22:20-25.

TABLE 71–7. Unemployment Rate in ACHD

Author, Year	Country	Unemployment Rate*
North America		
Samuel, 2019[52]	United States	23.6%
Sluman, 2019[53]	Canada	12.0%
Sluman, 2019[53]	United States	11.6%
South America		
Sluman, 2019[53]	Argentina	20.0%
Europe		
Areias, 2013[73]	Portugal	25.0%
Bygstad, 2012[55]	Denmark	25.0%
Kamphuis, 2002[54]	Netherlands	32.1%
Kronwitter, 2018[59]	Germany[a]	19.4%
Kronwitter, 2018[59]	Germany[b]	2.6%
Nieminen, 2003[56]	Finland	6.6%
Pfitzer, 2018[60]	Germany	13.2%
Sluman, 2019[53]	Belgium	2.8%
Sluman, 2019[53]	France	21.7%
Sluman, 2019[53]	Italy	14.5%
Sluman, 2019[53]	Malta	13.0%
Sluman, 2019[53]	Netherlands	3.7%
Sluman, 2019[53]	Norway	6.7%
Sluman, 2019[53]	Sweden	6.5%
Sluman, 2019[53]	Switzerland	5.1%
Asia		
Enomoto, 2015[18]	Japan	4.2%
Enomoto, 2020[18]	Japan	13.5%
Sluman, 2019[53]	India	41.4%
Sluman, 2019[53]	Japan	12.0%
Sluman, 2019[53]	Taiwan	9.5%
Oceania		
Sluman, 2019[53]	Australia	17.4%

*In the calculation of the unemployment rate, students, retired people, and persons with disability were excluded from the denominator.
[a]Status in 1995; [b]status in 2015

provided. During infancy and childhood, patients are typically managed and followed-up by pediatric cardiologists. When young persons with CHD are transitioning into adulthood, they are assumed to transfer from pediatric to adult-focused care or preferably into the care of an adult congenital heart disease cardiologist.

Transfer and transition are two related, albeit different concepts. Transfer is defined as "An event or series of events through which adolescents and young adults with chronic physical and medical conditions move their care from paediatric to an adult care environment."[68] A seamless transfer between pediatric and adult care assures that age- and developmental-appropriate care is provided, while assuring that patients remain under follow-up.[69] Nonetheless, research shows that 7% to 76% of patients with CHD present with care gaps.[70] Such care gaps are detrimental for the clinical status of the patients. Indeed, studies have reported that patients who presented for medical check-up after a care gap more often had a new diagnosis of hemodynamic significance and had a greater likelihood of needing an urgent surgical or catheter-based intervention.[71–73] Therefore, it is of great importance to identify patients at risk for care gaps and implement interventions that prevent such care gaps.[70]

Transition can be seen both as a developmental process and as a healthcare intervention.[74] As a developmental process, transitions are passages from one life phase, physical condition, or social role to another, resulting in a temporary

disconnectedness of the normal way of living, which demands an adjustment of the patient and the environment.[75,76] As a healthcare intervention, transition is defined as "a multifaceted, active process that attends to the medical, psychosocial, and educational/vocational needs of adolescents as they move from the child-focused to the adult-focused healthcare system."[77] In such an intervention, the adolescents are prepared to take charge of their lives and their health in adulthood.[68]

Transitional care should be provided in a comprehensive way, known as transition programs. Such transition programs comprise multiple components, each of which contribute to helping and supporting the young person to develop from a dependent child to an independent adult, and to become the manager of their own health. Several transition programs for CHD are in place.[78–81] The evidence base of the effectiveness of transitional care in CHD is growing. The CHAPTER 1 study, conducted in Canada, found that a 1-hour nurse-led transition intervention resulted in an improved self-management and cardiac knowledge.[82] This trial confirmed earlier findings that educational interventions are able to increase the level of knowledge in CHD patients.[83,84] In the CHAPTER 2 study, two nurse-led sessions were held with a 2-month interval.[85] This randomized controlled trial confirmed that the intervention improved knowledge and self-management skills in patients, and it also found that it reduced the likelihood of a delay in ACHD care.[85] The potential of transition programs to avoid or reduce discontinuity of care has been found in two non-randomized studies as well.[86,87] More randomized controlled

trials on transition programs in CHD are in progress.[88,89] A well-described transition program is developed in the STEP-STONES project (Swedish Transition Effects Projects Supporting Teenagers with chrONic mEdical conditionS).[88,90–93] The transition program is developed using the stringent methodology of intervention mapping,[90] and it comprises eight key components: (1) a transition coordinator; (2) a written person-centered transition plan; (3) provision of information and education about the condition, treatment, and health behaviors; (4) availability by telephone and email; (5) information about and contact with the ACHD clinic; (6) guidance of parents; (7) meeting with peers; and (8) the actual transfer to the ACHD clinic.[88] These components are implemented in five steps: (1) a first patient visit with the transition coordinator; (2) a second outpatient visit with the transition coordinator; (3) information

TABLE 71–8. Staged Implementation of Advance Care Planning

	Who	Action	Steps
Stage 1	**Anticipated life expectancy: decade(s)** Adult with CHD with any of the following • expressing interest in future health discussion (e.g. during transition to adulthood) • having unrealistic health expectations, particularly when confronted with important life planning decisions (e.g. family planning) • reduced life expectancy, such as - adults with Fontan procedure - adults with cyanotic heart disease - adults with a systemic right ventricle approaching 40 years of age	• Invite discussions about future health expectations and preferences • Explain the rationale and advantages of ACP • Discuss future health expectations, while acknowledging challenges with longer-term prognostication • Inquire about personal preferences, goals and personal values • Offer to include relatives or loved ones in the conversation	• Schedule dedicated outpatient visit(s) for the purpose, as appropriate • Provide written documentation in medical records of elements discussed • Share information with general practitioner and other healthcare professionals
Stage 2	**Anticipated life expectancy: years** Adult with CHD with any of the following • expressing interest in ACP discussion • before CRT or ICD implantation • at the time of diagnosis with advanced heart failure, particularly before heart transplant assessment[22] • requiring cardiac surgery, complex catheter-based therapeutic interventions	• Revisit the elements discussed at stage 1 and • Offer more comprehensive ACP discussion • Prepare or review advance directives including the nomination of a healthcare representative • Inform and discuss about POLST	• Schedule dedicated outpatient visit or facilitate ACP discussion during an inpatient stay • Provide an update of written documentation of ACP, if applicable • Document advance directives (including healthcare representative) and/or POLST and share this information with all stakeholders
Stage 3	**Anticipated life expectancy: weeks to months** Adult with CHD with any of the following • their provider would not be surprised if the patient died within the next year • refractory end-stage heart failure[21–22] (e.g. a failing Fontan circulation; repeated readmission for decompensated heart failure requiring inotropic support and/or ICU stay; if temporary or long-term mechanical circulatory support is considered or may arise in due management course)	• Revisit the elements discussed at stage 2 and • Discuss end-of-life preferences, including the location of death • Organize support for family members • Involve palliative care team as appropriate • As appropriate, discuss deactivation of implanted cardiac device functions	• Update written ACP documents as applicable • Consider organization of home care • Consider involvement of social work • Consider involvement of palliative care • Consider involvement of psychology and/or religious support providers
Stage 4	**Anticipated life expectancy: days** The dying adult with CHD	• Provide end-of-life care reflecting personal preferences and documented directives • Co-ordinate bereavement care for loved ones, as appropriate	• Consider involvement of social work • Consider involvement of palliative care • Consider involvement of psychology and/or religious support providers • Provide support to care team as necessary

Abbreviations: ACP, advance care planning; CHO, congenital heart disease; CRT, cardiac resynchronization therapy; ICD, implantable cardioverter defibrillator; ICU, intensive care unit; POLST, Physician Orders for Life-Sustaining Treatment.
Data from Denvir MA, Murray SA, Boyd KJ. Future care planning: a first step to palliative care for all patients with advanced heart disease. *Heart.* 2015 Jul;101(13):1002-1007.

day for adolescents and their parents; (4) a third outpatient visit with the transition coordinator; and (5) actual transfer to the ACHD clinic.[88] An effectiveness, process, and economic evaluation is in progress.

END-OF-LIFE DISCUSSION

Irrespective of the tremendous improvements in life expectancy, there is still premature mortality in ACHD. Death can occur suddenly or can be predicted after a slower period of deterioration of the clinical status. Whatever the mode of eventual death may be, issues that are associated with the end of life have to be discussed with patients and families well beforehand. An important feature in this respect is advance care planning, which is defined as "a process that supports and empowers individuals, at any stage of their lives or the disease process, to consider, communicate, and document preferences for future health care to their loved ones and healthcare providers. During this process, individuals have the opportunity to make decisions in advance about treatment they would and would not want should they be unable to express their wishes at that time."[94] Surveys among ACHD patients showed that 69% to 78% had a strong interest in advance care planning and advance care directives.[95-97] It was found that 78% of the patients even want to initiate advance care planning when they are still in good health.[97] Nonetheless, only 1% to 29% of the patients recall participating in advance care planning.[95,98]

There are multiple barriers to advance care planning communication. At patient level, there is minimal knowledge about advance care planning, reluctance to begin the discussion, avoidance to discuss health deterioration, and the desire to protect family and loved ones.[94] In healthcare providers, there is a fear of causing emotional distress in the patient, uncertainty about the prognosis, lack of confidence and skills in advance care planning, low familiarity with unique factors that require attention (eg, culture, religion), and personal discomfort with end-of-life discussions.[94] At an institutional level, it is often unclear who is responsible for initiating and maintaining the dialogue and there may be a lack of time.[94]

It is recommended that advance care planning is implemented in a staged way, throughout the life course of the patient.[94,99] Indeed, many patients may feel too healthy to develop advance care directives,[95] especially when the anticipated life expectancy is several decades.[94] However, in such patients, future health expectations or prognostication can be discussed. It is also important to get an understanding of the goals and personal values of the patients and their families. When the anticipated life expectancy is expressed in terms of years instead of decades, a more comprehensive discussion of advance care planning should be initiated.[94] **Table 71–8** describes the different stages in advance care planning that are recommended.[94]

SUMMARY

Psychosocial issues in ACHD are prevalent and require attention from healthcare professionals who are taking of these patients. The consequences of having a heart defect and required invasive treatments may impact on the psychological and social health of ACHD patients. Anxiety, depression, and PTSD are more prevalent in ACHD than in healthy counterparts. Employability and insurability is hampered in certain groups of ACHD patients. Although the exercise capacity in ACHD patients is reduced, the level of physical activities is largely in line with the general population. Nonetheless, only one-third of patients reach the recommended WHO level of physical activity. Lifelong expert care is warranted for people with CHD. Consequently, they need to transfer from pediatrics to adult-oriented care when they are growing into adulthood. Transition programs are developed to help and support young persons to develop independence, and to prepare for the imminent transfer to adult care providers. Evidence on the effectiveness and mechanism of effect are mounting. Irrespective of improvements in life expectancy, premature mortality still exists and requires that healthcare providers initiate end-of-life discussions. This can be done in a staged way, for which tools are available.

REFERENCES

1. Liu Y, Chen S, Zuhlke L, et al. Global birth prevalence of congenital heart defects 1970-2017: updated systematic review and meta-analysis of 260 studies. *Int J Epidemiol.* 2019;48:455-463. doi: 10.1093/ije/dyz009.

2. Mandalenakis Z, Rosengren A, Skoglund K, et al. Survivorship in children and young adults with congenital heart disease in Sweden. *JAMA Intern Med.* 2017;177:224-230. doi: 10.1001/jamainternmed.2016.7765.

3. Moons P, Bovijn L, Budts W, et al. Temporal trends in survival to adulthood among patients born with congenital heart disease from 1970 to 1992 in Belgium. *Circulation.* 2010;122:2264-2272. doi: 10.1161/CIRCULATIONAHA.110.946343.

4. Zigmond AS, Snaith RP. The hospital anxiety and depression scale. *Acta Psychiatr Scand.* 1983;67:361-370.

5. Moons P, Kovacs AH, Luyckx K, et al. Patient-reported outcomes in adults with congenital heart disease: inter-country variation, standard of living and healthcare system factors. *Int J Cardiol.* 2018;251:34-41. doi: 10.1016/j.ijcard.2017.10.064.

6. Ko JM, White KS, Kovacs AH, et al. Differential impact of physical activity type on depression in adults with congenital heart disease: a multi-center international study. *J Psychosom Res.* 2019;124:109762. doi: 10.1016/j.jpsychores.2019.109762.

7. Kovacs AH, Saidi AS, Kuhl EA, et al. Depression and anxiety in adult congenital heart disease: predictors and prevalence. *Int J Cardiol.* 2009;137:158-164.

8. Kasmi L, Calderon J, Montreuil M, et al. Neurocognitive and psychological outcomes in adults with dextro-transposition of the great arteries corrected by the arterial switch operation. *Ann Thorac Surg* 2018;105:830-836. doi: 10.1016/j.athoracsur.2017.06.055.

9. Westhoff-Bleck M, Briest J, Fraccarollo D, et al. Mental disorders in adults with congenital heart disease: unmet needs and impact on quality of life. *J Affect Disord.* 2016;204:180-186. doi: 10.1016/j.jad.2016.06.047.

10. Gierat-Haponiuk K, Haponiuk I, Chojnicki M, et al. Exercise capacity and the quality of life late after surgical correction of congenital heart defects. *Kardiol Pol.* 2011;69:810-815.

11. Pike NA, Evangelista LS, Doering LV, et al. Quality of life, health status, and depression: comparison between adolescents and adults after the Fontan procedure with healthy counterparts. *J Cardiovasc Nurs.* 2012;27:539-546. doi: 10.1097/JCN.0b013e31822ce5f6.

12. Pike NA, Woo MA, Poulsen MK, et al. Predictors of memory deficits in adolescents and young adults with congenital heart disease compared to healthy controls. *Front Pediatr.* 2016;4:117. doi: 10.3389/fped.2016.00117.

13. Yang HL, Chang NT, Wang JK, et al. Comorbidity as a mediator of depression in adults with congenital heart disease: a population-based

cohort study. *Eur J Cardiovasc Nurs.* 2020:1474515120923785. doi: 10.1177/1474515120923785.

14. Udholm S, Nyboe C, Dantoft TM, et al. Small atrial septal defects are associated with psychiatric diagnoses, emotional distress, and lower educational levels. *Congenit Heart Dis.* 2019;14:803-810. doi: 10.1111/chd.12808.

15. Muller J, Hess J, Hager A. Minor symptoms of depression in patients with congenital heart disease have a larger impact on quality of life than limited exercise capacity. *Int J Cardiol.* 2012;154:265-269. doi: 10.1016/j.ijcard.2010.09.029.

16. Eslami B, Sundin O, Macassa G, et al. Anxiety, depressive and somatic symptoms in adults with congenital heart disease. *J Psychosom Res.* 2013;74: 49-56. doi: 10.1016/j.jpsychores.2012.10.006.

17. Overgaard D, Schrader AM, Lisby KH, et al. Patient-reported outcomes in adult survivors with single-ventricle physiology. *Cardiology* 2011;120: 36-42. doi: 10.1159/000333112.

18. Enomoto J, Nakazawa M. Negative effect of aging on psychosocial functioning of adults with congenital heart disease. *Circ J.* 2015;79:185-192. doi: 10.1253/circj.CJ-14-0682.

19. Cohen M, Daniela M, Yalonetsky S, et al. Psychological functioning and health-related quality of life (HRQoL) in older patients following percutaneous closure of the secundum atrial septal defect (ASD). *Arch Gerontol Geriatr.* 2010;50:e5-e8. doi: 10.1016/j.archger.2009.04.003.

20. Bromberg JI, Beasley PJ, D'Angelo EJ, et al. Depression and anxiety in adults with congenital heart disease: a pilot study. *Heart Lung.* 2003;32:105-110.

21. Carazo MR, Kolodziej MS, DeWitt ES, et al. Prevalence and prognostic association of a clinical diagnosis of depression in adult congenital heart disease: results of the Boston Adult Congenital Heart Disease Biobank. *J Am Heart Assoc.* 2020;9:e014820. doi: 10.1161/JAHA.119.014820.

22. Diller GP, Brautigam A, Kempny A, et al. Depression requiring antidepressant drug therapy in adult congenital heart disease: prevalence, risk factors, and prognostic value. *Eur Heart J.* 2016;37:771-782. doi: 10.1093/eurheartj/ehv386.

23. Martínez-Quintana E, Girolimetti A, Jiménez-Rodríguez S, et al. Prevalence and predictors of psychological distress in congenital heart disease patients. *J Clin Psychol.* 2020. doi: 10.1002/jclp.22948.

24. Luyckx K, Rassart J, Goossens E, et al. Development and persistence of depressive symptoms in adolescents with CHD. *Cardiol Young.* 2016;26: 1115-1122. doi: 10.1017/S1047951115001882.

25. Muller J, Hess J, Hager A. General anxiety of adolescents and adults with congenital heart disease is comparable with that in healthy controls. *Int J Cardiol.* 2013;165:142-145. doi: 10.1016/j.ijcard.2011.08.005.

26. Karsdorp PA, Kindt M, Rietveld S, et al. Stress-induced heart symptoms and perceptual biases in patients with congenital heart disease. *Int J Cardiol.* 2007;114:352-357. doi: 10.1016/j.ijcard.2006.02.004.

27. Karsdorp PA, Kindt M, Rietveld S, et al. Interpretation bias for heart sensations in congenital heart disease and its relation to quality of life. *Int J Behav Med.* 2008;15:232-240. doi: 10.1080/10705500802212916.

28. Karsdorp PA, Kindt M, Rietveld S, et al. False heart rate feedback and the perception of heart symptoms in patients with congenital heart disease and anxiety. *Int J Behav Med.* 2009;16:81-88. doi: 10.1007/s12529-008-9001-9.

29. Raghuveer G, Hartz J, Lubans DR, et al. Cardiorespiratory fitness in youth: an important marker of health: a scientific statement from the American Heart Association. *Circulation.* 2020;142:e101-e118. doi: 10.1161/cir.0000000000000866.

30. Reybrouck T, Mertens L. Physical performance and physical activity in grown-up congenital heart disease. *Eur J Cardiovasc Prev Rehabil* 2005;12:498-502. doi: 10.1097/01.hjr.0000176510.84165.eb.

31. Schaan CW, Macedo ACP, Sbruzzi G, et al. Functional capacity in congenital heart disease: a systematic review and meta-analysis. *Arq Bras Cardiol.* 2017;109:357-367. doi: 10.5935/abc.20170125.

32. Kempny A, Dimopoulos K, Uebing A, et al. Reference values for exercise limitations among adults with congenital heart disease. Relation to activities of daily life—single centre experience and review of published data. *Eur Heart J.* 2012;33:1386-1396. doi: 10.1093/eurheartj/ehr461.

33. Moons P, Luyckx K, Thomet C, et al. Physical functioning, mental health, and quality of life in different congenital heart defects: comparative analysis in 3538 patients from 15 countries. *Can J Cardiol.* 2020. doi: 10.1016/j.cjca.2020.03.044.

34. Sandberg C, Thilen U, Wadell K, et al. Adults with complex congenital heart disease have impaired skeletal muscle function and reduced confidence in performing exercise training. *Eur J Prev Cardiol.* 2015;22: 1523-1530. doi: 10.1177/2047487314543076.

35. Sandberg C, Crenshaw AG, Elçadi GH, et al. Slower skeletal muscle oxygenation kinetics in adults with complex congenital heart disease. *Can J Cardiol.* 2019;35:1815-1823. doi: 10.1016/j.cjca.2019.05.001.

36. Li X, Chen N, Zhou X, et al. Exercise training in adults with congenital heart disease: a systematic review and meta-analysis. *J Cardiopulm Rehabil Prev.* 2019. doi: 10.1097/hcr.0000000000000420.

37. Meyer M, Brudy L, García-Cuenllas L, et al. Current state of home-based exercise interventions in patients with congenital heart disease: a systematic review. *Heart.* 2020;106:333. doi: 10.1136/heartjnl-2019-315680.

38. Dua JS, Cooper AR, Fox KR, et al. Exercise training in adults with congenital heart disease: feasibility and benefits. *Int J Cardiol.* 2010;138: 196-205.

39. Tran D, Maiorana A, Ayer J, et al. Recommendations for exercise in adolescents and adults with congenital heart disease. *Prog Cardiovasc Dis.* 2020;63:350-366. doi: 10.1016/j.pcad.2020.03.002.

40. Budts W, Börjesson M, Chessa M, et al. Physical activity in adolescents and adults with congenital heart defects: individualized exercise prescription. *Eur Heart J.* 2013;34:3669-3674. doi: 10.1093/eurheartj/eht433.

41. Budts W, Pieles GE, Roos-Hesselink JW, et al. Recommendations for participation in competitive sport in adolescent and adult athletes with Congenital Heart Disease (CHD): position statement of the Sports Cardiology & Exercise Section of the European Association of Preventive Cardiology (EAPC), the European Society of Cardiology (ESC) Working Group on Adult Congenital Heart Disease and the Sports Cardiology, Physical Activity and Prevention Working Group of the Association for European Paediatric and Congenital Cardiology (AEPC). *Eur Heart J.* 2020. doi: 10.1093/eurheartj/ehaa501.

42. Stout KK, Daniels CJ, Aboulhosn JA, et al. 2018 AHA/ACC guideline for the management of adults with congenital heart disease: a report of the American College of Cardiology/American Heart Association Task Force on Clinical Practice Guidelines. *J Am Coll Cardiol.* 2019;73:e81-e192. doi: 10.1016/j.jacc.2018.08.1029.

43. Holbein CE, Peugh J, Veldtman GR, et al. Health behaviours reported by adults with congenital heart disease across 15 countries. *Eur J Prev Cardiol.* 2020;27:1077-1087. doi: 10.1177/2047487319876231.

44. World Health Organization. *Global recommendations on physical activity for health.* 2010.

45. Larsson L, Johansson B, Sandberg C, et al. Geographical variation and predictors of physical activity level in adults with congenital heart disease. *Int J Cardiol Heart Vasc.* 2019;22:20-25. doi: 10.1016/j.ijcha.2018.11.004.

46. Larsson L, Johansson B, Wadell K, et al. Adults with congenital heart disease overestimate their physical activity level. *Int J Cardiol Heart Vasc.* 2019;22:13-17. doi: 10.1016/j.ijcha.2018.11.005.

47. Vigl M, Niggemeyer E, Hager A, et al. The importance of socio-demographic factors for the quality of life of adults with congenital heart disease. *Qual Life Res.* 2011;20:169-177. doi: 10.1007/s11136-010-9741-2.

48. Apers S, Kovacs AH, Luyckx K, et al. Quality of life of adults with congenital heart disease in 15 countries: evaluating country-specific characteristics. *J Am Coll Cardiol.* 2016;67:2237-2245. doi: 10.1016/j.jacc.2016.03.477.

49. Moons P, Van Deyk K, Marquet K, et al. Individual quality of life in adults with congenital heart disease: a paradigm shift. *Eur Heart J.* 2005;26: 298-307. doi: 10.1093/eurheartj/ehi054.

50. Moons P, Van Deyk K and Budts W. The NYHA classification, employment, and physical activities are poor indicators of quality of life after congenital cardiac surgery. *Ann Thorac Surg.* 2006;82:1167-1168; author reply 1168. doi: 10.1016/j.athoracsur.2006.01.077.

51. Enomoto J, Mizuno Y, Okajima Y, et al. Employment status and contributing factors among adults with congenital heart disease in Japan. *Pediatr Int.* 2020;62:390-398. doi: 10.1111/ped.14152.

52. Samuel BP, Marckini DN, Parker JL, et al. Complex determinants of work ability in adults with congenital heart disease and implications for clinical practice. *Can J Cardiol.* 2020;36:1098-1103. doi: 10.1016/j.cjca.2019.11.003.

53. Sluman MA, Apers S, Sluiter JK, et al. Education as important predictor for successful employment in adults with congenital heart disease worldwide. *Congenit Heart Dis.* 2019;14:362-371. doi: 10.1111/chd.12747.

54. Kamphuis M, Vogels T, Ottenkamp J, et al. Employment in adults with congenital heart disease. *Arch Pediatr Adolesc Med.* 2002;156:1143-1148.

55. Bygstad E, Pedersen LC, Pedersen TA, et al. Tetralogy of Fallot in men: quality of life, family, education, and employment. *Cardiol Young.* 2012;22:417-423. doi: 10.1017/S1047951111001934.

56. Nieminen H, Sairanen H, Tikanoja T, et al. Long-term results of pediatric cardiac surgery in Finland: education, employment, marital status, and parenthood. *Pediatrics.* 2003;112:1345-1350.

57. Mahoney LT, Skorton DJ. Insurability and employability. *J Am Coll Cardiol.* 1991;18:334-336.

58. Zomer AC, Vaartjes I, Uiterwaal CS, et al. Social burden and lifestyle in adults with congenital heart disease. *Am J Cardiol.* 2012;109:1657-1663. doi: 10.1016/j.amjcard.2012.01.397.

59. Kronwitter A, Mebus S, Neidenbach R, et al. Psychosocial situation in adults with congenital heart defects today and 20 years ago: any changes? *Int J Cardiol.* 2019;275:70-76. 2018/10/20. doi: 10.1016/j.ijcard.2018.10.030.

60. Pfitzer C, Helm PC, Rosenthal LM, et al. Educational level and employment status in adults with congenital heart disease. *Cardiol Young.* 2018;28:32-38. doi: 10.1017/S104795111700138x.

61. Hart EM, Garson A. Psychosocial concerns of adults with congenital heart disease. Employability and insurability. *Cardiol Clin.* 1993;11:711-715.

62. Truesdell SC and Clark EB. Health insurance status in a cohort of children and young adults with congenital cardiac diagnosis. *Circulation.* 1991;84:II-386.

63. Sluman MA, Apers S, Bouma BJ, et al. Uncertainties in insurances for adults with congenital heart disease. *Int J Cardiol.* 2015;186:93-95. doi: 10.1016/j.ijcard.2015.03.208.

64. Lin C-J, Novak E, Rich MW, et al. Insurance access in adults with congenital heart disease in the Affordable Care Act era. *Congenit Heart Dis.* 2018;13:384-391. doi: 10.1111/chd.12582.

65. Crossland DS, Jackson SP, Lyall R, et al. Life insurance and mortgage application in adults with congenital heart disease. *Eur J Cardiothorac Surg.* 2004;25:931-934.

66. Pickup L, Bowater S, Thorne S, et al. Travel insurance in adult congenital heart disease—Do they declare their condition? *Int J Cardiol.* 2016;223:316-317. doi: 10.1016/j.ijcard.2016.08.098.

67. Vonder Muhll I, Cumming G and Gatzoulis MA. Risky business: insuring adults with congenital heart disease. *Eur Heart J.* 2003;24:1595-1600.

68. Knauth A, Verstappen A, Reiss J, et al. Transition and transfer from pediatric to adult care of the young adult with complex congenital heart disease. *Cardiol Clin.* 2006;24:619-629. doi: 10.1016/j.ccl.2006.08.010.

69. Moons P, Hilderson D, Van Deyk K. Implementation of transition programs can prevent another lost generation of patients with congenital heart disease. *Eur J Cardiovasc Nurs.* 2008;7:259-263. doi: 10.1016/j.ejcnurse.2008.10.001.

70. Goossens E, Bovijn L, Gewillig M, et al. Predictors of care gaps in adolescents with complex chronic condition transitioning to adulthood. *Pediatrics* 2016;137:e20152413. doi: 10.1542/peds.2015-2413.

71. Iversen K, Vejlstrup NG, Sondergaard L, et al. Screening of adults with congenital cardiac disease lost for follow-up. *Cardiol Young.* 2007;17:601-608.

72. Yeung E, Kay J, Roosevelt GE, et al. Lapse of care as a predictor for morbidity in adults with congenital heart disease. *Int J Cardiol.* 2008;125:62-65.

73. Vis JC, van der Velde ET, Schuuring MJ, et al. Wanted! 8000 heart patients: identification of adult patients with a congenital heart defect lost to follow-up. *Int J Cardiol.* 2011;149:246-247. doi: 10.1016/j.ijcard.2011.02.019.

74. Moons P. Landmark lecture in nursing: a life-cycle perspective on CHD: what happens beyond your clinic? *Cardiol Young.* 2017;27:1954-1958. doi: 10.1017/s1047951117002104.

75. Meleis AI. *Transitions Theory: Middle-Range and Situation-Specific Theories in Nursing Research and Practice.* New York: Springer Publishing Company; 2010.

76. Schumacher KL, Meleis AI. Transitions: a central concept in nursing. *Image J Nurs Sch.* 1994;26:119-127.

77. Blum RW, Garell D, Hodgman CH, et al. Transition from child-centered to adult health-care systems for adolescents with chronic conditions. A position paper of the Society for Adolescent Medicine. *J Adolesc Health* 1993;14:570-576.

78. Berg SK, Hertz PG. Outpatient nursing clinic for congenital heart disease patients: Copenhagen Transition Program. *J Cardiovasc Nurs.* 2007;22:488-492. doi: 10.1097/01.JCN.0000297381.83507.08.

79. Thomet C, Lindenberg C, Schwerzmann M, et al. Adolescents' with congenital heart disease and their parents' experiences of a nurse-led transition program. An interpretive phenomenological study. *Pflege* 2018;31:9-18. doi: 10.1024/1012-5302/a000574.

80. de Hosson M, De Backer J, De Wolf D, et al. Development of a transition program for adolescents with congenital heart disease. *Eur J Pediatr.* 2020;179:339-348. doi: 10.1007/s00431-019-03515-4.

81. Ladouceur M, Calderon J, Traore M, et al. Educational needs of adolescents with congenital heart disease: impact of a transition intervention programme. *Arch Cardiovasc Dis.* 2017;110:317-324. doi: 10.1016/j.acvd.2017.02.001.

82. Mackie AS, Islam S, Magill-Evans J, et al. Healthcare transition for youth with heart disease: a clinical trial. *Heart.* 2014;100:1113-1118. doi: 10.1136/heartjnl-2014-305748.

83. Goossens E, Van Deyk K, Zupancic N, et al. Effectiveness of structured patient education on the knowledge level of adolescents and adults with congenital heart disease. *Eur J Cardiovasc Nurs.* 2014;13:63-70. doi: 10.1177/1474515113479231.

84. Goossens E, Fieuws S, Van Deyk K. Effectiveness of structured education on knowledge and health behaviors in patients with congenital heart disease. *J Pediatr.* 2015;166:1370-1376.e1371. doi: 10.1016/j.jpeds.2015.02.041.

85. Mackie AS, Rempel GR, Kovacs AH, et al. Transition intervention for adolescents with congenital heart disease. *J Am Coll Cardiol* 2018;71:1768-1777. doi: 10.1016/j.jacc.2018.02.043.

86. Hergenroeder AC, Moodie DS, Penny DJ, et al. Functional classification of heart failure before and after implementing a healthcare transition program for youth and young adults transferring from a pediatric to an adult congenital heart disease clinics. *Congenit Heart Dis.* 2018;13:548-553. doi: 10.1111/chd.12604.

87. Gaydos SS, Chowdhury SM, Judd RN, et al. A transition clinic intervention to improve follow-up rates in adolescents and young adults with congenital heart disease. *Cardiol Young.* 2020;30:633-640. doi: 10.1017/S1047951120000682.

88. Acuña Mora M, Sparud-Lundin C, Bratt E-L, et al. Person-centred transition programme to empower adolescents with congenital heart disease in the transition to adulthood: a study protocol for a hybrid randomised controlled trial (STEPSTONES project). *BMJ Open.* 2017;7:e014593. doi: 10.1136/bmjopen-2016-014593.

89. Werner O, Abassi H, Lavastre K, et al. Factors influencing the participation of adolescents and young adults with a congenital heart disease in a

transition education program: a prospective multicentre controlled study. *Patient Educ Couns.* 2019;102:2223-2230. doi: 10.1016/j.pec.2019.06.023.

90. Acuna Mora M, Saarijarvi M, Sparud-Lundin C, et al. Empowering young persons with congenital heart disease: using intervention mapping to develop a transition program—the STEPSTONES project. *J Pediatr Nurs.* 2020;50:e8-e17. 10.1016/j.pedn.2019.09.021.

91. Saarijarvi M, Wallin L, Moons P, et al. Transition program for adolescents with congenital heart disease in transition to adulthood: protocol for a mixed-method process evaluation study (the STEPSTONES project). *BMJ Open.* 2019;9:e028229. doi: 10.1136/bmjopen-2018-028229.

92. Saarijärvi M, Wallin L, Moons P, et al. Factors affecting adolescents' participation in randomized controlled trials evaluating the effectiveness of healthcare interventions: the case of the STEPSTONES project. *BMC Med Res Methodol.* 2020;20:205. doi: 10.1186/s12874-020-01088-7.

93. Brorsson AL, Bratt EL, Moons P, et al. Randomised controlled trial of a person-centred transition programme for adolescents with type 1 diabetes (STEPSTONES-DIAB): a study protocol. *BMJ Open.* 2020;10:e036496. doi: 10.1136/bmjopen-2019-036496.

94. Schwerzmann M, Goossens E, Gallego P, et al. Recommendations for advance care planning in adults with congenital heart disease: a position paper from the ESC Working Group of Adult Congenital Heart Disease, the Association of Cardiovascular Nursing and Allied Professions (ACNAP), the European Association for Palliative Care (EAPC), and the International Society for Adult Congenital Heart Disease (ISACHD). *Eur Heart J.* 2020. doi: 10.1093/eurheartj/ehaa614.

95. Steiner JM, Stout K, Soine L, et al. Perspectives on advance care planning and palliative care among adults with congenital heart disease. *Congenit Heart Dis.* 2019;14:403-409. doi: 10.1111/chd.12735.

96. Tobler D, Greutmann M, Colman JM, et al. Knowledge of and preference for advance care planning by adults with congenital heart disease. *Am J Cardiol.* 2012;109:1797-1800. doi: 10.1016/j.amjcard.2012.02.027.

97. Deng LX, Gleason LP, Khan AM, et al. Advance care planning in adults with congenital heart disease: a patient priority. *Int J Cardiol.* 2017;231: 105-109. doi: 10.1016/j.ijcard.2016.12.185.

98. Tobler D, Greutmann M, Colman JM, et al. End-of-life in adults with congenital heart disease: a call for early communication. *Int J Cardiol.* 2012;155:383-387. doi: 10.1016/j.ijcard.2010.10.050.

99. Troost E, Roggen L, Goossens E, et al. Advanced care planning in adult congenital heart disease: transitioning from repair to palliation and end-of-life care. *Int J Cardiol.* 2019;279:57-61. doi: 10.1016/j.ijcard.2018.10.078.

100. Gleason LP, Deng LX, Khan AM, et al. Psychological distress in adults with congenital heart disease: focus beyond depression. *Cardiol Young.* 2019; 29: 185-189. 2019/01/31. doi: 10.1017/s1047951118002068.

101. Leslie CE, Schofield K, Vannatta K, et al. Perceived health competence predicts anxiety and depressive symptoms after a three-year follow-up among adolescents and adults with congenital heart disease. *Eur J Cardiovasc Nurs.* 2020; 19: 283-290. 2019/11/15. doi: 10.1177/1474515119885858.

102. Bedair R, Babu-Narayan SV, Dimopoulos K, et al. Acceptance and psychological impact of implantable defibrillators amongst adults with congenital heart disease. *Int J Cardiol.* 2015; 181: 218-224. 2014/12/22. doi: 10.1016/j.ijcard.2014.12.028.

103. Berg SK, Rasmussen TB, Thrysoee L, et al. DenHeart: Differences in physical and mental health across cardiac diagnoses at hospital discharge. *J Psychosom Res.* 2017; 94: 1-9. doi: 10.1016/j.jpsychores.2017.01.003.

104. Martínez-Quintana E, Girolimetti A, Jiménez-Rodríguez S, et al. Prevalence and predictors of psychological distress in congenital heart disease patients. *J Clin Psychol.* 2020 2020/03/10. doi: 10.1002/jclp.22948.

105. Riley JP, Habibi H, Banya W, et al. Education and support needs of the older adult with congenital heart disease. *J Adv Nurs.* 2012; 68: 1050-1060. 2011/08/19. doi: 10.1111/j.1365-2648.2011.05809.x.

106. Amedro P, Basquin A, Gressin V, et al. Health-related quality of life of patients with pulmonary arterial hypertension associated with CHD: the multicentre cross-sectional ACHILLE study. *Cardiol Young.* 2016; 26: 1250-1259. 2016/03/17. doi: 10.1017/s1047951116000056.

107. Bordin G, Padalino MA, Perentaler S, et al. Clinical Profile and Quality of Life of Adult Patients After the Fontan Procedure. *Pediatr Cardiol.* 2015; 36: 1261-1269. 2015/04/02. doi: 10.1007/s00246-015-1156-y.

108. Horner T, Liberthson R and Jellinek MS. Psychosocial profile of adults with complex congenital heart disease. *Mayo ClinProc.* 2000; 75: 31-36.

109. Westhoff-Bleck M, Winter L, Aguirre Davila L, et al. Diagnostic evaluation of the hospital depression scale (HADS) and the Beck depression inventory II (BDI-II) in adults with congenital heart disease using a structured clinical interview: Impact of depression severity. *Eur J Prev Cardiol.* 2020; 27: 381-390. 2019/07/28. doi: 10.1177/2047487319865055.

110. Moon JR, Huh J, Song J, et al. The Center for Epidemiologic Studies Depression Scale is an adequate screening instrument for depression and anxiety disorder in adults with congenital heart disease. *Health Qual Life Outcomes.* 2017; 15: 176. 2017/09/07. doi: 10.1186/s12955-017-0747-0.

111. Deng LX, Khan AM, Drajpuch D, et al. *Prevalence* and Correlates of Post-traumatic Stress Disorder in Adults With Congenital Heart Disease. *Am J Cardiol.* 2016; 117: 853-857. 2016/01/25. doi: 10.1016/j.amjcard.2015.11.065.

112. Moreland P and Santacroce SJ. Illness Uncertainty and Posttraumatic Stress in Young Adults With Congenital Heart Disease. *J Cardiovasc Nurs.* 2018; 33: 356-362. 2018/03/31. doi: 10.1097/jcn.0000000000000471.

XII

SPECIAL POPULATIONS AND TOPICS IN CARDIOVASCULAR DISEASE

Perioperative Evaluation for Noncardiac Surgery

Daniel Alyesh, Prashant Vaishnava, and Kim A. Eagle

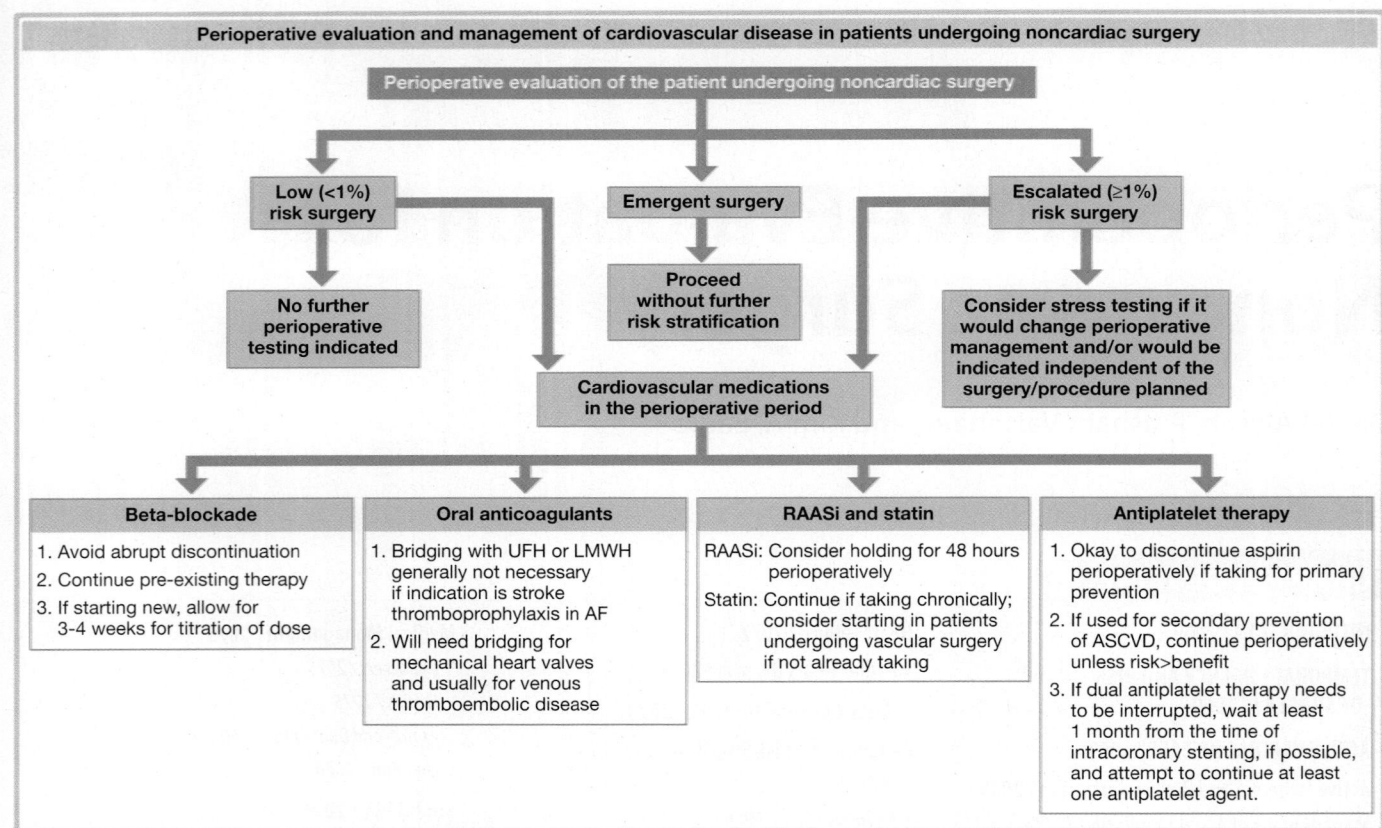

Chapter 72 Fuster and Hurst's Central Illustration. A thorough perioperative evaluation is a critical component of the preparation for noncardiac surgery and offers an opportunity to elucidate cardiac symptoms and optimize medical therapies in the context of the planned surgery. AF, atrial fibrillation; ASCVD, atherosclerotic cardiovascular disease; LMWH, low-molecular-weight heparin; RAASi, renin-angiotensin-aldosterone system inhibitors; UFH, unfractionated heparin.

CHAPTER SUMMARY

This chapter provides an overview of the perioperative evaluation of cardiovascular disease in patients undergoing noncardiac surgery. The cornerstone of this evaluation is a history and physical examination focused on establishing the temporal urgency of a procedure or surgery, a patient's functional status, and whether there are any signs or symptoms possibly of cardiac origin (see Fuster and Hurst's Central Illustration). Perioperative risk stratification depends on the inherent risk associated with a planned surgery and the risk ascribed to patient specific conditions. Risk stratification algorithms include the Revised Cardiac Risk Index and the National Surgical Quality Improvement Program (NSQIP) Surgical Risk Calculator. The underlying philosophy of preoperative testing should be guided by whether results of testing would change management outside of the context of the surgery planned. Prophylactic coronary revascularization has not been associated with improved outcomes. Considerations about medical therapy in the perioperative setting include decisions about ß-blockade, antiplatelet treatments, and statin medications. A thorough perioperative evaluation is a critical component of the preparation for noncardiac surgery and offers an opportunity to elucidate cardiac symptoms and optimize medical therapies in the context of the planned surgery.

INTRODUCTION

The perioperative evaluation of cardiovascular disease in patients undergoing noncardiac surgery remains a subject of much research and debate. The desire to optimally manage these patients is often confused with "cardiac clearance," but this term fails to capture the complexity of care. As with most clinical scenarios, the cornerstone of good perioperative management is a conscientious history and physical exam. Understanding a patient's functional status and carefully establishing whether a patient is experiencing any cardiac signs or symptoms are of paramount importance in guiding management decisions. As in the American College of Cardiology (ACC)/American Heart Association (AHA) and the European Society of Cardiology (ESC)/European Society of Anesthesiology (ESA) guidelines,[1,2] the best clinical approach to evaluating cardiac disease in patients prior to surgery is in the framework of whether the cardiac disease is active or stable while understanding the urgency and risk of the operation needed. A summary of our global approach to perioperative evaluation and management may be found in **Figs. 72–1 and 72–2.**[1]

TEMPORAL URGENCY AND RISK OF SURGERY

The urgency of a procedure or surgery is critically important in tailoring the perioperative evaluation for noncardiac surgery. This temporal urgency, in part, may dictate the extent of clinical evaluation and potential changes in management even potentially feasible prior to surgery. This is clearly reflected in the ACC/AHA clinical guideline writing group's taxonomy of temporal necessity of surgery into emergent, urgent, time-sensitive, and elective forms, as summarized in **Table 72–1.**[1]

ACTIVE CARDIAC DISEASE

Acute, or active, cardiovascular conditions typically require delay of nonemergent, nonurgent surgery. For patients undergoing elective surgery, management of acute cardiac conditions mirrors the management of such conditions were the patient not under consideration for surgery. Active cardiac disease can exist in the form of active ischemia, arrhythmia, heart failure (HF), and/or severe valve disease.

Active Ischemia and Revascularization

In acute coronary syndromes (ACSs), cardiac catheterization is generally recommended for the definition of coronary anatomy, risk stratification, and creation of the optimal treatment and revascularization strategy if appropriate. The optimal revascularization strategy is based upon the weight of existing evidence and recent clinical practice guidelines.[1,2] Patients with ST-segment elevation myocardial infarction (STEMI) may benefit from immediate reperfusion ideally with primary percutaneous coronary intervention (PCI), and appropriately selected patients with non-ST-segment elevation myocardial infarction-acute coronary syndrome (NSTEMI-ACS) may

benefit from an early invasive strategy within 72 hours. Following an ACS, the recommended duration of dual antiplatelet therapy (DAPT) is 12 months. The approach to PCI is not typically impacted by planned surgery. Third generation bioresorbable drug eluting stents (DES) present an opportunity for shorter duration DAPT as short as one month in patients of high bleeding risk, as approved by the FDA. Data for a one-month DAPT duration are not robust but do exist for a shorter three-month duration with similar rates of stent thrombosis with a shorter duration of DAPT in third generation DES.[3–5]

Management of Atrial Fibrillation

Atrial fibrillation (AF) is the most frequently encountered perioperative cardiac arrhythmia. A known history of clinically stable AF may not require modifications in perioperative clinical management other than acknowledgment of and planning for a strategy for interrupting and resuming anticoagulation. The calculus for perioperative anticoagulation involves careful balancing of the risks of bleeding associated with a procedure against those of systemic thromboembolism. In cases where operative bleeding is minimal, such as cataract surgery, or implantation of cardiac rhythm devices, anticoagulation with vitamin K antagonists may continue uninterrupted. Observational data indicates that when pursued, bridging anticoagulation can be done safely.[6–8] However, when concerns over operative bleeding are significant, recent randomized data indicate brief interruptions in vitamin K–factor dependent anticoagulation may be superior to bridging anticoagulation in low-risk patients. Published in 2015, the Perioperative Bridging Anticoagulation in Patients with Atrial Fibrillation (BRIDGE) trial randomized 1884 patients to perioperative interruption of anticoagulation versus bridging anticoagulation with dalteparin. At 30-day follow-up, there was no difference in the rate of transient ischemia or stroke between the two groups, but there were higher rates of major and minor bleeding in the group that received bridging anticoagulation.[9] These randomized data inform the discussion very well, but limitations of the study included poor representation of patients with CHA_2DS_2VASc scores of 5 and above, as well as a lack of representation of patients undergoing carotid endarterectomy or major oncologic surgery. On balance, the generally accepted paradigm for the management of anticoagulation in the perioperative period is interruption (for the minimal duration allowable, generally 5 days for vitamin K antagonists) of such therapy prior to a planned procedure or surgery, with resumption of anticoagulation as soon as feasible in the postoperative period. In those patients with particularly high thromboembolic risk or those patients with mechanical prosthetic valves (particularly in nonaortic positions), an informed discussion should take place and bridging therapy while oral anticoagulation is interrupted may be required. The recommended duration of interruption of direct oral anticoagulants (ie, direct thrombin inhibitors or factor Xa inhibitors) prior to a planned procedure or surgery is generally 48 hours, but may be impacted by patient age, comorbidities, and underlying renal function. Idarucizumab and andexanet alfa are FDA-approved reversal agents for the direct thrombin

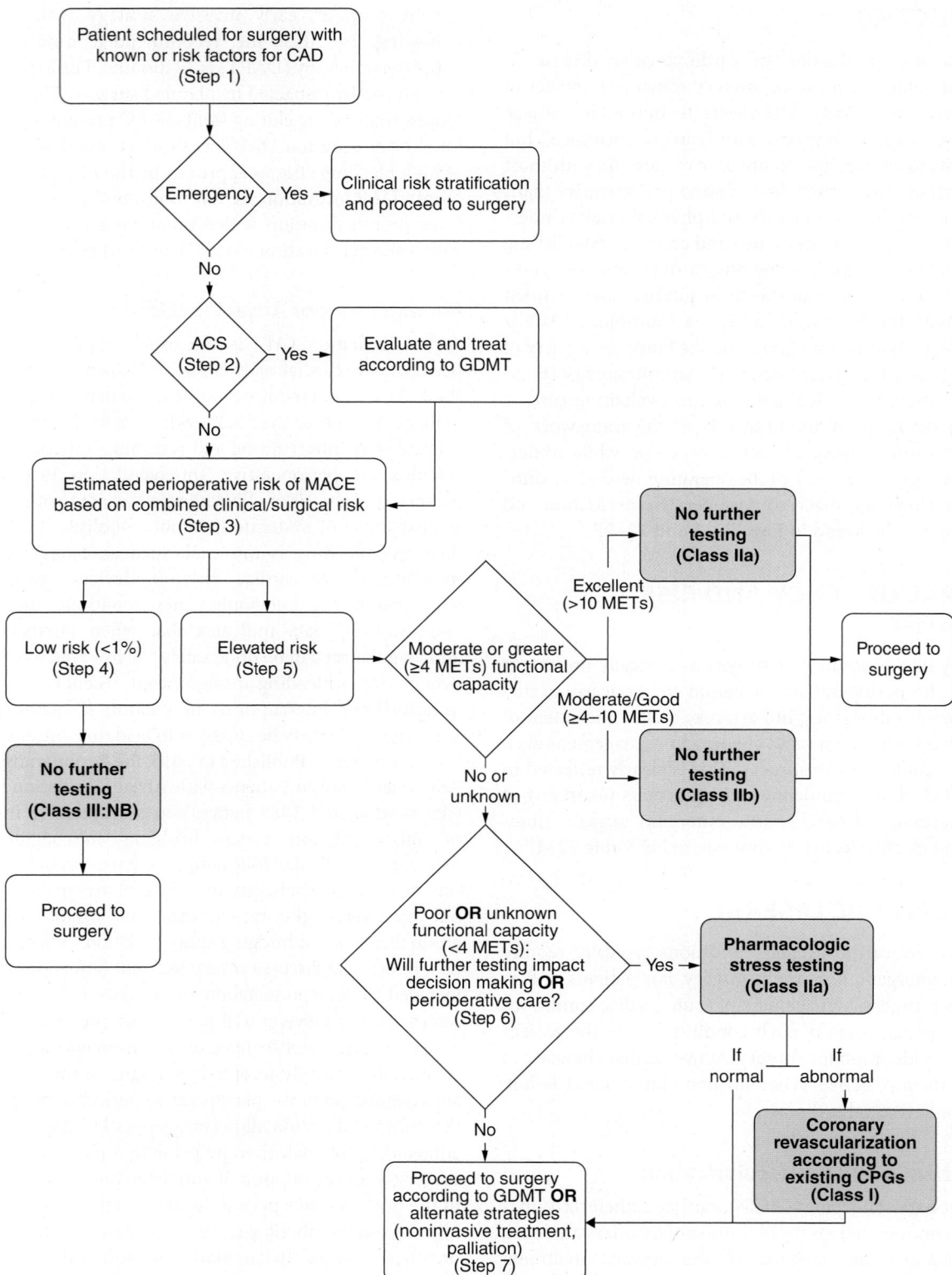

Figure 72–1. Summary algorithm for the cardiac evaluation and management of patients prior to noncardiac surgery from the 2014 ACC/AHA Clinical Practice Guidelines. ACS, acute coronary syndrome; CAD, coronary artery disease; CPGs, clinical practice guidelines; GDMT, guideline-directed medical therapy; MACE, major adverse cardiac event; METs, metabolic equivalents; NB, no benefit. Reproduced with permission from Fleisher LA, Fleischmann KE, Auerbach AD, et al. 2014 ACC/AHA guideline on perioperative cardiovascular evaluation and management of patients undergoing noncardiac surgery: a report of the American College of Cardiology/American Heart Association Task Force on Practice Guidelines. *Circulation.* 2014 Dec 9;130(24):e278-e333.

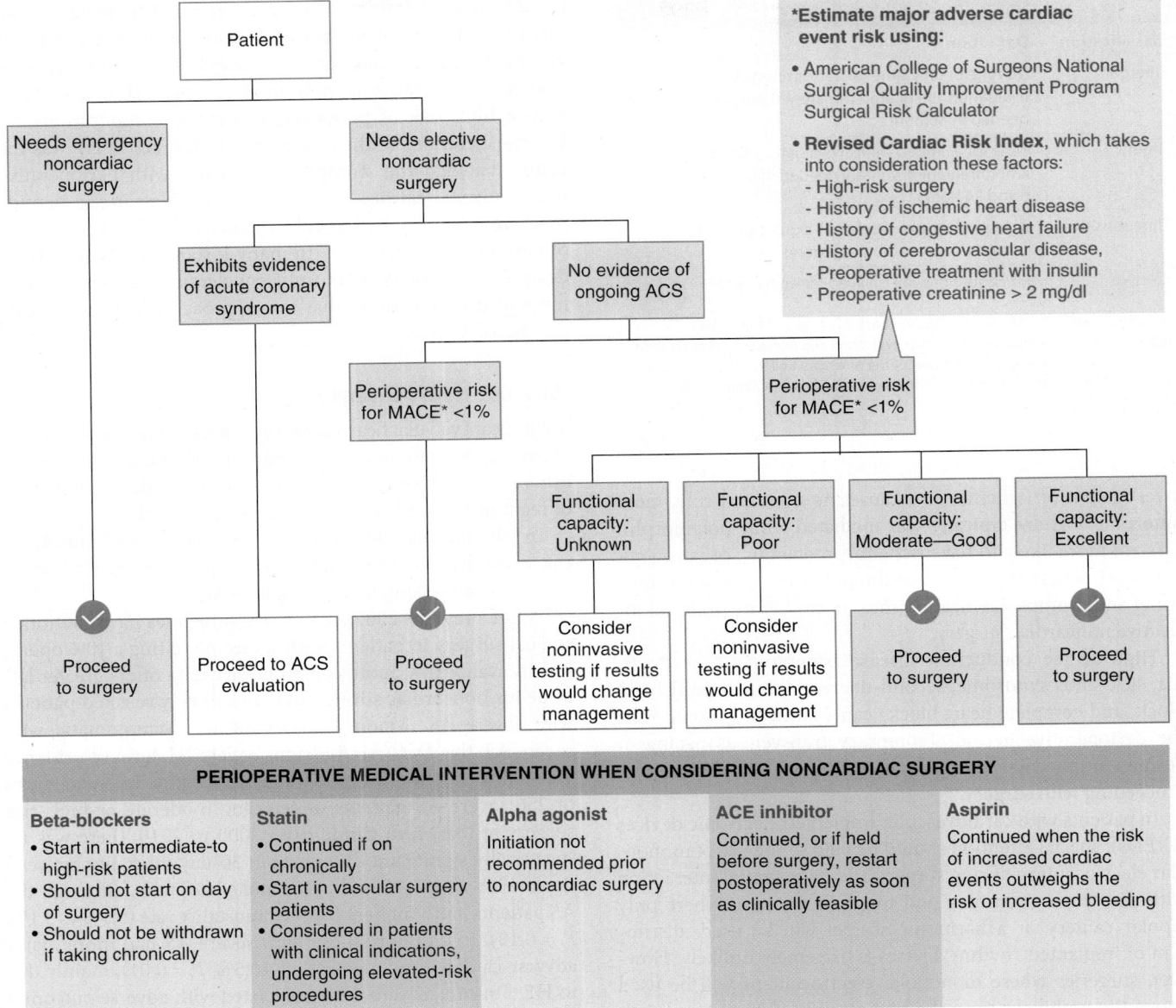

Figure 72–2. Summary of indication for noninvasive testing in the perioperative period and recommendations for continuation and initiation of different classes of medical therapies perioperatively. Reproduced with permission from Patel AY, Eagle KA, Vaishnava P. Cardiac risk of noncardiac surgery. *J Am Coll Cardiol.* 2015 Nov 10;66(19):2140-2148.

inhibitor dabigatran and the factor Xa inhibitors rivaroxaban and apixaban, respectively, and may be used if a surgery or procedure cannot be delayed in a patient with presumed therapeutic use/recent ingestion of one of these agents.

In the setting of AF with rapid ventricular rates (above a heart rate of 110 bpm), surgery may be delayed until either sinus rhythm is restored and/or ventricular rate is better controlled. Certainly, a supraventricular tachyarrhythmia associated with any hemodynamic instability requires termination with direct current cardioversion. Before selecting a rhythm or rate control management strategy in clinically stable patients, secondary causes of tachycardia such as sepsis, metabolic disturbances, venous thromboembolism, withdrawal from home medications (eg, atrioventricular-nodal slowing agents),

and volume derangements (particularly in patients who are fasting prior to surgery) should be excluded, as appropriate. Once the chosen management strategy has been successfully executed, surgery may again be reconsidered. With other forms of supraventricular tachycardia (SVT), arrhythmia termination by vagotonic maneuvers, atrioventricular nodal, or antiarrhythmic medications may be beneficial depending on the specific rhythm.

Uncontrolled Arrhythmias and High-Degree Conduction Disease

In the setting of sustained ventricular tachycardia (VT), prompt arrhythmia termination by chemical or electric means is critical. Cases of polymorphic and monomorphic VT necessitate

TABLE 72–1. Scheme for Classifying Surgical Urgency

Classification	Definition
Emergent	No time or only time for very limited clinical evaluation, life or limb threatened, surgery needed in <6 hours
Urgent	Time for a limited clinical evaluation, life or limb threatened, surgery needed in between 6 and 24 hours
Time sensitive	A delay of >1 to 6 weeks will significantly affect outcome (eg, oncologic surgery)
Elective	Procedure may be delayed for up to 1 year

Data from Fleisher LA, Fleischmann KE, Auerbach AD, et al. 2014 ACC/AHA guideline on perioperative cardiovascular evaluation and management of patients undergoing noncardiac surgery: a report of the American College of Cardiology/American Heart Association Task Force on Practice Guidelines. *Circulation*. 2014 Dec 9;130(24):e278-e333.

investigation of ischemia as a cause. As a general rule, monomorphic VTs are typically scar mediated while polymorphic VTs are more likely to have ischemic, metabolic, or iatrogenic etiologies. These rhythms have the potential to be life threatening and prompt stabilization must occur before undertaking elective noncardiac surgery.

High-degree conduction disease (symptomatic bradycardia, sick sinus syndrome, second-degree Mobitz type II heart block, and complete heart block) can significantly complicate the perioperative period. Temporary transvenous pacing or permanent pacemaker implantation may be necessary before proceeding with surgery.[11]

In patients with cardiovascular implanted electronic devices (CIEDs), special attention should be paid to the use of monopolar electrocautery during surgery and its potential interaction with device programming and function. In cases where only bipolar cautery or a harmonic scalpel will be used, disruption of implanted rhythm devices is extremely unlikely. However, surgeries where monopolar electrocautery will be used above the umbilicus pose the highest risk of interaction with implanted rhythm devices. In pacemaker-dependent patients, reprogramming to the DOO or VOO setting can minimize oversensing and failure to pace. In patients with implanted cardioverter-defibrillators (ICDs), turning off tachytherapies is helpful to avoid unnecessary patient shocks. These changes can be accomplished by magnet placement or device reprogramming. If ICD tachytherapies are disabled, connection to an external defibrillator until device reprogramming is highly advised. A dedicated discussion about rhythm device management should occur prior to surgery with a plan for immediate postoperative reprogramming to the device's original settings.[12]

Heart Failure

As the prevalence of HF increases, the need for perioperative management of HF becomes ever more common. It is important to discern whether HF is occurring with a reduced or preserved left ventricular ejection fraction (LVEF), or whether it is in the setting of hypertrophic cardiomyopathy

(HCM). Special care must be taken in HCM to avoid arterial dilation and overdiuresis, as such conditions can exacerbate left ventricular intracavitary obstructive gradients and potentially lead to perioperative complications. Active HF is associated with a high risk of perioperative cardiac complications.[13–15] In prior iterations of the cardiac risk index, active HF was the factor that had the strongest association with perioperative major adverse cardiac events (MACE).[14] Natriuretic peptide measurement may be helpful in management and prediction of perioperative events.[16–21] In many instances, it is optimal to delay surgery for diuresis until euvolemia is achieved. Prior investigation has found that this approach can help mitigate the risk of MACE.[22]

Valvular Heart Disease

If significant valvular heart disease is suspected based on symptoms of dyspnea or a new or changing murmur on exam, transthroracic echocardiography is critical for quantification of degree of stenosis or regurgitation and determination of surgical risk.

In patients with significant aortic stenosis (AS), anesthesia can cause hypotension, tachycardia, and decreased coronary perfusion, all potentially leading to MACE.[14]

While previous 2007 ACC/AHA guidelines have cautioned against surgery in patients with severe AS, citing a 10% operative mortality risk, more contemporary data offers greater latitude for noncardiac surgery in appropriately selected patients with severe AS. Among those who are asymptomatic with severe AS, the ACC/AHA assigns a class IIa, level of evidence C recommendation for moderate risk surgery. In one analysis of 256 severe AS patients undergoing moderate or high-risk surgery at the Mayo Clinic from 2000 to 2010, there was no statistically significant difference in 30-day mortality between those with severe AS and 256 matched controls, although the AS patients had a higher observed mortality rate (5.9% vs 3.1%, $P = 0.13$). In addition, those with severe AS had more major adverse cardiac events (18.8% vs 10.5%, $P = 0.01$), mainly due to HF.[23] In sum, severe AS is associated with adverse outcomes in patients undergoing noncardiac surgery; however, in contemporary cohorts, this risk may be less than has been historically stated. Balloon valvotomy is usually not recommended, but may serve a role in the minority of patients who need "bridging" to a necessary surgery or procedure; it is further limited by low long-term durability.

Although not specifically studied for the purposes of aortic valve intervention in perioperative patients undergoing noncardiac surgery, transcatheter aortic valve replacement (TAVR) may be considered for patients with severe symptomatic disease for whom open surgery is not an option or may prohibitively delay noncardiac surgery. Results of the Placement of Aortic Transcatheter Valves (PARTNER) trials have shown favorable outcomes in appropriate candidates, across the spectrum of risk.[26,27] If surgery is attempted without treatment of severe AS, meticulous cardiac anesthesia and perioperative monitoring are critical in the operative and postoperative settings.

Patients with severe mitral stenosis (MS) are prone to tachycardia, hypotension, and reduced cardiac output in the perioperative setting. Detection of MS, if present, is important in the perioperative setting. Symptomatic MS patients who are suitable candidates for balloon valvulotomy (ie, based on the echocardiographic features of valve thickening, subvalvular thickening, calcification, and leaflet mobility) or surgical commisurotomy should undergo intervention before elective surgery.[28]

As a general rule, left-sided regurgitant valve lesions are better tolerated than are stenotic lesions.[29,30] The main pathology of mitral regurgitation stems from left ventricular volume overload, and, medically, is best managed by maintaining preload and avoiding excessive afterload. Prior investigations have revealed that patients with moderate-to-severe and severe aortic regurgitation (AR) had higher in-hospital mortality than did case-matched patients without AR (9.0% vs 1.7%, $P = 0.008$). Predictors of mortality were a reduced LVEF (<55%) and renal dysfunction (creatinine >2.0).[29] In cases of asymptomatic moderate-to-severe or severe MR, noncardiac surgery may be considered with echocardiographic and selected invasive hemodynamic monitoring, as necessary.[1] Postoperatively, patients may need monitoring in an intensive care setting, although not necessarily. Prior investigation from a single tertiary care center of patients with moderate-to-severe or severe MR revealed worse outcomes in propensity matched cases (driven by 30-day mortality, myocardial infarction [MI], HF, and stroke) in the group with MR.[30] Important predictors of poor outcome were ischemic source of MR, diabetes mellitus, reduced LVEF <35%, and a history of carotid endarterectomy.

STABLE CARDIAC DISEASE

Understanding how best to manage stable patients involves a more nuanced and predictive approach. In this circumstance, management has become more conservative over time, with fewer patients needing further cardiac testing or revascularization than previously, largely because neither invasive nor medical therapies in otherwise stable patients have shown substantial benefit. Prior randomized investigations in stable coronary artery disease (CAD) patients have not proven that coronary revascularization is effective in patients without left main (LM) coronary disease for modifying the risk of perioperative events, even for patients undergoing high-risk surgery.[31] Risk-stratification methodologies, approaches to perioperative testing, and medical management are all important components of the perioperative evaluation of stable cardiac patients.

Perioperative Risk Stratification

Perioperative risk can generally be divided into two components: the inherent risk associated with an operation and the risk attributed to patient specific conditions. Three main risk-stratification algorithms exist: the revised cardiac risk index (RCRI), the American College of Surgeons National Surgical Quality Improvement Program Myocardial Infarction and Cardiac Arrest (NSQIP MICA), and the NSQIP Surgical Risk Calculator. Overall, the RCRI is most easily applied clinically and the NSQIP tools are more comprehensive. A comparison of the various tools is given in **Table 72–2**.

When assessing the inherent risk of an operation, typically low-stress surgeries with minimal fluid shifts are considered low risk (eg, cataracts, biopsies) and are associated with a <1% risk of MACE.[31] Vascular surgeries are considered the highest risk, but upfront risk can be tempered if an endovascular approach is taken, although conversion to open surgery remains a possibility even when an endovascular approach is anticipated or attempted. The intrinsic risk of an operation is multifactorial and sometimes difficult to predict; the ACC/AHA guidelines divide operations into low- and elevated-risk procedures.[1] In the ESC/ESA guidelines, operative risk is divided into low (<1%), intermediate (1%–5%), and high risk (>5%).[2]

RCRI

The RCRI is a simple and validated tool that assesses the risk of a major cardiac perioperative event defined as MI, pulmonary edema, ventricular fibrillation or primary cardiac arrest, or complete heart block.[13] The RCRI uses six factors (surgical risk, history of ischemic heart disease, HF, cerebrovascular disease, diabetes mellitus requiring insulin, and preoperative creatinine >2); only one of these is directly attributable to the inherent risk of the operation, where escalated surgical risk is assigned to any operation that is suprainguinal vascular, intraperitoneal, or intrathoracic. Based on the presence of none, one, two, three, or more of these clinical predictors, the rate of development of one of these four major cardiac events is estimated to be 0.4%, 0.9%, 7%, and 11%, respectively.

Biomarker testing with natriuretic peptide levels appears to independently predict the risk of cardiovascular events up to the first 30 days after vascular surgery and significantly improves the performance of the RCRI.[9–14,16–21] Further research is needed to validate whether measuring biomarkers leads to alterations in management that would improve patient outcomes.

NSQIP and NSQIP MICA

The NSQIP MICA and NSQIP risk calculators are based on data from over 1 million operations collected from 525 participating centers.[32] The NSQIP MICA score was created in 2011 in a large derivation and validation study. The inherent risk of surgery was derived from odds ratios based on surgical site, with inguinal hernias used as the reference. The primary outcomes were cardiac arrest (defined as a chaotic rhythm requiring basic or advanced life support) or MI. The NSQIP MICA appears to outperform the RCRI, particularly in cases of vascular surgery.

The NSQIP uses procedure specific terminology, including whether surgery is emergent, to assess the perioperative risk of MACE, death, or eight other outcomes. It requires 21 patient-specific variables for effective calculation and is likely the closest estimate of surgery specific risk of any of the risk calculators. The drawbacks are that it has not been validated in an external population, and it relies upon the American Society of Anesthesiologists classification, which may be subject to considerable interobserver variability.[33–35]

Perioperative Testing

Perioperative testing should be limited to circumstances that would change management independent of the surgery planned. Testing is not necessary for low-risk procedures, and

TABLE 72–2. Comparison of Perioperative Risk Calculators

	RCRI	NSQIP MICA	NSQIP

Criteria	• Creatinine ≥2 mg/mL
	• CHF
	• Insulin-dependent diabetes mellitus
	• Intrathoracic, intraabdominal, or suprainguinal vascular surgery
	• History of cerebrovascular accident or transient ischemic attack
	• Ischemic heart disease
		• Increasing age
		• Partially or completely dependent functional status
		• Surgery type:
		  • Anorectal
		  • Aortic
		  • Bariatric
		  • Brain
		  • Breast
		  • Cardiac
		  • ENT
		  • Foregut/hepatopancreatobiliary
		  • Gallbladder/adrenal/appendix/spleen
		  • Intestinal
		  • Neck
		  • Obstetric/gynecological
		  • Orthopedic
		  • Otherabdomen
		  • Peripheralvascular
		  • Skin
		  • Spine
		  • Thoracic
		  • Vein
		  • Urologic
			• Age
			• Acute renal failure
			• Functional status
			• Diabetes mellitus
			• Procedure (CPTcode)
			• American Society of Anesthesiologists physical status class
			• Wound class
			• Ascites
			• Systemic sepsis
			• Ventilator dependent
			• Disseminated cancer
			• Steroid use
			• Hypertension
			• Previous cardiac event
			• Sex
			• Dyspnea
			• Smoker
			• COPD
			• Dialysis
			• Acute kidney injury
			• Body mass index
			• Emergency case

Use outside original cohort	Yes	No	No
Sites	Most often single center, but findings correlate with multicenter	Multicenter	Multicenter
Calculation	Single point per risk factor	Web-based (http://www.surgicalriskcalculator.com/miorcardiacarrest)	Web-based (https://www.riskcalculator.facs.org)

Abbreviations: CHF, congestive heart failure; COPD, chronic obstructive pulmonary disease; CPT, Current Procedural Terminology; ENT, ear, nose, and throat; MICA, Myocardial Infarction and Cardiac Arrest; NSQIP, National Surgical Quality Improvement Program; RCRI, revised cardiac risk index.
Reproduced with permission from Fleisher LA, Fleischmann KE, Auerbach AD, et al. 2014 ACC/AHA guideline on perioperative cardiovascular evaluation and management of patients undergoing noncardiac surgery: a report of the American College of Cardiology/American Heart Association Task Force on Practice Guidelines. *Circulation*. 2014 Dec 9; 130(24):e278-e333.

in the current environment of overuse of perioperative testing, specialty societies have undertaken efforts to reduce unnecessary testing.[36,37] As has been previously noted, revascularization in stable coronary disease prior to surgery has not been associated with improved outcomes.[31] The cornerstone of determining the indication for further cardiac testing is assessment of a patient's symptoms, exercise status, and functional capacity. The risk of perioperative complications is indirectly proportional to functional status.[38] The conventional measurement standard for assessing functional status is metabolic equivalents (METs), where 1 MET is the basal oxygen consumption of a 40-year-old 70-kg man. If a patient has not had a recent exercise test, functional status can be estimated by performance during activities of daily living.[39] As an easy reference for functional status categories, METs and their examples may be found in **Table 72–3**.

Generally, formal functional testing is not indicated when a patient can easily and repetitively perform over 4 METs during activities of daily living, and an even stronger argument against testing can be made above 10 METs. Obtaining a 12-lead electrocardiogram (ECG) should generally be reserved for patients with known arrhythmia, CAD, peripheral vascular disease, and structural heart disease. Preoperative left ventricular function assessment is appropriate in patients with dyspnea of unknown origin, and patients with known left ventricular dysfunction and worsening or poorly controlled symptoms.

TABLE 72–3. Functional Status Categories with Associated Metabolic Equivalents (METs) and Examples

Classification	Quantification (METs)	Examples
Excellent	>10	Boxing, judo, cross-country skiing at least 10 kph
Good	7–10	Bicycling at 10–30 kph, fencing, kayaking at 12.5 kph
Moderate	4–6	Golf while carrying clubs, doubles tennis, walking 7 kph, walking up a hill, climbing a flight of stairs, heavy housework
Poor	<4	Driving, yoga, bowling, fishing from bank

Data from Jetté M, Sidney K, Blümchen G. Metabolic equivalents (METS) in exercise testing, exercise prescription, and evaluation of functional capacity. *Clin Cardiol*. 1990 Aug;13(8):555-565.

Functional Testing

Functional testing is potentially useful in patients with poor functional status when results will change management. Functional testing can be used to diagnose CAD; assess angina; and decide how to treat left ventricular dysfunction, dyspnea, or poor functional status. The evidence base for functional testing is fraught with limitations, including a heavy focus on vascular surgical patients, outdated stress protocols, and a lack of contemporary CAD management techniques. Nonetheless, the data confirm that patients able to achieve 7 to 10 METs are at low risk of perioperative cardiac events, and those that are unable to achieve 4 to 5 METs are at elevated risk.[40–43]

The available evidence regarding the role for preoperative functional testing is primarily from single centers using dobutamine stress echocardiography (DSE) or radionuclide myocardial perfusion imaging (MPI).[44–61] The predominant findings are summarized as follows:

1. Moderate to large areas of ischemia are associated with higher perioperative risk of MI and/or death.
2. Functional testing has a high negative predictive value.
3. Evidence of prior MI without inducible ischemia has little predictive value for perioperative events.
4. Prior studies have demonstrated clinical value and safety of either type of stress test.

The data are quite equivocal as to which technique performs best. We believe that these techniques should be viewed equally given variable institutional expertise and experience with either technique. Coronary computed tomography angiography (CCTA) may also have a role perioperatively, although has not been specifically studied in this setting.

Medical Management

After a thorough history, physical examination, and risk stratification, titration or addition of cardiac medications can be helpful in perioperative cardiac management. Most investigations and debate have centered on the role of β-blockers prior to surgery; there is still equipoise about the role of this therapy in the perioperative setting. Our discussion of perioperative medical management will focus on the role of β-blockade, statins, aspirin, DAPT, and clonidine.

β-Blockers

The debate around the use of perioperative β-blockade has nearly come full circle. Earlier, small randomized studies indicated possible benefit of β-blockers surrounding vascular surgery, findings that were subsequently confirmed in the Dutch Echocardiographic Cardiac Risk Evaluation Applying Stress Echocardiography (DECREASE) studies.[47,62,63] Unfortunately, all but the initial DECREASE family of studies, which previously formed the foundation of the guidelines supporting the use of perioperative β-blockade have been discredited and retracted due to concerns for research misconduct. Publications that followed DECREASE questioned β-blocker utility, which was the impetus for the large randomized Perioperative Ischemic Evaluation (POISE) trial.[64] POISE revealed that perioperative β-blockade improved perioperative cardiac events, but at the expense of more bradycardic and hypotensive episodes, strokes, and most importantly, deaths. Although some have criticized POISE for choices in β-blocker dosing and frequency that may exceed those used in clinical practice, further investigations have also confirmed equivocal findings with perioperative β-blockade.[66,67]

Based on the current literature, patients on longstanding stable β-blocker doses should have therapy continued at the time of surgery because of the risk of discontinuing β-blockade leading to subsequent withdrawal and related surges in heart rate and blood pressure.[66–69] β-blockers may help mitigate cardiac risk in moderate to high-risk patients, and specifically in patients with RCRI scores of ≥3.[70] Otherwise, β-blockers should be used only for appropriate clinical circumstances irrespective of upcoming surgery, because it is still unclear if they have any positive effects on perioperative outcomes for most patients. If β-blockade use is pursued, initiation and titration should occur several days or weeks (ideally at least 28 days) prior to surgery to avoid adverse events.

Statins

Statin therapy is effective for both primary and secondary prevention of cardiac events in patients with CAD, and statin indications are continuing to expand.[71,72] With regard to statin therapy's relationship to perioperative events, the randomized data are somewhat limited. A small trial of 100 patients randomized to either statin or placebo before vascular surgery found significantly lower MACE with statin use.[73] A Cochrane analysis revealed similar results, but again with a small sample size and most events attributed to a single study.[74] Statins may be helpful if started before surgery and present a great opportunity to improve long-term outcomes after surgery, but should be reserved for patients with established atherosclerosis. Both the ACC/AHA and ESC/ESA guidelines recommend statin therapy be continued at the time of surgery and that they may be of benefit in patients with peripheral arterial disease undergoing vascular surgery.[1,2] The ESC/ESA stipulates that statins are best initiated at least 2 weeks prior to vascular surgery.[2] The ACC/AHA guidelines further indicate that it might be reasonable to initiate statin therapy in patients without known atherosclerosis who have an indication for such therapy and are undergoing elevated risk surgery.[1]

Aspirin and Dual Antiplatelet Therapy

There appears to be uncertain benefit of aspirin for preventing cardiac events in the perioperative period in patients without any history of intracoronary stenting. Observational data have suggested an increased risk of thrombotic events associated with discontinuation of aspirin.[75] Large randomized studies have not shown benefit of taking aspirin. The Pulmonary Embolism Prevention (PEP) trial randomized 13,356 patients to either 160 mg aspirin or placebo with no difference in outcome.[76] The POISE-2 trial was a 2 × 2 factorial trial studying the effects of aspirin and clonidine on perioperative events. Over 10,000 patients undergoing orthopedic, general, urologic, and gynecological surgery were randomized to 200 mg of aspirin or placebo; there were few patients with CAD (23%) and those undergoing carotid endarterectomy were excluded. There was no difference in the primary outcomes between aspirin and placebo groups (7.0 vs 7.1%, respectively; hazard ratio, 0.99; 95% confidence interval, 0.86–1.15; P = 0.92). Major bleeding was more common in the aspirin group than in the placebo group (hazard ratio, 1.23; 95% confidence interval, 1.01–1.49; P = 0.04). Further study is needed to understand aspirin's impact on high-risk patient groups. It is worth noting that POISE-2 also included relatively few patients with intracoronary stents. In practice, for patients with coronary stents, aspirin is best continued during surgery (save those patients in whom bleeding would be catastrophic, eg, those undergoing neurologic or spine surgery) and should be reinitiated as soon can be done safely if discontinued perioperatively.[77] Consensus should be reached between the surgeon, anesthesiologist, and cardiologist regarding the risk benefit profile (thrombosis vs bleeding) of continuing aspirin therapy in individual patients.

Several important factors must be considered regarding the timing of noncardiac surgery after coronary stent implantation. These factors are the risk of stent thrombosis, the consequences of delaying surgery, and the risk of procedural associated bleeding related to DAPT. DAPT is known to significantly reduce the risk of stent thrombosis, and these affects are most profoundly noted in the first 4 to 6 weeks after stent implantation.[78–82] Mechanistically, stent thrombosis at the time of surgery is believed to result from endothelial disruption and the proinflammatory and prothrombotic effects throughout the coronary circulation.[83,84] Newer-generation DES are associated with a lower risk of stent thrombosis and often require a shorter duration of DAPT. Limitations aside, investigations of treating patients with newer-generation DES with 3 and 6 months of DAPT compared with longer durations after implantation did not reveal any significant difference in MACE.[85–89] Pooled analyses of these trials as well as data from the Patterns of Nonadherence to Antiplatelet Regimens in Stented Patients (PARIS) registry involving physician-initiated DAPT interruptions are all reassuring for shorter DAPT durations.[90,91] For patients treated with any type of stent for any indication, elective surgery should be delayed and DAPT should not be interrupted within 30 days of stent implantation. Elective, noncardiac surgery should be delayed for 5 days since the last dose of clopidogrel; 7 days, since the last dose of prasugrel; and 3 to 5 days, since the last dose of ticagrelor. The use of cangrelor, an intravenous reversible P2Y$_{12}$ receptor antagonist, may be an appealing bridging strategy (with an infusion given at a bridging dose of 0.75 μg/kg/min), although studies of its use in those undergoing cardiac and noncardiac surgery is limited.[92]

Clonidine

Initial investigations involving α-2 agonism at the time of surgery appeared to indicate that clonidine was beneficial. In 2004, randomized clinical data of 200 patients undergoing noncardiac surgery demonstrated a mortality benefit persisting to 2 years in patients receiving clonidine (15% vs 29%, P = 0.035).[93] Meta-analysis of 31 α-2 agonist trials also revealed promising effects, notably in vascular surgical patients.[94] However, the POISE-2 trial, which was orders of magnitude larger than prior investigations, failed to demonstrate these benefits and rather showed that clonidine increased the rate of nonfatal cardiac arrest and clinically important hypotension.[77] Therefore, clonidine is not recommended for mitigating cardiac risk at the time of noncardiac surgery.

SUMMARY

With all the intricacies of perioperative evaluation, the best preoperative cardiac test remains a careful history and physical directed at finding and grading CAD, left ventricular dysfunction, valve disease, rhythm disorders, or previously unsuspected vascular disease. Any testing or treatment should be justified by the patient's disease alone, because there is little evidence that treatments for the sole purpose of improving perioperative outcomes have any substantial benefit.

REFERENCES

1. Fleisher LA, Fleischmann KE, Auerbach AD, et al. 2014 ACC/AHA guideline on perioperative cardiovascular evaluation and management of patients undergoing noncardiac surgery: a report of the American College of Cardiology/American Heart Association Task Force on Practice Guidelines. *Circulation*. 2014;130:e278-e333.
2. Kristensen S, Knuuti J, Saraste A, et al. 2014 ESC/ESA Guidelines on noncardiac surgery: Cardiovascular assessment and management. The Joint Task Force on Non-cardiac Surgery: Cardiovascular Assessment and Management of the European Society of Cardiology (ESC) and the European Society of Anaesthesiology (ESA). *Eur Heart J*. 2014;35:2383-2431.
3. Kirtane AJ, Stoler R, Feldman R, Neumann FJ, Boutis L, Tahirkheli N, Toelg R, Othman I, Stein B, Choi JW, Windecker S, Yeh RW, Dauerman HL, Price MJ, Underwood P, Allocco D, Meredith I, Kereiakes DJ. Primary Results of the EVOLVE Short DAPT Study: Evaluation of 3-Month Dual Antiplatelet Therapy in High Bleeding Risk Patients Treated With a Bioabsorbable Polymer-Coated Everolimus-Eluting Stent. *Circ Cardiovasc Interv*. 2021 Mar;14(3):e010144.
4. Hawn M, Graham L, Richman J, Itani K, Henderson W, Maddox T. Risk of major adverse cardiac events following noncardiac surgery in patients with coronary stents. *JAMA*. 2013;310:1462-1472.
5. Levine G, Bates E, Bittl J, et al. 2016 ACC/AHA guideline focused update on duration of dual antiplatelet therapy in patients with coronary artery disease: a report of the American College of Cardiology/American Heart Association Task Force on Clinical Practice Guidelines. *J Am Coll Cardiol*. 2016;68(10):1082-1115.
6. Douketis J, Johnson J, Turpie A. Low-molecular-weight heparin as bridging anticoagulation during interruption of warfarin: AOF a standardized periprocedural anticoagulation regimen. *Arch Intern Med*. 2004;164:1319-1326.
7. Dunn A, Spyropoulos A, Turpie A. Bridging therapy in patients on long-term oral anticoagulants who require surgery: the Prospective Perioperative Enoxaparin Cohort Trial (PROSPECT). *J Thromb Haemost*. 2007;5:2211-2218.
8. Spyropoulos A, Turpie A, Dunn A, et al. Clinical outcomes with unfractionated heparin or low-molecular-weight heparin as bridging therapy in patients on long-term oral anticoagulants: the REGIMEN registry. *J Thromb Haemost*. 2006;4:1246-1252.
9. Douketis J, Spyropoulos A, Kaatz S, et al. Perioperative bridging anticoagulation in patients with atrial fibrillation. *N Engl J Med*. 2015;373:823-833.
10. January C, Wann L, Alpert J, et al. 2014 AHA/ACC/HRS guideline for the management of patients with atrial fibrillation: a Report of the American College of Cardiology/American Heart Association Task Force on Practice Guidelines and the Heart Rhythm Society. *Circulation*. 2014;130.

11. Gregoratos G, Abrams J, Epstein A, et al. American College of Cardiology/American Heart Association Task Force on Practice Guidelines/North American Society for Pacing and Electrophysiology Committee to Update the 1998 Pacemaker Guidelines. ACC/AHA/NASPE 2002 guideline update for implantation of cardiac pacemakers and antiarrhythmia devices: summary article. A Report of the American College of Cardiology/American Heart Association Task Force on Practice Guidelines (ACC/AHA/NASPE) Committee to Update the 1998 Pacemaker Guidelines). *Circulation*. 1998;106:2145-2161.

12. Crossley G, Poole J, Rozner M, et al. The Heart Rhythm Society (HRS)/American Society of Anesthesiologists (ASA) expert consensus statement on the perioperative management of patients with implantable defibrillators, pacemakers and arrhythmia monitors: facilities and patient management. *Heart Rhythm*. 2011;8:1114-1154.

13. Lee T, Marcantonio E, Mangione C, et al. Derivation and prospective validation of a simple index for prediction of cardiac risk of major noncardiac surgery. *Circulation*. 1999;100:1043-1049.

14. Goldman L, Caldera D, Nussbaum S, et al. Multifactorial index of cardiac risk in noncardiac surgical procedures. *N Engl J Med*. 1977;297:845-850.

15. Detsky A, Abrams H, McLaughlin J, et al. Predicting cardiac complications in patients undergoing non-cardiac surgery. *J Gen Intern Med*. 1986;1:211-219.

16. Rodseth RN LBG, Bolliger D, Burkhart CS, et al. The predictive ability of pre-operative B-type natriuretic peptide in vascular patients for major adverse cardiac events: an individual patient data meta-analysis. *J Am Coll Cardiol*. 2011;58:522-529.

17. Karthikeyan G, Moncur R, Levine O, et al. Is a pre-operative brain natriuretic peptide or N-terminal pro-B-type natriuretic peptide measurement an independent predictor of adverse cardiovascular outcomes within 30 days of noncardiac surgery? A systematic review and meta-analysis of observational studies. *J Am Coll Cardiol*. 2009;54:1599-1606.

18. Ryding A, Kumar S, Worthington A, Burgess D. Prognostic value of brain natriuretic peptide in noncardiac surgery: a meta-analysis. *Anesthesiology*. 2009;111:311-319.

19. Rajagopalan S, Croal B, Bachoo P, Hillis G, Cuthbertson B, Brittenden J. N-terminal pro B-type natriuretic peptide is an independent predictor of postoperative myocardial injury in patients undergoing major vascular surgery. *J Vasc Surg*. 2008;48:912-917.

20. Leibowitz D, Planer D, Rott D, Elitzur Y, Chajek-Shaul T, Weiss A. Brain natriuretic peptide levels predict perioperative events in cardiac patients undergoing noncardiac surgery: a prospective study. *Cardiology*. 2008;110:266-270.

21. Rodseth R, Biccard B, Le M, et al. The prognostic value of pre-operative and post-operative B-type natriuretic peptides in patients undergoing noncardiac surgery: B-type natriuretic peptide and N-terminal fragment of pro-B-type natriuretic peptide: a systematic review and individual patient data meta-analysis. *J Am Coll Cardiol*. 2013;63:170-180.

22. Xu-Cai Y, Brotman D, Phillips C, et al. Outcomes of patients with stable heart failure undergoing elective noncardiac surgery. *Mayo Clin Proc*. 2008;83:280-288.

23. Tashiro T, Pislaru S, Blustin J, et al. Perioperative risk of major non-cardiac surgery in patients with severe aortic stenosis: a reappraisal in contemporary practice. *Eur Heart J*. 2014;35:2372-2381.

24. Hayes S, Holmes D, Jr, Nishimura R, Reeder G. Palliative percutaneous aortic balloon valvuloplasty before noncardiac operations and invasive diagnostic procedures. *Mayo Clin Proc*. 1989;64:753-757.

25. Roth R, Palacios I, Block P. Percutaneous aortic balloon valvuloplasty: its role in the management of patients with aortic stenosis requiring major noncardiac surgery. *J Am Coll Cardiol*. 1989;13:1039-1041.

26. Leon M, Smith C, Mack M, et al. Transcatheter aortic-valve implantation for aortic stenosis in patients who cannot undergo surgery. *N Engl J Med*. 2010;363:1597-1607.

27. Smith C, Leon M, Mack M, et al. Transcatheter versus surgical aortic-valve replacement in high-risk patients. *N Engl J Med*. 2011;364:2187-2198.

28. Reyes V, Raju B, Wynne J, et al. Percutaneous balloon valvuloplasty compared with open surgical commissurotomy for mitral stenosis. *N Engl J Med*. 1994;331:961-967.

29. Lai H, Lai H, Lee W, et al. Impact of chronic advanced aortic regurgitation on the perioperative outcome of noncardiac surgery. *Acta Anaesth Scand*. 2010;54:580-588.

30. Bajaj N, Agarwal S, Rajamanickam A, et al. Impact of severe mitral regurgitation on postoperative outcomes after noncardiac surgery. *Am J Med*. 2013;126:529-535.

31. McFalls E, Ward H, Moritz T, et al. Coronary-artery revascularization before elective major vascular surgery. *N Engl J Med*. 2004;351:2795-2804.

32. Gupta P, Gupta H, Sundaram A, et al. Development and validation of a risk calculator for prediction of cardiac risk after surgery. *Circulation*. 2011;124:381-387.

33. Cohen M, Ko C, Bilimoria K, et al. Optimizing ACS NSQIP modeling for evaluation of surgical quality and risk: Patient risk adjustment, procedure mix adjustment, shrinkage adjustment, and surgical focus. *J Am Coll Surg*. 2013;217:336-346.

34. Aronson W, McAuliffe M, Miller K. Variability in the American Society of Anesthesiologists Physical Status Classification Scale. *AANA J*. 2003;71:265-274.

35. Mak P, Campbell R, Irwin M. American Society of Anesthesiologists. The ASA Physical Status Classification: inter-observer consistency. *Anaesth Intensive Care*. 2002;30:633-640.

36. Thilen S, Treggiari M, Lange J, Lowy E, Weaver E, Wijeysundera D. Pre-operative consultations for Medicare patients undergoing cataract surgery. *JAMA Intern Med*. 2014;174:380-388.

37. Choosing wisely: promoting conversations between patients and clinicians. *ABIM Foundation*. 2021. www.choosingwisely.org.

38. Crawford R, Cambria R, Abularrage C, et al. Preoperative functional status predicts perioperative outcomes after infrainguinal bypass surgery. *J Vasc Surg*. 2010;51:351-358.

39. Reilly D, McNeely M, Doerner D, et al. Self-reported exercise tolerance and the risk of serious perioperative complications. *Arch Intern Med*. 1999;159:2185-2192.

40. Leppo J, Plaja J, Gionet M, Tumolo J, Paraskos J, Cutler B. Noninvasive evaluation of cardiac risk before elective vascular surgery. *J Am Coll Cardiol*. 1987;9:269-276.

41. Carliner N, Fisher M, Plotnick G, et al. Routine preoperative exercise testing in patients undergoing major noncardiac surgery. *Am J Cardiol*. 1985;56:51-58.

42. Sgura F, Kopecky S, Grill J, Gibbons R. Supine exercise capacity identifies patients at low risk for perioperative cardiovascular events and predicts long-term survival. *Am J Med*. 2000;108.

43. McPhail N, Calvin J, Shariatmadar A, Barber G, Scobie T. The use of preoperative exercise testing to predict cardiac complications after arterial reconstruction. *J Vasc Surg*. 1988;7:60-68.

44. Lentine K, Costa S, Weir M, et al. American Heart Association Council on the Kidney in Cardiovascular Disease and Council on Peripheral Vascular Disease; American Heart Association; American College of Cardiology Foundation. Cardiac disease evaluation and management among kidney and liver transplantation candidates: A scientific statement from the American Heart Association and the American College of Cardiology Foundation. Endorsed by the American Society of Transplant Surgeons, American Society of Transplantation, and National Kidney Foundation. *Circulation*. 2012;126:617-663.

45. Douglas PS GM, Haines DE, Lai WW, et al. ACCF/ASE/AHA/ASNC/HFSA/HRS/SCAI/SCCM/SCCT/SCMR 2011 appropriate use criteria for echocardiography. A report of the American College of Cardiology Foundation Appropriate Use Criteria Task Force, American Society of Echocardiography, American Heart Association, American Society of Nuclear Cardiology, Heart Failure Society of America, Heart Rhythm Society, Society for Cardiovascular Angiography and Interventions, Society of Critical Care Medicine, Society of Cardiovascular Computed Tomography, and Society for

Cardiovascular Magnetic Resonance. Endorsed by the American College of Chest Physicians. *J Am Coll Cardiol.* 2011;57:1126-1166.

46. Baron J, Mundler O, Bertrand M, et al. Dipyridamole-thallium scintigraphy and gated radionuclide angiography to assess cardiac risk before abdominal aortic surgery. *N Engl J Med.* 1994;330:663-669.

47. Mangano D, London M, Tubau J, et al. Dipyridamole thallium-201 scintigraphy as a preoperative screening test. A reexamination of its predictive potential. Study of Perioperative Ischemia Research Group. *Circulation.* 1991;84:493-502.

48. Boucher C, Brewster D, Darling R, Okada R, Strauss H, Pohost G. Determination of cardiac risk by dipyridamole-thallium imaging before peripheral vascular surgery. *N Engl J Med.* 1985;1985:7.

49. McEnroe C, O'Donnell T Jr., Yeager A, Konstam M, Mackey W. Comparison of ejection fraction and Goldman risk factor analysis to dipyridamole-thallium 201 studies in the evaluation of cardiac morbidity after aortic aneurysm surgery. *J Vasc Surg.* 1990;11:497-504.

50. Fletcher J, Kershaw L. Outcome in patients with failed percutaneous transluminal angioplasty for peripheral vascular disease. *J Cardiovasc Surg.* 1988;29:733-735.

51. Sachs R, Tellier P, Larmignat P, et al. Assessment by dipyridamole-thallium-201 myocardial scintigraphy of coronary risk before peripheral vascular surgery. *Surgery.* 1988;103:584-587.

52. Younis L, Aguirre F, Byers S, et al. Perioperative and long-term prognostic value of intravenous dipyridamole thallium scintigraphy in patients with peripheral vascular disease. *Am Heart J.* 1990;119:1287-1292.

53. Strawn D, Guernsey J. Dipyridamole thallium scanning in the evaluation of coronary artery disease in elective abdominal aortic surgery. *Arch Surg.* 1991;126:880-884.

54. Watters T, Botvinick E, Dae M, et al. Comparison of the findings on preoperative dipyridamole perfusion scintigraphy and intraoperative transesophageal echocardiography: Implications regarding the identification of myocardium at ischemic risk. *J Am Coll Cardiol.* 1991;18:93-100.

55. Hendel R, Whitfield S, Villegas B, Cutler B, Leppo J. Prediction of late cardiac events by dipyridamole thallium imaging in patients undergoing elective vascular surgery. *Am J Cardiol.* 1992;70:1243-1249.

56. Madsen P, Vissing M, Munck O, Kelbaek H. A comparison of dipyridamole thallium 201 scintigraphy and clinical examination in the determination of cardiac risk before arterial reconstruction. *Angiology.* 1992;43:306-311.

57. Kresowik T, Bower T, Garner S, et al. Dipyridamole thallium imaging in patients being considered for vascular procedures. *Arch Surg.* 1993;128:299-302.

58. Bry J, Belkin M, O'Donnell T Jr, et al. An assessment of the positive predictive value and cost-effectiveness of dipyridamole myocardial scintigraphy in patients undergoing vascular surgery. *J Vasc Surg.* 1994;19:112-121.

59. Koutelou M, Asimacopoulos P, Mahmarian J, Kimball K, Verani M. Preoperative risk stratification by adenosine thallium 201 single-photon emission computed tomography in patients undergoing vascular surgery. *J Nucl Cardiol.* 1995;2:389-394.

60. Marshall E, Raichlen J, Forman S, Heyrich G, Keen W, Weitz H. Adenosine radionuclide perfusion imaging in the preoperative evaluation of patients undergoing peripheral vascular surgery. *Am J Cardiol.* 1995;76:817-821.

61. Van D, Piérard L, Gillain D, Benoit T, Rigo P, Limet R. Cardiac risk assessment before vascular surgery: a prospective study comparing clinical evaluation, dobutamine stress echocardiography, and dobutamine Tc-99m sestamibi tomoscintigraphy. *J Cardiovasc Surg.* 1997;5:54-64.

62. Poldermans D, Boersma E, Bax J, et al. The effect of bisoprolol on perioperative mortality and myocardial infarction in high-risk patients undergoing vascular surgery. Dutch Echocardiographic Cardiac Risk Evaluation Applying Stress Echocardiography Study Group. *N Engl J Med.* 1999;341:1789-1794.

63. Wallace A, Layug B, Tateo I, et al. Prophylactic atenolol reduces postoperative myocardial ischemia. *Anesthesiology.* 1998;88:7-17.

64. Devereaux P, Beattie W, Choi P, et al. How strong is the evidence for the use of perioperative beta blockers in non-cardiac surgery? Systematic

review and meta-analysis of randomised controlled trials. *BMJ.* 2005;331:313-321.

65. Chopra V, Eagle K. Perioperative mischief: The price of academic misconduct. *Am J Med.* 2012;125:953.

66. Lindenauer P, Pekow P, Wang K, Mamidi D, Gutierrez B, Benjamin E. Perioperative beta-blocker therapy and mortality after major noncardiac surgery. *N Engl J Med.* 2005;353:349-361.

67. London M, Hur K, Schwartz G, Henderson W. Association of perioperative β-blockade with mortality and cardiovascular morbidity following major noncardiac surgery. *JAMA.* 2013;309:1704-1713.

68. Andersson C, Mérie C, Jørgensen M, et al. Association of β-blocker therapy with risks of adverse cardiovascular events and deaths in patients with ischemic heart disease undergoing noncardiac surgery: a Danish nationwide cohort study. *JAMA Int Med.* 2014;174:336-344.

69. Hoeks S, Scholte O, Reimer WJ, et al. Increase of 1-year mortality after perioperative beta-blocker withdrawal in endovascular and vascular surgery patients. *Eur J Endovasc Surg.* 2006;33:13-19.

70. Boersma E, Poldermans D, Bax J, et al. DECREASE Study Group (Dutch Echocardiographic Cardiac Risk Evaluation Applying Stress Echocardiogrpahy). Predictors of cardiac events after major vascular surgery: Role of clinical characteristics, dobutamine echocardiography, and beta-blocker therapy. *JAMA.* 2001;285:1865-1873.

71. Ridker P, Wilson P. A trial-based approach to statin guidelines. *JAMA.* 2013;310:1123-1124.

72. Stone N, Robinson J, Lichtenstein A, et al. American College of Cardiology/American Heart Association Task Force on Practice Guidelines. 2013 ACC/AHA guideline on the treatment of blood cholesterol to reduce atherosclerotic cardiovascular risk in adults: a report of the American College of Cardiology/American Heart Association Task Force on Practice Guidelines. *J Am Coll Cardiol.* 2013;63:2889-2934.

73. Durazzo AE MF, Ikeoka DT, De Bernoche C, Monachini MC, Puech-Leão P, Caramelli B. Reduction in cardiovascular events after vascular surgery with atorvastatin: a randomized trial. *J Vasc Surg.* 2004;39:967-975.

74. Sanders R, Nicholson A, Lewis S, Smith A, Alderson P. Perioperative statin therapy for improving outcomes during and after noncardiac vascular surgery. *Cochrane Database Syst Rev.* 2013;3:9971.

75. Burger W, Chemnitius J, Kneissl G, Rücker G. Low-dose aspirin for secondary cardiovascular prevention: cardiovascular risks after its perioperative withdrawal versus bleeding risks with its continuation. Review and meta-analysis. *J Int Med.* 2005;257:399-414.

76. Prevention of pulmonary embolism and deep vein thrombosis with low dose aspirin: Pulmonary Embolism Prevention (PEP) trial. *Lancet.* 2000;355:1295-1302.

77. Devereaux P, Mrkobrada M, Sessler D, et al. Aspirin in patients undergoing noncardiac surgery. *N Engl J Med.* 2014;370:1494-1503.

78. Steinhubl S, Berger P, Mann J, et al. Clopidogrel for the reduction of events during observation. Early and sustained dual oral antiplatelet therapy following percutaneous coronary intervention: A randomized controlled trial. *JAMA.* 2002;288.

79. Yusuf S, Zhao F, Mehta S, Chrolavicius S, Tognoni G, Fox K. Clopidogrel in unstable angina to prevent recurrent events trial investigators. Effects of clopidogrel in addition to aspirin in patients with acute coronary syndromes without ST-segment elevation. *N Engl J Med.* 2001;345.

80. Leon M, Baim D, Popma J, et al. A clinical trial comparing three antithrombotic-drug regimens after coronary-artery stenting. Stent Anticoagulation Restenosis Study Investigators. *N Engl J Med.* 1998;339:1665-1671.

81. Schömig A, Neumann F, Kastrati A, et al. A randomized comparison of antiplatelet and anticoagulant therapy after the placement of coronary-artery stents. *N Engl J Med.* 1996;334:1084-1089.

82. Cutlip D, Baim D, Ho K, et al. Stent thrombosis in the modern era: a pooled analysis of multicenter coronary stent clinical trials. *Circulation.* 2001;103:1967-1971.

83. Rajagopalan S, Ford I, Bachoo P, et al. Platelet activation, myocardial ischemic events and postoperative non-response to aspirin in

patients undergoing major vascular surgery. *J Thromb Haemost.* 2007;5: 2028-2035.

84. Diamantis T, Tsiminikakis N, Skordylaki A, et al. Alterations of hemostasis after laparoscopic and open surgery. *Hematology.* 2007;12:561-570.

85. Colombo A, Chieffo A, Frasheri A, et al. Second-generation drug-eluting stent implantation followed by 6- versus 12-month dual antiplatelet therapy: The SECURITY randomized clinical trial. *J Am Coll Cardiol.* 2014;64: 2086-2097.

86. Gwon H, Hahn J, Park K, et al. Six-month versus 12-month dual antiplatelet therapy after implantation of drug-eluting stents: the Efficacy of Xience/ Promus Versus Cypher to Reduce Late Loss After Stenting (EXCELLENT) randomized, multicenter study. *Circulation.* 2012;125:505-513.

87. Kim B, Hong M, Shin D, et al. A new strategy for discontinuation of dual antiplatelet therapy: the RESET Trial (REal Safety and Efficacy of 3-month dual antiplatelet therapy following Endeavor zotarolimus-eluting stent implantation). *J Am Coll Cardiol.* 2012;60:1340-1348.

88. Feres F, Costa R, Abizaid A, et al. Three vs twelve months of dual antiplatelet therapy after zotarolimus-eluting stents: the OPTIMIZE randomized trial. *JAMA.* 2013;310:2510-2522.

89. Schulz-Schüpke S, Byrne R, Ten B, et al. Intracoronary stenting and antithrombotic regimen: Safety and Efficacy of 6 Months Dual Antiplatelet Therapy After Drug-Eluting Stenting (ISAR-SAFE) Trial Investigators. ISAR-SAFE: a randomized, double-blind, placebo-controlled trial of 6 vs. 12 months of clopidogrel therapy after drug-eluting stenting. *Eur Heart J.* 2015;36:1252-1263.

90. Palmerini T, Sangiorgi D, Valgimigli M, et al. Short- versus long-term dual antiplatelet therapy after drug-eluting stent implantation: An individual patient data pairwise and network meta-analysis. *J Am Coll Cardiol.* 2015;65:1092-1102.

91. Mehran R, Baber U, Steg P, et al. Cessation of dual antiplatelet treatment and cardiac events after percutaneous coronary intervention (PARIS): 2 year results from a prospective observational study. *Lancet.* 2013;382:1714-1722.

92. Angiolillo DJ, Firstenberg MS, Prince MJ, et al. Bridging antiplatelet therapy with cangrelor in patients undergoing cardiac surgery. *JAMA.* 2012;307(3):265-274.

93. Wallace A, Galindez D, Salahieh A, et al. Effect of clonidine on cardiovascular morbidity and mortality after noncardiac surgery. *Anesthesiology.* 2004;101:284-293.

94. Wijeysundera D, Naik J, Beattie W. Alpha-2 adrenergic agonists to prevent perioperative cardiovascular complications: a meta-analysis. *Am J Med.* 2003;114:742-752.

Anesthesia and the Patient with Cardiovascular Disease

David L. Reich, Elvera L. Baron, and Joel A. Kaplan

CHAPTER OUTLINE

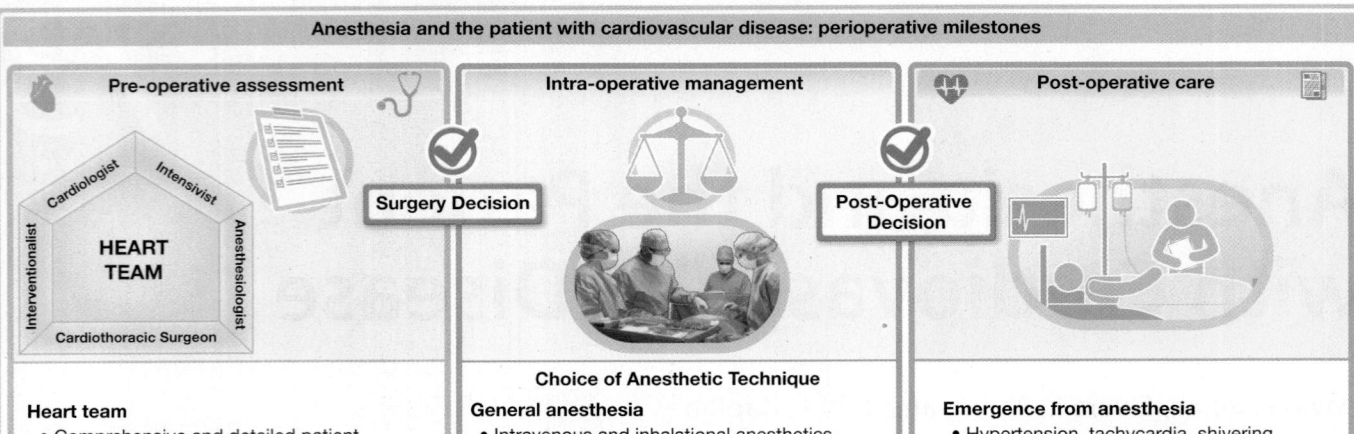

Anesthesia and the patient with cardiovascular disease: perioperative milestones

Pre-operative assessment

Cardiologist | Intensivist
Interventionalist | **HEART TEAM** | Anesthesiologist
Cardiothoracic Surgeon

Surgery Decision

Intra-operative management

Post-Operative Decision

Post-operative care

Heart team
- Comprehensive and detailed patient assessment
- Clear communication between providers, patient, and family
- Collaborative perioperative problem-solving

Cardiac risk assessment
- CRIS, NSQIP surgical risk calculator, RCRI, biomarker measurement

Preoperative optimization
- Timing of medications, including anticoagulant and antiplatelet therapy
- Summary of clinical, laboratory, radiologic, radionuclide, and catheterization data
- Cardiac anesthesiology consultation

Choice of Anesthetic Technique
General anesthesia
- Intravenous and inhalational anesthetics
- Neuromuscular blockade

Neuraxial and regional anesthesia
- Neuraxial: spinal and epidural anesthesia
- Neuraxial anesthesia and anticoagulation therapy
- Regional: nerve blocks and fascial plane blocks

Perioperative Monitoring
Non-invasive: heart rate, ECG, blood pressure, pulse oximetry, capnography, body temperature, cerebral oximetry, TTE

Invasive: Arterial line, CVP, PAC, TEE, cardiac output

Emergence from anesthesia
- Hypertension, tachycardia, shivering

Possible major complications
- Stroke, myocardial infarction, pulmonary edema, malignant ventricular arrhythmia, cardiac death

Other concerns
- Pain, AF, high catecholamine levels, hypercoagulability, discontinuation of antiplatelet therapy in patients with intra-coronary stents, hypovolemia, anemia, intravascular volume shifts, drug effects

Role of ERAS-C protocols
- Multidisciplinary and multimodal efforts to minimize physical and emotional stress during surgery or interventional procedure

Chapter 73 Fuster and Hurst's Central Illustration. As a member of the multidisciplinary heart team, the cardiac anesthesiologist plays a central role in perioperative planning. AF, atrial fibrillation; CRIS, Cardiac Risk Index Score; CVP, central venous pressure; ECG, electrocardiography; ERAS-C, enhanced recovery after surgery protocols specific to cardiac surgery; NSQIP, National Surgical Quality Improvement Program; PAC, pulmonary arterial catheter; RCRI, Revised Cardiac Risk Index; TEE, transesophageal echocardiography; TTE, transthoracic echocardiography.

CHAPTER SUMMARY

This chapter discusses the perioperative anesthetic management of patients with cardiovascular disease (CVD). Providing optimal perioperative care for CVD patients is a shared responsibility of cardiovascular clinicians, surgeons, and anesthesiologists. Any anesthetic agent or technique has the potential for producing adverse effects, and the margin of safety is reduced in CVD patients. As part of the multidisciplinary heart team, the cardiac anesthesiologist plays a central role in the shared decision-making regarding perioperative planning (see Fuster and Hurst's Central Illustration). This planning includes preoperative evaluation and risk assessment, creation of safe intraoperative monitoring and management plans, and development of postoperative pain control regimens and fast-track recovery pathways. Cardiovascular effects of general, neuraxial, and regional anesthetic techniques, as well as the risks and benefits of noninvasive and invasive perioperative monitoring methods, must be considered. An area of continued growth is nonoperating room anesthetizing locations, which have specific needs. As CVD remains highly prevalent in surgical populations, the need for effective communication among the specialties of cardiology, surgery, and anesthesiology will remain critical in assuring optimal patient outcomes.

INTRODUCTION

Providing safe anesthesia to patients with cardiovascular disease remains a great challenge. The constellation of anesthetic drug effects, the physiologic stresses of surgery, and underlying cardiovascular diseases can complicate and limit the choice of anesthetic techniques used for any specific procedure. The anesthesiologist's approach to the patient with cardiovascular disease is to select agents and techniques that will optimize the patient's cardiopulmonary function. The perioperative management of a patient with cardiovascular disease requires close cooperation between the cardiologist, interventionalist, intensivist, surgeon, and anesthesiologist. Each specialist has a unique knowledge base that complements that of the others. This multidisciplinary team approach should emphasize a continuum of care from the preoperative evaluation through the postoperative period.

Heart Team Concept

As the complexity of patients with cardiovascular disease requiring surgical interventions has increased over the last few decades, the concept of a hospital "Heart Team" has slowly emerged.[1-3] Specifically, it is a multidisciplinary decision-making team, tasked to select the most optimal treatment strategy for an individual patient.[3] Such an approach has been successfully utilized in other medical fields, including oncology and organ transplant medicine, with reported significant improvements in the quality of care.[4,5] Now this concept is emphasized in the context of treating patients with cardiovascular disease, becoming a standard of cardiovascular care worldwide.[1,2]

Although the exact composition of the Heart Team varies among institutions, in the cardiovascular arena, the noninvasive cardiologists, cardiac interventionalists, cardiac surgeons, and cardiac anesthesiologists are considered integral members of the institutional Heart Teams. In some cardiac subspecialties, such as myocardial revascularization, the Heart Team concept has recently become part of societies' guidelines recommendations.[6,7] Additionally, the Heart Team approach may increase research trial recruitment[8] and create robust collaborative clinical research opportunities.

A comprehensive and detailed patient assessment for medical versus interventional procedures, clear communication between medical providers, patient, and family, as well as collaborative perioperative problem-solving whenever the unexpected is encountered are at the center of a well-functioning and effective Heart Team.[1-3] In addition to providing clinical expertise by integrating and analyzing the available diagnostic evidence in the context of the given clinical condition, the individual patient's preferences are also considered in order to propose the most optimal treatment strategy.[3] The benefit of such shared decision-making has been shown in myocardial revascularization literature, for example, with improved survival outcomes.[9] Involvement of patients and their families has also been shown to increase patient satisfaction.[10]

The Anesthesiologist as Perioperative Consultant

Perioperative medicine is broadly defined as provision of medical care from the time of contemplation of surgery through the operative period to immediate postoperative recovery. In recent years, anesthesiologists' unique skillset, specifically the ability to seamlessly bridge the preoperative, intraoperative, and postoperative periods of a patient's medical care, has been increasingly recognized.[11] Consistent with that vision, a growing number of academic anesthesiology departments have amended their titles to include "perioperative medicine." As a member of the Heart Team, a cardiac anesthesiologist plays a central role in the shared decision-making perioperative planning: from preoperative evaluation and risk assessment to creation of a safe intraoperative monitoring and management plans to development of postoperative pain control regimen and fast-track recovery pathways.[11]

PREOPERATIVE EVALUATION

Classification Systems and Risk Scores

The assessment of cardiac risk and preoperative optimization of the patient's cardiovascular status are the traditional goals of the preoperative evaluation of patients with cardiovascular disease. In 1977, Goldman et al. initially introduced the Cardiac Risk Index Score (CRIS) to quantitatively guide the assignment of cardiac risk in patients undergoing noncardiac surgery.[12] The study had a major impact because clinicians concluded that preoperative improvements in heart failure symptoms and optimization of other comorbid conditions would decrease cardiac risk. The classification systems and risk scores continue to evolve and continue to help estimate perioperative risk.[13-17] The more recently developed scores include the Revised Cardiac Risk Index (RCRI), which is used to estimate a patient's risk of perioperative cardiac complications,[13,14] and the American College of Surgeons (ACS) NSQIP surgical risk calculator, used to estimate risk of any perioperative complications.[15] Specifically, the RCRI consists of six components, including presence of ischemic heart disease, cerebrovascular disease, chronic kidney disease with serum creatinine ≥ 2.0 mg/dL, heart failure, insulin-dependent diabetes, and high-risk surgery (vascular, or intraperitoneal, or intrathoracic); each of which is assigned one point toward the total score (0–6, 6 = worst).[13,18] Patients with an RCRI of 0 have an approximate risk of 0.4% for major cardiovascular complications, whereas those with an index of 3 or greater have an approximate risk of 10%.[17] The ACS NSQIP, on the other hand, is a more complex 21-component universal surgical risk calculator.[14,15]

Professional Society Guidelines

The American College of Cardiology (ACC)/American Heart Association (AHA) Task Force on Practice Guidelines published *Guidelines on Perioperative Cardiovascular Evaluation for Noncardiac Surgery*, last updated in 2014.[19] Similarly, the European Society of Cardiology (ESC) and European Society of Anaesthesiology (ESA) came out with guidelines on noncardiac surgery in 2014.[20] Although the algorithmic approach described in these guidelines has not yet been tested in any randomized clinical trial, it is nevertheless valuable in providing a consistent clinical approach to preoperative cardiovascular risk

---

BOX 73-1

Common Questions Asked During Preoperative Cardiac Evaluation (modified from ACC/AHA and ESC guidelines 2014)[19,20]

1. Is there a need for emergency noncardiac surgery?
2. Does the patient have signs of any cardiac conditions, including arrhythmias, symptomatic valvular abnormalities, ischemic heart disease, coronary stents, heart failure, systemic or pulmonary hypertension?
3. What is the patient's functional status? (Patients with adequate functional capacity should not have additional preoperative testing.)
4. If the patient's functional capacity is low, will further testing impact decision-making?
5. What is the patient's assessment of risk, based on either RCRI or NSQIP?
6. Based on the risk factors, what is the estimated combined surgical risk of major adverse cardiac events (MACE)?
7. Can nonsurgical treatments be considered as a viable alternative?
8. If patient proceeds with surgery, how can the risk of MACE be minimized? (Guideline-directed medical therapy, anesthetic technique, monitoring.)
9. Do patient's cardiac devices (such as pacemaker or implantable cardioverter-defibrillator) require interrogation or reprogramming pre- or intraoperatively?
10. Is the patient on anticoagulation or antiplatelet therapy that requires adjustment prior to surgery, or are there any contraindications for specific anesthetic techniques?

---

stratification. The information derived from the preoperative cardiac evaluation should provide answers to questions that are summarized in Box 73-1. Refer to Chapter 14 for additional details.

Biomarker Measurement

Perioperative risk assessment is a continuously evolving area of research and now includes preoperative measurement of biomarkers. There is some evidence that serum levels of several cardiac biomarkers, such as B-type natriuretic peptide (BNP), N-terminal pro-BNP (NT-ProBNP), cardiac troponin, or atrial stretch-induced polypeptide have been suggested to have a prognostic value for perioperative cardiovascular risk assessment.[19,21-23] However, the AHA/ACC guidelines do not yet recommend a BNP measurement as part of preoperative risk assessment, because biomarker-based perioperative management strategies have not yet been shown to reduce cardiovascular risk in the literature.[19] Furthermore, while the AHA/ACC guidelines recommend perioperative measurement of cardiac troponin levels whenever signs or symptoms are suggestive of myocardial ischemia or infarction,[19] a routine screening of cardiac troponin levels in asymptomatic patients is not recommended.

Anticoagulant and Antiplatelet Therapy

Cardiovascular disease management frequently includes anticoagulation therapy (eg, for stroke thromboprophylaxis

in patients with atrial fibrillation [AF]) or dual antiplatelet therapy (eg, following percutaneous coronary interventions [PCIs]). The surgical implications of such therapies include timing of surgery,[24] perioperative discontinuation of anticoagulation and/or antiplatelet regimen to minimize the risk of surgical bleeding without increasing the risk of stroke or coronary stent thrombosis, and postoperative reinstitution of these medications. Similarly, anticoagulant and antiplatelet therapies affect choice of anesthetic techniques. For example, administration of neuraxial anesthesia may need to be delayed or may be completely contraindicated. Potentially life-threatening complications may occur if current guidelines and recommendations are not followed (refer to section Neuraxial Anesthesia and Anticoagulation Therapy).

In patients with AF, anticoagulation has been typically interrupted 2 to 5 days prior to noncardiac surgery to reduce the risk of perioperative bleeding.[24] Douketis et al. randomly assigned patients with AF to either perioperative bridging therapy with low-molecular-weight heparin (after discontinuing warfarin 5 days before surgery) or placebo.[25] The authors found that the incidence of arterial thromboembolism was not different between the groups, but bridging anticoagulation patients had a statistically significant increased incidence of perioperative bleeding.[25]

The increased risk of perioperative cardiac events following PCI is related to perioperative hypercoagulability associated with surgical stress in the setting of nonendothelialized stent surfaces. The answers to when and if antiplatelet medications can be safely discontinued perioperatively is an ongoing process, as stent technology and drug therapies continue to evolve.[26-28] Ideally, elective noncardiac surgery should be delayed until the stent surface is fully endothelialized. The 2014 ACC/AHA guidelines do not recommend elective noncardiac surgery within 2 weeks of coronary balloon angioplasty, or 4 weeks after bare metal stent implantation.[19] Elective noncardiac surgery should be delayed for at least 6 months following drug-eluting stent (DES).[19,29] Such elective noncardiac surgery may be considered after 6 months or longer, if the risk of further delay is greater than the expected risks of myocardial infarction (MI) and stent thrombosis.[19,29] Yet, despite recommendations to delay noncardiac surgery after PCI,[29] approximately 3.5% of patients undergo noncardiac surgery within 6 months of stent placement.[30] For nonelective surgery, the task force encourages a consensus decision among the clinicians involved whether delaying surgery outweighs the risk of stent thrombosis. For urgent surgery that cannot be deferred and that necessitates interruption of thienopyridine therapy in the setting of recently placed coronary stents, aspirin should be continued if possible, and thienopyridine therapy should be restarted as soon as possible after the surgical procedure.[19] For a subset of high risk surgeries, such as neurosurgeries or ophthalmologic surgeries, temporary discontinuation of aspirin is also recommended after full discussion of the risks and benefits with the anesthesiologist, surgeon, and patient. In emergency procedures, patients on long-acting antiplatelet drugs have increased risk of hemorrhage, and platelet transfusions may be necessary to achieve hemostasis. Refer to Chapter 14 for additional details.

The American Society of Anesthesiologists (ASA) issued a Practice Alert for the perioperative management of patients with coronary artery stents in 2009.[29] Specifically, the alert reviewed published literature about the increased risk of perioperative MI and death, as well as relation between antiplatelet therapy and acute perioperative stent thrombosis.[29] The need for perioperative continuation of aspirin was emphasized, whenever possible, despite discontinuation of thienopyridine therapy in situations where surgery cannot be deferred in patients with recent coronary stents.[29]

More recent studies have emerged, focusing on perioperative management of patients on chronic antithrombotic therapy.[25,31] This is an emerging field that has seen introduction of new medications, such as novel oral anticoagulants, in the last decade. These agents introduce new issues and concerns with perioperative management.[32-34] Interruption of oral anticoagulant therapy may not be necessary in patients undergoing certain procedures with a low risk of bleeding risk, such as endodontal procedures, minor skin excisions, or cataract surgery.[31] However, interruption of such agents for moderate-high bleeding risk surgeries or invasive procedures is strongly recommended.[32-34] Those patients who are classified to have a moderate-to-high risk for thromboembolic complications raise greater concern for the possibility of a thromboembolic event during the period of time when their international normalized ratio (INR) may be subtherapeutic once anticoagulant therapy is paused. Unfractionated heparin may be used as a "bridge" for these patients in order to decrease the period of time when the patient is at an increased risk for thromboembolism.[25,31-34]

The selection and timing of short-acting agents are critical factors that affect the timing of surgery to avoid potential hemorrhaging or challenges with adequate hemostasis during the intraoperative and immediate postoperative periods. Additionally, recent studies have questioned the previously described dogmatic approach and currently there is no universal agreement on the specific withdrawal or reversal times for many anticoagulants.[32-34] The dilemma continues in the literature and interdisciplinary team discussions are warranted for each specific patient based on the evolving literature.[32-34]

Thus, a cogent summary of the pertinent clinical, laboratory, radiologic, echocardiographic, radionuclide, and cardiac catheterization data comprises the ideal cardiac consultation for the anesthesiologist. With the benefit of this information, the two specialties can make intelligent decisions regarding the patient's preoperative therapy and the optimal timing of surgery.

INTRAOPERATIVE ANESTHETIC MANAGEMENT

Risk assessment of perioperative cardiac complications, whether using RCRI or ACS NSQIP, informs the clinician's decision on whether surgery should proceed or if further medical optimization should be attempted prior to surgery. However, if surgery in a patient with significant risk is unavoidable, the anesthesiologist must choose an anesthetic technique, continue implementing guideline-directed medical therapy, and choose appropriate monitoring to further reduce the risk of perioperative cardiac complications.

Choice of Anesthetic Technique

The choice of anesthetic technique is inherently challenging because multiple factors must be considered. These include patient preferences, the requirements of the surgical procedure, and the patient's underlying medical condition(s). There is little scientific evidence that any specific anesthetic technique is superior to reasonable alternatives, or that anesthetic technique per se influences patient outcome. Published studies show controversial results,[35-37] with conflicting clinical evidence regarding the clear benefits of any one technique.

Recently, Leslie et al. analyzed patients registered in the PeriOperative ISchemic Evaluation-2 (POISE-2) trial regarding the effect of a neuraxial technique (spinal, lumbar epidural, or thoracic epidural) versus a general anesthetic on 30-day adverse cardiovascular outcomes (ie, death, stroke, MI).[38] In this post hoc subanalysis, 3986 patients with a neuraxial block were compared to 4938 control patients who received general anesthesia. Neuraxial anesthesia or postoperative epidural analgesia were not associated with death, MI, or stroke in high-risk noncardiac surgery patients.[38] Similarly, Poeran et al. retrospectively analyzed 98,290 elective colectomies, with general anesthesia used in the majority of cases (93.9%), while the remainder of patients received a combined anesthetic that included a neuraxial technique.[39] Although the addition of a neuraxial technique was associated with a decreased risk for thromboembolism and cerebrovascular events, MI, and other morbid outcomes, such as urinary tract infection, postoperative ileus, blood transfusion, and admission to the intensive care unit (ICU), were observed more frequently in the neuraxial group. Overall, the findings were inconsistent, showing no clear advantage for either anesthetic technique. In a systematic review, Guay et al.[40] inferred that there is a moderate level of evidence that the addition of a neuraxial technique to a general anesthetic may reduce 30-day mortality and the risk of pneumonia, but such addition does not impact rates of MI.

Overall, there are no definite recommendations for choosing a particular anesthetic to decrease the risk of perioperative cardiac complications. The most effective strategies remain preoperative optimization and vigilant perioperative monitoring to allow for early detection of hemodynamic compromise (refer to Chapter 14 for additional details).

In certain defined surgical procedures (eg, transurethral resection of prostate), a neuraxial technique may be advantageous in enabling early recognition of complications. This is not applicable to all circumstances, however, and clinical judgment must be exercised to make the best choices in individual circumstances. Regional anesthetics and monitored anesthesia care are sometimes converted to general anesthetics intraoperatively due to unexpectedly long surgery, patient discomfort, or changes in the surgical plan. No practitioner can be certain that a specific technique will be adequate for the surgical procedure, given the unpredictability of the situation, and a given anesthesiologist must have flexibility to alter the technique, as dictated by clinical needs. Therefore, communication among perioperative clinicians is essential; it is often not beneficial for the cardiologist or internist to recommend exclusion of specific anesthetic technique(s) during their preoperative consultation.

General Anesthesia

General anesthesia (GA) is defined as a reversible state consisting of amnesia, analgesia, anxiolysis, immobility, unconsciousness, and suppression of reflexes. The general anesthetics include many drugs, almost all of which have cardiovascular side effects. Intravenous agents are nearly always used for the induction of anesthesia in adults. Anesthesia is maintained using inhalational agents, intravenous agents, or a combination of the two.

Neuromuscular blocking drugs (muscle relaxants) are used to facilitate tracheal intubation, to lower the requirements for anesthetic agents, and to prevent involuntary muscular activity in surgical cases where complete paralysis is mandatory. In children, the induction of anesthesia is highly individualized according to patient needs, the practitioner's preferences, and institutional standards. With few exceptions, most general anesthetics include tracheal intubation and mechanical ventilation. As an alternative to tracheal intubation, supraglottic devices, such as the laryngeal mask airway, may be used to secure a patient's airway. Loss of consciousness is usually accompanied by a decrease in sympathetic tone. This, as well as the effects of positive pressure ventilation and the cardiac depressant properties of inhalational and most intravenous anesthetic agents, causes a moderate decrease in cardiac output.

General anesthesia masks many of the symptoms of cardiovascular decompensation, such as angina, dyspnea, dizziness, and palpitations. Other signs of cardiovascular disease, such as tachycardia or hypo- or hypertension, are nonspecific and may be misinterpreted as being caused by vasodilation, hypovolemia, pain, or inadequate depth of anesthesia. Depending on the type of surgery, large fluid shifts and decreased venous return may occur, sometimes unpredictably. It is for these reasons that

appropriate monitoring and selection of anesthetic agents is vital to the safe intraoperative management of the patient with cardiovascular disease.

Intravenous Anesthetics

Intravenous anesthetic induction medications are composed of lipophilic molecules that have an affinity for neuronal tissue or specific receptors. Their anesthetic actions (ie, hypnosis) are generally terminated by redistribution from the vessel-rich tissues (brain, heart, liver, and kidneys) to other tissues (muscle, fat, and skin). Elimination via hepatic metabolism and renal excretion is typically much slower and takes place over several hours. Most intravenous anesthetics exhibit some degree of cardiovascular depression in the form of reduced cardiac output or vasodilation. Reduced doses and slower injection of the drug (titrating to effect) will markedly decrease these cardiovascular effects. The use of synthetic opioids (ie, fentanyl, sufentanil, or remifentanil), etomidate, or ketamine may be indicated in patients with severely compromised cardiac function, since they tend to maintain hemodynamic stability. **Table 73–1** summarizes commonly used intravenous anesthetics.

Inhalational Anesthetics

Inhalational anesthetics include nitrous oxide and the potent volatile anesthetic agents, such as sevoflurane, desflurane, and isoflurane. Nitrous oxide has analgesic properties, but it is not a potent anesthetic. Concentrations up to 75% may be given safely (to maintain an adequate FiO_2), but incomplete amnesia, postoperative nausea, and movement in response to painful stimuli are likely. Thus, nitrous oxide is nearly always administered with other anesthetic agents, such as opioids or potent volatile anesthetics, and neuromuscular blockers. Many anesthesiologists opt to avoid nitrous oxide altogether, due to the minimal analgesic benefits and increasingly recognized undesirable side effects.

The use of inhalational anesthesia with potent volatile anesthetics is the most common anesthetic technique because of

		Cardiovascular Effects				
Generic Name	**Class**	**BP**	**HR**	**SVR**	**CO**	**Notes/Adverse Effects**
Midazolam	Benzodiazepine	–/↓	–/↑	–/↓	–/↓	Anxiolysis, sedation, amnesia
Morphine	Opioid	↓	↓	↓	–/↓	Histamine release
Fentanyl	Opioid	–/↓	↓	–/↓	–/↓	Chest wall rigidity
Sufentanil	Opioid	–/↓	↓	–/↓	–/↓	Chest wall rigidity
Remifentanil	Opioid	–/↓	↓	–/↓	–/↓	Chest wall rigidity
Meperidine	Opioid	↓	↑			Histamine release, anti-shivering
Ketamine	Phencyclidine	↑	↑	↑	↑	Dissociative anesthesia, analgesia
Etomidate	Imidazole derivative	–/↓	–/↓	–/↓	–	Adrenocortical suppression
Propofol	Phenol derivative	↓	–	↓	↓	Rapid recovery
Dexmedetomidine, clonidine	α_2-Agonist	↓	↓	↓	↓	Sedation, sympatholysis, anxiolysis, analgesia, bolus administration may cause transient increase in BP, dexmedetomidine more selective α_2-Agonist

TABLE 73–1. Intravenous Anesthetics

Abbreviations: BP, arterial blood pressure; CO, cardiac output; HR, heart rate; SVR, systemic vascular resistance; –, no or minimal change; ↓, decrease; ↑, increase.

its relatively low cost, ease of use, reliable amnesia, and over-all safety profile. The effect of these agents is rapidly changed when the inspiratory concentration is adjusted. The ability to easily titrate inhalational anesthetics is an advantage compared with intravenous drugs, because the duration of surgical procedures and the degree of surgical stimulation are often unpredictable. All volatile agents are myocardial depressants at higher doses and cause vasodilation resulting in some degree of hypotension. **Table 73–2** summarizes commonly used inhalational anesthetics in current practice.

There is evidence that potent volatile anesthetics offer some degree of myocardial protection from ischemic insult.[41] The mechanisms of anesthetic drug-induced protection from myocardial injury are complex, thought to be related to adaptive and protective cellular processes that confer protection to recurrent ischemic events. Myocardial preconditioning to ischemic events (ie, temporary coronary occlusion) elicits these processes; however, some volatile anesthetic agents and certain anesthetic drugs, such as opioids, mimic ischemic preconditioning.[41-45] Substantial literature has been published on this topic. In clinical practice, however, no meaningful differences in major outcome parameters have been found. The time course of administration of potent volatile agents (pre- vs. postconditioning), other comorbidities (eg, diabetes mellitus), and drugs that may abolish protective effects (eg, ketamine, β-blockers, and certain sulfonylureas) must be considered.[46-48] Currently, there are no conclusive data regarding which patients may benefit from anesthetic preconditioning or postconditioning.[42-48]

Neuromuscular Blockade

Two major classes of nondepolarizing neuromuscular blocking drugs are currently used: benzylisoquinolinium compounds (eg, cisatracurium) and aminosteroid derivates (eg, vecuronium and rocuronium). Cisatracurium undergoes a unique form of spontaneous degradation that is organ-independent (Hofmann elimination), and, therefore, is frequently used in patients with renal insufficiency or hepatic failure. Vecuronium is an aminosteroid nondepolarizing neuromuscular

blocking drug with an intermediate duration of action. Vecuronium does not have clinically significant cardiovascular adverse effects. Rocuronium has a more rapid onset of action, due to its lower potency and slightly increases heart rate. The modern aminosteroid compounds are mainly degraded by the liver. These nondepolarizing neuromuscular blocking drugs require reversal at the end of a procedure to restore normal muscle function and respiration. The pharmacologic reversal is usually produced with a combination of neostigmine and glycopyrrolate, which may lead to bradycardia, tachycardia, or other arrhythmias in patients with cardiovascular disease, and has been associated with cardiac arrest in patients with prior heart transplants. Recently, a new reversal agent, sugammadex, that traps aminosteroid molecules has been approved. It produces none of these adverse cardiovascular effects.[49,50]

Succinylcholine is a depolarizing short-acting neuromuscular blocker that is associated with rapid onset, and short duration of action. Its cardiovascular effects depend on whether nicotinic or muscarinic receptor effects predominate in a given patient. Thus, either tachycardia and hypertension or bradycardia and hypotension may occur. Vagal effects tend to predominate with repeated doses in children. In patients with various disorders (including neuromuscular diseases, recent burns, and massive trauma), hyperkalemic cardiac arrest may occur due to an exaggerated release of intracellular potassium from myocytes. It is, therefore, not recommended for routine use, particularly in children.

Neuraxial and Regional Anesthesia

Cushing coined the term *regional anesthesia* for operations where local anesthetics were used to operate on localized areas of the body without loss of consciousness. Regional anesthesia typically involves the use of a local anesthetic to block sensation and pain from one or several large peripheral nerves and associated area(s) of distribution. Neuraxial anesthesia infers placement of a local anesthetic around the nerves of the central nervous system (ie, spinal or epidural anesthesia).

The advantages of either technique include simplicity, low cost, and minimal equipment requirements. Many of the adverse effects of general anesthesia are avoided, such as myocardial and respiratory depression. There are many surgical procedures, however, that are not amenable to a regional or neuraxial anesthetic technique. Serious side effects, such as hypotension, may be long-lasting and not reversed as easily compared to a general anesthetic. Additional contraindications include use of systemic anticoagulation, use of select antiplatelet therapy, the patients' refusal to be awake in the operating room (OR), and local or systemic infections. The combination of a regional or neuraxial technique with a general anesthetic can be advantageous in providing adequate analgesia extending into the postoperative period with the added advantages of allowing for earlier mobilization and likely reducing thromboembolic risk.

Local Anesthetic Agents

Local anesthetics are classified based on their chemical structure as esters or amides. The esters are hydrolyzed by esterases in the plasma, and the amides are metabolized in the liver. The

TABLE 73–2. Inhalational Anesthetics

Inhalational Agent	Cardiovascular Effects				Notes
	BP	HR	SVR	CO	
Nitrous oxide	–	–	–	–	Rapidly diffuses into closed air spaces
Isoflurane	↓	↑	↓	–	Coronary steal clinically not significant
Desflurane	↓	–/↑	↓	–	Rapid induction and emergence, sympathomimetic during rapid induction
Sevoflurane	↓	–	↓	–	Preferred inhalational induction agent for children, nonpungent, potential nephrotoxicity

Abbreviations: BP, arterial blood pressure; CO, cardiac output; HR, heart rate; SVR, systemic vascular resistance; –, no or minimal change; ↓, decrease; ↑, increase.

duration of action of local anesthetic agents is affected by the protein-binding characteristics of the molecule. Epinephrine and phenylephrine, which produce local vasoconstriction, may be added in small doses to local anesthetic solutions to prolong their duration of action. The systemic absorption of epinephrine occurs very slowly, and the β-adrenergic effects predominate. This results in slight tachycardia and diastolic hypotension, which is undesirable in patients with certain cardiovascular diseases. Toxic reactions to local anesthetics are generally characterized by central nervous system excitation (seizures), which may be followed by central nervous system depression and cardiovascular collapse. **Table 73–3** provides an overview of commonly used local anesthetics in current practice.

Neuraxial: Spinal Anesthesia

The injection of a relatively small dose of local anesthetic into the subarachnoid space produces profound motor and sensory blockade. The level of the anesthetic block is usually controlled by the choice of local anesthetic, level of medication injection, and the position of the patient. Spinal anesthesia also produces blockade of preganglionic sympathetic fibers, resulting in a sympathetic blockade that is generally two dermatomal segments higher than the sensory dermatomal level. If the dermatomal level of sympathetic blockade reaches T1, then a complete sympathectomy is present until the block recedes. Higher levels of sympathetic blockade are associated with profound hypotension from arterial and venous vasodilatation, as well as bradycardia from the loss of cardiac accelerator fiber function. Blockade above a T2 level also produces respiratory insufficiency due to intercostal and phrenic nerve root blockade. Cardiovascular collapse and respiratory insufficiency (or apnea) are the signs of a "total spinal," a life-threatening situation that must be treated with tracheal intubation and aggressive vasoactive support. Because of the risk of sudden severe vasodilation and hypotension, spinal anesthesia is contraindicated in patients with preload dependent cardiovascular

diseases, such as severe valvular aortic stenosis or hypertrophic obstructive cardiomyopathy.

Neuraxial: Epidural Anesthesia

The epidural space lies immediately external to the dura mater and is filled with loose areolar tissue and a venous plexus. An indwelling catheter is usually placed percutaneously for intermittent bolus injections or continuous infusions of local anesthetic with or without opioids. The epidural space may be entered by thoracic, lumbar, or caudal approaches. The hemodynamic effects of epidural anesthesia are similar to those of spinal anesthesia, except that the onset of sympathetic blockade is more gradual. Thus, with appropriate monitoring, cautious administration of epidural anesthetics can be performed safely, even in patients with valvular aortic stenosis, or hypertrophic obstructive cardiomyopathy. In patients with cardiovascular disease, advanced monitoring techniques should be strongly considered. Beat-to-beat blood pressure monitoring via an intraarterial catheter, and a secure route of central drug administration, for example via a central venous catheter, allows the practitioner to monitor and promptly treat changes in hemodynamic parameters.

In patients with known coronary artery disease, epidural anesthesia and analgesia, especially thoracic epidural catheters, have been shown to reduce intraoperative and early postoperative ischemic events, lower hormonal stress response, and reduce the incidence of AF.[51,52] Patient outcome data, however, were inconclusive when epidural anesthesia was compared with general anesthesia in patients at risk for perioperative cardiac events undergoing vascular surgery.[53,54]

When compared with spinal anesthesia, epidural anesthesia requires higher doses of local anesthetic. This increases the potential for complications and adverse effects from inadvertent intravascular injection or absorption that can cause severe arrhythmias, including ventricular fibrillation and cardiovascular collapse. Potent local anesthetics such as bupivacaine and, to a lesser degree, ropivacaine are more cardiotoxic compared with lidocaine. The slower rate of recovery of fast sodium ion channels in the conduction system and myocardium seen with bupivacaine is frequently identified as the reason for its increased cardiotoxicity. Cardiac resuscitation following inadvertent intravenous administration and cardiac arrest is difficult. Intravenous lipid emulsion has been successfully used to reverse local anesthetic toxicity,[55,56] and is now recommended to treat cardiovascular collapse from local anesthetic toxicity.[57] The hemodynamic consequences of inadvertent intravenous injections of epinephrine-containing solutions may be significant for patients who cannot tolerate tachycardia. Epidural infusions of local anesthetic with or without opioids for postoperative analgesia may be complicated by pruritus, nausea, urinary retention, somnolence, and respiratory depression. Thus, appropriate monitoring and nursing care are required.

Neuraxial Anesthesia and Anticoagulation Therapy

Intraoperative central neuraxial anesthesia (eg, spinal and epidural) and postoperative neuraxial analgesia are contraindicated in patients with antithrombotic or thrombolytic therapy.[58]

TABLE 73–3. Local Anesthetics

Generic	Class	Uses	Notes/Adverse Effects
Cocaine	Ester	T	Central nervous system toxicity, arrhythmias, myocardial ischemia
Procaine	Ester	S, I	Vasoconstriction
Chloroprocaine	Ester	E, S, C, I	
Tetracaine	Ester	S, I, T	
Lidocaine	Amide	E, S, C, I, T	Antiarrhythmic properties
Mepivacaine	Amide	E, S, C, I	
Prilocaine	Amide	E, C, I	Methemoglobinemia
Bupivacaine	Amide	E, S, C, I	High cardiotoxicity, cardiovascular collapse
Levobupivacaine	Amide	E, S, C, I	Less cardiotoxicity compared with bupivacaine
Ropivacaine	Amide	E, S, C, I	Less cardiotoxicity compared with bupivacaine

Abbreviations: C, caudal; E, epidural; I, infiltration/field block; S, spinal; T, topical.

Appropriate patient selection is crucial to avoid potentially catastrophic complications, such as paraplegia from a spinal hematoma. A careful evaluation of medication history and bleeding diathesis provides essential information, since the risk of bleeding associated with many antithrombotic therapies will not be detected by standard preoperative coagulation tests.[58]

The establishment of guidelines for the use of neuraxial anesthesia and analgesia in patients who have or will receive anticoagulants is an evolving process. Recommendations from the American Society of Regional Anesthesia and Pain Medicine (ASRA) for appropriate withdrawal of anticoagulant and antiplatelet therapy prior to neuraxial anesthesia and can be found at https://www.asra.com.[58,59] **Table 73–4** summarizes these guidelines and the current literature. It is prudent to avoid neuraxial anesthesia in patients who are receiving potent antiplatelet drugs that include glycoprotein IIb/IIIa antagonists,

TABLE 73–4. Anticoagulation and Antiplatelet Therapy: Recommendations for Neuraxial Anesthesia (NA)[79-82]

Medication Class / Mechanism of Action	Medications (route of administration)	Clinical Test	Recommendations
Unfractionated Heparin (UH)	heparin (IV)	aPTT	1. UH IV: Neuraxial anesthetic is contraindicated in fully anticoagulated patients. 2. Prophylactic subcutaneous UH: no increased risk. 3. IV heparin infusion safe if started >1 h after needle placement; catheter removal 1 h before subsequent dose and 6-8 h following last heparin dose.
Low Molecular Weight Heparin (LMWH) and heparinoids; Xa indirect inhibitor	enoxaparin (SQ), fondaparinux (SQ)	Not useful	1. Increased risk for NA, especially when used in conjunction with antiplatelet therapy or NSAIDS. 2. Safe time interval between last administration and neuraxial manipulation varies depending on type and dosing interval. Enoxaparin >12-24 hrs, fondaparinux >36-42 hrs. 3. Administration with catheter in place is contraindicated. 4. Catheter removal 10-12 hrs after last LMWH dose; next dose 4-24 hrs after catheter removal depending on anticoagulant.
Vitamin K inhibitor	warfarin (PO)	PT	1. INR<1.5 before administration of neuraxial anesthesia. 2. Warfarin administration absolutely contraindicated while neuraxial catheter in place. 3. Neuraxial catheters should be removed when the INR is <1.5; wait 6 hrs after catheter removal before next dose administered.
Direct thrombin inhibitor (DTI)	lepirudin (IV), desirudin (IV), bivalirudin (IV), argatroban (IV), dabigatran (PO)	Thrombin time Ecarin clothing assays, aPTT, PT, and INR are unreliable	1. Significantly increased risk of spinal hematoma particularly with concomitant use of antiplatelet agents. 2. Safe time interval between last dose and safe neuraxial anesthesia not known. For dabigatran, at least 4-5 days and longer (up to 7 days) in renal insufficiency. 3. In patients taking argatroban or bivalirudin, neuraxial anesthesia is probably best avoided. 4. Dosing is contraindicated while catheter is in place. 5. In patients taking dabigatran, restart 2 hrs after catheter removal.
Direct factor Xa inhibitors (NOACs)	rivaroxaban (PO), apixaban (PO), edoxaban (PO)	Not useful	1. Safe time interval between last dose and safe neuraxial anesthesia 3 days. 2. 24 hours before neuraxial manipulation. Longer wait times in renal insufficiency.
COX inibitor	aspirin (PO)	Not useful	Very low risk unless used in conjunction with other antiplatelet or anticoagulant medications. No time restriction for catheter placement or removal.
Non-steroidal anti-inflammatory drugs (NSAIDs)	diclofenac (PO), ketorolac (PO), ibuprofen (PO), naproxen (PO)	Not useful	Very low risk unless used in conjunction with other antiplatelet or anticoagulant medications. No time restriction for catheter placement or removal.
Phosphodiesterase inhibitors	dipyridamole (IV or PO), cilostazol (PO)	Not useful	1. Minimum time between last dose and NA is 24 hrs for dipyridamole and 2 days for cilostazol. 2. Dosing is contraindicated while catheter is in place. 3. Minimum time between NA or catheter removal and next dose is 6 hrs for dipyrimadole and 6 hrs for cilostazol.
P2Y12 inhibitors	clopidogrel (PO), prasugrel (PO), ticagrelor (PO), cangrelor (IV)	Not useful	1. Clopidogrel is recommended to be discontinued for 7 days prior to NA, prasugrel discontinued for 10 days prior to NA, ticagrelor for 5 days prior to NA, and cangrelor for 3 hrs prior to NA. 2. Administration is contraindicated while catheter in place. 3. Minimum time between NA or catheter removal and when next dose can be given for clopidogrel 2 hrs, for prasugrel 6 hrs, for ticagrelor 6 hrs, and for cangrelor 8 hrs.
GP IIB/IIIA inhibitors	Abciximab (IV), eptifibatide (IV)		1. Minimum time between last dose and NA for abciximab is 48 hrs, for eptifibatide 8 hrs. 2. Dosing is contraindicated while catheter in place. 3. Minimum time between NA or catheter removal and next dose is 2 hrs.

direct-acting $P2Y_{12}$-receptor antagonists, adenosine diphosphate inhibitors, and low molecular weight heparins. There is currently very limited data on the safe use of the oral agent dabigatran, the intravenous thrombin inhibitors bivalirudin and argatroban, and the direct oral factor Xa inhibitors rivaroxaban, apixaban, and edoxaban, in patients considered for neuraxial anesthesia.[59,60] For patient safety, it is also crucial to monitor neurologic status carefully after administration of spinal or epidural anesthesia; rapid diagnosis and treatment of neuraxial hematoma probably improves outcome.[60]

Regional: Nerve Blocks and Infiltration of Local Anesthetic

Nerve blocks and local anesthetic infiltration may be performed to facilitate surgery of localized areas of the body. For upper extremity surgery, the brachial plexus can be blocked by various approaches. The lower extremity may be anesthetized by blocking the femoral, obturator, and sciatic nerves. Local anesthetic infiltration ("field block") is performed in defined regions, such as the inguinal area. These blocks, when properly performed, have minimal cardiovascular effects. They do, however, require large volumes of local anesthetic solution, which result in toxic reactions if inadvertent intravascular injection occurs. Intercostal blocks are associated with high blood concentrations even without intravascular injection, because the neurovascular bundle enhances absorption of the local anesthetic, and multiple blocks are required for clinical efficacy. Recently, thoracic paravertebral blocks have been used more frequently for patients having unilateral surgery to avoid the hemodynamic effects of epidural blockade.

Regional: New Fascial Blocks

An emergent area of regional anesthesia use includes its administration for sternal-sparing cardiac surgeries[61-63] and cardiovascular implantable electronic device (CIED) procedures.[64] The choices of specific anatomical placement of the fascial plane blocks is dictated by the location of the surgical incision[60] and includes: uni- or bilateral serratus anterior nerve block,[62,63,65] intercostal nerve block using the subpectoral interfascial plane approach,[66] pectoralis I and II nerve block,[65,67] erector spinae plane block,[65,68] and transverse thoracic muscle plane block.[69]

Few complications have been reported with administration of fascial blocks in the cardiothoracic population.[67,69] Theoretical complications include infection, pneumothorax, hematoma from vascular injury, intravascular local anesthetic injection, or local anesthetic systemic toxicity.[65]

These ultrasound-guided regional plane blocks have been administered preoperatively to serve as a primary intraoperative anesthetic, or postoperatively as an effective adjunct to a multimodal pain management strategy.[61-72] In this latter capacity, the regional technique allows for either overall decreased opioid use or generation of a completely opioid-sparing analgesic, without any pain relief worsening as compared to standard opioid-based perioperative pain management regimen.[70,71] Although few randomized controlled trials are available because the plane blocks are relatively new techniques, their role in a multimodal analgesic regimen is crucial. Furthermore, the relative safety and theoretically low risk in an anticoagulated

surgical patient may lead to improved postoperative pain management with these techniques.[72]

Perioperative Monitoring

Noninvasive Monitoring

Basic Hemodynamics: Perioperative monitoring has significantly contributed to attainment of the level of safety provided by modern anesthesia, allowing for more complex surgeries, even in the higher risk patients. The ASA established standards for basic intraoperative monitoring in 1986, with subsequent amendments most current of which was in 2015.[73] Intraoperative monitoring that is required based on these guidelines include the following: (1) heart rate, (2) electrocardiogram (ECG), (3) blood pressure, (4) pulse oximetry, (5) capnography, and (6) body temperature.

Cerebral Monitoring: Various "brain function" monitors using proprietary electroencephalographic analysis have been developed for the purpose of monitoring depth of sedation and level of consciousness.[74-78] Incomplete amnesia leading to intraoperative awareness is rare with current anesthetic techniques, with a reported incidence of 0.1% to 0.2%.[79,80] Although there is an ongoing discussion on whether the prevention of intraoperative awareness episodes should be a therapeutic goal for anesthesiologists, the ASA does not currently recommend routine brain function monitoring in patients undergoing general anesthesia.[80] Elevated risk of intraoperative awareness may be classified into three major groups: patient related, surgery related, and anesthetic technique related.[79] Specifically, intraoperative awareness has been associated with a prior history of intraoperative awareness, morbid obesity, substance abuse, chronic pain patients with opioid tolerance, and certain procedures (eg, trauma surgery, emergency surgery, obstetric surgery). Intraoperative brain function monitoring should thus be used on a case-by-case basis.

Near-infrared spectroscopy (NIRS) for measurement of cerebral oximetry has gained increasing popularity for monitoring the oxygen supply-demand ratio of the brain. The cerebral tissue saturations (derived from the outer cortex of the frontal lobes) mainly reflect the venous component, continuously, in real time. Thus, it can be viewed as a correlate of the jugular bulb saturation, with a constant bias toward higher readings due to the approximately 25% to 30% admixture of arterial blood in cerebral tissue.[81,82] Variables affecting cerebral saturations include cardiac output, cerebral perfusion pressure, oxygen carrying capacity, partial pressure of carbon dioxide ($PaCO_2$), anesthetic depth, and temperature.[82,83] Technical problems, such as cardiopulmonary bypass (CPB) cannula malpositioning in the superior vena cava or aorta could lead to acute changes. Trend monitoring, compared with baseline values obtained during hemodynamically stable conditions, as well as absolute lower thresholds have been recommended in clinical practice for decision-making.

Although there is increasing evidence that low cerebral saturations are associated with adverse outcomes, few studies show that interventions based on cerebral oximetry monitoring improve outcomes.[84-87] Murkin et al. monitored cerebral oximetry and targeted therapy to optimize cerebral tissue oxygenation in patients undergoing coronary artery bypass grafting.[84] They found that a composite measure of postoperative organ dysfunction was substantially improved in the treatment group, where goal-directed therapy aimed to maintain the cerebral tissue oxygen saturation values within 25% of the preinduction baseline.[84] More recently, in a prospective randomized controlled single blind trial, Kunst et al. examined the effect of cerebral oxygenation intraoperative optimization in elderly patients undergoing coronary artery bypass graft surgery on postoperative cognitive decline or delirium.[85] When the intervention group (bispectral index [BIS] target values 50 ± 10, regional cerebral tissue desaturations target values between −50% to +15% preinduction values) was compared to the control group (no adjustments based on BIS or regional cerebral tissue desaturation parameters), the incidence of cognitive function was found to be similar, yet postoperative delirium was observed to be significantly less in the intervention group.[85] Targeted therapy to optimize cerebral oxygenation was associated with better memory outcome in a group of cardiac surgical patients.[87]

One of the strengths of cerebral oximetry monitoring is the detection of catastrophic events, particularly during periods of nonpulsatile flow, such as during CPB, with certain left ventricular assist devices, or extracorporeal membrane oxygenation.[88,89] Additional clinical settings where this technology is increasingly deployed includes monitoring collateral cerebral blood flow during carotid endarterectomy or stenting,[90] ventricular tachycardia ablation in the electrophysiology lab,[91] real-time assessment of advanced cardiac life support/resuscitation efforts,[92,93] and pediatric cardiac surgery.[94] Cerebral oximetry combined with invasive blood pressure monitoring has been used to determine cerebral autoregulation blood pressure limits in real time, allowing individualized blood pressure treatment.[95,96]

Transthoracic Echocardiography:
Clinical applications of perioperative cardiac ultrasound have been expanding rapidly, and its use is becoming a standard of care in multiple clinical settings.[97-101] Although transthoracic echocardiography (TTE) has been traditionally used by cardiologists for diagnosis and management of patients with cardiac diseases, its clinical utility in the fields of anesthesiology and critical care medicine is increasingly recognized.[13,97-101] Specifically, benefits of point of care/focused TTE have been reported in various settings: perioperatively in emergency cases,[100] intraoperatively in cardiac procedures[99] and noncardiac surgeries,[98] and postoperatively in the ICUs.[101] Furthermore, perioperative ultrasound training, including basic TTE and lung ultrasound skills, has become part of a standard anesthesiology residency curriculum in the United States and is now specifically tested by the American Board of Anesthesiology as part of anesthesiology board exam.[102]

Invasive Monitoring
The indications for the use of more invasive monitors, such as intra-arterial and central venous monitoring, vary and depend

---

TABLE 73-5. Indications for Intra-Arterial Monitoring

- Major surgical procedures involving large fluid shifts and/or blood loss
- Surgery requiring cardiopulmonary bypass
- Major aortic surgery including surgery of the aorta requiring cross-clamping
- Patients with recent myocardial infarctions, unstable angina, or severe coronary artery disease
- Patients with decreased left ventricular function (congestive heart failure) or significant valvular heart disease
- Patients in hypovolemic, cardiogenic, or septic shock, or with multiple organ failure
- Procedures involving the use of deliberate hypotension or deliberate hypothermia
- Massive trauma
- Patients with right heart failure, chronic obstructive pulmonary disease, pulmonary hypertension, or pulmonary embolism
- Patients with electrolyte or metabolic disturbances requiring frequent blood samples
- Patients with pulmonary disease requiring frequent arterial blood gases
- Inability to measure arterial pressure noninvasively (eg, morbid obesity)

---

on patient and surgery specific factors, as well as institution and practitioner preferences (**Tables 73-5, 73-6, 73-7**).[103] It must be recognized though, that monitoring guidelines are almost entirely based on observational cohort analyses and expert opinion. Although adequate monitoring is essential for early detection of hemodynamic disturbances, a specific monitoring technique will not result in improved outcome unless timely and effective treatment is initiated and available.

Pulmonary Artery Catheter: The indications for pulmonary arterial catheter (PAC) monitoring are especially controversial. Large randomized prospective studies of PAC use in various clinical settings have failed to demonstrate improved patient outcomes.[104-108] As with all monitoring devices, the caregiver's competency in interpreting PAC-derived data and instituting appropriate treatment is essential to derive maximal benefit and avoid complications.[109-111] The ASA published practice parameters to guide practitioners in the appropriate use of the PAC.[112] The decision to use perioperative PAC monitoring should be based on a combination of patient risk factors, surgical risk, and the experience of the practitioner. Many clinicians believe

---

TABLE 73-6. Indications for Central Venous Line Placement

- Major operative procedures involving large fluid shifts and/or blood loss
- Major trauma
- Inadequate peripheral intravenous access
- Frequent venous blood sampling
- Rapid infusion of intravenous fluids (eg, major trauma, liver transplantation)
- Venous access for vasoactive or irritating drugs
- Chronic drug administration (eg, antibiotics, chemotherapy)
- Total parenteral nutrition
- Surgical procedures with a high risk of air embolism
- Intravascular volume assessment when urine output is not reliable or unavailable
- Patients with tricuspid stenosis

TABLE 73-7. Indications for Intraoperative Use of Transesophageal Echocardiography

- Major surgical procedures involving large fluid shifts and/or blood loss
- Surgery requiring cardiopulmonary bypass
- Major valvular surgery, including surgery of the aorta requiring cross-clamping
- Major transplant surgery, including heart, lung, liver transplantation
- Coronary artery bypass surgery, with or without cardiopulmonary bypass
- Congenital heart disease repair surgeries
- Surgery requiring resection of tumor invading major vasculature (renal cell)
- Surgery for blunt chest trauma
- Patients with recent myocardial infarctions, unstable angina, or severe coronary artery disease
- Patients with decreased left ventricular function (congestive heart failure) or significant valvular heart disease, undergoing major surgery
- Patients in hypovolemic, cardiogenic, or septic shock, or with multiple organ failure
- Structural heart procedures requiring echocardiographic guidance and those involving trans-septal puncture
- Patients with right heart failure, moderate to severe pulmonary hypertension, or pulmonary embolism

that certain patient groups benefit from PAC monitoring, such as selected patients undergoing cardiac surgery or liver transplantation, and patients with clinically significant right ventricular failure or severe pulmonary hypertension.[113]

Transesophageal Echocardiography: Transesophageal echocardiography (TEE) is less invasive compared to PAC and has become an integral part of perioperative management. The more widespread availability of these devices in the OR and ICU setting, and the development of newer modalities such as three-dimensional echocardiography and tissue Doppler, enhanced the ability of anesthesiologists, cardiologists, and surgeons to make intraoperative diagnoses, evaluate hemodynamic aberrations, and assess the quality and outcomes of cardiac surgical interventions.

TEE is now the most popular supplemental hemodynamic monitoring technology. As its clinical use has expanded, the standardized intraoperative examination guidelines for multiplane TEE[114,115] and training guidelines[116,117] have been published. The National Board of Echocardiography administers a certification process. The ASA and ACC have published practice guidelines that address perioperative TEE.[118,119] These guidelines focus on the use of TEE in surgical patients intraoperatively for cardiac and noncardiac surgeries, as well as postoperatively in the critical care setting, yet do not apply to nonsurgical or postdischarge patients.[118] The importance of physician proficiency in the use of perioperative TEE is highlighted by the Task Force, as risk of adverse outcomes is inherent from incorrect TEE interpretations.[118] These are guidelines only, and the practitioner should decide on intraoperative TEE monitoring based on their level of training and experience, as well as patient- and surgery-related factors. Significant updates have been provided on the use of TEE for critically ill patients and as an intraoperative TEE for ischemic heart disease, congestive heart failure, cardiomyopathies, and assessment of the LV function.[119,120]

Cardiac Output and Goal-Directed Therapy: Less invasive and noninvasive methods of cardiovascular monitoring are continually being developed. Cardiac output can be estimated using arterial pressure waveform analysis (pulse contour analysis), indicator dilution technique, electrical bioimpedance, and esophageal Doppler ultrasound. Parameters such as intrathoracic blood volume and extravascular lung water can also be estimated by some of these devices. One of the main limitations that remain with many newer cardiovascular monitoring technologies is the need for calibration against more invasive measurements. Additionally, several factors such as mechanical ventilation, stable hemodynamics, and regular rhythm are necessary for appropriate use of the new monitoring techniques.

Cardiac output as well as other monitoring modalities have been used in order to intervene and optimize target parameters early in the disease process.[121-126] This early goal-directed therapy has been suggested to improve outcomes in various clinical settings.[121-126] The lack of outcomes evidence in support of invasive monitoring and the established problems (eg, central line–associated bloodstream infections) give further impetus for improvements and innovations in less invasive and noninvasive monitoring.

THE POSTOPERATIVE PERIOD

Cardiac Complications

Emergence from anesthesia is frequently accompanied by hypertension and tachycardia, which may be due to incomplete analgesia, awakening with airway devices in the oropharynx or trachea, withdrawal from antihypertensive drugs, hypoxemia, hypercarbia, delirium, or bladder distension. In the postoperative period, hemodynamic parameters must be optimized, especially in patients at increased risk for major adverse cardiac events. If tachycardia, hypertension or hypotension persists, and an underlying modifiable cause is not identified, then intravenous drugs, such as nitroglycerin, labetalol, or esmolol, can be used to control hemodynamics in patients with cardiovascular disease. Shivering is another phenomenon that may occur due to hypothermia or emergence from volatile anesthetics. Shivering results in significant increases in oxygen consumption, which may be poorly tolerated by patients with cardiovascular disease. Although the mechanism is unknown, low doses of intravenous meperidine may decrease or eliminate shivering.

Patients with multiple risk factors are particularly prone to significant and devastating postoperative complications, such as stroke, MI, pulmonary edema, malignant ventricular arrhythmia, and cardiac death.[127-129] Myocardial injury, defined as an elevated troponin level above the 99th percentile, occurs in up to 20% of patients after noncardiac surgery.[130,131] Pain, high catecholamine levels, hypercoagulability, discontinuation of antiplatelet therapy in patients with intracoronary stents, hypovolemia, anemia, intravascular volume shifts, drug effects, and a decreased level of monitoring compared to the intraoperative period, likely contribute to the high incidence of complications in the postoperative period.

Another common adverse cardiac event, after either cardiac or noncardiac surgery, is postoperative AF. Its incidence has

TABLE 73-8. Strategies for prevention of perioperative atrial fibrillation (AF) in a cardiac surgical patient[132]

Patient Risk	Strategies to Prevent Perioperative AF	Phase of Care		
		Preoperative	Intraoperative	Postoperative
Normal				
	Continue β-blockers	x	x	x
	Administer β-blocker			x
Elevated				
	Continue β-blockers	x	x	x
	Prophylactic amiodarone	x	x	x
	Administer β-blocker			x

Risk Factors for Perioperative AF[132]
- Age >75
- History of AF
- Renal Failure
- Mitral valve surgery or disease
- Heart failure
- COPD

been reported 30% to 50% and is associated with increased morbidity, mortality, and hospital length of stay.[132] Recently, the Society of Cardiovascular Anesthesiologists and European Association of Cardiothoracic Anaesthetists generated a summary of current evidence-based best practices in an effort to improve perioperative management of AF.[132] Based on this practice advisory, **Table 73-8** reviews risk factors for perioperative AF and lists specific strategies for prevention of perioperative AF in cardiac surgical patients.

Enhanced Recovery After Surgery

Recently, anesthesiology and surgical services have been involved in the development of enhanced recovery after surgery (ERAS) protocols. By virtue of extensive training and experience with postprocedural care, anesthesiologists are often key members of the teams that design enhanced-recovery pathways. For example, epidural analgesia, catheter-based peripheral nerve blockade, patient-controlled analgesia, and multimodal therapies contribute to postoperative analgesia strategies as part of a comprehensive postoperative service.

The ERAS protocol is a multidisciplinary, multimodal, "bundled approach to perioperative care"[133]—a "perioperative patient management strategy"[134] where evidence-based efforts are made to minimize physical and emotional stresses during surgery or interventional procedure, with an ultimate goal to help return patients to their preoperative baseline as fast as possible.[133,134]

The ERAS protocols began in the field of colorectal surgery but have since been developed in most surgical subspecialties. Subsequently, an interest in developing ERAS specific in cardiac surgery (ERAS-C) has also grown.[133-140] The effects of ERAS on length of stay, costs, perioperative pain control, patient satisfaction, and postoperative complications have been examined by numerous studies with favorable results.[136-139] Consequently, central measures to any ERAS program include optimal patient education, presurgical psychological, nutritional and physical patient optimization, shortened preoperative fasting times, multimodal opioid-sparing analgesia, early return to oral diets, and mobilization.[133-140]

The development and implementation of a successful ERAS-C program requires an early identification of a patient who is a suitable ERAS-C candidate, preferably from the moment that the patient is scheduled for surgery. The approach mandates cultural and organizational changes within the medical community, shifting the focus toward patient-centered all-encompassing perioperative care while optimizing speed and completeness of recovery.[133-140] Salenger et al. suggested an organized methodical approach to create a strong ERAS program in a given institution. Similar to the multidisciplinary composition of the Heart Team (as aforementioned), the authors described the need for specific stakeholders to develop and implement the ERAS-C program.[133] The core team includes cardiac nurse manager, cardiac anesthesiologist, cardiac interventionalist, cardiac surgeon, intensivist, cardiac advance practitioner, physical therapist, respiratory therapist, pharmacist, information technology specialist, and the patient.[133] This core team is recommended to be small enough to meet regularly and communicate frequently, yet large enough to provide a breadth of expertise.[133] Additional individuals such as perfusionists, dietitians, clinical educators, social workers, and case managers also contribute to a successful sustainable ERAS-C program. The ERAS-C team determines which outcomes will be the focus of its program, identifies outcome metrics, and implements evidence-based clinical interventions to implement those targets.[134] Based on ERAS Cardiac Society's expert recommendations,[140] over 25 cardiac surgery bundles are currently available from which to choose for initial deployment in a given institution.[135,137,139,140] Currently, there are no national guidelines on which specific data elements should be tracked for every cardiac ERAS program.

ANESTHESIA IN NONOPERATING ROOM LOCATIONS

Multiple diagnostic and therapeutic procedures are now being performed outside the standard operating room locations. Provision of anesthesia for patients at these locations constitutes nonoperating room anesthesia (NORA),[141,142] with the proportion of cases performed there continuously increasing.[143] Recognizing a growing demand for anesthesiologists outside of the OR, the ASA released a "Statement on Non-Operating Room Anesthetizing Locations," with focus on periprocedural safety standards for NORA patients.[144]

Even though anesthesia for colonoscopy has been reported in 2017 as the most common procedure-specific type of NORA,[145] patients with cardiovascular disease also present for select cardiac catheterization procedures, electrophysiology interventions, and/or specialty noncardiac procedures.[142,145] Some of these procedures can be done with mild sedation, delivered by trained nonanesthesia personnel. Sedation is a continuum, however, and it is not always possible to predict the response of an individual patient.[146,147] Since patients who require these interventions may have complex cardiovascular diseases with multiple comorbidities, the presence of an anesthesiologist—who is ready and able to rescue the airway in those patients in whom the level of sedation becomes deeper than intended or the surgical circumstances require conversion from monitored anesthesia care (MAC) to general anesthesia—is essential in these cases.[145-150]

Delivery of a safe anesthetic in remote from the OR locations, such as in cardiac catheterization (CCL) or electrophysiology (EP) laboratories, potentially involving critically ill patients, poses specific challenges to an anesthesia provider.[141-143,145,148-150] Older patients and those with congenital heart disease patients are seen more frequently in CCLs and EP laboratories, with developed protocols to emergently transferring the patient from the CCL or EP suites to the OR in the event of complications. Some institutions, on the other hand, have moved toward hybrid operating rooms, which combine advanced imaging capability with a fully functioning operating room setup, integrating interventional cardiology capabilities with those of cardiac surgery and anesthesiology.[151]

A myriad of cardiovascular procedures is performed in these settings, such as cardiac catheterizations, percutaneous coronary interventions, catheter ablations, cardioversions, various CIED implantations, thrombectomies, transcatheter-based valvular interventions, percutaneous atrial septal defect, and left atrial appendage closures. The choice of anesthetic technique depends on the preoperative evaluation of the patient's comorbidities as well as the intervention planned, with many transcatheter-based valvular and EP procedures done under MAC sedation.[142,145,150,152] Recent studies have suggested decreased 30-day mortality, shorter ICU and overall hospital stay, reduced need for inotropes or vasopressors, and decreased incidence of postoperative delirium, without effects on procedural success or procedural complications, in patients under MAC sedation for transfemoral transcatheter aortic valve replacement (TAVR) as compared to those under general anesthesia.[153,154] No association has been reported between specific drug choices for MAC administration in TAVRs on perioperative outcomes or conversion rates to general anesthesia.[155] On the other hand, the use of general anesthesia for AF ablation procedures may be associated with better procedural success as compared to MAC administration.[156] Short-acting agents may be preferred to allow the patient to become more arousable for certain procedures, while controlled mechanical ventilation or paralysis maybe preferred for others. Therefore, close communication between anesthesiologist, interventionalist, and EP or CCL teams regarding the anesthetic plan is crucial for all interventions performed.

SUMMARY

The optimal perioperative care of patients with cardiovascular disease is the shared responsibility of internists, cardiologists, surgeons, and anesthesiologists. Any anesthetic agent or technique has the potential for producing adverse effects, and the margin of safety is reduced in patients with cardiovascular disease. It is the anesthesiologist's central role to aide in medical information synthesis and patient optimization preoperatively, in selection of a suitable anesthetic technique and appropriate location of intervention for the planned procedure and the condition of the individual patient, in utilization of pertinent monitoring technology and management of hemodynamic alterations intraoperatively, and in addressing patient's analgesic requirements perioperatively. As cardiovascular disease continues to become more prevalent in the surgical population, preoperative testing and intraoperative monitoring become more sophisticated, multidisciplinary ERAS-C protocols are widely implemented, and nonoperating room procedure locations continue to grow, the need for effective communication between the specialties of cardiology, surgery, and anesthesiology will become even more important.

1. **CV Monitoring during the Perioperative Period**
   A. Routine for all patients (ASA standard monitors):
      - heart rate
      - ECG
      - blood pressure
      - pulse oximetry
      - capnography
      - temperature

   B. Advanced monitoring for high-risk cardiovascular patients (in order of risk severity):
      - cerebral oximetry
      - direct arterial blood pressure via intra-arterial catheter
      - central venous catheter for monitoring via CVP and central drug administration
      - ultrasound: TTE or TEE
      - noninvasive cardiac output for goal-directed fluid and medication management
      - PAC for pulmonary hypertension or right ventricular problems

2. **Procedures performed in nonoperating rooms that have increased risk of anesthetic complications in patients with cardiac disease**
   A. Noncardiac procedures:
      - Endovascular aortic repair (EVAR)
      - Carotid artery stenting

- Interventional pulmonology procedures, such as ultrasound-guided biopsy
- Invasive radiologic procedures, such as transjugular intrahepatic portosystemic shunt (TIPS), liver biopsies, cerebral coiling, stenting, or embolization, vascular embolization procedures
- Endoscopic procedures, such as endoscopic retrograde cholangiopancreatography (ERCP), enteroscopies
- Psychiatric treatments, such as electroconvulsive therapy (ECT)

B. Cardiac procedures:
- Transcatheter aortic valve implantation (TAVI)
- Mitral valve repairs (TMVR)
- EP laboratory procedures, such as radiofrequency ablations, percutaneous left atrial appendage (LAA) device placements and atrial septal defect (ASD) closures
- CIEDs, such as wire removals or pacing systems implantation
- Minimally invasive procedures done in ICUs
- Cath lab procedures, such as cardiac biopsies, PCI placement
- Cardioversions with or without TEE

ACKNOWLEDGMENT

In previous editions, this chapter was co-written by Dr. Alexander J. C. Mittnacht, and portions of that chapter have been retained.

REFERENCES

1. Holmes DR, Rich JB, Zoghbi WA, Mack MJ, et al. The heart team of cardiovascular care. *J Am Coll Cardiol.* 2013;61:903-907.
2. Burlacu A, Covic A, Cinteza M, et al. Exploring current evidence on the past, the present, and the future of the heart team: a narrative review. *Cardiovasc Therap.* 2020. doi: 10.1155/2020/9241081
3. Head ST, Kaul S, Mack MJ, Serruys PW, Taggart DP, Holmes DR, et al. The rationale for heart team decision-making for patients with stable, complex coronary artery disease. *Eur Heart J.* 2013;34(32):2510-2518.
4. Kesson EM, Allardice GM, George WD, Burns HJ, Morrison DS. Effects of multidisciplinary team working on breast cancer survival: retrospective, comparative, interventional cohort study of 13 722 women. *BMJ* 2012;344:e2718.
5. van Hagen P, Spaander MC, van der Gaast A, van Rij CM, et al. Impact of a multidisciplinary tumour board meeting for upper-GI malignancies on clinical decision making: a prospective cohort study. *Int J Clin Oncol.* 2013;18(2):214-219.
6. Kolh P, Wijns W, Danchin N, Di Mario C, et al. Guidelines on myocardial revascularization. *Eur J Cardiothorac Surg.* 2010;38:S1-S52.
7. Hillis LD, Smith PK, Anderson JL, Bittl JA, et al. 2011 ACCF/AHA Guideline for Coronary Artery Bypass Graft Surgery: executive summary: a report of the American College of Cardiology Foundation/American Heart Association Task Force on Practice Guidelines. *Circulation* 2011;124:2610-2642.
8. Long J, Luckraz H, Thekkudan J, Maher A, Norell M. Heart team discussion in managing patients with coronary artery disease: outcome and reproducibility. *Interact Cardiovasc Thorac Surg.* 2012;14:594-598.
9. Feit F, Brooks MM, Sopko G, Keller NM, Rosen A, et al. Long-term clinical outcome in the Bypass Angioplasty Revascularization Investigation Registry: comparison with the randomized trial. BARI Investigators. *Circulation* 2000;101:2795-2802.
10. Shortell SM, Jones RH, Rademaker AW, Gillies RR, Dranove DS, Hughes EF, Budetti PP, Reynolds KS, Huang CF. Assessing the impact of total quality management and organizational culture on multiple outcomes of care for coronary artery bypass graft surgery patients. *Med Care* 2000;38:207-217.
11. Duhachek-Stapelman AL, Roberts EK, Schulte TE, Shillcutt SK. The cardiothoracic anesthesiologist as a perioperative consultant – echocardiography and beyond. *J Cardiothor Vasc Anesth.* 2019;33:744-754.
12. Goldman L, Caldera DL, Nussbaum SR, et al. Multifactorial index of cardiac risk in noncardiac surgical procedures. *N Engl J Med.* 1977;297:845-850.
13. Lee TH, Marcantonio ER, Mangione CM, et al. Derivation and prospective validation of a simple index for prediction of cardiac risk of major noncardiac surgery. *Circulation.* 1999;100(10):1043-1049.
14. Gupta PK, Gupta H, Sundaram A, et al. Development and validation of a risk calculator for prediction of cardiac risk after surgery. *Circulation.* 2011;124(4):381-387.
15. Bilimoria KY, Liu Y, Paruch JL, et al. Development and evaluation of the universal ACS NSQIP surgical risk calculator: a decision aid and informed consent tool for patients and surgeons. *J Am Coll Surg.* 2013;217(5):833-842, e1, e3.
16. Dakik HA, Chehab O, Eldirani M, et al. A new index for preoperative cardiovascular evaluation. *J Am Coll Cardiol.* 2019;73(24):3067-3078.
17. Smilowitz NR, Berger JS. Risk assessment and management for noncardiac surgery. *JAMA* 2020;324(3):279-290.
18. Ford MK, Beattie WS, Wijeysundera DN. Systematic review: prediction of perioperative cardiac complications and mortality by the revised cardiac risk index. *Ann Intern Med.* 2010;152(1):26-35.
19. Fleisher LA, Fleischmann KE, Auerbach AD, et al. American College of Cardiology; American Heart Association. 2014 ACC/AHA guideline on perioperative cardiovascular evaluation and management of patients undergoing noncardiac surgery: a report of the American College of Cardiology/American Heart Association Task Force on practice guidelines. *J Am Coll Cardiol.* 2014;64:e77-1373.
20. Kristensen SD, Knuuti J, Saraste A, Anker S, et al. 2014 ESC/ESA Guidelines on non-cardiac surgery: cardiovascular assessment and management. *Eur Heart J.* 2014;35:2383-2431.
21. Rodseth RN, Biccard BM, Le Manach Y, et al. The prognostic value of preoperative and postoperative B-type natriuretic peptides in patients undergoing noncardiac surgery: B-type natriuretic peptide and N-terminal fragment of pro-B-type natriuretic peptide: a systematic review and individual patient data meta-analysis. *J Am Coll Cardiol.* 2014;63(2):170-180.
22. Duceppe E, Patel A, Chan MTV, et al. Preoperative N-terminal pro-B-type natriuretic peptide and cardiovascular events after noncardiac surgery: a cohort study. *Ann Intern Med.* 2020;172(2):96-104.
23. De Hert SG, Buse GAL. Cardiac biomarkers for the prediction and detection of adverse cardiac events after noncardiac surgery: a narrative review. *Anesth Analg.* 2020;131(1):187-195.
24. Saia F, Belotti LM, Guastaroba P, et al. Risk of adverse cardiac and bleeding events following cardiac and noncardiac surgery in patients with coronary stent: how important is the interplay between stent type and time from stenting to surgery? *Circ Cardiovasc Qual Outcomes.* 2016;9(1):39-47.
25. Douketis JD, Spyropoulos AC, Kaatz S, et al. BRIDGE Investigators. Perioperative bridging anticoagulation in patients with atrial fibrillation. *N Engl J Med.* 2015;373(9):823-833.
26. Darvish-Kazem S, Gandhi M, Marcucci M, Douketis JD. Perioperative management of antiplatelet therapy in patients with a coronary stent who need noncardiac surgery: a systematic review of clinical practice guidelines. *Chest.* 2013;144:1848-1856.

27. Rossini R, Musumeci G, Capodanno D, et al. Perioperative management of oral antiplatelet therapy and clinical outcomes in coronary stent patients undergoing surgery: results of a multicentre registry. *Thromb Haemost*. 2015;113(2):272-282.

28. Albaladejo P, Marret E, Samama CM, et al. Non-cardiac surgery in patients with coronary stents: the RECO study. *Heart*. 2011;97(19):1566-1572.

29. American Society of Anesthesiologists Committee on Standards and Practice Parameters. Practice alert for the perioperative management of patients with coronary stents: a report by the American Society of Anesthesiologists Committee on Standards and Practice Parameters. *Anesthesiology*. 2009;110:22-23.

30. Berger PB, Kleiman NS, Pencina MJ, et al. EVENT Investigators. Frequency of major noncardiac surgery and subsequent adverse events in the year after drug-eluting stent placement: results from the EVENT (Evaluation of Drug-Eluting Stents and Ischemic Events) Registry. *JACC Cardiovasc Interv*. 2010;3(9):920-927.

31. Ortel, T. L. Perioperative management of patients on chronic antithrombotic therapy. *Blood*. 2012;120(24):4699-4705.

32. Capodanno D, Alfonso F, Levine G, et al. ACC/AHA versus ESC guidelines on dual antiplatelet therapy: Guideline Comparison. *JACC* 2018;72(23 Pt A):2915-2931.

33. Tomaselli G, Mahaffey K, Cuker A, et al. 2020 ACC expert consensus decision pathway on management of bleeding in patients on oral anticoagulants: a report of the American College of Cardiology Solution Set Oversight Committee. *JACC* 2020;76(5):594-622.

34. Erdoes G, Martinez Lopez De Arroyabe B, Bollinger D, et al. International consensus statement on the perioperative management of direct oral anticoagulants in cardiac surgery. *Anaesthesia* 2018;73(12):1535-1545.

35. Salata K, Abdallah FW, Hussain MA, de Mestral C, et al. Short-term outcomes of combine neuraxial and general anesthesia versus general anesthesia alone for elective open abdominal aortic aneurysm repair: retrospective population-based study. *Br J Anaesth*. 2020;124(5):544-552.

36. Barbosa FT, de Sousa Rodrigues CF, Castro AA, et al. Is there any benefit is associating neuraxial anesthesia to general anesthesia for coronary artery bypass graft surgery? *Braz J Anesthesiol*. 2016;66(3):304-309.

37. Pisano A, Torella M, Yavorovskiy A, Landoni G. The impact of anesthetic regimen on outcomes in adult cardiac surgery: a narrative review. *J Cardiothorac Vasc Anesth*. 2020;20:S1053-0770(20)30304-9.

38. Leslie K, McIlroy D, Kasza J, Forbes A, Kurz A, et al. Neuraxial block and postoperative epidural analgesia: effects on outcomes in the POISE-2 trial. *Br J Anaesth*. 2016;116(1):100-112.

39. Poeran J, Yeo H, Rasul R, Opperer M, Memtsoudis SG, Mazumdar M. Anesthesia type and perioperative outcome: open colectomies in the United States. *J Surg Res*. 2015;193:684-692.

40. Guay J, Choi PT, Suresh S, Albert N, Kopp S, Pace NL. Neuraxial anesthesia for the prevention of postoperative mortality and major morbidity: an overview of Cochrane systematic reviews. *Anesth Analg*. 2014;119:716-725.

41. Murphy GS, Szokol JW, Marymont JH, et al. Myocardial damage prevented by volatile anesthetics: a multicenter randomized controlled study. *J Cardiothorac Vasc Anesth*. 2006;20:477-483.

42. Kunst G, Klein, AA. Peri-operative anaesthetic myocardial preconditioning and protection - cellular mechanisms and clinical relevance in cardiac anaesthesia. *Anaesthesia*. 2015.70(4):467-482.

43. Zaugg M, Lucchinetti E, Uecker M, et al. Anaesthetics and cardiac preconditioning. Part I. Signaling and cytoprotective mechanisms. *Br J Anaesth*. 2003;91:551-565.

44. Chen Z, Li T, Zhang B. Morphine postconditioning protects against reperfusion injury in the isolated rat hearts. *J Surg Res*. 2008;145:287-294.

45. Landoni G, Biondi-Zoccai G, Zangrillo A, et al. Desflurane and sevoflurane in cardiac surgery: a meta-analysis of randomized clinical trials. *J Cardiothorac Vasc Anesth*. 2007;21:502-511.

46. Lange M, Smul TM, Blomeyer CA, et al. Role of the beta 1-adrenergic pathway in anesthetic and ischemic preconditioning against myocardial infarction in the rabbit heart in vivo. *Anesthesiology*. 2006;105:503-510.

47. Roleder T, Golba KS, Kunecki M, Malinowski M, et al. The co-application of hypoxic preconditioning and postconditioning abolishes their own protective effect on systolic function in human myocardium. *Cardiol J*. 2013;20(5):472-477.

48. Coverdale NS, Hamilton A, Petsikas D, McClure RS, et al. Remote ischemic preconditioning in high-risk cardiovascular surgery patients: a randomized-controlled trial. *Semin Thorac Cardiovasc Surg*. 2018;30(1):26-33.

49. Honin G, Martinini CH, Bom A, et al. Safety of sugammadex for reversal of neuromuscular block. *Expert Opin Drug Saf*. 2019;8(10):883-891.

50. Hristovska AM, Duch P, Allingstrup M, Afshari, A. The comparative efficacy and safety of sugammadex and neostigmine in reversing neuromuscular blockade in adults. A Cochrane systematic review with meta-analysis and trial sequential analysis. *Anaesthesia*. 2018;73(5):631-641.

51. Zawar BP, Mehta Y, Juneja R, et al. Nonanalgesic benefits of combined thoracic epidural analgesia with general anesthesia in high risk elderly off pump coronary artery bypass patients. *Ann Card Anaesth*. 2015;18:385-391.

52. Bakhtiary F, Therapidis P, Dzemali O, et al. Impact of high thoracic epidural anesthesia on incidence of perioperative atrial fibrillation in off-pump coronary bypass grafting: a prospective randomized study. *J Thorac Cardiovasc Surg*. 2007;134:460-464.

53. Wiis JT, Jensen-Gadegaard P, Altintas U, et al. One-week postoperative patency of lower enxtremity in situ bypass graft comparing epidural and general anesthesia: retrospective study of 822 patients. *Ann Vasc Surg*. 2014;28(2):295-300.

54. Sgroi MD, McFarland G, Mell MW. Utilization of regional versus general anesthesia and its impact on lower extremity bypass outcomes. *J Vasc Surg*. 2019;69(6):1874-1879.

55. Rosenblatt MA, Abel M, Fischer GW, et al. Successful use of a 20% lipid emulsion to resuscitate a patient after a presumed bupivacaine-related cardiac arrest. *Anesthesiology*. 2006;105:217-218.

56. Warren JA, Thoma RB, Georgescu A, et al. Intravenous lipid infusion in the successful resuscitation of local anesthetic-induced cardiovascular collapse after supraclavicular brachial plexus block. *Anesth Analg*. 2008;106:1578-1580.

57. Checklist for treatment of local anesthetic systemic toxicity. *ASRA*. November 1, 2020. https://www.asra.com/guidelines-articles/guidelines/guideline-item/guidelines/2020/11/01/checklist-for-treatment-of-local-anesthetic-systemic-toxicity. Accessed on July 16, 2021.

58. Horlocker TT, Vandermeulen E, Kopp, SL, et al. Regional anesthesia in the patient receiving antithrombotic or thrombolytic therapy: American Society of Regional Anesthesia and Pain Medicine Evidence-Based Guidelines (4th ed). *Reg Anesth Pain Med*. 2018;43:263-309.

59. ASRA. https://www.asra.com/advisory-guidelines/article/1/anticoagulation-3rd-edition. Accessed on July 1, 2020.

60. Kaye AD, Brunk AJ, Kaye AJ, Renschler JS, et al. Regional anesthesia in patients on anticoagulation therapies - evidence-based recommendations. *Curr Pain Headache Rep*. 2019;23(9):67.

61. Ayers B, Stahl R, Wood K, Bernstein W, et al. Regional nerve block decreases opioid use after complete sternal-sparing left ventricular assist device implantation. *J Card Surg*. 2019;34:250-255.

62. Berthoud V, Ellouze O, Nguyen M, et al. Serratus anterior plane block for minimal invasive heart surgery. *BMC Anesthesiol*. 2018;18(1):144.

63. Toscano A, Capuano P, Costamanga A, et al. The serratus anterior plane study: continuous deep serratus anterior plane block for mitral valve surgery performed in right minithoracotomy. *J Cardiothor Vasc Anesth*. 2020;27:S1053-0770(20)30482-1.

64. Mittnacht AJC, Shariat A, Weiner MM, et al. Regional techniques for cardiac and cardiac related procedures. *J Cardiothor Vasc Anesth*. 2019;33:532-546.

65. Kelava M, Alfirevic A, Bustamante S, Hargrave J, Marciniak D. Regional anesthesia in cardiac surgery: an overview of fascial plane chest wall blocks. *Anesth Analg*. 2020;131:127-135.

66. Raza I, Narayanan M, Venkataraju A, Ciocarlan A. Bilateral subpectoral interfascial plane catheters for analgesia for sternal fractures: a case report. *Reg Anesth Pain Med*. 2016;41(5):607-609.

67. Yalamuri S, Klinger RY, Bullock WM, Glower DD, Bottiger BA, Gadsden JC. Pectoral fascial (PECS) I and II blocks as rescue analgesia in a patient undergoing minimally invasive cardiac surgery. *Reg Anesth Pain Med.* 2017;42(6):764-766.

68. Leyva FM, Mendiola WE, Bonilla AJ, Cubillos J, Moreno DA, Chin KJ. Continuous erector spinae plane (ESP) block for postoperative analgesia after minimally invasive mitral valve surgery. *J Cardiothorac Vasc Anesth.* 2018;32(5):2271 2274.

69. Ueshima H, Otake H. Ultrasound-guided transversus thoracic muscle plane block: complication in 299 consecutive cases. *J Clin Anesth.* 2017;41:60.

70. Devlin JW, Skrobik Y, Gélinas C, et al. Clinical practice guidelines for the prevention and management of pain, agitation/sedation, delirium, immobility, and sleep disruption in adult patients in the ICU. *Crit Care Med.* 2018;46(9):e825-e873.

71. Khalil AE, Abdallah NM, Bashandy GM, Kaddah TA. Ultrasound-guided serratus anterior plane block versus thoracic epidural analgesia for thoracotomy pain. *J Cardiothorac Vasc Anesth.* 2017;31:152-158.

72. Mittnacht AJC. Fascial plane blocks in cardiac surgery: same but different. *J Cardiothorac Vasc Anesth.* 2019;33:426-427.

73. American Society of Anesthesiologists. Standards for basic intraoperative monitoring. Approved by House of Delegates on October 21, 1986 and last amended on October 28, 2015. Park Ridge, IL. https://www.asahq.org/standards-and-guidelines. Accessed on July 16, 2021.

74. Scheeren TWL, Kuizenga MH, Maurer H, Struys MMRF, Heringlake M. Electroencephalography and brain oxygenation monitoring in the perioperative period. *Anesth. Analg.* 2019;128(2):265-277.

75. Shoushtarian M, McGlade DP, Delacretaz LJ, Liley DT. Evaluation of the brain anaesthesia response monitor during anaesthesia for cardiac surgery: a double-blind, randomised controlled trial using two doses of fentanyl. *J Clin Monit Comput.* 2016;30:833-844.

76. Fahy BG, Chau DF. The technology of processed electroencephalogram monitoring devices for assessment of depth of anesthesia. *Anesth Analg.* 2018;126:111-117.

77. Chan MJ, Chung T, Glassford NJ, Bellomo R. Near-infrared spectroscopy in adult cardiac surgery patients: a systematic review and meta-analysis. *J Cardiothorac Vasc Anesth.* 2017;31:1155-1165.

78. Rogers CA, Stoica S, Ellis L. Randomized trial of near-infrared spectroscopy for personalized optimization of cerebral tissue oxygenation during cardiac surgery. *Br J Anaesth.* 2017;119:384-393.

79. Nunes RR, Porto VC, Miranda VT, et al. Risk factors for intraoperative awareness. *Rev Bras Anesthesiol.* 2012;62(3):365-374.

80. Practice advisory for intraoperative awareness and brain function monitoring. A report by the American Society of Anesthesiologists Task Force on intraoperative awareness. *Anesthesiology.* 2006;104:847-864.

81. Watzman HM, Kurth CD, Montenegro LM, et al. Arterial and venous contributions to near-infrared cerebral oximetry. *Anesthesiology* 2000; 93:947-953.

82. Salter BS, Baron EL. Chapter 3: Cerebral oximetry. In Leibowitz AB and Uysal S (eds). *Modern Monitoring in Anesthesiology and Perioperative Care.* Cambridge University Press;2020:20-29.

83. Jo YY, Shim JK, Soh S, Suh S, Kwak YL. Association between cerebral oxygenation saturation with outcome in cardiac surgery: brain as an index organ. *J Clin Med.* 2020;9(3):840.

84. Murkin JM, Adams SJ, Novick RJ, et al. Monitoring brain oxygen saturation during coronary bypass surgery: a randomized, prospective study. *Anesth Analg.* 2007;104:51-58.

85. Kunst G, Gauge N, Salaunkey K, et al. Intraoperative optimization of both depth of anesthesia and cerebral oxygenation in elderly patients undergoing coronary artery bypass graft surgery - a randomized controlled pilot trial. *J Cardiothorac Vasc Anesth.* 2020;34(5):1172-1181.

86. Holmgaard F, Vedel AG, Rasmussen LS, et al. The association between postoperative cognitive dysfunction and cerebral oximetry during cardiac surgery: a secondary analysis of a randomised trial. *Br J Aneaesth.* 2019;123(2):196-205.

87. Uysal S, Lin HM, Trinh M, Park CH, Reich DL. Optimizing cerebral oxygenation in cardiac surgery: A randomized controlled trial examining neurocognitive and perioperative outcomes. *J Thorac Cardiovasc Surg.* 2020;159:943-953.

88. Chan SK, Underwood MJ, Ho AM, et al. Cannula malposition during antegrade cerebral perfusion for aortic surgery: role of cerebral oximetry. *Can J Anaesth.* 2014;61:736-740.

89. Zheng F, Sheinberg R, Yee MS, Ono M, Zheng Y, Hogue CW. Cerebral near-infrared spectroscopy monitoring and neurologic outcomes in adult cardiac surgery patients: a systematic review. *Anesth Analg.* 2013;116:663-676.

90. Padhy SK, Ajayan N, Hrishi AP, et al. Novel application of near-infrared spectroscopy in detecting iatrogenic vasospasm during interventional neuroradiological procedures. *Brain Circ.* 2019;5(2):90-93.

91. Miller MA, Dukkipati SR, Mittnacht AJ, et al. Activation and entrainment mapping of hemodynamically unstable ventricular tachycardia using a percutaneous left ventricular assist device. *J Am Coll Cardiol.* 2011;58:1363-1371.

92. Yagi T, Kawamorita K, Tachibana E, Watanabe K, et al. Usefulness of new device to monitor cerebral blood oxygenation using NIRS during cardiopulmonary resuscitation in patients with cardiac arrest: a pilot study. *Adv Exp Med Biol.* 2020;1232:323-329.

93. Skrifvars MB, Aneman A. Near-infrared spectroscopy "under pressure" as a post-cardiac arrest monitoring technique of cerebral autoregulation. *Resuscitation* 2020;152:203-204.

94. Fletchet M, Guiza F, Vlasselaers D, et al. Near-infrared cerebral oximetry to predict outcome after pediatric cardiac surgery: a prospective observational study. *Pediatr Crit Care Med.* 2018;19(5):433-441.

95. Brady K, Joshi B, Zweifel C, et al. Real-time continuous monitoring of cerebral blood flow autoregulation using near-infrared spectroscopy in patients undergoing cardiopulmonary bypass. *Stroke.* 2010;41:1951-1956.

96. Rivera-Lara L, Zorrila-Vaca A, Healy R, et al. Determination of upper and lower limits of cerebral autoregulation with cerebral oximetry autoregulation curves: a case series. *Crit Care Med.* 2018;46(5):e473-e477.

97. Margale S, Marudhachalam K, Natani S. Clinical application of point of care transthoracic echocardiography in perioperative period. *Indian J Anaesth.* 2017;61(1):7-16.

98. Kratz T, Steinfeldt T, Exner M, et al. Impact of focused intraoperative transthoracic echocardiography by anesthesiologists on management of hemodynamically unstable high-risk noncardiac surgery patients. *J Cardiothor Vasc Anesth.* 2017;31:602-609.

99. Tamaka CY, Hartman KM, Patel PA, Neuburger PJ. Anesthesiologist can add value in transcatheter aortic valve replacement by performing transthoracic echocardiography. *J Cardiothor Vascul Anesth.* 2020;34:32-34.

100. Teran F, Prats MI, Nelson BP, Kessler R, Blaivas M, et al. Focused transesophageal echocardiography during cardiac arrest resuscitation: JACC review topic of the week. *JACC* 2020;76(6):745-754.

101. Shmidt S, Dieks J-K, Quintel M, Moerer O. Critical care echocardiography as a routine procedure for the detection and early treatment of cardiac pathologies. *Diagnostics (Basel)* 2020;10(9):E671.

102. The American Board of Anesthesiology. Objective Structured Clinical Exam (OSCE) content outline. https://www.theaba.org/pdfs/OSCE_Content_Outline.pdf. Accessed July 16, 2021.

103. Reich DL, Mittnacht AJ, London MJ, Kaplan JA. Chapter 9: Monitoring of the heart and vascular system. In: Kaplan JA, Augoustides JGT, Manecke GR, Mous T, Reich DL (eds.), Kaplan's Cardiac Anesthesia for Cardiac and Non-Cardiac Surgery (7th ed). Philadelphia, PA: Saunders Elsevier; 2017: 167-198.

104. Harvey S, Harrison DA, Singer M, et al. Assessment of the clinical effectiveness of pulmonary artery catheters in management of patients in intensive care (PAC-Man): a randomised controlled trial. *Lancet.* 2005;366:472-477.

105. Shah MR, Hasselblad V, Stevenson LW, et al. Impact of the pulmonary artery catheter in critically ill patients: meta-analysis of randomized clinical trials. *JAMA.* 2005;294:1664-1670.

106. Binanay C, Califf RM, Hasselblad V, et al. Evaluation study of congestive heart failure and pulmonary artery catheterization effectiveness: the ESCAPE trial. *JAMA*. 2005;294:1625-1633.

107. Schwann NM, Hillel Z, Hoeft, A, Barash, P, et al. Lack of effectiveness of the pulmonary artery catheter in cardiac surgery. *Anesth Analg*. 2011;113(5):994-1002.

108. Chen Y, Shlofmitz E, Khalid N, Bernardo NL, et al. Right-heart catheterization-related complications: a review of literature and best practices. *Cardiol Rev*. 2020;28(1):36-41.

109. Jacka M, Cohen MM, To T, et al. Pulmonary artery occlusion pressure estimation: how confident are anesthesiologists? *Crit Care Med*. 2002;30:1197-1203.

110. Joseph C, Garrubba M, Smith JA, Melder A. Does the use of a pulmonary artery catheter make a difference during or after cardiac surgery? *Heart Lung Circ*. 2018;27(8):952-960.

111. Rajaram SS, Desai NK, Kalra A, Gajera M, et al. Pulmonary artery catheters for adult patients in intensive care. *Cochrane Database Syst Rev*. 2013;2013(2):CD003408.

112. American Society of Anesthesiologists Task Force on Pulmonary Artery Catheterization. Practice guidelines for pulmonary artery catheterization: an updated report by the American Society of Anesthesiologists. *Anesthesiology*. 2003;99:988-1014.

113. Judge O, Ji F, Fleming N, Liu H. Current use of the pulmonary artery catheter in cardiac surgery: a survey study. *J Cardiothorac Vasc Anesth*. 2015;29:69-75.

114. Hahn RT, Abraham T, Adams MS, Bruce CJ, Glas KE, et al. Guidelines for performing a comprehensive transesophageal echocardiographic examination: recommendations from the American Society of Echocardiography and the Society of Cardiovascular Anesthesiologists. *J Am Soc Echocardiogr*. 2013;26:921-64.

115. Wheeler R, Steeds R, Rana B, Wharton G, et al. A minimum dataset for a standard transoesophageal echocardiogram: a guideline protocol from the British Society of Echocardiography. *Echo Res Pract*. 2015;2(4):G29-45.

116. Cahalan MK, Abel M, Goldman M, et al. American Society of Echocardiography and Society of Cardiovascular Anesthesiologists task force guidelines for training in perioperative echocardiography. *Anesth Analg*. 2002;94:1384-1388.

117. Mathew JP, Glas K, Troianos CA, Sears-Rogan P, Savage R, et al. American Society of Echocardiography/Society of Cardiovascular Anesthesiologists recommendations and guidelines for continuous quality improvement in perioperative echocardiography. American Society of Echocardiography; Society of Cardiovascular Anesthesiologists. *J Am Soc Echocardiogr*. 2006;19:1303-1313.

118. Thys DM, Brooker RF, Cahalan MK, et al. Practice guidelines for perioperative transesophageal echocardiography. An updated report by the American Society of Anesthesiologists and the Society of Cardiovascular Anesthesiologists Task Force on transesophageal echocardiography. *Anesthesiology*. 2010;112:1084-1096.

119. Cheitlin MD, Armstrong WF, Aurigemma GP, et al. ACC/AHA/ASE 2003 guideline update for the clinical application of echocardiography: summary article. A report of the American College of Cardiology/American Heart Association Task Force on Practice Guidelines (ACC/AHA/ASE Committee to Update the 1997 Guidelines for the Clinical Application of Echocardiography). *J Am SoEchocardiogr*. 2003;16:1091-1110.

120. Kahn R, Shernan SK, Konstadt SN, Weiss SJ, Savino JS. Chapter 10: Intraoperative Echocardiography. In: Kaplan's Cardiac Anesthesia Kaplan's Cardiac Anesthesia for Cardiac and Non-Cardiac Surgery (7th ed). Philadelphia, PA: Saunders Elsevier; 2017:167-198.

121. Mouncey PR, Osborn TM, Power GS, Harrison DA, Sadique MZ, et al. ProMISe Trial Investigators. Trial of early, goal-directed resuscitation for septic shock. *N Engl J Med*. 2015;372:1301-11.

122. Kapoor PM, Magoon R, Rawat R, Mehta Y. Perioperative utility of goal-directed therapy in high-risk cardiac patients undergoing cardiac artery bypass grafting: "A clinical outcome and biomarker-based study." *Ann Card Anaesth*. 2016;19(4):638-682.

123. Kapoor PM, Magoon R, Rawat RS, et al. Goal-directed therapy improves the outcome of high-risk cardiac patients undergoing off-pump coronary artery bypass. *Ann Card Anaesth*. 2017;20(1):83-89.

124. Lee S, Lee SH, Chang, B-C, Shim J-K. Efficacy of goal-directed therapy using bioreactance cardiac output monitoring after valvular heart surgery. *Yonsei Med J*. 2015;56(4):913-920.

125. Pestana D, Espinosa E, Eden A, et al. Perioperative goal-directed hemodynamic optimization using noninvasive cardiac output monitoring in major abdominal surgery: a prospective, randomized, multicenter, pragmatic trial: POEMAS Study (PeriOperative goal-directed thErapy in Major Abdominal Surgery). *Anesth Analg*. 2014;119(3):579-587.

126. Kendrick JB, Kaye AD, Tong Y, Belani K, et al. Goal-directed fluid therapy in the perioperative setting. *J Anaesthesiol Clin Pharmacol*. 2019;35(Suppl 1): S29-S34.

127. Thomas KN, Cotter JD, Williams MJ, van Rij AM. Diagnosis, incidence and clinical implications of perioperative myocardial injury in vascular surgery. *Vasc Endovascular Surg*. 2016;50(4):247-255.

128. Wagner BD, Grunwald GK, Hossein AG, et al. Factors associated with long-term survival in patients with stroke after coronary artery bypass grafting. *Int Med Res*. 2020;48(7):300060520920428.

129. Devereaux PJ, Szczeklik W. Myocardial injury after non-cardiac surgery: diagnosis and management. *Eur Heart J*. 2020;41(32):3083-3091.

130. Smilowitz NR, Redel-Traub G, Hausvater A, et al. Myocardial injury after noncardiac surgery: a systematic review and meta-analysis. *Cardiol Rev*. 2019;27(6):267-273.

131. Devereaux PJ, Biccard BM, Sigamani A, et al; Writing Committee for the VISION Study Investigators. Association of postoperative high-sensitivity troponin levels with myocardial injury and 30-day mortality among patients undergoing noncardiac surgery. *JAMA* 2017;317(16):1642-1651.

132. O'Brien B, Burrage PS, Ngai JY, Prutkin JM, et al. Society of Cardiovascular Anesthesiologists/European Association of Cardiothoracic Anaesthetists Practice Advisory for the Management of Perioperative Atrial Fibrillation in Patients Undergoing Cardiac Surgery. *J Cardiothorac Vasc Anesth*. 2019;33:12-26.

133. Salenger R, Morton-Bailey V, Grant M, et al. Cardiac enhanced recovery after surgery: a guide to team building and successful implementation. *Semin Thoracic Surg*. 2020;32:187-196.

134. Baxter R, Squiers J, Conner W, Kent M, et al. Enhanced recovery after surgery: a narrative review of its application in cardiac surgery. *Ann Thorac Surg*. 2020;109:1937-1945.

135. Borys M, Zurek S, Kurowicki A, Horeczy B, et al. Implementation of enhanced recovery after surgery (ERAS) protocol in off-pump coronary artery bypass graft surgery. A prospective cohort feasibility study. *Anaesthesiol Intensive Ther*. 2020;52(1):10-14.

136. Williams JB, McConnell G, Allender JE, Woltz P, et al. One-year results from the first US-based enhanced recovery after cardiac surgery (ERAS cardiac) program. *J Thorac Cardiovasc Surg*. 2019;157(5):1881-1888.

137. Grant MC, Isada TS, Ruzankin PJ, et al. Results from an enhanced recovery program for cardiac surgery. *J Thorac Cardiovasc Surg*. 2020;159(4): 1393-1402.

138. Markham T, Wegner R, Hernandez N, Lee JW, Choi W, et al. Assessment of a multimodal analgesia protocol to allow the implementation of enhanced recovery after surgery: retrospective analysis of patient outcomes. *J Clin Anesth*. 2019;54:76-80.

139. Li M, Zhang J, Gan TJ, Quin G, et al. Enhanced recovery after surgery pathway for patients undergoing cardiac surgery: a randomized clinical trial. *Eur J Cardiothorac Surg*. 2018;54(3):491-497.

140. Engelman DT, Ali WB, Williams JB, et al. Guidelines for perioperative care in cardiac surgery. *JAMA Surg*. 2019;154:755-766.

141. Reddy A, DiLorenzo A, Dority J. Non-operating room anesthesia. *Anesth Analg*. 2016;122:286-287.

142. Kozak M, Robertson B, Chambers CE. Chapter 2: The cardiac catheterization laboratory. In: Kaplan's Cardiac Anesthesia for Cardiac and Non-Cardiac Surgery (7th ed). Philadelphia, PA: Saunders Elsevier; 2017:167-198.

143. Nagrebetsky A, Gabriel RA, Dutton RP, Urman RD. Growth of nonoperating room anesthesia care in the United States: a contemporary trends analysis. *Anesth Analg.* 2017;124(4):1261-1267.

144. American Society of Anesthesiologists. Statement on Nonoperating Room Anesthetizing Locations. Standards and Practice Parameters Committee; 2013. Reaffirmed: October 17, 2018 (original approval: October 19, 1994). https://www.asahq.org/standards-and-guidelines/statement-on-nonoperating-room-anesthetizing-locations. Accessed July 16, 2021.

145. Lee DW, Masowicz M. Recent advances in nonoperating room anesthesia for cardiac procedures. *Curr Opin Anaesthesiol.* 2020;33(4):601-607.

146. Continuum of Depth of Sedation: Definition of General Anesthesia and Levels of Sedation/Analgesia. *American Society of Anesthesiologists (ASA).* October 23, 2019. https://www.asahq.org/standards-and-guidelines/continuum-of-depth-of-sedation-definition-ofgeneral-anesthesia-and-levels-of-sedationanalgesia. Accessed July 16, 2021.

147. Chapter 12: General, regional, or monitored anesthesia care for the cardiac patient undergoing non cardiac surgery. In: Kaplan JA, Cronin B, Mous TM. (Eds), *Essentials of Cardiac Anesthesia for Noncardiac Surgery: A Companion to Kaplan's Cardiac Anesthesia.* Elsevier; 2019.

148. Cheruku S, Boud TJ, Kulkarni N, Lynch IP. Demystifying the EP laboratory: anesthetic considerations for electrophysiology procedures. *Int Anesthesiol Clin.* 2018;56(4):98-119.

149. Yildiz M, Ak HY, Oksen D, Oral S. Anesthetic management in electrophysiology laboratory: a multidisciplinary review. *J Atr Fibrillation* 2018;10(5):1775-1783.

150. Whitehead NJ, Clark AL, Williams TD, Collins NJ, Boyle AJ. Sedation and analgesia for cardiac catheterization and coronary intervention. *Heart Lung Circ.* 2020;29(2):169-177.

151. Kaneko T, Davidson M. Use of the hybrid operating room in cardiovascular medicine. *Circulation* 2014;130:910-917.

152. Hyman MC, Vemulapalli S, Szeto WY, et al. Conscious sedation versus general anesthesia for transcatheter aortic valve replacement: insights from the National Cardiovascular Data Registry Society of Thoracic Surgeons/American College of Cardiology Transcatheter Valve Therapy Registry. *Circulation* 2017;136:2132-2140.

153. Villablanca PA, Mohananey D, Nikolic K, et al. Comparison of local versus general anesthesia in patients undergoing transcatheter aortic valve replacement: a meta-analysis. *Catheter Cardiovasc Interv.* 2018;91:330-342.

154. Tilley E, Psaltis PJ, Loetscher T, et al. Meta-analysis of prevalence and risk factors for delirium after transcatheter aortic valve implantation. *Am J Cardiol.* 2018;122:1917-1923.

155. Chen EY, Sukumar N, Dai F, et al. A pilot analysis of the association between types of monitored anesthesia care drugs and outcomes in transfemoral aortic valve replacement performed without general anesthesia. *J Cardiothorac Vasc Anesth.* 2018;32:666-671.

156. Di Biase L, Conti S, Mohanty P, et al. General anesthesia reduces the prevalence of pulmonary vein reconnection during repeat ablation when compared with conscious sedation: results from a randomized study. *Heart Rhythm* 2011;8:368-372.

74

Cardiovascular Disease in Patients with Cancer and Cardiovascular Complications of Cancer Therapies

Edward T. H. Yeh

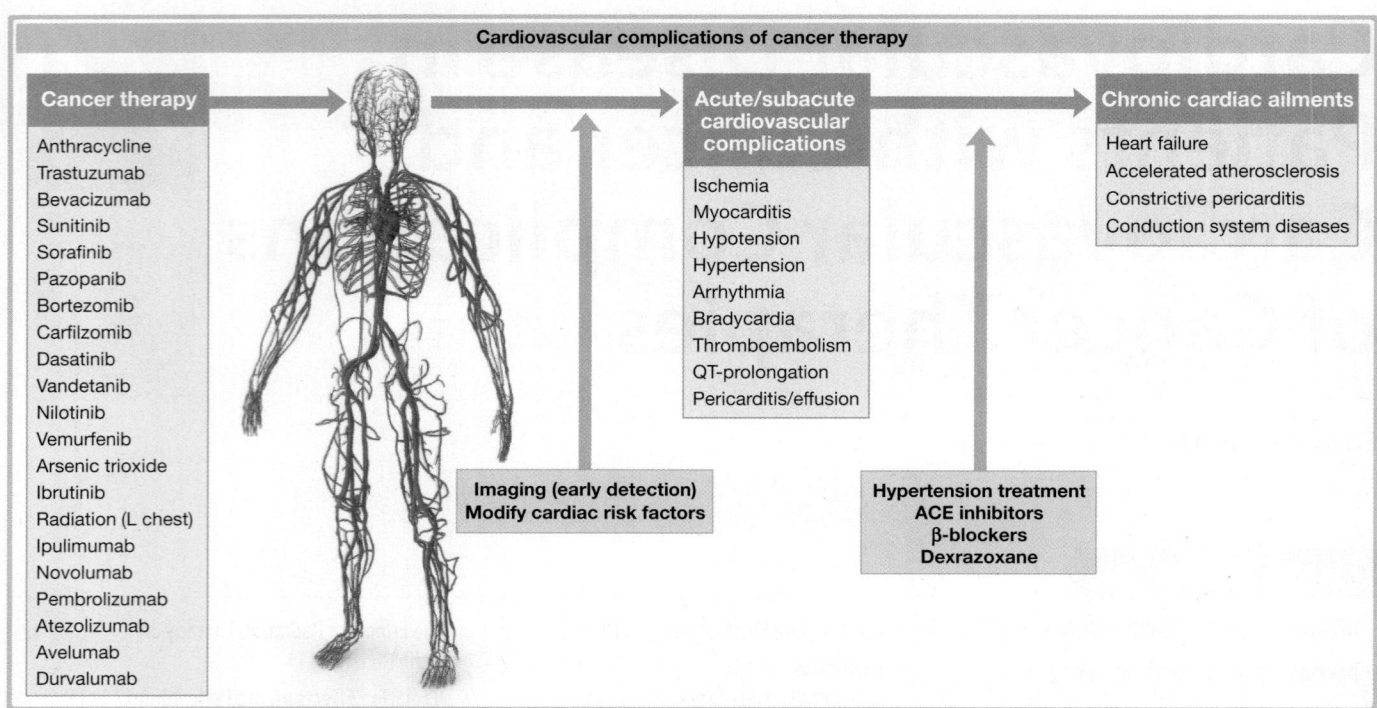

Chapter 74 Fuster and Hurst's Central Illustration. Cancer therapies, including chemotherapy, targeted therapy, immunotherapy, and radiation, can cause acute or subacute cardiovascular complications that can lead to development of chronic cardiac ailments, such as heart failure, accelerated atherosclerosis, conduction system diseases, and chronic pericarditis. Early detection and prompt intervention may prevent development of long-term sequelae, thus improving cancer survivorship. ACE, angiotensin-converting enzyme.

CHAPTER SUMMARY

This chapter discusses the cardiovascular complications of cancer therapies and tumors of the cardiovascular system. The treatment of cancer has undergone dramatic changes in this millennium. Many cancer patients have been cured, gone into remission, or have had their survival significantly extended by new therapies. Cancer therapies, including chemo- therapeutics, targeted therapy, cancer immunotherapy, and radiation treatment, can affect the cardiovascular system (see Fuster and Hurst's Central Illustration). Thus, it is important to identify risk factors, monitor potential cardiovascular compli- cations, and to administer cardioprotective treatments to cancer patients from the inception of diagnosis and throughout cancer therapy. New advances in deciphering the pathogenesis of anthracycline-induced cardiotoxicity may lead to the development of new cardioprotective strategies. Early identification and treatment of cardiovascular manifestations have been shown to prevent conversion of subclinical cardiotoxicity to heart failure or accelerated vascular diseases. With the introduction of novel cancer therapies, increased vigilance in detection of new cardiovascular complications is essential to improve delivery of optimal cancer therapy and to prevent long-term cardiovascular toxicity of cancer therapy.

INTRODUCTION AND EPIDEMIOLOGY

The treatment of cancer has undergone a dramatic change in this millennium. Many cancer patients have been cured, gone into remission, or have had their survival significantly extended by new therapies. As of January 1, 2016, more than 16.9 million Americans survived cancer and this number is expected to reach 22.1 million by 2230.[1]

Cancer patients may develop cardiovascular complications as a result of cancer therapy or as a result of progression of their underlying cardiac conditions. This may manifest during or immediately following cancer therapy. Damage to the cardiovascular system associated with cancer therapies can also be subclinical and manifest later in life. In the Childhood Cancer Survivor Study, 23,462 5-year cancer survivors were followed for more than 20 years.[2] Cumulative incidences of heart failure, coronary artery disease (CAD), pericardial disease, and arrhythmia are increased in cancer survivors compared to their siblings. Due to reductions in the dose of cardiac radiation, the cumulative incidence of CAD was lowered in patients treated after 1990 compared to earlier patient cohorts. However, new cardiovascular complications have been identified with the introduction of new cancer therapies.

The field of cardio-oncology, or onco-cardiology, has developed as a response to a rise in the incidence of cardiovascular complications caused by newer cancer therapies. Oncologists have faced the challenges of anthracycline-induced cardiotoxicity for more than 50 years, with only occasional cardiology consultation. However, cardiology services devoted to serving cancer patients emerged in the early 2000s. Many cancer centers and tertiary care hospitals have established cardio-oncology services where cardiologists work closely together with oncologists to manage cardiovascular complications during cancer treatments. Early detection of cardiotoxicity and optimal management of cardiotoxicity can improve the outcomes of cancer treatment. Prior to initiation of cancer therapy, cardiologists should work with cancer specialists to optimize management of preexisting cardiovascular conditions, including CAD, heart failure, hypertension, and arrhythmias. During treatment, cancer specialist should recognize and promptly refer suspected cardiovascular complications to cardiologists. There is also a role for cardiologists in the long-term follow-up for cancer survivors that developed cardiotoxicity during treatment or have accelerated progression of cardiovascular diseases after successful cancer therapy.

DEFINITION OF CARDIOTOXICITY

The Common Terminology Criteria for Adverse Events (CTCAE), developed by the National Cancer Institute,[3] recognizes a broad array of cardiovascular events and subclinical laboratory and imaging-based functional changes under the broad definition of cardiac and vascular disorders. These definitions should be used to report clinical or laboratory findings that resulted from cancer therapy.

Acute or subacute cardiotoxicity often manifests as chest pain, myocardial infarction (MI), hypertension, hypotension, myocarditis, pericarditis, thromboembolism, and supraventricular or ventricular arrhythmias according to the CTCAE criteria (**Tables 74–1** and **74–2**).[3-5] Chronic cardiotoxicity usually refers to cardiac disorders that manifest 1 year or more following cancer therapy. They include accelerated CAD, heart failure, conduction disorder, pericarditis, and valvular heart diseases. Injuries incurred at the time of cancer therapy may be subclinical and only manifest 1 year or more after successful cancer therapy.

FACTORS THAT CONTRIBUTE TO THE DEVELOPMENT OF CARDIOTOXICITY

Several risk factors are associated with the development of cardiotoxicity in patients being treated for cancer. These include age (older or younger), female sex, preexisting hypertension, CAD, metabolic syndrome, and past radiation therapy and chemotherapy.[4,5]

There also appears to be an important contribution of genetics to the development of cardiotoxicity, exemplified by genes associated with increase in the risk of developing anthracycline-induced cardiotoxicity.[6,7] There are also factors related to the pharmacokinetics of cancer therapy. For example, the dose of drug administered during each chemotherapy cycle, the cumulative dose, the schedule of delivery, the route of administration, concomitant use of other cardiotoxic drugs, and the sequence of administration of these drugs have been associated with relative risk of developing anthracycline-induced cardiotoxicity.[4] Cyclophosphamide causes cardiac dysfunction at doses exceeding 180 mg/kg and when given concomitantly with other cardiotoxic drugs. Similarly, ifosfamide can induce low-grade arrhythmias at doses of 1.2 to 2 g/m^2/d for 5 days, but may result in heart failure when administered at a higher dose of 10 to 18 g/m^2/d for 5 days. Interleukin (IL)-2, a T-cell growth factor, can cause body weight gain when given low dose as a continuous infusion at a rate of 9×10^6 IU/m^2/d and hypotension when given as a bolus at a dose of 600,000 IU/kg every 8 hours. Administering anthracyclines by continuous infusion over 24 to 96 hours rather than by rapid intravenous (IV) infusion reduces the risk of cardiotoxicity of these drugs in adults, but not pediatric patients.[4] Similarly, parenteral, although not oral, busulfan can result in tachyarrhythmias, hypertension, or hypotension, as well as left ventricular (LV) systolic dysfunction. Changing the sequence in which drugs are administered can also influence the risk or severity of cardiotoxicity. For example, the combination of IL-2 and interferon given simultaneously produces pronounced hypotension, but interferon treatment alone for 2 weeks followed by IL-2 treatment has less effect on blood pressure. Concomitant administration of anthracycline with trastuzumab caused heart failure in 18% of breast cancer patients in the initial trastuzumab clinical trials.

PATHOPHYSIOLOGY OF CARDIOTOXICITIES

Many cancer therapies can cardiotoxicities, including damage to the myocardium, vasculature, valves, or conduction system.[4,5] Damage to cardiovascular structures may be reversible or irreversible, depending on the nature and intensity of the damage and whether early remedial intervention has been

TABLE 74–1. Cardiotoxicity of Chemotherapy and Antibody-Based Therapy

Heart Failure	Ischemia	Hypotension	Hypertension	Bradycardia	QT Prolongation or Torsade de Pointes	Thromboembolism	Pericarditis/Pericardial Effusion
Anthracyclines	Bevacizumab (Avastin)	Alemtuzumab (Campath)	Bevacizumab (Avastin)	Paclitaxel (Taxol)	Asenic trioxide (Trisenox)	Bevacizumab (Avastin)	Doxorubicin (Adriamycin)
Mitoxantrone (Novantrone)	Capecitabine (Xeloda)	All-*trans*-retinoic acid (Atra; Tretinoin)	Sorafenib (Nexavar)	Thalidomide (Thalomid)	Dasatinib (Sprycel)	Cisplatin (Platinol-AQ)	Cyclophosphamide (Cytoxan)
Alkylating agents	Docetaxel (Taxotere)	Decitabine (Dacogen)	Sunitinib (Sutent)	Bortezomib (Velcade)	Lapatinib (Tykerb)	Erlotinib (Tarceva)	Busulphan (Myleran)
Cyclophosphamide (Cytoxan)	Erlotinib (Tarceva)	Denileukin (Ontak)	Imatinib (Gleevec)	Cisplatin (Platinol-AQ)	Nilotinib (Tasigna)	Lenalidomide (Revlimid)	Clofarabine (Clolar)
Ifosfamide (Ifex)	Fluorouracil (5-FU; Adrucil)	Etoposide (Vepsid)	Dasatinib (Sprycel)		Vorinostat (Zolinza)	Sunitinib (Sutent)	Dasatinib (Sprycel)
Antimicrotubule agent	Paclitaxel (Taxol)	Interferon-α	Mitoxantrone (Novantrone)		Pazopanib (Votrient)	Thalidomide (Thalomid)	Imatinib (Gleevec)
Docetaxel (Taxotere)	Sorafenib (Nexavar)	Interleukin-2				Vorinostat (Zolinza)	
Monoclonal antibody-based tyrosine kinase inhibitor	Sunitinib (Sutent)	Paclitaxel (Taxol)				Pomalidomide (Pomalyst)	
Bevacizumab (Avastin)	Lapatinib (Tykerb)	Rituximab (Rituxan)				Ponatinib (Iclusig)	
Trastuzumab (Herceptin)	Pazopanib (Votrient)						
Proteasome Inhibitor	Cytarabine (Depocyt)						
Bortezomib (Velcade)	Ifosfamide (Ifex)						
Carfilzomib (Krypolis)							
Small molecule tyrosine kinase inhibitors							
Dasatinib (Sprycel)							
Lapatinib (Tykerb)							
Imatinib (Gleevec)							
Sunitinib (Sutent)							
Antimetabolites							
Clofarabine (Clolar)							

TABLE 74–2. Cardiotoxicity of Immune Checkpoint Inhibitors

Immune Checkpoint Inhibitor	Target	CV complications
Ipulimumab	CTLA-4	Pericarditis, myocarditis
Novolumab	PD-1	Myocarditis, Cardiac arrhythmia
Pembrolizumab	PD-1	Heart failure
Atezolizumab	PDL-1	Myocardial infarction
Avelumab	PDL-1	Myocarditis
Durvalumab	PDL-1	Myocarditis

instituted. The anthracycline class of chemotherapy has long been known to cause a dose-dependent cardiotoxicity.[8] The old paradigm attributes anthracycline-induced cardiotoxicity to the chemical structure of anthracyclines, which can convert oxygen to superoxide and through an iron-dependent reaction to hydroxy radicals, leading to death of cardiomyocytes.[9,10] Dexrazoxane is the only FDA-approved drug that is effective in preventing anthracycline-induced cardiotoxicity. The efficacy was previously attributed to the antioxidative and iron-chelating property of dexrazoxane. However, recently studies showed that dexrazoxane is an inhibitor of topoisomerase 2 (Top 2), the molecular targets for anthracycline.[11] There are two Top 2 isoforms.[12] Top 2α is highly expressed in cancer cells and its inhibition causes DNA replication block and apoptosis.[13] However, the adult heart only expresses Top 2β and deletion of Top 2β in a murine model prevented doxorubicin-induced cardiotoxicity.[14] Furthermore, deletion of Top 2β also prevented doxorubicin-induced production of reactive oxygen-species and mitochondrial pathology due to inhibition of transcription of antioxidative and mitochondrial biogenesis genes (**Fig. 74–1**).

Thus, the Top 2β-based paradigm for anthracycline-induced cardiotoxicity explains three cardinal features including death of myocardial cells, generation of reactive oxygen species, and pathology of the mitochondria. This new paradigm does not exclude other contributory factors, such as iron-overload in hemochromatosis or proteins involved in the metabolism of anthracyclines.[15,16] The elucidation of the molecular basis of anthracycline-induced cardiotoxicity provides a rational approach to prevent anthracycline-induced cardiotoxicity (see section Prevention of Heart Failure).

Trastuzumab, antibody against HER2/Erb2 on the cell surface of cancer cells, is highly effective in treating HER2-poisitive tumors.[17] However, HER2 is also expressed at a lower level on the surface of the cardiomyocytes; binding neuregulin to HER2 promotes survival of cardiomyocytes. Deletion of HER2 on murine cardiomyocytes during development results in dilated cardiomyopathy and HER-2 negative cardiomyocytes are more sensitive to anthracycline-induced cardiotoxicity.[18] In early clinical trials, trastuzumab was used in conjunction with anthracyclines resulting a high incidence of heart failure. Newer studies, segregating the use of trastuzumab from anthracycline, resulted in a much lower incidence of heart failure.

Several multikinase inhibitors, such as sunitinib, induces hypertension through inhibition of the vascular endothelial growth factor/receptor (VEGF/VEGFR) and platelet-derived growth factor/receptor (PDGF/PDGFR) axis. Without prompt management of hypertension, these inhibitors can cause heart failure. PDGFR, expresses on cardiomyocytes, is important for survival of cardiomyocytes in response to load stress, such as hypertension. Furthermore, VEGF/VEGFR inhibition can also damage the endothelium and platelets leading to development of thromboembolism.

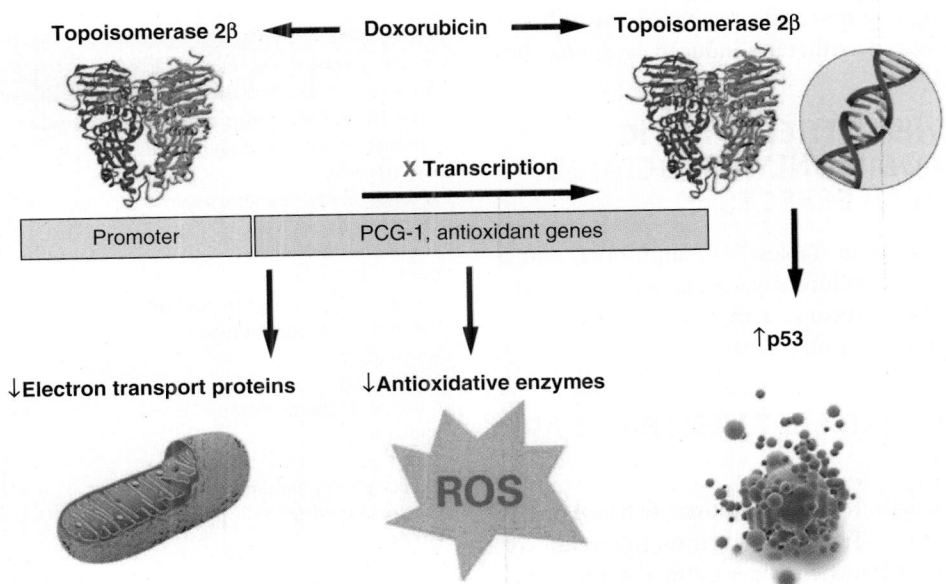

Figure 74–1. Mechanism of anthracycline-induced cardiotoxicity. Doxorubicin disrupts the normal catalytic cycle of Topoisomerase 2β, causing DNA double-stranded breaks leading to increase in p53 and death of cardiomyocytes. It also brings Topoisomerase 2β to the promoters of genes encoding electron transport proteins and antioxidative enzymes, leading to defective mitochondrial biogenesis and increase in reactive oxygen species (ROS). Thus, the Topoisomerase 2β hypothesis explained the three cardinal features of doxorubicin-induced cardiotoxicity.

Advances in cancer immunotherapy also introduced a new spectrum of cardiotoxicities that require close collaboration between cardiologists and oncologists. Immunotherapy typically targets tumors with an antibody against cancer surface receptor, such as HER-2, or receptors on the surface of immune cells. Of particular importance is the new class of immune checkpoint inhibitors that release "breaks" in the immune system by targeting cytotoxic T cell antigen 4 (CTLA-4), programmed cell death (PD-1), or programmed cell death ligand 1 (PDL-1) (see Table 73–2). CTLA-4 and PD-1 are expressed on T cells, whereas PDL-1 is expressed on tumor cells or dendritic cells and macrophages.[19] By activating T cells to kill cancer cells, these immune checkpoint inhibitors can also unleash the immune system to attack "self" organs, such as the heart. Cardiovascular complications of immune checkpoint therapy can range from myocarditis, pericarditis, cardiac arrhythmias, to MI.[20] The mechanisms whereby checkpoint therapies break immune tolerance leading to autoimmune response is not well understood. Another emerging immune therapy, chimeric antigen receptor (CAR) T-cell therapy, is delivered by autologous or allogenic T lymphocytes that stably expressed single-chain fragment variable region domain linked to the signaling domain of the T-cell receptor. The variable region domain is designed to recognize target-specific tumor antigens resulting in activation of strong T-cell immunity against tumors. A serious complication caused by hyper-activation of the immune response is the cytokine release syndrome (CRS). Cytokines are proteins produced by activated immune cells that further amplify the immune response resulting in hypotension, vascular leaks, thromboembolism, and respiratory failure. IL-6 is considered to be the central mediator of CRS, which can be treated with an antibody against soluble or membrane-bound IL-6 receptor.[21] Further understanding of the mechanisms whereby anticancer therapy causes cardiotoxicity is critical in designing more effective, mechanism-based intervention to prevent cancer therapy-induced cardiotoxicity.

CLASSES OF CHEMOTHERAPEUTIC AGENTS AND COMMONLY ASSOCIATED CARDIOVASCULAR EFFECTS

These classes are outlined in Tables 74–1 and 74–2, and a detailed discussion of heart failure, myocardial ischemia, myocarditis, changes in blood pressure, arrhythmias and QT prolongation, and thromboembolism follows.

HEART FAILURE AND LEFT VENTRICULAR DYSFUNCTION

There is no consensus definition of cardiotoxicity based on LV ejection fraction (LVEF).[22,23] Trials studying in anthracycline- or trastuzumab-induced cardiotoxicity have defined cardiac dysfunction as a ≥5% decline in LVEF to result in an LVEF <55% with symptoms of heart failure, or a ≥10% decline to result in an LVEF <55% without symptoms of heart failure.[24–26] The CTCAE by the National Cancer Institute defines three different

grades of decreased ejection fraction. Grade 2: EF 40% to 50% or 10% to 19% drop from baseline; Grade 3: EF 20% to 39% or ≥20% drop from baseline; Grade 4: EF <20%. The American Society of Echocardiography (ASE) defines chemotherapy-related cardiac dysfunction (CTRCD) as a decrease in the LVEF of greater than 10 percentage points, to a value <53%, which is deemed the normal reference value for two-dimensional (2D) echocardiography as per this society.[23] The European Society of Medical Oncology (ESMO) define CTRCD as a reduction in LVEF of 10% or more to <50% with or without symptoms.[22]

The basic pathophysiology of heart failure is essentially the same in both cancer and noncancer patients. The neurohormonal hypothesis that forms the basis of the diagnosis of heart failure and shapes the strategies for effective treatment is applicable in both groups of patients. Although the triggering event of the heart failure may be the chemotherapy, the contribution of preexisting and coexisting cardiovascular risk factors may be difficult to quantify separately. **Table 74-3** summarizes the typical causes of LV systolic dysfunction and heart failure in cancer patients. All of the major contributors to heart failure need to be investigated and treated appropriately to optimally affect the course of illness (see Chapters 48 and 50).

Strategies for Diagnosing Heart Failure and Left Ventricular Dysfunction

Physical examination remains important in detecting heart failure and LV systolic dysfunction in cancer patients, and is still the most reliable means of characterizing volume status. Physical findings such as a third heart sound or jugular venous distension can be highly predictive of heart failure (see Chapter 2).

Among basic laboratory studies, the electrocardiogram (ECG) does not discern heart failure or LV dysfunction, although it can confirm suspected abnormalities or indicate

TABLE 74–3. Causes of Left Ventricular Systolic Dysfunction or Heart Failure in Cancer Patients

Preexisting Risk Factors or Underlying Disease
Coronary artery disease and ischemia
Hypertension
Alcohol-related cardiomyopathy
Diabetes
Nutritional deficiencies
Cardiac cachexia
Thyrotoxicosis or hypothyroidism
Related to Cancer Diagnosis
Amyloidosis
Myocarditis
Cardiotoxic chemotherapy
Radiation
Sepsis
Capillary leak phenomenon
Carcinoid syndrome
Other
Arterial venous fistula
Endocarditis
Pericardial disease, including constrictive pericarditis
Pulmonary emboli
Pulmonary hypertension
Hemochromatosis and iron overload (frequent transfusions)

potential underlying cardiac disease, such as ischemia, conduction abnormalities, or chamber enlargement. Additional laboratory testing should include lipid panel to identify risk for vascular disease and blood glucose monitoring to screen for diabetes, both clinical predictors for heart failure. Anemia, especially common in cancer patients, has been directly correlated with outcomes in heart failure patients and should be part of a basic laboratory screen (see Chapter 48). Other specific biomarkers that are crucial in the evaluation of patients with suspected heart failure, especially those with cancer, include cardiac troponin I as well as B-type natriuretic peptide (BNP). Troponins may have value in screening for LV systolic dysfunction that develops during the course of chemotherapy.[4] The role of BNP levels to detect early cardiotoxicity, LV dysfunction, or to detect volume overload has been studied in this population.[27] However, it may be falsely elevated without the presence of LV dysfunction or heart failure in cancer patients.

LVEF, most commonly determined by echocardiography, is currently the mainstay of detecting heart failure or asymptomatic LV dysfunction during chemotherapy. Monitoring protocols for patients undergoing anthracycline-based chemotherapy in the 1970s and 1980s were developed and validated based on radionuclide multigated acquisition (MUGA) scans. These, although highly reproducible, have been largely replaced by echocardiography and, as such, the algorithms validated for MUGA may be applied to echocardiography imaging. Widespread availability, feasibility, lack of radiation exposure, and acquisition of additional cardiac imaging information (valvular, pericardial, and hemodynamic data) make echocardiography an attractive option for serial imaging. Echocardiographic strain imaging has recently emerged as a promising method for detection of early cardiotoxicity prior to LV dysfunction. Three-dimensional (3D) echo imaging has shown promising results with least inter- and intra-observer variability and reproducibility, which could be comparable to MUGA. However, there are certain circumstances in which one technique is favored over the other. In pediatric patients, echocardiography is preferred because of the lack of ionizing radiation. In obese patients, however, adequate echocardiographic windows may be difficult to attain. Furthermore, the usefulness of echocardiography is limited in other variations of thoracic anatomy, such as emphysema, tight intercostal spaces, and heavily calcified ribs. Three-dimensional echocardiography is dependent on patient's ability to hold the breath and requires a longer offline analysis. MUGA is less feasible in patients with arrhythmias as a result of poor electrocardiography-based triggering, which is more often seen in patients with heart failure. Often, the choice of technique is governed by the availability of local resources and personal experience, rather than which method is more accurate or more suitable for the individual patient. Therefore, all the described noninvasive techniques should be viewed as complementary.

Of particular interest in detecting early cardiotoxicity is the application of strain imaging, which is a measure of regional deformation of the myocardium. It is mainly obtained by angle-independent 2D speckle-tracking echocardiography, which can evaluate all three domains of myocardial mechanics (longitudinal, circumferential, and radial) and derive data for deformation and rate of deformation for each myocardial segment (**Fig. 74–2**). Two-dimensional speckle-tracking

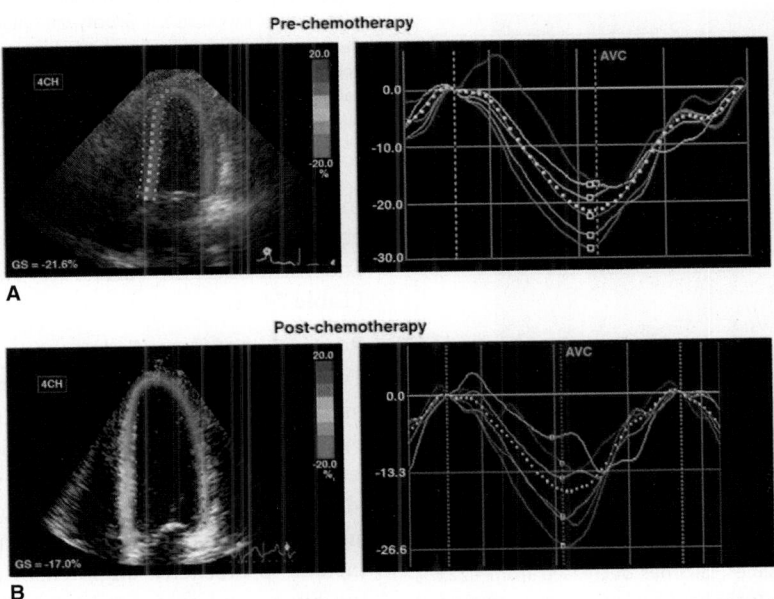

Figure 74–2. A 2D speckle-tracking echocardiogram-based strain in a patient with invasive ductal carcinoma. A patient with invasive ductal carcinoma (estrogen receptor negative, progesterone receptor negative, human epidermal growth factor receptor 2/neu positive), treated with the TCH regimen (docetaxel, carboplatin, and trastuzumab), had a baseline EF of 65%. The EF after 3 months of therapy was 58%. **(A)** and **(B)** utilize color to illustrate the global longitudinal strain (GLS) and regional strain values obtained at **(A)** baseline (prechemotherapy) and **(B)** 3 months after the initiation of trastuzumab-based regimen. The septal and anteroseptal segments exhibit abnormal regional strain after treatment. Reproduced with permission from Kongbundansuk S, Hundley WG. Noninvasive Imaging of Cardiovascular Injury Related to the Treatment of Cancer. *JACC Cardiovasc Imaging.* 2014 Aug;7(8):824-838.

echocardiography has been used in multiple independent studies, reporting changes in cardiac (mechanical) function before a decrease in LVEF and even before changes in diastolic function after chemotherapy.[23] Based on numerous studies of strain rate imaging during cancer chemotherapy, a greater than 10% change in global longitudinal strain (GLS) after completion of anthracycline-based chemotherapy relative to baseline is predictive of a future decrease in LVEF (**Fig. 74–3**). Conceivably, but subject to further studies, abnormal strain values before cancer therapy may signal higher baseline risk for chemotherapy-induced cardiotoxicity. Based on the above discussion, it seems appropriate to include strain imaging in monitoring algorithms for cardiotoxicity. Thereby, the ASE recommends strain rate imaging as an inherent part of a comprehensive echocardiogram for patients undergoing cancer chemotherapy. It also recommends 3D echocardiography as the preferred technique for monitoring of LV function and detecting CTRCD

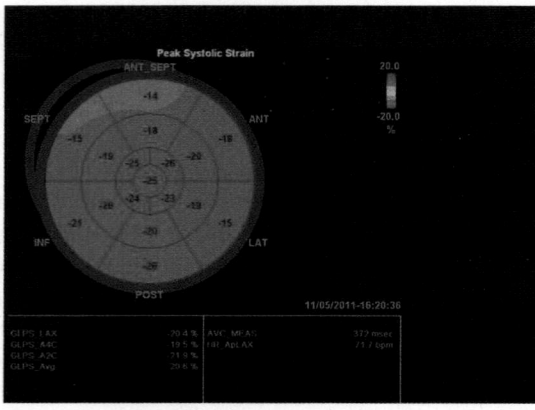

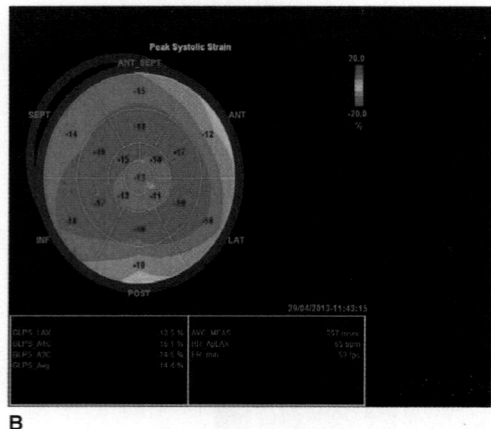

Figure 74–3. Bullseye plot showing global longitudinal strain (GLS) of a breast cancer patient. **(A)** GLS and regional longitudinal strain at baseline. **(B)** GLS and regional longitudinal strain 3 months during trastuzumab-based therapy after anthracyclines. GLS has decreased from −22.6% to −14.4% (30% decrease). The decrease in GLS is therefore considered of clinical significance (>15% vs baseline). Reproduced with permission from Plana JC, Galderisi M, Barac A, et al. Expert consensus for multimodality imaging evaluation of adult patients during and after cancer therapy: a report from the American Society of Echocardiography and the European Association of Cardiovascular Imaging. *Eur Heart J Cardiovasc Imaging.* 2014 Oct;15(10):1063-1093.

TABLE 74–4. Recommended Cardio-Oncology Echocardiogram Protocol
Standard transthoracic echocardiography
In accordance with ASE/EAE guidelines and IAC-Echo
2D strain imaging acquisition
Apical three-, four-, and two-chamber views
Acquire ≥3 cardiac cycles
Images obtained simultaneously maintaining the same 2D frame rate and imaging depth
Frame rate between 40 and 90 frames/sec or ≥40% of HR
Aortic VTI (aortic ejection time)
2D strain imaging analysis
Quantify segmental strain and GLS
Display the segmental strain curves from apical views in a quad format
Display the global strain in a bull's-eye plot
2D strain imaging pitfalls
Ectopy
Breathing translation
3D imaging acquisition
Apical four-chamber full volume to assess LV volumes and LVEF calculation
Single and multiple beats optimizing spatial and temporal resolution
Reporting
Timing of echocardiography with respect to the intravenous infusion (number of days before or after)
Vital signs (BP, HR)
3D LVEF/2D biplane Simpson's method
GLS (echocardiography machine, software, and version used)
In the absence of GLS, measurement of medial and lateral s' and MAPSE
RV: TAPSE, s', FAC

Abbreviations: ASE, American Society of Echocardiography; BP, blood pressure; EAE, European Association of Echocardiography; FAC, fractional area change; GLS, global longitudinal strain; HR, heart rate; IAC-Echo, Intersocietal Accreditation Commission Echocardiography; LV, left ventricular; LVEF, left ventricular ejection fraction; MAPSE, mitral annular plane systolic excursion; RV, right ventricle; TAPSE, tricuspid annular plane systolic excursion; VTI, velocity-time integral.

Reproduced with permission from Plana JC, Galderisi M, Barac A, et al. Expert consensus for multimodality imaging evaluation of adult patients during and after cancer therapy: a report from the American Society of Echocardiography and the European Association of Cardiovascular Imaging. *Eur Heart J Cardiovasc Imaging.* 2014 Oct;15(10):1063-1093.

in patients with cancer, because LVEF determination by 2D echocardiography, with or without contrast, has inherent inter- and intra-observer variability that may vary by up to 10% (**Table 74–4**).

Prevention of Heart Failure

Two approaches for primary prevention of anthracycline-induced cardiotoxicity are to (1) reduce cardiotoxic potency by administering via continuous infusion, liposome encapsulation, or using a less cardiotoxic derivative (eg, epirubicin or idarubicin); and (2) use a cardioprotective agent (eg, dexrazoxane) in conjunction with treatment. Other investigated agents include β-blockers, angiotensin-converting enzyme (ACE) inhibitors, and angiotensin receptor blockers (ARBs). Earlier trials, such as the OVERCOME trial,[28] have studied the role of carvedilol and enalapril in prevention of LV dysfunction in patients with hematological malignancies undergoing stem cell transplantation with high-dose chemotherapy, while newer trials such as PRADA[29] have demonstrated the role of ARBs such as valsartan in primary prevention of LV dysfunction in patients receiving anthracyclines for breast cancer.

Dexrazoxane, the only FDA-approved drug for prevention of anthracycline cardiotoxicity, is a potent Top 2β inhibitor.[11] The mechanism of dexrazoxane cardio-protection was originally attributed to the iron chelation properties of its EDTA-like hydrolysis product, leading to decreased levels of hydroxyl free radicals. This notion was challenged by subsequent studies documenting lack of protection against doxorubicin-induced cardiomyopathy provided by deferasirox (another iron chelator) and several other free radical scavengers.[30] More recently, it was shown that dexrazoxane-induced cardio-protection is related to its ability to antagonize the DNA damage caused by doxorubicin by means of interference with Top 2. Interestingly, dexrazoxane can degrade Top 2β, but not Top 2α, thus, removing the cardiotoxic Top 2β, but retaining the cancer killing Top 2α. In animal study, Top 2β is completely degraded 6 hours after administration of dexrazoxane and it takes 2 days for Top 2β to return to baseline level. A National Institute of Health–sponsored clinical trial will test this new strategy by administering dexrazoxane 8 hours before doxorubicin to determine whether cardiotoxicity can be ameliorated.

The Principles of Therapy for Heart Failure

The principles of therapy for heart failure and LV dysfunction in cancer patients are similar to those in patients without cancer. An often-overlooked management component is the education of both the patient and family members regarding early recognition of the symptoms of fluid overload and cardiac decompensation. Management of patients who develop heart failure from cardiotoxicity during or after cancer therapy should be in keeping with the American College of Cardiology/American Heart Association (ACC/AHA) and/or European Society of Cardiology (ESC) heart failure guidelines.[31,32]

ACE inhibitors and β-adrenergic blocking agents remain the cornerstone of therapy and have specifically been studied in cancer patients.[33] The timing from completion of anthracycline-based chemotherapy to initiation of heart failure therapy was identified as the crucial determinant of the response rate. Early initiation of these agents is key as the recovery of LV function is dependent on early initiation of heart failure treatment. The usefulness of ARBs, as alternatives to ACE inhibitors, for the treatment of heart failure can be extrapolated to the cancer population as well. The combination of nitrates and hydralazine may have specific efficacy in Black patients, as well as in patients with renal insufficiency not able to receive ACE inhibitors or ARBs. The precise role of aldosterone receptor antagonists (eg, spironolactone) in the treatment of chemotherapy-induced cardiomyopathy is currently unknown, but may be considered in those with New York Heart Association (NYHA) class >I symptoms and an LVEF of 35% or less. Moreover, the newer heart failure therapies such as Sacubitril/Valsartan and SGLT2 inhibitors have not been studied in chemo-induced cardiomyopathy.

Hemodynamic device support may be considered if medical therapy fails. Acute hemodynamic support can be temporarily lifesaving in situations such as acute myopericarditis owing to drugs such as cyclophosphamide. Alternatively, chronic LV assist device support may become a bridge to transplant or destination therapy in some cases.[34] The most severe heart failure may be observed in patients receiving both chemotherapy and radiation therapy.[35]

In addition, risk factors for heart failure should also be aggressively treated in cancer patients. For example, it is critical to treat tyrosine kinase inhibitor (TKI)–induced hypertension to avoid progression to overt heart failure. Moreover, the higher incidence of drug–drug interactions in cancer patients undergoing chemotherapy and heart failure therapy should be recognized. The addition of a potentially beneficial heart failure medications should be carefully weighed against the risk of possible interactions with anticancer agents.

Cardiac devices can be an integral part of heart failure management in cancer patients. Placement of an implantable cardioverter-defibrillator is reasonable in patients with LVEF of <30% to 35% of any origin with NYHA functional class II or III symptoms who are taking chronic optimal medical therapy and who have reasonable expectation of survival with good functional status of more than 1 year.[36] Similar considerations pertain to biventricular pacemaker implantation in appropriate cancer patients.

Surgical techniques may be appropriate in selected situations resulting in heart failure, such as pericardial stripping for constrictive pericarditis or removal of intracardiac masses. Ethical concerns are also important when deciding on the appropriate therapy for a cancer patient with heart failure. One must consider to what extent the two entities interplay and to what extent they affect the patient's overall prognosis. It is important to openly address end-of-life issues with patients so that the treatment approach incorporates the wishes of the patient as well as the reality of the clinical condition. The diagnosis of cancer should not imply that a patient's cardiovascular disease cannot or should not be aggressively treated. Treatment decisions should be individualized.

In addition to standard treatment of heart failure, key management of LV dysfunction resulting from cancer chemotherapy includes correction of risk factors, early detection, and regular surveillance. **Tables 74-5** and **74-6**, adapted from the ESMO guidelines,[22] include key points for consideration while evaluating patients before and during administration of potentially cardiotoxic chemotherapy.

Myocardial Ischemia

Chest pain is a common symptom in cancer patients who are undergoing various forms of anticancer therapy. Chest pain often necessitates the interruption of chemotherapy, while serial cardiac enzyme assessments and ECGs are performed. If non–ST-segment elevation MI or Q-wave MI is confirmed, patients should be managed according to the current ACC/AHA or ESC guidelines.[37] Thrombocytopenia and brain metastases pose a particular problem for cancer patients with acute coronary syndrome (ACS) because anticoagulant/antiplatelet therapies may be contraindicated under these circumstances. Similarly continuing dual antiplatelet therapy after

TABLE 74–5. Evaluation of Patients Before Initiation of Chemotherapy

Prechemotherapy

- All patients undergoing chemo- and/or radiation therapy should have careful clinical evaluation and assessment of cardiovascular risk factors and comorbidities
- Patients with pre-existing cardiovascular disease, especially cardiomyopathy, cardiac arrhythmias, or CAD, or significant modifiable cardiovascular risk factors, especially hypertension, should be adequately managed before and during therapy, preferably by a Cardio-Oncology consultation
- TTE and 12-lead ECG should be obtained in all patients before potential cardiotoxic cancer treatment
- In patients at high risk for cardiotoxicity (especially preexisting cardiomyopathy, heart failure, CAD, or hypertension, prior radiation or anthracycline therapy, age >60–65 years), cardioprotective agents should be considered; ACE inhibitors are first-line therapy including for those with BP >140/85 mm Hg, but recent data also support ARBs, carvedilol, or nebivolol
- Dexrazoxane is recommended as a cardioprotectant by the American Society of Clinical Oncology only for patients with metastatic breast cancer who have already received more than 300 mg/m² of doxorubicin
- If low or borderline LVEF, may consider a non-anthracycline-containing regimen

Abbreviations: ACE, angiotensin-converting enzyme; ARBs, angiotensin receptor blockers; BP, blood pressure; CAD, coronary artery disease; ECG, electrocardiogram; LVEF, left ventricular ejection fraction; TTE, transthoracic echocardiography.

Data from Curigliano G, Cardinale D, Suter T, et al. Cardiovascular toxicity induced by chemotherapy, targeted agents and radiotherapy: ESMO Clinical Practice Guidelines. *Ann Oncol.* 2012 Oct;23 Suppl 7:vii155-vii66.

TABLE 74–6. Evaluation of Patients during Chemotherapy

During chemotherapy

- If metastatic disease, LVEF should be monitored at baseline and then infrequently in the absence of symptoms
- Serial monitoring of cardiac function at baseline, 3, 6, and 9 months during treatment, and then at 12 and 18 months after the initiation of treatment, revised as indicated
- LVEF reduction ≥15% from baseline with normal function (LVEF ≥50%) is not an indication to discontinue chemotherapy
- In case of LVEF decline to <40% stop chemotherapy, discuss alternatives, and treat left ventricular dysfunction (standard guideline-based heart failure therapy)
- LVEF decline to <50% during chemotherapy necessitates reassessment after 3 weeks; if confirmed, hold chemotherapy, consider therapy for left ventricular dysfunction and further frequent clinical and echocardiographic checks
- Aggressive medical treatment of those patients, even asymptomatic, who show left ventricular dysfunction on echocardiography after anthracycline therapy is mandatory, especially if the neoplasia could have a long-term survival; it consists of angiotensin-converting enzyme inhibitor and β-blockers, and the earlier heart failure therapy is begun (within 2 months from the end of anthracycline therapy), the better the therapeutic response
- Patients who develop cardiac dysfunction during or following treatment with type II agents (trastuzumab) in the absence of anthracyclines can be observed if they remain asymptomatic and LVEF remains ≥40%

Abbreviation: LVEF, left ventricular ejection fraction. Data from Curigliano G, Cardinale D, Suter T, et al. Cardiovascular toxicity induced by chemotherapy, targeted agents and radiotherapy: ESMO Clinical Practice Guidelines. *Ann Oncol.* 2012 Oct;23 Suppl 7: vii155-vii66.

percutaneous coronary intervention in cancer patients with impending cancer surgery, active bleeding, or thrombocytopenia, or in those undergoing bone marrow transplant, poses a clinical challenge where risks for coronary thromboses have to be balanced against those for bleeding.

It is well established that radiation therapy to the mediastinum promotes an increased risk for future infarction, and it appears more prevalent in patients with left-sided chest radiation.[38] Additionally, several chemotherapy agents are known to precipitate or exacerbate myocardial ischemia. Cisplatin infusions can cause chest pain, palpitations, and, occasionally, elevated cardiac enzyme levels indicative of an MI.[4] Cisplatin is also implicated in cardiovascular complications such as hypertension, LV hypertrophy, myocardial ischemia, and MI as long as 10 to 20 years after the remission of metastatic testicular cancer. 5-Fluorouracil (5-FU) can also cause an ischemic syndrome that may range from subclinical myocardial ischemia to acute MI.[39] Subsequent re-challenge with 5-FU frequently reproduces the initial ischemic event. Nevertheless, ischemia is usually reversed when 5-FU treatment is stopped and anti-ischemic therapy implemented. In some patients, pretreatment with nitrates and calcium channel–blocking agents has allowed therapy deemed crucial to be continued. Capecitabine, which is currently used in the treatment of breast and gastrointestinal cancers, is believed to be less toxic than 5-FU, although its use has been associated with cardiotoxic effects including ischemic phenomena, arrhythmias, ECG changes, and (rarely) cardiomyopathy. Vinca alkaloids, such as vinorelbine, also have been reported to cause angina associated with ECG changes and arrhythmias, as well as MI. Angina and MI are serious, but relatively rare, consequences of interferon-α therapy. Fatal MI and thrombosis have also been noted after the use of all-*trans*-retinoic acid (ATRA). Bevacizumab, a recombinant humanized IgG$_1$ antibody that binds to and inhibits the activity of human VEGF, was recently shown to be associated with an increased risk of angina and MI, in addition to serious arterial thromboembolic events, including cerebrovascular accident and transient ischemic attacks.[40] It is used for the treatment of metastatic colon carcinoma and is generally used in combination with other agents. A new class of chemotherapy agents, termed *vascular disrupting agents*, is currently undergoing clinical evaluation. These agents have been noted to cause asymptomatic creatinine kinase-myocardial bound release and may be associated with ACS.

Blood Pressure Fluctuations

The classic malignancy causing hypertension, often paroxysmal or episodic in nature, is pheochromocytoma, a rare catecholamine-secreting tumor most commonly benign, although malignant in 10% of cases. Pheochromocytomas may be isolated tumors, but can also be associated with multiple endocrine neoplasia (MEN) syndromes of the type 2 variety, particularly the MEN 2A and MEN 2B syndromes. Bilateral pheochromocytomas are also associated with von Hippel–Lindau disease and neurofibromatosis. Benign pheochromocytomas usually can be resected surgically, but patients with such tumors require special anesthetic considerations, including pretreatment with phenoxybenzamine followed by the administration of a β-adrenergic blocking agent. Other tumors may also cause hypertension, including hyperthyroidism associated with thyroid tumors.

Several cancer therapies may cause hypertension or hypotension (Table 74–1).[5] Newer targeted cancer therapies, which inhibit angiogenesis, frequently cause hypertension in cancer patients. Sorafenib is a potent inhibitor of the VEGFR-2, VEGFR-3, FLT-3, c-kit, and platelet-derived growth factor receptor in vitro and may affect the regulation of endothelial cell proliferation and survival. In clinical trials, sorafenib increases blood pressure in 17% to 43% of patients, whereas sunitinib is associated with slightly less hypertension, seen in 5% to 24% of patients. Similarly, hypertension has been observed in 4% to 35% of bevacizumab-treated patients. The mechanism by which these agents induce hypertension is not fully understood; however, it is thought to be related to VEGF inhibition, which decreases nitric oxide production in the wall of the arterioles and other resistance vessels. When treating hypertension in these patients, some antihypertensive agents may be preferred over others, because each agent affects angiogenesis in different ways. ACE inhibitors may be selected as first-line therapy, because of their ability to prevent proteinuria and plasminogen activator inhibitor-1 expression. In addition, ACE inhibitors have demonstrated the potential to reduce microcirculatory changes, decrease the catabolism of bradykinin, and increase release of endothelial nitric oxide. Phosphodiesterase inhibitors and nitrates have also been suggested for the treatment of hypertension in these patients, because of their ability to increase nitric oxide levels. Lastly, the β-blocker, nebivolol, which has the unique mechanism of action of blocking β-adrenergic 1 receptor as well as causing vasodilation through the nitric oxide pathway, may also be beneficial in the treatment of hypertension caused by antiangiogenic cancer treatments. Antirejection regimen such as cyclosporine A, especially when used in conjunction with corticosteroids, are associated with hypertension; the incidence may be greater than 50%. The complex mechanism of cyclosporin-induced hypertension includes alterations in vascular reactivity that cause widespread vasoconstriction, vascular effects in the kidney leading to reduced glomerular filtration and impaired sodium excretion, stimulation of endothelin, and suppression of vasodilating prostaglandins. Effective therapy includes use of vasodilating agents, often calcium channel blockers.

Hypotension is the most common side effect of etoposide. The infusion of monoclonal antibodies commonly causes hypotension as a result of the massive release of cytokines (an acute transfusion reaction); these agents may also cause fever, dyspnea, hypoxia, and even death. Careful monitoring for hypotension is especially important for patients with preexisting cardiac disease. Cetuximab, a human/mouse chimeric monoclonal antibody that binds to the human epidermal growth factor receptor, may cause severe, potentially fatal infusion reactions characterized by hypotension, bronchospasm, and urticaria; this phenomenon occurs in approximately 3%

of patients. Rituximab, a chimeric murine/human monoclonal antibody directed against the CD20 antigen, may cause infusion-related side effects that occur within the first few hours of the start of infusion. Supportive measures that are usually effective include IV fluids, vasopressors, bronchodilators, diphenhydramine, and acetaminophen. Interferon-α usually causes acute symptoms during the first 2 to 8 hours after treatment; these include flulike symptoms, hypotension, tachycardia, and nausea, and vomiting. The retinoic acid syndrome appears in approximately 26% of patients who receive ATRA, typically within the first 21 days of treatment. This syndrome includes fever, dyspnea, hypotension, and pericardial and pleural effusions. High-dose treatment with IL-2 may result in adverse cardiovascular and hemodynamic effects similar to those of septic shock and may lead to hypotension, vascular leak syndrome (hypotension, edema, hypoalbuminemia), and respiratory insufficiency requiring pressor agents and mechanical ventilation support.

Blood pressure variations that are unrelated to chemotherapy are much more common in cancer patients; the combination of malnutrition and dehydration is one of the most common causes of hypotension. Other complications of malignancy, most notably sepsis, may be accompanied by profound and refractory hypotension.

Arrhythmias

Arrhythmia in cancer patients may be a consequence of cardiotoxic anticancer therapies, a response to an altered environment wherein the chemical, metabolic, or mechanical abnormalities promote abnormal impulse formation or propagation, exacerbation of underlying cardiac electrophysiologic abnormalities (unrelated to cancer or cancer treatment per se), or a manifestation of tumor spread. Cancer-related arrhythmias encompass the spectrum from trivial to life threatening.

Types of Arrhythmia

Supraventricular Arrhythmias: Supraventricular arrhythmias are a common occurrence in cancer patients. Atrial premature complexes are a well-recognized manifestation of early anthracycline cardiotoxicity and may be a harbinger of subsequent LV dysfunction. More sustained supraventricular arrhythmias are seen commonly in patients with a chest malignancy, especially lung cancer, which is often associated with increased pulmonary artery pressure. Pulmonary hypertension often precedes atrial flutter or fibrillation. Mechanical effects of an expanding tumor mass, as well as atelectasis or infection in areas distal to occluded bronchi, further increase right-sided pressures and cause arrhythmias. Hypoxia often confounds the problem. Supraventricular arrhythmias are especially frequent early in the postoperative period after lung resection. Supraventricular arrhythmias also occur in association with high-dose chemotherapy and stem cell transplantation. Various specific chemotherapeutic agents also have been associated with atrial fibrillation (AF) and include 5-FU, gemcitabine, docetaxel, and alemtuzumab. Radiation to the heart has a well-known association with arrhythmia; however, radiation to sites distant from the heart also has been associated with supraventricular arrhythmia. Other forms of sustained supraventricular tachycardia, including reentrant supraventricular tachycardia and multifocal atrial tachycardia, are also commonly seen in the cancer patient.

Ibrutinib, a Bruton kinase inhibitor used in the treatment of chronic lymphocytic leukemia, is significantly associated with AF. Three percent of patients receiving ibrutinib developed AF, whereas the other arm had no AF.[41] In a study of 56 patients, 76% of them developed AF within the first year on ibrutinib.[42] This complication can be managed with dose-reduction or anticoagulation in combination.[43]

Intracardiac masses, including benign tumors and malignant processes such as primary cardiac lymphomas and cardiac metastases from lung, breast, or melanoma, often present with supraventricular arrhythmias. AF is often associated with acute pulmonary embolism (PE) and pericarditis, conditions that may be encountered in cancer patients.

An important risk factor for significant supraventricular arrhythmias is intrinsic cardiac disease. In particular, conditions resulting in increased atrial size or that are associated with inflammation, such as increase in C-reactive protein,[44] contribute to elevated atrial pressure and result in atrial rhythm disturbances. Age, hypertension, lung disease, thyrotoxicosis, surgery, and other states that trigger increased catecholamine levels may all also contribute to elevated atrial pressure.

Ventricular Arrhythmias: Cancer patients are more prone to ventricular arrhythmias than the noncancer population.[45] Hypokalemia, alkalotic states, hypomagnesemia, thyrotoxicosis, pheochromocytomas, and the release of mediators such as serotonin and kinins associated with the carcinoid syndrome are all associated with potentially life-threatening ventricular tachycardia.

Prolonged QT Interval and Torsade de Pointes: Torsade de pointes, a form of ventricular tachycardia associated with prolongation of the QT interval, is related to an increasing list of medications, many of which are used in the management of malignancy and in their supportive care. Prolongation of the QT interval may also occur in association with the supplements that cancer patients sometimes ingest, among them cesium chloride, which is commonly used as an alternative therapy for various types of malignancies. Several anticancer agents may also lead to QT prolongation. Arsenic trioxide is associated with QT prolongation in more than 50% of treated patients.[46] Other cardiac side effects include sinus tachycardia, nonspecific ST-T changes, and torsade de pointes. In one study, the most common acute side effect was fluid retention with pleural and pericardial effusions. Complete heart block and sudden cardiac death have also been reported in patients receiving arsenic trioxide. Several newer cancer treatments such as dasatinib, lapatinib, nilotinib, and vorinostat have also been shown to prolong the QT interval. It is important to monitor the QT interval with serial ECGs, with particular attention to patients who are simultaneously receiving other drugs that have the potential to further prolong the QT interval.

Bradyarrhythmias and Atrioventricular Heart Block: Thalidomide may cause sinus bradycardia that may be mitigated by adjusting the dosage and is often asymptomatic, but occasionally permanent pacing may be required. Paclitaxel is used extensively in the treatment of many solid tumors and has been reported to cause sinus bradycardia, heart block, premature ventricular contractions, and ventricular tachycardia.

The conduction system of the heart can be interrupted at all levels by primary and metastatic tumors or by infiltrative processes such as amyloidosis. Pheochromocytomas, thymomas, high-dose chemotherapy, and stem cell transplantation are all associated with block at the level of the atrioventricular (AV) node. Individual chemotherapy agents associated with transient AV block include paclitaxel and octreotide.

Treatment of Arrhythmias

In managing arrhythmias in cancer patients, one must first consider possible cancer-related causes for the rhythm disturbance. In many instances, correcting metabolic abnormalities or removing arrhythmogenic agents is the most successful approach. The arrhythmia may be sufficiently serious that the permanent elimination of the offending agent from the treatment regimen must be recommended. In some settings, the arrhythmia may be controlled by the use of standard medications or procedures, thereby permitting completion of highly effective anticancer treatment. The use of implantable devices should not be denied to appropriate patients who have malignancy and who have reasonable expectation of survival with good functional status of more than 1 year, as per the ACC/AHA or ESC heart failure guidelines.[47]

Thromboembolism

General Considerations

The incidence of thrombosis is higher in patients with cancer than in the general population and portends a worse prognosis. The prevention, recognition, and treatment of thromboembolism are clinical challenges for physicians treating patients with cancer. Venous thromboembolism (VTE) occurs in 5% to 7% of patients with malignancy, an incidence that is much greater than that for the general population (approximately 0.1%). Patients with cancer constitute nearly 20% of all cases of thrombosis. Approximately 10% of all noncancer patients with VTE will be diagnosed with malignancy within 2 years.

The incidence of arterial thromboembolism is less than that of VTE in cancer patients, but occurs at a much higher incidence than in the general population. The source of arterial thromboembolism is most likely atherosclerosis, but the general inflammatory condition observed in patients with cancer and treatment with the new antiangiogenic agents are also important determinants. With the more widespread use of such agents, the incidence of arterial thrombosis likely will increase. Thrombotic events, such as deep venous thrombosis (DVT), PE, and arterial thrombosis have also been observed in approximately 11% of patients treated with IL-2.[48] The risk of death for cancer patients diagnosed with a DVT or PE is substantially higher than that in cancer patients without such an event. The same is true for arterial thrombi. The in-hospital mortality may approach 20% to 30%, especially in those with pulmonary emboli. Nonbacterial endocarditis (marantic endocarditis) and disseminated intravascular coagulation are additional examples of life-threatening thrombotic conditions associated with cancer.

Another agent most recently linked to increased risk of life-threatening arterial thrombotic events is ponatinib, a third-generation TKI, which was developed for the treatment of chronic myeloid leukemia (CML) and Philadelphia chromosome–positive (Ph+) acute lymphoblastic leukemia (ALL). Although ponatinib, similar to the other TKIs, acts as a platelet antagonist, paradoxically, in contrast to the bleeding side effects common to TKI chemotherapies, it can cause severe prothrombotic complications,[49] which resulted in the temporary suspension of the drug by the FDA in late 2013. The pathogenic mechanisms underlying the cardiovascular events observed in patients taking ponatinib remain poorly understood, but can cause arterial thrombosis in up to 20% of patients. The FDA has since lifted the suspension of ponatinib after issuing a "black box warning" regarding the risks of arterial thrombosis to be weighed against the oncological benefits.

Pathophysiology of Thrombosis

The triggers for venous and arterial thrombosis in the cancer patient are incompletely understood, and no single explanation pertains to all conditions in which thrombosis occurs (**Table 74–7**).

VTE in cancer patients most often occurs as a result of the classic triad of stasis, endothelial disruption, and hypercoagulability. In each situation, one component may predominate and, if identified, can be effectively treated. If, for example, a patient has an abdominal tumor that is compressing the inferior vena cava, causing stasis, and this tumor can be removed or reduced by chemotherapy or radiation, then the likelihood of VTE may be markedly reduced. Indwelling IV catheters may

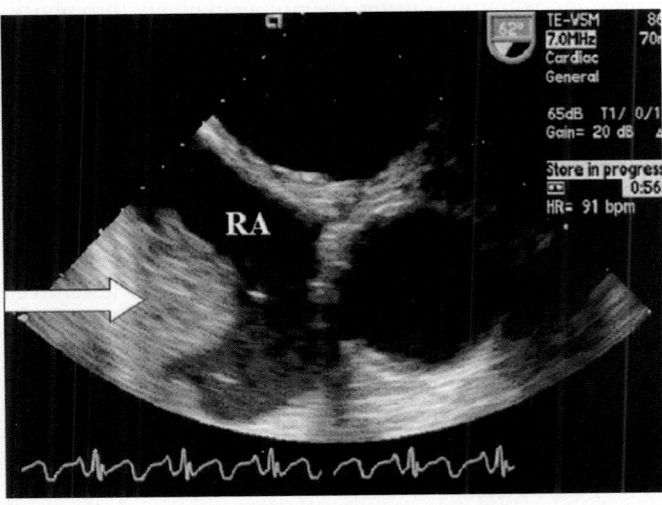

Figure 74–4. **(A)** and **(B)** Two views from a transesophageal echocardiogram showing a large thrombus in the right atrium (RA) associated with an indwelling catheter.

cause thrombus formation (**Fig. 74–4**). Removal of an indwelling central catheter is also likely to be effective in reducing the risk of subsequent recurrence or progression of a thrombus after the stimulus for hypercoagulability has been removed.

Arterial thrombosis in cancer patients is most commonly associated with platelet activation either in the presence or absence of atherosclerosis. The malignancy itself can lead to platelet activation. The exact mechanism also may include microvessel constriction and platelet activation.

Treatment of Thromboembolism

The optimal treatment of VTE is a challenge in cancer patients. Typically, these patients are at increased risk for bleeding and because they are often concurrently anemic, the consequences of bleeding are increased and disproportionate. Additional aggravating factors may be thrombocytopenia, hepatic failure, renal dysfunction, or development of a thrombus in a location that may predispose to bleeding complications. Antithrombotic

TABLE 74–7. Risks for Thrombotic Events in Cancer Patients
Immobilization
Genetic
Inherited coagulopathy
Polymorphism(s) at risk for thrombosis
Surgery
Trauma
Heart failure
Estrogen therapy
Prior thrombosis
Indwelling catheters
Chemotherapy or other agents
Tamoxifen
Thalidomide
Cisplatin (Platinol-AQ)
Erlotinib (Tarceva)
Lenalidomide (Revlimid)
Sunitinib (Sutent)
Vorinostat (Zolinza)
Bevacizumab
Ponatinib

therapy may consist of medications to prevent or limit the propagation of a thrombus or occasionally thrombolytic agents to promote thrombus dissolution. Furthermore, the risks associated with thrombus extension, distal embolization, or recurrence must be weighed against the risks of hemorrhage as part of the decision-making process.

Guidelines for antithrombotic therapy for VTE have been published by the Ninth American College of Chest Physicians Conference on Antithrombotic and Thrombolytic Therapy.[50] Standard treatment for VTE traditionally consists of low-molecular-weight heparin (LMWH), IV unfractionated heparin (UFH), or adjusted-dose subcutaneous heparin followed by long-term therapy with an oral anticoagulant. UFH has been superseded by LMWH as the initial treatment in most cancer patients with VTE in both inpatients and outpatients. Long-term treatment with warfarin may be complicated by several problems, including drug–drug interactions, malnutrition, nausea or vomiting during chemotherapy, and thrombocytopenia. Additionally, hepatic dysfunction in cancer patients may lead to unpredictable levels of anticoagulation and result in increased bleeding complications. LMWH is more effective than oral anticoagulant therapy with warfarin for the prevention of recurrent VTE in patients with cancer who have had acute, symptomatic proximal DVT, PE, or both (**Fig. 74–5**).[51] Further advantages of LMWH are that the doses are more easily adjusted, the pharmacokinetic properties are more predictable, laboratory monitoring is minimized, and fewer drug interactions occur than is the case with oral anticoagulants. Also in favor of heparin therapy in cancer patients are reports that the heparins have antiproliferative, antiangiogenetic, and antimetastatic effects and that LMWH may increase the response to chemotherapy, thereby prolonging the survival of cancer patients.[52] For these several reasons, secondary prophylaxis with LMWH may be more effective and feasible than oral anticoagulant therapy in cancer patients with VTE, although the risk of bleeding is the same for both treatment approaches. More recently, low-dose aspirin was safely used to prevent

thrombotic complications in patients with polycythemia vera and has been advocated as an alternative option in patients with cancer presenting with paraneoplastic thrombocytosis.

Newer oral antithrombotic agents or NOACs (novel oral anticoagulants) include thrombin inhibitors, such as dabigatran, and factor Xa inhibitors, such as rivaroxiban, edoxaban, and apixaban. These seem to be as effective and safe as conventional treatment of VTE in patients with cancer, as suggested in several clinical trials.[53] However, patients with primary brain tumors, brain metastasis, or acute leukemia should not receive apixaban.[54] LMWH is still preferred in patients at high risk for drug–drug interaction and for patients undergoing upper gastrointestinal track surgery.[53] Moreover, mechanical treatments, such as compression stockings used to prevent postthrombotic syndrome, have value in the treatment of cancer patients with thromboembolism, as do selected surgical techniques to treat venous ulceration. Venacaval filters may be used instead of anticoagulation in patients with recurrent PEs who also have a high risk of serious bleeding.

Prevention of Thromboembolism
Prompted by the high incidence of VTE in patients undergoing ambulatory chemotherapy, the 2013 American Society of Clinical Oncology (ASCO) guidelines recommend a scoring method (commonly called the Khorana score) as a risk calculator for chemotherapy-associated VTE in the ambulatory setting.[55] They recommend that patients with cancer be assessed for VTE risk at the time of chemotherapy initiation and periodically thereafter. The prophylactic anticoagulation of high-risk patients is feasible, safe, and effective as suggested by several randomized clinical trials, including the Prophylaxis of Thromboembolism During Chemotherapy Trial (PROTECHT) and the SAVE-ONCO investigation, the largest thromboprophylaxis study ever conducted in cancer patients.

RADIATION-INDUCED CARDIOVASCULAR DISEASE

The Effects of Radiation Therapy on the Heart
The basic mechanism of cardiotoxicity involves damage to blood vessels, mediated by generation of reactive oxygen species, which causes DNA strands breaks and inflammatory changes, resulting in extensive fibrosis. Common histologic changes observed in radiation-associated cardiotoxicity include diffuse interstitial fibrosis of the myocardium with significantly reduced ratio of capillaries to myocytes, leading to myocyte cell death, latent ischemia, and thrombosis; endothelial cell damage, triggering accelerated atherosclerosis; replacement of the pericardial fat with dense connective tissue, leading to pericardial fibrosis, effusion, or even tamponade; as well as fibrosis and calcification of valvular leaflets/cusps, more commonly left-sided, which suggests a mechanistic role of blood pressure levels in the pathogenesis of the lesions (**Fig. 74–6**).

Multiple predisposing factors facilitating the development of radiation-induced cardiotoxicity have been recognized thus far, including total radiation dose and dose per fraction, the volume of heart irradiated, and the concurrent administration

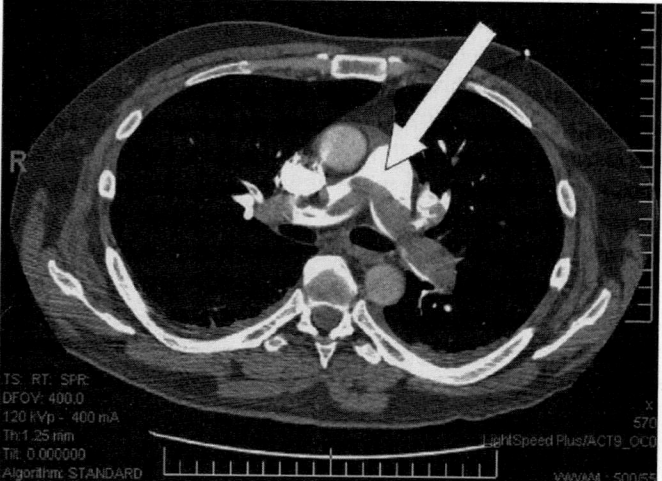

Figure 74–5. A contrast-enhanced computed tomography scan showing a massive pulmonary embolus (*arrow*).

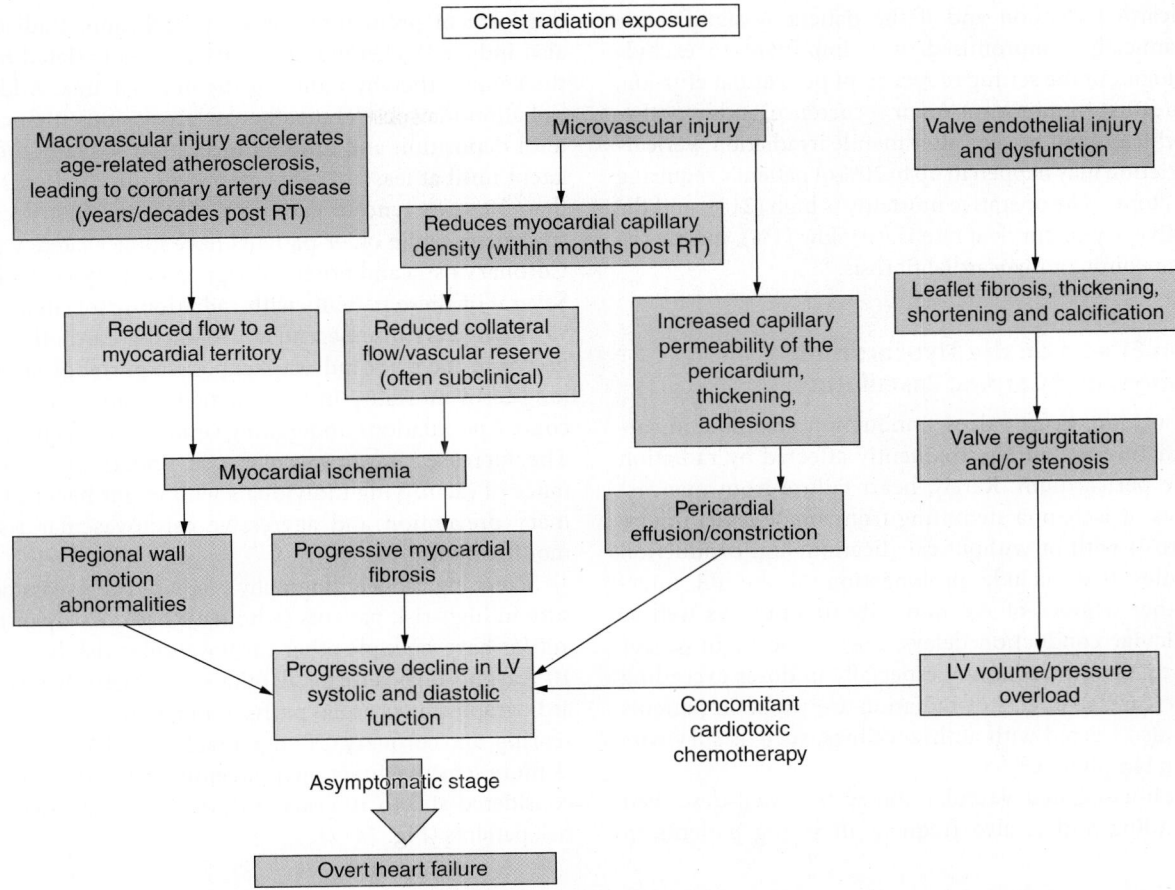

Figure 74–6. Pathophysiological manifestations of radiation-induced heart disease for different radiosensitive structures within the heart. LV, left ventricular; RT, radiotherapy. Reproduced with permission from Lancellotti P, Nkomo VT, Badano LP, et al. Expert consensus for multi-modality imaging evaluation of cardiovascular complications of radiotherapy in adults: a report from the European Association of Cardiovascular Imaging and the American Society of Echocardiography. *Eur Heart J Cardiovasc Imaging.* 2013 Aug;14(8):721-740.

of additional cardiotoxic agents, such as anthracyclines and trastuzumab. Younger age at the time of irradiation and the presence of other risk factors for coronary heart disease, such as hypertension, diabetes, and smoking, are patient-specific dynamics that may heighten the risk of radiation-induced cardiotoxicity.[56]

Cardiac manifestations of irradiation may be seen even before completion of the anticipated exposure or may occur years or decades later. Patients treated for both Hodgkin and non-Hodgkin lymphoma and patients treated for left-sided breast cancer are the most likely to show these manifestations, because treatment for these tumors sometimes involves portals that overlie the heart and as a result of incremental risks imposed by concomitant use of cardiotoxic drugs such as anthracyclines.[57]

Radiation Effects on the Pericardium

The pericardium is the most sensitive cardiac structure with regard to irradiation, because it consists of tissue with rapid cell turnover. Initially, exposure can cause an acute radiation-associated pericarditis presenting with signs and symptoms that are clinically undistinguishable from those associated with acute pericarditis from other causes. Sometimes, the symptoms

may be masked by the underlying disease or the applied chemotherapy.

Acute pericarditis used to be the most frequent complication, but advances reduced its incidence from 25% to 2%.[58] Chronic pericarditis still develops with a clinical incidence of 3% at 20 years and 12% at 30 years in those who underwent chest radiation at a dose of 35 Gy or greater. Fibrinous exudates, fibrous adhesions, and collagenous thickening (predominantly of the parietal pericardium) are characteristic features. The probability to develop radiation-induced pericarditis is influenced by the applied source, dose, its fractionation, duration, radiation exposed volume, form of mantle field therapy, and the age of the patients.

A normal ECG does not rule out acute radiation-associated pericarditis. The changes appear over a period of days and then dissipate. Imaging should start with echocardiography, followed by cardiac computed tomography (CT) or magnetic resonance imaging (MRI) if necessary, to rule out constriction. A chest radiograph is usually normal unless a large pericardial effusion is manifested as an increased cardiac silhouette.

Pericarditis without tamponade may be treated conservatively with the use of nonsteroidal anti-inflammatory agents. Pericardiocentesis might be indicated if there is an associated large pericardial effusion and if the patient is significantly hemodynamically compromised. It is important to exclude other etiologies in the setting of recurrent pericardial effusion, such as infection, tumor invasion or recurrence, and hypothyroidism, which might be seen after mantle irradiation. Pericardial constriction may happen in up to 20% of patients, requiring pericardiectomy. The operative mortality is high (21%) and the postoperative 5-year survival rate is very low (1%), mostly the result of concomitant myocardial fibrosis.[59]

Radiation Effects on the Myocardium, Heart Valves, and Cardiac Vasculature

The myocardium, heart valves, conduction system, and cardiac vasculature are all less frequently affected by radiation than is the pericardium. Rarely, heart failure from myocardial fibrosis or ischemia stemming from small vessel injury, valve sclerosis with or without calcification, and conduction abnormalities that include prolongation of the PR interval and other degrees of AV nodal dysfunction, as well as intraventricular conduction delays, may all occur in cancer patients treated with radiation, especially in doses exceeding 35 Gy. The cardiac effects of radiation are worse in patients who were also treated with anthracyclines, such as survivors of Hodgkin lymphoma.[57]

Radiation-associated vascular injury is a well-described autopsy finding and is also frequent in young patients in the form of premature coronary occlusion. Radiation may also induce thickening of the arterial wall related to intimal thickening, thereby reducing the luminal area. Additionally, radiation may accelerate atherosclerosis and enhance cholesterol deposition and luminal ulceration. Usually the CAD is latent until at least 10 years after exposure (patients younger than 50 years tend to develop CAD in the first decade after treatment, while older patients have longer latency periods). Coronary ostia and proximal segments are typically involved. Several of these patients with radiation-associated CAD and valvular heart disease end up requiring cardiothoracic surgery, and the prior radiation exposure portends an increased long-term mortality in these patients compared to matched control populations undergoing similar surgical procedures.[59] The increased cardiovascular risk underscores the importance of identifying individuals who might benefit from primary prevention and aggressive cardiovascular risk factor modification.

Screening echocardiography is advised at 5 years postexposure in high-risk patients (who have had >35 Gy of radiation and/or have multiple other cardiovascular risk factors) and at 10 years postexposure for all others. Alternatively, stress echocardiography, myocardial perfusion imaging, coronary calcium scoring, and coronary CT angiography (CCTA) have been used as more sensitive functional screening methods and should be considered at 5 to 10 years after radiation treatment in high-risk patients (**Fig. 74–7**).

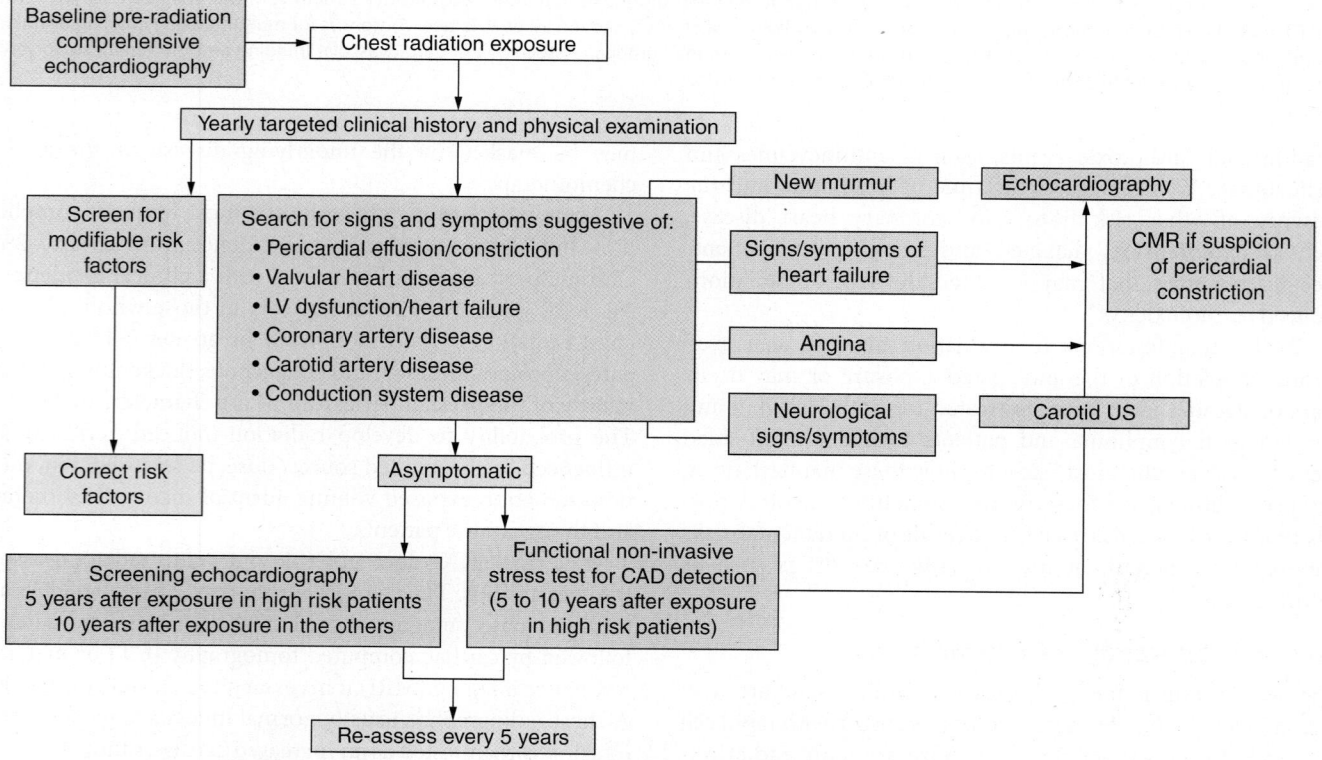

Figure 74–7. Algorithm for patient management after chest radiotherapy. CAD, coronary artery disease; CMR, cardiac magnetic resonance; LV, left ventricular; US, ultrasound. Reproduced with permission from Lancellotti P, Nkomo VT, Badano LP, et al. Expert consensus for multi-modality imaging evaluation of cardiovascular complications of radiotherapy in adults: a report from the European Association of Cardiovascular Imaging and the American Society of Echocardiography. *Eur Heart J Cardiovasc Imaging.* 2013 Aug;14(8):721-740.

TUMORS AND MALIGNANCIES OF THE CARDIOVASCULAR SYSTEM

Benign and Malignant Primary Pericardial Tumors

Both primary and metastatic tumors occur in the pericardium. Tumors are found to have spread to the pericardium in approximately 9% of cancer patients who come to autopsy. In the general population, approximately 7% of all patients who experience acute pericarditis either have a history of malignancy or are later found to have a malignancy related to their pericardial inflammation. Not surprisingly, 35% of invasive pericardial interventions are therefore performed on cancer patients. Among primary pericardial tumors, approximately 25% are malignant. Benign tumors present more frequently in infancy and childhood, and malignant tumors are more common after the age of 30 years; lipoma, a slow-growing benign tumor, is often seen later in life. Pericardial cysts, the most common pericardial tumor, are usually small and are most frequently seen along the right ventricular (RV) border. Pericardial cysts are often discovered as incidental findings at autopsy, but they may present with chest pain or arrhythmias or as a supplementary finding on chest radiography obtained for other purposes. Their presence can be confirmed by ultrasonography, CT scanning, or MRI. These lesions are not malignant, and patients have an excellent prognosis. **Table 74–8** enumerates the incidence of tumors (benign and malignant) and cysts of the heart and pericardium, and **Table 74–9** lists the general manifestations of neoplastic heart disease.

Pericardial teratomas are usually benign, usually occur in children, and are more common in girls. Compression of the right atrium is sometimes seen with these tumors, and large associated pericardial effusions are frequent. Surgery is the treatment of choice, and the prognosis is usually good when teratomas are benign.

The most common primary malignant tumor of the pericardium *is* mesothelioma; it usually presents in middle-aged adults, and men are afflicted more often than women. It is uncertain if this gender-related difference is linked to toxic exposure. Pericardial mesothelioma may present with pericardial effusion, pericarditis, constriction, and constitutional symptoms.

Angiosarcomas are the second most common primary pericardial malignancy; these tumors may originate in the right atrium or the pericardium, are usually seen in young adults, and are more common in young men. As with mesothelioma, the presentation may include pericarditis and pericardial effusion. Pericardial effusion is usually hemorrhagic; surgical treatment may be successful. When surgery is not possible, treatment options are limited; palliation with radiation and chemotherapy is suboptimal.

Pericardial lipomas are usually benign and surgically resectable; transformation to malignant liposarcoma is possible. These tumors may also be surgically resected, and repeated surgical resection is sometimes necessary. *Thymomas* may arise from the parietal pericardium without evidence of anterior mediastinal involvement and may be benign or malignant; they are not associated with myasthenia gravis.

TABLE 74–8. Tumors and Cysts of the Heart and Pericardium

Type	Number	Percentage
Benign		
Myxoma	130	24.4
Lipoma	45	8.4
Rhabdomyoma	36	6.8
Fibroma	17	3.2
Hemangioma	15	2.8
Teratoma	14	2.6
Mesothelioma of the atrioventricular node	12	2.3
Granular cell tumor	3	
Neurofibroma	3	
Lymphangioma	2	
Subtotal	319	59.8
Pericardial cyst	82	15.4
Bronchogenic cyst	7	1.3
Subtotal	89	16.7
Malignant		
Angiosarcoma	39	7.3
Rhabdomyosarcoma	26	4.9
Mesothelioma	19	3.6
Fibrosarcoma	14	2.6
Malignant lymphoma	7	1.3
Extraskeletal osteosarcoma	5	
Neurogenic sarcoma	4	
Malignant teratoma	4	
Thymoma	4	
Leiomyosarcoma	1	
Liposarcoma	1	
Synovial sarcoma	1	
Subtotal	125	23.5
Total	533	100.0

Reproduced with permission from McAllister H, Fenoglio JJ. *Tumors of the cardiovascular system. Fascicle 15, second series. Atlas of tumor pathology.* Washington, DC: Armed Forces Institute of Pathology, 1978.

Metastatic spread of tumors to the *pericardium* is common; it has been estimated that 10% of all malignancies spread to some portion of the heart, and 85% of these eventually involve the pericardium. Lung cancer, breast cancer, and hematologic malignancies together account for approximately two-thirds of the cases of metastatic disease to the pericardium. Melanoma is the tumor most likely to spread to the pericardium, with 70% of patients with metastatic melanoma having pericardial involvement at death. *Metastatic breast cancer* invades the pericardial space in approximately 21% of cases and lung cancer in approximately 19%.

The clinical presentation of metastatic disease to the pericardium is variable (**Fig. 74–8**). Sometimes pericardial involvement is an incidental finding at autopsy. It may also present as a

TABLE 74–9. General Manifestations of Neoplastic Heart Disease

Pericardial Involvement
Pericarditis and pain
Pericardial effusion
Radiographic enlargement
Arrhythmia, predominantly atrial
Tamponade
Constriction
Myocardial Involvement
Arrhythmias, ventricular and atrial
Electrocardiographic changes
Radiographic enlargement
    Generalized
    Localized
Conduction disturbances and heart block
Congestive heart failure
Coronary involvement
    Angina, infarction
Intracavitary tumor
    Cavity obliteration
    Valve obstruction and valve damage
    Embolic phenomena: systemic, neurologic, and coronary
    Constitutional manifestations

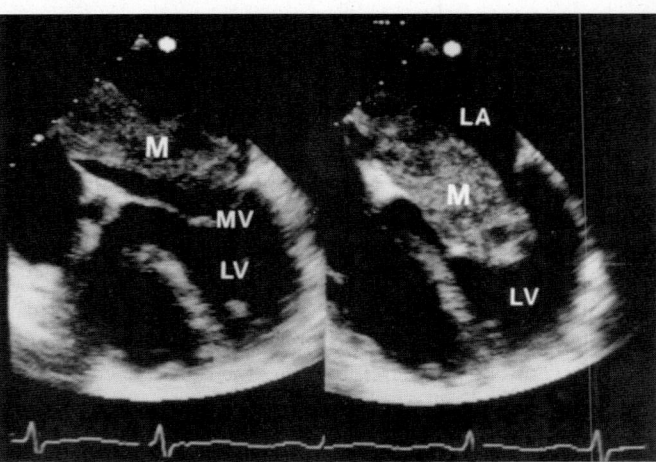

Figure 74–9. Transesophageal echocardiogram in the four-chamber view from a 50-year-old man who presented with exertional dyspnea and syncope. A large left atrial myxoma (M) attached to the interatrial septum is seen prolapsing across the mitral valve (MV) into the left ventricle (LV) in diastole (right panel). LA, left atrium. Reproduced with permission from Susan Wilansky, MD, Medical Director, Noninvasive Imaging, St. Luke's Episcopal Hospital, Houston, Texas.

catastrophic and life-threatening pericardial tamponade. More commonly, however, patients present with acute pericarditis, chronic effusion, and constrictive disease.

Echocardiography is the most helpful test for evaluating such patients (see Chapter 15), but CT scanning and MRI (see Chapter 3) are helpful adjuncts. The diagnosis is often confirmed by cytologic analysis of pericardial fluid removed for diagnostic or therapeutic pericardiocentesis; however, cytologic findings are not always positive in patients with malignant effusions, and not all pericardial effusions in cancer patients are malignant. Effusions in these patients may be the result of heart failure, renal failure, inflammation, interruption of lymphatic or venous drainage, infection, hypoalbuminemia, toxicities of chemotherapeutic agents, and chest irradiation.

Cardiac Myxomas

Intracardiac myxoma (**Fig. 74–9**) is the most frequent benign tumor of the heart. Although most (75%) are located in the left atrium, myxomas are also found in the right atrium (18%), right ventricle (4%), and left ventricle (3%). Cardiac myxomas usually originate from the region of the fossa ovalis, but may arise from a variety of locations within the atria. The DNA genotype of sporadic myxomas is normal in 80% of patients. Tumors are likely to be associated with other abnormal conditions and have a low recurrence rate. Approximately 5% of myxoma patients show a familial pattern of tumor development with autosomal dominant inheritance; 20% of those with sporadic myxoma have an abnormal DNA genotype chromosomal pattern. Carney complex, is characterized by cardiac and mucocutaneous myxomas, lentiginosis, and endocrine dysfunction including bilateral adrenal micronodular hyperplasia. The cardiac tumors are often multicentric, rarely metastasize and are amenable to surgical resection. There at least three different genetic loci with two identified genes for this complex. Most true myxomas arise only from the mural endocardium despite isolated reports that they arise from the cardiac valves, pulmonary vessels, and vena cava.

Pathology of Cardiac Myxomas

Attached to the endocardium by a broad base, myxomas are usually pedunculated, polypoid, and friable, although some may have a smooth surface and are rounded. A myxoma appears as a soft, gelatinous, mucoid, usually gray-white mass, often with areas of hemorrhage or thrombosis. Myxomas vary from 1 to 15 cm in diameter, with most measuring 5 to 6 cm.

On microscopic examination, the myxoma consists of an acid mucopolysaccharide myxoid matrix in which polygonal

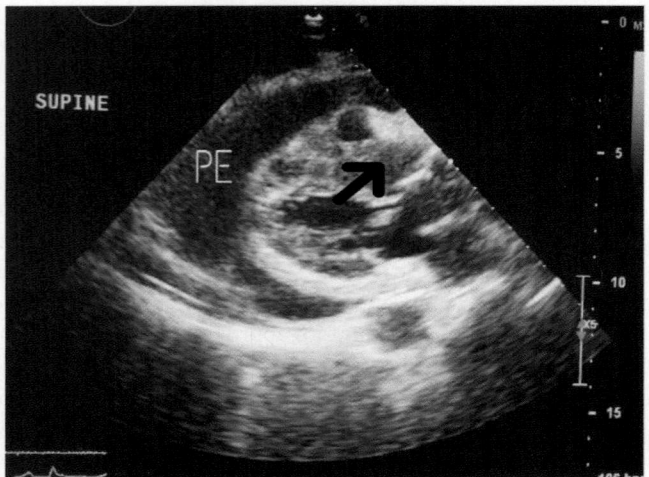

Figure 74–8. Parasternal long axis of a large circumferential pericardial effusion (PE) with involvement of the right ventricle with metastatic angiosarcoma (*arrow*) from the gluteal region. The right ventricular cavity and free wall have been infiltrated with the metastatic tumor. Reproduced with permission from Gagan Sahni, MD. Mount Sinai Hospital, New York.

cells and occasional blood vessels are embedded. Channels, often containing red blood cells, communicate from the surface to deep within the tumor and are lined by endothelial-like cells resembling multipurpose mesenchymal cells, from which the tumor is purported to arise. Similar endothelial cells line the surface of the tumor; however, fibrin, erythrocytes, and organized thrombi also may be present on the surface. Cystic areas; focal or gross hemorrhage; calcification; glandular elements; rarely, bone formation; and even hematopoietic tissue constitute the multiple, less common, variations.

Although asymptomatic patients with myxoma have been reported, most present with one or more effects of a *triad* of constitutional, embolic, and obstructive manifestations. Cardiac myxomas provoke systemic manifestations in 90% of the patients, characterized by weight loss, fatigue, fever, anemia (often hemolytic), elevated erythrocyte sedimentation rate, and elevated serum immunoglobulin concentration formed in response to tumor embolization, degenerative changes within the tumor, or overproduction of IL-6 by the tumor.

Constitutional manifestations and embolic potential are relatively common in patients with myxoma in any intracavitary location. The cardiac manifestations, symptoms, and physical findings are the consequence of the intracavitary mass and the particular location of the tumor. Myxomas of the left atrium may obstruct either the mitral or pulmonary venous orifices and produce pulmonary venous hypertension, secondary pulmonary hypertension, and right-sided heart failure. The clinical symptoms include dyspnea on exertion, orthopnea, paroxysmal nocturnal dyspnea, acute pulmonary edema, cough, and hemoptysis, along with palpitations, chest pain, fatigue, and peripheral edema. Episodes of syncope or dizziness are frequent, and sudden death may occur. A marked change in the severity of any symptom caused by a change in position of the patient, especially if recumbency relieves dyspnea, is suggestive of myxoma. On physical examination, the S_1 is loud and frequently split, with the second component corresponding to the tumor's expulsion from the mitral orifice in the case of left atrial myxoma (see Chapter 2). P_2 is accentuated, and an early diastolic sound, the "tumor plop," is usually heard 80 to 120 ms after the A_2, resembling an opening snap. The tumor plop may be confused with either an opening snap or a third heart sound and follows A_2 at an intermediate interval between these events.

The value of transthoracic echocardiography in the noninvasive diagnosis of intracavitary tumors is well documented (see Chapter 3). M-mode recordings in patients with a prolapsing left atrial myxoma typically demonstrate a diminished ejection fraction slope of the anterior leaflet of the mitral valve, behind which a dense array of wavy tumor echoes is seen (see Chapter 3). The tumor plop coincides with the completion of this anterior movement of tumor echoes. A similar array of tumor echoes may be seen in the left atrium during ventricular systole. Transthoracic echocardiography and transesophageal echocardiography identify the size, shape, point of attachment, and motion characteristics of left atrial myxomas. Transesophageal echocardiography permits superior imaging of the posterior cardiac structures and left atrial myxomas, especially their

point of attachment. Visualization of all four chambers permits recognition of multiple tumors, as well as tumors in less common locations. Doppler assessment of the flow patterns of the mitral valve and pulmonary vein provides further information regarding the hemodynamic consequences of left atrial myxomas (Fig. 74–9).

Surgical resection of a myxoma is the only effective therapy. For complete removal of left atrial myxoma, a full thickness of interatrial septum should be excised if the tumor is attached to the region of the fossa ovalis. Right atrial myxomas are commonly attached to the fossa ovalis, and with right-sided tumors, a full thickness of atrial septum should also be resected. If a large portion of the septum is removed, a patch of knitted Dacron cloth should be used for repair to avoid distortion, arrhythmias, or possible atrial septal defect. Ventricular standstill with cardioplegia solution is induced before manipulating the heart to reduce the possibility of fragmentation of the gelatinous tumor. Left atrial myxomas have been removed successfully during pregnancy, using cardiopulmonary bypass, with subsequent uncomplicated completion of a full-term pregnancy.

CANCER SURVIVORSHIP

Due to the success of modern cancer therapy, 22.1 million cancer patients are expected to become cancer survivors by 2230.[1] Although some of the cardiovascular complications caused by cancer therapy may be time limited, cancer therapy can cause subclinical damages to organs that will manifest later in life. Thus, specific cancer therapy discussed in this chapter should be considered as a risk factor for development of future cardiovascular diseases, including heart failure, hypertension, ischemic heart disease, and valvular heart disease. Optimal follow-up for cancer survivors should include optimal primary and secondary prevention strategies for cardiovascular disease.[60] The purpose of the increase in vigilance is to detect the earliest manifestation of cardiovascular diseases in cancer survivors that could be ameliorated by intense risk factor modifications or new therapy.

SUMMARY

Advances in cancer therapies that can have adverse cardiovascular adverse effects has led to the growing field of cardio-oncology. With this, the paradigm has shifted toward early recognition and treatment of cardiotoxicity and cardiovascular risk assessment, and modification even before cancer therapy. Key practical steps in a cardio-oncology approach, which reflect the topics discussed in this chapter, comprise the following:

1. A multidisciplinary approach with ongoing interaction between dedicated specialists comprising cardiologists, oncologists or hematologists, and radiation oncologists in a "cardio-oncology team" approach that evaluates potential cardiotoxic adverse effects of chemotherapeutic agents prior to the start of therapy.

2. Early and routine screening of cardiovascular diseases in cancer patients.

3. Risk stratification for the development of cardiotoxicity prior to the initiation of chemotherapy.

4. Institution-wide algorithms should be formulated based on current evidence-based medicine to guide use of cardiotoxic drugs and immune therapy.

5. Evolving imaging techniques such as longitudinal strain may establish themselves as a future modality for detection of early cardiotoxicity.

6. Awareness of cardiotoxic manifestations beyond LV dysfunction of various chemotherapeutic agents, immune therapy, and radiation therapy.

7. Monitoring of cardiovascular health and cardiac risk factor modification after successful cancer therapy should be a high priority for cancer survivors.

ACKNOWLEDGMENTS

This work is supported in part by a National Institute of Health RO1 grant (HL126916) awarded to Dr. Edward T. H. Yeh. The author would like to thank Drs. Gagan Sahni and Tiziano Scarabelli for their contributions to this chapter in the 14th edition.

REFERENCES

1. Miller KD, et al. Cancer treatment and survivorship statistics, 2019. *CA Cancer J Clin.* 2019;69(5):363-385.

2. Mulrooney DA, et al. Major cardiac events for adult survivors of childhood cancer diagnosed between 1970 and 1999: report from the Childhood Cancer Survivor Study cohort. *BMJ.* 2020;368:l6794.

3. Common terminology criteria for adverse events (CTCAE). 2017. https://ctep.cancer.gov/protocolDevelopment

4. Chang HM, et al. Cardiovascular complications of cancer therapy: best practices in diagnosis, prevention, and management: part 1. *J Am Coll Cardiol.* 2017;70(20):2536-2551.

5. Chang HM, et al. Cardiovascular complications of cancer therapy: best practices in diagnosis, prevention, and management: part 2. *J Am Coll Cardiol.* 2017;70(20):2552-2565.

6. Aminkeng F, et al. A coding variant in RARG confers susceptibility to anthracycline-induced cardiotoxicity in childhood cancer. *Nat Genet.* 2015;47(9):1079-1084.

7. Aminkeng F, et al. Recommendations for genetic testing to reduce the incidence of anthracycline-induced cardiotoxicity. *Br J Clin Pharmacol.* 2016;82(3):683-695.

8. Von Hoff DD, et al., Risk factors for doxorubicin-induced congestive heart failure. *Ann Intern Med.* 1979;91(5):710-717.

9. Doroshow JH. Doxorubicin-induced cardiac toxicity. *N Engl J Med.* 1991;324(12):843-845.

10. Minotti G, et al. Anthracyclines: molecular advances and pharmacologic developments in antitumor activity and cardiotoxicity. *Pharmacol Rev.* 2004;56(2):185-229.

11. Lyu YL, et al. Topoisomerase IIbeta mediated DNA double-strand breaks: implications in doxorubicin cardiotoxicity and prevention by dexrazoxane. *Cancer Res.* 2007;67(18):8839-8846.

12. Capranico G, et al. Different patterns of gene expression of topoisomerase II isoforms in differentiated tissues during murine development. *Biochim Biophys Acta.* 1992;1132(1):43-48.

13. Tewey KM, et al. Adriamycin-induced DNA damage mediated by mammalian DNA topoisomerase II. *Science.* 1984;226(4673):466-468.

14. Zhang S, et al. Identification of the molecular basis of doxorubicin-induced cardiotoxicity. *Nat Med.* 2012;18(11):1639-1642.

15. Olson LE, et al. Protection from doxorubicin-induced cardiac toxicity in mice with a null allele of carbonyl reductase 1. *Cancer Res.* 2003;63(20):6602-6606.

16. Lipshultz SE, et al. Impact of hemochromatosis gene mutations on cardiac status in doxorubicin-treated survivors of childhood high-risk leukemia. *Cancer.* 2013;119(19):3555-3562.

17. Pegram M, Slamon D. Biological rationale for HER2/neu (c-erbB2) as a target for monoclonal antibody therapy. *Semin Oncol.* 2000;27(5 Suppl 9):13-19.

18. Crone SA, et al. ErbB2 is essential in the prevention of dilated cardiomyopathy. *Nat Med.* 2002;8(5):459-465.

19. Wei SC, Duffy CR, Allison JP. Fundamental mechanisms of immune checkpoint blockade therapy. *Cancer Discov.* 2018;8(9):1069-1086.

20. Hu JR, et al. Cardiovascular toxicities associated with immune checkpoint inhibitors. *Cardiovasc Res.* 2019;115(5):854-868.

21. Maude SL, et al. Chimeric antigen receptor T cells for sustained remissions in leukemia. *N Engl J Med.* 2014;371(16):1507-1517.

22. Curigliano G, et al. Cardiovascular toxicity induced by chemotherapy, targeted agents and radiotherapy: ESMO Clinical Practice Guidelines. *Ann Oncol.* 2012;(23 Suppl 7):vii155-vii166.

23. Plana JC, et al. Expert consensus for multimodality imaging evaluation of adult patients during and after cancer therapy: a report from the American Society of Echocardiography and the European Association of Cardiovascular Imaging. *Eur Heart J Cardiovasc Imaging.* 2014;15(10):1063-1093.

24. Seidman A, et al. Cardiac dysfunction in the trastuzumab clinical trials experience. *J Clin Oncol.* 2002;20(5):1215-1221.

25. Swain SM, Whaley FS, Ewer MS. Congestive heart failure in patients treated with doxorubicin: a retrospective analysis of three trials. *Cancer.* 2003;97(11):2869-2879.

26. Tan-Chiu E, et al. Assessment of cardiac dysfunction in a randomized trial comparing doxorubicin and cyclophosphamide followed by paclitaxel, with or without trastuzumab as adjuvant therapy in node-positive, human epidermal growth factor receptor 2-overexpressing breast cancer: NSABP B-31. *J Clin Oncol.* 2005;23(31):7811-7819.

27. Lenihan DJ, et al. The utility of point-of-care biomarkers to detect cardiotoxicity during anthracycline chemotherapy: a feasibility study. *J Card Fail.* 2016;22(6):433-438.

28. Bosch X, et al. Enalapril and carvedilol for preventing chemotherapy-induced left ventricular systolic dysfunction in patients with malignant hemopathies: the OVERCOME trial (preventiOn of left Ventricular dysfunction with Enalapril and caRvedilol in patients submitted to intensive ChemOtherapy for the treatment of Malignant hEmopathies). *J Am Coll Cardiol.* 2013;61(23):2355-2362.

29. Gulati G, et al. Prevention of cardiac dysfunction during adjuvant breast cancer therapy (PRADA): a 2 × 2 factorial, randomized, placebo-controlled, double-blind clinical trial of candesartan and metoprolol. *Eur Heart J.* 2016;37(21):1671-1680.

30. Hasinoff BB, Patel D, Wu X. The oral iron chelator ICL670A (deferasirox) does not protect myocytes against doxorubicin. *Free Radic Biol Med.* 2003;35(11):1469-1479.

31. Yancy CW, et al. 2017 ACC/AHA/HFSA Focused Update of the 2013 ACCF/AHA guideline for the management of heart failure: a report of the American College of Cardiology/American Heart Association Task Force on Clinical Practice Guidelines and the Heart Failure Society of America. *J Am Coll Cardiol.* 2017;70(6):776-803.

32. Ponikowski P, et al. 2016 ESC Guidelines for the diagnosis and treatment of acute and chronic heart failure: the Task Force for the diagnosis and treatment of acute and chronic heart failure of the European Society of Cardiology (ESC). Developed with the special contribution of the Heart Failure Association (HFA) of the ESC. *Eur Heart J.* 2016;37(27):2129-2200.

33. Cardinale D, et al. Anthracycline-induced cardiomyopathy: clinical relevance and response to pharmacologic therapy. *J Am Coll Cardiol.* 2010;55(3):213-220.

34. Kurihara C, et al. Successful bridge to recovery with VAD implantation for anthracycline-induced cardiomyopathy. *J Artif Organs.* 2011;14(3):249-252.

35. Armstrong GT, Ross JD. Late cardiotoxicity in aging adult survivors of childhood cancer. *Prog Pediatr Cardiol.* 2014;36(1-2):19-26.

36. Kusumoto FM, et al. 2018 ACC/AHA/HRS guideline on the evaluation and management of patients with bradycardia and cardiac conduction delay: a report of the American College of Cardiology/American Heart Association Task Force on Clinical Practice Guidelines and the Heart Rhythm Society. *J Am Coll Cardiol.* 2019;74(7):e51-e156.

37. Thygesen K, et al. Fourth universal definition of myocardial infarction. *Eur Heart J.* 2019;40:237-269.

38. Darby SC, et al. Radiation-related heart disease: current knowledge and future prospects. *Int J Radiat Oncol Biol Phys.* 2010;76(3):656-665.

39. Rateesh S, et al. Myocardial infarction secondary to 5-fluorouracil: not an absolute contraindication to rechallenge? *Int J Cardiol.* 2014;172(2):e331-333.

40. Bair SM, Choueiri TK, Moslehi J. Cardiovascular complications associated with novel angiogenesis inhibitors: emerging evidence and evolving perspectives. *Trends Cardiovasc Med.* 2013;23(4):104-113.

41. Byrd JC, et al. Ibrutinib versus ofatumumab in previously treated chronic lymphoid leukemia. *N Engl J Med.* 2014;371(3):213-223.

42. Thompson PA, et al. Atrial fibrillation in CLL patients treated with ibrutinib. An international retrospective study. *Br J Haematol.* 2016;175(3):462-466.

43. Lee HJ, et al. Ibrutinib-related atrial fibrillation in patients with mantle cell lymphoma. *Leuk Lymphoma.* 2016;57(12):2914-2916.

44. Chung MK, et al. C-reactive protein elevation in patients with atrial arrhythmias: inflammatory mechanisms and persistence of atrial fibrillation. *Circulation.* 2001;104(24):2886-2891.

45. Enriquez A. et al. Increased incidence of ventricular arrhythmias in patients with advanced cancer and implantable cardioverter-defibrillators. *JACC Clin Electrophysiol.* 2017;3(1):50-56.

46. Barbey JT, Pezzullo JC, Soignet SL. Effect of arsenic trioxide on QT interval in patients with advanced malignancies. *J Clin Oncol.* 2003;21(19):3609-3615.

47. Al-Khatib SM, et al. 2017 AHA/ACC/HRS guideline for management of patients with ventricular arrhythmias and the prevention of sudden cardiac death: a report of the American College of Cardiology/American Heart Association Task Force on Clinical Practice Guidelines and the Heart Rhythm Society. *Circulation.* 2018;138(13):e272-e391.

48. Olsen E, et al. Pivotal phase III trial of two dose levels of denileukin diftitox for the treatment of cutaneous T-cell lymphoma. *J Clin Oncol.* 2001;19(2):376-388.

49. Cortes JE, et al. A phase 2 trial of ponatinib in Philadelphia chromosome-positive leukemias. *N Engl J Med.* 2013;369(19):1783-1796.

50. Weitz JI, Eikelboom JW, Samama MM. New antithrombotic drugs: Antithrombotic Therapy and Prevention of Thrombosis, 9th ed: American College of Chest Physicians Evidence-Based Clinical Practice Guidelines. *Chest.* 2012;141(2 Suppl):e120S-e151S.

51. Lee AY, et al. Low-molecular-weight heparin versus a coumarin for the prevention of recurrent venous thromboembolism in patients with cancer. *N Engl J Med.* 2003;349(2):146-153.

52. Smorenburg SM, Van Noorden CJ. The complex effects of heparins on cancer progression and metastasis in experimental studies. *Pharmacol Rev.* 2001;53(1):93-105.

53. Lee AYY. Anticoagulant therapy for venous thromboembolism in cancer. *N Engl J Med.* 2020;382(17):1650-1652.

54. Agnelli G. et al. Apixaban for the treatment of venous thromboembolism associated with cancer. *N Engl J Med.* 2020;382(17):1599-1607.

55. Lyman GH, et al. Venous thromboembolism prophylaxis and treatment in patients with cancer: American Society of Clinical Oncology clinical practice guideline update. *J Clin Oncol.* 2013;31(17):2189-2204.

56. Lancellotti P, et al. Expert consensus for multi-modality imaging evaluation of cardiovascular complications of radiotherapy in adults: a report from the European Association of Cardiovascular Imaging and the American Society of Echocardiography. *Eur Heart J Cardiovasc Imaging*, 2013;14(8):721-740.

57. Maraldo MV, et al. Cardiovascular disease after treatment for Hodgkin's lymphoma: an analysis of nine collaborative EORTC-LYSA trials. *Lancet Haematol.* 2015;2(11):e492-e502.

58. Jaworski C, et al. Cardiac complications of thoracic irradiation. *J Am Coll Cardiol.* 2013;61(23):2319-2328.

59. Wu W, et al. Long-term survival of patients with radiation heart disease undergoing cardiac surgery: a cohort study. *Circulation.* 2013;127(14):1476-1485.

60. Arnett DK, et al. 2019 ACC/AHA guideline on the primary prevention of cardiovascular disease: a report of the American College of Cardiology/American Heart Association Task Force on Clinical Practice Guidelines. *J Am Coll Cardiol.* 2019;74(10):e177-e232.

Heart Disease in Chronic Kidney Disease

Jared Hooker, Omar Baber, and Usman Baber

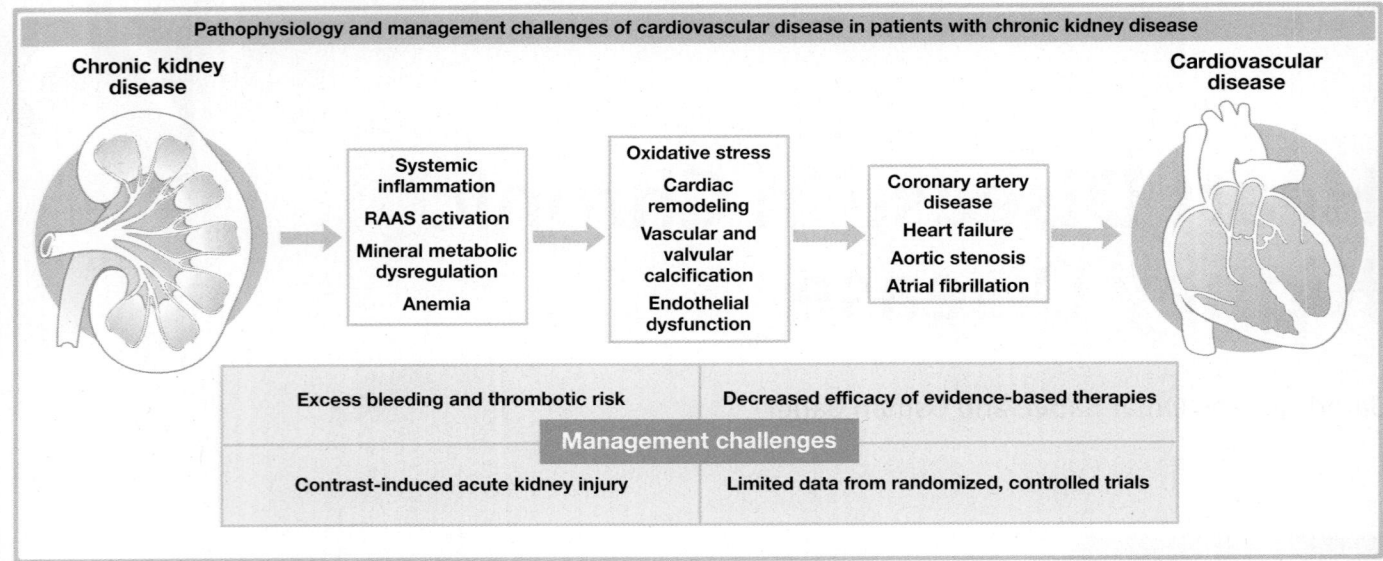

Chapter 75 Fuster and Hurst's Central Illustration. While traditional risk factors contribute to excess cardiac morbidity among patients with chronic kidney disease, the pathophysiology of cardiovascular disease is unique in this setting, and progressive as renal function worsens.

CHAPTER SUMMARY

This chapter examines the complex interplay between renal impairment and cardiovascular disease (CVD), with a focus on coronary artery disease, aortic stenosis, heart failure, atrial fibrillation and contrast-induced acute kidney injury. While traditional risk factors contribute to excess cardiac morbidity among patients with chronic kidney disease (CKD), the pathophysiology of CVD is unique in this setting, and is progressive as renal function worsens. Specifically, activation of the renin-angiotensin-aldosterone system, mineral metabolism dysregulation, oxidative stress, and inflammation promote a unique cardiovascular phenotype (see Fuster and Hurst's Central Illustration). These physiologic perturbations manifest as prevalent vascular and valvular calcification, along with cardiac structural and functional abnormalities. Management of CVD in patients with CKD is further complicated by greater risks associated with more intense or invasive approaches. Postprocedural complications, including heart failure, ischemic events, and bleeding, alter the risk–benefit ratio for commonly performed interventions. Moreover, robust evidence from large, randomized trials to inform clinical decisions in the setting of CVD and CKD remains limited. Reducing the burden of CVD in the growing CKD population has emerged as an increasingly important clinical and public health imperative.

INTRODUCTION

Chronic kidney disease (CKD) is defined as an abnormality of kidney structure or function that is present for at least 3 months.[1] Qualifying criteria include albuminuria, abnormalities of urine sediment or electrolytes, and structural abnormalities detected by imaging or prior kidney transplant. Renal function is usually expressed as estimated glomerular filtration rate (eGFR), quantified using validated equations[2,3] that incorporate age, sex, race, and serum creatinine (SCr) or serum cystatin. As endorsed by the National Kidney Foundation (NKF), patients may thus be categorized in relation to both eGFR category and degree of albuminuria, an important schema with prognostic implications (**Fig. 75-1**).

From an epidemiologic perspective, recent estimates indicate that 37 million United States adults (~13%) have CKD, with a large proportion unaware of this diagnosis.[4] The global burden of disease CKD Collaboration estimates that between 1990 and 2017, CKD mortality in the United States increased by 63%.[5] Overall CKD disease burden, expressed as disability adjusted life years (DALY), has also increased by 42.6% in the United States.[5] Healthcare costs attributable to CKD are substantial, with Medicare expenditures for end-stage renal disease (ESRD) or kidney failure approaching $36 billion in 2017.[6]

Risk factors for renal impairment include diabetes mellitus (DM), hypertension, and advanced age, which also contribute to the development of cardiovascular disease (CVD). Given this common pathologic substrate, CVD is highly prevalent among those with CKD and the presence of renal dysfunction augments cardiovascular risk. The prevalence of CKD, coupled with the substantial burden of CVD and associated costs related to this condition, reinforce the clinical and public health relevance of reducing cardiovascular risk in the presence of renal dysfunction. Importantly, the association between CKD and CVD risk is independent of traditional risk factors, highlighting the role of nontraditional mediators of cardiac risk. These include, but are not limited to, systemic inflammation, mineral metabolism dysregulation, oxidative stress, neurohormonal activation, dyslipidemia, vascular calcification, and anemia, among others (**Table 75-1**). In this chapter, we will examine the unique manifestations of CVD among those with CKD and focus specifically on common conditions: coronary artery disease, heart failure, aortic stenosis, atrial fibrillation, and contrast-induced acute kidney injury.

Prognosis of CKD by GFR and Albuminuria Category

Prognosis of CKD by GFR and Albuminuria Categories: KDIGO 2012				Persistent albuminuria categories Description and range		
				A1	**A2**	**A3**
				Normal to mildly increased	Moderately increased	Severely increased
				≤30 mg/g <30 mg/mmol	30-300 mg/g 3-30 mg/mmol	>300 mg/g >30 mg/mmol
GFR categories (ml/min/1.73 m²) Description and range	G1	Normal or high	≥90			
	G2	Mildly decreased	60-89			
	G3a	Mildly to moderately decreased	45-59			
	G3b	Moderately to severely decreased	30-44			
	G4	Severely decreased	15-29			
	G5	Kidney failure	<15			

Green: low risk (if no other markers of kidney disease, no CKD); Yellow: moderately increased risk; Orange: high risk; Red, very high risk.

Figure 75-1. Chart depicts prognosis in relation to estimated glomerular filtration rate (eGFR) category and degree of albuminuria. *Green* signifies favorable prognosis with *yellow, orange,* and *red* indicating progressive degradations in prognosis. Reproduced with permission from Levin A, Stevens PE. Summary of KDIGO 2012 CKD Guideline: behind the scenes, need for guidance, and a framework for moving forward. *Kidney Int.* 2014 Jan;85(1):49-61.

TABLE 75–1. Risk Factors for Atherosclerosis in the General Population and in CKD Patients

Classical Risk Factors	Risk Factors in CKD
Age	Mineral bone metabolism
Male gender	Vascular calcification
Left ventricular hypertrophy	Uremic toxins
Smoking	Inflammation
Diabetes mellitus	Oxidative stress
Dyslipidemia	Endothelial dysfunction
Physical inactivity	

Abbreviations: CKD, chronic kidney disease. Reproduced with permission from Valdivielso JM, Rodríguez-Puyol D, Pascual J, et al. Atherosclerosis in Chronic Kidney Disease: More, Less, or Just Different? *Arterioscler Thromb Vasc Biol.* 2019 Oct;39(10):1938-1966.

CORONARY ARTERY DISEASE

Epidemiology

In 1974, Lindner et al. postulated that "accelerated atherosclerosis" served as the etiologic mechanism for excess mortality observed in a cohort of 39 patients with ESRD treated with maintenance hemodialysis (HD).[7] Over a 13-year follow-up, the observed mortality rate in this cohort was 56%, with coronary heart disease (CHD) the most commonly cited cause of death. Numerous studies have since confirmed and extended these original observations, thus substantiating the strong link between renal impairment and both prevalent and incident CHD.

In this regard, a cross-sectional autopsy study of 126 decedents found that the burden of CHD at autopsy was inversely related to eGFR with advanced atherosclerotic disease observed in 33.6%, 41.7%, 52.3%, and 52.8% among those with eGFRs

≥60, 45 to 59, 30 to 44, and <30 mL/min/1.73 m[2], respectively.[8] Angiographic studies have also demonstrated that renal dysfunction predicts both the presence and severity of obstructive coronary artery disease; as eGFR declines, complex, multivessel disease is more common.[9] These perturbations appear most pronounced among those with advanced CKD or receiving HD. For example, a study of 30 asymptomatic patients at the time of initiation of renal replacement therapy found that 16 (53.3%) had at least 50% angiographic coronary stenosis.[10] In addition to prevalent CHD, numerous studies have also demonstrated a gradual and incremental risk for incident CHD as renal function declines. Among healthy community-dwelling adults, the risk for de novo atherosclerotic cardiovascular disease (ASCVD) increased by 7% for every 10 mL/min/1.73 m[2] reduction in eGFR (**Fig. 75–2**).[11] Importantly, similar patterns of risk persist when examining renal impairment based upon albuminuria, with or without concomitant reductions in glomerular filtration.[12]

Large, population-based studies have further characterized the associations between renal function, albuminuria, and risks for all-cause and cardiovascular death. Among adults within an integrated healthcare plan (n = 1.5 million; mean age 52 years), the adjusted hazard ratios (aHR) for all-cause death increased in an exponential fashion below eGFR <60 mL/min/1.73m[2].[13] Specifically, over 2.8 years, the aHR and 95% confidence intervals (CI) for all-cause mortality were 1.2 (95% CI, 1.1–1.2); 1.8 (95% CI, 1.7–1.9); 3.2 (95% CI, 3.1–3.4), and 5.9 (95% CI, 5.4–6.5) among those with eGFR 45 to 59, 30 to 44, 15 to 29, and <15 mL/min/1.73m[2], respectively. Similar patterns were observed for cardiovascular events and all-cause hospitalizations. A collaborative meta-analysis comprising 14 population-based cohorts (n = 105,872) found that albumin to creatinine ratio (ACR) displayed a monotonic, graded association with all-cause and cardiovascular mortality.[14] Moreover,

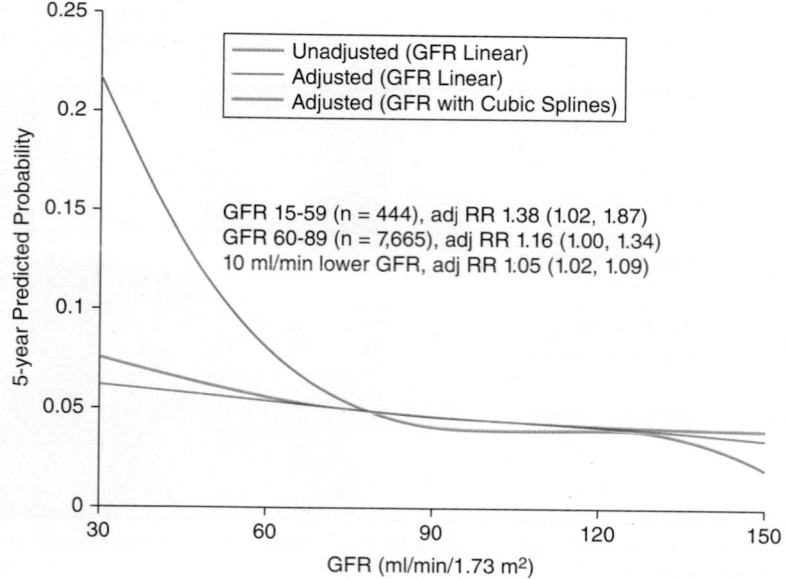

Figure 75–2. Probability of developing atherosclerotic cardiovascular disease (ASCVD) in the ARIC (Atherosclerosis Risk in Communities) study. adj, adjusted; GFR, glomerular filtration rate; RR, risk ratio. Adapted with permission from Manjunath G, Tighiouart H, Ibrahim H, et al: Level of kidney function as a risk factor for atherosclerotic cardiovascular outcomes in the community. *J Am Coll Cardiol.* 2003 Jan 1;41(1):47-55.

eGFR and ACR demonstrated a synergistic effect on mortality, highlighting the substantial risk for CVD among those with both abnormalities.

Excess cardiovascular risk associated with CKD persists among those presenting with acute coronary syndrome (ACS).[15,16] A multicenter cohort (n = 19,832) comprising ACS patients found that CKD was prevalent, observed in approximately 30% of patients. After multivariable adjustment, risks for recurrent myocardial infarction (MI) at 90 and 365 days were 25% and 36% higher among those with versus without CKD. Despite elevated ischemic risk, use of the potent antiplatelet agent prasugrel was 50% lower among those with renal impairment. Similar patterns have been observed with respect to use of invasive angiography or other evidence-based pharmacotherapy in relation to worsening renal function.[17]

Pathophysiology

An array of plausible mechanisms for accelerated atherogenesis in patients with CKD have been described including hypertension, endothelial dysfunction, impaired nitric oxide metabolism, oxidative stress, chronic inflammation, and dyslipidemia.[18,19] Hypertension is nearly universally present in this population and is potentiated by sodium retention, increased activity of the renin-angiotensin system, and increased sympathetic activation. Increased activity of the renin-angiotensin system is a compensatory mechanism for loss of functional renal mass, and activation of angiotensin I and II receptors increases formation of superoxide, a free radical, leading to increased oxidative stress.[20]

Endothelial dysfunction is an important factor in both the pathogenesis of renal impairment and in the development of atherosclerosis.[20] The Hoorn study was a population-based cohort study of 613 patients that demonstrated that increased markers of endothelial dysfunction in patients with mild renal dysfunction was associated with increased cardiovascular mortality.[21] Increased sympathetic activation[22] and diminished nitric oxide bioavailability have been demonstrated in patients with renal failure with both contributing to endothelial dysfunction and atherogenesis.[18,23] The etiology of diminished nitric oxide production in CKD patients is multifactorial, but increased asymmetric dimethylarginine (ADMA), a nitric oxide synthase inhibitor, is one important mechanism.[24]

Chronic inflammation and increased oxidative stress results in a unique, particularly atherogenic dyslipidemia characterized by dysfunctional high-density lipoproteins[25] and oxidized low-density lipoproteins (LDLs). Vascular calcification is more severe and progressive in CKD patients, owing at least in part to abnormalities in calcium and phosphorus balance in these patients;[26] degree of calcification has been demonstrated to correlate with mortality in ESRD patients.[27] Bone mineral metabolism involves a complex interplay including parathyroid hormone, calcium/phosphate balance, vitamin D homeostasis, and other factors that are not as clearly understood. CKD perturbs this process as phosphorus excretion and vitamin D conversion are impaired, resulting in increased parathyroid hormone excretion. Increases in circulating calcium and phosphorus with concomitant increased fibroblast growth factor 23 (FGF-23) and aberrations in its cofactors combine to activate calcium deposition processes within the arterial media.[28]

Histopathologic and in vivo imaging studies suggest the presence of a unique atherosclerotic phenotype in patients with CKD. Coronary plaques were characterized by more lipid and less fibrous volume among stable patients with versus without CKD undergoing percutaneous coronary intervention (PCI).[29] Analogous findings were observed in a larger ACS cohort using virtual histology intravascular ultrasound (VH-IVUS).[30] In this study, there was significantly higher necrotic core and reduced fibrous tissue associated with CKD (versus non-CKD) lesions. In a separate report, coronary plaque disruption based upon optical coherence tomography was observed more frequently among those with CKD.[31] In aggregate, these findings demonstrate that coronary atherosclerotic plaque vulnerability appears to increase as renal function declines, thus contributing to more diffuse atherosclerosis and coronary thrombosis.

Management

Diagnosis

Patients with CKD more commonly present with acute MI rather than angina as their initial manifestation of CHD.[32] This underscores the need for strong clinical suspicion and aggressive risk factor modification. However, the diagnostic performance of noninvasive modalities is reduced in CKD patients, with the most commonly used modalities (myocardial perfusion scintigraphy and stress echocardiography)[33] offering only moderate sensitivity at best. Given the high pretest probability of CAD in this population and limited diagnostic accuracy of traditional noninvasive tests, newer modalities may play an important role. In a study of renal transplant candidates, coronary computed tomography angiography (CTA) was significantly more sensitive than myocardial perfusion imaging (96% vs 56%) for the detection of 50% coronary stenoses; however, specificity was only 63%.[34]

Pharmacotherapy

Lipid Lowering: The foundation of modifying atherosclerotic risk in CKD patients, as in the general population, is lipid-lowering therapy. Available clinical practice guidelines from kidney-specific and cardiovascular societies support statin initiation for most adults with nondialysis-dependent CKD and continuation of statin therapy in patients who progress to dialysis.[35,36]

Although the data for statin therapy in CKD patients is not as robust as the general population, available evidence is supportive of broad statin use in this population. The Study of Heart and Renal Protection (SHARP) trial randomized 9270 patients with CKD (mean eGFR 26.6 mL/min/1.73m^2; 3023 were on renal replacement therapy) to simvastatin/ezetimibe therapy or placebo. Major atherosclerotic events including nonfatal MI, coronary death, ischemic stroke, and arterial revascularization procedures were reduced by 17% in the treatment arm over a mean follow-up of 4.9 years. This was largely driven by reduced rates of ischemic stroke and arterial revascularization.

Importantly, overall atherosclerotic event reduction was present in all subgroups, including patients on hemodialysis.[37]

Meta-analyses of CKD patients enrolled in statin trials have consistently demonstrated reductions in cardiovascular events, cardiovascular death, and all-cause mortality in CKD patients not on dialysis.[38] In contrast, randomized trials involving dialysis patients have not shown similar benefits. The 4D trial randomized 1255 patients with type 2 diabetes on hemodialysis to atorvastatin 20 mg daily or placebo; the primary endpoint was a composite of cardiovascular death, nonfatal MI, or stroke. Although atorvastatin significantly reduced LDL cholesterol by 42%, rates of the primary endpoint were similar between groups over a 4-year follow-up.[39] In the Use of Rosuvastatin in Subjects on Regular Hemodialysis: An Assessment of Survival and Cardiovascular Events (AURORA) trial, 2776 patients on hemodialysis were randomized to receive rosuvastatin 10 mg daily or placebo; primary outcome was a composite of cardiovascular death, nonfatal MI, or nonfatal stroke. At a median follow-up of 3.8 years, there was no significant difference in the primary outcome or any component of the primary outcome.[40] Reasons for lack of benefit in the setting of dialysis may reflect the presence of nonatherosclerotic mechanisms contributing to cardiovascular mortality, competing risks, and limited survival that precludes realization of statin-related benefit.

Antiplatelets: Dual antiplatelet therapy (DAPT) with aspirin (ASA) and an inhibitor of the platelet $P2Y_{12}$ receptor is recommended in all patients for at least 1 year following an index ACS event.[41] Prolonging DAPT exposure beyond 1 year may offer additional benefits in select patients.[42,43] Generalizing these results to the setting of CKD is challenging because renal dysfunction is strongly associated with both excess thrombosis and bleeding.[44,45] In a subgroup analysis of the Clopidogrel for the Reduction of Events During Observation (CREDO) trial, the safety and efficacy of adding a loading dose of clopidogrel at the time of elective PCI was examined in relation to renal function.[46] Although rates of 28-day adverse events increased in a graded fashion with worsening renal function, clopidogrel was associated with a clinical benefit only in the presence of normal renal function. In a separate analysis involving ACS patients, reductions in adverse events with use of clopidogrel and ASA versus ASA alone were attenuated as renal function worsened.[47] In the Study of Platelet Inhibition and Patient Outcomes (PLATO) trial, the safety and efficacy of ticagrelor versus clopidogrel was examined among high-risk ACS patients treated with ASA.[48] Among those with CKD (n = 3237), ticagrelor was associated with a significant 23% reduction in the primary end point of cardiovascular death, MI, and stroke over 12 months.[49] Analogous results were reported from a large clinical trial comparing ticagrelor and ASA versus ASA along among stable patients with prior history of MI.[50] Despite the salutary benefits of ticagrelor among those with CKD, clinical use of this agent decreases substantially as renal function worsens.[17] Similar findings were reported with respect to use of the potent $P2Y_{12}$ inhibitor prasugrel (**Fig. 75–3**).[15] Although reasons for such paradoxical use remain unclear, it is plausible that clinical concerns for bleeding may influence clinical decision-making to a stronger degree than the potential benefits of lowering thrombotic risk.

Coronary Revascularization

Among patients with stable ischemic heart disease (SIHD), coronary revascularization reduces anginal symptoms and improves quality of life as compared with medical therapy.[51,52] The choice of revascularization approach (surgical vs percutaneous) requires a comprehensive, patient-centric evaluation that integrates anatomic complexity, comorbid conditions, and patient values. The relative merits of coronary revascularization and optimal strategy in the setting of CKD is challenging because clinical trials that inform such decisions usually excluded patients with at least moderate-to-severe renal dysfunction (**Table 75–2**).

In a propensity-matched cohort comprising patients with at least moderate CKD (n = 5920) and multivessel CAD, 3-year mortality rates were comparable between patients treated with coronary artery bypass surgery (CABG) as compared with PCI.[53] However, CABG was associated with a reduced risk for MI, a benefit that was primarily driven by patients with

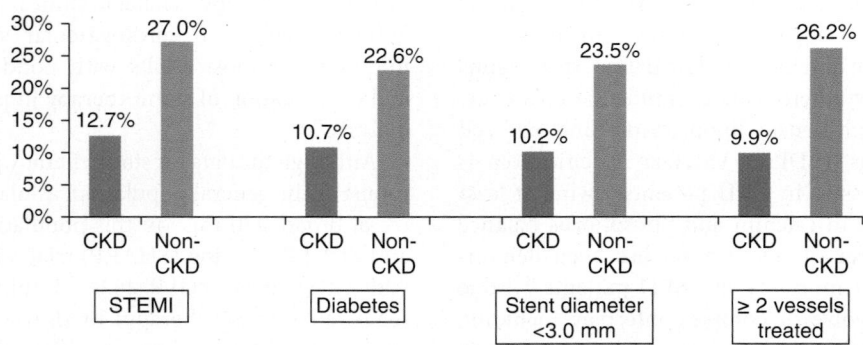

Figure 75–3. Frequency of prasugrel use among chronic kidney disease (CKD) and non-CKD patients with acute coronary syndrome undergoing percutaneous coronary intervention in relation to high-risk group: ST-segment elevation myocardial infarction; diabetes mellitus; stent diameter <3.0 mm, ≥2 vessels treated. Vertical bars represent frequency of prasugrel use in relation to CKD (*red*) and non-CKD (*blue*). Modified with permission from Baber U, Chandrasekhar J, Sartori S, et al. Associations Between Chronic Kidney Disease and Outcomes With Use of Prasugrel Versus Clopidogrel in Patients With Acute Coronary Syndrome Undergoing Percutaneous Coronary Intervention: A Report From the PROMETHEUS Study. *JACC Cardiovasc Interv.* 2017 Oct 23;10(20):2017-2025.

TABLE 75–2. Chronic Kidney Disease Inclusion in Clinical Trials Evaluating Coronary Revascularization

	ARTS	FREEDOM	EXCEL	SYNTAX	ISCHEMIA-CKD	COURAGE	BARI 2D
Sample size	1205	1900	1905	1638	777	2287	2368
Comparators	CABG vs PCI	CABG vs PCI	CABG vs PCI	CABG vs PCI	Early invasive vs medical therapy	Early invasive vs medical therapy	Early invasive vs medical therapy
Renal exclusion	SCr >1.7 mg/dL	eGFR <15 mL/min/1.73m²	None	None	N/A	None	SCr >2 mg/dL
CKD, n (%)	290 (25%)	451 (24.5%)	361 (19.3%)	309 (18.9%)	100%	320 (14%)	443 (18.7%)
Mean renal function	50 cc/min	47 mL/min/1.73m²	48.6 mL/min/1.73m²	47.6 mL/min/1.73m²	23 mL/min/1.73m²	SCr ~1.45	~50.5 mL/min/1.73m²

Abbreviations: ARTS, Arterial Revascularization Therapies Study; FREEDOM , Future Revascularization Evaluation in Patients with Diabetes Mellitus: Optimal Management of Multivessel Disease; EXCEL, Evaluation of XIENCE Versus Coronary Artery Bypass Surgery for Effectiveness of Left Main Revascularization; COURAGE, Clinical Outcomes Utilizing Revascularization and Aggressive Drug Evaluation; SYNTAX , Synergy between PCI with Taxus and Cardiac Surgery; BARI 2D, Bypass Angioplasty Revascularization Investigation 2 Diabetes; CKD, chronic kidney disease; CABG, coronary artery bypass graft; PCI, percutaneous coronary intervention; eGFR, estimated glomerular filtration rate.

3-vessel (6.1% vs 13.8%; $P < 0.001$) versus 2-vessel (6.3% vs 8.0%; $P = 0.37$) CAD. Repeat revascularization strongly favored surgical bypass whereas short and long-term risk for stroke was lower with PCI. Largely concordant results were reported in a subgroup analysis of the Future Revascularization Evaluation in Patients with Diabetes Mellitus: Optimal Management of Multivessel Disease (FREEDOM) trial that compared CABG versus PCI among patients with DM and multivessel CAD.[54] Among those with CKD randomized in the FREEDOM trial (n = 451; mean eGFR 47 mL/min/1.73m²), CABG significantly reduced MI and repeat revascularization over a median follow-up of 3.8 years. In contrast, rates of death were nonsignificantly different between groups and stroke risk was numerically higher among those with CKD (8.2% vs 3.8%; $P = 0.12$). These results suggest the risk-benefit calculus for choice of CABG versus PCI in the setting of mild-to-moderate CKD may warrant greater consideration of cerebrovascular risk as compared with non-CKD patients.

The role of coronary revascularization among those with more severe CKD is less clear. In the ISCHEMIA-CKD trial, patients with advanced CKD (n = 777; 53% receiving dialysis) and moderate-to-severe ischemia were randomized to an initial invasive strategy consisting of coronary angiography with revascularization or medical therapy.[55] Over a median follow-up of 2.2 years, rates of death or MI were nonsignificantly different between groups. Moreover, stroke risk was significantly increased among those allocated to an invasive strategy (aHR 3.76; 95% CI, 1.52–9.32). It is possible that the lack of benefit observed in this trial may reflect a true null effect, although a type II error is also plausible. For example, among patients randomized to an invasive strategy, coronary angiography and revascularization was only performed in 85% and 50%, respectively. The most common reason that revascularization was not performed was due to a lack of obstructive CAD at the time of angiography, highlighting the poor diagnostic accuracy of conventional tests in CKD patients. In addition, the majority of patients enrolled in ISCHEMIA-CKD presented with minimal symptoms (no angina in 48%). As a result, these findings are not generalizable to more symptomatic patients with a higher prevalence of obstructive CAD.

HEART FAILURE AND CHRONIC KIDNEY DISEASE

Epidemiology

As with other manifestations of cardiovascular disease, renal impairment is strongly associated with both prevalent and incident heart failure (HF). These epidemiologic links are not unexpected because the underlying substrates for both conditions (ie, hypertension, CAD, and DM) display substantial overlap. In a large cohort study of community-dwelling adults without prevalent HF (n = 14,857), Kottgen et al. found that the risk of incident HF was approximately 2-fold higher among those with an eGFR <60 mL/min/1.73m² as compared to those with eGFR >90 mL/min/1.73m².[56] Patterns of risk were unchanged in the absence of CHD, highlighting the putative role of nonatherosclerotic mediators as determinants of HF risk in the presence of CKD. Insights from the prospective Chronic Renal Insufficiency Cohort (CRIC) Study further demonstrate that HF hospitalization greatly increases risk for both progressive renal dysfunction and all-cause mortality among those with moderate CKD.[57] In aggregate, these studies highlight the consistent, strong, and durable associations between various measures of renal impairment and HF risk across different patient cohorts. The bidirectional links between progressive cardiac and renal deterioration may be characterized based upon acuity and *primum movens* as cardiorenal syndrome (CRS; **Table 75–3**).[58] Within this construct, type 1 and 2 CRS reflect acute and chronic cardiac failure resulting in kidney injury. In contrast, type 3 and 4 CRS are defined as acute or chronic

TABLE 75–3. Cardiorenal Syndromes

Type 1	Acute cardiac dysfunction resulting in acute kidney injury
Type 2	Chronic cardiac dysfunction resulting in CKD
Type 3	AKI resulting in acute cardiac dysfunction
Type 4	CKD of noncardiac etiology promotes cardiac disease
Type 5	Systemic disorder (not primarily cardiogenic or nephrogenic) results in simultaneous renal and cardiac dysfunction

Abbreviations: AKI, acute kidney injury; CKD, chronic kidney disease.

kidney disease with subsequent cardiac decompensation. Type 5 CRS is defined as systemic disorders culminating in cardiac and renal dysfunction (ie, amyloidosis).

Pathophysiology

Pathophysiologic links that appear most relevant in the setting of HF and concomitant CKD may be broadly categorized as hemodynamic, neurohormonal, or cardiac-related. A reduction in "forward flow" was presumed the primary driver of kidney injury in the setting of acute decompensated HF, or CRS 1. In this context, HF with reduced or preserved ejection fraction (HFrEF or HFpEF), reduces cardiac output ultimately compromising glomerular filtration once autoregulatory mechanisms have been overwhelmed. This could result in renal tubule hypoxia and acute tubular necrosis. However, results from several studies have demonstrated additional hemodynamic mechanisms contributing to renal injury in the setting of HF. In The Evaluation Study of Congestive Heart Failure and Pulmonary Artery Catheterization Effectiveness (ESCAPE) trial, for example, baseline renal function was associated with right atrial pressure, not cardiac index.[59] In a separate report, baseline central venous pressure emerged as a much stronger discriminator of worsening renal function as compared with cardiac index (c-statistic 0.73 vs 0.55; $P = 0.01$).[60] Elevations in right atrial pressure may compromise renal function by reducing renal blood flow via decreased transrenal perfusion pressure, increased intraglomerular hydrostatic pressure, and increased intratubular pressure. Increases in intrabdominal pressure, commonly observed in patients with HF, may also adversely affect renal function.

Neurohormones, sympathetic nervous activity, and filling status serve as key modulators of both cardiac and renal function. Activation of the renin-angiotensin-aldosterone system (RAAS) is an important pathologic hallmark of both cardiac failure and CKD. Specifically, increased levels of angiotensin II (Ang II) in the setting of HF exerts direct fibrotic effects on both cardiac myocytes and renal parenchyma. Aldosterone secretion leads to sodium and water retention thereby contributing to renal venous congestion and renal remodeling. Clinical and experimental studies demonstrate that sympathetic activation occurs early in the pathophysiology of CKD.[61-63] For example, noradrenaline secretion rates were increased among patients with nephrotic syndrome and autosomal dominant polycystic kidney disease despite normal renal function.[61,62] Among those with advanced CKD requiring dialysis, plasma catecholamine levels predict survival and cardiovascular events.[64] Moreover, sympathetic tone does not normalize following renal transplantation, suggesting a persistent role for renal afferent nerves in mediating sympathetic activity.[65] These findings are particularly germane for the development of HF because increased sympathetic activity can potentiate RAAS-mediated volume retention and systemic vasoconstriction.

Other pathologic mechanisms linking CKD and HF include chronic inflammation, anemia, and mineral metabolism dysregulation. Systemic inflammation is commonly observed in patients with either renal dysfunction or HF. Levels of inflammatory biomarkers, including C-reactive protein and interleukin-10, increase as renal function worsens. Moreover, inflammation is a predictor of cardiac and all-cause mortality in either disease state.[66,67] Inflammation may result from visceral edema, sympathetic activation, and oxidative stress among other pathways.[68] Direct effects of inflammatory mediators, such as T cells and monocytes, may promote vasculopathy and cardiac and renal remodeling.

Anemia is a common finding in advanced CKD that also links renal impairment with cardiac dysfunction and HF. Usually observed in more advanced CKD, anemia results from inadequate synthesis of erythropoietin (EPO). From a cardiac standpoint, persistent anemia is associated with functional and structural cardiac alterations, including left ventricular hypertrophy and dilatation.[69] Moreover, EPO may exert anti-apoptotic effects on cardiomyocytes.[70] These hypotheses are supported by clinical studies showing that anemia is a predictor of HF readmission and prognosis among those with both anemia and HF.[71] In addition, eryhropeoiesis-stimulating agents are associated with improved quality of life and exercise capacity in the setting of HF.[72]

The capacity of the kidney to excrete phosphate diminishes as renal function worsens, leading to a state of hyperphosphatemia thereby increasing levels of parathyroid hormone and FGF 23. Vitamin D deficiency also occurs in CKD, which reduces intestinal absorption of calcium thus lowering serum calcium levels. These pathologic alterations are observed even in mild-to-moderate CKD and are associated with left ventricular hypertrophy and cardiac fibrosis,[73,74] culminating in excess risk for development of HF.

Management

Decongestive therapies, particularly diuretics, are used almost universally among patients with acute symptomatic HF. Although not associated with reduction in mortality or rehospitalization, existing guidelines provide a class I recommendation for use of loop diuretics in the setting of HF.[75,76] Several studies have examined variable strategies of administering diuretics on renal and cardiac endpoints in the setting of HF.[77,78] The Diuretic Optimization Strategies Evaluation in Acute heart Failure (DOSE-AHF) trial compared bolus versus continuous furosemide infusion and low- versus high-dose regimen in a 2 × 2 factorial design. While no differences were observed between continuous and bolus administration, the high-dose strategy displayed a trend toward symptom improvement without compromising renal function. A pooled analysis from different clinical trials also found that a urine volume-guided diuretic algorithm demonstrated more weight and net fluid loss with an improvement in renal function as compared with standard diuretic therapy.[79]

In aggregate, these results suggest that high-dose furosemide boluses guided by urine volume appear effective and safe from a renal standpoint among patients hospitalized with symptomatic HF. Importantly, CKD is characterized by a reduced diuretic effect, or diuretic resistance, as compared to those without renal impairment. This is primarily attributable to reductions in the filtered load of sodium needed to achieve a diuretic effect. Achieving an adequate diuretic effect in the setting of CKD, therefore, may require more frequent dosing. Several studies have examined ultrafiltration as a nondiuretic-based approach toward decongestion in the setting of HF.[80,81] In a randomized comparison involving 200 patients with acute decompensated HF, ultrafiltration resulted in a greater weight loss at 48 hours as compared with loop diuretics without any differences in SCr at 90 days.[80] In contrast, among patients with acute HF and type 1 CRS ultrafiltration at a constant rate was associated with an increase in SCr and more adverse events as compared with conventional loop diuresis.[81]

RAAS inhibitors slow the progression of CKD and improve cardiovascular morbidity and mortality among those with HFrEF. However, the safety and efficacy of RAAS inhibition in the setting of CKD and HF is less clear because most clinical trials evaluating such therapeutics excluded patients with moderate-to-severe renal impairment. Nonetheless, subgroup analyses from clinical trials and other observational studies suggest that reductions in cardiovascular risk associated with RAAS inhibition are preserved among those with or without CKD in the presence of HF.

In the Studies of Left Ventricular Dysfunction (SOLVD), enalapril was compared to placebo among those with ambulatory HF and left ventricular ejection fraction <35%. Enalapril reduced mortality in a consistent fashion among those with (HR 0.88; 95% CI, 0.73–1.06) or without (HR 0.82; 95% CI, 0.69–0.98) CKD (P_{int} = 0.62).[82] Similar findings were reported in a propensity-matched analysis from the Digitalis Investigation Group (DIG) trial wherein angiotensin-converting enzyme I (ACE-I) use was associated with a 42% reduction in all-cause mortality as compared with no use among those with mild-to-moderate CKD.[83] The salutary benefits of RAAS inhibition are also apparent when achieved with either ACE-I or angiotensin receptor blockers (ARB).[84–86] Among patients hospitalized with HF use of either ACE-I or ARB was associated with reductions in mortality that increased in a graded fashion with worsening renal function.[86] Similar findings were observed in a separate report examining patients with CKD and HFpEF.[85] Despite these encouraging results, the addition of an ARB to ACE-I is discouraged due to an increased risk for adverse events.[87] Safety considerations may also account for reluctance in using such agents despite putative cardiovascular benefits.

The combination of neprilysin inhibition with RAAS inhibition has emerged a novel therapeutic strategy for HFrEF. In a pooled analysis comparing neprilysin/RAAS inhibition versus RAAS inhibition alone, combined therapy reduced death or HF hospitalization by 14%.[88] Importantly, combination therapy was associated with fewer adverse events defined as creatinine elevation or impaired renal function, although symptomatic hypotension was more commonly observed in all three trials. These results are corroborated by a more quantitative assessment of renal function decline, which was reduced among those receiving a neprilysin inhibitor and valsartan as compared with enalapril alone.[89]

Mineralocorticoid receptor antagonists (MRA) enhance RAAS suppression and reduce cardiovascular events among patients with HFrEF.[90–92] In the eplerenone in Mild Patients Hospitalization and Survival Study in Heart Failure (EMPHASIS-HF), the MRA eplerenone was compared to placebo in 2737 patients with mild symptoms and reduced ejection fraction.[91] Most patients (~95%) were already treated with ACE-I or ARB. Over a median follow-up of 21 months, eplerenone significantly reduced all-cause (12.5% vs 15.5%; P = 0.01) and cardiovascular mortality (10.8% vs 13.5%; P = 0.01). In a subgroup analysis among EMPHASIS-HF participants with CKD (n = 912, mean eGFR 48.6 mL/min/1.73m²), the benefits of eplerenone with respect to the primary efficacy outcome of cardiovascular death or HF hospitalization were preserved (24.4% vs 34.5%; P < 0.001).[93] However, hyperkalemia and drug discontinuation was more frequent among those with renal impairment. Moreover, the safety and efficacy profile of eplerenone among those with more advanced CKD and HFrEF may not be inferred from this analysis involving less severe CKD.

β-blockers are recommended with a Class I, level of evidence A for use in HFrEF due to reductions in mortality and HF hospitalization.[75,94] Subgroup analyses from clinical trials provide additional insights regarding the safety and efficacy of β-blockade in the presence of CKD and HFrEF.[95–97] Absolute reductions in all-cause mortality or HF hospitalization increased in a graded fashion with worsening renal function with use of extended release metoprolol as compared with placebo.[95] In a pooled analysis involving 6 randomized trials, β-blocker therapy was associated with a 28% and 34% relative reduction in all-cause and cardiovascular mortality as compared with placebo among those with CKD and HF.[96] However, bradycardia and hypotension were significantly increased with β-blocker use. Other reports have shown higher rates of β-blocker discontinuation in the setting of CKD, substantiating the increased risk for adverse side effects and/or less tolerance.[97]

Implantable cardioverter defibrillators (ICDs) provide a survival benefit in select patients with reduced EF. Extrapolation to the CKD population is challenging given the increased risk for procedural complications, noncardiac conditions that might impact survival, and increased risk for shocks due to nonfatal arrhythmias observed in such patients. In a patient-level pooled analysis of three randomized trials, Pun et al. examined the efficacy of ICD implantation for primary prevention of all-cause death[98] in relation to renal function. The study included 1040 patients with CKD with a mean eGFR 44.7 mL/min/1.73m². ICD therapy significantly lowered mortality among those with eGFR ≥60 mL/min/1.73m², whereas no benefit was observed among those with eGFR <60 mL/min/1.73m². Among those with advanced CKD requiring dialysis, the Implantable Cardioverter-Defibrillator in Dialysis Patients (ICD2) trial examined the efficacy of prophylactic ICD implantation among dialysis patients with an EF ≥35% (n = 200). While overall mortality over 5 years was high, there were no differences between groups with respect to all-cause mortality or sudden cardiac death.[99] Similar results were observed in a matched cohort study involving dialysis patients with reduced EF receiving ICD therapy.[100] In concert, these results suggest an attenuated or absent benefit with ICD therapy for purposes of primary prevention among patients with moderate-to-advanced CKD and HF. Thus, risk benefit calculations with respect to ICD use in such patients must consider other comorbidities that might impact survival, quality of life, and patient wishes.

AORTIC STENOSIS AND CHRONIC KIDNEY DISEASE

Epidemiology

The prevalence of aortic stenosis (AS) increases in a graded fashion as renal function worsens. Among patients referred for echocardiography at a large tertiary care center (n = 78,057), mild AS was detected in 1.9%, 4.4%, and 5.2% of those with an eGFR ≥60, 45 to 59, and <45 mL/min/1.73m², respectively.[101] The presence of renal impairment also associates with more rapid progression of AS. In a large observational cohort followed for a median of 5.1 years, the incidence rate (per 100 person-years) for AS was 0.34, 1.88, 4.61, 6.62, and 8.27 among those with an eGFR >90, 60 to 90, 45 to 59, 30 to 44, and <30 mL/min/1.73m², respectively.[102] Although attenuated, associations between renal dysfunction and AS remained significant after multivariable adjustment. The risk for AS displayed a nonlinear pattern with eGFR with an inflection point of ~44 mL/min/1.73m² below which the incidence of AS increased rapidly. Importantly, the presence of even mild AS confers a higher risk for mortality among those with versus without CKD. In one report, 5-year survival estimates for mild, moderate, and severe AS among those with CKD were 40%, 34%, and 42%, respectively, and 69%, 54%, and 67% in the absence of CKD (P_{int} < 0.001).[101]

Pathophysiology

Analogous to vascular calcification observed in the setting of renal impairment, calcification of aortic valve interstitial cells serves as an important pathologic substrate for progressive aortic stenosis in CKD and ESRD.[103] Mineral metabolism dysregulation leading to hyperphosphatemia, parathyroid hormone excess, and elevated calcium-phosphate product, each appear to play a role in this disease process. Furthermore, medications used in CKD and ESRD, such as calcitriol and calcium-containing phosphate binders may potentiate valvular calcification by increased calcium absorption and increased calcium-phosphate product.

Beyond the alterations in calcium and phosphate metabolism, there is also evidence of an atherogenic component to AS. This is evidenced by histopathologic evaluation of valves with "early" changes of degenerative aortic valve stenosis that showed findings similar to atherosclerotic lesions (lipid deposition, macrophage, and T-cell infiltration).[104] Renal dysfunction thus plays a synergistic role in this valvular atherogenic process via a chronic inflammatory state and increased oxidative stress.

The hemodynamic consequences of progressive renal impairment may also predispose to accelerated development of AS. Under normal conditions, repetitive opening and closure of the aortic valve leads to cyclic mechanical stress. In CKD and ESRD patients, anemia and atrioventricular fistulas may lead to high-output states, thus enhancing transvalvular turbulent flow. Subsequent development of valvular fibrosis and calcification leads to further reductions in valve mobility, more turbulent flow, and further calcification and stenosis in a self-perpetuating cycle.

Management

Aortic valve replacement (AVR), either surgical (SAVR) or transcatheter (TAVR), is the definitive treatment for severe AS. Although AS is highly prevalent among those with CKD,[101,103] AVR is not performed in a considerable proportion of such patients. These practice patterns may reflect concerns regarding operative risk, noncardiac morbidity, or postprocedure complications. Among patients undergoing TAVR, renal dysfunction is associated worse in-hospital outcomes (in-hospital mortality, length of stay, pacemaker implantation, bleeding complications) and reduced 30-day and 1-year survival.[105] Nonetheless, observational and retrospective data suggest a long-term mortality benefit from AVR versus conservative management in patients with severe AS and concomitant CKD or ESRD.[106-108] Based upon the results of large randomized trials, TAVR is recommended for patients with severe AS deemed prohibitive surgical risk and is considered a suitable alternative among those at intermediate or high risk.[109] With regards to TAVR versus SAVR in the subset of patients with CKD, results from the CoreValve US Pivotal High Risk Trial showed that TAVR resulted in lower major adverse cardiovascular and renal events (MACRE) at 3 years versus SAVR in patients with moderate-to-severe CKD (defined as eGFR <60 mL/min/1.73 m²).[110] Data comparing TAVR to SAVR in more advanced CKD and/or ESRD are limited given the exclusion of such patients from most pivotal studies.[111-113] However, a retrospective propensity score matched analysis of a cohort of patients with advanced CKD from the National Inpatient Sample showed TAVR was associated with lower in-hospital mortality and periprocedural complications as compared to SAVR.[114] Nonetheless, 1-year mortality rates were 31%, 40%, and 50% among TAVR recipients with Stage 3, 4, and 5 CKD, respectively, highlighting the significant risk associated with renal dysfunction following TAVR.[115] Accordingly, due to the significant risk of mortality and adverse outcomes, a multidisciplinary approach to patient selection and careful discussions about goals of care are important to address prior to proceeding with AVR.

ATRIAL FIBRILLATION AND CHRONIC KIDNEY DISEASE

Epidemiology

Atrial fibrillation (AF) is the most sustained arrhythmia found in clinical practice, with an estimated prevalence between 0.4% and 1% in the general population. Both prevalent[116,117] and incident[118] AF increase in a graded fashion as renal function worsens.

The presence of AF confers an increased risk for ischemic stroke, systemic embolism, and HF. Similar patterns are observed among those with CKD. In an observational cohort comprising CKD patients (n = 116,184; mean eGFR 51 mL/min/1.73m^2), incidence rates for AF (per 1000 person-years) were 29.4, 40.8, and 46.3 among those with eGFR 45 to 60 mL/min/1.73m^2, 30 to 45 mL/min/1.73m^2, and <30 mL/min/1.73m^2, respectively.[118] Over 4 years, the adjusted risks for all-cause death and ischemic stroke associated with AF were 1.76 and 2.11, respectively. Importantly, estimates remained large and significant after accounting for competing risks and persisted across eGFR categories. Among patients with CKD requiring dialysis, the overall burden and risk for AF increases substantially. In a large population-based cohort (n = 404,703) followed for 5.1 years, incident rates for AF (per 1000 person-years) were 5.0, 7.3, and 12.1 among those without CKD, non-dialysis-dependent CKD, and ESRD, respectively.[119]

Pathophysiology

There are multiple mechanisms by which CKD may predispose to the development of AF. Pathologic activation of the RAAS that occurs with declining renal function serves as a principal driver.[120] Signaling pathways mediated by the RAAS have been implicated in atrial remodeling and fibrosis, which predisposes to the development of AF. Beyond cardiac remodeling, modulation of membrane ion channels and gap junctions as well as alterations in intracellular calcium cycling mediated by the RAAS may also contribute to arrhythmogenesis.[121,122]

Left atrial enlargement is a known predictor of AF and is observed more frequently among those with versus without CKD.[123,124] Left atrial stretch represents a structural abnormality that may result from hemodynamic stressors observed in the early stages of CKD, such as hypertension and hypervolemia.[125–128] Furthermore, patients with CKD are frequently hypertensive, a known risk factor for the development of AF.

In addition to neurohormonal activation and hemodynamic factors, systemic inflammation appears to play a role in AF given its association with elevated inflammatory markers[129] as well as inflammatory changes found in atrial biopsies of AF patients.[130] These inflammatory changes may contribute to atrial remodeling, thereby contributing to a substrate with increased propensity for AF.[131] Kidney dysfunction, which associates with systemic inflammation and oxidative stress,[20] may thus contribute to this inflammatory milieu thereby increasing the risk for AF.

Management

Treatment considerations in patients with AF and concomitant renal impairment center around rate versus rhythm control and stroke prophylaxis. With regards to rate versus rhythm control strategies, data are limited with regards to the optimal approach in patients with CKD. Existing studies do not support an advantage of a rhythm control strategy and AF recurrence is more common among those with CKD following catheter ablation. Given the lack of clear evidence favoring either a rate or rhythm control approach, pharmacokinetic considerations and patient specific factors such as concurrent comorbidities, degree of renal dysfunction, and symptoms inform decision-making.[132,133]

Antithrombotic management among patients with CKD and concomitant AF is challenging given the dual risks for both ischemic events related to AF and bleeding risk associated with renal dysfunction. A systematic review of randomized trials comparing direct oral anticoagulants (DOACs) with warfarin comprising predominantly Stage 3 CKD participants (n = 12,545) found that DOACs reduced stroke or systemic embolism by 19% (risk ratio [RR] 0.81; 95% CI, 0.65–1.00) and intracranial hemorrhage by 57% (RR 0.43; 95% CI, 0.27–0.69; **Fig. 75–4**).[134] Rates of ischemic stroke and all-cause mortality were nonsignificantly different between groups. These results suggest DOACs demonstrate enhanced safety with comparable efficacy in at least moderate CKD, consistent with results in non-CKD patients.

Comparative data evaluating DOACs in the setting of ESRD are limited as these patients were excluded from pivotal trials leading to regulatory approval of these drugs. Off-label use of rivaroxaban and dabigatran in the setting of dialysis was associated with higher risks for major bleeding and death as compared with warfarin.[135] In contrast, results from an observational cohort of Medicare beneficiaries with ESRD and AF (n = 25,523) found that apixaban use was associated with lower risks for major bleeding as compared with warfarin while risks for stroke or systemic embolism were comparable.[136] Variable results across studies may reflect differences in the pharmacokinetic profile between agents because apixaban is the least renally cleared of the commercially available DOACs. Guidelines recommend DOACs at a reduced dose among those with nondialysis-dependent CKD and AF with an elevated risk for stroke while warfarin or apixaban is recommended in the setting of dialysis.[137]

CONTRAST-INDUCED ACUTE KIDNEY INJURY

Epidemiology

Contrast-induced acute kidney injury (CI-AKI) is defined by the Kidney Disease Improving Global Outcomes (KDIGO) working group as an increase in SCr of at least 0.3 mg/dL within 48 hours, or a 1.5-fold relative increase in SCr within 7 days after administration of intravascular contrast media, or a decrease in urine output to less than 0.5 mL/kg/hour for 6 hours after receipt of intravascular contrast media.[138] Other widely used criteria for AKI are shown in **Table 75–4**. The most common definition used in clinical trials is an increase in SCr of 0.5 mg/dL, or a 25% increase from the baseline value within 48 hours after contrast exposure. It should be noted that the terms "contrast-associated acute kidney injury" and "post-contrast acute kidney injury" are gaining favor due to difficulty in definitively ruling out alternative etiologies that may result in AKI concomitant with contrast exposure, such as atheroemboli or hemodynamic instability.[139]

The overall incidence of CI-AKI after contrast media exposure varies considerably based on patient population being studied, baseline risk factors and on the definition of AKI being used. Results from large cohorts undergoing coronary

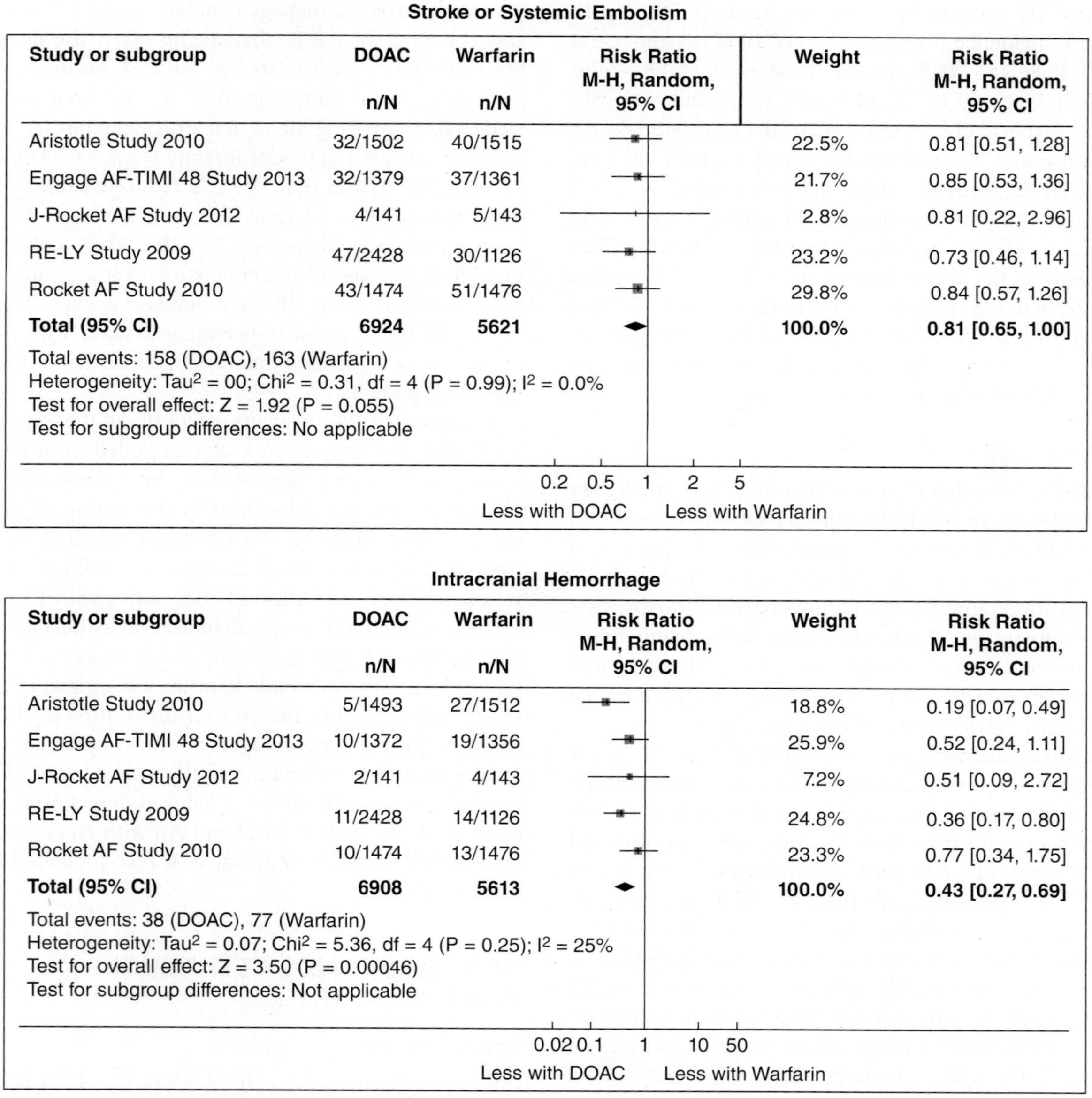

Stroke or Systemic Embolism

Study or subgroup	DOAC n/N	Warfarin n/N	Risk Ratio M-H, Random, 95% CI	Weight	Risk Ratio M-H, Random, 95% CI
Aristotle Study 2010	32/1502	40/1515		22.5%	0.81 [0.51, 1.28]
Engage AF-TIMI 48 Study 2013	32/1379	37/1361		21.7%	0.85 [0.53, 1.36]
J-Rocket AF Study 2012	4/141	5/143		2.8%	0.81 [0.22, 2.96]
RE-LY Study 2009	47/2428	30/1126		23.2%	0.73 [0.46, 1.14]
Rocket AF Study 2010	43/1474	51/1476		29.8%	0.84 [0.57, 1.26]
Total (95% CI)	**6924**	**5621**		**100.0%**	**0.81 [0.65, 1.00]**

Total events: 158 (DOAC), 163 (Warfarin)
Heterogeneity: Tau^2 = 00; Chi^2 = 0.31, df = 4 (P = 0.99); I^2 = 0.0%
Test for overall effect: Z = 1.92 (P = 0.055)
Test for subgroup differences: No applicable

0.2 0.5 1 2 5
Less with DOAC Less with Warfarin

Intracranial Hemorrhage

Study or subgroup	DOAC n/N	Warfarin n/N	Risk Ratio M-H, Random, 95% CI	Weight	Risk Ratio M-H, Random, 95% CI
Aristotle Study 2010	5/1493	27/1512		18.8%	0.19 [0.07, 0.49]
Engage AF-TIMI 48 Study 2013	10/1372	19/1356		25.9%	0.52 [0.24, 1.11]
J-Rocket AF Study 2012	2/141	4/143		7.2%	0.51 [0.09, 2.72]
RE-LY Study 2009	11/2428	14/1126		24.8%	0.36 [0.17, 0.80]
Rocket AF Study 2010	10/1474	13/1476		23.3%	0.77 [0.34, 1.75]
Total (95% CI)	**6908**	**5613**		**100.0%**	**0.43 [0.27, 0.69]**

Total events: 38 (DOAC), 77 (Warfarin)
Heterogeneity: Tau^2 = 0.07; Chi^2 = 5.36, df = 4 (P = 0.25); I^2 = 25%
Test for overall effect: Z = 3.50 (P = 0.00046)
Test for subgroup differences: Not applicable

0.02 0.1 1 10 50
Less with DOAC Less with Warfarin

Figure 75–4. Forest plots depicting risk ratios for stroke or systemic embolism and intracranial hemorrhage associated with direct oral anticoagulant (DOACs) versus warfarin use among patients with chronic kidney disease (CKD) enrolled in randomized trials. *Blue squares* represent point estimates and lines 95% confidence interval (CI). Reproduced with permission from Kimachi M, Furukawa TA, Kimachi K, et al. Direct oral anticoagulants versus warfarin for preventing stroke and systemic embolic events among atrial fibrillation patients with chronic kidney disease. *Cochrane Database Syst Rev.* 2017 Nov 6;11(11):CD011373.

angiography with or without intervention and utilizing similar AKI definitions to one another (KDIGO and/or Acute Kidney Injury Network [AKIN]), report an incidence of AKI post procedure of 7.1% to 13.9%.[140-142]

CI-AKI is strongly associated with an increased risk for both cardiovascular and renal adverse events. In a large retrospective analysis of patients undergoing PCI in the United States, in-hospital mortality rates were 0.5%, 9.7%, and 34% among those not developing AKI, with AKI and AKI requiring dialysis, respectively.[142] Similar patterns of risk were observed for other in-hospital complications, including bleeding and MI. The adverse prognosis associated with CI-AKI also is also durable over time. Among participants in a randomized trial undergoing PCI, postprocedure AKI was associated with

an approximate 2.4-fold higher risk for death and MI over 5 years.[143] Progression to ESRD may occur following an episode of CI-AKI, with risk increasing in a graded fashion with more acute renal injury. Among patients undergoing coronary angiography (n = 14,782; 55% PCI), rates of progression to ESRD over the ensuing 20 months (per 100 person-years) were 0.1, 1.6, and 11.5 among those without AKI, Stage 1, and Stage 2/3 AKI, respectively.[141] Associations remained significant after multivariable adjustment, highlighting the long-term adverse renal prognosis associated with CI-AKI. Underlying renal impairment is the strongest determinant of CI-AKI. Other risk factors include HF, advanced age, DM, hemodynamic instability, acuity of presentation, contrast media volume, and use of an intra-aortic balloon pump.[142,144]

TABLE 75-4. Classification of Acute Kidney Injury

RIFLE: Risk, Injury, and Heart Failure, Loss, and End-Stage Kidney Disease[158]

Stage	Assessments	
	Serum Creatinine Concentration/GFR	Urine Output
Risk	1.5-2.0 × baseline; or >25% reduction in GFR	<0.5 mL/kg/h for <6 h
Injury	2.0-3.0 × baseline; or >50% reduction in GFR	<0.5 mL/kg/h for >12 h
Failure	≥3.0 × baseline; or ≥4.0 mg/dL with an acute rise ≥0.5 mg/dL; or >75% reduction in GFR	<0.3 mL/kg/h for ≥24 h (oliguria); or anuria for ≥12 h

KDIGO

Stage	Assessments	
	Serum Creatinine Concentration	Urine Output
1	1.5-1.9 × baseline or ≥0.3 mg/dL	<0.5 mL/kg/h for 6-12 h
2	2.0-2.9 × baseline	<0.5 mL/kg/h for ≥24 h
3	≥3.0 × baseline, ≥4.0 mg/dL, or initiation of RRT	<0.3 mL/kg/h for ≥24 h or anuria for ≥12 h

AKIN

Stage	Assessments	
1	1.5-1.9 × baseline or ≥0.3 mg/dL within 48 h	<0.5 mL/kg/h for <6 h
2	2.0-2.9 × baseline	<0.5 mL/kg/h for >12 h
3	≥3.0 × baseline or baseline ≥4.0 mg/dL with increase ≥0.5 mg/dL	<0.3 mL/kg/h for ≥24 h (oliguria); or anuria for ≥12 h; or need for RRT

Abbreviations: AKIN, Acute Kidney Injury Network; GFR, glomerular filtration rate; KDIGO, Kidney Disease Improving Global Outcomes; RRT, renal replacement therapy.

Pathophysiology

The pathophysiology of CI-AKI remains incompletely understood, although putative mechanisms include direct cytotoxic effects of contrast media and altered renal perfusion.[139,145-147] Iodinated contrast modulates renal vasomotor tone leading to a decrease in renal blood flow and medullary hypoxia.[146,148,149] Renal vasoconstriction is mediated by alterations in the activity of vasoactive substances including nitric oxide, endothelin, and possibly adenosine.[145,148-151]

Radiocontrast media also exerts direct cytotoxic effects on renal tubular cells.[146,152] Elevated levels of tubular enzymes and proteins that are normally reabsorbed are found in urine after exposure to contrast media providing support to a cytotoxic mechanism.[152] Sloughing of cellular debris in the tubular space leads to contrast media stasis, further potentiating cellular toxicity as clearance of contrast media is impaired.[146] Generation of reactive oxygen species in the setting of intense vasoconstriction and cytotoxicity may also play a role in the pathophysiology of CI-AKI.[148-150] Specifically, free radicals may reduce the bioavailability of nitric oxide, impairing renal vasodilatory mechanisms.[148,150]

Management

The initial step in mitigating risk for CI-AKI is to identify at-risk patients. This may be achieved by calculating creatinine clearance or eGFR in all patients prior to coronary angiography or using established scoring systems. Beyond risk stratification, guidelines recommend use of intravascular hydration, minimizing the amount of contrast media exposure, use of low-osmolar or iso-osmolar contrast media, and consideration of high-dose statins.[153]

Although intravascular volume expansion appears beneficial in the prevention of CI-AKI, data regarding the ideal volume, type and route of administration remain limited. In the randomized POSEIDON (Prevention of Contrast Renal Injury with Different Hydration Strategies) trial, intravascular volume administration using normal saline and guided by left ventricular end-diastolic pressure was compared to a standard fluid administration protocol (1.5 mL/kg/hr) among 396 patients undergoing cardiac catheterization. The primary endpoint of CI-AKI was significantly lower in the guided versus conventional group (6.7% vs 16.3%; $P = 0.005$).[154] Pre- and postprocedure hydration, using a fixed or tailored approach, is a consistent recommendation for prevention of CI-AKI.[154,155]

Early administration of high-dose statins may also lower risk for CI-AKI. In a modest-sized randomized trial, the effect of rosuvastatin 40 mg given on admission followed by 20 mg daily was compared to no statin use among statin-naïve patients presenting with ACS undergoing an invasive strategy. The incidence of CI-AKI was significantly lower in the statin group (6.7% vs 15.1%; $P = 0.003$).[156] Recommendations from the European Society of Cardiology state it would be reasonable to consider starting a high dose statin to reduce the incidence of CI-AKI.[153]

Contrast media selection as well as volume administered influences CI-AKI risk. Low or iso-osmolar contrast media are preferred due to a lower risk for CI-AKI and a more favorable side effect profile. With respect to contrast media volume, calculating the contrast volume to calculated creatinine clearance (CV/CCC) ratio serves as useful metric that relates to CI-AKI risk and provides an "upper limit" for the amount of contrast volume that may be delivered without renal injury. Specifically, values that exceed 3 are associated with a marked increase in the risk for CI-AKI while values below 2 appear safe.[157] Avoiding nephrotoxic drugs and close monitoring of SCr levels postprocedurally are additional considerations in the management of patients with or at risk for CI-AKI (**Table 75–5**).

TABLE 75-5. Strategies to Reduce the Risk of Contrast-Induced Acute Kidney Injury

Assess the CI-AKI

Assess the need for contrast-enhancement, avoid unnecessary contrast administration

Avoid concomitant use of other nephrotoxic drugs

Hydrate the patient with isotonic saline and/or sodium bicarbonate before and after the procedure

N-acetyl-cysteine 1200 mg orally twice daily

Prefer iso-osmolal or hypo-osmolal contrast media

Use minimum amount of contrast media

REFERENCES

1. Levin A, Stevens PE, Bilous RW, et al. Kidney disease: Improving global outcomes (KDIGO) CKD work group. KDIGO 2012 clinical practice guideline for the evaluation and management of chronic kidney disease. *Kidney Int Suppl.* 2013;3:1-150.

2. Levey AS, Stevens LA. Estimating GFR using the CKD Epidemiology Collaboration (CKD-EPI) creatinine equation: more accurate GFR estimates, lower CKD prevalence estimates, and better risk predictions. *Am J Kidney Dis.* 2010;55:622-627.

3. Levey AS, Stevens LA, Schmid CH, et al. A new equation to estimate glomerular filtration rate. *Ann Intern Med.* 2009;150:604-612.

4. Chronic Kidney Disease Initiative. CDC. 2021. https://www.cdc.gov/kidneydisease/publications-resources/CKD-national-facts.html

5. Bikbov B, Purcell CA, Levey AS, et al. Global, regional, and national burden of chronic kidney disease, 1990-2013;2017: a systematic analysis for the Global Burden of Disease Study 2017. *Lancet.* 2020;395:709-733.

6. Chronic Kidney Disease Initiative: resources. CDC. 2021. https://www.cdc.gov/kidneydisease/pdf/CKD-common-serious-costly-h.pdf.

7. Lindner A, Charra B, Sherrard DJ, Scribner BH. Accelerated atherosclerosis in prolonged maintenance hemodialysis. *N Engl J Med.* 1974;290:697-701.

8. Nakano T, Ninomiya T, Sumiyoshi S, et al. Association of kidney function with coronary atherosclerosis and calcification in autopsy samples from Japanese elders: the Hisayama Study. *Am J Kidney Dis.* 2010;55:21-30.

9. Sarnak MJ, Amann K, Bangalore S, et al. Chronic kidney disease and coronary artery disease: JACC State-of-the-Art Review. *J Am Coll Cardiol.* 2019;74:1823-1838.

10. Ohtake T, Kobayashi S, Moriya H, et al. High prevalence of occult coronary artery stenosis in patients with chronic kidney disease at the initiation of renal replacement therapy: an angiographic examination. *J Am Soc Nephrol.* 2005;16:1141-1148.

11. Manjunath G, Tighiouart H, Ibrahim H, et al. Level of kidney function as a risk factor for atherosclerotic cardiovascular outcomes in the community. *J Am Coll Cardiol.* 2003;41:47-55.

12. Baber U, Gutierrez OM, Levitan EB, et al. Risk for recurrent coronary heart disease and all-cause mortality among individuals with chronic kidney disease compared with diabetes mellitus, metabolic syndrome, and cigarette smokers. *Am Heart J.* 2013;166:373-380.e2.

13. Go AS, Chertow GM, Fan D, McCulloch CE, Hsu C-y. Chronic kidney disease and the risks of death, cardiovascular events, and hospitalization. *N Eng J Med.* 2004;351:1296-1305.

14. Association of estimated glomerular filtration rate and albuminuria with all-cause and cardiovascular mortality in general population cohorts: a collaborative meta-analysis. *Lancet.* 2010;375:2073-2081.

15. Baber U, Chandrasekhar J, Sartori S, et al. Associations between chronic kidney disease and outcomes with use of prasugrel versus clopidogrel in patients with acute coronary syndrome undergoing percutaneous coronary intervention: a report from the PROMETHEUS Study. *JACC Cardiovasc Interv.* 2017;10:2017-2025.

16. Washam JB, Herzog CA, Beitelshees AL, et al. Pharmacotherapy in chronic kidney disease patients presenting with acute coronary syndrome: a scientific statement from the American Heart Association. *Circulation.* 2015;131:1123-1149.

17. Sahlén A, Varenhorst C, Lagerqvist B, et al. Contemporary use of ticagrelor in patients with acute coronary syndrome: insights from Swedish Web System for Enhancement and Development of Evidence-Based Care in Heart Disease Evaluated According to Recommended Therapies (SWE-DEHEART). *Eur Heart J: Cardiovasc Pharmacother.* 2015;2:5-12.

18. Gansevoort RT, Correa-Rotter R, Hemmelgarn BR, et al. Chronic kidney disease and cardiovascular risk: epidemiology, mechanisms, and prevention. *Lancet.* 2013;382:339-352.

19. Valdivielso JM, Rodríguez-Puyol D, Pascual J, et al. Atherosclerosis in chronic kidney disease. *Arterioscler Thromb Vasc Biol.* 2019;39:1938-1966.

20. Schiffrin EL, Lipman ML, Mann JFE. Chronic kidney disease. *Circulation.* 2007;116:85-97.

21. Stam F, van Guldener C, Becker A, et al. Endothelial dysfunction contributes to renal function–associated cardiovascular mortality in a population with mild renal insufficiency: the Hoorn Study. *J Am Soc Nephrol.* 2006;17:537-545.

22. Kaur J, Young BE, Fadel PJ. Sympathetic overactivity in chronic kidney disease: consequences and mechanisms. *Int J Mol Sci.* 2017;18:1682.

23. Förstermann U, Xia N, Li H. Roles of vascular oxidative stress and nitric oxide in the pathogenesis of atherosclerosis. *Circulation Res.* 2017;120:713-735.

24. Kielstein JT, Böger RH, Bode-Böger SM, et al. Marked increase of asymmetric dimethylarginine in patients with incipient primary chronic renal disease. *J Am Soc Nephrol.* 2002;13:170-176.

25. Rosenson RS, Brewer HB, Ansell BJ, et al. Dysfunctional HDL and atherosclerotic cardiovascular disease. *Nature Rev Cardiol.* 2016;13:48-60.

26. Kestenbaum BR, Adeney KL, de Boer IH, Ix JH, Shlipak MG, Siscovick DS. Incidence and progression of coronary calcification in chronic kidney disease: the Multi-Ethnic Study of Atherosclerosis. *Kidney Int.* 2009;76:991-998.

27. London GM, Guérin AP, Marchais SJ, Métivier F, Pannier B, Adda H. Arterial media calcification in end-stage renal disease: impact on all-cause and cardiovascular mortality. *Nephrol Dialysis Transplant.* 2003;18:1731-1740.

28. Reiss AB, Miyawaki N, Moon J, et al. CKD, arterial calcification, atherosclerosis and bone health: inter-relationships and controversies. *Atherosclerosis.* 2018;278:49-59.

29. Miyagi M, Ishii H, Murakami R, et al. Impact of renal function on coronary plaque composition. *Nephrol Dialysis Transplant.* 2009;25:175-181.

30. Baber U, Stone GW, Weisz G, et al. Coronary plaque composition, morphology, and outcomes in patients with and without chronic kidney disease presenting with acute coronary syndromes. *JACC: Cardiovasc Imaging.* 2012;5:S53-S61.

31. Kato K, Yonetsu T, Jia H, et al. Nonculprit coronary plaque characteristics of chronic kidney disease. *Circulation: Cardiovasc Imaging.* 2013;6:448-456.

32. Go AS, Bansal N, Chandra M, et al. Chronic kidney disease and risk for presenting with acute myocardial infarction versus stable exertional angina in adults with coronary heart disease. *J Am Coll Cardiol.* 2011;58:1600-1607.

33. Herzog CA, Natwick T, Li S, Charytan DM. Comparative utilization and temporal trends in cardiac stress testing in U.S. medicare beneficiaries with and without chronic kidney disease. *JACC Cardiovasc Imaging.* 2019;12:1420-1426.

34. Winther S, Svensson M, Jørgensen HS, et al. Diagnostic performance of coronary CT angiography and myocardial perfusion imaging in kidney transplantation candidates. *JACC: Cardiovasc Imaging.* 2015;8:553-562.

35. Lipid management in chronic kidney disease: synopsis of the kidney disease: Improving Global Outcomes 2013 Clinical Practice Guideline. *Ann Intern Med.* 2014;160:182-189.

36. Grundy SM, Stone NJ, Bailey AL, et al. 2018 AHA/ACC/AACVPR/AAPA/ABC/ACPM/ADA/AGS/APhA/ASPC/NLA/PCNA guideline on the management of blood cholesterol. A report of the American College of Cardiology/American Heart Association Task Force on Clinical Practice Guidelines. *Circulation.* 2019;73:e285-e350.

37. Baigent C, Landray MJ, Reith C, et al. The effects of lowering LDL cholesterol with simvastatin plus ezetimibe in patients with chronic kidney disease (study of heart and renal protection): a randomised placebo-controlled trial. *Lancet.* 2011;377:2181-2192.

38. Cholesterol Treatment Trialists C, Herrington WG, Emberson J, et al. Impact of renal function on the effects of LDL cholesterol lowering with statin-based regimens: a meta-analysis of individual participant data from 28 randomised trials. *Lancet Diabetes Endocrinol.* 2016;4:829-839.

39. Wanner C, Krane V, März W, et al. Atorvastatin in patients with type 2 diabetes mellitus undergoing hemodialysis. *N Eng J Med.* 2005;353:238-248.

40. Fellström BC, Jardine AG, Schmieder RE, et al. Rosuvastatin and cardiovascular events in patients undergoing hemodialysis. *N Eng J Med.* 2009;360:1395-1407.

41. Levine GN, Bates ER, Bittl JA, et al. 2016 ACC/AHA guideline focused update on duration of dual antiplatelet therapy in patients with coronary artery disease. a report of the American College of Cardiology/American Heart Association Task Force on Clinical Practice Guidelines. *Circulation* 2016;68:1082-1115.

42. Bonaca MP, Bhatt DL, Cohen M, et al. Long-term use of ticagrelor in patients with prior myocardial infarction. *N Eng J Med.* 2015;372:1791-1800.

43. Kereiakes DJ, Yeh RW, Massaro JM, et al. DAPT score utility for risk prediction in patients with or without previous myocardial infarction. *J Am Coll Cardiol.* 2016;67:2492-2502.

44. Baber U, Li SX, Pinnelas R, et al. Incidence, patterns, and impact of dual antiplatelet therapy cessation among patients with and without chronic kidney disease undergoing percutaneous coronary intervention. *Circu Cardiovasc Interv.* 2018;11:e006144.

45. Baber U, Mehran R, Kirtane AJ, et al. Prevalence and impact of high platelet reactivity in chronic kidney disease: results from the Assessment of Dual Antiplatelet Therapy with Drug-Eluting Stents registry. *Circ Cardiovasc Interv.* 2015;8:e001683.

46. Best PJM, Steinhubl SR, Berger PB, et al. The efficacy and safety of short- and long-term dual antiplatelet therapy in patients with mild or moderate chronic kidney disease: Results from the Clopidogrel for the Reduction of Events During Observation (CREDO) Trial. *Am Heart J.* 2008;155:687-693.

47. Keltai M, Tonelli M, Mann JF, et al. Renal function and outcomes in acute coronary syndrome: impact of clopidogrel. *Eur J Cardiovasc Prev Rehabil.* 2007;14:312-318.

48. Wallentin L, Becker RC, Budaj A, et al. Ticagrelor versus clopidogrel in patients with acute coronary syndromes. *N Eng J Med.* 2009;361:1045-1057.

49. James S, Budaj A, Aylward P, et al. Ticagrelor versus clopidogrel in acute coronary syndromes in relation to renal function. *Circulation* 2010;122:1056-1067.

50. Magnani G, Storey RF, Steg G, et al. Efficacy and safety of ticagrelor for long-term secondary prevention of atherothrombotic events in relation to renal function: insights from the PEGASUS-TIMI 54 trial. *Eur Heart J.* 2015;37:400-408.

51. Weintraub WS, Spertus JA, Kolm P, et al. Effect of PCI on quality of life in patients with stable coronary disease. *N Engl J Med.* 2008;359:677-687.

52. Spertus JA, Jones PG, Maron DJ, et al. Health-status outcomes with invasive or conservative care in coronary disease. *N Eng J Med.* 2020;382:1408-1419.

53. Bangalore S, Guo Y, Samadashvili Z, Blecker S, Xu J, Hannan EL. Revascularization in patients with multivessel coronary artery disease and chronic kidney disease: everolimus-eluting stents versus coronary artery bypass graft surgery. *J Am Coll Cardiol.* 2015;66:1209-1220.

54. Baber U, Farkouh ME, Arbel Y, et al. Comparative efficacy of coronary artery bypass surgery vs. percutaneous coronary intervention in patients with diabetes and multivessel coronary artery disease with or without chronic kidney disease. *Eur Heart J.* 2016;37:3440-3447.

55. Bangalore S, Maron DJ, O'Brien SM, et al. Management of coronary disease in patients with advanced kidney disease. *N Eng J Med.* 2020;382:1608-1618.

56. Kottgen A, Russell SD, Loehr LR, et al. Reduced kidney function as a risk factor for incident heart failure: the Atherosclerosis Risk in Communities (ARIC) Study. *J Am Soc Nephrol.* 2007;18:1307-1315.

57. Bansal N, Zelnick L, Bhat Z, et al. Burden and outcomes of heart failure hospitalizations in adults with chronic kidney disease. *J Am Coll Cardiol.* 2019;73:2691-2700.

58. Rangaswami J, Bhalla V, Blair JEA, et al. Cardiorenal syndrome: classification, pathophysiology, diagnosis, and treatment strategies: a scientific statement from the American Heart Association. *Circulation.* 2019;139:e840-e878.

59. Nohria A, Hasselblad V, Stebbins A, et al. Cardiorenal interactions: insights from the ESCAPE Trial. *J Am Coll Cardiol.* 2008;51:1268-1274.

60. Mullens W, Abrahams Z, Francis GS, et al. Importance of venous congestion for worsening of renal function in advanced decompensated heart failure. *J Am Coll Cardiol.* 2009;53:589-596.

61. Rahman SN, Abraham WT, Van Putten VJ, Hasbargen JA, Schrier RW. Increased norepinephrine secretion in patients with the nephrotic syndrome and normal glomerular filtration rates: evidence for primary sympathetic activation. *Am J Nephrol.* 1993;13:266-270.

62. Cerasola G, Vecchi M, Mulè G, et al. Sympathetic activity and blood pressure pattern in autosomal dominant polycystic kidney disease hypertensives. *Am J Nephrol.* 1998;18:391-398.

63. Johansson M, Elam M, Rundqvist B, et al. Increased sympathetic nerve activity in renovascular hypertension. *Circulation.* 1999;99:2537-2542.

64. Zoccali C, Mallamaci F, Parlongo S, et al. Plasma norepinephrine predicts survival and incident cardiovascular events in patients with end-stage renal disease. *Circulation.* 2002;105:1354-1359.

65. Hausberg M, Kosch M, Harmelink P, et al. Sympathetic nerve activity in end-stage renal disease. *Circulation.* 2002;106:1974-1979.

66. von Haehling S, Schefold JC, Lainscak M, Doehner W, Anker SD. Inflammatory biomarkers in heart failure revisited: much more than innocent bystanders. *Heart Fail Clin.* 2009;5:549-560.

67. Colombo PC, Ganda A, Lin J, et al. Inflammatory activation: cardiac, renal, and cardio-renal interactions in patients with the cardiorenal syndrome. *Heart Fail Rev.* 2012;17:177-190.

68. Schefold JC, Zeden J-P, Fotopoulou C, et al. Increased indoleamine 2,3-dioxygenase (IDO) activity and elevated serum levels of tryptophan catabolites in patients with chronic kidney disease: a possible link between chronic inflammation and uraemic symptoms. *Nephrol Dialysis Transplant.* 2009;24:1901-1908.

69. Levin A, Thompson CR, Ethier J, et al. Left ventricular mass index increase in early renal disease: Impact of decline in hemoglobin. *Am J Kidney Dis.* 1999;34:125-134.

70. Calvillo L, Latini R, Kajstura J, et al. Recombinant human erythropoietin protects the myocardium from ischemia-reperfusion injury and promotes beneficial remodeling. *Proc National Academy of Sciences.* 2003;100:4802-4806.

71. Young JB, Abraham WT, Albert NM, et al. Relation of low hemoglobin and anemia to morbidity and mortality in patients hospitalized with heart failure (insight from the OPTIMIZE-HF registry). *Am J Cardiol.* 2008;101:223-230.

72. van der Meer P, Groenveld HF, Januzzi JL, van Veldhuisen DJ. Erythropoietin treatment in patients with chronic heart failure: a meta-analysis. *Heart* 2009;95:1309-1314.

73. Achinger SG, Ayus JC. Left ventricular hypertrophy: is hyperphosphatemia among dialysis patients a risk factor? *J Am Soc Nephrol.* 2006;17:S255-S261.

74. Scialla JJ, Xie H, Rahman M, et al. Fibroblast growth factor-23 and cardiovascular events in CKD. *J Am Soc Nephrol.* 2014;25:349-360.

75. Yancy CW, Jessup M, Bozkurt B, et al. 2017 ACC/AHA/HFSA Focused Update of the 2013 ACCF/AHA guideline for the management of heart failure: a report of the American College of Cardiology/American Heart Association Task Force on Clinical Practice Guidelines and the Heart Failure Society of America. *J Am Coll Cardiol.* 2017;70:776-803.

76. Mullens W, Damman K, Harjola VP, et al. The use of diuretics in heart failure with congestion - a position statement from the Heart Failure Association of the European Society of Cardiology. *Eur J Heart Fail.* 2019;21:137-155.

77. Felker GM, Lee KL, Bull DA, et al. Diuretic strategies in patients with acute decompensated heart failure. *N Eng J Med.* 2011;364:797-805.

78. Palazzuoli A, Pellegrini M, Ruocco G, et al. Continuous versus bolus intermittent loop diuretic infusion in acutely decompensated heart failure: a prospective randomized trial. *Critical Care.* 2014;18:R134.

79. Grodin JL, Stevens SR, de las Fuentes L, et al. Intensification of medication therapy for cardiorenal syndrome in acute decompensated heart failure. *J Cardiac Fail*. 2016;22:26-32.

80. Costanzo MR, Guglin ME, Saltzberg MT, et al. Ultrafiltration versus intravenous diuretics for patients hospitalized for acute decompensated heart failure. *J Am Coll Cardiol*. 2007;49:675-683.

81. Bart BA, Goldsmith SR, Lee KL, et al. Ultrafiltration in decompensated heart failure with cardiorenal syndrome. *N Eng J Med*. 2012;367:2296-2304.

82. Bowling CB, Sanders PW, Allman RM, et al. Effects of enalapril in systolic heart failure patients with and without chronic kidney disease: insights from the SOLVD Treatment trial. *Int J Cardiol*. 2013;167:151-156.

83. Ahmed A, Love TE, Sui X, Rich MW. Effects of angiotensin-converting enzyme inhibitors in systolic heart failure patients with chronic kidney disease: a propensity score analysis. *J Cardiac Fail*. 2006;12:499-506.

84. Edner M, Benson L, Dahlström U, Lund LH. Association between renin–angiotensin system antagonist use and mortality in heart failure with severe renal insufficiency: a prospective propensity score-matched cohort study. *Eur Heart J*. 2015;36:2318-2326.

85. Ahmed A, Rich MW, Zile M, et al. Renin-angiotensin inhibition in diastolic heart failure and chronic kidney disease. *Am J Med*. 2013;126:150-161.

86. Berger AK, Duval S, Manske C, et al. Angiotensin-converting enzyme inhibitors and angiotensin receptor blockers in patients with congestive heart failure and chronic kidney disease. *Am Heart J*. 2007;153:1064-1073.

87. Yancy CW, Jessup M, Bozkurt B, et al. 2013 ACCF/AHA guideline for the management of heart failure: a report of the American College of Cardiology Foundation/American Heart Association Task Force on Practice Guidelines. *J Am Coll Cardiol*. 2013;62:e147-e239.

88. Solomon SD, Claggett B, McMurray JJV, Hernandez AF, Fonarow GC. Combined neprilysin and renin-angiotensin system inhibition in heart failure with reduced ejection fraction: a meta-analysis. *Eur J Heart Fail*. 2016;18:1238-1243.

89. Damman K, Gori M, Claggett B, et al. Renal effects and associated outcomes during angiotensin-neprilysin inhibition in heart failure. *JACC: Heart Fail*. 2018;6:489-498.

90. Pitt B, Remme W, Zannad F, et al. Eplerenone, a selective aldosterone blocker, in patients with left ventricular dysfunction after myocardial infarction. *N Eng J Med*. 2003;348:1309-1321.

91. Zannad F, McMurray JJV, Krum H, et al. Eplerenone in patients with systolic heart failure and mild symptoms. *N Eng J Med*. 2010;364:11-21.

92. Pitt B, Zannad F, Remme WJ, et al. The effect of spironolactone on morbidity and mortality in patients with severe heart failure. *N Eng J Med*. 1999;341:709-717.

93. Eschalier R, McMurray JJV, Swedberg K, et al. Safety and efficacy of eplerenone in patients at high risk for hyperkalemia and/or worsening renal function: analyses of the EMPHASIS-HF Study Subgroups (Eplerenone in Mild Patients Hospitalization And SurvIval Study in Heart Failure). *J Am Coll Cardiol*. 2013;62:1585-1593.

94. Ponikowski P, Voors AA, Anker SD, et al. 2016 ESC Guidelines for the diagnosis and treatment of acute and chronic heart failure: the Task Force for the diagnosis and treatment of acute and chronic heart failure of the European Society of Cardiology (ESC)Developed with the special contribution of the Heart Failure Association (HFA) of the ESC. *Eur Heart J*. 2016;37:2129-2200.

95. Ghali JK, Wikstrand J, Van Veldhuisen DJ, et al. The influence of renal function on clinical outcome and response to β-blockade in systolic heart failure: insights from Metoprolol CR/XL Randomized Intervention Trial in Chronic HF (MERIT-HF). *J Cardiac Fail*. 2009;15:310-318.

96. Badve SV, Roberts MA, Hawley CM, et al. Effects of beta-adrenergic antagonists in patients with chronic kidney disease: a systematic review and meta-analysis. *J Am Coll Cardiol*. 2011;58:1152-1161.

97. Castagno D, Jhund PS, McMurray JJV, et al. Improved survival with bisoprolol in patients with heart failure and renal impairment: an analysis of the cardiac insufficiency bisoprolol study II (CIBIS-II) trial. *Eur J Heart Fail*. 2010;12:607-616.

98. Pun PH, Al-Khatib SM, Han JY, et al. Implantable cardioverter-defibrillators for primary prevention of sudden cardiac death in CKD: a meta-analysis of patient-level data from 3 randomized trials. *Am J Kidney Dis*. 2014; 64:32-39.

99. Jukema JW, Timal RJ, Rotmans JI, et al. Prophylactic use of implantable cardioverter-defibrillators in the prevention of sudden cardiac death in dialysis patients. *Circulation*. 2019;139:2628-2638.

100. Pun PH, Hellkamp AS, Sanders GD, et al. Primary prevention implantable cardioverter defibrillators in end-stage kidney disease patients on dialysis: a matched cohort study. *Nephrol Dialysis Transplant*. 2014;30:829-835.

101. Samad Z, Sivak JA, Phelan M, Schulte PJ, Patel U, Velazquez EJ. Prevalence and outcomes of left-sided valvular heart disease associated with chronic kidney disease. *J Am Heart Assoc*. 2017;6.

102. Vavilis G, Bäck M, Occhino G, et al. Kidney dysfunction and the risk of developing aortic stenosis. *J Am Coll Cardiol*. 2019;73:305-314.

103. Marwick TH, Amann K, Bangalore S, et al. Chronic kidney disease and valvular heart disease: conclusions from a Kidney Disease: Improving Global Outcomes (KDIGO) Controversies Conference. *Kidney Int*. 2019;96:836-849.

104. Otto CM, Kuusisto J, Reichenbach DD, Gown AM, O'Brien KD. Characterization of the early lesion of "degenerative" valvular aortic stenosis. Histological and immunohistochemical studies. *Circulation*. 1994;90:844-853.

105. Mohananey D, Griffin BP, Svensson LG, et al. Comparative outcomes of patients with advanced renal dysfunction undergoing transcatheter aortic valve replacement in the United States From 2011 to 2014. *Circ Cardiovasc Interv*. 2017;10.

106. Patel KK, Shah SY, Arrigain S, et al. Characteristics and outcomes of patients with aortic stenosis and chronic kidney disease. *J Am Heart Assoc*. 2019;8:e009980.

107. Vollema EM, Prihadi EA, Ng ACT, et al. Prognostic implications of renal dysfunction in patients with aortic stenosis. *Am J Cardiol*. 2020;125:1108-1114.

108. Kawase Y, Taniguchi T, Morimoto T, et al. Severe aortic stenosis in dialysis patients. *J Am Heart Assoc*. 2017;6:e004961.

109. Nishimura RA, Otto CM, Bonow RO, et al. 2017 AHA/ACC Focused Update of the 2014 AHA/ACC guideline for the management of patients with valvular heart disease: a report of the American College of Cardiology/ American Heart Association Task Force on Clinical Practice Guidelines. *Circulation*. 2017;135:e1159-e1195.

110. Pineda AM, Kevin Harrison J, Kleiman NS, et al. Clinical impact of baseline chronic kidney disease in patients undergoing transcatheter or surgical aortic valve replacement. *Catheterizat Cardiovasc Intervent*. 2019;93:740-748.

111. Smith CR, Leon MB, Mack MJ, et al. Transcatheter versus surgical aortic-valve replacement in high-risk patients. *N Eng J Med*. 2011;364:2187-2198.

112. Leon MB, Smith CR, Mack MJ, et al. Transcatheter or surgical aortic-valve replacement in intermediate-risk patients. *N Eng J Med*. 2016;374:1609-1620.

113. Mack MJ, Leon MB, Thourani VH, et al. Transcatheter aortic-valve replacement with a balloon-expandable valve in low-risk patients. *N Eng J Med*. 2019;380:1695-1705.

114. Doshi R, Shah J, Patel V, Jauhar V, Meraj P. Transcatheter or surgical aortic valve replacement in patients with advanced kidney disease: A propensity score–matched analysis. *Clin Cardiol*. 2017;40:1156-1162.

115. Allende R, Webb JG, Munoz-Garcia AJ, et al. Advanced chronic kidney disease in patients undergoing transcatheter aortic valve implantation: insights on clinical outcomes and prognostic markers from a large cohort of patients. *Eur Heart J*. 2014;35:2685-2696.

116. Soliman EZ, Prineas RJ, Go AS, et al. Chronic kidney disease and prevalent atrial fibrillation: the Chronic Renal Insufficiency Cohort (CRIC). *Am Heart J*. 2010;159:1102-1107.

117. Baber U, Howard VJ, Halperin JL, et al. Association of chronic kidney disease with atrial fibrillation among adults in the United States. *Circ Arrhythm Electrophysiol*. 2011;4:26-32.

118. Carrero JJ, Trevisan M, Sood MM, et al. Incident atrial fibrillation and the risk of stroke in adults with chronic kidney disease: the Stockholm CREAtinine Measurements (SCREAM) Project. *Clin J Am Soc Nephrol.* 2018;13:1314-1320.

119. Liao JN, Chao TF, Liu CJ, et al. Incidence and risk factors for new-onset atrial fibrillation among patients with end-stage renal disease undergoing renal replacement therapy. *Kidney Int.* 2015;87:1209-1215.

120. Ding WY, Gupta D, Wong CF, Lip GYH. Pathophysiology of atrial fibrillation and chronic kidney disease. *Cardiovasc Res.* 2020.

121. Ehrlich JR, Hohnloser SH, Nattel S. Role of angiotensin system and effects of its inhibition in atrial fibrillation: clinical and experimental evidence. *Eur Heart J.* 2005;27:512-518.

122. Iravanian S, Dudley SC. The renin-angiotensin-aldosterone system (RAAS) and cardiac arrhythmias. *Heart Rhythm.* 2008;5:S12-S17.

123. Tripepi G, Benedetto FA, Mallamaci F, Tripepi R, Malatino L, Zoccali C. Left atrial volume in end-stage renal disease: a prospective cohort study. *J Hypertension.* 2006;24:1173-1180.

124. Hee L, Nguyen T, Whatmough M, et al. Left atrial volume and adverse cardiovascular outcomes in unselected patients with and without CKD. *Clin J Am Soc Nephrol.* 2014;9:1369-1376.

125. Kalantar-Zadeh K, Regidor DL, Kovesdy CP, et al. Fluid retention is associated with cardiovascular mortality in patients undergoing long-term hemodialysis. *Circulation.* 2009;119:671-679.

126. Essig M, Escoubet B, de Zuttere D, et al. Cardiovascular remodelling and extracellular fluid excess in early stages of chronic kidney disease. *Nephrol Dialysis Transplant.* 2007;23:239-248.

127. Hung S-C, Kuo K-L, Peng C-H, et al. Volume overload correlates with cardiovascular risk factors in patients with chronic kidney disease. *Kidney Int.* 2014;85:703-709.

128. Hung SC, Kuo KL, Peng CH, Wu CH, Wang YC, Tarng DC. Association of fluid retention with anemia and clinical outcomes among patients with chronic kidney disease. *J Am Heart Assoc.* 2015;4:e001480.

129. Wu N, Xu B, Xiang Y, et al. Association of inflammatory factors with occurrence and recurrence of atrial fibrillation: a meta-analysis. *Int J Cardiol.* 2013;169:62-72.

130. Frustaci A, Chimenti C, Bellocci F, Morgante E, Russo MA, Maseri A. Histological substrate of atrial biopsies in patients with lone atrial fibrillation. *Circulation.* 1997;96:1180-1184.

131. Chung MK, Martin DO, Sprecher D, et al. C-reactive protein elevation in patients with atrial arrhythmias. *Circulation.* 2001;104:2886-2891.

132. Washam JB, Holmes DN, Thomas LE, et al. Pharmacotherapy for atrial fibrillation in patients with chronic kidney disease: insights from ORBIT-AF. *J Am Heart Assoc.* 2018;7:e008928.

133. Potpara TS, Lenarczyk R, Larsen TB, et al. Management of atrial fibrillation in patients with chronic kidney disease in Europe Results of the European Heart Rhythm Association Survey. *EP Europace.* 2016;17: 1862-1867.

134. Kimachi M, Furukawa TA, Kimachi K, Goto Y, Fukuma S, Fukuhara S. Direct oral anticoagulants versus warfarin for preventing stroke and systemic embolic events among atrial fibrillation patients with chronic kidney disease. *Cochrane Database Syst Rev.* 2017;11(11):CD011373.

135. Chan KE, Edelman ER, Wenger JB, Thadhani RI, Maddux FW. Dabigatran and rivaroxaban use in atrial fibrillation patients on hemodialysis. *Circulation.* 2015;131:972-979.

136. Siontis KC, Zhang X, Eckard A, et al. Outcomes associated with apixaban use in patients with end-stage kidney disease and atrial fibrillation in the United States. *Circulation.* 2018;138:1519-1529.

137. January CT, Wann LS, Calkins H, et al. 2019 AHA/ACC/HRS focused update of the 2014 aha/acc/hrs guideline for the management of patients with atrial fibrillation: a report of the American College of Cardiology/ American Heart Association Task Force on Clinical Practice Guidelines and the Heart Rhythm Society in Collaboration with the Society of Thoracic Surgeons. *Circulation.* 2019;140:e125-e151.

138. Khwaja A. KDIGO clinical practice guidelines for acute kidney injury. *Nephron Clin Prac.* 2012;120:c179-c184.

139. Mehran R, Dangas GD, Weisbord SD. Contrast-associated acute kidney injury. *N Eng J Med.* 2019;380:2146-2155.

140. Brown JR, MacKenzie TA, Maddox TM, et al. Acute kidney injury risk prediction in patients undergoing coronary angiography in a national veterans health administration cohort with external validation. *J Am Heart Assoc.* 2015;4:e002136.

141. James MT, Ghali WA, Knudtson ML, et al. Associations between acute kidney injury and cardiovascular and renal outcomes after coronary angiography. *Circulation.* 2011;123:409-416.

142. Tsai TT, Patel UD, Chang TI, et al. Contemporary incidence, predictors, and outcomes of acute kidney injury in patients undergoing percutaneous coronary interventions: insights from the NCDR Cath-PCI Registry. *JACC: Cardiovasc Intervent.* 2014;7:1-9.

143. Arbel Y, Fuster V, Baber U, Hamza TH, Siami FS, Farkouh ME. Incidence, determinants and impact of acute kidney injury in patients with diabetes mellitus and multivessel disease undergoing coronary revascularization: results from the FREEDOM trial. *Int J Cardiol.* 2019;293:197-202.

144. Mehran R, Aymong ED, Nikolsky E, et al. A simple risk score for prediction of contrast-induced nephropathy after percutaneous coronary intervention: development and initial validation. *J Am Coll Cardiol.* 2004;44:1393-1399.

145. Azzalini L, Spagnoli V, Ly HQ. Contrast-induced nephropathy: from pathophysiology to preventive strategies. *Can J Cardiol.* 2016;32:247-255.

146. McCullough PA, Choi JP, Feghali GA, et al. Contrast-induced acute kidney injury. *J Am Coll Cardiol.* 2016;68:1465-1473.

147. Wong GTC, Irwin MG. Contrast-induced nephropathy. *Br J Anaest.* 2007;99:474-483.

148. Persson PB, Hansell P, Liss P. Pathophysiology of contrast medium-induced nephropathy. *Kidney Int.* 2005;68:14-22.

149. Detrenis S, Meschi M, Musini S, Savazzi G. Lights and shadows on the pathogenesis of contrast-induced nephropathy: state of the art. *Nephrol Dialysis Transplant.* 2005;20:1542-1550.

150. Tumlin J, Stacul F, Adam A, et al. Pathophysiology of contrast-induced nephropathy. *Am J Cardiol.* 2006;98:14-20.

151. Morcos SK, Dawson P, Pearson JD, et al. The haemodynamic effects of iodinated water soluble radiographic contrast media: a review. *Eur J Radiol.* 1998;29:31-46.

152. Solomon R. Contrast-medium-induced acute renal failure. *Kidney Int.* 1998;53:230-242.

153. Neumann FJ, Sousa-Uva M, Ahlsson A, et al. 2018 ESC/EACTS Guidelines on myocardial revascularization. *Eur Heart J.* 2019;40:87-165.

154. Brar SS, Aharonian V, Mansukhani P, et al. Haemodynamic-guided fluid administration for the prevention of contrast-induced acute kidney injury: the POSEIDON randomised controlled trial. *Lancet* 2014;383:1814-1823.

155. Riley RF, Henry TD, Mahmud E, et al. SCAI position statement on optimal percutaneous coronary interventional therapy for complex coronary artery disease. *Catheter Cardiovasc Interv.* 2020;96:346-362.

156. Leoncini M, Toso A, Maioli M, Tropeano F, Villani S, Bellandi F. Early high-dose rosuvastatin for contrast-induced nephropathy prevention in acute coronary syndrome: Results from the PRATO-ACS Study (Protective Effect of Rosuvastatin and Antiplatelet Therapy On contrast-induced acute kidney injury and myocardial damage in patients with Acute Coronary Syndrome). *J Am Coll Cardiol.* 2014;63:71-79.

157. Gurm HS, Dixon SR, Smith DE, et al. Renal function-based contrast dosing to define safe limits of radiographic contrast media in patients undergoing percutaneous coronary interventions. *J Am Coll Cardiol.* 2011;58:907-914.

158. Himmelfarb J, Ikizler TA. Acute kidney injury: changing lexicography, definitions, and epidemiology. *Kidney Int.* 2007;71:971-976.

Rheumatologic Disease and the Cardiovascular System

Emily Carroll and Yousaf Ali

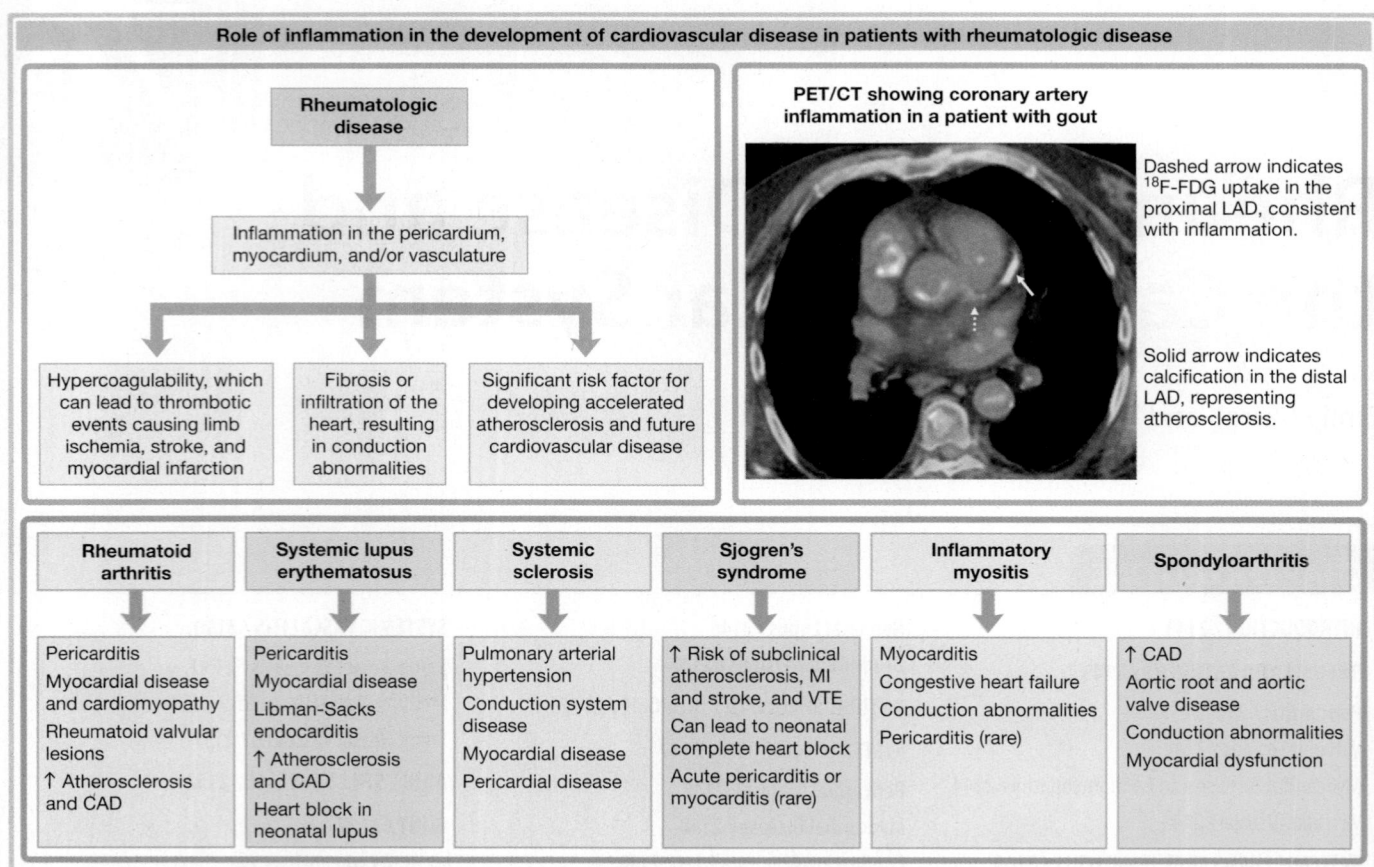

Chapter 76 Fuster and Hurst's Central Illustration. The increased level of inflammation in rheumatologic patients plays a large role in the development of associated cardiovascular disease. Early recognition and treatment of any underlying inflammatory process is vital for cardiovascular health. CAD, coronary artery disease; CT, computed tomography; ^{18}F-FDG, 2-[(18)F]-fluoro-2-deoxy-d-glucose; LAD, left anterior descending coronary artery; MI, myocardial infarction; PET, positron emission tomography; VTE, venous thromboembolism.

CHAPTER SUMMARY

This chapter covers the most common rheumatologic diseases encountered by cardiovascular clinicians, including connective tissue diseases, vasculitis, and crystalline arthritis. An overview of clinical presentations, diagnostic work-ups, and recommended treatments is provided, with special attention paid to the cardiovascular manifestations of these conditions. Increased levels of inflammation in rheumatologic patients are a primary driver of their symptoms and play a large role in the development of associated cardiovascular disease (see Fuster and Hurst's Central Illustration). Because of the systemic nature of rheumatologic illnesses, inflammation can be seen throughout the heart and its pericardial lining, as well as in various-sized blood vessels. Over time, this inflammation can lead to fibrosis, infiltrative disease, and cardiovascular dysfunction. Underlying inflammation also creates a hypercoagulable state, putting these patients at risk of thromboembolic events. Additionally, increased inflammation may be a significant risk factor for developing accelerated atherosclerosis and future cardiovascular disease. Early recognition and treatment of the underlying inflammatory process is vital for cardiovascular health.

INTRODUCTION

Rheumatologic diseases are notable for their widespread, multisystem involvement. The cardiovascular system plays a critical role in these diseases and can greatly impact the morbidity and mortality of patients living with rheumatologic conditions. The cardiovascular manifestations seen in rheumatologic diseases are wide-ranging in terms of their severity, when in the disease process they occur, and what aspects of the cardiovascular system they affect. There are three ways in which rheumatologic diseases affect the cardiovascular system: First, inflammation in the pericardium, myocardium, or vasculature, akin to that found in synovial tissue that causes the hallmark articular manifestations of many of these diseases; second, fibrosis or infiltration of the heart resulting in conduction abnormalities; and third, hypercoagulability that can lead to thrombotic events causing limb ischemia, stroke, and myocardial infarction (MI).

Even when there is no direct damage on the cardiovascular system, the heightened proinflammatory milieu that exists in these conditions may be a significant risk factor for atherosclerosis and cardiovascular disease (CVD). Elevated inflammatory markers such as CRP and IL-6 have been associated with increased risk for ischemic stroke and coronary heart disease (CAD).[1] Other markers of inflammation such as elevated erythrocyte sedimentation rate, tumor necrosis factor (TNF) alpha, and transforming growth factor (TGF) beta have also been linked with heightened risk of developing atherosclerosis.[1] Given the observed relationship between an elevated inflammatory state and cardiac disease, it is important that these rheumatologic diseases are recognized promptly and treated appropriately, in order to control inflammation and potentially mitigate deleterious effects on the cardiovascular system.

Patients with rheumatologic conditions frequently face a lengthy delay to diagnosis[2] and may seek out various doctors and specialists before the correct diagnosis is made. At times, the first presenting symptom may be cardiac involvement. Thus, it is important for cardiovascular clinicians to have a good understanding of, and high index of suspicion for, rheumatologic conditions, so that they can recognize and diagnose these patients and allow them to begin treatment earlier. This chapter will review the key features of the various rheumatologic conditions that cardiovascular clinicians can expect to encounter in their clinical practice, paying special attention to the potential cardiovascular manifestations that may arise and focusing on the screening, diagnosis, and evidence-based treatment of these conditions. A summary of these conditions (Table 76–1) is also provided for quick reference.

RHEUMATOID ARTHRITIS

Rheumatoid arthritis (RA) is a chronic, systemic inflammatory autoimmune disease. It is the most common systemic autoimmune disease with a prevalence of around 1% worldwide. RA affects women twice as often as men and most often presents in the third or fourth decade of life. The exact etiology of RA is unknown, but it is likely due to a complex interaction of predisposing genetic factors with lifestyle and environmental triggers. The diagnosis of RA is a clinical one, with patients demonstrating greater than 6 weeks of an inflammatory, symmetric polyarthritis with a predilection for the small joints of the hands and feet. This clinical diagnosis can be further supported by laboratory findings early in the disease and radiographs showing erosive changes late in the disease. The presence of rheumatoid factor (RF) or anticyclic citrullinated peptide antibodies

TABLE 76–1. Common Clinical and Cardiovascular Manifestations of Systemic Autoimmune Diseases

Disease	Epidemiology	Clinical and Diagnostic Features	Cardiovascular Manifestations
Rheumatoid arthritis	F > M, third and fourth decade of life	Symmetric, small joint polyarticular inflammatory arthritis. Erosive changes on hand and foot x-rays. Positive RF and anti-CCP.	Pericarditis. Cardiomyopathy. Rheumatoid valvular lesions. Increased rate of atherosclerosis and coronary artery disease.
Systemic lupus erythematosus	F > M, more common in Black and Hispanic patients	Malar rash. Photosensitivity. Nonerosive arthritis. Joint laxity. Renal involvement. Positive ANA and more specific serologies anti-dsDNA, anti-Smith. May also be associated with APS. Certain drugs can trigger drug-induced lupus.	Pericarditis. Libman–Sacks Endocarditis. Increased atherosclerosis and coronary artery disease. Heart block in neonatal lupus.
Systemic sclerosis	F > M	Limited (CREST) cutaneous form and Diffuse cutaneous form which has more proximal skin involvement and more often internal organ manifestations such as ILD, scleroderma renal crisis. Positive anti-SCl70 in diffuse and anticentromere in limited form.	PAH. Conduction system disease. Cardiomyopathy. Pericardial disease.
Sjogren's syndrome	F > M, more prevalent in Caucasians	Dry eyes and mouth. Often a secondary disorder with other systemic autoimmune diseases. Positive anti-Ro/SSA and anti-La/SSB.	Pericarditis. Increased atherosclerosis. Can lead to neonatal complete heart block.
Inflammatory myositis	F > M, fifth and sixth decade of life	Symmetric proximal muscle weakness. Skin rashes in dermatomyositis. Elevated muscle enzymes. Statins can cause immune-mediated necrotizing myositis.	Pericarditis. Myocarditis. Congestive heart failure. Conduction abnormalities.
Spondyloarthritis	M > F	Spine and sacroiliac joint arthritis. Dactylitis. Inflammatory eye disease. Can be associated with psoriasis, IBD. Positive HLA-B27	Aortic root and aortic valve disease. Conduction abnormalities.

(CCP) is seen in 70% to 80% of patients testing positive for RA, with the latter being more specific.

Although RA is primarily characterized by and diagnosed based on the presence of inflammatory joint disease, there are also extraarticular manifestations of RA. These include nonspecific complaints such as fever and fatigue, as well as multiorgan symptoms with skin, eye, lung, and cardiac involvement. Cardiovascular involvement, ranging from overt to subclinical disease, can be seen in up to half of patients with RA and is a frequent cause of morbidity and mortality in this population. The most well-recognized cardiovascular manifestations of RA are pericarditis, valvular lesions, myocardial disease and cardiomyopathy, and vascular disease.

Pericarditis

Symptomatic pericarditis is seen in 10% of patients with RA, although evidence of clinically insignificant pericardial effusions can be seen in up to one-third of patients on echocardiography and autopsy findings of pericardial involvement can be found in 30% to 50% of RA patients. RA patients with acute pericarditis are more likely to have a positive RF and to overall have very active disease with ongoing inflammatory arthritis and often other extraarticular manifestations such as rheumatoid nodules. Rarely, acute pericarditis has been the primary presentation of RA.[3] The pericarditis seen in RA is symptomatically indistinguishable from other causes of acute pericarditis, and presents with sharp, pleuritic, and positional chest pain. Imaging with an echocardiogram can assist in making this diagnosis, and in one case series, an associated pericardial effusion was found in 90% of RA patients with pericarditis.[4] Generally, these associated effusions do not cause hemodynamic compromise, although RA has been reported as a rare cause of cardiac tamponade.[5] If pericardiocentesis is performed for diagnostic or therapeutic purposes in the case of a large, hemodynamically significant pericardial effusion, it will show an exudative fluid with high lactate dehydrogenase, high protein, low glucose, and a neutrophilic predominance. Most patients with uncomplicated pericarditis respond to treatment with nonsteroidal anti-inflammatory drugs (NSAIDs), or corticosteroids for moderate-to-severe cases. In the much rarer case of constrictive pericarditis, procedures such as a pericardial window or pericardial stripping may be necessary.

Sometimes, pericarditis and pericardial effusions in RA patients are not due to the disease activity of the underlying RA, but rather the treatments that these patients are receiving. Drug-induced lupus (DIL), which will be discussed in further detail later on, can commonly result from anti-TNF therapy used in RA and can present with serositis, including pericardial involvement. Usually this will resolve within several weeks after the offending agent is discontinued. Because of this potential risk, in RA patients who already have a history of prior pericarditis, anti-TNFs are often eschewed in favor of other classes of biologics.

Valvular Lesions

Imaging-based studies have shown that valvular heart disease is more common in patients with RA compared to the general population.[6] This is thought to be due in large part to the presence of valvular rheumatoid nodules. Earlier autopsy studies found that valvular involvement in the form of rheumatoid nodules is relatively rare, occurring in under 5% of cases, but more recent imaging studies have reported a higher prevalence with valvular lesion found in over 30% of RA patients. When present, rheumatoid valvular nodules can be clinically significant leading to stroke and other embolic phenomena. On an echocardiogram, these rheumatoid nodules may mimic a vegetation or an atrial myxoma. Histologically, these nodules are identical to subcutaneous nodules seen in RA and have a central area of fibrinoid necrosis surrounded by an inflammatory cellular palisade.[7] These lesions tend to be larger than the nodules seen in acute rheumatic fever, and they also lack the pathognomonic Aschoff bodies that are seen in rheumatic heart disease. There is no evidence for using corticosteroids or disease-modifying antirheumatic drugs (DMARDs) in treating valvular lesions; instead, lesions resulting in severe, symptomatic disease require surgical intervention.

Myocardial Disease and Cardiomyopathy

The risk of heart failure in patients with RA is high, independent of the presence of traditional heart failure risk factors. Cardiomyopathy is one of the leading causes of mortality in patients with RA, especially male patients. Left ventricular (LV) dysfunction can be seen in patients with RA at rates 3 times higher than in the general population. Several processes can lead to myocardial dysfunction in RA including inflammation, fibrosis, and ischemia. Pancarditis and small-vessel vasculitis can lead to systolic failure. Secondary amyloidosis caused by long-standing inflammation can lead to impaired relaxation and diastolic dysfunction. RA can also cause a focal necrotizing or granulomatous myocarditis that can disrupt the conduction system and lead to various degrees of atrioventricular (AV) block. Confirming the diagnosis of myocarditis in RA can often be difficult. Endomyocardial biopsy is the gold standard diagnostic modality,[8] but owing to the patchy involvement, the sensitivity of endomyocardial biopsy is limited and on studies has been found to be as low as 35%. This procedure also carries risk of complications such as perforation. Instead, cardiac magnetic resonance (CMR) imaging can be a useful, noninvasive tool to differentiate between the different potential causes of cardiomyopathy in RA. T2-weighted CMR images showing focal areas of increased signal intensity can indicate granulomatous myocarditis in the appropriate clinical context, whereas CMR images with late gadolinium enhancement that shows diffuse endocardial hyperenhancement is suggestive of cardiac amyloidosis.

Vascular Disease

Overall, mortality in RA patients is increased compared to that of the general population and is largely attributable to CVD.[9] The presence of CVD in RA is equivalent to that in patients with diabetes mellitus. The increased cardiovascular mortality in patients with RA is in large part due to the risk of accelerated atherosclerosis and ischemic heart disease. Case-control studies have demonstrated a 2- to 3-fold risk in atherosclerosis due to the presence of RA as well as an increased risk of MI and sudden cardiac death. Chronic inflammation is the primary driver for accelerated atherosclerosis in patients with RA, with the duration and severity of the disease linked to cardiovascular risk. Even without the presence of atherosclerosis, RA can affect blood vessels by increasing arterial stiffness, which is an independent risk factor for adverse cardiovascular outcomes, and causing vasculitis, including coronary arteritis. Prior to effective therapies, as many as 20% of patients with RA showed evidence of coronary vasculitis on autopsy, but coronary arteritis and rheumatoid vasculitis as a whole have decreased in prevalence with the emergence of effective anti-inflammatory treatments.[10]

Despite these known risks, there are currently no evidence-based guidelines for preventive strategies for CVD in patients with RA. Expert consensus is that the goal should be to aggressively manage traditional cardiovascular risk factors including hyperlipidemia; although paradoxically, RA patients with low circulating low-density lipoprotein (LDL) concentration levels at baseline tend to have increased risk for cardiovascular events.[11] Studies have shown that low LDL concentration levels are related to higher coronary artery calcium scores in patients with RA,[12] suggesting that heightened screening may be considered in this subpopulation in particular. It is also important to tightly control other inflammatory manifestations of RA because studies have demonstrated that the use of treatments to control inflammation such as methotrexate and anti-TNF inhibitors also reduce rates of cardiovascular events and death.[13–15]

SYSTEMIC LUPUS ERYTHEMATOSUS

Systemic lupus erythematosus (SLE) is a chronic, systemic autoimmune disease that is far more common in women and in Hispanic and Black patients. Black women have the highest prevalence, 286.4 in 100,000, which is nearly double the prevalence in White women. Men and non-White patients tend to have more severe disease manifestations. There is an increased prevalence of renal and cardiac complications in non-White patients and these manifestations tend to occur at younger ages; there is also up to 3 times greater mortality rates in these patients.[16] These discrepancies in outcomes are, in part, explained by differences in socioeconomic status and other social determinants of disease susceptibility.[17]

In terms of diagnosis of SLE, antinuclear antibodies (ANA) are seen in 95% of patients with SLE, although the presence of a positive ANA is not diagnostic and can be seen in healthy individuals. More specific antibodies, like anti-Smith and anti-double-stranded DNA are more associated with SLE. Clinically, SLE can have variable presentations from mild joint and skin symptoms to life-threatening organ involvement. Cardiovascular involvement is very common and is found in over half of SLE patients.[18] The most frequently seen cardiac involvements include pericarditis, myocardial disease, Libman–Sacks valvular lesions, and accelerated atherosclerosis. Conduction abnormalities can also be seen in neonatal lupus. Lastly, DIL is an important entity to be aware of because not only can it present with pericarditis, but it can also be due to some medications prescribed by cardiovascular clinicians such as antiarrhythmics (procainamide and quinidine).

Pericardial Disease

Pericarditis is the most common cardiovascular complication of SLE, with between 20% and 50% of patients demonstrating some clinical manifestation. This pericarditis can rarely be associated with large pericardial effusions, although cardiac tamponade is rare unless the patient has concomitant renal disease. Patients with SLE are also at risk of infectious or malignant pericardial involvement, so alternative etiologies must be carefully considered. Unlike idiopathic or viral pericarditis where glucocorticoids are reserved for patients with symptoms refractory to NSAIDs and colchicine, in lupus pericarditis, glucocorticoids are much more commonly used. In very mild cases, NSAIDs may be sufficient, but many SLE patients have contraindications to NSAID use such as renal insufficiency. The dosage and route of glucocorticoids are dependent upon the severity of symptoms (**Table 76-2**). For mild cases refractory to NSAIDs, intramuscular (IM) triamcinolone or oral methylprednisolone are equally effective, although triamcinolone may lead to quicker symptom resolution.[19] In severe pericarditis or cardiac tamponade, intravenous (IV) methylprednisolone given as a bolus, usually 500 mg or 1 g for 3 days, is often used.[20] When hemodynamically significant effusion or tamponade physiology is present, additional intervention is also necessary, such as emergent pericardiocentesis or pericardial window or stripping procedures. In cases of recurrent pericarditis, or disease refractory to first-line therapy, additional immunosuppression with azathioprine, methotrexate, mycophenolate mofetil (MMF), or intravenous immunoglobulin (IVIG) may be required.[21] Belimumab has also been used effectively.[22]

Colchicine is also a useful adjunct therapy that has been shown to reduce the risk of recurrence after first episode of pericarditis.[23] Anakinra, an intraleukin-1 inhibitor whose efficacy for recurrent and refractory cases of idiopathic pericarditis has been well described,[24] is not well studied for lupus pericarditis, although there are data for its use in recurrent fevers and arthritis in SLE patients.[25]

Myocardial Disease

Myocardial dysfunction in SLE is most commonly due to ischemic heart disease, valvular disease, or hypertensive disease and in severe cases can lead to cardiomyopathy. Myocarditis is only

TABLE 76-2. Lupus Pericarditis Treatment Recommendations

Disease Severity	Treatment
Mild pericarditis	Oral or IM glucocorticoids + hydroxychloroquine
Severe pericarditis	IV solumedrol 500 mg–1 g × 3 days
Cardiac tamponade	Pericardiocentesis, pericardial window, or pericardial stripping
Recurrent pericarditis	Azathioprine, methotrexate, MMF, or IVIG

rarely seen but can be severe;[26] if present, it requires aggressive immunosuppression with high-dose glucocorticoids and usually cyclophosphamide or MMF to reverse wall motion abnormalities and depressed LV systolic function.[27,28]

Valvular Lesions

Valvular disease is common in SLE and the risk is increased in patients who also have antiphospholipid antibodies. Almost half of SLE patients have evidence of valvular disease on imaging, but only 22% of patients without antiphospholipid antibodies.[29] Valvular lesions seen in SLE are varied with nonspecific valve thickening, stenosis, and regurgitation commonly seen; however, the classic valvular pathology associated with SLE is Libman–Sacks endocarditis, which is defined as verrucous, noninfectious vegetations seen on heart valves and is seen in association with SLE, antiphospholipid syndrome, and some malignancies. Any of the heart valves may be affected, although mitral followed by aortic are the most common sites for valvular pathology in SLE, likely due to the more turbulent flow across these valves. The development of severe valvular regurgitation may be due to the presence of high anticardiolipin antibodies. Despite the high incidence of valve abnormality in lupus patients, the most recent guidelines from the American Heart Association do not recommend routine antibiotic prophylaxis for this population prior to dental procedures.[30]

For SLE patients with valvular disease, there is no clear consensus on conservative strategies with medical therapy, or surgical intervention due to the lack of large systemic studies in this population. In patients with Libman–Sacks endocarditis related to antiphospholipid syndrome (APS), titers of antiphospholipid serologies can fluctuate, and may even become transiently negative, so their monitoring has limited clinical utility when determining a treatment course. Glucocorticoids do not appear to prevent the formation of Libman–Sacks endocarditis, but by controlling inflammation they may promote healing of these lesions; therefore, some experts advocate for the use of prednisone 1 mg/kg/day in SLE patients with Libman–Sacks endocarditis.[31] However, glucocorticoids have also been reported to promote fibrosis and scarring, leading to additional valvular damage.[32] Usually, for significant disease, conservative therapy is insufficient and surgical intervention is necessary.

There are no standardized recommendations for when valvular surgery is indicated that are specific to patients with Libman–Sacks endocarditis. Standard guideline indications used for infective endocarditis are also applied to this noninfectious endocarditis, including symptoms of heart failure, severe valvular dysfunction, large vegetations, and recurrent embolization.[33] In general, mitral valve repair is favored over replacement when feasible owing to the lower operative mortality rates, higher overall survival rates, and better maintenance of LV function. Unlike in infective endocarditis when the entire valve must be removed and replaced, in Libman–Sacks endocarditis, it is possible to perform valvular repair. In select patients, with stable underlying disease and only localized valvular abnormalities, mitral repair has been shown to be a viable surgical option.[34] However, some studies report valve replacement is

superior in these patients if they do not have well-controlled underlying disease because, otherwise, the ongoing inflammation will lead to fibrosis and calcification, requiring early reintervention.[35] When mitral valve replacement is performed, the choice between mechanical and bioprosthetic valve is highly patient-specific. In patients with high bleeding risk, bioprosthetic valves are preferred, but bioprosthetic valves are more susceptible to calcification and degeneration, especially in SLE patients with underlying renal dysfunction, so a mechanical valve might be superior in certain instances.[36]

Other than valvular insufficiency, another important complication is thromboembolism. In the case of Libman–Sacks endocarditis in the setting of APS, long-term anticoagulation is advised. Even without the presence of APS, though, lifelong anticoagulation is recommended for patients with Libman–Sacks endocarditis who have suffered a previous thromboembolic event. Patients who undergo valve replacement with a mechanical valve will also require lifelong anticoagulation.

Atherosclerosis and Coronary Artery Disease

The premature onset of CAD and atherosclerosis is a well-reported phenomenon in patients with SLE. Independent of traditional risk factors, there is an increased risk of MI in patients with SLE, which is a significant cause of morbidity and mortality in this patient population. Older age at diagnosis of SLE, higher levels of homocysteine and LDL cholesterol, longer duration of SLE, and longer duration of steroid use are all associated with increased risk of CAD.[37] In patients with SLE, atherosclerosis progresses at twice the rate of the general population.[38] As a result of this increased risk, cardiovascular clinicians should have a low threshold to evaluate for CAD whenever for a patient with SLE presents with chest pain, dyspnea, or other atypical symptoms. Intermittent screening may also be warranted with stress testing in patients who have a long duration of SLE or concomitant traditional risk factors. In prospective imaging studies of SLE patients with no known CAD history, myocardial perfusion imaging was abnormal in 38% of patients with a mean duration of SLE of 8.7 years and the incidence of cardiac events was higher in those with an abnormal scan.[39] In addition to screening, other measures to reduce CVD risk should be undertaken such as minimizing glucocorticoid exposure, controlling hypertension and hyperlipidemia, and addressing modifiable risk factors like obesity, physical inactivity, and smoking. There is some data that hydroxychloroquine may have a cardioprotective effect in SLE patients and is associated with improved lipid profiles and blood glucose levels, as well as longer survival.[40] There may be a synergistic effect when low-dose aspirin is used with hydroxychloroquine, although this also carries a not insignificant risk of bleeding.[41]

Neonatal Lupus

Neonatal lupus is an autoimmune disease that is due to passive transplacental transfer of autoantibodies from the mother to the fetus. It occurs in infants of mothers with SLE and is more likely in mothers with anti-Ro/SSA and anti-La/SSB antibodies. Cutaneous manifestations and cardiac manifestations can occur in the newborn, with the most severe complications being complete heart block. Luckily, this is rare, with only 2% of infants demonstrating complete heart block. However, the probability of having subsequent children with congenital heart block is higher. If a prior pregnancy resulted in heart block, the risk that heart block will occur in a subsequent pregnancy is about 16%, and if a prior pregnancy resulted in a neonatal lupus skin rash, the risk that a heart block will occur in a subsequent pregnancy is 13%.[42] Given these risks, women with SLE should be followed by maternal-fetal medicine specialists during their pregnancies and should undergo frequent fetal echocardiographic surveillance because detection at earlier stages may improve outcomes in the neonate.

Drug-Induced Lupus

DIL is a rare side effect of certain medications, including hydralazine and the antiarrhythmics procainamide and quinidine. It can also be seen due to minocycline, isoniazid, phenytoin, and anti-TNFs. Unlike regular SLE, DIL affects men and women equally, and is more common in older, White patients. Antihistone antibodies are often present in DIL, although they can also be seen in SLE, and other auto-antibodies such as anti-double-stranded DNA and antineutrophil cytoplasmic antibodies (ANCAs) can also be found. Common symptoms are arthralgias, pericarditis, rash, and fever. Renal and other serious organ involvement from DIL is not typically seen. The syndrome will usually self-resolve upon discontinuation of the offending agent, although a short course of hydroxychloroquine or glucocorticoids may be required.

ANTIPHOSPHOLIPID SYNDROME

APS is a clinical autoimmune syndrome characterized by the presence of arterial and venous thrombosis and/or adverse pregnancy outcome in the presence of persistent antiphospholipid antibodies (anticardiolipin antibody, beta2 glycoprotein, and lupus anticoagulant). Positive serologic testing must occur on two separate occasions, at least 12 weeks apart, in order to confirm APS. APS can either occur as a primary disorder, or secondary to another autoimmune disorder such as SLE. In addition to pregnancy loss, the thrombotic complications of APS can also lead to widespread ischemic disease, including multiorgan failure known as catastrophic APS. The most common cardiac abnormality in APS is valvular disease, including valvular thickening and nodules (Libman–Sacks endocarditis, as aforementioned). Patients are also at increased risk of coronary thromboembolism and MI.[43] The annual risk of thrombosis in patients with secondary APS and SLE is 3%, compared with 1% for patients with primary APS.[44] Because of the thrombotic risk in APS, patients require both primary and secondary preventative treatment. The European Union League Against Rheumatism (EULAR) recommends primary prophylaxis with low-dose aspirin in patients with a high-risk APS serologic profile and for patients with a history of obstetric APS.[45] The treatment of acute thrombosis should be with heparin bridged to warfarin rather than a direct oral anticoagulant

(DOAC) based on recent evidence that DOACs are inferior to vitamin K antagonists in patients with APS.[46,47] Lifelong anticoagulation is recommended with a goal international normalized ratio (INR) of 2 to 3. There is ongoing debate over whether the addition of immunomodulatory agents is warranted in this population. There have been some case reports demonstrating benefit with rituximab in patients with APS and thrombocytopenia,[48,49] as well as showing reduced incidence in thrombotic events with hydroxychloroquine, but there are not sufficient data at this time to recommend its use for APS in the absence of concurrent SLE.[50]

SYSTEMIC SCLEROSIS

Systemic sclerosis (SSc) is an autoimmune disorder characterized by tissue fibrosis of various organ systems due to excessive accumulation of collagen and extracellular proteins. The exact etiology of SSc is unknown but several triggers have been posited including exposure to certain viruses and environmental agents that may cause the onset of symptoms in a genetically susceptible host. There is an increased risk of malignancy in patients with SSc and malignancy may serve as a trigger for disease onset, as well. The majority of patients with SSc are women, who more often present at younger ages and with limited systemic sclerosis, whereas men tend to have more diffuse involvement and increased cardiovascular manifestations.[51] In addition to the classic skin changes and hardening seen in SSc, a variety of internal organ manifestations can also be seen. There are two main clinical subtypes, limited and systemic cutaneous SSc, which present with different patterns of organ involvement. The diagnosis of SSc is clinical, but can be supported by positive serologies including ANA, anti-RNA polymerase III, anti-SCl70 (topoisomerase), and anticentromere antibody. Anti SCl70 is more often associated with diffuse systemic sclerosis and anticentromere with limited systemic sclerosis.

Limited systemic sclerosis, formerly called CREST syndrome, is notable for the presence of calcinosis cutis, Raynaud's phenomenon, esophageal dysmotility, sclerodactyly, and telangiectasias. Skin involvement is limited to the distal extremities. Conversely, in diffuse systemic sclerosis, the cutaneous manifestations are more widespread and there tends to be more significant, and earlier onset of, internal organ involvement. Cardiovascular complications occur in both forms of the disease and there can be involvement and fibrosis of the pericardium, myocardium, and conduction system, as well as pulmonary arterial hypertension (PAH). Compared to the general population, patients with SSc are at increased relative risk of developing CVD.[52]

Unlike with skin and pulmonary complications where there is good data, the role of immunosuppressive or antifibrotic treatment for the fibrotic cardiac complications of SSc is less clear, and the most recent EULAR guidelines for the treatment of SSc do not provide guidance for treatment of non-PAH cardiac manifestations.[53] A small, older study showed a slight decrease in arrythmias on 24-hour electrocardiograph monitoring in patients receiving plasmapheresis and immunosuppression with cyclophosphamide and azathioprine,[54] but in general, there is limited data showing that immunosuppression has a positive impact on cardiac outcomes in patients with SSc. What is known, though, is that high-dose glucocorticoids should be avoiding in treating cardiovascular manifestations of SSc due to their risk of precipitating scleroderma renal crisis.[55]

Pericardial Disease

Pericardial involvement is discovered not infrequently on autopsy studies in patients with SSc, but clinically significant pericardial effusion or pericarditis occurs in a minority of patients.[56] Pericardial effusions, when present, are typically small or moderate in size and rarely are associated with tamponade physiology. A new or worsening effusion in this population should prompt evaluation for scleroderma renal crisis.[57]

Myocardial Disease

Myocardial involvement tends to be more severe in patients with rapidly progressing skin involvement and positive anti-U3-RNP antibodies.[58] Myocardial fibrosis leads to stiffness and reduced ventricular compliance. Segmental wall motion abnormalities can be seen, as can increased LV wall thickness and diastolic dysfunction. Microvascular disease can contribute to myocardial ischemia, and increased vascular stiffness of small and large arteries has been reported.[59]

Conduction Abnormalities

In patients with SSc, conduction disease is common, with abnormalities seen on electrocardiogram (ECG) in 25% to 75% of patients.[60] Fibrosis of the AV node and bundle branches leads to diffuse conduction abnormalities and frequent arrhythmias,[61] with the most commonly encountered arrhythmia being premature ventricular contractions. This population also has an increased susceptibility to tachyarrhythmias such as atrial fibrillation, atrial flutter, paroxysmal supraventricular tachycardia, and ventricular tachycardia.[62] Arrythmias portend a poor prognosis and represent 6% of the mortality attributable to SSc.[63] There are no randomized trials looking at the treatment of various arrythmias specifically in patients with SSc, and therefore arrythmias are treated similar to those in patients without SSc. It is important to keep in mind, though, that certain medications may be contraindicated in this population. Nonselective β-blockers can exacerbate Raynaud's phenomenon[64] and in SSc patients with underlying pulmonary fibrosis, amiodarone should be used cautiously.[65] Ablation therapy and implantable pacemakers and cardioverter defibrillators should be used in SSc patients for the same indications as in the general population.

Pulmonary Arterial Hypertension

PAH is a serious cardiopulmonary manifestation of SSc, more commonly associated with the limited cutaneous variety. PAH due to SSc is included within the first group of the World Health Organization pulmonary hypertension classification system. PAH is found commonly at autopsy of SSc patients in up to 80%, but clinically apparent manifestations occur in only 10% of cases.[66] When PAH is present, patients with SSc have a markedly worse prognosis with a 50% mortality rate within 3 years of being diagnosed.[66] The SSc-associated form of PAH has a 3-fold higher mortality rate than idiopathic PAH, in part because the disease may be diagnosed later in SSc patients due to their other comorbidities that the PAH symptoms may be falsely attributed to, and also because SSc-associated PAH tends not to respond as well to conventional PAH therapies.[67]

Because of the increased mortality due to PAH, screening of patients with SSc is of utmost importance and most experts recommend that echocardiogram should be performed annually. However, there is some limitation in the ability of echocardiogram to accurate detect the presence and severity of PAH, because echocardiographic estimation of pulmonary arterial pressure relies upon the tricuspid regurgitant jet velocity, which is absent in 20% to 39%.[68] Therefore, if there is high clinical suspicion for PAH in a patient without signs of pulmonary hypertension on echocardiogram, a right heart catheterization should still be performed for a definitive answer.

In terms of treatment options for patients with SSc-associated PAH, the same general supportive measures such as inotropes, diuretics, and supplemental oxygen when needed, as are recommended for patients with idiopathic PAH. The one difference being that anticoagulation is not routinely advised for patients with SSc given the lack of demonstrable benefit in this population and potential for harm given increased bleeding risk from gastrointestinal telangiectasias and variable anticoagulation levels owing to inconsistent absorption of oral anticoagulants due to motility issues.[69] PAH-directed therapy with prostacyclin analogues, phosphodiesterase type 5 (PDE-5) inhibitors, and endothelin receptor antagonists that have been FDA approved for idiopathic PAH are also used in PAH associated with SSc.

SJOGREN'S SYNDROME

Sjogren's syndrome (SS) is a chronic autoimmune inflammatory disorder characterized by inflammation of the salivary and lacrimal glands that leads to decreased glandular function and resultant sicca symptoms of dry eyes and dry mouth. SS can occur as a primary disorder, but is also frequently seen as a secondary disorder with other systemic inflammatory connective tissue diseases. Diagnosis of SS is made based on objective findings of dry eyes or mouth and the presence of serologic or histopathologic evidence. The most commonly seen antibodies are anti-Ro/SSA and anti-La/SSB antibodies, although a positive RF and ANA are common. Biopsy of an affected salivary gland shows focal lymphocytic sialadenitis.

In addition to the classic sicca symptoms, many extraglandular manifestations of SS can occur, including CVD. SS is associated with an increased risk of subclinical atherosclerosis,[70] MI and stroke,[71] and venous thromboembolism.[72] Acute pericarditis and myocarditis can also rarely be seen in primary SS. Heart block is not commonly found in adult patients with SS, but similar to neonatal lupus, congenital heart block can develop in the fetus of a pregnant woman with SS due to transplacental passage of anti-Ro/SSA antibodies. Treatment of SS is based on a patient's specific organ involvement. In the case of cardiovascular complications like pericarditis, treatment is with colchicine and NSAIDs or glucocorticoids. In addition, the presence of cardiac manifestations should trigger an investigation for other systemic inflammatory autoimmune conditions such as SLE or overlap syndromes where cardiac involvement is more common.

INFLAMMATORY MYOSITIS

Dermatomyositis (DM) and polymyositis (PM) are two idiopathic inflammatory myopathies that often present with proximal muscle weakness, but can have multisystem involvement, including the cardiovascular system. There is a slight female predominance to inflammatory myopathies and the age of onset is most commonly in the fifth or sixth decade of life. The conditions are associated with elevated muscle enzymes like creatinine phosphokinase (CPK) and aldolase, as well as a wide array of serum auto-antibodies such as anti-Jo, antisynthetase, and antibodies against Mi-2, Ku, and signal recognition peptide antigens. Imaging with MRI can be suggestive of an inflammatory myopathy if it shows muscle inflammation and edema. Electromyography (EMG) findings may also assist in diagnosis. The gold standard for diagnosis is a muscle biopsy showing a perivascular infiltrate, or skin biopsy of a characteristic lesion in DM. When diagnosis of DM and PM is made, it is also important to evaluate for malignancy as this is a known trigger for the onset of these disorders, especially in the elderly.

The key distinction between DM and PM are the cutaneous manifestations seen in DM. The classic skin findings include Gottron's papules (violaceous papules over the extensor surface of joints, typically the metacarpophalangeal joints), heliotrope eruption (erythema and edema over the upper eyelids), and shawl or V-sign (hyperpigmentation over the upper chest and back). Both DM and PM also can have associated interstitial lung disease, bulbar weakness, and esophageal involvement. Cardiac manifestations are also well described in these diseases, including myocarditis, heart failure, and conduction abnormalities. Pericarditis is rarely seen.[73] The most frequent of these cardiovascular complications is cardiomyopathy.[74] The most common conduction abnormalities are AV block and bundle branch block, but other abnormal ECG findings including atrial and ventricular arrhythmias, abnormal Q waves, and ST segment changes can be seen.[75] Patients with PM and DM are also at a 3- to 4-fold increased risk for MI compared to the general population;[76] this may be due to the overall effects chronic inflammation has on accelerating atherosclerosis and promoting a hypercoagulable state, but also because the disease process can target the myocardium, in addition to skeletal muscle, and cause degeneration of cardiac myocytes.

Monitoring for inflammation or infarction of the myocardium can pose a challenge in these patients with concurrent myositis and elevated muscle enzymes, but cardiac troponin I has been found to be more specific for cardiac muscle involvement than CK-MB or cardiac troponin T.[77] Overall, cardiac involvement portends a poorer prognosis in patients with inflammatory myositis and complications such as heart failure and MI are the most common causes of mortality. Treatment of PM and DM involves high dose corticosteroids and initiation of steroid-sparing agents like methotrexate, azathioprine, or in severe cases IVIG and rituximab.

A third inflammatory myositis that cardiovascular clinicians should be aware of is immune-mediated necrotizing myopathy (IMNM). This is often associated with autoantibodies to HMG-CoA reductase and presents similarly to PM and DM, but is frequently triggered by recent statin use. Treatment requires prompt discontinuation of the statin, in addition to the above inflammatory myositis treatments.

SPONDYLOARTHRITIS

Spondyloarthritis (SpA) refers to a family of chronic, systemic inflammatory conditions including ankylosing spondylitis, psoriatic arthritis, inflammatory bowel disease-related arthritis, and reactive arthritis. They share common features such as spinal and sacroiliac arthritis, enthesitis, and extraarticular manifestations such as inflammatory eye disease and gastrointestinal involvement. There is a high incidence of HLA-B27 positivity seen in these patients, occurring in 90% of patients with ankylosing spondylitis and in 50% to 70% of patients with other types of SpA. It is important to note, though, that a negative HLA-B27 does not rule out these disorders and conversely, a positive HLA-B27 is not diagnostic as the vast majority of people who are HLA-B27 positive do not have spondyloarthritis. In contrast to other inflammatory arthritides like RA, SpA has a male predominance and the arthritis tends to affect the axial spine and larger joints in an asymmetric pattern.

Of the SpAs, ankylosing spondylitis and psoriatic arthritis are most strongly linked with cardiovascular manifestations. Patients with psoriatic arthritis have been shown to have accelerated coronary artery plaque formation.[78] In addition to coronary artery disease, the most common cardiac manifestations seen in SpA are disease of the aortic root and aortic valve leading to aortic regurgitation, conduction abnormalities, and myocardial dysfunction. Aortic valve disease is seen in roughly 10% of patients.[79] In SpA, there can be inflammation and sclerosis of the aortic root, aortic valve leaflets, and/or the interventricular septum leading to aortic regurgitation and conduction abnormalities. Conduction disease, which is predominantly AV blocks and bundle branch blocks, tends to occur in older, male patients with long-standing disease and higher disease activity.[80] Cardiovascular manifestations can occasionally be the presenting symptom of SpA, preceding articular findings.[81]

Treatment of SpA was previously limited to NSAIDs and physical therapy for mild disease and DMARDs such as sulfasalazine or methotrexate in patients with predominantly peripheral arthritis symptoms. However, more recent data has shown the efficacy of TNF antagonists in these conditions.[82] TNF antagonists also are associated with a decrease in major cardiovascular events when used for both psoriatic arthritis and ankylosing spondylitis.[83]

SYSTEMIC VASCULITIS

There is a wide variety of systemic vasculitides that are defined by an inflammatory infiltrate in blood vessel walls that results in systemic complications related to ischemia and necrosis of the affected downstream organs (**Table 76–3**). These diseases are categorized into large-, medium-, or small-vessel vasculitis based on the size of the involved vessel. The diagnosis is confirmed by biopsy, but there are also characteristic patterns of organ involvement and certain serologies that can help differentiate between the various systemic vasculitides.

Large-Vessel Vasculitis

The two forms of large-vessel vasculitis are giant cell arteritis (GCA) and Takayasu's arteritis. Clinically, there is significant overlap in the symptomatology of these two conditions, but the main distinguishing factor is their affected demographics. GCA, also referred to as temporal arteritis, is the most common vasculitis in patients greater than 50 years of age. It is more common in White patients, and has a female predominance. The hallmark symptoms are temporal headache, jaw claudication, and vision changes such as diplopia or amaurosis fugax. Constitutional symptoms like fever and fatigue are also seen frequently, and proximal joint pain in the form of polymyalgia rheumatica can occur in one-third of cases. Laboratory findings are nonspecific but ESR and CRP are usually markedly elevated, though can be normal in 10% of patients. Temporal artery biopsy is the gold standard diagnostic modality, with a positive biopsy showing granulomatous inflammation and destruction of the elastic lamina. However, the sensitivity of biopsy is limited because there is often patchy involvement of the affected artery and skip lesions that may be missed due to sampling error.[84] Doppler ultrasonography can provide noninvasive evidence of GCA with segmental, hypoechogenic thickening of the temporal artery wall, known as a "halo sign," showing a specificity of over 90% when used in experienced centers.[85] In addition to the temporal artery, GCA can also involve the large vessels and other peripheral arteries. Extremity claudication, diminished or absent peripheral pulses, and vascular bruits can all be seen in GCA, as can thoracic and abdominal aortic aneurysms and dissection.[86] Imaging modalities such as a CTA/MRA or FDG-PET scan can be useful for detecting large-vessel vasculitis because these sites are not easily amenable for biopsy.[87,88] Less commonly, CAD, aortic valve abnormalities, and LV dysfunction can also be seen in GCA.

Corticosteroids are the first line of treatment for GCA, with prompt recognition of the disease and initiation of treatment key to preventing life- and vision-threatening complications. Other immunosuppressive agents such as methotrexate are commonly added to help facilitate steroid taper, because long-term, high-dose steroids can have significant side effects, particularly in the elderly population most susceptible for developing GCA. There are also promising data for the use of tocilizumab, an IL-6 receptor antagonist, as a steroid-sparing agent.[89,90]

Takayasu arteritis (TA) is another large-vessel vasculitis that can be clinically indistinguishable from GCA as it also can present with extremity and jaw claudication, headache, vision changes, as well as systemic symptoms with fever, malaise, and weight loss. However, in TA, there is more common involvement of the aorta and its major branches than the temporal artery. TA is also often linked with hypertension due to renal artery stenosis. The patients afflicted with TA are much younger than those with GCA, with the average age of onset before 40.[91] It is also more common in patients of Asian or African descent.[92] Biopsy is often not performed in TA, given the inaccessibility of affected arteries, but imaging studies with CTA, MRA, or FDG-PET can be suggestive. If tissue is available following an aneurysm repair or revascularization procedure, the histopathology is indistinguishable from GCA with evidence of an active inflammatory infiltrate within the vessel wall along with giant cells and granulomas and destruction of the elastic lamina. Treatment of TA is often less successful than in GCA. The primary means of disease control is again

TABLE 76–3. Common Clinical and Cardiac Manifestations of Systemic Vasculitides

Disease	Vessel Size	Clinical and Diagnostic Features	Cardiovascular Manifestations
Giant cell arteritis	Large	Elderly patient with temporal headache, jaw claudication, vision loss, and PMR.	Aortitis. Large vessel aneurysm and dissection.
Takayasu arteritis	Large	Younger patient, often an Asian female, with limb claudication, peripheral pulse discrepancies, and headache.	Hypertension from renal artery stenosis. Aortic complications. Upper extremity limb claudication.
Kawasaki disease	Medium	Young child with fever, sore throat, lymphadenopathy, desquamating rash, and conjunctivitis.	Coronary artery aneurysms.
Polyarteritis nodosa	Medium	Multi-organ involvement but spares the lungs. Skin nodules. Renal involvement. Neuropathies. Abdominal vasculitis.	Angina. MI. Pericarditis. Cardiomyopathy.
GPA and MPA	Small	Lung and renal involvement. Sinusitis more common in GPA. Neuropathy more common in MPA. GPA with positive c-ANCA/anti-PR3. MPA with p-ANCA/anti-MPO.	Pericarditis. Coronary arteritis. Cardiomyopathy.
EGPA	Small	Asthma. Eosinophilia. Pulmonary infiltrates. associated with p-ANCA/MPO.	Cardiomyopathy. Pericarditis. Conduction abnormalities.
Behcet's disease	Variable	Genital and oral ulcers.	Aortitis. Aneurysms. Thrombosis.

Abbreviations: EGPA, eosinophilic granulomatosis with polyangiitis; GPA, granulomatosis with polyangiitis; MPA, microscopic polyangiitis.

with high-dose glucocorticoids, but glucocorticoids alone do not produce a lasting remission and more than half of patients require additional immunomodulatory agents.[93] There is evidence for the use of either methotrexate or azathioprine,[94] as well as data on the use of biologic therapy with TNF antagonists and tocilizumab.[95] Additionally, surgical intervention and revascularization are frequently required for management of stenosed or occluded arteries, and aortic valve surgery is often indicated in cases of worsening aortic regurgitation as a result of aortitis.[96]

Medium-Vessel Vasculitis

Kawasaki disease is a medium-vessel vasculitis of unknown etiology seen in children, often below the age of 5. Children present with fever, conjunctivitis, lymphadenopathy, and a desquamating rash. Many cardiovascular manifestations have been reporting during this acute phase including pericarditis, myocarditis, aortitis, valvular disease, heart failure, and arrhythmias. The most commonly reported manifestation is coronary artery vasculitis, which, if left untreated, can lead to the development of coronary aneurysms in 25% of patients.[97] If the aneurysms are large in size, greater than 8 mm, they are more likely to thrombose and potentially lead to MI.[98] The risk of MI is highest in the first 6 to 12 months, but continues into adulthood.[99] Prior to the widespread usage of IVIG, the incidence of sudden cardiac death in these patients was 1% to 2%.[100]

The acute treatment for Kawasaki disease is IVIG and aspirin. The use of a single infusion of high dose IVIG, in combination with aspirin, within 10 days after onset of fever decreases the risk of coronary aneurysm formation to 3% to 5%.[97] In patients who do form aneurysms, those who receive IVIG are more likely to have regression back to a normal lumen size within the first month.[101] Aneurysms regress in size up to 2 years from disease onset, but after that point, further regression is uncommon. Overall, 50% to 75% of aneurysms will regress back to a normal lumen size and the rest will persist in size, with or without developing stenosis.[102] The long-term outcome of coronary artery aneurysms is largely dependent on peak aneurysm size, with larger aneurysms less likely to regress. Because they can have lasting complications into adulthood, children who develop coronary artery aneurysms require long-term follow-up to assess for further cardiac complication. As adults, patients with a history of Kawasaki disease and persistent coronary artery aneurysm require long-term surveillance. They should undergo close monitoring with echocardiograms and stress testing, and, because they remain at chronic risk of thrombus, they require chronic low dose aspirin therapy, and consideration of systemic anticoagulation or dual antiplatelet therapy in patients with persistent large aneurysms.[103]

Polyarteritis nodosa (PAN) is a systemic, necrotizing vasculitis that predominantly affects the medium vessels without granuloma formation. PAN is most commonly diagnosed in the sixth decade of life, although it can be seen in children as well, and is slightly more common in men. Most cases are idiopathic, although PAN can also be seen in association with

hepatitis B and C infections, certain malignancies such as hairy cell leukemia, and drug use with amphetamines. Diagnosis is based on a biopsy of affected tissue, or alternatively arteriography or MRA/CTA can be diagnostic in the right clinical setting. The clinical presentation can be variable depending on the involved organ systems and virtually every organ system can be affected, although usually PAN spares the lungs. Cutaneous, renal, neurologic, and gastrointestinal manifestations are more often seen, but cardiac involvement also occurs in the form of heart failure, anginal pain, MI, and pericarditis.[104] Although, only 10% of patients with PAN report cardiac symptoms, on autopsy cardiovascular involvement can be seen in upward of 75% of patients.[105] Treatment is with glucocorticoids, plus the addition of other immunosuppressive agents like cyclophosphamide in cases of moderate or severe disease. PAN has a poor prognosis with a 7-year mortality of 25% and 50% of patients dying within 17 years;[106] even with treatment, relapse rates are higher than in many other systemic vasculitides.

Small-Vessel Vasculitis

The two main categories of small-vessel vasculitis are ANCA-Associated vasculitis (AAV) and immune-complex-mediated vasculitis, with the latter not often affecting the cardiovascular system. However, cardiac manifestations do occur in AAV. The three AAV that can have cardiovascular involvement are granulomatosis with polyangiitis (GPA), microscopic polyangiitis (MPA), and eosinophilic granulomatosis with polyangiitis (EGPA).

GPA is a systemic, necrotizing vasculitis that primarily involves the upper and lower airways and the kidneys, causing a pulmonary-renal syndrome, but it can affect any organ including the skin, eyes, nervous system, and cardiovascular system. There is usually a prodrome of nonspecific symptoms, with fever, malaise, decreased appetite commonly seen for weeks to months before specific organ symptoms emerge. It is classically associated with c-ANCA or anti-PR3 antibodies, although a minority of patients with GPA may have positive p-ANCA or anti-MPO antibodies, or will be ANCA-negative. Renal biopsy of these patients shows a pauci-immune, focal, segmental necrotizing glomerulonephritis and biopsy of an affected artery will show granulomatous inflammation. MPA is clinically similar to GPA, although may have more neurologic involvement and less upper airway, sinus and tracheal involvement. The key distinction is lack of granulomatous inflammation on biopsy and MPA is more commonly associated with p-ANCA or anti-MPO antibodies. GPA and MPA more commonly occur in White patients, and generally present at an older age than the average systemic autoimmune disease, although they can occur at any age. Both sexes are affected at equal rates. While cardiac involvement is not classic for either GPA or MPA, when it does occur it is usually in the form of pericarditis, myocarditis, or conduction abnormalities. In one case series of patients with GPA, cardiac findings were only seen in 3.3% of patients.[107] Even if no specific cardiac abnormality is found, though, patients with GPA and MPA are at higher risk for thrombotic events and may be at increased risk of ischemic heart disease.[108] Treatment for GPA and MPA when there is severe organ involvement, is induction therapy with high-dose glucocorticoids and either cyclophosphamide or rituximab,[109] with patients then continued on either rituximab maintenance therapy or switched to another immunomodulator such as azathioprine for maintenance following induction with cyclophosphamide.

EGPA, formerly called Churg–Strauss disease, is also a multisystem AAV that often presents with asthma, chronic rhinosinusitis, and peripheral eosinophilia. EGPA is the least common of the AAVs. Its average age of diagnosis is 40 years old and there is no sex predominance. ANCAs are found in 30% to 60% of patients, and more commonly EGPA is associated with p-ANCA or anti-MPO antibodies. If biopsy of involved tissue is obtained, it classically shows eosinophilic infiltrate with granuloma surrounding small vessels. EGPA can affect any organ system, with lung and skin involvement being the most common, but of all the AAVs, EGPA is the most likely to affect the cardiovascular system. Cardiac involvement is one of the most serious manifestations of EGPA. It accounts for up to half of the attributable mortality[110] and it is more commonly seen in EGPA patients who have higher eosinophil counts at initial presentation.[111] Cardiac manifestations include heart failure, pericarditis, and conduction abnormalities. Because cardiovascular complications can be severe in these patients, during the initial workup for EGPA, careful attention should be paid to cardiovascular symptoms and it is important to obtain a baseline ECG and echocardiogram. Even when patients are asymptomatic and have normal ECGs, up to 40% may have evidence of cardiac involvement on echocardiogram.[112] The most common findings on echocardiogram are wall motion abnormalities, with valvular abnormalities, pericardial effusion, and mural thrombi also seen. Abnormal findings on ECG or echocardiogram should prompt further evaluation with CMR, where evidence of gadolinium enhancement can be used to guide biopsy, because this CMR finding has been shown to correlate with endomyocardial biopsy evidence of eosinophilia.[113] Following a suggestive CMR, patients may also need to undergo further imaging with a PET scan to differentiate active disease from fibrosis.[114]

The primary treatment for EGPA is with glucocorticoids, and for cases with cardiac involvement an additional immunosuppressive agent is added, usually cyclophosphamide. However, there is also data that rituximab can also be used as induction for severe cases of EGPA.[115,116] Azathioprine and methotrexate can also be used in less severe disease.

There are also variable-vessel vasculitides that can affect vessels of differing sizes. The most well described is Behcet's disease. Behcet's disease is a systemic vasculitis of unknown etiology that is associated with HLA-B51 and is more commonly seen in patients of Mediterranean and Japanese descent. Clinically, it is characterized by recurrent oral and genital aphthous ulcers and patients can also have cutaneous, ocular, gastrointestinal, neurologic, joint, and cardiac involvement. Cardiac Behcet's disease is seen in up to 46% of patients and can present as thrombosis, valvular disease, and inflammation involving all layers of the heart including pericarditis,

myocarditis, and coronary arteritis.[117] Arterial involvement occurs in a minority of patients, but can cause severe complications including aortitis, pulmonary artery aneurysm, and coronary artery aneurysm and occlusion leading to MI.[118] Venous involvement is more common and can include Budd Chiari syndrome as well as dural sinus and vena cava thromboses.[119] The treatment is primarily with corticosteroids and immunomodulating agents like cyclophosphamide and azathioprine, and in patients with thrombotic disease, anticoagulation is also recommended.[120]

ADULT STILL'S DISEASE

Adult Still's disease is a rare inflammatory disorder characterized by daily fevers, polyarthritis, sore throat, and an evanescent rash that tends to occur with the fever. Adult Still's disease is similar in presentation to systemic juvenile inflammatory arthritis in children; however, it has a later onset, affecting younger adults usually <50 years old, although it can be seen at any age. Laboratory findings are characterized by markedly elevated ferritin, C-reactive protein (CRP), and erythrocyte sedimentation rate (ESR). Cardiac complications are a less well-recognized manifestation of the disease, but pericardial involvement can be seen. Pericarditis has been found to occur in up to a half of patients[121] and in rare instances there can be cardiac tamponade.[122] Initial treatment is with corticosteroids and additional steroid-sparing agents are added to facilitate steroid tapering. Methotrexate is often used, but more recent studies have shown promise for alternative agents like TNF inhibitors, tocilizumab, or anakinra (an IL-1 antagonist) in severe, refractory cases.[123,124]

GOUT

While gout does not have cardiac manifestations, per se, it may be the rheumatologic disease that cardiovascular clinicians see the most in their practice. Given the frequent usage of commonly implicated medication triggers like low-dose aspirin and thiazide and loop diuretics and the prevalence of chronic kidney disease in these patients, gout flares are a common occurrence in CVD populations. More importantly, hyperuricemia, which is the necessary precondition that, with the appropriate triggers, allows for the deposition of monosodium urate (MSU) crystals in joints and gives rise to the clinical syndrome of gout, is also a proven determinant of cardiovascular risk.

Many studies over the last few decades have demonstrated an association between elevated serum uric acid levels and various cardiovascular risk factors and diseases such as arterial hypertension, stroke, and heart failure, as well as cardiovascular mortality and reduced survival in patients with heart failure.[125] The effect of hyperuricemia on CAD seems to be particularly strong in women.[126] Recent data shows that patients with gout have MSU deposition not only in their joints but also within their vasculature, including coronary vessels, which could have implications for the increased rates of CVD seen in these patients.[127]

The treatment of gout with urate lowering therapies like allopurinol, a purine base analogue xanthine oxidase inhibitor, has been shown to reduce gout flares and is associated with better outcomes in heart failure and lower risk of major cardiovascular events.[128] It is important to note, though, that another urate lowering agent febuxostat (a nonpurine xanthine oxidase inhibitor) was associated with a significant increase in all cause and cardiovascular mortality, compared with allopurinol, when used in patients with gout and CVD.[129]

HEREDITARY CONNECTIVE TISSUE DISEASES

Heritable connective tissue diseases, while not rheumatologic or autoimmune in etiology, can be associated with significant cardiac manifestations. There are many heritable connective tissue diseases involving mutations of different genes that are key to the normal formation of connective tissue. Due to these mutations, there can be weakness of blood vessel walls leading to aneurysm formation and rupture. The two most common of these types of disorders are Marfan syndrome and Ehlers–Danlos. When there is concern for a heritable connective tissue disease, in addition to undergoing routine cardiovascular screening, these patients should also be referred to a medical geneticist.

The most prevalent heritable connective tissue disease is Marfan syndrome, which is due to a mutation in the fibrillin (*FBN1*) gene. The estimated prevalence is 1 in 3000 to 5000 persons. Patients have a Marfanoid habitus and appear tall and lanky, with high palatal arch, arachnodactyly, joint hypermobility, and chest wall abnormalities. Aortic root dilatation is common in this syndrome and is part of the diagnostic criteria. Mitral valve prolapse is the second most common cardiac manifestation. These patients can have significant morbidity and mortality from aortic dissection and heart failure secondary to severe aortic or mitral regurgitation. Patients are recommended to get annual screening echocardiograms and take β-blockers to reduce stress on the aortic walls, although there is evidence that angiotensin II receptor blockers may also be cardioprotective in these patients.[130] Elective repair of the aortic root is recommended if the diameter is greater than 50 mm or if the diameter is growing by more than 5 mm annually, if there is significant regurgitation, or a family history of dissection.[131]

Ehlers–Danlos syndrome is another heritable connective tissue disease that refers to a group of six clinical disorders related to mutations in collagen genes. The overall prevalence of Ehlers–Danlos syndrome is 1:5000 with type IV, the vascular type, accounting for 8% of cases.[132] Patients with this condition have marked skin flexibility, joint hypermobility, and easy bruising, and due to the fragility of their vascular walls they are prone to aneurysm formation and rupture.

ACKNOWLEDGMENTS

We would like to thank Dr Parisa Azizad-Pinto and Dr Victor F. Tapson, who contributed to the previous version of this chapter in the 14th edition.

REFERENCES

1. Valdes AM, Menni C. Inflammatory markers and mediators in heart disease. *Aging*. 2018;10(11):3061-3062.

2. Raciborski F, Kłak A, Kwiatkowska B, et al. Diagnostic delays in rheumatic diseases with associated arthritis. *Reumatologia*. 2017;55(4):169-176.

3. Movahedian M, Afzal W, Shoja T, Cervellione K, Nahar J, Teller K. Chest pain due to pericardial effusion as initial presenting feature of rheumatoid arthritis: case report and review of the literature. *Cardiol Res*. 2017;8(4):161-164.

4. Hara KS, Ballard DJ, Ilstrup DM, et al. Rheumatoid pericarditis: Clinical features and survival. *Medicine (Baltimore)*. 1990;69(2):81-91.

5. Yousuf T, Kramer J, Kopiec A, Bulwa Z, Sanyal S, Ziffra J. A rare case of cardiac tamponade induced by chronic rheumatoid arthritis. *J Clin Med Res*. 2015;7(9):720-723.

6. Buleu F, Sirbu E, Caraba A, Dragan S. heart involvement in inflammatory rheumatic diseases: a systematic literature review. *Medicina (Kaunas)*. 2019;55(6):249.

7. Vantrease A, Trabue C, Atkinson J, McNabb P. Large endocardial rheumatoid nodules: a case report and review of the literature. *J Community Hosp Intern Med Perspect*. 2017;7(3):175-177.

8. Caforio ALP, Adler Y, Agostini C, et al. Diagnosis and management of myocardial involvement in systemic immune-mediated diseases: a position statement of the European Society of Cardiology Working Group on Myocardial and Pericardial Disease. *Eur Heart J*. 2017 Sep 14; 38(35):2649-2662.

9. England BR, Thiele GM, Anderson DR, Mikuls TR. Increased cardiovascular risk in rheumatoid arthritis: mechanisms and implications. *BMJ*. 2018 Apr 23;361:k1036.

10. Kishore S, Maher L, Majithia V. Rheumatoid vasculitis: a diminishing yet devastating menace. *Curr Rheumatol Rep*. 2017;19(7):39.

11. Bag-Ozbek A, Giles JT. Inflammation, adiposity, and atherogenic dyslipidemia in rheumatoid arthritis: is there a paradoxical relationship? *Curr Allergy Asthma Rep*. 2015;15(2):497.

12. Giles JT, Wasko MCM, Chung CP, et al. Exploring the lipid paradox theory in rheumatoid arthritis: associations of low circulating low-density lipoprotein concentration with subclinical coronary atherosclerosis. *Arthritis Rheumatol*. 2019;71(9):1426-1436.

13. Ntusi NAB, Francis JM, Sever E, et al. Anti-TNF modulation reduces myocardial inflammation and improves cardiovascular function in systemic rheumatic diseases. *Int J Cardiol*. 2018;270:253-259.

14. Amigues I, Russo C, Giles JT, et al. Myocardial microvascular dysfunction in rheumatoid arthritis quantitation by 13N-ammonia positron emission tomography/computed tomography. *Circ Cardiovasc Imaging*. 2019;12(1):e007495.

15. De Vecchis R, Baldi C, Palmisani L. Protective effects of methotrexate against ischemic cardiovascular disorders in patients treated for rheumatoid arthritis or psoriasis: novel therapeutic insights coming from a meta-analysis of the literature data. *Anatol J Cardiol*. 2016 Jan;16(1):2-9.

16. Drenkard, Cristina; Lim, S. Sam. Update on lupus epidemiology: advancing health disparities research through the study of minority populations. *Curr Op Rheumatol*. 2019;31(6):689-696.

17. Chae DH, Drenkard CM, Lewis TT, Lim SS. Discrimination and cumulative disease damage among African American women with systemic lupus erythematosus. *Am J Public Health*. 2015;105(10):2099-2107.

18. Kreps A, Paltoo K, McFarlane I. Cardiac manifestations in systemic lupus erythematosus: a case report and review of the literature. *Am J Med Case Rep*. 2018;6(9):180-183.

19. Danowksi A, Madger L, Petri M. Flares in lupus: outcome assessment trial (FLOAT), a comparison between oral methylprednisolone and intramuscular triamcinolone. *J Rheumatol*. 2006;33:57-60.

20. Muangchan C, van Vollenhoven RF, Bernatsky SR, et al. Treatment algorithms in systemic lupus erythematosus. *Arthritis Care Res. (Hoboken)*. 2015;67(9):1237-1245.

21. Ward NKZ, Linares-Koloffon C, Posligua A, et al. Cardiac manifestations of systemic lupus erythematous: an overview of the incidence, risk factors, diagnostic criteria, pathophysiology and treatment options. *Cardiol Rev.* 2020. doi: 10.1097/CRD.0000000000000358

22. Carrión-Barberà I, Salman-Monte TC, Castell S, Castro-Domínguez F, Ojeda F, Monfort J. Successful treatment of systemic lupus erythematosus pleuropericarditis with belimumab. *Eur J Rheumatol.* 2019;6(3):150-152.

23. Papageorgiou N, Briasoulis A, Lazaros G, Imazio M, Tousoulis D. Colchicine for prevention and treatment of cardiac diseases: A meta-analysis. *Cardiovasc Ther.* 2017;35(1):10-18.

24. Jain S, Thongprayoon C, Espinosa RE, et al. Effectiveness and safety of anakinra for management of refractory pericarditis. *Am J Cardiol.* 2015;116(8):1277-1279.

25. Dein E, Ingolia A, Connolly C, Manno R, Timlin H. Anakinra for recurrent fevers in systemic lupus erythematosus. *Cureus.* 2018;10(12):e3782.

26. Tariq S, Garg A, Gass A, Aronow WS. Myocarditis due to systemic lupus erythematosus associated with cardiogenic shock. *Arch Med Sci.* 2018;14(2):460-462.

27. Zhang L, Zhu YL, Li MT, et al. Lupus myocarditis: a case-control study from China. *Chin Med J.* 2015;128:2588–2594.

28. Malhotra G, Chua S, Kodumuri V, Sivaraman S, Ramdass P. Rare presentation of lupus myocarditis with acute heart failure-a case report. *Am J Ther.* 2016;23(6):e1952-e1955.

29. Zuily S, Regnault V, Selton-Suty C, et al. Increased risk for heart valve disease associated with antiphospholipid antibodies in patients with systemic lupus erythematosus: meta-analysis of echocardiographic studies. *Circulation.* 2011;124(2):215-224.

30. Wilson W, Taubert KA, Gewitz M, et al. Prevention of infective endocarditis. *Circulation* 2007;116:1736-1754.

31. Ferreira E, Bettencourt PM, Moura LM. Valvular lesions in patients with systemic lupus erythematosus and antiphospholipid syndrome: an old disease but a persistent challenge. *Rev Port Cardiol.* 2012 Apr;31(4):295-299.

32. Hoffman R, Lethen H, Zunker U, Schöndube FA, Maurin N, Sieberth HG. Rapid appearance of severe mitral regurgitation under high-dosage corticosteroid therapy in a patient with systemic lupus erythematosus. *Eur Heart J.* 1994;15(1):138-139.

33. Keenan JB, Janardhanan R, Larsen BT, et al. Aortic valve replacement for Libman-Sacks endocarditis. *Case Reports.* 2016;2016:bcr2016215914.

34. Bouma W, Klinkenberg TJ, van der Horst IC, et al. Mitral valve surgery for mitral regurgitation caused by Libman-Sacks endocarditis: a report of four cases and a systematic review of the literature. *J Cardiothorac Surg.* 2010;5:13.

35. Hakim JP, Mehta A, Jain AC, Murray GF. Mitral valve replacement and repair. Report of 5 patients with systemic lupus erythematosus. *Tex Heart Inst J.* 2001;28:47-52.

36. Wartak S, Akkad I, Sadiq A, et al. Severe bioprosthetic mitral valve stenosis and heart failure in a young woman with systemic lupus erythematosus. *Case Rep Cardiol.* 2016;2016:3250845.

37. Teixeira V, Tam LS. Novel insights in systemic lupus erythematosus and atherosclerosis. *Front Med (Lausanne).* 2018;4:262.

38. Roman MJ, Crow MK, Lockshin MD, et al. Rate and determinants of progression of atherosclerosis in systemic lupus erythematosus. *Arthritis Rheum.* 2007;56:3412-3419.

39. Nikpour M, Gladman DD, Ibañez D, Bruce IN, Burns RJ, Urowitz MB. Myocardial perfusion imaging in assessing risk of coronary events in patients with systemic lupus erythematosus. *J Rheumatol.* 2009;36(2):288-294.

40. Alarcón GS, McGwin G, Bertoli AM, et al. Effect of hydroxychloroquine on the survival of patients with systemic lupus erythematosus: data from LUMINA, a multiethnic US cohort (LUMINA L). *Ann Rheum Dis.* 2007;66(9):1168-1172.

41. Fasano S, Pierro L, Pantano I, Iudici M, Valentini G. Longterm hydroxychloroquine therapy and low-dose aspirin may have an additive effectiveness in the primary prevention of cardiovascular events in patients with systemic lupus erythematosus. *J Rheumatol.* 2017;44(7):1032-1038.

42. Brito-Zerón P, Izmirly PM, Ramos-Casals M, Buyon JP, Khamashta MA. The clinical spectrum of autoimmune congenital heart block. *Nat Rev Rheumatol.* 2015;11(5):301-312.

43. Chighizola CB, Andreoli L, de Jesus GR, et al. The association between antiphospholipid antibodies and pregnancy morbidity, stroke, myocardial infarction, and deep vein thrombosis: a critical review of the literature. *Lupus.* 2015;24(9):980-984.

44. Lim W. Prevention of thrombosis in antiphospholipid syndrome. *Hematology Am Soc Hematol Educ Program.* 2016;2016(1):707-713.

45. Tektonidou MG, Andreoli L, Limper M, et al. EULAR recommendations for the management of antiphospholipid syndrome in adults. *Ann Rheum Dis.* 2019;78(10):1296-1304.

46. Pengo V, Denas G, Zoppellaro G, et al. Rivaroxaban vs warfarin in high-risk patients with antiphospholipid syndrome. *Blood.* 2018;132(13):1365-1371.

47. Ordi-Ros J, Sáez-Comet L, Pérez-Conesa M, et al. Rivaroxaban versus vitamin K antagonist in antiphospholipid syndrome: a randomized non-inferiority trial. *Ann Intern Med.* 2019;171(10):685-694.

48. Gamoudi D, Cutajar M, Gamoudi N, Camilleri DJ, Gatt A. Achieving a satisfactory clinical and biochemical response in antiphospholipid syndrome and severe thrombocytopenia with rituximab: two case reports. *Clin Case Rep.* 2017;5:845-848.

49. Wang CR, Weng CT, Liu MF. Monocentric experience of the rituximab therapy in systemic lupus erythematosus-associated antiphospholipid syndrome with warfarin therapy failure. *Semin Arthritis Rheum.* 2017;47:e7-e8.

50. Cohen H, Cuadrado MJ, Erkan D, et al. 16th International Congress on Antiphospholipid Antibodies Task Force report on antiphospholipid syndrome treatment trends. *Lupus.* 2020;29(12):1571-1593.

51. Peoples C, Medsger TA Jr, Lucas M, Rosario BL, Feghali-Bostwick CA. Gender differences in systemic sclerosis: relationship to clinical features, serologic status and outcomes. *J Scleroderma Relat Disord.* 2016;1(2):177-240.

52. Butt SA, Jeppesen JL, Torp-Pedersen C, et al. Cardiovascular manifestations of systemic sclerosis: a danish nationwide cohort study. *J Am Heart Assoc.* 2019;8(17):e013405.

53. Kowal-Bielecka O, Fransen J, Avouac J, EUSTAR Coauthors, et al. Update of EULAR recommendations for the treatment of systemic sclerosis. *Ann Rheumat Dis.* 2017;76:1327-1339.

54. Akesson A, Wollheim FA, Thysell H, et al. Visceral improvement following combined plasmapheresis and immunosuppressive drug therapy in progressive systemic sclerosis. *Scand J Rheumatol.* 1988;17(5):313-323.

55. Toescu SM, Mansell A, Dinneen E, Persey M. Steroid-induced scleroderma renal crisis in an at-risk patient. *BMJ Case Rep.* 2014;2014:bcr2014206675.

56. Fernández Morales A, Iniesta N, Fernández-Codina A, et al. Cardiac tamponade and severe pericardial effusion in systemic sclerosis: report of nine patients and review of the literature. *Int J Rheum Dis.* 2017;20(10):1582-1592.

57. Fujisawa Y, Hara S, Zoshima T, et al. THU0432 Pericardial effusion is an independent factor predictive of scleroderma renal crisis. *Ann Rheumat Dis.* 2018;77:428-429.

58. Bissell L, Yuzaiful M, Yusof M, Buch M, Primary myocardial disease in scleroderma—a comprehensive review of the literature to inform the UK Systemic Sclerosis Study Group cardiac working group, *Rheumatology.* 2017;56(6):882-889.

59. Kavian N, Batteux F. Macro- and microvascular disease in systemic sclerosis. *Vascul Pharmacol.* 2015;71:16-23.

60. Neskovic JS, Ristic A, Petronijevic M, Neskovic B, Gudelj O. Electrocardiographic findings in systemic sclerosis. *Serbian J Experiment Clin Res.* 2018.

61. Rodríguez-Reyna TS, Morelos-Guzman M, Hernández-Reyes P, et al. Assessment of myocardial fibrosis and microvascular damage in systemic sclerosis by magnetic resonance imaging and coronary angiotomography. *Rheumatology (Oxford).* 2015;54(4):647-654.

62. Nie LY, Wang XD, Zhang T, Xue J. Cardiac complications in systemic sclerosis: early diagnosis and treatment. *Chin Med J (Engl).* 2019;132(23):2865-2871.

63. Tyndall AJ, Bannert B, Vonk M, et al. Causes and risk factors for death in systemic sclerosis: a study from the EULAR Scleroderma Trials and Research (EUSTAR) database. *Ann Rheum Dis.* 2010;69:1809-1815.

64. Khouri C, Blaise S, Carpentier P, Villier C, Cracowski JL, Roustit M. Drug-induced Raynaud's phenomenon: beyond β-adrenoceptor blockers. *Br J Clin Pharmacol.* 2016;82(1):6-16.

65. Bissell LA, Anderson M, Burgess M, et al. Management of cardiac disease in systemic sclerosis. *Rheumatology.* 2017;56(6):912-921.

66. Launay D, Sobanski V, Hachulla E, Humbert M. Pulmonary hypertension in systemic sclerosis: different phenotypes. *Eur Respir Rev.* 2017;26(145):170056.

67. Morrisroe K, Stevens W, Huq M, et al. Survival and quality of life in incident systemic sclerosis-related pulmonary arterial hypertension. *Arthritis Res Ther.* 2017;19(1):122.

68. Hao Y, Thakkar V, Stevens W, et al. A comparison of the predictive accuracy of three screening models for pulmonary arterial hypertension in systemic sclerosis. *Arthritis Res Ther.* 2015;17(1):7.

69. Roldan T, Landzberg MJ, Deicicchi DJ, Atay JK, Waxman AB. Anticoagulation in patients with pulmonary arterial hypertension: an update on current knowledge. *J Heart Lung Transplant.* 2016;35(2):151-164.

70. Yong WC, Sanguankeo A, Upala S. Association between primary Sjogren's syndrome, arterial stiffness, and subclinical atherosclerosis: a systematic review and meta-analysis. *Clin Rheumatol.* 2019;38(2):447-455.

71. Bartoloni E, Baldini C, Schillaci G, et al. Cardiovascular disease risk burden in primary Sjögren's syndrome: results of a population-based multicentre cohort study. *J Intern Med.* 2015;278(2):185-192.

72. Mofors J, Holmqvist M, Westermark L, et al. Concomitant Ro/SSA and La/SSB antibodies are biomarkers for the risk of venous thromboembolism and cerebral infarction in primary Sjögren's syndrome. *J Intern Med.* 2019;286(4):458-468.

73. Parato VM, Corradini D, Di Matteo A, Scarano M. An unusual interventricular septal bounce in a patient with dermatomyositis: a case report. *Eur Heart J Case Rep.* 2019;3(2):ytz034.

74. Schwartz T, Diederichsen LP, Lundberg IE, Sjaastad I, Sanner H. Cardiac involvement in adult and juvenile idiopathic inflammatory myopathies. *RMD Open.* 2016;2(2):e000291.

75. Deveza LM, Miossi R, de Souza FH, et al. Electrocardiographic changes in dermatomyositis and polymyositis. *Rev Bras Reumatol Engl Ed.* 2016;56(2):95-100.

76. Rai SK, Choi HK, Sayre EC, Aviña-Zubieta JA. Risk of myocardial infarction and ischaemic stroke in adults with polymyositis and dermatomyositis: a general population-based study. *Rheumatology (Oxford).* 2016;55(3):461-469.

77. Hughes M, Lilleker JB, Herrick AL, Chinoy H. Cardiac troponin testing in idiopathic inflammatory myopathies and systemic sclerosis-spectrum disorders: biomarkers to distinguish between primary cardiac involvement and low-grade skeletal muscle disease activity. *Ann Rheum Dis.* 2015;74(5):795-798.

78. Szentpetery A, Healy GM, Brady D, et al. Higher coronary plaque burden in psoriatic arthritis is independent of metabolic syndrome and associated with underlying disease severity. *Arthritis Rheumatol.* 2018;70(3):396-407.

79. Balčiūnaitė A, Budrikis A, Rumbinaitė E, Sabaliauskienė J, Patamsytė V, Lesauskaitė V. ankylosing spondyloarthritis resulting severe aortic insufficiency and aortitis: exacerbation of ankylosing spondyloarthritis and stenosis of the main left coronary artery after mechanical aortic valve implantation with cardiopulmonary bypass. *Case Rep Rheumatol.* 2020;2020:9538527.

80. Bengtsson K, Klingberg E, Deminger A, et al. Cardiac conduction disturbances in patients with ankylosing spondylitis: results from a 5-year follow-up cohort study. *RMD Open.* 2019;5:e001053.

81. Ozkan Y. Cardiac involvement in ankylosing spondylitis. *J Clin Med Res.* 2016;8(6):427-430.

82. Callhoff J, Sieper J, Weiß A, Zink A, Listing J. Efficacy of TNFα blockers in patients with ankylosing spondylitis and non-radiographic axial spondyloarthritis: a meta-analysis. *Ann Rheum Dis.* 2015;74(6):1241-1248.

83. Lee JL, Sinnathurai P, Buchbinder R, Hill C, Lassere M, March L. Biologics and cardiovascular events in inflammatory arthritis: a prospective national cohort study. *Arthritis Res Ther.* 2018;20(1):171.

84. Bowling K, Rait J, Atkinson J, Srinivas G. Temporal artery biopsy in the diagnosis of giant cell arteritis: does the end justify the means? *Ann Med Surg. (Lond).* 2017;20:1-5.

85. Monti S, Floris A, Ponte C, et al. The use of ultrasound to assess giant cell arteritis: review of the current evidence and practical guide for the rheumatologist. *Rheumatology (Oxford).* 2018;57(2):227-235.

86. Koster MJ, Matteson EL, Warrington KJ. Large-vessel giant cell arteritis: diagnosis, monitoring and management. *Rheumatology.* 2018;57(2):ii32-ii42.

87. Hay B, Mariano-Goulart D, Bourdon A, et al. Diagnostic performance of 18F-FDG PET-CT for large vessel involvement assessment in patients with suspected giant cell arteritis and negative temporal artery biopsy. *Ann Nucl Med.* 2019;33(7):512-520.

88. Sammel AM, Hsiao E, Schembri G, et al. diagnostic accuracy of positron emission tomography/computed tomography of the head, neck, and chest for giant cell arteritis: a prospective, double-blind, cross-sectional study. *Arthritis Rheumatol.* 2019;71(8):1319-1328.

89. Stone JH, Tuckwell K, Dimonaco S, et al. Trial of tocilizumab in giant-cell arteritis. *N Engl J Med.* 2017;377(4):317-328.

90. Villiger PM, Adler S, Kuchen S, et al. Tocilizumab for induction and maintenance of remission in giant cell arteritis: a phase 2, randomised, double-blind, placebo-controlled trial. *Lancet.* 2016;387(10031):1921-1927.

91. Onen F, Akkoc N. Epidemiology of Takayasu arteritis. *Presse Med.* 2017;46(7-8 Pt 2):e197-e203.

92. Gudbrandsson B, Molberg Ø, Garen T, Palm Ø. Prevalence, incidence, and disease characteristics of Takayasu arteritis by ethnic background: data from a large, population-based cohort resident in Southern Norway. *Arthritis Care Res (Hoboken).* 2017;69(2):278-285.

93. Ohigashi H, Tamura N, Ebana Y, et al. Effects of immunosuppressive and biological agents on refractory Takayasu arteritis patients unresponsive to glucocorticoid treatment. *J Cardiol.* 2017;69(5):774-778.

94. Misra DP, Wakhlu A, Agarwal V, Danda D. Recent advances in the management of Takayasu arteritis. *Int J Rheum Dis.* 2019;22 Suppl 1:60-68.

95. Mekinian A, Comarmond C, Resche-Rigon M, et al. Efficacy of biological-targeted treatments in Takayasu arteritis: multicenter, retrospective study of 49 patients. *Circulation.* 2015;3;132(18):1693-1700.

96. Matsuura K, Ogino H, Kobayashi J, et al. Surgical treatment of aortic regurgitation due to Takayasu arteritis: long-term morbidity and mortality. *Circulation.* 2005;112(24):3707-3712.

97. Dionne A, Burns JC, Dahdah N, et al. Treatment intensification in patients with Kawasaki disease and coronary aneurysm at diagnosis. *Pediatrics.* 2019;143(6):e20183341.

98. Szymanski LJ, Huss-Bawab J, Ribe JK. Coronary artery aneurysms and thrombosis in Kawasaki disease. *Acad Forensic Pathol.* 2018;8(2):416-423.

99. Brogan P, Burns JC, Cornish J, et al. Lifetime cardiovascular management of patients with previous Kawasaki disease. *Heart.* 2020;106:411-420.

100. Kato H, Koike S, Yamamoto M, Ito Y, Yano E. Coronary aneurysms in infants and young children with acute febrile mucocutaneous lymph node syndrome. *J Pediatr.* 1975;86:892-898.

101. Friedman KG, Gauvreau K, Hamaoka-Okamoto A, et al. Coronary artery aneurysms in Kawasaki disease: risk factors for progressive disease and adverse cardiac events in the US population. *J Am Heart Assoc.* 2016;5(9):e003289.

102. Gordon JB, Kahn AM, Burns JC. When children with Kawasaki disease grow up: myocardial and vascular complications in adulthood. *J Am Coll Cardiol.* 2009;54(21):1911-1920.

103. McCrindle BW, Rowley AH, Newburger JW, et al. Diagnosis, treatment, and long-term management of Kawasaki disease: a scientific statement for health professionals from the American Heart Association. *Circulation.* 2017;135(17):e927-e999.

104. Peters B, von Spiczak J, Ruschitzka F, Distler O, Manka R, Alkadhi H. Cardiac manifestation of polyarteritis nodosa. *Eur Heart J.* 2018;39(27):2603.

105. Zimba O, Bagriy M THU0332 Cardiac involvement in polyarteritis nodosa: a retrospective pathological study of 37 autopsy cases. *Ann Rheumat Dis.* 2017;76:328-329.

106. Iaremenko O, Petelytska L. Long-term patient survival in polyarteritis nodosa. *Rheumatology* 2014;53(suppl_1):i187-i188.

107. McGeoch L, Carette S, Cuthbertson D, et al. Cardiac involvement in granulomatosis with polyangiitis. *J Rheumatol.* 2015;42(7):1209-1212.

108. Berti A, Matteson EL, Crowson CS, Specks U, Cornec D. Risk of cardiovascular disease and venous thromboembolism among patients with incident ANCA-associated vasculitis: a 20-year population-based cohort study. *Mayo Clin Proc.* 2018;93(5):597-606.

109. Stone JH, Merkel PA, Spiera R, et al. Rituximab versus cyclophosphamide for ANCA-associated vasculitis. *N Engl J Med.* 2010;363:221-232.

110. Mattsson G, Magnusson P. Eosinophilic granulomatosis with polyangiitis: myocardial thickening reversed by corticosteroids. *BMC Cardiovasc Disord.* 2017;17:299.

111. Pakbaz M, Pakbaz M. Cardiac involvement in eosinophilic granulomatosis with polyangiitis: a meta-analysis of 62 case reports. *J Tehran Heart Cent.* 2020;15(1):18-26.

112. Brucato A, Maestroni S, Masciocco G, Ammirati E, Bonacina E, Pedrotti P. Il coinvolgimento cardiaco nella sindrome di Churg-Strauss [Cardiac involvement in Churg-Strauss syndrome]. *G Ital Cardiol (Rome).* 2015;16(9):493-500.

113. Cereda AF, Pedrotti P, De Capitani L, Giannattasio C, Roghi A. Comprehensive evaluation of cardiac involvement in eosinophilic granulomatosis with polyangiitis (EGPA) with cardiac magnetic resonance. *Eur J Intern Med.* 2017;39:51-56.

114. Groh M, Pagnoux C, Baldini C, et al. Eosinophilic granulomatosis with polyangiitis (Churg-Strauss) (EGPA) Consensus Task Force recommendations for evaluation and management. *Eur J Intern Med.* 2015;26(7):545-553.

115. Thiel J, Troilo A, Salzer U, et al. Rituximab as induction therapy in eosinophilic granulomatosis with polyangiitis refractory to conventional immunosuppressive treatment: a 36-month follow-up analysis. *J Allergy Clin Immunol Pract.* 2017;5(6):1556-1563.

116. Jones RB, Ferraro AJ, Chaudhry AN, et al. A multicenter survey of rituximab therapy for refractory antineutrophil cytoplasmic antibody-associated vasculitis. *Arthritis Rheum.* 2009;60(7):2156-2168.

117. Demirelli S, Degirmenci H, Inci S, Arisoy A. Cardiac manifestations in Behcet's disease. *Intractable Rare Dis Res.* 2015;4(2):70-75.

118. Yanan G, Liang T, Jianjun T, Shenghua Z, Recurrent myocardial infarction due to coronary artery aneurysm in Behçet's syndrome: a case report. *Eur Heart J Case Rep.* 2019;3(4):1-4.

119. Güngen AC, Çoban H, Aydemir Y, Düzenli H. Consider Behcet's disease in young patients with deep vein thrombosis. *Respir Med Case Rep.* 2016;18:41-44.

120. Hatemi G, Christensen R, Bang D, et al. 2018 update of the EULAR recommendations for the management of Behçet's syndrome. *Ann Rheumat Dis.* 2018;77:808-818.

121. Jara Calabuig I, Sánchez Soriano RM, Marco Domingo TF, Pérez Ortiz C, Chamorro Fernández AJ, Chamorro Fernández CI. Recurrent pericarditis as the presenting form of adult Still's disease. *Rev Esp Cardiol (Engl Ed).* 2017;70(3):208-209.

122. Parvez N, Carpenter JL. Cardiac tamponade in Still disease: a review of the literature. *South Med J.* 2009;102(8):832-837.

123. Vercruysse F, Barnetche T, Lazaro E, et al. Adult-onset Still's disease biological treatment strategy may depend on the phenotypic dichotomy. *Arthritis Res Ther.* 2019;21(1):53.

124. Kaneko Y, Kameda H, Ikeda K, et al. Tocilizumab in patients with adult-onset still's disease refractory to glucocorticoid treatment: a randomized, double-blind, placebo-controlled phase III trial. *Ann Rheumat Dis.* 2018;77:1720-1729.

125. Muiesan ML, Agabiti-Rosei C, Paini A, Salvetti M. Uric acid and cardiovascular disease: an update. *Eur Cardiol.* 2016;11(1):54-59.

126. Wu J, Lei G, Wang X, et al. Asymptomatic hyperuricemia and coronary artery disease in elderly patients without comorbidities. *Oncotarget.* 2017;8(46):80688-80699.

127. Barazani SH, Chi WW, Pyzik R, et al. Quantification of uric acid in vasculature of patients with gout using dual-energy computed tomography. *World J Radiol.* 2020;12(8):184-194.

128. Larsen KS, Pottegård A, Lindegaard HM, Hallas J. Effect of allopurinol on cardiovascular outcomes in hyperuricemic patients: a cohort study. *Am J Med.* 2016;129:299-306.e2.

129. White WB, Saag KG, Becker MA, et al. Cardiovascular safety of febuxostat or allopurinol in patients with gout. *N Engl J Med.* 2018;378(13):1200-1210.

130. Kang YN, Chi SC, Wu MH, Chiu HH. The effects of losartan versus beta-blockers on cardiovascular protection in Marfan syndrome: a systematic review and meta-analysis. *J Formos Med Assoc.* 2020;119(1 Pt 1):182-190.

131. Hiratzka LF, Bakris GL, Beckman JA, et al. 2010 ACCF/AHA/AATS/ACR/ASA/SCA/ SCAI/SIR/STS/SVM guidelines for the diagnosis and management of patients with thoracic aortic disease. A report of the American College of Cardiology Foundation/American Heart Association Task Force on Practice Guidelines, American Association for Thoracic Surgery, American College of Radiology, American Stroke Association, Society of Cardiovascular Anesthesiologists, Society for Cardiovascular Angiography and Interventions, Society of Interventional Radiology, Society of Thoracic Surgeons, and Society for Vascular Medicine. *J Am Coll Cardiol.* 2010;55:e27-e129.

132. Busch A, Hoffjan S, Bergmann F, et al. Vascular type Ehlers-Danlos syndrome is associated with platelet dysfunction and low vitamin D serum concentration. *Orphanet J Rare Dis.* 2016;11:111.

Cardiovascular Disease in Patients with HIV

Pravin Manga, Keir McCutcheon, and Nqoba Tsabedze

CHAPTER OUTLINE

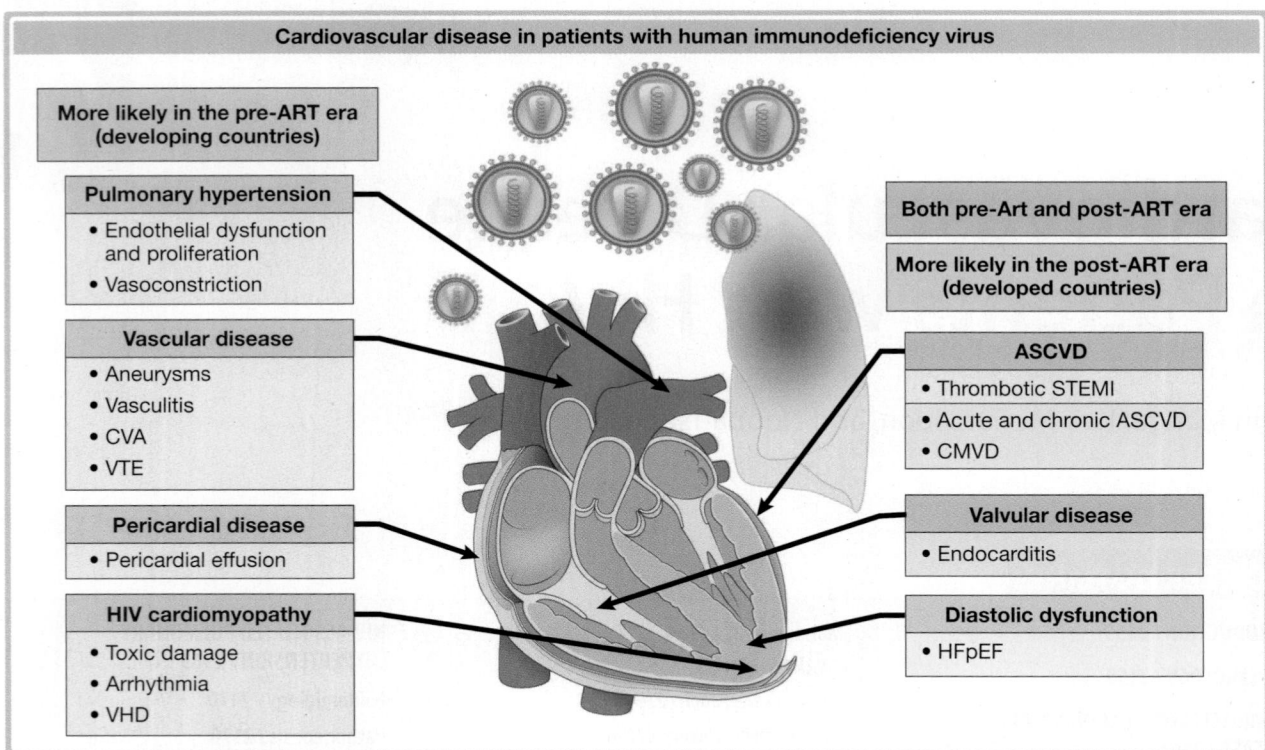

Cardiovascular disease in patients with human immunodeficiency virus

More likely in the pre-ART era (developing countries)

Pulmonary hypertension
- Endothelial dysfunction and proliferation
- Vasoconstriction

Vascular disease
- Aneurysms
- Vasculitis
- CVA
- VTE

Pericardial disease
- Pericardial effusion

HIV cardiomyopathy
- Toxic damage
- Arrhythmia
- VHD

Both pre-Art and post-ART era

More likely in the post-ART era (developed countries)

ASCVD
- Thrombotic STEMI
- Acute and chronic ASCVD
- CMVD

Valvular disease
- Endocarditis

Diastolic dysfunction
- HFpEF

Chapter 77 Fuster and Hurst's Central Illustration. Human immunodeficiency virus (HIV) affects most parts of the cardiovascular system. Certain pathologies are more prominent in patients who are not on combined antiretroviral (ART) therapy (yellow), whereas other diseases are becoming more frequent in patients who have access to ART (blue). Atherosclerotic cardiovascular disease (ASCVD) and valvular heart disease were seen in patients in the pre-ART era and are also seen in patients receiving ART (green). CMVD, coronary microvascular dysfunction; CVA, cerebrovascular accident; HFpEF, heart failure with preserved ejection fraction; STEMI, ST-segment elevation myocardial infarction; VHD, valvular hear disease; VTE, venous thromboembolism.

CHAPTER SUMMARY

This chapter focuses on current understanding of the pathogenesis and risk factors associated with heart disease in individuals with human immunodeficiency virus (HIV) infection, and discusses relevant advances in diagnosis and management. Heart disease associated with HIV infection encompasses a broad range of manifestations; infection with HIV may lead to involvement of the pericardium, myocardium, coronary arteries, cardiac valves, pulmonary vasculature, as well as the systemic vasculature (see Fuster and Hurst's Central Illustration). Depending on the level of viral suppression, patients may present with features of pericardial effusion, cardiomyopathy, ischemic heart disease, diastolic left ventricular dysfunction, pulmonary arterial hypertension, infective endocarditis, and manifestations of thrombotic events in the systemic or venous circulation. The availability of healthcare resources and combined antiretroviral therapy has had a major impact on both the prevalence and severity of cardiovascular disease as well as on short- and long-term outcomes. As many HIV infected persons are living much longer, the role of the cardiovascular specialist is increasingly important in the prevention and management of various cardiac manifestations that may develop in such patients.

INTRODUCTION

Infection with the human immunodeficiency virus (HIV) causes a number of structural and functional cardiac abnormalities as a result of persistent inflammation, drug toxicities, and opportunistic infections. The clinical scenarios are varied and dependent on levels of immunodeficiency and side effects of antiretroviral therapy (ART). Many patients with HIV, especially those in resource-rich countries, are now living longer as a result of effective combined antiretroviral therapy (cART). Thus, the cardiac presentation in these patients is now similar to that of patients without HIV. However, there remains a substantial number of patients with limited access to newer combination therapy who present with cardiac manifestations related to the acquired immunodeficiency syndrome (AIDS). The approach to the management of these two groups of people living with HIV (PLWH) is divergent and evolving. When considering the evidence presented in this chapter, it is important to differentiate data in the pre-cART era and in resource-poor settings from data obtained in the cART-era and in higher-income settings. The approach to the HIV patient is dependent on their socioeconomic background, and their management and prognosis will be determined by the ART regimen and follow-up that they receive.

EPIDEMIOLOGY

There are more than 37 million PLWH worldwide with an estimated 2 million new infections occurring annually.[1] Although the vast majority (70%) of PLWH reside in low- and middle-income countries, over 1 million people with HIV live in the United States, and more than 50% of these are over the age of 50 years (**Fig. 77-1**).[2] Based on data from over 10,000 Dutch patients, by 2030, 73% of HIV-positive patients will be older than 50 years of age and 78% of these will have cardiovascular disease (CVD).[3]

Over the last two decades, the relative risk of CVD in PLWH has decreased because of effective cART,[4] but as PLWH are living longer, the global burden of CVD has tripled (**Fig. 77-2**).[5] Compared to those patients without HIV, the increase in absolute CVD burden in PLWH on cART is due to higher rates of heart failure (HF) with and without reduced ejection fraction,[6-8] coronary artery disease (CAD),[4] and sudden cardiac death (SCD).[9]

ART has substantially changed the CVD profile in PLWH but the effects of cART on patient outcomes are complex and evolving as new, less toxic agents and combination therapies become available. Early evidence suggested a relationship between cART and CVD. One of the largest sources of cardiovascular (CV) data in HIV patients came from the Data Collection on Adverse Events of Anti-HIV Drugs (DAD) Study, which was initiated in 1999.[10] This was one of the first studies demonstrating that the incidence of myocardial infarction (MI) was increased with cumulative exposure to cART. However, it is possible that with improvements in the treatments for HIV with fewer drug–drug interactions, the risk of CVD due to cART may decline in future.[11]

Virological and immune status of individuals with HIV are important risk factors for CVD. There is substantial evidence

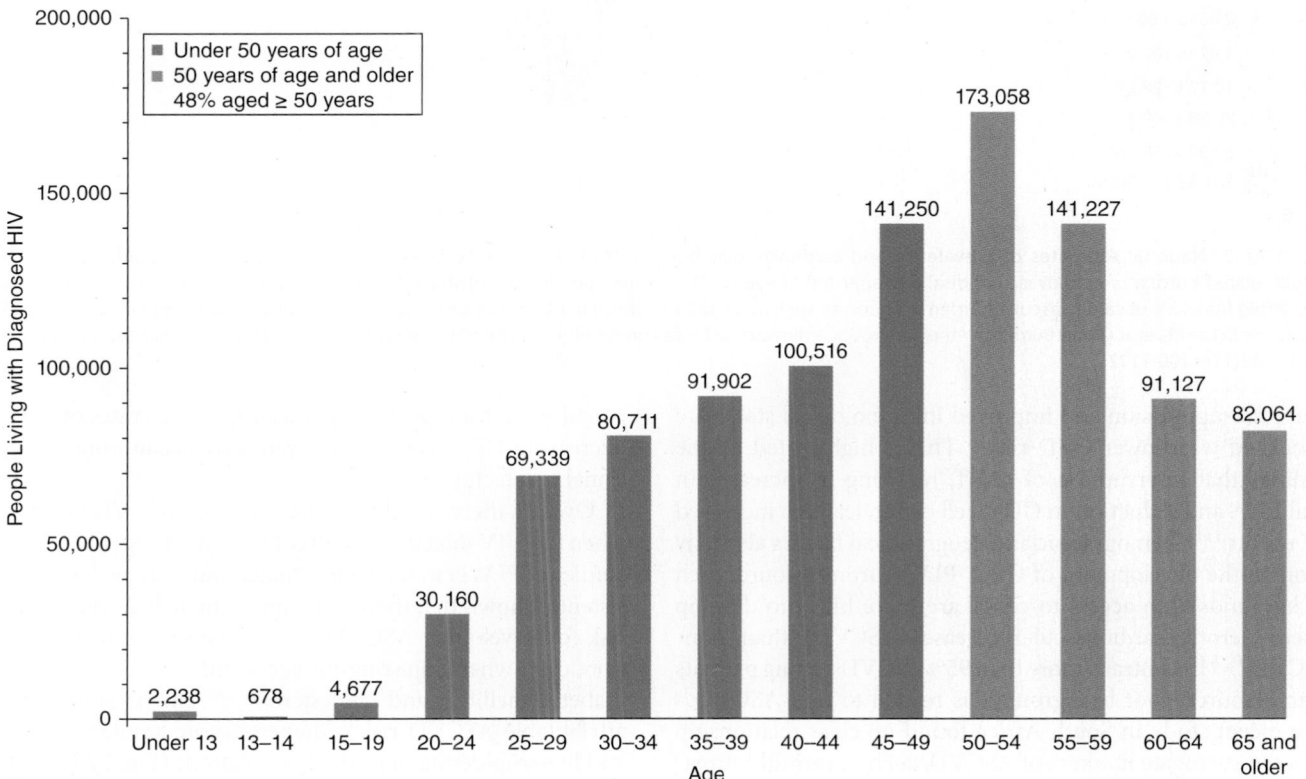

Figure 77-1. Number of PLWH in the United States per age group. Reproduced with permission from HIV Statistics. Center for Disease Control and Prevention, 2019.

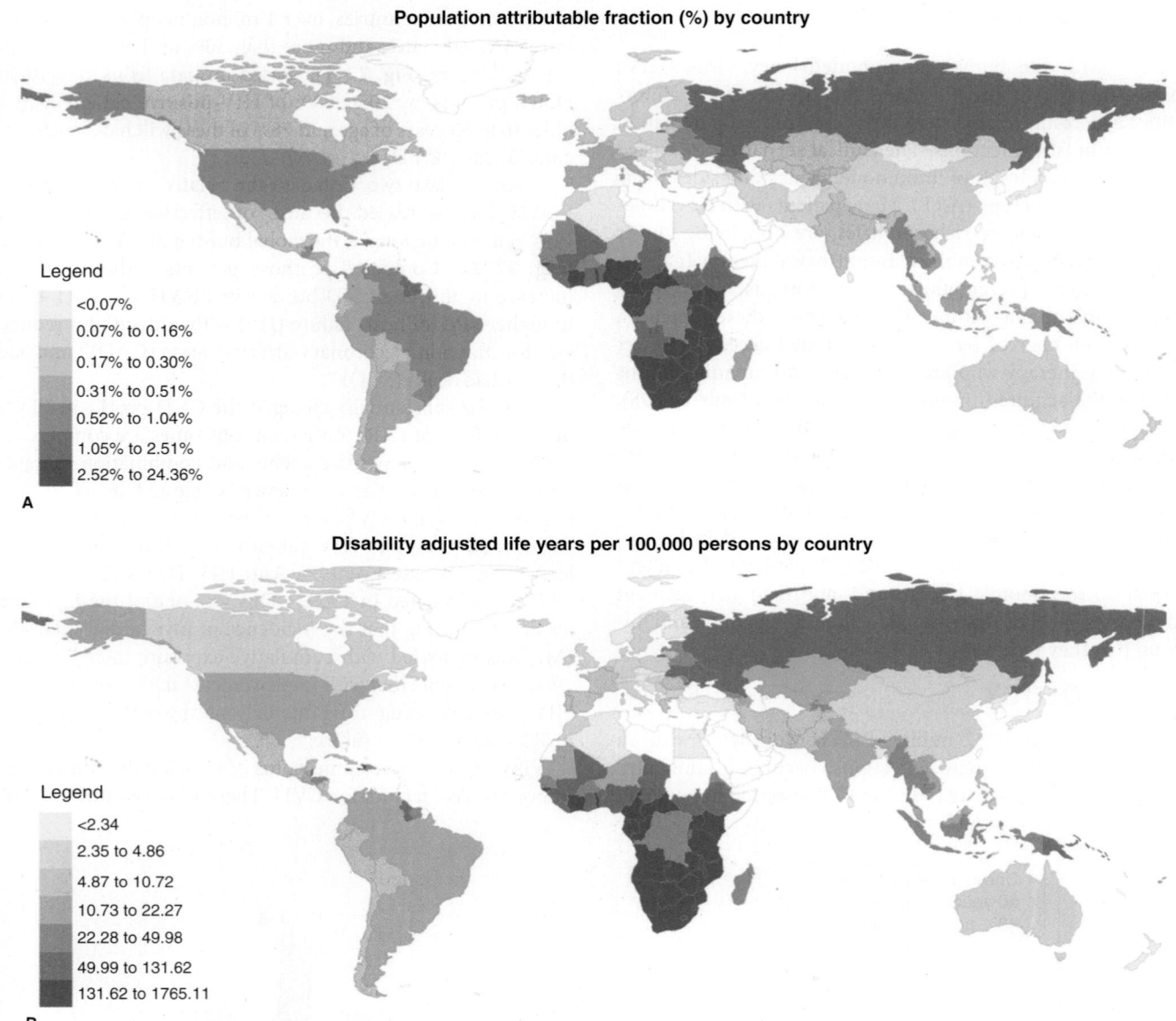

Figure 77-2. National estimates of prevalence and cardiovascular burden. (**A**) HIV-related cardiovascular burden (population-attributable fraction); (**B**) HIV-related burden of cardiovascular disability-adjusted life-years. The highest population-attributable fraction is observed in sub-Saharan countries, accounting for >15% of cardiovascular burden in countries such as Swaziland, Botswana, Lesotho, and South Africa. Reproduced with permission from Shah ASV, Stelzle D, Lee KK, et al. Global Burden of Atherosclerotic Cardiovascular Disease in People Living With HIV: Systematic Review and Meta-Analysis. *Circulation*. 2018 Sep 11;138(11):1100-1112.

that viral suppression and improved immunological status are associated with lower CVD risk.[12] This is highlighted by the findings that interruption of cART, resulting in increases in viral RNA and reduction in CD4+ cell count, leads to increased CV events.[13,14] Demographic and geographical factors also play a role in the development of CVD. PLWH from resource-rich backgrounds with access to cART are more likely to develop atherosclerotic cardiovascular disease (ASCVD) than non-ASCVD.[15,16] In contrast, more than 95% of CVD among patients from resource-poor backgrounds is related to non-ASCVD.[16] One recent study in South Africa found no clear relationship between surrogate markers of ASCVD, such as carotid intima-media thickness (CIMT) or carotid distensibility, and HIV or the use of ART,[17] whereas a large cohort study of PLWH from

North America reported significantly higher rates of MI with decreasing CD4+ cell counts even after accounting for traditional risk factors.[12]

Overall, there remains a substantial risk of CVD events even when the HIV infection is well controlled.[18] Large observational studies of PLWH in the United States and Europe, have all consistently shown that there is an approximately 2-fold increased risk for developing ASCVD-related events due to HIV infection, even when adjusting for age, gender, race, hypertension, diabetes mellitus, and cholesterol.[5,19,20] This is similar to the attributable ASCVD risk of hypertension, smoking, diabetes, and hyperlipidemia in normal populations (**Fig. 77-3**).

CVD is now an important cause of death in PLWH, contributing to 6.5% to 11.5% of overall mortality.[21,22] Moreover, PLWH

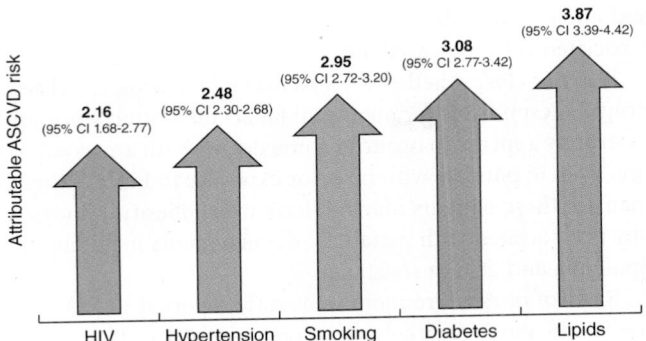

Figure 77–3. Cardiovascular risk of HIV compared with traditional risk factors. ASCVD, atherosclerotic cardiovascular disease. Data from Hsue PY, Waters DD. Time to Recognize HIV Infection as a Major Cardiovascular Risk Factor. *Circulation.* 2018 Sep 11;138(11):1113-1115.

who have CVD are generally treated less aggressively (fewer interventions than HIV-negative patients), have a greater risk of developing CV complications, and have higher CVD-related death rates compared with HIV-negative patients.

ATHEROSCLEROTIC CARDIOVASCULAR DISEASE

Risk Factors for ASCVD in PLWH

A number of studies indicate a high prevalence of traditional ASCVD risk factors in HIV-positive populations.[19] In combined data from the Women's Interagency HIV Study (WIHS) and the Multicenter AIDS Cohort Study (MACS), a high prevalence of modifiable risk factors were present in study participants.[23] However, prevalence estimates vary widely, due to differences in risk cutoffs, genetic background, geographic location, and access to cART. Many of the traditional risk factors, such as smoking, dyslipidemia, hypertension, and central obesity, are likely related to the socioeconomic factors in this population.

Smoking

In resource-rich countries, smoking rates are reported to be almost 2-fold higher in HIV-positive individuals.[10] In the United States, surveys have reported that more than 40% of PLWH are current smokers compared with 20% in the general population.[23,24] In the Danish HIV Cohort Study, nearly half of PLWH were smokers compared with only 20% in the general population.[25] Similar to HIV-negative populations, smoking was associated with an almost 3-fold increased risk of MI in active HIV-positive smokers compared with HIV-positive nonsmokers.[25]

Sex

HIV has a distinct effect on women with respect to CVD risk. Although observational studies have included predominantly male patients, data suggests that there is a higher risk of MI in HIV-infected women (relative risk [RR] 2.7–2.9 compared with the general population) versus the risk in HIV-infected men (RR 1.4).[20] The reasons for this higher risk is unclear but it may be related to higher levels of immune activation in women.[20]

Insulin Resistance and Diabetes Mellitus

Insulin resistance and diabetes mellitus are reported with increasing frequency in PLWH. In sub-Saharan Africa (SSA)

the prevalence of diabetes has been reported to be up to 26% in PLWH.[26] Risk factors in SSA for dysglycemia in PLWH include older age, male gender, and an elevated body mass index (BMI) in the overweight/obese range.[26] ARTs may also play a role in the development of diabetes. A recent report from SSA found a 2-fold prevalence of diabetes among PLWH who were on cART for more than 10 years, 90% of whom were on two nucleoside reverse transcriptase inhibitors (NRTIs) and one non-nucleoside reverse transcriptase inhibitor (NNRTI) regimen.[27] However, insulin resistance and diabetes mellitus were not increased among Danish HIV-positive patients using newer cART regimens compared with population-based age- and gender-matched controls.[28] Diabetes increases the risk of CVD events by over 2-fold in PLWH.[29]

Hypertension

HIV has been associated with an increased prevalence of arterial hypertension, but this is not a consistent association.[30] A meta-analysis of over 63,000 individuals living with HIV found that the prevalence of hypertension was 25% in the overall sample, 35% in those who were on cART, and 13% in those who were cART-naïve.[31] These rates increase to 42% in PLWH over the age of 50 years.[32] Hypertension is a well-established ASCVD risk factor and even prehypertension (130–139/85–89 mm Hg) in PLWH is associated with a 1.8-fold increased risk of MI.[33] Although it has been suggested that protease inhibitors (PIs) may predispose to hypertension, this has not been proven as findings from the DAD cohort failed to show an association between exposure to cART (including those on PIs) and the risk of hypertension.[34]

Lipid Derangements

There is a higher prevalence of dyslipidemia (elevated cholesterol and triglycerides) among PLWH, with and without cART.[23] A recent report found that women with HIV-infection status had a 2.9-fold risk of dyslipidemia as compared to HIV-negative controls.[35] The mechanism of increased LDL-C in PLWH, and associated adverse ASCVD outcomes, has been reported to be due to an increase in cholesterol absorption rather than an increase in cholesterol synthesis.[36] ART-related dyslipidemia is subsequently discussed in detail.

Antiretroviral Therapy

Certain cART agents have deleterious effects on lipid profile (**Table 77–1**), which in turn have an impact on the ASCVD risk in PLWH. This effect appears to be independent of socioeconomic background or gender. A meta-analysis of 14 trials from SSA of PLWH reported a 2.05-fold increased risk of hypertriglyceridemia after cART initiation.[37] Another smaller meta-analysis of participants from SSA showed that cART was associated with ASCVD risk in HIV-positive patients only through dyslipidemia but not through hypertension or diabetes.[38] cART use was associated with high total cholesterol (odds ratio [OR], 3.85; 95% confidence interval [CI], 2.45–6.07), high triglyceride (OR, 1.46; 95% CI, 1.21–1.75), and high low-density lipoprotein cholesterol (LDL-C) (OR, 2.38; 95% CI, 1.43–3.95) levels.[38]

Elevated total cholesterol and triglyceride levels have been specifically associated with PI use.[39] However, newer

TABLE 77–1. Effect of Anti-Retroviral Therapy on Lipid Parameters

cART	Effect	Comment
Protease inhibitors		
Lopinavir/ritonavir	↔/↑	Elevates TC and TG.
Fosamprenavir/ ritonavir	↑	Elevates TC and TG.
Atazanavir/ritonavir	↔	Protease inhibitor with best lipid profile.
Darunavir/ritonavir	↔/↑	May increase lipid levels.
NRTI		
Zidovudine	↑↑	Significant increase in TC and LDL.
Stavudine	↑↑	Significant increase in TC and TG.
Abacavir	↔/↑	TC/HDL ratio unchanged.
Tenofovir	↓	LDL and TC are reduced.
NNRTI		
Nevirapine	↓	May increase HDL level.
Efavirenz	↔/↑	May increase lipid levels slightly.
Etravirine	↔/↑	No significant effects on lipid levels.
Integrase inhibitor		
Raltegravir	↔	Low frequency of lipid abnormalities.
CCR5-inhibitor		
Maraviroc	↔	No significant effects on lipid levels.

NRTI, nucleoside reverse transcriptase inhibitor; NNRTI, non nucleoside reverse transcriptase inhibitor; TC, total cholesterol; TG, triglyceride; HDL, high-density lipoprotein; LCL, low-density lipoprotein; ↑, increases lipids; ↔, no effect on lipids; ↓, decreases lipids. Data from Vachiat A, McCutcheon K, Tsabedze N, et al: Atherosclerotic plaque in HIV-positive patients presenting with acute coronary syndromes. *Cardiovasc J Afr.* 2019 Jul/Aug 23;30(4):203-207.

combinations such as atazanavir-ritonavir have been associated with a more favorable lipid profile,[40] and switching from "boosted" PIs to raltegravir-based regimens improves total cholesterol, non–high-density lipoprotein cholesterol (HDL-C), and triglycerides.[41] The newer PI atazanavir is associated with more favorable lipid profiles and lower CV risk, whereas ASCVD risk still remains increased with darunavir.[42]

NRTIs have been associated with increased total LDL-C and HDL-C, whereas NNRTIs, integrase inhibitors, and chemokine receptor-5 antagonists do not adversely influence the lipid profile, with no increased risk of ASCVD. US guidelines caution against the use of the NRTI abacavir, in patients at high risk of CVD, because of emerging data showing an increase in ASCVD events with abacavir use.[43] In a US health-plan data set, including over 114,000 person-years of cART exposure, individuals using abacavir had a 1.43 hazard ratio (HR) of CV event compared with PLWH exposed to other cARTs.[44] At odds with this recommendation is the finding of a pooled analysis of 66 randomized controlled trials (RCTs), including over 13,000 low-CV risk PLWH on abacavir, which found no increased risk for MI or CV event.[45]

Lipodystrophy (abnormal fat redistribution with lipoatrophy and/or lipohypertrophy) can occur in some patients on cART. Lipohypertrophy, or visceral fat accumulation in the abdomen, is well described following cART initiation, and is associated with increased mortality in PLWH.

It is not clear whether a particular cART drug (or class of drug) is responsible for abnormal fat accumulation since lipodystrophy appears to occur to some degree with any combination even in patients with no prior exposure to PIs.[46] Although many of these patients may not have overt obesity, lipodystrophy is associated with metabolic derangements including dyslipidemia and insulin resistance.

Rates of obesity are more frequently reported in PLWH. In the WIHS and MACS cohorts, more than 40% of HIV-positive men and more than 60% of HIV-positive women were overweight or obese.[23] The increase in obesity is probably a function of cART-related immune reconstitution, and has been associated with an increase in noninvasive markers of ASCVD in PLWH.[47]

HIV as an Independent Risk Factor for ASCVD

HIV infection, through inflammation and immune dysfunction, is an independent predictor of ASCVD. PLWH have a stepwise increase in their risk of cardiac events, with a hazard ratio (HR) of 2.0 for those with one major ASCVD risk factor, increasing to 3.6 for those with 3 or more risk factors.[48] Ongoing viral replication may drive persistent inflammation, highlighting the importance of adherence to medication. HIV and attendant inflammation were important in conferring ASCVD risk in the Strategies for Management of Antiretroviral Therapy (SMART) trial,[13] and immunodeficiency (CD4+ cell counts <200 cells/mm^3 or a low CD4+/CD8+ ratio) is significantly associated with a higher risk of CAD.[19]

Co-Infections with Other Viruses

Coinfection with hepatitis B (HBV) or C (HCV) viruses and their influence on CVD risk in PLWH is unclear. HIV/HCV co infected patients are reported to be at elevated risk of metabolic syndrome.[49]

Pathogenesis of ASCVD in PLWH

Despite more than three decades of research in the field of HIV/AIDS, the underlying mechanisms of atherosclerotic disease in PLWH remain unclear. CAD in PLWH is thought to be the result of a number of complex interactions between inflammation, endothelial dysfunction, and coagulation disorders, which ultimately lead to atherosclerosis (**Fig. 77–4**).

Direct HIV Infection

Direct HIV infection of the coronary vascular wall appears to stimulate proliferation of vascular smooth muscle cells, and direct invasion of cardiomyocytes may lead to apoptosis.[50] However, there is no other mechanistic evidence that links direct infection of cardiac cells to the development of atherosclerosis. The endothelial dysfunction that potentially precedes coronary vascular dysfunction appears to be driven by the persistent inflammation and coagulopathy related to HIV infection.[51]

Inflammation

Rates of CV events are higher in patients with lower CD4+ counts and higher viral loads, suggesting that immunosuppression plays an important role in the pathogenesis of ASCVD.

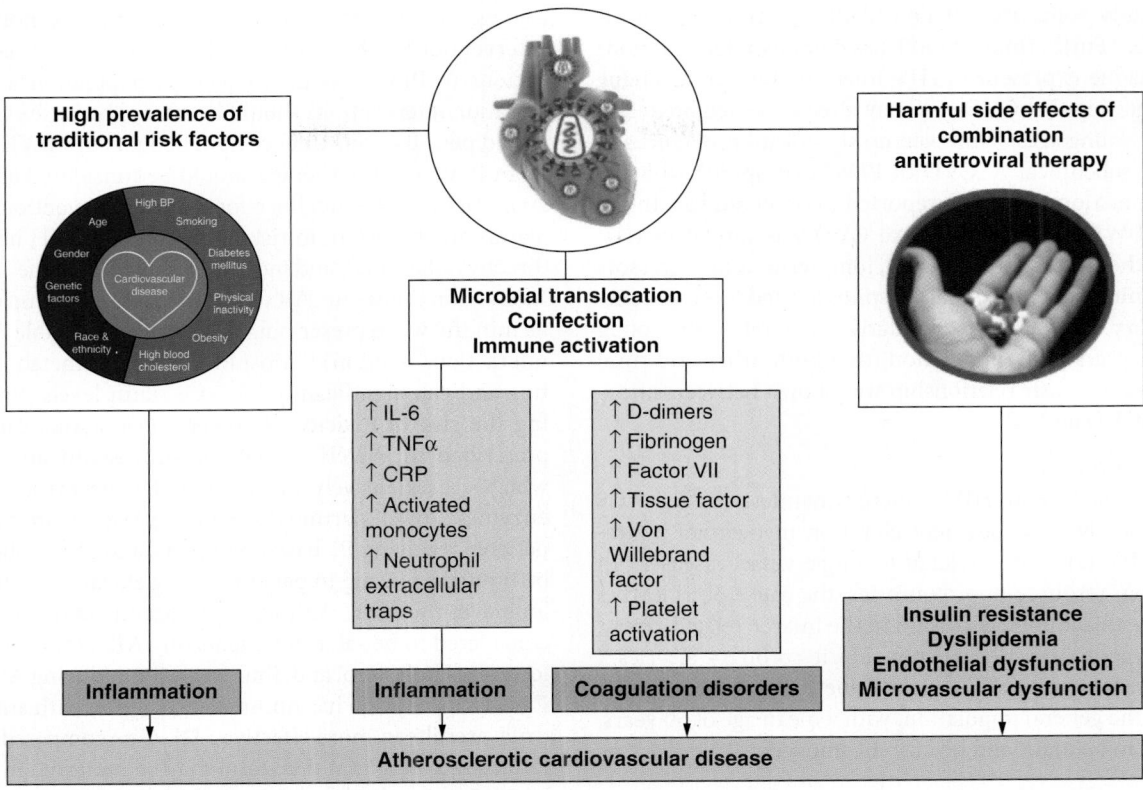

Figure 77–4. Proposed pathophysiological factors contributing to the development of ASCVD in PLWH.

Serum markers of inflammation such as IL-6, TNF-α1, and TNF-α2, and positron emission tomography-computed tomography (PET/CT) evidence for chronic inflammation are more prevalent in PLWH compared with HIV-negative individuals and have been shown to be associated with ASCVD.[52,53] Soluble CD163, CXCL10, CD14+, and CD16+ monocytes, markers of inflammation, are also increased in PLWH and have been found to be independent predictors of the presence of coronary plaque.[15] Continued viral replication, with the persistent production of viral proteins such as transactivator of transcription (Tat) and negative factor (Nef), has been implicated in stimulating vascular inflammation. However, many markers of inflammation remain elevated despite cART and viral suppression.[15,54]

Endothelial Dysfunction and Coronary Microvascular Dysfunction

Coronary microvascular dysfunction, which is predominantly caused by endothelial dysfunction, is an independent risk factor for CV events and mortality, and is a recognized complication of HIV infection.[51] Many diseases associated with chronic inflammation, such as obesity, diabetes, and rheumatoid arthritis, are associated with chronic systemic inflammation leading to endothelial dysfunction. Similarly, HIV infection causes persistent inflammation[53] and endothelial dysfunction.[55,56] Intercellular adhesion molecule-1 (ICAM-1) and vascular cell adhesion molecule-1 (VCAM-1), which are markers of endothelial dysfunction, are elevated in PLWH.[56] In a prospective study of 431 youths living with perinatally-acquired HIV, an

increased risk of endothelial dysfunction was reported, compared with age-matched controls, even after adjusting for physiologic differences.[57] Furthermore, PIs may contribute to persistent endothelial dysfunction.[51]

Coagulopathy

Abnormal elevation of D-dimers, fibrinogen, factor VII, von Willebrand factor, soluble thrombomodulin, and tissue factor levels are common in PLWH and are independently associated with the risk for ASCVD events.[15] Platelet activation, which contributes to inflammation and endothelial dysfunction, is reported to be elevated in PLWH, thus promoting hypercoagulability and thereby contributing to CV events.[58]

Presentation

Asymptomatic ASCVD

Evidence on subclinical ASCVD in PLWH is conflicting. Noninvasive imaging, such as CIMT and coronary computed tomography angiography (CCTA), has found an increased prevalence of subclinical atherosclerosis in PLWH compared with the general population.[59] Unlike atherosclerosis in the non-HIV population, the typical plaque in HIV-infected patients appears to be noncalcified atherosclerotic plaque. In a meta-analysis of 9 studies with 1229 PLWH and 1029 HIV-negative controls, the rates of noncalcified coronary plaques were higher in the HIV group (58% vs 17%).[59] A small prospective intravascular ultrasound (IVUS) study of coronary arteries in HIV patients presenting with an acute coronary syndrome (ACS), also found that atherosclerotic plaque was predominantly comprised of noncalcified fibrous and fibro-fatty plaque.[60] Furthermore, CIMT has demonstrated that non-calcified plaque is present in HIV-infected children receiving cART, suggesting that CVD risk may already be heightened in PLWH at a young age.[61] However, no significant differences in markers of subclinical ASCVD in PLWH compared with the general population have been reported in other studies. In the MACS and WIH Study, subclinical CVD was similar in HIV patients without detectable viremia, long-term nonprogressors and HIV-uninfected individuals despite elevated levels of some inflammatory biomarkers.[62] Similarly, in a relatively young (median 38 years) HIV population from both urban and rural South Africa, no clear relationship was shown between surrogates of ASCVD and HIV.[17]

Symptomatic ASCVD

Classically, ASCVD in HIV patients manifests as an ACS event, frequently as ST-segment elevation myocardial infarction (STEMI) most often related to single-vessel disease.[15] In patients from resource-poor countries, the cause of STEMI is often a large thrombotic occlusion in the infarct-related artery, with angiographically normal nonculprit coronary arteries.[63] PLWH presenting with STEMI tend to be younger than STEMI patients in the general population, with a mean age of 50 years, more likely to be male, and be current smokers.[63]

Management

Risk Assessment

Determining the risk of ASCVD in HIV patients is challenging because traditional risk calculators, such as the Framingham Risk Score, underestimate the risk in PLWH.[64] Furthermore, no long-term data in the modern ART era are yet available to identify risk patterns for PLWH on newer combinations of ART. Findings from the DAD study have been used to generate a CVD risk model for HIV patients.[29] This model incorporated traditional risks for ASCVD in addition to HIV-specific risks (such as CD4+ count, abacavir use, and exposure to PIs and nucleoside reverse transcriptase inhibitors) and was better able to predict ASCVD events than the Framingham risk score. However, HIV-specific risk calculators have not been widely validated. A recent scientific statement from the American Heart Association provides good guidance on risk stratification and management of CVD in PLWH (**Fig. 77–5**).[65]

Primary Prevention

There is no evidence from large-scale clinical trials to guide specific primary prevention for ASCVD in PLWH. Guidelines developed for the general population are of limited applicability in HIV populations in light of the exclusion of PLWH from many RCTs and lack of large-scale RCTs investigating ASCVD risk in PLWH. Nevertheless, lifestyle optimization including regular exercise is recommended in PLWH to reduce inflammation and improve cardiometabolic health.[65] Diabetes mellitus and hypertension should be managed according to current guidelines in the general population because there are insufficient data for a separate recommendation in PLWH.[65] Smoking cessation should be strongly advocated because the life expectancy of HIV-infected smokers has been found to be, on average, 8 years less than that of HIV-infected nonsmokers.[66] Interventions to help with smoking cessation are equally efficacious in PLWH as in the general population and tobacco cessation interventions should be offered because even nonsustained periods of abstinence have benefits in PLWH.[67]

In PLWH, statin therapy should be considered based on the 2019 ACC/AHA guidelines for primary prevention of CVD.[68] Statins are important in risk reduction in PLWH because they directly reduce LDL and indirectly reduce immune activation.[69] Interactions between cART and statins do exist, and one should be mindful when prescribing these drugs (see Table 77–3 "Drug interactions" section).[11] Most PIs inhibit the metabolism of statins and can significantly increase statin levels, thus increasing the risk of toxicity. However, most statins can be safely prescribed in PLWH except for simvastatin and lovastatin, which are extensively metabolized by the cytochrome P450 enzymes. Lower starting doses of atorvastatin are suggested in patients receiving PI-based regimens, and rosuvastatin should be limited to 10 mg in patients taking atazanavir-ritonavir and lopinavir-ritonavir. Although pravastatin and fluvastatin are considered to be safer in patients on cART, they are weaker in lowering cholesterol and, thus weaker at reducing ASCVD risk. Pitavastatin, which has minimal interaction with antiretroviral drugs, results in more effective LDL-C as compared to pravastatin, suggesting that this statin may be preferred in PLWH on cART. It is hoped that the Randomized Trial to Prevent Vascular Events in HIV (REPRIEVE, NCT02344290) study, which is the largest ongoing trial focusing on HIV-related CVD to date (>7500 participants and 6-year follow-up), will help clarify the benefit of pitavastatin in PLWH.

In PLWH on PIs who have hypercholesterolemia, statins could be trialed before changing the cART regimen. The addition of ezetimibe to statins has been shown to decrease LDL levels without concerns of drug interactions with cART, because it does not interact with cytochrome P450 3A4 (CYP3A4).[11] Proprotein convertase subtilisin/kexin type (PCSK9) inhibitors reduce LDL-C by approximately 60% in patients receiving standard lipid-lowering therapy. Whether PCSK9 inhibitors will prove equally effective in PLWH is currently being investigated in the EPIC-HIV study (Effect of PCSK9 inhibition on cardiovascular Risk in Treated HIV Infection; NCT 03207945). With regard to fibrates for the treatment of hypertriglyceridemia, fenofibrate is preferred over gemfibrozil due to fewer drug interactions.[11] In addition, a low carbohydrate and low alcohol diet is recommended to reduce the risk of pancreatitis.

Targeting the persistent inflammation and immune activation may lead to a reduction in the risk of ASCVD in PLWH.[70] Drawing on the CANTOS (The Canakinumab Anti-inflammatory Thrombosis Outcome Study) findings,[71] the monoclonal anti-IL-1B, canakinumab reduced plasma IL-6 and hsCRP after a single dose in ten suppressed HIV patients.[72] But larger studies with longer follow up will be required. In a phase 2 randomized, double-blind, multicenter trial in 176 PLWH, with CD4+ T-cell count ≥400 cells/μL at increased risk for ASCVD, low-dose methotrexate had no significant effect on endothelial function or inflammatory biomarkers, but was associated with a significant decrease in CD8+ T cells.[73] Several small

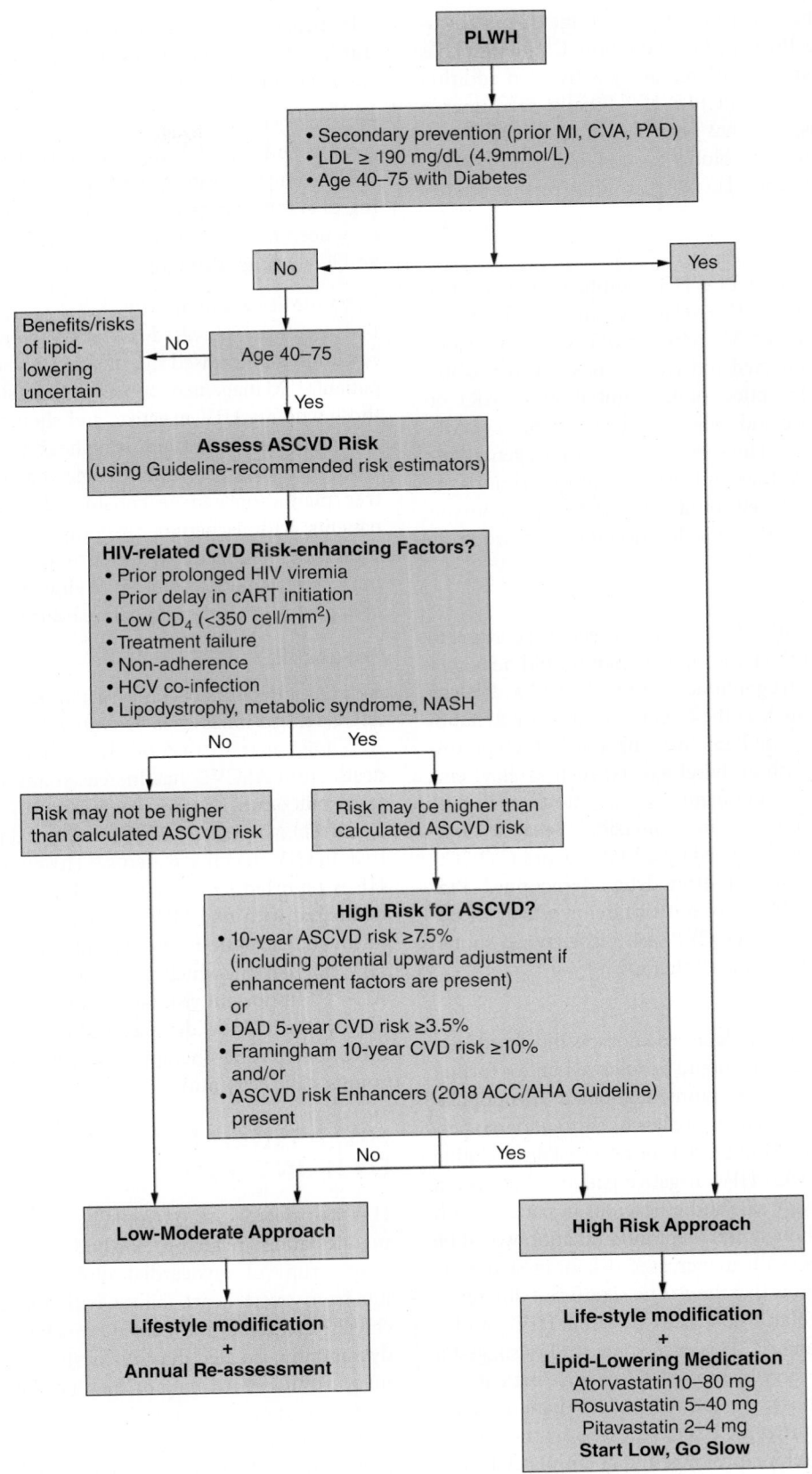

Figure 77–5. Approach to the management of atherosclerotic cardiovascular risk in PLWH.

trials are assessing the effect of antiplatelet agents on vascular surrogates, such as flow-mediated dilation. Clopidogrel has been shown to exhibit anti-inflammatory activity in addition to its antithrombotic effect in PLWH.[74] Finally, sevelamer, a drug that lowers phosphate, has been shown to reduce factors related to ASCVD, such as soluble tissue factor, and LDL-C, which may have cardiovascular benefits,[75] but further studies are warranted.

Antiretroviral Therapy

Early initiation of cART in PLWH is significantly associated with reduction of serious AIDS-related events and death at a mean follow-up of 3 years.[76] Therefore, cART is recommended for virtually all HIV-infected individuals as soon as possible after HIV diagnosis. The effect of early initiation of cART on ASCVD risk is unknown and long-term data with newer cART regimens is still needed. However, antiretroviral agents with more favorable lipid profiles and fewer drug interactions are recommended. The CD4+ cell count, HIV RNA level, genotype, and other laboratory tests should be monitored according to local guidelines.[43]

Acute Coronary Syndromes

HIV-positive patients with ACS should be treated according to current guidelines, but the treating physician should be cognizant of potential drug–drug interactions (see Table 77–4 "Drug interactions"). Agents such as the thienopyridines are metabolized by several cytochrome P450 liver enzymes, which predisposes to interactions with antiviral agents, such as efavirenz, and agents used to treat opportunistic infections, including azole antifungals, rifampicin, and isoniazid.[77] Because clopidogrel is significantly metabolized by CYP2C19 and CYP2C9, there are a number of potential drug–drug interactions.[11] Prasugrel is a reasonable alternative but ticagrelor, which is predominantly metabolized by the CYP3A4/5 isoenzyme, should be avoided in patients receiving PI therapy.[11,78]

Revascularization

Although revascularization guidelines do not specifically address PLWH, the recommendations should be followed unless further research supports alternative recommendations in this population. PLWH, in particular women, are less likely to undergo percutaneous coronary intervention (PCI) or receive a drug-eluting stent (DES) compared with HIV-negative patients.[79] However, DES appear to be similarly safe and efficacious in patients with and without HIV.[80] Although persistent inflammation would be expected to be associated with an increased risk for in-stent restenosis, several studies show that there is no significant difference in target vessel revascularization rates between HIV-positive and HIV-negative patients.[81,82] However, some studies suggest a higher rate of stent thrombosis among HIV-positive patients.[80,83] Certainly, stent thrombosis is expected in HIV patients since high platelet reactivity after PCI was reported in the EVER-E$_2$ST-HIV study.[58] Therefore, prolonged dual antiplatelet therapy (DAPT) or the use of more potent DAPT should strongly be considered after ACS in PLWH, unless contraindicated. Coronary artery bypass graft (CABG) surgery is feasible, and perioperative complications are no different from those in HIV-negative patients, even when CD4+ counts are <500 cells/mm^3. Indeed, CABG is now the most frequent cardiac surgery carried out in PLWH.[84]

Secondary Prevention

Aspirin and statin therapy are indicated in all patients after a CVD event.[68] However, as already discussed, selection and dosing of statins, antiplatelet agents, or novel oral anticoagulants may need to be adjusted depending on the background cART and likely drug–drug interactions.

Ischemic Cardiomyopathy

Because of the increased risk of CV events in PLWH, there is a concomitant increased risk of ischemic cardiomyopathy in these patients.[81] Management of such patients should be the same as for those who are HIV negative, and should follow recommended HF guidelines. Data supporting heart transplantation in PLWH are limited to case series and single-center experiences, but heart transplantation can be considered in selected HIV-positive patients with ischemic cardiomyopathy.[85] Preferably, PLWH should be compliant on cART, have CD4+ counts >450 cells/mm^3, have an undetectable HIV viral load, and have no evidence of opportunistic infection before heart transplantation.[84]

Prognosis

As HIV infection becomes a chronic disease, death due to AIDS-related illnesses is declining. In-hospital mortality from ACS is similar to that of HIV-negative patients.[15] However, death from ASCVD has increased among PLWH[86] and long-term outcomes remain worse for PLWH after a CV event. Recurrent MI post-ACS has been found to be higher in PLWH than in HIV-negative patients.[83] Hospitalization for episodes of HF is reported to be twice as likely in HIV-infected patients compared with non-HIV-infected patients.[81] This may be due to subclinical systolic and diastolic dysfunction in the broader HIV population, which only manifests after a first episode of ACS.[87,88] Important risk factors for death include the presence of chronic kidney disease, nucleoside reverse transcriptase inhibitor–sparing therapy, low ejection fraction, and CD4+ counts <200 cells/mm^3.[81,83]

HIV-ASSOCIATED MYOCARDIAL DYSFUNCTION

HIV-associated cardiomyopathy is one of the many cardiac manifestations related to chronic HIV infection. It represents a spectrum of myocardial diseases seen in PLWH, ranging from overt heart failure with reduced ejection fraction (HFrEF) (stage C–HF), asymptomatic left ventricular systolic dysfunction, isolated diastolic dysfunction (stage B–HF), focal myocarditis, which may or may not be associated with myocardial regional wall motion abnormalities, and heart failure with preserved ejection fraction (HFpEF).[88] The incidence and prevalence of these myocardial abnormalities in PLWH vary significantly between low-middle income countries (LMICs) and high-income countries, and have evolved from primarily systolic dysfunction to now reflect the growing recognition of isolated diastolic dysfunction.[89] The manner in which

HIV-associated myocardial dysfunction presents clinically is directly related to access to cART and its attendant maintenance of immune function and low HIV viral load.[16]

Epidemiology

The global adoption of the World Health Organization (WHO)-endorsed strategy of testing for HIV and treating all positive patients, has transformed HIV infection into a chronic disease, with PLWH having a near-normal life expectancy. Noncommunicable diseases have become the primary drivers of morbidity and mortality, with ischemic heart disease and HF dominating.[5]

The widespread use of cART has directly led to the decline of the incidence of HIV-associated cardiomyopathy from 25.6 to 3.9 cases per 1000 person-years.[90] However, this disease still remains an important cause of congestive HF in resource-poor settings where access to cART is restricted and a significant proportion of the population complicate with AIDS.[16] The Veterans Aging Cohort Study (VACS) found that PLWH have an elevated risk of HFrEF and HFpEF, ranging from 1.5 to 2-fold compared with uninfected individuals, even after adjusting for confounders and for ischemic heart disease (**Fig. 77–6**).[6] This study also showed that among PLWH, the most common incident forms of HIV-associated cardiomyopathy were HFrEF (37%), HFpEF (34%), and borderline HFpEF (15%).[6] A large administrative database of more than 36,000 PLWH found that although the absolute HF prevalence was higher in older PLWH, women and younger persons carried the highest relative risk.[91] Importantly, ischemic heart disease is now reported to be responsible for HF in two-thirds of PLWH.[15]

Although diminished immune status, with a high HIV viral load and a low CD4$^+$ cell count is associated with a greater HF risk, the VACS found that despite having less than 500 HIV viral RNA copies/mL and a CD4$^+$ count greater than 500 cells/mm^3, PLWH were still more likely to develop HIV-associated cardiomyopathy than uninfected individuals.[6,91]

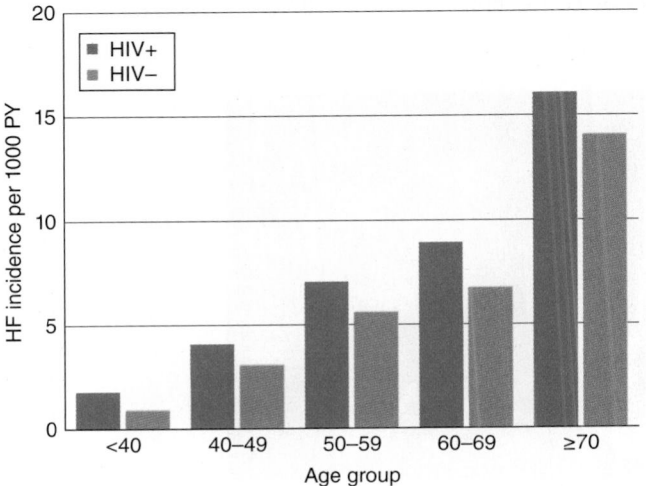

Figure 77–6. Incidence of heart failure in the Veterans Aging Cohort Study according to HIV status. PY, person-years. Reproduced with permission from Savvoulidis P, Butler J, Kalogeropoulos A. Cardiomyopathy and Heart Failure in Patients With HIV Infection. *Can J Cardiol.* 2019 Mar;35(3):299-309.

Etiology and Pathogenesis

Several hypotheses for the pathogenesis of HIV-associated cardiomyopathy have been postulated (**Fig. 77–7**).[16] Globally, a large proportion of PLWH are from SSA, and a significant number of these individuals from LMICs are not on optimal cART and live with uncontrolled HIV. This population remains at risk of HIV-driven myocardial inflammation, fibrosis, and apoptosis leading to congestive HF, features previously labeled as characteristic of AIDS cardiomyopathy.[16] For those on cART, HIV itself and possibly cART may also produce myocardial dysfunction by promoting inflammation, myocardial fibrosis, apoptosis, and steatosis.[92] Emerging data suggests that HIV-associated immune dysregulation, HIV-mediated chronic inflammation, and accelerated patchy myocardial fibrosis cause HIV-induced diastolic dysfunction.[88]

The increased incidence of ischemic heart disease seen in PLWH from economically developed countries also suggests that HIV-mediated ASCVD and increased thrombogenicity drives MI, which contributes to an increased incidence of ischemic cardiomyopathy.[93]

Recreational substance misuse is another potential etiology for HIV-associated cardiomyopathy. The misuse of alcohol, smoking, methamphetamine, and cocaine have been reported to be common in PLWH.[15,16] However, their true contribution to the burden of HIV-associated cardiomyopathy may be small based on the VACS analysis, given that the risk for HF in this study remained high after controlling for confounders such as substance abuse.[6]

Traditionally, the PI group of antiretroviral drugs has been associated with increased cardiovascular mortality and rehospitalisation for HF.[94] These group of drugs are no longer first line agents for cART. Old-generation antiretroviral drugs such as NRTIs raised concerns about the development of cardiomyopathy. These concerns have diminished with contemporary NRTIs such as abacavir.[95] To date, there are no data on the association of other antiretrovirals with HF. Furthermore, despite these hypothetical concerns, the benefits of early and sustained cART outweigh any potential antiretroviral drug-related harms.[76]

Clinical Presentation

Asymptomatic Manifestations (Stage B–HF)

A growing body of literature suggests that there is an increasing prevalence of subclinical myocardial disease among PLWH. In a meta-analysis of 2242 PLWH on cART, from economically developed countries, diastolic dysfunction was diagnosed in 43.4% and only 8.3% had systolic dysfunction.[96] A recent cardiac magnetic resonance (CMR) imaging study reported impaired radial, longitudinal, circumferential strain and strain rate in PLWH with preserved systolic function,[97] which has even been reported in younger PLWH.[96] However, the long-term consequences of these asymptomatic myocardial systolic and diastolic abnormalities remain unknown.

CMR imaging studies in asymptomatic HIV-positive patients on cART and without known CVD found that myocardial fibrosis and cardiac steatosis were prevalent in these patients (**Fig. 77–8**).[98,99] These myocardial tissue changes have

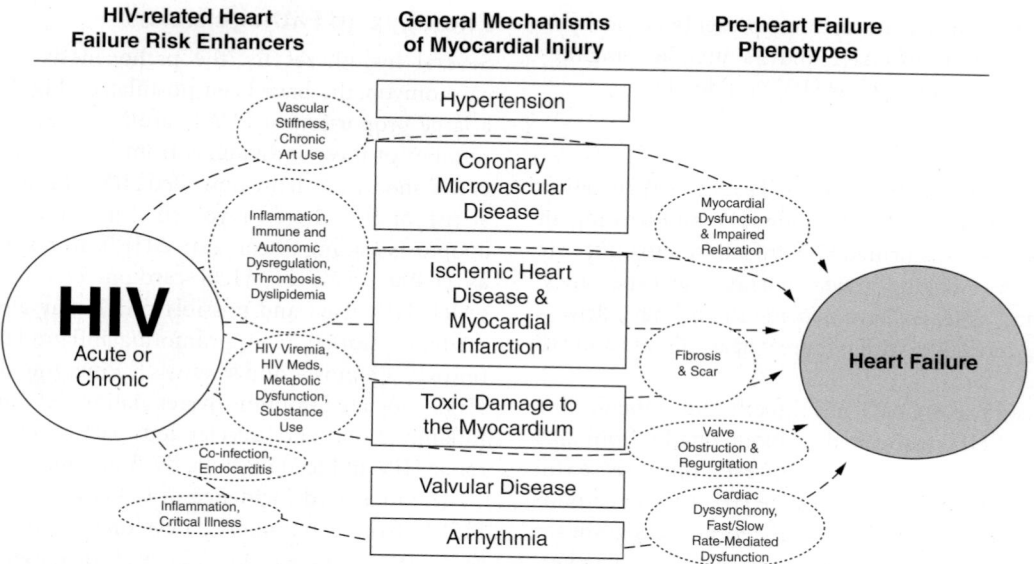

Figure 77–7. Proposed mechanisms of myocardial dysfunction and heart failure in PLWH. ART, anti-retroviral therapy. Reproduced with permission from Feinstein MJ, Hsue PY, Benjamin LA, et al.: Characteristics, Prevention, and Management of Cardiovascular Disease in People Living With HIV: A Scientific Statement From the American Heart Association. *Circulation.* 2019 Jul 9;140(2):e98-e124.

been postulated to underlie the myocardial dysfunction seen in this population. In one study, PLWH on cART had a 47% higher median myocardial lipid level compared with control subjects.[98] Furthermore, patchy myocardial fibrosis in the basal inferolateral wall of the left ventricle was noted in 76% of PLWH compared with 13% of control subjects.[98] The cardiac steatosis is hypothesized to be the sequel of chronic exposure to cART induced hyperlipidemia and dysglycaemia.[98,99]

PLWH on cART have been reported to have higher rates of diastolic dysfunction and at a younger age when compared with age-matched controls.[100] On CMR imaging with myocardial tagging, peak myocardial systolic and diastolic longitudinal strain has been found to be significantly lower in PLWH.[98] In the Characterizing Heart Function on Antiretroviral Therapy (CHART) study, PLWH with diastolic dysfunction had higher levels of fibrosis compared to PLWH and having no diastolic dysfunction.[101] The long-term consequences of diastolic dysfunction in PLWH are eagerly awaited as there is a growing concern about the link between diastolic dysfunction, HFpEF, and morbidity and mortality in PLWH.

Symptomatic Manifestations (Stage C–HF)

In the pre-ART era, cases of severe systolic dysfunction associated with a dilated cardiomyopathy were common in PLWH, with a reported prevalence ranging from 2% to 20%.[87] During this time, direct viral effects on the myocardium, opportunistic infections, nutritional deficiencies, and severe immunosuppression were presumed to be the causes of HIV-associated cardiomyopathy.[89,96] In the current cART era, there is a paucity of data on symptomatic HF in PLWH.

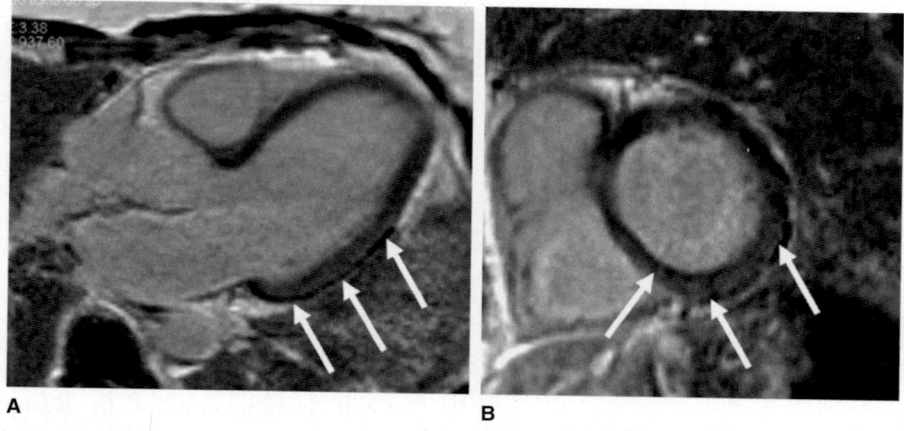

Figure 77–8. Cardiac MRI image demonstrating features of myocarditis in a HIV patient with heart failure. (A) Diffuse, patchy mid-wall late gadolinium enhancement in the basal-to-mid inferior wall and a small overlying pericardial effusion likely indicating prior myocarditis; **(B)** Short axis image of the same patient showing mid-wall enhancement in the inferior septum, basal inferior wall, and inferolateral wall (*white arrows*). Reproduced with permission from Dr. Ntobeko Ntusi, University of Cape Town.

Prognosis and Therapy

HIV-associated cardiomyopathy may portend a poor HF prognosis. A recent US healthcare system-based cohort study, which investigated the long-term outcomes of HF in women living with HIV, found higher rates of HF hospitalization, cardiovascular mortality, and all-cause mortality, compared with HIV-negative women with HF.[102] Furthermore, left ventricular dysfunction and a high viral load have been identified as predictors of SCD in PLWH.[103] These findings should motivate clinicians to have a high index of suspicion for HIV-associated cardiomyopathy in PLWH, and all PLWH presenting with signs and symptoms of HF should have assessment of their left ventricular function. This form of clinical screening should be eagerly pursued in those with a high cumulative viremia, low CD4+ cell count, and a history of substance abuse.

To date, there are no prospective randomized trial data guiding the management of HF in PLWH. Existing HF workup and management guidelines should be followed equally in PLWH as in uninfected HF patients. Despite the recommendation to follow current guidelines, prescribers should be aware of potential drug–drug interactions when prescribing multiple medications in PLWH who have HF (see section Drug Interactions). HF devices such as cardiac resynchronization therapy, implantable cardiac defibrillators, and left ventricular assist devices, and appropriate indication for their use, should all be considered in PLWH. Moreover, given the improved life expectancy that PLWH have when treated optimally with cART, heart transplantation is no longer contraindicated in these patients.

PERICARDIAL DISEASE IN HIV

Before the widespread introduction of cART, pericarditis and pericardial effusion were the most frequent cardiac manifestations in PLWH with prevalence estimates ranging from 11% to 40%.[104] In resource rich settings where there is almost universal coverage of cART the prevalence of pericarditis and pericardial effusion has diminished markedly.[105] In patients in whom pericardial effusion is found, it is generally small and patients are often asymptomatic.

Etiology

The etiology of pericardial effusion in the majority of patients is unknown but it may be a result of immune deficiency.[104] In those who are symptomatic, the majority are related to an infection or malignancy. Many HIV-positive patients are at heightened risk of numerous infections, which include bacterial infections as well as infections due to nocardia, cytomegalovirus, and cryptococcus. Malignancies such as Kaposi's sarcoma and lymphomas have been associated with pericardial effusion and pericardial tamponade in HIV-positive patients.[16]

In many resource-limited countries, tuberculosis is endemic. *Mycobacterium tuberculosis* has been reported to account for up to 90% of infections in patients who are HIV-positive presenting with pericardial effusion.[106] However, in developed countries, tuberculous pericarditis is very uncommon.

Clinical Presentation and Diagnosis

In the majority of HIV patients, the pericardial effusion is very small and thus most patients are asymptomatic. The effusion is often diagnosed incidentally on chest radiography or echocardiography. Those patients with much larger effusions will present most often with dyspnoea, fatigue, fever, or chest pain. About a third of these may develop cardiac tamponade with its attendant clinical features of raised jugular venous pressure, tachycardia, and diminished blood pressure. Myopericarditis, as defined by elevated creatine kinase myocardial band (CK-MB) or troponin T elevation and diminished left ventricular systolic dysfunction, was found to be present in 80% of HIV-positive patients presenting with tuberculous pericarditis.[107] Constrictive pericarditis is much less likely to occur in HIV-positive patients with pericardial effusion as compared with HIV-negative patients.[16]

The diagnostic evaluation should be dictated by geography and clinical presentation but would be similar to those of pericardial effusion in an HIV-negative patient. In moderate-to-large effusions, pericardiocentesis should be considered with appropriate analysis of pericardial fluid including cultures for bacteria and tuberculosis as well as cytological analysis. To improve diagnostic yield, pericardioscopy together with targeted pericardial biopsies with modern molecular biological tests should be considered because pericardial biopsies are more sensitive than pericardial fluid smears or cultures.

Prognosis and Management

The presence of pericardial effusion is associated with a poorer prognosis.[104] It is likely that the poor prognosis of pericardial effusion is related to diminished immune status associated with advanced HIV infection. In the pre cART era, in HIV-positive patients with AIDS and pericardial effusion, the mortality was almost nine-fold (64% vs 7 %) at the end of 6 months, as compared with HIV-positive patients with AIDS without pericardial effusion.[104] In developing regions, the mortality from tuberculous pericarditis in HIV-positive patients is twice as high as compared to HIV-negative patients with tuberculous pericarditis.[108]

In HIV-infected patients with pericardial effusion, the management is based on etiology and severity of the effusion. If the patient is not on cART at time of presentation, then this should be initiated. Asymptomatic patients with small effusions require no treatment other than regular observation. Patients with large effusions who are symptomatic will require pericardial drainage and appropriate diagnostic testing. Those with tamponade will require immediate drainage and diagnostic evaluation.

Bacterial or fungal infection should be treated with appropriate antimicrobial therapy. In HIV-positive patients with tuberculous pericarditis, treatment with oral prednisolone is contraindicated due to the 3-fold higher risk of HIV-associated malignancy.[109]

HIV-ASSOCIATED PULMONARY HYPERTENSION

HIV-associated pulmonary artery hypertension (HIV-PAH) is a well-defined clinical entity in PLWH, but the pathophysiology is unknown. It falls under the group 1 WHO classification of pulmonary hypertension together with idiopathic PAH.[110]

Epidemiology

HIV-PAH is an uncommon condition and reported to occur in 0.5% of HIV-positive patients in the pre-cART era, but surprisingly this prevalence has remained unchanged even after cART became the standard of care.[111] It is more common in men and, despite its overall low prevalence, it is still 6 to 12-fold higher as compared to PHT in HIV-negative patients.[111] Furthermore, the 2018 revised definition of PAH, in which the mean pulmonary pressure has been lowered from 25 to 20 mm Hg will clearly have an effect on the epidemiology and therapy of HIV-PAH in future.[112] The prevalence in developing nations is unclear, but a recent report suggested prevalence rates varying from 0.5% to 5%.[113]

Pathogenesis

The histology of HIV-PAH is identical to that found in idiopathic PAH. Several mechanisms have been postulated for the development of the characteristic plexiform lesions in HIV-PAH and these include induction of many mediators of inflammation, vasoconstrictors, and growth factors. HIV nucleic acids are absent in these plexiform lesions suggesting that HIV acts in an indirect way on the pulmonary vasculature with inflammatory pathways being the most likely trigger in susceptible individuals.[16] HIV-1 viral proteins, such as glycoprotein 120 (Gp 120), Tat, and Nef, contribute to HIV-PAH via a number of pathways leading to endothelial injury, promotion of smooth muscle cell proliferation, and induction of oxidative stress. Gp120, which induces entry of HIV into CD4+ lymphocytes and macrophages, targets human lung endothelial cells leading to secretion of endothelin-1, which in turn promotes vascular constriction.[114] Furthermore, there is induction of a proinflammatory and procoagulant state by stimulation of cytokines, such as IL-6, TNFα, and platelet-derived growth factor.[115]

Clinical Presentation and Diagnosis

Patients with HIV-PAH present with nonspecific and insidious symptoms that are indistinguishable from idiopathic PAH. Characteristic symptoms include progressive dyspnea, chest discomfort, fatigue, nonproductive cough, dizziness, and syncope.[111]

Echocardiography is the preferred initial investigation of choice, but its sensitivity is less than that of right heart catheterization. Until recently, screening for PAH in HIV-infected patients without symptoms in regions with low prevalence was not recommended.[111,116] However, this recommendation has been updated in 2018, in that for patients with risk factors such as female sex, co infection with hepatitis C, intravenous drug use such as cocaine, origin from a high HIV-prevalence country, and African American patients, screening by echocardiography is advised independent of symptoms.[117] Diagnosis of HIV-PAH is identical to that in a non-HIV patient. All potential causes of PAH need to be excluded. Following echocardiography, right heart catheterization is the gold standard for evaluation of the hemodynamics in HIV-PAH. Because of the very low rate (<2%) of positive pulmonary artery vasoreactivity in HIV-PAH, vasoreactivity testing is not recommended in these patients.[116]

Prognosis and Therapy

The diagnosis of HIV-PAH is associated with a poor survival rate. In the pre-cART era and absence of specific PAH therapy, the 1-year mortality rate was reported to be as high as 50%.[118] It is still not clear whether cART impacts on prognosis in patients with HIV-PAH. Although some early reports suggested that initiation of cART was associated with a fall in pulmonary artery pressures, a later study demonstrated no change in right heart pressures over a mean follow-up period of 37 months in those HIV-PAH patients who were treated with cART but did not receive specific PAH therapy.[119] A large prospective French cohort study also showed no change in prevalence of HIV-PAH after initiation of cART, suggesting that cART at the very least does not cause PAH.[111] Despite the lack of clarity on the benefits of introduction of cART to pulmonary artery pressures in patients with HIV-PAH, the overall survival has improved in the post cART era. A retrospective review of 77 patients who received guideline-mandated therapy for HIV and specific PAH therapy reported overall survival to be 88% at 1 year and 72% at 3 years.[119] In this study and consistent with other studies, survival was worse in patients who were in New York Heart Association in (NYHA) functional class IV.[119] Factors associated with inadequate or poor HIV control, such as low CD4+ lymphocyte counts and detectable viral loads were also found to be related to increased severity of HIV-PAH.[119] The REVEAL registry suggested that survival in HIV-PAH may in fact be slightly better than other forms of PAH with a reported 1-year survival rate of 93% for HIV-PAH versus 88% for idiopathic PAH.[120]

All patients with HIV should receive cART as per current guidelines. However, in patients with HIV-PAH, one has to be aware of potential drug interactions. In addition to cART, a similar treatment protocol used for patients with idiopathic PAH should also be considered for patients with HIV-PAH.[116] The current recommendation is to avoid anticoagulation in patients with HIV-PAH because there is insufficient evidence to support its use.[116] There is little benefit of calcium-channel blockers in patients with HIV-PAH, while prostanoids in HIV-PAH patients have shown improvements in symptoms and hemodynamics.[16] The use and benefit of sildenafil have only been reported in a few patients with HIV-PAH.[121] Combination of sildenafil with certain antiretroviral therapies such as indinavir, saquinavir, and ritonavir should be avoided because it may significantly increase the side effects of sildenafil. Tadalafil levels are only partially affected by ritonavir and guidelines recommend close monitoring once tadalafil treatment is commenced.[122] Treatment with an endothelin-1 receptor antagonist such as bosentan in HIV-PAH patients may be useful but in patients on ritonavir, bosentan should be started at lower doses because its level may be increased by ritonavir.[123] Newer endothelin receptor blockers such as macitentan and ambrisentan have replaced bosentan because they are associated with less liver derangements. Macitentan, a dual endothelin-receptor antagonist, has been shown to significantly reduce mortality and morbidity in patients with pulmonary artery hypertension of different etiologies, including HIV-PAH.[124]

VALVULAR AND VASCULAR DISEASE

Valvular Heart Disease

The prevalence of valvular diseases in PLWH is common with an echocardiographic study documenting up to 77% of patients having valvular regurgitation and the risk of valve disease was not related to CD4$^+$ cell counts or viral load.[125] In the majority of these patients, the regurgitation was documented as mild with only 4.7% having clinically significant regurgitation and only 0.4% having significant mitral stenosis.[125]

The risk of infective endocarditis in HIV-positive persons is similar to HIV-negative high-risk populations such as those who abuse drugs.[126] There is a 4-fold increase in the risk of developing infective endocarditis in HIV-positive patients with extremely low CD4$^+$ counts (<50 cells/mm^3) and high viral loads exceeding 100,000 copies/mL.[126] In developed countries, where most of the patients are on cART, infective endocarditis is found in restricted populations such as intravenous drug abusers, but in developing countries, rheumatic heart disease is frequently the underlying risk pathology.[126,127]

The clinical presentation of infective endocarditis and its management are identical to those of HIV-negative patients with infective endocarditis and are defined by the location of which valve is infected. In intravenous drug abusers the valve site is most commonly the tricuspid valve with *Staphylococcus aureas* the most common causative organism.[126] Resistance to penicillin is almost universal for *S. aureus* infections but even methicillin resistance to *S. aureus* infections in HIV-infected persons has been reported.[126,128] There is marked variability in the incidence of culture-negative infective endocarditis.

It is recommended that guideline-recommended therapy be followed for bacteriological as well surgical treatment. Prognosis is similar in patients with infective endocarditis whether patients are HIV-positive or HIV-negative.[127] Mortality in HIV-infected persons with infective endocarditis does appear to be higher in those who are immunocompromised with low CD4$^+$ cell counts (<200 cells mm^3).[16] A report from the United States found that that the rate of surgery for infective endocarditis in HIV-positive patients had fallen from 32% to 8% in a period of 10 years from 2000 to 2010 and at the end of the study period, HIV was no longer a risk predictor for operative mortality.[129]

VASCULAR DISEASE

Peripheral Arterial Disease

Risk factors for atherosclerotic cardiac disease such as smoking, hypertension, diabetes, and hyperlipidemia are more prevalent in HIV-positive individuals. The estimated prevalence of peripheral arterial disease (PAD) in PLWH is variable depending on age of study participants. The largest study to date, which assessed 91,953 participants from the VACS, with no PAD at baseline, found a cumulative PAD incident rate of 11.9 events per 1000 person-years as compared with 9.9 events per 1000 person-years in uninfected veterans.[130] More importantly, this study also found that HIV disease itself contributed to a 19% increased risk of developing PAD over the 9-year follow-up period, independent of traditional risk factors for PAD.[130] This study also found that once PAD has developed, HIV increases the risk of mortality compared with HIV-negative subjects. Immune deficiency plays a role in that the incident PAD risk was nearly double in those HIV-positive patients with sustained CD4$^+$ cell counts <200 cells mm^3 whereas those with sustained CD4$^+$ cell counts >500 cell mm^3 had no excess risk of PAD as compared with HIV-negative veterans.[130] This study clearly suggests that HIV together with immune deficiency is an independent risk factor for the development of PAD. This thesis is further supported by studies that have shown increased prevalence of noncalcified plaque on cardiac CT in HIV-positive individuals as compared to uninfected persons, even after adjusting for traditional cardiovascular risk factors.[131]

The underlying mechanisms that increase PAD risk are identical to those that increase atherosclerotic risk, and these have already been described. In an HIV-positive patient with PAD, the clinical presentation, diagnostic workup, and management are the same as that in the general population.

Vasculitis

HIV-associated vasculitis occurs rarely. HIV may cause direct vessel wall injury and it is found more commonly in young persons who are immunocompromised. It has also been postulated that an autoimmune response could be initiated by the interaction of the HIV envelope proteins with one or more vessel wall matrix specific antigenic proteins.[132] In HIV-infected patients, opportunistic infectious agents or drugs may also lead to vasculitis.[133] Histopathological studies have characterized large vessel vasculitis by occlusion of the vasa vasorum by an inflammatory cell infiltrate causing weakening of the vessel wall and subsequent aneurysm formation.[134] While large artery vasculopathy may affect any large artery the aneurysms typically are multiple, atypical in location, and more common in femoral, carotid, and popliteal arteries (**Fig. 77–9**).[134,135] There have been a few case reports of HIV-positive patients with aortitis presenting with aortic regurgitation.[136]

All patients should be started on cART if, at presentation, the patient is ART naïve. Management of HIV-associated vasculopathy should follow standard treatment guidelines for vasculopathy in HIV-negative patients.[135]

VENOUS THROMBOEMBOLIC DISEASE

Patients with HIV appear to have an increased risk of venous thromboembolic disease. Some studies have estimated that the risk is 2- to 10-fold higher than that in the general population, although the majority of thromboembolic events associated with patients with HIV were noted among those with CD4$^+$ cell counts <200 cells/ mm^3 or an AIDS-defining illness.[137] Factors that lead to a procoaguable state in HIV-positive patients include increased levels of D-dimers, lupus anticoagulant, antiphospholipid antibodies, Von Willebrand factor, and deficiencies of Protein C and S and antithrombin.[138] Other risk

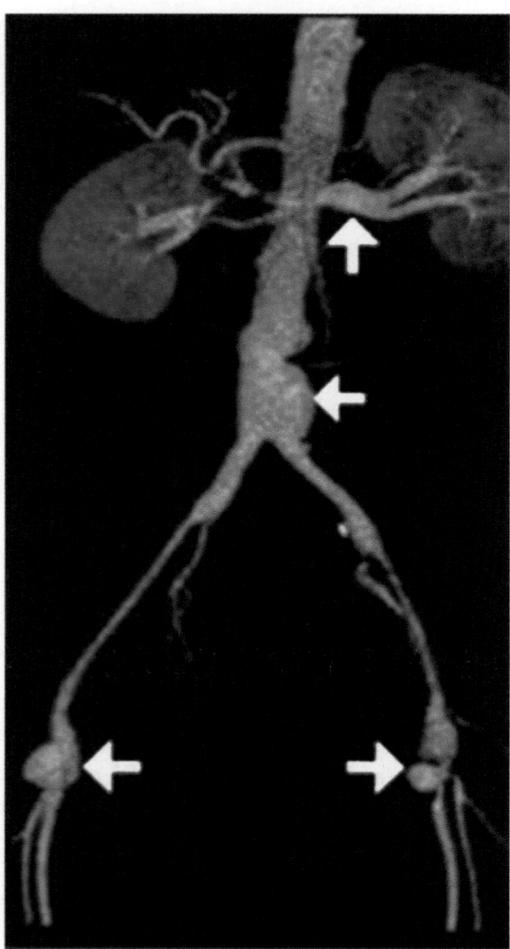

Figure 77–9. CT angiography showing multiple aneurysms in descending aorta, common iliac, and femoral arteries in a male HIV-positive patient. Reproduced with permission from Pillay B, Ramdial PK, Naidoo DP. HIV-associated large-vessel vasculopathy: a review of the current and emerging clinicopathological spectrum in vascular surgical practice. *Cardiovasc J Afr.* 2015 Mar-Apr;26(2):70-81.

factors include protease inhibitors, older age, and prolonged immobility.[139,140] The clinical presentation and management of HIV-associated venous thromoboembolic disease should follow that of standard clinical guidelines for patients without HIV.

CARDIAC RHYTHM DISTURBANCES IN HIV

PLWH have been reported to have a high arrhythmic burden compared to the general population. This is likely related to PLWH living longer and associated increasing prevalence of HIV-related CVDs such as ischemic heart disease and cardiomyopathy. Furthermore, these patients are also at risk of numerous drug–drug interactions, recreational substance abuse, and electrolyte imbalances.[141] HIV has also been directly implicated in the alteration of the electrophysiological properties of the heart leading to cardiac arrhythmias and SCD.[141,142]

Sudden Cardiac Death

SCD has been reported to be the third leading cause of mortality in PLWH.[143] In a retrospective study of 2860 PLWH with variable cART coverage, designed to determine the cause of death, SCD was responsible for 86% of cardiac deaths and was found to be 4.5 times higher than the general population.[143] SCD is more prevalent in those PLWH with more cardiovascular conditions such as hypertension, coronary heart disease, HF with low ejection fraction, cocaine use, and a spectrum of atrial and ventricular arrhythmias compared to those who died of other causes and AIDS.[143]

QTc Prolongation and Torsade de Pointes

Recently, a number of studies have demonstrated a higher prevalence of acquired long QTc in PLWH (**Table 77–2**).[144] Hospitalised HIV-positive patients were found to have prolonged QTc intervals that were 1.6 to 4 times that of their uninfected counterparts.[141,142] The majority of first-line cART have not been demonstrated to cause clinically significant QTc interval prolongation; however, the PIs have been identified as QTc interval-prolonging drugs. In vitro studies have demonstrated that protease inhibitors block the human ether-a-go-go- related gene (hERG), which codes for the rapidly activating delayed rectifier potassium current (I_{Kr}).[145] Despite these in vitro findings, a clinically significant risk for acquired long QT syndrome associated with PIs has not been shown.[146]

Non-cART drugs have also been implicated to cause acquired prolonged QTc in PLWH. Macrolides, antifungals, fluoroquinolones, pentamidine, and methadone may cause clinically relevant prolongation of the QT interval in this population.[148] Furthermore, accompanying end-organ dysfunction, such as acute kidney injury and hepatic dysfunction, may also exacerbate the risk of QTc prolongation by increasing the plasma concentration and half-life of implicated medication. Electrolyte disturbances such as hypokalemia, hypocalcemia, and hypomagnesemia are important risk factors for acquired QTc prolongation. These may occur due to multiple causes such as diarrhea, vomiting, and nutritional deficiencies, which are common in patients with AIDS.

Acquired QTc prolongation has also been associated with the HIV infection itself independent of polypharmacy and electrolyte imbalances. Comparing a cohort of asymptomatic PLWH with HIV-negative controls, the prevalence of QTc prolongation was 28% and 10%, respectively.[141] However, in the HIV-positive group, the prevalence of QTc prolongation increased from 28% to 45% when these participants were complicated with AIDS.[141] Similarly, in another study, the prevalence of QTc prolongation of 440 ms in men and 460 ms in women was 18.2% in PLWH on cART and 16.4% in cART-naïve patients and both cohorts

TABLE 77–2. Risk Factors for a Prolonged QTc Interval in PLWH Compared with the General Population

	Electrolyte imbalance	Cardiac disease	Poly-pharmacy
PLWH	19%	1.5x	24.4%
General population	<2%	1x	11.6%

Data from Brouillette J, Cyr S, Fiset C. Mechanisms of Arrhythmia and Sudden Cardiac Death in Patients With HIV Infection. *Can J Cardiol.* 2019 Mar;35(3):310-319.

had a higher prevalence of QTc prolongation compared with HIV-negative controls (10.5%).[142] These findings suggest that the cART-related QTc effects are not clinically significant, but rather that the HIV itself may directly interfere with electrical properties of the myocardium.[144]

Atrial Fibrillation

The incidence of atrial fibrillation has been shown to be significantly associated with advanced HIV infection. In a study of 30,533 HIV-infected veterans in the United States, the incidence of atrial fibrillation was 2.6% after a median follow-up duration of 6.8 years.[149] In this study, after adjusting for confounders, a low CD4+ cell count and a high HIV viral load were independently associated with new onset atrial fibrillation.[149] These study findings were later confirmed in a study of 5,052 PLWH compared to 10,121 uninfected controls. The incidence of atrial fibrillation/atrial flutter was 2.0% and 1.6%, respectively.[150] Similarly, a lower CD4+ cell count was associated with a 2-fold increased risk for atrial fibrillation/atrial flutter after adjusting for confounders.[150]

Atrial fibrillation should be managed according to current guidelines but, again, healthcare practitioners should be aware of potential drug–drug interactions with oral anticoagulants and direct oral anticoagulants (see section Drug Interactions).

DRUG INTERACTIONS

Drug–drug interactions are becoming less frequent with newer cART, making the treatment of HIV and cardiac comorbidities simpler. However, several HIV medications with important drug–drug interactions are still in use. The most important interactions involve drugs metabolized by the cytochrome (CYP) P450 system and/or drug transporters.[11] Some cART induce or inhibit these enzymes, which can affect serum concentrations of cardiac drugs metabolized by the CYP450 enzymes, while the efficacy of the cART may be affected by cardiac drugs that interact with these enzymes.

The most important interactions are those involving lipid-lowering agents (**Table 77–3**), antithrombotic agents

TABLE 77–3. Important Interactions between Lipid-Lowering Agents and ART

CV agent	ART with potential DDI	Effect on CV agent	Recommendations
STATINS			
Atorvastatin	ATV/r, DRV/r, DRV/c, LPV/r	↑↑	Start with lowest dose of statin and adjust dose based on clinical effect and toxicity. Do not exceed 20 mg/d atorvastatin.
Atorvastatin	EFV, ETR, NVP	↓	Monitor clinical effects and increase statin dose as needed.
Atorvastatin	ATV/c	↑↑↑	CONTRAINDICATED.
Fluvastatin	PI/r, PI/c, EVG/c	↑	Start with lowest dose of statin and adjust dose based on clinical effect and toxicity.
Lovastatin	PI/r, PI/c, EVG/c	↑↑↑	CONTRAINDICATED.
Lovastatin	EFV, ETR, NVP	↓	Monitor clinical effects and increase statin dose as needed.
Pitavastatin	None	NA	Use standard doses with all ARTs.
Pravastatin	PI/r, PI/c, EVG/c	Unlikely	Use standard doses with all ARTs; monitor for toxicity.
Pravastatin	EFV, ETR, NVP	↓	Monitor clinical effects and increase statin dose as needed.
Rosuvastatin	ATV/r, ATV/c, LPV/r	↑	Start with lowest dose of statin and adjust dose based on clinical effect and toxicity. Do not exceed 10 mg/d rosuvastatin.
Rosuvastatin	DRV/r, DRV/c, EVG/c	↑	Start with lowest dose of statin and adjust dose based on clinical effect and toxicity. Do not exceed 20 mg of rosuvastatin.
Simvastatin	PI/r, PI/c, EVG/c	↑↑↑	CONTRAINDICATED.
Simvastatin	EFV, ETR, NVP	↓	Monitor clinical effects and increase statin dose as needed.
BILE ACID SEQUESTRANTS			
Cholestyramine, colestipol	All	↓ absorption	Take ART at least 1 hour before or 4 to 6 hours after bile acid sequestrants.
Ezetimibe	PI/r	↓	Use standard doses and monitor clinical effects.
FIBRATES			
Bezafibrate, fenofibrate	None	NA	Use standard doses with all ARTs.
Gemfibrozil	PI/r	↓	Use standard doses and monitor clinical effects.
PCSK9 INHIBITORS			
Alirocumab evolocumab	None	NA	Use standard doses with all ARTs.

Abbreviations: CV, cardiovascular; ART, antiretroviral; DDI, drug-drug interaction; ↑, possible increased effect; ↑↑, strong effect; ↑↑↑, very strong effect; ↓, possible decreased effect; NA, not applicable; ATV, atazanavir; r, ritonavir; DRV, darunavir; c, cobicistat, LPV, lopinavir; EFV, efavirenz; ETR, etravirine; NVP, nevirapine; PI, protease inhibitor (ATV, DRV); EVG, elvitegravir; h, hour; CCB, calcium channel blocker; BB, β-blocker. Data from Giguère P, Nhean S, Tseng AL, et al: Getting to the Heart of the Matter: A Review of Drug Interactions Between HIV Antiretrovirals and Cardiology Medications. *Can J Cardiol.* 2019 Mar;35(3):326-340.

TABLE 77–4. Important Interactions between Anti-Thrombotic Agents and ART

CV agent	ART with potential DDI	Effect on CV agent	Recommendations
ANTI-PLATELETS			
Aspirin	None	NA	Use standard doses with all ARTs.
Clopidogrel	EFV, ETR	↓	Consider prasugrel.
Prasugrel	None	NA	Use standard doses with all ARTs.
Ticagrelor	PI/r, PI/c, EVG/c	↑	Consider prasugrel.
Ticagrelor	EFV, ETR, NVP	↓	Consider prasugrel.
Cangrelor	No data		No recommendation.
ANTICOAGULANTS			
Apixaban	PI/r, PI/c, EVG/c	↑	Change ART regimen, consider alternative or use 50% apixaban dose.
Apixaban	EFV, ETR, NVP	↓	Change ART regimen, consider alternative.
Dabigatran	DRV/c	NA	Use standard doses.
Dabigatran	PI/r	No change is given at same time; ↓ Dabigatran if given 2h before ritonavir	Consider alternative such as warfarin. If co-administered, should be taken at same time.
Dabigatran	ATV/c, EVG/c	↑ ↑	Consider alternatives or change ART regimen.
Edoxaban	PI/r	↑/↓	Consider alternatives or change ART regimen.
Edoxaban	ATV/c, EVG/c	↑	Consider alternatives or change ART regimen.
Rivaroxaban	PI/r, PI/c, EVG/c	↑	AVOID coadministration. Consider alternatives or change ART regimen.
Rivaroxaban	EFV, ETR, NVP	↓	AVOID coadministration. Consider alternatives or change ART regimen.
Warfarin	EFV, ETR, NVP, EVG/c, PI/c	↑/↓	Adjust warfarin dose as required.
Warfarin	PI/r	↓	Adjust warfarin dose as required.

Abbreviations: CV, cardiovascular; ART, antiretroviral; DDI, drug-drug interaction; ↑, possible increased effect; ↑ ↑, strong effect; ↑ ↑ ↑, very strong effect; ↓, possible decreased effect; NA, not applicable; ATV, atazanavir; r, ritonavir; DRV, darunavir; c, cobicistat, LPV, lopinavir; EFV, efavirenz; ETR, etravirine; NVP, nevirapine; PI, protease inhibitor (ATV, DRV); EVG, elvitegravir; h, hour; CCB, calcium channel blocker; BB, β-blocker. Data from Giguère P, Nhean S, Tseng AL, et al: Getting to the Heart of the Matter: A Review of Drug Interactions Between HIV Antiretrovirals and Cardiology Medications. *Can J Cardiol*. 2019 Mar;35(3):326-340.

(**Table 77–4**), and certain antiarrhythmic, antihypertensive, and HF medications (**Table 77–5**). Although most statins can safely be prescribed, simvastatin and lovastatin, which are extensively metabolized by the cytochrome P450 enzymes, should not be used in patients on PI-based or cobicistat-boosted elvitegravir regimens.[151] Lower starting doses of atorvastatin are suggested in patients receiving PI-based regimens, while atorvastatin is contraindicated in patients on cobicistat-boosted atazanavir regimens. Rosuvastatin should be limited to 10 mg in patients taking atazanavir-ritonavir and lopinavir-ritonavir.[65]

Because clopidogrel is significantly metabolized by CYP2C19 and CYP2C9, there are a number of potential drug interactions. Ticagrelor, which is predominantly metabolized by the CYP3A4/5 isoenzyme, should also be avoided in patients who are receiving PI therapy.[11] Prasugrel is a reasonable alternative and recommended with all antiretrovirals. Anticoagulation therapy in HIV patients poses several challenges. Since warfarin is metabolized by the CYP450 enzyme system, a higher mean warfarin maintenance dose is required in patients on cART compared with control patients receiving only warfarin. The international normalized ratio (INR) should be closely monitored during the initiation period after combining

ART and warfarin in PLWH. Rivaroxaban and apixaban are substrates of CYP3A4. In particular, rivaroxaban levels are likely to be increased when used with PIs and, therefore, this combination is strongly discouraged. Efavirenz, etravirine, and nevirapine might reduce the efficacy of rivaroxaban and an alternative combination is suggested.[11] No interaction is expected between NNRTIs and dabigatran. The integrase inhibitor, cobicistat, is a strong inhibitor of CYP3A4 and increases the risk of bleeding with rivaroxaban or apixaban, but not dabigatran. There are no expected interactions with other integrase inhibitors. Dabigatran is the recommended drug for patients on PIs, integrase inhibitor, and/or NNRTIs, but should ritonavir and dabigatran be co prescribed, they should be taken at least 2 hours apart to prevent any possible interaction.[11]

Caution is required with almost all combinations of antiarrhythmic agents and antiretrovirals.[11] Amiodarone is one of the most commonly used antiarrhythmic agents and is metabolized to its major metabolite, desethylamiodarone, by CYP3A4. It is also a substrate for CYP2C8 and inhibits CYP3A4, CYP2C9, CYP2D6, and P-glycoprotein. Levels of amiodarone may be increased by ritonavir- and cobicistat-boosted PIs and might be

TABLE 77–5. Important ART Drug–Drug Interactions with Anti-Arrhythmic, Anti-Hypertensive, Heart Failure Medications

CV agent	ART with potential DDI	Effect on CV agent	Recommendations
Amiodarone	PI/r, PI/c, EVG/c	↑	Use with caution and monitor for amiodarone toxicity.
Amiodarone	EFV, ETR, NVP	↓	Monitor clinical effects. Consider amiodarone serum level.
Bisoprolol	EFV, ETR, NVP	↓	Monitor clinical effects and increase dose if needed.
Carvedilol, metoprolol, bisoprolol	PI/r, PI/c, EVG/c	↑	Monitor clinical effects and decrease BB dose if needed.
Doxazosin, terazosin	EFV, ETR, NVP	↓	Monitor clinical effects and increase dose if needed.
Doxazosin, prazosin, terazosin	PI/r, PI/c, EVG/c	↑	Monitor clinical effects and decrease dose if needed.
Dronedarone	EVG/c	↑	Use with caution & monitor for dronedarone toxicity.
Dronedarone	EFV, ETR, NVP	↓	Monitor clinical effects. Consider dronedarone serum level.
Dronedarone	PI/r, PI/c	↑	CONTRAINDICATED.
Calcium channel blockers	PI/r, PI/c, EVG/c	↑	Monitor clinical effects and decrease CCB dose if necessary. ECG monitoring especially with ATV.
Calcium channel blockers	EFV, ETR, NVP	↓	Monitor efficacy and increase CCB dose if needed.
Digoxin	PI/r, PI/c, EVG/c, ETR	↑	Monitor digoxin levels closely and decrease digoxin dose if necessary.
Eplerenone	EFV, ETR, NVP	↓	Monitor clinical effects and increase eplerenone dose if needed.
Eplerenone	PI/r, PI/c, EVG/c	↑↑	CONTRAINDICATED.
Flecainide	PI/r, PI/c, EVG/c	↑	Not recommended. Monitor for flecainide toxicity.
Indapamide	PI/r, PI/c, EVG/c	↑	Monitor clinical effects and decrease indapmide dose if needed.
Irbesartan	r, EVG/c	↓	Monitor clinical effects and increase dose if needed.
Irbesartan	EFV, ETR	↑	Monitor clinical effects and decrease dose if needed.
Indapamide	EFV, ETR, NVP	↓	Monitor clinical effects and increase indapamide dose if needed.
Ivabradine	EFV, ETR, NVP	↓	Monitor clinical effects and increase ivabradine dose if needed.
Losartan	r, EVG/c	↑	Monitor clinical effects and decrease dose if needed.
Losartan	EFV, ETR	↓	Monitor clinical effects and increase dose if needed.
Ivabradine	PI/r, PI/c, EVG/c	↑↑	CONTRAINDICATED.
Mexiletine	PI/r, PI/c, EVG/c	↑	Not recommended. Monitor for mexiletine toxicity.
Propafenone	PI/r, PI/c, EVG/c	↑	Not recommended. Monitor for propafenone toxicity.
Propafenone	EFV, ETR, NVP	↓	Monitor clinical effects and consider propafenone serum levels if needed.
Sacubitril/valsartan	PI/r, PI/c	↑	Monitor clinical effects and decrease valsartan dose if needed.
Valsartan	PI/r, PI/c	↑	Monitor clinical effects and decrease dose if needed.

Abbreviations: CV, cardiovascular; ART, antiretroviral; DDI, drug-drug interaction; ↑, possible increased effect; ↑↑, strong effect; ↑↑↑, very strong effect; ↓, possible decreased effect; NA, not applicable; ATV, atazanavir; r, ritonavir; c, cobicistat; LPV, lopinavir; EFV, efavirenz; ETR, etravirine; NVP, nevirapine; PI, protease inhibitor (ATV, DRV); EVG, elvitegravir; CCB, calcium channel blocker; BB, β-blocker. Data from Giguère P, Nhean S, Tseng AL, et al: Getting to the Heart of the Matter: A Review of Drug Interactions Between HIV Antiretrovirals and Cardiology Medications. *Can J Cardiol.* 2019 Mar;35(3):326-340.

lowered by efavirenz, etravirine, and nevirapine, but no studies are yet available to confirm this.[11] Ivabradine and its major metabolite are metabolized by CYP3A4 and evidence shows that levels are increased by CYP3A4 inhibitors, which may lead to symptomatic bradycardia.[152]

Drug–drug interactions can be limited by either selecting agents that do not interfere with each other, adjusting the dose of agents, and/or close monitoring when the drug combination cannot be avoided. A multidisciplinary team including a cardiologist, HIV-specialist, and pharmacist is often required when choosing the best combination of medications for PLWH requiring cardiovascular medications.

REFERENCES

1. UNAIDS. Global HIV & AIDS statistics—2019 fact sheet. https://wwwunaidsorg/en/resources/fact-sheet. 2019. Accessed March 31, 2020.
2. CDC. HIV Statistics. https://wwwcdcgov/hiv/statistics/indexhtml. 2019.
3. Smit M, Brinkman K, Geerlings S, et al. Future challenges for clinical care of an ageing population infected with HIV: a modelling study. *Lancet Infect Dis.* 2015;15:810-818.
4. Klein DB, Leyden WA, Xu L, et al. Declining relative risk for myocardial infarction among HIV-positive compared with HIV-negative individuals with access to care. *Clinical Infect Dis.* 2015;60:1278-1280.
5. Shah ASV, Stelzle D, Lee KK, et al. Global burden of atherosclerotic cardiovascular disease in people living with HIV: systematic review and meta-analysis. *Circulation.* 2018;138:1100-1112.

6. Freiberg MS, Chang CH, Skanderson M, et al. Association between HIV infection and the risk of heart failure with reduced ejection fraction and preserved ejection fraction in the antiretroviral therapy era: results from the veterans aging cohort study. *JAMA Cardiol.* 2017;2:536-546.

7. Erqou S, Lodebo BT, Masri A, et al. Cardiac dysfunction among people living with HIV: a systematic review and meta-analysis. *JACC Heart Fail.* 2019;7:98-108.

8. Feinstein MJ, Steverson AB, Ning H, et al. Adjudicated heart failure in HIV-infected and uninfected men and women. *J Am Heart Assoc.* 2018;7:e009985.

9. Alvi RM, Neilan AM, Tariq N, et al. The risk for sudden cardiac death among patients living with heart failure and human immunodeficiency virus. *JACC Heart Fail.* 2019;7:759-767.

10. Friis-Moller N, Sabin CA, Weber R, et al. Combination antiretroviral therapy and the risk of myocardial infarction. *N Eng J Med.* 2003;349:1993-2003.

11. Giguere P, Nhean S, Tseng AL, Hughes CA, Angel JB. Getting to the heart of the matter: a review of drug interactions between HIV antiretrovirals and cardiology medications. *Canadian J Cardiol.* 2019;35:326-340.

12. Drozd DR, Kitahata MM, Althoff KN, et al. Increased risk of myocardial infarction in HIV-infected individuals in North America compared with the general population. *JAIDS (1999).* 2017;75:568-576.

13. El-Sadr WM, Lundgren J, Neaton JD, et al. CD4+ count-guided interruption of antiretroviral treatment. *N Eng J Med.* 2006;355:2283-2296.

14. Peyracchia M, De Lio G, Montrucchio C, et al. Evaluation of coronary features of HIV patients presenting with ACS: the CUORE, a multicenter study. *Atherosclerosis.* 2018;274:218-226.

15. Vachiat A, McCutcheon K, Tsabedze N, et al. HIV and ischemic heart disease. *J Am Coll Cardiol.* 2017;69:73-82.

16. Manga P, McCutcheon K, Tsabedze N, Vachiat A, Zachariah D. HIV and nonischemic heart disease. *J Am Coll Cardiol.* 2017;69:83-91.

17. Vos AG, Hoeve K, Barth RE, et al. Cardiovascular disease risk in an urban African population: a cross-sectional analysis on the role of HIV and antiretroviral treatment. *Retrovirology.* 2019;16:37.

18. Hsue PY, Waters DD. HIV infection and coronary heart disease: mechanisms and management. *Nature Rev Cardiol.* 2019;16:745-759.

19. Freiberg MS, Chang CC, Kuller LH, et al. HIV infection and the risk of acute myocardial infarction. *JAMA Int Med.* 2013;173:614-622.

20. Lang S, Mary-Krause M, Cotte L, Gilquin J, Partisani M, Simon A, Boccara F, Bingham A and Costagliola D. Increased risk of myocardial infarction in HIV-infected patients in France, relative to the general population. *AIDS (London, England).* 2010;24:1228-1230.

21. Goehringer F, Bonnet F, Salmon D, et al. Causes of death in HIV-infected individuals with immunovirologic success in a national prospective survey. *AIDS Res Human Retrovirus.* 2017;33:187-193.

22. Croxford S, Kitching A, Desai S, et al. Mortality and causes of death in people diagnosed with HIV in the era of highly active antiretroviral therapy compared with the general population: an analysis of a national observational cohort. *Lancet Public Health.* 2017;2:e35-e46.

23. Kaplan RC, Kingsley LA, Sharrett AR, et al. Ten-year predicted coronary heart disease risk in HIV-infected men and women. *Clin Infect.* 2007;45:1074-1081.

24. Mdodo R, Frazier EL, Dube SR, et al. Cigarette smoking prevalence among adults with HIV compared with the general adult population in the United States: cross-sectional surveys. *Ann Intern Med.* 2015;162:335-344.

25. Rasmussen LD, Helleberg M, May MT, et al. Myocardial infarction among Danish HIV-infected individuals: population-attributable fractions associated with smoking. *Clinical Infect Dis.* 2015;60:1415-1423.

26. Njuguna B, Kiplagat J, Bloomfield GS, Pastakia SD, Vedanthan R, Koethe JR. Prevalence, risk factors, and pathophysiology of dysglycemia among people living with HIV in Sub-Saharan Africa. *J Diabetes Res.* 2018:6916497.

27. Mathabire Rucker SC, Tayea A, Bitilinyu-Bangoh J, et al. High rates of hypertension, diabetes, elevated low-density lipoprotein cholesterol, and cardiovascular disease risk factors in HIV-infected patients in Malawi. *AIDS (London, England).* 2018;32:253-260.

28. Rasmussen LD, Mathiesen ER, Kronborg G, Pedersen C, Gerstoft J, Obel N. Risk of diabetes mellitus in persons with and without HIV: a Danish nationwide population-based cohort study. *PloS One.* 2012;7:e44575.

29. Friis-Moller N, Ryom L, Smith C, et al. An updated prediction model of the global risk of cardiovascular disease in HIV-positive persons: the Data-collection on Adverse Effects of Anti-HIV Drugs (D:A:D) study. *Eur J Prevent Cardiol.* 2016;23:214-223.

30. Brennan AT, Jamieson L, Crowther NJ, et al. Prevalence, incidence, predictors, treatment, and control of hypertension among HIV-positive adults on antiretroviral treatment in public sector treatment programs in South Africa. *PloS One.* 2018;13:e0204020.

31. Xu Y, Chen X, Wang K. Global prevalence of hypertension among people living with HIV: a systematic review and meta-analysis. *J Am Soc Hypertens.* 2017;11:530-540.

32. Dakum P, Kayode GA, Abimiku A, et al. Prevalence of hypertension among patients aged 50 and older living with human immunodeficiency virus. *Medicine.* 2019;98:e15024.

33. Armah KA, Chang CC, Baker JV, et al. Prehypertension, hypertension, and the risk of acute myocardial infarction in HIV-infected and -uninfected veterans. *Clin Infect Dis.;* 2014;58:121-129.

34. Hatleberg CI, Ryom L, d'Arminio Monforte A, et al. Association between exposure to antiretroviral drugs and the incidence of hypertension in HIV-positive persons: the Data Collection on Adverse Events of Anti-HIV Drugs (D:A:D) study. *HIV Med.* 2018;19:605-618.

35. Russell E, Albert A, Cote H, et al. Rate of dyslipidemia higher among women living with HIV: a comparison of metabolic and cardiovascular health in a cohort to sutdy aging in HIV. *HIV Med.* 2020;21(7):418-428.

36. Leyes P, Cofan M, Gonzalez-Cordon A, et al. Increased cholesterol absorption rather than synthesis is involved in boosted protease inhibitor-associated hypercholesterolaemia. *AIDS (London, England).* 2018;32:1309-1316.

37. Ekoru K, Young EH, Dillon DG, et al. HIV treatment is associated with a two-fold higher probability of raised triglycerides: pooled analyses in 21 023 individuals in sub-Saharan Africa. *Global Health Epidemiol Genom.* 2018;3:e7. doi: 10.1017/gheg.2018.7.

38. Dimala CA, Blencowe H, Choukem SP. The association between antiretroviral therapy and selected cardiovascular disease risk factors in sub-Saharan Africa: a systematic review and meta-analysis. *PloS One.* 2018;13:e0201404.

39. Worm SW, Sabin C, Weber R, et al. Risk of myocardial infarction in patients with HIV infection exposed to specific individual antiretroviral drugs from the 3 major drug classes: the data collection on adverse events of anti-HIV drugs (D:A:D) study. *J Infect Dis.* 2010;201:318-330.

40. Carey D, Amin J, Boyd M, Petoumenos K, Emery S. Lipid profiles in HIV-infected adults receiving atazanavir and atazanavir/ritonavir: systematic review and meta-analysis of randomized controlled trials. *J Antimicrobial Chemother.* 2010;65:1878-1888.

41. Eron JJ, Young B, Cooper DA, et al. Switch to a raltegravir-based regimen versus continuation of a lopinavir-ritonavir-based regimen in stable HIV-infected patients with suppressed viraemia (SWITCHMRK 1 and 2): two multicentre, double-blind, randomised controlled trials. *Lancet (London, England).* 2010;375:396-407.

42. Lundgren J, Mocroft A, Ryom L. Contemporary protease inhibitors and cardiovascular risk. *Curr Op Infect Dis.* 2018;31:8-13.

43. Saag MS, Benson CA, Gandhi RT, et al. Antiretroviral drugs for treatment and prevention of HIV infection in adults: 2018 recommendations of the International Antiviral Society-USA Panel. *JAMA.* 2018;320:379-396.

44. Dorjee K, Baxi SM, Reingold AL, Hubbard A. Risk of cardiovascular events from current, recent, and cumulative exposure to abacavir among persons living with HIV who were receiving antiretroviral therapy in the United States: a cohort study. *BMC infectious diseases.* 2017;17:708.

45. Nan C, Shaefer M, Urbaityte R, et al. Abacavir use and risk for myocardial infarction and cardiovascular events: pooled analysis of data from clinical trials. *Open Forum Infect Dis.* 2018;5:ofy086.

46. Lake JE, McComsey GA, Hulgan T, et al. Switch to raltegravir from protease inhibitor or nonnucleoside reverse-transcriptase inhibitor does not reduce visceral fat in human immunodeficiency virus-infected women with central adiposity. *Open Forum Infect Dis.* 2015;2:ofv059.

47. Glesby MJ, Hanna DB, Hoover DR, et al. abdominal fat depots and subclinical carotid artery atherosclerosis in women with and without HIV infection. *JAIDS (1999).* 2018;77:308-316.

48. Paisible AL, Chang CC, So-Armah KA, et al. HIV infection, cardiovascular disease risk factor profile, and risk for acute myocardial infarction. *JAIDS (1999).* 2015;68:209-216.

49. Collins LF, Adekunle RO, Cartwright EJ. Metabolic Syndrome in HIV/HCV co-infected patients. *Curr Treatm Opt Infect Dis.* 2019;11:351-371.

50. Lopes de Campos WR, Chirwa N, London G, et al. HIV-1 subtype C unproductively infects human cardiomyocytes in vitro and induces apoptosis mitigated by an anti-Gp120 aptamer. *PloS One.* 2014;9:e110930.

51. Rethy L, Feinstein MJ, Sinha A, Achenbach C, Shah SJ. Coronary microvascular dysfunction in HIV: a review. *J Am Heart Assoc.* 2020;9:e014018.

52. Bahrami H, Budoff M, Haberlen SA, et al. Inflammatory markers associated with subclinical coronary artery disease: the Multicenter AIDS Cohort Study. *J Am Heart Assoc.* 2016;5:1-13.

53. Hsu DC, Ma YF, Hur S, et al. Plasma IL-6 levels are independently associated with atherosclerosis and mortality in HIV-infected individuals on suppressive antiretroviral therapy. *AIDS (London, England).* 2016;30:2065-2074.

54. Lang S, Boccara F, Mary-Krause M, Cohen A. Epidemiology of coronary heart disease in HIV-infected versus uninfected individuals in developed countries. *Arch Cardiovasc Dis.* 2015;108:206-215.

55. Mosepele M, Mohammed T, Mupfumi L, et al. HIV disease is associated with increased biomarkers of endothelial dysfunction despite viral suppression on long-term antiretroviral therapy in Botswana. *Cardiovasc J Afr.* 2018;29:155-161.

56. Vachiat A, Dix-Peek T, Duarte R, Manga P. Endothelial dysfunction in HIV-positive patients with acute coronary syndromes. *Cardiovasc J Afr.* 2020;31:1-7.

57. Mahtab S, Zar HJ, Ntusi NAB, et al. Endothelial dysfunction in South African youth living with perinatally acquired HIV on antiretroviral therapy. *Clin Infect Dis.* 2020. doi: 10.1093/cid/ciaa396.

58. Hauguel-Moreau M, Boccara F, Boyd A, et al. Platelet reactivity in human immunodeficiency virus infected patients on dual antiplatelet therapy for an acute coronary syndrome: the EVERE2ST-HIV study. *Eur Heart J.* 2017;38:1676-1686.

59. D'Ascenzo F, Cerrato E, Calcagno A, et al. High prevalence at computed coronary tomography of non-calcified plaques in asymptomatic HIV patients treated with HAART: a meta-analysis. *Atherosclerosis.* 2015;240:197-204.

60. Vachiat A, McCutcheon K, Tsabedze N, Zachariah D, Manga P. Atherosclerotic plaque in HIV-positive patients presenting with acute coronary syndromes. *Cardiovasc J Afr.* 2019;30:203-207.

61. McComsey GA, O'Riordan M, Hazen SL, et al. Increased carotid intima media thickness and cardiac biomarkers in HIV infected children. *AIDS (London, England).* 2007;21:921-927.

62. Brusca RM, Hanna DB, Wada NI, et al. Subclinical cardiovascular disease in HIV controller and long-term nonprogressor populations. *HIV Med.* 2020;21:217-227.

63. Becker AC, Sliwa K, Stewart S, et al. Acute coronary syndromes in treatment-naive black South Africans with human immunodeficiency virus infection. *J Intervent Cardiol.* 2010;23:70-77.

64. Mooney S, Tracy R, Osler T, Grace C. Elevated biomarkers of inflammation and coagulation in patients with HIV are associated with higher Framingham and VACS risk index scores. *PloS One.* 2015;10:e0144312.

65. Feinstein MJ, Hsue PY, Benjamin LA, et al. Characteristics, prevention, and management of cardiovascular disease in people living with HIV: a scientific statement from the American Heart Association. *Circulation.* 2019;140:e98-e124.

66. Helleberg M, May MT, Ingle SM, et al. Smoking and life expectancy among HIV-infected individuals on antiretroviral therapy in Europe and North America. *AIDS (London, England).* 2015;29:221-229.

67. Pool ER, Dogar O, Lindsay RP, Weatherburn P, Siddiqi K. Interventions for tobacco use cessation in people living with HIV and AIDS. *Cochrane Database Syst Rev.* 2016:Cd011120.

68. Arnett DK, Blumenthal RS, Albert MA, et al. 2019 ACC/AHA guideline on the primary prevention of cardiovascular disease: a report of the American College of Cardiology/American Heart Association Task Force on Clinical Practice Guidelines. *J Am Coll Cardiol.* 2019;74:e177-e232.

69. Longenecker CT, Eckard AR, McComsey GA. Statins to improve cardiovascular outcomes in treated HIV infection. *Curr Op Infect Dis.* 2016;29:1-9.

70. Titanji B, Gavegnano C, Hsue P, Schinazi R, Marconi VC. Targeting inflammation to reduce atherosclerotic cardiovascular risk in people with HIV infection. *J Am Heart Assoc.* 2020;9:e014873.

71. Ridker PM, Everett BM, Thuren T, et al. antiinflammatory therapy with canakinumab for atherosclerotic disease. *N Eng J Med.* 2017;377:1119-1131.

72. Hsue PY, Li D, Ma Y, et al. IL-1beta inhibition reduces atherosclerotic inflammation in HIV infection. *J Am Coll Cardiol.* 2018;72:2809-2811.

73. Hsue PY, Ribaudo HJ, Deeks SG, et al. Safety and impact of low-dose methotrexate on endothelial function and inflammation in individuals with treated human immunodeficiency virus: AIDS clinical trials group study A5314. *Clin Infect Dis.* 2019;68:1877-1886.

74. O'Brien MP, Zafar MU, Rodriguez JC, et al. Targeting thrombogenicity and inflammation in chronic HIV infection. *Sci Advan.* 2019;5:eaav5463.

75. Sandler NG, Zhang X, Bosch RJ, et al. Sevelamer does not decrease lipopolysaccharide or soluble CD14 levels but decreases soluble tissue factor, low-density lipoprotein (LDL) cholesterol, and oxidized LDL cholesterol levels in individuals with untreated HIV infection. *J Infect Dis.* 2014;210:1549-1554.

76. Lundgren JD, Babiker AG, Gordin F, et al. Initiation of antiretroviral therapy in early asymptomatic HIV infection. *N Eng J Med.* 2015;373:795-807.

77. Wang ZY, Chen M, Zhu LL, et al. Pharmacokinetic drug interactions with clopidogrel: updated review and risk management in combination therapy. *Therapeut Clin Risk Manage.* 2015;11:449-467.

78. Zhou D, Andersson TB, Grimm SW. In vitro evaluation of potential drug-drug interactions with ticagrelor: cytochrome P450 reaction phenotyping, inhibition, induction, and differential kinetics. *Drug Metabol Disposition: Biol Fate Chem.* 2011;39:703-710.

79. Hatleberg CI, Ryom L, El-Sadr W, et al. Gender differences in the use of cardiovascular interventions in HIV-positive persons; the D:A:D Study. *J Int AIDS Soc.* 2018;21(3):e25083. doi: 10.1002/jia2.25083.

80. Peyracchia M, Verardi R, Rubin SR, et al. In-hospital and long-term outcomes of HIV-positive patients undergoing PCI according to kind of stent: a meta-analysis. *J Cardiovasc Med. (Hagerstown, Md).* 2019;20:321-326.

81. Lorgis L, Cottenet J, Molins G, et al. Outcomes after acute myocardial infarction in HIV-infected patients: analysis of data from a French nationwide hospital medical information database. *Circulation.* 2013;127:1767-1774.

82. Bundhun PK, Pursun M, Huang WQ. Does infection with human immunodeficiency virus have any impact on the cardiovascular outcomes following percutaneous coronary intervention?: a systematic review and meta-analysis. *BMC Cardiovasc Dis.* 2017;17:190.

83. D'Ascenzo F, Cerrato E, Appleton D, et al. Prognostic indicators for recurrent thrombotic events in HIV-infected patients with acute coronary syndromes: use of registry data from 12 sites in Europe, South Africa and the United States. *Thromb Res.* 2014;134:558-564.

84. Yanagawa B, Verma S, Dwivedi G, Ruel M. Cardiac surgery in HIV patients: state of the art. *Can J Cardiol.* 2019;35:320-325.

85. Koval CE, Farr M, Krisl J, et al. Heart or lung transplant outcomes in HIV-infected recipients. *J Heart Lung Transplant.* 2019;38:1296-1305.

86. Ingle SM, May MT, Gill MJ, et al. Impact of risk factors for specific causes of death in the first and subsequent years of antiretroviral therapy among HIV-infected patients. *Clin Infect Dis.* 2014;59:287-297.

87. Remick J, Georgiopoulou V, Marti C, et al. Heart failure in patients with human immunodeficiency virus infection: epidemiology, pathophysiology, treatment, and future research. *Circulation.* 2014;129:1781-1789.

88. Savvoulidis P, Butler J, Kalogeropoulos A. Cardiomyopathy and heart failure in patients with HIV infection. *Can J Cardiol.* 2019;35:299-309.

89. Bloomfield GS, Alenezi F, Barasa FA, Lumsden R, Mayosi BM, Velazquez EJ. Human immunodeficiency virus and heart failure in low- and middle-income countries. *JACC Heart Fail.* 2015;3:579-590.

90. Patel K, Van Dyke RB, Mittleman MA, et al. The impact of HAART on cardiomyopathy among children and adolescents perinatally infected with HIV-1. *AIDS (London, England).* 2012;26:2027-2037.

91. Al-Kindi SG, ElAmm C, Ginwalla M, et al. Heart failure in patients with human immunodeficiency virus infection: epidemiology and management disparities. *Int J Cardiol.* 2016;218:43-46.

92. Ntusi N, O'Dwyer E, Dorrell L, et al. HIV-1-related cardiovascular disease is associated with chronic inflammation, frequent pericardial effusions, and probable myocardial edema. *Circulation Cardiovasc Imaging.* 2016;9:e004430.

93. Feinstein MJ, Poole B, Engel Gonzalez P, et al. Differences by HIV serostatus in coronary artery disease severity and likelihood of percutaneous coronary intervention following stress testing. *J Nuclear Cardiol.* 2018;25:872-883.

94. Alvi RM, Neilan AM, Tariq N, et al. Protease inhibitors and cardiovascular outcomes in patients with HIV and heart failure. *J Am Coll Cardiol.* 2018;72:518-530.

95. Longenecker CT, Triant VA. Initiation of antiretroviral therapy at high CD4 cell counts: does it reduce the risk of cardiovascular disease? *Curr Op HIV AIDS.* 2014;9:54-62.

96. Cerrato E, D'Ascenzo F, Biondi-Zoccai G, et al. Cardiac dysfunction in pauci symptomatic human immunodeficiency virus patients: a meta-analysis in the highly active antiretroviral therapy era. *Eur Heart J.* 2013;34:1432-1436.

97. Luetkens JA, Doerner J, Schwarze-Zander C, et al. Cardiac magnetic resonance reveals signs of subclinical myocardial inflammation in asymptomatic HIV-infected patients. *Circulation Cardiovasc Imaging.* 2016;9:e004091.

98. Holloway CJ, Ntusi N, Suttie J, et al. Comprehensive cardiac magnetic resonance imaging and spectroscopy reveal a high burden of myocardial disease in HIV patients. *Circulation.* 2013;128:814-822.

99. Thiara DK, Liu CY, Raman F, et al. Abnormal myocardial function is related to myocardial steatosis and diffuse myocardial fibrosis in HIV-infected adults. *J Infect Dis.* 2015;212:1544-1551.

100. Lumsden RH, Bloomfield GS. The causes of HIV-associated cardiomyopathy: a tale of two worlds. *BioMed Res Int.* 2016;2016:8196560.

101. Butler J, Greene SJ, Shah SH, et al. Diastolic dysfunction in patients with human immunodeficiency virus receiving antiretroviral therapy: results from the CHART study. *J Cardiac Fail.* 2020;26:371-380.

102. Janjua SA, Triant VA, Addison D, et al. HIV infection and heart failure outcomes in women. *J Am Coll Cardiol.* 2017;69:107-108.

103. Moyers BS, Secemsky EA, Vittinghoff E, et al. Effect of left ventricular dysfunction and viral load on risk of sudden cardiac death in patients with human immunodeficiency virus. *Am J Cardiol.* 2014;113:1260-1265.

104. Heidenreich PA, Eisenberg MJ, Kee LL, et al. Pericardial effusion in AIDS. Incidence and survival. *Circulation.* 1995;92:3229-3234.

105. Lind A, Reinsch N, Neuhaus K, et al. Pericardial effusion of HIV-infected patients? Results of a prospective multicenter cohort study in the era of antiretroviral therapy. *Eur J Med Res.* 2011;16:480-483.

106. Reuter H, Burgess LJ, Doubell AF. Epidemiology of pericardial effusions at a large academic hospital in South Africa. *Epidemiol Infect.* 2005;133:393-399.

107. Syed FF, Ntsekhe M, Gumedze F, Badri M, Mayosi BM. Myopericarditis in tuberculous pericardial effusion: prevalence, predictors and outcome. *Heart (British Cardiac Society).* 2014;100:135-139.

108. Mayosi BM, Wiysonge CS, Ntsekhe M, et al. Mortality in patients treated for tuberculous pericarditis in sub-Saharan Africa. *S Afr Med J.* 2008;98:36-40.

109. Mayosi BM, Ntsekhe M, Bosch J, et al. Prednisolone and Mycobacterium indicus pranii in tuberculous pericarditis. *N Eng J Med.* 2014;371:1121-1130.

110. Simonneau G, Gatzoulis MA, Adatia I, et al. Updated clinical classification of pulmonary hypertension. *J Am Coll Cardiol.* 2013;62:D34-D41.

111. Sitbon O, Lascoux-Combe C, Delfraissy JF, et al. Prevalence of HIV-related pulmonary arterial hypertension in the current antiretroviral therapy era. *Am J Respirat Crit Care Med.* 2008;177:108-113.

112. Simonneau G, Montani D, Celermajer DS, et al. Haemodynamic definitions and updated clinical classification of pulmonary hypertension. *Eur Respirat J.* 2019;53:1801913.

113. Dzudie A, Dzekem BS, Ojji DB, et al. Pulmonary hypertension in low- and middle-income countries with focus on sub-Saharan Africa. *Cardiovasc Diag Ther.* 2020;10:316-324.

114. Kanmogne GD, Primeaux C, Grammas P. Induction of apoptosis and endothelin-1 secretion in primary human lung endothelial cells by HIV-1 gp120 proteins. *Biochem Biophys Res Comm.* 2005;333:1107-1115.

115. Pellicelli AM, Palmieri F, Cicalini S, Petrosillo N. Pathogenesis of HIV-related pulmonary hypertension. *Ann New York Academy Sciences.* 2001;946:82-94.

116. Galie N, Humbert M, Vachiery JL, et al. 2015 ESC/ERS Guidelines for the diagnosis and treatment of pulmonary hypertension: the Joint Task Force for the Diagnosis and Treatment of Pulmonary Hypertension of the European Society of Cardiology (ESC) and the European Respiratory Society (ERS): endorsed by: Association for European Paediatric and Congenital Cardiology (AEPC), International Society for Heart and Lung Transplantation (ISHLT). *Eur Heart J.* 2016;37:67-119.

117. Frost A, Badesch D, Gibbs JSR, et al. Diagnosis of pulmonary hypertension. *Eur Respirat J.* 2019;53:1801904.

118. Petitpretz P, Brenot F, Azarian R, et al. Pulmonary hypertension in patients with human immunodeficiency virus infection. Comparison with primary pulmonary hypertension. *Circulation.* 1994;89:2722-2727.

119. Degano B, Guillaume M, Savale L, et al. HIV-associated pulmonary arterial hypertension: survival and prognostic factors in the modern therapeutic era. *AIDS (London, England).* 2010;24:67-75.

120. Benza RL, Miller DP, Barst RJ, Badesch DB, Frost AE, McGoon MD. An evaluation of long-term survival from time of diagnosis in pulmonary arterial hypertension from the REVEAL Registry. *Chest.* 2012;142:448-456.

121. Schumacher YO, Zdebik A, Huonker M, Kreisel W. Sildenafil in HIV-related pulmonary hypertension. *AIDS (London, England).* 2001;15:1747-1748.

122. Garraffo R, Lavrut T, Ferrando S, et al. Effect of tipranavir/ritonavir combination on the pharmacokinetics of tadalafil in healthy volunteers. *J Clin Pharmacol.* 2011;51:1071-1078.

123. Dingemanse J, van Giersbergen PL, Patat A, Nilsson PN. Mutual pharmacokinetic interactions between bosentan and lopinavir/ritonavir in healthy participants. *Antiviral Ther.* 2010;15:157-163.

124. Pulido T, Adzerikho I, Channick RN, et al. Macitentan and morbidity and mortality in pulmonary arterial hypertension. *N Eng J Med.* 2013;369:809-818.

125. Reinsch N, Esser S, Gelbrich G, et al. Valvular manifestations of human immunodeficiency virus infection—results from the prospective, multicenter HIV-HEART study. *J Cardiovasc Med. (Hagerstown, Md).* 2013;14:733-739.

126. Gebo KA, Burkey MD, Lucas GM, Moore RD, Wilson LE. Incidence of, risk factors for, clinical presentation, and 1-year outcomes of infective endocarditis in an urban HIV cohort. *JAIDS.* 2006;43:426-32.

127. Nel SH, Naidoo DP. An echocardiographic study of infective endocarditis, with special reference to patients with HIV. *Cardiovasc J Afr.* 2014;25:50-57.

128. Furuno JP, Johnson JK, Schweizer ML, et al. Community-associated methicillin-resistant Staphylococcus aureus bacteremia and endocarditis among HIV patients: a cohort study. *BMC Infect Dis.* 2011;11:298.

129. Polanco A, Itagaki S, Chiang Y, Chikwe J. Changing prevalence, profile, and outcomes of patients with HIV undergoing cardiac surgery in the United States. *Am Heart J.* 2014;167:363-368.

130. Beckman JA, Duncan MS, Alcorn CW, et al. Association of human immunodeficiency virus infection and risk of peripheral artery disease. *Circulation.* 2018;138:255-265.

131. Post WS, Budoff M, Kingsley L, et al. Associations between HIV infection and subclinical coronary atherosclerosis. *Ann Intern Med.* 2014;160:458-467.

132. Tilson MD 3rd, Withers L. Arterial aneurysms in HIV patients: molecular mimicry versus direct infection? *Ann New York Academy of Sciences.* 2006;1085:387-391.

133. Ferfar Y, Savey L, Comarmond C, et al. Large-vessel vasculitis in human immunodeficiency virus-infected patients. *J Vasc Surg.* 2018;67:1501-1511.

134. Chetty R, Batitang S, Nair R. Large artery vasculopathy in HIV-positive patients: another vasculitic enigma. *Human Pathol.* 2000;31:374-379.

135. Pillay B, Ramdial PK, Naidoo DP. HIV-associated large-vessel vasculopathy: a review of the current and emerging clinicopathological spectrum in vascular surgical practice. *Cardiovasc J Afr.* 2015;26:70-81.

136. Javed MA, Sheppard MN, Pepper J. Aortic root dilation secondary to giant cell aortitis in a human immunodeficiency virus-positive patient. *Eur J Cardio-Thoracic Surg.* 2006;30:400-401.

137. Saber AA, Aboolian A, LaRaja RD, Baron H, Hanna K. HIV/AIDS and the risk of deep vein thrombosis: a study of 45 patients with lower extremity involvement. *Am Surgeon.* 2001;67:645-647.

138. Jackson BS, Pretorius E. Pathological clotting and deep vein thrombosis in patients with HIV. *Seminars Thromb Hemost.* 2019;45:132-140.

139. Vululi ST, Bugeza S, Zeridah M, et al. Prevalence of lower limb deep venous thrombosis among adult HIV positive patients attending an outpatient clinic at Mulago Hospital. *AIDS Res Ther.* 2018;15:3.

140. Alvaro-Meca A, Ryan P, Martinez-Larrull E, Micheloud D, Berenguer J, Resino S. Epidemiological trends of deep venous thrombosis in HIV-infected subjects (1997-2013): a nationwide population-based study in Spain. *Eur J Int Med.* 2018;48:69-74.

141. Sani MU, Okeahialam BN. QTc interval prolongation in patients with HIV and AIDS. *J Nat Med Assoc.* 2005;97:1657-1661.

142. Njoku PO, Ejim EC, Anisiuba BC, Ike SO, Onwubere BJ. Electrocardiographic findings in a cross-sectional study of human immunodeficiency virus (HIV) patients in Enugu, south-east Nigeria. *Cardiovasc J Afr.* 2016;27:252-257.

143. Tseng ZH, Secemsky EA, Dowdy D, et al. Sudden cardiac death in patients with human immunodeficiency virus infection. *J Am Coll Cardiol.* 2012;59:1891-1896.

144. Gili S, Mancone M, Ballocca F, et al. Prevalence and predictors of long corrected QT interval in HIV-positive patients: a multicenter study. *J Cardiovasc Med (Hagerstown).* 2017;18:539-544.

145. Kannankeril P, Roden DM, Darbar D. Drug-induced long QT syndrome. *Pharmacol Rev.* 2010;62:760-781.

146. Soliman EZ, Lundgren JD, Roediger MP, et al. Boosted protease inhibitors and the electrocardiographic measures of QT and PR durations. *AIDS.* 2011;25:367-377.

147. Brouillette J, Cyr S, Fiset C. Mechanisms of arrhythmia and sudden cardiac death in patients with HIV infection. *Can J Cardiol.* 2019;35:310-319.

148. Wisniowska B, Tylutki Z, Wyszogrodzka G, Polak S. Drug-drug interactions and QT prolongation as a commonly assessed cardiac effect-comprehensive overview of clinical trials. *BMC Pharmacol Toxicol.* 2016;17:12.

149. Hsu JC, Li Y, Marcus GM, et al. Atrial fibrillation and atrial flutter in human immunodeficiency virus-infected persons: incidence, risk factors, and association with markers of HIV disease severity. *J Am Coll Cardiol.* 2013;61:2288-2295.

150. Sanders JM, Steverson AB, Pawlowski AE, et al. Atrial arrhythmia prevalence and characteristics for human immunodeficiency virus-infected persons and matched uninfected controls. *PLoS One.* 2018;13:e0194754.

151. Feinstein MJ, Achenbach CJ, Stone NJ, Lloyd-Jones DM. A systematic review of the usefulness of statin therapy in HIV-infected patients. *Am J Cardiol.* 2015;115:1760-1766.

152. Yu J, Zhou Z, Tay-Sontheimer J, Levy RH, Ragueneau-Majlessi I. Risk of clinically relevant pharmacokinetic-based drug-drug interactions with drugs approved by the U.S. Food and Drug Administration Between 2013 and 2016. *Drug Metabol Disposit: Biologic Fate Chem.* 2018;46:835-845.

153. Hsue PY, Waters DD. Time to recognize HIV infection as a major cardiovascular risk factor. *Circulation.* 2018;138:1113-1115.

78

Heart Disease in Pregnancy

Dan G. Halpern, Amy Sarma, Katherine E. Economy, and Anne Marie Valente

Cardiovascular disease in pregnancy

- Most common cause of indirect maternal mortality, complicating 1-4% of pregnancies
- Rates of pregnancy associated complications are increasing due to advanced maternal age and increasing burden of cardiovascular disease risk factors (e.g., obesity, hypertension, diabetes)
- Most common etiologies: congenital heart disease (developed world), rheumatic heart disease (developing world)

Preconception evaluation

- **Counseling** on maternal and fetal risks and potential events during pregnancy
- **Complete workup** including vital signs, oxygen saturation, physical exam, ECG, appropriate cardiac imaging (e.g. echocardiogram, CT/MR angiography for aortic evaluation, consideration of stress testing
- Review of medications and adjustment as needed
- Performance of fetal echo at 20 weeks gestation with history of congenital heart disease
- Functional capacity of at least 80% compared to the general population is considered for a safe pregnancy

Pregnancy contraindicated

- Pulmonary arterial hypertension
- Severe systemic ventricular dysfunction (EF <30% or NYHA class III–IV)
- Previous peripartum cardio-myopathy with any residual left ventricular impairment
- Severe symptomatic aortic stenosis
- Systemic right ventricle with moderate or severely decreased ventricular function

- Severe aortic dilatation (>45 mm in Marfan syndrome or other HTAD, >50 mm in bicuspid aortic valve, Turner syndrome ASI >25 mm/m²)
- Severe mitral stenosis
- Vascular Ehlers–Danlos
- Severe (re)coarctation
- Fontan with any complication

Medications contraindicated during pregnancy

- ACE-I class
- ARB class
- Aldosterone antagonists

- Non-vitamin K oral antagonists
- ERAs (e.g., bosentan)
- Riociguat
- Nitroprusside should be used as last resort

- Statin class has mixed data and requires shared decision making
- Atenolol use requires shared decision making
- Amiodarone should be used as last resort

Cardiac conditions during pregnancy

- **Emergency:** In life-threatening conditions such as cardiac arrest, ACLS protocols should be followed and life-saving medications should not be withheld. Resuscitation should include the unique modification of manipulating the uterus left laterally by 1.5 cm to improve venous return.

- **Hypertension:** Complicates 10% of pregnancies, ≥ 140/90 (severe > 160/110 mmHg), may be associated with pre-eclampsia and end-organ damage. Nifedipine, labetolol and alpha-methyl-dopa are the first-line treatment regimen.

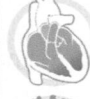

- **Peripartum cardiomyopathy** – newly diagnosed systolic cardiomyopathy (LVEF < 45%) without a reversible cause, presenting late in pregnancy or the early postpartum period. Bromocriptine use is being further studied.

- **Aortopathies:** risk of aortic dissections increases with connective tissue diseases. Pregestational counseling is imperative for risk stratification. Beta-blockade is advised when tolerated.

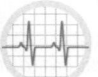

- **Arrhythmias:** Frequency of arrhythmias may increase during pregnancy. New onset of arrhythmia, especially ventricular, should prompt a structural evaluation. New onset atrial fibrillation should prompt a structural evaluation and consideration of a pulmonary embolus.

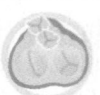

- **Valve disease:** Regurgitant lesions are better tolerated in pregnancy than stenotic lesions. Mechanical heart valves anticoagulant regimen is highly challenging as warfarin and heparin/enoxaparin portend higher fetal and maternal complications, respectively. Hemodynamic complications are commonly encountered in the early postpartum period as the systemic and pulmonary vascular resistance rise.

- **Ischemic heart disease:** Frequency of ischemic heart disease is rising, owing to the increase in cardiovascular risk factors and advanced maternal age. SCAD and coronary embolic events are the major causes. Invasive strategies should be limited to those with severe clinical decompensation and/or unresponsive to medical interventions.

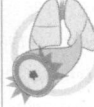

- **Pulmonary hypertension:** Pregnancy is contraindicated due to high maternal and fetal mortality. ERAs and riociguat are contraindicated in pregnancy. PGE-5 inhibitors (e.g., sildenafil) and prostanoids (e.g., epoprostenol, treprostinil) may be used.

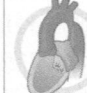

- **Non-cyanotic congenital heart disease:** majority tolerate pregnancy well, requires in-depth knowledge of the lesion and individualized care provided by ACHD experts.

Chapter 78 Fuster and Hurst's Central Illustration. ACE-I, angiotensin converting-enzyme inhibitors; ACHD, adult congenital heart disease; ACLS, advanced cardiovascular life-support; ARB, angiotensin receptor blockers; ASI, aortic size index; CT, computed tomography; ECG, electrocardiography; EF, ejection fraction; ERA, endothelin receptor antagonist; HTAD, hereditable thoracic aortic disease; LVEF, left ventricular ejection fraction; MR, magnetic resonance; NYHA, New York Heart Association; PGE-5, prostaglandin-5; SCAD, spontaneous coronary artery dissection.

CHAPTER SUMMARY

Cardiovascular disease (CVD) complicates 1% to 4% of pregnancies and is the primary cause of nonobstetric maternal mortality. Older maternal age, with associated increases in CVD risk factors such as obesity, hypertension, and diabetes, as well as improved survival of patients with congenital heart disease have increased the burden of CVD during pregnancy. Optimal patient care for the pregnant woman with CVD relies on an understanding of the unique hemodynamic changes of pregnancy and the pathophysiology, signs and symptoms, and natural history specific to each heart condition that may impact pregnancy. Preconception consultation of pregnant women with CVD is imperative and such individuals should be cared for by expert multidisciplinary teams in anticipation of possible complications that may arise during the antepartum, intrapartum, and postpartum periods. Pregnancy is not advised in several conditions and some medications are contraindicated during pregnancy (see Fuster and Hurst's Central Illustration).

INTRODUCTION

Preexisting and acquired cardiovascular disease (CVD) increases maternal and fetal morbidity and mortality during pregnancy.[1,2] CVD complicates 1% to 4% of pregnancies and according to a recent UK registry, accounts for 37% of non-obstetric maternal death and is the leading cause of indirect maternal mortality.[3,4] There is an increase in the burden of CVD during pregnancy related to advanced maternal age, increase in cardiovascular risk factors such as obesity, hypertension, and diabetes, and the improved survival of congenital heart disease (CHD) patients. CHD comprises the majority of cases of CVD during pregnancy in the Western world, whereas rheumatic heart disease is more common in developing countries;[5,6] other prevalent etiologies include connective tissue disease and cardiomyopathies.

There is evidence to suggest that most women with CVD may be able to tolerate pregnancy. However, careful preconception planning with providers experienced in high-risk pregnancy is needed. Risk stratification models summarizing maternal and fetal outcomes have been developed to counsel women with CVD desiring pregnancy. Optimal patient care for the pregnant woman with CVD relies on understanding of the unique hemodynamic changes of pregnancy and the pathophysiology, signs and symptoms, and natural history specific to each heart condition that may impact pregnancy. A multidisciplinary team (ie, pregnancy heart team) approach involving cardiologists, maternal fetal medicine specialists, and anesthesiologists in a center with experience is strongly advised for the care of pregnant women with heart disease.

PRECONCEPTION CONSIDERATIONS

Women with CVD should receive counseling regarding both maternal and fetal risks prior to conceiving a pregnancy. In addition, women with heart disease should be cared for at institutions with experience in treating CVD during pregnancy. There are certain high-risk conditions for which pregnancy is contraindicated including pulmonary arterial hypertension, congenital cyanotic lesions, severe systemic ventricular dysfunction, severe mitral stenosis, severe symptomatic aortic stenosis, certain aortopathies, and other conditions listed in **Table 78–1** as World Health Organization (WHO) class IV.[1] Women with CVD who are considering pregnancy should undergo a complete workup including a detailed medical and surgical history, physical exam including oxygen saturations, electrocardiogram (ECG), appropriate cardiac imaging, and consideration of cardiopulmonary stress testing for further risk stratification.[7] The European guidelines suggest that women with an exercise capacity that exceeds 80% have more favorable pregnancy outcomes.[1]

Genetic counseling is appropriate for patients with family members affected by congenital and inherited heart diseases (eg, hypertrophic cardiomyopathy, Marfan syndrome [MFS], long-QT syndromes). In nonsyndromic patients, CHD is present in about 0.8% of the population, yet for an affected individual, the risk of bearing children with CHD is increased to 2%

to 6%.[8,9] Further recurrences of CHD in the same family are higher. If there is a history of CHD in either biologic parent, fetal echocardiogram should be performed between 20 and 22 weeks of gestation.[10]

Preconceptual counseling will allow for careful planning for any anticipated or potential events during pregnancy. All prepregnancy medications should be reviewed to ensure their safety in pregnancy (see section Cardiovascular Medications Used in Pregnancy and Lactation).

HEMODYNAMIC CHANGES OF NORMAL PREGNANCY

The hemodynamic changes of pregnancy are marked and occur over a relatively condensed period of time (**Fig. 78–1**). While the healthy cardiovascular system adapts remarkably well, women with underlying cardiac conditions may not tolerate such intense hemodynamic changes. By 24 weeks of gestation, circulating plasma volume has increased by 40%, resulting in a 30% to 50% increase in cardiac output, which begins to rise as early as 5 weeks after the last menstrual cycle and steadily increases until 28 to 34 weeks.[1,11–17] A greater increase in plasma volume as compared to erythrocyte mass accounts for the physiologic anemia of pregnancy. In early pregnancy, the rise in cardiac output is primarily achieved through a 40% increase in stroke volume, which peaks at 28 to 31 weeks of gestation.[12,13] In the third trimester, the increase in heart rate primarily mediates cardiac output augmentation, with an average heart rate rise of 10 to 15 bpm.[1,16,18] Cardiac output begins to decline late in third trimester, but does not return to prepregnancy values until 2 to 4 week postpartum.[13] Systemic vascular resistance falls early in pregnancy, primarily due to maturation of placental circulation and the effects of endogenous hormones with a resulting 30% to 50% fall from prepregnancy values by the end of the second trimester, followed by an increase at the end of the third trimester.[11,13,18] In addition, local vasodilatory factors including prostacyclin and nitric oxide contribute to a fall in both systolic and diastolic blood pressure to 5 to 10 mm Hg below prepregnancy values, a change that begins as early as 6 to 8 weeks of gestation and nadirs in the second trimester before gradually increasing in the third trimester.[1,19] This increase in vascular compliance aids in accommodating the marked increase in plasma volume.[20,21]

The Hemodynamics of Labor and the Postpartum Period

Labor and delivery result in acute hemodynamic swings that place an additional stress on the maternal cardiovascular system. Cardiac output can increase by 15% to 25% in early labor, 50% during active labor, and up to 80% immediately postpartum as compared to prelabor values, primarily mediated by an increase in stroke volume.[22,23] In the immediate postpartum period, preload acutely rises from auto-transfusion from the utero-placental circulation and increased venous return in the setting of relief of uterine compression on the inferior vena cava.[11] Within 48 hours of delivery, the heart rate falls 14%,

TABLE 78–1. Predictors of Adverse Maternal Cardiovascular Events during Pregnancy

CARPREG	CARPREG II	ZAHARA	mWHO (modified WHO criteria)
(1) prior cardiovascular event (2) above class II New York heart association (NYHA) functional class symptoms or cyanosis (resting oxygen saturation <90% at rest) (3) left sided heart obstruction (peak left ventricular outflow tract gradient ≥30 mmHg, mitral valve area <2 cm², aortic valve area <1.5 cm²) and (4) systemic ventricular dysfunction, with an ejection fraction <40%. **Score:** 0 → 5% 1 → 27% >1 → 75%	1. Prior CV events or arrhythmia (3 points) 2. NYHA class >II or cyanosis (resting oxygen saturation <90% at rest) (3 points) 3. Mechanical valve (3 points) 4. Systemic ventricular dysfunction with LVEF <49% (2 points) 5. High-risk left-sided obstruction (peak LVOT >30 mmHg, mitral valve area <2 cm², aortic valve area <1.5 cm²; (2 points) 6. Pulmonary hypertension (RVSP > 49mmHg) (2 points) 7. Coronary artery disease (2 points) 8. High-risk aortopathy (2 points) 9. No prior cardiac intervention (1 point) 10. Later pregnancy assessment (2 points) Score: • 0–1 → 5% • 2 → 10% • 3 → 15% • 4 → 22% • ≥4 → 41%	(1) history of arrhythmia (1.5 points) (2) above II NYHA FC (0.75 points); (3) LVOT obstruction with a peak >50 mm Hg or aortic valve area < 1 cm² (2.5 points) (4) mechanical valve prosthesis (4.25 points) (5) moderate/severe systemic atrioventricular valve regurgitation (6) moderate/severe sub-pulmonary atrioventricular valve regurgitation (7) use of cardiac medications prepregnancy (8) repaired or unrepaired cyanotic heart disease (1 point) **Score:** **0–0.5 points → 2.9 %** **0.51–1.50 points →** **7.5 %–1.51–2.50 →** **17.5 %** **2.51–3.50 points →** **43.1 %** **≥3.51 points → 70.0**	**Class I—low risk** (2.5%–5% maternal cardiac event rate) mild pulmonic stenosis, small patent ductus arteriosus, mild mitral valve prolapse; successfully repaired simple lesions (atrial or ventricular septal defect, patent ductus arteriosus, or anomalous pulmonary venous drainage); and isolated atrial or ventricular ectopic beats. **Class II—moderate risk** (5.7%–10.5%) un-operated atrial or ventricular septal defect, repaired tetralogy of Fallot and most arrhythmia. **Class II-III—moderate to high risk** mild left ventricular impairment (LVEF >45%), hypertrophic cardiomyopathy, native or tissue heart valve disease not considered WHO I or IV, Marfan syndrome or other hereditary aortic disease without aortic dilatation and aorta <45 mm in aortic disease associated with bicuspid aortic valve; repaired coarctation, atrioventricular septal defect. **Class III—high risk** (10%–19%) Would change the whole list of class III to: "moderate left ventricular impairment (EF 30–45%), previous peripartum cardiomyopathy without any residual left ventricular impairment, systemic right ventricle with normal or mild impairment, uncomplicated Fontan, unrepaired cyanotic or other complex heart disease, moderate mitral stenosis, severe asymptomatic aortic stenosis, moderate aortic dilatation (40–45 mm in Marfan or other hereditary aortic disease; 45–50 mm in bicuspid aortic valve, Turner syndrome indexed size 20–25 mm/m²), ventricular tachycardia." **Class IV—extremely high risk, contraindicated** (40%–100%) pulmonary arterial hypertension of any cause, severe systemic ventricular dysfunction (LVEF <30%, NYHA III-IV), previous peripartum cardiomyopathy and any residual impairment of left ventricular function, severe mitral stenosis, severe symptomatic aortic stenosis, severe aortic dilatation (>45 mm in Marfan syndrome or other hereditary aortic disease, >50 mm in bicuspid aortic valve, Turner syndrome with index size > 25 mm/m², Vascular Ehlers-Danlos, severe (re)coarctation and Fontan with any complication.

followed by an additional 26% as compared to pregnancy values by 2 weeks postpartum.[17] While much of the hemodynamic changes of pregnancy have resolved by 2 weeks postpartum, full return to prepregnancy physiology occurs over the following 6 months.[17,24]

Structural Heart Adaptations of the Maternal Heart

In response to the hemodynamic demands of pregnancy, the maternal heart undergoes physiologic hypertrophy with an appreciable increase in left ventricular mass that reverses 8 to 14 weeks postpartum.[13,15,25,26] In addition, right ventricular (RV) mass can increase up to 40% as measured by cardiac magnetic resonance imaging (MRI).[27] Echocardiographic studies have revealed that while left ventricular ejection fraction remains stable, in parallel with the increase in stroke volume, left ventricular cavity dimensions and wall thickness, aortic size, and atrial dimensions all increase during pregnancy, with return to prepregnancy values in the postpartum period.[13,15,20,25,27–29] In addition, an increase in stroke work and decrease in left ventricular longitudinal strain has been observed in the later stages of pregnancy.[28] Increase in annular diameters resulting from chamber enlargement can result in physiologic mitral, tricuspid, and pulmonic regurgitation; the development of aortic insufficiency is rare given only a small (~5%) increase in left ventricular outflow tract diameter.[26,27,30] Despite the increase

in valvular regurgitation, women rarely are symptomatic from these changes.[31] In addition, pericardial effusions without hemodynamic significance develop in up to 40% of women and resolve by 6 weeks postpartum.[32,33]

CARDIOVASCULAR MEDICATIONS USED IN PREGNANCY AND LACTATION

The physiological changes of pregnancy may alter drug properties and can have an effect on the fetus.[34] Pharmacokinetic changes during pregnancy include delayed gastric emptying and motility with potential for decreased absorption, increased plasma volume and fat accumulation, increased volume of distribution, decrease in albumin and other protein binding, increased minute ventilation, and increased hepatic and renal clearance (Fig. 78–1). Commonly, the net effect of these changes is decreased drug effect; however, there are exceptions. Ideally, medications should be reviewed and switched prior to conception (see **Table 78–2** for a list of commonly considered cardiovascular medications during pregnancy). Close attention should be paid to the safety profile of each medication and a discussion of risks and benefits is essential, especially in the first trimester during organogenesis. Given that most of the medications do transfer to breast milk, consultation with the patient's obstetrician and pediatrician is advised. Use of regularly updated databases for medication safety is helpful.

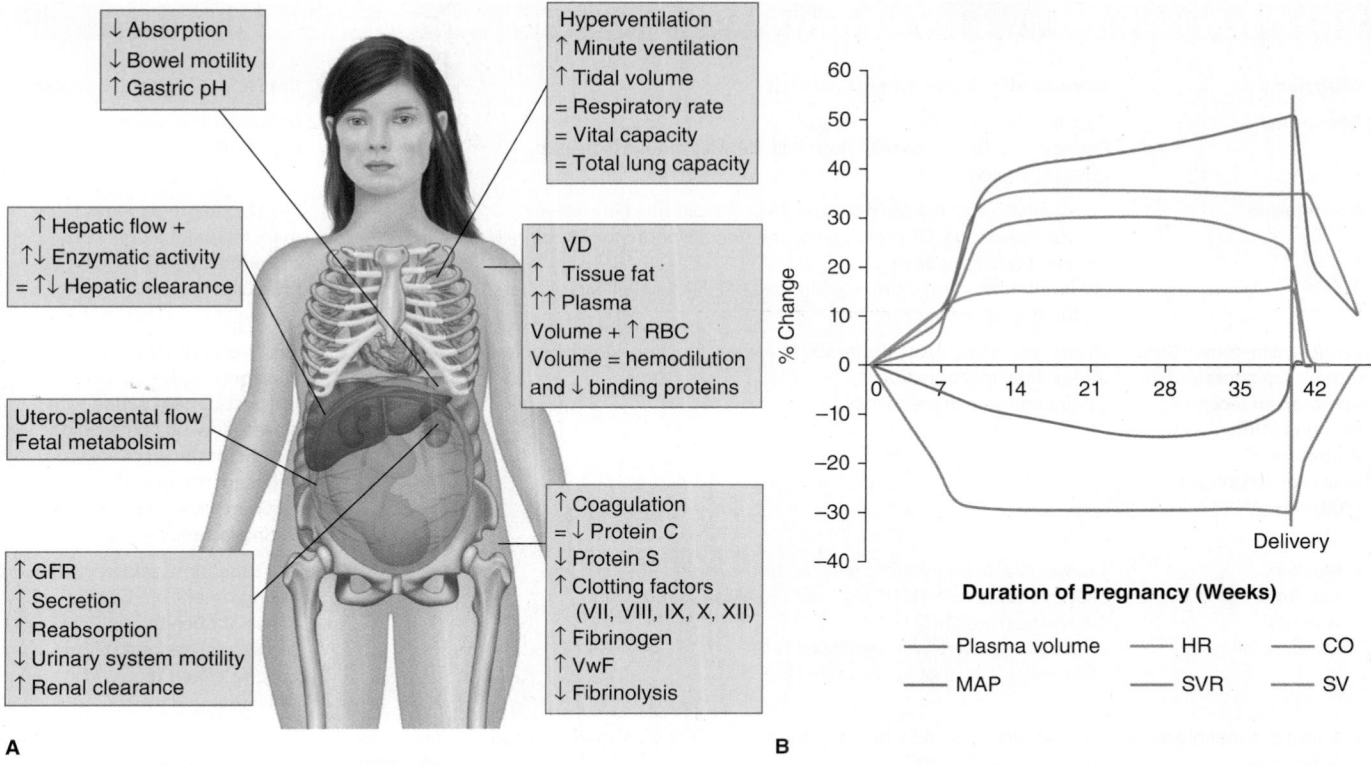

Figure 78–1. (A) Pharmacokinetic and (B) hemodynamic changes of pregnancy.

CO, cardiac output; GFR, glomerular filtration rate; HR, heart rate; MAP, mean arterial pressure; RBC, red blood cell; SvR, systemic vascular resistance; Vd, volume of distribution; VwF, Von Willebrand factor.

Fetal malformations have been a major concern since the 1960s after the effects of thalidomide were appreciated. It should be recognized that only a minority of medications have teratogenic effects. Warfarin is associated with facial, skeletal, and central nervous system malformation especially at a dose that exceeds 5 mg during the first trimester. Endothelin receptor antagonists (eg, bosentan, macitentan) are associated with mandibular malformations and cardiac defects.

Angiotensin converting enzyme inhibitors (ACEi), angiotensin receptor blockers (ARBs), and angiotensin receptor neprilysin inhibitors (ARNI) are contraindicated in pregnancy because they are associated with decreased fetal renal function, lung hypoplasia, and skeletal malformations. Aldosterone antagonists during pregnancy have anti-androgenic properties during the first trimester. Atenolol is considered a higher-risk β-blocker for fetal growth restriction. Data is mixed with regard to potential teratogenic effects of statin therapy, but their use and is currently contraindicated. Bile acid sequestrants such as cholestyramine are the only anti-lipemic agent currently acceptable to be used throughout pregnancy; however, they may reduce absorption of soluble vitamins that may affect fetal growth. Other anti-lipemics such as gemfibrozil and fenofibrate have teratogenic potential and should only be used in the second and their trimester for severe hypertriglyceridemia. Amiodarone treatment should be reserved for emergencies because it is associated with hypothyroidism and neurodevelopmental abnormalities in the fetus.

Women requiring anticoagulation must be advised of the challenges of managing anticoagulation during pregnancy and individualized strategies should be developed (which is subsequently discussed in this chapter). Non–vitamin K oral anticoagulants are contraindicated given the lack of data regarding their use in pregnancy.

Regardless, during a maternal emergency such as cardiac arrest, advanced cardiac life support (ACLS) protocols should be followed and lifesaving medications should not be withheld.

The FDA published the Pregnancy and Lactation Labeling Rule (PLLR) in 2014, which includes three subsections that provide details about the use of the drug in pregnancy and lactation in women and men of reproductive potential. These pregnancy subsections include potential risks to the developing fetus, known dosing alterations in pregnancy, effects of timing and duration of exposure during pregnancy, adverse maternal reactions, effects of the drug on labor and delivery, and information on pregnancy exposure registry for the drug if it exists.[35] This new labeling replaces the previous FDA ABCDX designation system.[1] Table 78–2 lists some of the common medications used in pregnancy and lactation and **Fig. 78–2** summarizes the medications according to use and risk.

CLINICAL EVALUATION OF THE PREGNANT PATIENT

During pregnancy, it is often challenging to distinguish between common symptoms related to the physiological changes of pregnancy and concerning cardiac manifestations.

TABLE 78–2. Medications Used in Pregnancy for Cardiovascular Disease: Adverse Effects, Comments, and Breast Feeding

Drug name	Adverse effects and other comments	Placenta crossing	Breast feeding drug transfer
Adenosine	Dyspnea, bradycardia. Endogenous substance with short half-life; May require increased dosages in pregnancy	No	Unknown, endogenous to breast milk
Amiodarone	Congenital goiter, thyroid disorders (hypothyroidism), neurodevelopmental retardation, QT prolongation, neurodevelopmental abnormalities and premature birth. Treats refractory arrhythmias, prolonged half-life, fetal effects unrelated to duration of use or dose	Yes	Yes. Due to prolonged half-life, manufacturer recommends discontinuation of nursing if drug use is needed
Angiotensin-converting enzyme inhibitors (ACE-I), angiotensin receptor blockers (ARB), Angiotensin Receptor-Neprilysin inhibitors (ARNi)	Oligohydramnios, IUGR, decreased fetal renal function, lung hypoplasia and skeletal malformations. Contraindicated in pregnancy.	Yes	Yes. Captopril, benazepril and enalapril may be considered in the post-partum period with close follow-up of the child's weight for the first 4 weeks. Other agents, manufacturers recommend against their use during lactation.
B-blockers Labetolol Atenolol Metoprolol	Bradycardia, hypoglycemia, reduced birth weight. Labetolol used for HTN (1st line), requires dose changes with GA and lean-weight. Atenolol associated with significant IUGR. Metoprolol is used as AAD and for HF	Yes	Yes. Labetolol – safe (reported asymptomatic bradycardia and Raynaud phenomenon). Metoprolol – acceptable, no adverse effects reported in a small trial.
Calcium channel blockers Nifedipine Verapamil Diltiazem Amlodipine	Pre-maturity, IUGR, fetal bradycardia in some CCB, suspected neonatal seizures if used in third trimester. Nifedipine used as HTN (1st line) and tocolysis (may create maternal hypotension and fetal hypoxemia when used with magnesium). Verapamil and diltiazem are used for SVT or HCM if used prior. Diltiazem associated with adverse fetal effect in animal studies. Amlodipine is probably safe for HTN.	Yes (no for diltiazem)	Yes. Minimal exposure. Nifedipine is acceptable to be used, whereas verapamil is not approved by some manufacturers, and there is limited data for diltiazem in regarding breast feeding.
Cholestyramine resin/colestipol	May lower fat-soluble vitamins	Unknown	No. May be used during lactation
Clonidine	May require shorting dosage intervals. May be used in a transdermal preparation for patients who cannot tolerate oral medications	Yes	Yes
Digoxin	Low birth weight. Used as 1st line for symptomatic SVT using the lowest effective dose; serum levels are unreliable throughout pregnancy	Yes	Yes. Minimal exposure.
Disopyramide	Uterine contraction, placental abruption, prolonged QT	Yes	Yes
Diuretics Loop diuretics (e.g. furosemide) Hydrochlorothiazide (HCTZ) Spironolactone/eplerenone	Oligohydramnios, fetal electrolyte abnormalities. Furosemide commonly used for edema and HF, associated with increased birth weight? Limited data about torsemide and bumetanide. HCTZ used for HTN if used prior, not recommended for routine diuretic purposes. May be associated with fetal/neonatal jaundice and thrombocytopenia and maternal bleeding diathesis and hyponatremia. Spironolactone has anti-androgenic (feminization) effect during first trimester. Eplerenone had adverse effects in animal reproduction studies.	Yes	Yes. Diuretics can suppress lactation. Both furosemide and HCTZ are acceptable, yet require infant follow up. Limited data on other diuretics. Spironolactone and eplerenone are not recommended for lactation.
Dopamine	Cardiac resuscitation drugs are used similarly as non-pregnancy state. May have vasoactive effect on fetus, animal reproduction studies had shown adverse effects	Unknown	Unknown.
Dobutamine	Cardiac resuscitation drugs are used similarly as non-pregnancy state. Not to be used in stress testing during pregnancy	Yes	Unknown.
Endothelin-receptor antagonists (bosentan, ambrisentan, macitentan)	Associated with birth defects including mandibular malformations and cardiac defects	Unknown	Limited data; ambrisentan has been associated with adverse outcomes.
Epinephrine	Cardiac resuscitation drugs are used similarly as non-pregnancy state. May cause uterine vasoconstriction and fetal hypoxia. Used for anaphylaxis state, severe asthma exacerbation and ACLS	Yes	Unknown.

(Continued)

TABLE 78–2. Medications Used in Pregnancy for Cardiovascular Disease: Adverse Effects, Comments, and Breast Feeding (Continued)

Drug name	Adverse effects and other comments	Placenta crossing	Breast feeding drug transfer
Ezetemibe	Associated with adverse fetal effect in animal studies. Not recommended	Unknown	Unknown
Fenofibrate	Limited data. Not recommended	Yes	Unknown
Flecainide	Maternal visual disturbances, acute interstitial nephritis, obstetric cholestasis, fetal bradycardia Used for maternal and fetal AAD	Yes	Yes
Fondaparinux	Used in allergies to heparin or heparin induced thrombocytopenia (HIT)	Yes	Unknown
Gemfibrozil	Associated with adverse fetal effect in animal studies. Not recommended		Unknown
Heparins Unfractionated heparin (UFH) LMWH - enoxaparin	Meticulous monitoring needed for anticoagulation in women with mechanical valves	No	Non excreted in milk
Hydralazine	Lupus-like syndrome, thrombocytopenia, reflex tachycardia Used for hypertension and heart failure	Yes	Yes
Ibutilide	Limited data	Unknown	Unknown
Iloprost	Limited data	Unknown	
Isosorbide Dinitrate	Animal reproduction studies had shown adverse effects Used for hypertension and heart failure	Unknown	Unknown
Lidocaine	CNS depression, cardiac and vascular tone effects Used for ventricular arrhythmia (1st line)	Yes	Yes
Methyldopa	Used for HTN (1st line). Fetal safe. 1% liver toxicity	Yes	Yes
Mexiletine	Used for ventricular arrhythmia. Limited data, but probably safe	Yes	Yes
Milrinone	Cardiac resuscitation drugs are used similarly as non-pregnancy state	Unknown	Unknown
Nitroprusside	Fetal cyanide and thiocyanate toxicity	Yes	Unknown
Norepinephrine	Cardiac resuscitation drugs are used similarly as non-pregnancy state	Yes	unknown
Phosphdiesterase 5 inhibitors (PDE-5i, sildenafil, tadalafil)	Limited data	-	Yes
Platelets aggregation inhibitors Aspirin Clopidogrel Prasugrel Ticagrelor	Aspirin is associated with IUGR, fetal bleeding, in first trimester. Neonatal acidosis and high dose (>325 mg) associated with premature closure of the ductus arteriosus.	Yes (aspirin) Unknown–clopidogrel, Ticagralor, prasugrel	Aspirin transfers, probably safe, yet manufacturer advises against. Unknown data for clopidogrel, prasugrel or ticagrelor
Procainamide	Lupus–like syndrome, prolonged QT Used for maternal and fetal AAD	Yes	Yes
Propafenone	Limited data. Probably safe	Yes	Yes
Quinidine	Fetal thrombocytopenia, prolonged QT	Yes	Yes
Sotalol	Higher risk for TdP (prolonged QT), Fetal bradycardia, hypoglycemia, reduced birth-weight. 1st line for fetal atrial flutter. Clearance increases in 3rd trimester	Yes	Yes
Statins	Limited data, congenital anomalies reported at a low risk – nevertheless should be avoided	Yes	Unknown
Warfarin	Crosses placenta, risk of embryopathy in first trimester (nasal and limb hypoplasia, stippled epiphyses), CNS abnormalities and hemorrhage risk remains throughout pregnancy. Risk of embryopathy is lessen with daily dose ≤ 5mg. Primary indication is mechanical valves	Yes	No transfer to minimal (up to 10%), yet monitor child for bruising.

Categories: A, no demonstrated risk to the fetus based on well controlled human studies; B, No demonstrated risk to the fetus based on animal studies; C, Animal studies have demonstrated fetal adverse effects, no human studies, potential benefits may warrant use of the drug; D, demonstrated human fetal risk, potential benefits may warrant use of the drug; X, demonstrated high risk for human fetal abnormalities outweighing potential benefit; N, nonclassified.

Abbreviations: AAD, anti-arrhythmic drug; ACLS, advanced cardiac life support; CNS, central nervous system; GA, gestation age; HCM, hypertrophic cardiomyopathy; HTN, hypertension; IUGR, intrauterine growth restriction; LMWH, low molecular weight heparin; SVT, supraventricular tachycardia; TdP, Torsades de Pointes.

Reproduced with permission from Halpern DG, Weinberg CR, Pinnelas R, et al. Use of Medication for Cardiovascular Disease During Pregnancy: JACC State-of-the-Art Review. *J Am Coll Cardiol.* 2019 Feb 5;73(4):457-476.

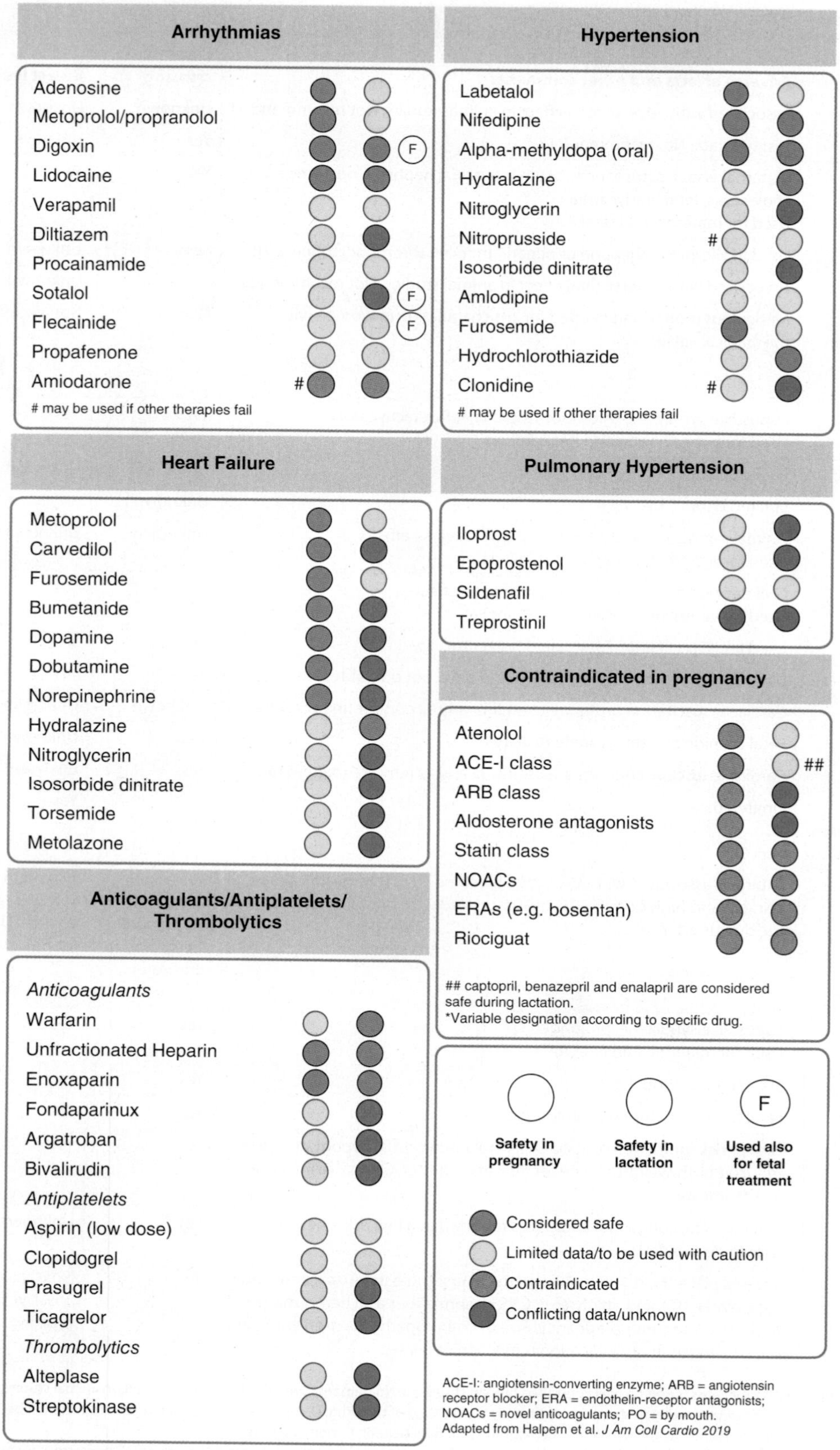

Arrhythmias

Adenosine		
Metoprolol/propranolol		
Digoxin		F
Lidocaine		
Verapamil		
Diltiazem		
Procainamide		
Sotalol		F
Flecainide		F
Propafenone		
Amiodarone	#	

may be used if other therapies fail

Hypertension

Labetalol		
Nifedipine		
Alpha-methyldopa (oral)		
Hydralazine		
Nitroglycerin		
Nitroprusside	#	
Isosorbide dinitrate		
Amlodipine		
Furosemide		
Hydrochlorothiazide		
Clonidine	#	

may be used if other therapies fail

Heart Failure

Metoprolol		
Carvedilol		
Furosemide		
Bumetanide		
Dopamine		
Dobutamine		
Norepinephrine		
Hydralazine		
Nitroglycerin		
Isosorbide dinitrate		
Torsemide		
Metolazone		

Pulmonary Hypertension

Iloprost		
Epoprostenol		
Sildenafil		
Treprostinil		

Contraindicated in pregnancy

Atenolol		
ACE-I class		##
ARB class		
Aldosterone antagonists		
Statin class		
NOACs		
ERAs (e.g. bosentan)		
Riociguat		

captopril, benazepril and enalapril are considered safe during lactation.
*Variable designation according to specific drug.

Anticoagulants/Antiplatelets/ Thrombolytics

Anticoagulants

Warfarin		
Unfractionated Heparin		
Enoxaparin		
Fondaparinux		
Argatroban		
Bivalirudin		

Antiplatelets

Aspirin (low dose)		
Clopidogrel		
Prasugrel		
Ticagrelor		

Thrombolytics

Alteplase		
Streptokinase		

Safety in pregnancy	Safety in lactation	F Used also for fetal treatment

- Considered safe
- Limited data/to be used with caution
- Contraindicated
- Conflicting data/unknown

ACE-I: angiotensin-converting enzyme; ARB = angiotensin receptor blocker; ERA = endothelin-receptor antagonists; NOACs = novel anticoagulants; PO = by mouth.
Adapted from Halpern et al. *J Am Coll Cardio 2019*

Figure 78–2. Cardiovascular medications used in pregnancy. Reproduced with permission from Halpern DG, Weinberg CR, Pinnelas R, et al. Use of Medication for Cardiovascular Disease During Pregnancy: JACC State-of-the-Art Review. *J Am Coll Cardiol.* 2019 Feb 5;73(4):457-476.

Women may sense dyspnea on exertion, decreased exercise capacity, hyperventilation, peripheral edema, and palpitations. Progesterone directly increases minute ventilation, causing a sense of dyspnea and is associated with the sensation of palpitations and increased arrhythmia burden. When these symptoms are mild and arise prior to 20 weeks, they are often attributable to the normal physiological changes of pregnancy. Worrisome symptoms during pregnancy include angina, significant resting dyspnea, paroxysmal nocturnal dyspnea, sustained palpitations, and syncope. Any symptoms that arise after 20 weeks and become progressively worse, or symptoms that significantly impair a woman from performing her daily activities, should prompt further evaluation. The cardiac exam reflects the increase in plasma volume and cardiac output in parallel to a decrease in systemic vascular resistance. Vital signs usually demonstrate an expected increase in heart rate and slight decrease blood pressures with a widened pulse pressure. Women may develop a sense of dyspnea due to progesterone-mediated increase in minute ventilation. Resting oxygen saturation should remain normal. As pregnancy progresses, women with tendency of postural orthostatic tachycardia may have their symptoms exacerbated. Examination of the cardiovascular system, particularly in later stages of gestation, may reveal elevated jugular venous pressures, mild lower extremity edema, and a bounding apical impulse that may be displaced leftward. A systolic flow murmur due to flow across the semilunar valves is common, and a third heart sound may be physiologic.[19,36] A mammary soufflé is a benign high-pitched continuous murmur best heard over the breasts during the third trimester and lactation representing superficial arterial flow. It is not affected by a Valsalva maneuver. Abnormal findings on cardiac exam include a holosystolic systolic murmur, any diastolic murmurs, fourth heart sound, or an exaggerated second heart sound suggesting pulmonary hypertension.[37]

ECG changes found in pregnancy may include sinus tachycardia, left axis deviation, shortened PR interval, increased R/S ration in leads V1 and V2, Q waves and inverted T waves in the inferior leads, and nonspecific transient ST-T changes.[1,38] Both atrial and ventricular premature beats are common in pregnant women.[39]

Echocardiography is very useful to assess ventricular function and valvular pathology during pregnancy.[26] Women should be referred for echocardiography if they present with unexplained symptoms, a history of CVD, unexpected ECG changes, or a new holosystolic or diastolic murmur.[40]

Exercise stress testing can be a useful objective tool for risk stratification of women with CVD prior to pregnancy. In a multicenter center trial of women with CHD, an abnormal chronotropic response correlated with adverse maternal cardiac outcomes.[41]

Cardiac MRI with gadolinium is generally avoided during pregnancy due to the concern of fetal exposure to the contrast agent.[42] Noncontrast MRI is thought to be safe during pregnancy. Concerns of magnetic field effects or local heat produced by the coils have not been documented. Placing the patient in the left recumbent position is advisable after 20 weeks to avoid aortocaval compression by the gravid uterus.[27]

Cardiac catheterization during pregnancy is rarely employed due to its invasive nature and the radiation involved. It should particularly be avoided during the first trimester.[43] Cardiac catheterization in pregnancy is primarily used for emergent hemodynamic evaluation, balloon valvuloplasty, and acute coronary syndrome assessment and treatment.[44-47] At the time of catheterization of any pregnant woman, abdominal shielding should be performed and when possible left lateral uterine displacement achieved by using a wedge or other device.

Natriuretic peptides (including B-type natriuretic peptide [BNP] and the inert N-terminal pro-B-type natriuretic peptide [NT-proBNP]) are emerging as useful tools for screening women for CVD and follow-up of women with cardiomyopathies and preeclampsia. A BNP value within normal range in women with CHD has a strong negative predictive value for adverse outcomes.[48] Nevertheless, this value should be read with caution since it is falsely decreased in obese patients and may be lower in gestational diabetes.[49] Further, the positive predictive value may be lower because a small study of healthy pregnant women found that 6.1% experienced elevations in BNP (>100 pg/mL) in the early postpartum period without associated clinical or echocardiographic evidence of cardiovascular dysfunction.[50]

RISK STRATIFICATION OF CARDIOVASCULAR DISEASE DURING PREGNANCY

Maternal Risk

There are several risk score models available to assess both maternal and fetal risks in the setting of cardiac disease in pregnancy (Table 78–1). These include CARPREG (CARdiac disease in PREGnancy) and now updated with CARPREG II,[51,52] ZAHARA,[53] and the modified WHO classification.[48,54]

The initial Cardiac Disease in Pregnancy (CARPREG) multicenter study pioneered prediction models for CVD in pregnancy. The recent CARPEG II risk score is now the most contemporary model incorporating risk factors identified from the previous models. CARPREG II followed 1938 pregnancies with a total of 16% complications, predominantly heart failure and arrhythmia. Maternal cardiac events rates ranged from 5% for 0 to 1 point to 41% with >4 points.[52] It should be noted that CARPREG II does not distinguish between systemic ventricular functional severity and includes MFS and bicuspid valve disease as high risk aortopathies, although they differ in aortic dissection prevalence.

The modified WHO classification is divided into four categories, listed in Table 78–1.[54] The recommended follow-up for women with WHO Class II is every trimester; women with WHO Class III and IV should be seen monthly or bimonthly.

The multinational Registry On Pregnancy and Cardiac disease (ROPAC) summarized outcomes from 1321 pregnancies of women with CVD from 28 countries between 2007 and 2011.[55] Modified WHO categories were strongly associated with maternal, obstetric, and fetal outcomes. Maternal death (1%), although rare, was significantly higher than that in the general population (0.007%) primarily from heart failure followed by thromboembolic complications and sepsis. Fetal and neonatal mortality were also higher in women with underlying CVD. The ROPAC investigators have since published articles on maternal and fetal outcomes for specific cardiac conditions.[56,57]

Overall, these models are helpful for initial stratification and counseling, yet each case requires a further in-depth lesion-specific evaluation and a tailored risk appraisal.

Obstetrical Risks and Delivery Planning

Obstetric complications appear to be higher in women with CVD. Historically, women with heart disease have been counseled to avoid the Valsalva maneuver during delivery; however, data from 113 pregnancies in 65 women with CHD suggested that women who were not allowed to Valsalva and had assisted second stage with either forceps or vacuum had increased rates of postpartum hemorrhage and vaginal lacerations.[2] Mode of delivery should generally be guided by obstetric indications. Most women with CVD will be able to undergo successful spontaneous vaginal delivery with careful monitoring.[58] Consideration of assisted second stage should take into account known risks of instrumented delivery such as hemorrhage and significant perineal trauma balanced against theoretic benefits of avoidance of Valsalva. In women who are likely to have a low tolerance for Valsalva, a passive second stage where the head is allowed to labor down to a very low fetal station is recommended. At that point, a trial of Valsalva may be attempted. For those women who become hemodynamically compromised with pushing in the second stage, forceps or vacuum instrumentation can be used to expedite delivery.

Neonatal Risk

There is a strong association between maternal morbidity and neonatal adverse events. Rate of neonatal complications and mortality have been reported between 20% and 37% and 1% and 4%, respectively. Risk factors for neonatal events included cyanosis, poor functional class, smoking, multiple gestations, use of anticoagulants during pregnancy, and mechanical valve prosthesis. Events included small for gestational age and prematurity with its associated complications such as respiratory distress syndrome and cerebral hemorrhage.[59]

SPECIFIC FORMS OF HEART DISEASE IN PREGNANCY

Hypertension and Related Disorders

Up to 10% of pregnancies are complicated by hypertensive diseases, which may complicate maternal and fetal health during pregnancy and portend an increased risk of CVD later in life.[60,61] The incidence of hypertensive disorders of pregnancy is increasing, with the rise occurring to a greater degree among Black women as compared with White women.[62,63] Further, independent of other comorbid and demographic risk, Black women with hypertensive disorders of pregnancy are at higher risk for adverse maternal and fetal outcomes.[64]

The American College of Obstetrics and Gynecology (ACOG) categorizes hypertensive disorders of pregnancy

(HDP) as (1) gestational hypertension (defined as new onset hypertension (≥140/90 mm Hg) after 20 weeks of gestation without features of preeclampsia), (2) preeclampsia (new onset hypertension after 20 weeks of gestation associated with significant proteinuria or evidence of end-organ dysfunction), (3) chronic hypertension (defined as hypertension that develops prior to 20 weeks of gestation or prior to conception), and (4) chronic hypertension with superimposed preeclampsia (chronic hypertension with either new-onset proteinuria or evidence of end-organ dysfunction) (**Table 78-3**).[65] Severe features of preeclampsia include severe hypertension (systolic blood pressure ≥160 mm Hg and/or diastolic blood pressure ≥110 mm Hg taken at least 4 hours apart), thrombocytopenia with a platelet count $<100 \times 10^9$/L, pulmonary edema, central nervous system symptoms (including persistent headaches and visual changes), renal insufficiency (serum creatinine >1.1 mg/dL or doubling of baseline serum creatinine) without another apparent cause, and liver dysfunction including persistent right upper quadrant or epigastric pain and/or liver function tests exceeding twice the upper limits of normal.[65] Approximately 10% of women with severe preeclampsia present with pulmonary edema.[66] Further, echocardiographic assessment in the acute setting has demonstrated an increased risk of adverse cardiac remodeling including evidence of diastolic dysfunction and abnormal RV strain among women with severe preeclampsia as compared with normotensive pregnant women.[66]

Treatment of high blood pressure in pregnancy is aimed at reducing periods of severe hypertension, defined as >160/110 mm Hg.[65] Concerns regarding decreased fetoplacental perfusion and consequent risk for fetal growth restriction have led to blood pressure goals of 120/80 mm Hg and less than 160/105 mm Hg in otherwise uncomplicated hypertensive pregnancies.[67-69] It is important to note that these recommendations are for women without underlying structural heart disease. Given that a 5 to 10 mm Hg drop in blood pressure is physiologic during pregnancy through the second trimester, antihypertensive therapies may actually require down-titration in early pregnancy for women with chronic prepregnancy hypertension. A prospective trial of tight control (target diastolic blood pressure 85 mm Hg) versus less-tight control (target diastolic 100 mm Hg) did not yield a difference in the composite primary outcome of pregnancy loss or need for high-level neonatal care or the secondary outcome of serious maternal complications despite a higher incidence of severe maternal hypertension (≥160/110 mm Hg) in the less-tight control group (40.6%) as compared to the tight-control group (27.5%, $P < 0.001$).[70] Further, antihypertensive therapy has not been demonstrated to reduce the risk of preeclampsia, placental abruption, or to improve fetal outcomes/reduce growth restriction.[68] Low-dose aspirin is recommended beginning in the second trimester (12–14 weeks gestation) for women with a history of chronic hypertension or hypertensive disease in a previous pregnancy.[71,72]

Blood Pressure Targets and Therapies

Guideline committees differ with respect to blood pressure limits that warrant antihypertensive therapy. Further, these

TABLE 78–3. Hypertensive Diseases of Pregnancy

Condition	Definition	Other features	Treatment
Chronic hypertension	Known preexisting hypertension or a blood pressure ≥140/90 mm Hg before the 20th week of gestation without proteinuria and/or persistence of hypertension >12 weeks postpartum	• 1%–5% incidence • Increased risk of superimposed preeclampsia, fetal growth restriction, placental abruption, preterm birth, and cesarean section	• Preconception evaluation for secondary causes of hypertension, counseling regarding pregnancy associated risks, and a 24-hour urine to evaluate for preexisting proteinuria • Recommendations for thresholds that merit antihypertensive therapy differ in the guidelines • First-line oral therapy: labetalol, nifedipine, methyldopa • Second-line oral therapy: β-blockers (excluding atenolol), calcium channel blockers • Intravenous therapy with labetalol, hydralazine, sodium nitropursside, or nitroglycerine is indicated for acute development of hypertension (SBP ≥ 160 or DBP ≥ 110) • Contraindicated: ACE inhibitors, ARBs, atenolol • Low-dose aspirin (60–150 mg/day) is recommended after the 12th week of gestation for preeclampsia prevention
Gestational hypertension	Development of new hypertension (SBP ≥140 or DBP ≥ 90) after the 20th week of gestation without proteinuria or end organ dysfunction	• 6%–7% incidence • This includes women who may develop preeclampsia later in gestation and those with previously undiagnosed chronic hypertension	Hypertensive management as in patients with chronic hypertension
Preeclampsia	Development of new hypertension (SBP ≥ 140 or DBP ≥ 90) after the 20th week of gestation with proteinuria of ≥ 300 mg in a 24-hour urine sample or end organ dysfunction	• 2%–5% incidence • Without proteinuria, preeclampsia is diagnosed by hypertension with at least one of the following: thrombocytopenia (<100,000/microliter), LFTs > 2x ULN, sCr > 1.1 mg/deciliter or 2x baseline sCr, pulmonary edema, cerebral or visual disturbances, or hemolysis	• Low-dose aspirin is recommended after the 12th week of gestation for women at high risk for preeclampsia, including those with ≥1 of the following: history of preeclampsia, chronic hypertension, type 1 or 2 diabetes, renal disease autoimmune disease, or carrying multiple gestations • When complicated by pulmonary edema, intravenous nitroglycerin should be used • Delivery is recommended for patients with severe preeclampsia • Close monitoring is recommended for patients with mild disease at <37 weeks of gestation • Delivery is recommended for all patients (even with mild disease) at ≥37 weeks of gestation • IV magnesium for eclampsia prophylaxis
Eclampsia	Features of preeclampsia plus seizures during pregnancy or the first 10 days postpartum	• <0.1% incidence	• IV magnesium • Delivery
Preeclampsia superimposed on chronic hypertension	Chronic hypertension with new onset proteinuria or an increase in proteinuria (if prepregnancy proteinuria was present) or worsening hypertension or the onset of HELLP syndrome	• Approximately 17%–25% of women with chronic hypertension develop superimposed preeclampsia	• Management as for patients with preeclampsia

Abbreviations: ACEi, angiotensin converting enzyme inhibitors; ARB, angiotensin receptor blockers; DBP, diastolic blood pressure; HELLP, hemolysis, elevated liver enzymes, low platelets; LFT, liver function tests; SBP, systolic blood pressure; sCr, serum creatinine; ULN, upper limit of normal.

recommendations do not apply to women with comorbid medical conditions or evidence of end-organ damage. Acute elevations in systolic blood pressure to greater than 160 mm Hg or diastolic blood pressure to greater than 110 mm Hg warrant prompt evaluation and treatment.

There are several choices for antihypertensive therapy in pregnant women. Some of the commonly used medications are included in Table 78–3. For acute management, intravenous labetalol, hydralazine, or oral nifedipine (for women lacking intravenous access) are most commonly used.[1] For women presenting with pulmonary edema in the context of preeclampsia, intravenous nitroglycerin should be considered.[73] For oral antihypertensive therapy, labetalol, nifedipine, and methyldopa are first-line agents, with hydrochlorothiazide being used as a second-line agent.[73–76] Concerns regarding associations between β-blocker use and fetal growth restriction stem from studies of atenolol use and thus atenolol use is discouraged in pregnancy.[69,77] Data regarding the safety of calcium channel blockers primarily stems from long-acting nifedipine, which has not been associated with adverse fetal or maternal outcomes.[78,79] Diuretics affect the normal volume expansion of pregnancy that is necessary to support uteroplacental blood flow, and should be used only when necessary to control pulmonary edema.[68,69,80] ACE-inhibitors and angiotensin receptor blockers have been associated with fetal renal dysfunction, oligohydramnios, growth abnormalities, skull hypoplasia, neonatal anuria, fetal and neonatal death, and are strictly contraindicated.[68,81–85]

Preeclampsia and Eclampsia

Preeclampsia is a multisystem disorder that affects 2% to 5% of pregnancies and is clinically characterized by the development of new onset hypertension after the 20th week of gestation accompanied by proteinuria exceeding 300 mg.[63] When proteinuria is absent, preeclampsia is identified by hypertension accompanied by end organ damage as manifested by thrombocytopenia, impaired liver function, renal insufficiency, pulmonary edema, or cerebral or visual disturbances.[72] Given that delivery is the mainstay of treatment for severe disease, preeclampsia is associated with an increased risk of iatrogenic preterm delivery, accounting for 15% of preterm births.[86] The term *eclampsia* is applied when the disorder is accompanied by seizures during pregnancy or in the first 10 postpartum days. It is a rare outcome, occurring in less than 0.1% of pregnancies.[87,88]

Together, preeclampsia and eclampsia account for over one-third of severe obstetrical complications, 12% of maternal mortality, and of the risk of perinatal mortality is doubled.[72,86] Among women at high risk for preeclampsia, low-dose aspirin initiated late in the first trimester is recommended to decrease risk for preeclampsia, growth restriction, and preterm delivery.[72,73] High-risk women are those with a history of preeclampsia, preterm delivery, chronic hypertension, diabetes, renal disease, autoimmune diseases, and those carrying multiple gestations.[72,73] In addition, regular exercise during pregnancy may play a role in preeclampsia prevention by improving vascular function.[73,89] Preeclampsia with severe clinical features should prompt delivery.[60] HELLP syndrome, a variant of severe preeclampsia, is defined by hemolysis, elevated liver enzymes, and low platelet count. Although delivery is the mainstay of treatment for severe preeclampsia, select women who are remote from term may be expectantly managed with close monitoring until 34 weeks of gestation provided that they remain clinically stable. Women with mild preeclampsia typically delivered at 37 weeks gestation.[60]

Hypertensive Disorders of Pregnancy and Future Cardiovascular Disease Risk

Women with a history of pregnancy-related hypertensive disorders—particularly preeclampsia—are at increased risk for future CVD.[90] The two may relate by overlapping risk profiles (including obesity, insulin resistance, hyperlipidemia, and renal disease) or through persistent endothelial dysfunction from hypertensive disorders of pregnancy increasing the risk for future CVD.[61,90–93] A recent analysis suggests that CVD risk is largely, although incompletely, mediated through the development of chronic hypertension, and increases a woman's risk of future CVD including coronary artery disease (CAD), heart failure, and valvular dysfunction including mitral regurgitation and aortic stenosis.[94] Further, CVD and chronic hypertension often develop as early as 10 years following a pregnancy complicated by a hypertensive disorder, with Black women being at highest risk.[95–97] Given this strong association, the American Heart Association has recently recognized hypertensive disorders of

pregnancy as important risk factors for the development of future CVD.[98] As such, all women should be asked about a history of adverse pregnancy outcomes—including hypertensive disorders of pregnancy, gestational diabetes, preterm delivery, and small for gestational age infants—when undergoing risk assessment for CVD.[99]

Cardiac Arrhythmias

Women both with and without a history of prior arrhythmia may be at increased risk for cardiac arrhythmias during pregnancy.[39,100–102] Potential mechanisms underlying this predisposition include myocyte stretch in the setting of increased plasma volume and hormonal changes, with some evidence for proarrhythmic properties of progesterone.[39,103,104] Among women with structural heart disease, maternal arrhythmias most commonly emerge in the second trimester.[52] Approximately 20% to 44% of women with preexisting tachyarrhythmias experience recurrence during pregnancy, and this may be associated with an increased risk of adverse fetal and neonatal complications (eg, prematurity, small for gestational age or fetal demise).[1,105] Nonetheless, while palpitations are a frequent complaint in pregnancy, most do not correlate with dangerous ectopy in women without structural heart disease.[100] Many women with structurally normal hearts experience premature atrial and ventricular ectopy during pregnancy,[100] yet sustained arrhythmias are rare, particularly outside of the context of structural heart disease, electrolyte disturbances, or thyroid dysfunction.[106] Women with CHD are at higher risk for developing arrhythmias requiring treatment during pregnancy.[1,107] Those with preexcitation are also more likely to experience arrhythmias during pregnancy, most commonly orthodromic atrioventricular reciprocating tachycardia.[39,108] When treatment is indicated, consideration should be made to avoid invasive procedures when possible, although many can now be performed with minimal or no radiation, and to use antiarrhythmic therapy sparingly given a lack of safety data with these agents, particularly in the first trimester. For hemodynamically unstable women, electrical cardioversion should be performed with close fetal monitoring, although the risk to the fetus has been low in prior studies.[39,101,109,110] It is advisable to involve a cardiac electrophysiologist with expertise in caring for pregnant women when considering arrhythmia management.

Supraventricular Tachycardias

Paroxysmal supraventricular tachycardias (SVTs) are the most common sustained arrhythmias in pregnancy, with a frequency of 24 in 100,000 among pregnancy-related hospitalizations.[106] While women with a history of SVT may experience recurrence, it is rare for a first episode of SVT to occur in pregnancy among women without structural heart disease, with an incidence of 3.9% among a cohort of women with symptomatic paroxysmal SVTs.[111] Among women who experience SVT in pregnancy, the most common arrhythmia is atrioventricular nodal reentrant tachycardia (AVNRT).[111] When possible, vagal maneuvers should first be attempted for arrhythmia termination (**Fig. 78–3**).[1,39,101] If ineffective, adenosine successfully terminates the majority of AVNRT without adverse effect on the fetus given the drug's short half-life.[39,101,112] For those refractory

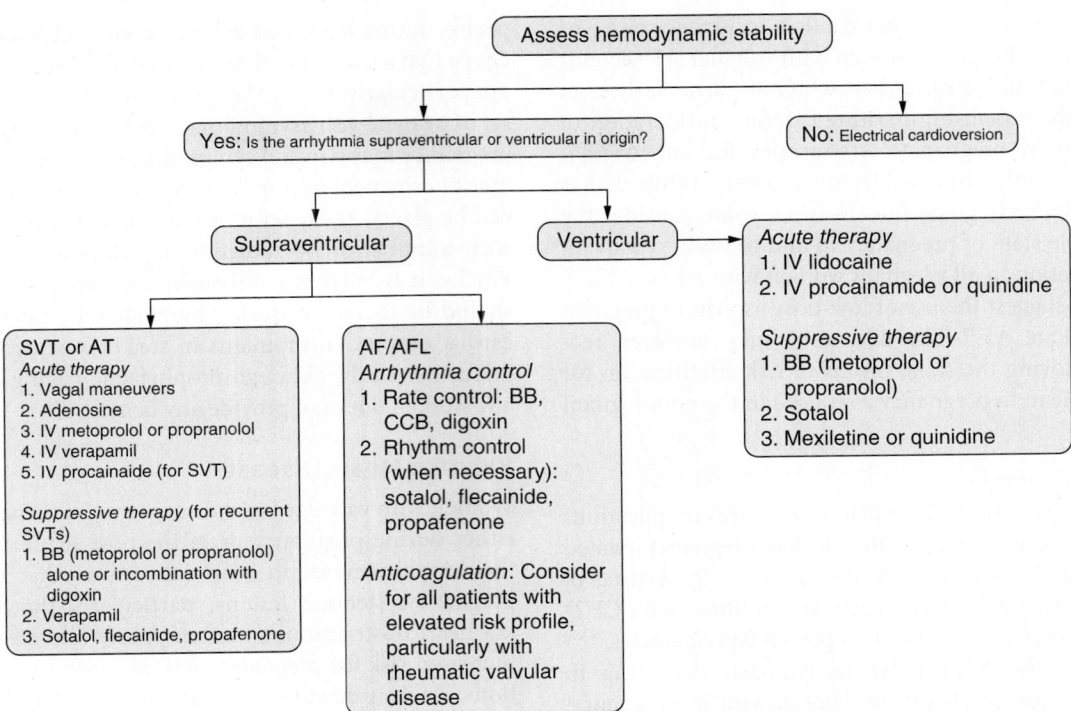

Figure 78–3. **Management of cardiac arrhythmias in pregnancy.** Recommendations are listed in order of highest to lowest utility and safety profile when applicable. AF, atrial fibrillation; AFL, atrial flutter; AT, atrial tachycardia; BB, β-blocker; CCB, calcium channel blocker; SVT, supraventricular tachycardia.

to adenosine, intravenous metoprolol or propranolol should be trialed before intravenous verapamil, which has a higher association with maternal hypotension.[101] Intravenous procainamide is a reasonable alternative agent in the acute setting.[1,101] In all instances, use of amiodarone should be avoided unless absolutely necessary given a high incidence of adverse fetal effects, most notably a 17% incidence of fetal hypothyroidism.[101]

For suppressive therapy in those with frequent symptomatic episodes, oral β-blockers (metoprolol or propranolol) and digoxin can be used as first-line therapy, with the addition of verapamil, sotalol, or flecainide or propafenone (in those without structural heart disease) if necessary.[39,101] As with all medications, antiarrhythmics should be avoided as much as possible in the first trimester and the lowest effective dose should be administered, with an understanding that uptitration may be necessary as the volume of distribution expands with pregnancy.[101] Older antiarrhythmic agents are preferred over newer agents (eg, dofetilide) given a lack of clinical experience in pregnancy with respect to safety.

Atrial tachycardias occur rarely in pregnancy, but are more likely to be resistant to medical therapy and more likely to recur after electrical cardioversion.[1] As with AVNRT, adenosine can be used acutely for diagnostic and therapeutic purposes and for those without response, β-blockers, calcium channel blockers, or digoxin can be used for rate control.[39] For those who fail nodal agents, sotalol, flecainide, or propafenone can be utilized.[1,39]

Atrial Fibrillation and Atrial Flutter

Atrial fibrillation (AF) and flutter (AFL) occur rarely in women without a prior history of these arrhythmias or structural heart disease, although more than half of women with a history of AF/AFL will experience recurrence with pregnancy.[39] In a registry of women with structural heart disease, the incidence of AF/AFL in pregnancy was 1.3%.[113] Risk factors for development of AF/AFL among women with structural heart disease include a prior history of AF/AFL, mitral and aortic valve diseases, and left ventricular cardiomyopathies, with the greatest risk for developing AF/AFL occurring in the second trimester.[113] Further, women with structural heart disease who experienced AF/AFL during pregnancy have a higher rate of maternal mortality and low birth weight as compared to those with structural heart disease who do not experience AF/AFL, although there were no differences between the two groups with respect to development of heart failure.[113]

As with other arrhythmias, women presenting with hemodynamic instability should undergo electrical cardioversion.[39] While experience with chemical cardioversion is limited, intravenous ibutilide or flecainide can also be considered for restoration of sinus rhythm.[1] In those tolerating the rhythm adequately, β-blockers, calcium channel blockers, and digoxin are options for both acute and chronic rate control.[1,39] In those with poor tolerance of AF/AFL in which a rhythm control strategy is necessary, sotalol is one potential option, or alternatively, flecainide, or propafenone can be trialed in women with structurally normal hearts.[1,39] Women with preexcitation who develop AF/AFL should receive intravenous procainamide acutely and should avoid verapamil or digoxin due to risk of rapid accessory pathway conduction.[39] Amiodarone, dronedarone, and dofetilide should be avoided due to lack of clinical experience and/or known adverse fetal effects.[39]

As with nonpregnant patients, thyroid function and the risk of thromboembolism should be assessed in pregnant women who have a history of or experience a first occurrence of AF or AFL in pregnancy. Pregnant women with valvular AF secondary to rheumatic mitral valve disease are at particularly high risk for thromboembolism, meriting careful consideration of anticoagulation in pregnancy[112] (strategies for anticoagulation are subsequently discussed in this chapter). While data is lacking to definitively guide this decision, some consider the hypercoagulable state of pregnancy in and of itself to warrant full anticoagulation in all pregnant women with AF or AFL.[112] Other authors suggest the use of low-dose aspirin in pregnant women with lone AF.[39] The ESC guidelines, however, recommend employing the same means of risk stratification for thromboembolism in pregnancy as is used in the nonpregnant population.[1]

Ventricular Arrhythmias

Ventricular tachycardia and fibrillation are rare complications of pregnancy, occurring in 2 in 100,000 pregnancy-related hospitalizations.[106] Most arrhythmias occur in the setting of structural abnormalities, particularly among those with CHD in which the prevalence is 4.5 to 18.9 per 1000 pregnancies.[39,114] However, idiopathic ventricular tachycardias occurring in structurally normal hearts can initially present in pregnancy, most frequently idiopathic RV outflow tract tachycardias.[1,112] When ventricular arrhythmias occur in the absence of known structural heart disease, particularly in late pregnancy or the early postpartum period, a diagnosis of peripartum cardiomyopathy should be considered.[1,39] Given that ventricular arrhythmias are frequently poorly tolerated from a hemodynamic perspective, these arrhythmias should be particularly carefully evaluated and followed during pregnancy in women with a potential predisposition to them. As in all circumstances, women presenting with hemodynamic instability should undergo electric cardioversion.[1] If the ventricular arrhythmia is hemodynamically tolerated, intravenous lidocaine or β-blockers are considered first-line agents, with procainamide, flecainide, and sotalol as second-line options. As for other arrhythmias, amiodarone should be avoided whenever possible given adverse fetal effects. For long-term suppression, metoprolol or propranolol should be considered first, with sotalol as an option for those refractory to beta blockade.[39] Mexiletine and quinidine can be considered for those who require further antiarrhythmic therapy. Given the length of most ventricular arrhythmia ablations, such procedures should be avoided in pregnancy given the risk of radiation to the fetus with long fluoroscopy times. Implantable cardioverter defibrillators (ICDs) in and of themselves do not pose an increased risk in pregnancy.[1,39] In a retrospective analysis of 44 women with ICDs who became pregnant, 11 received ICD therapy during pregnancy without adverse fetal outcomes, and the device itself did not pose addition complications to pregnancy or vaginal delivery.[115]

Bradyarrhythmias

Sinus node dysfunction and atrioventricular block occur rarely in pregnancy in the absence of structural heart disease.[1,39,106,116] Asymptomatic women with complete heart block can be managed expectantly and generally do not require temporary pacing during labor and delivery even with Valsalva.[1,39,102,112,116] Given that a rise in heart rate is needed to augment cardiac output particularly during the third trimester of pregnancy, a subset of women with asymptomatic complete heart block prior to pregnancy may develop symptoms during pregnancy that then merit permanent pacing.[116] If required, permanent pacemakers can be placed safely with use of echocardiographic guidance, with minimal or no radiation exposure to the fetus.[1,102,116,117] Finally, it is currently unknown whether pacemaker settings should be increased during pregnancy to aid in augmenting cardiac output. This remains an area of investigation that merits further study, although prophylactic pacing of asymptomatic women does not provide any benefit.[1,116]

Valvular Heart Disease

Women with valvular heart disease may experience challenges either during pregnancy or in the postpartum period. Given the natural increase in heart rate and cardiac output during pregnancy, stenotic lesions, particularly those resulting in left heart obstruction, are often poorly tolerated and pose an increased risk for pregnancy-related cardiovascular complications.[118] Likely due to impaired forward flow with severe mitral and aortic stenosis, there is an increased risk with these lesions of intrauterine growth restriction, preterm delivery, and low birth weight.[119] By contrast, the reduction in systemic vascular resistance and thus afterload during pregnancy results in better tolerance of chronic regurgitant lesions. However, such women are at risk for postpartum heart failure in the context of increased volume load and sudden increase in the systemic venous resistance with delivery of the placenta and fluid shifts. **Table 78–4** summarizes potential risks and proposed management strategies for valvular heart conditions during pregnancy. Please refer to the chapters on mitral and aortic valvular diseases for further discussion regarding diagnosis and management in the nonpregnant population.

Mitral Stenosis

Given the risk to mother and fetus, women with moderate or severe mitral stenosis should be counseled to undergo valvular intervention prior to pregnancy when the diagnosis is known prior to conception.[1] When possible, percutaneous balloon valvuloplasty should be considered in appropriately selected patients to obviate the complications of either prosthetic or mechanical valve replacement. However, women with mitral stenosis are often unaware of their disease, with symptoms emerging first in pregnancy. In the developing world, rheumatic disease results in a significant burden of often previously undiagnosed mitral stenosis during pregnancy. Given the tachycardia and volume load of pregnancy, women asymptomatic prior to pregnancy may develop heart failure, particularly in the second and third trimesters.[1,119–121] Heart rate control is essential to help mitigate symptoms. Heart failure should be treated with β1-selective blockers and diuretic therapy when needed for volume overload, with care to avoid overdiuresis.[1,122] The increased risk of thromboembolic events in the setting of concomitant AF mandates therapeutic anticoagulation in this particularly high-risk subset of women.[1,119,120,122] Even in

TABLE 78-4. Valvular Heart Disease in Pregnancy

Lesion	Common Etiologies in Pregnancy	Risk to Mother	Risk to Fetus	Possible Intervention
Mitral stenosis	Rheumatic	• Mild MS (area >1.5 cm²): low risk • Moderate-severe MS (area <1.5 cm², AF): risk of heart failure, mortality risk up to 3%	• Prematurity (20%–30%) • IUGR (5%–20%) • Still birth (1%–3%) • Higher risk in women NYHA class > II	• Prepregnancy: Consider intervention for moderate-severe MS • In pregnancy: BB, diuretics, digoxin (for AF). • Percutaneous mitral commissurotomy in NYHA III/IV or PAP >50 mm Hg on medical therapy
Aortic stenosis	Bicuspid	• *Severe asymptomatic AS on exercise testing: low risk • Severe symptomatic AS or drop in BP on exercise testing: 10% risk of heart failure and risk of arrhythmias	• Risk of preterm birth, IUGR, and low birth weight (in up to 25%) increase with AS severity	• Prepregnancy: Intervention for severe symptomatic AS or asymptomatic AS with LVEF <50% or aortic dilation >45 mm (for consideration of concomitant ascending aortic replacement) • In pregnancy: activity restriction. Consider percutaneous valvuloplasty with severely symptomatic patients despite bedrest and medical therapy
Mitral regurgitation	Rheumatic, congenital	• Moderate-severe MR with good LV function: low risk • Severe MR with LV dysfunction: high risk for heart failure or arrhythmia	• No increased fetal risk reported	• Prepregnancy: Surgery for patients with severe MR and symptoms or LVEF <60% or LVESD ≥40 mm • In pregnancy: Diuretics for volume overload.
Aortic regurgitation	Rheumatic, congenital, degenerative	• Moderate-severe AR with good LV function: low risk • Severe AR with LV dysfunction: high risk for heart failure or arrhythmia	• No increased fetal risk reported	• Prepregnancy: Surgery for patients with severe AR and symptoms or LVEF <50% or severe dilation (LVESD >50 mm, LVEDD >65 mm) • In pregnancy: Diuretics for volume overload
Tricuspid regurgitation	Functional, Ebstein anomaly, endocarditis	• Moderate-severe TR with good RV function: risk of arrhythmia • Moderate-severe TR with impaired RV function: risk of heart failure	• No increased fetal risk reported	• Prepregnancy: Surgery for patients with severe TR and symptoms or impaired LV or RV function or dilation • In pregnancy: Diuretics for volume overload
Pulmonary stenosis	Congenital, endocarditis	• Severe PS commonly well tolerated • Increased risk of pre-eclampsia • Risk of right ventricular failure and arrhythmia	• Preterm birth and higher offspring mortality	• Pre-pregnancy—balloon dilatation for severe PS (consideration of surgical/percutaneous PVR for mixed PS/PR per ACHD guidelines, RV/LV dysfunction) • Pregnancy—consideration of balloon dilatation for symptomatic severe PS without PI with fetal shielding (rarely needed)
Pulmonary regurgitation	Congenital, post-PS intervention (TOF, pulmonary valve stenosis), endocarditis	• Severe PR commonly well tolerated during pregnancy. • Increased right ventricular failure and arrhythmia, particularly with TOF and/or RV dysfunction	• No significant fetal risk reported for the isolated pulmonary valve disease. • TOF is associated with increased offspring complications including IUGR.	• Pre-pregnancy—transcutaneous or surgical pulmonary valve replacement for symptomatic severe PI with RV dysfunction (see ACHD guidelines) • In pregnancy—diuretics for volume overload

Abbreviations: ACHD, adult congenital heart disease; AF, atrial fibrillation; AR, aortic regurgitation; AS, aortic stenosis; BB, β-blockers; BP, blood pressure; HTN, hypertension; IUGR, intrauterine growth restriction; LV, left ventricular; LVEF, left ventricular ejection fraction; LVEDD, left ventricular end diastolic diameter; LVESD, left ventricular end systolic diameter; MR, mitral regurgitation; MS, mitral stenosis; NYHA, New York Heart Association; PAP, pulmonary arterial pressure; PS, pulmonary stenosis; RV, right ventricular; TOF, tetralogy of Fallot; TR, tricuspid regurgitation
Reproduced with permission from Sliwa K, Johnson MR, Zilla P, et al. Management of valvular disease in pregnancy: a global perspective. *Eur Heart J.* 2015 May 7;36(18):1078-1089.
*Severe aortic stenosis is defined as an aortic valve area ≤1.0 cm², aortic velocity ≥4.0 m/s, or mean pressure gradient ≥40 mm Hg.

sinus rhythm, anticoagulation should be considered in pregnant women with significant mitral stenosis, heart failure, left atrial enlargement (≥60 mL/m²), and evidence of spontaneous echocardiographic contrast in the left atrium.[1] Percutaneous mitral valvuloplasty is an option for women refractory to optimal medical therapy in whom the valvular anatomy is suitable to such an approach; ideally, it should be performed after 20 weeks of gestation with an experienced operator and measures to reduce fetal radiation exposure.[1,122] Given the exceptionally high risk of fetal demise with maternal cardiopulmonary bypass, maternal cardiac surgery should only be performed when other treatment strategies have been ineffective at stabilizing the mother.[1] Fetal risks are also high, with maternal mitral stenosis increasing the risk of fetal prematurity

(20%–30%), intrauterine growth retardation (5%–20%), and stillbirth (1%–3%).[1,119–121] While most women can be managed conservatively and delivered vaginally, planned caesarean section may be considered in women with severe disease with NYHA class III or IV symptoms with pulmonary hypertension that persists despite optimal medical and surgical therapy.[1] One study reported the outcomes of 273 women with rheumatic mitral stenosis and 23% were hospitalized during pregnancy with one antepartum maternal death and two deaths in the postpartum period.[57]

Aortic Stenosis

Congenital bicuspid aortic valve (BAV) disease, followed by rheumatic disease, are the primary etiologies of aortic stenosis during pregnancy and as with mitral stenosis, may be asymptomatic and/or undetected until pregnancy.[121,122] When the diagnosis is known prior to conception, transthoracic echocardiography should be performed to assess gradients across the aortic valve and exercise testing is recommended in asymptomatic women.[1] Even in the context of severe disease, those with a high exercise capacity who remain asymptomatic and have a normal blood pressure response with exercise testing may tolerate pregnancy without complications, provided their left ventricular function remains normal.[1,123] However, those with severe symptomatic aortic stenosis, rapid progression of stenosis, or concomitant impaired left ventricular function (with an ejection fraction <50%) should undergo valvular intervention prior to conception. Women with BAV may have associated dilatation of the ascending aorta and coarctation of the aorta with an increased risk of aortic dissection during pregnancy.[124,125] However, among those with an ascending aortic dimension <50 mm or <27 cc/m², the risk of dissection remains low.[1] Cardiac MRI prior to pregnancy may delineate baseline aortic dimensions and echocardiography is the modality of choice for follow-up of valve function and aortic dimensions during pregnancy.

As with mitral stenosis, women with aortic stenosis are at increased risk of heart failure (approximately 10%) and arrhythmias (up to 25%), with offspring at increased risk for preterm delivery, intrauterine growth retardation, and low birth weight (up to 35%).[1,56,126] Women who develop AF should be rate controlled with β-blockade, nondihydropyridine calcium channel antagonists, or digoxin when necessary. For women refractory to medical therapy, percutaneous balloon valvuloplasty remains an option in the absence of significant calcification or regurgitation, and should again be performed as late as possible in pregnancy and with measures to reduce fetal radiation exposure.[1] More recently, transcatheter aortic valve replacement has been explored on a case report level both for native aortic stenosis, as well as in women with prosthetic aortic stenosis, but has not yet been investigated in any larger studies.[127] Most women including those with severe aortic stenosis will be able to deliver vaginally. For women with severe symptomatic aortic stenosis, assisted second stage may be considered to shorten the duration of the second stage of labor. Cesarean delivery should be reserved for obstetric indications in all but the most critically ill women.

Pulmonic Stenosis

Congenital pulmonary stenosis (PS) is the most common cause of RV outflow tract obstruction in pregnant women. In a small sample of women with pulmonic stenosis, all women tolerated pregnancy without an increase in arrhythmia, need to initiate cardiovascular medications, maternal hospitalizations, or adverse fetal outcomes and thus this lesion is likely well tolerated during pregnancy in women without symptoms prior to pregnancy.[119] In symptomatic women with favorable valve anatomy and without significant pulmonary regurgitation, balloon valvuloplasty may be performed with adequate fetal shielding. Interestingly, there appears to be an increase incidence of preeclampsia and other hypertensive disorders in women with PS, although this association is not well understood.[128]

Regurgitant Lesions

Regurgitant lesions are better tolerated than stenotic lesions due to the decrease in systemic vascular resistance during pregnancy. As with mitral stenosis, rheumatic disease accounts for a large proportion of women with mitral regurgitation in pregnancy, with mitral valve prolapse representing another common etiology.[121,122] Common etiologies of aortic regurgitation include BAV, rheumatic disease, endocarditis, or aortic annular dilation.[122] With preserved left ventricular function, women with significant regurgitation usually tolerate pregnancy well, although they are at increased risk for the development of arrhythmias.[1,122] Those who develop AF during pregnancy are at particularly high risk for embolic events and anticoagulation should be considered. Women with severe regurgitation with left ventricular dysfunction or heart failure are at increased risk for adverse cardiovascular events during pregnancy and thus women who require repair or replacement should be intervened upon prior to conception.[1] The decision to proceed with prophylactic valve replacement for regurgitation prior to pregnancy is challenging in women who do not meet standard guidelines in anticipation of pregnancy, because prosthetic valves increase the risk for pregnancy-related complications.[122] Postpartum, women with regurgitant lesions may be at increased risk for development of heart failure in the context of a normalization of the systemic vascular resistance in the face of a continued volume load as compared to the pre-pregnancy state and thus women should be followed closely and treated with diuretic therapy if needed. Those who develop heart failure during pregnancy should be treated with diuretic therapy and afterload reduction with hydralazine and nitrate therapy.[122] As with other cardiac surgical procedures, surgical valve replacement should be avoided in pregnancy due to the high risk of fetal loss with cardiopulmonary bypass.[122]

Prosthetic Valves

While surgical techniques increasingly enable valve repair rather than replacement, in many instances valve characteristics or surgical expertise in a given center necessitates valve replacement in young patients. When valve replacements are required for treatment of valvular disease in a woman of childbearing age, there should be a discussion between the patient and cardiologist or cardiac surgeon regarding plans for future pregnancy, which may impact the choice of valve: bioprosthetic or mechanical. Women should be extensively counseled on the risks and benefits during pregnancy of each type of valve and understand that regardless of choice, prosthetic valves increase the potential for cardiovascular complications. In a prospective registry of women with CVD in pregnancy, maternal mortality occurred in 1.4% and 1.5% of women with a mechanical and bioprosthetic valve, respectively, as compared to a 0.2% mortality rate in women with CVD without a prosthetic valve, illustrating the high level of risk that pregnancy with a prosthetic valve carries even as compared to a high-risk population.[129] Further, only 79% of women with a bioprosthetic and 58% of women with a mechanical valve had pregnancies free of serious events, highlighting the risk that a prosthesis poses to the health of the mother and fetus in pregnancy and the need to carefully follow these women in a multidisciplinary fashion.[52,129] The AHA/ACC guidelines recommend use of low-dose aspirin for women in their second or third trimesters with any prosthetic valve, whereas the latest ESC guidelines specifically do not recommend aspirin due to the concern of increased hemorrhage.[1,130] However, beyond the risks of potential valve failure or thrombosis (see section Deep Vein Thrombosis and Pulmonary Embolism in Pregnancy), patients with prosthetic heart valves are at increased risk for development of infective endocarditis, regardless of pregnancy status. While current guidelines do not recommend antibiotic prophylaxis for delivery in women with prosthetic valves,[131] some authors report administering prophylactic antibiotics in women with prosthetic valves except in the instance of uncomplicated vaginal delivery.[132]

Bioprosthetic Valves

In light of persistent uncertainty regarding optimal management of anticoagulation in pregnancy—especially in women with mechanical valves—those desiring future pregnancy may elect to have a bioprosthesis.[1] While bioprosthetic valves do not require anticoagulation and have a lower risk of thrombosis, women should be aware that they have a higher rate of structural valve deterioration irrespective of pregnancy than do mechanical valves.[1,132,133] Thus, the decision to place a bioprosthesis in any young patient requires counseling on the near inevitability that they will require a repeat valve replacement in their lifetime, as well as careful periodic monitoring of their valve function. Potential modes of valve deterioration include calcification, degradation, and pannus overgrowth leading to leaflet immobility.[132] Whether pregnancy itself leads to accelerated valve deterioration remains unknown, with conflicting data in the existing literature and many postulating that deterioration during pregnancy may simply reflect the natural course of bioprosthetic valves as opposed to the increased demands of pregnancy.[1,132–136] However, in women with normal ventricular function with a well-functioning bioprosthetic valve, the risk of pregnancy is minimal and thus a desire for pregnancy is a class IIb indication for placing a bioprosthetic valve in a young woman as per the European Society of Cardiology guidelines.[1] Increasing numbers of women are undergoing transcatheter pulmonary valve replacement prior to pregnancy. Surveillance of valve function during pregnancy is important, as with increased maternal plasma volume, the peak gradient across the valve will increase; however, in most cases these gradients return to baseline in the postpartum period.[137]

Mechanical Valves

While mechanical prostheses have a longer durability than bioprosthetic valves that renders them the preference in young women who do not wish to become pregnant, they pose a significant challenge regarding management in pregnancy, mainly due to their highly thrombogenic nature that necessitates uninterrupted anticoagulation.[129] Mechanical valve thrombosis is a potentially devastating complication in any patient and has been reported to occur in 4.7% of pregnant women with mechanical valves in a prospective registry.[129] Hemorrhagic events occur significantly more commonly in women with mechanical valves (23.1%) as compared to those with bioprosthetic valves or those without prosthetic valves in pregnancy (5.1% and 4.9%, $P < 0.001$).[129] At present, there are inadequate studies to reassure women that any anticoagulation plan is completely safe during pregnancy and this issue should be discussed extensively prior to conception in any woman of reproductive age. In particular, the hypercoagulability of pregnancy heightens the risk of valve thrombosis, the increased volume of distribution often leads to vacillations in therapeutic doses that necessitate frequent monitoring and dose adjustments to ensure consistent therapeutic anticoagulation, and pregnancy itself carries an increased risk of bleeding—particularly around the time of delivery. Mechanical prostheses in the mitral or tricuspid position, concomitant AF, and a history of thromboembolic events increase the risk of thrombosis during pregnancy.[121,138] Further, much discussion regarding the risk of valve thrombosis derives from study of older valves, with a potentially lower risk profile among those receiving newer generation mechanical valves.[132]

Anticoagulation for Women with Mechanical Valves during Pregnancy: The optimal strategy for anticoagulation in pregnant women is controversial. While warfarin is often the preferred agent in nonpregnant women with mechanical prostheses, the risk of embryopathy exceeds 8% with doses over 5 mg.[1,130] The use of warfarin beyond the first trimester is associated with an increased risk of adverse fetal outcomes including miscarriage, hemorrhage, and fetal loss, an effect that in some studies appears to be dose dependent.[1,129,132,138–141] However, in a recent study, rates of miscarriage or fetal loss did not differ between women who took high versus low (≤5 mg) doses of warfarin.[129] Low-molecular-weight heparin (LMWH) does not cross the placenta and guidelines recommend switching from warfarin to LMWH in women whose warfarin dose exceeds 5 mg. Unfortunately, available data suggest that women are at high risk for valve thrombosis during the transition from warfarin to heparin products.[1,129,130] LMWH is the preferred method of anticoagulation during the first trimester, because heparin products do not cross the placenta, and remain an option throughout pregnancy. However, LMWH is associated with an increased risk of valve thrombosis in real-world practice.[132] While the factors responsible for this risk are incompletely understood, many authors postulate that inadequate monitoring rather than failure of the agent itself is responsible.[132] When LMWH is used during pregnancy, both peak and trough anti-Xa levels should be monitored weekly throughout to ensure consistent therapeutic anticoagulation, because the therapeutic dose required may significantly change with the increasing volume of distribution.[1,132,142–145] In one study of real-world use, however, anti-Xa levels were reported in only 57% of women treated with LMWH, suggesting inadequate monitoring of LMWH-use in global clinical practice.[129] Further, among those who did have anti-Xa levels checked, the number of levels reported per pregnancy ranged from 3 to 42, again reinforcing concerns regarding the use and monitoring of this anticoagulant.[129] While there is no universal recommendation for type of anticoagulation for women with mechanical valves during pregnancy, **Table 78–5** summarizes a proposed algorithm adapted from several strategies in the literature. While warfarin is the recommended strategy of anticoagulation in the second and third trimesters by guidelines, prospective studies of high quality and consistently therapeutic anticoagulation during pregnancy are required to more definitively recommend an anticoagulation strategy during pregnancy.[1,130] Steinberg et al.[146]

TABLE 78–5. Anticoagulation for Mechanical Valves during Pregnancy

Preconception:
- Discuss with the patient an anticoagulation strategy for pregnancy including a thorough discussion of the risks/benefits of each strategy and arrive at a preformed plan individualized based on patient preference and risk profile
- Counsel patient to monitor for pregnancy by tracking menstrual cycles and frequent pregnancy tests and contact patient's cardiologist as soon as pregnancy is known

Pregnancy: Conception to 12 weeks
- If the warfarin dose is <5 mg, it may be continued
- If the warfarin dose is ≥5 mg or if the patient prefers to avoid warfarin altogether during pregnancy, switch to weight-based LMWH BID and adjust dose based on weekly peak/trough monitoring for goal peak anti-Xa levels of 0.6–1.2 U/L mL 4 hours postdose. If trough levels are <0.6 IU/mL with therapeutic peaks, dose TID.

Pregnancy: Weeks 13–35
- All patients can be switched to warfarin
- For patients who prefer to avoid warfarin during pregnancy, LMWH can be continued with careful weekly monitoring as above

Pregnancy: Week 36
- Switch patients on warfarin to LMWH or IV UFH. LMWH should be monitored weekly, with a goal peak anti-Xa level of 0.7–1.2 U/L mL 4 hours postdose. If trough levels are <0.6 IU/mL with therapeutic peaks, dose TID

Labor and Postpartum:
- 36 hours prior to induction or cesarean section, all patients should be switched to IV UFH
- 6 hours prior to delivery, IV UFH should be stopped
- Restart IV UFH 4–6 hours after delivery (provided the risk of bleeding is not prohibitive from an obstetric perspective)
- Once safe to start long-term anticoagulation from a bleeding perspective, bridge with LMWH or IV UFH to warfarin with careful INR monitoring postpartum, especially in breastfeeding patients

Abbreviations: BID, twice daily; INR, international normalized ratio; IV, intravenous; LMWH, low molecular weight heparin; TID, three times per day; UFH, unfractionated heparin

Data from Pieper PG, Balci A, Van Dijk AP. Pregnancy in women with prosthetic heart valves. *Neth Heart J.* 2008 Dec;16(12):406-411.

---

have recently shown in a meta-analysis of 800 pregnancies with mechanical valves that warfarin was associated with the lowest risk of adverse maternal outcomes, whereas LMWH had the lowest risk of adverse fetal outcomes. Fetal risk was similar when administering warfarin dose of <5 mg and LMWH.[146] At present, there is no data to guide the use of non–vitamin K oral anticoagulants during pregnancy and thus their use cannot be recommended.

Unsurprisingly, women with mechanical valves are at highest risk of maternal hemorrhage at the time of delivery and thus they require careful monitoring peripartum.[129] Well before delivery, a multidisciplinary plan must be formulated in conjunction with cardiology, obstetrics, and anesthesia regarding the management of unexpected premature labor or emergency delivery and communicated to all physicians who may care for the patient in an emergent situation in order to minimize uncertainty. The 2018 ESC guidelines recommend planned delivery for women with mechanical prosthesis and transitioning warfarin to LMWH or unfractionated heparin at 36 weeks of gestation, in order to reduce the risk of fetal hemorrhage with vaginal delivery and delivery-associated maternal bleeding.[1,132,142] Women at increased risk for preterm labor and preterm birth should have their warfarin switched earlier based on clinical risk factors. For women who unexpectedly present in labor and require preterm emergent delivery, general anesthesia with use of blood products and reversal agents should be considered for Caesarian delivery, which is the advised mode of delivery among fully anticoagulated women with warfarin due to the risk of fetal hemorrhage, because warfarin also results in anticoagulation of the fetus. This is an extremely high-risk clinical scenario that requires significant surgical, anesthesia, and blood bank support. Prior to a scheduled induction or cesarean delivery, all women should be switched to unfractionated heparin and this should be stopped 6 hours prior to planned delivery.[132] Unfractionated heparin should be restarted 4 to 6 hours after delivery provided that the risk of bleeding from an obstetric perspective is not prohibitive.[132,142] Meticulous attention to hemostasis in operative deliveries and with significant vaginal lacerations is required. Use of pelvic and rectus-sheath drains may also be considered in women delivered by cesarean delivery.

There should remain a high suspicion for valve thrombosis in any woman with a mechanical valve during pregnancy or postpartum, especially with signs of new heart failure or an embolic event. A transthoracic echocardiogram should be used as the initial mode of investigation, although transesophageal echocardiography is often required for adequate visualization.[130] If unrevealing, fluoroscopy can and should be performed with minimal radiation for diagnosis.[1,130,132,147] For women with evidence of thrombosis but adequate valve function and clinical stability, optimization of anticoagulation can be trialed.[1,132,148] Critical valve thrombosis has been associated with a high rate of maternal mortality and should be treated with either fibrinolytics or surgically. As previously mentioned, the former strategy is associated with a high risk of bleeding and cardiac surgery during pregnancy is associated with an increased risk of fetal loss, with little experience with either strategy to guide recommendations during pregnancy.[1,132,149,150]

Deep Vein Thrombosis and Pulmonary Embolism in Pregnancy

Venous thromboembolic (VTE) complications are 5 times more prevalent during pregnancy and remain a diagnostic challenge as symptomatology overlaps with normal physiological changes.[73] Women with previous unprovoked VTE or estrogen-related VTE are considered high risk with an increased recurrence rate (up to 12%) and should be offered a prophylactic anticoagulation for the duration of pregnancy. Providers should have a low threshold for early suspicion of VTE and its investigation. The most vulnerable period is early postpartum with a rate of VTE in 0.5% of pregnancies.[1] Deep vein thrombosis (DVT) is estimated at 0.05% to 1.3% of pregnancies and is more commonly associated with the left-sided proximal vessels (ie, iliac, femoral).[1,151] PE is estimated at 0.03% to 0.3% of pregnancies with one-third of the patients asymptomatic, yet high mortality rates that reach 3.5%.[1,151] D-dimer levels physiologically increase during pregnancy and a higher cutoff is required for exclusion of PE, yet falsely negative normal range D-dimer levels have also been reported in patients with VTE during pregnancy. van der Pol et al. validated a useful approach for diagnosing and ruling out PE during pregnancy by incorporating the YEARS criteria (ie, clinical signs of DVT, hemoptysis and PE most likely diagnosis) together with a higher range of D-dimers (threshold of 1000 ng/mL if all YEARS questions are negatively answered, and 500 ng/mL if any is questioned is positively answered) as well as leg ultrasound in DVT suspected cases (**Fig. 78–4**).[152] This approach has shown to avert the need for CT angiogram in 40% to 60% of cases. The proposed algorithm is most effective in the first trimester and loses specificity as pregnancy progresses. Enoxaparin is the mainstay treatment for stable hemodynamics VTE and UFH is commonly reserved for unstable hemodynamics, peripartum diagnosis, and high clot burden. Thrombolytics and catheter-related lysis are reserved for patients in hemodynamic shock. Careful monitoring and follow-up is advised in the first 48 hours postpartum in any patient with PE because the pulmonary vascular resistance increases and may result in a pulmonary hypertensive crisis and ensuing right heart failure. Direct oral anticoagulants are not recommended in pregnancy.

Infectious Endocarditis in Pregnancy

Although extremely rare, infective endocarditis (IE) during pregnancy has high maternal and fetal mortality.[153,154] Risk factors for the development of IE include underlying valve disease (eg, rheumatic), CHD, intravenous drug use, and recent dental

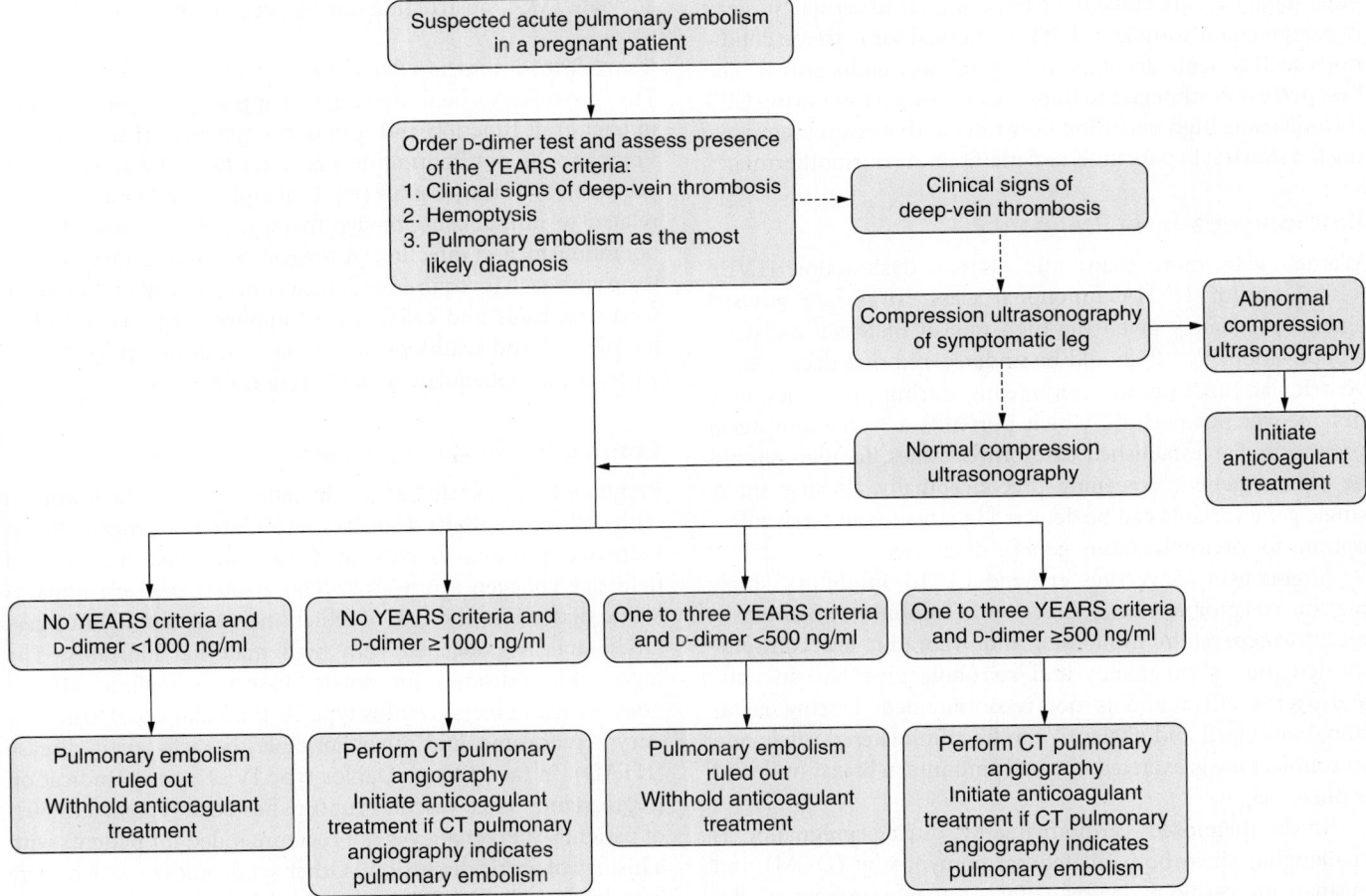

Figure 78–4. Pregnancy-adapted YEARS algorithm for diagnosis of pulmonary embolism. Reproduced with permission from van der Pol LM, Tromeur C, Bistervels IM, et al. Pregnancy-Adapted YEARS Algorithm for Diagnosis of Suspected Pulmonary Embolism. *N Engl J Med.* 2019 Mar 21;380(12):1139-1149.

work. The most common pathogen is *Streptococcus viridans* and the most commonly involved valve is the mitral valve followed by the aortic and tricuspid valves. Maternal morbidity is attributed to embolic events and valvulopathy-related heart failure.[155] Since IE in pregnancy is a life-threatening condition, intravenous antibiotics, close surveillance, and anticipation of valve surgery is mandated. Open-heart valve surgery during pregnancy is associated with high fetal mortality and prematurity as well as a high maternal complication rate. Clinical indications for surgery remain the same as in the general population.

Antibiotic prophylaxis is reasonable during vaginal delivery at the time of membrane rupture in women with prosthetic cardiac valves, presence of prosthetic material used for valve repair, or unrepaired or cyanotic heart disease.[7]

Cardiopulmonary Bypass in Pregnancy

Cardiopulmonary bypass (CPB) results in utero-placental hypoperfusion. The fetus experiences acidosis, hypoxemia, increased systemic vascular resistance, and decreased cardiac output. CPB may be associated with poor neonatal outcome (16%–33% mortality).[156,157] Other neonatal complications include premature deliveries, intra-uterine growth restriction (IUGR), respiratory distress syndrome, and developmental delay. Maternal outcomes are more reassuring and, contrary to older data, they are considered to be similar to cardiac surgery in nonpregnant women.[157] CPB is reserved for extreme conditions such as acute decompensating valvular endocarditis. The best perfusion strategies to improve fetal outcomes during CPB include using high perfusion flow rates and pressures, employing the shortest bypass time, and maintaining normothermia.[158]

Cardiomyopathy in Pregnancy

Women with more than mild systolic dysfunction (LVEF <40%) and/or NYHA functional class III/IV are advised against pregnancy given the high rate of maternal and fetal complications.[10,159] It should be underscored that decreases in ventricular function and remodeling during pregnancy may not recover postpartum, which portends a worse long-term prognosis. For established cardiomyopathies, families should be offered genetic screening preconceptually, because many single gene variants can be detected in advance and may allow options for preimplantation genetic diagnosis.

Angiotensin-converting enzyme (ACE) inhibitors, angiotensin receptor blockers, direct renin inhibitors, angiotensin receptor-neprysillin inhibitors, and ivabradin are contraindicated during pregnancy and spironolactone has an anti-androgenic effect and is not recommended. During lactation, benazepril and enalapril can be administered safely and spironolactone is excreted in small amounts in breast milk and is likely safe.

Newly diagnosed cardiomyopathy during pregnancy is challenging since both dilated cardiomyopathy (DCM) and peripartum cardiomyopathy (PPCM) may represent a disease within the spectrum of similar pathophysiology.[148] In both cases, it is important to exclude reversible causes of cardiomyopathy (eg, myocarditis, hypertension, underlying valve disease, toxin-induced, tachyarrhythmia or ischemia). A family history is useful to aid in the diagnosis of DCM.[159] There is evolving understanding of a shared genetic predisposition for DCM and PPCM with gene sequencing revealing common gene truncating variants. Women with variants in a titin gene have lower ventricular function at 1 year postpartum.[160] Preconceptual genetic screening can be offered because many single gene variants can be screened in advance and may allow options for preimplantation genetic diagnosis. The basic tenets of heart failure treatment during pregnancy include sodium and fluid restriction, afterload reduction (eg, nitrates, hydralazine), rhythm control (eg, β-blockers, digoxin), diuretics, and anticoagulation for thrombotic complications. See Chapter 52 for a detailed discussion of peripartum cardiomyopathy and Chapter 63 for the treatment of cardiogenic shock.

Hypertrophic Cardiomyopathy

Women with hypertrophic cardiomyopathy commonly tolerate pregnancy well. Maternal mortality is low (~1%) and morbidity is predominantly related to left ventricular outflow tract (LVOT) obstruction and arrhythmia.[161,162] In fact, the increased plasma volume during pregnancy may lessen the LVOT obstruction. Preconception evaluation includes NYHA assessment, degree of LVOT obstruction, and surveillance for arrhythmias. β-blockers remain the mainstay medication to alleviate LVOT obstruction during pregnancy.

Heart Transplantation Recipients

The physiologic hemodynamic changes of pregnancy may impact graft function and immunosuppressive therapy levels. Pregnancy is not contraindicated after heart transplantation, yet involves a risk for graft rejection and failure, teratogenicity related to immunosuppressive therapy, hypertension, thromboembolism, and infection. A pregestational multidisciplinary team approach is required to counsel the patient about the risks. Corticosteroids and calcineurin inhibitors (eg, cyclosporine, tacrolimus) and azathioprine can be used during pregnancies, whereas mycophenolate mofetil is contraindicated.

Connective Tissue Disorders

Pregnancy is associated with a dilatation of the aorta in women with connective tissue disorders secondary to estrogen effects, increased protease activity in the extracellular matrix, and defective collagen synthesis.[163] The greatest concern remains aortic dissection, the risk of which increases throughout gestation and is associated with high maternal mortality. The high-risk syndromes for aortic dissection include MFS,[164] Loeys–Dietz, Ehlers–Danlos type IV (vascular type), osteoaneurym syndrome, and other heritable thoracic aortic disease (HTAD). In fact, Ehlers–Danlos type IV is a contraindication to pregnancy since vascular rupture has been reported in 50% of patients.[165] Pregnancy is not recommended for patients with a history of aortic dissection.[1] Other syndromes in which there is an increased risk of dissection include BAV and Turner syndrome patients, who are now able to conceive through means of assisted reproduction. In women with MFS, the aortic root size may not return to the prepregnancy dimensions and there appears to be an increased risk of future aortic events or need for aortic root replacement after pregnancy.[166] Women interested in pregnancy should undergo preconception genetic counseling as these syndromes are commonly inherited in an autosomal dominant manner. Chest magnetic resonance angiography is advised to better delineate the baseline aortic dimensions. During pregnancy, echocardiogram surveillance of the aortic root is recommended. The frequency should be individualized but may be as often as monthly.[1] In MFS, normal aortic dimensions at baseline portend a low risk of dissection. Women with MFS considering pregnancy are counseled to undergo elective aortic root replacement and are counseled against pregnancy when the aortic root diameter exceeds 4.5 cm.[1,167] Those with aortic root size between 4.0 and 4.5 cm are at increased risk of an event, especially in the setting of a family history of dissection or rapid growth. Women with BAV commonly have dilated ascending aorta, yet have a significantly lower risk of dissection compared to those with MFS. For women with BAV considering pregnancy, surgical repair of the aorta should be recommended when the ascending aorta exceeds 5.0 cm (>2.7 cm/m^2) and pregnancy is not recommended beyond these dimensions.[1] Women with Turner syndrome are advised to undergo repair when the aortic diameter >2.5 cm/m^2. In Loeys-Dietz syndrome, aortic replacement is recommended with aortic dimensions above 4.0 cm or a rapidly expanding aneurysm >0.5 cm per year.[168] Medical management of aortic disease in pregnancy includes strict blood pressure control and β-blockers. Women who are taking ARBs prior to pregnancy should be transitioned to β-blockers. Vaginal delivery is the preferred mode of delivery and some authors recommend an expedited second stage as to avoid episodic hypertension that may promote dissections. Cesarean delivery is recommended for women with Ehlers–Danlos type IV syndrome, due to the risk of arterial, bowel, and uterine rupture.[169] Cesarean delivery should also be considered for aortic diameters exceeding 4.0 to 4.5 cm. Careful counseling and meticulous coordinated care is necessary in the delivery plan for all women with connective tissue disorders. Use of ergotamine is not recommended during delivery in women with enlarged aortas secondary to the risk of hypertension with these agents.

Ischemic Heart Disease during Pregnancy and Spontaneous Coronary Artery Dissections

Due to increasing maternal age and a higher prevalence of CVD risk factors, the incidence of ischemic heart disease complications during pregnancy is rising. In a review of 146 pregnancies associated with ischemic heart disease, 95% of women presented with chest pain, the majority of which occurred in the third trimester or postpartum period. Major causes of ischemia were found to be due to nonatherosclerotic causes such as spontaneous coronary artery dissections (SCAD) (35%) or thrombus/emboli (35%). Maternal mortality was 8% and the premature delivery rate was 56%.[170] CAD has been implicated in more than 20% of maternal cardiac deaths.[1] The clinical presentation is similar to the nonpregnant population with a non–ST-segment elevation myocardial infarction (NSTEMI) incidence slightly higher than STEMI (STEMI 45% and NSTEMI 55% in the postpartum period). Preexisting chronic CAD is associated with adverse outcomes and requires a thorough workup to rule out residual ischemia. As noted earlier, statin therapy is contraindicated during pregnancy.

SCAD refers to the spontaneous development of a hematoma between the intima and media of the coronary artery compressing the true lumen and causing downstream ischemia. Predominantly there is no dissection flap and no communication between the true and false lumens. Also thrombus formation is uncommon. Most cases of pregnancy-associated SCAD occur within the first week postpartum, yet should be considered until 6 weeks postpartum with a prevalence of 1.81 per 100,000 pregnancies. Since the majority of patients with SCAD are women, it is hypothesized that hormone levels or fluctuations in hormone levels may play a pathophysiological role. Pregnant women with SCAD tend to be older (>30 years) and multigravida. Additional risk factors for SCAD include systemic hypertension, diabetes, tobacco use, cocaine use, connective tissue diseases (eg, fibromuscular dysplasia), thrombophilia, and postpartum infections.[1,171] Beyond pregnancy as a stressor, physical and emotional stress have been implicated as triggers for development of SCAD.

SCAD-related myocardial infarction has more frequent involvement of the left main and left anterior descending arteries and multivessel disease, and a high incidence of shock and mortality presumably due to frequent involvement of the anterior wall.[172] SCAD-related cardiogenic shock has been reported in up to 20% of cases.

Cardiovascular invasive strategies in women during pregnancy should be limited to those with severe clinical decompensation and/or unresponsive to medical interventions. As significant amount of dissections do heal over the course of several months—conservative management is appropriate in most cases of a low-risk NSTEMI. Delineating the coronary anatomy with a coronary angiogram can be safely performed with appropriate fetal protection and should not be withheld due to concern of ionizing radiation risk. Primary percutaneous intervention (PCI) is the preferred re-perfusion strategy for STEMI and high risk NSTEMI during pregnancy. However, Havakuk et al. reviewed 120 cases of SCAD and reported a lower PCI success rate (50%), more cath-related complications and often the need for surgical coronary artery bypass.[173] Low-dose aspirin and heparin are considered safe and clopidogrel is added when primary PCI is performed. Paucity of data limits the use of other anti-platelet regimens. Tissue-plasminogen activator (t-PA) is not commonly used due to concern of hematoma propagation and other bleeding complications, although it does not cross the placenta. The choice for type of stent is evolving, because most experience surrounds bare-metal stents, yet second- and third-generation stents may be feasible with a shortened dual antiplatelet course. Specific pregnancy-related recommendations include utilizing left lateral recumbent position to improve venous return, fetal monitoring during the acute episode, consideration of corticosteroids when preterm delivery is anticipated within 7 days, and postponing delivery if possible by at least 2 weeks post event. In circumstances where the delivery cannot be postponed, a multidisciplinary team should stabilize the patient and plan on delivery under a controlled environment.[174] Extracorporeal membrane oxygenation (ECMO) has been successfully employed for respiratory failure in pregnancy.[175] In rare cases where cardiac bypass surgery is required in pregnancy, maternal survival is good; however, fetal loss remains high.[176] When cardiopulmonary bypass is needed, the use of high-flow, high-pressure, pulsatile, normothermic bypass with continuous fetal and uterine monitoring is recommended.[177]

Pulmonary Arterial Hypertension

Pulmonary arterial hypertension (PAH) refers to WHO group I pulmonary hypertension including idiopathic, heritable, congenital, and drug or toxin-induced PAH. Historically, PAH constitutes an extremely high-risk condition (Class IV WHO) with high maternal mortality ranging between 30% and 56% and fetal mortality between 10% and 28%. Pregnancy is generally contraindicated for women with PAH and preconception counseling should be provided.[178,179] Even though new advanced therapies for PAH have become available, outcomes remain guarded. A dedicated ROPAC registry for pulmonary hypertension in pregnancy showed a much lower incidence or mortality than classically reported (no deaths during pregnancy, 3.3% deaths in the first week postpartum, and 2.6% within the first 6 months postpartum), yet true PAH patients had much higher mortality rate (43%) compared to other forms of pulmonary hypertension.[180]

The vulnerable period for the development of a pulmonary hypertensive crisis and death occurs during the later stage of pregnancy, labor, and into the postpartum period. During pregnancy, women with PAH do not exhibit a physiological decrease in pulmonary vascular resistance (PVR) (similar to the fall in systemic vascular resistance) resulting in further RV dysfunction; this is then challenged by an increase in circulating plasma volume and stroke volume. During delivery, the increase in cardiac output together with blood loss and fluid shifts alters hemodynamics, and postpartum the acute return of systemic vascular resistance (SVR) to baseline promotes an acute deterioration. Risk factors associated with maternal mortality include late hospitalization, severity of pulmonary hypertension and general anesthesia. In terms of pregnancy planning, there is no known cutoff value of the pulmonary pressures to portend an increased risk of complications. Therefore, women with PAH should be counseled on appropriate forms of contraception and to avoid pregnancy. However, despite this, some women with PAH elect to proceed with pregnancy, and advanced pulmonary hypertension therapies may decrease the risk of complications;[181] although the experience is limited and certain agents such as the endothelin receptor antagonists (eg, bosentan, macitentan) and stimulator of soluble guanylate cyclase (eg, riociguat) are teratogenic. Calcium channel blockers may be continued for those who demonstrated vasoreactivity on cardiac catheterization and lack intracardiac shunts. Intravenous prostanoids (epoprostenol,

treprostinil) provide the best effect among agents and should be given to women with functional class (FC) IV symptoms and RV dysfunction. Attention should be given to their possible interference in platelet aggregation and possible bleeding. PDE-5-inhibitors (eg, sildenafil, tadalafil) cause both PVR and SVR decrease and may be used in women with normal RV function and FC WHO I and II symptoms. A combination of prostanoids and PDE-5 inhibitors may be beneficial.[182] Anticoagulation throughout pregnancy in women with PAH is advised in women who already have been on therapy prior to pregnancy with either only a short interruption during delivery or a transition to unfractionated heparin. Oxygen supplementation is often necessary. Meticulous intravenous (IV) care is imperative in the case of shunts using de-airing strategies and IV filters. Intensive maternal and fetal surveillance should be performed throughout pregnancy with repeated echocardiograms to assess RV function and pulmonary peak systolic pressures. A coordinated team effort is advised and delivery should be monitored in the ICU setting. Caution should be given to placement of a Swan-Ganz catheter due to the risk of vascular rupture and is not routinely recommended; however, a central line may aid in volume management. Intravenous prostanoids may be initiated in untreated women who show RV dysfunction or hemodynamic concerns. Vaginal delivery is preferred to cesarean section because of smaller volume shifts, although the latter may allow better timing and efficiency, yet with worse hemostasis. Slow epidural anesthesia causes less peripheral vasodilatation than general and spinal anesthesia and may provide the safest anesthesia.

Congenital Heart Disease in Pregnancy

Remarkable advancements in surgical and medical treatment of children with CHD have led to increasing numbers of women with CHD becoming pregnant. The hemodynamic changes of pregnancy may unmask previously unrecognized CHD or exacerbate residual hemodynamic lesions. Nonetheless, a majority of women will tolerate pregnancy well.[1] Meticulous knowledge of the congenital heart condition and potential complications is key for the management of CHD patients. Guidelines advise the referral of CHD patients to experienced centers where the full range of maternal fetal medicine and congenital heart expertise are available.[7] The modified WHO predictor model addresses specific lesion-related risk.

Shunt Lesions

Atrial septal defects (ASDs) are the most common congenital lesions encountered in women in the childbearing age. Unrepaired ASDs usually exhibit left-to-right shunting with subsequent right atrial and ventricular enlargement, potential RV dysfunction, arrhythmias, and in rare cases paradoxical emboli or pulmonary hypertension. Thromboembolic complications have been reported in up to 5% of these women and meticulous intravenous line care with filter placement is recommended during delivery and postpartum as well as DVT prophylaxis.[107] Unrepaired ASDs have been implicated in increased risk of preeclampsia, small for gestational age neonates, and increased neonatal mortality.[183] Women with repaired ASDs should tolerate pregnancy well, unless they have preexisting RV dysfunction. Meticulous IV de-airing maneuvers should be employed during delivery even in the setting of a clear left-to-right shunt. Device closure of secundum ASD is rarely required during pregnancy.

Hemodynamically significant VSDs cause left-sided heart volume overload, with potential ventricular dysfunction, arrhythmia, and rarely pulmonary hypertension. Large unrepaired VSDs in childhood may advance to Eisenmenger physiology and pregnancy is contraindicated in these women. Women with small, pressure-restrictive VSDs and normal left ventricular size are at low risk for complications during pregnancy; however, there is a reported increased risk of preeclampsia in women with unrepaired VSDs.[184]

A large patent ductus arteriosus (PDA) causes pulmonary artery enlargement, left-sided volume overload, and may lead to pulmonary hypertension.[7] Ductal flow decreases during pregnancy due to the decrease in systemic vascular resistance. However, small PDAs should not have hemodynamic significance during pregnancy.

Ebstein Anomaly

Outcomes in pregnancy in women with Ebstein anomaly are directly related to the degree of tricuspid valve displacement, degree of tricuspid regurgitation, RV dysfunction, cyanosis, and arrhythmia. In general, women with Ebstein anomaly tolerate pregnancy fairly well with overall risk of heart failure or arrhythmia in less than 5%.[107] Since many of these women have an atrial communication, embolic stroke and cyanosis may occur. Women are also at risk for atrial arrhythmias during pregnancy because Wolff–Parkinson-White syndrome is present in as many as 20% of women with Ebstein anomaly. Atrial arrhythmias in women with Ebstein anomaly may further deteriorate the RV function or result in life-threatening AF during pregnancy.[185,186] Neonatal outcomes include increased prematurity, fetal loss, and CHD.[187] Preconception counseling should focus on tricuspid valve function with repair or replacement consideration and arrhythmia evaluation and intervention when appropriate.

Transposition of the Great Arteries

Women with D-loop transposition of the great arteries who underwent an atrial switch (ie, Senning or Mustard operations) or those with physiologically corrected transposition of the great arteries (congenitally corrected TGA, cc-TGA, or L-TGA) have a morphological right ventricle functioning as the systemic ventricle. The long-standing volume and pressure overload affecting the systemic ventricle often leads to ventricular dysfunction. Systemic ventricular failure in pregnancy has been reported in 5% to 10% of these women.[107] Additional cardiovascular complications include tricuspid valve regurgitation, atrial arrhythmias, and cyanosis if there is an atrial level shunt present. Baseline systemic ventricular function and the burden of arrhythmia should be preemptively evaluated since both may worsen during pregnancy. In women with D-loop TGA who had previously undergone the Mustard procedure, it was shown that the increased systemic ventricular dimensions, decreased systolic function, and increased degree of tricuspid

regurgitation may persist after pregnancy and not return to baseline values.[188] Presently, children born with D-loop TGA will undergo an arterial switch procedure in the neonatal period. Data is scarce in this emerging population; however, a publication summarizing 17 pregnancies from 9 women reported two cardiac complications related to preexisting conditions (nonsustained ventricular arrhythmia in an impaired ventricle and a thrombosis of a mechanical valve).[189]

Coarctation of the Aorta

The most common complication encountered in women in pregnancy with coarctation of the aorta (CoA) is systemic hypertension, yet aortic wall complications, although rare, are of concern.[190] The increased flow across the narrowed isthmus coupled with hypertension may cause left ventricular failure and decreased fetal perfusion. Careful evaluation of the aortic dimensions prior to and during pregnancy and blood pressure control throughout gestation are imperative. Women with repaired CoA may have residual stenosis (peak-to-peak gradient on cardiac catheterization or mean Doppler gradient >20 mm Hg) or aneurysms at the repair site that should be adequately imaged and treated prior to pregnancy.[7] Aortic diameters <1.2 cm have been correlated with higher maternal cardiovascular events.[191] During pregnancy, women with CoA have increased incidence of hypertensive complications, cesarean section delivery, longer hospital stay, and higher hospital charges.[192] Although rarely necessary, placement of a covered stent within the narrowed isthmus is indicated for refractory hypertension or fetal or maternal complications related to CoA.[1]

Repaired Tetralogy of Fallot

The hemodynamic lesions of concern in repaired tetralogy of Fallot (TOF) during pregnancy are pulmonary regurgitation, RV dilation, and dysfunction. The volume overload of pregnancy exacerbates the degree of valve regurgitation and may cause further deterioration of RV function. The most common cardiac maternal events include heart failure and atrial arrhythmias.[107,193,194] It is important to consider pulmonary valve replacement prior to pregnancy in women with severe pulmonary regurgitation. There is evidence that women with repaired TOF who have undergone pregnancy have higher RV end-diastolic volumes than nulligravid women.[195] Additionally, changes in longitudinal strain occur during pregnancy in women with repaired TOF; however, these changes return to baseline after delivery and the global ejection fraction does not substantially change.[196]

Women with unrepaired TOF or those women palliated with only a systemic-to-pulmonary arterial shunt are counseled to avoid pregnancy due to the cyanosis and the risk of paradoxical emboli. Women with TOF should be offered genetic counseling to assess for 22q11 deletion, which is associated with conotruncal abnormalities.[7]

Cyanotic Conditions

In general, women with cyanotic heart conditions may be counseled to obtain a permanent form of sterilization as pregnancy is contraindicated due to the high prevalence of maternal and fetal mortality. Cyanosis secondary to right-to-left intracardiac shunting is increased during pregnancy due to the decrease in systemic vascular resistance. Cyanosis is associated with increased risk of thrombosis causing paradoxical emboli and hyperviscosity from erythrocytosis. In cyanotic patients without Eisenmenger syndrome, live births were reported at 43% with 37% prematurity and increased maternal complications when the maternal oxygen saturation is <85%.[197] Common maternal complications with cyanosis include heart failure, endocarditis, and thrombosis. Cyanosis associated with Eisenmenger syndrome carries an extremely high maternal mortality rate (at least 50%). Women with Eisenmenger syndrome are advised against pregnancy.

Single Ventricle with Fontan Palliation

Pregnancies in women with a single ventricle palliated with a Fontan circulation are associated with high maternal and neonatal risk.[198] There are high rate of miscarriages, with maternal complications such as supraventricular arrhythmias (most common), heart failure, and valve regurgitation.[199,200] Baseline functional capacity, arrhythmia burden, single ventricular function, and degree of cyanosis are the basic determinants of pregnancy risk. Women with cyanosis, ventricular dysfunction, moderate or more atrioventricular valve regurgitation, or the presence of protein-losing enteropathy should be advised against pregnancy.[1] Pregnancies in women with Fontan physiology have higher rates of miscarriage (30%), heart failure, arrhythmia, and bleeding.[198–200] Neonatal outcomes include prematurity and small for gestational age neonates.[201] Anticoagulation throughout pregnancy should be considered in the Fontan patient due the higher risk of thrombosis during pregnancy coupled with the inherent hypercoagulable state of the Fontan circulation.[202]

Cardiopulmonary Resuscitation during Pregnancy

Cardiac arrest during pregnancy has been reported in 1 in 30,000 pregnancies.[203,204] As delineated in a recent statement, maternal cardiac arrest requires a "bundled" emergency code with representatives from cardiology, maternal fetal medicine, neonatology, and anesthesia responding to the call. Management of cardiac arrest should be in accordance with the general ACLS protocols including life-saving medications and defibrillation with the unique modification of manipulating the uterus left laterally by 1.5 cm during the resuscitation, both to allow better venous return by relieving uterine compression off the inferior vena cava. Central intravenous access is also preferably placed above the umbilicus as not to be affected by the compressing uterus. Emergency cesarean section is advised if the cardiopulmonary resuscitation lasts more than 4 minutes or attempts to relieve the aorto-caval compression by the uterus are unsuccessful.[203]

SUMMARY

CVD complicates more than 1% to 4% of pregnancies and is the leading cause of indirect maternal mortality. Medical care begins in the preconception period with careful planning and anticipation of the possible complications that may arise during the antepartum, intrapartum, and the postpartum periods. Pregnant women with CVD should be cared for by a multidisciplinary team that understands the unique hemodynamic changes that occur and how these changes affect women and their offspring both during pregnancy and beyond.[205]

REFERENCES

1. Regitz-Zagrosek V, et al. 2018 ESC guidelines for the management of cardiovascular diseases during pregnancy. *Eur Heart J.* 2018;39(34):3165-3241.
2. Ouyang DW, et al. Obstetric outcomes in pregnant women with congenital heart disease. *Int J Cardiol.* 2010;144(2):195-199.
3. Draper ES, Gallimore ID, Smith LK, et al. MBRRACE-UK perinatal mortality surveillance report, UK perinatal deaths for births from January to December 2017. Leicester, UK: The Infant Mortality and Morbidity Studies, Department of Health Sciences, University of Leicester; 2019.
4. CDC Foundation. Building U.S. capacity to review and prevent maternal deaths. Report from maternal mortality review committees: a view into their critical role. 2017. https://www.cdcfoundation.org/sites/default/files/upload/pdf/MMRIAReport.pdf. Accessed July 25, 2021.
5. Kuklina E, Callaghan W. Chronic heart disease and severe obstetric morbidity among hospitalisations for pregnancy in the USA: 1995-2006. *BJOG.* 2011;118(3):345-352.
6. Gelson E, et al. Heart disease–why is maternal mortality increasing? *BJOG.* 2009;116(5):609-611.
7. Stout KK, et al. 2018 AHA/ACC guideline for the management of adults with congenital heart disease: a report of the American College of Cardiology/American Heart Association Task Force on Clinical Practice Guidelines. *J Am Coll Cardiol.* 2019;73(12):e81-e192.
8. Nora JJ, Nora AH. Maternal transmission of congenital heart diseases: new recurrence risk figures and the questions of cytoplasmic inheritance and vulnerability to teratogens. *Am J Cardiol.* 1987;59(5):459-463.
9. Romano-Zelekha O, et al. The risk for congenital heart defects in offspring of individuals with congenital heart defects. *Clin Genet.* 2001;59(5):325-329.
10. Baumgartner H, et al. 2020 ESC guidelines for the management of adult congenital heart disease. *Eur Heart J.* 2020;31.
11. Nanna M, Stergiopoulos K. Pregnancy complicated by valvular heart disease: an update. *J Am Heart Assoc.* 2014;3(3):e000712.
12. Easterling TR, et al. Maternal hemodynamics in normal and preeclamptic pregnancies: a longitudinal study. *Obstet Gynecol.* 1990;76(6):1061-1069.
13. Geva T, et al. Effects of physiologic load of pregnancy on left ventricular contractility and remodeling. *Am Heart J.* 1997;133(1):53-59.
14. Mabie WC, et al. A longitudinal study of cardiac output in normal human pregnancy. *Am J Obstet Gynecol.* 1994;170(3):849-856.
15. Mone SM, Sanders SP, Colan SD. Control mechanisms for physiological hypertrophy of pregnancy. *Circulation* 1996;94(4):667-672.
16. Robson SC, et al. Serial study of factors influencing changes in cardiac output during human pregnancy. *Am J Physiol.* 1989;256(4 Pt 2):H1060-1065.
17. Robson SC, Dunlop W, Hunter S. Haemodynamic changes during the early puerperium. *Br Med J (Clin Res Ed).* 1987;294(6579):1065.
18. Hunter S, Robson SC. Adaptation of the maternal heart in pregnancy. *Br Heart J.* 1992;68(6):540-543.
19. Sanghavi M, Rutherford JD. Cardiovascular physiology of pregnancy. *Circulation* 2014;130(12):1003-1008.
20. Gilson GJ, et al. Changes in hemodynamics, ventricular remodeling, and ventricular contractility during normal pregnancy: a longitudinal study. *Obstet Gynecol.* 1997;89(6):957-962.
21. Poppas A, et al. Serial assessment of the cardiovascular system in normal pregnancy. Role of arterial compliance and pulsatile arterial load. *Circulation.* 1997;95(10):2407-2415.

22. Robson SC, et al. Combined Doppler and echocardiographic measurement of cardiac output: theory and application in pregnancy. *Br J Obstet Gynaecol.* 1987;94(11):1014-1027.

23. Robson SC, et al. Cardiac output during labour. *Br Med J (Clin Res Ed).* 1987;295(6607):1169-1172.

24. Robson SC, et al. Haemodynamic changes during the puerperium: a Doppler and M-mode echocardiographic study. *Br J Obstet Gynaecol.* 1987;94(11):1028-1039.

25. Kametas NA, et al. Maternal left ventricular mass and diastolic function during pregnancy. *Ultrasound Obstet Gynecol.* 2001;18(5):460-466.

26. Tsiaras S, Poppas A. Cardiac disease in pregnancy: value of echocardiography. *Curr Cardiol Rep.* 2010;12(3):250-256.

27. Ducas RA, et al. Cardiovascular magnetic resonance in pregnancy: insights from the cardiac hemodynamic imaging and remodeling in pregnancy (CHIRP) study. *J Cardiovasc Magn Reson.* 2014;16:1.

28. Savu O, et al. Morphological and functional adaptation of the maternal heart during pregnancy. *Circ Cardiovasc Imaging.* 2012;5(3):289-297.

29. Easterling TR, et al. Maternal hemodynamics and aortic diameter in normal and hypertensive pregnancies. *Obstet Gynecol.* 1991;78(6):1073-1077.

30. Campos O, et al. Physiologic multivalvular regurgitation during pregnancy: a longitudinal Doppler echocardiographic study. *Int J Cardiol.* 1993;40(3):265-272.

31. Robson SC, et al. Incidence of Doppler regurgitant flow velocities during normal pregnancy. *Eur Heart J.* 1992;13(1):84-87.

32. Abduljabbar HS, et al. Pericardial effusion in normal pregnant women. *Acta Obstet Gynecol Scand.* 1991;70(4-5):291-294.

33. Ristic AD, et al. Pericardial disease in pregnancy. *Herz.* 2003;28(3):209-215.

34. Halpern DG, et al. Use of medication for cardiovascular disease during pregnancy: JACC State-of-the-Art Review. *J Am Coll Cardiol.* 2019;73(4):457-476.

35. Food and HHS Drug Administration. Content and format of labeling for human prescription drug and biological products; requirements for pregnancy and lactation labeling. Final rule. *Fed Regist.* 2014;79(233):72063-72103.

36. Cutforth R, MacDonald CB. Heart sounds and murmurs in pregnancy. *Am Heart J.* 1966;71(6):741-747.

37. Stout KK, Otto CM. Pregnancy in women with valvular heart disease. *Heart.* 2007;93(5):552-558.

38. Carruth JE, et al. The electrocardiogram in normal pregnancy. *Am Heart J.* 1981;102(6 Pt 1):1075-1078.

39. Enriquez AD, Economy KE, Tedrow UB. Contemporary management of arrhythmias during pregnancy. *Circ Arrhythm Electrophysiol.* 2014;7(5):961-967.

40. Mishra M, Chambers JB, Jackson G. Murmurs in pregnancy: an audit of echocardiography. *BMJ.* 1992;304(6839):1413-1414.

41. Lui GK, et al. Heart rate response during exercise and pregnancy outcome in women with congenital heart disease. *Circulation.* 2011;123(3):242-248.

42. Ray JG, et al. Association between MRI exposure during pregnancy and fetal and childhood outcomes. *JAMA.* 2016;316(9):952-961.

43. Chambers CE, et al. Radiation safety program for the cardiac catheterization laboratory. *Catheter Cardiovasc Interv.* 2011;77(4):546-556.

44. Joshi HS, et al. Study of effectiveness and safety of percutaneous balloon mitral valvulotomy for treatment of pregnant patients with severe mitral stenosis. *J Clin Diagn Res.* 2015;9(12):OC14-7.

45. Esteves CA, et al. Immediate and long-term follow-up of percutaneous balloon mitral valvuloplasty in pregnant patients with rheumatic mitral stenosis. *Am J Cardiol.* 2006;98(6):812-816.

46. Myerson SG, et al. What is the role of balloon dilatation for severe aortic stenosis during pregnancy? *J Heart Valve Dis.* 2005;14(2):147-150.

47. Hodson R. et al. Transcatheter aortic valve replacement during pregnancy. *Circ Cardiovasc Interv.* 2016;9(10).

48. Balci A, et al. Prospective validation and assessment of cardiovascular and offspring risk models for pregnant women with congenital heart disease. *Heart.* 2014;100(17):1373-1381.

49. Yuksel MA, et al. Maternal serum atrial natriuretic peptide (ANP) and brain-type natriuretic peptide (BNP) levels in gestational diabetes mellitus. *J Matern Fetal Neonatal Med.* 2015:1-4.

50. Mayama M, et al. Factors influencing brain natriuretic peptide levels in healthy pregnant women. *Int J Cardiol.* 2017;228:749-753.

51. Siu SC, et al. Risk and predictors for pregnancy-related complications in women with heart disease. *Circulation.* 1997;96(9):2789-2794.

52. Silversides CK, et al. Pregnancy outcomes in women with heart disease: the CARPREG II study. *J Am Coll Cardiol.* 2018;71(21):2419-2430.

53. Drenthen W, et al. Predictors of pregnancy complications in women with congenital heart disease. *Eur Heart J.* 2010;31(17):2124-2132.

54. Thorne S, MacGregor A, Nelson-Piercy C. Risks of contraception and pregnancy in heart disease. *Heart* 2006;92(10):1520-1525.

55. Greutmann M, Silversides CK. The ROPAC registry: a multicentre collaboration on pregnancy outcomes in women with heart disease. *Eur Heart J.* 2013;34(9):634-635.

56. Orwat S, et al. Risk of pregnancy in moderate and severe aortic stenosis: from the multinational ROPAC registry. *J Am Coll Cardiol.* 2016;68(16):1727-1737.

57. van Hagen IM, et al. Pregnancy outcomes in women with rheumatic mitral valve disease: results from the registry of pregnancy and cardiac disease. *Circulation.* 2018;137(8):806-816.

58. Easter SR, et al. Planned vaginal delivery and cardiovascular morbidity in pregnant women with heart disease. *Am J Obstet Gynecol.* 2020;222(1): 77 e1-e77.e11.

59. Siu SC, et al. Adverse neonatal and cardiac outcomes are more common in pregnant women with cardiac disease. *Circulation.* 2002;105(18):2179-2184.

60. Hypertension in pregnancy. Report of the American College of Obstetricians and Gynecologists' Task Force on Hypertension in Pregnancy. *Obstet Gynecol.* 2013;122(5):1122-1131.

61. Garovic VD, Hayman SR. Hypertension in pregnancy: an emerging risk factor for cardiovascular disease. *Nat Clin Pract Nephrol.* 2007;3(11):613-622.

62. Breathett K, et al. Differences in preeclampsia rates between African American and Caucasian women: trends from the National Hospital Discharge Survey. *J Womens Health (Larchmt).* 2014;23(11):886-893.

63. Ananth CV, Keyes KM, Wapner RJ. Pre-eclampsia rates in the United States, 1980-2010: age-period-cohort analysis. *BMJ.* 2013;347:f6564.

64. Shahul S. et al. Racial disparities in comorbidities, complications, and maternal and fetal outcomes in women with preeclampsia/eclampsia. *Hypertens Pregnancy.* 2015;34(4):506-515.

65. ACOG practice bulletin no. 202 summary: gestational hypertension and preeclampsia. *Obstet Gynecol.* 2019;133(1):211-214.

66. Vaught AJ, et al. Acute cardiac effects of severe pre-eclampsia. *J Am Coll Cardiol.* 2018;72(1):1-11.

67. von Dadelszen, et al. Fall in mean arterial pressure and fetal growth restriction in pregnancy hypertension: a meta-analysis. *Lancet.* 2000;355(9198):87-92.

68. Seely EW, Ecker J. Chronic hypertension in pregnancy. *Circulation* 2014;129(11):1254-1261.

69. ACOG practice bulletin. Diagnosis and management of preeclampsia and eclampsia. Number 33, January 2002. *Obstet Gynecol.* 2002;99(1):159-167.

70. Magee LA, et al. Less-tight versus tight control of hypertension in pregnancy. *N Engl J Med.* 2015;372(5):407-417.

71. Benigni A, et al. Effect of low-dose aspirin on fetal and maternal generation of thromboxane by platelets in women at risk for pregnancy-induced hypertension. *N Engl J Med.* 1989;321(6):357-362.

72. LeFevre ML, USPST Force. Low-dose aspirin use for the prevention of morbidity and mortality from preeclampsia: U.S. Preventive Services Task Force recommendation statement. *Ann Intern Med.* 2014;161(11):819-826.

73. Mehta LS, et al. Cardiovascular considerations in caring for pregnant patients: a scientific statement from the American Heart Association. *Circulation.* 2020;141(23):e884-e903.

74. Lindheimer MD, Taler SJ, Cunningham FJ. Hypertension in pregnancy. *J Am Soc Hypertens.* 2010;4(2):68-78.

75. Sibai BM, et al. A comparison of no medication versus methyldopa or labetalol in chronic hypertension during pregnancy. *Am J Obstet Gynecol.* 1990;162(4):960-966; discussion 966-967.

76. Xie RH, et al. Trends in using beta-blockers and methyldopa for hypertensive disorders during pregnancy in a Canadian population. *Eur J Obstet Gynecol Reprod Biol.* 2013;171(2):281-285.

77. Tabacova S, et al. Atenolol developmental toxicity: animal-to-human comparisons. *Birth Defects Res A Clin Mol Teratol.* 2003;67(3):181-192.

78. Nifedipine versus expectant management in mild to moderate hypertension in pregnancy. Gruppo di Studio Ipertensione in Gravidanza. *Br J Obstet Gynaecol.* 1998;105(7):718-722.

79. Magee LA, et al. The safety of calcium channel blockers in human pregnancy: a prospective, multicenter cohort study. *Am J Obstet Gynecol.* 1996;174(3):823-828.

80. Ferrer RL, et al. Management of mild chronic hypertension during pregnancy: a review. *Obstet Gynecol.* 2000;96(5 Pt 2):849-860.

81. Brent RL, Beckman DA. Angiotensin-converting enzyme inhibitors, an embryopathic class of drugs with unique properties: information for clinical teratology counselors. *Teratology.* 1991;43(6):543-546.

82. Barr M, Jr. Teratogen update: angiotensin-converting enzyme inhibitors. *Teratology.* 1994;50(6):399-409.

83. Serreau R, et al. Developmental toxicity of the angiotensin II type 1 receptor antagonists during human pregnancy: a report of 10 cases. *BJOG.* 2005;112(6):710-712.

84. Bos-Thompson MA, et al. Fetal toxic effects of angiotensin II receptor antagonists: case report and follow-up after birth. *Ann Pharmacother.* 2005;39(1):157-161.

85. Li DK, et al. Maternal exposure to angiotensin converting enzyme inhibitors in the first trimester and risk of malformations in offspring: a retrospective cohort study. *BMJ.* 2011;343:d5931.

86. Henderson JT, et al. Low-dose aspirin for prevention of morbidity and mortality from preeclampsia: a systematic evidence review for the U.S. Preventive Services Task Force. *Ann Intern Med.* 2014;160(10):695-703.

87. Schaap TP, et al. Eclampsia, a comparison within the International Network of Obstetric Survey Systems. *BJOG.* 2014;121(12):1521-1528.

88. Gold RA, et al. Effect of age, parity, and race on the incidence of pregnancy associated hypertension and eclampsia in the United States. *Pregnancy Hypertens.* 2014;4(1):46-53.

89. Meher S, Duley L. Exercise or other physical activity for preventing pre-eclampsia and its complications. *Cochrane Database Syst Rev.* 2006;2:CD005942.

90. Fraser A. et al. Associations of pregnancy complications with calculated cardiovascular disease risk and cardiovascular risk factors in middle age: the Avon Longitudinal Study of Parents and Children. *Circulation.* 2012;125(11):1367-1380.

91. Sibai BM, et al. Risk factors for preeclampsia in healthy nulliparous women: a prospective multicenter study. The National Institute of Child Health and Human Development Network of Maternal-Fetal Medicine Units. *Am J Obstet Gynecol.* 1995;172(2 Pt 1):642-648.

92. Sibai BM, et al. Risk factors associated with preeclampsia in healthy nulliparous women. The Calcium for Preeclampsia Prevention (CPEP) Study Group. *Am J Obstet Gynecol.* 1997;177(5):1003-1010.

93. Kaaja R. Insulin resistance syndrome in preeclampsia. *Semin Reprod Endocrinol.* 1998;16(1):41-46.

94. Honigberg MC, et al. Long-term cardiovascular risk in women with hypertension during pregnancy. *J Am Coll Cardiol.* 2019;74(22):2743-2754.

95. Ditisheim A. et al. Prevalence of hypertensive phenotypes after preeclampsia: a prospective cohort study. *Hypertension* 2018;71(1):103-109.

96. Jarvie JL. et al. Short-term risk of cardiovascular readmission following a hypertensive disorder of pregnancy. *Heart.* 2018;104(14):1187-1194.

97. Visser VS, et al. High blood pressure six weeks postpartum after hypertensive pregnancy disorders at term is associated with chronic hypertension. *Pregnancy Hypertens.* 2013;3(4):242-247.

98. Grundy SM, et al. 2018 AHA/ACC/AACVPR/AAPA/ABC/ACPM/ADA/AGS/APhA/ASPC/NLA/PCNA guideline on the management of blood cholesterol: a report of the American College of Cardiology/American Heart Association Task Force on Clinical Practice Guidelines. *Circulation.* 2019;139(25):e1082-e1143.

99. Valente AM, Bhatt DL, Lane-Cordova A. Pregnancy as a cardiac stress test: time to include obstetric history in cardiac risk assessment? *J Am Coll Cardiol.* 2020;76(1):68-71.

100. Shotan A, et al. Incidence of arrhythmias in normal pregnancy and relation to palpitations, dizziness, and syncope. *Am J Cardiol,* 1997;79(8):1061-1064.

101. Page RL, et al. 2015 ACC/AHA/HRS guideline for the management of adult patients with supraventricular tachycardia: a report of the American College of Cardiology/American Heart Association Task Force on Clinical Practice Guidelines and the Heart Rhythm Society. *Circulation* 2015.

102. Thaman R, et al. Cardiac outcome of pregnancy in women with a pacemaker and women with untreated atrioventricular conduction block. *Europace.* 2011;13(6):859-863.

103. Makhija A, et al. Hormone sensitive idiopathic ventricular tachycardia associated with pregnancy: successful induction with progesterone and radiofrequency ablation. *J Cardiovasc Electrophysiol.* 2011;22(1):95-98.

104. Rosano GM, et al. Cyclical variation in paroxysmal supraventricular tachycardia in women. *Lancet.* 1996;347(9004):786-788.

105. Silversides CK, et al. Recurrence rates of arrhythmias during pregnancy in women with previous tachyarrhythmia and impact on fetal and neonatal outcomes. *Am J Cardiol.* 2006;97(8):1206-1212.

106. Li JM, et al. Frequency and outcome of arrhythmias complicating admission during pregnancy: experience from a high-volume and ethnically-diverse obstetric service. *Clin Cardiol.* 2008;31(11):538-541.

107. Drenthen W, et al. Outcome of pregnancy in women with congenital heart disease: a literature review. *J Am Coll Cardiol.* 2007;49(24):2303-2311.

108. Gleicher N, et al. Wolff-Parkinson-White syndrome in pregnancy. *Obstet Gynecol.* 1981;58(6):748-752.

109. Wang YC, et al. The impact of maternal cardioversion on fetal haemodynamics. *Eur J Obstet Gynecol Reprod Biol.* 2006;126(2):268-269.

110. Barnes EJ, Eben F, Patterson D. Direct current cardioversion during pregnancy should be performed with facilities available for fetal monitoring and emergency caesarean section. *BJOG.* 2002;109(12):1406-1407.

111. Lee SH, et al. Effects of pregnancy on first onset and symptoms of paroxysmal supraventricular tachycardia. *Am J Cardiol.* 1995;76(10):675-678.

112. Joglar JA, Page RL. Management of arrhythmia syndromes during pregnancy. *Curr Opin Cardiol.* 2014;29(1):36-44.

113. Salam AM, et al. Atrial fibrillation or flutter during pregnancy in patients with structural heart disease. *JACC: Clin Electrophysiol.* 2015;1(4):284-292.

114. Tateno S, et al. Arrhythmia and conduction disturbances in patients with congenital heart disease during pregnancy: multicenter study. *Circ J.* 2003;67(12):992-997.

115. Natale A, et al. Implantable cardioverter-defibrillators and pregnancy: a safe combination? *Circulation.* 1997;96(9):2808-2812.

116. Hidaka N, et al. Pregnant women with complete atrioventricular block: perinatal risks and review of management. *Pacing Clin Electrophysiol.* 2011;34(9):1161-1176.

117. Antonelli D, Bloch L, Rosenfeld T. Implantation of permanent dual chamber pacemaker in a pregnant woman by transesophageal echocardiographic guidance. *Pacing Clin Electrophysiol.* 1999;22(3):534-535.

118. Safi LM, Tsiaras SV. Update on valvular heart disease in pregnancy. *Curr Treat Options Cardiovasc Med.* 2017;19(9):70.

119. Hameed A, et al. The effect of valvular heart disease on maternal and fetal outcome of pregnancy. *J Am Coll Cardiol.* 2001;37(3):893-899.

120. Silversides CK, et al. Cardiac risk in pregnant women with rheumatic mitral stenosis. *Am J Cardiol.* 2003;91(11):1382-1385.

121. Windram JD, et al. Valvular heart disease in pregnancy. *Best Pract Res Clin Obstet Gynaecol.* 2014;28(4):507-518.

122. Elkayam U, Bitar F. Valvular heart disease and pregnancy part I: native valves. *J Am Coll Cardiol.* 2005;46(2):223-230.

123. Silversides CK, et al. Early and intermediate-term outcomes of pregnancy with congenital aortic stenosis. *Am J Cardiol.* 2003;91(11):1386-1389.

124. Anderson RA, Fineron W. Aortic dissection in pregnancy: importance of pregnancy-induced changes in the vessel wall and bicuspid aortic valve in pathogenesis. *Br J Obstet Gynaecol.* 1994;101(12):1085-1088.

125. Immer FF, et al. Aortic dissection in pregnancy: analysis of risk factors and outcome. *Ann Thorac Surg.* 2003;76(1):309-314.

126. Yap SC, et al. Risk of complications during pregnancy in women with congenital aortic stenosis. *Int J Cardiol.* 2008;126(2):240-246.

127. Zhong C, et al. Pregnancy and transcatheter aortic valve replacement in a severely stenotic freestyle full aortic root stentless bioprosthesis. *Catheter Cardiovasc Interv.* 2020;95(6):1225-1229.

128. Drenthen W, et al. Non-cardiac complications during pregnancy in women with isolated congenital pulmonary valvar stenosis. *Heart.* 2006;92(12):1838-1843.

129. van Hagen IM, et al. Pregnancy in women with a mechanical heart valve: data of the European Society of Cardiology Registry of Pregnancy and Cardiac Disease (ROPAC). *Circulation.* 2015;132(2):132-142.

130. Nishimura RA, et al. 2014 AHA/ACC guideline for the management of patients with valvular heart disease: a report of the American College of Cardiology/American Heart Association Task Force on Practice Guidelines. *Circulation.* 2014;129(23):e521-e643.

131. Wilson W, et al. Prevention of infective endocarditis: guidelines from the American Heart Association: a guideline from the American Heart Association Rheumatic Fever, Endocarditis, and Kawasaki Disease Committee, Council on Cardiovascular Disease in the Young, and the Council on Clinical Cardiology, Council on Cardiovascular Surgery and Anesthesia, and the Quality of Care and Outcomes Research Interdisciplinary Working Group. *Circulation.* 2007;116(15):1736-1754.

132. Sliwa K, et al. Management of valvular disease in pregnancy: a global perspective. *Eur Heart J.* 2015;36(18):1078-1089.

133. North RA, et al. Long-term survival and valve-related complications in young women with cardiac valve replacements. *Circulation.* 1999;99(20):2669-2676.

134. Avila WS, et al. Influence of pregnancy after bioprosthetic valve replacement in young women: a prospective five-year study. *J Heart Valve Dis.* 2002;11(6):864-869.

135. Badduke BR, et al. Pregnancy and childbearing in a population with biologic valvular prostheses. *J Thorac Cardiovasc Surg.* 1991;102(2):179-186.

136. Jamieson WR, et al. Pregnancy and bioprostheses: influence on structural valve deterioration. *Ann Thorac Surg.* 1995;60(2 Suppl):S282-S286; discussion S287.

137. Duarte VE, Graf J, Marshall AC, Economy KE, Valente AM. Transcatheter pulmonary valve performance during pregnancy and the postpartum period. *J Am Coll Cardiol Case Rep.* 2020;2:847–851.

138. Ayad SW, et al. Maternal and fetal outcomes in pregnant women with a prosthetic mechanical heart valve. *Clin Med Insights Cardiol.* 2016;10:11-17.

139. Pieper G, Balci A, Van Dijk AP. Pregnancy in women with prosthetic heart valves. *Neth Heart J.* 2008;16(12):406-411.

140. Vitale N, et al. Dose-dependent fetal complications of warfarin in pregnant women with mechanical heart valves. *J Am Coll Cardiol.* 1999;33(6):1637-1641.

141. Cotrufo M, et al. Risk of warfarin during pregnancy with mechanical valve prostheses. *Obstet Gynecol.* 2002;99(1):35-40.

142. Elkayam U, Goland S. The search for a safe and effective anticoagulation regimen in pregnant women with mechanical prosthetic heart valves. *J Am Coll Cardiol.* 2012;59(12):1116-1118.

143. Kaneko T, Aranki SF. Anticoagulation for prosthetic valves. *Thrombosis.* 2013;2013:346752.

144. McLintock C, McCowan LM, North RA. Maternal complications and pregnancy outcome in women with mechanical prosthetic heart valves treated with enoxaparin. *BJOG.* 2009;116(12):1585-1592.

145. Yinon Y, et al. Use of low molecular weight heparin in pregnant women with mechanical heart valves. *Am J Cardiol.* 2009;104(9):1259-1263.

146. Steinberg ZL, et al. Maternal and fetal outcomes of anticoagulation in pregnant women with mechanical heart valves. *J Am Coll Cardiol.* 2017;69(22):2681-2691.

147. Montorsi P, et al. Role of cine-fluoroscopy, transthoracic, and transesophageal echocardiography in patients with suspected prosthetic heart valve thrombosis. *Am J Cardiol.* 2000;85(1):58-64.

148. Elkayam U, et al. Pregnancy-associated cardiomyopathy: clinical characteristics and a comparison between early and late presentation. *Circulation* 2005;111(16):2050-2055.

149. Ozkan M. et al. Thrombolytic therapy for the treatment of prosthetic heart valve thrombosis in pregnancy with low-dose, slow infusion of tissue-type plasminogen activator. *Circulation.* 2013;128(5):532-540.

150. Weiss BM, et al. Outcome of cardiovascular surgery and pregnancy: a systematic review of the period 1984-1996. *Am J Obstet Gynecol.* 1998;179 (6 Pt 1):1643-1653.

151. Meng K, et al. Incidence of venous thromboembolism during pregnancy and the puerperium: a systematic review and meta-analysis. *J Matern Fetal Neonatal Med.* 2015;28(3):245-253.

152. van der Pol LM, et al. Pregnancy-adapted YEARS algorithm for diagnosis of suspected pulmonary embolism. *N Engl J Med.* 2019;380(12):1139-1149.

153. Campuzano K, et al. Bacterial endocarditis complicating pregnancy: case report and systematic review of the literature. *Arch Gynecol Obstet.* 2003;268(4):251-255.

154. Montoya ME, Karnath BM, Ahmad M. Endocarditis during pregnancy. *South Med J.* 2003;96(11):1156-1157.

155. Kebed KY, et al. Pregnancy and postpartum infective endocarditis: a systematic review. *Mayo Clin Proc.* 2014;89(8):1143-1152.

156. Arnoni RT, et al. Risk factors associated with cardiac surgery during pregnancy. *Ann Thorac Surg.* 2003;76(5):1605-1608.

157. Chambers CE, Clark SL. Cardiac surgery during pregnancy. *Clin Obstet Gynecol.* 1994;37(2):316-323.

158. Kapoor MC. Cardiopulmonary bypass in pregnancy. *Ann Card Anaesth.* 2014;17(1):33-39.

159. Grewal J, et al. Pregnancy outcomes in women with dilated cardiomyopathy. *J Am Coll Cardiol.* 2009;55(1):45-52.

160. Ware JS, et al. Shared genetic predisposition in peripartum and dilated cardiomyopathies. *N Engl J Med.* 2016;374(3):233-241.

161. Autore C, et al. Risk associated with pregnancy in hypertrophic cardiomyopathy. *J Am Coll Cardiol.* 2002;40(10):1864-1869.

162. Thaman R, et al. Pregnancy related complications in women with hypertrophic cardiomyopathy. *Heart.* 2003;89(7):752-756.

163. Wu D, et al. Molecular mechanisms of thoracic aortic dissection. *J Surg Res.* 2013;184(2):907-924.

164. Elkayam U, et al. Cardiovascular problems in pregnant women with the Marfan syndrome. *Ann Intern Med.* 1995;123(2):117-122.

165. Rudd NL, et al. Pregnancy complications in type IV Ehlers-Danlos syndrome. *Lancet.* 1983;1(8314-8315):50-53.

166. Donnelly RT, et al. The immediate and long-term impact of pregnancy on aortic growth rate and mortality in women with Marfan syndrome. *J Am Coll Cardiol.* 2012;60(3):224-229.

167. Hiratzka LF, et al. 2010 ACCF/AHA/AATS/ACR/ASA/SCA/SCAI/SIR/STS/SVM guidelines for the diagnosis and management of patients with thoracic aortic disease: executive summary. A report of the American College of Cardiology Foundation/American Heart Association Task Force on Practice Guidelines, American Association for Thoracic Surgery, American College of Radiology, American Stroke Association,

Society of Cardiovascular Anesthesiologists, Society for Cardiovascular Angiography and Interventions, Society of Interventional Radiology, Society of Thoracic Surgeons, and Society for Vascular Medicine. *Catheter Cardiovasc Interv.* 2010;76(2):E43-E86.

168. MacCarrick G, et al. Loeys-Dietz syndrome: a primer for diagnosis and management. *Genet Med.* 2014;16(8):576-587.

169. Lurie S, Manor M, Hagay ZJ. The threat of type IV Ehlers-Danlos syndrome on maternal well-being during pregnancy: early delivery may make the difference. *J Obstet Gynaecol.* 1998;18(3):245-248.

170. Lameijer H, et al. Ischaemic heart disease during pregnancy or post-partum: systematic review and case series. *Neth Heart J.* 2015;23(5):249-257.

171. Ladner HE, Danielsen B, Gilbert WM. Acute myocardial infarction in pregnancy and the puerperium: a population-based study. *Obstet Gynecol.* 2005;105(3):480-484.

172. Elkayam U, et al. Pregnancy-associated acute myocardial infarction: a review of contemporary experience in 150 cases between 2006 and 2011. *Circulation* 2014;129(16):1695-1702.

173. Havakuk O, et al. Pregnancy and the risk of spontaneous coronary artery dissection: an analysis of 120 contemporary cases. *Circ Cardiovasc Interv.* 2017;10(3).

174. Hayes SN, et al. Spontaneous coronary artery dissection: JACC State-of-the-Art Review. *J Am Coll Cardiol.* 2020;76(8):961-984.

175. Anselmi A. et al. Extracorporeal membrane oxygenation in pregnancy. *J Card Surg.* 2015;30(10):781-786.

176. John AS, et al. Cardiopulmonary bypass during pregnancy. *Ann Thorac Surg.* 2011;91(4):1191-1196.

177. Sepehripour AH, et al. Can pregnant women be safely placed on cardiopulmonary bypass? *Interact Cardiovasc Thorac Surg.* 2012;15(6):1063-1070.

178. Hemnes AR, et al. Statement on pregnancy in pulmonary hypertension from the Pulmonary Vascular Research Institute. *Pulm Circ.* 2015;5(3):435-465.

179. Jais X, et al. Pregnancy outcomes in pulmonary arterial hypertension in the modern management era. *Eur Respir J.* 2012;40(4):881-885.

180. Sliwa K, et al. Pulmonary hypertension and pregnancy outcomes: data from the Registry Of Pregnancy and Cardiac Disease (ROPAC) of the European Society of Cardiology. *Eur J Heart Fail.* 2016;18(9):1119-1128.

181. Smith JS, Mueller J, Daniels CJ. Pulmonary arterial hypertension in the setting of pregnancy: a case series and standard treatment approach. *Lung.* 2012;190(2):155-160.

182. Goland S, et al. Favorable outcome of pregnancy with an elective use of epoprostenol and sildenafil in women with severe pulmonary hypertension. *Cardiology.* 2010;115(3):205-208.

183. Yap SC, et al. Comparison of pregnancy outcomes in women with repaired versus unrepaired atrial septal defect. *BJOG.* 2009;116(12):1593-1601.

184. Yap SC, et al. Pregnancy outcome in women with repaired versus unrepaired isolated ventricular septal defect. *BJOG.* 2010;117(6):683-689.

185. Kounis NG, et al. Pregnancy-induced increase of supraventricular arrhythmias in Wolff-Parkinson-White syndrome. *Clin Cardiol.* 1995;18(3):137-140.

186. Donnelly JE, Brown JM, Radford DJ. Pregnancy outcome and Ebstein's anomaly. *Br Heart J.* 1991;66(5):368-371.

187. Connolly HM, Warnes CA. Ebstein's anomaly: outcome of pregnancy. *J Am Coll Cardiol.* 1994;23(5):1194-1198.

188. Guedes A, et al. Impact of pregnancy on the systemic right ventricle after a Mustard operation for transposition of the great arteries. *J Am Coll Cardiol.* 2004;44(2):433-437.

189. Tobler D, et al. Pregnancy outcomes in women with transposition of the great arteries and arterial switch operation. *Am J Cardiol.* 2010;106(3):417-420.

190. Beauchesne LM, et al. Coarctation of the aorta: outcome of pregnancy. *J Am Coll Cardiol.* 2001;38(6):1728-1733.

191. Jimenez-Juan L, et al. Cardiovascular magnetic resonance imaging predictors of pregnancy outcomes in women with coarctation of the aorta. *Eur Heart J Cardiovasc Imaging.* 2014;15(3):299-306.

192. Krieger EV, et al. Comparison of risk of hypertensive complications of pregnancy among women with versus without coarctation of the aorta. *Am J Cardiol.* 2011;107(10):1529-1534.

193. Veldtman GR, et al. Outcomes of pregnancy in women with tetralogy of Fallot. *J Am Coll Cardiol.* 2004;44(1):174-180.

194. Balci A, et al. Pregnancy in women with corrected tetralogy of Fallot: occurrence and predictors of adverse events. *Am Heart J.* 2011;161(2):307-313.

195. Egidy Assenza G, et al. The effects of pregnancy on right ventricular remodeling in women with repaired tetralogy of Fallot. *Int J Cardiol.* 2013;168(3):1847-1852.

196. Duarte VE, et al. Impact of pregnancy on ventricular strain in women with repaired tetralogy of fallot. *Pediatr Cardiol.* 2020.

197. Presbitero P, et al. Pregnancy in cyanotic congenital heart disease. Outcome of mother and fetus. *Circulation.* 1994;89(6):2673-2676.

198. Drenthen W, et al. Pregnancy and delivery in women after Fontan palliation. *Heart.* 2006;92(9):1290-1294.

199. Canobbio MM, et al. Pregnancy outcomes after the Fontan repair. *J Am Coll Cardiol.* 1996;28(3):763-767.

200. Le Gloan L, et al. Pregnancy in women with Fontan physiology. *Expert Rev Cardiovasc Ther.* 2011;9(12):1547-1556.

201. Zentner D, et al. Fertility and pregnancy in the Fontan population. *Int J Cardiol.* 2016;208:97-101.

202. van den Bosch AE, et al. Long-term outcome and quality of life in adult patients after the Fontan operation. *Am J Cardiol.* 2004;93(9):1141-1145.

203. Jeejeebhoy FM, et al. Cardiac arrest in pregnancy: a scientific statement from the American Heart Association. *Circulation.* 2015;132(18):1747-1773.

204. Canobbio MM, et al. management of pregnancy in patients with complex congenital heart disease: a scientific statement for healthcare professionals from the American Heart Association. *Circulation.* 2017;135(8):e50-e87.

205. Easter SR, Valente AM, Economy KE. Creating a multidisciplinary pregnancy heart team. *Curr Treat Options Cardiovasc Med.* 2020;22(1):3.

79

Traumatic Heart Disease

T. Bruce Ferguson, Jr, Austin Rogers, and Robert Allman

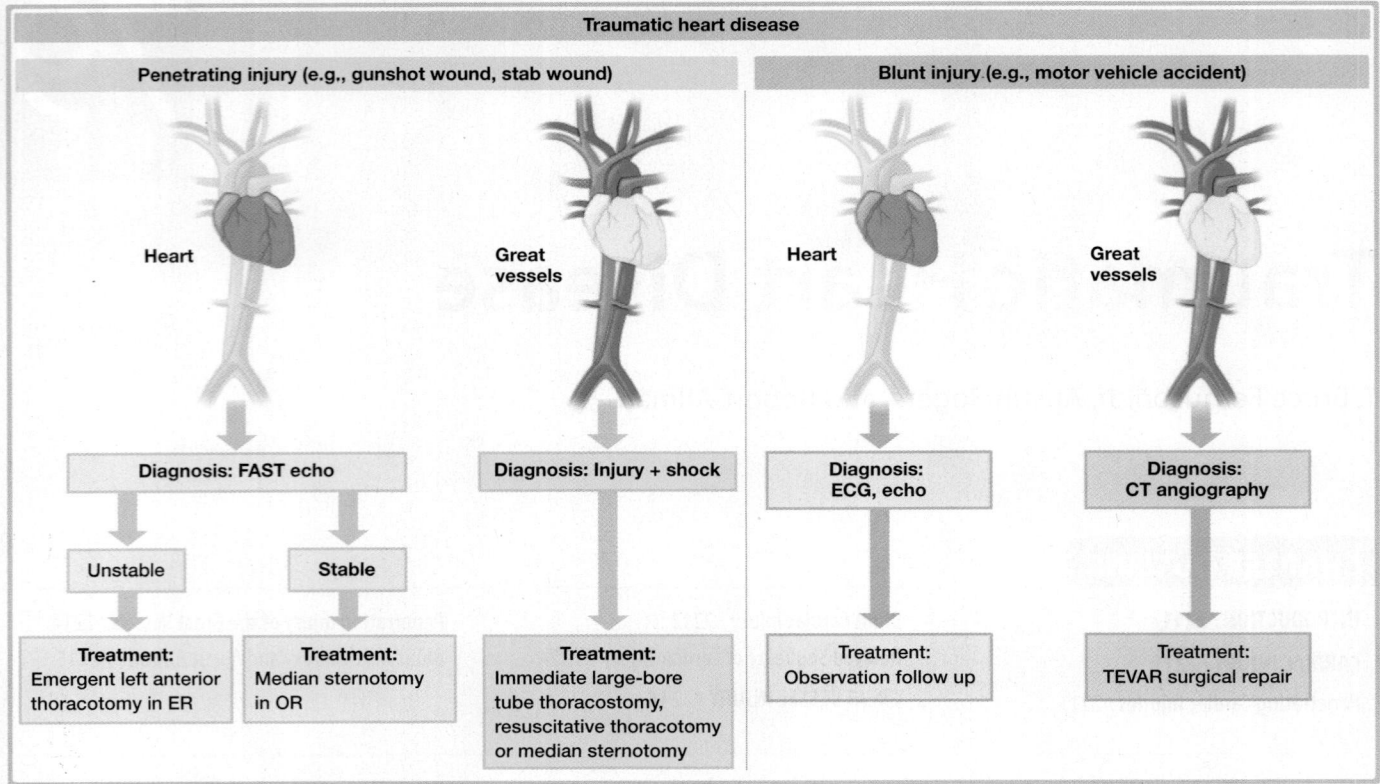

Chapter 79 Fuster and Hurst's Central Illustration. Traumatic thoracic injuries contribute to 75% of trauma-related deaths and primarily result from gunshot wounds and motor vehicle accidents. CT, computed tomography; ECG, electrocardiography; ER, emergency room; FAST, Focused Assessment by Sonography in Trauma; OR, operating room; TEVAR, thoracic endovascular aortic repair.

CHAPTER SUMMARY

This chapter discusses the diagnosis and management of traumatic heart disease. Traumatic thoracic injuries contribute to 75% of trauma-related deaths. These injuries are primarily from gunshot wounds and motor vehicle accidents. Penetrating cardiac injuries, in particular, are associated with high mortality. The American Association for the Surgery of Trauma Organ Injury Scale-Cardiac Surgery (AAST-OIS-CI) provides a description of cardiac injuries, where the increasing grade of injury is associated with increasing mortality. Echocardiography has replaced pericardial window as the gold standard for diagnosing cardiac injury (Focused Assessment by Sonography in Trauma [FAST]) (see Fuster and Hurst's Central Illustration). A left anterior thoracotomy in the emergency department is the approach of choice in hemodynamically unstable patients; stable patients are more appropriate for transport to the operating room for median sternotomy. The diagnosis of blunt cardiac injury is difficult. Electrocardiography may show nonspecific ST and T wave changes, and echocardiography may show regional wall motion abnormalities or structural defects. Management of these injuries is usually expectant. Long-term follow-up is required of significant cardiac injuries. Blunt aortic injury has a high death rate at the time of injury, but 70% of patients who survive to the hospital in stable condition can survive. Thoracic endovascular aortic repair has become the standard of care for treating blunt aortic injury.

INTRODUCTION

Trauma is the leading cause of death and disability among young people in the United States,[1-4] and the third leading cause of death across all age groups, accounting for 20% of all deaths.[5] Thoracic injuries account for 20% to 25% of deaths due to trauma, and contribute to 25% to 50% of the remaining deaths. Thus, thoracic injuries are a contributing factor in up to 75% of all trauma-related deaths.[6]

The two prinicipal causes of thoracic injuries are gunshot wounds and motor vehicle accidents.[7,8] Cardiac injury is present in a significant proportion of thoracic injuries that lead to death. Causes of thoracic injuries to the heart and great vessels can both be broadly divided into penetrating or blunt mechanisms. According to an analysis from the Oklahoma Trauma Registry, the mortality of patients with cardiac injury in the setting of trauma has increased, correlating with an increase in penetrating trauma.[5]

CARDIAC INJURY

The American Association for the Surgery of Trauma Organ Injury Scale: Cardiac Injury (AAST OIS-CI) describes cardiac injuries in six grades (**Table 79–1**).[9] Asensio et al. correlated AAST-OIS for cardiac injuries with mortality rate; 94% of deaths occurred in grades IV–VI.[10]

Penetrating Cardiac Injuries

Penetrating injury to the heart must be suspected with any missile (typically gunshot) or knife wound to the thorax or upper abdomen. The mechanism of injury may be categorized as low, medium, or high velocity. Knife wounds are low velocity, shotgun injuries are medium velocity, and high-velocity injuries include bullet wounds caused by rifles and wounds resulting from military and civilian weapons. The amount of tissue damage is directly related to the amount of energy exchange between the penetrating object and the body part.[6]

Penetrating cardiac injury accounts for only 0.1% of all trauma admissions,[11] and is therefore seen infrequently, even at busy trauma centers. These wounds can result in death from cardiac tamponade or exsanguination. Early diagnosis of the injured organ(s) is difficult. Unlike other forms of trauma, preoperative resuscitation can be of limited benefit.[7] Despite tremendous progress in other fields of trauma care, up to 90% of victims with penetrating cardiac trauma die before reaching the hospital.[12,13]

Table 79–2 shows the spectrum of penetrating cardiac injury by anatomic location.[14] Multiple chambers are injured in 18% of cases, but direct coronary artery injury occurs in <5%.[11] Other potentially injured structures include the interatrial or interventricular septum, valves, subvalvular apparatus, and conduction system.[12] In a series analyzing the LA County-USC trauma registry, among 202 patients with isolated cardiac injury, 93.1% had a single chamber injury, with a survival rate of 46.6%. In contrast, multiple chamber injury conveyed a 95.6% mortality.[20] High-velocity missiles produce injury beyond the region of myocardial penetration secondary to concussive

effects and are more frequently lethal. Low-velocity injuries, such as stab wounds, produce damage commensurate to the structure penetrated and size of the defect.[15-18] In the United States, gunshot wounds outnumber stab wounds almost 2:1, unlike the rest of the world.[11-19]

Beyond the primary manifestations of cardiac penetration of hemorrhage and tamponade, valve or coronary injury may produce acute valvular incompetence or myocardial infarction. Stab victims often present with tamponade when clot and surrounding pericardial fat partially seal the pericardial defect. Injuries to the left ventricle more commonly result in overt hemorrhage. Patients presenting with tamponade may have a

TABLE 79–1. AAST Injury Scale: Cardiac Injuries[9]

Grade I:
1. blunt cardiac injury with minor EKG abnormality (nonspecific ST- or T-wave changes, premature atrial or ventricular contractions, or persistent sinus tachycardia
2. blunt or penetrating pericardial wound without cardiac injury, tamponade, or cardiac herniation

Grade II:
1. blunt cardiac injury with heart block or ischemic changes without cardiac failure
2. penetrating tangential cardiac wound, up to but not extending through endocardium, without tamponade

Grade III:
1. blunt cardiac injury with sustained or multifocal ventricular contractions
2. blunt or penetrating cardiac injury with septal rupture, pulmonary or tricuspid incompetence, papillary muscle dysfunction, or distal coronary artery occlusion without cardiac failure
3. blunt pericardial laceration with cardiac herniation
4. blunt cardiac injury with cardiac failure
5. penetrating tangential myocardial wound, up to but not through endocardium, with tamponade

Grade IV:
1. blunt or penetrating cardiac injury with septal rupture, pulmonary or tricuspid incompetence, papillary muscle dysfunction, or distal coronary artery occlusion producing cardiac failure
2. blunt or penetrating cardiac injury with aortic or mitral incompetence
3. blunt or penetrating cardiac injury of the right ventricle, right or left atrium

Grade V:
1. blunt or penetrating cardiac injury with proximal coronary artery occlusion
2. blunt or penetrating left ventricular perforation
3. stellate injuries, less than 50% tissue loss of the right ventricle, right or left atrium

Grade VI:
1. blunt avulsion of the heart
2. penetrating wound producing more than 50% tissue loss of a chamber

TABLE 79–2. Spectrum of Penetrating Cardiac Injury by Anatomic Location[14]

Right ventricle:	37%–67%
Left ventricle:	19%–40%
Right atrium:	5%–20%
Left atrium:	2%–12%

survival advantage, with mortality rates as low as 8% in experienced trauma centers.[15] This is likely due to the relatively early clinical signs of tamponade in Beck's triad: hypotension, jugular venous distension, and muffled heart sounds. Early diagnosis is critical to survival, and this is only possible with a high index of suspicion, bearing in mind that patients with potentially fatal wounds can be stable at presentation. Echocardiography as part of the Focused Assessment by Sonography in Trauma (FAST) is currently the most widely practiced method for diagnosing traumatic hemopericardium, and this has replaced a pericardial window as the gold standard for diagnosis of penetrating cardiac trauma with some reports of 100% sensitivity, 97% specificity, and 97% accuracy.[20,21] Pericardiocentesis is too unreliable as a diagnostic test in this situation. With echocardiography, however, the lack of an effusion does not disprove cardiac or other anatomic injury.

Management of penetrating wounds to the heart depends on the stability of the patient. If the patient presents with a recent loss of vital signs or in a moribund state, a left anterior thoracotomy performed in the emergency department is potentially lifesaving.[22] Emergent thoracotomy may salvage as many as 20% of unstable or pulseless patients who have isolated penetrating trauma to the heart, but results are less favorable with missile wounds.[10,23] Most cardiac wounds can be repaired through a left thoracotomy. Additionally, the thoracic aorta can be compressed or clamped to improve cerebral and cardiac perfusion while volume is restored.[24] More stable patients are transported to the operating room, where a median sternotomy is the preferred approach. Depending upon the injury and after stabilization, the patient can be transferred to the operating room for a median sternotomy that allows adequate exposure of all cardiac structures and permits rapid institution of cardiopulmonary bypass when required. Most injuries are repaired with simple sutures using finger control to stop bleeding once identified. If a coronary artery injury is identified, the surgeon must use their judgment regarding coronary artery bypass versus ligation. An effort should be made to bypass large epicardial vessels, whereas smaller terminal branches or side branches can be ligated. The principal objective is to relieve tamponade and stop life-threatening hemorrhage. Further procedures, once again, require individualized surgical judgment based on the severity of the lesion and the physiologic significance on echocardiogram.[10]

In general, surgical repair techniques must be individualized for the immediate circumstances. Recently, investigators have provided preliminary evidence for intraoperative adjunct therapeutics to facilitate rapid control and establish the basis for surgical repair of the injury. Kokotsakis et al. reported on intravenous administration of adenosine for surgical management of penetrating heart wounds in three patients. Adenosine enabled the accurate placement of simple sutures with or without Teflon felt pledgets. All three injuries were repaired without the need for cardiopulmonary bypass in these severe trauma patients.[25] This technique has also been used in off-pump coronary artery bypass surgery.[26] Ingraham and Sperry reported on several series using BioGlue (CryoLife, Inc, Kennesaw, GA) to repair and/or reinforce surgical repair of traumatic heart wounds.[20]

TABLE 79-3. Spectrum of Blunt Cardiac Injury by Anatomy Location[27]

Right atrium:	8%–65%
Right ventricle:	17%–32%
Left ventricle:	8%–15%
Left atrium:	0%–31%
Coronary artery:	0%–5%
LAD most common	
Valve injury:	0%–5%
Aortic valve most common	
Blunt pericardial rupture:	0%–3%

Abbreviation: LAD, left anterior descending artery.

Blunt Cardiac Injury

The reported incidence of blunt cardiac trauma varies widely in the literature, but blunt injury is involved in up to 20% of all motor vehicle collision deaths.[27] The Centers for Disease Control and Prevention estimates 30,000 cases per year of blunt cardiac injury (BCI) in the United States.[28] Establishing a firm definition of BCI is difficult, ranging from a mild myocardial contusion to valve disruption and conduction abnormalities[29] to frank cardiac chamber rupture.[10] BCI results from either a rapid deceleration mechanism or a direct blow to the precordium; in all cases, BCI requires significant force, such as occurs in motor vehicle crashes, pedestrians struck by motor vehicles, falls from heights, and sports-related injuries. Severe sudden abdominal compression can acutely increase pressure and blood flow to the heart, resulting in right-sided rupture. The absence of a clear definition and rapid laboratory testing makes the diagnosis of BCI difficult.

Resulting injuries include cardiac contusion, valve disruption, atrial or ventricular septal defects, or frank cardiac rupture. These injuries vary by anatomic location (**Table 79-3**). Once again, because of its anterior position, the right ventricle is the chamber most frequently involved. Cardiac rupture is a common mechanism of death in blunt trauma, with survival being uncommon.[27,28,30] In patients reaching medical care with vital signs, however, a reasonable survival rate can be expected if cardiac injury is promptly recognized and operated on.[31] Those surviving cardiac rupture more frequently have right heart injury versus left heart injury.[32] A case of traumatic left ventricular intramural dissection has recently been reported (**Fig. 79–1**).[33,41]

Myocardial contusion encompasses a spectrum of injuries. In its mildest form, cardiac contusion results in mild epicardial ecchymosis without functional significance. More severe contusion can cause muscular injury, dysfunction, and infarction. The true incidence of myocardial contusion following blunt trauma is difficult to discern. It is important to note that severe myocardial injury can occur with little evidence of external chest trauma.

A high index of suspicion along with careful evaluation of mechanism should accompany all trauma patients from these

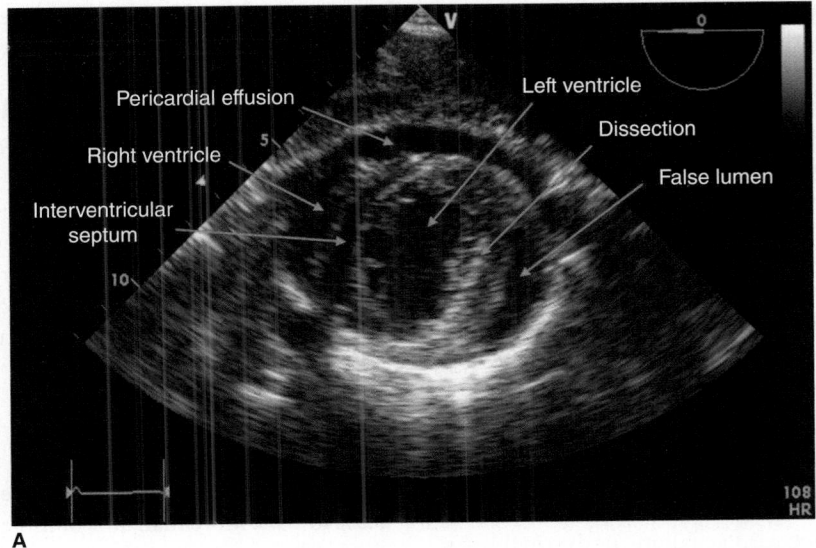

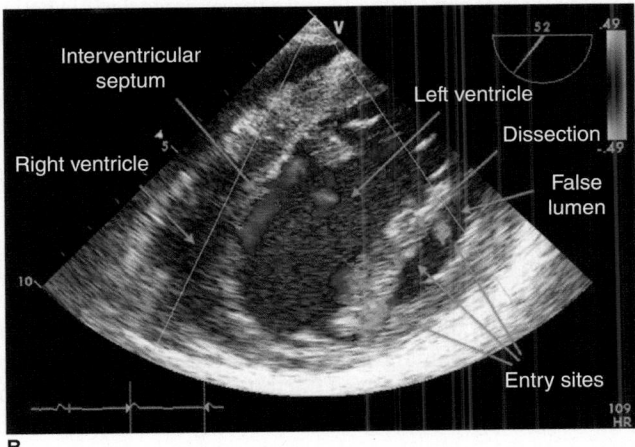

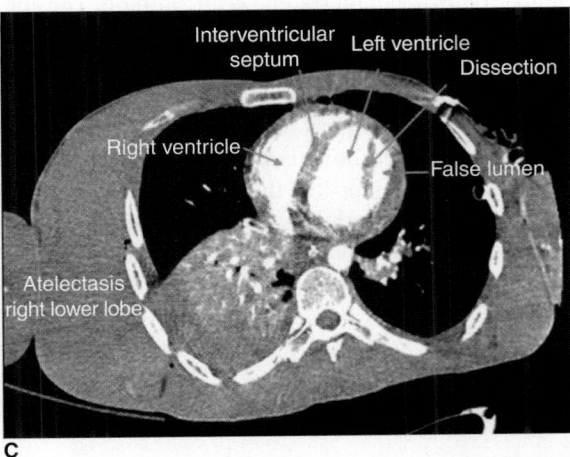

Figure 79–1. Traumatic left ventricular intramural dissection. A 30-year-old male sustained severe blunt chest injury from a hydraulic pipe thruster. He required high-dose vasopressors and inotropes. Transesophageal echocardiography (TEE) revealed a small pericardial effusion (**A**) and an extended intramural dissection (**A–C**) of the left ventricle involving the anterolateral papillary muscle and the apical and mid-segments of the anterior and lateral ventricular walls. An epicardial patch was placed over a severely thinned part of the anterolateral wall to prevent apical rupture. Reproduced with permission from Groves DS, Schmidt C. Traumatic left ventricular intramural dissection. *Eur Heart J.* 2010 Oct;31(20):2481.

accident scenarios, because many patients with blunt cardiac trauma are asymptomatic. All patients who have a significant mechanism of injury should have a screening electrocardiogram (ECG). However, diagnostic testing including chest x-rays, ECG, Holter monitoring, cardiac markers (CPK, CK-MB, troponin T, Troponin I), transthoracic and transesophageal echocardiography, cardiac computed tomography (CT), or magnetic resonance imaging (MRI) imaging may be needed to make the diagnosis.[6] On ECG, findings suggestive of cardiac contusion include nonspecific ST- and T-wave changes. Arrhythmias such as atrial fibrillation, atrial flutter, and premature ventricular complexes are also common and are usually self-limiting. Ventricular tachycardia and fibrillation are uncommon in patients surviving to the hospital. With a normal ECG in an otherwise uninjured patient, the risk of complications is low. Serial cardiac enzyme measurements are nonspecific for the diagnosis of myocardial contusion in the blunt injury patient.[34]

More recently, the role of serum cardiac troponin I (cTnI) and ECG was evaluated to identify patients at risk after BCI. In this prospective study by Salim et al., this combination of ECG (50% abnormal) and troponin I (admission, 4 hours, 8 hours; 23.5% abnormal) reliably identified the presence or absence of significant BCI.[35] In the patient who remains unstable or responds poorly to standard resuscitative efforts, echocardiography is indicated to look for regional wall motion abnormalities, pericardial effusion, or structural defects.

Clinically, BCI can be divided into two types: acute and subacute.[10] The management of myocardial contusion is often expectant, particularly in the patient who remains hemodynamically stable after treatment of concurrent injuries. Arrhythmias are treated with standard agents for rate control and/or rhythm control, as indicated, as well as optimization of electrolytes. In patients with hemodynamic instability, a complete echocardiographic study should be obtained. In cases of severe ventricular dysfunction and low cardiac output, inotropic support is appropriate, with perhaps less concern for extension of injury than with a primary ischemic event. If inotropic support does not produce satisfactory improvement, intraaortic balloon counterpulsation or other forms of mechanical left ventricular support may be considered.

Pericardial injury may result from direct high-energy impact of acute increase in intraabdominal pressure. The presence of absence of a sternal fracture is not diagnostic. The pericardium may rupture along the diaphragmatic or pleural surface parallel to the phrenic nerve, resulting in evisceration of the heart and/or torsion of the great vessels. Pneumopericardium, abnormal gas pattern, or displacement of the cardiac silhouette may be present. Emergency surgical intervention via sternotomy is mandatory.

Direct coronary artery blunt injury may cause arterial thrombosis, resulting in myocardial infarction, post–myocardial infarction ventricular septal defect, cardiac failure, or dysrhythmias.

Valve injury following blunt trauma is uncommon. The aortic valve is most frequently involved and can result from commissural avulsion, leaflet tears, or aortic dissection, all resulting in acute aortic insufficiency.[36,37] Isolated injury of the mitral valve is less common and most frequently involves rupture of the papillary muscle or chordal apparatus. Tricuspid valve injury is more commonly reported than mitral injury perhaps because the latter is frequently fatal. **Figure 79–2** shows the two-dimensional transthoracic echocardiogram in a female patient who was kicked in the anterior chest wall by her horse.[38]

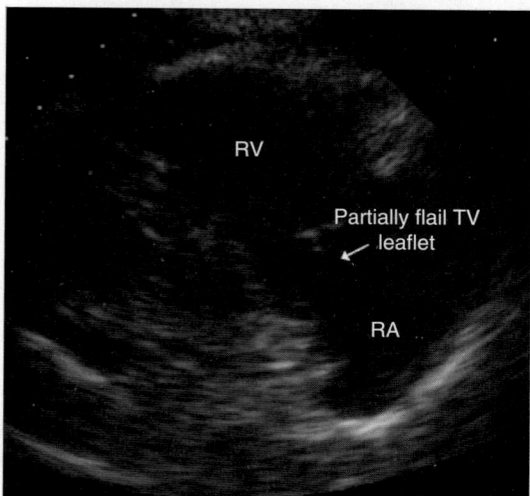

Figure 79–2. A 53-year-old woman was kicked by her horse, with the hoof striking her in the center of the chest. She developed severe chest pain. Cardiac auscultation was normal. Rib radiographs did not show any rib fractures, and chest x-rays showed clear lung fields and a normal cardiac silhouette. ECG (12-lead) demonstrated sinus tachycardia with a minor right ventricular conduction delay and no ischemic changes. Troponin I was elevated. Two-dimensional echocardiogram demonstrated a partially flail septal leaflet of the tricuspid valve (*white arrow*); RA, right atrium; RV, right ventricle. Reproduced with permission from Morsli H, Weissman G, Cooper HA. Images in cardiovascular medicine. Blunt cardiac injury: a case report. *Circulation.* 2008 May 13;117(19):e333-e335.

Tricuspid valve injury may become evident at a time remote from the injury as right heart failure develops.[8,39–41]

Delayed Sequelae of Cardiac Injury

Patients sustaining significant blunt or penetrating cardiac injuries require long-term follow-up. Injuries may not be appreciated at the time of trauma. In survivors, long-term outcomes can be excellent.[42] However, possible late sequelae include evolving atrial or ventricular septal defects, progressive valvular incompetence, aortocardiac or aortopulmonary fistulas, coronary artery fistulas, ventricular aneurysms, and post-traumatic pericarditis.[43–45]

GREAT VESSEL INJURY

The prevalence of great vessel injuries with trauma ranges from 0.3% to 10%. More than 90% of thoracic great vessel injuries are caused by penetrating trauma.[6,27] Thoracic vascular injury in trauma victims can be divided into three categories: (1) patients who die at the scene due to exsanguination; (2) patients who become unstable en route to medical care, where the majority (>96%) die secondary to multisystem trauma; and (3) patients who survive the initial trauma and remain relatively stable. The chance of survival in this group goes up to 705 to 95%.[10,46]

Penetrating Injury of the Great Vessels

The great vessels of the chest include the aorta, its major branches at the arch (innominate, carotid, subclavian), and the major pulmonary arteries. The primary venous conduits include the superior and inferior vena cavae, their main tributaries (eg, azygous vein), and the pulmonary veins. The pathophysiology of penetrating wounds to the great vessels is similar to penetrating wounds of the heart, with the extent of injury being determined by the specific structures injured and the velocity of the weapon. Cardiac tamponade may develop if the wound is below the pericardial reflection. Delayed sequelae of great vessel injury include pseudoaneurysm formation with delayed rupture and arteriovenous malformation with development of congestive heart failure.

Penetrating injuries of the great vessels have an extremely high mortality rate. The incidence varies based on geographic location, predominantly in urban areas, those prone to interpersonal violence, and areas of conflict.[46] In military and civilian studies, 95% of persons with penetrating injuries to the arch and great vessels are male, and single projectile firearms are the leading cause of injury (69%) followed by stab (18%) and shotgun (12%).[7] The majority of patients present in shock (82%), requiring immediate surgical intervention in the form of large-bore tube thoracostomy, resuscitative thoracotomy, or median sternotomy. The trauma surgeon must resuscitate, diagnose, and treat the patient within minutes following admission to the trauma emergency unit. Through an emergent left thoracotomy, operative repair of thoracic aortic injuries is virtually always possible by direct aortic repair with short cross-clamp times.[10,47] Only rarely is an interposition graft required, and adjunctive measures of cardiopulmonary bypass, bypass shunts, or active aortic shunts (eg, a centrifugal pump) are usually not described for penetrating injuries but are almost exclusively used for blunt injury. Paraplegia following successful repair of penetrating aortic injuries is rare, even with prolonged aortic clamping following emergency thoracotomy.[6]

Blunt Aortic Injury and Aortic Rupture

In thoracic trauma, the thoracic aorta is the most commonly injured vessel (84% of injuries). Eighty-one percent of these occur as an isolated injury, while the nonaortic great vessels are injured in 16% and a combined aortic and branch great vessel injury occurs in 35%.[48] Thoracic aortic injury occurs in 2% of cases with blunt aortic injury (BAI), and is predominantly life-threatening. The degree of aortic wall injury is proportional to the energy imparted to the structures. Over 90% of patients die at the scene, but approximately 70% of patients who arrive at the emergency room in a stable condition can survive.[49] Historically, aortic injury (predominantly [96%] located at the isthmus) is the second most common cause of death in blunt trauma, after closed head neurologic injury.[48] More than 80% of BAIs are due to motor vehicle accidents.[47]

BAI with some form of transection results in an estimated 8000 deaths in the United States annually.[50-52] It is believed that approximately 20% of patients sustaining descending aortic transections survive to reach medical care.[51] The injury mechanism involves any type of severe deceleration, most commonly a motor vehicle accident or a fall from more than 4 to 5 meters. Tears are most often encountered at the aortic isthmus just beyond the subclavian artery where the aorta is tethered by the ligamentum arteriosum.[52,53] The grading system used for assessing thoracic BAI is (I) intimal tear; (II) intramural hematoma; (III) pseudoaneurysm; and (IV) rupture. Patients acutely surviving aortic injury have partial or complete transections contained by adventitia and surrounding structures forming a false aneurysm. Avulsion of the innominate, carotid, or subclavian arteries occurs less frequently.[54,55]

Aortic transection must be suspected based on the mechanism of injury. Patients may have multiple other injuries or have remarkably few other manifestations of severe trauma. The classic findings of a widened mediastinum, apical capping, or depression of the left main stem bronchus may not be evident on plain films of the chest in a patient with an aortic injury. Aortography has previously been the definitive means of diagnosis, but advancements in multidetector computed tomography (MDCT) have made CT angiography a more commonly used tool to identify aortic injury in major trauma centers. Transesophageal echocardiography can be performed at the bedside or in the operating room in the patient too unstable for the CT scanner. In skilled hands, this has a sensitivity similar to that of helical CT scanning.[56,57]

Modern treatments strategies of BAI following three principles. The first is aggressive pharmacologic blood pressure control with intravenous β-blockade and alpha-blockers, the second is appropriate selection and prioritization of repair, and the final is the utilization of therapeutic interventions.[10,47,49] Once a diagnosis of aortic transection from blunt aortic

trauma is made, several emergent/urgent treatment options are available.[4] Historically, immediate repair through a left thoracotomy was considered the principal treatment option, depending on the patient's stability and other injuries.[6,47] Delayed repair is appropriate in the multiply injured patient requiring ongoing resuscitation, and this management strategy has grown in popularity.[49] Nonoperative management is not risk free, however, with as many as 4% of patients thought to be candidates for delayed repair experiencing rupture within a week of injury in some series.[58,59]

In the last decade, the emergence of thoracic endovascular aortic repair (TEVAR) has revolutionized therapeutic intervention for injury grade III and IV BAI. Initially, expanded application of abdominal EVAR techniques to the thoracic yielded promising results (**Fig. 79–3**) when compared with traditional repair.[59-65] A study based on the Society for Vascular Surgery database documented endovascular treatment for acute aortic transections, 97% of which were due to motor vehicle accident. Sixty symptomatic patients were treated with an aortic endograft, with an all-cause mortality rate of 9.1% at 30 days, and a

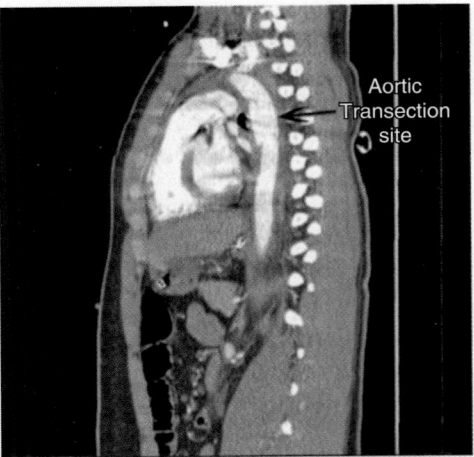

A

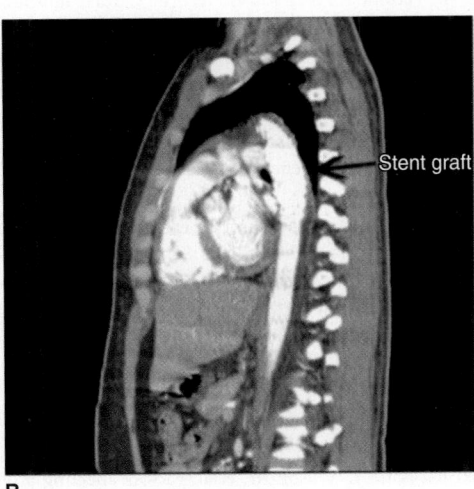

B

Figure 79–3. (A) CT angiogram of a patient who sustained an aortic transection following a motor vehicle accident. (B) CT angiogram of the same patient following insertion of a thoracic stent graft with successful exclusion of the false aneurysm.

mean operative time of 125 minutes, and a stroke rate less than surgical intervention.[66]

The 1-year and 5-year results from the Performance of the Valiant Thoracic Stent-Graft With the Captivia Delivery System [Medtronic, Inc. Minneapolis, MN] for the Endovascular Treatment of BTI) RESCUE trial have solidified the effectiveness of TEVAR in this patient population.[67] Thirty-day mortality was 8% and with a survival rate at 85.2% through 5 years.[68] These excellent 5-year results support the approach that thoracic endovascular repair with TEVAR is the safe and effective treatment of choice for most patients with BAI, and is the first option of choice in these trauma patients who often have multiple other concomitant injuries.

REFERENCES

1. Symbas PN. *Cardiothoracic Trauma*. Philadelphia, PA: Saunders; 1989.
2. Center for Disease Control and Prevention. National Centers for Injury Prevention and Control Web-Based Injury Statistics Query and Reporting System (WISQARS). https://www.cdc.gov/injury/wisquars. Accessed August 20, 2020.
3. Rfhee P, Joseph B, Pandit V, et al. Increasing trauma deaths in the United States. *Ann Surg.* 2014;260:13-21.
4. Price PR, Mackenzie EJ. Cost of injury—United States: a report to Congress. *JAMA.* 1989;262:2803-2804.
5. Tran H-V, Charles M, Garrett RC, Kempe PW, Howard A, Khorgami Z. Ten-year trends in traumatic cardiac injury and outcomes: a trauma registry analysis. *Ann Thorac Surg.* 2020:110(3):844-848.
6. Shahani R. Penetrating chest trauma treatment & management. *Medscape.* Updated July 1, 2021. https://emedicine.medscape.com/article/425698-treatment. Accessed July 18, 2021.
7. Markov NP, Rasumssen TE. Penetrating injuries to the aortic arch and intrathoracic great vessels. In: Stanley JC, Veith FJ, Wakefield TW, eds. *Current Therapy in Vascular and Endovascular Surgery*, 5th ed. Philadelphia, PA: Saunders; 2014.
8. Kemmerer WT, Eckert WG, Gathwright JB, et al. Patterns of thoracic injuries in fatal traffic accidents. *J Trauma.* 1961;1:595-599.
9. Moore EE, Malangoni MA, Cogbill TH, et al. Organ injury scaling IV: Thoracic, vascular, lung, cardiac, and diaphragm. *J Trauma.* 1994;36:229-300.
10. Asensio JA, Petrone P, Perez-Alonso A, et al. Cardiac injuries, in thoracic injuries. In: Asensio JA, Trunkey DD, eds. *Current Therapy of Trauma and Surgical Critical Care*. Philadelphia, PA: Elsevier, Inc.; 2016.
11. Kang N, Hsee L, Rizoli S, Alison P. Penetrating cardiac injury: overcoming the limits set by nature. *Injury, Int. J Care Injured.* 2009;40:919-927.
12. Karrel R, Shaffer MA, Franaszek JB. Emergency diagnosis, resuscitation, and treatment of acute penetrating cardiac trauma. *Ann Emerg Med.* 1982;11:504-517.
13. Campbell NC, Thomso SR, Muckart DJ, et al. Review of 1198 cases of penetrating cardiac trauma. *Br J Surg.* 1997;84:1737-1740.
14. Dynamed [Internet]. Ipswich (MA): EBSCO Information Services. 1995—Record No. T905587, Penetrating Cardiac Injury–Emergency Management. Updated Nov 30, 2018. https://www.dynamed.com/topics/dmp~AN~T905587. Cited August 20, 2020. Registration and login required.
15. Degiannis E, Loogna P, Doll D, et al. Penetrating cardiac injuries: recent experience in South Africa. *World J Surg.* 2006;30:1258-1264.
16. Tyburski JG, Astra L, Wilson RF, et al. Factors affecting prognosis with penetrating wounds of the heart. *J Trauma.* 2000;48:587-591.
17. Mittal V, McAleese P, Young S, et al. Penetrating cardiac injuries. *Am Surg.* 1999;65:444-448.
18. Thourani VH, Filiciano DV, Cooper WA, et al. Penetrating cardiac trauma at an urban trauma center: a 22-year experience. *Am Surg.* 1999;65:811-818.
19. Morse BC, Mina MJ, Carr JA, et al. Penetrating cardiac injuries: a 36-year perspective at an urban, Level 1 trauma center. *J Trauma Acute Care Surg.* 2016;81:623-631.
20. Ingraham A, Sperry J. Operative management of cardiac injuries: diagnosis, technique and postoperative complications. *Curr Trauma Rep.* 2015;1:225-231.
21. Rozycki GS, Feliciano DV, Pchsner MG, et al. The role of ultrasound in patients with possible penetrating cardiac wounds: a prospective multicenter study. *J Trauma.* 1999;46:543-551.
22. Topaloglu S, Aras D, Cagli K, et al. Penetrating trauma to the mitral valve and ventricular septum. *Tex Heart Inst J.* 2006;33:392-395.
23. Molina EJ, Gaughan JP, Kulp H, et al. Outcomes after emergency department thoracotomy for penetrating cardiac injuries: a new perspective. *Interact Cardiovasc Thorac Surg.* 2008;7:845-848.
24. Biocina B, Sultic Z, Husedzinovic I, et al. Penetrating cardiothoracic war wounds. *Eur J Cardiothorc Surg.* 1997;11:399-405.
25. Kokotsakis J, Hountis P, Antonopoulos N, Skoutell E, Athanasiou T, Lioulias A. Intravenous adenosine for surgical management of penetrating heart wounds. *Tex Heart Inst J.* 2007;34:80-81.
26. Robinson MC, Theilmeier KA, Hill BB. Persistent ventricular asystole using adenosine during minimally invasive and open sternotomy coronary artery bypass grafting. *Ann Thorac Surg.* 1997;63:S30-4.
27. Ottosen J, Guo WA. Blunt cardiac injury. *AAST.* 2012. https://www.aast.org/resources-detail/blunt-cardiac-injury. Accessed July 18, 2021.
28. Elie MC. Blunt cardiac injury. *Mt. Sinai J Med.* 2006;73:542-552.
29. Thors A, Guarneri R, Costantini EN, et al. Atrial septal rupture, flail tricuspid valve and complete heart block due to nonpenetrating chest trauma. *Ann Thorac Surg.* 2007;83:2207-2210.
30. Tanabe T, Hashimoto M, Nishibe M, et al. Statistical analysis of deaths due to cardiovascular injuries. *Kyukyuigaku.* 1984;8:361-367.
31. Namai A, Sakurai M, Fujiwara H. Five cases of blunt traumatic cardiac rupture: success and failure in surgical management. *Gen Thorac Cardiovasc Surg.* 2007;55:200-204.
32. Pevec WC, Udekwu AO, Peitzman AB. Blunt rupture of the myocardium. *Ann Thorac Surg.* 1989;48:139-142.
33. Groves DS, Schmidt C. Traumatic left ventricular intramural dissection. *Eur Heart J.* 2010. doi: 10.1093/eurheartj/ehq196.
34. Biffl WL, Moore FA, Moore EE, et al. Cardiac enzymes are irrelevant in the patient with suspected myocardial contusion. *Am J Surg.* 1994;168:523-528.
35. Salim A, Velmahos GC, Jindal A, et al. Clinically significant blunt cardiac trauma. Role of serum troponin levels combined with electrocardiographic findings. *J Trauma* 2001;50:237-243.
36. Asbach S, Siegenthaler MP, Bode C, et al. Aortic valve rupture after blunt chest trauma. *Clin Res Cardiol.* 2006;95:675-679.
37. Aris A, Delgado LJ, Montiel J, et al. Multiple intracardiac lesions after blunt chest trauma. *Ann Thorac Surg.* 2000;70:1692-1694.
38. Morsli H, Weissman G, Cooper HA. Images in cardiovascular medicine. Blunt cardiac injury- a case report. *Circulation.* 2008;117:e333-e335.
39. Caparrelli DJ, Cattaneo SM, Brock MV, et al. Aortic and mitral valve disruption following nonpenetrating chest trauma. *J Trauma.* 2002;52:377-379.
40. Dounis G, Matssakas E, Poularas J, et al. Traumatic tricuspid insufficiency: a case report with review of the literature. *Eur J Emerg Med.* 2002;9:258-261.
41. Kulik A, Al-Saigh M, Yelle J, et al. Subacute tricuspid valve rupture after traumatic cardiac and pulmonary contusions. *Ann Thorac Surg.* 2006;81:1111-1112.
42. Kaljusto M-L, Skaga NO, Pillgram-Larsen J, Tonnessen T. Survival predictor for penetrating cardiac injury: a 10-year consecutive cohort from a Scandinavian trauma center. *Scandinavial J Trauma Resuscitat Emerg Med.* 2015:23:41.
43. Symbas PN, DiOrio DA, Tyras DH, et al. Penetrating cardiac wounds: significant residual and delayed sequelae. *J Thorac Cardiovasc Surg.* 1973;6:526-532.

44. Demetriades D, Charalambides C, Sareli P, et al. Late sequelae of penetrating cardiac injuries. *Br J Surg*. 1990;77:813-814.

45. Jeganathan R, Irwin G, Johnston PW, Jones JM. Traumatic left anterior descending artery-to-pulmonary artery fistula with delayed pericardial tamponade. *Ann Thorac Surg*. 2007;84:276-278.

46. Edgecombe L, Sigmon DF, Galuska MA, Angus LD. Thoracic trauma. *StatPearls*. 2020. https://www.ncbi.nlm.nih.gov/books/NBK534843. Accessed October 9, 2020.

47. Ayad MT, Gillespie DL. Surgical and endovascular management of vascular trauma including aortic transection. In: Moore WS, Lawrence PE, Oderich GS, eds. *Moore's Vascular and Endovascular Surgery*, 9th ed. Philadelphia, PA: Elsevier; 2019.

48. McPherson SJ. Thoracic aortic and great vessel trauma and its management. *Semin Intervent Radiol*. 2007;24:180-196.

49. Buczkowski P, Puslecki M, Stefaniak S, et al. Post-traumatic acute thoracic aortic injury (TAI)—a single center experience. *J Thorac Dis*. 2017;9(11):4477-4485.

50. Wall MJ, Mattox KL, Chen CD, et al. Acute management of complex cardiac injuries. *J Trauma*. 1997;42:905-912.

51. Fabian TC, Richardson JD, Croce MA, et al. Prospective study of blunt aortic injury: multicenter trial of the American Association for the Surgery of Trauma. *J Trauma*. 1997;42:374-380.

52. Asensio JA, et al. Trauma to the heart. In: Feliciano DV, Mattox KL, Moore EE, eds. *Trauma*, 6th ed. New York: McGraw Hill; 2008.

53. Nagy K, Fabian T, Rodman G, et al. Guidelines for the diagnosis and management of blunt aortic injury: an EAST Practice Management Guidelines Work Group. *J Trauma*. 2000;48:1128-1143.

54. Chu MW, Myers ML. Traumatic innominate artery disruption and aortic valve rupture. *Ann Thorac Surg*. 2006;82:1095-1097.

55. Karmy-Jones R, DuBose R, King S. Traumatic rupture of the innominate artery. *Eur J Cardiothorac Surg*. 2003;23:782-787.

56. Wintermark M, Wicky S, Schnyder P. Imaging of acute traumatic injuries of the thoracic aorta. *Eur Radiol*. 2002;12:431-442.

57. Vignon P, Martaille JF, Francois B, et al. Transesophageal echocardiography and therapeutic management of patients sustaining blunt aortic injuries. *J Trauma*. 2005;58:1150-1158.

58. Holmes JH, Bloch RD, Hall RA, et al. Natural history of traumatic rupture of the thoracic aorta managed nonoperatively: a longitudinal analysis. *Ann Thorac Surg*. 2002;73:1149-1154.

59. Jahromi AS, Kazemi K, Safar HA, et al. Traumatic rupture of the thoracic aorta: cohort study and systematic review. *J Vasc Surg*. 2001;34:1029-1034.

60. Ott MC, Stewart TC, Lawlor DK, et al. Management of blunt thoracic aortic injuries: endovascular stents versus open repair. *J Trauma*. 2004;56:565-570.

61. Peterson BG, Matsumura JS, Morasch MD, et al. Percutaneous endovascular repair of blunt thoracic aortic transection. *J Trauma*. 2005;59:1062-1065.

62. Kokitsakis J, Kaskarelis I, Misthos P, et al. Endovascular versus open repair of blunt thoracic aortic injury: short-term results. *Ann Thorac Surg*. 2007;84:1965-1970.

63. Moainie SL, Neschis DG, Gammie JS, et al. Endovascular stenting for traumatic aortic injury: an emerging new standard of care. *Ann Thorac Surg*. 2008;85:1625-1630.

64. Saratzis NA, Saratzis AN, Melas N, et al. Endovascular repair of traumatic rupture of the thoracic aorta: single-center experience. *Cardiovasc Intervent Radiol*. 2007;30:370-375.

65. Azizzadeh A, Keyhani K, Miller C, et al. Blunt traumatic aortic injury: initial experience with endovascular repair. *J Vasc Surg*. 2009;49:1403-1408.

66. Dake MD, White RA, Diethrich EB, et al. Report on endograft management of traumatic thoracic aortic transections at 30 days and 1 year from a multidisciplinary subcommittee of the Society for Vascular Surgery Outcomes Committee. *J Vasc Surg*. 2011;53(4):1091-1096.

67. Khoynezhad A, Donayre CD, Azizzadeh A, White R, on behalf of the RESCUE Investigators. One-year results of thoracic endovascular arotic repair for blunt thoracic aortic injury (RESCUE trial). *J Thorac Cardiovasc Surg*. 2015;149:155-161.

68. Patel HJ, Azizzadeh A, Matsumoto AH, et al. Five-year outcomes from the United States pivotal trial of valiant Captiva stent graft for blunt aortic injury. *Ann Thorac Surg*. 2020;110:815-820.

Women and Ischemic Heart Disease

Leslee J. Shaw, Viviany R. Taqueti, and Nanette K. Wenger

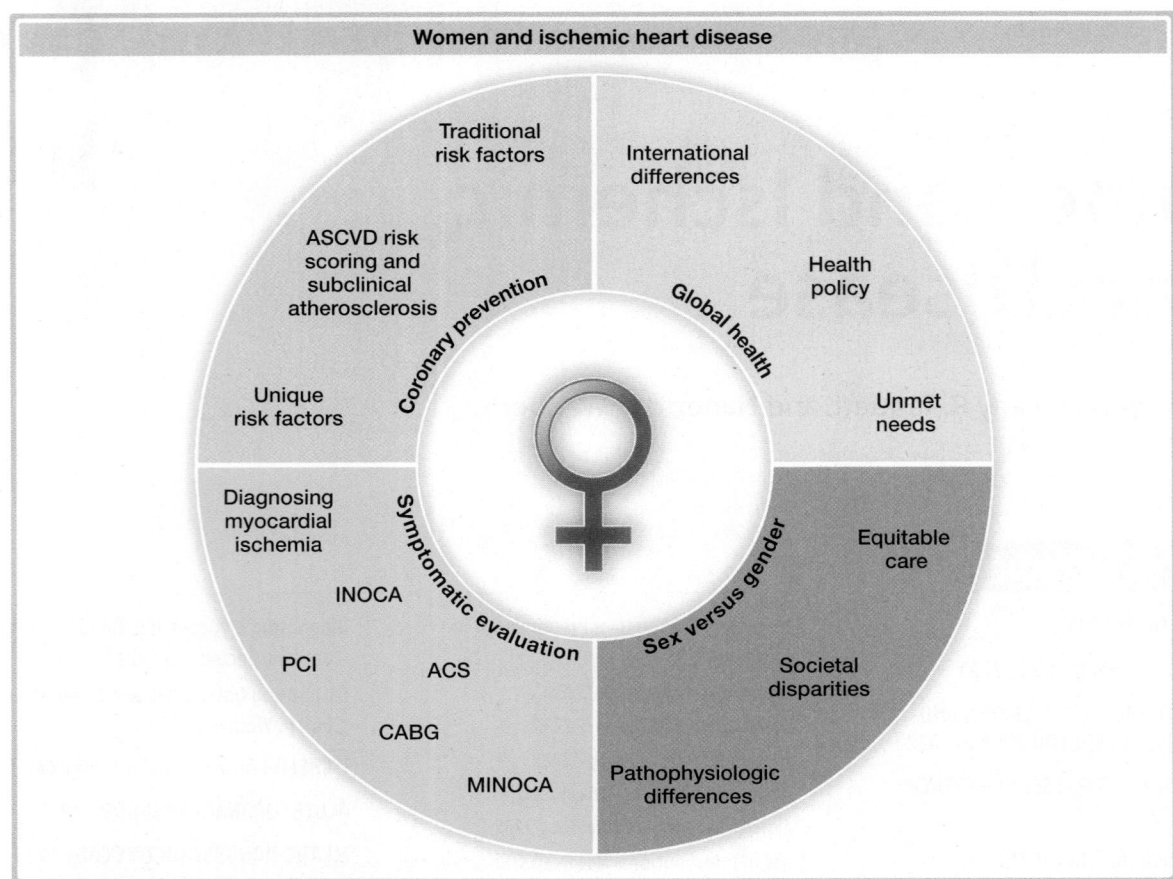

Chapter 80 Fuster and Hurst's Central Illustration. Burgeoning evidence now exists on sex differences in pathophysiology, prevention, presentation, diagnostic evaluation, management, and clinical outcomes of women as compared to men at risk for and living with known ischemic heart disease. ACS, acute coronary syndrome; ASCVD, atherosclerotic cardiovascular disease; CABG, coronary artery bypass grafting; INOCA, ischemia and nonobstructive coronary artery disease; MINOCA, myocardial infarction and nonobstructive coronary artery disease; PCI, percutaneous coronary intervention.

CHAPTER SUMMARY

This chapter highlights the evidence on sex differences in the pathophysiology and clinical presentations of ischemic heart disease (IHD), and identifies significant disparities in primary prevention and both stable and acute management strategies contributing to the often-reported high adverse risk for women. Throughout the 20th century, atherosclerotic cardiovascular disease (ASCVD) was viewed as predominantly a disease of older-aged men, and little information was available regarding its impact on women. Recent decades have witnessed emerging attention to ASCVD in women, with consequent research hypotheses focused on data specific to women. Today, there exists growing evidence on sex differences in prevention, presentation, diagnostic evaluation, management, and clinical outcomes of women compared with men with suspected and known IHD. The gamut of cultural, social, and financial differences among women and men profoundly impact prompt diagnosis, clinical management, and outcomes of at-risk women. Goals for reducing ASCVD risk tailored to women remain underexplored. The role of biology, clinical and population needs of women, and the socioeconomic disparities of females remain sizeable hurdles to effecting changes to the large population of young to older women at risk for ASCVD (see Fuster and Hurst's Central Illustration).

INTRODUCTION

Throughout the 20th century, atherosclerotic cardiovascular disease (ASCVD) was viewed predominantly as a disease affecting older men, and limited information was available regarding its impact on women. Recent decades have witnessed emerging attention to ASCVD in women, with consequent research hypotheses focused on data specific to women. Today, there exists burgeoning evidence on sex differences in the prevention, presentation, diagnostic evaluation, management, and clinical outcomes of patients with suspected and known ischemic heart disease (IHD).[1-8] This evidence has evolved rapidly but remains incomplete with regard to understanding the biologic basis for sex differences, distinct pathophysiologic alterations, and variability in diagnostic and treatment effectiveness that contribute to the risk for morbid and fatal outcomes of ASCVD among women as compared to men. The gamut of cultural, social, and financial differences among at-risk women and men profoundly impact their prompt diagnosis, clinical management, and outcomes. In this chapter, we will highlight recent research findings on IHD prevention, diagnosis, management, and clinical outcomes for women with stable or acute IHD.

DEFINING SEX DIFFERENCES

Sex differences are biologic differences such as genetic and hormonal, and are increasingly acknowledged to exist even at the cellular level.[6,9,10] Sex differences in IHD are wide-ranging and include anatomic (eg, size of coronary blood vessels), physiologic (eg, rate of resting coronary blood flow), age-related hormonal, and comorbid factors uniquely impacting women versus men. Importantly, these differences contribute to variations in disease susceptibility and resilience throughout the lifespan of women and men. Although many have used the term sex dimorphism to define one biologic trait for women that varies from another in men, others have proposed more complex or structural differences that interact across varied disease states.[11] For definitional purposes, the term "gender" relates to self-identification, behavior, and interactions with societal roles and expectations, which also uniquely affect all facets of IHD detection, risk, and treatment in women as compared to men. In many cases, as we review the evidence on IHD in women, there will be a complex interplay between sex and gender that impacts clinical care and outcomes of women.

ASCVD EPIDEMIOLOGY: OVERVIEW AND DISPARITIES IN CARE FOR WOMEN

Over the years, substantial declines in ASCVD mortality have been reported, yet declines for women are far less than those reported for men (**Fig. 80–1**).[8] Moreover, since 2010, data from the National Center for Health Statistics reveal an increase in case fatality rates in the United States for both women and men, which is often attributed to the high rate of obesity and diabetes.[12-14] Despite the progress and with more recent setbacks, ASCVD remains the leading cause of death for nearly 1 in 5 women.[15]

Over half of the nearly 10 million patients in the United States with chronic stable angina are women.[16] Compared to men, women have a higher age-adjusted prevalence of angina, the main symptom of IHD. At all ages, including among elderly individuals, women have a lower prevalence of coronary artery disease (CAD). However, once clinical manifestations of IHD

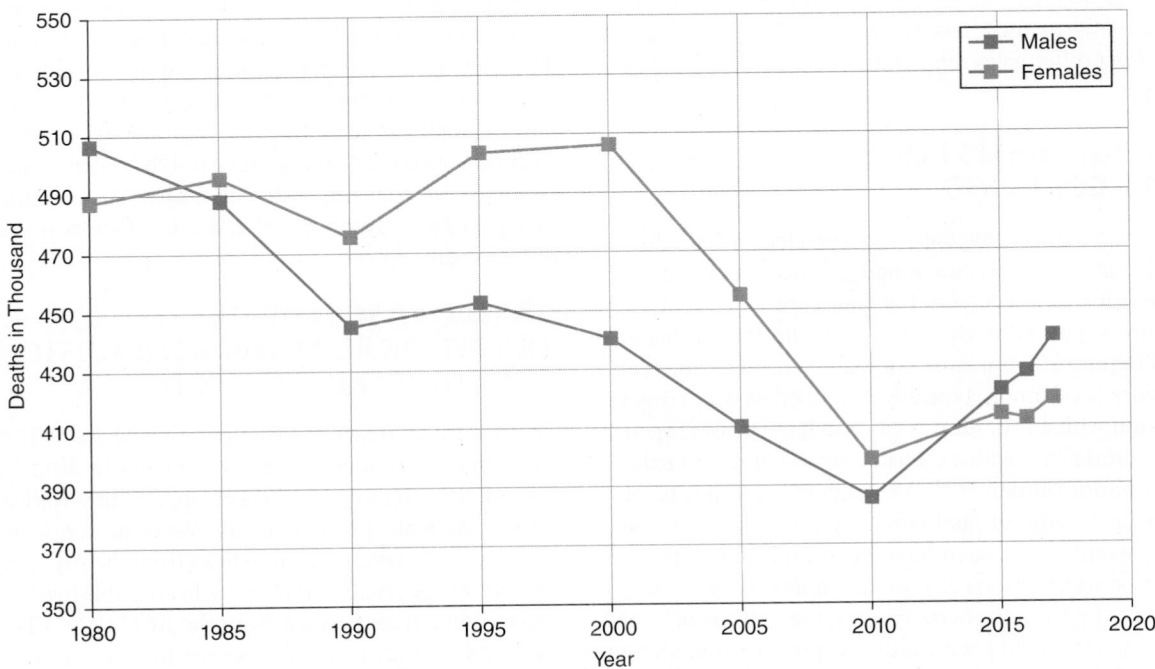

Figure 80–1. CVD mortality trends for males and females, United States: 1980–2017. Reproduced with permission from National Center for Health Statistics. National Vital Statistics System: public use data file documentation: mortality multiple cause-of-death microdata files, 2017. Centers for Disease Control and Prevention website.

develop, women have a less favorable outcome than their male peers in the setting of stable IHD, acute coronary syndromes (ACSs), and coronary revascularization.

In the acute setting, more than one-quarter of a million women are hospitalized each year with an ACS,[12] and the rate of unrecognized myocardial infarction (MI)[17] is higher for women as compared to men. Women hospitalized with acute MI experience longer lengths of stay, elevated in-hospital mortality, higher readmission rates, and persistently higher death rates over 5 to 10 years of follow-up when compared to men.[18–20] Sex-differences for in-hospital outcomes related to ACS have been attributed to variability in comorbidity, clinical presentation, and the severity and extent of CAD; yet these observed patterns have persisted over decades of treatment advances.[21]

Sex-related differences in morbid and fatal outcomes have persisted over the last few decades despite advances in treatment and guideline-directed management of IHD.[22] Extensive literature documents the reduced use of risk-factor modifying and anti-ischemic treatments in at-risk women as compared to men, with lower referrals for noninvasive and invasive procedures including coronary revascularization, as well as cardiac rehabilitation and other lifestyle recommendations.[23,24] This less intensive pattern of care for women has impacted not only on their quality of care but also on their worsening clinical outcomes. Disparities in detection and treatment of ASCVD affect large sectors of our female population who are now characterized as a priority population targeted for appropriate care consistent with guideline-directed strategies.[25] Improvements in care for women may be realized with increased awareness from public health campaigns, the application of guideline-directed strategies of care, and also focused clinical research on sex-related differences,[26] While the underuse of guideline-based preventive and therapeutic strategies for women has contributed substantially to their less favorable IHD outcomes, the spectrum of sex differences reflects a combination of both bias and biology.[24]

PATHOLOGIC BASIS FOR SEX DIFFERENCES IN IHD

Pathologic and angiographic data have revealed varied atherosclerotic plaque characteristics ranging from plaque rupture to plaque erosion as precursors for fatal coronary events.[27–29] This evidence supports mechanisms for acute events that are uniquely different in women as compared to men. For men, plaque rupture is common, typically described as occurring in a culprit lesion with a thin fibrous cap and large thrombogenic lipid-rich necrotic core with expansive remodeling and extensive atherosclerotic burden.[28,30,31] Although plaque rupture may account for up to 76% of fatal coronary events among men, only half of events in women have been ascribed to plaque rupture.[32] In contrast, plaque erosion is a more common mechanism of ACS in women, occurring in the setting of more fibrous lesions (P <0.001) with reduced positive remodeling (P = 0.003) and a smaller plaque burden (P = 0.003) that is often not calcified.[30,33–36] Pathologic data also suggest age variability in the occurrence of plaque erosion, which occurs more

often in younger women while older women have an increased frequency of plaque rupture.[37]

MI in the absence of obstructive CAD is more common among women at younger ages.[21] The rarity of plaque rupture in premenopausal women may be related to a protective effect of estrogen.[38] Up to one-third of women with documented ACS have no angiographically obstructive CAD, such that their MI may be related to alternative mechanisms including plaque erosion, vasospasm, or embolism.[21,39] Despite the high prevalence of nonobstructive CAD, plaque disruption is evident in almost 40% of women with ACS.[40] In a recent report addressing mechanisms of MI among women without obstructive CAD, there was evidence of plaque erosion with distal embolization of atherosclerotic debris and/or vasospasm.[21,39]

Contemporary in vivo invasive imaging of atherosclerotic plaque has also contributed important evidence on sex-specific patterns that are concordant with previously described pathologic findings.[31] Culprit plaques identified using intravascular ultrasound (IVUS) include those with features of echolucency (ie, with a lipid-rich necrotic core), large plaque burden, and positive remodeling.[31,41] The Providing Regional Observations to Study Predictors of Events in the Coronary Tree (PROSPECT) registry included 697 patients (n = 168 women) who underwent 3-vessel IVUS and were followed for approximately 3 years for documentation of major CAD events.[42] From PROSPECT, culprit lesions more often had a higher plaque burden, smaller minimal luminal area, and thin cap fibroatheroma (all P <0.001).[42] In a secondary analysis from PROSPECT, women as compared with men less often had documented plaque rupture (P = 0.002) despite having more comorbid risk factors.[27]

These data support sex-specific differences in atherosclerotic plaque progression that may underlie the varying presentation and clinical outcomes between women and men commonly observed in ACS registries and treatment trials. The varying plaque features may require development of sex-specific targeted treatment strategies yet to be elucidated in current stable or acute IHD trials. Moreover, additional investigation is also needed to understand the potential contribution of smaller arterial size, differential shear stress conditions, coronary vascular dysfunction, and other factors on sex-specific outcome differences.

CARDIOVASCULAR PREVENTION— TRADITIONAL AND NONTRADITIONAL CORONARY RISK FACTORS

The American Heart Association's (AHA) ASCVD prevention guidelines for women were last updated in 2011[23] and highlighted that markedly different approaches were needed to assure adequate preventive interventions for women. Since 2011, several prevention guidelines from the American College of Cardiology (ACC)/AHA have been published[43–45] and synthesized in a recent review from the ACC's ASCVD in Women committee.[46] Cardiovascular prevention remains key when one considers that two-thirds of US women have at least one major coronary risk factor, with this percentage increasing with age.[47] During the last two decades, increasing Framingham Risk

Scores have been observed and are likely the result of the epidemic of obesity and sedentary lifestyle.[48,49] Additionally, for women aged 35 to 54 years, in contrast to the total population of women, ASCVD mortality has increased, reversing the favorable trend of the last four decades. Substantial data now underscore that nontraditional ASCVD risk factors unique to or predominant in women also impart differential risk for women and men.[50] These characteristics support the importance of providing preventive ASCVD screening for women.

Although women represent 46% of the US population with ASCVD, they have constituted only 25% of participants in ASCVD prevention trials, with sex-specific data cited in only 31% of primary trial publications.[51] It must be appreciated that women are not a homogeneous group. Almost half of Black American women have some form of ASCVD, with a 44% prevalence of hypertension that is earlier in onset than their White counterparts, also with higher rates of metabolic syndrome, ASCVD, and mortality; and in all studies receive less guideline-directed therapies. In contrast, although Hispanic women have double the occurrence of diabetes compared with non-Hispanic White women (12.6% vs 6.5%), they experience lower mortality as compared with non-Hispanic White women.[52,53]

Traditional ASCVD Risk Factors

Hypertension

Hypertension is a leading cause of ASCVD worldwide, with a 2-fold higher mortality in women as compared with men (29.0% vs 14.9%). It is also more strongly associated with MI in women than in men.[54] Although women are less likely than men to have hypertension before 45 years of age, hypertension becomes a predominant risk factor in women relative to men after age 65 years. Whereas 80% of US women aged 75 years and older have hypertension, only 29% of elderly women in the United States have adequate blood pressure control compared with 41% of men.[52,54–57] In addition, there is a strong correlation between elevated systolic blood pressure and body mass index in women, indicating a potentially important consideration for their hypertension management.

Controversy remains in both women and men as to appropriate blood pressure targets. In the Systolic Blood Pressure Intervention Trial (SPRINT), treating to a systolic blood pressure target of <120 mm Hg compared with <140 mm Hg resulted in a 25% lower risk of fatal and nonfatal ASCVD events and all-cause death.[58] However, women were underrepresented in this trial and the age range of 50 to 80 years excluded young as well as many elderly women with hypertension and, by design, diabetic patients.[59] As such, goal blood pressure for older adults remains uncertain. In 2017, the ACC/AHA recommended a goal of <130/80 mm Hg, whereas the European Society of Cardiology/European Society of Hypertension (ESC/ESH) in 2018 proposed a goal of 130 to 139/70 mm Hg.[43,60]

Cigarette Smoking

Smoking is an important preventable cause of MI in women.[61] Although cigarette smoking rates have decreased over all, the decline is less for women than men, particularly in developing countries where the number of female smokers has increased. Nearly 1 in 5 women in the United States still smoke cigarettes, with smoking among younger women more common than among younger men. The ASCVD risk for female smokers is 25% higher than that for male smokers, with cigarette smoking tripling the MI risk for women. Moreover, smoking in association with oral contraceptive use increases the risk of acute MI, stroke, and venous thromboembolism.[62] Smoking cessation is the most cost-effective of risk modifying programs.[52,63]

Diabetes Mellitus

The 2015 AHA Scientific Statement on Sex Differences in the ASCVD Consequences of Diabetes Mellitus noted that the prevalence of diabetes is increasing rapidly in the United States, currently at 9.3% of the population.[64] Overall, the prevalence of type 2 diabetes is similar for women and men, with about 12.6 million women over age 20 years estimated to have type 2 diabetes. Yet at hospitalization for acute MI, women are more likely than men to have diabetes mellitus, with a rate of 25.5% versus 16.2% for women and men, respectively. ASCVD is the leading cause of morbidity and mortality among type 2 diabetics, accounting for more than 75% of hospitalizations and 50% of all deaths.[65] Although nondiabetic women have fewer ASCVD events than comparably aged nondiabetic men, this sex-specific advantage is lost once type 2 diabetes develops.[66,67]

Diabetes confers greater risk for ASCVD death in women compared with men, and the rate of diabetes in Hispanic women is more than double that of non-Hispanic White women. Women with diabetes have a 3-fold excess risk of cardiovascular mortality as compared with nondiabetic women and a higher adjusted hazard for cardiovascular death when compared to men. A meta-analysis of 850,000 individuals showed that the relative risk of ASCVD was 44% greater in diabetic women than in diabetic men.[68] Based on a comprehensive population survey, diabetic women are the sole group without a documented mortality reduction from 1971 to 2000.[69] Diabetic women have a worse ASCVD risk profile than their male peers, with higher rates of impaired endothelium-dependent vasodilation, hypercoagulability, dyslipidemia, and the metabolic syndrome.[64]

The reasons for these sex differences are not well understood but likely related to inherent physiological differences (ie, the impact of sex hormones on adiposity and insulin resistance), differences in ASCVD risk factors, and differences in the treatment of women and men with diabetes and ASCVD.[70] In all studies, diabetic women receive less treatment and are less likely to have control of their ASCVD risk factors than diabetic men.[71–74] Women with diabetes are less likely to be treated appropriately than men, and this contributes to worsening outcomes.[75]

Hypercholesterolemia

Hypercholesterolemia imparts a high population-adjusted risk for women, with all studies showing similar statin benefit for women and for men. In the US population, however, fewer than half of adults eligible for cholesterol medications may actually take them,[76] with women less likely to be prescribed statin therapy[77,78] and with variable adherence.[79] The 2013 ACC/AHA guidelines for cholesterol management promulgated significant change in the management of dyslipidemia.[80] First, they introduced the use of the ASCVD risk score, which includes sex-specific calculations.[81] Lifestyle guidelines are offered for diet, physical activity, and risk factor optimization. Lifestyle modifications, particularly diet and exercise, are important for primary and secondary prevention of ASCVD. Pharmacologic therapy for secondary prevention is equally effective among women and men for the reduction of recurrent CAD events and mortality. Fixed-dose statin therapy for women is based on their risk categorization by the ASCVD risk score, without use of target low-density lipoprotein cholesterol (LDL-C) levels. Nonstatin therapies are generally not recommended. Beyond 75 years of age, moderate rather than high-intensity dose statins are recommended due to altered statin metabolism in the elderly.[82–86] Recommendations for ezetimibe and proprotein convertase subtilisin kexin 9 (PCSK9) inhibitors were not included in these guidelines because the clinical trial results were not available by 2013. Ezetimibe added to statin decreases LDL-C by ~15% and has been associated with a decrease in ASCVD events,[87] and PCSK9 inhibitors have resulted in even more dramatic lowering of LDL-C.[88–91] Women appear to have a greater likelihood than men of developing diabetes on statins.[92]

The 2018 AHA/ACC Guideline on the Management of Blood Cholesterol[44] addresses cholesterol management in very high-risk ASCVD patients and those with severe primary hypercholesterolemia. It considers reasonable the addition of ezetimibe to maximally tolerated statin therapy when the LDL level remains > 70 mg/dL and adding a PCSK9 inhibitor when this combination results in suboptimal LDL-C levels.[90,91] The Guideline further addresses issues specific to women, including considering premature menopause, pregnancy-associated disorders when discussing lifestyle interventions and the benefit of statin therapy, recommending reliable contraception for sexually active women of childbearing age treated with statin therapy, and recommending discontinuation of statin therapy 1 to 2 months before oral contraception is discontinued and pregnancy is attempted (and discontinuing statin use immediately if pregnancy occurs while on a statin).

Not yet included in any guideline, but FDA-approved and in several scientific statements[93] is icosapent ethyl (pure EPA) based on the REDUCE-IT trial.[94] In statin-treated patients with high ASCVD risk, it reduced the composite endpoint of MACE by 25%. Both first and total events were decreased over 5 years.[95] Data from REDUCE-IT demonstrate that women benefit similarly to men with respect to icosapent ethyl, a novel therapy for the prevention of ASCVD.[96]

Obesity/Overweight

Two-thirds of women in the United States are either obese or overweight, and obesity is closely associated with physical inactivity, hypertension, dyslipidemia, and insulin resistance. In the Framingham Heart Study, obesity was associated with an increase in ASCVD risk by 64% in women compared with 46% in men.[97] Obesity is a major risk factor for MI in women,

increasing their risk nearly 3-fold.[98] Whereas the prevalence of obesity is equivalent among women and men in higher income countries, it is double in women as compared to men in low- to middle-income nations.[99] Detailed guidelines released by the ACC/AHA are available for the management of obesity.[99]

Physical Inactivity

Nearly one-third of adults in the United States, including 32.2% of women and 29.9% of men, are physically inactive. In the INTERHEART study, the protective effects of exercise were more prominent for women than for men. Physical inactivity is the most prevalent risk factor for women, with one-quarter of US women reporting no regular physical activity and three-quarters reporting less than the recommended amount of activity.[54] Moreover, the development of diabetes and risk of ASCVD events is decreased for women who exercise regularly. The recommended levels in the physical activity guidelines for adult Americans are at least 150 minutes per week of moderate-intensity aerobic activity such as walking, 75 minutes of vigorous-intensity aerobic activity such as jogging, or a combination of both, with muscle strength training activity recommended on 2 or more days of the week.[100] Higher levels of physical activity are associated with lower rates of ASCVD.[101]

Psychosocial Issues: Depression and Stress

Psychosocial issues, particularly depression, preferentially disadvantage women. In the INTERHEART study, psychosocial factors increased ASCVD mortality by 45% for women as compared to 23% for men.[54] These factors include stress at work or home, financial stress, and major life events.[54] There is growing evidence that psychological factors and emotional stress influence the onset and clinical course of IHD, particularly for women. From the Variation in Recovery: Role of Gender on Outcomes of Young AMI Patients (VIRGO) registry, young women compared with young men had significantly higher stress scores and were more likely to have a history of depression.[102] Depression among women appears to be a powerful predictor of early onset MI[103] and is a risk factor for adverse outcomes with ACS.[104–107] Depression following MI occurs with increased frequency in women, with the greatest risk in younger women.[108] Depression may be a component of the increased ASCVD event risk of younger women following both MI and coronary artery bypass graft (CABG) procedures.[109,110]

Increased mortality has also been reported among depressed young women (<65 years of age) with established CAD. Depression is associated with a 1.6-fold increase in ASCVD mortality independent of the severity of depression. Likely contributors are the high-risk behaviors and nonadherence to therapies associated with depression.

Aspirin Therapy

Recommendations for the preventive use of aspirin for ASCVD previously varied by sex. Aspirin was routinely recommended for primary prevention in men but not women, based on the Women's Health Study.[111] In this study, 38,876 healthy low-risk women older than 45 years old were randomized to 100 mg of aspirin every other day versus placebo. Aspirin prevented stroke but not MI or ASCVD death among those <65 years of age, with a sizeable risk for gastrointestinal bleeding. For older women, aspirin prevented stroke, MI, and ASCVD death but at an increased risk of gastrointestinal bleeding, which was comparable to the preventive benefits, thus mandating treatment individualization.

Based on a meta-analysis of three recent trials, the 2019 ACC/AHA Guideline on the Primary Prevention of ASCVD[45] identified that low-dose aspirin might be considered for primary prevention in select adults 40 to 70 years who are at increased ASCVD but not bleeding risk, and that low-dose aspirin should not be routinely administered for primary prevention of ASCVD events among adults >70 years. The Guideline further addresses that low-dose aspirin should not be administered for primary prevention among adults at any age who are at increased bleeding risk. Comparable sex-specific recommendations for aspirin use are routine in all clinical practice guidelines for secondary prevention.[112]

Risk Factors Unique to or Predominant in Women

Pregnancy Complications

Pregnancy complications, including preeclampsia, gestational diabetes, pregnancy-induced hypertension, preterm delivery, and small for gestational age at birth are all early indicators of future ASCVD risk and may occur in 10% to 20% of pregnancies.[113] Preterm delivery (<34 weeks gestation) appears to be an independent risk factor for subsequent long-term ASCVD morbidity and hospitalizations.[114] These data support that a detailed pregnancy history is an integral component of risk assessment for all women. It has been suggested that pregnancy is the first "stress test" that a woman undergoes, in that the cardiovascular and metabolic stresses of pregnancy have the potential for early prediction of future ASCVD risk. It is likely that preeclampsia and ASCVD share risk factors that are unmasked by pregnancy. Preeclampsia and gestational hypertension increase by 3- to 6-fold the risk for subsequent hypertension and double the risk for subsequent ASCVD events including stroke. Further, gestational diabetes increases by 7-fold the risk of subsequent development of type 2 diabetes.[115–117] It has traditionally been taught that preeclampsia subsides with the delivery of the placenta. However, residual endothelial dysfunction may persist, which has been associated with an increase in coronary artery calcium (CAC), a marker of atherosclerosis. Regrettably, these adverse pregnancy outcomes are often not included in the electronic health record, even if delivery occurred at the same institution where the woman receives primary care.[118–120] The importance of collaboration of internists/cardiologists with obstetricians/gynecologists is pivotal in promoting risk identification and reduction of ASCVD in women.

Oral Contraceptive Therapy

There is no apparent increase in ASCVD risk for healthy women without risk factors receiving oral contraceptive therapy. However, smoking increases their risk by 7-fold and there may be an increase in blood pressure for women with hypertension.[121,122] There is also a nearly 2-fold increase in stroke risk which increases with older age at oral contraceptive therapy use. There are differences among the oral contraceptives, with earlier formulations, particularly Levonorgestrel, increasing MI risk, and more recent oral contraceptives associated with a lesser increase in blood pressure or even a decrease, but all with an elevated risk of venous thromboembolism. The recommendations are for precise risk factor ascertainment and management in women using oral contraceptive preparations.[121,122]

Hormonal Fertility Therapy

A new area of potential risk involves the response to hormonal fertility therapy. From a Canadian population cohort, women with successful fertility therapy experienced a decreased risk of all-cause mortality, stroke, thromboembolism, and heart failure that was evident across age and income subsets.[123] In contrast, unsuccessful fertility therapy in the same cohort was associated with an increase in adverse ASCVD events.[124]

Menopausal Hormone Therapy

Menopausal hormone therapy is an area where clinical trial data have dramatically altered clinical recommendations and practice.[125] Based on data from the Women's Health Initiative (in healthy women) and the Heart and Estrogen Progestin Replacement Study (in women with ASCVD) respectively, menopausal hormone therapy is not recommended for primary or secondary prevention of ASCVD. The US Preventive Services Task Force recommendations also state that menopausal hormone therapy should not be recommended for the primary prevention of chronic conditions such as ASCVD.[126,127]

Systemic Autoimmune Disorders

Systemic autoimmune disorders are highly prevalent among women and have adverse consequences, increasing the risk of ASCVD and stroke. ASCVD is the leading cause of both morbidity and mortality in women with systemic lupus erythematosus. There is a 2- to 3-fold increase in MI and ASCVD mortality among women with rheumatoid arthritis. Increased ASCVD risk has also been reported among women with psoriasis.[23,128,129] Detailed screening for ASCVD risk factors and prompt risk intervention are recommended for women with systemic autoimmune disorders.

Class III Interventions: Not Useful/Effective and May Be Harmful for ASCVD Prevention in Women

Menopausal Hormone Therapy

The Heart and Estrogen/progestin Replacement Study[130] and the Women's Health Initiative Hormone trials[131] documented that menopausal hormone therapy did not prevent incident or recurrent ASCVD in women but increased their risk of stroke. These trials displaced menopausal hormone therapy as the ubiquitous solution to women's ASCVD risk, refocusing attention on established cardiovascular preventive therapy. In summary, hormone therapy and selective estrogen receptor modulators should not be used for the primary or secondary prevention of ASCVD, in keeping with recommendations from the US Preventive Services Taskforce.[125,126]

Antioxidant Supplements and Folic Acid

The Women's Antioxidant ASCVD and the Women's Antioxidant and Folic Acid ASCVD studies identified that vitamins E,

C, and beta carotene and folic acid and B vitamin supplements, respectively, did not prevent incident or recurrent ASCVD in women. Antioxidant supplements (eg, vitamins E, C, and beta carotene) should not be used for the primary or secondary prevention of ASCVD.[132,133] As well, folic acid, with or without vitamin B6 and B12 supplementation, should not be used for the primary or secondary prevention of ASCVD.[134]

ASCVD RISK SCORES AND SUBCLINICAL CORONARY ATHEROSCLEROTIC PLAQUE

The 2019 ACC/AHA Guideline for the Primary Prevention of Cardiovascular Disease[45] recommends the use of the ASCVD risk score for adults aged 40 to 75 as the basis for clinician/patient risk discussion prior to starting pharmacologic therapy. Nonetheless, the ASCVD risk score, which guides preventive care, is reported to be imprecise in women, especially those of diverse race/ethnicity and in non-US populations.[135-137] Use of ASCVD risk scores and a threshold of >7.5% results in fewer women recommended for statin therapy as compared to men (33% vs 63%; *P* <0.001).[138] As such, the 2019 primary prevention guidelines also recognize the importance of assessing other risk-enhancing factors highly relevant to women, including the metabolic syndrome, chronic inflammatory conditions, and a history of premature menopause or pregnancy-associated conditions such as preeclampsia, which increase future ASCVD risk. High-risk race/ethnicity (eg, South Asian, East Asian, Native American, and Middle Eastern ancestry) is also addressed.

Use of Coronary Artery Calcium Scoring

Ample prognostic evidence from contemporary cohorts suggest that adjunctive imaging, particularly with quantification of CAC, improves risk detection with ample prognostic evidence from contemporary cohorts of women undergoing CAC scoring.[139,140] The CAC score may be helpful to guide preventive management, especially for women in whom global risk scores may be imprecise. From the CAC Consortium, the prevalence of CAC ranged from 26% to 72% for women aged 50 to 70 years old (**Fig. 80–2**).[139] Also, women with multivessel CAC involvement have a nearly 2-fold higher long-term ASCVD mortality risk as compared to men.[139] These data suggest that, in addition to advanced age, the burden of CAC layered onto smaller epicardial vessels may disproportionately worsen risk for women as compared to men. For the many women with a CAC score of 0, their long-term ASCVD risk reveals a 12-year event rate well below the 7.5% ASCVD risk threshold for statin recommendation.[140] Thus, the use of CAC scoring may help to define a woman's risk and guide preventive management.

SYMPTOMATIC EVALUATION OF STABLE IHD IN WOMEN

Women report higher rates of suspected angina as compared to men.[141,142] From a meta-analysis of 13,331 women and 11,511 men, the prevalence of angina was 20% higher among women as compared to men (*P* <0.0001).[142] Evidence supports a variable symptom profile for women versus men.[141] Women with angina frequently report symptoms following emotional stress occurring at rest, which differs from the typical exertional pattern of symptoms triggered during physical work that is classically described in male patients.[141] Moreover, a consistent pattern among women presenting with chest pain, even in younger females (<55 years of age),[143] is that of increased angina frequency along with reduced quality of life.[144,145] This can complicate the index evaluation for ASCVD and potentially contribute to the high rates of persistent symptoms reported among women, which are 2-fold higher than that in men.[146,147]

Adequate assessment of CAD risk requires the synthesis of multiple risk factors and clinical history, including a detailed

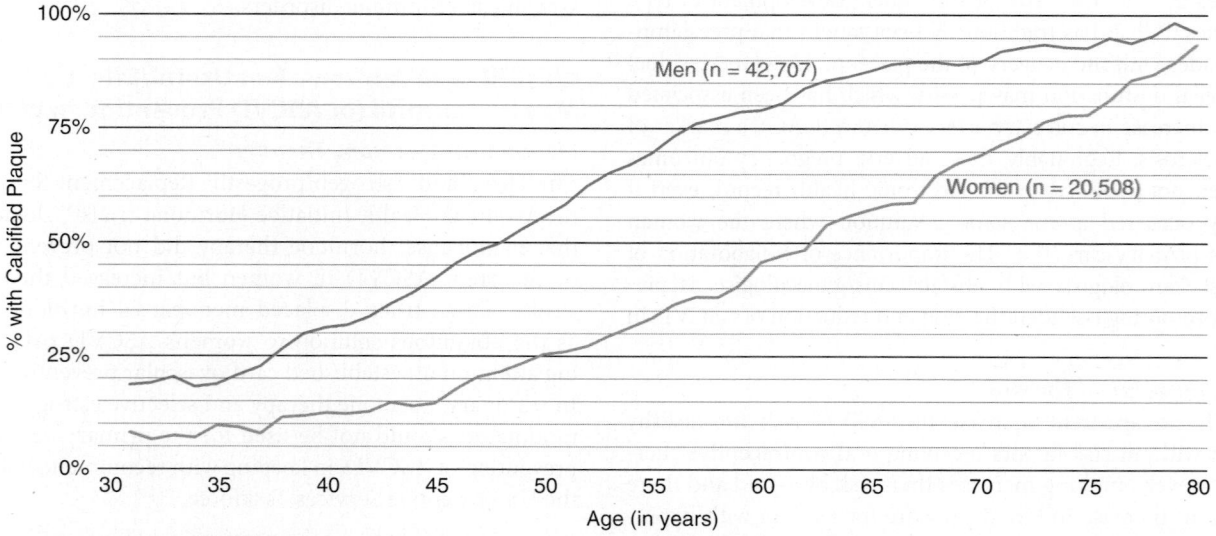

Figure 80–2. **Prevalence of atherosclerotic plaque, defined as detectable CAC, in women and men enrolled in the CAC Consortium.** Reproduced with permission from Shaw LJ, Min JK, Nasir K, et al. Sex differences in calcified plaque and long-term cardiovascular mortality: observations from the CAC Consortium. *Eur Heart J.* 2018 Nov 1;39(41):3727-3735.

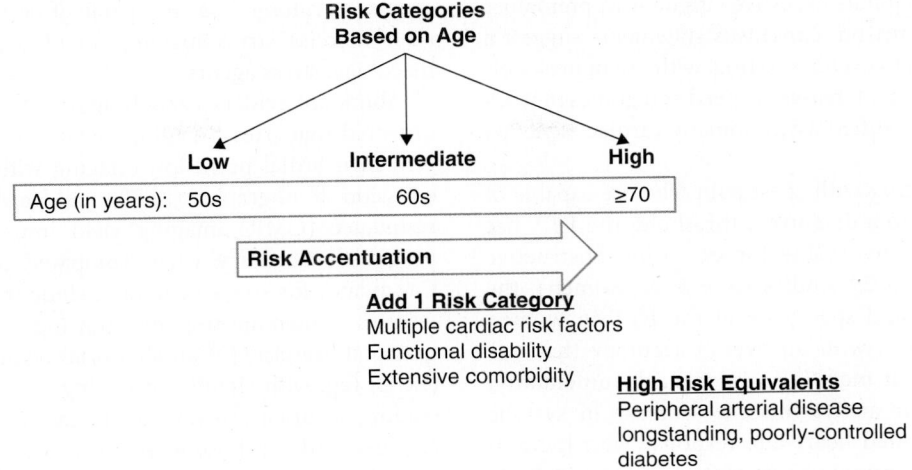

Figure 80-3. A simplified approach to categorize risk in women presenting with stable symptoms from the 2014 AHA Consensus Statement on the diagnostic evaluation of IHD in women details. Reproduced with permission from Mieres JH, Gulati M, Bairey Merz N, et al. Role of noninvasive testing in the clinical evaluation of women with suspected ischemic heart disease: a consensus statement from the American Heart Association. *Circulation.* 2014 Jul 22;130(4):350-379.

assessment of activities of daily living and features of symptom frequency and stability.[141] Many conventional scores estimate likelihood of obstructive CAD with the highest estimates for patients with typical chest pain symptoms. However, because symptomatic women frequently manifest fewer exertional symptoms and lower rates of obstructive CAD, these likelihood estimates result in their categorization as uniformly lower risk.[141] McSweeney and colleagues identified five prominent prodromal symptoms in women presenting with IHD, which include discomfort in the jaw or teeth, unusual fatigue, arm discomfort, shortness of breath, and general chest discomfort.[148] The relative hazard for CAD events (at 2-years of follow-up) was elevated 4-fold for women reporting more than one of these symptoms.[148] The 2014 AHA Consensus Statement on the diagnostic evaluation of IHD in women presented a simplified approach to categorize risk (**Fig. 80-3**).[141] For women with stable symptoms, risk is broadly categorized as low, intermediate, and high risk, respectively, for those in their fifties, sixties, and seventies or older.[141] Risk may be accentuated by one category (eg, low-to-intermediate risk) for those with multiple CAD risk factors, functional disability, or extensive comorbidity. Additionally, high-risk equivalent women are those with long-standing or poorly controlled diabetes, or those with peripheral arterial disease. This approach provides a means to define risk in women and captures the prominent impact of age as driving clinical outcomes and CAD prevalence. Women allocated to low risk status are less likely to benefit from immediate diagnostic testing; optimal candidates for noninvasive functional or anatomic testing include women at intermediate-high CAD risk.[141]

Diagnosing Myocardial Ischemia in Women with Suspected IHD

There has long been a misperception that documented ischemic or other stress test abnormalities in women, particularly without accompanying anatomic findings of obstructive CAD,

represented false positive results.[149,150] These misperceptions led to a pattern of less intensive posttest changes in clinical management. In one trial, less than 10% of women with abnormal stress test findings received any intensification or initiation of antiischemic therapies or referral to invasive coronary angiography.[149] However, an evolution in thought regarding the role of ischemia as elevating risk in women has occurred over the last decade. A landmark population registry reported that coronary mortality was significantly elevated for women with ischemic findings on noninvasive testing, particularly for those <75 years of age where the relative hazard for CAD death was higher among women as compared to similarly aged men.[151] Although issues remain with potential technical artifacts confounding interpretation of imaging results (eg, breast tissue attenuation artifact in stress myocardial perfusion single photon emission computed tomography [SPECT]), extensive contemporary evidence now documents the prognostic accuracy of ischemic findings among women.[152-155] This issue highlights the importance of recognizing functional, not simply anatomic, abnormalities as potentiating adverse outcomes in ASCVD, particularly in women. Thus, we recommend the term IHD to identify myocardial ischemia as the culprit for symptom burden among women, with emphasis on the importance of the prognostic risk associated with ischemia severity also in the setting of ischemia and no obstructive CAD (INOCA) and coronary microvascular dysfunction (CMD).

The mainstay of functional or stress testing has been the exercise tolerance test (ETT), with strong evidence for its diagnostic and prognostic accuracy in women.[141,156,157] The ETT is indicated for intermediate risk women who are capable of performing activities of daily living (approximately five metabolic equivalents [METs] of exercise or higher).[1] Given the predominance of limitations in physical functioning among female patient cohorts, the candidate pool of women capable of maximal levels of exercise is less than that of men. However, the commonly applied Bruce protocol may be too rigorous for many women and precipitate excessive fatigue with premature termination. For this reason, consensus statements suggest a personalized approach to exercise testing, with use of protocols with smaller incremental increases in speed and grades of work when indicated (eg, modified asymptomatic cardiac ischemia pilot protocol).[141,158]

For women presenting with chest pain who are capable of exercising maximally to a diagnostic threshold, the ETT has a high negative predictive value for excluding obstructive CAD.[141] However, from 29 studies (n = 3392 women), the diagnostic sensitivity and specificity of the ETT in women was only 62% and 68%, with an overall accuracy that was decidedly lower than in men.[159] As in men, documentation of frequent ventricular arrhythmias, a decrease in systolic blood pressure or blunted heart rate response with increasing physical work, a 1-minute heart rate recovery <12 beats from peak exercise, and the occurrence of diagnostic ST segment changes of ≥2 mm all signify high-risk findings on the ETT.[158,160] Older reports highlight the prognostic accuracy of the Duke treadmill score (exercise time – [5 × maximum ST segment change] – [4 × angina index]) in women as well as men, stratifying patient risk by categories of low (score ≥+5) to high risk (score ≤–11).[141,161] Those with intermediate-high risk (score ≤+4) are generally considered candidates for further risk assessment with noninvasive imaging and, in select high-risk cases, coronary angiography.

In a younger, lower risk cohort, the What is the Optimal Method for Ischemia Evaluation in Women (WOMEN) trial revealed similar 2-year outcomes (ie, cardiac death or hospitalization for heart failure or an ACS) for women randomized to an ETT as compared to exercise myocardial perfusion SPECT (P = 0.59).[149] Based in part on this trial, an AHA consensus statement introduced the concept of an ETT-first strategy whereby selective imaging is performed in women whose index ETT identifies indeterminate or positive findings.[141] Women incapable of performing five or more METs of exercise are at elevated risk of all-cause mortality and other major CAD

events.[141] Among those incapable of performing adequate levels of exercise, stress imaging should be performed with pharmacologic stress agents.

Abundant evidence spanning decades in women have documented that stress imaging, including stress echocardiography, myocardial perfusion imaging with SPECT or positron emission tomography (PET), and cardiovascular magnetic resonance (CMR) imaging yield improved diagnostic and prognostic accuracy when compared to ETT alone.[141,162,163] Candidates for stress imaging include intermediate-high pretest risk women meeting the following criteria: (1) incapable of maximal exercise; (2) an abnormal resting electrocardiogram (ECG) (eg, with significant resting ST-T wave changes), precluding accurate assessment of exercise-induced ST segment changes; and (3) those with known CAD.[1,141] With regards to the latter, this may also include women with nonobstructive CAD where evidence of a functionally abnormal stenosis may guide clinical decision-making.

Stress echocardiography is useful for ruling out wall motion abnormalities with a high diagnostic accuracy (sensitivity = 79% and specificity = 83%) in women, and may be particularly helpful for younger and lower-risk women.[2,159] Image quality, particularly for the obese or those with lung disease, may be improved with the use of intravenous contrast.[141] For women capable of exercising, absence of an inducible wall motion abnormality in the setting of maximal exercise identifies those at low risk of future CAD events.[164] Following the principles of demand ischemia, an inducible wall motion abnormality is more likely to be elicited in the setting of more severely flow-limiting stenosis and, thus, a failure to document a new wall motion abnormality may occur in a woman with nonobstructive or single vessel obstructive CAD.[165] Recent evidence from the NHLBI-sponsored International Study of Comparative Health Effectiveness with Medical and Invasive Approaches (ISCHEMIA) trial revealed that only 62% of women with inducible ischemia on stress echocardiography had obstructive CAD as compared to 92% of men (**Fig. 80–4**;

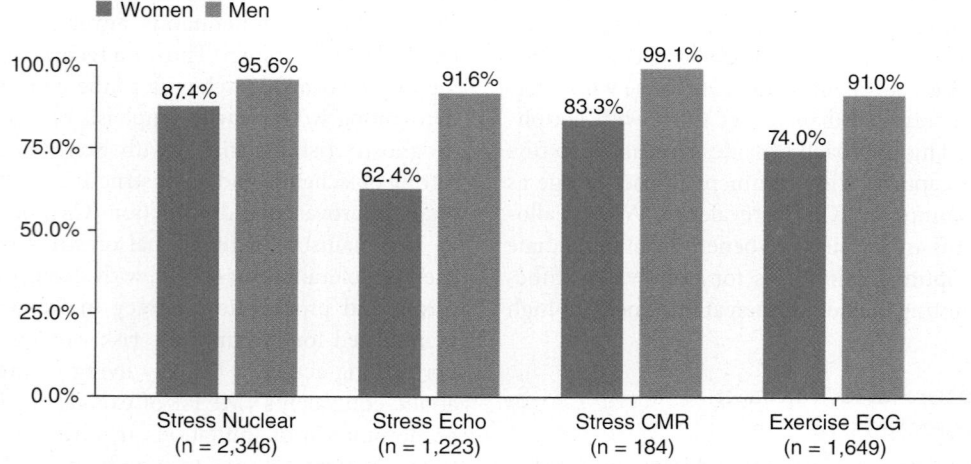

Figure 80–4. Rates of obstructive CAD among women and men presenting with stress-induced myocardial ischemia enrolled in the ISCHEMIA trial. Data from Reynolds HR, Shaw LJ, Min JK, et al. Association of Sex With Severity of Coronary Artery Disease, Ischemia, and Symptom Burden in Patients With Moderate or Severe Ischemia: Secondary Analysis of the ISCHEMIA Randomized Clinical Trial. *JAMA Cardiol.* 2020 Jul 1;5(7):773-786.

P <0.001).[145] This apparently lower diagnostic accuracy in women was not observed in other stress imaging modalities and may be related to diverse etiology for inducible wall motion abnormalities including factors such as hypertensive heart disease.[166] Nonimaging stress parameters may help to improve risk detection in select women and men. For example, a hypertensive response to exercise has been identified as a potential cause for stress-induced echocardiographic wall motion abnormalities absent obstructive CAD.[167] Echocardiography can also be helpful in assessing noncoronary etiologies for symptoms such as diastolic dysfunction, abnormal filling pressures, or abnormal myocardial mechanics using tissue Doppler or speckle tracking.[2]

There is also a robust evidence base for the utility of stress myocardial perfusion SPECT and PET in women.[1] From the ISCHEMIA trial, 87% of women and 96% of men with ischemia on cardiac stress SPECT and PET had obstructive CAD on CCTA, supporting a similarly high diagnostic accuracy in both sexes (Fig. 80–4).[145] Myocardial perfusion imaging allows for effective risk stratification in women by defining the extent and severity of rest and stress abnormalities (ie, MI and ischemia, respectively, as a gradient relationship with % abnormal myocardium).[141,168–171] Breast tissue attenuation artifact reduces the diagnostic accuracy of SPECT for women who are obese and/or for those with large breasts, but may be overcome by using attenuation correction algorithms or use of two-position supine/prone imaging.[172–174] The evidence base is expansive on the prognostic utility of SPECT imaging in women undergoing exercise or pharmacologic stress, including for those who are obese, diabetic, and of diverse race and ethnicity.[175,176]

An important limitation with the use of conventional myocardial perfusion SPECT imaging is that the overall radiation burden is higher than that for cardiac PET imaging, with a typical effective dose of 10 to 15 mSv for rest and stress technetium-99m SPECT.[177,178] Over the last decade, there has been substantial focus on optimization of dose reduction techniques in nuclear cardiology, including the expanded use of stress-only imaging, high resolution solid-state detectors, and/or PET imaging. For many women, stress imaging should be performed first and, if normal, elimination of the resting scan will reduce radiation exposure considerably (ie, stress-only imaging).[178] There should be limited use of SPECT imaging for younger women (ie, <50 years of age) but if clinical indications warrant, these patients should undergo testing with low dose exposure (eg, with stress-only imaging or, preferably, PET).

Relative to conventional SPECT, PET myocardial perfusion imaging has markedly improved spatial resolution, substantially lower radiation exposure (~3 mSv), and robust capabilities for quantifying absolute myocardial blood flow at rest and post-stress. Use of cardiac PET allows for superior image quality (ie, reduced breast tissue artifact) which translates into high diagnostic accuracy for women, particularly for the obese.[179] For stress myocardial perfusion PET, the diagnostic accuracy is higher as compared to SPECT (88% vs 67%; $P = 0.009$).[155,179] As with SPECT imaging, risk stratification with PET based on the rest and stress % abnormal or ischemic myocardium appears to similarly risk stratify women and men.[154,155,180–183]

One clear advantage of PET is the added contribution of myocardial blood flow reserve (MBFR) measures documenting the ratio of stress/rest absolute myocardial blood flow.[2,184] MBFR has been extensively applied to quantify global and regional myocardial blood flow and reserve, which further refine cardiovascular prognosis and allow for the detection of CMD. An interesting finding is that up to 50% of patients with normal or low risk cardiac PET perfusion imaging also have reduced MBFR (≤2), which is associated with worse cardiovascular outcomes, including death.[185–187] A reduced MBFR combined with increasing ischemia severity is associated with a higher rate of cardiovascular events.[186,188] Reductions in MBFR are proportional to stenosis severity, but in the patient with angiographically normal or nonobstructive coronary arteries may reflect dysfunction in the microvasculature, or CMD.[154,189] **Figure 80–5** reveals that women with severely impaired MBFR

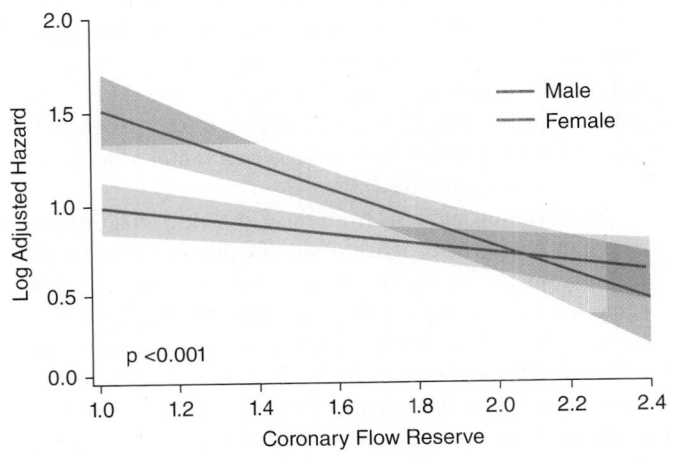
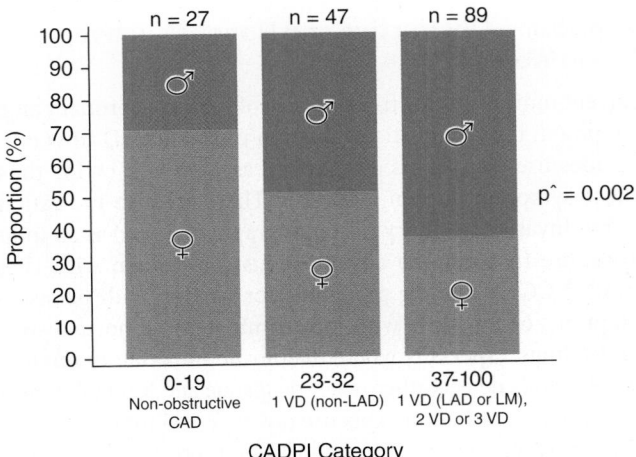

Figure 80–5. Women with reduced PET MBFR have a higher risk of CVD events as compared to men, despite the lower prevalence of obstructive CAD. Reproduced with permission from Taqueti VR, Shaw LJ, Cook NR, et al. Excess Cardiovascular Risk in Women Relative to Men Referred for Coronary Angiography Is Associated With Severely Impaired Coronary Flow Reserve, Not Obstructive Disease. *Circulation.* 2017 Feb 7;135(6):566-577.

(<1.6) have a higher rate of cardiovascular events as compared to men with similarly impaired MBFR, and yet are less likely to have severely obstructive CAD. These data suggest that the etiology of impaired MBFR in women may differ from that in men, and is less related to anatomically obstructive CAD, the historic gatekeeper for IHD management. Rather, in these female patients, a severely impaired MBFR is more likely related to diffuse atherosclerosis and CMD, for which novel therapeutic strategies beyond revascularization of obstructive CAD are needed.[180] These data support a role of CMD and nonobstructive CAD in the pathophysiology of ASCVD events in women.[4,154,183] Additionally, an understanding of impaired flow and ischemic abnormalities in relation to high-risk atherosclerotic plaque features may improve detection of at-risk women and guide future treatment strategies.[190–192]

Stress CMR imaging is another functional testing modality with demonstrated utility in evaluating women with suspected IHD.[2,193] The development of rapid high-spatial resolution techniques has bolstered the use of CMR perfusion imaging, particularly for the evaluation of women, and overcomes issues related to breast attenuation common to SPECT imaging.[2,194] A subset analysis of the single center Clinical Evaluation of Magnetic Resonance Imaging in Coronary Heart Disease (CE-MARC) trial compared women who were randomized to a multiparametric CMR evaluation including angiography, function, perfusion, and scar imaging as compared to myocardial perfusion SPECT.[193] In this subset analysis, CMR outperformed SPECT for diagnosis of IHD with a higher diagnostic accuracy (P <0.0001); sensitivity in women was significantly higher for CMR than SPECT (89% vs 51%), with comparable specificity (84% for both). Recently, outcomes data with CMR perfusion also demonstrated that women with ischemia have worsened prognosis (P <0.001).[194] Additionally, CMR techniques to measure myocardial perfusion reserve (MPR) with vasodilator stress may allow detection of CMD in symptomatic women.[195] A final important consideration is the value of late gadolinium enhancement CMR imaging to improve detection of infarcted or scarred myocardium and identify women with previously undocumented MI.[196,197]

Diagnosing Obstructive and Nonobstructive CAD in Women

Current indications for frontline use of invasive coronary angiography in the diagnostic evaluation of stable IHD in women includes use in patients categorized as high risk or for those whose symptom burden is severe.[1] There are also indications for noninvasive coronary CT angiography (CCTA) as an index procedure that may be advantageous for women with chest pain.[1,198] CCTA may be preferable for women with persistent symptoms or for those with indeterminate or abnormal stress test findings, especially where diagnostic uncertainty remains. CCTA readily detects atherosclerotic plaque and luminal stenosis with minimal radiation exposure (average 3–5 mSv).[199,200]

For invasive angiography and CCTA, there is a proportional increase in the risk of major CAD events with increasing number of vessels with obstructive CAD.[201] As with men, women have a higher risk of major CAD events with more severe and extensive multivessel CAD.[201] A remarkably consistent finding across all female patient cohorts undergoing invasive coronary angiography for evaluation of acute and stable IHD is their higher frequency of nonobstructive CAD as compared to male patients.[4,170,202] Approximately half of women referred for angiography do not have obstructive CAD, including women of diverse race and ethnicity.[4,170,171] Similarly, women have more nonobstructive CAD on CCTA as compared to men, although the overall prevalence of obstructive CAD using this noninvasive modality is much lower at 10% to 20%.[199,203–205] Secondary analysis by sex was recently reported in the NHLBI-sponsored Prospective Multicenter Imaging Study for Evaluation of Chest Pain (PROMISE) trial.[206,207] From PROMISE (n = 8966), women had less documented obstructive CAD (8%) on CCTA as compared to positive stress test findings (12%; P <0.001), while men had a similar rate of positive findings on CCTA and stress testing (14%–16%; P = 0.046). Women with obstructive CAD on CCTA had a nearly 10-fold higher (P <0.001) hazard of death, MI, or unstable angina hospitalization, while females with a positive stress test had a 5-fold (P = 0.002) hazard for the clinical outcome—resulting in a significantly higher risk noted with CCTA versus stress testing for women (P = 0.043). These data suggest that CCTA may aid in the evaluation of symptomatic women due to its ability to detect risk and provide details on nonobstructive and obstructive CAD.

The updated approach to diagnosis of CAD now includes an understanding of the prognostic significance of nonobstructive CAD as well as obstructive CAD, especially in women. Nonobstructive CAD with luminal narrowing of 1% to 49% is associated with worsening event-free survival in women undergoing CCTA and invasive coronary angiography.[4,171,208,209] From the Coronary CT Angiography Evaluation For Clinical Outcomes: An International Multicenter Registry (CONFIRM) registry of patients with suspected IHD, the presence of nonobstructive CAD on CCTA was associated with worsening mortality[201] and a ~2-fold increase in major CAD events.[210] Five-year incidence of death or MI was significantly higher among women as compared to men with nonobstructive left main stenosis (**Fig. 80–6**).[211] As well, from the CONFIRM registry, age modified risk associated with nonobstructive CAD where women >60 years of age had a higher risk than men in the setting of nonobstructive CAD.[212] Moreover, in patients with nonobstructive CAD, prognosis also worsens among those with diffuse segmental atherosclerosis (ie, >4 segments involved).[213]

An intriguing analysis from the PROMISE trial involved an examination of the prognostic significance of high-risk plaque features on CCTA including low attenuation plaque, positive remodeling, or a napkin ring sign (**Fig. 80–7**).[214] All three of these features have been reported as precursors to incident ACS.[29,215] The presence of high-risk plaque increased the relative hazard for CAD events by nearly 3-fold.[214] However, the presence of high-risk plaque features was predictive in women (hazard ratio 2.4, 1.3–4.6) but not men (hazard ratio 1.4, 0.8–2.4).

Several recent randomized trials compared CCTA versus ETT for 1-year CAD outcomes and costs of care in suspected

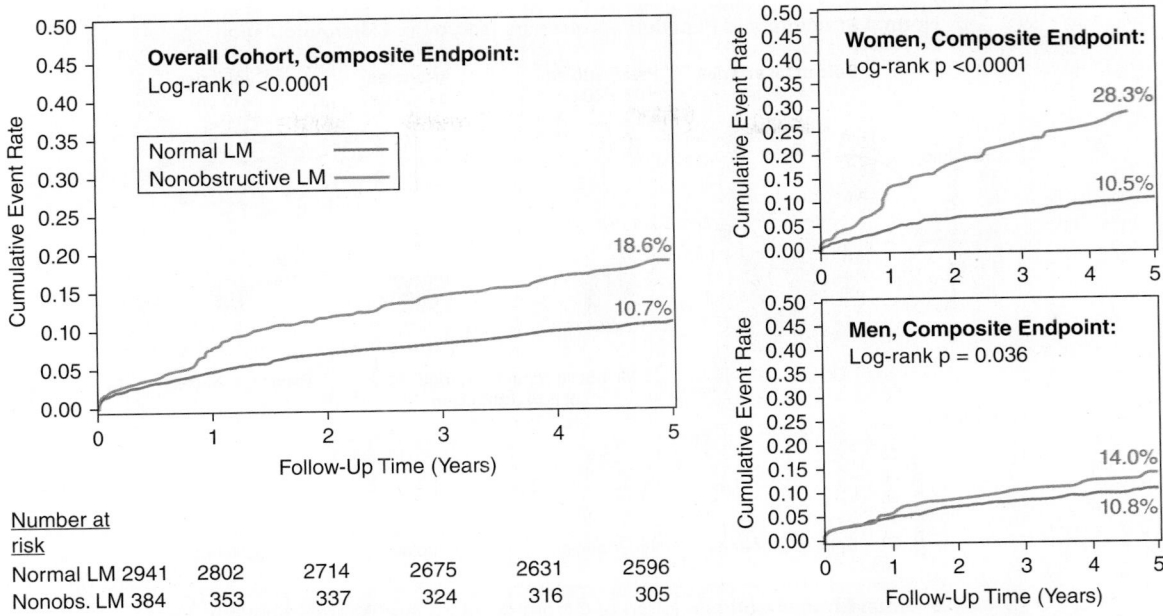

Figure 80-6. Five-year rates of death or MI are higher for women than men with nonobstructive left main stenosis (1%–49%). Reproduced with permission from Xie JX, Eshtehardi P, Varghese T, et al. Prognostic Significance of Nonobstructive Left Main Coronary Artery Disease in Women Versus Men: Long-Term Outcomes From the CONFIRM (Coronary CT Angiography Evaluation For Clinical Outcomes: An International Multicenter) Registry. *Circ Cardiovasc Imaging.* 2017 Aug;10(8):e006246.

IHD patients.[216,217] In both trials, 1-year CAD outcomes were improved, angina was more often reduced, and costs of care were lower for CCTA versus ETT, although no subset analysis was performed in women. Given the lower diagnostic accuracy of isolated ETT, these data suggest that CCTA may be a favorable option in selected patients. In the Computed Tomography versus Exercise Testing in Suspected Coronary Artery Disease (CRESCENT) trial, a CAC score was initially performed and CCTA was limited to patients with detectable plaque.[216,218] This approach of applying CAC scoring either as the index approach or together with the exercise ECG may be one alternative to improve detection of women with underlying atherosclerosis. Importantly in the CRESCENT trial, no events were documented in the 40% of patients without detectable CAC. In a secondary analysis, nearly half of women enrolled in the CRESCENT trial had a CAC score of 0 while only 15% had

obstructive CAD or a CAC score of 400 or higher.[218] Women enrolled in CRESCENT with a CAC-guided care approach had greater angina relief ($P = 0.02$) with similar event-free survival ($P = 0.061$) as compared to those in the stress testing arm.

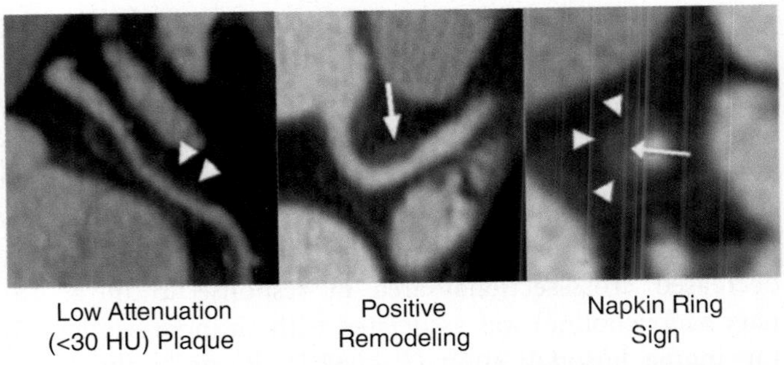

ISCHEMIA AND NO OBSTRUCTIVE CAD

INOCA is common with estimates that nearly 1 in 3 individuals, usually women, with an abnormal stress test lack coronary stenosis of 50% or higher.[145,219,220] The structure and function of normal and abnormal coronary micro- and macrocirculation is detailed in **Fig. 80-8**. A focus of the literature has been on identifying CMD as the underlying mechanism causing ischemia, yet many also have a burden of atherosclerotic plaque whereby intensification of preventive care may influence clinical outcomes (**Fig. 80-9**). Important for this discussion is that CMD as a mechanism for ischemia often coexists with epicardial atherosclerosis and, thus, is not an either/or diagnosis.[221] CMD may co-occur with or without atherosclerosis of varying stenosis severity in the epicardial coronary arteries, thus complicating the INOCA evaluation. From the recent *Computed TomogRaphic Evaluation of Atherosclerotic DEtermiNants of Myocardial IsChEmia* (CREDENCE) trial, factors associated with vessel-specific ischemia on fractional flow reserve but nonobstructive CAD included vessel size, presence of serial or tandem mild stenosis, the burden of noncalcified plaque, and features such as positive remodeling.[222] The combination of these CCTA factors in a model estimating reduced FFR was associated with a high area under the receiver operating characteristics curve for women (0.88) and men (0.82). The defining of epicardial atherosclerotic plaque, particularly if extensive

Low Attenuation
(<30 HU) Plaque

Positive
Remodeling

Napkin Ring
Sign

Figure 80-7. High risk atherosclerotic plaque features, including low attenuation plaque, positive remodeling, and the napkin ring sign. The presence of any high risk plaque feature is associated with a higher relative hazard for events in women as compared to men.

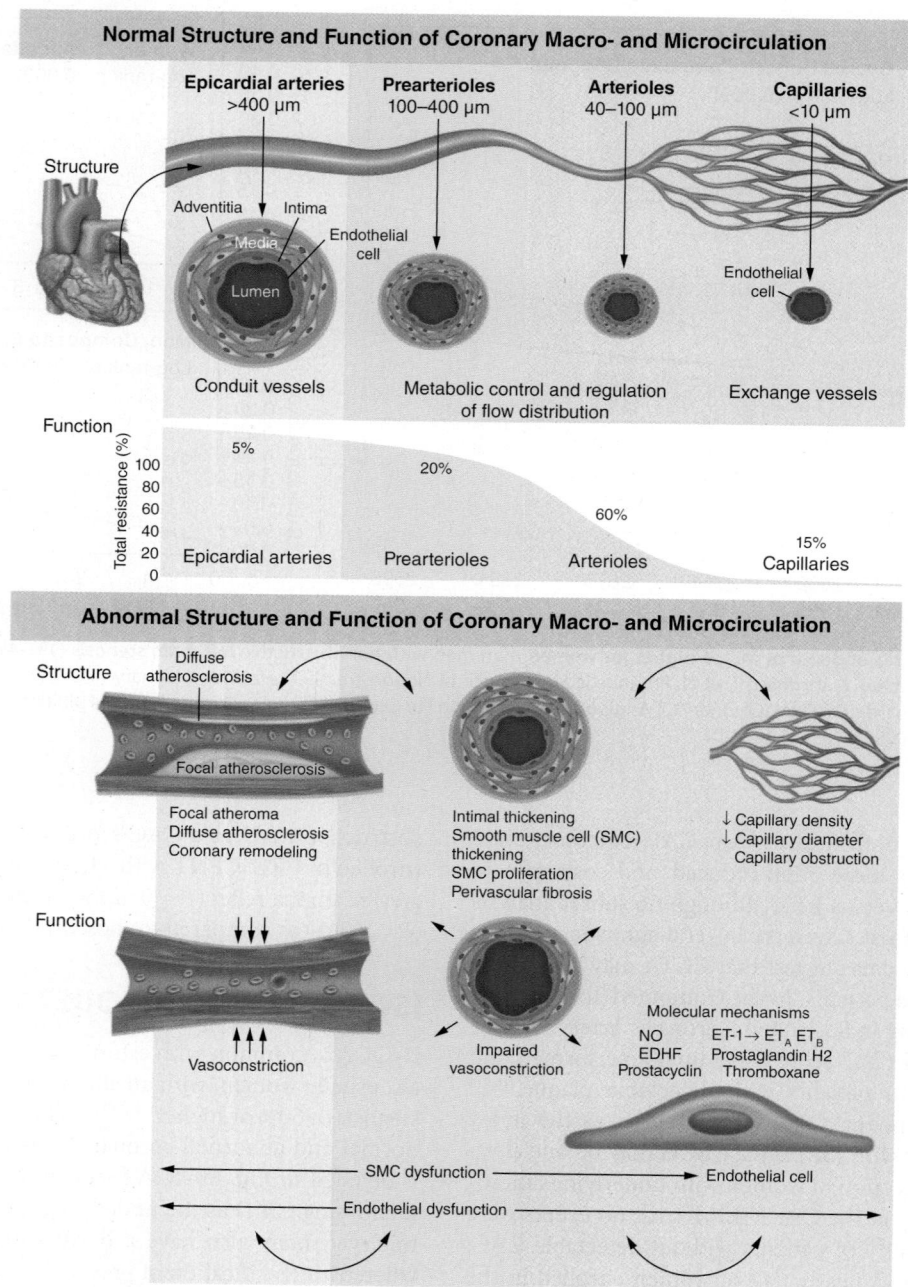

Figure 80–8. Structure and function of normal and abnormal coronary micro- and macro-circulation. Reproduced with permission from Taqueti VR, Di Carli MF. Coronary Microvascular Disease Pathogenic Mechanisms and Therapeutic Options: JACC State-of-the-Art Review. *J Am Coll Cardiol.* 2018 Nov 27;72(21):2625-2641.

or with high-risk features, may improve IHD risk detection and facilitate targeted treatment strategies for this large group of patients with CMD and nonobstructive CAD.[4]

Potential mechanisms for INOCA include CMD, vaso-spastic angina, or their combination.[223] The varying INOCA endotypes may be categorized using invasive coronary function testing with adenosine-induced hyperemia to measure fractional flow reserve, coronary flow reserve, and the index of microcirculatory resistance, followed by vasoreactivity testing with acetylcholine.[223-225] From the NHLBI-sponsored Women's Ischemia Syndrome Evaluation (WISE), coronary

reactivity testing was employed in 224 symptomatic women with no obstructive CAD.[226] A reduced coronary flow reserve <2.32 was associated with an elevated 10-year risk of major adverse CAD events ($P = 0.021$) and mortality ($P = 0.038$). In addition, impaired epicardial coronary reactivity (ie, decreased cross-sectional area in response to intracoronary acetylcholine) was associated with an increased hazard for angina hospitalization ($P <0.001$). Recently, the Coronary Microvascular Angina (CorMicA) trial randomized 151 patients (74% women) to treatment guided by invasive functional testing (intervention group) versus a blinded

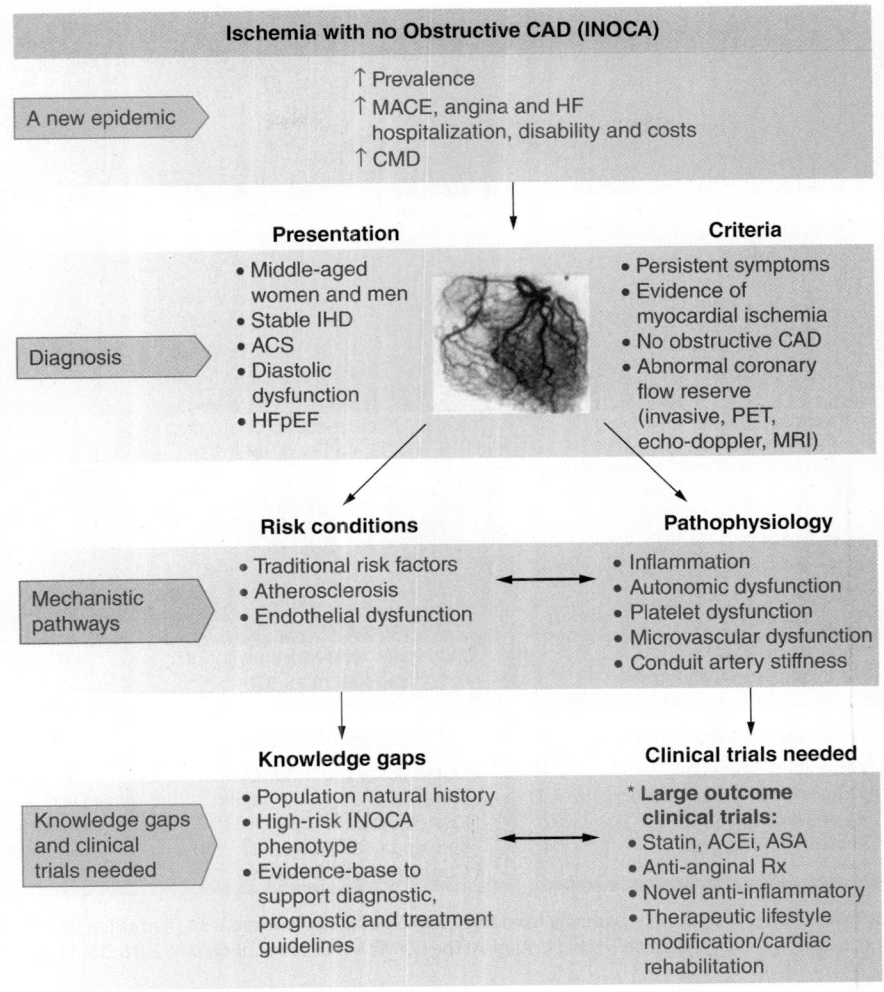

Figure 80–9. Diagnostic criteria, mechanistic pathways, and knowledge gaps for women with INOCA from a Consensus Statement published by the ACC's CVD in Women Committee, NIH-NHLBI, AHA, and European Society of Cardiology. Reproduced with permission from Bairey Merz CN, Pepine CJ, Walsh MN, et al. Ischemia and No Obstructive Coronary Artery Disease (INOCA): Developing Evidence-Based Therapies and Research Agenda for the Next Decade. *Circulation.* 2017 Mar 14;135(11):1075-1092.

control group.[227,228] The testing and treatment algorithm is detailed in **Fig. 80–10.** At 6 months, angina (measured using the summary Seattle Angina Questionnaire Score) was significantly improved ($P = 0.001$) as was overall quality of life ($P = 0.024$), and no differences in major CAD events were observed by treatment group ($P = 1.0$). These findings remained consistent at 1 year of follow-up.[229,230]

ACUTE CORONARY SYNDROME

Relative to men, women have different clinical profiles, presentations, and outcomes with ACS. There are multiple reasons why MI may preferentially disadvantage women, and these are likely a consequence of both biology and bias.[231] A review of 59 studies challenged whether a classical chest pain presentation for ACS was truly "typical" for either sex.[232] In this review, 37% of women as compared with 27% of men had no chest pain or discomfort, with absence of chest pain more common with advancing age. In the Gender and Sex Determinants of Cardiovascular Disease: From Bench to Beyond Premature ACS

(GENESIS PRAXY) registry, although chest pain was the most prevalent symptom in both sexes, women were less likely than men to experience chest pain and more likely to have additional symptoms, including back, neck and jaw pain; dyspnea; paroxysmal nocturnal dyspnea; nausea; indigestion; and weakness or fatigue.[233] This multiplicity of other symptoms may lead to diagnostic challenges for the clinician[234] including misdiagnosis, delayed revascularization and increased ACS mortality rates.[235] Women experience greater delays than men in seeking emergency care which may worsen their in-hospital mortality,[236] potentially due to insufficient awareness or inaccurate symptom attribution.[237,238]

Age and comorbidities are major covariates interacting with sex and impacting outcomes. Women with ACS are older, with more diabetes, hypertension, and heart failure. This often results in a greater rate of in-hospital mortality for women with ACS.[239,240] From an analysis of international randomized trials in ACS, 30-day mortality was higher among women as compared to men presenting with ST-segment elevation MI (STEMI), and lower for females presenting with unstable

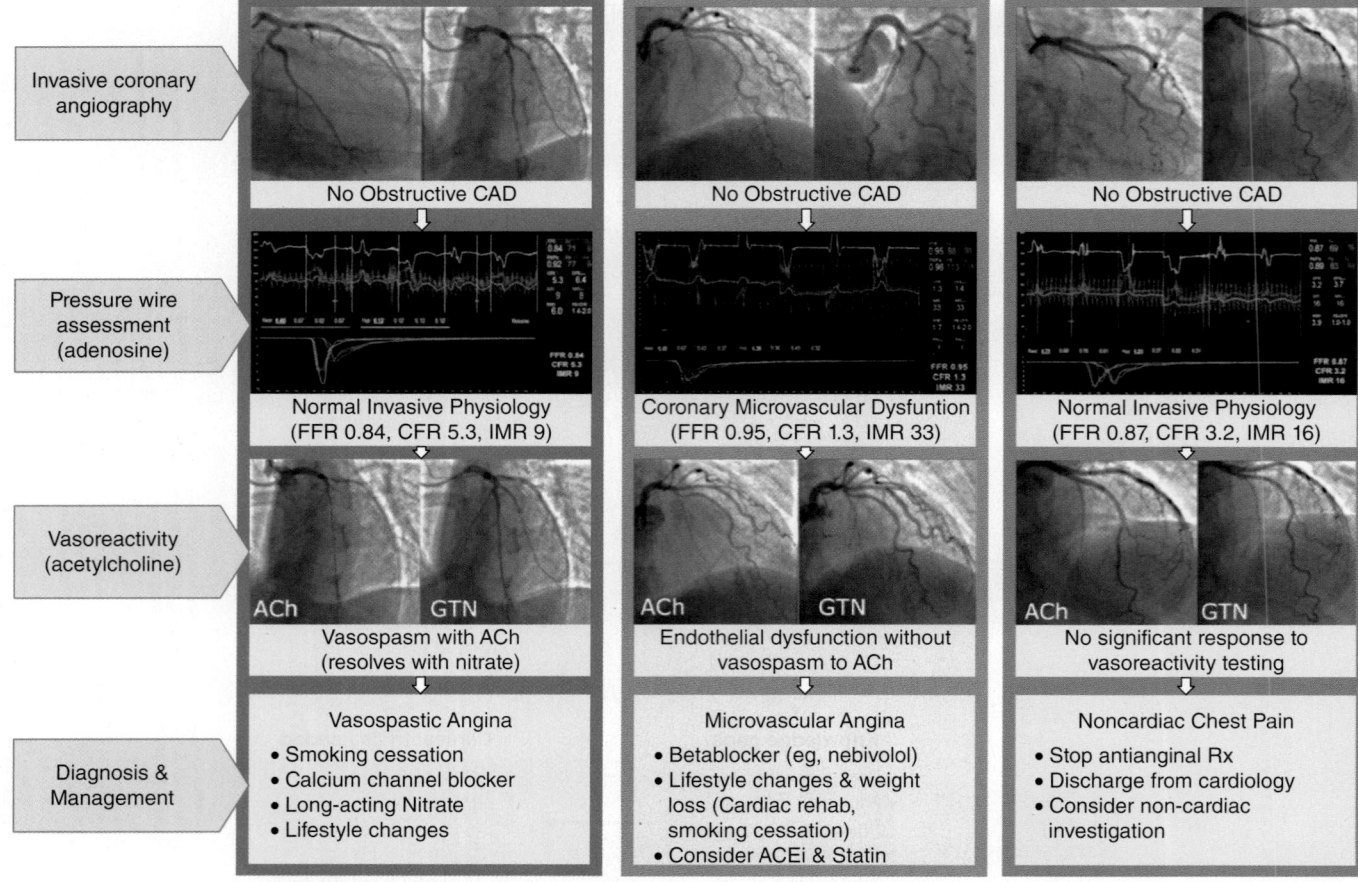

Figure 80–10. The diagnostic evaluation and treatment pathway from the CorMicA trial. Reproduced with permission from Ford TJ, Stanley B, Good R, et al. Stratified Medical Therapy Using Invasive Coronary Function Testing in Angina: The CorMicA Trial. *J Am Coll Cardiol*. 2018 Dec 11;72(23 Pt A):2841-2855.

angina or non-STEMI (NSTEMI).[21] However, after adjustment for angiographic disease severity, sex differences in mortality by ACS type disappeared. From the National Inpatient Sample, declines in fatal MI between 2001 and 2010 were observed for women overall, yet mortality remained higher for females <55 years as compared to similarly aged men.[241] Over a similar time period, a population survey reported increasing MI prevalence among midlife women compared with declines among men.[49] Women with MI are more likely than men to have recurrent MI and be subsequently disabled by heart failure.[242]

At angiography, more women than men have nonobstructive CAD, and therefore a lower need for mechanical reperfusion with percutaneous coronary intervention (PCI).[243] Nonetheless, there are no sex-specific guideline recommendations for PCI.[244-247] PCI for NSTEMI reduces mortality and recurrent MI in high-risk women undergoing an early invasive strategy.[246,247] Early invasive management of ACS remains an effective treatment strategy for women, however, bleeding risk is an important consideration and major bleeding independently predicts 30-day mortality. As women are at increased risk of procedural bleeding complications, an early invasive management strategy showed benefit only in the higher risk women with ACS. Thus, the ACC/AHA Guidelines recommend an initial conservative strategy for low risk women with ACS, as an early invasive strategy for such women affords no benefit.[248,249] Women with STEMI undergoing CABG have an increased in-hospital mortality compared with men, but no sex-specific guideline recommendations are available.

Complication rates following MI are higher in women than men, despite similar success rates with treatment. Following NSTEMI, these include bleeding, heart failure, shock, renal failure, reinfarction, stroke, and readmission.[243] Mechanical complications such as acute severe mitral regurgitation, septal rupture, free wall rupture, and heart failure are also more likely to occur in women, whereas ventricular arrhythmias do not differ by sex. Data from the Global Registry of Acute Coronary Events reported that women had a 43% increased risk of bleeding during hospitalization.[250] Women undergoing PCI also incurred more in-hospital major bleeding, including access-related complications,[251] in part due to inappropriate dosing of antithrombotic therapies.

Regarding additional medical management, antithrombotic drugs such as antiplatelet and anticoagulant therapies reduce the risk of thrombotic complications and recurrent ischemic events. However, women have an increased bleeding risk with antiplatelet and antithrombotic agents, mandating careful attention to weight and renal calculation of doses.[249] Despite this, women with ACS are recommended to receive the same pharmacologic therapy as men, including aspirin and other antiplatelet agents, anticoagulants, statins, β-blockers, and angiotensin-converting enzyme (ACE) inhibitors, both in the acute and chronic setting for secondary prevention. Statin therapy is an effective secondary prevention intervention for both women and men, but women had no benefit for reduced stroke or all-cause mortality.[252]

A post hoc analysis from the Metabolic Efficiency with Ranolazine for Less Ischemia in Non-ST-Elevation Acute Coronary Syndromes (MERLIN)-TIMI 36 trial evaluating ranolazine in the management of ACS[253] showed striking sex differences.[254] In MERLIN, a total of 6,650 patients with NSTEMI were randomized to ranolazine versus placebo, with no effect on the primary endpoint (ASCVD death, MI, or recurrent ischemia). However, the primary endpoint in women was significant ($P = 0.03$), with a marked difference in the component endpoint of reduced recurrent ischemia ($P = 0.002$). Furthermore, women in the MERLIN trial had more ischemic episodes on continuous ECG recording during the hospitalization, with ECG ischemia predictive of an unfavorable outcome.[254]

Women with both STEMI and NSTEMI are recommended to receive behavioral interventions including smoking cessation and referral to a comprehensive cardiac rehabilitation program.[244,249] Cardiac rehabilitation is an essential component of comprehensive care following ACS with unquestionable morbidity and mortality benefits.[255] Nonetheless, women are 55% less likely to participate in cardiac rehabilitation than men, with one contributor being the lack of referral by the treating physician.[256,257] Women especially at risk of not participating in cardiac rehabilitation include the uninsured, unmarried, socioeconomically disadvantaged, smokers, depressed, obese, sedentary, elderly, and non-White and also those with less education, social support, and competing family obligations. Home-based cardiac rehabilitation may prove effective for women with significant barriers to attending structured outpatient programs.[258]

A uniform finding across the years is that women with ACS are less likely to be treated with guideline-directed medical therapies and less likely to undergo cardiac catheterization and coronary revascularization.[259-261] Data from the Get with the Guidelines CAD registry encompassing 78,254 patients with acute MI in 420 hospitals between 2001 and 2006 highlighted important sex differences.[261] Compared to men, women were older, more likely to have comorbidities, and less likely to experience STEMI. However, although there were no sex differences in hospital mortality, women with STEMI had higher adjusted mortality rates, 10.2% versus 5.5%, with increased STEMI mortality evident very early and within the initial 24 hours. This was associated with a lower likelihood of early aspirin and β-blocker use, reperfusion therapy, and timely reperfusion. Underuse of evidence-based treatment for women and delayed reperfusion represent opportunities to decrease sex disparities in the care and outcomes of women with STEMI.[261] Also in this

registry in a subset of 49,358 patients aged 65 years and older, women were less likely than men to receive optimal care at discharge. The authors concluded that approximately 69% of the sex disparity may potentially be reduced by providing optimal quality of care to women. In contrast, the higher mortality in Black American patients observed in both sexes could not be accounted for by differences in the quality of care as measured in this study.[262] In the VIRGO registry of women and men aged 18 to 55 with acute MI,[263,264] women were less likely to return to work after MI than were men.[265] The Canadian ACS registry assessed the factors influencing the underutilization of evidence-based therapies in women.[266] Women in this ACS cohort had higher death rates than men but lower use of ACE inhibitors, β-blockers, and statins. There was apparent lower assessment of patient risk, as evidenced by the clinical decision not to investigate further with cardiac catheterization. Despite adjustment for confounders, female sex remained associated with underutilization of therapy with lipid modifying agents and ACE inhibitors.

MI AND NONOBSTRUCTIVE CAD

MI and nonobstructive CAD (MINOCA) occurs in 6% of patients where the diagnosis is initially considered at the time of invasive coronary angiography.[267,268] Nearly half of MINOCA patients are women.[267] There are assorted clinical conditions that are causative and additional evaluation is required to guide clinical management of MINOCA patients. MINOCA patients may present with STEMI or NSTEMI but generally have a lower troponin elevation and overall have an improved prognosis when compared to other acute MI patients.[267,269] A key to management is the detection of nonischemic (eg, myocarditis) from ischemic mechanisms of myocardial injury. CMR imaging demonstration of myocardial necrosis is useful to examine alternative etiologies such as nonischemic cardiomyopathy or myocarditis.[270-273] In the largest series of 388 patients (48% women), CMR was able to identify the cause of the troponin elevation in 75% of patients including those with myocarditis (25%), cardiomyopathy (25%), and MI (25%).[271] Over 3.5 years of follow-up, mortality was worse for those with cardiomyopathy (19%) and MI (4%) as compared to those with myocarditis (2%) or for those with a normal CMR.

Other noteworthy but underdiagnosed causes of ACS in women include spontaneous coronary artery dissection (SCAD), spasm, and Takotsubo cardiomyopathy.[37,274-277] SCAD is defined as a spontaneous separation of the coronary artery wall (unrelated to iatrogenic catheter use or trauma) and its prevalence in ACS is estimated at 1% to 4%.[276,277] A case of SCAD in a 69-year-old woman with a baseline CCTA and an invasive coronary angiogram following incident MI at 3 years of follow-up is presented in **Fig 80–11**.[278] Those with SCAD present with ACS and troponin elevation, with varied proportions categorized as STEMI.[276] Angiographic features of diffusivity, tortuosity, and multiple radiolucent lumens are characteristic of SCAD. Importantly, SCAD is much more prevalent among women than men, especially in those ≤50 years of age.[276,277,279,280]

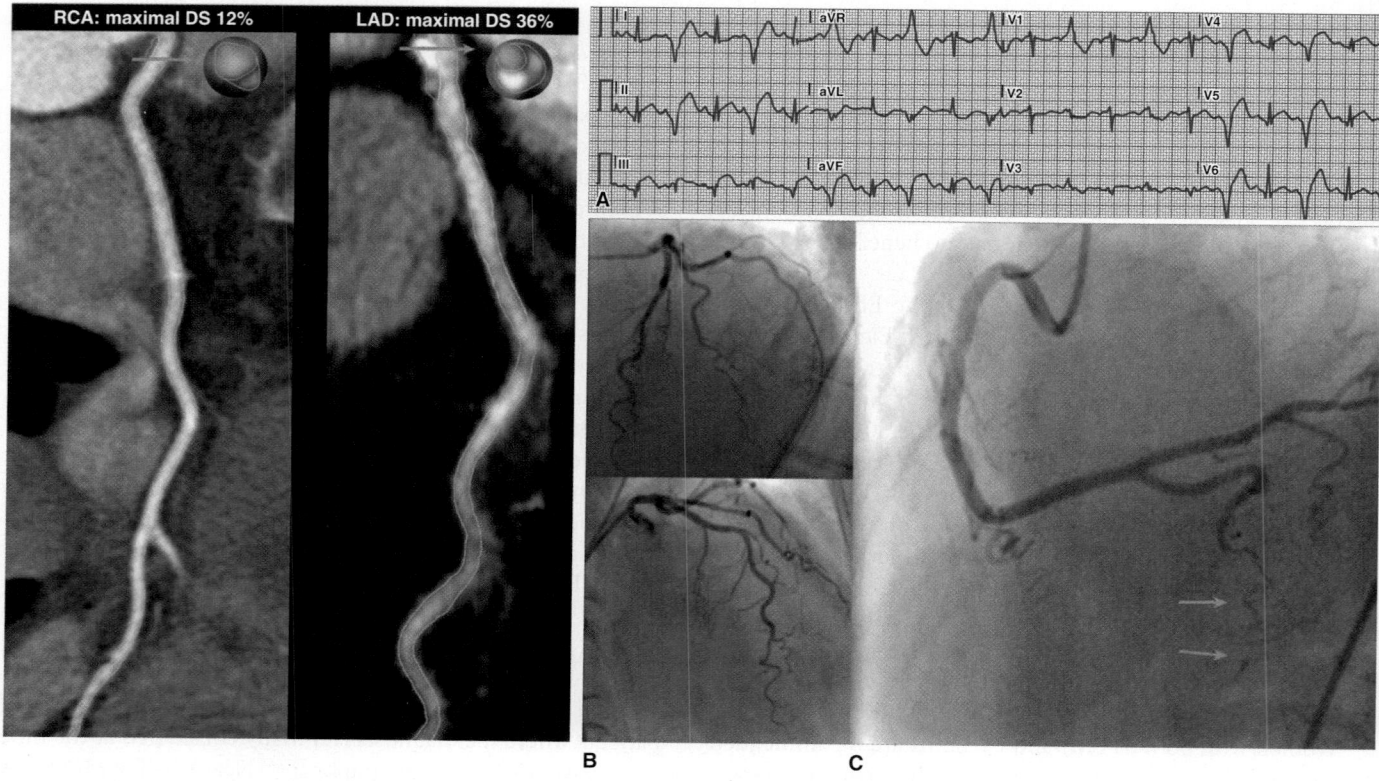

Figure 80–11. A case of SCAD in a 69-year-old woman with a baseline CCTA and an invasive coronary angiogram following incident MI at 3 years of follow-up. *Orange arrows* indicate cross section of maximal diameter stenosis. On the cross section, *light green* indicates fibrofatty plaque 31–130 Hounsfield units (HU); *dark green* indicates fibrous plaque 131 to 350 HU; and *gray* indicates calcified plaque >350 HU. (**A**) ECG showing an STEMI. (**B**) Invasive coronary angiography (ICA) showing minimal CAD in the left anterior descending artery and left circumflex artery. (**C**) ICA showing a SCAD of the right posterior descending artery, classified as a type 2B due to a long diffuse and smooth stenosis that extends to the distal tip of the artery (*orange arrows*). LAD, left anterior descending artery; RCA, right coronary artery. Reproduced with permission from van den Hoogen IJ, Gianni U, Wood MJ, et al. The Clinical Spectrum of Myocardial Infarction and Ischemia With Nonobstructive Coronary Arteries in Women. *JACC Cardiovasc Imaging*. 2021 May;14(5):1053-1062.

Fibromuscular dysplasia is the most commonly associated condition.[277] SCAD is also the most common cause of pregnancy-related MI, with risk increasing with multiparity.[281] Precipitating physical or emotional stress is commonly reported.[280] Nearly 1 in 10 patients (91% women) have recurrent SCAD over ~3 years of follow-up.[282] The 10-year mortality is also high at 7.7%, with a very high incidence of major CAD events at 47%.[279] Despite the overall low early mortality rate with SCAD, complications are high in PCI-treated patients, because PCI may propagate the dissection.[279]

Coronary vasospasm remains an important consideration despite unclear evidence as to varied occurrence in women versus men.[283] Nearly 1 in 4 ACS patients do not have an identifiable culprit lesion.[284] From the Coronary Artery Spasm in Patients With Acute Coronary Syndrome (CASPAR) registry including ACS patients with nonobstructive CAD, nearly half of patients had verified spasm following acetylcholine provocation.[284]

Finally, Takotsubo cardiomyopathy is characterized by stress-induced left ventricular dysfunction, often presenting with apical ballooning, that is transient and typically resolves within 1 to 2 months.[285,286] Nearly 90% of Takotsubo cardiomyopathy cases are women. Emotional or physical stress may be identified as common triggers resulting in catecholamine excess stimulation causing left ventricular dysfunction. In-hospital complications are common, including acute heart failure, mitral regurgitation, and cardiogenic shock.[285]

CORONARY REVASCULARIZATION

Percutaneous Coronary Interventions

Across both elective and urgent cases undergoing PCI, women are older and have more comorbidities.[287] In the NHLBI Dynamic Registry of PCI, women were more likely to have high-risk characteristics than men, including older age, diabetes, hypertension, hypercholesterolemia, heart failure, and unstable angina.[288] Over time, improvement in outcomes for women have been reported, perhaps related to better appreciation of pathophysiologic variables specific to women.[289] From the large German Society of Cardiology registry including all indications for PCI, primary PCI success was identical between the sexes (94%).[290] From a patient-level pooled analysis, women receiving drug eluting stents had a reduced 3-year rate of death or MI when compared to those receiving bare metal stents (10.9% vs 12.8%; *P* = 0.001).[291] By comparison, a recent analysis of long-term, 5-year major adverse CAD events (defined as

CAD death, MI, or ischemia-driven target lesion revascularization), women had higher rates of MACE compared with men (18.9% vs 17.7% for women and men, respectively, P = 0.003) and this difference persisted in multivariable models.

When considering procedural complications, women are at an increased risk of bleeding, transfusion, vascular complications, and post-PCI renal failure.[292,293] From a large PCI registry, women had twice the access-related complications as men.[290] Results from several large contemporary registries of coronary stenting show that women experienced higher procedural risk than men, but improved near and long-term survival.[19,294] Although women have almost twice the rate of bleeding after PCI as men,[295] the registry-based randomized Study of Access Site for Enhancement of PCI for Women trial showed reductions in bleeding or vascular complications with radial access.[296]

In the acute setting, young women less than 50 years of age demonstrated an increased risk of target vessel and target lesion failure despite less severe angiographic CAD when compared to men.[297] Moreover, from the Nationwide Inpatient Sample of 6,601,526 patients (33% women) undergoing PCI from 2004 to 2014,[287] women as compared to men were more often older, with increased rates of comorbidities and NSTEMI. Consequently, women had higher rates of in-hospital mortality (2.0% vs 1.4% in men) and complications (11.1% vs 7.0% for men), even in models controlling for varied clinical and procedural variables. Women with STEMI experienced a 20% higher age-adjusted risk of in-hospital death and other ischemic events.[290]

Numerous trials in patients with stable CAD have compared the effectiveness of PCI with optimal medical therapy (OMT) versus OMT alone. The Clinical Outcomes Utilizing Revascularization and Aggressive Drug Evaluation (COURAGE) trial reported no differences in treatment effectiveness by sex (P = 0.07).[298] There was, however, a significant interaction between women and men with regards to hospitalization for heart failure (P = 0.02). The relative hazard for PCI with OMT versus OMT alone was 0.59 for women (P <0.001) and 0.86 for men (P = 0.47). Recently, the results from the NHLBI-sponsored ISCHEMIA trial reported on 5179 patients with stable CAD and moderate-severe ischemia who were randomized to an invasive versus conservative strategy of care revealing similar outcomes through 3.2 years of follow-up.[219] A secondary analysis revealed that women in ISCHEMIA had more frequent angina, independent of less severe ischemia and less extensive CAD than men.[145]

CABG Surgery

Women constitute 20% to 30% of the CABG surgical population, about 180,000 procedures annually. Mortality is greater for women than for men,[299] especially among younger women.[300] It is estimated that an excess of nearly 400 deaths occur each year within 30 days of isolated CABG surgery among women when compared to men.[301] Contributing factors may be an increase in nonelective surgery or late referral, reduced use of an arterial conduit, and an excess of procedural complications. Worse outcomes have also been attributed to smaller coronary arteries with more diffuse CAD.[302] From the Society of Thoracic Surgeons registry[303] comprising 344,913 patients (28% women), female patients were older and more likely to have diabetes, hypertension, peripheral vascular disease, and to undergo nonelective procedures. Operative mortality was 4.5% for women versus 2.6% for men. Women had increased operative mortality for every risk factor examined univariately. In a review of 23 CABG studies that reported data stratified by sex,[304] women were older and sicker at the time of CABG. Adjustment for baseline differences reduced but did not eliminate the increased in-hospital mortality observed for women. Women were less likely to receive an internal mammary artery graft and had more postoperative complications including renal failure, neurological complications, and postoperative MI.[304]

Data from the National CVD Network registry (n = 51,187 patients with 30% women) also reported that women were at greater risk following CABG surgery as compared to men.[109] For women younger than age 50, there was a 3-fold increase in hospital mortality, with sex differences decreasing with advancing age.[109] Despite these findings, women versus men of all ages had better left ventricular function and fewer diseased vessels at surgery. In the Northern New England CVD registry of 26,725 CABG patients, hospital mortality rate was 4.1% for women and 2.1% for men.[305] The majority of excess mortality in women was related to diabetes or to an urgent/emergent presentation. Women as compared to men less than 50 years of age had a greater burden of comorbidities and were more likely to have emergency surgery and decreased use of arterial grafts, the latter possibly explaining the excess mortality observed among younger women. In a case-control study of CABG, women had higher perioperative risk in all comorbidity categories compared with matched male controls.[303] As with all other coronary presentations, women undergoing CABG had an excess of bleeding complications, and it remains unclear if sex differences in blood vessels or blood factors underlie the increased bleeding risk. In a recent report, women received less complete multiple arterial coronary revascularization than men, and were less likely to receive bilateral internal thoracic artery or three arterial grafts.[306] In contrast, a recent analysis of 1,863,719 Medicare beneficiaries revealed some favorable trends in mortality among women undergoing CABG from 1999 to 2014 with declines occurring in in-hospital, 30-day, and 1-year mortality.[307]

The Synergy Between PCI with Taxus and Cardiac Surgery (SYNTAX) trial, which enrolled patients with multivessel CAD, reported a higher 4-year mortality for women treated with PCI as compared to men, while women and men undergoing CABG had similar outcomes.[308] Recently, the Evaluation of XIENCE Versus CABG for Effectiveness of Left Main Revascularization (EXCEL) trial reported that near-term results at 30 days were worse for women undergoing PCI (P <0.001) as compared to other groups undergoing CABG or for men treated with PCI.[309] This higher risk status for women treated with PCI was of borderline significance at 3 years of follow-up (P = 0.06).

GLOBAL PERSPECTIVES

In the United States, declines in ASCVD burden have been reported over the last 30 years, yet the rate of decline has been significantly less for women as compared to men.[310] Around the world, the largest number of deaths from noncommunicable diseases is from ASCVD including nearly 18 million deaths, increasing by 21% since 2007 and including 8.5 million women.[311-314] Overall, more than 200 million women are living with ASCVD worldwide, including 46.1 million with IHD.[314] The burden of ASCVD is attributable to progressive urbanization resulting in unfavorable changes in ASCVD lifestyles in developing nations including increasing rates of obesity, hypertension, dyslipidemia, and diabetes. From 1990 to 2020, there was a 120% increase in ASCVD mortality among women in developing countries, contrasted with a 29% increase for females within industrialized countries. In the INTERHEART study, modifiable risk factors accounted for 94% of the population-adjusted ASCVD mortality in women.[54,315-317]

In 2018, the United Nations held its Third Summit on Noncommunicable Diseases where they set goals for reducing premature deaths by 45%.[318] A series of these health summits have been held and highlight sex disparities in prognosis and access to diagnostic and treatment services, establishing compelling linkages with the empowerment of women. The vulnerability of women was highlighted in these summits by the finding that 60% of the world's poor are women and two-thirds of illiterate adults are women.[319] Women are often a focal point of a majority of households throughout the world, with the matriarch of the family central to understanding and adapting habits of a heart-healthy lifestyle.[315] Because women often serve as role models in the lives of others, their examples of good ASCVD health (eg, exercising, not smoking, limiting alcohol, managing high blood pressure and diabetes, managing stress, and eating well) have the potential to improve not only their own personal health, but to positively influence others to do the same.[320] Key global goals are to educate women about ASCVD risk factors, specifically modifiable behavioral risk factors. Prominent among these are smoking cessation, a diet decreased in sodium and saturated fats and increased in fresh fruits and vegetables, as well increased physical activity.[315,321]

UNMET NEEDS

Despite the continued focus on sex differences in ASCVD, inequities of care profoundly impact the lives of millions of women of diverse race and ethnicity around the world.[24] Given that suboptimal care of women has been reported for decades, the relative lack of substantive progress and potential for indifference on the part of physicians, scientists, and other stakeholders regarding the importance of reducing the gap in cardiovascular care for women as compared to men.[24] Throughout the years, there have been calls for a more thorough examination of clinical detection and care gaps that disproportionately impact women. In 2015, the First National Policy and Science Summit on Women's ASCVD Health[322]

highlighted several unanswered research questions likely to positively impact ASCVD outcomes for women including: (1) the identification of unique biological variables most influential for the development of adverse sequelae of ASCVD, (2) the development of effective preventive strategies, and (3) the understanding of causal factors which impact disparities in care between women and men. More recently, *The Lancet* convened a clinical commission on women and ASCVD. The goals of this commission were to summarize the evidence and devise specific recommendations to improve gaps in research and care, and generate global awareness regarding the needs and issues that specifically impact women.[323] Throughout the world, women are uniquely vulnerable and disadvantaged both in society and in the clinical care setting.[324] A woman's vulnerabilities impact ASCVD in varied ways such that age, race, ethnicity, and socioeconomic status compound our abilities to define sex-specific phenotypes. Certainly, any concept of a single defining signature of risk is overly simplistic and likely many phenotypic variations exist. However, until we seek to engage across multiple dimensions of gender (culture/society) and sex (biology), our abilities to reduce the impact of ASCVD on women will be diminished.[325] Women's awareness of IHD is a critical variable. In the decade from 2009 to 2019, awareness of heart disease as the leading cause of death declined from 65% to 44%, particularly among Hispanic and Black women and in younger women, in whom primary prevention may be most effective.[326] Thus, women's cardiovascular health is not solely a medical issue. Eradication or lessening of the burden of ASCVD requires a multifaceted approach and involvement from the community, government, social advocates, and others in order to support social change meeting the unique needs of women. Both in developed and developing nations, a focus on preventive care should not only target high-risk populations, but create population programs to globally reduce the burden of ASCVD in a manner that is also optimized for women.

SUMMARY

This chapter highlights the evidence on sex differences in the pathophysiology and clinical presentations of IHD, and identifies significant disparities in the management of ASCVD, from primary prevention to the treatment of stable and acute coronary syndromes, resulting in an elevated risk of adverse events in women. The greater risk factor and comorbidity burden as well as advanced age of women presenting for cardiovascular care compounds the challenges of their appropriate management and further accelerates their ASCVD risk.[171,327] Women often present with variable symptom characteristics and with a reduced frequency of obstructive CAD that may confound traditional methods of risk assessment and management, yet likely reflect varying manifestations of sex-specific atherosclerotic plaque biology.[4,328] A working model of female-specific angina is detailed in **Fig. 80-12**. While substantive progress has been made in understanding the role of vascular dysfunction and coronary blood flow abnormalities with CMD as a driver for worsening clinical outcomes,

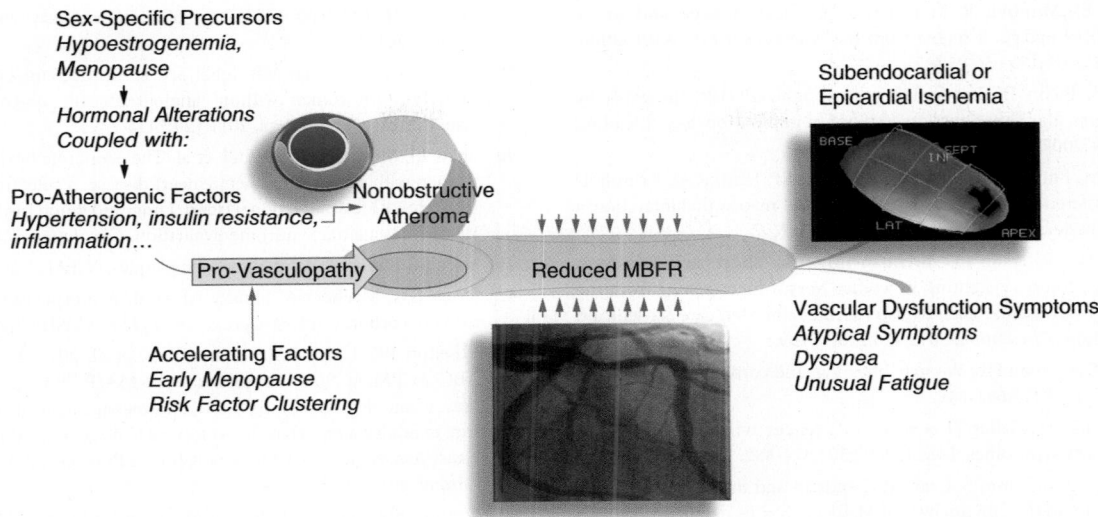

Figure 80–12. Hypothetical model of female-specific angina. Reproduced with permission from Shaw LJ, Bugiardini R, Merz CN. Women and ischemic heart disease: evolving knowledge. *J Am Coll Cardiol.* 2009 Oct 20;54(17):1561-1575.

much work remains to be done in this area.[4] There is growing evidence to suggest that diffuse nonobstructive atherosclerosis inclusive of high-risk plaque features, such as low attenuation plaque and positive remodeling, may act as a precursor to future CVD events in women. Ongoing investigations correlating pathologic and in vivo imaging evidence may profoundly impact clinical diagnosis of at-risk women. Currently, guideline-directed strategies for nonobstructive CAD remain ill-defined. However, considerable research has focused on strategies to improve the elevated risk status of women referred for coronary revascularization with some success. There remains in general considerable unmet needs of women at risk for ASCVD. Without concentrated population health and point of care strategies tailored for women, it remains unlikely that marked reductions in the observed high rates of adverse cardiovascular outcomes in women will be realized in the near future. Timely reduction of ASCVD risk specifically in women will depend on the generation and application of evidence-based approaches targeting the role of sex differences in biology, unique clinical and population needs of women, and persistent gender-based socioeconomic disparities. Only by systematically targeting these sizeable hurdles can we hope to effect meaningful change in outcomes for the large and growing population of young and older women at risk for ASCVD.

REFERENCES

1. Fihn SD, Gardin JM, Abrams J, et al. 2012 ACCF/AHA/ACP/AATS/PCNA/SCAI/STS Guideline for the diagnosis and management of patients with stable ischemic heart disease: a report of the American College of Cardiology Foundation/American Heart Association Task Force on Practice Guidelines, and the American College of Physicians, American Association for Thoracic Surgery, Preventive Cardiovascular Nurses Association, Society for Cardiovascular Angiography and Interventions, and Society of Thoracic Surgeons. *J Am Coll Cardiol.* 2012;60:e44-e164.

2. Baldassarre LA, Raman SV, Min JK, et al. Noninvasive imaging to evaluate women with stable ischemic heart disease. *JACC Cardiovasc Imaging.* 2016;9:421-435.

3. Agrawal S, Mehta PK, Bairey Merz CN. Cardiac syndrome X: update. *Heart Fail Clin.* 2016;12:141-156.

4. Pepine CJ, Ferdinand KC, Shaw LJ, et al. Emergence of nonobstructive coronary artery disease: a woman's problem and need for change in definition on angiography. *J Am Coll Cardiol.* 2015;66:1918-1933.

5. Bairey Merz CN, Regitz-Zagrosek V. The case for sex- and gender-specific medicine. *JAMA Intern Med.* 2014;174:1348-1349.

6. Ouyang P, Wenger NK, Taylor D, et al. Strategies and methods to study female-specific cardiovascular health and disease: a guide for clinical scientists. *Biol Sex Differences.* 2016;7:19.

7. Ma J, Ward EM, Siegel RL, Jemal A. Temporal trends in mortality in the United States, 1969-2013. *JAMA.* 2015;314:1731-1739.

8. Wilmot KA, O'Flaherty M, Capewell S, Ford ES, Vaccarino V. Coronary heart disease mortality declines in the United States from 1979 through 2011: evidence for stagnation in young adults, especially women. *Circulation.* 2015;132:997-1002.

9. Miller VM, Reckelhoff JF. Sex as a biological variable: now what?! *Physiology (Bethesda).* 2016;31:78-80.

10. Miller VM, Rocca WA, Faubion SS. Sex differences research, precision medicine, and the future of women's health. *J Womens Health (Larchmt).* 2015;24:969-971.

11. Becker JB, Arnold AP, Berkley KJ, et al. Strategies and methods for research on sex differences in brain and behavior. *Endocrinology.* 2005;146:1650-1673.

12. Writing Group M, Mozaffarian D, Benjamin EJ, et al. Heart disease and stroke statistics-2016 update: a report from the American Heart Association. *Circulation.* 2016;133:e38-e60.

13. Hartley A, Marshall DC, Salciccioli JD, Sikkel MB, Maruthappu M, Shalhoub J. Trends in mortality from ischemic heart disease and cerebrovascular disease in Europe: 1980 to 2009. *Circulation.* 2016;133:1916-1926.

14. Virani SS, Alonso A, Benjamin EJ, et al. Heart disease and stroke statistics-2020 update: a report from the American Heart Association. *Circulation.* 2020;141:e139-e596.

15. Center for Disease Control and Prevention NCfHS. Underlying Cause of Death 1999-2017 on CDC WONDER Online Database, released December 2018.

16. Benjamin EJ, Muntner P, Alonso A, et al. Heart disease and stroke statistics-2019 update: a report from the American Heart Association. *Circulation.* 2019;139:e56-e528.

17. Owens DS, Plehn JF. Recognizing unrecognized risk: the evolving role of ventricular functional assessment in population-based studies. *Circulation.* 2007;116:126-130.

18. Bucholz EM, Butala NM, Rathore SS, Dreyer RP, Lansky AJ, Krumholz HM. Sex differences in long-term mortality after myocardial infarction: a systematic review. *Circulation.* 2014;130:757-767.

19. Anderson ML, Peterson ED, Brennan JM, et al. Short- and long-term outcomes of coronary stenting in women versus men: results from the National Cardiovascular Data Registry Centers for Medicare & Medicaid services cohort. *Circulation.* 2012;126:2190-2199.

20. Ahmed B, Dauerman HL. Women, bleeding, and coronary intervention. *Circulation.* 2013;127:641-649.

21. Berger JS, Elliott L, Gallup D, et al. Sex differences in mortality following acute coronary syndromes. *JAMA.* 2009;302:874-882.

22. Singh JA, Lu X, Ibrahim S, Cram P. Trends in and disparities for acute myocardial infarction: an analysis of Medicare claims data from 1992 to 2010. *BMC Med.* 2014;12:190.

23. Mosca L, Benjamin EJ, Berra K, et al. Effectiveness-based guidelines for the prevention of cardiovascular disease in women–2011 update: a guideline from the American Heart Association. *Circulation.* 2011;123:1243-1262.

24. Shaw LJ, Pepine CJ, Xie J, et al. Quality and equitable health care gaps for women: attributions to sex differences in cardiovascular medicine. *J Am Coll Cardiol.* 2017;70:373-388.

25. Shaw LJ, Butler J. Targeting priority populations to reduce disparities in cardiovascular care: health equity for all. *J Am Coll Cardiol.* 2014;64:346-348.

26. Mehta LS, Beckie TM, DeVon HA, et al. Acute myocardial infarction in women: a scientific statement from the American Heart Association. *Circulation.* 2016;133:916-947.

27. Lansky AJ, Ng VG, Maehara A, et al. Gender and the extent of coronary atherosclerosis, plaque composition, and clinical outcomes in acute coronary syndromes. *JACC Cardiovasc Imaging* 2012;5:S62-72.

28. Virmani R, Burke AP, Farb A, Kolodgie FD. Pathology of the vulnerable plaque. *J Am Coll Cardiol.* 2006;47:C13-C18.

29. Chang HJ, Lin FY, Lee SE, et al. Coronary atherosclerotic precursors of acute coronary syndromes. *J Am Coll Cardiol.* 2018;71:2511-2522.

30. Jia H, Abtahian F, Aguirre AD, et al. In vivo diagnosis of plaque erosion and calcified nodule in patients with acute coronary syndrome by intravascular optical coherence tomography. *J Am Coll Cardiol.* 2013;62:1748-1758.

31. Osborn EA, Jaffer FA. Imaging atherosclerosis and risk of plaque rupture. *Current Atheroscler Rep.* 2013;15:359.

32. Falk E, Nakano M, Bentzon JF, Finn AV, Virmani R. Update on acute coronary syndromes: the pathologists' view. *Eur Heart J.* 2013;34:719-728.

33. Higuma T, Soeda T, Abe N, et al. A combined optical coherence tomography and intravascular ultrasound study on plaque rupture, plaque erosion, and calcified nodule in patients with ST-segment elevation myocardial infarction: incidence, morphologic characteristics, and outcomes after percutaneous coronary intervention. *JACC Cardiovasc Intervent.* 2015;8:1166-1176.

34. Lafont A. Basic aspects of plaque vulnerability. *Heart.* 2003;89:1262-1267.

35. Sheifer SE, Canos MR, Weinfurt KP, et al. Sex differences in coronary artery size assessed by intravascular ultrasound. *Am Heart J.* 2000;139:649-653.

36. Han SH, Bae JH, Holmes DR, Jr. et al. Sex differences in atheroma burden and endothelial function in patients with early coronary atherosclerosis. *Eur Heart J.* 2008;29:1359-1369.

37. Yahagi K, Davis HR, Arbustini E, Virmani R. Sex differences in coronary artery disease: pathological observations. *Atherosclerosis.* 2015;239:260-267.

38. Davies MJ. The pathophysiology of acute coronary syndromes. *Heart.* 2000;83:361-366.

39. Reynolds HR, Srichai MB, Iqbal SN, et al. Mechanisms of myocardial infarction in women without angiographically obstructive coronary artery disease. *Circulation.* 2011;124:1414-1425.

40. Shaw LJ, Merz CN, Pepine CJ, et al. The economic burden of angina in women with suspected ischemic heart disease: results from the National Institutes of Health–National Heart, Lung, and Blood Institute–sponsored Women's Ischemia Syndrome Evaluation. *Circulation.* 2006;114:894-904.

41. Narula J, Strauss HW. The popcorn plaques. *Nat Med.* 2007;13:532-534.

42. Stone GW, Maehara A, Lansky AJ, et al. A prospective natural-history study of coronary atherosclerosis. *N Engl J Med.* 2011;364:226-235.

43. Whelton PK, Carey RM, Aronow WS, et al. 2017 ACC/AHA/AAPA/ABC/ACPM/AGS/APhA/ASH/ASPC/NMA/PCNA guideline for the prevention, detection, evaluation, and management of high blood pressure in adults: a report of the American College of Cardiology/American Heart Association Task Force on Clinical Practice Guidelines. *J Am Coll Cardiol.* 2018;71:e127-e248.

44. Grundy SM, Stone NJ, Bailey AL, et al. 2018 AHA/ACC/AACVPR/AAPA/ABC/ACPM/ADA/AGS/APhA/ASPC/NLA/PCNA guideline on the management of blood cholesterol: a report of the American College of Cardiology/American Heart Association Task Force on Clinical Practice Guidelines. *J Am Coll Cardiol.* 2019;73:e285-e350.

45. Arnett DK, Blumenthal RS, Albert MA, et al. 2019 ACC/AHA guideline on the primary prevention of cardiovascular disease: a report of the American College of Cardiology/American Heart Association Task Force on Clinical Practice Guidelines. *J Am Coll Cardiol.* 2019;74:e177-e232.

46. Cho L, Davis M, Elgendy I, et al. Summary of updated recommendations for primary prevention of cardiovascular disease in women: JACC State-of-the-Art Review. *J Am Coll Cardiol.* 2020;75:2602-2618.

47. Mosca L, Benjamin EJ, Berra K, et al. Effectiveness-based guidelines for the prevention of cardiovascular disease in women–2011 update: a guideline from the American Heart Association. *J Am Coll Cardiol.* 2011;57:1404-1423.

48. Ford I, Murray H, Packard CJ, et al. Long-term follow-up of the West of Scotland Coronary Prevention Study. *N Engl J Med.* 2007;357:1477-1486.

49. Towfighi A, Zheng L, Ovbiagele B. Sex-specific trends in midlife coronary heart disease risk and prevalence. *Arch Int Med.* 2009;169:1762-1766.

50. Brown HL, Warner JJ, Gianos E, et al. Promoting risk identification and reduction of cardiovascular disease in women through collaboration with obstetricians and gynecologists: a presidential advisory from the American Heart Association and the American College of Obstetricians and Gynecologists. *Circulation.* 2018;137:e843-e852.

51. Melloni C, Berger JS, Wang TY, et al. Representation of women in randomized clinical trials of cardiovascular disease prevention. *Circ Cardiovasc Qual Outcomes.* 2010;3:135-142.

52. Go AS, Mozaffarian D, Roger VL, et al. Heart disease and stroke statistics–2014 update: a report from the American Heart Association. *Circulation.* 2014;129:e28-e292.

53. Leifheit-Limson EC, Spertus JA, Reid KJ, et al. Prevalence of traditional cardiac risk factors and secondary prevention among patients hospitalized for acute myocardial infarction (AMI): variation by age, sex, and race. *J Womens Health (Larchmt).* 2013;22:659-666.

54. Yusuf S, Hawken S, Ounpuu S, et al. Effect of potentially modifiable risk factors associated with myocardial infarction in 52 countries (the INTERHEART study): case-control study. *Lancet.* 2004;364:937-952.

55. Chobanian AV, Bakris GL, Black HR, et al. The seventh report of the Joint National Committee on prevention, detection, evaluation, and treatment of high blood pressure: the JNC 7 report. *JAMA.* 2003;289:2560-2572.

56. Hajjar I, Kotchen JM, Kotchen TA. Hypertension: trends in prevalence, incidence, and control. *Annu Rev Public Health.* 2006;27:465-490.

57. Wolf HK, Tuomilehto J, Kuulasmaa K, et al. Blood pressure levels in the 41 populations of the WHO MONICA Project. *J Human Hypertens.* 1997;11:733-742.

58. Group SR, Wright JT, Jr., Williamson JD, et al. A randomized trial of intensive versus standard blood-pressure control. *N Engl J Med.* 2015;373:2103-2116.

59. Wenger NK, Ferdinand KC, Merz CN, et al. Women, hypertension, and the SPRINT. *Am J Med.* 2016.

60. Williams B, Mancia G, Spiering W, et al. 2018 ESC/ESH guidelines for the management of arterial hypertension: the Task Force for the management of arterial hypertension of the European Society of Cardiology and the European Society of Hypertension. *J Hypertens.* 2018;36:1953-2041.

61. Njolstad I, Arnesen E, Lund-Larsen PG. Smoking, serum lipids, blood pressure, and sex differences in myocardial infarction. A 12-year follow-up of the Finnmark Study. *Circulation.* 1996;93:450-456.

62. Pomp ER, Rosendaal FR, Doggen CJ. Smoking increases the risk of venous thrombosis and acts synergistically with oral contraceptive use. *Am J Hematol.* 2008;83:97-102.

63. Huxley RR, Woodward M. Cigarette smoking as a risk factor for coronary heart disease in women compared with men: a systematic review and meta-analysis of prospective cohort studies. *Lancet.* 2011;378: 1297-1305.

64. Regensteiner JG, Golden S, Huebschmann AG, et al. Sex differences in the cardiovascular consequences of diabetes mellitus: a scientific statement from the American Heart Association. *Circulation.* 2015;132: 2424-2447.

65. National Institutes of Health NIoDaDaKD. Diabetes in America. 1995.

66. Kannel WB, Wilson PW. Risk factors that attenuate the female coronary disease advantage. *Arch Intern Med.* 1995;155:57-61.

67. Hu G, Jousilahti P, Qiao Q, Katoh S, Tuomilehto J. Sex differences in cardiovascular and total mortality among diabetic and non-diabetic individuals with or without history of myocardial infarction. *Diabetologia.* 2005;48:856-861.

68. Huxley R, Barzi F, Woodward M. Excess risk of fatal coronary heart disease associated with diabetes in men and women: meta-analysis of 37 prospective cohort studies. *BMJ.* 2006;332:73-78.

69. Gregg EW, Gu Q, Cheng YJ, Narayan KM, Cowie CC. Mortality trends in men and women with diabetes, 1971 to 2000. *Ann Intern Med.* 2007;147:149-155.

70. Gouni-Berthold I, Berthold HK, Mantzoros CS, Bohm M, Krone W. Sex disparities in the treatment and control of cardiovascular risk factors in type 2 diabetes. *Diabetes Care.* 2008;31:1389-1391.

71. Kalyani RR, Lazo M, Ouyang P, et al. Sex differences in diabetes and risk of incident coronary artery disease in healthy young and middle-aged adults. *Diabetes Care.* 2014;37:830-838.

72. Wannamethee SG, Papacosta O, Lawlor DA, et al. Do women exhibit greater differences in established and novel risk factors between diabetes and non-diabetes than men? The British Regional Heart Study and British Women's Heart Health Study. *Diabetologia.* 2012;55:80-87.

73. Peters SA, Yang L, Guo Y, et al. Parenthood and the risk of diabetes in men and women: a 7 year prospective study of 0.5 million individuals. *Diabetologia.* 2016;59:1675-1682.

74. Peters SA, Huxley RR, Woodward M. Diabetes as a risk factor for stroke in women compared with men: a systematic review and meta-analysis of 64 cohorts, including 775,385 individuals and 12,539 strokes. *Lancet.* 2014;383:1973-1980.

75. Bird CE, Fremont AM, Bierman AS, et al. Does quality of care for cardiovascular disease and diabetes differ by gender for enrollees in managed care plans? *Womens Health Issues.* 2007;17:131-138.

76. Mercado C, DeSimone AK, Odom E, Gillespie C, Ayala C, Loustalot F. Prevalence of cholesterol treatment eligibility and medication use among adults–United States, 2005-2012. *MMWR.* 2015;64:1305-1311.

77. Virani SS, Woodard LD, Ramsey DJ, et al. Gender disparities in evidence-based statin therapy in patients with cardiovascular disease. *Am J Cardiol.* 2015;115:21-26.

78. Safford MM, Gamboa CM, Durant RW, et al. Race-sex differences in the management of hyperlipidemia: the REasons for Geographic and Racial Differences in Stroke study. *Am J Prevent Med.* 2015;48:520-527.

79. Parris ES, Lawrence DB, Mohn LA, Long LB. Adherence to statin therapy and LDL cholesterol goal attainment by patients with diabetes and dyslipidemia. *Diabetes Care.* 2005;28:595-599.

80. Stone NJ, Robinson JG, Lichtenstein AH, et al. 2013 ACC/AHA guideline on the treatment of blood cholesterol to reduce atherosclerotic cardiovascular risk in adults: a report of the American College of Cardiology/ American Heart Association Task Force on Practice Guidelines. *J Am Coll Cardiol.* 2014;63:2889-2934.

81. Karmali KN, Goff DC, Jr., Ning H, Lloyd-Jones DM. A systematic examination of the 2013 ACC/AHA pooled cohort risk assessment tool for atherosclerotic cardiovascular disease. *J Am Coll Cardiol.* 2014;64: 959-968.

82. Goff DC, Jr., Lloyd-Jones DM, Bennett G, et al. 2013 ACC/AHA guideline on the assessment of cardiovascular risk: a report of the American College of Cardiology/American Heart Association Task Force on Practice Guidelines. *Circulation.* 2014;129:S49-S73.

83. Go AS, Bauman MA, Coleman King SM, et al. An effective approach to high blood pressure control: a science advisory from the American Heart Association, the American College of Cardiology, and the Centers for Disease Control and Prevention. *Hypertension.* 2014;63:878-885.

84. Eckel RH, Jakicic JM, Ard JD, et al. 2013 AHA/ACC guideline on lifestyle management to reduce cardiovascular risk: a report of the American College of Cardiology/American Heart Association Task Force on Practice Guidelines. *Circulation.* 2014;129:S76-S99.

85. Eckel RH. LDL cholesterol as a predictor of mortality, and beyond: to fast or not to fast, that is the question? *Circulation.* 2014;130:528-529.

86. Kostis WJ, Cheng JQ, Dobrzynski JM, Cabrera J, Kostis JB. Meta-analysis of statin effects in women versus men. *J Am Coll Cardiol.* 2012;59: 572-582.

87. Cannon CP, Blazing MA, Braunwald E. Ezetimibe plus a statin after acute coronary syndromes. *N Engl J Med.* 2015;373:1476-1477.

88. Everett BM, Smith RJ, Hiatt WR. Reducing LDL with PCSK9 inhibitors–the clinical benefit of lipid drugs. *N Engl J Med.* 2015;373:1588-1591.

89. Joseph L, Robinson JG. Proprotein convertase subtilisin/kexin type 9 (PCSK9) inhibition and the future of lipid lowering therapy. *Progress Cardiovasc Dis.* 2015;58:19-31.

90. Sabatine MS, Giugliano RP, Keech AC, et al. Evolocumab and clinical outcomes in patients with cardiovascular disease. *N Engl J Med.* 2017;376:1713-1722.

91. Schwartz GG, Steg PG, Szarek M, Bhatt DL, et al. Alirocumab and cardiovascular outcomes after acute coronary syndrome. *N Engl J Med.* 2018;379:2097-2107.

92. Aiman U, Najmi A, Khan RA. Statin induced diabetes and its clinical implications. *J Pharmacol Pharmacother.* 2014;5:181-185.

93. Arnold SV, Bhatt DL, Barsness GW, et al. Clinical management of stable coronary artery disease in patients with type 2 diabetes mellitus: a scientific statement from the American Heart Association. *Circulation.* 2020;141:e779-e806.

94. Bhatt DL, Steg PG, Brinton EA, et al. Rationale and design of REDUCE-IT: Reduction of Cardiovascular Events with Icosapent Ethyl-Intervention Trial. *Clin Cardiol.* 2017;40:138-148.

95. Bhatt DL, Steg PG, Miller M, et al. Effects of icosapent ethyl on total ischemic events: From REDUCE-IT. *J Am Coll Cardiol.* 2019;73:2791-2802.

96. Mosca L, Navar AM, Kass Wenger N. Reducing cardiovascular disease risk in women beyond statin therapy: new insights 2020. *J Womens Health (Larchmt).* 2020.

97. Wilson PW, D'Agostino RB, Sullivan L, Parise H, Kannel WB. Overweight and obesity as determinants of cardiovascular risk: the Framingham experience. *Arch Intern Med.* 2002;162:1867-1872.

98. Kanaya AM, Grady D, Barrett-Connor E. Explaining the sex difference in coronary heart disease mortality among patients with type 2 diabetes mellitus: a meta-analysis. *Arch Intern Med.* 2002;162:1737-1745.

99. Jensen MD, Ryan DH, Apovian CM, et al. 2013 AHA/ACC/TOS guideline for the management of overweight and obesity in adults: a report

of the American College of Cardiology/American Heart Association Task Force on Practice Guidelines and The Obesity Society. *Circulation.* 2014;129:S102-S138.

100. Go AS, Mozaffarian D, Roger VL, et al. Heart disease and stroke statistics–2013 update: a report from the American Heart Association. *Circulation.* 2013;127:e6-e245.

101. Shiroma EJ, Lee IM. Physical activity and cardiovascular health: lessons learned from epidemiological studies across age, gender, and race/ethnicity. *Circulation.* 2010;122:743-752.

102. Xu X, Bao H, Strait K, et al. Sex differences in perceived stress and early recovery in young and middle-aged patients with acute myocardial infarction. *Circulation.* 2015;131:614-623.

103. Smolderen KG, Strait KM, Dreyer RP, et al. Depressive symptoms in younger women and men with acute myocardial infarction: insights from the VIRGO study. *J Am Heart Assoc.* 2015;4.

104. Shah AJ, Ghasemzadeh N, Zaragoza-Macias E, et al. Sex and age differences in the association of depression with obstructive coronary artery disease and adverse cardiovascular events. *J Am Heart Assoc.* 2014;3:e000741.

105. Lichtman JH, Froelicher ES, Blumenthal JA, et al. Depression as a risk factor for poor prognosis among patients with acute coronary syndrome: systematic review and recommendations: a scientific statement from the American Heart Association. *Circulation.* 2014;129:1350-1369.

106. Rutledge T, Linke SE, Johnson BD, et al. Relationships between cardiovascular disease risk factors and depressive symptoms as predictors of cardiovascular disease events in women. *J Womens Health (Larchmt).* 2012;21:133-139.

107. Varghese T, Hayek SS, Shekiladze N, Schultz WM, Wenger NK. Psychosocial risk factors related to ischemic heart disease in women. *Curr Pharmaceut Design.* 2016.

108. Mallik S, Spertus JA, Reid KJ, et al. Depressive symptoms after acute myocardial infarction: evidence for highest rates in younger women. *Arch Intern Med.* 2006;166:876-883.

109. Vaccarino V, Abramson JL, Veledar E, Weintraub WS. Sex differences in hospital mortality after coronary artery bypass surgery: evidence for a higher mortality in younger women. *Circulation.* 2002;105:1176-1181.

110. Vaccarino V, Parsons L, Every NR, Barron HV, Krumholz HM. Sex-based differences in early mortality after myocardial infarction. National Registry of Myocardial Infarction 2 Participants. *N Engl J Med.* 1999;341: 217-225.

111. Cook NR, Lee IM, Gaziano JM, et al. Low-dose aspirin in the primary prevention of cancer: the Women's Health Study: a randomized controlled trial. *JAMA.* 2005;294:47-55.

112. Berger JS, Roncaglioni MC, Avanzini F, Pangrazzi I, Tognoni G, Brown DL. Aspirin for the primary prevention of cardiovascular events in women and men: a sex-specific meta-analysis of randomized controlled trials. *JAMA.* 2006;295:306-313.

113. Valente AM, Bhatt DL, Lane-Cordova A. Pregnancy as a cardiac stress test: time to include obstetric history in cardiac risk assessment? *J Am Coll Cardiol.* 2020;76:68-71.

114. Kessous R, Shoham-Vardi I, Pariente G, Holcberg G, Sheiner E. An association between preterm delivery and long-term maternal cardiovascular morbidity. *Am J Obstetrics Gynecol.* 2013;209:368.e1-e8.

115. Fraser A, Nelson SM, Macdonald-Wallis C, et al. Associations of pregnancy complications with calculated cardiovascular disease risk and cardiovascular risk factors in middle age: the Avon Longitudinal Study of Parents and Children. *Circulation.* 2012;125:1367-1380.

116. Wenger NK. Recognizing pregnancy-associated cardiovascular risk factors. *Am J Cardiol.* 2014;113:406-409.

117. Ahmed R, Dunford J, Mehran R, Robson S, Kunadian V. Pre-eclampsia and future cardiovascular risk among women: a review. *J Am Coll Cardiol.* 2014;63:1815-1822.

118. Theilen LH, Fraser A, Hollingshaus MS, et al. All-cause and cause-specific mortality after hypertensive disease of pregnancy. *Obstet Gynecol.* 2016;128:238-244.

119. Stuart JJ, Tanz LJ, Cook NR, et al. Hypertensive disorders of pregnancy and 10-year cardiovascular risk prediction. *J Am Coll Cardiol.* 2018;72:1252-1263.

120. Stuart JJ, Tanz LJ, Missmer SA, et al. Hypertensive disorders of pregnancy and maternal cardiovascular disease risk factor development: an observational cohort study. *Ann Intern Med.* 2018;169:224-232.

121. Shufelt CL, Bairey Merz CN. Contraceptive hormone use and cardiovascular disease. *J Am Coll Cardiol.* 2009;53:221-231.

122. Bushnell C, McCullough L. Stroke prevention in women: synopsis of the 2014 American Heart Association/American Stroke Association guideline. *Ann Intern Med.* 2014;160:853-857.

123. Udell JA, Lu H, Redelmeier DA. Long-term cardiovascular risk in women prescribed fertility therapy. *J Am Coll Cardiol.* 2013;62:1704-1712.

124. Dayan N, Laskin CA, Spitzer K, et al. Pregnancy complications in women with heart disease conceiving with fertility therapy. *J Am Coll Cardiol.* 2014;64:1862-1864.

125. Lundberg G, Wu P, Wenger NK. Menopausal hormone therapy: a comprehensive review. *Curr Atheroscler Rep.* 2020.

126. Moyer VA and Force USPST. Menopausal hormone therapy for the primary prevention of chronic conditions: U.S. Preventive Services Task Force recommendation statement. *Ann Intern Med.* 2013;158:47-54.

127. Nelson HD, Walker M, Zakher B, Mitchell J. Menopausal hormone therapy for the primary prevention of chronic conditions: a systematic review to update the U.S. Preventive Services Task Force recommendations. *Ann Intern Med.* 2012;157:104-113.

128. Salmon JE, Roman MJ. Subclinical atherosclerosis in rheumatoid arthritis and systemic lupus erythematosus. *Am J Med.* 2008;121:S3-8.

129. Zhang J, Chen L, Delzell E, et al. The association between inflammatory markers, serum lipids and the risk of cardiovascular events in patients with rheumatoid arthritis. *Ann Rheumat Dis.* 2014;73:1301-1308.

130. Hulley S, Grady D, Bush T, et al. Randomized trial of estrogen plus progestin for secondary prevention of coronary heart disease in postmenopausal women. Heart and Estrogen/progestin Replacement Study (HERS) Research Group. *JAMA.* 1998;280:605-613.

131. Rossouw JE, Anderson GL, Prentice RL, et al. Risks and benefits of estrogen plus progestin in healthy postmenopausal women: principal results From the Women's Health Initiative randomized controlled trial. *JAMA.* 2002;288:321-333.

132. Lee IM, Cook NR, Gaziano JM, et al. Vitamin E in the primary prevention of cardiovascular disease and cancer: the Women's Health Study: a randomized controlled trial. *JAMA.* 2005;294:56-65.

133. Cook NR, Albert CM, Gaziano JM, et al. A randomized factorial trial of vitamins C and E and beta carotene in the secondary prevention of cardiovascular events in women: results from the Women's Antioxidant Cardiovascular Study. *Arch Intern Med.* 2007;167:1610-1618.

134. Bonaa KH, Njolstad I, Ueland PM, et al. Homocysteine lowering and cardiovascular events after acute myocardial infarction. *N Engl J Med.* 2006;354:1578-1588.

135. Santos-Ferreira C, Baptista R, Oliveira-Santos M, Moura JP, Goncalves L. A 10- and 15-year performance analysis of ESC/EAS and ACC/AHA cardiovascular risk scores in a Southern European cohort. *BMC Cardiovasc Disord.* 2020;20:301.

136. Kelkar AA, Schultz WM, Khosa F, et al. Long-term prognosis after coronary artery calcium scoring among low-intermediate risk women and men. *Circ Cardiovasc Imaging.* 2016;9:e003742.

137. DeFilippis AP, Young R, McEvoy JW, et al. Risk score overestimation: the impact of individual cardiovascular risk factors and preventive therapies on the performance of the American Heart Association-American College of Cardiology-Atherosclerotic Cardiovascular Disease risk score in a modern multi-ethnic cohort. *Eur Heart J.* 2017;38:598-608.

138. Navar-Boggan AM, Peterson ED, D'Agostino RB, Sr., Pencina MJ, Sniderman AD. Using age- and sex-specific risk thresholds to guide statin therapy: one size may not fit all. *J Am Coll Cardiol.* 2015;65: 1633-1639.

139. Shaw LJ, Min JK, Nasir K, et al. Sex differences in calcified plaque and long-term cardiovascular mortality: observations from the CAC Consortium. *Eur Heart J.* 2018;39:3727-3735.

140. Budoff MJ, Young R, Burke G, et al. Ten-year association of coronary artery calcium with atherosclerotic cardiovascular disease (ASCVD) events: the multi-ethnic study of atherosclerosis (MESA). *Eur Heart J.* 2018;39:2401-2408.

141. Mieres JH, Gulati M, Bairey Merz N, et al. Role of noninvasive testing in the clinical evaluation of women with suspected ischemic heart disease: a consensus statement from the American Heart Association. *Circulation.* 2014;130:350-379.

142. Hemingway H, Langenberg C, Damant J, Frost C, Pyorala K, Barrett-Connor E. Prevalence of angina in women versus men: a systematic review and meta-analysis of international variations across 31 countries. *Circulation.* 2008;117:1526-1536.

143. Dreyer RP, Wang Y, Strait KM, et al. Gender differences in the trajectory of recovery in health status among young patients with acute myocardial infarction: results from the variation in recovery: role of gender on outcomes of young AMI patients (VIRGO) study. *Circulation.* 2015;131:1971-1980.

144. Norris CM, Saunders LD, Ghali WA, et al. Health-related quality of life outcomes of patients with coronary artery disease treated with cardiac surgery, percutaneous coronary intervention or medical management. *Can J Cardiol.* 2004;20:1259-1266.

145. Reynolds HR, Shaw LJ, Min JK, et al. Association of sex with severity of coronary artery disease, ischemia, and symptom burden in patients with moderate or severe ischemia: secondary analysis of the ISCHEMIA randomized clinical trial. *JAMA Cardiol.* 2020.

146. Johnson BD, Shaw LJ, Pepine CJ, et al. Persistent chest pain predicts cardiovascular events in women without obstructive coronary artery disease: results from the NIH-NHLBI-sponsored Women's Ischaemia Syndrome Evaluation (WISE) study. *Eur Heart J.* 2006;27:1408-1415.

147. Figueras J, Domingo E, Ferreira I, Lidon RM, Garcia-Dorado D. Persistent angina pectoris, cardiac mortality and myocardial infarction during a 12 year follow-up in 273 variant angina patients without significant fixed coronary stenosis. *Am J Cardiol.* 2012;110:1249-1255.

148. McSweeney J, Cleves MA, Fischer EP, et al. Predicting coronary heart disease events in women: a longitudinal cohort study. *J Cardiovasc Nursing* 2014;29:482-492.

149. Shaw LJ, Mieres JH, Hendel RH, et al. Comparative effectiveness of exercise electrocardiography with or without myocardial perfusion single photon emission computed tomography in women with suspected coronary artery disease: results from the What Is the Optimal Method for Ischemia Evaluation in Women (WOMEN) trial. *Circulation.* 2011;124:1239-1249.

150. Shaw LJ, Miller DD, Romeis JC, Kargl D, Younis LT, Chaitman BR. Gender differences in the noninvasive evaluation and management of patients with suspected coronary artery disease. *Ann Intern Med.* 1994;120:559-566.

151. Hemingway H, McCallum A, Shipley M, Manderbacka K, Martikainen P, Keskimaki I. Incidence and prognostic implications of stable angina pectoris among women and men. *JAMA.* 2006;295:1404-1411.

152. Taqueti VR, Di Carli MF. Coronary microvascular disease pathogenic mechanisms and therapeutic options: JACC State-of-the-Art Review. *J Am Coll Cardiol.* 2018;72:2625-2641.

153. Taqueti VR, Dorbala S, Wolinsky D, et al. Myocardial perfusion imaging in women for the evaluation of stable ischemic heart disease-state-of-the-evidence and clinical recommendations. *J Nucl Cardiol.* 2017;24:1402-1426.

154. Taqueti VR, Shaw LJ, Cook NR, et al. Excess cardiovascular risk in women relative to men referred for coronary angiography is associated with severely impaired coronary flow reserve, not obstructive disease. *Circulation.* 2017;135:566-577.

155. Kay J, Dorbala S, Goyal A, et al. Influence of sex on risk stratification with stress myocardial perfusion Rb-82 positron emission tomography: results from the PET (Positron Emission Tomography) Prognosis Multicenter Registry. *J Am Coll Cardiol.* 2013;62:1866-1876.

156. Gulati M, Shaw LJ, Thisted RA, Black HR, Bairey Merz CN, Arnsdorf MF. Heart rate response to exercise stress testing in asymptomatic women: the St. James women take heart project. *Circulation.* 2010;122:130-137.

157. Gulati M, Black HR, Shaw LJ, et al. The prognostic value of a nomogram for exercise capacity in women. *N Engl J Med.* 2005;353:468-475.

158. Shaw LJ, Xie JX, Phillips LM, et al. Optimising diagnostic accuracy with the exercise ECG: opportunities for women and men with stable ischaemic heart disease. *Heart Asia.* 2016;8:1-7.

159. Sanders GD, Patel MR, Chatterjee R, et al. *Noninvasive Technologies for the Diagnosis of Coronary Artery Disease in Women: Future Research Needs: Identification of Future Research Needs From Comparative Effectiveness Review No 58.* Rockville, MD; 2013.

160. Lauer MS, Pothier CE, Magid DJ, Smith SS, Kattan MW. An externally validated model for predicting long-term survival after exercise treadmill testing in patients with suspected coronary artery disease and a normal electrocardiogram. *Ann Intern Med.* 2007;147:821-828.

161. Alexander KP, Shaw LJ, Shaw LK, Delong ER, Mark DB, Peterson ED. Value of exercise treadmill testing in women. *J Am Coll Cardiol.* 1998;32:1657-1664.

162. Shaw LJ. Sex Differences in Cardiovascular Imaging. *JACC Cardiovasc Imaging.* 2016;9:494-497.

163. Shaw LJ, Kohli P, Chandrashekhar Y, Narula J. Cardiovascular imaging of women: we have come a long way but still have a ways to go. *JACC Cardiovasc Imaging.* 2016;9:502-503.

164. Arruda-Olson AM, Juracan EM, Mahoney DW, McCully RB, Roger VL, Pellikka PA. Prognostic value of exercise echocardiography in 5,798 patients: is there a gender difference? *J Am Coll Cardiol.* 2002;39:625-631.

165. Mieres JH, Shaw LJ, Arai A, et al. Role of noninvasive testing in the clinical evaluation of women with suspected coronary artery disease: consensus statement from the Cardiac Imaging Committee, Council on Clinical Cardiology, and the Cardiovascular Imaging and Intervention Committee, Council on Cardiovascular Radiology and Intervention, American Heart Association. *Circulation.* 2005;111:682-696.

166. Radico F, Cicchitti V, Zimarino M, De Caterina R. Angina pectoris and myocardial ischemia in the absence of obstructive coronary artery disease: practical considerations for diagnostic tests. *JACC Cardiovasc Interv.* 2014;7:453-463.

167. Ha JW, Juracan EM, Mahoney DW, et al. Hypertensive response to exercise: a potential cause for new wall motion abnormality in the absence of coronary artery disease. *J Am Coll Cardiol.* 2002;39:323-327.

168. Shaw LJ, Berman DS, Picard MH, et al. Comparative definitions for moderate-severe ischemia in stress nuclear, echocardiography, and magnetic resonance imaging. *JACC Cardiovasc Imaging.* 2014;7:593-604.

169. Santos MT, Parker MW, Heller GV. Evaluating gender differences in prognosis following SPECT myocardial perfusion imaging among patients with diabetes and known or suspected coronary disease in the modern era. *J Nucl Cardiol.* 2013;20:1021-1029.

170. Shaw LJ, Shaw RE, Merz CN, et al. Impact of ethnicity and gender differences on angiographic coronary artery disease prevalence and in-hospital mortality in the American College of Cardiology-National Cardiovascular Data Registry. *Circulation.* 2008;117:1787-1801.

171. Shaw LJ, Bugiardini R, Merz CN. Women and ischemic heart disease: evolving knowledge. *J Am Coll Cardiol.* 2009;54:1561-1575.

172. Arsanjani R, Hayes SW, Fish M, et al. Two-position supine/prone myocardial perfusion SPECT (MPS) imaging improves visual inter-observer correlation and agreement. *J Nuclear Cardiol.* 2014;21:703-711.

173. Berman DS, Kang X, Nishina H, et al. Diagnostic accuracy of gated Tc-99m sestamibi stress myocardial perfusion SPECT with combined supine and prone acquisitions to detect coronary artery disease in obese and nonobese patients. *J Nuclear Cardiol.* 2006;13:191-201.

174. Duvall WL, Croft LB, Corriel JS, et al. SPECT myocardial perfusion imaging in morbidly obese patients: image quality, hemodynamic response to pharmacologic stress, and diagnostic and prognostic value. *J Nuclear Cardiol.* 2006;13:202-209.

175. Shaw LJ, Hendel RC, Cerquiera M, et al. Ethnic differences in the prognostic value of stress technetium-99m tetrofosmin gated single-photon emission computed tomography myocardial perfusion imaging. *J Am Coll Cardiol.* 2005;45:1494-1504.

176. Cerci MS, Cerci JJ, Cerci RJ, et al. Myocardial perfusion imaging is a strong predictor of death in women. *JACC Cardiovasc Imaging.* 2011;4:880-888.

177. Einstein AJ, Berman DS, Min JK, Patient-centered imaging: shared decision making for cardiac imaging procedures with exposure to ionizing radiation. *Journal of the American College of Cardiology.* 2014;63:1480-9.

178. Einstein AJ. Effects of radiation exposure from cardiac imaging: how good are the data? *J Am Coll Cardiol.* 2012;59:553-565.

179. Bateman TM, Heller GV, McGhie AI, et al. Diagnostic accuracy of rest/stress ECG-gated Rb-82 myocardial perfusion PET: comparison with ECG-gated Tc-99m sestamibi SPECT. *J Nuclear Cardiol.* 2006;13:24-33.

180. Taqueti VR, Everett BM, Murthy VL, et al. Interaction of impaired coronary flow reserve and cardiomyocyte injury on adverse cardiovascular outcomes in patients without overt coronary artery disease. *Circulation.* 2015;131:528-535.

181. Taqueti VR, Blankstein R. Understanding sex differences in coronary artery disease risk: is coronary anatomy sufficient? *Circ Cardiovasc Imaging.* 2017;10.

182. Taqueti VR, Hachamovitch R, Murthy VL, et al. Global coronary flow reserve is associated with adverse cardiovascular events independently of luminal angiographic severity and modifies the effect of early revascularization. *Circulation.* 2015;131:19-27.

183. Taqueti VR, Solomon SD, Shah AM, et al. Coronary microvascular dysfunction and future risk of heart failure with preserved ejection fraction. *Eur Heart J.* 2018;39:840-849.

184. Danad I, Raijmakers PG, Harms HJ, et al. Impact of anatomical and functional severity of coronary atherosclerotic plaques on the transmural perfusion gradient: a [15O]H2O PET study. *Eur Heart J.* 2014;35:2094-2105.

185. Gould KL, Johnson NP, Bateman TM, et al. Anatomic versus physiologic assessment of coronary artery disease. Role of coronary flow reserve, fractional flow reserve, and positron emission tomography imaging in revascularization decision-making. *J Am Coll Cardiol.* 2013;62:1639-1653.

186. Murthy VL, Lee BC, Sitek A, et al. Comparison and prognostic validation of multiple methods of quantification of myocardial blood flow with 82Rb PET. *J Nuclear Med.* 2014;55:1952-1958.

187. Lin F, Shaw LJ, Berman DS, et al. Multidetector computed tomography coronary artery plaque predictors of stress-induced myocardial ischemia by SPECT. *Atherosclerosis.* 2008;197:700-709.

188. Murthy VL, Naya M, Foster CR, et al. Improved cardiac risk assessment with noninvasive measures of coronary flow reserve. *Circulation.* 2011;124:2215-2224.

189. Kaufmann PA, Camici PG. Myocardial blood flow measurement by PET: technical aspects and clinical applications. *J Nuclear Med.* 2005;46:75-88.

190. Camici PG, Crea F. Coronary microvascular dysfunction. *N Engl J Med.* 2007;356:830-840.

191. Khuddus MA, Pepine CJ, Handberg EM, et al. An intravascular ultrasound analysis in women experiencing chest pain in the absence of obstructive coronary artery disease: a substudy from the National Heart, Lung and Blood Institute-Sponsored Women's Ischemia Syndrome Evaluation (WISE). *J Intervention Cardiol.* 2010;23:511-519.

192. Lee BK, Lim HS, Fearon WF, et al. Invasive evaluation of patients with angina in the absence of obstructive coronary artery disease. *Circulation.* 2015;131:1054-1060.

193. Greenwood JP, Motwani M, Maredia N, et al. Comparison of cardiovascular magnetic resonance and single-photon emission computed tomography in women with suspected coronary artery disease from the Clinical Evaluation of Magnetic Resonance Imaging in Coronary Heart Disease (CE-MARC) Trial. *Circulation.* 2014;129:1129-1138.

194. Coelho-Filho OR, Seabra LF, Mongeon FP, et al. Stress myocardial perfusion imaging by CMR provides strong prognostic value to cardiac events regardless of patient's sex. *JACC Cardiovasc Imaging.* 2011;4:850-861.

195. Zorach B, Shaw PW, Bourque J, et al. Quantitative cardiovascular magnetic resonance perfusion imaging identifies reduced flow reserve in microvascular coronary artery disease. *J Cardiovasc Magn Reson.* 2018;20:14.

196. Kim HW, Klem I, Shah DJ, et al. Unrecognized non-Q-wave myocardial infarction: prevalence and prognostic significance in patients with suspected coronary disease. *PLoS Med.* 2009;6:e1000057.

197. Schelbert EB, Cao JJ, Sigurdsson S, et al. Prevalence and prognosis of unrecognized myocardial infarction determined by cardiac magnetic resonance in older adults. *JAMA.* 2012;308:890-896.

198. Wolk MJ, Bailey SR, Doherty JU, et al. ACCF/AHA/ASE/ASNC/HFSA/HRS/SCAI/SCCT/SCMR/STS 2013 multimodality appropriate use criteria for the detection and risk assessment of stable ischemic heart disease: a report of the American College of Cardiology Foundation Appropriate Use Criteria Task Force, American Heart Association, American Society of Echocardiography, American Society of Nuclear Cardiology, Heart Failure Society of America, Heart Rhythm Society, Society for Cardiovascular Angiography and Interventions, Society of Cardiovascular Computed Tomography, Society for Cardiovascular Magnetic Resonance, and Society of Thoracic Surgeons. *J Am Coll Cardiol.* 2014;63:380-406.

199. Douglas PS, Hoffmann U, Patel MR, et al. Outcomes of anatomical versus functional testing for coronary artery disease. *N Engl J Med.* 2015;372:1291-1300.

200. Chinnaiyan KM, Peyser P, Goraya T, et al. Impact of a continuous quality improvement initiative on appropriate use of coronary computed tomography angiography. Results from a multicenter, statewide registry, the Advanced Cardiovascular Imaging Consortium. *J Am Coll Cardiol.* 2012;60:1185-1191.

201. Min JK, Dunning A, Lin FY, et al. Age- and sex-related differences in all-cause mortality risk based on coronary computed tomography angiography findings results from the International Multicenter CONFIRM (Coronary CT Angiography Evaluation for Clinical Outcomes: An International Multicenter Registry) of 23,854 patients without known coronary artery disease. *J Am Coll Cardiol.* 2011;58:849-860.

202. Jespersen L, Hvelplund A, Abildstrom SZ, et al. Stable angina pectoris with no obstructive coronary artery disease is associated with increased risks of major adverse cardiovascular events. *Eur Heart J.* 2012;33:734-744.

203. Grunau GL, Ahmadi A, Rezazadeh S, et al. Assessment of sex differences in plaque morphology by coronary computed tomography angiography–are men and women the same? *J Womens Health (Larchmt).* 2014;23:146-150.

204. Cheng VY, Berman DS, Rozanski A, et al. Performance of the traditional age, sex, and angina typicality-based approach for estimating pretest probability of angiographically significant coronary artery disease in patients undergoing coronary computed tomographic angiography: results from the multinational coronary CT angiography evaluation for clinical outcomes: an international multicenter registry (CONFIRM). *Circulation.* 2011;124:2423-32, 1-8.

205. Otaki Y, Gransar H, Cheng VY, Dey D, et al. Gender differences in the prevalence, severity, and composition of coronary artery disease in the young: a study of 1635 individuals undergoing coronary CT angiography from the prospective, multinational confirm registry. *Eur Heart J Cardiovasc Imaging.* 2015;16:490-499.

206. Pagidipati NJ, Hemal K, Coles A, et al. Sex differences in functional and CT angiography testing in patients with suspected coronary artery disease. *J Am Coll Cardiol.* 2016;67:2607-2616.

207. Hemal K, Pagidipati NJ, Coles A, et al. Sex differences in demographics, risk factors, presentation, and noninvasive testing in stable outpatients with suspected coronary artery disease: insights from the PROMISE Trial. *JACC Cardiovasc Imaging.* 2016.

208. Schulman-Marcus J, Hartaigh BO, Gransar H, et al. Sex-specific associations between coronary artery plaque extent and risk of major adverse cardiovascular events: the CONFIRM long-term registry. *JACC Cardiovasc Imaging*. 2016;9:364-372.

209. Maddox TM, Stanislawski MA, Grunwald GK, et al. Nonobstructive coronary artery disease and risk of myocardial infarction. *JAMA*. 2014;312:1754-1763.

210. Leipsic J, Taylor CM, Gransar H, et al. Sex-based prognostic implications of nonobstructive coronary artery disease: results from the international multicenter CONFIRM study. *Radiology*. 2014;273:393-400.

211. Xie JX, Eshtehardi P, Varghese T, et al. Prognostic significance of nonobstructive left main coronary artery disease in women versus men: long-term outcomes from the CONFIRM (Coronary CT Angiography Evaluation For Clinical Outcomes: An International Multicenter) Registry. *Circ Cardiovasc Imaging*. 2017;10.

212. Plank F, Beyer C, Friedrich G, Wildauer M, Feuchtner G. Sex differences in coronary artery plaque composition detected by coronary computed tomography: quantitative and qualitative analysis. *Neth Heart J*. 2019;27:272-280.

213. Bittencourt MS, Hulten E, Ghoshhajra B, et al. Prognostic value of nonobstructive and obstructive coronary artery disease detected by coronary computed tomography angiography to identify cardiovascular events. *Circ Cardiovasc Imaging*. 2014;7:282-291.

214. Ferencik M, Mayrhofer T, Bittner DO, et al. Use of high-risk coronary atherosclerotic plaque detection for risk stratification of patients with stable chest pain: a secondary analysis of the PROMISE randomized clinical trial. *JAMA Cardiol*. 2018;3:144-152.

215. Puchner SB, Liu T, Mayrhofer T, et al. High-risk plaque detected on coronary CT angiography predicts acute coronary syndromes independent of significant stenosis in acute chest pain: results from the ROMICAT-II trial. *J Am Coll Cardiol*. 2014;64:684-692.

216. Lubbers M, Dedic A, Coenen A, et al. Calcium imaging and selective computed tomography angiography in comparison to functional testing for suspected coronary artery disease: the multicentre, randomized CRESCENT trial. *Eur Heart J*. 2016;37:1232-1243.

217. McKavanagh P, Lusk L, Ball PA, et al. A comparison of cardiac computerized tomography and exercise stress electrocardiogram test for the investigation of stable chest pain: the clinical results of the CAPP randomized prospective trial. *Eur Heart J Cardiovasc Imaging*. 2015;16:441-448.

218. Lubbers M, Coenen A, Bruning T, et al. Sex differences in the performance of cardiac computed tomography compared with functional testing in evaluating stable chest pain: subanalysis of the multicenter, randomized CRESCENT Trial (Calcium Imaging and Selective CT Angiography in Comparison to Functional Testing for Suspected Coronary Artery Disease). *Circ Cardiovasc Imaging*. 2017;10.

219. Maron DJ, Hochman JS, Reynolds HR, et al. Initial invasive or conservative strategy for stable coronary disease. *N Engl J Med*. 2020;382:1395-1407.

220. Hochman JS, Reynolds HR, Bangalore S, et al. Baseline characteristics and risk profiles of participants in the ISCHEMIA randomized clinical trial. *JAMA Cardiology*. 2019;4:273-286.

221. Crea F, Camici PG, Bairey Merz CN. Coronary microvascular dysfunction: an update. *Eur Heart J*. 2014;35:1101-1111.

222. Stuijfzand WJ, van Rosendael AR, Lin FY, et al. Stress myocardial perfusion imaging vs coronary computed tomographic angiography for diagnosis of invasive vessel-specific coronary physiology: predictive modeling results from the Computed Tomographic Evaluation of Atherosclerotic Determinants of Myocardial Ischemia (CREDENCE) Trial. *JAMA Cardiol*. 2020.

223. Kunadian V, Chieffo A, Camici PG, et al. An EAPCI expert consensus document on ischaemia with non-obstructive coronary arteries in collaboration with European Society of Cardiology Working Group on Coronary Pathophysiology & Microcirculation Endorsed by Coronary Vasomotor Disorders International Study Group. *Eur Heart J*. 2020.

224. Lanza GA, Crea F. Primary coronary microvascular dysfunction: clinical presentation, pathophysiology, and management. *Circulation*. 2010;121:2317-2325.

225. Melikian N, Vercauteren S, Fearon WF, et al. Quantitative assessment of coronary microvascular function in patients with and without epicardial atherosclerosis. *EuroIntervention*. 2010;5:939-945.

226. AlBadri A, Bairey Merz CN, Johnson BD, et al. Impact of abnormal coronary reactivity on long-term clinical outcomes in women. *J Am Coll Cardiol*. 2019;73:684-693.

227. Ford TJ, Stanley B, Good R, et al. Stratified medical therapy using invasive coronary function testing in angina: the CorMicA trial. *J Am Coll Cardiol*. 2018;72:2841-2855.

228. Taqueti VR. Coronary microvascular dysfunction in vasospastic angina: provocative role for the microcirculation in macrovessel disease prognosis. *J Am Coll Cardiol*. 2019;74:2361-2364.

229. Ford TJ, Stanley B, Sidik N, et al. 1-year outcomes of angina management guided by invasive coronary function testing (CorMicA). *JACC Cardiovasc Interventions*. 2020;13:33-45.

230. Taqueti VR. Treating coronary microvascular dysfunction as the "culprit" lesion in patients with refractory angina: lessons from CorMicA at 1 year. *JACC Cardiovasc Interventions*. 2020;13:46-48.

231. Wenger NK. Why does myocardial infarction preferentially disadvantage women? *J Am Coll Cardiol*. 2020;76:1761-1762.

232. Canto JG, Goldberg RJ, Hand MM, et al. Symptom presentation of women with acute coronary syndromes: myth vs reality. *Arch Intern Med*. 2007;167:2405-2413.

233. Khan NA, Daskalopoulou SS, Karp I, et al. Sex differences in acute coronary syndrome symptom presentation in young patients. *JAMA Intern Med*. 2013;173:1863-1871.

234. Wenger NK. Angina in women. *Current cardiology reports*. 2010;12:307-314.

235. Devon HA, Rosenfeld A, Steffen AD, Daya M. Sensitivity, specificity, and sex differences in symptoms reported on the 13-item acute coronary syndrome checklist. *J Am Heart Assoc*. 2014;3:e000586.

236. Ting HH, Bradley EH, Wang Y, et al. Factors associated with longer time from symptom onset to hospital presentation for patients with ST-elevation myocardial infarction. *Arch Intern Med*. 2008;168:959-968.

237. DeVon HA, Saban KL, Garrett DK. Recognizing and responding to symptoms of acute coronary syndromes and stroke in women. *J Obs Gynecol Neonat Nurs*. 2011;40:372-382.

238. DeVon HA. Promoting cardiovascular health in women across the life span. *J Obs Gynecol Neonat Nurs*. 2011;40:335-336.

239. Canto JG, Rogers WJ, Goldberg RJ, et al. Association of age and sex with myocardial infarction symptom presentation and in-hospital mortality. *JAMA*. 2012;307:813-822.

240. Izadnegahdar M, Mackay M, Lee MK, et al. Sex and ethnic differences in outcomes of acute coronary syndrome and stable angina patients with obstructive coronary artery disease. *Circ Cardiovasc Qual Outcomes* 2016;9:S26-S35.

241. Gupta A, Wang Y, Spertus JA, et al. Trends in acute myocardial infarction in young patients and differences by sex and race, 2001 to 2010. *J Am Coll Cardiol*. 2014;64:337-345.

242. Wenger NK. Coronary heart disease: the female heart is vulnerable. *Prog Cardiovasc Dis*. 2003;46:199-229.

243. Ricci B, Cenko E, Vasiljevic Z, et al. Acute coronary syndrome: the risk to young women. *J Am Heart Assoc*. 2017;6.

244. O'Gara PT, Kushner FG, Ascheim DD, et al. 2013 ACCF/AHA guideline for the management of ST-elevation myocardial infarction: a report of the American College of Cardiology Foundation/American Heart Association Task Force on Practice Guidelines. *Circulation*. 2013;127:e362-e425.

245. O'Gara PT, Kushner FG, Ascheim DD, et al. 2013 ACCF/AHA guideline for the management of ST-elevation myocardial infarction: executive summary: a report of the American College of Cardiology Foundation/American Heart Association Task Force on Practice Guidelines. *Circulation*. 2013;127:529-555.

246. Amsterdam EA, Wenger NK, Brindis RG, et al. 2014 AHA/ACC guideline for the management of patients with non-ST-elevation acute coronary syndromes: executive summary: a report of the American College of

Cardiology/American Heart Association Task Force on Practice Guidelines. *Circulation*. 2014;130:2354-2394.

247. Amsterdam EA, Wenger NK, Brindis RG, et al. 2014 AHA/ACC guideline for the management of patients with non-ST-elevation acute coronary syndromes: a report of the American College of Cardiology/American Heart Association Task Force on Practice Guidelines. *Circulation*. 2014;130:e344-e426.

248. Manoukian SV, Feit F, Mehran R, et al. Impact of major bleeding on 30-day mortality and clinical outcomes in patients with acute coronary syndromes: an analysis from the ACUITY Trial. *J Am Coll Cardiol*. 2007;49:1362-1368.

249. Amsterdam EA, Wenger NK, Brindis RG, et al. 2014 AHA/ACC Guideline for the Management of Patients with Non-ST-Elevation Acute Coronary Syndromes: a report of the American College of Cardiology/American Heart Association Task Force on Practice Guidelines. *J Am Coll Cardiol*. 2014;64:e139-e228.

250. Moscucci M, Fox KA, Cannon CP, et al. Predictors of major bleeding in acute coronary syndromes: the Global Registry of Acute Coronary Events (GRACE). *Eur Heart J*. 2003;24:1815-1823.

251. Alexander KP, Chen AY, Newby LK, et al. Sex differences in major bleeding with glycoprotein IIb/IIIa inhibitors: results from the CRUSADE (Can Rapid risk stratification of Unstable angina patients Suppress ADverse outcomes with Early implementation of the ACC/AHA guidelines) initiative. *Circulation*. 2006;114:1380-1387.

252. Gutierrez J, Ramirez G, Rundek T, Sacco RL. Statin therapy in the prevention of recurrent cardiovascular events: a sex-based meta-analysis. *Arch Intern Med*. 2012;172:909-919.

253. Morrow DA, Scirica BM, Karwatowska-Prokopczuk E, et al. Effects of ranolazine on recurrent cardiovascular events in patients with non-ST-elevation acute coronary syndromes: the MERLIN-TIMI 36 randomized trial. *JAMA*. 2007;297:1775-1783.

254. Mega JL, Hochman JS, Scirica BM, et al. Clinical features and outcomes of women with unstable ischemic heart disease: observations from metabolic efficiency with ranolazine for less ischemia in non-ST-elevation acute coronary syndromes-thrombolysis in myocardial infarction 36 (MERLIN-TIMI 36). *Circulation*. 2010;121:1809-1817.

255. Kwan G, Balady GJ. Cardiac rehabilitation 2012: advancing the field through emerging science. *Circulation*. 2012;125:e369-373.

256. Suaya JA, Shepard DS, Normand SL, Ades PA, Prottas J, Stason WB. Use of cardiac rehabilitation by Medicare beneficiaries after myocardial infarction or coronary bypass surgery. *Circulation*. 2007;116:1653-1662.

257. Ghisi GL, Polyzotis P, Oh P, Pakosh M, Grace SL. Physician factors affecting cardiac rehabilitation referral and patient enrollment: a systematic review. *Clin Cardiol*. 2013;36:323-335.

258. Thomas RJ, Beatty AL, Beckie TM, et al. Home-based cardiac rehabilitation: a scientific statement from the American Association of Cardiovascular and Pulmonary Rehabilitation, the American Heart Association, and the American College of Cardiology. *Circulation*. 2019;140:e69-e89.

259. Blomkalns AL, Chen AY, Hochman JS, et al. Gender disparities in the diagnosis and treatment of non-ST-segment elevation acute coronary syndromes: large-scale observations from the CRUSADE (Can Rapid Risk Stratification of Unstable Angina Patients Suppress Adverse Outcomes With Early Implementation of the American College of Cardiology/American Heart Association Guidelines) National Quality Improvement Initiative. *J Am Coll Cardiol*. 2005;45:832-837.

260. Radovanovic D, Erne P, Urban P, et al. Gender differences in management and outcomes in patients with acute coronary syndromes: results on 20,290 patients from the AMIS Plus Registry. *Heart*. 2007;93:1369-1375.

261. Jneid H, Fonarow GC, Cannon CP, et al. Sex differences in medical care and early death after acute myocardial infarction. *Circulation*. 2008;118:2803-2810.

262. Li S, Fonarow GC, Mukamal KJ, et al. Sex and race/ethnicity-related disparities in care and outcomes after hospitalization for coronary artery disease among older adults. *Circ Cardiovasc Qual Outcomes*. 2016;9:S36-S44.

263. Lichtman JH, Leifheit-Limson EC, Watanabe E, et al. Symptom recognition and healthcare experiences of young women with acute myocardial infarction. *Circ Cardiovasc Qual Outcomes*. 2015;8:S31-S38.

264. Dreyer RP, Smolderen KG, Strait KM, et al. Gender differences in pre-event health status of young patients with acute myocardial infarction: a VIRGO study analysis. *Eur Heart J Acute Cardiovasc Care*. 2016;5:43-54.

265. Dreyer RP, Xu X, Zhang W, et al. Return to work after acute myocardial infarction: comparison between young women and men. *Circ Cardiovasc Qual Outcomes*. 2016;9:S45-S52.

266. Bugiardini R, Yan AT, Yan RT, et al. Factors influencing underutilization of evidence-based therapies in women. *Eur Heart J*. 2011;32:1337-1344.

267. Pasupathy S, Air T, Dreyer RP, Tavella R, Beltrame JF. Systematic review of patients presenting with suspected myocardial infarction and nonobstructive coronary arteries. *Circulation*. 2015;131:861-870.

268. Tamis-Holland JE, Jneid H, Reynolds HR, et al. Contemporary diagnosis and management of patients with myocardial infarction in the absence of obstructive coronary artery disease: a scientific statement from the American Heart Association. *Circulation*. 2019;139:e891-e908.

269. Safdar B, Spatz ES, Dreyer RP, et al. Presentation, clinical profile, and prognosis of young patients with myocardial infarction with nonobstructive coronary arteries (MINOCA): results from the VIRGO study. *J Am Heart Assoc*. 2018;7.

270. Pathik B, Raman B, Mohd Amin NH, et al. Troponin-positive chest pain with unobstructed coronary arteries: incremental diagnostic value of cardiovascular magnetic resonance imaging. *Eur Heart J Cardiovasc Imaging*. 2016;17:1146-1152.

271. Dastidar AG, Rodrigues JCL, Johnson TW, et al. Myocardial infarction with nonobstructed coronary arteries: impact of CMR early after presentation. *JACC Cardiovasc Imaging*. 2017;10:1204-1206.

272. Assomull RG, Lyne JC, Keenan N, et al. The role of cardiovascular magnetic resonance in patients presenting with chest pain, raised troponin, and unobstructed coronary arteries. *Eur Heart J*. 2007;28:1242-1249.

273. Tornvall P, Gerbaud E, Behaghel A, et al. Myocarditis or "true" infarction by cardiac magnetic resonance in patients with a clinical diagnosis of myocardial infarction without obstructive coronary disease: a meta-analysis of individual patient data. *Atherosclerosis*. 2015;241:87-91.

274. Nef HM, Mollmann H, Akashi YJ, Hamm CW. Mechanisms of stress (Takotsubo) cardiomyopathy. *Nat Rev Cardiol*. 2010;7:187-193.

275. Vrints CJ. Spontaneous coronary artery dissection. *Heart*. 2010;96:801-808.

276. Saw J, Mancini GBJ, Humphries KH. Contemporary review on spontaneous coronary artery dissection. *J Am Coll Cardiol*. 2016;68:297-312.

277. Hayes SN, Kim ESH, Saw J, et al. Spontaneous coronary artery dissection: current state of the science: a scientific statement From the American Heart Association. *Circulation*. 2018;137:e523-e557.

278. van den Hoogen IJ, Gianni U, Wood MJ, et al. The clinical spectrum of myocardial infarction and ischemia with nonobstructive coronary arteries in women. *JACC Cardiovasc Imaging*. 2021;14(5):1053-1062.

279. Tweet MS, Hayes SN, Pitta SR, et al. Clinical features, management, and prognosis of spontaneous coronary artery dissection. *Circulation*. 2012;126:579-588.

280. Saw J, Aymong E, Sedlak T, et al. Spontaneous coronary artery dissection: association with predisposing arteriopathies and precipitating stressors and cardiovascular outcomes. *Circ Cardiovasc Interv*. 2014;7:645-655.

281. Elkayam U, Jalnapurkar S, Barakkat MN, et al. Pregnancy-associated acute myocardial infarction: a review of contemporary experience in 150 cases between 2006 and 2011. *Circulation*. 2014;129:1695-1702.

282. Saw J, Humphries K, Aymong E, et al. Spontaneous coronary artery dissection: clinical outcomes and risk of recurrence. *J Am Coll Cardiol*. 2017;70:1148-1158.

283. Ahmed B, Creager MA. Alternative causes of myocardial ischemia in women: an update on spontaneous coronary artery dissection, vasospastic angina and coronary microvascular dysfunction. *Vasc Med*. 2017;22:146-160.

284. Ong P, Athanasiadis A, Hill S, Vogelsberg H, Voehringer M, Sechtem U. Coronary artery spasm as a frequent cause of acute coronary syndrome: the CASPAR (Coronary Artery Spasm in Patients With Acute Coronary Syndrome) study. *J Am Coll Cardiol.* 2008;52:523-527.

285. Ghadri JR, Wittstein IS, Prasad A, et al. International Expert Consensus document on Takotsubo syndrome (part I): clinical characteristics, diagnostic criteria, and pathophysiology. *Eur Heart J.* 2018;39:2032-2046.

286. Ghadri JR, Wittstein IS, Prasad A, et al. International Expert Consensus document on Takotsubo syndrome (part II): diagnostic workup, outcome, and management. *Eur Heart J.* 2018;39:2047-2062.

287. Potts J, Sirker A, Martinez SC, et al. Persistent sex disparities in clinical outcomes with percutaneous coronary intervention: Insights from 6.6 million PCI procedures in the United States. *PLoS One.* 2018;13:e0203325.

288. Jacobs AK, Johnston JM, Haviland A, et al. Improved outcomes for women undergoing contemporary percutaneous coronary intervention: a report from the National Heart, Lung, and Blood Institute Dynamic registry. *J Am Coll Cardiol.* 2002;39:1608-1614.

289. Lansky AJ, Pietras C, Costa RA, et al. Gender differences in outcomes after primary angioplasty versus primary stenting with and without abciximab for acute myocardial infarction: results of the Controlled Abciximab and Device Investigation to Lower Late Angioplasty Complications (CADILLAC) trial. *Circulation.* 2005;111:1611-1618.

290. Heer T, Hochadel M, Schmidt K, et al. Sex differences in percutaneous coronary intervention-insights from the coronary angiography and PCI registry of the German Society of Cardiology. *J Am Heart Assoc.* 2017;6.

291. Stefanini GG, Baber U, Windecker S, et al. Safety and efficacy of drug-eluting stents in women: a patient-level pooled analysis of randomised trials. *Lancet.* 2013;382:1879-1888.

292. Levit RD, Reynolds HR, Hochman JS. Cardiovascular disease in young women: a population at risk. *Cardiology Rev.* 2011;19:60-65.

293. Alkhouli M, Alqahtani F, Elsisy MF, Kawsara A, Alasnag M. Incidence and outcomes of acute ischemic stroke following percutaneous coronary interventions in men versus women. *Am J Cardiol.* 2020;125:336-340.

294. Davis MB, Maddox TM, Langner P, Plomondon ME, Rumsfeld JS, Duvernoy CS. Characteristics and outcomes of women veterans undergoing cardiac catheterization in the Veterans Affairs Healthcare System: insights from the VA CART Program. *Circ Cardiovasc Qual Outcomes.* 2015;8:S39-S47.

295. Hess CN, McCoy LA, Duggirala HJ, et al. Sex-based differences in outcomes after percutaneous coronary intervention for acute myocardial infarction: a report from TRANSLATE-ACS. *J Am Heart Assoc.* 2014;3:e000523.

296. Rao SV, Hess CN, Barham B, et al. A registry-based randomized trial comparing radial and femoral approaches in women undergoing percutaneous coronary intervention: the SAFE-PCI for Women (Study of Access Site for Enhancement of PCI for Women) trial. *JACC Cardiovasc Intervent.* 2014;7:857-867.

297. Epps KC, Holper EM, Selzer F, et al. Sex differences in outcomes following percutaneous coronary intervention according to age. *Circ Cardiovasc Qual Outcomes.* 2016;9:S16-S25.

298. Acharjee S, Teo KK, Jacobs AK, et al. Optimal medical therapy with or without percutaneous coronary intervention in women with stable coronary disease: a pre-specified subset analysis of the Clinical Outcomes Utilizing Revascularization and Aggressive druG Evaluation (COURAGE) trial. *Am Heart J.* 2016;173:108-117.

299. Blankstein R, Ward RP, Arnsdorf M, Jones B, Lou YB, Pine M. Female gender is an independent predictor of operative mortality after coronary artery bypass graft surgery: contemporary analysis of 31 Midwestern hospitals. *Circulation.* 2005;112:I323-I327.

300. Dalen M, Nielsen S, Ivert T, Holzmann MJ, Sartipy U. Coronary artery bypass grafting in women 50 years or younger. *J Am Heart Assoc.* 2019;8:e013211.

301. Filardo G, Hamman BL, Pollock BD, et al. Excess short-term mortality in women after isolated coronary artery bypass graft surgery. *Open Heart.* 2016;3:e000386.

302. Mannacio VA, Mannacio L. Sex and mortality associated with coronary artery bypass graft. *J Thorac Dis.* 2018;10:S2157-S2159.

303. Edwards FH, Carey JS, Grover FL, Bero JW, Hartz RS. Impact of gender on coronary bypass operative mortality. *Ann Thoracic Surg.* 1998;66:125-131.

304. Bukkapatnam RN, Yeo KK, Li Z, Amsterdam EA. Operative mortality in women and men undergoing coronary artery bypass grafting (from the California Coronary Artery Bypass Grafting Outcomes Reporting Program). *Am J Cardiol.* 2010;105:339-342.

305. O'Connor GT, Morton JR, Diehl MJ, et al. Differences between men and women in hospital mortality associated with coronary artery bypass graft surgery. The Northern New England Cardiovascular Disease Study Group. *Circulation.* 1993;88:2104-2110.

306. Jabagi H, Tran DT, Hessian R, Glineur D, Rubens FD. Impact of gender on arterial revascularization strategies for coronary artery bypass grafting. *Ann Thorac Surg.* 2018;105:62-68.

307. Angraal S, Khera R, Wang Y, et al. Sex and race differences in the utilization and outcomes of coronary artery bypass grafting among Medicare beneficiaries, 1999-2014. *J Am Heart Assoc.* 2018;7.

308. Farooq V, Serruys PW, Bourantas C, et al. Incidence and multivariable correlates of long-term mortality in patients treated with surgical or percutaneous revascularization in the synergy between percutaneous coronary intervention with taxus and cardiac surgery (SYNTAX) trial. *Eur Heart J.* 2012;33:3105-3113.

309. Serruys PW, Cavalcante R, Collet C, et al. Outcomes after coronary stenting or bypass surgery for men and women with unprotected left main disease: the EXCEL trial. *JACC Cardiovasc Interv.* 2018;11:1234-1243.

310. Rosamond WD. Geographic variation in cardiovascular disease burden: clues and questions. *JAMA Cardiol.* 2018;3:366-368.

311. Mensah GA, Roth GA, Fuster V. The global burden of cardiovascular diseases and risk factors: 2020 and beyond. *J Am Coll Cardiol.* 2019;74:2529-2532.

312. Collaborators GBDCoD. Global, regional, and national age-sex-specific mortality for 282 causes of death in 195 countries and territories, 1980-2017: a systematic analysis for the Global Burden of Disease Study 2017. *Lancet.* 2018;392:1736-1788.

313. Collaborators GBDM. Global, regional, and national age-sex-specific mortality and life expectancy, 1950-2017: a systematic analysis for the Global Burden of Disease Study 2017. *Lancet.* 2018;392:1684-1735.

314. Roth GA, Johnson C, Abajobir A, et al. Global, regional, and national burden of cardiovascular diseases for 10 causes, 1990 to 2015. *J Am Coll Cardiol.* 2017;70:1-25.

315. Gupta D, Wenger NK. Guidelines for the prevention of cardiovascular disease in women: international challenges and opportunities. *Expert Rev Cardiovasc Ther.* 2012;10:379-385.

316. Yusuf S, Reddy S, Ounpuu S, Anand S. Global burden of cardiovascular diseases: Part II: variations in cardiovascular disease by specific ethnic groups and geographic regions and prevention strategies. *Circulation.* 2001;104:2855-2864.

317. Yusuf S, Reddy S, Ounpuu S, Anand S. Global burden of cardiovascular diseases: part I: general considerations, the epidemiologic transition, risk factors, and impact of urbanization. *Circulation.* 2001;104:2746-2753.

318. Secretary-General's remarks at third high-level meeting of the United Nations General Assembly on the prevention and control of non-communicable diseases. *United Nations.* September 27, 2018. https://www.un.org/sg/en/content/sg/statement/2018-09-27/secretary-generals-remarks-third-high-level-meeting-united-nations. Accessed July 21, 2021.

319. http://www.wineuseF.

320. Peters SA, Huxley RR, Sattar N, Woodward M. Sex differences in the excess risk of cardiovascular diseases associated with type 2 diabetes: potential explanations and clinical implications. *Curr Cardiovasc Risk Rep.* 2015;9:36.

321. Chiuve SE, Fung TT, Rexrode KM, et al. Adherence to a low-risk, healthy lifestyle and risk of sudden cardiac death among women. *JAMA.* 2011;306:62-69.

322. Wood SF, Mieres JH, Campbell SM, Wenger NK, Hayes SN, Scientific Advisory Council of WomenHeart: The National Coalition for Women with Heart Disease. Advancing women's heart health through policy and science: highlights from the first national policy and science summit on women's cardiovascular health. *Women's Health Issues* 2016;26: 251-255.

323. Mehran R, Vogel B, Ortega R, Cooney R, Horton R. The Lancet Commission on women and cardiovascular disease: time for a shift in women's health. *Lancet*. 2019;393:967-968.

324. Kandasamy S, Anand SS. Cardiovascular disease among women from vulnerable populations: a review. *Can J Cardiol*. 2018;34:450-457.

325. Aggarwal NR, Patel HN, Mehta LS, et al. Sex differences in ischemic heart disease: advances, obstacles, and next steps. *Circ Cardiovasc Qual Outcomes*. 2018;11:e004437.

326. Cushman M, Shay CM, Howard VJ, et al. Ten-year differences in women's awareness related to coronary heart disease: results of the 2019 American Heart Association national survey: a special report from the American Heart Association. *Circulation*. 2020:CIR0000000000000907.

327. Shaw LJ, Bairey Merz CN, Pepine CJ, et al. Insights from the NHLBI-Sponsored Women's Ischemia Syndrome Evaluation (WISE) Study: Part I: gender differences in traditional and novel risk factors, symptom evaluation, and gender-optimized diagnostic strategies. *J Am Coll Cardiol*. 2006;47:S4-S20.

328. Pepine CJ, Anderson RD, Sharaf BL, et al. Coronary microvascular reactivity to adenosine predicts adverse outcome in women evaluated for suspected ischemia results from the National Heart, Lung and Blood Institute WISE (Women's Ischemia Syndrome Evaluation) study. *J Am Coll Cardiol*. 2010;55:2825-2832.

329. Bairey Merz CN, Pepine CJ, Walsh MN, Fleg JL. Ischemia and no obstructive coronary artery disease (INOCA): developing evidence-based therapies and research agenda for the next decade. *Circulation*. 2017;135:1075-1092.

330. Ford TJ, Corcoran D, Sidik N, McEntegart M, Berry C. Coronary microvascular dysfunction: assessment of both structure and function. *J Am Coll Cardiol*. 2018;72:584-586.

81

Race, Ethnicity, Disparities, Diversity, and Heart Disease

Clyde W. Yancy

Disproportionate burden of cardiovascular disease in racial/ethnic minorities

Black individuals

Hypertension, diabetes, and obesity:
↑ Prevalence

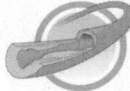

Coronary heart disease:
Smaller decline in incidence, ↑ mortality due to CHD

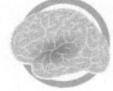

Stroke:
↑ Stroke mortality, ↑ rate of intracerebral hemorrhage in those aged ≤ 75 years

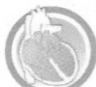

Heart failure:
Earlier age of onset, more-frequent hospitalization, ↑ risk of death due to heart failure

Sudden cardiac death:
↑ Rate, younger age at onset, ↓ survival to discharge if resuscitated and hospitalized

Peripheral vascular disease:
↑ Rate of peripheral arterial occlusive disease, ↑ risk of limb amputation

Chronic renal disease:
↑ Incidence

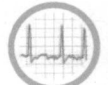

Atrial fibrillation:
↓ Incidence but stronger association of AF with CVD outcomes

Critical aortic stenosis:
Less likely to undergo transcatheter aortic valve replacement

Allostatic load:
↑ Environmental, societal, personal stress contributes to somatic aging and risk factors

Hispanic individuals

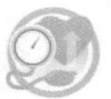

Cardiovascular disease:
↓ Incidence than in non-Hispanic white individuals

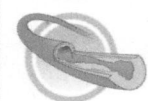

Hypertension, diabetes, and obesity:
↑ Incidence

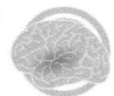

Coronary artery disease:
↓ Incidence than in non-Hispanic white individuals

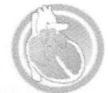

Stroke:
↑ Incidence of intracranial atherothrombosis & lacunar infarcts, ↓ incidence of cardioembolic strokes

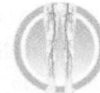

Heart failure:
↑ Incidence than white individuals but ↓ incidence than black individuals

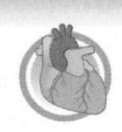

Peripheral vascular disease:
↓ Rate, ↑ rate of limb amputation

South Asian individuals

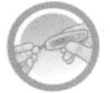

Cardiovascular disease:
↑ Risk when compared to Asians defined as Chinese, Filipino, Japanese, Korean and Vietnamese

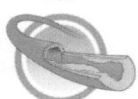

Type 2 diabetes:
↑ Incidence

Atherosclerotic cardiovascular disease:
↑ Risk, earlier age of onset, ↑ hospitalization rates, ↑ mortality

Chapter 81 Fuster and Hurst's Central Illustration. Race is not a proxy for the biology of disease and is more significant as an approximation of the life and living circumstances of groups of people. In all racial and ethnic minorities the disproportionate burden of cardiovascular disease is potentially amplified by subconscious bias with resultant health disparities. AF, atrial fibrillation; CHD, coronary heart disease; CVD, cardiovascular disease.

CHAPTER SUMMARY

This chapter defines the taxonomy and historical context of race, ethnicity, diversity, and bias and sets the root causes of disparities impacting cardiovascular disease. The epidemiology and consistently higher burden of cardiovascular disease are described according to race, ethnicity, indigenous, and immigrant status. By understanding that race is a social and not a biologic construct, the chapter suggests a more plausible reframing around genetics and ancestry. Racial and ethnic minorities experience a disproportionate burden of cardiovascular disease (see Fuster and Hurst's Central Illustration), which is strongly associated with the social condition and further amplified by subconscious bias with resultant health disparities. It has become increasingly clear that social determinants of health drive outcomes. Emerging science links life and living circumstances to an increased burden of cardiovascular risk, plausibly mediated via inflammatory pathways and subsequently yielding an increased burden of cardiovascular disease. As such, addressing the still evident race/ethnicity-based health disparities in cardiovascular disease will require a longitudinal committed and multifaceted approach that raises awareness, reduces the influence of bias, introduces more diversity in the healthcare workforce, involves more genetic discovery, targets more equity in the built environment, and roots out racism in medicine.

TAXONOMY

Race can be described as a grouping of humans based on shared physical, cultural, and social qualities in categories viewed as distinct by others.[1] Most scientists, however, assert that race is not biological and rather they define race as a social construct, meaning that race congregates humans according to shared life and living experiences. Moreover, race is a political construct where, especially in the United States, the designation of race evolved from a history that emanates from slavery and that still fuels racism. Racial categorization allows for broad generalizations and stereotyping, which can be counterproductive in cardiovascular medicine.

The correct ascertainment of race per se is by self assignment. The greater question is why is the ascertainment of racial status important in contemporary medicine? The social context, inferred by race, is of great importance in the attainment of health and access to health care, but for conditions, including cardiovascular conditions, presumed to be inherited or to have a genetic basis, ancestry is the more appropriate biologically based clinical inquiry. Race is not a proxy for genetics, but ancestry does serve as a surrogate for familial or shared inherited genetics that not only define groups of people but inform the likelihood for certain conditions and/or the response to certain therapeutics. Even ancestry is complicated because the ancestry of Black people in the Americas can be traced to the period from 1619 to 1850 when millions of indigenous West and Central Africans from seven African coastal regions were kidnapped and transported to the Americas.[1,2] The subsequent genetic admixture from comingling of populations and non-African parentage has yielded sufficient heterogeneity in individual genetics that race is fully obviated as a marker of inherited conditions.

Nevertheless, we must recognize that 13% of the US population self-identifies as Black and do share similar health and cardiovascular disease (CVD) characteristics.[3] And especially when race is queried in clinical medicine, it is often a binary question: Black or White? By convention, racial data are routinely captured and both health status and disease are currently presented as a function of race. These data continue to inform our understanding of health disparities and importantly any progress in minimizing those disparities. As the ease with which genomic data and especially genetic admixture analyses can be ascertained and the precision with which there is an alignment of genetics and disease, the use of race to infer biological descriptions of disease in clinical medicine should dissipate—but the role that race plays in capturing shared social experiences that implicate health status will continue.

Ethnicity is more easily defined but is often conflated with race, therefore resulting in marked confusion in clinical medicine.[4] By definition, ethnicity is consistently defined as a category of people who identify with each other on the basis of similarities in language, history, society, culture, religion, and race. A simpler definition is that ethnicity recognizes differences between people mostly based on language and shared custom. Ethnicity is derived from the Spanish term *ethnicidad* and entered US lexicon in 1970 when the US Census adopted the term to capture those who self-identify as Hispanic.[5] Hispanic was intended to capture any individual of any race with origins in Mexico, the Caribbean, Central America, or other Spanish-speaking countries. Today, the Hispanic population are the largest minority group in the United States, constituting 17% of the population or approximately 50 million people. By 2050, that number will approach 30% of the US population. Genetic admixture has also impacted Hispanic individuals, resulting in variations depending upon the extent of African, European, and Amerindian ancestry.

Discussions about race and ethnicity are not limited to Black versus White or Hispanic versus non-Hispanic. Many self-identify ethnicity as Asian but in multiple iterations. Some self-describe aptly as South Asian descent. The countries of origin for this group includes Bangladesh, Bhutan, India, the Maldives, Nepal, Pakistan, and Sri Lanka. Asian also captures those with origin from China, Japan, and other prototypical Asian countries. Asian Pacific Islanders note Samoa, Guam, and other Pacific Island countries or territories as their origin.[6] Most importantly, Native Americans or Indigenous Americans captures those with origin from one of 574 recognized tribes with habitats in North America, some of which date to 15,000 years prior to European colonization of North America.

For all of the foregoing groups, race and ethnicity serve as the basis upon which disease descriptions are offered and also serve as the basis for bias, explicit and implicit, and stereotyping in medical decision-making. These powerful influences drive outcomes that may result in disparate care and are in part responsible for health inequities.

DIVERSITY AND INCLUSION, BIAS, AND DISPARITIES

Diversity describes the heterogeneity within groups and captures the distribution of individuals in a targeted domain as a function of race and ethnicity (although sex and gender are appropriate attributes of consideration in certain domains, particularly professional cohorts). In many professions and especially in medicine, including cardiovascular medicine, there is an absence of diversity. Inclusion is an overt intentionality to fully incorporate all members of a group in shared governance, responsibility, and ownership. Ostensibly, more diversity in medicine is expected to result in more equitable decision-making, although this premise remains unproven. *Diversity and inclusion* entered the lexicon within the last several decades. The origin of diversity and inclusion was driven by the recognition of striking differences by race/ethnicity/sex and gender for inexplicable reasons and mostly heralded by various social movements (eg, suffrage, civil rights, and gay rights). The evolution of diversity and inclusion led to targeted programs to achieve greater representation, many of which initially failed. The current iteration, now aptly described as "diversity, equity and inclusion" is considered a pathway toward a greater good with the intent of capturing more diversity of thought to be associated with a goal in medicine, and in turn cardiovascular medicine, of achieving better health outcomes and higher quality.[7] The driver for these efforts has been the still evident disparate health outcomes as a function of race/ethnicity driven, at least in part by the pernicious influence of bias—both overt and especially subconscious bias.

Bias is an automatic preference (or dislike) for a social group that is often subconscious (ie, not operative in the cognitive awareness of an individual). Bias is informed by lived experiences and is heavily influenced by culture. Rigorous testing of implicit bias in medicine demonstrates a consistent 70% preference for men of European descent *by medical students irrespective of their own race/ethnicity/gender/sex.*[8] The function of these automatic responses is to introduce a thought economy that allows for the rapid assessment of circumstances, particularly threats followed by a patterned response. Not all biases are negative, some are positive—physical appearance, personality, intellect—but it is in this "sorting" process that some are subjected to less than fair or equitable decision-making. This in part leads to health disparities.

The definition of a health disparity was codified in a seminal Institute of Medicine (now the National Academy of Medicine) report, "Unequal Treatment."[9] This treatise on the state of inequitable and biased care in the United States continues to stand as the reference point for healthcare disparities. In the setting where there is equal access to care by race, a persistent difference in health quality is consistently noted. Where those differences are attributable to clinical appropriateness and patient preference, the differences are simply that—differences. However, those differences in health outcomes that are attributable to circumstances in healthcare delivery systems, differences in the built environment, social determinants of health (SDOH), and especially when biased decision-making is at play, become not just differences, but disparities (**Fig. 81–1**).

The COVID-19 pandemic will for some time stand as the most substantial example of healthcare disparities to date. Black individuals experienced a 3-fold greater rate of death and Hispanic people experienced a nearly 3-fold greater rate of death than White individuals. (https://www.apmresearchlab.org/covid/deaths-by-race)

The known risk factors for SARS-CoV-2 infection including hypertension, CVD including heart failure, obesity, and diabetes were all disproportionately represented in Black and Hispanic populations but a particular onerous risk variable was the community of residence with remarkable evidence of clustered infection and death in those communities known to have the highest vulnerability, measured as the Social Vulnerability Index (SVI) (https://svi.cdc.gov/), to calamitous events. The impact of longitudinal disinvestment in marginalized communities and the subsequent vulnerability became evident in the COVID-19 pandemic as a dramatic burden of illness and death uniquely impacting Black and Hispanic people.[10]

EPIDEMIOLOGY OF CARDIOVASCULAR DISEASE BY RACE/ETHNICITY

Despite a decade-long decline in the incidence of coronary heart disease and a corresponding decrease in the incidence of death due to coronary heart disease, those declines have been much less noteworthy in the Black population. The decline for Black men has been ~3% per year versus 6.5% per year for White men; and 4% per year versus 5% per year for Black women versus White women. Death rates due to fatal coronary heart disease for both Black men and women are 2-fold higher than for White men and women.[11]

Variations by race in heart failure have been well described. Black individuals experience heart failure at an earlier age

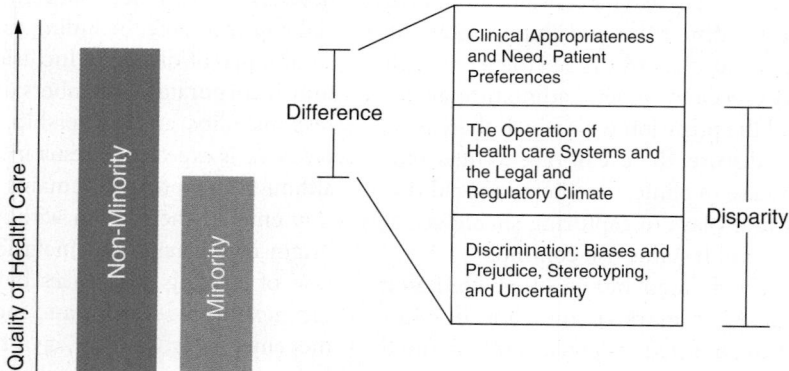

IOM Report: Differences, Disparities, and Discrimination

Disparities: racial or ethnic differences in health care that are not due to access related factors, clinical needs, patient preferences, or the appropriateness of the intervention.

Quality of Health Care

Non-Minority

Minority

Difference

Clinical Appropriateness and Need, Patient Preferences

The Operation of Health care Systems and the Legal and Regulatory Climate

Discrimination: Biases and Prejudice, Stereotyping, and Uncertainty

Disparity

Populations with Equal Access to Health Care

Figure 81–1. Differences, disparities, and discrimination: Populations with equal access to health care. Reproduced with permission from Smedley BD, Stith AY, Nelson AR, et al. *Unequal Treatment: Confronting Racial and Ethnic Disparities in Healthcare.* Washington, DC: The Institute of Medicine, National Academies Press; 2002.

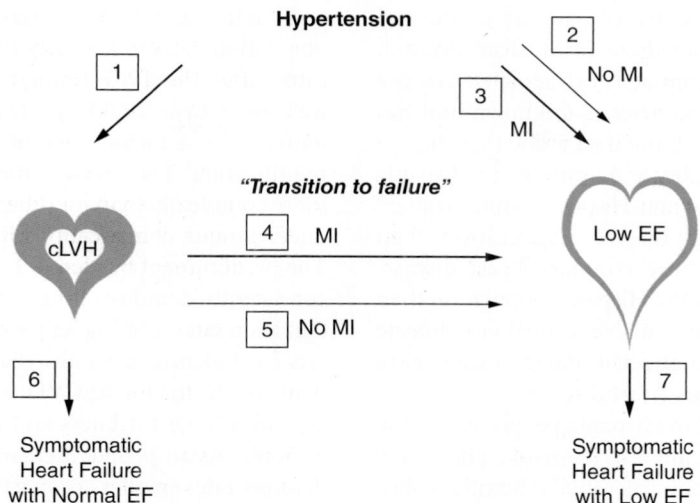

Figure 81–2. The 7 pathways in the progression from hypertension to heart failure. Hypertension progresses to concentric (thick-walled) LVH (cLVH; pathway 1). The direct pathway from hypertension to dilated cardiac failure (increased LV volume with reduced LV ejection fraction [LVEF]) can occur without (pathway 2) or with (pathway 3) an interval myocardial infarction (MI). Concentric hypertrophy progresses to dilated cardiac failure (transition to failure) most commonly via an interval MI (pathway 4). Recent data suggest that it is not common for concentric hypertrophy to progress to dilated cardiac failure without interval MI (pathway 5). Patients with concentric LVH can develop symptomatic heart failure with a preserved LVEF (pathway 6), and patients with dilated cardiac failure can develop symptomatic heart failure with reduced LVEF (pathway 7). The influences of other important modulators of the progression of hypertensive heart disease, including obesity, diabetes mellitus, age, environmental exposures, and genetic factors, are not shown to simplify the diagram. A *thicker arrow* depicts a more common pathway compared with a *thinner arrow*. Reproduced with permission from Drazner MH. The transition from hypertrophy to failure: how certain are we? *Circulation.* 2005 Aug 16;112(7):936-938.

and experience more frequent hospitalization. A presumed nonischemic etiology remains a well-described observation.[12] Hypertension and hypertensive heart disease are the presumed culprit etiologies, although ongoing research continues to evolve biological mechanisms that connect hypertension, left ventricular hypertrophy (LVH), and ventricular remodeling with reduced ejection fraction (**Fig. 81–2**).[13] Recent data now demonstrate a disturbing increase in the risk of death due to heart failure in the Black population, especially younger Black men. For the period from 1999 through 2012, age-adjusted rates for heart failure–related cardiovascular deaths declined but began to increase in 2017 and especially so in Black versus White populations: 1.43/1.54-fold higher in Black men and women respectively compared to White men and women. Especially in those 35 to 64 years of age, there were 2.6/2.9-fold higher death rates for Black versus White men and women, respectively.[14] Whether these new data describing death rates due to heart failure can be attributed to the burden of heart failure risk factors, access to care, or health policy is not clear.

Sudden cardiac arrest also varies by race as the rate of sudden cardiac death is twice as high for Black versus White populations and the age at onset is 6 years younger. If resuscitated and hospitalized, survival to discharge is less for Black versus White patients, 25% versus 37%.[15]

In parallel with the prevalence of hypertension in the Black population, stroke is a major concern. As with death due to coronary heart disease, multiple public health initiatives, increased detection and treatment for hypertension, and the evolution of effective acute stroke interventions have resulted

in an 80% decrement in stroke mortality. This public health triumph has not however been fully shared by the Black population because the stroke mortality rates for the Black versus White population remains 4- to 5-fold higher. Stronger public health initiatives targeting detection and control of hypertension in Black individuals are needed.[16] This difference is driven in part by the regionalization of risk as those in the traditional "Stroke Belt" do carry a disproportionate stroke-related morbidity (possibly greater vulnerability) and mortality. Intracerebral hemorrhage is an especially onerous stroke phenotype and impacts the Black population more than the White population, especially at younger ages where the rate is doubled in the 45 to 64 age group but falls to unity in those >75.[17]

Peripheral vascular disease impacts the Black population disproportionately. The rate of peripheral arterial occlusive disease is 2-fold higher.[18] This is in part due to the burden of risk factors, especially smoking but remarkably, even after adjusting for all known risk factors, there is persistent evidence of a greater incidence of peripheral vascular disease in the Black population. Among the first descriptions of disparate care was the differential incidence of limb amputation for peripheral vascular disease in Black versus White populations. Even contemporary analyses have identified Black race as a risk factor for limb amputation with Black individuals experiencing a 37% higher amputation risk than White individuals, even after controlling for socioeconomic status.[19]

The epidemiology of CVD for the Hispanic population is in variance from that described for the Black population. Data describing the epidemiology of CVD in the Hispanic population are rarely subdivided by country of origin and the majority contribution is from those of Mexican descent. Whether or not data can be appropriately extrapolated to those from other Spanish speaking countries is unknown and has been called into question. Overall, the data argue that though CVD is a leading cause of morbidity and mortality in Hispanic people, the incidence is *less* than in non-Hispanic White people.[20] The incidence of coronary artery disease is again lower than in non-Hispanic people. Premature coronary heart disease, age <40, is substantially lower in the Hispanic population than all other groups. Where data are available to further delineate which Hispanic people are most affected, Puerto Ricans have the highest prevalence of coronary heart disease.[21]

Stroke incidence is increased in Hispanic people, especially in those of Mexican origin.[22] Of interest, the stroke phenotype varies with a greater incidence of intracranial atherothrombosis and lacunar infarcts and a lesser incidence of cardioembolic strokes. Data for heart failure events position the Hispanic population between the Black (highest incidence) and White population (lower incidence) for heart failure. A similar burden of risk factors for heart failure is noted with a higher incidence of diabetes, obesity, and hypertension. Like all other groups, heart failure with preserved ejection fraction represents at least 50% of all persons affected. Peripheral vascular disease occurs at a lower rate in Hispanic than White individuals and a much lower rate in Hispanic than Black individuals (about one-half that is seen in Black individuals); but limb amputation rates are higher than in White individuals.[23] This is presumed to represent an evident healthcare disparity but further study is required.

Given the surfeit of risk factors for coronary artery disease, heart failure, and stroke—especially obesity, hypertension, and diabetes, the findings of a lesser incidence of CVD has been designated the *Hispanic Paradox*.[24] The paradox extends beyond heart disease and incorporates a 24% lower all-cause mortality risk. These data have not been disaggregated as a function of country of origin and explanations are lacking. Hispanic people are presumed to be healthier at the time of immigration, and are known to have lower smoking rates and stronger social networks. Some have argued the existence of a "salmon bias" hypothesis where Hispanic people return to their country of origin to die, which would result in gross underestimation of mortality rates in the United States.[25] No biologically plausible data have been posited to otherwise explain these observations and in more contemporary data sets, it may no longer be true and moreover may not be applicable for all Hispanic groups. In carefully acquired data according to country of origin, only Mexican and Central American Hispanic groups experience a lesser incidence of all-cause mortality. Additionally, as a function of time spent living in the United States, the paradox narrows, likely due to acculturation of Western lifestyles.

South Asian people constitute a growing percent of the US population and bear a higher risk of atherosclerotic cardiovascular disease (ASCVD) as well as a higher burden of ASCVD risk factors. The risk of CVD is decidedly increased compared to Asian people defined as Chinese, Filipino, Japanese, Korean,

and Vietnamese.[26] The presence of a significant South Asian population dates to the early 20th century, but the largest influx came after the 1965 Immigration and Nationality Act that welcomed over 20,000 professionals and 25,000 physicians followed by a major wave of immigration leading to family reunification. The several different languages spoken leads to more complexity than for other racial/ethnic groups and introduces unique complications in healthcare seeking behaviors. The predominant burden of CVD has been ASCVD with data consistently demonstrating earlier age of onset, higher hospitalization rates, and higher mortality rates. Multiple cohort data sets have identified South Asian race/ethnicity as an independent risk factor for ASCVD. Markers of early atherosclerosis, carotid intimal thickness and coronary calcium are increased in South Asian people. Remarkably, angiography consistently demonstrates smaller coronary artery luminal diameters and a greater likelihood of multivessel coronary disease present at the time of diagnosis even after adjustment for known risk factors for coronary artery disease.[27,28]

The disproportionate burden of coronary artery disease may be attributable to the cardiometabolic burden of impaired glucose tolerance, insulin resistance, and the metabolic syndrome. Lower insulin-like growth factor-binding protein and higher plasma leptin levels have also been described. As a result, South Asian people have a 200% higher incidence of type 2 diabetes mellitus with over 120 million South Asian people expected to have diabetes by 2030.[29] Obesity is yet another risk factor of importance. The World Health Organization has identified different waist circumference measurements in the definition of obesity in South Asian individuals so as to more accurately capture those at risk. This re-calibration is important because South Asian individuals have lower body mass index (BMI) and even body weight compared with most other race/ethnic groups but higher levels of visceral, hepatic, and pericardial fat. The variation in obesity extends to higher percent of body fat and higher waist-to-hip ratio. Lipid profiles also differ. Lower levels of high-density lipoprotein cholesterol and hypertriglyceridemia are consistently noted. Lipoprotein(a) elevations have been described in South Asian people and have been associated with the burden of atherosclerosis. As lipoprotein(a) is likely genetically determined, this finding would add credence to an inherited tendency for increased ASCVD in the South Asian population. There are additional concerns that South Asian people may experience more ASCVD due to a prothrombotic risk as earmarked by higher homocysteine, plasminogen activator inhibitor-1, and a higher inflammatory burden characterized by increased C-reactive protein, interleukin-6, and tumor necrosis factor alpha (TNF-a). These prothrombotic and proinflammatory markers when combined with predominant cardiometabolic disease create a milieu that leads to increased ASCVD. The likelihood for genetic factors contributing to the increased risk of ASCVD is supported by recent genome-wide association studies (GWASs) with common variants associated with diabetes described in South Asian people.[30] Fully elucidating the genetic underpinning of ASCVD in South Asian people will require much more work given the heterogeneity of the cohort and the multiple epigenetic factors at play.

THE UNIQUE BURDEN OF CARDIOVASCULAR DISEASE RISK IN THE BLACK POPULATION

Traditional risk factors for CVD are well described and include hypertension, diabetes, dyslipidemia, obesity, smoking, and physical inactivity. Importantly, all of these risk factors and risk behaviors are disproportionately represented in the Black population.

Hypertension is the most compelling risk factor for CVD in the Black population and impacts over 40% of Black men and women over the age of 20.[31] This prevalence is among the highest in the world and varies according to the percent African ancestry. Differences in the pattern of hypertension emerge in childhood and remain evident throughout the lifespan, up to a 1.5 times higher risk of hypertension.[32] The consequences of hypertension are also greater in Black people with the association of systolic blood pressure levels and stroke 3 times higher, even after treatment for hypertension.[33] LVH is an important substrate that results in CVD events and all-cause mortality.

Important data make clear the greater incidence, up to 3-fold, of LVH in Black people even after controlling for systolic blood pressure (**Fig. 81–3**).[34] Even when LVH is not present, Black people manifest a higher incidence of greater LV mass when indexed to height and weight otherwise known as inappropriate left ventricular mass (iLVM). The presence of iLVM, like LVH, associates with an increased risk of CVD events (2.5-fold higher) and an increased risk for all-cause mortality (1.24-fold higher).[35]

Diabetes mirrors a similar pattern in Black individuals with a higher prevalence noted in Black versus non-Hispanic White individuals (21% vs 11%).[36] The prevalence of prediabetes is also elevated and the disproportionate burden of diabetes persists through the life course. One in three Black individuals with diabetes is not diagnosed and the consequences of the disease evolve unchecked. Over the lifespan, Black men develop diabetes 1.5 times as often and Black women 2.4 times as often as White men and women. Even establishing the diagnosis of diabetes requires re-calibration in Black individuals because Hgb A1c can be lower, especially in those with the sickle cell

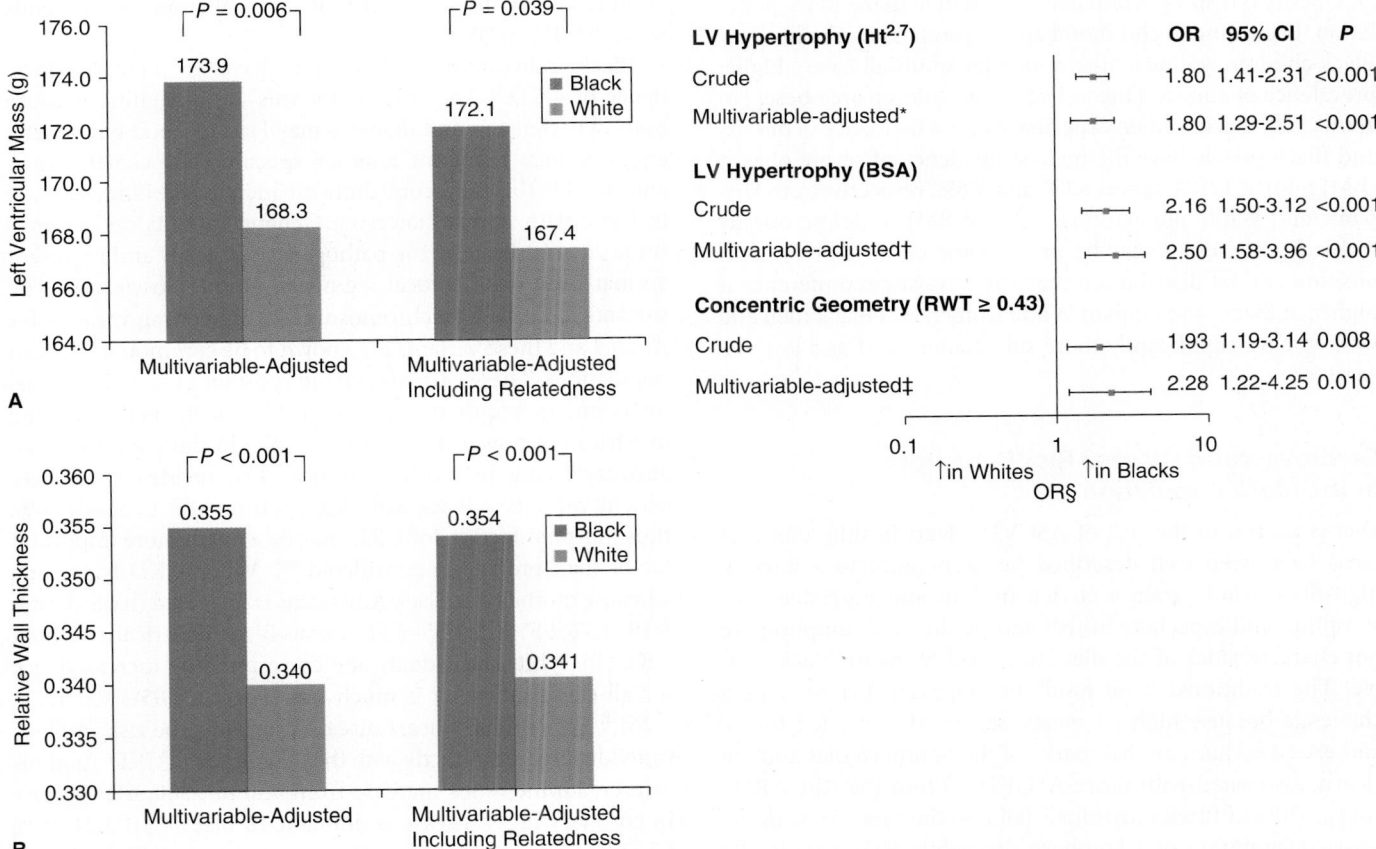

Figure 81–3. LVH is thought to be detrimental end-organ manifestation of hypertension. Black Americans are at higher risk. HYPERGEN is an NHLBI cohort study of >2000 Black and White hypertensive individuals aimed at studying genetic determinants of hypertension. **(A)** LV mass by race after multivariable adjustment and after multivariable adjustment including relatedness. **(B)** Relative wall thickness by race after multivariable adjustment and after multivariable adjustment including relatedness. These findings confirm the strong association between Black ethnicity and increased LV mass and relative wall thickness in hypertensive adults and demonstrate that these differences are independent of standard clinical and hemodynamic parameters. Reproduced with permission from Kizer JR, Arnett DK, Bella JN, et al. Differences in left ventricular structure between black and white hypertensive adults: the Hypertension Genetic Epidemiology Network study, *Hypertension*. 2004 Jun;43(6):1182-1188.

trait. Once diagnosed with diabetes, Black individuals are less likely to experience control and microvascular complications thus proliferate—four times as likely to have ophthalmological disease and nearly four times as likely to experience diabetes-related end-stage renal disease.[37]

Dyslipidemia does not appear to follow the same lines of racial differences. The prevalence of increased cholesterol levels is about the same in Black versus White populations (~32%–37%), but this is despite the known higher incidence of ASCVD in Black versus White populations. In older persons, age >45, the incidence of dyslipidemia is higher in Black men (risk ratio [RR] 1.15; 95% confidence interval [CI], 1.04–1.28) and women (RR 1.17; 95% CI, 1.08–1.28) compared to White men and women. These differences continue to widen with advancing age: Black men (RR 1.26; 95% CI, 1.06–1.51) and women (RR 1.39; 95% CI, 1.00–1.95) versus White men and women >75.[38] What is perhaps more revealing is the awareness of dyslipidemia and thus the opportunity to initiate disease modifying therapy. In both the Reasons for Geographic And Racial Differences in Stroke (REGARDS) study and in the Multi-Ethnic Study of Atherosclerosis (MESA) cohort study, Black individuals were less likely to be aware of dyslipidemia and experienced the lowest rates of control.[39]

Obesity is disproportionately represented in the Black population. Beginning in childhood and encompassing the lifespan, Black children, young adults, and older adults all have a higher prevalence of obesity. One in five Black children are obese. For adults >20, Black women experience a 58% incidence of obesity and Black people have the highest incidence of severe obesity (BMI >40) at 12.1% versus 5.8% and 5.6%, respectively, in Hispanic and White populations.[40] Use of BMI to define obesity in Black individuals may be problematic because body composition and fat distribution may vary. Waist circumference is higher in Black women than White women and Black men and women have significantly more subcutaneous fat and less visceral fat.

Cardiovascular Disease Risk Behaviors in the Black Population

Diet is central in the risk of ASCVD. Heart healthy diet patterns have been well described but adherence to a low-fat, high-fiber, whole grain diet rich in fruit and vegetable consumption and especially in fish and poultry consumption are not characteristics of the diet consumed by many Black people. The traditional "soul food" or Southern diet remains a challenge because high-fat meats, saturated fats, fried foods, and excess sodium are hallmarks of the Southern diet and are clearly associated with more ASCVD.[41] From the REGARDS study, ~10% of Black individuals fall into the category with the least consumption of a Southern diet while 60% were in the uppermost quartile for dietary consumption of a Southern diet. In the REGARDS study, adjustment for this behavior alone (ie, the Southern diet), mediated 63% of the risk for stroke.[42]

Very few Americans engage in sufficient physical activity and Black individuals are no different. Only 1 in 5 Black men and 1 in 6 Black women engage in the recommended levels of physical activity. Time spent in sedentary activities is on par with other groups. Whether or not there are unique barriers to physical activity remains under investigation but income limitations, work expectations, and predilections for certain activities and biases against other activities may be responsible in part for the high level of physical inactivity observed in Black individuals.

Smoking is a major concern because the risk of cigarette smoking is the same regardless of race/ethnicity. Younger White people have a higher incidence of smoking behaviors but Black people have a greater exposure to secondhand smoke and have a lower quit rate. A particularly vexing problem is the increased use of addiction enhancing mentholated tobacco products in Black neighborhoods that appears to be aligned with marketing strategies unique to Black neighborhoods. The use of mentholated products among adults who smoke is 71% in Black, 28% in Hispanic, and 21% in White populations. Correspondingly, quit rates are lowest in the Black population.[43]

Important Comorbidities in the Black Population

In the evaluation of the Black population with ASCVD, it is important to account for common comorbidities including chronic kidney disease (CKD), atrial fibrillation, aortic stenosis, and HIV/AIDS.

Black individuals are known to have an increased incidence of CKD.[44] The reasons for this are intriguing because both hypertension and diabetes may lead to CKD but genetic ancestry may represent another specific risk. Genetic variants in APOL1 may contribute to increased kidney disease in those with African ancestry. Genetic variants on chromosome 22 contribute to the pathogenesis of CKD and represent an increased risk for focal segmental glomerulosclerosis. The variants identified on chromosome 22 are coding variants for APOL1 and these variants are known to be common in African populations. These variants expand resistance to trypanosomal infection, an acquired mutation of benefit for persons living in Africa but now a risk factor for CKD in those with African ancestry living in North America. The incidence of these genetic variants in Black Americans is from ~8% to nearly 20%, thus this predilection for CKD may be a much more important factor than previously considered.[45,46] When CKD is present, all-cause mortality in Black Americans is increased (hazard ratio [HR] 1.76; 95% CI, 1.35–2.31) versus Black Americans without CKD. In White individuals, the corresponding increased risk for all-cause mortality is much less (HR 1.13; 95% CI, 1.02–1.26).[47] For coronary heart disease mortality, the risk in Black individuals varies directly with the magnitude of CKD. As albumin/creatinine ratios increase from <30 to >300, the increase in coronary heart disease is dramatic in Black (HR 3.21; 95% CI, 2.02–5.09) compared to White individuals (HR 1.49; 95% CI, 0.80–2.76). The corresponding increase in the risk of stroke was HR 2.70 (95% CI, 1.58–4.61) versus no increase in stroke risk for White individuals.[48]

Conversely, atrial fibrillation is less likely to occur in the Black population despite the preponderance of risk factors for atrial fibrillation including obesity, hypertension, and heart failure. Over a 20-year follow-up in the Atherosclerosis Risk in Communities (ARIC) cohort study, the incidence rate per 1000 person-years was 8.1 (95% CI, 7.7–8.5) in White and 5.8 (95% CI; 5.2–6.3) in Black individuals.[49] This observation has led to consideration of an "atrial fibrillation" paradox in the Black population. Even with advancing age, the increase in incidence of atrial fibrillation remains less in Black than White populations. This differential burden of atrial fibrillation may be driven in part by genetic factors. A recent genome wide admixture study of nine candidate single nucleotide polymorphisms yielded rs10824026 on chromosome 10 as a mediator for the higher risk of atrial fibrillation (AF) in White versus Black populations.[50] Despite the lesser incidence, the clinical outcomes are more worrisome in Black versus White individuals. In ARIC, the association of AF with CVD outcomes including stroke, heart failure, and coronary heart disease was stronger in Black versus White individuals, about 1.5- to 2.0-fold higher risk.[51] The strong association of AF with the risk of stroke requires appropriate preemptive treatment to mitigate the onset of stroke. An important observational study from the Outcomes Registry for Better Informed Treatment of Atrial Fibrillation II (ORBIT II), assessing the use of oral anticoagulation in those patients with adequate access to care demonstrated that even after controlling for socioeconomic factors, Black patients were less likely to receive the most effect guideline directed therapy to prevent stroke and the overall quality of anticoagulant therapy, regardless of choice, was lower in Black and Hispanic patients.[52]

Transcatheter aortic valve replacement (TAVR) has reduced the traditional risk of valve replacement and has increased longevity in those undergoing TAVR for critical aortic stenosis. For Black patients who experience critical aortic stenosis, the experience with TAVR is decidedly disparate. Among 70,221 patients undergoing TAVR and entered into the Transcatheter Valve Therapy registry, 91.3% were White, while only 3.8% were Black and 3.4% were Hispanic.[53] There were no differences in periprocedural outcomes and there is no evidence of higher referral for SAVR or surgical aortic valve replacement. This apparent disparity is under intense study beginning with a better understanding of the natural history of trileaflet calcific aortic stenosis in Black patients but assuming the natural history is not dissimilar, the focus will necessarily shift to root causes of this potential disparity.

Despite advances in our understanding of HIV/AIDS and more importantly in the treatment of HIV/AIDS, Black individuals continue to represent a disproportionate percentage of those with HIV infection now accounting for ~40% of those living with HIV/AIDS. It is known that HIV/AIDS is associated with a higher CVD risk but it is not clear that the increased risk varies as a function of race/ethnicity.

GENETICS AND ANCESTRY IN LIEU OF RACE

As previously stated, race is an insufficient proxy for genetics. But genetic predisposition to diseases and the response to therapeutic interventions have been described as the consequence of African ancestry. The best-described genetic variations address fibrinogen, C-reactive protein, Na+/K+/Ca++ exchanger, PCSK9, and SCN5A. Early descriptions of genetic differences in CVD burden as a function of race focused on single nucleotide polymorphisms (SNPs). Although informative, few if any SNPs are responsible for sufficient genetic variability alone to account uniquely for the differential expression of diseases. GWASs have greatly enabled the exploration of genetic-based descriptions of disease and disease burden. Using SNPs, the entire genome is searched in a large number of individuals to identify if the candidate SNP is consistently identified and maps to a gene of interest. When the populations studied carry the traits of interest or the disease under investigation the GWAS becomes a phenotype driven study; alternatively, a genotype study of carriers of a known SNP allows for association of that SNP with clinical disease. GWASs typically report allele frequency and effect size. Allele frequency varies as "mutation," rare, low frequency, and common variants while effect size is intuitively expressed as small, moderate, or large.

Fibrinogen is integral in clot formation and higher fibrinogen levels track with CVD. Up to 50% of the fibrinogen level may reflect heritability. African ancestry is associated with increased fibrinogen levels. GWASs have identified several genetic loci associated with fibrinogen but no more than 5% of the variance in Black Americans has been attributed to these variations. This continues to be an ongoing field of study.[54]

Twin studies suggest that hypertension may be heritable and perhaps up to 35% is genetic. Given the known excess burden of hypertension in the Black population, the presumption is that a genetic association, likely polygenic, must be present. Although candidate genes including those encoding the Na+/K+/Ca++ exchanger have been studied, no association has yet achieved statistical significance in GWASs. When African ancestry has been uniquely studied in genetic admixture mapping analyses, loci have been found on chromosome 5 (rs7726475) that are associated with systolic and diastolic blood pressure.[55] However, additional analyses have not been able to replicate these provocative findings. Studies are ongoing to further evaluate genetic associations in Black Americans with systolic and diastolic blood pressure.

GWASs focused on dyslipidemia have yielded SNPs in 13 candidate genes affecting all races.[56] Among these candidate genes: APOC3, APOL1 (previously described), and PCSK9. GWASs have identified variants in the PCSK9 gene that associate with large effects on low-density lipoprotein (LDL) in persons of African ancestry. This too remains an area of ongoing intense investigation.

Remarkably, the discovery story of proprotein convertase subtilisin/kexin type 9 inhibitors (PCSK9i) intersects with race-based science. Investigators leading the Dallas Heart Study identified common mutations in the coding region of the PCSK9 gene—Y142X and C679X—associated with a 40% reduction in plasma levels of LDL cholesterol. In seminal work, these mutations were tested in a different population (ARIC), and in 3363 Black individuals, the mutation was present in 2.6%, led to a nearly 30% reduction in mean LDL cholesterol, and an 88% reduction in the risk of coronary heart disease.

These discoveries led to the development of the PCSK9i now firmly established as evidence-based disease modifying therapy that reduces the risk of ASCVD.[57,58]

Great interest resides in the *SCN5A* gene that is important in cardiac conduction. A common variant is now well described in persons of African ancestry—*SCN5A-1103Y* allele. This variant may be present in 15% of Black Americans. An interaction has been described with QT prolongation and hypokalemia raising concerns for a predisposition to sudden cardiac death, particularly in diuretic associated hypokalemia.[59]

Heart failure in Black individuals appears to be a separate and distinct phenotype. Both the genetic predisposition to progression of disease and the pharmacogenomics of the response to medical therapy are important. Variations in nitric oxide homeostasis and increased oxidative stress have been implicated in the evolution of nonischemic LV dysfunction (**Fig. 81–4**). Candidate SNPs impacting nitric oxide synthase,[60] aldosterone synthase, and G-protein beta-3 subunit (GNB3)[61] have been implicated in the response to the combination of nitrates and hydralazine. Additionally, variations in beta-adrenergic receptor expression have been described as a function of race. Yet, the search for a genetic profile of heart failure in Black Americans remains a work in progress.[62] Despite the promise of personalized medicine, to date, there has been no effective implementation of a personalized pharmacogenomic approach in the treatment of heart failure.

The discovery of the benefit of the combination of nitrates and hydralazine in addition to angiotensin-converting enzyme (ACE) inhibitor/angiotensin receptor blocker (ARB) and evidence-based β-blocker therapy is yet another foray into race-based science. The Veterans Administration Cooperative Study (V-HeFT I) was amongst the earliest randomized double-blind placebo-controlled trials in cardiovascular medicine and tested the benefit of nitrates plus hydralazine versus placebo in patients with chronic heart failure. In post hoc analysis, a remarkable signal of benefit emerged among the small number of Black participants. This benefit was later tested prospectively in the African American Heart Failure Trial (AHeFT), a trial which included a Black-only study cohort (the signal was not present in the White cohort in V-HeFT I). The study was halted early for benefit with a 44% relative risk reduction in a composite of death, hospitalization, and quality of life. The US Food and Drug Administration (FDA) approval of fixed dose hydralazine plus isosorbide dinitrate remains the only race-based cardiovascular therapeutic. Uptake of this regimen in clinical practice has been minimal despite guideline prompted care. Reasons for lesser use include polypharmacy, the aura of race-based medicine, and most importantly the imprecision of the indication—which patient actually responds to nitric oxide enhancement? Ongoing research is exploring both genetic and admixture studies to elucidate more precise markers of benefit other than race.[63]

Thus, there is evidence for a genetic basis of disproportionate CVD in Black Americans. However, these signals have not yet yielded any definitive candidate genes or SNPs that convincingly describe disease risk and response to medical therapy, and have sufficient utility to impact clinical cardiovascular medicine. However, the *APOL1* story is the prototype and there

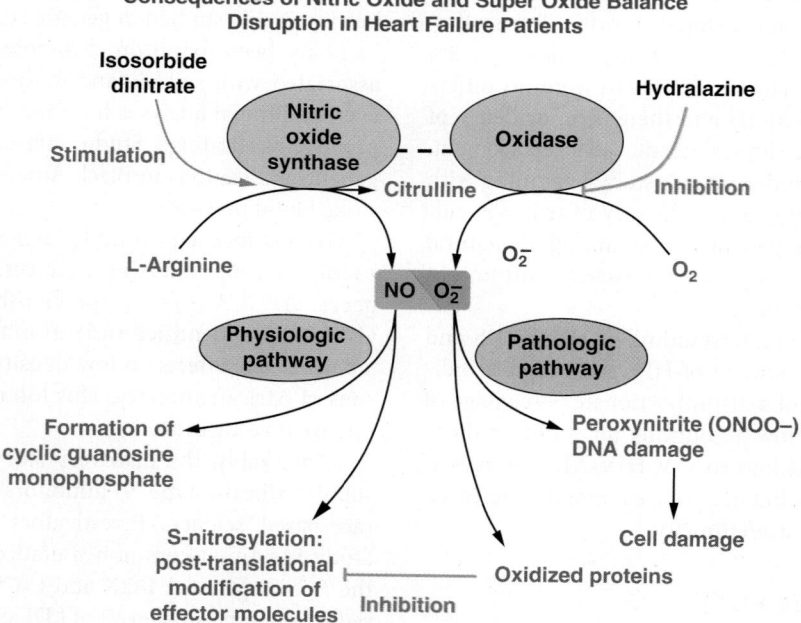

Consequences of Nitric Oxide and Super Oxide Balance Disruption in Heart Failure Patients

Figure 81–4. The interaction between nitric oxide (NO) and superoxide (O₂⁻), or the nitroso-redox balance, which has fundamental roles in cell and organ failure at key sites in the cardiovascular system. Isosorbide dinitrate, which stimulates the NO pathway, and hydralazine, an antioxidant that inhibits superoxide synthesis, may restore the balance of NO and superoxide production. Reproduced with permission from Hare JM. Nitroso-redox balance in the cardiovascular system. *N Engl J Med.* 2004 Nov 11;351(20):2112-2114.

are likely to be other examples that will emerge based on ongoing research. As such, we must return to an insistent position that race not be approximated to genetics and moreover maintain that race does not represent a biological construct.

RACE AS A SOCIAL CONSTRUCT

Where continued incorporation of race as a descriptor of health and disease matters is as a proxy for the social experience. It has become increasingly clear that the social conditions faced by many people drive health outcomes. In particular, the decided decrements in death due to coronary heart disease mentioned in the foregoing text are now beginning to plateau and may well start to increase being driven mostly by surges in hypertension, obesity, and diabetes. The close interdigitation of societal conditions and the built environment with these predominant cardiovascular risk factors requires a careful consideration of the influence of the social circumstance on CVD. The way in which the social circumstance exercises that influence has been articulated through the SDOH. Specifically, these determinants include (1) socioeconomic position (SEP), (2) race/ethnicity, (3) social support, (4) culture and language, (5) access to care, and (6) residential environment.[64] The SEP captures characteristics of importance including wealth, income, education, employment (**Table 81–1**). SEP defines access to and control of resources and defines social status—a variable that relates directly with health and life expectancy. Lower SEP in the United States is associated with CVD outcomes. Education is a clear marker of SEP and lower thresholds of attained education are associated with higher CVD mortality. The education-based differences observed between groups of people, especially as a function of race, account for nearly 20% of the gap in life expectancy between those same groups. The perverse influence of poor education attainment is again seen in health literacy and leads to an inability to navigate healthcare systems and manage complex medical conditions.[65]

Beyond education, there is evidence associating an increase in family income with a decrease in mortality and weakly associating higher status employment with lower levels of hypertension. However, job loss is clearly associated with CVD, including an increased incidence of myocardial infarction.[66]

A recently explored factor impacting CVD has been racism. Ambulatory blood pressure monitoring studies have identified an association between hypertension and self-reports of racism and discrimination.[67] Those reporting the highest levels of self-reported racism and hostility were more likely to exhibit an absence of nocturnal blood pressure dipping, a known marker for hypertension-related CVD.[68] Additional evidence demonstrates greater blood pressure variability (increase) during the recall of hostile experiences in Black versus White *normotensive* adults.[69] Beyond overt racism, the entry of bias into patient encounters may lead to lower quality care and lesser use of guideline directed therapies; and may also introduce "stereotype threat" where individuals fear being judged negatively according to racial stereotypes.[70]

The "weathering" hypothesis attempts to explain the effect of racism and hostility on health outcomes via an argument that the result of chronic exposure to social and economic disadvantage leads to acceleration of normal aging and predisposition to unfavorable health conditions. This hypothesis has been studied among young mothers and has been associated with low birth weight infants. Direct associations of weathering and CVD remain inconclusive but studies evaluating allostatic load (ie, wear and tear) have been associated with clear evidence of premature cellular aging as characterized by shorter telomere length and increased telomerase activity (TA). Men, especially Black men, having shorter telomeres with high TA show monocyte chemoattractant protein-1, reduced responsivity in diastolic BP, heart rate, and cortisol, when challenged with mental stress versus men with longer telomeres. Shorter telomeres with high TA are associated with reduced social support, lower optimism, higher hostility, and greater early life adversity. In aggregate, these provocative data suggest that cellular stress is associated with impaired proinflammatory and prothrombotic physiological stress responses and impoverished psychosocial resources. These observations on weathering and allostatic load offer an intriguing connection between psychological and physiological stress.[71]

Social support, defined as a network of others who provide care for a given individual, has been strongly associated with CVD outcomes. For those experiencing myocardial infarction, the absence of social support is associated with worse outcomes, and for those experiencing cardiac events as unmarried adults without an evident support network, the adjusted HR for survival is increased by up to 3-fold.[72]

A concept of increasing importance is that of "place" or residential environment. Striking differences in the burden of CVD have been associated with living in disadvantaged neighborhoods. The seminal work in this field identified US Census block groups based on a portfolio of socioeconomic factors and discovered neighborhoods with a 40% to 90% higher risk of coronary heart disease in both White and Black populations independent of any other characteristics including known ASCVD risk factors.[73] Besides US Census blocks, determination of the SVI, Social Deprivation Index, and inferences from geocoding also qualify place as a contribution to disease burden. Characteristics of the built environment have been associated with an independent risk of type 2 diabetes, obesity, and stroke. In the

---

TABLE 81–1. Social Determinants of Health

Socioeconomic Position
Race/Ethnicity
Social Support
Culture and Language
Access to Affordable Quality Care
Built/Residential Environment
Socioeconomic Position (SEP)
    Income
    Education
    Employment

Data from Havranek EP, Mujahid MS, Barr DA, et al. Social Determinants of Risk and Outcomes for Cardiovascular Disease: A Scientific Statement From the American Heart Association. *Circulation.* 2015 Sep 1;132(9):873-898.

only study of its kind, "Moving to Opportunity Study," women living in high-poverty neighborhoods who received housing vouchers to move to a low-poverty neighborhood were significantly less likely to have a BMI >35 or a HgbA1c >6.5.[74]

The link between SDOH and biology remains under investigation but there is an emerging science that chronic exposure to stress is associated with systemic inflammation. Lines of evidence now argue that activation of the sympathetic nervous system and the hypothalamic–pituitary–adrenal (HPA) axis initiate the stress immune response. Beginning in childhood, exposure to adverse childhood experiences (ACEs) defined as traumatic childhood events, may lead to an increase in CVD risk through several immune mediated pathways.[75] These traumatic childhood events include abuse, household dysfunction, poverty, and neglect. When the burden of exposure to these early life stress (ELS) events is high, evidence demonstrates an association with both the metabolic syndrome as an adult and an increased incidence of ischemic heart disease. The burden of ACEs is especially notable in Black children and has been associated with chronic exposure to corticosteroids and hypertension.[76] The exposure to stress leads to dysregulation of the HPA axis and in turn a proliferation of markers of inflammation including C-reactive protein, circulating peripheral blood mononuclear cells, and TNF-alpha.[77] A remarkable and consistent finding has been activation of the amygdala via this same cascade of chronic stress in children.[78] This in turn further exacerbates sympathetic nervous system activation and is identified by increased salivary alpha-amylase, a marker of sympathetic

nervous system activity.[79] Additional consequences of ACEs include increased vasoreactivty with increases in plasma endothelin-1 levels and increased leptin activity. Corroboration of these mechanisms is seen in animal data evaluating ELS. Dysregulation of the HPA axis is consistently noted among animals deprived of maternal bonding and exhibiting anxiety-like behavior (**Fig. 81–5**).

These phenomena have now been described in adults. A recent 10-year study identified stress-associated neurobiological pathways linking socioeconomic disparities and CVD. Median income (lowest quartile) was associated with amygdalar activity and arterial inflammation as determined by whole body positron emission tomography (PET) imaging.[80] Neighborhood crime rate similarly varied with amygdalar activity and arterial inflammation. Survival free of major adverse cardiovascular events varied directly with quartiles of income after adjustment for known risk factors. A mediation analysis associated low socioeconomic status with amygdalar activity, bone marrow activity, arterial inflammation, and major adverse cardiovascular events (**Fig. 81–6**). These remarkable data serve as a provocative link between the burden of SDOH and CVD and potentially offer insight regarding the disproportionate burden of CVD as a function of the life and living circumstances impacting groups of people.

What matters most about the emerging science linking the life and living circumstances to an increased burden of cardiovascular risk and subsequently an increased burden of CVD is the awareness that addressing the still evident racial disparities

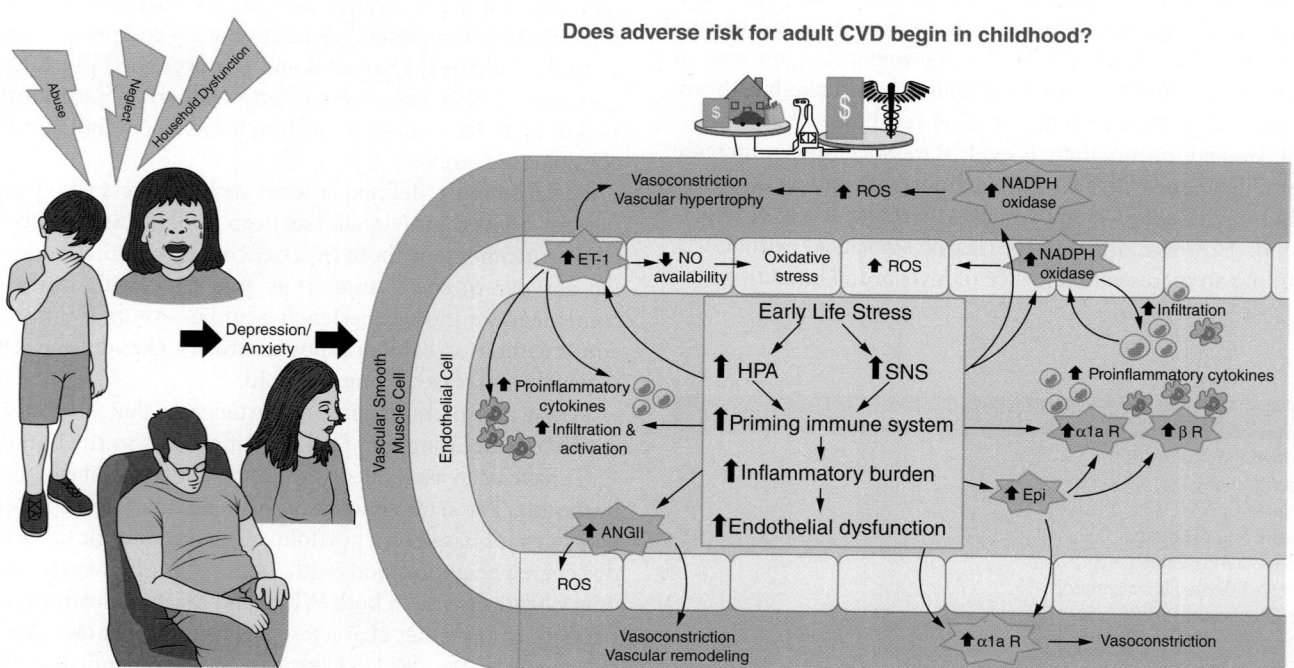

Figure 81–5. A diagram of potential molecular mechanisms involved in ACE exposure-induced, immune-mediated, vascular dysfunction. Studies using rodent models of ELS have indicated activation of inflammatory pathways that can contribute to the development of hypertension and CVD. Additionally, increased activation and/or sensitivity of vasoactive pathways such as ET 1, renin-angiotensin-aldosterone system, oxidative stress, and SNS promote vascular dysfunction. *Green cells*, T cells; *purple cells*, macrophages; α1aR, α-adrenoceptor; β R, β-adrenoceptor; NA, noradrenaline; ADR, adrenaline.

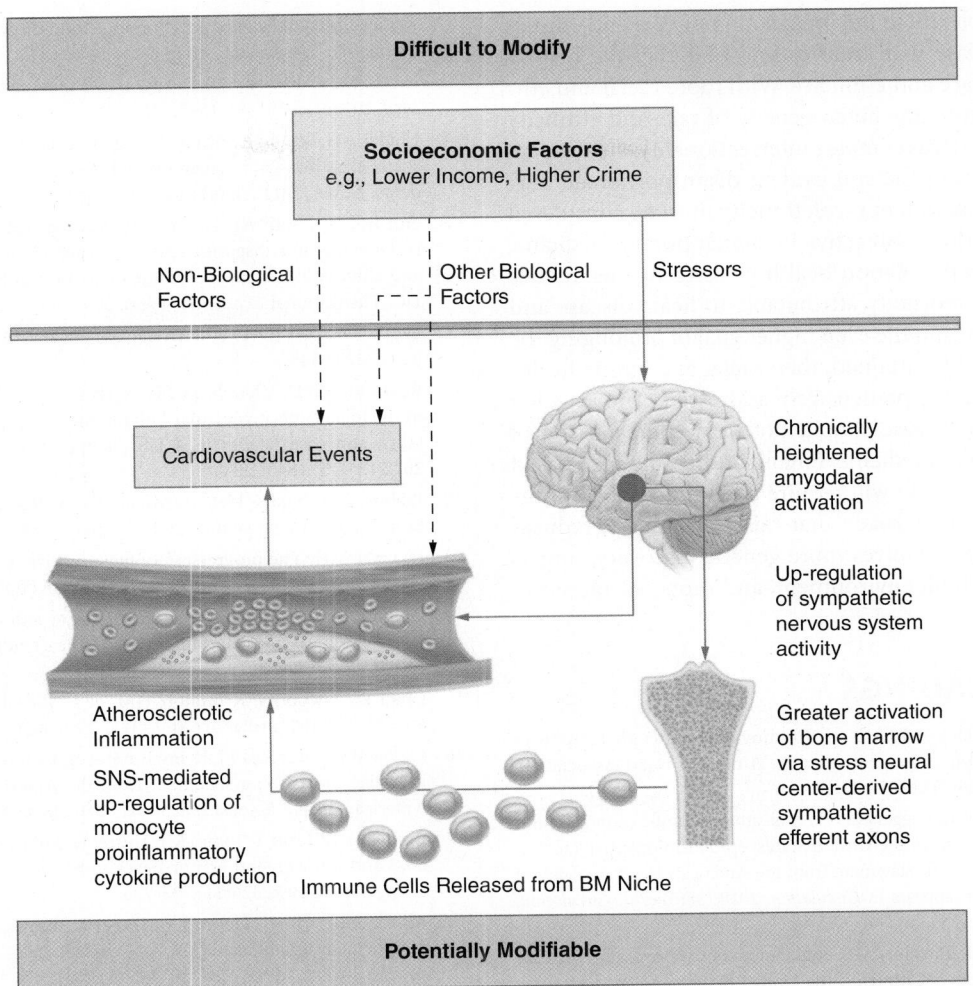

Figure 81–6. Prior data have demonstrated a link between low socioeconomic status and higher rate of cardiovascular disease. This study suggests that a biological pathway contributes to this link, involving, in series, higher amygdalar activation, increased activation of the bone marrow (with release of inflammatory cells), which in turn leads to increased atherosclerotic inflammation and its atherothrombotic manifestations. Nonbiological (and likely other biological) paths also exist. Although the social variables involved in this pathway are notoriously difficult to change, the biological factors are potentially more modifiable. BM, bone marrow. Reproduced with permission from Tawakol A, Osborne MT, Wang Y, et al. Stress-Associated Neurobiological Pathway Linking Socioeconomic Disparities to Cardiovascular Disease. *J Am Coll Cardiol.* 2019 Jul 2;73(25):3243-3255.

will require a broad lens. Simply treating hypertension and diabetes will not be sufficient. Risk mitigation not only involves an elevated awareness of the unique burden of CVD as a function of race/ethnicity but also a sharp focus on known CVD risk factors and an increasing emphasis on health and public policy initiatives that address the social determinants of health. It is clear from this emerging body of work that *place* may matter as much as, and possibly even more than, race as we deconstruct this disproportionate burden of disease.

SUMMARY

Defining race is less important as a biological marker of disease and is more significant as an approximation of the life and living circumstances of groups of people. The SDOH capture the burden of the life and living circumstances and help to illuminate some, but not all of the disproportionate burden of CVD. Genetics and more importantly ancestry will over time better inform true biological risk of disease and response to treatments. The entire portfolio of risk for CVD is heightened in Hispanic and South Asian populations and especially exaggerated in the Black population. In all racial and ethnic minorities, the disproportionate burden of CVD is potentially amplified by subconscious bias and the resultant health disparities. Those disparities are now better elucidated when the lifespan of Black people is considered recognizing that the nidus for disproportionate CVD begins with exposure to early life stress or ACEs. The link between these experiences and CVD appears to propagate through a dysregulated HPA axis inciting proinflammatory stimuli and potentially resulting in a greater burden of CVD. That dysregulation is driven in part by ACEs, stress, the pernicious influence of racism, and the origin of the race construct in the United States.

There is a complexity to the intersection of race and ethnicity with heart disease that requires knowledge of the history and taxonomy of race and ethnicity. With more racial and ethnic genetic admixture, the heterogeneity of race and ethnicity will only expand and this complex intersectionality will deepen. Elevating awareness of the still evident disproportionate burden of CVD as a function of race/ethnicity must be considered a necessary high priority objective in contemporary medicine. Particularly if lofty population health goals to further reduce the morbidity and mortality attributable to heart disease and stroke are to be met, and the even higher goal of prolonging the healthy lifespan will be attained, then racial and ethnic health disparities must be comprehensively addressed. The ongoing unequal burden of disease should not be a characteristic of today's cardiovascular medicine. Finally, addressing race-based health disparities in CVD will require a longitudinal committed and multifaceted approach that raises awareness, reduces the influence of bias, involves more genetic discovery, targets more equity in the built environment, and roots out racism in medicine.

SELECTED READINGS

Carnethon MR, Pu J, Howard G, et al. Cardiovascular health in African Americans: a scientific statement from the American Heart Association. *Circulation.* 2017;136(21):e393-e423.

Volgman AS, Palaniappan LS, Aggarwal NT, et al. atherosclerotic cardiovascular disease in South Asians in the United States: epidemiology, risk factors, and treatments: a scientific statement from the American Heart Association [published correction appears in *Circulation.* 2018;138(5):e76]. *Circulation.* 2018;138(1):e1-e34.

Rodriguez CJ, Allison M, Daviglus ML, et al. Status of cardiovascular disease and stroke in Hispanics/Latinos in the United States: a science advisory from the American Heart Association. *Circulation.* 2014;130(7):593-625.

Havranek EP, Mujahid MS, Barr DA, et al. Social determinants of risk and outcomes for cardiovascular disease: a scientific statement from the American Heart Association. *Circulation.* 2015;132(9):873-898.

Tawakol A, Osborne MT, Wang Y, et al. Stress-associated neurobiological pathway linking socioeconomic disparities to cardiovascular disease. *J Am Coll Cardiol.* 2019;73(25):3243-3255.

REFERENCES

1. Carnethon MR, Pu J, Howard G, et al. Cardiovascular health in African Americans: a scientific statement from the American Heart Association. *Circulation.* 2017;136(21):e393-e423.
2. Baharian S, Barakatt M, Gignoux CR, et al. The great migration and African-American genomic diversity. *PLoS Genet.* 2016;12(5):e1006059.
3. Vespa J, Medina L, Armstrong DM. Demographic turning points for the United States: population projections for 2020 to 2060. United States Census Bureau. 2020. https://www.census.gov/content/dam/Census/library/publications/2020/demo/p25-1144.pdf
4. Bryce E. This question reveals something much deeper about the ways we understand—and misunderstand—race. *Live Science.* February 8, 2020. https://www.livescience.com/difference-between-race-ethnicity.html
5. Rodriguez CJ, Allison M, Daviglus ML, et al. Status of cardiovascular disease and stroke in Hispanics/Latinos in the United States: a science advisory from the American Heart Association. *Circulation.* 2014;130(7):593-625.
6. Volgman AS, Palaniappan LS, Aggarwal NT, et al. Atherosclerotic cardiovascular disease in South Asians in the United States: epidemiology, risk factors, and treatments: a scientific statement from the American Heart
Association [published correction appears in *Circulation.* 2018;138(5):e76]. *Circulation.* 2018;138(1):e1-e34.
7. Nivet MA. A diversity 3.0 update: are we moving the needle enough? *Acad Med.* 2015;90(12):1591-1593.
8. Haider AH, Sexton J, Sriram N, et al. Association of unconscious race and social class bias with vignette-based clinical assessments by medical students. *JAMA.* 2011;306(9):942-951.
9. Smedley BD, Stith AY, Nelson AR, eds. Unequal treatment; confronting racial and ethnic disparities in health care. committee on understanding and eliminating racial and ethnic disparities in health care. Washington DC: The National Academies Press; 2003.
10. Yancy CW. COVID-19 and African Americans. *JAMA.* 2020. doi: 10.1001/jama.2020.6548.
11. Rosamond WD, Chambless LE, Heiss G, et al. Twenty-two-year trends in incidence of myocardial infarction, coronary heart disease mortality, and case fatality in 4 US communities, 1987-2008. *Circulation.* 2012;125(15):1848-1857.
12. Bibbins-Domingo K, Pletcher MJ, Lin F, et al. Racial differences in incident heart failure among young adults. *N Engl J Med.* 2009;360(12):1179-1190.
13. Drazner MH. The progression of hypertensive heart disease. *Circulation.* 2011;123(3):327-334. doi: 10.1161/CIRCULATIONAHA.108.845792
14. Glynn P, Lloyd-Jones DM, Feinstein MJ, Carnethon M, Khan SS. Disparities in cardiovascular mortality related to heart failure in the United States. *J Am Coll Cardiol.* 2019;73(18):2354-2355.
15. Chan PS, Nichol G, Krumholz HM, et al. Racial differences in survival after in-hospital cardiac arrest. *JAMA.* 2009;302(11):1195-1201.
16. Lackland DT, Roccella EJ, Deutsch AF, et al. Factors influencing the decline in stroke mortality: a statement from the American Heart Association/American Stroke Association. *Stroke.* 2014;45(1):315-353.
17. Broderick JP, Brott T, Tomsick T, Huster G, Miller R. The risk of subarachnoid and intracerebral hemorrhages in blacks as compared with whites. *N Engl J Med.* 1992;326(11):733-736.
18. Allison MA, Ho E, Denenberg JO, et al. Ethnic-specific prevalence of peripheral arterial disease in the United States [published correction appears in *Am J Prev Med.* 2014;47(1):103]. *Am J Prev Med.* 2007;32(4):328-333.
19. Arya S, Binney Z, Khakharia A, et al. Race and socioeconomic status independently affect risk of major amputation in perheral artery disease. *J Am Heart Assoc.* 2018;7(2):e007425.
20. Mozaffarian D, Benjamin EJ, Go AS, et al. Heart disease and stroke statistics–2015 update: a report from the American Heart Association [published correction appears in *Circulation.* 2015;131(24):e535] [published correction appears in *Circulation.* 2016;133(8):e417].
21. Daviglus ML, Talavera GA, Avilés-Santa ML, et al. Prevalence of major cardiovascular risk factors and cardiovascular diseases among Hispanic/Latino individuals of diverse backgrounds in the United States. *JAMA.* 2012;308(17):1775-1784.
22. Smith MA, Risser JM, Lisabeth LD, Moyé LA, Morgenstern LB. Access to care, acculturation, and risk factors for stroke in Mexican Americans: the Brain Attack Surveillance in Corpus Christi (BASIC) project. *Stroke.* 2003;34(11):2671-2675.
23. Morrissey NJ, Giacovelli J, Egorova N, et al. Disparities in the treatment and outcomes of vascular disease in Hispanic patients. *J Vasc Surg.* 2007;46(5):971-978.
24. Borrell LN, Lancet EA. Race/ethnicity and all-cause mortality in US adults: revisiting the Hispanic paradox. *Am J Public Health.* 2012;102(5):836-843.
25. Pablos-Méndez A. Mortality among Hispanics. *JAMA.* 1994;271(16):1237.
26. Volgman AS, Palaniappan LS, Aggarwal NT, et al. Atherosclerotic cardiovascular disease in South Asians in the United States: epidemiology, risk factors, and treatments: a scientific statement from the American Heart Association [published correction appears in *Circulation.* 2018;138(5):e76]. *Circulation.* 2018;138(1):e1-e34.
27. Hasan RK, Ginwala NT, Shah RY, Kumbhani DJ, Wilensky RL, Mehta NN. Quantitative angiography in South Asians reveals differences in vessel size

and coronary artery disease severity compared to Caucasians. *Am J Cardiovasc Dis.* 2011;1:31-37.

28. Jose PO, Frank AT, Kapphahn KI, et al. Cardiovascular disease mortality in Asian Americans. *J Am Coll Cardiol.* 2014;64:2486-2494.

29. Gujral UP, Pradeepa R, Weber MB, Narayan KM, Mohan V. Type 2 diabetes in South Asians: similarities and differences with white Caucasian and other populations. *Ann N Y Acad Sci.* 2013;1281:51-63.

30. Kooner JS, Saleheen D, Sim X, et al. Genome-wide association study in individuals of South Asian ancestry identifies six new type 2 diabetes susceptibility loci. *Nat Genet.* 2011;43(10):984-989.

31. National Center for Health Statistics (US). *Health, United States, 2015: With Special Feature on Racial and Ethnic Health Disparities.* Hyattsville (MD): National Center for Health Statistics (US); May 2016.

32. Carson AP, Howard G, Burke GL, Shea S, Levitan EB, Muntner P. Ethnic differences in hypertension incidence among middle-aged and older adults: the multi-ethnic study of atherosclerosis. *Hypertension.* 2011;57(6):1101-1110.

33. Howard G, Banach M, Cushman M, et al. Is blood pressure control for stroke prevention the correct goal? The lost opportunity of preventing hypertension. *Stroke.* 2015;46(6):1595-1600.

34. Kizer JR, Arnett DK, Bella JN, et al. Differences in left ventricular structure between black and white hypertensive adults: the Hypertension Genetic Epidemiology Network study. *Hypertension.* 2004;43(6):1182-1188.

35. Anstey DE, Tanner RM, Booth JN 3rd, et al. Inappropriate left ventricular mass and cardiovascular disease events and mortality in blacks: The Jackson Heart Study. *J Am Heart Assoc.* 2019;8(16):e011897.

36. Menke A, Casagrande S, Geiss L, Cowie CC. Prevalence of and trends in diabetes among adults in the United States, 1988-2012. *JAMA.* 2015;314(10):1021-1029.

37. Narres M, Claessen H, Droste S, et al. The incidence of end-stage renal disease in the diabetic (compared to the non-diabetic) population: a systematic review. *PLoS One.* 2016;11(1):e0147329.

38. Howard G, Safford MM, Moy CS, et al. Racial differences in the incidence of cardiovascular risk factors in older black and white adults. *J Am Geriatr Soc.* 2017;65(1):83-90.

39. Taylor HA Jr, Akylbekova EL, Garrison RJ, et al. Dyslipidemia and the treatment of lipid disorders in African Americans. *Am J Med.* 2009;122(5):454-463.

40. Ogden CL, Carroll MD, Lawman HG, et al. Trends in obesity prevalence among children and adolescents in the United States, 1988-1994 through 2013-2014. *JAMA.* 2016;315(21):2292-2299.

41. Shikany JM, Safford MM, Newby PK, Durant RW, Brown TM, Judd SE. Southern dietary pattern is associated with hazard of acute coronary heart disease in the reasons for geographic and racial differences in stroke (REGARDS) study. *Circulation.* 2015;132(9):804-814.

42. Judd SE, Gutiérrez OM, Newby PK, et al. Dietary patterns are associated with incident stroke and contribute to excess risk of stroke in black Americans. *Stroke.* 2013;44(12):3305-3311.

43. Delnevo CD, Gundersen DA, Hrywna M, Echeverria SE, Steinberg MB. Smoking-cessation prevalence among U.S. smokers of menthol versus non-menthol cigarettes. *Am J Prev Med.* 2011;41(4):357-365.

44. Muntner P, Newsome B, Kramer H, et al. Racial differences in the incidence of chronic kidney disease. *Clin J Am Soc Nephrol.* 2012;7(1):101-107.

45. Dummer PD, Limou S, Rosenberg AZ, et al. APOL1 kidney disease risk variants: an evolving landscape. *Semin Nephrol.* 2015;35(3):222-236. doi:10.1016/j.semnephrol.2015.04.008

46. Friedman DJ, Pollak MR. *APOL1* and kidney disease: from genetics to biology. *Annu Rev Physiol.* 2020;82:323-342.

47. Weiner DE, Tighiouart H, Amin MG, et al. Chronic kidney disease as a risk factor for cardiovascular disease and all-cause mortality: a pooled analysis of community-based studies. *J Am Soc Nephrol.* 2004;15(5):1307-1315.

48. Gutiérrez OM, Khodneva YA, Muntner P, et al. Association between urinary albumin excretion and coronary heart disease in black vs white adults. *JAMA.* 2013;10(7):706-714.

49. Mou L, Norby FL, Chen LY, et al. Lifetime risk of atrial fibrillation by race and socioeconomic status: ARIC study (Atherosclerosis Risk in Communities). *Circ Arrhythm Electrophysiol.* 2018;11(7):e006350.

50. Roberts JD, Hu D, Heckbert SR, et al. genetic investigation into the differential risk of atrial fibrillation among black and white individuals. *JAMA Cardiol.* 2016;1(4):442-450.

51. Magnani JW, Norby FL, Agarwal SK, et al. Racial differences in atrial fibrillation-related cardiovascular disease and mortality: The Atherosclerosis Risk in Communities (ARIC) sStudy. *JAMA Cardiol.* 2016;1(4):433-441.

52. Essien UR, Holmes DN, Jackson LR 2nd, et al. Association of race/ethnicity with oral anticoagulant use in patients with atrial fibrillation: findings from the Outcomes Registry for Better Informed Treatment of Atrial Fibrillation II. *JAMA Cardiol.* 2018;3(12):1174-1182.

53. Alkhouli M, Alqahtani F, Holmes DR, Berzingi C. Racial disparities in the utilization and outcomes of structural heart disease interventions in the United States. *J Am Heart Assoc.* 2019;8(15):e012125.

54. Dehghan A, Yang Q, Peters A, et al. Association of novel genetic Loci with circulating fibrinogen levels: a genome-wide association study in 6 population-based cohorts. *Circ Cardiovasc Genet.* 2009;2(2):125-133.

55. Zhu X, Young JH, Fox E, et al. Combined admixture mapping and association analysis identifies a novel blood pressure genetic locus on 5p13: contributions from the CARe consortium. *Hum Mol Genet.* 2011;20(11):2285-2295.

56. Chang MH, Yesupriya A, Ned RM, Mueller PW, Dowling NF. Genetic variants associated with fasting blood lipids in the U.S. population: Third National Health and Nutrition Examination Survey. *BMC Med Genet.* 2010;11:62. Published 2010 Apr 20.

57. Cohen J, Pertsemlidis A, Kotowski IK, Graham R, Garcia CK, Hobbs HH. Low LDL cholesterol in individuals of African descent resulting from frequent nonsense mutations in PCSK9 [published correction appears in *Nat Genet.* 2005 Mar;37(3):328]. *Nat Genet.* 2005;37(2):161-165.

58. Cohen JC, Boerwinkle E, Mosley TH Jr, Hobbs HH. Sequence variations in PCSK9, low LDL, and protection against coronary heart disease. *N Engl J Med.* 2006;354(12):1264-1272.

59. Akylbekova EL, Payne JP, Newton-Cheh C, et al. Gene-environment interaction between SCN5A-1103Y and hypokalemia influences QT interval prolongation in African Americans: the Jackson Heart Study. *Am Heart J.* 2014;167(1):116-122.e1.

60. McNamara DM, Tam SW, Sabolinski ML, et al. Endothelial nitric oxide synthase (NOS3) polymorphisms in African Americans with heart failure: results from the A-HeFT trial. *J Card Fail.* 2009;15(3):191-198.

61. McNamara DM, Taylor AL, Tam SW, et al. G-protein beta-3 subunit genotype predicts enhanced benefit of fixed-dose isosorbide dinitrate and hydralazine: results of A-HeFT. *JACC Heart Fail.* 2014;2(6):551-557.

62. Johnson AE, Hanley-Yanez K, Yancy CW, Taylor AL, Feldman AM, McNamara DM. Adrenergic polymorphisms and survival in African Americans with heart failure: results from A-HeFT. *J Card Fail.* 2019;25(7):553-560.

63. Taylor AL, Ziesche S, Yancy C, et al. Combination of isosorbide dinitrate and hydralazine in blacks with heart failure [published correction appears in *N Engl J Med.* 2005 Mar 24;352(12):1276]. *N Engl J Med.* 2004;351(20):2049-2057.

64. Havranek EP, Mujahid MS, Barr DA, et al. Social determinants of risk and outcomes for cardiovascular disease: a scientific statement from the American Heart Association. *Circulation.* 2015;132(9):873-898.

65. Evangelista LS, Rasmusson KD, Laramee AS, et al. Health literacy and the patient with heart failure: implications for patient care and research: a consensus statement of the Heart Failure Society of America. *J Card Fail.* 2010;16(1):9-16.

66. Dupre ME, George LK, Liu G, Peterson ED. The cumulative effect of unemployment on risks for acute myocardial infarction. *Arch Intern Med.* 2012;172:1731-1737.

67. Brondolo E, Rieppi R, Kelly KP, Gerin W. Perceived racism and blood pressure: a review of the literature and conceptual and methodological critique. *Ann Behav Med.* 2003;25:55-65.

68. Brondolo E, Libby DJ, Denton EG, et al. Thompson S, Beatty DL, Schwartz J, Sweeney M, Tobin JN, Cassells A, Pickering TG, Gerin W. Racism and ambulatory blood pressure in a community sample. *Psychosom Med.* 2008;70:49-56.

69. Williams DR, Mohammed SA. Discrimination and racial disparities in health: evidence and needed research. *J Behav Med.* 2009;32:20-47.

70. Burgess DJ, Warren J, Phelan S, Dovidio J, van Ryn M. Stereotype threat and health disparities: what medical educators and future physicians need to know. *J Gen Intern Med.* 2010;25(suppl 2):S169-S177.

71. Zalli A, Carvalho LA, Lin J, et al. Shorter telomeres with high telomerase activity are associated with raised allostatic load and impoverished psychosocial resources. *Proc Natl Acad Sci U S A.* 2014;111(12):4519-4524.

72. Dhindsa DS, Khambhati J, Schultz WM, Tahhan AS, QAuyyumi AA. Marital status and outcomes in patients with cardiovascular disease. *Trends in Cardiovascular Medicine.* 2020;30(4):215-220.

73. Diez Roux AV, Merkin SS, Arnett D, et al. Neighborhood of residence and incidence of coronary heart disease. *N Engl J Med.* 2001;345: 99-106.

74. Ludwig J, Sanbonmatsu L, Gennetian L, et al. Neighborhoods, obesity, and diabetes: a randomized social experiment. *N Engl J Med.* 2011;365: 1509-1519.

75. Obi IE, McPherson KC, Pollock JS. Childhood adversity and mechanistic links to hypertension risk in adulthood. *Br J Pharmacol.* 2019;176(12):1932-1950.

76. Duru OK, Harawa NT, Kermah D, Norris KC. Allostatic load burden and racial disparities in mortality. *J Natl Med Assoc.* 2012;104(1-2):89-95.

77. Baumeister D, Akhtar R, Ciufolini S, Pariante CM, Mondelli V. Childhood trauma and adulthood inflammation: a meta-analysis of peripheral C-reactive protein, interleukin-6 and tumour necrosis factor-α. *Mol Psychiatry.* 2016;21(5):642-649.

78. Tottenham N, Hare TA, Millner A, Gilhooly T, Zevin JD, Casey BJ. Elevated amygdala response to faces following early deprivation. *Dev Sci.* 2011;14(2):190-204.

79. Kuras YI, McInnis CM, Thoma MV, et al. Increased alpha-amylase response to an acute psychosocial stress challenge in healthy adults with childhood adversity. *Dev Psychobiol.* 2017;59(1):91-98.

80. Tawakol A, Osborne MT, Wang Y, et al. Stress-associated neurobiological pathway linking socioeconomic disparities to cardiovascular disease. *J Am Coll Cardiol.* 2019;73(25):3243-3255.

Cardiovascular Disease and Ageing: Cellular and Molecular Mechanisms

Zoltan Ungvari, Dao-Fu Dai, Bela Merkely, and Anna Csiszar

CHAPTER OUTLINE

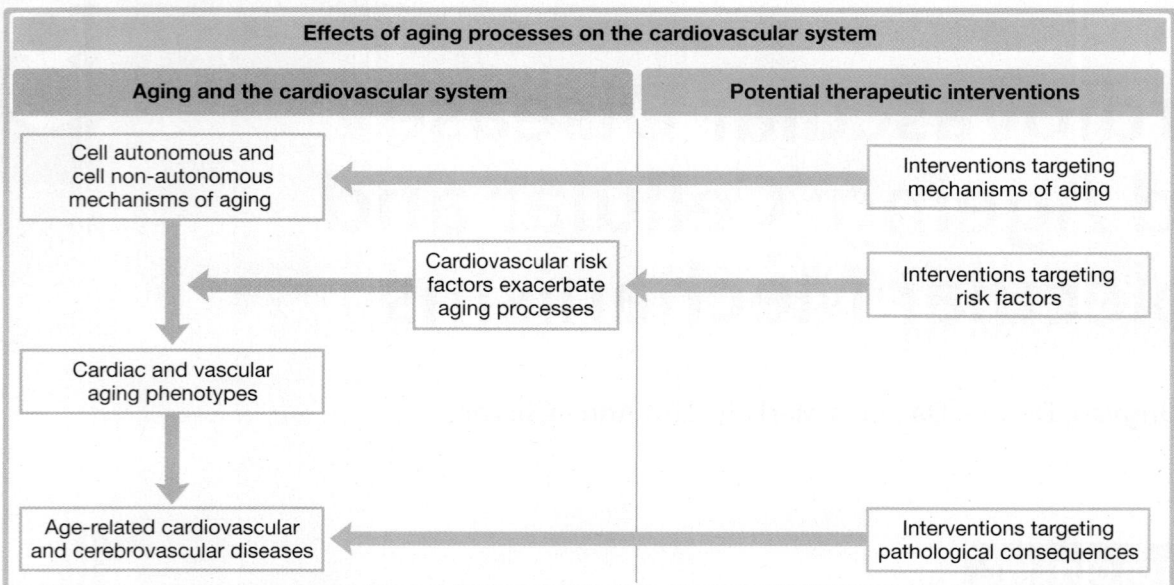

Chapter 82 Fuster and Hurst's Central Illustration. Fundamental aging processes contribute to cardiac and vascular aging phenotypes and the pathogenesis of age-related cardiovascular and cerebrovascular diseases. Understanding of the aging processes enables the identification of targets for therapeutic intervention to reverse the deleterious consequences of cardiovascular aging and to improve cardiovascular and cerebrovascular health in older adults.

CHAPTER SUMMARY

This chapter discusses the pathophysiology of the aging processes in relation to the cardiovascular system. Epidemiological studies demonstrate that the impact of conventional cardiovascular risk factors (eg, diabetes, hypertension, dyslipidemia, lifestyle factors, etc.) on the prevalence of cardiovascular and cerebrovascular diseases are dwarfed by the magnitude of effect of advanced aging in relation to these diseases. Both cell autonomous and cell nonautonomous mechanisms of aging contribute to the pathogenesis of these diseases, including age-related oxidative stress, mitochondrial dysfunction, NAD^+ depletion and dysregulation of sirtuin-regulated pathways, impaired proteostasis and autophagy, low-grade sterile inflammation, and cellular senescence (see Fuster and Hurst's Central Illustration). Emerging experimental evidence also supports the existence and significance of diverse secreted/circulatory factors derived from distal organs that modulate cardiac and vascular aging processes (including endocrine regulation). Emerging understanding of cardiac and vascular aging processes can enable the identification of novel targets for therapeutic intervention to reverse the deleterious consequences of cardiovascular aging and to improve cardiovascular and cerebrovascular health in older adults.

INTRODUCTION

Significant increases in expected lifespan in previous decades have led to the rapid growth of the older population (aged ≥65 years) across the world and in the United States.[1] In 2015, 617.1 million people (9% of the total world population) were aged 65 and older. By 2050, this number will increase to 1.6 billion (17% of the total world population).[1] In 2016, 19.2% of the population of the European Union was aged 65 or over and it is projected that by 2050, a quarter of the European Union's total population will be comprised of older individuals. In the United States, the population aged 65 and over is projected to reach 83.7 million by 2050, almost double its estimated population of 43.1 million in 2012.[1] Governments and other stakeholders (healthcare systems, policymakers, nongovernmental organizations, funding agencies, clinicians, and researchers) have realized the importance of reducing the prevalence of chronic disease and disability associated with aging, to prevent a substantial strain on healthcare resources and the economy.

The famous 17th-century physician Thomas Sydenham (1624–1689), known as the "English Hippocrates," observed, "a man is as old as his arteries." Modern cardiovascular medicine concurs: Diseases of the circulatory system are the leading causes of morbidity, serious long-term disability, and mortality among older adults in the developed world.[2,3] Cardiovascular and cerebrovascular diseases account for approximately one-third of all deaths in the United States at the age of 65 and nearly two-thirds at the age of 85.[4] Addressing age-related cardiovascular and cerebrovascular diseases is of critical importance because the annual cost to care for these older patients are projected to more than double over the next 30 years.[5]

A wide range of diseases affecting the heart and the vascular system increase in prevalence and severity with advanced aging.[3] In the United States, nearly 70% of all adults ≥60 years old and more than 85% of those ≥80 years old have known cardiovascular disease (CVD).[3] The prevalence of coronary heart disease (CHD; **Fig. 82–1A**), stroke (**Fig. 82–1B**), and peripheral artery disease (**Fig. 82–1C**) increases exponentially with age.[3] Pathological studies confirm that the prevalence of obstructive atherosclerosis in the coronary circulation increases significantly with age, from 10% to 20% in patients in their forties to 50% to 70% among patients in their 80.[6] Similar trends for a significant age-related increase in morbidity are also evident for other diseases of the circulatory system, ranging from heart failure (HF), valvular heart disease, and arrhythmias to vascular cognitive impairment.[3] Accordingly, in the United States, approximately 10% of all US adults aged ≥80 years have an established diagnosis of HF and half of the HF-related hospitalizations occur in adults aged ≥75 years.[3] Also, >75% of pacemakers are implanted in older adults.[3] Further, the prevalence of symptomatic aortic stenosis (AS) also increases with advanced age, from 0.2% in individuals aged <60 years to close to 10% in patients ≥80 years of age.[7]

Importantly, epidemiological studies demonstrate that the impact of conventional cardiovascular risk factors (eg diabetes, hypertension, dyslipidemia, lifestyle factors, etc) on the prevalence of cardiovascular and cerebrovascular diseases are

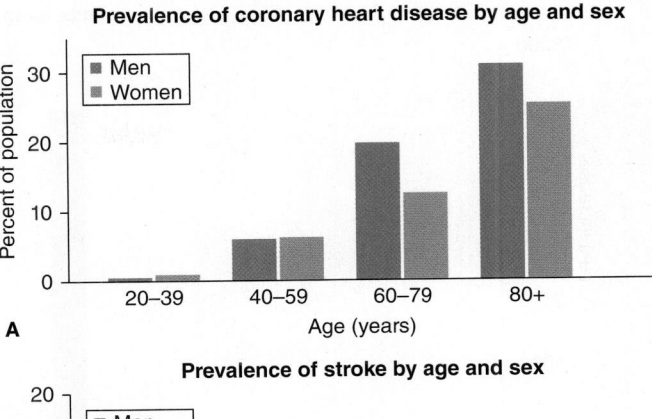

Prevalence of coronary heart disease by age and sex

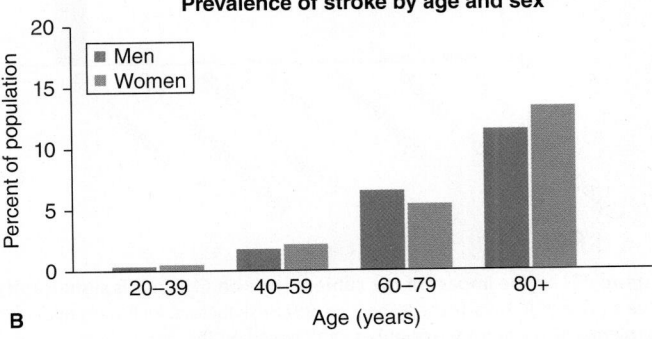

Prevalence of stroke by age and sex

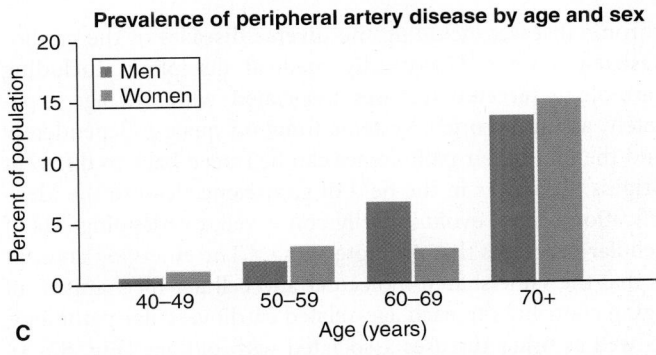

Prevalence of peripheral artery disease by age and sex

Figure 82–1. The prevalence of cardiovascular and cerebrovascular diseases increases with age. Bar charts show that the prevalence of (**A**) coronary heart disease, (**B**) stroke, and (**C**) peripheral artery disease in the United States by age and sex. Data from references 3, 432, 433 based on the results of the National Health and Nutrition Examination Survey.

dwarfed by the single most important risk factor for these diseases: advanced aging.[2] For instance, advanced age is the strongest predictor of ischemic heart disease-related events in the Framingham Risk Score.[8,9] The impact of the subject's age on ischemic heart disease risk is significantly greater than that of other conventional risk factors, such as hypertension, smoking, lipid profiles, or diabetes (**Fig. 82–2**). In the Reynolds Risk Score and similar advanced algorithms, which are designed to predict an individual's risk of having a future heart attack, stroke, or other major heart diseases in the next 10 years, age provides several-fold more statistical weight to the risk estimate than all the other conventional risk factors.[10,11]

The central message of this chapter is that "aging" is not simply one of the several "nonmodifiable risk factors." Rather, evolutionarily conserved cellular and molecular processes of aging play a fundamental role in the pathogenesis of each age-related

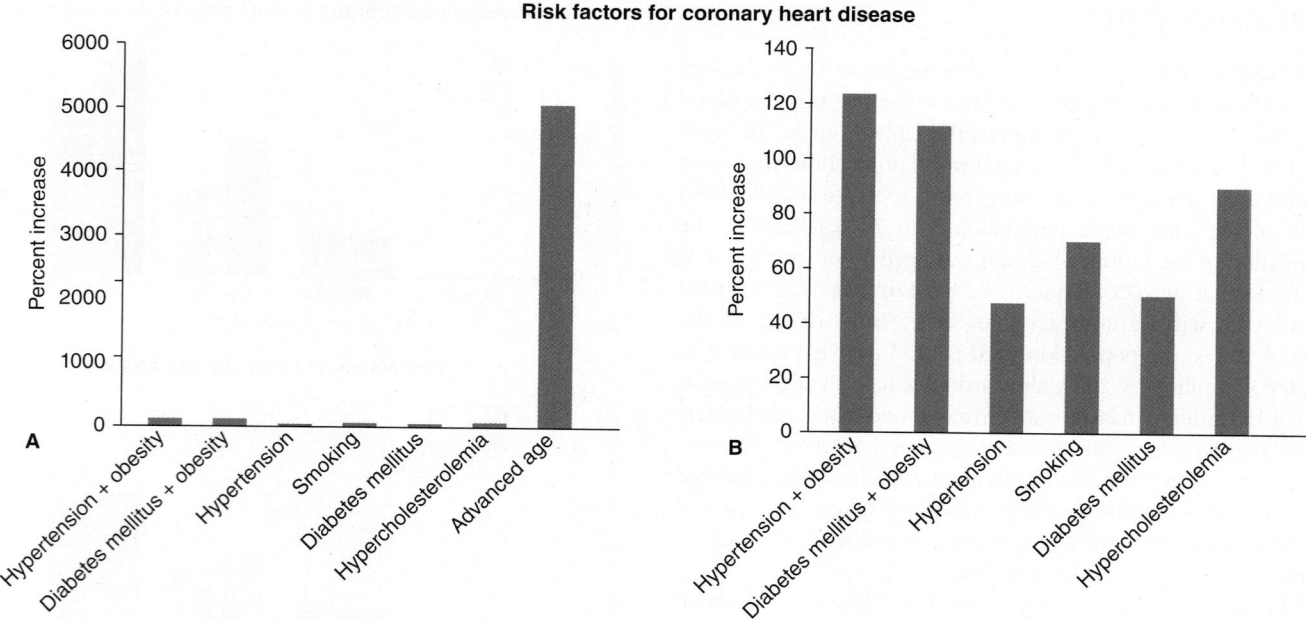

Figure 82–2. **The impact of the subject's age on CHD risk is significantly greater than that of any other conventional risk factor.** Increased risk for CHD due to aging (**A**) dwarfs the impact of other risk factors, including hypertension (w/wo obesity), diabetes mellitus (w/wo obesity), smoking, or hypercholesterolemia (**B**). Data from references [434–438] based on the results from the Framingham Heart Study.

chronic disease, including the diverse diseases of the cardiovascular system. Historically medical disciplines including cardiology targeted diseases associated with old age separately, assuming organ systems function quasi-independently and therefore their pathologies can be traced back to different origins. Advances in the field of geroscience lead to the identification of key, evolutionarily conserved, overlapping sets of cellular processes that promote aging.[12] The emerging concept is that the same shared molecular and cellular mechanisms of aging contribute to each age-related cardiovascular pathology, as well as other diseases associated with old age (**Fig. 82–3**). This constitutes a paradigm shift, this chapter argues, because these processes are inherently "modifiable."

In this chapter, the pathophysiological roles of these fundamental aging processes in the cardiovascular system are considered in terms of their contribution to both cardiac and vascular aging phenotypes and the pathogenesis of age-related cardiac and vascular diseases. Both cell-autonomous and cell nonautonomous mechanisms of aging are discussed. We describe the cumulative effects of deleterious changes that occur during aging and demonstrate how they are exacerbated by exogenous factors (cardiovascular "risk factors"). We also provide an overview of emerging experimental evidence, which supports the existence and significance of diverse secreted/circulatory factors derived from distal organs that modulate cardiac and vascular aging processes (including endocrine regulation). Our emerging understanding of cardiac and vascular aging processes enables the identification of novel targets for therapeutic intervention to reverse the deleterious consequences of cardiovascular aging and to improve cardiovascular and cerebrovascular health in older adults (**Fig. 82–3**). Finally, the potential therapeutic benefits of such emerging experimental treatments are also discussed.

PATHOPHYSIOLOGY OF CARDIOVASCULAR AGING AND AGE-RELATED CARDIOVASCULAR DISEASES

Changes in Cardiac Structure and Function

The Framingham Heart Study (FHS) reported that echocardiographic left ventricular hypertrophy (LVH) significantly increased with age for both men and women. The age-dependent increases in the prevalence of LVH are observed in individuals across all systolic blood pressure groups from normal (<110 mm Hg), mild to stage II hypertension (>140 mm Hg). In addition, FHS also reported exponential increases in the prevalence of HF and atrial fibrillation (AF).[2,13,14] The Baltimore Longitudinal Study on Aging (BLSA) demonstrated that the left ventricular (LV) wall thickness measured by echocardiography progressively increases with age in apparently healthy adult men and women,[15] indicating age-dependent LVH. Postmortem studies show an age-dependent increase in normal human heart weight index (heart weight/body surface area) and septal wall thickness.[16] In aged rodent hearts, the histopathology demonstrates lipofuscin accumulation, cytoplasmic vacuolization, enlarged myocardial fibers and cardiomyocyte nuclei sizes (cardiomyocyte hypertrophy), mineralization, arteriosclerosis and arteriolosclerosis,[17] interstitial fibrosis and remodeling of extracellular matrix,[18] and increased deposition of senile amyloid.[19,20]

Both FHS and BLSA reported a progressive decline in diastolic function with age, evidenced by reduced LV filling in early diastole and measured as decreased peak E wave by Doppler echocardiography and increased dependency on atrial contraction (increased A wave) to maintain LV filling. The LV ejection fraction (EF), the most commonly used clinical measure of LV systolic performance, is relatively preserved at rest

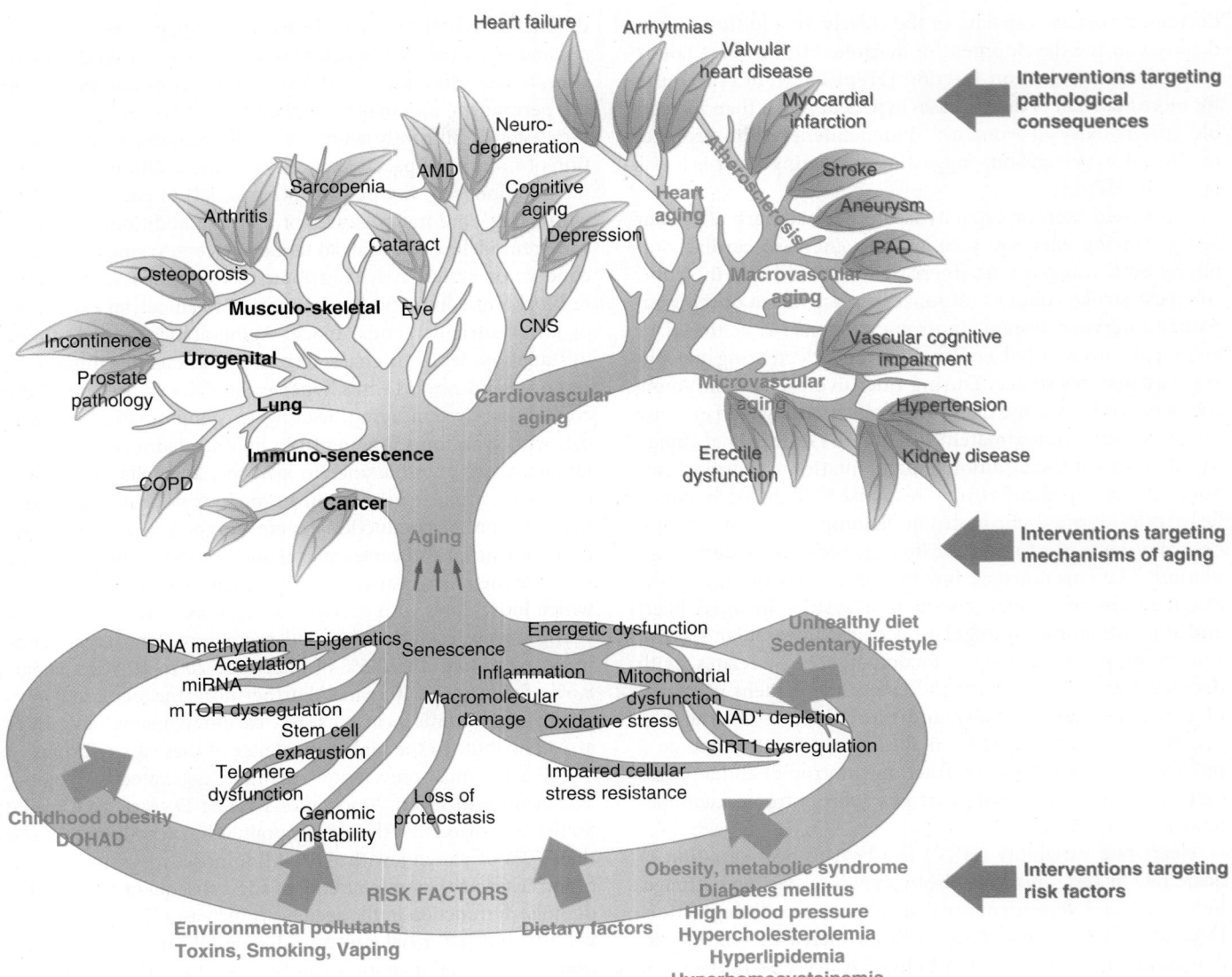

Figure 82–3. Conceptual model illustrating that multiple shared mechanisms of aging contribute to the pathogenesis of diverse age-related diseases in each organ system, including the heart and the vasculature, simultaneously. Consequences of cardiovascular aging lead to the genesis of heart diseases and micro- and macrovascular pathologies, ranging from ischemic heart disease and HF to erectile dysfunction and vascular cognitive impairment. The model illustrates that the same age-related pathologies (endothelial cell dysfunction, chronic inflammation, cellular energetic dysfunction) contribute to the organ-specific manifestations of age-related CVDs. Conventional risk factors (*purple*) promote age-related cardiovascular pathologies by exacerbating one or more fundamental molecular and cellular aging processes (*roots*). Clinical disciplines (including cardiology and vascular medicine), biogerontology, and preventive medicine/public health research separately focus on the individual age-related diseases (*leaves*), the biological mechanisms of aging (*roots*), and the risk factors, respectively. Geroscience is an integrative scientific field that considers the interaction of all of these levels, promoting interdisciplinary collaboration. Current interventions aim to treat pathological consequences of cardiovascular aging individually (manifestation of age-related CVDs) or reduce/eliminate the risk factors that modulate aging processes (*green arrows*). Future interventions are expected to target causal cellular and molecular mechanisms of aging. Of note, both interventions that prevent exacerbation of aging processes (eg, lifestyle interventions) and targeted antiaging interventions that delay molecular and cellular aging processes are expected to prevent/delay a wide range of age-related diseases simultaneously. Adapted with permission from Ungvari Z, Tarantini S, Sorond F, et al. Mechanisms of Vascular Aging, A Geroscience Perspective: JACC Focus Seminar. *J Am Coll Cardiol.* 2020 Mar 3;75(8):931-941.

during aging. However, the maximal EF during exhausting exercise decreases with age in healthy volunteers in the BLSA study.

Diastolic dysfunction is highly prevalent in the geriatric population, especially in elderly women.[21] There are several contributors to diastolic dysfunction in aging. Reduced rates of calcium reuptake by myocardial sarcoplasmic reticulum ATPase (SERCA2a) delay ventricular relaxation, thus

compromise LV filling during early diastole. Decreased ventricular elasticity and compliance due to LVH and increased ventricular fibrosis further impaired LV filling, which together with decreased SERCA2 can lead to diastolic dysfunction. Increased dependency on atrial contraction during late diastole causes elevated left atrial pressure and inadvertently cause atrial hypertrophy and fibrosis, which predisposes to the development of AF. Diastolic dysfunction also contributes to decreased exercise capacity in the elderly. In addition, it predisposes to the development of diastolic HF, or heart failure with preserved ejection fraction (HFpEF). HFpEF accounts for more than half of the HF cases in patients older than 75 years old (particularly in women),[22] independent of the presence of clinical hypertension, suggesting that aging itself is a risk factor for HFpEF.

Decreased exercise capacity is another hallmark of cardiac aging. During exercise, young adults increase cardiac output by both chronotropic (increase heart rate) and inotropic (increase stroke volume) responses via activation of the sympathetic nervous system. Inotropic response is achieved by enhancing myocardial contractility and decreasing peripheral vascular resistance. During intensive exercise in young subjects, stroke volume increases proportionally with exercise intensity until approximately 40% to 50% of maximal capacity, after which the additional augmentation of cardiac output is driven by chronotropic response.[23] Reduced maximal heart rate—termed chronotropic incompetence—is a major contributing factor to exercise intolerance in the elderly population. The chronotropic incompetence may be due to the degeneration of cardiac conduction system in aged heart and the autonomic dysregulation of cardiovascular system. Interestingly, chronotropic incompetence correlates with decreased exercise capacity and is an independent predictor of cardiovascular mortality and morbidity.[24,25] Overall, the decreased exercise capacity in the elderly is attributed to a modest decrease in ejection fraction (inotropic) and a prominent decline in maximal heart rate (chronotropic incompetence) at peak exercise.

Heart rate variability (HRV) is a beat-to-beat variation of heart rate at rest, and it has been shown to decline with age, indicating age-dependent cardiac autonomic dysregulation. Decreased HRV is associated with an increased risk of cardiovascular mortality and morbidity.[26] A decrease in the postsynaptic beta-adrenergic signaling efficiency is a feature of age-dependent autonomic dysfunction.[15] It is evidenced by decreased cardiovascular responses to beta-adrenergic agonist infusions at rest. Interestingly, the deficits in sympathetic (adrenergic) modulation of cardiac and arterial functions with aging occur in the presence of exaggerated neurotransmitter levels. Plasma levels of norepinephrine and epinephrine during any perturbation from the supine basal state increase to a greater extent in older compared with younger healthy individuals.[14] The age-associated increase in plasma levels of norepinephrine results from an increased spillover into the circulation and, to a lesser extent, reduced plasma clearance.[27] Aged hearts demonstrate increased catecholamine spillover during strenuous exercise, due to deficient norepinephrine reuptake at nerve endings. During prolonged exercise, however, diminished neurotransmitter reuptake might also be associated with depletion and reduced release and spillover.[28]

Rhythm Changes

Aging predisposes to various cardiac arrhythmia and conduction system diseases, attributable to age-dependent degeneration of the cardiac electrical system, progressive fibrosis, and scattered foci of calcification. Sick sinus syndrome or sinus node dysfunction (SND) is the most common indication for permanent pacemaker implantation,[29] and its prevalence increased significantly with age.[30] The progressive degeneration of sinus node pacemaker cells and the declining ion channel functions (eg, L-type calcium channel) in pacemaker cells with aging[31] are major causes of SND. In addition, the structural remodeling of the atrial tissue adjacent to sinus node and conduction system may contribute to voltage loss and slowing or block[32] of conduction, predisposing to sinoatrial exit block, or atrioventricular nodal block. Aging-associated autonomic dysfunction, which is characterized by deficits in sympathetic response and carotid sinus hypersensitivity, can precipitate the conduction system aging, leading to symptomatic bradycardia, with symptoms ranging from lightheadedness, confusion, fatigue, exercise intolerance to syncope, and falls. As a result of slowing impulse generation from sinus node and propagation through the conduction system, competing impulses from nonnodal atrial and ventricular tissues as premature beats may increase the risk of various tachyarrhythmias. In the BLSA, in which individuals with exercise-induced ischemic ST-segment changes were excluded, isolated premature ventricular complexes were found in 0.5% of men aged 20 to 40 years versus 8.6% of men aged ≥60 years.[33] Furthermore, the increased prevalence of ischemic heart disease, cardiomyopathy, and LVH also contribute to the higher incidence of these arrhythmias.

AF is the most prevalent arrhythmia associated with aging. The American Heart Association's Heart Disease and Stroke Statistics showed that the elderly population accounts for more than 70% of patients with AF.[34] AF imposes a significant risk of intracardiac thromboembolism and subsequent stroke.[35] LV diastolic dysfunction in the aged heart increases LV end-diastolic volume and left atrial pressure. Increased left atrial pressure induces left atrial dilatation and fibrosis. Age-dependent myxomatous changes of the mitral valve may cause mitral regurgitation, which also results in left atrial enlargement. Left atrial enlargement, together with SND and ectopic atrial beats, predispose to AF, which further induces extensive atrial remodeling, fibrosis, and dilation, contributing to a vicious cycle and the notion of "AF begets AF" in the setting of aged hearts.

Valvular Changes

Valvular changes in aged hearts involve myxomatous degeneration and collagen deposition, called valvular sclerosis. Aortic valve sclerosis is present in approximately 30% to 80% of elderly individuals,[36-38] including calcification of aortic valve leaflets and the aortic annulus.[39,40] At earlier stages, aortic valve sclerosis is asymptomatic and subclinical, but it can progress into clinical AS when severe thickening, stiffening, and calcification of the leaflet results in obstruction of the aortic output. Increased leaflet calcification and decreased leaflet mobility may serve as early signs of this progression. Approximately 10% of the elderly ≥80 years of age develop symptomatic AS.[7] AS is the most common valvular abnormality requiring procedural intervention and over 70% of all aortic valve procedures are performed in the geriatric population. The risk factors of aortic sclerosis include chronic hypertension, LV hypertrophy, hyperlipidemia, smoking, end-stage renal disease, and congenital bicuspid aortic valves.[41] In addition to AS, aortic regurgitation is also related to the calcification of the aortic cusps and annulus and it also increases with age and is present in 13% to 16% of the elderly population.[36]

Mitral annular calcification (MAC) is a degenerative process involving the fibrous annulus of the mitral valve during aging. MAC occurs when calcium deposits along and beneath the mitral valve annulus,[42] resulting in mitral sclerosis.[43,44] MAC increased the risks of mitral stenosis and regurgitation, HF, AF, conduction system diseases, stroke, coronary and vascular diseases, mortality, and adverse cardiovascular events.[37] MAC is frequently associated with hypertension, end-stage renal disease, AS, as well as mitral valve prolapse. Mitral regurgitation is also increased in the elderly population, predominantly due to age-dependent myxomatous degeneration of the valve and ischemic heart disease.[45] Chronic mitral valve regurgitation is one of the most common indications for valve surgery in elderly patients.[46]

Vascular Changes

Thickening of arterial intimal media thickness (IMT) is a hallmark of vascular aging, even in the absence of other cardiovascular risk factors. Measurements of carotid artery IMT in apparently healthy adults in BLSA show progressive thickening of carotid artery IMT, with an approximately 2- to 3-fold increase in IMT between 20 and 90 years of age. Postmortem studies demonstrate the thickening of aortic wall in the elderly subjects, even in individuals without clinical atherosclerosis. Increases in arterial IMT are a risk factor of atherosclerosis and it predicts future adverse cardiovascular events. In addition to increased IMT, fraying of medial elastic fibers and increased collagen deposition in the *tunica media* of the arteries reduces arterial distensibility, leading to stiffening of the arteries.[47] This may lead to increased systolic blood pressure (SBP). In contrast, diastolic blood pressure (DBP) tends to increase until the sixth decade and then decline thereafter, due to the reduced elastic recoil and stiffer arteries.[47] The differential effect of aging on SBP and DBP typically manifests as isolated systolic hypertension. The pulse pressure, the difference between SBP and DBP, becomes widened with aging, augmenting the perceived pulses. Indeed, studies in the elderly suggest that widening or increased pulse pressure is a more potent predictor of cardiovascular events than either SBP or DBP.[48] The pulse wave velocity (PWV), the velocity of arterial pulse propagation along the arteries, is another sensitive index of arterial stiffness. Aortofemoral PWV, measured between the carotid and femoral arteries, increases 2- to 3-fold from young to old in normotensive subjects. Elevated PWV also predicts future cardiovascular events in both healthy individuals and those with CVD, independent of the blood pressure.

Generalized endothelial dysfunction in aging vessels manifests as decreased endothelial nitric oxide (NO)–mediated vasodilation.[49] This contributes to the pathogenesis of age-related

ischemic diseases of the heart, brain (stroke, vascular cognitive impairment), and lower extremities (peripheral artery disease).

In addition to the large arteries, aging also has a profound impact on the microcirculation. As the microcirculation is pervasive, being present in every tissue in the body, its age-related alterations have a unique ability to influence the local environment of the majority of tissues and organs. As such, aging-induced functional and structural alterations of the microcirculation contribute to the pathogenesis of a wide range of age-related diseases including vascular cognitive impairment, Alzheimer's disease, sarcopenia, and kidney and eye diseases. Aging is known to reduce microvascular density (termed "microvascular rarefaction") in the heart, skeletal muscle, and the brain, which contributes to tissue ischemia.[49] The dynamic balance between processes of angiogenesis and vascular regression is critical for maintenance of the microvascular network in the heart and in other organs, including the brain. Advanced aging is associated with a progressive deterioration of microvascular homeostasis, at least in part, due to age-related impairment of angiogenic processes.[50-55] In the heart, capillary rarefaction may promote coronary ischemia and compromise cardiac systolic and diastolic function, particularly during stress or exercise. Indeed, microcirculatory failure has been proposed as an important mechanism causing HFpEF[56] and exercise intolerance in the elderly. Aging also alters the barrier function of the microvascular endothelial cells, which results in an age-related disruption of the blood–brain barrier, contributing to the pathogenesis of neurodegenerative diseases.[57,58]

Decreased Cardiovascular Reserve in Aging

Ventricular, valvular, rhythm, and vascular changes in cardiovascular aging can result in compromise in the cardiovascular functional reserve capacity, lowering the threshold for the development of HF and cardiovascular complications.[59] Together with increased exposure to other cardiovascular risk factors, this makes the aged cardiovascular system much more susceptible to stresses and disease-related challenges, thus contributing to increased HF and cardiovascular mortality in the elderly. The age-dependent structural and functional changes in the cardiovascular system, along with the increasing prevalence of most atherosclerotic and cardiometabolic risk factors, all contribute to the increasing severity of CHD, arrhythmia, and chronic HF. HF is the most common and costly reason for acute hospitalization in elderly populations. Although HF in elderly patients is partly due to the sequela of acute myocardial infarction (MI) and other CVDs, aging-induced ventricular, valvular, rhythm, macro- and microvascular changes contribute significantly to the development of HF. These also include long-standing hypertension (which is present in 75% of patients with HF and in >60% in the elderly older than 80), vascular stiffness, LV diastolic dysfunction, SND, progressive valvular heart disease, coronary ischemia and decreased coronary flow reserve, reduced responsiveness to β-adrenergic stimulation, and decreased mitochondrial response to increased demand for adenosine triphosphate (ATP) production.[60] The increased exposure time to CVD risks as well as declining cardiovascular reserve with age leads to an exponential increase in HF in the elderly population.

SHARED MECHANISMS OF CARDIOVASCULAR AGING

A proposed integrative model for aging-induced diseases predicts that a range of shared and interconnected molecular and cellular mechanisms of aging contribute both to the genesis of cardiovascular aging phenotypes promoting age-related CVDs and to age-related pathologies of other organ systems (**Fig. 82–3**). Important cellular and molecular mechanisms of cardiovascular aging identified are listed in **Table 82–1**. The goal of geroscience research in the 21st century is to develop novel drugs and therapeutic interventions (including dietary interventions) for prevention and treatment of a range of chronic diseases of old age as a class, by targeting these shared mechanisms of aging.[12] It is expected that this strategy will also result in revolutionary novel interventions preventing, attenuating, and/or reversing age-related diseases of the heart and the vascular system.[61]

The relative contribution of cell-autonomous and non-autonomous mechanisms to systemic aging in humans is hotly debated. Scientific progress in the last two decades has led to a comprehensive understanding of evolutionarily conserved cell-autonomous mechanisms of aging, which include both coordinated changes in the expression of genes and pathways (eg, through epigenetic regulation) and changes in

TABLE 82–1. Shared Cellular and Molecular Mechanisms of Cardiovascular Aging

Cellular and molecular mechanisms of aging	Putative role in cardiac and vascular pathologies[60]	Potential target for intervention[59]
Oxidative and nitrative stress	Heart failure, atherogenesis, inflammation, endothelial dysfunction,[72,79] blood flow↓, ECM remodeling, hypertension, microhemorrhages, aneurysm formation	yes (dietary interventions/Mediterranean diet, antioxidants, peroxynitrite scavengers, upstream activators of antioxidant pathways)
Impaired oxidative stress resistance (including Nrf2 dysfunction)[86]	Impaired response to injury, heart failure, exacerbated effects of cardiovascular risk factors (hypertension, metabolic diseases, smoking), inflammation, atherogenesis, aneurysm formation, microvascular damage, impaired angiogenesis[86,88–90,437]	yes (Nrf2 activators, dietary interventions/Mediterranean diet, caloric restriction)
Chronic low-grade sterile inflammation (NF-κB activation,[438] cytokine dysregulation, DAMPs)	Atherogenesis, paracrine effects on tissue function (including stem cell niche impairment), barrier dysfunction, white blood cell extravasation	Yes (inhibitors of NF-κB, upstream activators of anti-inflammatory pathways)
Mitochondrial dysfunction, mtDNA damage	Impaired endothelial vasomotor,[427] transport and barrier functions,[67] inflammation,[77] atherogenesis[439,440]	yes (mitochondria-targeted antioxidants[427])
NAD+ depletion[103]	Endothelial dysfunction,[212,214] cellular energetics↓, impaired angiogenesis, atherogenesis (?), cardiac dysfunction[218]	yes (nicotinamide mononucleotide,[212] nicotinamide riboside, nicotinamide; dietary interventions, PARP1 inhibitors[109])
SIRT1 dysregulation	Endothelial dysfunction,[228] inflammation, atherogenesis, microvascular dysfunction[227,228]	yes (sirtuin activator compounds,[228] dietary interventions)
mTOR dysregulation	Heart failure,[441] microvascular rarefaction, inflammation, atherosclerosis, vasomotor dysfunction,[429,442] blood–brain barrier disruption[443]	yes (rapamycin, rapalogs[429])
AMPK dysregulation	Endothelial dysfunction,[444] vascular inflammation	yes (metformin[428])
Δ DNA methylation	Vascular inflammation, aneurysm formation[445]	Uncertain
miRNA dysregulation	Angiogenesis↓, atherogenesis[60]	Uncertain
Loss of proteostasis (ubiquitin-proteasome↓, lysosome-autophagy system↓)	Heart failure,[446] Atherosclerosis,[318] vascular inflammation,[447,448] Alzheimer's disease, amyloidosis, endothelial dysfunction[449]	Uncertain
Apoptosis↑, necroptosis↑	Heart failure,[450] inflammation (?),[226] aneurysms (?), microvascular rarefaction	Uncertain
Progenitor cell exhaustion	Microvascular rarefaction (?), impaired angiogenesis and collateralization(?),[451] impaired cardiac repair	Uncertain
Genomic instability	Endothelial dysfunction, increased vascular stiffness, increased presence of senescence cells, hypertension,[452] atherosclerosis[453]	Uncertain
Cellular senescence↑[309,315]	Impaired cardiac regeneration,[313] heart failure,[317] aortic aneurysm,[319] atherogenesis,[309,318] angiogenesis↓, endothelial dysfunction,[315] inflammation↑, blood brain–barrier dysfunction, microvascular rarefaction	yes (senolytics, dietary interventions, exercise[315])

biomolecules and organelles involved in the aging process. In general, many of the later mechanisms are related to spontaneous, stochastic damage to macromolecules and organelles that activate evolutionarily conserved cellular programs (eg senescence, inflammatory responses, etc) and the pathways determining the resilience of the cells to such damage/stress (eg, loss of proteostasis, impaired Nrf2-driven antioxidant response and DNA repair, etc).[62] In this chapter, the role of oxidative stress and its consequences (including sterile low-grade inflammation), mitochondrial dysfunction, NAD+ depletion and dysregulation of sirtuin-regulated survival pathways, impairment of autophagy and macromolecular degradation pathways, and increased cellular senescence in cardiovascular aging, and their potential therapeutic considerations, are discussed in more detail.

It is also evident that in multicellular organisms, cell-autonomous mechanisms per se are inadequate to explain aging at a tissue or organismal level. In fact, emerging evidence in recent years from parabiosis, serum transfer, and cell ablation studies suggest that cell nonautonomous mechanisms also play critical roles in driving organismal aging, including age-related degeneration of the cardiovascular system. Understanding these nonautonomous factors, which are still unknown for the most part, represents one of the most exciting frontiers of research at the interface of biogerontology and cardiovascular research. In this chapter, a conceptual framework is presented that informs future mechanistic research into the role of circulating progeronic factors (whose production increases with age and which impair cardiovascular homeostasis) and antigeronic factors (which reverse/prevent the development of aging phenotypes) in the regulation of cardiovascular aging.

Role of Oxidative Stress and Impaired Oxidative Stress Resilience

The free radical theory of aging, originally proposed by Denham Harman in 1956,[63] postulates that the oxidative damage to cellular organelles and cells caused by free radicals is a causal factor in the aging process. During the previous decades, the theory has evolved to reconcile it with experimental observations (disconnect between the beneficial effects of antioxidative treatments on healthspan and lack of effect of these treatments on lifespan in experimental animals) and to answer a number of questions regarding the biological actions of reactive oxygen species (ROS). In particular, a vast body of data implicates increased oxidative stress in aging processes in the heart and the vasculature. Accordingly, increased production of ROS by upregulated NAD(P)H oxidases (including NOX1, NOX2, and NOX4)[64-68] and dysfunctional mitochondria[69-74] was shown to contribute to endothelial dysfunction, microvascular impairment, pathological vascular remodeling, and/or atherogenesis with advancing age both in laboratory animals[64,65,75-79] and humans.[66,80,81] Age-related upregulation of NAD(P)H oxidase-[82,83] and mitochondria-derived ROS production in cardiac myocytes has also been causally linked to impaired myocyte contractility, dysregulation of calcium signaling,[84] and pathological remodeling of the extracellular matrix in the heart,[85] all of which contribute to age-related cardiac dysfunction.

Equally as important as increased ROS production per se is the ability of the cardiomyocytes and vascular cells to activate adaptive stress response mechanisms and scavenge/eliminate excess ROS and repair or otherwise cope with the oxidative damage. This "oxidative stress resilience" is progressively diminished in cardiac and vascular tissues with advanced aging. As a consequence, in the aged heart and vascular system, the same pathological stressors (including hypertension, metabolic stressors, etc) elicit exacerbated oxidative stress as compared to young tissues.[86,87] Current understanding is that this age-related loss of cardiac and vascular oxidative stress resilience importantly contributes to the increased propensity of the aged heart and vasculature to ROS-mediated damage. A critical mechanism responsible for impaired oxidative stress resilience is an age-related deterioration of Nrf2 (nuclear factor-erythroid-2–related factor 2)/ARE (antioxidant response element)-dependent antioxidative defense pathways.[71,88–90] Nrf2 is an evolutionarily highly conserved transcription factor, which serves as a master regulator of the transcription of hundreds of antioxidants, prosurvival, anti-inflammatory, and macromolecular damage repair genes involved in the cytoprotective response against oxidative stressors. Classical Nrf2 target genes encode antioxidant proteins (eg, catalase, heme oxygenase 1, glutathione peroxidases, NAD(P)H quinone dehydrogenase (NQO1), glutathione-S-transferases, peroxiredoxins, thioredoxins, thioredoxin reductases, and glutamate-cysteine ligase, which is the rate-limiting enzyme for glutathione synthesis). Nrf2 also regulates expression of genes involved in autophagy, the proteasome, and DNA repair pathways, limiting macromolecular damage induced by oxidative stressors. Genetic Nrf2 depletion in mice results in accelerated cardiovascular aging, including the increased propensity for endothelial dysfunction, vascular senescence, cerebrovascular impairment, and HF.[89,91,92]

One of the most potent effects of increased ROS in the aged vasculature is the inactivation of endothelium-derived NO. Decreased bioavailability of NO is responsible for aging-induced impairment of endothelium-dependent dilation in the coronary circulation promoting myocardial ischemia.[64] Endothelial dysfunction caused by aging-induced increased oxidative stress also contributes significantly to impairment of neurovascular coupling responses,[69,93,94] decreasing cerebral blood flow and promoting vascular cognitive impairment. Generalized age-related endothelial dysfunction also contributes both to skeletal muscle ischemia in peripheral artery disease (PAD) and to erectile dysfunction. In addition to the inactivation of NO by increased ROS, changes in eNOS activation status and substrate (L-arginine) and cofactor (BH4) availability and/or downregulation of eNOS[95–97] may also contribute to impaired bioavailability of NO in aging. As NO confers potent anti-inflammatory and antithrombotic cellular effects, endothelial dysfunction also favors atherogenesis in the aging vasculature.[98–100]

Many of the consequences of increased age-related cellular oxidative stress are mediated via generation of the highly reactive oxidant and nitrating agent peroxynitrite ($ONOO^-$), formed by the combination of NO and superoxide.[101,102] Increased presence of

3-nitrotyrosine (a biochemically detectable product of tyrosine nitration mediated by peroxynitrite), a biomarker of increased production of peroxynitrite, has been well documented in the aged vasculature and the myocardium.[64,75,77,82,103,104] There is evidence that treatment with a peroxynitrite decomposition catalyst can rescue aging-associated cardiac dysfunction and improve endothelial function in the aorta of rats.[104] The mechanisms by which peroxynitrite contributes to cardiovascular aging are multifaceted and include direct cytotoxic effects, damage to nuclear and mitochondrial DNA, adverse effects on mitochondrial function, and activation of inflammatory pathways.[101] Importantly, peroxynitrite-induced DNA damage promotes overactivation of NAD$^+$ utilizing poly (ADP-ribose) polymerase (PARPs, including PARP-1) enzymes.[105] PARP-1 is a constitutive factor of the DNA damage surveillance network responsible for maintenance of genome integrity, which is activated upon oxidative/nitrative stress-induced DNA damage in aged cells.[106–110] PARP-1 cleaves NAD$^+$ and transfers the resulting ADP-ribose moiety onto target nuclear proteins and onto subsequent polymers of ADP-ribose, thereby depleting cellular NAD$^+$ pools in oxidatively stressed cells. NAD$^+$ depletion is an important mechanism involved in age-related cardiovascular dysfunction (see section Role of NAD$^+$ Depletion and Sirtuin-Regulated Pathways). The findings that pharmacological inhibition of PARP-1 rescues endothelial function in the aorta as well as the cerebral microcirculation and improves cardiac function in aged rodents[109–113] is consistent with the hypothesis that peroxynitrite-mediated overactivation of PARP-1 and consequential NAD$^+$ depletion is an important mechanism contributing to cardiovascular aging. Increased oxidative/nitrative stress-mediated PARP-1 activation has also been causally linked to endothelial impairment and cardiac dysfunction associated with accelerated cardiovascular aging in hypertension[109] and diabetes mellitus.[114,115]

Increased levels of reactive oxygen and nitrogen species in the aged cardiovascular system cause oxidative modification of cellular macromolecules, including DNA, lipids, proteins, and carbohydrates. Due to the oxidative environment within the mitochondria in the aged heart and vasculature, the mtDNA, mitochondrial proteins, and lipids are the most susceptible to sustaining oxidative damage. Oxidative modifications of proteins (eg, protein carbonylation, nitration[103]) are known to alter their function. Lipid peroxidation alters membrane lipids, leading to the formation of reactive aldehydes. In the aging heart and vasculature increased levels of biomarkers of lipid peroxidation (eg, trans-4-hydroxy-2-nonenal [4-HNE],[116–118] malondialdehyde [MDA], and isoprostanes[119]) are evident. Aldehydes generated from the peroxidation of polyunsaturated fatty acids (eg, 4-HNE) form adducts with cellular proteins, impairing their function and modifying cellular signaling pathways.[120] Isoprostane, derived from lipid peroxidation of arachidonic acid, can activate the TxA$_2$ prostanoid receptor (TP), affecting endothelial function, promoting vasoconstriction, and conferring prothrombotic effects. Oxidative damage to nuclear and mitochondrial DNA results in mutations (eg, 8-oxo-7,8-dihydro-guanine, 8-oxo-7,8-dihydro-2′deoxyguanosine), strand breaks, and/or deletions. Oxidative damage

to cardiac mtDNA was shown to significantly increase both in humans[121,122] and experimental animals.[123] Oxidative damage to nuclear DNA in the heart also increases with age albeit its level is lower than damage to mtDNA.[124] Oxidative DNA damage has also been demonstrated in the aorta of older adults.[118] Accumulation of oxidative DNA damage is a common trigger for cellular senescence (see section Role of Cellular Senescence), which has emerged as a critical mechanism of cardiovascular aging in recent years.

ROS also serve important signaling functions. In the aged heart and vasculature increased ROS were shown to activate redox-sensitive cellular signaling pathways, including NF-kB, which are implicated in chronic low-grade sterile inflammation.[66,79,90,125] In the aged heart, NF-kB activation has been linked to heightened cardiac inflammatory status and increased fibrosis.[126] In the aged vasculature, NF-kB-mediated inflammatory processes promote endothelial activation[127] and lead to pro-atherogenic changes in the cellular gene expression profile.[71,128,129]

Increased oxidative stress in the aged heart and the vasculature has also been linked to upregulation and activation of matrix metalloproteinases (MMPs) and consequential remodeling of the extracellular matrix.[85,130–132] In the aged heart, MMP activation and adverse ventricular remodeling may contribute to impaired cardiac function and alter outcomes after acute MI.[131] Age-related, oxidative stress-mediated increases in MMP activation/expression[132,133] in the aorta likely contribute to the genesis of aneurysms.[134,135] In the aged cerebral circulation, ROS-dependent activation and upregulation of MMPs was causally linked to increased microvascular fragility and the development of cerebral microhemorrhages,[87] which are known to contribute to cognitive decline, geriatric psychiatric syndromes, and gait disorders in older adults.[136] In preclinical animal models, similar antioxidative treatments were shown to prevent stiffening of large arteries,[137] formation of cerebral microhemorrhages,[87] and progression of aortic aneurysms,[134] providing additional evidence for shared pathogenic mechanisms. Importantly, MMPs are also abundantly expressed and secreted by senescent cells in the aged cardiovascular system (see section Role of Cellular Senescence).

Taken together, there is convincing experimental evidence that oxidative stress contributes to cardiovascular aging and is involved in the pathogenesis of atherosclerosis, which, in turn, provides a compelling argument that antioxidant treatments may effectively decrease the risk of age-related CVDs. The epidemiological data, in general, support an association between intake of dietary antioxidants (α-tocopherol, ascorbic acid) and decreased risk of CVD and coronary artery disease.[138–142] However, in spite of the abundance of experimental and observational study evidence suggesting that antioxidants should help prevent age-related CVDs, the results from large-scale randomized clinical trials have been disappointing.[143]

After two decades of clinical trials that investigated the impacts of α-tocopherol or ascorbic acid treatments on the incident of CVD, there is no data to indicate that these interventions alone are effective.[144] Several theories attempt to explain the apparent disconnect between experimental studies and clinical trials. A likely explanation is that ROS production and ROS-mediated macromolecular damage is highly compartmentalized within cells. Different localization and transport of antioxidants (ascorbic acid is water soluble; α-tocopherol is localized to lipid membranes) may result in inefficient antioxidant activity in critical compartments (eg, mitochondria). Based on emerging evidence, it is plausible that there will be a role for targeted antioxidative therapies in the prevention of age-related CVD. It is expected that future studies will test the effects of antioxidative treatments targeted to mitochondria or designed to activate endogenous antioxidant defenses (eg, pharmacological Nrf2 activators) on cardiovascular endpoints.

As oxidative stress is only one cellular mechanism of aging, future studies should also consider combination treatments, targeting several aging processes simultaneously. Dietary intervention studies also assessed the beneficial effects of increased consumption of foods high in antioxidants on CVD risk.[145] Complex antioxidative dietary interventions likely have the advantage that some ingredients (eg, dietary polyphenols) may induce endogenous antioxidant defense mechanisms effective in different cellular/subcellular compartments. There can also be cooperation and compensation between different antioxidant systems targeting different cellular/subcellular compartments. The PREvención con DIeta MEDiterránea (PREDIMED) study, a multicenter, randomized, controlled, clinical trial evaluated the protective effects of consumption of a Mediterranean diet supplemented with mixed nuts or extra-virgin olive oil on cardiovascular outcomes.[146] After a median follow-up of 4.8 years, a 28% to 30% reduction in major adverse cardiovascular events was reported in participants randomized to consume the Mediterranean diet,[146] which was attributed to the decreased oxidative stress.[147] Although some aspects of the study have been criticized and biomarkers of cardiovascular aging were not directly tested, the results are encouraging and warrant further studies.

Role of Mitochondria in Cardiovascular Aging

Aging is associated with mitochondrial derangement, which is characterized by increased mitochondrial oxidative stress and declining oxidative phosphorylation due to impaired electron transport chain activities in old age, especially the mitochondrial respiratory complexes I and IV.[148] As a highly metabolic active organ, the heart has numerous mitochondria that are susceptible to oxidative damage. Evidence showing the accumulation of oxidative damage to mitochondrial proteins and DNA in aged mouse hearts[149,150] suggest that damaged cardiac mitochondria produce more ROS. Respiratory complexes with oxidative damage or defective subunits due to mutant mitochondrial DNA (especially complex I, III, and IV) cause increased mitochondrial ROS production. This may lead to a vicious cycle of ROS amplification within cardiac mitochondria.[151,152] Direct evidence supporting the critical role of mitochondrial ROS in cardiac aging was shown in mice overexpressing catalase targeted to the mitochondria (mCAT), which mitigate mitochondrial oxidative damage,[149] in parallel with amelioration of LVH and fibrosis and diastolic dysfunction in aged hearts. The crucial role of mitochondria

in aging is further supported by mice with proofreading-deficient homozygous mutation of mitochondrial polymerase gamma (Polg$^{D257A/D257A}$), which induces a substantial increase in mitochondrial DNA mutations and deletions.[153,154] These mice display an age-dependent accumulation of mt-DNA mutations, shortened lifespan,[154] and several "accelerated aging" phenotypes, including an age-dependent cardiomyopathy.[150,153] The observations that mitochondrial damage and cardiomyopathy can be partially rescued by mCAT suggests that mitochondrial ROS and mt-DNA damage are part of a vicious cycle of ROS-induced ROS release.[150] The accelerated aging phenotypes in both skeletal and cardiac muscles in Polg$^{D257A/D257A}$ mice are also ameliorated by endurance exercise.[155] Exercise may induce augmentation of mitochondrial biogenesis, which helps to maintain the overall mitochondrial function in these muscles with mitochondrial DNA mutations. Since the accumulation of mitochondrial DNA damages are also documented in aged human hearts,[156,157] the benefit of endurance exercise in Polg$^{D257A/D257A}$ mice is consistent with the well-known benefit of regular aerobic exercise for human hearts.

Mitochondria are dynamic organelles undergoing fusion and fission as an important quality control process to maintain normal shape, number, and function of the mitochondria.[158] Cardiomyocyte mitochondria show morphological changes in old age and heart disease,[159,160] suggesting that the derangement of fusion and fission may also play roles in cardiac aging. For example, excessive mitochondrial fission results in fragmented mitochondria with poor oxidative phosphorylation activity, low membrane potential, and are the target for degradation.[161] Mitochondrial fusion is physiologically essential to maintain mitochondrial integrity and function in cardiomyocytes. Mitofusin1 (Mfn1), mitofusins2 (Mfn2), and OPA1 are key proteins in mitochondrial fusion. The dysregulation of these proteins leads to abnormal mitochondrial structure and function, with loss of efficiency of cellular respiration in many tissues,[162–164] including the aging heart.[165,166] In cardiomyocytes, partial suppression of Mfn2 and OPA1 caused altered mitochondrial morphology, resulting in large pleomorphic and irregular mitochondria with disrupted cristae structure.[166,167] Deficiency of both Mfn1 and 2 in mice results in mitochondrial fragmentation, impaired mitochondrial respiration, and fatal cardiomyopathy.[168] Deletion of Mfn1 leads to mitochondrial fragmentation and may result in cardiac hypertrophy and dysfunction.[166] Mfn2 deficiency in cardiomyocytes is associated with disruption of cell cycle progression, cardiac hypertrophy, reduced oxidative metabolism, and altered mitochondrial permeability transition, which leads to systolic dysfunction.[166] Consistent with this, the downregulation of Mfn2 expression has been reported in several experimental models of HF.[169]

Mitophagy is a special form of autophagy that degrades damaged mitochondria. The best-studied mechanism of mitophagy involves a PTEN-induced putative kinase 1 (PINK1)-Parkin-mitofusin 2 (Mfn2) complex, which marks a damage/depolarized mitochondria to be engulfed by autophagosomes through an LC3-receptor–dependent mechanism.[170] PINK1 induces phosphorylation of ubiquitin, which recruits LC3 receptor proteins and other autophagy factors to mitochondria.[171]

Deletion of Parkin led to the accumulation of disorganized mitochondria in aged mouse cardiomyocytes[172] and exacerbated cardiac injury in the MI mouse model.[173] These studies emphasize the role of Parkin-mediated mitophagy in cardiac aging[174] and MI. In addition to mitophagy, other mechanisms of mitochondrial quality control may include mitochondrial proteases, ubiquitin proteasome-dependent mechanisms. As mitochondrial quality declines with age, it is expected that many of these quality control mechanisms are impaired in old age.

The defect in mitochondrial function and energetics is well documented in human HF.[175] The mechanisms by which mitochondrial dysfunction aggravate HF progression may include mitochondrial biogenesis that does not keep up with the increasing demand in cardiac hypertrophy,[176] mitochondrial uncoupling and decreased substrate availability,[177] increased mitochondrial DNA deletions,[178] and altered mitochondrial bioenergetics. Vascular mitochondrial alterations were shown to contribute to endothelial dysfunction and dysregulation of cerebral blood flow.[69,179]

Preliminary mechanistic studies of mitochondrial-targeted antioxidants in murine models show the potential for mitigating several aspects of CVD,[69,178,180,181] and this is reinforced by the aforementioned genetic model of mitochondrial-targeted catalase (mCAT). One commonly used strategy for targeting mitochondria is using positively charged Triphenylphosphonium ions (TPP^+), which can effectively target the mitochondria because of the potential gradient across the mitochondrial membrane. Mitochondrial membrane potential is regulated between -100 and -200 mV in normal cells, depending on cell types and the activity of oxidative phosphorylation. The potential-dependent targeting method by TPP^+ can concentrate the molecules within mitochondria up to 1000-fold higher concentration than that within the cytosol.[182] Some examples of antioxidants conjugated with TTP^+ for mitochondrial targeting are coenzyme Q (MitoQ),[183] TEMPOL (Mito-TEMPOL), and Plastoquinone (SkQ1). MitoQ and other TPP^+ antioxidant conjugates reduce systolic blood pressure and cardiac hypertrophy in spontaneously hypertensive rats,[184,185] prolong lifespan in $SOD^{-/-}$ *Dropsophila*,[186] and attenuate the neurodegenerative phenotypes in rodent models with Alzheimer's or Parkinson diseases.[187,188] SkQ1 has been shown to reduce intracellular ROS and improve lifespan.[189,190] Although both MitoQ and SkQ1 have some protective effect against mitochondrial oxidative damage, such as in the context of ischemia-reperfusion injury, yet they may also inhibit oxidative phosphorylation and ATP production.[191] The latter may counteract the beneficial effect of reducing mitochondrial ROS. Elamipretide (also known as SS-31 and Bendavia), a tetrapeptide of alternating aromatic and positively charged amino-acid, H-D-Arg-Dmt-Lys-Phe-NH$_2$, is another small molecule previously developed as a mitochondrial antioxidant. Elamipretide targets mitochondria by direct interaction with cardiolipin,[191] which is highly enriched in the mitochondrial inner membrane. Cardiolipin assists in maintaining the ultrastructure of mitochondrial cristae, the docking sites of mitochondrial electron transport supercomplexes.[192,193] The interaction of Elamipretide with cardiolipin inhibits the peroxidase activity of cytochrome c,[194] thereby preserving

mitochondrial cristae ultrastructure, enhancing the electron transfer efficiency, and indirectly decreasing mitochondrial ROS production. Elamipretide has been shown to improve cardiac function in rodents and dog model of MI, chronic hypertension, and pressure-overload induced HF, in parallel with better preservation of mitochondrial functions and mitochondrial proteome.[195-197] A recent study shows that Elamipretide ameliorates cardiac aging in mice.[198] However, phase II clinical trials for Elamipretide in ST-elevation MI and HFrEF have shown only modest benefit,[199-201] despite the report that Elamipretide significantly improved failing mitochondrial function in cardiac explants from patients with end-stage HF.[202]

Role of NAD⁺ Depletion and Sirtuin-Regulated Pathways

Advanced age is associated with decreased availability of cellular NAD⁺,[108,203,204] which is likely a common contributor to aging processes in the heart, the vasculature,[105] and other tissues. NAD⁺ and its phosphorylated form NADP⁺ have central roles in cellular metabolism, energy production, anabolic processes, and survival. Over 400 enzymes require NAD⁺ and NADP⁺, predominantly to accept or donate electrons for redox reactions. NAD⁺ is also the substrate for at least four classes of enzymes that play important roles in the regulation of aging processes, cellular survival, and normal physiological function. These include enzymes with mono-ADP ribosyltransferase and poly (ADP-ribose) polymerase (PARP) activities, which catalyze ADP-ribosyl transfer reactions. NAD⁺ is a rate-limiting cosubstrate for sirtuin ("Sir2-like") enzymes (SIRT1-SIRT7), which are key regulators of cellular metabolism, mitochondrial function, prosurvival pathways, and inflammatory processes, and catalyze the removal of acyl groups from acylated proteins. As histone deacetylases, sirtuins play critical roles in epigenetic regulation of aging processes. Both PARP enzymes and sirtuins are involved in DNA repair pathways. Additionally, ADP-ribosyl cyclases such as CD38, which have relevance for calcium signaling and regulation of endothelial NO-mediated vasodilation,[205] also require NAD⁺. Age-related NAD⁺ depletion may impact many of the aforementioned pathways, compromising multiple cellular functions in parallel.

The mechanisms underlying the age-related decline in NAD⁺ in the cardiovascular system are likely multifaceted[206] and likely include increased utilization of NAD⁺ by activated PARP-1.[111,207] Importantly, cardiovascular risk factors (eg, obesity,[208,209] high homocysteine levels,[210] diabetes mellitus[114,211]) that promote accelerated vascular aging by increasing oxidative stress and oxidative stress-mediated PARP-1 activation also result in cellular NAD⁺ depletion.

Growing evidence shows that restoration of cellular NAD⁺ levels by treatment with NAD⁺ precursors (including nicotinamide mononucleotide [NMN] and nicotinamide riboside [NR]) exerts multifaceted antiaging effects, improving both general health and longevity in mice.[212,213] Restoration of youthful NAD⁺ levels in the aged murine vasculature by treatment with NAD⁺ boosters was shown to rescue endothelial function, attenuate oxidative stress, and improve endothelial mitochondrial bioenergetics.[214-216] It also reverses age-related capillary rarefaction and improves blood flow in the skeletal muscle,[215] likely by reversing age-related impairment of endothelial angiogenic capacity.[215,217,218] Treatment of aged mice with NMN also rescues cerebromicrovascular function, improves neurovascular coupling responses, increases cerebral blood flow, and reverses age-related changes in endothelial gene expression profile.[214,219] Of note, treatment with NAD$^+$ boosters was also shown to restore NAD$^+$ levels and improve cardiac function in mouse models of HF,[220] illustrating the concept that shared mechanisms of aging contribute to the pathogenesis of diverse age-related CVDs. Age-related NAD$^+$ depletion is known to impair the activity of sirtuin enzymes, which confer multifaceted cardiovascular protective effects (including regulation of eNOS activity, mitochondrial function and mitochondrial ROS production, and NADPH oxidase activity). A key mechanism underlying the antiaging action of NAD$^+$ booster treatments is sirtuin activation, which has been causally linked to improved cellular energetics, restoration of mitochondrial function and attenuation of mitochondrial oxidative stress.[203,214] Importantly, dietary/caloric restriction was also shown to activate sirtuins, which contributes to its antiaging[221-223] and cardiovascular protective effects.[128,129,224,225] Similar to the effects of NAD$^+$ boosters, sirtuin-activating compounds (STACs), including the naturally occurring polyphenol resveratrol and the synthetic compound SRT1720, have also been demonstrated to exert significant cardiac and vasoprotective effects in models of aging and pathological conditions associated with accelerated cardiovascular aging.[226-233] Similar to NAD$^+$ booster treatments, STACs also attenuate mitochondrial oxidative stress in the aged vasculature.[71,87,234] STACs were also demonstrated to restore endothelial function, improve blood flow regulation, increase capillarization, and prevent microvascular fragility in the aged mouse brain.[87,93,235] STACS were also shown to confer vasoprotective effects in nonhuman primate models.[236,237]

Role of Proteostasis and Autophagy

Protein homeostasis (proteostasis) is an equilibrium state between protein synthesis, maintenance, and degradation and it is essential to maintain cellular health. Autophagy is a major protein degradation system that acts through the digestion of macromolecules by lysosomal enzymes.[238] The delivery of intracellular components to the lysosome for degradation includes three major autophagic pathways. Microautophagy works through invaginations of the lysosomal membrane, which directly engulf portions of cytoplasm into a lysosomal lumen lined by single membrane vesicles, resulting in the degradation of cytoplasmic material.[239,240] Chaperone-mediated autophagy is a targeted process, in which cytosolic proteins containing a pentapeptide KFERQ motif are targeted and translocated across the lysosomal membrane, resulting in degradation of specific proteins.[241] The third pathway, macroautophagy, involves phagophores, small vesicular sacs that enclose cytosolic proteins and organelles, resulting in the formation of autophagosomes, which fuse with lysosomes, leading to the degradation of the sequestered cellular contents by lysosomal enzymes.[242,243] Macroautophagy is the most extensively studied in the context of aging and cell survival and has been shown to be an important

determinant of longevity. The lifespan extension observed in model organisms with overexpression of autophagy-related 8a (Atg8a)[244] and overexpression of Atg5 in mice[245] provide direct evidence for the role of autophagy in aging. These key autophagic proteins are involved in autophagosome formation and their overexpression has been shown to extend lifespan and maintain youthful phenotypes in aged organisms. The beneficial effect of autophagy is mediated through the removal of toxic protein aggregates and damaged mitochondria, including those containing harmful levels of ROS. These harmful molecules or organelles are removed by autophagy in normal conditions. However, the capacity of autophagy is exhausted in aging due to excessive ROS production, increased oxidative damage, and misfolded proteins. If not removed, these harmful macromolecules can trigger cell death, organ dysfunction, and eventually lead to mortality.

The ubiquitin-proteasome system (UPS) is the other major protein degradation pathway in the cells. In contrast to autophagy, which nonspecifically degrades macromolecules or organelles through fusion with lysosomes, the UPS pathway is more specific to particular proteins. Whereas autophagy often degrades a complex mixture of cytoplasmic biomolecules within the vesicles using lysosomal hydrolases, the UPS specifically targets ubiquitinated proteins. Poly-ubiquitin tagging of proteins is destined for degradation by proteasomal proteases.[238,246,247] This targeted degradation is regulated by sophisticated mechanisms having a high spatial and temporal precision.[238,246-249] The UPS is also essential for cellular proteostasis. Disrupting UPS function can cause accumulation of abnormal protein inclusions, leading to severe toxicity and cell death.[249,250] For example, genetic depletion of proteasome subunits in the brains of mice has been shown to induce neuronal protein inclusions, and the mice display phenotypes of neurodegenerative diseases.[250] Although previous studies show that proteasomal activity decline with aging and are restored by calorie restriction,[246,249] the overall role of UPS in aging remains unclear.

Accumulation of damaged proteins and inefficient proteostasis is observed in the aged hearts as protein aggregates, such as in senile amyloid deposition and lipofuscin.[251] Lipofuscin is yellow-brown pigment granules composed of lipid-containing remnants of lysosomal digestion. It has been conventionally known as an aging or "wear-and-tear" pigment, although its biological role remains elusive. Studies using a novel sensitive method of deuterated leucine labeling proteomics reported that proteome turnover is either unchanged or only modestly increased during aging in various mouse tissues, including heart,[252] skeletal muscle,[253] and liver.[254] Increased protein oxidative damage in aged tissues should predict a significant increase in proteolysis and proteome turnover. The absence of increased proteome turnover in aged tissues[255,256] suggests a decline in the efficiency of protein degradation machinery with advanced age, contributing to the accumulation of macromolecular aggregates.

As already discussed, mice with Atg5 overexpression demonstrate enhanced autophagy and extended longevity. In contrast, mice with cardiac-specific knockdown of Atg5 displayed accelerated cardiac aging phenotypes, including LVH, decreased fractional shortening, and premature death.[257] These findings indicate that autophagy plays an important role in maintaining normal heart function during aging. While the mechanism by which autophagy maintains cardiac function is not fully understood, an accumulation of ubiquitinated proteins and p62 in Atg5 mutants suggests that the removal of damaged proteins is an important protective mechanism.[257,258] Another study in cardiomyocyte cell lines also found that induction of autophagy mitigated oxidative stress-induced protein aggregation, reduced levels of protein ubiquitination, improved mitochondrial function, and reduced cell death, suggesting that autophagy has an important role in maintaining quality mitochondria.[259]

Calorie restriction and rapamycin treatment, two antiaging interventions that act in part via inhibition of mTOR complex I pathway, have been shown to activate autophagy pathways.[260] Shorter-term calorie restriction or rapamycin treatment (10–12 weeks) initiated at middle age significantly rejuvenated age-associated cardiac hypertrophy, diastolic dysfunction, and inflammation.[252,261] These are in parallel with the amelioration of age-related cardiac proteomic remodeling.[252] Activation of autophagic markers was observed only during the initial period of rapamycin treatment, indicating a transient induction of autophagy to remove damaged macromolecules and organelles (eg, mitochondria) and an induction of biogenesis to replenish and rejuvenate mitochondria as part of homeostasis. Despite transient autophagic induction, the beneficial effect of rapamycin was sustained even after cessation of treatment. These findings imply that rejuvenation of autophagy and proteostasis pathways are critical in maintaining youthful hearts.

Taken together, evidence suggest that perturbation of proteostasis may have some causative role in aging and restoration of protein homeostasis (especially autophagy) may be protective against aging and age-related disease. As the major mechanisms controlling proteostasis, both autophagy and the UPS are expected to work in synchrony to regulate protein degradation. A study has shown that poly-ubiquitination can also promote the clearance of such proteins through autophagy.[262] However, the interactions between various mechanisms of autophagy and ubiquitin-proteasome systems remain largely unknown. Further studies are needed to investigate the mechanisms underlying the protective effects of enhancing proteostasis by autophagy and UPS on lifespan and healthspan benefits.

Inflammaging

Aging is associated with immune dysregulation and chronic low-grade sterile inflammation, characterized by higher circulating and paracrine levels of proinflammatory factors,[263] such as IL-1, IL-1 receptor antagonist (IL-1RN), IL-6, IL-8, IL-13, IL-18, C-reactive protein (CRP), interferon α and β, transforming growth factor-β (TGFβ), TNFα and its soluble receptors (TNF receptor superfamily), and serum amyloid A. This inflammaging state predispose the elderly to a range of chronic diseases, disability, frailty, and death.[264,265] Potential contributors to inflammaging include cellular senescence, oxidative stress (eg, from dysfunctional mitochondria) and NF-κB

activation, immune cell dysregulation, as well as changes in the microbiome and chronic infections.

Genetic susceptibility of inflammatory genes has been reported in several large population studies, which identify various genetic polymorphisms that affect circulating levels of inflammatory mediators.[266–268] A few examples include *IL1RN* 1018 haplotype that correlates with higher concentrations of IL-1β and IFNγ[269] *IL6* 174G > C allele that magnifies IL-6 production in response to inflammatory stimuli,[270] multiple SNPs in the CRP gene (alleles C at rs3093059 and G at rs1205) that associate with higher CRP levels.[268,271] The carriers of these proinflammatory variants have increased susceptibility to CVDs and related comorbidities.[272,273] Some genetic variants are protective and associated with lower levels of inflammatory markers, such as *IL1RN* rs4251961 minor allele, CRP 1059 CC allele, and *IL6* rs2069837.[269,274] The latter has been associated with extreme longevity in a genome-wide association study of more than 2000 Chinese centenarians, suggesting a critical role of inflammation in aging and longevity.[275]

Intrinsic defects in immune cells have been reported in aging. For instance, the elderly have CD4[+] lymphocytes with elevated NF-κB activity compared with CD4[+] cells from young adults.[276] This phenomenon may be due to the intrinsic aging of immune cells or related to chronic infection. Chronic infection can stimulate immune response and increase proinflammatory markers. Serological examinations have shown a high prevalence of anti-CMV IgG in the elderly populations, suggesting a latent infection.[277] Intermittent reactivation of CMV may occur several times throughout life and may lead to enhanced inflammatory signals in old age. This is further supported by the report that CMV-specific memory T cells can comprise up to 50% of the total memory T cell compartment in the elderly.[278,279] Thus, chronic CMV infection with intermittent reactivation has been proposed to play critical roles in immunosenescence and inflammaging. Some studies suggest that CMV infection in the elderly is associated with increased risk of CVD and mortality, in association with inflammaging.[280–283] However, the association between CMV infection, inflammaging, and CVD and mortality remains controversial.[284,285] Some chronic infections may cause the release of pathogen-associated molecular patterns into the circulation, which can elicit a proinflammatory state that increases the risk of CVD. As an example, there is strong evidence to support an association between chronic periodontitis and atherosclerotic CVDs.[286]

Microbiome alterations have been reported in aging, characterized by a reduction in beneficial commensal microorganisms, such as *Coprococcus, Faecalibacterium,* and *Lactobacillus.*[287,288] These beneficial microbiomes normally counteract the expansion of pathogenic microbes and maintain intestinal barrier integrity.[288] The decline in these beneficial microbiomes with aging increases the permeability of the mucosal barrier, thereby allowing pathogenic bacteria and their associated molecular patterns to get into the circulatory system, leading to activation of innate immunity, exacerbating systemic proinflammatory state.[289] Understanding the role of age-related changes in the microbiome in low-grade sterile inflammation in the cardiovascular system is a focus of ongoing investigations.

Conventional cardiovascular risk factors can exacerbate age-related chronic sterile inflammation in the cardiovascular system. For example, abdominal obesity and metabolic syndrome are strongly associated with a proinflammatory state, and predict worse coronary atherosclerosis and cardiometabolic prognosis.[284,290,291] Adipocytes, particularly from visceral fat, may secrete proinflammatory cytokines and chemokines, such as IL-6, IL-1β, TNF, and C-C motif chemokine 2 (CCL2). Furthermore, visceral adipose tissue from obese subjects demonstrates the infiltration of T lymphocytes, macrophages, and monocytes. T lymphocytes secrete IFNγ, which stimulates the secretion of several chemokines from adipocytes, including CCL2, CCL5, C-X-C motif chemokine 9 (CXCL9), and CXCL10, which further amplify tissue T cell migration. Besides, B lymphocytes and macrophages are also increased and are well correlated with body mass index.[292] In experimental old mice, there is an accumulation of a specific subset of B cells producing TNF, IFNγ, and granzyme B.[293] Cytokines secreted by B cells contribute to the phenotypic switch of adipocytes in the visceral cavity, stimulating the release of proinflammatory adipokines.[294] In contrast, weight loss by diet control or bariatric surgery has been associated with decreased proinflammatory markers, which may be attributable to decreased proinflammatory state in white adipose tissue and downregulation of the NLRP3 inflammasome.[295–297] Calorie restriction as the most reproducible antiaging intervention, has been shown to inhibit inflammation in rodents and nonobese humans.[298] The combination of weight loss and aerobic exercise significantly improves functional status and reduces frailty in older obese individuals, which further improves the risk of CVD.[299–301]

Several epidemiological and clinical studies support that inflammation is a risk factor, or at least a risk marker, for CVD. Elevated serum inflammatory markers, such as CRP and IL-6, are independently associated with the risk of CVD.[272,302–304] Whether the relationship of inflammations and CVD is a causal effect or merely a bystander association as reactive markers of underlying pathology has been controversial, although an increasing number of studies have suggested that inflammatory cells, cytokines, and acute phase reactant (eg, CRP) may have a direct contribution to the pathogenesis of CVD, particularly atherosclerosis. One of the best clinical evidence of the direct roles of inflammatory processes in atherosclerotic CVD is the CANTOS trial. CANTOS is a randomized controlled trial of canakinumab, a therapeutic monoclonal antibody targeting IL-1β as secondary prevention in patients with prior MI and elevated CRP of 2 mg/L or more. CANTOS reported that canakinumab significantly reduced recurrent cardiovascular events in >10,000 stable patients who had residual inflammation after MI, independent of lowered lipid levels.[273,305]

Inflammation plays a critical role in the initiation of atherogenesis and progression of atherosclerosis, from early endothelial dysfunction to the development of acute thrombotic complications triggered by plaque rupture.[306–308] Atherogenesis initiates from injured endothelium that allows the accumulation of cholesterol-containing oxidized low-density lipoprotein (LDL) particles in the arterial wall, which are phagocytosed by macrophages, later transformed into foam cells, which triggers further inflammatory response. Cholesterol crystals and various molecular patterns within the atherosclerotic lesion activate the inflammasomes within macrophages, leading to the release of proinflammatory cytokines (eg, IL-1β, IL-18, etc.), which attract T cells and B cells, driving the progression of atherosclerosis.[309,310] Progression of atheroma is characterized by extensive cell death and accumulation of numerous senescent cells, which further secrete proinflammatory molecules (collectively called senescent-associated secretory phenotypes [SASPs]), leading to the formation of a necrotic core. The lipid-rich necrotic cores within the atheroma are soft and fragile and are prone to rupture. Senescent cells can produce metalloproteinases that facilitate plaques rupture, which subsequently activates platelets and coagulation cascades leading to the formation of thromboemboli and eventually cause acute vascular occlusion.

Role of Cellular Senescence

Cellular senescence (defined as irreversible cell cycle arrest) is regarded as a fundamental aging process characterized by functional impairment and profound disease-promoting changes to the cellular secretome.[311] Various endogenous and exogenous stressors linked to cellular damage (eg, reactive oxygen and nitrogen species, DNA damage, mitochondrial dysfunction, telomere dysfunction, and paracrine signals) can exacerbate cellular senescence in aging.[312,313] There is strong preclinical evidence that depletion of p16^{INK4A} expressing senescent cells can significantly extend lifespan and promote healthspan in mouse models of aging.[312] These findings provide proof-of-concept that increased senescent cells contribute to the age-related physiological decline and promote the pathogenesis of diverse age-related diseases, ranging from chronic kidney disease, cataracts, and cancer to osteoporosis, osteoarthritis, and neurodegenerative diseases.[314] There is also strong evidence that aging associates with an increased presence of senescent cells in the heart[312,315] and the vasculature.[316–318] Multiple cell types, including endothelial cells, smooth muscle cells, fibroblasts, pericytes, and resident cardiac progenitor cells[315] are affected by age-related senescence. Accumulating evidence from pathological examination of human samples and preclinical models indicates a causal role for senescent cells in the genesis of age-related cardiovascular pathologies, including HF,[319] advanced atherosclerosis,[311,320] and abdominal aortic aneurysm.[321] Pathophysiological conditions that exacerbate cardiovascular aging (eg, diabetes mellitus) also associate with an increased presence of senescent cells in the vasculature.[322] Although the fraction of senescent cells is usually low, multiple mechanisms have been identified by which they may impair tissue function and promote the pathogenesis of age-related CVDs.

Senescent cells acquire a SASP, which is characterized by altered production of secreted proteins and peptides, including an upregulation of inflammatory cytokines and chemokines, growth factors, proteases (eg, MMPs), dysregulated synthesis of lipid mediators,[323] and altered shedding of exosomes and ectosomes containing enzymes, microRNA, DNA fragments, and other bioactive factors.[324] Through the secretion of the

SASP factors, senescence cells modify the tissue microenvironment and disrupt the normal function of cardiac myocytes and vascular cells by promoting chronic inflammation, induction of fibrosis, and inhibition of stem cells function.[325] SASP factors can also promote oxidative stress and reduce NAD^+ levels in neighboring nonsenescent cells. In senescent cells, the biosynthesis of components of the extracellular matrix (ECM), secretion of ECM degrading proteases (eg, MMPs), and expression of growth factors that regulate remodeling of the ECM are also altered. SASP factors alter ECM homeostasis in the neighboring tissue. The secretion of SASP factors may also induce proliferating neighbor cells to undergo senescence (termed paracrine senescence). This later mechanism appears particularly important for cardiac progenitor cell dysfunction.[315] Endothelial cells are connected by gap junctions and function as a syncytium. Thus, it is possible that the vasculature signals that induce endothelial senescence may be transmitted between cells.[325] Paracrine senescence may be potentially important for age-related impairment of regenerative and angiogenic capacity of the microvascular endothelial cells. Through the aforementioned mechanisms, the increased presence of senescent cells in the aged vasculature may contribute to endothelial dysfunction,[316] impaired barrier function, chronic sterile vascular inflammation, and pathological remodeling of arteries and the microcirculatory network.[326] Increase in senescent cells in the aged heart likely contributes to pathological remodeling of the ventricles and impaired regeneration in the heart.[315,327] The role of senescent cells in vascular aging is also supported by experimental observations that in mouse models of accelerated DNA damage-dependent vascular senescence (including mouse models of γ-irradiation-induced senescence,[323] hypomorphic BubR1 mutant [BubR1$^{H/H}$] mice[328]), induction of senescence in cells of the neurovascular unit associates with blood–brain barrier disruption,[328] dysregulation of cerebral blood flow,[329] and microvascular rarefaction,[330] mimicking the cerebrovascular aging phenotype. Both BubR1$^{H/H}$ mice[331] and γ-irradiated mice exhibit aging-like phenotypic changes both in large arteries (including endothelial dysfunction and ECM alterations) and the heart.[332,333]

It is expected that antiaging therapeutic strategies, which improve cellular stress resilience, would also prevent the induction of senescence. The Nrf2-dependent homeostatic antioxidant defense pathway plays a critical role in oxidative stress resilience in the cardiovascular system by regulating both DNA repair mechanisms and detoxification of ROS. Accordingly, genetic disruption of Nrf2 signaling exacerbates aging-induced senescence in the vasculature.[91] Nrf2 dysfunction has also been causally linked to increased oxidative stress-mediated senescence of endothelial progenitor cells.[334] Future studies should determine whether chronic treatment with pharmacological activators of Nrf2 (eg, dietary polyphenols), which attenuate ROS-mediated DNA damage, can prevent cellular senescence in the aging heart and vasculature.

Recent advances in geroscience research have enabled the development of targeted senolytic drugs for selective pharmacological elimination of senescent cells.[335] Several experimental senolytic strategies have been developed and tested in preclinical animal models. These include treatment with dasatinib (a selective tyrosine kinase receptor inhibitor that is used in the therapy of chronic myelogenous leukemia), the polyphenols quercetin and fisetin, and the Bcl-2/Bcl-XL inhibitor navitoclax (ABT263), which effectively eliminate senescent cells in various organs, including the blood vessels.[311,335] There are studies extant showing that senolytic treatments may prevent atherogenesis[311] and improve endothelial function in aged mice.[316] Senolytic treatment with navitoclax was also shown to prevent HF[336] and improve myocardial remodeling and rescue diastolic function following MI in mouse models of aging.[337] Elimination of senescent cells in aged mice (transgenic INK-ATTAC mice, which permits targeted elimination of p16^{INK4A}-positive senescent cells, or wild-type mice treated with desitanib plus quercetin) was also shown to rescue the function of resident cardiac progenitor cells.[315] Based on these promising preclinical findings, it is reasonable to expect that translationally relevant senolytic strategies can be developed in the future to eliminate senescent cells in older adults to improve cardiovascular healthspan and prevent multiple age-related diseases simultaneously.

Regulation of Cardiovascular Aging by Progeronic and Antigeronic Circulating Factors

It is evident that cell-autonomous mechanisms alone[12] are inadequate to explain all aspects of cardiovascular aging. There is compelling evidence that the hierarchical regulatory cascade for cardiovascular aging also involves modulation of cellular and molecular aging processes in the heart and the vasculature by systemic/circulating factors.[62] Critical evidence to demonstrate a key role of circulating antigeronic factors regulating cardiovascular aging processes is derived from preclinical studies of calorie restriction, a dietary regimen that extends healthspan and/or lifespan. Calorie restriction in rodents is associated with cardiac[225,252,338] and vascular[62] rejuvenation, including a youthful transcriptional reprogramming, prevention of pathological remodeling, improved myocardial contractility, the rescue of endothelial function, and attenuation of oxidative stress and inflammation. Critically, in vitro treatment of detector endothelial cells in culture with complement-inactivated sera obtained from calorie-restricted rodent and nonhuman primate models can recapitulate fundamental cellular rejuvenating effects (eg, anti-inflammatory, pro-angiogenic effects, activation of SIRT1) observed in vivo in caloric restricted animals.[129,224] Sera derived from calorie-restricted animals was also shown to promote mitochondrial protective effects and oxidative stress resilience.[339,340] Initial studies demonstrate that sera obtained from humans on a calorie-restricted diet also confer cytoprotective effects.[341] Ongoing research efforts are directed toward the identification of pharmacological interventions (calorie restriction mimetics) that convey cardiovascular health benefits similar to the circulating factors induced by calorie restriction.[228,252,342]

The fundamental role of systemic pro- and antigeronic factors in the regulation of cellular aging phenotypes was also demonstrated by studies using murine models of heterochronic parabiosis (when a young mouse is surgically joined to an aged mouse connecting their circulatory systems[343]) and mice with heterochronic blood apheresis[344] (which enables heterochronic blood exchange between young and old mice without sharing other organ systems and free from adaptations to being surgically joined for several weeks). The existing evidence shows that circulating antigeronic factors derived from young parabiont mice can improve cardiac function[345] and rejuvenate both endothelial function in the aorta[346] and microvascular network architecture in aged heterochronic parabionts.[343] Young blood factors were also shown to attenuate vascular oxidative stress and reverse age-related changes in the vascular transcriptome.[346] Specifically, it was reported that out of 347 differentially expressed genes in the aged mouse aorta, the expression of 212 genes was shifted back toward the young phenotype by the presence of young blood in aged heterochronic parabiont animals.[346] Pathway analysis revealed that vascular protective effects mediated by young blood-regulated genes include mitochondrial rejuvenation.[346] Old blood factors may also contribute to the exacerbation of cardiovascular aging processes.[344]

The exact nature of the young blood factors and old blood factors responsible for the modulation of cardiovascular aging processes and transposition of cardiovascular aging

phenotypes observed in the aforementioned studies is a focus of intense investigations. **Figure 82–4** depicts potential young blood factor candidates whose role can be inferred from preclinical parabiosis experiments, serum treatment studies, and indirect evidence. Proteomics studies identified the TGF-β superfamily member GDF11 as a putative circulating antigeronic factor that regulates cardiac aging,[345] although the results were disputed. Other candidates young blood-borne factors that have been linked to rejuvenation of other organs (eg, brain) include thrombospondin-4 (THBS4), SPARC-like protein 1 (SPARCL1),[347] tissue inhibitor of metalloproteinases 2 (TIMP2),[348] GnRH,[349] and oxytocin.[350]

Epidemiological and experimental studies provide multiple layers of evidence in support of the concept that circulating insulin-like growth factor-1 (IGF-1) acts as a young blood factor. IGF-1 is a pleiotropic anabolic hormone that confers multifaceted antiaging effects in the cardiovascular system.[351] Circulating levels of IGF-1 are high in young adults and significantly decrease with age.[352] Additionally, levels of IGF binding protein (IGFBP)-1,[353,354] IGFBP-2, and/or IGFBP-3[352] increase in older adults, further reducing free IGF-1 levels. Age-related IGF-1 deficiency was reported to predict increased cardiovascular mortality in older adults.[354,355] High IGFBP levels also increase the risk for CVDs, including HF.[356] Preclinical studies

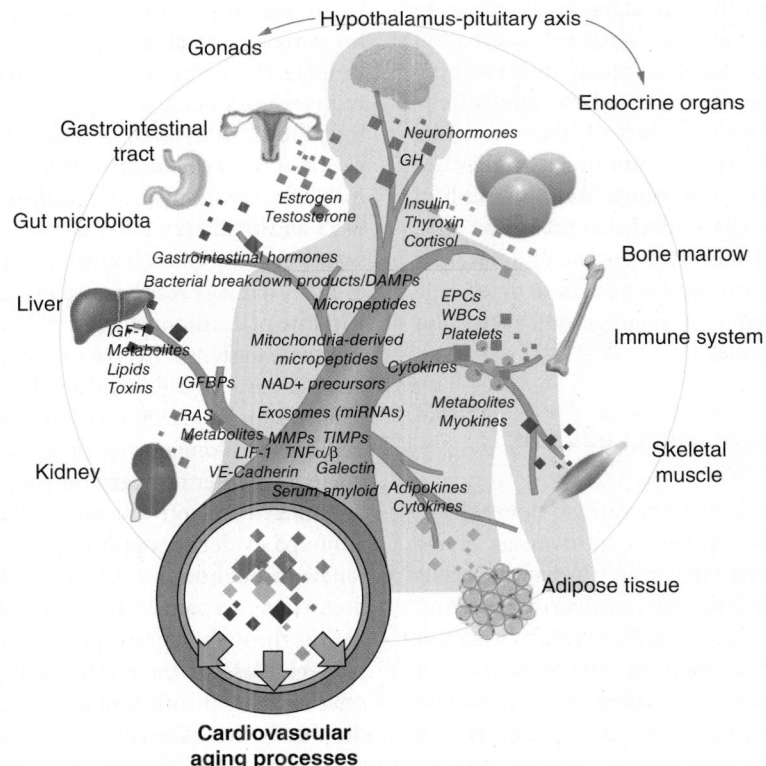

Figure 82–4. Regulation of cardiovascular aging processes by progeronic and antigeronic circulating factors. The model depicts the role of altered interorgan communication in the hierarchical regulatory cascade for cardiovascular aging. Cell-autonomous cellular and molecular processes of aging in the cardiac myocytes and the vasculature are modulated by the systemic milieu. Circulating progeronic factors and antigeronic factors derived from the central nervous system, endocrine organs, the immune system, the adipose tissue, and other organs (including the gastrointestinal tract) orchestrate cardiac and vascular aging processes. Age-related changes in the balance of these circulating factors result in generalized functional and phenotypic alterations in the heart and the vasculature, promoting the pathogenesis diverse age-related cardiovascular diseases. RAS, renin-angiotensin system; MMPs, matrix metalloproteinases; DAMPs, damage-associated molecular patterns; EPCs, endothelial progenitor cells; GH, growth hormone. Adapted with permission from Ungvari Z, Tarantini S, Sorond F, et al. Mechanisms of Vascular Aging, A Geroscience Perspective: JACC Focus Seminar. *J Am Coll Cardiol.* 2020 Mar 3;75(8):931-941.

confirm that IGF-1 deficiency promotes atherogenesis,[357,358] endothelial dysfunction,[359,360] pathological vascular remodeling,[361,362] impaired cellular oxidative stress resilience,[363,364] impaired angiogenic processes, and microvascular rarefaction.[365,366] IGF-1 deficiency has also been linked to accelerated cardiac aging, promoting cardiac mitochondrial oxidative stress,[367,368] cardiomyocyte apoptosis,[369] and contractile dysfunction.[370,371] Importantly, in a recent parabiosis study, IGF1R signaling was identified as a likely upstream regulator involved in young blood-mediated vascular transcriptomic rejuvenation in aged heterochronic parabionts.[346]

In addition to the role of young blood-borne proteins and peptides, the contribution of steroid hormones and other lipid mediators, micropeptides, metabolites, NAD$^+$ precursors,[372] and circulating exosomes, which contain many types of biomolecules, including cellular proteins, miRNAs, and mRNAs, should also be elucidated in future studies. It has been proposed that dilution of old blood factors with young blood may also contribute to organ rejuvenation.[373] The existing evidence suggest that inflammatory cytokines (eg, TNFα) may act as circulating progeronic factors.[62] Of note, many of these factors are derived from senescent cells residing in the adipose tissue and other organs.[313,314] Further, age-related increases in intestinal permeability ("leaky gut") results in an increased presence of bacterial breakdown products in the circulation, which may also contribute to the heightened inflammatory status of the cardiovascular system (see section Exacerbation of Vascular Aging Processes by Cardiovascular Risk Factors). Future studies should also identify the cellular origins of circulating progeronic and antigeronic factors that modulate cardiac and vascular aging processes. Additional studies are warranted to better characterize the contribution of youthful circulating cells (white blood cells, endothelial precursor cells, and platelets) in young blood-mediated cardiac and vascular rejuvenation. Epidemiological studies are needed to determine the effects of circulating progeronic and antigeronic factors on cardiovascular risk in older adults.

The Role of Resident Cardiac Stem Cells and Cardiomyocytes Proliferation

Since its initial report,[374] the role of adult cardiac stem cells in cardiac physiology and disease has been controversial. A few independent laboratories reported that c-kit$^+$ cardiac stem cells are necessary and sufficient for functional cardiac regeneration and repair in the adult heart,[375] however, these results were not reproducible by several other laboratories. The application of various lineage-tracing methods had failed to demonstrate the significance of c-kit$^+$ cells in cardiac regeneration. In one study, c-kit$^+$ stem cells showed minimal contribution to cardiomyocytes regeneration during development, aging, or in response to injury.[376] Another study reported that c-kit cells predominantly express endothelial cell markers in developing and adult hearts[377] and only rarely coexpress cardiac progenitor marker Nkx2.5, or the cardiac troponin T (cTnT) marker. Another population of resident stem cells marked by stem cell antigen 1 (Sca-1), a surface marker of murine hematopoietic

stem cells, has been initially reported to contribute to the generation of adult cardiomyocytes,[378,379] yet a later fate-mapping study demonstrated that endogenous Sca-1$^+$ cells predominantly mark CD31$^+$ endothelial cells and minimally mark troponin positive cardiomyocytes (<0.01%) under physiological and after MI.[380]

According to a consensus statement on cardiomyocyte regeneration by the American Heart Association (AHA) in 2018, de novo cardiomyocyte turnover is approximately 1% per year in the adult mammalian heart.[381] This estimation came from the analysis of the human cardiac DNA turnover rate derived from the environmental ^{14}C of human tissue data. There were increases in atmospheric ^{14}C following the atomic bomb testing of the mid-20th century. Using mathematical modeling of ^{14}C decay to estimate the rate of cardiomyocyte turnover, they estimated that cardiomyocyte turnover is approximately 1% per year at the age of 25, and the turnover rate decrease to 0.45% per year at the age of 75 in adult human hearts,[382] indicating an aging effect on spontaneous cardiomyocyte renewal in human hearts. They further reported that cardiomyocyte turnover is highest in early childhood, until the hearts have the final number of cardiomyocytes ($\sim 3.2 \times 10^9 \pm 0.75 \times 10^9$ cells) at approximately 1 month of age. The number of cardiomyocytes remain constant over the lifetime.[383] These observations are supported by the findings in rodent hearts. The rodent heart continues to grow by means of cardiomyocyte proliferation only during the early postnatal period, up to a postnatal window of 7 days in mice.[384] During the first postnatal week, myocardial injury induces a regenerative response, resulting in the replacement of lost cardiomyocytes by new ones.[384] Fate-mapping studies suggest that this type of myocardial regeneration is mediated primarily by cardiomyocyte proliferation,[384,385] which is limited by ROS and oxidative DNA damage. Postnatal hypoxemia, ROS scavenging by mitochondrial-targeted catalase, or inhibition of DNA damage response all extend the postnatal proliferative window of cardiomyocytes.[386] Interestingly, gradual exposure to severe systemic hypoxemia may inhibit oxidative metabolism, decreasing ROS and oxidative DNA damage, leading to reactivation of cardiomyocyte regeneration from previously existing cardiomyocytes in adult mouse hearts.[387] It is still unclear whether this cardiomyocyte regenerative potential can be induced in large animals or humans. It is noteworthy that although evidence supporting the cardiomyocytes' potential to renew throughout life, this happens at a very low rate and the dominant mechanism of postnatal heart growth in the mammals is through hypertrophy mechanism, not by proliferation.

Regardless of their role during normal physiology, these c-kit$^+$ cells are insufficient to prevent the progression of CVD in the elderly, evidenced by the absence of cardiomyocyte regeneration following acute ischemic events in humans. Even though c-kit$^+$ or Sca-1$^+$ cells may not regenerate cardiomyocytes during physiological or pathological conditions, they are indeed resident stem cells within the hearts that give rise to endothelial cells. Intrinsic aging of these resident stem cells is supported by experiments in rodents, which show that c-kit$^+$ stem cells in the older hearts had a higher rate of apoptosis and shorter telomeres.[388] In a rodent model of diabetic cardiomyopathy, c-kit+ cells display telomere shortening, increased expression of senescence markers p53 and p16INK4a, and increased apoptosis. All of the above changes in diabetic cardiomyopathy were attenuated by the ablation of the p66Shc gene,[389] suggesting a central role of mitochondrial ROS in the aging of resident c-kit+ stem cells. Studies using cardiosphere-derived cells, another type of resident cardiac stem cells, also demonstrate a significant age-dependent decline in the number and function of such stem cells derived from aged mouse atrial explant.[390]

Intrinsic aging of stem cells has been widely documented in various organ systems.[391–393] For regenerative therapeutics, studies using other types of stem cells also show that the age of the stem cell donor is crucial. For instance, mesenchymal stem cells from old donors were more susceptible to ROS-induced damage when transplanted into rats with a myocardial infarct.[394] Antiaging interventions, such as SIRT1 overexpression, ameliorate aged mesenchymal stem cells senescent phenotypes and improve their regenerative efficacy in experimental myocardial infarcts.[395] Finally, an extrinsic hostile microenvironment and persistent adverse stimuli associated with advanced age may also impair regenerative capacity in aged hearts and warrants future investigation.

Role of the Microbiome

As already discussed, the alterations of the intestinal microbiome in aging promote a systemic proinflammatory state due to declining beneficial commensal microbes and the expansion of pathogenic microbes.[288] As the most reproducible antiaging intervention, calorie restriction has been shown to ameliorate microbiomes in aging, thereby decreasing inflammation and improving gut barrier integrity.[396] Some emerging evidence has shown that administration of probiotics and/or prebiotics[397] may reduce systemic inflammation and thus has potential to slow progression of cardiometabolic diseases, presumably due to the anti-inflammatory effect. However, more evidence is needed. In turn, this suggests that promoting a healthy intestinal tract flora may have beneficial effects on cardiometabolic health.[398] In addition to the direct effect on gut inflammation, healthy gut microbiome produce numerous metabolites, some of which are absorbed into the systemic circulation and are biologically active circulating factors, whereas others are metabolized by host enzymes to mediate the cardiovascular health benefit.[399,400] Gut microbiome interacts with the host through several pathways. One example is the trimethylamine (TMA)/trimethylamine N-oxide (TMAO) pathway.[401] TMAO is the hepatic oxidation product of the microbial metabolite TMA that has been shown to contribute to the progression of atherosclerosis and cardiometabolic diseases.[402,403] This remains an area in need of additional investigation.

EXACERBATION OF VASCULAR AGING PROCESSES BY CARDIOVASCULAR RISK FACTORS

From the perspective of geroscience, conventional risk factors promote cardiovascular and cerebrovascular pathologies by inducing "accelerated aging" phenotypes in the heart and vasculature (**Figs. 82–1A** to **82–1C**), which contribute to the interindividual variability in the rate of development and progression of age-related CVDs.[325] These dietary, social, environmental, and lifestyle factors can exacerbate one or more shared cellular and molecular aging processes in the cardiovascular system.[325] Accordingly, hypertension, consumption of a high-fat, high-calorie Western diet, obesity, diabetes mellitus, hypercholesterolemia, and hyperhomocysteinemia promote inflammation, endothelial apoptosis, increase oxidative/nitrosative stress, macromolecular damage and mitochondrial dysfunction, and/or promote cellular senescence in the heart and vasculature.[62,92,228,404–408] Smoking, vaping, environmental pollutants (eg, diesel exhaust particles, polycyclic aromatic hydrocarbons, and heavy metals), and other toxicants promote oxidative/nitrosative stress, mitochondrial dysfunction, inflammation, induce DNA damage, and/or promote cellular senescence in the heart and the vascular system.[232,404,409,410] A sedentary lifestyle and its metabolic (eg, insulin resistance) and hemodynamic consequences (eg, decreased wall shear stress) are associated with heightened inflammatory status, increased oxidative stress,[411,412] and increased vascular senescence.[317] Ionizing radiation (eg, radiation therapy of tumor patients) and genotoxic drugs (eg, chemotherapy) promote DNA damage and induce cellular senescence in proliferating cells, including endothelial cells and cardiac progenitor cells, contributing to the genesis of HF[413,414] and vascular cognitive impairment.[330,415–418]

Preventive measures are available to lower cardiovascular risk, presumably by reducing the impact of these factors on shared cellular and molecular mechanisms of aging. A healthy diet rich in fish, fruit, and vegetables, and low in dairy products and red meat, was shown to reduce inflammatory status[419] and attenuate oxidative stress, improving endothelial function[419] and lowering the incidence of CVD.[420–422] Pharmacological treatment of hypertension, diabetes mellitus, and normalization of lipid profiles also likely reduce oxidative stress and inflammation, improve endothelial function, and may decrease cellular senescence.[423–425] Physical exercise, reduction of calorie intake, and weight loss exert multifaceted cardiovascular protective effects, including attenuation of oxidative stress and rescue of NO production, attenuation of inflammation, prevention of cellular senescence, rescue of stem cell function, and mitochondrial protection.[317,412,426–428] Smoking cessation and reducing and managing environmental pollution decrease the impact of genotoxic stressors. It is expected that in the future, the aforementioned preventive measures will be combined with interventions that target shared mechanisms of aging, increasing the stress resilience of the heart and the vascular system, limiting the impact of cardiovascular risk factors (eg, by boosting endogenous cell survival pathways, including SIRT1[230] and Nrf2-regulated pathways[228]).

SUMMARY

Studies in the last two decades have established the paradigm of the plasticity of cardiovascular aging, showing that cardiac and vascular aging phenotypes can be slowed or reversed.[228,316,317,428]

The concept presented here (**Table 82–1, Figs. 82–1A to 82–1C**) implies that several interrelated cell-autonomous cellular and molecular aging processes, which are also modulated by circulating/systemic factors, contribute to the development of age-related cardiovascular and cerebrovascular diseases. We predict that effective future strategies for delaying cardiovascular aging and prevention of these diseases will use multimodal treatment paradigms, combining diet and exercise therapy with pharmacological interventions targeting diverse cellular aging processes simultaneously. It is likely that in the future, senolytic strategies[316] can be combined with interventions that prevent induction of cellular senescence (eg, ROS and peroxynitrite scavengers, Nrf2 activators[228]), confer anti-inflammatory effects mitigating the impact of the SASP factors,[428] rescue mitochondrial function,[429] activate AMPK[430] and sirtuin pathways,[230] inhibit mTOR,[431] and/or restore cellular NAD^+ levels.[111,214] As our population continues to age, substantial additional clinical research into the role of such antiaging treatment paradigms in CVD prevention in older adults is imperative.

REFERENCES

1. Ortman JM, Velkoff VA, Hogan H. *An aging nation: the older population in the United States, current population reports 2014.* Washington, DC: U.S. Census Bureau; 2014:25-1140.

2. Lakatta EG, Levy D. Arterial and cardiac aging: major shareholders in cardiovascular disease enterprises: part I: aging arteries: a "set up" for vascular disease. *Circulation.* 2003;107:139-146.

3. Virani SS, Alonso A, Benjamin EJ, et al. Heart disease and stroke statistics-2020 update: a report from the American Heart Association. *Circulation.* 2020;141:e139-e596.

4. National Center for Health Statistics. *Health, United States, 2016: with chartbook on long-term trends in health.* Hyattsville, MD: NCHS; 2017.

5. Heidenreich PA, Trogdon JG, Khavjou OA, et al. Forecasting the future of cardiovascular disease in the United States: a policy statement from the American Heart Association. *Circulation.* 2011;123:933-944.

6. Elveback L, Lie JT. Continued high incidence of coronary artery disease at autopsy in Olmsted county, Minnesota, 1950 to 1979. *Circulation.* 1984;70:345-349

7. Otto CM, Prendergast B. Aortic-valve stenosis–from patients at risk to severe valve obstruction. *N Engl J Med.* 2014;371:744-756.

8. D'Agostino RB, Sr., Vasan RS, Pencina MJ, et al. General cardiovascular risk profile for use in primary care: the Framingham Heart Study. *Circulation.* 2008;117:743-753.

9. Pencina MJ, D'Agostino RB, Sr., Larson MG, Massaro JM, Vasan RS. Predicting the 30-year risk of cardiovascular disease: the Framingham Heart Study. *Circulation.* 2009;119:3078-3084.

10. Ridker PM, Buring JE, Rifai N, Cook NR. Development and validation of improved algorithms for the assessment of global cardiovascular risk in women: the Reynolds risk score. *JAMA.* 2007;297:611-619.

11. Ridker PM, Paynter NP, Rifai N, Gaziano JM, Cook NR. C-reactive protein and parental history improve global cardiovascular risk prediction: the Reynolds risk score for men. *Circulation.* 2008;118:2243-2251, 2244p following 2251.

12. Lopez-Otin C, Blasco MA, Partridge L, Serrano M, Kroemer G. The hallmarks of aging. *Cell.* 2013;153:1194-1217.

13. Lakatta EG. Arterial and cardiac aging: major shareholders in cardiovascular disease enterprises: part III: cellular and molecular clues to heart and arterial aging. *Circulation.* 2003;107:490-497.

14. Lakatta EG, Levy D. Arterial and cardiac aging: major shareholders in cardiovascular disease enterprises: part II: the aging heart in health: links to heart disease. *Circulation.* 2003;107:346-354.

15. Gerstenblith G, Frederiksen J, Yin FC, Fortuin NJ, Lakatta EG, Weisfeldt ML. Echocardiographic assessment of a normal adult aging population. *Circulation.* 1977;56:273-278

16. Kitzman DW, Scholz DG, Hagen PT, Ilstrup DM, Edwards WD. Age-related changes in normal human hearts during the first 10 decades of life. Part II (maturity): a quantitative anatomic study of 765 specimens from subjects 20 to 99 years old. *Mayo Clin Proc.* 1988;63:137-146.

17. Treuting PM, Linford NJ, Knoblaugh SE, et al. Reduction of age-associated pathology in old mice by overexpression of catalase in mitochondria. *J Gerontol A Biol Sci Med Sci.* 2008;63:813-822.

18. Horn MA, Trafford AW. Aging and the cardiac collagen matrix: novel mediators of fibrotic remodelling. *J Mol Cell Cardiol.* 2016;93:175-185

19. Mohammed SF, Mirzoyev SA, Edwards WD, et al. Left ventricular amyloid deposition in patients with heart failure and preserved ejection fraction. *JACC Heart Fail.* 2014;2:113-122.

20. Westermark P, Johansson B, Natvig JB. Senile cardiac amyloidosis: evidence of two different amyloid substances in the ageing heart. *Scand J Immunol.* 1979;10:303-308.

21. Bursi F, Weston SA, Redfield MM, et al. Systolic and diastolic heart failure in the community. *JAMA.* 2006;296:2209-2216

22. Upadhya B, Kitzman DW. Heart failure with preserved ejection fraction in older adults. *Heart Fail Clin.* 2017;13:485-502.

23. Vella CA, Robergs RA. A review of the stroke volume response to upright exercise in healthy subjects. *Br J Sports Med.* 2005;39:190-195.

24. Lauer MS, Francis GS, Okin PM, Pashkow FJ, Snader CE, Marwick TH. Impaired chronotropic response to exercise stress testing as a predictor of mortality. *JAMA.* 1999;281:524-529.

25. Bhatheja R, Francis GS, Pothier CE, Lauer MS. Heart rate response during dipyridamole stress as a predictor of mortality in patients with normal myocardial perfusion and normal electrocardiograms. *Am J Cardiol.* 2005;95:1159-1164.

26. Stein PK, Barzilay JI, Chaves PH, et al. Novel measures of heart rate variability predict cardiovascular mortality in older adults independent of traditional cardiovascular risk factors: the cardiovascular health study (chs). *J Cardiovasc Electrophysiol.* 2008;19:1169-1174.

27. Esler MD, Turner AG, Kaye DM, et al. Aging effects on human sympathetic neuronal function. *Am J Physiol.* 1995;268:R278-R285.

28. Seals DR, Taylor JA, Ng AV, Esler MD. Exercise and aging: autonomic control of the circulation. *Med Sci Sports Exerc.* 1994;26:568-576.

29. Kusumoto FM, Goldschlager N. Cardiac pacing. *N Engl J Med.* 1996;334:89-97.

30. Jensen PN, Gronroos NN, Chen LY, et al. Incidence of and risk factors for sick sinus syndrome in the general population. *J Am Coll Cardiol.* 2014;64:531-538.

31. Jones SA, Boyett MR, Lancaster MK. Declining into failure: the age-dependent loss of the l-type calcium channel within the sinoatrial node. *Circulation.* 2007;115:1183-1190.

32. Kistler PM, Sanders P, Fynn SP, et al. Electrophysiologic and electroanatomic changes in the human atrium associated with age. *J Am Coll Cardiol.* 2004;44:109-116.

33. Fleg JL, Kennedy HL. Cardiac arrhythmias in a healthy elderly population: detection by 24-hour ambulatory electrocardiography. *Chest.* 1982;81:302-307.

34. Rosamond W, Flegal K, Friday G, et al. Heart disease and stroke statistics–2007 update: a report from the American Heart Association statistics committee and stroke statistics subcommittee. *Circulation.* 2007;115:e69-e171.

35. Wolf PA, Abbott RD, Kannel WB. Atrial fibrillation as an independent risk factor for stroke: the Framingham Study. *Stroke.* 1991;22:983-988.

36. Nassimiha D, Aronow WS, Ahn C, Goldman ME. Association of coronary risk factors with progression of valvular aortic stenosis in older persons. *Am J Cardiol.* 2001;87:1313-1314.

37. Karavidas A, Lazaros G, Tsiachris D, Pyrgakis V. Aging and the cardiovascular system. *Hellenic J Cardiol.* 2010;51:421-427.

38. Stewart BF, Siscovick D, Lind BK, et al. Clinical factors associated with calcific aortic valve disease. Cardiovascular health study. *J Am Coll Cardiol.* 1997;29:630-634.

39. Freeman RV, Otto CM. Spectrum of calcific aortic valve disease: pathogenesis, disease progression, and treatment strategies. *Circulation.* 2005;111:3316-3326.

40. Otto CM, Lind BK, Kitzman DW, Gersh BJ, Siscovick DS. Association of aortic-valve sclerosis with cardiovascular mortality and morbidity in the elderly. *N Engl J Med.* 1999;341:142-147.

41. Olsen MH, Wachtell K, Bella JN, et al. Aortic valve sclerosis relates to cardiovascular events in patients with hypertension (a life substudy). *Am J Cardiol.* 2005;95:132-136.

42. Fulkerson PK, Beaver BM, Auseon JC, Graber HL. Calcification of the mitral annulus: etiology, clinical associations, complications and therapy. *Am J Med.* 1979;66:967-977.

43. Jeon DS, Atar S, Brasch AV, et al. Association of mitral annulus calcification, aortic valve sclerosis and aortic root calcification with abnormal myocardial perfusion single photon emission tomography in subjects age < or =65 years old. *J Am Coll Cardiol.* 2001;38:1988-1993.

44. Faggiano P, Antonini-Canterin F, Erlicher A, et al. Progression of aortic valve sclerosis to aortic stenosis. *Am J Cardiol.* 2003;91:99-101.

45. Jebara VA, Dervanian P, Acar C, et al. Mitral valve repair using Carpentier techniques in patients more than 70 years old. Early and late results. *Circulation.* 1992;86:II53-II59.

46. Akins CW, Daggett WM, Vlahakes GJ, et al. Cardiac operations in patients 80 years old and older. *Ann Thorac Surg.* 1997;64:606-614; discussion 614-605.

47. Aronow WS, Fleg JL, Pepine CJ, et al. Accf/aha 2011 expert consensus document on hypertension in the elderly: a report of the American College of Cardiology Foundation Task Force on Clinical Expert Consensus Documents. *Circulation.* 2011;123:2434-2506.

48. Fleg JL, Strait J. Age-associated changes in cardiovascular structure and function: a fertile milieu for future disease. *Heart Fail Rev.* 2012;17:545-554.

49. Ungvari Z, Tarantini S, Kiss T, et al. Endothelial dysfunction and angiogenesis impairment in the ageing vasculature. *Nat Rev Cardiol.* 2018;15:555-565.

50. Tarnawski AS, Pai R, Tanigawa T, Matysiak-Budnik T, Ahluwalia A. Pten silencing reverses aging-related impairment of angiogenesis in microvascular endothelial cells. *Biochem Biophys Res Commun.* 2010;394:291-296.

51. Bach MH, Sadoun E, Reed MJ. Defects in activation of nitric oxide synthases occur during delayed angiogenesis in aging. *Mech Ageing Dev.* 2005;126:467-473.

52. Sadoun E, Reed MJ. Impaired angiogenesis in aging is associated with alterations in vessel density, matrix composition, inflammatory response, and growth factor expression. *J Histochem Cytochem.* 2003;51:1119-1130.

53. Ungvari Z, Kaley G, de Cabo R, Sonntag WE, Csiszar A. Mechanisms of vascular aging: new perspectives. *J Gerontol A Biol Sci Med Sci.* 2010;65:1028-1041.

54. Ahluwalia A, Tarnawski AS. Activation of the metabolic sensor—amp activated protein kinase reverses impairment of angiogenesis in aging myocardial microvascular endothelial cells. Implications for the aging heart. *J Physiol Pharmacol.* 2011;62:583-587.

55. Lahteenvuo J, Rosenzweig A. Effects of aging on angiogenesis. *Circ Res.* 2012;110:1252-1264.

56. Franssen C, Chen S, Unger A, et al. Myocardial microvascular inflammatory endothelial activation in heart failure with preserved ejection fraction. *JACC Heart Fail.* 2016;4:312-324.

57. Sweeney MD, Sagare AP, Zlokovic BV. Blood-brain barrier breakdown in Alzheimer disease and other neurodegenerative disorders. *Nat Rev Neurol.* 2018;14:133-150.

58. Montagne A, Barnes SR, Sweeney MD, et al. Blood-brain barrier breakdown in the aging human hippocampus. *Neuron.* 2015;85:296-302.

59. Correia LC, Lakatta EG, O'Connor FC, et al. Attenuated cardiovascular reserve during prolonged submaximal cycle exercise in healthy older subjects. *J Am Coll Cardiol.* 2002;40:1290-1297.

60. Rich MW. Heart failure in the 21st century: a cardiogeriatric syndrome. *J Gerontol A Biol Sci Med Sci.* 2001;56:M88-M96.

61. Alfaras I, Di Germanio C, Bernier M, et al. Pharmacological strategies to retard cardiovascular aging. *Circ Res.* 2016;118:1626-1642.

62. Ungvari Z, Tarantini S, Donato AJ, Galvan V, Csiszar A. Mechanisms of vascular aging. *Circ Res.* 2018;123:849-867.

63. Harman D. Aging: a theory based on free radical and radiation chemistry. *J Gerontol.* 1956:298-300.

64. Csiszar A, Ungvari Z, Edwards JG, et al. Aging-induced phenotypic changes and oxidative stress impair coronary arteriolar function. *Circ Res.* 2002;90:1159-1166.

65. van der Loo B, Labugger R, Skepper JN, et al. Enhanced peroxynitrite formation is associated with vascular aging. *J Exp Med.* 2000;192:1731-1744.

66. Donato AJ, Eskurza I, Silver AE, et al. Direct evidence of endothelial oxidative stress with aging in humans: relation to impaired endothelium-dependent dilation and upregulation of nuclear factor-kappaB. *Circulation research.* 2007;100:1659-1666.

67. Jacobson A, Yan C, Gao Q, et al. Aging enhances pressure-induced arterial superoxide formation. *Am J Physiol Heart Circ Physiol.* 2007;293:H1344-H1350.

68. Fan LM, Geng L, Cahill-Smith S, et al. Nox2 contributes to age-related oxidative damage to neurons and the cerebral vasculature. *J Clin Invest.* 2019;129:3374-3386.

69. Tarantini S, Valcarcel-Ares NM, Yabluchanskiy A, et al. Treatment with the mitochondrial-targeted antioxidant peptide ss-31 rescues neurovascular coupling responses and cerebrovascular endothelial function and improves cognition in aged mice. *Aging Cell.* 2018;17.

70. Vendrov AE, Vendrov KC, Smith A, et al. Nox4 nadph oxidase-dependent mitochondrial oxidative stress in aging-associated cardiovascular disease. *Antioxid Redox Signal.* 2015;23:1389-1409.

71. Csiszar A, Sosnowska D, Wang M, Lakatta EG, Sonntag WE, Ungvari Z. Age-associated proinflammatory secretory phenotype in vascular smooth muscle cells from the non-human primate macaca mulatta: reversal by resveratrol treatment. *J Gerontol A Biol Sci Med Sci.* 2012;67:811-820.

72. Canugovi C, Stevenson MD, Vendrov AE, et al. Increased mitochondrial nadph oxidase 4 (nox4) expression in aging is a causative factor in aortic stiffening. *Redox Biol.* 2019;26:101288.

73. Zhou RH, Vendrov AE, Tchivilev I, et al. Mitochondrial oxidative stress in aortic stiffening with age: the role of smooth muscle cell function. *Arterioscler Thromb Vasc Biol.* 2012;32:745-755.

74. Gioscia-Ryan RA, LaRocca TJ, Sindler AL, Zigler MC, Murphy MP, Seals DR. Mitochondria-targeted antioxidant (mitoq) ameliorates age-related arterial endothelial dysfunction in mice. *J Physiol.* 2014;592:2549-2561.

75. Sun D, Huang A, Yan EH, et al. Reduced release of nitric oxide to shear stress in mesenteric arteries of aged rats. *Am J Physiol Heart Circ Physiol.* 2004;286:H2249-H2256.

76. Hamilton CA, Brosnan MJ, McIntyre M, Graham D, Dominiczak AF. Superoxide excess in hypertension and aging: a common cause of endothelial dysfunction. *Hypertension.* 2001;37:529-534.

77. Francia P, delli Gatti C, Bachschmid M, et al. Deletion of p66shc gene protects against age-related endothelial dysfunction. *Circulation.* 2004;110:2889-2895.

78. Csiszar A, Labinskyy N, Orosz Z, et al. Vascular aging in the longest-living rodent, the naked mole-rat. *Am J Physiol.* 2007;293:H919-H927.

79. Ungvari ZI, Orosz Z, Labinskyy N, et al. Increased mitochondrial h2o2 production promotes endothelial nf-kb activation in aged rat arteries. *Am J Physiol Heart Circ Physiol.* 2007;293:H37-H47.

80. Jablonski KL, Seals DR, Eskurza I, Monahan KD, Donato AJ. High-dose ascorbic acid infusion abolishes chronic vasoconstriction and restores resting leg blood flow in healthy older men. *J Appl Physiol.* 2007;103:1715-1721.

81. Fleenor BS, Seals DR, Zigler ML, Sindler AL. Superoxide-lowering therapy with tempol reverses arterial dysfunction with aging in mice. *Aging Cell.* 2012;11:269-276.

82. Adler A, Messina E, Sherman B, et al. Nad(p)h oxidase-generated superoxide anion accounts for reduced control of myocardial o2 consumption by no in old Fischer 344 rats. *Am J Physiol Heart Circ Physiol.* 2003;285:H1015-H1022.

83. Ago T, Matsushima S, Kuroda J, Zablocki D, Kitazono T, Sadoshima J. The nadph oxidase nox4 and aging in the heart. *Aging (Albany NY).* 2010;2:1012-1016.

84. Rueckschloss U, Villmow M, Klockner U. Nadph oxidase-derived superoxide impairs calcium transients and contraction in aged murine ventricular myocytes. *Exp Gerontol.* 2010;45:788-796.

85. Wang M, Zhang J, Walker SJ, Dworakowski R, Lakatta EG, Shah AM. Involvement of nadph oxidase in age-associated cardiac remodeling. *J Mol Cell Cardiol.* 2010;48:765-772.

86. Springo Z, Tarantini S, Toth P, et al. Aging exacerbates pressure-induced mitochondrial oxidative stress in mouse cerebral arteries. *J Gerontol A Biol Sci Med Sci.* 2015;70:1355-1359.

87. Toth P, Tarantini S, Springo Z, et al. Aging exacerbates hypertension-induced cerebral microhemorrhages in mice: role of resveratrol treatment in vasoprotection. *Aging Cell.* 2015;14:400-408.

88. Ungvari Z, Bailey-Downs L, Sosnowska D, et al. Vascular oxidative stress in aging: A homeostatic failure due to dysregulation of nrf2-mediated antioxidant response *Am J Physiol Heart Circ Physiol.* 2011;301:H363-H372.

89. Silva-Palacios A, Konigsberg M, Zazueta C. Nrf2 signaling and redox homeostasis in the aging heart: a potential target to prevent cardiovascular diseases? *Ageing Res Rev.* 2016;26:81-95.

90. Ungvari Z, Bailey-Downs L, Gautam T, et al. Age-associated vascular oxidative stress, nrf2 dysfunction and nf-kb activation in the non-human primate macaca mulatta *J Gerontol A Biol Sci Med Sci.* 2011;66:866-875.

91. Fulop GA, Kiss T, Tarantini S, et al. Nrf2 deficiency in aged mice exacerbates cellular senescence promoting cerebrovascular inflammation. *Geroscience.* 2018;40:513-521.

92. Tarantini S, Valcarcel-Ares MN, Yabluchanskiy A, et al. Nrf2 deficiency exacerbates obesity-induced oxidative stress, neurovascular dysfunction, blood brain barrier disruption, neuroinflammation, amyloidogenic gene expression and cognitive decline in mice, mimicking the aging phenotype. *J Gerontol A Biol Sci Med Sci.* 2018;73(7):853-863.

93. Toth P, Tarantini S, Tucsek Z, et al. Resveratrol treatment rescues neurovascular coupling in aged mice: role of improved cerebromicrovascular endothelial function and down-regulation of nadph oxidas. *Am J Physiol Heart Circ Physiol.* 2014;306:H299-H308.

94. Park L, Anrather J, Girouard H, Zhou P, Iadecola C. Nox2-derived reactive oxygen species mediate neurovascular dysregulation in the aging mouse brain. *J Cereb Blood Flow Metab.* 2007;27:1908-1918.

95. Cernadas MR, Sanchez de Miguel L, Garcia-Duran M, et al. Expression of constitutive and inducible nitric oxide synthases in the vascular wall of young and aging rats. *Circ Res.* 1998;83:279-286.

96. Chou TC, Yen MH, Li CY, Ding YA. Alterations of nitric oxide synthase expression with aging and hypertension in rats. *Hypertension.* 1998;31:643-648.

97. Csiszar A, Labinskyy N, Smith K, Rivera A, Orosz Z, Ungvari Z. Vasculoprotective effects of anti-tumor necrosis factor-alpha treatment in aging. *Am J Pathol.* 2007;170:388-398.

98. Ganz P, Vita JA. Testing endothelial vasomotor function: nitric oxide, a multipotent molecule. *Circulation.* 2003;108:2049-2053.

99. Moncada S, Higgs A. The l-arginine-nitric oxide pathway. *N Engl J Med.* 1993;329:2002-2012.

100. Moncada S, Palmer RM, Higgs EA. Nitric oxide: physiology, pathophysiology, and pharmacology. *Pharmacol Rev.* 1991;43:109-142.

101. Pacher P, Beckman JS, Liaudet L. Nitric oxide and peroxynitrite in health and disease. *Physiological Rev.* 2007;87:315-424.

102. Csiszar A, Podlutsky A, Wolin MS, Losonczy G, Pacher P, Ungvari Z. Oxidative stress and accelerated vascular aging: implications for cigarette smoking. *Front Biosci.* 2009;14:3128-3144.

103. Kanski J, Behring A, Pelling J, Schoneich C. Proteomic identification of 3-nitrotyrosine-containing rat cardiac proteins: effect of biological aging. *Am J Physiol Heart Circ Physiol.* 2004.

104. Radovits T, Seres L, Gero D, et al. The peroxynitrite decomposition catalyst fp15 improves ageing-associated cardiac and vascular dysfunction. *Mech Ageing Dev.* 2007;128:173-181.

105. Csiszar A, Tarantini S, Yabluchanskiy A, et al. Role of endothelial NAD+ deficiency in age-related vascular dysfunction. *Am J Physiol Heart Circ Physiol.* 2019;316(6):H1253-H1266.

106. Braidy N, Guillemin GJ, Mansour H, Chan-Ling T, Poljak A, Grant R. Age related changes in NAD+ metabolism oxidative stress and SIRT1 activity in wistar rats. *PLoS One.* 2011;6:e19194.

107. Jagtap P, Szabo C. Poly(adp-ribose) polymerase and the therapeutic effects of its inhibitors. *Nat Rev Drug Discov.* 2005;4:421-440.

108. Massudi H, Grant R, Braidy N, Guest J, Farnsworth B, Guillemin GJ. Age-associated changes in oxidative stress and NAD+ metabolism in human tissue. *PLoS One.* 2012;7:e42357.

109. Pacher P, Mabley JG, Soriano FG, Liaudet L, Szabo C. Activation of poly(adp-ribose) polymerase contributes to the endothelial dysfunction associated with hypertension and aging. *Int J Mol Med.* 2002;9:659-664.

110. Pacher P, Vaslin A, Benko R, et al. A new, potent poly(adp-ribose) polymerase inhibitor improves cardiac and vascular dysfunction associated with advanced aging. *J Pharmacol Exp Ther.* 2004;311:485-491.

111. Pacher P, Mabley JG, Soriano FG, et al. Endothelial dysfunction in aging animals: the role of poly(adp-ribose) polymerase activation. *Br J Pharmacol.* 2002;135:1347-1350.

112. Radovits T, Seres L, Gero D, et al. Single dose treatment with parp-inhibitor ino-1001 improves aging-associated cardiac and vascular dysfunction. *Exp Gerontol.* 2007;42:676-685.

113. Tarantini S, Yabluchanskiy A, Csipo T, et al. Treatment with the poly(adp-ribose) polymerase inhibitor pj-34 improves cerebromicrovascular endothelial function, neurovascular coupling responses and cognitive performance in aged mice, supporting the NAD+ depletion hypothesis of neurovascular aging. *Geroscience.* 2019;41:533-542.

114. Soriano FG, Pacher P, Mabley J, Liaudet L, Szabo C. Rapid reversal of the diabetic endothelial dysfunction by pharmacological inhibition of poly(adp-ribose) polymerase. *Circ Res.* 2001;89:684-691.

115. Szabo C, Zanchi A, Komjati K, et al. Poly(adp-ribose) polymerase is activated in subjects at risk of developing type 2 diabetes and is associated with impaired vascular reactivity. *Circulation.* 2002;106:2680-2686.

116. Asano S, Rice KM, Kakarla S, et al. Aging influences multiple indices of oxidative stress in the heart of the Fischer 344/nnia x brown Norway/binia rat. *Redox Rep.* 2007;12:167-180.

117. Zarkovic K, Larroque-Cardoso P, Pucelle M, et al. Elastin aging and lipid oxidation products in human aorta. *Redox Biol.* 2015;4:109-117.

118. Miura Y, Tsumoto H, Iwamoto M, et al. Age-associated proteomic alterations in human aortic media. *Geriatr Gerontol Int.* 2019;19:1054-1062.

119. Kwak HB, Lee Y, Kim JH, et al. Mnsod overexpression reduces fibrosis and pro-apoptotic signaling in the aging mouse heart. *J Gerontol A Biol Sci Med Sci.* 2015;70:533-544.

120. Zhang H, Forman HJ. 4-hydroxynonenal-mediated signaling and aging. *Free Radic Biol Med.* 2017;111:219-225.

121. Mohamed SA, Hanke T, Erasmi AW, et al. Mitochondrial DNA deletions and the aging heart. *Exp Gerontol.* 2006;41:508-517.

122. Corral-Debrinski M, Shoffner JM, Lott MT, Wallace DC. Association of mitochondrial DNA damage with aging and coronary atherosclerotic heart disease. *Mutat Res.* 1992;275:169-180.

123. Muscari C, Giaccari A, Stefanelli C, et al. Presence of a DNA-4236 bp deletion and 8-hydroxy-deoxyguanosine in mouse cardiac mitochondrial DNA during aging. *Aging (Milano).* 1996;8:429-433.

124. Herrero A, Barja G. Effect of aging on mitochondrial and nuclear DNA oxidative damage in the heart and brain throughout the life-span of the rat. *J Am Aging Assoc.* 2001;24:45-50.

125. Helenius M, Hanninen M, Lehtinen SK, Salminen A. Aging-induced up-regulation of nuclear binding activities of oxidative stress responsive nf-kb transcription factor in mouse cardiac muscle. *J Mol Cell Cardiol.* 1996;28:487-498.

126. Castello L, Froio T, Maina M, et al. Alternate-day fasting protects the rat heart against age-induced inflammation and fibrosis by inhibiting oxidative damage and nf-kb activation. *Free Radic Biol Med.* 2010;48:47-54.

127. Csiszar A, Wang M, Lakatta EG, Ungvari ZI. Inflammation and endothelial dysfunction during aging: role of nf-{kappa}b. *J Appl Physiol.* 2008;105:1333-1341.

128. Csiszar A, Gautam T, Sosnowska D, et al. Caloric restriction confers persistent anti-oxidative, pro-angiogenic, and anti-inflammatory effects and promotes anti-aging miRNA expression profile in cerebromicrovascular endothelial cells of aged rats. *Am J Physiol Heart Circ Physiol.* 2014;307:H292-H306.

129. Csiszar A, Labinskyy N, Jimenez R, et al. Anti-oxidative and anti-inflammatory vasoprotective effects of caloric restriction in aging: role of circulating factors and SIRT1. *Mech Ageing Dev.* 2009;130:518-527.

130. Moreau KL, Gavin KM, Plum AE, Seals DR. Ascorbic acid selectively improves large elastic artery compliance in postmenopausal women. *Hypertension* %R 10.1161/01.HYP.0000165678.63373.8c. 2005;45:1107-1112.

131. Meschiari CA, Ero OK, Pan H, Finkel T, Lindsey ML. The impact of aging on cardiac extracellular matrix. *Geroscience.* 2017;39:7-18.

132. Wang M, Takagi G, Asai K, et al. Aging increases aortic mmp-2 activity and angiotensin ii in nonhuman primates. *Hypertension.* 2003;41:1308-1316.

133. McNulty M, Spiers P, McGovern E, Feely J. Aging is associated with increased matrix metalloproteinase-2 activity in the human aorta. *Am J Hypertens.* 2005;18:504-509.

134. Kaneko H, Anzai T, Morisawa M, et al. Resveratrol prevents the development of abdominal aortic aneurysm through attenuation of inflammation, oxidative stress, and neovascularization. *Atherosclerosis.* 2011;217:350-357.

135. Liu Y, Wang TT, Zhang R, et al. Calorie restriction protects against experimental abdominal aortic aneurysms in mice. *J Exp Med.* 2016;213:2473-2488.

136. Ungvari Z, Tarantini S, Kirkpatrick AC, Csiszar A, Prodan CI. Cerebral microhemorrhages: mechanisms, consequences, and prevention. *Am J Physiol Heart Circ Physiol.* 2017;312:H1128-H1143.

137. Fleenor BS, Eng JS, Sindler AL, Pham BT, Kloor JD, Seals DR. Superoxide signaling in perivascular adipose tissue promotes age-related artery stiffness. *Aging Cell.* 2014;13:576-578.

138. Rimm EB, Stampfer MJ, Ascherio A, Giovannucci E, Colditz GA, Willett WC. Vitamin e consumption and the risk of coronary heart disease in men. *N Engl J Med.* 1993;328:1450-1456.

139. Simon JA, Hudes ES. Serum ascorbic acid and cardiovascular disease prevalence in u.S. Adults: The third national health and nutrition examination survey (nhanes iii). *Ann Epidemiol.* 1999;9:358-365.

140. Nyyssonen K, Parviainen MT, Salonen R, Tuomilehto J, Salonen JT. Vitamin c deficiency and risk of myocardial infarction: prospective population study of men from eastern Finland. *BMJ.* 1997;314:634-638.

141. Klipstein-Grobusch K, den Breeijen JH, Grobbee DE, Boeing H, Hofman A, Witteman JC. Dietary antioxidants and peripheral arterial disease: the Rotterdam study. *Am J Epidemiol.* 2001;154:145-149.

142. Kritchevsky SB, Shimakawa T, Tell GS, et al. Dietary antioxidants and carotid artery wall thickness. The Aric study. Atherosclerosis risk in communities study. *Circulation.* 1995;92:2142-2150.

143. Myung SK, Ju W, Cho B, et al. Efficacy of vitamin and antioxidant supplements in prevention of cardiovascular disease: Systematic review and meta-analysis of randomised controlled trials. *BMJ.* 2013;346:f10.

144. Leopold JA. Antioxidants and coronary artery disease: from pathophysiology to preventive therapy. *Coron Artery Dis.* 2015;26:176-183.

145. Rees K, Takeda A, Martin N, et al. Mediterranean-style diet for the primary and secondary prevention of cardiovascular disease. *Cochrane Database Syst Rev.* 2019;3:CD009825.

146. Estruch R, Ros E, Salas-Salvado J, et al. Primary prevention of cardiovascular disease with a Mediterranean diet supplemented with extra-virgin olive oil or nuts. *N Engl J Med.* 2018;378:e34.

147. Fito M, Guxens M, Corella D, et al. Effect of a traditional mediterranean diet on lipoprotein oxidation: a randomized controlled trial. *Arch Intern Med.* 2007;167:1195-1203.

148. Navarro A, Boveris A. The mitochondrial energy transduction system and the aging process. *Am J Physiol Cell Physiol.* 2007;292:C670-C686.

149. Dai DF, Santana LF, Vermulst M, et al. Overexpression of catalase targeted to mitochondria attenuates murine cardiac aging. *Circulation.* 2009;119:2789-2797.

150. Dai DF, Chen T, Wanagat J, et al. Age-dependent cardiomyopathy in mitochondrial mutator mice is attenuated by overexpression of catalase targeted to mitochondria. *Aging Cell.* 2010;9:536-544.

151. Dai DF, Chen T, Johnson SC, Szeto H, Rabinovitch PS. Cardiac aging: from molecular mechanisms to significance in human health and disease. *Antioxid Redox Signal.* 2012;16:1492-1526.

152. Dai DF, Rabinovitch PS, Ungvari Z. Mitochondria and cardiovascular aging. *Circ Res.* 2012;110:1109-1124.

153. Trifunovic A, Wredenberg A, Falkenberg M, et al. Premature ageing in mice expressing defective mitochondrial DNA polymerase. *Nature.* 2004;429:417-423.

154. Kujoth GC, Hiona A, Pugh TD, et al. Mitochondrial DNA mutations, oxidative stress, and apoptosis in mammalian aging. *Science.* 2005;309:481-484.

155. Safdar A, Bourgeois JM, Ogborn DI, et al. Endurance exercise rescues progeroid aging and induces systemic mitochondrial rejuvenation in mtDNA mutator mice. *Proc Natl Acad Sci U S A.* 2011.

156. Corral-Debrinski M, Stepien G, Shoffner JM, et al. Hypoxemia is associated with mitochondrial DNA damage and gene induction. Implications for cardiac disease. *JAMA.* 1991;266:1812-1816.

157. Zhang C, Bills M, Quigley A, et al. Varied prevalence of age-associated mitochondrial DNA deletions in different species and tissues: a comparison between human and rat. *Biochem Biophys Res Commun.* 1997;230: 630-635.

158. Bereiter-Hahn J, Voth M. Dynamics of mitochondria in living cells: shape changes, dislocations, fusion, and fission of mitochondria. *Microsc Res Tech.* 1994;27:198-219.

159. Hom J, Sheu SS. Morphological dynamics of mitochondria—a special emphasis on cardiac muscle cells. *J Mol Cell Cardiol.* 2009;46:811-820.

160. Ong SB, Hausenloy DJ. Mitochondrial morphology and cardiovascular disease. *Cardiovasc Res.* 2010;88:16-29.

161. Matsuda N, Sato S, Shiba K, et al. Pink1 stabilized by mitochondrial depolarization recruits Parkin to damaged mitochondria and activates latent Parkin for mitophagy. *J Cell Biol.* 2010;189:211-221.

162. Chen H, Chomyn A, Chan DC. Disruption of fusion results in mitochondrial heterogeneity and dysfunction. *J Biol Chem.* 2005;280:26185-26192.

163. Szabadkai G, Simoni AM, Chami M, Wieckowski MR, Youle RJ, Rizzuto R. Drp-1-dependent division of the mitochondrial network blocks intraorganellar Ca2+ waves and protects against Ca2+-mediated apoptosis. *Mol Cell.* 2004;16:59-68.

164. Westermann B. Mitochondrial fusion and fission in cell life and death. *Nat Rev Mol Cell Biol.* 2010;11:872-884.

165. Bossy-Wetzel E, Barsoum MJ, Godzik A, Schwarzenbacher R, Lipton SA. Mitochondrial fission in apoptosis, neurodegeneration and aging. *Curr Opin Cell Biol.* 2003;15:706-716.

166. Papanicolaou KN, Khairallah RJ, Ngoh GA, et al. Mitofusin-2 maintains mitochondrial structure and contributes to stress-induced permeability transition in cardiac myocytes. *Mol Cell Biol.* 2011;31:1309-1328.

167. Piquereau J, Caffin F, Novotova M, et al. Down-regulation of opa1 alters mouse mitochondrial morphology, ptp function, and cardiac adaptation to pressure overload. *Cardiovasc Res.* 2012;94:408-417.

168. Chen Y, Liu Y, Dorn GW, 2nd. Mitochondrial fusion is essential for organelle function and cardiac homeostasis. *Circ Res.* 2011;109:1327-1331.

169. Fang L, Moore XL, Gao XM, Dart AM, Lim YL, Du XJ. Down-regulation of mitofusin-2 expression in cardiac hypertrophy in vitro and in vivo. *Life Sci.* 2007;80:2154-2160.

170. Chen Y, Dorn GW, 2nd. Pink1-phosphorylated mitofusin 2 is a Parkin receptor for culling damaged mitochondria. *Science.* 2013;340:471-475.

171. Lazarou M, Sliter DA, Kane LA, et al. The ubiquitin kinase pink1 recruits autophagy receptors to induce mitophagy. *Nature.* 2015;524:309-314.

172. Kubli DA, Quinsay MN, Gustafsson AB. Parkin deficiency results in accumulation of abnormal mitochondria in aging myocytes. *Commun Integr Biol.* 2013;6:e24511.

173. Kubli DA, Zhang X, Lee Y, et al. Parkin protein deficiency exacerbates cardiac injury and reduces survival following myocardial infarction. *J Biol Chem.* 2013;288:915-926.

174. Leon LJ, Gustafsson AB. Staying young at heart: autophagy and adaptation to cardiac aging. *J Mol Cell Cardiol.* 2016;95:78-85.

175. Ventura-Clapier R, Garnier A, Veksler V. Transcriptional control of mitochondrial biogenesis: the central role of pgc-1alpha. *Cardiovasc Res.* 2008;79:208-217.

176. Goffart S, von Kleist-Retzow J-C, Wiesner RJ. Regulation of mitochondrial proliferation in the heart: power-plant failure contributes to cardiac failure in hypertrophy. *Cardiovasc Res.* 2004;64:198-207.

177. Murray AJ, Anderson RE, Watson GC, Radda GK, Clarke K. Uncoupling proteins in human heart. *Lancet.* 2004;364:1786-1788.

178. Dai DF, Johnson SC, Villarin JJ, et al. Mitochondrial oxidative stress mediates angiotensin ii-induced cardiac hypertrophy and g{alpha}q overexpression-induced heart failure. *Circ Res.* 2011;108:837-846.

179. Csiszar A, Yabluchanskiy A, Ungvari A, Ungvari Z, Tarantini S. Overexpression of catalase targeted to mitochondria improves neurovascular coupling responses in aged mice. *Geroscience.* 2019;41:609-617.

180. Dai DF, Johnson SC, Villarin JJ, et al. Mitochondrial oxidative stress mediates angiotensin ii-induced cardiac hypertrophy and g{alpha}q overexpression-induced heart failure. *Circ Res.* 2011.

181. Dai DF, Hsieh EJ, Liu Y, Chen T, et al. Mitochondrial proteome remodelling in pressure overload-induced heart failure: the role of mitochondrial oxidative stress. *Cardiovasc Res.* 2012;93:79-88.

182. Murphy MP, Smith RA. Targeting antioxidants to mitochondria by conjugation to lipophilic cations. *Annu Rev Pharmacol Toxicol.* 2007;47:629-656.

183. Smith RA, Hartley RC, Cocheme HM, Murphy MP. Mitochondrial pharmacology. *Trends Pharmacol Sci.* 2012;33:341-352.

184. Graham D, Huynh NN, Hamilton CA, et al. Mitochondria-targeted antioxidant mitoq10 improves endothelial function and attenuates cardiac hypertrophy. *Hypertension.* 2009;54:322-328.

185. Dikalova AE, Bikineyeva AT, Budzyn K, et al. Therapeutic targeting of mitochondrial superoxide in hypertension. *Circ Res.* 2010;107:106-116.

186. Magwere T, West M, Riyahi K, Murphy MP, Smith RA, Partridge L. The effects of exogenous antioxidants on lifespan and oxidative stress resistance in drosophila melanogaster. *Mech Ageing Dev.* 2006;127:356-370.

187. Manczak M, Mao P, Calkins MJ, et al. Mitochondria-targeted antioxidants protect against amyloid-beta toxicity in Alzheimer's disease neurons. *J Alzheimers Dis.* 2010;20 (Suppl 2):S609-631.

188. Ghosh A, Chandran K, Kalivendi SV, et al. Neuroprotection by a mitochondria-targeted drug in a Parkinson's disease model. *Free Radic Biol Med.* 2010;49:1674-1684.

189. Skulachev VP, Anisimov VN, Antonenko YN, et al. An attempt to prevent senescence: a mitochondrial approach. *Biochim Biophys Acta.* 2009;1787:437-461.

190. Skulachev VP. Cationic antioxidants as a powerful tool against mitochondrial oxidative stress. *Biochem Biophys Res Commun.* 2013;441:275-279.

191. Szeto HH. First-in-class cardiolipin-protective compound as a therapeutic agent to restore mitochondrial bioenergetics. *Br J Pharmacol.* 2014;171:2029-2050.

192. Zhang M, Mileykovskaya E, Dowhan W. Gluing the respiratory chain together. Cardiolipin is required for supercomplex formation in the inner mitochondrial membrane. *J Biol Chem.* 2002;277:43553-43556.

193. Pfeiffer K, Gohil V, Stuart RA, et al. Cardiolipin stabilizes respiratory chain supercomplexes. *J Biol Chem.* 2003;278:52873-52880.

194. Birk AV, Chao WM, Bracken C, Warren JD, Szeto HH. Targeting mitochondrial cardiolipin and the cytochrome c/cardiolipin complex to promote electron transport and optimize mitochondrial atp synthesis. *Br J Pharmacol.* 2014;171:2017-2028.

195. Dai W, Shi J, Gupta RC, Sabbah HN, Hale SL, Kloner RA. Bendavia, a mitochondria-targeting peptide, improves post-infarction cardiac function, prevents adverse left ventricular remodeling and restores mitochondria-related gene expression in rats. *J Cardiovasc Pharmacol.* 2014.

196. Dai DF, Chen T, Szeto H, et al. Mitochondrial targeted antioxidant peptide ameliorates hypertensive cardiomyopathy. *J Am Coll Cardiol.* 2011;58:73-82.

197. Dai DF, Hsieh EJ, Chen T, et al. Global proteomics and pathway analysis of pressure-overload-induced heart failure and its attenuation by mitochondrial-targeted peptides. *Circ Heart Fail.* 2013;6:1067-1076.

198. Whitson JA, Bitto A, Zhang H, et al. Ss-31 and nmn: two paths to improve metabolism and function in aged hearts. *Aging Cell.* 2020:e13213.

199. Gibson CM, Giugliano RP, Kloner RA, et al. Embrace stemi study: a phase 2a trial to evaluate the safety, tolerability, and efficacy of intravenous mtp-131 on reperfusion injury in patients undergoing primary percutaneous coronary intervention. *Eur Heart J.* 2016;37:1296-1303.

200. Daaboul Y, Korjian S, Weaver WD, et al. Relation of left ventricular mass and infarct size in anterior wall ST-segment elevation acute myocardial infarction (from the embrace stemi clinical trial). *Am J Cardiol.* 2016;118:625-631.

201. Daubert MA, Yow E, Dunn G, et al. Novel mitochondria-targeting peptide in heart failure treatment: a randomized, placebo-controlled trial of elamipretide. *Circ Heart Fail.* 2017;10.

202. Chatfield KC, Sparagna GC, Chau S, et al. Elamipretide improves mitochondrial function in the failing human heart. *JACC Basic Transl Sci.* 2019;4:147-157.

203. Gomes AP, Price NL, Ling AJ, et al. Declining NAD(+) induces a pseudohypoxic state disrupting nuclear-mitochondrial communication during aging. *Cell.* 2013;155:1624-1638.

204. Yoshino J, Baur JA, Imai SI. NAD(+) intermediates: the biology and therapeutic potential of NMN and NR. *Cell Metab.* 2018;27:513-528.

205. Zhang G, Teggatz EG, Zhang AY, et al. Cyclic adp ribose-mediated Ca2+ signaling in mediating endothelial nitric oxide production in bovine coronary arteries. *Am J Physiol Heart Circ Physiol.* 2006;290:H1172-H1181.

206. Schultz MB, Sinclair DA. Why NAD(+) declines during aging: it's destroyed. *Cell Metab.* 2016;23:965-966.

207. Tarantini S, Yabluchanskiy A, Csipo T, et al. Treatment with the poly(ADP-ribose) polymerase inhibitor PJ-34 improves cerebromicrovascular endothelial function, neurovascular coupling responses and cognitive performance in aged mice, supporting the NAD+ depletion hypothesis of neurovascular aging. *Geroscience.* 2019.

208. Canto C, Houtkooper RH, Pirinen E, et al. The NAD(+) precursor nicotinamide riboside enhances oxidative metabolism and protects against high-fat diet-induced obesity. *Cell Metab.* 2012;15:838-847.

209. Gariani K, Menzies KJ, Ryu D, et al. Eliciting the mitochondrial unfolded protein response by nicotinamide adenine dinucleotide repletion reverses fatty liver disease in mice. *Hepatology.* 2016;63:1190-1204.

210. Blundell G, Jones BG, Rose FA, Tudball N. Homocysteine mediated endothelial cell toxicity and its amelioration. *Atherosclerosis.* 1996;122:163-172.

211. Soriano FG, Virag L, Szabo C. Diabetic endothelial dysfunction: role of reactive oxygen and nitrogen species production and poly(ADP-ribose) polymerase activation. *J Mol Med (Berl).* 2001;79:437-448.

212. Zhang H, Ryu D, Wu Y, et al. NAD(+) repletion improves mitochondrial and stem cell function and enhances life span in mice. *Science.* 2016;352:1436-1443.

213. Mills KF, Yoshida S, Stein LR, et al. Long-term administration of nicotinamide mononucleotide mitigates age-associated physiological decline in mice. *Cell Metab.* 2016;24:795-806.

214. Tarantini S, Valcarcel-Ares MN, Toth P, et al. Nicotinamide mononucleotide (nmn) supplementation rescues cerebromicrovascular endothelial function and neurovascular coupling responses and improves cognitive function in aged mice. *Redox Biol.* 2019;24:101192.

215. Das A, Huang GX, Bonkowski MS, et al. Impairment of an endothelial NAD(+)-h2s signaling network is a reversible cause of vascular aging. *Cell.* 2018;173:74-89;e20.

216. de Picciotto NE, Gano LB, Johnson LC, et al. Nicotinamide mononucleotide supplementation reverses vascular dysfunction and oxidative stress with aging in mice. *Aging Cell.* 2016;15:522-530.

217. Borradaile NM, Pickering JG. Nicotinamide phosphoribosyltransferase imparts human endothelial cells with extended replicative lifespan and enhanced angiogenic capacity in a high glucose environment. *Aging Cell.* 2009;8:100-112.

218. Kiss T, Balasubramanian P, Valcarcel-Ares MN, et al. Nicotinamide mononucleotide (NMN) treatment attenuates oxidative stress and rescues angiogenic capacity in aged cerebromicrovascular endothelial cells: a potential mechanism for the prevention of vascular cognitive impairment. *Geroscience.* 2019;41:619-630.

219. Kiss T, Nyul-Toth A, Balasubramanian P, et al. Nicotinamide mononucleotide (NMN) supplementation promotes neurovascular rejuvenation in aged mice: transcriptional footprint of SIRT1 activation, mitochondrial protection, anti-inflammatory, and anti-apoptotic effects. *Geroscience.* 2020;42:527-546.

220. Diguet N, Trammell SAJ, Tannous C, et al. Nicotinamide riboside preserves cardiac function in a mouse model of dilated cardiomyopathy. *Circulation.* 2018;137:2256-2273.

221. Cohen HY, Miller C, Bitterman KJ, et al. Calorie restriction promotes mammalian cell survival by inducing the SIRT1 deacetylase. *Science.* 2004;305:390-392.

222. Moroz N, Carmona JJ, Anderson E, Hart AC, Sinclair DA, Blackwell TK. Dietary restriction involves NAD(+)-dependent mechanisms and a shift toward oxidative metabolism. *Aging Cell.* 2014;13:1075-1085.

223. Wood JG, Rogina B, Lavu S, et al. Sirtuin activators mimic caloric restriction and delay ageing in metazoans. *Nature.* 2004;430:686-689.

224. Csiszar A, Sosnowska D, Tucsek Z, et al. Circulating factors induced by caloric restriction in the nonhuman primate macaca mulatta activate angiogenic processes in endothelial cells. *J Gerontol A Biol Sci Med Sci.* 2013;68:235-249.

225. Yamamoto T, Tamaki K, Shirakawa K, et al. Cardiac SIRT1 mediates the cardioprotective effect of caloric restriction by suppressing local complement system activation after ischemia-reperfusion. *Am J Physiol Heart Circ Physiol.* 2016;310:H1003-H1014.

226. Sulaiman M, Matta MJ, Sunderesan NR, Gupta MP, Periasamy M, Gupta M. Resveratrol, an activator of SIRT1, upregulates sarcoplasmic calcium ATPase and improves cardiac function in diabetic cardiomyopathy. *Am J Physiol Heart Circ Physiol.* 2010;298:H833-H843.

227. Danz ED, Skramsted J, Henry N, Bennett JA, Keller RS. Resveratrol prevents doxorubicin cardiotoxicity through mitochondrial stabilization and the SIRT1 pathway. *Free Radic Biol Med.* 2009;46:1589-1597.

228. Pearson KJ, Baur JA, Lewis KN, et al. Resveratrol delays age-related deterioration and mimics transcriptional aspects of dietary restriction without extending life span. *Cell Metab.* 2008;8:157-168.

229. Chen YX, Zhang M, Cai Y, Zhao Q, Dai W. The SIRT1 activator srt1720 attenuates angiotensin ii-induced atherosclerosis in apoe(-)/(-) mice through inhibiting vascular inflammatory response. *Biochem Biophys Res Commun.* 2015;465:732-738.

230. Gano LB, Donato AJ, Pasha HM, et al. The SIRT1 activator srt1720 reverses vascular endothelial dysfunction, excessive superoxide production, and inflammation with aging in mice. *Am J Physiol Heart Circ Physiol.* 2014;307:H1754-H1763.

231. Minor RK, Baur JA, Gomes AP, et al. Srt1720 improves survival and healthspan of obese mice. *Sci Rep.* 2011;1.doi:10.1038/srep00070.

232. Csiszar A, Labinskyy N, Podlutsky A, et al. Vasoprotective effects of resveratrol and SIRT1: attenuation of cigarette smoke-induced oxidative stress and proinflammatory phenotypic alterations. *Am J Physiol Heart Circ Physiol.* 2008;294:H2721-H2735.

233. Tong C, Morrison A, Mattison S, et al. Impaired SIRT1 nucleocytoplasmic shuttling in the senescent heart during ischemic stress. *FASEB J.* 2013;27:4332-4342.

234. Ungvari Z, Labinskyy N, Mukhopadhyay P, et al. Resveratrol attenuates mitochondrial oxidative stress in coronary arterial endothelial cells. *Am J Physiol Heart Circ Physiol.* 2009;297:H1876-H1881.

235. Oomen CA, Farkas E, Roman V, van der Beek EM, Luiten PG, Meerlo P. Resveratrol preserves cerebrovascular density and cognitive function in aging mice. *Front Aging Neurosci.* 2009;1:4.

236. Bernier M, Wahl D, Ali A, et al. Resveratrol supplementation confers neuroprotection in cortical brain tissue of nonhuman primates fed a high-fat/sucrose diet. *Aging (Albany NY).* 2016;8:899-916.

237. Mattison JA, Wang M, Bernier M, et al. Resveratrol prevents high fat/sucrose diet-induced central arterial wall inflammation and stiffening in nonhuman primates. *Cell Metab.* 2014;20:183-190.

238. Morimoto RI, Cuervo AM. Protein homeostasis and aging: taking care of proteins from the cradle to the grave. *J Gerontol A Biol Sci Med Sci.* 2009;64:167-170.

239. Schneider JL, Cuervo AM. Autophagy and human disease: emerging themes. *Curr Opin Genet Dev.* 2014;26:16-23.

240. Mijaljica D, Prescott M, Devenish RJ. Different fates of mitochondria: alternative ways for degradation? *Autophagy.* 2007;3:4-9.

241. Dice JF, Terlecky SR, Chiang HL, et al. A selective pathway for degradation of cytosolic proteins by lysosomes. *Semin Cell Biol.* 1990;1:449-455.

242. Levine B, Kroemer G. Autophagy in the pathogenesis of disease. *Cell.* 2008;132:27-42.

243. Gatica D, Chiong M, Lavandero S, Klionsky DJ. Molecular mechanisms of autophagy in the cardiovascular system. *Circ Res.* 2015;116:456-467.

244. Simonsen A, Cumming RC, Brech A, Isakson P, Schubert DR, Finley KD. Promoting basal levels of autophagy in the nervous system enhances longevity and oxidant resistance in adult drosophila. *Autophagy.* 2008;4:176-184.

245. Pyo JO, Yoo SM, Ahn HH, et al. Overexpression of atg5 in mice activates autophagy and extends lifespan. *Nat Commun.* 2013;4:2300.

246. Koga H, Kaushik S, Cuervo AM. Protein homeostasis and aging: the importance of exquisite quality control. *Ageing Res Rev.* 2011;10:205-215.

247. Wong E, Cuervo AM. Integration of clearance mechanisms: the proteasome and autophagy. *Cold Spring Harb Perspect Biol.* 2010;2:a006734.

248. Douglas PM, Dillin A. Protein homeostasis and aging in neurodegeneration. *J Cell Biol.* 2010;190:719-729.

249. Jana NR. Protein homeostasis and aging: role of ubiquitin protein ligases. *Neurochem Int.* 2012;60:443-447.

250. Bedford L, Hay D, Devoy A, et al. Depletion of 26s proteasomes in mouse brain neurons causes neurodegeneration and lewy-like inclusions resembling human pale bodies. *J Neurosci.* 2008;28:8189-8198.

251. Brunk UT, Terman A. Lipofuscin: mechanisms of age-related accumulation and influence on cell function. *Free Radic Biol Med.* 2002;33:611-619.

252. Dai DF, Karunadharma PP, Chiao YA, et al. Altered proteome turnover and remodeling by short-term caloric restriction or rapamycin rejuvenate the aging heart. *Aging Cell.* 2014;13:529-539.

253. Kruse SE, Karunadharma PP, Basisty N, et al. Age modifies respiratory complex I and protein homeostasis in a muscle type-specific manner. *Aging Cell.* 2016;15:89-99.

254. Karunadharma PP, Basisty N, Dai DF, et al. Subacute calorie restriction and rapamycin discordantly alter mouse liver proteome homeostasis and reverse aging effects. *Aging Cell.* 2015;14:547-557.

255. Miller BF, Robinson MM, Bruss MD, Hellerstein M, Hamilton KL. A comprehensive assessment of mitochondrial protein synthesis and cellular proliferation with age and caloric restriction. *Aging Cell.* 2012;11:150-161.

256. Price JC, Guan S, Burlingame A, Prusiner SB, Ghaemmaghami S. Analysis of proteome dynamics in the mouse brain. *Proc Natl Acad Sci U S A.* 2010;107:14508-14513.

257. Taneike M, Yamaguchi O, Nakai A, et al. Inhibition of autophagy in the heart induces age-related cardiomyopathy. *Autophagy.* 2010;6:600-606.

258. Wohlgemuth SE, Calvani R, Marzetti E. The interplay between autophagy and mitochondrial dysfunction in oxidative stress-induced cardiac aging and pathology. *J Mol Cell Cardiol.* 2014;71:62-70.

259. Dutta D, Xu J, Kim JS, Dunn WA, Leeuwenburgh C. Upregulated autophagy protects cardiomyocytes from oxidative stress-induced toxicity. *Autophagy.* 2013;9:328-344.

260. Han X, Turdi S, Hu N, Guo R, Zhang Y, Ren J. Influence of long-term caloric restriction on myocardial and cardiomyocyte contractile function and autophagy in mice. *J Nutr Biochem.* 2012;23:1592-1599.

261. Flynn JM, O'Leary MN, Zambataro CA, et al. Late-life rapamycin treatment reverses age-related heart dysfunction. *Aging Cell.* 2013;12:851-862.

262. Tan JM, Wong ES, Kirkpatrick DS, et al. Lysine 63-linked ubiquitination promotes the formation and autophagic clearance of protein inclusions associated with neurodegenerative diseases. *Hum Mol Genet.* 2008;17:431-439.

263. Rea IM, Gibson DS, McGilligan V, McNerlan SE, Alexander HD, Ross OA. Age and age-related diseases: role of inflammation triggers and cytokines. *Front Immunol.* 2018;9:586.

264. Fabbri E, An Y, Zoli M, S, et al. Aging and the burden of multimorbidity: associations with inflammatory and anabolic hormonal biomarkers. *J Gerontol A Biol Sci Med Sci.* 2015;70:63-70.

265. Soysal P, Stubbs B, Lucato P, et al. Inflammation and frailty in the elderly: a systematic review and meta-analysis. *Ageing Res Rev.* 2016;31:1-8.

266. Smith AJ, Humphries SE. Cytokine and cytokine receptor gene polymorphisms and their functionality. *Cytokine Growth Factor Rev.* 2009;20:43-59.

267. Sarwar N, Butterworth AS, Freitag DF, et al. Interleukin-6 receptor pathways in coronary heart disease: a collaborative meta-analysis of 82 studies. *Lancet.* 2012;379:1205-1213.

268. Dehghan A, Dupuis J, Barbalic M, et al. Meta-analysis of genome-wide association studies in >80 000 subjects identifies multiple loci for c-reactive protein levels. *Circulation.* 2011;123:731-738.

269. Rafiq S, Stevens K, Hurst AJ, et al. Common genetic variation in the gene encoding interleukin-1-receptor antagonist (IL-1ra) is associated with altered circulating IL-1ra levels. *Genes Immun.* 2007;8:344-351.

270. Hou H, Wang C, Sun F, Zhao L, Dun A, Sun Z. Association of interleukin-6 gene polymorphism with coronary artery disease: an updated systematic review and cumulative meta-analysis. *Inflamm Res.* 2015;64:707-720.

271. Sheu WH, Wang WC, Wu KD, et al. Crp-level-associated polymorphism rs1205 within the crp gene is associated with 2-hour glucose level: the sapphire study. *Sci Rep.* 2017;7:7987.

272. Ridker PM, Cushman M, Stampfer MJ, Tracy RP, Hennekens CH. Inflammation, aspirin, and the risk of cardiovascular disease in apparently healthy men. *N Engl J Med.* 1997;336:973-979.

273. Ridker PM, Everett BM, Thuren T, et al. Antiinflammatory therapy with canakinumab for atherosclerotic disease. *N Engl J Med.* 2017;377:1119-1131.

274. Dai DF, Chiang FT, Lin JL, et al. Human c-reactive protein (CRP) gene 1059g>c polymorphism is associated with plasma CRP concentration in patients receiving coronary angiography. *J Formos Med Assoc.* 2007;106:347-354.

275. Zeng Y, Nie C, Min J, et al. Novel loci and pathways significantly associated with longevity. *Sci Rep.* 2016;6:21243.

276. Bektas A, Zhang Y, Wood WH, 3rd, et al. Age-associated alterations in inducible gene transcription in human CD4+ t lymphocytes. *Aging (Albany NY).* 2013;5:18-36.

277. Cannon MJ, Schmid DS, Hyde TB. Review of cytomegalovirus seroprevalence and demographic characteristics associated with infection. *Rev Med Virol.* 2010;20:202-213.

278. Vescovini R, Biasini C, Fagnoni FF, et al. Massive load of functional effector CD4+ and CD8+ t cells against cytomegalovirus in very old subjects. *J Immunol.* 2007;179:4283-4291.

279. Simon CO, Holtappels R, Tervo HM, et al. CD8 t cells control cytomegalovirus latency by epitope-specific sensing of transcriptional reactivation. *J Virol.* 2006;80:10436-10456.

280. Roberts ET, Haan MN, Dowd JB, Aiello AE. Cytomegalovirus antibody levels, inflammation, and mortality among elderly Latinos over 9 years of follow-up. *Am J Epidemiol.* 2010;172:363-371.

281. Spyridopoulos I, Martin-Ruiz C, Hilkens C, et al. CMV seropositivity and T-cell senescence predict increased cardiovascular mortality in octogenarians: results from the Newcastle 85+ study. *Aging Cell.* 2016;15:389-392.

282. Brodin P, Jojic V, Gao T, et al. Variation in the human immune system is largely driven by non-heritable influences. *Cell.* 2015;160:37-47.

283. Aiello AE, Chiu YL, Frasca D. How does cytomegalovirus factor into diseases of aging and vaccine responses, and by what mechanisms? *Geroscience.* 2017;39:261-271.

284. Dai DF, Lin JW, Kao JH, et al. The effects of metabolic syndrome versus infectious burden on inflammation, severity of coronary atherosclerosis, and major adverse cardiovascular events. *J Clin Endocrinol Metab.* 2007;92:2532-2537.

285. Goldeck D, Pawelec G, Norman K, et al. No strong correlations between serum cytokine levels, CMV serostatus and hand-grip strength in older subjects in the berlin base-II cohort. *Biogerontology.* 2016;17:189-198.

286. Dietrich T, Webb I, Stenhouse L, et al. Evidence summary: the relationship between oral and cardiovascular disease. *Br Dent J.* 2017;222:381-385.

287. Mariat D, Firmesse O, Levenez F, et al. The firmicutes/bacteroidetes ratio of the human microbiota changes with age. *BMC Microbiol.* 2009;9:123.

288. Biagi E, Franceschi C, Rampelli S, et al. Gut microbiota and extreme longevity. *Curr Biol.* 2016;26:1480-1485.

289. Zapata HJ, Quagliarello VJ. The microbiota and microbiome in aging: potential implications in health and age-related diseases. *J Am Geriatr Soc.* 2015;63:776-781.

290. Rocha VZ, Libby P. Obesity, inflammation, and atherosclerosis. *Nat Rev Cardiol.* 2009;6:399-409.

291. Vandanmagsar B, Youm YH, Ravussin A, et al. The nlrp3 inflammasome instigates obesity-induced inflammation and insulin resistance. *Nat Med.* 2011;17:179-188.

292. Frasca D, Blomberg BB. Adipose tissue inflammation induces b cell inflammation and decreases B cell function in aging. *Front Immunol.* 2017;8:1003.

293. Lee-Chang C, Bodogai M, Moritoh K, et al. Accumulation of 4-1BBL+ B cells in the elderly induces the generation of granzyme-B+ CD8+ T cells with potential antitumor activity. *Blood.* 2014;124:1450-1459.

294. Frasca D, Blomberg BB, Paganelli R. Aging, obesity, and inflammatory age-related diseases. *Front Immunol.* 2017;8:1745.

295. Panagiotakos DB, Pitsavos C, Yannakoulia M, Chrysohoou C, Stefanadis C. The implication of obesity and central fat on markers of chronic inflammation: the attica study. *Atherosclerosis.* 2005;183:308-315.

296. Clément K, Viguerie N, Poitou C, et al. Weight loss regulates inflammation-related genes in white adipose tissue of obese subjects. *Faseb J.* 2004;18:1657-1669.

297. Illán-Gómez F, Gonzálvez-Ortega M, Orea-Soler I, et al. Obesity and inflammation: change in adiponectin, c-reactive protein, tumour necrosis factor-alpha and interleukin-6 after bariatric surgery. *Obes Surg.* 2012;22:950-955.

298. Meydani SN, Das SK, Pieper CF, et al. Long-term moderate calorie restriction inhibits inflammation without impairing cell-mediated immunity: a randomized controlled trial in non-obese humans. *Aging (Albany NY).* 2016;8:1416-1431.

299. Zomer E, Gurusamy K, Leach R, et al. Interventions that cause weight loss and the impact on cardiovascular risk factors: a systematic review and meta-analysis. *Obes Rev.* 2016;17:1001-1011.

300. Ma C, Avenell A, Bolland M, et al. Effects of weight loss interventions for adults who are obese on mortality, cardiovascular disease, and cancer: systematic review and meta-analysis. *BMJ.* 2017;359:j4849.

301. Villareal DT, Aguirre L, Gurney AB, et al. Aerobic or resistance exercise, or both, in dieting obese older adults. *N Engl J Med.* 2017;376:1943-1955.

302. Ridker PM, Hennekens CH, Buring JE, Rifai N. C-reactive protein and other markers of inflammation in the prediction of cardiovascular disease in women. *N Engl J Med.* 2000;342:836-843.

303. Cushman M, Arnold AM, Psaty BM, et al. C-reactive protein and the 10-year incidence of coronary heart disease in older men and women: the cardiovascular health study. *Circulation.* 2005;112:25-31.

304. Cesari M, Penninx BW, Newman AB, et al. Inflammatory markers and onset of cardiovascular events: results from the Health ABC study. *Circulation.* 2003;108:2317-2322.

305. Ridker PM, Howard CP, Walter V, et al. Effects of interleukin-1β inhibition with canakinumab on hemoglobin a1c, lipids, c-reactive protein, interleukin-6, and fibrinogen: a phase IIb randomized, placebo-controlled trial. *Circulation.* 2012;126:2739-2748.

306. Hansson GK. Inflammation, atherosclerosis, and coronary artery disease. *N Engl J Med.* 2005;352:1685-1695.

307. Libby P, Ridker PM, Hansson GK. Inflammation in atherosclerosis: from pathophysiology to practice. *J Am Coll Cardiol.* 2009;54:2129-2138.

308. De Caterina R, D'Ugo E, Libby P. Inflammation and thrombosis—testing the hypothesis with anti-inflammatory drug trials. *Thromb Haemost.* 2016;116:1012-1021.

309. Libby P, Ridker PM, Hansson GK. Progress and challenges in translating the biology of atherosclerosis. *Nature.* 2011;473:317-325.

310. Warnatsch A, Ioannou M, Wang Q, Papayannopoulos V. Inflammation. Neutrophil extracellular traps license macrophages for cytokine production in atherosclerosis. *Science.* 2015;349:316-320.

311. Childs BG, Baker DJ, Wijshake T, Conover CA, Campisi J, van Deursen JM. Senescent intimal foam cells are deleterious at all stages of atherosclerosis. *Science.* 2016;354:472-477.

312. Baker DJ, Childs BG, Durik M, et al. Naturally occurring p16(ink4a)-positive cells shorten healthy lifespan. *Nature.* 2016;530:184-189.

313. Baker DJ, Wijshake T, Tchkonia T, et al. Clearance of p16ink4a-positive senescent cells delays ageing-associated disorders. *Nature.* 2011;479:232-236.

314. Tchkonia T, Zhu Y, van Deursen J, Campisi J, Kirkland JL. Cellular senescence and the senescent secretory phenotype: therapeutic opportunities. *J Clin Invest.* 2013;123:966-972.

315. Lewis-McDougall FC, Ruchaya PJ, Domenjo-Vila E, et al. Aged-senescent cells contribute to impaired heart regeneration. *Aging Cell.* 2019;18:e12931.

316. Roos CM, Zhang B, Palmer AK, et al. Chronic senolytic treatment alleviates established vasomotor dysfunction in aged or atherosclerotic mice. *Aging Cell.* 2016;15:973-977.

317. Rossman MJ, Kaplon RE, Hill SD, et al. Endothelial cell senescence with aging in healthy humans: prevention by habitual exercise and relation to vascular endothelial function. *Am J Physiol Heart Circ Physiol.* 2017;313:H890-H895.

318. Kiss T, Nyul-Toth A, Balasubramanian P, et al. Single-cell RNA sequencing identifies senescent cerebromicrovascular endothelial cells in the aged mouse brain. *Geroscience.* 2020;42:429-444.

319. Gevaert AB, Shakeri H, Leloup AJ, et al. Endothelial senescence contributes to heart failure with preserved ejection fraction in an aging mouse model. *Circ Heart Fail.* 2017;10.

320. Grootaert MOJ, Moulis M, Roth L, et al. Vascular smooth muscle cell death, autophagy and senescence in atherosclerosis. *Cardiovasc Res.* 2018;114:622-634.

321. Chen HZ, Wang F, Gao P, et al. Age-associated sirtuin 1 reduction in vascular smooth muscle links vascular senescence and inflammation to abdominal aortic aneurysm. *Circ Res.* 2016;119:1076-1088.

322. Hayashi T, Kotani H, Yamaguchi T, et al. Endothelial cellular senescence is inhibited by liver x receptor activation with an additional mechanism for its atheroprotection in diabetes. *Proc Natl Acad Sci U S A.* 2014;111:1168-1173.

323. Ungvari Z, Podlutsky A, Sosnowska D, et al. Ionizing radiation promotes the acquisition of a senescence-associated secretory phenotype and impairs angiogenic capacity in cerebromicrovascular endothelial cells: role of increased DNA damage and decreased DNA repair capacity in microvascular radiosensitivity. *J Gerontol A Biol Sci Med Sci.* 2013;68:1443-1457.

324. Borghesan M, Fafian-Labora J, Eleftheriadou O, et al. Small extracellular vesicles are key regulators of non-cell autonomous intercellular communication in senescence via the interferon protein IFITM3. *Cell Rep.* 2019;27:3956-3971;e3956.

325. Ungvari Z, Tarantini S, Sorond F, Merkely B, Csiszar A. Mechanisms of vascular aging, a geroscience perspective: JACC focus seminar. *J Am Coll Cardiol.* 2020;75:931-941.

326. Morgan RG, Ives SJ, Lesniewski LA, et al. Age-related telomere uncapping is associated with cellular senescence and inflammation independent of telomere shortening in human arteries. *Am J Physiol Heart Circ Physiol.* 2013;305:H251-H258.

327. Gude NA, Broughton KM, Firouzi F, Sussman MA. Cardiac ageing: extrinsic and intrinsic factors in cellular renewal and senescence. *Nat Rev Cardiol.* 2018;15:523-542.

328. Yamazaki Y, Baker DJ, Tachibana M, et al. Vascular cell senescence contributes to blood-brain barrier breakdown. *Stroke.* 2016;47:1068-1077.

329. Yabluchanskiy A, Tarantini S, Balasubramanian P, et al. Pharmacological or genetic depletion of senescent astrocytes prevents whole brain irradiation-induced impairment of neurovascular coupling responses protecting cognitive function in mice. *Geroscience.* 2020;42:409-428.

330. Warrington JP, Ashpole N, Csiszar A, Lee YW, Ungvari Z, Sonntag WE. Whole brain radiation-induced vascular cognitive impairment: mechanisms and implications. *J Vasc Res.* 2013;50:445-457.

331. Matsumoto T, Baker DJ, d'Uscio LV, Mozammel G, Katusic ZS, van Deursen JM. Aging-associated vascular phenotype in mutant mice with low levels of BubR1. *Stroke.* 2007;38:1050-1056.

332. Wijshake T, Malureanu LA, Baker DJ, Jeganathan KB, van de Sluis B, van Deursen JM. Reduced life- and healthspan in mice carrying a mono-allelic BubR1 MVA mutation. *PLoS Genet.* 2012;8:e1003138

333. Benderitter M, Maingon P, Abadie C, et al. Effect of in vivo heart irradiation on the development of antioxidant defenses and cardiac functions in the rat. *Radiat Res.* 1995;144:64-72.

334. Wang R, Liu L, Liu H, et al. Reduced nrf2 expression suppresses endothelial progenitor cell function and induces senescence during aging. *Aging (Albany NY).* 2019;11:7021-7035.

335. Xu M, Pirtskhalava T, Farr JN, et al. Senolytics improve physical function and increase lifespan in old age. *Nat Med.* 2018;24:1246-1256.

336. Jia K, Dai Y, Liu A, et al. The senolytic agent navitoclax inhibits angiotensin II-induced heart failure in mice navitoclax inhibits heart failure. *J Cardiovasc Pharmacol.* 2020.

337. Walaszczyk A, Dookun E, Redgrave R, et al. Pharmacological clearance of senescent cells improves survival and recovery in aged mice following acute myocardial infarction. *Aging Cell.* 2019;18:e12945.

338. Lee CK, Klopp RG, Weindruch R, Prolla TA. Gene expression profile of aging and its retardation by caloric restriction. *Science.* 1999;285:1390-1393.

339. de Cabo R, Furer-Galban S, Anson RM, Gilman C, Gorospe M, Lane MA. An in vitro model of caloric restriction. *Experiment Gerontol.* 2003;38:631-639.

340. Cerqueira FM, Chausse B, Baranovski BM, et al. Diluted serum from calorie-restricted animals promotes mitochondrial beta-cell adaptations and protect against glucolipotoxicity. *FEBS J.* 2016;283:822-833.

341. Allard JS, Heilbronn LK, Smith C, et al. In vitro cellular adaptations of indicators of longevity in response to treatment with serum collected from humans on calorie restricted diets. *PLoS ONE.* 2008;3:e3211.

342. Barger JL, Vann JM, Cray NL, et al. Identification of tissue-specific transcriptional markers of caloric restriction in the mouse and their use to evaluate caloric restriction mimetics. *Aging Cell.* 2017;16:750-760.

343. Katsimpardi L, Litterman NK, Schein PA, et al. Vascular and neurogenic rejuvenation of the aging mouse brain by young systemic factors. *Science.* 2014;344:630-634.

344. Rebo J, Mehdipour M, Gathwala R, et al. A single heterochronic blood exchange reveals rapid inhibition of multiple tissues by old blood. *Nat Commun.* 2016;7:13363.

345. Loffredo FS, Steinhauser ML, Jay SM, et al. Growth differentiation factor 11 is a circulating factor that reverses age-related cardiac hypertrophy. *Cell.* 2013;153:828-839.

346. Kiss T, Tarantini S, Csipo T, et al. Circulating anti-geronic factors from heterochonic parabionts promote vascular rejuvenation in aged mice: transcriptional footprint of mitochondrial protection, attenuation of oxidative stress, and rescue of endothelial function by young blood. *Geroscience.* 2020.

347. Gan KJ, Sudhof TC. Specific factors in blood from young but not old mice directly promote synapse formation and nmda-receptor recruitment. *Proc Natl Acad Sci U S A.* 2019;116:12524-12533.

348. Castellano JM, Mosher KI, Abbey RJ, et al. Human umbilical cord plasma proteins revitalize hippocampal function in aged mice. *Nature.* 2017;544:488-492.

349. Zhang G, Li J, Purkayastha S, et al. Hypothalamic programming of systemic ageing involving IKK-beta, NF-KAPPAB and GNRH. *Nature.* 2013;497:211-216.

350. Elabd C, Cousin W, Upadhyayula P, et al. Oxytocin is an age-specific circulating hormone that is necessary for muscle maintenance and regeneration. *Nat Commun.* 2014;5:4082

351. Higashi Y, Sukhanov S, Anwar A, Shai SY, Delafontaine P. Aging, atherosclerosis, and IGF-1. *J Gerontol A Biol Sci Med Sci.* 2012;67:626-639.

352. Wennberg AMV, Hagen CE, Petersen RC, Mielke MM. Trajectories of plasma IGF-1, IGFBP-3, and their ratio in the Mayo Clinic Study of Aging. *Exp Gerontol.* 2018;106:67-73.

353. Benbassat CA, Maki KC, Unterman TG. Circulating levels of insulin-like growth factor (IGF) binding protein-1 and -3 in aging men: relationships to insulin, glucose, IGF, and dehydroepiandrosterone sulfate levels and anthropometric measures. *J Clin Endocrinol Metab.* 1997;82:1484-1491.

354. Kaplan RC, Buzkova P, Cappola AR, et al. Decline in circulating insulin-like growth factors and mortality in older adults: cardiovascular health study all-stars study. *J Clin Endocrinol Metab.* 2012;97:1970-1976.

355. Sanders JL, Guo W, O'Meara ES, et al. Trajectories of IGF-I predict mortality in older adults: the cardiovascular health study. *J Gerontol A Biol Sci Med Sci.* 2018;73:953-959.

356. Kaplan RC, McGinn AP, Pollak MN, et al. High insulinlike growth factor binding protein 1 level predicts incident congestive heart failure in the elderly. *Am Heart J.* 2008;155:1006-1012.

357. Shai SY, Sukhanov S, Higashi Y, Vaughn C, Rosen CJ, Delafontaine P. Low circulating insulin-like growth factor I increases atherosclerosis in apoe-deficient mice. *Am J Physiol Heart Circ Physiol.* 2011.

358. Sukhanov S, Higashi Y, Shai SY, et al. IGF-1 reduces inflammatory responses, suppresses oxidative stress, and decreases atherosclerosis progression in apoe-deficient mice. *Arterioscler Thromb Vasc Biol.* 2007;27:2684-2690.

359. Napoli R, Guardasole V, Matarazzo M, et al. Growth hormone corrects vascular dysfunction in patients with chronic heart failure. *J Am Coll Cardiol.* 2002;39:90-95.

360. Toth P, Tarantini S, Ashpole NM, et al. IGF-1 deficiency impairs neurovascular coupling in mice: implications for cerebromicrovascular aging. *Aging Cell.* 2015;14:1034-1044.

361. Tarantini S, Valcarcel-Ares NM, Yabluchanskiy A, et al. Insulin-like growth factor 1 deficiency exacerbates hypertension-induced cerebral microhemorrhages in mice, mimicking the aging phenotype. *Aging Cell.* 2017;16:469-479.

362. Fulop GA, Ramirez-Perez FI, Kiss T, et al. IGF-1 deficiency promotes pathological remodeling of cerebral arteries: a potential mechanism contributing to the pathogenesis of intracerebral hemorrhages in aging. *J Gerontol A Biol Sci Med Sci.* 2018.

363. Bailey-Downs LC, Mitschelen M, Sosnowska D, et al. Liver-specific knockdown of IGF-1 decreases vascular oxidative stress resistance by impairing the NRF2-dependent antioxidant response: a novel model of vascular aging. *J Gerontol A Biol Sci Med Sci.* 2012;67:313-329.

364. Higashi Y, Pandey A, Goodwin B, Delafontaine P. Insulin-like growth factor-1 regulates glutathione peroxidase expression and activity in vascular endothelial cells: implications for atheroprotective actions of insulin-like growth factor-1. *Biochim Biophys Acta.* 2013;1832:391-399.

365. Lopez-Lopez C, LeRoith D, Torres-Aleman I. Insulin-like growth factor I is required for vessel remodeling in the adult brain. *Proc Natl Acad Sci U S A.* 2004;101:9833-9838.

366. Tarantini S, Tucsek Z, Valcarcel-Ares MN, et al. Circulating IGF-1 deficiency exacerbates hypertension-induced microvascular rarefaction in the mouse hippocampus and retrosplenial cortex: implications for cerebromicrovascular and brain aging. *Age (Dordr).* 2016;38:273-289.

367. Zhang Y, Yuan M, Bradley KM, Dong F, Anversa P, Ren J. Insulin-like growth factor 1 alleviates high-fat diet-induced myocardial contractile dysfunction: role of insulin signaling and mitochondrial function. *Hypertension.* 2012;59:680-693.

368. Csiszar A, Labinskyy N, Perez V, et al. Endothelial function and vascular oxidative stress in long-lived GH/IGF-deficient Ames dwarf mice. *Am J Physiol Heart Circ Physiol.* 2008;295:H1882-H1894.

369. Torella D, Rota M, Nurzynska D, et al. Cardiac stem cell and myocyte aging, heart failure, and insulin-like growth factor-1 overexpression. *Circ Res.* 2004;94:514-524.

370. Reddy AK, Amador-Noguez D, Darlington GJ, et al. Cardiac function in young and old little mice. *J Gerontol A Biol Sci Med Sci.* 2007;62:1319-1325.

371. Li Q, Wu S, Li SY, Lopez FL, et al. Cardiac-specific overexpression of insulin-like growth factor 1 attenuates aging-associated cardiac diastolic contractile dysfunction and protein damage. *American J Physiol.* 2007;292:H1398-H1403.

372. Imai S. The NAD world: a new systemic regulatory network for metabolism and aging--SIRT1, systemic NAD biosynthesis, and their importance. *Cell Biochem Biophys.* 2009;53:65-74.

373. Mehdipour M, Skinner C, Wong N, et al. Rejuvenation of three germ layers tissues by exchanging old blood plasma with saline-albumin. *Aging (Albany NY).* 2020;12:8790-8819.

374. Beltrami AP, Barlucchi L, Torella D, et al. Adult cardiac stem cells are multipotent and support myocardial regeneration. *Cell.* 2003;114:763-776.

375. Ellison GM, Vicinanza C, Smith AJ, et al. Adult c-kit(pos) cardiac stem cells are necessary and sufficient for functional cardiac regeneration and repair. *Cell.* 2013;154:827-842.

376. van Berlo JH, Kanisicak O, Maillet M, et al. C-kit+ cells minimally contribute cardiomyocytes to the heart. *Nature.* 2014;509:337-341.

377. Sultana N, Zhang L, Yan J, et al. Resident c-kit(+) cells in the heart are not cardiac stem cells. *Nat Commun.* 2015;6:8701.

378. Uchida S, De Gaspari P, Kostin S, et al. Sca1-derived cells are a source of myocardial renewal in the murine adult heart. *Stem Cell Reports.* 2013;1:397-410.

379. Oh H, Bradfute SB, Gallardo TD, et al. Cardiac progenitor cells from adult myocardium: homing, differentiation, and fusion after infarction. *Proc Natl Acad Sci U S A.* 2003;100:12313-12318.

380. Neidig LE, Weinberger F, Palpant NJ, et al. Evidence for minimal cardiogenic potential of stem cell antigen 1-positive cells in the adult mouse heart. *Circulation.* 2018;138:2960-2962.

381. Eschenhagen T, Bolli R, Braun T, et al. Cardiomyocyte regeneration: a consensus statement. *Circulation.* 2017;136:680-686.

382. Bergmann O, Bhardwaj RD, Bernard S, et al. Evidence for cardiomyocyte renewal in humans. *Science.* 2009;324:98-102.

383. Bergmann O, Zdunek S, Felker A, et al. Dynamics of cell generation and turnover in the human heart. *Cell.* 2015;161:1566-1575.

384. Porrello ER, Mahmoud AI, Simpson E, et al. Transient regenerative potential of the neonatal mouse heart. *Science.* 2011;331:1078-1080.

385. Senyo SE, Steinhauser ML, Pizzimenti CL, et al. Mammalian heart renewal by pre-existing cardiomyocytes. *Nature.* 2013;493:433-436.

386. Puente BN, Kimura W, Muralidhar SA, et al. The oxygen-rich postnatal environment induces cardiomyocyte cell-cycle arrest through DNA damage response. *Cell.* 2014;157:565-579.

387. Nakada Y, Canseco DC, Thet S, et al. Hypoxia induces heart regeneration in adult mice. *Nature.* 2017;541:222-227.

388. Anversa P, Rota M, Urbanek K, et al. Myocardial aging—a stem cell problem. *Basic Res Cardiol.* 2005;100:482-493.

389. Rota M, LeCapitaine N, Hosoda T, et al. Diabetes promotes cardiac stem cell aging and heart failure, which are prevented by deletion of the P66SHC gene. *Circ Res.* 2006;99:42-52.

390. Hsiao LC, Perbellini F, Gomes RS, et al. Murine cardiosphere-derived cells are impaired by age but not by cardiac dystrophic dysfunction. *Stem Cells Dev.* 2014;23:1027-1036.

391. Geiger H, Denkinger M, Schirmbeck R. Hematopoietic stem cell aging. *Curr Opin Immunol.* 2014;29:86-92.

392. Oh J, Lee YD, Wagers AJ. Stem cell aging: mechanisms, regulators and therapeutic opportunities. *Nat Med.* 2014;20:870-880.

393. Liang R, Ghaffari S. Stem cells, redox signaling, and stem cell aging. *Antioxid Redox Signal.* 2014;20:1902-1916.

394. Li L, Guo Y, Zhai H, et al. Aging increases the susceptivity of MSCs to reactive oxygen species and impairs their therapeutic potency for myocardial infarction. *PLoS One.* 2014;9:e111850.

395. Liu X, Chen H, Zhu W, et al. Transplantation of SIRT1-engineered aged mesenchymal stem cells improves cardiac function in a rat myocardial infarction model. *J Heart Lung Transplant.* 2014;33:1083-1092.

396. Ott B, Skurk T, Hastreiter L, Lagkouvardos I. Effect of caloric restriction on gut permeability, inflammation markers, and fecal microbiota in obese women. 2017;7:11955.

397. Liu Y, Gibson GR, Walton GE. An in vitro approach to study effects of prebiotics and probiotics on the faecal microbiota and selected immune parameters relevant to the elderly. *PLoS One.* 2016;11:e0162604.

398. Turchet P, Laurenzano M, Auboiron S, Antoine JM. Effect of fermented milk containing the probiotic lactobacillus casei DN-114001 on winter infections in free-living elderly subjects: a randomised, controlled pilot study. *J Nutr Health Aging.* 2003;7:75-77.

399. Wang Z, Klipfell E, Bennett BJ, et al. Gut flora metabolism of phosphatidylcholine promotes cardiovascular disease. *Nature.* 2011;472:57-63.

400. Koeth RA, Wang Z, Levison BS, et al. Intestinal microbiota metabolism of l-carnitine, a nutrient in red meat, promotes atherosclerosis. *Nat Med.* 2013;19:576-585.

401. Zhu W, Gregory JC, Org E, et al. Gut microbial metabolite tmao enhances platelet hyperreactivity and thrombosis risk. *Cell.* 2016;165:111-124.

402. Tang WH, Hazen SL. The contributory role of gut microbiota in cardiovascular disease. *J Clin Invest.* 2014;124:4204-4211.

403. Brown JM, Hazen SL. The gut microbial endocrine organ: bacterially derived signals driving cardiometabolic diseases. *Annu Rev Med.* 2015;66:343-359.

404. Niemann B, Rohrbach S, Miller MR, Newby DE, Fuster V, Kovacic JC. Oxidative stress and cardiovascular risk: obesity, diabetes, smoking, and pollution: part 3 of a 3-part series. *J Am Coll Cardiol.* 2017;70:230-251.

405. Ungvari Z, Csiszar A, Edwards JG, et al. Increased superoxide production in coronary arteries in hyperhomocysteinemia: role of tumor

406. necrosis factor-alpha, NAD(p)h oxidase, and inducible nitric oxide synthase. *Arterioscler Thromb Vasc Biol.* 2003;23:418-424.

406. Tucsek Z, Toth P, Sosnowsk D, et al. Obesity in aging exacerbates blood brain barrier disruption, neuroinflammation and oxidative stress in the mouse hippocampus: effects on expression of genes involved in beta-amyloid generation and Alzheimer's disease *J Gerontol A Biol Sci Med Sci.* 2014;69:1212-1226.

407. Wang CY, Kim HH, Hiroi Y, et al. Obesity increases vascular senescence and susceptibility to ischemic injury through chronic activation of Akt and mTOR. *Sci Signal.* 2009;2:ra11.

408. Brodsky SV, Gealekman O, Chen J, et al. Prevention and reversal of premature endothelial cell senescence and vasculopathy in obesity-induced diabetes by ebselen. *Circ Res.* 2004;94:377-384.

409. Dikalov S, Itani H, Richmond B, et al. Tobacco smoking induces cardiovascular mitochondrial oxidative stress, promotes endothelial dysfunction, and enhances hypertension. *Am J Physiol Heart Circ Physiol.* 2019;316:H639-H646.

410. Wilson SJ, Miller MR, Newby DE. Effects of diesel exhaust on cardiovascular function and oxidative stress. *Antioxid Redox Signal.* 2018;28:819-836.

411. Eskurza I, Monahan KD, Robinson JA, Seals DR. Effect of acute and chronic ascorbic acid on flow-mediated dilatation with sedentary and physically active human ageing. *J Physiol.* 2004;556:315-324.

412. DeSouza CA, Shapiro LF, Clevenger CM, et al. Regular aerobic exercise prevents and restores age-related declines in endothelium-dependent vasodilation in healthy men. *Circulation.* 2000;102:1351-1357.

413. Luscher TF. Tumours and the heart: common risk factors, chemotherapy, and radiation. *Eur Heart J.* 2016;37:2737-2738.

414. Boerma M, Sridharan V, Mao XW, et al. Effects of ionizing radiation on the heart. *Mutat Res.* 2016;770:319-327.

415. Ungvari Z, Tarantini S, Hertelendy P, et al. Cerebromicrovascular dysfunction predicts cognitive decline and gait abnormalities in a mouse model of whole brain irradiation-induced accelerated brain senescence. *Geroscience.* 2017;39:33-42.

416. Carlson BW, Craft MA, Carlson JR, Razaq W, Deardeuff KK, Benbrook DM. Accelerated vascular aging and persistent cognitive impairment in older female breast cancer survivors. *Geroscience.* 2018;40:325-336.

417. Brown PD, Jaeckle K, Ballman KV, et al. Effect of radiosurgery alone vs radiosurgery with whole brain radiation therapy on cognitive function in patients with 1 to 3 brain metastases: a randomized clinical trial. *JAMA.* 2016;316:401-409.

418. Brown WR, Blair RM, Moody DM, et al. Capillary loss precedes the cognitive impairment induced by fractionated whole-brain irradiation: a potential rat model of vascular dementia. *J Neurol Sci.* 2007;257:67-71.

419. van Bussel BC, Henry RM, Ferreira I, et al. A healthy diet is associated with less endothelial dysfunction and less low-grade inflammation over a 7-year period in adults at risk of cardiovascular disease. *J Nutr.* 2015;145:532-540.

420. Knoops KT, de Groot LC, Kromhout D, et al. Mediterranean diet, lifestyle factors, and 10-year mortality in elderly European men and women: the Hale project. *JAMA.* 2004;292:1433-1439.

421. Mitrou PN, Kipnis V, Thiebaut AC, et al. Mediterranean dietary pattern and prediction of all-cause mortality in a us population: results from the nih-aarp diet and health study. *Arch Intern Med.* 2007;167:2461-2468.

422. Hu FB, Rimm EB, Stampfer MJ, Ascherio A, Spiegelman D, Willett WC. Prospective study of major dietary patterns and risk of coronary heart disease in men. *Am J Clin Nutr.* 2000;72:912-921.

423. Sack MN, Fyhrquist FY, Saijonmaa OJ, Fuster V, Kovacic JC. Basic biology of oxidative stress and the cardiovascular system: part 1 of a 3-part series. *J Am Coll Cardiol.* 2017;70:196-211.

424. Napoli C, Bruzzese G, Ignarro LJ, et al. Long-term treatment with sulfhydryl angiotensin-converting enzyme inhibition reduces carotid intima-media thickening and improves the nitric oxide/oxidative stress pathways

in newly diagnosed patients with mild to moderate primary hypertension. *Am Heart J.* 2008;156:1154;e18.

425. Meaney E, Vela A, Samaniego V, et al. Metformin, arterial function, intima-media thickness and nitroxidation in metabolic syndrome: the mefisto study. *Clin Exp Pharmacol Physiol.* 2008;35:895-903.

426. Donato AJ, Walker AE, Magerko KA, et al. Life-long caloric restriction reduces oxidative stress and preserves nitric oxide bioavailability and function in arteries of old mice. *Aging Cell.* 2013;12:772-783.

427. Seals DR, Desouza CA, Donato AJ, Tanaka H. Habitual exercise and arterial aging. *J Appl Physiol.* 2008;105:1323-1332.

428. Wang M, Zhang L, Zhu W, et al. Calorie restriction curbs proinflammation that accompanies arterial aging, preserving a youthful phenotype. *J Am Heart Assoc.* 2018;7:e009112.

429. Rossman MJ, Santos-Parker JR, Steward CAC, et al. Chronic supplementation with a mitochondrial antioxidant (MITOQ) improves vascular function in healthy older adults. *Hypertension.* 2018;71:1056-1063.

430. Sardu C, Paolisso P, Sacra C, et al. Effects of metformin therapy on coronary endothelial dysfunction in patients with prediabetes with stable angina and nonobstructive coronary artery stenosis: the codyce multicenter prospective study. *Diabetes Care.* 2019;42:1946-1955.

431. Lin AL, Zheng W, Halloran JJ, et al. Chronic rapamycin restores brain vascular integrity and function through no synthase activation and improves memory in symptomatic mice modeling Alzheimer's disease. *J Cereb Blood Flow Metab.* 2013;33:1412-1421.

432. Selvin E, Erlinger TP. Prevalence of and risk factors for peripheral arterial disease in the United States: results from the national health and nutrition examination survey, 1999-2000. *Circulation.* 2004;110:738-743.

433. Mozaffarian D, Benjamin EJ, Go AS, et al. Heart disease and stroke statistics–2015 update: a report from the American Heart Association. *Circulation.* 2015;131:e29-322.

434. Wilson PW, D'Agostino RB, Sullivan L, Parise H, Kannel WB. Overweight and obesity as determinants of cardiovascular risk: the Framingham experience. *Arch Intern Med.* 2002;162:1867-1872.

435. Kannel WB, D'Agostino RB, Wilson PW, Belanger AJ, Gagnon DR. Diabetes, fibrinogen, and risk of cardiovascular disease: the Framingham experience. *Am Heart J.* 1990;120:672-676

436. Wilson PW, D'Agostino RB, Levy D, Belanger AM, Silbershatz H, Kannel WB. Prediction of coronary heart disease using risk factor categories. *Circulation.* 1998;97:1837-1847.

437. Kannel WB. Framingham study insights into hypertensive risk of cardiovascular disease. *Hypertens Res.* 1995;18:181-196.

438. Burke GM, Genuardi M, Shappell H, D'Agostino RB, Sr., Magnani JW. Temporal associations between smoking and cardiovascular disease, 1971 to 2006 (from the Framingham heart study). *Am J Cardiol.* 2017;120:1787-1791.

Artificial Intelligence and Cardiovascular Care

John S. Rumsfeld, Bobak J. Mortazavi, and Harlan M. Krumholz

CHAPTER OUTLINE

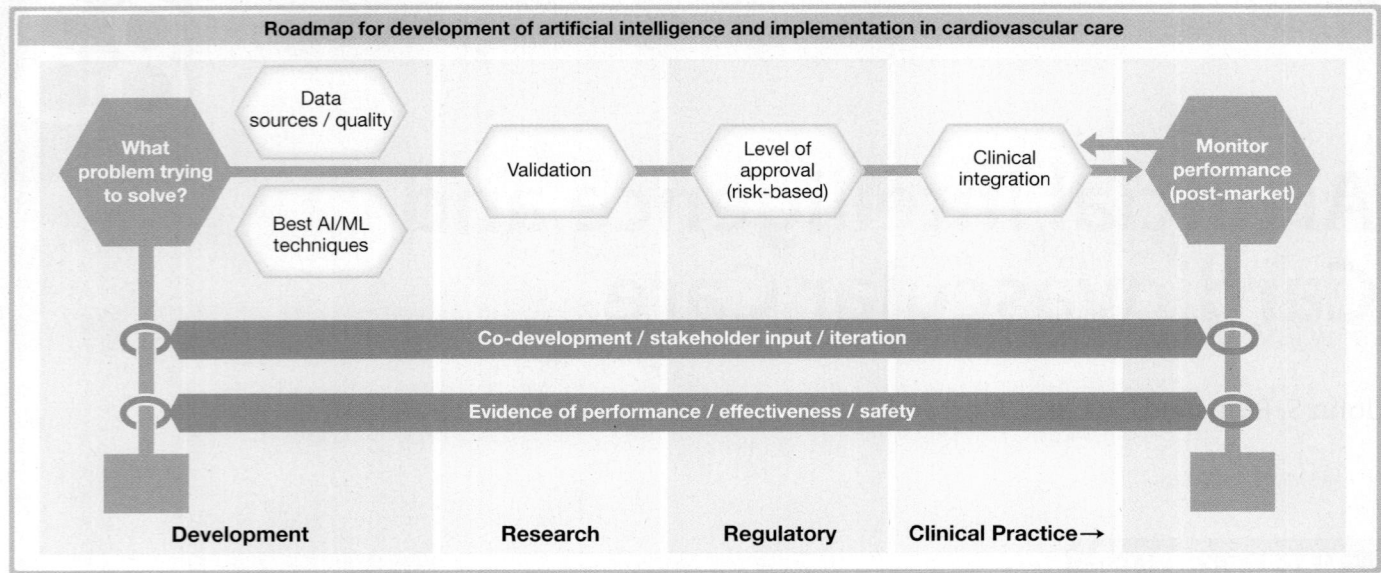

Chapter 83 Fuster and Hurst's Central Illustration. Artificial intelligence (AI) is more likely to achieve success in cardiovascular care if development and clinical adoption follow the roadmap depicted here. Key concepts for consideration throughout development and clinical deployment include the importance of co-development (e.g. clinicians working closely with data scientists), relevant stakeholder input at all steps, and iteration to improve AI solutions over time. Evidence for — and monitoring of — performance, effectiveness and safety of AI solutions for use in cardiovascular care during development as well as after integration into clinical practice is essential. ML, machine learning.

CHAPTER SUMMARY

This chapter provides an overview of the current and potential applications for artificial intelligence (AI) in cardiovascular care. AI techniques can mimic human thought processes, learning capacity, and knowledge storage. Current AI applications do not have independent reasoning or abstraction; instead they are focused on specific tasks such as automation, risk prediction, and pattern recognition. Most current AI techniques involve some form of machine learning methods. AI holds substantial promise for cardiovascular care, given the variety of ever-growing digital data becoming available. Because pattern recognition is a particularly good application for AI, cardiovascular imaging is a high-yield area for its use. The use of AI in risk prediction has also grown rapidly, as has the interpretation of digital health data (eg, from wearable or nonwearable biosensors). However, the evidence base for AI solutions for cardiovascular care so far has been limited, and deployment of AI in routine cardiovascular clinical practice has been minimal to date. Current challenges must be successfully navigated before wide adoption of AI takes place in our field, with careful development and adoption in clinical practice (see Fuster and Hurst's Central Illustration). With this approach, AI has the potential to advance the concepts of both precision health and population health management. Ultimately, AI is best developed and deployed as "augmented intelligence"—that is, to enhance human intelligence—in support of cardiovascular clinicians and health systems in achieving higher quality of care and improved health outcomes.

INTRODUCTION

Artificial intelligence (AI) applications in health care carry great promise. If successfully developed and deployed, AI has the potential to improve efficiency and reduce waste in health-care delivery; provide novel insights on patient risk and disease trajectory, improving diagnosis and treatment decisions; and improve patient health engagement and outcomes.[1–7] AI can be applied to large and diverse data sets, such as omics, imaging, or electronic health records (EHRs), and in conjunction with other emerging technologies such as wearable and nonwearable biosensors, voice or optical technologies, robotics, or any combination. These represent just a partial list of potential data sources and technologies for AI in cardiovascular (CV) care.

Despite all of this potential, the evidence base for AI solutions for CV care has been limited to date and there is minimal deployment of AI in routine CV clinical practice. Accordingly, the goals of this chapter are to discuss why now for AI and CV care; provide an overview of several AI methods; focus on two key areas for application with specific examples reflecting a spectrum of CV conditions and modalities; and discuss key challenges and mitigation strategies for AI to fulfill its potential for CV care. We conclude with the concept of augmented intelligence as a likely success factor for AI in CV care.

WHY NOW FOR AI AND CV CARE?

AI is a computer science field that aims to mimic human thought processes, learning capacity, and knowledge storage.[4] Comprised of an array of data science analytic methods, most of which involve machine learning (ML) techniques, AI can execute statistical automation, iterative pattern matching, and predictive analytics on massive, diverse data sources.[1–5] Exponential growth in computing power, digital data availability, and a mode for transmitting such data (the Internet) over the last 20 years have fueled the development and adoption of AI in many sectors.

Health care, however, has thus far lagged in the utilization of AI. In part, this reflects the fact that health care did not previously have significant amounts of digital data on which to apply AI techniques. Even as digital data in health care has rapidly grown, several factors have impeded adoption. These are further considered in the section Challenges for AI in CV Care, but include a lack of data standards and interoperability in health care, complexity of integration of new technology solutions into health-care delivery, issues of data privacy and security, the potential for bias in AI algorithms, and lack of evidence base to date demonstrating improved efficiency, effectiveness, and safety of AI solutions. Health care is different from other fields, because utilization of AI may directly influence diagnosis and treatment and thus impact patients' health and outcomes. As such, these challenges, including potential hazards, must be successfully navigated before wide adoption of AI in CV care.

At the same time, AI has substantial promise for health care. First, there is continued, exponential growth in digital health and health-care data. Health-care data approaches a zettabyte (10^{21} bytes, or a billion terabytes) of data annually, and is estimated to double approximately every 2 years.[5,8] This greatly exceeds the capacity for meaningful assessment by individual humans. Similarly, while traditional biostatistical methods remain highly useful in many instances, they have limitations with regard to the analysis of massive, diverse data sets.

Cardiology is a particularly data-rich field, ranging across omics, imaging, biomarker, EHR, clinical registry, and research data sources, in addition to administrative (claims) and Internet data.[5] Increasingly, data is also available from digital health and remote monitoring data sources including mobile applications, wearable and nonwearable biosensors, voice and optical data, and so on. Cardiology also arguably has the largest scientific evidence base than any other medical field, with journal publications far beyond the ability for individual CV clinicians to read. AI carries the potential to serve as a tool to ingest data from multiple such data sources and identify meaningful patterns and outputs. This capability can be relevant to all aspects of CV care, ranging from CV prevention to CV imaging modalities to CV procedures to diagnosis and management of all CV conditions, acute and chronic. Select examples are provided in the section Key Applications in CV Care.

At the same time, there continues to be rising health-care costs, unexplained variation in the quality of care, and suboptimal prevention and patient health outcomes. These concerns are global health and health-care issues, and are particularly problematic in the current US health-care system. CV care costs, in particular, are among the highest in US health care, estimated to exceed $1 trillion dollars over the next 15 years.[9] AI carries the promise of improving efficiency and reducing waste in health-care delivery. It also has the potential to provide novel information to better inform risk assessment, diagnostic and treatment decisions, and preventive and chronic care management. Cardiology stands to benefit as much as any field in medicine from this potential.

Finally, AI carries the potential to advance the concepts of both precision health and population health management. Leveraging the ability of AI to analyze diverse data sources simultaneously, individualized patient phenotypes and risk estimates can be developed and analyzed over time. This approach closely relates to the concept of "digital phenotypes," where data from digital sources, ranging from Internet to apps to wearable biosensors, is used to identify personalized health status and trajectory.[10] These may be combined with more traditional data sources such as imaging, biomarker, or EHRs, to yield novel data patterns at the individual level. In theory, this can enhance risk prediction and inform both diagnosis and treatment that is more precise for a given individual. To date, there is little proof of concept for this. However, initial studies on "phenomapping" or "phenogrouping" are starting to appear in the literature, for example in heart failure and aortic stenosis.[11–14]

Population health management can be defined as active assessment and management of health for patient populations, such as for a given CV practice or for specific cohorts (heart failure, diabetes, atrial fibrillation, etc). Leveraging digital health tools such as biosensors for remote patient monitoring, it is not surprising that there can quickly be a massive data burden to effectively monitor patient populations. AI is well-suited for the task of ingesting such data to inform the detection of decompensation or alert clinicians to signals within the data. Such signals may be preset by clinical teams (eg, an alert for a low pulse oximetry reading or downward trend) or AI may help identify novel patterns of data that correlate with clinical change. While many technology companies are focused on aspects of remote patient monitoring coupled with AI analytics to achieve population health management, evidence proving this concept remains nascent.

Ultimately, there is a balance of tremendous promise and substantial challenge for AI to positively transform CV care. There is little doubt, however, that AI will increasingly be utilized in CV research as well as technology, medical device, and pharmaceutical development, and will increasingly become part of CV care. Accordingly, it will be essential for CV clinicians and researchers to have at least basic knowledge of AI methods, potential applications, and barriers to overcome.

AI METHODS: AN OVERVIEW

CV clinicians should have basic knowledge about the data science methods that support AI applications, including general concepts, semantics, and examples of techniques. Collaboration between data scientists and CV clinicians and researchers will continue to grow, and relevant informatics and data science methods should increasingly be incorporated into medical training. This knowledge provides a foundation to evaluate new tools and innovations leveraging AI. As such, clinicians should have some working knowledge of the data science techniques and semantics as utilized in AI analytics.

AI analytic techniques are used to develop models to execute tasks usually considered part of human intelligence, such as pattern recognition and problem solving.[1-4] In general, the goal for AI analytics in health care is to utilize computational programs to extract novel information from data—often large, diverse data sets—in support of clinical decision-making. Nonetheless, AI techniques do not have independent reasoning or abstraction. While some people predict that in the (distant) future, there may be "generalized AI," including independent reasoning, current AI is "narrow," focused on specific tasks or applications.[15]

Machine Learning

The vast majority of current AI techniques involve ML.[1-3,15,16] In fact, these terms are often used interchangeably or together (AI/ML). ML can identify patterns in data sets and performance can improve with more "training" of the model (ie, with iterative modeling or on additional data). The improvement in performance by ML models is usually referred to as "learning," for which there are three main approaches: supervised, unsupervised, and reinforcement. Each approach provides different advantages and one is not inherently better than another; they are suited to different purposes.

Supervised Learning

In supervised learning, humans guide the modeling via notation of data inputs and outputs.[1,3,15,16] This approach includes both independent—or predictor—variables, which are referred to in the data science world as features; and outcome variables, which may be referred to as labels, or responses. Supervised ML models optimize patterns of data to predict an outcome of interest. A large number of ML techniques, such as those based on decision trees (eg, Random Forests, Gradient Descent Boosted Decision Trees, etc), can model a number of feature types (continuous, binary, and categorical), and response labels (regression or classification). This ability supports feature (predictor variable) selection and model training together in one step, to find linear and nonlinear relationships between the features and labels, or outcomes.

In the current era, many ML techniques utilize artificial neural networks.[15,17] These techniques are so-named because data is deployed in the modeling process in layers of input data (features), which may have multiple nodes (akin to neurons), and an output layer. Modeling optimizes the patterns of input within and across layers, akin to a neural system, where weighting of data patterns is analogous to synaptic pathways.

These AI modeling techniques can be quite complex, and those that utilize multiple neural network layers are often referred to as deep learning.[15,18,19] Deep learning techniques are more and more common in health-care/CV applications of AI. For example, CV clinicians may increasingly encounter convolutional neural networks, a form of deep learning highly suited to image interpretation because of its ability to extract features/patterns in data local to each other, as is the case in images.[20,21,22] As another example, recurrent neural networks identify relationships in data over time. They can support natural language processing applications, such as AI interpretation of unstructured text in EHR notes. They can also be applied to time-series signals, looking for recurrent patterns in biomedical variables that are repeatedly captured over time. A key advantage to these deep learning techniques is their automatic ability to identify important features. Deep neural networks are often used with supervised learning but can also be utilized with unsupervised or reinforcement learning.

Unsupervised Learning

Unsupervised learning does not try to fit data for an outcome and does not have a priori notations for patterns in the data.[1,3,15,16,23] Instead, the ML models optimize pattern matching, or clustering, driven solely by the data set characteristics. In other words, unsupervised learning is data exploration to identify patterns. Cluster analysis identifies related groups by analyzing patterns within data sets without a priori classification of the data. It can be applied, for example, to diverse data sets such as EHR and imaging to identify new potential disease phenotypes. Several examples of cluster analysis techniques that CV clinicians may encounter are k-means, hierarchical clustering, and Gaussian mixture modeling (GMM). Unsupervised learning approaches may inform hypothesis generation about new disease phenotypes or may be used to inform supervised modeling (ie, using the patterns found in unsupervised learning to then predict an outcome via supervised learning).

Reinforcement Learning

Reinforcement learning techniques are a method to train models on decision-making tasks.[1,3,15,16] These algorithms take as inputs the current state (eg, patient health status) and a series of available actions, and then iterate through a series of choices of applying or not applying these actions to evaluate eventual outcomes. When provided with a score of how well or how poorly they performed, they learn which actions to take and which to avoid. These methods have been used in data science fields to evaluate game-playing strategies. They can potentially be useful for treatment decision support, and there are a few emerging examples in medicine.[24,25] Because of obvious limitations of choosing actions that could cause harm when applied in health care, they are currently limited to off-policy (retrospective) analysis, which may not properly model new potential actions.

APPLICATIONS IN CV CARE

There are myriad potential uses of AI in CV care. Here, we focus on two exemplar areas—imaging and risk prediction—with associated recent examples from the literature. Other application areas such as drug development and clinical research are also important, but the areas presented here are relevant to other AI applications and are most proximal to clinical practice. Of note, AI models may be deployed in any number of "vehicles" (apps/smartphone, digital health technologies, Internet, EHR, robotics, etc) and/or may be utilized in different CV care settings (procedural, hospital, clinic, patient home, etc).

Imaging

Pattern recognition is a particularly good application for AI. Thus, CV imaging is a high yield area for the use of AI/ML, and is likely to be first to become part of routine CV clinical practice.[26–28] In fact, AI/ML techniques are already used in software packages for some common imaging applications, such as echocardiography (echo).[29] To date, these are deployed in the background; for example, for image optimization, edge detection, or statistical automation of measurements. However, there is very active research and technology development that will propel AI in CV imaging, including direct interpretation of imaging studies and risk estimation, diagnosis, and therapeutic guidance.[26–28] In other words, not only will AI likely interpret images, at least as a "preread" for CV clinicians, it can also recognize patterns in imaging beyond human perception that may portend risk of subsequent events, support new diagnosis, and/or suggest therapeutic interventions. While not CV imaging, the case of retinography serves as a good example of this spectrum and has relevance for CV risk (**Box 83–1**).[30,31]

Publications are rapidly growing across the spectrum of AI applied to CV imaging. Any type of CV imaging can lend itself to modern AI/ML methods such as deep learning. Within the last 5 years, there has been particular growth in publications related to echo, cardiac magnetic resonance imaging (CMR),

---

BOX 83–1. AI APPLIED TO RETINOGRAPHY

Recent publications on AI/ML methods applied to retinographic images help demonstrate the potential for AI in relation to imaging:

- In an initial study led by Google scientists, a deep learning algorithm was trained on 128,175 retinal fundus photographs. Subsequent validation was performed on two separate data sets and included grading by board-certified ophthalmologists. The deep learning model had >90% sensitivity and specificity for diabetic retionopathy.[30]
- Subsequently, Google/Verily scientists utilized retinograph data to infer CV risk. Utilizing a training data set of ~285,000 patients, with validation on another ~13,000 patients, they were able to infer from the retinographs patient gender, smoking status, systolic blood pressure, and major cardiac events, with degrees of accuracy comparable to or higher than traditional CV risk prediction models.[31]

These AI algorithms to assess retinographs for diabetic retinopathy and to estimate CV risk have not yet been adopted in routine clinical practice. However, they demonstrate the promise of AI in medical imaging, to potentially improve efficiency and accuracy, including reductions in inter-rater variance.

A challenge remains to demonstrate the value of the predictive risk information for the patient, and the degree to which this information adds to what is known from other sources.

They do, however, demonstrate the potential that images contain more information than humans perceive, and thus could improve risk assessment, diagnosis (eg, case-finding), and potentially treatment decision support (eg, earlier prevention interventions).

All of this will require additional evidence and consideration of integration into clinical practice, as well as other factors considered in the section Challenges for AI in CV Care.

---

cardiac computed tomography (CT)/coronary CT angiography (CTA), and electrocardiography (ECG).[26–28,32–47] There have been publications on AI/ML applied to other CV imaging modalities to a lesser degree to date (eg, coronary angiography, myocardial perfusion imaging, intravascular ultrasound, optical coherence tomography, implantable cardioverter-defibrillator electrograms, etc).[48–54]

A number of these studies focus on specific aspects of CV imaging such as image segmentation, view classification, lumen detection, or tissue/plaque analysis. An increasing number of studies focus on automated measurements such as coronary stenosis, left ventricular/right ventricular (LV/RV) chamber size and function estimates, fractional flow reserve, and so on. As the body of literature grows, initial publications on automated imaging study interpretation (eg, echo, CTA, CMR) are starting to emerge. Analogous to the retinopathy example (**Box 83–1**), AI is also being applied to cardiac imaging for patient risk prediction, disease phenotyping, and diagnosis.[55–57] It is expected that studies will increasingly combine imaging data with other data sources (biomarker, EHR, wearable devices, etc), particularly with regard to predicting outcomes.

Echocardiography is an especially rapid growth area for AI research and application development. Therefore, several recent representative examples, intended to provide a sense of the "state of play" of AI and echo research to date, are listed here:

- Madani and colleagues demonstrated the feasibility for rapid, accurate view classification for echocardiograms using deep learning.[32]
- Sengupta and colleagues published a pilot study of differentiating restrictive cardiomyopathy versus constrictive pericarditis using ML applied to echo studies.[33]
- Casaclang-Verzosa and colleagues applied ML to develop phenotypic patterns of LV responses during the progression of aortic stenosis. While a pilot study, one implication is the potential for personalization of individual patient risk of more rapid progression of aortic stenosis.[13]
- Asch and colleagues developed and trained a ML algorithm to assess left ventricular ejection fraction (LVEF) on an echo data set of >50,000 studies. The automated algorithm had >90% sensitivity and specificity for detecting LVEF ≤0.35.[34]
- Zhang and colleagues applied deep learning to >14,000 echocardiograms, and were able to successfully train models to recognize standard echo views, assess LVEF and longitudinal strain, and identify cases of hypertrophic cardiomyopathy, cardiac amyloidosis, and pulmonary hypertension with c-indices ≥0.85.[35] This study thereby advances the foundation for AI-guided echocardiogram interpretation.

Surface ECG (eg, single lead, Holter/event monitors, 12-lead) has also become a particularly rapid growth area for AI applications. Several recent examples of AI/ML applied to single or 12-lead ECGs are listed here:

- Galloway and colleagues developed a deep learning model to screen for hyperkalemia on 12-lead ECG.[41]
- Kwon and colleagues have applied deep learning algorithms to accurately diagnose heart failure with reduced ejection fraction and LV hypertrophy on 12-lead ECG.[45,46]
- Attia and colleagues have a series of publications on AI applied to 12-lead ECGs, including screening for LV dysfunction and identification of patients with prior atrial fibrillation on sinus rhythm 12-lead ECGs.[43,44]
- Kagiyama and colleagues utilized ML methods to assess myocardial relaxation and thus detect LV diastolic dysfunction via 12-lead ECG prior to echocardiography.[47]
- Hannun and colleagues applied deep learning to >91,000 single lead ECGs from >53,000 patients, with a goal of assessing a wide variety of dysrhythmias (atrial and ventricular, heart block, etc).[42] Validated against a separate data set with annotation by expert electrocardiologists, the deep learning model had an average c-index of 0.97 for discrimination of dysrhythmias.

Risk Prediction

Similar to the application of AI/ML to CV imaging, risk prediction is an area of rapid growth in publications and development of AI solutions for potential use by CV clinicians. The potential for AI/ML risk prediction models for use in health

care in general is immense, because of advances in risk modeling techniques and the ability for these techniques to utilize large, diverse data sets.[5,58,59] However, this arena also presents particular challenges for AI in order to fulfill its potential. These include addressing: (1) transparency, or interpretability, limiting clinical insights and trust in AI risk prediction models; (2) evidence that AI/ML models are superior to existing risk models or risk scores (ie, what is gained by using AI/ML?); (3) the need to develop AI/ML risk models that yield actionable information; (4) the need for clinical validation and stable model performance when applied in practice; (5) potential bias in models depending on underlying data quality used to develop the algorithms; and (6) the need for clinical integration to support adoption in CV practice.

Despite these impediments, there are a growing number of publications that demonstrate the potential for AI risk models in CV care. For instance, demonstrating predictive accuracy for meaningful clinical outcomes and/or higher performance than existing risk models and/or utilizing imaging to develop risk models that could improve CV diagnosis. Moreover, publications of AI risk models are increasingly accompanied by methods to identify or display which features are contributing most to risk prediction, including in higher order interaction with each other, helping support clinical interpretation. There is still a need to demonstrate that deployment of such models in clinical practice can improve health outcomes.

Examples of AI/ML risk prediction publications relevant to aspects of CV care are provided here:

- Kwon and colleagues developed a deep learning model to predict in-hospital mortality for CV patients based on echo data; they conclude that the echo-derived AI model was more accurate than established risk scores for coronary artery disease and heart failure patients.[55]
- Samad and colleagues utilized ML models that combined clinical data sources (including EHR) with echo variables to predict 5-year survival in a cohort of >170,000 patients; the ML models had higher predictive accuracy than logistic regression or standard risk scores.[57]
- Motwani and colleagues also leveraged ML to combine clinical and CTA data to predict 5-year survival in a cohort of >10,000 patients; they concluded that ML prediction models were more accurate than either clinical or CTA variable models alone.[56]
- Mortazavi and colleagues used ML techniques to predict heart failure readmissions, an outcome which has traditionally been difficult to predict; the best performing ML models had c-indices ~20% higher than logistic regression and with more predictive range.[60]
- Huang and colleagues used ML to develop models to predict acute kidney injury following percutaneous coronary intervention based on patient factors and contrast dose. ML models accounted for nonlinearity and heterogeneity of risk, suggesting that these models could be used for personalized risk assessment in percutaneous coronary intervention decision-making.[61]

- Rajkomar and colleagues applied deep learning methods to EHR data from two hospitals on >215,000 patients, which yielded >46 billion data points for analysis. They developed risk models to predict length of stay (c-index ~0.85), in-hospital mortality (c-index ~0.93), and readmission (c-index ~0.75).[62]
- In contrast, Loring and colleagues assessed outcomes (death, major bleeding stroke) in >74,000 patients with atrial fibrillation from two large clinical registries. They concluded that ML methods, including multilayer neural networks, did not improve prediction of outcome compared to logistic regression.[63]

Most of these example publications underscore the potential for AI for improving risk prediction in CV care. However, AI/ML may not be superior to existing risk models or risk scores in some use cases. In fact, hundreds of risk models already exist in the field of cardiology and are rarely deployed in clinical decision-making. In order for AI-based risk models to transform CV care, the challenges discussed in the next section must be successfully navigated.

CHALLENGES FOR AI IN CV CARE

To deliver on the promise of AI for CV care, a number of challenges, including some potential hazards, need to be overcome (**Table 83–1**).[64–70] These challenges reflect, in part, the unique context of health care, where effectiveness and safety of AI applications are essential in order to avoid unintended consequences, including patient harm. All health-care stakeholders, specifically including developers of AI/ML solutions, should be aware of the challenges and associated mitigation factors. Such awareness can yield an AI development and implementation roadmap to optimize chances of success (Central Illustration).[2,69,70]

A couple of aspects of Central Illustration, also noted in Table 83–1, are worth additional emphasis. First, successful development and implementation of AI models, or solutions, in CV care should be anchored by clear articulation of what clinical problems are being addressed, what information would be actionable for clinical decision-making, and what monitoring of performance is necessary once integrated into clinical practice. Monitoring of performance includes assessment of how AI solutions may improve efficiency and effectiveness of care, stability of performance over time and in different clinical settings, and also safety monitoring for potential unintended consequences. Monitoring of performance in clinical practice should be an extension of evidence across the process of clinical validation, regulatory approval, and clinical integration.

Second, engagement of "end-users" (eg, patients, clinicians) across the spectrum from development to implementation is critical. This may include codevelopment and stakeholder input or feedback at each stage. Such engagement should be iterative, not just at one stage, and should continue even after clinical deployment since AI solutions inherently can continue to "learn" (improve) over time.

THE WAY FORWARD: AUGMENTED INTELLIGENCE

The challenges for successful adoption in CV care (**Table 83–1**) have impeded the rapid adoption of AI that has occurred in other sectors of the economy. However, AI still carries high potential to improve the efficiency and effectiveness of CV care in an era of nonsustainable health-care costs and desire to optimize health and health outcomes. Rapid growth in scientific literature on AI/ML, coupled with estimates that AI in health care will be a >$6 billion market as of 2021 and may exceed $45 billion by 2026, suggest that we are in the era of AI in health care.[82,83] There is widespread expectation that the use of AI in various aspects of CV care, and more generally in health care, will continue to accelerate.

Amid varying degrees of enthusiasm, skepticism, or concern about AI, the concept of "augmented intelligence" suggests a promising way forward for CV clinicians.[65,68,84–87] Rather than thinking that AI may assume human intelligence, or at an extreme replace CV clinicians, augmented intelligence is the use of AI/ML to enhance human intelligence. Also referred to as "intelligence augmentation," if properly developed and deployed in clinical practice, AI/ML can be used to improve CV clinician efficiency and effectiveness by providing a "clinician-in-the-loop" decision-support system.

At the least, AI can be utilized for statistical automation—replacing low-value, repetitive tasks for CV clinicians and other health-care workers, such as clerical functions. AI algorithms can also save time for things like image processing, optimization (eg, edge detection), and calculations (eg, LVEF), even if these applications run "in the background" in software packages deployed in imaging, cath or EP labs, the CCU, and so on. Examples of published studies presented earlier in this chapter further help demonstrate potential for increased efficiency and accuracy for CV clinicians using AI applications for image interpretation or risk prediction.

Deep learning natural language processing may support voice/audio applications (so-called "ambient clinical intelligence") such as automated dictation and documentation of clinical encounters; or as "clinician extenders" to interact with patients and support higher engagement and health education. AI solutions may help with case-finding or earlier diagnosis of CV risk or disease through various data source inputs, leading to earlier prevention of CV disease and or optimal timing of therapeutics or procedures.

AI solutions may be applied to increasingly diverse data sources (ranging from omics/biomarkers to EHR to imaging to digital health tools such as wearable or nonwearable biosensors) to support disease management, diagnostic, or therapeutic recommendations. These latter applications speak both to the concept of precision medicine and population health management, augmenting individual clinician and care team efficiency and capacity. They also can support the "digital transformation of health care," where CV care is increasingly centered on virtual care (telehealth) with aspects of remote monitoring (mobile, biosensors).[6,88]

TABLE 83-1. Challenges and Mitigation Strategies for Successful AI Adoption in CV Care

Challenge	Mitigation
Clinically important problems and information ------------ Too many current AI solutions on the market are "technology solutions in search of a problem." That is, not specifically designed and developed to help solve important clinical issues. Moreover, too many yield large amounts of data but not necessarily clinically actionable information.	A strong emphasis on defining the problem(s) to be addressed by a given AI solution before model development. This should include consideration of use cases (eg, CV risk or condition scenarios), and what clinically actionable knowledge may be yielded by a given solution. Then, the utility/performance should be monitored once deployed in clinical practice, with ongoing input from end-users on what outputs yield clinically actionable information.
Data sources and quality ------------ AI analytics are highly sensitive to underlying data quality. Larger amounts of data do not obviate this; data sets carry the limitations and potential biases of underlying data source(s).[5,69,71] For example, when AI is applied to EHR data, it carries all potential biases that may be inherent in such data, including missing data which is often not missing at random. Ultimately, any underlying data quality issues can negatively impact the performance of AI models, including introducing learning bias.[69,72]	Clinicians (and health systems) need to be aware that AI solutions are only as good as the quality of their underlying data sources. As such, there should generally be more skepticism of AI models derived from sources with data quality issues (eg, current EHRs), whereas higher quality data sources (imaging, wearable or nonwearable biosensors) are more likely to yield valid bases for AI models. Rigorous assessment of underlying data quality is thus an essential success factor. The best AI/ML methods, or techniques for the problem being addressed and data sources can then be determined (and in some cases more traditional methods may suffice). If data quality is insufficient, the process should be stopped.
Algorithmic bias ------------ An aspect of data quality, when models are developed on data that do not include underrepresented groups (eg, low socioeconomic status, racial/ethnic, gender), the model may have systematic bias in its outputs.[69,70,72,73]	There must be vigilance on what data sources are used to train AI models to avoid potential bias. Awareness of potential bias and striving to include data sources from underrepresented groups are essential. Issues such as bias in AI algorithms have led to calls for ethical guidance in the development and use of AI/ML models.[69,70,72–74] It is hoped that evolving digital/mobile technologies—such as wearable or nonwearable biosensors—hold promise for unbiased data, and could potentially replace data sources more prone to bias (eg, EHR or claims data). However, attention is needed on facilitators and barriers to use of digital health tools in low-income populations.[75]
Lack of data standards/interoperability ------------ Because health-care data is highly heterogeneous in nature, lacking in data standards often interoperable between sites (hospitals, clinics, etc), AI models developed on one health-care data set may not be valid when applied in other settings. This also creates a challenge for patient outcomes assessment. For example, it can be difficult to capture relevant outcomes in health systems like that of the United States, because a patient may be seen in different care settings and the outcome data is not necessarily available at the site where an AI model may be deployed.	A continued push by all health-care stakeholders, ranging from patients/consumers to hospitals/health systems to professional organizations to government, to pursue health-care data standards, is essential. The topic of interoperability of health-care data goes far beyond AI alone, but will also benefit AI applications. There should also be continued efforts to capture patient outcome data in a standard way, to inform accurate outcomes assessment and prediction (with appropriate data security and privacy: see below).
Overfitting and replication ------------ AI models may become optimized for one data set but then perform poorly (lack of replication) when applied to another data set. This is often because the initial model optimizes specific features of the original dataset, some of which may not be of clinical importance. This is also due to the lack of standard, interoperable health-care data or suboptimal approaches to model development and validation.	In addition to health-care data standardization, approaches to AI model development and validation are critical. Importantly, separate data should be used for model development ("training") and validation ("testing") on additional data.[3,16,26] Data used for training should not be used for testing. The same data set may be divided for this purpose for initial validation, but ultimately if AI solutions are to be more broadly adopted in CV care, they must have additional, external validation. Even with initial validation, model performance may not hold when applied in other settings; thus, initial validation is necessary but not sufficient for clinical adoption. There are emerging recommendations for optimal reporting of AI/ML analyses.[76–78]
Evidence base ------------ Clinicians rightfully look to the supporting evidence (or, where available, clinical practice guidelines that synthesize evidence) base for a given clinical tool. Where AI analytic solutions are intended to support or replace aspects of clinical decision-making, there must be evidence of validity, effectiveness, and safety. To date, the published evidence supporting AI solutions for CV care is limited. In part, this just reflects that it is still early in the "AI era," and the literature on AI/ML and health care is rapidly growing. However, much of what has been published to date reflects initial development or validation, or limited application of AI models. Robust clinical studies demonstrating effectiveness and safety, are largely lacking to date. Moreover, the proprietary nature of AI analytics for companies may preclude transparency of supporting evidence.	The scientific literature on AI/ML and cardiology/CV care is growing exponentially, suggesting that the evidence base will rapidly grow. At the same time, there is debate about "how much evidence" is needed for specific AI applications, and how much evidence is needed for initial approval/clinical deployment versus "postmarket surveillance." In general, there should be publication of, or access to, initial validation of AI models, to ensure proof of concept that they can perform as intended. Where there is independent clinical judgment (eg, image interpretation, provision of data trends from wearable biosensors, etc), AI models may be deployed as decision support, with assessment of performance in clinical practice. However, any AI solutions that will yield independent diagnostic or therapeutic information should be subject to rigorous clinical studies before clinical adoption.

(Continued)

TABLE 83–1. Challenges and Mitigation Strategies for Successful AI Adoption in CV Care (Continued)

Challenge	Mitigation
Regulatory The complex, iterative, and often nontransparent nature of AI analytic models creates new challenges for medical regulatory approvals. Unlike traditional biostatistical models—which may be static in their programming when deployed in software in, for example, a medical device—AI analytics are intended to change over time as new data is ingested and algorithms "learn." Traditional regulatory approval pathways are ill-suited for the "iterative modification" inherent in AI/ML models.	Many global regulatory bodies are developing pathways for health-care AI solutions/software as a medical device (SaMD).[70,79–81] For example, the US Food and Drug Administration has released guidance documents speaking to matching level of regulation/regulatory approval to the risk of a given AI solution, assessing AI companies versus specific products (given their iterative nature), etc.[80,81] In general, the more a given AI solution will influence diagnosis and treatment, a higher the level of evidence of performance, higher degree of assessment for approval, and more rigorous monitoring of performance in clinical practice will be needed. CV clinicians, health systems, and professional organizations can help support assessment of performance of AI solutions when deployed in care. These entities can also encourage international collaboration among regulatory bodies to help support the ethical use of health-care AI solutions globally.
Data security and privacy While not specific to AI, as digital health-care data sources continue to grow exponentially and many stakeholders (industry, researchers, hospitals/health systems, governments, etc) look to apply AI analytics to such data sources, concerns about data security and privacy grow in parallel. There are specific concerns about data ownership and access, particularly in regard to identified patient data (eg, personal identifiers, images, etc).	Similar to interoperability, health-care data security and privacy are a topic far beyond AI alone. However, there is also unfortunate potential for nefarious use of AI (eg, risk profiling); thus, data security and privacy are essential to the ethical use of AI in health care. Ethical standards and surveillance by health-care stakeholders as AI is increasingly deployed in health care are essential.
Interpretability and performance As opposed to most traditional CV risk models or risk scores, AI models can be "black box" in nature. That is, AI/ML modeling optimizes risk prediction in a way that may precludes straightforward identification of which variables, or features, are contributing to the outcome. This can limit clinical interpretation or understanding of which patient factors are contributing to predictions. Moreover, AI analytics are iterative—changing over time as data changes. This may limit the ability of clinicians to know when model performance has changed.	While not directly analogous to traditional biostatistical models, AI models can yield outputs to enhance transparency. For example, they can indicate which features are most predictive for outcomes. Clinicians (and health systems) considering deploying AI solutions should insist on transparency where AI will help inform diagnostic or treatment decisions or predict outcomes. Companies with proprietary AI solutions are more likely to be successful with such a commitment to transparency. Once deployed, AI solutions should have ongoing monitoring of performance (postmarket) in clinical practice. How this will be done should be overtly considered before clinical adoption, as a failure to monitor performance may have unintended consequences. As noted above, there are existing recommendations for optimal documentation of AI methods.[76–78]
Clinical integration An underappreciated—and often overlooked—barrier to success for AI in CV care (and health care in general) is clinical integration. This has several aspects, including: (1) education and training of the CV clinical workforce, to gain sufficient familiarity with AI applications in order to adopt them in clinical care; (2) matching AI "solutions" with clinical use cases, or clinical problems that need to be solved; (3) changes in clinical workflow that will follow the adoption of AI solutions; and (4) surveillance, or monitoring, of the impact of AI solutions on health outcomes in clinical practice. Without addressing these aspects, the adoption of AI in CV care is likely to be unsuccessful and slow; AI solutions may not improve care efficiency or outcomes (eg, predictive models alone do not change care and outcomes); and/or AI solutions deployed in care could have unintended consequences.	CV clinicians, working with health systems and CV professional organizations, should advocate for education and training of the CV clinical workforce on the essentials of AI methods and applications. These same entities should help guide the appropriate deployment of AI solutions in CV care and ongoing monitoring of performance, including changes in clinical workflow and optimization of clinician-patient/family interfaces. Where possible, AI solutions should be codeveloped with CV clinicians and patients, to help ensure they will be clinically useful, improve efficiency and outcomes, and minimize potential for unintended consequences. Consideration of how AI solutions will be deployed for use in clinical practice is critical. How will they be integrated into current clinical workflow and/or to what degree will clinical workflow need to change? How will the outputs of a given AI solution be accessed and acted upon by CV clinical teams?

This potential range of application of AI for CV care is already feasible, and some health systems in the United States and globally have started to implement "AI-based tools" for disease management, remote monitoring, image interpretation, and risk prediction. It is likely that in the very near future, CV clinicians that utilize AI solutions to augment their intelligence will be superior to those that do not. This should not ever replace clinical decision-making, and must be founded on scientific rigor, in keeping with the tenants of evidence-based medicine that have guided the field of cardiology.

AI that is developed and deployed as augmented intelligence, however, can support CV clinicians and health systems in achieving higher quality of care and improved health outcomes. The highest chance of success for this will be if CV clinicians and researchers are involved in development, validation, clinical integration, and monitoring in clinical practice of AI tools.

ACKNOWLEDGMENT

The authors thank Jai Nahar, MD FACC (Attending, Division of Cardiology, Children's National Hospital, Associate Professor of Pediatrics, George Washington University School of Medicine and Health Sciences, Washington DC; JNahar@childrensnational.org) for his expert review of this chapter.

REFERENCES

1. Yan Y, Zhang JW, Zang GY, Pu J. The primary use of artificial intelligence in cardiovascular diseases: what kind of potential role does artificial intelligence play in future medicine? *J Geriatr Cardiol.* 2019;16(8):585-591. doi: 10.11909/j.issn.1671-5411.2019.08.010

2. He J, Baxter SL, Xu J, Xu J, Zhou X, Zhang K. The practical implementation of artificial intelligence technologies in medicine. *Nat Med.* 2019;25(1):30-36. doi: 10.1038/s41591-018-0307-0.

3. Johnson KW, Torres Soto J, Glicksberg BS, et al. Artificial intelligence in cardiology. *J Am Coll Cardiol.* 2018 Jun 12;71(23):2668-2679. doi: 10.1016/j.jacc.2018.03.521.

4. Krittanawong C, Zhang H, Wang Z, et al. Artificial intelligence in precision cardiovascular medicine. *J Am Coll Cardiol.* 2017;69:2657–2664.

5. Rumsfeld JS, Joynt KE, Maddox TM. Big data analytics to improve cardiovascular care: promise and challenges. *Nature Rev Cardiol.* 2016;13(6):350-359.

6. Bhavnani SP, Parakh K, Atreja A, et al. 2017 roadmap for innovation-ACC health policy statement on healthcare transformation in the era of digital health, big data, and precision health. *J Am Coll Cardiol.* 2017;70(21):2696-2718. doi: 10.1016/j.jacc.2017.10.018

7. Dobkowski, D. AI can benefit care of patients with CVD, diabetes. *Cardiology Today.* August 25, 2020. https://www.healio.com/news/cardiology/20200825/ai-can-benefit-care-of-patients-with-cvd-diabetes. Accessed September 1, 2020.

8. May T. The fragmentation of health data. *Datavant.* 2018. https://datavant.com/2018/08/01/the-fragmentation-of-health-data/. Accessed August 20, 2020.

9. American Heart Association. *Cardiovascular Disease: A Costly Burden for America. Projections Through 2035.* Washington, DC: American Heart Association; 2017. http://www.heart.org/idc/groups/heart-public/@wcm/@adv/documents/downloadable/ucm_491543.pdf.

10. Jain SH, Powers BW, Hawkins JB, Brownstein JS. The digital phenotype. *Nat Biotechnol* ;33(5):462-463. doi: 10.1038/nbt.3223.

11. Shah SJ, Katz DH, Selvaraj S, et al. Phenomapping for novel classification of heart failure with preserved ejection fraction. *Circulation.* 2015;131(3):269-79. doi: 10.1161/CIRCULATIONAHA.114.010637.

12. Cikes M, Sanchez-Martinez S, Claggett B, et al. Machine learning-based phenogrouping in heart failure to identify responders to cardiac resynchronization therapy. *Eur J Heart Fail.* 2019;21(1):74-85. doi: 10.1002/ejhf.1333

13. Casaclang-Verzosa G, Shrestha S, Khalil MJ, et al. Network tomography for understanding phenotypic presentations in aortic stenosis. *JACC Cardiovasc Imaging.* 2019;12(2):236-248. doi: 10.1016/j.jcmg.2018.11.025

14. Ghaffar YA, Osman M, Shrestha S, et al. Usefulness of semi-supervised machine learning-based phenogrouping to improve risk assessment for patients undergoing transcatheter aortic valve implantation. *Am J Cardiol.* 2020. doi: 10.1016/j.amjcard.2020.048.

15. A Brief Taxonomy of AI. *Sharper AI.* October 10, 2018. https://www.sharper.ai/taxonomy-ai/. Accessed August 25, 2020.

16. Krittanawong C, Johnson KW, Rosenson RS, et al. Deep learning for cardiovascular medicine: a practical primer. *Eur Heart J.* 2019;40(25):2058-2073. doi:10.1093/eurheartj/ehz056

17. Shahid N, Rappon T, Berta W. Applications of artificial neural networks in health care organizational decision-making: a scoping review. *PLoS One.* 2019;14(2). doi:10.1371/journal.pone.0212356

18. Camacho DM, Collins KM, Powers RK, Costello JC, Collins JJ. Next-generation machine learning for biological networks. *Cell.* 2018;173(7):1581-1592. doi: 10.1016/j.cell.2018.05.015.

19. LeCun Y, Bengio Y, Hinton G. Deep learning. *Nature.* 2015;521(7553):436-44. doi: 10.1038/nature14539.

20. Betancur J, Commandeur F, Motlagh M, et al. Deep learning for prediction of obstructive disease from fast myocardial perfusion SPECT: a multicenter study. *JACC Cardiovasc Imaging.* 2018;11(11):1654-1663. doi: 10.1016/j.jcmg.2018.01.020.

21. Madani A, Ong JR, Tibrewal A, et al. Deep echocardiography: data-efficient supervised and semi-supervised deep learning towards automated diagnosis of cardiac disease. *NPJ Digit Med.* 2018;1(59). doi: 10.1038/s41746-018-0065-x

22. Ghorbani A, Ouyang D, Abid A, et al. Deep learning interpretation of echocardiograms. *NPJ Digit Med.* 2020;3(10). doi: 10.1038/s41746-019-0216-8

23. Loh BCS, Fong AYY, Ong TK, Then PHH. P203 unsupervised one-class classification and anomaly detection of stress echocardiograms with deep denoising spatio-temporal autoencoders, *Eur Heart J.* 2020;41(S1). doi: 10.1093/ehjci/ehz872.074

24. Komorowski M, Celi LA, Badawi O, et al. The artificial intelligence clinician learns optimal treatment strategies for sepsis in intensive care. *Nat Med.* 2018;24:1716–1720 doi: 10.1038/s41591-018-0213-5

25. Liu S, See KC, Ngiam KY, Celi LA, Sun X, Feng M. Reinforcement learning for clinical decision support in critical care: comprehensive review. *J Med Internet Res.* 2020;22(7):e18477.

26. Dey D, Slomka PJ, Leeson P, et al. Artificial intelligence in cardiovascular imaging: JACC state-of-the-art review. *J Am Coll Cardiol.* 2019;73(11):1317-1335. doi: 10.1016/j.jacc.2018.12.054

27. Slomka PJ, Dey D, Sitek A, Motwani M, Berman DS, Germano G. Cardiac imaging: working towards fully-automated machine analysis & interpretation. *Expert Rev Med Devices.* 2017;14(3):197-212. doi: 10.1080/17434440.2017.1300057

28. Leiner T, Rueckert D, Suinesiaputra A, et al. Machine learning in cardiovascular magnetic resonance: basic concepts and applications. *J Cardiovasc Magn Reson.* 2019;21(1):61. doi: 10.1186/s12968-019-0575-y.

29. Bandura, O. Use of artificial intelligence to locate standard echo heart views. Diagnostic and interventional cardiology. *DAIC.* July 17, 2017. https://www.dicardiology.com/article/use-artificial-intelligence-locate-standard-echo-heart-views. Accessed August 22, 2020.

30. Gulshan V, Peng L, Coram M, et al. Development and validation of a deep learning algorithm for detection of diabetic retinopathy in retinal fundus photographs. *JAMA.* 2016;316(22):2402-2410. doi: 10.1001/jama.2016.17216

31. Poplin R, Varadarajan AV, Blumer K, et al. Prediction of cardiovascular risk factors from retinal fundus photographs via deep learning. *Nat Biomed Eng.* 2018;2:158–164. doi: 10.1038/s41551-018-0195-0

32. Madani A, Arnaout R, Mofrad M, Arnaout R. Fast and accurate view classification of echocardiograms using deep learning. *NPJ Digit Med.* 2018;1:6. doi:10.1038/s41746-017-0013-1

33. Sengupta PP, Huang YM, Bansal M, et al. Cognitive machine-learning algorithm for cardiac imaging a pilot study for differentiating constrictive pericarditis from restrictive cardiomyopathy. *Circ Cardiovas Imag.* 2016;9(6):e004330.

34. Asch FM, Poilvert N, Abraham T, et al. Automated echocardiographic quantification of left ventricular ejection fraction without volume measurements using a machine learning algorithm mimicking a human expert. *Circ Cardiovasc Imaging.* 2019;12. doi: 10.1161/CIRCIMAGING.119.009303

35. Zhang J, Gajjala S, Agrawal P, et al. Fully automated echocardiogram interpretation in clinical practice. *Circulation.* 2018;138(16):1623-1635. doi:10.1161/CIRCULATIONAHA.118.034338

36. Tran PV. A fully convolutional neural network for cardiac segmentation in short-axis MRI. 2016. https://arxiv.org/abs/1604.00494. Accessed April 27, 2017.

37. Lin DJ, Johnson PM, Knoll F, Lui YW. Artificial intelligence for MR image reconstruction: an overview for clinicians. *J Magn Reson Imaging.* 2020. doi:10.1002/jmri.27078

38. Bai W, Sinclair M, Tarroni G, et al. Automated cardiovascular magnetic resonance image analysis with fully convolutional networks. *J Cardiovasc Magn Reson.* 2018;20(1):65. doi:10.1186/s12968-018-0471-x

39. van den Oever LB, Vonder M, van Assen M, et al. Application of artificial intelligence in cardiac CT: from basics to clinical practice. *Eur J Radiol.* 2020. doi:10.1016/j.ejrad.2020.108969

40. Hampe N, Wolterink JM, van Velzen SGM, Leiner T, Išgum I. Machine learning for assessment of coronary artery disease in cardiac CT: a survey. *Front Cardiovasc Med.* 2019;6:172. doi:10.3389/fcvm.2019.00172

41. Galloway CD, Valys AV, Shreibati JB, et al. Development and validation of a deep-learning model to screen for hyperkalemia from the electrocardiogram. *JAMA Cardiol.* 2019;4(5):428-436. doi:10.1001/jamacardio.2019.0640

42. Hannun AY, Rajpurkar P, Haghpanahi M, et al. Cardiologist-level arrhythmia detection and classification in ambulatory electrocardiograms using a deep neural network. *Nat Med.* 2019;25(1):65-69. doi:10.1038/s41591-018-0268-3 [published correction appears in *Nat Med.* 2019 Mar;25(3):530]

43. Attia ZI, Noseworthy PA, Lopez-Jimenez F, et al. An artificial intelligence-enabled ECG algorithm for the identification of patients with atrial fibrillation during sinus rhythm: a retrospective analysis of outcome prediction. *Lancet.* 2019;394(10201):861-867. doi:10.1016/S0140-6736(19)31721-0

44. Attia ZI, Kapa S, Lopez-Jimenez F, et al. Screening for cardiac contractile dysfunction using an artificial intelligence-enabled electrocardiogram. *Nat Med.* 2019;25(1):70-74. doi:10.1038/s41591-018-0240-2

45. Kwon JM, Jeon KH, Kim HM, et al. Comparing the performance of artificial intelligence and conventional diagnosis criteria for detecting left ventricular hypertrophy using electrocardiography. *Europace.* 2020;22(3):412-419. doi:10.1093/europace/euz324

46. Kwon JM, Kim KH, Jeon KH, et al. Development and validation of deep-learning algorithm for electrocardiography-based heart failure identification. *Korean Circ J.* 2019;49(7):629-639. doi:10.4070/kcj.2018.0446

47. Kagiyama N, Piccirilli M, Yanamala N, et al. Machine learning assessment of left ventricular diastolic function based on electrocardiographic features. *J Am Coll Cardiol.* 2020;76(8):930-941. doi:10.1016/j.jacc.2020.06.061

48. Cho H, Lee JG, Kang SJ, et al. Angiography-based machine learning for predicting fractional flow reserve in intermediate coronary artery lesions. *J Am Heart Assoc.* 2019;8(4):e011685. doi:10.1161/JAHA.118.011685

49. Nakajima K, Kudo T, Nakata T, et al. Diagnostic accuracy of an artificial neural network compared with statistical quantitation of myocardial perfusion images: a Japanese multicenter study. *Eur J Nucl Med Mol Imaging.* 2017;44:2280–2289.

50. Betancur J, Commandeur F, Motlagh M, et al. Deep learning for prediction of obstructive disease from fast myocardial perfusion SPECT: a multicenter study. *JACC Cardiovasc Imaging.* 2018;11:1654–1663.

51. Su S, Hu Z, Lin Q, et al. An artificial neural network method for lumen and media-adventitia border detection in IVUS. *Comput Med Imaging Graph.* 2017;57:29–39.

52. Abdolmanafi A, Duong L, Dahdah N, et al. Deep feature learning for automatic tissue classification of coronary artery using optical coherence tomography. *Biomed Opt Express.* 2017;8:1203–1220

53. Au-Yeung WM, Reinhall PG, Bardy GH, Brunton SL. Development and validation of warning system of ventricular tachyarrhythmia in patients with heart failure with heart rate variability data. *PloS One.* 2018;13(11). doi:10.1371/journal.pone.0207215

54. Shakibfar S, Krause O, Lund-Andersen C, et al. Predicting electrical storms by remote monitoring of implantable cardioverter-defibrillator patients using machine learning. *Europace.* 2019;21(2):268-274. doi:10.1093/europace/euy257

55. Kwon JM, Kim KH, Jeon KH, Park J. Deep learning for predicting in-hospital mortality among heart disease patients based on echocardiography. *Echocardiography.* 2019;36(2):213-218. doi:10.1111/echo.14220

56. Motwani M, Dey D, Berman DS, et al. Machine learning for prediction of all-cause mortality in patients with suspected coronary artery disease: a 5-year multicentre prospective registry analysis. *Eur Heart J.* 2017;38(7):500-507. doi:10.1093/eurheartj/ehw188

57. Samad MD, Ulloa A, Wehner GJ, et al. Predicting survival from large echocardiography and electronic health record datasets: optimization with machine learning. *JACC Cardiovasc Imaging.* 2019;12(4):681-689. doi:10.1016/j.jcmg.2018.04.026

58. Wiens J, Horvitz E, Guttag JV. Patient risk stratification for hospital-associated C. diff as a time-series classification task. In: *Advances in Neural Information Processing Systems 25 (NIPS 2012).* http://papers.nips.cc/paper/4525-patient-risk-stratification-for-hospital-associated-c-diff-as-a-time-series-classification-task. Accessed September 24, 2020.

59. Henry KE, Hager DN, Pronovost PJ, Saria S. A targeted real-time early warning score (TREWScore) for septic shock. *Sci Translation Med.* 2015;7(299):299ra122. doi: 10.1126/scitranslmed.aab3719.

60. Mortazavi BJ, Downing NS, Bucholz EM, et al. Analysis of machine learning techniques for heart failure readmissions. *Circ Cardiovasc Qual Outcomes.* 2016;9:629–640.

61. Huang C, Li SX, Mahajan S, et al. Development and validation of a model for predicting the risk of acute kidney injury associated with contrast volume levels during percutaneous coronary intervention. *JAMA Netw Open.* 2019;2(11):e1916021. doi:10.1001/jamanetworkopen.2019.16021

62. Rajkomar A, Oren E, Chen K, et al. Scalable and accurate deep learning with electronic health records. *NPJ Digit Med.* 2018;1:18. doi:10.1038/s41746-018-0029-1

63. Loring Z, Mehrotra S, Piccini JP, et al. Machine learning does not improve upon traditional regression in predicting outcomes in atrial fibrillation: an analysis of the ORBIT-AF and GARFIELD-AF registries. *Europace.* 2020. doi:10.1093/europace/euaa172

64. Krumholz HM. The promise of big data: opportunities and challenges. *Circ Cardiovasc Qual Outcomes.* 2016;9(6):616-617. doi:10.1161/CIRCOUTCOMES.116.003366

65. Chen JH, Asch SM. Machine learning and prediction in medicine-beyond the peak of inflated expectations. *N Engl J Med.* 2017;376:2507–2509.

66. Shah RU, Rumsfeld JS. Big data in cardiology: will big data lead to big improvements in cardiovascular care? *Eur Heart J.* 2017;38(24):1865-1867. doi: https://doi.org/10.1093/eurheartj/ehx284

67. Stead WW. Clinical implications and challenges of artificial intelligence and deep learning. *JAMA.* 2018;320(11):1107-1108. doi:10.1001/jama.2018.11029

68. Maddox TM, Rumsfeld JS, Payne PRO. Questions for artificial intelligence in health care. *JAMA.* 2019;321(1):31-32. doi: 10.1001/jama.2018.18932

69. Wiens J, Saria S, Sendak M, et al. Do no harm: a roadmap for responsible machine learning for health care. *Nat Med.* 2019;25(9):1337-1340. doi: 10.1038/s41591-019-0548-6. [Erratum in: *Nat Med.* 2019 Oct;25(10):1627]

70. Reddy S, Allan S, Coghlan S, Cooper P. A governance model for the application of AI in health care. *J Am Med Informat Assoc.* 2000;27(3):491-497. doi: 10.1093/jamia/ocz192

71. Harrell F. Is medicine mesmerized by machine learning? *Statistical Thinking.* February 1, 2018. https://www.fharrell.com/post/medml/. Accessed September 15, 2020.

72. Char DS, Shah NH, Magnus D. Implementing machine learning in health care – addressing ethical challenges. *N Engl J Med.* 2018;378(11):981-983. doi: 10.1056/NEJMp1714229

73. Gianfrancesco MA, Tamang S, Yazdany J, Schmajuk G. Potential biases in machine learning algorithms using electronic health record data. *JAMA Intern Med.* 2018;178(11):1544-1547. doi: 10 .1001/jamainternmed.2018.3763

74. Ramesh S. A checklist to protect human rights in artificial-intelligence research. *Nature.* 2017;552:334–334

75. Liu P, Astudillo K, Velez D, et al. Use of mobile health applications in low-income populations: a prospective study of facilitators and barriers. *Circ Cardiovasc Qual Outcomes.* 2020;13. doi: 10.1161/CIRCOUTCOMES.120.007031

76. Yusuf M, Atal I, Li J, et al. Reporting quality of studies using machine learning models for medical diagnosis: a systematic review. *BMJ Open* 2020;10. doi:10.1136/ bmjopen-2019-034568

77. Sengupta PP, Shrestha S, Berthon B, et al. Proposed requirements for cardiovascular imaging-related machine learning evaluation (PRIME): a checklist: reviewed by the American College of Cardiology Healthcare Innovation Council. *JACC Cardiovasc Imaging.* 2020;13(9):2017-2035. doi: 10.1016/j.jcmg.2020.07.015.

78. Stevens LM, Mortazavi BJ, Deo RC, Curtis L, Kao DP. Recommendations for reporting machine learning analyses in clinical research. *Circ Cardiovasc Qual Outcomes.* 2020;13(10). doi: 10.1161/CIRCOUTCOMES.120.006556

79. Software as a Medical Device Working Group. *Software as a Medical Device (SaMD): Clinical Evaluation.* International Medical Device Regulators Forum (IMDRF); 2017. http://www.imdrf.org/docs/imdrf/final/technical/imdrf-tech-170921-samd-n41-clinical-evaluation_1.pdf

80. US Food and Drug Administration and Center for Devices and Radiologic Health Digital Health Program. *Digital Health Action Plan.* Maryland: FDA; 2018. https://www.fda.gov/media/106331/download

81. US Food and Drug Administration. *Proposed Regulatory Framework for Modifications to Artificial Intelligence/Machine Learning (AI/ML)-Based Software as a Medical Device (SaMD).* Maryland: FDA; 2020. https://www.fda.gov/medical-devices/software-medical-device-samd/artificial-intelligence-and-machine-learning-software-medical-device

82. Japsen, B. Healthcare's artificial intelligence market may hit $6 Billion. *Forbes.* March 6, 2018. https://www.forbes.com/sites/brucejapsen/2018/03/06/healthcares-artificial-intelligence-market-may-hit-6-billion/#57295d25292a. Accessed September 1, 2020.

83. Markets and Markets. Artificial intelligence in healthcare market worth $45.2 billion by 2026. *Cision PR Newswire.* June 9, 2020. https://www.prnewswire.com/news-releases/artificial-intelligence-in-healthcare-market-worth-45-2-billion-by-2026---exclusive-report-by-marketsandmarkets-301072636.html. Accessed September 1, 2020.

84. Verghese A, Shah NH, Harrington RA. What this computer needs is a physician: humanism and artificial intelligence. *JAMA.* 2018;319(1):19-20. doi: 10.1001/jama.2017.19198

85. Topol EJ. High-performance medicine: the convergence of human and artificial intelligence. *Nat Med.* 2019;25:44–56. doi: 10.1038/s41591-018-0300-7

86. Leeson P, Fletcher AJ. Combining artificial intelligence with human insight to automate echocardiography. *Circ Cardiovasc Imaging.* 2019;12(9). doi: 10.1161/CIRCIMAGING.119.009727

87. Sengupta PP, Adjeroh DA. Will artificial intelligence replace the human echocardiographer? *Circulation.* 2018;138(16):1639-1642. doi: 10.1161/CIRCULATIONAHA.118.037095

88. Walsh MN, Rumsfeld JS. Leading the digital transformation of healthcare: the ACC Innovation Strategy. *J Am Coll Cardiol.* 2017;70(21):2719-2722. doi: 10.1016/j.jacc.2017.10.020

84

Cardiovascular Manifestations of COVID-19

Sean P. Pinney, Gennaro Giustino, and Jeffrey I. Mechanick

Cardiovascular manifestations of COVID-19

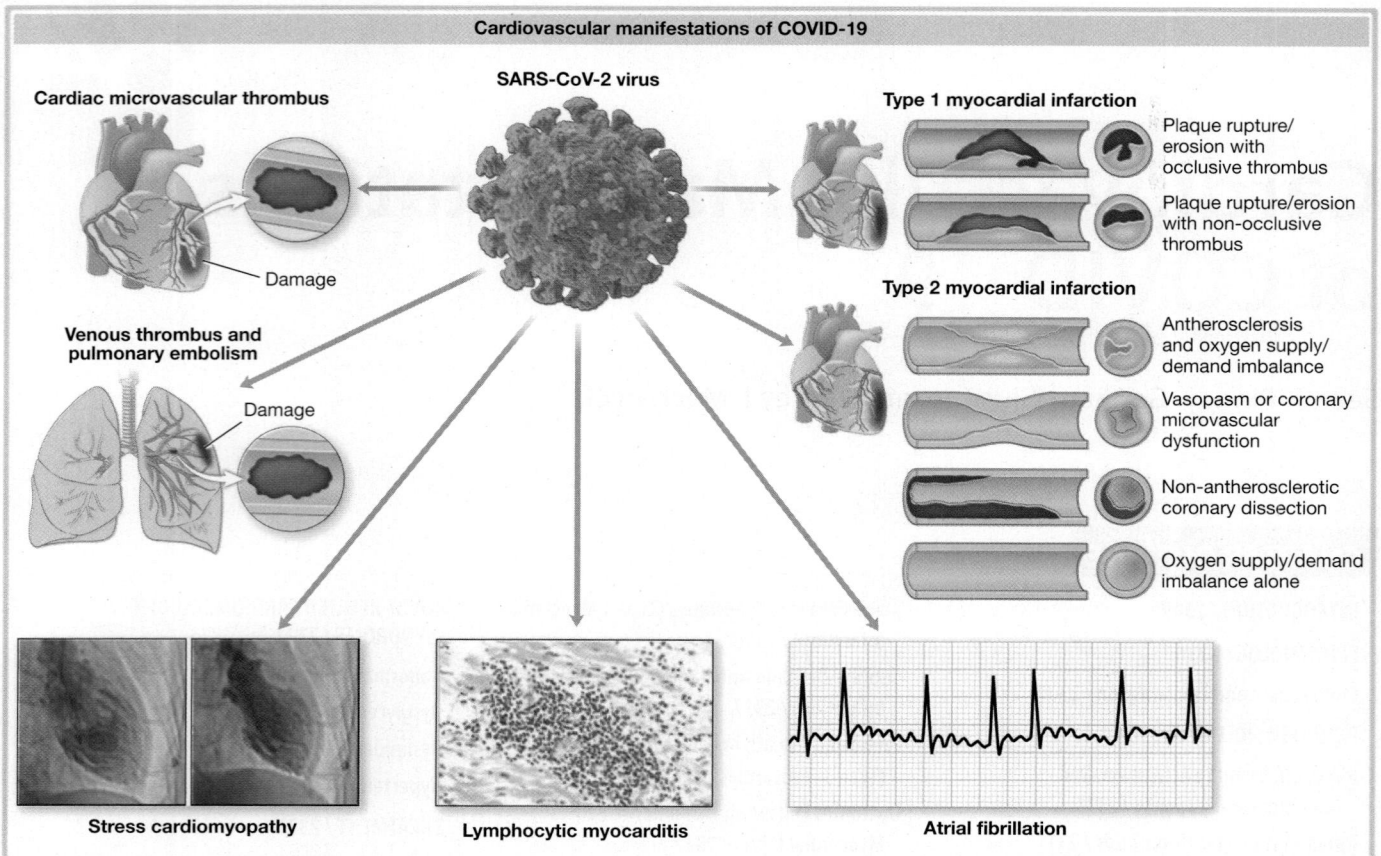

Cardiac microvascular thrombus

Damage

Venous thrombus and pulmonary embolism

Damage

SARS-CoV-2 virus

Type 1 myocardial infarction

Plaque rupture/erosion with occlusive thrombus

Plaque rupture/erosion with non-occlusive thrombus

Type 2 myocardial infarction

Antherosclerosis and oxygen supply/demand imbalance

Vasopasm or coronary microvascular dysfunction

Non-antherosclerotic coronary dissection

Oxygen supply/demand imbalance alone

Stress cardiomyopathy

Lymphocytic myocarditis

Atrial fibrillation

Chapter 84 Fuster and Hurst's Central Illustration. Primarily a respiratory virus, SARS-CoV-2 can produce an inflammatory and hypercoaguable state that broadly impacts the cardiovascular system. Cardiovascular manifestations of COVID-19 include myocardial infarction (Type 2 > Type 1), cardiac arrhythmias, venous thromboembolic disease and microvascular thrombosis resulting in multi-organ failure. Lymphocytic myocarditis and stress cardiomyopathy (Takotsubo) have been reported but are not a common feature of COVID-19. The stress cardiomyopathy and lymphocytic myocarditis images were reproduced with permission from Giustino G, Pinney SP, Lala A, et al. Coronavirus and Cardiovascular Disease, Myocardial Injury, and Arrhythmia, JACC Focus Seminar. *J Am Coll Cardiol*. 2020 Oct 27;76(17):2011-2023.

CHAPTER SUMMARY

This chapter reviews the current understanding of cardiovascular manifestations of COVID-19. Although primarily a respiratory virus, SARS-CoV-2 can produce an inflammatory reaction manifested by cytokine storm, endothelial activation, and hypercoaguability that can broadly affect the cardiovascular system (see Fuster and Hurst's Central Illustration). Initial binding of the virus's spike protein to the angiotensin-converting enzyme 2 (ACE-2) receptor on vascular endothelium sets off a chain of events resulting in loss of ACE-2 receptor density, down-regulation of ACE-2 activity, and accumulation of angiotensin II leading to a vasoactive state that is profibrotic, hypertrophic, and vasoconstrictive. Evidence of myocardial injury (eg, elevated troponin) is common in hospitalized patients. It is usually minor in degree but is associated with more severe illness and higher mortality. Venous thromboembolism, arterial thrombosis, and microvascular thrombi occur more commonly in severe COVID-19 and may result in multiorgan failure. Epidemiological and mechanistic associations of cardiometabolic-based chronic disease with COVID-19 substantiate a COVID-related cardiometabolic syndrome (CIRCS) spanning the pre-, acute-, and postinfection stages propelled by four key metabolic drivers: abnormal adiposity, dysglycemia, dyslipidemia, and hypertension. Treatment with anticoagulants, antiviral agents, and corticosteroids have some demonstrated efficacy, with additional clinical trial evidence forthcoming.

INTRODUCTION

In December 2019, a cluster of pneumonia cases from an unknown etiology emerged in Wuhan, China.[1] Originating from a wet market, the source of these infections was later identified as SARS-CoV-2 and the clinical syndrome it produced became labeled as COVID-19. What started as a local cluster spread rapidly from Asia to Europe and the United States. The World Health Organization declared a global pandemic on March 11, 2020, and 9 months later there were more than 70 million reported cases and 1.5 million deaths worldwide. Although initial attention was focused on its pulmonary involvement, it soon became apparent that COVID-19 was a multisystem inflammatory and thrombotic disorder that both directly and indirectly affected the cardiovascular system.[2,3] This chapter will focus on the cardiovascular manifestations of COVID-19 by discussing its epidemiology, pathophysiology, clinical manifestations, and reported outcomes. The full extent and impact of postacute sequelae of COVID-19 (PASC) are not yet known, but are expected to have lasting implications for cardiovascular health.

EPIDEMIOLOGY

Global Cases and Transmission

As of November 2021, more than 250 million cases of COVID-19 infection and 5.1 million deaths related to COVID-19 were reported worldwide, across all continents (Figs. 84–1A and 84–1B). However, it should be noted the reported case counts underestimate the overall burden of COVID-19, because only a fraction of acute infections was diagnosed and reported particularly at the beginning of the pandemic in part due to the lack of universal testing and access to healthcare systems.[4] In addition, it is likely that a large number of individuals with asymptomatic COVID-19 infection have remained undiagnosed. In fact, seroprevalence surveys in the United States and Europe have suggested that the rate of prior exposure to SARS-CoV-2, as reflected by the presence of detectable anti-SARS-CoV-2 antibodies, exceeds the incidence of reported cases by 10-fold or more.[4-6]

The detailed mechanisms and patterns of transmission of COVID-19 are still unclear. Direct person-to-person respiratory transmission is the primary means of transmission of the virus mostly through close-range contact (eg, within 2 m) via respiratory droplets from an infected person.[7,8] Infection might also occur if a person's hands are contaminated by droplets or by touching contaminated surfaces and then they touch their eyes, nose, or mouth. Transmission can also occur via direct contact by touching contaminated surfaces and then mucous membranes. SARS-CoV-2 can also be transmitted longer distances through the airborne route (through inhalation of particles smaller than droplets that remain in the air over time and distance) but the contribution of this route to the overall transmission burden is unclear.[7,8] Several studies have the potential for longer distance airborne transmission in enclosed, poorly ventilated spaces, as well as hospital ventilation systems.[8] SARS-CoV-2 has also been detected in nonrespiratory

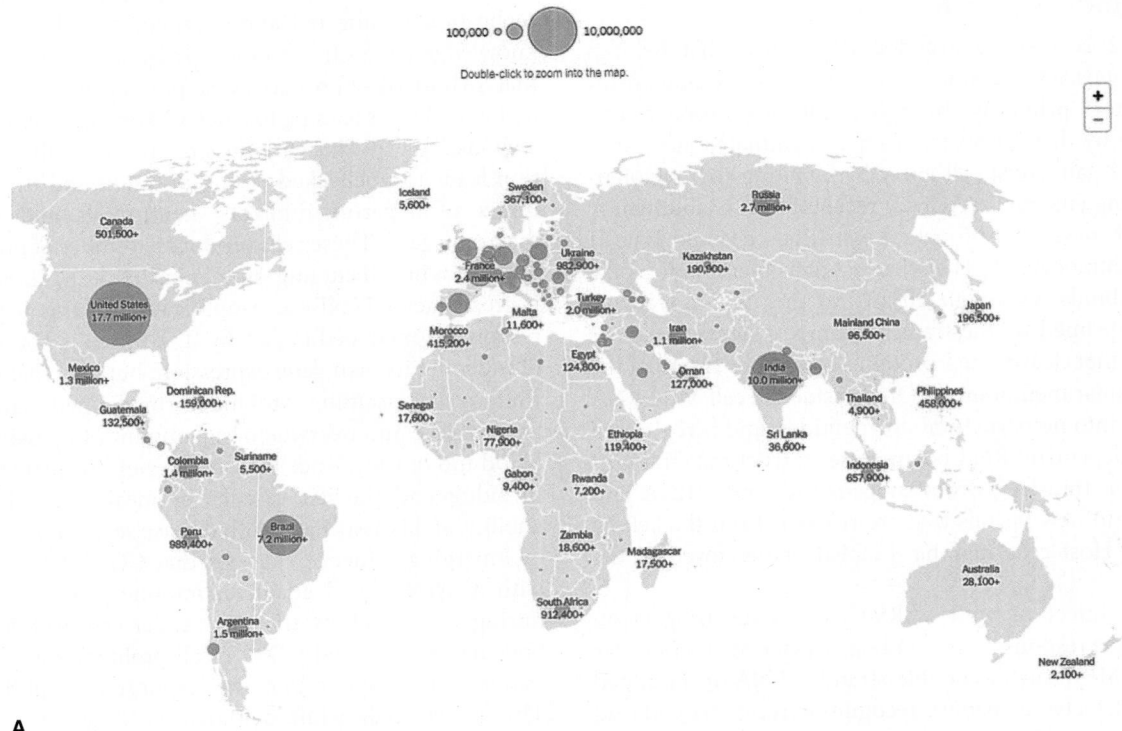

A

Figure 84–1. (A) Confirmed cases and (B) mortalities from COVID-19 as per March 2021.

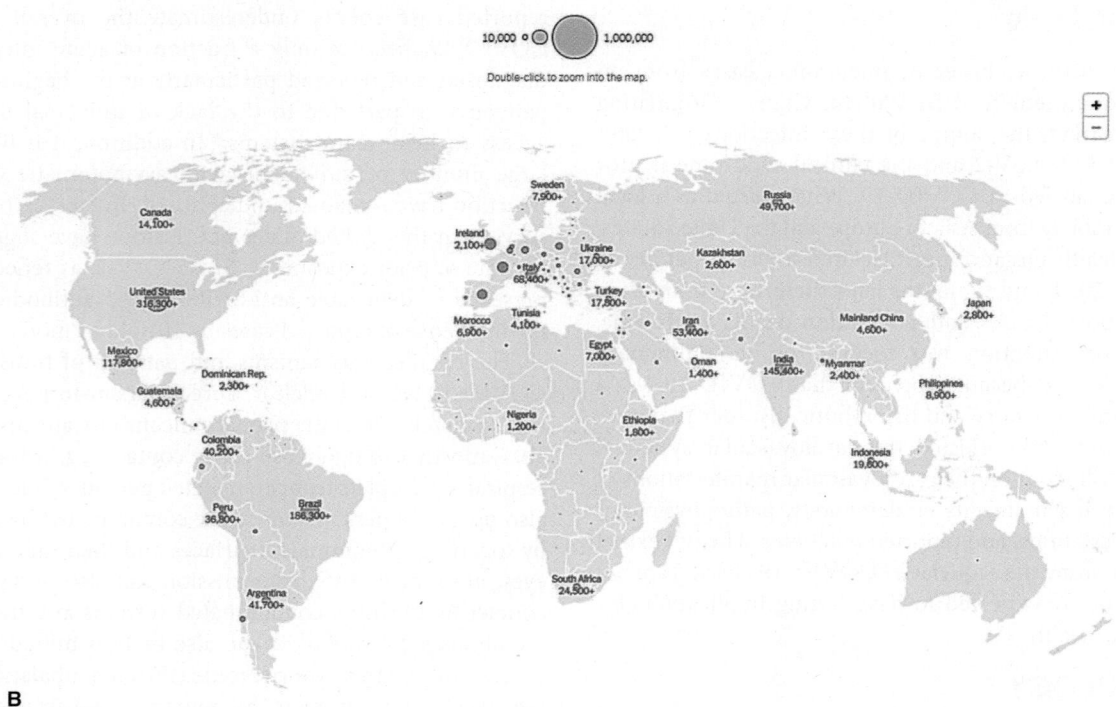

B

Figure 84–1. (Continued)

specimens such as stool, blood, or ocular secretions but the role of these sites in transmission is uncertain.[9,10]

PATHOPHYSIOLOGY

Infection, Immune Activation, and Inflammatory Response

SARS-CoV-2 is a single-stranded RNA virus that belongs to the *Coronaviridae* family. It can be spread by human-to-human contact primarily through respiratory droplets, and occasionally by direct transfer from contaminated surfaces.[11] SARS-CoV-2 gains host cell entry by targeting the angiotensin-converting enzyme 2 (ACE-2) receptor that is abundantly expressed on nasal and bronchial epithelial cells and type II alveolar pneumocytes.[12] The virus's outer membrane spike protein (S) binds with high affinity to the ACE-2 receptor and is then primed by the transmembrane protease serine 2 (TMPRSS2) that cleaves the S protein allowing for fusion of the viral and cellular membranes.[13] Once inside the cell, viral RNA is translated into nonstructural polypeptides, and is replicated by an RNA-dependent RNA polymerase.[14] Structural viral proteins are then translated from subgenomic viral mRNA and assembled into new virions that are released from the cell by exocytosis.[14] Host cells may be disabled or destroyed in the process.[15]

Host cell infection with SARS-CoV-2 virus triggers an innate immune response. Viral pathogen-associated molecular patterns (PAMPs), such as double-stranded RNA or uncapped mRNA, are detected by pattern recognition receptors and lead to the production of type 1 interferon (IFN) and other proinflammatory cytokines.[16,17] Type I IFNs signal through IFNα/β

receptor and downstream molecules, such as signal transducer and activator of transcription (STAT) proteins, to stimulate the production of antiviral proteins that are encoded by interferon stimulated genes (ISGs). This type 1 IFN response, consisting of the production of proinflammatory cytokines, IFN and antiviral proteins, is responsible for limiting viral replication in infected and neighboring cells.[16] Based upon knowledge from other *Coronaviridae* infections, it is thought that SARS-CoV-2 produces viral proteins that inhibit host signaling pathways leading to a delayed or suppressed type 1 IFN response.[12,14,16,17] This early loss of control at the site of infection leads to unchecked viral replication and the subsequent influx of hyperinflammatory neutrophils and monocytes/macrophages.[17] These cells produce a number of proinflammatory cytokines including interleukin (IL)-1β, IL-6, and tissue necrosis factor (TNF)-α. Amplification of this hyperimmune response is mediated in part by IL-1 which is not only capable of inducing its own gene expression, but also that of IL-6 and TNF-α.[3] The resulting cytokine storm, defined as the release of an excessive and overwhelming amount of cytokines into the blood too quickly, leads to a number of downstream sequelae including endotheliitis, vascular permeability, and hypercoaguability, and is associated with disease severity and death.[4,18]

Emerging evidence suggests that COVID-19 is associated with a dysregulated adaptive immune response.[19] Typically, during acute viral infections, viral-derived peptides stimulate both naïve CD8+ and CD4+ T-cell proliferation and differentiation. This adaptive immune response is amplified by Th1/Th17 CD4+ cells while cytotoxic CD8+ are responsible for killing viral-infected cells. Antigen presenting cells expressing MHC II, such as macrophages and some lung endothelial cells, activate CD4+ cells, which in turn induce B-cells into antibody-producing plasma cells. In the case of SARS-CoV-2, detectable levels of neutralizing IgM and IgG are typically present within 2 weeks of infection.[17] In cases of chronic viral infection, evasion or suppression of adaptive immune responses must be present for the virus to persist.[19] Given its subacute presentation and the frequent finding of lymphopenia, it is thought that SARS-CoV-2 infection exhibits features suggestive of both immune suppression and exhaustion.[19] Lung-infiltrating T-cells have gene expression patterns and molecular transcripts that mirror that of exhausted CD8+ cells while immune senescence is postulated to be one of the reasons why COVID-19 is more often severe and fatal in elderly persons.[19] Younger patients are advantaged over the elderly not only because they are thought to have more robust innate immune responses, but also because older persons have fewer naïve T-cells with proliferative capacity.[20]

The critical linkage between SARS-CoV-2 infection and severe COVID-19 is provided by the vascular endothelium.[3,21] This monolayer that lines arteries, veins, and capillaries performs a number of homeostatic functions including the maintenance of vascular integrity, promotion of vasomotion, and avoidance of thrombosis. These homeostatic functions are disrupted when the endothelium becomes activated by exposure to inflammatory cytokines, damage-associated molecular patterns (DAMPs) from necrotic cells, or PAMPs from viral or bacterial invasion. Following SARS-CoV-2 infection and subsequent cytokine storm, lung endothelial cells contribute to the development and propagation of acute respiratory distress syndrome (ARDS) by increasing vascular permeability and leakage. This occurs through viral-induced cell death and lysis; reduced ACE-2 activity and indirect activation of the kallikrein–bradykinin pathway, increasing vascular permeability; recruitment of reactive oxygen species by activated neutrophils recruited by inflamed endothelial cells; enhanced endothelial cell contractility and loosened inter-endothelial junctions; and IL-1β and TNF-α induced activation of glucuronidases that degrade the glycocalyx and upregulate hyaluronic acid synthase culminating in the deposition of hyaluronic acid in the extracellular space and the promotion of fluid retention.[21]

Inflammation and Thrombosis

In its homeostatic state, the endothelium rarely tilts toward thrombosis. When activated by inflammatory cytokines, PAMPs, or neutrophil extracellular traps (NETs), the endothelial surface becomes procoagulant.[22,23] It releases tissue factor, thromboxane, and preformed von Willebrand factor from Weibel–Palade bodies. The activated endothelium also antagonizes various antifibrinolytic activities by releasing plasminogen activator inhibitor (PAI)-1. Not only does SARS-CoV-2 infection create a prothrombotic endothelium, but is also produces to a systemic hypercoaguable state. Amplified IL-6 production, in part spurred on by IL-1, leads to enhanced hepatocyte production of both fibrinogen and PAI-1 in concert with CRP.[24] Pathologic evidence of endotheliitis across multiple vascular beds with mononuclear cell infiltrates invading the vascular endothelium triggering apoptosis and producing end-organ damage have been provided by autopsy studies.[25]

Central Role of ACE-2 in COVID-19

ACE-2 is expressed extensively throughout the circulatory system. Vascular smooth muscle coexpresses the ACE-2 receptor and TMPRSS2.[15] Similarly, both arterial and venous endothelial cells are characterized by high levels of ACE-2 receptor expression.[26] In the setting of SARS-CoV-2 infection, membrane-bound ACE-2 is internalized, leading to decreased receptor density. Because ACE-2 is primarily responsible for the conversion of angiotensin II (Ang II) to angiotensin-(1-7), there is a reduction in the amount of this protective, vasodilating peptide. Furthermore, the loss of ACE-2 receptor density and down-regulation of ACE-2 activity leads to an accumulation of Ang II leading to a vasoactive state that is profibrotic, hypertrophic, and vasoconstrictive[27] (**Fig. 84–2**). Increased binding of Ang II to the Ang II type 1 receptor (AT_1R) triggers a signaling cascade that leads to a disintegrin and metalloproteinase domain 17 (ADAM-17) phosphorylation and enhanced catalytic activity.[27,28] Activated ADAM-17 cleaves the ACE-2 receptor from its membrane bound domain thereby increasing ACE-2 shedding and further reducing Ang II clearance. This vicious positive feedback loop is further enhanced by additional ADAM-17 activities including the cleavage of TNF-α from its transmembrane domain. The resulting release of soluble TNF-α works in both an auto- and paracrine fashion to amplify the inflammatory cascade. After binding to its primary receptor, TNF-α itself stimulates ADAM-17 activity. The additional release of soluble TNF-α into the circulation, in combination with circulating cytokines IL-1 and -6, together contribute to the cytokine storm.

Early concern for the ongoing use of ACE inhibitors and angiotensin receptor blockers (ARBs) was centered on the uncertain role that these drugs may play in disease progression recognizing that SARS-CoV-2 gains cell entry after first binding to ACE-2, the expression of which may be indirectly enhanced by antagonizing the renin-angiotensin system.[29] Guidance provided by professional societies in the absence of outcomes data was to continue ACE inhibitors and ARBs believing that their antagonism of Ang II in the ongoing treatment of cardiovascular disorders likely produced a benefit that outweighed the theoretical risk of enhanced SARS-CoV-2 binding.[30,31] This advice was later underscored by observational and case control studies that failed to show an association between ACE inhibitor or ARB use and an increased likelihood of COVID-19–related hospitalization or mortality.[32-35] Whether ACE inhibitors or ARBs affect outcomes in patients hospitalized with COVID-19 was tested in a prospective, randomized clinical trial.[36] One hundred fifty-two patients were enrolled from 20 centers worldwide and randomized to either continuation or discontinuation of ACE inhibitor or ARB therapy. There was no difference in the global rank score outcome consisting of time to death, duration of mechanical ventilation, time on renal replacement or vasopressor therapy, and multiorgan dysfunction during the hospitalization. Currently, the

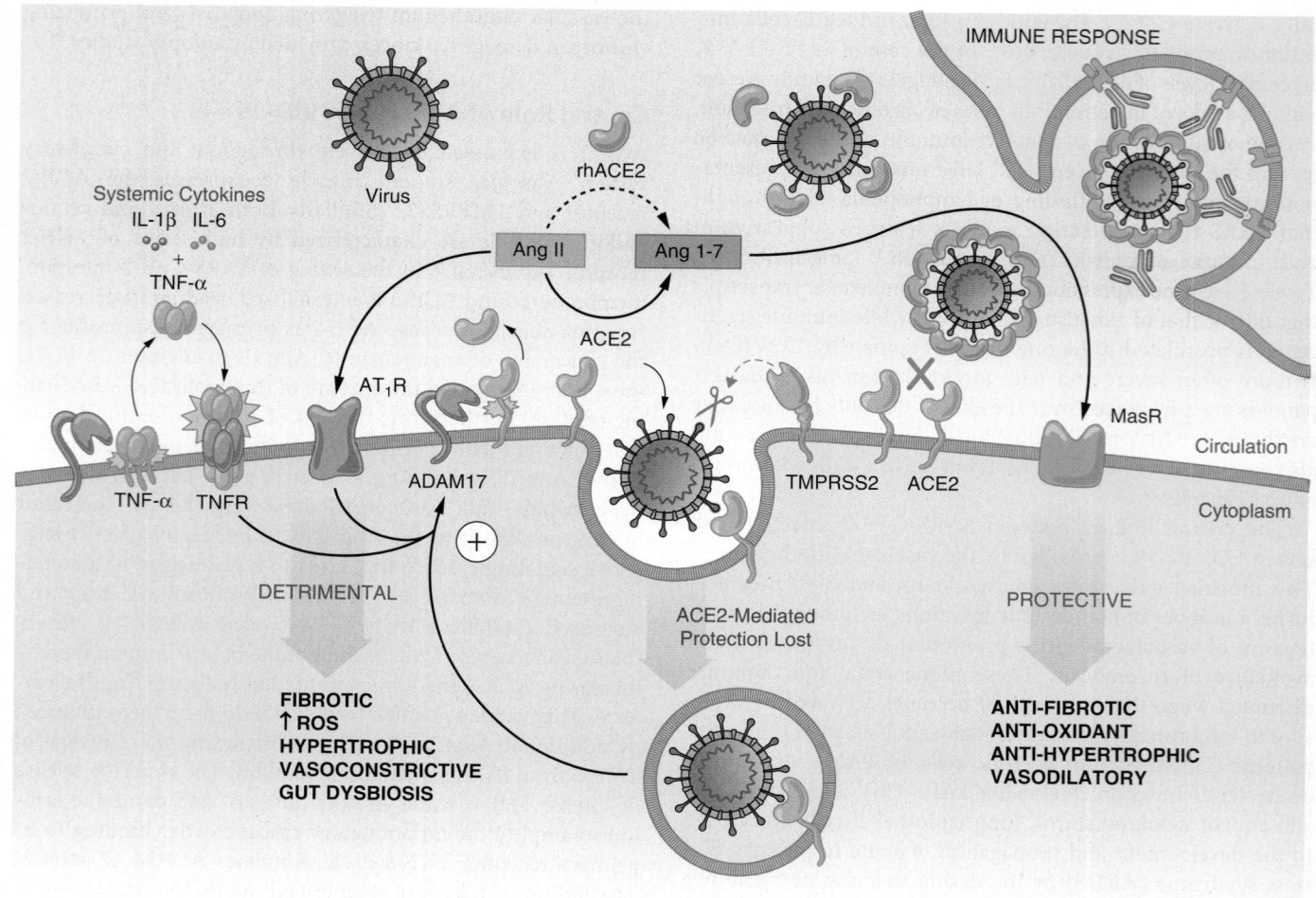

Figure 84–2. Central role of ACE-2, ADAM-17, inflammation, and thrombosis. Reproduced with permission from Gheblawi M, Wang K, Viveiros A, et al: Angiotensin-Converting Enzyme 2: SARS-CoV-2 Receptor and Regulator of the Renin-Angiotensin System: Celebrating the 20th Anniversary of the Discovery of ACE2. *Circ Res.* 2020 May 8;126(10):1456-1474.

weight of evidence supports continuing ACE inhibitor and ARB therapy in patients receiving these therapies for appropriate cardiovascular indications.

CLINICAL MANIFESTATIONS

Risk Factors

The risk of transmission from an individual with SARS-CoV-2 infection is influenced by different factors such as the type and duration of exposure, use of preventive measures, and patient-related factors (eg, the amount of viral shedding).[4,37–39] The risk of transmission after contact with an individual with COVID-19 increases with the closeness and duration of contact and appears highest with prolonged contact in indoor settings. In fact, most of the cases of infection have been described among household contacts followed by other congregate settings where individuals are residing or working closely.[40] Of course, workers in healthcare settings are also at high risk of exposure particularly if personal protective equipment or appropriate isolation measures are not used.[41]

Among individuals that get infected with SARS-CoV-2, development of severe COVID-19 infection predominantly occurs in individuals of advanced age and/or with preexisting comorbidities.[4,37–39] A summary of the recognized demographic, clinical, and laboratory risk factors for severe COVID-19 is reported in **Table 84–1**.[42–48] Age is one of the strongest risk factors for mortality associated with COVID-19. Based on data from the Chinese Center for Disease Control and Prevention Report that included 44,500 patients, the overall COVID-19 case-fatality rate was around 2.3%. This rate increases to 8.0% in patients 70 to 79 years, 14.8% in patients aged ≥80 years, and 49.0% in critically ill patients. Mild disease was observed in 81% of cases, severe disease (eg, dyspnea, hypoxia, or radiologic abnormalities) in 14% of cases, and critical disease in 5%. Similar mortality trends have been reported in Europe and the United States, with progressively higher case fatality rates per increase in age range with most deaths occurring in patients aged 60 years or more. Comorbidities and other conditions that have been associated with severe illness and mortality include cardiovascular diseases, diabetes mellitus, chronic

TABLE 84–1. Risk Factors of Severe COVID-19 Infection and In-Hospital Mortality

Demographic	• Advanced age • Male sex • Non-White race or ethnicity
Clinical	• Cardiovascular disease (eg, coronary artery disease, heart failure) • Chronic lung disease • Obesity • Chronic kidney disease • Solid or hematologic malignancy • Diabetes mellitus • Current smoking
Laboratory	• Elevated inflammatory markers (eg, C-reactive protein [CRP], ferritin) and inflammatory cytokines (ie, interleukin 6) • Elevated D-dimer • Elevated cardiac troponin (myocardial injury) • Elevate creatinine (acute kidney injury) • Elevated liver enzymes (liver injury) • Thrombocytopenia • Lymphopenia • Elevated lactate dehydrogenase

kidney disease, chronic lung disease, solid or hematological malignancies, obesity, and active smoking.[42-48] Among patients with both advanced age and medical comorbidities, COVID-19 infections are frequently severe and associated with a very high mortality rate. For example, in a SARS-CoV-2 outbreak across several long-term care facilities in Washington state, the median age was 83 years, and 94% had a chronic underlying condition.[49] The hospitalization and case fatality rates were 55% and 34%, respectively, higher than other reports.

Demographic and socioeconomic risk factors also play an important role. Male sex has been shown to be a risk factor for in-hospital mortality in many different cohorts across the globe. In unadjusted analyses, individuals of Black, Hispanic, and South Asian race or ethnicity had a higher number of infections and deaths related to COVID-19 in the United States, possibly due to preexisting health disparities.[50] For example, the Bronx (one of the five boroughs of New York City), which has the highest proportion of racial/ethnic minorities, the most persons living in poverty, and the lowest levels of educational attainment, had higher rates of hospitalization and death related to COVID-19 than the other four boroughs.[51] In contrast, the rates for hospitalizations and deaths were lowest among residents of the most affluent borough, Manhattan, which is composed of a predominately White population.[51] However, other studies have not found an association between Black race and worse COVID-19 outcomes when adjusting for baseline confounders.[52]

Symptoms and Disease Manifestation

The clinical manifestations of COVID-19 encompass a broad clinical spectrum from asymptomatic infection, to mild non-specific symptoms to severe disease requiring hospitalization.[42-48] A summary of the symptoms at the time of clinical presentation,

laboratory characteristics, and in-hospital outcomes across large observational studies is reported in **Table 84–2** and a proposed staging system is illustrated in **Fig. 84–3**. The exact prevalence of asymptomatic COVID-19 infection is still unclear but has been estimated that asymptomatic cases account for approximately 40% to 45% of SARS-CoV-2 infections. Subjects with asymptomatic COVID-19 can transmit the virus to others similarly to symptomatic COVID-19. In a cohort study of symptomatic and asymptomatic patients with SARS-CoV-2 infection who were isolated in a community treatment center in Cheonan, Republic of Korea, the cycle threshold (Ct) values in RT-PCR for SARS-CoV-2 detection were similar between symptomatic and asymptomatic individuals, suggesting that the viral load and shedding is not influenced by the presence of symptoms and underscoring the importance of social distancing and universal masking in order to reduce the spread.

Subjects with mild COVID-19 may experience symptoms similar to other respiratory viral diseases including fever or chills, cough, shortness of breath, palpitations, fatigue, muscle or body aches, headache, new anosmia or dysgeusia, sore throat, nausea or vomiting, and diarrhea.[42-48] In a multicenter registry from China including 1099 patients from 552 hospitals, the most common presenting symptoms included cough (67.8%), fever (43.8%), and fatigue (38.1%).[13] The estimated median incubation period for COVID-19 is 5 days from exposure. Both mild symptomatic and asymptomatic infections may be associated with subclinical lung abnormalities, as detected by computed tomography (CT). Most patients with mild symptomatic will resolve their symptoms in 5 to 10 days with only supportive care without requiring hospitalization.

Severe Disease

Around 10% of all patients with COVID-19 infection will progress to a more severe disease stage requiring medical care and/or hospitalization.[42-48] Patients who progress to more severe stages of the disease are more likely to have preexisting medical conditions including chronic obstructive pulmonary disease, diabetes mellitus, hypertension, and coronary artery disease. More severe manifestations of the infection include worsening shortness of breath or dyspnea on exertion, fever that is refractory to antipyretic therapy, failure to thrive, and altered mental status. Most of the patients presenting with severe COVID-19 infection have signs of respiratory compromise including hypoxemia requiring supplemental oxygen therapy and bilateral infiltrates on chest x-ray or chest CT scan. In registry studies, the most frequent findings included bilateral multifocal opacities on chest radiography and ground-glass opacities on chest CT imaging (56.4%); however, some patients with COVID-19 may not have radiological abnormalities. The extent of radiological abnormalities has been shown to correlate with the severity of clinical presentation. On laboratory work-up, these patients will typically have leukopenia with lymphopenia and elevations in inflammatory biomarkers (eg, erythrocyte sedimentation rate, C-reactive protein, or interleukin-6) and D-dimer. Less frequently, patients may initially

TABLE 84–2. Clinical Characteristics and In-Hospital Outcomes in Selected Reports of Patients with COVID-19

	Guan et al. (42) (n = 1099)	Zhou et al. (43) (n = 191)	Bhatraju et al. (44) (n = 24)	Goyal et al. (45) (n = 393)	Richardson et al. (46) (n = 5700)	Cummings et al. (47) (n = 257)	Paranjpe et al. (2) (n = 2199)
Geographic region	China	China	Washington (US)	New York (US)	New York (US)	New York (US)	New York (US)
Demographics							
Age, years	47	56	64.0	62.2	63.0	62.0	65
Male sex	58.1%	62%	63.0%	60.6%	60.3%	67.0%	58.8%
Symptoms at presentation							
Fever	43.8%	94%	50.0%	77.1%	30.7%	71.0%	25%
Cough	67.8%	79%	88.0%	79.4%	-	66.0%	-
Fatigue	38.1%	23%	-	-	-	-	-
Shortness of breath	18.7%	-	88.0%	56.5%	-	74.0%	-
Nausea and/or vomiting	5.0%	4%	-	19.1%	-	-	-
Diarrhea	3.8%	5%	-	23.7%	-	12.0%	-
Myalgia or arthralgia	14.9%	15%	-	27.2%	-	26.0%	-
Chills	11.5%	-	-	-	-	-	-
Headache	13.6%	-	8.0%	-	-	4.0%	-
Time from symptoms to admission	-	11.0	7.0	5.0	-	5.0	-
Past medical history							
Hypertension	15.0%	30%	-	50.1%	56.6%	63.0%	37%
Diabetes mellitus	7.4%	19%	58.0%	25.2%	33.8%	36.0%	26.5%
Current or former smoker	14.5%	6%	22.0%	5.1%	15.6%	13.0%	-
Coronary artery disease	2.5%	8%	-	13.7%	11.1%	19.0%	15.6%
Cerebrovascular disease	1.4%	-	-	-	-	-	7%
Chronic kidney disease	0.7%	1%	21.0%	4.6%	5.0%	14.0%	9.4%
Asthma	-	-	14.0%	12.5%	9.0%	8.0%	8.2%
COPD	1.1%	3%	4.0%	5.1%	5.4%	9.0%	5.1%
Cancer	0.9%	1%	-	5.9%	6.0%	7.0%	6.9%
Immunodeficiency	0.2%	-	-	5.4%	1.8%	7.0%	-
Laboratory findings			-				
Leukocytosis	5.9%	21%	38.0%	13.0%	-	-	25%
Lymphopenia	83.2%	40%	75.0%	90.0%	60.0%	-	11%
Thrombocytopenia	36.2%	7%	-	27.0%	-	-	-
Elevated troponin	-	17.0%	-	4.5%	22.6%	-	-
Elevated creatinine	1.6%	4.0%	-	16.0%	-	-	-
Elevated c-reactive protein	60.7%	-	-	43.5%	-	-	-
Elevated ferritin	-	80.0%	-	66.2%	-	-	-
Elevated interleukin 6	-	9.0%	-	-	-	-	-
Elevated lactate dehydrogenase	41.0%	67.0%	-	-	-	-	-
Elevated D-dimer	46.4%	42.0%	-	36.4%	-	-	33%
Elevated procalcitonin	5.5%	9.0%	-	16.9%	-	-	28%
Elevated lactate	41.0%	67%	53.0%	-	-	-	51%
Elevated alanine aminotransferase	21.3%	31.0%	32.0%	32.0%	58.4%	-	-
Elevated aspartate aminotransferase	22.2%	-	41.0%	46.5%	39.0%	-	-

(Continued)

TABLE 84–2. Clinical Characteristics and In-Hospital Outcomes in Selected Reports of Patients with COVID-19 (Continued)

	Guan et al. (42) (n = 1099)	Zhou et al. (43) (n = 191)	Bhatraju et al. (44) (n = 24)	Goyal et al. (45) (n = 393)	Richardson et al. (46) (n = 5700)	Cummings et al. (47) (n = 257)	Paranjpe et al. (2) (n = 2199)
In-hospital outcomes							
Death	1.4%	28.3%	50.0%	10.2%	21.0%	39.0%	29%
ICU admission	5.0%	26.0%	100.0%	-	14.2%	100.0%	36%
Acute respiratory distress syndrome	3.4%	31.0%	75.0%	-	-	-	-
Mechanical ventilation	6.1%	17.0%	75.0%	33.1%	12.2%	79.0%	-
Shock	1.1%	20.0%	-	-	-	-	-
Acute kidney injury	0.5%	15.0%	-	-	22.2%	31.0%	-
Cardiac injury	-	17.0%	-	-	22.6%	-	-
Arrhythmias	-	-	-	7.4%	-	-	-
Use of ECMO	0.5%	2.0%	0.0%	-	-	3.0%	-

Abbreviations: COPD, chronic obstructive pulmonary disease; ECMO, extracorporeal membrane oxygenation; ICU, intensive care unit.

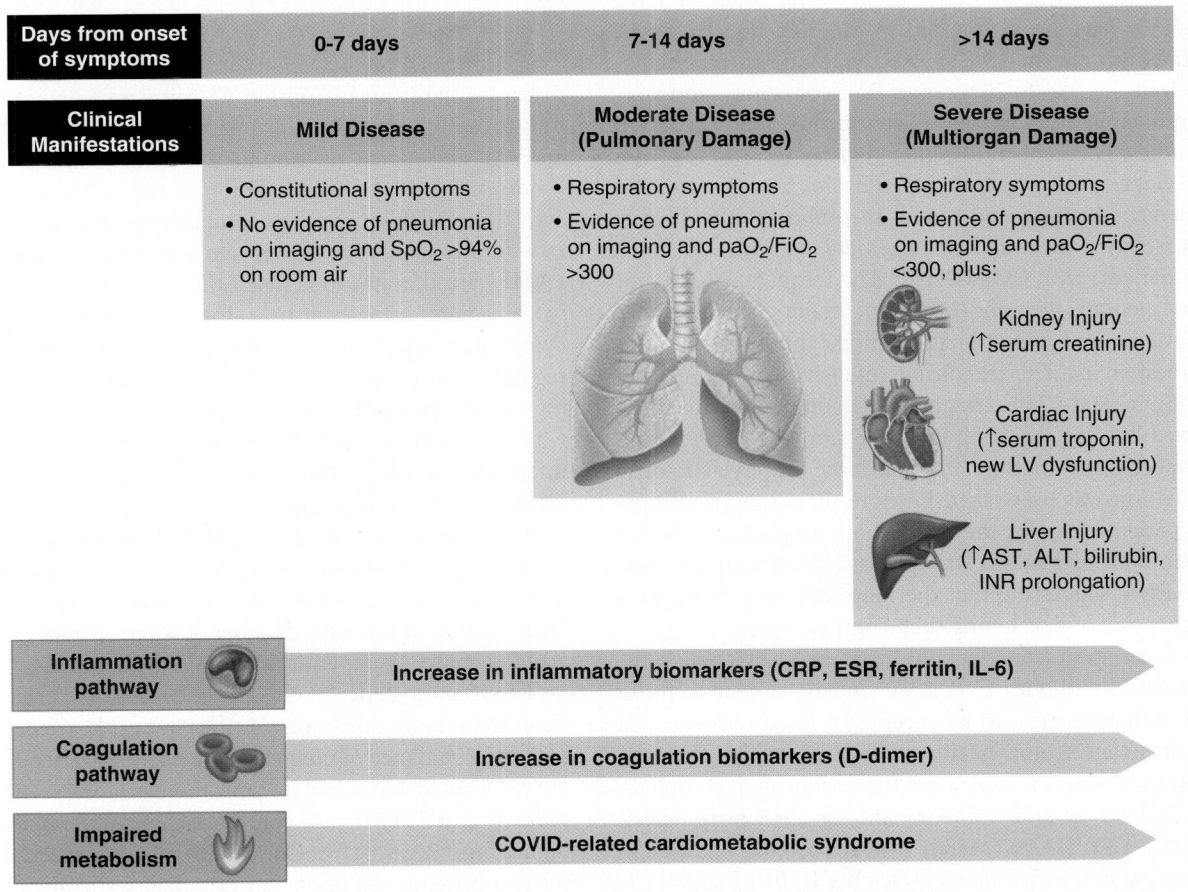

Figure 84–3. COVID-2019 produces a spectrum of clinical illness ranging from mild respiratory and constitutional symptoms to pneumonia with severe hypoxia and respiratory failure. Severe illness is associated with systemic inflammation and disturbances in coagulation leading to small- and large-vessel thrombosis. Myocardial injury when present is usually mild but associated with worse outcomes. ALT, alanine aminotransferase; AST, aspartate aminotransferase; CRP, C-reactive protein; ESR, erythrocyte sedimentation rate; FiO_2, fraction of inspired oxygen; IL, interleukin; INR, international normalized ratio; LV, left ventricular; paO_2, partial pressure of oxygen; SpO_2, blood oxygen saturation. Reproduced with permission from Pinney SP, Giustino G, Halperin JL, et al: Coronavirus Historical Perspective, Disease Mechanisms, and Clinical Outcomes: JACC Focus Seminar. *J Am Coll Cardiol.* 2020 Oct 27;76(17):1999-2010.

present with secondary COVID-19 complications, including thromboembolic events (eg, stroke, peripheral limb ischemia, pulmonary embolism), or end-organ damage, including myocardial injury, liver injury, and acute kidney injury, even in absence of predominant respiratory symptoms. Presence of these particular laboratory abnormalities at the time of clinical presentation have been associated with worse outcomes in multiple studies.

Clinical Outcomes

In-hospital mortality rates and need for intensive care are variable across published reports reflecting differences in demographic factors and the prevalence of preexisting comorbidities.[42–48] Acute respiratory distress syndrome (ARDS) is the most frequent COVID-19 complication ranging between 20% and 40% among hospitalized patients, and is strongly associated with higher risk of in-hospital mortality. Patients who require mechanical ventilation are at higher mortality risk compared with those managed with noninvasive ventilation, with very poor survival rates reported in the early studies (in-hospital mortality >90%).[42–48] The rates of other in-hospital complications associated with COVID-19 are also variable across studies, reflecting the different study populations. Rates of acute kidney injury have been reported in the 20% to 30% range, myocardial injury in the 15% to 30% range, and cardiocirculatory shock in the 10% to 20% range. Rates of venous and arterial thromboembolic events have been inconsistently reported across studies. A recent multicenter registry (n = 1114) from the Mass General Brigham integrated health network assessed the frequency of arterial and venous thromboembolic disease, risk factors, prevention and management patterns, and outcomes in patients with COVID-19.[53] The frequencies of major arterial or venous thromboembolism, major cardiovascular adverse events, and symptomatic venous thromboembolism were highest in patients requiring intensive care admission (35.3%, 45.9%, and 27.0%, respectively) compared with those hospitalized but not requiring intensive care (2.6%, 6.1%, and 2.2%, respectively). In this study, at least prophylactic-dose anticoagulation was prescribed in more than 80% of all hospitalized patients. Finally, the risk of both arterial and venous thromboembolic events was strongly associated with the presence of ARDS, suggesting that the more critically ill patients are at higher risk of developing such complications.

It has been speculated that the rates of in-hospital complications associated with COVID-19 maybe similar to those observed with influenza. More recently, a large retrospective analysis using electronic health records from the Veterans Health Administration compared the in-hospital complications of COVID-19 and influenza among 3948 hospitalized patients with COVID-19 (March 1–May 31, 2020) and 5453 hospitalized patients with influenza (October 1, 2018–February 1, 2020).[54] Patients with COVID-19 had almost 19 times the risk for ARDS than did patients with influenza, (adjusted risk ratio [aRR], 18.60; 95% confidence interval [CI], 12.40–28.00), and more than twice the risk for myocarditis, deep vein thrombosis, pulmonary embolism, intracranial hemorrhage, acute hepatitis/

liver failure, bacteremia, and pressure ulcers. The percentage of COVID-19 patients who died while hospitalized (21.0%) was more than 5 times that of influenza patients (3.8%), and the duration of hospitalization was almost 3 times longer for COVID-19 patients. These findings highlight the higher risk for most complications associated with COVID-19 compared with influenza and might aid clinicians and researchers in recognizing, monitoring, and managing the spectrum of COVID-19 manifestations.

CARDIOVASCULAR MANIFESTATIONS

COVID-19 can impact the cardiovascular system, and may produce complex and protean clinical presentations. Chest pain is a frequent complaint and may be a symptom of ischemic heart disease, pericarditis, myocarditis, stress cardiomyopathy, or coronary spasm.[55] Two particular challenges have emerged during this pandemic. The first is the need to appropriately manage patients presenting with cardiovascular disease and the second is overcoming the public's concern for safety in seeking care for heart disease.

Acute Coronary Syndromes (Type 1 Myocardial Infarction)

Type 1 myocardial infarction (MI) is caused by atherosclerotic disease with plaque disruption.[56] Several potential mechanisms link together systemic viral infection with plaque disruption and the subsequent development of acute coronary ischemic syndromes.[57] Viral PAMPs entering the systemic circulation activate cellular immune receptors expressed on existing atherosclerotic plaques and predispose to plaque rupture.[58] Such PAMPs are thought to activate the inflammasome and result in conversion of nascent procytokines into biologically active cytokines.[59] Infection and inflammation can also lead to dysregulation of coronary vascular endothelial function producing vasoconstriction and thrombosis.[60] In patients presenting with concomitant COVID-19 and ST-elevation myocardial infarction (STEMI), there has been a signal toward higher thrombus burden and poorer clinical outcomes.[61] Investigators from a single-center observational study reported higher levels of troponin T, D-dimer, and C-reactive protein in addition to higher rates of multivessel thrombosis and stent thrombosis. Such patients also required higher doses of unfractionated heparin to achieve therapeutic activated clotting times.[61]

The true incidence of COVID-related STEMI has been difficult to measure due to disruptions in healthcare delivery and patients' avoidance of medical centers.[62–67] In general, throughout the United States and Europe, there has been a 40% to 50% reduction in STEMI case volume with a corresponding 3-fold higher mortality rate.[62–67] Contributing to this uncertainty is the relative infrequency of performing diagnostic angiography in the setting of COVID-19 due to concerns regarding the safety of healthcare workers. To minimize viral transmission, cardiac catheterization with coronary angiography has been performed in a relatively small proportion of patients with symptoms and electrocardiographic evidence of acute myocardial injury.

One European registry study reported that 6609 patients underwent primary percutaneous coronary intervention (PCI) for STEMI in 2020 during the pandemic, representing a 19% reduction compared with preceding year.[68] Delays in PCI delivery characterized by late hospital presentation and prolonged door to balloon times may have contributed to the increased mortality observed during the pandemic. Recognizing the patient and provider challenges posed by providing STEMI care in a pandemic, professional societies have reaffirmed the primacy of PCI as the standard of care for STEMI patients at PCI-capable hospitals, assuming it can be provided in a timely fashion, with an expert team outfitted with personal protective equipment in a dedicated cardiac catheterization laboratory.[55,69,70] A fibrinolysis-based strategy may be entertained at non–PCI-capable referral hospitals or in specific situations where primary PCI cannot be executed or is not deemed the best option.[55]

Supply–Demand Imbalance (Type 2 Myocardial Infarction)

MI resulting from an imbalance between myocardial oxygen supply and demand is classified as Type 2 MI.[56] In particular, four specific mechanisms in the context of COVID-19 appear relevant: fixed coronary atherosclerosis limiting myocardial perfusion, endothelial dysfunction within the coronary microcirculation, severe systemic hypertension resulting from elevated circulating angiotensin II levels and intense arteriolar vasoconstriction, and hypoxemia resulting from ARDS or from in situ pulmonary vascular thrombosis. In the setting of sepsis, lung injury, and respiratory failure, severe physiological stress can be associated with elevations in biomarkers of myocardial strain and injury.[71–73] Individuals with atherosclerosis are susceptible to myocardial ischemia and infarction in the setting of systemic inflammatory states and severe infections, including H1N1 influenza and coronavirus pneumonia.[74–76] Infection in general, and pneumonia in particular, can disrupt the balance between myocardial oxygen supply and demand. The physiological demands triggered by systemic infection may be so great that this supply–demand imbalance may exist even in the absence of atherothrombotic plaques. It is challenging to distinguish patients with non-ST elevation myocardial infarction (NSTEMI) from those with myocarditis or demand-based myocardial injury in the setting of fever, tachycardia, or hypoxemia due to ARDS. It is very likely that multiple concurrent mechanisms of myocardial injury overlap within individual patients.

Similar to patients with STEMI, those presenting with NSTEMI during the pandemic were more likely to delay care, present later, and suffer higher rates of complications and death.[77,78] In one study from Berlin, time from symptom onset until first medical contact exceeded 72 hours in more than 28% of NSTEMI patients compared to only 6% in a comparable period prior to the pandemic.[78] Similarly, time from first medical contact to revascularization was significantly delayed in NSTEMI patients and was associated with lower left ventricular ejection fraction (LVEF) and higher levels of NT-proBNP at hospital discharge.

Prehospital Death in Cardiovascular Disease (Type 3 Myocardial Infarction)

Suspicion of MI without the ability to obtain biomarker confirmation is termed Type 3 MI. Sudden death and unexplained death at home in persons with known coronary heart disease suspected of having COVID-19 may very well be due Type 3 MI. During the surge of cases in New York and Italy, patients avoided hospital-based care out of fear of contracting COVID-19.[63,79] Observational studies have now recorded that almost half of the excess number of cardiovascular deaths attributed to the pandemic occurred in the community and many of which were not associated with COVID-19, further suggesting that persons delayed or avoided seeking medical attention.[80,81]

Outcomes Following Ischemic Myocardial Injury

Generally speaking, a few conclusions can be drawn about the impact of myocardial injury in the context of COVID-19. First, myocardial injury is prevalent among hospitalized COVID-19 patients. Second, troponin concentrations are generally present in low levels. Third, troponin elevation is associated with higher mortality for patients hospitalized with COVID-19.[82–85] An observational study of over 2700 hospitalized patients in New York City found that more than one-third (36%) had an elevated troponin level at the time of presentation.[82] Cardiovascular risk factors such as hypertension and diabetes were more prevalent in patients experiencing myocardial injury as was established cardiovascular disease including atrial fibrillation, coronary artery disease, and heart failure. After controlling for disease severity and the presence of cardiovascular disease, even small elevations of troponin were associated with a 75% increased risk of hospital mortality while higher admission levels (troponin I >0.09 ng/dL) were associated with a 3-fold higher risk.[82] The prevalence of myocardial injury and associated mortality are even greater for those patients with severe or critical COVID-19. Half of the patients requiring intubation and mechanical ventilation in one report from the Johns Hopkins Healthcare System had elevated troponin levels.[83] Those with levels exceeding 10 times the upper limit of normal had a mortality rate nearly 3 times higher than those without myocardial injury (61.5% vs 22.7%). After controlling for age, sex, and multisystem organ dysfunction, this association was no longer statistically different. Furthermore, and somewhat unexpectedly, the risk associated with COVID-19 myocardial injury appeared to be less significant than that associated with other forms of ARDS.[83] Among patients with COVID-19 who underwent transthoracic echocardiogram (TTE), cardiac structural abnormalities were present in nearly two-thirds of patients with myocardial injury.[84] Rates of in-hospital mortality were 5.2%, 18.6%, and 31.7% in patients without myocardial injury, with myocardial injury without TTE abnormalities, and with myocardial injury and TTE abnormalities. These findings help explain the observation that increased deaths in the early portion of the COVID-19 pandemic were attributable to ischemic heart disease and hypertensive diseases, even though deaths due to heart failure were unaffected.[85]

Additional insights into the etiology of myocardial injury are provided by an early study from Tel Aviv that sampled troponin levels and performed echocardiograms in 100 consecutive patients hospitalized with COVID-19.[86] Similar to other reports, 20% of these patients had elevated troponin levels consistent with myocardial injury. Rather than identify left ventricular (LV) dysfunction, investigators noted right ventricular (RV) enlargement or dysfunction in 39%. Ten percent had LV systolic dysfunction, another 16% had LV diastolic dysfunction, and 32% had a completely normal echocardiogram. Twenty percent of patients experienced significant clinical worsening and subsequent echocardiograms within this subgroup showed further worsening of RV function, perhaps reflecting the cumulative burden of increased RV afterload posed by ARDS or pulmonary thromboembolism.

Myocarditis and Heart Failure

Lymphocytic myocarditis is not a common feature of COVID-19. Even though individual case reports and some autopsy series have identified lymphocytes, macrophages, and occasionally eosinophils in myocardial samples, the prevalence of myocarditis is estimated to be only around 3% among hospitalized patients.[87-94] Endomyocardial biopsy samples and postmortem examinations have confirmed that SARS-CoV-2 virus replicates within myocardial tissue.[92,93] This is consistent with the understanding that the virus gains cell entry by binding to the ACE-2 receptor that is expressed in myocardial tissue. In an autopsy series from Germany, investigators confirmed the presence of SARS-CoV-2 viral genome within myocardial tissue.[93] Using in situ hybridization, they showed that virus was located within the interstitial cells or in macrophages invading myocardial tissue rather than within myocytes. Five of the 39 hearts sampled in this series had a viral load above 1000 copies, a level considered to be clinically significant and indicative of ongoing viral replication. Cytokine expression in these five hearts was increased, but neither these nor the other remaining hearts had evidence of an inflammatory infiltrate. Notably, the patients in this series did not have clinical evidence of myocarditis. The long-term consequences of having cardiac viral infection even in absence of clinical myocarditis remains uncertain.

Other autopsy series have identified myocarditis as defined by the presence of an inflammatory infiltrate associated with myocyte injury.[87-89] In an international, multi-institutional study that included cardiac samples from 21 consecutive autopsies in patients with confirmed COVID-19, lymphocytic myocarditis was present in 3 (14%) of the cases.[87] The myocarditis was multifocal in all three cases and involved both the left and right ventricles **(Fig. 84-4)**. In two cases, the lymphocytes were predominantly CD4+, and in the other, CD8+ lymphocytes predominated. Six additional cases without myocyte necrosis had focally increased interstitial T-lymphocytes within the myocardium. Similar to the study by Lindner et al., increased interstitial macrophage infiltration was present in 18 (86%) of the cases.[87,93] An autopsy series from New York City reported on 25 cases where the heart was examined.[88] In 15 (60%) of these cases, there was a patchy epicardial mononuclear infiltrate with CD4+ lymphocytes predominating over CD8+ cells **(Fig. 84-5)**. There was no associated myonecrosis. Also noted in three cases were small vessel thrombi proximal to areas of epicardial inflammatory infiltrates. Hemophagocytosis was noted in one area of epicardial inflammation. Finally, in an autopsy series from Washington state, only one of 14 (7%) patients had microscopic evidence of myocarditis.[90] Aggregates of lymphocytes were seen in association with necrotic myocytes, but SARS-CoV-2 spike protein could not be identified by immunohistochemistry in that patient's myocardial tissue samples. Viral particles could not be identified in any of the cardiac samples from the 14 patients in this series. Taken together, these autopsy series demonstrate a low occurrence of proven myocarditis. More common abnormalities include myocyte hypertrophy and interstitial fibrosis, nonspecific changes that are more likely reflective of preexisting cardiovascular disease.

Cardiac magnetic resonance imaging (CMR) studies are revealing that cardiac inflammation persists following clinical recovery from COVID-19.[95-97] Among 100 patients recently recovered from COVID-19, 78% had cardiac abnormalities

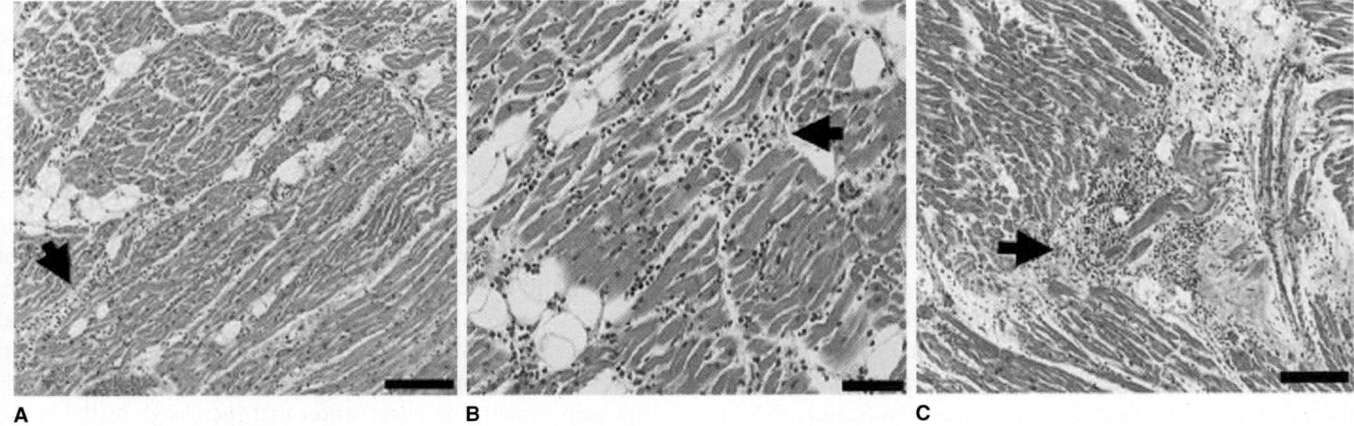

Figure 84-4. Biventricular multifocal lymphocytic myocarditis (*arrows*) with myocyte injury in a 64-year-old man who developed atrial fibrillation 2 days before death. **(A)** H&E X 100; **(B)** H&E X 200; **(C)** H&E X 100. H&E, hematoxylin and eosin staining. Reproduced with permission from Basso C, Leone O, Rizzo S, et al: Pathological features of COVID-19-associated myocardial injury: a multicentre cardiovascular pathology study. *Eur Heart J.* 2020 Oct 14;41(39):3827-3835.

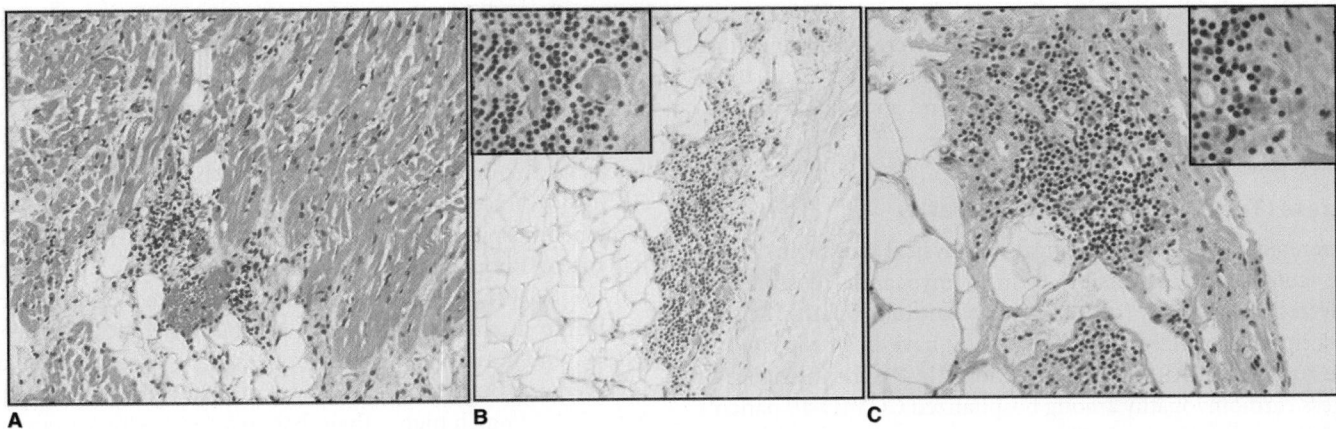

Figure 84–5. Hematoxylin and eosin staining of the heart. **(A)** (10×) Patchy mild interstitial chronic inflammation within the myocardium without myonecrosis. **(B)** (10×) Epicardial mononuclear cell infiltrate with small vessel thrombi (inset at 40×). **(C)** (20×) Epicardial inflammation with focal hemophago-cytosis (inset at 40×). Reproduced with permission from Bryce C, Grimes Z, Pujadas E, et al: Pathophysiology of SARS-CoV-2: targeting of endothelial cells renders a complex disease with thrombotic microangiopathy and aberrant immune response. The Mount Sinai COVID-19 autopsy experience. *medRxiv.*

detected by CMR with 60% showing signs of ongoing myocardial inflammation (increased T1 and T2 signal) **(Fig. 84–6)**.[95] These findings were independent of preexisting conditions, the severity of COVID-19, time from diagnosis, or presence of cardiac symptoms. Typical indices of myocardial structure and function, such as LV end-diastolic volume index and ejection fraction, were only slightly abnormal compared to matched controls. Among the patients who recovered from COVID-19 in the hospital as compared to home, native T1 signal values and high sensitivity troponin T levels were higher, but T2 signal values were similar. These results from Germany were extended by two studies of college athletes in the United States.[96,97] In the first, athletes from the Ohio State University who tested positive for coronavirus underwent CMR.[96] None of the 26 athletes were hospitalized or received specific antiviral treatment. Four athletes (15%) had CMR findings (increased T2 signal and late gadolinium enhancement [LGE]) suggestive of myocarditis and 8 additional athletes (30.8%) exhibited LGE alone suggestive

of prior myocardial injury. None of the athletes had elevated troponin I levels, and half (2 out of 4) of those with myocarditis were asymptomatic. In a separate study, 54 athletes testing positive for SARS-CoV-2 completed imaging studies including echocardiography in all and CMR in 48.[97] Although none of the athletes had CMR evidence of myocarditis (increased native T2 signal), 19 (39.5%) had pericardial enhancement and 6 of these had reduced global longitudinal strain and/or increased native T1 signal. The long-term implications for these studies are not yet clear.

A preceding history of heart failure appears to be a risk factor for adverse clinical outcomes for patients hospitalized with COVID-19.[98–100] A registry study from New York City reported that approximately 7% of patients hospitalized in one of several urban hospitals had a history of heart failure and this was associated with a doubling in the risk of death, 3-fold higher risk of needing mechanical ventilation, and longer hospital length of stay.[100] Outcomes were similar among heart failure patients

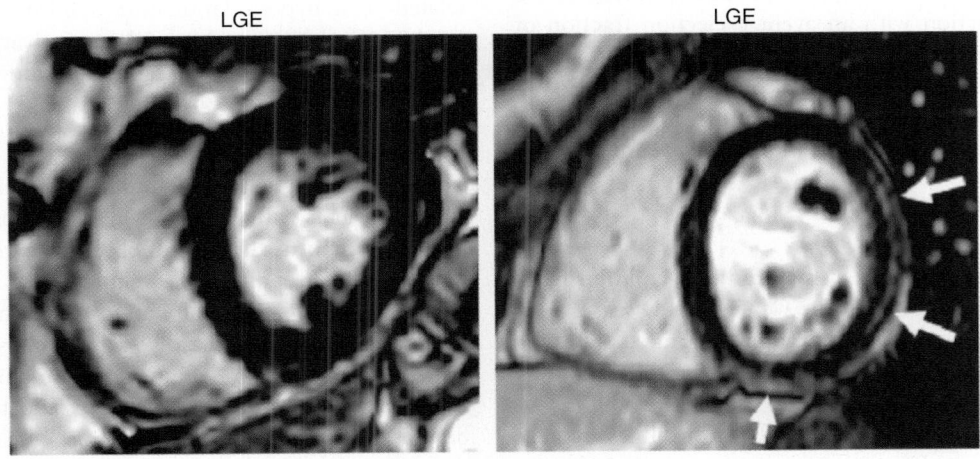

LGE: median 0% [IQR 0%-2%]

Figure 84–6. Representative CMR images of two patients with COVID-19 -related myocarditis. The image on the left has no late gadolinium enhancement (LGE). The image on the right shows a thin stripe of LGE in the lateral wall occupying about 3% of the myocardium. Reproduced with permission from Esposito A, Palmisano A, Natale L, et al. Cardiac Magnetic Resonance Characterization of Myocarditis-Like Acute Cardiac Syndrome in COVID-19. *JACC Cardiovasc Imaging.* 2020 Nov;13(11):2462-2465.

regardless of ejection fraction, except for rates of cardiogenic shock and 30-day rehospitalization that were higher for those with reduced ejection fraction heart failure. Race and treatment with renin-angiotensin-aldosterone antagonists had no impact on outcome.

Stress (Takotsubo) Cardiomyopathy

Severe emotional, psychological, or physical stress can trigger an acute, usually reversible form of myocardial dysfunction referred to as stress (or Takotsubo) cardiomyopathy. Several descriptions of stress cardiomyopathy have been reported in the context of SARS-CoV-2 infection.[94,101–105] The incidence of stress cardiomyopathy among hospitalized COVID-19 patients is estimated to be about 2% among those patients undergoing echocardiography.[94] In a single-center study from New York City, 118 consecutive laboratory-confirmed COVID-19 patients underwent a clinically indicated TTE, of which 5 (4.2%) patients were diagnosed with stress cardiomyopathy.[103] These patients had higher peak concentration of troponin I than those with other forms of COVID-19 myocardial injury and lower levels of inflammatory and prothrombotic biomarkers such as IL-6 and D-dimer.[103] The outcomes for these patients, all of whom were men, were mixed. Two patients had improved LVEF on repeat imaging and were discharged, a third was discharged home clinically improved, and two died in hospital, one on mechanical ventilatory support and the other on venoarterial extracorporeal membrane oxygenation (VA-ECMO). The emotional stress of the pandemic seems to have increased the incidence of stress cardiomyopathy in the general population. A community study from two catheterization laboratories in Northeast Ohio reported an incidence of stress cardiomyopathy during the COVID-19 period of 7.8% compared with a prepandemic incidence of 1.5% to 1.8%.[104] More consistent with previous reports of stress cardiomyopathy, the majority of these patients were women (65%), with highly prevalent cardiovascular risk factors including hypertension (95%), hyperlipidemia (70%), and diabetes (15%). In spite of having severe ventricular dysfunction with an average ejection fraction of 30%, these patients had low levels of troponin and better hospital survival (95%) than those with confirmed SARS-CoV-2 infection.[103,104] Hospital length of stay and readmission rates were generally higher in this population.

Hyperinflammatory Syndrome and Cardiogenic Shock

Reports of a hyperinflammatory syndrome in children from the United Kingdom prompted the Centers for Disease Control to initiate surveillance of children in the United States for the emergence of a Kawasaki-like illness now referred to as Multisystem Inflammatory Syndrome in Children (MIS-C).[106–108] The case definition included six criteria: serious illness requiring hospitalization, age less than 21, fever for at least 24 hours, elevated inflammatory markers, multisystem involvement, and SARS-CoV-2 infection.[108] Although the gastrointestinal system was most frequently involved, cardiovascular involvement was very common (149 out of 186, 80%). Half of the patients

required treatment with vasoactive medications. Most had elevated levels of brain natriuretic peptide (73%) and troponin (50%). More than 90% had an echocardiogram with coronary artery aneurysms documented in 9%. Outcomes for these children were mixed. The majority (80%) received care in an intensive care unit and 20% required mechanical ventilation or ECMO (4%). Most had been discharged (70%), but many (28%) remained hospitalized at the time of publication. Only 4 (2%) had died. Although these case series call attention to the potential for COVID-19 to produce a multisystem inflammatory syndrome in children, there are notable differences between MIS-C and Kawasaki disease. Both can have cardiovascular involvement, but the observed rates of cardiogenic shock with MIS-C were much higher than that associated with Kawasaki's disease (50% vs 5%) whereas coronary artery aneurysm formation was lower (9% vs 25%).[108] The impact of treatment with IV immune globulin or other immunomodulators is uncertain as are the long-term health consequences in survivors.

One additional case series highlights the potential for COVID-19 to produce a steroid-responsive hyperinflammatory multisystem disorder in young adults.[109] Seven men (aged 20–42) without cardiovascular risk factors were hospitalized at a single center in New York City with high-grade fever, multisystem involvement, severe LV dysfunction, and vasoplegia. All had CMR performed, four had nonspecific LGE, and none had increased native T2 signal. They were treated with methylprednisolone (1 mg/kg daily) and therapeutic anticoagulation with unfractionated or low-molecular-weight heparin. All were successfully titrated off pharmacological and mechanical hemodynamic support within 3.7 days (2.5–7.0 days). Inflammatory markers (IL-6, C-reactive protein) and lymphopenia improved as did end-organ function at time of hospital discharge 7 to 18 days after admission. Several patients did have nonspecific rashes and other overlapping features of Kawasaki's disease, although none had clinical vasculitis on coronary angiograms. Whether this represents a unique subset of COVID-19 in men manifested by combined cardiogenic and vasodilatory shock related to a hyperinflammatory syndrome, elevated SARS-CoV-2 IgG Ab titers and steroid responsiveness will need to be confirmed by additional observational studies.

Cardiac Arrythmias

The incidence of tachyarrhythmias and conduction system disease in patients with COVID-19 varies across studies. In most published reports, the type of observed cardiac arrhythmia is not accurately reported. In a clinical case series of hospitalized patients in China, palpitations were an initial presenting symptom in 7.3%, and cardiac arrhythmias were reported in 16.7%, including 44.4% of intensive care unit (ICU) patients.[41] A study of 323 hospitalized patients reported arrhythmias to be present in 30.3% of the full cohort, and occurred in more than 90% of cases in critically-ill patients.[110] Sinus tachycardia is the most commonly observed arrhythmia overall in patients with COVID-19 and reflects the degree of respiratory and systemic illness. Other commonly observed arrhythmias include supraventricular tachyarrhythmias (including atrial fibrillation and atrial flutter) and bradyarrhythmias including sinus bradycardia.

Malignant arrhythmias in the setting of COVID-19 have been evaluated in several studies. In one single-center study of 187 patients with detailed telemetry data review, malignant arrhythmias occurred in 5.9% of hospitalized COVID-19 patients including ventricular tachycardia lasting more than 30 seconds, inducing hemodynamic instability, or ventricular fibrillation.[111] Among patients with severe COVID-19 who experience cardiac arrest, pulseless electrical activity (PEA)/asystole is the most commonly reported cardiac rhythm at the time of the arrest. In another single-center study from the United States of 700 patients admitted with COVID-19, 9 patients experienced cardiac arrest, although only 1 patient had a shockable rhythm of torsades de pointes (8 patients had PEA/asystole). No patients experienced sustained monomorphic ventricular tachycardia, ventricular fibrillation, or complete heart block. Finally, among a cohort of 136 Chinese patients with severe pneumonia due to COVID-19 who experienced in-hospital cardiac arrest and attempted resuscitation, most arrests were deemed respiratory in origin, and the initial rhythm was nonshockable in more than 90% of patients. Survival in this cohort has been reported to be extremely poor (close to 0% at 30 days).

Multiple mechanisms can explain the occurrence of arrhythmias in the setting of COVID-19 including hypoxia, systemic hyperinflammatory status with or without shock, electrolyte disturbances, myocardial injury or ischemia, administration of QT-prolonging therapies, and preexisting cardiac conditions.

Thromboembolic Events

Venous thromboembolism (VTE), including extensive deep vein thrombosis (DVT) and pulmonary embolism (PE), are very common in critically ill patients with COVID-19, even when prophylactic anticoagulation is used.[53,112–114] In a large study of more than 3000 hospitalized patients with COVID-19, any thrombotic event occurred in 533 (16.0%) patients of which 207 (6.2%) were venous (3.2% PE and 3.9% DVT) and 365 (11.1%) were arterial (1.6% ischemic stroke, 8.9% MI, and 1.0% systemic thromboembolism).[115] Of note, these rates were higher among patients who required ICU admission. By multivariate analysis predictors of thrombotic events were older age, male sex, Hispanic ethnicity, coronary artery disease, prior myocardial infarction, and higher D-dimer (>500 ng/mL) at hospital presentation. In addition, any thrombotic event was independently associated with increased risk of in-hospital mortality (adjusted hazard ratio [aHR], 1.82; 95% CI, 1.54–2.15; P <0.001), including both venous (aHR, 1.37; 95% CI, 1.02–1.86) and arterial events (aHR, 1.99; 95% CI, 1.65–2.40).

Arterial thrombotic events, including stroke, have also been observed in patients with COVID-19; however, data estimating its incidence are limited. In a report from the Mount Sinai Health System, five cases of acute ischemic stroke associated with COVID-19 were identified over a 2-week period, with symptoms suggesting large-vessel occlusion; of note all patients were under 50 years of age.[116,117] In comparison, the same institution treated every 2 weeks over the previous 12 months, on average, 0.73 patients <50 years of age with large-vessel stroke. Acute limb ischemia has also been observed among critically-ill patients with COVID-19; however, data is also limited. In the largest case series, which included 42 patients with acute limb ischemia, most of the events were in the lower extremities (71%). Other events included upper limb ischemia (14%), mesenteric ischemia (4%), cerebral ischemia (10%), and some had multiple locations involved.

COVID-19-associated thromboembolic events still seem to occur among patients receiving thromboprophylaxis. In the CORONA-VTE registry that included a cohort of 1114 patients from the Mass General Brigham integrated health network, prophylactic anticoagulation was prescribed in 89.4% of patients with COVID-19 in the intensive care cohort and 84.7% of those in the hospitalized nonintensive care setting.[53] Despite these high rates of usage of prophylactic anticoagulation, the frequencies of major arterial or venous thromboembolism, major cardiovascular adverse events, and symptomatic venous thromboembolism were high in the intensive care cohort (35.3%, 45.9%, and 27.0%, respectively) as well as in the hospitalized nonintensive care cohort (2.6%, 6.1%, and 2.2%, respectively).

Rates of thromboembolic events among outpatients with COVID-19 are currently unclear and some advocate for empiric outpatient anticoagulation to prevent thromboembolism among nonhospitalized patients. In the CORONA-VTE registry that also included 715 outpatients with COVID-19, there were no diagnosed cases of arterial or venous thromboembolic events.[53]

Pathological Correlates

Several autopsy studies have evaluated the role of hypercoagulability and thrombo-inflammation as important contributors of death in patients with COVID-19. A postmortem examination of 21 individuals with COVID-19 found prominent PE in 4 patients, with microthrombi in alveolar capillaries in 5 of 11 who had available histology.[118] In this series, 3 patients also had evidence of thrombotic microangiopathy with fibrin thrombi in glomerular capillaries. In a separate postmortem study of 12 individuals, DVT was present among 7 out of 12. Of note, this was often associated with undiagnosed PE.[119] Finally, in an autopsy study that compared pulmonary pathology from individuals who died from COVID-19 versus influenza or other causes, those who died from COVID-19 had evidence of severe endothelial injury (endotheliitis), widespread thrombosis with microangiopathy, and alveolar capillary microthrombi supporting the role of severe endothelial damage as mechanism of microvascular thrombosis in COVID-19.[120]

COVID-RELATED CARDIOMETABOLIC SYNDROME

Cardiometabolic-based chronic disease (CMBCD) results from primary (genetic, environmental, and behavioral) and metabolic drivers (abnormal adiposity, dysglycemia, and other metabolic syndrome traits).[121–122] Epidemiological/mechanistic associations of CMBCD with COVID-19 substantiate a postulated COVID-related cardiometabolic syndrome (CIRCS) spanning the pre-, acute, and postinfection stages. In a case series of 5700 patients admitted to 12 hospitals in New York City metropolitan area, the most common comorbidities were hypertension (56.6%), obesity (41.7%), and diabetes (33.8%).[46] In a meta-analysis, cardiovascular disease (CVD) (odds ratios [OR], 2.93; P <0.001), diabetes (OR, 2.47; P <0.001), and hypertension (OR, 2.29; P <0.001) were identified as predictors of COVID-19 symptoms or ICU admission.[123] The role of healthy lifestyles and pharmacotherapy targeting metabolic drivers to reduce cardiovascular risk in the pre–COVID-19 stage is well established.[121,122] However, lessons learned from the COVID-19 pandemic support short-lived benefits of these interventions, similar to observed benefits on acute CVD outcomes.[124] Therefore, a cardiometabolic prevention program for patients of all ages should be developed to prevent severe acute COVID-19, CVD complications and related mortality during acute COVID-19, and morbidity and mortality from chronic CIRCS. Effective management of CIRCS should be principally directed at four key metabolic drivers: abnormal adiposity, dysglycemia, dyslipidemia, and hypertension.

Abnormal Adiposity

Whereas overweight and obesity are strictly defined in terms of body mass index alone, adiposity-based chronic disease (ABCD) has been developed as a new framework incorporating abnormal adiposity amount, distribution, and function, with interventions based on clinical complication severity.[124] Not surprisingly, ABCD not only leads to obesity-related complications, but also insulin resistance, inflammation, type 2 diabetes (T2D), and CVD.[121,122,125] Epidemiologically, older age is a risk factor for severe COVID-19, and although abnormal adiposity increases with age, there were 71.6% of US adults ≥20 years old with overweight/obesity during 2015 to 2016, emphasizing the magnitude of this risk factor.[126] Physiologically, ABCD can promote inflammatory pericardial/epicardial fat,[121] increasing the risk for arrhythmia; vascular inflammation, atherosclerosis, and arterial stiffness; cardiomyocyte fibrosis/apoptosis, and LV hypertrophy; and aortic valve sclerosis.[121,127] In several studies,[128–131] patients with COVID-19 and obesity were more likely to be admitted to the ICU and have higher mortality rates than those without obesity. Possible mechanisms include dysregulated immunity with high leptin/adiponectin ratios[132] and sedentariness,[133] increased ACE-2 expression in epicardial adipose tissue,[134] concurrent cardiopulmonary disease,[121,135] and lipotoxic adiposity.[121]

Prudent recommendations can be made based on the high prevalence of overweight/obesity and unhealthy lifestyle in the general population. Formal programs should implement evidence-based algorithms that incorporate lifestyle medicine, pharmacotherapy, and bariatric procedures in the context of social distancing and resource limitations.[136,137] Specifically, with school and lunch program closings,[138] and new work- or stay-at-home routines,[139] the risks of weight gain and

deconditioning need to be countered by planned home physical activities.

Dysglycemia

Diabetes is characterized by abnormally high blood glucose levels sufficient to cause end-organ damage and falls within a dysglycemia-based chronic disease (DBCD) spectrum, consisting of insulin resistance, prediabetes, T2D, and vascular complications.[121,140] There are higher prevalence rates of obesity, hypertension (HTN), dyslipidemia, and CVD with DBCD, intensifying risks for CMBCD progression. Of note, 50.1% of those with diabetes, and 88.4% with prediabetes, are unaware of their condition,[141,142] necessitating case finding strategies for dysglycemia. COVID-19 incidence and disease severity markers are increased in patients with diabetes.[42,44,143–149] COVID-19 is also associated with worse outcomes in patients with T2D, but less so when the hyperglycemia is better controlled.[150] Potential mechanisms accounting for worse outcomes with DBCD include cytokine-mediated aggravation of insulin resistance[151] and hypercoagulability;[152] increased expression of the SARS-CoV-2 receptor (ACE-2) with renin-angiotensin system (RAS) agents;[153] effects of SARS-CoV-2 on pancreatic ACE-2 with decreased β-cell insulin reserve;[154] immunosuppression; glycosylation of viral spike protein and ACE-2 with increased viral binding/entry;[155] decreased viral clearance and increased viral replication;[156,157] and comorbidities.[44] Adverse outcomes with diabetes have also been reported with Pandemic Influenza A 2009 (H1N1) and Middle-East Respiratory Syndrome coronavirus (MERS-CoV).[158]

Patients with T2D should restructure their routines due to potential disruptions in work, sleep, and meal times. Diabetes practice preparedness includes patient access to telemedicine technology. Over-prescribing is dissuaded to avoid hoarding and patients are reassured about ready accessibility to medications and supplies. Continuous glucose monitoring should be considered in patients checking levels multiple times a day, especially with type 1 diabetes (T1D), to alleviate burdens of maintaining supplies. Notwithstanding secondary CVD prevention goals, healthcare professionals (HCPs) should (1) avoid sodium-glucose cotransporter-2 inhibitors (SGLT2i) in patients with acute COVID-19, and (2) consider holding outpatient SGLT2i in patients at risk for COVID-19, especially with poor or variable oral intake, to lower the risk for diabetic ketoacidosis (euglycemic and hyperglycemic) and avoidable non–COVID-19 hospitalizations. Of note, however, the SGT2i dapagliflozin is being evaluated as a potential treatment of COVID-19 for organ protection (Clinical Trials: NCT04350593 and NCT04393246). Practically, HCPs should determine if patients have diabetes or take a "sugar medicine." The glucose and hemoglobin A1c levels should be checked in all patients upon presentation. All oral and noninsulin injectable diabetes medication are stopped in the hospital, and only standing + correction insulin is used according to established protocols. Endocrinologists should be consulted for patients with T1D or those with recalcitrant hyperglycemia. Both ICU and non-ICU glycemic targets are 140 to

180 mg/dL, prioritizing the avoidance of severe hyperglycemia and hypoglycemia. Despite the adverse effects of undernutrition in COVID-19,[159] nutrition support should not be started until severe hyperglycemia is controlled, especially with concurrent or planned glucocorticoid use. If hyperglycemia is recalcitrant on nutrition support, then hold (or significantly reduce) the nutrition support until glycemic control is reestablished. Also, to limit HCP exposures, it may be necessary to manage patients without IV insulin and/or with less frequent monitoring; in this case by using sq NPH q 6 to 8 hours for basal insulinization, and rapid-acting insulin q 3 to 6 hours for correction, depending on when personnel are already in the room. Lastly, insulin requirements need to be preemptively increased when steroids are administered, and decreased as steroids are tapered.

Dyslipidemia

Statins have cholesterol-lowering and anti-inflammatory properties that mitigate the risk of CVD events. Notably, statins diminish inflammatory responses and possibly improve survival in a hyperinflammatory subphenotype of acute respiratory distress syndrome.[160] Although many patients with COVID-19 take a statin, the use of statins to specifically manage viral illnesses remains unclear due to a lack of clinical studies. In vitro, suppression of sterol biosynthesis with simvastatin reduces viral replication and cytokine production at a farnesylation step.[161] In a rabbit atherosclerosis model, atorvastatin mediates epigenetic histone modifications and ACE-2 upregulation.[162] Nevertheless, in mice, combined treatment with simvastatin does not enhance the efficacy of the antiviral, neuraminidase inhibitor oseltamivir.[163] Patients with familial hypercholesterolemia represent another challenge with COVID-19 due to increased risk for premature coronary heart disease, LDL-receptor variants modulating the immune response to SARS-CoV-2, and higher lipoprotein(a) and risk for atherothrombosis.[164,165]

Continuation of statin therapy is recommended in high-/very high-risk patients with COVID-19 who have increased susceptibility to a CVD event with hypercytokinemia. The safety of continued statin therapy must be considered because 5% to 20% of patients taking a statin report adverse muscle events,[166] mimicking viral-induced muscle symptoms. In addition, drug interactions and tissue organ failure may adversely impair statin elimination, increasing the risk of muscle injury. Certain immunomodulatory bioactive lipids (eg, arachidonic acid and other unsaturated fatty acids) may confer anti-SARS-CoV-2 activity and should be investigated.[167] Ruxo-Sim-20 is an open-label, randomized trial investigating whether combined ruxolitinib with simvastatin has a synergistic effect on viral entry and reduced inflammation with confirmed SARS-Cov-2 (NCT04348695). C-19 ACS is a prospective, multicenter clinical trial investigating multiple cardioprotective therapies on all-cause mortality at 30 days after admission with acute coronary syndrome (NCT04333407). The intervention includes aspirin 75 mg or clopidogrel 75 mg, rivaroxaban 2.5 mg for patients not receiving an anticoagulant, atorvastatin 40 mg if not taking a statin, and omeprazole 20 mg daily.

Hypertension

Among patients with HTN, 49.5% have obesity, 63.2% hypercholesterolemia, and 27.2% diabetes.[168] Among patients with COVID-19, HTN is associated with frequent cardiovascular morbidities (24.3%), diabetes (15.2%), cardiac disease (6.2%), and high mortality risk.[169] In another study, HTN is associated with a ~2.5-fold increased risk of COVID-19 severity and mortality, mainly in those patients over >60 years old.[170] The renin-angiotensin-aldosterone system (RAAS) is a key driver for HTN. ACE-2 is a master regulator that converts angiotensin I and II into angiotensin-(1-9) and (1-7), respectively.[171] With SARS-CoV-2 binding to ACE-2 and subsequent entry into the epithelium, ACE-2 and dependent counter-regulatory RAAS pathways steps are down regulated, compromising cardioprotection and leading to CVD. However, based on the evidence, the risk of SARS-CoV-2 infection does not appear affected with RAAS inhibitors.[33,34]

Although still controversial, there is consensus among professional medical societies to continue RAAS antagonists in those currently prescribed these agents.[172,173] Of note, inpatient use of ACE inhibitors/ARB in patients with hypertension and COVID-19 was associated with lower disease severity and interleukin-6 levels, peak viral load, and increased CD3 and CD8 T-cell counts in peripheral blood, compared with other antihypertensive drugs.[174] In another inpatient study, there was lower mortality with ACE inhibitor/ARB use compared with those not on ACE inhibitor/ARB therapy.[175] Spironolactone has also been proposed as an alternative therapy due to theoretical advantages of avoiding ACE inhibitor/ARB withdraw.[176]

TREATMENT

A complete description of the therapeutic management of COVID-19 is beyond the scope of this chapter. Clinical guidance regarding infection control, oxygenation and ventilation, including the use of proning, hemodynamic resuscitation, and the management of acute kidney injury has been provided by several governmental health organizations.[177–179] Recommendations regarding the therapeutic management of COVID-19 continue to evolve as clinical evidence accumulates regarding the safety and efficacy of various antiviral and adjunctive therapies. Guidelines incorporating these therapeutics are tailored to the five identified clinical stages of COVID-19 ranging from asymptomatic infection to critical illness (**Table 84–3**).

Antiviral Therapy

Remdesivir is the only US Food and Drug Administration (FDA)-approved drug for the treatment of COVID-19. Remdesivir is a prodrug that is metabolized to an analogue of adenosine triphosphate and inhibits viral RNA polymerases. It has shown in vitro activity against filoviruses (eg, Ebola) and coronaviruses (eg, SARS-CoV-1, SARSCoV-2, MERS-CoV) and has been well tolerated in clinical use.[180] Results from a National Institutes of Health (NIH)–sponsored multinational clinical trial led to the emergency use authorization (EUA) by the FDA for remdesivir in patients hospitalized with severe

TABLE 84–3. Summary of the Illness Severity Classification for COVID-19

Asymptomatic/Presymptomatic Infection	Mild Illness	Moderate Illness	Severe Illness	Critical Illness
Individuals who test positive for SARS-CoV-2 using a virologic test (ie, a nucleic acid amplification test or an antigen test) but who have no symptoms that are consistent with COVID-19	Individuals who have any of the various signs and symptoms of COVID-19 (eg, fever, cough, sore throat, malaise, headache, muscle pain, nausea, vomiting, diarrhea, loss of taste and smell) but who do not have shortness of breath, dyspnea, or abnormal chest imaging	Individuals who show evidence of lower respiratory disease during clinical assessment or imaging and who have saturation of oxygen (SpO_2) ≥94% on room air at sea level	Individuals who have SpO_2 <94% on room air at sea level, a ratio of arterial partial pressure of oxygen to fraction of inspired oxygen (PaO_2/FiO_2) <300 mm Hg, respiratory frequency >30 breaths/min, or lung infiltrates >50%	Individuals who have respiratory failure, septic shock, and/or multiple organ dysfunction

disease.[181] This trial enrolled 1062 patients with a mean age of 58.9 years, 55.2% of whom had two or more comorbidities, with a median time from symptom onset to randomization of 9 days. Remdesivir significantly reduced time to recovery compared with placebo (10 days vs 15 days), with the clearest benefit observed in the subgroup who had lower respiratory tract infection at study enrollment. Mortality at 15 days was lower for remdesivir-treated patients (6.7% vs 11.9% with placebo), but the difference failed to reach statistical significance. There was no observed benefit in patients with mild disease (small enrollment numbers), nor for those requiring mechanical ventilation or extracorporeal membrane oxygenation. Serious adverse events were reported less frequently in remdesivir-treated patients. Recommendations endorse the use of remdesivir in moderate and severe COVID-19[177] (**Fig. 84–7**).

Baricitinib is an oral Janus kinase (JAK) inhibitor that is approved to treat severe rheumatoid arthritis. It was predicted through the use of artificial intelligence to be effective against SARS-CoV-2 infection by preventing viral cell entry and disrupting the intracellular signaling pathway of cytokines implicated in COVID-19.[182,183] Baricitinib was tested in a randomized trial of 1033 patients hospitalized with COVID-19, all of whom were receiving remdesivir.[184] Patients receiving baricitinib had a median time of recovery of 7 days versus 8 days with placebo. This benefit was more pronounced for patients receiving high-flow oxygen or noninvasive ventilation at enrollment who had a time to recovery of 10 days with combination treatment versus 18 days with control. The 28-day mortality rate was lower in baricitinib-treated patients (5.1% vs 7.8%), but the difference failed to reach statistical significance. On November 19, 2020, the FDA issued an EUA for the use of baricitinib in combination with remdesivir in hospitalized adults and children aged ≥2 years with COVID-19 who require supplemental oxygen, invasive mechanical ventilation, or ECMO. Guidance from the NIH prioritizes the combination of corticosteroids with remdesivir in hospitalized, nonintubated patients who require supplemental oxygen and reserves the use of baricitinib plus remdesivir for the rare circumstances where corticosteroids cannot be used[177] (Fig. 84–7).

Other agents with antiviral activity have been tested in patients with COVID-19, but none are currently endorsed for routine use. Lopinavir-ritonavir is a protease inhibitor that has shown activity against SARS-CoV-2 replication in vitro and has been tested in a randomized, clinical trial of hospitalized patients with severe COVID-19.[185] Because it failed to demonstrate efficacy, and due to ongoing concerns about the safety and tolerability of this protease inhibitor at concentrations needed to inhibit activity in vivo, its use is not currently supported.[177] The antimalarial drugs chloroquine and hydroxychloroquine were believed to be effective against SARS-CoV-2 because they increase endosomal pH and inhibit fusion of the virus with host cell membranes.[186] Furthermore, chloroquine inhibits glycosylation of the ACE-2 receptor that may interfere with viral receptor binding.[187] In spite of the promising results from early clinical trials with noted methodologic flaws, subsequent prospective, randomized studies have repeatedly demonstrated no benefit of these drugs with or without the use of azithromycin.[188–191] Ivermectin is an antiparasitic drug that is postulated to have salutary effects in COVID-19. It interferes with a host nuclear transport protein (importin α/β-1) that the virus hijacks to suppress a host antiviral response.[192] Some clinical studies showed no worsening of clinical disease with ivermectin use, but its use is not currently supported by clinical guidelines.[177,193,194]

Immunomodulators

Corticosteroids appear to be effective in targeting the hyperimmune and inflammatory response to SARS-CoV-2 viral infection that leads to tissue damage. Steroids dampen nuclear factor-kB production of TNF-α, IL-1, and IL-6 but have previously not improved outcomes in ARDS.[195] Initial clinical evaluation of their use in the most severe COVID-19 cases showed a decreased rate of viral clearance, increased mortality, greater bacterial superinfections, and prolonged hospital stay.[196] These concerns were quelled by RECOVERY, a randomized open-label trial conducted in the United Kingdom in which 2104 hospitalized patients with COVID-19 were assigned to receive intravenous or oral dexamethasone (6 mg once daily) and were compared to those receiving standard care.[197] Overall, treatment with dexamethasone resulted in significantly lower rates of all-cause mortality at 28 days (22.9% vs 25.7% with usual care), reducing mortality by one-third in ventilated patients (29.3% vs 41.4%) and by one-fifth in those requiring oxygen only (23.3% vs 26.2%). Results varied depending on the extent of respiratory support, with no benefit observed for those patients not requiring oxygen or mechanical ventilation. Based on these findings, the NIH strongly recommends the use of dexamethasone in patients hospitalized with moderate, severe, or critical COVID-19[177] (Fig. 84–7).

DISEASE SEVERITY	PANEL'S RECOMMENDATIONS
Not Hospitalized, Mild to Moderate COVID-19	There are insufficient data to recommend either for or against any specific antiviral or antibody therapy. SARS-CoV-2 neutralizing antibodies (**bamlanivimab** or **casirivimab plus imdevimab**) are available through EUAs for outpatients who are at high risk of disease progression.[a] These EUAs do not authorize use in hospitalized patients. **Dexamethasone** should not be used (**AIII**).
Hospitalized[a] but Dose Not Require Supplemental Oxygen	**Dexamethasone** should not be used (**AIIa**). There are insufficient data to recommend either for or against the routine use of **remdesivir**. For patients at high risk of disease progression, the use of remdesivir may be appropriate.
Hospitalized[a] and Requires Supplemental Oxygen (But Does Not Require Oxygen Delivery through a High-Flow Device, Noninvasive Ventilation, Invasive Mechanical Ventilation, or ECMO)	Use one of the following options: • **Remdesivir**[b,c] (eg, for patients who require minimal supplemental oxygen) (**BIIa**) • **Dexamethasone**[d] plus **remdesivir**[b,c] (eg, for patients who require increasing amounts of supplemental oxygen) (**BIII**)[e,f] • **Dexamethasone**[d] (eg, when combination therapy with remdesivir cannot be used or is not available) (**BI**)
Hospitalized[a] and Requires Oxygen Delivery through a High-Flow Device or Noninvasive Ventilation	Use one of the following options: • **Dexamethasone**[d,f] (**AI**) • **Dexamethasone**[d] plus **remdesivir**[b,c] (**BIII**)[e,f]
Hospitalized[a] and Requires Invasive Mechanical Ventilation or ECMO	**Dexamethasone**[d] (**AI**)[g]

Rating of Recommendations: A = Strong; B = Moderate; C = Optional
Rating of Evidence: I = One or more randomized trials without major limitations; IIa = Other randomized trials or subgroup analyses of randomized trials; IIb = Nonrandomized trials or observational cohort studies; III = Expert opinion

[a]See the Panel's statements on the FDA EUAs for bamlanivimab and casirivimab plus imdevimab. These EUAs do not authorize use in hospitalized patients.
[b]The remdesivir dose is 200 mg IV for one dose, followed by 100 mg IV once daily for 4 days or until hospital discharge (unless the patient is in a health care setting that can provide acute care that is similar to inpatient hospital care). Treatment duration may be extended to up to 10 days if there is no substantial clinical improvement by Day 5.
[c]For patients who are receiving remdesivir but progress to requiring oxygen through a high-flow device, noninvasive ventilation, invasive mechanical ventilation, or ECMO, remdesivir should be continued until the treatment course is completed.
[d]The dexamethasone dose is 6 mg IV or PO once daily for 10 days or until hospital discharge. If dexamethasone is not available, equivalent doses of other corticosteroids, such as prednisone, methylprednisolone, or hydrocortisone, may be used. See the Corticosteroids section for more information.
[e]The combination of dexamethasone and remdesivir has not been studied in clinical trials.
[f] In the rare circumstances where corticosteroids cannot be used, baricitinib plus remdesivir can be used (**BIIa**). The FDA has issued an EUA for baricitinib use in combination with remdesivir. The dose for baricitinib is 4 mg PO once daily for 14 days or until hospital discharge.
[g]The combination of dexamethasone and remdesivir may be considered for patients who have recently been intubated (**CIII**). Remdesivir alone **is not recommended.**

Key: ECMO = extracorporeal membrane oxygenation; EUA = Emergency Use Authorization; FDA = Food and Drug Administration; IV = intravenous; the Panel = the COVID-19 Treatment Guidelines Panel; PO = orally; SARS-CoV-2 = severe acute respiratory syndrome coronavirus 2

Figure 84–7. Summary of FDA treatment guidelines current as of February 1, 2021.

Anakinra is a recombinant human IL-1 receptor antagonist that is currently FDA approved for the treatment of rheumatoid arthritis. Its potential role in treating the cytokine storm associated with COVID-19 is drawn from the experience gained from using Anakinra off label to treat severe chimeric antigen receptor T-cell (CAR T-cell)-mediated cytokine release syndrome. To date, small case-control and retrospective studies have yielded inconclusive results about its efficacy in treating COVID-19 in part due to study design, low numbers of patients treated, and therapeutic confounding.[198–200] The use of Anakinra is not endorsed by NIH guidelines.[177]

IL-6 is a key inflammatory cytokine known to contribute to thrombo-inflammatory responses associated with acute and chronic inflammation.[201] Elevated levels of IL-6 have been associated with increased immature platelet production, platelet adhesion, and thrombotic responses. IL-6 is produced by a variety of cell types including T-lymphocytes, macrophages, and, in the case of COVID-19, bronchial epithelial cells.[202] Monoclonal antibodies targeting the IL-6 receptor, such as tocilizumab and sarilumab, are approved for rheumatoid arthritis treatment while others targeting IL-6 itself, such as siltuximab, are approved for the treatment of some metastatic cancers and Castleman's disease. To date, the use of these IL-6 antagonists has yielded inconsistent results.[203–207] Although there was a signal in some instances of tocilizumab preventing clinical worsening, these randomized trials when taken as a whole failed to demonstrate any mortality benefit in hospitalized patients with COVID-19 pneumonia. As of this writing, the NIH updated its recommendation to include the use of select IL-6 antagonists (eg, tocilizumab, sarilumab) in combination with IV dexamethasone for hospitalized patients who require supplemental oxygen, high-flow oxygen, non-invasive ventilation or invasive mechanical ventilation.[177]

Although regarded almost exclusively as a treatment for gout and pericarditis, colchicine has a number of pleiotropic immunomodulatory effects.[208] Notably, it disrupts inflammasome assembly, reduces IL-1β production, and inhibits neutrophil chemotaxis and activity in response to vascular injury.[208] One small, hypothesis-exploring clinical trial in patients hospitalized with COVID-19, colchicine appeared to improve the time to clinical worsening.[209] There is currently insufficient evidence to recommend colchicine for treating COVID-19.

Antibody-Based Therapies

Use of passive immunotherapy has been used in medicine for over a century.[210] Including during the 1918 influenza pandemic, serum from convalescent patients was used to treat influenza, with some success.[210] More recently, passive immunotherapy has been evaluated for severe SARS, MERS, and Ebola virus disease.[210] The use of convalescent plasma against SARS-CoV-2 has been proposed as a therapeutic option to treat COVID-19. The evidence supporting the routine use of convalescent plasma in COVID-19 has been mixed, with some studies concluding lack of efficacy while others supporting its effectiveness. Initial randomized trials of convalescent plasma in patients with COVID-19 focused on hospitalized patients who were already moderately to severely ill, and these trials provided weak evidence of clinical efficacy.[211–213] Importantly, early trials were heterogeneous with respect to the characteristics of the convalescent plasma used (eg, its antibody titer) and the type of patients enrolled. For example, in the PlasmAr trial, a double-blind, placebo-controlled, multicenter trial conducted at 12 clinical sites in Argentina, 228 hospitalized adult patients with severe COVID-19 pneumonia were randomized in a 2:1 ratio to receive convalescent plasma or placebo.[214] The infused convalescent plasma had a median titer of 1:3200 of total SARS-CoV-2 antibodies (interquartile range, 1:800 to 1:3200). At 30 days, there were no significant differences between the convalescent plasma group and the placebo group in terms of all-cause mortality or clinical recovery. Conversely, more recently, in another randomized, double-blind, placebo-controlled trial convalescent plasma with high IgG titers against SARS-CoV-2

was used.[113] This trial enrolled 160 older adult patients within 72 hours after the onset of mild COVID-19 symptoms. The primary end point was the development of severe respiratory disease, defined as a respiratory rate of 30 breaths per minute or more, an oxygen saturation of less than 93% while the patient was breathing ambient air, or both. In this trial, use of convalescent plasma with high IgG titers (>1:1000) resulted in significantly lower risk of progression to severe respiratory disease compared with placebo (RR, 0.52; 95% CI, 0.29 to 0.94; $P = 0.03$). Of note, a dose-dependent effect relative to the antibody titers after infusion was observed suggesting that higher antibody titers in convalescent plasma may account for its efficacy. A separate study based on a US national registry evaluated whether the anti–SARS-CoV-2 IgG antibody levels in convalescent plasma used to treat hospitalized adults with COVID-19 were associated with improved or worse clinical outcomes among 3082 patients.[215] In this study, death within 30 days after plasma transfusion occurred in 22.3% of patients in the high-titer group, 27.4% in the medium-titer group, and 29.6% in the low-titer group. Of note, a lower risk of death within 30 days in the high-titer group than in the low-titer group was observed among patients who had not received mechanical ventilation before transfusion, suggesting that early plasma administration is beneficial in the setting of COVID-19. Of note, in none of the aforementioned trials a higher rates of safety adverse events related to plasma administration was noted.

Considering this evidence, the FDA concluded that the totality of the evidence suggests that the benefits of convalescent plasma outweighs its risks, and given the lack of effective treatments, the FDA granted an Emergency Use Authorization and provided guidance on the manufacture and use of convalescent plasma in hospitalized patients with signs of progressive infection.[210] Conversely, the Infectious Diseases Society of America and the American Association of Blood Banks recommend that the use of convalescent plasma be limited to clinical trials, that critically ill patients and those in the ICU are unlikely to benefit from transfusions of convalescent plasma, and that convalescent plasma should be used as early as possible in the course of infection (preferably within 3 days after diagnosis) in order to achieve the best clinical outcomes.

Finally, monoclonal antibodies targeting the SARS-CoV-2 spike protein and preventing viral cell entry are being currently evaluated. However, so far, the only available randomized controlled trial testing bamlanivimab (LY-CoV555), a neutralizing monoclonal antibody, did not demonstrate efficacy among hospitalized patients who had COVID-19 without end-organ failure when co-administered with remdesivir.[216] Conversely, promising data has been reported with REGN-COV2 an antibody cocktail containing two SARS-CoV-2–neutralizing antibodies casirivimab (REGN10933) and imdevimab (REGN10987) that bind to nonoverlapping epitopes of the spike protein receptor binding domain of SARS-CoV-2. In an ongoing, double-blind, phase 1–3 trial involving nonhospitalized patients with COVID-19, REGN-COV2 significantly reduced viral load, with a greater effect in patients whose immune response had not yet been initiated or who had a high viral load at baseline.[217]

Antithrombotics

Given the high frequency of thromboembolic events observed in patients with COVID-19 despite the use of prophylactic-dose anticoagulation, full-dose anticoagulation has been advocated to be used routinely among hospitalized patients.[4,37,116,117] However, antithrombotic treatments also increase the risk of hemorrhagic complications, therefore the balance between thrombotic and bleeding risk needs to be taken into account. As stated by the American Society of Hematology and the Global COVID-19 Thrombosis Collaborative Group, empiric full-dose anticoagulation for individuals who do not have an indication to be fully anticoagulated remains controversial, since data demonstrating improved outcomes are lacking and observational studies have produced mixed results.[116,117] Currently, therapeutic-dose anticoagulation (eg, enoxaparin 1 mg/kg every 12 hours) can be considered appropriate in documented or strongly suspected venous or arterial thromboembolisms and patients with clotting of vascular access devices (which has been frequently observed particularly in patients admitted to the ICU), unless there is a contraindication to anticoagulation. At the present time, there are currently insufficient data to recommend for or against the use of thrombolytic agents or increasing anticoagulant doses for VTE prophylaxis in hospitalized COVID-19 patients outside the setting of a clinical trial.

Promising results were recently released by the NIH-sponsored ACTIV-4, REMAP-CAP and ATTACC trials being conducted worldwide. Based on the interim results of more than 1000 moderately ill hospitalized patients, treatment-dose anticoagulation appeared to result in lower rates of clinical deterioration or the need for ventilation compared with usual care. Of note, this trial platform also stopped enrollment in the critically-ill cohort due to safety issues related to treatment-dose anticoagulation. Full trial results are expected in 2021. Another large trial evaluating anticoagulation strategies is the FREEDOM-COVID trial in which 3600 hospitalized patients with COVID-19 who are not admitted to the ICU are randomized to prophylactic-dose enoxaparin, full-dose enoxaparin, or apixaban 5 mg twice-daily. The primary endpoint is the 30-day event rate of all-cause death, intubation requiring mechanical ventilation or systemic thromboembolism. Results were expected in 2021, but were not available as of the submission date for this chapter.

Tissue plasminogen activator (tPA) has also been proposed in the treatment of severe COVID-19 given the high frequency of pulmonary microvascular and macrovascular thrombi. Small case series (three to five patients) have described administration of tPA to individuals with ARDS associated with COVID-19 and have reported nonsustained improvement in partial arterial pressure of oxygen/fraction of inspired oxygen ratios.[116] At the present time, the use of tPA in absence of a clear indication (eg, massive PE, acute stroke, or life-threatening DVT) is not recommended.

Vaccination

Vaccines to prevent the spread of SARS-CoV-2 infection have the potential to control the COVID-19 pandemic. The development of vaccines for COVID-19 has been unprecedented in terms of the resources invested and the pace of development, testing, and approval of the currently available agents. The primary antigenic target for COVID-19 vaccines is the large surface spike protein that binds to the ACE-2 receptor on host cells and induces membrane fusion. COVID-19 vaccines have been developed using multiple biotechnologies. Some of these are the traditional inactivated virus or live-attenuated virus platforms, other include newer approaches such as recombinant proteins or RNA-based vaccines. In the United States, the messenger RNA (mRNA) vaccines BNT162b2 (Pfizer-BioNTech COVID-19 Vaccine) and mRNA-1273 (Moderna COVID-19 Vaccine) have been granted the emergency use authorization for use based on very positive results from randomized controlled trials reporting more than 90% efficacy in preventing COVID-19 infection compared with placebo and close to 100% efficacy in preventing severe COVID-19 cases.[218,219] Both vaccines leverage the mRNA technology. Once administered, the mRNA enters in the cell cytosol and is translated into the target protein that is intended to elicit an immune response. Of note, the mRNA remains in the cell cytosol and does not enter into the cell nucleus, thus it does not interfere with the recipient's DNA. Other vaccines were under active investigation as of the submission of this chapter.

POSTACUTE SEQUELAE OF COVID-19

The COVID-19 pandemic has resulted in a growing population of patients that have recovered from the infection but have broad range of persistent symptoms. These symptoms are very heterogeneous and include fatigue, dyspnea, chest pain, palpitations, and cough. Less common persistent physical symptoms include anosmia, joint pain, headache, dysgeusia, sweating, and diarrhea. Patients may also experience psychological or cognitive complaints including posttraumatic stress disorder, anxiety, and depression. These manifestations can be considered part of a post–COVID-19 syndrome when they continue for at least 3 to 4 months following recovery and are not explained by an alternative diagnosis. The mechanisms underlying these manifestations are currently unclear and are subject to active investigation but its prevalence seems to be high. In a follow-up study from Italy, 179 patients underwent comprehensive evaluation at a mean of 60 days after onset of the first COVID-19 symptom.[114] At the time of the evaluation, only 18 (12.6%) were completely free of any COVID-19–related symptom, while 32% had one or two symptoms and 55% had three or more. Worsened quality of life was observed among 44.1% of patients and a high proportion of individuals still reported fatigue (53.1%), dyspnea (43.4%), joint pain, (27.3%), and chest pain (21.7%). In another study of 1600 patients from the United States who were hospitalized for moderate or severe COVID-19, at 60 days after discharge, 33% reported persistent symptoms and 19% reported new or worsening symptoms.[220] The most common reported symptom was dyspnea on exertion. Data on detailed cardiopulmonary testing after COVID-19 is currently evolving. In several retrospective modest-size studies of patients who were hospitalized for COVID-19, persistent pulmonary function and radiologic abnormalities were common and still detected around 6 weeks after discharge. It has also postulated that COVID-19 infection may have important sequelae also on cardiac function given the high incidence of myocardial injury observed in hospitalized patients with COVID-19. In a German study of 100 patients who recently recovered from COVID-19, CMR imaging (performed a median of 71 days after the diagnosis) revealed cardiac involvement in 78% and ongoing myocardial inflammation in 60%. In another study of 26 competitive college athletes who had COVID-19 infection, none of whom required hospitalization and the majority without reported symptoms, 12 (46%) had evidence of myocardial inflammation by CMR imaging. The consequences and clinical relevance of these findings is currently unclear and longer-term follow-up studies are needed to evaluate the long-term health consequences of COVID-19 on a population level.

SUMMARY

The global COVID-19 pandemic has sickened millions of people worldwide. SARS-CoV-2 broadly impacts the cardiovascular resulting in thrombosis, myocardial injury, and an increased likelihood of death for hospitalized patients. Many evidence gaps remain regarding SARS-CoV-2 infection, cardiovascular involvement and, in particular, its long-term sequelae on cardiovascular health. The effectiveness of vaccination efforts to stem the spread of the global pandemic are currently being assessed and are being tempered by viral genetic variants and the acquisition of more effective transmission. The strongest recommendation for patients with cardiovascular disease is to remain vigilant and not neglect their cardiovascular health during the pandemic.

REFERENCES

1. Zhu N, Zhang D, Wang W, et al. China Novel Coronavirus Investigating and Research Team. A novel coronavirus from patients with pneumonia in China, 2019. *N Engl J Med.* 2020;382:727-733.
2. Paranjpe I, Fuster V, Lala A, et al. Association of treatment dose anticoagulation with in-hospital survival among hospitalized patients with COVID-19. *J Am Coll Cardiol.* 2020;76:122-124.
3. Libby P, Luscher T. COVID-19 is, in the end, an endothelial disease. *Eur Heart J.* 2020;41:3038–3044.
4. Pinney SP, Giustino G, Halperin JL, et al. Coronavirus historical perspective, disease mechanisms, and clinical outcomes: JACC Focus Seminar. *J Am Coll Cardiol.* 2020;76:1999-2010.
5. Stringhini S, Wisniak A, Piumatti G et al. Seroprevalence of anti-SARS-CoV-2 IgG antibodies in Geneva, Switzerland (SEROCoV-POP): a population-based study. *Lancet.* 2020;396:313-319.
6. Havers FP, Reed C, Lim T et al. Seroprevalence of antibodies to SARS-CoV-2 in 10 sites in the United States, March 23-May 12, 2020. *JAMA Intern Med.* 2020 Jul 21.
7. Meyerowitz EA, Richterman A, Gandhi RT, Sax PE. Transmission of SARS-CoV-2: a review of viral, host, and environmental factors. *Ann Intern Med.* 2021;174:69-79.
8. Klompas M, Baker MA, Rhee C. Airborne transmission of SARS-CoV-2: theoretical considerations and available evidence. *JAMA.* 2020 Jul 13.
9. Bwire GM, Majigo MV, Njiro BJ, Mawazo A. Detection profile of SARS-CoV-2 using RT-PCR in different types of clinical specimens: a systematic review and meta-analysis. *J Med Virol.* 2021;93:719-725.
10. Wang W, Xu Y, Gao R, et al. Detection of SARS-CoV-2 in different types of clinical specimens. *JAMA.* 2020;323:1843-1844.
11. Chu DK, Akl EA, Duda S, et al. COVID-19 Systematic Urgent Review Group Effort (SURGE) study authors. Physical distancing, face masks, and eye protection to prevent person-to-person transmission of SARS-CoV-2 and COVID-19: a systematic review and meta-analysis. *Lancet.* 2020;395:1973-1987.
12. Wiersinga WJ, Rhodes A, Cheng AC, et al. Pathophysiology, transmission, diagnosis, and treatment of coronavirus disease 2019 (COVID-19) a review. *JAMA.* 2020;324:782-793.
13. Hoffmann M, Kleine-Weber H, Schroeder S, et al. SARS-CoV-2 cell entry depends on ACE2 and TMPRSS2 and is blocked by a clinically proven protease inhibitor. *Cell.* 2020;181:271-280.
14. Oberfeld B, Achanta A, Chen P, et al. SnapShot: Covid-19. *Cell.* 2020;181:954.e1.
15. Liu PP, Blet A, Smyth D, Li H. The science underlying COVID-19: implications for the cardio- vascular system. *Circulation.* 2020;142:68-78.
16. de Wit E, van Doremalen N, Falzarano D, Munster VJ. SARS and MERS: recent insights into emerging coronaviruses. *Nat Rev Microbiol.* 2016;14:523-534.
17. Prompetchara E, Ketloy C, Palaga T. Immune responses in COVID-19 and potential vaccines: Lessons learned from SARS and MERS epidemic. *Asian Pac J Allergy Immunol.* 2020;38:1-9.
18. Merad, M., Martin, J.C. Pathological inflammation in patients with COVID-19: a key role for monocytes and macrophages. *Nat Rev Immunol.* 2020;20:355-362.
19. Vardhana SA, Wolchok JD. The many faces of the anti-COVID immune response. *J Exp Med.* 2020;217(6):e20200678.
20. Xu Y, Li X, Zhu B, et al. Characteristics of pediatric SARS-CoV-2 infection and potential evidence for persistent fecal viral shedding. *Nat Med.* 2020;26:502-505.
21. Teuwen LA, Geldhof V, Pasut A, Carmeliet P. COVID-19: the vasculature unleashed. *Nat Rev Immunol.* 2020;20(7):389-391.
22. Croce K, Libby P. Intertwining of thrombosis and inflammation in atherosclerosis. *Curr Opin Hematol.* 2007;14:55-61.
23. Folco EJ, Mawson TL, Vromman A, et al. Neutrophil extracellular traps induce endothelial cell activation and tissue factor production through interleukin-1a and cathepsin G. *Arterioscler Thromb Vasc Biol.* 2018;38:1901-1912.
24. Wright FL, Vogler TO, Moore EE, et al. Fibrinolysis shutdown correlates to thromboembolic events in severe COVID-19 infection. *J Am Coll Surg.* 2020;231(2):193-203.e1.
25. Varga Z, Flammer AJ, Steiger P, et al. Endothelial cell infection and endotheliitis in COVID-19. *Lancet.* 2020;395:1417-1418.
26. Hamming I, Cooper ME, Haagmans BL, et al. The emerging role of ACE2 in physiology and disease. *J Pathol.* 2007;212:1-11.
27. Gheblawi M, Wang K, Viveiros A, et al. Angiotensin-converting enzyme 2: SARS-CoV-2 receptor and regulator of the renin-angiotensin system: celebrating the 20th anniversary of the discovery of ACE2. *Circ Res.* 2020;126:1456-1474.
28. Scott AJ, O'Dea KP, O'Callaghan D, et al. Reactive oxygen species and p38 mitogen activated protein kinase mediate tumor necrosis factor alpha-converting enzyme (TACE/ADAM-17) activation in primary human monocytes. *J Biol Chem.* 2011;286:35466-35476.
29. Ferrario CM, Jessup J, Chappell MC, et al. Effect of angiotensin-converting enzyme inhibition and angiotensin II receptor blockers on cardiac angiotensin-converting enzyme 2. *Circulation.* 2005;111:2605-2610.
30. HFSA/ACC/AHA statement addresses concerns re: using RAAS antagonists in COVID-19. *American College of Cardiology.* March 17, 2020. https://

www.acc.org/latest-in-cardiology/articles/2020/03/17/08/59/hfsa-acc-aha-statement-addresses-concerns-re-using-raas-antagonists-in-covid-19.

31. Considerations for certain concomitant medications in patients with COVID-19. *National Institutes of Health.* July 20, 2020. https://www.covid19treatmentguidelines.nih.gov/concomitant-medications.

32. Mehta N, Kalra A, Nowacki AS, et al. Association of use of angiotensin-converting enzyme inhibitors and angiotensin II receptor blockers with testing positive for coronavirus disease 2019 (COVID-19). *JAMA Cardiol.* 2020;5:1020-1026.

33. Mancia G, Rea F, Ludergnani M, Apolone G, Corrao G. Renin-angiotensin-aldosterone system blockers and the risk of COVID-19. *N Engl J Med.* 2020;382:2431-2440.

34. Reynolds HR, Adhikari S, Pulgarin C, et al. Renin-angiotensin-aldosterone system inhibitors and risk of COVID-19. *N Engl J Med.* 2020;382:2441-2448.

35. de Abajo FJ, Rodríguez-Martín S, Lerma V, et al. Use of renin-angiotensin-aldosterone system inhibitors and risk of COVID-19 requiring admission to hospital: a case-population study. *Lancet.* 2020;395:1705-1714.

36. Cohen JB, Hanff TC, William P, et al. Continuation versus discontinuation of renin-angiotensin system inhibitors in patients admitted to hospital with COVID-19: a prospective, randomised, open-label trial. *Lancet Respir Med.* 202:S2213-2600(20)30558-0.

37. Driggin E, Madhavan MV, Bikdeli B et al. Cardiovascular considerations for patients, health care workers, and health systems during the COVID-19 pandemic. *J Am Coll Cardiol.* 2020;75:2352-2371.

38. Wynants L, Van Calster B, Collins GS et al. Prediction models for diagnosis and prognosis of covid-19 infection: systematic review and critical appraisal. *BMJ.* 2020;369:m1328.

39. Huang C, Wang Y, Li X et al. Clinical features of patients infected with 2019 novel coronavirus in Wuhan, China. *Lancet.* 2020;395:497-506.

40. Madewell ZJ, Yang Y, Longini IM, Jr., Halloran ME, Dean NE. Household transmission of SARS-CoV-2: a systematic review and meta-analysis. *JAMA Netw Open.* 2020;3:e2031756.

41. Wang D, Hu B, Hu C et al. Clinical characteristics of 138 hospitalized patients with 2019 novel coronavirus-infected pneumonia in Wuhan, China. *JAMA.* 2020;323:1061-1069.

42. Guan WJ, Ni ZY, Hu Y et al. Clinical characteristics of coronavirus disease 2019 in China. *N Engl J Med.* 2020;382:1708-1720.

43. Zhou F, Yu T, Du R et al. Clinical course and risk factors for mortality of adult inpatients with COVID-19 in Wuhan, China: a retrospective cohort study. *Lancet.* 2020;395:1054-1062.

44. Bhatraju PK, Ghassemieh BJ, Nichols M et al. Covid-19 in critically ill patients in the Seattle region—case series. *N Engl J Med.* 2020;382:2012-2022.

45. Goyal P, Choi JJ, Pinheiro LC et al. Clinical characteristics of Covid-19 in New York City. *N Engl J Med.* 2020;382:2372-2374.

46. Richardson S, Hirsch JS, Narasimhan M et al. Presenting characteristics, comorbidities, and outcomes among 5700 patients hospitalized with COVID-19 in the New York City area. *JAMA.* 2020;323:2052-2059.

47. Cummings MJ, Baldwin MR, Abrams D et al. Epidemiology, clinical course, and outcomes of critically ill adults with COVID-19 in New York City: a prospective cohort study. *Lancet.* 2020;395:1763-1770.

48. Grasselli G, Zangrillo A, Zanella A et al. Baseline characteristics and outcomes of 1591 patients infected with SARS-CoV-2 admitted to ICUs of the Lombardy region, Italy. *JAMA.* 2020;323:1574-1581.

49. McMichael TM, Currie DW, Clark S et al. Epidemiology of Covid-19 in a long-term care facility in King County, Washington. *N Engl J Med.* 2020;382:2005-2011.

50. Ogedegbe G, Ravenell J, Adhikari S, et al. Assessment of racial/ethnic disparities in hospitalization and mortality in patients with COVID-19 in New York City. *JAMA Netw Open.* 2020;3:e2026881.

51. Wadhera RK, Wadhera P, Gaba P et al. Variation in COVID-19 hospitalizations and deaths across New York City boroughs. *JAMA.* 2020;323:2192-2195.

52. Price-Haywood EG, Burton J, Fort D, Seoane L. Hospitalization and mortality among black patients and white patients with Covid-19. *N Engl J Med.* 2020;382:2534-2543.

53. Piazza G, Campia U, Hurwitz S et al. Registry of arterial and venous thromboembolic complications in patients with COVID-19. *J Am Coll Cardiol.* 2020;76:2060-2072.

54. Cates J, Lucero-Obusan C, Dahl RM et al. Risk for in-hospital complications associated with COVID-19 and influenza—veterans health administration, United States, October 1, 2018-May 31, 2020. *MMWR Morb Mortal Wkly Rep.* 2020;69:1528-1534.

55. Mahmud E, Dauerman HL, Welt FGP, et al. Management of acute myocardial infarction during the COVID-19 pandemic: a position statement from the Society for Cardiovascular Angiography and Interventions (SCAI), the American College of Cardiology (ACC), and the American College of Emergency Physicians (ACEP). *J Am Coll Cardiol.* 2020;76:1375-1384.

56. Thygesen K, Alpert JS, Jaffe AS et al. Fourth Universal Definition of Myocardial Infarction (2018). *J Am Coll Cardiol.* 2018;72:2231-2264.

57. Libby P, Loscalzo J, Ridker PM et al. Inflammation, immunity, and infection in atherothrombosis: JACC Review Topic of the Week. *J Am Coll Cardiol.* 2018;72:2071-2081.

58. Mogensen TH. Pathogen recognition and inflammatory signaling in innate immune defenses. *Clin Microbiol Rev.* 2009;22:240-273.

59. van de Veerdonk FL, Netea MG, Dinarello CA, Joosten LA. Inflammasome activation and IL-1beta and IL-18 processing during infection. *Trends Immunol.* 2011;32:110-116.

60. Vallance P, Collier J, Bhagat K. Infection, inflammation, and infarction: does acute endothelial dysfunction provide a link? *Lancet.* 1997;349:1391-1392.

61. Choudry FA, Hamshere SM, Rathod KS, et al. High thrombus burden in patients with COVID-19 presenting with ST-segment elevation myocardial infarction. *J Am Coll Cardiol.* 2020;76:1168-1176.

62. Mafham MM, Spata E, Goldacre R, et al. COVID-19 pandemic and admission rates for and management of acute coronary syndromes in England. *Lancet.* 2020;396:381-389.

63. De Rosa S, Spaccarotella C, Basso C, et al. Reduction of hospitalizations for myocardialinfarction in Italy in the COVID-19 era. *Eur Heart J.* 2020;41:2083-2088.

64. Metzler B, Siostrzonek P, Binder RK, et al. Decline of acute coronary syndrome admissions in Austria since the outbreak of COVID-19: the pandemic response causescardiac collateral damage. *Eur Heart J.* 2020;41:1852-1853.

65. Garcia S, Albaghdadi MS, Meraj PM, et al. Reduction in ST-segment elevation cardiac catheterization laboratory activations in the United States during COVID-19 pandemic. *J Am Coll Cardiol.* 2020;75:2871-2872.

66. Solomon MD, McNulty EJ, Rana JS, et al. The COVID-19 pandemic and the incidence of acute myocardial infarction. *N Engl J Med.* 2020;383:691-693.

67. De Filippo O, D'Ascenzo F, Angelini F, et al. Reduced rate of hospital admissions for ACS during COVID-19 outbreak in Northern Italy. *N Engl J Med.* 2020;383:88-89.

68. De Luca G, Verdoia M, Cercek M, et al. Impact of COVID-19 pandemic on mechanical reperfusion for patients with STEMI. *J Am Coll Cardiol.* 2020;76:2321-2330.

69. Welt FGP, Shah PB, Aronow HD, et al. Catheterization laboratory considerations during the coronavirus (COVID-19) pandemic: from the ACC's Interventional Council and SCAI. *J Am Coll Cardiol.* 2020;75:2372-2375.

70. Szerlip M, Anwaruddin S, Aronow HD, et al. Considerations for cardiac catheterization laboratory procedures during the COVID-19 pandemic perspectives from the Society for Cardiovascular Angiography and Interventions Emerging Leader Mentorship (SCAI ELM) Members and Graduates. *Catheter Cardiovasc Interv.* 2020;96:586-597.

71. Lim W, Qushmaq I, Devereaux PJ, et al. Elevated cardiac troponin measurements in critically ill patients. *Arch Intern Med.* 2006;166:2446-2454.

72. Sarkisian L, Saaby L, Poulsen TS, et al. Prognostic impact of myocardial injury related to various cardiac and noncardiac conditions. *Am J Med.* 2016;129:506-514.e1.

73. Sarkisian L, Saaby L, Poulsen TS, et al. Clinical characteristics and outcomes of patients with myocardial infarction, myocardial injury, and nonelevated troponins. *Am J Med.* 2016;129:446.e5-e446.e21.

74. Smeeth L, Thomas SL, Hall AJ, et al. Risk of myocardial infarction and stroke after acute infection or vaccination. *N Engl J Med.* 2004;351:2611-2618.

75. Harrington RA. Targeting inflammation in coronary artery disease. *N Engl J Med.* 2017;377:1197-1198.

76. Kwong JC, Schwartz KL, Campitelli MA, et al. Acute myocardial infarction after laboratory-confirmed influenza infection. *N Engl J Med.* 2018;378:345-353.

77. Gluckman TJ, Wilson MA, Chiu ST, et al. Case rates, treatment approaches, and outcomes in acute myocardial infarction during the coronavirus disease 2019 pandemic. *JAMA Cardiol.* 2020;5:1419-1424.

78. Primessnig U, Pieske BM, Sherif M. Increased mortality and worse cardiac outcome of acute myocardial infarction during the early COVID-19 pandemic. *ESC Heart Fail.* 2020;8:333-343.

79. Krumholz HM. Where have all the heart attacks gone? *New York Times.* April 6, 2020.

80. Wu J, Mamas MA, Mohamed MO, et al. Place and causes of acute cardiovascular mortality during the COVID-19 pandemic. *Heart.* 2021;107: 113-119.

81. Faust JS, Krumholz HM, Du C, et al. All-cause excess mortality and COVID-19-related mortality among US Adults aged 25–44 years, March-July 2020. *JAMA.* 2020:e2024243. doi: 10.1001/jama.2020.24243.

82. Lala A, Johnson KW, Januzzi JL, et al. Prevalence and impact of myocardial injury in patients hospitalized with COVID-19 infection. *J Am Coll Cardiol.* 2020;76:533-546.

83. Metkus TS, Sokoll LJ, Barth AS, et al. Myocardial injury in severe COVID-19 compared to non-COVID acute respiratory distress syndrome. *Circulation.* 2020 Nov 13. doi: 10.1161/CIRCULATIONAHA.120.050543.

84. Giustino G, Croft LB, Stefanini GG, et al. Characterization of myocardial injury in patients with COVID-19. *J Am Coll Cardiol.* 2020;76: 2043-2055.

85. Wadhera RK, Shen C, Gondi S, et al. Cardiovascular deaths during the COVID-19 pandemic in the United States. *J Am Coll Cardiol.* 2021;77:159-169.

86. Szekely Y, Lichter Y, Taieb P, et al. Spectrum of cardiac manifestations in COVID-19: a systematic echocardiographic study. *Circulation.* 2020;142:342-353.

87. Basso C, Leone O, V Rizzo S, et al. Pathological features of COVID-19-associated myocardial injury: a multicentre cardiovascular pathology study. *Eur Heart J.* 2020;41:3827-3835.

88. Bryce C, Grimes Z, Pujadas E, et al. Pathophysiology of SARS-CoV-2: targeting of endothelial cells renders a complex disease with thrombotic microangiopathy and aberrant immune response. The Mount Sinai COVID-19 autopsy experience. *medRxiv.* 2020 May 22. doi: 10.1101/2020.05.18.20099960.

89. Satturwar S, Fowkes M, Farver C, et al. Postmortem findings associated with SARS-CoV-2 systematic review and meta-analysis. *Am J Surg Pathol.* 2021 Jan 20. doi: 10.1097/PAS.0000000000001650.

90. Bradley BT, Maioli H, Johnson R, et al. Histopathology and ultrastructural findings of fatal COVID-19 infections in Washington State: a case series. *Lancet.* 2020;396:320-332.

91. Craver R, Huber S, Sandomirsky M, et al. Fatal eosinophilic myocarditis in a healthy 17-year-old male with severe acute respiratory syndrome coronavirus 2 (SARS-CoV-2c). *Fetal Pediatr Pathol.* 2020;39:263-268.

92. Escher F, Pietsch H, Aleshcheva G, et al. Detection of viral SARS-CoV-2 genomes and histopathological changes in endomyocardial biopsies. *ESC Heart Fail.* 2020;7:2440-2447.

93. Lindner D, Fitzek A, Bräuninger H, et al. Association of cardiac infection with SARS-CoV-2 in confirmed COVID-19 autopsy cases. *JAMA Cardiol.* 2020;5(11):1281-1285.

94. Dweck MR, Bularga A, Hahn RT, et al. Global evaluation of echocardiography in patients with COVID-19. *Eur Heart J Cardiovasc Imaging.* 2020;21:949-958.

95. Puntmann VO, Carerj ML, Wieters I, et al. Outcomes of cardiovascular magnetic resonance imaging in patients recently recovered from coronavirus disease 2019 (COVID-19). *JAMA Cardiol.* 2020;5:1265-1273.

96. Rajpal S, Tong MS, Borchers J, et al. Cardiovascular magnetic resonance findings in competitive athletes recovering from COVID-19 infection. *JAMA Cardiol.* 2021;6:116-118.

97. Brito D, Meester S, Yanamala N, et al. High prevalence of pericardial involvement in college student athletes recovering from COVID-19. *JACC Cardiovasc Imaging.* 2020 Nov 4:S1936-878X(20)30946-3.

98. Inciardi RM, Adamo M, Lupi L, et al. Characteristics and outcomes of patients hospitalized for COVID-19 and cardiac disease in Northern Italy. *Eur Heart J.* 2020;41:1821-1829.

99. Andersson C, Andersson C, Gerds T, et al. Incidence of new-onset and worsening heart failure before and after the COVID-19 epidemic lockdown in Denmark: a nationwide cohort study. *Circ Hear Fail.* 2020;13:e007274.

100. Alvarez-Garcia J, Lee S, Gupta A, et al. Prognostic impact of prior heart failure in patients hospitalized with COVID-19. *J Am Coll Cardiol.* 2020;76:2334-2348.

101. Meyer P, Degrauwe S, Van Delden C, et al. Typical takotsubo syndrome triggered by SARS-CoV-2 infection. *Eur Heart J.* 2020;41:1860.

102. Minhas AS, Scheel P, Garibaldi B, et al. Takotsubo syndrome in the setting of COVID-19. *JACC Case Rep.* 2020;2:1321-1325.

103. Giustino G, Croft LB, Oates CP, et al. Takotsubo cardiomyopathy in COVID-19. *J Am Coll Cardiol.* 2020;76:628-629.

104. Jabri A, Kalra A, Kumar A, et al. Incidence of stress cardiomyopathy during the coronavirus disease 2019 pandemic. *JAMA Netw Open.* 2020;3:e2014780.

105. Tsao CW, Strom JB, Chang JD, Manning WJ. COVID-19-associated stress (Takotsubo) cardiomyopathy. *Circ Cardiovasc Imaging.* 2020;13:e011222.

106. Riphagen S, Gomez X, Gonzalez-Martinez C, et al. Hyperinflammatory shock in children during COVID-19 pandemic. *Lancet.* 2020;395:1607-1608.

107. Dufort EM, Koumans EH, Chow EJ, et al. Multisystem inflammatory syndrome in children in New York State. *N Engl J Med.* 2020;383:347-358.

108. Feldstein LR, Rose EB, Horwitz SM, et al. Multisystem inflammatory syndrome in U.S. children and adolescents. *N Engl J Med.* 2020;383:334-346.

109. Chau VQ, Giustino G, Mahmood K, et al. Cardiogenic shock and hyperinflammatory syndrome in young males with COVID-19. *Circ Heart Fail.* 2020;13:e007485.

110. Hu L, Chen S, Fu Y et al. Risk factors associated with clinical outcomes in 323 COVID-19 hospitalized patients in Wuhan, China. *Clin Infect Dis.* 2020;71(16):2089-2098.

111. Guo T, Fan Y, Chen M et al. Cardiovascular implications of fatal outcomes of patients with coronavirus disease 2019 (COVID-19). *JAMA Cardiol.* 2020.

112. Malas MB, Naazie IN, Elsayed N, Mathlouthi A, Marmor R, Clary B. Thromboembolism risk of COVID-19 is high and associated with a higher risk of mortality: a systematic review and meta-analysis. *EClinicalMedicine.* 2020;29:100639.

113. Libster R, Perez Marc G, Wappner D et al. Early high-titer plasma therapy to prevent severe Covid-19 in older adults. *N Engl J Med.* 2021 Jan 6.

114. Carfi A, Bernabei R, Landi F, Gemelli Against C-P-ACSG. Persistent symptoms in patients after acute COVID-19. *JAMA.* 2020;324:603-605.

115. Bilaloglu S, Aphinyanaphongs Y, Jones S, Iturrate E, Hochman J, Berger JS. Thrombosis in hospitalized patients with COVID-19 in a New York City health system. *JAMA.* 2020;324:799-801.

116. Giustino G, Pinney SP, Lala A et al. Coronavirus and cardiovascular disease, myocardial injury, and arrhythmia: JACC focus seminar. *J Am Coll Cardiol.* 2020;76:2011-2023.

117. Bikdeli B, Madhavan MV, Jimenez D et al. COVID-19 and thrombotic or thromboembolic disease: implications for prevention, antithrombotic

therapy, and follow-up: JACC State-of-the-Art Review. *J Am Coll Cardiol.* 2020;75:2950-2973.

118. Menter T, Haslbauer JD, Nienhold R et al. Postmortem examination of COVID-19 patients reveals diffuse alveolar damage with severe capillary congestion and variegated findings in lungs and other organs suggesting vascular dysfunction. *Histopathology.* 2020;77:198-209.

119. Wichmann D, Sperhake J-P, Lutgehetmann M, et al. Autopsy findings and venous thromboembolism in patients with COVID-19: a prospective cohort study. *Ann Intern Med.* 2020;173:268-277.

120. Ackermann M, Verleden SE, Kuehnel M, et al. Pulmonary vascular endothelialitis, thrombosis, and angiogenesis in Covid-19. *N Engl J Med.* 2020;383:120-128.

121. Mechanick JI, Farkouh ME, Newman JD, et al. Cardiometabolic-based chronic disease—adiposity and dysglycemia drivers. *J Am Coll Cardiol.* 2020;75:525-538.

122. Mechanick JI, Farkouh ME, Newman JD, et al. Cardiometabolic-based chronic disease—addressing knowledge and clinical practice gaps in the preventive care plan. *J Am Coll Cardiol.* 2020;75:539-555.

123. Wang B, Li R, Lu Z, et al. Does comorbidity increase the risk of patients with COVID-19: evidence from meta-analysis. *Aging.* 2020;12:6049-6057.

124. Lee YM, Kim RB, Lee HJ, et al. Relationships among medication adherence, lifestyle modification, and health-related quality of life in patients with acute myocardial infarction: a cross-sectional study. *Health Qual Life Outcomes.* 2018;16:100.

125. Mechanick JI, Hurley DL, Garvey WT. Adiposity-based chronic disease as a new diagnostic term: American Association of Clinical Endocrinologists and the American College of Endocrinology position statement. *Endocr Pract.* 2017;23:372-378.

126. Centers for Disease Control and Prevention. National Center for Health Statistics, Obesity and Overweight. https://www.cdc.gov/nchs/fastats/obesity-overweight.htm. Accessed on April 3, 2020.

127. Dutour A, Achard V, Sell H, et al. Secretory type II phospholipase A2 is produced and secreted by epicardial adipose tissue and overexpressed in patients with coronary artery disease. *J Clin Endocrinol Metab.* 2010;95:963-967.

128. Simonnet A, Chetboun M, Poissy J, et al. High prevalence of obesity in severe acute respiratory syndrome coronavirus-2 (SARSCoV-2) requiring invasive mechanical ventilation. *Obesity.* 2020. doi:10.1002/oby.22831.

129. Lighter J, Phillips M, Hochman S, et al. Obesity in patients younger than 60 years is a risk factor for Covid-19 hospital admission. *Clin Infect Dis.* 2020. doi:10.1093/cid/ciaa415.

130. *Audit I 2020 ICNARC Report on COVID-19 in Critical Care.* London, UK: ICNARC; April 10, 2020.

131. Wu J, Li W, Shi X, et al. Early antiviral treatment contributes to alleviate the severity and improve the prognosis of patients with novel coronavirus disease (COVID-19). *J Intern Med.* 2020. doi:10.1111/joim.13063.

132. Richard C, Wadowski M, Goruk S, et al. Individuals with obesity and type 2 diabetes have additional immune dysfunction compared with obese individuals who are metabolically healthy. *BMJ Open Diabetes Res Care.* 2017;5:e000379.

133. Zheng Q, Cui G, Chen J et al. Regular exercise enhances the immune response against microbial antigens through upregulation of toll-like receptor signaling pathways. *Cell Physiol Biochem.* 2015;37:735-746.

134. Patel VB, Mori J, McLean BA, et al. ACE2 deficiency worsens epicardial adipose tissue inflammation and cardiac dysfunction in response to diet-induced obesity. *Diabetes.* 2016;65:85–95. doi:10.2337/db15-0399.

135. Jose RJ, Manuel A. Does COVID-19 disprove the obesity paradox in ARDS? *Obesity.* 2020. doi:10.1002/oby.22835.

136. Garvey WT, Mechanick JI, Brett EM, et al.; Reviewers of the AACE/ACE Obesity Clinical Practice Guidelines. American Association of Clinical Endocrinologists and American College of Endocrinology Clinical Practice Guidelines for comprisive medical care of patients with obesity—executive summary. *Endocr Pract.* 2016;22:842-884.

137. Rubino F, Cohen RV, Mingrone G, et al. Bariatric and metabolic surgery during and after the COVID-19 pandemic: DSS recommendations for management of surgical candidates and postoperative patients and prioritization of access to surgery. *Lancet Diabetes Endocrinol.* 2020 May 7: S2213-8587(20)30157-1.

138. Rundle AG, Park Y, Herbstman JB, et al. COVID-19 related school closings and risk of weight gain among children. *Obesity.* 2020. doi:10.1002/oby.22813.

139. Chen P, Mao L, Nassis GP, et al. Coronavirus disease (COVID-19): the need to maintain regular physical activity while taking precautions. *J Sport Health Sci.* 2020;9:103-104.

140. Mechanick JI, Garber AJ, Grunberger G, et al. Dysglycemia-based chronic disease: an American Association of Clinical Endocrinologists position statement. *Endocr Pract.* 2018;24:995-1011.

141. International Diabetes Federation. *IDF Diabetes Atlas, Ninth Edition.* 2019. https://www.diabetesatlas.org/en. Accessed on April 2, 2020.

142. *2020 National Diabetes Statistics Report.* Atlanta, GA: Centers for Disease Control and Prevention; 2020.

143. Zhang JJ, Dong X, Cao YY, et al. Clinical characteristics of 140 patients infected by SARS-CoV-2 in Wuhan, China. *Allergy.* 2020. doi:10.1111/all.14238.

144. Bode B, Garrett V, Messler J, et al. Glycemic characteristics and clinical outcomes of COVID-19 patients hospitalized in the United States. *J Diabetes Sci Technol.* 2020 May 9;1932296820924469. doi:10.1177/1932296820924469.

145. Yang X, Yu Y, Xu J, et al. Clinical course and outcomes of critically ill patients with SARS-CoV-2 pneumonia in Wuhan, China: a single-centered, retrospective, observational study. *Lancet Respir Med.* 2020. doi:10.1016/S2213-2600(20)30079-5.

146. Wu Z, McGoogan JM. Characteristics of and important lessons from the coronavirus disease 2019 (COVID-19) outbreak in China: summary of a report of 72 314 cases from the Chinese center for disease control and prevention. *J Am Med Assoc.* 2020. doi:10.1001/jama.2020.2648.

147. Deng SQ, Peng HJ. Characteristics of and public health responses to the coronavirus disease 2019 outbreak in China. *J Clin Med.* 2020;9. doi:10.3390/jcm9020575.

148. Ruan Q, Yang K, Wang W, et al. Clinical predictors of mortality due to COVID-19 based on an analysis of data of 150 patients from Wuhan, China. *Intensive Care Med.* 2020. doi:10.1007/s00134-020-05991-x.

149. Guan WJ, Liang WH, Zhao Y, et al. Comorbidity and its impact on 1590 patients with Covid-19 in China: a nationwide analysis. *Eur Respir J.* 2020. doi:10.1183/13993003.00547-2020.

150. Zhu L, She ZG, Cheng X, et al. Association of blood glucose control and outcomes in patients with COVID-19 and pre-existing type 2 diabetes. *Cell Metab.* 2020;31:1068-1077.

151. Rehman K, Akash MS. Mechanisms of inflammatory responses and development of insulin resistance: how are they linked? *J Biomed Sci.* 2016;23:87.

152. Guo W, Li M, Dong Y, et al. Diabetes is a risk factor for the progression and prognosis of COVID-19. *Diabetes Metab Res Rev.* 2020;e3319. doi:10.1002/dmrr.3319.

153. Wan Y, Shang J, Graham R, et al. Receptor recognition by novel coronavirus from Wuhan: an analysis based on decade long structural studies of SARS. *J Virology.* 2020. doi:10.1128/ JVI.00127-20.

154. Liu F, Long X, Zou W, et al. Highly ACE2 expression in pancreas may cause pancreas damage after SARS-CoV-2 infection. *medRxiv* 2020 Mar 3. doi:10.1101/2020.02.28.20029181.

155. Fernandez C, Rysa J, Almgren P, et al. Plasma levels of the proprotein convertase furin and incidence of diabetes and mortality. *J Intern Med.* 2018;284:377-387.

156. Philips BJ, Meguer JX, Redman J, et al. Factors determining the appearance of glucose in upper and lower respiratory tract secretions. *Intensive Care Med.* 2003;12:2204-2210.

157. Walls AC, Park Y-J, Tortorici MA, et al. Structure, function, and antigenicity of the SARS-CoV-2 spike glycoprotein. *Cell.* 2020. doi:10.1016/j.cell.2020.02.058.

158. Badawi A, Ryoo SG. Prevalence of diabetes in the 2009 influenza A (H1N1) and the Middle East respiratory syndrome coronavirus: a systematic review and meta-analysis. *J Public Health Res.* 2016;5:733.

159. Caccialanza R, Laviano A, Lobascio F, et al. Early nutritional supplementation in non-critically ill patients hospitalized for the 2019 novel coronavirus disease (COVID-19): rationale and feasibility of a shared pragmatic protocol. *Nutrition.* 2020;110835. doi: 10.1016/j.nut.2020.110835.

160. Calfee CS, Delucchi KL, Sinha P, et al. ARDS subphenotypes and differential response to simvastatin: secondary analysis of a randomized controlled trial. *Lancet Respir Med.* 2018;6:691-698.

161. Mehrbod P, hair-Bejo M, Ibrahim TAT, et al. Simvastatin modulates cellular components in influenza A virus-infected cells. *Int J Mol Med.* 2014;34:61-73.

162. Tikoo K, Patel G, Kuman S, et al. Tissue specific up regulation of ACE2 in rabbit model of atherosclerosis by atorvastatin: role of epigenetic histone modifications. *Biochem Pharmacol.* 2015;93:343-351.

163. Belser JA, Szretter KJ, Katz JM, et al. Simvastatin and oseltamivir combination therapy does not improve the effectiveness of oseltamivir alone following highly pathogenic avian H5N1 influenza virus infection in mice. *Virology.* 2013;439:42-46.

164. Hennig BJW, Hellier S, Frodsham AJ et al. Association of low-density lipoprotein receptor polymorphisms and outcome of hepatitis C infection. *Genes Immun.* 2002;3:359-367. [Erratum in *Genes Immun.* 2007;8:707.]

165. Vuorio A, Watts GF, Schneider WJ, Tsimikas S, Kovanen PT. Familial hypercholesterolemia and elevated lipoprotein(a): double heritable risk and new therapeutic opportunities. *J Int Med.* 2020;287:2-18.

166. Rosenson RS, Baker S, Banach M, et al. Optimizing cholesterol treatment in patients with muscle complaints. *J Am Coll Cardiol.* 2017;70:1290-1301.

167. Das UN. Can bioactive lipids inactivate coronavirus (COVID-19)? *Arch Med Res.* 2020;51:282-286.

168. Whelton PK, Carey RM, Aranow WS, et al. 2017 ACC/AHA/AAPA/ABC/ACPM/AGS/AphA/ASH/ASPC/NMA/PCNA guideline for the prevention, detection, evaluation, and amangement of high blood pressure in adults. *J Am Coll Cardiol.* 2018;71:e127-e248.

169. Zuin M, Rigatelli G, Zuliani G, et al. Arterial hypertension and risk of death in patients with COVID-19 infection: systematic review and emta-analysis. *J Infect.* 2020. doi: 10.1016/j.jinf.2020.03.059.

170. Lippi G, Wong J, Henry BM. Hypertension and its severity or mortality in coronavirus disease 2019 (COVID-19): a pooled analysis. *Pol Arch Intern Med.* 2020. doi: 10.20452/pamw.15272.

171. Paz Ocaranza M, Riquelme JA, Garcia L, et al. Counter-regulatory renin-angiotensin system in cardiovascular disease. *Nat Rev Cardiol.* 2020;17:116-129.

172. Bavishi C, Maddox TM, Messerli FH. Coronavirus disease 2019 (COVID-19) infection and renin angiotensin system blockers. *JAMA Cardiol.* 2020. doi: 10.1001/jamacardio.2020.1282.

173. Vaduganathan M, Vardeny O, Michel T, et al. Renin-angiotensin-aldosterone system inhibitors in patients with Covid-19. *N Engl J Med.* 2020. doi: 10.1056/NEJMsr2005760.

174. Meng J, Xiao G, Zhang J, et al. Renin-angiotensin system inhibitors improve the clinical outcomes of COVID-19 patients with hypertension. *Emerg Microbes Infect.* 2020;9:757-760.

175. Zhang P, Zhu L, Cai J, et al. Association of inpatient use of angiotensin converting enzyme inhibitors and antiotensin II receptor blockers with mortality among patients with hypertension hospitalized with COVID-19. *Circulation Res.* 2020. doi: 10.1161/CIRCRESAHA.120.317134.

176. Cadegiani FA. Can spironolactone be used to prevent COVID-19-induced actue respiratory distress syndrome in patients with hypertension? *Am J Physiol Endocrinol Metab.* 2020;318:e587-e588.

177. Coronavirus Disease 2019 (COVID-19) Treatment Guidelines. https://www.covid19treatmentguidelines.nih.gov. Accessed January 4, 2021.

178. World Health Organization Clinical Management of COVID-19. https://www.who.int/publications/i/item/clinical-management-of-covid-19. Accessed January 4, 2021.

179. European Centre for Disease Prevention and Control: COVID-19 pandemic. https://www.ecdc.europa.eu/en/covid-19/latest-evidence/vaccines-and-treatment. Accessed January 4, 2021.

180. Mulangu S, Dodd LE, Davey RT Jr., et al. A randomized, controlled trial of Ebola virus disease therapeutics. *N Engl J Med.* 2019;381:2293-2303.

181. Beigel JH, Tomashek KM, Dodd LE, et al. Remdesivir for the treatment of COVID-19—Final report. *N Engl J Med.* 2020;383:1813-1826.

182. Richardson P, Griffin I, Tucker C, et al. Baricitinib as potential treatment for 2019-nCoV acute respiratory disease. *Lancet.* 2020;395(10223):e30-e31.

183. Stebbing J, Phelan A, Griffin I, et al. COVID-19: combining antiviral and anti-inflammatory treatments. *Lancet Infect Dis.* 2020;20:400-402.

184. Kalil AC, Patterson TF, Mehta AK, et al. Baricitinib plus remdesivir for hospitalized adults with Covid-19. *N Engl J Med.* 2020. doi: 10.1056/NEJMoa2031994.

185. Cao B, Wang Y, Wen D, et al. A trial of lopinavir-ritonavir in adults hospitalized with severe COVID-19. *N Engl J Med.* 2020;382(19):1787-1799.

186. Wang M, Cao R, Zhang L, et al. Remdesivir and chloroquine effectively inhibit the recently emerged novel coronavirus (2019-nCoV) in vitro. *Cell Res.* 2020;30(3):269-271.

187. Vincent MJ, Bergeron E, Benjannet S, et al. Chloroquine is a potent inhibitor of SARS coronavirus infection and spread. *Virol J.* 2005;2:69.

188. The RECOVERY Collaborative Group. Effect of hydroxychloroquine in hospitalized patients with Covid-19. *N Engl J Med.* 2020;383(21):2030-2040.

189. Cavalcanti AB, Zampieri FG, Rosa RG, et al. Hydroxychloroquine with or without azithromycin in mild-to-moderate Covid-19. *N Engl J Med.* 2020;383:2041-2052.

190. Skipper CP, Pastick KA, Engen NW, et al. Hydroxychloroquine in non-hospitalized adults with early COVID-19: a randomized trial. *Ann Intern Med.* 2020;173(8):623-631.

191. Boulware DR, Pullen MF, Bangdiwala AS, et al. A randomized trial of hydroxychloroquine as postexposure prophylaxis for Covid-19. *N Engl J Med.* 2020;383(6):517-525.

192. Yang SNY, Atkinson SC, Wang C, et al. The broad spectrum antiviral ivermectin targets the host nuclear transport importin alpha/beta1 heterodimer. *Antiviral Res.* 2020;177:104760.

193. Ahmed S, Karim MM, Ross AG, et al. A five-day course of ivermectin for the treatment of COVID-19 may reduce the duration of illness. *Int J Infect Dis.* 2020;103:214-216.

194. Chachar AZK, Khan KA, Asif M, et al. Effectiveness of ivermectin in SARS-COV-2/COVID-19 Patients. *Int J of Sci.* 2020;9:31-35.

195. Steinberg KP, Hudson LD, Goodman RB, et al. Efficacy and safety of corticosteroids for persistent acute respiratory distress syndrome. *N Engl J Med.* 2006;354:1671-1684.

196. Yang Z, Liu J, Zhou Y, et al. The effect of corticosteroid treatment on patients with coronavirus infection: a systemic review and metaanalysis. *J Infect.* 2020;81:e13-e20.

197. RECOVERY Collaborative Group, Horby P, Lim WS, Emberson JR, et al. Dexamethasone in hospitalized patients with COVID-19—Preliminary report. *N Engl J Med.* 2020 Jul 17:NEJMoa2021436.

198. Huet T, Beaussier H, Voisin O, et al. Anakinra for severe forms of COVID-19: a cohort study. *Lancet Rheumatol.* 2020;2(7):e393-e400.

199. Cavalli G, De Luca G, Campochiaro C, et al. Interleukin-1 blockade with high-dose anakinra in patients with COVID-19, acute respiratory distress syndrome, and hyperinflammation: a retrospective cohort study. *Lancet Rheumatol.* 2020;2(6):e325-e331.

200. Aouba A, Baldolli A, Geffray L, et al. Targeting the inflammatory cascade with anakinra in moderate to severe COVID-19 pneumonia: case series. *Ann Rheum Dis.* 2020;79(10):1381-1382.

201. Senchenkova EY, Russell J, Yildirim A, et al. Novel role of T cells and IL-6 (interleukin-6) in angiotensin II–induced microvascular dysfunction. *Hypertension.* 2019;73:829-838.

202. Yoshikawa T, Hill T, Li K, et al. Severe acute respiratory syndrome (SARS) coronavirus-induced lung epithelial cytokines exacerbate SARS pathogenesis by modulating intrinsic functions of monocyte-derived macrophages and dendritic cells. *J Virol.* 2009;83:3039-3048.

203. Sanofi. Sanofi and Regeneron provide update on Kevzara® (sarilumab) Phase 3 U.S. trial in COVID-19 patients. 2020. https://www.sanofi.com/en/media-room/press-releases/2020/2020-07-02-22-30-00. Accessed January 11, 2021.

204. Salvarani C, Dolci G, Massari M, et al. Effect of tocilizumab vs standard care on clinical worsening in patients hospitalized with COVID-19 pneumonia: a randomized clinical trial. *JAMA Intern Med.* 2021;181:24-31.

205. Hermine O, Mariette X, Tharaux PL, et al. Effect of tocilizumab vs usual care in adults hospitalized with COVID-19 and moderate or severe pneumonia: a randomized clinical trial. *JAMA Intern Med.* 2021;181:32-40.

206. Stone JH, Frigault MJ, Serling-Boyd NJ, et al. Efficacy of tocilizumab in patients hospitalized with Covid-19. *N Engl J Med.* 2020;383:2333-2344.

207. Salama C, Han J, Yau L, et al. Tocilizumab in patients hospitalized with Covid-19 pneumonia. *N Engl J Med.* 2021;384:20-30.

208. Leung YY, Yao Hui LL, Kraus VB. Colchicine—update on mechanisms of action and therapeutic uses. *Semin Arthritis Rheum.* 2015;45(3):341-350.

209. Deftereos SG, Giannopoulos G, Vrachatis DA, et al. Effect of colchicine vs standard care on cardiac and inflammatory biomarkers and clinical outcomes in patients hospitalized with coronavirus disease 2019: the GRECCO-19 randomized clinical trial. *JAMA Netw Open.* 2020;3:e2013136.

210. Katz LM. (A little) clarity on convalescent plasma for Covid-19. *N Engl J Med.* 2021 Feb 18. doi: 10.1056/NEJMe2035678

211. Chai KL, Valk SJ, Piechotta V et al. Convalescent plasma or hyperimmune immunoglobulin for people with COVID-19: a living systematic review. *Cochrane Database Syst Rev.* 2020;10:CD013600.

212. Li L, Zhang W, Hu Y et al. Effect of convalescent plasma therapy on time to clinical improvement in patients with severe and life-threatening COVID-19: a randomized clinical trial. *JAMA.* 2020;324:460-470.

213. Agarwal A, Mukherjee A, Kumar G et al. Convalescent plasma in the management of moderate covid-19 in adults in India: open label phase II multicentre randomised controlled trial (PLACID Trial). *BMJ.* 2020; 371:m3939.

214. Simonovich VA, Burgos Pratx LD, Scibona P et al. A randomized trial of convalescent plasma in Covid-19 severe pneumonia. *N Engl J Med.* 2021;384(7):619-629.

215. Joyner MJ, Carter RE, Senefeld JW et al. Convalescent plasma antibody levels and the risk of death from Covid-19. *N Engl J Med.* 2021 Mar 18. doi: 10.1056/NEJMoa2031893

216. Group A-TL-CS, Lundgren JD, Grund B et al. A neutralizing monoclonal antibody for hospitalized patients with covid-19. *N Engl J Med.* 2021;384(10):905-914.

217. Weinreich DM, Sivapalasingam S, Norton T et al. REGN-COV2, a neutralizing antibody cocktail, in outpatients with Covid-19. *N Engl J Med.* 2021;384:238-251.

218. Baden LR, El Sahly HM, Essink B et al. Efficacy and safety of the mRNA-1273 SARS-CoV-2 vaccine. *N Engl J Med.* 2021;384:403-416.

219. Polack FP, Thomas SJ, Kitchin N et al. Safety and efficacy of the BNT162b2 mRNA Covid-19 vaccine. *N Engl J Med.* 2020;383:2603-2615.

220. Chopra V, Flanders SA, O'Malley M, Malani AN, Prescott HC. Sixty-day outcomes among patients hospitalized with COVID-19. *Ann Intern Med.* 2021;174(4):576-578.

Index

Note: Page numbers followed by *b* indicate boxed material; those followed by *f* indicate figures; and those followed by *t* indicate tables.